MW00710170

Taber's®

CYCLOPEDIC MEDICAL DICTIONARY

Editor
Donald Venes, M.D., M.S.J.
(*In loving memory of Victoria Webb, MD*)

Coeditor
Clayton L. Thomas, M.D., M.P.H.
Director Emeritus of Medical Affairs
Tambrands Inc.

Managing Editor
Elizabeth J. Egan

Assistant Editors
Nancee A. Morelli
Alison D. Nell

Copy Editor
Ann Houska

Proofreaders
Joy Matkowski
Christopher Muldor

Dictionary Illustrator
Beth Anne Willert, M.S.

EDITION

19

ILLUSTRATED IN FULL COLOR

Taber's®

CYCLOPEDIC MEDICAL DICTIONARY

F. A. DAVIS COMPANY

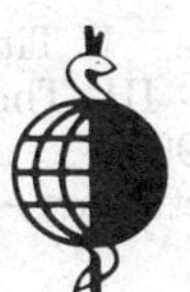

PHILADELPHIA

PRINTED IN THE UNITED STATES OF AMERICA

Last digit indicates print number 10 9 8 7 6 5 4 3

NOTE: As new scientific information becomes available through basic and clinical research, recommended treatments and drug therapies undergo changes. The author and publisher have done everything possible to make Taber's accurate, up to date, and in accord with accepted standards at the time of publication. The author, editors, and publisher are not responsible for errors or omissions or for consequences from application of the book, and make no warranty, expressed or implied, in regard to the contents of the book. Any practice described in this book should be applied by the reader in accordance with professional standards of care used in regard to the unique circumstances that may apply in each situation. The reader is advised always to check product information (package inserts) for changes and new information regarding dose and contraindications before administering any drug. Caution is especially urged when using new or infrequently ordered drugs.

Library of Congress Cataloging in Publication Data

Taber's cyclopedic medical dictionary.—Ed. 19, illustrated in full color / editor, Donald Venes; coeditor, Clayton L. Thomas
p. ; cm.
Includes bibliographical references and index.
ISBN 0-8036-0654-0 (index)—ISBN 0-8036-0655-9 (non index)—ISBN 0-8036-0656-7 (deluxe)
1. Medicine—Dictionaries. I. Title: Cyclopedic medical dictionary. II. Venes, Donald, 1952- III. Thomas, Clayton L., 1921-IV. Taber, Clarence Wilbur, 1870-1968
[DNLM: 1. Medicine—Dictionary—English. W 13 T113d 2001]
R121.T18 2001
610′.3—dc21
ISSN 1065-1357 00-064688
ISBN 0-8036-0655-9
ISBN 0-8036-0654-0 (indexed)
ISBN 0-8036-0656-7 (deluxe)
ISBN 0-8036-0657-5 (CD-ROM)

DISTRIBUTORS

United States of America

F. A. DAVIS COMPANY
1915 Arch St.
Philadelphia, PA 19103

Atlanta, Georgia

J. A. MAJORS COMPANY
4004 Tradeport Blvd.
P.O. Box 82686, 30354

Houston, Texas

J. A. MAJORS COMPANY
9464 Kirby Drive, 77054

Lewisville, Texas

J. A. MAJORS COMPANY
P.O. Box 819074
1401 Lake Drive, 75057

Los Angeles, California

J. A. MAJORS COMPANY
1220 West Walnut St.
Compton, CA 90220

Philadelphia, Pennsylvania

RITTENHOUSE BOOK DISTRIBUTORS, INC.
511 Feheley Drive
King of Prussia, PA 19406

St. Louis, Missouri

MATTHEWS BOOK COMPANY
11559 Rock Island Court
Maryland Heights, MO 63043

Canada

LOGIN BROTHERS CANADA
324 Saulteaux Crescent
Winnipeg, Manitoba R3J 3T2

Europe

MEDICUS MEDIA
Ferry Lane
Shepperton, Middlesex TW17 9LH
England

Australia & New Zealand

MACLENNAN AND PETTY, PTY. LTD.
Suite 405
152 Bunnerong Rd.
Eastgardens NSW 2036
Australia

Mexico & Central America

LIBRERIA INTERNACIONAL, S. A. DE C.V.
A. Sonora 206
Col. Hipodromo
06100 Mexico, D.F.

Brazil

ERNESTO REICHMANN, DISTRIBUIDORA DE LIVROS
Rua Coronel Marques, 335
Tatuape
Sao Paolo—SP 03440-0000

Panama & South America

INTER-BOOK MARKETING SERVICE
Rua das Palmeiras, 32-Apt. 701
22270 Rio de Janeiro
Brazil

India

JAYPEE BROTHERS MEDICAL PUBLISHERS
G/16 EMCA House
23/23 B, Ansari Rd.
Darya Ganj, New Delhi 110 002
India

Middle East

INTERNATIONAL PUBLISHERS REPRESENTATIVES LIMITED
4 Michalakis Karaolis St.
P.O. Box 5731
Engomi, Nicosia
Cyprus

Southeast Asia

CHOICETEXTS (ASIA) PTE. LTD
31 Kaki Bukit Road 3, #06–07
Techlink, Singapore 417818

CONTENTS

INTRODUCTION TO EDITION 19

About a third of a century ago I became the medical editor of *Taber's Cyclopedic Medical Dictionary*. That had been my task until the editing process for the 19th edition began. For this edition Dr. Donald Venes and I have shared the assignment, with Dr. Venes having the major responsibility.

After publication of the 19th edition, I will no longer be involved as a medical editor for *Taber's*. I would have expected this to cause personal sadness, but this is not the case due to my confidence in the future of *Taber's*. This conviction is based on my admiration for the quality and quantity of the intellectual effort brought to *Taber's* by Dr. Venes and on my faith in the continuing excellence of the leadership provided by the managing editor, Elizabeth Egan, and her talented associates.

The *sine qua non* for *Taber's* record of leadership was the continued support of the F. A. Davis Company through the admirable direction of the principals, Robert H. Craven and Robert H. Craven, Jr.

Finally, my association with the lexicographic icon, known to its millions of users as *Taber's,* would have been impossible without the support of myriad individuals, but especially of my wife of 50 years, Peggy.

Clayton Lay Thomas, M.D., M.P.H.

About 3 years ago, with encouragement from my wife, Victoria Webb, and the mentoring of Clayton Thomas, I took on the awesome task of editing this 19th edition of *Taber's Cyclopedic Medical Dictionary*. It has been a labor of love.

Since the last edition of *Taber's* was published, the health professions and the vocabulary of health care have taken some surprising new directions. The art and science of complementary medical practices have burgeoned, the economics of managed care has transformed the landscape, and the scientific and technical underpinnings of patient care have taken startling new turns. Working together, Dr. Thomas, the consultants, the editorial staff at F. A. Davis, and I have tried to capture these changes in this edition. As a result, you will find definitions for *black cohosh, copayment, DNA vaccine, ghost surgeon, grab sample, jazz ballet bottom, jet injection, kava, LASIK, magic syndrome, paleolithic diet, qi gong, ultrafast computerized tomography, transmyocardial revascularization, viator,* and many other remarkable new concepts and terms in this edition of the dictionary.

Together, the *Taber's* editorial team has rewritten or revised more than 12,000 entries, added more than 2000 new words to the text, and included dozens of new images and tables to this edition. We have added more useful details about patient care and updated nearly every encyclopedic entry and appendix in the book. We have also made the text easier to understand, more topical, and more available to students and educators, nurses, allied health professionals, mid-level practitioners, complementary medical providers, administrators, physicians, and patients alike.

Dozens of people helped us in the compilation of *Taber's* 19th edition, and we are grateful for their contributions. I would like to offer special thanks to those readers who took the time to write or call us with suggestions for the text. Thank you, one and all, for your suggestions, corrections, and helpful comments.

I hope that after you leaf through the 19th edition of *Taber's* you will find this new edition to be an indispensable addition to your health care reference library.

Donald Venes, M.D.

CONSULTANTS

Tonia Dandry Aiken, RN, BSN, JD
Joea E. Bierchen, RN, MSN, EdD
Carroll Conner Bouman, RN, PhD
Richard R. Carlton, MS, RT(R), FAERS
Charles Christiansen, EdD, OTR, OTC, FAOTA
Marilynn E. Doenges, RN, BSN, MA, CS
Janet Duffey, MS, RN, CS
Robert Elling, MPA, REMT-P
Jacqueline Fawcett, PhD, FAAN
Rose S. Fife, MD
Maxine Goldman, BSHC, RN
Paul C. Good, DPM
Barbara A. Gylys, MEd, CMA-A
Bruce E. Hirsch, MD, FACP
Christopher Holmes, MD, MSPH
Donna Ignatavicius, MS, RN, Cm
Elizabeth Ikeda, PT, MS, OCS
Jeanette G. Kernicki, RN, PhD, ANP
Ruth Lipman, PhD
Judith E. Meissner, RN, BSN, MSN
Mary Frances Moorhouse, RN, CRRN, CLNC
Robert F. Moran, MS, PhD, FCCM, FAIC
Thomas J. Rahilly, PhD, EMT-CC
Betty J. Reynard, EdD, RDH
Valerie C. Scanlon, PhD
Chad Starkey, PhD, ATC
Victoria Webb, MD *(Deceased)*
Mary Ann Wharton, PT, MS
Robert L. Wilkins, PhD, RRT

(Material supplied by the consultants has been reviewed and edited by Donald Venes, MD, MSJ and Clayton L. Thomas, MD, MPH, editors, with whom final responsibility rests for the accuracy of the content.)

Taber's Feature Finder

MAIN ENTRY — **abduction** (ăb-dŭk´shŭn) **1.** Lateral movement of the limbs away from the median plane of the body, or lateral bending of the head or trunk. SEE: illus. **2.** Movement of the digits away from the axial line of a limb. **3.** Outward rotation of the eyes. — ILLUSTRATION CROSS REFERENCE

acetaminophen (ă-sĕt″ă-mĭn´ō-fĕn) A drug with antipyretic and analgesic effects similar to those of aspirin, but with limited anti-inflammatory or antirheumatic effects.

Caution: Acute overdose may cause fatal hepatic necrosis. — CAUTION

ABBREVIATION — **ACH** *adrenocortical hormone.*

PRONUNCIATION — **achloropsia** (ă-klō-rŏp´sē-ă) [″+ *chloros,* green, + *opsis,* vision] Color blindness in which green cannot be distinguished. SYN: *deuteranopia.* — ETYMOLOGY — SYNONYM

Addison's disease [Thomas Addison, Brit. physician, 1793–1860] A rare illness marked by gradual and progressive failure of the adrenal glands and insufficient production of steroid hormones. — BIOGRAPHICAL INFORMATION

ETIOLOGY — ETIOLOGY: Adrenal failure typically results from autoimmune destruction of the adrenal glands, chronic infections, or cancers that metastasize to the adrenal glands from other organs.

SYMPTOMS — SYMPTOMS: The patient may be symptom-free until the majority of adrenal tissue is destroyed. Early complaints are usually nonspecific: a feeling of weakness or fatigue, lack of appetite, weight loss, nausea, vomiting, abdominal pain, and dizziness.

TREATMENT — TREATMENT: Chronic adrenal insufficiency is managed with corticosteroids, such as prednisone, usually taken twice a day. SEE: *adrenal crisis.* — CROSS REFERENCE

PROGNOSIS — PROGNOSIS: If untreated, the disease will continue a chronic course with progressive but usually relatively slow deterioration; in some patients the deterioration may be rapid. Patients treated properly have an excellent prognosis.

PATIENT CARE — PATIENT CARE: Patients with primary adrenal insufficiency who are suffering other acute conditions are assessed frequently for hypotension, tachycardia, fluid balance, and electrolyte and glucose levels. SEE: Nursing Diagnoses Appendix. — NURSING DIAGNOSES CROSS REFERENCE

adenoma (ăd″ĕ-nō´mă) *pl.* **adenomata** [″+ *oma*, tumor] A benign tumor made of epithelial cells. **adenomatous** (-nō´mă-tŭs), *adj.* — PLURAL — ADJECTIVAL FORM

SUBENTRY — ***chromophobe a.*** Tumor of the pituitary gland composed of cells that do not stain readily. It may cause pituitary deficiency or diabetes insipidus.

follicular a. Adenoma of the thyroid.

Not an actual page.

FEATURES AND THEIR USE

This section describes the major features found in *Taber's* and provides information that may help you use the dictionary more efficiently. The Feature Finder on page xiii, is a graphic representation of many of the features described below.

1. **Vocabulary:** The extensive vocabulary defined in *Taber's* has been updated to meet the ongoing needs of students, educators, and clinicians in the health sciences as well as interested consumers. The medical editor and the nursing and allied health consultants have researched and written new entries, revised existing entries, and deleted obsolete ones, reflecting the many changes in health care technology, clinical practice, and patient care. American, rather than British, spellings are preferred.

2. **Entry format:** *Taber's* entries are organized according to a main entry–subentry format, which makes it easier—especially for students—to find and compare medical terms that share a common element or classification. All single-word terms (e.g., **cell**) are main entries, and most compound, or multiple-word, terms (e.g., **stem cell**) are subentries under the main entry (or headword)—in this case, **cell.** However, some compound terms (e.g., eponyms, such as **Parkinson's disease,** and the names of individuals and organizations) are listed as main entries. An especially important compound term may be listed as both a main entry and a subentry, with one of the terms serving as a cross-reference to the other. All main entries are printed in bold type; subentries are indented under the main entry and are printed in bold italic type. All entries are listed and defined in the singular whenever possible.

3. **Alphabetization:**

   Main entries are alphabetized letter by letter, regardless of spaces or hyphens that occur between the words; a comma marks the end of a main entry for alphabetical purposes (e.g., **skin, tenting of** precedes **skin cancer**). In eponyms the **'s** is ignored in alphabetizing (e.g., **Albini's nodules** precedes **albinism**).

   Subentries are listed in straight-ahead order following the same letter-by-letter alphabetization used for main entries; a comma marks the end of a subentry for alphabetical purposes. The headword is abbreviated in all subentries (such as ***premature l.*** under **labor** or ***emergency medical t.*** under **technician**).

4. **Eponyms:** Included as main entries are the names of individuals who were the first to discover, describe, or popularize a concept, a microorganism, a disease, a syndrome, or an anatomical structure. A brief biography appears in brackets after the pronunciation. Bio-

graphical information includes the person's medical designation, the country in which the person was born or worked, and the date of birth and death if known.

5. **Definitions:** The text that occurs before the first period in an entry constitutes the definition for that entry. Many entries are written in encyclopedic style, offering a comprehensive understanding of the disease, condition, or concept defined. See "Encyclopedic entries" for further information.

6. **Pronunciations:** Most main entries are spelled phonetically. Phonetic pronunciations, which appear in parentheses after the boldface main entry, are given as simply as possible with most long and short vowels marked diacritically and secondary accents indicated. *Diacritics* are marks over or under vowels. Only two diacritics are used in *Taber's:* the macron ¯ showing the long sound of vowels, as the *a* in rate, *e* in rebirth, *i* in isle, *o* in over, and *u* in unite; and the breve ˘ showing the short sound of vowels, as the *a* in apple, *e* in ever, *i* in it, *o* in not, and *u* in cut. *Accents* are marks used to indicate stress upon certain syllables. A single accent ′ is called a primary accent. A double accent ″ is called a secondary accent; it indicates less stress upon a syllable than that given by a primary accent. This difference in stress can be seen in the word *an″es-the′si-a.*

7. **Singular/Plural forms:** When the spelling of an entry's singular or plural form is a nonstandard formation (e.g., **villus** *pl.* **villi,** or **viscera** *sing.* **viscus**), the spelling of the singular or plural form appears in boldface after the pronunciation for the main entry. Nonstandard singular and plural forms appear as entries themselves at their normal alphabetical positions.

8. **Etymologies:** An etymology indicates the origin and historical development of a term. For most medical terms the origin is Latin or Greek. An etymology is given for most main entries and appears in brackets following the pronunciation.

9. **Abbreviations:** Standard abbreviations for entries are included with the definition and also are listed alphabetically throughout the text. Additional abbreviations used for charting and prescription writing are listed in the Appendices. A list of nonmedical abbreviations used in text appears on page xxxiii.

10. **Encyclopedic entries:** Detailed, comprehensive information is included with entries that require additional coverage because of their importance or complexity. Often this information is organized into several subsections, each with its own subheading. The most frequently used subheadings are Patient Care, Symptoms, Etiology, Treatment, Caution, Diagnosis, and Prognosis.

11. **Illustrations:** This edition of *Taber's* includes 630 illustrations, 150 of which are new to this edition. More than three fourths of the images are four-color photographs and line drawings. The images were carefully chosen to complement the text of the entries with which they are associated. Each illustration is cross-referenced from its associated entry. A complete list of illustrations begins on page xix.

12. **Tables:** This edition contains 88 color-screened tables located appropriately throughout the Vocabulary section. A list of tables appears on page xxxi.

13. **Adjectives:** The adjectival forms of many noun main entries appear at the end of the definition of the noun form or, if the entry is long, at the end of the first paragraph. Pronunciations for most of the adjectival forms are included. Many common adjectives appear as main entries themselves.

14. **Caution statements:** This notation is used to draw particular attention to clinically important information. The information is of more than routine interest and should be considered when delivering health care. These statements are further emphasized by colored rules above and below the text.

15. **Synonyms:** Synonyms are listed at the end of the entry or, in encyclopedic entries, at the end of the first paragraph. The abbreviation SYN: precedes the synonymous term(s). Terms listed as synonyms have their own entries in the Vocabulary, which generally carry a cross-reference to the entry at which the definition appears.

16. **Cross-references:** Illustrations, tables, appendices, or other relevant vocabulary entries may be given as cross-references. These are indicated by SEE: followed by the name(s) of the appropriate element(s) in italics. Cross-references to the Nursing Diagnoses Appendix are highlighted in color at the end of the entry as SEE: *Nursing Diagnoses Appendix.* Entries at which an illustration appears carry the color-highlighted SEE: illus.

17. **Appendices:** The Appendices contain detailed information that could be organized or presented more easily in one section rather than interspersed throughout the Vocabulary. This edition features several new appendices: Integrative Therapies: Complementary and Alternative Medicine, Nursing Interventions Classification, Nursing Outcomes Classification, Omaha Classification System, and Home Health Care Classification System. Among the revised appendices are Nursing Diagnoses, Standard and Universal Precautions, Medical Abbreviations, Prefixes, Suffixes, and Combining Forms, the Computer Glossary, Conceptual Models and Theories of Nursing, Medical Emergencies, and Nutrition.

18. **Nursing Diagnoses Appendix:** This appendix has been updated through the 14th NANDA (North American Nursing Diagnosis Association) Conference. It is divided into several sections, including two lists of NANDA's nursing diagnoses organized into Doenges and Moorhouse's Diagnostic Divisions and Gordon's Functional Health Patterns; an at-a-glance look at the most recent diagnoses approved by NANDA; nursing diagnoses commonly associated with almost 300 diseases/disorders (cross-referenced from the body of the dictionary); and a complete description of all NANDA-approved diagnoses through the 14th conference (in 2000) in alphabetical order. Included are the diagnostic division, definition, related factors, and defining characteristics for each nursing diagnosis. See the *Quick View of Contents* on page 2641 for further explanation.

LIST OF ILLUSTRATIONS

Illustrations are listed according to the main entry or subentry they accompany. Information in parentheses indicates the source of the illustration; a list of sources appears at the end of the list.

ILLUSTRATION SOURCES

Bartelt, MA: Diagnostic Bacteriology: A Study Guide. FA Davis, Philadelphia, 1999.

Berkow, R (ed): The Merck Manual, ed 13. Merck & Co., Inc., Rahway, NJ, 1977.

Brown, KR and Jacobson, S: Mastering Dysrhythmias: A Problem Solving Guide. FA Davis, Philadelphia, 1988.

Colyar, MR and Ehrhardt, CR: Ambulatory Care Procedures for the Nurse Practitioner. FA Davis, Philadelphia, 1999.

Doenges, ME, Moorhouse, MF and Geissler, AC: Nursing Care Plans: Guidelines for Individualizing Patient Care, ed 5. FA Davis, Philadelphia, 1999.

Gilman, S and Newman, SW: Manter & Gatz's Essentials of Clinical Neuroanatomy and Neurophysiology, ed 9. FA Davis, Philadelphia, 1996.

Goldsmith, LA, Lazarus, GS and Tharp, MD: Adult and Pediatric Dermatology: A Color Guide to Diagnosis and Treatment, FA Davis, Philadelphia, 1997.

Hatch, H, Gold Beach, OR.

Harmening, DM: Clinical Hematology and Fundamentals of Hemostasis, ed 3. FA Davis, Philadelphia, 1997.

Hillman, RS and Finch, CA: Red Cell Manual, ed 7. FA Davis, Philadelphia, 1996.

Kern, ME and Blevins, KS: Medical Mycology: A Self-Instructional Text, ed 2. FA Davis, Philadelphia, 1997.

Kozol, RA, Fromm, D and Konen, JC: When to Call the Surgeon: Decision Making for Primary Care Providers. FA Davis, Philadelphia, 1999.

Lentner, C (ed): Geigy Scientific Tables, ed 8. Ciba Geigy, Basle, Switzerland, 1981.

Leventhal, R and Cheadle, RF: Medical Parasitology: A Self-Instructional Text, ed 4. FA Davis, Philadelphia, 1996.

Luckmann, J, Fonteyne, M and Hopkins, T: Medical Surgical Nursing for Evidence-Based Practice. FA Davis, Forthcoming.

Mazziotta, JC, and Gilman, S: Clinical Brain Imaging: Principles and Applications. Oxford University Press, New York, 1992. Used by Permission of Oxford University Press, Inc.

Morton, PG: Health Assessment in Nursing, ed 2. FA Davis, Philadelphia, 1993

McKinnis, L: Fundamentals of Orthopedic Radiology, FA Davis, Philadelphia, 1997.

Perry, LP: "Perry's Perenials." http://www.uvm.edu/pass/perry (August 2000).

Reeves, JRT and Maibach, HI: Clinical Dermatology Illustrated: A Regional Approach, ed 3. MacLennan & Petty Pty Ltd, Sydney, Australia, 1998 (distributed in North America by FA Davis, Philadelphia).

Sacher, RA, McPherson, RA with Campos, JM: Widmann's Clinical Interpretation of Laboratory Tests, ed 11. FA Davis, Philadelphia, 2000.

Scanlon, VC and Sanders, T: Essentials of Anatomy and Physiology, ed 3. FA Davis, Philadelphia, 1999.

Starkey, C and Ryan, JL: Evaluation of Orthopedic and Athletic Injuries. FA Davis, Philadelphia, 1996.

Stevens, CD: Clinical Immunology and Serology: A Laboratory Perspective. FA Davis, Philadelphia, 1996.

Strasinger, SK: Urinalysis and Body Fluids, ed 3. FA Davis, Philadelphia, 1994.

Wallace, JE: Radiographic Exposure: Principals and Practice. FA Davis, Philadelphia, 1995.

Williams, LS and Hopper, PD (eds): Understanding Medical-Surgical Nursing. FA Davis, Philadelphia, 1999.

LIST OF TABLES

ABBREVIATIONS USED IN TEXT*

ABBR	abbreviation
Amerind	American Indian
approx.	approximately
AS	Anglo-Saxon
at. no.	atomic number
at. wt.	atomic weight
Brit.	British
C	centigrade
CNS	central nervous system
D.	Dutch
e.g.	exempli gratia (for example)
esp.	especially
F	Fahrenheit
Fr.	French
fr.	from
Ger.	German
Gr.	Greek
i.e.	id est (that is)
illus.	illustration
L.	Latin
LL.	Late Latin
MD.	Middle Dutch
ME.	Middle English
Med. L.	Medieval Latin
NL	New Latin
O.Fr.	Old French
pert.	pertaining
pl.	plural
rel.	related; relating
sing.	singular
Sp.	Spanish
sp. gr.	specific gravity
SYMB	symbol
SYN	synonym

*Additional abbreviations are listed in the Units of Measurement Appendix and the Medical Abbreviations Appendix.

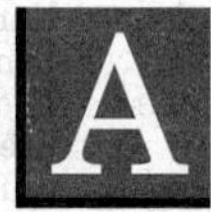

α Alpha, the first letter of the Greek alphabet.
Å *angstrom unit.*
A_2 *aortic second sound.*
a *accommodation; ampere; anode; anterior; aqua; area; artery.*
ā [L.] *ante,* before.
a-, an- [Gr., not] Prefix meaning *without, away from, not* (a- is usually used before a consonant; an- is usually used before a vowel).
A.A., a.a. *achievement age; Alcoholics Anonymous; amino acid; arteriae.*
a̅a̅ [Gr. *ana,* of each] Prescription notation meaning *the stated amount of each of the substances is to be used in compounding the prescription.*
AAA *American Ambulance Association.*
A.A.A. *American Academy of Allergists; American Association of Anatomists.*
A.A.A.S. *American Association for the Advancement of Science.*
AABB *American Association of Blood Banks.*
AACC *American Association for Clinical Chemistry.*
A.A.C.N. *American Association of Critical-Care Nurses; American Association of Colleges of Nursing.*
A.A.F.P. *American Academy of Family Physicians.*
AAHN *American Association for the History of Nursing.*
AAL *anterior axillary line.*
A.A.M.A. *American Association of Medical Assistants.*
A.A.M.I. *Association for the Advancement of Medical Instrumentation.*
AAMS *Association of Air Medical Services.*
AAMT *American Association for Medical Transcription.*
A.A.N. *American Academy of Nursing.*
A.A.N.A. *American Association of Nurse Anesthetists.*
A.A.N.N. *American Association of Neuroscience Nurses.*
A.A.O.H.N. *American Association of Occupational Health Nurses.*
A.A.O.S. *American Academy of Orthopedic Surgeons.*
A.A.P. *American Academy of Pediatrics; American Association of Pathologists.*
A.A.P.A. *American Academy of Physician Assistants.*
AAPMR *American Academy of Physical Medicine and Rehabilitation.*
A.A.R.C. *American Association for Respiratory Care.*
AARP *American Association of Retired Persons.*
AAS *atomic absorption spectroscopy.*
AASECT *American Association of Sex Educators, Counselors, and Therapists.*
Ab *antibody.*
ab- [L. *ab,* from] Prefix meaning *from, away from, negative, absent.*
abacavir (ă-băk′ă-vēr) A nucleoside analogue reverse transcriptase inhibitor used in the treatment of HIV-1.
Abadie's sign (ă-bă-dēz′) [Charles A. Abadie, Fr. ophthalmologist, 1842–1932] In exophthalmic goiter, spasm of the levator palpebrae superioris.
Abadie's sign (ă-bă-dēz′) [Jean Abadie, Fr. neurologist, 1873–1946] In tabes dorsalis, insensibility to pressure over the Achilles tendon.
A band A dark-staining area in the center of a sarcomere in skeletal or cardiac muscle, composed of overlapping myosin and actin filaments. SYN: *anisotropic disk.*
abandonment A premature termination of the professional treatment relationship by the health care provider without adequate notice or the patient's consent.
abaptiston (ă″băp-tĭs′tŏn) [Gr. *abaptistos,* not dipped] Trephine that cannot slip and injure the brain.
abarognosis (ăb″ăr-ŏg-nō′sĭs) [Gr. *a-,* not, + *baros,* weight, + *gnosis,* knowledge] Loss of ability to sense weight. SEE: *baragnosis.*
abarthrosis (ăb-ăr-thrō′sĭs) [L. *ab,* from, + Gr. *arthron,* joint, + *osis,* condition] A movable joint or point at which bones move freely against each other. SYN: *diarthrosis.*
abarticular [″ + *articulus,* joint] At a distance from a joint.
abarticulation **1.** Ambiguous term meaning dislocation of a joint. **2.** Diarthrosis. SYN: *abarthrosis.*
abasia (ă-bā′zē-ă) [Gr. *a-,* not, + *basis,* step] **1.** Motor incoordination in walking. **2.** Inability to walk due to impairment of coordination. **abasic, abatic,** *adj.*

a.-astasia Lack of motor coordination with inability to stand or walk. SYN: *astasia-abasia.*

paralytic a. Abasia in which the leg muscles are paralyzed.

paroxysmal trepidant a. Abasia caused by trembling and sudden stiffening of legs on standing, making walking impossible. It may be related to hysteria.

abate (ă-bāt′) [L. *ab,* from, + *battere,* to beat] **1.** To lessen or decrease. **2.** To cease or cause to cease.
abatement (ă-bāt′mĕnt) Decrease in severity of pain or symptoms.

abaxial, abaxile (ăb-ăk′sē-al, -sĭl) [L. *ab*, from, + *axis*, axis] **1.** Not within the axis of a body or part. **2.** At the opposite end of the axis of a part.

Abbe-Wharton-McIndoe operation, McIndoe operation (ă′bē-whăr′tŏn-măk′-ĭn-dō) A surgical procedure performed to create a new vagina in patients who do not have one. This is achieved by creating adequate space between the rectum and bladder; the inlaying of a split-thickness graft; and most importantly, continuous and prolonged dilatation during the healing stage when tissues are most likely to contract.

PATIENT CARE: The health care team supports the patient medically and psychologically, by helping the patient learn about her condition and the procedure, by answering questions, and by alleviating anxiety.

Abbott's method [Edville G. Abbott, U.S. orthopedic surgeon, 1871–1938] A treatment for scoliosis that is no longer used, in which a series of plaster jackets were applied to straighten the spine.

ABC *antigen-binding capacity; airway, breathing, circulation* (mnemonic for assessing status of emergency patients).

ABCD A mnemonic to aid health care providers in the recognition of malignant melanoma. The letters represent "asymmetry," "border," "color," and "diameter." Pigmented lesions on the skin with irregularities of growth and color and diameters greater than 0.7 mm have a considerable likelihood of being melanomas and should be professionally examined. Additional characteristics of melanomas include the sudden change of an existing mole or sudden appearance of pigmented moles. In some cases an existing mole that was flat elevates above the skin. SEE: *melanoma*.

abciximab (ăb-sĭx′ĭ-măb) A monoclonal antibody that inhibits platelet aggregation and prevents blood clots from forming. It is used esp. to treat and prevent clots in the coronary arteries, for example, in acute myocardial infarction, and after stent placements.

abdomen (ăb-dō′mĕn, ăb′dō-mĕn) [L., belly] The portion of the trunk lying between the thorax and the pelvis. It contains the stomach, lower part of the esophagus, small and large intestines, liver, gallbladder, spleen, and internal genitalia. The peritoneum, a serous membrane, lines the abdomen but envelops all of the organs in it. The kidneys, adrenal glands, ureters, prostate, seminal vesicles, and greater vascular structures are located behind the peritoneum (retroperitoneal or extraperitoneal). SEE: *abdominal quadrants* for illus.

INSPECTION: Visual examination of the abdomen is best done while the patient is supine with the knees slightly bent. In a healthy person the abdomen is oval shaped, with elevations and depressions corresponding to abdominal muscles, umbilicus, and to some degree the forms of underlying viscera. Relative to chest size, it is larger in children than in adults; it is more rotund and broader inferiorly in males than in females.

Disease can alter the shape of the abdomen. A general, symmetrical enlargement may result from ascites; a partial and irregular enlargement may result from tumors, hypertrophy of organs such as the liver or spleen, or intestinal distention caused by gas. Retraction of the abdomen may occur in extreme emaciation and in several forms of cerebral disease, esp. tubercular meningitis of children.

The respiratory movements of the abdominal walls are related to movements of the thorax and are often increased when the latter are arrested and vice versa; thus, abdominal movements are increased in pleurisy, pneumonia, and pericarditis, but are decreased or wholly suspended in peritonitis and disease-caused abdominal pain.

The superficial abdominal veins are sometimes visibly enlarged, indicating an obstruction of blood flow in either the portal system (as in cirrhosis) or the inferior vena cava.

AUSCULTATION: Listening to sounds produced in abdominal organs provides useful diagnostic information. Absent or diminished bowel sounds may indicate paralytic ileus or peritonitis. High-pitched tinkling sounds are associated with intestinal obstruction. Bruits may indicate atherosclerosis, or an abdominal aortic aneurysm. During pregnancy, auscultation enables identification and evaluation of the fetal heart rate and vascular sounds from the placenta.

PERCUSSION: For the practitioner to obtain the greatest amount of information, the patient should be supine with the head slightly raised and knees slightly flexed. Percussion should be carried out in a systematic fashion over the anterior surface of the abdomen. A combination of audible or tactile sensation will be perceived by the examiner according to underlying structures (e.g., gaseous distended organs versus solid organs). A large abdominal aneurysm gives dullness or flatness over it unless a distended intestine lies above it.

PALPATION: The abdomen may be palpated with fingertips, the whole hand, or both hands; pressure may be slight or forceful, continuous or intermittent. The head is supported to relax the abdominal wall. On occasion, the patient may be examined in a standing position (e.g., palpation of groin hernias that might not be palpable in the supine position).

Palpation is helpful in detecting the size, consistency, and position of viscera, the existence of tumors and swellings, and whether the tumors change position with respiration or are movable. It is necessary to ascertain whether tenderness exists in any portion of the abdominal cavity, whether pain is increased or relieved by firm pressure, and whether pain is accentuated by sudden release of firm pressure (i.e., rebound tenderness).

An arterial impulse, if one exists, is systolic and expansive. A thrill accompanying a bruit may occasionally be palpated. A tumor's surface is usually firm and smooth but may be nodular. Inflammatory masses are typically firm and reproducibly tender. Effusion of blood into tissues (e.g., hematoma) may produce a palpable mass.

acute a. An abnormal condition of the abdomen in which there is a sudden, abrupt onset of severe pain. It requires urgent evaluation and diagnosis, as it may indicate a need for immediate surgical intervention. SYN: *surgical a.*

pendulous a. A condition in which the excessively relaxed anterior abdominal wall hangs down over the pubis.

scaphoid a. A condition in which the anterior wall is hollowed, presenting a sunken appearance as in emaciation.

surgical a. Acute a.

abdomin- SEE: *abdomino-*.

abdominal (ăb-dŏm′ĭ-năl) Pert. to the abdomen.

abdominal decompression A technique used in obstetrics to facilitate childbirth. The abdominal area is surrounded by an airtight chamber in which pressure may be intermittently decreased below atmospheric pressure. During labor pains, the pressure is decreased and the uterus is permitted to work more efficiently because the abdominal muscles are elevated away from the uterus.

abdominalgia (ăb-dŏm-ĭn-ăl′jē-ă) [L. *abdomen*, belly, + Gr. *algos*, pain] Pain in the abdomen.

abdominal muscles The group of four muscles that make up the abdominal wall, consisting of: 1. the external oblique (the most superficial of the four), whose fibers are directed downward and medially from the lower ribs to the linea alba and pelvis; 2. the internal oblique, whose fibers are directed upward and medially from the iliac crest and lumbodorsal fascia to the lower ribs; 3. the rectus abdominis, a vertically oriented muscle from the crest of the pubis to the cartilages of the fifth, sixth, and seventh ribs and xiphoid process; and 4. the transversus abdominis, whose fibers are oriented transversely. These muscles participate in a variety of functions, including flexion, side bending and rotation of the trunk, stabilization of the trunk in the upright posture, the expiratory phase of respiration, coughing, and Valsalva's maneuver.

abdominal quadrants Four parts or divisions of the abdomen determined by drawing imaginary vertical and horizontal lines through the umbilicus. The quadrants and their contents are:

Right upper quadrant (RUQ): right lobe of liver, gallbladder, part of transverse colon, part of pylorus, hepatic flexure, right kidney, and duodenum; *Right lower q. (RLQ):* cecum, ascending colon, small intestine, appendix, bladder if distended, right ureter, right spermatic duct in the male; right ovary and right tube, and uterus if enlarged, in the female; *Left upper q. (LUQ):* left lobe of liver, stomach, transverse colon, splenic flexure, pancreas, left kidney, and spleen; *Left lower q. (LLQ):* small intestine, left ureter, sigmoid flexure, descending colon, bladder if distended, left spermatic duct in the male; left ovary and left tube, and uterus if enlarged, in the female. SEE: illus.

abdominal reflexes Contraction of the muscles of the abdominal wall on stimulation of the overlying skin. Absence of these reflexes indicates damage to the pyramidal tract.

abdominal regions The abdomen and its external surface, divided into nine regions by four imaginary planes: two horizontal, one at the level of the ninth costal cartilage (or the lowest point of the costal arch) and the other at the level of the highest point of the iliac crest; two vertical, through the centers of the inguinal ligaments (or through the nipples or through the centers of the clavicles) or curved and coinciding with the lateral borders of the two abdominal rectus muscles. SEE: illus.

abdominal rescue Emergency cesarean delivery of a fetus jeopardized during labor or failed vaginal birth. Indications for surgical intervention include fetal distress associated with dystocia, arrested descent, abruptio placentae, or umbilical cord prolapse.

abdominal rings The apertures in the abdominal wall. *External inguinal* or *superficial*: An interval in the aponeurosis of the external oblique muscle, just above and to the outer side of the crest of the pubic bone. *Triangular:* About 1 in. (2.5 cm) from base to apex and ½ in. (1.3 cm) transversely; provides passage for the spermatic cord in the male and the round ligament in the female. *Internal inguinal* or *deep:* Situated in the transversalis fascia, midway between the anterior superior spine of the ilium and the symphysis pubis, ½ in. (1.3 cm) above Poupart's ligament; oval form,

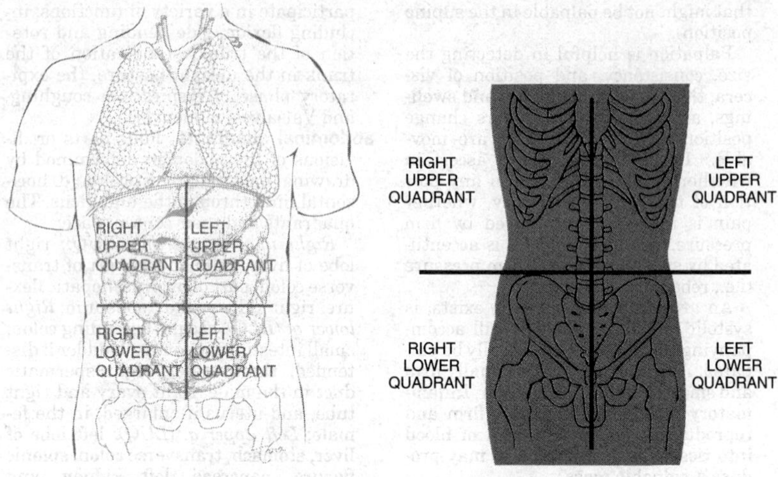

ABDOMINAL QUADRANTS

larger in the male; surrounds spermatic cord in the male and round ligament in the female.

abdomino-, abdomin- (ăb-dŏm′ĭ-nō) Combining form meaning *abdomen.*

abdominocentesis (ăb-dŏm″ĭ-nō-sĕn-tē′sĭs) [L. *abdomen*, belly, + Gr. *kentesis*, puncture] Puncture of the abdomen with an instrument for withdrawal of fluid from the abdominal cavity. SYN: *abdominal paracentesis.*

abdominocyesis (ăb-dŏm″ĭn-ō-sī-ēs′ĭs) Abdominal pregnancy.

abdominocystic [″ + Gr. *kystis*, bladder] Pert. to the abdomen and bladder.

abdominodiaphragmatic breathing A controlled breathing pattern using reciprocal action of the abdominal muscles for expiration and the diaphragm for inspiration; used to maintain control during exertion or to regain control in dyspnea.

abdominogenital (ăb-dŏm″ĭ-nō-jĕn′ĭ-tăl) Pert. to the abdomen and genital organs.

abdominohysterectomy [L. *abdomen*, belly, + Gr. *hystera*, womb, + *ektome*, excision] Removal of the uterus through abdominal incision.

abdominohysterotomy (ăb-dŏm″ĭ-nō-hĭs-tĕr-ŏt′ō-mē) [″ + ″ + *tome*, inci-

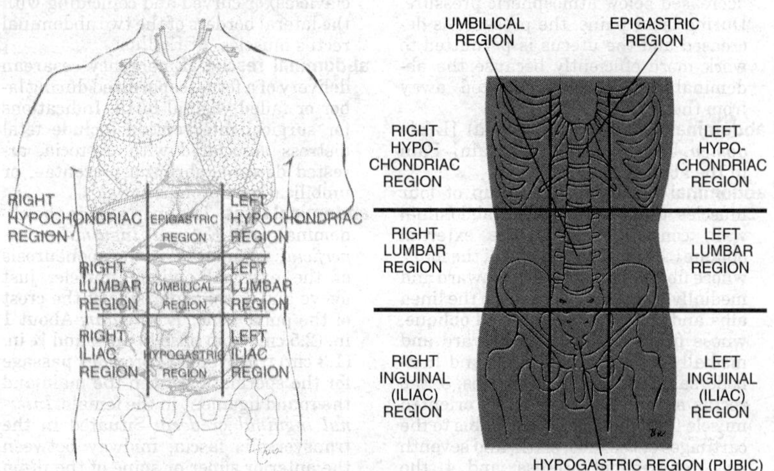

ABDOMINAL REGIONS

sion] Incision of the uterus through a surgical opening in the abdomen.

abdominoperineal Pert. to the abdomen and perineal area.

abdominoplasty (ăb-dŏm″ĭ-nō′plăs-tē) Plastic surgery on the abdomen.

abdominoscopy (ăb-dŏm″ĭ-nŏs′kō-pē) [L. *abdomen*, belly, + Gr. *skopein*, to examine] An outdated term for laparoscopy.

abdominoscrotal [″ + *scrotum*, bag] Pert. to the abdomen and scrotum.

abdominoscrotal muscle Cremaster.

abdominothoracic (ăb-dŏm″ĭ-nō-thō-ră′sĭk) [L. *abdomen*, belly, + Gr. *thorax*, chest] Pert. to the abdomen and thorax.

abdominouterotomy (ăb-dŏm″ĭ-nō-ū-tĕr-ŏt′ō-mē) [L. *abdomen*, belly, + *uterus*, womb, + Gr. *tome*, incision] Abdominohysterotomy.

abdominovaginal (ăb-dŏm″ĭ-nō-văj′ĭ-năl) [″ + *vagina*, sheath] Pert. to the abdomen and vagina.

abdominovesical (ăb-dŏm″ĭ-nō-vĕs′ĭ-kăl) [″ + *vesica*, bladder] Pert. to the abdomen and urinary bladder.

abducens (ăb-dū′sĕnz) [L., drawing away] Pert. to drawing away from the midline of the body.

a. labiorum The muscle that elevates the angle of the mouth. Also called *caninus muscle* and *levator anguli oris muscle*.

a. oculi Musculus rectus lateralis bulbi.

abducens muscle Rectus lateralis muscle of the eye; it moves the eyeball outward.

abducens nerve The sixth cranial nerve; it innervates the lateral rectus muscle of the eye. SEE: *cranial nerve*.

abducent (ăb-dū′sĕnt) [L. *abducens*, drawing away] **1.** Abducting; leading away. **2.** Abducens.

abducent nerve Abducens nerve.

abduct (ăb-dŭkt′) [L. *abductus*, led away] To draw away from the median plane of the body or one of its parts.

abduction (ăb-dŭk′shŭn) **1.** Lateral movement of the limbs away from the median plane of the body, or lateral bending of the head or trunk. SEE: illus. **2.** Movement of the digits away from the axial line of a limb. **3.** Outward rotation of the eyes.

abductor (ăb-dŭk′tor) A muscle that on contraction draws a part away from the median plane of the body or the axial line of an extremity. Opposite of adductor.

abenteric (ăb-ĕn-tĕr′ĭk) [L. *ab*, from, + Gr. *enteron*, intestine] Rel. to or involving organs located outside the intestines.

Abernethy's fascia (ăb′ĕr-nē″thē) [John Abernethy, Brit. surgeon, 1764–1831] A layer of areolar tissue separating the external iliac artery from the iliac fascia over the psoas muscle.

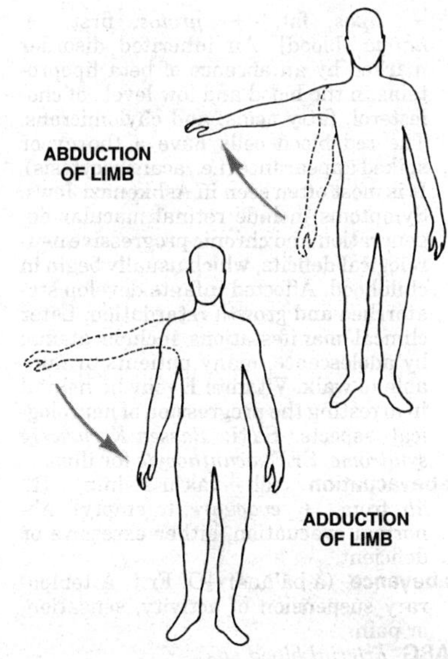

aberrant (ăb-ĕr′ănt) [L. *ab*, from, + *errare*, to wander] Deviating from the normal. SYN: *abnormal*.

aberrant conduction In the electrical conduction system of the heart, the passage of the electrical stimulus via an abnormal pathway, diagnosed by examination of the electrocardiogram.

aberratio (ăb-ĕr-ā′shē-ō) [L.] Aberration.

a. testis Location of a testis in a position away from the path of normal descent.

aberration (ăb-ĕr-ā′shŭn) [L. *ab*, from, + *errare*, to wander] **1.** Deviation from the normal. **2.** Imperfect refraction of light rays.

chromatic a. Unequal refraction of different wavelengths of light through a lens, producing a colored image.

chromosomal a. An abnormality in chromosomes regarding number (aneuploidy, polyploidy) or chromosomal material (translocation, deletion, duplication).

dioptric a. Spherical a.

lateral a. Deviation of a ray from the focus measured on a line perpendicular to the axis.

longitudinal a. Deviation of a ray from the direction parallel to the optic axis.

spherical a. Aberration or distortion of an image due to rays entering the peripheral portion of a spherical mirror or lens being refracted differently from those closer to the center. Thus the peripheral rays are focused on the optical axis at a different point from the central rays.

abetalipoproteinemia (ā-bā″tă-lĭp″ō-prō″tēn-ē′mē-ă) [Gr. *a-*, not, + *beta*

+ *lipos*, fat, + *protos*, first, + *haima*, blood] An inherited disorder marked by an absence of beta lipoproteins in the blood and low levels of cholesterol, fatty acids, and chylomicrons. The red blood cells have a thorny or spiked appearance (i.e., acanthocytosis). It is most often seen in Ashkenazi Jews. Symptoms include retinal macular degeneration and chronic progressive neurological deficits, which usually begin in childhood. Affected infants develop steatorrhea and growth retardation. Later clinical manifestations include ataxia; by adolescence, many patients are unable to walk. Vitamin E may be helpful in arresting the progression of neurological aspects. SYN: *Bassen-Kornzweig syndrome*. SEE: *acanthocyte* for illus.

abevacuation (ăb-ē-văk″ū-ā′shŭn) [L. *ab*, from, + *evacuare*, to empty] Abnormal evacuation, either excessive or deficient.

abeyance (ă-bā′ăns) [O. Fr.] A temporary suspension of activity, sensation, or pain.

ABG *arterial blood gas*.

ability An individual's performance capability for a given task, based on genetic makeup and learning.

cognitive a. The ability of the brain to process, retrieve, and store information. Impairment of these brain functions is common in patients with dementia, drug intoxication, or head injury.

constructional a. The ability to copy or draw shapes, figures, or lines (e.g., with a pen and paper). This nonverbal ability depends on the integration of several higher brain functions including perception, planning, and motor coordination. It is lost in organic brain syndromes.

functional a. The ability to perform activities of daily living, including bathing, dressing, and other independent living skills, such as shopping and housework. Many functional assessment tools are available to quantify functional ability. SEE: *activities of daily living*.

impaired transfer a. Limitation of independent movement between two nearby surfaces. This nursing diagnosis was approved at the NANDA 13th Conference, 1998. SEE: *Nursing Diagnoses Appendix*.

verbal a. The ability to use words, spoken or written, to communicate.

abiogenesis (ăb-ē-ō-jĕn′ĕ-sĭs) [Gr. *a*-, not, + *bios*, life, + *genesis*, generation, birth] Spontaneous generation of life; theoretical production of living organisms from nonliving matter. **abiogenetic, abiogenous** (-jĕ-nĕt′ĭk, ăb-ē-ŏj′ĭ-nŭs), *adj.*

abiosis (ăb-ē-ō′sĭs) [Gr. *a*-, not, + *bios*, life, + *osis*, condition] Absence of life. **abiotic,** *adj.*

abiotrophy (ăb-ē-ŏt′rō-fē) [″ + ″ + *trophe*, nourishment] Premature loss of vitality or degeneration of tissues and cells with consequent loss of endurance and resistance.

ablactation (ăb-lăk-tā′shŭn) [L. *ab*, from, + *lactatio*, suckling] **1.** The cessation of milk secretion. **2.** Weaning.

ablate (ăb-lāt′) [L. *ablatus*, taken away] To remove.

ablatio (ăb-lā′shē-ō) [L., carrying away] Ablation, removal, detachment.

a. placentae Abruptio placentae.

a. retinae Detachment of the retina. SEE: *retina*.

ablation (ăb-lā′shŭn) [L. *ab*, from, + *latus*, carried] Removal of a part, pathway, or function by surgery, chemical destruction, electrocautery, or radiofrequency.

endometrial a. Removal or destruction of the whole thickness of the endometrium and some superficial myometrium. The purpose is to remove all of the endometrial glandular material. This is done to treat benign disturbances of menstrual bleeding in women who do not wish to preserve fertility. Ablation may be done by use of the following: *Laser or electrosurgical*: YAG laser or high-powered "rollerball" electrocoagulation is used to destroy the uterine endometrium and 2 to 3 cm of myometrium. *Thermal*: A balloon catheter containing a heating element that delivers temperatures to 188°F (87°C) and a controller that monitors, displays, and regulates pressure, time, and temperature is used for heat-mediated endometrial destruction.

radiofrequency a. Ablation in which an electrode delivers a low-voltage, high-frequency current to cauterize and destroy abnormal tissues. Destruction of electrical conduction pathways in the heart with an intracardiac catheter removing the abnormal conducting tissues has been used to treat Wolff-Parkinson-White syndrome, atrioventricular reentrant tachycardia, and other cardiac arrhythmias.

ABLEDATA (ā′bul-dā-tah) A searchable Internet database of assistive technology information maintained by the National Institute on Disability and Rehabilitation Research of the U.S. Department of Education. The website address is www.abledata.com.

ablepharia (ăb-lĕ-fā′rē-ă) [Gr. *a*-, not, + *blepharon*, eyelid] Congenital absence of or reduction in the size of the eyelids. **ablepharous** (ă-blĕf′ă-rŭs), *adj.*

ablepsia (ă-blĕp′sē-ă) [Gr. *a*-, not, + *blepein*, to see] Blindness.

ablution (ăb-lū′shŭn) A cleansing or washing.

abnormal (ăb-nor′măl) [L. *ab*, from, + *norma*, rule] **1.** Diverging from a known standard or mean; exceptional. SYN: *aberrant*. **2.** Unexpected.

abnormality (ăb″nor-măl′ĭ-tē) Deviation from the normal. SYN: *aberration*.

Abnormal Involuntary Movement Scale test ABBR: AIMS test. A system used to assess abnormal involuntary movements, such as hand tremors or rhythmic movements of the tongue and jaw, that may result from the long-term administration of psychotropic drugs. The test is often given before patients are started on antipsychotic drugs and then readministered periodically to monitor side effects.

abocclusion (ăb″ŏ-kloo′zhŭn) Dentition in which the teeth of the mandible and the maxilla are not in contact.

aborad (ăb-ō′răd) [L. *ab*, from, + *oris*, mouth] Away from the mouth.

aboral (ăb-ō′răl) Opposite to, or away from, the mouth.

abort (ă-bort′) [L. *abortare*, to miscarry] **1.** To expel an embryo or fetus prior to viability. **2.** To arrest the progress of disease. **3.** To arrest growth or development. **4.** To discontinue an effort or project before its completion.

abortifacient (ă-bor-tĭ-fā′shĕnt) [L. *abortio*, abortion, + *facere*, to make] Anything used to cause or induce an abortion. SEE: *mifepristone*.

abortion (ă-bor′shŭn) [L. *abortio*] The spontaneous or induced termination of pregnancy before the fetus reaches a viable age. The legal definition of viability—usually 20 to 24 weeks—differs from state to state. Some premature neonates of fewer than 24 weeks or 500 g are viable. Symptoms of spontaneous abortion include abdominal cramps and vaginal bleeding, sometimes with the passage of clots or bits of membrane or tissue.

ETIOLOGY: Among the most common causes are faulty development of the embryo, abnormalities of the placenta, endocrine disturbances, acute infectious diseases, severe trauma, and shock. Other causes include problems related to the uterus, genetic factors, immunologic factors, and use of certain drugs.

PATIENT CARE: Assessment includes monitoring vital signs, fluid balance, and abortion status and progress. Historical data must include duration of pregnancy; Rh status; and time of onset, type, and intensity of abortion symptoms. Character and amount of vaginal bleeding are noted, and any passed tissue (embryonic or fetal) is preserved for laboratory examination. The patient is evaluated for shock, sepsis, and disseminated intravascular coagulation.

The patient's knowledge of her condition and any misconceptions are determined, and appropriate written and verbal information is provided. The patient's psychological status is assessed. A health care professional remains with the patient as much as possible to help allay anxiety, is aware of the patient's coping mechanisms, and is alert for responses such as grief, anger, guilt, sadness, depression, relief, or happiness.

If an elective abortion or surgical completion of the abortion is needed, the procedure and expected sensations are explained, and general preoperative and postoperative care are provided. If the patient is Rh negative and Coombs negative (not isoimmune), and if the pregnancy exceeded 8 weeks' gestation, Rho(D) is administered as prescribed within 72 hr of the abortion. Prescribed fluids, oxytocics, antibiotics, and transfusions are administered as required.

After abortion, the patient is instructed to report excessive bleeding, pain, inflammation, or fever and to avoid intercourse, tampon use, and douching until after the follow-up examination in 2 weeks.

complete a. An abortion in which the total products of conception have been expelled.

elective a. Voluntary termination of a pregnancy for other than medical reasons. The procedure may be recommended when the mother's mental or physical state would be endangered by continuation of the pregnancy or when the fetus has a condition incompatible with life. It may also be performed at the mother's request.

habitual a. Three or more consecutive spontaneous abortions.

imminent a. Impending abortion characterized by bleeding and colicky pains that increase. The cervix is usually effaced and patulous.

incomplete a. An abortion in which part of the products of conception has been retained in the uterus.

induced a. The intentional termination of a pregnancy by means of dilating the cervix and evacuating the uterus. Methods used during the first trimester include cervical dilation and surgical, suction, or vacuum curettage (D&C). In the second trimester, hypertonic saline may be instilled into the uterus or intrauterine and systemic prostaglandins may be used to generate labor and expulsion of the products of conception. SEE: *curettage, uterine; mifepristone*.

inevitable a. An abortion that cannot be halted.

infected a. Abortion accompanied by infection of retained material with resultant febrile reaction.

missed a. Abortion in which the fetus has died before completion of the 20th week of gestation but the products of conception are retained in the uterus for 8 weeks or longer.

partial-birth a. A lay term for a second- or third-trimester abortion, sometimes referred to medically as "dilation and extraction." The cranial contents of the fetus are evacuated prior to the removal of the fetus from the uterus.

septic a. Abortion in which there is an infection of the products of conception and the endometrial lining of the uterus.

spontaneous a. Abortion occurring without apparent cause. SYN: *miscarriage*. SEE: *Nursing Diagnoses Appendix*.

therapeutic a. Abortion performed when the pregnancy endangers the mother's mental or physical health or when the fetus has a known condition incompatible with life.

threatened a. The appearance of signs and symptoms of possible loss of the fetus. Vaginal bleeding with or without intermittent pain is usually the first sign. If the fetus is still alive and attachment to the uterus has not been interrupted, the pregnancy may continue. Absolute bedrest and sedation are recommended, with avoidance of coitus, douches, stress, or cathartics.

tubal a. **1.** A spontaneous abortion in which the fetus has been expelled through the distal end of the uterine tube. **2.** The escape of the products of conception into the peritoneal cavity by way of the uterine tube.

abortionist (ă-bor′shŭn-ĭst) One who performs an abortion.

abortive (ă-bor′tĭv) [L. *abortivus*] **1.** Preventing the completion of something. **2.** Abortifacient; that which prevents the normal continuation of pregnancy.

abortus (ă-bor′tŭs) [L.] A fetus born before 20 weeks' gestation or weighing less than 500 g.

aboulia SEE: *abulia*.

ABP *arterial blood pressure*.

abrachia (ă-brā′kē-ă) [Gr. *a-*, not, + *brachium*, arm] Congenital absence of arms.

abrachiocephalia (ă-brā″kē-ō-sĕ-fā′lē-ă) [″ + ″ + *kephale*, head] Congenital absence of arms and head.

abradant (ă-brād′ĕnt) An abrasive.

abrade (ă-brād′) [L. *ab*, from, + *radere*, to scrape] **1.** To chafe. **2.** To roughen or remove by friction.

abrasion (ă-brā′zhŭn) [″ + *radere*, to scrape] **1.** A scraping away of skin or mucous membrane as a result of injury or by mechanical means, as in dermabrasion for cosmetic purposes. SEE: *avulsion; bruise*. **2.** The wearing away of the substance of a tooth. It usually results from mastication, but may be done by mechanical or chemical means.

abrasive **1.** Producing abrasion. **2.** That which abrades.

abreaction (ăb″rē-ăk′shŭn) [L. *ab*, from, + *re*, again, + *actus*, acting] In psychoanalysis, the release of emotion by consciously recalling or acting out a painful experience that had been forgotten or repressed. The painful or consciously intolerable experience may become bearable as a result of the insight gained during this process. SEE: *catharsis* (2).

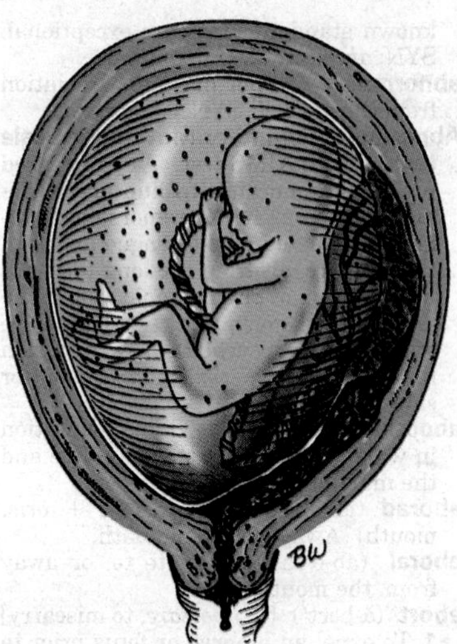

PARTIAL SEPARATION (APPARENT HEMORRHAGE)

ABRUPTIO PLACENTAE

abruptio (ă-brŭp′shē-ō) [L. *abruptus*] A tearing away from.

PATHOLOGY: Three types of abruption occur: *a. centralis:* a partial central detachment with hidden bleeding between the placenta and the uterine wall; occasionally, blood will invade the myometrium (Couvelaire uterus); *a. complete:* total placental detachment, marked by profuse vaginal bleeding, profound fetal distress, and rapid fetal demise; *a. marginalis:* partial separation of an edge of the placenta, as evidenced by vaginal bleeding. The large amount of circulating thromboplastin may cause a coagulation defect to occur, resulting in hypofibrinogenemia. SEE: *Couvelaire uterus; disseminated intravascular coagulation*.

PROGNOSIS: Prognoses varies with the type, extent, and immediacy of diagnosis, associated complications, and treatment. Although maternal mortality is unusual, other than as noted, the perinatal mortality is between 20% and 30%.

a. placentae The sudden premature detachment of the placenta from a normal uterine site of implantation. The incidence of abruptio is 1:120 births, and the risk of recurrence in later pregnancies is much higher than that for cohorts. SYN: *ablatio placentae*. SEE: illus; *placenta*.

ETIOLOGY: The cause is unknown; however, the condition often is associated with toxemia and may be related to current cocaine abuse.

SYMPTOMS: These vary with the type and extent of placental detachment; however, severe, unremitting pain is characteristic of central and complete abruptions. The abdomen is taut, the uterus is extremely tender, and fetal heart tones may or may not be present. If detachment is extensive and the bleeding profuse, the woman exhibits signs of hypovolemic shock.

PATHOLOGY: Extravasation of blood occurs between the placenta and the uterine wall, occasionally between muscle fibers of the uterus.

TREATMENT: This varies with the type and extent of abruption. Women experiencing only a small marginal separation from the uterine wall may be confined to bed and monitored closely for signs of further threat to maternal or fetal status. If prematurity also is a factor, the woman may be given betamethasone to expedite development of fetal pulmonary surfactant. If the woman is at or near term, induction of labor and vaginal delivery may be an option. SEE: *betamethasone*.

Supportive treatment and prompt surgical intervention is indicated for women who have moderate to severe abruptions. Complete detachment calls for immediate cesarean delivery, concomitant treatment of shock and, sometimes, management of a coagulation defect. The massive loss of blood jeopardizes the mother's survival; fetal mortality is 100%. If the uterus fails to contract after the surgical delivery, immediate hysterectomy may be necessary. SEE: *Couvelaire uterus*.

PATIENT CARE: Early recognition and prompt management of the event and any associated complications are vital. The woman's vital signs, fundal height, uterine contractions, labor progress, and fetal status data are monitored, including heart rate and rhythm. Any changes are noted, such as prolonged decelerations in fetal heart rate or alterations in baseline variability; uterine tetany; complaints of sudden, severe abdominal pain; and the advent of or increase in vaginal bleeding. Vaginal blood loss is estimated by weighing perineal pads and subtracting the known weight of dry pads. The interval between pad changes, the character and amount of the bleeding, and the degree of pad saturation are noted. Prescribed IV fluids and medications are administered through a large-bore catheter. A central venous pressure line may be placed to provide access to the venous circulation, and an indwelling catheter is inserted to monitor urinary output and fluid balance. A calm atmosphere is maintained, and the patient's verbalization is encouraged. The patient is assisted in coping with her fears and anxiety. Questions are answered truthfully, comfort measures are implemented, and reassurance is provided as possible and consistent with the current situation and prognosis. All procedures are explained, and the woman and her family are prepared for induction of labor, vaginal delivery, or cesarean birth as appropriate. The possibility of neonatal death should be tactfully mentioned; the neonate's survival depends primarily on gestational age, blood loss, and associated hypertensive disorders. SEE: *Nursing Diagnoses Appendix*.

abscess (ăb′sĕs) [L. *abscessus*, a going away] A localized collection of pus in any body part that results from invasion of a pyogenic bacterium or other pathogen. *Staphylococcus aureus* is a common cause. The abscess is surrounded by a membrane of variable strength created by macrophages, fibrin, and granulation tissue. Abscesses can disrupt function in adjacent tissues and can be life threatening if the swelling interferes with breathing or vital organ function. SEE: illus; *inflammation; pus; suppuration; Standard and Universal Precautions Appendix*.

acute a. An abscess associated with significant inflammation, producing intense heat, redness, swelling, and throbbing pain. The tissue over the abscess becomes elevated, soft, and eventually unstable (fluctuant) and discolored as the abscess comes to a head (points). An abscess can rupture spontaneously or be drained via an incision. If it is left untreated, the pathogens may spread to adjacent tissues or to other parts of the body via the bloodstream. Appearance of or increase in fever may indicate sepsis.

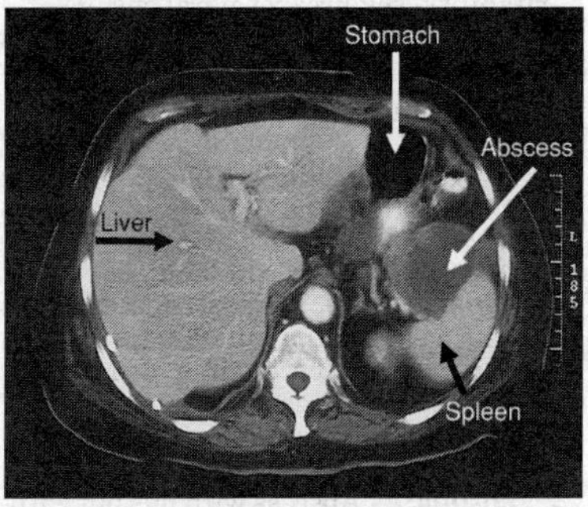

INTRA-ABDOMINAL ABSCESS

CT scan shows abscess between stomach and spleen (Courtesy of Harvey Hatch, MD, Curry General Hospital)

alveolar a. Abscess about the root of a tooth in the alveolar cavity. It is usually the result of necrosis and infection of dental pulp following dental caries. SEE: *periapical a.*

amebic a. An abscess caused by *Entamoeba histolytica.* SYN: *endamebic a.*

anorectal a. Abscess in the ischiorectal fossa. SYN: *ischiorectal a.*

apical a. **1.** Abscess at the apex of a lung. **2.** Periapical a.

appendicular a. Pus formation around an inflamed vermiform appendix.

axillary a. Abscess or multiple abscesses in the axilla.

Bartholin a. Abscess of Bartholin's gland.

bicameral a. Abscess with two pockets.

bile duct a. Abscess of the bile duct. SYN: *cholangitic a.*

biliary a. Abscess of the gallbladder.

bone a. Brodie's a.

brain a. An intracranial abscess involving the brain or its membranes. It is seldom primary but usually occurs secondary to infections of the middle ear, nasal sinuses, face, or skull or from contamination from penetrating wounds or skull fractures. It may also have a metastatic origin arising from septic foci in the lungs (bronchiectasis, empyema, lung abscess), in bone (osteomyelitis), or in the heart (endocarditis). Infection of nerve tissue by the invading organism results in necrosis and liquefaction of the tissue, with edema of surrounding tissues. Brain abscesses may be acute, subacute, or chronic. Their clinical manifestations depend on the part of the brain involved, the size of the abscess, the virulence of the infecting organism, and other factors. SYN: *cerebral a.; intracranial a.* SEE: *Nursing Diagnoses Appendix.*

SYMPTOMS: Symptoms may include headache, fever, vomiting, malaise, irritability, seizures, or paralysis.

TREATMENT: The usual treatment is chemotherapy. Surgical intervention may be required.

breast a. Mammary a.

Brodie's a. Suppuration of the articular end of a bone, esp. the tibia. SYN: *bone a.*

bursal a. Abscess in a bursa.

canalicular a. Breast abscess that discharges into the milk ducts.

caseous a. Abscess in which the pus has a cheesy appearance.

cerebral a. Brain a.

cholangitic a. Bile duct a.

chronic a. Abscess with pus but without signs of inflammation. It usually develops slowly as a result of liquefaction of tuberculous tissue. It may occur anywhere in or on the body but occurs more frequently in the spine, hips, genitourinary tract, and lymph glands. Symptoms may be very mild. Pain when present is caused by pressure on surrounding parts; tenderness is often absent. Chronic septic changes accompanied by afternoon fever may occur. Amyloid disease may develop if the abscess persists for a prolonged period. SYN: *cold a.*

circumtonsillar a. Peritonsillar a.

cold a. Chronic a.

collar-button a. Two pus-containing cavities, one larger than the other, connected by a narrow channel.

dental a. Acute inflammatory infection within the maxilla or mandible. Infections are classified as periapical or periodontal. SEE: *periapical a.; periodontal a.*

dentoalveolar a. Abscess in the alveolar process surrounding the root of a tooth.

diffuse a. A collection of pus not circumscribed by a well-defined capsule.

dry a. Abscess that disappears without pointing or breaking.

embolic a. Abscess due to movement of infectious material from the site of an infection to another site.

emphysematous a. Abscess containing air or gas, produced by organisms such as *Clostridium perfringens.* SYN: *gas a.; tympanitic a.*

endamebic a. Amebic a.

epidural a. Extradural a.

extradural a. Abscess on the dura mater. SYN: *epidural a.*

fecal a. Abscess containing feces. SYN: *stercoral a.*

filarial a. Abscess caused by filaria.

follicular a. Abscess in a follicle.

fungal a. Abscess caused by a fungus.

gas a. Emphysematous a.

gingival a. Abscess of the gum.

helminthic a. Worm a.

hemorrhagic a. Abscess containing blood.

hepatic a. Abscess of the liver, either a pyrogenic or amebic abscess. SYN: *liver a.*

hot a. Acute a.

hypostatic a. Wandering a.

idiopathic a. Abscess due to an unknown cause.

iliac a. Abscess in the iliac region.

iliopsoas a. An abscess in the psoas and iliacus muscles.

intracranial a. Brain a.

intradural a. Abscess within the layers of the dura mater.

intraperitoneal a. Peritoneal a.

ischiorectal a. Anorectal a.

kidney a. One or more abscesses arising in the kidney, typically following pyelonephritis or a blood-borne infection. The most common causative organisms are gram-negative bacteria from the lower urinary tract that spread to the kidneys and *Staphylococcus aureus* from a blood-borne infection. Immunocompromised patients may develop abscesses caused by *Nocardia, Candida,* or *Aspergillus.* Occasionally, mycobacterium tuberculosis and *Echinococcus* are responsible agents. SYN: *renal a.*

TREATMENT: Antimicrobial agents are used in combination with surgical drainage. Occasionally, nephrectomy or retroperitoneal exploration are required.

lacrimal a. Suppuration of a lacrimal gland or in a lacrimal duct.

lateral alveolar a. Abscess in periodontal tissue.

liver a. Hepatic a.

lumbar a. Abscess in the lumbar region.

lung a. Pulmonary a.

lymphatic a. Abscess of a lymph node.

mammary a. Abscess in the female breast, esp. one involving the glandular tissue. It usually occurs during lactation or weaning. SYN: *breast a.*

mastoid a. Suppuration of the mastoid portion of the temporal bone.

metastatic a. Secondary abscess at a distance from the focus of infection.

miliary a. Multiple small embolic abscesses.

milk a. Mammary abscess during lactation.

mycotic a. Abscess caused by fungi.

nocardial a. Abscess caused by *Nocardia.*

orbital a. Suppuration in the orbit.

palatal a. Abscess in a maxillary tooth, erupting toward the palate.

palmar a. Purulent effusion into the tissues of the palm of the hand.

pancreatic a. Abscess of pancreatic tissue, usually as a complication of acute pancreatitis or abdominal surgery.

parafrenal a. Abscess on the side of the frenulum of the penis. It usually involves Tyson's gland.

parametric a. Abscess between the folds of the broad ligaments of the uterus.

paranephric a. Abscess in the tissues around the kidney.

parapancreatic a. Abscess in the tissues adjacent to the pancreas.

parietal a. Periodontal abscess arising in the periodontal tissue other than the orifice through which the vascular supply enters the dental pulp.

parotid a. Abscess of the parotid gland.

pelvic a. Abscess of the pelvic peritoneum, esp. in Douglas' pouch.

perianal a. Abscess of the skin around the anus.

periapical a. An accumulation of acute inflammatory cells at the apex of a tooth, usually resulting from dental caries or tooth trauma. It may be classified further as an acute periapical abscess, a chronic periapical abscess, a periapical granuloma, or a radicular cyst. SYN: *apical a.* (2); *root a.*

pericemental a. Alveolar abscess not involving the apex of a tooth.

pericoronal a. Abscess around the crown of an unerupted molar tooth.

peridental a. Abscess of periodontal tissue.

perinephric a. Abscess in tissue around the kidney.

periodontal a. A localized area of acute or chronic inflammation with pus formation found in the gingiva, periodontal pockets, or periodontal ligament.

peripleuritic a. Abscess in the tissue surrounding the parietal pleura.

periproctic a. Abscess in the areolar tissue about the anus.

peritoneal a. Abscess within the peritoneal cavity usually following peritonitis. SYN: *intraperitoneal a.*

peritonsillar a. Abscess of the tissue around the tonsillar capsule. Needle aspiration of the abscess, with subsequent antibiotic therapy, is an effective treatment in 90% of cases. SYN: *circumtonsillar a.*

periureteral a. Abscess in the area around a ureter.

periurethral a. Abscess in tissue surrounding the urethra.

perivesical a. Abscess in tissue around the urinary bladder.

pneumococcic a. Abscess due to infection with pneumococci.

prelacrimal a. Abscess of the lacrimal bone producing a swelling at the inner canthus of the eye.

premammary a. Subcutaneous or subareolar abscess of the mammary gland.

prostatic a. Abscess within the prostate gland.

protozoal a. Abscess caused by a protozoon.

psoas a. Abscess with pus descending in the sheath of the psoas muscle due to vertebral disease, usually of tuberculous origin.

pulmonary a. Abscess of the lungs; suppuration of lung tissue with one or more localized areas of necrosis, resulting in pulmonary cavitation. SYN: *lung a.; empyema.*

pulp a. **1.** A cavity discharging pus formed in the pulp of a tooth. **2.** Abscess of the tissues of the pulp of a finger.

pyemic a. A metastatic abscess, usually multiple, due to pyogenic organisms.

rectal a. Abscess in the rectum.

renal a. Kidney a.

retrocecal a. An abscess located behind the cecum.

retromammary a. Abscess between the mammary gland and the chest wall.

retroperitoneal a. Abscess located

between the peritoneum and the posterior abdominal wall.

retropharyngeal a. Abscess of the lymph nodes in the walls of the pharynx. It sometimes simulates diphtheritic pharyngitis.

ETIOLOGY: *Staphylococcus aureus* and group A hemolytic streptococcus are the most common pathogens.

SYMPTOMS: Typically, a history of pharyngitis is elicited. This is is followed by high fever, dysphagia, and refusal to eat. The condition progresses to respiratory distress with hyperextension of the head ("sniffing position"), tachypnea, labored breathing, and drooling. An exquisitely tender bulge in the pharyngeal wall is usually evident.

TREATMENT: A retropharyngeal abscess, if fluctuant, should be treated with incision and drainage. If recognized before it becomes fluctuant, the abscess should be treated with antibiotics, intravenously administered if the patient is unable to swallow.

retrovesical a. Abscess behind the bladder.

root a. Periapical a.

sacrococcygeal a. Abscess over the sacrum and coccyx.

septicemic a. Abscess resulting from septicemia.

spermatic a. Abscess of the seminiferous tubules.

spinal a. Abscess due to necrosis of a vertebra.

splenic a. Abscess of the spleen.

stercoraceous a. Fecal a.

sterile a. Abscess from which microorganisms cannot be cultivated.

stitch a. Abscess formed about a stitch or suture.

streptococcal a. Abscess caused by streptococci.

subaponeurotic a. Abscess beneath an aponeurosis or fascia.

subarachnoid a. Abscess of the midlayer of the covering of the brain and spinal cord.

subareolar a. Abscess underneath the areola of the mammary gland, sometimes draining through the nipple.

subdiaphragmatic a. Abscess beneath the diaphragm. SYN: *subphrenic a.*

subdural a. Abscess beneath the dura of the brain or spinal cord.

subfascial a. Abscess beneath the fascia.

subgaleal a. Abscess beneath the galea aponeurotica (i.e., the epicranial aponeurosis).

subpectoral a. Abscess beneath the pectoral muscles.

subperiosteal a. Bone abscess below the periosteum.

subperitoneal a. Abscess between the parietal peritoneum and the abdominal wall.

subphrenic a. Subdiaphragmatic a.

subscapular a. Abscess between the serratus anterior and the posterior thoracic wall.

subungual a. Abscess beneath the fingernail. It may follow injury from a pin, needle, or splinter.

sudoriparous a. Abscess of a sweat gland.

suprahepatic a. Abscess in the suspensory ligament between the liver and the diaphragm.

syphilitic a. Abscess occurring in the tertiary stage of syphilis, esp. in bone.

thecal a. Abscess in a tendon sheath.

thymus a. Abscess of the thymus.

tonsillar a. Acute suppurative tonsillitis.

tooth a. Alveolar a.

tropical a. Amebic abscess of the liver.

tuberculous a. Chronic a.

tubo-ovarian a. Abscess involving both the fallopian tube and the ovary.

tympanitic a. Emphysematous a.

tympanocervical a. Abscess arising in the tympanum and extending to the neck.

tympanomastoid a. A combined abscess of the tympanum and mastoid.

urethral a. Abscess in the urethra.

urinary a. Abscess caused by escape of urine into the tissues.

urinous a. Abscess that contains pus and urine.

verminous a. Worm a.

wandering a. Abscess at a distance from the focus of disease with pus along fascial sheaths of muscles. SYN: *hypostatic a.*

warm a. Acute a.

worm a. An abscess caused by or containing insect larvae, worms, or other animal parasites. SYN: *helminthic a.; verminous a.*

abscissa (ăb-sĭs′ă) [L. *abscindere*, to cut off] The horizontal line, or x-axis, in a graph of a two-dimensional coordinate system wherein horizontal and perpendicular lines are crossed in order to provide a frame of reference. The ordinate is the vertical line, or y-axis. SEE: illus.

abscission (ăb-sĭ′zhŭn) [L. *abscindere*, to cut off] Removal by excision.

abscopal (ăb-skō′păl) Concerning the effect of radiation on tissues at some distance from the actual radiation site or target.

absence (ăb′sĕnz) **1.** Brief temporary loss of consciousness, as may occur in petit mal epilepsy. SYN: *absentia epileptica*. **2.** Lack of development of a structure.

absenteeism Prolonged or repeated absence from work, school, or assigned duties.

absentia epileptica (ăb-sĕn′shē-ă) [L., absence] Momentary loss of consciousness. There is no convulsion but there

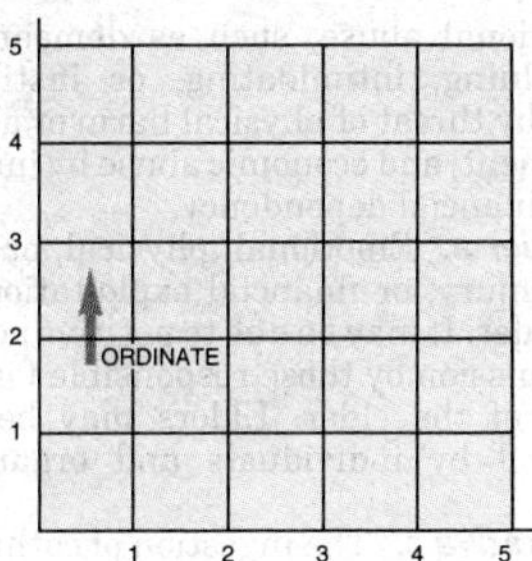

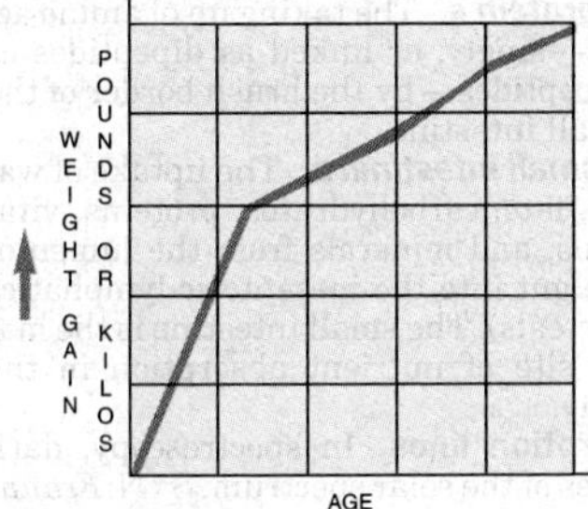

ABSCISSA (HORIZONTAL AXIS)

may be transient stereotyped muscle movement. SEE: *absence seizure; epilepsy.*

abs. feb. [L.] *absente febre,* in the absence of fever.

Absidia (ăb-sĭd′ē-ă) Genus of pathogenic fungi of the order Phycomycetes and the family Mucoraceae.

absinthe, absinth (ăb′sĭnth) [L. *absinthium*, wormwood] A liquor containing oil of wormwood, anise, and other herbs. It is highly toxic, esp. to the nervous system.

absinthism (ăb′sĭn-thĭzm) Deterioration of the nervous system following excessive use of absinthe.

absolute Unrestricted, complete.

absorb (ăb-sorb′) [L. *absorbere*, to suck in] To take in, suck up, or imbibe. SEE: *absorption; adsorb; adsorption.*

absorbance (ăb-sor′băns) The ability of a material or tissue to absorb radiation.

absorbefacient (ăb-sor″bĕ-fā′shĕnt) [L. *absorbere*, to suck in, + *facere*, to make] **1.** Causing absorption. **2.** An agent that causes absorption.

absorbent (ăb-sor′bĕnt) **1.** A substance that absorbs. **2.** Having the power to absorb.

absorptiometer (ăb-sorp″shē-ŏm′ĕ-tĕr) [L. *absorptio*, absorption, + Gr. *metron*, measure] **1.** An instrument that measures the thickness of a layer of liquid, drawn by capillary attraction, between glass plates. **2.** An instrument that measures the absorption of gas by a liquid.

absorptiometry A radiographic technique for measuring the dissipation of x-ray energy as the beam goes through tissue.

dual beam a. A radiographic technique to measure tissue density by measuring the amount of absorbed radiation. One use is to detect bone loss in the spine and hips.

dual photon a. A dual-energy x-ray examination, used to measure bone mass in patients suspected of having osteoporosis. SEE: *bone densitometry.*

absorption (ăb-sorp′shŭn) [L. *absorptio*] **1.** The taking up of liquids by solids, or of gases by solids or liquids. **2.** The taking up of light or of its rays by black or colored rays. **3.** The taking up by the body of radiant heat, causing a rise in body temperature. **4.** The reduction in intensity of an x-ray photon as it passes through a substance or a beam of light as it passes through a solution (used in clinical photometry as well as nuclear methods). **5.** The passage of a substance through some surface of the body into body fluids and tissues, such as the passage of ether through the respiratory epithelium of the lungs into the blood during anesthesia or the passage of oil of wintergreen through the skin (which is the result of several processes: diffusion, filtration, and osmosis).

carbohydrate a. The taking up of fructose, galactose, and glucose—the monosaccharides—by the brush border of the small intestine.

colonic a. The normal absorption of water (important in the conservation of body fluids) and byproducts of bacterial metabolism, esp. in the ascending colon. Some nutrients and drugs are absorbed by the lower bowel.

cutaneous a. Absorption through the skin. SYN: *percutaneous a.*

external a. Absorption of material by the skin and mucous membrane.

fat a. The taking up of glycerols and fatty acids, suspended in bile salts, into the villi of the small intestine.

gastric a. Absorption of water, alcohol, and some salts through the gastric mucosa.

mouth a. Oral absorption of material. Some substances, but no nutrients, can be absorbed from the mouth; some drugs, esp. alkaloids, can be absorbed through the oral mucosa.

parenteral a. Absorption from a site other than the gastrointestinal tract.

pathological a. Absorption of a substance normally excreted (e.g., urine) or of a product of disease processes (e.g., pus) into the blood or lymph.

percutaneous a. Cutaneous a.

protein a. The taking up of amino acids—singly, or linked as dipeptides or tripeptides—by the brush border of the small intestine.

small intestinal a. The uptake of water, fats, carbohydrates, proteins, vitamins, and minerals from the lumen of the gut into the mesenteric lymphatics (lacteals). The small intestine is the major site of nutrient absorption in the body.

absorption lines In spectroscopy, dark lines of the solar spectrum. SYN: *Fraunhofer's lines.*

absorptive (ăb-sorp'tĭv) Absorbent.

abstinence (ăb'stĭ-nĕns) [L. *abstinere*, to abstain] Going without something voluntarily, esp. refraining from indulgence in food, alcoholic beverages, or sexual intercourse.

abstract (ăb'străkt, ăb-străkt') [L. *abstrahere*, to draw away] **1.** A preparation containing the soluble principles of a drug concentrated and mixed with lactose. **2.** A summary or abridgment of an article, book, or address.

discharge a. A summary of a patient's record from a health care facility that is prepared after the time of discharge.

abstraction (ăb-străk'shŭn) **1.** Removal or separation of a constituent from a mixture or compound. **2.** Distraction of the mind; inattention or absent-mindedness. **3.** The process whereby thoughts and ideas are generalized and dissociated from particular concrete instances or material objects.

abterminal (ăb-tĕr'mĭ-năl) [L. *ab*, from, + *terminus*, end] Away from an end and toward the center, said of electric currents in muscles.

abulia (ă-bū'lē-ă) [Gr. *a*-, not, + *boule*, will] **1.** Absence of or decreased ability to exercise willpower (or initiative) or to make decisions. **2.** Syndrome of slow reaction, lack of spontaneity, and brief spoken responses. It may be part of the clinical picture that accompanies injuries to or diseases of the internal capsules, basal ganglia, or frontal lobes of the brain.

abuse (ă-būs') [L. *abusus*, using up] **1.** Misuse; excessive or improper use (e.g., abuse of alcohol or other agents). **2.** Injurious, pathological, or malignant treatment of another person or living thing, for example by verbal, physical, or sexual assault; by depriving others of the means to maintain their own health, nutrition, or safety; or by exposing others to unnecessary risks.

domestic a. The mistreatment or injury of individuals in a domestic setting. Forms include physical violence, such as striking or forcibly restraining a family member; passive abuse, such as withholding access to resources needed to maintain health; psychological or emotional abuse, such as demeaning, devaluing, intimidating, or instilling fear by threat of physical harm or abandonment; and economic abuse by imposing financial dependency.

elder a. Emotional, physical, or sexual injury, or financial exploitation, of an elder. It may be due to positive action or omission by those responsible for the care of the elder. Elders may be exploited by individuals and organizations.

laxative a. The ingestion of cathartic drugs to relieve perceived constipation (when none is present), or to prevent the absorption of nutrients (e.g., in bulimia). Patients who consume excessive quantities of laxatives may complain of chronic diarrhea or may present with illnesses caused by electrolyte deficiencies.

sexual a. **Fondling, rape, sexual assault, or sexual molestation. The abuser may be a male or female adult or child. The victim may be of the same sex as the abuser or of the opposite sex. SEE:** *incest; rape.*

spouse a. Emotional, physical, or sexual mistreatment of one's spouse.

substance a. Abuse of drugs, alcohol, or other substances that alter mood or behavior. SEE: *Nursing Diagnoses Appendix.*

abutment (ă-bŭt'mĕnt) [Fr. *abouter*, to place end to end] A structure that provides support for fixed restorations and prosthetic devices. Examples of dental abutments include natural teeth and implants.

ABVD *Adriamycin, bleomycin, vinblastine,* and *dacarbazine*, a combination of chemotherapy drugs.

A.C. *acromioclavicular; adrenal cortex; air conduction; alternating current; anodal closure; atriocarotid; auriculocarotid; axiocervical.*

Ac Symbol for the element actinium.

a.c. L. *ante cibum*, before meals.

acacia (ă-kā'shē-ă) Gum arabic. A dried gummy exudation from the tree *Acacia senegal*. It is used as a suspending agent in pharmaceutical products.

acalculia (ă-kăl-kū'lē-ă) [Gr. *a*-, not, + L. *calculare*, to reckon] A learning or speech disorder characterized by the inability to perform simple arithmetic operations.

acampsia (ă-kămp'sē-ă) [" + *kamptein*, to bend] Inflexibility of a limb; rigidity; ankylosis.

acanth- SEE: *acantho-.*

acantha [Gr. *akantha*, thorn] **1.** The spine. **2.** A vertebral spinous process.

acanthamebiasis (ă-kăn"thă-mē-bī'ă-sĭs) A rare disease of the brain and meninges caused by free-living amebae. The organisms invade the nasal mucosa of persons swimming in fresh water, the natural habitat of *Acanthamoeba* and

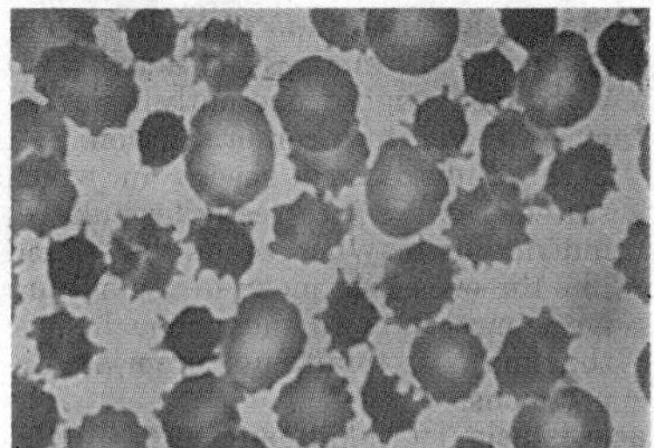

ACANTHOCYTES IN PATIENT WITH ABETALIPOPROTENEMIA (X6400)

Naegleria fowleri. The organisms invade the central nervous system through the olfactory foramina. The symptoms begin after an incubation period of 2 to 15 days and are those of acute meningitis. Debilitated or immunocompromised persons are esp. susceptible. Diagnosis is made by finding the amebae in the spinal fluid. Treatment is virtually ineffective and most patients die within a week of onset. Swimming pools adequately treated with chlorine are not a source of the amebae. SEE: *meningoencephalitis, primary amebic.*

acanthesthesia (ă-kăn″thĕs-thē′zē-ă) [Gr. *akantha*, thorn, + *aisthesis*, sensation] A sensation as of a pinprick; a form of paresthesia.

Acanthia lectularia (ă-kăn′thē-ă lĕk-tū-lă′rē-ă) Cimex lectularius.

acanthiomeatal line An imaginary line through the acanthion and external auditory meatus.

acanthion [Gr. *akanthion*, little thorn] The tip of the anterior nasal spine.

acantho-, acanth- [Gr. *akantha*, thorn] Combining forms meaning *thorn, spine.*

Acanthocephala (ă-kăn″thō-sĕf′ă-lă) [″ + *kephale*, head] A class of wormlike entozoa related to the Platyhelminthes, including a few species parasitic in humans.

acanthocephaliasis (ă-kăn″thō-sĕf-ă-lī′ă-sĭs) An infestation with Acanthocephala.

Acanthocheilonema perstans (ă-kăn″thō-kī″lō-nē′mă pĕr′stăns) *Dipetalonema perstans.* A species of filaria that infects wild or domestic animals and occasionally humans. In humans, the adult worm migrates to the subcutaneous tissue and produces a nodule. Rarely, the adult worm may be seen beneath the conjunctiva.

acanthocyte (ă-kăn′thō-sīt″) [Gr. *akantha*, thorn, + *kytos*, cell] An abnormal erythrocyte that in wet preparations has cytoplasmic projections so that the cell appears to be covered with thorns. SEE: illus.; *abetalipoproteinemia.*

acanthocytosis (ă-kăn″thō-sī-tō′sĭs) [″ + ″ + *osis*, condition] Acanthocytes in the blood.

acanthoid (ă-kăn′thoyd) [″ + *eidos*, form, shape] Thorny; spiny; of a spinous nature.

acanthokeratodermia (ă-kăn″thō-kĕr″ă-tō-dĕr′mē-ă) [″ + *keras*, horn, + *derma*, skin] Hypertrophy of the horny portion of the skin of the palms of the hands and soles of the feet, and thickening of the nails.

acantholysis (ă-kăn-thŏl′ĭ-sĭs) [″ + *lysis*, dissolution] Any disease of the skin accompanied by degeneration of the cohesive elements of the cells of the outer or horny layer of the skin.

a. bullosa Obsolete term for epidermolysis bullosa.

acanthoma (ăk″ăn-thō′mă) [″ + *oma*, tumor] A benign tumor of the skin. It was previously used to denote skin cancer.

a. adenoides cysticum A cystic tumor, often familial, occurring on the chest and face and in the axillary regions. The tumor contains tissues resembling sweat glands and hair follicles. SYN: *epithelioma adenoides cysticum.*

acanthopelvis, acanthopelyx (ă-kăn″thō-pĕl′vĭs, -pĕl′ĭks) [″ + *pelyx*, pelvis] A prominent and sharp pubic spine on a rachitic pelvis.

acanthosis (ăk″ăn-thō′sĭs) [″ + *osis*, condition] Increased thickness of the prickle cell layer of the skin. **acanthotic** (ăk″ăn-thŏt′ĭk), *adj.*

a. nigricans A skin disorder in which dark brown or gray velvety plaques appear on the skin, typically under the arms, in the groin or upper thighs, on the neck, or near the genitalia. They usually appear in patients with relative insulin excess, such as adults with obesity, type 2 diabetes mellitus, or polycystic ovaries. The condition may rarely be associated with internal malignancy. SYN: *keratosis nigricans.*

acapnia (ă-kăp′nē-ă) [Gr. *akapnos*, smokeless] Literally, the absence of carbon dioxide. The term is incorrectly used to indicate less than the normal amount of carbon dioxide in blood and tissues (e.g., after overbreathing). SYN: *hypocapnia.* **acapnial** (ă-căp′nē-ăl), *adj.*

acarbia (ă-kăr′bē-ă) Decrease of bicarbonate in the blood.

acarbose (ăk′ăr-bōz) An oral antidiabetic drug that delays the absorption of glucose from the gastrointestinal tract. It can be used to treat type 2 (adult-onset) diabetes mellitus. Many patients treated with this agent develop abdominal bloating and gas.

acardia (ă-kăr′dē-ă) [Gr. *a-*, not, + *kardia*, heart] Congenital absence of the heart. **acardiac** (ă-kăr′dē-ăk), *adj.*

acardiacus (ă-kăr-dī′ă-kŭs) A parasitic twin without a heart, therefore using the circulation of its twin. SYN: *acardius.*

acardiotrophia (ă-kăr″dē-ō-trō′fē-a) [Gr. *a-*, not, + *kardia*, heart + *trophe*, nutrition] Atrophy of the heart.

acardius Acardiacus.

acariasis (ăk″ă-rī′ă-sĭs) [L. *acarus*, mite, + Gr. *-iasis*, condition] Any disease caused by a mite or acarid. SYN: *acarinosis; acaridiasis.*

demodectic a. Infection of hair follicles with *Demodex folliculorum.*

sarcoptic a. Infestation with a burrowing mite, *Sarcoptes scabiei,* which deposits its eggs in the burrows. SEE: *scabies.*

acaricide (ă-kăr′ĭ-sīd) [″ + *caedere*, to kill] **1.** An agent that destroys acarids. **2.** Destroying a member of the order Acarina.

acarid, acaridan (ăk′ă-rĭd, ă-kăr′ĭ-dăn) [L. *acarus*, mite] A tick or mite of the order Acarina.

Acaridae A family of mites that irritate the skin. SEE: *itch, grain; itch, grocer's.*

acaridiasis (ă-kăr″ĭ-dī′ă-sĭs) [″ + Gr. *-iasis*, condition] Acariasis.

Acarina (ăk″ă-rī′nă) An order of the class Arachnida that includes a large number of species of minute animals known as mites or ticks. Most are skin parasites, with infestation causing local dermatitis with pruritus and sometimes systemic reactions. They are vectors of a number of diseases. SEE: *Ixodidae; Lyme disease; Sarcoptidae; scabies; tick.*

acarinosis (ă-kăr″ĭ-nō′sĭs) [L. *acarus*, mite, + Gr. *osis*, condition] Acariasis.

acarodermatitis (ăk″ă-rō-dĕr″mă-tī′tĭs) [″ + Gr. *derma*, skin, + *itis*, inflammation] Skin inflammation caused by a mite.

acaroid (ăk′ă-royd) [″ + Gr. *eidos*, form, shape] Resembling a mite.

acarology (ăk″ă-rŏl′ō-jē) [″ + Gr. *logos*, word, reason] The study of mites and ticks.

acarophobia (ăk″ăr-ō-fō′bē-ă) [″ + Gr. *phobos*, fear] Abnormal fear of small objects such as pins, needles, worms, mites, and other small insects. This may include fear of parasites crawling under the skin.

Acarus (ăk′ăr-ŭs) [L., mite] A genus of mites.

A. folliculorum Demodex folliculorum.

A. scabiei *Sarcoptes scabiei.* SEE: *scabies; Sarcoptidae.*

acarus [L.] Any mite or tick.

acaryote (ă-kăr′ē-ōt) [Gr. *a-*, not, + *karyon*, nucleus] Without a nucleus. SEE: *eukaryote; prokaryote.*

acatalasemia Acatalasia.

acatalasia (ă″kăt-ă-lā′zē-ă) A rare inherited disease in which there is an absence of the enzyme catalase. The gingival and oral tissues are particularly susceptible to bacterial invasion with subsequent gangrenous changes and alveolar bone destruction. SYN: *acatalasemia.*

acataphasia (ă-kăt″ă-fā′zē-ă) [″ + *kataphasis*, affirmation] **1.** Inability to verbalize thoughts coherently. This condition is due to a cerebral lesion. **2.** A form of disordered speech in which statements are incorrectly formulated; individuals may use words that sound like the ones they mean to use but are not appropriate to their thoughts, or they may use totally inappropriate expressions.

acatastasia (ă-kăt-ăs-tā′zē-ă) [Gr. *akatastasis*, disorder] Irregularity; deviation from the normal.

acathexis (ă″kă-thĕks′ĭs) [Gr. *a-*, not, + *kathexis*, retention] In psychoanalysis, a lack of emotion toward something that is unconsciously important to the individual.

acathisia (ă″kă-thĭz′ē-ă) [″ + *kathisis*, sitting] Akathisia.

acaudal, acaudate (ā-kaw′dăl, -dāt) [″ + L. *cauda*, tail] Having no tail.

ACC *anodal closure contraction.*

acc *accommodation.*

accelerated idioventricular rhythm ABBR: AIVR. An abnormal ectopic cardiac rhythm originating in the ventricular conducting system. This may occur intermittently after myocardial infarction at a rate of 60 to 100 beats per minute.

acceleration (ăk-sĕl″ĕr-ā′shŭn) [L. *accelerans*, hastening] **1.** An increase in the speed of an action or function, such as pulse or respiration. **2.** The rate of change in velocity for a given unit of time.

angular a. Rate of change in velocity per unit of time during circular movement.

central a. Centripetal a.

centripetal a. Rate of change in velocity per unit of time while on a circular or curved course. SYN: *central a.*

fetal heart rate a. **1.** The increase in heart rate associated with fetal movement. It may indicate a need for a reactive nonstress test. **2.** A reassuring sign during labor that the fetus is not experiencing intrauterine hypoxemia.

linear a. Rate of change in velocity per unit of time while on a straight course.

negative a. Decrease in the rate of change in velocity per unit of time.

positive a. Increase in the rate of change in velocity per unit of time.

standard a. of free fall The rate of change in velocity of a freely falling body as it is acted on by gravity to travel to the earth. It is 9.81 m (or 32.17 ft)/sec^2.

acceleration injury Head injury caused when the head remains stationary and is hit by a moving object, such as a batter being hit in the head by a baseball.

acceleration-deceleration injury An injury caused when the body at motion abruptly comes to a stop and the body structures are contused from within (e.g., whiplash or brain contusion, rupture of the splenic or hepatic capsules).

accelerator (ăk-sĕl′ĕr-ā″tor) **1.** Anything that increases action or function. **2.** In chemistry, a catalyst. **3.** A device that speeds up charged particles to high energy levels to produce x-radiation and neutrons.

accelerometer An instrument that detects a change in the velocity of the object to which it is attached. The device may be designed to record the changes and indicate the direction(s) of the acceleration.

acceptance **1.** According to Dr. Elisabeth Kübler-Ross, the fifth and final stage of dying. Individuals who reach this stage (not all do) come to terms with impending death and await the end with quiet expectation. **2.** In organ transplantation, the harmonious integration of grafted tissue into the body of the transplant recipient. **3.** Approval or acquiescence (e.g., of a recommended treatment or a functional impairment produced by an illness).

acceptor (ăk-sĕp′tor) [L. *accipere*, to accept] A compound that unites with a substance freed by another compound, called a donor.

hydrogen a. A substance that combines with hydrogen and is reduced when a substrate is oxidized by an enzyme.

oxygen a. A substance that combines with oxygen and is oxidized when a substrate is reduced by an enzyme.

access, medical SEE: *medical access*.

access, vascular A portal of entry into the circulation, for example, by way of a dialysis catheter.

accessorius (ăk″sĕs-ō′rē-ŭs) [L., supplementary] Accessory or supplementary, as in some muscles, glands, and nerves.

accessory (ăk-sĕs′ō-rē) Auxiliary; assisting. This term is applied to a lesser structure that resembles in structure and function a similar organ, as the accessory pancreatic duct (of Santorini) or accessory suprarenal glands.

accessory motion Passive movement that accompanies active voluntary range of motion in synovial and secondary cartilaginous joints and is necessary for full painless joint range of motion and function. These relatively small rolling and gliding movements, also called accessory movements or joint play, cannot be isolated voluntarily.

accessory muscles of respiration Muscles that are recruited to increase ventilation by patients with labored breathing. The intercostal abdominal muscles and the platysma may be used. Their use represents an abnormal or labored breathing pattern and is a sign of respiratory distress.

accessory nerve The eleventh cranial nerve, one of a pair of motor nerves made up of a cranial part and a spinal part that supplies the trapezius and sternomastoid muscles and the pharynx. The accessory portion joins the vagus to supply motor fibers to the pharynx, larynx. SYN: *spinal accessory nerve*. SEE: *cranial nerve* for illus.

accident (ăk′sĭ-dĕnt) [L. *accidens*, happening] **1.** An unforeseen occurrence of an unfortunate nature; a mishap. **2.** An unexpected complicating event in the course of a disease or following surgery. **accidental** (-dĕn′tăl), *adj.*

cerebrovascular a. ABBR: CVA. Stroke.

radiation a. Undesired excessive exposure to ionizing radiation.

accident-prone Said of persons having an unusually high rate of accidents. The validity of this concept is questionable.

accipiter (ăk-sĭp′ĭ-tĕr) [L., a hawk] A nose bandage with clawlike ends that spread over the facc.

acclimation, acclimatization (ăk-lĭ-mā′shŭn, ă-klī″mă-tĭ-zā′shŭn) [Fr. *acclimater*, acclimate] The act of becoming accustomed to a different environment.

acclimatize (ăk-klī′mă-tīz) To become accustomed to a different environment.

accommodation (ă-kŏm″ō-dā′shŭn) [L. *accommodare*, to suit] ABBR: a; acc. **1.** Adjustment or adaptation. **2.** In ophthalmology, a phenomenon noted in receptors in which continued stimulation fails to elicit a sensation or response. **3.** The adjustment of the eye for various distances whereby it is able to focus the image of an object on the retina by changing the curvature of the lens. In accommodation for near vision, the ciliary muscle contracts, causing increased rounding of the lens, the pupil contracts, and the optic axes converge. These three actions constitute the accommodation reflex. The ability of the eye to accommodate decreases with age. **4.** In the learning theory of Jean Piaget, the process through which a person's schema of understanding incorporates new experiences that do not fit existing ways of understanding the world. SEE: illus.; *adaptation*.

absolute a. Accommodation of one eye independently of the other.

amplitude of a. The difference in the refractive power of the eye when accommodating for near and far vision. It is measured in diopters (D) and normally diminishes progressively from childhood to old age. It is approx. 16 D at age 12, 6.5 D at age 30, and 1 D at age 50.

binocular a. Coordinated accommodation of both eyes jointly.

excessive a. Greater-than-needed accommodation of the eye.

mechanism a. Method by which cur-

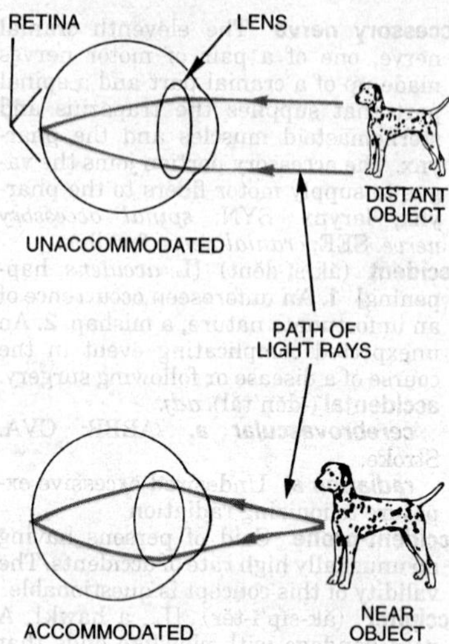

VISUAL ACCOMMODATION

vature of the eye lens is changed in order to focus close objects on the retina.

negative a. Relaxation of the ciliary muscle to adjust for distant vision.

positive a. Contraction of the ciliary muscle to adjust for near vision.

range of a. Distance of vision from its closest to its most remote points.

reasonable a. An employer's responsibility to provide necessary workplace changes, reassignment, equipment modification, devices, training materials, interpreters, and other reasonable adjustments for disabled employees.

relative a. The extent to which accommodation is possible for any specific state of convergence of the eyes.

spasm of a. A spasm of the ciliary muscle, usually the result of excessive strain from overuse; it is common in myopia.

subnormal a. Insufficient accommodation.

accoucheur, accoucheuse (ă-koo-shŭr′, ă-koo-shĕz′) [Fr.] An obstetrician or midwife.

accountability Responsibility of health care professionals for the actions and judgments involved in patient care.

ACCP *American College of Chest Physicians.*

accreditation The voluntary process of recognizing that a facility or institution has met established standards. In the U.S. there are two types of educational accreditation: institutional and specialized. The former recognizes the institution for having facilities, policies, and procedures that meet accepted standards. The latter recognizes specific programs of study within institutions for having met established standards.

Accreditation Commission for Acupuncture and Oriental Medicine ABBR: ACAOM. An organization that monitors, accredits, and sets curriculum standards for acupuncture training programs in the U.S.

Accredited Record Technician ABBR: A.R.T. A person who, as a result of training and experience, is competent to process, maintain in a secure place, compile, and report information in a patient's medical record. This is done according to rules set by the health care facility to comply with medical, administrative, ethical, legal, and accreditation considerations.

accrementition (ăk″rĕ-mĕn-tĭsh′ŭn) [L. *accrescere*, to increase] Growth of tissues by addition of similar tissue.

accretio (ă-krē′shē-ō) [L.] Adhesion of parts normally separate from each other.

a. cordis The extension of fibrous bands from the external pericardium to surrounding structures, resulting in angulation and torsion of the heart.

accretion (ă-krē′shŭn) [L. *accrescere*, accrue] **1.** An increase by external addition; accumulation. **2.** The growing together of parts naturally separate. **3.** Accumulation of foreign matter in a cavity.

acculturation The process by which a member of one culture assumes the values, attitudes, and behavior of a second culture.

accuracy **1.** The ratio of the error of measurement to the true value. **2.** State of being free of error.

ACD *absolute cardiac dullness.*

ACD sol Citric acid, trisodium citrate, dextrose solution; an anticoagulant used in collecting blood.

ACE *angiotensin-converting enzyme.*

acedia (ă-sē′dē-ă) [Gr. *a*-, not, + *kedos*, care] Mental state of indifference, insensibility, and/or lack of energy or emotion. SYN: *apathy.*

acellular Not containing cells.

acenesthesia (ă-sĕn″ĕs-thē′zē-ă) [Gr. *a*-, not, + *koinos*, common, + *aisthesis*, sensation] Absence of a feeling of well-being. It occurs in somatoform disorders.

acentric (ă-sĕn′trĭk) [″ + L. *centrum*, center] Not central; peripheral.

A.C.E.P. *American College of Emergency Physicians.*

acephalia, acephalism (ă-sĕ-fā′lē-ă, ă-sĕf′ă-lĭzm) [Gr. *a*-, not, + *kephale*, head] Congenital absence of the head.

acephalobrachia (ă-sĕf″ă-lō-brā′kē-ă) [″ + ″ + *brachion*, arm] Congenital absence of the head and arms.

acephalocardia (ă-sĕf″ă-lō-kăr′dē-ă) [″ + ″ + *kardia*, heart] Congenital absence of the head and heart.

acephalochiria (ă-sĕf″ă-lō-kī′rē-ă) [″ +

" + *cheir*, hand] Congenital absence of the head and hands.

acephalocyst (ă-sĕf′ă-lō-sĭst) [" + " + *kystis*, bag] A sterile hydatid cyst.

acephalogastria (ă-sĕf″ă-lō-găs′trē-ă) [" + " + *gaster*, stomach] Congenital absence of the head, chest, and upper abdomen.

acephalopodia (ă-sĕf″ă-lō-pō′dē-ă) [" + " + *pous*, foot] Congenital absence of the head and feet.

acephalorhachia (ă-sĕf″ă-lō-rā′kē-ă) [" + " + *rhachis*, spine] Congenital absence of the head and vertebral column.

acephalostomia (ă-sĕf″ă-lō-stō′mē-ă) [" + " + *stoma*, mouth] Congenital absence of the head; however, an opening resembling a mouth is present on the superior portion of the body.

acephalothoracia (ă-sĕf″ă-lō-thō-rā′sē-ă) [" + " + *thorax*, chest] Congenital absence of the head and chest.

acephalus (ă-sĕf′ă-lŭs) A fetus lacking a head.

acervulus (ă-sĕr′vū-lŭs) [L.] Sandy, gritty, sabulous.

acetabular (ăs″ĕ-tăb′ū-lăr) Pert. to the acetabulum.

acetabulectomy (ăs″ĕ-tăb″ū-lĕk′tō-mē) [L. *acetabulum*, a little saucer for vinegar, + Gr. *ektome*, excision] Surgical removal of the acetabulum.

acetabuloplasty (ăs″ĕ-tăb′ū-lō-plăs″tē) [" + Gr. *plassein*, to form] Surgical repair and reconstruction of the acetabulum.

acetabulum (ăs″ĕ-tăb′ū-lŭm) [L., a little saucer for vinegar] The cavity or depression on the lateral surface of the innominate bone (hip bone) that provides the socket into which the head of the femur fits. SEE: illus.

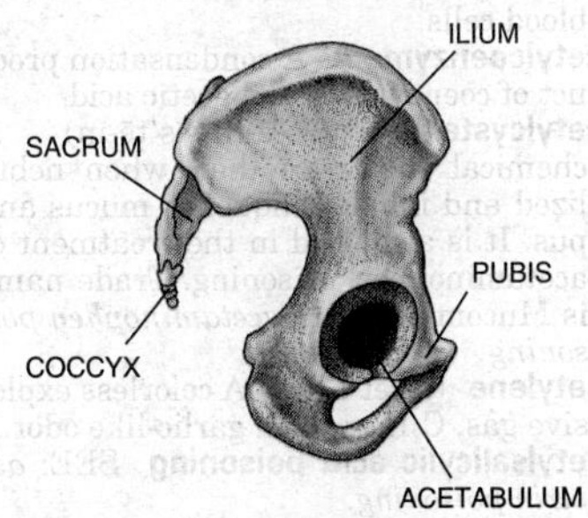

ACETABULUM OF RIGHT HIP BONE (FEMALE)

acetal (ăs′ĕ-tăl) Chemical combination of an aldehyde with alcohol.

acetaldehyde (ăs″ĕt-ăl′dĕ-hīd″) CH_3CHO; an intermediate in yeast fermentation and alcohol metabolism. SYN: *acetic aldehyde*.

acetamide (ăs″ĕt-ăm′īd) Acetic acid amide, CH_3CONH_2, used in industry for synthesis of chemicals and as a solvent.

acetaminophen (ă-sēt″ă-mĭn′ō-fĕn) A drug with antipyretic and analgesic effects similar to those of aspirin, but with limited anti-inflammatory or antirheumatic effects. It is used to treat mild to moderate pain. Unlike aspirin and related drugs, it is not irritating to the stomach.

CAUTION: Acute overdose may cause fatal hepatic necrosis.

acetaminophen poisoning Liver injury, necrosis, or failure resulting from an overdose of acetaminophen. In emergency departments and hospitals, this is one of the most common poisonings encountered. **If a reliable history of the amount of drug can be obtained, ingestions that exceed 7.5 g in the adult or about 150mg/kg in children should always be considered potentially toxic. In most cases, however, historical data about overdoses are not reliable, and** plasma levels of acetaminophen concentration are routinely measured and compared with standard nomograms to decide whether a patient will need antidotal therapy with N-acetylcysteine.

CLINICAL COURSE: Shortly after ingestion, patients may suffer nausea, vomiting, and malaise. If appropriate treatment is not instituted, hepatitis develops, with elevated liver enzymes in the first day, and jaundice and coagulation disorders by about 36 hr. Encephalopathy (altered mentation, drowsiness, or coma) may follow. A prolonged course of recovery or complete liver failure may result, depending on the amount of drug ingested and the severity of the liver injury.

TREATMENT: Gastric lavage should be done immediately (the airway must be protected). This is most effective if done within 4 hr of ingestion of the drug. A specific antidote, *N*-acetylcysteine, is given orally within 8 to 10 hr after ingestion in an initial dose of 140 mg/kg and then in 70 mg/kg doses every 4 hr for 17 doses if acetaminophen levels are toxic. SEE: *Poisons and Poisoning Appendix; Rumack nomogram*.

acetanilid (ăs″ĕ-tăn′ĭ-lĭd) A white powder or crystalline substance obtained by interaction of glacial acetic acid and aniline.

ACTION/USES: Acetanilid has analgesic, antipyretic, and anti-inflammatory effects. Acute or chronic poisoning may develop as a result of prolonged administration or drug idiosyncrasy. Because of its toxicity, it is rarely used.

acetanilid poisoning Toxicity caused by acetanilid ingestion. Symptoms are cyanosis due to formation of methemoglobin; cold sweat; irregular pulse; dyspnea; and unconsciousness. Sudden cardiac failure may occur.

FIRST AID: Irrigate exposed skin with soap and water, for example, in the safety shower. Support breathing and oxygenation. Notify the local poison control center. SEE: *Poisons and Poisoning Appendix.*

acetarsol, acetarsone (ăs″ĕ-tăr′sŏl, -sōn) An arsenic compound, acetylaminohydroxy-phenylarsonic acid, that contains 27% arsenic. It formerly was used to treat amebiasis and *Trichomonas vaginalis* infections.

acetate (ăs′ĕ-tāt) A salt of acetic acid.

acetazolamide (ăs″ĕt-ă-zŏl′ă-mīd) A drug that inhibits the enzyme carbonic anhydrase. At one time it was used as a diuretic, but more effective drugs are now available. It has been used to treat epilepsy and to reduce intraocular pressure in managing glaucoma. Trade name is Diamox.

acetic (ă-sē′tĭk) [L. *acetum*, vinegar] Pert. to vinegar; sour.

acetic aldehyde Acetaldehyde.

acetify (ă-sĕt′ĭ-fī) [L. *acetum*, vinegar, + *fieri*, to become] To produce acetic fermentation or vinegar.

Acetobacter (ă-sē″tō-băk′tĕr) [L. *acetum*, vinegar, + Gr. *bakterion*, little rod] A genus of nonpathogenic bacteria of the family Pseudomonadaceae.

acetohexamide (ăs″ĕ-tō-hĕks′ă-mīd) An orally administered hypoglycemic agent used to treat Type 2 diabetes mellitus.

acetoin (ă-sĕt′ō-ĭn) The substance formed when glucose is fermented by *Enterobacter aerogenes.*

acetone (ăs′ĕ-tōn) Dimethyl ketone, C_3H_6O, a colorless, volatile, flammable liquid used as a solvent. It has a sweet, fruity, ethereal odor and is found in the blood and urine in diabetes, in other metabolic disorders, and after lengthy fasting. It is produced when fats are not properly oxidized due to inability to oxidize glucose in the blood. SEE: *ketone; ketonuria; ketosis; test, acetone.*

a. in urine, test for A simple urine screening test, used principally in monitoring patients with type 1 diabetes mellitus, to determine the presence of ketoacidosis. To perform the test, the patient wets a specially treated paper or dipstick with urine. If ketones are present, the paper will change color within a specified time.

acetonemia (ăs″ĕ-tō-nē′mē-ă) [*acetone* + Gr. *haima*, blood] Large amounts of acetone in the blood. The symptoms are altered mental status, abdominal pain, and anorexia.

acetonitrile (ăs″ĕ-tō-nī′trĭl) Methyl cyanide, CH_3CN, an ingredient of some commercially available nail care products. When ingested, it produces a toxic reaction similar to cyanide poisoning. The onset is delayed 9 to 12 hr or more. It is also found in the urine of cigarette smokers. Treatment for poisoning is the same as for cyanide poisoning. SEE: *cotinine; cyanide poisoning.*

acetonuria (ăs″ĕ-tō-nū′rē-ă) [*acetone* + Gr. *ouron*, urine] Ketonuria.

acetophenazine maleate (ăs″ĕ-tō-fĕn′ă-zēn măl′ē-āt) An antipsychotic drug of the phenothiazine group. Trade name is Tindal.

acetophenetidin (ăs″ĕ-tō-fĕ-nĕt′ĭ-dĭn) Former name for phenacetin.

acetous (ăs′ĕ-tŭs) [L. *acetum*, vinegar] **1.** Pert. to vinegar. **2.** Sour in taste.

acetum (ă-sē′tŭm) *pl.* **aceta** [L.] **1.** Vinegar. **2.** A drug dissolved in a weak vinegar solution.

acetyl (ăs′ĕ-tĭl, ă-sēt′ĭl) [″ + Gr. *hyle*, matter] CH_3CO, a univalent radical.

a. CoA Acetylcoenzyme A.

acetylation (ă-sĕt″ĭ-lā′shŭn) The introduction of one or more acetyl groups into an organic compound.

acetylcholine (ăs″ĕ-tĭl-kō′lēn) ABBR: ACh. An ester of choline that is the neurotransmitter at somatic neuromuscular junctions, the entire parasympathetic nervous system, sympathetic preganglionic fibers (cholinergic fibers), and at some synapses in the central nervous system. It is inactivated by the enzyme cholinesterase. SEE: *cholinergic fiber.*

a. chloride A salt solution of acetylcholine used in irrigation of the iris to produce contraction of the pupil after cataract surgery. The sterile solution is instilled in the anterior chamber of the eye before suturing. Trade name is Miochol.

acetylcholinesterase (ăs″ĕ-tĭl-kō″lĭn-ĕs′tĕr-ās) ABBR: AChE. An enzyme that stops the action of acetylcholine. It is present in various body tissues, including muscles, nerve cells, and red blood cells.

acetylcoenzyme A A condensation product of coenzyme A and acetic acid.

acetylcysteine (ăs″ĕ-tĭl-sĭs′tē-ĭn) A chemical substance that, when nebulized and inhaled, liquefies mucus and pus. It is also used in the treatment of acetaminophen poisoning. Trade name is Mucomyst. SEE: *acetaminophen poisoning.*

acetylene (ă-sĕt′ĭ-lēn) A colorless explosive gas, C_2H_2, with a garlic-like odor.

acetylsalicylic acid poisoning SEE: *aspirin poisoning.*

acetyltransferase (ăs″ĕ-tĭl-trăns′fĕr-ās) Enzyme that is effective in the transfer of an acetyl group from one compound to another.

ACH *adrenocortical hormone.*

ACh *acetylcholine.*

achalasia (ăk″ă-lā′zē-ă) [Gr. *a-*, not, + *chalasis*, relaxation] Failure to relax; said of muscles, such as sphincters, the normal function of which is a persistent contraction with periods of relaxation. SEE: *Nursing Diagnoses Appendix.*

a. of the cardia Failure of the cardiac sphincter to relax, restricting the passage of food to the stomach. In advanced cases, dysphagia is marked and dilation of the esophagus may occur. SYN: *cardiospasm.*

cricopharyngeal a. Failure of the lower pharyngeal muscles to relax during swallowing. The condition may cause dysphagia or aspiration of food.

pelvirectal a. Congenital absence of ganglion cells in the distal large bowel, resulting in failure of the colon to relax.

sphincteral a. Failure of the intestinal sphincters to relax.

AChE *acetylcholinesterase.*

ache (āk) [AS. *acan*] **1.** Pain that is persistent rather than sudden or spasmodic. It may be dull or severe. **2.** To suffer persistent pain.

acheilia (ă-kī′lē-ă) [Gr. *a-*, not, + *cheilos*, lip] Congenital absence of one or both lips.

acheiria (ă-kī′rē-ă) [″ + *cheir*, hand] **1.** Congenital absence of one or both hands. **2.** A loss of sensation in one or both hands. This may result from temporary or permanent injury or malfunction of the sensory mechanism, or it may occur in hysteria. **3.** Inability to determine to which side of the body a stimulus has been applied. SYN: *achiria.*

acheiropodia (ă-kī″rō-pō′dē-ă) [″ + ″ + *pous*, foot] Congenital absence of the hands and feet.

Achilles jerk (ă-kĭl′ēz) [Achilles, hero of the *Iliad*, whose vulnerable spot was his heel] Achilles tendon reflex.

Achilles tendon The tendon of the gastrocnemius and soleus muscles of the leg. SYN: *calcaneal tendon.*

Achilles tendon reflex Plantar flexion, also called extension of the ankle, resulting from contraction of the calf muscles after a sharp blow to the Achilles tendon. The variations and their significance correspond closely to those of the knee jerk. It is exaggerated in upper motor neuron disease and diminished or absent in lower motor neuron disease.

achillobursitis (ă-kĭl″ō-bŭr-sī′tĭs) [*Achilles* + L. *bursa*, a pouch, + Gr. *itis*, inflammation] Inflammation of the bursa lying over the Achilles tendon. SYN: *Albert's disease.*

achillodynia (ă-kĭl″ō-dĭn′ē-ă) [″ + Gr. *odyne*, pain] Pain caused by inflammation between the Achilles tendon and bursa.

achillorrhaphy (ă-kĭl-or′ă-fē) [″ + Gr. *rhaphe*, seam, ridge] Suture of the Achilles tendon.

achillotenotomy (ă-kĭl″ō-tĕn-ŏt′ō-mē) [″ + Gr. *tenon*, tendon, + *tome*, incision] Achillotomy.

achillotomy (ă-kĭl-ŏt′ō-mē) [″ + *tome*, incision] Division of the Achilles tendon. SYN: *achillotenotomy.*

achiria (ă-kī′rē-ă) [Gr. *a-*, not, + *cheir*, hand] Acheiria.

achlorhydria (ă″klor-hī′drē-ă) [″ + *chloros*, green, + *hydor*, water] Absence of free hydrochloric acid in the stomach; may be associated with gastric carcinoma, gastric ulcer, pernicious anemia, adrenal insufficiency, or chronic gastritis. SEE: *achylia.*

histamine-proved a. Absence of free acid in gastric secretion even after subcutaneous injection of histamine hydrochloride.

achloropsia (ă-klō-rŏp′sē-ă) [″ + *chloros*, green, + *opsis*, vision] Color blindness in which green cannot be distinguished. SYN: *deuteranopia.*

acholuria (ă-kō-lū′rē-ă) [″ + *chole*, bile, + *ouron*, urine] Absence of bile pigments in the urine in some forms of jaundice.

achondrogenesis (ă-kŏn″drō-jĕn′ĕ-sĭs) [Gr. *a-*, not, + *chondros*, cartilage, + *genesis*, generation, birth] Failure of bone to grow, esp. the bones of the extremities.

achondroplasia (ă-kŏn″drō-plā′sē-ă) [″ + ″ + *plasis*, a molding] Defect in the formation of cartilage at the epiphyses of long bones, producing a form of dwarfism; sometimes seen in rickets. SYN: *chondrodystrophy.*

achroma (ă-krō′mă) [″ + *chroma*, color] An absence of color or normal pigmentation as in leukoderma, albinism, and vitiligo.

achromasia (ăk″rō-mā′zē-ă) [Gr. *achromatos*, without color] **1.** Absence of normal pigmentation of the skin as in albinism, vitiligo, or leukoderma. **2.** Pallor. **3.** Inability of cells or tissues to be stained.

achromate (ă-krō′māt) [Gr. *a-*, not, + *chroma*, color] A person who is colorblind.

achromatic (ăk″rō-măt′ĭk) [Gr. *achromatos*, without color] **1.** Colorless. **2.** Not dispersing light into constituent components. **3.** Not containing chromatin. **4.** Difficult to stain, with reference to cells and tissues.

achromatin (ă-krō′mă-tĭn) The weakly staining substance of a cell nucleus.

achromatism (ă-krō′mă-tĭzm″) [Gr. *a-*, not, + *chroma*, color, + *-ismos*, condition] Colorlessness.

achromatocyte (ăk″rō-măt′ō-sīt) [Gr. *achromatos*, without color, + *kytos*, cell] Achromocyte.

achromatolysis (ă-krō″mă-tŏl′ĭ-sĭs) [″ + *lysis*, dissolution] Dissolution of cell achromatin.

achromatophil (ă″krō-măt′ō-fĭl) [″ + *philos*, love] A cell or tissue not stainable in the usual manner. SYN: *achromophil.*

achromatopsia (ă-krō″mă-tŏp′sē-ă) [″ + *opsis*, vision] Complete color blindness.

achromatosis (ă-krō″mă-tō′sĭs) [″ + *osis*, condition] The condition of being without natural pigmentation. SEE: *achroma*.

achromatous (ă-krō′mă-tŭs) Without color.

achromaturia (ă-krō″mă-tū′rē-ă) [Gr. *achromatos*, without color, + *ouron*, urine] Colorless or nearly colorless urine.

achromia (ă-krō′mē-ă) [Gr. *a-*, not, + *chroma*, color] **1.** Absence of color; pallor. **2.** Achromatosis. **3.** Condition in which erythrocytes have large central pale areas; hypochromia.

congenital a. Albinism.

achromic (ă-krō′mĭk) Lacking color.

Achromobacter A genus of gram-negative bacilli that may inhabit the lower gastrointestinal tract; may cause nosocomial infections.

achromocyte (ă-krō′mō-sīt) [Gr. *a-*, not, + *chroma*, color + *kytos*, cell] In a blood smear, a large, pale, crescent-shaped cell produced from fragile red cells as the bloodfilm preparation is being made. SYN: *achromatocyte; crescent body; selenoid cell*.

achromophil (ă-krō′mō-fĭl) [″ + ″ + *philos*, love] Achromatophil.

achromotrichia (ă-krō″mō-trĭk′ē-ă) [″ + ″ + *trichia*, condition of the hair] Lack of color or graying of the hair. SYN: *canities*.

nutritional a. Grayness of the hair due to dietary deficiency.

achylia (ă-kī′lē-ă) [Gr. *a-*, not, + *chylos*, juice] Absence of chyle or other digestive enzymes. SYN: *achylosis*.

a. gastrica Complete absence or marked decrease in the amount of gastric juice. SEE: *achlorhydria*.

a. pancreatica Absence or deficiency of pancreatic secretion; usually a sign of chronic pancreatitis.

achylosis (ă″kī-lō′sĭs) Achylia.

achylous (ă-kī′lŭs) [Gr. *achylos*, without chyle] **1.** Lacking in any kind of digestive secretion. **2.** Without chyle.

acicular (ă-sĭk′ū-lăr) [L. *aciculus*, little needle] Needle-shaped.

acid [L. *acidum*, acid] **1.** Any substance that liberates hydrogen ions (protons) in solution; a hydrogen ion donor (Bronsted acid). An acid reacts with a metal to form a salt, neutralizes bases, and turns litmus paper red. **2.** A substance that can accept a pair of electrons (Lewis acid). SEE: *alkali; base; indicator; pH*. **3.** A sour substance. **4.** Slang term for LSD.

acetic a. The substance, CH_3COOH, that gives the sour taste to vinegar; also used as a reagent. Glacial acetic acid contains at least 99.5% acetic acid by weight.

acetoacetic a. A ketone body, CH_3COCH_2COOH, formed when fats are incompletely oxidized; appears in urine in abnormal amounts in starvation and in inadequately treated diabetes. SYN: *acetylacetic a*.

acetylacetic a. Acetoacetic a.

acetylsalicylic a. Aspirin.

adenylic a. Adenosine monophosphate.

amino a. SEE: *amino acid*.

aminoacetic a. Glycine.

aminobenzoic a. Para-aminobenzoic a.

aminocaproic a. $H_2N(CH_2)_5COOH$; a hemostatic drug. It is a specific antidote for an overdose of a fibrinolytic agent. Trade name is Amicar.

aminoglutaric a. Glutamic a.

aminosalicylic a. Para-aminosalicylic a.

aminosuccinic a. Aspartic a.

arachidonic a. $C_{20}H_{32}O_2$; an essential fatty acid formed by the action of enzymes on phospholipids in cell membranes. It is metabolized primarily by the cyclo-oxygenase or 5-lipoxygenase pathways to produce prostaglandins and leukotrienes, which are important mediators of inflammation. Corticosteroids inhibit formation of arachidonic acid from phospholipids when cell membranes are damaged. Nonsteroidal anti-inflammatory agents such as salicylates, indomethacin, and ibuprofen inhibit the synthesis of prostaglandins and leukotrienes. Arachidonic acid is found in many foods.

ascorbic a. Vitamin C, $C_6H_8O_6$, a vitamin that occurs naturally in fresh fruits, esp. citrus, and vegetables, and can also be synthesized. It is essential in maintenance of collagen formation, osteoid tissue of bones, and formation and maintenance of dentin. This essential vitamin is used as a dietary supplement and in the prevention and treatment of scurvy. Scurvy develops after approx. 3 mo. of ascorbic acid deficiency in the diet. Large daily doses (1 to 5 g/day) of vitamin C are purported to prevent or treat the common cold, but this has not been established. Continual consumption of large doses can cause kidney stones. SYN: *antiscorbutic vitamin; vitamin C*.

aspartic a. A nonessential amino acid, $HOOC \cdot CH_2 \cdot CH(NH_2) \cdot COOH$. It is a product of pancreatic digestion. SYN: *aminosuccinic a*.

barbituric a. A crystalline compound, $C_4H_4N_2O_3$, from which phenobarbital and other barbiturates are derived. SYN: *malonylurea*.

benzoic a. A white crystalline material, $C_7H_6O_2$, having a slight odor. It is used in keratolytic ointments and as a food preservative. Saccharin is a derivative of this acid.

bile a. Any one of the complex acids that occur as salts in bile (e.g., cholic, glycocholic, and taurocholic acids). They give bile its foamy character, are important in the digestion of fats in the intestine, and are reabsorbed from the intestine to be used again by the liver.

boric a. A white crystalline substance, H_3BO_3, that in water forms a very weak acid solution poisonous to plants and animals. It is soluble in water, alcohol, and glycerin. SEE: *boric acid poisoning*.

CAUTION: Because of its toxicity, boric acid should be used rarely. It is particularly dangerous because it can be accidentally swallowed by children or used in food because of its resemblance to sugar.

butyric a. A fatty acid, C_3H_7COOH, derived from butter but rare in most fats. It is a viscid liquid with a rancid odor; it is used in disinfectants, emulsifying agents, and pharmaceuticals.

carbolic a. Phenol.

carbonic a. H_2CO_3; an acid formed when carbon dioxide is dissolved in water.

carboxylic a. Any acid containing the group -COOH. The simplest examples are formic and acetic acids.

cholic a. $C_{24}H_{40}O_5$; an acid formed in the liver by hydrolysis of other bile acids. It is important in digestion.

citric a. An acid, $C_6H_8O_7$, found naturally in citrus fruits or prepared synthetically. It acts as a sequestrant, helping to preserve food quality.

deoxyribonucleic a. ABBR: DNA. A complex nucleic acid of high molecular weight consisting of deoxyribose, phosphoric acid, and four bases (two purines, adenine and guanine, and two pyrimidines, thymine and cytosine). These are arranged as two long chains that twist around each other to form a double helix joined by bonds between the complementary components. Nucleic acid, present in chromosomes of the nuclei of cells, is the chemical basis of heredity and the carrier of genetic information for all organisms except the RNA viruses. Formerly spelled desoxyribonucleic acid. SEE: *chromosome; gene; ribonucleic acid; virus; Watson-Crick helix*.

desoxyribonucleic a. Former spelling of deoxyribonucleic acid.

eicosapenteanoic a. ABBR: EPA. One of a group of fatty acids containing 20 carbons and five double bonds that are prevalent in fish oils. SEE: *omega-3 (ω3) fatty a.*

essential fatty a. A fatty acid (alpha-linoleic and linoleic) that must be present in the diet, as it cannot be synthesized in the body and is essential to maintaining health. SEE: *digestion*.

ethylenediaminetetraacetic a. ABBR: EDTA. A chelating agent that, in the form of its calcium or sodium salts, is used to remove metallic ions such as lead and cadmium from the body. SEE: *chelation*.

fatty a. A hydrocarbon in which one of the hydrogen atoms has been replaced by a carboxyl (COOH) group; a monobasic aliphatic acid made up of an alkyl radical attached to a carboxyl group.

Saturated fatty acids have single bonds in their carbon chain with the general formula $C_{n+1}H_{2n+3}-COOH$. They include acetic, butyric, capric, caproic, caprylic, formic, lauric, myristic, palmitic, and stearic acids. Unsaturated fatty acids have one or more double or triple bonds in the carbon chain. They include those of the oleic series (oleic, tiglic, hypogeic, and palmitoleic) and the linoleic or linolic series (linoleic, linolenic, clupanodonic, arachidonic, hydrocarpic, and chaulmoogric). Fatty acids are insoluble in water. This would prevent their absorption from the intestines if the action of bile salts on the fatty acids did not enable them to be absorbed. SEE: *fat*.

folic a. A water-soluble B complex vitamin needed for DNA synthesis and occurring naturally in green leafy vegetables, beans, and yeast. It is used in the treatment of megaloblastic and macrocytic anemias. It is used to prevent neural tube defects (NTDs) as well as cardiovascular disease in adults. The U.S. Public Health Service recommends that all women of childbearing age in the U.S. who are capable of becoming pregnant should consume 0.4 mg of folic acid per day to reduce their risk of having a child affected with spina bifida or other NTDs. SEE: *neural tube defect*.

CAUTION: Folic acid should not be used to treat pernicious anemia (a vitamin B_{12} deficiency) because it does not protect patients against the development of changes in the central nervous system that accompany this type of anemia.

formic a. HCOOH; the first and strongest member of the monobasic fatty acid series. It occurs naturally in certain animal secretions and in muscle, but it may also be prepared synthetically. It is one of the irritants present in the sting of insects such as bees and ants.

formiminoglutamic a. $C_6N_2O_4H_{10}$; an intermediate product in the metabolism of histidine. Its increase in the urine after administration of histidine in patients with folic acid deficiency is the basis for the FIGLU excretion test.

free fatty a. ABBR: FFA. The form in which a fatty acid leaves the cell to be transported for use in another part of the body. These acids are not esterified and may be unbound (i.e., not bound to protein). In the plasma, the nonesterified fatty acids released immediately combine with albumin to form bound, free fatty acids.

gadolinium-diethylenetriamine pentaacetic a. ABBR: GD-DTPA. A radiographic contrast agent, used in magnetic resonance imaging to enhance the appearance of blood vessels.

gallic a. A colorless crystalline acid, $C_6H_2(OH)_3COOH$. It occurs naturally as an excrescence on the twigs of trees, esp. oaks, as a reaction to the deposition of gall wasp eggs. It is used as a skin astringent and in the manufacture of writing inks and dyes.

gammalinoleic a. An essential fatty acid promoted by alternative medicine practitioners as a treatment for skin and inflammatory disorders, cystic breast disease, and hyperlipidemia.

glucuronic a. $CHO(CHOH)_4COOH$; an oxidation product of glucose that is present in the urine. Toxic products (such as salicylic acid, menthol, and phenol) that have entered the body through the intestinal tract are detoxified in the liver by conjugation with glucuronic acid.

glutamic a. $HOOC \cdot (CH_2)_2 \cdot CH(NH_2) \cdot COOH$; an amino acid formed in protein hydrolysis and an excitatory neurotransmitter in the central nervous system. SYN: *aminoglutaric a.*

glyceric a. $CH_2OH \cdot CHOH \cdot COOH$; an intermediate product of the oxidation of fats.

glycocholic a. A bile acid, $C_{26}H_{43}NO_6$, yielding glycine and cholic acid on hydrolysis.

homogentisic a. An intermediate product of tyrosine catabolism; found in the urine in alkaptonuria. SYN: *alkapton(e).*

hyaluronic a. An acid mucopolysaccharide found in the extracellular matrix of connective tissue that acts as a binding and protective agent. It is found, for example, in the synovial fluid and vitreous and aqueous humors of the eye.

hydriodic a. SYMB: HI. An acid used in solution in various forms of chemical analyses. SYN: *hydrogen iodide.*

hydrochloric a. HCl; an inorganic acid that is normally present in gastric juice. It destroys fermenting bacteria that might cause intestinal tract disturbances. Five to 10 ml of a 10% solution of hydrochloric acid in 125 to 250 ml of water is used in treating hypoacidity or achlorhydria.

CAUTION: When so used, it must be diluted accurately and sipped through a drinking straw. This will prevent the acid from damaging the teeth.

---

hydrocyanic a. HCN; a colorless, extremely poisonous, highly volatile liquid that occurs naturally in plants but can be produced synthetically. It has many industrial uses: electroplating, fumigation, and production of dyes, pigments, synthetic fibers, and plastic. Exposure of humans to 200 to 500 parts of hydrocyanic acid per 1,000,000 parts of air for 30 min is fatal. It acts by preventing cellular respiration. SYN: *hydrogen cyanide.* SEE: *cyanide in Poisons and Poisoning Appendix.*

hydroxy a. An acid containing one or more hydroxyl (-OH) groups in addition to the carboxyl (-COOH) group (e.g., lactic acid, $CH_3COHCOOH$).

hydroxybutyric a. An acid present in the urine, esp. in diabetic ketoacidosis, when fatty acid conversion to ketones increases.

hydroxycitric a. An herbal extract promoted by alternative medicine practitioners for the treatment of weight loss. Placebo-controlled studies have not found any benefit to the treatment.

hypochlorous a. An acid, HClO, used as a disinfectant and bleaching agent. It is usually used in the form of one of its salts.

imino a. An acid formed as a result of oxidation of amino acids in the body.

inorganic a. An acid containing no carbon atoms.

keto a. Any organic acid containing the ketone CO (carbonyl radical).

lactic a. An organic acid, $C_3H_6O_3$, that is formed in muscles during the anaerobic cell respiration that occurs during strenuous exercise. It is also formed during anaerobic muscle activity when glucose cannot be changed to pyruvic acid in glycolysis. It contributes to muscle aches and fatigue.

linoleic a. $C_{18}H_{32}O_2$; an unsaturated fatty acid that is a dietary essential. It was first isolated from linseed oil but is also found in corn oil. It is required for the synthesis of prostaglandins.

linolenic a. $C_{18}H_{30}O_2$; a major omega-6 essential fatty acid.

lysergic a. A crystalline substance, $C_{16}H_{16}N_2O_2$, derived from ergot. Its derivative, lysergic acid diethylamide (LSD), is a potent hallucinogen. SEE: *LSD.*

lysophosphatidic a. ABBR: LPA. A diverse group of substances purified from the ascitic fluid of patients with ovarian cancer. It stimulates the growth of ovarian cancer and may be a useful screening test for the disease.

malic a. $C_4H_6O_5$; a substance found in certain sour fruits such as apples and apricots and active in the aerobic metabolism of carbohydrates.

malonic a. A dibasic acid, $C_3H_4O_4$, formed by the oxidation of malic acid and active in the tricarboxylic acid cycle in carbohydrate metabolism. Its inhibition of succinic dehydrogenase is the classic example of competitive inhibition. Malonic acid is found in beets.

mandelic a. $C_8H_8O_3$; a colorless hydroxy acid. Its salt is used to treat urinary tract infections.

monounsaturated fatty a. A fatty acid containing one double bond between carbon atoms. This type of fatty acid is found in olive oil. It is thought to reduce low-density lipoprotein levels without affecting high-density lipoprotein levels. It is the predominant fat in what has been called the Mediterranean diet. SEE: *Mediterranean diet.*

nicotinic a. $C_6H_5NO_2$; a member of the vitamin B complex; used for the prevention and treatment of pellagra. It occurs naturally in liver, yeast, milk, cheese, and cereals. SYN: *niacin.*

nitric a. A strong corrosive acid, HNO_3, prepared from sulfuric acid and a nitrate. It is used in the manufacture of explosives and dyes.

nucleic a. Any one of a group of high-molecular-weight substances found in the cells of all living things. They have a complex chemical structure formed of sugars (pentoses), phosphoric acid, and nitrogen bases (purines and pyrimidines). Most important are ribonucleic acid and deoxyribonucleic acid.

oleic a. $C_{18}H_{34}O_2$; an unsaturated fatty acid found in most organic fats and oils.

omega-3 (ω3) fatty a. A group of fatty acids found in the oils of some saltwater fish. They have been used to attempt to reduce levels of very-low-density lipoproteins and chylomicrons in plasma. People whose diets are rich in these substances are associated with a decreased risk of cardiovascular disease.

omega-6 (ω6) fatty a. Fatty acids, such as linoleic and arachidonic, thought to influence cardiovascular and growth function when balanced with omega-3 fatty acids in eicosanoid production.

organic a. An acid containing the carboxyl radical, -COOH. Acetic acid, formic acid, lactic acid, and all fatty acids are organic.

orotic a. Uracil-6-carboxylic acid. It is a precursor in the formation of pyrimidine nucleotides.

oxalic a. $C_2H_2O_4$; the simplest dibasic organic acid. Its potassium or calcium salt occurs naturally in rhubarb, wood sorrel, and many other plants. It is the strongest organic acid and is poisonous. When properly diluted, it removes ink or rust stains from cloth. It is used also as a reagent.

palmitic a. $C_{16}H_{32}O_2$; a saturated fatty acid occurring as esters in most natural fats and oils.

pantothenic a. $C_9H_{17}NO_5$; one of the B-complex vitamins.

para-aminobenzoic a. ABBR: PABA. $NH_2C_6H_4COOH$; a B-complex vitamin used as a dietary supplement, an antirickettsial drug, a reagent, and a sunscreen agent. It should not be used in persons known to be sensitive to sulfonamides. It inhibits the bacteriostatic action of sulfonamides, so all but topical use is contraindicated during sulfonamide therapy. SYN: *aminobenzoic a.*

para-aminosalicylic a. ABBR: PAS. An antituberculosis drug, $C_7H_7NO_3$, the effectiveness of which is greatly enhanced when it is combined with other drugs such as isoniazid; a white and practically odorless powder that darkens when exposed to air or light. SYN: *aminosalicylic a.*

pentanoic a. Valeric a.

perchloric a. $HClO_4$, a colorless unstable liquid compound. It is the highest oxygen-containing acid of chlorine.

phenylglycolic a. Mandelic a.

phosphoric a. An acid formed by oxidation of phosphorus. The phosphoric acids are orthophosphoric acid, H_3PO_4; pyrophosphoric acid, $H_4P_2O_7$; metaphosphoric acid, HPO_3; and hypophosphoric acid, $H_4P_2O_6$. The salts of these acids are phosphates. Orthophosphoric acid, a tribasic acid, is used as a 30% to 50% solution to etch enamel of teeth in preparation for bonding of resin dental restorations.

phosphorous a. An oxygen acid of phosphorus. The phosphorous acids are orthophosphorous acid, $H_2(HPO_3)$; pyrophosphorous acid, $H_4P_2O_5$; metaphosphorous acid, HPO_2; and hypophosphorous acid, $H(H_2PO_2)$. The salts of these acids are phosphites.

picric a. $C_6H_2(NO_2)_3OH$; a yellow crystalline substance that precipitates proteins and explodes when heated or charged. Salts of picric acid are used in the Juffee reaction for determination of serum creatinine. Picric acid is used as a dye and a reagent. SYN: *trinitrophenol.*

pyruvic a. An organic acid, $CH_3CO \cdot COOH$, that plays an important role in the Krebs cycle. It is an intermediate product in the metabolism of carbohydrates, fats, and amino acids. Its quantity in the blood and tissues increases in thiamine deficiency because thiamine is essential for its oxidation.

ribonucleic a. ABBR: RNA. A nucleic acid that controls protein synthesis in all living cells and is the sole nucleic acid in certain viruses. It differs from DNA in that its sugar is ribose and the pyrimidine base uracil rather than thymine is present. RNA occurs in several forms that are determined by the number of nucleotides. SEE: illus.; *deoxyribonucleic acid.*

Messenger RNA (mRNA) carries the

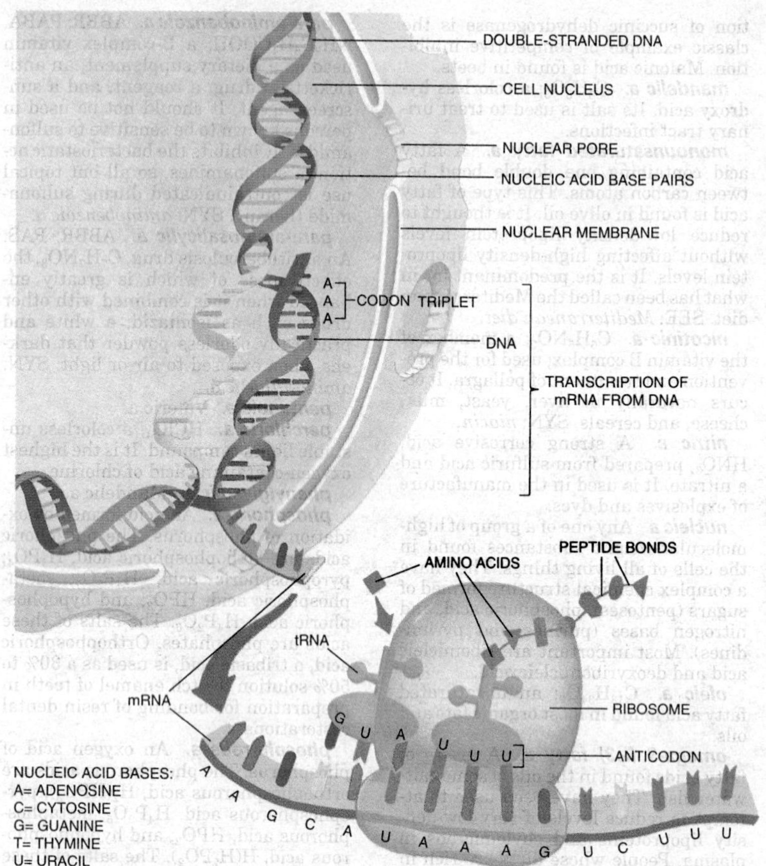

RIBONUCLEIC ACID
Roles in protein synthesis

code for specific amino acid sequences from the DNA to the cytoplasm for protein synthesis.

Transfer RNA (tRNA) carries the amino acid groups to the ribosome for protein synthesis.

Ribosomal RNA exists within the ribosomes and assists in protein synthesis.

salicylic a. $C_7H_6O_3$; a white crystalline powder used as a local antiseptic or keratolytic agent.

saturated fatty a. Fatty acid in which the carbon atoms are linked to other carbon atoms by single bonds. SEE: *fatty a.; unsaturated fatty a.*

silicic a. An acid containing silica, as H_2SiO_3, H_2SiO_4, or H_2SiO_6. When silicic acid is precipitated, silica gel is obtained.

stearic a. A monobasic fatty acid, $C_{18}H_{36}O_2$, occurring naturally in plants and animals. It is used in the manufacture of soap and pharmaceutical products such as glycerin suppositories.

succinic a. $HOOC(CH_2)_2COOH$; an intermediate in carbohydrate metabolism.

sulfonic a. An organic compound of the general formula SO_2OH derived from sulfuric acid by replacement of a hydrogen atom.

sulfosalicylic a. A crystalline acid soluble in water or alcohol; used as a reagent for precipitating proteins, as in testing for albumin in urine.

sulfuric a. H_2SO_4; a colorless, corrosive, heavy liquid prepared from sulfur and used in the production of a great number of industrial products. It is rarely used in medicine.

sulfurous a. An inorganic acid, H_2SO_3. It is a powerful chemical reducing agent that is used commercially, esp. for its bleaching properties.

tannic a. A mixture of digallic acid esters of D(+) glucose prepared from oak galls and sumac. It yields gallic acid and glucose on hydrolysis.

tartaric a. $C_4H_6O_6$; a substance obtained from byproducts of wine fermentation. It is widely used in industry in the manufacture of carbonated drinks, flavored gelatins, dyes, and metals. It is also used as a reagent.

taurocholic a. A bile acid that yields cholic acid and taurine on hydrolysis.

trans fatty a. The solid fat produced by heating liquid vegetable oils in the presence of hydrogen and certain metal catalysts. This process of partial hydrogenation changes some of the unsaturated bonds to saturated ones. The more trans fatty acids in the diet, the higher the serum cholesterol and low density lipoprotein cholesterol.

trichloroacetic a. A caustic drug used to destroy certain types of warts, condylomata, keratoses, and hyperplastic tissue. This reagent is also used to precipitate proteins.

unsaturated fatty a. Organic acid in which some of the carbon atoms are linked to other carbon atoms by double bonds, thus containing less than the maximum possible number of hydrogen atoms; for example, unsaturated oleic and linoleic acids as compared with the saturated stearic acid. SEE: *fatty a.; saturated fatty a.*

uric a. $C_5H_4N_4O_3$; an organic constituent of normal urine and plasma. It usually occurs in form of salts (urates). Uric acid crystals that precipitate in joints are the cause of gouty arthritis.

valeric a. $C_5H_{10}O_2$; an oily liquid of the fatty acid series, existing in four isomeric forms and having a distinctly disagreeable odor. SYN: *pentanoic a.*

valproic a. A drug used to treat seizure disorders.

acidaminuria (ăs″ĭd-ăm″ĭ-nū′rē-ă) [L. *acidum*, acid, + *amine* + Gr. *ouron*, urine] An excess of amino acids in urine. SYN: ***hyperacidaminuria.***

acidemia (ăs-ĭ-dē′mē-ă) [L. *acidum*, acid, + Gr. *haima*, blood] A decrease in the arterial blood pH below 7.35. The hydrogen ion concentration of the blood increases, as reflected by a lowering of serum pH values. SEE: *acid-base balance; acidity; acidosis.*

acid-fast Not decolorized easily by acids after staining; pert. to bacteria that after staining are decolorized by a mixture of acid and alcohol. The acid-fast bacteria retain the red dyes, but the surrounding tissues are decolorized. An example of this type of organism is *Mycobacterium tuberculosis.*

acidifiable (ă-sĭd′ĭ-fī″ă-bl) [L. *acidum*, acid, + *fieri*, to be made, + *habilis*, able] Capable of being transformed to produce an acid reaction.

acidification (ă-sĭd″ĭ-fĭ-kā′shŭn) [″ + *factus*, made] Conversion into an acid or acidic conditions.

acidifier (ă-sĭd′ĭ-fī″ĕr) [″ + *fieri*, to be made] A substance that causes acidity.

acidify **1.** To make a substance acid. **2.** To become acid.

acidity (ă-sĭd′ĭ-tē) **1.** The quality of possessing hydrogen ions (protons). SEE: *acid; hydrogen ion; pH.* **2.** Sourness.

a. of the stomach The lowered pH of the gastric contents, due to hydrogen ion release by parietal cells.

titratable a. The amount of hydrogen ion excreted in the urine in a dihydrogen form.

acidophil(e) (ă-sĭd′ō-fĭl, -fīl) [″ + Gr. *philos*, love] **1.** Acidophilic. **2.** An acid-staining cell of the anterior pituitary. **3.** A bacterial organism that grows well in an acid medium.

acidophilic (ă-sĭd″ō-fĭl′ĭk) **1.** Having affinity for acid or pert. to certain tissues and cell granules. **2.** Pert. to a cell capable of being stained by acid dyes.

acidoresistant (ăs″ĭ-dō-rē-zĭs′tănt) Acid-resisting; said about bacteria.

acidosis (ăs″ĭ-dō′sĭs) [L. *acidum*, acid, + Gr. *osis*, condition] An actual or relative increase in the acidity of blood due to an accumulation of acids (as in diabetic acidosis or renal disease) or an excessive loss of bicarbonate (as in renal disease). The hydrogen ion concentration of the fluid is increased, lowering the pH. SEE: *acid-base balance; acidemia; buffer; pH.* **acidotic** (ăs″ĭ-dŏt′ĭk), *adj.*

carbon dioxide a. Respiratory a.

compensated a. Acidosis in which the pH of body fluids has returned to normal. Compensatory mechanisms maintain the normal ratio of bicarbonate to carbonic acid (approx. 20 : 1) in blood plasma, even though the bicarbonate level is decreased or the carbon dioxide level is elevated.

diabetic a. Diabetic ketoacidosis.

hypercapnic a. Respiratory a.

hyperchloremic a. Acidosis in which there is an abnormally high level of chloride in the blood serum.

lactic a. An accumulation of lactic acid in the blood, often as a result of the inadequate perfusion and oxygenation of vital organs (such as occurs in cardiogenic, ischemic, or septic shock), drug overdoses (commonly, salicylates or ethanol), skeletal muscle overuse (e.g., after heavy exercise or seizures), or other serious illnesses (some cancers; diabetes mellitus). Lactic acid is produced more quickly than normal when there is inadequate oxygenation of skeletal muscle and other tissues. Thus, any disease that leads to tissue hypoxia, exercise, hyperventilation, or some drugs (e.g., oral hypoglycemic agents) may cause this condition. In general, when blood pH is less than 7.35 and lactate is greater than 5 to 6 mmol/L (5 to 6 mEq/L), lactic acidosis is present.

metabolic a. Any process that causes a decrease in the pH of the body as a result of the retention of acids, or the loss of bicarbonate buffers. Metabolic acidosis is usually categorized by the presence or absence of an abnormal anion gap. The anion gap metabolic acidoses include diabetic, alcoholic, and lactic acidoses; the acidosis of renal failure; and acidoses that result from the consumption of excess acids, such as salicylates, methanol, or ethanol. Non-anion gap metabolic acidoses occur in diarrhea, renal tubular acidosis, and multiple myeloma, among other conditions.

ETIOLOGY: Possible causes include excessive ingestion of acids, salicylates, methanol, or ethylene glycol; failure of the kidneys to excrete acids (e.g., in renal failure or renal tubular acidosis); ketoacidosis (diabetic, alcoholic, owing to starvation) severe dehydration; diarrhea; rhabdomyolysis; seizures; and shock.

PATIENT CARE: A history is obtained, focusing on the patient's urine output, fluid intake, dietary habits (including recent fasting), associated disorders (such as diabetes mellitus and kidney or liver dysfunction), and the use of medications (including aspirin) and alcohol. Arterial blood gas values, serum potassium level, and fluid balance are monitored. The patient is assessed for lethargy, drowsiness, and headache, and for diminished muscle tone and deep tendon reflexes. The patient is also evaluated for hyperventilation, cardiac dysrhythmias, muscle weakness, and flaccidity, and for gastrointestinal distress such as nausea, vomiting, diarrhea, and abdominal pain. Prescribed intravenous fluids, medications such as sodium bicarbonate or insulin, and other therapies such as oxygen or mechanical ventilation are administered. The patient is positioned to promote chest expansion and repositioned frequently. Frequent oral hygiene with sodium bicarbonate rinses will neutralize mouth acids and a water-soluble lubricant will prevent lip dryness. A safe environment with minimal stimulation is provided, and preparations should be available if seizures occur. Both patient and family are given verbal and written information about managing related disease processes and prescribed medications. SEE: *Nursing Diagnoses Appendix.*

renal a. Acidosis caused either by kidney failure, in which phosphoric and sulfuric acids and inorganic anions accumulate in the body, or by renal tubular diseases. The acidosis is induced by urinary wasting of bicarbonate and inability to excrete phosphoric and sulfuric acids.

PATIENT CARE: Renal acidosis resulting from one of the renal tubular acidoses responds to treatment either with sodium bicarbonate or with citrated salts (e.g., potassium citrate). The acidosis of chronic renal failure may require therapy with sodium bicarbonate or may be treated with dialysis using a bicarbonate-rich dialysate. Diets are adjusted for patients with renal failure to limit the metabolic production of acids—these usually rely on limitations of daily dietary protein. Foods that are rich in potassium and phosphate are also restricted. Patients with renal failure should be monitored for signs and symptoms of renal acidosis, including loss of appetite changes in levels of consciousness, or alterations in respiratory rate or effort. Laboratory monitoring may include frequent assessments of arterial blood gas values, serum electrolytes, carbon dioxide levels, and blood urea nitrogen and creatinine. Prescribed intravenous fluids are given to maintain hydration.

respiratory a. Acidosis caused by inadequate ventilation and the subsequent retention of carbon dioxide. SYN: *carbon dioxide a.*

PATIENT CARE: The patient suspected of developing acute respiratory acidosis is monitored using arterial blood gases, level of consciousness, and orientation to time, place, and person. The patient is also evaluated for diaphoresis, a fine or flapping tremor (asterixis), depressed reflexes, and cardiac dysrhythmias. Vital signs and ventilatory effort are monitored, and ventilatory difficulties such as dyspnea documented. Prescribed intravenous fluids are given to maintain hydration. The patient is oriented as often as necessary, and information and reassurance are given to allay the patient's and family's fears and concerns. Prescribed therapies for associated hypoxemia and underlying conditions are provided, responses are evaluated, and related patient education is given.

The respiratory therapist (RT) works with the attending physician to determine when to intubate and mechanically ventilate the patient with acute respiratory acidosis. Once the patient is intubated and receiving mechanical ventilation, the RT monitors and maintains the patient's airway and tolerance of the positive pressure ventilation. This requires the respiratory therapist to perform frequent (Q1-Q2) assessments of the patient and the ventilator and report side effects to the attending physician.

CAUTION: Acute respiratory acidosis is a medical emergency in which immediate efforts to improve ventilation are required.

acid poisoning Ingestion of a toxic acid. SEE: *acids in Poisons and Poisoning in Appendix.*

FIRST AID: Dilute with large volumes of water. Give demulcents and morphine for pain. Treat as a chemical burn.

CAUTION: The use of emetics and stomach tubes is contraindicated.

---

acid-proof Acid-fast.

acid rain Rain that, in passing through the atmosphere, is contaminated with acid substances, esp. sulfur dioxide and nitrogen oxide. These pollutants are oxidized in the atmosphere to sulfuric acid and nitric acid. Rainwater is considered abnormally acid if the pH is below 5.6. It may damage ecosystems or individual plants and animal species.

acid-reflux disorder gastroesophageal reflux disease.

acid-reflux test Test for reflux of acid into the esophagus from the stomach. An electrode for detecting the pH is placed in the stomach and a reading is taken; then the electrode is withdrawn until it is in the esophagus. Normally, the pH will become more alkaline (i.e., rise) as the electrode is moved from the stomach into the esophagus. If there is acid reflux, the pH will be acid in both the stomach and esophagus.

acidulate [L. *acidulus*, slightly acid] To make somewhat sour or acid.

acidulous (ă-sĭd′ū-lŭs) Slightly sour or acid.

acidum (ăs′ĭ-dŭm) [L.] Acid.

aciduria (ăs-ĭd-ū′rē-ă) [L. *acidum*, acid, + Gr. *ouron*, urine] The condition of excessive acid in the urine.

glutaric a. An inherited disorder marked by multiple neurological deficits in childhood, including motor dysfunction, developmental delay, and brain atrophy. It is caused by defective manufacture of glutaryl-coenzyme A dehydrogenase.

orotic a. An inherited disorder of pyrimidine metabolism in which orotic acid accumulates in the body. Clinically, children fail to grow and have megaloblastic anemia and leukopenia. The disease responds to administration of uridine or cytidine.

aciduric (ăs″ĭ-dū′rĭk) [″ + *durare*, to endure] Capable of growing in an acid medium, but preferring a slightly alkaline one.

acinar (ăs′ĭ-năr) [L. *acinus*, grape] Pert. to an acinus.

Acinetobacter (ăs″ĭ-nĕt″ō-băk′tĕr) [Gr. *akinetos*, immovable, + *bakterion*, rod] A genus of microorganisms widely distributed in nature that are usually nonpathogenic. *Acinetobacter lwoffi* was previously known as *Mima polymorpha*, and *Acinetobacter anitratus* was previously known as *Herellea vaginicula*.

acini (ăs′ĭ-nī) Pl. of acinus.

aciniform (ă-sĭn′ĭ-form) [L. *acinus*, grape, + *forma*, shape] Resembling grapes. SYN: *acinous*.

acinitis (ăs″ĭ-nī′tĭs) [″ + Gr. *itis*, inflammation] Inflammation of glandular acini.

acinose (ăs′ĭ-nōs) [L. *acinosus*, grape-like] Composed of acini.

acinous (ăs′ĭ-nŭs) Pert. to glands resembling a bunch of grapes, such as acini and alveolar glands. SYN: *aciniform*.

acinus (ăs′ĭ-nŭs) *pl.* **acini** [L., grape] **1.** The smallest division of a gland; a group of secretory cells surrounding a cavity. **2.** The terminal respiratory gas exchange unit of the lung, composed of airways and alveoli distal to a terminal bronchiole.

ACIP *The Advisory Committee on Immunization Practices of the U.S. Public Health Service.*

A.C. joint *acromioclavicular joint.*

ackee (ă′kē) Akee.

acladiosis (ăk-lăd″ē-ŏ′sĭs) An ulcerative skin disease believed to be caused by fungi of the genus *Acladium*.

aclasis, aclasia (ăk′lă-sĭs, ă-klā′zē-ă) [Gr. *a-*, not, + *klasis*, a breaking away] Abnormal tissue arising from and continuous with a normal structure, as in achondroplasia.

diaphyseal a. Imperfect formation of cancellous bone in cartilage between diaphysis and epiphysis.

acleistocardia (ă-klĭs″tō-kăr′dē-ă) [Gr. *akleistos*, not closed, + *kardia*, heart] Patent foramen ovale of the heart.

ACLS *Advanced Cardiac Life Support.*

acme (ăk′mē) [Gr. *akme*, point] **1.** The highest point; peak. **2.** The time of greatest intensity of a symptom or disease process. **3.** The segment of uterine labor contraction during which muscle tension is greatest.

acne (ăk′nē) [Gr. *akme*, point] **1.** An inflammatory disease of the sebaceous follicles of the skin, marked by comedones, papules, and pustules. It is exceptionally common in puberty and adolescence. Acne usually affects the face, chest, back, and shoulders. In severe cases, cysts, nodules, and scarring occur.

ETIOLOGY: The cause is unknown, but predisposing factors include hereditary tendencies and disturbances in the androgen-estrogen balance. Acne begins at puberty, when the increased secretion of androgen in both males and females increases the size and activity of the pilosebaceous glands. Specific inciting factors may include food allergies, endocrine disorders, therapy with adrenal corticosteroid hormones, and psychogenic factors. Vitamin deficiencies, ingestion of halogens, and contact with chemicals such as tar and chlorinated hydrocarbons may be specific causative factors. The fact that bacteria are important once the disease is present is indicated by the successful results following antibiotic therapy. The lesions may become worse in women and girls before the menstrual period.

SYMPTOMS: Acne vulgaris is marked by either papules about comedones with black centers (pustules) or hypertrophied nodules caused by overgrowth of connective tissue. In the indurative type, the lesions are deep-seated and cause scarring. The face, neck, and shoulders are common sites. Acne may be obstinate and recurrent.

TREATMENT: Treatments include skin cleansing, topical agents (e.g., benzoyl peroxide or vitamin A derivatives), oral or topical antibacterial drugs, and oral isotretinoin, among others.

PATIENT CARE: The patient is instructed to wash the skin thoroughly but gently, avoiding intense scrubbing and skin abrasion; to keep hands away from the face and other sites of lesions; to limit the use of cosmetics; and to observe for, recognize, and avoid or modify predisposing factors that may cause exacerbations. The need to reduce sun exposure is explained, and the patient is advised to use a sunscreen agent when vitamin A acid or tetracycline is prescribed. Information is provided to fill knowledge gaps or correct misconceptions, and emotional support and understanding are offered, particularly if the patient is an adolescent.

2. Acne vulgaris.

a. atrophica Acne with residual pitting and scarring.

bromide a. Characteristic acne caused by bromide.

a. ciliaris Acne that affects the edges of the eyelids.

a. conglobata Acne vulgaris with abscesses, cysts, and sinuses that leave scars.

cystic a. Acne with cysts containing keratin and sebum. SEE: illus.

TREATMENT: Isotretinoin, a vitamin A derivative, has been effective in treating this condition. For Caution concerning its use, SEE: *isotretinoin*.

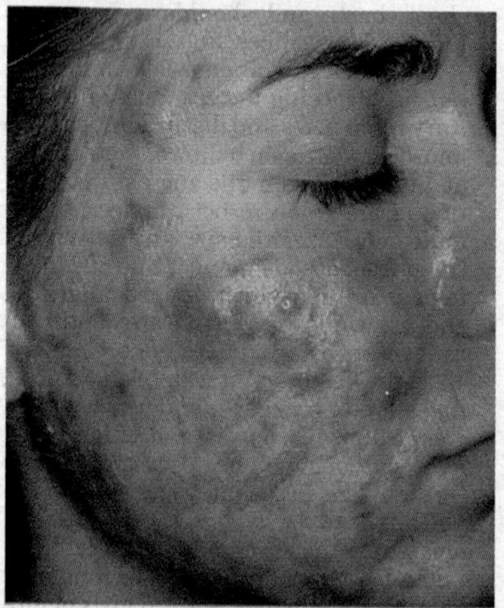

CYSTIC ACNE

a. fulminans A rare type of acne in teenage boys, marked by inflamed, tender, ulcerative, and crusting lesions of the upper trunk and face. It has a sudden onset and is accompanied by fever, leukocytosis, and an elevated sedimentation rate. About half of the cases have inflammation of several joints.

halogen a. Acne due to exposure to halogens such as bromine, chlorine, or iodine.

a. indurata Acne vulgaris with chronic, discolored, indurated surfaces.

keloid a. Infection about the hair follicles at the back of the neck, causing scars and thickening of the skin.

a. keratosa Acne vulgaris in which suppurating nodules crust over to form horny plugs. These occur at the corners of the mouth.

a. neonatorum Newborn, or neonatal acne. Acne in the newborn is a common occurrence, appearing about the second to fourth week of life. Comedones, inflamed papules, and pustules may be seen (the latter yield staphylococcal species when cultured). The rash resolves spontaneously in most cases by the third or fourth month of life; usually no treatment is required.

a. papulosa Acne characterized by formation of papules with very little inflammation. SEE: illus.

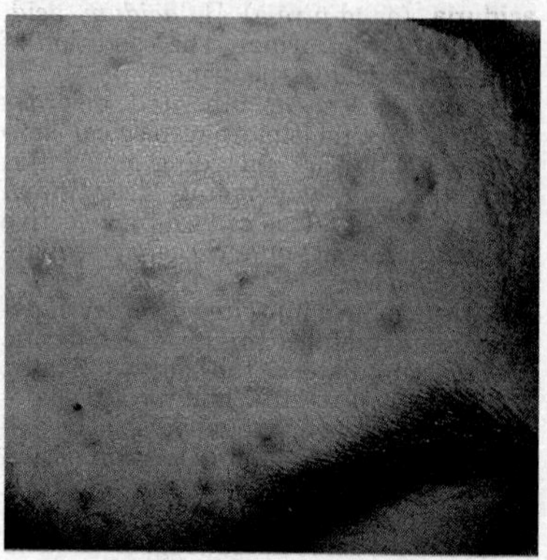

ACNE PAPULOSA

petroleum a. Acne that may occur in those who work with petroleum and oils.

a. pustulosa Acne with pustule formation and subsequent deep scars.

a. rosacea Rosacea.

steroid a. Acne caused by systemic or topical use of corticosteroid drugs.

summer a. Acne that appears only in hot, humid weather or that is much worse in such weather. Although the exact cause is unknown, the condition is not caused by increased exposure to the sun's rays.

tropical a. Severe acne caused by or aggravated by living in a hot, humid climate. The skin of the thorax, back, and legs is most commonly affected.

a. urticaria An acneiform eruption of itching wheals.

a. varioliformis Vesiculopustular folliculitis that occurs mostly on the temples and frontal margins of the scalp but may be seen on the chest, back, or nose.

a. vulgaris Common acne. SEE: *acne.*

acnegenic (ăk″nē-jĕn′ĭk) [Gr. *akme,* point, + *gennan,* to produce] Causing acne.

acneiform (ăk-nē′ĭ-form) [″ + L. *forma,* shape] Resembling acne; also spelled *acneform.*

acnemia (ăk-nē′mē-ă) [Gr. *a-,* not, + *kneme,* lower leg] Wasting of the calves of the legs.

A.C.N.M. *American College of Nurse Midwives.*

A.C.O.G. *American College of Obstetricians and Gynecologists.*

aconite (ăk′ō-nīt) [Gr. *akoniton*] The dried tuberous root of *Aconitum,* esp. *A. napellus* (monkshood) and *A. lycoctonum* (wolfsbane); a poisonous alkaloid that may cause life-threatening cardiac arrhythmias. Aconite is believed to have been used as an arrow poison early in Chinese history and perhaps also by the inhabitants of ancient Gaul. It was also used as an herbal remedy in traditional Chinese medicine.

aconitine (ă-kŏn′ĭ-tĭn) The active ingredient in aconite.

acorea (ă-kō-rē′ă) [Gr. *a-,* not, + *kore,* pupil] Absence of the pupil of the eye.

acoria (ă-kō′rē-ă) [″ + *koros,* satiety] Lacking in satisfaction after eating but not from hunger.

acormus (ă-kor′mŭs) [″ + *kormos,* trunk] **1.** Lack of a trunk. **2.** A fetal abnormality consisting of a head and extremities without a trunk.

ACOTE *Accreditation Council for Occupational Therapy Education.*

acous- SEE: *acousto-.*

acousia (ă-koo′zē-ă) [Gr. *akousis,* hearing] The hearing faculty. SYN: *acusis.*

acousmatamnesia [″ + *amnesia,* forgetfulness] Inability to recall and identify sounds.

acoust- SEE: *acosuto-.*

acoustic (ă-koos′tĭk) [Gr. *akoustikos*] Pert. to sound or to the sense of hearing.

acoustic center The hearing center in the brain; located in the temporal lobe of the cerebrum.

acoustic meatus The opening to the external or internal auditory canal.

acoustic nerve The eighth cranial nerve; it consists of two separate parts: the vestibular and cochlear nerves, with superficial origin at the junction of the pons and medulla.

PHYSIOLOGY: The acoustic nerve relays impulses for the special senses of hearing and equilibrium. The vestibular and cochlear nerves consist of somatic afferent fibers. Cells of origin of the vestibular nerve are bipolar and lie in the vestibular ganglion, peripheral branches terminating in receptors of semicircular ducts, saccule, and utricle. Cells of origin of the cochlear nerve are bipolar and lie in the spiral ganglion, peripheral branches terminating in the spiral organ of Corti. The two nerves become joined, enter the internal acoustic meatus with the facial nerve, and then separate. SYN: *auditory nerve; eighth cranial nerve; vestibulocochlear nerve.*

acousticophobia (ă-koos″tĭ-kō-fō′bē-ă) [Gr. *akoustos,* heard, + *phobos,* fear] Abnormal fear of loud sounds.

acoustic reflectometry Diagnostic technique for the detection of middle ear effusion. It measures the level of sound transmitted and reflected from the middle ear to a microphone located in a probe tip placed against the ear canal opening and directed toward the tympanic membrane.

acoustics (ă-koos′tĭks) The science of sound, its production, transmission, and effects.

acoustic trauma Injury to hearing by noise, esp. loud noise.

acousto-, acoust-, acous- [Gr. *akouenin,* hear] Combining forms meaning *hearing.*

A.C.P. *American College of Physicians; American College of Pathologists.*

acquired (ă-kwīrd′) [L. *acquirere,* to get] Not hereditary or innate.

acquired immunodeficiency syndrome AIDS.

acquisitus (ă-kwĭs′ĭ-tŭs) [L.] Acquired.

A.C.R. *American College of Radiology.*

acral (ăk′răl) [Gr. *akron,* extremity] Pert. to extremities.

acrania (ă-krā′nē-ă) [Gr. *a-,* not, + *kranion,* skull] Partial or complete congenital absence of the cranium.

acrid (ăk′rĭd) [L. *acer,* sharp] Burning, bitter, irritating.

acridine (ăk′rĭ-dĭn) A coal tar hydrocarbon from which certain dyes are prepared.

acrimony (ăk′rĭ-mō″nē) Quality of being pungent, acrid, irritating, rancorous, or caustic.

acritical (ă-krĭt′ĭ-kăl) [Gr. *a-,* not, + *kritikos,* critical] Not marked by a crisis.

ACRM *American Congress of Rehabilitation Medicine.*

acro- (ăk′rō) [Gr. *akron,* extremity] Combining form meaning *extremity, top, extreme point.*

acroagnosis (ăk″rō-ăg-nō′sĭs) [″ + *gnosis*, knowledge] Absence of feeling of one's limb.

acroanesthesia (ăk″rō-ăn-ĕs-thē′zē-ă) [″ + *an-*, not, + *aisthesis*, sensation] Lack of sensation in one or more of the extremities.

acroasphyxia (ăk″rō-ăs-fĭk′sē-ă) [″ + *asphyxia*, pulse stoppage] Cold, pale condition of hands and feet; symptom of Raynaud's disease.

acroblast (ăk′rō-blăst) [″ + *blastos*, germ] A part of the Golgi apparatus in the spermatid from which the acrosome arises.

acrobrachycephaly (ăk″rō-brăk″ĭ-sĕf′ă-lē) [″ + *brachys*, short, + *kephale*, head] The condition of having an abnormally short head in the anterior-posterior diameter due to fusion of the coronal suture.

acrocentric (ăk″rō-sĕn′trĭk) [Gr. *akron*, extremity + L. *centrum*, center] Pert. to a chromosome in which the centromere is located near one end. At metaphase it has the appearance of a wishbone.

acrocephalia (ăk″rō-sĕf-ā′lē-ă) [″ + *kephale*, head] Acrocephaly.

acrocephalosyndactylia, acrocephalosyndactyly (ăk″rō-sĕf″ă-lō-sĭn-dăk-tĭl′ē-ă, -sĭn-dăk′tĭl-ē) [″ + ″ + *syn*, together, + *daktylos*, a finger] A congenital condition marked by a peaked head and webbed fingers and toes. SYN: *Apert's syndrome*.

acrocephaly (ăk″rō-sĕf′ă-lē) [″ + *kephale*, head] The condition of having a malformed cranial vault with a high or peaked appearance and a vertical index above 77. It is caused by premature closure of the coronal, sagittal, and lambdoidal sutures. SYN: *acrocephalia; oxycephaly*. **acrocephalic** (-sĕ-făl′ĭk), *adj.*

acrochordon (ăk″rō-kor′dŏn) [″ + *chorde*, cord] A small, benign, polyp-shaped growth composed of skin and subcutaneous tissue; typically found on the neck, in the axilla, or near the eyelids. SYN: *fibroepithelial polyp; skin tag*.

acrocontracture [″ + L. *contrahere*, to draw together] Contracture of the hands or feet.

acrocyanosis (ăk″rō-sī-ă-nō′sĭs) [″ + *kyanosis*, dark-blue color] A blue or purple mottled discoloration of the extremities, esp. the fingers, toes, and/or nose. This physical finding is associated with many diseases and conditions, such as anorexia nervosa, autoimmune diseases, cold agglutinins, or Raynaud's disease or phenomenon. Cyanosis of the extremities may be commonly observed in newborns and in others after exposure to cold temperatures, and in those patients with reduced cardiac output. In patients with suspected hypoxemia, it is an unreliable sign of diminished oxygenation. (Instead of relying on this physical sign, pulse oximetry or arterial blood gases should be measured.)

acrodermatitis (ăk″rō-dĕr-mă-tī′tĭs) [″ + *derma*, skin, + *itis*, inflammation] Dermatitis of the extremities.

a. chronica atrophicans Dermatitis of the hands and feet that progresses slowly upward on the affected limbs.

a. continua An obstinate eczematous eruption confined to the extremities.

a. enteropathica Rare disease in children aged 3 weeks to 18 months that may be fatal if untreated. The genetically determined cause is malabsorption of zinc. Onset is insidious with failure to thrive, diarrhea, loss of hair, and development of vesiculobullous lesions, particularly around body orifices.

TREATMENT: Zinc sulfate given orally will abolish all clinical manifestations of the disease within a few days.

a. hiemalis Dermatitis that occurs in winter and affects the extremities. It tends to disappear spontaneously.

a. perstans A. continua.

acrodermatosis (ăk″rō-dĕr″mă-tō′sĭs) [Gr. *akron*, extremity, + *derma*, skin, + *osis*, condition] Any skin disease that affects the hands and feet.

acrodolichomelia (ăk″rō-dŏl″ĭ-kō-mē′lē-ă) [″ + *dolichos*, long, + *melos*, limb] A condition in which the hands and feet are abnormally long.

acrodynia (ăk″rō-dĭn′ē-ă) [″ + *odyne*, pain] A disease of infants and young children caused by chronic mercury poisoning. It has a prolonged clinical course with various grades of severity. The child is listless, irritable, and no longer interested in play. The rash has several variations. Initially, the tips of the fingers and toes become pink; the hands and feet become pink but color shades off at the wrists and ankles. As the disease progresses, the skin of the extremities desquamates, there are profuse sweating and pruritus, and pain is excruciating in the hands and feet. Neurological symptoms with neuritis and mental apathy develop. SYN: *pink disease*.

TREATMENT: Treatment consists of removing the source of the mercury, administering dimercaprol (BAL) antidote, and providing supportive therapy.

acrodysesthesia (ăk″rō-dĭs″ĕs-thē′zē-ă) [″ + *dys*, bad, + *aisthesis*, sensation] Dysesthesia in the arms and legs.

acroesthesia (ăk″rō-ĕs-thē′zē-ă) [″ + *aisthesis*, sensation] **1.** Abnormal sensitivity of the extremities. **2.** Pain in the extremities.

acrogeria (ăk″rō-jĕr′ē-ă) [″ + *geron*, old man] A condition in which the skin of the hands and feet shows signs of premature aging.

acrognosis (ăk″rŏg-nō′sĭs) [″ + *gnosis*, knowledge] Sensory perception of limbs.

acrohyperhidrosis (ăk″rō-hī″pĕr-hī-drō′sĭs) [″ + *hyper*, excessive, + *hidrosis*, sweating] Excessive perspiration of the hands and feet.

acrohypothermy (ăk″rō-hī″pō-thĕr′mē) [″ + *hypo*, below, + *therme*, heat] Abnormal coldness of the extremities.

acrokeratosis verruciformis (ăk″rō-kĕr″ă-tō′sĭs vĕ-roo′sĭ-for″mĭs) [″ + *keras*, horn, + *osis*, condition; L. *verruca*, wart, + *forma*, form] Hereditary disease of the skin characterized by warty growths on the extremities, principally on the backs of the hands and on the feet.

acrokinesia (ăk″rō-kĭn-ē′sē-ă) [″ + *kinesis*, movement] Excessive motion of the extremities.

acromacria (ăk″rō-măk′rē-ă) [Gr. *akron*, extremity, + *makros*, long] Abnormal length of the fingers. SYN: *arachnodactyly*. SEE: *Marfan's syndrome*.

acromastitis (ăk″rō-măs-tī′tĭs) [″ + *mastos*, breast, + *itis*, inflammation] Inflammation of the nipple. SYN: *thelitis*.

acromegaly (ăk″rō-mĕg′ă-lē) [″ + *megas*, big] A chronic syndrome of growth hormone excess, most often caused by a pituitary macroadenoma. It is characterized by gradual coarsening and enlargement of bones and facial features. The diagnosis is suggested by a growth hormone level that does not suppress after glucose administration. It is confirmed by radiologic imaging of the pituitary gland. SYN: *Marie's disease*.

ETIOLOGY: Overproduction of growth hormone by somatotroph cells of the anterior pituitary is responsible for most cases.

SYMPTOMS: The onset is often so gradual that patients and their close associates may not notice a change in appearance or function. Increased sweating, decreased libido, somnolence, mood disorders, muscular pain, weakness, and loss of vision may occur eventually. Signs include a thickening of facial features, enlargement of hands and feet, deepening voice, and separation of the teeth. A quarter of patients develop diabetes mellitus.

TREATMENT: Transsphenoidal resection of a growth-hormone secreting adenoma is the primary method of therapy. When this fails, medications, such as bromocriptine or octreotide, or radiotherapy may provide some relief.

acromelalgia (ăk″rō-mĕl-ăl′jē-ă) [Gr. *akron*, extremity, + *melos*, limb, + *algos*, pain] Erythromelalgia.

acromelic (ăk″rō-mĕl′ĭk) [″ + *melos*, limb] Pert. to the end of the extremities.

acrometagenesis (ăk″rō-mĕt″ă-jĕn′ĕ-sĭs) [″ + *meta*, beyond, + *genesis*, generation, birth] Abnormal growth of the extremities.

acromial (ăk-rō′mē-ăl) [″ + *omos*, shoulder] Rel. to the acromion.

acromial process Acromion.

acromial reflex Forearm flexion with internal rotation of the hand as a result of a quick blow to the acromion; elicited in hyperreflexic states.

acromicria (ăk″rō-mĭk′rē-ă) [Gr. *akron*, extremity, + *mikros*, small] Congenital shortness or smallness of the extremities and face.

acromioclavicular joint (ă-krō″mē-ŏ-klă-vĭk′ū-lăr) [″ + *omos*, shoulder, + L. *clavicula*, small key] ABBR: AC joint. A gliding or plane joint between the acromion and the acromial end of the clavicle.

acromiocoracoid (ă-krō″mē-ŏ-kor′ă-koyd) [″ + ″ + *korax*, crow, + *eidos*, form, shape] Pert. to the acromion and coracoid process.

acromiohumeral (ăk-rō″mē-ŏ-hū′mĕr-ăl) [″ + ″ + L. *humerus*, shoulder] Pert. to the acromion and humerus.

acromion (ă-krō′mē-ŏn) [Gr. *akron*, extremity, + *omos*, shoulder] The lateral triangular projection of the spine of the scapula that forms the point of the shoulder and articulates with the clavicle. SYN: *acromial process*. SEE: *acromioclavicular joint*.

acromioplasty The surgical removal of the distal inferior acromion process of the scapula to relieve impingement of soft tissues in the subacromial space. This is usually performed with release of the coracoacromial ligament, arthroscopically or through open incision.

acromioscapular (ă-krō″mē-ŏ-skăp′ū-lăr) [″ + ″ + L. *scapula*, shoulder blade] Pert. to the acromion and scapula.

acromiothoracic (ă-krō″mē-ŏ-thō-răs′ĭk) [″ + ″ + *thorax*, chest] Pert. to the acromion and thorax.

acromphalus (ăk-rŏm′făl-ŭs) [″ + *omphalos*, umbilicus] **1.** Center of the navel. **2.** Projection of the umbilicus, as in the beginning of an umbilical hernia.

acromyotonia, acromyotonus (ăk″rō-mī-ō-tō′nē-ă, -ŏt′ō-nŭs) [″ + *mys*, muscle, + *tonos*, tension] Myotonia of the extremities, causing spasmodic deformity.

acroneurosis (ăk″rō-nŭ-rō′sĭs) [Gr. *akron*, extremity, + *neuron*, nerve, + *osis*, condition] Nerve disease in the extremities.

acro-osteolysis (ăk″rō-ŏs″tē-ŏl′ĭ-sĭs) [Gr. *akron*, extremity, + *osteon*, bone, + *lysis*, dissolution] **1.** A familial disease causing dissolution of the tips of the bones in the extremities of young children. There is no history of trauma, and spontaneous amputation does not occur. The etiology is unknown. **2.** An occupational disease seen in workers who come in contact with vinyl chloride polymerization processes. It is marked by Raynaud's phenomenon, scleroderma-like skin changes, and radiological evidence of bone destruction of the distal phalanges of the hands. Recovery follows removal from exposure. SEE: *Raynaud's disease*.

acropachyderma (ăk″rō-păk″ē-dĕr′mă) [″ + ″ + *derma*, skin] Clubbing of the fingers, deformed long bones, and thickening of the skin of the scalp, face, and extremities.

acroparalysis (ăk″rō-pă-răl′ĭ-sĭs) [″ + *paralyein*, to disable] Paralysis of one or more extremities.

acroparesthesia (ăk″rō-păr-ĕs-thē′zē-ă) [″ + *para*, abnormal, + *aisthesis*, sensation] Sensation of prickling, tingling, or numbness in the extremities.

acropathology (ăk″rō-pă-thŏl′ō-jē) [″ + *pathos*, disease, suffering, + *logos*, word, reason] Pathology of disease of the extremities.

acrophobia (ăk-rō-fō′bē-ă) [″ + *phobos*, fear] Morbid fear of high places. SYN: *hypsophobia*.

acroposthitis (ăk″rō-pŏs-thī′tĭs) [Gr. *akroposthis*, prepuce, + *itis*, inflammation] Inflammation of the prepuce of the penis. SYN: *posthitis*.

acropustulosis, infantile Cyclical eruption of pustules on the soles and feet of infants 2 to 10 months of age. The pustules become vesicopapular, crust over, and heal in 7 to 10 days. A new crop appears in 2 to 3 weeks and they also heal. Periodic outbreaks occur for about 2 years and then stop. The cause is unknown; symptomatic therapy is all that is required.

acroscleroderma (ăk″rō-sklĕr-ō-dĕr′mă) [Gr. *akron*, extremity, + *scleros*, hard, + *derma*, skin] Hard, thickened skin condition of toes and fingers. SYN: *sclerodactylia*.

acrosclerosis (ăk″rō-sklĕr-ō′sĭs) [″ + ″ + *osis*, condition] A scleroderma of the upper extremities, sometimes extending to the neck and face, that usually follows Raynaud's disease.

acrosome (ăk′rō-sōm) [″ + *soma*, body] A specialized lysosome on the head of a sperm cell that contains enzymes to digest the membrane of an egg cell. SEE: *spermatozoon* for illus.

acroteric (ăk″rō-tĕr′ĭk) [Gr. *akroterion*, summit] Pert. to the outermost parts of the extremities, as the tips of the fingers.

acrotism (ăk′rō-tĭzm) [Gr. *a-*, not, + *krotos*, striking, + *-ismos*, condition] Imperceptibility of the pulse.

acrotrophoneurosis (ăk″rō-trŏf″ō-nū-rō′sĭs) [Gr. *akron*, extremity, + *trophe*, nourishment, + *neuron*, nerve, + *osis*, condition] Trophoneurosis of the extremities with trophic, neuritic, and vascular changes. It is usually caused by prolonged immersion in water.

acrylamide (ă-krĭl′ă-mīd) The amide of acrylic acid, C_3H_5NO. Acrylamide is used in many types of gel electrophoresis to separate and to identify proteins.

acrylate (ăk′rĭ-lāt) A salt or ester of acrylic acid.

acrylic acid (ă-krĭl′ĭk) CH_2:CH·COOH; a colorless corrosive liquid used in making acrylic polymers and resins.

acrylonitrile (ăk″rĭ-lō-nī′trĭl) C_3H_3N; a toxic compound used in making plastics. SYN: *vinyl cyanide*.

A.C.S., ACS *American Cancer Society; American Chemical Society; American College of Surgeons; acute confusional state; anodal closing sound.*

A.C.S.M. *American College of Sports Medicine.*

act (ăkt) **1.** To accomplish a function. **2.** The accomplishment of a function. **3.** Legislation that has been passed and made law; also referred to as legislative act and statutory law.

compulsive a. The repetitive, ritualistic performance of an act. This may be done despite the individual's attempts to resist the act.

impulsive a. Sudden action caused by an abnormal impulse or desire.

ACTH *adrenocorticotropic hormone*, a pituitary hormone that stimulates the cortex of the adrenal glands to produce adrenal cortical hormones.

actin (ăk′tĭn) One of the contractile proteins that make up the sarcomeres of muscle tissue. During contraction, the actin filaments are pulled toward the center of the sarcomere by the action of myosin filaments, and the sarcomere shortens.

actin- SEE: *actino-*.

acting out Expressing oneself through actions rather than speech.

neurotic a.o. **1.** A form of transference, in which tension is relieved when one responds to a situation as if it were the same situation that originally gave rise to the tension; a displacement of behavioral response from one situation to another. **2.** In psychoanalysis, a form of displacement, in which the patient relives memories rather than expressing them verbally.

actinic (ăk-tĭn′ĭk) [Gr. *aktis*, ray] **1.** Pert. to radiant energy, such as x-rays, ultraviolet light, and sunlight, esp. the photochemical effects. **2.** Pert. to the ability of radiant energy to produce chemical changes.

actinic burns Burns caused by ultraviolet or sun rays. Treatment is the same as for dry heat burns. SEE: *burn.*

actinism (ăk′tĭn-ĭzm) The property of radiant energy that produces chemical changes, as in photography or heliotherapy.

actinium (ăk-tĭn′ē-ŭm) [Gr. *aktis*, ray] SYMB: Ac. A radioactive element; atomic weight 227; atomic number 89.

actino-, actin- (ăk′tĭ-nō) [Gr. *aktis*, ray] Combining forms meaning *ray* or *radiation.*

Actinobacillus (ăk″tĭ-nō-bă-sĭl′lŭs) Small gram-negative coccobacilli that affect domestic animals mostly; however, *Actinobacillus actinomycetem comitans* has been implicated in endocarditis in humans.

actinodermatitis (ăk″tĭn-ō-dĕr-mă-tī′tĭs) [″ + *derma*, skin, + *itis*, inflammation] Dermatitis caused by exposure to radiation.

actinogenic (ăk″tĭn-ō-jĕ′nĭk) Radiogenic.

Actinomyces (ăk″tĭn-ō-mī′sēz) [″ + *mykes*, fungus] A genus of bacteria of the family Actinomycetaceae that contain gram-positive staining filaments. These bacteria cause various diseases in humans and animals.

A. antibioticus A species of *Actinomyces* from which the antibiotic actinomycin is obtained.

A. bovis A species of *Actinomyces* that causes actinomycosis in cattle.

A. israelii A species of *Actinomyces* that causes actinomycosis in humans. One clinical form is called lumpy jaw due to the characteristic appearance of the swollen jaw produced by the infection. Prolonged therapy with very large doses of penicillin G is required.

Actinomycetales (ăk″tĭ-nō-mī″sĕ-tā′lēz) An order of bacteria that includes the families Mycobacteriaceae, Actinomycetaceae, Actinoplanaceae, Dermatophilaceae, Micromonosporaceae, Nocardiaceae, and Streptomycetaceae.

actinomycete (ăk″tĭ-nō-mī′sēt) Any bacterium of the order Actinomycetales. **actinomycetic** (-mī-sēt′ĭk), *adj.*

actinomycetin (ăk″tĭn-ō-mī-sēt′ĭn) A lytic substance obtained from *Actinomyces;* it destroys some gram-positive and gram-negative organisms.

actinomycin A (ăk″tĭn-ō-mī′sĭn) A highly toxic antibiotic obtained from *Actinomyces antibioticus* that is effective against gram-positive organisms. This orange-colored heat-stable antibiotic is soluble in alcohol and ether.

actinomycin B An antibiotic similar to actinomycin A but not soluble in alcohol. Because of its toxicity, it is not used clinically.

actinomycoma (ăk″tĭ-nō-mī-kō′ma) [Gr. *aktis*, ray, + *mykes*, fungus, + *oma*, tumor] A tumor produced by actinomycosis.

actinomycosis (ăk″tĭn-ō-mī-kō′sĭs) [″ + ″ + *osis*, condition] An infectious bacterial disease in animals and humans. Infection may be of the cervicofacial, thoracic, or abdominal regions, or it may be generalized. **actinomycotic** (-kŏt′ĭk), *adj.*

ETIOLOGY: Causative organisms are *Actinomyces bovis* in cattle and *Actinomyces israelii* (which is normally present in the mouth) in humans. SEE: *nocardiosis.*

SYMPTOMS: Slow-growing granulomas form and later break down, discharging viscid pus containing minute yellowish (sulfur) granules.

TREATMENT: Prolonged administration of penicillin is usually effective. Tetracyclines are the second choice. Surgical incision and drainage of accessible lesions is helpful when combined with chemotherapy.

actinon (ăk′tĭn-ŏn) [Gr. *aktis*, ray] A radioactive isotope of actinium.

actinoneuritis (ăk″tĭn-ō-nū-rī′tĭs) [″ + *neuron*, nerve, + *itis*, inflammation] Inflammation of a nerve or nerves resulting from exposure to radium or x-rays.

actinophytosis (ăk″tĭ-nō-fī-tō′sĭs) [″ + *phyton*, plant, + *osis*, condition] Infection due to *Actinomyces.*

actinotherapy (ăk″tĭn-ō-thĕr′ă-pē) [″ + *therapeia*, treatment] Treatment of disease by rays of light, esp. actinic or photochemically active rays, or by x-rays or radium.

action (ăk′shŭn) [L. *actio*] Performance of a function or process; in pathology, a morbid process.

antagonistic a. The ability of a drug or muscle to oppose or resist the action or effect of another drug or muscle; opposite of synergistic action.

bacteriocidal a. Action that kills bacteria.

bacteriostatic a. Action that stops or prevents the growth of bacteria without killing them.

ball-valve a. Intermittent obstruction of a passageway or opening so that the flow of fluid or air is prevented from moving in and out in equal amounts.

calorigenic a. Heat produced by the metabolism of food.

capillary a. A surface tension effect shown by the elevation or depression of a liquid at the point of contact with a solid, as in capillary tubes. SYN: *capillarity.*

cumulative a. Sudden increased action of a drug after several doses have been given.

drug a. The function of a drug in various body systems.

Local: When the drug is applied locally or directly to a tissue or organ, it may combine with the cells' membrane or penetrate the cell. Its action may be (1) astringent when the drug causes the cell or tissue to contract, (2) corrosive when the drug is strong enough to destroy cells, or (3) irritating when too much of the drug combines with cells and impairs them.

General, or systemic: This type of action occurs when the drug enters the bloodstream by absorption or direct injection, affecting tissues and organs not near the site of entry. Systemic action may be (1) specific, when it cures a certain disease; (2) substitutive or replenishing, when it supplies substances deficient in the body; (3) physical, when some cell constituents are dissolved by the action of the drug in the bloodstream; (4) chemical, when the drug or some of its principles combine with the constituents of cells or organs to form a new chemical combination; (5) active by osmosis, caused by dilution of salt (also acids, sugars, and alkalies) in the stomach or intestines by fluid withdrawn from the blood and tissues; or by diffusion, when water is absorbed by cells from the lymph; (6) selective, when action is produced by drugs that affect only certain tissues or organs; (7) synergistic, when one drug increases the action of another; (8) antagonistic, when one drug counteracts another; (9) physiological, when the drug exerts a potentially beneficial effect similar to that which the body normally produces; (10) therapeutic, when the effect is to treat or repair diseased organs or tissues; (11) side active, creating an undesired effect; (12) empiric, producing results not proved by clinical or laboratory tests to be effective; or (13) toxicological, having a toxic or undesired effect, generally the result of overdose or long-term usage.

Cumulative: Some drugs are slowly excreted or absorbed so that with repeated doses an accumulation in the body produces a toxic effect. Such drugs should not be administered continuously.

Incompatible: Undesired side effects occur when some drugs are administered together. This may be due to the antagonistic action of one drug to others, or to a physical interaction of the drugs that inactivates one of them (e.g., precipitation of some drugs mixed in intravenous fluids).

reflex a. Involuntary movement produced by sensory nerve stimulation.

sparing a. The effect of a nonessential nutrient in the diet such that it decreases the requirement for an essential nutrient. For example, protein is esp. important for tissue growth and development in children. If protein intake is sufficient but caloric intake is inadequate, a protein deficiency will develop. In this situation, the addition of sufficient carbohydrates to the diet is said to spare the protein.

specific a. The particular action of a drug on another substance or on an organism or part of that organism.

specific dynamic a. Stimulation of the metabolic rate by ingestion of certain foods, esp. proteins.

synergistic a. The ability of a drug or muscle to aid or enhance the action or effect of another drug or muscle; opposite of antagonistic action.

thermogenic a. Action of a food, drug, or physical agent to cause a rise in output of body heat.

trigger a. The initiation of activity, physiological or pathological, that may have no relation to the action that started it.

activate (ăk′tĭ-vāt) To make active.

activated partial thromboplastin time ABBR: APTT. The time required for a fibrin clot to form after the activating factor, calcium, and a specific phospholipid mix have been added to the blood or plasma sample. The normal value ranges from about 16 to 40 sec. A prolonged time indicates any one of several diseases or medications (such as heparin). This test is used most often to monitor patients receiving heparin anticoagulation.

activation The process that stimulates resting, or nonfunctional, white blood cells to assume their role in the immune response. The process involves recognition of an antigen or a response to cytokines. SEE: *antigen processing; cytokine; immune response.*

activator (ăk′tĭ-vā″tor) **1.** A substance in the body that converts an inactive molecule into an active agent, such as the conversion of pepsinogen into pepsin by hydrogen ions. **2.** Any substance that specifically induces an activity, such as an inductor or organizer in embryonic development or a trophic hormone. **3.** A removable orthodontic appliance that transmits force passively from muscles to the teeth and alveolar process in contact with it. Also called *myofunctional appliance.*

active assistive range of motion ABBR: AAROM. An exercise in which an external force assists specific muscles and joints to move through their available excursion. AAROM exercises are used when the patient has difficulty moving or when tissue forces need to be reduced.

active plate activator A removable orthodontic appliance equipped to provide the force for tooth movement. It may be used continuously or intermittently.

active range of motion ABBR: AROM. The range of movement of a joint that is produced when a patient actively contracts without assistance the muscles that cross that joint.

Activities of Daily Living and Factors Affecting Them

Category	Activities	Affecting Factors
Personal care	Climbing stairs, moving into and out of chair or bed, feeding self, opening containers, dressing, using toilet, maintaining hygiene, taking medication	Altered mobility, physical or emotional illness, elimination problems
Family responsibilities	Shopping, cooking, doing laundry, cleaning, caring for yard, caring for family and pets, managing money	Altered mobility, heavy work schedule, insomnia, physical or emotional illness
Work or school	Fulfilling work responsibilities or school assignments, getting to and from work or school	Altered mobility, stress, heavy family demands, job dissatisfaction, difficulties in school, physical or emotional illness
Recreation	Pursuing hobbies and interests, exercising, reading, watching television	Altered mobility, physical or emotional illness
Socialization	Using the telephone, traveling, visiting family and friends, joining group activities, expressing sexuality	Altered mobility, physical or emotional illness, relocation

activins A family of polypeptide growth factors which help regulate various biological functions, esp. fertility. SEE: *inhibin.*

activities of daily living ABBR: ADL. Tasks performed by individuals in a typical day that allow independent living. Basic activities of daily living (BADL) include feeding, dressing, hygiene, and physical mobility. Instrumental activities of daily living (IADL) include more advanced skills such as managing personal finances, using transportation, telephoning, cooking, performing household chores, doing laundry, and shopping.

The ability to perform activities of daily living may be hampered by illness or accident resulting in physical or mental disability. Health care rehabilitation workers play a significant role in teaching individuals to maintain or relearn these skills so that the individual may achieve the highest possible degree of independence.

PATIENT CARE: The nurse and other members of the rehabilitation team, including occupational and physical therapists, assess the patient's ability to perform ADLs. The rehabilitation team instructs and trains the patient in techniques to relearn the skill, or to accommodate for inability to perform the task, with a goal of achieving the maximum possible independence. Where appropriate family members are involved in the rehabilitation program. referrals to community agencies are arranged when specific tasks cannot be performed independently. SEE: table.

instrumental a.d.l. ABBR: IADL. Those activities and tasks of living beyond basic self-care that are necessary for living independently, such as mobility, communication, cooking, shopping, cleaning the house, and doing laundry. M. Powell Lawton, U.S. gerontologist, identified these complex tasks. Other tasks considered necessary for living independently in the community include using the telephone, managing medications, and banking. SEE: *activities of daily living; self-care.*

activities of daily living, index of An assessment tool developed by American gerontologist S. Katz and his colleagues. It assesses self-maintenance in the elderly and focuses on the unaided performance of six basic personal care activities: eating, toileting, dressing, bathing, transferring, and continence.

activity (ăk-tĭv′ĭ-tē) The production of energy or motion; the state of being active. The word *activity* describes various conditions: enzyme activity describes the rate of influence of an enzyme on a particular system; extravehicular activity indicates the actions of space travelers while outside a space vehicle; radiation activity indicates the energy produced by a source of radiation.

graded a. In occupational therapy, a principle of therapeutic intervention in which tasks are classified and presented gradually according to the individual's level of function and the challenge or degree of skill (physical, social, or cognitive) required by the task.

leisure a. Activities chosen because they are pleasurable, relaxing, or in other ways emotionally satisfying, typically after work and other responsibilities are done.

optical a. In chemistry, the rotation of the plane of polarized light when the light passes through a chemical solution. Measurement of this property, called polarimetry, is useful in the determination of optically active substances such as dextrose. Sugars are classified according to this criterion. Optical activity of a substance in solution can be detected by placing it between polarizing and analyzing prisms.

pulseless electrical a. ABBR: PEA. A clinical condition in which the patient's heart is beating, as shown on the electrocardiogram, but the pulse cannot be felt or palpated.

purposeful a. The goal-directed use of time, energy, or attention that involves the active participation of the doer. Purposeful activity by humans often involves a social environment (others), a physical environment (objects, tools, and materials), and a process, which often culminates in a product.

activity analysis The process used by occupational therapists to determine the social, symbolic, physical, cognitive, and developmental characteristics of a task or activity and thus its therapeutic potential. Typical characteristics of interest include safety, cost, gradability, required space, tools or supplies, complexity, and social or cultural significance.

activity intolerance Inadequate mental or physical energy to accomplish daily activities. Risk factors include debilitating physical conditions such as anemia, obesity, musculoskeletal disorders, neurological deficits (such as those following stroke), severe heart disease, chronic pulmonary disease, metabolic disorders, and prolonged sedentary lifestyle. SEE: *Nursing Diagnoses Appendix.*

activity intolerance, risk for A state in which an individual is at risk of experiencing insufficient physiological or psychological energy to endure or complete required or desired daily activities. SEE: *Nursing Diagnoses Appendix.*

activity theory A social theory of aging that asserts that the more active older persons are, the higher their life satisfaction and morale. According to this theory, individuals who are aging successfully cultivate substitutes for former societal roles that they may have had to relinquish.

actomyosin (ăk″tō-mī′ō-sĭn) The combination of actin and myosin in a muscle.

actual (ăk′chū-ăl) [L. *actus*, doing] Real, existent.

actual cautery Cautery acting by heat and not chemically.

actuator (ăk′chū-ā-tŏr) A component of a mechanical or electronic device that initiates a given action.

acufilopressure (ăk″ū-fī′lō-prĕsh″ŭr) [L. *acus*, needle, + *filum*, thread, + *pressura*, pressure] Acupressure increased by a ligature.

acuity (ă-kū′ĭ-tē) [L. *acuere*, to sharpen] **1.** Clearness, sharpness of a sensory function (i.e., visual acuity). **2.** In emergency and critical care medicine, the severity of a patient's illness, and the level of attention or service he or she will need from professional staff.

visual a. Sharpness of vision.

acuminate (ă-kū′mĭn-āt) [L. *acuminatus*, sharpened] Conical or pointed.

acupressure (ăk′ū-prĕsh″ŭr) [L. *acus*, needle, + *pressura*, pressure] Finger pressure applied therapeutically at selected points on the body. In traditional Chinese medicine, the pressure points follow lines along the body called meridians. Techniques include shiatsu, tsubo, jin shin yutsu, and jon shin do.

acupressure forceps Spring-handled forceps for compressing blood vessels.

acupressure needles Elastic needles for compressing blood vessels.

acupuncture (ăk′ū-pŭngk″chūr) [L. *acus*, needle, + *punctura*, puncture] Technique for treating certain painful conditions and for producing regional anesthesia by passing long thin needles through the skin to specific points. The free ends of the needles are twirled or in some cases used to conduct a weak electric current. Anesthesia sufficient to permit abdominal, thoracic, and head and neck surgery has been produced by the use of acupuncture alone. The patient is fully conscious during the surgery. Acupuncture has been known in the Far East for centuries but received little attention in Western cultures until the early 1970s.

CAUTION: It is important that the acupuncturist use sterile or disposable needles and that care be taken to prevent puncturing adjacent organs.

---

acusis SEE: *presbycusis.*

acute (ă-kūt′) [L. *acutus*, sharp] **1.** Sharp, severe. **2.** Having rapid onset, severe symptoms, and a short course; not chronic.

acute care Health care delivered to patients experiencing sudden illness or trauma. Acute care generally occurs in the prehospital, hospital, or emergency department and is usually short-term rather than long-term or chronic care.

acute confusional state SEE: *confusional state, acute.*

acute mountain sickness ABBR: AMS. altitude sickness.

acute phase reaction The release of physiologically active proteins by the liver into the blood in response to interleukin-6 or other cytokines that participate in the destruction of pathogens and promote healing during inflammation. SYN: *acute phase response.* SEE: *cytokine; inflammation; interleukin-6; protein, acute phase.*

acute respiratory distress syndrome ABBR: ARDS. Respiratory insufficiency marked by progressive hypoxemia, due to severe inflammatory damage causing abnormal permeability of the alveolar-capillary membrane. The alveoli fill with fluid, which interferes with gas exchange. SEE: *disseminated intravascular coagulation; sepsis; systemic inflammatory response syndrome; Nursing Diagnoses Appendix.*

SYMPTOMS: Dyspnea and tachypnea are followed by a progressive hypoxemia that, despite oxygen therapy, is the hallmark of ARDS. Diffuse, fluffy infiltrates can be seen on chest radiographs.

DIAGNOSIS: Based on a history of a recent event associated with the onset of ARDS, the presence of non-cardiogenic pulmonary edema on the chest radiograph, and persistent hypoxemia on arterial blood gases.

ETIOLOGY: Acute respiratory distress syndrome may result from direct trauma to the lungs (e.g., near drowning, aspiration of gastric acids, severe lung infection) or systemic disorders such as shock, septicemia, disseminated intravascular coagulation (DIC), cardiopulmonary bypass, and reaction to multiple blood transfusions. Widespread damage to the alveolar-capillary membranes is initiated through the aggregation and activity of neutrophils and macrophages and the activation of complement. Cytokines, oxygen free radicals, and other inflammatory mediators damage the walls of capillaries and alveoli, producing diffuse inflammatory interstitial and alveolar edema, fibrin exudates, and hyaline membranes that block oxygen delivery to the blood.

TREATMENT: Endotracheal intubation and the use of mechanical ventilation with positive end-expiratory pressure (PEEP) are required along with high concentrations of oxygen, prevention or treatment of pneumonia, and drugs to maintain blood pressure and organ perfusion. Fluid restriction and a diuretic may be used to reduce pulmonary edema. The patient should be carefully monitored for hypoxia-induced cardiac arrhythmias, oxygen toxicity, renal failure, thrombocytopenia, sepsis, and DIC.

PROGNOSIS: Mortality is high, approx. 60% to 70% depending on the amount of lung tissue involved and the ability to maintain adequate oxygen flow to vital organs. After resolution of the inflammation, the damaged lung tissue becomes fibrotic and can cause chronic restrictive lung disease. Prolonged use of more than 50% oxygen increases the risk of residual lung damage.

PATIENT CARE: To avert ARDS, respiratory status is monitored in at-risk patients. Recognizing and treating early signs and symptoms can be crucial to a patient's survival. Ventilatory rate, depth, and rhythm are monitored, and subtle changes are noted; the onset of ARDS is marked by the onset of a rapid and shallow breathing pattern. The patient also is observed for chest wall retractions on inspiration, use of accessory breathing muscles, and level of dyspnea. The patient's consciousness level, cardiac rate and rhythm, blood pressure, arterial blood gas (ABG) values, serum electrolyte levels, and chest radiograph results are monitored. Fluid balance is closely watched by measuring intravenous (IV) fluid intake and urinary output, central venous pressure, and pulmonary artery wedge pressure; by weighing the patient daily; and by assessing for peripheral edema. A patent airway is maintained, and oxygen therapy with continuous positive airway pressure or mechanical ventilation with positive end-expiratory pressure (PEEP) is provided by the respiratory therapist as prescribed by the attending physician. Routine management of a mechanically ventilated patient includes monitoring breath sounds, chest wall movement, vital signs and comfort, and ventilator settings and function; suctioning the endotracheal tube and oropharynx; and assessing changes in pulse oximetry and ABG values.

Cardiac output may be decreased because PEEP increases intrathoracic pressure and reduces venous return. For this reason, health care professional staff monitor blood pressure, urine output, mental status, peripheral pulses, and pulmonary capillary wedge pressure to determine the effects of positive pressure ventilation on hemodynamics. Inotropic drugs are administered as prescribed if cardiac output falls. Hemoglobin levels and oxygen saturation values also are monitored closely, as packed red blood cell transfusion may be required if hemoglobin is inadequate for oxygen delivery. The nurse and respiratory therapist observe for signs and symptoms of barotrauma such as subcutaneous emphysema, pneumothorax, and pneumomediastinum (air leaks resulting from alveolar rupture caused by high airway pressures). If mechanical ventilation is used, sedation may help to calm the patient and reduce the incidence of poor synchronization between the patient and the ventilator. Enteral and parenteral nutrition and prescribed IV fluids to maintain fluid volume are administered. Nursing measures are used to prevent problems of immobility. Strict asepsis is observed in dressing changes, suctioning, handwashing, and oral care. The patient is routinely assessed for fever, sputum color changes, and elevated WBC count. Response to therapy is evaluated and adverse reactions are noted. The family is encouraged to talk to the patient even though he or she may not respond verbally.

The respiratory therapist plays a key role in the care of patients with ARDS. He or she initiates mechanical ventilation as prescribed by the attending physician and monitors arterial blood gases and pulse oximetry to assure adequate oxygenation. The respiratory therapist adjusts the tidal volume, respiratory rate, and PEEP levels to optimize tissue oxygenation. He or she also helps determine when the patient may be ready for weaning from mechanical ventilation by periodic assessment of the patient's cardiopulmonary status.

acute respiratory failure SEE: *respiratory failure, acute.*

acute tubular necrosis ABBR: ATN. Acute damage to the renal tubules; usually due to ischemia associated with shock. SEE: *renal failure, acute.*

acute urethral syndrome Syndrome experienced by women, marked by acute dysuria, urinary frequency, and lack of significant bacteriuria; pyuria may or may not be present. The cause is unknown, but it is important to determine whether a specific bacterial infection of the bladder or vagina is present to ensure that appropriate drugs are given as needed. The syndrome is referred to colloquially as "honeymoon cystitis" because it may occur during periods of increased sexual activity.

PATIENT CARE: A history of the illness, including events that increase or decrease symptoms, is obtained. The degree and nature of the patient's pain, its location and possible radiation, and its frequency and duration are ascertained. The patient is instructed in the procedure for collecting a clean-catch, midstream urine specimen and is prepared for vaginal examination. If a bladder or vaginal bacterial infection is diagnosed, prescribed treatment measures are explained and demonstrated.

acyanoblepsia (ă-sī″ă-nō-blĕp′sē-ă) [Gr. *a-*, not, + *kyanos*, blue, + *blepsis*, vision] Inability to discern blue colors. Also called *acyanopsia.*

acyanotic (ă-sī″ă-nŏt′ĭk) [″ + *kyanos*, blue] Pert. to the absence of cyanosis.

acyclic (ă-sī′klĭk) **1.** Without a cycle. **2.** In chemistry, aliphatic.

acyclovir (ă-sī′klō-vĭr) An antiviral drug approved for use in herpes simplex infections of the genitals, face, and central nervous system. Trade name is Zovirax.

acyl (ăs′ĭl) General formula RC=O; in organic chemistry, the radical derived from an organic acid when the hydroxyl group (OH) is removed.

acylation (ăs″ĭ-lā′shŭn) Incorporation of an acid radical into a chemical.

acystia (ă-sĭs′tē-ă) [Gr. *a-*, not, + *kystis*, bladder] Congenital absence of the bladder.

acystinervia, acystineuria (ă-sĭs″tĭ-nĕr′vē-ă, -nū′rē-ă) [″ + ″ + *neuron*, nerve] Defective nerve supply to or paralysis of the bladder.

AD *anodal duration; average deviation.*

ad [L., to] In prescription writing, an indication that a substance should be added to the formulation up to a specified volume.

ad- [L., to] Prefix indicating *adherence, increase, toward,* as in adduct.

-ad [L., to] Suffix meaning *toward* or *in the direction of*, as in cephalad.

a.d. [L.] *auris dextra,* right ear.

A.D.A. *American Dental Association; American Diabetes Association; American Dietetic Association; Americans with Disabilities Act.*

A.D.A.A. *American Dental Assistants Association.*

adactylia, adactylism, adactyly (ă″dăk-tĭl′ē-ă, ā-dăk′tĭ-lĭzm, -lē) [Gr. *a-*, not, + *daktylos*, finger] Congenital absence of digits of the hand or foot.

adamantine (ăd″ă-măn′tĭn) [Gr. *adamantinos*] Very hard; said of enamel of teeth.

adamantinoma (ăd″ă-măn″tĭ-nō′mă) [″ + *oma*, tumor] A tumor of the jaw, esp. of the lower one, that arises from enamel-forming cells and may be partly cystic, partly solid. It may be benign or of low-grade malignancy. SYN: *ameloblastoma.*

adamantoblast (ăd″ă-măn′tō-blăst) [Gr. *adamas*, hard surface, + *blastos*, germ] An enamel-forming cell present only during tooth formation. SYN: *ameloblast.*

adamantoblastoma (ăd″ă-măn″tō-blăs-tō′mă) [″ + ″ + *oma*, tumor] Overgrowth of an adamantoblast.

adamantoma (ăd″ă-măn-tō′mă) [Gr. *adamas*, hard surface, + *oma*, tumor] Adamantinoma.

Adam's apple The laryngeal prominence formed by the two laminae of the thyroid cartilage. SYN: *pomum adami; prominentia laryngea.*

Adams-Stokes syndrome SEE: *Stokes-Adams syndrome.*

Adams test A measurement of lateral spinal curvature (scoliosis) after the patient bends forward at the waist. A scoliometer is used to measure the degree of curvature.

adaptation (ăd″ăp-tā′shŭn) [L. *adaptare*, to adjust] **1.** Adjustment of an organism to a change in internal or external conditions or circumstances. **2.** Adjustment of the eye to various intensities of light, accomplished by changing the size of the pupil and accompanied by chemical changes occurring in the rods. **3.** In psychology, a change in quality, intensity, or distinctness of a sensation that occurs after continuous stimulation of constant intensity. **4.** In dentistry, the proper fitting of dentures or bands to the teeth, or closeness of a filling to walls of a cavity.

chromatic a. A change in hue or saturation, or both, resulting from pre-exposure to light of other wavelengths.

color a. The fading of intensity of color perception after prolonged visual stimulation.

dark a. Adjustment of the eyes for vision in dim light. SYN: *scotopia*.

light a. Adjustment of the eyes for vision in bright light. SYN: *photopia*.

retinal a. Adjustment of the rods and cones of the retina to ambient light.

Adaptation Model A conceptual model of nursing developed by nursing theorist Sister Callista Roy that is based on the individual's adaptation to environmental stimuli. In this model the goal of nursing is to promote adaptive physiological, self-concept, role function, and interdependent responses. SEE: Nursing Theory Appendix.

adapted clothing Garments designed with special features, such as Velcro closures, to enable persons with disabilities to dress themselves without assistance.

adapter (ă-dăp′tĕr) **1.** Device for joining one part of an apparatus to another part. **2.** Device to facilitate connecting electrical supply cords to different receptacles. **3.** Device for adapting one type of electrical supply source to the specific requirements of an instrument.

adaptive capacity, intracranial, decreased A clinical state in which intracranial fluid dynamic mechanisms that normally compensate for increases in intracranial volumes are compromised, resulting in repeated disproportionate increases in intracranial pressure in response to a variety of noxious and nonnoxious stimuli. SEE: *Nursing Diagnoses Appendix.*

adaptometer A device for determining the time required for retinal adaptation.

adaxial (ăd-ăk′sē-ăl) [L. *ad*, toward, + *axis*, axis] Toward the main axis; opposite of abaxial.

add Prescription abbreviation meaning *let there be added.*

adde (ăd′ē) [L.] *Add,* used as a direction in writing prescriptions.

addict (ăd′ĭkt) [L. *addictus*, given over] **1.** An individual who cannot control his or her need or craving for a substance or a behavior. **2.** To make someone dependent or to become dependent on a substance or behavior.

addiction (ă-dĭk′shŭn) A compulsive and maladaptive dependence on a substance (e.g., alcohol, cocaine, opiates, or tobacco) or a behavior (e.g., gambling). The dependence typically produces adverse psychological, physical, economic, social, or legal ramifications.

Addis count method (ăd′ĭs) [Thomas Addis, Scot.-born U.S. physician, 1881–1949] Method for counting the sediment (casts and cells) in a 12-hr urine sample.

Addison's disease [Thomas Addison, Brit. physician, 1793–1860] A rare illness marked by gradual and progressive failure of the adrenal glands and insufficient production of steroid hormones. Patients with Addison's disease make inadequate amounts of both glucocorticoids and mineralocorticoids.

ETIOLOGY: Adrenal failure typically results from autoimmune destruction of the adrenal glands, chronic infections (e.g., tuberculosis, cytomegalovirus, or histoplasmosis), or cancers that metastasize to the adrenal glands from other organs (e.g., the lungs or breast).

SYMPTOMS: The patient may be symptom-free until the majority of adrenal tissue is destroyed. Early complaints are usually nonspecific: a feeling of weakness or fatigue. Subsequently, patients may notice lack of appetite, weight loss, nausea, vomiting, abdominal pain, and dizziness. Physical findings may include postural hypotension and increased skin pigmentation. Laboratory studies may reveal hyponatremia and hyperkalemia. If these findings are present, a cosyntropin stimulation test may be performed to establish the diagnosis.

TREATMENT: Chronic adrenal insufficiency is managed with corticosteroids, such as prednisone, usually taken twice a day. During episodic illnesses or stresses (e.g., surgeries) the maintenance dose of these medications is increased, then tapered over several days back to baseline levels. SEE: *adrenal crisis.*

PROGNOSIS: If untreated, the disease will continue a chronic course with progressive but usually relatively slow deterioration; in some patients the deterioration may be rapid. Patients treated properly have an excellent prognosis.

PATIENT CARE: Patients with primary adrenal insufficiency who are suffering other acute conditions are assessed frequently for hypotension, tachycardia, fluid balance, and electrolyte and glucose levels. Prescribed adrenocortical steroids, with sodium and fluid replacement, are administered. The patient is protected from stressors such as infection, noise, and light and temperature changes. Extra time for rest and relaxation is planned.

For chronic maintenance therapy: Both patient and family are taught about the need for lifelong replacement therapy and medical supervision. Patients are taught about self-administration of steroid therapy (typically two thirds of the dose is given in the a.m., and one third in the p.m.). Symptoms of overdosage and underdosage and the course of action if either occurs are explained. The patient is instructed to increase fluid and salt replacement if perspiring and to follow a diet high in sodium, carbohydrates, and protein, with small, frequent meals if hypoglycemia or anorexia occurs. Measures to help prevent infection include getting adequate rest, avoiding fatigue, eating a balanced diet, and avoiding people with infections. Verbalization of feelings and concerns is encouraged. The patient is assisted to develop coping strategies and is referred for further mental health or stress management counseling if warranted. SEE: *Nursing Diagnoses Appendix.*

addisonism (ăd'ĭ-sŭn-ĭzm") Symptom complex resembling Addison's disease caused by adrenal glands, destruction by infectious agents such as *Mycobacterium tuberculosis* or *Cytomegalovirus*.

Addison's planes Imaginary planes that divide the abdomen into nine regions to aid in the location of internal structures. SEE: *abdominal regions*.

addition (ă-dĭ'shŭn) In chemistry, a reaction in which two substances unite without loss of atoms or valence.

additive (ăd'ĭ-tĭv) In pharmacology, the effect that one drug or substance contributes to the action of another drug or substance.

food a. Substance added to food to maintain or impart a certain consistency, to improve or maintain nutritive value, to enhance palatability or flavor, to produce a light texture, or to control pH. Food additives are used to help bread rise during baking, to keep bread mold-free, to color margarine, to prevent discoloration of some fruits, and to prevent fats and oils from becoming rancid. The U.S. Food and Drug Administration regulates the use of food additives.

adducent (ă-dū'sĕnt) [L. *adducere*, to bring toward] Causing adduction.

adduct (ă-dŭkt') [L. *adductus*, brought toward] To draw toward the main axis of the body or a limb.

adduction (ă-dŭk'shŭn) Movement of a limb or eye toward the median plane of the body or, in the case of digits, toward the axial line of a limb. SEE: *abduction* for illus.

convergent-stimulus a. Convergence of the eyes when the gaze is fixed on an object at the near point of vision.

adductor (ă-dŭk'tor) A muscle that draws toward the medial line of the body or to a common center.

adductor reflex Contraction of the adductor muscles of the thigh on applying pressure to, or tapping, the medial surface of the thigh or knee.

adelomorphous (ă-dĕl"ō-mor'fŭs) [Gr. *adelos*, not seen, + *morphe*, shape] Having undefined form, as in the central cells of the gastric glands.

aden- SEE: *adeno-*.

adenalgia (ăd"ĕn-ăl'jē-ă) [Gr. *aden*, gland, + *algos*, pain] Pain in a gland. SYN: *adenodynia*.

adenase (ăd'ĕ-nāz) [" + *-ase*, enzyme] Enzyme secreted by the pancreas, spleen, and liver that converts adenine into hypoxanthine. SEE: *enzyme*.

adendric, adendritic (ă-dĕn'drĭk, ă"dĕn-drĭt'ĭk) [Gr. *a-*, not, + *dendrites*, rel. to a tree] Without dendrites, as in certain cells in the spinal ganglia.

adenectomy (ăd"ĕn-ĕk'tō-mē) [Gr. *aden*, gland, + *ektome*, excision] Excision of a gland.

adenectopia (ăd"ĕ-nĕk-tō'pē-ă) [" + " + *topos*, place] Malposition of a gland; a gland in a position that is other than its normal position.

adenia (ă-dē'nē-ă) Chronic inflammation and enlargement of a lymph gland.

adeniform (ă-dĕn'ĭ-form) [Gr. *aden*, gland, + L. *forma*, shape] Glandlike in form.

adenine (ăd'ĕ-nĭn) A purine base, $C_5H_5N_5$, that is part of the genetic code of DNA and RNA. In DNA it is paired with thymine and in RNA, with uracil.

adenitis (ăd"ĕ-nī'tĭs) [Gr. *aden*, gland, + *itis*, inflammation] Inflammation of lymph nodes or a gland.

adenization (ăd"ĕ-nĭ-zā'shŭn) Abnormal change into a glandlike structure.

adeno-, aden- [Gr. *aden*, gland] Combining form meaning *gland*.

adenoacanthoma (ăd"ĕ-nō-ăk"ăn-thō'mă) [" + *akantha*, thorn, + *oma*, tumor] Adenocarcinoma in which some cells have undergone squamous metaplasia.

adenoameloblastoma (ăd"ĕ-nō-ă-mĕl"ō-blăs-tō'mă) [" + O. Fr. *amel*, enamel, + Gr. *blastos*, germ, + *oma*, tumor] Benign tumor of the jaw, originating from ameloblast cells of forming teeth; an odontogenic tumor.

adenoblast (ăd'ĕ-nō-blăst) [" + *blastos*, germ] **1.** Embryonic cells that produce glandular tissue. **2.** Any tissue that produces secretory or glandular activity.

adenocarcinoma (ăd"ĕ-nō-kăr"sĭn-ō'mă) [" + *karkinos*, crab, + *oma*, tumor]

A malignant tumor arising from a glandular organ.

acinar a. Adenocarcinoma in which the cells are in the shape of alveoli. SYN: *alveolar a.*

alveolar a. Acinar a.

adenocele (ăd′ĕ-nō-sēl″) [″ + *kele*, tumor, swelling] **1.** A cystic tumor arising from a gland. **2.** A tumor of glandular structure.

adenocellulitis (ăd″ĕ-nō-sĕl″ū-lī′tĭs) [″ + L. *cella*, small chamber, + Gr. *itis*, inflammation] Inflammation of a gland and adjacent cellular tissue.

adenocyst (ăd′ĕ-nō-sĭst″) [″ + *kystis*, sac] A cystic tumor arising from a gland.

adenocystoma (ăd″ĕ-nō-sĭs-tō′mă) [″ + *kystis*, sac, + *oma*, tumor] Cystic adenoma.

adenodynia (ăd″ĕ-nō-dĭn′ē-ă) [″ + *odyne*, pain] Pain in a gland. SYN: *adenalgia.*

adenoepithelioma (ăd″ĕ-nō-ĕp″ĭ-thēl-ē-ō′mă) [″ + *epi*, on, + *thele*, nipple, + *oma*, tumor] A tumor consisting of glandular and epithelial elements.

adenofibroma (ăd″ĕ-nō-fī-brō′mă) [″ + L. *fibra*, fiber, + Gr. *oma*, tumor] A tumor of fibrous and glandular tissue (connective tissue); frequently found in the uterus or breast.

adenofibrosis (ăd″ĕ-nō-fī-brō′sĭs) [″ + ″ + Gr. *osis*, condition] Degeneration of a tumor that contains fibrous connective tissue.

adenogenous (ăd″ĕ-nŏj′ĕ-nŭs) [″ + *gennan*, to produce] Originating in glandular tissue.

adenohypophysis (ăd″ĕ-nō-hī-pŏf′ĭ-sĭs) [″ + *hypo*, under, + *phyein*, to grow] The anterior lobe of the pituitary gland.

adenoid (ăd′ĕ-noyd) [″ + Gr. *eidos*, form, shape] Lymphoid; having the appearance of a gland.

adenoidectomy (ăd″ĕ-noyd-ĕk′tō-mē) [″ + ″ + *ektome*, excision] Excision of the adenoids. SEE: *tonsillectomy; Nursing Diagnoses Appendix.*

PATIENT CARE: Vital signs are monitored, and the patient is observed for signs of shock. The mouth and pharynx are checked for bleeding, large clot formation, or oozing; the patient is observed for frequent swallowing, which indicates bleeding or large clot formation. Clots should be prevented from obstructing the oropharnyx. The patient is placed in either a prone position with the head turned to the side or in a lateral recumbent position to promote drainage. When the operative wound has healed sufficiently, the oral intake of cool (not hot or iced) fluids and soft foods is encouraged. The patient is also advised not to gargle until the surgical site has healed.

Young patients: The child is reassured concerning care routines and procedures. Emotional support is provided, and parental presence is encouraged. The child is evaluated for vomiting swallowed blood, and is monitored for ability to swallow fluids.

adenoid hypertrophy Enlargement of the pharyngeal tonsil. It occurs commonly in children and may be congenital or result from infection of Waldeyer's ring.

adenoiditis (ăd″ĕ-noyd-ī′tĭs) [Gr. *aden*, gland, + *eidos*, form, + *itis*, inflammation] Inflammation of adenoid tissue.

adenoids (ăd′ĕ-noyds) Lymphatic tissue forming a prominence on the wall of the pharyngeal recess of the nasopharynx. SEE: *pharyngeal tonsil.*

adenolipoma (ăd″ĕ-nō-lĭp-ō′mă) [Gr. *aden*, gland, + *lipos*, fat, + *oma*, tumor] A benign tumor having glandular characteristics but composed of fat.

adenolymphocele (ăd″ĕ-nō-lĭm′fō-sēl) [″ + ″ + Gr. *kele*, tumor, swelling] Cystic dilatation of a lymph node from obstruction.

adenolymphoma (ăd″ĕ-nō-lĭm-fō′mă) [″ + ″ + Gr. *oma*, tumor] A lymph gland adenoma.

adenoma (ăd″ĕ-nō′mă) *pl.* **adenomata** [″ + *oma*, tumor] A benign (not malignant) tumor made of epithelial cells, usually arranged like a gland. **adenomatous** (-nō′mă-tŭs), *adj.*

acidophil(ic) a. Tumor of the pituitary gland in which cells stain with acid dyes. It usually produces growth hormones and causes acromegaly and gigantism. SYN: *eosinophil(ic) a.; somatotroph a.*

adrenocorticotrophin-secreting a. A pituitary tumor that secretes adrenocorticotropic hormone, the substance responsible for Cushing's syndrome.

basophil(ic) a. Tumor of the pituitary gland in which cells stain with basic dyes. It usually produces adrenocorticotrophin and causes Cushing's syndrome.

chromophobe a. Tumor of the pituitary gland composed of cells that do not stain readily. It may cause pituitary deficiency or diabetes insipidus.

eosinophil(ic) a. Acidophil(ic) a.

fibroid a. Fibroadenoma.

follicular a. Adenoma of the thyroid.

gonadotroph-cell a. The most common macroadenoma of the pituitary gland. Because it does not cause endocrine disorders it is considered a nonfunctioning tumor.

Hürthle cell a. Tumor of the thyroid that contains mostly eosinophil-staining cells; occasionally found in diseases such as Hashimoto's thyroiditis.

malignant a. Adenocarcinoma.

nonfunctioning pituitary a. Gonadotroph-cell a.

papillary a. Adenoma with nipple-shaped glands.

pituitary a. Adenoma of the pituitary gland.

prolactin-secreting a. Prolactinoma.

sebaceous a. Enlarged sebaceous glands, esp. of the face. SYN: *a. sebaceum.*

a. sebaceum sebaceous a.

somatotroph a. A growth-hormone-secreting tumor of the anterior pituitary that causes acromegaly or giantism.

villous a. Large polyp of the mucosal surface of the large intestine.

adenomatome (ăd″ĕ-nō′mă-tōm) [″ + *oma*, tumor, + *tome*, incision] An instrument for removing adenoids.

adenomatosis (ăd″ĕ-nō-mă-tō′sĭs) [″ + *oma*, tumor, + *osis*, condition] The condition of multiple glandular tissue overgrowths.

adenomere (ăd′ĕ-nō-mēr″) [″ + *meros*, part] The functional part of a gland.

adenomyoma (ăd″ĕ-nō-mī-ō′mă) [″ + *mys*, muscle, + *oma*, tumor] Tumor containing glandular and smooth muscular tissue.

adenomyometritis (ăd″ĕ-nō-mī″ō-mĕ-trī′tĭs) [″ + ″ + *metra*, womb, + *itis*, inflammation] A hyperplastic condition of the uterus caused by pelvic inflammation; it grossly resembles an adenomyoma.

adenomyosarcoma (ăd″ĕ-nō-mī″ō-săr-kō′mă) [″ + ″ + *sarx*, flesh, + *oma*, tumor] Adenosarcoma that includes muscle tissue.

adenomyosis (ăd″ĕ-nō-mī-ō′sĭs) [″ + *mys*, muscle, + *osis*, condition] Benign invasive growth of the endometrium into the muscular layer of the uterus. SEE: *endometriosis* for illus.

adenopathy (ăd-ĕ-nŏp′ă-thē) [″ + *pathos*, disease, suffering] Swelling and morbid change in lymph nodes; glandular disease.

adenopharyngitis (ăd″ĕ-nō-făr″ĭn-jī′tĭs) [″ + *pharynx*, throat, + *itis*, inflammation] Inflammation of tonsils and pharyngeal mucous membrane.

adenophthalmia (ăd″ĕ-nŏf-thăl′mē-ă) [″ + *ophthalmos*, eye] Inflammation of the meibomian gland.

adenosarcoma (ăd″ĕ-nō-săr-kō′mă) [″ + *sarx*, flesh, + *oma*, tumor] A tumor with adenomatous and sarcomatous characteristics.

adenosclerosis (ăd″ĕ-nō-sklĕ-rō′sĭs) [″ + *sklerosis*, hardening] Glandular hardening.

adenose (ăd′ĕ-nōs) Glandlike.

adenosine (ă-dĕn′ō-sēn) A nucleotide containing adenine and ribose.

a. 3′,5′-cyclic monophosphate ABBR: AMP. A cyclic form of adenosine. Its synthesis from adenosine triphosphate (ATP) is stimulated by an enzyme, adenylate cyclase (also called cyclic AMP synthetase). Adenosine 3′,5′-cyclic monophosphate is important in a wide variety of metabolic responses to cell stimuli.

a. deaminase conjugated with polyethylene glycol ABBR: PEG-ADA. A cytoplasmic enzyme used to treat severe combined immunodeficiency disease (SCID) due to adenosine deaminase deficiency. Trade name is Adagen. SEE: *severe combined immunodeficiency disease.*

a. diphosphate ABBR: ADP. A compound of adenosine containing two phosphoric acid groups. ADP is used to synthesize ATP with the energy released in cell respiration. When ATP is used for cellular functions such as protein synthesis, ADP is reformed.

a. monophosphate ABBR: AMP; 5′-AMP. Substance formed by condensation of adenosine and phosphoric acid. It is one of the hydrolytic products of nucleic acids and is present in muscle, red blood cells, yeast, and other nuclear material. SYN: *adenylic acid.*

a. triphosphatase ABBR: ATPase. Enzyme that splits adenosine triphosphate to yield phosphate and energy.

a. triphosphate ABBR: ATP. A compound of adenosine containing three phosphoric acid groups. ATP is present in all cells; it is formed when energy is released from food molecules during cell respiration. Cells contain enzymes to split ATP into ADP, phosphate, and energy, which is then available for cellular functions such as mitosis.

adenosis (ăd″ĕ-nō′sĭs) [Gr. *aden*, gland, + *osis*, condition] Any disease of a gland, or of glandular tissue.

adenotome (ăd′ĕ-nō-tōm) [″ + *tome*, incision] Device for excising a gland, esp. the adenoid glands.

adenotonsillectomy (ăd″ĕ-nō-tŏn″sĭl-lĕk′tō-mē) [″ + L. *tonsilla*, almond, + Gr. *ektome*, excision] Surgical removal of the tonsils and adenoids.

adenous (ăd′ĕ-nŭs) Like a gland.

adenovirus (ăd′ĕ-nō-vī′rŭs) One of a group of closely related viruses that can cause infections of the upper respiratory tract. A large number have been isolated. SEE: illus.

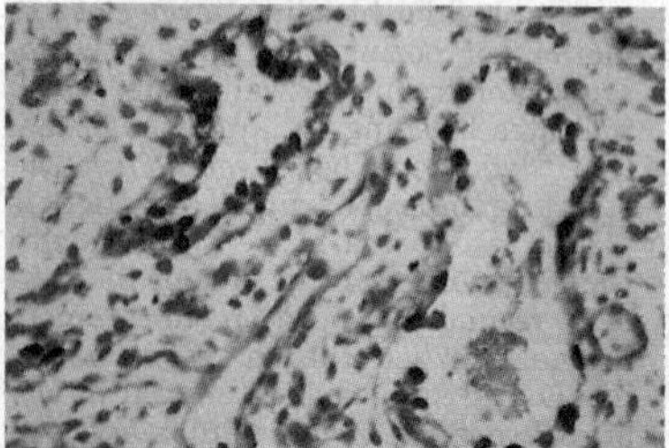

ADENOVIRUS

Adenovirus inclusions (stained blue-black) in the cells lining a bronchiole

adenyl (ăd′ĕ-nĭl) The radical $C_5H_4N_5$; present in adenine.

a. cyclase An enzyme that catalyzes the production of cyclic AMP (adenosine 3′,5′-cyclic monophosphate) from ATP (adenosine triphosphate). It is present on most cell surfaces.

adenylate cyclase (ă-dĕn′ĭ-lāt sī′klās) An enzyme important in the synthesis of cyclic AMP (adenosine 3′,5′-cyclic monophosphate) from adenosine triphosphate. SYN: *cyclic AMP synthetase.*

adermia (ă-dĕr′mē-ă) [Gr. *a*-, not, + *derma*, skin] Congenital or acquired defect of or lack of skin.

adermogenesis (ă-dĕr″mō-jĕn′ĕ-sĭs) [″ + ″ + *genesis*, generation, birth] Imperfect development of skin.

ADH *antidiuretic hormone* (vasopressin).

A.D.H.A. *American Dental Hygienists' Association.*

adherence (ăd′hēr-ĕns) **1.** Stickiness **2.** Compliance.

bacterial a. [ăd-hēr′ĕns] The ability of bacteria to adhere to specific receptors that are present on some cells but not on others. If bacteria normally present in the intestinal tract did not have this ability, they would be washed out of the intestines.

adherent (ăd-hē′rĕnt) [L. *adhaerere*, to stick to] Attached to, as of two surfaces.

adhesin **1.** In conjugation of some bacteria, a protein on the cell surface that causes aggregation of cells. **2.** A protein found on the cell wall of bacteria such as *Escherichia coli* that enables the bacteria to bind to the host's cells.

adhesion (ăd-hē′zhŭn) [L. *adhaesio*, stuck to] **1.** A holding together or uniting of two surfaces or parts, as in wound healing. **2.** A fibrous band holding parts together that are normally separated. **3.** An attraction to another substance: thus, molecules or blood platelets adhere to each other or to dissimilar materials.

abdominal a. Adhesion in the abdominal cavity, usually involving the intestines; caused by inflammation or trauma. If adhesions cause great pain or intestinal obstruction, they are treated surgically.

pericardial a. Adhesion of the pericardium. If extensive, adhesions may lead to restriction of the normal movement of the heart. SEE: *pericarditis.*

adhesiotomy (ăd-hē″zē-ŏt′ō-mē) [L. *adhaesio*, stuck to, + Gr. *tome*, incision] Surgical division of adhesions.

adhesive (ăd-hē′sĭv) [L. *adhaesio*, stuck to] **1.** Causing adhesion. **2.** Sticky; adhering. **3.** A substance that causes two bodies to adhere.

adhesive capsulitis Adherence of folds causing inflammatory thickening in an articular (joint) capsule, esp. the shoulder, thereby restricting movement.

adhesive inflammation Inflammation of the serous membrane, enhancing the likelihood of adhesions.

adiadochokinesia, adiadochokinesis (ă-dī″ă-dō″kō-kĭ-nē′sē-ă, -nē′sĭs) [Gr. *a*-, not, + *diadochas*, successive, + *kinesis*, movement] Inability to make rapid alternating movements.

adiaphoresis (ă-dī″ă-fō-rē′sĭs) [″ + *diaphorein*, to perspire] Deficiency or absence of sweat.

adiastole (ă″dī-ăs′tō-lē) [″ + *diastole*, dilatation] Imperceptibility of diastole.

Adie's syndrome (ā′dēz) [William John Adie, Brit. neurologist, 1886–1935] A syndrome marked by a tonic pupil that responds slowly or not at all to light, with impaired accommodation and slow constriction and relaxation in the change from near to distant vision. The affected pupil is frequently larger than the normal pupil. Loss of certain deep tendon reflexes may also be present, but there are no other signs of central nervous system disease. SEE: *pupil, tonic.*

adip- SEE: *adipo-.*

adipectomy (ăd″ĭ-pĕk′tō-mē) [L. *adeps*, fat, + Gr. *ektome*, excision] Excision of fat or adipose tissue, usually a large quantity. SEE: *liposuction.*

adipic (ă-dĭp′ĭk) Rel. to adipose tissue.

adipo-, adip- [L. *adeps*, fat] Combining form meaning fat. See also *lipo-, steato-.*

adipocele (ăd′ĭ-pō-sēl″) [L. *adeps*, fat, + Gr. *kele*, tumor] A hernia that contains fat or fatty tissue. SYN: *lipocele.*

adipocellular (ăd″ĭ-pō-sĕl′ū-lăr) Containing fat and cellular tissue.

adipocere (ăd′ĭ-pō-sēr″) [L. *adeps*, fat, + *cera*, wax] A brown, waxlike substance composed of fatty acids and calcium soaps. It is formed in animal tissues post-mortem.

adipocyte SEE: *fat cell.*

adipofibroma [″ + *fibra*, fiber, + Gr. *oma*, tumor] A fibroma and adipoma.

adipogenous, adipogenic (ăd″ĭ-pŏj′ĕn-ŭs, -pō-jĕn′ĭk) [″ + Gr. *gennan*, to produce] Inducing the formation of fat.

adipoid (ăd′ĭ-poyd) [L. *adeps*, fat, + Gr. *eidos*, form, shape] Fatlike; lipoid.

adipokinesis (ăd″ĭ-pō-kĭ-nē′sĭs) [″ + Gr. *kinesis*, movement] **1.** Metabolism of fat with production of free fatty acids. **2.** Mobilization and metabolism of body fat.

adipokinetic action The action of substances to promote formation of free fatty acids from body fat stores.

adiponecrosis (ăd″ĭ-pō-nĕ-krō′sĭs) [″ + Gr. *nekrosis*, state of death] Necrosis affecting fatty tissue.

adipose [L. *adiposus*, fatty] Fatty; pert. to fat.

adiposis (ăd″ĭ-pō′sĭs) [L. *adeps*, fat, + Gr. *osis*, condition] Abnormal accumulation of fat in the body. SYN: *corpulence; liposis; obesity.*

a. cerebralis Obesity due to intracranial disease, esp. of the pituitary.

a. dolorosa Dercum's disease.

a. hepatica Fatty degeneration or infiltration of the liver.

adipositis (ăd″ĭ-pō-sī′tĭs) [L. *adiposus*, fatty, + Gr. *itis*, inflammation] Infiltration of an inflammatory nature in and beneath subcutaneous adipose tissue.

adiposity (ăd″ĭ-pŏs′ĭ-tē) Excessive fat in the body. SYN: *adiposis; corpulence; obesity*.

adiposuria (ăd″ĭ-pō-sū′rē-ă) [″ + Gr. *ouron*, urine] Fat in the urine. SYN: *lipuria*.

adipsia, adipsy (ă-dĭp′sē-ă, -sē) [Gr. *a*-, not, + *dipsa*, thirst] Absence of thirst.

aditus (ăd′ĭ-tŭs) [L.] An approach; an entrance.

a. ad antrum The recess of the tympanic cavity that leads from the epitympanic recess to the tympanic antrum.

a. laryngis Upper aperture of the larynx.

adjunct (ăd′jŭnkt) An addition to the principal procedure or course of therapy.

adjuster A device for holding together the ends of the wire forming a suture.

adjustment [L. *adjuxtare*, to bring together] **1.** Adaptation to a different environment; a person's relation to his or her environment and self. **2.** A change made to improve function or condition. **3.** A modification made to a tooth or a dental prosthesis to enhance fit, function, or patient acceptance. SEE: *occlusal adjustment*.

cost of living a. ABBR: COLA. In determining social security payments and other financial benefits, a change in compensation based on the rate of inflation, as demonstrated by the U.S. Consumer Price Index.

adjustment disorder A maladaptive reaction to an identifiable psychological or social stress that occurs within 3 months of the onset of the stressful situation. The reaction is characterized by impaired function or symptoms in excess of what would be considered normal for that stress. The symptoms are expected to remit when the stress ceases; if the stress continues, a new level of adaptation is achieved.

adjustment, impaired Inability to modify lifestyle/behavior in a manner consistent with a change in health status. SEE: *Nursing Diagnoses Appendix*.

adjuvant (ăd′jū-vănt) [L. *adjuvans*, aiding] **1.** That which assists, esp. a drug added to a prescription to hasten or increase the action of a principal ingredient. **2.** In immunology, chemicals such as aluminum hydroxide and aluminum phosphate that are added to an antigen to increase the body's immunologic response. The adjuvants increase the size of the antigen, making it easier for B lymphocytes and phagocytes to recognize it, promote chemotaxis, and stimulate the release of cytokines. Adjuvants are not effective with all antigens and do not stimulate T lymphocyte activity.

Freund's complete a. A water-in-oil emulsion in which an antigen solution is emulsified in mineral oil with killed mycobacteria to enhance antigenicity. The intense inflammatory response produced by this emulsion makes it unsuitable for use in humans.

Freund's incomplete a. A water-in-oil emulsion in which an antigen solution without mycobacteria is emulsified in mineral oil. On injection, this mixture induces a strong persistent antibody formation.

ADL *activities of daily living*.

Adler, Alfred Austrian psychiatrist (1870–1937) who founded the school of individual psychology. SEE: *psychology, individual*.

ad lib [L. *ad libitum*] Prescription abbreviation meaning *as desired*.

ad libitum [NL] As desired.

administration The giving of a therapeutic agent.

Administration on Aging ABBR: AOA. An agency of the U.S. Department of Health and Human Services that conducts research in the field of aging and assists federal, state, and local agencies in planning and developing programs for the aged. It is responsible for implementing the Older Americans Act of 1965.

admission of fact Written requests to accept or deny mutually agreed upon deeds, statements, or assertions of a lawsuit.

A.D.N. *Associate Degree in Nursing*.

ad nauseam (ăd naw′sē-ăm) [L.] Of such degree or extent as to produce nausea.

adneural (ăd-nū′răl) [L. *ad*, to, + Gr. *neuron*, nerve] Near or toward a nerve.

adnexa (ăd-nĕk′să) [L.] Accessory parts of a structure.

dental a. Tissues surrounding the tooth (i.e., periodontal ligament and alveolar bone proper).

a. oculi Lacrimal gland.

a. uteri Ovaries and fallopian tubes.

adnexal (ăd-nĕk′săl) Adjacent or appending.

adnexitis (ăd″nĕk-sī′tĭs) [L. *adnexa*, appendages, + Gr. *itis*, inflammation] Inflammation of the adnexa uteri.

adolescence (ăd″ō-lĕs′ĕns) [L. *adolescens*] The period from the beginning of puberty until maturity. Because the onset of puberty and maturity is a gradual process and varies among individuals, it is not practical to set exact age or chronological limits in defining the adolescent period.

adolescent (ăd″ō-lĕs′ĕnt) **1.** Pert. to adolescence. **2.** A young man or woman not fully grown.

adolescent turmoil In psychoanalytic theory, the belief that adolescence is invariably accompanied by behavioral or psychological upheaval. This is no longer thought to be inevitable, or even the usual case.

adoption (ă-dŏp′shŭn) [L. *ad*, to, + *optare*, to choose] Assumption of responsibility for the care of a child by a person or persons who are not the biological parents. This usually requires a legal procedure.

adoral (ăd-ō′răl) [″ + *os*, mouth] Toward or near the mouth.

ADP *adenosine diphosphate.*

ADR *Adverse drug reaction.*

adren- SEE: *adrenalo-*.

adrenal (ăd-rē′năl) [L. *ad*, to, + *ren*, kidney] Originally used to indicate nearness to the kidney; now used in reference to the adrenal gland or its secretions.

adrenal- SEE: *adrenalo-*.

adrenal crisis Acute adrenocortical insufficiency. SEE: *Addison's disease; Waterhouse-Friderichsen syndrome.*

adrenalectomy (ăd-rē″năl-ĕk′tō-mē) [L. *ad*, to, + *ren*, kidney, + Gr. *ektome*, excision] Excision of one or both adrenal glands.

Patient Care: Vital signs, central venous pressure, and urine output are monitored frequently. Signs and symptoms of hypocorticism are assessed hourly for the first 24 hr; significant changes are reported to the surgeon immediately. Additional IV glucocorticoids are given as prescribed. The patient is monitored for early indications of shock or infection, and for alterations in blood glucose and electrolyte levels. To counteract shock, IV fluids and vasopressors are administered as prescribed, and the patient's response is evaluated every 3 to 5 min. Increased steroids to meet metabolic demands are needed if additional stress (e.g., infection) occurs. Other medications, including analgesics, are given as prescribed, and the patient's response is evaluated. The room is kept cool and the patient's clothing and bedding are changed often if he or she perspires profusely (a side effect of surgery on the adrenal gland). The abdomen is assessed for distention and return of bowel sounds. Physical and psychological stresses are kept to a minimum. Medications may be discontinued in a few months to a year after unilateral adrenalectomy, but lifelong replacement therapy will be needed after bilateral adrenalectomy. The patient must learn to recognize the signs of adrenal insufficiency, that sudden withdrawal of steroids can precipitate adrenal crisis, and that continued medical follow-up will be needed so that steroid dosage can be adjusted during stress or illness. Patients should take steroids in a two-thirds A.M. and one-third P.M. dosing pattern to mimic diurnal adrenal activity, with meals or antacids to minimize gastric irritation. Adverse reactions to steroids (e.g., weight gain, acne, headaches, diabetes, and osteoporosis) are explained. SEE: *Nursing Diagnoses Appendix.*

adrenal hyperplasia, congenital ABBR: CAH. An inherited disorder marked by congenital deficiency or absence of one or more enzymes essential to the production of adrenal cortical hormones. CAH is one of the adrenogenital syndromes. It is transmitted as an autosomal recessive trait, most often in Ashkenazi Jews and Mediterranean peoples. The enzyme involved most commonly is 21-hydroxylase (21-OHD). The inability to synthesize mineralocorticoids or glucocorticoids results in an overproduction of adrenal androgens. A severe deficiency or absence of 21-OHD also affects aldosterone synthesis. Symptoms of CAH include ambiguous genitalia or pseudohermaphroditism in infant girls. In other forms of CAH, decreased secretion of corticosterones and increased production of ACTH may cause a variety of clinical changes. Newborns who have salt-losing CAH develop vomiting, fluid and electrolyte imbalances (hyponatremia, hypokalemia), and hypotension within 2 weeks of birth. Treatment consists of hormonal therapy and surgery to correct genital abnormalities.

Adrenalin (ă-drĕn′ă-lĭn) Trade name for epinephrine.

adrenaline (ă-drĕn′ă-lēn) British designation for epinephrine.

adrenalinemia (ă-drĕn″ă-lĭn-ē′mē-ă) [L. *ad*, to, + *ren*, kidney, + Gr. *haima*, blood] Epinephrine in the blood.

adrenalinuria (ă-drĕn″ă-lĭn-ū′rē-ă) [″ + ″ + Gr. *ouron*, urine] Epinephrine in the urine.

adrenalo-, adrenal-, adreno-, adren- [L. *ad*, toward + ren, kidney] Combining form meaning adrenal glands.

adrenarche (ăd″rĕn-ăr′kē) [″ + ″ + Gr. *arche*, beginning] Changes that occur at puberty as a result of increased secretion of adrenocortical hormones. SEE: *menarche; pubarche.*

adrenergic (ăd-rĕn-ĕr′jĭk) [″ + ″ + Gr. *ergon*, work] Relating to nerve fibers that release norepinephrine or epinephrine at synapses. SEE: *sympathomimetic.*

adrenergic agonist Any one of a group of therapeutic agents that mimic or stimulate the sympathetic nervous system.

adrenergic neuron-blocking agents Substances that inhibit transmission of sympathetic nerve stimuli regardless of whether alpha- or beta-adrenergic receptors are involved. SEE: *alpha-adrenergic receptor; beta-adrenergic receptor.*

adrenitis (ăd″rē-nī′tĭs) [L. *ad*, to, + *ren*, kidney, + Gr. *itis*, inflammation] Inflammation of the adrenal glands.

adreno- SEE: *adrenalo-*.

adrenoceptive (ă-drē″nō-sĕp′tĭv) [″ + ″ + *recipere*, to receive] Concerning the sites in organs or tissues that are acted on by adrenergic transmitters.

adrenochrome (ăd″rē′nō-krōm) [″ + ″ + Gr. *chroma*, color] $C_9H_9NO_3$; a red pigment obtained by oxidation of epinephrine.

adrenocortical (ăd-rē″nō-kor′tĭ-kăl) Pert. to the adrenal cortex.

adrenocortical hormones A group of hormones secreted by the adrenal cortex that are classified by biological activity into glucocorticoids, mineralocorticoids, androgens, estrogens, and progestins. SEE: *adrenal gland.*

adrenocortical insufficiency, acute Sudden deficiency of adrenocortical hormone brought on by sepsis, surgical stress, or acute hemorrhagic destruction of both adrenal glands (i.e., Waterhouse-Friderichsen syndrome). A frequent cause is sudden withdrawal of adrenal corticosteroids from patients with adrenal atrophy secondary to chronic steroid administration. SYN: *Addisonian crisis; adrenal crisis.*

adrenocorticosteroid A hormone produced by the adrenal cortex; any synthetic derivative of such a hormone.

adrenocorticotropic (ăd-rē″nō-kor″tĭ-kō-trŏp′ĭk) [L. *ad*, to, + *ren*, kidney, + *cortex*, bark, + Gr. *tropikos*, turning] Having a stimulating effect on the adrenal cortex.

adrenocorticotropic hormone ABBR: ACTH. A hormone secreted by the anterior lobe of the pituitary that controls the development and functioning of the adrenal cortex, including its secretion of glucocorticoids and androgens. SYN: *corticotropin.*

adrenocorticotropin (ăd-rē″nō-kor″tĭ-kō-trŏp′ĭn) Adrenocorticotropic hormone.

adrenogenital (ăd-rē-nō-jĕn′ĭ-tăl) [L. *ad*, to, + *ren*, kidney, + *genitalis*, genital] Pert. to the adrenal glands and the genitalia.

adrenogenous (ăd″rĕn-ŏj′ĕ-nŭs) [L. *ad*, to, + *ren*, kidney, + Gr. *gennan*, to produce] Originating in or produced by the adrenal gland.

adrenoleukodystrophy (ă-drē″nō-loo″kō-dĭs′trō-fē) [″ + ″ + Gr. *leukos*, white, + *dys*, bad, + *trephein*, to nourish] A hereditary disease of children, transmitted as a sex-linked recessive trait. There is an abnormality of the white matter of the brain and atrophy of the adrenal glands. The mental and physical deterioration progresses to dementia, aphasia, apraxia, dysarthria, and blindness.

adrenolytic (ăd″rēn-ō-lĭt′ĭk) [L. *ad*, to, + *ren*, kidney, + Gr. *lysis*, dissolution] sympathicolytic.

adrenomegaly (ăd-rēn″ō-mĕg′ă-lē) [″ + ″ + Gr. *megas*, large] Enlarged adrenal gland(s).

adrenomimetic (ă-drē″nō-mĭ-mĕt′ĭk) [″ + ″ + Gr. *mimetikos*, imitating] Sympathomimetic.

adrenopathy (ăd″rĕn-ŏp′ă-thē) [″ + ″ + Gr. *pathos*, disease, suffering] Any disease of the adrenal glands.

adrenosterone (ăd″rĕ-nŏs′tĕ-rōn) An androgenic hormone secreted by the adrenal cortex.

adrenotoxin (ăd-rē″nō-tŏk′sĭn) [″ + ″ + *Gr. toxikon*, poison] A substance toxic to the adrenal glands.

adrenotropic (ăd-rē″nō-trŏp′ĭk) [″ + ″ + Gr. *tropikos*, turning] Nourishing or stimulating to the adrenal glands, with reference esp. to hormones that stimulate adrenal gland function.

Adson's maneuver [Alfred W. Adson, U.S. neurosurgeon, 1887–1951] A test for thoracic outlet syndrome. The patient's arm is moved back into extension and external rotation with the elbow extended and forearm supinated. The radial pulse is palpated while the patient is asked to tuck the chin, side bend the head toward the opposite side, and rotate the chin toward the side of the extended arm. The patient is then asked to inhale. A positive sign of numbness or tingling in the hand or diminished pulse indicates the brachial plexus or blood vessels are compromised at the site of the scalene muscle.

adsorb Attachment of a substance to the surface of another material. SEE: *absorb; absorption.*

adsorbate (ăd-sor′bāt) Anything that is adsorbed.

adsorbent (ăd-sor′bĕnt) **1.** Pert. to adsorption. **2.** A substance that leads readily to adsorption, such as activated charcoal or magnesia.

adsorption (ăd-sorp′shŭn) [L. *ad*, to, + *sorbere*, to suck in] Adhesion by a gas or liquid to the surface of a solid.

adsternal (ăd-stĕr′năl) [″ + Gr. *sternon*, chest] Near or toward the sternum.

adterminal (ăd-tĕr′mĭ-năl) [″ + *terminus*, boundary] Toward the extremity of any structure, such as the end of a nerve or muscle.

adtorsion (ăd-tor′shŭn) [″ + *torsio*, twisted] Convergent squint; inward rotation of both eyes.

adult (ă-dŭlt′) [L. *adultus*, grown up] The fully grown and mature organism.

adulteration (ă-dŭl″tĕr-ā′shŭn) [L. *adulterare*, to pollute] The addition or substitution of an impure, weaker, cheaper, or possibly toxic substance in a formulation or product.

adult-onset gangliosidosis A rare, slowly progressing dementing illness caused by the gradual accumulation of the GM ganglioside in neurons. It is marked clinically by impaired learning and social interactions, altered emotional expressions, psychosis, muscle atrophy, and clumsiness.

adult respiratory distress syndrome SEE: *acute respiratory distress syndrome.*

advance (ăd-văns′) [Fr. *avancer*, to set forth] To carry out the surgical procedure of advancement.

advanced cardiac life support ABBR: ACLS. SEE: *cardiopulmonary resuscitation; life support*.

advance directive A written document in the form of a living will or durable power of attorney prepared by a competent individual that specifies what, if any, extraordinary procedures, surgeries, medications, or treatments the patient desires in the future, when he or she can no longer make such decisions about medical treatment. SEE: *living will; power of attorney, durable, for health care.*

advancement (ăd-văns′mĕnt) [Fr. *avancer*, to set forth] Surgical detachment of a segment of tissue (e.g., skin, muscle, tendon) with reattachment to a position beyond the initial site. An example would be an operation to remedy strabismus in which an extrinsic occular muscle is severed and reattached farther from its origin.

capsular a. Attachment of the capsule of Tenon in front of its normal position.

adventitia (ăd″vĕn-tĭsh′ē-ă) [L. *adventicius*, coming from abroad] The outermost part or layer of a structure or organ, such as the tunica adventitia or outer layer of an artery.

adventitious (ăd″vĕn-tĭsh′ŭs) **1.** Acquired; accidental. **2.** Arising sporadically. **3.** Pert. to adventitia.

adventitious breath sounds Abnormal breath sounds heard when listening to the chest as the person breathes. These may be wheezes, crackles (rales), or stridor. They do not include sounds produced by muscular activity in the chest wall or friction of the stethoscope on the chest.

adverse reaction In pharmacology and therapeutics, an undesired side effect or toxicity caused by the administration of drugs. Onset may be sudden or take days to develop. Early detection by use of laboratory tests is sometimes possible in the case of drugs that might adversely affect the blood-forming organs, liver, or kidneys. It is important for health care personnel to be aware of the specific potential for adverse reactions of each and every drug. SYN: *drug reaction*. SEE: *drug interaction*.

advocacy (ăd′vō-kă-sē) In health care, pleading or representation for a desired goal or interest group, such as patients, staff, providers, biomedical researchers, or others.

adynamia (ăd″ĭ-nā′mē-ă) [Gr. *a-*, not, + *dynamis*, strength] Weakness or loss of strength, esp. due to muscular or cerebellar disease. SYN: *asthenia; debility*. **adynamic** (ā-dī-năm′ĭk), *adj.*

A.E. *above elbow;* term refers to the site of amputation of an upper extremity.

AED *Automatic external defibrillator*.

Aedes (ă-ē′dēs) [Gr. *aedes*, unpleasant] A genus of mosquitoes belonging to the family Culicidae. Many species are troublesome pests and some transmit disease.

A. aegypti A species of *Aedes* that transmits yellow fever and dengue among many other diseases.

A. triseriatus A species that transmits Jamestown Canyon virus, La Crosse virus, and other California encephalitis viruses.

aer- SEE: *aero-*.

aerated (ĕr′ā″tĕd) Containing air or gas.

aeration (ĕr″ā′shŭn) **1.** Act of airing. **2.** Process whereby carbon dioxide is exchanged for oxygen in blood in the lungs. **3.** Saturating or charging a fluid with gases.

aero-, aer- (ĕr′ō) Combining forms meaning *air* or *gas*.

aerobe (ĕr′ōb) *pl.* **aerobes** [″ + *bios*, life] A microorganism that is able to live and grow in the presence of oxygen.

facultative a. A microorganism that prefers an environment devoid of oxygen but has adapted so that it can live and grow in the presence of oxygen.

obligate a. A microorganism that can live and grow only in the presence of oxygen.

aerobic (ĕr-ō′bĭk) **1.** Living only in the presence of oxygen. **2.** Concerning an organism living only in the presence of oxygen.

aerobic exercise Exercise during which oxygen is metabolized to produce energy. Aerobic exercise is required for sustained periods of hard work and vigorous athletic activity. SEE: *anaerobic exercise*.

aerobic training Exercise training for the purpose of attaining aerobic conditioning. Although no formula should be slavishly applied, a general guideline is that aerobic conditioning will be obtained by normal, healthy persons who exercise three to five times a week for 30 min or more and at an intensity that produces a heart rate of 220 minus the age of the individual.

aerobiosis (ĕr″ō-bī-ō′sĭs) [Gr. *aer*, air, + *biosis*, mode of living] Living in an atmosphere containing oxygen.

aerocele (ĕr′ō-sēl) [″ + *kele*, tumor, swelling] Distention of a cavity with gas.

aerocoly (ĕr″ŏk′ō-lē) [″ + *kolon*, colon] Distention of the colon with gas.

aerocystoscopy (ĕr″ō-sĭs-tŏs′kō-pē) [″ + *kystis*, bladder, + *skopein*, to examine] Examination with a cystoscope of the bladder distended by air.

aerodontalgia (ĕr″ō-dŏnt-ăl′jē-ă) [″ + *odous*, tooth, + *algos*, pain] Pain in the teeth resulting from a change in atmospheric pressure.

aerodontia (ĕr″ō-dŏn′shē-ă) Branch of dentistry concerned with the effect of changes in atmospheric pressure on the teeth.

aerodynamics (ĕr″ō-dī-năm′ĭks) [Gr. *aer*, air, + *dynamis*, force] The science of air or gases in motion.

aeroembolism (ĕr″ō-ĕm′bō-lĭzm) [″ + *embolos*, plug, + *-ismos*, condition] A condition in which nitrogen bubbles form in body fluids and tissues during rapid ascent to high altitudes; can also occur in scuba diving or in hyperbaric oxygen therapy if return to sea level atmospheric pressure is too rapid. SEE: *bends*.

SYMPTOMS: Symptoms include boring, gnawing pain in the joints, itching of skin and eyelids, unconsciousness, convulsions, and paralysis. Symptoms are relieved by recompression (i.e., return to lower altitudes or placement of the patient in a hyperbaric pressure chamber). Even though oxygen by mask may be available, ascents above 25,000 ft should be avoided except in planes with pressurized cabins.

aerogenesis (ĕr″ō-jĕn′ĕ-sĭs) [″ + *genesis*, generation, birth] Formation of gas. **aerogenic, aerogenous** (ĕr″ō-jĕn′ĭk, -ŏj′ĕn-ŭs), *adj.*

aerometer (ĕr-ŏm′ĕ-tĕr) [Gr. *aer*, air, + *metron*, measure] A device for measuring gas density.

Aeromonas (ĕr″ō-mō′năs) A genus of bacteria found in natural water sources and soil. It is a gram-negative, nonspore-forming, motile bacillus. Aeromonads are commonly pathogenic for cold-blooded marine animals. Their importance in serious human diseases has been increasing, esp. in immunocompromised hosts. As opportunistic infections, *Aeromonas* infections may occur in otherwise healthy hosts.

A. hydrophilia A type of *Aeromonas* that is pathogenic for humans; it is sensitive to chloramphenicol, trimethoprim-sulfamethoxazole, and some quinolones.

aero-otitis aerotitis.

aeroparotitis Swelling of one or both parotid glands due to introduction of air into the glands. This may occur in those who play wind instruments; it also occurs in nose blowing and Valsalva's maneuver if done too vigorously.

aeroperitoneum, aeroperitonia (ĕr″ō-pĕr″ĭ-tō-nē′ŭm, -tō′nē-ă) [″ + *peritonaion*, peritoneum] Distention of the peritoneal cavity caused by gas.

aerophagia, aerophagy (ĕr″ō-fā′jē-ă, ĕr″ŏf′ă-jē) [″ + *phagein*, to eat] Swallowing of air.

aerophilic, aerophilous (ĕr″ō-fĭl′ĭk, -ŏf′ĭ-lŭs) [″ + *philein*, to love] Requiring air for growth and development. SYN: *aerobic*.

aerophobia (ĕr-ō-fō′bē-ă) [″ + *phobos*, fear] Morbid fear of a draft or of fresh air.

aerosinusitis (ĕr″ō-sī″nŭs-ī′tĭs) [″ + L. *sinus*, a hollow, + Gr. *itis*, inflammation] Chronic inflammation of nasal sinuses due to changes in atmospheric pressure.

aerosol (ĕr′ō-sŏl) [″ + L. *solutio*, solution] **1.** A solution dispensed as a mist. **2.** Any suspension of particles in air or gas.

aerosolization (ĕr″ō-sŏl″ĭ-zā′shŭn) Production of an aerosol.

aerosol therapy The inhalation of aerosolized medicines, such as corticosteroids or mucolytic agents, in the treatment of pulmonary conditions such as asthma, bronchitis, and emphysema. SEE: *inhalation therapy*.

aerotherapy (ĕr″ō-thĕr′ă-pē) [″ + *therapeia*, treatment] The use of air in the treatment of disease, using changes in composition and density. SEE: *hyperbaric oxygen*.

aerothermotherapy (ĕr″ō-thĕr″mō-thĕr′ă-pē) [″ + *thermos*, heat, + *therapeia*, treatment] Therapeutic use of hot air.

aerotitis (ĕr-ō-tī′tĭs) [″ + *ot-*, ear, + *itis*, inflammation] Inflammation of the ear, esp. the middle ear, due to failure of the eustachian tube to remain open during sudden changes in barometric pressure, as may occur during flying, diving, or working in a pressure chamber. SYN: *aero-otitis; barotitis*.

aerotropism (ĕr-ŏt′rō-pĭzm) [″ + *trope*, a turn, + *-ismos*, condition] The tendency of organisms, esp. bacteria and protozoa, to move toward air (positive aerotropism) or away from it (negative aerotropism).

aerourethroscope (ĕr-ō-ū″rē′thrō-skōp″) [″ + *ourethra*, urethra, + *skopein*, to examine] An apparatus for visual examination of the urethra after dilatation by air.

aerourethroscopy (ĕr″ō-ū″rē-thrŏs′kō-pē) Visual examination of the urethra when distended with air.

Aesculapius (ĕs″kū-lā′pē-ŭs) The Roman name for the god of medicine; son of Apollo and the nymph Coronis.

staff of A. A rod or crude stick with a snake wound around it, used to signify the art of healing and adopted as the emblem of some medical organizations (e.g., American Medical Association). Snakes were sacred to Aesculapius because they were believed to have the power to renew their youth by shedding their old skin and growing a new one. SEE: *caduceus*.

aesthetics (ĕs-thĕt'ĭks) [Gr. *aisthesis*, sensation] The philosophy or the theory of beauty and the fine arts. These concepts are esp. important in dental restorations and in plastic and cosmetic surgery. Also spelled *esthetics*.

dental a. The application of aesthetics to natural or artificial teeth or restorations, usually with regard to form and color.

afebrile (ă-fĕb'rĭl) [Gr. *a-*, not, + L. *febris*, fever] Without fever.

affect (ăf'fĕkt) [L. *affectus*, exerting influence on] In psychology, the emotional reaction associated with an experience. SEE: *mood*.

blunted a. Greatly diminished emotional response to a situation or condition.

flat a. Virtual absence of emotional response to a situation or condition.

affection (ă-fĕk'shŭn) **1.** Love, feeling. **2.** Physical or mental disease.

affective (ă-fĕk'tĭv) Pert. to an emotion or mental state.

affective disorder A group of disorders marked by a disturbance of mood accompanied by a full or partial manic or depressive syndrome that is not caused by any other physical or mental disorder. SEE: *Nursing Diagnoses Appendix*.

afferent (ăf'ĕr-ĕnt) [L. *ad*, to, + *ferre*, to bear] Transporting toward a center, such as a sensory nerve that carries impulses toward the central nervous system; opposite of efferent. Certain blood vessels and lymphatic vessels are also said to be afferent.

afferent loop syndrome A group of gastrointestinal symptoms that occur in some patients who have had partial gastric resection with gastrojejunostomy. The condition is caused by partial obstruction of an incompletely draining segment of bowel. In some cases there is bacterial overgrowth in the afferent loop. Symptoms include abdominal bloating, nausea, vomiting, and pain after eating.

affidavit A voluntary written or printed statement of facts that is confirmed by the person's oath or affirmation.

affiliation (ă-fĭl-ē-ā'shŭn) [L. *affiliare*, to take to oneself as a son] **1.** Membership in a larger organization. **2.** Association. In nursing or medical education, the administrative merger of two hospitals or schools of nursing. This enables students to obtain specialized training and experience that might not otherwise be available to them.

affinity (ă-fĭn'ĭ-tē) [L. *affinis*, neighboring] Attraction.

chemical a. Force causing certain atoms to combine with others to form molecules. SEE: *chemoreceptor*.

A fiber A heavily myelinated, fast-conducting nerve fiber.

afibrinogenemia (ă-fī"brĭn-ō-jĕ-nē'mē-ă) [Gr. *a-*, not, + L. *fibra*, fiber, + Gr. *gennan*, to produce, + *haima*, blood] Absence or deficiency of fibrinogen in the bloodstream.

aflatoxicosis (ăf'lă-tŏk"sĭ-kō'sĭs) Poisoning caused by ingestion of peanuts or peanut products contaminated with *Aspergillus flavus* or other *Aspergillus* strains that produce aflatoxin. Farm animals and humans are susceptible to this toxicosis. SYN: *x-disease*.

aflatoxin (ăf'lă-tŏk'sĭn) A toxin produced by some strains of *Aspergillus flavus* and *A. parasiticus* that causes cancer in laboratory animals. It may be present in peanuts and other seeds contaminated with *Aspergillus* molds. It is not practical to try to remove aflatoxin from contaminated foods in order to make them edible.

AFO *ankle-foot orthosis*.

AFP *alpha-fetoprotein*.

afteraction Continued reaction for some time after the stimulus ceases, esp. in nerve centers. In the sensory centers this action gives rise to aftersensations.

afterbirth The placenta and membranes expelled from the uterus after the birth of a child.

aftercare **1.** Care of a convalescent after conclusion of treatment in a hospital or mental institution. **2.** A continuing program of rehabilitation designed to reinforce the effects of therapy and to help patients adjust to their environment.

aftercataract **1.** Secondary cataract. **2.** An opacity of the lens capsule that develops after cataract removal.

aftercurrent Current produced in a tissue after electrical stimulation has ceased.

afterdamp A gaseous mixture formed by the explosion of methane and air in a mine; contains a large percentage of carbon dioxide, nitrogen, and carbon monoxide.

afterdepolarization (ăf"tĕr-dē-pō"lăr-ĭ-ză'shŭn) Abnormal electrical activity that occurs during repolarization of the pacemaker cells of the heart. This activity may prolong the action potential and trigger abnormal atrial or ventricular rhythms.

afterdischarge The discharge of impulses from a reflex center after stimulation of the receptor has ceased. It results in prolongation of the response.

aftereffect A response occurring some time after the original stimulus or condition has produced its primary effect.

afterhearing Perception of sound after the stimulus producing it has ceased to act.

afterimage Image that persists subjectively after cessation of the stimulus. If colors are the same as those of the object, it is called positive; it is called negative if complementary colors are seen.

In the former case, the image is seen in its natural bright colors without any alteration; in the latter, the bright parts become dark, while dark parts are light.

negative a. Afterimage in which the colors and light intensity are reversed.

positive a. Afterimage in which the colors and light intensity are unchanged.

afterimpression Aftersensation.

afterload In cardiac physiology, the forces that impede the flow of blood out of the heart. The heart contracts against a resistance primarily composed of the pressure in the peripheral vasculature, the compliance of the aorta, and the mass and viscosity of blood. SEE: *preload.*

afterloading In brachytherapy, the insertion of the radioactive source after the placement of the applicator has been confirmed.

aftermovement Persistent and spontaneous contraction of a muscle after a strong contraction against resistance has ceased. This is easily seen when a person forcibly pushes an arm against a wall while standing with the frontal plane perpendicular to the wall. When this is stopped and the person moves away from the wall, the arm abducts involuntarily and is elevated by the deltoid muscle. SYN: *Kohnstamm's phenomenon.*

afterpains Uterine cramps caused by contraction of the uterus and commonly seen in multiparas during the first few days after childbirth. The pains, which are more severe during nursing, rarely last longer than 48 hr postpartum.

TREATMENT: Analgesics provide relief, but aspirin should not be given if there is a bleeding tendency. The sooner an analgesic is given, the less is needed.

afterperception Perception of a sensation after cessation of the stimulus.

afterpotential wave The wave produced after the action potential wave passes along a nerve. On the recording of the electrical activity, it will be either a negative or positive wave smaller than the main spike.

afterpressure A feeling of pressure that remains for a few seconds after removal of a weight or other pressure.

aftersensation A sensation that persists after the stimulus causing it has ceased.

aftertaste Persistence of gustatory sensations after cessation of the stimulus.

aftertreatment Secondary treatment or that which follows the primary treatment regimen. SEE: *aftercare.*

aftervision Afterimage.

Ag [L. *argentum*] Symbol for the element silver.

AGA *Appropriate for gestational age.*

against medical advice ABBR: AMA. Referring to a patient's refusal of medically recommended treatments, esp. in the hospital. Dropping out of care, or leaving a hospital AMA, typically occurs when patients are dissatisfied with the pace or course of their care, carry substance abuse diagnoses, or have a history of multiple hospitalizations. The action may result in an increase in both morbidity and rehospitalization.

PATIENT CARE: The patient is asked to sign a release form indicating that the health care facility and those responsible for medical care are not liable for any adverse outcome that may result from the termination of care.

agamic (ă-găm'ĭk) [Gr. *a-*, not, + *gamos*, marriage] **1.** Reproducing asexually. **2.** Asexual.

agammaglobulinemia (ă-găm"ă-glŏb"ū-lĭn-ē'mē-ă) [" + *gamma globulin* + Gr. *haima*, blood] A broad term pert. to disorders marked by an almost complete lack of immunoglobulins or antibodies. The cause is abnormal B lymphocyte function. Agammaglobulinemias cause severe immunodeficiencies, with recurrent infections. Treatments include immuneglobulins, antibiotics, and bone marrow transplantation.

agamogenesis (ăg"ă-mō-jĕn'ĕ-sĭs) [" + *gamos*, marriage, + *genesis*, generation, birth] **1.** Asexual reproduction. **2.** Parthenogenesis.

agar (ā'găr, ăg'ăr) [Malay, gelatin] **1.** A dried mucilaginous product obtained from certain species of algae, esp. of the genus *Gelidium.* Because it is unaffected by bacterial enzymes, it is widely used as a solidifying agent for bacterial culture media; it is also used as a laxative because of its great increase in bulk on absorption of water. **2.** A culture medium containing agar.

agar-agar Agar.

agaric (ă-găr'ĭk) [Gr. *agarikon*, a sort of fungus] A toxic or hallucinogenic mushroom, esp. species of the genus *Agaricus.*

agastria (ă-găs'trē-ă) [Gr. *a-*, not, + *gaster*, stomach] Absence of the stomach. **agastric** (ă-găst'rĭk), *adj.*

AgCl Symbol for silver chloride.

age [Fr. *age*, L. *aetas*] **1.** The time from birth to the present for a living individual measured in days, months, or years. **2.** A particular period of life (e.g., middle age or old age). **3.** To grow old. **4.** In psychology, the degree of development of an individual expressed in terms of the age of an average individual of comparable development or accomplishment.

achievement a. ABBR: A.A. The age of a person with regard to level of acquired learning; determined by a proficiency test and expressed in terms of the chronological age of the average person showing the same level of attainment.

anatomical a. An estimate of age as

judged by the stage of development or deterioration of the body or tissue as compared with persons or tissues of known age.

biological a. One's present position in regard to the probability of survival. Determination of biological age requires assessment and measurment of the functional capacities of the life-limiting organ system (e.g., the cardiovascular system).

bone a. An estimate of biological age based on radiological studies of the developmental stage of ossification centers of the long bones of the extremities. SEE: *epiphysis*.

chronological a. ABBR: C.A. Age as determined by years since birth.

conceptional a. The estimated gestational age as referenced from the actual time of conception. It is usually considered to be at least 14 days after the first day of the last menstrual period. SYN: *ovulation a.*

developmental a. An index of maturation expressed in months or years, which represents a value obtained by comparing performance with scaled norms for a particular age group. SEE: *age, achievement*.

emotional a. Judgment of age with respect to the stage of emotional development.

functional a. Age defined in terms of physical or functional capacity; frequently applied to the elderly.

gestational a. The age of an embryo or fetus as timed from the date of onset of the last menstrual period.

menarcheal a. Elapsed time expressed in years from menarche.

mental a. ABBR: M.A. The age of a person with regard to mental ability, determined by a series of mental tests devised by Binet and expressed in terms of the chronological age of the average person showing the same level of attainment.

ovulation a. Conceptional a.

physiological a. The relative age of a person, esp. when comparing that individual's physical status with those of other persons of the same chronological age.

age of consent The age at which a minor may legally engage in voluntary sexual intercourse or no longer require parental consent for marriage. It varies among states, but is usually between ages 13 and 18.

aged (ājd′, ā′jĕd) **1.** To have grown older or more mature. **2.** Persons who have grown old. SEE: *aging*.

Age Discrimination Act Also known as Age Discrimination in Employment Act, 29 U.S.C. subsection 621 (1967), a law that prohibits unfair and discriminatory treatment by an employer against anyone forty (40) years old or older. In health care, this act has been used to challenge the termination of mature employees.

ageism (āj′ĭzm) [Robert Butler, U.S. physician, who coined the term in 1968] Discrimination against aged persons.

Agency for Healthcare Research and Quality ABBR: AHRQ. An office of the U.S. Department of Health and Human Services dedicated to supporting, conducting, and disseminating research; promoting improvements in clinical practice; and enhancing the quality, organization, financing, and delivery of health care services. Formerly called the Agency for Health Care Policy and Research; the name was changed in December 1999.

agenesia, agenesis (ă″jĕn-ē′sē-ă, ă-jĕn′ĕ-sis) [Gr. *a*-, not, + *genesis*, generation, birth] **1.** Failure of an organ or part to develop or grow. **2.** Lack of potency.

agenitalism (ă-jĕn′ĭ-tăl-ĭzm) [″ + L. *genitalis*, genital, + Gr. *-ismos*, condition] Absence of genitals.

agent (ā′jĕnt) [L. *agere*, to do] Something that causes an effect; thus, bacteria that cause disease are said to be agents of the specific diseases they cause. A medicine is considered a therapeutic agent.

buffering a. Buffer.

chelating a. A drug, such as calcium disodium edetate, that is used to chelate substances, esp. toxic chemicals in the body.

fixing a. SEE: *clearing agent*.

immunosuppressive a. SEE: *immunotherapy*.

oral hypoglycemic a. ABBR: OHA. A drug taken by mouth to help control hyperglycemia in type 2 diabetes mellitus.

riot control a. A class of chemicals used by law enforcement personnel to disable people, esp. those felt to be violent or potentially violent. The most commonly used chemicals are tear gas and pepper spray (oleoresin capsicum). Toxic effects of riot control agents include tearing of the eyes, irritation of the mucus membranes, asthma, coughing, and dermatitis, among others.

sclerosing a. A substance used to cause sclerosis, esp. of the lining of a vein. SEE: *varicose vein*.

surface-active a. Surfactant.

wetting a. In radiographic wet film processing, a solution used after washing to reduce surface tension and accelerate water flow from the film to speed drying.

Agent Orange A defoliant that U.S. military forces used extensively in the Vietnam War. It contained the toxic chemical dioxin as an unwanted and undesired contaminant. SEE: *dioxin*.

agerasia (ā-jĕr-ā′sē-ă) [Gr. *a*-, not, +

geras, old age] Healthy, vigorous old age; youthful appearance of an old person.

age-specific Pert. to data, esp. in vital statistics and epidemiology, that are related to age.

ageusia, ageustia (ă-gū′sē-ă, ă-goos′tē-ă) [Gr. *a*-, not + *geusis*, taste] Absence, partial loss, or impairment of the sense of taste. SEE: *dysgeusia; hypergeusesthesia; hypogeusia.*

ETIOLOGY: Ageusia may be caused by disease of the chorda tympani or of the gustatory fibers, excessive use of condiments, the effect of certain drugs, aging, or lesions involving sensory pathways or taste centers in the brain.

central a. Ageusia due to a cerebral lesion.

conduction a. Ageusia due to a lesion involving sensory nerves of taste.

peripheral a. Ageusia due to a disorder of taste buds of the mucous membrane of tongue.

agglomerate (ă-glŏm′ĕ-rāt) [L. *ad*, to, + *glomerare*, to wind into a ball] To congregate; to form a mass.

agglutinable (ă-gloo′tĭ-nă-bl) [L. *agglutinans*, gluing] Capable of agglutination.

agglutinant (ă-gloo′tĭ-nănt) **1.** Substance causing adhesion. **2.** Causing union by adhesion, as in the healing of a wound. **3.** Agglutinin.

agglutination (ă-gloo″tĭ-nā′shŭn) **1.** A type of antigen-antibody reaction in which a solid cell or particle coated with antigens drops out of solution when it is exposed to a previously soluble antibody. The particles involved commonly include red blood cells, bacteria, and inert carriers such as latex. Agglutination also refers to laboratory tests used to detect specific antigens or antibodies in disease states. When agglutination involves red blood cells, it is called hemagglutination. **2.** Adhesion of surfaces of a wound.

direct a. The formation of an insoluble network of antigens and their antibodies, when the antigen is mixed with specific antiserum. Direct agglutination reactions are used, for example, in typing blood or in assessing the presence of antibodies against microorganisms.

passive a. A test for the presence of a specific antibody in which inert particles or cells with no foreign antigenic markers are coated with a known soluble antigen and mixed with serum. If clumping occurs, the patient's blood contains antibodies specific to the antigen. In the past, red blood cells were used as the carriers after they are washed to remove any known antibodies; currently, latex, bentonite, and charcoal also are used.

platelet a. Clumping of platelets in response to immunological reactions.

agglutinative (ă-gloo′tĭ-nā″tĭv) Causing or capable of causing agglutination.

agglutinin (ă-gloo′tĭ-nĭn) [L. *agglutinans*, gluing] An antibody present in the blood that attaches to an antigen present on cells or solid particles, causing them to agglutinate or clump together; used primarily in reference to laboratory tests of agglutination. Agglutinins cause transfusion reactions when blood from a different group is given. These antibodies are present at birth and require no exposure to an antigen to be created, since they are genetically determined.

anti-Rh a. An antibody produced by persons with Rh-negative blood who are exposed to blood containing the Rh antigen. This antibody develops in Rh-negative individuals who receive Rh-positive blood and in Rh-negative women carrying an Rh-positive fetus. The antibody may cause lysis of fetal red blood cells (hemolytic disease of the newborn) in subsequent Rh-positive pregnancies.

cold a. The agglutination of erythrocytes (usually from sheep) at low temperatures by the serum of patients with certain diseases.

warm a. An agglutinin effective only at body temperature, 98.6°F (37°C).

agglutinogen (ă-gloo-tĭn′ō-jĕn) [L. *agglutinans*, gluing, + Gr. *gennan*, to produce] The specific antigen that stimulates the recognition of an agglutinin, or antibody; used primarily in reference to laboratory testing for antibodies against specific blood types. SEE: *blood group*. **agglutinogenic, agglutogenic** (ă-gloo″tĭ-nō-jen′ĭk, ă-gloo″tō-jĕn′ĭk), *adj.*

A and B a. Antigenic substances discovered by Karl Landsteiner in 1901 that are found on the membranes of red blood cells in humans and that react with the alpha (anti-A) and beta (anti-B) isoagglutinins in mismatched blood. The red corpuscles may contain A or B, both A and B, or neither A nor B agglutinogens. The four resulting blood groups are A, B, AB, and O, respectively. Blood groups are inherited according to Mendel's laws. SEE: *blood group; ABO incompatibility.*

M and N a. Antigenic substances found on the membranes of red blood cells in humans. Anti-M and anti-N agglutinins are rarely found in normal serum. The red blood cells may contain M or N, or both M and N agglutinogens, resulting in blood types M, N, or MN, respectively. SEE: *blood group.*

Rh a. A specific substance called the Rh factor, which is found on the membranes of the red blood cells. It was discovered in 1940 by Landsteiner and Wiener, who prepared anti-Rh serum by injecting red cells from Rhesus monkeys into rabbits or other animals. They found that the red cells of 85% of people of the Caucasian race will be agglutinated when in contact with anti-Rh serum. These people are called Rh-positive. The remaining 15%, whose red cells are not agglutinated by anti-Rh serum, are termed Rh-negative. More than 25 blood factors are known to belong to the Rh system. Their importance in blood typing and blood type incompatibility between mother and fetus makes this blood group system second in importance only to the ABO group. SEE: *blood group; Rh blood group; Rh factor*.

agglutinophilic (ă-gloo″tĭn-ō-fĭl′ĭk) [″ + Gr. *philos*, fond] Readily agglutinating.

aggrecan (ăg-grē′căn) A large glycoprotein that provides stiffness and structural strength to many tissues including joint cartilage, tendons, and the aorta.

aggregate (ăg′rĕ-gāt) [L. *aggregatus*, collect] **1.** Total substances making up a mass. **2.** To cluster or come together.

aggregation (ăg″rĕ-gā′shŭn) A clustering or coming together of substances.

cell a. Clumping together of blood cells, esp. platelets or red cells.

familial a. A cluster of the same disease in closely related families.

aggression (ă-grĕsh′ŭn) [L. *aggredi*, to approach with hostility] **1.** A forceful physical, verbal, or symbolic action. It may be appropriate and self-protective, indicating healthy self-assertiveness, or it may be inappropriate. The behavior may be directed outward toward the environment or inward toward the self. **2.** Activity performed in a forceful manner.

aging (āj′ĭng) **1.** Growing older. There is no precise method for determining the rate or degree of aging. In a study of 1500 persons aged 100 years or more, the following were determined: longevity is not inheritable; sexual activity is both good and feasible for the aged; the strain of child rearing does not shorten life; the older person's offspring need not love him or her; and one should work hard all during life, however long.

The physiological changes occurring with age (diminished neurotransmitters, circulatory capacity, sensory acuity, and perception) affect the brain. These changes do not indicate a loss of cognitive function. There is evidence of slower reaction time and information processing, but the majority of functioning and intelligence remains intact and sufficient.

Emotional trauma and multiple losses occurring in older age often lead to a diminished investment in life, causing professionals to misdiagnose cognitive dysfunction. The stress of demanding situations often contributes to what appears to be an organic disorder. Validation by a team of specialists is important in the diagnosis and treatment of any disorder affecting older persons. SEE: *Alzheimer's disease; dementia*.

2. Maturing. **3.** Any physiological, cellular, or biochemical change that occurs with the passage of time, and not because of injury or disease.

agitated depression Depression accompanied by restlessness and increased psychomotor activity.

agitation (ăj″ĭ-tā′shŭn) [L. *agitare*, to drive] **1.** Excessive restlessness, increased mental and physical activity, esp. the latter. **2.** Tremor. **3.** Severe motor restlessness, usually nonpurposeful, associated with anxiety. **4.** Shaking of a container so that the contents are rapidly moved and mixed.

agitographia (ăj″ĭ-tō-grăf′ē-ă) [″ + Gr. *graphein*, to write] Writing with excessive rapidity, with unconscious omission of words and syllables.

agitophasia (ăj″ĭ-tō-fā′zē-ă) [″ + Gr. *phasis*, speech] Excessive rapidity of speech, with slurring, omission, and distortion of sounds.

aglaucopsia, aglaukopsia (ă″glaw-kŏp′sē-ă) [Gr. *a-*, not, + *glaukos*, green, + *opsis*, vision] Green blindness; color blindness in which there is a defect in the perception of green. SEE: *color blindness*.

aglossia (ă-glŏs′ē-ă) [″ + *glossa*, tongue] Congenital absence of the tongue.

aglossostomia (ă″glōs-ō-stō′mē-ă) [″ + ″ + *stoma*, mouth] Congenital absence of the tongue and mouth opening.

aglutition (ă-gloo-tĭsh′ŭn) [″ + L. *glutire*, to swallow] Difficulty in swallowing or inability to swallow.

aglycemia (ă″glī-sē′mē-ă) [″ + *glykys*, sweet, + *haima*, blood] Lack of sugar in the blood.

aglycon, aglycone The substance attached to the chemical structure of digitalis glycosides. It is responsible for the cardiotonic activity of those agents.

aglycosuric (ă-glī″kō-sū′rĭk) [″ + ″ + *ouron*, urine] Free from glycosuria.

agminate(d) (ăg′mĭ-nāt) [L. *agmen*, a crowd] Aggregated; grouped in clusters.

agminated follicle Aggregation of a solitary follicle or a group of lymph nodes, principally in the lower portion of the small intestine. SYN: *Peyer's patch*.

agnathia (ăg-nā′thē-ă) [Gr. *a-*, not, + *gnathos*, jaw] Absence of the lower jaw.

agnea (ăg′nē-ă) [″ + *gnosis*, knowledge] Inability to recognize objects.

$AgNO_3$ Symbol for silver nitrate.

agnogenic (ăg-nō-jĕn′ĭk) [″ + *gnosis*, knowledge, + *gennan*, to produce] Of unknown origin or etiology.

agnosia (ăg-nō′zē-ă) [″ + *gnosis*, knowledge] Loss of comprehension of auditory, visual, or other sensations although the sensory sphere is intact.

auditory a. Mental inability to interpret sounds.

color a. An inability to recognize or name specific colors.

finger a. Inability to identify fingers of one's own hands or of others.

optic a. Mental inability to interpret images that are seen.

tactile a. Inability to distinguish objects by sense of touch.

time a. Unawareness of the sequence and duration of events.

unilateral spatial a. SEE: *inattention, unilateral.*

visual object a. SEE: *visual object agnosia.*

-agogue (ă-gŏg) [Gr. *agogos*, leading, inducing] Suffix meaning *producer, secretor, or promoter of the excretion of a specific substance.*

agonad, agonadal (ā-gō′năd, ā-gŏn′ă-dăl) [Gr. *a*-, not, + *gone*, seed] Lacking gonads.

agonal (ăg′ō-năl) [Gr. *agon*, a contest] Rel. to death or dying.

agonist (ăg′ŏn-ĭst) **1.** The muscle directly engaged in contraction as distinguished from muscles that have to relax at the same time; thus, in bending the elbow, the biceps brachii is the agonist and the triceps the antagonist. **2.** In pharmacology, a drug that binds to the receptor and stimulates the receptor's function. Drugs that mimic the body's own regulatory function are called agonists.

beta a. A drug that stimulates adrenergic receptors in the lungs, heart, uterus, and other organs. Beta agonists are used to treat asthma and chronic obstructive lung diseases and to manage pregnancy.

beta-2 a. A medication that stimulates bronchodilation. Examples include albuterol, salmeterol, terbutaline, and many others. SYN: *bronchodilator.*

PATIENT CARE: Beta-2 agonists are used to treat patients with asthma or any pulmonary disease associated with bronchospasm. Patients given such medications need to be monitored for side effects such as tremor, tachycardia, and nausea.

agony (ăg′ō-nē) **1.** Extreme mental or physical suffering. **2.** Death struggle.

agoraphobia (ăg″ō-ră-fō′bē-ă) [Gr. *agora*, marketplace, + *phobos*, fear] Overwhelming symptoms of anxiety that occur on leaving home; a form of social phobia. The attack may occur in a variety of everyday situations (e.g., standing in line, eating in public, in crowds of people, on bridges or in tunnels; while driving) in which a person may be unable to escape or get help and may be embarrassed. Symptoms often include rapid heartbeat, chest pain, difficulty breathing, gastrointestinal distress, faintness, dizziness, weakness, sweating, fear of losing control or going crazy, and fear of dying or impending doom. People with these symptoms often avoid phobic situations by rarely, if ever, leaving home.

-agra [Gr. *agra*, a seizure] Suffix indicating sudden severe pain.

agranulocyte (ă-grăn′ū-lō-sīt) [Gr. *a*-, not, + L. *granulum*, granule, + Gr. *kytos*, cell] A nongranular leukocyte.

agranulocytosis (ă-grăn″ū-lō-sī-tō′sĭs) [″ + ″ + ″ + *osis*, condition] An acute disease marked by a deficit or absolute lack of granulocytic white blood cells (neutrophils, basophils, and eosinophils). SYN: *granulocytopenia.* **agranulocytic** (-sĭt′ĭk), *adj.*

agranuloplastic (ă-grăn″ū-lō-plăs′tĭk) [″ + L. *granulum*, granule, + Gr. *plastikos*, formative] Unable to form granular cells.

agranulosis (ă-grăn″ū-lō′sĭs) Agranulocytosis.

agraphesthesia Inability to recognize letters or numbers drawn by the examiner on skin. Patients' eyes are closed if this is done on skin visible to them. SEE: *graphesthesia.*

agraphia (ă-grăf′ē-ă) [Gr. *a*-, not, + *graphein*, to write] Loss of the ability to write. SYN: *logagraphia*. SEE: *aphasia, motor.*

absolute a. Complete inability to write.

acoustic a. Inability to write words that are heard.

amnemonic a. Inability to write sentences, although letters or words can be written.

cerebral a. Inability to express thoughts in writing.

motor a. Inability to write due to muscular incoordination.

optic a. Inability to copy words.

verbal a. Inability to write words although letters can be written.

agrypnocoma (ă-grĭp″nō-kō′mă) [Gr. *agrypnos*, sleepless, + *koma*, a deep sleep] Coma in which the individual is partially awake as if in an extreme lethargic state; may be associated with muttering, delirium, and lack of sleep.

agrypnotic (ă″grĭp-nŏt′ĭk) **1.** Afflicted with insomnia. **2.** Causing wakefulness.

AGS *American Geriatrics Society.*

agyria (ă-jī′rē-ă) [Gr. *a*-, not, + *gyros*, circle] Incompletely developed convolutions of the cerebral cortex. **agyric** (-rĭk), *adj.*

ah *hypermetropic astigmatism.*

A.H.A. *American Heart Association; American Hospital Association.*

AHF *antihemophilic factor*, coagulation factor VIII. SEE: *coagulation factor.*

AHG *antihemophilic globulin,* coagulation factor VIII. SEE: *coagulation factor.*

AHIMA *American Health Information Management Association.*

Ahlfeld's sign (ăl′fĕlts) [Friedrich Ahlfeld, Ger. obstetrician, 1843–1929] Irregular uterine contractions after the third month of pregnancy. It is a presumptive sign of pregnancy.

AHRQ *Agency for Healthcare Research and Quality.*

A.I. *aortic insufficiency; artificial insemination; artificial intelligence; axioincisal.*

aichmophobia (āk″mō-fō′bē-ă) [Gr. *aichme*, point, + *phobos*, fear] Morbid fear of being touched by pointed objects or fingers.

A.I.D. *Agency for International Development; artificial insemination by donor* (heterologous insemination).

aid (ād) Assistance provided to a person, esp. one who is sick, injured, or troubled. SEE: *first aid.*

hearing a. A sound-amplifying apparatus used by those with impaired hearing. The modern electronic hearing aid may simply amplify sound or may be designed to attenuate certain portions of the sound signal and amplify others. The cost may vary from several hundred dollars to more than a thousand dollars. As a variety of hearing aids are available, it is important that patients buy the type most suitable for their needs and comfort. Patients should have a trial period prior to making the final decision to purchase the device.

robotic a. A mechanical device guided remotely by a person with a disability to assist with or enable daily living tasks.

aide (ād) Assistant.

certified medicine a. ABBR: CMA. An unlicensed caregiver who can hand out oral and topical medications in long-term or chronic care facilities after successfully completing a state-approved medication administration course.

physical therapy a. A person who is trained by a physical therapist or physical therapist assistant to provide support services, such as tasks that do not require clinical decision making or problem solving, in physical therapy. Physical therapy aides should function with continuous on-site supervision.

AIDS *Acquired immunodeficiency syndrome,* a late stage of infection with the human immunodeficiency virus (HIV). Criteria for the diagnosis include HIV infection with 1) a CD4+ helper T-cell count of less than 200 cells/mm^3, plus 2) infection with an opportunistic pathogen, and/or 3) the presence of an AIDS-defining malignancy. Although AIDS was unknown before 1982, it is now a worldwide epidemic that affects tens of millions of people. The majority of people with AIDS are between the ages of 15 and 44, poor, and heterosexual; have limited access to optimal care; and live in developing nations in Africa and Asia. SEE: *Nursing Diagnoses Appendix.*

AIDS is the leading cause of death among Americans between the ages of 25 and 44. More than 688,000 cases of AIDS have been reported in the U.S., primarily among injection drug users, men who have sex with men, and recipients of tainted blood products. In addition, about 7000 American children are born to HIV-infected mothers each year. About 47,000 new cases are reported annually in the U.S. SEE: *human immunodeficiency virus; opportunistic infection.*

ETIOLOGY: Two human immunodeficiency viruses, HIV-1 and HIV-2, have been identified. Both cause AIDS, but infection with HIV-2 has been primarily limited to West Africa. Infection occurs when a viral envelope glycoprotein (gp120) binds to CD4 receptors and co-receptors (called CXCR4 and CCR5) on lymphocytes, macrophages, and other immune system cells, causing viral uptake and cellular destruction. HIV is a retrovirus that uses an enzyme called reverse transcriptase to convert its viral RNA to viral DNA, using the host cell DNA to do so. The viral DNA then becomes incorporated into the host cell DNA. About 100 billion virions, many with minor but protective mutations, are created during each reproductive cycle of HIV. Most newborn viruses quickly infect circulating immune cells or take up residence in body reservoirs that are relatively inaccessible to drug therapy. HIV's ability to change and evade treatment has made drug management of the disease complicated and has hindered vaccine development. Nonetheless, decreasing the viral load with combinations of drugs decreases the body's viral burden and the development of drug-resistant mutant clones, while prolonging disease-free survival.

In the U.S., common opportunistic infections that infect AIDS patients include *Pneumocystis carinii* pneumonia, *Mycobacterium avium intracellulare* (MAI), cytomegalovirus, *Toxoplasma gondii*, *Candida albicans*, *Cryptosporidium*, and *Histoplasma capsulatum*. AIDS patients also are subject to nonopportunistic infections (e.g., tuberculosis, syphilis, herpesviruses, papillomaviruses, and streptococcus pneumonia) at rates and with a virulence far exceeding those in the general population.

SYMPTOMS: The opportunistic infections that accompany AIDS cause fatigue, fevers, chills, sweats, breathlessness, oral ulceration, swallowing difficulties, pneumonia, diarrhea, skin rashes, anorexia, weight loss, confusion, dementia, strokelike symptoms, and many other illnesses. Initial infection with HIV-1 sometimes causes a mono-

Clinical Conditions and Opportunistic Infections Indicating AIDS

Candida infections (candidiasis) of the trachea, bronchi, or lungs	Kaposi's sarcoma
Candidiasis of the esophagus	Lymphoma, Burkitt's
Cervical cancer, invasive	Lymphoma, immunoblastic
Coccidioides immitis: Extrapulmonary infections or disseminated	Lymphoma, primary brain
Cryptococcus neoformans: Infections outside the lung	*Mycobacterium avium* complex or *M. kansasii:* Extrapulmonary infections or disseminated
Cryptosporidium: Chronic infections of the gastrointestinal tract[1]	*Mycobacterium tuberculosis*: Pulmonary or extrapulmonary infections
Cytomegalovirus: Infections other than liver, spleen, or lymph nodes	*Mycobacterium*, other species: Extrapulmonary infections or disseminated
Cytomegalovirus retinitis with loss of vision	*Pneumocystis carinii*: Pneumonia
Herpes simplex: Chronic oral ulcers, bronchitis, pneumonitis, or esophagitis	Pneumonia, recurrent
Histoplasma capsulatum: Infections outside of lung or disseminated	Progressive multifocal leukoencephalopathy
HIV-related encephalopathy	*Salmonella*: Septicemia, recurrent
Isosporiasis, chronic intestinal	*Toxoplasma*: Brain infections
	Wasting syndrome of HIV

1. Chronic—more than 1 month's duration
SOURCE: CDC:MMWR 41 (RR-17):2-3, 15, 1992.

nucleosis-like syndrome, with fevers, sore throat, swollen glands, and muscle and joint aches. SEE: table.DIAGNOSIS: The presence of antibodies to HIV in the blood is a marker of HIV infection; when these are detected in a patient with low T helper cell counts and related illnesses, AIDS is diagnosed. Enzyme-linked immunosorbent assays (ELISA) are the primary tests used in screening for HIV antibodies. If these antibodies are detected, the Western blot test is used for confirmation. The polymerase chain reaction can also be used to detect the presence of HIV nucleic acid in the blood. Measurement of the absolute levels of T helper cells and the level of HIV viremia (also called the viral load) are the principal tests used to monitor the course of established infection and the effectiveness of administered therapies.

NATURAL HISTORY: Research in the late 1990s showed that 60% to 80% of HIV-infected individuals developed AIDS within 10 years of seroconversion.

PREVENTION: The public should be educated about HIV infection and its mode of transmission. Condom use and other safe sexual behaviors should be encouraged, esp. among teenagers and young adults. The sharing of contaminated needles should be strongly discouraged. Abstinence from risky behaviors prevents the spread of the disease.

Transfusion-associated HIV infection is now extremely rare, as a result of careful screening of the blood supply. All pregnant women should be counseled about testing for the presence of HIV antibodies because the use of antiretroviral therapies during and immediately after pregnancy reduces the incidence of HIV infection in infants.

TREATMENT: The use of highly active antiretroviral therapies (HAART), typically including a drug that inhibits HIV-1 protease and two antiretroviral drugs, has revolutionized the treatment of AIDS. Combination drug cocktails can decrease viral loads to undetectable levels and restore a level of immunological function to AIDS patients that, although imperfect, defends against most opportunistic infections. Since the introduction of HAART in the U.S. (1997), the numbers of hospitalizations for and deaths due to AIDS have dropped. The promise of these therapies is realized only when patients strictly comply with their prescription regimens and avoid risky behaviors. Even while taking highly active therapies, patients can infect others with HIV.

Treatments for AIDS patients are also directed against the opportunistic infections of AIDS. These include drugs such as trimethoprim/sulfamethoxazole or pentamidine for *Pneumocystis carinii*; clarithromycin and other agents for MAI; ganciclovir for cytomegalovirus; amphotericin B for *Histoplasmosis*; and many others.

Treatment for AIDS-related malignancies includes interferon-α for Kaposi's sarcoma and combination chemotherapies for non-Hodgkin's lymphoma.

PATIENT CARE: HIV infection is spread by direct contact with the blood or bodily secretions of infected persons, usually through a break in the skin or across mucous membranes. In most instances, it has been transmitted from person to person by one of three modes: sexually, by injection or transfusion of blood products, or from mother to fetus or infant. Health care providers are not at an increased risk for AIDS or HIV infection as long as they follow standard precautions. Individuals engaging in unsafe sexual behaviors and those who engage in injection drug use with contaminated needles are at the greatest risk for contracting the disease. Occupational exposures to body fluids from AIDS patients is common in health care, but the transmission of disease is rare. The risk of HIV infection after a puncture wound from a contaminated needle is 0.3%; the risk of seroconversion after mucous membranes are splashed with contaminated blood is 0.09%. The virus does not proliferate or survive outside the body (i.e., on counters or other surfaces).

Health care professionals should contribute actively to the education of patients about prevention of the spread of HIV. Affected patients are encouraged to adhere to complicated drug regimens because failure to do so may result in the evolution of drug-resistant viruses. In addition, patients are encouraged to maintain as much physical activity as is tolerable, allowing time for exercise and rest. Supportive care is provided for fatigue, anorexia, and fever. Meticulous skin and oral care is provided, esp. for debilitated patients. Caloric intake is recorded, and the need for small, frequent meals, nutritional supplements, or parenteral nutrition is assessed. Mothers with HIV or AIDS are strongly discouraged from breastfeeding. The patient is assisted in getting social service support; information about the disease; funds for housing, food, and medication; as well as inpatient, outpatient, and hospice care when appropriate.

perinatal AIDS Infection with the human immunodeficiency virus (HIV) as a result of vertical transmission of the virus from an infected mother. Worldwide, 22 million infants were infected in 1996, 90% of whom were in developing nations. In the U.S. between 1992 and 1997, testing pregnant women to identify HIV infection and treating affected individuals with zidovudine decreased the risk of perinatal AIDS by about 70%.

TRANSMISSION: Transmission of HIV to infants occurs in utero, during labor and delivery, and through breastfeeding. Approx. 50% to 70% are infected during childbirth (esp. preterm birth with prolonged rupture of membranes), and 30% to 50% are infected in utero; 20% of HIV-positive mothers can transmit the infection through breastfeeding.

DIAGNOSIS: The diagnosis is made through two positive blood test results for the presence of HIV or the growth of HIV in culture. Transmission is unlikely to occur in women whose viral load of HIV RNA has been reduced by effective antiretroviral therapy.

SYMPTOMS: Infants may be asymptomatic even when infected with HIV. Infection is monitored by measuring the absolute CD4+ T-cell count, measuring the amount of virus in the blood (viral load), and assessing for the presence of opportunistic infections in infancy or early childhood. Over time, the infected infant may present with *Pneumocystis carinii* (PCP) pneumonia, chronic diarrhea, recurrent bacterial infections, failure to thrive, developmental delays, and recurrent *Candida* and herpes simplex infections. The majority of perinatally infected children develop an AIDS-defining illness by the age of 4. Anemia and neutropenia may occur as side effects of drug therapy.

TREATMENT: Zidovudine (AZT) is given for 6 weeks to all infants born of HIV-positive mothers. Prophylaxis for *P. carinii* pneumonia with trimethoprim-sulfamethoxazole begins at 6 weeks and continues for 6 months in children whose HIV test results are negative and for 1 year in infected infants. The use of highly active antiretroviral therapy (HAART) is being studied. Breastfeeding is contraindicated for all HIV-infected mothers, to minimize the risk of transmission of the virus.

PATIENT CARE: Women in the childbearing years who engage in high-risk behaviors should be counseled to be tested for HIV before becoming pregnant, or as soon as they know they are pregnant, to reduce the baby's risk of infection. For women who are HIV-positive, antiretroviral therapy should begin immediately. Universal precautions are used with babies born of HIV-positive mothers until diagnostic tests indicate that they are not infected. Mothers and other care providers must be instructed in the use of universal precautions and to watch for and quickly report respiratory infections.

AIDS-dementia complex ABBR: ADC. Encephalopathy caused by direct infection of brain tissue by the human immunodeficiency virus (HIV). This condition affects as many as 15% of AIDS patients, but in 1997 its incidence decreased to approx. 30% of its previous occurrence because of the effectiveness of highly active antiretroviral therapy (HAART). Central nervous system HIV infections in children tend to be more pronounced than those in adults.

ETIOLOGY: The exact cause of AIDS

dementia is unknown, but current theories suggest that it results from HIV infection of macrophages in the brain (microglia) and the destructive release of cytokines that disrupt neurotransmitter function.

SYMPTOMS: AIDS dementia is characterized by slow onset of memory loss, decreased ability to concentrate, a general slowing of cognitive processes, and mood disorders, all of which progress over time. Motor dysfunction may also be present, including ataxia, bowel and bladder incontinence, and seizures. Higher levels of HIV RNA in the cerebrospinal fluid (CSF viral load) are correlated with increased problems.

TREATMENT: Treatment options may include zidovudine and highly active antiretroviral therapies, although the efficacy of these treatments is limited.

PATIENT CARE: The patient's mental status and level of consciousness must be assessed and documented. Clear documentation is essential to track a patient's changes over time. Orientation to person, place, and time; thought processes (cognition); verbal communication skills; and memory losses can be determined through simple conversations that reveal the patient's ability to recall normal details of the day and previous teaching. Particular attention is paid to patients' abilities to comply with their complex medication regimen; inability to do so requires another person to assume responsibility for this task. The patient's affect and mood; the presence of agitated, restless, or lethargic behavior; and the extent to which clothing is clean and appropriate for the weather—all may reveal progressing dementia when compared with previously documented mental status assessments.

Interventions are based on clear communication. As patients develop dementia, they may become frightened, so a consistently gentle approach with positive feedback is essential. Clocks, calendars, and memory aids help the patient become reoriented. Step-by-step written instructions should be given to augment verbal instructions. Caregivers need to learn how to reorient the patient, how to recognize and treat hallucinations, how to create a safe environment, how to ensure that basic hygiene needs are met, and how to document medication schedules and intake, as patients may forget to eat or drink adequately.

AIDS peripheral neuropathies Direct infection of peripheral nerves by the human immunodeficiency virus (HIV) resulting in sensory and motor changes due to destruction of axons or their myelin covering. Acute or chronic inflammatory myelin damage may be the first sign of peripheral nerve involvement. Patients display gradual or abrupt onset of motor weakness and diminished or absent reflexes. Diagnostic biopsies of peripheral nerves show inflammatory changes and loss of myelin. Distal sensory neuropathy occurs in up to 30% of patients with AIDS, usually late in the disease. There is increased risk in older patients and those with diabetes mellitus, nutritional deficiencies, low CD4 cell counts, and vitamin B_{12} deficiencies. Patients report sharp pain, numbness, or burning in the feet. Destruction of dorsal root ganglions and degeneration of central peripheral axons is seen on autopsy. Some antiretroviral drugs (ddI, ddC, and d4T) also cause a reversible peripheral neuropathy in about 20% of patients. SEE: *AIDS; Guillain-Barré syndrome; polyneuropathy, chronic inflammatory demyelinating*.

TREATMENT: NSAIDs, opioids, gabapentin anticonvulsants, and topical agents have all been used, with variable success, to treat the pain of AIDS-related sensory neuropathy. Acupuncture is not effective. Human nerve growth factor (NGF), which stimulates regeneration of damaged nerve fibers, is being studied, esp. to minimize the neuropathy that antiretroviral drugs cause.

AIDS-related complex ABBR: ARC. The symptomatic stage of infection with human immunodeficiency virus (HIV) before the onset of AIDS. Its clinical signs include fatigue, intermittent fevers, weight loss greater than 10%, chronic or persistent intermittent diarrhea, night sweats, diminished delayed hypersensitivity (skin test) response to common allergens, presence of HIV antibodies in blood, and decreased CD4+ T-lymphocyte count. The term is not used extensively. SEE: *AIDS*.

AIDS wasting syndrome Malnutrition in the HIV-infected patient, including both starvation (weight loss from lack of food) and cachexia (loss of lean body mass). SEE: *cachexia; cytokine; Food Guide Pyramid; starvation*.

PATHOPHYSIOLOGY: The mechanisms by which HIV causes malnutrition include decreased nutritional intake, metabolic abnormalities, and the combination of diarrhea and malabsorption. Decreased oral intake may be related to loss of appetite, oral or esophageal ulcers (esp. from *Candida* or herpes simplex virus), difficulty chewing, fatigue, changes in mental status, or inadequate finances. Metabolic abnormalities include elevated serum cortisol, decreased anabolism, micronutrient deficiencies (vitamin B_{12}, pyridoxine, and vitamin A, zinc, and selenium), and decreased antioxidants. Malabsorption and diarrhea affect 60% to 100% of patients with AIDS. Primary gastrointestinal pathogens that contribute to malnutrition include *Cryptospor-*

idia, *Microsporidia*, and *Mycobacterium avium intracellulare*. Concerns about diarrhea and fecal incontinence may underlie a patient's decreased oral intake.

PATIENT CARE: Assessment and education of patients must begin as soon as they are diagnosed as having HIV infection. Obtaining a careful history of the patient's normal nutritional intake and activity level provides the baseline for nutritional instruction. Patients are encouraged to maintain the recommended daily allowance (RDA) for all foods by following the Food Guide Pyramid; protein intake of 1 to 2 g/kg of ideal body weight and vitamin and mineral intake three to four times the RDA are also encouraged. Small frequent feedings, good oral hygiene, limited fluids with meals, and the use of preferred foods are helpful strategies in countering anorexia. A written schedule may help the patient adhere to the recommended plan for intake. Any increase in exercise or activity must be accompanied by an increase in food intake. As opportunistic infections develop, the health care team must work together with the patient to limit the problems that inhibit good nutritional intake.

A.I.H. *artificial insemination by husband* (homologous insemination).

ailment A mild illness.

ailurophobia (ă-lū″rō-fō′bē-ă) [Gr. *ailouros*, cat, + *phobos*, fear] Morbid fear of cats.

ainhum (ān′hŭm) [East African, to saw] A fissured constriction around a digit; the cause is unknown. Due to the constriction, the digit will eventually require amputation. The fourth or fifth toe is usually affected and less commonly other digits of the feet or hands. It occurs primarily in people of color. There is no specific treatment.

air (ār) [Gr. *aer*, air] The invisible, tasteless, odorless mixture of gases surrounding the Earth. Clean air at sea level comprises approx. 78% nitrogen and 21% oxygen by volume. The remaining constituents are water vapor, carbon dioxide, and traces of ammonia, argon, helium, neon, krypton, xenon, and other rare gases.

alveolar a. Air in the alveoli; that involved in the pulmonary exchange of gases between air and the blood. Its content is determined by sampling the last portion of a maximal expiration.

complemental a. An old term for the volume of air that can be inspired over and above the tidal air by deepest possible inspiration. SYN: *inspiratory reserve volume*.

dead space a. The volume of air that fills the respiratory passageways and is not available for exchange of gases with the blood.

functional residual a. An old term for functional residual capacity.

liquid a. Air liquefied by great pressure and/or low temperature. It produces intense cold on evaporation.

mechanical dead space a. Dead space air provided by artificial means, as with mechanical ventilation or the addition of plastic tubing to a ventilator circuit.

minimal a. The small volume of air trapped in the alveoli when lungs collapse.

reserve a. Expiratory reserve volume.

residual a. An old term for reserve volume.

supplemental a. An old term for expiratory reserve volume.

tidal a. An old term for tidal volume.

air bronchogram sign Radiographic appearance of an air-filled bronchus as it passes through an area of increased anatomic density as in pulmonary edema and pneumonia.

air cell Air vesicle.

air conduction The conduction of sound to the inner ear via the pathway provided by the air in the ear canal.

air curtain A current of air directed around a patient to block the air that would normally circulate around and contaminate the patient; used in isolating patients from dustborne bacteria or allergens. SEE: *laminar air flow*.

air evacuation Transport of patients from one location to another by specially equipped helicopters or other aircraft. Indications for air transport include severe trauma, burns, and other conditions requiring immediate skilled care and treatment.

air flow, laminar SEE: *laminar air flow*.

air gap principle A procedure used to decrease the amount of scattered radiation reaching the radiographic film by increasing the object-image receptor distance.

air medical services Air medical transportation.

air medical transportation The use of helicopters or fixed-wing aircraft to transport patients from the scene of an incident or local hospital to a regional trauma or specialty care center.

airplane splint An appliance usually used on ambulatory patients in the treatment of fractures of the humerus. It takes its name from the elevated (abducted) position in which it holds the arm suspended in air.

airsickness A form of motion sickness marked by dizziness, nausea, vomiting, headache, and often drowsiness that occurs during travel in aircraft. SEE: *motion sickness; seasickness*.

air swallowing Voluntary or involuntary swallowing of air. It occurs involuntarily in infants as a result of improper feeding. Adults may swallow air during eating or drinking.

air syringe A syringe on a dental unit that delivers compressed air, water, or both through a fine nozzle to clear or dry an area or to evacuate debris from an operative field.

CAUTION: Use of high pressure may injure the tissues.

air vesicle An obsolete term for pulmonary alveolus.

airway **1.** A natural passageway for air to enter and exit the lungs. **2.** A device used to prevent or correct an obstructed respiratory passage, esp. during anesthesia and cardiopulmonary resuscitation. Maintaining the airway is essential to the life of the patient. In an emergency situation, esp. when the patient is unconscious or has a bilateral fracture of the lower jaw, there is a good possibility that the tongue will close the oropharyngeal airway. Methods for opening the airway are described in the entries for cardiopulmonary resuscitation; chin-lift airway technique, head tilt; jaw-thrust technique, and tracheostomy. SEE: illus.; *jaw thrust*.

CAUTION: If a patient is unconscious or has an injury to the head and upper neck, one should assume there is spinal injury. In these situations, the airway should be opened using techniques that avoid cervical spinal trauma.

esophageal gastric tube a. ABBR: EGTA. An esophageal airway with a 37-cm-long, large-bore tube attached to a mask that makes an airtight seal with the patient's face. A balloon at the distal end of the tube is inflated following insertion into the esophagus. This improves ventilation and eliminates the possibility of regurgitation. The EGTA has an opening at the distal end of the tube for decompression of the stomach.

esophageal obturator a. ABBR: EOA. An airway device (primarily used in emergency medical service systems) in which the tube is blindly inserted into the esophagus, thereby blocking vomitus and permitting lung ventilation.

laryngeal mask a. ABBR: LMA. A device shaped like a miniature mask used in inhalation anesthesia. It is inserted blindly into the hypopharynx and forms a seal around the glottic opening to the larynx. Because laryngoscopy is not necessary in order to properly position the mask, establishing an airway is facilitated even when used by persons with no prior experience in resuscitation. Anesthetic gases may be administered through the device.

CAUTION: Guidelines concerning the risk of aspiration should be followed.

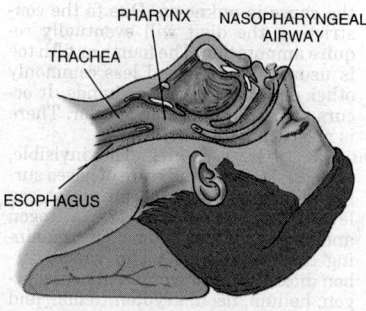

NASOPHARYNGEAL AIRWAY

PHARYNX

NASOPHARYNGEAL AIRWAY

TRACHEA

ESOPHAGUS

TILT HEAD BACK BEFORE INSERTING NASOPHARYNGEAL AIRWAY. INSERT THROUGH NOSTRIL, PAST THE PHARYNX INTO THE LARYNX AND TRACHEA TO MAINTAIN PATENCY OF AIRWAY

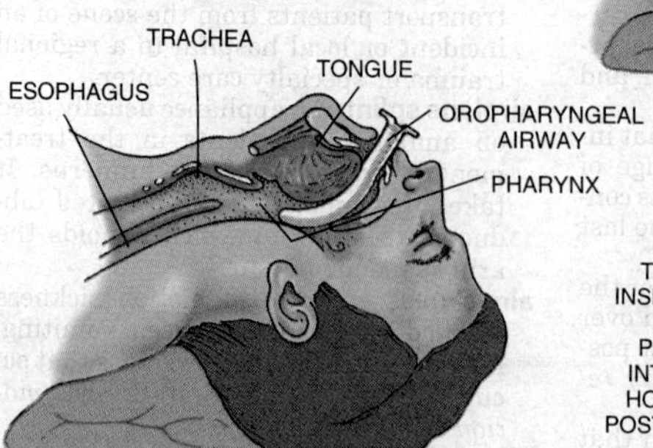

TILT HEAD BACK BEFORE INSERTING OROPHARYNGEAL AIRWAY. TO MAINTAIN PATENCY INSERT DEVICE INTO PROPER POSITION TO HOLD TONGUE AWAY FROM POSTERIOR WALL OF PHARYNX

NASOPHARYNGEAL/OROPHARYNGEAL AIRWAY

nasopharyngeal a. ABBR: NPA. A soft, flexible uncuffed tube placed through the nasal passages into the nasopharynx. It is used to maintain the free passage of air to and from the lungs in patients with facial trauma or lockjaw or in nearly comatose patients who are breathing spontaneously. The tube should be long enough to extend from the tip of the patient's nose to the earlobe. The diameter should match that of the patient's smallest finger. SEE: *Standard and Universal Precautions Appendix.*

oropharyngeal a. A curved plastic device used to establish an airway in a patient by displacing the tongue from the posterior wall of the oropharynx. The device should be equal in length to the distance from either the corner of the mouth to the earlobe or the center of the mouth to the angle of the jaw. It has a flange on the end remaining outside the mouth to keep it from sliding into the pharynx too far. This device is reserved for unconscious patients who do not have a gag reflex. SEE: *cardiopulmonary resuscitation; Standard and Universal Precautions Appendix.*

CAUTION: The head of an unconscious patient should be stabilized before the airway is inserted to prevent paralysis.

airway clearance, ineffective Inability to clear secretions or obstructions from the respiratory tract to maintain a patent airway. SEE: *Nursing Diagnoses Appendix.*

A.K. *above knee;* term used to refer to the site of amputation of a lower extremity.

akaryocyte (ă-kăr′ē-ō-sīt″) [Gr. *a-*, not, + *karyon*, kernel, + *kytos*, cell] A cell without a nucleus (e.g., an erythrocyte).

akaryote (ă-kăr′ē-ōt) [″ + *karyon*, kernel] Akaryocyte.

akathisia, acathisia (ăk″ă-thĭ′zē-ă) [″ + *kathisis*, sitting] Motor restlessness; intolerance of inactivity. This symptom may appear as a side effect of antipsychotic drug therapy (e.g., treatment with phenothiazines).

SYMPTOMS: Affected persons cannot sit still, are jumpy, and may appear distracted.

TREATMENT: The urge to move resolves when the offending drug is withdrawn. Propranolol is also used to reduce motor restlessness.

akee (ăk′ē, ă-kē′) [Liberian] The tropical tree *Blighia sapida.* Ingestion of the unripe fruit can cause severe hypoglycemia. Also spelled *ackee.*

akinesia (ă″kĭ-nē′zē-ă) [Gr. *a-*, not, + *kinesis*, movement] Complete or partial loss of muscle movement; also spelled *acinesia.* **akinetic** (-nĕt′ĭk), *adj.*

a. algera Akinesia with intense pain caused by voluntary movement.

Al Symbol for the element aluminum (British: aluminium).

-al [L.] **1.** Suffix meaning *relating to*, as in abdominal, intestinal. **2.** In chemistry, suffix indicating an aldehyde.

ala (ā′lă) *pl.* **alae** [L., wing] **1.** An expanded or winglike structure or appendage. **2.** Axilla.

a. auris Protruding portion of the external ear. SYN: *auricle; pinna.*

a. cerebelli Winglike projection of the central lobule of the cerebellum. SYN: *a. lobuli centralis.*

a. cinerea Gray triangular prominence on the floor of the fourth ventricle. The autonomic fibers of the vagus nerve arise from the cells of the nucleus of this area. Also called *triangle of the vagus nerve* and *trigonum nervi vagi.*

a. cristae galli Small projection on each side of the crista galli of the ethmoid bone.

a. lobuli centralis A. cerebelli.

a. major ossis sphenoidalis Greater wing of the sphenoid bone.

a. minor ossis sphenoidalis Lesser wing of the sphenoid bone.

a. nasi Wing of the nose; broad portion forming the lateral wall of each nostril.

a. of ethmoid Small projection on each side of the ethmoid bone.

a. of ilium Broad, upper portion of the iliac bone.

a. of sacrum Broad projection on each side of the base of the sacrum.

a. vomeris Wing of the vomer; projection on each side of the superior border of the vomer.

alacrima (ā-lăk′rĭ-mă) [Gr. *a-*, not, + L. *lacrima*, tear] Deficiency of or absence of tears. SYN: *dry eye.* SEE: *Sjögren's syndrome.*

Alagille syndrome [Daniel Alagille, Fr. physician, b. 1925] Arteriohepatic dysplasia with bile duct hypoplasia or paucity.

alalia (ă-lā′lē-ă) [″ + *lalein*, to talk] Inability to speak due to defect or paralysis of the vocal organs; aphasia. An organic brain disease is usually responsible.

alanine (ăl′ă-nēn) A naturally occurring amino acid, $C_3H_7NO_2$, considered nonessential in human nutrition.

alanine aminotransferase ABBR: ALT. An intracellular enzyme involved in amino acid and carbohydrate metabolism. It is present in high concentrations in muscle, liver, and brain. An increased level of this enzyme in the blood indicates necrosis or disease in these tissues. Its measurement is most commonly used as part of the differential diagnosis of liver disease (e.g., hepatitis) and in the tracking of the course of the disease process. This enzyme was formerly called serum glutamic pyruvic transaminase (SGPT) or glutamic-pyruvic transaminase.

Al-Anon A nonprofit organization that provides group support for the family and close friends of alcoholics. SEE: *Alcoholics Anonymous.*

alar (ā'lăr) [L. *ala*, wing] **1.** Pert. to or like a wing. **2.** Axillary.

ALARA *as low as reasonably achievable.*

alar artery Branch of the angular artery that supplies the tissues of the ala nasi.

alar cartilage Cartilage forming the broad lateral wall of each nostril.

Alateen A nonprofit organization that provides support for children of alcoholics. SEE: *Alcoholics Anonymous.*

alba [L. *albus*, white] **1.** White. **2.** White matter of the brain.

albedo (ăl-bē'dō) [L.] Whiteness. Reflection of light from a surface.

a. retinae Reflections associated with retinal edema.

a. unguium White semilunar area near the nail root. SYN: *lunula.*

Albers-Schönberg disease (ăl-bārs-shĕrn'bārg) [Heinrich Ernst Albers-Schönberg, Ger. roentgenologist, 1865–1921] Hereditary condition marked by excessive calcification of bones causing spontaneous fractures and marblelike appearance. SYN: *marble bone; osteopetrosis.*

Albert's disease [Eduard Albert, Austrian surgeon, 1841–1900] Inflammation of the bursae lying over the Achilles tendon. SYN: *achillobursitis.*

albicans [L.] White; whitish.

Albini's nodules (ăl-bē'nēz) [Giuseppe Albini, It. physiologist, 1830–1911] Minute nodules on the margins of the mitral and tricuspid valves of the heart; sometimes seen in newborns.

albinism (ăl'bĭn-ĭzm) [L. *albus*, white, + Gr. *-ismos*, condition] Genetic, nonpathological, partial or total absence of pigment in skin, hair, and eyes. It is often accompanied by astigmatism, photophobia, and nystagmus because the choroid is not sufficiently protected from light as a result of lack of pigment.

albino (ăl-bī'nō) A person afflicted with albinism.

albinuria (ăl″bĭ-nū'rē-ă) [L. *albus*, white, + Gr. *ouron*, urine] Passing of white or colorless urine of low specific gravity. SYN: *achromaturia.*

Albright's disease [Fuller Albright, U.S. physician, 1900–1969] Polyostotic fibrous dysplasia accompanied by café au lait macules and endocrine disorders, esp. precocious puberty in girls. The patient is fracture prone, and deformity and shortening of bones may develop. SEE: *dysplasia, polyostotic fibrous.*

albuginea (ăl-bū-jĭn'ē-ă) [L. from *albus*, white] A layer of firm white fibrous tissue forming the investment of an organ or part, as of the eye, testicle, ovary, or spleen. SYN: *tunica albuginea.*

a. corporum cavernosorum A strong, very elastic, white fibrous sheath of both corpora cavernosa of the penis.

a. oculi The sclera, or fibrous connective tissue outer layer of the eyeball.

a. ovarii The layer of firm fibrous tissue lying beneath the epithelial ovarian covering.

a. testis The thick, unyielding layer of white fibrous tissue lying under the tunica vaginalis.

albugineotomy (ăl″bū-jĭn″ē-ŏt'ō-mē) [*albuginea* + Gr. *tome*, incision] Incision of tunica albuginea, esp. of the testis.

albugineous (ăl″bū-jĭn'ē-ŭs) Pert. to or resembling the tunica albuginea.

albuginitis (ăl″bū-jĭn-ī'tĭs) [″+ Gr. *itis*, inflammation] Inflammation of the tunica albuginea.

albumin (ăl-bū'mĭn) [L. *albumen*, white of egg] One of a group of simple proteins widely distributed in plant and animal tissues; it is found in the blood as serum albumin, in milk as lactalbumin, and in the white of egg as ovalbumin. In the blood, albumin acts as a carrier molecule and helps to maintain blood volume and blood pressure. In humans, the principal function of albumin is to provide colloid osmotic pressure, preventing plasma loss from the capillaries. Albumin, like all the plasma proteins, can act as a source for rapid replacement of tissue proteins. It is soluble in cold water; when coagulated by heat it is no longer dissolved by cold or hot water. In the stomach, coagulated albumins are made soluble by peptidases, which breaks them down to smaller polypeptides and amino acids. In general, albumins from animal sources are of higher nutritional quality than those from vegetable sources because animal proteins contain greater quantities of essential amino acids. SEE: *amino acid; peptone.*

blood a. Serum a.

circulating a. Albumin present in body fluids.

egg a. Ovalbumin.

human a. A sterile solution of serum albumin obtained from healthy blood donors. It is administered intravenously to restore blood volume.

serum a. The main protein found in the blood. SYN: *blood a.* SEE: *blood; simple protein.*

urinary a. Albumin in urine, a finding in glomerular diseases.

vegetable a. Albumin in, or derived from, plant tissue.

albuminate (ăl-bū'mĭ-nāt) The compound formed when albumin combines with an acid or alkali (base).

albuminaturia (ăl-bū″mĭ-nă-tū′rē-ă) [L. *albumen*, white of egg, + Gr. *ouron*, urine] Presence of albuminates in urine.

albuminiferous (ăl-bū″mĭn-ĭf′ĕ-rŭs) [″ + *ferre*, to bear] Producing albumin.

albuminimeter (ăl-bū″mĭn-ĭm′ĕ-tĕr) [″ + Gr. *metron*, measure] Instrument for measuring the amount of albumin in urine.

albuminiparous (ăl-bū″mĭn-ĭp′ă-rŭs) [″ + *parere*, to bring forth, to bear] Yielding albumin.

albuminocholia (ăl-bū″mĭ-nō-kō′lē-ă) [″ + Gr. *chole*, bile] Albumin in the bile.

albuminogenous (ăl-bū″mĭn-ŏj′ĕ-nŭs) [″ + Gr. *gennan*, to produce] Producing albumin.

albuminoid (ăl-bū′mĭ-noyd″) [″ + Gr. *eidos*, form, shape] Resembling albumin.

albuminolysis (ăl-bū″mĭn-ŏl′ĭ-sĭs) [″ + Gr. *lysis*, dissolution] Proteolysis; decomposition of protein.

albuminoreaction (ăl-bū″mĭ-nō-rē-ăk′shŭn) [″ + *re*, again, + *agere*, to act] The presence (positive reaction) or absence (negative reaction) of albumin in the sputum. A positive reaction was formerly used to indicate inflammation of the lungs.

albuminorrhea (ăl-bū″mĭ-nō-rē′ă) [″ + Gr. *rhoia*, flow] The presence of albumin in urine. SYN: *albuminuria*.

albuminose (ăl-bū′mĭn-ōs) Albuminous.

albuminosis (ăl-bū″mĭ-nō′sĭs) [″ + Gr. *osis*, condition] An abnormal increase of albumin in blood plasma.

albuminous (ăl-bū′mĭ-nŭs) Pert. to, resembling, or containing albumin.

albumin test Any chemical test for the presence of albumin, usually with electrophoresis, chromatography, spectrophotometry, spectrometry, or immunoassay, and sometimes by simple chemical reactions on dipsticks.

albuminuretic [L. *albumen*, white of egg, + Gr. *ouretikos*, causing urine to flow] Pert. to or causing albuminuria.

albuminuria (ăl-bū-mĭ-nū′rē-ă) [″ + Gr. *ouron*, urine] The presence of readily detectable amounts of serum protein, esp. serum albumin but also serum globulin and others, in the urine. Albuminuria is a common sign of renal impairment (nephrotic syndrome and other kidney disorders); it also occurs in fever, malignant hypertension, and in healthy people after vigorous exercise among other conditions. SYN: *proteinuria*. SEE: *nephritis; nephrosis*. **albuminuric** (-nū′rĭk), *adj.*

cyclic a. Presence of small amounts of albumin in the urine at regular diurnal intervals, esp. in childhood and adolescence.

digestive a. Albuminuria following ingestion of certain foods.

extrarenal a. Albuminuria due to contamination of urine with pus, chyle, or blood.

functional a. Intermittent or temporary albuminuria not associated with a pathological condition. SYN: *physiological a.*

intrinsic a. Albuminuria resulting from intrinsic renal disease. SYN: *true a.*

orthostatic a. Postural a.

pathological a. Albuminuria caused by a disease.

physiological a. Functional a.

postural a. Transient albuminuria in normal individuals who have been erect for a long period. SYN: *orthostatic a.*

renal a. Albuminuria caused by defective renal function, esp. of the glomeruli.

toxic a. Albuminuria caused by internal or external toxins.

true a. Intrinsic a.

albumoscope (ăl-bū′mō-skōp) [L. *albumen*, white of egg, + Gr. *skopein*, to examine] An instrument for determining the presence of albumin in the urine.

albus [L.] White.

Albuterol Bronchodilator administered by inhalation or tablet.

Alcaligenes (ăl″kă-lĭj′ĭ-nēz) A genus of rod-shaped, gram-negative bacteria found in the intestinal tract of humans, in dairy products, and in soil.

A. faecalis A species of bacteria normally found in the intestinal tract of humans. It has been associated with septicemia and epidemics of urinary tract infections.

Alcock's canal [Benjamin Alcock, Irish anatomist, b. 1801] Pudendal canal. SYN: *Pudendal c.*

alcohol (ăl′kō-hŏl) [Arabic *al-koh'l*, something subtle] **1.** A class of organic compounds that are hydroxyl derivatives of hydrocarbons. **2.** Ethyl alcohol (C_2H_5OH), a colorless, volatile, flammable liquid. Its molecular weight is 46.07; its boiling point is 78.5°C. It is present in fermented or distilled liquors and is obtained, in its pure form, from grain by fermentation and fractionation distillation. SYN: *ethanol; grain a.*

ACTION/USES: Taken in excessive amounts, alcohol acts as a depressant to the nervous system. Because it arrests the growth of bacteria, it is useful in preserving biological specimens and in some patent medicines. It is also used in preparing essences, tinctures, and extracts; in the manufacture of ether, ethylene, and other industrial products; as a rubbing compound; and as an antiseptic in 70% solution. SEE: *alcoholism; fetal alcohol syndrome*.

absolute a. A solution that contains 99% alcohol and not more than 1% by weight of water.

cetyl a. A white insoluble solid substance, $C_{16}H_{34}O$, used in the manufacture of ointments.

dehydrated a. Alcohol containing not less than 99.2% by weight of ethyl alcohol. This corresponds to 99.5% by volume of ethyl alcohol.

denatured a. Alcohol rendered unfit for use as a beverage or medicine by the addition of toxic ingredients; used commercially as a solvent.

diluted a. Alcohol containing not less than 41% and not more than 42% by weight of ethyl alcohol; used as a solvent. Also called diluted ethanol.

ethyl a. C_2H_6O; grain alcohol. SEE: *alcohol*(2); *Poisons and Poisoning Appendix.*

grain a. Ethyl a. SEE: *alcohol*(2).

isopropyl a. C_3H_8O; a clear flammable liquid similar to ethyl alcohol and propyl alcohol. It is used in medical preparations for external use, antifreeze, cosmetics, and solvents. SEE: *Poisons and Poisoning Appendix.*

CAUTION: Isopropyl alcohol is toxic when taken internally.

---

methyl a. CH_4O; a colorless, volatile, flammable liquid obtained from distillation of wood. Even though its physical properties are similar to those of ethyl alcohol, it is not fit for human consumption. Ingestion of methyl alcohol can lead to blindness and death. It is used as a solvent, for fuel, as an additive for denaturing ethyl alcohol, as an antifreeze agent, and in the preparation of formaldehyde. SYN: *methanol; wood alcohol.* SEE: *methyl alcohol in Poisons and Poisoning Appendix.*

pathological reaction to a. An exceedingly severe reaction to ingestion of alcohol, esp. to small amounts. It is manifested by irrational violent behavior followed by exhaustion, sleep, and loss of recall of the event. The patient may not be intoxicated. The etiology is unknown but is associated with hypoglycemia, exhaustion, and stress. SEE: *alcoholism.*

rubbing a. A preparation containing not less than 68.5% and not more than 71.5% dehydrated alcohol by volume. The remainder consists of water and denaturants and may or may not contain color additives and perfume oils. It is used as a rubefacient. Rubbing alcohol is packaged, labeled, and sold in accordance with the regulations issued by the U.S. Treasury Department, Bureau of Alcohol, Tobacco and Firearms.

CAUTION: Because of the added denaturant, it is poisonous if taken internally.

---

wood a. Methyl a.

Alcohol, Drug Abuse, and Mental Health Administration ABBR: ADAMHA. A U.S. government agency that is part of the National Institutes of Health within the Department of Health and Human Services. The agency administers grant programs supporting research, training, and service programs in alcoholism, drug abuse, and mental health.

alcoholic (ăl-kō-hŏl′ĭk) [L. *alcoholicus*] **1.** Pert. to alcohol. **2.** One afflicted with alcoholism.

alcoholic blackout An episode of forgetting all or part of what occurred during or following a period of alcohol intake.

Alcoholics Anonymous ABBR: A.A. An organization consisting of alcoholics and recovering alcoholics who are trying to help themselves and others abstain from alcohol by offering encouragement and discussing experiences, problems, feelings, techniques, and so on. The organization has groups in most U.S. cities; local chapters are listed in the telephone directory. SEE: *Al-Anon; Alateen.*

alcoholism (ăl′kō-hŏl-ĭzm) [Arabic *alkoh'l*, something subtle, + Gr. *-ismos*, condition] A chronic, frequently progressive and sometimes fatal disease marked by impaired control over alcohol use despite adverse effects from its consumption. Dependence on alcohol, tolerance of its effects, and remissions and relapses are common. Psychological features include preoccupation with alcohol use and denial of addiction, even when strong evidence to the contrary exists.

Alcohol abuse is one of the major threats to health in the U.S; each year 10% of all deaths are related to alcohol use. Chronic alcoholism and alcohol-related disorders can be physically, psychologically, and economically devastating to patients and their families. SEE: *fetal alcohol syndrome; substance abuse.*

ETIOLOGY: Psychological, physiological, genetic, familial, and cultural factors play a part in alcoholism. Family members of alcoholics and males are most likely to be predisposed to the disease.

SYMPTOMS: Pathological effects of alcoholism can be found in almost any organ of the body but are most commonly identified in the nervous system, bone marrow, liver, pancreas, stomach, and the other organs of the gastrointestinal tract. Symptoms arise both from organ-specific damage and from the psychological effects of the drug. Alcoholics are more likely than nonalcoholics to suffer falls, fractures, automotive accidents, job loss, imprisonment, and other legal difficulties. In addition, they have hypertension, gastritis, pancreatitis, hepatitis, cirrhosis, portal hypertension, memory disturbances, and oropharyngeal cancers at rates that exceed those in the general population. In severe alcoholism, abstinence results in withdrawal symptoms and, occasionally, hallucinosis, delirium tremens, or withdrawal seizures. The life expectancy of alcoholics is shorter than that of nonalcoholics. SEE: *alcohol withdrawal syndrome; cirrhosis; delirium tremens.*

DIAGNOSIS: Alcoholism is diagnosed clinically. Although some alcoholics have many abnormal laboratory findings, none of these is definitively diagnostic of the disease. In severe hepatic disease, BUN is elevated and serum glucose is decreased. Elevated liver function studies may indicate liver damage, and elevated serum amylase levels acute pancreatitis. Anemia, thrombocytopenia, increased prothrombin time, and increased partial thromboplastin time may be noted from hematologic studies.

Screening for alcoholism is best undertaken with questionnaires, like the Michigan Alcohol Screening Test (MAST) and the Alcohol Use Disorders Identification Test (AUDIT). CAGE, a widely used screening questionnaire, asks the questions: Do you feel the need to *c*ut down on drinking? Are you *an*noyed by people who complain about your drinking? Do you feel *g*uilty about your drinking? Do you need an *e*ye-opener when you wake up? These tests are designed to determine when alcohol use has become physically, behaviorally, or emotionally problematic for patients. Denial is a major concern, and patients may give false information in their health histories and deny physical problems associated with alcoholism. The usefulness of the assessment instrument depends upon the patient's honesty. The assessor should be aware, however, that indirect information obtained from the history and physical examination often reveals more than does direct questioning.

TREATMENT: Abstinence from alcohol remains the cornerstone of treatment for alcoholism. Support groups for alcoholics, such as Alcoholics Anonymous (AA), have reported the highest rates of treatment success. SEE: *Alcoholics Anonymous.*

PATIENT CARE: During acute intoxication or withdrawal, the patient is carefully monitored. Assessments should include mental status, temperature, heart rate, breath sounds, and blood pressure. Medications prescribed for symptom relief are administered, and desired and undesired effects are evaluated. Evaluation for signs of inadequate nutrition and dehydration is also necessary. The patient requires orientation to reality because he or she may have hallucinations or may try to harm self or others. A calm environment with minimal noise and shadows reduces the incidence of delusions and hallucinations. Seizure precautions are instituted, with mechanical restraint avoided. Health care professionals should approach the patient in a nonthreatening way, limit sustained eye contact, and explain all procedures. Even if the patient is verbally abusive, care providers should listen attentively and reply with empathy. The patient also is monitored for signs of depression or impending suicide.

In long-term care of alcoholism, the patient is assisted to accept his or her drinking problem and the need for abstinence. The patient should be confronted about alcohol-related behaviors and urged to examine actions. If the patient is taking disulfiram (or has taken it within the last 2 weeks), he or she is warned of the effects of alcohol ingestion, which may last from 30 minutes to 3 hours or longer. Even a small amount of alcohol will induce adverse reactions (e.g., nausea, vomiting, facial flushing, headache, shortness of breath, red eyes, blurred vision, sweating, tachycardia, hypotension, and fainting). The longer the patient takes the drug, the greater his or her sensitivity will be. Therefore, the patient must be warned to avoid medicinal or hygienic sources of alcohol (e.g., cough syrups, cold remedies, liquid vitamins, and mouthwashes).

The entire family is assisted to develop a long-term plan for follow-up and relapse prevention, including referral to organizations such as AA, Al-Anon, and Alateen. Family involvement in rehabilitation helps reduce family stressors and tensions. If the alcoholic patient has lost contact with family and friends and has a long history of unemployment, trouble with the law, or financial difficulties, social services or other appropriate agencies may assist with rehabilitation efforts. These may involve job training, sheltered workshops, halfway houses, and other supervised facilities.

acute a. intoxication (2).

chronic a. Alcoholism.

alcoholuria (ăl″kō-hŏl-ū′rē-ă) [″ + Gr. *ouron*, urine] The presence of alcohol in the urine.

alcohol withdrawal syndrome The neurological, psychiatric, and cardiovascular signs and symptoms that result when a person accustomed to consuming large quantities of alcohol suddenly becomes abstinent. Alcohol withdrawal usually follows a predictable pattern. In the first hours of abstinence, patients are often irritable, anxious, tremulous, and easily startled. Their blood pressure and pulse rises, but they remain alert and oriented. If they do not consume alcohol (or receive drug treatment) in the first 12 to 48 hours, they may suffer an alcohol withdrawal seizure. Abstinence for 72 to 96 hours may result in severe agitation, hallucinations, and marked fluctuations in blood pressure and pulse. This stage of withdrawal is known as delirium tremens, or alcoholic delirium; it may prove fatal in as many as 15% of patients. SEE: *alcoholism, chronic; delirium tremens.*

TREATMENT: Benzodiazepines (e.g., chlordiazepoxide) remain the preferred agents for the management of alcohol withdrawal, although other agents, such as carbamazepine, may be useful in treating mild cases.

aldehyde (ăl′dĕ-hīd) [*al*cohol *dehyd*rogenatum] **1.** Oxidation product of a primary alcohol; it has the characteristic group —CHO. **2.** Acetaldehyde, CH_3CHO; an intermediate in yeast fermentation and alcohol metabolism.

Alder-Reilly anomaly [Albert von Alder, Ger. physician, b. 1888; William Anthony Reilly, U.S. pediatrician, b. 1901] Large dark leukocyte granules that stain lilac. They consist of mucopolysaccharide deposits and are indicative of mucopolysaccharidosis.

aldolase (ăl′dō-lās) An enzyme present in skeletal and heart muscle and the liver; important in converting glycogen into lactic acid. Its serum level is increased in certain muscle diseases and in hepatitis.

aldopentose (ăl″dō-pĕn′tōs) A five-carbon sugar with the aldehyde group, —CHO, at the end. Arabinose is an aldopentose.

aldose A carbohydrate of the aldehyde group (—CHO).

aldosterone (ăl-dŏs′tĕr-ōn, ăl″dō-stēr′ōn) The most biologically active mineralocorticoid hormone secreted by the adrenal cortex. Aldosterone increases sodium reabsorption by the kidneys, thereby indirectly regulating blood levels of potassium, chloride, and bicarbonate, as well as pH, blood volume, and blood pressure. SEE: *adrenal gland.*

aldosteronism (ăl″dŏ-stĕr′ōn-ĭzm″) An uncommon cause of hypertension, in which the blood contains abnormally high levels of aldosterone, a mineralocorticoid usually produced by the adrenal glands. The syndrome results from sodium retention and excretion of potassium by the kidneys. Although it is frequently asymptomatic, occasionally patients may have frequent urination, nocturia, or headache. If potassium losses are severe, muscular weakness, cramps, tetany, or cardiac arrhythmias may occur. SYN: *hyperaldosteronism.*

primary a. Aldosteronism due to excess secretion of mineralocorticoid by the adrenal gland. An aldosterone-secreting adenoma frequently is responsible. Removal of the adenoma will cure hypertension in some affected patients. SYN: *Conn's syndrome.* SEE: *Nursing Diagnoses Appendix.*

secondary a. Aldosteronism due to extra-adrenal disorders.

aldrin (ăl′drĭn) A derivative of chlorinated naphthalene used as an insecticide. SEE: *dieldrin in Poisons and Poisoning Appendix.*

alemmal (ă-lĕm′ăl) [Gr. *a-*, not, + *lemma*, husk] Without a neurilemma, as in a nerve fiber.

alendronate (ă-lĕn′drō-nāt) A drug that stops osteoclasts from absorbing bone; it increases the density of bone, and is used to treat and prevent osteoporosis and the fractures it causes. Trade name is Fosamax.

CAUTION: To prevent the drug from lodging in the upper gastrointestinal tract, and causing esophagitis, the pill should be given to patients with a large glass of water. Patients should also maintain an upright posture for at least a half hour after taking this medicine.

Aleppo boil Cutaneous leishmaniasis, caused by infection with the parasite *Leishmania tropica* and marked by one or multiple ulcerations of the skin. SYN: *Delhi boil; Oriental sore.*

aleukemia (ă-loo-kē′mē-ă) [″ + *leukos*, white, + *haima*, blood] A deficiency of leukocytes in the blood; the existence of leukopenia or aleukocytosis.

aleukemic leukemia SEE: *acute nonlymphocytic l.*

aleukocytosis (ă-loo″kō-sī-tō′sĭs) [Gr. *a-*, not, + *leukos*, white, + *kytos*, cell, + *osis*, condition] Absence or extreme decrease of leukocytes in the blood.

aleurone (ăl-oo′rōn) [Gr. *aleuron*, flour] The protein granules present in the outer layer of the endosperm of cereal grain.

Alexander-Adams operation [William Alexander, Brit. surgeon, 1844–1919; James A. Adams, Scot. gynecologist, 1857–1930] Surgery in which the round ligaments of the uterus are shortened and their ends sutured to the exterior abdominal ring; used in treating uterine displacement.

Alexander technique (ăl-ĕks-ăn′dĕr) [Frederick Matthias Alexander, Australian actor, 1869–1955] A form of body work that promotes postural health, particularly of the spine, head, and neck.

alexia [Gr. *a-*, not, + *lexis*, word] Inability to read, or word blindness, caused by a lesion of the central nervous system.

motor a. Inability to read aloud while remaining able to understand what is written or printed.

musical a. Inability to read music. It may be sensory, optic, or visual, but not motor.

optic a. Inability to understand what is written or printed.

alexithymia A clinical feature common in posttraumatic stress disorder (PTSD) characterized by the inability to identify and articulate feelings. Often feelings are reported to the health care worker in the form of physical symptoms. Patients suffering from chemical dependency and somatoform disorders may also display alexithymia.

ALG *antilymphocyte globulin.* SEE: *globulin, antilymphocyte.*

algae (ăl′jē) [L. *alga*, seaweed] Photosynthetic organisms of several phyla in the kingdom Protista. They are nonparasitic and lack roots, stems, or leaves; they contain chlorophyll and vary in size from microscopic forms to massive seaweeds. They live in fresh or salt water and in moist places. Some serve as a source of food. Examples are kelp and Irish moss.

blue-green a. Cyanobacteria; photosynthetic organisms in the kingdom Monera. Some members of this kingdom are responsible for epidemic diarrhea.

algefacient Refrigerant.

algesia (ăl-jē′zē-ă) [Gr. *algesis*, sense of pain] Supersensitivity to pain; a form of hyperesthesia. SYN: *algesthesia.* **algesic, algetic** (ăl-jēz′ĭk, ăl-jĕt′ĭk), *adj.*

algesthesia (ăl″jĕs-thē′zē-ă) [Gr. *algos*, pain, + *aisthesis*, sensation] **1.** Perception of pain. **2.** Algesia.

-algia (ăl′jē-ă) [Gr.] Suffix meaning *pain.* SEE: *-dynia.*

algicide (ăl′jĭ-sīd) [L. *alga*, seaweed, + *caedere*, to kill] A substance that kills algae.

algid (ăl′jĭd) [L. *algidus*, cold] Cold; chilly.

alginate (ăl′jĭ-nāt) Any salt of alginic acid. It is derived from kelp, a type of seaweed, and is used as a thickener in foods and as a pharmaceutical aid. In dentistry, this irreversible hydrocolloid is used as a material for taking impressions.

algiomotor (ăl″jē-ō-mō′tor) [Gr. *algos*, pain, + L. *motor*, a mover] Causing painful contraction of muscles, particularly pain during peristalsis. SYN: *algiomuscular.*

algiomuscular (ăl″jē-ō-mŭs′kū-lăr) [″ + L. *musculus*, muscle] Algiomotor.

alglucerase A drug prepared from human placental tissue. It is used in treating type I Gaucher's disease.

algolagnia (ăl″gō-lăg′nē-ă) [Gr. *algos*, pain, + *lagneia*, lust] Sexual satisfaction derived by experiencing pain or by inflicting pain on others.

active a. Sadism.

passive a. Masochism.

algolagnist (ăl-gō-lăg′nĭst) One who practices algolagnia.

algometer [″ + *metron*, measure] An instrument for measuring the degree of sensitivity to pain.

algophobia (ăl″gō-fō′bē-ă) [Gr. *algos*, pain, + *phobos*, fear] Morbid fear of pain.

algorithm (ăl′gŏ-rĭthm) A formula or set of rules for solving a particular problem. In medicine, a set of steps used in diagnosing and treating a disease. Appropriate use of algorithms in medicine may lead to more efficient and accurate patient care as well as reduced costs.

Alice in Wonderland syndrome [Alice, from Lewis Carroll's *Alice in Wonderland*] Perceptual distortions of space and size. This may be a symptom of neurological involvement in infectious mononucleosis, and may be caused by hallucinogenic drugs.

alicyclic (ăl-ĭ-sī′klĭk) Having properties of both aliphatic (open-chain) and cyclic (closed-chain) compounds.

alienate (āl′yĕn-āt) To isolate, estrange, or dissociate.

alienation (āl″yĕn-ā′shŭn) [L. *alienare*, to make strange] Isolation, estrangement, or dissociation, esp. from society.

aliform (ăl′ĭ-form) [L. *ala*, wing, + *forma*, shape] Wing-shaped.

aliform process Wing of the sphenoid bone.

alignment (ă-līn′mĕnt) [Fr. *aligner*, to put in a straight line] **1.** The act of arranging in a straight line. **2.** The state of being arranged in a straight line. **3.** In orthopedics, the placing of portions of a fractured bone into correct anatomical position. **4.** In dentistry, bringing teeth into correct position. **5.** In radiography, the positioning of the body part in correct relation to the radiographic film and x-ray tube to enable proper visualization.

aliment (ăl′ĭ-mĕnt) [L. *alimentum*, nourishment] Nutriment; food.

alimentary (ăl″ĭ-mĕn′tăr-ē) [L. *alimentum*, nourishment] Pert. to food or nutrition, or the digestive tract.

alimentary duct An outdated term for the thoracic duct.

alimentation (ăl″ĭ-mĕn-tā′shŭn) The process of nourishing the body, including mastication, swallowing, digestion, absorption, and assimilation. SEE: *hyperalimentation*; *total parenteral nutrition.*

artificial a. Provision of nutrition, usually intravenously or via a tube passed into the gastrointestinal tract of a patient unable to take or utilize normal nourishment. SEE: *total parenteral nutrition.*

forced a. **1.** Feeding of a patient unwilling to eat. **2.** Forcing of a person to eat a greater quantity than desired.

rectal a. Feeding by means of nutrient enemas.

alimentotherapy (ăl″ĭ-mĕn″tō-thĕr′ă-pē) [L. *alimentum*, nourishment, + Gr.

therapeia, treatment] Treatment of disease by dietary regulation. SYN: *dietotherapy*. SEE: *dietetics*.

alinasal [L. *ala*, wing, + *nasus*, nose] Pert. to the alae nasi, or wings of the nose.

alinement (ă-līn′mĕnt) [Fr. *aligner*, to put in a straight line] Alignment.

aliphatic (ăl″ĭ-făt′ĭk) [Gr. *aleiphar*, *aleiphatos*, fat, oil] Belonging to that series of organic chemical compounds characterized by open chains of carbon atoms rather than by rings.

aliquot (ăl′ĭ-kwŏt) [L. *alius*, other, + *quot*, how many] A portion that represents a known quantitative relationship to the whole or to other portions.

alisphenoid (ăl-ĭ-sfē′noyd) [L. *ala*, wing, + Gr. *sphen*, wedge, + *eidos*, form, shape] Pert. to the greater wing of the sphenoid bone.

alizarin (ă-lĭz′ă-rĭn) [Arabic *ala sara*, extract] A red dye obtained from coal tar or madder.

alkalemia (ăl″kă-lē′mē-ă) [Arabic *al-qaliy*, ashes of salt wort, + Gr. *haima*, blood] An increase in the arterial blood pH above 7.45 due to a decrease in the hydrogen ion concentration or an increase in hydroxyl ions. The blood is normally slightly alkaline (pH 7.35 to 7.45).

alkali (ăl′kă-lī) *pl.* **alkalis, alkalies** [Arabic *al-qaliy*, ashes of salt wort] A strong base, esp. the metallic hydroxides. Alkalies combine with acids to form salts, combine with fatty acids to form soap, neutralize acids, and turn litmus paper blue. SEE: *acid; base; pH;* words beginning with *alkal-*.

corrosive a. A strongly corrosive metallic hydroxide most commonly of sodium, ammonium, and potassium, as well as carbonates. Because of their great combining power with water and their action on the fatty tissues, they cause rapid and deep tissue destruction. They have a tendency to gelatinize tissue, turning it a somewhat grayish color and forming a soapy, slippery surface, accompanied by pain and burning. SEE: *corrosion; corrosive poisoning*.

alkalimetry (ăl″kă-lĭm′ĕ-trē) Measurement of the alkalinity of a mixture.

alkaline (ăl′kă-lĭn) Pert. to or having the reactions of an alkali.

alkaline salts SEE: *hydrogen sulfide in Poisons and Poisoning Appendix.*

alkalinity (ăl″kă-lĭn′ĭ-tē) The state of being alkaline. SEE: *hydrogen ion*.

alkalinize (ăl′kă-lĭn-īz″) To make alkaline. SYN: *alkalize*.

alkalinuria (ăl″kă-lĭn-ū′rē-ă) [*alkali* + Gr. *ouron*, urine] Alkaline urine.

alkali poisoning Ingestion of an alkali.

TREATMENT: Large amounts of water are given by mouth. Consultation with an ear, nose, and throat specialist is often advisable. Tracheostomy or intubation is performed if necessary to protect the airway. Morphine is useful to allay pain. Rest, heat, quiet, and adequate fluid intake are imperative.

CAUTION: Emetics, strong acids, and lavage should be avoided. Fluid balance and electrolytes should be carefully monitored.

alkalization (ă″kă-lĭ-zā′shŭn) The process of making something alkaline.

alkalize (ăl′kă-līz) To make alkaline. SYN: *alkalinize*.

alkaloid (ăl′kă-loyd) [*alkali* + Gr. *eidos*, form, shape] One of a group of organic alkaline substances (such as morphine or nicotine) obtained from plants. Alkaloids react with acids to form salts that are used for medical purposes.

vinca a. A drug made from vinca plants and used in cancer therapy.

alkalosis (ăl″kă-lō′sĭs) [″ + Gr. *osis*, condition] An actual or relative increase in blood alkalinity due to an accumulation of alkalies or reduction of acids. SEE: *acid-base balance*. **alkalotic** (-lŏt′ĭk), *adj*.

altitude a. Alkalosis resulting from the increased respiratory rate associated with exposure to the decreased oxygen content of air at high altitudes. This causes respiratory alkalosis. SEE: *respiratory alkalosis*.

compensated a. Alkalosis in which the pH of body fluids has been returned to normal. Compensatory mechanisms maintain the normal ratio of bicarbonate to carbonic acid (approx. 20 : 1) even though the bicarbonate level is increased.

hypochloremic a. Metabolic alkalosis due to loss of chloride; produced by severe vomiting, gastric tube drainage, or massive diuresis.

hypokalemic a. Metabolic alkalosis associated with an excessive loss of potassium. It may be caused by diuretic therapy.

metabolic a. Any process in which plasma bicarbonate is increased. This is usually the result of increased loss of acid from the stomach or kidney, potassium depletion accompanying diuretic therapy, excessive alkali intake, or severe adrenal gland hyperactivity. SEE: *acid-base balance*.

SYMPTOMS: There are no specific signs or symptoms, but if the alkalosis is severe, there may be apathy, confusion, stupor, and tetany as evidenced by a positive Chvostek's sign.

TREATMENT: Therapy for the primary disorder is essential. Saline solution should be administered intravenously and, in patients with hypokalemia due to diuretic therapy, potassium. Only rarely will it be necessary to administer acidifying agents IV.

PATIENT CARE: Arterial blood gas values, serum potassium level, and fluid balance are monitored. The patient is assessed for anorexia, nausea and vomiting, tremors, muscle hypertonicity, muscle cramps, tetany, Chvostek's sign, seizures, mental confusion progressing to stupor and coma, cardiac dysrhythmias due to hypokalemia, and compensatory hypoventilation with resulting hypoxia. Prescribed oxygen, oral or IV fluids, sodium chloride or ammonium chloride, and potassium chloride if hypokalemia is a factor, along with therapy prescribed to correct the cause, are administered. Seizure precautions are observed; a safe environment and reorientation as needed are provided for the patient with altered thought processes. The patient's response to therapy is evaluated, and the patient is taught about the dangers of excess sodium bicarbonate intake if that is a factor. The ulcer patient is taught to recognize signs of metabolic alkalosis, including anorexia, weakness, lethargy, and a distaste for milk. If potassium-wasting diuretics or potassium chloride supplements are prescribed, the patient's understanding of the regimen's purpose, dosage, and possible adverse effects is ascertained.

respiratory a. Alkalosis with an acute reduction of carbon dioxide followed by a proportionate reduction in plasma bicarbonate.

ETIOLOGY: Hyperventilation (whether it is caused by hypoxia, anxiety, panic attacks, fever, salicylate intoxication, exercise, or excessive mechanical ven tilation) is the primary cause of respiratory alkalosis.

SYMPTOMS: Patients may develop paresthesias; air hunger; dry oral mucosa; numbness or tingling of the nose, circumoral area, or extremities; muscle twitching; tetany and hyperreflexia; lightheadedness; inability to concentrate; mental confusion and agitation; lethargy; or coma.

TREATMENT: Therapy is given for the underlying cause. In acute hyperventilation produced by panic or anxiety, treatment includes coaching a patient to breathe in a slow, controlled, and relaxed fashion by providing reassurance and support.

PATIENT CARE: Preventive measures are taken, such as having the hyperventilating patient breathe in a slow controlled fashion, using cues provided by caregivers. The respiratory therapist prevents or corrects respiratory alkalosis in patients receiving mechanical ventilation by increasing deadspace or decreasing volume. Arterial blood gas values, vital signs, and neurological status are monitored. In severe cases, serum potassium level is monitored for hypokalemia and cardiac status for dysrhythmias. Prescribed therapy is administered to treat the cause. The patient is reassured, and a calm, quiet environment is maintained during periods of extreme stress and anxiety. The patient is helped to identify stressors and to learn coping mechanisms and anxiety-reducing techniques, such as guided imagery, controlled breathing, or meditation.

alkalotherapy (ăl″kă-lō-thĕr′ă-pē) [*alkali* + Gr. *therapeia*, treatment] Therapeutic use of alkalies.

alkapton(e) (ăl-kăp′tōn) [″ + Gr. *hapto*, to bind to] $C_8H_8O_4$ homogentisic acid; a yellowish-red substance sometimes occurring in urine as the result of the incomplete oxidation of tyrosine and phenylalanine.

alkaptonuria (ăl″kăp-tō-nū′rē-ă) [*alkapton* + Gr. *ouron*, urine] A rare inherited disorder marked by the excretion of large amounts of homogentisic acid in the urine, a result of incomplete metabolism of the amino acids tyrosine and phenylalanine. Presence of the acid is indicated by the darkening of urine on standing or when alkalinated and the dark staining of diapers or other linen. SEE: *ochronosis*.

alkene (ăl′kēn) A bivalent aliphatic hydrocarbon containing one double bond.

alkyl (ăl′kĭl) Any hydrocarbon radical with the general formula C_nH_{2n+1}. The resulting substances are called alkyl groups or alkyl radicals.

alkylate (ăl′kĭ-lāt) To provide therapy involving the use of an alkylating agent.

alkylating agent A substance that introduces an alkyl radical into a compound in place of a hydrogen atom. Because these substances have the ability to interfere with cell metabolism and growth, they are used in treating certain types of malignancies.

alkylation (ăl″kĭ-lā′shŭn) A chemical process in which an alkyl radical replaces a hydrogen atom.

ALL *acute lymphocytic leukemia.*

all- [Gr. *allos*, other] SEE: *allo-*.

allachesthesia (ăl″ă-kĕs-thē′zē-ă) [Gr. *allache*, elsewhere, + *aisthesis*, sensation] Perception of tactile sensation as being remote from the actual point of stimulation.

allantochorion (ă-lăn″tō-kō′rē-ŏn) Fusion of the allantois and chorion into one structure.

allantoic (ăl″ăn-tō′ĭk) Pert. to the allantois.

allantoid [Gr. *allantos*, sausage, + *eidos*, form, shape] **1.** Sausage-shaped. **2.** Pert. to the allantois.

allantoin (ă-lăn′tō-ĭn) $C_4H_6N_4O_3$; a white crystalline substance in allantoic and amniotic fluids and the end product of purine metabolism in mammals other than primates. It is produced synthetically by the oxidation of uric acid. At one time allantoin was used to promote wound healing.

allantoinuria (ă-lăn″tō-ĭn-ū′rē-ă) [*allantoin* + Gr. *ouron*, urine] Allantoin in the urine.

allantois (ă-lăn′tō-ĭs) [Gr. *allantos*, sausage, + *eidos*, form, shape] An elongated bladder developing from the hindgut of the fetus in mammals, birds, and reptiles. In mammals, it contributes to the development of the umbilicus and placenta. In birds and reptiles, it provides for the exchange of gases through the shell.

allayed (ă-lād′) Mitigated.

allele (ă-lēl′, ă-lĕl′) [Gr. *allelon*, of one another] One of two or more different genes containing specific inheritable characteristics that occupy corresponding positions (loci) on paired chromosomes. A pair of alleles is usually indicated by a capital letter for the dominant and a lowercase letter for the recessive. An individual with a pair of identical alleles, either dominant or recessive, is said to be homozygous for this gene. The union of a dominant gene and its recessive allele produces a heterozygous individual for that characteristic. Some traits may have multiple alleles, that is, more than two possibilities, but an individual has only two of those alleles (e.g., the genes for blood type, A, B, and O, are at the same position on the chromosome pair, but an individual has only two of these genes, which may be the same or different). SYN: *allelic gene; allelomorph*. **allelic** (ă-lĕl′ĭk), *adj*.

histocompatibility a. One of many different forms of the histocompatibility gene. Each allele creates specific cell surface antigenic markers on cells. SEE: *histocompatibility locus antigen*.

allelic gene Allele.

allelomorph (ă-lē′lō-morf, ă-lĕl′ō-morf) [″ + *morphe*, form] Allele.

allelotaxis (ă-lē″lō-tăk′sĭs) [″ + *taxis*, order] Development of a part from several embryonic structures.

Allen Cognitive Level Test A standardized method of assessing information processing based on a theory that postulates six levels of cognitive function. It is used widely by occupational therapists.

Allen-Doisy test (ăl′ĕn-doy′sē) [Edgar V. Allen, U.S. endocrinologist, 1892–1943; Edward A. Doisy, U.S. biochemist and physiologist, b. 1893] A test used to determine estrogen content. A spayed mouse is injected with the material being tested. The appearance of cornified cells on a vaginal smear constitutes a positive reaction.

Allen-Doisy unit The smallest amount of estrogen that will produce a characteristic change (appearance of cornified cells) in the vaginal epithelium of a spayed mouse. SYN: *mouse unit*.

Allen test A bedside test used to evaluate the patency of the arteries of the hand before arterial puncture. The patient elevates the hand and repeatedly makes a fist while the examiner places digital occlusive pressure over the radial and ulnar arteries at the wrist. The hand will lose its normal pink color. Digital pressure is released from one artery (usually the ulnar) while the other (i.e., the radial) remains compressed. If there is normal blood flow through the unobstructed artery, color should return to the hand within 10 sec. The return of color indicates that the hand has a good collateral supply of blood, and that arterial puncture of the compressed artery can be safely performed.

allergen (ăl′ĕr-jĕn) [Gr. *allos*, other, + *ergon*, work, + *gennan*, to produce] Any substance that causes a hypersensitivity reaction. It may or may not be a protein. Among common allergens are inhalants (dusts, pollens, fungi, smoke, perfumes, odors of plastics), foods (wheat, eggs, milk, chocolate, strawberries), drugs (aspirin, antibiotics, serums), infectious agents (bacteria, viruses, fungi, animal parasites), contactants (chemicals, animals, plants, metals), and physical agents (heat, cold, light, pressure, radiations). SEE: *allergy; antigen; irritation; sensitization*.

allergenic (ăl″ĕr-jĕn′ĭk) Producing allergy.

allergic (ă-lĕr′jĭk) Pert. to, sensitive to, or caused by an allergen.

allergist A physician who specializes in diagnosing and treating allergies.

allergy (ăl′ĕr-jē) [Gr. *allos*, other, + *ergon*, work] An immune response to a foreign antigen that results in inflammation and organ dysfunction. Allergies range from the life-threatening to the annoying, and include systemic anaphylaxis, laryngeal edema, transfusion reactions, bronchospasm, vasculitis, angioedema, urticaria, eczematous dermatitis, hay fever, rhinitis, and conjunctivitis. They affect about 20% of the American public and can be triggered by inhalation (e.g., pollens or dust mites), direct contact (e.g., poison ivy or oak), ingestion (e.g., drugs or foods), or injection (e.g., stinging insects and many drugs). Allergic responses may be initiated and sustained by occupational exposures to allergens, by foods, animals, fungal spores, metals, rubber products, and other agents. The most severe cases are often associated with Hymenoptera stings, penicillin products, radiological contrast media, and latex. SYN: *hypersensitivity reaction*. SEE: *atopy*.

ETIOLOGY: The immune system has two main functions: first, to identify germs and parasites that may cause damage to the body and second, to repel attacks by these organisms with toxic defenses. Allergic reactions can occur when immune functions are turned on by any agent—infectious or not—that is richly endowed with alien antigens.

Once the immune system has been sensitized, subsequent exposures result in the binding of specific immunoglobulins (esp. IgE) or the activation of immunologically active cells (including mast cells, basophils, or T cells). These can release inflammatory chemicals such as histamines, kinins, leukotrienes, and interleukins that, acting locally or systemically, create allergic symptoms.

SYMPTOMS: Nasal inflammation, mucus production, watery eyes, itching, rashes, tissue swelling, bronchospasm, stridor, and shock are all potential symptoms of allergy.

DIAGNOSIS: A history of exposure and reaction is crucial to the diagnosis of allergy. Tests for specific allergies include skin prick tests, intradermal injections, bronchial provocation tests, or blood tests (e.g., measurements of antigen-specific immunoglobulins).

TREATMENT: Avoiding allergens is the first step in treatment. Effective drugs for allergic symptoms include antihistamines, cromolyn, corticosteroids, and epinephrine. Which of these is given depends on the severity of the reaction. Antigen desensitization (immunotherapy) may be used by experienced professionals; however, this technique may occasionally trigger severe systemic reactions.

PATIENT CARE: Before any drug is given, the health care provider should determine if the patient has any history of allergy. Patients receiving any injected drugs or blood products are closely observed for rash, itch, wheezing, stridor, or hypotension. If an allergic reaction begins, medications prescribed for immediate management are given to the patient. Patients are taught how to identify and avoid common allergens and how to identify an allergic reaction. The use of drugs for the chronic management of allergies is explained. If a patient needs injectable epinephrine for emergency outpatient treatment of anaphylaxis, both the patient and family are instructed in its use.

atopic a. atopy.

contact a. A type IV hypersensitivity reaction following direct contact with an allergen; most frequently involves the skin. SEE: *contact dermatitis*.

drug a. A type I hypersensitivity reaction to a drug.

food a. An immunologic reaction to food to which a patient has become sensitized. It requires a first exposure (sensitization), which stimulates the production of IgE antibodies; subsequent exposures produce symptoms. Sensitivity to almost any food may develop, but it develops most frequently to milk, eggs, wheat, shellfish, and chocolate. Because food allergies are type I reactions, symptoms can appear within minutes. Mild symptoms, such as urticaria, eczema, abdominal cramps, and gastrointestinal upset, are most common, but food allergies also can cause life-threatening systemic anaphylaxis.

Food allergies are identified by eliminating any foods suspected of causing symptoms and reintroducing them one at a time. Blood tests for IgE are useful in separating food allergies from abnormal metabolic or digestive responses to food. Desensitization to food allergies is not possible, and use of antihistamines, epinephrine, and corticosteroids, the most common treatments for symptoms, cannot be used for prophylaxis. Many adverse reactions to foods are not allergic in nature, but may be caused by toxic, metabolic, or pharmacological reactions. SEE: *anaphylaxis; desensitization; hypersensitivity reaction*.

latex a. An immune reaction resulting from contact with products derived from the rubber tree, *Hevea brasiliensis*. Latex antigens can be absorbed through the skin or inhaled. The allergic reaction may be relatively mild (marked by rashes or reddened skin) or more severe (rhinitis, hives, bronchospasm, or anaphylaxis). In health care workplaces, where universal precautions against contact with blood and body fluids have made the wearing of protective latex gloves common, non-latex products have been substituted for latex barriers to reduce exposure.

latex a. response An allergic response to natural latex rubber products. SEE: *Nursing Diagnoses Appendix*.

This diagnosis was approved at the NANDA 13th Conference, 1998.

risk for latex a. response At risk for allergic response to natural latex rubber products. SEE: *Nursing Diagnoses Appendix*.

This diagnosis was approved at the NANDA 13th Conference, 1998.

allesthesia (ăl″ĕs-thē′sē-ă) [″ + *aisthesis*, sensation] Perception of stimulus in the limb opposite the one stimulated. SYN: *allochesthesia; allochiria*.

alleviate To lessen the effect of.

alliaceous (ăl″ē-ā′shŭs) [L. *allium*, garlic, + *-aceus*, of a specific kind] Tasting like garlic or onions.

allied health professional An individual who has received special training in an allied health field, such as clinical laboratory science, radiology, emergency medical services, physical therapy, respiratory therapy, medical assisting, athletic training, dental hygiene, or occupational therapy.

alliesthesia (ăl″ē-ĕs-thē′sē-ă) [Gr. *allios*, changed, + *aisthesis*, sensation] The perception of an external stimulus as pleasant or unpleasant depending upon internal stimuli. A particular stimulus may be perceived as pleasant at one time and unpleasant at another.

alliteration (ă-lĭt″ĕr-ā′shŭn) [L. *ad*, to, + *litera*, letter] A speech disorder in which words beginning with the same consonant sound are used to excess.

allo-, all- [Gr. *allos*, other] Combining form indicating *divergence, difference from,* or *opposition to the normal.*

alloantigen (ăl″lō-ăn′tĭ-jĕn) [″ + *anti*, against, + *gennan*, to produce] An antigen in the blood or tissue of a donor that is not present in the recipient, which can therefore trigger an immune response.

allochesthesia (ăl″ō-kĕs-thē′zē-ă) [Gr. *allache*, elsewhere, + *aisthesis*, sensation] Allesthesia.

allochezia, allochetia (ăl″ō-kē′zē-ă, ăl″ō-kē′shē-ă) [Gr. *allos*, other, + *chezein*, to defecate] The excretion of feces through an abnormal opening.

allochiria, allocheiria (ăl″ō-kī′rē-ă) [″ + *cheir*, hand] Allesthesia.

allochroism (ăl-ōk′rō-ĭzm, ăl″ō-krō′ĭzm) [″ + *chroa*, color, + *-ismos*, condition] A change in color.

allochromasia (ăl″ō-krō-mā′sē-ă) A change in the color of hair or skin.

allocinesia (ăl″ō-sĭn-ē′sē-ă) [Gr. *allos*, other, + *kinesis*, movement] Movement on the side of the body opposite the one the patient was asked to move. SEE: *allokinesis*.

allodiploidy (ăl″ō-dĭp′loy-dē) [″ + *diploe*, fold, + *eidos*, form, shape] Possession of two sets of chromosomes, each from a different species. A hybrid is allodiploid.

allodynia (ăl″ō-dĭn′ē-ă) The condition in which an ordinarily painless stimulus, once perceived, is experienced as being painful.

alloeroticism, alloerotism (ăl″ō-ē-rŏt′ĭ-sĭzm, -ĕr′ō-tĭzm) [″ + *Eros*, god of love] Sexual urges stimulated by and directed toward another person. Opposite of autoerotism.

alloesthesia Allesthesia.

allogeneic, allogenic (ăl″ō-jĕ-nē′ĭk, ăl″ō-jĕn′ĭk) Having a different genetic constitution but belonging to the same species. SEE: *isogeneic*.

allograft (ăl′ō-grăft) [″ + L. *graphium*, grafting knife] Transplant tissue obtained from a member of one's species. Commonly transplanted organs include cornea, bone, artery, cartilage, kidney, liver, lung, heart, and pancreas. Recipients of allografts take immunosuppressive drugs to prevent tissue rejection. SYN: *homograft*. SEE: *autograft; heterograft; transplantation*.

alloimmune (ăl″ō-ĭm-ūn′) [″ + L. *immunis*, safe] The lack of an immune response to antigens on blood or tissue cells received from a donor of the same species.

allokinesis (ăl″ō-kĭ-nē′sĭs) [″ + *kinesis*, movement] Passive or reflex movement; involuntary movement. **allokinetic** (-kĭ-nĕt′ĭk), *adj.*

allolalia (ăl″ō-lā′lē-ă) [″ + *lalia*, talk] A speech defect or impairment, esp. due to a brain lesion, in which words are spoken unintentionally or inappropriate words are substituted for appropriate ones.

allomerism (ă-lŏm′ĕr-ĭzm) [″ + *meros*, part, + *-ismos*, condition] A change in chemical constitution without a change in form. SEE: *allomorphism*.

allomorphism (ăl″ō-mor′fĭzm) [″ + *morphe*, form, + *-ismos*, condition] A change in form without a change in chemical constitution. SEE: *allomerism*.

allopath (ăl′ō-păth) One who practices allopathy.

allopathy (ăl″ŏp′ă-thē) [Gr. *allos*, other, + *pathos*, disease, suffering] **1.** A system of treating disease by inducing a pathological reaction that is antagonistic to the disease being treated. **2.** A term erroneously used for the regular practice of medicine to differentiate it from homeopathy.

allophasis (ăl-ŏf′ă-sĭs) [Gr. *allos*, other, + *phasis*, speech] Incoherent speech.

alloplasia (ăl″ō-plā′zē-ă) [″ + *plasis*, a molding] The development of tissue at a location where that type of tissue would not normally occur. SYN: *heteroplasia*.

alloplasty (ăl′ō-plăs-tē) [″ + *plasis*, a molding] **1.** Plastic surgery using inert materials or those obtained from a tissue bank (e.g., cornea, bone). **2.** In psychiatry, adaptation by altering the external environment rather than changing oneself. SEE: *autoplasty*.

alloploidy (ăl″ō-ploy′dē) [″ + *ploos*, fold, + *eidos*, form, shape] The state of having two or more sets of chromosomes derived from different ancestral species.

allopolyploidy (ăl″ō-pŏl′ē-ploy-dē) [″ + *polys*, many, + *ploos*, fold, + *eidos*, form, shape] The state of having more than two sets of chromosomes derived from different ancestral species.

allopsychic (ăl-ō-sī′kĭk) [″ + *psyche*, mind] Pert. to mental processes in relation to the external environment.

allopurinol (ăl″ō-pū′rĭn-ōl) A drug that inhibits the enzyme xanthine oxidase. Because its action causes a reduction in both serum and urine levels of uric acid, allopurinol is used in the treatment of gout and of renal calculi caused by uric acid.

A rare but important side effect of allopurinol is a potentially fatal rash.

allostery (ăl-ŏ′stĕr-ē) [Gr. *allos*, other + *stereos*, shape] In bacteria, alteration of a regulatory site on a protein that changes its shape and activity. This change is important in altering the way the organism responds to its molecular environment.

allotherm (ăl′ō-thĕrm) [″ + *therme*, heat] An animal whose body temperature varies according to the temperature of the environment. SYN: *poikilotherm*. SEE: *homotherm*.

allotransplantation (ăl″ō-trăns″plăn-tā′shŭn) [″ + L. *trans*, through, +

plantare, to plant] Grafting or transplantation of tissue from one individual into another of the same species. SYN: *homeotransplantation*.

allotriogeustia (ă-lŏt″rē-ŏ-jŭst′ē-ă, -gū′stē-ă) [Gr. *allotrios*, strange, + *geusis*, taste] Perverted appetite or sense of taste. SEE: *parageusia*.

allotriophagy (ă-lŏt″rē-ŏf′ă-jē) [″ + *phagein*, to eat] A perversion of appetite with ingestion of material not suitable as food, such as starch, clay, ashes, or plaster. SYN: *pica*.

allotriosmia heterosmia.

allotropic (ăl″ō-trŏp′ĭk) [Gr. *allos*, other, + *tropos*, direction] **1.** Pert. to the existence of an element in two or more distinct forms with different physical properties. **2.** Altered by digestion so as to be changed in its nutritive value. **3.** Indicating one who is concerned with the welfare and interests of others (i.e., not self-centered).

allotropism, allotropy (ă-lŏt′rō-pĭzm, -pē) [″ + *trope*, a turn, + *-ismos*, condition] The existence of an element in two or more distinct forms with different physical properties.

allotype Any one of the genetic variants of protein that occur in a single species. The serum from a person with one form of allotype could be antigenic to another person.

alloxan (ăl-ŏk′săn) [*all*antoin + *ox*alic] $C_2H_2N_2O_4$; an oxidation product of uric acid. In laboratory animals, it causes diabetes by destroying the islet cells of the pancreas.

alloy (ăl′oy, ă-loy′) [Fr. *aloyer*, to combine] A metallic substance (e.g., brass) resulting from the fusion or mixture of two or more metals; also, a substance (e.g., steel) formed from the fusion or mixture of a metal and a nonmetal. In dentistry, several alloys are commonly used to restore teeth. Alloys used to construct cast restorations are often gold- and copper-based alloys. Common "silver fillings" are alloys of silver, copper, tin, and mercury. The silver-tin-mercury alloys are called amalgam.

allyl (ăl′ĭl) [L. *allium*, garlic, + Gr. *hyle*, matter] C_3H_5; a univalent unsaturated radical found in garlic and mustard.

Alma-Ata Declaration A declaration made in 1978 at the Conference on Primary Health Care in Alma-Ata, Russia. It stated that primary health care is the key to attaining health for all by the year 2000. Defined as essential to this were eight elements: education, food supply, safe water, maternal and child health, including family planning, immunization, prevention and control of endemic diseases, appropriate treatment of common diseases and injuries, and provision of essential drugs.

ALOC *altered level of consciousness*.

alochia (ă-lō′kē-ă) [Gr. *a-*, not, + *lokhos*, pert. to childbirth] Absence of lochia, the vaginal discharge following childbirth.

aloe (ăl′ō) The dried juice of one of several species of plants of the genus *Aloe*, used to heal skin conditions.

alogia Inability to speak.

aloin (ăl′ō-ĭn) A yellow crystalline substance obtained from aloe.

alopecia (al″ō-pē′shē-ă) [Gr. *alopekia*, fox mange] Absence or loss of hair, esp. of the head.

ETIOLOGY: Alopecia may result from serious illness, drugs, endocrine disorders, certain forms of dermatitis, hereditary factors, radiation, or physiological changes as a part of the aging process.

TREATMENT: Treatments may include drugs, such as minoxidil or finasteride; surgeries, such as hair transplantation; or prostheses (wigs).

a. areata Loss of hair in sharply defined patches usually involving the scalp or beard. SEE: illus.

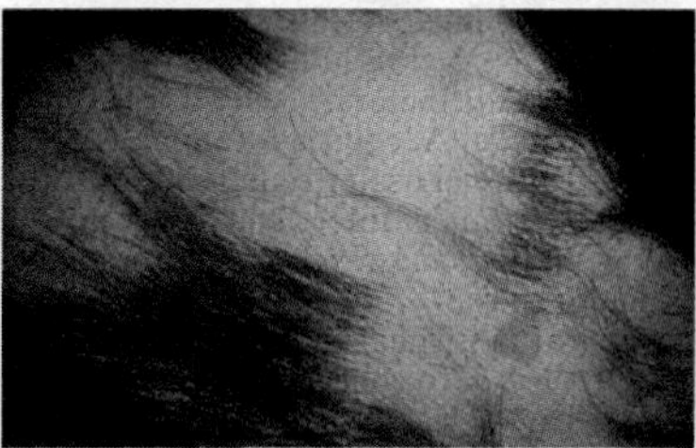

ALOPECIA AREATA OF SCALP

a. capitis totalis Complete or near complete loss of hair on the scalp. SEE: illus.

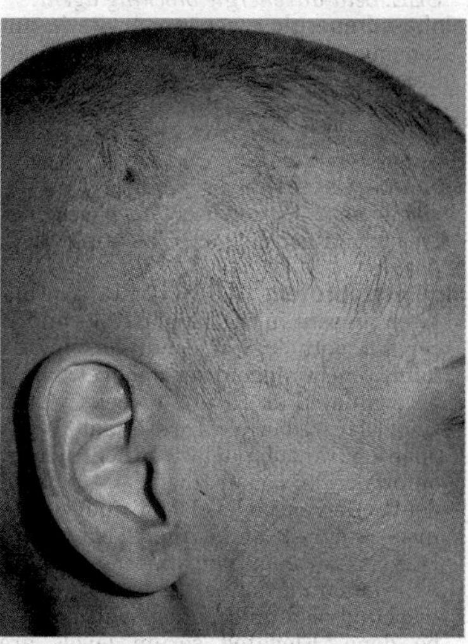

ALOPECIA CAPITIS TOTALIS

cicatricial a. Loss of hair due to formation of scar tissue.

a. congenitalis Baldness due to absence of hair bulbs at birth.

a. follicularis Baldness due to inflammation of the hair follicles of the scalp.

a. liminaris Loss of hair along the hairline, both front and back, of the scalp.

male pattern a. Typical hair loss pattern of males in which the alopecia begins in the frontal area and proceeds until only a horseshoe area of hair remains in the back and temples. This loss is dependent on the presence of the androgenic hormone testosterone.

a. medicamentosa Loss of hair due to administration of certain medicines, esp. those containing cytotoxic agents.

a. pityroides Loss of both scalp and body hair accompanied by desquamation of branlike scales.

a. prematura Premature baldness.

a. symptomatica Loss of hair after prolonged fevers or during the course of a disease; may result from systemic or psychogenic factors.

a. totalis A. capitis totalis.

a. toxica Loss of hair thought to be due to toxins of infectious disease.

a. universalis Loss of hair from the entire body.

alpha (ăl′fă) The first letter of the Greek alphabet, α. In chemistry, it denotes the first in a series of isomeric compounds or the position adjacent to a carboxyl group.

alpha-adrenergic blocking agent A substance that interferes with the transmission of stimuli through pathways that normally allow sympathetic nervous excitatory stimuli to be effective. SEE: *beta-adrenergic blocking agent*.

alpha-adrenergic receptor A site in autonomic nerve pathways at which excitatory responses occur when adrenergic agents such as norepinephrine and epinephrine are released. SEE: *beta-adrenergic receptor*.

alpha-D-galactosidase An enzyme, derived from *Aspergillus niger*, used in treating intestinal gas or bloating. SEE: *flatus*.

alpha-fetoprotein ABBR: AFP. An antigen present in the human fetus and in certain pathological conditions in the adult. The maternal serum level should be evaluated at 15 to 20 weeks' gestation. Elevated levels are associated with open neural tube defects; anencephaly; omphalocele; gastrochisis; and fetal death. Decreased levels may indicate an increased risk of having a baby with Down syndrome. If an abnormal level of AFP is found, further tests such as ultrasound or amniocentesis will need to be done. Elevated serum levels are found in adults with certain hepatic carcinomas or chemical injuries. Test results also may be abnormal in persons with diabetes, multiple pregnancies, or obesity.

alpha-globulin One of the serum globulins. SEE: *globulin, serum*.

alpha particles, alpha rays Radioactive, positively charged particles, two protons and two neutrons, ejected at high speeds in certain atomic reactions.

alpha-rhythm In electroencephalography, rhythmic oscillations in electric potential occurring at an average rate of 10/sec. SYN: *alpha-wave*.

alpha-tocopherol The most active form of vitamin E found in food.

alpha-wave Alpha-rhythm.

Alport's syndrome [Arthur Cecil Alport, S. African physician, 1880–1959] Congenital glomerulonephritis associated with deafness and a decrease in large thrombocytes. Occasionally there are eye abnormalities such as cataracts. There is no specific treatment for this disease, but renal dialysis or kidney transplantation may be beneficial. SEE: *macrothrombocyte*.

alprostadil (ăl-prŏs′tă-dēl) A synthetic prostaglandin used to treat erectile dysfunction.

ALS *amyotrophic lateral sclerosis*.

ALT *alanine aminotransferase*.

alternans (awl-tĕr′nănz) [L. *alternare*, to alternate] Alternation.

pulsus a. Regular heart rhythm in which strong beats alternate with weak ones.

Alternaria (awl″tĕr-nā′rē-ă) A genus of fungi of the Dematiaceae family. The fungus can cause pneumonitis and may cause wound or skin infections in immunocompromised patients. It has been implicated as the cause of pulmonary disease in wood pulp workers. SEE: illus.

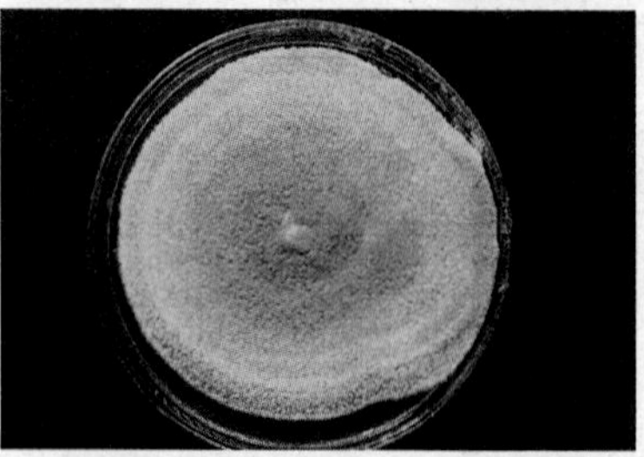

ALTERNARIA IN CULTURE

alternator An electrical generator that produces alternating current.

alt. hor. L. *alternis horis*, every other hour.

altitude sickness Symptoms produced by decreased oxygen in the environment. The symptoms may come on abruptly, as when an airplane ascends quickly to high altitude, or slowly, as in mountain climbing. The deficiency of oxygen causes headache, shortness of breath, malaise, decreased ability to concentrate, lack of judgment, lightheadedness, fainting and, if severe, death. The initial symptom may be euphoria so that the individual is unaware of the cause of the difficulty. Adaptation to living at high altitudes is best done over a period of weeks and months. SYN: *acute mountain sickness; mountain sickness.* SEE: *bends; altitude hypoxia.*

altretamine A drug used for treating persistent or recurrent ovarian cancer.

altricious (ăl-trĭsh′ŭs) [L. *altrix*, nourisher] **1.** Slow in developing. **2.** Requiring long-term nursing care.

alum (ăl′ŭm) [L. *alumen*] **1.** A double sulfate of aluminum and potassium or aluminum and ammonia; used as an astringent and styptic. **2.** Any of a group of double sulfates of a trivalent metal and a univalent metal.

ammonia a. Aluminum ammonia sulfate.

potassium a. Aluminum potassium sulfate.

aluminosis (ă-loo″mĭn-ō′sĭs) [″ + Gr. *osis*, condition of] Chronic inflammation of the lungs in alum workers due to alum particles in inspired air.

aluminum SYMB: Al. A silver-whitish metal used to filter low-energy radiation out of the x-ray beam; atomic mass 26.9815, atomic number 13.

a. acetate A salt formed by the reaction between aluminum sulfate and lead acetate. Its aqueous solution (Burow's solution) is used as a local astringent.

a. ammonia sulfate An astringent. SYN: *ammonia alum.*

a. chloride A chemical substance used as an astringent and antiperspirant.

a. phosphate gel An aqueous suspension of aluminum phosphate used as an astringent and antacid.

a. potassium sulfate An astringent and styptic. SYN: *potassium alum.*

a. sulfate A chemical substance used topically as an antiperspirant.

alveoalgia [L. *alveolus*, small cavity, + Gr. *algos*, pain] Pain in the socket of a tooth.

alveobronchiolitis, alveobronchitis (ăl″vē-ō-brŏng″kē-ŏ-lī′tĭs, -brŏng-kī′tĭs) [L. *alveolus*, small hollow or cavity, + Gr. *bronchos*, windpipe, + *itis*, inflammation] Inflammation of the bronchioles and pulmonary alveoli. SYN: *bronchopneumonia.*

alveolalgia (ăl″vē-ŏ-lăl′jē-ă) [″ + Gr. *algos*, pain] Pain in the alveolus of a tooth.

alveolar (ăl-vē′ō-lăr) Pert. to an alveolus.

alveolar-capillary block Impaired ability of gases to pass through the pulmonary alveolar-capillary membrane.

alveolar proteinosis Pulmonary alveolar proteinosis.

alveolate (ăl-vē′ō-lāt) Honeycombed; pitted.

alveolectomy (ăl″vē-ŏ-lĕk′tō-mē) [L. *alveolus*, small hollow or cavity, + Gr. *ektome*, excision] Surgical removal of all or part of the alveolar process of the mandible or maxilla; usually performed in treatment of neoplasms.

alveoli (ăl-vē′ō-lī) [L.] Pl. of alveolus.

a. breast The glandular structures that comprise the mammary lobules and are the site of milk synthesis.

a. dentales Tooth sockets.

a. pulmonis Air sacs of the lungs.

alveolitis (ăl″vē-ŏ-lī′tĭs) [″ + Gr. *itis*, inflammation] Inflammation of the alveoli.

allergic a. Inflammation of the bronchial tree, interstitial tissue, and alveoli of the lung caused by a hypersensitivity reaction to an inhaled antigen. With repeated exposure, large numbers of macrophages, the primary white blood cell in the lungs, form granulomas, which damage and scar lung tissue. Inhaled allergens are most often bacteria or fungi found in grains, fertilizer, grasses, and compost. Farmer's lung and bagassosis are two common names for forms of allergic alveolitis. SYN: *hypersensitivity pneumonitis.*

alveoloclasia (ăl-vē″ō-lō-klā′sē-ă) [″ + Gr. *klasis*, fracture] Destruction of a tooth socket.

alveolodental (ăl-vē″ō-lō-dĕn′tăl) [″ + *dens*, tooth] Pert. to the alveolus of the tooth and to the tooth itself.

alveololingual (ăl-vē″lō-lĭng′gwăl) [″ + *lingua*, tongue] Concerning the alveolar process and tongue.

alveoloplasty (ăl-vē″ō-lō-plăs′tē) [″ + Gr. *plassein*, to form] Surgical reconstruction of the alveolus.

alveolotomy (ăl″vē-ŏ-lŏt′ō-mē) [″ + Gr. *tome*, incision] Surgical incision of the alveolus of a tooth.

alveolus (ăl-vē′ō-lŭs) *pl.* **alveoli** [L., small hollow or cavity] **1.** A small hollow. **2.** The socket of a tooth. **3.** An air sac of the lungs. SEE: illus.; *c.of Lambert; pores of Kohn.* **4.** One of the honeycombed depressions of the gastric mucous membrane. **5.** A follicle of a racemose gland.

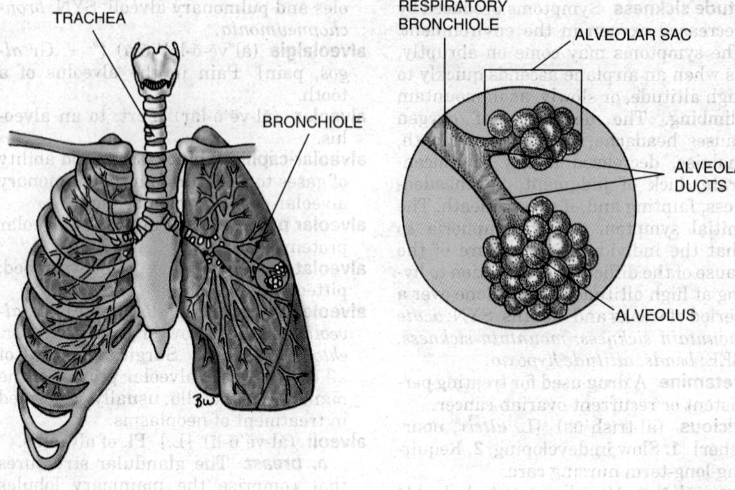

ALVEOLUS OF LUNGS

a. dentalis Tooth socket.

pulmonary a. One of the terminal epithelial sacs of an alveolar duct where gases are exchanged in respiration. SYN: *air sac; air vesicle.*

alveus (ăl′vē-ŭs) [L.] A channel or groove.

a. hippocampi A layer of white matter covering the ventricular surface of the hippocampus.

alymphia (ă-lĭm′fē-ă) [Gr. *a-*, not, + L. *lympha*, lymph] Complete or partial deficiency of lymph.

alymphocytosis (ă-lĭm″fō-sī-tō′sĭs) [″ + ″ + Gr. *kytos*, cell, + *osis*, condition] Decreased number or absence of lymphocytes in the blood.

alymphoplasia (ă″lĭm-fō-plā′zē-ă) [″ + ″ + Gr. *plasis*, a developing] Failure of lymphatic tissue to develop.

thymic a. Thymic aplasia.

Alzheimer's disease (ălts′hī-mĕrz) [Alois Alzheimer, Ger. neurologist, 1864–1915] ABBR: AD. A chronic, progressive, degenerative cognitive disorder that accounts for more than 60% of all dementias. The most common form occurs in people over 65 (senile dementia of the Alzheimer's type [SDAT]), but the presenile form can begin between the ages of 40 and 60. The illness causes significant functional disability, and costs more than $33 billion for health care and lost wages in the U.S. every year. SEE: *dementia, senile; tomography, positron emission* for illus.; *Nursing Diagnoses Appendix.*

ETIOLOGY: There are probably multiple interacting causes, including some genetic risk factors. These include the presence of the apolipoprotein epsilon 4 allele in late-onset disease and presenilin genes in early onset AD. People with Down syndrome are at increased risk for the disease. Environmental agents, especially viruses and aluminum toxicity, previous head trauma, and immunological factors are possible etiologies.

SYMPTOMS: The disease begins with a mild memory loss (Stage I), which then progresses to deterioration of intellectual functions, personality changes, and speech and language problems (Stage II). In the terminal stage (Stage III), patients depend on others for activities of daily living. Seizures, hallucinations, delusions, paranoia, or depression can occur in either Stage II or III. SEE: table.

DIAGNOSIS: The diagnosis is usually made by ruling out other causes of cognitive dysfunction, although a variety of laboratory tests also are employed in some settings.

PATHOPHYSIOLOGY: Characteristic pathophysiological changes in the brain are neuritic plaques, neurofibrillary tangles, and marked cerebral atrophy. In addition to structural changes, abnormalities in the cranial neurotransmitters may also occur. Acetylcholine, for example, may be reduced by as much as 75%, contributing to cognitive impairment.

TREATMENT: The treatment of Alzheimer's disease includes environmental structuring and drug therapy.

Stages of Alzheimer's Disease

Stage	Common Behaviors
Stage I (early stage, mild dementia)	Loss of short-term memory Decreased judgment (safety concern) Inability to perform mathematical calculations Inability to comprehend abstract ideas
Stage II (middle stage, moderate dementia)	Difficulty with speech and language (aphasia, anomia) Labile personality changes Changes in usual grooming habits Inability to remember purpose of items (apraxia) Urinary incontinence Wandering Seizures Psychotic behaviors, such as hallucinations and paranoia Depression
Stage III (late stage, severe dementia)	Inability to perform activities of daily living, such as eating, dressing, and bathing; requires total care Unable to remember how to walk, toilet, swallow Minimal or no communication Eventually becomes bedridden and develops complications of immobility, such as pneumonia, pressure ulcers, and constipation

Environmental structuring involves providing a safe, nonstimulating milieu that provides consistency and comfort for the patient. Drug therapy is aimed at improving memory rather than curing the disease. Several cholinergic drugs, such as donepezil HCl (Aricept) and physostigmine salicylate (Antilirium), are anticholinesterase inhibitors that prevent the breakdown of acetylcholine to enhance cognitive function. Antidepressants and psychotropic medications should be reserved for patients who have secondary diagnoses such as depression and hallucinations.

PATIENT CARE: Reality orientation is helpful for patients in Stage I of the disease. Validation therapy is most appropriate for patients in Stage II or III. These patients are unable to be reoriented and need reassurance and affirmation of their feelings and thoughts. Validation therapy is a form of communication in which the patient's feelings are valued and supported by all members of the health care team, rather than refuted.

In collaboration with the physical and occupational therapists, the nurse assesses the patient's need for assistance with activities of daily living. Self-care, exercise, and other activities are encouraged to the fullest extent possible. If sleep disturbances occur, the patient should rest between daytime activities, but sleeping during daytime hours is discouraged. Neurological function, including mental and emotional states and motor capabilities, is monitored for further deterioration. Vital signs and respiratory status are assessed for signs and symptoms of pneumonia and other infections. The patient is evaluated for indications of gastrointestinal or urinary problems (anorexia, dysphagia, and urinary or fecal incontinence), and fluid and food intake is monitored to detect imbalances. The nurse or assistive nursing personnel takes the patient to the bathroom or bedside commode before and after meals and every 2 hr in between. Skin is inspected for evidence of trauma, such as bruises, abrasions, or other breakdown. The occupational therapist, home health nurse, or case manager assesses the patient's living environment to eliminate hazards, and teaches the family to monitor the patient's activity to prevent falls, burns, and other injuries. Expectations should not exceed the patient's ability to perform tasks. Because the patient may misperceive the environment, health professionals should speak softly and calmly and allow sufficient time for answers, given the patient's slowed thought processes and impaired ability to communicate verbally. The case manager or nurse evaluates the caregiver's ability to manage the patient at home and makes the appropriate referrals to available local resources such as counseling, support groups, and respite care as indicated.

The local chapter of the Alzheimer's Disease and Related Disorders Association (ADRDA), sometimes simply referred to as the Alzheimer's Association, is an excellent resource. A list of local chapters can be found through the national ADRDA at 919 N. Michigan Avenue, Suite 1000, Chicago, IL 60611-1676 or at their web site at www.alz.org.

Am **1.** *mixed astigmatism.* **2.** *ametropia.* **3.** Symbol for the element americium.

A.M.A. *American Medical Association.*

AMA *against medical advice.*

amaas (ă′măs) A mild form of smallpox. SYN: *variola minor.*

amacrine (ăm′ă-krĭn) [Gr. *a-*, not, + *makros*, long, + *is, inos*, fiber] Lacking a long process.

amacrine cell A modified nerve cell in the retina that has short branches (dendrites) but no long process (axon). SEE: *neuron.*

amalgam (ă-măl′găm) [Gr. *malagma*, soft mass] Any alloy containing mercury.

dental a. A dental restorative material made by mixing approx. equal parts of elemental liquid mercury (43% to 54%) and an alloy powder (57% to 46%) composed of silver, tin, copper, and sometimes smaller amounts of zinc, palladium, or indium. It has been used for more than 150 years in dental restorations; only gold has been used longer for this purpose. It is known that a fraction of the mercury in amalgam is absorbed by the body and that people with amalgam restorations in their teeth have higher concentrations of mercury in various tissues (including the blood, urine, kidneys, and brain) than those without amalgam fillings. In 1993 the Public Health Service of the U.S. Department of Health and Human Services published a report acknowledging that scientific data are insufficient to conclude that amalgam fillings have compromised health. Furthermore, there is no evidence that removal of amalgam fillings has a beneficial effect on health.

amalgamate (ă-măl′gă-māt″) The combining of mercury with silver, tin, and copper to produce a dental restorative alloy called amalgam.

amalgamation (ă-măl″gă-mā′shŭn) The process of combining mercury with silver, tin, and copper to produce a dental restorative alloy called amalgam.

amalgamator (ă-măl′gă-mā″tor) A device that provides a mechanical means of amalgamation. This can also be done by hand using a mortar and pestle.

amanita (ăm″ă-nī′tă, -nē′tă) [Gr. *amanitai*, mushrooms] Any of various mushrooms of the genus *Amanita* (e.g., *A. muscaria* and *A. phalloides*). Most are extremely poisonous. SEE: *Poisons and Poisoning Appendix.*

amantadine hydochloride (ă-măn′tă-dēn hī″drō-klor′īd) An antiviral agent used for prophylaxis against influenza A virus and to treat Parkinson's disease. Trade name is Symmetrel.

amastia (ă-măs′tē-ă) [″ + *mastos*, breast] Absence of breast tissue. SYN: *amazia.*

amaurosis (ăm″aw-rō′sĭs) [Gr., darkening] Complete loss of vision, esp. that in which there is no apparent pathological condition of the eye. **amaurotic** (ăm-aw-rŏt′ĭk), *adj.*

albuminuric a. Amaurosis caused by kidney disease.

congenital a. Amaurosis present at birth.

diabetic a. Amaurosis associated with diabetes.

epileptoid a. Sudden blindness following an epileptic seizure and lasting up to 2 weeks.

a. fugax Temporary loss of vision (lasting less than a day) and usually affecting a single eye. Patients often describe a dark shade descending into the field of vision. In mature adults, esp. those with diabetes mellitus, hypertension, or tobacco abuse, the symptom is usually caused by atheroembolic disease. In younger adults, the symptom may be caused by migraine. SYN: *blindness, transient.*

TREATMENT: Patients suspected of having atheroemboli should be treated with antiplatelet drugs (e.g., aspirin, clopidogrel, or ticlopidine) and referred for studies of the carotid arteries.

lead a. Amaurosis caused by lead poisoning.

a. partialis fugax Sudden transitory blindness with symptoms similar to those of migraine: nausea; vomiting; dizziness; and disturbances of vision.

reflex a. Amaurosis due to reflex action caused by irritation of a remote part.

saburral a. Amaurosis in conjunction with acute gastritis.

toxic a. Amaurosis from optic neuritis caused by toxins that may be endogenous (as in diabetes) or exogenous (as in alcohol or tobacco).

uremic a. Amaurosis caused by acute renal failure.

amaxophobia [Gr. *amaxa*, a carriage, + *phobos*, fear] Fear of riding in a vehicle.

amazia (ă-mā′zē-ă) [Gr. *a-*, not, + *mazos*, breast] Amastia.

ambi- [L. *ambi-*, on both sides] Prefix indicating *both, both sides, around,* or *about.*

ambidextrous (ăm″bĭ-dĕk′strŭs) [″ + *dexter*, right] Having the ability to work effectively with either hand.

ambient (ăm′bē-ĕnt) [L. *ambiens*, going around] Surrounding.

ambient noise The total noise from all sources in a given environment.

ambiguous [L. *ambiguus*, to be uncertain] To have several meanings or interpretations. In anatomy, being difficult to classify.

ambilateral (ăm″bĭ-lăt′ĕr-ăl) [L. *ambi-*, on both sides, + *latus*, side] Pert. to both sides.

ambilevous (ăm-bĭ-lē′vŭs) [″ + *laevus*,

lefthanded] Awkward in the use of either hand. SYN: *ambisinister*.

ambiopia (ăm″bē-ō′pē-ă) [″ + Gr. *ops*, eye] Double vision. SYN: *diplopia*.

ambisexual (ăm″bĭ-sĕks′ū-ăl) [″ + *sexus*, sex] Pert. to both sexes. SEE: *bisexual*.

ambisinister (ăm″bĭ-sĭn′ĭs-tĕr) [″ + *sinister*, left] Ambilevous.

ambitendency (ăm″bĭ-tĕn′dĕn-sē) [″ + *tendere*, to stretch] Ambivalence of the will. SEE: *ambivalence*.

ambivalence (ăm-bĭv′ă-lĕns) [″ + *valentia*, strength] Coexistence of contradictory feelings about an object, person, or idea. **ambivalent** (ăm-bĭv′ă-lĕnt), *adj.*

ambivert (ăm′bĭ-vĕrt) [″ + *vertere*, to turn] An individual whose personality type falls between introversion and extroversion, having tendencies of each.

amblyacousia (ăm″blē-ă-koo′sē-ă) [Gr. *amblys*, dull, + *akousis*, hearing] Dullness of hearing.

amblychromasia (ăm″blē-krō-mă′sē-ă) [″ + *chroma*, color] The state in which the cell nucleus stains faintly.

amblychromatic (ăm″blē-krō-măt′ĭk) Staining faintly.

Amblyomma (ăm′blē-ō-mă) A genus of ticks that includes the Lone Star tick (*A. americanum*) and the Gulf Coast tick (*A. maculatum*). Some ticks from this genus are vectors of tularemia, human ehrlichiosis, and tick bite paralysis.

amblyopia (ăm″blē-ō′pē-ă) [″ + *ops*, eye] Reduction or dimness of vision, esp. that in which there is no apparent pathologic condition of the eye. **amblyopic** (-ō′ĭk), *adj.*

crossed a. Amblyopia of one eye with hemianesthesia of the opposite side of the face. SYN: *a. cruciata*.

a. cruciata Crossed a.

deprivation a. Amblyopia resulting from nonuse of the eye. It is usually secondary to an organic problem such as cataract or ptosis.

a. ex anopsia Amblyopia resulting from disuse. It usually occurs in one eye and is associated with convergent squint or very poor visual acuity.

reflex a. Amblyopia due to irritation of the peripheral area.

strabismic a. Amblyopia secondary to malalignment of the eyes. In this condition, the brain suppresses the visual image from the deviating eye to prevent double vision. About 50% of childhood amblyopia is strabismic.

toxic a. Amblyopia due to the effect of alcohol, tobacco, lead, drugs, or other toxic substances.

uremic a. Dimness or loss of vision during a uremic attack.

amblyoscope (ăm′blē-ŏ-skōp″) [″ + ″ + *skopein*, to examine] An instrument for measuring binocular vision; used to stimulate vision in an amblyopic eye.

ambon (ăm′bŏn) [Gr., edge of a dish] The elevated ring of fibrocartilage around the edge of a bone socket.

ambos (ăm′bōs) [Ger.] Incus or anvil bone of the middle ear.

Ambu bag (ăm′bū) Proprietary name for a bag used to assist in providing artificial ventilation of the lungs. SEE: *bag-valve-mask resuscitator* for illus.

ambulance [L. *ambulare*, to move about] A vehicle for transporting the sick or injured, staffed with appropriately certified or licensed personnel and equipped with prehospital emergency medical care supplies and equipment such as oxygen, defibrillator, splints, bandages, adjunctive airway devices, and patient-carrying devices.

ambulant, ambulatory (ăm′bū-lănt, -lă-tō″rē) Able to walk; not confined to bed.

ambulate (ăm′bū-lāt) To walk or move above freely.

ambulation (ăm-bū-lā′shun) The action of walking or moving above freely.

ameba (ă-mē′ba) *pl.* **amebas, amebae** [Gr. *amoibe*, change] A unicellular organism of the genus *Amoeba* in the kingdom Protista, found in water and soil. It constantly changes shape by sending out fingerlike processes of cytoplasm (pseudopods), through which it moves about and obtains nourishment. It feeds by surrounding its food with pseudopods, forming a food vacuole in which digestion takes place. Oxygen and carbon dioxide are exchanged by simple diffusion through the cell membrane. Reproduction is by binary fission. Some species of *Entamoeba* are parasitic in humans. **amebic** (ă-mē′bĭk), *adj.*

amebapore A pore-forming protein released on a cell membrane by *Entamoeba histolytica*. This forms large pores in the target cell membrane (i.e., the cell the ameba is attacking).

amebiasis, amoebiasis (am″ĕ-bī′ă-sĭs) [″ + *-iasis*, state] Infection or colonization with amebas, esp. *Entamoeba histolytica*. Approx. 500 million people in tropical countries are infected. The infection typically begins in the colon but may spread to other organs, such as the liver or, less often, the skin or lungs. SYN: *amebic dysentery*. SEE: *amebapore; cyst; dysentery*.

ETIOLOGY: Amebiasis is acquired by ingesting contaminated food or drink that contains *E. histolytica* cysts, which gastric acid does not destroy. The cysts enter the intestines, where they release trophozoites, the feeding form of the organism, which may invade the walls of the colon or spread to the liver via the portal vein. Trophozoites divide to form new cysts, which may subsequently be excreted in stool.

DIAGNOSIS: The diagnosis of amebiasis is based on the detection of cysts or trophozoites of *E. histolytica* in stools and the presence of antibodies to the amebae in the blood. Antiamebic antibodies appear by the seventh day of infection. A colonoscopy may be performed to obtain tissue samples to differentiate amebiasis from inflammatory bowel disease. A liver abscess is diagnosed when a patient has right upper quadrant pain, jaundice, and fever; a mass in the liver (found by ultrasonography or computed tomography); and positive serological tests for *E. histolytica*.

SYMPTOMS: Most infected patients have no tissue invasion and, thus, are asymptomatic. Acute colitis, when it occurs, is marked by bloody diarrhea, abdominal pain, tenesmus, and weakness. The symptoms may be confused with those of ulcerative colitis. The dysentery lasts 3 to 4 weeks. Complications occasionally include toxic megacolon and ulcer perforation. Patients who develop liver abscesses present with severe upper right quadrant pain and fever; massive diarrhea is usually not present.

TREATMENT: Asymptomatic patients are treated with paromomycin (500 mg PO tid for 7 days) or iodoquinol (650 mg PO tid for 20 days). Dysentery and liver abscess are treated with metronidazole (750 mg PO tid for 10 days), followed by iodoquinol (650 mg PO tid for 20 days).

PATIENT CARE: People traveling to developing countries, esp. India and Mexico, should be taught to avoid unboiled water, ice, and fresh fruits and vegetables, all of which may be infected with amebic cysts.

hepatic a. Infection of the liver by *Entamoeba histolytica*, resulting in hepatitis and abscess formation; usually a sequel to amebic dysentery.

amebic carrier state State in which an individual harbors a form of pathogenic ameba but has no clinical signs of the disease.

amebicide, amebacide (ă-mē′bĭ-sīd) [Gr. *amoibe*, change, + L. *caedere*, to kill] An agent that kills amebas.

amebiform (ă-mē′bĭ-form) [″ + L. *forma*, shape] Shaped like an ameba.

amebocyte (ă-mē′bō-sīt″) [″ + *kytos*, cell] A cell showing ameboid movements.

ameboid (ă-mē′boyd) [″ + *eidos*, form, shape] Resembling an ameba.

ameboidism (ă-mē′boyd-ĭzm) **1.** Ameba-like movements. **2.** Denoting a condition shown by certain white blood cells.

ameboma (ăm″ē-bō′mă) [″ + *oma*, tumor] A tumor composed of inflammatory tissue caused by amebiasis.

ameburia (ăm″ē-bū′rē-ă) [Gr. *amoibe*, change, + *ouron*, urine] The presence of amebas in the urine.

amelanotic (ă″mĕl-ă-nŏt′ĭk) Lacking melanin; unpigmented.

amelia (ă-mē′lē-ă) [Gr. *a*-, not, + *melos*, limb] Congenital absence of one or more limbs. SEE: *phocomelia*.

amelification (ă-mĕl″ĭ-fĭ-kā′shŭn) [O. Fr. *amel*, enamel, + L. *facere*, to make] Formation of dental enamel by ameloblasts.

amelioration (ă-mēl″yō-rā′shŭn) [L. *ad*, to, + *melior*, better] Improvement; moderation of a condition.

ameloblast (ă-mĕl′ō-blăst) [O. Fr. *amel*, enamel, + Gr. *blastos*, germ] A cell from which tooth enamel is formed.

ameloblastoma (ă-mĕl″ō-blăs-tō′mă) [″ + ″ + *oma*, tumor] A tumor of the jaw, esp. the lower one, arising from enamel-forming cells and having low-grade malignancy. It may be partly cystic and partly solid and may become large. SYN: *adamantinoma*.

amelodentinal [O. Fr. *amel*, enamel, + L. *dens*, *dent*-, tooth] Pert. to both enamel and dentin.

amelogenesis (ăm″ĕ-lō-jĕn′ĕ-sĭs) [″ + Gr. *genesis*, generation, birth] The formation of dental enamel by ameloblasts.

amelus (ăm′ĕ-lŭs) [Gr. *a*-, not, + *melos*, limb] An individual with congenitally absent arms and legs.

amenorrhea (ă-mĕn″ō-rē′ă) [″ + ″ + *rhoia*, flow] Absence of menstruation, either as a result of lack of menarche (i.e., lack of menstruation by age 16) or absence of menstruation for more than 3 months in women who had previously experienced menstruation and who are not pregnant. Amenorrhea may be classed as physiological, or primary, when it occurs during pregnancy, early lactation, or after menopause. Pathological, or secondary, amenorrhea is caused by several conditions.

ETIOLOGY: The primary causes of abnormal amenorrhea are related either to an underlying hypothalamic-pituitary-endocrine dysfunction or to congenital or acquired abnormalities of the reproductive tract. Common abnormal diagnoses include metabolic disorders, such as diabetes, malnutrition, or obesity; emotional and stress-related disorders, such as anorexia nervosa; and systemic diseases, such as cancer, lupus, or tuberculosis.

TREATMENT: The underlying cause should be determined and corrected. If hormone deficiencies exist, substitutional therapy is recommended.

PATIENT CARE: The patient is assessed for other symptoms and is encouraged to seek medical attention if absence of menses is not related to pregnancy, menopause, or hormonal therapy.

dietary a. Cessation of menses due to voluntary or involuntary (as in starvation) dietary restriction.

emotional a. Amenorrhea resulting from shock, fright, or hysteria.

exercise a. A form of stress-related

failure to menstruate, often seen in women who participate in esp. intensive workouts or exercise programs. SEE: *hypothalamic a.*

hyperprolactinemic a. Amenorrhea due to an excessive secretion of prolactin by the pituitary. SEE: *prolactin*.

hypothalamic a. Absence of menstruation related to interference with release of gonadotropin-releasing hormone (GnRH) or with pituitary release of follicle-stimulating hormone or luteinizing hormone. Hypothalamic dysfunction may be drug-induced (e.g., related to abuse of marijuana or tranquilizers); psychogenic (e.g., related to chronic anxiety); functional (e.g., related to excessive exercise, anorexia, or obesity); or related to chronic medical illness, head injuries, or cancer.

lactational a. Suppression of normal cyclic hormonal changes, resulting from breastfeeding. The advent of postpartum ovulation and menses is related to the amount of time the mother breastfeeds. Even after the resumption of menses, 50% of initial cycles are anovulatory. Women who stop nursing within 30 days usually experience the return of menstruation between 6 and 10 weeks after delivery; among those who continue to nurse, ovulation usually occurs between postpartum weeks 17 and 28, with menstruation 30 to 36 weeks after the birth.

pathological a. Inability to menstruate related to organic damage, disease, or dysfunction. Common causes include hypothalamic-pituitary dysfunction; ovarian dysfunction; alteration or obstruction of the genital outflow tract; congenital abnormalities; neoplasms; and injuries. Examples of inability to menstruate related to disease include Ascherman syndrome, Blizzard syndrome, Savage syndrome, Sheehan's syndrome, and Turner's syndrome.

physiological a. Absence of menstruation related to normal aspects of body function in response to age, such as immaturity in the prepubescent girl and aging in the postmenopausal woman, or to hormonal interruptions in the gonadotropic feedback loop, such as occur during pregnancy and lactation. It is not related to organic disease.

postpartum a. Amenorrhea following childbirth that may last for only a month or two and thus would be within normal limits; or it may be permanent and thus abnormal. *NOTE:* The onset of menstruation after childbirth may be delayed by continued breastfeeding. SEE: *Sheehan's syndrome*.

primary a. Delay of menarche until after age 16 or the absence of secondary sex characteristics after age 14. Typical causes include congenital abnormalities of reproductive structures, such as the mullerian ducts; absence of the uterus and/or vagina; imperforate hymen; or ovarian failure secondary to chromosomal abnormalities, such as occurs in Turner's syndrome.

secondary a. Cessation of menses in women who have menstruated previously but have not had a period in 6 months. Pregnancy is the single most common cause of secondary amenorrhea. It should be excluded before other causes are sought.

stress a. Cessation of menses secondary to extreme mental or physical stress. The condition was first identified in women incarcerated in prisoner-of-war camps and has been observed in some female athletes and others undergoing intensive, rigorous training. It may be related to hormonal changes caused by stress or to the concomitant alteration in the ratio of muscle to fat as training intensity increases. SEE: *pseudocyesis*. **amenorrheic** (-rē′ĭk), *adj.*

amentia (ă-mĕn′shē-ă) [L. *ab*, from, + *mens*, mind] **1.** Congenital mental deficiency; mental retardation. **2.** Mental disorder characterized by confusion, disorientation, and occasionally stupor. SEE: *dementia*.

nevoid a. Sturge-Weber syndrome; a congenital syndrome marked by port-wine nevi along the trigeminal nerve distribution, angiomas of the leptomeninges and choroid, intracranial calcifications, mental retardation, epileptic seizures, and glaucoma.

phenylpyruvic a. Mental retardation due to phenylketonuria.

American Academy of Nursing An organization formed by the American Nurses' Association. Membership in this honorary association indicates that the person selected has contributed significantly to nursing. A member is titled Fellow of the American Academy of Nursing, abbreviated F.A.A.N.

American Association of Blood Banks ABBR: AABB. A professional organization whose mission is to promulgate standard practices in immunohematology.

American Association for Clinical Chemistry ABBR: AACC. A U.S.-based association of clinical laboratory scientists including clinical chemists, microbiologists, pathologists, hematologists, and medical technologists.

American Association for Respiratory Care ABBR: AARC. The primary professional association for respiratory care practitioners in the U.S.

American Association of Retired Persons ABBR: AARP. The largest voluntary association of older adults (retired or not) in the U.S., with a membership of more than 30 million. The association lobbies on behalf of its members, sponsors research on aging, operates a mail-order pharmaceutical service, and publishes magazines and other literature for older adults.

American College of Toxicology The current name of the American Board of Medical Toxicology.

American Federation for Aging Research ABBR: AFAR. An association of physicians, scientists, and other individuals involved or interested in research on aging and associated diseases. Its purpose is to encourage and fund research on aging.

American Geriatrics Society ABBR: AGS. An association of health care professionals interested in the problems of the elderly. It enourages and promotes the study of geriatrics and stresses the importance of medical research in the field of aging.

American Medical Records Association ABBR: AMRA. A professional organization of individuals trained in health information management, including patient records, particularly in medical care facilities.

American Nurses Association ABBR: A.N.A. The only full-service professional organization representing the 2.2 million registered nurses in the U.S. It comprises 53 State Nurses Associations. The organization fosters high standards of nursing practice, promotes the economic and general welfare of nurses in the work environment, projects a realistic, positive view of nursing, and lobbies Congress and regulatory agencies about health care issues affecting nurses and the public. SEE: *Code for Nurses*.

American Nurses Association Network ABBR: ANA*NET. A wide-area computer network linking the 53 constituent State Nurses Associations with the national headquarters. It provides databases pert. to workplace and practice issues, and various databases and services related to nursing practice. Future plans include subscriber service for all nurses, nursing organizations, and nursing schools.

American Occupational Therapy Association ABBR: AOTA. A national professional organization concerned with establishing and enforcing standards of practice for occupational therapists.

American Psychiatric Nurses Association ABBR: APNA. An organization that provides leadership to advance psychiatric-mental health nursing practice; improve mental health care for individuals, families, groups, and communities; and shape health policy for the delivery of mental health services.

American Red Cross A branch of the international philanthropic organization Red Cross Society. It provides emergency aid during civil disasters such as floods and earthquakes, offers humanitarian services for armed forces personnel and their families, and operates centers for collecting and processing blood and blood products.

American Sign Language ABBR: ASL. A nonverbal method of communicating by deaf or speech-impaired people in which the hands and fingers are used to indicate words and concepts.

American Standard Association rating ABBR: ASA rating. A measure of photographic film speed, created by the American Standard Association.

Americans with Disabilities Act ABBR: ADA. Legislation passed by the U.S. Congress in 1990 to ensure the rights of persons with disabilities. It provides enforceable standards to ensure access and prohibit discrimination in employment, public services, transportation, public accommodation, communications, and other areas. Also called *Public Law 101-336*.

americium (ăm-ĕr-ĭsh′ē-ŭm) SYMB: Am. A metallic radioactive element, atomic number 95. The atomic weight of the longest-lived isotope is 243.

Ames test [Bruce Nathan Ames, U.S. biochemist, b. 1928] A laboratory test of the mutagenicity of chemicals. Special strains of organisms are incubated with the test chemical and their growth is an indicator of the mutagenicity of the substance. Most chemicals that test positive are carcinogens. Use of the test has helped reduce the use of mammals for tests of mutagenicity.

ametria (ă-mē′trē-ă) [Gr. *a*-, not, + *metra*, uterus] Congenital absence of the uterus.

ametrometer (ăm″ĕ-trŏm′ĕ-tĕr) [*ametropia* + Gr. *metron*, measure] An instrument for measuring the degree of ametropia.

ametropia (ă″mĕ-trō′pē-ă) [Gr. *ametros*, disproportionate, + *ops*, eye] Imperfect refractive powers of the eye in which the principal focus does not lie on the retina, as in hyperopia, myopia, or astigmatism. **ametropic,** *adj.*

AMI *acute myocardial infarction.*

amicrobic (ă″mī-krō′bĭk) [Gr. *a*-, not, + *mikros*, small, + *bios*, life] **1.** Lacking microbes. **2.** Not caused by microbes.

amidase (ăm′ĭ-dās) A deamidizing enzyme; one that catalyzes the hydrolysis of amides.

amide (ăm′ĭd) Any organic substance that contains the monovalent radical $—CONH_2$. It is usually formed by replacing the hydroxyl (—OH) group of the —COOH by the $—NH_2$ group.

amido- A prefix indicating the presence of the radical $CONH_2$.

amidulin (ă-mĭd′ū-lĭn) [Fr. *amidon*, starch] Soluble starch.

amikacin sulfate An aminoglycoside antibiotic. Trade name is Amikin.

amimia (ă-mĭm′ē-ă) [Gr. *a*-, not, + *mi*-

SERINE	TYROSINE	GLYCINE
ASPARTIC ACID	ARGININE	HISTIDINE

EXAMPLES OF AMINO ACIDS

mos, mimic] Loss of power to express ideas by signs or gestures.

amnesic a. Amimia in which signs and gestures can be made but their meaning is not remembered.

amine (ă-mēn′, ăm′ĭn) Any one of a group of nitrogen-containing organic compounds that are formed when one or more of the hydrogens of ammonia have been replaced by one or more hydrocarbon radicals.

amino- (ă-mē′nō, ăm′ĭ-nō) Prefix denoting the presence of an amino group (NH_2).

amino acid One of a large group of organic compounds marked by the presence of both an amino (NH_2) group and a carboxyl (COOH) group. Amino acids are the building blocks of proteins and the end products of protein digestion.

Approx. 80 amino acids are found in nature, but only 20 are necessary for human metabolism or growth. Of these, some can be produced by the liver; the rest—called essential amino acids—must be supplied by food. These are histidine, isoleucine, leucine, lysine, methionine, cysteine, phenylalanine, tyrosine, threonine, tryptophan, and valine. The nonessential amino acids are alanine, aspartic acid, arginine, citrulline, glutamic acid, glycine, hydroxyglutamic acid, hydroxyproline, norleucine, proline, and serine. Oral preparations of amino acids may be used as dietary supplements.

Arginine, while nonessential for the adult, cannot be formed quickly enough to supply the demand in infants and thus is classed as essential in early life.

Some proteins contain all the essential amino acids and are called complete proteins. Examples are milk, cheese, eggs, and meat. Proteins that do not contain all the essential amino acids are called incomplete proteins. Examples are vegetables and grains. Amino acids pass unchanged through the intestinal wall into the blood, then through the portal vein to the liver and into the general circulation, from which they are absorbed by the tissues according to the specific amino acid needed by that tissue to make its own protein. Amino acids if not otherwise metabolized may be converted into urea. SEE: illus.; *deamination; digestion; protein.*

branched-chain a.a. ABBR: BCAA. The essential amino acids, leucine, isoleucine, and valine. "Branched-chain" refers to their chemical structure. Therapeutically, they are valuable because they bypass the liver and are available for cellular uptake from the circulation. Parenteral administration, alone or mixed with other amino acids, is thought to be beneficial whenever catabolism due to physiological stress occurs. The skeletal muscle can use these amino acids for energy.

conditionally dispensable a.a. An amino acid that becomes essential when a specific clinical condition is present.

essential a.a. An amino acid that is required for growth and development but that cannot be produced by the body and must be obtained from food.

nonessential a.a. An amino acid that can be produced by the body and is not required in the diet.

semi-essential a.a. An amino acid of which an adequate amount must be consumed in the diet to prevent the use of essential amino acids to synthesize it. An example is tyrosine. Without adequate dietary intake, the essential amino acid, phenylalanine, is used to make tyrosine.

aminoacidemia (ă-mē″nō-, ăm″ĭ-nō-ăs″ĭ-dē′mē-ă) [*amino acid* + Gr. *haima*, blood] Excess of amino acids in the blood.

amino acid group The NH_2 group that characterizes the amines.

aminoacidopathies (ăm″ĭ-nō-ăs″ĭ-dŏp′ă-thēz) [″ + Gr. *pathos*, disease, suffering] Various disorders of amino acid metabolism, of which there are nearly 100, including cystinuria, alkaptonuria, and albinism.

aminoaciduria (ă-mē″nō-, ăm″ĭ-nō-ăs″ĭ-dū′rē-ă) [″ + Gr. *ouron*, urine] Excess amino acids in the urine.

aminobenzene (ă-mē″nō-, ăm″ĭ-nō-bĕn′zēn) The simplest aromatic amine, C_6H_7N; an oily liquid derived from benzene. It is used in the manufacture of medical and industrial dyes. SYN: *phenylamine*.

aminoglutethimide (ăm″ĭ-nō-gloo-tĕth′ĭ-mīd) A chemical that interferes with the production of adrenocortical hormone. It has been used to decrease the hypersecretion of cortisol by adrenal tumors and to treat cancer of the adrenal gland and breast cancer that is sensitive to adrenal hormone stimulation.

aminoglycoside A class of antibiotics, including gentamicin and tobramycin, some of which are derived from microorganisms while others are produced synthetically.

aminohippuric acid, sodium The sodium salt of aminohippuric acid. It is given intravenously to test renal blood flow and the excretory capacity of the renal tubules.

aminolysis (ăm″ĭ-nŏl′ĭ-sĭs) [*amine* + Gr. *lysis*, dissolution] Metabolic transformation of amino-containing compounds by removal of the amino group.

aminophylline (ăm-ĭ-nŏf′ĭ-lĭn, ăm″ĭ-nō-fĭl′ĭn) A mixture of theophylline and ethylenediamine, used esp. to treat patients with reactive airway disease that does not respond to safer medications such as beta-agonist drugs, other bronchodilators, or inhaled or injected corticosteroids. Besides stimulating diaphragmatic movement, it is a bronchodilator and increases heart rate. Common side effects include gastrointestinal upset and tachycardia. SYN: *theophylline ethylenediamine*.

aminophylline poisoning SEE: *Poisons and Poisoning Appendix*.

aminopterin (ăm-ĭ-nŏp′tĕr-ĭn) A folic acid antagonist used to treat acute leukemia.

aminopurine (ăm″ĭ-nō-pū′rĭn) An oxidation product of purine; includes adenine and guanine. SEE: *methyl purine; oxypurine*.

aminopyrine (ăm″ĭn-ō-pī′rĭn) An antipyretic and analgesic drug. It is not approved for use in the U.S.

CAUTION: Because this drug may cause fatal agranulocytosis, it should not be used.

aminuria (ăm-ĭ-nū′rē-ă) [*amine* + Gr. *ouron*, urine] Presence of amines in urine.

amiodarone (ă-mē-ō′dă-rōn) An antiarrhythmic drug with a complex pharmacology that is effective in the treatment of both atrial and ventricular rhythm disturbances. Its side effects include pulmonary fibrosis and thyroid dysfunction, among others.

amitosis (ăm″ĭ-tō′sĭs) [Gr. *a-*, not, + *mitos*, a thread, + *osis*, condition] Direct cell division; simple division of the nucleus and cell without the changes in the nucleus that characterize mitosis. **amitotic** (-tŏt′ik), *adj.*

amitryptyline hydrochloride (ăm″ĭ-trĭp′tĭ-lēn) A tricyclic antidepressant administered orally or intramuscularly. Common side effects are drowsiness, sedation, and dry mouth.

AML *acanthiomeatal line; acute myelocytic leukemia.*

amlodipine (ăm-lō′dĭ-pēn) An antihypertensive drug that is primarily excreted by the liver, and therefore often used in patients with kidney failure. It is a calcium channel blocker. Trade name is Norvasc.

ammeter (ăm′mē-tĕr) [*ampere* + Gr. *metron*, measure] An instrument, calibrated in amperes, that measures the quantity (number of electrons) in an electric current. SEE: *milliammeter*.

ammoaciduria (ăm″ō-ăs″ĭ-dū′rē-ă) [*ammonia* + *amino acid* + Gr. *ouron*, urine] An abnormal amount of ammonia and amino acids in the urine.

ammonia (ă-mō′nē-ă) [*Ammo*, Egyptian deity near whose temple it was originally obtained] An alkaline gas, NH_3, formed by decomposition of nitrogen-containing substances such as proteins and amino acids. Ammonia is converted into urea in the liver. It is related to many poisonous substances but also to the proteins and many useful chemicals. Dissolved in water, it neutralizes acids and turns litmus paper blue.

aromatic spirit of a. A pungent solution of approx. 4% ammonium carbonate in 70% alcohol flavored with lemon, lavender, and myristica oil. It is used to elicit reflex stimulation of respiration and as "smelling salts" to stimulate people who have fainted.

blood a. SEE: *ammoniemia.*

ammoniacal (ăm″ō-nī′ă-kăl) Having the characteristics of or pert. to ammonia.

ammonia intoxication SEE: *ammonia toxicity.*

ammonia solution, diluted A solution containing approx. 10 g of ammonia per 100 ml of water.

ammonia solution, strong A solution containing approx. 28% ammonia in water.

ammoniated (ă-mō′nē-āt′d) Containing ammonia.

ammonia toxicity Poisoning caused by an excess of ammonia. Ammonia is produced in the intestinal tract by bacterial action. After absorption it is transported to the liver, where it is converted to the less toxic urea. In diseases such as cirrhosis of the liver, the ammonia absorbed may be shunted past the liver. This results in an accumulation of ammonia in the blood (ammoniemia). Alterations in consciousness (including impaired concentration, distractibility, and amnesia) and a flapping tremor (asterixis) may be due in part to the toxic effects of ammonia on the brain, or may be caused by metabolic changes that accompany high serum ammonia levels. SEE: *hepatic encephalopathy; Poisons and Poisoning Appendix.*

TREATMENT: Treatment is aimed at preventing production and absorption of ammonia in the intestinal tract. Laxatives, such as lactulose, and antibiotics, such as neomycin, are used to reduce the production and absorption of ammonia from the intestines. Dietary protein should be limited.

ammonia water Ammonium hydroxide.

ammoniemia (a-mō″nĭ-ē′mē-ă) [*ammonia* + Gr. *haima*, blood] Excessive ammonia in the blood. Normally only faint traces of ammonia are found in the blood. Increased amounts are due to a pathological condition such as impaired liver function. Also spelled *ammonemia.* SEE: *ammonia toxicity.*

ammonium (ă-mō′nē-ŭm) A radical, NH_4^+, that forms salts analogous to those of alkaline metals.

a. alum Aluminum ammonium sulfate, an astringent. SEE: *alum.*

a. carbonate A compound used in preparing aromatic ammonia spirit; $(NH_4)_2CO_3$.

a. chloride A compound used as an expectorant and as an acidifier in treating acid-base balance; NH_4Cl.

a. hydroxide A solution of ammonia in water, used as a household cleaner and a refrigerant; NH_4OH. SEE: *ammonia in Poisons and Poisoning Appendix.*

a. thiosulfate The chemical in fixing solution that removes unexposed silver bromide crystals from radiographic film during the development process.

ammoniuria (ă-mō″nē-ū′rē-ă) [″ + Gr. *ouron*, urine] Excessive ammonia in the urine.

amnesia (ăm-nē′zē-ă) [Gr.] A loss of memory. The term is often applied to episodes during which patients forget recent events, although they may conduct themselves properly enough, and following which no memory of the period persists. Such episodes often are caused by strokes, seizures, trauma, senility, alcoholism, or intoxication. Often the cause is unknown. **amnesiac, amnesic, amnestic** (-nē′zē-ăk, -nē′sĭk, nĕs′tĭk), *adj.*

anterograde a. Amnesia for events that occurred after a precipitating event or medication.

CAUTION: This type of short-term memory loss may be induced in people who use benzodiazepine drugs (e.g., triazolam, lorazepam, or flurazepam).

---

auditory a. Loss of memory for the meanings of sounds or spoken words. SYN: *auditory aphasia; word deafness.*

dissociative a. Inability to recall important personal information, usually of a traumatic or stressful nature, that is too extensive to be explained by ordinary forgetfulness. This was formerly called psychogenic amnesia.

lacunar a. Loss of memory for isolated evnts.

posttraumatic a. ABBR: PTA. A state of agitation, confusion, and memory loss that the patient with traumatic brain injury (TBI) enters soon after the injury or on awakening from coma. Edema, hemorrhage, contusions, shearing of axons, and metabolic disturbances impair the brain's ability to process information accurately, resulting in unusual behaviors that often are difficult to manage. Trauma patients with normal brain scans may have a mild TBI and display some of the symptoms of PTA. Posttraumatic amnesia can last for months but usually resolves within a few weeks. During PTA, the patient moves from a cognitive level of internal confusion to a level of confusion about the environment. SEE: *Rancho Los Amigos Guide to Cognitive Levels.*

SYMPTOMS: Symptoms include restlessness, moaning or crying out, uninhibited behavior (often sexual or angry), hallucinations (often paranoid), lack of continuous memory, story fabrication to replace memory (confabulation), combative behavior, confused language, disorientation, repetition of movements or thoughts (perseveration), and sleep disturbances. Deficits in attention and memory may persist, and communication and other cognitive weaknesses may become more apparent, such as difficulty with problem solving, reasoning, organizing thoughts, sequencing, word finding, and carrying out planned motor movements (as in activities of daily living).

PATIENT CARE: The patient is evaluated for symptoms of PTA. The patient is continually reoriented by keeping a large calendar and clock within sight; each interaction with the patient begins with a repetition of who is in attendance, why the attendant is present, and what activity is planned; and the patient is kept safe and comfortable and is allowed as much freedom of movement as possible. At a cognitive level of internal confusion, the patient does not understand what is happening and becomes agitated. Health care professionals can limit agitation and confusion by speaking softly in simple phrases, using gestures as necessary, allowing time for the patient to respond, and avoiding towering over the patient. Regular visits from family are important; they should be prepared for the patient's appearance and behavior, and their participation in assisting the patient with activities of daily living should be encouraged. The patient may respond best to the person he or she cares about most. Stimulation is limited, and frequent rest periods are scheduled. Equipment designed for agitated patients is used; wrist restraints are avoided if possible. Urinary catheters may increase agitation due to physical discomfort (incontinence briefs can be used during the training period of a toileting program). The patient's swallowing function is evaluated as soon as possible to avoid feeding tubes, but swallowing precautions are observed. A list of stimulations that increase or decrease the patient's agitation is posted for the use of everyone in contact with the patient. Distance is maintained during aggressive outbursts; the aggression is waited out and a soft speaking voice is used. The patient's personal space should not be invaded without warning (e.g., the patient should be told in advance that his or her genitals are to be washed). The patient should be approached from the front, and items should be placed in positions where the patient can best see them. Hallucinations or confabulation are not encouraged, and the patient's attention is redirected when he or she becomes argumentative. As the patient progresses, his or her self-awareness will be limited and variable. Health care professionals should watch closely for impulsive movement that can jeopardize the patient. They should warn others that the patient cannot monitor behavior, and that words and actions will occur without awareness or forethought. All possible independence and self-care are encouraged. The patient is engaged in short activities with a motor component. One behavior at a time should be monitored if the patient displays several that interfere with treatment. To promote abstract reasoning, humor should be used if the patient understands it. A consistent daily schedule continues to be used and the patient is taught to use compensatory cues (a watch or written activity schedule) to aid memory. The patient is also assessed for posttraumatic headache, which is treated with prescribed nonnarcotic analgesics.

psychogenic a. Dissociative a.

retrograde a. Amnesia for events that occurred before the precipitating trauma.

selective a. Inability to remember events that occurred at the same time as other experiences that are recalled.

tactile a. Inability to distinguish objects by sense of touch. SYN: *astereognosis*.

transient global a. Short-term memory loss that occurs in otherwise healthy people; remote memory is retained. Onset is usually sudden and may last for a few hours. Recovery is usually rapid. The memory loss in this syndrome is believed to be caused by a temporary loss of blood flow to the temporal lobes of the brain.

traumatic a. Amnesia caused by sudden physical injury.

visual a. Inability to remember the appearance of objects or to be cognizant of printed words.

amnesiac, amnesic A person who has amnesia.

amniocentesis (ăm″nē-ō-sĕn-tē′sĭs) [Gr. *amnion*, lamb, + *kentesis*, puncture] Transabdominal puncture of the amniotic sac under ultasound guidance using a needle and syringe in order to remove amniotic fluid. The sample obtained is studied chemically and cytologically to detect genetic and biochemical disorders and maternal-fetal blood incompatibility and, later in the pregnancy, to determine fetal maturity. The procedure also allows for transfusion of the fetus with platelets or blood and instillation of drugs for treating the fetus.

This procedure is usually performed no earlier than at 14 weeks' gestation. It is important that the analysis be done by experts in chemistry, cytogenetics, and cell culture. Cell cultures may require 30 days, and if the test has to be repeated, the time required may be insufficient to allow corrective action. SEE: illus.

CAUTION: The procedure can cause abortion or trauma to the fetus.

PATIENT CARE: The patient's knowledge about the procedure is evaluated. The patient learns about sensations that she may experience, and signs a consent form. The amniocentesis equipment is assembled; amber-colored test

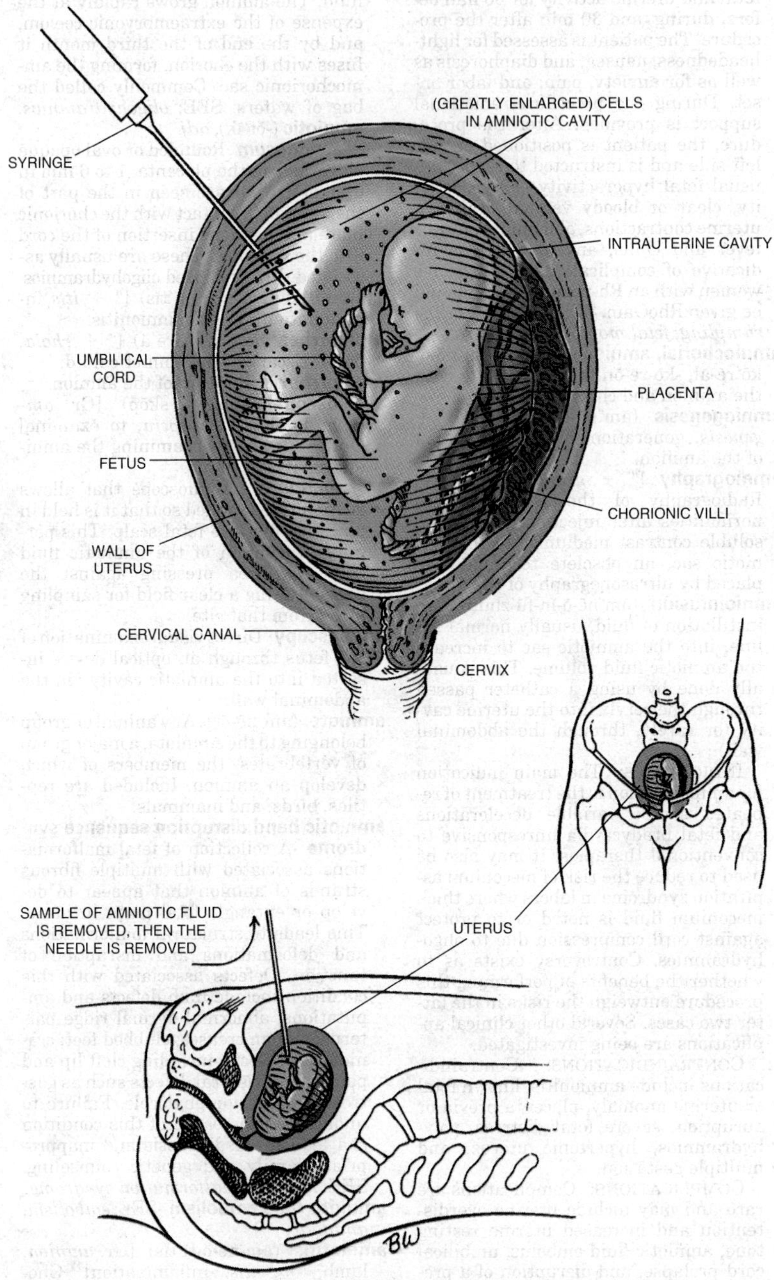

AMNIOCENTESIS

tubes are used (or clear test tubes are covered with aluminum foil) to shield the fluid from light, which could break down bilirubin. Baseline vital signs and fetal heart rate are obtained, and the fundus is palpated for fetal position and fetal and uterine activity for 30 min before, during, and 30 min after the procedure. The patient is assessed for lightheadedness, nausea, and diaphoresis as well as for anxiety, pain, and labor onset. During the procedure, emotional support is provided. After the procedure, the patient is positioned on her left side and is instructed to report unusual fetal hyperactivity or hypoactivity, clear or bloody vaginal drainage, uterine contractions, abdominal pain, or fever and chills, any of which is indicative of complications. Rh-negative women with an Rh-positive fetus should be given RhoGam. SEE: *chorionic villus sampling; fetal monitoring in utero.*

amniochorial, amniochorionic (ăm″nē-ō-kō′rē-ăl, -kō-rē-ŏn′ĭk) Relating to both the amnion and chorion.

amniogenesis (ăm″nē-ō-jĕn′ĕ-sĭs) [″ + *genesis*, generation, birth] Formation of the amnion.

amniography [″ + *graphein*, to write] Radiography of the fetus for abnormalities after injection of a water-soluble contrast medium into the amniotic sac, an obsolete technique replaced by ultrasonography of the fetus.

amnioinfusion (ăm″nē-ō-ĭn-fū′zhŭn) The instillation of fluid, usually normal saline, into the amniotic sac to increase the amniotic fluid volume. This is usually done by using a catheter passed through the cervix into the uterine cavity (or rarely, through the abdominal wall).

INDICATIONS: The main indication for amnioinfusion is the treatment of repeated severe variable decelerations and fetal bradycardia unresponsive to conventional therapies. It may also be used to reduce the risk of meconium aspiration syndrome in labors where thick meconium fluid is noted or to protect against cord compression due to oligohydramnios. Controversy exists as to whether the benefits of performing this procedure outweigh the risks in the latter two cases. Several other clinical applications are being investigated.

CONTRAINDICATIONS: Contraindications include amnionitis, known fetal or uterine anomaly, placenta previa or abruption, severe fetal distress, polyhydramnios, hypertonic uterus, and multiple gestation.

COMPLICATIONS: Complications are rare and may include uterine overdistention and increased uterine resting tone, amniotic fluid embolus, umbilical cord prolapse, and disruption of a previous uterine scar.

PATIENT CARE: Consult local protocols for amnioinfusion, as these may vary from hospital to hospital.

amnion (ăm′nē-ŏn) [Gr. *amnion*, lamb] The innermost fetal membrane; a thin, transparent sac that holds the fetus suspended in the liquor amnii, or amniotic fluid. The amnion grows rapidly at the expense of the extraembryonic coelom, and by the end of the third month it fuses with the chorion, forming the amniochorionic sac. Commonly called the bag of waters. SEE: *oligohydramnios.*

amniotic (-ŏt′ĭk), *adj.*

a. nodosum Rounded or oval opaque elevations in the placenta, 1 to 6 mm in diameter, that are seen in the part of the amnion in contact with the chorionic plate and near the insertion of the cord into the placenta. These are usually associated with prolonged oligohydramnios.

amnionitis (ăm″nē-ō-nī′tĭs) [″ + *itis*, inflammation] Chorioamnionitis.

amniorrhea (ăm″nē-or-rē′ă) [″ + *rhoia*, flow] Escape of the amniotic fluid.

amniorrhexis Rupture of the amnion.

amnioscope (ăm′nē-ŏ-skōp) [Gr. *amnion*, lamb, + *skopein*, to examine] Optical device for examining the amniotic cavity.

suction a. Amnioscope that allows suction to be applied so that it is held in place against the fetal scalp. This permits evacuation of the amniotic fluid from the area pressing against the scalp, leaving a clear field for sampling blood from that site.

amnioscopy Direct visual examination of the fetus through an optical device inserted into the amniotic cavity via the abdominal wall.

amniote (ăm′nē-ōt) Any animal or group belonging to the Amniota, a major group of vertebrates, the members of which develop an amnion. Included are reptiles, birds, and mammals.

amniotic band disruption sequence syndrome A collection of fetal malformations associated with multiple fibrous strands of amnion that appear to develop or entangle fetal parts in utero. This leads to structural malformations and deformations and disruption of function. Defects associated with this condition include limb defects and amputations; abnormal dermal ridge patterns; simian creases; clubbed feet; craniofacial defects, including cleft lip and palate; and visceral defects such as gastroschisis and omphalocele. Failure to understand the cause of this condition can lead to misdiagnosis and inappropriate family and genetic counseling. SEE: *multiple malformation syndrome.*

amniotic fluid embolism SEE: *embolism, amniotic.*

amniotitis (ăm-nē-ŏ-tī′tĭs) [Gr. *amnion*, lamb, + *itis*, inflammation] Chorioamnionitis.

amniotome (ăm′nē-ŏ-tōm) [″ + Gr.

tome, incision] Instrument for puncturing fetal membranes.

amniotomy (ăm″nē-ŏt′ō-mē) Intentionally breaking the amniotic sac with a sterile amniohook, allis forceps, or amniotome to stimulate or augment labor. SYN: *artificial rupture of membranes.*

PATIENT CARE: Explanation of the procedure is reinforced. The patient is positioned and draped correctly, and the perineum is thoroughly cleansed. Before the procedure, baseline information is obtained on fetal heart rate (FHR) and uterine contractions, and these are monitored during and after the procedure. Immediately after the amniotomy, the electronic recording of FHR is auscultated or checked, because the procedure increases the risk of cord compression or prolapse. The color, odor, consistency, and approximate amount of amniotic fluid expelled are assessed and documented. If any question exists as to its origin (amniotic fluid versus urine), the fluid's pH is tested with nitrazine paper, which will turn blue (demonstrating alkalinity) in the presence of amniotic fluid. Bloody show or insufficient amniotic fluid can cause a false test result. The patient is evaluated for onset of labor, which should begin within 12 hr of rupture, and for fever or other signs of infection in prolonged rupture. Oxytocin induction often is used with amniotomy to limit this potential.

amnitis (ăm-nī′tĭs) Inflammation of the amnion. SYN: *amniotitis; amnionitis.*

amobarbital (ăm″ō-bar′bĭ-tăl) An odorless white crystalline powder used as a sedative; $C_{11}H_{18}N_2O_3$.

a. sodium An odorless white granular powder used as a sedative; $C_{11}H_{17}N_2NaO_3$. It is absorbed and inactivated rapidly in the liver.

A-mode (amplitude modulation) display SEE: *ultrasound, A-mode.*

amodiaquine hydrochloride (ăm″ō-dī′ă-kwĭn) An antimalarial drug similar in action to chloroquine. Trade name is Camoquin Hydrochloride.

Amoeba (ă-mē′ba) [Gr. *amoibe*, change] A genus of protozoa of the class Sarcodina; commonly called amebas. Some are parasitic in humans but most of the parasitic species have been reclassified in the genus *Entamoeba.*

amoeba (ă-mē′ba) *pl.* **amoebas, amoebae** SEE: *ameba.*

amok (ă-mŏk′, ă-mŭk′) [Malay, to engage furiously in battle] A state of murderous frenzy. Also spelled *amuck.*

amoxicillin (ă-mŏks″ĭ-sĭl′ĭn) A semisynthetic penicillin. Trade names include Amoxil, Polymox, and Trimox.

AMP *adenosine monophosphate.*

amperage (ăm-pĕr′ĭj) The measure of the number of electrons in an electrical circuit, expressed in amperes.

ampere (ăm′pēr) ABBR: amp. The basic unit of current, defined as the flow of 6.25×10^{-18} electrons per sec (1 coulomb of charge flowing per sec). SEE: *electromotive force.*

amph- SEE: *ampho-.*

amphetamine (ăm-fĕt′ă-mēn, -mĭn) A colorless liquid that volatilizes slowly at room temperature. It is a central nervous system stimulant. The preparation most commonly used is the sulfate form, marketed as tablets or capsules. SEE: *a. sulfate.*

a. sulfate A synthetic white crystalline substance that acts as a central nervous system stimulant; $(C_9H_{13}N)_2SO_4$. It is used to treat narcolepsy and certain types of mental depression. Use of amphetamine sulfate to control appetite is contraindicated. Large doses are toxic, and prolonged use may cause drug dependence. It's trade name is Benzadrine.

amphetamine poisoning SEE: *Poisons and Poisoning Appendix.*

amphi- [Gr. *amphi*, on both sides] Prefix indicating *on both sides, on all sides, double.* In chemistry, it denotes certain positions or configurations of molecules.

amphiarthrosis (ăm″fē-ăr-thrō′sĭs) [″ + *arthrosis*, joint] A form of articulation in which the body surfaces are connected by cartilage; mobility is slight but may be exerted in all directions. The articulations of the bodies of the vertebrae are examples.

amphiaster (ăm″fē-ăs′tĕr) [″ + *aster*, star] Double star figure formed during mitosis. SYN: *diaster.*

Amphibia (ăm-fĭb′ē-ă) [Gr. *amphibios*, double life] A class of cold-blooded animals that live on land and in water; includes salamanders, frogs, and toads. They breathe through gills during their aquatic larval stage but through lungs in their adult stage.

amphibious (ăm-fĭb′ē-ŭs) Able to live both on land and in water.

amphiblastula (ăm″fē-blăs′tū-lă) [Gr. *amphi*, on both sides, + *blastula*, little sprout] A form of blastula in which the blastomeres are of unequal size; seen in sponges.

amphibolism (ăm-fĭb′ŏ-lĭzm) Metabolic pathways that lead to both catabolic and anabolic outcomes, such as beta-oxidation of fatty acids by the liver. The resulting acetyl groups may enter the citric acid cycle for energy production, or may be used for the synthesis of other lipids or steroids.

amphichroic, amphichromatic (ăm″fē-krō′ĭk, -krō-măt′ĭk) [″ + *chroma*, color] **1.** Turning red litmus paper blue, and blue litmus paper red. **2.** Reacting as both an acid and an alkali. **3.** Capable of exhibiting two colors.

amphicyte SEE: *cell, satellite.*

amphidiarthrosis (ăm″fē-dī-ăr-thrō′sĭs) [″ + *diarthrosis*, articulation] An articulation containing an amphiarthrosis and a diarthrosis, such as that of the lower jaw.

amphipathic (ăm-fē-păth′ĭk) In chemistry, having polar and nonpolar (water-soluble and water-insoluble) regions within a single molecule. This two-part structure allows these chemicals to link, or to segregate, oils and water. Phospholipids, bile salts, and detergents are examples of amphipathic molecules.

amphitheater (ăm″fĭ-thē′ă-tĕr) [″ + *theatron*, theater] An operating room or auditorium with tiers of seats around it for students and other observers.

amphitrichate, amphitrichous (ăm-fĭt′rĭ-kāt, -kŭs) [″ + *thrichos*, hair] Having a flagellum or flagella at both ends, said of microorganisms.

ampho-, amph- [Gr. *ampho*, both] Prefix indicating *both, both sides, on all sides,* or *double.*

amphocyte (ăm′fō-sīt) [″ + *kytos*, cell] A cell that stains with either acid or basic stains.

amphodiplopia (ăm-fō-dĭ-plō′pē-ă) [″ + *diploos*, double, + *ops*, vision] Double vision in each eye. SYN: *amphoterodiplopia.*

ampholyte (ăm′fō-līt) [″ + *electrolyte*] A substance that acts as a base or an acid, depending on the pH of the solution into which it is introduced.

amphophil (ăm′fō-fĭl) Amphocyte.

amphoric (ăm-for′ĭk) [L. *amphoricus*] Pert. to a sound such as that caused by blowing across the mouth of a bottle; a resonance; a cavernous sound on percussion of a pulmonary cavity.

amphoricity (ăm″for-ĭs′ĭ-tē) The condition of producing amphoric sounds.

amphoriloquy (ăm″for-ĭl′ō-kwē) [L. *amphora*, jar, + *loqui*, to speak] The presence of amphoric sounds in speaking.

amphorophony (ăm″for-ŏf′ō-nē) [Gr. *amphoreus*, jar, + *phone*, voice] Amphoric voice sound.

amphoteric, amphoterous (ăm-fō-tĕr′ĭk, ăm-fŏt′ĕr-ŭs) [Gr. *amphoteros*, both] Being able to react as both an acid and a base.

amphoteric compound A compound that reacts as both an acid and a base.

amphotericin B (ăm″fō-tĕr′ĭ-sĭn) An antibiotic agent obtained from a strain of *Streptomyces nodosus*. It is used to treat deep-seated fungal infections. The drug usually is administered intravenously. Premedication with antipyretics, antihistamines, or corticosteroids is often necessary to decrease febrile hypersensitivity reactions. Patients must be monitored for hypokalemia or renal failure.

amphoteric reaction Reaction in which a compound reacts as both an acid and a base.

amphoterism (ăm-fō′tĕr-ĭzm) State of reacting as both an acid and a base.

amphoterodiplopia (ăm-fŏt″ĕr-ō-dĭ-plō′pē-ă) [″ + *diploos*, double, + *ops*, vision] Double vision in each eye. SYN: *amphodiplopia*.

ampicillin (ămp″ĭ-sĭl′ĭn) A semisynthetic penicillin. Trade names include Amcill, Omnipen, Polycillin, and Principen.

a. sodium Monosodium salt of ampicillin. Trade names include Omnipen-N and Principen/N.

amplification (ăm″plĭ-fĭ-kā′shŭn) [L. *amplificatio*, making larger] Enlargement, magnification, expansion.

amplifier (ăm′plĭ-fī″ĕr) **1.** That which enlarges, extends, increases, or makes more powerful. **2.** In electronics, a device for increasing the electric current or signal.

amplitude (ăm′plĭ-tūd) [L. *amplitudo*] **1.** Amount, extent, size, abundance, or fullness. **2.** In physics, the extent of movement, as of a pendulum or sound wave. The maximum displacement of a particle, as that of a string vibrating, as measured from the mean to the extreme. **3.** Magnitude of an action potential. **4.** In radiography, the extent of tube travel during tomography.

amplitude modulation Modification of the amplitude, esp. of a current used for muscle stimulation.

ampule (ăm′pūl) [Fr. *ampoule*] A small glass container that can be sealed and its contents sterilized. This is a French invention for containing hypodermic solutions.

ampulla (ăm-pŭl′lă) *pl.* **ampullae** [L., little jar] Saclike dilatation of a canal or duct.

a. ductus deferentis An irregular and nodular dilatation of the vas deferens just before its junction with the secretory duct of the seminal vesicle.

hepatopancreatic a. The entry of the common bile duct and main pancreatic duct into the duodenum. SYN: *a. of Vater; papilla of Vater*.

a. of lacrimal duct Slight dilatation of the lacrimal duct medial to the punctum.

a. of rectum Slight dilatation of the rectum proper just before continuing as the anal canal. Also called *infraperitoneal portion of rectum proper.*

a. of semicircular canal A dilatation at the end of the semicircular canal that houses an ampulla of a semicircular duct.

a. of semicircular ducts Dilatation of semicircular ducts near their junction with the utricle. In their walls are the cristae ampullares.

a. of uterine fallopian tube The dilated distal end of a uterine tube terminating in a funnel-like infundibulum.

a. of vas deferens A. ductus deferentis.

a. of Vater Hepatopancreatic a.

ampullitis (ăm″pŭl-lī′tĭs) [″ + Gr. *itis*, inflammation] Inflammation of any ampulla, esp. of the ductus deferens.

ampullula (ăm-pŭl′ū-lă) [dim. of L. *ampulla*] A small dilatation, esp. of a lymph or blood vessel.

amputation (ăm″pū-tā′shŭn) [L. *amputare*, to cut around] Removal, usually by surgery, of a limb, part, or organ. Amputation also may be secondary to accidental trauma or spontaneously as in certain vascular disorders.

PATIENT CARE: In the immediate postoperative period, vital signs are assessed, the dressing is observed for bleeding at least every 2 hr, drain patency is checked, and the amount and character of drainage are documented. Limb circulation is ascertained by checking proximal pulses, skin color, and temperature. Postoperative pain is managed by parenteral, and later, oral analgesics. To prevent contracture formation, the patient is encouraged to ambulate, change position, rest in proper body alignment with the residual limb in extension rather than in flexion, do range-of-motion exercises (esp. extension), and do muscle-strengthening exercises as soon as these are prescribed postoperatively. Residual limb-conditioning exercises and correct residual limb bandaging (applying graded, moderate pressure to mold the residual limb into a cone shape that allows a good prosthesis fit) assist limb shrinkage. The residual limb may initially have a rigid plaster dressing; care for this type of cast is the same as for any plaster cast. The patient is instructed in skin hygiene techniques; to massage the limb; to examine the entire limb daily, using a mirror to visualize hidden areas; and to report symptoms such as swelling, redness, excessive drainage, increased pain, and residual limb skin changes (rashes, blisters, or abrasions). The patient is taught how to bandage the residual limb or, when it is dry, to apply a residual limb shrinker (a custom-fitted elastic stocking that fits over the residual limb) and is advised against applying body oil or lotion because it can interfere with proper fit of a prosthesis. The need for constant bandaging until edema subsides and the prosthesis is properly fitted, and the use of a residual limb sock and proper prosthesis care, are explained. The patient is encouraged to verbalize anger and frustration; to cope with grief, self-image, and lifestyle adjustments; and to deal with phantom limb sensation (itching, numbness, or pain perceived in the area of amputation even though the limb is no longer there) if this occurs. The patient may require referral to a local support group or for further psychological counseling. SEE: *Nursing Diagnoses Appendix*.

congenital a. Amputation of parts of the fetus in utero, formerly believed to be caused by constricting bands but now believed to be a developmental defect.

double-flap a. Amputation in which two flaps of soft tissue are formed to cover the end of the bone.

a. in contiguity Amputation at a joint.

a. in continuity Amputation at a site other than a joint.

primary a. Amputation performed before inflammation or infection sets in.

secondary a. Amputation performed after onset of infection.

spontaneous a. Nonsurgical separation of an extremity or digit. SEE: *ainhum*.

traumatic a. The sudden amputation of some part of the body due to an accidental injury.

amputee (ăm″pū-tē′) A person who has had one or more amputations of an extremity; it may be congenital or acquired through trauma or surgery.

Amsler grid [Marc Amsler, Swiss ophthalmologist, 1891–1968] A grid of lines used in testing for macular degeneration. The grid is observed with each eye separately.

A.M.T. *American Medical Technologists.*

amuck (ă-mŭk′) Amok.

amusia (ă-mū′sē-ă) [Gr. *amousos*, unmusical] Music deafness; inability to produce or appreciate musical sounds.

motor a. Inability to produce musical sounds.

sensory a. Music deafness; inability to appreciate musical sounds.

vocal a. Inability to sing.

Amussat's operation (ăm′ū-săz) [Jean Z. Amussat, Fr. surgeon, 1796–1856] Surgical formation of an artificial anus, by lumbar colotomy in ascending colon.

amychophobia (ă-mī″kō-fō′bē-ă) [Gr. *amyche*, scratch, + *phobos*, fear] Morbid fear of being scratched; fear of the claws of any animal.

amyelencephaly (ă-mī″ĕl-ĕn-sĕf′ă′lē) [Gr. *a-*, not, + *myelos*, marrow, + *enkephalos*, brain] Congenital absence of the brain and spinal cord.

amyelia (ă-mī-ē′lē-ă) [″ + *myelos*, marrow] Congenital absence of the spinal cord.

amyelinic (ă-mī″ĕ-lĭn′ĭk) Not possessing a myelin sheath.

amyelus (ă-mī′ĕ-lŭs) An individual with congenital absence of the spinal cord.

amygdala (ă-mĭg′dă-lă) *pl.* **amygdalae** [L., almond] A mass of gray matter in the anterior portion of the temporal lobe. It is believed to play an important role in arousal and emotional states.

amygdalin (ă-mĭg′dă-lĭn) A bitter-tasting glycoside derived from the pit or other seed parts of several plants, including almonds and apricots. Amygdalin, from which the poisonous hydrocyanic acid can be produced by enzymatic action, is the substance known in the U.S. as Laetrile. Amygdalin has no therapeutic or nutritional value. SEE: *Laetrile*.

amygdaline (ă-mĭg′dă-līn, -lĭn) [L. *amygdalinus*] **1.** Pert. to a tonsil. **2.** Pert. to or shaped like an almond. SYN: *amygdaloid*.

amygdaloid (ă-mĭg′dă-loyd) [Gr. *amygdale*, almond, + *eidos*, form, shape] Resembling an almond.

amygdaloid tubercle A projection from the middle cornu of the lateral ventricle, marking the area of the amygdaloid nucleus.

amygdalolith (ă-mĭg′dă-lō-lĭth″) [″ + *lithos*, stone] Stone in a distended crypt of a tonsil.

amygdalopathy (ă-mĭg″dă-lŏp′ă-thē) [″ + *pathos*, disease, suffering] Any disease of a tonsil.

amygdalotome (ă-mĭg′dă-lō-tōm″) [″ + *tome*, incision] An instrument for excision of a tonsil.

amyl (ăm′ĭl) [Gr. *amylon*, starch] A hypothetical univalent radical, C_5H_{11}, nonexistent in a free state.

a. nitrite $C_5H_{11}NO_2$; a volatile and highly flammable clear liquid used as a vasodilator, esp. in the past for anginal pain.

amylaceous (ăm″ĭ-lā′shē-ŭs) Starchy.

amylase (ăm′ĭ-lās) [″ + *-asis*, colloid enzyme] A class of enzymes that split or hydrolyze starch. Those found in animals are called alpha-amylases; those in plants are called beta-amylases. SEE: *enzyme; macroamylase*.

pancreatic a. Amylopsin.

salivary a. Ptyalin.

vegetable a. Diastase.

amylasuria (ăm″ĭ-lās-ū′rē-ă) [″ + *ouron*, urine] Increased amount of amylase in the urine; occurs in pancreatitis.

amylodextrin [″ + *dexter*, right] Soluble substance produced during the hydrolysis of starch into sugar.

amylodyspepsia (ăm″ĭ-lō-dĭs-pĕp′sē-ă) [″ + *dys*, bad, + *pepsis*, digestion] Inability to digest starchy foods.

amylogenesis (ăm″ĭ-lō-jĕn′ĕ-sĭs) [″ + *genesis*, generation, birth] The production of starch. **amylogenic** (-jĕn′ĭk), *adj.*

amyloid (ăm′ĭ-loyd) [Gr. *amylon*, starch, + *eidos*, form, shape] **1.** Resembling starch; starchlike. **2.** A protein-polysaccharide complex produced and deposited in tissues during some chronic infections, malignancies, and rheumatological disorders. It is a homogeneous substance staining readily with Congo red. It is associated with a variety of chronic diseases, particularly tuberculosis, osteomyelitis, leprosy, Hodgkin's disease, and carcinoma. SEE: *amyloidosis*.

amyloid degeneration Degeneration of organs or tissues from amyloid deposits, which are waxy and translucent and have a hyaline appearance. The liver, spleen, and kidneys are usually involved, but any tissue may be infiltrated.

amyloid disease Amyloidosis.

amyloid nephrosis A nephrotic syndrome from amyloid deposits in the kidney.

amyloidosis (ăm″ĭ-loy-dō′sĭs) [Gr. *amylon*, starch, + *eidos*, form, shape, + *osis*, condition] A group of incompletely understood metabolic disorders resulting from the insidious deposition of protein-containing fibrils (amyloid) in tissues. The disease may cause localized or widespread organ failure. Amyloid may infiltrate many organs, including the heart and blood vessels, brain and peripheral nerves, kidneys, liver, spleen, skin, endocrine glands, or intestines. As a result, the clinical manifestations of amyloidosis are enormously varied, and the disease may mimic many other conditions ranging from nephrotic syndrome (when kidneys are infiltrated) to dementias (brain involvement) or congestive heart failure (myocardial deposition). Amyloidosis of the tongue may cause this organ to become markedly enlarged, interfering with speech or swallowing. Amyloid infiltration of endocrine organs can cause pituitary, thyroid, or pancreatic dysfunction, among others.

Primary amyloidosis is said to be present when amyloid proteins are deposited throughout the body as a result of their overproduction by malignant clones of immune cells. Multiple myeloma and B-cell lymphoma are the two hematologic malignancies associated with primary amyloidosis.

Secondary amyloidosis is the production and deposition of amyloid in patients with chronic inflammatory conditions (e.g., chronic tuberculosis or rheumatoid arthritis). This category of amyloidosis is also known as *reactive, systemic amyloidosis.*

Localized amyloidosis is present when amyloid infiltrates an isolated organ (e.g., the brain or the pancreas).

DIAGNOSIS: Amyloid in tissues can be demonstrated by its characteristically green appearance when stained with Congo Red stain and viewed under a polarizing microscope.

TREATMENT: Corticosteroids and melphalan are somewhat helpful in treating primary amyloidosis. In secondary amyloidosis, controlling the primary inflammatory illness may arrest the progress of the disease. In general, the prognosis in systemic amyloidosis is poor—most patients with the disease live less than 3 years.

lichen a. A form of amyloidosis limited to the skin.

localized a. Amyloidosis in which

isolated amyloid tumors are formed. SEE: *amyloidosis.*

primary a. Amyloidosis not associated with a chronic disease. SEE: *amyloidosis.*

secondary a. Amyloidosis associated with a chronic disease, such as tuberculosis, syphilis, Hodgkin's disease, or rheumatoid arthritis, and with extensive tissue destruction. The spleen, liver, kidneys, and adrenal cortex are most frequently involved. SEE: *amyloidosis.*

amylolysis (ăm″ĭl-ŏl′ĭ-sĭs) [″ + *lysis,* dissolution] Hydrolysis of starch into sugar in the process of digestion. **amylolytic** (-ō-lĭt′ĭk), *adj.*

amylopectin (ăm″ĭl-ō-pĕk′tĭn) The insoluble component of starch. The soluble component is amidin.

amylophagia (ăm″ĭ-lō-fā′jē-ă) [″ + *phagein,* to eat] Abnormal craving for starch.

amylopsin (ăm″ĭ-lŏp′sĭn) [″ + *opsis,* appearance] An enzyme in pancreatic juice that hydrolyzes starch into achroodextrin and maltose. SYN: *pancreatic amylase.* SEE: *digestion; duodenum; enzyme.*

amylose (ăm′ĭ-lōs) [Gr. *amylon,* starch] A group of carbohydrates that includes starch, cellulose, and dextrin.

amylosuria (ăm″ĭ-lō-sū′rē-ă) [″ + *ouron,* urine] Amylose in the urine.

amyluria [″ + Gr. *ouron,* urine] Starch in the urine.

amyosthenia (ă-mī″ŏs-thē′nē-ă) [Gr. *a-,* not, + *mys,* muscle, + *sthenos,* strength] Muscular weakness. SEE: *myasthenia.* **amyosthenic, amyasthenic,** *adj.*

amyotonia (ă-mī″ō-tō′nē-ă) [″ + ″ + *tonos,* tone] Deficiency or lack of muscular tone.

a. congenita SEE: *m. congenita.*

amyotrophia, amyotrophy (ă-mī″ō-trō′fē-ă, ă-mī-ŏt′rō-fē) [″ + ″ + *trophe,* nourishment] Muscular atrophy. **amyotrophic** (-trŏf′ĭk), *adj.*

progressive spinal a. Progressive muscular atrophy.

amyxia (ă-mĭks′ē-ă) [″ + *myxa,* mucus] Absence or deficiency of mucus.

amyxorrhea (ă-mĭks-ō-rē′ă) [″ + ″ + *rhoia,* flow] Lack of normal secretion of mucus.

An 1. Symbol for actinon. **2.** *anisometropia.* **3.** *anode.* **4.** *antigen.*

an- [Gr.] SEE: *a-.*

A.N.A. *American Nurses' Association.*

ana (ăn′ă) ABBR: $\overline{aa}$. **1.** Prescription term meaning *so much of each.* **2.** *antinuclear antibody.*

ana- Prefix used in words derived from Greek. It indicates *up, against,* or *back.*

anabolic agent Testosterone, or a steroid hormone resembling testosterone, which stimulates the growth or manufacturing of body tissues. Anabolic steroids have been used, sometimes in large doses, by male and female athletes to improve performance, esp. in events requiring strength. This use has been judged to be illegal by various organizations that supervise sports, including the International Olympic Committee and the U.S. Olympic Committee. They also are used to treat patients with wasting illnesses. SEE: *doping; ergonomic aid.*

CAUTION: Indiscriminate use of anabolic agents is inadvisable because of the undesirable side effects they may produce (e.g., in women, hirsutism, masculinization, and clitoral hypertrophy; in men, aggressiveness, testicular atrophy, and other conditions).

---

anabolism (ă-năb′ō-lĭzm) [Gr. *anabole,* a building up, + *-ismos,* condition] The building of body tissues; the constructive phase of metabolism by which cells take from the blood nutrients required for repair or growth, and convert these inorganic chemicals into cell products or parts of living cells. Anabolism is the opposite of catabolism, the destructive phase of metabolism. **anabolic** (ăn″ă-bŏl′ĭk), *adj.*

anabolite (ă-năb′ō-līt″) Any product of anabolism.

anacamptometer (ăn″ă-kămp-tŏm′ĕ-tĕr) [Gr. *ana,* up, + *kamptos,* bent, + *metron,* to measure] A device for measuring the intensity of deep reflexes.

anacatesthesia (ăn″ă-kăt″ĕs-thē′zē-ă) [″ + ″ + *aisthesis,* sensation] A sensation of hovering.

anacidity (ăn″ă-sĭd′ĭ-tē) [Gr. *an-,* not, + L. *acidum,* acid] Abnormal deficiency of acidity, esp. of hydrochloric acid in the gastric juice.

anaclasis (ă-năk′lă-sĭs) [Gr. *anaklasis,* reflection] **1.** Refraction or reflection of light. **2.** Refraction of light in the interior of the eye. **3.** Reflex action. **4.** Refraction for therapeutic reasons. **5.** Forcible movement of a joint in order to treat fibrous ankylosis.

anaclitic (ăn″ă-klĭt′ĭk) Leaning or depending on. In psychoanalysis, pert. to the dependence of an infant on the mother figure for care.

anacrotic (ăn″ă-krŏt′ĭk) [Gr. *ana,* up, + *krotos,* stroke] **1.** Pert. to the ascending or vertical upstroke of a sphygmogram. **2.** Pert. to a pulse with more than one expansion of the artery. **3.** Pert. to two heartbeats traced on the ascending line of a sphygmogram. SEE: *pulse.*

anacrotism (ă-năk′rō-tĭzm) Existence of a double beat on the ascending line of a sphygmogram. SYN: *anadicrotism.*

anacusia, anacusis, anakusis (ăn-ă-kū′sē-ă, -sĭs) [Gr. *an-,* not, + *akouein,* to hear] Total deafness.

anadicrotism (ăn-ă-dĭk′rō-tĭzm) [Gr. *ana*, up, + *dikrotos*, double beating] Anacrotism. **anadicrotic** (ăn-ă-dī-krŏt′ĭk), *adj.*

anadidymus (ăn″ă-dĭd′ĭ-mŭs) [″ + *didymos*, twin] A developmental abnormality in which the upper parts of the bodies of twins are fused, but the buttocks and legs are free.

anadipsia (ăn″ă-dĭp′sē-ă) [Gr. *ana*, intensive, + *dipsa*, thirst] Intense thirst.

anadrenalism (ăn″ă-drē′năl-ĭzm) [Gr. *an-*, not, + *adrenal* + Gr. *-ismos*, condition] Failure of the adrenal gland to function.

anadromous [Gr. *anadromos*, running upward] Descriptive of fish that migrate from sea water to fresh water.

anaerobe (ăn′ĕr-ōb) [Gr. *an-*, not, + *aer*, air, + *bios*, life] A microorganism that can live and grow in the absence of oxygen.

facultative a. An organism that can live and grow with or without oxygen.

obligatory a. An organism that can live and grow only in the absence of oxygen.

anaerobic (ăn″ĕr-ō′bĭk) **1.** Pert. to an anaerobe. **2.** Able to live without oxygen.

anaerobic exercise Exercise during which the energy needed is provided without use of inspired oxygen. This type of exercise is limited to short bursts of vigorous activity. SEE: *aerobic exercise.*

anaerobiosis (ăn″ĕr-ō-bī-ō′sĭs) [″ + *aer*, air, + *bios*, life, + *osis*, condition] **1.** Life in an oxygen-free atmosphere. **2.** Functioning of an organ or tissue in the absence of free oxygen.

anagen (ăn′ă-jĕn) [Gr. *ana*, up, + *genesis*, generation, birth] The growth stage of hair development. SEE: *catagen; telogen.*

anakatadidymus (ăn″ă-kăt″ă-dĭd′ĭ-mŭs) [Gr. *ana*, up, + *kala*, down, + *didymos*, twin] A congenital anomaly in which twins are separated above and below but joined at the trunk.

anakré [African, big nose] Goundou.

anal (ā′năl) [L. *analis*] Rel. to the anus or outer rectal opening.

anal continence plug A device to prevent fecal soilage. It was used in incontinence involving both liquid and solid fecal material. Neither the subcutaneously implanted magnetic (Maclet) ring nor disposable balloon-tipped plugs are effective in most applications. SEE: *anal dynamic graciloplasty.*

anal dynamic graciloplasty The construction of a "new" anal sphincter to treat severe intractable fecal incontinence. The gracilis muscle tendon is detached at its insertion, mobilized, and reattached wrapped about the sphincter. Some patients can be trained to make the sphincter functional. If necessary a sustained contraction can be stimulated by implanted electrodes, closing the anus. Additional procedures have been employed as gluteal muscle mobilization. An implantable artificial sphincter has been employed. The functional result of all of these procedures is variable.

analeptic (ăn″ă-lĕp′tĭk) [Gr. *analeptikos*, restorative] **1.** A drug that stimulates the central nervous system. **2.** A restorative agent.

anal erotism Localization of the libido in the anal region. SEE: *anal stage.*

analgesia (ăn-ăl-jē′zē-ă) [Gr. *an-*, not, + *algos*, pain] Absence of a normal sense of pain.

a. algera Spontaneous pain with loss of sensibility in a part.

continuous caudal a. Analgesia to reduce the pain of childbirth. The anesthetic is injected continuously into the epidural space at the sacral hiatus.

epidural a. A postoperative pain management technique in which narcotics are infused into the peridural space through an indwelling catheter. Administration may be at a continuous basal infusion rate or self-administered within programmed limits.

infiltration a. Anesthesia produced in a local area by injecting an anesthetic agent into the nerve endings.

paretic a. Complete analgesia of an upper limb in conjunction with partial paralysis.

patient-controlled a. ABBR: PCA. A drug administration method that permits the patient to control the rate of drug delivery for the control of pain. It is usually accomplished by the use of an infusion pump. The patient must have complete understanding of the system and be willing to use it. The system should be designed so that the patient will be unable to administer an overdose of the analgesic; also, as with all narcotics, the system has to be designed to prevent its theft.

pre-emptive a. The administration of anesthetic before surgery in an attempt to abort postoperative pain and disability.

analgesic (ăn″ăl-jē′sĭk) **1.** Relieving pain. **2.** A drug that relieves pain. Analgesic drugs include nonprescription drugs, such as aspirin and other nonsteroidal anti-inflammatory agents, and those classified as controlled substances and available only by prescription. SYN: *analgetic.*

analgetic (ăn″ăl-jĕt′ĭk) Analgesic.

analgia (ăn-ăl′jē-ă) [″ + *algos*, pain] State of being without pain.

anal incontinence Failure of the anal sphincter to prevent involuntary expulsion of gas, liquid, or solids from the lower bowel.

analog, analogue (ăn′ă-lŏg) [Gr. *analo-*

gos, analogy, proportion] **1.** One of two organs in different species that are similar in function but different in structure. **2.** In chemistry, a compound that is structurally similar to another.

estrogen a. A compound that mimics the effects of estrogens.

analogous (ă-năl′ō-gŭs) Similar in function but different in origin or structure.

analogy (ă-năl′ō-jē) [Gr. *analogos*, analogy, proportion] **1.** Likeness or similarity between two things that are otherwise unalike. **2.** In biology, similarity in function, but difference in structure or origin; opposite of homology.

anal personality In Freudian psychology, a personality disorder marked by excessive orderliness, stinginess, and obstinacy. If carried to an extreme, these qualities lead to the development of obsessive-compulsive behavior.

anal stage In Freudian psychology, the second phase of sexual development, from infancy to childhood, in which the libido is concentrated in the anal region. In order of appearance, the phases of sexual development are oral, anal, phallic, and genital.

anal wink Contraction of the anal sphincter in response to pinprick stimulus of the perineum.

analysand (ăn-ăl′ĭ-zănd) A patient who is being psychoanalyzed.

analysis (ă-năl′ĭ-sĭs) *pl.* **analyses** [LL. *ana*, up, back, + Gr. *lysis*, dissolution] **1.** Separation of anything into its constituent parts. **2.** In chemistry, determination of or separation into constituent parts of a substance or compound. **3.** Psychoanalysis.

batch a. An automated analysis in which all of the samples collected for a specific, nonemergent assay undergo the same testing process at the same time. By contrast, samples collected for stat analyses are not saved in batches. These analyses are performed instead whenever individual specimens are received.

chromatographic a. Analysis of substances on the basis of color reaction of the constituents as they are differentially absorbed on one of a variety of materials such as filter paper.

cohort a. The tabulation and analysis of morbidity or mortality in relation to the ages of a specific group of people (cohort), identified at a particular period of time and followed as they pass through different ages during part or all of their life span.

colorimetric a. **1.** Analysis by adsorption of a compound and the identification of its components by color. **2.** Analysis of the amount of a substance present in a sample, based on the amount of light absorbed by the substance (or a derivative of the substance). SEE: *Beer's law*.

continuous-flow a. Analysis using a type of laboratory instrument that separates samples and appropriate reagents before specimens are analyzed, by placing air bubbles between individual specimens and the reagents as they are injected into a tube. Specimens are then analyzed using various analytical principles (colorimetry, electrochemistry) as they flow along the tube.

densimetric a. Analysis by determination of the specific gravity (density) of a solution and estimation of the amount of solids.

discrete a. An automated methodology in which samples are held in separate containers to be assayed. In a continuous flow system, all samples flow through the same tubing.

gastric a. Analysis of the stomach contents to determine the concentration of free hydrochloric acid and combined (total) acid and the presence of lactic acid, occult blood, pus, and excessive mucus, and the amount and types of bacteria.

hair a. Investigation of the chemical composition of hair. It is used in studying exposure to toxic chemicals in the environment, in poisoning investigations, in nutritional studies, and in monitoring the course of certain diseases. The sample should be obtained from new-growth hair within 5 cm of the scalp to reduce the chance of contamination of the hair by air pollutants.

immunoprecipitin a. An immunoassay in which the antibody-antigen reaction forms a visible substance that drops out of solution. This is most commonly represented by turbidity in a liquid matrix or a band of turbidity in a gel matrix. The amount of turbidity or the size of the band allows quantification.

least squares a. A technique for statistical assessment of data that minimizes the sum of the squares of the distances from each data point to a line or plane. As part of the process, the slope, intercept, and correlation coefficient are also usually calculated. Once this is done, various statistical and analytical inferences can be made, so that the quality of the analytical process can be assessed.

qualitative a. Determination of the presence of a substance in a test sample or of the physicochemical characteristics of a substance in a sample.

quantitative a. Determination of the amount of a substance in a specified material. The amount may be represented in various ways: "x" grams, "x" g/L, kPa (i.e., an absolute quantity, a concentrational quantity, an intensive quantity).

spectrophotometric a. Determination of materials in a compound by measuring the amount of light they absorb in the infrared, visible, or ultraviolet region of the spectrum.

volumetric a. Quantitative analysis performed by the measurement of the volume of solutions or liquids. **analytic** (ăn-ă-lĭt′ĭk), *adj.*

analysis of variance ABBR: ANOVA. A statistical technique for defining and segregating the causes of variability affecting a set of observations. Use of this technique provides a basis for analyzing the effects of various treatments or variables on the subjects or patients being investigated. In an experimental design in which several samples or groups are drawn from the same population, estimates of population variance between samples should differ from each other only by chance. ANOVA provides a method for testing the hypothesis that several random and independent samples are from a common, normal population.

analyst (ăn′ă-lĭst) [Fr. *analyse*, analysis] **1.** One who analyzes. **2.** A practitioner of psychoanalysis. SYN: *psychoanalyst.*

analyte A substance being analyzed, esp. a chemical analysis.

analyze (ăn′ă-līz) [Fr. *analyse*, analysis] To separate into parts or principles in order to determine the nature of the whole; to examine methodically.

analyzer (ăn′ă-lī″zĕr) **1.** A device used to determine the optical rotation produced when polarized light passes through a solution. **2.** An oxygen device used to monitor delivered oxygen concentration by the measurement of partial pressure or concentration. Analyzers are physical, electric, and electrochemical and use paramagnetic, thermal conductive polarographic, and galvanic cells, respectively. **3.** Any device that determines some characteristic of the object, chemical, or action being investigated. There are devices for analyzing a voice; the breath for presence of certain chemicals such as alcohol; images; cells in a solution; and chemicals.

automated a. A chemical instrument system designed to perform assays that were done, and may still be done, manually.

batch a. A discrete automated chemical analyzer in which the instrument system sequentially performs a single test on each of a group of samples.

continuous flow a. An automated chemical analyzer in which the samples and reagents are pumped continuously through a system of modules interconnected by tubing.

discrete a. An automated chemical analyzer in which the instrument performs tests on samples that are kept in "discrete containers," in contrast to a continuous flow analyzer.

parallel a. A discrete automated chemical analyzer that performs a single test on a group of samples at practically the same time (actually, within milliseconds).

pulse height a. ABBR: PHA. A circuit that differentiates between pulses of varying sizes. It is used in scintillation, blood cell, and particle counters.

anamnesis (ăn″ăm-nē′sĭs) [Gr. *anamnesis*, recalling] **1.** Recollection; the faculty of remembering. **2.** That which is remembered. **3.** The medical history of a patient. SEE: *catamnesis.*

anamnestic (ăn″ăm-nĕs′tĭk) **1.** Pert. to the medical history of a patient. **2.** Assisting the memory.

anamniotic (an″am-ne-ot′ik) [Gr. *an-*, not, + *amnion*, amnion] (an″am-ne-ot′ik) Without an amnion.

ANA*NET *American Nurses Association Network.*

anangioplasia (ăn-ăn″jē-ō-plā′sē-ă) [Gr. *an-*, not, + *angeion*, vessel, + *plassein*, to form] Imperfect vascularization of a part. **anangioplastic** (-plăs′tĭk), *adj.*

anaphase (ăn′ă-fāz) [″ + *phainein*, to appear] The third stage in meiosis, and mitosis (between metaphase and telophase), in which there is longitudinal bisection of chromosomes (the chromatids), which separate and move toward their respective poles.

anaphoresis (ăn″ă-fō-rē′sĭs) [″ + *phoresis*, bearing] The flow of electropositive particles toward the anode (positive pole) in electrophoresis.

anaphoria (ăn″ă-for′ē-ă) [Gr. *ana*, up, + *phorein*, to carry] The tendency of the eyeballs to turn upward. SYN: *anatropia.*

anaphrodisia (ăn-ăf″rō-dĭz′ē-ă) [Gr. *an-*, not, + *aphrodisia*, sexual desire] Diminished or absent desire for sex. SEE: *aphrodisiac.*

anaphrodisiac (ăn″ăf-rō-dĭz′ē-ăk) **1.** Repressing sexual desire. **2.** An agent that represses sexual desire.

anaphrodite (ăn-ăf′rō-dīt) A person with impaired or absent sexual desire.

anaphylactogenic (ăn″ă-fĭ-lăk″tō-jĕn′ĭk) **1.** Producing anaphylaxis. **2.** The agent producing anaphylactic reactions.

anaphylatoxin (ăn″ă-fĭ-lă-tŏk′sĭn) Complement components C3a, C4a, and C5a, which cause degranulation of mast cells and release of chemical mediators that promote the smooth muscle spasm, increased vascular permeability, increased mucous secretion, and attraction of neutrophils and eosinophils associated with systemic anaphylaxis.

anaphylaxis (ăn″ă-fĭ-lăk′sĭs) [″ + *phylaxis*, protection] A type I hypersensitivity (allergic) reaction between an allergenic antigen and immunoglobulin E (IgE) bound to mast cells, which stimulates the sudden release of immunological mediators locally or throughout the body. The first symptoms occur within minutes, and a recurrence may follow hours later (late-stage response). Anaphylaxis can only occur in an individual previously sensitized to an allergen, as it is the initial exposure that causes immunoglobulin E (IgE) to bind to mast cells. It is categorized as local or systemic. Local anaphylactic reactions include hay fever, hives, and allergic gastroenteritis. Systemic anaphylaxis, which produces peripheral vasodilation, bronchospasm, and laryngeal edema, can be life-threatening. **anaphylactic** (-lăk′tĭk), *adj.*

ETIOLOGY: IgE antibodies bound to mast cells throughout the body as the result of previous exposure to an allergenic antigen (sensitization) react when the allergen is introduced a second time. The mast cells release packets containing chemical mediators (degranulation) that attract neutrophils and eosinophils and also stimulate urticaria, vasodilation, increased vascular permeability, and smooth muscle spasm, esp. in the bronchi and gastrointestinal tract. Chemical mediators involved in anaphylaxis include histamine, proteases, chemotactic factors, leukotrienes, prostaglandin D, and cytokines (e.g., TNF-α and interleukins 1, 3, 4, 5, and 6). The most common agents triggering anaphylaxis are drugs, food, and insect stings. Local anaphylactic reactions are also commonly triggered by pollens (e.g., hay fever, allergic rhinitis, allergic asthma). SEE: *anaphylactic shock*.

SYMPTOMS: Local anaphylaxis causes signs to appear at the site of allergen-antibody interaction including urticaria (hives), edema, warmth, and erythema. In systemic anaphylaxis the respiratory tract, cardiovascular system, skin, and gastrointestinal system are involved. The primary signs are urticaria, angioedema, flushing, wheezing, dyspnea, increased mucous production, nausea and vomiting, and feelings of generalized anxiety. Systemic anaphylaxis may be mild or severe enough to cause shock when massive vasodilation is present.

TREATMENT: Local anaphylaxis is treated with antihistamines and occasionally epinephrine, if the reaction is severe. Treatment for systemic anaphylaxis includes protection of the airway and administration of oxygen; antihistamines (e.g., diphenhydramine or cimetidine to block histamine H1 and H2 receptors); IV fluids to support blood pressure) and vasopressors (e.g., epinephrine or dopamine) to prevent or treat shock. Epinephrine also is used to treat bronchospasm. Generally, drugs are given intravenously; drugs may also be given intramuscularly (e.g., diphenhydramine) or endotracheally (e.g., epinephrine). In mild cases they may be given subcutaneously. Corticosteroids may be used to prevent recurrence of bronchospasm and increased vascular permeability.

PATIENT CARE: *Prevention:* A history of allergic reactions, particularly to drugs, blood, or contrast media, is obtained. The at-risk patient is observed for reaction during and immediately after administration of any of these agents. The patient is taught to identify and avoid common allergens and to recognize an allergic reaction.

Patients also should be taught to wear tags identifying allergies to medications, food, or insect venom at all times to prevent inappropriate treatment during an emergency. Individuals who have had an anaphylactic reaction and are unable to avoid future exposure to allergens should carry a kit containing a syringe of epinephrine and be taught how to administer it. Patients who are allergic to the venom of Hymenoptera insects (bees, wasps, hornets) can receive desensitization.

active a. Anaphylaxis resulting from injection of an antigen.

exercise-induced a. anaphylactoid reaction.

local a. A reaction between IgE antibodies bound to mast cells and an allergen that is limited to a small part of the body. Localized edema and urticaria (hives) result and may vary in intensity. SEE: *anaphylaxis*. SYN: *Arthus reaction*.

passive a. Anaphylaxis induced by injection of serum from a sensitized animal into a normal one. After a few hours the latter becomes sensitized.

passive cutaneous a. ABBR: PCA. A laboratory test of antibody levels in which serum from a sensitized individual is injected into the skin. Intravenous injection of an antigen accompanied by Evans blue dye at a later time reacts with the antibodies produced in response to the antigen, creating a wheal and blue spot at the site, indicating local anaphylaxis.

systemic a. A reaction between IgE antibodies bound to mast cells and an allergen that causes the sudden release of immunological mediators in the skin, respiratory, cardiovascular, and gastrointestinal systems. The consequences may range from mild (e.g., itching, hives) to life-threatening (airway obstruction and shock). SEE: *allergy; anaphylaxis; anaphylactic shock*.

anaplasia (ăn″ă-plā′zē-ă) [″ + *plassein*, to form] Loss of cellular differentiation and function, characteristic of most malignancies. **anaplastic** (-plăs′tĭk), *adj.*

anapnea (ăn″ăp-nē′ă) [Gr. *anapnein*, to breathe again] **1.** Respiration. **2.** Regaining the breath.

anapneic (ăn″ăp-nē′ĭk) Pert. to anapnea or relieving dyspnea.

anapophysis (ăn″ă-pŏf′ĭ-sĭs) [Gr. *ana*,

back, + *apophysis*, offshoot] An accessory spinal process of a vertebra, esp. a thoracic or lumbar vertebra.

anarthria (ăn-ăr′thrē-ă) [Gr. *an-*, not, + *arthron*, joint] Loss of motor power to speak distinctly. It may result from a neural lesion or a muscular defect.

a. literalis Stammering.

anasarca (ăn″ă-săr′kă) [Gr. *ana*, through, + *sarkos*, flesh] Severe generalized edema. SYN: *dropsy*. **anasarcous** (-săr′kŭs), *adj.*

anaspadias (ăn″ă-spā′dē-ăs) [″ + *spadon*, a rent] Congenital opening of the urethra on the dorsum of the penis; or opening by separation of the labia minora and a fissure of the clitoris. SYN: *epispadias*.

anastole (ăn-ăs′tō-lē) [Gr.] Shrinking away or retraction of the edges of a wound.

anastomose (ă-năs′tō-mōs) [Gr. *anastomosis*, opening] **1.** To communicate directly or by means of connecting two parts together, esp. nerves or blood vessels. **2.** To make such a connection surgically.

anastomosis (ă-năs″tō-mō′sĭs) *pl.* **anastomoses** [Gr., opening] **1.** A natural communication between two vessels; may be direct or by means of connecting channels. **2.** The surgical or pathological connection of two tubular structures. **anastomotic** (-mŏt′ĭk), *adj.*

antiperistaltic a. Anastomosis between two parts of the intestine such that the peristaltic flow in one part is the opposite of that in the other.

arteriovenous a. Anastomosis between an artery and a vein by which the capillary bed is bypassed.

biofragmentable a. ring ABBR: BFR; BAR. An absorbable (i.e., temporary) surgical implant used to join resected loops of bowel. The ring is composed of two parts polyglycolic acid (Dexon) and one part barium sulfate. It dissolves, or “fragments,” about 3 weeks after implantation, when major tissue healing has occurred. The ring is easy to use; postoperative complications may include constipation, leakage, and rarely, intestinal stricture.

PATIENT CARE: Vital signs and fluid intake and output are recorded. If a nasogastric tube was used, it should be checked. The patient is taught to observe stools for ring fragments or bleeding. The patient should return gradually to a normal diet, as prescribed.

crucial a. An arterial anastomosis on the back of the thigh, formed by the medial femoral circumflex, inferior gluteal, lateral femoral circumflex, and first perforating arteries.

end-to-end a. Anastomosis in which the ends of two structures are joined.

Galen's a. Anastomosis between the superior and inferior laryngeal nerves.

heterocladic a. Anastomosis between branches of different arteries.

homocladic a. Anastomosis between branches of the same artery.

Hyrtl's a. An occasional looplike anastomosis between the right and left hypoglossal nerves in geniohyoid muscle.

intestinal a. Surgical connection of two portions of the intestines. SYN: *enteroenterostomy*.

isoperistaltic a. Anastomosis between two parts of the intestine such that the peristaltic flow in both parts is in the same direction.

magnetic ring a. A surgical instrument that holds two segments of resected bowel together with progressively increasing magnetic force. It is used to help restore bowel continuity in patients who have had colonic resection. It consists of two cobalt magnetic circles embedded in polyester and applied to the bowel so that the submucosal layers of the resected bowel segments are brought into tight apposition. After 7 to 12 days of intestinal healing, the submucosal and intermediate layers of bowel necrose, and the intestines expel the magnets by peristalsis.

PATIENT CARE: The patient is observed for evidence of dehiscence. Stools are examined for unusual amounts of bleeding and for the passage of the magnetic ring.

precapillary a. Anastomosis between small arteries just before they become capillaries.

Schmiedel's a. Abnormal communications between the vena cava and the portal system.

side-to-side a. Anastomosis between two structures lying or positioned beside each other.

terminoterminal a. Anastomosis between the peripheral end of an artery and the central end of the corresponding vein and between the distal end of the artery and the terminal end of the vein.

ureterotubal a. Anastomosis between the uterus and fallopian tube.

ureteroureteral a. Anastomosis between two parts of the same ureter.

anatomic, anatomical (ăn″ă-tŏm′ĭk, -tŏm′ĭ-kăl) [Gr. *anatome*, dissection] Rel. to the anatomy of an organism.

anatomical snuffbox Tabatière anatomique.

anatomist (ă-năt′ō-mĭst) A specialist in the field of anatomy.

anatomy (ă-năt′ō-mē) [Gr. *anatome*, dissection] **1.** The structure of an organism. **2.** The branch of science dealing with the structure of organisms.

applied a. Application of anatomy to diagnosis and treatment, esp. surgical treatment.

comparative a. Comparison of homologous structures of different animals.

descriptive a. Description of individual parts of the body. SYN: *systematic anatomy.*

developmental a. Embryology of the organism from the time of egg fertilization until adulthood is attained.

gross a. Study of structures able to be seen with the naked eye. SYN: *macroscopic a.*

macroscopic a. Gross a.

microscopic a. Study of structure by use of a microscope. SYN: *histology.*

morbid a. Pathological a.

pathological a. Study of the structure of abnormal, diseased, or injured tissue. SYN: *morbid a.*

radiological a. Anatomical study based on the radiological appearance of tissues and organs. SYN: *x-ray a.*

sectional a. Study of anatomy from transverse, sagittal, coronal, or oblique sections. Many digital imaging systems present only sectional images.

surface a. Study of form and markings of the surface of the body, esp. as they relate to underlying structures.

systematic a. Descriptive a.

topographic a. Study of the structure and form of a portion of the body with particular emphasis on the relationships of the parts to each other.

x-ray a. Radiological a.

anatoxin (ăn″ă-tŏks′ĭn) [Gr. *ana*, backward, + *toxikon*, poison] A toxin that has been deactivated so that it can no longer destroy cells but can still stimulate the production of antibodies when injected. SYN: *toxoid.* **anatoxic** (-tŏks′ĭk), *adj.*

anatricrotism (ăn″ă-trĭk′rō-tĭzm) [Gr. *ana*, up, + *tresis*, three, + *krotos*, stroke] The existence of three beats on the ascending line of a sphygmogram. **anatricrotic** (-trī-krŏt′ĭk), *adj.*

anatripsis (ăn″ă-trĭp′sĭs) [″ + *tripsis*, friction] Therapeutic use of rubbing or friction massage.

anatriptic (ăn″ă-trĭp′tĭk) [″ + *tripsis*, friction] **1.** Pert to anatripsis. **2.** An agent applied by rubbing.

anatropia (ăn″ă-trō′pē-ă) [″ + *trope*, a turning] Tendency of eyeballs to turn upward. SYN: *anaphoria.*

anaxon(e) (ăn-ăk′sŏn) [Gr. *an*-, not, + *axon*, axis] A nerve cell, as of the retina, having no axon.

ANC *absolute neutrophil count.*

A.N.C. *Army Nurse Corps.*

anchor (ăng′ker) [Gr. *ankyra*, anchor] **1.** Any structure that provides stability for a prosthetic dental appliance such as a crown, bridge, or denture. The anchor may be a metal or ceramic implant; a cast restoration, such as a crown; or a natural tooth. **2.** In emergency medicine, to tie or attach a rope or sling so it will not move and can support the weight of the rescuers, basket, and patient. **3.** A tree, rock, door casing, or other strong stable device that will not move when a rescuer and patient's weight are attached to it. **4.** In cell biology, a scaffold within the cell or its membranes, on which enzymes or other important molecules are suspended.

anchorage (ăng′kĕr-ĭj) **1.** Surgical fixation, as of prolapsed abdominal organs. **2.** The fixation of a prosthesis to a fixed support structure or anchor.

ancillary (ăn′sĭl-lār″ē) [L. *ancillaris*, handmaid] **1.** Subordinate, secondary. **2.** Auxiliary, supplementary.

anconad (ăn′kō-năd) [Gr. *ankon*, elbow, + L. *ad*, to] Toward the elbow.

anconagra (ăn″kŏn-ăg′ră) [″ + *agra*, a seizure] Gout of the elbow.

anconal, anconeal (ăn′kō-năl, ăn-kō′nē-ăl) Pert. to the elbow.

anconal fossa, anconeal fossa Fossa olecrani; the hollow on the distal end of the humerus, in which the olecranon rests when the elbow is extended.

anconeus (ăn-kō′nē-ŭs) [Gr. *ankon*, elbow] The short extensor muscle of the forearm, located on the back of the elbow. It arises from the back portion of the lateral epicondyle of the humerus, and its fibers insert on the side of the olecranon and upper fourth of the shaft of the ulna. It extends the forearm and abducts the ulna in pronation of the wrist.

anconitis (ăn″kō-nī′tĭs) [″ + *itis*, inflammation] Inflammation of the elbow joint.

ancrod An enzyme purified from the venom of a Malayan pit viper and used as an anticoagulant.

Ancylostoma (ăn″sĭl-ŏs′tō-mă) [Gr. *ankylos*, crooked, + *stoma*, mouth] A genus of nematodes of the family Ancylostomatidae whose members are intestinal parasites and include the hookworms.

A. braziliense Species of hookworm that infests dogs and cats and may cause cutaneous larva migrans in humans. SEE: *larva migrans, cutaneous.*

A. caninum Species of hookworm that infests dogs and cats and may cause cutaneous larva migrans in humans. SEE: *larva migrans, cutaneous.*

A. duodenale Species of hookworm that commonly infests humans, causing ancylostomiasis; widely found in temperate regions. SEE: *Necator americanus.*

Ancylostomatidae (ăn″sĭ-lŏs″tō-măt′ĭ-dē) A family of nematodes belonging to the suborder Strongylata. It includes the genera *Ancylostoma* and *Necator*, common hookworms of humans.

ancylostomiasis (ăn″sĭ-lŏs-tō-mī′ă-sĭs) [Gr. *ankylos*, crooked, + *stoma*, mouth, + *-iasis*, condition] Hookworm.

ancyroid (ăn′sĭ-royd) [Gr. *ankyra*, anchor, + *eidos*, form, shape] Shaped like the fluke of an anchor.

Andernach's ossicles (ŏn′dĕr-nŏks) [Johann Winther von Andernach, Ger. physician, 1487–1574] A rarely used term for wormian, or sutural bones.

Andersen's disease [Dorothy H. Andersen, U.S. pediatrician, 1901–1963] Glycogen storage disease, type IV. SEE: *glycogen storage disease*.

andro- [Gr. *andros*, man] Combining form meaning *man, male*, or *masculine*.

androgalactozemia (ăn″drō-găl-ăk″tō-zē′mē-ă) [″ + *gala*, milk, + *zemia*, loss] Oozing of milk from a man's breast.

androstenedione A precursor of testosterone used orally by some athletes to enhance performance or increase body bulk.

androgen (ăn′drō-jĕn) [Gr. *andros*, man, + *gennan*, to produce] A substance producing or stimulating the development of male characteristics (masculinization), such as the hormones testosterone and androsterone.

androgenic (ăn″drō-jĕn′ĭk) Causing masculinization. SYN: *andromimetic*.

androgyne (ăn′drō-jīn) [″ + *gyne*, woman] A female pseudohermaphrodite. SYN: *androgynus*.

androgynoid (ăn-drŏj′ĭ-noyd) [″ + ″ + *eidos*, form, shape] A person possessing female gonads (ovaries) but secondary sex characteristics of a male (a female pseudohermaphrodite). Term is less commonly used for a person possessing male gonads (testes) but secondary sex characteristics of a female (a male pseudohermaphrodite).

androgynous (ăn-drŏj′ĭ-nŭs) [″ + *gyne*, woman] **1.** Resembling or pert. to an androgynoid. **2.** Without definite sexual characteristics.

androgynus (ăn-drŏj′ĭ-nŭs) A female pseudohermaphrodite. SYN: *androgyne*.

android (ăn′droyd) [″ + *eidos*, form, shape] Resembling a male; manlike.

andromimetic (ăn″drō-mĭ-mĕt′ĭk) [″ + *mimetikos*, imitative] Androgenic.

andromorphous (ăn″drō-mor′fŭs) [″ + *morphe*, form] Resembling a male in physical structure and appearance.

androphobia (ăn″drō-fō′bē-ă) [″ + *phobos*, fear] Morbid fear of the male sex.

androstane (ăn′drō-stān) A steroid hydrocarbon, $C_{19}H_{32}$, that is the precursor of androgenic hormones.

androsterone (ăn″drō-stĕr′ōn, ăn-drŏs′tĕr-ōn) $C_{19}H_{30}O_2$; an androgenic steroid found in the urine. It is a metabolite of testosterone and androstenedione. It has been synthesized. As one of the androgens (male sex hormones), androsterone contributes to the characteristic changes of growth and development of the genitals and axillary and pubic hair, deepening of the voice, and development of the sweat glands in the male.

-ane In chemistry, a suffix indicating a saturated hydrocarbon.

anecdotal evidence (ăn″ĭk-dōt′l) [Gr. *an*, not, + *ekdotos*, given out] Clinical lore based on the analysis of individual cases, rather than the study of scientifically randomized groups of patients.

anecdotal records Notes used in nursing education to document observed incidents of a student's clinical behavior related to attainment of clinical learning objectives. Such anecdotal notes have been upheld in court as documented evidence for failing a student; the notes have not been treated as hearsay evidence.

anechoic room A room in which the boundaries are made so that all sound produced in the room is absorbed (i.e., not reflected).

Anel's operation (ă-nĕlz′) [Dominique Anel, Fr. surgeon, 1679–1725] Ligation of an artery immediately above and on the proximal side of an aneurysm.

anemia (ă-nē′mē-ă) [Gr. *an-*, not, + *haima*, blood] A reduction in the mass of circulating red blood cells. Generally, people are considered anemic when their hemoglobin levels are more than two standard deviations below the mean level in their hospital's laboratory. The diagnosis of anemia is influenced by variables such as the patient's age (neonates are anemic at levels of hemoglobin that would be considered polycythemic in some adults), gender (men have higher hemoglobin levels than women), pregnancy status (hemodilution in pregnancy lowers measured hemoglobin), residential altitude, and ethnic or racial background.

Symptomatic anemia exists when hemoglobin content is less than that required to meet the oxygen-carrying demands of the body. If anemia develops slowly, however, there may be no functional impairment even though the hemoglobin is less than 7 g/100 ml of blood.

Anemia is not a disease but rather a symptom of other illnesses. Commonly, it is classified on the basis of mean corpuscular volume as microcytic (<80), normocytic (80–94), and macrocytic (94); on the basis of mean corpuscular hemoglobin as hypochromic (<27), normochromic (27–32), and hyperchromic (>32); and on the basis of etiological factors.

ETIOLOGY: Anemia may be caused by bleeding (e.g., from the gastrointestinal tract or the uterus); vitamin or mineral deficiencies (esp. vitamin B_{12}, folate, or iron deficiencies); decreases in red blood cell production (e.g., bone marrow suppression in kidney failure or bone marrow failure in myelodysplastic syndromes); increases in red blood cell destruction (e.g., hemolysis due to sickle cell disease); or increases in red blood cell sequestration by the spleen (e.g., portal hypertension).

SYMPTOMS: Anemic patients may experience weakness, fatigue, lightheadedness, breathlessness, palpitations, angina pectoris, and headache. Signs of anemia may include a rapid pulse or rapid breathing if blood loss occurs rapidly. Chronically anemic persons may have pale skin, mucous membranes, or nailbeds; fissures at the corners of the mouth; among other signs.

TREATMENT: Treatment of anemia must be specific for the cause. The prognosis for recovery from anemia is excellent if the underlying cause is treatable.

Anemia due to excessive blood loss: For acute blood loss, immediate measures should be taken to stop the bleeding, to restore blood volume by transfusion, and to combat shock. Chronic blood loss usually produces iron-deficiency anemia.

Anemia due to excessive blood cell destruction: The specific hemolytic disorder should be treated.

Anemia due to decreased blood cell formation: For deficiency states, replacement therapy is used to combat the specific deficiency (e.g., iron, vitamin B_{12}, folic acid, ascorbic acid). For bone marrow disorders, if anemia is due to a toxic state, removal of the toxic agent may result in spontaneous recovery.

Anemia due to renal failure: Erythropoietin injections are helpful.

PATIENT CARE: The patient is evaluated for signs and symptoms, and the results of laboratory studies are reviewed for evidence of inadequate erythropoiesis or premature erythrocyte destruction. Prescribed diagnostic studies are scheduled and carried out. *Rest*: The patient is evaluated for fatigue; care and activities are planned and regular rest periods are scheduled. *Mouth care*: The patient's mouth is inspected daily for glossitis, mouth lesions, or ulcers. The sponge stick is recommended for oral care, and alkaline mouthwashes are suggested if mouth ulcers are present. A dental consultation may be required. *Diet*: The patient is encouraged to eat small portions at frequent intervals. Mouth care is provided before meals. The nurse or a nutritionist provides counseling based on type of anemia. *Medications*: Health care professionals teach the patient about medication actions, desired effects, adverse reactions, and correct dosing and administration. *Patient education*: The cause of the anemia and the rationale for prescribed treatment are explained to the patient and family. Teaching should cover the prescribed rest and activity regimen, diet, prevention of infection including the need for frequent temperature checks, and the continuing need for periodic blood testing and medical evaluation. SEE: *Nursing Diagnoses Appendix.*

achlorhydric a. A hypochromic, microcytic anemia associated with a lack of free hydrochloric acid in gastric juice.

aplastic a. Anemia caused by deficient red cell production due to bone marrow disorders. SEE: illus; *marrow* for illus. of normal marrow.

ETIOLOGY: Idiopathic cases range from 40% to 70% and are most common in adolescents and young adults. Exposure to chemical and antineoplastic agents and ionizing radiation can result in aplastic anemia and chronic renal failure; and infiltration of the bone marrow by cells that are not normally present there can interfere with normal blood production. Examples are metastatic carcinoma, miliary tuberculosis. A congenital form has been described.

TREATMENT: Most patients can be treated effectively with bone marrow transplantation or immunosuppressive drugs.

PATIENT CARE: The patient and family are educated about the cause and treatment of the illness. Measures to prevent infection are explained, and the importance of adequate rest is emphasized. In the acute phase, prescribed treatment is carried out, the side effects of drugs and transfusions are explained, and a restful environment is ensured. If the patient's platelet count is low (less than 20,000/cu mm), the following steps are taken to prevent hemorrhage: avoiding parenteral injections, suggesting the use of an electric razor, humidifying oxygen to prevent dry mucous membranes, and promoting regular bowel movements with stool softeners and dietary measures. Pressure is applied to all venipuncture sites until bleeding has stopped, and bleeding is detected early by checking for occult blood in urine and stools and by assessing the skin for pe-

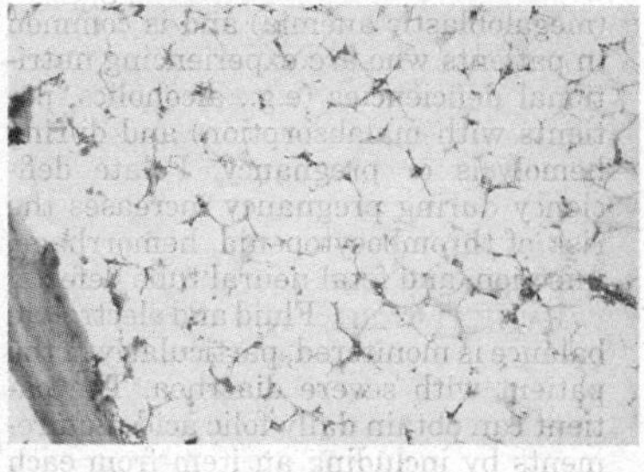

APLASTIC ANEMIA

Normal blood-forming cells are absent (×200)

techiae and ecchymoses. Universal precautions and careful handwashing (and protective isolation if necessary) are used, a diet high in vitamins and protein is provided, and meticulous oral and perianal care are provided. The patient is assessed for life-threatening hemorrhage, infection, adverse effects of drug therapy, or blood transfusion reactions. Throat, urine, and blood cultures are done regularly. SEE: *protective isolation.*

autoimmune hemolytic a. ABBR: AIHA. Anemia caused by antibodies produced by the patient's own immune system that destroy red blood cells. They are classified by the thermal properties of the antibody involved; the "warm" form is most common and may be associated with viral infections. Drug-induced hemolytic anemias are clinically indistinguishable from AIHA; for that reason, they are classified with this disorder.

congenital hemolytic a. A group of inherited chronic diseases marked by disintegration of red blood cells, jaundice, splenomegaly, and gallstones. Hereditary spherocytosis is the most common of these hemolytic diseases. Other congenital hemolytic anemias include congenital elliptocytosis and hereditary stomatocytosis, and hemolytic anemias due to enzymatic defects of the red cell, of which G-6-PD and pyruvate kinase deficiency are the most important. SYN: *hemolytic icterus; hemolytic jaundice.* SEE: *glucose-6-phosphate dehydrogenase.*

Cooley's a. Erythroblastic a.

deficiency a. Condition resulting from lack of an essential ingredient, such as iron or vitamins, in the diet or the inability of the intestine to absorb them. SYN: *nutritional a.*

erythroblastic a. Anemia resulting from inheritance of a recessive trait responsible for interference with hemoglobin synthesis. SYN: *Cooley's a.; thalassemia major.*

folic acid deficiency a. Anemia resulting from a deficiency of folic acid. It is a cause of red blood cell enlargement (megaloblastic anemia) and is common in patients who are experiencing nutritional deficiencies (e.g., alcoholics, patients with malabsorption) and during hemolysis or pregnancy. Folate deficiency during pregnancy increases the risk of thrombocytopenia, hemorrhage, infection, and fetal neural tube defects.

PATIENT CARE: Fluid and electrolyte balance is monitored, particularly in the patient with severe diarrhea. The patient can obtain daily folic acid requirements by including an item from each food group in every meal; a list of foods rich in folic acid (green leafy vegetables, asparagus, broccoli, liver, organ meats, milk, eggs, yeast, wheat germ, kidney beans, beef, potatoes, dried peas and beans, whole-grain cereals, nuts, bananas, cantaloupe, lemons, and strawberries) is provided. The rationale for replacement therapy is explained, and the patient is advised not to stop treatment until test results return to normal.

hemolytic a. Anemia as the result of the destruction of red blood cells (RBCs) by drugs, artificial heart valves, toxins, snake venoms, infections, and antibodies. Drugs may either destroy the RBC membrane directly or may stimulate production of autoantibodies that lyse (kill) the RBCs. Children may develop hemolytic anemia in response to destruction of RBCs by viral and bacterial organisms. Artificial valves cause physical damage to the RBC membrane during the circulation of blood through the heart. SEE: *hemolytic uremic syndrome.*

hyperchromic a. Anemia in which mean corpuscular hemoglobin concentration (MCHC) is greater than normal. The red blood cells are darker staining than normal.

hypochromic a. Anemia in which hemoglobin is deficient and mean corpuscular hemoglobin concentration is less than normal.

hypoplastic a. Term that has been used to describe aplastic anemia. If anemia due to failure of formation of red blood cells is meant, pure red blood cell aplasia is the term of choice.

iron-deficiency a. Anemia resulting from a greater demand on stored iron than can be supplied. The red blood cell count may sometimes be normal, but there will be insufficient hemoglobin. Erythrocytes will be pale (hypochromia) and have abnormal shapes (poikilocytosis). This condition is present in about 8% of men and 14% of women aged 3 to 74 years in U.S.

ETIOLOGY: The condition is caused by inadequate iron intake, malabsorption of iron, blood loss, pregnancy and lactation, intravascular hemolysis, or a combination of these factors.

SYMPTOMS: Chronically anemic patients often complain of fatigue and dyspnea on exertion. Iron deficiency resulting from rapid bleeding may produce palpitations, orthostatic dizziness, or syncope.

DIAGNOSIS: Laboratory studies reveal decreased iron levels in the blood, with elevated iron-binding capacity, and a diminished transferrin saturation. Ferritin levels are low. The bone marrow does not show stainable iron.

ADDITIONAL DIAGNOSTIC STUDIES: Adult nonmenstruating patients with iron-deficiency anemia should be evaluated to rule out a source of bleeding in the gastrointestinal tract.

TREATMENT: Dietary iron intake is supplemented with oral ferrous sulfate or ferrous gluconate (with vitamin C to increase iron absorption). When underlying lesions are found in the gastrointestinal tract (e.g. ulcers, esophagitis, cancer of the colon) they are treated with medications or surgery.

macrocytic a. Anemia marked by abnormally large erythrocytes.

Mediterranean a. SEE: *thalassemia.*

megaloblastic a. Anemia in which megaloblasts are found in the blood.

microcytic a. Anemia marked by abnormally small red blood cells.

milk a. In a young child, iron-deficiency anemia caused by consistent consumption of milk in amounts greater than 1 qt daily. This excessive milk intake displaces iron-rich foods in the diet.

a. of the newborn Hemoglobin levels less than 14 g/dl in term newborns. Common causes include: peripartum bleeding, hemolytic disease of the newborn, and impaired red cell manufacture caused by glucose-6-phosphate dehydrogenase deficiency.

normochromic a. Anemia in which the red blood cells contain the normal amount of hemoglobin.

normocytic a. Anemia in which the size and hemoglobin content of red blood cells remain normal.

nutritional a. Deficiency a.

pernicious a. A chronic, macrocytic anemia marked by achlorhydria. It occurs most often in 40- to 80-year-old northern Europeans of fair skin, but has been reported in other races and ethnic groups. It is rare in blacks and Asians.

ETIOLOGY: Pernicious anemia is an autoimmune disease. The parietal cells of the stomach lining fail to secrete enough intrinsic factor to ensure intestinal absorption of vitamin B_{12}, the extrinsic factor. This is due to atrophy of the glandular mucosa of the fundus of the stomach and is associated with absence of hydrochloric acid.

SYMPTOMS: Symptoms include weakness, sore tongue, paresthesias (tingling and numbness) of extremities, and gastrointestinal symptoms such as diarrhea, nausea, vomiting, and pain; in severe anemia, there may be signs of cardiac failure.

TREATMENT: Vitamin B_{12} is given parenterally or, in patients who respond, orally.

physiological a. of pregnancy Pseudoanemia of pregnancy.

pure red cell aplasia a. Anemia due to decreased production of red cells.

runner's a. Mild hemolysis with hematuria, hemoglobinemia, and hemoglobinuria produced by strenuous exercise including running. Blood may be lost in the feces, presumably due to transient ischemia of the gut during vigorous exercise.

septic a. Anemia due to severe infection.

sickle cell a. An inherited disorder transmitted as an autosomal recessive trait that causes an abnormality of the globin genes in hemoglobin. The frequency of the genetic defect responsible for this chronic anemia disorder is highest among African-American, native African, and Mediterranean populations. Approximately 75,000 people in the U.S. have sickle cell anemia. The illness affects one of every 500 African-American babies. Roughly 8% of the African-American population carries the sickle cell trait. Sickle cell anemia during pregnancy increases the risk of crisis, pre-eclampsia, urinary tract infection, congestive heart failure, and pulmonary infarction. Use of supplemental oxygen during labor is recommended. SEE: *hemoglobin S disease;* illus.; *Nursing Diagnoses Appendix.*

ETIOLOGY: When both parental genes carry the same defect, the person is homozygous for hemoglobin S, that is, HbSS, and manifests the disorder. When exposed to a decrease in oxygen, hemoglobin S becomes viscous. This causes the red cells to become crescent-shaped (sickling), rigid, sticky, and fragile. When they clump together, circulation through the capillaries is impeded, causing obstruction, tissue hypoxia, and further sickling. In infants younger than 5 months old, high levels of fetal hemoglobin inhibit the reaction of the hemoglobin S molecule to decreased oxygen.

SYMPTOMS: The shortened lifespan of the abnormal red cells (10 to 20 days) results in a chronic anemia; pallor, weakness, and fatigue are common. Jaundice may result from the hemolysis of red cells. Crisis may occur as a result of sickling, thrombi formation, vascular occlusion, tissue hypoxia, and infarction. SEE: *sickle cell crisis*.

TREATMENT: Supportive therapy includes supplemental iron and blood transfusion. Administration of hydroxyurea stimulates the production of hemoglobin S and decreases the need for blood transfusions and painful crises. Prophylactic daily doses of penicillin have demonstrated effectiveness in reducing the incidence of acute bacterial infections in children.

PATIENT CARE: Sickle cell crisis should be suspected in the sickle cell patient with pale lips, tongue, palms, or nailbeds; lethargy; listlessness; difficulty awakening; irritability; severe pain; or temperature over 104°F (37.8°C) lasting at least 2 days. During a crisis, warm compresses are applied to

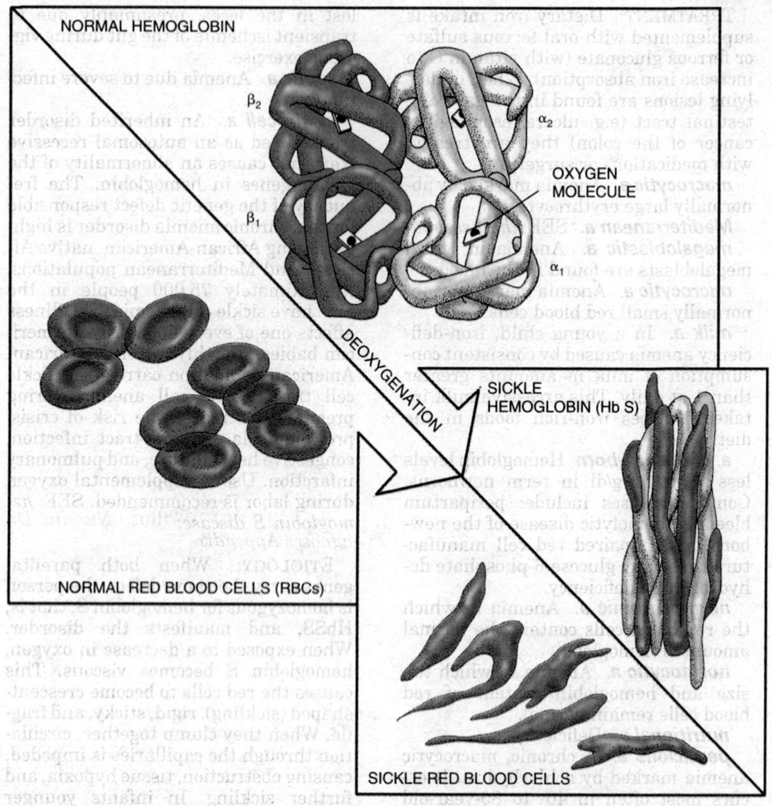

SICKLE CELL ANEMIA

Structure of hemoglobin A and hemoglobin S and their effect on erythrocytes

the painful areas, and the patient is covered with a blanket. (Cold compresses aggravate the condition.) Prescribed analgesic-antipyretics such as aspirin or acetaminophen are given. Bedrest is encouraged, with the patient in a sitting position. Dehydration and severe pain are the two chief reasons for hospitalization; the patient should increase fluid intake to prevent dehydration that may result from impaired urine-concentrating ability. During remission, the patient can prevent exacerbations by avoiding tight clothing that restricts circulation; strenuous exercise; vasoconstricting drugs; cold temperatures; and unpressurized aircraft, high altitudes, and other hypoxia-provoking conditions. Parents are warned against being overprotective. The child must avoid strenuous exercise and body-contact sports but can still enjoy most activities. Parents are referred for genetic counseling regarding risks to future children, and screening of family members is recommended to determine heterozygote carriers. Both parents and patients are referred to community-based support groups; parents may also require psychological counseling to cope with guilt feelings.

splenic a. Enlargement of the spleen due to portal or splenic hypertension with accompanying anemia, leukopenia, thrombocytopenia, and gastric hemorrhage. SYN: *Banti's syndrome; congestive splenomegalia.*

transfusion-dependent a. Anemia for which the only effective therapy is repeated blood transfusions.

anemic (ă-nē′mĭk) Pert. to anemia; deficient in red blood cells, in hemoglobin, or in volume of blood.

anemometer In pulmonary function studies, a device for measuring the rate of air flow through a tube. The rate at which air flows into or out of the lung may be measured by using a calibrated anemometer.

anemophobia (ăn″ĕ-mō-fō′bē-ă) [Gr. *anemos*, wind, + *phobos*, fear] Morbid fear of drafts or of the wind.

anencephalus (ăn″ĕn-sĕf′ă-lŭs) [Gr. *an-*, not, + *enkephalos*, the brain] Congenital absence of the brain and cranial vault, with the cerebral hemispheres missing or reduced to small masses. This condition is incompatible with life. SEE: *neural tube defect.*

anephric Without kidneys.

anephrogenesis (ă-nĕf″rō-jĕn′ĕ-sĭs) [Gr. *a-*, not, + *nephros*, kidney, + *genesis*, generation, birth] Congenital absence of the kidneys.

anergasia (ăn″ĕr-gā′sē-ă) [Gr. *an-*, not + *ergon*, work] Anergia; functional inactivity resulting from a structural lesion of the central nervous system.

anergastic reaction (ăn″ĕr-găs′tĭk) Disorder involving cerebral lesions or organic psychoses; marked by loss of memory and impairment of mental activity, function, or judgment.

anergia (ăn-ĕr′jē-ă) [″ + *ergon*, work] Inactivity; lack of energy.

anergy (ăn′ĕr-jē) **1.** Impaired or absent ability to react to common antigens administered through skin testing. **2.** Lack of energy. **anergic** (ăn-ĕr′jĭk), *adj.*

aneroid (ăn′ĕr-ŏyd) [Gr. *a-*, not, + *neron*, water, + *eidos*, form, shape] Operating without fluid, such as an aneroid barometer that uses atmospheric pressure instead of a liquid such as mercury.

anerythroplasia (ăn″ĕ-rĭth″rō-plā′zē-ă) [Gr. *an-*, not, + *erythros*, red, + *plasis*, a molding] Absence of red blood cell formation in the bone marrow. **anerythroplastic** (-plăs′tĭk), *adj.*

anerythropsia (ăn″ĕ-rĭ-thrŏp′sē-ă) [″ + ″ + *opsis*, vision] Inability to distinguish clearly the color red.

anesthecinesia, anesthekinesia (ăn-ĕs-thē″sĭn-ē′zē-ă, -kĭ-nē′zē-ă) [″ + *aisthesis*, sensation, + *kinesis*, movement] Sensory and motor paralysis.

anesthesia (ăn″ĕs-thē′zē-ă) [″ + *aisthesis*, sensation] **1.** Partial or complete loss of sensation, with or without loss of consciousness, as a result of disease, injury, or administration of an anesthetic agent, usually by injection or inhalation.

SIGNS: The signs of depth of anesthesia, based on pupillary size, eye motion, and the character of respirations as originally described for ether, have been found to be unreliable and poorly correlated with the alveolar concentration of anesthetic. The types of medicines used for premedication as well as the type of anesthetic employed will influence the signs of anesthesia.

PATIENT CARE: *Preoperative:* Before induction of anesthesia, hearing aids, dentures, wristwatch, and jewelry are removed. If a menstruating female is using a tampon, it is removed and replaced with a perineal pad.

Postoperative: During emergence from general anesthesia, the patient's airway is protected and vital signs monitored. Level of consciousness, status of protective reflexes, motor activity, and emotional state are evaluated. The patient is reoriented to person, place, and time; this information is repeated as often as necessary. For patients who have received ketamine, a quiet area with minimal stimulation is provided. Before nerve block anesthesia, an intravenous infusion is established to ensure hydration. The patient is protected with side rails and other safety measures, and the anesthetized body part is protected from prolonged pressure. For regional anesthesia, sympathetic blockade is assessed by monitoring sensory levels along with vital signs (the block will wear off from head to toe, except for the sacrum and perineum, which wear off last). In obstetrics, maternal hypotension results in diminished placental perfusion and potential fetal compromise. Outcomes indicating returned sympathetic innervation include stable vital signs and temperature, ability to vasoconstrict, perianal pinprick sensations ("anal wink"), plantar flexion of the foot against resistance, and ability to sense whether the great toe is flexed or extended. It is ensured that the patient can urinate, and that the patient with postanesthesia headache remains flat in bed. Prescribed analgesics are administered, comfort measures, abdominal support, and position changes are provided, and fluids are offered to increase hydration.

2. The science and practice of anesthesiology.

audio a. Anesthesia produced by sound; used by dentists to inhibit pain perception.

basal a. A level of unconsciousness that is just above the level of complete surgical anesthesia. The patient does not respond to verbal stimuli but does react to noxious stimuli, such as a pinprick. Basal anesthesia is useful in combination with local or regional anesthesia, making the patient unaware of the surgical experience.

block a. A regional anesthetic injected into a nerve (intraneural) or immediately around it (paraneural). SYN: *conduction a.; neural a.*

bulbar a. Anesthesia produced by a lesion of the pons.

caudal a. Anesthesia produced by insertion of a needle into the sacrococcygeal notch and injection of a local anesthetic into the epidural space.

central a. Pathological anesthesia due to a lesion of the central nervous system.

closed a. Inhalation anesthesia tech-

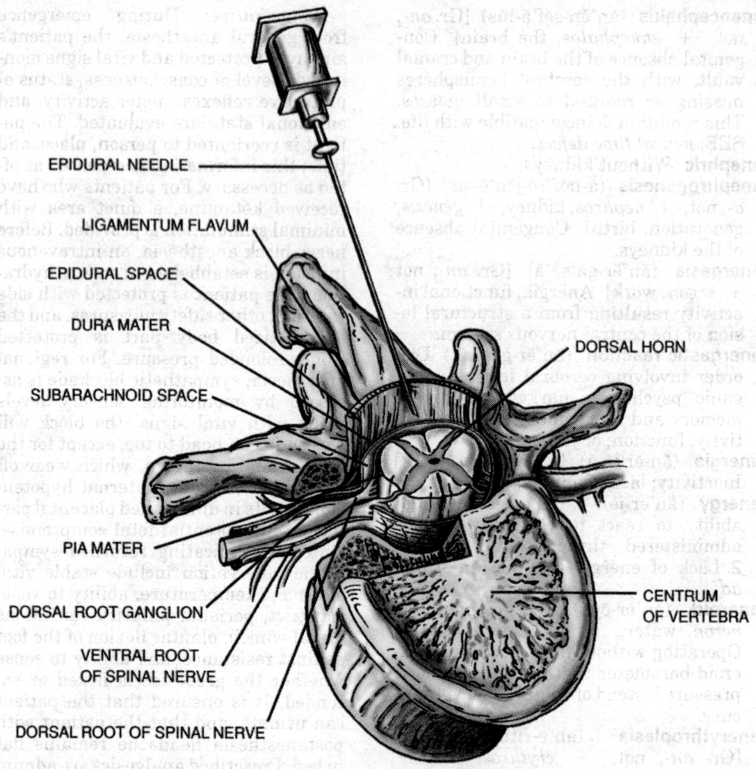

EPIDURAL ANESTHESIA

Injection of epidural needle into epidural space

nique in which the gases are rebreathed. This requires appropriate treatment of the exhaled gas in order to absorb the expired carbon dioxide and to replenish the oxygen and the anesthetic.

conduction a. Block a.

crossed a. Anesthesia of the side opposite to the site of a central nervous system lesion.

dissociative a. A type of anesthesia marked by catalepsy, amnesia, and marked analgesia. The patient experiences a strong feeling of dissociation from the environment.

a. dolorosa Pain in an anesthetized zone, as in thalamic lesions.

electric a. Anesthesia induced by the use of an electric current.

endotracheal a. Anesthesia in which gases are administered via a tube inserted into the trachea.

epidural a. Anesthesia produced by injection of a local anesthetic into the peridural space of the spinal cord. SYN: *peridural a.* SEE: illus.

general a. Anesthesia that is complete and affects the entire body with loss of consciousness when the anesthetic acts on the brain. This type of anesthesia is usually accomplished following administration of inhalation or intravenous anesthetics. It is commonly used for surgical procedures.

Gwathmey's a. Anesthesia induced by injection of an olive oil and ether solution into the rectum.

hypotensive a. Anesthesia during which the blood pressure is lowered.

hypothermic a. General anesthesia during which the body temperature is lowered.

hysterical a. Bodily anesthesia occurring in conversion disorders.

ice a. Refrigeration a.

infiltration a. Local anesthesia produced by injection of the local anesthetic solution directly into the tissues, such as injection of procaine solution into the gums for dental procedures.

inhalation a. General anesthesia produced by the inhalation of vapor or gaseous anesthetics such as ether, nitrous oxide, and methoxyflurane.

insufflation a. Instillation of gaseous anesthetics into the inhaled air.

intratracheal a. Anesthesia administered through a catheter passed to the level of the trachea.

local a. The pharmacological inhibition of nerve impulses in a body part, typically to make it easier to treat a small lesion or laceration or to perform minor surgery. Commonly used agents include lidocaine, bupivacaine, or novocaine. All local anesthetic agents work by decreasing the flow of sodium ions into nerve cells, thereby blocking the action potential of the cells. SEE: *block anesthesia; infiltration anesthesia.*

mixed a. General anesthesia produced by more than one drug, such as propofol, for induction followed by an inhaled drug for maintenance of anesthesia.

neural a. Block a.

neuroleptic a. General anesthesia produced by a neuroleptic agent such as droperidol.

open a. Application, usually by dropping, of a volatile anesthetic agent onto gauze held over the nose and mouth.

peridural a. Epidural a.

peripheral a. Local anesthesia produced when a nerve is blocked with an appropriate agent.

primary a. The first stage of anesthesia, before unconsciousness.

pudendal a. A type of local anesthesia used in obstetrics. The pudendal nerve on each side, near the spinous process of the ischium, is blocked.

rectal a. General anesthesia produced by introduction of an anesthetic agent into the rectum, used esp. in managing pediatric patients.

refrigeration a. Anesthesia induced by lowering the temperature of a body part to near freezing either by spraying it with ethyl chloride or by immersing it in a container of finely cracked ice.

regional a. Nerve or field blocking, causing loss of sensation over a particular area. SEE: *block anesthesia; infiltration anesthesia.*

saddle block a. A type of anesthesia produced by introducing the anesthetic agent into the fourth lumbar interspace. This anesthetizes the perineum and the buttocks area.

segmental a. Anesthesia due to a pathological or surgically induced lesion of a nerve root.

sexual a. Loss of genital sensation, with accompanying secondary sexual dysfunction.

spinal a. **1.** Anesthesia resulting from disease or injury to conduction pathways of the spinal cord. **2.** Anesthesia produced by injection of anesthetic into the subarachnoid space of the spinal cord.

splanchnic a. Anesthesia produced by injection of an anesthetic into the splanchnic ganglion.

stages of a. The distinct series of steps through which anesthesia progresses. The first stage of pharmacologically induced general anesthesia includes preliminary excitement until voluntary control is lost. Because hearing is the last sense to be lost, the conversation of operating room staff should be guarded during this stage. The second stage consists of loss of voluntary control. In the third stage there is entire relaxation, no muscular rigidity, and deep regular breathing.

surgical a. Depth of anesthesia at which relaxation of muscles and loss of sensation and consciousness are adequate for the performance of surgery.

tactile a. Loss of sense of touch.

topical a. Local anesthesia induced by application of an anesthetic directly to the surface of the area to be anesthetized.

traumatic a. Loss of sensation resulting from nerve injury.

tumescent a. The injection of large volumes of diluted lidocaine, bicarbonate, and epinephrine subcutaneously for use in local anesthesia. This procedure is most often used prior to liposuction to limit blood loss and pain.

twilight a. State of light anesthesia. SEE: *twilight sleep.*

anesthesiologist (ăn″ĕs-thē″zē-ŏl′ō-jĭst) A physician specializing in anesthesiology.

anesthesiology (ăn″ĕs-thē″zē-ŏl′ō-jē) [″ + ″ + *logos*, word, reason] The branch of medicine concerned with the control of acute or chronic pain; the use of sedative, analgesic, hypnotic, antiemetic, respiratory, and cardiovascular drugs; preoperative assessment, intraoperative patient management, and postoperative care; and autonomic, neuromuscular, cardiac, and respiratory physiology.

anesthetic (ăn″ĕs-thĕt′ĭk) **1.** Pert. to or producing anesthesia. **2.** An agent that produces anesthesia; subdivided into inhaled, intravenous, general, or local, according to its action and administration. SEE: *anesthesia.*

anesthetist (ă-nĕs′thĕ-tĭst) One who administers anesthetics, esp. for general anesthesia; may be an anesthesiologist or specially trained nurse.

anesthetization (ă-nĕs″thĕ-tĭ-zā′shŭn) Induction of anesthesia.

anesthetize (ă-nĕs′thĕ-tīz) To induce anesthesia.

anetoderma (ăn″ĕt-ō-dĕr′mă) [Gr. *anetos*, relaxed, + *derma*, skin] Localized laxity of the skin with protruding, saclike areas. These lesions are due to loss of normal skin elasticity. They may be excised. SYN: *macular atrophy.*

aneuploidy (ăn″ū-ploy′dē) [Gr. *an-*, not, + *eu*, well, + *ploos*, fold, + *eidos*, form, shape] Condition of having an abnormal number of chromosomes for the species indicated. **aneuploid** (ăn′ū-ployd), *adj.*

aneurysm (ăn′ū-rĭzm) [Gr. *aneurysma*, a widening] Localized abnormal dilatation of a blood vessel, usually an artery; due to a congenital defect or weakness in the wall of the vessel. SEE: illus.

ETIOLOGY: In the aorta, atherosclerosis is the most common cause. Syphilitic aneurysms occasionally are seen in the ascending aorta. Bacterial or mycotic infection and trauma are common causes of aneurysms in peripheral arteries.

abdominal aortic a. ABBR: AAA. A localized dilatation (saccular, fusiform, or dissecting) of the wall of the abdominal aorta (the portion of the descending aorta that passes from the aortic hiatus of the diaphragm into the abdomen, descending ventral to the vertebral column, and ending at the fourth lumbar vertebra where it divides into the two common iliac arteries). It is generally found to involve the renal arteries and frequently the iliac arteries. Occasionally the dilatation can extend upward through the diaphragm.

SYMPTOMS: Symptoms, when present, include generalized abdominal pain, low back pain unaffected by movement, sensations of gastric or abdominal fullness, sudden lumbar or abdominal pain radiating to the flank and groin. Signs can include a pulsating mass in the periumbilical area, and a systolic bruit over the aorta.

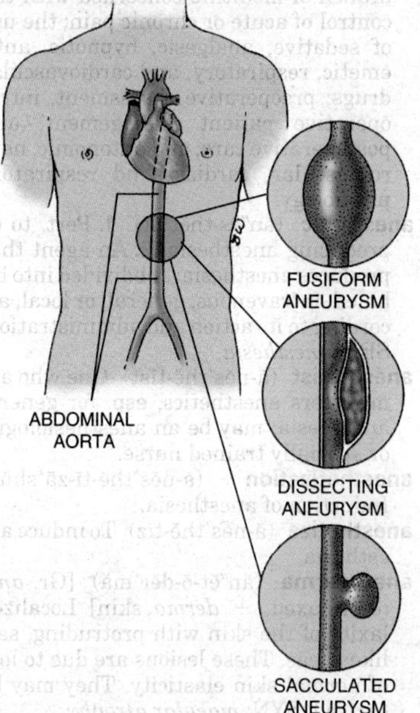

AORTIC ANEURYSMS

TREATMENT: If untreated, most abdominal aneurysms will continue to enlarge and may rupture. Surgical repair is recommended for all aneurysms 6 cm or greater in size. If an aneurysm is tender and known to be enlarging rapidly (no matter what its size), surgery is strongly recommended. Surgical therapy consists of replacing the aneurysmal segment with a synthetic fabric graft. Immediate surgery is indicated for ruptured aortic abdominal aneurysm.

PATIENT CARE: In acute situations, arterial blood gas values and cardiac rhythm are monitored, and a pulmonary artery line is inserted to monitor hemodynamics. The patient is observed for signs of rupture, which may be fatal; these include acute blood loss and shock; increasing pulse and respiratory rates; cool, clammy skin; restlessness; and decreased sensorium. Palpation of the abdomen for a mass is avoided if abdominal aortic aneurysm has been diagnosed or is suspected, because deep palpation may precipitate rupture.

Prescribed medications are administered, and the patient is instructed in their use. In acute situations, admission to the intensive care unit is arranged, a blood sample is obtained for typing and crossmatching, and a large-bore (14G) venous catheter is inserted to facilitate blood replacement. The patient is prepared for, and informed about, elective surgery if indicated or emergency surgery if rupture occurs.

Desired outcomes include the patient's ability to express anxiety, use support systems, and perform stress reduction techniques that assist with coping; demonstrated abatement of physical signs of anxiety; avoidance of activities that increase the risk of rupture; understanding of and cooperation with the prescribed treatment regimen; ability to identify indications of rupture and to institute emergency measures; maintenance of normal fluid and blood volume in acute situations; and recovery from elective or emergency surgery with no complications.

PREVENTION: Because of the relatively high incidence of AAA in men over age 60 (esp. those with hypertension), screening for AAA is recommended in this population.

aortic a. An aneurysm affecting any part of the aorta from the aortic valve to the iliac arteries. The dilated artery usually is asymptomatic and often identified by chance.

arteriovenous a. An aneurysm of congenital or traumatic origin in which an artery and vein become connected. Symptoms may include pain, expansive pulsation, and bruits, or occasionally, high output heart failure.

atherosclerotic a. Aneurysm due to degeneration or weakening of the arterial wall caused by atherosclerosis.

berry a. A small saccular congenital aneurysm of a cerebral vessel. It communicates with the vessel by a small opening. Rupture of this type of aneurysm may cause subarachnoid hemorrhage, a devastating form of stroke.

cerebral a. Aneurysm of a blood vessel in the brain.

cirsoid a. A dilatation of a network of vessels commonly occurring on the scalp. The mass may form a pulsating subcutaneous tumor. SYN: *racemose a.*

compound a. Aneurysm in which some of the layers of the vessel are ruptured and others dilated.

dissecting a. Aneurysm in which the blood makes its way between the layers of a blood vessel wall, separating them; a result of necrosis of the medial portion of the arterial wall. SEE: *aneurysm* for illus.

fusiform a. Aneurysm in which all the walls of a blood vessel dilate more or less equally, creating a tubular swelling. SEE: *aneurysm* for illus.

mycotic a. Aneurysm due to bacterial infection.

racemose a. Cirsoid a.

sacculated a. Aneurysm in which there is weakness on one side of the vessel; usually due to trauma. It is attached to the artery by a narrow neck. SEE: *aneurysm* for illus.

varicose a. Aneurysm forming a blood-filled sac between an artery and a vein.

venous a. Aneurysm of a vein. **aneurysmal** (ăn″ū-rĭz′măl), *adj.*

aneurysmectomy (ăn″ū-rĭz-mĕk′tō-mē) [″ + *ektome*, excision] Surgical removal of the sac of an aneurysm.

aneurysmoplasty (ăn″ū-rĭz′mō-plăs″tē) [″ + *plassein*, to form] Surgical repair of an aneurysm.

aneurysmorrhaphy (ăn″ū-rĭz-mor′ă-fē) [″ + *rhaphe*, seam, ridge] Surgical closure of the sac of an aneurysm.

aneurysmotomy (ăn″ū-rĭz-mŏt′ō-mē) [″ + *tome*, incision] Incision of the sac of an aneurysm, allowing it to heal by granulation.

A.N.F. *American Nurses' Foundation.*

angel dust Phencyclidine hydrochloride.

angel's trumpet [*Datura ruaveolens*] A flowering shrub native to the southeastern U.S. Portions of the plant are used for hallucinogenic effects. The flowers are made into a stew or tea, and the leaves are eaten. The flowers contain large quantities of the alkaloids atropine, hyoscyamine, and hyoscine. Ingestion of the plant produces intense thirst, visual disturbances, flushing, central nervous system hyperexcitability, sensory flooding, delirium and paranoia. This is followed by hyperthermia, tachycardia, hypertension, visual hallucinations, disturbed consciousness, clonus, and subsequent convulsions. If the condition is untreated, death may occur.

TREATMENT: Treatment consists of gastric lavage, followed by 1 to 4 mg of intravenous physostigmine sulfate. This dosage should reverse the acute delirious state in 1 to 2 hr, but it may need to be repeated several times.

angel's wing Posterior projection of the scapula; usually caused by paralysis of the serratus anterior muscle. SYN: *winged scapula.*

Angelucci's syndrome (ăn″jĕ-loo′chēz) [Arnaldo Angelucci, It. ophthalmologist, 1854–1934] Great excitability, palpitation, and vasomotor disturbance associated with vernal conjunctivitis.

anger (ăng′er) [L. *angere*, anguish] The basic emotion of extreme displeasure or exasperation in reaction to a person, a situation, or an object. Anger is instrumental in mobilizing and enhancing the ability to respond to adverse situations; for that reason, it may be essential to survival in some situations. Occasionally, anger may be a reaction to disease or dying and may be directed toward friends or family and those responsible for a patient's medical care.

angi- (ăn′jē) [Gr. *angeion*, vessel] SEE: *angio-*.

angiasthenia (ăn″jē-ăs-thē′nē-ă) [″ + *a-*, not, + *sthenos*, strength] Loss of vascular tone.

angiectomy (ăn″jē-ĕk′tō-mē) [″ + *ektome*, excision] Excision or resection of a blood vessel.

angiectopia (ăn″jē-ĕk′tō′pē-ă) [″ + *ektopos*, out of place] Displacement of a vessel.

angiemphraxis (ăn″jē-ĕm-frăk′sĭs) [″ + *emphraxis*, stoppage] Obstruction of a vessel.

angiitis (ăn″jē-ī′tĭs) [″ + *itis*, inflammation] Inflammation of blood vessels. SYN: *vasculitis.*

angina (ăn-jī′nă, ăn′jĭ-nă) [L. *angina*, quinsy, from *angere*, to choke] **1.** Angina pectoris. **2.** Acute sore throat. **anginal** (ăn′jĭ-nal), *adj.*

abdominal a. Abdominal pain that occurs after meals, caused by insufficient blood flow to the mesenteric arteries. This symptom typically occurs in patients with extensive atherosclerotic vascular disease and is often associated with significant weight loss. SYN: *intestinal a.*

a. decubitus Attacks of angina pectoris occurring while an individual is in a recumbent position.

a. of effort Angina pectoris with onset during exercise. SYN: *exertion a.*

exertion a. A. of effort.

intestinal a. Abdominal a.

Ludwig's a. Submaxillary cellulitis;

a deep infection of the tissues of the floor of the mouth.

a. pectoris An oppressive pain or pressure in the chest caused by inadequate blood flow and oxygenation to heart muscle. It is usually produced by atherosclerosis of the coronary arteries, and in Western cultures is one of the most common emergent complaints bringing adult patients to medical attention. It typically occurs after (or during) events that increase the heart's need for oxygen, such as increased physical activity, a large meal, exposure to cold weather, or increased psychological stress. SEE: illus; table.

SYMPTOMS: Patients typically describe a pain of pressure located behind the sternum, that may have a "tight" or binding quality; the sensation may radiate into the neck, jaw, shoulders, or arms, and be associated with difficulty breathing, nausea or vomiting, sweating, anxiety, or fear. The pain is not usually described by patients as "sharp," or "stabbing," and is usually not worsened by deep breathing, coughing, swallowing, or twisting or turning the muscles of the trunk, shoulders, or arms.

TREATMENT: In health care settings, oxygen, nitroglycerin, and aspirin are provided, and the patient is placed at rest. At home, patients typically rest and use short-acting nitroglycerin. Morphine sulfate is given for pain that does not resolve after about 15 minutes of treatment with that regimen. Beta blocking drugs (e.g. propranolol, metoprolol, atenolol, and others) are used to slow the heart rate and decrease blood pressure. They provide the mainstay for chronic treatment of coronary insufficiency, and are indispensable when treating unstable angina or acute myocardial infarction. Patients with chronic or recurring angina pectoris may get symptomatic relief from long-acting nitrates or calcium channel blockers.

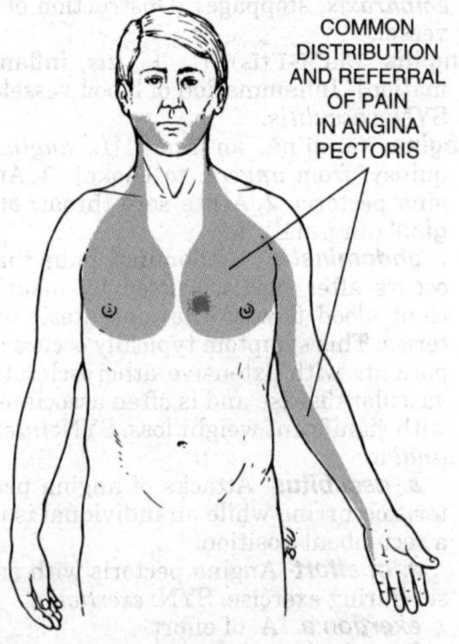

ANGINA PECTORIS

PATIENT CARE: The pattern of pain, including OPQRST (onset, provocation, quality, region, radiation, referral, severity, and time) is monitored and documented. Cardiopulmonary status is evaluated for evidence of tachypnea, dyspnea, diaphoresis, pulmonary crackles (rales), bradycardia or tachycardia, altered pulse strength, the appearance of a systolic third or fourth heart sound or mid- to late-systolic murmurs over the apex on auscultation, pallor, hypotension or hypertension, gastrointestinal distress, or nausea and vomiting. The 12-lead electrocardiogram is monitored for ST-segment elevation or depression, T-wave inversion, and cardiac dysrhythmias. Prescribed medication, such as sublingual nitroglycerin if the patient remains hypertensive or normotensive, and high concentration oxygen are administered, and the patient's response is noted. A health care provider should remain with the patient and provide emotional support throughout the episode. The patient is taught how to use the prescribed form of nitroglycerin for anginal attacks and about the importance of seeking medical attention if prescribed dosing does not provide relief. When appropriate the patient also is taught about prescribed beta-adrenergic or calcium channel blockers, clotbusters, cardiac catheterization diagnostic tests, and needed interventions to ensure the patient's understanding of these procedures should they become necessary. SEE: *Nursing Diagnoses Appendix.*

preinfarction a. Angina pectoris occurring in the days or weeks before a myocardial infarction. The symptoms may be unrecognized by patients without a history of coronary artery disease.

Prinzmetal's a. Variant a.

silent a. Unrecognized angina pectoris, that is, coronary insufficiency that presents with symptoms other than chest pain or pressure. The patient may experience dyspnea on exertion, heartburn, nausea, arm pain, or other atypical symptoms. Silent angina pectoris occurs most often in the elderly, in women, in post-operative patients who are heavily medicated, or in patients with diabetic neuropathy.

stable a. Angina that occurs with exercise and is predictable; usually promptly relieved by rest or nitroglycerin.

unstable a. Angina that has changed to a more frequent and more severe form. It can occur during rest and may be an indication of impending myocardial infarction. Unstable angina should be treated as

Stages of Angina Pectoris

Class	Description
I	Ordinary physical activity, such as walking or climbing stairs, does not cause angina. Angina occurs with strenuous, rapid, or prolonged exertion at work or recreation.
II	Slight limitation of ordinary activity. Angina occurs on walking or climbing stairs rapidly, walking uphill, walking or stair climbing after meals, in cold, or in wind, under emotional stress, only during the few hours after awakening, or walking more than two level blocks and climbing more than one flight of stairs at a normal pace and in normal conditions.
III	Marked limitation of ordinary physical activity. Angina occurs on walking one to two level blocks and climbing one flight of stairs in normal conditions at a normal pace.
IV	Inability to carry on any physical activity without discomfort—angina symptoms may be present at rest.

SOURCE: Campeau, L: Grading of Angina Pectoris [letter]. Circulation 54(3), 522. Copyright 1976, American Heart Association.

a medical emergency and the patient hospitalized without delay.

variant a. Chest pain that results from the spasm of coronary arteries, rather than from exertion or other increased demands on the heart. The pain typically occurs at rest. During coronary catheterization, the spasm is usually found near an atherosclerotic plaque, often in the right coronary artery. Infusions of ergonovine may provoke it. On the electrocardiogram, the diagnostic hallmark is elevation of the ST segments during episodes of resting pain. Treatments include nitrates and calcium channel blocking drugs. Beta-blocking drugs, frequently used as first-line therapy in typical angina pectoris, are often ineffective in this form of angina. SYN: *Prinzmetal's a.*

Vincent's a. acute necrotizing ulcerative gingivitis.

anginoid (ăn′jĭ-noyd) [″ + Gr. *eidos*, form, shape] Resembling angina, esp. angina pectoris.

anginophobia (ăn″jĭ-nō-fō′bē-ă) [″ + Gr. *phobos*, fear] Morbid fear of an attack of angina pectoris.

anginose, anginous (ăn′jĭ-nōs, -nŭs) [L. *angina*, quinsy] Pert. to or resembling angina.

angio-, angi- (ăn′jē-ō) [Gr. *angeion*, vessel] Combining form denoting *lymph* or *blood vessels*.

angioataxia (ăn″jē-ō-ă-tăk′sē-ă) [″ + *ataktos*, out of order] Variability in arterial tonus.

angioblast (ăn′jē-ō-blăst) [″ + *blastos*, germ] **1.** The earliest tissue arising from the mesenchymal cells of the embryo, from which blood vessels develop. **2.** A cell that participates in vessel formation.

angioblastoma (ăn″jē-ō-blăs-tō′mă) [″ + ″ + *oma*, tumor] A tumor of blood vessels of the brain or of the meninges.

angiocardiogram (ăn″jē-ō-kăr′dē-ō-grăm) [″ + *kardia*, heart, + *gramma*, something written] The image of the heart and great blood vessels obtained by angiocardiography.

angiocardiography (ăn″jē-ō-kăr″dē-ŏg′ră-fē) [″ + ″ + *graphein*, to write] Serial imaging, usually cineradiography, of the heart and great blood vessels after intravascular or intracardiac injection of a water-soluble contrast medium.

angiocardiopathy (ăn″jē-ō-kăr″dē-ŏp′ă-thē) [″ + ″ + *pathos*, disease, suffering] Disease of the blood vessels of the heart.

angiocarditis (ăn″jē-ō-kăr-dī′tĭs) [″ + ″ + *itis*, inflammation] Inflammation of the heart and large blood vessels.

angiocavernous (ăn″jē-ō-kăv′ĕr-nŭs) [″ + L. *caverna*, cavern] Rel. to angioma cavernosum.

angiocholecystitis (ăn″jē-ō-kō″lē-sĭs-tī′tĭs) [″ + *chole*, bile, + *kystis*, bladder, + *itis*, inflammation] Inflammation of the gallbladder and bile vessels.

angiocholitis (ăn″jē-ō-kō-lī′tĭs) [″ + ″ + *itis*, inflammation] Inflammation of the biliary vessels. SYN: *cholangitis*.

angiodysplasia (ăn″jē-ō-dĭs-plā′zē-ă) Vascular ectasis in the mucosa of the intestine, usually the cecum, an occasional cause of lower gastrointestinal bleeding. Lesions increase with advancing age and can cause occult or obvious blood loss.

angioedema (ăn″jē-ō-ĕ-dē′mă) [″ + *oidema*, swelling] A condition marked by the development of edematous areas of skin, mucous membranes, or internal organs. It is frequently associated with urticaria (hives), which is benign when limited to the skin but can cause respiratory distress when present in the mouth, pharynx, or larynx. It is usually the result of a type I hypersensitivity reaction. Histamine released during an immunoglobin E antibody reaction to ingested allergens such as food or drugs causes vasodilation and increased vascular permeability producing the characteristic nonpitting, nondependent swelling that distinguishes it from regular edema. The nonallergic forms of angioedema are hereditary angioedema, which is caused by a complement deficiency, and anaphylactoid reactions. SYN: *angioneurotic edema.* SEE: *urticaria.*

TREATMENT: Antihistamines are used first for immediate relief. Epinephrine is used if swelling of the upper airways compromises breathing.

hereditary a. ABBR: HAE. A rare autosomal dominant disease marked by episodic bouts of subcutaneous and submucosal edema, especially of the gastrointestinal tract or the upper airways. It is caused by the hereditary lack of a protein (C1 INH) that inactivates complement or by the malfunction of this protein. Physical trauma or psychological stress may precipitate attacks. The symptoms usually worsen after puberty Anabolic steroids are typically used to treat HAE.

angioendothelioma (ăn″jē-ō-ĕn″dō-thē″lē-ō′mă) *pl.* **angioendotheliomas, -mata** [″ + *endon*, within, + *thele*, nipple, + *oma*, tumor] A tumor consisting of endothelial cells, commonly occurring as single or multiple tumors of bone.

angiofibroma (ăn″jē-ō-fī-brō′mă) *pl.* **angiofibromas, -mata** [″ + L. *fibra*, fiber, + Gr. *oma*, tumor] A tumor consisting of vascular and fibrous tissue.

angiogenesis (ăn″jē-ō-jĕn′ĕ-sĭs) [″ + *genesis*, generation, birth] Development of blood vessels. **angiogenic** (-jĕn′ĭk), *adj.*

angiogenic growth factors A group of polypeptides that stimulate the formation of new blood vessels. They include agents like vascular endothelial growth factor (VEGF) and blood vessel fibroblastic growth factor (bFGF). These factors are active in healing wounds, chronic inflammatory conditions, retrolental fibroplasia, and malignant tumors, which require new blood vessels for continued growth.

angioglioma (ăn″jē-ō-glī-ō′mă) [Gr. *angeion*, vessel, + *glia*, glue, + *oma*, tumor] A mixed angioma and glioma.

angiogram (ăn′jē-ō-grăm) [″ + *gramma*, something written] A radiographic record of the size, shape, and location of the heart and blood vessels after introduction of a radiopaque contrast medium. A catheter is usually inserted into a peripheral vessel and guided to the affected area by use of the Seldinger technique. The recording can be either serial film or digital imaging.

aortic a. Angiogram of the aorta; used in diagnosing aneurysms or tumors that contact and deform the aorta.

cardiac a. Angiogram of the heart; used to determine the size and shape of the cavities of the heart and the condition of the valves.

cerebral a. Angiogram of blood vessels of the brain.

angiograph (ăn′jē-ō-grăf″) [″ + *graphein*, to write] A variety of sphygmograph.

angiography (ăn″jē-ŏg′ră-fē) **1.** A description of blood vessels and lymphatics. **2.** Diagnostic or therapeutic radiography of the heart and blood vessels using a radiopaque contrast medium. Types include magnetic resonance angiography, interventional radiology, and computed tomography. **3.** Recording of arterial pulse movements by use of a sphygmograph.

aortic a. Angiography of the aorta and its branches.

cardiac a. Angiography of the heart and coronary arteries.

cerebral a. Angiography of the vascular system of the brain.

coronary a. Angiography of the coronary arteries, to determine any pathological obstructions to blood flow to the heart muscle.

digital subtraction a. Use of a computer technique to investigate arterial blood circulation. A reference image is obtained by fluoroscopy. Then a contrast medium is injected intravenously. Another film is produced from the fluoroscopic image, and then the computer technique "subtracts" the image produced by surrounding tissues. The third image is an enhanced view of the arteries.

pulmonary a. Angiography of the pulmonary vessels (e.g., in the diagnosis of pulmonary embolism).

selective a. Angiography in which a catheter is introduced directly into the vessel to be visualized.

angiohyalinosis (ăn″jē-ō-hī″ă-lĭn-ō′sĭs) [Gr. *angeion*, vessel, + *hyalos*, glass, + *osis*, condition] Hyaline degeneration of blood vessel walls.

angiohypertonia (ăn″jē-ō-hī″pĕr-tō′nē-ă) [″ + *hyper*, over, + *tonos*, act of stretching, tension] Spasm of blood vessels, esp. arteries. SYN: *angiospasm; vasospasm.*

angiohypotonia (ăn″jē-ō-hī″pō-tō′nē-ă) [″ + *hypo*, under, + *tonos*, act of stretching, tension] Angioparalysis; angioparesis; vascular dilatation.

angioid (ăn′jē-oyd) [″ + *eidos*, form, shape] Resembling a blood vessel.

angioid streaks Dark, wavy, anastomosing striae lying beneath retinal vessels.

angiokeratoma (ăn″jē-ō-kĕr″ă-tō′mă) [″ + *keras*, horn, + *oma*, tumor] A skin disorder occurring chiefly on the feet and legs, marked by formation of telangiectases or warty growths accompanied by thickening of the epidermis along the course of dilated capillaries.

angiokinetic (ăn″jē-ō-kĭ-nĕt′ĭk) [″ + *ki-*

nesis, movement] Pert. to constriction and dilation of blood vessels. SYN: *vasomotor*.

angioleukitis (ăn″jē-ō-loo-kī′tĭs) [″ + *leukos*, white, + *itis*, inflammation] Inflammation of lymphatics.

angiolipoma (ăn′jē-ō-lĭp-ō′mă) [″ + *lipos*, fat, + *oma*, tumor] A mixed angioma and lipoma.

angiolith (ăn′jē-ō-lĭth) [″ + *lithos*, stone] Calcareous deposit in the wall of a blood vessel.

angiology (ăn″jē-ŏl′ō-jē) [″ + *logos*, word, reason] The study of blood vessels and lymphatics.

angiolymphitis (ăn″jē-ō-lĭm-fī′tĭs) [″ + L. *lympha*, lymph, + *itis*, inflammation] Inflammation of the lymphatics. SYN: *lymphangitis*.

angiolysis (ăn″jē-ŏl′ĭ-sĭs) [″ + *lysis*, dissolution] Obliteration of blood vessels, as in the umbilical cord when it is tied just after birth.

angioma (ăn″jē-ō′mă) [″ + *oma*, tumor] A form of tumor, usually benign, consisting principally of blood vessels (hemangioma) or lymph vessels (lymphangioma). It is considered to represent remnants of fetal tissue misplaced or undergoing disordered development. SEE: *choristoma; epithelioma; hamartoma; nevus*. **angiomatous** (-ō′mă-tŭs), *adj.*

capillary a. Congenital, superficial hemangioma appearing as an irregularly shaped, red discoloration of otherwise normal skin; due to overgrowth of capillaries. SYN: *a. simplex*.

a. cavernosum Congenital hemangioma appearing as an elevated dark red benign tumor, ranging in size from a few millimeters to several centimeters. It may pulsate. It commonly involves the subcutaneous or submucous tissue and consists of blood-filled vascular spaces. Small ones may disappear without therapy.

cherry a. A benign 0.5-mm to 6.0-mm dome-shaped cherry-red papule on the trunk, esp. in persons over age 30. It consists of a compressible mass of blood vessels. SYN: *ruby spot; senile a.*

senile a. Cherry a.

serpiginous a. A skin disorder marked by the appearance of small red vascular dots arranged in rings; due to proliferation of capillaries.

a. simplex Capillary a.

spider a. SYN: *spider nevus*.

stellate a. Skin lesion in which numerous telangiectatic vessels radiate from a central point; commonly associated with liver disease, hypertension, or pregnancy. SYN: *spider nevus*.

telangiectatic a. Angioma composed of abnormally dilated blood vessels.

a. venosum racemosum Swelling associated with severe varicosities of superficial veins.

angiomalacia (ăn″jē-ō-mă-lā′sē-ă) [Gr. *angeion*, vessel, + *malakia*, softness] Softening of blood vessel walls.

angiomatosis (ăn″jē-ō-mă-tō′sĭs) [″ + *oma*, tumor, + *osis*, condition] Condition of having multiple angiomas.

bacillary a. An acute infectious disease caused by *Bartonella quintana*. It is characterized by skin lesions that may vary from small papules to pyogenic granulomas or pedunculated masses. These occur anywhere on the skin and may involve mucous membranes. If the lesions ulcerate, they can extend to and destroy underlying bone. In addition, the organisms are disseminated to the liver, spleen, bone marrow, and lymph nodes. In the liver there may be painful, multiple, cystic, blood-filled spaces (peliosis hepatitis). Most patients with this disease are immunocompromised or infected with human immunodeficiency virus (HIV). In the untreated immunocompetent patient, recovery may be prolonged but is usually complete. In the untreated immunocompromised patient, death is the likely outcome. When the organisms are disseminated, treatment for several months with oral doxycycline or oral erythromycin will be of benefit in altering the course of the disease. Culture of the organism provides diagnosis. SEE: *cat scratch disease; trench fever*.

angiomegaly (ăn″jē-ō-mĕg′ă-lē) [″ + *megas*, large] Enlargement of blood vessels, esp. in the eyelid.

angiomyocardiac (ăn″jē-ō-mī″ō-kăr′dē-ăk) [″ + *mys*, muscle, + *kardia*, heart] Pert. to blood vessels and cardiac muscle.

angiomyolipoma (ăn″jē-ō-mī″ō-lĭ-pō′mă) [″ + ″ + *lipos*, fat, + *oma*, tumor] A benign tumor containing vascular, fatty, and muscular tissue.

angiomyoma (ăn″jē-ō-mī-ō′mă) [″ + ″ + *oma*, tumor] A tumor composed of blood vessels and muscle tissue. SYN: *myoma telangiectodes*.

angiomyoneuroma (ăn″jē-ō-mī″ō-nū-rō′mă) [″ + ″ + *neuron*, nerve, + *oma*, tumor] A painful, benign tumor of the arteriovenous anastomoses of the skin. SYN: *glomangioma*.

angiomyosarcoma (ăn″jē-ō-mī″ō-săr-kō′mă) [″ + ″ + *sarx*, flesh, + *oma*, tumor] A tumor composed of blood vessels, muscle tissue, and connective tissue.

angioneurectomy (ăn″jē-ō-nū-rĕk′tō-mē) [″ + *neuron*, nerve, + *ektome*, excision] Excision of vessels and nerves.

angioneuromyoma Angiomyoneuroma.

angioneurotomy (ăn″jē-ō-nū-rŏt′ō-mē) [″ + ″ + *tome*, incision] Cutting of vessels and nerves.

angionoma (ăn″jē-ō-nō′mă) [Gr. *angeion*, vessel, + *nome*, ulcer] Ulceration of a vessel.

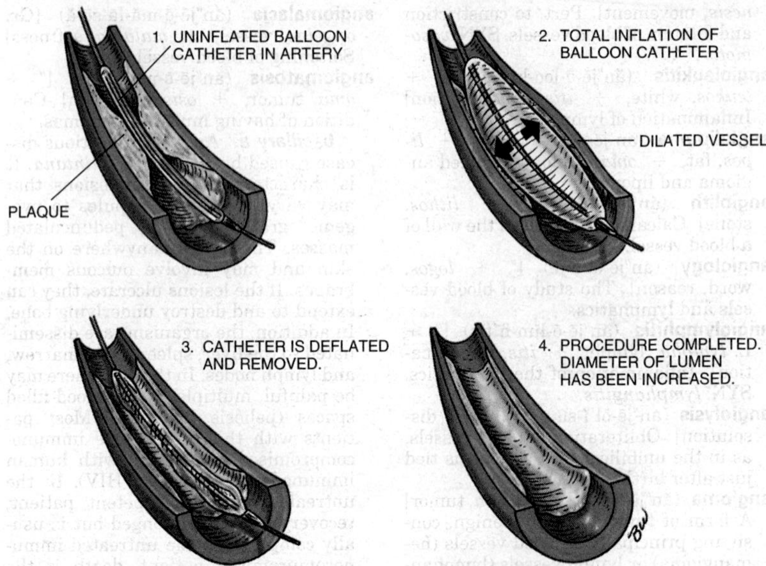
1. UNINFLATED BALLOON CATHETER IN ARTERY
PLAQUE
2. TOTAL INFLATION OF BALLOON CATHETER
DILATED VESSEL
3. CATHETER IS DEFLATED AND REMOVED.
4. PROCEDURE COMPLETED. DIAMETER OF LUMEN HAS BEEN INCREASED.

ARTERIAL BALLOON ANGIOPLASTY

angioparalysis (ăn″jē-ō-pă-răl′ĭ-sĭs) [″ + *paralyein*, loosen, dissolve] Vasomotor relaxation of blood vessel tone.

angiopathology (ăn″jē-ō-pă-thŏl′ō-jē) [″ + *pathos*, disease, suffering, + *logos*, word, reason] Morbid changes in diseases of the blood vessels.

angiopathy (ăn-jē-ŏp′ă-thē) Any disease of blood or lymph vessels. SYN: *angiosis*.

amyloid a. An abnormality of cerebral blood vessels in which amyloid is deposited in the walls of small arteries and arterioles. These changes are a common cause of intracerebral hemorrhage in the elderly.

angiophacomatosis, angiophakomatosis (ăn″jē-ō-făk″ō-mă-tō′sis) [″ + *phakos*, lens, + *oma*, tumor, + *osis*, condition] Hippel's disease.

angioplasty (ăn′jē-ō-plăs″tē) [″ + *plassein*, to form] Any endovascular procedure that reopens narrowed blood vessels and restores forward blood flow. Most often angioplasties are performed on coronary, carotid, or peripheral arteries occluded by atherosclerosis. Some common angioplasty techniques include the following: *atherectomy*, which opens occluded, scarred, or calcified vessels by removing atherosclerotic plaques with rapidly rotating drills; *balloon angioplasty*, which relies on the inflation of high-pressure balloons within blocked arteries to force them open; *laser and radiofrequency angioplasties*, which vaporize or ablate atherosclerotic plaques; *endovascular stents*, which hold vessels open with expandable lattices inserted across the narrowed section of the artery SEE: illus.; *percutaneous transluminal coronary a.*

laser coronary a. The use of laser energy to vaporize an atherosclerotic plaque in a diseased coronary vessel. SEE: *percutaneous transluminal coronary a.*

percutaneous transluminal coronary a. ABBR: PTCA. A method of treating localized coronary artery narrowing. A special double-lumen catheter is designed so that a cylindrical balloon surrounds a portion of it. After the catheter is inserted transcutaneously in the artery, inflation of the balloon with pressure between between 9 and 15 atmospheres (approximately 135 to 225 psi) dilates the narrowed vessel. This technique may be used on narrowed arteries other than the coronaries.

In the U.S. alone, more than 400,000 coronary angioplasties are performed each year. Modifications in this technique may be used to open blocked arteries in many regions of the circulation (e.g., renal, iliac, or femoral arteries).

PATIENT CARE: *Preoperative*: The cardiologist's explanation of the procedure is reinforced. The patient is encouraged to verbalize feelings and concerns, and misconceptions are clarified. The patient is prepared physically for the procedure according to the surgeon's orders. Baseline data needed for comparison with postoperative assessment data are gathered.

Postoperative: Vital signs, cardiac rate and rhythm, and neurovascular status distal to the catheter insertion site are monitored. A Doppler stethoscope should be used if peripheral pulses are difficult to palpate. The catheter site is inspected periodically for hematoma formation, ecchymosis, or hemorrhage. The dressing is marked, and the health care provider is notified of any rapid progression. If bleeding occurs, direct pressure is applied to the catheter site. The patient should keep the leg straight and limit head elevation to no more than 15 degrees to prevent hip flexion and potential catheter migration. The patient is assessed for chest pain, which may indicate vasospasm or reocclusion of the ballooned vessel. Intravenous fluids are administered as prescribed to promote excretion of contrast medium. The patient is assessed for signs and symptoms of fluid overload (i.e., dyspnea, pulmonary crackles, distended neck veins, tachycardia, bounding pulse, hypertension, gallop rhythms). Pharmacological therapy is continued as prescribed (I.V. nitroglycerin, heparin). Catheter removal is explained to the patient, and direct pressure is applied to the insertion site for 30 min and then pressure dressing. Vital signs continue to be monitored until it is certain that no occult hemorrhage is occurring. Discharge instructions are provided to the patient and family regarding the scheduled return visit with the cardiologist, follow-up exercise, thallium stress testing or angiography, and any exercise prescriptions or activity restrictions (usually patients can walk 24 hr after the procedure and return to work in 2 wk). The importance of drug regimens, including desired effects and potential adverse reactions, is reinforced.

rescue a. The use of angioplasty to open coronary arteries that remain occluded after intravenous thrombolytic therapy for acute myocardial infarction.

angiopoiesis (ăn″jē-ō-poy-ē′sĭs) [″ + *poiein*, to make] The formation of blood vessels. **angiopoietic** (-poy-ĕt′ĭk), *adj.*

angiopressure (ăn′jē-ō-prĕsh″ŭr) Pressure applied to a blood vessel to arrest hemorrhage.

angiorrhaphy (ăn″jē-or′ă-fē) [″ + *rhaphe*, seam, ridge] Suture of a vessel, esp. a blood vessel.

angiorrhexis (ăn″jē-or-ĕk′sĭs) [″ + *rhexis*, rupture] Rupture of a vessel, esp. a blood vessel.

angiosarcoma (ăn″jē-ō-săr-kō′mă) [″ + *sarx*, flesh, + *oma*, tumor] Malignant neoplasm originating from blood vessels. SYN: *hemangiosarcoma*.

angiosclerosis (ăn″jē-ō-sklĕ-rō′sĭs) [″ + *sklerosis*, hardening] Hardening of the walls of the vascular system.

angioscotoma (ăn″jē-ō-skō-tō′mă) [″ + *skotoma*, darkness] The defect produced in the visual field by the shadows of the retinal blood vessels.

angiosis (ăn″jē-ō′sĭs) [Gr. *angeion*, vessel, + *osis*, condition] Any disease of blood vessels or lymph vessels. SYN: *angiopathy*.

angiospasm (ăn′jē-ō-spăzm) [″ + *spasmos*, a convulsion] Spasmodic contraction of blood vessels; may cause cramping of muscles or intermittent claudication. **angiospastic** (ăn″jē-ō-spăs′tĭk), *adj.*

angiostatin (ăn″jē-ō-stăt′ĭn) A protein fragment of plasminogen that inhibits the growth of blood vessels, possibly by blocking the enzyme ATP synthetase on the endothelium. It may shrink malignant tumors by decreasing their blood supply.

angiostenosis (ăn″jē-ō-stĕ-nō′sĭs) [″ + *stenoein*, to make narrow, + *osis*, condition] Narrowing of a vessel, esp. a blood vessel.

angiosteosis (ăn″jē-ŏs″tē-ō′sĭs) [″ + *osteon*, bone, + *osis*, condition] Calcification of a vessel.

angiostomy (ăn″jē-ŏs′tō-mē) [″ + *stoma*, mouth] An operation that makes an artificial fistulous opening into a blood vessel.

angiostrophy (ăn″jē-ŏs′trō-fē) [″ + *strophe*, twist] The twisting of the cut end of a blood vessel to arrest bleeding.

angiotelectasis (ăn″jē-ō-tĕl-ĕk′tă-sĭs) [″ + *telos*, end, + *ektasis*, stretching out] Dilatation of terminal arterioles.

angiotensin (ăn″jē-ō-tĕn′sĭn) A vasopressor produced when renin is released from the kidney. Renin is formed by the juxtaglomerular apparatus of the kidney. SEE: *apparatus, juxtaglomerular*.

a. I Physiologically inactive form of angiotensin; converted to angiotensin II in the lungs.

a. II Physiologically active form of angiotensin; a powerful vasopressor and stimulator of aldosterone production and secretion.

a. amide A vasoconstricting compound of angiotensin.

angiotensin-converting enzyme inhibitor Any of the therapeutic agents that inhibit conversion of angiotensin I to angiotensin II. As a result, blood pressure falls. ACE inhibitors are used to treat hypertension, heart failure, and other diseases.

angiotensinogen (ăn″jē-ō-tĕn-sĭn′ō-jĕn) A serum globulin fraction formed in the liver; converted to angiotensin as a result of hydrolysis by renin.

angiotitis (ăn″jē-ō-tī′tĭs) [″ + *otos*, ear, + *itis*, inflammation] Inflammation of the blood vessels of the ear.

angiotome (ăn′jē-ō-tōm″) [Gr. *angeion*, vessel, + *tome*, incision] Any segment of the embryonic vascular system.

angiotomy (ăn″jē-ŏt″ō-mē) Sectioning of blood vessels.

angiotonic (ăn″jē-ō-tŏn′ĭk) [″ + *tonos*, tension] Increasing arterial tension.

angiotribe [″ + Gr. *tribein*, to crush] A forceps designed for application of a strong, crushing force to a tissue containing an artery. This is done to control hemorrhage.

angiotrophic (ăn″jē-ō-trŏf′ĭk) [″ + *trophe*, nourishment] Pert. to nutrition of blood vessels or lymph vessels.

angle (ăng′gl) [L. *angulus*] **1.** The figure or space outlined by the diverging of two lines from a common point or by the meeting of two planes. **2.** A projecting or sharp corner.

acromial a. The angle formed by the junction of the lateral and posterior borders of the acromion.

acute a. An angle less than 90°.

alpha a. The angle formed by intersection of the visual line with the optic axis.

alveolar a. The angle between the horizontal plane and a line drawn through the base of the nasal spine and the middle point of the alveolus of the upper jaw.

biorbital a. The angle formed by the meeting of the axes of the orbits.

cardiophrenic a. The medial, inferior corner of the pulmonary cavity bordered by the heart and diaphragm.

carrying a. The angle made at the elbow by extending the long axis of the forearm and the upper arm. This obtuse angle is more pronounced in women than in men.

caudal a. In radiology, angulation of the central ray toward the patient's feet.

cavity a. The angle formed by two or more walls of a cavity preparation in restorative dentistry.

cephalic a. In radiology, angulation of the central ray toward the patient's head.

cephalometric a. The angle formed by intersecting anthropometric lines used in studies of the skull and for diagnosis of orthodontic problems.

cerebellopontine a. The angle formed by the junction of the cerebellum and the pons. SYN: *pontine a.*

Cobb a. The degree of lateral curvature of the spine, measured from a standing x-ray film of the spine. This angle is used in the diagnosis of scoliosis. SEE: *scoliosis.*

a. of convergence The angle between the visual axis and the median line when an object is looked at.

costal a. The meeting point of the lower border of the false ribs with the axis of the sternum.

costophrenic a. The lateral, inferior corner of the pulmonary cavity bordered by the ribs and diaphragm.

costovertebral a. The angle formed on each side of the trunk by the junction of the last rib with the lumbar vertebrae.

craniofacial a. The angle formed by the basifacial and basicranial axes at the midpoint of the sphenoethmoidal suture.

facial a. The angle made by lines from the nasal spine and external auditory meatus meeting between the upper middle incisor teeth.

flat a. The angle between two lines that join at an angle of almost 180°.

gamma a. The angle between the line of vision and the optic axis.

gonial a. A. of jaw.

a. of incidence The angle between a ray striking a surface and a line drawn perpendicular to the surface at the point of incidence.

a. of iris The angle between the cornea and iris at the periphery of the anterior chamber of the eye.

a. of jaw The angle formed by the junction of the posterior edge of the ramus of the mandible and the lower surface of the body of the mandible. SYN: *gonial a.; a. of mandible.*

a. of mandible A. of jaw.

metafacial a. The angle between the base of the skull and the pterygoid process.

obtuse a. An angle greater than 90°.

occipital a. The angle formed at the opisthion by the intersection of lines from the basion and from the lower border of the orbit.

ophryospinal a. The angle formed at the anterior nasal spine by the intersection of lines drawn from the auricular point and the glabella.

parietal a. The angle formed by the meeting of a line drawn tangent to the maximum curve of the zygomatic arch and a line drawn tangent to the end of the maximum frontal diameter of the skull. If these lines are parallel, the angle is zero; if they diverge, a negative angle is formed.

pontine a. Cerebellopontine a.

pubic a. The angle formed by the junction of the rami of the pubes.

right a. An angle of 90°.

sphenoid a. The angle formed at the top of the sella turcica by the intersection of lines drawn from the nasal point and the tip of the rostrum of the sphenoid.

sternal a. The angle formed by the junction of the manubrium and the body of the sternum.

a. of Treitz Sharp curve at the duodenojejunal junction.

venous a. The angle formed by the junction of the internal jugular and subclavian veins.

visual a. The angle formed by lines drawn from the nodal point of the eye to the edges of the object viewed.

Angle's classification SEE: *malocclusion.*

angor (ăng′gor) [L., strangling] Violent distress, as in angina pectoris.

angor animi (ăng′gor ăn′ĭ-mē) [″ + L. *animus*, soul] The feeling that one is dying, as may occur in connection with angina pectoris.

angstrom unit (ŏng′strŭm) [Anders J. Ångström, Swedish physicist, 1814–1874] ABBR: A. SYMB: Å. U. An internationally adopted unit of length equal to 10^{-10} m, or 0.1 nm; used esp. to measure radiation wavelengths.

angular (ăng′gū-lăr) [L.] Having corners or angles.

angular artery The artery at the inner canthus of the eye; the facial artery.

angulation (ăng″ū-lā′shŭn) **1.** Abnormal formation of angles by tubular structures such as the intestines, blood vessels, or ureter. **2.** In radiology, the direction of the primary beam in relation to the film and the object being imaged.

anhedonia (ăn″hē-dō′nē-ă) [Gr. *an-*, not, + *hedone*, pleasure] Lack of pleasure in acts that are normally pleasurable. SEE: *hedonism*. **anhedonic** (-dŏn′ĭk), *adj.*

anhidrosis (ăn″hī-drō′sĭs) [″ + *hidros*, sweat] Diminished or complete absence of secretion of sweat. It may be generalized or localized, temporary or permanent, disease related or congenital. SYN: *anidrosis*.

TREATMENT: Treatment consists of therapy for the cause or accompanying conditions. The patient should wear soft, nonirritating clothing and use bland, soothing skin ointments and lubricants. Air conditioning provides comfort in most instances.

anhidrotic (ăn″hī-drŏt′ĭk) **1.** Inhibiting or preventing perspiration. **2.** An agent that inhibits or prevents perspiration. SYN: *anidrotic; antihidrotic; antiperspirant; antisudorific*.

anhydrase (ăn″hī′drās) [″ + *hydor*, water, + *-ase*, enzyme] An enzyme that promotes the removal of water from a chemical compound.

anhydration (ăn-hī′drā′shŭn) [″ + *hydor*, water] Removal of water from a substance. SYN: *dehydration*.

anhydride (ăn-hī′drīd) [Gr. *an-*, not, + *hydor*, water] A compound formed by removal of water from a substance, esp. from an acid.

anhydrochloric (ăn-hī-drō-klō′rĭk) [″ + ″ + *chloros*, green] Lacking hydrochloric acid.

anhydrous (ăn-hī′drŭs) [″ + *hydor*, water] Lacking water.

anianthinopsy (ăn-ē-ăn′thĭn-ŏp″sē) [″ + *ianthinos*, violet, + *opsis*, vision] Inability to recognize violet or purple.

anicteric (ăn″ĭk-tĕr′ĭk) [″ + *ikteros*, jaundice] Without jaundice.

anidrosis (ăn-ĭ-drō′sĭs) Anhidrosis.

anidrotic (ăn-ĭ-drŏt′ĭk) Anhidrotic.

aniline (ăn′ĭ-lĭn) [Arabic *an-nil*, the indigo plant] The simplest aromatic amine, C_6H_7N; an oily liquid derived from benzene. It is used in the manufacture of medical and industrial dyes. Aniline has antipyretic action but is too toxic to use as a medicine.

aniline poisoning SEE: *Poisons and Poisoning Appendix*.

anilingus [L. *anus* + *lingere*, to lick] Oral stimulation of the anus by use of the tongue or lips. SEE: *cunnilingus*.

anilism (ăn′ĭl-ĭzm) [Arabic *an-nil*, the indigo plant, + Gr. *-ismos*, condition] Chronic aniline poisoning. Symptoms include cardiac block, weakness, intermittent pulse, vertigo, muscular depression, and cyanosis.

anima (ăn′ĭ-mă) [L., soul] **1.** Soul. **2.** According to Carl Jung, an individual's inner self as distinguished from the external personality (persona). **3.** Jung's term for the feminine inner personality present in men. SEE: *animus*.

animal (ăn′ĭ-măl) [L. *animalis*, living] **1.** A living organism that requires oxygen and organic foods, is incapable of photosynthesis, has limited growth, and is capable of voluntary movement and sensation. **2.** Any animal other than humans. **3.** Pert. to or from an animal.

cold-blooded a. An animal whose body temperature varies according to the temperature of the environment.

control a. In medical research involving the use of animals, an animal that is not treated, but is housed and cared for under the same conditions as the treated animal(s). SEE: *control*(2).

warm-blooded a. An animal whose body temperature remains constant regardless of the temperature of the environment. SYN: *homotherm*.

animation (ăn-ĭ-mā′shŭn) [L. *animus*, soul] State of being alive or active.

suspended a. Temporary cessation of vital functions with loss of consciousness; state of apparent death.

animatism (ăn′ĭ-mă-tĭzm) The belief that everything in nature, animate and inanimate, contains a spirit or soul.

animi agitatio (ăn′ĭ-mē ă-jĭ-tā′shē-ō) [″ + *agitare*, to turn over] Mental agitation.

animism (ăn′ĭ-mĭzm) Attribution of spiritual qualities and mental capabilities to inanimate objects.

animus [L., breath, mind, soul] **1.** An animating or energizing motive or intention. **2.** A feeling of bitter hostility; a grudge. **3.** According to Carl Jung, the masculine inner personality present in women. SEE: *anima*.

anion (ăn′ī-ŏn) [Gr. *ana*, up, + *ion*, going] An ion carrying a negative charge; the opposite of cation. An anion is attracted by, and travels to, the anode (positive pole). Examples are acid radicals and corresponding radicals of their salts. SEE: *electrolyte; ion*. **anionic** (ăn″ī-ŏn′ĭk), *adj.*

anion channel Channels in red blood cells that cross the cell membrane. Chloride ions (Cl^-) and bicarbonate ions (HCO_3^-) are exchanged via these channels.

anion exchange SEE: *resin, ion-exchange*.

anion gap The difference between the measured cations sodium (Na^+) and potassium (K^+) and the measured anions chloride (Cl^-) and bicarbonate (HCO_3^-). In accordance with the principle of electroneutrality, in any body fluid the number of net positive charges contributed by cations must equal the number of net negative charges contributed by anions. The apparent difference is accounted for by the unmeasured anions present (the *anion gap*); these include lactate, sulfates, phosphates, proteins, ketones, and other organic acids. In general, an anion gap of 8 to 18 mmol/L is normal. An increased value is present in some forms of metabolic acidosis.

anionic detergent A natural or synthetic chemical substance with disinfectant properties due to the presence of an active, negatively charged chemical group.

aniridia (ăn″ĭ-rĭd′ē-ă) [Gr. *an-*, not, + *iris*, rainbow, iris] Congenital absence of all or part of the iris. SYN: *irideremia*.

anisakiasis (ăn″ĭs-să-kī′ă-sĭs) Disease of the gastrointestinal tract accompanied by intestinal colic, fever, and abscesses; caused by eating uncooked fish containing larval nematodes of the family Anisakidae.

anise (ăn″ĭs) An annual herb, *Pimpinella anisum*, cultivated for its licorice-flavored seeds; used as a culinary herb, an aromatic, and a digestive aid.

aniseikonia (ăn-ĭs-ī-kō′nē-ă) [Gr. *anisos*, unequal, + *eikon*, image] A condition in which the size and shape of the ocular image of one eye differ from those of the other. SYN: *anisoiconia*.

anismus Excessive contraction of the external sphincter of the rectum.

aniso- (ăn-ī′sō) [Gr. *anisos*, unequal] Combining form meaning *unequal, asymmetrical,* or *dissimilar*.

anisoaccommodation (ăn-ī″sōă-kŏm″mŏ-dā′shŭn) [″ + L. *accommodare*, to suit] Difference in the ability of the eyes to accommodate. SEE: *accommodation*.

anisochromatic (ăn-ī″sō-krō-măt′ĭk) [″ + *chroma*, color] Not of uniform color.

anisocoria (ăn-ī″sō-kō′rē-ă) [″ + *kore*, pupil] Inequality of the size of the pupils; may be congenital or associated with aneurysms, head trauma, diseases of the nervous system, brain lesion, paresis, or locomotor ataxia.

anisocytosis (ăn-ī″sō-sī-tō′sĭs) [″ + *kytos*, cell, + *osis*, condition] Condition in which there is excessive inequality in the size of cells, esp. erythrocytes.

anisogamy (ăn″ī-sŏg′ă-mē) [″ + *gamos*, marriage] Sexual fusion of two gametes of different form and size.

anisognathous (ăn″ī-sŏg′nă-thŭs) [″ + *gnathos*, jaw] Having an upper jaw wider than the lower one.

anisoiconia (ăn-ī″sō-ī-kō′nē-ă) [″ + *eikon*, image] Aniseikonia.

anisokaryosis (ăn-ī″sō-kăr″ē-ō′sĭs) [″ + *karyon*, nucleus, + *osis*, condition] Unequal size of the cell nuclei.

anisomastia (ăn-ī-sō-măs′tē-ă) [″ + *mastos*, breast] Condition in which the breasts are markedly unequal in size.

anisomelia (ăn-ī″sō-mē′lē-ă) [″ + *melos*, limb] Condition in which paired limbs are noticeably unequal.

anisometrope (ăn-ī″sō-mĕt′rōp) [Gr. *anisos*, unequal, + *metron*, measure, + *ops*, vision] One afflicted with anisometropia.

anisometropia (ăn-ī″sō-mĕ-trō′pē-ă) Condition in which the refractive power of the eyes is unequal. **anisometropic** (-trŏp′ĭk), *adj.*

anisonormocytosis (ăn-ī″sō-nor″mō-sī-tō′sĭs) [″ + L. *norma*, rule, + Gr. *kytos*, cell, + *osis*, condition] Condition in which the total number of leukocytes is normal but the proportion of different types is abnormal.

anisophoria (ăn″ī-sō-fō′rē-ă) [″ + *phoros*, bearing] Eye muscle imbalance so that the horizontal visual plane of one eye is different from that of the other.

anisopia (ăn″ī-sō′pē-ă) [″ + *ops*, vision] Condition in which the visual power of the eyes is unequal.

anisosthenic (ăn-ī″sŏs-thĕn′ĭk) [″ + *sthenos*, strength] Of unequal strength; used of paired muscles.

anisotonic (ăn-ī″sō-tŏn′ĭk) [″ + *tonos*, act of stretching, tension] Pert. to a solution not isotonic as compared with another.

anisotropal (ăn″ī-sŏt′rō-păl) [″ + *tropos*, a turning] **1.** Not equal in every direction. **2.** Unequal in power of refraction. SYN: *anisotropous*.

anisotropic (ăn-ī″sō-trŏp′ĭk) **1.** Having different optical properties in different directions, as with certain crystals. **2.** Having double polarizing power.

anisotropous (ăn-ī-sŏt′rō-pŭs) Anisotropal.

ankle (ăng′kl) [AS. *ancleow*] **1.** The joint between the leg and foot; the articulation of the tibia, fibula, and talus. The ankle is a hinge joint. **2.** In popular usage, the region of this joint, including the tarsus and lower end of the leg. SEE: *foot* for illus.

ankle clonus Repetitive extension-flexion movement of the ankle muscles, associated with increased muscle tonus; a common symptom of corticospinal disease.

PATIENT CARE: The patient's foot is maintained at a right angle to the horizontal plane of the body, usually with a foot splint. When the splint is removed, dorsiflexion of the foot should be avoided to prevent ankle movement, clonus, or spasm. Correct movement of the involved joint, which should be slow and even, with the extremity supported on the palms rather than grasped, is demonstrated. Exercise should be performed when the joint is warm and relaxed.

a.c. reflex A reflex elicited by quick, vigorous dorsiflexion of the foot while the knee is held in a flexed position, resulting in repeated clonic movement of the foot as long as it is maintained in dorsiflexion. In women with pregnancy-induced hypertension, this reflects hyperirritability of the central nervous system and increased risk for eclamptic convulsions.

ankle-foot orthosis ABBR: AFO. Any of a class of external orthopedic appliance, brace, or splint devised to control, limit, or assist foot and ankle motion, and provide leg support. Typically, orthotics are made of lightweight thermoplastic material, but may be constructed of metal uprights with single or double-axis ankle joints. These devices provide some measure of foot and leg support, typically by preventing dorsiflexion and inversion-eversion.

ankle joint Ankle.

ankylo-, ankyl- (ăng′kĭ-lō) [Gr. *ankylos*, crooked] Combining form meaning *crooked, bent,* or *a fusion or growing together of parts.*

ankyloblepharon (ăng″kĭ-lō-blĕf′ăr-ŏn) [″ + *blepharon*, eyelid] Blepharosynechia.

ankylochilia (ăng″kĭ-lō-kī′lē-a) [″ + *cheilos*, lip] Adhesion of the upper and lower lips.

ankylodactylia (ăng-kĭ-lō-dăk-tĭl′ē-a) [″ + *daktylos*, finger] Adhesion of two or more fingers or toes.

ankyloglossia (ăng″kĭ-lō-glŏs′sē-ă) [″ + *glossa*, tongue] Abnormal shortness of the frenulum of the tongue. SYN: *lingua frenata; tongue-tie.*

ankylopoietic (ăng″kĭ-lō-poy-ĕt′ĭk) [Gr. *ankyle*, stiff joint, + *poiein*, to form] **1.** Indicating the presence of ankylosis. **2.** Causing ankylosis.

ankyloproctia (ăng″kĭ-lō-prŏk′shē-ă) [Gr. *ankylos*, crooked, + *proktos*, anus] Stricture or imperforation of the anus.

ankylosed **1.** Fixed; stiffened; held by adhesions. **2.** Affected with ankylosis.

ankylosis (ăng″kĭ-lō′sĭs) [Gr. *ankyle*, stiff joint, + *osis*, condition] Immobility of a joint. The condition may be congenital (sometimes hereditary), or it may be the result of disease, trauma, surgery, or contractures resulting from immobility.

PATIENT CARE: Immobility-induced contractures that can result in ankylosis can be prevented by putting joints through their normal range of motion passively whenever they cannot be exercised actively. If a nonsurgical ankylosis is present, the joint is maintained in a functional position, splints are used for patients with spastic muscles, passive range-of-motion exercises to affected joints are initiated, and physical therapy or orthopedic intervention may be appropriate. If an ankylosis is surgically created, the joint is immobilized until the bone has healed (usually in 6 to 12 weeks), and correct body alignment is maintained.

artificial a. The surgical fixation of a joint.

bony a. The abnormal union of the bones of a joint. SYN: *True a.*

dental a. A condition marked by the loss of tooth movement due to the fusion of the root cementum with the adjacent alveolar bone.

extracapsular a. Ankylosis caused by rigidity of parts outside a joint.

false a. Fibrous a.

fibrous a. Ankylosis due to the formation of fibrous bands within a joint. SYN: *false a.; ligamentous a.*

intracapsular a. Ankylosis due to undue rigidity of structures within a joint.

ligamentous a. Fibrous a.

true a. Bony a.

Ankylostoma (ăng″kĭ-lŏs′tō-mă) Ancylostoma.

ankylostomiasis (ăng″kĭ-lō-stō-mī′ă-sĭs) Hookworm.

ankylotia (ăng″kĭ-lō′shē-ă) [Gr. *ankylos*, crooked, + *ot-*, ear] Stricture or imperforation of the external auditory meatus of the ear.

ankylotome (ăng′kĭl-ō-tōm, ăng-kĭl′ō-tōm) [″ + *tome*, incision] An instrument for cutting the frenulum of the tongue in tongue-tie.

ankylurethria (ăng″kĭl-ū-rē′thrē-ă) [″ + *ourethra*, urethra] Stricture or imperforation of the urethra.

anlage (ŏn′lŏ-jhă) [Ger., a laying on] The first accumulation of cells in an embryo; the beginning of an organized tissue, organ, or part. SYN: *primordium.*

A.N.N.A. *American Nephrology Nurses' Association.*

anneal (an-nēl′) [AS. *anaelan*, to burn] To soften a material, such as glass, metal, or wax, by heating and cooling to remove internal stresses and to make it more easily adapted or swaged, as in preparation of materials for restorative dentistry.

annectant, annectent (ă-nĕk′tĕnt) [L. *annectens*, tying or binding to] Linking; connecting.

Annelida (ă-nĕl′ĭ-dă) The phylum that includes earthworms, leeches, and other segmented worms. Some annelids serve as intermediate hosts for parasitic worms. Leeches are ectoparasites. The medicinal leech, *Hirudo medicinalis*, is the source of an anticoagulant that is used to treat myocardial infarction and other conditions caused by blood clots.

annexa (ă-nĕks′ă) [L. *annectere*, to tie or bind to] Accessory parts of a structure. SYN: *adnexa*.

annexitis (ă-nĕks-ī′tĭs) [″ + Gr. *itis*, inflammation] Inflammation of the adnexa uteri. SYN: *adnexitis*.

annular (ăn′ū-lăr) [L. *annulus*, ring] Circular; ring-shaped (e.g., annular ligament of the elbow).

annulorrhaphy (ăn″ū-lor′ă-fē) [″ + Gr. *rhaphe*, seam, ridge] Closure of a hernial ring by suture.

annulus (ăn′ū-lŭs) *pl.* **annuli** [L.] A ring-shaped structure; a ring. Also spelled *anulus*.

anococcygeal (ā″nō-kŏk-sĭ′jē-al) [L. *anus*, anus, + Gr. *kokkyx*, coccyx] Rel. to both the anus and coccyx.

anococcygeal body The muscle and fibrous tissue lying between the coccyx and the anus.

anococcygeal ligament A band of fibrous tissue joining the tip of the coccyx with the external sphincter ani.

anodal closure contraction ABBR: ACC. Contraction of the muscles at the anode on closure of the circuit.

anodal opening contraction ABBR: AOC. Contraction of the muscles at the anode when the electrical circuit is open.

anode (ăn′ōd) [Gr. *ana*, up, + *hodos*, way] **1.** The positive pole of an electrical source. **2.** In radiography, the target of the x-ray tube. SEE: *cathode*. **anodal** (ăn-ō′dăl), *adj.*

anodmia (ăn-ŏd′mē-ă) [Gr. *an-*, not, + *odme*, stench] Anosmia.

anodontia (ăn″ŏ-dŏn′shē-ă) [″ + *odous*, tooth] Absence of the teeth. SYN: *edentia*.

anodyne (ăn′ō-dīn) [″ + *odyne*, pain] A drug that relieves pain. SYN: *analgesic*.

anodynia (ăn″ō-dĭn′ē-ă) Cessation or absence of pain.

anogenital Concerning the anal and genital areas.

anoikis (ăn-ŏy′ē-kĭs) Programmed cell death (apoptosis) occurring in epithelial cells. It is associated with loss of the normal ability to establish contacts between the cell and the extracellular matrix. SYN: *apoptosis*.

anomaloscope (ă-nŏm′ă-lō-skōp″) [Gr. *anomalos*, irregular, + *skopein*, to examine] A device for detecting color blindness.

anomalous (ă-nŏm′ă-lŭs) [Gr. *anomalos*, uneven] Irregular; deviating from or contrary to normal.

anomaly (ă-nŏm′ă-lē) [Gr. *anomalia*, irregularity] Deviation from normal.

congenital a. Intrauterine development of an organ or structure that is abnormal in form, structure, or position. SYN: *birth defect*.

anomia (ă-nō′mē-ă) [Gr. *a-*, not, + *onoma*, name] Inability to remember names of objects.

anomie (ăn′ŏ-mē) [Fr. from Gr. *anomia*, lawlessness] A term coined by the French sociologist Emile Durkheim (1858–1917) to indicate a condition similar to alienation. The individual feels there has been a disintegration of his or her norms and values. Durkheim felt such individuals were prone to take their lives because of the anxiety, isolation, and alienation that they experience.

anonychia (ăn-ō-nĭk′ē-ă) [Gr. *an-*, not, + *onyx*, nail] Absence of the nails.

anoperineal (ā″nō-pĕr-ĭ-nē′ăl) Rel. to both the anus and perineum.

Anopheles (ă-nŏf′ĕ-lēz) [Gr. *anopheles*, harmful, useless] A genus of mosquitoes belonging to the family Culicidae, order Diptera. It is a vector of *Plasmodium,* the causative agent of malaria, and may be involved in transmitting the causative agent of dengue, filariasis, and many other diseases. Of the almost 100 species of Anopheles, only a few are capable of transmitting the causative organism of malaria. SEE: *malaria*.

anophoria Hyperphoria.

anophthalmia (ăn-ŏf-thăl′mē-ă) [Gr. *an-*, not, + *ophthalmos*, eye] Congenital absence of one or both eyes. SYN: *anopia*(1).

anopia (an-ō′pē-ă) [″ + *ops*, eye] **1.** Anophthalmia. **2.** Anophoria.

anoplasty (ā′nō-plăs″tē) [L. *anus*, anus, + Gr. *plassein*, to form] Reconstructive surgery of the anus.

Anoplura (an-ō-ploo′ră) [Gr. *anoplos*, unarmed, + *oura*, tail] An order of insects composed of the sucking lice. SEE: *louse; pediculosis*.

anopsia (ăn-ŏp′sē-ă) [Gr. *an-*, not, + *opsis*, sight] **1.** Hyperphoria. **2.** Inability to use the vision, as occurs in strabismus, cataract, or refractive errors or in those confined in the dark.

anorchia Anorchidism.

anorchidism, anorchism (ăn-or′kĭ-dĭzm″, ăn-or′kĭzm) [″ + *orchis*, testicle, + *-ismos*, condition] Congenital absence of one or both testes. SYN: *anorchia*.

anorectal (ā-nō-rĕk′tăl) Pert. to both the anus and rectum.

anorectic, anorectous (ăn-ō-rĕk′tĭc, -tŭs) [Gr. *anorektos*, without appetite for] Having no appetite.

anorexia (ăn-ō-rĕk′sē-ă) [Gr. *an-*, not, + *orexis*, appetite] Loss of appetite. Anorexia is seen in depression, malaise, commencement of fevers and illnesses, disorders of the alimentary tract (esp. the stomach), and alcoholism and drug addiction (esp. cocaine). Many medicines and medical procedures have the undesired side effect of causing the suppression of appetite. **anorexic** (-rĕk′sĭk), *adj.*

PATIENT CARE: Oral hygiene is provided before and after eating. The patient's food preferences are determined, and only preferred foods are offered. Small, frequent meals or smaller meals with between-meal and bedtime nutritional snacks are provided. The patient area is kept free of odors, and a quiet atmosphere is provided for meals. Family and friends are encouraged to bring favorite home-cooked meals and to join the patient for meals. Mealtime conversation should focus on pleasant topics and should not involve the patient's food intake. Actual intake is documented, indicating food types, amounts eaten, and approximate caloric and nutrient intake.

a. nervosa An eating disorder marked by weight loss, emaciation, a disturbance in body image, and a fear of weight gain. Patients with the disorder lose weight either by excessive dieting or by purging themselves of calories they have ingested. The illness is typically found in industrialized nations and usually begins in the teen years. Young women are 10 to 20 times more likely than men to suffer from the disorder. Weight loss of greater than 15% of body weight is typical, often with significant metabolic consequences. These may include severe electrolyte disturbances, hypoproteinemia, and endocrine dysfunction. Immune disturbances, anemia, and secondary cardiac arrhythmias may occur. In women, amenorrhea is also characteristic. The disease often resists therapy.

Diagnosis is made by the following criteria: Intense fear of becoming obese. This does not diminish as weight loss progresses. The patient claims to feel fat even when emaciated. A loss of 25% of original weight may occur. No known physical illness accounts for the weight loss. There is a refusal to maintain body weight over a minimal normal weight for age and height.

Psychiatric therapy in a hospital is usually required if the patient refuses to eat. The patient may need to be fed parenterally. SEE: *bulimia; Nursing Diagnoses Appendix.*

PATIENT CARE: The nurse, nutritionist, and physician monitor the patient's vital signs and electrolyte balance; daily fluid intake and output; food types, amounts, and approximate nutrient intake; and laboratory values. The patient is weighed daily or weekly as prescribed. As necessary, the patient's body orifices, underarm area, and hair are checked for hidden weight before weighing. Small, frequent meals and nutritionally complete fluids are provided; the patient may accept the latter more readily. If tube feeding or parenteral nutrition is required, the procedure is explained to the patient and family. Edema or bloating, if present, is also explained, and the patient is reassured of its temporary nature. The patient's activities are strictly monitored as a precaution against vomiting, catharsis, or excessive exercise. The patient is taught that improved nutrition can correct abnormal laboratory findings. Arguments about food or related subjects are avoided. The patient is encouraged to recognize and express feelings; assertive behavior is supported. Assistance is offered to the family and close friends in dealing with their feelings about the patient and the patient's behavior, and they are instructed not to discuss food or weight with the patient. The patient and family are encouraged to seek professional counseling, and are referred to local and national support and information organizations. Stable weight and eating patterns, the ability to express feelings, and the establishment of healthier patient-family relationships are good indicators of successful intervention.

anorexiant (ăn-ō-rĕks′ē-ănt) An appetite suppressor. Examples include amphetamines, fenfluramine, phentermine, and related drugs.

anorexic (ăn-ō-rĕk′sĭk) **1.** Of or relating to anorexia; anorectic. **2.** One who is affected with anorexia.

anorexigenic (ăn″ō-rĕk″sĭ-jĕn′ĭk) [″ + ″ + *gennan*, to produce] Causing loss of appetite.

anorgasmic Relating to the inability to experience orgasm.

anorgasmy (ăn-or-găz′mē) [″ + *orgasmos*, swelling] Failure to reach orgasm during sexual intercourse or masturbation.

anorthopia (ăn″or-thō′pē-ă) [″ + ″ + *ops*, eye] **1.** Vision in which straight lines do not appear straight; symmetry and parallelism not properly perceived. **2.** Strabismus.

anoscope (ā′nō-skōp) [L. *anus*, anus, + Gr. *skopein*, to examine] Speculum for examining the anus and lower rectum.

anosigmoidoscopy (ā″nō-sĭg″moy-dŏs′kō-pē) [″ + Gr. *sigmoeides*, shaped like Greek S, + *skopein*, to examine] Proctosigmoidoscopy.

anosmatic (ăn-ŏz-măt′ĭk) [Gr. *an-*, not, + *osme*, smell] Lacking the sense of smell.

anosmia (ăn-ŏz′mē-ă) Loss of the sense of smell. SYN: *anodmia*.

anosmic, anosmous (ăn-ŏz′mĭk, -mŭs) **1.** Lacking the sense of smell. **2.** Odorless.

anosognosia (ăn-ō-sŏg-nō′zē-ă) [″ + ″ + *gnosis*, knowledge] The apparent denial or unawareness of one's own neurological defect.

visual a. A neurological syndrome in

which patients who cannot see deny that they are blind. An excuse such as "I lost my glasses" may be offered. The lesion is in the visual association areas of the cortex of the brain. SYN: *Anton's syndrome*.

anosphrasia (ăn-ŏs-frā′zē-ă) [Gr. *an-*, not, + *osphresis*, smell] Absence of or imperfect sense of smell.

anospinal (ā″nō-spī′năl) [L. *anus* + *spina*, thorn] Pert. to the anus and spinal cord or to the center in the spinal cord that controls the contraction of the anal sphincter.

anostosis (ăn-ŏs-tō′sĭs) [Gr. *an-*, not, + *osteon*, bone, + *osis*, condition] A defective formation or development of bone; failure to ossify.

anotia (ăn-ō′shē-ă) [″ + *ours*, ear] Congenital malformation with absence of the ears.

anotropia (ăn″ō-trō′pē-ă) [Gr. *ana*, up, + *trope*, a turning] Tendency of the eyes to turn upward and away from the visual axis.

ANOVA Term used in statistics for *an*alysis *o*f *va*riance. SEE: *analysis of variance.*

anovaginal (ā″nō-văj′ĭ-năl) Pert. to the anus and vagina.

anovarism (ăn-ō′văr-ĭzm) [Gr. *an-*, not, + LL. *ovarium*, ovary, + Gr. *-ismos*, condition] Absence of ovaries.

anovesical (ā″nō-vĕs′ĭ-kl) [L. *anus*, anus, + *vesica*, bladder] Rel. to both the anus and urinary bladder.

anovular, anovulatory (ăn-ŏv′ū-lăr, ăn-ŏv′ū-lă-tō″rē) [Gr. *an-*, not, + LL. *ovarium*, ovary] Without ovulation.

anovular cycle Menstrual cycle in which ovulation is absent.

anoxemia (ăn-ŏk-sē′mē-ă) [″ + *oxygen* + Gr. *haima*, blood] Insufficient oxygenation of the blood. SEE: *hypoxemia; respiration.*

anoxia (ăn-ŏk′sē-ă) [″ + *oxygen*] Absence of oxygen. This term is often used incorrectly to indicate hypoxia. **anoxic** (ăn-ŏks′ĭk), *adj.*

ANP *advanced nurse practitioner.*

ANS *autonomic nervous system.*

ansa (ăn′să) *pl.* **ansae** [L., a handle] In anatomy, any structure in the form of a loop or arc.

a. cervicalis A nerve loop in the neck formed by fibers from the first three cervical nerves. Formerly called *ansa hypoglossi.*

a. hypoglossi A. cervicalis.

a. lenticularis Tortuous fiber tract from the globus pallidus, extending around the internal capsule, to the ventral thalamic nucleus.

a. nervorum spinalium Connecting loops of nerve fibers between the anterior spinal nerves.

a. peduncularis Complex fiber tract from the anterior temporal lobe, extending around the internal capsule to the mediodorsal thalamic nucleus.

a. sacralis Nerve loop connecting the sympathetic trunk with the coccygeal ganglion.

a. subclavia Nerve loop that passes anterior and inferior to the subclavian artery, connecting the middle and inferior cervical sympathetic ganglia.

ANSER system A group of questionnaires for evaluating developmental dysfunction in children.

A.N.S.I. *American National Standards Institute.*

ansiform (ăn′sĭ-form) [L. *ansa*, a handle, + *forma*, shape] Shaped like a loop.

ant- SEE: *anti-*.

ant Small social insect of the order Hymenoptera and family Formicidae, distributed worldwide. Ants live in highly organized colonies whose members specialize in performing specific tasks. Because some ants secrete formic acid their bite can be painful.

Antabuse (ăn′tă-būs″) Proprietary name for disulfiram; administered orally in treatment of alcoholism. Drinking alcohol after taking this drug causes severe reactions, including nausea and vomiting, and may endanger the life of the patient. SEE: *Poisons and Poisoning Appendix.*

antacid (ănt-ăs′ĭd) [Gr. *anti*, against, + L. *acidum*, acid] An agent that neutralizes acidity, esp. in the stomach and duodenum. Examples are aluminum hydroxide and magnesium oxide.

antagonism (ăn-tăg′ō-nĭzm″) [Gr. *antagonizesthai*, to struggle against] Mutual opposition or contrary action, as between muscles or medicines.

microbial a. The inhibition of one bacterial organism by another. This is a function of the normal bacterial flora and is one of the most important host defenses against microbial pathogens. SEE: *opportunistic infection.*

antagonist (ăn-tăg′ō-nĭst) That which counteracts the action of something else, such as a muscle or drug; opposite of synergist.

dental a. The tooth in the opposite arch with which a tooth occludes in function.

drug a. A drug that prevents receptor stimulation. An antagonist drug has an affinity for a cell receptor and, by binding to it, prevents the cell from responding to an agonist.

endothelin-receptor a. A medicine that lowers blood pressure by opposing the vasoconstricting effects of endothelins.

leukotriene-receptor a. Any of several medications (e.g., zafirlukast and montelukast) that block the inflammatory effects of leukotrienes and are used to treat patients with asthma. These medications help to reduce the dependence of asthmatic patients on corticosteroids and beta agonist inhalers.

muscular a. A muscle that opposes the action of the prime mover and produces a smooth movement by balancing the opposite forces.

narcotic a. A drug that prevents or reverses the action of a narcotic. SEE: *nalorphine hydrochloride*.

serotonin a. A class of medications used to treat or prevent severe nausea. The antiemetics in this drug class have markedly improved the experience of undergoing chemotherapy. Examples are ondansetron (Zofran) and granisetron (Kytril.)

antalkaline (ănt-ăl′kă-līn, -lĭn) [″ + *alkaline*] An agent that neutralizes alkalinity.

antaphrodisiac (ănt″ăf-rō-dĭz′ē-ăk) [″ + *aphrodisiakos*, sexual] An agent that depresses sexual desire. SYN: *anaphrodisiac*.

antasthenic (ănt″ăs-thĕn′ĭk) [″ + *astheneia*, weakness] Relieving weakness; strengthening, invigorating.

antatrophic (ănt″ă-trō′fĭk) [″ + *atrophia*, atrophy] Preventing or curing atrophy.

antazoline phosphate (ăn-tăz′ō-lēn) An antihistamine used in dilute solution to treat allergic conjunctivitis. A component of the trade name preparation Vasocon-A.

ante- [L.] Prefix meaning *before*.

antebrachium (ăn″tē-brā′kē-ŭm) [L. *ante*, before, + *brachium*, arm] The forearm. **antebrachial** (-ăl), *adj*.

antecardium (ăn″tē-kăr′dē-ŭm) [″ + Gr. *kardia*, heart] The area on the anterior surface of the body overlying the heart and the lower part of the thorax; also spelled *anticardium*. SYN: *precordia; precordium*.

antecedent (ăn″tē-sē′dĕnt) [L. *antecedere*, to precede] Something that comes before something else; a precursor.

plasma thromboplastin a. ABBR: PTA. Blood coagulation factor XI. SYN: *Christmas factor*. SEE: *coagulation factor*.

ante cibum (ăn′tē sē′bŭm) [L.] ABBR: a.c. Used in prescription writing to indicate *before meals*.

antecubital (ăn″tē-kū′bĭ-tăl) [″ + *cubitum*, elbow] In front of the elbow; at the bend of the elbow.

antecubital fossa Triangular area lying anterior to and below the elbow, bounded medially by the pronator teres and laterally by the brachioradialis muscles. SYN: *cubital fossa*.

antecurvature (ăn″tē-kŭr′vă-tŭr″) [″ + *curvatura*, bend] Bending forward abnormally. SYN: *anteflexion*.

antefebrile (an″tē-fē′brĭl, -fē′brīl, -fĕb′rĭl) [L. *ante*, before, + *febris*, fever] Before the development of fever. SYN: *antepyretic*.

anteflect (ăn′tē-flĕkt) [″ + *flectere*, to bend] To bend or cause to bend forward.

anteflexion (ăn″tē-flĕk′shŭn) The abnormal bending forward of part of an organ, esp. of the uterus at its body and neck. SEE: *anteversion*.

antegrade (ăn′tē-grād) Moving forward or in the same direction as the flow.

antelocation (ăn″tē-lō-kā′shŭn) [″ + *locare*, to place] Forward displacement of an organ.

antemortem (ăn′tē-mor′tĕm) [L.] Before death.

antemortem statement Declaration made by an individual immediately preceding death. SYN: *deathbed statement*.

antenatal (ăn″tē-nā′tăl) [″ + *natus*, born] Before birth. SYN: *prenatal*.

antenatal surgery Surgical procedure done on the fetus prior to delivery. This type of surgery is done only at certain medical centers. SEE: *amnioscopy; embryoscopy*.

antepartal, antepartum (ăn″tē-păr′tăl, -tŭm) [L.] Period of pregnancy between conception and onset of labor, used with reference to the mother.

antepyretic (ăn″tē-pī-rĕt′ik) [L. *ante*, before, + Gr. *pyretos*, fever] Before the development of fever. SYN: *antefebrile*.

anterior (ăn-tĭr′ē-or) [L.] Before or in front of; in anatomical nomenclature, refers to the ventral or abdominal side of the body.

anterior drawer test, anterior drawer sign **1.** *Knee:* A test for anterior cruciate ligament rupture. It is positive if anterior glide of the tibia is increased. **2.** *Ankle:* A test for stability of the anterior talofibular ligament of the ankle. It is positive if movement is increased as the examiner grasps the heel with one hand and the distal tibia with the other and draws the heel forward.

anterior horn cell A somatic motor neuron with its cell body in the ventral (anterior) horn of the gray matter of the spinal cord, and an axon that innervates skeletal muscle.

antero- [L.] Prefix denoting *anterior, front, before*.

anteroexternal (ăn″tĕr-ō-ĕks-tĕr′năl) [L. *antero*, anterior, + *externus*, outside] In anatomy, located to the front and laterally. This is not a preferred term.

anterograde [″ + *gradior*, to step] Moving frontward.

anteroinferior [″ + *inferior*, below] In front and below.

anterointernal (ăn″tĕr-ō-ĭn-tĕr′năl) [″ + *internus*, within] In anatomy, located to the front and to the inner side.

anterolateral [″ + *latus*, side] In front and to one side.

anteromedial [″ + *medius*, middle] In front and toward the center.

anteroposterior (ăn″tĕr-ō-pō′stĭr-ē-or) [″ + *posterior*, rear] Passing from front to rear.

anterosuperior [″ + *superior*, above] In front and above.

anteversion (ăn″tē-vĕr′zhŭn) [″ + *vertere*, to turn] **1.** A tipping forward of an organ as a whole, without bending. SEE: *anteflexion*. **2.** Excessive anterior angulation of the neck of the femur (i.e., femoral neck anteversion), leading to excessive internal rotation of the femur. The normal value for femoral neck anteversion is approx. 15°. Any increase in this anterior angulation is called femoral anteversion.

anteverted (ăn″tē-vĕrt′ĕd) Tipped forward.

anthelix (ănt′hē-lĭks, ăn′thē-lĭks) [Gr. *anti*, against, + *helix*, coil] Antihelix.

anthelmintic, anthelminthic (ănt″hĕl-mĭn′tĭk, -thĭk) [″ + *helmins*, worm] An agent that treats or destroys parasitic worms. SYN: *helminthagogue; vermicide*.

Anthemis (ăn′thĕm-ĭs) **1.** A genus of aromatic flowering plants. **2.** Chamomile; dried blossoms of *Anthemis nobilis*; a bitter tonic and antispasmodic.

anthemorrhagic (ănt″hĕm-ō-răj′ĭk) [″ + *haima*, blood, + *rhegnynai*, to burst forth] Antihemorrhagic.

anthocyanin (ăn″thō-sī′ă-nĭn) [Gr. *anthos*, flower, + *kyanos*, a blue substance] Any one of a group of reddish-purple pigments occurring in flowers.

Anthomyia (ăn″thō-mī′yă) [″ + *myia*, fly] A genus of fly of the order Diptera, related to the housefly. Larvae sometimes infest humans.

A. canicularis A small black housefly, whose larvae may infest the human intestine after accidental ingestion, often resulting in gastrointestinal disturbances.

anthophobia (ăn″thō-fō′bē-ă) [″ + *phobos*, fear] Morbid dislike or fear of flowers.

anthracene (ăn′thră-sēn) $C_{14}H_{10}$; a hydrocarbon obtained from distilling coal tar. It is used in manufacturing dyes.

anthracoid (an′thră-koyd) [″ + *eidos*, form, shape] Resembling or pert. to anthrax.

anthracosilicosis (ăn″thră-kō-sĭl″ĭ-kō′sĭs) [″ + L. *silex*, flint, + Gr. *osis*, condition] A form of pneumoconiosis in which carbon and silica deposits accumulate in the lungs due to coal dust inhalation. SYN: *coal worker's pneumoconiosis*. SEE: *anthracosis; silicosis*.

anthracosis (ăn-thră-kō′sĭs) [″ + *osis*, condition] Accumulation of carbon deposits in the lungs due to inhalation of smoke or coal dust. SYN: *black lung*.

anthracycline (ăn-thră-sī′klēn) Any of several antibiotic-based drugs that block DNA synthesis in tumors. They are used in the treatment of solid organ cancers and leukemias. Examples include doxorubicin and daunorubicin.

anthralin (ăn′thră-lĭn) A synthetic hydrocarbon used in ointment form for treating various skin diseases, including fungal infections and eczema.

anthrax (ăn′thrăks) [Gr., coal, carbuncle] Acute, infectious disease caused by inhaling the spores of *Bacillus anthracis*, a large, Gram-positive, nonmotile, spore-forming bacterial rod, or by eating contaminated meat. People who work with contaminated textiles or animal products usually contract it from skin contact with animal hair, hides, or waste (the most common form of the disease, accounting for 95% of cases), but the bacilli may cause a fatal pneumonia if they are inhaled. SEE: illus.

IMMUNIZATION: The anthrax bacillus has been prepared in aerosol form for use in biological warfare. As a result, millions of American troops are now vaccinated against the disease during their military training with one of several evolving vaccines. Their effectiveness in disease prevention remains uncertain. Vaccination is also given to patients affected by active anthrax to prevent relapses. SEE: *biological warfare; Standard and Universal Precautions Appendix*.

SYMPTOMS: Cutaneous anthrax presents with large painless boils ("malignant pustules"), vesicles, or skin ulcers and surrounding brawny edema usually on an exposed body surface, such as the skin of the hand. Inhalation anthrax (also called pulmonary anthrax or "Woolsorter's disease") is marked by fevers, cough, weakness, respiratory failure, and often, rapidly developing symptoms of septic shock or meningitis.

TREATMENT: Treatment for cutaneous anthrax consists of penicillin G parenterally, given usually until the swelling around the skin ulcer resolves (about 7 to 14 days). Therapy for anthrax pneumonia includes penicillin G, plus an anthrax vaccine. For penicillin-sensitive adults, doxycycline, ciprofloxacin, erythromycin, streptomycin, tetracycline, or chloramphenicol may be used.

PATIENT CARE: Health supervision is provided to at-risk employees, along with prompt medical care of all lesions. Terminal disinfection of textile mills contaminated with *B. anthracis* is supervised, using vaporized formaldehyde or other recommended treatment. All

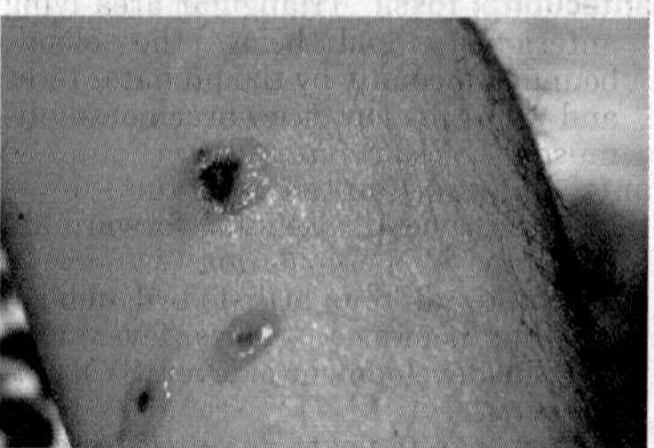

ANTHRAX

cases of anthrax are reported to local health authorities. Isolation procedures (mask, gown, gloves, handwashing, and incineration of contaminated materials) are maintained to protect against drainage and secretions for the duration of illness in both inhalation and cutaneous anthrax. For patients with inhalation anthrax, vital signs are monitored and respiratory support is provided. For patients with cutaneous anthrax, lesions are kept clean and covered with sterile dressings. Prescribed antibiotics are administered. Frequent oral hygiene and skin care are provided. Oral fluid intake and frequent small, nutritious meals are encouraged.

anthropo- [Gr. *anthropos*, man] Prefix denoting relationship to *human beings* or *human life*.

anthropobiology (ăn″thrō-pō-bī-ŏl′ō-jē) [″ + *bios*, life, + *logos*, word, reason] Study of the biology of humans and the great apes.

anthropoid (ăn′thrō-poyd) [″ + *eidos*, form, shape] **1.** Resembling humans. **2.** An ape.

anthropological baseline An imaginary line that passes from the lower border of the orbit to the superior margin of the external auditory meatus.

anthropology (ăn″thrō-pŏl′ō-jē) [″ + *logos*, word, reason] The scientific study of humans. It includes the investigation of human origin and the development of the physical, cultural, religious, and social attributes.

physical a. The branch of anthropology concerned with physical measurement of human beings (as living subjects or skeletal remains).

anthropometer (ăn″thrō-pŏm′ĕ-tĕr) [″ + *metron*, measure] A device for measuring the human body and its parts.

anthropometry (ăn-thrō-pŏm′ĕt-rē) The science of measuring the human body, including craniometry, osteometry, and skin fold evaluation for subcutaneous fat estimation, and height and weight measurements; usually performed by an anthropologist. **anthropometric** (-pō-mĕt′rĭk), *adj.*

anthropomorphism (ăn″thrō-pō-mor′fĭzm) [″ + *morphe*, form, + *-ismos*, condition] Attributing human qualities to nonhuman organisms or objects.

anthropophilic (ăn″thrō-pō-fĭl′ĭk) [″ + *philein*, to love] Preferring humans, said of parasites that prefer a human host to an animal.

anthropozoonosis (ăn″thrō-pō-zō″ō-nō′sĭs) [″ + *zoon*, animal, + *nosis*, disease] An infectious disease acquired by humans from vertebrate hosts of the causative agents. Examples are rabies and trichinosis.

anti-, ant- [Gr.] Prefix meaning *against, opposing, counteracting*.

antiadrenergic (ăn″tē-ă-drĕn-ĕr′jĭk) [Gr. *anti*, against, + L. *ad*, to, + *ren*, kidney, + Gr. *ergon*, work] Preventing or counteracting adrenergic action.

antiagglutinin (ăn″tē-ă-gloo′tĭ-nĭn) A specific antibody opposing the action of an agglutinin.

antiaggregant, platelet A medicine, such as aspirin, that interferes with the aggregation or clumping of platelets.

antiamebic (ăn″tē-ă-mē′bĭk) [″ + *amoibe*, change] A medicine used to prevent or treat amebiasis.

antianaphylaxis (ăn″tē-ăn-ă-fĭ-lăks′ĭs) [″ + *ana*, away from, + *phylaxis*, protection] Desensitization.

antiandrogen (ăn″tē-ăn′drō-jĕn) [″ + *androgen*] A substance that inhibits or prevents the action of an androgen.

antianemic (ăn″tē-ă-nē′mĭk) Preventing or curing anemia.

antiangiogenesis (ăn″tē-ăn″jē-ō-jĕn′ĕ-sĭs) The blocking of the formation of new blood vessels, esp. the blood vessels that grow under the influence of malignant tumors. Numerous agents have such activity, including angiostatin, endostatin, tetracyclines, and paclitaxel, among others. They are useful in the treatment of cancer. SEE: *angiogenesis*.

antiantibody (ăn″tē-ăn′tĭ-bŏd-ē) [″ + *antibody*] An antibody that blocks the binding site of another antibody. Blocking the site inhibits antibody-antigen binding since the antigen must compete with the antiantibody for the binding site.

antiantitoxin (ăn″tē-ăn″tĭ-tŏk′sin) [″ + *antitoxin*] An antibody that acts against an antitoxin, which is an antibody that binds with and destroys a bacterial toxin. SEE: *antibody; antitoxin*.

antiarrhythmic (ăn″tē-ă-rĭth′mĭk) [″ + *a-*, not, + *rhythmos*, rhythm] A drug or physical force that acts to control or prevent cardiac arrhythmias.

antiarthritic (ăn″tē-ăr-thrĭt′ĭk) [″ + *arthritikos*, gouty] Relieving arthritis.

antiasthmatic (ănt″ăz-măt′ĭk) [″ + Gr. *asthma*, panting] **1.** Preventing or relieving asthma. **2.** An agent that prevents or relieves an asthma attack.

antibacterial (ăn″tĭ-băk-tē′rē-ăl) **1.** Destroying or stopping the growth of bacteria. **2.** An agent that destroys or stops the growth of bacteria.

antibiosis (an″tĭ-bī-ō′sĭs) [″ + *bios*, life] An association or relationship between two organisms in which one is harmful to the other.

antibiotic (ăn″tĭ-bī-ŏt′ĭk) **1.** Destructive to life. **2.** Pert. to antibiosis. **3.** A natural or synthetic substance that destroys microorganisms or inhibits their growth. Antibiotics are used extensively to treat infectious diseases in plants, animals, and humans. SEE: *antimicrobial drug; bacterium*.

bactericidal a. An antibiotic that kills microorganisms.

bacteriostatic a. An antibiotic that inhibits the growth of microorganisms.

beta-lactam a. Any of the antimicrobial drugs, such as penicillins or cephalosporins, that kill germs by interfering with the synthesis of bacterial cell walls.

***broad-spectrum* a.** An antibiotic that is effective against a wide variety of microorganisms.

***narrow-spectrum* a.** An antibiotic that is specifically effective against a limited group of microorganisms.

antibiotic-impregnated polymethacrylate beads Vehicles for delivering high-concentration antibiotic therapy to a specific area. The antibiotic-impregnated beads are implanted in open wounds with loss of tissue substance, such as open fractures.

antibiotic resistant Having the ability to resist the action of antibiotics.

antibody (ăn′tĭ-bŏd″ē) ABBR: Ab. An immunoglobulin produced by B lymphocytes in response to a unique antigen. Each Ab molecule combines with a specific antigen to destroy or control it. All antibodies, except natural antibodies (e.g., antibodies to different blood types), are created by B cells linking with a foreign antigen, typically a foreign protein, polysaccharide, or nucleic acid. SYN: *immunoglobulin*. SEE: illus.; *antigen; autoantibody; cytokine*.

Antibodies neutralize or destroy antigens in several ways. They can initiate lysis of the antigen by activating the complement system, neutralizing toxins released by bacteria, coating (opsonizing) the antigen or forming a complex to stimulate phagocytosis, promoting antigen clumping (agglutination), or preventing the antigen from adhering to host cells.

An antibody molecule consists of four polypeptide chains (two light and two heavy), which are joined by disulfide bonds. The heavy chains form the complement-binding site, and the light and heavy chains form the site that binds the antigen.

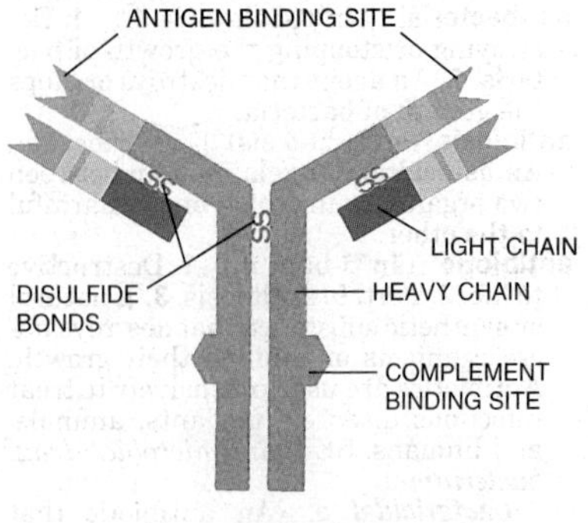

ANTIBODY

Schematic structure of immunoglobulin G antibody

***antiphospholipid* a.** Antibodies against the phospholipids contained in cell membranes. They are occasionally responsible for catastrophic coagulation disorders, which result in cerebral infarction (stroke), placental infarction (with loss of pregnancy), or blood clotting in other organs.

***antireceptor* a.** An antibody that reacts with the antigen receptor on a cell rather than with an antigen itself.

***blocking* a.** An antibody that prevents an antigen from binding with a cell.

***cross-reacting* a.** An antibody that reacts with antigens other than its specific antigen, because they contain binding sites that are structurally similar to its specific antigen. SEE: *antigenic determinant*.

***cytotoxic* a.** An antibody that lyses cells by binding to a cellular antigen and activating complement or killer cells.

***fluorescent* a.** ABBR: FA. An antibody that has been stained or marked by a fluorescent material. The fluorescent antibody technique permits rapid diagnosis of various infections.

***immune* a.** An antibody produced by immunization or as a result of transfusion of incompatible blood.

***maternal* a.** An antibody produced by the mother and transferred to the fetus in utero or during breastfeeding.

***monoclonal* a.** SEE: *hybridoma; monoclonal antibody*.

***natural* a.** An antibody present in a person without known exposure to the specific antigen, such as an anti-A antibody in a person with B blood type.

***polyclonal* a.** An antibody that reacts with many different antigens.

***protective* a.** An antibody produced in response to an infectious disease. SEE: *immunity*.

***warm* a.** Warm autoagglutinin.

antibody combining site The particular area on an antibody molecule to which part of an antigen links, creating an antigen-antibody reaction. SEE: *antibody; antigen; antigenic determinant*.

antibody-dependent cellular cytotoxicity ABBR: ADCC. The process by which phagocytes and natural killer cells bind with receptors on antibodies to destroy the antigens to which the antibodies are bound. SEE: *natural killer cell*.

antibody therapy The creation of antibodies that target specific antigens; used to treat immunological deficiencies, some cancers, and organ transplant rejection. The antibodies are given by injection. SEE: *monoclonal antibody*.

antibrachium (ăn″tĭ-brā′kē-ŭm) Antebrachium; the forearm.

antibromic (ăn″tĭ-brō′mĭk) [Gr. *anti*,

against, + *bromos*, smell] **1.** Deodorizing. **2.** A deodorant.

anti–burn scar garment A carefully fitted garment of material with calibrated stretch characteristics worn to provide uniform pressure over burn graft sites in order to reduce scarring during healing.

anticarcinogenic **1.** Tending to delay or prevent tumor formation. **2.** A substance or action that prevents or delays tumor formation.

anticariogenic A substance or action that interferes with the development of dental caries.

anticarious (ăn″tĭ-kā′rē-ŭs) [″ + *caries*, decay] Preventing decay of teeth.

anticholinergic (ăn″tĭ-kō″lĭn-ĕr′jĭk) **1.** Impeding the impulses of cholinergic, esp. parasympathetic, nerve fibers. **2.** An agent that blocks parasympathetic nerve impulses. The side effects, which include dry mouth and blurred vision, are seen in phenothiazine and tricyclic antidepressant drug therapy. SYN: *parasympatholytic*.

anticholinesterase (ăn″tĭ-kō-lĭn-ĕs′tĕr-ās) A chemical (e.g., an enzyme or drug) that opposes the action of cholinesterase.

anticipate (ăn-tĭs′ĭ-pāt) [L. *ante*, before, + *capere*, to take] **1.** To occur prior to the usual time of onset of a particular illness or disease, said of an event, sign, or symptom. **2.** In nursing and medicine, to prepare for other than the routine or fully expected.

anticipation, genetic anticipation (ăn-tĭs″ĭ-pā′shŭn) In congenital illnesses, the progressive worsening of the expression of a trait as it is passed from generation to generation.

anticipatory grief Mental anguish caused by the impending loss of a body part, a function, or a loved one.

anticipatory guidance Information concerning normal expectations of an age group or disease entity in order to provide support for coping with problems before they arise.

anticlinal (ăn″tĭ-klī′năl) [Gr. *anti*, against, + *klinein*, to incline] Inclined in opposite directions.

anticoagulant (ăn″tĭ-kō-ăg′ū-lănt) [″ + L. *coagulans*, forming clots] **1.** Delaying or preventing blood coagulation. **2.** An agent that prevents or delays blood coagulation. Anticoagulants used for storing whole blood include anticoagulant citrate dextrose solution, anticoagulant citrate phosphate dextrose solution, anticoagulant heparin solution, and anticoagulant sodium citrate solution.

warfarin sodium a. SEE: *warfarin sodium*.

anticodon (ăn″tĭ-kō′dŏn) A triplet (codon) of bases on tRNA (transfer RNA) that complements the corresponding codon on mRNA (messenger RNA), which ensures the proper sequence of amino acids in the protein being synthesized.

anticonvulsant (ăn″tĭ-kŏn-vŭl′sănt) [″ + L. *convulsio*, pulling together] **1.** Preventing or relieving convulsions. **2.** An agent that prevents or relieves convulsions.

anticytotoxin Something that opposes the action of a cytotoxin. SEE: *cytotoxin*.

antidepressant (ăn″tĭ-dē-prĕs′sănt) Any medicine or other mode of therapy that acts to prevent, cure, or alleviate mental depression.

tricyclic and tetracyclic a. A class of antidepressant agents whose chemical structure has three fused rings. These drugs block the reuptake of norepinephrine and serotonin at the nerve endings.

antidiabetic (ăn″tĭ-dī″ă-bĕt′ĭk) **1.** Preventing or relieving diabetes. **2.** An agent that prevents or relieves diabetes. SEE: *oral hypoglycemic agent*.

antidiarrheal (ăn″tĭ-dī-ă-rē′ăl) A substance used to prevent or treat diarrhea.

antidiuretic (ăn″tĭ-dī-ū-rĕt′ĭk) [″ + *dia*, intensive, + *ouresis*, urination] **1.** Lessening urine formation. **2.** A drug that decreases urine formation.

antidotal (ăn″tĭ-dō′tăl) Acting as or pert. to an antidote.

antidote (ăn′tĭ-dōt) [Gr. *antidoton*, given against] A substance that neutralizes poisons or their effects. **antidotal,** *adj.*

chemical a. An antidote that reacts with the poison to produce a harmless chemical compound. For example, table salt precipitates silver nitrate and forms the much less toxic silver chloride. Chemical antidotes should be used sparingly and, after their use, should be removed from the stomach by gastric lavage because they may produce serious results if allowed to remain there.

mechanical a. An antidote that prevents absorption of the poison. Examples are fats, oils, milk (casein coagulum), whites of eggs, finely divided charcoal, fuller's earth, and mineral oil. (Fats and oils are not to be used in treating phosphorus, camphor, aspidium, and cantharides poisonings.)

physiologic a. An antidote that produces physiological effects opposite to the effects of the poison; e.g., sedatives are given for convulsants and stimulants are given for hypnotics. These should not be given without a physician's definite instructions.

universal a. An idealized antidote that is effective against many poisons (there is no known antidote that is literally universal).

antidromic (ăn″tĭ-drŏm′ĭk) [Gr. *anti*, against, + *dromos*, running] Denoting nerve impulses traveling in the opposite direction from normal.

antiemetic (ăn″tĭ-ē-mĕt′ĭk) [″ + *emetikos*, inclined to vomit] **1.** Preventing or relieving nausea and vomiting. **2.** An agent that prevents or relieves nausea and vomiting.

antienzyme (an″tĭ-ĕn′zīm) A substance that opposes the action of an enzyme.

antiepileptic (ăn″tĭ-ĕp″ĭ-lĕp′tĭk) **1.** Opposing epilepsy. **2.** Any procedure or therapy that combats epilepsy.

antiestrogen (ăn″tĭ-ĕs′trō-jĕn) A substance that blocks or modifies the action of estrogen.

antifebrile (ăn″tĭ-fē′brĭl, -fē′brīl, -fĕb′rĭl) [″ + L. *febris*, fever] **1.** Reducing fever. **2.** An agent that reduces fever. SYN: *antipyretic*.

antifibrinolysin (ăn″tĭ-fī″brĭ-nŏl′ĭ-sĭn) [″ + L. *fibra*, fiber, + Gr. *lysis*, dissolution] A substance that counteracts fibrinolysis.

antifungal (ăn″tĭ-fŭng′găl) **1.** Destroying or inhibiting the growth of fungi. **2.** An agent that destroys or inhibits the growth of fungi.

antigalactic (ăn″tĭ-gă-lăk′tĭk) **1.** Preventing or diminishing the secretion of milk. **2.** An agent that prevents or diminishes the secretion of milk.

antigen (ăn′tĭ-jĕn) [Gr. *anti*, against, + *gennan*, to produce] A protein or oligosaccharide marker on the surface of cells that identifies the cell as *self* or *non-self;* identifies the type of cell, e.g., skin, kidney; stimulates the production of antibodies, by B lymphocytes, that will neutralize or destroy the cell if necessary; and stimulates cytotoxic responses by granulocytes, monocytes, and lymphocytes.

Antigens on the body's own cells are called autoantigens. Antigens on all other cells are called foreign antigens. Matching certain types of tissue antigens is important for the success of an organ transplant. Inflammation occurs when neutrophils, monocytes, and macrophages encounter an antigen from any source during bodily injury. The antigen may be foreign or may be an autoantigen that has been damaged and, therefore, appears to be foreign. Reactions to antigens by T and B cells are part of the specific immune response. SEE: *autoantigen; cytokine; histocompatibility locus antigen*.

allogeneic a. An antigen that occurs in some individuals of the same species. Examples are the human blood group antigens.

alpha-fetoprotein a. SEE: *alpha-fetoprotein*.

carcinoembryonic a. ABBR: CEA. A molecular marker found on normal fetal cells and in the bloodstream of patients with cancers of the colon, breast, lung, and other organs. Assays for CEA are used both to monitor the effectiveness of treatments for cancer and to provide prognostic information to patients.

CD a. Cell surface molecules, also known as cluster of differentiation antigens, that determine the immunological ancestry, functional development, or stage of maturity of a cell. They are designated CD1, CD2, and so on. The markers may be identified by specific monoclonal antibodies and used to designate cell populations (e.g., the CD4 lymphocyte is the major target for HIV, the virus that causes AIDS).

CD4 a. A cell surface molecule present on T cells, monocytes, and macrophages that identifies them. It is the receptor for the human immunodeficiency virus associated with AIDS. SEE: *cluster of differentiation*.

class I a. One of the major histocompatibility molecules present on almost all cells except human red blood cells. These antigens are important in the rejection of grafts and transplanted organs.

class II a. One of the major histocompatibility molecules present on immunocompetent cells.

cross-reacting a. An antigen having the ability to react with more than one specific antibody.

D a. The protein marker in the Rh group of antigens that stimulates the greatest immune response. SEE: *Rh blood group*.

H a. A flagellar protein present on the surface of some enteric bacilli such as *Escherichia coli*. The antigen is important in classifying these bacilli.

histocompatibility locus a. ABBR: HLA. One of the multiple antigens present on all nucleated cells in the body that identify the cells as "self." Immune cells compare these antigens to foreign antigens, which do not match the "self" and which therefore trigger an immune response. These markers determine the compatibility of tissue for transplantation.

They are derived from genes at seven sites (loci) on chromosome 6, in an area called the major histocompatibility complex (MHC) and each histocompatibility antigen is divided into one of two MHC classes.

In humans, the proteins created in the MHC are called human leukocyte antigens (HLA) because these markers were originally found on lymphocytes. Each gene in the MHC has several forms or alleles. Therefore, the number of different histocompatibility antigens is huge, making it necessary to identify and match HLAs in donors and recipients involved in tissue and organ transplantation. The identification of HLAs is called tissue typing.

The identification of HLA sites on chromosome 6 has enabled researchers to correlate the presence of specific histocompatibility and certain autoimmune diseases including insulin-dependent diabetes mellitus, multiple sclerosis, some forms of myasthenia gravis, rheumatoid arthritis, and ankylosing spondylitis. SYN: *human leukocyte antigen*. SEE: *major histocompatibility complex*.

human leukocyte a. SEE: *histocompatibility locus antigen*.

H-Y a. A histocompatibility antigen located on the cell membrane. It has a primary role in determining the sexual differentiation of the male embryo.

K a. A capsular antigen present on the surface of some enteric bacilli. The antigen is important in classifying these bacilli.

O a. A surface antigen of some enteric bacilli. The antigen is important in classifying these bacilli.

oncofetal a. An antigen normally expressed in the fetus that may reappear in the adult in association with certain tumors. Examples include alpha-fetoprotein and carcinoembryonic antigens.

p24 a. The core protein of the human immunodeficiency virus (HIV). The presence of p24 antigen in the blood is a marker of uncontrolled HIV replication. p24 antigenemia is encountered in the acute retroviral syndrome before host immune response and in advanced acquired immunodeficiency syndrome when the immune system has been destroyed. When p24 antigen is detected in the blood, the HIV viral load is high and the person is highly infectious to others.

prostate-specific a. ABBR: PSA. A marker for cancer of the prostate, found in the blood. It is secreted by both benign and malignant prostate tumors, but cancerous prostate cells secrete it at much higher levels. Prostate-specific antigen is used as a screening test for cancer of the prostate and as a means of following the results of treatment in patients with known prostate cancer. SEE: *prostate cancer*.

soluble a. An antigen present in a liquid (aqueous) substance. A soluble antigen is recognized by B lymphocytes but cannot be detected by T lymphocytes until it has been processed by an antigen-presenting cell. SEE: *T cell*.

T-dependent a. An antigen that can stimulate an antibody response only in the presence of helper T cells.

T independent a. One of two types of antigens that stimulate B cell production of antibodies without the presence of T cells. TI-1 antigens, such as lipopolysaccharides from gram-negative organisms, stimulate production of both specific (monoclonal) and nonspecific (polyclonal) antibodies and promote the release of cytokines from macrophages that enhance the immune response. TI-2 antigens, which result in monoclonal antibody production, may require the presence of cytokines. SEE: *B cell; T cell*.

tumor-specific a. An antigen produced by certain tumors. It appears on the tumor cells but not on normal cells derived from the same tissue.

antigen binding site Antigenic determinant.

antigenemia (ăn″tĭ-jĕ-nē′mē-ă) The presence of an antigen in the bloodstream.

antigenic (ăn-tĭ-jĕn′ĭk) Capable of causing the production of an antibody.

antigenic determinant The specific area of an antigen that binds with an antibody combining site and determines the specificity of the antigen-antibody reaction. SEE: *antigen*.

epitope a.d. The simplest form of an antigenic determinant within a complex antigenic marker. The epitope links with a paratope, one area of an antibody combining site.

antigenic drift A minor change in the protein marker or antigen on an organism. Small changes in the antigenic surface markers of some microorganisms (such as the influenza virus) occur from year to year. Vaccinations against the virus are adapted annually to combat these changes and prevent epidemic infection.

antigenic specificity The property of mature B and T lymphocytes that enables them to respond to specific foreign antigens entering the body. Antigen specificity requires mature B and T cells that have been previously exposed to the antigen and, therefore, are able to recognize it again and respond by neutralizing or destroying it. The exact process by which B lymphocytes become capable of recognizing and responding to antigens is unknown. Development of antigen specificity by T cells requires macrophage processing of the antigen for recognition.

antigenicity The condition of being able to produce an immune response to an antibody. **antigenic,** *adj*.

antigen-presenting cell ABBR: APC. A cell that breaks down antigens and displays their fragments on surface receptors next to major histocompatibility complex molecules. This presentation is necessary for some T lymphocytes that are unable to recognize soluble antigens. Macrophages are the primary antigen-presenting cells, but B cells and dendritic cells also can act as APCs. SEE: *cell, T; macrophage processing.*

antigen processing The mechanism by which foreign antigens are taken into antigen-presenting cells (APCs) and broken up. Part of the antigen is then displayed (presented) on the surface of the APC next to a histocompatibility or "self" antigen, activating T lymphocytes and cell-mediated immunity. T lymphocytes are unable to recognize or respond to most antigens without APC assistance. The most active APCs are macrophages, B cells, and dendritic cells. SEE: *antigen; macrophage processing; self.*

antiglobulin (ăn″tĭ-glŏb′ū-lĭn) An antibody that binds with globulin and makes it precipitate out of solution. Antiglobulins are used in Coombs' test to detect the presence of a particular antibody or to type blood groups.

antiglobulin test A test for the presence in human blood of antibodies. The antibodies present in the blood do not, themselves, cause agglutination. It is the addition of an antibody made in animals (antiglobulin) that stimulates red blood cell clumping. The direct antiglobulin test (DAT) is used to diagnose autoimmune hemolytic anemia and hemolytic disease of the newborn. The indirect antiglobulin test (IAT), or Coombs' test, is used to identify blood types. SYN: *Coombs' test.*

direct a. t. ABBR: DAT. A laboratory test for the presence of complement or an antibody that are bound to a patient's red blood cells (RBCs). The test is used in patients with autoimmune hemolytic anemia, hemolytic disease of the newborn, and transfusion reactions. After the patient's RBCs are washed to remove unbound antibodies, they are mixed with antihuman globulin serum containing polyvalent antibodies that bind with the antibody or complement on the RBCs and cause them to agglutinate (clump). Monoclonal antibodies can be used to identify the specific class of antibody or complement component causing RBC destruction. SEE: *Coombs' test.*

antigoitrogenic (ăn″tĭ-goy″trō-jĕn′ĭk) [″ + L. *guttur*, throat, + Gr. *gennan*, to produce] Preventing the formation of a goiter.

antihelix (ăn″tĭ-hē′lĭks) [″ + Gr. *helix*, coil] The inner curved ridge of the external ear parallel to the helix. SYN: *anthelix.*

antihemolysin (ăn″tĭ-hĕ-mŏl′ĭ-sĭn) A substance that opposes the action of hemolysin.

antihemorrhagic (ăn″tĭ-hĕm-ō-răj′ĭk) [″ + *haima*, blood, + *rhegnynai*, to burst forth] **1.** Preventing or arresting hemorrhage. **2.** An agent that prevents or arrests hemorrhage.

antihidrotic (ăn″tĭ-hī-drŏt′ĭk) [″ + *hidrotikos*, sweating] Antiperspirant.

antihistamine (ăn″tĭ-hĭs′tă-mēn, -mĭn) A drug that opposes the action of histamine. Although there are two classes of histamine-blocking drugs, the term *antihistamine* is typically used to describe agents that block the action of histamines on H_1 receptors. These agents are used to treat allergies, hives, and other local and systemic hypersensitivity (allergic) reactions. Side effects of first-generation antihistamines (e.g, chlorpheniramine) include sedation, drying of mucous membranes, and urinary retention. Some first-generation antihistamines can also be used to treat insomnia, motion sickness, or vertigo. Second-generation agents (e.g., loratadine) tend to be less sedating, but still have beneficial effects in the treatment of allergies. SYN: *histamine blocking agent.* SEE: *histamine.*

antihistamine poisoning SEE: *Poisons and Poisoning Appendix.*

antihistaminic (ăn″tĭ-hĭs″tă-mĭn′ĭk) **1.** Opposing the action of histamine. **2.** An agent that opposes the action of histamine.

antihormone A substance that interferes with the action of a hormone.

antihypercholesterolemic (ăn″tĭ-hī″pĕr-kō-lĕs″tĕr-ŏl-ē′mĭk) [″ + *hyper*, above, + *chole*, bile, + *stereos*, solid, + *haima*, blood] **1.** Preventing or controlling elevation of the serum cholesterol level. **2.** An agent that prevents or controls elevation of the serum cholesterol level.

antihypertensive (ăn″tĭ-hī″pĕr-tĕn′sĭv) [″ + ″ + L. *tensio*, tension] **1.** Preventing or controlling high blood pressure. **2.** An agent that prevents or controls high blood pressure.

antihypnotic (ăn″tĭ-hĭp-nŏt′ĭk) **1.** Preventing or inhibiting sleep. **2.** An agent that prevents or inhibits sleep.

anti-icteric (ăn″tĭ-ĭk-tĕr′ĭk) [″ + *ikteros*, jaundice] **1.** Preventing or relieving jaundice. **2.** An agent that prevents or relieves jaundice.

anti-inflammatory (ăn″tĭ-ĭn-flăm′ă-tō-rē) **1.** Counteracting inflammation. **2.** An agent that counteracts inflammation.

antiketogenesis (ăn″tĭ-kē-tō-jĕn′ĕ-sĭs) [″ + *ketone* + Gr. *gennan*, to produce] The prevention or inhibition of formation of ketone bodies. In starvation, diabetes, and certain other conditions, production of ketones is increased, but they accumulate in the blood because cells do not use them as rapidly as they would carbohydrate energy sources. Increased carbohydrate intake will help to prevent or treat this. Carbohydrates are therefore antiketogenic. In ketonemia due to diabetes, both insulin and carbohydrates are needed to allow carbohydrate metabolism to proceed at a rate that would control ketone formation. **antiketogenetic, antiketogenic** (-jĕ-nĕt′ĭk, -jĕn′ĭk), *adj.*

antilactase (ăn″tĭ-lăk′tās) [″ + *lac*, milk, + *-ase*, enzyme] A substance that opposes the action of lactase.

antilipemic (ăn″tĭ-lī-pē′mĭk) **1.** Preventing or counteracting the accumulation of fatty substances in the blood. **2.** An agent that prevents or counteracts the accumulation of fatty substances in the blood.

antilithic (ăn″tĭ-lĭth′ĭk) [″ + *lithos*, stone] **1.** Preventing or relieving calculi. **2.** An agent that prevents or relieves calculi.

antilymphocyte serum (ăn″tĭ-lĭm″fō-sīt′) ABBR: ALS. An antibody-containing serum that is used to reduce rejection of transplanted organs and tissues. Its immunosuppressive effects are directed against B and T lymphocytes, the cells that promote the formation of antibodies and of cell-mediated immunity. SYN: *antilymphocyte globulin.* SEE: *monoclonal antibody.*

antilysin (ăn-tĭ-lī′sĭn) Antibody that opposes the action of lysin.

antilysis (ăn-tĭ-lī′sĭs) [″ + *lysis*, dissolution] Prevention of lysis (death) of a cell. **antilytic** (-lĭt′ĭk), *adj.*

antilyssic (ăn-tĭ-lĭs′ĭk) [″ + *lyssa*, frenzy] Preventing rabies.

antimalarial (ăn″tĭ-mă-lā′rē-ăl) **1.** Preventing or relieving malaria. **2.** An agent that prevents or relieves malaria.

antimere (ăn′tĭ-mēr) [″ + *meros*, a part] One of corresponding parts of the body on opposite sides of the long axis.

antimetabolite (ăn″tĭ-mĕ-tăb′ō-līt) **1.** A substance that opposes the action of or replaces a metabolite and is structurally similar to it. Certain antibiotics are effective because they act as antimetabolites. **2.** A class of antineoplastic drugs used to treat cancer. Antimetabolites are structurally similar to vitamins, coenzymes, or other substances essential for growth and division of normal and neoplastic cells. These drugs are most effective against rapidly growing tumors. A drug-induced block of DNA synthesis occurs when the cells take in the antimetabolite rather than the necessary nutrient or enzyme.

antimetropia (ăn″tĭ-mĕ-trō′pē-ă) [″ + *metron*, measure, + *ops*, eye] An ocular disorder in which each eye has a different error of refraction (e.g., one eye may be hyperopic; the other, myopic).

antimicrobial (ăn″tĭ-mī-krō′bē-ăl) **1.** Destructive to or preventing the development of microorganisms. **2.** An agent that destroys or prevents the development of microorganisms.

antimicrobial drug A chemical substance that either kills microorganisms or prevents their growth.

antimicrobic (ăn″tĭ-mī-krō′bĭk) [″ + *mikros*, small, + *bios*, life] Antimicrobial.

antimitotic (ăn″tĭ-mī-tŏt′ĭk) Interfering with or preventing mitosis.

antimonial (ăn″tĭ-mō′nē-ăl) Pert. to or containing antimony.

antimony (ăn′tĭ-mō″nē) SYMB: Sb. Stibium; a crystalline metallic element, atomic weight 121.75, atomic number 51. Its compounds are used in alloys and medicines and may form poisons.

antimony poisoning Toxicity caused by ingestion of antimony. Symptoms include an acrid metallic taste; cardiac failure; sweating and vomiting about 30 min after ingestion. In large doses, it causes irritation of the lining of the alimentary tract, resembling arsenic poisoning.

FIRST AID: British antilewisite (BAL) can be used as an antidote. SEE: *arsenic in Poisons and Poisoning Appendix.*

antimuscarinic Opposing the action of muscarine or agents that act like muscarinics. Atropine and scopolamine are antimuscarinic drugs.

antimycotic (ăn″tĭ-mī-kŏt′ĭk) [Gr. *anti*, against, + *mykes*, fungus] Inhibiting or preventing the growth of fungi.

antinarcotic (ăn″tĭ-năr-kŏt′ĭk) [″ + *narkotikos*, benumbing] **1.** Opposing the action of a narcotic. **2.** An agent that opposes the action of a narcotic. Naloxone is an antinarcotic medication that is used in the reversal of narcotic overdose.

antinatriuresis (ăn″tĭ-nā″trĭ-ū-rē′sĭs) [″ + L. *natrium*, sodium, + Gr. *ouresis*, making water] Decreasing the excretion of sodium in the urine.

antinauseant (ăn″tĭ-naw′sē-ănt) **1.** Preventing or relieving nausea. **2.** An agent that prevents or relieves nausea.

antineoplastic (ăn″tĭ-nē″ō-plăs′tĭk) **1.** Preventing the development, growth, or proliferation of malignant cells. **2.** An agent that prevents the development, growth, or proliferation of malignant cells.

antinephritic (ăn″tĭ-nĕ-frĭt′ĭk) **1.** Preventing or relieving inflammation of the kidneys. **2.** An agent that prevents or relieves inflammation of the kidneys.

antineuralgic (ăn″tĭ-nū-răl′jĭk) [″ + *neuron*, nerve, + *algos*, pain] **1.** Relieving neuralgia. **2.** An agent that relieves neuralgia.

antineuritic (ăn″tĭ-nū-rĭt′ĭk) **1.** Preventing or relieving inflammation of a nerve. **2.** An agent that prevents or relieves inflammation of a nerve.

antinuclear (ăn″tĭ-nū′klē-ăr) Reacting with or destroying the nucleus of a cell.

antinuclear antibodies ABBR: ANA. A group of autoantibodies that react against normal components of the cell nucleus. These antibodies are present in a variety of immunologic diseases, including systemic lupus erythematosus, progressive systemic sclerosis, Sjögren's syndrome, scleroderma, polymyositis, and dermatomyositis, and in some persons taking hydralazine, procainamide, or isoniazid. In addition, ANA is present in some normal individuals. Tests for ANAs are used in the diagnosis and management of autoimmune diseases.

antiodontalgic (ăn″tē-ō″dŏn-tăl′jĭk) [″ + *odous*, tooth, + *algos*, pain] **1.** Relieving toothache. **2.** An agent that relieves toothache.

anti-oncogene A gene that inhibits or prevents the growth of tumor cells. SEE: *oncogene*.

antiovulatory (ăn″tē-ŏv′ū-lă-tō″rē) Inhibiting or preventing ovulation.

antioxidant (ăn″tē-ŏk′sĭ-dănt) An agent that prevents or inhibits oxidation. Antioxidants are substances that may protect cells from the damaging effects of oxygen radicals, highly reactive chemicals that play a part in atherosclerosis, some forms of cancer, and reperfusion injuries.

antiparallel (ăn″tĭ-păr′ă-lĕl) The characteristic sequencing of the deoxyribonucleotides on one strand of the DNA helix, which is matched by the opposite sequencing on the other strand.

antiparalytic (ăn″tĭ-păr-ă-lĭt′ĭk) Relieving paralysis.

antiparkinsonian **1.** Pert. to any effective therapy for parkinsonism. **2.** An agent effective against parkinsonism.

antiparasitic (ăn″tĭ-păr-ă-sĭt′ĭk) **1.** Destructive to parasites. **2.** An agent that destroys parasites.

antipathy (ăn-tĭp′ă-thē) **1.** Feeling of strong aversion. **2.** Antagonism. **antipathic** (ăn″tĭ-păth′ĭk), *adj.*

antipedicular (ăn″tĭ-pĕ-dĭk′ū-lăr) Effective against pediculosis, said of a medicine or procedure.

antiperistalsis (ăn″tĭ-pĕr″ĭ-stăl′sĭs) [″ + *peri*, around, + *stalsis*, constriction] Reversed peristalsis; a wave of contraction in the gastrointestinal tract moving toward the oral end. In the duodenum it is associated with vomiting; in the ascending colon it occurs normally. SEE: *peristalsis*. **antiperistaltic** (-stăl′tĭk), *adj.*

antiperspirant (ăn″tĭ-pĕr′spĭ-rănt) **1.** Inhibiting perspiration. **2.** A substance that inhibits perspiration. SYN: *anhidrotic; antihidrotic; antisudorific*.

antiphagocytic (ăn″tĭ-făg-ō-sĭt′ĭk) Preventing or inhibiting phagocytosis.

antiplastic (ăn″tĭ-plăs′tĭk) [″ + *plassein*, to form] **1.** Preventing or inhibiting wound healing. **2.** An agent that prevents or inhibits wound healing by preventing formation of granulation tissue.

antiplatelet (ăn″tĭ-plāt′lĕt) **1.** Destructive to platelets. **2.** An agent that destroys platelets.

antipodal (ăn-tĭp′ō-dăl) [Gr. *antipous*, with feet opposite] Located at opposite positions.

antiporter (ăn′tē-por″tĕr) A cell membrane protein that moves two substances in opposite directions through the membrane; the opposite of symporter.

antiprostaglandin (ăn″tĭ-prŏs″tă-glăn′dĭn) Any agent that blocks the release or action of prostaglandins. Antagonists of prostaglandins are primarily used to relieve pain and inflammation. SEE: *nonsteroidal anti-inflammatory drug*.

antiprostatitis (ăn″tĭ-prŏs″tă-tī′tĭs) Inflammation of Cowper's gland.

antiprotease (ăn″tĭ-prō′tē-ās) A chemical that interferes with the hydrolysis of proteins by a protease enzyme.

antiprotozoal (ăn″tĭ-prō″tō-zō′ăl) Destructive to protozoa.

antipruritic (ăn″tĭ-proo-rĭt′ĭk) **1.** Preventing or relieving itching. **2.** An agent that prevents or relieves itching.

antipsoriatic (ăn″tĭ-sō″rē-ăt′ĭk) [Gr. *anti*, against, + *psora*, itch] **1.** Preventing or relieving psoriasis. **2.** An agent that prevents or relieves psoriasis.

antipyresis (ăn″tĭ-pī-rē′sĭs) [″ + *pyretos*, fever] Use of antipyretics.

antipyretic (ăn-tĭ-pī-rĕt′ĭk) **1.** Reducing fever. **2.** An agent that reduces fever. SYN: *antifebrile*.

antipyrotic (ăn″tĭ-pī-rŏt′ĭk) [″ + *pyrotikos, burning*] **1.** Promoting the healing of burns. **2.** An agent that promotes the healing of burns.

antirachitic (ăn″tĭ-ră-kĭt′ĭk) [″ + *rachitis*, rickets] **1.** Helping to cure rickets. **2.** An agent for treating rickets.

antiretroviral (ăn″tĭ-rĕt″rō-vī′răl) Any agent that acts against retroviruses such as the human immunodeficiency virus, the virus that causes the acquired immunodeficiency syndrome.

antirheumatic (ăn″tĭ-roo-măt′ĭk) **1.** Preventing or relieving rheumatism. **2.** An agent that prevents or relieves rheumatism.

antiscabietic (ăn″tĭ-skā″bē-ĕt′ĭk) [Gr. *anti*, against, + L. *scabies*, itch] **1.** Preventing or relieving scabies. **2.** An agent that prevents or relieves scabies.

antiscorbutic (ăn″tĭ-skor-bū′tĭk) [″ + L. *scorbutus*, scurvy] **1.** Preventing or relieving scurvy. **2.** An agent that prevents or relieves scurvy.

antiseborrheic (ăn″tĭ-sĕb″ō-rē′ĭk) **1.** Counteracting or effectively treating seborrhea. **2.** An agent that counteracts or relieves seborrhea.

antisecretory (ăn″tĭ-sē-krē′tō-rē) **1.** Inhibiting secretion of a gland or organ. **2.** An agent that inhibits secretion of a gland or organ.

antiself The reaction of antibodies or lymphocytes with antigens present in the host. SEE: *autoantibody; autoimmune disease.*

antisense compounds Manufactured compounds that may alter disease processes by blocking the production of harmful proteins by diseased cells. These molecules seek out and impede the functioning of a diseased cell's messenger RNA (i.e., a "sense" strand). Without this intervention, the RNA would carry basic directions for the production of disease-causing proteins.

antisepsis (ăn″tĭ-sĕp′sĭs) [″ + *sepsis*, putrefaction] The prevention of sepsis by preventing or inhibiting the growth of causative microorganisms.

antiseptic (ăn″tĭ-sĕp′tĭk) **1.** Rel. to antisepsis. **2.** An agent capable of producing antisepsis.

Chemically, antiseptics may be inorganic, such as the mercury preparations, or organic, such as carbolic acid (phenol). Oxidizing disinfectants liberate oxygen when in contact with pus or organic substances. When in use they should be washed away and replaced frequently to help remove pus, blood, and other substances. Different types of bacteria are sensitive to different antiseptics. SEE: *disinfectant* for table.

antiserum (ăn″tĭ-sē′rŭm) A serum that contains antibodies for a specific antigen. It may be of human or animal origin. SYN: *immune serum.*

monovalent a. Antiserum containing antibodies specific for one antigen.

polyvalent a. Antiserum containing antibodies specific for more than one antigen.

antishock garment A special garment that can be placed quickly on a patient in hypovolemic shock. The device contains inflatable compartments that, when filled with air, compress the lower extremities and abdominal area. This compression helps to prevent pooling of blood and fluids in the tissues. The value of this garment in treating shock is questionable. Also known as MAST *(military antishock trousers).*

CAUTION: This garment is contraindicated in congestive heart failure, cardiogenic shock, and penetrating chest trauma.

PATIENT CARE: Inflatable compartments are filled to appropriate pressure (approximately 104 mm Hg or until the pop-off valves begin to leak), from the bottom up, and inflation is maintained until venous access and fluid resuscitation are initiated. Compartments are then deflated from top to bottom; the patient's blood pressure and pulse are monitored frequently for evidence of hypotension. SEE: *anti-G suit.*

antisialagogue (ăn″tĭ-sī-ăl′ă-gŏg) [Gr. *anti*, against, + *sialon*, saliva, + *agogos*, drawing forth] An agent, such as atropine, that lessens or prevents production of saliva.

antisialic (ăn″tĭ-sī-ăl′ĭk) **1.** Inhibiting the secretion of saliva. **2.** An agent that inhibits the secretion of saliva.

antisocial (ăn″tĭ-sō′shăl) Pert. to a person whose outlook and actions are socially negative and whose behavior is repeatedly in conflict with what society perceives as the norm. SEE: *asocial.*

antispasmodic [″ + *spasmos*, convulsion] **1.** Preventing or relieving spasm. **2.** An agent that prevents or relieves spasm. SEE: *spasm.*

antistaphylococcic (ăn″tĭ-stăf″ĭ-lō-kŏk′sĭk) [Gr. *anti*, against, + *staphyle*, bunch of grapes, + *cocci*, bacteria] Destructive to staphylococci.

antistreptococcic (ăn″tĭ-strĕp″tō-kŏk′sĭk) Destructive to streptococci.

antistreptolysin (ăn″tĭ-strĕp-tŏl′ĭ-sĭn) Antibody that opposes the action of streptolysin, a hemolysin produced by streptococci.

antisudorific (ăn″tĭ-soo″dor-ĭf′ĭk) Antiperspirant.

antisyphilitic (ăn″tĭ-sĭf″ĭ-lĭt′ĭk) [″ + L. *syphiliticus*, pert. to syphilis] **1.** Curing or relieving syphilis. **2.** An agent that cures or relieves syphilis.

antithenar (ăn-tĭth′ĕn-ăr) [″ + *thenar*, palm] The eminence on the ulnar side of the palm, formed by the muscles of the little finger. SYN: *hypothenar eminence.*

antithrombin Any agent that prevents the action of thrombin.

a. III A plasma protein that inactivates thrombin and inhibits coagulation factors IX, X, XI, and XII, preventing abnormal clotting.

antithrombotic (ăn″tĭ-thrŏm-bŏt′ĭk) Interfering with or preventing thrombosis or blood coagulation.

antithyroid (ăn″tĭ-thī′royd) [″ + *thyreoeides*, thyroid] **1.** Preventing or inhibiting the functioning of the thyroid gland. **2.** An agent that prevents or inhibits the functioning of the thyroid gland.

antitoxigen (ăn″tĭ-tŏk′sĭ-gĕn) [″ + ″ + *gennan*, to produce] Antitoxinogen.

antitoxin (ăn″tĭ-tŏk′sĭn) An antibody produced in response to and capable of neutralizing a specific biologic toxin such as those that cause diphtheria, gas-gangrene, or tetanus. Antitoxins are used for prophylactic and therapeutic purposes. SEE: *antivenin.* **antitoxic** (-tŏk′sĭk), *adj.*

antitoxinogen (ăn″tĭ-tŏk-sĭn′ō-jĕn) [Gr. *anti*, against, + *toxikon*, poison, + *gennan*, to produce] An antigen that stimulates production of antitoxin. SYN: *antitoxigen.*

antitragicus (ăn″tĭ-trăj′ĭ-kŭs) A small muscle in the pinna of the ear.
antitragus (ăn″tĭ-trā′gŭs) [″ + L. *tragus*, goat] A projection on the ear of the cartilage of the auricle in front of the tail of the helix, posterior to the tragus.
antitrichomonal **1.** Resistant to or lethal to trichomonads. **2.** A medicine effective in treating trichomonal infections.
antitrismus (ăn″tĭ-trĭs′mŭs) [″ + *trismos*, grinding] A condition in which the mouth cannot close because of tonic spasm. SEE: *trismus*.
antitrypsin (ăn″tĭ-trĭp′sĭn) A substance that inhibits the action of trypsin.
alpha-1-a. A low-molecular-weight glycoprotein that inhibits proteolytic enzymes. Deficiency of this enzyme is associated with early-onset emphysema in some patients and liver disease in others. Replacement therapy for patients with this enzyme deficiency became available in the 1990s.
antitryptic (ăn″tĭ-trĭp′tĭk) Inhibiting the action of trypsin.
antituberculotic (ăn″tĭ-too-bĕr′kū-lŏt″ĭk) Inhibiting the spread or progress of tuberculosis in the body.
antitussive (ăn″tĭ-tŭs′ĭv) [Gr. *anti*, against, + L. *tussis*, cough] **1.** Preventing or relieving coughing. **2.** An agent that prevents or relieves coughing.
centrally acting a. An agent that depresses medullary centers, suppressing the cough reflex.
antivenene (ăn″tĭ-vĕn′ēn) Antivenin.
antivenereal (ăn″tĭ-vĕ-nē′rē-ăl) Preventing or curing sexually transmitted diseases.
antivenin (ăn″tĭ-vĕn′ĭn) A serum that contains antitoxin specific for an animal or insect venom. Antivenin is prepared from immunized animal sera and is used in the treatment of poisoning by animal or insect venom. SYN: *antivenene*.
black widow spider a. Antitoxic serum obtained from horses immunized against the venom of the black widow spider *(Latrodectus mactans)* and used specifically to treat bites of the black widow spider. The serum is available from Merck & Co., Inc., West Point, PA 19486.
(Crotalidae) polyvalent a. Antisnakebite serum obtained from serum of horses immunized against venom of four types of pit vipers: *Crotalus atrox, C. adamanteus, C. terrificus,* and *Bothrops atrox* (family Crotalidae). The serum is used specifically to treat bites of these snakes.
antivenomous (ăn″tĭ-vĕn′ŏ-mŭs) Opposing the action of venom.
antiviral (ăn″tĭ-vī′răl) Opposing the action of a virus.
antiviral resistance The developed resistance of a virus to specific antiviral therapy.
antivitamin A vitamin antagonist; a substance that makes a vitamin ineffective.
antivivisection (ăn″tĭ-vĭv″ĭ-sĕk′shŭn) Opposition to the use of live animals in experimentation. SEE: *vivisection*.
antixerotic (ăn″tĭ-zē-rŏt′ĭk) [″ + *xerosis*, dryness] Preventing dryness of the skin.
antizymotic (ăn″tĭ-zī-mŏt′ĭk) [″ + *zymosis*, fermentation] An agent that prevents or arrests fermentation (e.g., alcohol or salicylic acid).
Anton's syndrome [Gabriel Anton, Ger. psychiatrist, 1858–1933] SEE: *anosognosia, visual*.
antro-, antr- [L. *antrum*, cavity] Combining form denoting *relationship to an antrum*.
antra (ăn′tră) [L.] Pl. of antrum.
antrectomy (ăn-trĕk′tō-mē) [L. *antrum*, cavity, + Gr. *ektome*, excision] Excision of the walls of an antrum.
antritis (ăn″trī′tĭs) [″ + Gr. *itis*, inflammation] Inflammation of an antrum, esp. the maxillary sinus.
antroatticotomy (ăn″trō-ăt″ĭ-kŏt′ō-mē) [″ + *atticus*, attic, + Gr. *tome*, incision] Operation to open the maxillary sinus and the attic of the tympanum.
antrobuccal (ăn″trō-bŭk′ăl) [″ + *bucca*, cheek] Concerning the maxillary sinus and the cheek.
antrocele (ăn′trō-sēl) [″ + Gr. *kele*, tumor, swelling] Fluid accumulation in a cyst in the maxillary sinus.
antroduodenectomy (ăn″trō-dū″ō-dĕ-nĕk′tō-mē) [″ + *duodeni*, twelve, + Gr. *ektome*, excision] Surgical removal of the pyloric antrum and the upper portion of the duodenum.
antronasal (ăn″trō-nā′zăl) [″ + *nasalis*, nasal] Rel. to the maxillary sinus and nasal fossa.
antroscope (ăn′trō-skōp) [″ + Gr. *skopein*, to examine] An instrument for visual examination of a cavity, esp. the maxillary sinus.
antrostomy (ăn-trŏs′tō-mē) [″ + Gr. *stoma*, mouth] Operation to form an opening in an antrum.
antrotomy (ăn″trŏt′ō-mē) Cutting through an antral wall.
antrotympanic (ăn″trō-tĭm-păn′ĭk) [L. *antrum*, cavity, + Gr. *tympanon*, drum] Rel. to the mastoid antrum and the tympanic cavity.
antrotympanitis (ăn″trō-tĭm″păn-ī′tĭs) [″ + ″ + *itis*, inflammation] Chronic inflammation of the tympanic cavity and mastoid antrum.
antrum (ăn′trŭm) *pl.* **antra** [L., cavity] Any nearly closed cavity or chamber, esp. in a bone. **antral** (-trăl), *adj.*
a. auris External acoustic meatus.
a. cardiacum A Latin term for the portion of the esophagus lying below the diaphragm that abuts the cardia of the stomach.

duodenal a. The duodenal cap; a dilatation of the duodenum near the pylorus. It is seen during digestion.

gastric a. Distal non–acid-secreting segment of the stomach or pyloric gland region that produces the hormone gastrin.

a. of Highmore Maxillary a.

mastoid a. A cavity in the mastoid portion of the temporal bone. SYN: *tympanic a.*

maxillary a. The maxillary sinus; a cavity in the maxillary bone communicating with the middle meatus of the nasal cavity. SYN: *a. of Highmore.*

puncture of the a. Puncture of the maxillary sinus by insertion of a trocar through the sinus wall in order to drain fluid. The instrument is inserted near the floor of the nose, approx. 1½ in. (3.8 cm) from the nasal opening. SYN: *antrotomy.*

PATIENT CARE: The antrum is irrigated with the prescribed solution (often warm normal saline solution) according to protocol. The character and volume of the returned solution and the patient's response to treatment are carefully monitored and documented. Ice packs are applied as prescribed for edema and pain; these are replaced by warm compresses as healing progresses. Assessments are made for chills, fever, nausea, vomiting, facial or periorbital edema, visual disturbances, and personality changes, which may indicate the development of complications.

pyloric a. A bulge in the pyloric portion of the stomach along the greater curvature on distention.

tympanic a. Mastoid a.

ANTU Alpha-naphthylthiourea, a powerful rat poison.

anuclear (ă-nū′klē-ăr) Lacking a nucleus, said of erythrocytes.

ANUG *acute necrotizing ulcerative gingivitis.* SEE: under *gingivitis.*

anulus (ăn′ū-lŭs) *pl.* **anuli** [L.] A ring-shaped structure; a ring. Also spelled *annulus.*

a. abdominalis A. inguinalis profundus.

a. femoralis Femoral ring; the abdominal opening of the femoral canal.

a. fibrosus The outer portion of the intervertebral disk, consisting of concentric rings of collagen fibers (lamellae) oriented in varying directions and designed to withstand tensile and compressive loads on the spine as it transmits weight.

a. inguinalis profundus Deep inguinal ring; the opening in the fascia transversalis for the ductus deferens in the male and the round ligament in the female. SYN: *a. abdominalis.*

a. inguinalis superficialis Superficial inguinal ring; the opening in the external oblique muscle for the ductus deferens in the male and the round ligament in the female.

a. tympanicus Tympanic ring; the part of the temporal bone forming a ring at the inner end of the external auditory canal.

a. umbilicalis An opening in the abdominal wall of a fetus through which the umbilical vessels pass.

a. urethralis Elevated muscular ring surrounding the opening of the bladder into the urethra. SYN: *bladder sphincter.*

anuresis (ăn-ū-rē′sĭs) [Gr. *an-*, not, + *ouresis*, urination] Absence of urination. SEE: *anuria.* **anuretic** (-rĕt′ĭk), *adj.*

anuria (ăn-ū′rē-ă) [″ + *ouron*, urine] Absence of urine formation. SEE: *anuresis.* **anuric,** *adj.*

anus (ā′nŭs) [L.] The outlet of the rectum lying in the fold between the buttocks.

artificial a. An opening into the bowel formed by colostomy.

imperforate a. Condition in which the anus is closed.

vulvovaginal a. Congenital anomaly in a female in which the anus is imperforate but there is an opening from the rectum to the vagina.

anvil (ăn′vĭl) [AS. *anfilt*] A common name for the incus, the second of the three bones in the middle ear. SYN: *incus.* SEE: *ear* for illus.

anxiety (ăng-zī′ĕ-tē) A vague uneasy feeling of discomfort or dread accompanied by an autonomic response; the source is often nonspecific or unknown to the individual; a feeling of apprehension caused by anticipation of danger. It is an altering signal that warns of impending danger and enables the individual to take measures to deal with threat. SEE: *neurosis, anxiety; Nursing Diagnoses Appendix.*

PATIENT CARE: Health care providers evaluate the patient's level of anxiety and document related behaviors and physical characteristics, such as sympathetic nervous system arousal and effects on the patient's perceptual field and ability to learn and solve problems. Coping and defense mechanisms, avoidance behaviors, and surrounding circumstances are also assessed. A calm, caring, quiet, and controlled atmosphere can prevent progression of the patient's anxiety and even reduce it by lessening feelings of isolation and instability. Patients with mild anxiety are assisted to identify and eliminate stressors, if possible. Appropriate outlets are provided for excess energy. Health care providers establish a trusting relationship with the patient, encouraging the patient to express feelings and concerns. False reassurance is never offered. Care for patients with severe anxiety is focused on reducing environmental and other stimuli. Clear, simple validating statements are used to communicate with the patient and are repeated as often as necessary, and reality is reinforced if distortion is evident. The patient's physical needs are addressed, and activity is encouraged to help the patient discharge excess energy and relieve stress.

death a. The apprehension, worry, or fear related to death or dying. SEE: *Nursing Diagnoses Appendix.*

This diagnosis was approved at the NANDA 13th Conference, 1998.

free-floating a. Anxiety unrelated to an identifiable condition, situation, or cause.

separation a. Distress, agitation, or apprehension expressed by toddlers or others when they are removed from mother, family, home, or other familiar surroundings.

anxiety attack An imprecise term for sudden onset of anxiety, sometimes accompanied by a sense of imminent danger or impending doom and an urge to escape. SEE: *panic attack.*

anxiety disorder Any of a group of mental conditions that include panic disorder with or without agoraphobia, agoraphobia without panic disorder, simple (specific) phobia, social phobia, obsessive-compulsive disorder, posttraumatic stress disorder, acute stress disorder, generalized anxiety disorder, anxiety caused by a general medical condition, and substance-induced anxiety disorder. The symptoms vary widely but interfere significantly with normal functioning. SEE: *Nursing Diagnoses Appendix.*

generalized a.d. Excessive anxiety and worry predominating for at least 6 mo. Restlessness, easy fatigability, difficulty in concentrating, irritability, muscle tension, and disturbed sleep may be present. Adults with this disorder often worry about everyday, routine circumstances such as job responsibilities, finances, the health of family members, misfortune to their children, or minor matters such as being late or completing household chores. Frequently they experience cold, clammy hands; dry mouth; sweating; nausea or diarrhea; urinary frequency; trouble swallowing or a "lump in the throat"; an exaggerated startle response; or depressive symptoms. The intensity, duration, or frequency of the anxiety and worry is far out of proportion to the actual likelihood or impact of the feared event.

anxiolytic (ăng″zī-ō-lĭt′ĭk) [L. *anxietas*, anxiety, + Gr. *lysis*, dissolution] **1.** Counteracting or relieving anxiety. **2.** A drug that relieves anxiety.

A.O.A. *Alpha Omega Alpha,* an honorary medical fraternity in the U.S.; *American Osteopathic Association.*

AoA *Administration on Aging.*

A.O.C. *anodal opening contraction.*

A.O.R.N. *Association of Operating Room Nurses.*

aorta (ā-or′tă) *pl.* **aortas, aortae** [L. from Gr. *aorte*] The main trunk of the arterial system of the body.

The aorta is about 3 cm in diameter at its origin in the upper surface of the left ventricle. It passes upward as the ascending aorta, turns backward and to the left (arch of the aorta) at about the level of the fourth thoracic vertebra, and then passes downward as the descending aorta, which is divided into the thoracic and abdominal aorta. The latter terminates at its division into the two common iliac arteries. At the junction of the aorta and the left ventricle is the aortic semilunar valve, which contains three cusps. This valve opens when the ventricle contracts and is closed by the backup of blood when the ventricle relaxes. SEE: illus.

The divisions of the aorta are as follows:

Ascending aorta (two branches): Two coronary arteries (right and left) provide blood supply to the myocardium.

Aortic arch (three branches): The brachiocephalic artery divides into the right subclavian artery, which provides blood to the right arm and other areas, and right common carotid artery, which supplies the right side of the head and neck. The left common carotid artery supplies the left side of the head and neck. The left subclavian artery provides blood for the left arm and portion of the thoracic area.

Thoracic aorta: Two or more bronchial arteries provide blood for bronchi. Esophageal arteries provide blood to the esophagus. Pericardial arteries supply the pericardium. Nine pairs of intercostal arteries supply blood for intercostal areas. Mediastinal branches supply lymph glands and the posterior mediastinum. Superior phrenic arteries supply the diaphragm.

Abdominal aorta: The celiac artery supplies the stomach, liver, and spleen. The superior mesenteric artery supplies all of the small intestine except the superior portion of the duodenum. The inferior mesenteric artery supplies all of the colon and rectum except the right half of the transverse colon. The middle suprarenal branches supply the adrenal (suprarenal) glands. The renal arteries supply the kidneys, ureters, and adrenals. The testicular arteries supply the testicles and ureter. The ovarian arteries (which correspond to internal spermatic arteries of the male) supply the ovaries, part of the ureters, and the

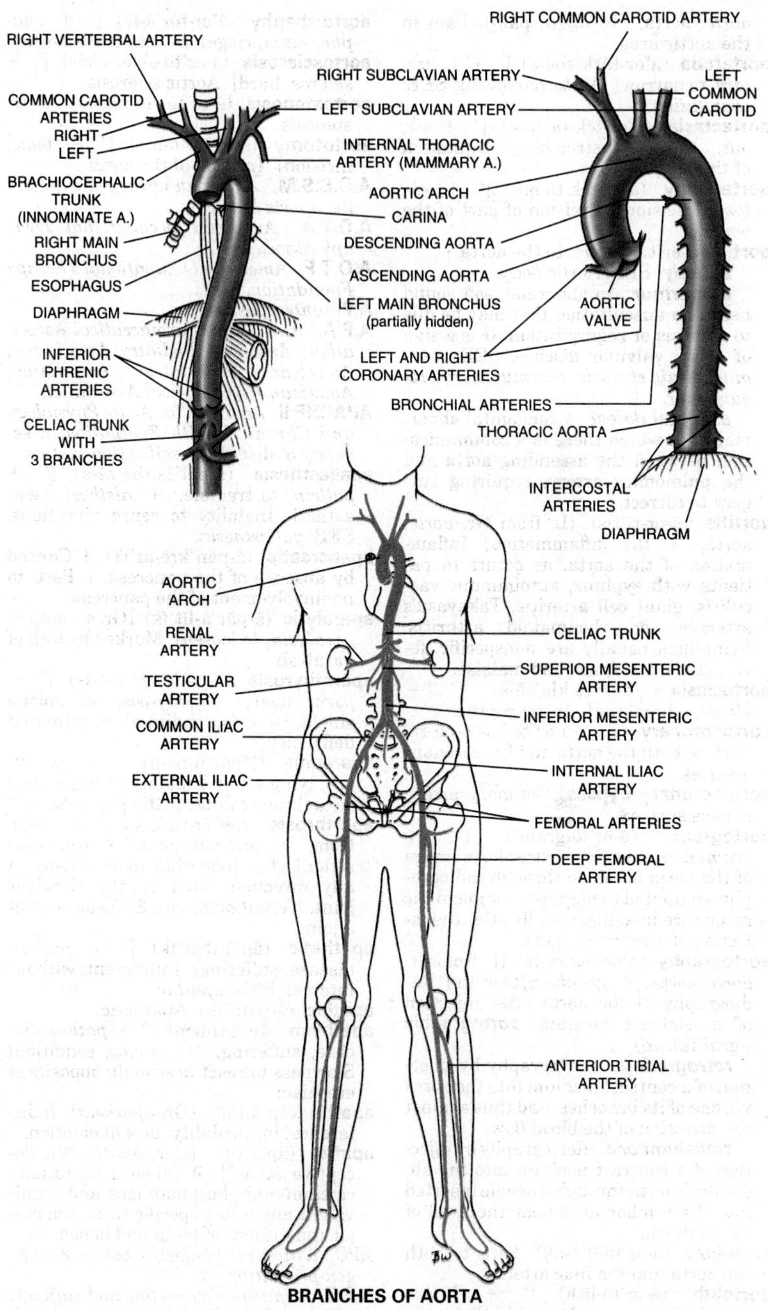

BRANCHES OF AORTA

uterine tubes. The inferior phrenic arteries supply the diaphragm and esophagus. The lumbar arteries supply the lumbar and psoas muscles and part of the abdominal wall musculature. The middle sacral artery supplies the sacrum and coccyx. The right and left common iliac arteries supply the lower pelvic and abdominal areas and the lower extremities. **aortal, aortic** (ā-or′tăl, -tĭk), *adj.*

aortalgia (ā″or-tăl′jē-ă) [L. from Gr.

aorte, aorta, + *algos*, pain] Pain in the aortic area.

aortarctia (ā″or-tărk′shē-ă) [″ + L. *arctare*, to narrow] Aortic narrowing. SEE: *coarctation*.

aortectasia (ā″or-tĕk-tā′zē-ă) [″ + *ek*, out, + *tasis*, a stretching] Dilatation of the aorta.

aortectomy (ā″or-tĕk′tō-mē) [″ + *ektome*, excision] Excision of part of the aorta.

aortic (ā-or′tĭk) Pert. to the aorta.

a. body SEE: *Aortic body*.

a. murmur An abnormal, soft sound heard on auscultation that may be due to stenosis or regurgitation. It is a sign of aortic valvular disease. SEE: *murmur, aortic stenosis; murmur, aortic regurgitant*.

a. septal defect A congenital abnormality in which there is a communication between the ascending aorta and the pulmonary artery, requiring surgery to correct.

aortitis (ā-or-tī′tĭs) [L. from Gr. *aorte*, aorta, + *itis*, inflammation] Inflammation of the aorta, as occurs in patients with syphilis, autoimmune vasculitis, giant cell arteritis, Takayasu's arteritis, or rheumatoid arthritis. Symptoms usually are nonspecific: fever, chills, myalgias, and malaise.

aortoclasia (ā″or-tō-klā′zē-ă) [″ + *klasis*, a breaking] Aortic rupture.

aortocoronary (ā-or″tō-kor′ŏ-nā-rē) Pert. to both the aorta and the coronary arteries.

aortocoronary bypass Coronary artery bypass surgery.

aortogram (ā-or′tō-grăm″) [″ + *gramma*, something written] An image of the aorta obtained through radiography, computed tomography, or magnetic resonance imaging, usually after the injection of a contrast agent.

aortography (ā″or-tog′ră-fē) [L. from Gr. *aorte*, aorta, + *graphein*, to write] Radiography of the aorta after injection of a contrast medium. **aortographic** (-grăf′ĭk), *adj*.

retrograde a. Aortography by injection of a contrast medium into the aorta via one of its branches, and thus against the direction of the blood flow.

translumbar a. Aortography by injection of a contrast medium into the abdominal aorta through a needle inserted into the lumbar area near the level of the 12th rib.

aortoiliac (ā-or″tō-ĭl′ē-ăk) Pert. to both the aorta and the iliac arteries.

aortolith (ă-or′tō-lĭth) [″ + *lithos*, stone] Calcareous deposit in the aortic wall.

aortomalacia (ā-or″tō-mă-lā′shē-ă) [″ + *malakia*, softness] Softening of the walls of the aorta.

aortoplasty (ā-or″tō-plăs′tē) Surgical repair of the aorta, frequently requiring a graft.

aortorrhaphy (ā″or-tor′ă-fē) [″ + *rhaphe*, seam, ridge] Suture of the aorta.

aortosclerosis (ā-or″tō-sklĕr-ō′sĭs) [″ + *skleros*, hard] Aortic sclerosis.

aortostenosis (ā-or″tō-stĕ-nō′sĭs) Aortic stenosis.

aortotomy (ā″or-tŏt′ō-mē) [″ + *tome*, incision] Incision of the aorta.

A.O.S.S.M. *American Orthopedic Society for Sports Medicine*.

A.O.T.A. *American Occupational Therapy Association*.

A.O.T.F. *American Occupational Therapy Foundation*.

A.P. *anteroposterior*.

A.P.A. *American Pharmaceutical Association; American Podiatry Association; American Psychiatric Association; American Psychological Association*.

APACHE II Acronym for *Acute Physiology and Chronic Health Evaluation*, a severity of disease classification system.

apallesthesia (ă-păl″ĕs-thē′zē-ă) [″ + *pallein*, to tremble, + *aisthesis*, sensation] Inability to sense vibrations. SEE: *pallesthesia*.

apancreatic (ă-păn″krē-ăt′ĭk) **1.** Caused by absence of the pancreas. **2.** Pert. to noninvolvement of the pancreas.

aparalytic (ă-păr″ă-lĭt′ĭk) [Gr. *a-*, not, + *paralyein*, to loosen] Marked by lack of paralysis.

aparathyrosis (ă-păr″ă-thī-rō′sĭs) [″ + *para*, near, + *thyreos*, an oblong shield, + *osis*, condition] Parathyroid deficiency.

apareunia (ă″păr-ū′nē-ă) [″ + *pareunos*, lying with] Inability to accomplish sexual intercourse. SEE: *dyspareunia*.

aparthrosis (ăp″ăr-thrō′sĭs) [Gr. *apo*, from, + *arthron*, joint, + *osis*, condition] **1.** A joint that moves freely in any direction, such as the shoulder joint. SYN: *diarthrosis*. **2.** Dislocation of a joint.

apathetic (ăp″ă-thĕt′ĭk) [″ + *pathos*, disease, suffering] Indifferent; without interest. SYN: *apathic*.

apathic (ă-păth′ĭk) Apathetic.

apathism (ăp′ă-thĭzm) [″ + *pathos*, disease, suffering, + *-ismos*, condition] Slowness to react to stimuli; opposite of erethism.

apathy (ăp′ă-thē) [Gr. *apatheia*] Indifference; insensibility; lack of emotion.

apatite (ăp′ă-tīt″) [Ger. *Apatit*, "the deceptive stone"] A mineral containing calcium and phosphate ions and a univalent anion in a specific ratio; the major constituent of teeth and bones.

APC **1.** *absolute phagocyte count*. **2.** *antigen-presenting cell*.

A.P.C. *aspirin, phenacetin,* and *caffeine,* common ingredients in various headache and cold tablets. Phenacetin is no longer considered suitable for use in any form.

APE *anterior pituitary extract*.

apellous (ă-pĕl′ŭs) [Gr. *a-*, not, + L. *pellis*, skin] **1.** Lacking skin. **2.** Lacking foreskin; circumcised.

Apgar Score

Sign	SCORE 0	1	2
Heart rate	Absent	Slow (less than 100)	Greater than 100
Respiratory effort	Absent	Slow, irregular	Good; crying
Muscle tone	Limp	Some flexion of extremities	Active motion
Reflex irritability	No response	Grimace	Cry
Color*	Blue, pale	Body pink; extremities blue	Completely pink

* Skin color or its absence may not be a reliable guide in infants with dark complexions although melanin is less apparent at birth than later.

apepsia (ă-pĕp′sē-ă) [Gr. *a-*, not, + *pepsis*, digesting] Cessation of digestion.

apepsinia (ă″pĕp-sĭn′ē-ă) Absence of pepsin in the gastric juice.

aperient (ă-pĕr′ē-ĕnt) [L. *aperiens*, opening] **1.** Having a mild laxative effect. **2.** A mild laxative.

aperiodic Occurring other than periodically.

aperistalsis (ă″pĕr-ĭ-stăl′sĭs) [Gr. *a-*, not, + *peri*, around, + *stalsis*, constriction] Absence of peristalsis.

apéritif (ă-pĕr″ĭ-tēf′) [L. *aperire*, to open] An alcoholic beverage, such as wine, taken before a meal to stimulate the appetite.

aperitive (ă-pĕr′ĭ-tĭv) **1.** Stimulating the appetite. **2.** Aperient.

Apert's syndrome (ă-pārz′) [Eugene Apert, Fr. pediatrician, 1868–1940] A congenital condition marked by a peaked head and webbed fingers and toes. Oral manifestations include cleft palate or uvula, a prognathic mandible, and maxillary hypoplasia, resulting in extreme malocclusion.

apertura (ăp″ĕr-tū′ră) *pl.* **aperturae** [L.] An opening.

aperture (ăp′ĕr-chūr″) An orifice or opening, esp. to anatomical or bony spaces or canals.

apex (ā′pĕks) *pl.* **apexes, apices** [L., tip] The pointed extremity of a conical structure. **apical** (ăp′ĭ-kal, ā′pĭ-kal), *adj.*

a. of the lung The superior, subclavicular portion of the lung.

root a. The end of the root of a tooth. The anatomical landmark in the apical region is the apical foramen.

apexcardiogram A graphic record of chest wall movements produced by the apex beat.

apexigraph, apexograph (ā-pĕks′ĭ-grăf, -ō-grăf) [L. *apex*, tip, + Gr. *graphein*, to write] An instrument for determining the location and size of the apex of a tooth root.

Apgar score [Virginia Apgar, U.S. anesthesiologist, 1909–1974] A system for evaluating an infant's physical condition at birth. The infant's heart rate, respiration, muscle tone, response to stimuli, and color are rated at 1 min, and again at 5 min after birth. Each factor is scored 0, 1, or 2; the maximum total score is 10. *Interpretation of scores:* 7 to 10, good to excellent; 4 to 6, fair; less than 4, poor condition. A low score at 1 min is a sign of perinatal asphyxia and the need for immediate assisted ventilation. Infants with scores below 7 at 5 min should be assessed again in 5 more min; scores less than 6 at any time may indicate need for resuscitation. In depressed infants, a more accurate determination of the degree of fetal hypoxia may be obtained by direct measures of umbilical cord oxygen, carbon dioxide partial pressure, and pH. SEE: table.

A.P.H.A. *American Public Health Association.*

aphacia, aphakia (ă-fā′sē-ă, -kē-ă) [″ + *phakos*, lentil] Absence of the crystalline lens of the eye. **aphacic, aphakic** (ă-fā′sĭk, -kĭk), *adj.*

aphagia (ă-fā′jē-ă) [Gr. *a-*, not, + *phagein*, to eat] Inability to swallow.

aphalangia (ă″fă-lăn′jē-ă) [″ + *phalanx*, closely knit row] Absence of fingers or toes.

aphanisis (ă-făn′ĭ-sĭs) [Gr. *aphaneia*, disappearance] Fear or apprehension that sexual potency will be lost.

aphasia (ă-fā′zē-ă) [Gr. *a-*, not, + *phasis*, speaking] Absence or impairment of the ability to communicate through speech, writing, or signs because of brain dysfunction. It is considered complete or total when both sensory and motor areas are involved. SEE: *alalia*. **aphasic** (-zĭk), *adj.*

amnesic a. Anomic a.

anomic a. Inability to name objects; loss of memory for words.

auditory a. Inability to understand spoken words. SYN: *word deafness*.

Broca's a. Motor a.

conduction a. A speech deficit whose hallmarks are an inability to repeat what one has heard and impairments in writing and word finding.

crossed a. Aphasia that develops paradoxically in a right-handed person after a stroke or lesions affecting the right hemisphere.

executive a. Motor a.

fluent a. Aphasia in which words are easily spoken but those used are incorrect and may be unrelated to the content of the other words spoken.

gibberish a. Utterance of meaningless phrases.

global a. Total aphasia involving failure of all forms of communication.

jargon a. Communication that results in the use of jargon or disconnected words.

mixed a. Combined sensory and motor aphasia.

motor a. Aphasia in which patients know what they want to say but cannot say it; inability to coordinate the muscles controlling speech. It may be complete or partial. Broca's area is disordered or diseased. SYN: *executive a.*

nominal a. Inability to name objects.

optic a. Inability to name an object recognized by sight without the aid of sound, taste, or touch; a form of agnosia.

semantic a. Inability to understand the meaning of words.

sensory a. Inability to understand spoken words if the auditory word center is involved (auditory aphasia) or written words if the visual word center is affected (visual aphasia). If both centers are involved, the patient will not understand spoken or written words.

syntactic a. Loss of the ability to use proper grammatical construction.

transcortical a. A speech impairment in which the ability to repeat words is preserved, but other language functions are absent.

traumatic a. Aphasia caused by head injury.

visual a. Inability to understand the written word. SYN: *alexia*; *word blindness.*

Wernicke's a. An injury to Wernicke's area in the temporal lobe of the dominant hemisphere of the brain, resulting in an inability to comprehend the spoken or written word. Visual and auditory pathways are unaffected; however, patients are unable to differentiate between words and interpret their meaning. Although patients speak fluently, they are unable to function socially because their ability to communicate effectively is impaired by a disordered speech pattern called paraphasia (i.e., inserting inappropriate syllables into words or substituting one word for another). They also may be unable to repeat spoken words.

aphasiac (ă-fā'zē-ăk) An individual affected with aphasia.

aphasic (ă-fā"zĭk) **1.** Pert. to aphasia. **2.** An individual affected with aphasia.

aphasiologist (ă-fā"zē-ŏl'ō-jĭst) [Gr. *a-*, not, + *phasis*, speaking, + *logos*, word, reason] A person who studies the pathology of language and the production of speech and written language.

aphemia (ă-fē'mē-ă) [" + *pheme*, speech] **1.** Loss of the power to speak. SYN: *motor aphasia.* **2.** Loss of the power to speak distinctly. SYN: *anarthria.*

aphephobia (af"ĕ-fō'bē-ă) [Gr. *haphe*, touch, + *phobos*, fear] Morbid fear of being touched.

apheresis, therapeutic (ă-fĕr'ē-sĭs) [Gr. *aphairesis*, separation] Removal of unwanted or pathological components from a patient's blood by means of a continuous-flow separator; the process is similar to hemodialysis, as treated blood is returned to the patient. The removal of cellular material is termed cytapheresis; leukapheresis describes the removal of leukocytes only. Plasmapheresis, also called plasma exchange, involves removal of noncellular materials. Therapeutic apheresis has been used to treat blood hyperviscosity, cold agglutinin hemolytic anemia, posttransfusion purpura, thrombotic thrombocytopenic purpura, myasthenia gravis, sickle cell anemia, Guillain-Barré syndrome, familial hypercholesterolemia, and certain drug overdoses.

aphonia (ă-fō'nē-ă) [Gr. *a-*, not, + *phone*, voice] Loss of speech sounds from the larynx, as may occur in chronic laryngitis. It is not caused by a brain lesion. The condition may be caused by disease of the vocal cords, paralysis of the laryngeal nerves, or pressure on the recurrent laryngeal nerve; or it may be functional (due to psychiatric causes).

hysterical a. Aphonia due to somatoform disorders. There is no organic defect.

a. paranoica Obstinate silence in the mentally ill.

postoperative a. Loss of speech following laryngectomy. Restoration of speech is accomplished with speech synthesizers and speech therapy.

spastic a. Aphonia resulting from spasm of the vocal muscles, esp. that initiated by efforts to speak.

aphonogelia (ă-fō"nō-jē'lē-ă) [" + *phone*, voice, + *gelos*, laughter] Inability to laugh out loud.

aphose (ăf'ōz) [" + *phos*, light] A subjective visual perception of darkness or of a shadow.

aphrasia (ă-frā'zē-ă) [" + *phrasis*, speech] Inability to speak or understand phrases.

aphrodisiac (ăf"rō-dĭz'ē-ăk) **1.** Stimulating sexual desire. **2.** A drug, food, environment, or other agent that arouses sexual desire.

aphtha (ăf'thah) *pl.* **aphthae** [Gr. *aphtha*, small ulcer] A small ulcer on a mucous membrane of the mouth, as in thrush. **aphthic** (-thik), *adj.*

Bednar's a. SEE: *Bednar's aphthae.*

cachectic a. A lesion formed beneath the tongue and accompanied by severe constitutional symptoms.

aphthoid (ăf′thoyd) Resembling aphthae.

aphthongia (ăf-thŏn′jē-ă) [Gr. *a-*, not, + *phthongos*, voice] Inability to speak due to spasm of muscles controlling speech.

aphthosis (ăf-thō′sĭs) [Gr. *aphtha*, small ulcer, + *osis*, condition] Any condition characterized by aphthae.

aphthous (ăf′thŭs) [Gr. *aphtha*, small ulcer] Pert. to, or characterized by, aphthae.

apical (ăp′ĭ-kal, ā′pĭ-kal) [L. *apex*, tip] Pert. to the apex of a structure.

apical heave Visible heaving of the chest over the apex of the heart. This usually indicates left ventricular hypertrophy. SEE: *substernal thrust.*

apicectomy (ăp″ĭ-sĕk′tō-mē) [L. *apex*, tip, + Gr. *ektome*, excision] Excision of the apex of the petrous portion of the temporal bone.

apices (ā′pĭ-sēz, ăp′ĭ-sēz) [L.] Pl. of apex.

apicitis (ăp-ĭ-sī′tĭs) [L. *apices*, tips, + Gr. *itis*, inflammation] Inflammation of an apex, esp. that of a lung or tooth root.

apicoectomy (ăp-ĭ-kō-ĕk′tō-mē) [L. *apex*, tip, + Gr. *ektome*, excision] Excision of the apex of the root of a tooth.

apicolocator (ă″pĭ-kō-lō′kā-tor) [″ + *locare*, to place] An instrument for locating the apex of the root of a tooth.

apicolysis (ăp″ĭ-kŏl′ĭ-sĭs) [″ + Gr. *lysis*, dissolution] Artificial collapse of the apex of a lung by creation of an opening through the anterior chest wall. The technique is sometimes used to treat multidrug-resistant tuberculosis.

PATIENT CARE: The patient's understanding of the procedure is determined, and misinformation is corrected. At the same time, the patient is evaluated for symptoms of anxiety, and emotional support is provided. During and after the procedure, the patient is assessed for symptoms of tension pneumothorax (increased pulse and respirations, cyanosis, and marked dyspnea, along with severe sharp pain, tympanic resonance to percussion, and absent breath sounds on auscultation of the affected side) and for symptoms of a mediastinal shift (cyanosis, severe dyspnea, distended neck veins, increased pulse and respiratory rate, and excessive, uncontrollable coughing). After the procedure, the patient is positioned as prescribed, usually on the affected side.

Apicomplexa A phylum of the kingdom Protista (formerly a division of protozoa called *Sporozoa;* named for a complex of cell organelles (apical microtubule complex) at the apex of the sporozoite form that can penetrate host cells. It includes the medically important genera *Plasmodium*, *Toxoplasma*, *Cryptosporidium*, and *Isospora*.

apicostomy (āp″ĭ-kŏs′tō-mē) [L. *apex*, tip, + Gr. *stoma*, mouth] Surgical removal of the mucoperiosteum and bone in order to expose the apex of the root of a tooth.

apicotomy (ăp″ĭ-kŏt′ō-mē) [L. *apex*, tip, + Gr. *tome*, incision] Incision of an apical structure.

apinealism (ă-pĭn′ē-ăl-ĭzm) [Gr. *a-*, not, + L. *pinea*, pine cone, + Gr. *-ismos*, condition] Absence of the pineal gland.

apiphobia [L. *apis*, bee, + phobia] Unrealistic fear of bees.

apitherapy In alternative medicine, the application of bee stings or their chemical constituents for their putative anti-inflammatory effects.

A.P.L. Trade name for chorionic gonadotropin, human.

aplanatic (ă″plă-năt′ĭk) [Gr. *a-*, not, + *planetos*, wandering] Free from or correcting spherical aberration.

aplasia (ă-plā′zē-ă) [″ + *plasis*, a developing] Failure of an organ or tissue to develop normally. **aplastic** (ă-plăs′tĭk), *adj.*

a. axialis extracorticalis congenita Congenital defect of the axon formation on the surface of the cerebral cortex.

a. cutis congenita Defective development of a localized area of the skin, usually on the scalp. The area is usually covered by a thin, translucent membrane.

thymic a. A sometimes fatal disorder in which the thymus fails to develop, causing a deficiency of gamma globulin. There is a deficiency of lymph tissue throughout the body. SYN: *thymic alymphoplasia.*

aplastic crisis, transient ABBR: TAC. A serious complication of infection with human parvovirus B-19 infection in patients with chronic hemolytic anemia such as sickle cell disease. This virus causes erythema infectiosum. SEE: *erythema infectiosum.*

Apley's scratch test A test to functionally assess range of motion of the shoulders. The patient reaches over the head with one hand and behind the back with the other hand and is then asked to scratch the back. This is a quick method of testing abduction and lateral rotation of one shoulder and adduction and medial rotation of the other shoulder.

A.P.M.A. *American Podiatric Medical Association.* Formerly called the American Podiatry Association.

apnea (ăp-nē′ă) [″ + *pnoe*, breathing] Temporary cessation of breathing and, therefore, of the body's intake of oxygen and release of carbon dioxide. It is a serious symptom, esp. in patients with other potentially life-threatening conditions. SEE: *apnea monitoring; Cheyne-Stokes respiration; sleep apnea; sudden infant death syndrome.*

central a. Absence of breathing during sleep that occurs when the respiratory center of the brainstem does not send normal periodic signals to the muscles of respiration. Observation of the patient reveals no respiratory effort, that is, no movement of the chest, and no breath sounds.

deglutition a. Cessation of breathing while swallowing.

a.–hypopnea index The number of episodes of reduced or absent respiratory effort per hour.

mixed a. Dysfunctional breathing that combines elements of obstructive and central sleep apneas.

obstructive a. Absent or dysfunctional breathing that occurs when the upper airway is intermittently blocked during sleep. Observation of the patient reveals vigorous but ineffective respiratory efforts, often with loud snoring or snorting.

a. of prematurity ABBR: AOP. A condition of the premature newborn, marked by repeated episodes of apnea lasting longer than 20 sec. The diagnosis of AOP is one of exclusion, made when no treatable cause can be found. Increased frequency of apneic episodes directly relates to the degree of prematurity. AOP is not an independent risk factor for sudden infant death syndrome. Apneic episodes may result in bradycardia, hypoxia, and respiratory acidosis.

TREATMENT: There is no specific treatment. Any infant who has experienced an episode needs to be closely monitored. Methylxanthines such as theophylline are helpful.

PATIENT CARE: Care should include maintenance of a neutral thermal environment, avoidance of prolonged oral feedings, use of tactile stimulation early in the apneic episode, and ventilatory support as needed. The infant who has experienced and survived an episode of apnea is maintained on cardiac and respiratory monitoring devices. Before discharge, parents are taught cardiopulmonary resuscitation, use of monitoring equipment, and how to recognize signs of medication toxicity if medications are used.

sleep a. The temporary absence of breathing during sleep. This common disorder, which affects about a quarter of all middle-aged men in the U.S., and about 10% of middle-aged women, is classified according to the mechanism involved and by whether or not it is associated with daytime sleepiness.

In obstructive sleep apnea, vigorous respiratory efforts are present during sleep but the flow of air in and out of the airways is blocked by upper airway obstruction. Patients with obstructive apnea are usually middle-aged, obese men who make loud snorting, snoring, and gasping sounds during sleep. By contrast, central sleep apnea is marked by absence of respiratory muscle activity. Patients with central apnea may exhibit excessive daytime sleepiness, but snorting and gasping during sleep are absent. Occasionally life-threatening central apneas occur as a result of strokes.

Mixed apnea begins with absence of respiratory effort, followed by upper airway obstruction. Whenever apneas are prolonged, oxygenation drops and carbon dioxide blood levels rise. Patients often awaken many times during the night or have fragmented sleep architecture. In the morning, many patients complain of headache, fatigue, drowsiness, or an unsatisfying night's rest. In addition, these individuals often have hypertension, arrhythmias, type 2 diabetes mellitus, or signs and symptoms of right-sided heart failure. Although these findings may suggest the diagnosis, formal sleep studies in a laboratory are needed to document the disorder and to measure the effects of apneas on oxygenation and other physical parameters.

SYMPTOMS: Partners of patients with sleep apnea are often the first to notice the patient's disordered breathing during sleep. Occasionally patients present to their health care providers because of hypersomnolence: they may report falling asleep during the daytime in unusual circumstances (e.g., at traffic lights or whenever seated in a quiet room).

TREATMENT: Optimal therapy of obstructive sleep apnea is to assist breathing with continuous positive airway pressure (CPAP) if the patient cannot correct the condition by losing weight. CPAP provides a pneumatic splint that maintains airway patency during sleep. Palatal obstruction, a finding in a small number of patients, can be surgically corrected. Medroxyprogesterone may be of some benefit but is clearly less effective than CPAP.

apnea alarm mattress A mattress that is designed to sound an alarm when the infant lying on it ceases to breathe. SEE: *apnea monitoring; sudden infant death syndrome.*

apnea monitoring Monitoring the respiratory movements, esp. of infants. This may be done by use of an apnea alarm mattress, or devices to measure the infant's thoracic and abdominal movements and heart rate. SEE: *sudden infant death syndrome.*

apneic oxygenation The supplying of oxygen to the upper airway of patients who are not breathing.

apneumatic (ăp″nū-măt′ĭk) [Gr. *a-*, not, + *pneuma*, air] **1.** Free of air, as in a collapsed lung. **2.** Pert. to a procedure done in the absence of air.

apneumatosis (ăp″nū-mă-tō′sĭs) [″ + ″ + *osis*, condition] Noninflation of air cells of the lung; congenital atelectasis.

apneumia (ăp-nū′mē-ă) [″ + *pneumon*, lung] Congenital absence of the lungs.

apneusis (ăp-nū′sĭs) Abnormal respiration marked by sustained inspiratory effort; caused by surgical removal of the upper portion of the pons.

apo- (ăp′ō) [Gr. *apo*, from] Combining form meaning *separated from* or *derived from.*

apo(a) Abbreviation for apolipoprotein(a).

apocamnosis (ăp″ō-kăm-nō′sĭs) [Gr. *apokamnein*, to grow weary] Weariness; easily induced fatigue.

apochromatic (ăp″ō-krō-măt′ĭk) Free from spherical and chromatic aberrations.

apocrine (ăp′ō-krēn, -krīn, -krĭn) [Gr. *apo*, from, + *krinein*, to separate] Denoting secretory cells that contribute part of their protoplasm to the material secreted. SEE: *eccrine; holocrine; merocrine.*

apocrine sweat glands Sweat glands located in the axillae and pubic region that open into hair follicles rather than directly onto the surface of the skin as do eccrine sweat glands. They appear after puberty and are better developed in women than in men. The characteristic odor of perspiration is produced by the action of bacteria on the material secreted by the apocrine sweat glands. SEE: *sweat glands.*

apodal (ă-pō′dăl) [Gr. *a-*, not, + *pous*, foot] Lacking feet.

apodia (ă-pō′dē-ă) [Gr. *a-*, not, + *pous*, foot] Congenital absence of one or both feet.

apoenzyme (ăp-ō-ĕn′zīm) The protein portion of an enzyme. SEE: *holoenzyme; prosthetic group.*

apoferritin (ăp″ō-fĕr′ĭ-tĭn) A protein that combines with iron to form ferritin. In the body, it is always bound to iron.

apogee (ăp′ō-jē) [Gr. *apo*, from, + *gaia*, earth] The climax or period of greatest severity of a disease.

apolar (ă-pō′lăr) [Gr. *a-*, not, + *polos*, pole] Without poles or processes. Some nerve cells are apolar.

apolipoprotein Proteins imbedded in the outer shell of lipoproteins. The apolipoproteins (Apo) are designated ApoAI, ApoAII, ApoAIV; ApoB48 and B100; ApoCI, ApoCII, ApoCIII; and ApoE. Except for ApoII and ApoAIV, the metabolic functions are concerned with metabolizing and transporting lipoproteins. The functions of ApoAII and ApoAIV are not fully understood. All are synthesized in the liver; ApoE is synthesized also in macrophages, neurons, and glial cells. SEE: *lipoprotein.*

apolipoprotein E ABBR: ApoE. A protein that regulates lipid concentrations in plasma and repairs neuronal damage in the central nervous system. ApoE4 allele is associated with early-onset Alzheimer's disease, probably because it protects neurons less effectively than other ApoE alleles.

apomorphine (ăp″ō-mor′fēn) [Gr. *apo*, from, + *morphine*] A morphine derivative prepared by removal of one molecule of water from the morphine molecule.

a. hydrochloride A grayish white powder that becomes green on exposure to water or air. An emetic, apomorphine hydrochloride formerly was used to treat oral overdoses. In small doses it may be used as an expectorant.

aponeurology (ăp″ō-nū-rŏl′ō-jē) [″ + *neuron*, nerve, tendon, + *logos*, word, reason] The branch of anatomy dealing with aponeuroses.

aponeurorrhaphy (ăp″ō-nū-ror′ă-fē) [″ + ″ + *rhaphe*, seam, ridge] Suture of an aponeurosis.

aponeurosis (ăp″ō-nū-rō′sĭs) *pl.* **aponeuroses** [″ + *neuron*, nerve, tendon] A flat fibrous sheet of connective tissue that attaches muscle to bone or other tissues; may sometimes serve as a fascia. **aponeurotic** (-rŏt′ĭk), *adj.*

epicranial a. Fibrous membrane connecting the occipital and frontal muscles. SYN: *galea aponeurotica.*

lingual a. Connective tissue sheet of the tongue to which lingual muscles attach.

palatine a. Connective tissue sheet of the soft palate to which palatal muscles attach.

pharyngeal a. Sheet of connective tissue lying between the mucosal and muscular layers of the pharyngeal wall. SYN: *pharyngobasilar fascia.*

plantar a. Sheet of connective tissue investing the muscles of the sole of the foot. SYN: *plantar fascia.*

aponeurositis (ăp″ō-nū-rō-sī′tĭs) [″ + ″ + *itis*, inflammation] Inflammation of an aponeurosis.

aponeurotome (ăp″ō-nū′rō-tōm) [″ + ″ + *tome*, incision] Surgical instrument for cutting an aponeurosis.

aponeurotomy (ăp″ō-nū-rŏt′ō-mē) Incision of an aponeurosis.

apophysis (ă-pŏf′ĭ-sĭs) *pl.* **apophyses** [Gr. *apophysis*, off-shoot] A projection, esp. from a bone (e.g., a tubercle); an outgrowth without an independent center of ossification. **apophyseal, apophysial** (ăp″ō-fĭz′ē-ăl), *adj.*

basilar a. Basilar process of the occipital bone.

a. of Ingrassia Smaller wing of the sphenoid bone.

lenticular a. Lenticular process of the incus, which articulates with the stapes.

a. raviana Anterior process of the malleus.

temporal a. Mastoid process of the temporal bone.

apophysitis (ă-pŏf″ĭ-sī′tĭs) [Gr. *apo*, from, + *physis*, growth, + *itis*, inflammation] Inflammation of an apophysis.

apoplectic (ăp″ō-plĕk′tĭk) [Gr. *apoplektikos*, crippled by stroke] Pert. to apoplexy.

apoplectiform (ăp″ō-plĕk′tĭ-form) [Gr. *apoplexia*, stroke, + L. *forma*, form] Resembling apoplexy. SYN: *apoplectoid*.

apoplectoid (ăp″ō-plĕk′toyd) [″ + *eidos*, form, shape] Apoplectiform.

apoplexia (ăp″ō-plĕk′sē-ă) [Gr. *apoplessein*, to cripple by a stroke] Apoplexy.

a. uteri Sudden hemorrhage from the uterus.

apoplexy (ăp′ō-plĕk″sē) [Gr. *apoplessein*, to cripple by a stroke] **1.** Copious effusion of blood into an organ, as in abdominal apoplexy or pulmonary apoplexy. **2.** An outmoded term for stroke, esp. a stroke in which a blood vessel in the brain ruptures.

pituitary a. Hemorrhage into or necrosis of the pituitary gland. The symptoms are sudden headache, vision loss, and circulatory collapse. Treatment usually includes prompt administration of adrenal steroids. Sometimes neurosurgery is attempted to prevent permanent blindness.

apoptosis (ă-pŏp-tō′sĭs, ă-pō-tō′sĭs) [Gr. *apo*, from, + *ptosis*, a dropping] **1.** Programmed cell death; genetic limitation of the lifespan of cells. The process may be important in limiting growth of tumors. **2.** Programmed death of cells.

aporepressor (ăp″ō-rē-prĕs′or) A protein, the synthesis of which is directed by a regulator gene, that functions only when bound with specific low-molecular-weight compounds called corepressors.

aposia (ă-pō′zē-ă) [Gr. *a-*, not, + *posis*, drink] Absence of thirst. SYN: *adipsia*.

apotemnophilia (ăp″ō-tĕm″nō-fēl′ē-ă) [Gr. *apo*, away, + *temnein*, to cut, + *philein*, to love] A form of paraphilia characterized by the individual requesting amputation of an extremity for erotic reasons.

apothecaries' weights and measures An outdated and obsolete system of weights and measures formerly used by physicians and pharmacists; based on 480 grains to 1 oz and 12 oz to 1 lb. It has been replaced by the metric system. SEE: Weights and Measures Appendix.

apothecary (ă-pŏth′ĕ-kā-rē) [Gr. *apotheke*, storing place] A druggist or pharmacist. In England and Ireland, one licensed by the Society of Apothecaries of London or the Apothecaries' Hall of Ireland as an authorized physician and dispenser of drugs.

apothem, apotheme (ăp′ō-thĕm, -thēm) [Gr. *apo*, from, + *thema*, deposit] The brown precipitate that appears when vegetable decoctions or infusions are exposed to the air or are boiled a long time.

apotripsis (ăp″ō-trĭp′sĭs) [Gr. *apotribein*, to abrade] Removal of a corneal scar or opacity.

apparatus (ăp″ă-rā′tŭs, -răt′ŭs) [L. *apparare*, to prepare] **1.** A number of parts that act together to perform a special function. **2.** A group of structures or organs that work together to perform a common function. **3.** A mechanical device or appliance used in operations and experiments.

acoustic a. Auditory apparatus; the anatomical structures essential for hearing.

attachment a. The cementum, periodontal ligament, and alveolar bone that serve to attach the tooth to the bone.

biliary a. Structures concerned with secretion and excretion of bile; includes liver, gallbladder, and hepatic, cystic, and common bile ducts.

dental a. The tooth and its supporting tissues.

Golgi a. SEE: *Golgi apparatus*.

juxtaglomerular a. The juxtaglomerular cells of the afferent arteriole and the macula densa of the distal tubule. This structure initiates the renin-angiotensin mechanism to elevate blood pressure and increase sodium retention.

kite a. An apparatus for the reeducation of weak muscles and for assistance in overcoming contractures of the forearm, wrist, and fingers.

lacrimal a. SEE: *lacrimal apparatus*.

masticatory a. The teeth, jaws, muscles of mastication, and the temporomandibular joints; used for chewing.

respiratory a. Respiratory system.

sound-conducting a. Those parts of the acoustic apparatus that transmit sound.

vocal a. The organs that produce sounds and speech.

apparent [L. *apparens*, appearing] **1.** Obvious and easily seen; not disguised or hidden. **2.** Appearing to the senses to be obvious and clear based on evidence that, with greater knowledge or closer examination, may or may not be valid.

appearance The visible presentation of an object.

appendage (ă-pĕn′dĭj) Anything attached to a larger or major body part, such as a tail or a limb. SEE: *appendix*.

atrial a. A small muscular pouch attached to each atrium of the heart.

auricular a. **1.** Atrial appendage. **2.** Additional tissue attached to the ear.

a. of the eye The eyelid, eyelashes, eyebrow, lacrimal apparatus, and conjunctiva.

Some Severe Illnesses That May Mimic Appendicitis

Disease	Clinical Findings That May Suggest the Diagnosis
Abdominal aortic aneurysm, rupture	Pulsatile abdominal mass; abdominal bruits; mature patient; imaging studies
Colic caused by kidney stone	Blood present in the urine; visualization of stone by pyelography
Crohn's disease, flare	History of inflammatory bowel disease; pus or blood in stools
Diverticulitis, right-sided	May be difficult to distinguish without imaging studies, laparotomy, or laparoscopy
Ectopic pregnancy	Positive pregnancy test; abdominal ultrasound
Gastroenteritis	Others at home also ill; recent travel abroad; vomiting and diarrhea present
Ischemia of the GI tract	Pain more notable than physical findings; metabolic acidosis; blood in stools; mature patient; smoker
Perforation of an internal organ	Abdominal rigidity; free air under the diaphragm on abdominal x-ray studies
Pyelonephritis	Leukocytes and bacteria in catheterized urine specimen
Salpingitis	Sexually active woman; cervical purulence; tenderness of pelvic organs on examination
Typhlitis	History of leukemia

NOTE: Surgical consultation and abdominal imaging (e.g., with computerized tomography) will lower the likelihood of missed diagnoses or inappropriate surgery.

a. of the fetus The amnion, chorion, and umbilical cord.

a. of the skin The nails, hair, and the sebaceous and sweat glands.

uterine a. The ovaries, fallopian tubes, and uterine ligaments.

appendectomy (ăp″ĕn-dĕk′tō-mē) [″ + Gr. *ektome*, excision] Surgical removal of the vermiform appendix.

incidental a. Removal of the appendix during another surgical procedure in the abdominal cavity.

appendical, appendiceal (ă-pĕn′dĭ-kăl, ăp-ĕn-dĭs′ē-ăl) Pert. to an appendix.

appendicectasis (ă-pĕn″dĭ-sĕk′tă-sĭs) [L. *appendere*, hang to, + Gr. *ektasis*, a stretching] Dilatation of the vermiform appendix.

appendicectomy (ă-pĕn″dĭ-sĕk′tō-mē) Appendectomy.

appendicitis (ă-pĕn″dĭ-sī′tĭs) [L. *appendere*, hang to, + Gr. *itis*, inflammation] Inflammation of the vermiform appendix, caused by blockage of the lumen of the appendix and followed by infection. It may be acute, subacute, or chronic and occasionally is difficult to diagnose because many other illnesses may cause acute abdominal pain. SEE: *acute a.*and other subentries; *Nursing Diagnoses Appendix.*

TREATMENT: Surgery is typically required. Preoperative intravenous hydration and antibiotics are given in most instances.

acute a. A common presentation of appendiceal inflammation. Classic presentations, which occur about 60% of the time, include abdominal pain (initially diffuse, gradually localizing to the right lower quadrant), loss of appetite, nausea, fever, and an elevated white blood cell count. The disease is more common in males and generally occurs in the young, usually between the ages of 10 and 20, but rarely before age 2 and less often after age 50.

DIAGNOSIS: Diagnosis is simple when pain eventually localizes to the right lower quadrant, with rebound tenderness and rigidity over the right rectus muscle or McBurney's point. Diagnostic difficulties may arise because the anatomical location of the appendix can vary; as a result, pain may be present in the pelvis, in the right upper quadrant, or in other locations. Tachycardia and moderate to severe discomfort are common. The differential diagnosis of this presentation includes flares of inflammatory bowel disease, mesenteric adenitis, pelvic inflammation, and many other illnesses. When this diagnosis is considered in a woman, it must be differentiated from pain associated with ovulation (mittelschmerz), ruptured ectopic pregnancy, torsion of the ovary, and pelvic inflammatory disease.To aid preoperative diagnosis, imaging studies, such as helical computed tomography scanning of the abdomen, are often performed to avoid unnecessary surgeries. SEE: table.

The greater the delay in diagnosis, the higher the incidence of complications, such as abscess formation, appendiceal rupture, sepsis, and death.

PATIENT CARE: *Preoperative:* The patient is assessed for signs and symptoms of appendicitis, such as elevated temperature; nausea or vomiting; onset, location, quality, and intensity of pain; rebound tenderness; constipation or diarrhea; and an elevated white blood cell count. The patient is positioned for comfort and prepared physically and emotionally for surgery.

CAUTION: To prevent possible rupture of an inflamed appendix, cathartics or enemas should not be used, nor should heating pads, for a patient with suspected appendicitis.

Postoperative: Vital signs, the status of bowel sounds, abdominal flatus, lung sounds, and intake and output, including prescribed intravenous fluids, are monitored and documented. The patient is positioned comfortably (Fowler's position in the case of a ruptured appendix or peritonitis). Prescribed analgesics and noninvasive comfort measures are provided. Position changes, deep breathing and coughing, and early ambulation are encouraged. The patient's ability to urinate is ascertained and documented. If required, antibiotics are administered as prescribed. The dressing is inspected for any bleeding or drainage and the findings documented. The patient is prepared for return to home, work, and other activities.

chronic a. Appendicitis that may follow an acute but untreated attack, leaving fibrosis and narrowing of the lumen of the appendix. Some authorities question the existence of this entity, as those pathological changes can result from other inflammatory conditions or simply from a gradual narrowing of the lumen.

gangrenous a. Appendicitis in which inflammation is extreme, blood vessels are blocked in the mesentery, circulation to the appendix is cut off, and diffuse peritonitis ensues.

appendicoenterostomy (ă-pĕn″dĭk-ō-ĕn″tĕr-ŏs′tō-mē) [L. *appendere*, hang to, + Gr. *enteron*, intestine, + *stoma*, mouth] **1.** Appendicostomy. **2.** The establishment of an anastomosis between the appendix and intestine.

appendicolysis (ă-pĕn″dĭ-kŏl′ĭ-sĭs) [″ + Gr. *lysis*, dissolution] Surgery to free the appendix from adhesions. This is done by slitting the serosa at its base.

appendicopathy (ă-pĕn″dĭ-kŏp′ă-thē) [″ + Gr. *pathos*, disease, suffering] Any disease of the vermiform appendix.

a. oxyurica A lesion of the appendical mucosa supposedly due to oxyurids (intestinal parasitic worms).

appendicostomy (ă-pĕn″dĭ-kŏs′tō-mē) Surgical opening and fixation of the appendix onto the skin. The opening is employed as a vent to an obstructed colon (it is less efficient than a colostomy or cecostomy). Through the appendiceal lumen a tube can be passed to either instill medication (as in cases of colitis) or fluids (e.g., to relieve fecal impaction in infants with Hirschsprung's disease or in the infirm elderly patient). The opening can also be used to remove foreign bodies from the intestinal lumen.

Patient Care: Emotional support is given to the patient and family members. Ostomy care is taught.

appendicular (ăp″ĕn-dĭk′ū-lăr) [L. *appendere*, to hang to] **1.** Pert. to an appendix. SYN: *appendical; appendiceal.* **2.** Pert. to the limbs.

appendix (ă-pĕn′dĭks) *pl.* **appendixes** *pl.* **appendices** [L.] An appendage, esp. the appendix vermiformis. SYN: *appendage.* SEE: *digestive system* and *omentum* for illus.

atrial a. A small muscular pouch attached to each atrium of the heart.

auricular a. Atrial a.

ensiform a. A term formerly used to indicate the xiphoid process of the sternum.

a. epididymidis A cystic structure attached to the epididymis, a vestigial remnant of the mesonephric duct.

a. epiploica One of numerous pouches of the peritoneum, filled with fat and attached to the colon.

a. testis A small bladder-like structure at the upper end of the testis, a vestigial remnant of the cephalic portion of the müllerian duct.

ventricular a. SEE: *saccule, laryngeal.*

a. vermiformis A worm-shaped process projecting from the blind end of the cecum and lined with a continuation of the mucous membrane of the cecum. SEE: *vermiform appendix.*

vesicular a. A cystic structure attached to the fimbriated end of the uterine tube. It is a vestigial remnant of the mesonephric duct.

xiphoid a. Xiphoid process. SYN: *ensiform a.*

apperception (ăp″ĕr-sĕp′shŭn) [L. *ad*, to, + *percipere*, to perceive] The perception and interpretation of sensory stimuli; awareness of the meaning and significance of a particular sensory stimulus as modified by one's own experiences, knowledge, thoughts, and emotions. **apperceptive** (-tĭv), *adj.*

appestat (ăp′ĕ-stăt) [L. *appetitus*, longing for, + Gr. *states*, stand] The area of the brain (probably in the hypothalamus) that is thought to control appetite and food intake.

appetite (ăp′ĕ-tīt) [L. *appetitus*, longing for] A strong desire, esp. for food. Appetite differs from hunger in that the latter is an uncomfortable sensation caused by lack of food, whereas appetite is a pleasant sensation based on previous experience that causes one to seek food for the purpose of tasting and enjoying.

perverted a. Pica.

appetizer (ăp′ĕ-tī″zĕr) That which promotes appetite.

applanation (ăp″lă-nā′shŭn) [L. *ad*, toward, + *planare*, to flatten] Abnormal flattening, esp. of the corneal surface.

applanometer (ăp″lă-nŏm′ĕ-tĕr) [″ + *planum*, plane, + Gr. *metron*, measure] A device for measuring intraocular pressure. SEE: *tonometer*.

apple packer's epistaxis Nosebleed due to handling packing trays containing certain dyes.

apple picker's disease Bronchitis resulting from a fungicide used on apples.

apple sorter's disease Contact dermatitis caused by chemicals used in washing apples.

appliance (ă-plī′ăns) **1.** In dentistry, a device to provide or facilitate a particular function, such as artificial dentures or a device used to correct bite. SEE: *dental prosthesis*. **2.** A device for influencing a specific function (e.g., a cane, crutch, or walker to assist walking or an appliance to discourage thumb sucking). SEE: *prosthesis*.

applicator (ăp′lĭ-kā″tor) [L. *applicare*, to attach] A device, usually a slender rod with a pledget of cotton on the end, for making local applications.

apposition (ăp″ō-zĭ′shŭn) [L. *ad*, toward, + *ponere*, to place] **1.** Condition of being positioned side by side or fitted together. SYN: *contiguity*. **2.** Addition of one substance to another, as one layer of tissue upon another. **3.** Development by means of accretion, as in the formation of bone or dental cementum.

approach (ă-prōch′) The surgical procedure for exposing an organ or tissue.

appropriate (ăp-prō′prē-āt) **1.** In psychiatry, relating to a behavior that is suitable and congruent. **2.** In medical practice, relating to care that is expected to yield health benefits that considerably exceed risk.

approximal (ă-prŏk′sĭ-măl) [″ + *proximus*, nearest] Contiguous; next to.

approximate (ă-prŏk′sĭ-māt) [″ + *proximare*, to come near] To place or bring objects close together.

apractagnosia Agnosia marked by the inability to use common instruments or tools whether they are being used on the individual's body or in the environment. This is usually due to a lesion in the parietal area of the brain.

apraxia (ă-prăk′sē-ă) [Gr. *a-*, not, + *praxis*, action] **1.** Inability to perform purposive movements although there is no sensory or motor impairment. **2.** Inability to use objects properly. **apraxic** (ă-prăk′sĭk), *adj.*

akinetic a. Inability to carry out spontaneous movements.

amnesic a. Inability to produce a movement on command because the command is forgotten, although the ability to perform the movement is present.

buccofacial a. Inability to use the muscles of the face or mouth (e.g., to whistle a tune or suck liquids through a straw).

constructional a. Inability to draw or construct two- or three-dimensional forms or figures and impairment in the ability to integrate perception into kinesthetic images.

developmental a. Disorder of motor planning and execution occurring in developing children; thought to be due to central nervous system immaturity.

dressing a. Inability to dress due to patient's deficient knowledge of the spatial relations of his or her body.

ideational a. Misuse of objects due to inability to perceive their correct use. SYN: *sensory a.*

limb a. The inability to use the arms or legs to perform previously learned movements, such as combing one's hair or kicking a ball, despite having normal muscle strength in those body parts.

motor a. Inability to perform movements necessary to use objects properly, although the names and purposes of the objects are known and understood.

sensory a. Ideational a.

verbal a. The inability to form words or speak, despite the ability to use oral and facial muscles to make sounds.

aproctia (ă-prŏk′shē-ă) [Gr. *a-*, not, + *proktos*, anus] Absence or imperforation of anus.

apron (ā′prŏn) [O. Fr. *naperon*, cloth] **1.** Outer garment covering the front of the body for protection of clothing during surgery or certain nursing procedures. **2.** Part of the body resembling an apron.

Hottentot a. SEE: *Hottentot apron*.

lead a. An apron that contains lead or equivalent material and is sufficiently pliable to wear as protection from ionizing radiation. It is used to shield patients and personnel during radiological procedures.

aprosody (ă-prŏs′ō-dē) [Gr. *a-*, not, + *prosodia*, voice modulation] Absence of normal variations of pitch, rhythm, and stress in the speech.

aprosopia (ăp″rō-sō′pē-ă) [″ + *prosopon*, face] Congenital defect in which part or all of the face is absent.

aprotes Chemical substances that are either cations such as sodium, calcium, potassium, and magnesium that carry a positive charge, or anions such as chloride and sulfate that carry a negative charge. These chemicals are unable to donate or accept protons; thus they are not acids, bases, or buffers. SEE: *buffer*.

aprotinin A serine protease inhibitor obtained from bovine pancreas. Its action is believed to be inhibition of plasmin and kallikrein. It is used to decre blood loss and thus transfusion requirements during surgery.

APRV *airway pressure release ventilation.*

APT *alum-precipitated toxoid.*

A.P.T.A. *American Physical Therapy Association.*

aptitude (ăp′tĭ-tūd) Inherent ability or skill in learning or performing physical or mental endeavors.

APT test In infants, a method of differentiating swallowed maternal blood in the stool from gastrointestinal bleeding from the infant. The blood could be swallowed during delivery or from a bleeding nipple fissure. To test: 1. A bloody stool or diaper is rinsed until a pink supernatant is obtained. 2. The supernatant is centrifuged and the top fluid is removed. 3. To 5 parts of the removed solution, 1 part of 0.25 normal (1%) sodium hydroxide is added. Within 1 to 2 min, a color reaction takes place. A yellow-brown color indicates the blood originated from the mother; a persistent pink color indicates the blood is from the infant. It is advisable to test control specimens from both the mother and the infant. SYN: *swallowed blood syndrome.*

aptyalia, aptyalism (ăp″tē-ā′lē-ă, ă-tī′ă-lĭzm) [″ + *ptyalon,* saliva] Absence of or deficiency in secretion of saliva. The condition may be caused by disease (mumps, typhoid fever), dehydration, drugs, radiation therapy to the salivary glands, old age, obstruction of salivary ducts, or Sjögren's syndrome, in which there is deficient function of lacrimal, salivary, and other glands.

APUD cells *amine precursor uptake and decarboxylation* cells. A class of cells, derived from the neural crest of the embryo, that produce hormones (such as insulin, ACTH, glucagon, and thyroxine) and amines (such as dopamine, serotonin, and histamine). These cells are involved in multiple endocrine neoplasia, types I and II.

apudoma [from *APUD cells*] A tumor of APUD cells.

apulmonism (ă-pool′mŏn-ĭzm) [Gr. *a-,* not, + L. *pulmo,* lung, + Gr. *-ismos,* condition] Congenital absence of part or all of a lung.

apus (ā′pŭs) [″ + *pous,* foot] A person who has apodia, congenital absence of the feet.

apyknomorphous (ă-pĭk″nō-mor′fŭs) [″ + *pyknos,* thick, + *morphe,* form] Not pyknomorphous; pert. to a cell that does not stain deeply because its stainable material is not compact.

apyogenous (ā-pī-ŏj′ĕn-ŭs) [″ + *pyon,* pus, + *genos,* origin] Not producing pus.

apyretic (ā-pī-rĕt′ĭk) [″ + *pyretos,* fever] Without fever. SYN: *afebrile.*

apyrexia (ā-pī-rĕks′ē-ă) [″ + *pyrexis,* feverishness] Absence of fever.

apyrogenetic, apyrogenic (ā″pī-rō-jĕ-nĕt′ĭk, -jĕn′ĭk) [″ + ″ + *genos,* origin] Not causing fever.

AQ *achievement quotient.*

aq L. *aqua,* water.

aqua (awk′wă) *pl.* **aquae** [L. *aqua*] ABBR: a; aq. Water.

medicated a. An aqueous solution of a volatile substance. It usually contains only a comparatively small percentage of the active drug. Some of these solutions are merely water saturated with a volatile oil. They are used mostly as vehicles to give odor and taste to solutions.

aquaphobia (ăk″wă-fō′bē-ă) [″ + Gr. *phobos,* fear] An abnormal fear of water. SYN: *hydrophobia.*

aquapuncture (ăk″wă-pŭngk′chūr) [″ + *punctura,* puncture] Subcutaneous injection of water, as to produce counterirritation.

aquatic **1.** Pert. to water. **2.** Inhabiting water.

aqueduct (ăk′wĕ-dŭkt″) [″ + *ductus,* duct] Canal or channel. SYN: *aqueductus.*

cerebral a. Canal in the midbrain connecting the third and fourth ventricles. SYN: *aqueductus cerebri.*

vestibular a. Small passage reaching from the vestibule to the posterior surface of the temporal bone's petrous section.

aqueductus (ăk″wĕ-dŭk′tŭs) A canal or channel. SYN: *aqueduct.*

a. cerebri Canal in the midbrain connecting the third and fourth ventricles. SYN: *cerebral aqueduct.*

a. cochleae Canal connecting subarachnoid space and the perilymphatic space of the cochlea.

a. Fallopii Canal for facial nerve in the temporal bone.

a. vestibuli Small passage reaching from the vestibule to the posterior surface of the temporal bone's petrous section.

aqueous (ā′kwē-ŭs) [L. *aqua,* water] **1.** Of the nature of water; watery. **2.** Aqueous humor.

aqueous chambers Anterior and posterior chambers of the eye, which contain the aqueous humor.

aquiparous (ăk-wĭp′ă-rŭs) [″ + *parere,* to bring forth, to bear] Producing water.

AR **1.** *achievement ratio.* **2.** *alarm reaction.*

Ar Symbol for the element argon.

ara-A Vidarabine.

arabinose (ă-răb′ĭ-nōs) Gum sugar, a pentose obtained from plants; sometimes found in urine.

arabinosuria (ă-răb″ĭ-nō-sū′rē-ă) [*arabinose* + Gr. *ouron,* urine] Arabinose in the urine.

Ara-C Cytarabine, an antineoplastic drug of the antimetabolite class.

arachnid (ă-răk′nĭd) A member of the class Arachnida.

Arachnida (ă-răk′nĭ-dă) [Gr. *arachne*, spider] A class of the Arthropoda, including the spiders, scorpions, ticks, and mites.

arachnidism (ă-răk′nĭd-ĭzm) [″ + *eidos*, form, shape, + *-ismos*, condition of] Systemic poisoning from a spider bite. SYN: *arachnoidism*. SEE: *spider bite*.

arachnitis (ă″răk-nī′tĭs) Arachnoiditis.

arachnodactyly (ă-răk″nō-dăk′tĭl-ē) [″ + *dactylos*, finger] Spider fingers; a state in which fingers and sometimes toes are abnormally long and slender. SYN: *acromacria*. SEE: *Marfan's syndrome*.

arachnoid (ă-răk′noyd) [″ + *eidos*, form, shape] **1.** Resembling a web. **2.** Arachnoid membrane.

cranial a. Arachnoidea encephali.

spinal a. Arachnoidea spinalis.

arachnoidea (ă-răk-noyd′ē-ă) Arachnoid membrane.

a. encephali The part of the arachnoidea enclosing the brain. SYN: *cranial arachnoid*.

a. spinalis The part of the arachnoidea enclosing the spinal cord. SYN: *spinal arachnoid*.

arachnoidism (ă-răk′noyd-ĭzm) Arachnidism.

arachnoiditis (ă-răk″noyd-ī′tĭs) [″ + *eidos*, form, shape, + *itis*, inflammation] Inflammation of the arachnoid membrane. SYN: *arachnitis*.

arachnolysin (ă-răk-nŏl′ĭ-sĭn) [″ + *lysis*, dissolution] The hemolysin present in spider venom.

arachnophobia (ă-răk″nō-fō′bē-ă) [″ + *phobos*, fear] Morbid fear of spiders.

Aran-Duchenne disease Spinal muscular atrophy.

Arantius' body, Arantius' nodule (ăr-ăn′shē-ŭs) *pl.* **Arantii** [Julius Caesar Arantius, It. anatomist and physician, 1530–1589] A small nodule at the center of each of the aortic valve cusps.

ARB *Angiotensin II receptor blocker*.

arbitration A process of dispute resolution in which both sides select a neutral third party who has technical knowledge in the area of contention to listen to the arguments presented by the disputing parties and render a decision. The decision can be binding or nonbinding.

arbor A structure resembling a tree with branches.

arborescent (ăr″bor-ĕs′ĕnt) [L. *arborescere*, to become a tree] Branching; treelike.

arborization (ăr″bor-ĭ-zā′shŭn) [L. *arbor*, tree] Ramification; branching, esp. terminal branching of nerve fibers and capillaries. SEE: *nerve*.

arbor vitae (ăr′bor vī′tē) [L. *arbor*, tree, + *vita*, life] **1.** A treelike structure; a treelike outline seen in a section of the cerebellum. **2.** A tree or shrub of the genus *Thuja* or *Thujopsis*. **3.** A series of branching ridges within the cervix of the uterus. SYN: *palmate plica*.

arbovirus (ăr″bō-vī′rŭs) [*ar*thropod-*bo*rne *virus*] Any of a large group of viruses that multiply in both vertebrates and arthropods such as mosquitoes and ticks. Arboviruses cause diseases such as yellow fever and viral encephalitis. SEE: *arenaviruses; Togaviridae*.

ARC *AIDS-related complex*. SEE: *AIDS*.

arc (ărk) [L. *arcus*, bow] A curved line; a portion of a circle.

reflex a. The path followed by a nerve impulse to produce a reflex action. The impulse originates in a receptor at the point of stimulation, passes through an afferent neuron or neurons to a reflex center in the brain or spinal cord, and from the center out through efferent neurons to the effector organ, where the response occurs. SEE: illus.

arcade (ăr-kād) Any anatomic structure composed of a series of arches.

Flint's a. The arteriovenous anastomoses at the bases of the pyramids of the kidney.

arcanum (ăr-kā′nŭm) *pl.* **arcana** [L. *arcanum*, a secret] Secret remedy.

arcate (ăr′kăt) [L. *arcatus*, bow-shaped] Arched; bow-shaped.

arc eyes Eye burn caused when welders fail to wear protective eye shields while welding or following extended periods of welding even though protective eye gear was worn. Irrigation of the eyes with copious amounts of sterile saline may be necessary for several hours in addition to pain medication and instillation of anti-inflammatory eye drops and other medications.

arch [L. *arcus*, a bow] Any anatomical structure having a curved or bowlike outline. SYN: *arcus*.

abdominothoracic a. The costal arch; the anterior and lateral boundary between the line dividing the thorax and the abdomen.

alveolar a. Arch of the alveolar process of either jaw.

aortic a. Proximal curved part of the aorta, at about the level of the fourth thoracic vertebra. The brachiocephalic, left common carotid, and left subclavian arteries arise from the aortic arch.

aortic a. A series of six pairs of vessels that develop in the embryo and connect the aortic sac with the dorsal aorta. During the fifth to seventh weeks of gestation, the arches undergo transformation, some persisting as functional vessels, others persisting as rudimentary structures, and some disappearing entirely.

axillary a. An anomalous muscular slip across the axilla, between the pectoralis major and latissimus dorsi muscles. SYN: *Langer's muscle*.

branchial a. Five pairs of arched structures that form the lateral and ventral walls of the pharynx of the embryo. The first is the mandibular arch; the second is the hyoid arch; the third, fourth, and fifth arches are transitory. They are partially separated from each other externally by the branchial clefts and internally by the pharyngeal pouches. They are important in the formation of structures of the face and neck. SYN: *pharyngeal a.*

carotid a. The third aortic arch, which provides the common carotid artery.

a. of Corti A series of arches made up of the rods of Corti in the inner ear.

costal a. Arch formed by the ribs.

crural a. The inguinal ligament, which extends from the anterior superior iliac spine to the pubic tubercle. SYN: *Poupart's ligament*.

deep crural a. A band of fibers arching in front of the sheath of femoral vessels; the downward extension of the transversalis fascia.

deep palmar a. An arch formed in the palm by the communicating branch of the ulnar and the radial artery.

dental a. The arch formed by the alveolar process and teeth in each jaw.

glossopalatine a. The anterior pillar of the fauces; one of two folds of mucous membrane extending from the soft palate to the sides of the tongue.

hemal a. **1.** Arch formed by the body and processes of a vertebra, such as a pair of ribs and the sternum; also the sum of all such arches. **2.** In lower vertebrates, extensions from the lateral areas of the caudal vertebrae that fuse to enclose the caudal artery and vein. In humans these are represented by the costal processes of the vertebrae.

hyoid a. The second branchial arch, which gives rise to the styloid process, the stylohyoid ligament, and the lesser cornu of the hyoid bone.

inferior tarsal a. The arch of the median palpebral artery that supplies the lower eyelid.

longitudinal a. The anteroposterior arch of the foot; the medial portion is formed by the calcaneus, talus, navicular, cuneiforms, and first three metatarsals; the lateral portion is formed by the calcaneus, cuboid, and fourth and fifth metatarsals.

mandibular a. **1.** The first branchial arch, from which the upper and lower jawbones and associated structures develop. It also gives rise to the malleus and incus. **2.** The curved composite structure of natural dentition and supporting tissues of the lower jaw; the residual bony ridge after teeth have been lost from the lower jaw.

maxillary a. The curved composite structure of the natural dentition and supporting tissues of the upper jaw; the residual bony ridge after teeth have been lost from the upper jaw.

nasal a. Arch formed by the nasal bones and by the nasal processes of the maxilla.

neural a. Vertebral a.

palmar a. SEE: *deep palmar a.; superficial palmar a.*

pharyngeal a. Branchial a.

pharyngopalatine a. The posterior pillar of the fauces; one of two folds of mucous membrane extending from the pharynx to the sides of the pharynx.

plantar a. The arch formed by the external plantar artery and the deep branch of the dorsalis pedis artery.

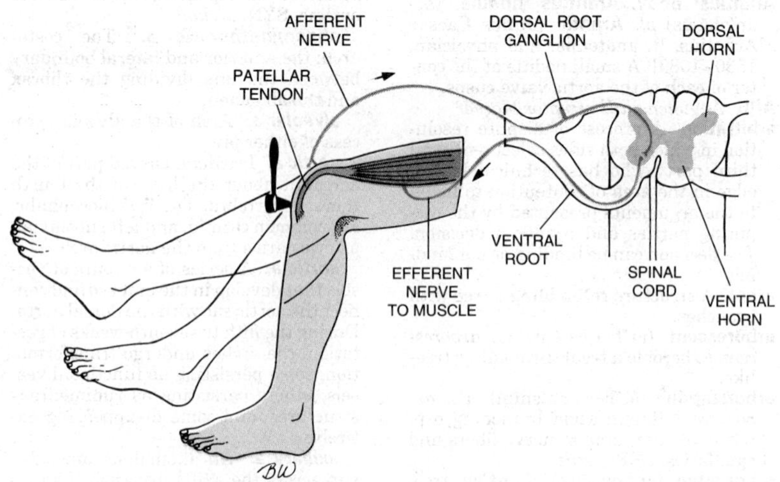

REFLEX ARC FOR PATELLAR TENDON REFLEX

pubic a. The arch formed by the rami of the ischia and pubic bones. It forms the anterior portion of the pelvic outlet.

pulmonary a. The fifth aortic arch on the left side. It becomes the pulmonary artery.

superciliary a. A curved process of the frontal bone lying just above the orbit and subjacent to the eyebrow.

superficial palmar a. An arch in the palm forming the termination of the ulnar artery.

superior tarsal a. The arch of the median palpebral artery that supplies the upper eyelid.

supraorbital a. A bony arch formed by the upper margin of the orbit.

tarsal a. SEE: *inferior tarsal a.; superior tarsal a.*

thyrohyoid a. The third branchial arch, which gives rise to the greater cornu of the hyoid bone.

transverse a. The transverse arch of the foot formed by the navicular, cuboid, cuneiform, and metatarsal bones.

vertebral a. The arch formed by the posterior projection of a vertebra that, with the body, encloses the vertebral foramen. SYN: *neural a.*

zygomatic a. The arch formed by the malar and temporal bones.

arch- SEE: *archi-*.

arche- SEE: *archi-*.

archenteron (ărk-ĕn′tĕr-ŏn) [Gr. *arche*, beginning, + *enteron*, intestine] The primitive digestive cavity of the gastrula, which is lined with endoderm. Its opening to the outside is the blastopore. SYN: *gastrocoele*.

archeokinetic (ăr″kē-ō-kĭ-nĕt′ĭk) [″ + *kinetikos*, concerning movement] Pert. to a low and primitive type of motor nerve mechanism as found in the peripheral and ganglionic nervous systems. SEE: *paleokinetic*.

archetype (ăr′kĕ-tīp) [″ + *typos*, model] **1.** The original type, from which other forms have developed by differentiation. **2.** An ideal or perfect anatomical type; used as a theoretical standard in judging other individuals.

ARCF *American Respiratory Care Foundation.*

archi-, arche-, arch- [Gr. *arche*, beginning] Combining form meaning *first, principal, beginning,* or *original*.

archiblast (ăr′kĭ-blăst) [″ + *blastos*, a germ, bud] The outer layer that surrounds the germinal vesicle.

archiblastic (ăr″kĭ-blăs′tĭk) Derived from or pert. to the archiblast.

archiblastoma (ăr″kĭ-blăs-tō′mă) [″ + *blastos*, germ, + *oma*, tumor] A tumor of archiblastic tissue.

archigaster (ăr′kĭ-găs″tĕr) [″ + *gaster*, belly] The primitive embryonic alimentary canal.

archinephron (ăr″kĭ-nĕf′rŏn) Mesonephros.

archipallium (ăr″kĭ-păl′ē-ŭm) [″ + L. *pallium*, a cloak] Olfactory cortex; phylogenetically older than the neopallium.

archistome (ăr′kĭ-stōm) Blastopore.

architectural barrier Any limitation in the design of facilities that restricts the access of persons with disabilities and limited mobility, including those using wheelchairs.

architis (ăr-kī′tĭs) [Gr. *archos*, anus, + *itis*, inflammation] Inflammation of the anus; proctitis.

arch width The measured distance between the canines, bicuspids, and the first molars. These distances establish the shape and size of the dental arch.

arciform (ăr′sĭ-form) Arcuate.

arctation (ărk-tā′shŭn) [L. *arctatus*, pressing together] Stricture of any canal opening.

arcuate (ăr′kū-āt) [L. *arcuatus*, bowed] Bowed; shaped like an arc. SYN: *arciform*.

arcuation (ăr-kū-ā′shŭn) A bending; curvature.

arcus (ăr′kŭs) *pl.* **arcus** [L. *arcus*, a bow] Arch.

a. alveolaris mandibulae The arch formed by the alveolar process of the body of the mandible.

a. alveolaris maxillae The arch formed by the alveolar process of the maxilla.

a. dentalis Dental arch.

a. juvenilis Opaque ring about the periphery of the cornea similar to arcus senilis but occurring in young individuals; may be due to hypercholesterolemia, corneal irritation or inflammation, or a congenital anomaly.

a. plantaris Plantar arch.

a. senilis Opaque white ring about the periphery of the cornea, seen in aged persons; caused by the deposit of fat granules in the cornea or by hyaline degeneration.

ARD *acute respiratory distress.*

ardor (ăr′dor) [L., heat] Burning; great heat.

ARDS *acute respiratory distress syndrome.*

area (ā′rē-ă) *pl.* **areae, areas** [L. *area*, an open space] **1.** A circumscribed space; one having definite boundaries. **2.** Part of an organ that performs a specialized function.

acoustic a. A part of the brain that lies over the vestibular and cochlear nuclei.

association a. Area of the cerebral cortex connected to motor and sensory areas of the same side, to similar areas on the other side, and to other regions of the brain (e.g., the thalamus). It integrates the simpler motor and sensory functions.

auditory a. The hearing center of the cerebral cortex; located in the floor of the lateral fissure and surfacing on the dorsal surface of the superior temporal gyrus. It receives auditory fibers from the medial geniculate body.

body surface a. The surface area of the body expressed in square meters. Body surface area is an important measure in calculating pediatric dosages, drug dosages in chemotherapy, in managing burn patients, and in determining radiation doses. Nomograms for accurately determining body surface area are available for both pediatric and adult patients. SEE: illus.; *burn; rule of nines.*

Broca's a. SEE: *Broca's area.*

Brodmann's a. SEE: *Brodmann's areas.*

Nomogram for the Assessment of Body Surface Area*

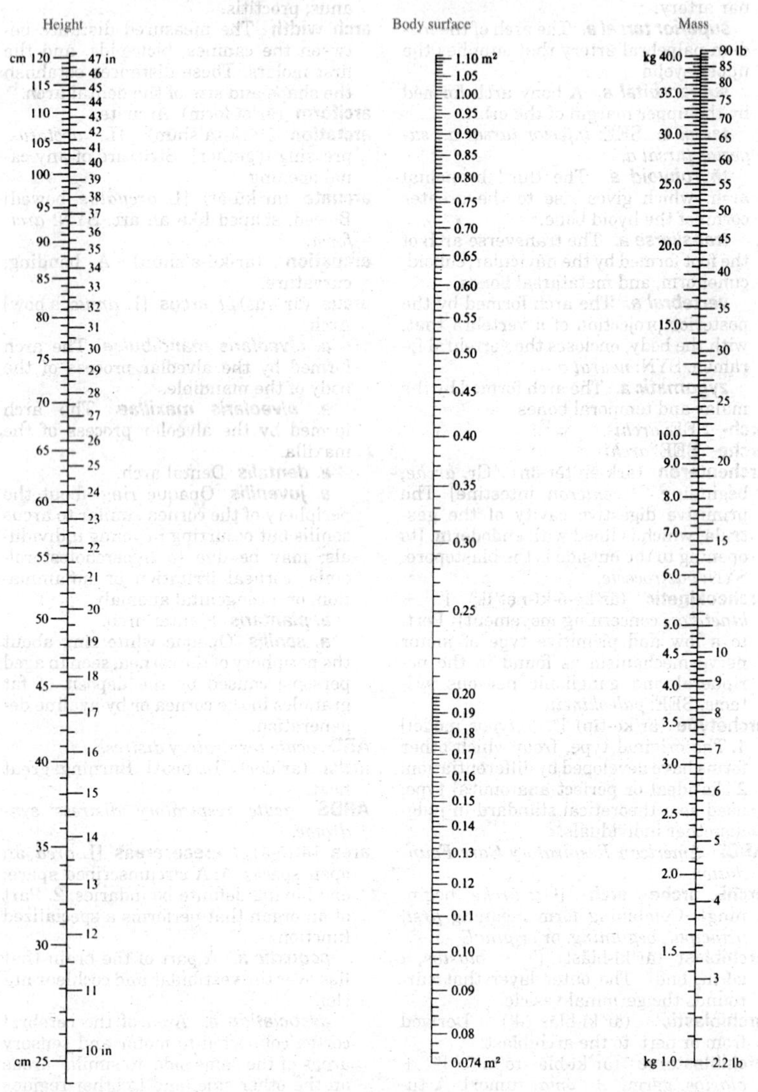

Source: Lentner, C (ed): Geigy Scientific Tables, ed 8. Ciba Geigy, Basle, Switzerland, 1981.

*The body surface area is given by the point of intersection with the middle scale of a straight line joining height and weight.

catchment a. a geographical area defining the portion of a population served by a designated medical facility.

controlled a. An area in which a protection officer oversees the occupational exposure of personnel to ionizing radiation. Controlled access, occupancy, and working conditions are necessary for radiation protection.

effective radiating a. ABBR: ERA. The area of a therapeutic ultrasound head that produces useful ultrasonic energy, measured in square centimeters (cm^2). The effective radiating area is calculated by identifying all points where the ultrasonic energy is at least 5% of the maximum measured intensity at the transducer's surface.

Nomogram for the Assessment of Body Surface Area* (Continued)

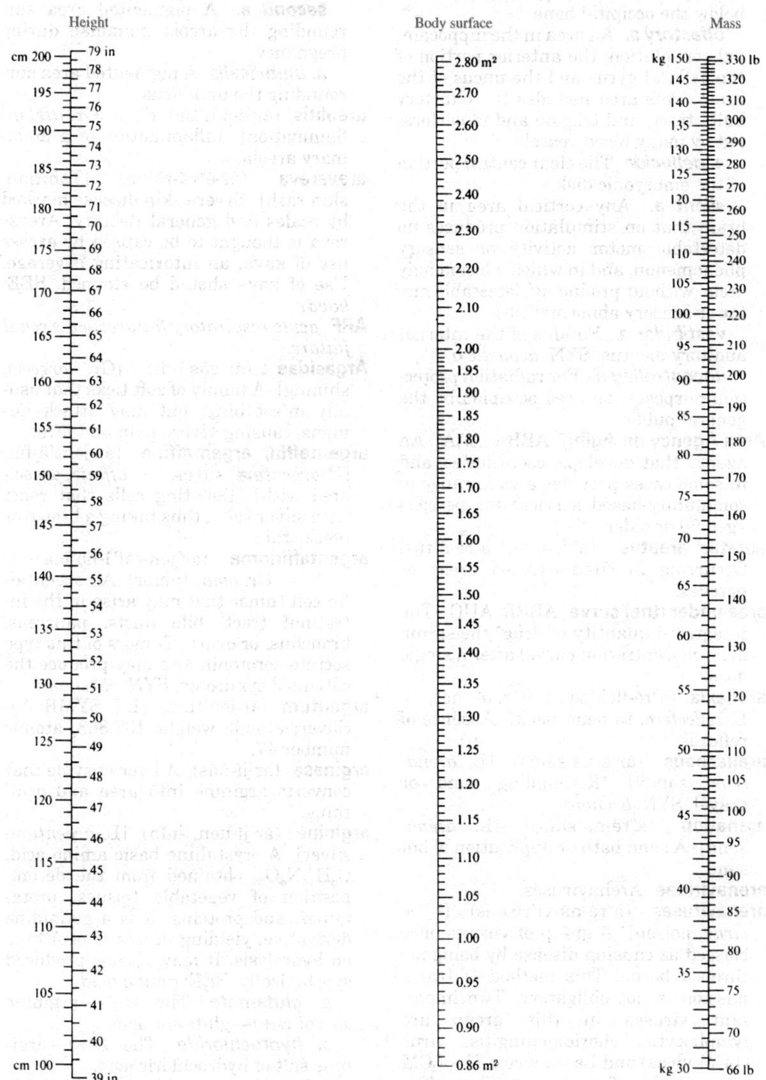

*The body surface area is given by the point of intersection with the middle scale of a straight line joining height and weight.

Kiesselbach's a. SEE: *Kiesselbach's area.*

macular a. Area of the retina that provides central vision.

mitral a. Area over the apex of the heart where mitral valve sounds are heard.

motor a. Posterior part of frontal lobe anterior to the central sulcus, from which impulses for volitional movement arise.

occipital a. The portion of the brain below the occipital bone.

olfactory a. An area in the hippocampal convolution; the anterior portion of the callosal gyrus and the uncus of the brain. This area includes the olfactory bulb, tract, and trigone and is perforated by many blood vessels.

a. pellucida The clear central portion of the embryonic disk.

silent a. Any cortical area in the brain that on stimulation produces no detectable motor activity or sensory phenomenon, and in which a lesion may occur without producing detectable motor or sensory abnormalities.

vestibular a. Fundus of the internal auditory meatus. SYN: *acoustic a.*

uncontrolled a. For radiation protection purposes, an area occupied by the general public.

Area Agency on Aging ABBR: AAA. An agency that develops, coordinates, and in some cases provides a wide range of community-based services for persons aged 60 or older.

areata, areatus (ă″rē-ā′tă, ă″rē-ā′tŭs) Occurring in circumscribed areas or patches.

area under (the) curve ABBR: AUC. The integrated quantity of drug (the serum drug concentration curve) after a single dose.

areflexia (ă″rē-flĕk′sē-ă) [Gr. *a-*, not, + L. *reflectere*, to bend back] Absence of reflexes.

arenaceous (ăr″ĕ-nā′sē-ŭs) [L. *arenaceus*, sandy] Resembling sand or gravel. SYN: *arenoid.*

arenation (ă″rĕ-nā′shŭn) [L. *arena*, sand] A sand bath or application of hot sand.

arenaviridae Arenaviruses.

arenaviruses (ă″rē-nă-vī′rŭs-ĕs) [″ + *virus*, poison] A group of viruses once classed as causing disease by being arthropod borne. This method of transmission is not obligatory. Two important viruses in this group are lymphocytic choriomeningitis virus (LCM virus) and Lassa virus. The LCM virus rarely infects humans, but when it does, the disease is usually a mild form of meningitis. The Lassa virus causes a highly contagious, severe febrile illness and may be fatal. SEE: *Lassa fever.*

arenoid (ăr′ĕ-noyd) Arenaceous.

areola (ă-rē′ō-lă) *pl.* **areolae, areolas** [L. *areola*, a small space] **1.** A small space or cavity in a tissue. **2.** A circular area of different pigmentation, as around a wheal, around the nipple of the breast, or the part of the iris around the pupil. **areolar** (-lăr), *adj.*

a. mammae The pigmented area surrounding the nipple. SYN: *a. papillaris.*

a. papillaris A. mammae.

second a. A pigmented area surrounding the areola mammae during pregnancy.

a. umbilicalis A pigmented area surrounding the umbilicus.

areolitis (ăr″ē-ō-lī′tĭs) [″ + Gr. *itis*, inflammation] Inflammation of a mammary areola.

arevareva (ăr-ē″vă-rā′vă) [Tahitian, skin rash] Severe skin disease marked by scales and general debility. Arevareva is thought to be caused by excess use of kava, an intoxicating beverage. Use of kava should be stopped. SEE: *kava.*

ARF *acute respiratory failure; acute renal failure.*

Argasidae (ăr-găs′ĭ-dī) [Gr. *argeeis*, shining] A family of soft ticks that usually infest birds but may attack humans, causing severe pain and fever.

argentaffin, argentaffine (ăr-jĕnt′ă-fĭn) [L. *argentum*, silver, + *affinis*, associated with] Denoting cells that react with silver salts, thus taking a brown or black stain.

argentaffinoma (ăr″jĕn-tăf″ĭ-nō′mă) [″ + ″ + Gr. *oma*, tumor] An argentaffin cell tumor that may arise in the intestinal tract, bile ducts, pancreas, bronchus, or ovary. Tumors of this type secrete serotonin and may produce the carcinoid syndrome. SYN: *carcinoid.*

argentum (ăr-jĕn′tŭm) [L.] SYMB: Ag. Silver; atomic weight 107.868, atomic number 47.

arginase (ăr′jĭ-nās) A liver enzyme that converts arginine into urea and ornithine.

arginine (ăr′jĭ-nēn, -nĭn) [L. *argentum*, silver] A crystalline basic amino acid, $C_6H_{14}N_4O_2$, obtained from the decomposition of vegetable tissues, protamines, and proteins. It is a guanidine derivative, yielding urea and ornithine on hydrolysis. It may also be produced synthetically. SEE: *amino acid.*

a. glutamate The L(+)—arginine salt of L(+)—glutamic acid.

a. hydrochloride The L(+)—arginine salt of hydrochloric acid.

suberyl a. A combination of suberic acid and arginine. It forms a portion of the molecule of various bufotoxins (toad poisons).

argininosuccinic acid (ăr″jĭ-nĭ″nō-sŭk-sĭn′ĭk) A compound intermediate in the synthesis of arginine; formed from citrulline and aspartic acid.

argininosuccinicaciduria (ăr″jĭn-ĭn-ō-sŭk-sĭn″ĭk-ăs-ĭ-dū′rē-ă) A hereditary metabolic disease caused by excessive excretion, and thus deficiency, of argininosuccinase, an enzyme required to metabolize argininosuccinic acid. Presentation of this defect includes mental retardation, friable tufted hair, convulsions, ataxia, liver disease, and epilepsy.

argon (ăr′gŏn) [Gr. *argos*, inactive] SYMB: Ar. An inert gas; atomic weight 39.948, atomic number 18. It composes approx. 1% of the atmosphere.

Argyll Robertson pupil (ăr-gīl′ rŏb′ĕrt-sŏn) [Douglas Argyll Robertson, Scottish ophthalmologist, 1837–1909] More properly the name of a symptom often present in paralysis and locomotor ataxia (due to syphilis), in which the light reflex is absent but there is no change in the power of contraction during accommodation. Usually bilateral. SYN: *Robertson's pupil*.

argyria, argyriasis (ăr-jĭr′ē-ă, ăr″jĭ-rī′ă-sĭs) [Gr. *argyros*, silver] Bluish discoloration of the skin and mucous membranes as a result of prolonged administration of silver. SYN: *argyrosis*.

argyric (ăr-jĭr′ĭk) Pert. to silver.

argyrophil (ăr-jī′rō-fĭl) [″ + *philos*, fond] Denoting cells that bind with silver salts, which can then be reduced to produce a brown or black stain.

argyrosis (ăr″jĭ-rō′sĭs) Argyria.

arhinia Arrhinia.

arhythmia Arrhythmia.

Arias-Stella reaction [Javier Arias-Stella, Peruvian pathologist, b. 1924] An endometrial gland cell abnormality consisting of hyperchromatic nuclei, which may be present in normal or ectopic pregnancy. It is not a sign of endometrial adenocarcinoma.

ariboflavinosis (ă-rī″bō-flā″vĭn-ō′sĭs) [Gr. *a*-, not, + *riboflavin* + Gr. *osis*, condition] Condition arising from a deficiency of riboflavin in the diet. Symptoms include lesions on the lips, stomatitis and, later, fissures in the angles of the mouth, seborrhea around the nose, and vascularization of the cornea. Riboflavin is given orally.

arm [AS] **1.** In anatomy, the upper extremity from shoulder to elbow. **2.** In popular usage, the entire upper extremity, from shoulder to hand. SEE: illus.

articulated a. A jointed instrument used in imaging and in therapeutic procedures (e.g., to permit stereotactic localization of deep anatomical structures; to guide the collection of ultrasonic images; or to focus or direct laser energy).

PATIENT CARE: Care involves general support, answering questions, and giving explanations regarding the procedure. All equipment is checked and regulations observed. The surgeon is assisted as necessary, and the procedure is recorded in the laser log.

CAUTION: Laser safety precautions must be observed. There is a special coating on the lens, which must be cared for according to manufacturer's directions.

---

brawny a. Hard, swollen arm caused by lymphedema after mastectomy.

Saturday-night a. A form of paralysis of the brachial plexus, sometimes seen in intoxicated persons. It may be caused by sleeping in a chair, with the arm hanging over the back of the chair while the head rests on the shoulder or arm.

arm, carrying angle of The angle between the long axes of the upper and lower arm. This angle is nearly straight in the male and is increased in the female (i.e., in the female the lower part of the arm will deviate away from the body more than is the case in the male). This is a secondary sex characteristic.

armamentarium (ăr″mă-mĕn-tā′rē-ŭm) [L. *armamentum*, implement] The total equipment of a physician or institution, such as instruments, drugs, books, and supplies.

armature (ăr′mă-tūr) [L. *armatura*, equipment] **1.** In biology, a structure that serves to protect or is used to attack a predator (e.g., a stinger). **2.** A part of an electrical generator, consisting of a coil of insulated wire mounted around a soft iron core.

arm board **1.** A board placed under and attached to the arm for stabilization during intravenous administration. **2.** A device attached to the sides of a wheelchair to permit support or positioning of the arm, esp. for persons with upper-extremity paralysis.

armpit Axilla.

Arndt-Schultz principle Therapeutically applied energy (e.g., thermal agents, ultrasonic energy) must be of the proper intensity to stimulate the desired physiological response. Energy that lacks the needed intensity will not produce useful therapeutic effects. Energy that is applied at too great an intensity will destroy otherwise healthy biological tissue. The Arndt-Schultz principle is used to determine appropriate treatment dosages.

Arneth, Joseph (ăr′nāt) German physician, 1873–1955.

A.'s classification of neutrophils A classification of polymorphonuclear neutrophils based on the number of lobes (one to five) in the nucleus, termed stages one to five, respectively.

A.'s formula The normal ratio of various types of polymorphonuclear neu-

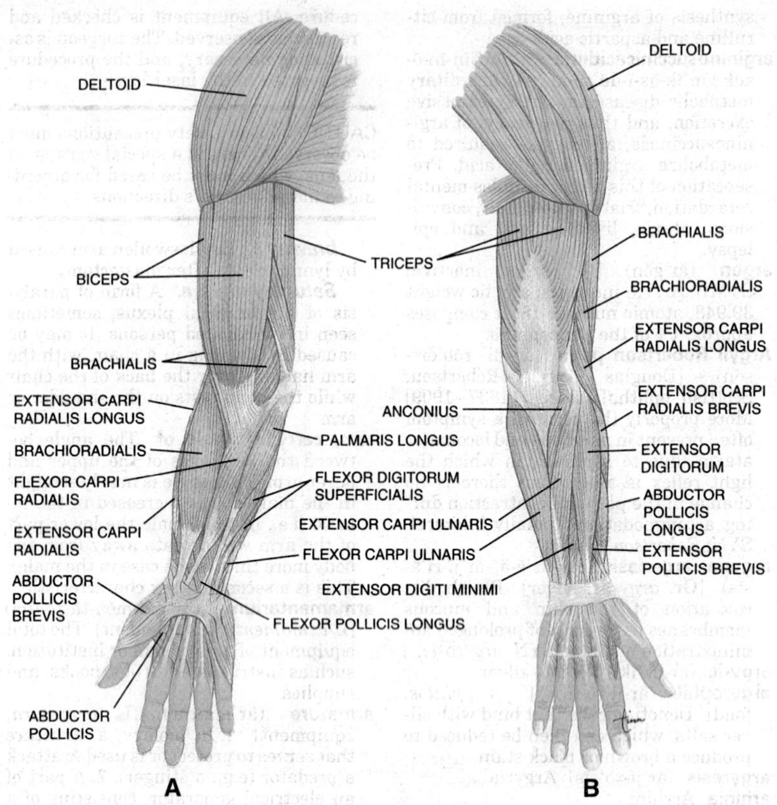

MUSCLES OF THE ARM

(A) anterior view, (B) posterior view

trophils based on the number of lobes (one to five) in the nucleus.

arnica (ar'ni-căh) A perennial herb, *Arnica montana*, used in ointments as a homeopathic remedy for pain, inflammation, and bacterial infection.

Arnold, Friedrich German anatomist, 1803–1890.

A.'s canal Passage in the temporal bone for the lesser superficial petrosal nerve.

A.'s ganglion Otic ganglion.

A.'s nerve Auricular branch of the vagus nerve. SEE: *cough, reflex*.

Arnold-Chiari deformity (ăr'nōlt-kē'ă-rē) [Julius Arnold, Ger. pathologist, 1835–1915; Hans Chiari, Austrian pathologist, 1851–1916] A condition in which the inferior poles of the cerebellar hemispheres and the medulla protrude through the foramen magnum into the spinal canal. It is one of the causes of hydrocephalus and is usually accompanied by spina bifida cystica and meningomyelocele.

AROM **1.** *active range of motion.* **2.** *artificial rupture of membranes*

aroma (ă-rō'mă) [Gr. *aroma*, spice] An agreeable odor.

aromatherapy The use of fragrant oils in baths, as inhalants, or during massage to relieve stress and to treat skin conditions.

aromatic (ăr"ō-măt'ĭk) **1.** Having an agreeable odor. **2.** Denoting an organic chemical compound in which the carbon atoms form closed rings (as in benzene).

a. ammonia spirit A solution consisting of 34 g of ammonium carbonate in 1000 ml of diluted ammonia solution, fragrant oils, alcohol, and purified water; used as an antacid and carminative. It acts as a reflex stimulant when its vapor is inhaled.

a. compounds Ring or cyclic compounds related to benzene, many having a fragrant odor.

a. elixir A flavoring agent used in preparing medicines.

arousal **1.** Alertness; the state of being prepared to act. **2.** Erotic excitement.

a. level An individual's degree of alertness or responsiveness to stimuli. In testing a newborn's behavior, the level of arousal is important. These levels are deep sleep; sleep with rapid eye movements; drowsy state; a quiet, alert state; an awake and active state; and a state of active, intense crying. The infant is capable of the most responsive and complex interactions with the environment in the quiet and alert states. SEE: *psychomotor and physical development of infant*.

arraignment (ah-rān′měnt) A procedure whereby an accused person is brought

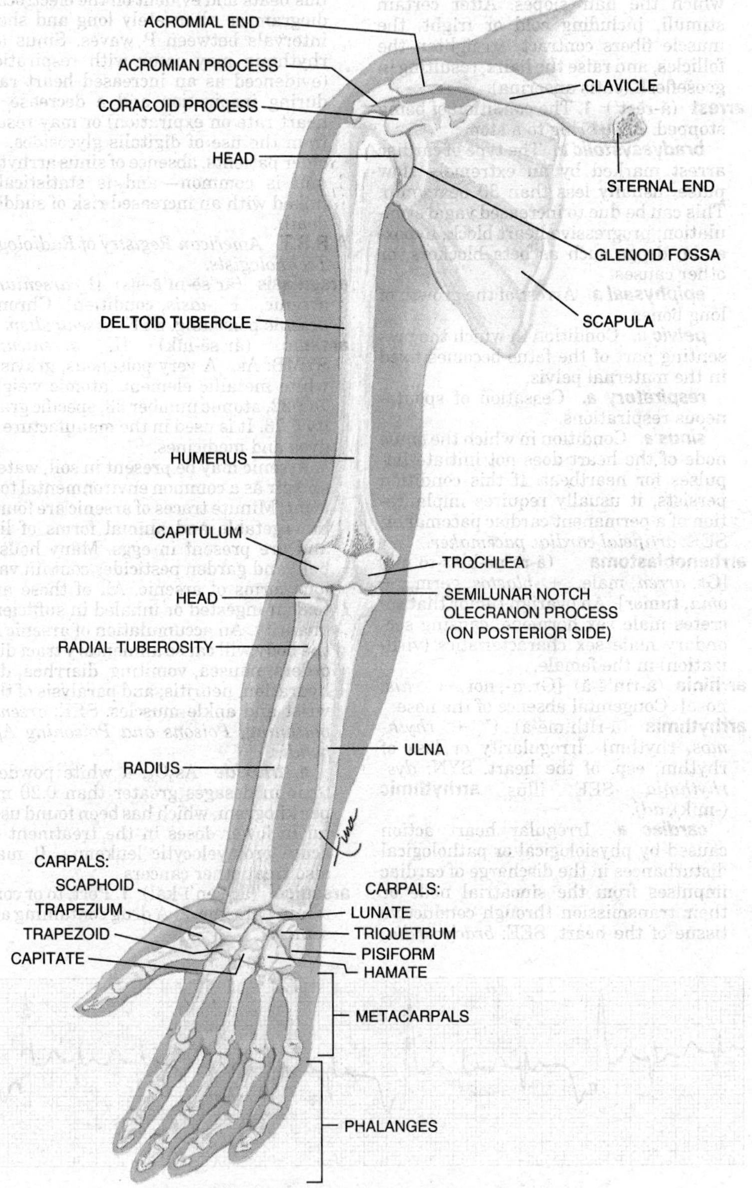

BONES OF THE ARM AND SHOULDER GIRDLE

Bones of the arm and shoulder girdle

before the court to plead to a criminal charge. A person may plead guilty, not guilty, or nolo contendere ("no contest"). The judge then sets bail.

arrector pili *pl.* **arrectores pilorum** [L. *arrectores*, raisers, + *pilus*, hair] One of the involuntary muscle fibers arising in the skin and extending down to connect with the hair follicles on the side toward which the hair slopes. After certain stimuli, including cold or fright, the muscle fibers contract, straighten the follicles, and raise the hairs, resulting in gooseflesh (cutis anserina).

arrest (ă-rĕst′) **1.** The condition of being stopped. **2.** To bring to a stop.

bradyasystolic a. The type of cardiac arrest marked by an extremely slow pulse, usually less than 30 beats/min. This can be due to increased vagal stimulation, progressive heart block, hypoxemia, drugs such as beta blockers, or other causes.

epiphyseal a. Arrest of the growth of long bones.

pelvic a. Condition in which the presenting part of the fetus becomes fixed in the maternal pelvis.

respiratory a. Cessation of spontaneous respirations.

sinus a. Condition in which the sinus node of the heart does not initiate impulses for heartbeat. If this condition persists, it usually requires implantation of a permanent cardiac pacemaker. SEE: *artificial cardiac pacemaker*.

arrhenoblastoma (ă-rē″nō-blăs-tō′mă) [Gr. *arren*, male, + *blastos*, germ, + *oma*, tumor] An ovarian tumor that secretes male sex hormone, causing secondary male sex characteristics (virilization) in the female.

arrhinia (ă-rĭn′ē-ă) [Gr. *a-*, not, + *rhis*, nose] Congenital absence of the nose.

arrhythmia (ă-rĭth′mē-ă) [″ + *rhythmos*, rhythm] Irregularity or loss of rhythm, esp. of the heart. SYN: *dysrhythmia*. SEE: illus. **arrhythmic** (-mĭk), *adj.*

cardiac a. Irregular heart action caused by physiological or pathological disturbances in the discharge of cardiac impulses from the sinoatrial node or their transmission through conductive tissue of the heart. SEE: *bradycardia; cardioversion; artificial cardiac p.; sick sinus syndrome; tachycardia; Nursing Diagnoses Appendix.*

reperfusion a. Cardiac arrhythmia that occurs as the infarcted heart is resupplied with blood following angioplasty or thrombolysis.

sinus a. Cardiac irregularity marked by variation in the interval between sinus beats and evident on the electrocardiogram as alternately long and short intervals between P waves. Sinus arrhythmia may occur with respiration (evidenced as an increased heart rate during inspiration and a decrease in heart rate on expiration) or may result from the use of digitalis glycosides. In older patients, absence of sinus arrhythmia is common—and is statistically linked with an increased risk of sudden death.

A.R.R.T. *American Registry of Radiologic Technologists.*

arseniasis (ăr″sĕ-nī′ă-sĭs) [L. *arsenium*, arsenic, + *-iasis*, condition] Chronic arsenic poisoning. SYN: *arsenicalism*.

arsenic (ăr′sĕ-nĭk) [L. *arsenicum*] SYMB: As. A very poisonous, grayish-white metallic element, atomic weight 74.922, atomic number 33, specific gravity 5.73. It is used in the manufacture of dyes and medicines.

Arsenic may be present in soil, water, and air as a common environmental toxicant. Minute traces of arsenic are found in vegetable and animal forms of life and are present in eggs. Many household and garden pesticides contain various forms of arsenic. All of these are toxic if ingested or inhaled in sufficient quantity. An accumulation of arsenic in the body will cause alimentary tract disorders, nausea, vomiting, diarrhea, dehydration, neuritis, and paralysis of the wrist and ankle muscles. SEE: *arsenic poisoning; Poisons and Poisoning Appendix.*

a. trioxide As_2O_3; a white powder, toxic in dosages greater than 0.20 mg per kilogram, which has been found useful in lower doses in the treatment of acute promyelocytic leukemia. It may also treat other cancers.

arsenical (ăr-sĕn′ĭ-kăl) **1.** Pert. to or containing arsenic. **2.** A drug containing arsenic.

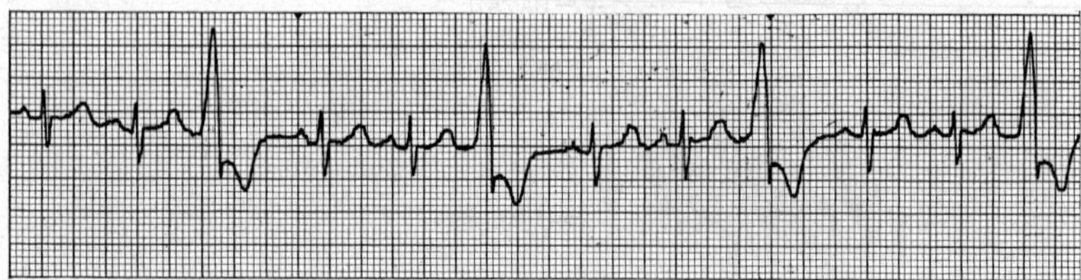

VENTRICULAR ARRHYTHMIA

Ventricular trigeminy

arsenicalism (ăr-sĕn′ĭ-kăl-ĭzm) [L. *arsenicum*, arsenic, + Gr. *-ismos*, condition of] Chronic arsenic poisoning. SYN: *arseniasis*.

arsenicophagy (ăr″sĕn-ĭ-kŏf′ă-jē) [″ + *phagein*, to eat] Habitual eating of arsenic.

arsenium (ăr-sē′nē-ŭm) [L.] Arsenic.

arsine (ăr′sĭn) A very poisonous gas used in chemical warfare.

arsphenamine (ărs-fĕn′ă-mēn) A light yellow powder containing about 30% arsenic; formerly used in the treatment of syphilis. SYN: *salvarsan*.

ART *assisted reproductive technology*.

A.R.T. *Accredited Record Technician*.

artefact SEE: *artifact*.

arterectomy (ăr″tĕ-rĕk′tō-mē) [Gr. *arteria*, artery, + *ektome*, excision] Excision of an artery or arteries.

arteri- SEE: *arterio-*.

arteria (ăr″tē′rē-ă) *pl.* **arteriae** The Latin word for artery.

arterial (ăr-tē′rē-ăl) Pert. to one or more arteries.

arterial blood gas ABBR: ABG. Literally, any of the gases present in blood; operationally and clinically, they include the determination of levels of pH, oxygen (O_2), and carbon dioxide (CO_2) in the blood. ABGs are important in the diagnosis and treatment of disturbances of acid-base balance, pulmonary disease, electrolyte balance, and oxygen delivery. Values of the gases themselves are usually expressed as the partial pressure of carbon dioxide or oxygen, although derived values are reported in other units. Several other blood chemistry values are important in managing acid-base disturbances, including the levels of the bicarbonate ion, HCO_3, blood pH, sodium, potassium, and chloride.

arterial circulation Movement of blood through the arteries. It is maintained by the pumping of the heart and influenced by the elasticity and extensibility of arterial walls, peripheral resistance in the areas of small arteries, and the quantity of blood in the body. SEE: *circulation*.

arterial line A hemodynamic monitoring system consisting of a catheter in an artery connected to pressure tubing, a transducer, and an electronic monitor. It is used to measure systemic blood pressure and to provide ease of access for the drawing of blood (e.g., in intensive care, when regular monitoring of blood gases is necessary.

arteriectasis, arteriectasia (ăr″tĕ-rē-ĕk′tă-sĭs, -ĕk-tā′zē-ă) [″ + *ektasis*, a stretching out] Arterial dilatation.

arteriectomy (ăr″tĕ-rē-ĕk′tō-mē) [″ + *ektome*, excision] Surgical removal of part of an artery.

arterio-, arteri- [Gr. *arteria*, artery] Combining form indicating *relationship to an artery*.

arteriocapillary (ăr-tē″rē-ō-kăp′ĭ-lăr″ē) [″ + L. *capillus*, like hair] Pert. to both arteries and capillaries.

arteriofibrosis (ăr-tē″rē-ō-fī-brō′sĭs) [″ + L. *fibra*, fiber, + Gr. *osis*, condition] Arteriocapillary fibrosis.

arteriogram (ăr-tē′rē-ō-grăm″) [″ + *gramma*, something written] A radiograph of an artery after injection of a radiopaque contrast medium, usually directly into the artery or near its origin. SEE: *angiogram*.

arteriography (ăr″tē-rē-ŏg′ră-fē) [″ + *graphein*, to write] **1.** A radiographic procedure for obtaining an arteriogram. SEE: *angiography*. **2.** Description of arteries.

arteriola (ăr-tē″rē-ō′lă) *pl.* **arteriolae** [L.] A small artery; an arteriole.

a. macularis inferior The inferior macular arteriole, which supplies the macula retinae of the eye.

a. macularis superior The superior macular arteriole, which supplies the macula retinae of the eye.

a. medialis retinae The medial arteriole of the retina.

a. nasalis retinae inferior The inferior nasal arteriole of the retina.

a. nasalis retinae superior The superior nasal arteriole of the retina.

a. recta One of the small arteries of the kidney that supply the renal pyramids.

a. temporalis retinae inferior The inferior temporal artery of the retina.

a. temporalis retinae superior The superior temporal artery of the retina.

arteriole (ăr-tē′rē-ōl) *pl.* **arterioles** [L. *arteriola*] A minute artery, esp. one that, at its distal end, leads into a capillary. SYN: *arteriola*. **arteriolar** (ăr-tē-rē-ō′lăr), *adj.*

arteriolith (ăr-tē′rē-ō-lĭth) [″ + Gr. *lithos*, stone] An arterial calculus.

arteriolitis (ăr-tēr″ē-ō-lī′tĭs) [″ + Gr. *itis*, inflammation] Inflammation of the arteriolar wall.

arteriolonecrosis (ăr-tē″rē-ō″lō-nĕ-krō′sĭs) [″ + Gr. *nekros*, corpse, + *osis*, condition] Destruction of an arteriole.

arteriolosclerosis (ăr-tē″rē-ō″lō-sklĕ-rō′sĭs) [L. *arteriola*, small artery, + Gr. *sklerosis*, hardening] Thickening of the walls of the arterioles, with loss of elasticity and contractility. **arteriolosclerotic** (-rŏt′ĭk), *adj.*

arteriomotor (ăr-tē″rē-ō-mō′tor) [Gr. *arteria*, artery, + L. *movere*, to move] Causing changes in the interior diameter of arteries by dilatation and constriction.

arteriomyomatosis (ăr-tē″rē-ō-mī″ō-mă-tō′sĭs) [″ + *mys*, muscle, + *oma*, tumor, + *osis*, condition] Thickening of arterial walls due to overgrowth of muscle fibers.

arterionecrosis (ăr-tē″rē-ō-nĕ-krō′sĭs) [″ + *nekros*, corpse, + *osis*, condition] Arterial necrosis.

arteriopathy (ăr″tē-rē-ŏp′ă-thē) [″ + *pathos*, disease, suffering] Any disease of the arteries.

obliterative a. In cardiac transplantation, diffuse concentric stenosis of the coronary arteries resulting from immunologic rejection.

arterioplasty (ăr-tē″rē-ō-plăs′tē) [″ + *plassein*, to form] Repair or reconstruction of an artery.

arteriopressor (ăr-tē″rē-ō-prĕs′or) [″ + L. *pressura*, force] Causing increased arterial blood pressure.

arteriorrhaphy (ăr-tē″rē-or′ă-fē) [″ + *rhaphe*, seam, ridge] Arterial suture.

arteriorrhexis (ăr-tē″rē-ō-rĕk′sĭs) [″ + *rhexis*, rupture] Rupture of an artery.

arteriosclerosis (ăr-tē″rē-ō-sklĕ-rō′sĭs) [″ + *sklerosis*, to harden] A disease of the arterial vessels marked by thickening, hardening, and loss of elasticity in the arterial walls. Three forms of arteriosclerosis are generally recognized: atherosclerosis, sclerosis of arterioles, and calcific sclerosis of the medial layer of arteries (Mönckeberg's calcification). Atherosclerosis is the single most important cause of disease and death in Western societies.

SEE: *atherosclerosis*.

a. obliterans Arteriosclerosis in which the lumen of the artery is completely occluded. **arteriosclerotic** (-rŏt′ĭk), *adj.*

arteriospasm (ăr-tē′rē-ō-spăzm″) [Gr. *arteria*, artery, + *spasmos*, a convulsion] Arterial spasm.

arteriostenosis (ăr-tē″rē-ō-stĕ-nō′sĭs) [″ + *stenosis*, act of narrowing] Narrowing of the lumen of an artery; may be temporary or permanent.

arteriostosis (ăr-tē″rē-ŏs-tō′sĭs) [″ + *osteon*, bone, + *osis*, condition] Calcification of an artery.

arteriostrepsis (ăr-tē″rē-ō-strĕp′sĭs) [″ + *strepsis*, a twisting] Twisting of the divided end of an artery to arrest hemorrhage.

arteriosympathectomy (ăr-tē″rē-ō-sĭm″pă-thĕk′tō-mē) [″ + *sympatheia*, suffer with, + *ektome*, excision] Removal of the arterial sheath containing fibers of the sympathetic nerve.

arteriotomy (ăr″tē-rē-ŏt′ō-mē) Surgical division or opening of an artery.

arteriovenous (ăr-tē″rē-ō-vē′nŭs) [″ + L. *vena*, a vein] ABBR: A-V. Rel. to both arteries and veins.

arteriovenous access Use of a shunt to connect an artery to a vein. This may be used in renal dialysis.

arterioversion (ăr-tē″rē-ō-vĕr′shŭn) [″ + L. *versio*, a turning] Eversion of an arterial wall to arrest hemorrhage from the open end.

arteritis (ăr″tĕ-rī′tĭs) [″ + *itis*, inflammation] Inflammation of an artery. SEE: *endarteritis*.

giant cell a. temporal a.

a. nodosa Widespread inflammation of adventitia of small and medium-sized arteries with impaired function of the involved organs. SYN: *periarteritis nodosa; polyarteritis nodosa*.

a. obliterans Inflammation of the intima of an artery, causing occlusion of the lumen. SYN: *endarteritis obliterans*.

rheumatic a. Arachaic term for inflammation of small arteries as a result of rheumatic fever.

Takayasu's a. SEE: *Takayasu's arteritis*.

temporal a. A relatively common chronic inflammation of large arteries, usually the temporal, occipital, or ophthalmic arteries, identified on pathological specimens by the presence of giant cells. It causes thickening of the intima, with narrowing and eventual occlusion of the lumen. It typically occurs after age 50. Symptoms include headache, tenderness over the affected artery, loss of vision, and facial pain. The cause is unknown, but there may be a genetic predisposition in some families. Corticosteroids usually are administered. **arteritic** (-rĭt′ĭk), *adj.*

artery (ăr′tĕr-ē) *pl.* **arteries** [Gr. *arteria*, windpipe] One of the vessels carrying blood from the heart to the tissues. There are two divisions, pulmonary and systemic. The pulmonary arteries carry deoxygenated blood from the right ventricle to the lungs. The systemic arteries carry oxygenated blood from the left ventricle to the rest of the body. SEE: illus. (Systemic Arteries); ***aorta*** and *coronary artery disease* for illus.

ANATOMY: An arterial wall has three layers: the inner layer (tunica intima) is endothelial tissue; the middle layer (tunica media) is smooth muscle and elastic connective tissue; and the outer layer (tunica externa) is white fibrous connective tissue. SEE: illus. (Structure of an Artery).

brachiocephalic a. Innominate a.

celiac a. The first branch of the abdominal aorta. Its branches supply the stomach, liver, spleen, duodenum, and pancreas.

coiled a. Spiral a.

conducting a. Elastic a.

dominant a. In cardiology, the coronary artery that supplies the major posterior descending artery (PDA) of the heart. The coronary circulation is said to be "right dominant" when the PDA receives its blood flow from the right coronary artery, and "left dominant" when its flow comes from the circumflex artery.

elastic a. A large artery in which elastic connective tissue is predominant in the middle layer (tunica media). Elastic arteries include the aorta and its larger branches (innominate, common carotid, subclavian, and common iliac), which conduct blood to the muscular arteries. SYN: *conducting a.*

end a. An artery whose branches do not anastomose with those of other arteries (e.g., arteries to the brain and spinal cord). SYN: *terminal a.*

hyaloid a. A fetal artery that supplies nutrition to the lens. It disappears in the later months of gestation.

innominate a. The right artery arising from the arch of the aorta, and dividing into the right subclavian and right common carotid arteries. SYN: *brachiocephalic a.*

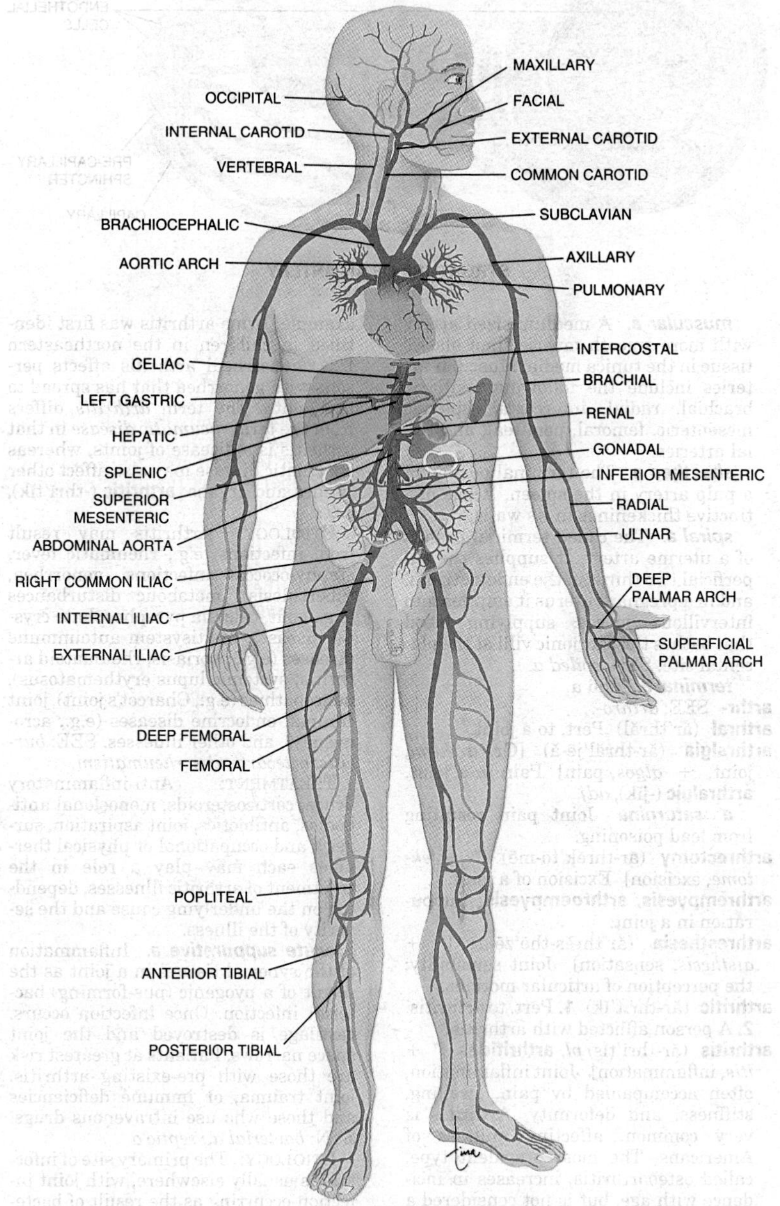

SYSTEMIC ARTERIES

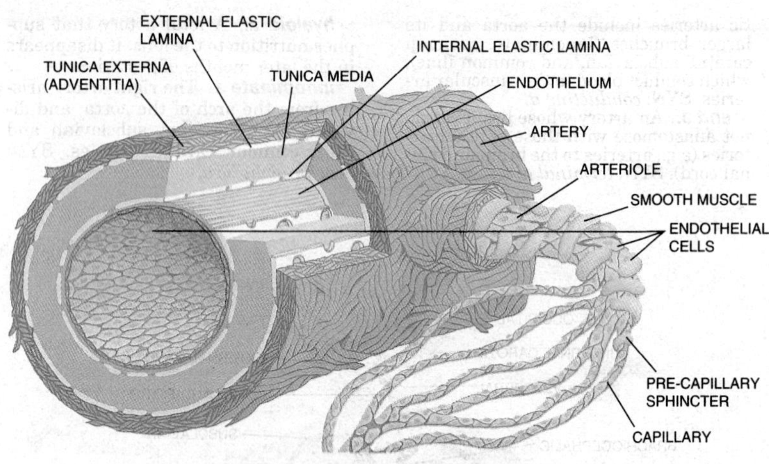

STRUCTURE OF AN ARTERY

muscular a. A medium-sized artery with more smooth muscle than elastic tissue in the tunica media. Muscular arteries include the following: axillary, brachial, radial, intercostal, splenic, mesenteric, femoral, popliteal, and tibial arteries.

sheathed a. The terminal portion of a pulp artery in the spleen. It has distinctive thickenings in its walls.

spiral a. The coiled terminal branch of a uterine artery. It supplies the superficial two thirds of the endometrium, and in a pregnant uterus it empties into intervillous spaces, supplying blood that bathes the chorionic villi at the placental site. SYN: *coiled a.*

terminal a. End a.

arthr- SEE: *arthro-.*

arthral (ăr′thrăl) Pert. to a joint.

arthralgia (ăr-thrăl′jē-ă) [Gr. *arthron*, joint, + *algos*, pain] Pain in a joint. **arthralgic** (-jĭk), *adj.*

a. saturnina Joint pain resulting from lead poisoning.

arthrectomy (ăr-thrĕk′tō-mē) [″ + *ektome*, excision] Excision of a joint.

arthrempyesis, arthroempyesis Suppuration in a joint.

arthresthesia (ăr″thrĕs-thē′zē-ă) [″ + *aisthesis*, sensation] Joint sensibility; the perception of articular motions.

arthritic (ăr-thrĭt′ĭk) **1.** Pert. to arthritis. **2.** A person afflicted with arthritis.

arthritis (ăr-thrī′tĭs) *pl.* **arthritides** [″ + *itis*, inflammation] Joint inflammation, often accompanied by pain, swelling, stiffness, and deformity. Arthritis is very common, affecting millions of Americans. The most prevalent type, called osteoarthritis, increases in incidence with age, but is not considered a part of normal aging. Other forms of arthritis affect specific populations. For example, Lyme arthritis was first identified in children in the northeastern U.S.; gonorrheal arthritis affects persons with gonorrhea that has spread to the joints. The term *arthritis* differs from the term *rheumatic disease* in that arthritis is a disease of joints, whereas rheumatic disease may also affect other tissues and organs. **arthritic** (-thrĭ′tĭk), *adj.*

ETIOLOGY: Arthritis may result from infections (e.g., rheumatic fever, staphylococcal infections, gonorrhea, tuberculosis), metabolic disturbances (e.g., gout, calcium pyrophosphate crystal disease), multisystem autoimmune diseases (e.g., psoriasis, rheumatoid arthritis, systemic lupus erythematosus), neuropathies (e.g., Charcot's joint), joint trauma, endocrine diseases (e.g., acromegaly), and other illnesses. SEE: *bursitis; osteoarthritis; rheumatism.*

TREATMENT: Anti-inflammatory drugs, corticosteroids, monoclonal antibodies, antibiotics, joint aspiration, surgery, and occupational or physical therapies each may play a role in the treatment of arthritic illnesses, depending on the underlying cause and the severity of the illness.

acute suppurative a. Inflammation of the synovial tissues in a joint as the result of a pyogenic (pus-forming) bacterial infection. Once infection occurs, cartilage is destroyed and the joint space narrows. Patients at greatest risk are those with pre-existing arthritis, joint trauma, or immune deficiencies and those who use intravenous drugs. SYN: *bacterial a.; septic a.*

ETIOLOGY: The primary site of infection is usually elsewhere, with joint infection occurring as the result of bacteremia or spread from osteomyelitis in an adjacent bone. The most common pathogen for those 16 to 40 years old is *Neisseria gonorrhoeae;* other common bacteria include *Staphylococcus aureus*, group B streptococci, and gram-negative bacilli such as *Escherichia coli* and *Salmonella* sp.

SYMPTOMS: Suppurative arthritis is marked by an acutely painful, warm, swollen joint with limited range of motion and fever; the white blood cell count and erythrocyte sedimentation rates are increased. Except in gonococcal arthritis, only one joint is affected, most commonly the knee, hip, or shoulder.

TREATMENT: Prompt treatment is necessary, including drainage of the joint and antimicrobial drug therapy (intravenous penicillinase-resistant penicillins and third-generation cephalosporins). The affected joint is supported with a sling or pillows, and the patient's pain is treated with mild opioids and nonsteroidal anti-inflammatory agents. Without vigorous treatment, significant joint destruction can occur.

adjuvant a. ABBR: AA. An experimental model of arthritis in rodents induced by injection of foreign substance, such as Freund's adjuvant, into the tail vein or paw. This model can be used to study new agents for human arthritis treatment. SYN: *experimental a.* SEE: *rheumatoid a.*

allergic a. Arthritis occurring in serum sickness or, rarely, as a result of food allergies.

bacterial a. Infection of joints associated with fever and other systemic symptoms. Joint destruction occurs if the infection is not treated expeditiously. Removal of pus from the joint is necessary. In older or immunosuppressed patients, the most common causative organism is *Staphylococcus aureus*. Staphylococci, anaerobes, or gram-negative bacteria are found in prosthetic joint infections. Gonococci and *Borrelia burgdorferi*, the spirochete that causes Lyme disease, differ from other forms of bacteria that cause joint infection in that they tend to affect younger and more active individuals. SYN: *acute suppurative a.; septic a.*

cricoarytenoid a. One of the causes of dysphonia and vocal fold immobility that does not involve laryngeal nerve damage. It is caused by degenerative changes of the cricoarytenoid joints.

degenerative a. Osteoarthritis.

enteropathic a. Joint disease associated with inflammatory bowel disease.

experimental a. Adjuvant a.

gonococcal a. Arthritis, often with tenosynovitis and/or rash, caused by disseminated gonococcal infection. The joints of the knees, wrists, and hands are most commonly affected. The disease may affect any sexually active person, and is relatively common in inner-city populations and people who attend sexually transmitted disease clinics, and may follow infection of a mucous membrane by gonorrhea.

TREATMENT: It is treated with penicillinase-resistant penicillins and third-generation cephalosporins.

gouty a. Arthritis caused by gout.

hypertrophic a. Osteoarthritis.

infectious a. Joint inflammation caused by a germ, usually a bacterium, and occasionally a virus or a fungus. SEE: *bacterial a.; gonorrheal a.; Lyme disease; syphilitic a.*

juvenile rheumatoid a. ABBR: JRA. A group of chronic, inflammatory diseases involving the joints and other organs in juveniles and children under age 16. The age of onset is variable, as are the extra-articular manifestations. JRA affects about 1 in 1000 children and is the most common form of arthritis in childhood. At least five subgroups are recognized. SYN: *Still's disease*. SEE: *Nursing Diagnoses Appendix.*

TREATMENT: Anti-inflammatory agents are the mainstay of drug treatment. Corticosteroids should rarely be used. Methotrexate is an alternative treatment for patients who do not respond to NSAIDs, and hematopoietic stem cell transplantation may be used in specialized treatment centers. Physical and occupational therapy are needed to maintain muscle strength and range of joint motion. Iridocyclitis should be managed by an ophthalmologist. Other extra-articular manifestations should be referred to experienced medical and surgical specialists.

PATIENT CARE: The child and family are instructed about the disease process and treatment and coping strategies, and are encouraged to express concerns. A well-balanced diet, regular rest periods, and avoidance of excessive fatigue and overexertion are encouraged. Moist heat helps to relieve pain and stiffness. Placing the child in a warm bath, immersing painful hands and feet in pans of warm water for 10 min two to three times daily, or using daily whirlpool baths, a paraffin bath, or hot packs provides temporary relief of acute swelling and pain. Swimming is recommended to strengthen muscles and maintain mobility. Good posture and body mechanics are important; sleeping on a firm mattress without a pillow or with only a thin pillow is recommended to maintain proper body alignment. The patient should lie prone to straighten the hips and knees when resting or watching television. If braces or splints are required, their use is explained and demonstrated. Activities of daily living and the child's natural affinity for play provide opportunities to maintain mobility and incorporate therapeutic exercises using assistive and safety devices. The child with photophobia due to iridocyclitis should wear sunglasses. The child and family are referred to local and national support and information groups like the Arthritis Foundation (404-872-7100) (www.arthritis.org). Desired outcomes include the child's ability to achieve and maintain optimal health with joints that are movable, flexible, and free of deformity, to move with minimal or no discomfort, to engage in activities suitable to his or her interests, capabilities, and developmental level, and to perform self-care activities to maximum capabilities.

Lyme a. The large-joint arthritis that develops in approx. 35% to 80% of patients with Lyme disease, caused by the spirochete *Borrelia burgdorferi*. It appears 2 weeks to 2 years after infection and is marked by periodic episodes of pain that move among different joints; the shoulders, knees, elbows, and ankles are involved most commonly. Approx. 10% of patients develop permanent deformities. The likelihood of chronic arthritic complaints is markedly diminished if patients are treated with amoxicillin or other appropriate antibiotics. SEE: *Lyme disease*.

neuropathic a. Arthritis associated with diseases of the nervous system. It occurs most commonly as a result of diabetes but can occur in tabes dorsalis, syphilis, and syringomyelia. SEE: *Charcot's joint*.

palindromic a. Transient recurrent arthritis, of unknown etiology, usually affecting large joints, such as the knees and elbows.

pauciarticular type I juvenile rheumatoid a. A form of JRA that accounts for about 33% of all JRA cases; 80% of cases occur in girls, usually presenting in early childhood. As the name implies, few joints are involved, typically the large joints of the knee, ankle, or elbow. One third of cases develop chronic iridocyclitis. Results of rheumatoid factor evaluation are usually negative. Ultimately, 10% of these children develop ocular damage, and 20% go on to develop polyarthritis.

pauciarticular type II juvenile rheumatoid a. A form of JRA that 90% of the time occurs in boys. As with type I, few joints are involved in this form of JRA; the hip girdle is usually the one involved. Sacroilitis and acute iridocyclitis are the important extra-articular manifestations; an unknown percentage of children develop chronic spondyloarthropathy.

polyarticular juvenile rheumatoid a., rheumatoid factor–negative A form of JRA that accounts for about 25% of all JRA cases, 90% of cases occur in girls. It may involve multiple joints. Iridocyclitis, its most severe extra-articular manifestation, is rare. Severe arthritis develops in 10% to 15% of these children.

polyarticular juvenile rheumatoid a., rheumatoid factor–positive A form of JRA that accounts for 5% to 10% of all JRA cases; 80% of cases occur in girls. Typically presenting later in childhood, this form may affect multiple joints. There are few extra-articular manifestations but 50% or more of these children develop severe arthritis.

psoriatic a. Arthritis associated with psoriasis. The exacerbations and remissions of arthritic symptoms do not always parallel those of psoriasis. "Sausage-shaped" deformities of the fingers and toes are often present.

reactive a. Joint inflammation that occurs after an infection of another organ, possibly as a result of immunological mimicry.

rheumatoid a. A chronic systemic disease marked by inflammation of multiple synovial joints (often the proximal interphalangeal joints of the hands). The disease usually affects similar groups of joints on both sides of the body, creating bony erosions that can be seen radiographically. Subcutaneous nodule formation and elevated serum rheumatoid factor levels are common. Patients typically complain of joint stiffness in the morning rather than after activities. Women are affected 3 times more often than men. Members of some ethnic groups, such as American Indians, have higher rates of this disease than the general population. The illness usually begins in mid-life, but any age group can be affected. SEE: illus.

ETIOLOGY: The etiology is unknown but autoimmune mechanisms are implicated.

SYMPTOMS: Joint pains, morning stiffness, gelling (stiffness that returns after the patient sits or rests), malaise, and fatigue are often present. Systemic disease marked by pleural effusions, pericarditis, pulmonary fibrosis, neuropathies, and ocular disorders can lead to symptoms from each of these organs. Symptoms usually develop gradually over the course of several months but may begin abruptly in some patients.

TREATMENT: Most rheumatologists now recommend aggressive therapy with disease-modifying antirheumatic drugs (DMARDs) early in the course of the illness to prevent bony erosions and loss of joint function. Drugs in this class include agents like hydroxychloroquine and methotrexate, both of which may take several months to achieve symptomatic benefits. Other agents such as monoclonal antibodies to tumor necrosis factor, nonsteroidal anti-inflammatory drugs (e.g., ibuprofen), or cortico-

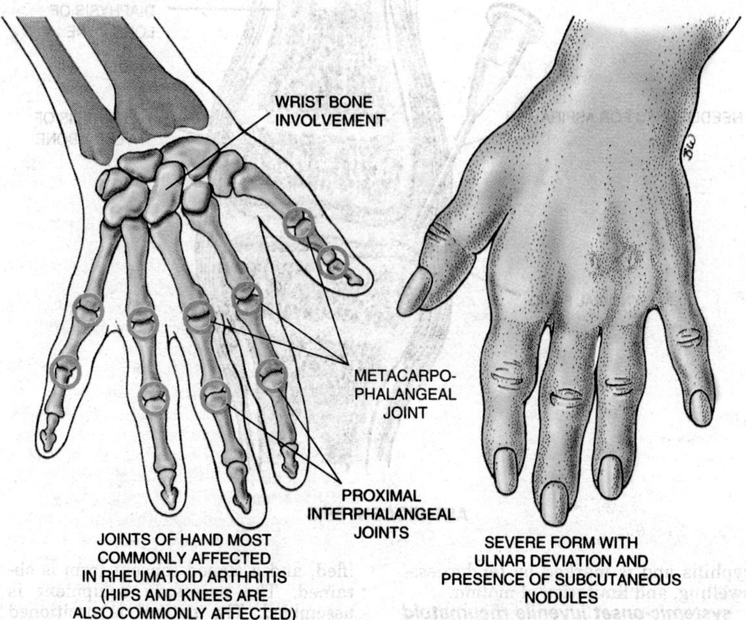

RHEUMATOID ARTHRITIS

steroids also are typically prescribed. Many patients may continue to take low-dose corticosteroids for years, but the benefits of long-term steroid use have to be weighed against the risks, such as diabetes, osteoporosis, and adrenal suppression. Gold compounds can be used, but they are weaker than DMARDs and newer agents. Powerful immunosuppressive agents like cyclosporine, azathioprine, and mycophenolate may also be used. Combination therapies involving several agents from different classes often are used. Joint replacement surgery can be helpful for some patients.

PATIENT CARE: All joints are assessed for inflammation, deformities, and contractures. The patient's ability to perform activities of daily living (ADL) is evaluated. The patient is assessed for fatigue, irritability, and temperature elevation; vital signs are monitored; and weight changes, sensory disturbances, pain (location, quality, severity, inciting and relieving factors), and morning stiffness (esp. duration) are documented. Use of moist heat is encouraged to relieve stiffness and pain. Prescribed anti-inflammatory and analgesic drug therapy is administered and evaluated; the patient is taught about the use of these medications. Inflamed joints occasionally are splinted in extension as prescribed to prevent contractures. Pressure areas are noted, and range of motion is maintained with gentle, passive exercise, if the patient cannot comfortably perform active movement. Once inflammation has subsided, the patient is instructed about active range-of-motion exercise for specific joints. Warm baths or soaks are encouraged before or during exercise. Cleansing lotions or oils should be used for dry skin. The patient is encouraged to perform ADL, if possible, allowing extra time as needed. Assistive and safety devices may be recommended for some patients. The patient should pace activities, alternate sitting and standing, and take short rest periods. The patient should sleep on a firm mattress, preferably in a supine position. Referral to an occupational or physical therapist may be needed. Both patient and family should be referred to local and national support and information groups. Desired outcomes include cooperation with prescribed medication and exercise regimens, ability to perform ADL, slowed progression of debilitating effects, pain control, and proper use of assistive devices. For more information, contact the Arthritis Foundation (404-872-7100) (www.arthritis.org). SEE: *Nursing Diagnoses Appendix.*

septic a. acute suppurative a.

syphilitic a. Arthritis that occurs in the secondary and tertiary stages of

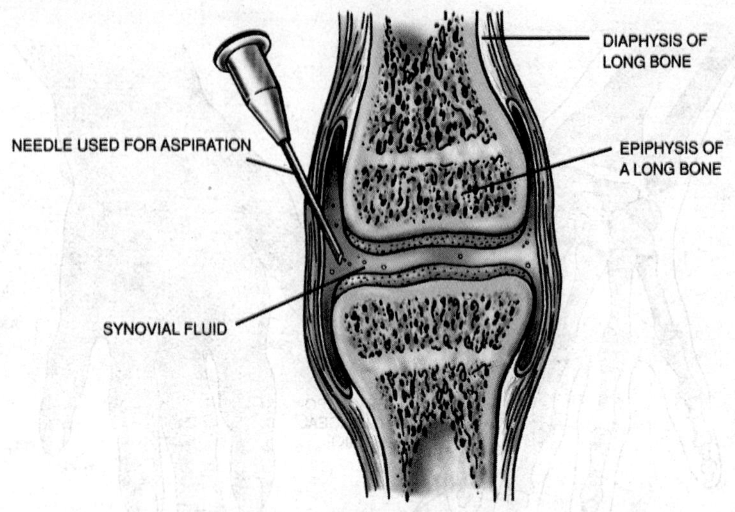

ARTHROCENTESIS

syphilis and is marked by tenderness, swelling, and limitation of motion.

systemic-onset juvenile rheumatoid a. A form of JRA that accounts for 20% of all JRA cases; boys are affected 60% of the time. Fever and rash may be the presenting symptoms, either with or without joint involvement. Ultimately, 25% of these children develop severe arthritis.

tuberculous a. Chronic, slowly progressive infection of joints (such as hips, knees, ankles, or intervertebral disks) by *Mycobacterium tuberculosis*. The organism usually spreads via the blood or from osteomyelitis in an adjacent bone. The macrophage and lymphocyte response to the mycobacterium destroys the bone along the joint margins, resulting in progressive pain, fibrosis, and restricted movement. SEE: *granuloma*.

arthritogenic (ăr-thrī′tō-jĕn″ĭk) An agent that can cause or accelerate arthritis. Some bacteria such as *Chlamydia spp.*, *Shigella*, and *Pseudomonas*, and some drugs are thought to produce arthritis.

arthro-, arthr- [Gr. *arthron*, joint] Combining forms meaning *joint*.

arthrocele (ăr′thrō-sēl) [″ + *kele*, tumor, swelling] **1.** Hernia of a synovial membrane, penetrating the capsule of a joint. **2.** Any joint swelling.

arthrocentesis (ăr″thrō-sĕn-tē′sĭs) [″ + *kentesis*, a puncture] Puncture of a joint space with a needle to remove accumulated fluid from the joint. SEE: illus.

Patient Care: The patient is prepared for the procedure; the operator's explanation of the procedure and expected sensations is reinforced and clarified, and a signed consent form is obtained. The necessary equipment is assembled. The patient is positioned and draped, the surgical site is cleansed and anesthetized, specimens are collected, and medications are administered. A dressing is applied to the surgical site; the site is monitored for excessive bleeding, and bleeding is controlled should it occur. Follow-up care includes elevating the affected limb and applying ice or cold packs to the joint for 24 to 36 hr to decrease pain and swelling; reporting symptoms such as fever and increased joint pain, redness, or swelling; and avoiding overuse of the affected joint for several days.

arthrochondritis (ăr″thrō-kŏn-drī′tĭs) [″ + *chondros*, cartilage, + *itis*, inflammation] Inflammation of an articular cartilage.

arthroclasia (ăr″thrō-klā′zē-ă) [″ + *klasis*, a breaking] Artificial breaking of adhesions of an ankylosed joint to provide movement.

arthrodesis (ăr-thrō-dē′sĭs) [″ + *desis*, binding] The surgical immobilization of a joint; artificial ankylosis.

arthrodia (ăr-thrō′dē-ă) [Gr.] A type of synovial joint that permits only simple gliding movement within narrow limits imposed by ligaments.

arthrodynia (ăr″thrō-dĭn′ē-ă) [Gr. *arthron*, joint, + *odyne*, pain] Pain in a joint.

arthrodysplasia (ăr″thrō-dĭs-plā′zē-ă) [″ + *dys*, bad, + *plassein*, to form] A hereditary condition marked by deformity of various joints.

arthroendoscopy (ăr″thrō-ĕn-dŏs′kō-pē) [″ + *endon*, within, + *skopein*, to examine] Inspection of the interior of a joint with an endoscope. SEE: *arthroscopy*.

arthrogram (ăr′thrō-grăm) [″ + *gramma*, something written] Visualization of a joint by radiographic study after injection of a contrast medium into the joint space.

arthrography (ăr-thrŏg′ră-fē) [″ + *graphein*, to write] **1.** Radiography of a joint. **2.** Radiography of a synovial joint after injection of a contrast medium. The medium may be radiolucent (air), radiopaque, or both.

arthrogryposis (ăr″thrō-grĭ-pō′sĭs) [″ + *grypos*, curved, + *osis*, condition] Fixation of a joint in a flexed or contracted position; may be due to adhesions in or around the joint.

a. multiplex congenita Congenital generalized fixation or ankylosis of joints; may be due to a variety of changes in the spinal cord, muscles, or connective tissue.

arthrokinematics Description of the movement of the joint surfaces when a bone moves through a range of motion. Terms used to describe arthrokinematics include roll, spin, and glide. These movements are a necessary component of osteokinematic (bone) movement. They are accessory motions that are not under the voluntary control of the patient.

arthrokleisis (ăr″thrō-klī′sĭs) [″ + *kleisis*, a closure] Ankylosis produced naturally or surgically.

arthrolith (ăr′thrō-lĭth) [″ + *lithos*, stone] Calculous deposit in a joint.

arthrology (ăr-thrŏl′ō-jē) [Gr. *arthron*, joint, + *logos*, word, reason] The scientific study of joints.

arthrolysis (ăr-thrŏl′ĭ-sĭs) [″ + *lysis*, dissolution] The operation of restoring mobility to an ankylosed joint.

arthrometer (ăr-thrŏm′ĕ-tĕr) [Gr. *arthron*, joint, + *metron*, measure] An instrument that measures the degree of movement of a joint. SYN: *goniometer*.

arthroneuralgia (ăr″thrō-nū-răl′jē-ă) [″ + *neuron*, nerve, + *algos*, pain] Pain in or around a joint.

arthropathology (ăr″thrō-pă-thol′ō-jē) [″ + *pathos*, disease, + *logos*, word, reason] The pathology of joint disease.

arthropathy (ăr-thrŏp′ă-thē) [″ + *pathos*, disease, suffering] Any joint disease.

Charcot's a. SEE: *Charcot's joint*.

inflammatory a. An inflammatory joint disease, such as rheumatoid arthritis.

arthrophyte (ăr′thrō-fīt) [Gr. *arthron*, joint, + *phyton*, growth] Abnormal growth in a joint cavity.

arthroplasty (ăr′thrō-plăs″tē) [″ + *plassein*, to form] Plastic surgery to reshape or reconstruct a diseased joint. This may be done to alleviate pain, to permit normal function, or to correct a developmental or hereditary joint defect. The procedure may require use of an artificial joint.

PATIENT CARE: *Preoperative*: The patient is prepared physically and emotionally for the procedure. Baseline data are gathered.

Postoperative: The surgeon may prescribe traction or other immobilization devices, such as splints, pillows, or casts, or a continuous passive motion device. Bedrest is maintained for the prescribed period, and the patient is positioned as prescribed. The affected joint is maintained in proper alignment, immobilization devices are inspected for pressure, and frequent neurovascular and motor checks are performed on the involved extremity distal to the operative site. Prescribed analgesics are administered, and the patient is taught about self-administration. Noninvasive measures are employed to reduce pain and anxiety. Vital signs are monitored for hypovolemic shock due to blood loss, and the patient is assessed for other complications such as thromboembolism, fat embolism, and infection. The incision is dressed according to protocol and assessed for local signs of infection. Deep breathing and coughing, frequent position changes, and adequate fluid intake are encouraged. The patient is assisted with prescribed exercise and activity, with appropriate measures taken to prevent dislocation of the prosthesis and to reinforce prescribed activity restrictions. The patient is taught to report symptoms such as fever, pain, and increased joint stiffness and is referred for home care and outpatient physical therapy. SEE: *Nursing Diagnoses Appendix*.

arthropneumoradiography (ăr″thrō-nū″mō-rā-dē-ŏg′ră-fē) [″ + *pneuma*, air, + *radiography*] Radiography of a synovial joint after injection of a radiolucent contrast medium such as air or helium. SEE: *arthrogram*.

arthropod (ăr′thrō-pŏd) A member of the phylum Arthropoda.

Arthropoda (ăr-thrŏp′ō-dă) [″ + *pous*, foot] A phylum of invertebrate animals marked by bilateral symmetry, a hard, jointed exoskeleton, segmented bodies, and jointed paired appendages. It includes the crustaceans, insects, myriapods, arachnids, and similar forms. It is the largest animal phylum, containing over 900,000 species. Many have medical importance as causative agents of disease, as vectors, or as parasites.

arthropyosis (ăr″thrō-pī-ō′sĭs) [″ + *pyosis*, suppuration] Suppuration of a joint.

arthrosclerosis [Gr. *arthron*, joint, + *sklerosis*, a hardening] Stiffening or hardening of the joints, esp. in the aged.

arthroscope (ăr′thrō-skōp) [″ + *sko-*

pein, to examine] An endoscope for examining the interior of a joint.

arthroscopy (ăr-thrŏs′kō-pē) Direct joint visualization by means of an arthroscope, usually to remove tissue, such as cartilage fragments or torn ligaments, or to anneal injured tissues.

PATIENT CARE: *Preoperative*: The patient is prepared physically and emotionally for the procedure. Baseline data (e.g., range of motion, girth measurements) are gathered. The operative site is prepared according to protocol and type of anesthesia.

Postoperative: Vital signs are monitored until stable, and intravenous or oral fluids are provided depending on the type of anesthesia used. The surgical dressing is inspected for drainage, and the presence of any drainage devices and their contents are documented. The dressing is reinforced or replaced under strict asepsis according to protocol. Postoperative teaching stresses expected sensations, such as joint soreness and grinding; the application of ice to relieve pain and swelling; analgesic use; activity or ambulation restrictions; weight-bearing exercises; and use of crutches or other assistive devices. The patient is instructed to report any unusual drainage, redness, joint swelling, unusual softness in the joint, severe or persistent pain, or fever, because these may indicate infection, effusion, hemarthrosis, or a synovial cyst. The patient is referred for outpatient follow-up care as necessary. SEE: *Nursing Diagnoses Appendix*.

arthrosis (ăr-thrō′sĭs) [″ + *osis*, condition] **1.** Joint. **2.** A joint disorder caused by trophic degeneration.

arthrospore (ăr′thrō-spor) [″ + *sporos*, a seed] A bacterial spore formed by segmentation.

arthrosteitis (ăr″thrŏs-tē-ī′tĭs) [″ + *osteon*, bone, + *itis*, inflammation] Inflammation of the bony structures of a joint.

arthrostenosis (ăr″-thrō-stĕ-nō′sĭs) [″ + *stenos*, narrow] Pathological narrowing of a joint.

arthrostomy (ăr-thrŏs′tō-mē) [″ + *stoma*, mouth] The surgical formation of a temporary opening into a joint for drainage purposes.

arthrosynovitis (ăr″thrō-sĭn″ō-vī′tĭs) [″ + L. *synovia*, joint fluid, + Gr. *itis*, inflammation] Inflammation of the synovial membrane of a joint.

arthrotome (ăr′thrō-tōm) [″ + *tome*, incision] A knife for making incisions into a joint.

arthrotomy (ăr-thrŏt′ō-mē) Cutting into a joint.

arthrous (ăr′thrŭs) [Gr. *arthron*, joint] Jointed or pert. to a joint.

arthroxesis (ăr-thrŏk′sĭ-sĭs) [″ + *xexis*, scraping] Scraping of diseased tissue from a joint.

Arthus reaction, Arthus phenomenon (ăr-toos′) [Nicholas Maurice Arthus, Fr. bacteriologist, 1862–1945] A severe local inflammatory reaction that occurs at the site of injection of an antigen in a previously sensitized individual. Arthus reactions are a form of type III hypersensitivity reactions producing an antigen-antibody immune complex.

articulate (ăr-tĭk′ū-lāt) [L. *articulatus*, jointed] **1.** To join together as a joint. **2.** In dentistry, to arrange teeth on a denture. **3.** To speak clearly.

Articaine (ăr-tĭ-kān′) An amide local anesthetic that has more potency and tissue penetration than lidocaine or procaine, and fewer adverse effects when used in appropriately selected patients. It should not be used in patients with methemoglobinemia, anemia, cardiac or respiratory failure with hypoxia.

articulatio (ăr-tĭk″ū-lā′shē-ō) [L.] The Latin term for a joint (an articulation): the site of union or junction of two bones.

articulation (ăr-tĭk″ū-lā′shŭn) **1.** A joint; the site of close approximation of two or more bones. It may be immovable (as in synarthrosis), slightly movable (amphiarthrosis), or freely movable (diarthrosis). Cartilage or fibrous connective tissue lines the opposing surfaces of all joints. **2.** The relative position of the tongue and palate necessary to produce a given sound. **3.** Enunciation of words and sentences. **4.** The movement of articulating surfaces through their available joint play or range of motion, used to determine joint mobility or to treat joint pain. **articular** (ăr-tĭk′ū-lăr), *adj.*

apophyseal a. The joint between the superior and the inferior articulating processes of the vertebrae.

articulator a. The use of a mechanical device to simulate the action of the temporomandibular joint when placing teeth in complete dentures or partial removable dentures so that they articulate properly.

confluent a. Speech in which syllables are run together.

dental a. The contact relationship between upper and lower teeth when moving against each other or into or out of centric position.

working a. The occlusion of teeth on the side toward which the mandible is moved. *Also called* working bite.

articulator (ăr-tĭk′ū-lā″tor) In dentistry, a device for maintaining casts of the teeth in a precise and natural relationship.

articulo mortis (ăr-tĭk′ū-lō″ mor′tĭs) [L.] At the time of death.

articulus (ăr-tĭk′ū-lŭs) [L.] **1.** A knuckle or a joint. **2.** A segment.

artifact (ăr′tĭ-făkt) [L. *ars*, art, + *facere*, to make] **1.** Anything artificially produced. **2.** In histology and radiography any structure or feature produced by the technique used and not occurring naturally. **3.** In electronics, the appearance of a spurious signal not consistent with results expected from the signal being studied. For example, an electrocardiogram may contain artifacts produced by a defective machine, electrical interference, patient movement, or loose electrodes.

motion a. Blurring of a radiographic image, produced by respiratory or muscular movement of the patient.

artificial (ăr″tĭ-fĭsh′ăl) Not natural; formed in imitation of nature.

artificial hyperemia Bringing of blood to the superficial tissues by means of counterirritation, such as may be produced by cupping or acupuncture.

artificial kidney transplant The implantation of a device to take over kidney function. Efforts to perfect such a device are experimental.

artificial rupture of membranes ABBR: AROM. Amniotomy.

artisan's cramp A muscle spasm induced by prolonged work requiring delicate coordination; most likely to occur in writing, piano playing, sewing, and typing. SEE: *writer's cramp.*

arum family poisoning Poisoning caused by ingestion of plants of the genus *Arum* (e.g., dieffenbachia, caladium, and philodendron), which contain poisonous calcium oxalate crystals. Symptoms include irritation, pain, burning, and swelling of the affected areas. The affected area should be washed with water, and ice should be applied. If pain is severe, corticosteroids are of benefit.

aryepiglottic (ăr″ē-ĕp″ĭ-glŏt′ĭk) [Gr. *arytaina*, ladle, + *epi*, upon, + *glottis*, back of tongue] Pert. to the arytenoid cartilage and epiglottis.

aryl- Prefix denoting a radical derived from an aromatic hydrocarbon.

a. group In chemistry, a radical group of the aromatic or benzene series.

arytenoid (ăr″ĭ-tē′noyd) [Gr. *arytaina*, ladle, + *eidos*, form, shape] **1.** Resembling a ladle or pitcher mouth. **2.** Pert. to the arytenoid cartilages or muscles of the larynx. SEE: *larynx* for illus.

arytenoidectomy (ăr″ĭ-tē″noyd-ĕk′tō-mē) [″ + ″ + *ektome*, excision] Excision of arytenoid cartilage.

arytenoiditis (ăr-ĭt″ē-noy-dī′tĭs) [″ + ″ + *itis*, inflammation] Inflammation of arytenoid cartilage or muscles.

arytenoidopexy (ăr″ĭ-tē-noy′dō-pĕk″sē) [″ + ″ + *pexis*, fixation] Surgical fixation of the arytenoid muscle or cartilage.

AS *ankylosing spondylitis; aortic stenosis;* L., *auris sinistra,* left ear.

As **1.** *astigmatic.* **2.** *astigmatism.* **3.** Symbol for the element arsenic.

ASA *acetylsalicylic acid.*

asafetida, asafoetida (ăs-ă-fĕt′ĭd-ă) [L. *asa*, gum, + *foetida*, smelly] A gum resin, obtained from the roots of *Ferula asafoetida,* with a characteristic strong odor and garlic taste. Although this substance is no longer used in medicine, it has historical interest. In the early 20th century, it was used as a carminative and as an amulet to ward off disease. It is used in Asia as a condiment and food flavoring and as an animal repellent in veterinary medicine.

ASAHP *Association of Schools of Allied Health Professions.*

asana (ă′să-nă) Any yoga posture employed in traditional Indian healing for flexibility, strength, relaxation, and mental discipline.

ASAP *as soon as possible.* SEE: *stat.*

asaphia (ă-săf′ē-ă, ă-să′fē-ă) [Gr. *asapheia*, obscurity] Inability to speak distinctly.

asbestiform (ăs-bĕs′tĭ-form) [Gr. *asbestos*, unquenchable, + L. *forma*, appearance] Having a structure similar to that of asbestos.

asbestos (ăs-bĕs′tŏs) [Gr. *asbestos*, unquenchable] A fibrous, incombustible form of magnesium and calcium silicate used to make insulating materials. Although asbestos fibers are commercially useful, they have been implicated in several human diseases, including fibrosis of the lung and cancers of the respiratory and gastrointestinal systems. Because of these health hazards they are no longer sold or manufactured in the U.S.

asbestos bodies A beaded, dumbbell-shaped body formed when a macrophage engulfs asbestos fibers.

asbestosis (ăs″bĕ-stō′sĭs) [″ + *osis*, condition] Lung disease, a form of pneumoconiosis resulting from protracted inhalation of asbestos particles. Exposure to asbestos has been linked with lung cancer, including bronchogenic carcinoma and esp. mesothelioma. The latency period may be 20 years or more.

SYMPTOMS: Symptoms include exertional dyspnea or, with extensive fibrosis, dyspnea at rest. In advanced disease, the patient may complain of a dry cough (productive in smokers), chest pain (often pleuritic), and recurrent respiratory tract infections. Tachypnea, crackles, and clubbing may be present.

PATIENT CARE: A history of occupational, family, or neighborhood exposure to asbestos fibers is obtained. The chest is auscultated for tachypnea and fine crackles in the lung bases, and the fingers are inspected for clubbing. Changes in sputum quality and quantity, restlessness, increased tachypnea, and changes in breath sounds are monitored and documented. Complications such as cor pulmonale or pulmonary hypertension are noted.

Oxygen is administered when arterial blood gas levels or pulse oximetry indicate hypoxemia on room air. Mucolytics and chest physical therapy usually are not needed unless the patient develops a secondary lung infection with excessive secretions.

The patient is advised to avoid persons with known respiratory infections and to obtain influenza and pneumococcal immunizations. Instruction by the respiratory therapist is given in the use and care of required oxygen and aerosol equipment, inhalers, or transtracheal catheters. Patients often require home use of oxygen, requiring education by the respiratory therapist on the safe and effective use of needed equipment. Patients who smoke tobacco are encouraged to join smoking cessation programs because cigarettes and asbestos both damage the lungs and the damage from the combined exposures to these agents is more than additive.

ascariasis (ăs″kă-rī′ă-sĭs) [Gr. *askaris*, pinworm, + *-iasis*, condition of] Condition resulting from infestation by *Ascaris lumbricoides*.

ascaricide (ăs-kăr′ĭ-sīd) [″ + L. *cidus*, killing] An agent that kills ascarids. **ascaricidal** (ăs-kăr-ĭ-sī′dăl), *adj.*

ascarid (ăs′kă-rĭd) A nematode worm of the family Ascaridae.

Ascaris (ăs′kă-rĭs) A genus of nematode worms belonging to the family Ascaridae. They inhabit the intestines of vertebrates.

A. lumbricoides A species of *Ascaris* that lives in the human intestine; adults may grow to 12 in. long. Eggs are passed with the feces and require at least 2 weeks' incubation in the soil before they become infective. After being swallowed, the eggs hatch in the intestinal tract and the larvae enter the venous circulation and pass to the lungs. From there they migrate up the respiratory passages, are swallowed, and reach their site of continued residence, the jejunum. In a 1- to 2-year life span, the female is capable of producing 200,000 eggs per day. The eggs are passed with the feces, and a new cycle is started. Children up to the ages of 12 to 14 are likely to be infected. Intestinal obstruction may be a complication in children under 6 years of age. SEE: illus.

TREATMENT: Pyrantel pamoate is the drug of choice. Mebendazole is also effective. No drug is useful during the pulmonary phase of the infection.

ascaris *pl.* **ascarides** A worm of the genus *Ascaris.*

Aschner's phenomenon (ăsh′nĕrz) [Bernhard Aschner, Austrian gynecologist, 1883–1960] Slowing of the pulse after pressure is applied to the eyeball or the carotid sinus. It may be used to slow the heart during attacks of supraventricular tachycardia or as a diagnostic test for angina pectoris. Slowing of the heart produced by this reflex may relieve anginal pain. Also called *Aschner's reflex* and *sign.* SYN: *oculocardiac reflex.*

Aschoff, Ludwig (ăsh′ŏf) German pathologist, 1866–1942.

A.'s cells Large cells with basophilic cytoplasm and a large vesicular nucleus, often multinucleated. They are characteristic of Aschoff's nodules.

A.'s nodules Small nodules composed of cells and leukocytes found in the interstitial tissues of the heart in rheumatic myocarditis.

asci (ăs′ī) Pl. of ascus.

ascia (ăs′ē-ă, ăs′kē-ă) [L. *ascia*, ax] A form of spiral bandage with each turn overlapping the previous one for a third of its width.

ascites (ă-sī′tēz) [Gr. *askitēs* from *askos*, a leather bag] The accumulation of serous fluid in the peritoneal cavity. SEE: *edema; peritonitis.*

ETIOLOGY: Ascites may be caused by interference in venous return as occurs

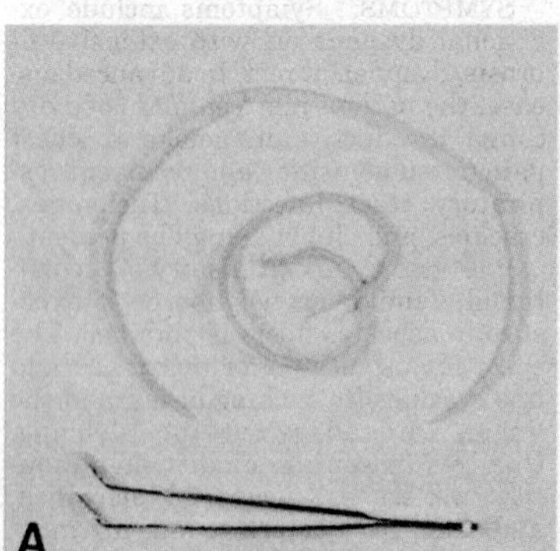

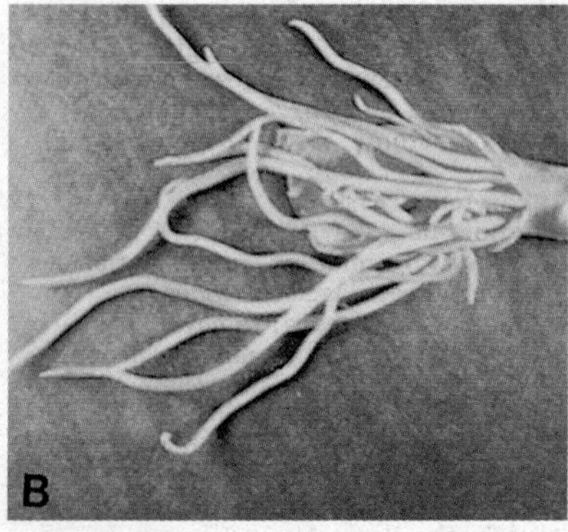

ASCARIS LUMBRICOIDES

(A) Smaller male encircled by female, (B) mass of worms removed from the intestine

in congestive heart failure; obstruction of flow in the vena cava or portal vein; obstruction in lymphatic drainage; disturbance in electrolyte balance as occurs in sodium retention; depletion of plasma proteins; cirrhosis of the liver; malignancies; or infections within the peritoneum.

PATIENT CARE: Ventilatory effort, appetite and food intake, fluid intake and output, and weight are assessed. Abdominal girth is measured at the largest point, and the site marked for future measurements. Paracentesis if necessary is explained to the patient. Preparation necessary for the paracentesis include assembling the equipment; preparing the site; monitoring vital signs, weight, and girth; and obtaining serum protein, albumin, sodium, and potassium levels before and after the procedure. Emotional and physical support are provided to the patient throughout the procedure. Desired outcomes include eased ventilatory effort, improved appetite, improved general comfort, and identification of the cause of the accumulated fluid.

a. chylosus Chyle in the ascitic fluid, usually resulting from rupture of the thoracic duct.

hemorrhagic a. Bloody ascites, usually caused by malignancy or occasionally by tuberculosis. **ascitic** (-sĭt′ĭk), *adj.*

ascitic fluid Clear and pale straw-colored fluid occurring in ascites. Specific gravity is 1.005 to 1.015.

A.S.C.L.S. *American Society for Clinical Laboratory Science,* formerly American Society for Medical Technology.

Ascoli's reaction (ăs-kō′lēz) [Alberto Ascoli, It. serologist, 1877–1957] Precipitation test for anthrax; used for detection of anthrax bacilli in animal hides and meat. Also called *Ascoli's test.*

Ascomycetes (ăs″kō-mī-sē′tēz) [Gr. *askos,* leather bag, + *mykes,* fungus] The largest class of Eumycetes (or true fungi) of the phylum Thallophyta; the sac fungi, which includes the true yeasts, blue molds, and penicillin. Organisms in this group are characterized by possession of a saclike sporangium (or ascus), in which ascospores are developed.

ascospore (ăs′kō-spor) [Gr. *askos,* leather bag, + *sporos,* seed] A spore produced within an ascus or spore sac.

ascus (ăs′kŭs) *pl.* **asci** [Gr. *askos,* leather bag] A saclike spore case in which ascospores, typically eight, are formed; characteristic of the Ascomycetes.

-ase A suffix used in forming the name of an enzyme. It is added to the name of the substance upon which it acts (e.g., lipase, which acts on lipids).

asemia Asymbolia.

asepsis (ā-sĕp′sĭs) [Gr. *a-,* not, + *sepesthai,* to decay] A condition free from germs, infection, and any form of life. SEE: *antisepsis; sterilization.* **aseptic** (-tĭk), *adj.*

aseptic-antiseptic [Gr. *a-,* not, + *sepsis,* decay, + *anti,* against, + *sepsis,* decay] Both aseptic and antiseptic.

aseptic technique A method used in surgery to prevent contamination of the wound and operative site. All instruments used are sterilized, and physicians and nurses wear caps, masks, shoe coverings, sterile gowns, and gloves. The technique is adapted at the bedside (e.g., during procedures) and in emergency and treatment rooms. SEE: *Standard and Universal Precautions Appendix.*

asexual (ā-sĕk′shū-ăl) [″ + L. *sexualis,* having sex] Without sex; nonsexual.

asexualization (ā-sĕk″shū-ăl-ĭ-zā′shŭn) Sterilization by ablation of the ovaries or testes.

ash (ăsh) [AS. *aesc,* ash] Incombustible powdery residue of a substance that has been incinerated.

ASHD *atherosclerotic heart disease.*

Asherman's syndrome [Joseph G. Asherman, Czech. physician, b. 1889] Secondary amenorrhea related to endometrial scarring. Causes include endometritis and aggressive curettage for purposes of removing the products of conception, such as in abortion or removal of retained placental fragments.

asialia (ă″sī-ā′lē-ă, ā″sē-ā′lē-ă) [Gr. *a-,* not, + *sialon,* spittle] Absence or deficiency of saliva. SYN: *aptyalia.*

Asiatic cholera SEE: *cholera.*

asiderosis (ă″sĭd-ĕ-rō′sĭs) [″ + *sideros,* iron, + *osis,* condition] Deficiency of iron reserve in the body.

ASIS *anterior superior iliac spine.* Radiographic palpation point on the skin on each side of the front of the pelvis.

-asis Suffix meaning *condition, state.*

ASLO *antistreptolysin-O.*

as low as reasonably achievable ABBR: ALARA. A philosophy of radiation protection advocated by many agencies, including government regulators and voluntary accrediting agencies.

asocial (ā-sō′shĭl) **1.** Withdrawn from society. **2.** Inconsiderate of the needs of others.

asoma (ā-sō′mă) [Gr. *a-,* not, + *soma,* body] A deformed fetus with an imperfectly formed trunk and head.

asonia (ă-sō′nē-ă) [″ + L. *sonus,* sound] Tone deafness.

asparaginase (ăs-păr′ă-jĭn-āz) An antineoplastic agent derived from the bacterium *Escherichia coli.*

asparagine (ăs-păr′ă-jĭn) Aminosuccinic acid, a nonessential amino acid.

Asparagus (ă-spăr′ă-gŭs) [Gr. *asparagos*] A genus of liliaceous herbs.

aspartame (ă-spăr′tām) A low calorie artificial sweetener made of aspartic acid and phenylalanine. It should not be consumed by individuals with phenylketonuria, and is unsuitable for cooking because its flavor is changed when heated. Trade names are Equal and NutraSweet.

aspartate aminotransferase ABBR: AST. An intracellular enzyme involved in amino acid and carbohydrate metabolism. It is present in high concentrations in muscle, liver, and brain. An increased level of this enzyme in the blood indicates necrosis or disease in these tissues. Formerly called serum glutamic-oxaloacetic transaminase (SGOT) or glutamic-oxaloacetic transaminase.

aspastic (ă-spăs′tĭk) [Gr. *a-*, not, + *spastikos*, having spasms] Nonspastic.

aspecific (ă-spĕ-sĭf′ĭk) Not specific.

aspect (ăs′pĕkt) [L. *aspectus*, a view] **1.** The part of a surface facing in any designated direction. **2.** Appearance, looks.

A.S.P.E.N. *American Society for Parenteral and Enteral Nutrition.*

Asperger's disorder A severe and sustained impairment of social interaction and functioning. In contrast to autism, there are no clinically significant delays in language, cognitive, or developmental age-appropriate skills.

aspergillin (ăs″pĕr-jĭl′ĭn) A pigment produced by *Aspergillus niger*.

aspergillosis (ăs″pĕr-jĭl-ō′sĭs) [*aspergillus* + Gr. *osis*, condition] Infection caused by the *Aspergillus* fungus or one of its mold species, of which *A. fumigatus* is the most common. Colonizing aspergillosis involves growth of the fungus within the body, without tissue invasion. Invasive aspergillosis is an opportunistic infection that affects people with immunodeficiencies; the primary infection is usually pneumonia, but the brain, kidney, and heart valves may also be affected. It is treated with intravenous amphotericin B or long-term oral itraconazole. SEE: illus; *allergic alveolitis*.

TREATMENT: Amphotericin B is administered.

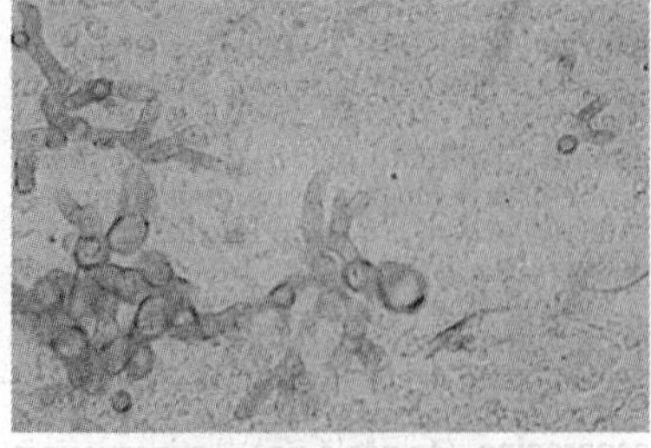

ASPERGILLOSIS OF LUNG
Growth of fungus (purple) fills the alveoli (×450)

allergic bronchopulmonary a. A disease in which a patient with asthmatic bronchitis develops a hypersensitivity to *Aspergillus* colonizing (not invading) the airways.

SYMPTOMS: Worsening of asthma, fleeting infiltrates, eosinophilia, and positive aspergillus precipitants are clues to diagnosis.

TREATMENT: The mainstay of therapy is the use of steroids to suppress the hypersensitivity.

aural a. A form of otomycosis caused by *Aspergillus*.

pulmonary a. Lung disease caused by *Aspergillus*.

Aspergillus (ăs″pĕr-jĭl′ŭs) [L. *aspergere*, to sprinkle] A genus of Ascomycetes fungi, including several mold species, some of which are pathogenic. The principal pathogen is *Aspergillus fumigatus*, although others (*A. flavus, A. nidulans*, and *A. niger*) may be pathogenic. SEE: *aspergillosis*.

A. clavatus A species found in soil and manure.

A. concentricus A species once thought to be the cause of tinea imbricata ringworm.

A. flavus A mold found on corn, peanuts, and grain.

A. fumigatus The fungus that is the common cause of aspergillosis in humans and birds. It is found in soil and manure.

A. glaucus A bluish mold found on dried fruit.

A. nidulans A species common in soil, causing one form of white mycetoma.

A. niger A pathogenic form with black spores, frequently present in the external auditory meatus. It may cause otomycosis. SEE: illus.

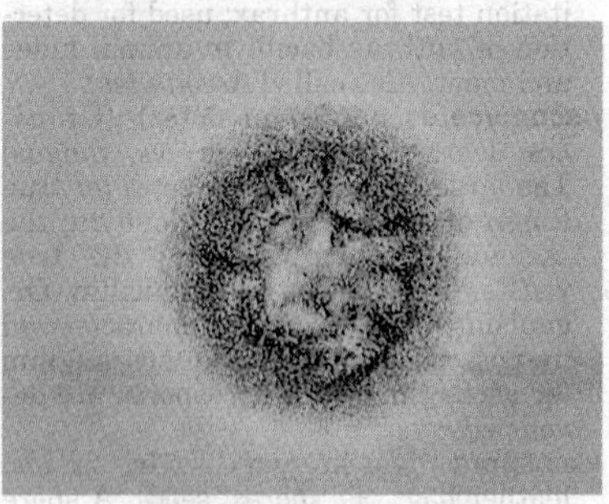

ASPERGILLUS NIGER **IN CULTURE**

A. ochraceus A species that produces the characteristic odor of brewing coffee.

A. versicolor A species that produces a toxin similar to aflatoxin.

aspermatogenesis (ă-spĕr″mă-tō-jĕn′ĕ-sĭs) [″ + ″ + *genesis*, generation, birth] Nonfunction of the sperm-producing system of the testicles.

aspermia (ă-spĕr′mē-ă) [″ + *sperma*,

seed] Failure to form semen or to ejaculate. **aspermic** (-mĭk), *adj.*

aspersion (ăs-pĕr′zhŭn) [L. *aspersio*, sprinkling] Sprinkling an affected part with water; a form of hydrotherapy.

asphalgesia (ăs″făl-jē′zē-ă) [Gr. *asphe-*, self, + *algos*, pain] A burning sensation sometimes felt on touching certain articles during hypnosis.

asphyctic, asphyctous (ăs-fĭk′tĭk, -tŭs) [Gr. *a-*, not, + *sphyxis*, pulse] **1.** Pert. to, or affected with, asphyxia. **2.** Without pulse.

asphyxia (ăs-fĭk′sē-ă) [″ + *sphyxis*, pulse] Condition caused by insufficient intake of oxygen. **asphyxial** (-sē-ăl), *adj.*

ETIOLOGY: Extrinsic causes include choking, toxic gases, exhaust gas (principally carbon monoxide), electric shock, drugs, anesthesia, trauma, crushing injuries of the chest, compression of the chest, injury of the respiratory nerves or centers, diminished environmental oxygenation, and drowning.

Intrinsic causes include hemorrhage into the lungs or pleural cavity, foreign bodies in the throat, swelling of the airways, diseases of the airways, ruptured aneurysm or abscess, edema of the lung, cardiac deficiency, tumors such as goiter, and pharyngeal and retropharyngeal abscesses. Other causes include paralysis of the respiratory center or of respiratory muscles, anesthesia, pneumothorax, narcotic drugs, electrocution, and child abuse.

SYMPTOMS: In general, symptoms range in severity from dyspnea, palpitations, and impairment of consciousness, to coma, seizures, permanent brain injury, and death.

FIRST AID: Artificial respiration should be given.

autoerotic a. Autoerotic hypoxia.

a. carbonica Suffocation from inhalation of coal or water gas or of carbon monoxide.

fetal a. Asphyxia occurring in a fetus; results from interference in placental circulation, umbilical cord compression, or from premature separation of the placenta, as in abruptio placentae.

a. livida Asphyxia in which the skin is cyanotic from lack of oxygen in the blood.

local a. Asphyxia affecting a limited portion of the body (e.g., fingers, hands, toes, or feet) due to insufficient blood supply; a symptom usually associated with Raynaud's disease.

a. neonatorum Respiratory failure in the newborn.

a. pallida Asphyxia in which difficulty in breathing is accompanied by weak and thready pulse, pale skin, and absence of reflexes.

sexual a. Autoerotic hypoxia.

asphyxiant (ăs-fĭk′sē-ănt) An agent, esp. any gas, that will produce asphyxia.

asphyxiate (ăs-fĭk′sē-āt) To cause asphyxiation or asphyxia.

asphyxiation (ăs-fĭk″sē-ā′shŭn) **1.** A state of asphyxia or suffocation. **2.** The act of producing asphyxia.

asphyxiophilia Dependence on self-strangulation for production of cerebral hypoxia. This act may intensify enjoyment of orgasm, but if continued too long may result in death. SEE: *autoerotic hypoxia.*

aspidium (ăs-pĭd′ē-ŭm) [Gr. *aspidion*, little shield] The root and stalk of *Dryopteris filixmas* (male fern) or *D. marginalis* (marginal fern); used medicinally in the form of oleoresin.

a. oleoresin Extract of the male fern; male fern oleoresin; formerly used as an anthelmintic in the treatment of tapeworm infestation of the intestines.

aspirate (ăs′pĭ-rāt) [L. *ad*, to, + *spirare*, to breathe] **1.** To draw in or out by suction. **2.** To make a sound like that of the letter *h*.

aspiration (ăs-pĭ-rā′shŭn) **1.** Drawing in or out by suction. Foreign bodies may be aspirated into the nose, throat, or lungs on inspiration. **2.** Withdrawal of fluid from a cavity by suctioning with an aspirator. The purpose of aspiration is to remove fluid or air from an affected area (as in pleural effusion, pneumothorax, ascites, or an abscess) or to obtain specimens (such as blood from a vein or serum from the spinal canal).

EQUIPMENT: Aspiration equipment includes disinfecting solution for the skin; local anesthetic; two aspirating needles with the aspirating apparatus as indicated; a utensil for receiving the fluid and a sterile receptacle for the specimen; sterile sponges, towels, basins; sterile gloves, face masks, and gowns; sterile forceps; surgical dressings as the case may require; a stimulant ordered if the indication arises.

PATIENT CARE: Pathological respiratory aspiration is prevented by placing the unconscious patient (or any other patient without a gag reflex) in a head-low position to protect the airway, to prevent silent regurgitation, and to promote evacuation of mucus or vomitus; and by suctioning the nasopharynx as necessary. The nurse assists with the aspiration procedures by assembling necessary equipment, by explaining the procedure and expected sensations to the patient, and by ascertaining that a consent form has been signed. The patient is draped to ensure privacy and warmth as well as emotional comfort. Emotional support is provided throughout the procedure. The operator is assisted in obtaining and processing specimens. The type and amount of any drainage or aspirated material is observed and documented. The operative site is dressed, and patient outcomes and any complications are monitored.

The respiratory therapist often is involved in aspirating (suctioning) excessive airway secretions. This procedure may be done as a therapeutic maneuver to ease breathing or as a diagnostic procedure to collect a sputum sample for analysis of the microbes associated with the infection.

fetal meconium a. Aspiration by the fetus of the first stool, occurring either in utero during episodes of severe fetal hypoxia or with the first few breaths after birth. SYN: *meconium aspiration syndrome.*

aspiration, risk for The state in which an individual is at risk for entry of gastric secretions, oropharyngeal secretions, or exogenous food or fluids into tracheobronchial passages due to dysfunction or absence of normal protective mechanisms. SEE: *Nursing Diagnoses Appendix.*

aspirator (ăs′pĭ-rā-tor) An apparatus for evacuating the fluid contents of a cavity. Varieties are piston pump, compressible rubber tube, rubber bulb, and siphon, a trocar and cannula, and hypodermic needle and syringe.

dental a. An aspirator that suctions water, saliva, blood, or tissue debris from the oral cavity.

aspirin (ăs′pĕr-ĭn) ABBR: ASA. Acetylsalicylic acid, $C_9H_8O_4$, a nonsteroidal anti-inflammatory drug that is a derivative of salicylic acid. It occurs as white crystals or powder. It is one of the most widely used and prescribed analgesic-antipyretic and anti-inflammatory agents. Because of its ability to bind irreversibly to blood platelets and inhibit platelet aggregration, aspirin in a dose of 80 to 325 mg/day is used prophylactically to prevent coronary artery disease, transient ischemic attacks, and thromboembolic disease of the cerebral vessels. Aspirin causes prolongation of the bleeding time. A single dose of 65 mg approx. doubles the bleeding time of normal persons for a period of 4 to 7 days. This same antiplatelet effect can cause the undesired effects of intestinal bleeding and peptic ulceration.

CAUTION: Children with viral infections such as varicella or influenza should not be given aspirin because of the possibility of increasing their risk of developing Reye's syndrome.

---

aspirin poisoning Toxicity caused by ingesting an excessive amount of aspirin. In acute poisoning, signs vary with increasing doses from mild lethargy and hyperpnea to coma and convulsions. Sweating, dehydration, hyperpnea, hyperthermia, and restlessness may be present with moderate doses. In chronic poisoning, tinnitus, skin rash, bleeding tendency, weight loss, and mental symptoms may be present. Aspirin poisoning in very young infants may produce very few signs and symptoms other than dehydration or hyperpnea.

TREATMENT: Activated charcoal is given by mouth. Intravenous (IV) fluids are given for dehydration, but must not be overloaded. Enough IV fluids should be given to establish 3 to 4 ml/kg/hr of urine flow. Alkalinization of urine is achieved by administering bicarbonate. The goal is a urine pH of 8 or higher. After urine flow is established, potassium 30 mEq/L of administered fluid should be added. After serum potassium levels reach 5 mEq/L, potassium should be discontinued. If alkalinization of the urine is not accomplished, hemodialysis may be needed. SEE: *salicylates in Poisons and Poisoning Appendix.*

asplenia (ă-splē′nē-ă) [Gr. *a-*, not, + L. *splen*, spleen] Absence of the spleen.

asplenia syndrome A rare disorder of fetal development that occurs before the fifth gestational week and results in congenital anomalies of the left hemibody, including absence of the spleen.

asporogenic (ăs″pō-rō-jĕn′ĭk) [″ + *sporos*, seed, + *gennan*, to produce] Not reproducing by spores.

asporous (ă-spō′rŭs) Having no spores.

A.S.R.T. *American Society of Radiologic Technologists.*

assault (ă-sawlt′) [L. *assultus*, having assailed] **1.** The threat of unlawful touching of another. **2.** The willful attempt to harm someone. SEE: *battery.*

sexual a. Actual or attempted oral, anal, or vaginal penetration against the victim's will. This includes sexual intercourse and forced entry of the orifices with an object and grasping of the victim's breasts, buttocks, or genitals. SEE: *rape.*

assay (ă-sā′, ăs′ā) [O. Fr. *assai*, trial] The analysis of a substance or mixture to determine its constituents and the relative proportion of each.

biological a. Bioassay.

fetal fibronectin a. ABBR: fFN. A screening test that identifies the probability of preterm labor. Fibronectin, a cold insoluble globulin, is usually found in cervicovaginal fluid during the first 20 weeks of pregnancy. It is then undetectable until about gestational week 37. A positive fFN test result in women with symptoms of threatened preterm labor indicates the probability of delivery within 1 week. Aggressive treatment of threatened preterm labor with tocolytics and corticosteroids increases potential for fetal survival.

gel mobility shift a. Electrophoretic study in a gel that permits the identification of interactions between DNA and other molecules, such as receptor proteins, based on their differential movement.

hormone a. A blood test to assess endocrine system status.

immunoradiometric a. ABBR: IRMA. Radioassay in which the antibody rather than the antigen is labeled. This offers an advantage in that antibodies are generally more stable than antibodies when a label is attached.

intracellular killing a. A laboratory test of bacterial ingestion by phagocytes. Neutrophils or macrophages are placed in a culture with bacteria. After 30 min, the remaining bacteria are killed with an antibiotic and the phagocytes are stained and examined for the number of bacteria they have ingested. This assay is only accurate if the phagocytes have been tested previously for the ability to ingest bacteria. SYN: *neutrophil microbicidal a.*

neutrophil microbicidal a. Intracellular killing a.

assessment **1.** An appraisal or evaluation of a patient's condition by a physician or nurse, based on clinical and laboratory data, medical history, and the patient's account of symptoms. **2.** The process by which a patient's condition is appraised or evaluated.

comprehensive a. A detailed, systematic physical examination of a patient.

comprehensive geriatric a. ABBR: CGA. A multidisciplinary process to evaluate the medical, functional, psychiatric, and social strengths and limitations in older patients. CGA provides a focus on the interrelated factors that contribute to illness. By addressing the complexity of needs, in some studies CGA improves survival and decreases the frequency of acute care hospitalization.

external quality a. ABBR: EQA. Proficiency testing.

functional a. In rehabilitation, the determination of a person's ability to perform everyday tasks and requirements of living. Functional assessment scales vary greatly with respect to the number, type, and scoring of the tasks used to determine performance levels, their degree of standardization, and their predictive validity. SEE: *activities of daily living.*

gestational age a. **1.** Estimation of the prenatal age of the fetus, typically by reviewing the pregnant woman's menstrual history, making measurements of fundal height, or by making ultrasonic measurements of fetal parts. This information is essential so that appropriately timed obstetrical care can be provided and the pregnancy's progress can be compared with normal standards. SEE: *amniocentesis; fundal height.* **2.** Estimation of newborn maturity; comparison of newborn assessment findings against the expected physical and neuromuscular characteristics consistent with a given point in gestation. SEE: *Dubowitz tool; large for gestational age; small for gestational age.*

initial a. The first evaluation of the patient in the field, conducted after it is clear that the scene is safe. This preliminary evaluation is designed to locate and manage life-threatening injuries or illness, and to determine the patient's triage priority. The initial assessment follows the sequence of mental status, airway, breathing, and circulation.

nursing a. SEE: *nursing assessment.*

ongoing a. The evaluation and care of patients recovered from the field, performed en route to the hospital. It includes reassessments of mental status, airway, breathing, circulation, vital signs, chief complaints, and the effectiveness of initial treatments.

rapid trauma a. The evaluation of a trauma patient's head, neck, chest, abdomen, pelvis, extremities, and posterior, conducted after the initial assessment in patients with a forceful mechanism of injury, such as a car crash.

Assessment of Motor and Process Skills ABBR: AMPS. A performance test of complex tasks required for activities of daily living, used in rehabilitation. It is one of the first of a generation of functional performance assessments designed to accommodate differences in settings and raters through statistical mechanisms. SEE: *functional assessment.*

assignment (ăs-sīn′mĕnt) The amount of money Medicare approves for specific health care services. Health care providers who "accept assignment" from Medicare agree to provide medical services in exchange for Medicare's monetary reimbursement and do not seek additional payments from patients.

assimilable (ă-sĭm′ĭ-lă-bl) [L. *ad*, to, + *similare*, to make like] Capable of assimilation.

assimilate (ă-sĭm′ĭ-lāt) **1.** To absorb digested food. **2.** In psychology, to absorb newly perceived information into the existing subjective conscious structure.

assimilation (ă-sĭm″ĭ-lā′shŭn) **1.** The transformation of food into living tissue; the constructive phase of metabolism (i.e., anabolism). **2.** In psychology, the absorption of newly perceived information into the existing subjective conscious structure.

assistant One who aids or supports. SYN: *aide.*

dental a. One who assists in the care and treatment of dental patients. The responsibilities vary according to the needs of the dentist, the training and capability of the individual, and the state regulations of duties.

physician a. ABBR: PA. A specially trained and (when necessary) licensed individual who performs tasks usually done by physicians and works under the direction of a supervising physician. PA training programs are accredited by the American Medical Association. Nearly all states require PAs to pass the certification examination of the National Commission on Certification of Physician Assistants.

assisted circulation Use of a mechanical device to augment or replace the action of the heart in pumping blood.

assisted death Help that enables an individual who wants to die to do so. This may take the form of counseling or actually providing the means and instruments for allowing the person to commit suicide. The legal and moral questions concerning such acts, esp. if the assisting person is a physician or someone involved in medical care, are topics of active debate. SEE: *assisted suicide; euthanasia.*

assisted living A group residence for adults, in which tenants live in individual apartments but receive some group services, including shared meals, day and night supervision, assistance with prescriptions, and other benefits.

assisted reproduction technologies ABBR: ART. Techniques to assist infertile women to conceive and give birth. These include hormonal stimulation of ovulation, and operative techniques such as in vitro fertilization with embryonic transfer, zygote intrafallopian transfer for women whose infertility results from tubal factors, and gamete intrafallopian transfer for couples whose infertility stems from semen inadequacy. In 1996, fewer than one-third of attempted ART procedures succeeded in either generating in vitro fertilization or returning an egg fertilized in vitro to infertile women.

assisted suicide, physician-assisted suicide The rendering of assistance to a person who wants to end his or her life but is not able to do this alone. This may be due to a physical disability or due to lack of knowledge of how to accomplish suicide. Whether physicians should become involved in helping patients commit suicide is a topic of active debate. Physicians or other medical care personnel who do assist a patient who wishes to take his or her life may be considered in the U.S. legal system to have committed murder. However, some state governments have legalized this procedure. SEE: *assisted death; euthanasia.*

assistor A ventilation system in which the patient initiates the inspiration cycle.

association [L. *ad*, to, + *socius*, companion] **1.** The act of joining or uniting; coordination with another idea or structure; relationship. In psychiatry, association refers in particular to the interrelationship of the conscious and unconscious ideas. **2.** In genetics, the occurrence together of two characteristics at a frequency greater than would be predicted by chance. **3.** In clinical epidemiology, the relationship of the occurrence of two events, without evidence that the event being investigated actually causes the second condition (e.g., malaria occurs in warm climates with proper breeding conditions for certain types of mosquitoes, but those conditions are *associations*). The actual *cause* is the malaria parasite.

controlled a. Induced a.

free a. **1.** The trend of thoughts when one is not under mental restraint or direction. **2.** The procedure in psychoanalysis that requires the patient to speak his or her thought flow aloud, word for word, without censorship.

induced a. The idea suggested when the examiner gives a stimulus word. SYN: *controlled a.* SEE: *association test.*

association center Center controlling associated movements.

Association for Gerontology in Higher Education ABBR: AGHE. An agency that promotes the education and training of persons preparing for research or careers in gerontology. It is committed to the development of education, research, and public service, and works to increase public awareness of the needs of gerontological education.

association neuron A neuron of the central nervous system that transmits impulses from sensory to motor neurons or to other association neurons. SYN: *interneuron.*

association of ideas The linking together in a memory chain of two or more ideas because of their similarity, relationship, or timing.

association time SEE: *association test.*

assonance (ăs′ō-năns) [L. *assonans*, answering with same sound] **1.** Similarity of sounds in words or syllables. **2.** Abnormal tendency to use alliteration.

assumption (ă-sŭmp′shŭn) A supposition; an idea that is not subjected to logical or empirical study.

assumption of risk A doctrine of law whereby the plaintiff assumes the risk of medical treatment or procedures and may not recover damages for injuries sustained as a result of the known and described dangers.

AST *aspartate aminotransferase.*

Ast *astigmatism.*

astasia (ă-stā′zē-ă) [Gr. *a-*, not, + *stasis*, stand] Inability to stand or sit erect due to motor incoordination.

astasia-abasia A form of hysterical ataxia, with incoordination and inability to stand or walk although all leg movements can be performed while sitting or lying down.

astatine (ăs′tă-tēn, -tīn) [Gr. *astatos*, unstable] SYMB: At. A radioactive element, atomic number 85, atomic weight 210.

asteatosis (ăs″tē-ă-tō′sĭs) [Gr. *a-*, not, + *stear*, tallow, + *osis*, condition] Any disease condition in which there is persistent scaling of the skin, suggesting deficiency or absence of sebaceous secretion.

a. cutis winter itch

aster (ăs′tĕr) [Gr., star] The stellate rays forming around the dividing centrosome during mitosis.

astereognosis (ă-stĕr″ē-ŏg-nō′sĭs) [Gr. *a-*, not, + *stereos*, solid, + *gnosis*, knowledge] Inability to recognize objects or forms by touch.

asterion (ăs-tē′rē-ŏn) *pl.* **asteria** [Gr., starlike] A craniometric point at the junction of the lambdoid, occipitomastoid, and parietomastoid sutures.

asterixis (ăs″tĕr-ĭk′sĭs) [Gr. *a-*, not, + *sterixis*, fixed position] Abnormal muscle tremor consisting of involuntary jerking movements, esp. in the hands, but also seen in the tongue and feet. It may be due to various diseases, but is usually found in patients with diseases of the liver. SYN: *flapping tremor*. SEE: *alcoholism; hepatic encephalopathy*.

asternal (ā-stĕr′năl) [″ + *sternon*, chest] **1.** Not connected with the sternum. **2.** Having no sternum.

asternia (ă-stĕr′nē-ă) Congenital absence of the sternum.

asteroid (ăs′tĕr-oyd) [Gr. *aster*, star, + *eidos*, form, shape] Star-shaped.

asthenia (ăs-thē′nē-ă) [Gr. *asthenes*, without strength] Lack or loss of strength; debility; any weakness, but esp. one originating in muscular or cerebellar disease. SYN: *adynamia*.

neurocirculatory a. A somatoform disorder marked by mental and physical fatigue, dyspnea, giddiness, precordial pain, and palpitation, esp. on exertion. The cause is unknown but the condition occurs in those under stress. It is common among soldiers in combat. Psychotherapy and removal of the stress situation are needed. SYN: *cardiac neurosis*. SEE: *chronic fatigue syndrome; post-traumatic stress disorder*.

asthenic (ăs-thĕn′ĭk) **1.** Weak; pert. to asthenia. **2.** Pert. to a body habitus marked by a narrow, shallow thorax, a long thoracic cavity, and a short abdominal cavity.

asthenobiosis (ăs-thĕ″nō-bī-ō′sĭs) [Gr. *asthenes*, without strength, + *bios*, life, + *osis*, condition] Condition of reduced biological activity of an animal, resembling hibernation but not related to temperature or humidity.

asthenocoria (ăs-thē″nō-kō′rē-ă) [″ + *kore*, pupil] A sluggish pupillary light reflex.

asthenometer (ăs″thĕ-nŏm′ĕ-ter) [″ + *metron*, measure] An instrument for determining muscular strength or weakness.

asthenope (ăs′thĕ-nōp) [″ + *opsis*, power of sight] An individual who is affected with asthenopia.

asthenopia (ăs″thĕ-nō′pē-ă) Weakness or tiring of the eyes accompanied by pain, headache, and dimness of vision. Symptoms include pain in or around the eyes; headache, usually aggravated by use of the eyes for close work; fatigue; vertigo; reflex symptoms such as nausea, twitching of facial muscles, or migraine. **asthenopic** (-nŏp′ĭk), *adj.*

accommodative a. Asthenopia due to strain of the ciliary muscles.

muscular a. Asthenopia caused by weakness of the extrinsic ocular muscles.

nervous a. Asthenopia of hysteric or neurasthenic origin.

asthenospermia (ăs″thĕ-nō-spĕr′mē-ă) [″ + *sperma*, seed] Loss or reduction of motility of spermatozoa in semen; associated with infertility.

asthma (ăz′mă) [Gr., panting] A disease caused by increased responsiveness of the tracheobronchial tree to various stimuli, which results in episodic narrowing and inflammation of the airways.

Clinically, most patients present with wheezing and shortness of breath. Cough is also a common symptom. Between attacks the patient may have normal respiratory function. Although most asthmatics have mild disease, in some cases the attacks become continuous. This condition, called *status asthmaticus*, may be fatal.

ETIOLOGY: The recurrence and severity of attacks is influenced by a variety of triggers, including allergens, dust, fumes, medicines, dyes, odors, exercise, or occupational exposures. Autonomic and inflammatory mediators (esp. arachidonic acid derivatives, such as leukotrienes) play important roles. The role of emotional disturbance in asthmatic attacks has been difficult to quantify.

TREATMENT: Mild episodic asthma is well managed with intermittent use of beta-agonists, such as albuterol. Patients with more severe disease often rely on multiple medications, including short-acting and long-acting beta agonists, corticosteroids, mast cell-stabilizing drugs (e.g., cromolyn), and inhibitors of leukotrienes. Theophylline use, which may produce toxicity, has diminished in recent years. Patients who receive theophylline must be carefully monitored for safe dosing and to avoid drug-drug interactions.

Acute asthmatic attacks may require high doses or frequent dosing of beta agonists and steroids. Oxygen therapy is an important part of treatment in most asthma attacks. For persistent asthma, hospitalization with monitoring of peak air flow, oxygen saturation, blood gases, and cardiac rhythm is often indicated. Intubation and mechanical ventilation are needed in severe attacks. Antibiotics are used for bacterial infection only.

EPIDEMIOLOGY: Asthma occurs most often in childhood or early adulthood but may plague adults and the elderly as well. Before puberty, twice as many boys as girls have asthma; in adults, the disease is equally distributed between the sexes.

PREVENTION: Limiting exposure to indoor inhalants such as house dust, cockroach antigen, dander, molds, tobacco smoke, and strong odors can help prevent asthmatic attacks. Asthmatics with outdoor allergies may benefit from relocation to new climates or judicious use of medications. Regular use of drugs such as cromolyn sodium is effective in preventing asthmatic attacks and respiratory decompensation. Immunization and desensitization to allergens is often desirable.

PATIENT CARE: The patient is observed closely to see how well he or she adapts to the demands imposed by airway obstruction. Key elements of the patient's response are subjective sense of breathlessness, fatigue experienced during breathing, and whether the attack is worsening or improving with treatment. How well the patient tolerates any administered medications should also be noted.

Assessments best made by the nurse, respiratory therapist, and physician are whether respiratory rate, adventitious sounds such as inspiratory and expiratory wheezes and rhonchi, respiratory muscle use, air movement, mental status, oxygen saturation, and arterial blood gases are improving or deteriorating. Exhaustion or altered mental status may be signs of impending respiratory failure, which might warrant close monitoring or endotracheal intubation.

The patient who is experiencing labored breathing should be closely monitored and reassured. He or she should be seated in an upright (high-Fowler's) position to ease ventilatory effort and given low-flow oxygen and other prescribed medications per instructions. Elevating the patient's arms on pillows at his sides or on a pillow placed on an over-bed table may ease ventilatory effort. If the patient is coughing, his or her ability to clear secretions and the character of the sputum should be noted. Purulent sputum should be sent to the laboratory for culture and sensitivity, gram stain, or other ordered studies. When the acute attack subsides, the nurse or respiratory therapist instructs the patient in the proper use of inhaled medications, paying special attention to how well the patient manages the metered dose inhalers and adding a spacer device as necessary to improve utilization.

The health care provider educates the patient about eliminating exposure to allergens or irritants (e.g., second-hand smoke, cold air) and teaches home measures to prevent or decrease the severity of future attacks. Caregivers ascertain that patient and family understand the prescribed maintenance regimen, including the rationale for the order in which inhalers are to be used and any adverse effects to be reported, as well as the use of emergency treatment if an attack threatens. Preventive therapies (such as vaccinations against the influenza virus and pneumococcal pneumonia and desensitization to specific allergens in children) are administered if they have not already been given. Follow-up is arranged with home health and/or the primary care provider so that the patient can be carefully re-evaluated and any questions or concerns that the patient or family may have can be addressed. SEE: *Nursing Diagnoses Appendix*.

bronchial a. Allergic asthma; a common form of asthma due to hypersensitivity to an allergen.

cardiac a. Wheezing that results from heart disease, esp. acute or chronic heart failure.

exercise-induced a. Asthmatic attacks that occur during physical exertion.

extrinsic a. Reactive airway disease triggered by an allergic (hypersensitivity) response to an antigen.

intrinsic a. Asthma assumed to be due to some endogenous cause because no external cause can be found.

nocturnal a. An increase in asthmatic symptoms during sleep. Nocturnal asthma may be caused by a variety of conditions, including gastroesophageal reflux, allergens in the bedroom, circadian variations in circulating hormone levels, or inadequate doses of antiasthmatic medications at night. Treatment is tailored to the underlying cause.

occupational a. Airway narrowing resulting from exposures in the workplace to environmental dusts, fibers, gases, smoke, sprays, or vapors.

stable a. Asthma in which there has been no increase in symptoms or need for additional medication for at least the past 4 weeks.

unstable a. An increase in asthmatic symptoms during the past 4 weeks.

TREATMENT: Usually the dosage of the patient's bronchodilator or other medications needs to be increased.

PATIENT CARE: The patient must be monitored closely for signs of respiratory failure such as abnormal sensorium and severe tachypnea and tachycardia. **asthmatic** (ăz-măt′ĭk), *adj.*

asthmagenic Producing asthma.

astigmatism (ă-stĭg′mă-tĭzm) [Gr. *a*-, not, + *stigma*, point, + *-ismos*, condition of] ABBR: As; Ast. A form of ametropia in which the refraction of a ray of light is spread over a diffuse area rather than sharply focused on the retina. It is due to differences in the curvature in various meridians of the cornea and lens of the eye. The exact cause is unknown. Some types show a familial pattern. **astigmatic** (ăs″tĭg-măt′ĭk), *adj.*

compound a. Astigmatism in which both horizontal and vertical curvatures are involved.

index a. Astigmatism resulting from inequalities in the refractive indices of different parts of the lens.

mixed a. Astigmatism in which one meridian is myopic and the other hyperopic.

simple a. Astigmatism along one meridian only.

astigmatometer, astigmometer (ăs″tĭg-mă-tŏm′ĕ-tĕr, -mŏm′ĕ-tĕr) [″ + *stigma*, point, + *metron*, measure] An instrument for measuring astigmatism.

astigmia (ă-stĭg′mē-ă) Astigmatism.

astomatous, astomous (ăs-tōm′ă-tŭs, ăs′tō-mŭs) [Gr. *a*-, not, + *stoma*, mouth] Without a mouth or oral aperture; as certain protozoa.

astomia (ă-stō′mē-ă) Congenital absence of the mouth.

astragalectomy (ăs″trăg-ă-lĕk′tō-mē) [*astragalus* + Gr. *ektome*, excision] Surgical removal of the talus (astragalus).

astragalus (ă-străg′ă-lŭs) [Gr. *astragalos*, ball of the ankle joint] Obsolete term for the talus of the ankle. SEE: *talus*.

Astragalus membranaceus An herbal remedy recommended by alternative medical practitioners as a treatment for respiratory infections and flu.

astraphobia (ăs-tră-fō′bē-ă) [Gr. *astrape*, the heavens, + *phobos*, fear] Fear of thunder and lightening.

astriction (ă-strĭk′shŭn) Action of an astringent.

astringent (ă-strĭn′jĕnt) [L. *astringere*, to bind fast] **1.** Drawing together, constricting, binding. **2.** An agent that has a constricting or binding effect (i.e., one that checks hemorrhages or secretions by coagulation of proteins on a cell surface). The principal astringents are salts of metals such as lead, iron, zinc (ferric chloride, zinc oxide); permanganates; and tannic acid. SEE: *styptic*.

astro- [Gr. *astron*, star] Combining form indicating relationship to a *star*, or *star-shaped*.

astrobiology Study of extraterrestrial life.

astroblast (ăs′trō-blăst) [″ + Gr. *blastos*, germ] A cell that gives rise to an astrocyte. It develops from spongioblasts derived from embryonic neuroepithelium.

astroblastoma (ăs″trō-blăs-tō′mă) [″ + ″ + *oma*, tumor] A grade II astrocytoma, composed of cells with abundant cytoplasm and two or three nuclei.

astrocyte (ăs′trō-sīt) [″ + *kytos*, cell] A neuroglial cell of the central nervous system that supports neurons and contributes to the blood-brain barrier. SYN: *Spider cell*.

astrocytoma (ăs″trō-sī-tō′mă) [″ + ″ + *oma*, tumor] Tumor of the brian or spinal cord composed of astrocytes. They are graded according to the prognosis.

malignant a. A tumor of the brainstem, cerebellum, spinal cord, or the white matter of the cerebral hemispheres. Onset is typically in the fifth decade of life. Prognosis after treatment by surgery, radiation, or other means is poor; few survive more than 2 years.

astroglia (ăs-trŏg′lē-ă) [″ + *glia*, glue] Astrocytes making up neuroglial tissue.

astrokinetic motions (ăs″trō-kĭ-nĕt′ĭk) [″ + *kinesis*, movement] Pert. to movements of the centrosome.

astrophobia (ăs″trō-fō′bē-ă) [″ + *phobos*, fear] Morbid fear of stars and celestial space.

astrosphere (ăs′trō-sfĕr) [″ + *sphaira*, sphere] A group of fibrils or fine rays that radiate from the centrosome (microcentrum) of a dividing cell. SYN: *aster*.

astrostatic (ăs″trō-stăt′ĭk) [″ + *statikos*, standing] Pert. to an astrosphere in its resting condition.

Astroviridae A virus family that causes epidemic viral gastroenteritis in adults and children. The incubation period has been estimated to be 3 to 4 days. The outbreaks are self-limiting and in the absence of coexisting pathogens, the intestinal signs and symptoms last 5 days or less. Treatment, if required, is supportive and directed to maintaining hydration and electrolyte balance. SEE: *Caliciviridae*.

astrovirus (ăs′trō-vī″rŭs) An adenovirus with worldwide distribution that causes gastroenteritis in children. Clinical symptoms include anorexia, headache, fever, diarrhea, and vomiting.

ASV *Anodic stripping voltammetry*.

asyllabia (ă″sĭl-ā′bē-ă) [Gr. *a*-, not, + *syllabe*, syllable] A form of alexia, in which the patient recognizes letters but cannot form syllables or words.

asymbolia (ā-, ă-sĭm-bō′lē-ă) [Gr. *a*-, not, + *symbolon*, a sign] Inability to comprehend words, gestures, or any type of symbol. SYN: *asemia*. SEE: *aphasia*.

asymmetry (ā-sĭm′ĕ-trē) [″ + *symme-*

tria, symmetry] Lack of symmetry. **asymmetric, asymmetrical** (ā-sĭ-mĕ′trĭk, -trĭ-kăl), *adj.*

asymphytous (ă-sĭm′fĭ-tŭs) [″ + *symphysis*, a growing together] Separate or distinct; not grown together.

asymptomatic (ā″sĭmp-tō-măt′ĭk) [″ + *symptoma*, occurrence] Without symptoms.

asynchronism (ă-sĭn′krō-nĭzm) [″ + *syn*, together, + *chronos*, time, + *-ismos*, condition of] **1.** The failure of events to occur in time with each other as they usually do. **2.** Incoordination. **asynchronous** (-nŭs), *adj.*

asynclitism (ă-sĭn′klĭ-tĭzm) [″ + *synklinein*, to lean together, + *-ismos*, condition of] An oblique presentation of the fetal head in labor. SEE: *presentation* for illus.

anterior a. Anterior parietal presentation. SYN: *Naegele's obliquity*.

posterior a. Posterior parietal presentation. SYN: *Litzmann's obliquity*.

asyndesis (ă-sĭn′dĕ-sĭs) [Gr. *a-*, not, + *syn*, together, + *desis*, binding] Mental defect in which related thoughts cannot be assembled to form a comprehensive concept.

asynechia (ă″sĭ-nĕk′ē-ă) [″ + *synecheia*, continuity] Lack of continuity of structure in an organ or tissue.

asynergia, asynergy (ă-sĭn-ĕr′jē-ă, ă-sĭn′ĕr-jē) [″ + Gr. *synergia*, cooperation] Lack of coordination among parts or organs normally acting in unison; in neurology, lack of coordination between muscle groups. Movements are jerky and in sequence instead of being made together. It is seen in cerebellar diseases. **asynergic** (ā-sĭ-nĕr′gĭk), *adj.*

asynovia (ă-sĭn-ō′vē-ă) [″ + *syn*, with, + *oon*, egg] Lack or insufficient secretion of synovial fluid of a joint.

asyntaxia (ă″sĭn-tăk′sē-ă) [″ + *syntaxis*, orderly arrangement] Failure of the embryo to develop properly.

asystematic (ă-sĭs″tĕ-măt′ĭk) [″ + LL. *systema*, arrangement] Not systematic; not limited to one system or set of organs.

asystole, asystolia (ă-sĭs′tō-lē, ă″sĭs-tō′lē-ă) [″ + *systole*, contraction] Cardiac standstill; absence of electrical activity and contractions of the heart evidenced on the surface electrocardiogram as a flat (isoelectric) line during cardiac arrest.

At Symbol for the element astatine.

atactiform (ă-tăk′tĭ-form) [″ + L. *forma*, form] Similar to ataxia.

ataractic (ăt″ă-răk′tĭk) [Gr. *ataraktos*, quiet] **1.** Of or pert. to ataraxia. **2.** A tranquilizer.

ataraxia, ataraxy (ăt″ă-răk′sē-ă, -sē) [Gr. *ataraktos*, quiet] A state of complete mental calm and tranquility, esp. without depression of mental faculties or clouding of consciousness.

atavism (ăt′ă-vĭzm) [L. *atavus*, ancestor, + Gr. *-ismos*, condition] The appearance of a characteristic presumed to have been present in some remote ancestor; due to chance recombination of genes or environmental conditions favorable to their expression in the embryo. **atavistic** (ăt-ă-vĭs′tĭk), *adj.*

ataxia (ă-tăk′sē-ă) [Gr., lack of order] Defective muscular coordination, esp. that manifested when voluntary muscular movements are attempted. **atactic, ataxic** (ă-tăk′tĭk, -tăk′sĭk), *adj.*

alcoholic a. In chronic alcoholism, ataxia due to a loss of proprioception.

bulbar a. Ataxia due to a lesion in the medulla oblongata or pons.

cerebellar a. Ataxia due to cerebellar disease.

choreic a. Lack of muscular coordination seen in patients with chorea.

Friedreich's a. An inherited degenerative disease with sclerosis of the dorsal and lateral columns of the spinal cord, accompanied by ataxia, speech impairment, lateral curvature of the spinal column, and peculiar swaying and irregular movements, with paralysis of the muscles, esp. of the lower extremities. Onset occurs in childhood or adolescence.

hysterical a. Ataxia of leg muscles due to somatoform disorders.

locomotor a. Tabes dorsalis.

motor a. Inability to perform coordinated muscle movements.

optic a. Loss of hand-eye coordination in reaching for an object one has seen, as a result of damage to visually dedicated regions of the cerebral cortex.

sensory a. Ataxia resulting from interference in conduction of sensory responses, esp. proprioceptive impulses from muscles. The condition becomes aggravated when the eyes are closed. SEE: *Romberg's sign; spinal a.*

spinal a. Ataxia due to spinal cord disease.

static a. Loss of deep sensibility, causing inability to preserve equilibrium in standing.

ataxiagram (ă-tăk′sē-ă-grăm) [Gr. *ataxia*, lack of order, + *gramma*, something written] A record or tracing produced by an ataxiagraph.

ataxiagraph (ă-tăk′sē-ă-grăf) [″ + *graphein*, to write] Instrument for measuring the degree and direction of swaying in ataxia.

ataxiameter (ă-tăk″sē-ăm′ĕ-tĕr) [″ + *metron*, measure] Apparatus measuring ataxia.

ataxiamnesia (ă-tăk″sē-ăm-nē′zē-ă) [″ + *amnesia*, forgetfulness] Condition marked by ataxia and amnesia.

ataxiaphasia (ă-tăk″sē-ă-fā′zē-ă) [″ + *phasis*, speech] Inability to arrange words into sentences. Also spelled *ataxaphasia*.

ataxia-telangiectasia A degenerative brain disease of children, marked by cellular and humoral immunodeficiency, progressive cerebellar degeneration, telangiectasis of the bulbar conjunctiva, and increased risk of malignancy. It is transmitted as an autosomal recessive trait. Death usually occurs in adolescence or early adulthood. Parents should be informed that subsequent children have a 25% risk of having this condition. SYN: *Louis-Bar syndrome*.

ataxophobia (ă-tăk″sō-fō′bē-ă) [″ + *phobos*, fear] Fear of disorder or untidiness.

A.T.B.C.B. *Architectural and Transportation Barriers Compliance Board,* a federal agency charged with enforcing legislation requiring that federal buildings and transportation facilities be accessible to the disabled.

ATC *Athletic Trainer, Certified.*

ATCC *American Type Culture Collection.*

atelectasis (ăt″ĕ-lĕk′tă-sĭs) [Gr. *ateles*, imperfect, + *ektasis*, expansion] **1.** A collapsed or airless condition of the lung. **2.** A condition in which the lungs of a fetus remain partially or totally unexpanded at birth.

ETIOLOGY: It may be caused by obstruction of one or more airways with mucus plugs; by hypoventilation secondary to pain (e.g., from fractured ribs) or to ventilation with inadequate tidal volumes; by inadequate surfactant production; or by compression of the lung or the bronchi by tumors, aneurysms, or enlarged lymph nodes. It is sometimes a complication following abdominal or thoracic surgery, caused by splinting. Chronic atelectasis, called *middle lobe syndrome*, results from compression of the middle lobe bronchus by surrounding lymph nodes.

SYMPTOMS: Symptoms may not be present if the atelectasis is minor and the patient has previously healthy lungs. Dyspnea is common when the atelectasis is severe.

TREATMENT: Treatment varies with the etiology. The patient with atelectasis due to persistent ventilation with small tidal volumes is given lung expansion therapy such as incentive spirometry. The patient with atelectasis due to mucus plugging needs bronchial hygiene therapy to assist with mucus removal. Artificial surfactant may be useful for the infant with premature lungs and atelectasis.

PATIENT CARE: Patients at risk are evaluated for dyspnea, decreased chest wall movement, inspiratory substernal or intercostal retractions, diaphoresis, tachypnea, tachycardia, and pleuritic chest pain. Lung fields are percussed for decreased resonance, and the chest is auscultated for abnormal breath sounds. Pulse oximetry and arterial blood gas values are monitored for evidence of hypoxemia. Bronchial hygiene therapies are useful for the patient with atelectasis due to retained pulmonary secretions. The nurse or respiratory therapist instructs and monitors the patient on the use of incentive spirometry to prevent or correct existing atelectasis.

Atelectasis can be prevented in at-risk patients by encouraging deep breathing and coughing exercises every 1 to 2 hr, by repositioning the patient often, and by administering prescribed analgesics. Adequate fluid intake is encouraged, inspired air is humidified as necessary, and the patient is assisted to mobilize and clear secretions. Intubated or obtunded patients are suctioned as necessary. If the patient is being mechanically ventilated, tidal volume is maintained at 10 to 15 cc/kg of body weight to ensure adequate lung expansion when appropriate.

absorption a. Lung collapse associated with high alveolar oxygen concentrations.

passive a. Collapse of a portion of the distal lung units owing to persistent breathing with small tidal volumes.

TREATMENT: The patient must be stimulated to breathe deeply and ambulate when possible.

resorption a. Collapse of distal lung units resulting from plugging of the airway with mucus.

TREATMENT: The patient needs clearing of the airways (with suctioning or chest physiotherapy).

atelencephalia (ăt-ĕl″ĕn-sĕ-fā′lē-ă) [Gr. *ateleia*, incompleteness, + *enkephalos*, brain] Congenital anomaly with imperfect development of the brain. Also spelled *ateloencephalia.*

atelia (ă-tē′lē-ă) [Gr. *ateleia*, incompleteness] Imperfect or incomplete development.

ateliosis [Gr. *a*-, not, + *teleios*, complete, + *osis*, condition] A form of infantilism due to pituitary insufficiency, in which there is arrested growth but no deformity. The voice and face may resemble those of a child. **ateliotic** (-ŏt′ĭk), *adj.*

atelo- (ăt′ĕ-lō) [Gr. *ateles*, imperfect] Combining form meaning *imperfect* or *incomplete*.

atelocardia (ăt″ĕ-lō-kăr′dē-ă) [″ + *kardia*, heart] Congenital incomplete development of the heart.

atelocephaly (ăt″ĕ-lō-sĕf′ă-lē) [″ + *kephale*, head] Incomplete development of the head.

atelocheilia (ăt″ĕ-lō-kī′lē-ă) [″ + *cheilos*, lip] Incomplete development of the lip.

atelocheiria (ăt″ĕ-lō-kī′rē-ă) [″ + *cheir*, hand] Incomplete development of the hand.

ateloglossia (ăt″ĕ-lō-glŏs′ē-ă) [″ + *glossa*, tongue] Incomplete development of the tongue.

atelognathia (ăt″ĕ-lŏg-nā′thē-ă) [″ + *gnathos*, jaw] Incomplete development of the jaw.

atelomyelia (ăt″ĕ-lō-mī-ē′lē-ă) [″ + *myelos*, marrow] Incomplete development of the spinal cord.

atelopodia (ăt″ĕ-lō-pō′dē-ă) [″ + *pous*, foot] Incomplete development of the foot.

ateloprosopia (ăt″ĕ-lō-prō-sō′pē-ă) [″ + *prosopon*, face] Incomplete development of the face.

atelorhachidia (ăt″ĕ-lō-ră-kĭd′ē-ă) [″ + *rhachis*, spine] Incomplete development of the spinal cord.

atelostomia (ăt″ĕ-lō-stō′mē-ă) [″ + *stoma*, mouth] Incomplete development of the mouth.

atenolol (ă-tĕn′ō-lŏl) A beta-blocking agent. Trade name is Tenormin.

athelia (ă-thē′lē-ă) [Gr. *a-*, not, + *thele*, nipple] Congenital absence of the nipples.

atherectomy A technique using high speed drills to remove atheromatous plaques from arteries.

ather- SEE: *athero-*.

athero-, ather- [Gr. *athere*, gruel, porridge] Combining form meaning *fatty plaque*.

atherogenesis (ăth″ĕr-ō-jĕn′ĕ-sĭs) [Gr. *athere*, porridge, + *genesis*, generation, birth] Formation of atheromata in the walls of arteries.

atheroma (ăth″ĕr-ō′mă) *pl.* **atheromata** [″ + *oma*, tumor] Fatty degeneration or thickening of the walls of the larger arteries occurring in atherosclerosis. SEE: *arteriosclerosis*. **atheromatous** (-ō′mă-tŭs), *adj.*

atheromatosis (ăth″ĕr-ō″mă-tō′sĭs) Generalized atheromatous disease of the arteries.

atheronecrosis (ăth″ĕr-ō″nĕ-krō′sĭs) [″ + *nekros*, corpse, + *osis*, condition] Necrosis or degeneration accompanying arteriosclerosis.

atherosclerosis (ăth″ĕr-ō″sklĕ-rō′sĭs) [″ + Gr. *sklerosis*, hardness] The most common form of arteriosclerosis, marked by cholesterol-lipid-calcium deposits in the walls of arteries. SEE: *coronary artery disease* for illus.

PATHOLOGY: The initial pathological changes, called fatty streaks, are visible on the endothelial surfaces of major blood vessels by the age of 10. These lesions may progress to thickening of the lining of arteries (a process called intimal thickening) if risk factors for atherosclerosis are not addressed. Whether these lesions in turn progress to advanced lesions, called fibrous plaques, depends on hemodynamic forces (such as hypertension) and abnormal plasma levels of lipoproteins (e.g., high levels of total and LDL cholesterol; low levels of HDL cholesterol). Ultimately, arteries affected by the disease may become nearly completely blocked, a condition that causes insufficient blood flow (ischemia). If a plaque within a blood vessel suddenly ruptures, the blood vessel can close and organs or tissues may infarct. SEE: *myocardial infarction; peripheral vascular disease; stroke.*

ETIOLOGY: Risk factors for atherosclerosis include tobacco abuse, diabetes mellitus, abnormal blood lipid concentrations, hypertension, family history, male gender, increased age, sedentary lifestyle, and obesity. The role of vascular inflammation due to chronic infections (e.g., with chlamydia or cytomegalovirus) and the part played by elevated homocysteine levels are topics of active research.

SYMPTOMS: Symptoms may develop in any organ system with a blood supply diminished by atherosclerosis. Commonly these symptoms include angina pectoris, intermittent claudication, strokes, transient ischemic attacks, and renal insufficiency.

TREATMENT: Treatment includes regular exercise, smoking cessation, and a dietary regimen of low-cholesterol and low-fat foods. Medical treatment of hypertension, lipid disorders, and diabetes mellitus is also helpful. Angioplasty, atherectomy, or arterial bypass graft operations are beneficial for selected patients.

PATIENT CARE: The patient and family are taught about risk factors associated with atherosclerosis, and the health care professionals help the patient modify these factors. Patients who smoke cigarettes are encouraged to enroll in smoking cessation programs. Community-based plans and programs to change sedentary activity patterns, reduce stress, control obesity, and decrease saturated fat intake to control triglyceride and cholesterol levels are explored with the patient. The nurse or other health care professionals refers the patient for medical treatment to control hypertension and diabetes mellitus and supports the patient's efforts to cooperate with lifestyle and health care changes. Regular exercise of a type and extent appropriate for the patient's health and adequate rest are prescribed. The patient is informed of the need for long-term follow-up care to prevent a variety of body system complications.

athetoid (ăth′ĕ-toyd) [Gr. *athetos*, unfixed, changeable, + *eidos*, form, shape] Resembling or affected with athetosis.

athetosis (ăth-ĕ-tō′sĭs) [″ + *osis*, condition] A condition in which slow, irregular, twisting, snakelike movements occur in the upper extremities, esp. in the hands and fingers. These involuntary movements prevent sustaining the body, esp. the extremities, in one position. All four limbs may be affected or the involvement may be unilateral. The symptoms may be due to encephalitis, cerebral palsy, hepatic encephalopathy, drug toxicity, or Huntington's chorea or may be an undesired side effect of prolonged treatment of parkinsonism with levodopa.

There are several types of athetosis. In *athetosis with spasticity,* muscle tone fluctuates between normal and hypertonic; often there is moderate spasticity in the proximal parts and athetosis more distally. Modified primitive spinal reflex patterns are often present. In *athetosis with tonic spasms,* muscle tone fluctuates between hypotonic and hypertonic. Excessive extension or flexion is evident. There are strong postural asymmetry and frequent spinal or hip abnormalities or deformities.

In *choreoathetosis,* muscle tone fluctuates from hypotonic to normal or hypertonic. There are extreme ranges of motion. Deformities are rare, but subluxation of the shoulder and finger joints often occurs. *Pure athetosis* is much rarer than the others. Muscle tone fluctuates between hypotonic and normal. Deformities are rare. Twitches and jerks of muscles or individual muscle fibers are seen, along with slow, writhing, involuntary movements that are more proximal than distal.

PATIENT CARE: Muscle tone and joint range of motion are assessed; joints are inspected for involuntary movements, spasticity, and joint deformities and subluxations. Degree of interference with activities of daily living and self-image is evaluated. Prescribed therapies (based on the etiology) are administered and evaluated for desired effects and adverse reactions. Emotional support and acceptance are provided, and the patient is informed about local and national groups and services offering support and information.

athletic trainer A person who has completed educational and clinical experiences and is capable of working with athletes and their environment to help prevent injuries, advise them concerning appropriate equipment, recognize and evaluate injuries, administer emergency treatment, determine if specialized medical care is required, and rehabilitate those with sports injuries. In many instances, the first member of the health care team an injured athlete encounters is an athletic trainer, who must be able to provide the best possible treatment. Athletic trainers work under the supervision of trained physicians. In most states, athletic trainers must be licensed to practice. SEE: *training, athletic*.

athrepsia, athrepsy (ă-thrĕp'sē-ă, -sē) [Gr. *a-*, not, + *threpsis*, nourishment] Marasmus. **athreptic** (-thrĕp'tĭk), *adj.*

athyroidemia (ath"ĭ-roy-, ă-thī"roy-dē'mē-ă) [" + " + " + *haima*, blood] Absence of thyroid hormone in the blood.

athyroidism (ă-thī'roy-dĭzm) [" + " + " + *-ismos*, condition of] Suppression of thyroid secretions, or absence of the thyroid gland. SEE: *hypothyroidism*.

atlantad (ăt-lăn'tăd) Toward the atlas.

atlantal (ăt-lăn'tăl) Pert. to the atlas.

atlantoaxial (ăt-lăn"tō-ăk'sē-ăl) [Gr. *atlas*, a support, + L. *axis*, a pivot] Pert. to the atlas (first cervical vertebra) and the axis (second cervical vertebra).

atlantodidymus (ăt-lăn"tō-dĭd'ĭ-mŭs) [" + *didymus*, twin] Atlodidymus.

atlanto-occipital (ăt-lăn"tō-ŏk-sĭp'ĭ-tăl) [" + L. *occipitalis*, occipital] Pert. to the atlas and the occipital bones.

atlas (ăt'lăs) [Gr.] The first cervical vertebra by which the spine articulates with the occipital bone of the head; named for Atlas, the Greek god who was supposed to support the world on his shoulders.

atloaxoid (ăt"lō-ăk'soyd) [" + L. *axis*, a pivot, + Gr. *eidos*, form, shape] Pert. to the atlas and axis.

atlodidymus (ăt-lō-dĭd'ĭ-mŭs) [" + Gr. *didymos*, twin] A malformed fetus with one body and two heads.

ATLS *advanced trauma life support.*

atm *atmosphere; atmospheric.*

atmosphere (ăt'mŏs-fēr) [" + *sphaira*, sphere] **1.** The gases surrounding the earth. **2.** Climatic condition of a locality. **3.** In physics, the pressure of the air on the earth at mean sea level, approx. 14.7 lb/sq in. (101,325 pascals or 760 torr). **4.** In chemistry, any gaseous medium around a body. **atmospheric** (ăt"mŏs-fēr'ĭk), *adj.*

standard a. The pressure of air at sea level when the temperature is 0°C (32°F). This is equal to 14.7 lb/sq in., or 760 torr, or 101,325 pascals (newtons per square meter).

ATN *acute tubular necrosis.*

ATNR *asymmetrical tonic neck reflex.*

atom (ăt'ŏm) [Gr. *atomos*, indivisible] The smallest part of an element. An atom consists of a nucleus (which contains protons and neutrons) and surrounding electrons. The nucleus is positively charged, and this determines the atomic number of an element. A large number of entities in the atomic nucleus have been identified, and the search for others continues. Dimensions of atoms are of the order of 10^{-8} cm. SEE: *atomic theory; electron*. **atomic** (ă-tŏm'ĭk), *adj.*

tagged a. Tracer.

atomic theory **1.** The theory that all matter is composed of atoms. **2.** Theories pert. to the structure, properties, and behavior of the atom.

atomization (ăt″ŏm-ĭ-zā′shŭn) Converting a fluid into spray or vapor form. SEE: *nebulizer; vaporizer*.

atomize (ăt′ŏm-īz) To convert a liquid to a spray or vapor.

atomizer (ăt′ŏm-ī-zĕr) An apparatus for converting a jet of liquid to a spray.

atonicity (ăt-ō-nĭs′ĭ-tē) [Gr. *a-*, not, + *tonos*, stretching] State of being atonic or without tone.

atony (ăt′ō-nē) [″ + *tonos*, stretching] Debility; lack of normal tone or strength. **atonic** (ă-tŏn′ĭk), *adj.*

gastric a. Lack of muscle tone in the stomach and failure to contract normally, causing a delay in movement of food out of the stomach.

atopen (ăt′ō-pĕn) [″ + *topos*, place] An infrequently used synonym for allergen.

atopic (ă-tŏp′ĭk) **1.** Pert. to atopy. **2.** Displaced; malpositioned.

atopognosis (ă-tŏp″ŏg-nō′sĭs) [″ + *topos*, place, + *gnosis*, knowledge] Inability to locate a sensation of touch or feeling.

atopy (ăt′ō-pē) [Gr. *atopia*, strangeness] A type I hypersensitivity or allergic reaction for which there is a genetic predisposition. It differs from normal hypersensitivity reactions to allergies that are not genetically determined. The basis for the predisposition lies in the histocompatibility genes. The child of two parents with the atopic allergy has a 75% chance of developing similar symptoms; if one parent is affected, the child has a 50% chance of developing the atopy. Hay fever and asthma are two of the most commonly inherited allergies; contact dermatitis and gastrointestinal reactions may also be inherited. As with all type I hypersensitivity reactions, IgE is the primary antibody involved. SYN: *atopic allergy*. SEE: *allergy; immunity; reagin*.

atorvastatin (ăh-tŏr″vă-stă′-tĭn) A lipid-lowering drug used to treat elevated serum cholesterol and LDL cholesterol levels.

atoxic [Gr. *a-*, not, + *toxikon*, poison] Nonpoisonous.

ATP *adenosine triphosphate*.

ATPase *adenosine triphosphatase*.

ATPS *ambient temperature and pressure* (saturated with water vapor).

atraumatic (ā″traw-măt′ĭk) [Gr. *a-*, not, + *traumatikos*, relating to injury] Not causing trauma or injury. SEE: *needle, atraumatic*.

atresia (ă-trē′zē-ă) [″ + *tresis*, a perforation] Congenital absence or closure of a normal body opening or tubular structure. **atresic, atretic** (-zĭk, -trĕ-tĭk), *adj.*

anal a. Imperforate anus.

aortic a. Congenital closure of the aortic valvular opening into the aorta.

biliary a. Closure or absence of some or all of the major bile ducts.

choanal a. A congenital occlusion of the passage between the nose and pharynx by a bony or membranous structure.

congenital aural a. Failure of the external ear canal to develop in utero. When this condition affects both ears, the child may suffer permanent hearing loss and have difficulty speaking and acquiring language skills. Unilateral cases require no specific therapy.

duodenal a. Congenital closure of a portion of the duodenum.

esophageal a. Congenital failure of the esophagus to develop.

follicular a. Normal death of the ovarian follicle following failure of the ovum to be fertilized.

intestinal a. Congenital closure of any part of the intestine.

mitral a. Congenital closure of the mitral valve opening between the left atrium and ventricle.

prepyloric a. Congenital closure of the pyloric end of the stomach.

pulmonary a. Congenital closure of the pulmonary valve between the right ventricle and the pulmonary artery.

tricuspid a. Congenital closure of the tricuspid valve between the right atrium and ventricle.

urethral a. Absence or closure of the urethral orifice or canal.

vaginal a. Congenital closure or absence of the vagina.

atria (ā′trē-ă) Pl. of atrium.

atrial (ā′trē-ăl) Pert. to the atrium.

atrial natriuretic factor A peptide secreted by the atrial tissue of the heart in response to an increase in blood pressure. It influences blood pressure, blood volume, and cardiac output. It increases the excretion of sodium and water in urine, thereby lowering blood volume and blood pressure and influencing cardiac output. Its secretion rate depends on glomerular filtration rate and inhibits sodium reabsorption in distal tubules. These actions reduce the workload of the heart. Also called *atrial natriuretic hormone* or *atrial natriuretic peptide*.

atrial septal defect A congenital heart defect in which there is an opening between the atria.

atrichia (ă-trĭk′ē-ă) [Gr. *a-*, not, + *thrix*, hair] **1.** Absence of hair. **2.** Lack of cilia or flagella.

atrichosis (ă-trĭ-kō′sĭs) [″ + ″ + *osis*, condition] Congenital absence of hair.

atrichous (ă-trĭk′ŭs) **1.** Without flagella. **2.** Without hair.

atrionector (ăt″rē-ō-nĕk′tor) [L. *atrium*, corridor, + *nector*, connector] Sinoatrial node.

atriopeptin (āt′rē-ō-pĕp″tĭn) Atrial natriuretic factor.

atrioseptopexy (ā″trē-ō-sĕp′tō-pĕk″sē) [″ + *saeptum*, a partition, + Gr. *pexis*, fixation] Plastic surgical repair of an interatrial septal defect.

atriotome (ā′trē-ō-tōm) [″ + Gr. *tome*, incision] Instrument used in surgically opening the cardiac atrium.

atrioventricular (ā″trē-ō-vĕn-trĭk′ū-lăr) [″ + *ventriculus*, ventricle] Pert. to both the atrium and the ventricle.

atrioventricularis communis (ā″trē-ō-vĕn-trĭk″ū-lā′rĭs kŏ-mū′nĭs) Persistence of the common atrioventricular canal. In this congenital anomaly of the heart, the division of the common atrioventricular canal in the embryo fails to occur. This causes atrial septal defect and atrioventricular valve incompetence.

atriplicism (ă-trĭp′lĭ-sĭzm) Poisoning due to eating one form of spinach, *Atriplex littoralis*.

atrium (ā′trē-ŭm) *pl.* **atria** [L., corridor] A chamber or cavity communicating with another structure.

a. of the ear The portion of the tympanic cavity lying below the malleus; the tympanic cavity proper.

a. of the heart The upper chamber of each half of the heart. The right atrium receives deoxygenated blood from the entire body (except lungs) through the superior and inferior venae cavae and coronary sinus; the left atrium receives oxygenated blood from the lungs through the pulmonary veins. Blood passes from the atria to the ventricles through the atrioventricular valves. In the embryo, the atrium is a single chamber that lies between the sinus venosus and the ventricle.

a. of the lungs The space at the end of an alveolar duct that opens into the alveoli, or air sacs, of the lungs.

atrophoderma (ăt″rō-fō-dĕr′mă) [Gr. *a*-, not, + *trophe*, nourishment, + *derma*, skin] Atrophy of the skin.

atrophy (ăt′rō-fē) [Gr. *atrophia*] **1.** A wasting; a decrease in size of an organ or tissue. Atrophy may result from death and resorption of cells, diminished cellular proliferation, pressure, ischemia, malnutrition, decreased activity, or hormonal changes. **2.** To undergo or cause atrophy. **atrophic** (ā-trō′fĭk), *adj.*

acute yellow a. An outdated term for fulminant hepatic failure.

brown a. Atrophic tissue that is yellowish-brown rather than its normal color. It is seen principally in the heart and liver of the aged. The pigmentation is due to the presence of lipofuscin, the "wear and tear" pigment that may be associated with aging. Its presence in tissue is a sign of injury from free radicals. SEE: *lipofuscin; free radical*.

compression a. Atrophy due to constant pressure on a part.

correlated a. Wasting of a part following destruction of a correlated part.

Cruveilhier's a. Spinal muscular a.

disuse a. Atrophy from immobilization or failure to exercise a body part.

group a. A change in the appearance of muscle fibers that have lost their nerve supply; marked by an increase in the size of the motor unit and a decrease in the fibers within to a uniformly small size.

healed yellow a. Postnecrotic cirrhosis of the liver.

Hoffmann's a. SEE: *Werdnig-Hoffmann disease*.

Landouzy-Déjérine a. Landouzy-Déjérine dystrophy.

macular a. Anetoderma.

multiple systems a. A neurological syndrome marked by Parkinson's disease, autonomic failure (loss of sweating, urinary incontinence, dizziness or syncope on arising, miosis), and unsteady gait (ataxia).

muscular a. Atrophy of muscle tissue, esp. due to lack of use or denervation.

myelopathic a. Muscular atrophy resulting from a lesion of the spinal cord.

myotonic a. Myotonia congenita.

optic a. Atrophy of the optic disk as a result of degeneration of the second cranial (optic) nerve.

pathological a. Atrophy that results from the effects of disease processes.

peroneal muscular a. Charcot-Marie-Tooth disease.

physiological a. Atrophy caused by the normal aging processes in the body. Examples are atrophy of embryonic structures; atrophy of childhood structures on reaching maturity, as the thymus; atrophy of structures in cyclic phases of activity, as the corpus luteum; atrophy of structures following cessation of functional activity, as the ovary and mammary glands; and atrophy of structures with aging.

postmenopausal vaginal a. SEE: *vaginal atrophy, postmenopausal*.

progressive muscular a. Spinal muscular a.

spinal muscular a. An autosomal recessive hereditary disorder in which motor neurons in the spinal cord die, leading to muscle paralysis. The type 1 form usually is fatal by age 4; the cause of death is respiratory paralysis. Types 2 and 3 are slower to progress. Treatments aim to prevent nutritional deficiencies, orthopedic deformities, and respiratory infections. SYN: *Werdnig-Hoffmann disease*.

Sudeck's a. Acute atrophy of a bone at the site of injury; probably due to reflex local vasospasm.

trophoneurotic a. Atrophy due to disease of the nerves or nerve centers supplying the affected muscles.

unilateral facial a. Progressive atrophy of one side of the facial tissues.

atropine sulfate (ăt′rō-pēn sŭl′fāt) Salt of an alkaloid obtained from belladonna. A parasympatholytic agent, it counteracts the effects of parasympathetic stimulation. It is used primarily to treat potentially life-threatening bradycardias and heart blocks.

atropine sulfate poisoning Anticholinergic side effects of atropine exposure, including restlessness, dry mouth, fever, hot and dry skin, pupillary dilation, tachycardia, hallucinations, delirium, and coma. SYN: *atropinism.*

PATIENT CARE: Oxygen is given; a cardiac monitor, oximeter, and automated blood pressure cuff are applied; and intravenous fluids are administered. Patients who are experiencing restlessness may respond to the administration of a benzodiazepine such as lorazepam or diazepam. If the atropine has been ingested orally, gastric lavage with activated charcoal may absorb some of the toxin from the gastrointestinal tract. Severe neurological side effects, such as seizures, may be treated with physostigmine. SEE: *Poisons and Poisoning Appendix.*

atropinism, atropism (ăt′rō-pĭn-ĭzm, -pĭzm) Atropine sulfate poisoning.

atropinization (ăt-rō″pĭn-ĭ-zā′shŭn) Administration of atropine until desired pharmacologic effect is achieved.

ATS *American Thoracic Society.*

attachment (ă-tăch′mĕnt) **1.** A device or other material affixed to something else. **2.** In dentistry, a plastic or metal device used for retention or stabilization of a dental prosthesis, such as a partial denture. **3.** An enduring psychological bond of affection.

epithelial a. The link between the reflection of the junctional (gingival) epithelium and the enamel, cementum, or dentin of the tooth.

parent-newborn a. Unconscious incorporation of the infant into the family unit. Characteristic parental claiming behaviors include seeking mutual eye contact with the infant, initiating touch with their fingertips, calling the infant by name, and expressing recognition of physical and behavioral similarities with other family members. Attachment is enhanced or impeded by the infant's responses. SEE: *bonding, mother-infant; engrossment; position, en face.*

attack (ă-tăk′) [Fr. *attaquer*, join] **1.** The onset of an illness or symptom, usually dramatic (e.g., a heart attack or an attack of gout). **2.** An assault.

attendant A paramedical hospital employee who assists in the care of patients.

attending The person having primary responsibility for a patient.

attention (ă-tĕn′shŭn) The directing of consciousness to a person, thing, perception, or thought.

attention-deficit hyperactivity disorder ABBR: ADHD. A persistent pattern of inattention, and hyperactivity, and impulsivity or both, occurring more frequently and severely than is typical in individuals at a comparable level of development. The illness may begin in early childhood, but may not be diagnosed until after the symptoms have been present for many years. The prevalence is estimated to be 3% to 5% in children; data for adults are not available.

ETIOLOGY: The origin is unknown; however, the disorder may reflect a deficiency in neurochemicals that influence functions of the brain's reticular activating system.

SYMPTOMS: Signs may be minimal or absent when the person is under strict control or is engaged in esp. interesting or challenging situations. They are more likely to occur in group situations. Although behaviors vary widely, children usually exhibit low frustration levels, marked intolerance for changes in their immediate environments, and failure to respond to discipline. Young children commonly exhibit temper tantrums, excessive large muscle activity, and negativity. Older children frequently display restlessness, carelessness, stubbornness, rapid mood swings, and low self-esteem.

DIAGNOSIS: The disorder is difficult to diagnose in children under age 5. It is important to distinguish this illness from age-appropriate behaviors in active children, and from disorders such as mental retardation, alteration of mood, anxiety, or personality changes caused by illness or drugs. The criteria determined by the American Psychiatric Association now include specific limits concerning the duration and severity of symptoms of inattention and hyperactivity-impulsivity. The findings must be severe enough to be maladaptive and inconsistent with specified levels of development.

TREATMENT: In both children and adults, the domestic, school, social, and occupational environments are evaluated to determine contributing factors and their relative importance. The drug of choice for use in children is methylphenidate. Dextroamphetamine may be used for those who do not tolerate methylphenidate. Pemoline, although weaker, also may be used.

attention reflex Change in the size of the pupil when attention is suddenly fixed. SYN: *Piltz's reflex.*

attenuate (ă-tĕn′ū-āt) To render thin or make less virulent. In radiology, to make less intense. **attenuated,** *adj.*

attenuation (ă-tĕn″ū-ā′shŭn) **1.** Dilution. **2.** The lessening of virulence. Bacteria and viruses are made less virulent by being heated, dried, treated with chemicals, passed through another organism, or cultured under unfavorable conditions. **3.** The decrease in intensity (quantity and quality) of an x-ray beam as it passes through matter. **4.** In acoustics, the reduction in sound intensity of the initial sound source as compared with the sound intensity at a point away from the source. **5.** The reduction of amplitude, magnitude, or strength of an electrical signal. In electronics, it is the opposite of amplification.

attic (ăt'ĭk) [L. *atticus*] The cavity of the middle ear or the portion lying above the tympanic cavity proper. It contains the head of the malleus and the short limb of the incus. SYN: *epitympanic recess*. SEE: *ear; tympanum*.

attic disease Chronic suppurative inflammation of the attic of the ear.

atticitis (ăt"ĭ-sī'tĭs) [L. *atticus*, attic, + Gr. *itis*, inflammation] Inflammation of the attic of the ear.

atticoantrotomy (ăt"ĭ-kō-ăn-trŏt'ō-mē) [" + Gr. *antron*, cave, + *tome*, incision] Surgical opening of the attic and mastoid antrum of the ear.

atticotomy (ăt"ĭ-kŏt'ō-mē) [" + Gr. *tome*, incision] Surgical opening of the tympanic attic of the ear.

attitude [LL. *aptitudo*, fitness] **1.** Bodily posture or position, esp. the position of the limbs. A particular attitude is often a symptom of disease or abnormal mental state (e.g., the stereotyped position assumed by catatonics or the theatrical expression seen in hysteria). **2.** Behavior based on conscious or unconscious mental views developed through cumulative experience.

crucifixion a. Position in which the body is rigid with the arms at right angles to the long axis of the body; seen in catatonia.

defense a. Position automatically assumed to avert pain.

fetal a. Relationship of the fetal parts to one another, such as the head and extremities flexed against the body.

forced a. Abnormal position due to disease or contractures.

frozen a. Stiffness of gait, seen in amyotrophic lateral sclerosis.

stereotyped a. Position taken and held for a long period, seen frequently in mental diseases.

atto [Danish, *atten*, eighteen] Symbol: a. In SI units, a prefix indicating 10^{-18}.

attolens (ă-tōl'ĕnz) [L.] Raising or lifting up.

attraction (ă-trăk'shŭn) [L. *attrahere*, to draw toward] A force that causes particles of matter to be drawn to each other.

chemical a. The tendency of atoms of one element to unite with those of another to form compounds.

molecular a. The tendency of molecules with unlike electrical charges to attract each other. SEE: *adhesion; cohesion*.

attrahens To bring toward.

attribute [L. *attributus*, character, reputation] A quality or characteristic of animate or inanimate objects (e.g., adaptability is an attribute of living organisms).

attrition (ă-trĭsh'ŭn) [L. *attritio*, a rubbing against] **1.** The act of wearing away by friction or rubbing. **2.** Any friction that breaks the skin. **3.** The process of wearing away, as of teeth, in the course of normal use.

atypia (ā-tĭp'ē-ă) [Gr. *a-*, not, + *typos*, type] Deviation from a standard or regular type.

atypical (ā-tĭp'ĭ-kăl) [" + *typikos*, pert. to type] Deviating from the normal; not conforming to type.

A.U. *angstrom unit; aures unitas,* both ears; *auris uterque,* each ear.

Au [L. *aurum*] Symbol for the element gold.

Aub-Dubois table (awb-dū-boy') [Joseph C. Aub, U.S. physician, 1890–1973; Eugene F. Dubois, U.S. physician, 1882–1959] Table of normal basal metabolic rates according to age.

AUC *Area under (the) curve.*

audible Capable of being heard.

audible sound Sound containing frequency components between 15 and 15,000 Hz (cycles per second).

audile (aw'dĭl) **1.** Pert. to hearing; auditory. **2.** A person who retains more auditory information than information received through other senses. **3.** In psychoanalysis, one whose mental perceptions are auditory. SEE: *motile; visile*.

audioanesthesia (aw"dē-ō-ăn"ĕs-thē'zē-ă) [L. *audire*, to hear, + Gr. *an-*, not, + *aisthesis*, sensation] Anesthesia or analgesia produced by sound; used by dentists to help prevent perception of pain.

audiogenic (aw-dē-ō-jĕn'ĭk) [" + Gr. *genesis*, generation, birth] Originating in sound.

audiogram (aw'dē-ō-grăm") [" + Gr. *gramma*, something written] A graphic record produced by an audiometer. SEE: illus.

audiologist A specialist in audiology.

audiology (aw"dē-ŏl'ō-jē) [" + Gr. *logos*, word, reason] The study of hearing disorders through identification and evaluation of hearing loss, and the rehabilitation of those with hearing loss, esp. that which cannot be improved by medical or surgical means.

audiometer (aw"dē-ŏm'ĕ-tĕr) [" + Gr. *metron*, measure] An instrument for testing hearing.

audiometry (aw"dē-ŏm'ĕ-trē) Testing of the hearing sense. SEE: *spondee threshold*.

averaged electroencephalic a. A

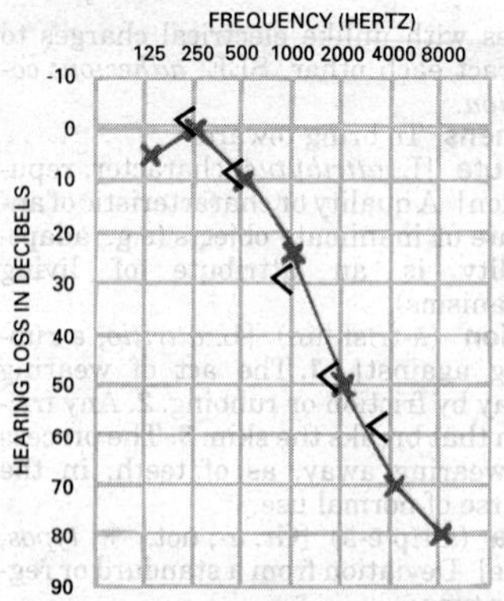

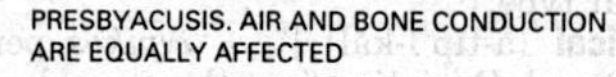

A PRESBYACUSIS. AIR AND BONE CONDUCTION ARE EQUALLY AFFECTED

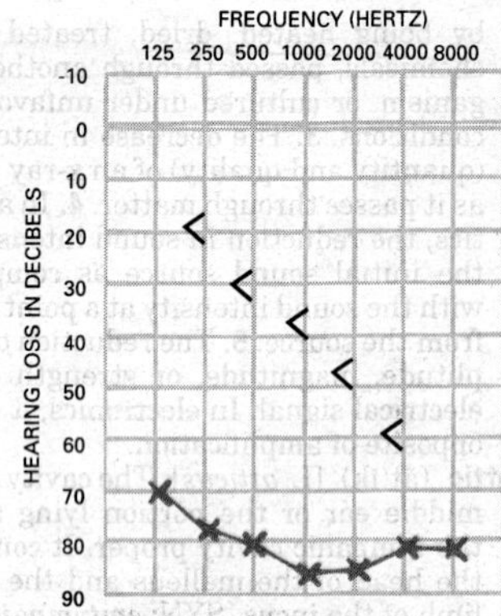

B SEVERE MIXED HEARING LOSS

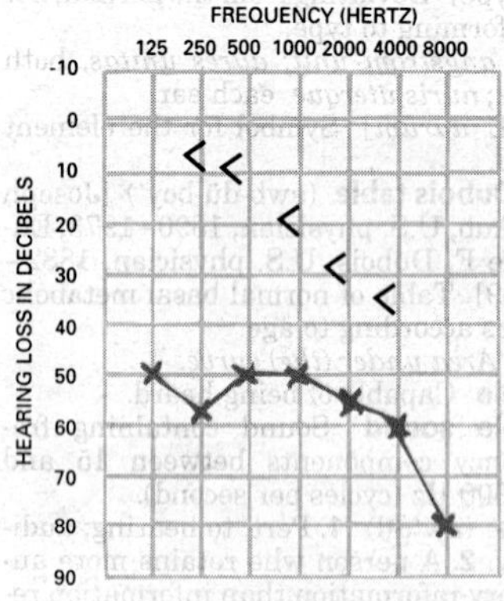

C MODERATELY SEVERE MIXED HEARING LOSS

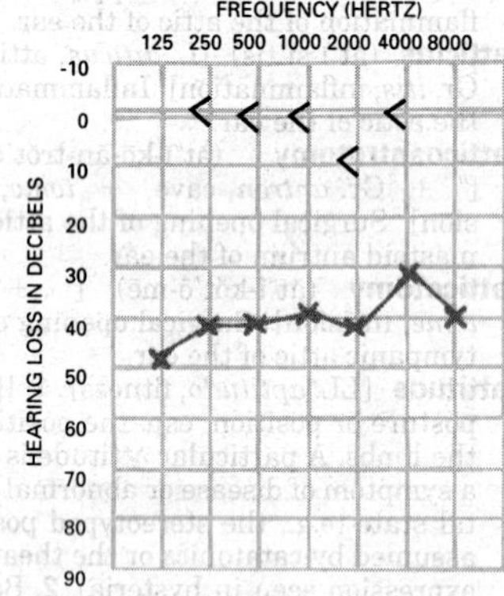

D PURE AIR CONDUCTION LOSS BECAUSE OF UNCOMPLICATED OTOSCLEROSIS

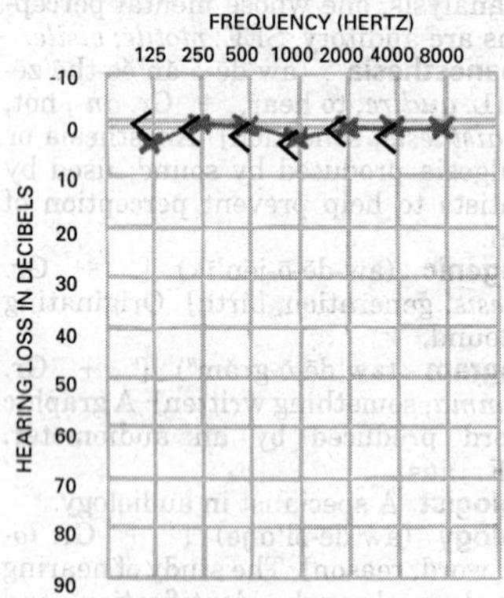

E NORMAL AUDIOGRAM

< LEFT EAR BONE CONDUCTION, RIGHT EAR MASKED

✖ LEFT EAR CONDUCTION

AUDIOGRAM LEFT EAR

Left ear

method of testing the hearing of children who cannot be adequately tested by conventional means. The test is based on the electroencephalogram's being altered by perceived sound without the need for a behavioral response, so the test may be done on an autistic, severely retarded, or hyperkinetic child who is asleep or sedated. SEE: *auditory evoked response*.

evoked response a. Use of computer-aided technique to average the brain's response to latency of auditory stimuli. Auditory brainstem evoked response (ABER) is one form of this type of audiometry. This method is used to test the hearing of individuals, esp. children, who cannot be tested in the usual manner.

pure tone a. Measurement of hearing using pure tones, which are almost completely free of extraneous noise.

speech a. Test of the ability to hear and understand speech. The threshold of detection is measured in decibels.

audit In medical care facilities, an official examination of the record of all aspects of patient care. This is done by trained staff who are not usually affiliated with the institution. The purpose of an audit is to compare and evaluate the quality of care provided with accepted standards.

audition (aw-dĭ′shŭn) [L. *auditio*, hearing] Hearing.

chromatic a. Condition in which certain color sensations are aroused by sound stimuli. SYN: *colored a.*

colored a. Chromatic a.

gustatory a. Condition in which certain taste sensations are aroused by sound stimuli.

mental a. Recollection of a sound based on previous auditory impressions.

audito-oculogyric reflex (aw″dĭt-ō-ŏk″ū-lō-jī′rĭk) The sudden turning of the head and eyes toward an alarming sound.

auditory (aw′dĭ-tō″rē) [L. *auditorius*] Pert. to the sense of hearing.

a. defensiveness Excessive attention to sounds that do not disturb others. This behavior is thought to indicate a sensory processing disorder.

auditory bulb The membranous labyrinth and cochlea.

auditory epilepsy Epilepsy triggered by certain sounds. SEE: *epilepsy*.

auditory evoked response Response to auditory stimuli as determined by a method independent of the individual's subjective response. The electroencephalogram has been used to record response to sound. By measuring intensity of sound and presence of response, one can test the acuity of hearing of psychiatric patients, persons who are asleep, and children too young to cooperate in a standard hearing test.

auditory muscles The tensor tympani and stapedius muscles.

auditory nerve The eighth cranial nerve; a sensory nerve with two sets of fibers: cochlear nerve (hearing) and vestibular nerve (equilibrium), the latter having three branches, the superior, inferior, and middle branches. SYN: *vestibulocochlear nerve*.

Auenbrugger's sign (ow-ĕn-broog′ĕrz) [Leopold Joseph Auenbrugger, Austrian physician, 1722–1809] Epigastric prominence due to marked pericardial effusion.

Auerbach's plexus (ow′ĕr-băks) [Leopold Auerbach, Ger. anatomist, 1828–1897] An autonomic nerve plexus between the circular and longitudinal fibers of the muscular layer of the stomach and intestines. SYN: *myenteric plexus*.

Auer bodies (ow′ĕr) [John Auer, U.S. physician, 1875–1948] Rod-shaped structures, present in the cytoplasm of myeloblasts, myelocytes, and monoblasts, found in leukemia. Also called *Auer rods*. SEE: illus.

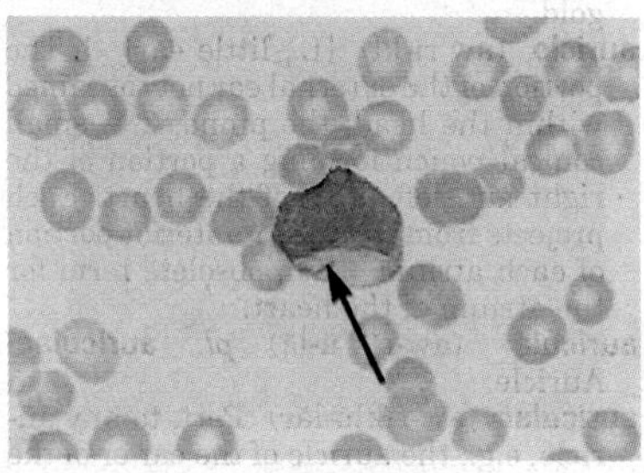

AUER BODY

Auer body (arrow) in myeloblast in acute leukemia (×640)

Aufrecht's sign (owf′rĕkhts) [Emanuel Aufrecht, Ger. physician, 1844–1933] Diminished breathing sound that is heard above the jugular fossa, which is indicative of tracheal stenosis.

augmentation (awg″mĕn-tā′shŭn) **1.** The act of adding to or increasing the size, function, or strength of something. **2.** In obstetrics, the use of pharmacological or surgical interventions to help the progression of a previously dysfunctional labor.

bladder a. Surgical enlargement of the urinary bladder with a segment of bowel. The technique enlarges the reservoir of the bladder and enhances the compliance of the detrusor muscles. It is used esp. in patients with neurogenic bladder problems that are refractory to medical therapy. When a major portion of the bladder is resected (malignancy), an isolated intestinal pouch is used as a substitute for the bladder (neoenterocystoplasty). SYN: *enterocystoplasty*.

breast a. SEE: *mammaplasty, augmentation*.

augnathus (awg-nā′thŭs) [Gr. *au*, again, + *gnathos*, jaw] Fetus with a double lower jaw.

aura (aw′ră) [L., breeze] A subjective, but recognizable sensation that precedes and signals the onset of a convulsion or migraine headache. In epilepsy the aura may precede the attack by several hours or only a few seconds. An epileptic aura may be psychic, or it may be sensory with olfactory, visual, auditory, or taste hallucinations. In migraine the aura immediately precedes the attack and consists of ocular sensory phenomena.

aural (aw'răl) [L. *auris*, the ear] **1.** Pert. to the ear. **2.** Pert. to an aura.

aurantiasis cutis (aw"răn-tī'ă-sĭs kū'tĭs) [L. *aurantium*, orange, + Gr. *-iasis*, condition of; L. *cutis*, skin] Yellow pigmentation of skin due to ingestion of excessive amounts of food that contain carotene, such as carrots, oranges, and squash. SEE: *carotenemia*.

auriasis (aw-rī'ă-sĭs) Chrysiasis.

auric (aw'rĭk) [L. *aurum*, gold] Pert. to gold.

auricle (aw'rĭ-kl) [L., little ear] **1.** The portion of the external ear not contained within the head; the pinna. **2.** A small conical pouch forming a portion of the right and left atria of the heart. Each projects from the upper anterior portion of each atrium. **3.** An obsolete term for the atrium of the heart.

auricula (aw-rĭk'ū-lă) *pl.* **auriculae** Auricle.

auricular (aw-rĭk'ū-lăr) Pert. to any auricle, e.g., the auricle of the ear or of the cardiac atria.

auriculare (aw-rĭk"ū-lā'rē) *pl.* **auricularia** A craniometric point at the center of the opening of the external auditory canal.

auriculocervical nerve reflex (aw-rĭk"ū-lō-sĕr'vĭk'l) [L. *auricula*, little ear, + *cervicalis*, pert. to the neck] Snellen's reflex.

auriculocranial (aw-rĭk"ū-lō-krā'nē-ăl) [" + *cranialis*, pert. to the skull] Pert. to the ear and the cranium.

auriculopalpebral reflex (aw-rĭk"ū-lō-păl'pĕb-răl) [" + *palpebra*, eyelid] Kisch's reflex.

auriculotemporal (aw-rĭk"ū-lō-tĕm'pŏ-răl) [" + *temporalis*, pert. to the temples] Pert. to the ear and area of the temple.

auriform (aw'rĭ-form) [L. *auris*, ear, + *forma*, shape] Ear-shaped.

auris (aw'rĭs) [L.] Ear.

a. dextra Right ear.

a. externa External ear (pinna and external auditory meatus).

a. interna Internal ear (semicircular canals, vestibule, cochlea).

a. media Middle ear (eardrum and auditory bones).

a. sinistra Left ear.

aurotherapy (aw"rō-thĕr'ă-pē) [L. *aurum*, gold, + Gr. *therapeia*, treatment] Treatment of disease by administration of gold salts; used in the treatment of rheumatoid arthritis, autoimmune bullous disease, esp. pemphigus vulgaris. The advisability of using gold in treating rheumatoid arthritis is controversial. SYN: *chrysotherapy*.

CAUTION: Side effects, including toxicity to the kidneys and bone marrow, are significant. The patient will need frequent monitoring of blood and urine.

aurum (aw'rŭm) [L.] Gold.

auscult (aws-kŭlt') Auscultate.

auscultate (aws'kŭl-tāt) [L. *auscultare*, listen to] To examine by auscultation. SYN: *auscult*.

auscultation (aws"kŭl-tā'shŭn) Listening for sounds within the body, esp. from the chest, neck, or abdomen. A stethoscope is typically used. It is applied to the patient's skin surface gently but firmly, to eliminate any environmental noises that may be present. Auscultation is used to detect heart rate and rhythm and any cardiac murmurs, rubs, or gallops; crackles or wheezes in the lungs; pleural rubs; movement of gas or food through the intestines; vascular or thyroid bruits; fetal heart tones; and other physiological phenomena.

immediate a. Auscultation in which the ear is applied directly to the skin.

mediate a. Auscultation in which sounds are conducted from the surface to the ear through an instrument such as a stethoscope.

auscultatory (aws-kŭl'tă-tō"rē) Pert. to auscultation.

Austin Flint murmur [Austin Flint, U.S. physician, 1812–1886] A presystolic or late diastolic heart murmur best heard at the apex of the heart. It is present in some cases of aortic insufficiency. It is thought to be due to the vibration of the mitral valve caused by the backward-flowing blood from the aorta meeting the blood flowing in from the left atrium.

Australia antigen, Australian antigen An antigen present in the sera of patients with hepatitis B, but rarely in patients with other forms of hepatitis. This antigen is also found in normal populations in the Tropics and southeast Asia. It was first isolated in the serum of an Australian aborigine. SYN: *hepatitis B surface antigen*.

autacoid (aw'tă-koyd) [Gr. *autos*, self, + *akos*, remedy, + *eidos*, form, shape] **1.** A term originally used by the British physiologists Edward Shäfer and Sharpey-Shafer as a substitute for the word *hormone*. **2.** A term used to describe prostaglandins and related compounds that form rapidly, act, and then decay or are destroyed enzymatically.

autism (aw'tĭzm) [Gr. *autos*, self, + *-ismos*, condition] **1.** In classic psychiatry, mental introversion in which the attention or interest is thought to be focused on the ego. Objective validation of this concept is lacking. **2.** Withdrawal from communication with others, often accompanied by repetitive or primitive behaviors. SEE: *Nursing Diagnoses Appendix*.

infantile a. A syndrome appearing in childhood with symptoms of self-absorption, inaccessibility, aloneness, inability to relate, highly repetitive play and rage reactions if interrupted, predilection for rhythmical movements, and many language disturbances. The cause is unknown.

auto- [Gr. *autos*, self] Combining form meaning *self*.

autoactivation (aw″tō-ăk″tĭ-vā′shŭn) [″ + L. *agere*, to act] Gland activation by its own secretion.

autoagglutination (aw″tō-ă-gloo″tĭ-nā′shŭn) [″ + L. *agglutinare*, adhere to] Agglutination, or clumping of red blood cells, in response to an autotransfusion (e.g., the transfusion of a person's own blood that has been removed by phlebotomy or during surgery).

autoagglutinin (aw″tō-ă-glū′tĭ-nĭn) A substance present in an individual's blood that agglutinates that person's red blood cells.

cold a. An IgM class autoantibody that is activated only when the temperature falls below 100°C. These antibodies may destroy the patient's red blood cells and are one cause of autoimmune hemolytic anemia. They are found in the serum of patients (esp. those older than 50 years) with atypical (e.g., mycoplasma) pneumonia, infectious mononucleosis, cytomegalovirus infections, mumps, and certain blood diseases. The complement-mediated, autoimmune hemolysis that results is an example of a type II hypersensitivity reaction. SYN: *cold agglutinin*. SEE: *autoantibody; hemolytic anemia*.

warm a. An IgG class autoantibody that is activated at a temperature of 37°C. These antibodies damage the membranes on the patient's own red blood cells, which results in their destruction by the spleen, producing an autoimmune hemolytic anemia. The source of the autoantibodies is unclear in 50% of the cases. In the other 50% of patients, they are related to a drug reaction, autoimmune diseases, esp. systemic lupus erythematosus, or malignancies. SYN: *warm antibody*. SEE: *autoantibody; hemolytic anemia*.

autoamputation (aw″tō-ăm″pū-tā′shŭn) Spontaneous amputation of a part or limb. SEE: *ainhum*.

autoanalysis (aw″tō-ă-năl′ĭ-sĭs) [″ + *analyein*, break down] A patient's own analysis of the mental state underlying his or her mental disorder.

autoantibody (aw″tō-ăn′tĭ-bŏd″ē) [″ + *anti*, against, + AS *bodig*, body] ABBR: AAb. An antibody, produced by B cells in response to an altered "self" antigen on one type of the body's own cells, that attacks and destroys these cells. Autoantibodies are the basis for autoimmune diseases such as rheumatoid arthritis and diabetes mellitus. Several theories exist as to why autoantibodies are formed. The most commonly accepted theory proposes that AAbs develop as the result of a combination of hereditary and environmental risk factors that cause a "self" antigen to be seen as foreign by B cells; as a result, antibodies are produced for its destruction. SEE: *antibody; antigen; autoimmune disease; autoimmunity; immunoglobulin*.

autoantigen (aw″tō-ăn′tĭ-jĕn) [″ + ″ + *gennan*, to produce] A "self" antigen in autoimmune disease. Autoantigens on the cell surface of body tissues are part of the process in which an immune response by B lymphocytes or self-reacting T lymphocytes causes damage to the tissues with the autoantigen.

autoantitoxin (aw″tō-ăn″tĭ-tŏk′sĭn) [″ + ″ + *toxikon*, poison] Antitoxin produced by the body itself.

autocatalysis (aw″tō-kă-tăl′ĭ-sĭs) [″ + *katalysis*, dissolution] Increase in the rate of a chemical reaction resulting from products that are produced in the reaction acting as catalysts. SEE: *catalyst*.

autocatharsis (aw-tō-kă-thăr′sĭs) [″ + *katharsis*, a cleansing] A form of psychotherapy in which patients in discussing their own problems gain an insight into their mental difficulties.

autocatheterization Catheterization of oneself, esp. urinary catheterization.

autochthonous (aw-tŏk′thō-nŭs) [Gr. *autos*, self, + *chthon*, earth] **1.** Found where developed, as in the case of a blood clot or a calculus. **2.** Pert. to a tissue graft to a new site on the same individual.

autochthonous infection Infection due to organisms normally present in the patient's body. It may occur when host defenses are compromised, or when resistant flora are introduced into an abnormal site.

autocinesia, autocinesis (aw″tō-sĭ-nē′sē-ă, -nē′sĭs) Autokinesis.

autoclasis (aw″tŏk′lă-sĭs) [″ + *klasis*, a breaking] Destruction of a part from internal causes.

autoclave (aw′tō-klāv) [″ + L. *clavis*, a key] A device that sterilizes by steam pressure, usually at 250°F (121°C) for a specified length of time. SEE: *sterilization*.

autocrine factor A growth factor produced by the cell that stimulates the same cell to grow.

autocrine system Secretion of cells that act to influence only their own growth; a local hormone. SEE: *paracrine*.

autocystoplasty (aw″tō-sĭs′tō-plăs″tē) [″ + *kystis*, bladder, + *plassein*, to mold] Plastic repair of the bladder with grafts from one's own body.

autocytolysis (aw″tō-sī-tŏl′ĭ-sĭs) Self-digestion or self-destruction of cells.

autodermic (aw″tō-dĕr′mĭk) [″ + *derma*, skin] Pert. to one's own skin, esp. pert. to dermatoplasty with a patient's own skin.

autodigestion (aw″tō-dī-jĕs′chŭn) [″ + L. *dis*, apart, + *gerere*, to carry] Digestion of tissues by their own secretions, such as the digestion of the pancreas during severe pancreatitis.

autodiploid (aw″tō-dĭp′loyd) [″ + *diploe*, fold, + *eidos*, form, shape] Having two sets of chromosomes; caused by redoubling the chromosomes of the haploid cell.

autodrainage (aw″tō-drān′ĭj) [″ + AS *dreahnian*, drain] Drainage of a cavity by the fluid passing through a channel in one's own tissues or to the outside of the body.

autoecholalia (aw″tō-ĕk-ō-lā′lē-ă) [″ + *echo*, echo, + *lalia*, babble] Repetition of the last portion of one's own statements.

autoecic (aw-tē′sĭk) [″ + *oikos*, house] Pert. to a parasite that spends its entire life cycle in one organism.

autoerotic hypoxia Cerebral oxygen deprivation that a person self-induces (e.g., by hanging oneself or by tying a constricting device around the neck) during masturbation. The practice of limiting cerebral blood flow during masturbation has been thought to intensify pleasure during orgasm. It has occasionally resulted in brain damage or death from hypoxia. SYN: *autoerotic asphyxia; sexual asphyxia*. SEE: *asphyxiophilia*.

autoeroticism Autoerotism.

autoerotism (aw″tō-ē-rŏt′ĭsm) [Gr. *autos*, self, + *erotikos*, rel. to love] **1.** Self-gratification of the sexual instinct, usually by manual stimulation of erogenous areas, esp. the penis or clitoris. SEE: *masturbation; autoerotic hypoxia; urolagnia*. **2.** Self-admiration combined with sexual emotion, such as that obtained from viewing one's naked body or one's genitals. SYN: *autoeroticism*. **autoerotic** (-ē-rŏt′ĭk), *adj.*

autoexamination (aw″tō-ĕg-zăm″ĭ-nā′shŭn) [″ + L. *examinare*, to examine] Self-examination. SEE: *breast self-examination*.

autofundoscope (aw″tō-fŭn′dō-skōp) [″ + L. *fundus*, bottom, + Gr. *skopein*, to examine] Apparatus for autoexamination of retinal vessels of the eye.

autogenesis (aw-tō-jĕn′ĕ-sĭs) [″ + *genesis*, generation, birth] Self-generation. SYN: *abiogenesis*. **autogenetic** (-jĕ-nĕt′ĭk), *adj.*

autogenous (aw-tŏj′ĕ-nŭs) **1.** Self-producing; originating within the body. **2.** Denoting a vaccine from a culture of the patient's own bacteria.

autograft (aw′tō-grăft) [″ + L. *graphium*, grafting knife] A graft transferred from one part of a patient's body to another.

limbal cell a. Limbal stem cell a.

limbal stem cell a. The transfer of healthy limbal tissue from a patient's donor eye to repair damaged ocular epithelium in the other eye, esp. after that caused by a chemical burn or congenital defect. SYN: *limbal cell a.; stem cell a.*

stem cell a. Limbal stem cell a.

autohemagglutination (aw″tō-hĕm″ă-glū″tĭ-nā′shŭn) Agglutination of one's own red cells.

autohemic (aw″tō-hē′mĭk) [″ + *haima*, blood] Done with one's own blood.

autohemolysin (aw″tō-hē-mŏl′ĭ-sĭn) [″ + ″ + *lysis*, dissolution] An antibody that acts on the corpuscles of the individual in whose blood it is formed.

autohemolysis (aw″tō-hē-mŏl′ĭ-sĭs) Hemolysis of one's blood cells by one's own serum.

autohemotherapy (aw″tō-hē″mō-thĕr′ă-pē) [″ + *haima*, blood, + *therapeia*, treatment] Treatment by withdrawal and injection intramuscularly of one's own blood.

autohypnosis (aw″tō-hĭp-nō′sĭs) Self-induced hypnosis.

autoimmune theory of aging A theory of aging, originally proposed by Dr. Ray Walford, in which aging is thought to occur because antibodies develop, attack, and destroy the normal cells in the body. According to this theory, a progressive deficiency in immunological tolerance results in the inability to distinguish self from foreign structures.

autoimmunity (aw″tō-ĭm-mū′nĭ-tē) The body's tolerance of the antigens present on its own cells (i.e., self- or autoantigens). It is theorized that self-reactive T lymphocytes (those with receptors that react to self-antigens) are destroyed in the thymus by negative selection. Self-reactive T cells that escape destruction in the thymus may become tolerant because they are exposed to thousands of self-antigens as they circulate in the blood.

The loss of self-tolerance is believed to be the result of multiple hereditary and environmental factors and occurs when self-antigens are damaged, when they link with a foreign antigen, when the structure of a self-antigen is very similar to that of a foreign antigen (molecular mimicry), or when self-reactive T cells are not adequately controlled or are activated by nonspecific antigens. The changes in the appearance of the self-antigen or activation of self-reactive T-cells result in "self" antigens being perceived as foreign. Inflammation and destruction of the tissues bearing the antigen occur because of the production of autoantibodies by B cells or the cytotoxicity of self-reactive T cells, which attack the self-antigens. SEE: *antigen; autoantibody*.

autoinfusion (aw″tō-ĭn-fū′zhŭn) [Gr. *autos*, self, + L. *in*, into, + *fundere*, to pour] Forcing of blood from extremities to the body core by applying Esmarch bandages.

autoinjector (aw″tō-ĭn-jĕk′tor) A syringe that contains a spring-loaded needle with a preloaded dose of medication. When placed against the body with a stabbing motion, the device activates and administers a calculated dose of medication. Commonly used for self-administration of epinephrine (to mitigate anaphylaxis); by migraine sufferers (to achieve prompt relief of headache); or by military and emergency services workers to combat the effects of nerve agents.

autoinoculation (aw″tō-ĭn-ŏk″ū-lā′shŭn) [″ + L. *inoculare*, to ingraft] Inoculation with organisms obtained from one's own body.

autointoxication (aw″tō-ĭn-tŏk″sĭ-kā′shŭn) [″ + L. *in*, into, + Gr. *toxikon*, poison] A condition caused by toxic substances produced within the body. SYN: *autotoxemia; endogenic toxicosis.*

autoisolysin (aw″tō-ī-sŏl′ĭ-sĭn) [″ + *isos*, equal, + *lysis*, dissolution] An antibody that causes dissolution of cells of the individual from which it was obtained and of other individuals of the same species.

autokeratoplasty (aw″tō-kĕr′ă-tō-plăs″tē) [″ + *keras*, horn, + *plassein*, to form] Grafting of corneal tissue taken from the patient's other eye.

autokinesis (aw″tō-kĭ-nē′sĭs) [″ + *kinesis*, movement] Voluntary movement. SYN: *autocinesia*. **autokinetic** (-nĕt′ĭk), *adj.*

visual a. The illusion that an object in space, esp. at night, moves as one continues to look at it. Thus, an aviator looking at a distant light may perceive that the light has moved even though it is stationary.

autolesion (aw′tō-lē″zhŭn) [″ + L. *laedere*, to wound] Self-inflicted injury.

autologous (aw-tŏl′ō-gŭs) [″ + *logos*, word, reason] Originating within an individual, esp. a factor present in tissues or fluids.

a. endometrial co-culture An assisted reproduction technique in which a zygote created by in vitro fertilization is incubated in endometrial tissue harvested from an infertile woman's uterus through the pre-embryonic period before transfer.

autolysate (aw-tŏl′ĭ-sāt) [″ + *lysis*, dissolution] Specific product of autolysis.

autolysis (aw-tŏl′ĭ-sĭs) **1.** The self-dissolution or self-digestion that occurs in tissues or cells by enzymes in the cells themselves, such as occurs after death and in some pathological conditions. **2.** Hemolysis. **autolytic** (aw″tō-lĭt′ĭk), *adj.*

autolysosomes The lysosomes that enable digestion of injured portions of the cell in which they are located.

automatic [Gr. *automatos*, self-acting] Spontaneous; involuntary.

automatic implanted ventricular defibrillator Cardioverter surgically implanted in patients at high risk for sudden cardiac death from ventricular arrhythmias. This device is capable of automatically restoring normal heartbeat.

automaticity The unique property of cardiac muscle tissue to contract without nervous stimulation.

automation, laboratory The use of clinical laboratory instruments that assay large numbers of samples mechanically.

automatism (aw-tŏm′ă-tĭzm) [″ + *-ismos*, condition of] **1.** Automatic actions or behavior without conscious volition or knowledge. **2.** The spontaneous activity of cells or tissues, as the movement of cilia or the contraction of smooth muscles in tissues or organs removed from the body.

autonomic (aw-tō-nŏm′ĭk) [Gr. *autos*, self, + *nomos*, law] **1.** Self-controlling; functioning independently. **2.** Rel. to the autonomic nervous system.

autonomic hyperreflexia A condition commonly seen in patients with injury to the upper spinal cord. It is caused by massive sympathetic discharge of stimuli from the autonomic nervous system. It may be triggered by distention of the bladder or colon, catheterization of or irrigation of the bladder, cystoscopy, or transurethral resection. Symptoms include sudden hypertension, bradycardia, sweating, severe headache, and gooseflesh.

PATIENT CARE: Vital signs and symptoms are assessed with the patient seated (to decrease blood pressure), and are monitored until the episode resolves. The urinary bladder is drained by catheterization. The indwelling catheter is checked for kinking or other obstruction and irrigated with no more than 30 ml of sterile normal saline solution if necessary. If the catheter remains obstructed, it is removed, and a new catheter is inserted immediately. The patient's rectum is checked for impaction; a local anesthetic ointment is used for lubrication and for anesthesia if removal of an impaction is necessary. Any other stimuli that may be triggering the response are also removed. A urine specimen is obtained for culture because infection may be a cause. Prescribed medications to reduce blood pressure are administered, and the patient's response is evaluated. A calm atmosphere is created, and emotional support is offered throughout the episode. The patient is educated about this complication, and actions are explained to prevent and alleviate it.

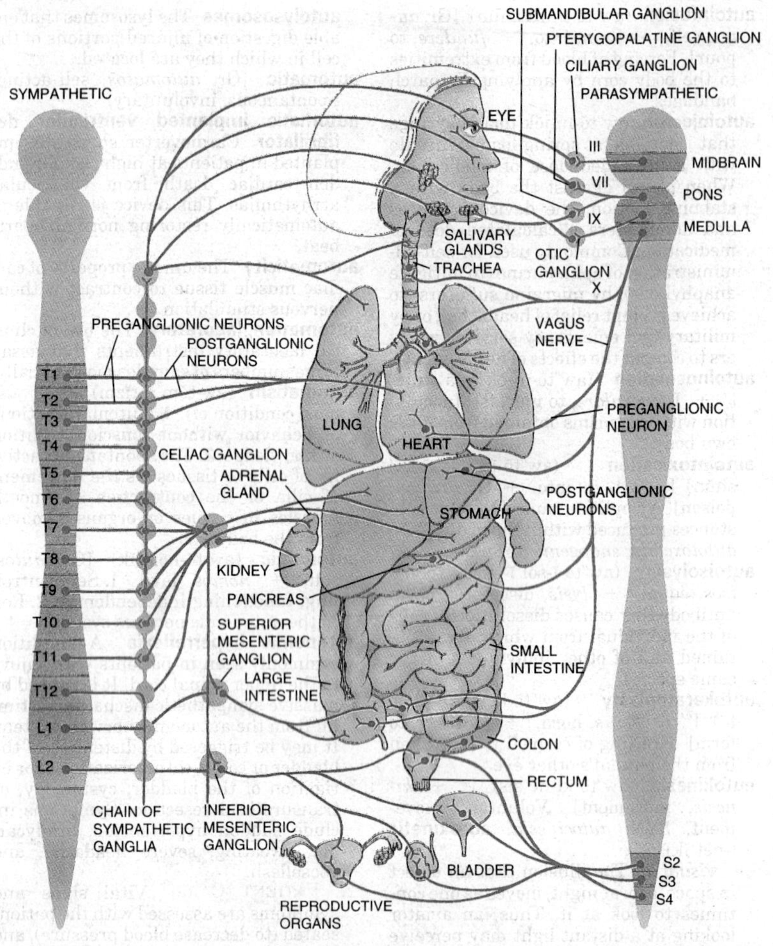

AUTONOMIC NERVOUS SYSTEM

autonomic nervous system ABBR: ANS. The part of the nervous system that controls involuntary bodily functions. It is inappropriately named because rather than being truly "autonomic," it is intimately responsive to changes in somatic activities. The ANS consists of motor nerves to visceral effectors: smooth muscle, cardiac muscle, glands such as the salivary, gastric, and sweat glands, and the adrenal medullae.

The two divisions of the ANS are the sympathetic or thoracolumbar division and the parasympathetic or craniosacral division. The sympathetic division consists of the paired chains of ganglia on either side of the backbone, their connections (rami communicantes) with the thoracic and lumbar segments of the spinal cord, the splanchnic nerves, and the celiac and mesenteric ganglia in the abdomen and their axons to visceral effectors. The parasympathetic division consists of some fibers of cranial nerves 3, 7, 9, and 10; the fibers of some sacral spinal nerves and ganglia; and short axons near or in the visceral effectors. SEE: illus.

FUNCTION: Sympathetic impulses have the following effects: vasodilation in skeletal muscle and vasoconstriction in the skin and viscera occur; heart rate and force are increased; the bronchioles dilate; the liver changes glycogen to glucose; sweat glands become more active; peristalsis and gastrointestinal secretions decrease; the pupils dilate; the salivary glands secrete small amounts of thick saliva; and the hair stands on end (gooseflesh). The sympathetic division dominates during stressful situations such as anger or fright, and the body responses contribute to fight or flight, with unimportant activities such as digestion markedly slowed. Most sympathetic neurons release the neurotransmitter norepinephrine at the visceral effector.

The parasympathetic division dominates during nonstressful situations, with the following effects: the heart slows to normal, the bronchioles constrict to normal, peristalsis and gastrointestinal secretion increase for normal digestion, the pupils constrict to normal, secretion of thin saliva increases, and the urinary bladder constricts normally. If parasympathetic supply to the bladder is impaired, there will be incomplete emptying and urinary retention. All parasympathetic neurons release the transmitter acetylcholine at the visceral effector. SEE: *nervous system*.

EXAMINATION: The following tests are helpful in evaluating the state of the autonomic nervous system: Blood pressure and body temperature may be measured serially with respect to diurnal variation. Sweating by painting an area of the skin may be tested with iodine and dusting the area with starch; the areas without autonomic function will fail to turn dark. Parasympathetic function may be tested by instilling a 2% solution of methacholine into one conjunctival sac. This produces constriction of the pupil in patients with parasympathetic disorders.

autonomous (aw-tŏn'ō-mŭs) Independent of external influences.

autonomy (aw-tŏn'ō-mē) [Gr. *autos*, self, + *nomos*, law] Independent functioning. The concept of autonomy varies with cultural practices and thought. This is important when communicating with persons from different cultural backgrounds.

AutoPap An automated (computerized) method of screening and analyzing Pap smears for abnormal cells.

auto-PEEP The inadvertent application of positive end-expiratory pressure (PEEP) to the lungs of a patient receiving mechanical ventilation. It occurs most often in patients with obstructive lung disease whose mechanical ventilator is set at an insufficient expiratory time.

ETIOLOGY: Auto-PEEP is caused by air-trapping during mechanical ventilation.

PATIENT CARE: It may cause the patient to "fight" the ventilator, breathing at the wrong time in the respiratory cycle. It is treated by reducing tidal volume and increasing the expiratory time during ventilation.

autophagia, autophagy (aw"tō-fā'jē-ă, aw-tŏf'ă-jē) [" + *phagein*, to eat] **1.** Biting oneself. **2.** Self-consumption by a cell.

autophagocytosis In a cell, the digestion of portions of cell organelles or mitochondria injured or atrophied. This digestive process is essential to the survival of the cell. SEE: *endocytosis; phagocytosis; pinocytosis*.

autophil (aw'tō-fĭl) [" + *philein*, to love] A person who has a sensitive autonomic nervous system.

autophilia (aw-tō-fĭl'ē-ă) Narcissism; self-love.

autophobia (aw"tō-fō'bē-ă) [" + *phobos*, fear] **1.** A psychoneurotic fear of being alone. **2.** Abnormal fear of being egotistical.

autophony (aw-tŏf'ō-nē) [" + *phone*, voice] The vibration and echolike reproduction of one's own voice, breath sounds, and murmurs; usually due to diseases of the middle ear and auditory tube.

autoplasmotherapy (aw"tō-plăs"mō-thĕr'ă-pē) [" + LL. *plasma*, form, mold, + *therapeia*, treatment] Treatment that consists of injection of the patient's own blood plasma.

autoplasty (aw'tō-plăs"tē) Plastic surgery using grafts from the patient's body. **autoplastic** (aw"tō-plăs'tĭk), *adj.*

autopolyploidy (aw"tō-pŏl'ē-ploy"dē) [" + *polys*, many, + *ploos*, fold, + *eidos*, form, shape] The condition of having more than two complete sets of chromosomes.

autoprecipitin (aw"tō-prē-sĭp'ĭ-tĭn) [Gr. *autos*, self, + L. *praecipitare*, to cast down] Precipitin active against the serum of the animal in which it was formed.

autopsy (aw'tŏp-sē) Postmortem examination of the organs and tissues of a body to determine the cause of death or pathological conditions. SYN: *necropsy; necroscopy*.

psychological a. An attempt to determine what, if any, emotional or psychological factors caused or contributed to an individual's suicide.

autopsychic (aw"tō-sī'kĭk) [" + *psyche*, soul] Aware of one's own personality.

autopsychosis (aw"tō-sī-kō'sĭs) [" + *psyche*, soul] Mental disease in which patients' ideas about themselves are disordered.

autoradiogram Autoradiograph.

autoradiograph (aw"tō-rā'dē-ō-grăf)The radiograph formed by radioactive materials present in the tissue or individual. This is made possible by injecting radiochemicals into the person or tissue and then exposing x-ray film by placing the individual or tissue adjacent to the film. SYN: *autoradiogram; radioautograph*.

autoradiography Use of autoradiographs in investigating certain diseases.

autoregulation (aw"tō-rĕg"ū-lā'shŭn) Control of an event such as blood flow through a tissue (e.g., cardiac muscle) by alteration of the tissue. If not enough blood is flowing through a tissue, certain changes cause an increase; if the flow is too great, another type of change causes a decrease.

autoreinfusion (aw″tō-rē″ĭn-fū′zhŭn) [″ + L. *re*, back, + *in*, into, + *fundere*, to pour] Intravenous injection of a patient's blood that has been collected from a site in which bleeding had occurred, such as the abdominal or pleural cavity. SEE: *autologous blood transfusion*.

autosensitization (aw″tō-sĕn″sĭ-tĭ-zā′shŭn) Sensitivity to one's own cells, fluids, or tissues.

autosepticemia (aw″tō-sĕp″tĭ-sē′mē-ă) [″ + *septos*, rotten, + *haima*, blood] Septicemia from resident bacterial flora or their toxins.

autoserodiagnosis (aw″tō-sē″rō-dī-ăg-nō′sĭs) [″ + L. *serum*, whey, + Gr. *dia*, through, + *gnosis*, knowledge] Diagnosis through serum from the patient's blood.

autoserotherapy (aw″tō-sē″rō-thĕr′ă-pē) [″ + ″ + Gr. *therapeia*, treatment] Treatment by hypodermic injection of the patient's own blood serum.

autoserum (aw″tō-sē′rŭm) Serum obtained from the patient's own blood or cerebrospinal fluid to be reinjected into the patient.

autosite (aw′tō-sīt) [Gr. *autos*, self, + *sitos*, food] The fairly normal member of asymmetrical conjoined twins, the other twin being dependent on the autosite for its nutrition.

autosmia (aw-tŏz′mē-ă) [″ + *osme*, smell] Awareness of the odor of one's own body.

autosomatognosis (aw″tō-sō″mă-tŏg-nō′sĭs) [″ + *soma*, body, + *gnosis*, knowledge] The feeling that a part of the body that has been removed is still present. SEE: *phantom limb*.

autosome (aw′tō-sōm) [″ + *soma*, body] Any chromosome other than the sex (X and Y) chromosomes. SEE: *chromosome*.

autosplenectomy (aw″tō-splĕn-ĕk′tō-mē) [″ + *splen*, spleen, + *ektome*, excision] Multiple infarcts of the spleen that cause it to become fibrotic and nonfunctioning; seen in sickle cell anemia.

autostimulation (aw″tō-stĭm″ū-lā′shŭn) **1.** In immunology, stimulation by antigens present in the organism. **2.** Stimulation or motivation of oneself.

autosuggestibility (aw″tō-sŭg-jĕs″tĭ-bĭl′ĭ-tē) [″ + L. *suggerere*, to suggest] Peculiar lack of resistance to any suggestion originating in one's own mind.

autosuggestion (aw″tō-sŭg-jĕs′chŭn) The acceptance of an idea or thought arising from within one's own mind, bringing about some physical or mental action or change.

autotemnous (aw″tō-tĕm′nŭs) [″ + *temnein*, to divide] Pert. to cells propagating by spontaneous division.

autotomography (aw″tō-tō-mŏg′ră-fē) [″ + Gr. *tome*, incision, + *graphein*, to write] Radiographic tomography in which the patient rather than the x-ray tube is moved.

autotopagnosia (aw″tō-tŏp-ăg-nō′zē-ă) [″ + *topos*, place, + *a-*, not, + *gnosis*, knowledge] Inability to orient various parts of the body correctly; occurs in lesions of the thalamoparietal pathways of the cortex.

autotoxemia, autotoxicosis (aw″tō-tŏk-sē′mē-ă, aw″tō-tŏk″sĭ-kō′sĭs) Autointoxication.

autotoxin (aw″tō-tŏk′sĭn) Poison generated within the body on which it acts.

autotransfusion (aw″tō-trăns-fū′zhŭn) [″ + L. *trans*, across, + *fundere*, pour] A method of returning the patient's own extravasated blood to the circulation. Blood shed during surgery, e.g., during the repair of a ruptured spleen, is collected during the operation and returned intravenously into the circulation of the patient.

autotransplantation (aw″tō-trăns″plăn-tā′shŭn) [″ + ″ + *plantare*, to plant] Surgical transfer of tissue from one part of the body to another part.

autotrophic (aw″tō-trō′fĭk) [″ + *trophe*, nourishment] Self-nourishing; capable of growing in the absence of organic compounds; pert. to green plants and bacteria, which form protein and carbohydrate from inorganic salts and carbon dioxide.

autovaccination (aw″tō-văk″sĭ-nā′shŭn) [″ + *vacca*, cow] **1.** Vaccination with autogenous vaccine or autovaccine. **2.** A vaccination resulting from virus or bacteria from a sore of a previous vaccination, as may occur when a smallpox vaccination sore is scratched and the virus is subsequently transferred to a break in the skin elsewhere.

autovaccine (aw″tō-văk′sēn) Vaccine prepared from a virus in the patient's own body.

auxiliary (ăwg-zĭl′ē-ăr-ē) [L. *auxiliarius*, help] **1.** Providing additional aid. **2.** A person who aids.

dental a. A person who assists in the care and treatment of dental patients. Responsibilities vary according to the needs of the dentist, training and capabilities of the individual, and state regulations. Common dental auxiliaries include receptionist, dental assistant, dental hygienist, and dental lab technician.

auxin [Gr. *auxe*, increase] A substance that promotes growth in plant cells and tissues.

auxotroph (awk′sō-trōf) [″ + *trophe*, nutrition] An auxotrophic organism.

auxotrophic (awk-sō-trō′fĭk) Requiring

a growth factor that is different from that required by the parent organism.

A-V **1.** *arteriovenous*. **2.** *atrioventricular*.

A-V access *Arteriovenous access*.

availability In nutrition, the extent to which a nutrient is present in a form that can be absorbed and used by the body.

avalanche theory [Fr. *avaler*, to descend] The theory that nervous impulses are reinforced and thereby become more intense as they travel peripherally.

avalvular (ă-văl′vū-lăr) Without valves.

avascular (ă-văs′kū-lăr) [Gr. *a*-, not, + L. *vasculum*, little vessel] Lacking in blood vessels or having a poor blood supply, said of tissues such as cartilage.

avascularization (ă-văs″kū-lăr-ĭ-zā′shŭn) Expulsion of blood from tissues, esp. the extremities, as in the use of Esmarch's bandage.

Avellis' paralysis syndrome [Georg Avellis, Ger. laryngologist, 1864–1916] Paralysis of half of the soft palate, pharynx, and larynx and loss of pain, heat, and cold sensations on the opposite side.

average Arithmetic mean.

aversion therapy A form of behavior therapy designed to reduce or extinguish unwanted or hazardous behaviors. The goal of aversion therapy is to have the patient associate the undesirable behavior with something noxious, such as a foul taste, a headache, a hot flash, nausea or vomiting, or profuse sweating. In chemical aversion therapy, for example, a patient may be treated with a drug that makes the consumption of another substance, such as alcohol, extremely unpleasant. The use of chemical aversion therapy is controversial because in some cases it produces side effects that may themselves be injurious or life-threatening. Aversion therapy also has been used to treat other forms of drug dependence, eating disorders, paraphilias, self-mutilation, and tobacco abuse. SEE: *disulfiram*.

avian Concerning birds.

aviation medicine Aerospace medicine.

aviation physiology The branch of physiology that deals with conditions encountered by humans in flying, mountain climbing, or space flight. The conditions studied are hypoxia, extreme temperature and radiation, effects of acceleration and deceleration, weightlessness, motion sickness, enforced inactivity, mental stress, acclimatization, and disturbance of biological rhythm.

avidin (ăv′ĭ-dĭn) [L. *avidus*, greedy] A protein in egg whites that binds biotin and inhibits its absorption. Avidin is destroyed by cooking.

avidity **1.** Eagerness; a strong attraction for something. **2.** The ability of antibodies to bind to antigens; the net affinity of all binding sites of antibodies.

avirulent (ă-vĭr′ū-lĕnt) [Gr. *a*- not, + L. *virus*, poison] Without virulence.

avitaminosis (ā-vī″tă-mĭ-nō′sĭs) [″ + *vitamin* + *osis*, condition] Disease caused by vitamin deficiency. SEE: *vitamin*. **avitaminotic** (-mĭ-nŏt′ĭk), *adj.*

avivement (ă-vēv-mŏn′) [Fr.] Surgical trimming of wound edges before suturing them.

Avogadro's law (ŏv-ō-gŏd′rōs) [Amadeo Avogadro, It. physicist, 1776–1856] Equal volumes of gases at the same pressure and temperature contain equal numbers of molecules.

Avogadro's number Number of molecules, 6.0221367×10^{23}, in one gram-molecular weight of a compound.

avoidance (ă-voyd′ăns) The conscious or unconscious effort to escape from situations or events perceived by the individual to be threatening to personal comfort, safety, or well-being.

avoirdupois measure (ăv″ĕr-dĕ-poyz′) [Fr., to have weight] A system of weighing or measuring articles in which 7000 grains equal 1 lb. SEE: Weights and Measures Appendix.

AVPU An acronym used to remind health care providers of the worsening stages of a patient's mental status. It stands for **a**lert; responds to **v**erbal stimuli; responds to **p**ainful stimuli; and **u**nresponsive.

avulsion (ă-vŭl′shŭn) [Gr. *a*-, not, + L. *vellere*, to pull] **1.** A tearing away forcibly of a part or structure. If surgical repair is necessary, a sterile dressing may be applied while surgery is awaited. If fingers, toes, feet, or even entire limbs are completely avulsed and separated, members are recovered. **2.** The complete separation of a tooth from its alveolus, which under appropriate conditions may be reimplanted. The term usually refers to dental injuries resulting from acute trauma. SYN: *evulsion*.

phrenic nerve a. Elevation of a side of the diaphragm and semicollapse of the corresponding lung by excision of part of the phrenic nerve.

awareness, fertility The identification of the days during a woman's menstrual cycle when her potential for conception is highest. SEE: *basal temperature chart; mucus, cervical; mittelschmerz*.

A.W.H.O.N.N. *Association of Women's Health, Obstetric, and Neonatal Nurses*. Formerly Nurses' Association of the American College of Obstetrics and Gynecology (NAACOG).

axanthopsia (ăk″săn-thŏp′sē-ă) [″ + *xanthos*, yellow, + *opsis*, vision] Yellow blindness.

axenic (ă-zĕn′ĭk) [″ + *xenos*, stranger] Germ free, as pert. to animals, or pure, as pert. to cultures or microorganisms; sterile.

axial (ăk′sē-ăl) [L. *axis*, axle] Situated in or pert. to an axis.

axifugal (ăks-ĭf′ū-găl) Centifugal.

axilemma (ăk″sĭ-lĕm′ă) [″ + Gr. *lemma*, husk] Axolemma.

axilla (ăk-sĭl′ă) *pl.* **axillae** [L. *axilla*] The armpit.

axilla conformer A splint designed to prevent adduction contractures after severe burns to the axillary region.

axillary (ăk′sĭ-lār-ē) Pert. to the axilla.

axillofemoral bypass graft (ăk″sĭl-ō-fĕm′or-ăl) The surgical establishment of a connector between the axillary artery and the common femoral arteries. A synthetic artery graft is used and implanted subcutaneously. This technique is used in treating patients with insufficient blood flow to the legs (peripheral vascular disease).

axio- (ăk′sē-ō) [L. *axis*, axle] Combining form meaning *relating to an axis;* in dentistry, the long axis of the tooth.

axiobuccal (ăk″sē-ō-bŭk′kăl) [L. *axis*, axle, + *bucca*, cheek] Concerning the angle formed by the long axis of the tooth and the buccal walls of a cavity of the tooth.

axioincisal (ăk″sē-ō-ĭn-sī′zăl) [″ + *incisor*, a cutter] Concerning the angle formed by the long axis of the tooth and the incisal walls of a cavity in the tooth.

axiolabial (ăk″sē-ō-lā′bē-ăl) [″ + *labialis*, pert. to the lips] Concerning the angle formed by the long axis of the tooth with the labial walls of a cavity in the tooth.

axiolingual (ăk″sē-ō-lĭng′gwăl) [″ + *lingua*, tongue] Concerning the angle formed by the long axis of the tooth and the lingual walls of a cavity in the tooth.

axiomesial (ăk″sē-ō-mē′zē-ăl) [″ + Gr. *mesos*, middle] Concerning the angle formed by the long axis of a tooth and the mesial walls of a cavity in the tooth.

axio-occlusal (ăk″sē-ō-ŏ-klū′zăl) [″ + *occlusio*, closure] Concerning the angle formed by the long axis of the tooth and the occlusal walls of a cavity in the tooth.

axioplasm (ăk′sē-ō-plăzm) [″ + LL. *plasma*, form, mold] The cytoplasm of an axon.

axiopulpal (ăk″sē-ō-pŭl′păl) [″ + *pulpa*, pulp] Concerning the angle formed by the long axis of a tooth and the pulpal walls of a cavity in the tooth.

axipetal (ăk-sĭp′ĕt-ăl) Centripetal.

axis [L.] **1.** A real or imaginary line that runs through the center of a body or about which a part revolves. **2.** The second cervical vertebra, or epistropheus; it bears the odontoid process (dens), about which the atlas rotates.

basicranial a. Axis connecting the basion and gonion.

basifacial a. Axis from the subnasal point to the gonion.

binauricular a. Axis between the two auricular points.

cardiac a. A graphic representation of the main conduction vector of the heart, determined through measurements of direction and amplitude of the complexes in several leads on a 12-lead electrocardiogram. Normal axis is zero to +90°.

celiac a. Axis between the celiac artery and the abdominal aorta.

condylar a. A projected line connecting the condyles of the mandible. Movement of the mandible is rotation around this imaginary line. SYN: *mandibular a.*

frontal a. An imaginary line, running from side to side in the frontal plane, about which the anterior to posterior movement occurs. Also called *coronal axis.*

hinge a. Condylar a.

mandibular a. Condylar a.

neural a. Central nervous system.

optic a. A line that connects the anterior and posterior poles of the eye.

principal a. In optics, a line that passes through the optical center or nodal point of a lens perpendicular to the surface of the lens.

sagittal a. Imaginary line running anterior-posterior, about which frontal plane motion occurs.

transverse mandibular a. Condylar a.

visual a. A line passing from the object of vision directly through the center of the cornea and lens to the fovea.

axis cylinder Axon (2).

axis deviation A shift of the normal electrical vectors of the heart, seen sometimes as a result of conduction disease, enlargement of the chambers of the heart, obstructive lung disease, or other conditions.

axo- [Gr. *axon*, axis] Combining form meaning *axis* or *axon.*

axofugal (ăk-sŏf′ū-găl) Axifugal.

axolemma (ăk″sō-lĕm′ă) [″ + *lemma*, husk] The cell membrane of an axon. SYN: *axilemma.*

axolysis (ăk-sŏl′ĭ-sĭs) [″ + *lysis*, dissolution] Destruction of the axis cylinder of a nerve.

axometer (ăk-sŏm′ĕ-tĕr) [″ + *metron*, measure] Measuring device for adjusting eyeglasses so that the lenses are suitable for the optic axes of the eyes.

axon, axone (ăk′sŏn, -sōn) [Gr. *axon*, axis] **1.** A process of a neuron that conducts impulses away from the cell body. Typically, it arises from a portion of the cell devoid of Nissl granules, the axon hillock. Axons may possess either or both of two sheaths (myelin sheath and neurilemma) or neither. Axons are usually long and straight, and most end in synapses in the central nervous system or ganglia or in effector organs (e.g., motor neurons). They may give off side branches or collaterals. An axon with its sheath(s) constitutes a nerve fiber. **2.** A nerve cell process that resembles an axon in structure; specifically, the peripheral process of a dorsal root ganglion cell (sensory neuron) that functionally and embryologically is a dendrite, but structurally is indistin-

guishable from an axon. SYN: *axis cylinder; neuraxon.* SEE: *nerve; neuron.*
axonal (ăk′sŏn-ăl), *adj.*

axoneme (ăk′sŏn-nēm) [″ + *nema*, a thread] Axial thread of a chromosome.

axonometer (ăk-sō-nŏm′ĕ-tĕr) [″ + *metron*, measure] Device for determining the axis of astigmatism.

axonotmesis (ăk″sŏn-ŏt-mē′sĭs) [″ + *tmesis*, incision] Nerve injury that damages the nerve tissue without actually severing the nerve.

axopetal (ăk-sŏp′ĕ-tăl) [″ + L. *petere*, to seek] Conducted along an axon toward a cell body of a neuron.

axoplasm (ăk′sō-plăzm) [″ + LL. *plasma*, form, mold] The cytoplasm (neuroplasm) of an axon that encloses the neurofibrils.

ayurvedic medicine (ă″yŭr-vă′dĭc) [Sanskrit *ayus*, lifespan, life, + *veda*, knowledge, science] An ancient Hindu medical system, promoted by alternative medical practitioners as a means of restoring balance and health by harmonizing mind and body. It uses herbal remedies, massage therapy, yoga, and pulse diagnosis.

azalein (ă-zā′lē-ĭn) [L. *azalea*, azalea] A red dye.

azathioprine (ā″ză-thī′ō-prēn) A cytotoxic chemical substance used for immunosuppression. Trade name is Imuran.

azidothymidine Zidovudine.

azithromycin (ā-zĭth′rō-mī-sĭn) A macrolide antibiotic related to erythromycin. It is used primarily to treat infections caused by respiratory pathogens, such as *Haemophilus influenzae*, *Moraxella catarrhalis*, *Streptococcus pneumoniae*, and *Legionella pneumophila*, and urethritis caused by gonococci and chlamydia. Trade name is Zithromax.

azo- Prefix indicating the presence of —N:N— group in a chemical structure. This group is usually connected at both ends to carbon atoms. SEE: *azo compounds.*

azo compounds Organic substances that contain the azo group. An example is azobenzene, $C_6H_5N:NC_6H_5$. They are related to aniline and include important dyes and indicators. SEE: *indicator* for table.

azoospermia (ă-zō-ō-spĕr′mē-ă) [″ + *zoon*, animal, + *sperma*, seed] Absence of spermatozoa in the semen.

Azorean disease (ā-zor′ē-ăn) A form of hereditary ataxia present in Portuguese families whose ancestors lived in the Azores. It is a degenerative disease of the nervous system. Symptoms vary but may include gait ataxia, limitation of eye movements, widespread muscle fasciculations, mild cerebellar tremor, loss of reflexes in lower limbs, and extensor plantar reflex response.

azotemia (ăz″ō-tē′mē-ă) [″ + ″ + *haima*, blood] Presence of nitrogenous bodies, esp. urea in increased amounts, in the blood. SEE: *uremia.*

Azotobacter (ă-zō″tō-băk′tĕr) Rod-shaped, gram-negative, nonpathogenic soil and water bacteria that fix atmospheric nitrogen; the single genus of the family Azotobacteraceae.

azoturia (ăz″ō-tū′rē-ă) [″ + ″ + *ouron*, urine] An increase in nitrogenous compounds, esp. urea, in urine.

AZT *Azidothymidine*, the former name for zidovudine.

azure lunulae (ăz′ŭr loo′nū-lē) [O.Fr. *azur*, blue, + L. *lunula*, little moon] Blue discoloration of the base, or lunulae, of the fingernails. It may be seen in patients with hepatolenticular degeneration (Wilson's disease). Blue discoloration of the entire nail may be present in argyria and following therapy with quinacrine hydrochloride.

azurophil(e) (ăz-ū′rō-fĭl) [″ + Gr. *philein*, to love] Staining readily with azure dye.

azurophilia (ăz″ū-rō-fĭl′ē-ă) Condition in which some blood cells have azurophil granules.

azygography (ăz″ĭ-gŏg′ră-fē) [Gr. *a*-, not, + *zygon*, yoke, + *graphein*, to write] Radiography of the azygos veins by the use of an intravenous contrast medium.

azygos (ăz′ĭ-gŏs) [″ + *zygon*, yoke] **1.** Occurring singly, not in pairs. **2.** An unpaired anatomical part. **azygos, azygous** (ăz′ĭ-gŭs), *adj.*

azygos vein A single vein arising in the abdomen as a branch of the ascending lumbar vein. It passes upward through the aortic hiatus of the diaphragm into the thorax, then along the right side of the vertebral column to the level of the fourth thoracic vertebra, where it turns and enters the superior vena cava. In the thorax, it receives the hemiazygos, accessory azygos, and bronchial veins, as well as the right intercostal and subcostal veins. If the inferior vena cava is obstructed, the azygos vein is the principal vein by which blood can return to the heart.

azymia (ă-zĭ′mē-ă) [″ + *zyme*, ferment] Condition of absence of an enzyme.

B

β Beta, second letter of the Greek alphabet. SEE: *beta*.

B **1.** Symbol for the element boron. **2.** *Bacillus; Balantidium; barometric; base; bath; behavior; buccal.*

B.A. *Bachelor of Arts.*

Ba Symbol for the element barium.

BAAM *Beck airway airflow monitor.*

Babbitt metal (băb′ĭt) [Isaac Babbitt, U.S. inventor, 1799–1862] An antifriction alloy of copper, antimony, and tin used occasionally in dentistry.

Babcock's operation (băb′kŏks) [William Wayne Babcock, U.S. surgeon, 1872–1963] Extirpation of the saphenous vein; a treatment for varicose veins.

Babesia (bă-bē′zē-ă) [Victor Babès] A genus of the family Babesiidae that consists of tick-borne parasites, which invade the red blood cells of cattle, sheep, horses, dogs, and other vertebrate animals. Destruction of the red blood cells by the parasite causes hemolytic anemia.

B. bigemina The causative organism of Texas fever in cattle.

B. bovis The causative organism of hemoglobinuria and jaundice (redwater fever) in cattle.

babesiosis (bă-bē-zē-ō′sĭs) A rare, usually self-limited disease caused by an intraerythrocytic protozoan, *Babesia microti,* and perhaps other Babesia species. The disease is transmitted by deer ticks, and occurs most often in New England in the U.S. It has also been reported elsewhere. Severe forms are most likely to occur in elderly people and in people without functioning spleens. Rarely, the infection is transmitted by blood transfusion from an asymptomatic carrier. The incubation period may last from weeks to months.

SYMPTOMS: Symptoms include fever, chills, headache, sweats, myalgia, arthralgia, and nausea and vomiting.

DIAGNOSIS: The diagnosis is suggested when a patient with an appropriate outdoor exposure presents with typical symptoms, plus hemolytic anemia. Thick and thin blood smears and other laboratory techniques (e.g., the polymerase chain reaction) may be used *for definitive confirmation.*

PREVENTION: The skin should be protected from tick exposure. Asplenic persons should avoid endemic areas. After possible exposure, removal of ticks or their nymphs may prevent infection.

TREATMENT: Drugs used include atovaquone and quinine plus clindamycin or azithromycin, both given orally. Asplenic patients may require exchange transfusion.

Babinski's reflex (bă-bĭn′skēz) [Joseph Babinski, Fr. neurologist, 1857–1932] Dorsiflexion of the great toe when the sole of the foot is stimulated. Normally, when the lateral aspect of the sole of the relaxed foot is stroked, the great toe flexes. If the toe extends instead of flexes and the outer toes spread out, Babinski's reflex is present. It is a normal reflex in infants under the age of 6 months but indicates a lesion of the pyramidal (corticospinal) tract in older individuals. Care must be taken to avoid interpreting voluntary extension of the toe as Babinski's reflex.

Babinski's sign Loss of or diminished Achilles tendon reflex in sciatica.

baby [ME. *babie*] Infant.

battered b. A baby or child whose body provides evidence of physical abuse such as bruises, cuts, scars, fractures, or abdominal visceral injuries that have occurred at various times in the past. SEE: *battered child syndrome.*

blue b. An infant born with cyanosis, which may be caused by anything that prevents proper oxygenation of the blood, esp. a congenital anomaly that permits blood to go directly from the right to the left side of the heart without going through the lungs. The most common cyanotic congenital heart defects are tetralogy of Fallot, transposition of the great vessels, and hypoplastic left heart syndrome.

collodion b. A newborn covered with a collodion-like layer of desquamated skin; may be due to ichthyosis vulgaris.

baby bottle syndrome Decay of primary teeth in older infants and toddlers related to taking a bottle of punch or other sweet liquid to bed and retaining the liquid. This creates massive caries. SYN: *bottle mouth caries; nursing-bottle syndrome.*

Baby Doe regulations Federal, state, and hospital policies insuring that handicapped infants will receive nourishment, warmth, and life-saving treatment without regard to the quality of life.

BAC *blood alcohol concentration.*

bacciform (băk′sĭ-form) [″ + *forma,* form] Berry-shaped; coccal.

Bacillaceae (băs-ĭ-lā′sē-ē) A family of rod-shaped, usually gram-positive bacteria of the order Eubacteriales that produce endospores and are commonly found in soil. Genera of this family include *Bacillus* and *Clostridium.*

bacillar, bacillary (băs′ĭl-ăr, băs′ĭl-ăr-ē) **1.** Pert. to or caused by bacilli. **2.** Rod-like.

bacille Calmette-Guérin (bă-sēl′) An organism of the strain *Mycobacterium bovis,* weakened (attenuated) by long-term cultivation on bile-glycero-potato medium. SEE: *BCG vaccine.*

bacillemia (băs-ĭ-lē′mē-ă) [L. *bacillus,* rod, + Gr. *haima,* blood] The presence of bacilli in the blood.

bacilli (bă-sĭl′ī) Pl. of bacillus.

bacilliform (bă-sĭl′ĭ-form) [″ + *forma,* form] Resembling a bacillus in shape.

bacillophobia (băs″ĭ-lō-fō′bē-ă) [″ + Gr. *phobos,* fear] Morbid fear of bacilli.

bacillosis (băs″ĭ-lō′sĭs) [″ + Gr. *osis,* infection] Infection by bacilli.

bacilluria (băs″ĭ-lū′rē-ă) [″ + Gr. *ouron,* urine] Bacilli in the urine. SEE: *clean-catch method.*

Bacillus (bă-sĭl′ŭs) [L.] A genus of bacteria of the family Bacillaceae. All species are rod-shaped, sometimes occurring in chains. They are spore-bearing, aerobic, motile or nonmotile; most are gram-positive and nonpathogenic. A well-known species pathogenic to humans is *Bacillus anthracis,* which causes anthrax. SEE: illus.; *bacterium.*

bacillus *pl.* **bacilli 1.** Any rod-shaped microorganism. **2.** A rod-shaped microorganism belonging to the class Schizomycetes. SEE: *Bacillus; bacterium.*

acid-fast b. ABBR: AFB. A bacillus not readily decolorized by acids or other means when stained. *Mycobacterium tuberculosis* is one example of an acid-fast bacillus.

Bacillus species ABBR: Bacillus spp. All of the species of *Bacillus.*

bacitracin (băs-ĭ-trā′sĭn) An antibiotic substance obtained from a strain of *Bacillus subtilis.* Its antibacterial actions are similar to those of penicillin, including gram-positive cocci and bacilli and some gram-negative organisms. Because of its toxicity when used parenterally, bacitracin is usually applied topically in ointment form.

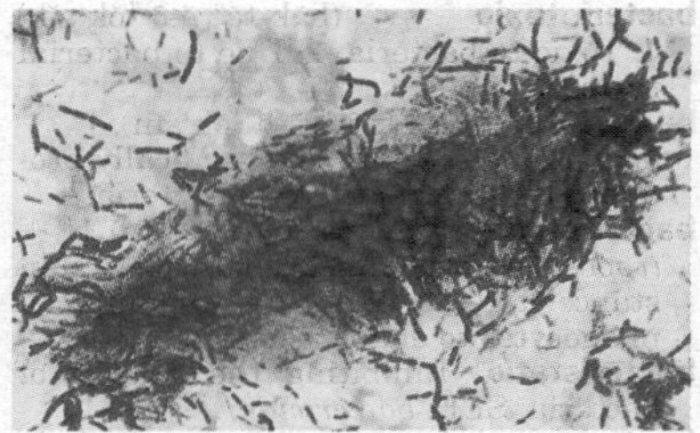

BACILLUS

Gram stain of *Bacillus* species (spores visible in upper left quadrant)

zinc b. The zinc salt of bacitracin, used in topical antibacterial ointments.

back 1. The dorsum. **2.** The posterior region of the trunk from neck to pelvis.

Misuse of the back is common among those who care for the sick. Therefore, it is important to learn basic concepts in back care. SEE: illus.; *back pain.*

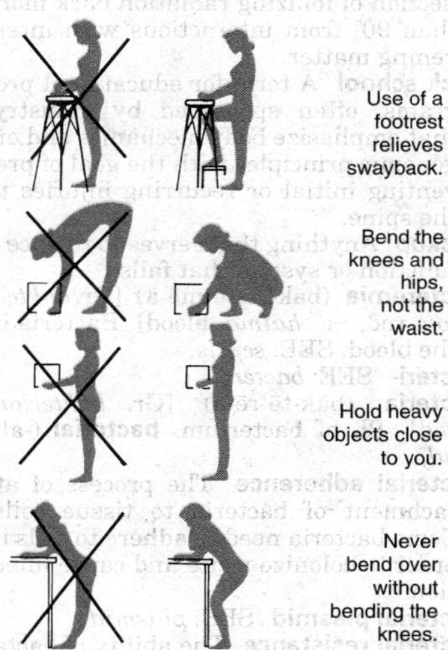

Use of a footrest relieves swayback.
Bend the knees and hips, not the waist.
Hold heavy objects close to you.
Never bend over without bending the knees.

HOW TO STAY ON YOUR FEET WITHOUT TIRING YOUR BACK

back board A stiff board on which a spine-injured patient is secured so that the patient's back, neck, and head are maintained in-line during transport to the hospital. This device should be used with a head immobilization device and a cervical collar.

long b.b. A long, flat board approx. 6 ft long and 2 ft wide, often made of wood, fiberglass, or plastic, used to immobilize a patient with a potential head and/or spine injury. This device should be used with a head immobilization device and a cervical collar.

short b.b. A flat board, approx. 3 ft long and 2 ft wide, used to immobilize a seated patient with a potential spinal injury. The short backboard is often used to remove an injured patient from a vehicle, after which the long backboard is used for full immobilization. This device should be used with a cervical collar.

backbone The vertebral column; spinal column. SEE: *vertebra.*

backcross In genetics the pairing of a first filial generation hybrid with an organism whose genotype is identical to the parental strain.

backflow Abnormal backward flow of fluids.

background radiation Total radioactivity from cosmic rays, natural radioactive materials, and other radiation that may be in a specific area.

back pain SEE: *pain, back*.

backrest An adjustable device that supports the back in bed.

backscatter In radiation physics, the deflection of ionizing radiation back more than 90° from interactions with intervening matter.

back school A term for educational programs, often sponsored by industry, that emphasize body mechanics and ergonomic principles with the goal of preventing initial or recurring injuries to the spine.

backup Anything that serves to replace a function or system that fails.

bacteremia (băk-tĕr-ē′mē-ă) [Gr. *bakterion,* rod, + *haima,* blood] Bacteria in the blood. SEE: *sepsis*.

bacteri- SEE: *bacterio-*.

bacteria (băk-tē′rē-ă) [Gr. *bakterion,* rod] Pl. of bacterium. **bacterial** (-ăl), *adj.*

bacterial adherence The process of attachment of bacteria to tissue cells. Some bacteria need to adhere to cells in order to colonize a site and cause infection.

bacterial plasmid SEE: *plasmid*.

bacterial resistance The ability of bacteria to survive and cause continuous infection in the presence of antibiotics. SEE: *antiviral resistance; antibiotic resistance; multidrug resistance; transfer factor.*

bacterial synergism The interaction of indigenous flora to allow a strain of bacteria to become pathogenic when it would normally be harmless.

bactericidal (băk″tĕr-ĭ-sī′dăl) Capable of killing bacteria.

bactericide (băk-tĕr′ĭ-sīd) [Gr. *bakterion,* rod, + L. *caedere,* to kill] An agent that destroys bacteria, but not necessarily their spores.

bactericidin Anything lethal to bacteria.

bacteriemia (băk-tĕr-ē-ē′mē-ă) Bacteremia.

bacterio-, bacteri- (băk-tē′rē-ō) Combining form meaning *bacteria*.

bacterioagglutinin (băk-tē″rē-ō-ă-gloo′tĭ-nĭn) [″ + L. *agglutinans,* gluing] An antibody in serum that causes agglutination, or clumping, of bacteria in vitro.

bacteriocidal (băk″tĕr-ē-ō-sī′dăl) Bactericidal.

bacteriocin (băk-tē′rē-ō-sĭn) Protein produced by certain bacteria that exerts a lethal effect on closely related bacteria. In general, bacteriocins are more potent but have a narrower range of activity than antibiotics. SEE: *colicin*.

bacteriogenic (băk-tē″rē-ō-jĕn′ĭk) [″ + *gennan,* to produce] **1.** Caused by bacteria. **2.** Producing bacteria.

bacteriohemagglutinin (băk-tē″rē-ō-hĕm″ă-gloo′tĭ-nĭn) [″ + *haima,* blood, + L. *agglutinans,* gluing] A hemagglutinin formed in the body by bacterial action.

bacteriohemolysin (băk-tē″rē-ō-hē-mŏl′ĭ-sĭn) [″ + ″ + *lysis,* dissolution] A hemolysin formed in the body by bacterial action.

bacteriologic, bacteriological [″ + *logos,* word, reason] Pert. to bacteriology.

bacteriologist An individual trained in the field of bacteriology.

bacteriology Scientific study of bacteria.

bacteriolysin (băk-tē″rē-ŏl′ĭ-sĭn) [″ + *lysis,* dissolution] A substance, esp. an antibody produced within the body of an animal, that is capable of bringing about the lysis of bacteria.

bacteriolysis (băk-tē″rē-ŏl′ĭ-sĭs) The destruction or dissolution of bacteria. **bacteriolytic** (-ō-lĭt′ĭk), *adj.*

bacteriophage (băk-tē′rē-ō-fāj″) [Gr. *bakterion,* rod, + *phagein,* to eat] A virus that infects bacteria. Bacteriophages are widely distributed in nature, having been isolated from feces, sewage, and polluted surface waters. They are regarded as bacterial viruses, the phage particle consisting of a head composed of either RNA or DNA and a tail by which it attaches to host cells. SYN: *phage*.

bacteriophytoma (băk-tē″rē-ō-fī-tō′mă) [″ + *phyton,* plant, + *oma,* tumor] A tumor-like growth caused by bacteria.

bacterioprecipitin (băk-tē″rē-ō-prē-sĭp′ĭ-tĭn) Precipitin produced in the body by the action of bacteria.

bacterioprotein (băk-tē″rē-ō-prō′tē-ĭn) Any of the proteins within the cells of bacteria.

bacteriopsonin (băk-tē″rē-ŏp′sō-nĭn) An opsonin, acting on bacteria.

bacteriosis (băk-tē″rē-ō′sĭs) [″ + *osis,* condition] Any disease caused by bacteria.

bacteriostasis (băk-tē″rē-ŏs′tă-sĭs) [″ + *stasis,* standing still] The arrest of bacterial growth.

bacteriostatic (băk-tē-rē-ō-stăt′ĭk) Inhibiting or retarding bacterial growth.

bacteriotoxic (băk-tē″rē-ō-tŏk′sĭk) **1.** Toxic to bacteria. **2.** Due to bacterial toxins.

bacteriotoxin (băk-tē″rē-ō-tŏk′sĭn) [″ + *toxikon,* poison] Toxin specifically produced by or destructive to bacteria.

bacteriotropin (băk-tē″rē-ŏt′rō-pĭn) [″ + *tropos,* a turn] An opsonin or a substance that enhances the ability of phagocytes to engulf bacteria.

bacteristatic Inhibiting the growth of bacteria. SEE: *bactericidal*.

bacterium *pl.* **bacteria** A one-celled organism without a true nucleus or cell organelles, belonging to the kingdom Procaryotae (Monera). The cytoplasm is surrounded by a rigid cell wall com-

Common Bacterial Infections

Organism	Type of and/or Site of Infection
Gram-Positive Bacteria	
Clostridium difficile	Pseudomembranous colitis
Staphylococcus aureus	Pneumonia, cellulitis, boils, toxic shock, postoperative bone/joints, eyes, peritonitis
Staphylococcus epidermidis	Postoperative bone/joints, IV line–related phlebitis
Streptococcus pneumoniae (pneumococcus)	Pneumonia, meningitis, otitis media, sinusitis, septicemia
Streptococcus pyogenes	Scarlet fever, pharyngitis, impetigo, rheumatic fever, erysipelas
Streptococcus viridans	Endocarditis
Gram-Negative Bacteria	
Campylobacter jejuni	Diarrhea (most common worldwide cause)
Escherichia coli	Urinary tract, pyelonephritis, septicemia, gastroenteritis, peritonitis
Haemophilus influenzae	Pneumonia, meningitis, otitis media, epiglottitis
Klebsiella pneumoniae	Pneumonia, wounds
Legionella pneumophilia	Pneumonia
Neisseria gonorrhoeae	Gonorrhea
Neisseria meningitidis (meningococcus)	Meningitis
Pseudomonas aeruginosa	Wounds, urinary tract, pneumonia, IV lines
Salmonella enteritidis	Gastroenteritis, food poisoning
Salmonella typhi	Typhoid fever
Shigella dysenteriae	Dysentery
Vibrio cholerae	Cholera

posed of carbohydrates and other chemicals that provide the basis for the Gram stain. Some bacteria also produce a polysaccharide or polypeptide capsule for additional protection, particularly from phagocytosis by white blood cells. Bacteria synthesize DNA, RNA, and proteins, and they can reproduce independently but may need a host to provide food and a favorable environment. Millions of nonpathogenic bacteria live on human skin and mucous membranes; these are called *normal flora*. Bacteria that cause disease are called *pathogens*. SEE: table.

CHARACTERISTICS: *Shape:* There are three principal forms of bacteria. *Spherical* or *ovoid* bacteria occur as single cells (micrococci) or in pairs (diplococci), clusters (staphylococci), chains (streptococci), or cubical groups (sarcinae). *Rod-shaped* bacteria are called bacilli, more oval ones are called coccobacilli, and those forming a chain are called streptobacilli. *Spiral* bacteria are rigid (spirilla), flexible (spirochetes), or curved (vibrios). SEE: illus.

Size: On average, bacilli measure about 1 μm in diameter by 4 μm in length. They range in size from less than 0.5 to 1.0 μm in diameter to 10 to 20 μm in length for some of the spirilla.

Reproduction: Binary fission is the usual method of reproduction, but some bacteria exchange genetic material with members of the same species or different species. Reproductive rate is affected by changes in temperature, nutrition, and pH. If the environment becomes unfavorable, some bacilli form spores, in which their genetic material is condensed and surrounded by a thick wall. Spores are highly resistant to heat, drying, and disinfectants. When the environment again becomes favorable, the spores germinate.

Mutation: Bacteria, like all living things, undergo mutations, and the environment determines which mutations are beneficial and have survival value. Certainly beneficial to bacteria, though not at all to humans, are the mutations that provide resistance to the potentially lethal effects of antibiotics.

Motility: None of the cocci are capable of moving, but most bacilli and spiral forms can move independently. Locomotion depends on the possession of one or more flagella, slender whiplike appendages that work like propellers.

Food and oxygen requirements: Most bacteria are heterotrophic (require organic material as food). If they feed on living organisms, they are called *parasites;* if they feed on nonliving organic material, they are called *saprophytes*. Bacteria that obtain their energy from inorganic substances, including many

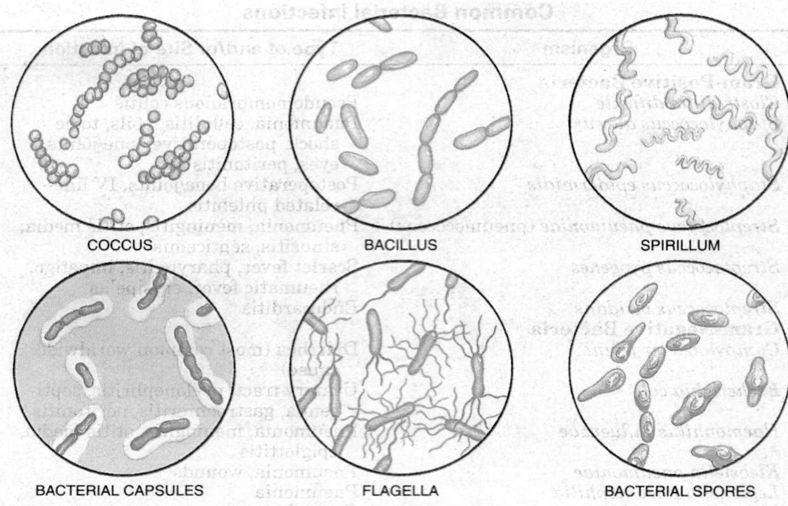

BACTERIA

Bacterial shapes and specialized structures (×1000)

of the soil bacteria, are called *autotrophic* (self-nourishing). Bacteria that require oxygen are called aerobes; those that grow only in the absence of oxygen are called anaerobes. Bacteria that grow both with and without oxygen are facultative anaerobes. Most bacteria in the human intestines are anaerobic. SEE: *infection, opportunistic*.

Temperature requirements: Although some bacteria live at very low or very high temperatures, the optimum temperature for most human pathogens is 97° to 99°F (36° to 38°C).

ACTIVITIES: *Enzyme production:* Bacteria produce enzymes that act on complex food molecules, breaking them down into simpler materials; they are the principal agents of decay and putrefaction. Putrefaction, the decomposition of nitrogenous and other organic materials in the absence of air, produces foul odors. Decay is the gradual decomposition of organic matter exposed to air by bacteria and fungi.

Toxin production: Special molecules called *adhesins* bind bacteria to the host cells. Once attached, the bacteria may produce poisonous substances called toxins. There are two types: exotoxins, enzymes that are released by bacteria into their host, and endotoxins, which are parts of the cell walls of gram-negative bacteria and are toxic even after the death of the cell. Endotoxins stimulate production of cytokines that can produce widespread vasodilation and shock. SEE: *endotoxin; sepsis*.

Miscellaneous: Some bacteria produce pigments; some produce light, thus appearing luminescent in the dark. Many chemicals are produced as a result of bacterial activity, among them acids, gases, alcohol, aldehydes, ammonia, carbohydrates, and indole. Pathogenic forms produce hemolysins, leukocidins, coagulases, and fibrinolysins. Soil bacteria play an important role in various phases of the nitrogen cycle (nitrification, nitrogen fixation, and denitrification).

IDENTIFICATION: Several methods are used to identify bacteria in the laboratory: SEE: illus.

Culture: Bacteria are grown on various culture media; a visible colony containing millions of cells may be visible within several hours. A colony is usually composed of the descendants of a single cell. Each species of bacteria grows in colonies with a characteristic color, shape, size, texture, type of margin or edge, and particular chemical features. Groups of cells can then be examined under a microscope, usually with Gram's stain. In addition, colonies can be separated and antibiotics applied to assess their sensitivity to different drugs.

Hanging drop: Unstained bacteria in a drop of liquid are examined under ordinary or dark-field illumination.

Gram's stain: Gram-positive bacteria retain dye, turning purple; gram-negative bacteria can be decolorized by alcohol and colored red by a second dye;

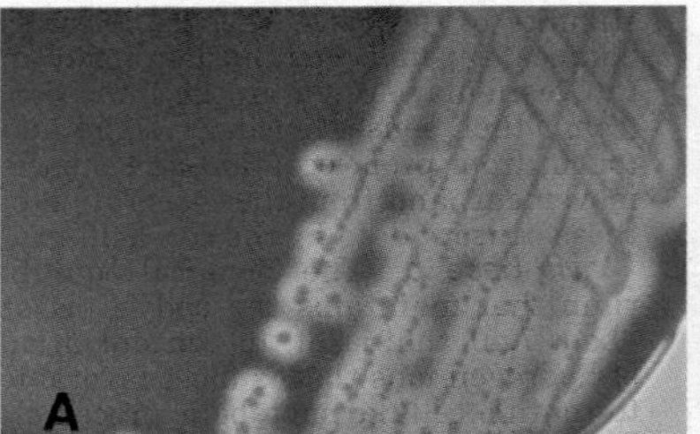

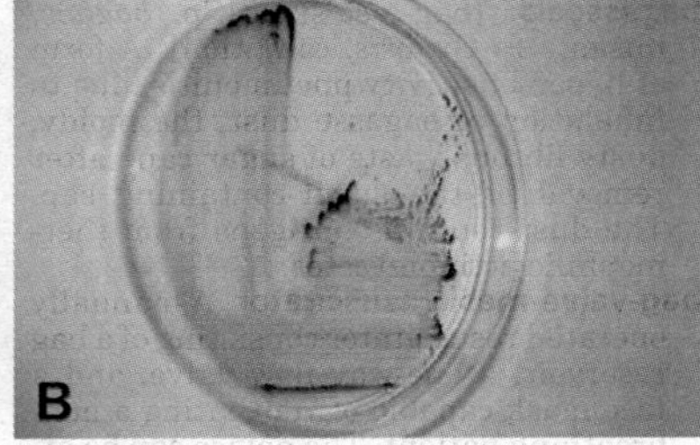

BACTERIA

(A) Group A streptococci; beta-hemolysis on blood agar; (B) salmonella; H2S production (black) on SS (*Salmonella-Shigella*) agar

acid-fast bacteria retain the dye even when treated with an acid. Bacteria are often described by a combination of their response to Gram's stain and their appearance. For example, "gram-positive staphylococcus" indicates a cluster of spheres that stain purple, whereas gram-negative bacilli are rod-shaped and pink.

Immunofluorescence: Bacteria stained with fluorescein and examined under a microscope equipped with fluorescent light appear yellow-green.

antibody-coated b. **1.** A bacterium coated with an antibody that acts as an opsonin to make the bacterium more susceptible to phagocytosis. **2.** A laboratory test using fluorescein-labeled antibodies to locate antigens with which the antibody links. SEE: *opsonin.*

flesh-eating b. A colloquial name given in the popular press to a rare invasive infection of the skin and underlying soft tissue by group A streptococcus. The infection is very difficult to treat with antibiotics alone because it progresses rapidly through tissue planes. Emergency surgical debridement is required. SEE: *necrotizing fasciitis.*

bacteriuria (băk-tē″rē-ū′rē-ă) [Gr. *bakterion,* rod, + *ouron,* urine] The presence of bacteria in the urine.

asymptomatic b. Bacteria in the urine without symptoms of urinary tract infection or pyelonephritis. This condition may occasionally precede symptomatic urinary tract infection. It is common in elderly women and in patients with indwelling urinary catheters. In children, it may be a sign of underlying urinary tract abnormalities. Screening for asymptomatic bacteriuria is recommended for pregnant women at 12 to 16 weeks' gestation. Screening school-age children is not beneficial.

significant b. Concentration of pathogenic bacteria in the urine of 10^5 per ml or greater. Concentrations above this level have been thought to represent evidence of urinary tract infection, although infection may be present at much lower levels.

bacteroid (băk′tĕr-oyd) [″ + *eidos,* form, shape] **1.** Resembling a bacterium. **2.** A structurally modified bacterium.

Bacteroides (băk-tĕr-oyd′ēz) A genus of non-spore-forming, gram-negative, rod-shaped, anaerobic bacteria that occur normally in digestive, respiratory, and genital tracts and are often found in necrotic tissue and in the blood after an infection. Some species are pathogenic and may be implicated in peritonitis and peritoneal abscesses. *Bacteroides* are the most common bacteria in the colon, where they outnumber *Escherichia coli* by at least 100 to 1; the species most commonly encountered is *B. fragilis.*

bad breath Offensive odor of the breath. Its origin may be in the mouth or nose, lungs, blood, or digestive tract. Many individuals have bad breath due to drying of the oral mucosa. On awakening, those who snore or sleep with their mouths open may have particularly noticeable bad breath. If bad breath is due to an ingested food, such as onions or garlic, local therapy with a mouthwash will be of no benefit because the odor is present in the blood and is excreted from the lungs. Other causes are respiratory infections such as bronchiectasis or lung abscess, acute necrotizing gingivitis, herpetic gingivostomatitis, periodontal disease, dental caries, cigarette smoking, hepatic failure, or diabetic ketoacidosis. SYN: *halitosis.* SEE: *hepatic coma.*

baffle In respiratory care, a component of a nebulizer designed to remove large airborne particles.

bag [ME. *bagge*] A sack or pouch.

colostomy b. A watertight receptacle that holds the discharge from a colostomy site.

Douglas b. SEE: *Douglas bag.*

b.of waters Amnion.

Politzer b. SEE: *Politzer bag.*

bagassosis (băg-ă-sō′sĭs) [Sp. *bagazo,* husks, + Gr. *osis,* condition] A form of hypersensitivity pneumonitis, due to inhalation of bagasse dust, the moldy, dusty fibrous waste of sugar cane after removal of the sugar-containing sap. The dust contains antigens from thermophilic actinomycetes.

bag-valve-mask resuscitator A manually operated resuscitator consisting of a bag reservoir, a one-way flow valve, and a face mask capable of ventilating a nonbreathing patient. The device can be attached to an oxygen source to increase the oxygen concentration delivered to the patient. SEE: illus.

Bailey, Harriet [U.S. nurse educator, b. 1875] The first nurse educator to write a textbook on psychiatric nursing. *Nursing Mental Diseases* was published by Macmillan in 1920 and was the standard text for psychiatric nursing for two decades.

baker [AS. *bacan,* cook by dry heat] Two or more electric lamps mounted in semicircular containers used for applying heat to various parts of the body. They are also called *electric light bakers*.

Baker's cyst [William M. Baker, Brit. surgeon, 1839–1896] A synovial cyst (pouch) arising from the synovial lining of the knee. It occurs in the popliteal fossa.

BAL *British anti-lewisite.*

balance (băl′ăns) [L. *bilanx*] **1.** Scale; a device for measuring weight. **2.** A state of equilibrium; condition in which the intake and output of substances such as water and nutrients are approx. equal. SEE: *homeostasis*. **3.** Coordination and stability of the body in space. Normal balance depends on information from the vestibular system in the inner ear, from other senses such as sight and touch, from proprioception and muscle movement, and from the integration of these sensory data by the cerebellum.

acid-base b. The chemical equilibrium that maintains the body's pH at about 7.40; that is, at the concentration of hydrogen ions that is most favorable to routine cellular metabolic processes. The equilibrium is maintained by the action of buffer systems of the blood and the regulatory (homeostatic) functions of the respiratory and urinary systems. Disturbances in acid-base balance result in acidosis or alkalosis. SEE: *pH*.

analytical b. A very sensitive scale used in chemical analysis.

fluid b. The balance between intake and output (excretion) of fluids, esp. water, in the body.

metabolic b. Comparison of the intake and excretion of a specific nutrient. The balance may be negative when an excess of the nutrient is excreted or positive when more is taken in than excreted.

nitrogen b. The body state in which intake of nitrogen in protein foods is equal to nitrogen output, principally through loss of nitrogenous substances in the urine and feces.

balance beam In occupational and physical therapy, a device used to assess and improve balance and motor coordination; usually consists of a narrow beam elevated several inches from the floor.

balance board A device usually consisting of a padded platform mounted on a

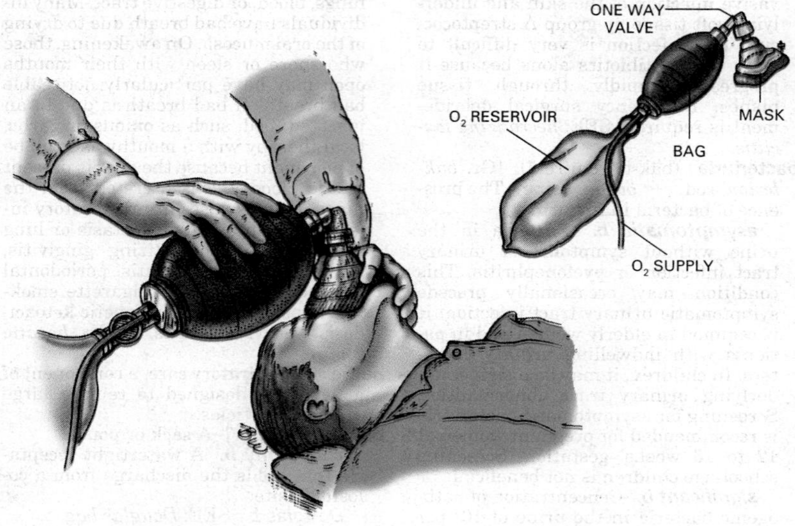

BAG–VALVE–MASK RESUSCITATOR

curved base. It is commonly used in therapy with children having central nervous system deficits to facilitate the development of appropriate equilibrium-related postural reflexes. It is also used in patients/clients of all ages to stimulate lower extremity and trunk proprioception and kinesthetic sense.

balan- SEE: *balano-*.

balanic (bă-lăn′ĭk) [Gr. *balanos,* glans] Pert. to the glans clitoridis or glans penis.

balanitis (băl-ă-nī′tĭs) [″ + *itis,* inflammation] Inflammation of the skin covering the glans penis.

b. xerotica obliterans Sclerotic and atrophic patches on the skin of the penis that can cause narrowing of the urinary meatus and phimosis. The cause is chronic balanoposthitis, and the condition is associated with penile lichen sclerosis (e.g., circumcision for phimosis).

TREATMENT: High-dose topical steroids or long courses of antibiotics are given.

balano-, balan- (băl′ă-nō) [Gr. *balanos,* glans] Combining form meaning *glans penis* or *glans clitoridis*.

balanocele (băl′ă-nō-sēl″) [″ + *kele,* tumor, swelling] Protrusion of the glans penis through a rupture of the prepuce.

balanoplasty (băl′ă-nō-plăs″tē) [″ + *plassein,* to form] Plastic surgery of the glans penis.

balanoposthitis (băl″ă-nō-pŏs-thī′tĭs) [″ + *posthe,* prepuce, + *itis,* inflammation] Balanitis.

balanopreputial (băl″ă-nō-prē-pū′shē-ăl) Pert. to the glans penis and prepuce.

balanorrhagia (băl″ă-nŏ-rā′jē-ă) [″ + *rhegnynai,* burst forth] Balanitis with pus formation.

balantidial (băl-ăn-tĭd′ē-ăl) Pert. to *Balantidium,* a genus of protozoa.

balantidiasis (băl″ăn-tĭ-dī′ă-sĭs) Infection caused by infestation with *Balantidium coli.*

SYMPTOMS: Symptoms include abdominal pain, diarrhea, vomiting, weakness, and weight loss.

TREATMENT: Treatment consists of tetracyclines, metronidazole, or paromomycin.

Balantidium (băl-ăn-tĭd′ē-ŭm) [Gr. *balantidion,* a bag] A genus of ciliated protozoa. A number of species are found in the intestines of both vertebrates and invertebrates.

B. coli A normal parasite of swine and the largest protozoan parasitic of humans. It causes balantidiasis. SEE: illus.

balanus (băl′ă-nŭs) [Gr. *balanos,* glans] The glans penis or glans clitoridis.

baldness [ME. *ballede,* without hair] Lack of or partial loss of hair on the head. SEE: *alopecia*.

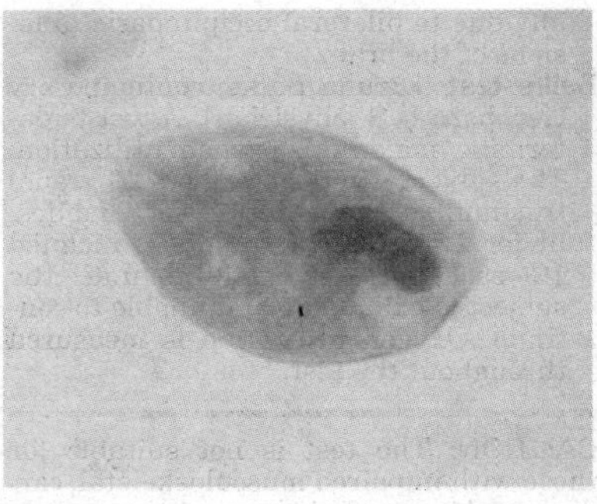

BALANTIDIUM COLI **(X400)**

Edge of cell appears indistinct because of cilia (×400)

male pattern b. Baldness in the male due to influence of the male hormone testosterone. Genetic predisposition is also a factor, and baldness does not usually occur in males having no familial tendency to become bald. Minoxidil or finasteride have helped stimulate growth of hair in some individuals. SEE: illus.

Balint's syndrome [Rudolph Balint, Hungarian physician, 1874–1929] Inability to scan the peripheral visual field and to grasp an object under visual guidance, and visual inattention; usu-

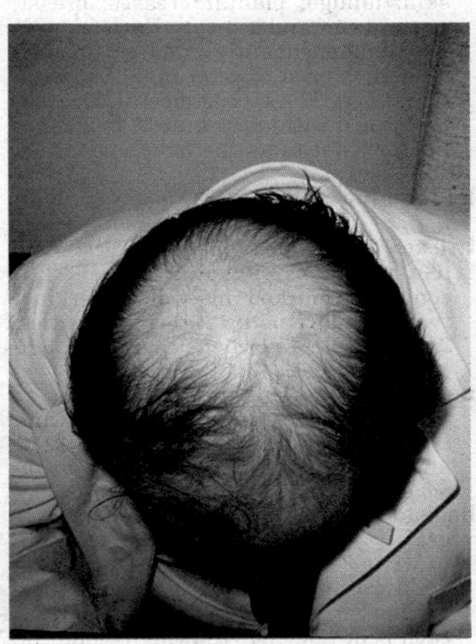

MALE PATTERN BALDNESS

ally due to bilateral occipitoparietal lesions of the brain.

Balke test [Bruno Balke, contemporary Ger.-born U.S. physician] A test to determine maximum oxygen utilization. The subject walks on a flat (0% grade) treadmill at a constant rate of 3.5 miles/hr for 2 min. The treadmill is inclined 1% each successive minute until the subject is exhausted and unable to continue. Oxygen utilization is measured throughout the test.

CAUTION: The test is not suitable for those with impaired musculoskeletal, cardiovascular, or respiratory systems.

ball A spherical object.

b. of the foot The padded portion of the anterior extremity of the sole of the foot.

b. of the thumb The thenar eminence of the thumb.

Ballard tool, Ballard score [Jeanne Ballard, American neonatologist] A system for estimating newborn gestational age by rating physical and neuromuscular characteristics of maturity. For infants born between 20 and 28 weeks' gestation, Ballard tools are more accurate than other systems of estimating gestational age. Five neuromuscular markers are assessed: posture, square window (degree of wrist flexion), arm recoil, popliteal angle (degree of knee flexion); scarf sign (ability to extend infant's arm across the chest past the midline); and heel-to-ear extension. Seven physical characteristics are also evaluated: skin; lanugo; plantar creases; breast; eye and ear; and genitals. Each factor is scored independently, and then an overall sum is used to determine the gestational age. The tool is most accurate if performed within the first 12 to 20 hr of life, or as soon as the baby's condition stabilizes.

ball bearing feeder SEE: *mobile arm support.*

ballism, ballismus (băl'ĭzm, bă-lĭz'mŭs) [Gr. *ballismos,* jumping about] **1.** A condition marked by violent jerking, twisting movements of the extremities. **2.** An obsolete term for paralysis agitans.

ballistics (bă-lĭs'tĭks) [Gr. *ballein,* to throw] The science of the motion and trajectory of bullets, bombs, rockets, and guided missiles. SEE: *gunshot wound.*

ballistocardiograph (bă-lĭs″tō-kăr'dē-ō-grăf) [″ + *kardia,* heart, + *graphein,* to write] A mechanism for measuring and recording the impact caused by the discharge of blood from the heart at each beat and the resulting recoil. The minute movements of the body with each heartbeat are recorded as they are transmitted to the special platform that supports the subject.

balloon [Fr. *ballon,* great ball] **1.** To expand, dilate, or distend, as to expand a cavity by filling it with air or water in a bag. **2.** A flexible, expandable object that can be placed inside a vessel or cavity to expand it or at the end of a catheter to prevent its removal. SEE: *catheter; percutaneous transluminal coronary angioplasty.*

balloon tamponade, nasal SEE: *nosebleed* for illus.; *epistaxis.*

ballottable (bă-lŏt'ă-bl) Capable of identification by ballottement.

ballottement (băl-ŏt-mŏn') [Fr. *balloter,* to toss about] **1.** A palpatory technique used to detect or examine a floating object in the body, such as an organ. It is used in examining the abdomen esp. when ascites is present, and joint effusions. **2.** A diagnostic maneuver in pregnancy. The fetus or a fetal part rebounds when displaced by a light tap of the examining finger through the vagina.

balm [Gr. *balsamon,* balsam] **1.** Balsam. **2.** A soothing or healing ointment.

b. of Gilead **1.** Mecca balsam from *Commiphora opobalsamum,* probably biblical myrrh. **2.** Balsam fir, source of Canadian balsam. **3.** Poplar bud resin.

balneology (băl-nē-ŏl'ō-jē) [L. *balneum,* bath, + Gr. *logos,* word, reason] The science of baths and bathing.

balneotherapy, balneotherapeutics (băl″nē-ō-thĕr'ă-pē, -thĕr″ă-pū'tĭks) [″ + Gr. *therapeia,* treatment] The use of baths in treatment of disease.

balsam (bawl'săm) [Gr. *balsamon,* balsam] A fragrant, resinous, oily exudate from various trees and plants. It is used in topical preparations to treat irritated skin or mucous membrane.

b. of Peru A dark brown, viscid, resinous liquid obtained from the bark of the tree *Myroxylon perierae* or *M. balsamum.*

BALT *bronchus-associated lymphoid tissue.*

bamboo spine In ankylosing spondylitis, a spinal column that on a radiograph resembles a bamboo stalk.

Bancroft's filariasis [Joseph Bancroft, Brit. physician, 1836–1894] A filarial infection caused by *Wuchereria bancrofti.* SEE: *elephantiasis.*

band **1.** A cord or tapelike tissue that connects or holds structures together. SEE: *bundle; ligament; tract.* **2.** Any appliance that encircles or binds the body or a limb. **3.** A segment of a myofibril. **4.** A metal strip or seamless band for attaching orthodontic appliances to teeth. **5.** An immature, unsegmented neutrophil in the differential section of a complete blood count. An increase in bands indicates that all mature neutrophils have been released from the bone marrow, usually during severe inflammation or infection, and that the marrow is releasing immature cells.

H b. A narrow band in the center of the A band of a sarcomere; it contains only thick (myosin) filaments and is bisected by the M line. SYN: *Engelmann's disk; H zone*.

I b. In muscle fibers, the light band segment of a sarcomere, containing lateral ends of thin (actin) filaments. There is one to either side of the medial A band. SYN: *isotropic b.*

iliotibial b. A thick, wide fascial layer from the iliac crest along the lateral thigh to the fascia around the lateral aspect of the knee joint. Fibers from the tensor fascia lata and gluteus maximus insert into the proximal band.

isotropic b. I b.

bandage [ME. *bande,* a band] **1.** A piece of soft, usually absorbent gauze or other material applied to a limb or other part of the body as a dressing. **2.** To cover by wrapping with a piece of gauze or other material.

Bandages are used to hold dressings in place, apply pressure to a part, immobilize a part, obliterate cavities, support an injured area, and check hemorrhages. Types of bandages include roller, triangular, four-tailed, many-tailed (Scultetus), quadrangular, elastic (elastic knit, rubber, synthetic, or combinations of these), adhesive, elastic adhesive, newer cohesive bandages under various proprietary names, impregnated bandages (plaster of paris, waterglass [silica], starch), and stockinet. Use of a self-adhering, form-fitting roller bandage facilitates bandaging by eliminating the special techniques needed when ordinary gauze roller bandages are used. SEE: illus.; *sling*.

CAUTION: Skin-to-skin contact will, if continuous, cause ulceration or infection.

abdomen b. A single wide cravat or several narrow ones used to hold a dressing in place or to exert a moderate pressure.

Ace b. Trade name for a woven elastic bandage available in various widths and lengths. It provides uniform support, yet permits joint movement without loosening the bandage.

adhesive b. A bandage made of adhesive tape.

amputation-stump b. An elastic bandage applied to an amputation stump to control postoperative edema and to shape the stump. The elastic bandage is applied in a recurrent or figure-of-eight fashion with more pressure applied to the distal, rather than the proximal, portion of the limb.

ankle b. Bandage in which one loop is brought around the sole of foot and the other around the ankle; it is secured in front or on the side.

axilla b. A bandage with a spica-type turn starting under the affected axilla, crossing over the shoulder of the affected side, and making the long loop under the opposite armpit.

back b. Open bandage to the back; applied the same as a chest bandage, the point being placed above the scapula of the injured side.

Barton b. A double figure-of-eight bandage for the lower jaw.

breast b. Suspensory bandage and compress for the breasts.

butterfly b. An adhesive bandage formerly used in place of sutures to hold wound edges together. The application of filmy sterile adhesive strips has replaced this entity (e.g., Steri-Strips™)

buttocks b. T or double-T bandage or open triangular bandage for the buttocks.

capeline b. A bandage applied to the head or shoulder or to a stump like a cap or hood.

chest b. Figure-of-eight (spica), many-tailed (Scultetus), or triangular (open-chest) bandage for the chest.

circular b. A bandage applied in circular turns about a part.

cohesive b. A bandage made of material that sticks to itself but not to other substances; used to bandage fingers and extremities or to build up pads.

cravat b. A triangular bandage folded to form a band around an injured part.

cravat elbow b. A bandage in which the elbow is bent about 45° and the center of the bandage is placed over the point of the elbow. One end is brought around the forearm and the other end around the upper arm; the bandage is pulled tight and tied.

cravat b. for clenched fist A hand bandage to arrest bleeding or to produce pressure. The wrist is placed on the center of the cravat, one end is brought around over the fist and back to the starting point, and the same procedure is then repeated with the other end. The two ends are pulled tight, twisted, and carried around the fist again so that pressure is placed on the flexed fingers.

cravat b. for fracture of clavicle Bandage in which one first puts a soft pad 2 × 4 in. (5.1 × 10.2 cm) in the forepart of the axilla. A sling is made by placing the point of the open bandage on the affected shoulder, the hand and wrist laid on it and directed toward the opposite shoulder, the point brought over and tucked underneath the wrist and hand. The ends are then lifted and the bandage is laid flat on the chest, the covered hand is carried up on the shoulder, the ends are brought together in the back and tied, the tightness being

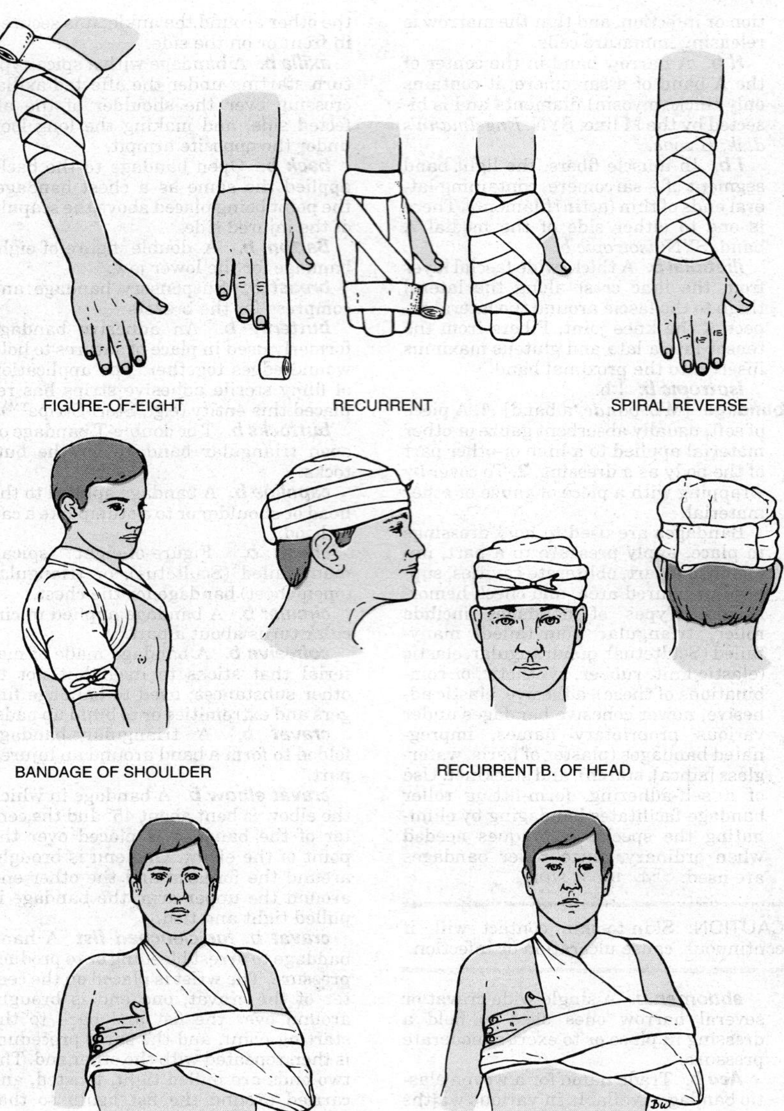

TYPES OF BANDAGES

decided by how high the shoulder should be carried. A cravat bandage is then applied horizontally above the broad part of the elbow and tied over a pad on the opposite side of the chest. Tightening this cravat pushes out the shoulder.

cravat b. sling A bandage used for support of the hand or a fractured upper arm. The wrist is laid upon the center of the cravat bandage, the forearm being held at right angle, and the two ends are carried around the neck and tied. SEE: *binder*.

crucial b. SEE: *T b.*

demigauntlet b. A bandage that covers the hand but leaves the fingers uncovered.

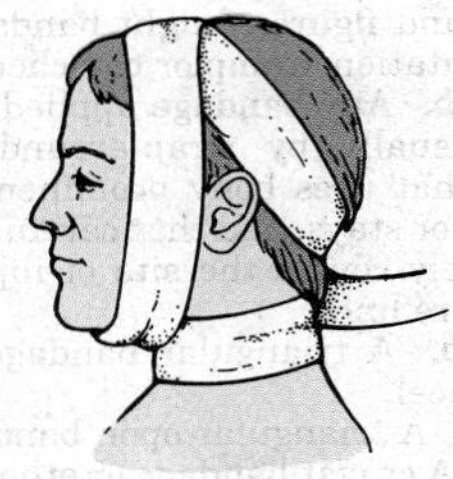

BARTON

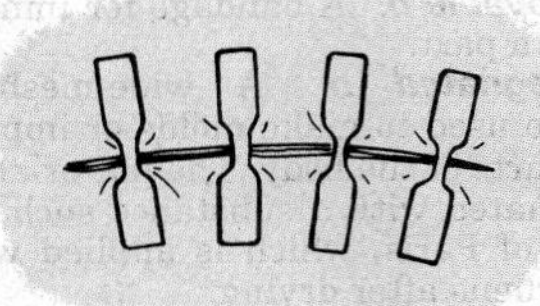

BUTTERFLY STRIPS

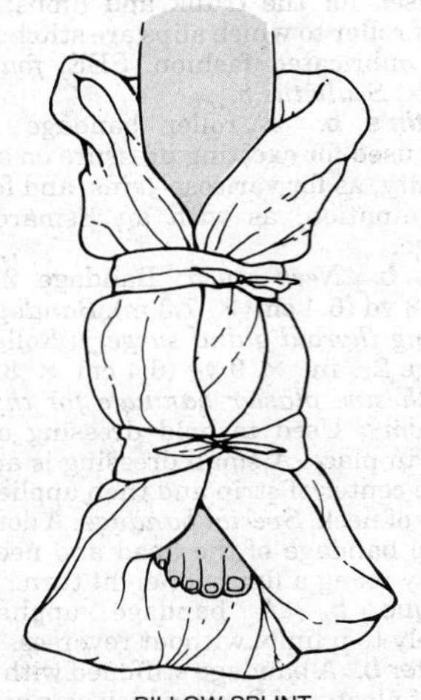

PILLOW SPLINT

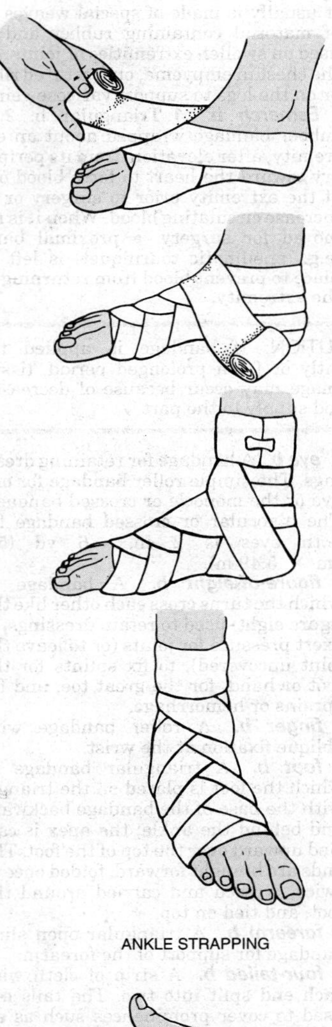

ANKLE STRAPPING

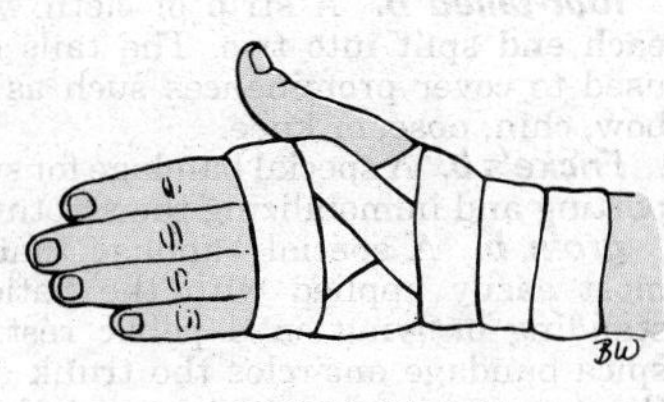

WRIST BANDAGE

TYPES OF BANDAGES

ear b. T bandage for the ear. A piece is sewn across the right angle of the T bandage.

elastic b. A bandage that can be stretched to exert continuous pressure. It usually is made of special weaves or of material containing rubber and is used on swollen extremities or joints, on the chest in empyema, on fractured ribs, or on the legs to support varicose veins.

Esmarch b. **1.** Triangular b. **2.** A rubber bandage wrapped about an extremity, after elevation, from its periphery toward the heart to force blood out of the extremity prior to surgery or to increase circulating blood. When it is removed for surgery, a proximal band (e.g., pneumatic tourniquet) is left in place to prevent blood from returning to the extremity.

CAUTION: If bandage is applied too tightly or for a prolonged period, tissue damage may occur because of decreased blood supply to the part.

---

eye b. A bandage for retaining dressings. The simple roller bandage for one eye or the monocle or crossed bandage. The binocular or crossed bandage for both eyes is 2 in. × 6 yd (5.1 cm × 5.49 m).

figure-of-eight b. A bandage in which the turns cross each other like the figure eight; used to retain dressings, to exert pressure for joints (or to leave the joint uncovered), to fix splints for the foot or hand, for the great toe, and for sprains or hemorrhage.

finger b. A roller bandage with oblique fixation at the wrist.

foot b. A triangular bandage in which the foot is placed on the triangle with the base of the bandage backward and behind the ankle; the apex is carried upward over the top of the foot. The ends are brought forward, folded once or twice, crossed and carried around the foot, and tied on top.

forearm b. A triangular open sling bandage for support of the forearm.

four-tailed b. A strip of cloth with each end split into two. The tails are used to cover prominences such as elbow, chin, nose, or knee.

Fricke's b. A special bandage for supporting and immobilizing the scrotum.

groin b. A special bandage that is most easily applied with the patient standing or lying on a pelvic rest. A spica bandage encircles the trunk and the crossing is placed either anteriorly or laterally. To bandage both groins, the double spica is used. Such a double bandage is used principally in applying a plaster cast.

hand b. A demigauntlet bandage that secures a dressing on the back of the hand. For thumb and hand, the ascending spica of the thumb, with spiral of the hand, is used. A triangular bandage is used for an open bandage of the hand. A descending spica is used for the thumb and figure-of-eight bandage for an amputation stump or clenched fist.

head b. Any bandage applied to the head, usually by wrap-around technique, that uses bony prominences as anchors or stays, and that carefully and completely covers the site of injury or the suture line.

heel b. A triangular bandage used for the heel.

hip b. A triangular open bandage of the hip. A cravat bandage or other band is tied around the waist; the point of another bandage is slipped under and rolled or pinned directly above the position of the wound. The base is rolled up and the ends are carried around the thigh, crossed, and tied.

immovable b. A bandage for immobilizing a part.

impregnated b. A wide-meshed bandage used to make molds or immobilize parts of the body. The material is impregnated with a substance such as plaster of Paris, which is applied wet and hardens after drying.

knee b. The knee cravat; triangular and the figure-of-eight bandages are used.

leg b. A bandage applied by fixing the initial end by a circular or oblique fixation at the ankle or with a figure-of-eight of the foot and ankle.

many-tailed b. A bandage with split ends used for the trunk and limbs; a piece of roller to which slips are stitched in an imbricated fashion. SEE: *four-tailed b.; Scultetus b.*

Martin's b. A roller bandage of rubber used for exerting pressure on an extremity, as for varicose veins, and for exsanguination, as with an Esmarch bandage.

neck b. *Neck spica*: Bandage 2½ in. × 8 yd (6.4 cm × 7.3 m). *Bandage following thyroid gland surgery*: Roller bandage 2½ in. × 9 yd (6.4 cm × 8.2 m). *Adhesive plaster bandage for thyroidectomy*: Used to hold dressing on wound in place. A small dressing is applied to center of strip and then applied to back of neck. *Special bandage*: A double-loop bandage of the head and neck made by using a figure-of-eight turn.

oblique b. A bandage applied obliquely to a limb, without reverses.

plaster b. A bandage stiffened with a paste of plaster of Paris, which sets and becomes very hard.

pressure b. A bandage for applying pressure; usually used to stop hemorrhage or prevent edema.

protective b. A bandage that covers a part or keeps dressings in place.

***quadrangular* b.** A towel or large handkerchief, folded variously and applied as a bandage of head, chest, breast, or abdomen.

***recurrent* b.** A bandage over the end of a stump.

***reversed* b.** A bandage applied to a limb in such a way that the roller is inverted or half twisted at each turn so as to make it fit smoothly and resist slipping off the limb. SEE: *spiral reverse b.*

***roller* b.** A long strip of soft material, usually from ½ to 6 in. (1.3 to 15.2 cm) wide and 2 to 5 yd (1.83 to 4.57 m) long, rolled on its short axis. When rolled from both ends to meet at the center, it is called a double-headed roller.

***rubber* b.** A rubber roller bandage used to apply pressure to prevent swelling or hemorrhage of a limb. SEE: *Esmarch bandage.*

***Scultetus* b.** A many-tailed bandage; a succession of interlocking, overlapping bands originally used to enclose a rigid support against a fractured extremity but now used without the splint or impregnated as a supporting bandage of the abdomen or lower extremity. SEE: *Scultetus binder* for illus.

***shoulder* b.** An open bandage of the shoulder (spica bandage); a shawl bandage of both shoulders and neck.

***spica* b.** A bandage in which a number of figure-of-eight turns are applied, each a little higher or lower, overlapping a portion of each preceding turn so as to give an imbricated appearance. This type of bandage is used to support, to exert pressure, or to retain dressings on the breast, shoulder, limbs, thumb, great toe, and hernia at the groin.

***spiral reverse* b.** A technique of twisting, in its long axis, a roller bandage on itself at intervals during application to make it fit more uniformly. These reverse folds may be necessary every turn or less, depending on the contour of the part being bandaged.

***suspensory* b.** A bandage for supporting any part but esp. the breast or scrotum.

***T* b.** A bandage shaped like the letter T and used for the perineum and, in certain cases, the head.

***tailed* b.** A bandage split at the end.

***triangular* b.** A 36- to 42-in. (232- to 271-cm) square of material, usually muslin, that is cut diagonally, making two triangular bandages; frequently used in first aid. SYN: *Esmarch bandage* (1). SEE: *triangular bandage* for illus.

***Velpeau* b.** A special immobilizing roller bandage that incorporates the shoulder, arm, and forearm.

bandage roller A device for rolling bandages.

banding The use of chemicals to stain chromosomes so that the characteristic bands may be visualized.

Bandl's ring (băn′d'ls) [Ludwig Bandl, Ger. obstetrician, 1842–1892] Ringlike thickening and indentation at the junction of the upper and lower uterine segments that obstructs delivery of the fetus. SEE: *pathologic retraction ring.*

bandpass, photometric The wavelength selectivity of a laboratory photometer.

bandwidth In electronics the range of frequencies within which performance with respect to some characteristic falls within specified limits.

bank A stored supply of body fluids or tissues for use in another individual (e.g., blood bank, eye bank, kidney bank, tissue bank).

***sperm* b.** A repository for the storage of semen used for artificial insemination. In some banks the specimen is frozen. SEE: *Standard and Universal Precautions Appendix.*

Bankart lesion An avulsion injury of the capsule and labrum from the glenoid rim of the glenohumeral joint. This lesion is the most common reason for recurrent shoulder dislocations.

Banting, Sir Frederick Grant Canadian scientist, 1891–1941; co-discoverer of insulin, with Charles Herbert Best and John J. R. Macleod in 1922; Nobel laureate 1923.

Banti's syndrome (băn′tēz) [Guido Banti, It. physician, 1852–1925] A syndrome combining anemia, splenic enlargement, hemorrhages, and ultimately cirrhosis of the liver; secondary to portal hypertension.

bar **1.** A metal piece attaching two or more units of a removable dental prosthesis. **2.** A rigid component of a splint or brace. **3.** A section of tissue that connects two similar structures.

***lumbrical* b.** A component of a hand splint that rests on the dorsal surface of the proximal phalanges to prevent hyperextension of the metacarpophalangeal joints.

***median* b.** Contracture or constriction of the vesical neck of the bladder caused by benign hypertrophy or fibrosis of the prostate. It may obstruct the flow of urine from the bladder.

bar- SEE: *baro-.*

baragnosis (băr-ăg-nō′sĭs) [Gr. *baros,* weight, + *a-,* not, + *gnosis,* knowledge] The inability to estimate weights; the opposite of barognosis. It is indicative of a parietal lobe lesion. SYN: *abarognosis.*

Bárány's caloric test [Robert Bárány, Austrian physician and physiologist, 1876–1936. Awarded Nobel Prize in medicine in 1914] Evaluation of vestibular function by irrigation of the ear canal with either warm or cold water. Normally when warm water is used, rotatory nystagmus toward the irrigated ear is observed; with cold water, the normal response is rotatory nystagmus away from the irrigated ear. If vestibular function is impaired, the response may be absent or diminished. If one ear is normal and the other is not, a comparison between the two may be made.

barbiturates (băr-bĭt′ū-rāts, băr-bĭ-tū′rāts) A group of organic compounds derived from barbituric acid (e.g., amobarbital, phenobarbital, secobarbital) that are used to treat and prevent convulsions, relieve anxiety, or aid sleep. Side effects include drowsiness, depressed respirations, decreased blood pressure, and decreased body temperature. These drugs can also cause tolerance and dependence. SEE: *Poisons and Poisoning Appendix.*

barbotage (băr-bō-tŏzh′) [Fr. *barboter,* to dabble] Repeated injection and withdrawal of fluid, as in gastric lavage, or the administration of an anesthetic into the subarachnoid space by alternate injection of anesthetic and withdrawal of cerebrospinal fluid into the syringe.

barbula hirci (băr′bū-lă hĭr′sī) [L. *barbula,* little beard, + *hircus,* goat] **1.** Hairs present on the ears. **2.** Axillary hair.

bar code A parallel array of alternately spaced black bars and white spaces representing a coded number, numbers, or letters, depending on the format employed. It is used clinically for patient sample identification.

baresthesia (băr-ĕs-thē′zē-ă) [Gr. *baros,* weight, + *aisthesis,* sensation] Sense of weight or pressure; pressure sense.

bariatrics (băr″ē-ă′trĭks) [″ + *iatrike,* medical treatment] The branch of medicine that deals with prevention, control, and treatment of obesity.

baritosis Pneumoconiosis caused by inhalation of barium dust.

barium (bă′rē-ŭm) SYMB: Ba. A soft metallic element of the alkaline earth group; atomic mass 137.373, atomic number 56.

b. sulfate A radiopaque contrast medium used in radiographic studies of the gastrointestinal tract.

barium compounds Compounds containing barium and suitable diluents or additives. They are used in the form of insoluble barium sulfate, to visualize, that is, to outline, the hollow viscera in roentgenography. Poisoning occasionally occurs when the soluble salts are used accidentally in place of the insoluble sulfate. SEE: *Poisons and Poisoning Appendix.*

barium meal The ingestion of barium sulfate to outline the esophagus, stomach, and small intestines during x-ray or fluoroscopic examination. The exam may be used as an alternative to endoscopy to diagnose reflux, dysphagia, peptic disease, or other upper gastrointestinal conditions. Also called *upper G.I. series.*

PROCEDURE: If the exam or procedure does not follow a barium enema, the patient should receive nothing by mouth after midnight on the night before the test. No food or liquids should be taken by mouth until the last image is produced. If the test is done within a few days after a barium enema examination, it is important to be sure the colon is free of barium, which could interfere with visualization of the stomach and intestines. A cleansing enema the evening before the test may remove residual barium from the colon.

barium swallow Radiographic examination of the esophagus during and after introduction of a contrast medium consisting of barium sulfate. Structural abnormalities of the esophagus (such as strictures or tumors) and vessels (such as esophageal varices) may be demonstrated.

barium test Nonspecific term for any exam involving use of barium sulfate as a radiopaque material for outlining anatomical areas such as the esophagus and other portions of the intestinal tract by use of radiographic or fluoroscopic examinations. SEE: *barium enema; barium meal.*

Barlow's disease [Sir Thomas Barlow, Brit. physician, 1845–1945] A deficiency disease due to lack of vitamin C (ascorbic acid). It occurs in both breast-fed and bottle-fed babies—usually between 6 and 12 months of age—who fail to receive adequate supplements of vitamin C. SEE: *scurvy, infantile.*

TREATMENT: Therapy includes vitamin C and adequate daily intake of fruit juices (orange, grapefruit, tomato).

Barlow's test A maneuver designed to detect subluxation or dislocation of the hip. The examiner adducts and then extends the legs. The examiner keeps his or her fingers over the heads of the femurs. A dysplastic joint will be felt to dislocate as the femur leaves the acetabulum.

baro-, bar- [Gr. *baros,* weight] Combining form meaning *weight* or *pressure.*

barognosis (băr-ŏg-nō′sĭs) [″ + *gnosis,* knowledge] The ability to estimate weights; the opposite of baragnosis.

barograph A device used to measure and record changes in atmospheric pressure.

baroreceptor (băr″ō-rē-sĕp′tor) A sensory nerve ending that is stimulated by changes in pressure. Baroreceptors are found in the walls of the atria of the heart, vena cava, aortic arch, and carotid sinus. SYN: *pressoreceptor.*

baroreflexes (băr″ō-rē′flĕk-sĕs) [″ + L. *reflexus,* bent back] Reflexes mediated or activated through a group of nerves located in various blood vessels in the intrathoracic and cervical areas and in the heart and its great vessels. They are sensitive to mechanical changes produced when the pressure inside the vessel to which they are attached is altered. The response is called a baroreflex. Because the nerve groups are stimulated by mechanical rather than chemical means, they are called mechanoreceptors.

baroscope (băr′ō-skōp) [″ + *skopein,* to examine] An instrument that registers changes in the density of air.

barostat A receptor that is sensitive to changes in pressure and provides feedback stimuli to counteract the changes. Such a feedback system is present in the part of the carotid sinus sensitive to changes in blood pressure.

barotitis (băr″ō-tī′tĭs) Aerotitis.

barotrauma (băr″ō-traw′mă) [″ + *trauma,* wound] Any injury caused by a change in atmospheric pressure between a potentially closed space and the surrounding area. SEE: *aerotitis; barotitis; bends.*

Barr body [Murray L. Barr, Canadian anatomist, b. 1908] Sex chromatin mass seen within the nuclei of normal female somatic cells. According to the Lyon hypothesis, one of the two X chromosomes in each somatic cell of the female is genetically inactivated. The Barr body represents the inactivated X chromosome.

barratry The practice of encouraging or sponsoring legal actions, esp. frivolous or unnecessary lawsuits.

barrel chest An increased anteroposterior chest diameter caused by increased functional residual capacity due to loss of elastic recoil in the lung. It is most often seen in patients with chronic obstructive pulmonary disease (i.e., chronic bronchitis and emphysema).

barren [O. Fr. *barhaine,* unproductive] Sterile; incapable of producing offspring.

Barrett's esophagus [Norman R. Barrett, Brit. surgeon, 1903–1979] Replacement of the squamous epithelium of the distal esophagus with metaplastic columnar epithelium as a result of chronic exposure of the esophagus to stomach acid. The pathological changes usually occur after many years of gastroesophageal reflux disease and are occasionally followed by adenocarcinoma of the distal esophagus. SEE: *gastroesophageal reflux disease.*

barrier [O. Fr. *barriere*] An obstacle, impediment, obstruction, boundary, or separation.

blood-brain b. ABBR: BBB. Special characteristics of the capillary walls of the brain that prevent potentially harmful substances (including many medications) from moving out of the bloodstream into the brain or cerebrospinal fluid. It consists of either the perivascular glial membrane or the vascular endothelium or both.

placental b. The selective ability of the placental membranes to limit the exchange of substances between the maternal and fetal circulations. Although water, oxygen and other gases, drugs, needed nutrients (e.g., glucose and amino acids), maternal antibodies, and viruses cross the barrier unimpaired, large molecules, red blood cells, bacteria, and protozoa cross it only through breaks in placental integrity.

primary radiation b. A wall or partition that shields the radiographer and others from direct exposure to x-rays. It must be capable of adequate lead equivalency to reduce the maximum possible x-ray beam strength to the level of background exposure.

secondary radiation b. A wall or partition that shields against scattering or leakage of x-rays.

barrier-free design The planning and arrangement of living environments that emphasize accessibility and use by persons with functional limitations.

Barthel index A widely used functional assessment of activities of daily living. It assesses a person's ability to perform feeding, transfers, personal grooming and hygiene, toileting, walking, negotiating stairs, and controlling bowel and bladder functions.

Bartholin's abscess (băr′tō-lĭnz) [Caspar Bartholin, Danish anatomist, 1655–1738] An abscess that develops when Bartholin's glands become occluded in an acute inflammatory process.

Bartholin's cyst Cyst commonly formed in chronic inflammation of Bartholin's glands.

Bartholin's ducts Large ducts of the sublingual salivary gland. They parallel Wharton's duct.

Bartholin's gland One of two small compound mucous glands located one in each lateral wall of the vestibule of the vagina, near the vaginal opening at the base of the labia majora.

bartholinitis (băr″tō-lĭn-ī′tĭs) [*Bartholin* + Gr. *itis,* inflammation] Inflammation of Bartholin's gland.

Barton, Clara U.S. nurse, 1821–1912. Founder of the American National Red Cross. She aided the wounded in the Civil War and was a contemporary of Florence Nightingale.

Bartonella (băr″tō-nĕl′ă) [A. L. Barton, S. Amer. physician, 1871–1950] A genus of bacteria of the family Bartonellaceae.

B. bacilliformis Motile gram-negative bacillus that causes bartonellosis.

B. elizabethae The organism previously known as *Rochalimaea elizabethae.* It causes an infection that has been identified most often in immunocompromised patients with HIV infection. It has been implicated as a cause of bacteremia and endocarditis.

B. henselae A gram-negative rod of the family Bartonellaceae that, together with *B. quintana,* causes acute and persistent bacteremia and localized tissue infection, which may lead to bacillary angiomatosis, bacillary peliosis, and other inflammatory responses. This infection can occur in immunocompromised and immunocompetent individuals but is seen most frequently in patients with HIV infection. *B. henselae,* previously named *Rochalimaea henselae,* is the causative agent of cat scratch disease. Therapy for bacillary angiomatosis is oral antibiotics. SEE: *bacillary angiomatosis; disease, cat scratch; peliosis, bacillary.*

B. quintana The organism previously known as *Rochalimaea quintana* or *Rickettsia quintana.* During World War I, it caused trench fever, a debilitating febrile illness, in battlefield troops. Together with *B. henselae,* it may cause bacillary angiomatosis, bacillary peliosis, and other inflammatory diseases. Treatment includes oral antibiotics.

bartonellosis (băr″tō-nĕl-ō′sĭs) [*Bartonella* + Gr. *osis,* condition] A disease caused by infection with *Bartonella bacilliformis,* transmitted by female sandflies *(Phlebotomus).* It occurs in the valleys of the Andes Mountains in Peru, Chile, Bolivia, and Colombia. The first clinical stage is noneruptive and is called Oroya fever, a severe, febrile, hemolytic anemia. The second stage, called verruga peruana, is eruptive and is marked by the appearance of small tumors on the skin and mucous membranes. SYN: *Carrion's disease.*

TREATMENT: The causative organism responds to several antibiotics, but ampicillin or chloramphenicol has the advantage of being effective against *Salmonella,* which may be present as a secondary infection.

Bartter's syndrome [Frederic Crosby Bartter, U.S. physician, 1914–1983] Hyperplasia of the juxtaglomerular cells of the kidney, hypokalemic alkalosis, and hyperaldosteronism without a rise in blood pressure. It usually occurs in children and may be accompanied by growth retardation. Etiology is unknown. Affected patients are treated with potassium supplements and angiotensin-converting enzyme inhibitors or potassium-sparing diuretics.

Baruch's law (băr′ooks) [Simon Baruch, Ger.-born U.S. physician, 1840–1921] The theory that water has a sedative effect when its temperature is the same as that of the skin and a stimulating effect when it is below or above the skin temperature.

bary- [Gr. *barys,* heavy] Prefix indicating *heavy, dull, hard.*

baryglossia (băr-ĭ-glŏs′ē-ă) [Gr. *barys,* heavy, + *glossa,* tongue] Slow, thick utterance of speech.

barylalia (băr-ĭ-lā′lē-ă) [″ + *lalia,* speech] Indistinct, husky speech due to imperfect articulation. SYN: *baryphonia* (2).

baryophobia The unreasonable fear that one's child will become obese. The allowed diet may be insufficient to support the child's growth and development needs.

baryphonia (băr″ĭ-fō′nē-ă) [″ + *phone,* voice] **1.** Heavy, thick quality of the voice. **2.** Barylalia.

basad (bā′săd) [Gr. *basis,* base, + L. *ad,* toward] Toward the base.

basal (bā′săl) **1.** Pert. to the base. **2.** Of primary importance.

basal ganglia Four masses of gray matter located deep in the cerebral hemispheres—caudate, lentiform, and amygdaloid nuclei and the claustrum. The caudate and lentiform nuclei and the fibers of the internal capsule that separate them constitute the corpus striatum. The function of the basal ganglia is complex. They contribute to some of the subconscious aspects of voluntary movement such as accessory movements and inhibiting tremor. They do not initiate movement but rather provide coordination of complex motor circuits. Neurotransmitters that affect the basal ganglia are acetylcholine, dopamine, gamma-aminobutyric acid (GABA), and serotonin.

basal metabolic rate ABBR: BMR. The metabolic rate as measured 12 hr after eating, after a restful sleep, no exercise or activity preceding test, elimination of emotional excitement, and in a comfortable temperature. It is usually expressed in terms of kilocalories per square meter of body surface per hour. It increases, for example, in hyperthyroidism.

basal ridge An eminence on the lingual surface of the incisor teeth, esp. the upper ones. It is situated near the gum. SYN: *cingulum* (2).

base [Gr. *basis,* base] **1.** The lower part of anything; the supporting part. **2.** The principal substance in a mixture. **3.** Any substance that combines with hydrogen ions (protons); a hydrogen ion acceptor (Bronsted base). Strong bases (such as sodium hydroxide, or lye) are corrosive to human tissues. Whether an unknown chemical compound is a base or an acid may be determined by the color produced when it is added to a solution containing an indicator. SYN: *alkali.* SEE: *acid; pH.* **4.** A substance that can donate a pair of electrons (Lewis base).

cavity b. In dentistry, the lining material placed in a cavity preparation, such as zinc phosphate, zinc oxide-eugenol, or calcium hydroxide along with small amounts of other medicinal or adhesive materials.

denture b. That part of the denture made of metal or resin, or both, that supports the artificial teeth and rests on abutment teeth or the residual alveolar ridge.

nucleic b. In molecular biology, a ring-shaped chemical—either a purine or a pyrimidine—that specifies the coded genetic structure of DNA and RNA. DNA is made up of the bases adenosine, cytosine, thymine, and guanine; RNA contains uracil, in place of thymine.

b. of radiographic film A layer of polyester or other suitable material that supports the film emulsion.

Basedow's disease (băz′ē-dōz) [Karl A. von Basedow, Ger. physician, 1799–1854] Graves' disease.

baseline (bās′līn) A known or initial value with which subsequent determinations of what is being measured can be compared (e.g., baseline temperature or blood pressure).

basement lamina [Gr. *basis,* base, + L. *lamina,* thin plate] The preferred term for a thin layer of delicate noncellular material of a fine filamentous texture underlying the epithelium. Its principal component is collagen. SYN: *basal lamina; basement membrane; hyaline membrane.*

baseplate (bās′plāt) A temporary, preformed shape made of wax, metal, or acrylic resin that represents the base of a denture; used in assessing the relations of maxillary-mandibular teeth or for placement of artificial teeth in denture preparation.

basi- [Gr. *basis,* base] SEE: *basio-.*

basial (bā′sē-ăl) [L. *basialis*] Pert. to the basion.

basiarachnoiditis (bā″sē-ă-răk″noy-dī′tĭs) [Gr. *basis,* base, + *arachne,* spider, + *eidos,* form, shape, + *itis,* inflammation] Inflammation of the arachnoid membrane at the base of the brain.

basic **1.** In chemistry, possessing the properties of a base. **2.** Fundamental.

Basic Trauma Life Support ABBR: BTLS. A continuing education course sponsored by the American College of Emergency Physicians for emergency medical providers to develop the skills of rapid initial assessment, management of life-threatening injuries, and early transport of the traumatized patient to the most appropriate facility.

Basidiomycetes (bă-sĭd″ē-ō-mī-sē′tēz) One of the four major classes of true fungi of the division Eumycetes, which includes toadstools, mushrooms, and tree fungi. This type of fungus is distinguished by basidiospores, sexual spores that form on a specialized structure called a basidium. Basidiomycetes cause plant diseases, and their toxins may be lethal to humans when eaten. Basidiospores have been implicated as a cause of allergic asthma.

basihyal (bā″sē-hī′ăl) [″ + *oeides,* hyoid] The body of the hyoid bone.

basilar (băs′ĭ-lăr) [L. *basilaris*] Basal (1).

basilateral (bā″sē-lăt′ĕr-ăl) [″ + L. *lateralis,* pert. to the side] Both lateral and basilar.

basilic (bă-sĭl′ĭk) [L. *basilicus*] Prominent, important.

b. vein The large vein on the inner side of the biceps just above the elbow. It is usually chosen for intravenous injection or withdrawal of blood.

basin An open, bowl-like container for holding liquids. It may be shaped to fit around a structure.

emesis b. A kidney-shaped basin that can fit close to the neck so vomitus may be collected.

basio-, basi- [Gr. *basis,* base] Combining form meaning *base* or *foundation.*

basioccipital bone (bā″sē-ŏk-sĭp′ĭ-tăl) [″ + L. *occiput,* head] The basilar process of the occipital bone.

basion (bā′sē-ŏn) The midpoint of the anterior border of the foramen magnum.

basiphobia (bā″sē-fō′bē-ă) [Gr. *basis,* a stepping, + *phobos,* fear] Fear of walking.

basirhinal (bā-sē-rī′năl) [Gr. *basis,* base, + *rhis,* nose] Pert. to the base of the brain and the nose.

basis (bā′sĭs) *pl.* **bases** [L., Gr.] The base of a structure or organ.

basisphenoid (bā-sē-sfē′noyd) [Gr. *basis,* base, + *sphen,* wedge, + *eidos,* form, shape] An embryonic bone that becomes the lower portion of the sphenoid bone.

basket [ME.] A netlike terminal arborization of an axon (or its collateral) of a basket cell that forms a network about the cell body of a Purkinje cell.

Basle Nomina Anatomica ABBR: BNA. An official anatomical nomenclature adopted by the German Anatomical Society in 1895, at Basel, Switzerland. It includes some 4500 terms. Revisions were published until 1955, when the Congress of Anatomists modified the nomenclature and applied the name Nomina Anatomica. SEE: *Nomina Anatomica.*

basophil(e) (bā′sō-fĭl, -fīl) [Gr. *basis,* base, + *philein,* to love] **1.** A cell or part of a cell that stains readily with basic dyes such as methylene blue. **2.** A type of cell found in the anterior lobe of the pituitary gland. It usually produces corticotropin, the substance that stimulates the adrenal cortex to secrete cortisol. **3.** One type of granulocytic white blood cell. Basophils make up less than 1% of all leukocytes but are essential to the nonspecific immune response to inflammation because of their role in releasing histamine and other chemicals that dilate blood vessels. SEE: *blood* for illus.

basophilia (bā-sō-fĭl′ē-ă) **1.** A pathological condition in which basophilic erythrocytes are found in the blood. **2.** A condition marked by a high number of basophilic leukocytes in the blood.

basophilic (bā-sō-fĭl′ĭk) Pert. to the staining characteristics of various cells.

basophilism (bā-sŏf′ĭ-lĭzm) A condition marked by an excessive number of basophils in the blood.

pituitary b. Cushing's syndrome.

basophobia (bās-ō-fō′bē-ă) [Gr. *basis,* a stepping, + *phobos,* fear] **1.** Abnormal fear of walking. **2.** Emotional inability to stand or walk in the absence of muscle disease.

Bassen-Kornzweig syndrome [Frank A. Bassen, U.S. physician, b. 1903; Abraham L. Kornzweig, U.S. physician, b. 1900] Abetalipoproteinemia.

Bassini's operation (bă-sē′nēz)[Edoardo Bassini, It. surgeon, 1844–1924] A specific surgical procedure for inguinal hernia.

BAT *brown adipose tissue.*

Bates exercises [William H. Bates, U.S. ophthalmologist, 1881–1931] A series of systematic vision exercises devised in the 19th century to relax, tone, and strengthen the eye muscles.

bath [AS. *baeth*] The medium and method of cleansing the body or any part of it, or treating it therapeutically as with air, light, vapor, or water. The temperature of the cleansing bath for a bed patient should be about 95°F (35°C) with a room temperature of 75° to 80°F (23.9° to 26.7°C).

THERAPEUTIC EFFECT: Warm and hot baths and applications soothe both the mind and the body. Gradually elevated hot tub and vapor baths relax all the muscles of the body. Hot baths promote vasodilation in the skin, drawing blood from the deeper tissues, and also help to relieve pain and stimulate nerves. Cold baths and applications abstract heat and stimulate reaction, esp. if followed by brisk rubbing of the skin. Cold constricts small blood vessels when applied locally. SEE: *hydrotherapy.*

air b. The therapeutic use of air, warmed or vaporized, on the nude body.

alcohol b. Application of a diluted alcohol solution to the skin as a stimulant and defervescent.

alkaline b. A bath in which 8 oz (227 g) of sodium bicarbonate or washing soda is added to 30 gal (114 L) of water.

alum b. A bath using alum in washing solution as an astringent.

antipyretic b. A cool water bath (65° to 75°F or 18.3° to 28.9°C). The patient should not be cooled to the point of shivering, as this indicates excessive heat loss.

aromatic b. A bath to which some volatile oil, perfume, or some herb is added.

astringent b. Bathing in liquid containing an astringent.

bed b. A bath for a patient confined to bed.

PATIENT CARE: All necessary equipment is assembled, the room temperature is adjusted to a comfortable level, and the room is checked for drafts. While shielding the patient, the health care provider removes the top covers and replaces them with a bath blanket for the patient's physical warmth. The patient's ability to bathe independently is assessed, and the patient is encouraged to do so to the extent possible and permitted. Bath water should be comfortably warm, 110° to 120°F (43.3° to 48.1°C), and the water should be changed as often as necessary to maintain the desired temperature and to permit thorough rinsing. The entire body, including the perineal area and genitalia, is washed, rinsed, and dried thoroughly, one area at a time. The patient remains covered except for the area being bathed. After the bath, lotion is applied to the skin (if not contraindicated), a clean gown is applied, the bed is remade with clean linens, and the patient's hair is combed or brushed. Oral hygiene is performed in conjunction with bathing; the health care provider helps if the patient requires assistance. When bathing obese patients, drying of crevices may be facilitated by using a hand-held hair dryer. Additional hair care (shampoo, dry shampoo, styling) is provided as necessary, following protocols.

bland b. Bath containing substances such as starch, bran, or oatmeal for the relief of skin irritation; an emollient bath.

brine b. Saline b.

bubble b. A bath in which the water contains many small bubbles produced mechanically as by an air pump or chemically by bubble bath preparations.

CAUTION: Perfumes used in bubble baths are frequently the cause of vaginitis and skin irritation, esp. in children.

---

carbon dioxide b. An effervescent saline bath consisting of water, salts, and carbon dioxide (CO_2). The natural CO_2 baths are known as Nauheim baths.

cold b. A bath in water at a temperature below 65°F (18.3°C).

colloid b. Emollient b.

continuous b. A bath administered for an extended period but seldom for longer than several hours. It is used in treating hypothermia or hyperthermia and certain skin diseases.

contrast b. Alternate immersion of hands or feet in hot water (1 min) then cold water (30 sec) for a prescribed length of time to promote circulation. The initial water temperature should be maintained throughout the bath, and the bath should end with immersion in cold water.

emollient b. A bath used for irritation and inflammation of skin and after erysipelas. SYN: *colloid b.* SEE: *glycerin b.; oatmeal b.; powdered borax b.; starch b.*

foam b. A tub bath to which an extract of a saponin-containing vegetable fiber has been added. Oxygen or carbon dioxide is driven through this mixture to create foam.

foot b. Immersion of the feet and legs to a depth of 4 in. (10 cm) above the ankles in water at 98°F (36.7°C).

full b. A bath in which the whole body except the head is immersed in water. It is sometimes called *complete bed bath,* implying that the caregiver bathes the patient.

glycerin b. A bath consisting of 10 oz (300 ml) of glycerin added to 30 gal (114 L) water.

herb b. A full bath to which is added a mixture of 1 to 2 lb (454 to 907 g) of herbs such as chamomile, wild thyme, or spearmint tied in a bag and boiled with 1 gal (3.8 L) of water.

hip b. Sitz b.

hot b. A tub bath with the water covering the body to slightly above the nipple level. The temperature is gradually raised from 98°F (36.7°C) to the desired degree, usually to 108°F (42.2°C).

hot air b. Exposure of the entire body except the head to hot air in a bath cabinet.

hyperthermal b. A bath in which the whole body except the head is immersed in water from 105° to 120°F (40.6° to 48.9°C) for 1 to 2 min.

kinetotherapeutic b. A bath given for underwater exercises of weak or partially paralyzed muscles.

lukewarm b. A bath in which the patient's body except the head is immersed in water from 94° to 96°F (34.4° to 35.6°C) for 15 to 60 min.

medicated b. A bath to which substances such as bran, oatmeal, starch, sodium bicarbonate, Epsom salts, pine products, tar, sulfur, potassium permanganate, and salt are added.

milk b. A bath taken in milk for emollient purposes.

mud b. The use of mud in order to apply moist heat.

mustard b. A stimulative hot foot bath consisting of a mixture of 1 tablespoon (15 ml) of dry mustard in a quart (946 ml) of hot water added to a pail or large basin filled with water of 100° to 104°F (37.8° to 40°C).

Nauheim b. A bath in which the body is immersed in warm water through which carbon dioxide is bubbled.

needle b. A bath in which water is forced at high speeds through small jets or openings onto the body. It is generally used for débridement.

neutral b. A bath in which no circulatory or thermic reaction occurs, temperature 92° to 97°F (33.3° to 36.1°C).

neutral sitz b. Same as sitz bath, except temperature is 92° to 97°F (33.3° to 36.1°C) or for foot bath 104° to 110°F (37.8° to 40°C), duration 15 to 60 min.

oatmeal b. A bath consisting of 2 to 3 lb (907 g to 1.4 kg) oatmeal added to 30 gal (114 L) water.

oxygen b. A bath given by introducing oxygen into the water through a special device that is connected to an oxygen tank.

paraffin b. A bath used to apply topical heat to traumatized or inflamed limbs. The limb is repeatedly immersed in warm paraffin, 104° to 150°F (37.8° to 65.6°C), and quickly withdrawn until it is encased in layers of the material. Paraffin may be applied with a paintbrush for larger joints.

powdered borax b. Bath consisting of ½ lb (227 g) added to 30 gal (114 L) water; 5 oz (150 ml) glycerin may be added.

saline b. Bath given in artificial seawater made by dissolving 8 lb (3.6 kg) of sea salt or a mixture of 7 lb (3.2 kg) of sodium chloride and ½ lb (227 g) of magnesium sulfate in 30 gal (114 L) of water. SYN: *brine b.; salt b.; seawater b.*

salt b. Saline b.

sauna b. A hot, humid atmosphere created in a small enclosed area by pouring water on heated rocks.

seawater b. Saline b.

sedative b. A prolonged warm bath. A continuous flow of water as well as an air cushion or back rest may be used.

sheet b. A bath given by wrapping the patient in a sheet previously dipped in water 80° to 90°F (26.7° to 32.2°C), and by rubbing the whole body with vigorous strokes on the sheet.

shower b. Water sprayed down upon the body from an overhead source.

sitz b. The immersion of thighs, buttocks, and abdomen below the umbilicus in water. In a hot sitz bath the water is first 92°F (33.3°C) and then elevated to 106°F (41.1°C). SYN: *hip b.*

sponge b. A bath in which the patient is not immersed in a tub but washed with a washcloth or sponge.

starch b. A bath consisting of 1 lb (454 g) of starch mixed into cold water, with boiling water added to make a solution of gluelike consistency, then added to 30 gal (114 L) of water.

stimulating b. A bath that increases cutaneous blood flow. SEE: *cold b.; mustard b.; saline b.*

sun b. Exposure of all or part of the nude body to sunlight.

sweat b. A bath given to induce perspiration.

towel b. A bath given by applying towels dipped in water 60° to 70°F (15.6° to 21.1°C) to the arms, legs, and anterior and posterior surfaces of trunk, and then removing the towels and drying the parts.

whirlpool b. A therapeutic stainless steel, fiberglass, or plastic tank that uses turbines to agitate and aerate water into which the body, or part of it, is immersed. Tanks come in various sizes to accommodate treatment of different body parts (Hubbard and 'low boy' tanks for full-body treatments, or extremity tanks for arm or leg treatments). Water temperature selection will vary depending on the condition of the patient, and the desired therapeutic outcome. Cold whirlpools (ranging from 32°–79°F) are useful in treating acute inflammation. Tepid whirlpools (79°–92°F) are used to facilitate exercise. Neutral temperatures (92°–96°F) are generally indicated for treatment of wounds or with patients who present with circulatory, cardiac, or sensory disorders or with neurological changes in muscle tone. Hot whirlpools (99°–110°F) are beneficial in relieving pain, increasing soft tissue extensibility, and in treating chronic conditions such as arthritis. In general, whirlpool temperatures should not exceed 110° to 115°F because of risk of burns.

bathophobia (băth″ō-fō′bē-ă) [Gr. *bathos,* deep, + *phobos,* fear] Abnormal fear of depths; commonly refers to fear of height or of looking down from a high place.

bathyanesthesia (băth-ē-ăn″ĕs-thē′zē-ă) [″ + *an-,* not, + *aisthesis,* sensation] Loss of deep sensibility.

bathyesthesia (băth″ē-ĕs-thē′zē-ă) [″ + *aisthesis,* sensation] A consciousness or sensibility of parts of the body beneath the skin.

bathyhyperesthesia (băth-ē-hī″pĕr-ĕs-thē′zē-ă) [″ + *hyper,* above, + *aisthesis,* sensation] Excessive sensitivity of muscles and other deep body structures.

bathyhypesthesia (băth″ē-hīp″ĕs-thē′zē-ă) [″ + *hypo,* under, + *aisthesis,* sensation] Impairment of sensitivity in muscles and other deep body structures.

Batten disease [Frederick E. Batten, English ophthalmologist, 1865–1918] A hereditary disturbance of metabolism that results in blindness and mental retardation. SYN: *Spielmeyer-Vogt disease.* SEE: *sphingolipidosis.*

battered child syndrome Physical abuse of a child by an adult, often under circumstances that make it appear that the injury was accidental. The child may exhibit bruises, scratches, burns, hematomas, or fractures of the long bones, ribs, or skull. Poor skin hygiene and some degree of malnutrition also may be present. SEE: *child abuse; shaken baby syndrome; Nursing Diagnoses Appendix.*

ETIOLOGY: The abuser is usually a parent or guardian who was abused when he or she was a child.

DIAGNOSIS: The most distinguishing features are the location of the injuries (e.g., the ocular area), the fracture patterns, and the variation in the stages of healing of bone lesions seen in radiographic images, indicating the injuries were incurred at different times.

PROGNOSIS: Prognosis is variable. The death rate is high, and surviving children often suffer from long-term physical and mental injuries and may become abusive parents. If a child has been abused by parents, it is important to examine the child's siblings without delay because in about 20% of cases the battered child's siblings will also show signs of physical abuse.

battered woman A woman who has been physically or sexually assaulted by her husband, partner, or former partner. Typically verbal abuse precedes physical violence. An escalating pattern of intimidation and injury often results, sometimes culminating in death. Frequently women are reluctant to report this type of abuse because they feel trapped or isolated. Women from any socioeconomic level may be affected. Shelters and support for battered women are available in many locations.

battery [Fr. *battre,* to beat] **1.** A device for generating electric current by chemical action. **2.** A series of tests, procedures, or diagnostic examinations given to or done on a patient. **3.** The unlawful touching of another without consent, justification, or excuse. In legal medicine, battery occurs if a medical or surgical procedure is performed without proper consent. SEE: *assault; sexual harassment.*

Battle sign [William Henry Battle, Brit. surgeon, 1855–1936] Ecchymosis behind the ear; a physical finding in patients with basilar skull fracture.

Baudelocque's diameter (bōd-lŏks′) [Jean Louis Baudelocque, Sr., Fr. obstetrician, 1746–1810] The distance between the depression beneath the last lumbar vertebra and the margin of the symphysis pubis; the external conjugate diameter of the pelvis. SYN: *Baudelocque's line.*

Baudelocque's method In obstetrics, manipulation to convert a fetal face presentation into a vertex presentation.

Baumé scales (bō-mā′) [Antoine Baumé, Fr. chemist, 1728–1805] Hydrometer scales for determination of the specific gravity of liquids.

bay (bā) An anatomical recess or depression filled with liquid.

Bayes' theorem [Thomas Bayes, Brit. mathematician, 1702–1761] A statistical theorem concerned with analyzing the probability that a patient may have a specific condition after diagnostic testing. The theorem states that if a disease is very rare (the pretest probability is low), the patient is unlikely to have that condition even with a positive diagnostic test. Conversely, when the pretest probability of a specific condition is very high, a negative test result does not rule out the condition.

Bayley Scales of Infant Development A standardized battery of tests used to provide information about the developmental status of children aged 2 to 30 months. The battery is designed to indicate motor, mental, and behavioral levels based on performance and parental reports.

Bazin's disease (bă-zănz′) [Antoine P. E. Bazin, Fr. dermatologist, 1807–1878] A chronic skin disease occurring in young adult females; characterized by hard cutaneous nodules that break down to form necrotic ulcers that leave atrophic scars. The disease is almost invariably preceded by tuberculosis, but the etiological relationship to that disease is debated. SYN: *erythema induratum.*

BBT *basal body temperature.*

BCAA *branched-chain amino acids.*

B-cell–mediated immunity SEE: *immunity, humoral.*

BCG vaccine Bacille Calmette-Guérin vaccine, a preparation of a dried, living but attenuated culture of *Mycobacterium bovis.* In areas with a high incidence of tuberculosis (TB), it is used to provide passive TB immunity to infants and to protect adults who have an unavoidable risk of TB infection. The vaccine cannot be used in pregnant women or in immunosuppressed individuals. A disadvantage of the use of the vaccine is that it produces hypersensitivity to TB skin tests, making them unreliable for several years. The vaccine can also be used in cancer chemotherapy, e.g., in the treatment of multiple myeloma and cancer of the colon. It is also used as a bladder wash in patients with carcinoma of the bladder. SEE: *bacille Calmette-Guérin.*

bcl-2 Member of a family of oncogenes that is involved in tumor suppression. *Bcl-2* is an oncogene that is responsible for some of the ability of certain tumors to elude the host organism's defenses. *Bcl-2* suppresses apoptosis, permitting the metastasis of tumors. When referring to the protein product of the gene, the term "Bcl-2" is used. SEE: *apoptosis; oncogene.*

BCLS *Basic cardiac life support.*

b.d. L. *bis die,* twice a day.

Bdellovibrio [Gr. *bdello,* leech, + *vibrio*] A genus of gram-negative bacteria that parasitize other bacteria by living and reproducing inside them.

B.E. *below elbow,* referring to the site of amputation of an arm; *barium enema.*

Be Symbol for the element beryllium.

beaded (bēd′ĕd) Referring to disjointed colonies along the inoculation line in a streak or stab culture.

beads, rachitic Visible swelling where the ribs join the cartilage, seen in rickets. SYN: *rachitic rosary.*

beaker (bē′kĕr) A widemouthed glass vessel for mixing or holding liquids.

beam **1.** In nuclear medicine and radiology, a group of atomic particles traveling a parallel course. **2.** The part of an analytical balance to which the weighing pans are attached. **3.** A long, slender piece of wood, metal, or plastic resin that acts as a support in a dental appliance.

beard The hair on the face and throat.

bearing down The expulsive effort of a parturient woman in the second stage of labor. Valsalva's maneuver is used, causing increased pressure against the uterus by increasing intra-abdominal pressure.

beat [AS. *beatan,* to strike] A pulsation or throb as in contraction of the heart or the passage of blood through a vessel.

apex b. The impulse of the heartbeat felt by the hand when held over the fifth or sixth intercostal space in the left midclavicular line.

artificially paced b. A heartbeat stimulated by an artificial pacemaker.

capture b. A ventricular contraction responding to an impulse from the sinus that reaches the atrioventricular node at a time at which the node is nonrefractory.

dropped b. The absence of a ventricular contraction of the heart.

ectopic b. A heartbeat beginning at a place other than the sinoatrial node.

escape b. A heartbeat that occurs after a prolonged pause, or failure of the sinus node to stimulate the heart to contract.

forced b. Extrasystole brought on by artificial heart stimulation.

premature b. A heartbeat that arises from a site other than the sinus node and occurs early in the cardiac cycle before the expected sinus beat.

Beau's lines (bōz) [Joseph Honoré Simon Beau, Fr. physician, 1806–1865] White lines across the fingernails, usually a sign of systemic disease. They may be due to trauma, coronary occlusion, hypercalcemia, or skin disease. The lines are visible until the affected area of the nail has grown out and been trimmed away.

Bechterew's reflex, Bekhterev's reflex (běk′tĕr-ĕvs) [Vladimir Mikhailovich von Bechterew, Russ. neurologist, 1857–1927] **1.** Contraction of the facial muscles due to irritation of the nasal mucosa. **2.** Dilatation of the pupil on exposure to light. **3.** Contraction of the lower abdominal muscles when the skin on the inner thigh is stroked.

Beck's triad The signs seen with pericardial tamponade, consisting of hypotension, distended neck veins, and muffled heart sounds.

beclomethasone dipropionate A corticosteroid drug. Trade names are Vancenase and Beclovent.

becquerel (běk′rěl) [Antoine Henri Becquerel, Fr. physicist, 1852–1908] SYMB: Bq. An SI-derived unit of activity of a radionuclide equal to the quantity of the material having one spontaneous nuclear transition, i.e., disintegrations, per second. One curie has 3.7×10^{10} transitions per second. Thus, one curie is equivalent to 3.7×10^{10} becquerels. SEE: *curie; SI Units Appendix.*

bed [AS. *bedd*] **1.** A supporting structure or tissue. **2.** A couch or support for the body during sleep.

air b. **1.** Large inflated cushion used as a mattress. **2.** Air-fluidized bed.

air-fluidized b. A bed consisting of a mattress filled with approx. 100 billion ceramic spheres that are suspended by a continuous flow of warm air at the rate of approx. 40 cu ft/min. This creates a surface that feels like a liquid, having a specific gravity of 1.3. The patient "floats" on the mattress with only minimal penetration. Because of the even distribution of weight, the bed is particularly useful in treating patients with burns or decubitus ulcers. Nursing care of the patient is simplified because the patient can be moved by fingertip pressure.

b. blocks Blocks of sturdy material, usually wood, placed under the legs of a bed to elevate one end of it. Raising the foot of the bed may be useful in treatment of shock, inguinal hernia, bleeding from the lower limbs, or edema of the lower limbs, vulva, or scrotum. It may also be helpful when weight is used on the lower limbs or when a patient has difficulty with enema retention. Raising the head of the bed may be used to drain the abdomen or pelvis, to treat congestive heart failure, to aid respiration, or to treat bleeding from the head, neck, or upper chest. It is also recommended while taking certain medications that may be irritating to the esophagus (e.g., alendronate [Fosamax]).

b. board A firm board placed beneath a mattress to keep it from sagging. It is used to treat some persons with back difficulties. It is also used in cardiopulmonary resuscitation to improve the effectiveness of chest compressions.

capillary b. A network of capillaries.

circular b. A bed that allows a patient to be turned end-over-end while held between two frames. This permits turning the patients without disturbing them by turning the two frames inside a circular apparatus that holds the ends of the frames. It is useful in treating paralyzed or immobilized patients. SYN: *Circ-O-Lectric bed.*

float b. A bed in which the patient is supported either on a water mattress or on minute ceramic beads with air flowing through them. This type of bed is useful for patients with decubitus ulcers or burns.

flotation b. A bed in which the patient reclines in a hollow, flexible, mattress-shaped device filled with water. This enables equal distribution of pressure on the body. It is used to treat and prevent decubiti.

fracture b. A bed for patients who have fractures.

Gatch b. An adjustable bed that provides elevation of the back and the knees.

hydrostatic b. Water b.

kinetic b. A bed that constantly turns patients side to side through 270°. It is used to prevent the hazards of immobility in patients requiring prolonged bedrest, as in multiple trauma and some neuromuscular diseases. Trademark is Roto-Bed.

low air-loss b. A mattress composed of inflatable air cushions that is used to relieve pressure on body parts, esp. in patients who are being hospitalized for a long time or who have skin breakdown.

metabolic b. A bed arranged to facilitate collection of feces and urine of a patient so that metabolic studies can be done.

nail b. The skin that lies beneath a nail at the tip of a digit.

open b. A bed available for assignment to a patient.

recovery b. A bed, usually a portable bed or stretcher, prepared to receive a patient immediately after surgery. It may also be a standard bed in the Postanesthesia Recovery Room.

rocking b. A device used to create abdominal displacement ventilation in patients with respiratory failure.

surgical b. A bed equipped with mechanisms that can elevate or lower the entire bed platform, flex or extend individual components of the platform, or raise or lower the head or the feet of the patient independently.

tilt b. SEE: *table, tilt.*

water b. A water-filled rubber mattress used for prevention of bedsores. SYN: *hydrostatic b.* SEE: *flotation b.*

bedbug An insect, *Cimex lectularius* of the family *Cimicidae,* the saliva of which contains an irritating substance that causes a purpuric reaction or an urticarial wheal. The adult bugs are about 4 to 5 mm in length and survive for up to a year without feeding and at low temperature. The female ingests 0.0185 ml of blood each feeding, and the male 0.015 ml. Bedbugs can be a cause of anemia in infants. There is much speculation but no proof that bedbugs transmit bloodborne infections (such as hepatitis B) to humans, either through bites or infected feces. Treatment for bites consists of application of antipruritic lotions. In heavy infestations, an appropriate insecticide should be used to spray furniture, mattresses, floors, baseboards, and walls. The use of wooden frames for beds should be avoided, as this provides a nesting and breeding site for these insects.

bedfast Unable or unwilling to leave the bed; bedridden.

bedlam [From Hospital of St. Mary of Bethlehem, pronounced Bedlem in Middle English.] **1.** An asylum for the insane. **2.** Any place or situation characterized by a noisy uproar.

bed mobility, impaired Limitation of independent movement from one bed position to another. SEE: *Nursing Diagnoses Appendix.*

Bednar's aphthae [Alois Bednar, physician in Vienna, 1816–1888] Infected, traumatic ulcers appearing on the hard palate of infants; usually caused by sucking infected objects.

bedpan [AS. *bedd,* bed, + *panna,* flat vessel] A pan-shaped device placed under a bedridden patient for collecting fecal and urinary excreta.

NOTE: In general, because bedpan use is uncomfortable and awkward, it requires more exertion on the patient's part than using a bedside toilet. Patients, esp. those recovering from myocardial infarction, should not be forced to use a bedpan if it is possible for them to use a bedside toilet.

bedrest **1.** A device for propping up patients in bed. **2.** The confining of a patient to bed for rest.

bedridden Unable or unwilling to leave the bed; bedfast.

bedsore [AS. *bedd,* bed, + *sare,* open wound] Pressure sore.

bedwetting Enuresis.

BEE *basal energy expenditure.*

bee [AS. *beo,* bee] An insect of the order Hymenoptera and superfamily Apoidea. Included is the common honeybee, *Apis mellifera,* which produces honey and beeswax.

b. sting Injury resulting from bee venom and causing pain, redness, and swelling. The stinger of the honeybee has multiple barbs that usually anchor it in the skin. The stinger, if present, should be removed and the area cooled as quickly and efficiently as possible to prevent the venom from entering the general circulation. To prevent further injection of venom, the stinger should be grasped gently by fingernails or forceps. Antihistamines help to relieve discomfort.

CAUTION: Some individuals are hypersensitive to bee venom and may suffer severe anaphylactic reactions leading to death. In such cases immediate subcutaneous or intravenous administration of epinephrine is indicated.

bee sting therapy Apitherapy.

Beer's law [August Beer, Ger. physicist, 1825–1863] The basic law that is the foundation for all absorption photometry. It predicts the linear relationship between the monochromatic light absorbance (A) of a solution and its concentration (c). The law is given as $A = \epsilon lc$, where A = absorbance, ϵ = molar absorptivity, l = path distance, and c = concentration. It is also known as the Beer-Lamber or Bougher-Beer law.

Beer's operation [Georg Joseph Beer, Ger. ophthalmologist, 1763–1821] A flap operation for cataract or artificial pupil.

beeswax (bēz′wăks) Yellow wax obtained from the honeycomb of bees. A purified form is used in ointments.

beeturia (bēt-ū′rē-ă) Deep red or pink coloration of urine caused by betanin, the pigment in beets. This condition is common in iron-deficient adults and children and can occur after ingestion of even one beet.

behavior [ME. *behaven,* to hold oneself in a certain way] **1.** The manner in which one acts; the actions or reactions of individuals under specific circumstances. **2.** Any response elicited from an organism.

self-consoling b. The self-quieting actions of infants, such as sucking on their fists and watching mobiles and other moving objects.

self-injurious b. ABBR: SIB. Maladaptive behaviors of various types, sometimes exhibited by persons with mental retardation; they include self-scratching, repeated head banging, and other potentially dangerous acts. The cause is unknown, but one theory is that the behaviors are self-stimulatory.

type A b. A behavior pattern marked by the characteristics of competitiveness, aggressiveness, easily aroused hostility, and an overdeveloped sense of urgency. Although some studies have suggested that this behavior pattern is important in coronary artery disease and hypertension, the evidence supporting this claim is controversial. The risk of accidents, suicide, and murder is higher in type A individuals.

type B b. A behavior pattern marked by the lack of competitiveness, hostility, and time pressure.

behavioral science The science concerned with all aspects of behavior.

behavioral system model A conceptual model of nursing developed by Dorothy Johnson. The person is regarded as a behavioral system with seven subsystems—attachment, dependency, ingestion, elimination, sexuality, aggression, achievement. The goal of nursing is to restore, maintain, or attain behavioral system balance and stability. SEE: Nursing Theory Appendix.

behaviorism A theory of conduct that regards normal and abnormal behavior as the result of conditioned reflexes quite apart from the concept of will. It does not apply to conditions resulting from organic disease.

Behçet's syndrome (bā′sĕts) [Hulusi Behçet, Turkish dermatologist, 1889–1948] A rare, multisystem, chronic, recurrent disease of unknown cause, marked by ulceration of the mouth and genitalia and by uveitis. The central nervous system, blood vessels, joints, and intestinal tract may be involved. It is genetically associated with HLA-B51. The disease occurs worldwide, but is most common in the eastern Mediterranean area and eastern Asia. In these areas it occurs mostly in young men and is a leading cause of blindness. In the Western world, where the disease is less severe, it affects men twice as frequently as it does women but is not a leading cause of blindness. The period between attacks is irregular, but may be as short as days or as long as years. The syndrome is also known as Behçet's disease, or cutaneomucouveal syndrome.

TREATMENT: Therapy depends on the severity of the clinical findings. Mild disease of skin and joints may be treated with topical steroids or nonsteroidal anti-inflammatory drugs. Involvement of the central nervous system or gastrointestinal tract may require high dose steroids or cytotoxic drugs, such as chlorambucil, cyclophosphamide, or methotrexate.

bejel (bĕj′ĕl) A nonvenereal form of syphilis endemic in Arab countries; children are especially susceptible.

bel (bĕl) SYMB: B. A unit of measurement of the intensity of sound. It is expressed as a logarithm of the ratio of two sounds of acoustic intensity, one of which is fixed or standard; the ratio is expressed in decibels.

belay (bĕ-lāy′) To fasten with a rope.

belch [AS. *baelcan,* to eructate] **1.** To expel gas from the stomach through the mouth; to eructate. **2.** An act of belching; eructation.

belching Raising of gas from the stomach and expelling it through the mouth and nose. For belching to occur, there is first an increase in gastric pressure; then the lower esophagus sphincter relaxes to allow equalization of pressure in the stomach and esophagus. Relaxation of the upper esophagus sphincter allows the gas to escape through the pharynx and mouth. SEE: *water brash*.

ETIOLOGY: Belching may be caused by gastric fermentation, air swallowing, or ingestion of carbonated drinks or gas-producing foods.

belemnoid (bē-lĕm′noyd) [Gr. *belemnon,* dart, + *eidos,* form, shape] Dart-shaped. SYN: *styloid*.

Bell, Sir Charles Scottish physiologist and surgeon, 1774–1842.

B.'s law, Bell-Magendie's law The fact that anterior spinal nerve roots contain only motor fibers and posterior roots only sensory fibers.

B.'s nerve Long thoracic nerve; nervus thoracicus longus.

B.'s palsy Unilateral facial paralysis of sudden onset. The paralysis involves both the upper and lower halves of the face, distinguishing it from the facial paralysis associated with some strokes, which affect the muscles of the mouth more than those of the eye or forehead. Bell's palsy is usually caused by a reactivation of herpes simplex virus, although other infections (e.g., syphilis or Lyme disease) are sometimes implicated. Complications may include corneal drying and ulceration and mild dysarthria. Either side of the face may be affected. Attacks recur in about 10% of cases.

SYMPTOMS: The paralysis distorts smiling, eye closure, salivation, and tear formation on the affected side.

TREATMENT: Tapering doses of prednisone along with an antiviral drug, such as acyclovir, provide the most effective results. In addition, the affected eye should be protected from drying with artificial tears or unmedicated ointments. Some practitioners advise wearing sunglasses during the palsy or patching the eye to protect it from foreign bodies or drying.

PROGNOSIS: Partial facial paralysis is usually resolved within several months. The likelihood of complete recovery after total paralysis varies from 20% to 90%.

B.'s phenomenon Rolling of the eyeball upward and outward when an attempt is made to close the eye on the side of the face affected in peripheral facial paralysis.

belladonna (bĕl″ă-dŏn′ă) [It., beautiful lady] An anticholinergic derived from *Atropa belladonna,* a poisonous plant with reddish flowers and shiny black berries. Belladonna is the source of various alkaloids (stramonium, hyoscyamus, scopolamine, and atropine) and is used mainly for its sedative and spasmolytic effects on the gastrointestinal tract. All alkaloids derived from belladonna are highly toxic. SEE: *atropine in Poisons and Poisoning Appendix.*

b. leaf Powder from the dried leaf and flowering top of *Atropa belladonna Linné* or *A. belladonna acuminata.* An anticholinergic agent, it is used generally in tincture form though the dry extract in tablet form may be used.

Bellini's tubule (bĕ-lē′nēz) [Lorenzo Bellini, It. anatomist, 1643–1704] The straight connecting tubule of the kidney.

Bellocq's cannula (bĕl-ŏks′) [Jean Jacques Bellocq, Fr. surgeon, 1732–1807] An instrument for drawing in a plug through the nostril and mouth to control epistaxis.

belly [AS. *baelg,* bag] **1.** The abdomen or abdominal cavity. **2.** The fleshy, central portion of a muscle.

bellyache Gastralgia.

belly button Umbilicus.

belonephobia (bĕl″ō-nĕ-fō′bē-ă) [Gr. *belone,* needle, + *phobos,* fear] Morbid fear of sharp-pointed objects.

belonoskiascopy (bĕl″ō-nō-skī-ăs′kō-pē) [″ + *skia,* shadow, + *skopein,* to examine] Subjective retinoscopy by means of shadows and movements to determine refraction.

Bence Jones protein [Henry Bence Jones, Brit. physician, 1814–1873] The light chain portion of immunoglobulin molecules that may be deposited in the renal tubules and excreted in the urine of patients with multiple myeloma. The protein is involved in renal amyloidosis and renal failure.

benchmark (bĕnch′mărk) A criterion of quality or service in health care, usually expressed as a measurable standard.

Bender's Visual Motor Gestalt test [Lauretta Bender, U.S. psychiatrist, 1897–1987] A test in which the subject copies a series of patterns. The results vary with the type of psychiatric disorder present.

bendroflumethiazide (bĕn″drō-floo″mĕthī′ă-zīd) A rarely used thiazide-type diuretic.

bends Pain in the limbs and abdomen caused by bubbles of nitrogen in blood and tissues as a result of rapid reduction of atmospheric pressure. This condition may also develop when a person ascends too rapidly after being exposed to increased pressure while deep sea diving. Pressure should be restored by placing the patient in a hyperbaric chamber and slowly returning to ambient pressure. SEE: *decompression illness; hyperbaric chamber.*

benediction hand Condition of the hand in which there is flexion of some of the fingers, especially of the terminal phalanges. The hand at the wrist may be extended. The condition may be caused by paralysis of the ulnar and median nerves.

Benedict's solution (bĕn′ĕ-dĭkts) [Stanley R. Benedict, U.S. chemist, 1844–1936] A solution used to test for the presence of sugar. To 173 g sodium or potassium citrate and 100 g anhydrous sodium carbonate (dissolved in 700 ml water) is added 17.3 g crystalline copper sulfate that has been dissolved in 100 ml of water. Sufficient water is added to the mixture to make 1000 ml. SEE: *Benedict's test.*

Benedict's test A test to determine the presence of sugar in the urine by adding 8 drops of clear urine (filtered if necessary) to a test tube containing 5 ml of Benedict's solution. The mixture is boiled then allowed to cool. This test is performed rarely in clinical medicine owing to the advent of simpler, more specific tests for glycosuria.

Benedikt's syndrome [Moritz Benedikt, Austrian physician, 1835–1920] Hemiplegia with oculomotor paralysis and clonic spasm or tremor on the opposite side. Benedikt's syndrome is caused by lesions that damage the third nerve and involve the nucleus ruber and corticospinal tract.

beneficence (bĕn-ĕf′ă-sĕns) **1.** An ethical principle that emphasizes doing what is best for the patient. **2.** Choosing to do good; acting kindly or charitably.

benefit **1.** Something that promotes health. **2.** A term for service stipulations of an insurance policy, esp. a medical policy.

benign (bē-nīn′) [L. *benignus,* mild] Not recurrent or progressive; nonmalignant.

benign forgetfulness A memory defect marked by the inability to immediately recall a name or date. The item, whether recent or remote, is eventually recalled.

benign senescent forgetfulness Minor, nonprogressive memory loss that does not interfere with daily living. This generally is a normal age-related cognitive change.

Bennett double-ring splint A metal splint that slips on the finger and limits hyperextension of the proximal interphalangeal joint.

bentonite (bĕn′tŏn-īt) [Fort Benton, U.S.] A hydrated aluminosilicate that forms a thick, slippery substance when water is added. It is used as a suspending and clarifying agent. It may be heat-sterilized.

benzaldehyde (bĕn-zăl′dĕ-hīd) A pharmaceutical flavoring agent derived from oil of bitter almond.

benzalkonium chloride (bĕnz″ăl-kō′nē-ŭm klō′rīd) An antimicrobial preservative with viricidal properties, used as a detergent, contact lens cleaner, and vaginal microbicide.

benzene, benzin, benzine (bĕn′zēn, bĕn-zēn′, bĕn′zĭn) [*benz*(oin) + Gr. *ene,* suffix used in chemistry to denote unsaturated compound] C_6H_6; a highly flammable, volatile liquid that is the simplest member of the aromatic series of hydrocarbons. It is immiscible with water, and it dissolves fats. It is used as a solvent and in the synthesis of dyes and drugs. The phenyl radical, C_6H_6, will be recognized in the formulae for phenol, dimethylaminoazobenzene (see under *azo compounds*), and benzoic acid. SYN: *benzol*. SEE: *Poisons and Poisoning Appendix*.

benzidine (bĕn′zĭ-dĭn) $C_{12}H_{12}O_{12}$; compound formerly used as a test to determine traces of blood in feces. A diet free of iron-containing foods should be followed for at least 48 hr before any test for occult blood in stool. This clears the intestinal tract of iron-containing foods and helps to prevent a false-positive test for iron. It has been reported that benzidine is a carcinogen.

benzoate (bĕn′zō-āt) A salt of benzoic acid.

benzocaine (bĕn′zō-kān) Ethyl aminobenzoate, a local anesthetic used topically. Trade name is Americaine.

benzodiazepine (bĕn″zō-dī-ăz′ĕ-pēn) Any of a group of chemically similar psychotropic drugs with potent hypnotic and sedative action; used predominantly as antianxiety and sleep-inducing drugs. Side effects of these drugs may include impairment of psychomotor performance; amnesia; euphoria; dependence; and rebound (i.e., the return of symptoms) transiently worse than before treatment, upon discontinuation of the drug.

benzoic acid $C_7H_6O_2$; a white crystalline material having a slight odor. It is used in keratolytic ointments and in food preservation. Saccharin is a derivative of this acid.

benzoin (bĕn′zoyn, -zō-ĭn) [Fr. *benjoin*] A balsamic resin obtained from trees of various species of *Styrax,* esp. *S. benzoin* or *S. paralleloneuris*. It is used as a stimulant expectorant, as an inhalant in laryngitis and bronchitis, and as a protective coating for ulcers. It also is used as a solution applied to the skin to prepare it for application of adhesives, esp. adhesive tape.

benzol Benzene.

benzonatate (bĕn-zō′nă-tāt) A substance chemically related to procaine; used in anticough preparations. Trade name is Tessalon.

benzoylecgonine (bĕn-zoyl-ĕk′gō-nīn) The principal metabolite of cocaine. Screening tests for cocaine determine its presence or absence.

benzoyl peroxide A topical agent used for the treatment of acne vulgaris. It is usually considered as a first-line treatment for mild to moderate acne. Common side effects include drying of the skin and skin discomfort.

benztropine mesylate (bĕnz′trō-pēn) An antiparasympathomimetic agent usually used with other drugs in treating parkinsonism. Trade name is Cogentin.

benzyl $C_6H_5COOCH_2C_6H_5$; the hydrocarbon radical of benzyl alcohol and various other compounds.

b. benzoate An aromatic, clear, colorless oily liquid with a sharp, burning taste. It is used as a topical scabicide. Trade name is Benylate.

benzylpenicillin procaine (bĕn″zĭl-pĕn-ĭ-sĭl′ĭn) Penicillin G procaine.

Bérard's aneurysm (bā-rărz′) [Auguste Bérard, Fr. surgeon, 1802–1846] An arteriovenous aneurysm in the tissues surrounding the injured vein.

Béraud's valve (bā-rōz′) [Bruno J. J. Béraud, Fr. surgeon, 1823–1865] A fold of mucous membrane of the lacrimal sac at the junction of the lacrimal duct. SYN: *Krause's valve*.

berdache (bĕr-dăsh′) [Fr.] An individual of a definite sex, male or female, who assumes the status and role of the opposite sex and who is viewed by the community as being of one physiologic sex but as having assumed the status and role of the opposite sex. Transvestism is not synonymous with berdache, nor is homosexual behavior necessarily a component of this condition.

bereavement The expected reactions of grief and sadness upon learning of the loss of a loved one. The period of bereavement is associated with increased mortality. It is important for those who care for the bereaved to emphasize human resilience and the power of life rather than the stress that accompanies bereavement.

Berg balance test A physical performance evaluation of fourteen activities including; sit-to-stand, reaching, turning, and single leg stance. The activities are rated on a 0 to 4 scale. This test has been shown to be highly predictive of patient falls.

beriberi (bĕr′ē-bĕr′ē) [Singhalese *beri,* weakness] A disease marked by peripheral neurologic, cerebral, and cardiovascular abnormalities and caused by a lack of thiamine. Early deficiency produces fatigue, irritation, poor memory, sleep disturbances, precordial pain, anorexia, abdominal discomfort, and constipation. Beriberi is endemic in Asia, the Philippines, and other islands of the Pacific. SYN: *kakke*.

ETIOLOGY: Deficiency is caused by subsistence on highly polished rice, which has lost all thiamine content through the milling process. Secondary deficiency can arise from decreased absorption, impaired absorption, or impaired utilization of thiamine.

TREATMENT: Treatment consists of oral or parenteral administration of thiamine and eating a balanced diet.

Berkefeld filter (bĕr′kē-fĕld) [Wilhelm Berkefeld, Ger. manufacturer, 1836–1897] A filter of diatomaceous earth designed to allow virus-size particles to pass through.

berkelium (bĕrk′lē-ŭm) [U. of California at Berkeley, where first produced] SYMB: Bk. A transuranium element; atomic weight 247, atomic number 97.

berloque dermatitis SEE: *dermatitis, berlock.*

Bernard's glandular layer The inner layer of cells lining the acini of the pancreas.

Bernard-Soulier syndrome [Jean A. Bernard, Fr. hematologist, b. 1907; Jean-Pierre Soulier, Fr. hematologist, b. 1915] An autosomal recessive bleeding disorder marked by an inherited deficiency of a platelet glycoprotein. The platelets are large. Bleeding results from defective adhesion of platelets to subendothelial collagen and is disproportionate to the reduction in platelets.

Bernoulli effect [Jakob Bernoulli, Swiss mathematician, 1654–1705] In pulmonology, the inverse variation in pressure with gas velocity in tubal air flow.

Bernstein test [Lionel Bernstein, U.S. physician, b. 1923] Test to reproduce the pain of heartburn. This is done by swallowing a dilute solution (0.1 N) hydrochloric acid. This is compared with a placebo infusion of normal saline into the esophagus. The latter does not cause heartburn.

Bertin, column of (bĕr′tăn) [Exupère Joseph Bertin, Fr. anatomist, 1712–1781] Any of the renal cortical columns that support the blood vessels in the kidneys and separate the medullary pyramids.

Bertin's ligament Iliofemoral ligament.

berylliosis (bĕr″ĭl-lē-ō′sĭs) [*beryllium* + Gr. *osis,* condition] Beryllium poisoning, usually of the lungs. The beryllium particles cause fibrosis and granulomata at any site, whether inhaled or accidentally introduced into or under the skin.

beryllium (bĕ-rĭl′ē-ŭm) [Gr. *beryllos,* beryl] A metallic element, symbol Be, atomic weight 9.0122, atomic number 4, specific gravity 1.848. It is used as a window in some x-ray tubes to produce a soft (low kilovoltage) beam appropriate for imaging soft tissue (mammography or specimen radiography) or for forensic and industrial radiography of extremely thin objects (e.g., a postage stamp or fingerprint).

bestiality (bĕs-tē-ăl′ĭ-tē) [L. *bestia,* beast] The use of animals (e.g., snakes, poultry, and nonhuman mammals) for the purpose of sexual enjoyment.

beta (bā′tă) **1.** Second letter of Gr. alphabet, written β. **2.** In chemistry, a prefix to denote isomeric variety or position in compounds of substituted groups.

beta-adrenergic agent A synthetic or natural drug that stimulates beta (sympathetic) receptors.

beta-adrenergic blocking agent Any drug that inhibits the activity of the sympathetic nervous system and of adrenergic hormones.

Members of this class of drugs are used to treat hypertension, angina pectoris, myocardial infarction, aortic dissection, arrhythmias, glaucoma, and other conditions. Commonly prescribed beta blockers include atenolol, carvedilol, metoprolol, nadolol, propranolol, and pindolol. Side effects of these medications include worsening of asthma, blunting of the cardiovascular symptoms of hypoglycemia, bradycardia, and heart block. Rapid withdrawal from a beta-blocking drug in a patient who has become accustomed to its use may produce tachycardia or other arrhythmias, rebound hypertension, or myocardial ischemia or infarction. SYN: *beta blocker.*

beta-adrenergic receptor A site in autonomic nerve pathways wherein inhibitory responses occur when adrenergic agents such as norepinephrine and epinephrine are released.

beta blocker Beta-adrenergic blocking agent.

beta carotene A yellow-orange pigment found in fruits and vegetables; it is the most common precursor of vitamin A. The daily human requirement for vitamin A can be met by dietary intake of beta carotene.

TOXICITY: Ingestion of large doses of vitamin A either acutely or chronically causes skin and liver damage, among other injuries. Beta carotene supplements increase the risk of death among smokers and have no known beneficial effects on nonsmokers.

BENEFITS: A diet rich in beta carotene has been associated with a decreased risk of certain cancers.

DOSING: Vitamin A activity in foods is expressed as retinol equivalents (RE). Six mg of beta carotene equals 1 μg of retinol or 1 RE. SEE: *vitamin A; retinol.*

beta cells **1.** Basophilic cells in the anterior lobe of pituitary that give a positive periodic acid stain reaction. **2.** Insulin-secreting cells of the islets of Langerhans of the pancreas.

betacism (bā′tă-sĭzm) [Gr. *beta,* the letter b, + *-ismos,* condition] A speech defect giving the *b* sound to other consonants.

betaine hydrochloride (bē′tă-ĭn) [L. *beta,* beet] A colorless crystalline substance containing 23% hydrochloric acid. It is obtained from an alkaloid found in the beet and other plants and is used orally as a source of hydrochloric acid in treating hypochlorhydria.

beta lactamase (bā-tă lăk'tă-māz) An enzyme that destroys the beta lactam ring of penicillin-like antibiotics and makes them ineffective.

beta-lactamase resistance The ability of microorganisms that produce the enzyme beta-lactamase, also called penicillinase, to resist the action of certain types of antibiotics, including some but not all forms of penicillin.

extended-spectrum b.l.r. ABBR: ESBL. An enzymatically mediated type of antibiotic resistance found in gram-negative bacilli (e.g., *Klebsiella pneumoniae, Enterobacter cloacae,* and *Pseudomonas aeruginosa*), that make these bacteria resistant to cephalosporins and penicillin antibiotics.

betamethasone (bā"tă-mĕth'ă-sōn) A powerful, synthetic glucocorticoid used to treat many conditions including dermatitis, arthritis, inflammatory bowel disease, reactive airways disease, and respiratory distress syndrome in preterm infants, among others.

beta$_2$ microglobulin ABBR: β_2-m. A polypeptide that is one of the class I major histocompatibility markers on cell surfaces; it is grouped into chains of low molecular weight called light chains. The β_2-m chain may be affected by the *nef* gene in HIV, preventing CD8+ T lymphocytes from recognizing the virus. SEE: *acquired immunodeficiency syndrome; major histocompatibility complex.*

beta subunit Glycoprotein hormones containing two different polypeptide subunits designated α and β chains. Analysis of the units of these hormones (e.g., follicle-stimulating, luteinizing, chorionic gonadotropin, and thyrotropin) enables early diagnosis of such conditions as pregnancy and ectopic pregnancy.

betatron (bā'tă-trŏn) A circular electron accelerator that produces either high-energy electrons or x-ray photons.

betazole hydrochloride (bā'tă-zōl) An isomer of histamine used intramuscularly to stimulate gastric secretion. It is contraindicated in those with atopic allergy. Trade name is Histalog.

bethanechol chloride (bĕ-thā'nĕ-kŏl) A cholinergic drug used to treat paralytic ileus and also urinary retention not caused by organic disease. Trade names are Urecholine and Duvoid.

Bethesda System, The ABBR: TBS. A system for reporting cervical or vaginal cytologic diagnoses. Use of TBS replaces the numerical designations (Class 1 through 5) of the Papanicolaou smear with descriptive diagnoses of cellular changes. Cellular changes are identified as benign; reactive, such as those due to inflammation, atrophy, radiation, or use of an intrauterine device; or malignant. Hormonal evaluation of vaginal smears is provided. Low-grade squamous intraepithelial lesions include what was previously called grade 1 cervical intraepithelial neoplasia (CIN 1) and cellular changes due to human papilloma virus, that is, koilocytosis. High-grade squamous intraepithelial neoplasia includes what was once identified as CIN 2 and CIN 3. SEE: *cervix, cancer of; cervical intraepithelial neoplasia.*

Betz cells [Vladimir A. Betz, Russ. anatomist, 1834–1894] A type of giant pyramidal cell in the cortical motor area of the brain. The axons of these cells are included in the pyramidal tract.

bevel (bĕv'ĕl) **1.** A surface slanting from the horizontal or vertical. **2.** In dentistry, to produce a slanting surface in the enamel margins of a cavity preparation, named according to the surface resulting.

bezoar (bē'zor) [Arabic *bazahr,* protecting against poison] A hard mass of entangled material sometimes found in the stomachs and intestines of animals and humans, such as a hairball (trichobezoar), a hair and vegetable fiberball (trichophytobezoar), or a vegetable foodball (phytobezoar).

BFP *biologically false positive.*

Bi Symbol for the element bismuth.

bi- (bī) [L. *bis,* twice] Prefix meaning *two, double, twice.*

biarticular (bī"ăr-tĭk'ū-lăr) [" + *articulus,* joint] Pert. to two joints; diarthric (e.g., temporomandibular joints).

bias (bī'ŭs) In experimental medicine, statistics, and epidemiology, any effect or interference at any stage of an investigation tending to produce results that depart systematically from the true value.

bibasic (bī-bā'sĭk) [" + Gr. *basis,* foundation] Pert. to an acid with two hydrogen atoms replaceable by bases to form salts.

bibasilar (bī-băs'ĭ-lăr) Pertaining to both lung bases.

bibliomania (bĭb"lē-ō-mā'nē-ă) [Gr. *biblion,* book, + *mania,* madness] An obsession with the collecting of books.

bibliotherapy (bĭb"lē-ō-thĕr'ă-pē) [" + *therapeia,* treatment] A nonphysical, psychotherapeutic technique in which the patient is induced to read books. Formerly used in treating mental illness.

bibulous (bĭb'ū-lŭs) [L. *bibulus,* from *bibere,* to drink] Absorbent. SYN: *hydrophilous; hygroscopic.*

bicameral (bī-kăm'ĕr-ăl) [L. *bis,* twice, + *camera,* a chamber] Having two cavities or chambers.

bicapsular (bī-kăp'sū-lăr) [" + *capsula,* container] Having two capsules.

bicarbonate (bī-kăr′bō-nāt) Any salt containing the HCO_3^- (bicarbonate) anion. SEE: *carbonic acid.*

blood b. Measured HCO_3^- in the blood. The amount present is an indicator of the alkali reserve and is best understood when comparison is made of the blood bicarbonate, pH, PCO_2 and base excess, using the Henderson-Hasselbalch equation.

b. of soda Sodium bicarbonate.

bicellular (bī-sĕl′ū-lăr) [″ + *cellularis,* little cell] **1.** Composed of two cells. **2.** Having two chambers or compartments.

biceps (bī′sĕps) [″ + *caput,* head] A muscle with two heads.

b. brachii The muscle of the upper arm that flexes the arm and forearm and supinates the hand.

b. femoris One of the hamstring muscles lying on the posterior lateral side of the thigh. It flexes the leg and rotates it outward.

Bichat, Marie François X. (bē-shă′) French physiologist and anatomist, 1771–1802; founder of scientific histology and pathological anatomy.

B.'s canal The subarachnoid canal, which extends from the third ventricle to the middle of Bichat's fissure and carries the veins of Galen.

B.'s fat ball The mass of fat behind the buccinator muscle. SYN: *fat pad* (1); *sucking pad.*

B.'s fissure The horseshoe fissure separating the cerebrum from the cerebellum.

B.'s ligament The lower fasciculus of the posterior sacroiliac ligament.

B.'s tunic Tunica intima.

bichloride of mercury (bī-klō′rīd) $HgCl_2$; corrosive mercuric chloride; a crystalline salt. SEE: *mercuric chloride; mercuric chloride poisoning; mercuric chloride in Poisons and Poisoning Appendix.*

bicipital (bī-sĭp′ĭ-tăl) [L. *biceps,* two heads] **1.** Pert. to a biceps muscle. **2.** Having two heads.

biconcave (bī-kŏn′kāv) [L. *bis,* twice, + *concavus,* concave] Concave on each side, esp. as a type of lens. SEE: illus.

biconvex (bī-kŏn′vĕks) [″ + *convexus,* rounded raised surface] Convex on two sides, esp. as a type of lens. SEE: *biconcave* for illus.

bicornate, bicornis (bī-kor′nāt, -nĭs) [″ + *cornutus,* horned] Having two processes or hornlike projections.

bicoronal (bī″kō-rō′năl) [″ + Gr. *korone,* crown] Pert. to the two coronas.

bicorporate (bī-kor′pŏ-rāt) [″ + *corpus,* body] Having two bodies.

bicuspid (bī-kŭs′pĭd) [″ + *cuspis,* point] Having two cusps or projections or having two cusps or leaflets.

b. tooth A premolar tooth; a permanent tooth with two cusps on the grinding surface and a flattened root. There are four premolars in each jaw, two on each side between the canines and the molars. SEE: *tooth.*

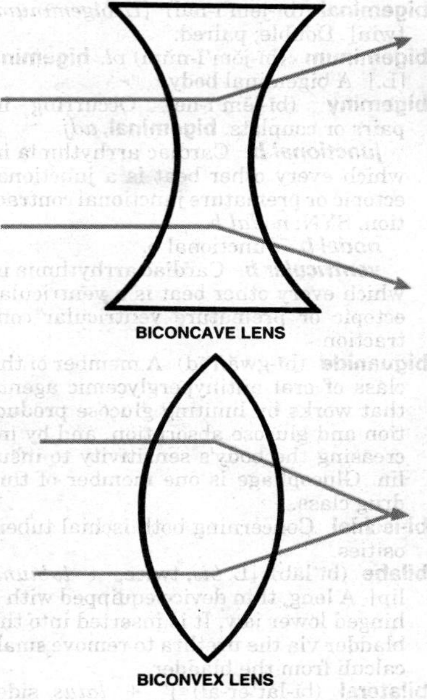
BICONCAVE LENS

BICONVEX LENS

b.i.d. L. *bis in die,* twice daily.

bidet (bē-dā′) [Fr., a small horse] A basin used for cleaning the perineum.

bidi (bē′dē) A hand-rolled and often flavored cigarette imported from India or Southeast Asia. It is popular with young smokers, but has a higher nicotine and tar content than most commercially available cigarettes in the U.S. Like other brands of tobacco in the U.S., it causes cancers, an increased risk of fetal death during pregnancy, heart disease, peripheral vascular disease, chronic obstructive lung disease, and genetic mutations.

Bielschowsky disease (bē″ĕl-shō′skē) [Max Bielschowsky, Ger. neuropathologist, 1869–1940] An early juvenile type of cerebral sphingolipidosis.

bifacial (bī-fā′shē-ăl) [″ + *facies,* face] Having similar opposite surfaces.

bifid (bī′fĭd) [″ + *findere,* to cleave] Cleft or split into two parts.

bifocal (bī-fō′kăl) [″ + *focus,* hearth] Having two foci, as in bifocal eyeglasses.

bifurcate, bifurcated (bī′fŭr-kāt, bī-fŭr′kāt′d) [″ + *furca,* fork] Having two branches or divisions; forked.

bifurcation (bī-fŭr-kā′shŭn) **1.** A separation into two branches; the point of forking. **2.** The branch point where roots divide in a double-rooted tooth.

bigemina (bī-jĕm′ĭ-nă) [L.] Pl. of bigeminum.

bigeminal (bī-jĕm′ĭ-năl) [L. *bigeminum,* twin] Double; paired.

bigeminum (bī-jĕm′ĭ-nŭm) *pl.* **bigemina** [L.] A bigeminal body.

bigeminy (bī-jĕm′ĭ-nē) Occurring in pairs or couplets. **bigeminal,** *adj.*

junctional b. Cardiac arrhythmia in which every other beat is a junctional ectopic or premature junctional contraction. SYN: *nodal b.*

nodal b. Junctional b.

ventricular b. Cardiac arrhythmia in which every other beat is a ventricular ectopic or premature ventricular contraction.

biguanide (bī-gwăn′ĭd) A member of the class of oral antihyperglycemic agents that works by limiting glucose production and glucose absorption, and by increasing the body's sensitivity to insulin. Glucophage is one member of this drug class.

bi-ischial Concerning both ischial tuberosities.

bilabe (bī′lāb) [L. *bis,* twice, + *labium,* lip] A long, thin device equipped with a hinged lower jaw. It is inserted into the bladder via the urethra to remove small calculi from the bladder.

bilateral (bī-lăt′ĕr-ăl) [″ + *latus,* side] Pert. to, affecting, or relating to two sides.

b. carotid body resection ABBR: BCBR. A rarely used method of treating carotid sinus syncope that relies on the bilateral surgical removal of the carotid bodies. SEE: *carotid body; carotid sinus syncope.*

bilateralism (bī-lăt′ĕr-ăl-ĭzm) [″ + ″ + Gr. *-ismos,* condition] Bilateral symmetry.

bilayer A two-component layer.

lipid b. The outer membrane of most cells includes two layers of phospholipid molecules. These layers are arranged so their two hydrophilic (water-soluble) sides face the interior and the exterior of the cell, and their hydrophobic (nonpolar) core is in between. The membrane is relatively impermeable to molecules such as glucose and amino acids but very permeable to lipid-soluble molecules such as oxygen, carbon dioxide, and alcohol. SEE: *cell* for illus.

bile (bīl) [L. *bilis,* bile] A thick, viscid, bitter-tasting fluid secreted by the liver. It passes from the bile duct of the liver into the common bile duct and then into the duodenum as needed. The bile from the liver is straw colored, while that from the gallbladder varies from yellow to brown or green.

Bile also is stored in the gallbladder, where it is concentrated, drawn upon as needed, and discharged into the duodenum. Contraction of the gallbladder is brought about by cholecystokinin-pancreozymin, a hormone produced by the duodenum; its secretion is stimulated by the entrance of fatty foods into the duodenum. Added to water, bile decreases surface tension, giving a foamy solution favoring the emulsification of fats and oils; this action is due to the bile salts, mainly sodium glycocholate and taurocholate.

COMPOSITION: Bile pigments (principally bilirubin and biliverdin) are responsible for the variety of colors observed. In addition, bile contains cholesterol, lecithin, mucin, and other organic and inorganic substances.

FUNCTION: Bile's importance as a digestive fluid is due to its emulsifying action, which facilitates the digestion of fats in the small intestine by pancreatic lipase. Bile also stimulates peristalsis. Normally the ejection of bile occurs only during duodenal digestion. Bile is both an antiseptic and a purgative. About 800 to 1000 ml/24 hr are secreted in the normal adult. SEE: *gallbladder.*

PATHOLOGY: Interference with the flow of bile produces jaundice and results in the presence of unabsorbed fats in the feces. In such instances, fats should be restricted in the diet. A restricted flow of bile may also produce gallstones in the gallbladder. SEE: *jaundice.*

b. acids Complex acids, of which cholic, glycocholic, and taurocholic acids are examples, and which occur as salts in bile. They give bile its foamy character, are important in the digestion of fats in the intestine, and are reabsorbed from the intestine to be used again by the liver. This circulation of bile acids is called the enterohepatic circulation.

cystic b. Bile stored in the gallbladder. It is concentrated as compared with hepatic bile.

b. ducts Intercellular passages that convey bile from the liver to the hepatic duct, which joins the duct from the gallbladder (cystic duct) to form the common bile duct (ductus choledochus), and which enters the duodenum about 3 in. (7.6 cm) below the pylorus. SEE: illus.

hepatic b. Bile secreted by the liver cells. It is collected in the bile ducts and flows to the gallbladder.

lithogenic b. Bile that favors gallstone production. This may be associated with several conditions; the most important is increased secretion of cholesterol in the bile as occurs with obesity, high-caloric diets, or drugs such as clofibrate.

b. pigments Complex, highly colored substances (e.g., bilirubin and biliverdin) found in bile derived from hemoglobin. They impart brown color to intestinal contents and feces. Van den Bergh's test is used to detect the type of bilirubin in the blood serum.

b. salts Alkali salts of bile sodium glycocholate and sodium taurocholate.

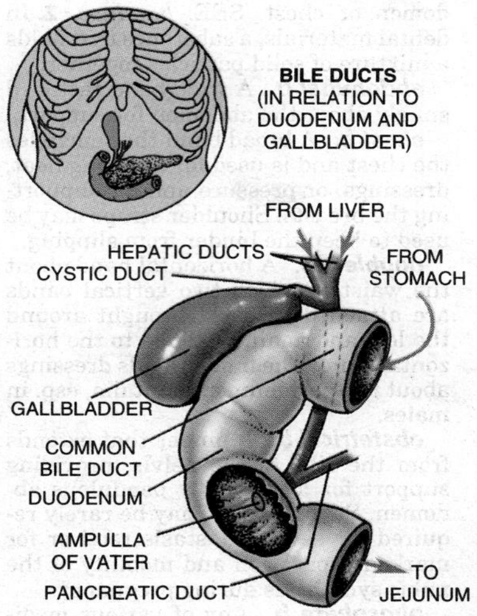

BILE DUCTS

Bilharzia (bĭl-hăr′zē-ă) [Theodor Maximilian Bilharz, Ger. helminthologist, 1825–1862] Former name for *Schistosoma,* the human blood fluke. SEE: *Schistosoma*.

bilharzial, bilharzic (bĭl-hăr′zē-ăl, -zĭk) Pert. to *Bilharzia* (*Schistosoma*).

bilharziasis (bĭl″hăr-zī′ă-sĭs) Schistosomiasis. SEE: *Bilharzia*.

bili- [L. *bilis*] Combining form meaning *bile*.

biliary (bĭl′ē-ār-ē) Pert. to bile.

biliblanket (bĭl′ē-blănk-ĕt) A phototherapy device for treating hyperbilirubinemia in newborns. It consists of an illuminator and a fiber-optic pad with a disposable cover.

bilicyanin (bĭl″ĭ-sī′ă-nĭn) [L. *bilis,* bile, + *cyaneus,* blue] A blue or purple pigment, an oxidation product of biliverdin.

biliflavin (bĭl″ĭ-flā′vĭn) [″ + *flavus,* yellow] A yellow pigment derived from biliverdin.

bilifuscin (bĭl″ĭ-fŭs′ĭn) [″ + *fuscus,* brown] A dark brown pigment from bile and gallstones.

biligenesis (bĭl″ĭ-jĕn′ĕ-sĭs) [″ + Gr. *genesis,* generation, birth] The formation of bile.

biligenetic, biligenic (bĭl″ĭ-jĕn-ĕt′ĭk, -jĕn′ĭk) [″ + Gr. *gennan,* to produce] Forming bile.

bilious (bĭl′yŭs) [L. *bilosus*] **1.** Pert. to bile. **2.** Afflicted with biliousness.

biliousness (bĭl′yŭs-nĕs) **1.** A symptom of a disorder of the liver causing constipation, headache, loss of appetite, and vomiting of bile. **2.** An excess of bile.

bilirubin (bĭl-ĭ-roo′bĭn) [″ + *ruber,* red] $C_{33}H_{36}O_6N_4$; the orange-colored or yellowish pigment in bile. It is derived from hemoglobin of red blood cells that have completed their life span and are destroyed and ingested by the macrophage system of the liver, spleen, and red bone marrow. When produced elsewhere, it is carried to the liver by the blood. It is changed chemically in the liver and excreted in the bile via the duodenum. As it passes through the intestines, it is converted into urobilinogen by bacterial enzymes, most of it being excreted through the feces. If urobilinogen passes into the circulation, it is excreted through the urine or re-excreted in the bile. The pathological accumulation of bilirubin leads to jaundice in many cases, such as physiologic jaundice of the newborn. SEE: illus.

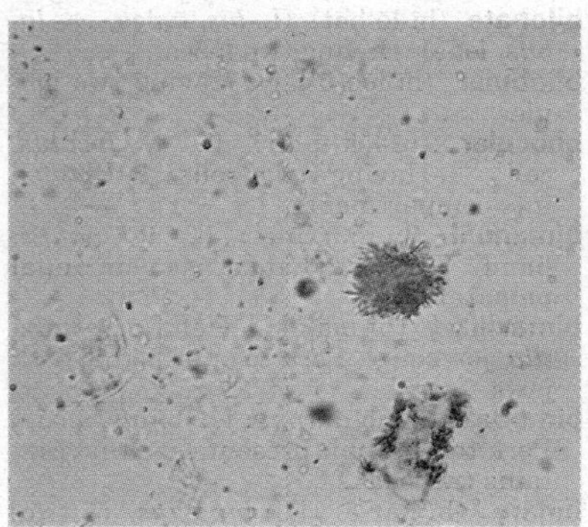

BILIRUBIN CRYSTALS (X400)

direct b. Bilirubin conjugated by the liver cells to form bilirubin diglucuronide, which is water-soluble and excreted in urine.

indirect b. Unconjugated bilirubin that is present in the blood. It is fat-soluble.

bilirubinate (bĭl-ĭ-roo′bĭn-āt) A salt of bilirubin.

bilirubinemia (bĭl″ĭ-roo-bĭn-ē′mē-ă) [″ + *ruber,* red, + Gr. *haima,* blood] Bilirubin in the blood, usually in excessive amounts. Bilirubin normally is present in the blood in small amounts. It increases, however, in diseases in which there is excessive destruction of red blood cells or interference with bile excretion; the amount is also increased when the liver is diseased or damaged. Also called *hyperbilirubinemia*. SEE: *jaundice*.

bilirubinometry (bĭl″ĭ-roo-bĭn-ŏm′ĭ-trē) The laboratory technique of measuring bilirubin levels in blood, skin, cerebrospinal fluid, or urine. These measurements are used esp. in the treatment of hyperbilirubinemia in neonates. SEE: *hyperbilirubinemia; kernicterus*.

bilirubinuria (bĭl″ĭ-roo-bĭn-ū′rē-ă) [″ + ″ + Gr. *ouron,* urine] Presence of bilirubin in urine.

biliuria (bĭl-ĭ-ū′rē-ă) The presence of bile in the urine.

biliverdin (bĭl-ĭ-vĕr′dĭn) [″ + *viridis,* green] $C_{33}H_{34}O_6N_4$; a greenish pigment in bile formed by the oxidation of bilirubin.

billion [Fr. *bi,* two, + *million,* million] **1.** In the U.S., billion is a number equal to 1 followed by 9 zeros (1,000,000,000) or (10^9). **2.** In Europe, billion is a number equal to 1 followed by 12 zeros (10^{12}), that is, bi-million, or twice the number of zeros in a million (10^6).

Billroth, Christian A.T. Austrian surgeon, 1829–1894.

B. I operation Gastroduodenostomy.

B. II operation Gastrojejunostomy.

bilobate (bī-lō′bāt) [L. *bis,* twice, + *lobus,* lobe] Having two lobes.

bilobular (bī-lŏb′ū-lăr) Having two lobules.

bilocular (bī-lŏk′ū-lăr) [″ + *loculus,* cell] **1.** Having two cells. **2.** Divided into compartments.

bimanual (bī-măn′ū-ăl) [″ + *manus,* hand] With both hands, as in bimanual palpation.

bimaxillary (bī-măk′sĭ-lĕr″ē) [″ + *maxilla,* jawbone] Pert. to or afflicting both jaws.

bimodal (bī-mō′dăl) [″ + *modus,* mode] Pert. to a graphic presentation that contains two peaks.

binary (bī′năr-ē) [L. *binarius,* of two] **1.** Composed of two elements. **2.** Separating into two branches.

b. acid An acid containing hydrogen and one other element.

b. code SEE: *b. system*.

b. digit One of two digits, usually 0 or 1, used in a binary system of enumeration.

b. system A numbering system particularly well suited to use by computers. All of the information placed into a computer is in binary form, that is, numbers made up of zeros and ones (0's and 1's). In this system each "place" in a binary number represents a power of 2 (i.e., the number of times 2 is to be multiplied by itself).

binaural (bĭn-aw′răl) [L. *bis,* twice, + *auris,* ear] Pert. to both ears.

binauricular (bĭn″aw-rĭk′ū-lăr) [″ + *auricula,* little ear] Binaural; pert. to both auricles of the ear.

bind **1.** To fasten, wrap, or encircle with a bandage. **2.** In chemistry and immunology, the uniting or adherence (i.e., bonding) of one molecule or chemical entity to another (e.g., the joining of a toxin to an antitoxin or of a hormone to its receptor on a cell surface).

binder (bīnd′ĕr) [AS. *bindan,* to tie up] **1.** A broad bandage most commonly used as an encircling support of the abdomen or chest. SEE: *bandage*. **2.** In dental materials, a substance that holds a mixture of solid particles together.

abdominal b. A wide band fastened snugly about the abdomen for support.

chest b. A broad band that encircles the chest and is used for applying heat, dressings, or pressure and for supporting the breasts. Shoulder straps may be used to keep the binder from slipping.

double-T b. A horizontal band about the waist to which two vertical bands are attached in back, brought around the leg, and again fastened to the horizontal band. The binder holds dressings about the perineum or genitalia, esp. in males.

obstetrical b. A binder that extends from the ribs to the pelvis, providing support for a markedly pendulous abdomen. Such support may be rarely required for severe diastasis recti or for marked separation and mobility of the pubic symphysis during pregnancy.

phosphate b. Any of various medications used to prevent hyperphosphatemia in patients with end-stage renal disease. Calcium carbonate taken with meals is the most commonly employed agent. In the past aluminum-containing antacids were used for this purpose, but this practice is now avoided because of the toxic accumulation of aluminum in patients with renal failure.

Scultetus b. [Johann Schultes (Scultetus), German surgeon, 1595–1645] A many-tailed binder or bandage, applied around the abdomen so that the ends overlap each other as if they were roof shingles. The binder holds dressings in place and supports abdominal muscles postoperatively. SEE: illus.

T b. Two strips of material fastened together resembling a T, used as a bandage to hold a dressing on the perineum of women.

towel b. A towel that encircles the abdomen or chest and whose ends are pinned together.

Binder's syndrome A syndrome related to facial growth, with hypoplasia of the maxillae and nasal bones resulting in a flattened face, elongated nose, and

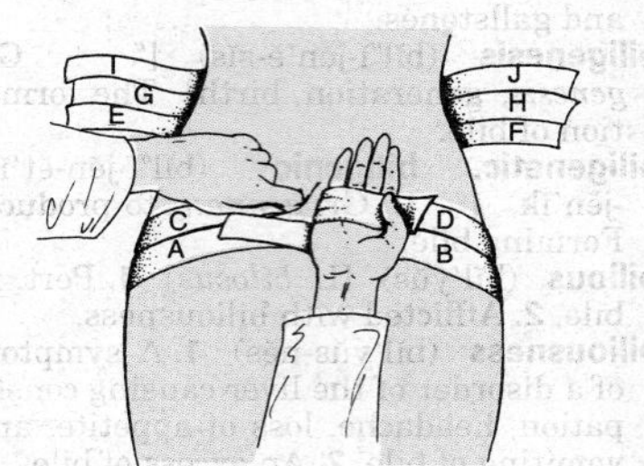

SCULTETUS BINDER

smaller maxillary arch with crowding of the teeth and malocclusions.

binge drinking (bĭnj) The consumption of more than four or five alcoholic drinks in a row (the lower number applies to women; the higher number applies to men). The behavioral consequences of this practice include impaired driving, sexual assaults, and other forms of violence. SEE: *alcoholism*.

binge eating An eating disorder marked by rapid consumption of large amounts of food in a short period of time. SEE: *bulimia*.

binocular (bĭn-ŏk′ū-lăr) [L. *bis,* twice, + *oculus,* eye] Pert. to both eyes.

binomial (bī-nō′mē-ăl) [″ + *nomen,* name] In mathematics and statistics, an equation containing two variables.

binotic (bĭn-ŏt′ĭk) [″ + Gr. *ous,* ear] Pert. to or having two ears.

binovular (bĭn-ŏv′ū-lăr) Biovular.

binuclear, binucleate (bī-nū′klē-ăr, -āt) [″ + *nucleus,* kernel] Having two nuclei.

bio- [Gr. *bios,* life] Combining form indicating *relationship to life*.

bioactive Affecting living tissues.

bioassay (bī″ō-ăs′ā) [″ + O. Fr. *asaier,* to try] In pharmacology, the determination of the strength of a drug or substance by comparing its effect on a live animal or an isolated organ preparation with that of a standard preparation.

bioastronautics (bī″ō-ăs″trō-naw′tĭks) The study of the effects of space travel on living plants and animals.

bioavailability (bī″ō-ă-văl″ă-bĭl′ĭ-tē) The rate and extent to which an active drug or metabolite enters the general circulation, permitting access to the site of action. Bioavailability is determined either by measurement of the concentration of the drug in body fluids or by the magnitude of the pharmacologic response.

biocatalyst (bī-ō-kăt′ă-lĭst) [″ + *katalyein,* to dissolve] An enzyme; a biochemical catalyzer.

biocenosis (bī″ō-sĕn-ō′sĭs) [″ + *koinos,* shared in common, + *osis,* condition] An ecological unit or community.

biochemical (bī-ō-kĕm′ĭ-kăl) Of or rel. to biochemistry.

b. marker Any biochemical compound such as an antigen, antibody, abnormal enzyme, or hormone that is sufficiently altered in a disease to serve as an aid in diagnosing or in predicting susceptibility to the disease.

biochemistry [″ + *chemeia,* chemistry] The chemistry of living things; the science of the chemical changes accompanying the vital functions of plants and animals.

biochemorphology (bī″ō-kĕ-mor-fŏl′ō-jē) [″ + ″ + *morphe,* shape, + *logos,* word, reason] The science of the relationship between chemical structure and biological action. SEE: *stereochemistry*.

biocide (bī′ō-sīd) [″ + L. *caedere,* to kill] A substance, esp. a pesticide or an antibiotic, that destroys living organisms.

bioclimatology (bī″ō-klī-mă-tŏl′ō-jē) [″ + *klima,* climate, + *logos,* word, reason] Study of the relationship of climate to life.

biocolloid (bī″ō-kŏl′oyd) [″ + *kollodes,* glutinous] A colloid from animal, vegetable, or microbial tissue.

biocompatibility The condition of being harmonious with living systems.

biocontainment In infectious disease laboratories, the process and procedures used to confine harmful microorganisms to the areas in which they are being investigated. The precise regulations vary with the pathogenicity of the organisms. SEE: *biosafety levels*.

biodegradable Susceptible to degradation by biological processes, such as bacterial or enzymatic action.

biodegradation (bī″ō-dĕg″rĕ-dā′shŭn) The breakdown of organic materials into simple chemicals by biochemical processes. Also called *biological degradation*.

biodynamics (bī″ō-dī-năm′ĭks) [Gr. *bios,* life, + *dynamis,* force] The science of the force or energy of living matter.

bioelectronics (bī″ō-ē″lĕk-trŏn′ĭks) The study of the transfer of electrons between molecules in biological systems.

bioenergetics (bī″ō-ĕn″ĕr-jĕt′ĭks) Study of energy transfer and relationships between all living systems.

bioengineering The application of engineering concepts, equipment, skills, and techniques to solving medical problems. SEE: *biomedical engineering*.

bioequivalence (bī″ō-ĭ-kwĭv′ă-lĕnts) The property of having the same biological effects of that to which a medicine was compared.

bioequivalent **1.** Of or relating to bioequivalence. **2.** A bioequivalent drug.

biofeedback A training program designed to develop one's ability to control the autonomic (involuntary) nervous system. After learning the technique, the patient may be able to control heart rate, blood pressure, and skin temperature or to relax certain muscles. The patient learns by using monitoring devices that sound a tone when changes in pulse, blood pressure, brain waves, and muscle contractions occur. Then the patient attempts to reproduce the conditions that caused the desired changes.

biofilm A moist film that covers surfaces, esp. those of implanted devices, including catheters. This film consists of bacteria imbedded in a film of an adhesive biopolymer. Bacteria within the film may be protected from the action of antibiotics. The film may be seen with a scanning electron microscope.

biogenesis (bī″ō-jĕn′ĕ-sĭs) [″ + *genesis,* generation, birth] The accepted theory that life can originate only from pre-existing life and never from nonliving material. **biogenetic** (-jĕ-nĕt′ĭk), *adj.*

biogenic (bī-ō-jĕn′ĭk) Produced by living organisms.

b. amines A group of chemical compounds, most of which are important in neurotransmission. Included are norepinephrine, histamine, serotonin, and dopamine.

biohazard Anything that is harmful or potentially harmful to humans, other species, or the environment. SEE: *biosafety levels*.

bioinequivalent Not being equivalent to that to which a drug is compared.

bioinstrument A device placed in the body to record or transmit data from the individual.

biokinetics (bī″ō-kĭ-nĕt′ĭks) [″ + *kinetikos,* moving] The study of growth changes and movements in developing organisms.

biologic [″ + *logos,* word, reason] Pert. to biology.

b. half-life The time required to reduce the concentration of a drug in the blood, plasma, or serum by 50%. This is a measure of the rate of drug distribution and elimination. SEE: *half-life; pharmacokinetics*.

biological [″ + *logos,* word, reason] **1.** Pert. to biology. **2.** A medicinal compound (such as a serum, vaccine, antigen, or antitoxin) prepared from living organisms and their products.

b. armature SEE: *armature (1)*.

b. degradation The breakdown of organic materials into simple chemicals by biochemical processes.

b. fitness SEE: *fitness, biological*.

b. warfare ABBR: BW. Warfare in which disease-producing microorganisms, toxins, or organic biocides (e.g., anthrax, brucellosis, plague) are deliberately used to destroy, injure, or immobilize livestock, vegetation, or human life. SYN: *biowar*. SEE: *chemical warfare*.

biologist A specialist in biology.

biology (bī-ŏl′ō-jē) [Gr. *bios,* life, + *logos,* word, reason] The science of life and living things.

molecular b. The branch of biology dealing with analysis of the structure and development of biological systems with respect to the chemistry and physics of their molecular constituents.

radiation b. The scientific study of the effects of radiation on living organisms.

bioluminescence (bī″ō-loo″mĭ-nĕs′ĕns) [″ + L. *lumen,* light] Emission of visible light from living organisms. The best known example is the cold light produced by fireflies. SEE: *luciferase*.

biolysis (bī-ŏl′ĭ-sĭs) [″ + *lysis,* dissolution] The chemical decomposition of living tissue by the action of living organisms. **biolytic** (bī-ō-lĭt′ĭk), *adj.*

biomarker **1.** A signal that serves as an indicator of the state of a living organism. **2.** A biochemical, genetic, or molecular indicator that can be used to screen diseases, such as cancer. An example of a simple biomarker is body temperature. Hormonal or enzymatic changes in response to toxic substances also serve as biomarkers.

biomass (bī′ō-măs) [″ + L. *massa,* mass] All of the living organisms in a specified area.

biome (bī′ōm) [″ + *oma,* mass] A major type of environment, such as tundra, forest, or swamp, marked by its climate, flora, fauna, and unique diseases.

biomechanics (bī″ō-mĕ-kăn′ĭks) The application of mechanical forces to living organisms and the investigation of the effects of the interaction of force and the body or system. Includes forces that arise from within and outside the body. SEE: *kinesiology*.

biomedical Biological and medical; pert. to application of natural sciences to the study of medicine.

b. engineer A certified design engineer, usually with a Bachelor of Science degree and employed in a hospital or a commercial company to design and/or maintain medical equipment. Also referred to as a *clinical engineer*.

b. engineering Application of the principles and practices of engineering science to biomedical research and health care, as seen in the development of devices such as cardiac pacemakers, hearing aids, and sophisticated artificial limbs and joints.

b. engineering technologist A certified repair specialist usually with an AAS degree usually employed in a hospital or commercial company to repair and maintain medical equipment.

biomedicalization of aging The treatment of aging as a biological or medical problem that must be combatted or cured.

biometeorology (bī″ō-mē″tē-or-ŏl′ŏ-jē) [″ + *meteoros,* raised from off the ground, + *logos,* word, reason] Study of the effects of meteorology on all forms of life.

biometrics (bī″ō-mĕt′rĭks) The study of the application of mathematics and statistics to the analysis and solution of problems in the fields of biology and other life sciences.

biometry (bī-ŏm′ĕ-trē) [″ + *metron,* measure] **1.** The application of statistics to biological science. **2.** The computation of life expectancy.

ophthalmic b. Measurement of any part of the eye, from the cornea to the retina, using ophthalmic ultrasound.

biomicroscope (bī″ō-mī′krŏ-skōp) A microscope used with a slit lamp for viewing segments of the eye.

bion (bī′ŏn) [Gr. *bios*, life] Any living organism.

bionics (bī-ŏn′ĭks) The study of biological functions and mechanisms and the application of these findings to the design of machines, esp. computers.

biophysics (bī″ō-fĭz′ĭks) [″ + *physikos*, natural] Application of physical laws to biological processes and functions. **biophysical** (-ĭ-kăl), *adj.*

biopsy (bī′ŏp-sē) [″ + *opsis*, vision] The obtaining of a representative tissue sample for microscopic examination, usually to establish a diagnosis. The tissue may be obtained surgically or by using a syringe and needle. The procedure can be guided by computed tomography, ultrasonography, magnetic resonance imaging, ultrasound, or radiography, or it can be performed without imaging (i.e., "blindly").

aspiration b. The removal of tissue by use of a needle and syringe, for example, from a cyst or the bone marrow.

brush b. The removal of tissue for investigation by use of a brush.

cone b. The removal of a cone-shaped piece of tissue for examination, esp. from the uterine cervix.

endometrial b. The removal of a sample of uterine endometrium for subsequent microscopic study. The procedure is commonly used in fertility assessment to confirm ovulation and as a diagnostic tool to determine the cause of dysfunctional and postmenopausal bleeding.

fine needle aspiration b. ABBR: FNA biopsy. The removal of tissue through a long needle with or without guidance.

liver b. The removal of tissue from the liver by use of a large-bore needle that permits removal of a core of tissue.

muscle b. The removal of muscle tissue for microscopic examination and chemical analysis.

needle b. The removal of tissue by use of a needle. It may be attached to a syringe or to mechanized systems guided by ultrasound, computed tomography, or other technologies.

percutaneous breast b. Use of a directional, high-speed, rotating cutter attached to a vacuum source to gather multiple contiguous core samples of breast tissue through a single point of insertion. This minimally invasive procedure is usually performed under local anesthesia, using stereotactic imaging or real-time ultrasonography.

percutaneous transthoracic needle aspiration b. Use of a fluoroscopically guided aspiration needle to obtain a sample of tissue in cases of suspected pulmonary malignancies or other unknown lesions. Because of the risk of pneumothorax, the procedure is usually contraindicated in patients receiving mechanical ventilation.

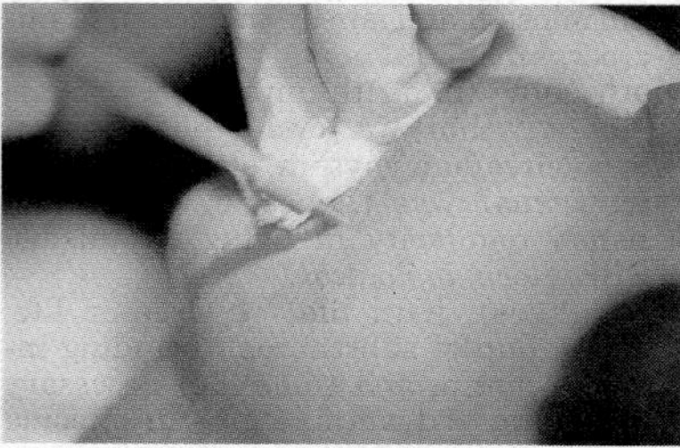
(A) SCREWING PUNCH INTO SKIN

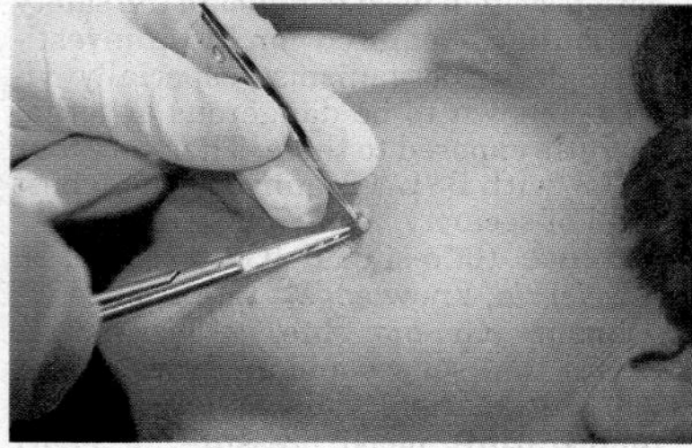
(B) REMOVING THE BIOPSY SPECIMEN

PUNCH BIOPSY

punch b. The removal of a small piece of tissue (usually of the skin) with a hollow, round cutting tool. SEE: illus.

sentinel node b. Technique for identifying the initial site of cancer metastasis. After injection of a radioactive tracer directly into the tumor mass, the tissue is massaged to encourage uptake of tracer by lymphatic vessels. A negative biopsy of the first node infiltrated by the tracer suggests that the malignancy has not yet spread to neighboring regional lymph nodes.

biopsychosocial Biological, psychological, and social; pert. to the application of knowledge from the biological and behavioral sciences to solve human problems.

biopterin (bī-ŏp′tĕr-ĭn) The chemical 2-amino-4-hydroxy-6-(1,2-hydroxypropyl) pteridine, important in metabolizing phenylalanine. A deficiency of biopterin is a rare cause of phenylketonuria.

bioptome (bī-ŏp′tōm) A tool used to obtain biopsies of the endomyocardium. It consists of a forceps (with small tissue-cutting jaws) that is advanced into the ventricle along a catheter or guidewire.

bioremediation The conversion of hazardous wastes and pollutants into harmless materials by the action of microorganisms.

biorhythm (bī-ō-rĭth″ŭm) [″ + *rhythmos,* rhythm] A cyclic phenomenon (e.g., circadian rhythm, sleep cycle, and menstrual cycle) that occurs with established regularity in living organisms. SEE: *clock, biological*.

bios (bī′ŏs) [Gr., life] **1.** Organic life. **2.** A group of substances (including inositol, biotin, and thiamine) necessary for the most favorable growth of some yeasts.

biosafety levels ABBR: BSL. A classification system used to indicate the safety precautions required for those investigating microorganisms, especially viruses known to be dangerous or lethal to those exposed to them. There are four BSLs, with BSL-4 requiring the highest level of security.

bioscience (bī″ō-sī′ĕns) [Gr. *bios,* life, + L. *scientia,* knowledge] Life science.

biosensor [Gr. *bios,* life, + sensor] A device that senses and analyzes biological information. This may be simple temperature, blood pressure, or heart rate or more sophisticated determination of chemicals and enzymes in body fluids. The device may be used in the laboratory or placed within the body.

biospectrometry (bī″ō-spĕk-trŏm′ĕ-trē) [″ + L. *spectrum,* image, + Gr. *metron,* measure] Use of a spectroscope to determine the amounts and kinds of substances in tissues.

biospectroscopy (bī″ō-spĕk-trŏs′kō-pē) [″ + ″ + Gr. *skopein,* to examine] Examination of tissue by use of a spectroscope.

biosphere (bī′ō-sfēr″) [″ + *sphaira,* ball] The parts of earth's land, water, and atmosphere in which living organisms can exist.

biostatistics The application of statistical processes and methods to the analysis of biological data. SEE: *life table; morbidity rate; vital statistics*.

biosynthesis (bī″ō-sĭn′thĕ-sĭs) [″ + *synthesis,* a putting together] The formation of chemical compounds by a living organism.

biota (bī-ō′tă) [Gr. *bios,* life] The combined animal and plant life in an area.

biotaxis, biotaxy (bī″ō-tăk′sĭs, -sē) [″ + *taxis,* arrangement] **1.** The selecting and arranging activity of living cells. **2.** Systematic classification of living organisms.

Biot's breathing (bē-ōz′) [Camille Biot, Fr. physician, b. 1878] Breathing marked by several short breaths followed by long, irregular periods of apnea. It is seen in patients with increased intracranial pressure. SEE: *Cheyne-Stokes respiration*.

biotechnology The application of biological systems and organisms to technical and industrial processes. This broad definition includes such ancient endeavors as the use of yeast in preparing bread for baking, and such modern concepts as genetic engineering. SEE: *molecular biology*.

biotelemetry (bī″ō-tĕl-ĕm′ĕ-trē) [Gr. *bios,* life, + *tele,* distant, + *metron,* measure] Recording biological events such as temperature, heart rate, ECG, and EEG in subjects remote from the investigator. This is done by transmitting and receiving by telephone or other electronic methods.

biotherapy In complementary medicine, the use of biological response modifiers, such as phytochemicals and phytonutrients, enzymes, and botanicals, to enhance the immune response, alter hormone levels, or assist in the treatment of cancer.

biotics (bī-ŏt′ĭks) [Gr. *biotikos,* living] The science that deals with the functions of life.

biotin (bī′ō-tĭn) A B vitamin that is a coenzyme involved in gluconeogenesis and fat synthesis. It is commonly found in egg yolks, peanut butter, liver, kidney, cauliflower, and yeast. Deficiencies occur when people consume large amounts of raw egg white, which contains avidin, a chemical that binds biotin with great affinity. Deficiency is also common among alcoholics. Children with biotin deficiency have retarded mental and physical development, alopecia, impaired immunity, and anemia.

biotoxin (bī-ō-tŏk′sĭn) [Gr. *bios,* life, + *toxikon,* poison] A toxin produced by or found in a living organism.

biotransformation The chemical alteration that a substance undergoes in the body.

biotype (bī′ō-tīp) [″ + *typos,* mark] **1.** Individuals possessing the same genotype. **2.** In microbiology, the former name for biovar. SEE: *biovar*.

biovar [*bio*logical *var*iation] In microbiology, a term for variants within a species. These are usually distinguished by certain biochemical or physiological characteristics. SEE: *morphovar; serovar*.

biovular (bī-ŏv′ū-lăr) [L. *bis,* twice, + *ovum,* egg] Derived from or pert. to two ova. SYN: *binovular*.

biowar (bī-ō-wăr′) Biological warfare.

BiPAP A type of continuous positive airway pressure in which both inspiratory and expiratory pressures are set above atmospheric levels. This type of ventilatory support assists patients with sleep apnea, congestive heart failure, hypoventilation, and other forms of respiratory insufficiency.

bipara (bĭp′ă-ră) [″ + *parere,* to bring forth, to bear] A woman who has given birth for the second time to an infant or infants, alive or dead, weighing 500 g or more. SYN: *secundipara*.

biparental (bī″pă-rĕn′tăl) [″ + *parere,* to bring forth, to bear] Derived from two parents, male and female.

biparietal (bī″pă-rī′ĕ-tăl) Concerning the parietal bones or their eminences.

biparous (bĭp′ă-rŭs) Producing two ova or offspring at one time.

biped (bī′pĕd) [″ + *pes,* foot] An animal with two feet.

bipenniform (bī-pĕn′ĭ-form) [″ + *penna,* feather, + *forma,* shape] Muscle fibers that come from each side of a tendon in the manner in which barbs come from the central shaft of a feather.

biperforate (bī-pĕr′fō-rāt) [″ + *perforatus,* pierced with holes] Having two openings or perforations.

biperiden (bī-pĕr′ĭ-dĕn) An anticholinergic drug used in treating parkinsonism. Trade name is Akineton.

biphasic (bī-fāz′ĭk) Consisting of two phases.

bipolar (bī-pōl′ăr) [″ + *polus,* a pole] **1.** Having two poles or processes. **2.** Pert. to the use of two poles in electrotherapeutic treatments. The term *biterminal* should be used when referring to an alternating current. **3.** A two-poled nerve cell.

biramous (bī-rā′mŭs) [″ + *ramus,* a branch] Possessing two branches.

bird breeder's lung An allergic (hypersensitivity) inflammation of the lung caused by exposure to bird excreta. In some patients the onset is slow rather than acute. Symptoms, which include chills, fever, cough, and shortness of breath, usually subside when exposure to the antigen ceases. SYN: *pigeon breeder's disease*. SEE: *psittacosis*.

birefractive (bī″rē-frăk′tĭv) [″ + *refrangere,* to break up] Pert. to or having birefringence.

birefringence (bī″rē-frĭn′jĕns) The splitting of a ray of light in two. **birefringent** (-jĕnt), *adj.*

birth [Old Norse *burdhr*] The act of being born; passage of a child from the uterus.

complete b. The instant of complete separation of the body of the infant from that of the mother, regardless of whether the cord or placenta is detached.

cross b. Crossbirth.

dry b. A birth following premature rupture of the fetal membranes.

live b. An infant showing one of the three evidences of life (breathing, heart action, movements of a voluntary muscle) after complete birth. In some countries a live birth is considered not to have occurred if the infant dies during the 24 hr following delivery. Obviously, which of these two definitions is used has considerable effect on various vital statistics concerned with the viability of the fetus at time of delivery.

multiple b. The birth of two or more offspring produced in the same gestation period.

premature b. Preterm b.

preterm b. The delivery of a fetus anytime after the date of defined viability and before completion of 37 weeks' gestation. SYN: *premature b.*

birth canal The canal, comprising the cervix, vagina, and vulva, through which the products of conception, including the fetus, pass during labor and birth.

birth center An alternative nonhospital facility that provides family-oriented maternity care for women judged to be at low risk of experiencing obstetrical complications.

birth certificate A legal written record of the birth of a child, as required by U.S. law.

birth control Prevention of conception or implantation of the fertilized ovum, or termination of pregnancy. Methods of birth control may be temporary and reversible, or permanent. Temporary methods to avoid conception include physical barriers (e.g., male and female condoms, diaphragm, cervical cap, and vaginal sponge) that are most effective when used in conjunction with chemical barriers, such as spermicidal vaginal suppositories, creams, jellies, or foams. Hormonal methods include oral contraceptive pills and progestin implants to suppress ovulation. Fertility awareness methods, such as rhythm, involve identification of and abstinence during ovulation, graphing basal body temperature and changes in cervical mucus consistency, and estimation of the day of ovulation. Intrauterine devices (IUD) prevent zygote implantation. Sterilization techniques include male vasectomy and female tubal ligation. Sterilization usually is permanent, but may be reversible. SEE: *abortion; contraceptive; family planning; infanticide; mifepristone*.

birth control pill A class of medicines taken orally to control conception. They contain synthetic forms of estrogen and progesterone or synthetic progesterone alone. SEE: *contraceptive*.

birth defect A congenital anomaly. Birth defects are a leading cause of infant mortality in the U.S. and most developed countries. Each year in the U.S. about 150,000 babies are born with serious birth defects. Known causes include human teratogens, chromosomal defects, and single-gene defects. The cause is unknown in about two thirds of the cases.

birthing chair A chair designed for use during childbirth. The mother is in a sitting or semireclining position, which facilitates the labor process and is more comfortable than the usual supine position.

birth injury Injury sustained by the neonate during the birth process.

birthmark Nevus (1).

birth mother The woman who actually gives birth to a child, whether or not she is the biological mother (i.e., provided the ovum that developed into that child). SEE: *surrogate parenting*.

birth parent(s) The biological parent(s) of a child. SEE: *surrogate parenting*.

birth weight The weight of the newborn. Normal weight of the newborn is between 5.5 lb (2.5 kg) and 10 lb (4.5 kg). Birth weight is an important index of maturation and chance for survival. Weight of less than 2.5 kg is associated with an increased chance of death in the perinatal period. Medical advances have increased the chance of survival of newborns of 2.0 kg or more. SEE: *large for gestational age; small for gestational age*.

birth weight, low SEE: *low birth weight*.

bisacodyl (bĭs-ăk′ō-dĭl; bĭs″ă-kō′dĭl) A cathartic drug that acts by its direct effect on the colon. It may be administered orally or by rectal suppository. Trade names are Dulcolax and Theralax.

bisacromial (bĭs″ă-krō′mē-ăl) [L. *bis,* twice, + Gr. *akron,* point, + *omos,* shoulder] Pert. to the two acromial processes.

bisection (bī-sĕk′shŭn) [″ + *sectio,* a cutting] Division into two parts by cutting.

bisexual (bī-sĕks′ū-ăl) [″ + *sexus,* sex] **1.** Hermaphroditic; having imperfect genitalia of both sexes in one person. **2.** An individual who is sexually active with others of either sex. SEE: *heterosexual; homosexual; lesbian*.

bisferious (bĭs-fĕr′ē-ŭs) [″ + *ferire,* to beat] Having two beats. SYN: *dicrotic*.

Bishop's score A system for evaluating the potential for successful elective induction of labor. Factors assessed include fetal station, cervical position, effacement, dilation, and consistency. Each factor receives a score of 0, 1, 2, or 3, so the maximum predictive total score is 15. The lower the score, the greater the possibility that labor induction will fail.

bisiliac (bĭs-ĭl′ē-ăk) [″ + *ilium,* ilium] Pert. to the two iliac crests or any corresponding iliac structures.

bis in die [L.] ABBR: b.d.; b.i.d. Twice in a day.

bismuth (bĭz′mŭth) [Ger. *Wismuth,* white mass] SYMB: Bi. A silvery metallic element; atomic weight 208.980, atomic number 83. Its compounds are used as a protective for inflamed surfaces. Its salts are used as an astringent and as a treatment for diarrhea.

b. subcarbonate An odorless, tasteless powder used as an antacid, astringent, and protective.

INCOMPATIBILITY: Sulfides, acids, acid salts.

b. subgallate A bright yellow powder without odor or taste. It was first used for treatment of skin diseases. General use is the same as for bismuth subnitrate.

b. subnitrate A heavy white odorless powder; used as an astringent, protective, and antiseptic.

INCOMPATIBILITY: Acids, tannins, and sulfides.

b. subsalicylate ABBR: BSS. BSS has antisecretory and antimicrobial effects in vitro. Its unlabeled use is for prevention of travelers' diarrhea due to enterotoxigenic *Escherichia coli*. It also relieves abdominal cramps. Trade name is Pepto-Bismol.

bismuth colloids Several bismuth compounds that are effective in treating peptic ulcers. They act in an acid medium by inhibiting the action of pepsin and reacting with the proteins in the ulcer crater to form a barrier that prevents the diffusion of acid into the area. SEE: *peptic ulcer*.

bismuth poisoning Poisoning due to ingestion of bismuth.

SYMPTOMS: Symptoms include metallic taste, foul breath, fever, gastrointestinal irritation, a bluish line at the gum margin, ulcerative process of the gums and mouth, headache, and renal tubular damage.

FIRST AID: The source of bismuth is removed; gastric lavage and high enemas are performed; respiratory support and chelation therapy with BAL are provided.

bisphosphonate (bĭs-fŏs′fō-nāt) Any of a class of medications that inhibit the resorption of bones by osteoclasts. Medications in this class are used to treat osteoporosis, hypercalcemia, and metastatic bone cancers. Examples include pamidronate, etidronate, clodronate, and alendronate.

bisulfate (bī-sŭl′fāt) An acid sulfate in which a monovalent metal and a hydrogen ion are combined with the sulfate radical. SEE: *disulfate*.

bite (bīt) [AS. *bitan,* to bite] **1.** To cut with the teeth. **2.** An injury in which the body surface is torn by an insect or animal, resulting in abrasions, punctures, or lacerated wounds. There may be evidence of a wound, usually surrounded by a zone of redness and swelling, often accompanied by pain, itching, or throbbing. This type of wound often becomes infected and may contain specific noxious materials such as bacteria, toxins, viruses, or venom. SEE: *sting*. **3.** In dentistry, the angle and manner in which the maxillary and mandibular teeth occlude. SEE: *occlusion*.

balanced b. Balanced occlusion of the teeth.

cat b. A wound inflicted by the teeth of a cat; typically a puncture wound on the hand or the arm. A cat bite is usually infected with multiple aerobic and anaerobic organisms, including *Pasteurella multocida*. Broad-spectrum antibiotics are required. About 20% of the time, the wound does not respond to antibiotic therapy and needs incision and drainage or débridement.

closed b. A bite in which the lower incisors lie behind the upper incisors.

dog b. A lacerated or punctured wound made by the teeth of a dog. The dog should be observed for 10 days to determine the presence of rabies. SEE: *Capnocytophaga canimorsus; rabies*.

TREATMENT: The wound must be cleansed thoroughly. It should be washed vigorously with soap and water for at least 10 min to remove saliva. Flushing with a viricidal agent should be followed with a clear rinse. Unless massive, bleeding should not be stopped because blood flow helps to cleanse the wound. Routine tetanus prophylaxis should be provided and information obtained about the animal, its location, and its owner. These data should be included in a report to public health authorities. Appropriate antirabies therapy must be initiated if the animal is known to have rabies.

end-to-end b. A bite in which the incisors of both jaws meet along the cutting edge when the jaw is closed.

fire ant b. Injury caused by fire ant venom, resulting in local redness and tenderness, and occasional episodes of life-threatening anaphylaxis.

TREATMENT: The area, which may contain multiple bites, should be washed with soap and water. Epinephrine, 0.3 to 0.5 ml of a 1:1000 aqueous solution, should be given subcutaneously every 20 to 30 min. This may be life saving. Use of a tourniquet slows absorption of the venom. Application of ice packs to the area relieves pain. Oxygen, endotracheal intubation, and vasopressors, as well as corticosteroids and antibiotics, may be required.

flea b. SEE: under *flea*.

human b. A laceration or puncture wound caused by the teeth of a human. The aerobic and anaerobic organisms transmitted from the mouth may cause a cellulitis, and, occasionally, infections of other soft tissues and bones.

TREATMENT: The wound should be irrigated thoroughly and may require surgical débridement. A moist dressing should be applied and tetanus prophylaxis administered. A penicillin with a beta-lactamase inhibitor usually provides adequate antibiotic coverage.

insect b. An injury in which the body surface is torn by an insect, resulting in abrasions, punctures, or lacerated wounds. Insect bites cause more deaths than do snake bites. For more information, see entries for individual insects.

SYMPTOMS: The reaction of a previously sensitized person is a potentially life-threatening medical emergency that requires prompt, effective therapy. Symptoms may include hives, itching and swelling in areas other than the site of the bite, tightness in the chest and difficulty in breathing, hoarse voice, swelling of the tongue, dizziness or hypotension, unconsciousness, and cardiac arrest.

FIRST AID: If the wound is suspected of containing venom, a bandage sufficiently tight to prevent venous return is applied if the bite is on an extremity. The wound is washed with saline solution thoroughly and a dry sterile dressing is applied. Appropriate antitetanus therapy is applied. Treatment for shock may be needed.

Some insect bites contain an acid substance resembling formic acid and consequently are relieved by topically applied alkalies, such as ammonia water or baking soda paste. For intense local pain, injection of local anesthetic may be required. Systemic medication may be needed for generalized pain.

Individuals who have had an allergic reaction to an insect bite may benefit from venom immunotherapy. This treatment involves administration of very small amounts of the insect venom over several weeks until immunity develops. Immunity is then maintained by periodic venom boosters.

Persons who have a history of an anaphylactic reaction to insect bites should avoid exposure to insects by wearing protective clothing, gloves, and shoes. Cosmetics, perfumes, and hair sprays should be avoided because they attract some insects, as do brightly colored and white clothing. Because foods and odor attract insects, care should be taken when cooking and eating outdoors.

mosquito b. SEE: under *mosquito*.

open b. A bite in which a space exists between the upper and lower incisors when the mouth is closed.

snake b. SEE: under *snake*.

spider b. SEE: under *spider*.

stork b. Colloquial term for telangiectasia.

tick b. SEE: under *tick*.

bitelock A device used in dentistry for retaining bite rims outside the mouth in the same position as they were inside the mouth.

bitemporal (bī-tĕm′pō-răl) [L. *bis,* twice, + *temporalis,* pert. to a temple] Pert. to both temples or temporal bones.

biteplate (bīt′plāt) A dental device used to correct or diagnose malocclusion. It is worn in the palate, usually on a temporary basis.

Bitot's spots (bē′tōz) [Pierre A. Bitot, Fr. physician, 1822–1888] Triangular shiny gray spots on the conjunctiva seen in vitamin A deficiency.

bitrochanteric (bī″trō-kăn-tĕr′ĭk) Concerning both greater trochanters of the two femurs.

bitter (bĭt′ĕr) [AS. *biter,* strong] Having a disagreeable taste.

biuret (bī′ū-rĕt) [L. *bis,* twice, + *urea*] $NH_2CONHCONH_2$; a crystalline decomposition derivative of urea.

biuret test A method for measuring protein in the serum. The presence of biuret can be detected by the addition of sodium hydroxide and copper sulfate solutions to the sample. A rose to violet color indicates the presence of protein, and a pink and finally blue color indicates the presence of urea.

bivalent (bī-vā′lĕnt) [″ + *valens,* powerful] **1.** Divalent. **2.** In cytology, a structure consisting of two paired homologous chromosomes, each split into two sister chromatids during meiosis.

biventer (bī-vĕn′tĕr) [″ + *venter,* belly] A muscle with two bellies.

biventral (bī-vĕn′trăl) Digastric.

bizygomatic (bī″zī-gō-măt′ĭk) Concerning the most prominent point on each of the two zygomatic arches.

Bjerrum's screen (byĕr′oomz) [Jannik P. Bjerrum, Danish ophthalmologist, 1827–1892] A 1-m square planar surface viewed from a distance of 1 m and consisting of a large square of black cloth with a central mark for fixation. It is used to plot the physiological blind spot, the central and paracentral scotomata, and other visual field defects. SYN: *tangent screen.*

Bjerrum's sign A sickle- or comet-shaped blind spot usually found in the central zone of the visual field; seen in glaucoma.

B.K. *below knee,* a term used to refer to the site of amputation of a lower extremity.

Bk Symbol for the element berkelium.

black (blăk) [AS. *blaec*] **1.** Devoid of color or reflecting no light. **2.** Marked by dark pigmentation.

black cohosh *Cimicifuga racemosa,* a perennial herb whose rootstock preparations are believed by alternative medicine practitioners to relieve menstrual and menopausal discomforts. Black cohosh is also known as *black snakeroot* and *bugbane.*

blackdamp In a coal mine, an atmosphere formed by the slow absorption of oxygen and the release of carbon dioxide from coal.

blackhead An open comedo. SEE: *comedo.*

black lung Lay term for the chronic lung disease or pneumoconiosis found in coal miners. SYN: *coal worker's pneumoconiosis.*

blackout Sudden loss of consciousness. SYN: *syncope.* SEE: *alcoholic blackout; red-out.*

blackwater fever Bloody urine (hemoglobinuria) that occurs as a complication of falciparum malaria infection. It is the result of red blood cell destruction and the release of hemoglobin. It occurs most commonly in patients who have been treated with drugs derived from quinine. SEE: *falciparum malaria.*

SYMPTOMS: The illness is marked by high fevers, dark urine, epigastric pain, vomiting, jaundice, and shock. Physical findings include enlargement of the liver and spleen. Laboratory hallmarks include severe anemia, and, occasionally, renal failure.

bladder (blăd′dĕr) [AS. *blaedre*] A membranous sac or receptacle for a secretion, as the gallbladder; commonly used to designate the urinary bladder. SEE: *bladder, urinary; genitourinary system.*

atony of b. Inability to urinate due to lack of muscle tone. It is frequently seen after traumatic deliveries or after the use of epidural anesthesia.

autonomous b. A bladder in which there is interruption in both the afferent and efferent limbs of the reflex arcs. Bladder sensation is absent; dribbling is constant; residual urine amount is large.

exstrophy of b. Congenital eversion of the urinary bladder. The abdominal wall fails to close and the inside of the bladder may protrude through the abdominal wall.

hypertonic b. **1.** A bladder with excessive muscle tone. **2.** Increased muscular activity of the bladder.

irritable b. Bladder condition marked by increased frequency of contraction with an associated desire to urinate.

motor paralytic b. A neurogenic bladder caused by defective nerve supply to the bladder. In the acute form urination is not possible. In the chronic form there is difficulty in urinating, which may lead to recurrent urinary tract infections.

nervous b. A condition marked by the repeated desire to urinate, but doing so fails to empty the bladder.

neurogenic b. Any dysfunction of the urinary bladder caused by lesions of the central nervous system or nerves supplying the bladder.

spastic b. Neurogenic bladder due to complete transection of the spinal cord above the sacral segments.

urinary b. A muscular, membranous, distensible reservoir that holds urine situated in the pelvic cavity. It receives urine from the kidneys through the ureters and discharges it from the body through the urethra. SYN: *vesica urinaria*. SEE: illus.; *urinary system*.

ANATOMY: The bladder is situated in the anterior inferior portion of the pelvic cavity. In the female it lies in front of the anterior wall of the vagina and the uterus; in the male it lies in front of the rectum. The lower portion of the bladder, continuous with the urethra, is called the neck; its upper tip, connected with the umbilicus by the median umbilical ligament, is called the apex. The region between the openings of the two ureters and the urethra is the trigone. The wall of the bladder has three major layers. The mucous membrane lining is transitional epithelium. The middle layer is three sheets (longitudinal, circular, longitudinal) of smooth muscle, called the detrusor muscle. The outer layer on the superior surface is the visceral peritoneum; on the lateral and inferior surfaces it is areolar connective tissue. The bladder is supported by numerous ligaments; it is supplied with blood by the superior, middle, and inferior vesical arteries, and drained by numerous veins and lymphatics; and it is innervated by branches of the third and fourth sacral nerves by way of the hypogastric plexus.

The bladder has a normal storage capacity of 500 ml (about 34 oz) or more. In disease states it may be greatly distended. A frequent cause of distention of the bladder in elderly men is interference with urination due to hypertrophy of the prostate gland, which surrounds the urethra and neck of the bladder.

PHYSIOLOGY: An average of 40 to 50 oz (about 1.2 to 1.5 L) of urine is secreted in a 24-hr period, but this varies with the amount of fluid ingested and the amount lost through exhalation, sweat, and the bowels. Inability to empty the bladder is known as retention and may require catheterization. Sphincter muscles are part of the mechanism that controls retention within the bladder.

For patients who need help in managing bladder elimination problems there are a variety of options: indwelling urethral catheters, Kegel exercises, intermittent catheterization, suprapubic indwelling catheters, external collecting devices (urinals and specially designed bedpans), medications for promoting bladder emptying (such as bethanechol, phenoxybenzamine, diazepam, dantrolene, or baclofen), and medicines to promote bladder storage (such as imipramine, oxybutynin, propanthelene, pseudoephedrine, or phenylpropanolamine). For men, a condom designed to collect and contain urine is available. SEE: *bladder drill*.

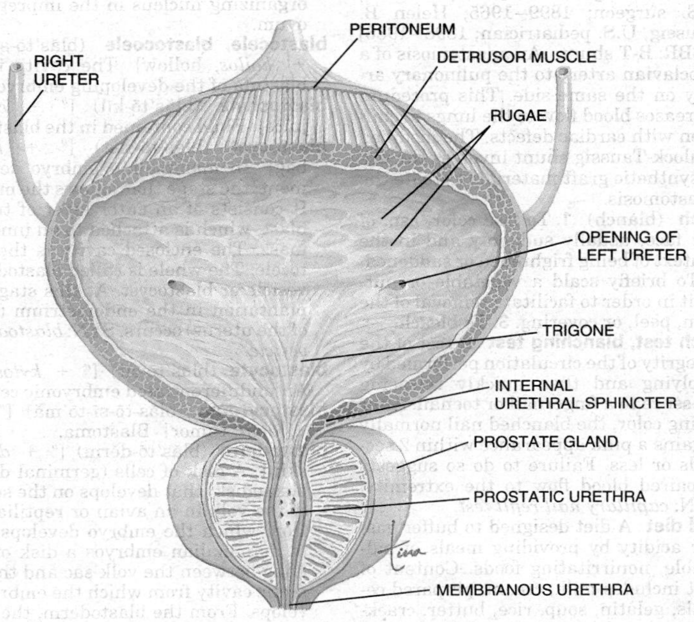

URINARY BLADDER

The force of urination is much greater in a child than in an adult because in the child the bladder is more an abdominal organ than a pelvic one. The child's abdominal muscles help to expel the urine.

EXAMINATION: *Palpation:* The bladder cannot be palpated when empty. When full it appears as a tumor in the suprapubic region that is smooth and oval on palpation.

Percussion: When it is distended with urine, the rounded superior margin is easily made out by observing the tympanic sound of the intestines on one hand and dull sound of the bladder on the other.

bladder drill A technique used to treat stress urinary incontinence in women in which the patient charts the number of urinations, the intervals between urination, and the volume of urine passed. She also notes the degree and frequency of incontinence. The intervals between urinations are gradually increased. Also called *bladder training*.

bladder worm Cysticercus.

Blalock-Hanlon procedure [Alfred Blalock, U.S. surgeon, 1899–1965; C. Rollins Hanlon, U.S. surgeon, b. 1915] The surgical creation of an atrial septal defect or enlargement of the foramen ovale in an infant with transposition of the great arteries. This procedure helps to improve oxygenation until total repair is undertaken.

Blalock-Taussig shunt [Alfred Blalock, U.S. surgeon; 1899–1965; Helen B. Taussig, U.S. pediatrician; 1898–1986] ABBR: B-T shunt. An anastomosis of a subclavian artery to the pulmonary artery on the same side. This procedure increases blood flow to the lungs in children with cardiac defects. The modified Blalock-Taussig shunt involves the use of synthetic graft material to create the anastomosis.

blanch (blănch) **1.** To lose color, esp. of the face, usually suddenly and in the context of being frightened or saddened. **2.** To briefly scald a vegetable or nut-fruit in order to facilitate removal of the skin, peel, or covering. **3.** To bleach.

blanch test, blanching test A test of the integrity of the circulation performed by applying and then quickly releasing pressure to a fingernail or toenail. After losing color, the blanched nail normally regains a pink appearance within 2 seconds or less. Failure to do so suggests impaired blood flow to the extremity. SYN: *capillary nail refill test*.

bland diet A diet designed to buffer gastric acidity by providing meals of palatable, nonirritating foods. Content of diet includes milk, cream, prepared cereals, gelatin, soup, rice, butter, crackers, eggs, lean meats, fish, cottage cheese, custards, tapioca, cookies, and plain cake. Multivitamins may be a necessary adjunct. A bland diet may be indicated in treatment of gastritis, peptic ulcer, and hiatal hernia.

Blandin's glands (blŏn-dănz') [Philippe F. Blandin, Fr. surgeon, 1798–1849] Small glands situated deep on each side of the frenulum of the tongue near the apex. SYN: *Nuhn's glands*.

blank (blănk) A surrogate analytical sample that either has no analyte present or is subject to only part of the analytical process. The purpose of the blank is to assess the contribution of nonspecific effects on the final reaction, and thus be able to eliminate those effects from the final analytical results. The term "blank" may be modified by a word indicating the type of effect being evaluated, with the resultant complete term being, for example, "reagent blank," a blank containing only reagents.

blast [AS. *bloest,* a puff of wind] A violent movement of air such as accompanies the explosion of a shell or bomb; a violent sound, as the blast of a horn.

-blast [Gr. *blastos,* germ] Combining form used as a suffix indicating *an embryonic state of development*.

blast A cell that produces something (e.g., osteoblast, fibroblast).

blastema (blăs-tē'mă) [Gr. *blastema,* sprout] The immature material from which cells and tissues are formed.

blastid (blăs'tĭd) [Gr. *blastos,* germ] The clear space marking the site of the organizing nucleus in the impregnated ovum.

blastocele, blastocoele (blăs'tō-sēl) [" + *koilos,* hollow] The cavity in the blastula of the developing embryo.

blastochyle (blăs'tō-kīl) [" + *chylos,* juice] Fluid contained in the blastocele.

blastocyst (blăs'tō-sĭst) [" + *kystis,* bag] In mammalian embryo development, the stage that follows the morula. It consists of an outer layer of trophoblast, which is attached to an inner cell mass. The enclosed cavity is the blastocele. The whole is called blastodermic vesicle or blastocyst. At this stage, implantation in the endometrium (lining of the uterus) occurs. SYN: *blastodermic vesicle*.

blastocyte (blăs'tō-sīt) [" + *kytos,* cell] An undifferentiated embryonic cell.

blastocytoma (blăs-tō-sī-tō'mă) [" + " + *oma,* tumor] Blastoma.

blastoderm (blăs'tō-dĕrm) [" + *derma,* skin] A disk of cells (germinal disk or blastodisk) that develops on the surface of the yolk in an avian or reptilian egg from which the embryo develops; also, in mammalian embryos a disk of cells lying between the yolk sac and the amniotic cavity from which the embryo develops. From the blastoderm, the three germ layers (ectoderm, mesoderm, and endoderm) arise.

blastodisk (blăs′tō-dĭsk) [″ + *diskos,* disk] A flat disk of embryonic cells on the surface of the yolk of the ovum. It forms from the blastomeres.

blastogenesis (blăs″tō-jĕn′ĕ-sĭs) [″ + *genesis,* generation, birth] **1.** Multiplication by budding. **2.** Transmission of characteristics by the germ plasm.

blastokinin (blăs″tō-kī′nĭn) A globulin found in the uterine lumen of some mammals near the time of blastocyst implantation.

blastolysis (blăs-tŏl′ĭ-sĭs) [″ + *lysis,* dissolution] Lysis or destruction of a germ cell or a blastoderm.

blastoma (blăs-tō′mă) *pl.* **blastomata** [″ + *oma,* tumor] A neoplasm composed of immature, undifferentiated cells derived from the blastema of an organ or tissue. SYN: *blastocytoma.* SEE: *blastema.*

blastomere (blăs′tō-mēr) [″ + *meros,* a part] One of the cells resulting from the cleavage of a fertilized ovum.

blastomerotomy (blăs″tō-mēr-ŏt′ō-mē) [″ + ″ + *tome,* incision] Destruction of blastomeres.

Blastomyces (blăst-ō-mī′sēz) [Gr. *blastos,* germ, + *mykes,* fungus] A genus of yeastlike budding fungi pathogenic to humans. At room temperature the genus grows as a mycelial (fungal) form and at body temperature as a yeastlike form.

B. brasiliensis The fungus that causes South American blastomycosis. This organism and disease are also called *Paracoccidioides brasiliensis* and paracoccidioidomycosis, respectively.

B. dermatitidis The fungus that causes North American blastomycosis, a rare fungal infection in humans. SEE: illus.

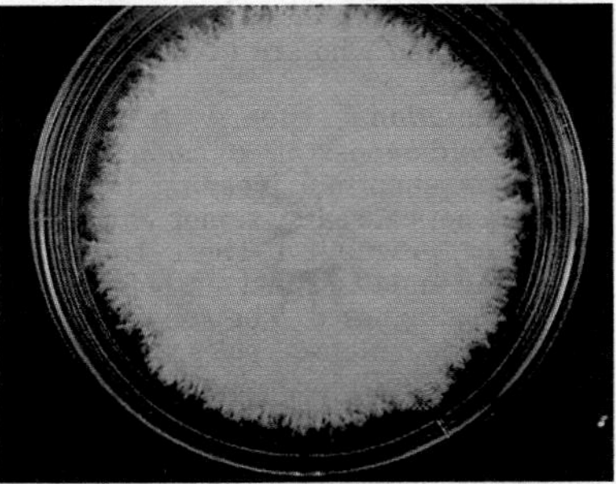

***BLASTOMYCES DERMATITIDIS* IN CULTURE**

Fungal form at room temperature

blastomycete (blăs″tō-mī′sēt) Any organism of the genus *Blastomyces.*

blastomycosis (blăs″tō-mī-kō′sĭs) [″ + *mykes,* fungus, + *osis,* condition] Infection caused by inhalation of the conidia of *Blastomyces dermatitidis.* This rare fungal infection may produce inflammatory lesions of the skin (cutaneous form) or lungs or a generalized invasion of the skin, lungs, bones, central nervous system, kidneys, liver, and spleen. SYN: *North American b.; Gilchrist's disease.*

TREATMENT: Treatment consists of amphotericin B or ketoconazole.

North American b. Blastomycosis.

South American b. Paracoccidioidomycosis.

blastopore (blăs′tō-por) [″ + *poros,* passageway] In the embryo of mammals, the small opening into the archenteron made by invagination of the blastula.

blastospore (blăs′tō-spor) [″ + *sporos,* seed] A spore formed by budding from a hypha, as in yeast.

blastula (blăs′tū-lă) *pl.* **blastulae** [L.] An early stage in the development of an ovum, consisting of a hollow sphere of cells enclosing a cavity, the blastocele. In large-yolked eggs, the blastocele is reduced to a narrow slit. In mammalian development, the blastocyst corresponds to the blastula of lower forms.

Blatta (blăt′ă) [L.] A genus of insects (that includes the cockroaches) of the order Orthoptera.

B. germanica The German cockroach or croton bug.

B. orientalis The Oriental cockroach, also known as the black beetle, a common European house pest.

bleaching Use of an oxidizing chemical to remove stain or discoloration from a tooth. Bleaching techniques vary according to the vitality of the pulp.

at-home b. The lightening or whitening of discolored teeth, using a bleaching gel. Carbamide peroxide and hydrogen peroxide are common bleaching agents used for this purpose in concentrations ranging from 3% to 25%. Treatment must be carefully monitored to avoid over-bleaching and damage to surrounding soft tissue.

CAUTION: Bleaching agents must not be placed on exposed root surfaces or soft tissue.

bleaching powder Chlorinated lime or calcium hypochlorite.

bleb (blĕb) An irregularly shaped elevation of the epidermis; a blister or a bulla. Blebs may vary in size from less than 1 cm to as much as 5 to 10 cm; they may contain serous, seropurulent, or bloody fluid. Blebs are a primary skin lesion that may occur in many disorders, including dermatitis herpetiformis, pemphigus, and syphilis. SEE: *bulla.*

Control of Arterial Bleeding

Artery	Course	Bone Involved	Spot to Apply Pressure
For Wounds of the Face			
Temporal	Upward ½ in. (13 mm) in front of ear	Temporal bone	Against bony prominence immediately in front of ear or on temple
Facial	Upward across jaw diagonally	Lower part of lower maxilla	1 in. (2.5 cm) in front of angle of lower jaw
For Wounds of the Upper Extremity			
Axillary	Downward across outer side of armpit to inside of humerus	Head of humerus	High up in armpit against upper part of humerus
Brachial	Along inner side of humerus under edge of biceps muscle	Shaft of humerus	Against shaft of humerus by pulling aside and gripping biceps, pressing tips of fingers deep down against bone
For Wounds of the Lower Extremity			
Femoral	Down thigh from pelvis to knee from a point midway between iliac spine and symphysis pubis to inner side of end of femur at knee joint	Brim of pelvis	Against brim of pelvis, midway between iliac spine and symphysis pubis
Femoral		Shaft of femur	High up on inner side of thigh, about 3 in. (7.6 cm) below brim of pelvis, over line given in direction of knee
Posterior tibial	Downward to foot in hollow just behind prominence of inner ankle	Inner side of tibia, low down above ankle	For wounds in sole of foot, against tibia in center of hollow behind inner ankle

bleeder [AS. *bledan,* to bleed] **1.** One whose ability to coagulate blood is either deficient or absent, so that small cuts and injuries lead to prolonged bleeding. SEE: *hemophilia*. **2.** A small artery that has been cut or torn.

bleeding [AS. *bledan,* to bleed] **1.** Emitting blood, as from an injured vessel. **2.** The process of emitting blood, as a hemorrhage or the operation of letting blood.

Normally, when blood is exposed to air, it changes to allow fibrin to form. This entangles the cells and forms a blood clot. SEE: *coagulation, blood; coagulation factor; hemorrhage*.

arterial b. Bleeding in spurts of bright red blood, from an artery.

FIRST AID: Arterial bleeding may be controlled by applying pressure with the fingers at the nearest pressure point between it and the heart. The artery is located and digital pressure is applied above it until bleeding stops or until the artery is ligated. A tourniquet should not be used. SEE: table.

breakthrough b. Intermenstrual spotting or bleeding experienced by some women who are taking oral contraceptives.

dysfunctional uterine b. ABBR: DUB. A diagnosis of exclusion in which there is abnormal bleeding from the uterus not caused by tumor, inflammation, or pregnancy. These causes of bleeding must be ruled out before DUB may be diagnosed. The condition may occur with ovulatory cycles, but most often occurs with anovulation. It is common in women with polycystic ovary syndrome. Endometrial hyperplasia followed by sloughing of the endometrium may occur in women with repeated anovulatory cycles.

ETIOLOGY: The absence of the luteal progesterone phase interferes with normal endometrial preparation for implantation or menstruation. Prolonged constant levels of estrogen stimulate uneven endometrial hypertrophy so that some areas slough and bleed before others, causing intermittent bleeding.

herald b. Spontaneous hemorrhage from the gastrointestinal tract in a patient with an aortic bypass graft. The hemorrhage typically stops suddenly, only to recur massively days or weeks later. Many practitioners believe that this type of hemorrhage is a clinical hallmark of bleeding from an aortoenteric fistula.

internal b. Hemorrhage from an internal organ or site, esp. the gastrointestinal tract.

menstrual b. SEE: *menstruation.*

occult b. Inapparent bleeding, esp. that which occurs into the intestines and can be detected only by chemical tests of the feces.

venous b. A continuous flow of dark red blood.

FIRST AID: Venous bleeding may be controlled by firm, continuous pressure applied directly to the bleeding site. If bleeding is from an area over soft tissues, a large, compress bandage should be held firmly against the site.

CAUTION: A tourniquet should not be used. If the bleeding is over a bony area, as in the case of a ruptured varicose vein of the leg, pressure held firmly against the vein will provide immediate control of the blood loss. The patient should be taken to a health care provider as soon as possible if bleeding does not stop.

blenn- SEE: *blenno-.*

blennadenitis (blĕn″ăd-ĕ-nī′tĭs) [″ + *aden,* gland, + *itis,* inflammation] Inflammation of the mucous glands.

blennemesis (blĕn-ĕm′ĕ-sĭs) [″ + *emesis,* vomiting] Vomiting of mucus.

blenno-, blenn- [Gr. *blennos,* mucus] Combining form meaning *mucus.*

blennogenic, blennogenous (blĕn″ō-jĕn′ĭk, blĕn-ŏj′ĕ-nŭs) [″ + *gennan,* to produce] Secreting mucus.

blennoid (blĕn′oyd) [″ + *eidos,* form, shape] Like mucus. SYN: *mucoid (2).*

blennophthalmia (blĕn″ŏf-thăl′mē-ă) [″ + *ophthalmos,* eye] **1.** Catarrhal conjunctivitis. **2.** Gonorrheal ophthalmia.

blennorrhagia (blĕn″ō-rā′jē-ă) [″ + *rhegnynai,* to break forth] Blennorrhea.

blennorrhea (blĕn″ō-rē′ă) [Gr. *blennos,* mucus, + *rhoia,* flow] Any discharge from mucous membranes. SYN: *blennorrhagia.*

inclusion b. Inflammation of the conjunctiva in newborns. It is caused by *Chlamydia trachomatis,* a bacterium that forms cytoplasmic inclusion bodies in the epithelial cells. SYN: *ophthalmia neonatorum.*

blennothorax (blĕn″ō-thō′răks) [″ + *thorax,* chest] The accumulation of mucus in the bronchial tubes or alveoli.

blennuria (blĕn-ū′rē-ă) [″ + *ouron,* urine] The presence of mucus in the urine.

bleomycin (blē-ō-mī′sĭn) Any one of a group of antitumor agents produced by *Streptomyces verticillus.*

sterile sulfate b. Bleomycin used in treating various carcinomas of the skin, head, neck, and lungs, as well as testicular tumors. Trade name is Blenoxane.

blephar- SEE: *blepharo-.*

blepharadenitis (blĕf″ăr-ăd-ĕ-nī′tĭs) [Gr. *blepharon,* eyelid, + *aden,* gland, + *itis,* inflammation] Inflammation of the meibomian glands.

blepharal (blĕf′ăr-ăl) Pert. to an eyelid.

blepharectomy (blĕf″ă-rĕk′tō-mē) [″ + *ektome,* excision] Surgical excision of all or part of an eyelid.

blepharedema (blĕf″ăr-ĕ-dē′mă) [″ + *oidema,* swelling] Edema of the eyelids, causing swelling and a baggy appearance.

blepharism [″ + *-ismos,* condition] Twitching or blinking of the eyelids. SEE: *blepharospasm.*

blepharitis (blĕf″ăr-ī′tĭs) [″ + *itis,* inflammation] Ulcerative or nonulcerative inflammation of the hair follicles and glands along the edges of the eyelids.

SYMPTOMS: The eyelids become red, tender, and sore with sticky exudate and scales on the edges; the eyelids may become inverted; there may be watering of the eyes and loss of eyelashes. Styes and meibomian cysts are associated with the condition.

ETIOLOGY: The ulcerative type is usually caused by infection with staphylococci. The cause of the nonulcerative type is often unknown; it may be due to allergy or exposure to dust, smoke, or irritating chemicals.

PATIENT CARE: Patients are taught how to keep their scalp, eyebrows, and eyelids clean and to avoid rubbing their eyes with their hands. The need to wash hands and then eyelids before providing care and to wash hands afterwards to prevent the spread of infection is emphasized. Drainage or crusts can be softened with warm, saline compresses before being removed with a soft, wet cloth. Antibiotic ointments are applied to the lid margins in a narrow ribbon, beginning at the inner and working toward the outer canthus of the eye. The ointment container should not touch the lid or eye surface.

b. angularis Blepharitis in which the medial angle of the eye is involved with blocking of openings of lacrimal ducts.

b. ciliaris Inflammation affecting the ciliary margins of the eyelids. SYN: *b. marginalis.*

b. marginalis B. ciliaris.

b. parasitica Blepharitis caused by parasites such as mites or lice.

seborrheic b. A nonulcerative form of blepharitis in which waxy scales form on the eyelids. It is usually associated with seborrheic dermatitis of the surrounding skin.

b. squamosa Chronic blepharitis with scaling.

b. ulcerosa Blepharitis with ulceration.

blepharo-, blephar- [Gr. *blepharon,* eyelid] Combining form meaning *eyelid.*

blepharoadenitis SEE: *blepharadenitis.*

blepharoadenoma (blĕf″ăr-ō-ăd-ĕ-nō′mă) [″ + ″ + *oma,* tumor] A glandular tumor of the eyelid.

blepharoatheroma (blĕf″ăr-ō-ăth″ĕ-rō′mă) [″ + *athere,* thick fluid, + *oma,* tumor] A sebaceous cyst of the eyelid.

blepharochalasis (blĕf″ăr-ō-kăl′ă-sĭs) [″ + *chalasis,* relaxation] Hypertrophy of the skin of the upper eyelid due to loss of elasticity following edematous swellings as in recurrent angioneurotic edema of the lids. The skin may droop over the edge of the eyelid when the eyes are open.

blepharoclonus (blĕf″ă-rŏk′lō-nŭs) [″ + *klonos,* tumult] Clonic spasm of the muscles that close the eyelids (orbicularis oculi).

blepharoconjunctivitis (blĕf″ă-rō-kŏn-jŭnk″tĭ-vī′tĭs) [″ + L. *conjungere,* to join together, + Gr. *itis,* inflammation] Inflammation of the eyelids and conjunctiva.

blepharodiastasis (blĕf-ă-rō-dī-ăs′tă-sĭs) [″ + *diastasis,* separation] Excessive separation of the eyelids, causing the eyes to open wide.

blepharoncus (blĕf″ă-rŏn′kŭs) [″ + *onkos,* tumor] A tumor of the eyelid.

blepharopachynsis (blĕf″ă-rō-pă-kĭn′sĭs) [″ + *pachynsis,* thickening] Abnormal thickening of the eyelid.

blepharophimosis (blĕf″ă-rō-fī-mō′sĭs) [″ + *phimosis,* narrowing] Blepharostenosis.

blepharoplast (blĕf′ă-rō-plăst) Basal body.

blepharoplasty (blĕf′ă-rō-plăs″tē) Plastic surgery upon the eyelid.

blepharoplegia (blĕf″ă-rō-plē′jē-ă) [Gr. *blepharon,* eyelid, + *plege,* a stroke] Paralysis of an eyelid.

blepharoptosis (blĕf″ă-rō-tō′sĭs) [″ + *ptosis,* a dropping] Drooping of the upper eyelid.

blepharopyorrhea (blĕf″ă-rō-pī-ō-rē′ă) [″ + *pyon,* pus, + *rhoia,* flow] Purulent discharge from the eyelid.

blepharorrhaphy (blĕf″ă-ror′ă-fē) [″ + *rhaphe,* seam, ridge] Tarsorrhaphy.

blepharorrhea (blĕf″ă-rō-rē′ă) [″ + *rhoia,* flow] Discharge from the eyelid.

blepharospasm (blĕf′ă-rō-spăsm) [″ + *spasmos,* a convulsion] A twitching or spasmodic contraction of the orbicularis oculi muscle due to tics, eyestrain, or nervous irritability. SEE: *Marcus Gunn syndrome.*

essential b. Blepharospasm of unknown cause. It may be so severe as to be debilitating. Surgery has helped some patients. Botulinum toxin A injected into the muscles that control the spasm has been of benefit. This treatment will need to be repeated after 2 to 3 months.

blepharosphincterectomy (blĕf″ă-rō-sfĭnk″tĕr-ĕk′tō-mē) [″ + *sphinkter,* a constrictor, + *ektome,* excision] Excision of part of the orbicularis palpebrarum to relieve pressure of the eyelid on the cornea.

blepharostat (blĕf′ă-rō-stăt) [″ + *histanai,* cause to stand] A device for separating the eyelids during an operation.

blepharostenosis (blĕf″ă-rō-stĕn-ō′sĭs) [″ + *stenosis,* act of narrowing] Narrowing of the palpebral slit due to an inability to open the eye normally. SYN: *blepharophimosis.*

blepharosynechia (blĕf″ă-rō-sĭ-nē′kē-ă) [″ + *synecheia,* a holding together] Adhesion of the edges of the upper eyelid to the lower one. SYN: *ankyloblepharon.*

blepharotomy (blĕf-ă-rŏt′ō-mē) [″ + *tome,* incision] Surgical incision of the eyelid.

Bleuler, Eugen [1857–1939] Swiss psychiatrist known for studies on schizophrenia.

blind [AS.] **1.** Without sight. **2.** In research, a study in which the subjects and/or the researchers are unaware of which group is receiving active treatment and which is receiving a placebo. Blinding reduces the potential for bias.

blind loop syndrome A condition caused by intraluminal growth of bacteria in the upper portion of the small intestine. Conditions associated with this syndrome are anatomical lesions that lead to stasis such as diverticula or surgically created blind loops; diseases associated with motor function of the small intestine; and any condition that decreases gastric acid secretion. The syndrome is diagnosed by the clinical signs and symptoms of malabsorption and the use of breath tests for detecting overgrowth of bacteria in the intestine.

TREATMENT: Antimicrobial therapy and nutritional support are needed. Tetracyclines may be ineffective due to bacterial resistance.

blindness Inability to see. The leading causes of blindness in the U.S. are cataracts, glaucoma, age-related macular degeneration, diabetes mellitus, and trauma to the eye.

Blindness may be caused by diseases of the lens, the retina, or the eye structures; diseases of the optic nerve; or lesions of the visual cortex or pathways of the brain. A small number of infants are born blind, but far more people become blind during life. In the U.S., blindness due to infection is rare, but worldwide diseases like trachoma and onchocerciasis are relatively common causes of severe visual impairment. In malnourished persons, vitamin A deficiency is another important cause of blindness.

A variety of free services are available for the blind and physically handicapped. Talking Books Topics published bimonthly in large-print, cassette, and disc formats is distributed free to blind and physically handicapped individuals who participate in the Library of Congress free reading program. It lists recorded books and magazines available though a national network of cooperating libraries and provides news of developments and activities in library services. Subscription requests may be sent to Talking Books Topics, CMLS, P.O. Box 9150, Melbourne, FL 32902-9150.

amnesic color b. An inability to remember the names of colors.

color b. SEE: *color blindness*.

cortical b. Blindness due to lesions in the left and right occipital lobes of the brain. The eyes are still able to move and the pupillary light reflexes remain, but the blindness is as if the optic nerves had been severed. The usual cause is occlusion of the posterior cerebral arteries. Transitory cortical blindness may follow head injury.

day b. An inability to see in daylight; hemeralopia.

eclipse b. Blindness due to burning the macula while viewing an eclipse without using protective lenses. Looking directly at the sun anytime can damage the eyes. SYN: *solar b.*

hysterical b. An inaccurate term for functional blindness (i.e., blindness caused by psychological disorders rather than demonstrable organic pathology).

legal b. A degree of loss of visual acuity that prevents a person from performing work requiring eyesight. In the U.S. this is defined as corrected visual acuity of 20/200 or less, or a visual field of 20° or less in the better eye. In the U.S. there are about three quarters of a million blind people, and about 8 or 9 million people with significant visual impairment.

letter b. An inability to understand the meaning of letters; a form of aphasia.

night b. An inability to see at night; nyctalopia.

object b. A disorder in which the brain fails to recognize things even though the eyes are functioning normally. SEE: *apraxia*.

psychic b. Sight without recognition due to a brain lesion.

river b. SEE: *onchocerciasis*.

snow b. Blindness, usually temporary, resulting from the glare of sunlight on snow. It may result in photophobia and conjunctivitis, the latter resulting from effects of ultraviolet radiation.

solar b. Eclipse b.

transient b. Temporary blindness in one or both eyes. The onset is usually sudden. It may be caused in both eyes by any condition that temporarily interferes with blood flow to the ophthalmic arteries, such as migraine; carotid artery insufficiency; emboli; temporal arteritis; retinal artery spasm caused by hypertensive encephalopathy, uremia, or eclampsia; optic neuritis; glaucoma; and conversion disorders. SYN: *amaurosis fugax*.

word b. An inability to understand written or printed words.

blink To open and close the eyes involuntarily; to wink rapidly. Blinking, which normally occurs about 12 to 20 times a minute, helps protect the cornea against microscopic injury. It occurs less often in neurodegenerative diseases, such as Parkinson's disease, and more often in meningitis and corneal irritation. SEE: *blink reflex*.

blink reflex Sudden closing of the eyelids in response to head turning, loud noises, bright lights, or visual threats. Absence of this reflex occurs in blindness and in injuries to cranial nerves III, V, and VII.

blister [MD. *bluyster,* a swelling] **1.** A collection of fluid below or within the epidermis. **2.** To form a blister.

TREATMENT: The area should be cleansed with mild soap and a protective dressing applied. Unless a blister is painful or interferes with function due to its size, it should not be punctured. If puncturing is needed, it should be done aseptically, with the skin left in place. A sterile pressure bandage should be applied. SEE: *Standard and Universal Precautions Appendix*.

CAUTION: If infection develops, treatment is the same as for any other wound, including tetanus prophylaxis or booster as required.

blood b. A small subcutaneous or intracutaneous extravasation of blood due to the rupture of blood vessels.

TREATMENT: A firm dressing should be applied with moderate pressure to prevent extravasation and hasten absorption. In some cases it is desirable to puncture aseptically and aspirate.

fever b. A vesicular rash usually appearing on the lips or mucous membrane of the mouth during another infectious illness. The rash is caused by herpes simplex virus. SYN: *cold sore*.

fly b. A blister produced by application of cantharides to the skin.

Blizzard syndrome, Johanson-Blizzard syndrome Amenorrhea related to autoimmune ovarian failure.

bloated (blōt′ĕd) [AS. *blout*] Swollen or distended beyond normal size as by serum, water, or gas.

bloating Abdominal discomfort related to disorders of intestinal motility and intestinal sensitivity to distention. This symptom is often presumed to be related to the retention of fluid or gas in the bowel, but it also may be produced by disorders of the ovaries or other genitourinary organs.

block [MD. *blok,* trunk of a tree] **1.** An obstruction or stoppage. **2.** A method of regional anesthesia used to stop the passage of sensory impulses in a nerve, a nerve trunk, the dorsal root of a spinal nerve, or the spinal cord, thus depriving a patient of sensation in the area involved. SEE: *anesthesia*. **3.** To obstruct any passageway or opening.

air b. Leakage of air from the respiratory passageways and its accumulation in connective tissues of the lungs, forming an obstruction to the normal flow of air.

atrioventricular b. A condition in which the depolarization impulse is delayed or blocked at the atrioventricular (A-V) node or a more distal site, as in the A-V bundle or bundle branches. A-V block can be partial or complete. There are several degrees of A-V block. *First-degree* block is due to prolonged A-V conduction; electrocardiograms show a characteristic prolonged PR interval. *Second-degree* blocks are intermittent (i.e., some, but not all, A-V impulses are transmitted to the ventricles). *Third degree* block, also known as complete A-V block, is present when no atrial impulses are conducted to the ventricles.

A-V b. Atrioventricular b.

bite b. **1.** A wedge of sturdy material used to maintain space between the two jaws. **2.** A film holder held between the teeth for stable retention of the film packet during dental radiology.

digital b. The injection of a regional anesthetic into the proximal portion of a finger or toe.

ear b. Blockage of the auditory tube to the middle ear. It may result from trauma, infection, or an accumulation of cerumen. SEE: *aerotitis; otitis media*.

epidural b. SEE: *anesthesia, epidural*.

field b. Regional anesthesia in which a limited operative area is walled off by an anesthetic.

mandibular b. Regional anesthesia of the lower face and mandibular tissues by infiltration of the mandibular division of the trigeminal nerve.

maxillary b. Second division b.

nerve b. The induction of regional anesthesia by preventing sensory nerve impulses from reaching the central nervous system. This is usually done on a temporary basis, by using chemical or electrical means. In the former case, it is accomplished by injecting an anesthetic solution, such as lidocaine.

neuromuscular b. A disturbance in the transmission of impulses from a motor endplate to a muscle. It may be caused by an excess or deficiency of acetylcholine or by drugs that inhibit or destroy acetylcholine.

paravertebral b. Infiltration of the stellate ganglion with a local anesthetic.

saddle b. SEE: under *anesthesia*.

second division b. Regional anesthesia of the upper face and maxillary tissues by infiltration of the maxillary division of the trigeminal nerve. SYN: *maxillary b.*

sinoatrial b. Heart block in which there is interference in the passage of impulses between the sinus node and the atria.

spinal b. Blockage in the flow of cerebrospinal fluid within the spinal canal.

ventricular b. Interference in the flow of cerebrospinal fluid between the ventricles or from the ventricles through the foramina to the subarachnoid space.

blockade (blŏk-ād′) Prevention of the action of something, such as a drug or a body function.

adrenergic b. Inhibition of responses to adrenergic sympathetic nerve impulses and to agents such as epinephrine.

cholinergic b. Inhibition of cholinergic nerve stimuli or cholinergic agents.

lymphatic b. A local defense mechanism in which minute bits of material, such as fibrinous exudate from injured tissue, enter local lymphatic vessels, obstructing them and preventing foreign substances, esp. bacteria, from passing through them.

blocker A drug that prevents the normal action of a system or cell receptor. SEE: *antagonist; blockade; inhibitor*.

blocking **1.** Obstructing. **2.** In psychoanalysis, a sudden break in free association as a defense against unpleasant ideas.

blood [AS. *blod*] The cell-containing fluid that circulates through the heart, arteries, veins, and capillaries, carrying nourishment, electrolytes, hormones, vitamins, antibodies, heat, and oxygen to the tissues and taking away waste matter and carbon dioxide. SEE: *erythropoietin*.

CHARACTERISTICS: Blood has a distinctive, somewhat metallic, odor. Arterial blood is bright red or scarlet and usually pulsates if the artery has been

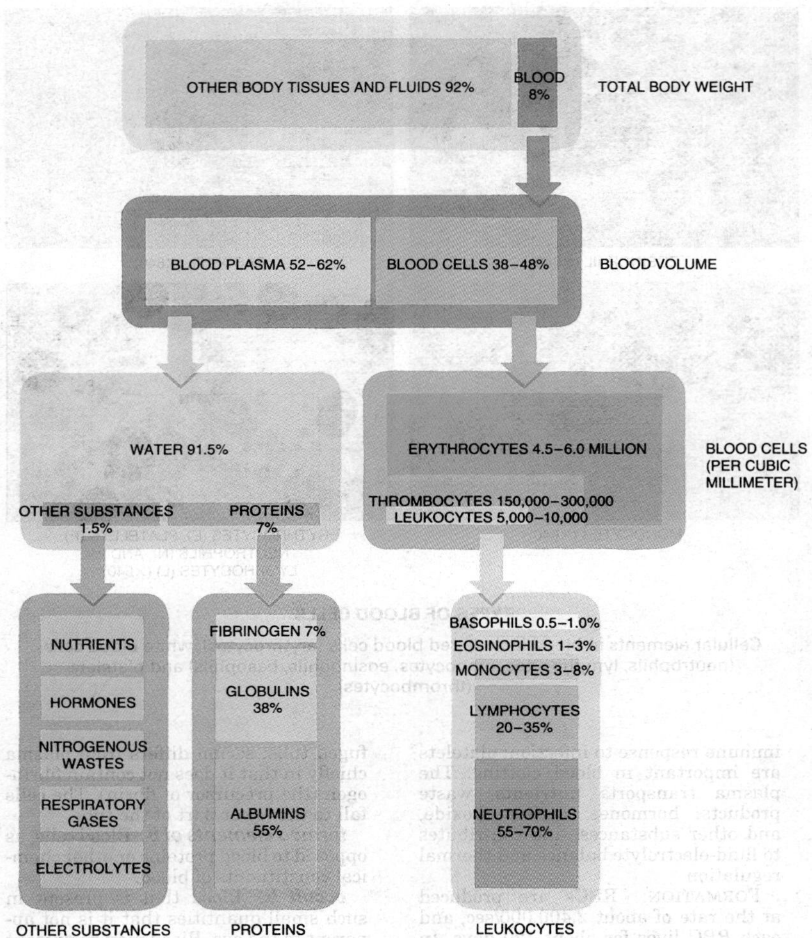

BLOOD COMPOSITION

Components of blood and relationship to other body tissues

cut. Venous blood is dark red or crimson and flows steadily from a cut vein.

COMPOSITION: Human blood is about 52% to 62% plasma and 38% to 48% cells. The plasma is mostly water, ions, proteins, hormones, and lipids. The cellular components are the erythrocytes (red blood cells [RBCs]), leukocytes (white blood cells [WBCs]), and thrombocytes (platelets). The leukocytes comprise neutrophils, eosinophils, basophils, lymphocytes, and monocytes. SEE: illus.; *buffy coat; plasma; serum*.

An adult weighing 70 kg has a blood volume of about 5 L or 70 ml/kg of body weight. Blood constitutes about 7% to 8% of the body weight. The pH of the blood is from 7.35 to 7.45. The specific gravity of blood varies from 1.048 to 1.066, the cells being heavier and plasma lighter than this. Blood is of slightly higher specific gravity in men than in women. Specific gravity is higher after exercise and at night. SEE: *blood count; cell; erythrocyte; leukocyte; plasma; platelet*.

FUNCTION: In passing through the lungs, the blood gives up carbon dioxide and absorbs oxygen; after leaving the heart, it is carried to the tissues as arterial blood and then returned to the heart in the venous system. It moves in the aorta at an average speed of 30 cm/sec, and it makes the circuit of the vascular system in about 20 sec. RBCs carry oxygen; WBCs participate in the

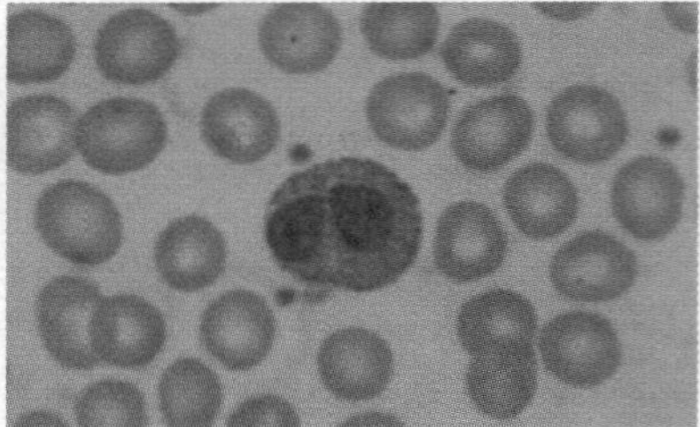
EOSINOPHIL (×640)

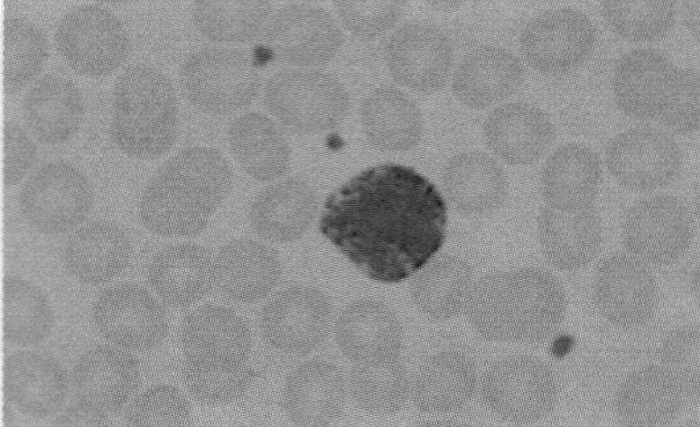
BASOPHIL (×640)

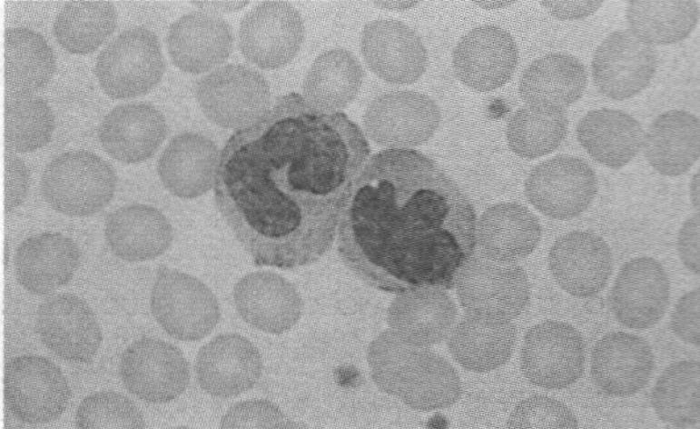
MONOCYTES (×640)

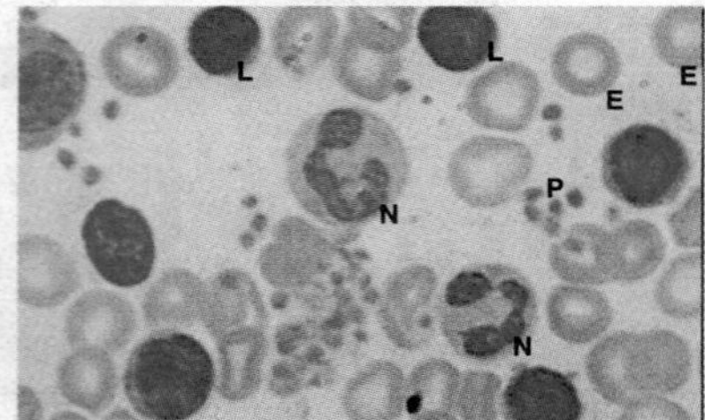

ERYTHROCYTES (E), PLATELETS (P), NEUTROPHILS (N), AND LYMPHOCYTES (L) (×640)

TYPES OF BLOOD CELLS

Cellular elements in blood include red blood cells (erythrocytes), white blood cells (neutrophils, lymphocytes, monocytes, eosinophils, basophils) and platelets (thrombocytes).

immune response to infection; platelets are important in blood clotting. The plasma transports nutrients, waste products, hormones, carbon dioxide, and other substances, and contributes to fluid-electrolyte balance and thermal regulation.

FORMATION: RBCs are produced at the rate of about 2,400,000/sec, and each RBC lives for about 120 days. In healthy individuals, the concentration of RBCs in the blood remains stable over time.

arteriolized b. Blood that has been exposed to oxygen in the lung.

clotting of b. SEE: *coagulation, blood.*

cord b. The blood present in the umbilical vessels connecting the placenta to the fetus. Because cord blood is immunologically immature, it is esp. useful in transfusion therapy and hematological transplantation.

defibrinated b. Whole blood from which fibrin was separated during the clotting process. If whole blood is stirred, the stringy elastic fibrin comes out on the stirrer; the fibrin can be washed until white. The remaining thick red blood, called defibrinated blood, can no longer clot. If it is centrifuged, a clear liquid called serum appears in the upper half of the centrifuged tube; serum differs from plasma chiefly in that it does not contain fibrinogen (the precursor of fibrin). The cells fall to the lower part of the tube.

formed elements of b. Blood cells, as opposed to blood proteins or other chemical constituents of blood.

occult b. Blood that is present in such small quantities that it is not apparent to the eye. Blood may be present in feces but of such color and consistency as to be unnoticed by the patient. Occult blood is usually detected only by chemical tests or by microscopic or spectroscopic examination. SEE: table.

predonation of b. The collection of a patient's own blood before surgery, to be used if the patient needs a transfusion during or after the surgery, to reduce the possibility of needing banked blood, and with it the risk of having a transfusion reaction or contracting a transmissible infection.

PATIENT CARE: The usual blood transfusion checks are performed: 1. The patient's armband name and number are verified by comparing them with those on the chart. 2. The number and blood type of the unit of blood are checked against those of the patient. 3. The number and blood type of the unit of blood should match that information on all the paperwork.

Diagnostic Tests for Occult Bleeding

Diagnostic Test	Purpose/Considerations
Hemoglobin and hematocrit levels	Essential for ongoing assessment. Results are unreliable during or immediately after acute hemorrhage–levels may not accurately reflect early blood loss. Low baseline levels may indicate preexisting anemia.
A coagulation profile	Detects actual or potential abnormalities, especially in a patient taking an anticoagulant or drugs that affect platelet function. Factor assay may reveal clotting disorders such as hemophilia; low platelet count or elevated prothrombin time, activated partial thromboplastin time, or international normalized ratio indicates coagulopathy.
Serum lactate level and arterial blood gases	Evaluate tissue perfusion. A rising lactate level signals insufficient perfusion. An arterial pH less than 7.35 and a falling bicarbonate level indicate impaired perfusion and metabolic acidosis.
A computed tomography scan	May reveal fluid collections or injury to solid organs; free fluid may indicate bleeding into organs or spaces.
X-rays	May reveal fluid in the thorax or hemothorax, aortic injury, pelvic fracture, or fracture of other large bones, such as the femur, which can cause significant blood loss.
Arteriography	Helps detect arterial disruption caused by trauma or vascular abnormality. It may be used to guide injection of a clot-forming substance into the bleeding vessel. Aortic imaging helps rule out traumatic disruption or dissecting thoracic aneurysm.
Ultrasound	Helps detect bleeding in the peritoneal cavity, thorax, pericardium, retroperitoneum, pelvis, or uterus. It permits simultaneous procedures, such as placing I.V. lines or an endotracheal tube.
Endoscopy	Allows visualization of a gastrointestinal bleeding source and may allow the physician to sclerose bleeders.
Diagnostic peritoneal lavage	May be performed at the bedside to rapidly identify intraperitoneal hemorrhage in an unstable or critical patient. It doesn't identify retroperitoneal bleeding or pinpoint hemorrhage site. If results are positive, the patient may require laparotomy.
Laparoscopy	May help rule out intra-abdominal hemorrhage. It is not appropriate for acute hemorrhage because setup is time-consuming and surgical access is limited.
Transesophageal echocardiography	May be performed at the bedside to detect cardiac injury, such as aortic dissection. It is contraindicated in esophageal trauma.

SOURCE: Used with permission from *Nursing 97*, 27(9):38, © Springhouse Corporation/Springnet.com.

sludged b. Blood in which red cells have massed together in the smaller blood vessels, and block or slow the blood flowing through the vessels.

unit of b. Approx. 1 pint (473 ml) of blood, the usual amount available for use in transfusion.

blood alcohol concentration ABBR: BAC. The amount of alcohol in the blood, usually expressed as g/dl. Persons with BACs equal to or greater than 0.10 mg/dl are considered intoxicated. The National Highway Transportation Safety Administration considers a fatal crash to be alcohol-related if the individual—driver or pedestrian—has a BAC equal to or greater than 0.10 mg/dl. Blood alcohol levels of 400–500 mg/dl may be deadly. They often are associated with coma and respiratory failure.

blood bank A place in which whole blood and certain derived components are processed, typed, and stored until needed for transfusion. Blood is mixed with adenine-supplemented citrate phosphate dextrose and is stored at 4°C (39°F). Heparin may be used as a preservative. Banked blood should be used as soon as possible because the longer it is stored, the fewer red blood cells survive in usable form. Ninety percent of the red cells survive up to 14 days of storage, but only 70% remain after 24 days.

CAUTION: It is mandatory that appropriate quality assurance measures are undertaken to ensure that patients are properly identified at the bedside and at the blood bank, to prevent the transfusion of mismatched blood. Blood banking measures are designed to minimize the risk of communicable illnesses, including hepatitis viruses and the human immunodeficiency virus.

---

blood cell casts Masses of red cells molded by the renal tubules, the blood originating from the glomeruli. Abnormal microscopic body in the urine composed of coagulated serum covered with red blood cells.

blood component therapy Transfusion of one or more of the components of whole blood. The blood components may have been taken from the patient previously (autologous transfusion) or donated by someone else (homologous transfusion). Except in the case of acute hemorrhage, the transfusion of whole blood is rarely needed. Use of a component rather than whole blood permits several patients to benefit from a single blood donation. Components used in clinical medicine include packed red blood cells; leukocyte-poor red blood cells; frozen glycerolized red blood cells (RBCs); thawed deglycerolized RBCs; washed RBCs; whole blood; heparinized whole blood; granulocytes; platelets; plasma and plasma fractions. The latter include antihemophilic factor (factor VIII), prothrombin complex (factors VII, IX, and X), gamma globulin, and albumin. SEE: *blood transfusion; Standard and Universal Precautions Appendix.*

blood corpuscle An old term for any blood cell.

blood count The number of red cells and leukocytes per microliter (μl) of whole blood. Normally, the number of erythrocytes in men averages 5 million/μl; in women, 4.5 million/μl. Prolonged exposure to high altitude increases the number. Leukocytes average 5,000 to 10,000/μl. Platelets range from 140,000 to 400,000/μl. Hemoglobin and hematocrit are determined from samples of whole blood.

differential b.c. The number and type of white blood cells as determined by microscopic examination of a thin layer of blood on a glass slide after it has been suitably stained to show the morphology of the various cells. The number and variety of white cells in a sample of a given size are obtained. Even though the red cells are not counted by this method, their shape, size, and color can be evaluated. Some blood diseases and inflammatory conditions may be recognized in this way. In a differential count, the varieties of the leukocytes and their percentages normally should be: neutrophils (segmented), 40% to 60%; eosinophils, 1% to 3%; basophils, 0.5% to 1%; lymphocytes, 20% to 40%; monocytes, 4% to 8%.

blood crossmatching The process of mixing a sample of the donor's red blood cells with the recipient's serum (major crossmatching), and mixing a sample of the recipient's blood with the donor's serum (minor crossmatching). It is done before transfusion to determine compatibility of blood.

blood donation, preoperative The preoperative collection of autologous blood from a patient for the purpose of reinfusing it at the time of elective surgery.

blood donor One who gives blood to be used for transfusion.

blood gas analysis Chemical analysis of the pH, carbon dioxide and oxygen concentrations, and oxygen saturation of the blood. This analysis is used to diagnose serious metabolic and respiratory disorders. It may be performed using arterial or venous blood although only arterial blood gas analysis evaluates lung function; the specimen may be obtained from numerous sites. Mixed venous samples may be obtained from the right atrium of the heart. The blood sample is usually collected in a heparinized syringe, with care being taken to ensure that the specimen is immediately placed on ice (to avoid misinterpretations caused by temperature) and not exposed to air (to prevent oxygenation of the sample).

CAUTION: Occasionally, arterial punctures taken from the wrist may damage the radial artery or compromise the blood supply of the hand.

SEE: *Allen test; blood gases.*

blood gases The oxygen used and carbon dioxide produced during metabolic processes. Levels of these gases vary in response to many diseases that affect respiration, such as asthma, chronic obstructive lung disease, congestive heart failure, and ketoacidosis (to name just a few). SEE: *acidosis; alkalosis; arterial blood gas; blood gas analysis.*

blood group A genetically determined system of antigens located on the surface of the erythrocyte. There are a number of human blood group systems; each system is determined by a series of two or more genes that are allelic or closely linked on a single autosomal chromosome. The ABO system (discovered in 1901 by Karl Landsteiner) is of prime importance in blood transfusions. The Rhesus (Rh) system is esp. important in obstetrics. There are about 30 Rh antigens. SEE: illus.; *Rh factor.*

The population can be phenotypically divided into four ABO blood groups: A, B, AB, and O. Individuals in the A group have the A antigen on the surface of their red cells; B group has the B antigen on red cells; AB group has A and B

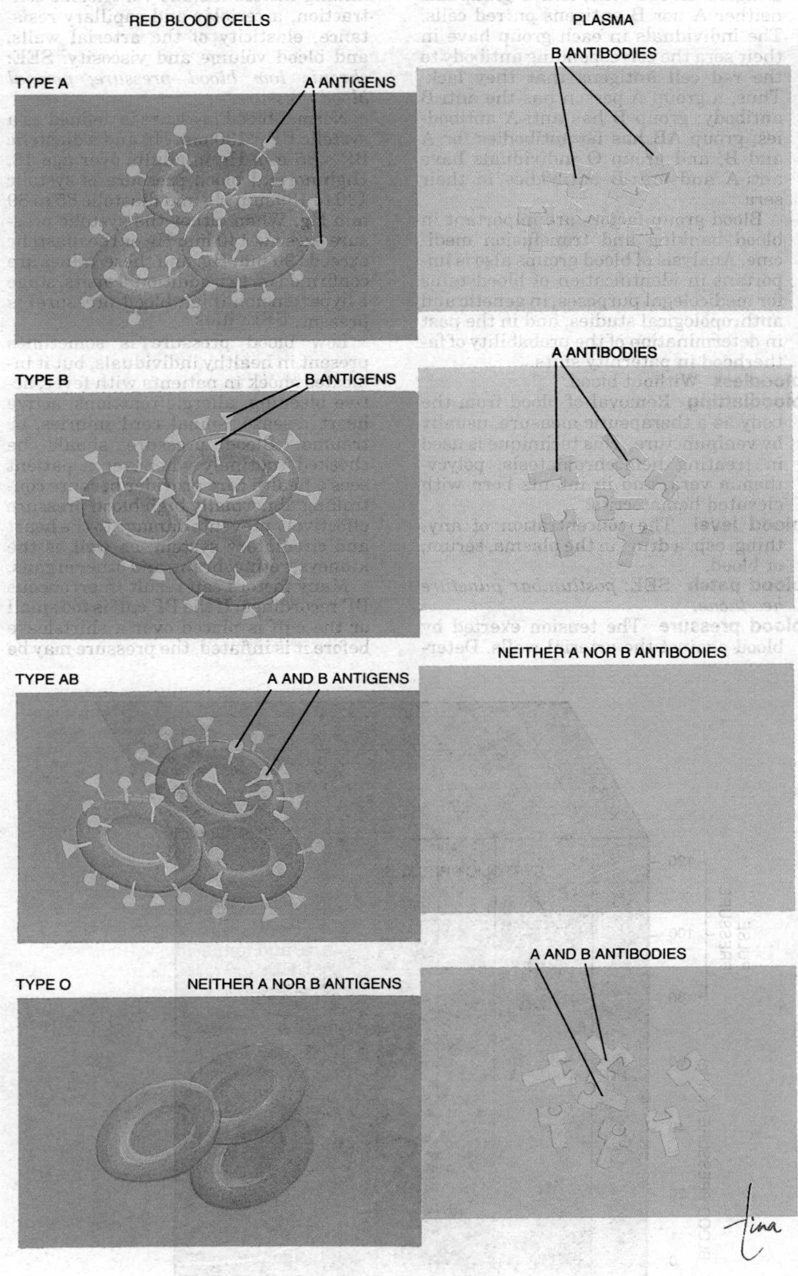

ABO BLOOD TYPES

Schematic representation of antigens on RBCs and antibodies in plasma

antigens on red cells; and O group has neither A nor B antigens on red cells. The individuals in each group have in their sera the corresponding antibody to the red cell antigens that they lack. Thus, a group A person has the anti-B antibody; group B has anti-A antibodies; group AB has no antibodies for A and B; and group O individuals have anti-A and anti-B antibodies in their sera.

Blood group factors are important in blood banking and transfusion medicine. Analysis of blood groups also is important in identification of bloodstains for medicolegal purposes, in genetic and anthropological studies, and in the past in determination of the probability of fatherhood in paternity suits.

bloodless Without blood.

bloodletting Removal of blood from the body as a therapeutic measure, usually by venipuncture. This technique is used in treating hemochromatosis, polycythemia vera, and in infants born with elevated hematocrits.

blood level The concentration of anything, esp. a drug, in the plasma, serum, or blood.

blood patch SEE: *postlumbar puncture headache*.

blood pressure The tension exerted by blood against the arterial walls. Determining factors include ventricular contraction, arteriolar and capillary resistance, elasticity of the arterial walls, and blood volume and viscosity. SEE: *chronic low blood pressure; normal blood pressure*.

Normal blood pressure is defined as a systolic BP <130 mm Hg and a diastolic BP <85 mm Hg in adults over age 18. High-normal blood pressure is systolic 130 to 139 mm Hg and diastolic 85 to 89 mm Hg. When either the systolic pressure exceeds 140 mm Hg or the diastolic exceeds 90 mm Hg, and these values are confirmed on two additional visits, stage I hypertension (high blood pressure) is present. SEE: illus.

Low blood pressure is sometimes present in healthy individuals, but it indicates shock in patients with fever, active bleeding, allergic reactions, active heart disease, spinal cord injuries, or trauma. Blood pressure should be checked routinely whenever a patient sees a health care provider because controlling abnormally high blood pressure effectively prevents damage to the heart and circulatory system, as well as the kidneys, retina, brain, and other organs.

Many factors can result in erroneous BP recordings. If the BP cuff is too small or the cuff is placed over a shirtsleeve before it is inflated, the pressure may be

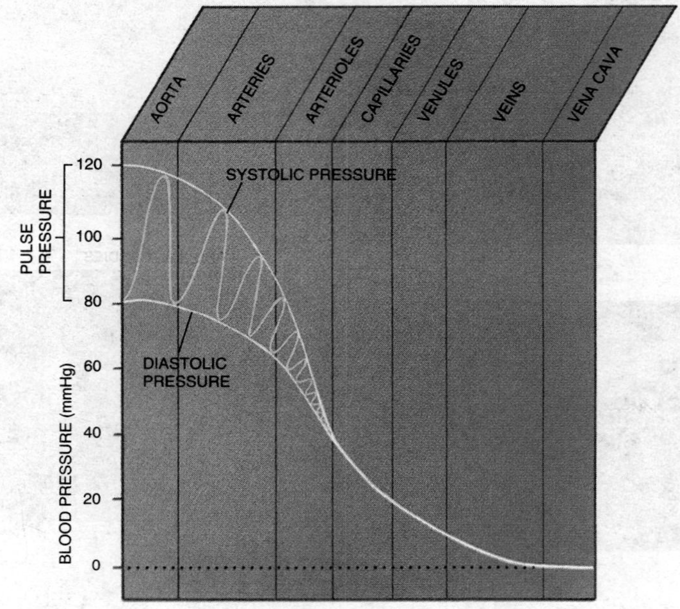

SYSTEMIC BLOOD PRESSURE

Systemic BP changes through the vascular system; systolic and diastolic pressures merge as blood enters capillaries

falsely elevated. If the BP is checked in only one arm, falsely high or low values may be recorded (the pressure in the arms may differ because of subclavian artery atherosclerosis). The BP may be increased if measured while the patient is talking or just after the patient has had coffee, or smoked a cigarette. When the pressure is taken in a clinic or by a physician, it may be temporarily elevated owing to patient anxiety. This phenomenon, called "white coat hypertension," resolves when the patient measures his or her own pressure in a less-stressful setting. Devices for ambulatory BP monitoring are available for home use by patients suspected of having this problem, as well as for patients in whom detailed BP records are needed. They are easy to use, and the information they provide is valuable to patients and health care providers in guiding therapy. SEE: *hypertension; shock*.

TREATMENT: Elevated blood pressures should first be addressed by giving advice to patients about lifestyle modifications, such as limiting the intake of alcohol, following a diet approved by the American Heart Association, and increasing the level of physical exercise. Weight loss in obese patients is also advisable. Medications are added to lifestyle instructions most of the time. Antihypertensive medications are used according to evidence-based guidelines and the side effects these drugs may cause in particular patients. Diuretics, for example, are esp. helpful in blacks and elderly patients (but may be inadvisable in patients with gout); beta blockers are the drugs of choice in patients with a history of myocardial infarction (but would be contraindicated in patients with advanced heart block); alpha blockers are well-suited for men with prostatic hypertrophy; angiotensin-converting enzyme inhibitors prevent kidney disease in patients with diabetes mellitus. Other antihypertensive drug classes include the angiotensin II receptor antagonists, centrally active alpha antagonists, and calcium channel blockers. Low blood pressure is not treated in healthy patients; in patients with acute illnesses, it is often corrected with hydration or pressor agents.

augmented diastolic b.p. An increase in diastolic pressure, usually by an artificial device, such as an intra-aortic balloon pump. SEE: *intra-aortic balloon counterpulsation*.

central b.p. Blood pressure in the heart chambers, in a great vein, or close to the heart. If determined in a vein, it is termed central venous pressure; if in the aorta or a similar large artery close to the heart, it is designated central arterial pressure.

chronic low b.p. A condition in which the systolic blood pressure is consistently less than 100 mm Hg. In the absence of associated disease, low blood pressure is often a predictor of longevity and continued health. SEE: *hypotension; orthostatic hypotension*.

diastolic b.p. The arterial blood pressure when the ventricles of the heart are refilling with blood. In healthy people, this equals about 60 mm Hg to 85 mm Hg.

direct measurement of b.p. Determination of the blood pressure in one of several arteries. It is done by placing a sterile needle or small catheter inside an artery and having the blood pressure transmitted through that system to a suitable recorder. As the blood pressure fluctuates, the changes are recorded graphically.

high b.p. Blood pressure that is above the normal range. The person making this diagnostic judgment must consider the person's age, body build, previous blood pressure, and state of mental and physical health at the time the blood pressure is measured. Generally it is inadvisable to declare that a person has elevated blood pressure if the opinion is based on one blood pressure measurement. SYN: *hypertension*.

indirect measurement of b.p. A simple external method for measuring blood pressure.

Palpation method: The same arm, usually the right, should be used each time the pressure is measured. The arm should be raised to heart level if the patient is sitting, or kept parallel to the body if the patient is recumbent. The patient's arm should be relaxed and supported in a resting position. Exertion during the examination could result in a higher blood pressure reading. Either a mercury-gravity or aneroid-manometer type of blood pressure apparatus may be used. The blood compression cuff should be the width and length appropriate for the size of the subject's arm: narrow (2.5 to 6 cm) for infants and children and wide (13 cm) for adults. The inflatable bag encased in the cuff should be 20% wider than one third the circumference of the limb used. The deflated cuff is placed evenly and snugly around the upper arm so that its lower edge is about 1 in. above the point of the brachial artery where the bell of the stethoscope will be applied. While feeling the radial pulse, inflate the cuff until the pressure is about 30 mm above the point where the radial pulse was no longer felt. Deflate the cuff slowly and record as accurately as possible the pressure at which the pulse returns to the radial artery. Systolic blood pressure is determined by this method; diastolic blood pressure cannot be determined by this method.

Auscultatory method: Begin as above. After inflating the cuff until the pressure is about 30 mm above the point where the radial pulse disappears, place the bell of the stethoscope over the brachial artery just below the blood pressure cuff. Then deflate the cuff slowly, about 2 to 3 mm Hg per heartbeat. The first sound heard from the artery is recorded as the systolic pressure. The point at which sounds are no longer heard is recorded as the diastolic pressure. For convenience the blood pressure is recorded as figures separated by a slash. The systolic value is recorded first.

Sounds heard over the brachial artery change in quality at some point prior to the point the sounds disappear. Some physicians consider this the diastolic pressure. This value should be noted when recording the blood pressure by placing it between the systolic pressure and the pressure noted when the sound disappears. Thus, 120/90/80 indicates a systolic pressure of 120 with a first diastolic sound change at a pressure of 90 and a final diastolic pressure of 80. The latter pressure is the point of disappearance of all sounds from the artery. When the values are so recorded, the physician may use either of the last two figures as the diastolic pressure. When the change in sound and the disappearance of all sound coincide, the result should be written as follows: 120/80/80.

mean b.p. The sum of twice the diastolic blood pressure plus the systolic blood pressure, all divided by 3. The normal value is <100 mm Hg.

negative b.p. Blood pressure that is less than atmospheric pressure, as in the great veins near the heart.

normal b.p. In healthy young persons, a blood pressure reading of 100 to 139 mm Hg systolic and 60 to 89 mm Hg diastolic. Loss of resilience in the vascular tree and physiological changes of age must be considered when levels above 140 systolic or above 90 diastolic are obtained in apparently healthy older persons.

systolic b.p. Blood pressure during contraction of the ventricles; systemic pressure is normally 90 to 135 mm Hg.

blood pressure monitoring, ambulatory The measurement of blood pressure by outpatients using a portable blood pressure monitor. These monitors are used to record the patient's diastolic and systolic pressures during activity and rest throughout the day.

blood salvage During surgery, a collection of the siphoned blood that has escaped from the operative site in noncontaminated surgeries so that after appropriate filtration it may be returned to the patient. SEE: *autologous blood transfusion; cell saver.*

bloodshot Local congestion of the smaller blood vessels of a part, as when the vessels of the conjunctiva are dilated and visible.

blood shunting A condition in which blood, by going through an abnormal pathway or bypass, does not travel its normal route. It may occur when an arteriovenous fistula forms or in congenital anomalies of the heart in which the blood passes from the right atrium or ventricle directly to the left atrium or ventricle respectively, through a defect in the wall (septum) that normally separates the atria and ventricles.

bloodstream The blood that flows through the circulatory system of an organism.

blood test A test to determine the chemical, physical, or serological characteristics of the blood or some portion of it.

blood thinner A popular but erroneous name for an anticoagulant.

blood transfusion The replacement of blood or one of its components. Effective and safe transfusion therapy requires a thorough understanding of the clinical condition being treated. Most patients require blood components rather than whole blood. SEE: *blood component therapy; autologous blood transfusion; exchange transfusion; transfusion reaction; Standard and Universal Precautions Appendix.*

The following measures should be taken during transfusion therapy:

1. Screen donors for transmissible diseases
2. Test blood for pathogens
3. Ensure that cross-matched blood products are given to correctly identified patients
4. Intervene promptly in transfusion reactions
5. Avoid unnecessary transfusions
6. Avoid volume overload during transfusions
7. Avoid hypothermia, electrolyte, and clotting disorders.

Administration of a single unit may be indicated in young or old surgical patients, in persons with coronary disease, and in patients who have an acute blood loss of several units but whose blood pressure, pulse, and oxygen are stabilized by use of one unit.

The risk of HIV, HBV, or HCV on blood collected and distributed in the U.S. is very low but finite. The risk in Australia/New Zealand and Canada approaches that in the U.S. Outside of the geographical areas noted, the blood supply may be suspect, to the extent that most U.S. embassies have their own supply or a specific procedure for dealing with the need for obtaining safe blood.

Patient Care: The patient is identified from both the hospital identification band and blood bank band. Two health-care professionals (one the administering nurse) verify the patient's ABO and Rh blood type and its compatibility with the unit of blood or packed cells to be administered, as well as the unit's expiration date and time. Outdated blood is not used; it is returned to the blood bank for disposal. The blood or blood product is retrieved from the blood bank refrigerator immediately before administration, because blood should not be stored in other than approved refrigerators. Also, it cannot be returned to blood bank storage if the unit's temperature exceeds 50°F (10°C), a change that will occur within about 30 min of removal from storage.

Before the transfusion is started, the patient's vital signs (including temperature) are checked and documented. The blood is inspected visually for clots or discoloration, and then the transfusion is administered through an approved line containing a blood filter, preferably piggybacked through physiological saline solution on a Y-type blood administration set. No other IV solutions or drugs may be infused with blood (unless specifically prescribed) because of potential incompatibility. In the first 15 min, the blood flow rate is slowed to limit intake to no more than 50 ml. A health care professional remains with the patient during this time and instructs the patient to report any adverse reactions, such as back or chest pain, hypotension, fever, increase in temperature of more than 1.8°F (1°C), chills, pain at the infusion site, tachycardia, tachypnea, wheezing, cyanosis, urticaria, or rashes. If any of these occurs, the transfusion is stopped immediately, the vein is kept open with physiological saline solution, and the patient's physician and the blood bank are notified. If incompatibility is suspected, the blood and set are returned to the blood bank; samples of the patient's blood and urine are obtained for laboratory analysis; and the data are recorded from the unit. If no symptoms occur in the first 15 min and vital signs remain stable, the transfusion rate is increased to complete the tranfusion within the prescribed time, or (if necessary) the transfusion is administered as fast as the patient's overall condition permits. Once the transfusion begins, the blood is administered within a maximum of 4 hr to maintain biological effectiveness and limit the risk of bacterial growth. (If the patient's condition does not permit transfusing the prescribed amount within this time frame, arrangements are made to have the blood bank split the unit and properly store the second portion.) The patient's vital signs and response are monitored every 30 min throughout the transfusion and 30 min afterward; stated precautions are observed, and caregivers monitor for indications of volume overload (distended neck veins, bounding pulse, hypertension, dyspnea). Blood should not be administered through a central line unless an approved in-line warming device is used. A warmer also should be used whenever multiple transfusions place the patient at risk for hypothermia, which can lead to dysrhythmias and cardiac arrest.

blood urea nitrogen ABBR: BUN. Nitrogen in the blood in the form of urea, the metabolic product of the breakdown of amino acids used for energy production. The normal concentration is about 8 to 18 mg/dl. The level of urea in the blood provides a rough estimate of kidney function. Blood urea nitrogen levels may be increased in the presence of dehydration, decreased renal function, upper gastrointestinal bleeding, or treatment with drugs such as steroids or tetracyclines. SEE: *creatinine*.

blood vessels The veins, arteries, and capillaries.

blood warmer A device for warming banked blood to body temperature before it is transfused.

bloody weeping Hemorrhage from the conjunctiva.

blotch A blemish, spot, or area of discoloration on the skin.

blotting method A technique for analyzing a tiny portion of the primary structure of genomic material (DNA or RNA).

Northern b.m. A blot analysis technique for analyzing a small portion of RNA. Operationally, this test is identical to Southern blotting except for the target (RNA) and the specific reagents used.

Southern b.m. A technique used in molecular genetics to analyze a small portion of DNA first by purifying it, then by controlled fragmentation, electrophoretic separation, and fixing the fragment identity using specific DNA probes. It is used most commonly for G cell and T cell rearrangement analysis, bcr gene rearrangement analysis, and fragile X syndrome analysis.

Western b.m. A technique for analyzing protein antigens.

Blount's disease [W. P. Blount, Am. surgeon, b. 1900] A pathological bowing of the leg (genu varum). Unlike the physiological bowlegs of the infant and toddler, the bowing in Blount's disease progressively worsens after the first 2 years of life and is often unilateral. The condition is more common in girls than in boys and more common in blacks than in European Americans. Most cases occur in the first 2 or 3 years of life, but a juvenile form (onset at age 4 to 10 years) and an adolescent form (onset at 11 years or older) are recognized. SYN: *tibia vara*.

DIAGNOSIS: Diagnosis is based on clinical presentation and x-ray of the leg.

TREATMENT: In the early stages, simple bracing and splinting may be all that is necessary. If the disease has gone undetected or untreated, or if it is one of the later-onset forms, surgery may be required.

blowfly One of the flies belonging to the family Calliphoridae. Most blowflies are scavengers. Their larvae live in decaying flesh or meat, although occasionally they may live in decaying or suppurating tissue. However, one species, the screw-worm fly, *Callitroga hominivorax,* attacks living tissue, laying its eggs in the nostrils or open wounds of its domestic animal or human host, giving rise to myiasis. SEE: *Calliphora vomitoria; myiasis*.

blowpipe A tube through which a gas or current of air is passed under pressure and directed upon a flame to concentrate and intensify the heat.

BLS *basic life support.*

blue [O. Fr. *bleu*] **1.** A primary color of the spectrum; sky color; azure. **2.** Cyanotic.

blue bloater A person with chronic bronchitis who demonstrates evidence of cyanosis and pedal edema. SEE: *chronic bronchitis*.

ETIOLOGY: It is most often the result of long-term cigarette smoking.

TREATMENT: The patient often benefits from oxygen therapy, bronchial hygiene (e.g., clearing of the lungs), and smoking cessation.

bluebottle fly A fly of the family Calliphoridae. It breeds in dung or the flesh of dead animals.

Blue Cross A nonprofit medical care insurer in the U.S. The insurance is mostly for hospital services. SEE: *Blue Shield*.

Blue Shield A nonprofit medical care insurer in the U.S. The insurance is for that part of medical care provided by health care professionals. SEE: *Blue Cross*.

Blumberg's sign (blŭm'bĕrgs) [Jacob Moritz Blumberg, Ger. surgeon and gynecologist, 1873–1955] The occurrence of a sharp acute pain when the examiner presses his or her hand over McBurney's point and then releases the hand pressure suddenly. This sign is indicative of peritonitis. SYN: *rebound tenderness*.

Blumenbach's clivus (bloo'mĕn-bŏks) [Johann F. Blumenbach, Ger. physiologist and anthropologist, 1752–1840] The sloping part of the sphenoid bone behind the posterior clinoid processes.

blush [AS. *blyscan,* to be red] Redness of the face and neck due to vasodilation caused by emotion or heat. Blushing may also be associated with certain diseases, including carcinoid syndrome, pheochromocytoma, and Zollinger-Ellison syndrome.

B.M.A. *British Medical Association.*

B.M.E *Biomedical Engineer.*

B.M.E.T *Biomedical Engineering Technologist.*

BMI *Body mass index.*

B-mode (brightness mode) display In ultrasonography, imaging dots on the screen indicate echoes. The brighter the dot relative to the background, the greater the strength of the echo.

B.M.R. *basal metabolic rate.*

B.M.S. *Bachelor of Medical Science.*

BMT *bone marrow transplant.*

BNA *Basle Nomina Anatomica.*

board **1.** A long, flat piece of a substance such as wood or firm plastic. SEE: *bed board*. **2.** A corporate or governmental body, such as a board of directors or board of health.

board certification In medicine, a process that ensures that an individual has met standards beyond those of admission to licensure and has passed specialty examinations in the field. The various medical professional organizations establish their own standards and administer their own board certification examinations. Individuals successfully completing all requirements are called Fellows, such as Fellow of the American College of Surgeons (F.A.C.S.) or Fellow of the American College of Physicians (F.A.C.P.). Board certification may be required by a hospital for admission to the medical staff or for determination of a staff member's rank (e.g., general staff, associate staff, or full attending status).

board eligible In medicine, a designation that signifies that a physician has completed all the requirements for admission to the medical specialty board certification examination but has not yet taken and passed the examination. SEE: *board certification*.

boarder baby An infant kept in a hospital nursery until status permits discharge to family care or transfer to another agency for maintenance or adoption.

Boas' point (bō'ăz) [Ismar I. Boas, Ger. physician, 1858–1938] A tender spot left of the 12th dorsal vertebra in patients with gastric ulcer.

Bochdalek's ganglion (bŏk'dăl-ĕks) [Victor Bochdalek, Czech. anatomist, 1801–1883] A ganglion of the plexus of the dental nerve in the maxilla above the canine tooth.

Bodo (bō'dō) A genus of nonpathogenic, flagellate protozoa of the family Bodonidae often found in stale feces or urine and sometimes in the urinary bladder.

body [AS. *bodig*] **1.** The physical part of the human as distinguished from mind and spirit. SYN: *soma* (1). **2.** Trunk (1). **3.** The principal mass of any structure. **4.** The largest or most important part of any organ.

EXAMINATION: The nude body is examined and both sides are compared. Physical examination is made by inspection, palpation, manipulation, mensuration, auscultation, and use of the sense of smell. It should also include observation of the body as the person walks and goes through the various ranges of motion of the trunk, neck, and extremities. Chemical and microscopic examination may be made of the blood, sputum, feces, urine, cerebrospinal fluids, and other bodily fluids. Radiological studies also may be used.

acetone b. Ketone b.

amygdaloid b. An almond-shaped mass of gray matter in the lateral wall and roof of the third ventricle of the brain.

aortic b. A chemoreceptor in the wall of the arch of the aorta that detects changes in blood gases (esp. oxygen) and pH. It stimulates reflex changes in heart rate, respiration, and blood pressure that restore normal blood oxygen levels. It is innervated by the vagus nerve.

asbestosis b. One of the minute bodies formed by the deposition of various salts and minerals around an asbestos particle. These may be found in the sputum, lung, or feces.

Aschoff b. Microscopic foci of fibrinoid degeneration and granulomatous inflammation found in the interstitial tissues of the heart in rheumatic fever.

Barr b. SEE: *Barr body*.

basal b. A small granule usually present at the base of a flagellum or cilium in protozoa. SYN: *basal granule; blepharoplast*.

carotid b. The chemoreceptors at the bifurcation of each common carotid artery, which detect changes in blood gases (esp. oxygen) and pH. They stimulate reflex changes in heart rate, respiration, and blood pressure that restore normal blood oxygen levels. They are innervated by the glossopharyngeal nerves.

chromaffin b. One of a number of bodies composed principally of chromaffin cells, arranged serially along both sides of the dorsal aorta and in the kidney, liver, and gonads. They are ectodermal in origin, having the same origin as cells of the sympathetic ganglia. SYN: *paraganglion*.

ciliary b. A structure directly behind the iris of the eye. It secretes the aqueous humor and contains the ciliary muscle that changes the shape, and thus the refractive power, of the lens by tightening and relaxing the tension on the lens zonule. SEE: *eye* for illus.

coccygeal b. An arteriovenous anastomosis at the tip of the coccyx formed by the middle sacral artery. SYN: *glomus coccygeum*.

Donovan b. The common name for *Calymmatobacterium granulomatis,* which causes granuloma inguinale.

foreign b. SEE: *foreign body*.

Heinz b. SEE: under *Heinz*.

Hensen's b. A modified Golgi net found in the hair cells of the organ of Corti.

hyaline b. A homogeneous substance resulting from colloid degeneration; found in degenerated cells. SEE: *degeneration, hyaline*.

inclusion b. Microscopic structures (made of a dense, occasionally infective core surrounded by an envelope) seen in the cytoplasm and nuclei of cells infected with some intracellular pathogens. Inclusion bodies are seen in cells infected with herpesviruses (esp. cytomegalovirus), smallpox, lymphogranuloma venereum, psittacosis, and other organisms.

ketone b. One of a number of substances that increase in the blood as a result of faulty carbohydrate metabolism. Among them are β-hydroxybutyric acid, acetoacetic acid, and acetone. They increase in persons with untreated or inadequately controlled diabetes mellitus and are the primary cause of acidosis. They may also occur in other metabolic disturbances. SYN: *acetone b.*

lateral geniculate b. One of two bodies forming elevations on the lateral portion of the posterior part of the thalamus. Each is the termination of afferent fibers from the retina, which it receives through the optic nerves and tracts.

Leishman-Donovan b. Small bodies found in the spleen and liver of victims of kala-azar or dum-dum fever; now known as *Leishmania donovani,* the causative organism of the disease. They are found both within and outside living cells and in circulating blood.

loose b. A fragment of bone or cartilage within the joint of a patient with severe degenerative or neuropathic arthritis.

malpighian b. **1.** A historically important but out-of-date term for splenic lymph nodules or renal cells. **2.** A lymph nodule found in the spleen.

mammillary b. A rounded body of gray matter found in the diencephalon. It forms a rounded eminence projecting into the anterior portion of the interpeduncular fossa, and its nucleus constitutes an important relay station for olfactory impulses.

medial geniculate b. One of two bodies lying in the posterior part of the dorsal thalamus. Each receives fibers from the acoustic tract of the pons and the inferior colliculus through the brachium.

medullary b. The deeper white matter of the cerebellum enclosed within the cortex.

Negri b. SEE: *Negri bodies.*

Nissl b. SEE: *Nissl bodies.*

olivary b. A rounded mass in the anterolateral portion of the medulla oblongata. It consists of a convoluted sheet of gray matter enclosing white matter. SYN: *oliva.*

pacchionian b. arachnoid granulation.

perineal b. A mass of tissue that separates the anus from the vestibule and the lower part of the vagina. SEE: *perineum* for illus.

pineal b. SEE: *pineal gland.*

pituitary b. Obsolete term for the pituitary gland.

polar b. A small nonfunctional cell produced in oogenesis resulting from the divisions of the primary and secondary oocytes.

postbranchial b. One of two bodies that develop from the posterior wall of the fourth pharyngeal pouch and become incorporated into the thyroid gland. SYN: *ultimobranchial b.*

psammoma b. A laminated calcareous body seen in certain types of tumors and sometimes associated with chronic inflammation.

quadrigeminal b. Four rounded projections from the roof of the midbrain. SEE: *colliculus inferior; colliculus superior.*

restiform b. One of the inferior cerebellar peduncles of the brain, found along the lateral border of the fourth ventricle. These two bands of fibers, principally ascending, connect the medulla oblongata with the cerebellum.

striate b. The corpus striatum, composed of the cordate and lenticular nuclei of the brain.

trachoma b. A mass of cells present as an inclusion body in the conjunctival epithelial cells of individuals with trachoma.

ultimobranchial b. Postbranchial b.

vertebral b. A short column of bone forming the weight-supporting portion of a vertebra. From its dorsolateral surfaces project the roots of the arch of a vertebra.

vitreous b. A jellylike substance within the eye that fills the space between the lens and the retina. It is colorless, structureless, and transparent. It may contain minute particles called "floaters."

wolffian b. Mesonephros.

body composition Quantitation of the various components of the body, esp. of the fat, water, protein, and bone. Determination of the specific gravity of the body is done to estimate the percentage of fat. This may be calculated by various methods, including underwater weighing, which determines the density of the individual; use of radioactive potassium, ^{40}K; measuring the total body water by dilution of tritium; and use of various anthropometric measurements such as height, weight, and skin fold thickness at various sites. None of these methods is free of the potential for error. Underwater weighing is useful but may provide misleading information when used in analyzing body composition of highly trained athletes. The obese person has a lower body density than does the lean person, because the specific gravity of fat tissue is less than that of muscle tissue. The fat content for young men will vary from about 5% to 27% and for women from about 18% to 35%.

body fluid A fluid found in one of the fluid compartments of the body. The principal fluid compartments are intracellular and extracellular. A much smaller segment, the transcellular, includes fluid in the tracheobronchial tree, the gastrointestinal tract, and the bladder; cerebrospinal fluid; and the aqueous humor of the eye. The chemical composition of fluids in the various compartments is carefully regulated. In a normal 154 lb (70 kg) adult human male, 60% of total body weight (i.e., 42 L) is water; a similar female is 55% water (39 L). SEE: *acid-base balance; fluid replacement; fluid balance.*

body image disturbance Disruption in the way one perceives one's body image (e.g., after an injury or illness) or an incongruity between one's actual appearance and the way one perceives it (e.g., in anorexia nervosa). SEE: *Nursing Diagnoses Appendix.*

body language The unconscious use of posture, gestures, or other nonverbal expression in communication. SEE: *kinesics.*

body mechanics Application of kinesiology to use of the body in daily life activities and to the prevention and correction of problems related to posture and lifting.

body odor The aroma or fragrance emanating from the human body. It may be derived from sweat gland secretions, urine, feces, expiration, saliva, breasts, skin, and sex organs. The major sources are the eccrine and apocrine sweat glands. Sebaceous gland secretions from the skin contribute to these odors. Eating garlic or onions or taking certain drugs may add to the odors produced by sweat glands, but the major sources of body sweat odor are the volatile fatty acids, steroids, and amines emitted by apocrine glands. Bacteria and fungi in and around these glands can intensify the odors. The secretions increase at puberty and decrease after menopause, are enhanced by stress, and are partially genetically controlled. SEE: *halitosis*.

body packer syndrome Drug overdose as a result of the ingestion of multiple small packages, usually containing drugs of abuse (esp. cocaine), to transport them illegally. Inadvertent overdose may occur if the packages rupture.

body rocking Rhythmic, purposeless body movement seen in individuals, whether adults or infants, who are bored, lonely, cognitively impaired, or disturbed. It is also seen in some blind children.

body scheme Knowledge of one's body parts and their relative positions. SEE: *proprioception*.

body section radiography Tomography.

body snatching Robbing a grave of its body, which was done in the past to obtain bodies for anatomical study in medical schools.

body temperature, altered, risk for The state in which the individual is at risk for failure to maintain body temperature within normal range. SEE: *Nursing Diagnoses Appendix*.

body type Classification of the human body according to muscle and fat distribution. SEE: *ectomorph; endomorph; mesomorph; somatotype*.

body work Musculoskeletal manipulations such as massage, stretching, postural alignment, and breathing exercises that are used to relieve stress and promote a sense of wellness.

Boeck's sarcoid (bĕks) [Caesar P. M. Boeck, Norwegian dermatologist, 1845–1917] Former name for sarcoidosis.

Boerhaave syndrome (boor'hă-vĕ) [Hermann Boerhaave, Dutch physician, 1668–1738] Spontaneous rupture of the esophagus usually associated with violent retching or vomiting. SEE: *Mallory-Weiss syndrome*.

Bohr effect [Christian Bohr, Danish physiologist, 1855–1911] The effect of an acid environment on hemoglobin; hydrogen ions alter the structure of hemoglobin and increase the release of oxygen. It is esp. important in active tissues producing carbon dioxide and lactic acid.

boil [AS. *byl*, a swelling] A tender, dome-shaped skin lesion, typically caused by infection around a hair follicle with *Staphylococcus aureus*. Boils usually arise on the face, neck, axilla, or buttocks (i.e., on body surfaces that frequently perspire and chafe). When they first appear they are often superficial, but as they mature they form localized abscesses with pus and necrotic debris at their core. On rare occasions they spread to deeper tissues, sometimes with tragic consequences (e.g., a boil on the neck or face may spread to the brain or meninges). SYN: *furuncle*. SEE: *carbuncle*.

TREATMENT: Warm moist compresses relieve pain and encourage drainage of the infected nodule to the skin surface. Oral antistaphylococcal antibiotics, such as dicloxacillin or clindamycin, are given when the lesion is surrounded by local cellulitis. Incision and drainage is sometimes needed.

boiling Process of vaporizing a liquid. Boiling water destroys most microorganisms (but may not kill spores and some viruses); toughens and hardens albumin in eggs; toughens (i.e., denatures) fibrin and dissolves tissues in meat; bursts starch granules; and softens cellulose in cereals and vegetables.

bolometer (bō-lŏm'ĕ-tĕr) [Gr. *bole*, a ray, + *metron*, measure] An instrument for measuring small amounts of radiated heat.

bolus (bō'lŭs) [L., from Gr. *bolos*, a lump] **1.** A mass of masticated food ready to be swallowed. **2.** A rounded preparation of medicine for oral ingestion. **3.** A concentrated mass of a diagnostic substance given rapidly intravenously, such as an opaque contrast medium, or an intravenous medication. **4.** In radiology, a tissue-equivalent material placed on the surface of the body to minimize the effects of an irregularly shaped body surface. The dose at the skin surface tends to increase, minimizing the skin-sparing effect of megavoltage radiation.

alimentary b. A mass of masticated food in the esophagus that is ready to be passed into the stomach.

bombesin (bŏm'bĕ-sĭn) A neuropeptide present in the gut and brain tissue of humans. It is also present in increased concentrations in cell cultures of small-cell carcinomas of the lung.

bona fide [L.] Carried out in good faith; honest, without fraud or deception, real, legal, and valid.

bond **1.** A force that binds ions or atoms together. It is represented by a line drawn from one molecule or atom to another as in H—O—H. **2.** An interpersonal connection or tie.

covalent b. Chemical bond formed when atoms share one, two, or three pairs of electrons. This is the type of bond found in organic molecules.

disulfide b. A covalent bond between two sulfur-containing amino acids, which helps maintain the shape of proteins such as insulin, keratin, and antibodies. SYN: *disulfide bridge*.

hydrogen b. The weak attraction of a covalently bonded hydrogen to nearby oxygen or nitrogen atoms in the same or a different molecule. Hydrogen bonds give water its cohesiveness and its surface tension. These bonds also help maintain the three-dimensional shape of proteins and nucleic acids; such shape is essential to their functioning.

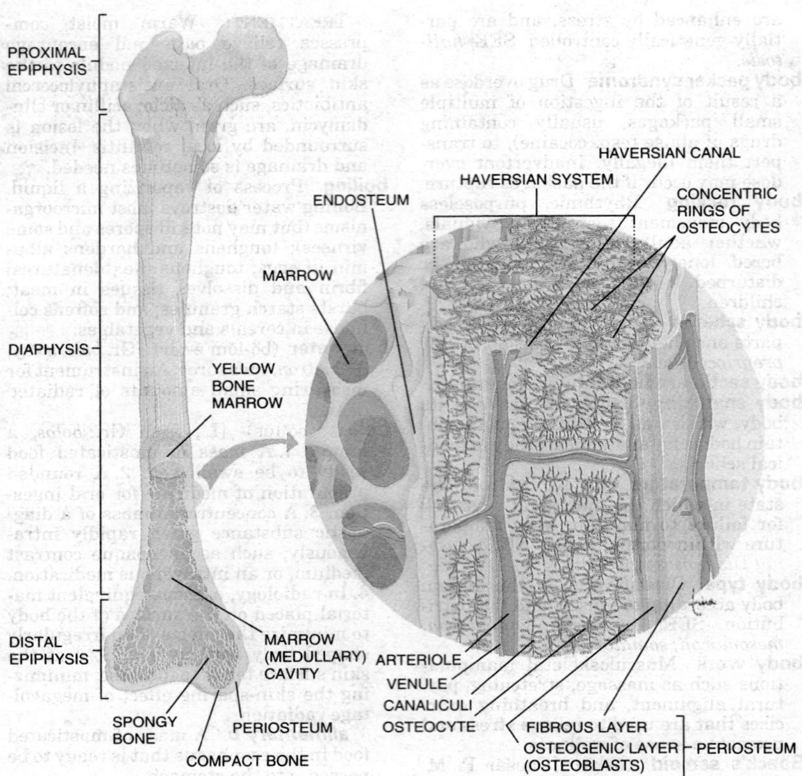

BONE TISSUE

(A) Femur with distal end sectioned; (B) compact bone with haversian systems

ionic b. A chemical bond formed by the loss and gain of electrons between atoms. This type of bond is found in inorganic acids, bases, and salts.

nonpolar covalent b. A covalent bond in which the pair of electrons is shared equally between two atoms.

polar covalent b. A covalent bond in which one atom attracts the shared pair of electrons more strongly than does the other atom, and thus has a slightly negative charge. The atom with the weaker attraction has a slightly positive charge.

bonding **1.** In dentistry, the use of a low-viscosity polymerizable adhesive to provide mechanical retention of cast restorations, autopolymerizing restorations, and orthodontic appliances. **2.** Development of a strong emotional attachment between individuals (e.g., a mother and child) after frequent or prolonged close contact.

mother-infant b. The emotional and physical attachment between infant and mother that is initiated in the first hour or two after normal delivery of a baby who has not been dulled by anesthetic agents or drugs. It is believed that the stronger this bond, the greater the chances of a mentally healthy infant-mother relationship in both the short- and long-term periods after childbirth. For that reason, the initial contact between mother and infant should be in the delivery room and the contact should continue for as long as possible in the first hours after birth.

bone [AS. *ban,* bone] **1.** Osseous tissue, a specialized form of dense connective tissue consisting of bone cells (osteocytes) embedded in a matrix of calcified intercellular substance. Bone matrix contains collagen fibers and the minerals calcium phosphate and calcium carbonate. SEE: illus. (Bone Tissue). **2.** A unit of the skeleton; the human skeleton has 206 bones. Bones surround and protect some vital organs, and give points of attachment for the muscles, serving as levers and making movement possi-

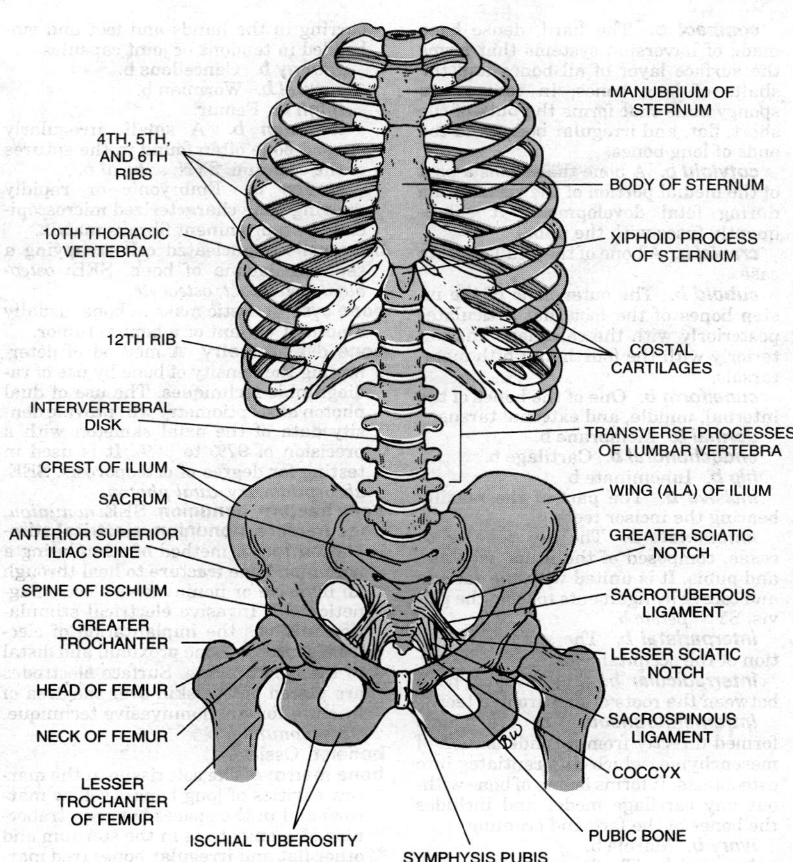

BONY STRUCTURES OF THE THORAX, ABDOMEN, AND PELVIS

ble. In the embryo, the bones of the skull are first made of fibrous connective tissue, which is gradually replaced by bone matrix. The remainder of the skeleton is first made of hyaline cartilage, which is also replaced by bone matrix, also beginning during the third month of gestation. The outer surface of a bone is compact bone, and the inner more porous portion is cancellous (spongy) bone. The shafts of long bones are made of compact bone that surrounds a marrow canal. Compact bone is made of haversian systems, which are precise arrangements of osteocytes, blood vessels, and lymphatics within the bony matrix. All of these contribute to the maintenance and repair of bone. The periosteum is the fibrous connective tissue membrane that covers a bone. It has blood vessels that enter the bone, and it provides a site of attachment for tendons and ligaments. Bones are classified according to shape as long, short, flat, or irregular. In the elderly, esp. women, osteoporosis may develop, a condition in which bones become brittle and break easily. SEE: illus. (Bony Structures of the Thorax, Abdomen, and Pelvis); *skeleton* for names of principal bones.

alveolar b. The bony tissue or process of the maxilla or mandible that supports the teeth. SYN: *alveolar process*.

breast b. Sternum.

brittle b. Bone that is abnormally fragile, as in osteogenesis imperfecta.

cancellous b. A spongy bone in which the matrix forms connecting bars and plates, partially enclosing many intercommunicating spaces filled with bone marrow. SYN: *spongy b.*

cartilage b. A bone formed by endochondral ossification developing from the primary centers of bone formation. SYN: *endochondral b.*

cavalry b. Rider's b.

compact b. The hard, dense bone made of haversian systems that forms the surface layer of all bones and the shafts of long bones, in contrast to spongy bone that forms the bulk of the short, flat, and irregular bones and the ends of long bones.

cotyloid b. A bone that forms a part of the medial portion of the acetabulum during fetal development. It subsequently fuses with the pubis.

cranial b. A bone of the skull or brain case.

cuboid b. The outer bone of the instep bones of the foot that articulates posteriorly with the calcaneus and anteriorly with the fourth and fifth metatarsals.

cuneiform b. One of the bones of the internal, middle, and external tarsus.

dermal b. Membrane b.

endochondral b. Cartilage b.

hip b. Innominate b.

incisive b. The part of the maxilla bearing the incisor teeth.

innominate b. The hip bone or os coxae, composed of the ilium, ischium, and pubis. It is united with the sacrum and coccyx by ligaments to form the pelvis. SYN: *pelvic b.*

interparietal b. The squamous portion of the occipital bone.

interradicular b. The alveolar bone between the roots of multirooted teeth.

intramembraneous b. A bone formed directly from a condensation of mesenchyme, which differentiates into osteoblasts. It forms layers of bone without any cartilage model and includes the bones of the face and cranium.

ivory b. Marble b.

lacrimal b. The bone at the medial side of the orbital cavity.

marble b. An abnormally calcified bone with a spotted appearance on a radiograph. SYN: *ivory b.* SEE: *Albers-Schönberg disease; osteopetrosis.*

membrane b. Bone that is formed within fibrous connective tissue in the embryo (e.g., most of the skull bones). SYN: *dermal b.*

mosaic b. Bone appearing as small pieces fitted together, characteristic of Paget's disease.

pelvic b. Innominate b.

perichondrial b. Bone formed beneath the perichondrium.

periosteal b. Bone formed by osteoblasts of the periosteum.

ping pong b. A thin shell of osseous tissue covering a giant-cell sarcoma in a bone.

replacement b. Any bone that develops within cartilage.

rider's b. Ossification of the distal end of the adductor muscles of the thigh, as may be seen in horseback riders. SYN: *cavalry b.*

sesamoid b. A type of short bone occurring in the hands and feet and embedded in tendons or joint capsules.

spongy b. Cancellous b.

sutural b. Wormian b.

thigh b. Femur.

wormian b. A small, irregularly shaped bone often found in the sutures of the cranium. SYN: *sutural b.*

woven b. Embryonic or rapidly growing bone characterized microscopically by a prominent fibrous matrix.

bone cell A nucleated cell occupying a separate lacuna of bone. SEE: *osteoblast; osteoclast; osteocyte.*

bone cyst A cystic mass in bone, usually a normal variant or a benign tumor.

bone densitometry A method of determining the density of bone by use of radiographic techniques. The use of dual photon absorptiometry will provide density data of the axial skeleton with a precision of 97% to 98%. It is used in testing for degree of osteoporosis. SEE: *absorptiometry, dual photon.*

bone fracture, nonunion SEE: *nonunion.*

bone fracture, nonunion, electrical stimulation for A method of stimulating a nonunion bone fracture to heal through an invasive or noninvasive electromagnetic field. Invasive electrical stimulation involves the implantation of electrodes into the bone proximal and distal to the fracture site. Surface electrodes are placed on the skin over the area of fracture for the noninvasive technique. SEE: *nonunion.*

bonelet Ossicle.

bone marrow The soft tissue in the marrow cavities of long bones (yellow marrow) and in the spaces between trabeculae of spongy bone in the sternum and other flat and irregular bones (red marrow). Yellow marrow is mostly fat, stored energy. Red marrow produces all the types of blood cells.

bone paste One of several composite materials that can be used to repair defects in bones during orthopedic surgery.

bone remodeling The process in which bone is resorbed and new bone formed at the same site. This process keeps the bone tissue in dynamic equilibrium.

bone scan The use of short half-life radiopharmaceutical agents to visualize bones. This is esp. useful in delineating osteomyelitis and metastases to the bone.

bony Resembling or of the nature of bone. SYN: *osseous.*

booster (boo′stĕr) An additional dose of an immunizing agent to increase the protection afforded by the original series of injections. The booster is given some months or years after the initial immunization.

boot A special shoe or bandage for covering the foot, ankle, and lower leg.

borate (bō′rāt) Any basic salt of boric acid. SEE: *Poisons and Poisoning Appendix.*

borated Mixed with borax.

borax (bor′ăks) [L., from Arabic, from Persian *burah*] Sodium borate, used as a detergent, a water softener, and a weak antiseptic.

borborygmus (bor″bō-rĭg′mŭs) *pl.* **borborygmi** [Gr. *borborygmos,* rumbling in the bowels] A gurgling, splashing sound normally heard over the large intestine; it is caused by passage of gas through the liquid contents of the intestine. Its absence may indicate paralytic ileus or obstruction of the bowels due to torsion, volvulus, or strangulated hernia.

border (bor′dĕr) The outer part or edge; boundary.

brush b. The microvilli on the free surface of the cells lining the small intestine and the proximal convoluted portion of the renal tubules. Microvilli are folds of the cell membrane and greatly increase the surface area for absorption.

vermilion b. The red boundary of the lips that represents the highly vascular, hyalinized, keratinized epithelial covering between the outer skin and the moist oral mucosa of the mouth.

borderline An incomplete state, as in a borderline diagnosis, in a patient who has some of the requirements for a definite diagnosis but not enough for certainty; a condition judged numerically (e.g., high blood pressure in which the value is close to a hypertensive level but not at a diagnostic level).

Bordetella (bor″dĕ-tĕl′lă) [Jules Bordet, Belg. physician, bacteriologist, and physiologist, 1870–1961] A genus of hemolytic gram-negative coccobacilli of the family Brucellaceae. Some species are parasitic and pathogenic in warm-blooded animals, including humans.

B. pertussis The causative agent of whooping cough; formerly called *Haemophilus pertussis.* SEE: *pertussis.*

bore The internal diameter of a tube.

boredom A feeling of tiredness or depression because of lack of activity or challenging, meaningful stimuli. SEE: *apathy.*

Borg's dyspnea scale A system used to document the severity of the patient's shortness of breath using numbers anchored with verbal descriptions (e.g., 10 = completely out of breath; 5 = somewhat breathless; 1 = breathing easily). The patient or athlete chooses the number that best corresponds to his or her current perceived respiratory effort.

boric acid poisoning Intoxication caused by the consumption of or exposure to boric acid.

SYMPTOMS: Symptoms may include nausea, vomiting, diarrhea, convulsions, weakness, central nervous system depression, livid skin rash characterized as "boiled lobster rash," and shock. Acute renal failure and cardiac failure may result from large ingestions.

TREATMENT: Activated charcoal may prevent absorption of boric acid from the gastrointestinal tract. Hemodialysis is sometimes required for severe intoxications. SEE: *Poisons and Poisoning Appendix.*

borism The symptoms caused by the internal use of borax or boron compounds. These include dry skin, eruptions, and gastric disturbances.

Bornholm disease (born′hōm) [named for the Danish island Bornholm] An epidemic disease marked by sudden intense pleuritic or abdominal pain and fever. It is caused by various coxsackie viruses. SYN: *devil's grip; epidemic pleurodynia.*

TREATMENT: Nonsteroidal anti-inflammatory agents and local application of heat may control symptoms.

boron [*bor*ax + carb*on*] SYMB: B. A nonmetallic element found only as a compound such as boric acid or borax; atomic weight 10.81, atomic number 5.

Borrelia (bor-rē′lē-ă) A genus of spirochetes, some of which are causative agents for relapsing fevers and Lyme disease in humans.

B. burgdorferi The causative agent of Lyme disease.

B. duttonii The causative agent for tick-borne relapsing fever in Central and South America.

B. recurrentis The causative agent of louse-borne relapsing fever.

borreliosis Any of several arthropod-borne diseases caused by spirochetes of the genus *Borrelia.*

boss [O. Fr. *boce,* a swelling] A round circumscribed swelling or growth (e.g., a tumor) that becomes large enough to produce swelling.

bosselated (bŏs′ĕ-lāt-ĕd) Marked by numerous bosses.

bossing Protuberance of the frontal areas of the skull.

Boston arm A myoelectric prosthesis for above-the-elbow amputations. The elbow is powered by a small battery-driven motor, activated in proportion to the strength of contraction detected in the control muscle. SYN: *Boston elbow; Liberty Mutual elbow.*

Boston brace A low-profile plastic thoracolumbosacral orthosis (spinal jacket) with no metal suprastructure, used to treat mild to moderate lower thoracic and lumbar scoliosis.

Boston elbow Boston arm.

Botallo's duct (bō-tăl′ōz) [Leonardo Botallo, It. anatomist, 1530–1600] Ductus arteriosus.

botanical (bō-tă′nĭ-kl) **1.** Relating to botany or plants. **2.** A plant extract used to maintain health or prevent illness.

botany (bŏt′n-ē) [Gr. *botanikos,* pert. to plants] The study of plants; a division of biology.

botfly (bŏt′flī) *pl.* **botflies** An insect that belongs to the family Oestridae of the order Diptera and is parasitic to mammals, esp. horses and sheep. Human infestation is rare.

botryoid (bŏt′rē-oyd) [Gr. *botrys,* bunch of grapes, + *eidos,* form, shape] Resembling a bunch of grapes. SYN: *staphyline.*

botuliform (bŏt-ū′lĭ-form) [L. *botulus,* sausage, + *forma,* shape] Shaped like a sausage.

botulin (bŏt′chū-lĭn) The neurotoxin responsible for botulism. It is not destroyed by the action of gastric or intestinal secretions.

botulinic acid A toxin found in putrid sausage.

botulism (bŏt′ū-lĭzm) [″ + Gr. *-ismos,* condition] A paralytic and occasionally fatal illness caused by exposure to toxins released from *Clostridium botulinum,* an anaerobic, gram-positive bacillus. In adults, the disease usually occurs after food contaminated by the toxin is eaten, after gastrointestinal surgery, or after the toxin is released into an infected wound. In infants, the illness results from intestinal colonization by clostridial spores. Because the toxin is extraordinarily lethal and easy to manufacture and distribute, concern has been raised regarding its use as an agent of biological warfare.

Foodborne botulism may result from consumption of improperly cooked and canned meals, in which the spores of the bacillus survive and reproduce. Wound botulism may begin in abscesses, where an anaerobic environment promotes the proliferation of the germ and absorption of its poison. In either case cranial nerve paralysis and failure of the autonomic and respiratory systems may occur; however, gastrointestinal symptoms are likely only in foodborne outbreaks.

The poison responsible for botulism damages the nervous system by blocking the release of acetylcholine at the neuromuscular junction. This is the cause of the paralysis associated with the illness.

SYMPTOMS: Nausea, diarrhea, vomiting, double vision, slurred speech, and swallowing difficulties are all common in adults. Constipation, poor feeding, and flaccidity may occur in children. The spectrum of illness is broad; some patients suffer other complications, including generalized paralysis and respiratory failure.

DIAGNOSIS: Positive stool cultures for botulinum toxin, or a positive mouse inoculation test (using samples from suspected food sources), will make the diagnosis in patients in whom other neurological evaluations are negative. Because the clinical presentation is similar to stroke and Guillain-Barré and Eaton-Lambert syndromes, neural imaging and spinal fluid analysis are generally performed; results are negative in botulism.

TREATMENT: Trivalent antitoxin (ABE), an antitoxin made from horses, should be administered early in patients suspected of having botulism. Early usage decreases mortality and morbidity associated with the illness. Antitoxin is available from the Centers for Disease Control and Prevention by calling (404) 639-2206 (daytime) or (404) 639-2888 (evening). SEE: *Poisons and Poisoning Appendix.*

PATIENT CARE: Patients who have ingested tainted foods may benefit from gastrointestinal decontamination. Very close monitoring of affected patients, preferably in intensive care units, is indicated so that prompt intubation and mechanical ventilation can begin if respiratory failure develops. Vital signs, respiratory effort, and respiratory distress are documented and reported. Arterial blood gases are monitored. Motor function is carefully and repeatedly assessed. Before botulinum antitoxin is administered, a history of the patient's allergies, esp. to horse serum, is obtained.

If relatives or other close contacts of the patient have eaten similar foods or shown similar symptoms, they should be carefully assessed and treated.

infant b. A form of botulism first recognized in 1976 that affects infants less than 1 year old who ingest soil or food (esp. honey) containing *Clostridium botulinum* spores. The infant's protective intestinal flora is not yet established, and the spores germinate into active bacteria that produce the neurotoxin. It is treated with oral amoxicillin.

SYMPTOMS: The symptoms include constipation, lethargy, listlessness, poor feeding, ptosis, loss of head control, difficulty in swallowing, hypotonia, generalized weakness, and respiratory insufficiency. The disease may be mild or severe.

wound b. Botulism acquired when spores of the bacteria contaminate an anaerobic wound, germinate, and produce the neurotoxin.

Bouchard's nodes Bony enlargements or nodules, located at the proximal interphalangeal joints, that result from osteoarthritis or degenerative joint disease.

Bouchut's respiration (boo-shooz′) [Jean A. E. Bouchut, Fr. physician, 1818–1891] Respiration in which expiration is longer than inspiration, as seen in children with bronchopneumonia and asthma.

Bouchut's tubes [Jean Antoine E. Bouchut, French physician, 1818–1891] A set of tubes used for intubation of the larynx.

bougie (boo'zhē) [Fr. *bougie,* candle] A slender, flexible instrument for exploring and dilating tubal organs, esp. the male urethra.

bouillon (boo-, bool-yŏn') [Fr.] A clear broth made from meat. It may be used as a culture medium for bacteria.

Bouin's fluid (boo-ăns') [Paul Bouin, Fr. anatomist, 1870–1962] A fixative for embryological and histological tissue. It consists of formaldehyde, glacial acetic acid, trinitrophenol (picric acid), and water.

bound **1.** In chemistry, the holding in combination of one molecule by another. SEE: *bind* (2). **2.** Contained, not free.

bouquet (boo-kā') [Fr., nosegay] A cluster or bunch of structures, esp. blood vessels.

Bourdon gauge A low-pressure flow metering device.

boutonnière (boo-tŏn-yār') [Fr., buttonhole] **1.** Incision through the perineum behind an impervious stricture. **2.** A surgically produced buttonhole-like opening in a membrane.

boutonnière deformity Contracture of hand musculature marked by proximal interphalangeal joint flexion and distal interphalangeal joint hyperextension.

boutons terminaux (boo-tŏn' tĕr-mĭ-nō') [Fr., terminal buttons] The bulblike expansions at the tips of axons that come into synaptic contact with the cell bodies of other neurons.

bovine (bō'vīn) [L. *bovinus*] Pert. to cattle; derived from cattle.

bovine somatotropin A ABBR: BST A. A growth hormone used to increase milk production in cows.

bowel [O. Fr. *boel,* intestine] Intestine.

bowel incontinence Change in normal bowel habits characterized by involuntary passage of stool. SEE: *Nursing Diagnoses Appendix.*

bowel movement Evacuation of feces. The number of bowel movements varies in healthy individuals, some having a movement after each meal, others one in the morning and one at night, and still others only one in several days. Thus, to say that the healthy person must have at least one bowel movement a day in order to maintain health is unreasonable and not based on factual evidence. SYN: *defecation.*

CAUTION: A persistent change in bowel habits should be investigated thoroughly because it may be a sign of a malignant growth in the gastrointestinal tract.

PATIENT CARE: A history is obtained of the patient's usual bowel habits, and any change is documented. The patient is questioned and the stool is inspected for color, shape, odor, consistency, and other characteristics, as well as the presence of any unusual coatings or contents (mucus, blood, fat, parasites). Privacy is provided for the patient when he or she is using a bed pan, toilet, or bedside commode. The area should be ventilated or a deodorant spray used after the bowel movement to limit the patient's embarrassment and to reduce the discomfort of others sharing the area. The patient is taught the use of diet and activity to help prevent constipation, and the rationale for testing the stool for occult blood, if this is required, is explained.

bowel sounds The normal sounds associated with movement of the intestinal contents through the lower alimentary tract. Auscultation of the abdomen for bowel sounds may provide valuable diagnostic information. Absent or diminished sounds may indicate paralytic ileus or peritonitis. High-pitched tinkling sounds are associated with intestinal obstruction.

bowel training A program for assisting adult patients to reestablish regular bowel habits. Patients with chronic constipation, colostomies, or spinal cord injuries affecting the muscles involved in defecation may benefit from bowel training. Assessments include determining the etiology and duration of the bowel problem (e.g., a patient complaining of chronic constipation also should be queried regarding the usual normal pattern and the use of enemas, suppositories, or laxatives to promote bowel evacuation). Interventions include dietary changes, supervised training to elicit evacuation at convenient times, biofeedback, and psychotherapy.

PATIENT CARE: The patient is encouraged to increase the dietary intake of fresh fruits and vegetables and whole grains, and to drink 3000 ml of fluid each day. The need to heed normal evacuatory urges is emphasized. Use of laxatives is discouraged, and the actions of stool softeners are explained. The advantages of generating evacuation 30 min after meals to enlist normal peristaltic action are communicated to the patient. Digital anal stimulation or insertion of suppository, if indicated, is demonstrated.

bowleg (bō'lĕg) A bending outward of the leg. SYN: *bandy leg; genu varum.*

Bowman's capsule (bō'măns) [Sir William Bowman, Brit. physician, 1816–1892] Part of the renal corpuscle. It consists of a visceral layer closely applied to the glomerulus and an outer parietal layer. It is a filter in the formation of urine. SEE: *kidney* for illus.

Bowman's glands The olfactory glands, or branched tubuloalveolar glands located in the lamina propria of the olfactory membrane. Mucus from these glands keeps the olfactory surface moist.

Bowman's membrane The thin homogeneous membrane separating the corneal epithelium from the corneal substance. SYN: *anterior elastic lamina*.

boxing In dentistry, the building up of vertical walls, usually in wax, around an impression to produce the desired size and form of the base of the cast and to preserve certain landmarks of the impression.

box-note In emphysema, a hollow sound heard on percussion.

Boyden chamber A chamber used to measure chemotaxis. Cells are placed on one side of a membrane and chemotactic material on the other. The number of cells migrating to the filter quantitates the chemotactic effect.

Boyer's bursa (bwă-yāz') [Baron Alexis de Boyer, Fr. surgeon, 1757–1833] A bursa anterior to the thyrohyoid membrane.

Boyer's cyst A painless and gradual enlargement of the subhyoid bursa.

Boyle's law [Robert Boyle, Brit. physicist, 1627–1691] A law stating that at a constant temperature, the volume of a gas varies inversely with the pressure. SEE: *Charles' law; Gay-Lussac's law*.

Bozeman-Fritsch catheter (bōz'măn-frĭtch) [Nathan Bozeman, U.S. surgeon, 1825–1905; Heinrich Fritsch, Ger. gynecologist, 1844–1915] A double-lumen uterine catheter with several openings at the tip.

B.P. *blood pressure; British Pharmacopoeia.*

b.p. *boiling point.*

BPD *biparietal diameter; bronchopulmonary dysplasia.*

BPH *benign prostatic hypertrophy.*

Bq *becquerel.*

Br **1.** Symbol for the element bromine. **2.** *Brucella.*

brace (brās) *pl.* **braces 1.** Any of a variety of devices used in orthopedics for holding joints or limbs in place. **2.** A colloquial term for temporary dental prostheses used to align or reposition teeth.

brachi- SEE: *brachio-*.

brachial (brā'kē-ăl) [L. *brachialis*] Pert. to the arm.

brachial artery The main artery of the arm; a continuation of the axillary artery on the inside of the arm. SEE: illus.

brachialgia (brā"kē-ăl'jē-ă) [L. *brachialis,* brachial, + Gr. *algos,* pain] Intense pain in the arm.

brachialis (brā"kē-ăl'ĭs) [L. *brachialis,* brachial] A muscle of the arm lying immediately under the biceps brachii.

brachial plexus A network of the last four cervical and the first thoracic spinal nerves supplying the arm, forearm, and hand.

brachial veins The veins that accompany the brachial artery.

brachio-, brachi- [L. *bracchium,* arm] Combining form meaning *arm.*

brachiocephalic (brā"kē-ō-sĕ-făl'ĭk) [L. *brachium,* arm, + Gr. *kephale,* head] Pert. to the arm and head.

brachiocrural (brā"kē-ō-kroo'răl) [" + *cruralis,* pert. to the leg] Pert. to the arm and thigh.

brachiocubital (brā"kē-ō-kū'bĭ-tăl) [" + *cubitus,* forearm] Pert. to the arm and forearm.

brachiocyllosis (brā"kē-ō-sĭl-ō'sĭs) [" + Gr. *kyllosis,* a crooking] Abnormal curvature of the arm.

brachioradialis (brā"kē-ō-rā"dē-ă'lĭs) [" + *radialis,* radius] A muscle lying on the lateral side of the forearm.

brachium (brā'kē-ŭm) *pl.* **brachia** [L., arm, from Gr. *brakhion,* shorter, hence "upper arm" as opposed to longer forearm] **1.** The upper arm from shoulder to elbow. **2.** Anatomical structure resembling an arm.

b. conjunctivum Superior cerebellar peduncle.

b. pontis Middle cerebellar peduncle.

brachy- [Gr. *brachys,* short] Combining form meaning *short.*

brachybasia (brăk-ē-bā'sē-ă) [" + *basis,* walking] A slow, shuffling gait seen in partial paraplegia.

brachycardia (brăk-ē-kăr'dē-ă) [" + *kardia,* heart] Bradycardia.

brachycephalic, brachycephalous (brăk"ē-sĕ-făl'ĭk, -sĕf'ă-lŭs) [" + *kephale,* head] Having a cephalic index of 81.0 to 85.4. This is considered a short head but not necessarily abnormal, as this index falls within the standard range of variation among humans.

brachycheilia (brăk"ē-kī'lē-ă) [" + *cheilos,* lip] Abnormal shortness of the lips.

brachydactylia (brăk"ē-dăk-tĭl'ē-ă) [" + *daktylos,* finger] Abnormal shortness of the fingers and toes.

brachygnathia (brăk-ĭg-nā'thē-ă) [" + *gnathos,* jaw] Abnormal shortness of the lower jaw.

brachymorphic (brăk"ē-mor'fĭk) [" + *morphe,* form] Shorter and broader than usual, with reference to body type.

brachyphalangia (brăk"ē-fă-lăn'jē-ă) [" + *phalanx,* closely knit row] Shortness of a bone or bones of a finger or toe.

brachytherapy (brăk"ē-thĕr'ă-pē) [" + *therapeia,* treatment] In radiation therapy, the use of implants of radioactive materials such as radium, cesium, iridium, or gold at the treatment site (e.g., an internal organ with a malignant lesion).

CAUTION: The treated patient can emit radiation and can endanger others. If the radiation source is dislodged, it is removed by a radiation safety officer using special long-handled tongs and is placed in a lead container. All linens and dressings are considered contaminated. Pregnant women and children younger than 16 should not visit the patient.

bracket A support of wood, metal, or some durable material. In dentistry, a variety of specific brackets used in orthodontic appliances.

Braden scale A commonly used assessment tool that quantifies the degree to which a person is at risk for developing a pressure ulcer. Each assessment parameter is measured on a scale from a low of 1 to a high of 4, including the individual's sensory perception, moisture,

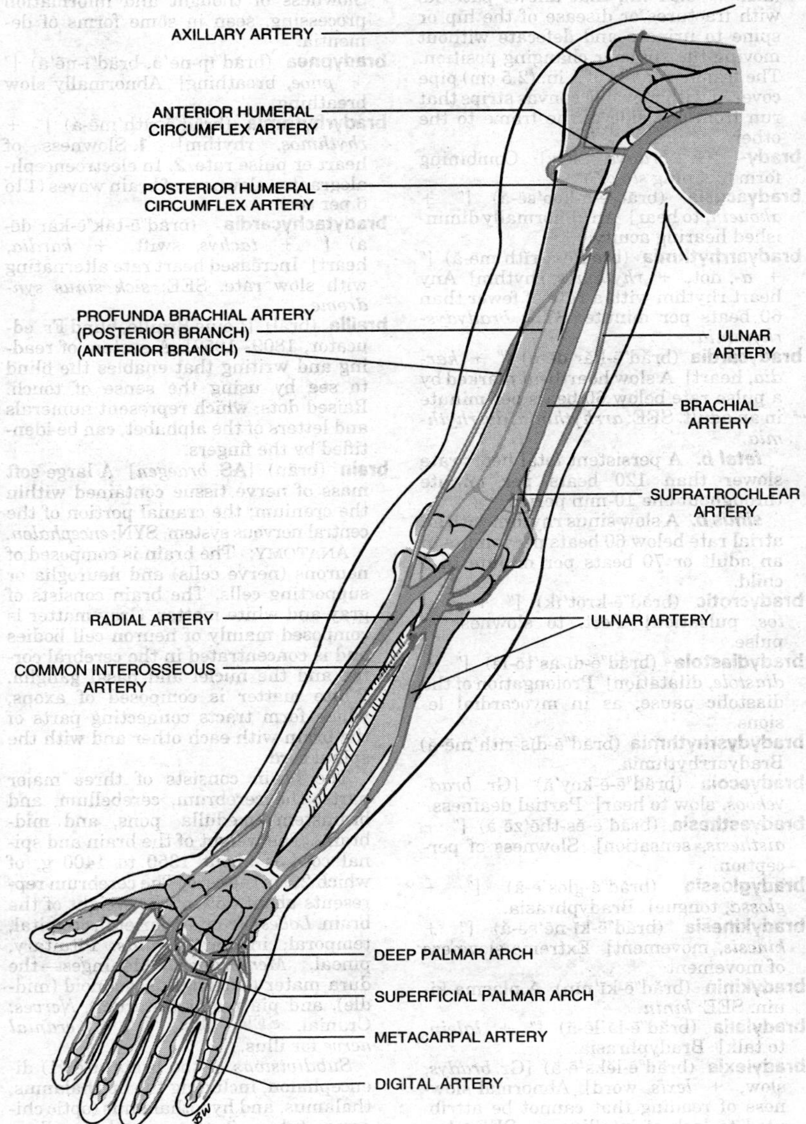

RIGHT ANTERIOR ARM

BRACHIAL ARTERY

activity, mobility, nutrition, and friction and shear. The lower the number, the higher the risk for pressure ulcer development. Individuals are at risk for developing pressure ulcers if the total score is less than 17.

Bradford frame [Edward H. Bradford, U.S. orthopedic surgeon, 1848–1926] An oblong frame, about 7 × 3 ft (2.13 × 0.91 m), that allows patients with fractures or disease of the hip or spine to urinate and defecate without moving the spine or changing position. The frame is made of 1 in. (2.5 cm) pipe covered with movable canvas strips that run from one side of the frame to the other.

brady- [Gr. *bradys,* slow] Combining form meaning *slow.*

bradyacusia (brăd″ē-ă-koo′sē-ă) [″ + *akouein,* to hear] An abnormally diminished hearing acuity.

bradyarrhythmia (brăd″ē-ă-rĭth′mē-ă) [″ + *a-,* not, + *rhythmos,* rhythm] Any heart rhythm with a rate of fewer than 60 beats per minute. SYN: *bradydysrhythmia.*

bradycardia (brăd″ē-kăr′dē-ă) [″ + *kardia,* heart] A slow heartbeat marked by a pulse rate below 60 beats per minute in an adult. SEE: *arrhythmia; dysrhythmia.*

fetal b. A persistent fetal heart rate slower than 120 beats per minute throughout one 10-min period.

sinus b. A slow sinus rhythm with an atrial rate below 60 beats per minute in an adult or 70 beats per minute in a child.

bradycrotic (brăd″ē-krŏt′ĭk) [″ + *krotos,* pulsation] Pert. to slowness of pulse.

bradydiastole (brăd″ē-dī-ăs′tō-lē) [″ + *diastole,* dilatation] Prolongation of the diastolic pause, as in myocardial lesions.

bradydysrhythmia (brăd″ē-dĭs-rĭth′mē-ă) Bradyarrhythmia.

bradyecoia (brăd″ē-ē-koy′ă) [Gr. *bradyekoos,* slow to hear] Partial deafness.

bradyesthesia (brăd″ē-ĕs-thē′zē-ă) [″ + *aisthesis,* sensation] Slowness of perception.

bradyglossia (brăd″ē-glŏs′ē-ă) [″ + *glossa,* tongue] Bradyphrasia.

bradykinesia (brăd″ē-kĭ-nē′sē-ă) [″ + *kinesis,* movement] Extreme slowness of movement.

bradykinin (brăd″ē-kī′nĭn) A plasma kinin. SEE: *kinin.*

bradylalia (brăd″ē-lā′lē-ă) [″ + *lalein,* to talk] Bradyphrasia.

bradylexia (brăd″ē-lĕks′ē-ă) [Gr. *bradys,* slow, + *lexis,* word] Abnormal slowness of reading that cannot be attributed to lack of intelligence. SEE: *dyslexia.*

bradylogia (brăd″ē-lō′jē-ă) [″ + *logos,* word, reason] Slow speech due to mental impairment.

bradyphagia (brăd″ē-fā′jē-ă) [″ + *phagein,* to eat] Abnormal slowness in eating.

bradyphrasia (brăd″ē-frā′zē-ă) [″ + *phrasis,* utterance] Slowness of speech; seen in some types of mental disease. SYN: *bradyglossia; bradylalia.* SEE: *speech.*

bradyphrenia [″ + Gr. *phren,* mind] Slowness of thought and information processing, seen in some forms of dementia.

bradypnea (brăd″ĭp-nē′ă, brăd″ĭ-nē′ă) [″ + *pnoe,* breathing] Abnormally slow breathing.

bradyrhythmia (brăd″ē-rĭth′mē-ă) [″ + *rhythmos,* rhythm] **1.** Slowness of heart or pulse rate. **2.** In electroencephalography, slowness of brain waves (1 to 6 per sec).

bradytachycardia (brăd″ē-tăk″ē-kăr′dē-ă) [″ + *tachys,* swift, + *kardia,* heart] Increased heart rate alternating with slow rate. SEE: *sick sinus syndrome.*

braille (brāl) [Louis Braille, blind Fr. educator, 1809–1852] A system of reading and writing that enables the blind to see by using the sense of touch. Raised dots, which represent numerals and letters of the alphabet, can be identified by the fingers.

brain (brān) [AS. *braegen*] A large soft mass of nerve tissue contained within the cranium; the cranial portion of the central nervous system. SYN: *encephalon.*

ANATOMY: The brain is composed of neurons (nerve cells) and neuroglia or supporting cells. The brain consists of gray and white matter. Gray matter is composed mainly of neuron cell bodies and is concentrated in the cerebral cortex and the nuclei and basal ganglia. White matter is composed of axons, which form tracts connecting parts of the brain with each other and with the spinal cord.

The brain consists of three major parts: the cerebrum, cerebellum, and brainstem (medulla, pons, and midbrain). The weight of the brain and spinal cord is about 1350 to 1400 g, of which 2% is the cord. The cerebrum represents about 85% of the weight of the brain. *Lobes:* Frontal, parietal, occipital, temporal, insular. *Glands:* Pituitary, pineal. *Membranes:* Meninges—the dura mater (external), arachnoid (middle), and pia mater (internal). *Nerves:* Cranial. SEE: illus. (Brain); *cranial nerve* for illus.

Subdivisions of the brain are (1) diencephalon, including the epithalamus, thalamus, and hypothalamus (optic chiasma, tuber cinereum, and maxillary bodies); (2) myelencephalon, including the corpora quadrigemina, tegmentum, crura cerebri, and the medulla oblongata; (3) metencephalon, including the cerebellum and pons; (4) telencephalon, including the rhinencephalon, corpora striata, and cerebrum (cerebral cortex).

Ventricles: The cavities of the brain are the first and second lateral ventricles, which lie in the cerebral hemispheres, the third ventricle of the diencephalon, and the fourth ventricle posterior to the medulla and pons. The first and second communicate with the third by the interventricular foramina, the third with the fourth by the cerebral aqueduct (of Sylvius), the fourth with the subarachnoid spaces by the two foramina of Luschka and the foramen of Magendie. The ventricles are filled with cerebrospinal fluid, which is formed by the choroid plexuses in the walls and roofs of the ventricles. SEE: illus. (Vascular Anatomy of Brain).

PHYSIOLOGY: The brain is the primary center for regulating and coordinating body activities. Sensory impulses are received through afferent nerves and register as sensations, the basis for perception. It is the seat of consciousness, thought, memory, reason, judgment, and emotion. Motor impulses are discharged through efferent nerves to muscles and glands initiating activities. Through reflex centers automatic control of body activities is maintained. The most important reflex centers are the cardiac, vasomotor, and respiratory centers, which regulate circulation and respiration. SEE: *central nervous system; spinal cord.*

brain attack A term proposed by the National Stroke Association to describe the sudden loss of neurological function that constitutes a stroke. The term was designed to be similar to “heart attack” to convey the emergent nature of strokes and the need for affected patients to seek care immediately, when treatments may do the most good in improving outcomes.

brain fever Meningitis.

brain graft An experimental technique in which brain cells are transplanted into the brain.

Brain's reflex [Walter Russell Brain, Brit. physician, 1895–1966] Extension of the flexed arm when the quadrupedal posture is assumed.

brain scan The use of radioactive isotopes injected into the circulation to detect abnormalities in the structure and function of the brain.

brainstem The stemlike part of the brain that connects the cerebral hemispheres with the spinal cord. It comprises the medulla oblongata, the pons, and the midbrain. SEE: illus.

brainstem auditory evoked potential ABBR: BAEP. The study of brain (ECG) waves during sound stimuli. It is used to determine the threshold of sound required to produce a brainstem response. This provides an objective measure of hearing acuity. SEE: *auditory evoked response; evoked response; somatosensory evoked response; visual evoked response*.

brain swelling Brain edema.

brainwashing Intense psychological indoctrination for the purpose of displacing the individual's previous thoughts

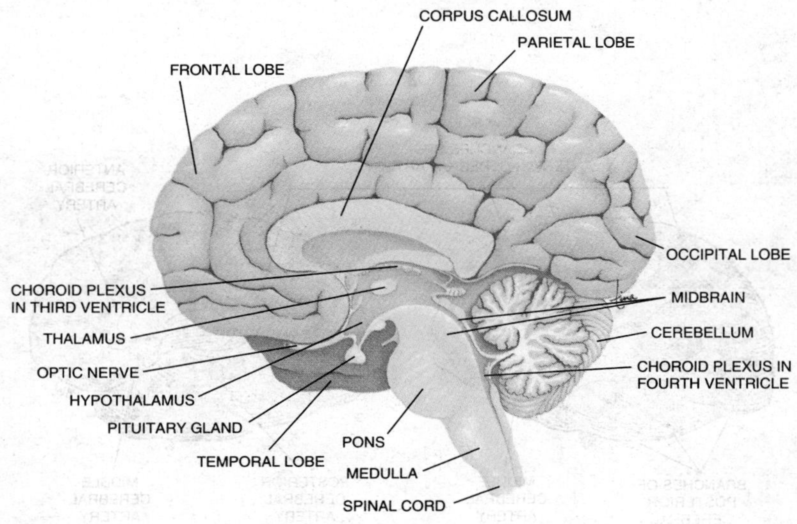

BRAIN

Midsagittal section of brain as seen from left

and attitudes with those selected by the regime or person inflicting the indoctrination.

bran The outer covering of cereal grains, such as wheat, oats, and rice, which are rich in hemicellulose. Some of this fiber is insoluble and may be used to add bulk to the diet to help prevent or treat constipation. SEE: *dietary fiber*.

branch In anatomy, a subdivision arising from a main or larger portion, esp. of an artery, vein, nerve, or lymphatic vessel.

branchial (brăng′kē-ăl) [L. *branchia*, gills] Pert. to or resembling gills of a fish or a homologous structure in higher animals.

branchiogenic, branchiogenous (brăng″kē-ō-jĕn′ĭk, brăng″kē-ŏj′ĕ-nŭs) [L.

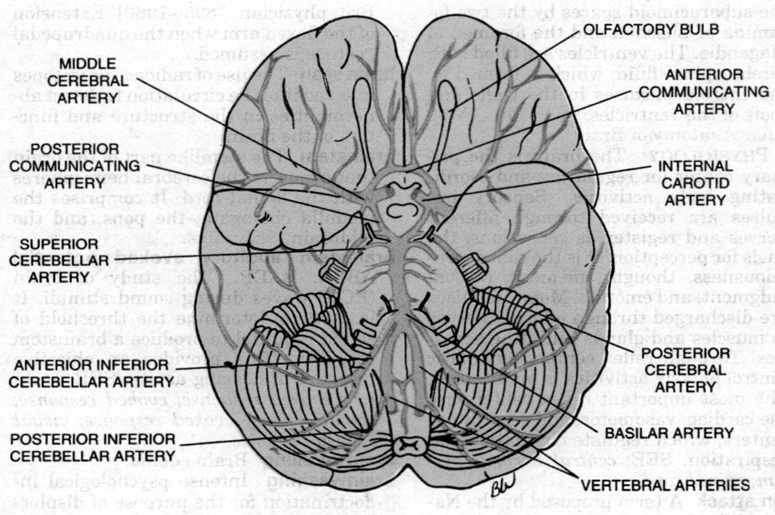

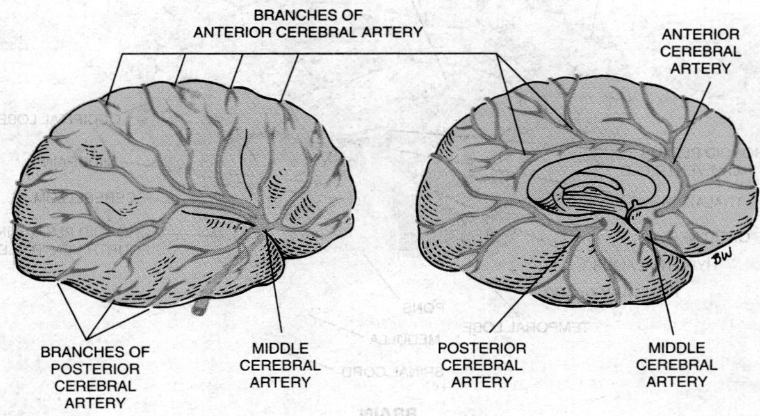

VASCULAR ANATOMY OF BRAIN

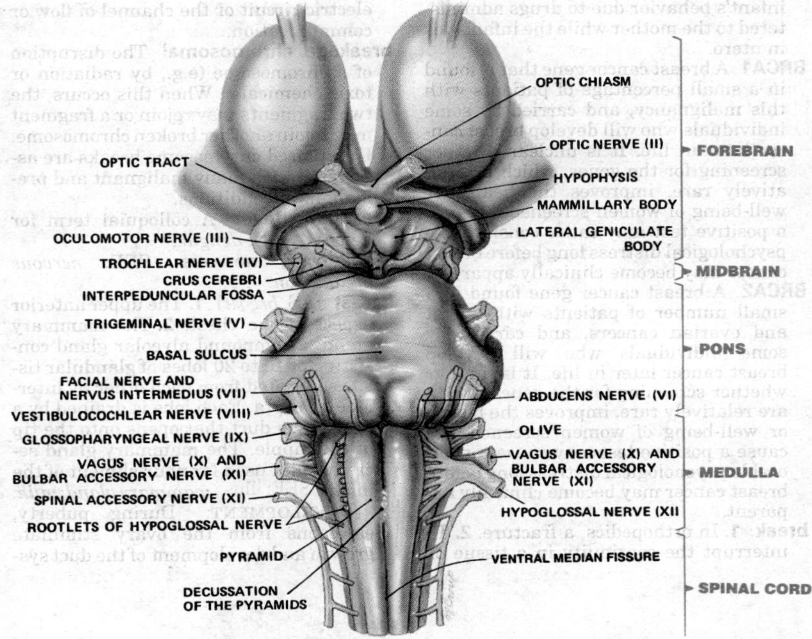

BRAINSTEM

Ventral surface of the brainstem and surrounding structures

branchia, gills, + Gr. *gennan,* to produce] Having origin in a branchial cleft.

branchioma (brăng″kē-ō′mă) [″ + Gr. *oma,* tumor] A tumor derived from the branchial epithelium.

branchiomeric (brăng″kē-ō-mĕr′ĭk) [″ + Gr. *meros,* part] Pert. to the branchial arches.

Brandt-Andrews maneuver A technique for expressing the placenta from the uterus during the third stage of labor. One hand puts gentle traction on the cord while the other presses the anterior surface of the uterus backward. SEE: *Credé's method.*

Branham's sign (brăn′hămz sīn) In a patient with an arteriovenous fistula, the slowing of the heart rate that occurs when the fistula is compressed.

brash A burning sensation in the stomach sometimes accompanied by belching of sour fluid. SYN: *heartburn; pyrosis.*

water b. Reflex salivary hypersecretion in response to peptic esophagitis.

brass chills SEE: *metal fume fever.*

brass poisoning Poisoning due to the inhalation of fumes of zinc and zinc oxide, causing destruction of tissue in the respiratory passage. It is rarely fatal. Symptoms include dryness and burning in respiratory tract, coughing, headache, and chills.

CAUTION: Call the nearest poison control center to determine proper therapy.

brawny induration Pathological hardening and thickening of tissues, usually due to inflammation.

Braxton Hicks contractions [John Braxton Hicks, Brit. gynecologist, 1823–1897] Intermittent painless uterine contractions that may occur every 10 to 20 min. They occur after the third month of pregnancy. These contractions are not true labor pains but are often interpreted as such. They are not present in every pregnancy. SYN: *Hicks sign.*

Brazelton Neonatal Assessment Scale [T. Berry Brazelton, American pediatrician, b. 1918] A scale for evaluating the behavior and responses of the newborn infant. It is based on four dimensions: interaction with the environment; motor processes, including motor responses, general activity level, and reflexes; control of physiological state as determined by reaction to a distinct stimulus such as a rattle, bell, light, or a pinprick; and response to stress as judged by tremulousness, startle reaction, and change in skin coloration. The test has been used as late as 1 week after birth to demonstrate alteration in an infant's behavior due to drugs administered to the mother while the infant was in utero.

BRCA1 A breast cancer gene that is found in a small percentage of patients with this malignancy, and carried by some individuals who will develop breast cancer later in life. It is unclear whether screening for the genes, which are relatively rare, improves the health or well-being of women screened, because a positive test may cause considerable psychological distress long before breast cancer may become clinically apparent.

BRCA2 A breast cancer gene found in a small number of patients with breast and ovarian cancers, and carried by some individuals who will develop breast cancer later in life. It is unclear whether screening for the genes, which are relatively rare, improves the health or well-being of women screened, because a positive test may cause considerable psychological distress long before breast cancer may become clinically apparent.

break **1.** In orthopedics, a fracture. **2.** To interrupt the continuity in a tissue or electric circuit or the channel of flow or communication.

breakage, chromosomal The disruption of a chromosome (e.g., by radiation or toxic chemicals). When this occurs, the two fragments may rejoin or a fragment may rejoin another broken chromosome. Unrepaired chromosome breaks are associated with many malignant and premalignant conditions.

breakbone fever A colloquial term for dengue. SYN: *dengue*.

breakdown, nervous SEE: *nervous breakdown*.

breast [AS. *breost*] **1.** The upper anterior aspect of the chest. **2.** The mammary gland, a compound alveolar gland consisting of 15 to 20 lobes of glandular tissue separated from each other by interlobular septa. Each lobe is drained by a lactiferous duct that opens onto the tip of the nipple. The mammary gland secretes milk used for nourishment of the infant. SEE: illus.; *mammary gland; milk*.

DEVELOPMENT: During puberty, estrogens from the ovary stimulate growth and development of the duct sys-

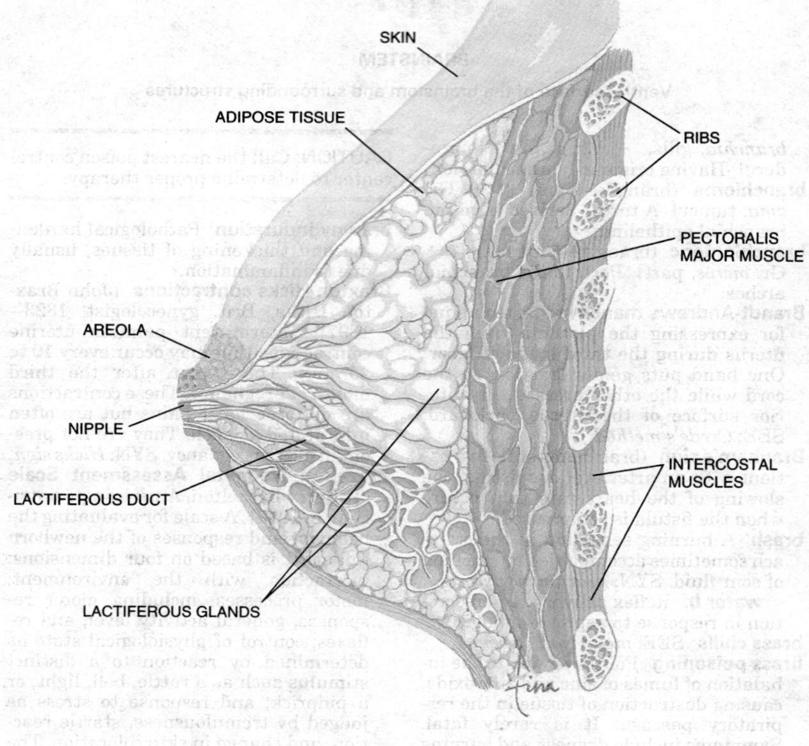

BREAST
Mammary gland in midsagittal section

tem. During pregnancy, progesterone secreted by the corpus luteum and placenta acts synergistically with estrogens to bring the alveoli to complete development. Following parturition, prolactin in conjunction with adrenal steroids initiates lactation, and oxytocin from the posterior pituitary induces ejection of milk. Sucking or milking reflexly stimulates both milk secretion and discharge of milk.

CHANGES IN PREGNANCY: During the first 6 to 12 weeks, there is fullness and tenderness, erectile tissue develop in the nipples, nodules are felt, pigment is deposited around the nipple (primary areola) (in blondes the areolae and nipples become darker pink and in brunettes they become dark brown and in some cases even black), and a few drops of fluid may be squeezed out. During the next 16 to 20 weeks, the secondary areola shows small whitish spots in pigmentation due to hypertrophy of the sebaceous glands (glands of Montgomery).

chicken b. A deformity in which the sternum projects anteriorly; caused by rickets or obstructed respiration in childhood. SYN: *pigeon b.*

ductal carcinoma in situ of the b. ABBR: DCIS. A cluster of malignant cells in the mammary ducts. If left untreated, as many as 50% of patients with DCIS will develop invasive cancer. Because these cells grow in the ducts they develop without forming a palpable mass. In their early stage they are diagnosed through the use of mammography. SEE: *breast cancer; mammography.*

pigeon b. Chicken b.

b. self-examination ABBR: BSE. A technique that enables a woman to detect changes in her breasts. The accompanying illustration explains the specific steps to be followed. The examination should be done each month soon after the menstrual period ends, as normal physiological changes that may confuse results occur in the premenstrual period. This method of self-examination is useful in the early detection of breast cancer, esp. when combined with regular professional examinations and mammography. SEE: illus.; *mammography.*

breast cancer A malignant neoplasm (usually an adenocarcinoma) of the breast; the most common malignancy of American women and the leading cause of death in American women aged 40 to 55. In their lifetimes, American women have a 12% incidence of breast cancer, but more than two thirds of women affected by it are now cured. Breast cancer usually presents as a dominant mass in one breast, although it may first become evident when nipple discharge, nipple retraction, skin dimpling, or asymmetric swelling of the breast occurs. In most cases, breast cancers are first identified by women performing breast self-examination. A smaller but considerable number are detected by professional examination or mammography. About 1000 men are diagnosed with breast cancer annually. Breast cancer has several pathological variants. Ductal carcinoma in situ, the most localized form of the disease, represents a preinvasive stage of breast cancer that will spread if left untreated. Other presentations include lobular carcinoma, infiltrating ductal carcinoma, inflammatory carcinoma, and Paget's disease of the nipple. SEE: illus.

ETIOLOGY: There are several known risk factors for breast cancer. The relationship between risk of breast cancer and a high-fat diet is not well-established. SEE: table.

SYMPTOMS: A dominant breast mass; bloody, brown, or serous discharge from a nipple; and/or breast nodularity or lumpiness are the most common symptoms of breast cancer.

DIAGNOSIS: Regular breast self-examination, professional breast examination, and mammography are the keys to screening for breast cancer. All these screenings identify many more benign lesions than malignant ones, esp. in younger patients, and none of these techniques can definitively exclude breast cancer. More than 70% of mammographically detected lesions, for example, are benign, and about 15% of the time mammography will fail to detect lesions that are truly malignant. If a suspicious mass is identified, fine needle aspiration, core biopsy, or excisional biopsy must be used to obtain tissue for analysis. Ultrasonography can be used before biopsy to identify solid masses and cysts. Solid masses have a much greater chance of being malignant than cysts. SEE: *breast self-examination; double reading; mammography.*

STAGING: The size of tumors and their possible metastasis to the chest wall, skin, axilla, or distant sites all determine the stage of breast cancer. Lymphatic mapping during cancer surgery can be used to find metastases to sentinel lymph nodes and guide therapies. Staging provides important information about the need for particular forms of therapy and the prognosis.

CAUTION: A biopsy is usually recommended for any breast mass that does not resolve spontaneously within one or two menstrual cycles. Negative results from mammography and ultrasonography are not always accurate enough to rule out a malignant diagnosis.

TREATMENT: Combined modalities (including surgery, radiation, or drug therapies) are offered to many women with breast cancer, depending on their menopausal status and the stage of their disease at the time of diagnosis. Patients with stage I or II disease are offered either modified radical mastectomy or lumpectomy with axillary dissection and radiotherapy, provided they have no contraindications to either of these choices. In premenopausal women with tumors larger than a centimeter, adjuvant chemotherapy prolongs survival, probably by eliminating microscopic metastases. Chemotherapeutic regimens commonly used include CMF (cyclophosphamide, methotrexate, and fluorouracil) or CA (cyclophosphamide and doxorubicin [Adriamycin]). These same regimens are offered to vigorous postmenopausal women whose cancer has spread to axillary lymph nodes. Hormonal therapies like tamoxifen are also beneficial, esp. in patients with estrogen-receptor positive tumors and in

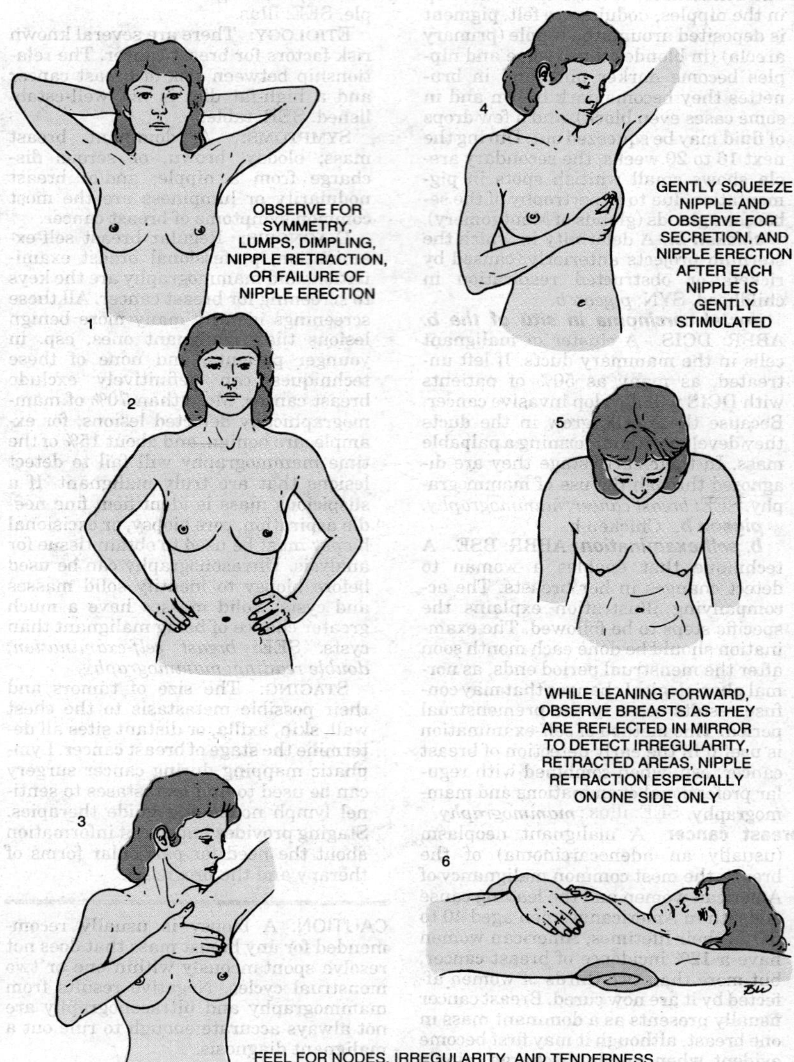
1
OBSERVE FOR SYMMETRY, LUMPS, DIMPLING, NIPPLE RETRACTION, OR FAILURE OF NIPPLE ERECTION
2
3
4
GENTLY SQUEEZE NIPPLE AND OBSERVE FOR SECRETION, AND NIPPLE ERECTION AFTER EACH NIPPLE IS GENTLY STIMULATED
5
WHILE LEANING FORWARD, OBSERVE BREASTS AS THEY ARE REFLECTED IN MIRROR TO DETECT IRREGULARITY, RETRACTED AREAS, NIPPLE RETRACTION ESPECIALLY ON ONE SIDE ONLY
6
FEEL FOR NODES, IRREGULARITY, AND TENDERNESS BOTH IN BREASTS AND AXILLARY AREAS

BREAST SELF EXAMINATION

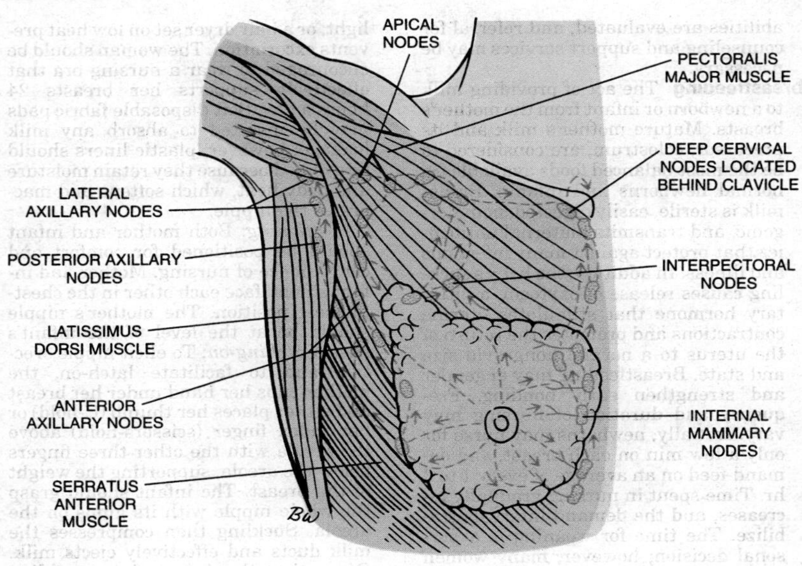

BREAST CANCER

Possible paths of lymphatic spread

older women who may not tolerate intensive chemotherapeutic regimens. After breast surgery, some women choose to have cosmetic restoration of the breast, either with implants or with tissue reconstructions made from the abdominal muscles. If breast cancer recurs after treatment, very high-dose chemotherapies and peripheral stem cell transplantation are occasionally considered, although their value is as yet unproven. SEE: *breast, ductal carcinoma in situ of*.

Risk Factors for Breast Cancer

- A personal history of breast cancer
- Age (the risk increases with age)
- Family history of breast cancer (in a mother, sister, daughter, or two or more close relatives, such as cousins)
- Age at first live birth (women who had their first child after age 30 and women who have never given birth are at higher risk)
- Age at first menstrual period (women who had their first period before age 12 are at slightly higher risk)
- Benign breast changes (atypical hyperplasia) or two or more breast biopsies even if no atypical cells were found
- Race (white women are more likely to develop breast cancer than black women, but blacks are more likely than whites to die of it; Hispanic and Asian women have a lower risk of developing the disease)

SOURCE: National Cancer Institute, National Institutes of Health

PATIENT CARE: The patient's feelings and level of knowledge about her disease are determined. She is encouraged to express fears and concerns, and her family, supporters, or health care professionals stay with her during periods of anxiety or anguish. If surgery is planned, the procedure, postoperative care, and expected outcomes are explained.

Prescribed chemotherapy is administered, and the patient is monitored for adverse reactions, such as nausea, vomiting, anorexia, stomatitis, GI ulceration, leukopenia, thrombocytopenia, and bleeding, so that they can be managed early. Weight and nutrition status are evaluated. Skin is inspected for redness, irritation, or breakdown if radiation therapy is prescribed. Prescribed analgesics are administered, and noninvasive nursing measures to relieve pain are instituted and taught to the patient. Comfort measures are used to promote relaxation and rest and to relieve anxiety. If immobility develops late in the disease, careful repositioning, excellent skin care, respiratory toilet, and low-pressure mattresses are used to prevent complications (skin breakdown, respiratory problems, pathological fractures). The patient's and family's coping abilities are evaluated, and referral for counseling and support services may be necessary.

breastfeeding The act of providing milk to a newborn or infant from the mother's breasts. Mature mother's milk and its precursor, colostrum, are considered to be the most balanced foods available for normal newborns and infants. Breast milk is sterile, easily digested, nonallergenic, and transmits maternal antibodies that protect against many infections and illness. In addition, the baby's suckling causes release of oxytocin, a pituitary hormone that stimulates uterine contractions and promotes the return of the uterus to a normal nongravid size and state. Breastfeeding may engender and strengthen early bonding. Frequency and duration of nursing may vary. Initially, newborns may nurse for only a few min on each breast, and demand-feed on an average of every 1 to 3 hr. Time spent in nursing gradually increases, and the demand intervals stabilize. The time for weaning is a personal decision; however, many women choose to breastfeed until solid foods are introduced and well-accepted by the infant.

PATIENT CARE: *Prenatal preparations*: During the last trimester of pregnancy, techniques that increase the potential for successful breastfeeding are discussed with women who have selected that infant-feeding option. Lactation consultants commonly encourage nipple-rolling. The woman is instructed to cup her breast in one hand, supporting the weight with three fingers while grasping the nipple with the thumb and forefinger, and gently rolling it between the two fingers. She should implement ten to 20 repetitions of these actions several times daily. Precoital suckling by the woman's partner also helps in preparing the nipples for breastfeeding. Nipple shields are recommended for women whose nipples are either flat or inverted. Women who are at high-risk for preterm labor are discouraged from engaging in prenatal nipple stimulation.

Postpartum breastfeeding: A successful breastfeeding experience is potentiated by assisting the woman to develop confidence, comfort, and skill in using techniques for appropriate infant latch-on, feeding, and disengagement. Basic breast care is described, discussed, and demonstrated to minimize the potential for discomforts that interfere with successful breastfeeding, such as nipple soreness. Washing the breasts and nipples with clear water and avoiding the use of soap, which removes the natural breast lubricants that protect the nipples against drying and cracking, are recommended. Drying the nipples thoroughly by exposing them to air, sunlight, or a hair dryer set on low heat prevents excoriation. The woman should be encouraged to wear a nursing bra that effectively supports her breasts 24 hours a day. Soft disposable fabric pads may be inserted to absorb any milk leakage; however, plastic liners should be avoided because they retain moisture and body heat, which softens and macerates the nipple.

Positioning: Both mother and infant should be positioned for comfort and convenience of nursing. Mother and infant should face each other in the chest-to-chest position. The mother's nipple should be at the level of the infant's nose. *Latching-on*: To elicit nipple erection and to facilitate latch-on, the mother cups her hand under her breast and either places her thumb (C-hold) or her index finger (scissors-hold) above the areola with the other three fingers below the areola, supporting the weight of the breast. The infant should grasp the whole nipple with its gums on the areola. Suckling then compresses the milk ducts and effectively ejects milk. Preventing the infant from suckling only on the end of the nipple reduces potential for nipple soreness, erosion, and cracking. *Feeding*: Infants should be allowed to feed until they exhibit signs of satisfaction. Feeding from a single breast is allowable as long as the infant nurses approximately every 2 hours and feeds until satisfied; this encourages the intake of the higher calorie, high fat hind milk. *Disengaging*: The mother should gently insert her fingers between the infant's gums to break the suction and withdraw the breast from the baby's mouth. *Engorgement*: Feeding the newborn on demand usually prevents the development of engorgement. Should it occur, the mother either may apply warm wet compresses or stand beneath a shower of warm water to stimulate the let-down reflex and manually express enough milk to relieve the pressure and soften the areola to encourage latch-on when feeding.

Nipple soreness: Some discomfort is common during the first few breastfeeding days. The mother's first actions should be to check the infant's feeding position and grasp of the nipple. Altering her position for feeding also alters the stress points on the nipple as the infant suckles and enhances breast emptying. If soreness is related to the newborn's vigorous sucking because of hunger, the mother may elect to nurse more frequently. The mother is encouraged to continue with breastfeeding; however, if the suggested measures prove ineffective and discomfort persists throughout the feeding interval or does not subside by the end of the first postpartum week, the mother should seek consultation.

breastfeeding, effective The state in which the mother and infant exhibit appropriate proficiency and satisfaction with breastfeeding. Expected outcomes include maternal nipple trauma and soreness related to breastfeeding are minimized. Infant weight gain proceeds within expected parameters. SEE: *Nursing Diagnoses Appendix.*

breastfeeding, ineffective The state in which a mother, infant, or child experiences dissatisfaction or difficulty with the breastfeeding process. SEE: *Nursing Diagnoses Appendix.*

breast implant A surgical alteration in the size and/or contour of the breast or chest wall, using the patient's own adipose tissue (e.g., pedicle graft) or a prosthesis.

breastfeeding, interrupted A break in the continuity of the breastfeeding process as a result of inability or inadvisability to put a baby to breast for feeding. SEE: *Nursing Diagnoses Appendix.*

breast stimulation In pregnancy, nipple rolling or the application of heat to the breasts to elicit release of endogenous oxytocin and to generate uterine contractions. The procedure also has been used to evaluate placental sufficiency in the third trimester and to increase contractions in patients with ruptured membranes and when contractions are absent, rare, irregular, or of poor quality. SEE: *oxytocin challenge test.*

breath (brĕth) [AS. *braeth,* odor] The air inhaled and exhaled in respiration.

liver b. The characteristic odor of the breath that accompanies severe liver disease. It has been described as "mousy." SEE: *hepatic coma.*

uremic b. The "fishy" or ammoniacal breath odor characteristic of individuals with uremia.

breath-holding The voluntary or involuntary stopping of breathing may be seen in children who use this to attempt to control the behavior of their parents.

breath-holding attacks A benign condition that always has its onset with crying. The young child stops breathing and becomes cyanotic, the limbs become rigid and extended, and consciousness may be lost. This is followed by the body becoming limp, resumption of respirations and, after a few seconds, full alertness. This pattern of behavior usually disappears spontaneously prior to school age.

breathing The act of inhaling and exhaling air. SEE: *chest; respiration.*

abdominodiaphragmatic b. A controlled method of breathing in which the diaphragm is used for inspiration and the abdominal muscles for expiration; this technique improves exertional dyspnea, esp. in patients with chronic pulmonary disease. SYN: *diaphragmatic b.*

apneustic b. An abnormal breathing pattern marked by prolonged inspiratory pauses. This is usually associated with brainstem injuries.

asthmatic b. Harsh breathing with prolonged wheezing heard throughout during expiration.

ataxic b. An irregular, uncoordinated breathing pattern common in infants.

bronchial b. Harsh breath sounds with a tubular quality. It is heard when consolidated lung tissue is present.

Cheyne-Stokes b. SEE: *Cheyne-Stokes respiration.*

continuous positive-pressure b. A method of mechanically assisted pulmonary inflation. A device administers air or oxygen to the lungs under a continuous pressure that is always greater than zero. SYN: *continuous positive-pressure ventilation.*

diaphragmatic b. Abdominodiaphragmatic b.

frog b. A respiratory pattern in which the air in the mouth and pharynx is forced into the lungs by gulping and swallowing it. This may be observed in patients whose respiratory muscles are weak or paralyzed.

inspiratory resistive b. Inspiration with an added workload to increase the strength and endurance of the inspiratory muscles.

intermittent positive-pressure b. ABBR: IPPB. A mechanical method for assisting pulmonary ventilation employing a device that administers air or oxygen for the inflation of the lungs under positive pressure. Exhalation is usually passive. SYN: *intermittent positive-pressure ventilation.*

Kussmaul b. A very deep, repetitive, gasping respiratory pattern associated with profound acidosis (e.g., diabetic ketoacidosis). Kussmaul's respiration may be a sign of impending death.

periodic b. An irregular respiratory pattern marked by alternating periods of rapid and slow respirations and by apneic periods lasting 15 sec or less.

pursed-lip b. An expiratory maneuver in which the patient exhales through puckered lips to slow expiratory flow and to create slight back pressure. This action may prevent premature closure of intrapulmonary airways, esp. in the patient with chronic obstructive lung disease.

shallow b. Breathing in which the volume of inspired and expired air is diminished (e.g., $<$200 ml per breath in adults). It is common in elderly patients, patients with rib or pleural pain, or obstructive lung diseases.

vesicular b. Normal breathing.

breathing pattern, ineffective Inspiration and/or expiration that does not provide adequate ventilation. SEE: *Nursing Diagnoses Appendix.*

breathlessness dyspnea.

breath test A test that may be used to detect a specific substance in the breath to help explain metabolic changes. Breath tests are used, for example, to detect evidence of bacterial overgrowth in the intestines, to investigate the causes of malabsorption, and to detect *Helicobacter pylori* in the stomach.

carbon-urea b.t. A diagnostic test in which the patient ingests 13C-labeled or 14C-labeled urea, which binds to and can be measured in exhaled carbon dioxide. It is used to diagnose infection with *Helicobacter pylori,* a common cause of peptic ulcer. SEE: *Helicobacter pylori; peptic ulcer*.

breath test for lactase deficiency The measurement of hydrogen in the breath after ingestion of 50 g of lactase. SEE: *lactase deficiency syndrome*.

breech [AS. *brec,* buttocks] The nates, or buttocks.

bregma (brĕg′mă) *pl.* **bregmata** [Gr., front of head] The point on the skull where the coronal and sagittal sutures join. The anterior fontanel in the fetus and young infant. **bregmatic** (-măt′ĭk), *adj.*

bregmocardiac reflex (brĕg″mō-kăr′dē-ăk) [Gr. *bregma,* front of head, + *kardia,* heart] A reduced heart rate following pressure on the anterior fontanel.

Brenner's tumor [Fritz Brenner, Ger. pathologist, 1877–1969] A benign fibroepithelioma of the ovary.

bretylium tosylate (brĕ-tĭ′lē-ŭm tŏs′ĭ-lāt) An antiarrhythmic and antihypertensive drug used primarily in the management of refractory ventricular fibrillation and ventricular tachycardia.

brevicollis (brĕv″ĭ-kŏl′ĭs) [L. *brevis,* short, + *collum,* neck] Shortness of the neck.

brevilineal (brĕv-ĭ-lĭn′ē-ăl) [L. *brevis,* short, + *linea,* line] Having a body build that is shorter and broader than usual. SYN: *brachymorphic*.

bridge (brĭj) [AS. *brycg*] **1.** A narrow band of tissue. **2.** A cast dental restoration that replaces missing teeth. The restoration is usually made of gold alloy, with or without a porcelain exterior, and is attached to adjacent or abutment teeth for support. Lay persons often call such a restoration a "bridge." SYN: *fixed partial denture*.

disulfide b. disulfide bond.

b. of nose The upper part of the external nose formed by the junction of the nasal bones.

bridging (brĭj′ĭng) A treatment activity used to activate abdominal and hip extensor muscles. To bridge, a person lies in a supine position with knees flexed and feet flat against a horizontal surface, such as a floor, bed, or plinth (treatment table). The hips are then lifted, while the feet, shoulders, and head maintain contact with the surface.

bridgework (brĭj′work) A partial denture held in place by attachments other than clasps.

fixed b. A partial plate held by crowns or inlays cemented to the natural teeth.

removable b. A partial plate held by clasps that permit its removal.

bridle (brī′dl) In anatomy, a frenum.

Bright's disease [Richard Bright, Brit. physician, 1789–1858] A vague and obsolete term for kidney disease. It usually refers to nonsuppurative inflammatory or degenerative kidney disease marked by proteinuria and hematuria and sometimes by edema, hypertension, and nitrogen retention. SEE: *nephritis*.

brightness gain The increase in the intensity of a fluoroscopic image by the use of an image intensifier.

brim **1.** An edge or margin. **2.** The brim of the pelvis; the superior aperture of the lesser or true pelvis; the inlet. It is formed by the iliopectineal line of the innominate bone and the sacral promontory. It is oval-shaped in the female, heart-shaped in the male.

Briquet's syndrome [Paul Briquet, Fr. physician, 1796–1881] A personality disorder in which alcoholism and somatization disorder occur.

Brissaud's reflex (brĭs-sōz′) [Edouard Brissaud, Fr. physician, 1852–1909] Contraction of the tensor fasciae latae muscle when the sole of the foot is stroked or tickled; a component of the extensor plantar response.

British antilewisite ABBR: BAL. Trade name for dimercaprol, a compound used as an antidote in poisoning due to heavy metals such as arsenic, gold, and mercury.

British Pharmacopoeia ABBR: B.P. The standard reference on drugs and their preparations used in Great Britain.

brittle diabetes diabetes, brittle.

broach (brōch) [ME. *broche,* pointed rod] **1.** A dental instrument used for enlarging a root canal or removing the pulp. **2.** A technique used for preparing the intramedullary canal of a bone by using a cutting device. This is done in preparation for a prosthetic replacement.

Broadbent's sign [Sir William Henry Broadbent, Brit. physician, 1835–1907] A visible retraction of the left side and back in the region of the 11th and 12th ribs synchronous with the cardiac systole in adhesive pericarditis.

Broca's area (brō′kăs) [Pierre Paul Broca, Fr. anatomist, anthropologist, neurologist, and surgeon, 1824–1880] The area of the left hemisphere of the brain at the posterior end of the inferior frontal gyrus. It contains the motor speech area and controls movements of tongue, lips, and vocal cords. Loss of speech may follow any stroke affecting this area. SYN: *motor speech area; speech center*. SEE: *motor aphasia*.

Brodie's abscess [Sir Benjamin Collins Brodie, Brit. surgeon, 1783–1862] A small collection of pus that occurs in pyogenic osteomyelitis; it is usually walled off by new bone formation. SEE: *osteomyelitis*.

SYMPTOMS: There may be aching pain in the affected area, followed by slight swelling and tenderness on movement. The symptoms are similar to those of osteomyelitis but are less acute.

Brodmann's areas [Korbinian Brodmann, Ger. neurologist, 1868–1918] The division of the cerebral cortex into 47 areas. This was originally done on the basis of cytoarchitectural characteristics, but the areas are now classified according to their functions.

brom-, bromo- [Gr. *bromos,* stench] Combining form indicating the presence of bromine.

bromelain (brō′mĕ-lān) A proteolytic enzyme present in the pineapple plant.

bromide (brō′mīd) [Gr. *bromos,* stench] A binary compound of bromine combined with an element or a radical. It is a central nervous system depressant, and overdosage can cause serious mental disturbance.

bromide poisoning Poisoning due to an overdose of bromide.

SYMPTOMS: Symptoms include vomiting; abdominal pain; respiratory and eye irritation if inhaled; corrosion of the mouth and intestinal tract if swallowed; cyanosis; tachycardia; and shock.

FIRST AID: If bromide is inhaled, oxygen is administered, respiratory support provided, and pulmonary edema treated. If bromide is swallowed, gastric lavage may reduce intestinal absorption. SEE: *Poisons and Poisoning Appendix*.

bromidrosiphobia (brō″mĭ-drō-sĭ-fō′bē-ă) [″ + *hidros,* sweat, + *phobos,* fear] An abnormal fear of personal odors, accompanied by hallucinations.

bromidrosis, bromhidrosis (brō″mĭ-drō′sĭs) Sweat that is fetid or offensive due to bacterial decomposition. It occurs mostly on the feet, in the groin, and under the arms.

PATIENT CARE: The axillae, groin, and feet should be cleansed daily with soap and water, rinsing well and drying thoroughly. Deodorant preparations should be used; and clothing and shoes changed, aired, and cleaned frequently. SYN: *kakidrosis*.

bromine (brō′mēn, -mĭn) [Gr. *bromos,* stench] SYMB: Br. A liquid nonmetallic element obtained from natural brines from wells and sea water; atomic mass 79.904, atomic number 35. Its compounds are used in medicine and photography. SEE: *bromide*.

bromism, brominism (brō′mĭzm, brō′mĭn-ĭzm) [″ + *-ismos,* condition] Poisoning that results from prolonged use of bromides. SEE: *bromides in Poisons and Poisoning Appendix.*

bromocriptine mesylate (brō″mō-krĭp′tēn) An ergot derivative that suppresses secretion of prolactin. It has been used to treat patients with hyperprolactinemia (e.g., in those with pituitary adenomas); to stimulate ovulation in patients with amenorrhea; to treat patients with acromegaly; and to treat patients with parkinsonism, as an adjunct to levodopa. Common side effects include nausea, dizziness, and headache.

bromoderma (brō″mō-dĕr′mă) [″ + *derma,* skin] An acnelike eruption due to allergic sensitivity to bromides.

bromodiphenhydramine hydrochloride (brō″mō-dī″fĕn-hī′dră-mēn) An antihistamine. It also has sedative properties.

bromoiodism (brō″mō-ī′ō-dĭzm) [″ + *ioeides,* violet colored, + *-ismos,* condition] Poisoning from bromine and iodine or their compounds.

bromomenorrhea (brō″mō-mĕn-ō-rē′ă) [″ + *men,* month, + *rhoia,* flow] Menstrual discharge marked by an offensive odor.

brompheniramine maleate (brōm″fĕn-ĭr′ă-mēn) An antihistamine. Its primary side effect is sedation.

Brompton's cocktail [Brompton Chest Hospital, England] A mixture of cocaine, morphine, and antiemetics, formerly used to alleviate pain and induce euphoria, esp. in patients with cancer.

bromsulphalein ABBR: BSP. Trade name for sulfobromophthalein sodium, a dye used for testing liver function in nonjaundiced patients.

bronch- SEE: *broncho-*.

bronchi- SEE: *broncho-*.

bronchi (brŏng′kī) *sing.,* **bronchus** [L.] The two main branches leading from the trachea to the lungs, providing a passageway for air. The trachea divides opposite the third thoracic vertebra into the right and left main bronchi. The point of division, called the carina trachea, is the site where foreign bodies too large to enter either bronchus would rest after passing through the trachea. The right bronchus is shorter and more vertical than the left one. After entering the lung each bronchus divides further and terminates in bronchioles. SEE: *bronchus* for illus.

foreign bodies in b. Any materials that are aspirated into the lower airways, such as beans, nuts, seeds, or coins. These items, which usually lodge in the right bronchus because of its anatomical relation to the trachea, may cause pneumonia, airway inflammation, abscess formation, or atelectasis.

TREATMENT: They can be removed with postural drainage or bronchoscopy.

bronchial (brŏng′kē-ăl) Pert. to the bronchi or bronchioles.

bronchial breath sounds SEE: under *sound*.

bronchial crisis A paroxysm of coughing in persons with locomotor ataxia due to syphilis.

bronchial tube One of the smaller divisions of the bronchi.

bronchial washing Irrigation of one or both bronchi to collect cells for cytologic study or to help cleanse the bronchi.

bronchiectasis (brŏng″kē-ĕk′tă-sĭs) [″ + *ektasis,* dilatation] Chronic dilation of a bronchus or bronchi, usually in the lower portions of the lung, caused by the damaging effects of a long-standing infection.

SYMPTOMS: Symptoms include coughing, dyspnea, and expectoration of foul sputum, esp. in the morning or when the individual changes position.

ETIOLOGY: The condition may be acquired or congenital and may occur in one or both lungs. Acquired bronchiectasis usually occurs secondary to an obstruction or an infection such as bronchopneumonia, chronic bronchitis, tuberculosis, cystic fibrosis, or whooping cough.

TREATMENT: Therapy consists of antibiotics, prophylaxis, and postural drainage. Resection of affected areas may be done in selected patients. Aerosols may be useful for bronchodilation if bronchospasm is present. SEE: *postural drainage*.

PATIENT CARE: The patient is assessed for the presence or increased severity of respiratory distress. Ventilatory rate, pattern, and effort are observed, breath sounds are auscultated, and sputum is inspected for changes in quantity, color, or viscosity. The respiratory therapist evaluates gas exchange by monitoring arterial blood gas values, and administers oxygen according to protocol or as prescribed. The patient is observed for complications such as cor pulmonale. The patient should increase oral fluid intake and be shown how to use a humidifier or nebulizer to help thin inspissated secretions. The patient also is taught to breathe deeply and cough effectively. Chest physiotherapy is most effective and least disruptive if carried out in the morning, ½ hr before meals, and at bedtime. The nurse or respiratory therapist suctions the oropharynx if the patient is unable to clear the airway and teaches the patient and family how to do this. The need for frequent oral hygiene to remove foul-smelling secretions and to help prevent anorexia is explained. The patient is taught to dispose of secretions, to cleanse items contaminated by secretions, and to wash hands thoroughly to avoid spreading infections. Air pollutants and people with upper respiratory infections should be avoided. If the patient smokes, he or she may need referral to a smoking cessation program or nicotine patch therapy. Prescribed medications, such as antibiotics, bronchodilators, and expectorants, are given, and both patient and family are instructed in their use, action, and side effects. The patient is advised not to take over-the-counter drugs without the health care provider's approval. Supportive care is provided to help the patient adjust to the lifestyle changes that irreversible lung damage requires. If surgery is scheduled, the patient is prepared physically and emotionally. Preoperative and postoperative teaching and care are conducted, and the patient's status is monitored to prevent complications.

saccular b. Dilated bronchi that are of saccular or irregular shape. The proximal third to fourth branches of the bronchi are severely dilated and end blindly with extensive collapse.

varicose b. Dilated bronchi that resemble varicose veins; irregular dilatation and constriction as seen in cystic fibrosis.

bronchiloquy (brŏng-kĭl′ō-kwē) [″ + L. *loqui,* to speak] Unusual vocal resonance over a bronchus covered with consolidated lung tissue.

bronchiocele (brŏng′kē-ō-sēl) [″ + *kele,* tumor, swelling] Circumscribed dilatation of a bronchus.

bronchiogenic (brŏng″kē-ō-jĕn′ĭk) [″ + *gennan,* to produce] Having origin in the bronchi.

bronchiol- SEE: *bronchiolo-*.

bronchiole (brŏng′kē-ōl) *pl.* **bronchioles** [L. *bronchiolus,* air passage] One of the smaller subdivisions of the bronchial tubes.

respiratory b. The last division of the bronchial tree. Respiratory bronchioles are branches of terminal bronchioles and continue to the alveolar ducts, which lead to the alveoli.

terminal b. The next-to-last subdivision of a bronchiole, leading to the respiratory bronchioles.

bronchiolectasis (brŏng″kē-ō-lĕk′tă-sĭs) [″ + Gr. *ektasis,* dilatation] Dilatation of the bronchioles; capillary bronchiectasis.

bronchiolitis (brŏng″kē-ō-lī′tĭs) [″ + Gr. *itis,* inflammation] Inflammation of the bronchioles, particularly as an acute process in children during the first 2 years of life, with peak incidence around 6 months of age. Most cases occur during the winter and early spring months.

ETIOLOGY: The respiratory syncytial virus (RSV) accounts for 50% of cases. Other viruses (parainfluenza, adenoviruses) and mycoplasma species make up the remaining cases. There is no evidence that bacteria cause the illness, or that antibiotics cure it.

SYMPTOMS: URI symptoms (runny

nose, sneezing) appear first, quickly replaced by the hallmarks of the disease, respiratory distress with tachypnea and wheezing. The wheezing is what gives the disease its commonly used name, "baby asthma." Some infants, especially those a few months old, develop severe respiratory distress with hypoxia and gasping respirations, requiring hospitalization, oxygen, and assisted ventilation. Chest x-ray films show hyperinflation of the lungs with scattered areas of pneumonia and/or atelectasis.

TREATMENT: Infants with moderate or worse respiratory distress should be admitted to the hospital for observation, ventilation therapy, and oxygen. Whether bronchodilators such as nebulized albuterol have any value in the treatment is still debated, but they are often used. Ribavirin, a nebulized antiviral agent, is used in severe cases of bronchiolitis due to proven RSV infection in children under age 2.

PROGNOSIS: The case fatality rate is less than 1%, but a significant proportion of affected infants develop reactive airway disease (i.e., asthma) in later childhood.

PREVENTION: Preventive drugs have been developed for infants with bronchopulmonary dysplasia and other congenital cardiac or pulmonary diseases. These include palivizumab, a monoclonal antibody, and an RSV immune globulin.

PATIENT CARE: The infant requires close observation regarding the demands imposed by airway obstruction at the bronchiolar level. The infant is observed for gradually increasing respiratory distress, paroxysmal cough, dypsnea and irritability, as well as for tachypnea with flaring nostrils and intercostal and subcostal retractions, and shallow respiratory excursion.

The infant should be percussed for hyperresonance and scattered consolidation and auscultated for fine crackles, prolonged expiratory phase, and diminished breath sounds by the nurse, respiratory therapist, and physician. Audible or auscultatory wheezing may be present, as well as hyperinflation leading to emphysema with barrel chest and depressed diaphragm.

The parents are educated regarding the need for hospitalization, and treatments that will be employed are explained. The use of a mist tent and oxygen are discussed, also assisted ventilation if this becomes necessary, and the parents are taught how to maintain contact with their infant. The parents also need to understand that tachypnea, weakness, and fatigue limit the infant's ability to obtain fluids in sufficient amounts to provide adequate hydration, thus intravenous fluids will be used until symptoms abate. Since parents expect medications to be prescribed for their infant, the nurse explains why various drugs (antibiotics, bronchodilators, corticosteroids, cough suppressants, and expectorants) are not employed and helps them to understand why sedatives are contraindicated although rest is an important part of therapy. Hospitalization of an infant is traumatic to parents and to the child depending on his or her age and severity of illness, so emotional support is provided to all throughout this crisis. The parents are helped to provide love, touch, and care for their infant, are instructed how they can contact the nurse if they must be absent from the cribside, and are assisted to understand and deal with behavioral regression that may occur.

b. exudativa Bronchiolitis with fibrinous exudation and grayish sputum; often associated with asthma.

b. obliterans Bronchiolitis in which the bronchioles and, occasionally, some of the smaller bronchi are partly or completely obliterated by nodular masses that contain granulation and fibrotic tissue.

bronchiolo-, bronchiol- [L. *bronchiolus,* air passage] Combining forms meaning *bronchiole.*

bronchiolus (brŏng-kē′ō-lŭs) *pl.* **bronchioli** [L.] Bronchiole.

bronchiospasm (brŏng′kē-ō-spăzm) [Gr. *bronchos,* windpipe, + *spasmos,* a convulsion] Bronchospasm.

bronchiostenosis (brŏng″kē-ō-stĕn-ō′sĭs) [″ + *stenosis,* act of narrowing] Narrowing of the bronchial tubes.

bronchitis (brŏng-kī′tĭs) [″ + *itis,* inflammation] Inflammation of the mucous membranes of the bronchial airways, caused by irritation or infection, or both, by pathogen. Bronchitis can be acute or chronic. SEE: *Nursing Diagnoses Appendix.*

ETIOLOGY: Bronchitis is caused by infectious agents such as viruses (esp. rhinoviruses, influenza A and B, parainfluenza, adenoviruses, and respiratory syncytial virus) or, less often, mycoplasma, chlamydia, streptococcus, haemophilus, bramhamella, or staphylococcus. Infection is often indistinguishable from the common cold and is usually treated as such unless pneumonia is also present. Acute bronchial irritation (noninfectious bronchitis) may also be caused by exposure to various physical and chemical agents such as dust, fumes, or pollens. Allergies and pre-existing conditions such as asthma or chronic obstructive lung disease may be important cofactors.

PATIENT CARE: A history is obtained documenting tobacco use, including type, duration, and frequency. Calculation of pack-year history gives useful information. The health care provider assesses for other known respiratory irritants and allergens, exertional or worsening dyspnea, and productive cough. The patient is evaluated for changes in baseline respiratory function such as the use of accessory muscles in breathing, cyanosis, neck vein distention, pedal edema, prolonged expiratory time, tachypnea, and wheezes or rales. The color and characteristics of sputum are often documented (but may have little diagnostic value). Tests such as arterial blood gas analysis, chest x-rays, oximetry, peak flow measurements, pulmonary function testing, and sputum gram stain are occasionally employed. They are explained to the patient if they have been ordered. Prescribed antihistamines, bronchodilators, corticosteroids, decongestants, expectorants, and other medications are administered and the response is documented. Antibiotics are rarely indicated. Daily activities are interspersed with rest periods to conserve energy and to prevent fatigue. Adequate fluids are given to loosen secretions (unless otherwise restricted), and fluid intake is monitored should patients with comorbid conditions be hospitalized. Patients needing help to quit smoking are given counseling and support, and are referred to smoking cessation programs and for adjunctive drug therapy when prescribed.

acute b. **1.** An infection of the bronchi that may be indistinguishable from the common cold, often associated with repetitive coughing or sputum production. It is usually caused by viruses (esp. rhinoviruses, influenza A or B, parainfluenza, adenoviruses, or respiratory syncytial virus) or less often by *Mycoplasma pneumoniae,* Chlamydia, streptococci, *Haemophilus spp, Moraxella lacunata, Bordetella pertussis,* or staphylococci. **2.** Noninfectious inflammation of the bronchi caused by exposure to such irritants as dusts, fumes, or pollens.

TREATMENT: Patients are treated with bedrest, increased fluid intake, and antipyretics and analgesics for comfort. Vaporizers may be used to decrease bronchial irritation. Antibiotics are rarely indicated (even if purulent sputum is present), unless the symptoms continue for more than 10 days or there is an underlying disease such as congestive heart failure, chronic obstructive lung disease, bronchitis, or an immunodeficiency. Some prolonged cases of acute bronchitis will eventually prove to be caused by pertussis, which will respond to erythromycin-based drugs. A chest x-ray examination to check for pneumonia is indicated when clinically suspected (e.g., if severe respiratory symptoms, fever, tachycardia, hypoxia, or abnormal lung sounds are present).

asthmatic b. Bronchitis compounded by wheezing, caused by spasm of hyperreactive airways.

chronic b. Bronchitis marked by increased mucus secretion by the tracheobronchial tree. A productive cough must be present for at least 3 months in two consecutive years for the clinical diagnosis of chronic bronchitis to be made; also, other bronchopulmonary diseases (e.g., bronchiectasis, tuberculosis, tumor) must be excluded. SEE: *chronic obstructive pulmonary disease.*

ETIOLOGY: Chronic irritation by inhaled irritants (esp. cigarette smoking) and repeated infections are the primary risk factors. Chronic bronchitis is 4 to 10 times more common in heavy smokers; cigarette smoke interferes with the movement of cilia and inhibits the activity of white blood cells in the bronchi and alveoli. The predominant pathological changes are hypertrophy and hyperplasia of the mucus-secreting glands of the large and small airways. Some patients also have hyperreactive airways. The changes in the respiratory epithelium may increase the risk of lung cancer.

SYMPTOMS: Although the disease begins earlier, signs and symptoms may not appear until patients are 40 to 50 years old. A chronic cough producing copious amounts of sputum occurs early, and patients have frequent respiratory problems, often as a result of acute bronchopulmonary infections. Dyspnea is generally moderate and occurs relatively late in the disease process. Over time, right-sided heart failure (cor pulmonale) develops, marked by dependent edema, distended neck veins, pulmonary hypertension, and an enlarged right ventricle.

TREATMENT: Bronchodilators, inhaled steroids, and other drugs are used to prevent bronchospasm, improve airflow, and aid in the removal of secretions. Increased fluid intake (about 3 L/day) may be needed to help remove secretions. Acute respiratory infections are treated with empirical antibiotics such as amoxicillin/clavulanate or trimethoprim/sulfamethoxazole, among others. Patients with underlying chronic bronchitis should receive pneumococcal and influenza vaccines. Other treatments are symptom based. Cessation of smoking is an important part of the overall treatment.

PATIENT CARE: The initial history and assessment covers tobacco use, presence of other known respiratory irritants and allergens, degree of dyspnea, use of accessory muscles for breathing, presence of wheezes or rhonchi, color, sputum characteristics, nutritional status, and the effect of the disease on desired activity. Patients who smoke are referred to a smoking cessation program. The patient's lungs are auscultated before and after aerosol therapy to assess the effectiveness of bronchodilators.

The patient/family need extensive education and ongoing psychosocial support to cope with this chronic disease. Simple pathophysiology of the disease process is taught and used as a basis for explanations about diagnostic tests (e.g., pulmonary function tests) and all interventions to increase patient cooperation in the complex care regimen. Written materials usually augment verbal instruction. Patients and families are taught how to ensure and document adequate fluid intake (about 3 L/day unless otherwise restricted) to loosen secretions; to schedule small, frequent, high-protein meals to combat anorexia and weight loss; to use pursed-lip breathing and controlled cough to increase airflow and prevent fatigue from coughing spasms; to provide oral care frequently to minimize anorexia and the risk of infection; and to maintain muscle strength by continuing to exercise, but with a plan to pace activities to avoid fatigue. They also are taught to watch for and report signs of possible heart failure (e.g., dependent edema, rales, or weight gain of more than 1 kg/day) or acute respiratory infection (e.g., increased dyspnea and changes in sputum characteristics such as color or amount). As the disease progresses, the family is assisted to make decisions about how routines may be modified to best meet individual needs.

The respiratory therapist delivers bronchodilators and humidity therapy as indicated by the presence of wheezing or evidence of retained airway secretions. Chest physical therapy may prove useful when the patient cannot easily cough them out. The patient with acute bronchitis may need oxygen therapy temporarily if oxygenation is found to be inadequate.

plastic b. Bronchitis marked by violent cough and paroxysms of dyspnea in which casts of the bronchial tubes are expectorated.

putrid b. A chronic form of bronchitis with foul-smelling sputum.

vegetal b. Bronchitis resulting from lodging of foods of vegetable origin in the bronchus.

bronchium (brŏng′kē-ŭm) *pl.* **bronchia** [Gr. *bronchos*] One of the subdivisions of the bronchus. It is smaller than a bronchus and larger than a bronchiole.

broncho-, bronch-, bronchi- [Gr. *bronchos,* windpipe] Combining form meaning *airway.*

bronchoalveolar (brŏn″kō-ăl-vē′ō-lăr) [″ + *alveolus,* small hollow] Concerning the bronchi and alveoli.

bronchoalveolar lavage The removal of secretions, cells, and protein from the lower respiratory tract by insertion of sterile saline solution into the airways through a fiberoptic bronchoscope. The fluid may be used to treat cystic fibrosis, pulmonary alveolar proteinosis, or bronchial obstruction due to mucus plugging, or to obtain specimens for diagnostic purposes.

bronchoblennorrhea (brŏng″kō-blĕn″ō-rē′ă) [″ + *blennos,* mucus, + *rhoia,* flow] Chronic bronchitis in which sputum is copious and thin.

bronchocele (brŏng′kō-sēl) [″ + *kele,* tumor, swelling] A localized dilatation of a bronchus.

bronchoconstriction (brŏng″kō-kŏn-strĭk′shŭn) [″ + L. *constringere,* to draw together] Constriction of the bronchial tubes.

bronchodilatation (brŏng″kō-dĭl-ă-tā′shŭn) [″ + L. *dilatare,* to open] Dilatation of a bronchus.

bronchodilator A drug that expands the bronchi by relaxing bronchial muscle. There are three classes of bronchodilators: $\beta_2$adrenergic-receptor agonists, methylxanthines, and anticholinergic agents. The β_2 adrenergic-receptor agonists produce the greatest bronchodilation in patients with bronchial asthma. The beta$_2$ adrenergic-receptor agonists are the best drugs for patients with mild, intermittent asthma and for acute attacks of reactive airway disease. SEE: table for features of bronchodilator drugs.

bronchoedema (brŏng″kō-ĕ-dē′mă) [″ + *oidema,* swelling] Edematous swelling of the mucosa of the bronchial tubes, reducing the size of air passageways and inducing dyspnea.

bronchoesophageal (brŏng″kō-ĕ-sŏf″ă-jē′ăl) [″ + *oisophagos,* esophagus] Concerning the bronchus and the esophagus.

bronchofiberscope (brŏng″kō-fī′bĕr-skōp) [″ + L. *fibra,* fiber, + Gr. *skopein,* to examine] An old term for bronchoscope.

bronchogenic (brŏng-kō-jĕn′ĭk) [″ + *gennan,* to produce] Having origin in a bronchus.

bronchogram (brŏng′kō-grăm) [″ + *gramma,* something written] Previously used term for a radiograph of the lung obtained during bronchography, an obsolete technique.

bronchography (brŏng-kŏg′ră-fē) [″ + *graphein,* to write] An obsolete radiographic technique for imaging the tracheobronchial tree after instillation of an oil-based contrast medium. This examination has been replaced by bronchoscopy and computed tomography.

broncholith (brŏng′kō-lĭth) [″ + *lithos,* stone] A calculus in a bronchus.

Features of Bronchodilator Drugs

Drug Class	Route	Uses	Common Side Effects
$Beta_2$ agonists (e.g., albuterol)	Orally or by inhalation	Intermittent attacks of wheezing; exercise-induced asthma	Palpitations, tachycardia, nervousness
Methylxanthines (e.g., theophylline)	Orally, intravenously	Asthma; COPD	Palpitations, tachycardias, nausea, vomiting, seizures
Anticholinergics (e.g., ipratropium)	By inhalation	COPD; acute asthma (when combined with beta-agonist drug)	Dry mouth, cough, nausea

broncholithiasis (brŏng″kō-lĭth-ī′ă-sĭs) [″ + *lithos,* stone, + *-iasis,* state] Bronchial inflammation or obstruction caused by calculi in the bronchi.

bronchomotor (brŏng″kō-mō′tor) [″ + L. *motus,* moving] Causing dilation or constriction of the bronchi.

bronchomycosis (brŏng″kō-mī-kō′sĭs) [″ + *mykes,* fungus, + *osis,* condition] Any fungal infection of the bronchi or bronchial tubes, usually caused by fungi of the genus *Candida.*

bronchopathy (brŏng-kŏp′ă-thē) [″ + *pathos,* disease, suffering] Any pathological condition involving the bronchi or bronchioles.

bronchophony (brŏng-kŏf′ō-nē) [″ + *phone,* voice] An abnormal increase in tone or clarity in vocal resonance.

bronchoplasty (brŏng′kō-plăs″tē) [″ + *plassein,* to form] Surgical repair of a bronchial defect.

bronchopleural (brŏng″kō-ploor′ăl) [″ + *pleura,* side, rib] Pert. to the bronchi and the pleural cavity.

bronchopneumonia (brŏng″kō-nū-mō′nē-ă) [″ + *pneumonia,* lung inflammation] A type of pneumonia marked by scattered consolidation (areas filled with inflammatory exudate) in one or more lobes of the lung. It occurs primarily in infants and in elderly persons, both of whom have decreased resistance to bacterial and viral infections. It is often a complication of bronchitis.

bronchopulmonary (brŏng″kō-pŭl′mō-nă-rē) [Gr. *bronchos,* windpipe, + L. *pulmonarius,* pert. to lung] Pert. to the bronchi and lungs.

bronchopulmonary lavage Bronchoalveolar lavage.

bronchorrhagia (brŏng″kor-ā′jē-ă) [″ + *rhegnynai,* to break forth] A bronchial hemorrhage.

bronchorrhaphy (brŏng-kor′ă-fē) [″ + *rhaphe,* seam, ridge] The suturing of a bronchial wound.

bronchorrhea (brŏng-kō-rē′ă) [″ + *rhoia,* flow] An abnormal secretion from the bronchial mucous membranes.

bronchorrhoncus (brŏng″kor-ŏn′kŭs) [″ + *rhonchos,* snore] A bronchial crackle.

bronchoscope (brŏng′kō-skōp) [″ + *skopein,* to examine] An endoscope designed to pass through the trachea for visual inspection of the tracheobronchial tree. The device can be used for lavage, or to remove tissue for biopsy or foreign bodies from the tracheobronchial tree.

bronchoscopy (brŏng-kŏs′kō-pē) Examination of the bronchi through a bronchoscope.

bronchosinusitis (brŏng″kō-sī″nŭs-ī′tĭs) [″ + L. *sinus,* a hollow, + Gr. *itis,* inflammation] Infection of a bronchus and a sinus at the same time.

bronchospasm (brŏng′kō-spăzm) [″ + *spasmos,* a convulsion] An abnormal narrowing with partial obstruction of the lumen of the bronchi due to spasm of the peribronchial smooth muscle. Clinically this is accompanied by coughing and wheezing. Bronchospasm occurs in reactive airway diseases such as asthma and bronchitis. Treatment may include bronchodilators and corticosteroids. SEE: *asthma.*

bronchospirometer (brŏng″kō-spĭ-rŏm′ĕ-tĕr) [″ + L. *spirare,* to breathe, + Gr. *metron,* measure] An instrument for determining the volume of air inspired from one lung and for collecting air for analysis.

bronchostaxis (brŏng″kō-stăk′sĭs) [″ + *staxis,* dripping] Hemorrhage from the walls of a bronchus.

bronchostenosis (brŏng″kō-stĕn-ō′sĭs) [″ + *stenosis,* act of narrowing] Stenosis of a bronchus.

bronchostomy (brŏng-kŏs′tō-mē) [″ + *stoma,* mouth] The surgical formation of an opening into a bronchus.

bronchotomy (brŏng-kŏt′ō-mē) [″ + *tome,* incision] Surgical incision of a bronchus, the larynx, or the trachea.

bronchotracheal (brŏng″kō-trā′kē-ăl) [″ + *trachea,* rough] Pert. to the bronchi and trachea.

bronchovesicular (brŏng″kō-vĕ-sĭk′ū-lăr) [″ + L. *vesicula,* a tiny bladder] Pert. to bronchial tubes and alveoli with special reference to sounds intermediate between bronchial or tracheal sounds and alveolar sounds.

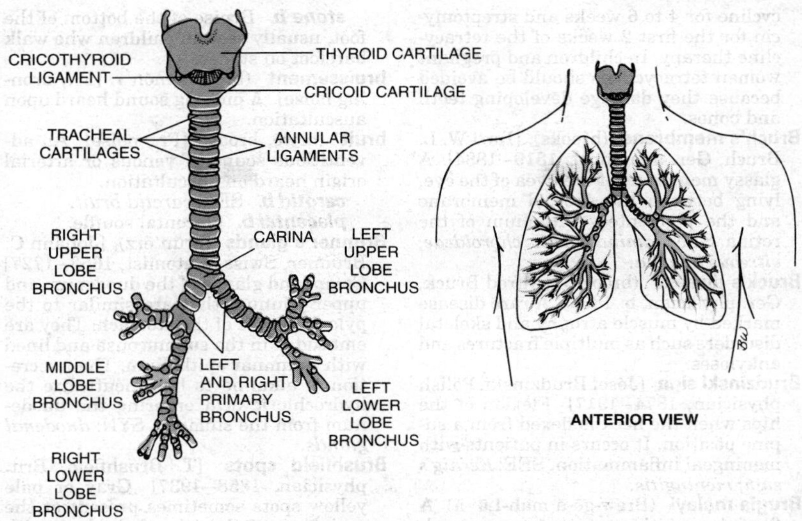

TRACHEA AND BRONCHI

b. breath sounds SEE: under *sound*.

bronchus (brŏng′kŭs) *pl.* **bronchi** [Gr. *bronchos,* windpipe] One of the two large branches of the trachea. The trachea proper terminates at the level of the fourth thoracic vertebra. SEE: illus.; *bronchi.*

brontophobia (brŏn″tō-fō′bē-ă) [Gr. *bronte,* thunder, + *phobos,* fear] An abnormal fear of thunder.

bronzed skin A condition seen in chronic adrenocortical insufficiency (Addison's disease), and in hemochromatosis, some cases of diabetes mellitus, and cirrhosis of the liver.

brood To worry or ponder anxiously.

brood capsule A cystlike body that develops within a hydatid cyst of *Echinococcus granulosus.*

broth [ME.] **1.** A nutrient drink made from meat (e.g., bouillon) usually served hot. **2.** A liquid medium made from meat, used in making bacterial culture media.

brow The forehead.

brown baby syndrome The dark grayish brown skin color seen in infants undergoing extensive phototherapy for hyperbilirubinemia. The condition may last for months but is not known to produce permanent harm.

brownian movement (brow′nē-ăn) [Robert Brown, Brit. botanist, 1773–1858] The oscillatory movement of particles resulting from chance bombardment by molecules moving at high velocities.

Brown-Séquard's syndrome (brown′sā-kărz′) [Charles E. Brown-Séquard, Fr. physician, 1817–1894] Hemisection of the spinal cord with the following neurological changes: paralysis on the same side as the lesion, loss of position and vibratory sense, and ataxia; loss of pain and temperature sensitivity on the side opposite the lesion.

Brucella (broo-sĕl′ă) [Sir David Bruce, Brit. physician and bacteriologist, 1855–1931] A genus of nonmotile, aerobic, gram-negative coccobacilli that are pathogenic to humans and cause undulant fever and abortion in cattle, hogs, and goats. SEE: *brucellosis.*

brucella *pl.* **brucellae** *pl.* **brucellas** Any bacterium of the genus *Brucella.* **brucellar** (broo-sĕl′ĕr), *adj.*

brucellin (broo-sĕl′ĭn) An extract of any species of *Brucella.* It formerly was used in skin tests to diagnose brucellosis. Agglutination tests and cultures are now used.

brucellosis (broo″sĕl-ō′sĭs) [*Brucella* + Gr. *osis,* condition] A widespread infectious febrile disease affecting principally cattle, swine, and goats, and sometimes other animals and humans. It is caused by bacteria of several *Brucella* species. *B. melitensis* and *B. suis* cause brucellosis in goats and swine, respectively, and *B. abortus* causes contagious abortion in cattle, dogs, and other domestic animals. The organisms are intracellular parasites. In humans it is called brucellosis, Malta fever, and Gibraltar fever and is caused by any of the three species. SYN: *Gibraltar fever*.

TREATMENT: In adult humans, treatment consists of combined tetracycline for 4 to 6 weeks and streptomycin for the first 2 weeks of the tetracycline therapy. In children and pregnant women tetracyclines should be avoided because they damage developing teeth and bones.

Bruch's membrane (brooks) [Karl W. L. Bruch, Ger. anatomist, 1819–1884] A glassy membrane of the uvea of the eye, lying between the choroid membrane and the pigmented epithelium of the retina. SYN: *lamina basalis choroideae; vitreous lamella.*

Bruck's disease (brooks) [Alfred Bruck, Ger. physician, b. 1865] A rare disease marked by muscle atrophy and skeletal disorders such as multiple fractures and ankyloses.

Brudzinski sign [Jósef Brudzinski, Polish physician, 1874–1917] Flexion of the hips when the neck is flexed from a supine position. It occurs in patients with meningeal inflammation. SEE: *Kernig's sign; meningitis.*

Brugia malayi (Brew-gē-ă mah-Lā'-ă) A filarial parasitic worm that can cause elephantiasis. SEE: *elephantiasis; Wuchereria.*

Bruininks-Oseretsky Test of Motor Proficiency ABBR: BOTMP. A standardized test of gross and fine motor performance for children from 4 to 14 years of age.

bruise (brooz) [O. Fr. *bruiser,* to break] A traumatic injury (usually to the skin but sometimes to internal organs) in which blood vessels are broken but tissue surfaces remain intact. Discoloration, swelling, inflammation, and pain are typical signs and symptoms. Fresh bruises on the skin are usually red or purple. Older bruises turn green and then yellow or brown, as the blood products within them age and are resorbed. SYN: *ecchymosis.*

FIRST AID: Cold applications are needed first, followed by application of a firm bandage to prevent swelling. Twenty-four to 48 hr later, application of heat is desirable, followed by gentle massage.

b. of head, chest, and abdomen A bruise that may be associated with internal injuries. SEE: *ecchymosis.*

SYMPTOMS: Symptoms include pain, swelling, tenderness, and discoloration.

PATIENT CARE: Historical data are collected regarding the exact cause and location of the injury. The bruised area is inspected, and the location, color, size, discomfort, and other pertinent characteristics are documented. The patient is assessed for other injuries dependent on the specific location and severity of the original injury. Related skin abrasions are cleansed thoroughly. Neurological status (AVPU) is monitored hourly or as needed for any patient with a suspected head injury.

stone b. Bruise of the bottom of the foot, usually seen in children who walk barefoot on stones.

bruissement (broo-ēs-mŏn') [Fr., droning noise] A purring sound heard upon auscultation.

bruit (brwē, broot) [Fr., noise] An adventitious sound of venous or arterial origin heard on auscultation.

carotid b. SEE: *carotid bruit.*

placental b. placental souffle.

Brunner's glands (brŭn'ĕrz) [Johann C. Brunner, Swiss anatomist, 1653–1727] Compound glands of the duodenum and upper jejunum that are similar to the pyloric glands of the stomach. They are embedded in the submucousa and lined with columnar epithelium. Their secretion is alkaline to help neutralize the hydrochloric acid entering the duodenum from the stomach. SYN: *duodenal glands.*

Brushfield spots [T. Brushfield, Brit. physician, 1858–1937] Gray or pale yellow spots sometimes present at the periphery of the iris of children with Down syndrome.

brushing **1.** A technique of tactile stimulation using small, electrically rotated brushes over selected dermatomes to elicit muscular responses in the rehabilitation of persons with central nervous system damage. **2.** Cleaning with a brush, as in toothbrushing.

bruxism (brŭk'sĭzm) [Gr. *brychein,* to grind the teeth, + *-ismos,* condition] The grinding of the teeth, esp. in children, during sleep. If untreated, it can damage teeth and the temporomandibular joint. In severe cases the teeth are worn down due to attrition.

ETIOLOGY: Psychological stress or abnormalities of tooth occlusion are the principal causes.

TREATMENT: If the condition is due to psychological causes, tension, anxiety, and stress should be reduced. The teeth should be treated for caries, malocclusion, or periodontal disease. Occlusal guards for the teeth may be of benefit.

Bryant's traction [Sir Thomas Bryant, Brit. surgeon, 1828–1914] Traction applied to the lower legs with the force pulling vertically. It is used esp. in treating fractures of the femur in children.

B.S. *Bachelor of Science; Bachelor of Surgery.*

BSE **1.** *breast self-examination.* **2.** *bovine spongiform encephalopathy.*

BSI *Body substance isolation.*

B.S.N. *Bachelor of Science in Nursing.* The individual who earns this degree may apply to take the registered nurse (R.N.) licensing examination.

BSP *Bromsulphalein.*

BTPS *body temperature and pressure* (saturated with water vapor).

BTU *British thermal unit.*

bubo (boo′bō) *pl.* **buboes** [Gr. *boubon,* groin, swollen gland] An inflamed, swollen, or enlarged lymph node often exhibiting suppuration, occurring commonly after infective disease due to absorption of infective material. The nodes most commonly affected are those of the groin and axilla.

axillary b. A bubo in the armpit.

indolent b. A bubo in which suppuration does not occur.

inguinal b. A bubo in the region of the groin. SYN: *buboadenitis.*

venereal b. A bubo resulting from a venereal disease. SEE: *lymphogranuloma venereum.*

bubonadenitis (boo-bŏn-ăd-ĕ-nī′tĭs) [″ + *aden,* gland, + *itis,* inflammation] inguinal bubo.

bucca (bŭk′ă) *pl.* **buccae** [L., cheek] The cheek.

buccal (bŭk′ăl) Relating to the cheek or mouth.

b. fat pad An encapsulated mass of fat lying superficial to the buccinator muscle. It is well developed in infants and is thought to aid in the act of sucking. SYN: *B.'s fat ball; fat p.* (1); *sucking pad.*

buccinatolabialis (bŭk″sĭn-ā-tō-lā″bē-ă′lĭs) [L. *buccinator,* trumpeter, + *labialis,* pert. to the lips] The buccinator and orbicularis oris considered as a single muscle.

buccinator (bŭk′sĭn-ā-tor) The muscle of the cheek.

bucco- [L. *bucca,* mouth] Combining form meaning *cheek.*

buccoaxiocervical (bŭk″kō-ăk″sē-ō-sĕr′vĭ-kăl) The angle formed by the intersection of the buccal, axial, and cervical walls of a cavity in a tooth.

buccocervical (bŭk″kō-sĕr′vĭ-kăl) Concerning the buccal surface and cervical margin of a tooth.

buccodistal (bŭk″kō-dĭs′tăl) Concerning the buccal and distal surfaces of a tooth.

buccogingival (bŭk″kō-jĭn′jĭ-văl) Concerning the buccal and gingival surfaces of a tooth.

buccolabial (bŭk″kō-lā′bē-ăl) Concerning the buccal and labial surfaces of a tooth.

buccolingual (bŭk″kō-lĭng′gwăl) Concerning the buccal and lingual surfaces of a tooth.

buccomesial (bŭk″kō-mē′zē-ăl) Concerning the buccal and mesial surfaces of a tooth.

bucco-occlusal (bŭk″kō-ŏ-kloo′săl) Concerning the buccal and occlusal surfaces of a tooth.

buccopharyngeal (bŭk″kō-fă-rĭn′jē-ăl) Concerning the mouth and pharynx.

buccopulpal (bŭk″kō-pŭl′păl) Concerning the buccal and pulpal surfaces of a tooth.

buccoversion (bŭk″kō-vĕr′zhŭn) [L. *bucca,* cheek, + *versio,* turning] A tooth that twists in a buccal direction.

buccula (bŭk′ū-lă) [L., a little cheek] A fold of fatty tissue under the chin.

Buck's extension [Gurdon Buck, U.S. surgeon, 1807–1877] SEE: *extension.*

Bucky diaphragm, Potter-Bucky diaphragm [Gustav P. Bucky, Ger.-born U.S. radiologist, 1880–1963; Hollis Potter, U.S. radiologist, 1880–1964] A specialized film holder with a moving grid located immediately beneath the radiographic table or upright apparatus. It decreases the effects of scatter and secondary radiation during a radiographic exposure.

Bucky factor A measure of the amount of radiation absorbed by the Bucky diaphragm. This indicates the amount by which to increase the technical factors when a grid is being used.

bud [ME. *budde,* to swell] **1.** In anatomy, a small structure resembling a bud of a plant. **2.** In embryology, a small protuberance or outgrowth that is the anlage or primordium of an organ or structure.

taste b. An ovoid body embedded in the stratified epithelium of the tongue and also found sparingly on the epiglottis and soft palate. Buds contain the sensory receptors for taste.

tooth b. The earliest evidence of tooth development. SEE: *enamel organ.*

Budd-Chiari syndrome SEE: *thrombosis, hepatic vein.*

budding A method of asexual reproduction in which a small offshoot or sprout grows from the side or end of the parent and develops into a new organism, which in some cases remains attached and in others separates and lives an independent existence. Budding is common in lower animals (e.g., sponges and coelenterates) and plants (e.g., yeasts and molds).

Buerger's disease (bŭr′gĕrz) [Leo Buerger, U.S. physician, 1879–1943] A chronic, recurring, inflammatory, vascular occlusive disease, chiefly of the peripheral arteries and veins of the extremities. The disease is seen most commonly in males 20 to 40 years of age who smoke cigarettes. SYN: *thromboangiitis obliterans.*

SYMPTOMS: Symptoms include paresthesias of the foot, easy fatigability, and leg cramps. The legs tire quickly, esp. during walking. Ulceration or moist gangrene may set in; amputation may be necessary.

TREATMENT: Absolute and continued abstinence from tobacco in all forms is extremely important. The patient should avoid excessive use of the affected limb, exposure to temperature extremes, use of drugs that diminish the blood supply to extremities, trauma, and fungus infections. If gangrene, pain, or ulceration is present, complete bedrest is advised; if these are absent, the patient should walk at a comfortable pace for 30 min twice daily. For arterial spasm, blocking of the sympathetic nervous system by injection of various drugs or by sympathectomy may be done.

PATIENT CARE: The history should document occurrences of painful, intermittent claudication of the instep, calf, or thigh, which exercise aggravates and rest relieves; the patient's walking ability (distance, time, and rest required); the patient's foot response to exposure to cold temperatures (initially cold, numb, and cyanotic; later reddened, hot, and tingling); and any involvement of the hands, such as digital ischemia, trophic nail changes, painful fingertip ulcerations, or gangrene. Peripheral pulses are palpated, and absent or diminished radial, ulnar, or tibial pulses documented. Feet and legs are inspected for superficial vein thrombophlebitis, muscle atrophy, peripheral ulcerations, and gangrene, which occur late in the disease. Soft padding is used to protect the feet, which are washed gently with a mild soap and tepid water, rinsed thoroughly, and patted dry with a soft towel. The patient is instructed in this and advised to inspect tissues for injury such as cuts, abrasions, and signs of skin breakdown (redness or soreness) and to report all injuries to the health care provider for treatment. The patient is advised to avoid wearing tight or restrictive clothing, sitting or standing in one position for long periods, and walking barefoot; also, shoes and stockings should be carefully fitted, but stockings should not be tight enough to hinder venous return from the legs. Extremities must be protected from temperature extremes, esp. cold. The patient is taught Buerger's postural exercises if prescribed. Prescribed medications are administered, the patient's response is evaluated, desired and adverse reactions are explained, and the patient is cautioned to avoid use of over-the-counter drugs without the attending health care provider's approval. The patient who smokes is referred to a smoking cessation program, but nicotine patch therapy would not be prescribed given the patient's associated hypersensitivity to nicotine. Both patient and family should receive emotional support and psychological counseling if necessary to help them cope with this chronic disease. For the patient with ulcers and gangrene, bedrest is prescribed, and a padded footboard or cradle used to prevent pressure from bed linens. If amputation has been done, rehabilitative needs are considered, esp. regarding changes in body image, and the patient is referred for physical and occupational therapy and for social services as appropriate. SEE: *exercise, Buerger's postural.*

buffalo hump A deposit of fat in the lower midcervical and upper thoracic area of the back. It is usually caused by excessive adrenocortical hormone production or therapy.

buffer (bŭf′ĕr) [ME. *buffe,* to deaden shock of] **1.** A substance, esp. a salt of the blood, tending to preserve original hydrogen-ion concentration of its solution, upon adding an acid or base. **2.** A substance tending to offset reaction of an agent administered in conjunction with it.

blood b. A buffer present in the blood. The principal buffers are carbonic acid, carbonates and bicarbonates, monobasic and dibasic phosphates, and proteins. Hemoglobin is an important protein buffer.

buffy coat A light stratum of blood seen when the blood is centrifuged or allowed to stand in a test tube. The red blood cells settle to the bottom and, between the plasma and the red blood cells, a light-colored layer contains mostly white blood cells. Platelets are at the top of this coat; the next layers, in order, are lymphocytes and monocytes; granulocytes; and reticulocytes. In normal blood, the buffy coat is barely visible; in leukemia and leukemoid reactions, it is much larger. SEE: illus.

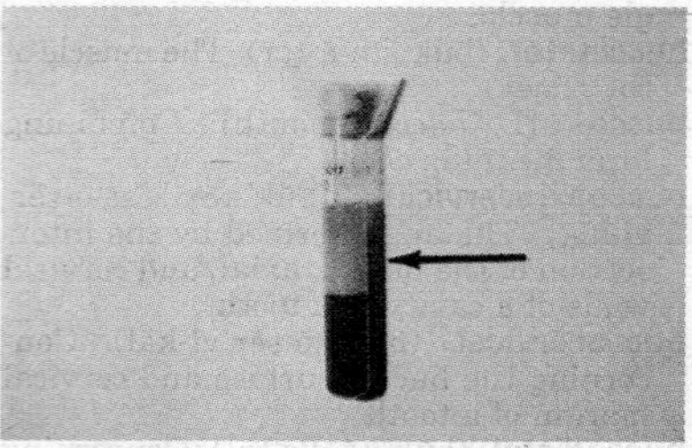

BUFFY COAT

bufotoxin [L. *bufo,* toad, + Gr. *toxikon,* poison] A general term for any toxin present in the skin of a toad.

bug A term applied loosely to any small insect or arthropod, esp. of the order Hemiptera, that has sucking mouth parts, incomplete metamorphosis, and two pairs of wings, the fore pair being half membranous. SEE: *bedbug; chiggers.*

assassin b. A member of the family Reduviidae. Many are predaceous; others are blood-sucking. *Panstrongylus, Triatoma,* and *Rhodnius* are vectors of trypanosome diseases (Chagas' disease) in humans. SEE: *trypanosomiasis.*

kissing b. Several species of the family Reduviidae. *Melanolestes picipes* is the common kissing bug, or black corsair.

red b. Chiggers.

buggery Sodomy.

bulb [L. *bulbus,* bulbous root; Gr. *bolbos*] Any rounded or globular structure.

aortic b. The dilated portion of the truncus arteriosus in the embryo that gives rise to the roots of the aorta and pulmonary arteries.

duodenal b. The upper duodenal area just beyond the pylorus.

hair b. The expanded portion at the lower end of the hair root. The growth of a hair results from the proliferation of cells of the hair bulb.

b. of the eye Eyeball.

b. of the urethra The posterior portion of the corpus spongiosum found between the two crura of the penis.

b. of the vestibule Bulbus vestibuli.

olfactory b. An anterior enlargement of the olfactory tract.

terminal b. of Krause An encapsulated sensory nerve ending similar in structure to the corpuscles of Pacini. SYN: *Golgi-Mazzoni corpuscle.*

bulbar Pert. to or shaped like a bulb.

bulbiform (bŭl′bĭ-form) [″ + *forma,* shape] Shaped like a bulb.

bulbitis (bŭl-bī′tĭs) [″ + Gr. *itis,* inflammation] Inflammation of the urethra in its bulbous portion.

bulbocavernosus (bŭl″bō-kăv″ĕr-nō′sŭs) [″ + *cavernosus,* hollow] A muscle ensheathing the bulb of the penis in the male or covering the bulbus vestibuli in the female. It is also called *ejaculator urinae* or *accelerator urinae* in males and *sphincter vaginae* in females.

bulbocavernosus reflex Contraction of bulbocavernosus muscle on percussing the dorsum of the penis.

bulboid (bŭl′boyd) [″ + Gr. *eidos,* form, shape] Shaped like a bulb.

bulbomimic reflex (bŭl″bō-mĭm′ĭk) [″ + Gr. *mimikos,* imitator] In coma, contraction of facial muscles following pressure on the eyeball. SYN: *facial reflex; Mondonesi's reflex.*

bulbonuclear (bŭl″bō-nū′klē-ăr) [″ + *nucleus,* kernel] Pert. to the nuclei in the medulla oblongata.

bulbospongiosus (bŭl″bō-spŏn″jē-ō′sŭs) One of the three voluntary muscles of the penis. It acts to empty the canal of the urethra after urination and to assist in erection of the corpus cavernosum urethrae. The anterior fibers contribute to penile erection by contracting to compress the deep dorsal vein of the penis.

bulbospongiosus reflex Contraction of bulbospongiosus muscle on percussing the dorsum of the penis.

bulbourethral gland (bŭl″bō-ū-rē′thrăl) [″ + Gr. *ourethra,* urethra] Either of two small, yellow glands, one on each side of the prostate gland, each with a duct about 1 in. (2.5 cm) long, terminating in the wall of the urethra. They secrete a viscid fluid forming part of the seminal fluid. They correspond to the Bartholin glands in the female. SYN: *Cowper's glands.* SEE: *prostate; urethra.*

bulbous (bŭl′bŭs) [L. *bulbus*] Bulb-shaped; swollen; terminating in an enlargement.

bulbus [L.; Gr. *bolbos*] Bulb.

b. corpus spongiosum Bulb of the urethra. A bulbous swelling of the corpus spongiosum penis at the base of the penis.

b. vestibuli Either of two oval masses of erectile tissue lying beneath the vestibule and resting on the urogenital diaphragm. In the female they are homologous to the bulbus spongiosum of the penis.

bulimarexia (bū-lĭm″ă-rĕk′sē-ă) Binge eating followed by self-induced vomiting.

bulimia (bū-lĭm′ē-ă) [L.] Excessive and insatiable appetite. **bulimic** (-ĭk), *adj.*

b. nervosa A disorder marked by recurrent episodes of binge eating, self-induced vomiting and diarrhea, excessive exercise, strict dieting or fasting, and an exaggerated concern about body shape and weight. SEE: *anorexia nervosa.*

PATIENT CARE: Early recognition and intervention can prevent an eating disorder from increasing in severity and duration. Risk factors that should ring a warning bell for further assessment include individuals considering or involved in careers requiring low weight; individuals who have been sexually abused or who come from families with a history of eating, affective, or substance abuse disorders; and individuals with low self-esteem, feelings of not being "in control," or communication and emotional difficulties.

Health history includes a weight history (frequency of weighing, premorbid weight, menstrual threshold, history of weight fluctuations). Changes are graphed to help identify stress-related patterns. The patient's facial expressions and body language may, on rare occasions help health care professionals to assess weight-associated anxiety levels. The patient should be questioned regarding perceptions of ideal weight and total body appearance, as well as specific areas (e.g., hips, thighs, abdomen). Having the patient draw pictures of self-perception may help to communicate this information. Any dieting behaviors are determined, including onset, type, frequency, and duration, what prompted them, and the presence of external influences, such as peer pressure.

A comprehensive physical examination includes mental status, with assessments of systemic findings that may indicate an eating disorder. The Beck depression inventory may identify coexisting depression. Laboratory testing includes serum electrolyte studies and complete blood count.

Assessments for psychologic, sexual, and physiologic manifestations of bulimia, including depression, suicidal ideation, and substance abuse, are important. Family history should include information concerning psychiatric problems, existence of physical or sexual abuse, communication patterns, and quality of relationships.

The patient with bulimia nervosa should be referred for counseling, with emphasis placed on ways to break the binge/purge cycle and to regain control over eating behaviors. The patient and family must recognize and understand the need for inpatient or outpatient therapy, including behavior modification, structured group therapy, and family therapy. If antidepressants are used as adjunctive therapy, the dosing schedule and desired and adverse effects are explained.

In an inpatient setting, the patient is supervised during mealtimes and for an hour afterward, with time limits set for each meal and a pleasant environment provided throughout. Contracts may be employed regarding amounts and types of foods to be eaten, and rewards established for satisfactory weight gain. The patient is encouraged to recognize and verbalize feelings about eating behaviors. Assertiveness training is provided to help the patient regain control over behavior and to achieve a realistic, positive self-image. The risks of vomiting behaviors, as well as emetic, diuretic, and laxative abuse, are described. Self-help groups and associations such as the American Anorexia/Bulimia Association are sources for additional support and information.

bulk In nutrition, a substance that absorbs water in the intestinal tract. The increased mass helps to stimulate peristalsis. Bulk materials, such as psyllium, are used to prevent constipation.

bulla (bŭl′lă) *pl.* **bullae** [L., a bubble] A large blister or skin vesicle filled with fluid; a bleb. SEE: illus.; *pompholyx*.

b. ethmoidalis A rounded projection into the middle meatus of the nose underneath the middle turbinated bone, formed by an anterior ethmoid sinus.

b. ossea The dilated portion of the bony external meatus of the ear.

bullous (bŭl′ŭs) [L. *bulla,* bubble] Like a blister or vesicle.

BUN *blood urea nitrogen.*

bundle A group of fibers. SYN: *fasciculus; fasciola.*

Arnold's b. The frontopontile tract. It passes from the cerebral cortex of the frontal lobe through the internal capsule and cerebral peduncle to the pons.

atrioventricular b. A bundle of fibers of the impulse-conducting system of the heart. From its origin in the atrioventricular node, it enters the interventricular septum, where it divides into two branches whose fibers pass to the right and left ventricles respectively, the fibers of each trunk becoming continuous with the Purkinje fibers of the ventricles. SYN: *A-V bundle; bundle of His.* SEE: *heart block.*

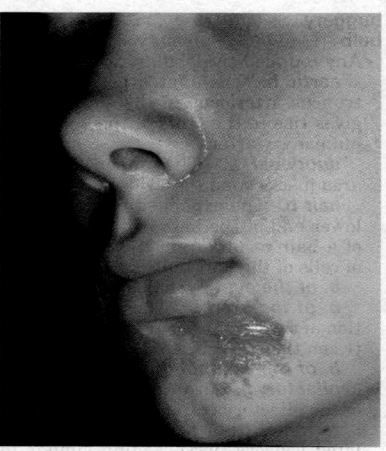

BULLAE OF IMPETIGO

A-V b. Atrioventricular b.

b. of His Atrioventricular b.

b. of Kent Kent's bundles.

b. of Türck The temporopontinus tract. Fibers pass from the cerebral cortex of the temporal lobe and terminate in the pons.

bundle branch block ABBR: BBB. Defect in the heart's electrical conduction system in which there is failure of conduction down one of the main branches of the bundle of His. On the surface electrocardiogram, the QRS complex is >0.12 sec. and its shape is altered. SEE: *heart block.*

left b.b.b. ABBR: LBBB. Defect in the conduction system of the heart in which electrical conduction down the left bundle branch is delayed. On the 12-lead EKG, it gives the QRS complex a widened QS complex in lead V_1 (0.12 sec.).

right b.b.b. ABBR: RBBB. Defect in the conductive system of the heart in which electrical conduction down the right bundle branch is delayed. On the 12-lead EKG, it gives the widened QRS complex an RSR appearance in leads V_1 and V_2.

bundling A mandatory system of drug distribution involving monitoring and reporting side effects to the U.S. Food and Drug Administration.

bunion (bŭn′yŭn) Inflammation and thickening of the first metatarsal joint of the great toe, usually associated with marked enlargement of the joint and lateral displacement of the toe.

ETIOLOGY: Bunions may be caused by heredity, degenerative bone or joint diseases such as arthritis, but most often are produced by tight-fitting shoes and high heels that force toes together and displace weight onto the forefoot.

Bunnell block An orthotic device used after surgical repair of flexor tendon hand injuries. It prevents flexion at joints proximal to the one being exercised during the rehabilitation regimen.

Bunsen burner (bŭn′sĕn) [Robert W. E. von Bunsen, Ger. chemist, 1811–1899] A gas burner in which air holes at the bottom of the tube can be closed or opened. If the holes are closed, the flame burns yellow and gives light but a relatively small amount of heat. If the air intake is adjusted, a blue flame is produced. This is the hottest, most efficient, smokeless flame that can be produced by the burner.

Bunyaviridae (bŭn″yă-vĭr′ĭ-dē) A family of viruses that includes a large group of arthropod-borne viruses. Diseases caused by these viruses include certain types of encephalitis, some types of hemorrhagic fevers, phlebotomus fever, and Rift Valley fever.

buphthalmia, buphthalmos (būf-thăl′mē-ă, -mōs) [Gr. *bous,* ox, + *ophthalmos,* eye] Infantile glaucoma resulting in uniform enlargement of the eye, particularly the cornea. The disease may stop spontaneously or continue until it produces blindness. Treatment is surgical. SEE: *glaucoma; hydrophthalmos.*

buprenorphine An opioid agonist/antagonist used to manage moderate or severe pain.

bupropion (bū-prŏp′ē-ŏn) An antidepressant medication that is also moderately effective in aiding smoking cessation, esp. when used along with cognitive and behavioral therapies. Trade names are Zyban and Wellbutrin.

Burch procedure, Burch colposuspension Surgery in which a sling is sutured around the urethra and neck of the bladder to the iliopectineal ligament. It is used to alleviate stress urinary incontinence in women.

PATIENT CARE: Vital signs, suprapubic catheter, and wound drainage are checked. The patient is helped to void as needed. Fluid intake and output is measured and recorded.

Burkholderia cepacia An aerobic gram-negative bacillus that thrives in liquids. This species commonly causes infections in hospitalized patients, esp. those in intensive care units and those receiving mechanical ventilation, and in persons with cystic fibrosis or chronic granulomatous disease. It is resistant to aminoglycosides and many cephalosporin antibiotics.

burp **1.** To belch. **2.** To hold a baby against the chest and pat it on the back to induce belching.

bur, burr (bŭr) A device that is held and powered by a hand-held dental motor. The bur rotates at high speed to cut or abrade tooth structure, bone, restorative materials, and other dental materials.

Burdach's tract (boor′dăks) [Karl F. Burdach, Ger. physiologist, 1776–1847] Continuation of the dorsolateral column of the spinal cord into the medulla oblongata. SYN: *fasciculus cuneatus.*

buret, burette (bū-rĕt′) [Fr.] **1.** A special hollow glass tube usually with a stopcock at the lower end. It is used in chemical analysis to measure the amount of liquid reagent used. **2.** A calibrated chamber used to ensure accurate measurement of small amounts of intravenous fluid and to prevent fluid infusion overload. The chamber is usually connected to a larger container of fluid.

Burkitt's lymphoma [Denis P. Burkitt, Ugandan physician, 1911–1993] A relatively undifferentiated lymphoblastic lymphoma that involves sites other than the lymph nodes and reticuloendothelial system. It is rare in the U.S but common in Central Africa, where the distribution suggests that environmental and climatic factors, such as insect vectors, are determinants. There is a strong association of this disease with the Epstein-Barr virus.

Bureau of Medical Devices ABBR: BMD. A branch of the U.S. Food and Drug Administration that regulates medical devices.

burn [AS. *baernan,* to burn] Tissue injury resulting from excessive exposure to thermal, chemical, electrical, or radioactive agents. The effects may be local, resulting in cell injury or death, or both local and systemic, involving primary shock (which occurs immediately after the injury and is rarely fatal) or secondary shock (which develops insidiously following severe burns and is often fatal). Burns are usually classified as:

First degree A superficial burn in which damage is limited to the outer layer of the epidermis and is marked by redness, tenderness, and mild pain. Blisters do not form and the burn heals without scar formation. A common example is sunburn.

Second degree A burn that damages epidermal and some dermal tissues but does not damage the lower-lying hair follicles, sweat, or sebaceous glands. The burn is painful and red; blisters form, and wounds may heal with a scar.

Third degree A burn that extends through the full thickness of the skin layer and often into underlying tissues. The skin has a pale, brown, gray, or

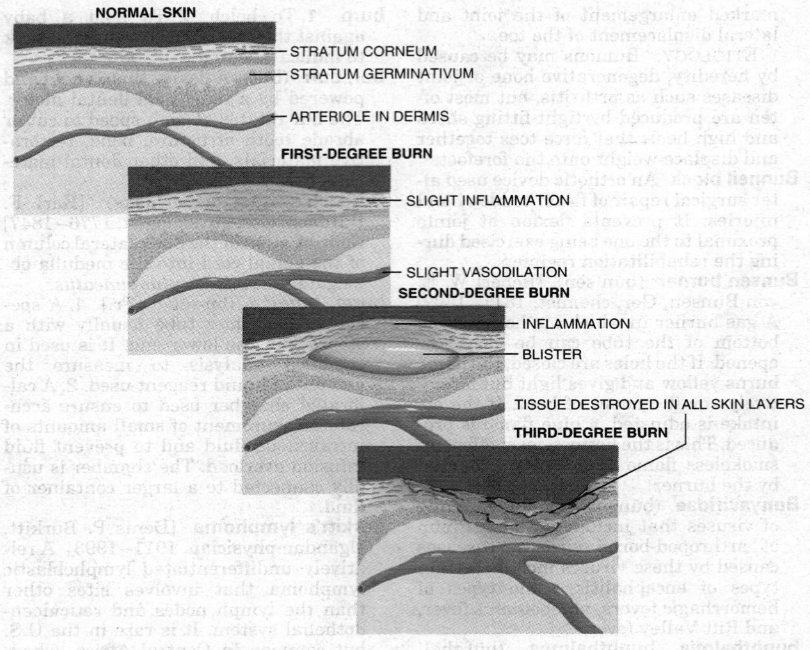

BURNS

blackened appearance. The burn is painless because it destroys nerves in the skin. Scar formation is likely. SEE: illus.

COMPLICATIONS: Sloughing of skin, gangrene, scarring, erysipelas, nephritis, pneumonia, immune system impairment, or intestinal disturbances are possible complications. Shock and infection must always be anticipated with higher-degree or larger burns. The risk of complication is greatest when more than 25% of the body surface is burned.

ETIOLOGY: Burns may result from ultraviolet radiation, bursts of steam, heated liquids and metals, chemical fires, electrocution, or direct contact with flame or flammable clothing.

PRECAUTIONS: A person in burning clothing should never be allowed to run. The individual should lie down and roll. A rug, blanket, or anything within reach can be used to smother the flames. Care must be taken so that the individual does not inhale the smoke. The clothing should be cut off carefully so that the skin is not pulled away. Blisters should not be opened, as this increases the chance for infection. All burned patients must receive appropriate tetanus prophylaxis.

NOTE: In severe, widespread burns, the patient must be transferred to a burn center as soon as is practical.

TREATMENT: The first responsibility in the care of the burn patient is to assess the patency of the airway and to ensure that breathing is unimpaired. If smoke inhalation or airway injury is suspected, intubation should be performed before edema makes this impossible. Airway injury is most likely to occur after facial burns or smoke inhalation in closed spaces. A cough productive of soot or charred material increases the likelihood of inhalational injury.

The second task in burn care is to ensure cardiac output and tissue perfusion. Volume resuscitation with crystalloid is given per standard protocols; at the same time, urinary output, blood pressure and pulse, body weights, and renal function are closely monitored to ensure adequate hydration.

The care of the burn itself involves the removal of any overlying clothing and the irrigation of the affected tissues, taking care to avoid excessively cooling the body. Gentle tissue débridement should be followed by application of nonadherent dressings, skin substitutes, topical antiseptics, or autografts, as dictated by circumstances. Tetanus prophylaxis is routinely given, usually with both tetanus toxoid and tetanus immune globulin.

In specific circumstances, additional interventions such as hyperbaric oxygen therapy for carbon monoxide intoxication, escharotomy for circumferential burns, antibiotic therapy for infections, pressor support for hypotension, or nutritional support may be needed.

Patients with large or complex burn injuries should be transferred to regional burn centers or to the care of surgeons with special interest in burn management.

PATIENT CARE: In the emergency care of the burn patient, the nurse actively participates in the assessment and management of the airway, breathing, and circulation; removes patient clothing; irrigates the burn wound; establishes intravenous access; sets up noninvasive oxygen and blood pressure monitors; and places Foley catheters (to monitor urinary output) and nasogastric suction (to decompress the stomach).

During the next stages of burn care, devitalized tissue is débrided, with care taken not to disturb blisters. Débridement is performed with aseptic technique. Appropriate antimicrobial ointments may be applied, and the wound is dressed with nonadhesive, bulky dressings. Prescribed tetanus prophylaxis, antibiotic therapy, and intravenous analgesics are administered, and the patient's response is evaluated. All procedures are explained, and noninvasive pain relief is provided.

Fluid balance is carefully monitored, as is nutritional therapy. Emotional support is offered to help the patient cope with altered body image or lifestyle concerns. Burned tissues are positioned per protocols to minimize edema and contractures. Therapies are instituted to prevent venous thrombosis, pneumonia, and complications resulting from immobility.

During rehabilitation, individually fitted elastic garments are applied to prevent hypertrophic scar formation, and joints are exercised to promote a full range of motion. The patient is encouraged to increase activity tolerance, obtain adequate rest, strive for physical and emotional independence, and resume vocational and social functioning. Referrals for occupational therapy, psychological counseling, support groups, or social services are often necessary. Reconstructive and cosmetic surgery may be required. Support groups and services are available to assist the patient with life adjustments. SEE: *Nursing Diagnoses Appendix.*

acid b. A burn caused by exposure to corrosive acids such as sulfuric, hydrochloric, and nitric.

FIRST AID: The burn area should be washed with large volumes of water. For further details of definitive treatment, see under *sulfuric acid poisoning.*

b. of aerodigestive tract Necrosis of the oral mucosa, trachea, or esophagus due to the ingestion of caustic substances. After an assessment of the patient's airway, breathing, and circulation, the medical team determines the severity of the exposure by physical examination or laryngoscopy. Some patients may require hospitalization for local care and the administration of intravenous steroids, histamine antagonists, and antibiotics. Late complications may include strictures of the affected internal organs.

alkali b. A burn caused by caustic alkalies such as lye, caustic potash (potassium hydroxide), and caustic soda (sodium hydroxide), and marked by a painful skin lesion, often associated with gelatinization of tissue.

TREATMENT: The burn is irrigated with large volumes of water and dressed.

CAUTION: Be careful to brush dry powder off the skin before applying water, as some chemicals, such as lye, react with water.

---

brush b. A combined burn and abrasion resulting from friction.

TREATMENT: Loose dirt is carefully brushed away and the area is cleansed with soap and water. An antiseptic solution or ointment is applied and covered with a dressing. Tetanus toxoid or antitoxin is given if required.

chemical b. Tissue destruction caused by corrosive or irritating chemicals such as strong acids or bases, phenols, pesticides, disinfectants, fertilizers, or chemical warfare agents.

electric b. Tissue destruction caused by the passage of electrical current through the body, usually as a result of industrial accidents or lightning exposures. Entry and exit wounds are usually present; significant internal organ damage may be found along the path of the current through the body.

fireworks b. Injury from explosives; usually a burn, often with embedded foreign bodies and a high incidence of infection and tetanus, which should be prevented by meticulous care of injury and use of antitetanus toxoid and immune globulin.

flash b. A burn resulting from an explosive blast such as occurs from ignition of highly inflammable fluids, or in war from a high-explosive shell or a nuclear blast.

gunpowder b. A burn resulting from exploding gunpowder, usually at very close range. It is often followed by tetanus, which should be prevented by administration of antitetanus toxoid and immune globulin and meticulous care of the injury area.

inhalation b. A burn caused by inhalation of flames or very hot gases.

This type of burn is suspected in all patients with facial burns or with singed nose hairs or elevated carboxyhemoglobin greater than 5–10 torr in arterial blood gases. A major complication is airway obstruction from edema of the air passages. SYN: *respiratory b.*

TREATMENT: The usual treatment is early intubation and ventilatory management with high oxygen levels.

b. of eye A burn of the eyeball due to contact with chemical, thermal, electrical, or radioactive agents.

FIRST AID: The eye should be washed immediately with the nearest available supply of water, even if it is not sterile. Irrigation may need to be continued for hours if burn is due to lye. Care must be taken to prevent runoff from draining into the uninjured eye.

radiation b. A burn resulting from over-exposure to radiant energy as from x-rays, radium or other radioactive elements, sunlight, or nuclear blast.

respiratory b. Inhalation b.

thermal b. A burn resulting from contact with fire, hot objects, or fluids.

x-ray b. SEE: *radiation burn.*

burner Trauma to the brachial plexus, marked by a fiery sensation in the neck that radiates down the arm, esp. when the neck is deviated from the involved side and the contralateral shoulder is depressed. This condition, which is esp. prevalent in contact sports, causes the cervical nerve root to become compressed between two vertebrae. Weakness and numbness follow the burning sensation but are usually transient. Repeated brachial plexus trauma can result in permanent neuropathy. SYN: *stinger.*

CAUTION: The presence of a vertebral fracture should be ruled out (e.g., with x-rays) before testing for brachial plexus trauma.

Burnett's syndrome [Charles Hoyt Burnett, U.S. physician, 1913–1967] Milk-alkali syndrome.

burning foot syndrome A painful sensation in the sole of the foot, usually caused by a peripheral neuropathy or myopathy. It occurs in certain vitamin deficiencies and in patients with chronic renal failure, due to build-up of uremic waste products.

burning mouth syndrome A burning sensation in one or several parts of the mouth. It occurs in the elderly and is generally related to menopausal or psychological factors. Identified causes are denture irritation, yeast infection, decreased salivary production, systemic factors such as nutritional and estrogen deficiencies, and sensory neuropathies. It is also called *oral dysesthesia*. Treatment consists of therapy for the causative condition.

burnish (bĕr′nĭsh) To condense or polish a metal surface with a smooth metal instrument.

burnisher (bĕr′nĭsh-ĕr) An instrument with a blade or nib for smoothing the margins of a dental restoration.

burnout **1.** Rendering unserviceable by excessive heat. **2.** A condition resulting from chronic job stress. It is characterized by physical and emotional exhaustion and sometimes physical illness. Frustration from a perceived inability to end the stresses and problems associated with this lack of power in the job contribute to the individual's loss of concern for patients or good job performance. Nurses are esp. prone to burnout, particularly those working in highly stressful conditions.

inlay b. Wax b.

wax b. Removal of an invested wax pattern from a mold by heating, thereby preparing the mold for casting metal. SYN: *inlay burnout.*

Burow's solution [Karl August von Burow, Ger. surgeon, 1809–1874] A solution of aluminum acetate; used in dermatology as a drying agent for weeping skin lesions.

burr SEE: *bur.*

burrow (bŭr′rō) A tunnel made in or under the skin (e.g., by an insect or a parasite). SEE: *cutaneous larva migrans*; *scabies.*

burrowing The formation of a subcutaneous tunnel made by a parasite or of a fistula or sinus containing pus.

bursa (bŭr′să) *pl.* **bursae** [Gr., a leather sack] **1.** A padlike sac or cavity found in connective tissue usually in the vicinity of joints. It is lined with synovial membrane and contains a fluid (synovia) that reduces friction between tendon and bone, tendon and ligament, or between other structures where friction is likely to occur. **2.** A blind sac or cavity.

Achilles b. A bursa located between the tendon of Achilles and the calcaneus.

adventitious b. A bursa not usually present but developing in response to friction or pressure.

olecranon b. A bursa at the elbow joint lying between the olecranon process and the skin.

omental b. The lesser peritoneal cavity; the cavity of the great omentum. It communicates with the greater or true peritoneal cavity via the vestibule and epiploic foramen.

patellar b. One of several bursae located in the region of the patella; includes the suprapatellar, infrapatellar, and prepatellar bursae. Some communicate with the cavity of the knee joint.

pharyngeal b. A small, median, blind

sac found in the lower portion of the pharyngeal tonsil.

subacromial b. The large bursa lying between the acromion and the coracoacromial ligament above and the insertion of the supraspinatus muscle below. It is also known as the subdeltoid bursa.

bursae (bŭr′sē) Pl. of bursa.

bursal (bŭr′săl) Pert. to a bursa.

bursalis (bŭr-săl′ĭs) [L., pert. to a bursa] Obturator internus muscle.

bursectomy (bŭr-sĕk′tō-mē) [Gr. *bursa,* a leather sack, + *ektome,* excision] Excision of a bursa.

bursitis (bŭr-sī′tĭs) [″ + *itis,* inflammation] Inflammation of a bursa, esp. between bony prominences and muscle or tendon, as in the shoulder and knee. Common forms include rotator cuff, miner's or tennis elbow, housemaid's knee (prepatellar bursitis), and bunion. SEE: *Nursing Diagnoses Appendix.*

TREATMENT: Therapy includes rest and immobilization of the affected part during the acute stage. Active mobilization as soon as acute symptoms subside will help to reduce the likelihood of adhesions. Analgesics, heat, and diathermy are helpful. Injection of local anesthetics or cortisone into bursae may be required. In chronic bursitis, surgery may be necessary.

PATIENT CARE: Rest is prescribed, and movement of the affected part is restricted during the acute phase if pain and limited range of joint motion are present. If pain and loss of function are severe and do not improve with rest, the patient is referred for medical evaluation; physical therapy may also be needed.

anserine b. Inflammation of the sartorius bursa located over the medial side of the tibia just below the knee. This causes pain upon climbing stairs.

bursolith (bŭr′sō-lĭth) [″ + *lithos,* stone] A calculus formed in a bursa.

bursopathy (bŭr-sŏp′ă-thē) [″ + *pathos,* disease, suffering] Any pathological condition of a bursa.

bursotomy (bŭr-sŏt′ō-mē) [″ + *tome,* incision] Incision of a bursa.

bursula (bŭr′sū-lă) [L., little sack] A small bursa.

b. testium The scrotum.

Burton's line (bŭr′tŏns) [Henry Burton, Brit. physician, 1799–1849] A blue line along the margin of the gingiva visible in chronic lead poisoning.

Buschke's scleredema [Abraham Buschke, Ger. dermatologist, 1868–1943] Generalized nonpitting edema that begins on the head or neck and spreads to the body. This lasts a year or less and leaves no sequelae. The cause is unknown. SYN: *scleredema adultorum.*

bush tea disease Veno-occlusive disease of the liver due to ingestion of highly toxic alkaloids present in some herbal teas.

buspirone (byu′ spī-rōn) An anxiety reducing medication that binds to serotonin receptors in the brain. It differs from other anxiolytics, in that it is nonaddictive, and is neither a benzodiazepine, a barbiturate, nor an alcohol. Common side effects of the drug include dizziness and drowsiness. Trade name is Buspar. SEE: *buspirone hydrochloride.*

buspirone hydrochloride An antianxiety agent that is neither a benzodiazepine nor a barbiturate. It has minimal central nervous system depressant actions, produces minimal sedation, and does not enhance the depressant effects of alcohol and other central nervous system depressants. The drug is used in treating short-term anxiety.

busulfan (bū-sŭl′făn) An antineoplastic agent used in treating chronic granulocytic leukemia.

butacaine sulfate (bū′tă-kān) A topical local anesthetic.

butane (bū′tān) C_4H_{10}; a gaseous, inflammable hydrocarbon derived from petroleum.

butt [ME. *butte,* end] To join the ends of two objects together.

butterfly 1. Anything shaped like a butterfly. **2.** An adhesive bandage used in place of sutures to hold wound edges together.

buttocks (bŭt′ŭks) [AS. *buttuc,* end] The external prominences posterior to the hips; formed by the gluteal muscles and underlying structures. SYN: *nates.*

button (bŭt′n) An anatomical or pathological structure that resembles a button.

button aid An adaptive device permitting button closure by persons with the functional use of only one extremity.

buttonhole An incision (sometimes inadvertent) into the wall of a cavity or membrane. This term may be applied to surgical procedures on hollow organ systems such as the gastrointestinal, urinary tract, and cardiovascular systems and to some of myocutaneous grafts.

butylene (bū′tĭ-lēn) A hydrocarbon gas, C_4H_8.

butyraceous (bū″tĭ-rā′shŭs) [L. *butyrum,* butter] Containing or resembling butter.

butyrate (bū′tĭ-rāt) A salt of butyric acid.

butyrin (bū′tĭr-ĭn) A soft, yellow semiliquid fat that is present in butter.

butyroid (bū′tĭ-royd) [″ + Gr. *eidos,* form, shape] Having the appearance or consistency of butter.

butyrometer (bū″tĭ-rŏm′ĕ-tĕr) [″ + Gr. *metron,* measure] A device for estimating the amount of butterfat in milk.

butyrophenone (bū″tĭ-rō-fē′nōn) A class of drugs, some of which are used to treat

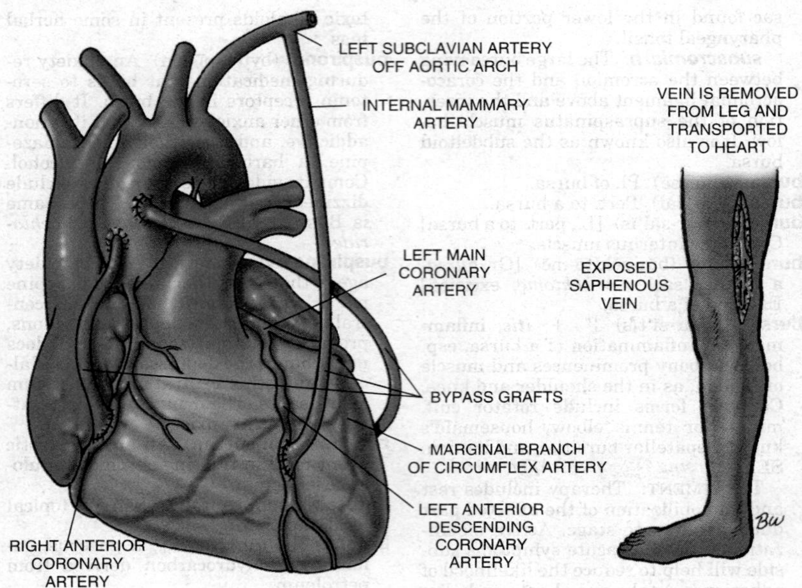

CORONARY ARTERY BYPASS

Anterior view of heart with sites of saphenous vein bypass grafts

psychoses, acute agitation, Tourette's syndrome, and other disorders. Tardive dyskinesia may be a side effect of prolonged use.

Byler's disease An inherited disorder in which infants develop cholestatic jaundice and, gradually, cirrhosis. A high incidence of retinitis pigmentosa is associated with this disease, and mental retardation is frequently seen in the children. Death from liver disease occurs by adolescence.

bypass A means of circumvention; a shunt. It is used surgically to install an alternate route for the blood to bypass an obstruction if a main or vital artery such as the abdominal aorta or a coronary artery becomes obstructed. The various procedures are named according to the arteries involved (e.g., coronary artery, aortoiliac, or femoropopliteal bypasses). The circulation of the heart may be bypassed by providing an extracorporeal device to pump blood while a surgical procedure is being done on the coronary arteries or cardiac valves. SEE: illus.

extra-anatomic vascular b. Surgical revascularization for peripheral vascular disease of the limbs, using a prosthetic graft (e.g., axillofemorally or femorofemorally) to divert blood to a site distal to an arterial obstruction.

PATIENT CARE: Postoperatively, it is important to monitor the patient's vital signs for changes, esp. of pulse and rhythm, and to assess the patient for symptoms of angina pectoris or arrhythmias. Cardiac monitoring and frequent ECGs are routine aspects of care. The surgical wound is checked for bleeding or hematoma formation, or signs of infection or dehiscence. Peripheral pulses are palpated using a doppler, if necessary, to determine peripheral perfusion.

jejunoileal b. A surgical procedure for decreasing absorption of nutrients from the small intestine by anastomosing the proximal jejunum to the distal ileum. Although it can be used to treat obesity, jejunoileal bypass has been replaced by gastric bypass procedures because of the significant complications of jejunoileal bypass surgery.

byssinosis (bĭs″ĭ-nō′sĭs) [Gr. *byssos,* cotton, + *osis,* condition] Reactive airways disease of cotton, flax, and hemp workers. Byssinosis is caused by the inhalation of dust and foreign materials, including bacteria, mold, and fungi. The disease does not occur in textile workers who work with cotton after it is bleached. It is marked by symptomatic wheezing and tightness in the chest. Symptoms are usually more pronounced at the beginning of each work week than later on. SEE: *pneumonoconiosis*.

byssocausis (bĭs″ō-kaw′sĭs) [″ + *kausis,* burning] Moxibustion.

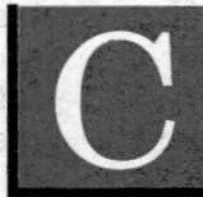

C **1.** Symbol for the element carbon. **2.** *Celsius; centigrade; cervical vertebra* (C1 to C7); *kilocalorie* (large calorie).

^{14}C Carbon-14.

c *calorie; centum* (a hundred); *circa* (about); *clonus; closure; compound; congius* (gallon).

c̄ [L.] *cum,* with.

CA 125 An antigen produced by tissues derived from coelomic epithelium. It is associated with various epithelial cancers, including ovarian cancer. It may be used to assess response to treatment in women with known ovarian cancer.

Ca Symbol for the element calcium.

CAAHEP *Commission on Accreditation for Allied Health Educational Programs.*

CABG *coronary artery bypass graft.*

Cabot's rings (kăb′ŏts) [Richard C. Cabot, U.S. physician, 1868–1939] Blue-staining threadlike inclusions of unknown origin, found in the red blood cells in severe anemia. They may appear as rings, figures-of-eight, or twisted. They seem to be parts of the nucleus, with histones and iron but no DNA. SEE: illus.

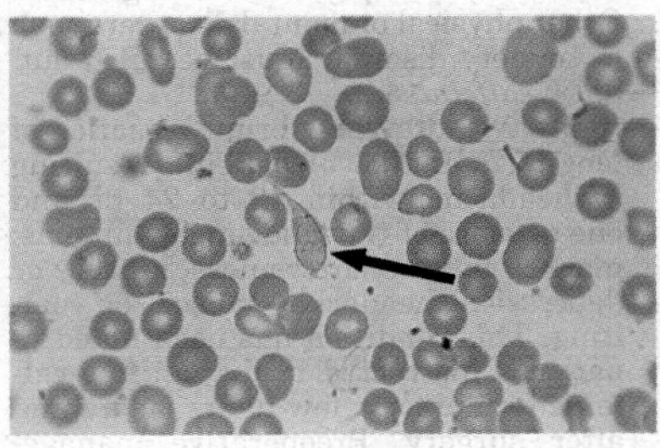

CABOT'S RING

(Orig. mag. ×640)

cac-, caci- [Gr. *kakos,* bad] SEE: *caco-.*

CaC_2 Calcium carbide.

cacao (kă-kā′ō, kă-kaw′ō) [Mex.-Sp. from Nahuatl *cacahuatl,* cacao beans] **1.** The seed of *Theobroma cacao* used to prepare cacao butter (theobroma oil), chocolate, and cocoa. **2.** A reddish to brown powder prepared from the roasted ripe seeds of *Theobroma cacao* (family Sterculiaceae), having a chocolate odor and taste. It is used as a syrup base, as a flavoring for certain medications, and in beverages and confections.

cachectin (kă-kĕk′tĭn) Tumor necrosis factor alpha.

cachexia (kă-kĕks′ē-ă) [Gr. *kakos,* bad, + *hexis,* condition] A state of ill health, malnutrition, and wasting. It may occur in many chronic diseases, malignancies, and infections. **cachectic** (-kĕk′tĭk), *adj.*

PATIENT CARE: Activities should be interspersed with frequent rest periods, and the patient's response to activity monitored to prevent fatigue. Oral hygiene is provided before and after eating. Small, frequent meals of high-calorie, high-nutrient, concentrated soft foods are offered along with fluids to reduce the effort required in eating. The patient is repositioned frequently to promote ventilatory excursions, to mobilize secretions, and to prevent skin breakdown. The skin is inspected for breakdown, and tissues are protected from pressure with flotation pads or mattresses and other assistive devices. When moved, the patient is handled gently and the joints are supported to prevent pain and pathological fractures. Assisted passive or active range-of-motion exercises are provided to maintain joint mobility. Elimination is monitored to prevent retention of urine or stools, and the patient is assisted with toileting. If incontinence occurs, steps are taken to protect skin integrity and to preserve the patient's self-esteem. Assistance is offered to the patient and family in coping with feelings about change in body image, illness state, and approaching death.

cancerous c. Wasting caused by cancer.

c. hypophysiopriva Panhypopituitarism.

malarial c. Wasting due to chronic malaria.

pituitary c. Panhypopituitarism.

cachinnation (kăk-ĭ-nā′shŭn) [L. *cachinnare,* to laugh aloud] Excessive, inappropriate, loud laughter. It may be associated with schizophrenia.

$CaCl_2$ Calcium chloride.

caco-, caci-, cac- [Gr. *kakos,* bad] Combining form denoting *bad* or *ill.*

$CaCO_3$ Calcium carbonate, precipitated.

CaC_2O_4 Calcium oxalate.

cacodylate (kăk′ō-dĭl-āt) A salt of cacodylic acid.

cacogeusia (kăk″ō-gū′sē-ă) [″ + *geusis,* taste] An unpleasant taste that may be associated with foods that normally taste good.

cacosmia (kă-kŏz′mē-ă) [″ + *osme,* smell] **1.** An unpleasant odor. **2.** Subjective perception of a disagreeable odor. SYN: *kakosmia.* SEE: *hallucination, olfactory; parosmia.*

cacumen (kăk-ū′mĕn) *pl.* **cacumina** [L. *cacumen,* summit] **1.** The anterior portion of the superior vermis of the cerebellum. SYN: *culmen.* **2.** The top or apex of a plant.

CAD *coronary artery disease; computer-assisted design; computer-aided dispatch.*

cadaver (kă-dăv′ĕr) *pl.* **cadavera** [L. *cadere,* to fall, die] A dead body, a corpse; usually applied to a body used for dissection.

cadaveric (kă-dăv′ĕr-ĭk) Pert. to or derived from a dead body (e.g., an organ for transplantation).

cadaverous (kă-dăv′ĕr-ŭs) Resembling, esp. having the color or appearance of, a corpse.

cadmiosis (kăd-mē-ō′sĭs) A form of pneumoconiosis caused by inhalation of and tissue reaction to cadmium dust.

cadmium (kăd′mē-ŭm) [Gr. *kadmia,* earth] SYMB: Cd. A soft bluish-white metal present in zinc ores; atomic number 48, atomic weight 112.40, specific gravity 8.65. It is used industrially in electroplating and in atomic reactors. Its salts are poisonous. SEE: *Poisons and Poisoning Appendix.*

caduceus (kă-dū′sē-ŭs) [L., a herald's wand] In mythology, the wand or staff that belonged to Apollo and was given to Hermes, or Mercury. It consists of two serpents entwined around a staff, surmounted by two wings, and is used as the medical insignia of certain groups such as the U.S. Army Medical Corps. Although the caduceus is sometimes used to symbolize the medical profession, the staff of Aesculapius is usually considered the more appropriate symbol.

caecum Cecum.

caelotherapy (sē″lō-thĕr′ă-pē) [L. *caelum,* heaven, + Gr. *therapeia,* treatment] Therapy using religion or religious symbols.

Caenorhabditis elegans A roundworm, about 1 mm long. It is the first multicellular organism for which the full genome was sequenced.

café au lait macules Pale brown areas of increased melanin in the skin. The sites are usually 0.8 to 8 in. (2 to 20 cm) in diameter with irregular borders. They appear in infancy and tend to disappear with age. These macules are occasionally markers for systemic disease including neurofibromatosis.

caffeine (kăf′ēn, kă-fēn′) $C_8H_{10}N_4O_2$; an alkaloid present in coffee, chocolate, tea, many cola drinks, cocoa, and some over-the-counter medicines. The amount of caffeine in these beverages varies from 40 to 180 mg in 6 oz (180 ml) of coffee, from 2 to 5 mg in decaffeinated coffee, and from 20 to 110 mg in 5 oz (150 ml) of tea. The caffeine in cola drinks ranges from 30 to 90 mg in a 360-ml (12-oz) serving. The pharmacological action of caffeine includes stimulation of the central nervous system and of gastric acid and pepsin secretion, elevation of free fatty acids in plasma, diuresis, basal metabolic rate increase, total sleep time decrease, and possible blood glucose level increase. Caffeine is considered an ergogenic aid in athletics because it tends to enhance endurance and improves reaction time. Adverse effects include drug dependence and withdrawal in some habitual users. SEE: *caffeine intoxication; caffeine withdrawal.*

c. and sodium benzoate A mixture of equal parts of caffeine and sodium benzoate. It is used as a central nervous system stimulant and headache treatment.

c. and sodium salicylate A mixture of caffeine with sodium salicylate, now rarely used, containing about 52% caffeine. It combines the actions of caffeine and salicylate. SEE: *sodium salicylate.*

citrate c. A mixture of equal parts of caffeine and citric acid; used as a respiratory and central nervous system stimulant.

caffeine intoxication The reaction that follows the ingestion of excessive caffeine, usually more than 250 mg. At least five of the following side effects are experienced: restlessness, nervousness, excitement, insomnia, flushed face, gastrointestinal disturbance, muscle twitching, diuresis, rambling flow of thought and speech, tachycardia or arrhythmia, and psychomotor agitation. Other physical or mental disorders such as anxiety disorder must be ruled out. SYN: *caffeinism.*

caffeine withdrawal Abrupt cessation of long-term intake of caffeine resulting in headache within 12 to 24 hr and one or more of the following symptoms: marked fatigue, drowsiness, anxiety or depression, headache, nausea, or vomiting. This condition has been noted in patients instructed to discontinue caffeine intake for a few hours before and after surgery. Preoperative management of persons at risk of developing these withdrawal signs should include either gradual withdrawal beginning several days prior to surgery or, if possible, continuation of caffeine intake preoperatively and postoperatively. SEE: *caffeine; coffee; tea.*

caffeinism (kăf′ēn-ĭzm) Caffeine intoxication.

Caffey, John (kăf′ē) U.S. pediatrician, 1895–1966.

C.'s disease Infantile cortical hyperostosis.

cage, Faraday A room or space entirely enclosed within a wire mesh to prevent electromagnetic interference with electronic devices.

cage, thoracic The soft tissue and bones enclosing the thoracic cavity.

CAH *congenital adrenal hyperplasia.*

CAI *computer-assisted instruction.*

cainotophobia (kī-nō″tō-fō′bē-ă) [Gr. *kainotes,* novelty, + *phobos,* fear] Cenotophobia.

caked breast Accumulation of milk in the secreting ducts of the breast following delivery. SEE: *breast.*

Cal large *calorie.*

cal small *calorie.*

calamine (kăl′ă-mīn) A pink powder, containing zinc oxide with a small amount of ferric oxide. It is used externally in various skin conditions as a protective and astringent, an ointment, or a lotion.

calamus scriptorius [L.] The inferior portion of the floor of the fourth ventricle of the brain. It is shaped like a pen and lies between the restiform bodies.

calcaneoapophysitis (kăl-kā′nē-ō-ă-pŏf″ĕ-zī′tĭs) [L. *calcaneus,* heel, + Gr. *apophysis,* offshoot, + *itis,* inflammation] Pain and inflammation of the posterior portion of the calcaneus at the place of insertion of the Achilles tendon.

calcaneocuboid (kăl-kā″nē-ō-kū′boyd) [″ + Gr. *kubos,* cube, + *eidos,* form, shape] Pert. to the calcaneus and cuboid bone.

calcaneodynia (kăl-kā″nē-ō-dĭn′ē-ă) [″ + Gr. *odyne,* pain] Pain in the heel.

calcaneofibular (kăl-kā″nē-ō-fĭb′ū-lăr) [″ + *fibula,* pin] Pert. to the calcaneus and fibula.

calcaneonavicular (kăl-kā″nē-ō-nă-vĭk′ū-lăr) [″ + *navicula,* boat] Pert. to the calcaneus and navicular bone.

calcaneoscaphoid (kăl-kā″nē-ō-skă′foyd) [″ + Gr. *skaphe,* skiff, + *eidos,* form, shape] Pert. to the calcaneus and scaphoid bone.

calcaneotibial (kăl-kā″nē-ō-tĭb′ē-ăl) [″ + *tibia,* shinbone] Pert. to the calcaneus and tibia.

calcaneum (kăl-kā′nē-ŭm) *pl.* **calcanea** [L. *calcaneus,* heel] Calcaneus.

calcaneus (kăl-kā′nē-ŭs) *pl.* **calcanei** [L.] The heel bone, or os calcis. It articulates with the cuboid bone and with the talus. SEE: *leg* for illus. **calcaneal, calcanean** (-kā′nē-ăl, -ăn), *adj.*

calcanodynia (kăl″kăn-ō-dĭn′ē-ă) [″ + Gr. *odyne,* pain] Pain in the heel when standing or walking; calcaneodynia.

calcar (kăl′kăr) [L., a spur] A spurlike process.

c. avis Hippocampus minor.

c. femorale A bony spur that strengthens the femoral neck.

c. pedis The heel.

calcareous (kăl-kā′rē-ŭs) [L. *calcarius,* of lime] Having the nature of lime; chalky.

calcarine (kăl′kăr-ĭn) [L. *calcar,* spur] Spur-shaped.

calcariuria (kăl-kăr″ē-ū′rē-ă) [L. *calcarius,* of lime, + Gr. *ouron,* urine] The presence of calcium salts in the urine.

calcemia (kăl-sē′mē-ă) [L. *calx,* lime, + Gr. *haima,* blood] Hypercalcemia.

calcic (kăl′sĭk) [L. *calcarius*] Pert. to calcium or lime.

calcicosis (kăl″sĭ-kō′sĭs) [L. *calx,* lime, + Gr. *osis,* infection] Pneumoconiosis caused by inhaling dust from limestone (marble).

calciferol (kăl-sĭf′ĕr-ŏl) Vitamin D_2. A synthetic vitamin D. It has the most vitamin D activity of those substances derived from ergosterol. It is used for prophylaxis and treatment of vitamin D deficiency, rickets, and hypocalcemic tetany. SYN: *ergocalciferol.*

calciferous (kăl-sĭf′ĕr-ŭs) [″ + *ferre,* to carry] Containing calcium, chalk, or lime.

calcific (kăl-sĭf′ĭk) [″ + *facere,* to make] Forming or composed of lime.

calcification (kăl″sĭ-fĭ-kā′shŭn) The process in which organic tissue becomes hardened by the deposition of calcium salts in the tissues.

arterial c. Calcium deposition in the arterial walls.

dystrophic c. The deposition of calcium salts in dead, dying, or necrotic tissues.

metastatic c. Calcification of soft tissue with transference of calcium from bone, as in osteomalacia and disease of the parathyroid glands.

Mönckeberg's c. Calcium deposition in the media of arteries.

placental c. The deposition of calcium in the placenta as a result of placental abruption, infarction, or aging. This form of placental degeneration may contribute to preterm labor and fetal distress. SEE: *abruptio placentae; infarction.*

calcific tendinitis Calcium deposition in a chronically inflamed tendon, esp. a tendon of the shoulder.

calcigerous (kăl-sĭj′ĕr-ŭs) [″ + *gerere,* to bear] Containing calcium or lime salts.

calcination (kăl″sĭ-nā′shŭn) [L. *calcinare,* to char] Drying by roasting to produce a powder.

calcine (kăl′sĭn) **1.** To expel water and volatile materials by heating to a high temperature. Lime is formed from limestone in this way by the removal of carbon dioxide. **2.** A powder produced by roasting.

calcinosis (kăl″sĭ-nō′sĭs) [L. *calx,* lime, + Gr. *osis,* condition] A condition marked by abnormal deposition of calcium salts in tissues.

c. circumscripta Subcutaneous calcification.

calcipenia (kăl″sĭ-pē′nē-ă) [″ + Gr. *penia,* poverty] Calcium deficiency in body tissues and fluids.

calcipexis, calcipexy (kăl″sĭ-pĕk′sĭs, -pĕk′sē) [″ + Gr. *pexis,* fixation] Fixation of calcium in body tissues. **calcipectic** (-pĕk′tĭk), *adj.*

calciphylaxis (kăl″sĭ-fĭ-lăk′sĭs) [″ + Gr.

phylaxis, protection] A state of induced tissue sensitivity marked by calcification of tissue when challenged by an appropriate stimulus.

calciprivia (kăl″sĭ-prĭv′ē-ă) [″ + *privus,* without] Deficiency or absence of calcium.

calcitonin (kăl″sĭ-tō′nĭn) A hormone produced by the human thyroid gland that is important for maintaining a dense, strong bone matrix and regulating the blood calcium level. In patients with medullary carcinoma of the thyroid, calcitonin levels are markedly increased and serve as a tumor marker. Given nasally, salmon calcitonin can be used to treat osteoporosis. SYN: *calcitonin hormone*. SEE: illus.

calcitriol The active hormone form of vitamin D that promotes the absorption of calcium and phosphate in the intestines, decreases calcium excretion by the kidneys, and acts along with parathyroid hormone to maintain bone homeostasis.

calcium (kăl′sē-ŭm) [L. *calx,* lime] SYMB: Ca. A silver-white metallic element; atomic number 20, atomic weight 40.08. It is a major component of limestone. Lime, CaO, is its oxide. Calcium phosphate constitutes 75% of body ash and about 85% of mineral matter in bones.

FUNCTION: Calcium is important for blood clotting, enzyme activation, and acid-base balance; it gives firmness and rigidity to bones and teeth; and it is essential for lactation, the function of nerves and muscles including heart muscle, and maintenance of membrane permeability. Most absorption of calcium occurs in the duodenum and is dependent on the presence of calcitriol. Dietary factors affecting calcium absorption include phytic acids found in grains, excess phosphorus consumption, and polyphenols found in teas. Approximately 40% of the calcium consumed is absorbed. Blood levels of calcium are regulated by parathyroid hormone; deficiency of this hormone produces hypocalcemia. Its serum level is normally about 8.5 to 10.5 mg/dl. Low blood calcium causes tetany, that is, muscular twitching, spasms, and convulsions. Blood deprived of its calcium will not clot. Calcium is deposited in the bones but can be mobilized from them to keep

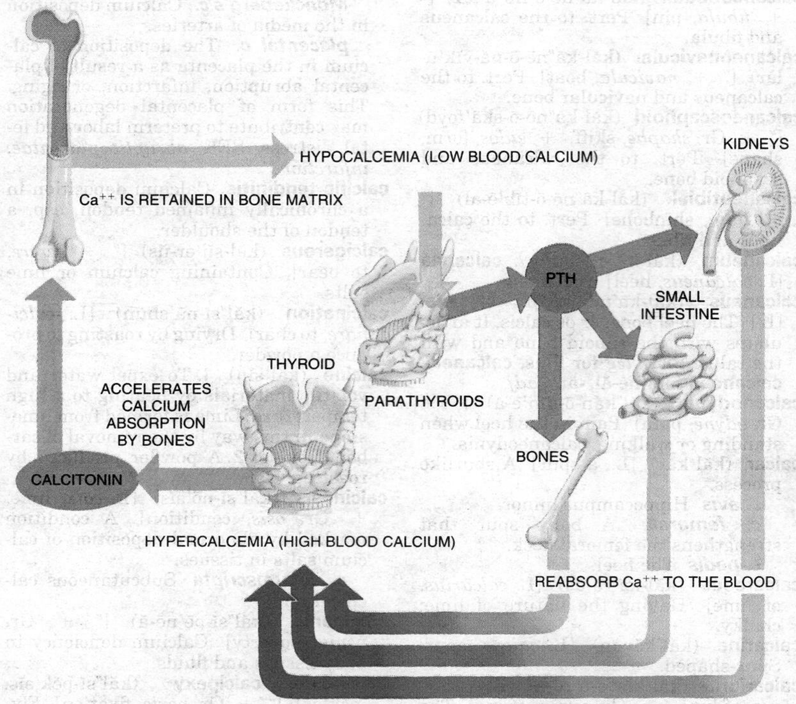

CALCITONIN

Complementary functions of calcitonin and parathyroid hormone the blood level constant when dietary intake is inadequate. At any given time the body of an adult contains about 700 g of calcium phosphate; of this, 120 g is the element calcium. Adults should consume at least 1 g of calcium daily. Pregnant, lactating and postmenopausal women should consume 1.2–1.5 g of calcium per day.

SOURCES: Excellent calcium sources include milk, yogurt, cheese (but not cottage cheese), calcium-fortified orange juice, and ice cream. Good sources include canned salmon and sardines, broccoli, tofu, rhubarb, almonds, figs, and turnip greens.

DEFICIENCY: The consequences of calcium deficiency include poor development of bones and teeth, osteoporosis, dental caries, rickets, and excessive bleeding. SEE: *osteoporosis; Recommended Daily Dietary Allowances Appendix.*

CAUTION: Laboratory error and variation may sometimes cause inaccurate or inconsistent values in evaluating the calcium level.

EXCESS: Hypercalcemia can cause constipation, renal stones, cardiac arrhythmias, cardiac arrest, and depressed brain function (e.g., lethargy or coma). High serum calcium levels are usually the result of either hyperparathyroidism or metastatic cancer and may be reduced with hydration, diuresis, corticosteroids, or biphosphonate drugs like pamidronate.

c. carbonate, precipitated $CaCO_3$; precipitated chalk, a fine, white, tasteless, and odorless powder used as an antacid and, in the past, as an antidote to corrosive acid poisoning.

c. chloride $CaCl_2 \cdot 2H_2O$; a deliquescent salt used to raise the calcium content of the blood in disorders such as in hypocalcemic tetany, calcium channel blocker, or beta blocker overdose. It is used in solution and administered intravenously. It is incompatible with epinephrine.

c. cyclamate An artificial sweetening agent. SEE: *cyclamate*.

c. disodium edetate A substance used to bind metallic ions, such as lead or zinc. It is used to treat poisoning caused by those metals.

c. gluconate A granular or white powder without odor or flavor used, for example, to treat hypocalcemia, calcium channel blocker, or beta blocker overdose.

c. glycerophosphate The calcium salt of glycerophosphoric acid. It is used as a dietary supplement and in formulating drugs.

c. hydroxide $Ca(OH)_2$; a white powder used as an astringent applied to the skin and mucous membranes and in dentistry as cavity liner or a pulp-capping material under a layer of zinc phosphate. It induces tertiary dentin formation for bridging or root closure, but may be related to a chronic pulpitis and pulp necrosis after pulp capping. SYN: *slaked lime*.

c. lactate A white, odorless, and nearly tasteless powder, less irritating than calcium chloride. It is used orally or parenterally as an alternative to calcium gluconate.

c. levulinate A soluble white powder formerly used to replenish serum calcium levels.

c. mandelate The calcium salt of mandelic acid formerly used to treat urinary tract infections.

c. oxalate A calcium-containing substance present in urine in crystalline form. It is a constituent of some kidney stones. SEE: illus.

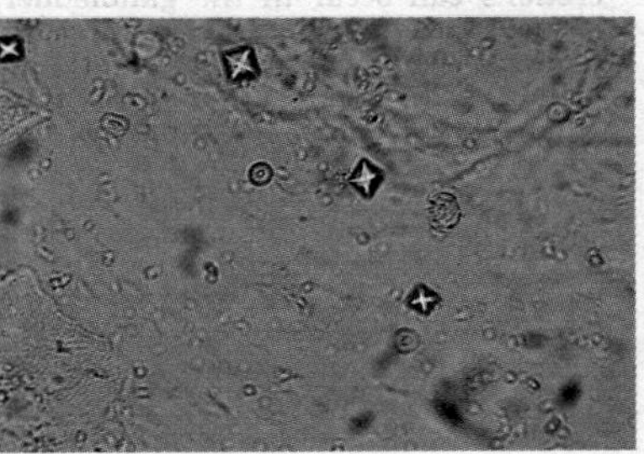

CALCIUM OXALATE CRYSTALS IN URINE

(Orig. mag. ×400)

c. oxide A corrosive and easily pulverized mineral occurring as a hard white or grayish-white mass. It is has been used as a germicide and disinfectant.

c. pantothenate One of the B complex vitamins. SEE: *vitamin B complex*.

c. phosphate, precipitated A white, amorphous powder used as an antacid.

c. saccharin An artificial sweetening agent. SEE: *saccharin*.

c. sulfate A white powder that absorbs water. It is used in making plaster of Paris.

total serum c. The sum of the soluble and protein-bound calcium in the blood.

c. tungstate A fluorescent material used for radiological imaging. It is used in intensifying screens to amplify the image, thereby reducing the radiation exposure to the patient.

calcium-45 (^{45}Ca) A radioactive isotope of calcium. It has a half-life of 164 days.

calcium channel blocker Any of a group of drugs that slow the influx of calcium ions into smooth muscle cells, resulting in decreased arterial resistance and oxygen demand. These drugs are used to treat angina, hypertension, vascular spasm, intracranial bleeding, congestive heart failure, and supraventricular tachycardia. Because hypotension occurs as both an intended and occasionally an unwelcome effect, blood pressure must be monitored especially closely during the initial treatment period.

calciuria (kăl″sē-ū′rē-ă) [″ + Gr. *ouron,* urine] Calcium in the urine.

calcospherite (kăl″kō-sfē′rīt) [″ + Gr. *sphaira,* sphere] One of many small calcareous bodies found in tumors, nervous tissue, the thyroid, and the prostate.

calculogenesis (kăl″kū-lō-jĕn′ĕ-sĭs) [″ + Gr. *genesis,* generation, birth] The formation of calculi.

calculous (kăl′kū-lŭs) Like a calculus.

calculus (kăl′kū-lŭs) *pl.* **calculi** [L., pebble] Any abnormal concretion, commonly called a stone, within the animal body. A calculus is usually composed of mineral salts. These pathological concretions can occur in the gallbladder, kidneys, ureters, bladder, or urethra, and are usually formed of crystalline urinary salts held together by viscid organic matter. SEE: *gallstone; kidney stone.*

ETIOLOGY: Renal calculi can be caused by abnormal function of the parathyroid glands, disordered uric acid metabolism as in gout, or excessive intake of milk, oxalates, and alkali. The cause of many kidney stones is unknown.

biliary c. Gallstone.

dental c. Mineralized dental plaque, located above or below the gums.

hemic c. A calculus formed from coagulated blood.

pancreatic c. A calculus in the pancreas, formed of calcium carbonate with other salts and inorganic materials.

renal c. A calculus in the kidney that may block urine flow. If the ureter is blocked by the stone, there is sudden, severe, and paroxysmal renal colic often with chills, fever, hematuria, and frequency of urination. If stones do not pass spontaneously, they should be removed.

TREATMENT: Pain relief should be a priority, as should forcing fluids unless passage is completely blocked by the calculus. Smooth muscle relaxants help in passing the stone and relieving pain. If the stone is preventing urine flow or continues to grow and cause infection, surgery must be performed. Alternatively, the stone may be disintegrated ultrasonically. SEE: *extracorporeal shock-wave lithotriptor; kidney stone removal, laser treatment for.*

salivary c. A calculus in the salivary duct. It usually affects the duct of the submandibular gland. The calculus obstructs the flow of saliva, causing severe pain and swelling of the gland, esp. during eating. Surgical removal of the stone is the treatment.

urinary c. SEE: *kidney stone; Nursing Diagnoses Appendix.*

vesical c. A calculus in the bladder, marked by increased frequency of urination, pain, and diurnal hematuria increased by exercise.

TREATMENT: An analgesic and antispasmodic should be used if necessary, and fluid intake should be adequate. Special urological, ultrasonic, or surgical procedures should be performed if the stone is large or impacted. These stones are usually small enough to pass through the urethra.

calefacient (kăl″ĕ-fā′shĕnt) [L. *calere,* to be warm, + *facere,* to make] Conveying a sense of warmth when applied to a part of the body; something that conveys such a sense.

calf (kăf) [AS. *cealf*] The fleshy muscular back part of the leg below the knee, formed by the gastrocnemius and soleus muscles.

caliber (kăl′ĭ-bĕr) [Fr. *calibre,* diameter of bore of gun] The diameter of any orifice, canal, or tube.

calibration (kăl-ĭ-brā′shŭn) **1.** Determination of the accuracy of an instrument by comparing its output with that of a known standard or an instrument known to be accurate. **2.** Measuring of size, esp. the diameter of vessels or the caliber of an orifice.

c. of instruments A procedure in which the mechanical functioning or electrical circuitry of a device is brought into alignment with a known standard. SEE: *calibration; calibrator.*

calibrator (kăl′ĭ-brā-tor) **1.** An instrument for measuring the inside diameter of tubes or orifices. **2.** A tool used to ensure that a laboratory device, test specimen, or sample matches known standards and performs accurately and precisely.

caliceal (kăl″ĭ-sē′ăl) [Gr. *kalyx,* cup of a flower] Pert. to a calix.

calicectasis (kăl″ĭ-sĕk′tă-sĭs) [″ + *ektasis,* dilatation] Dilatation of the renal calyx. SYN: *caliectasis.*

calices Pl. of calix.

Caliciviridae (kăl-ĭ-sē-vĭ′rĭ-dā) [L. *chalice, calyx,* "cuplike" appearance of viral particles under electron microscopy] A virus family that was previously classed as a genus in the family of picornaviruses. SEE: *Astroviridae; Calicivirus.*

Calicivirus (kăl-ĭs′ĭ-vī″rŭs) A genus of the family Caliciviridae that causes epidemic viral gastroenteritis in adults and children. Genera are classed in accordance with the geographic areas in which they have been identified. SEE: *Norwalk agent.*

caliculus (kă-lĭk′ū-lŭs) [L., small cup] A cup-shaped structure.

c. gustatorius Taste bud.

c. ophthalmicus Optic cup.

caliectasis (kăl″ē-ĕk′tă-sĭs) [Gr. *kalyx,*

cup of a flower, + *ektasis,* dilatation] Dilatation of the renal calyx. SYN: *calicectasis.*

californium (kăl″ĭ-for′nē-ŭm) [Named for California, the state and university where it was first discovered in 1950] SYMB: Cf. A chemical element prepared by bombardment of curium with alpha particles; atomic weight 251, atomic number 98. It has properties similar to dysprosium.

caligo (kă-lī′gō) [L., darkness] Dimness of vision.

caliper(s) (kăl′ĭ-pĕr) [Fr. *calibre,* diameter of bore of gun] A hinged instrument for measuring thickness or diameter.

calisthenics (kăl″ĭs-thĕn′ĭks) [Gr. *kalos,* beautiful, + *sthenos,* strength] An exercise program that emphasizes development of gracefulness, suppleness, and range of motion and the strength required for such movement.

Calliphora vomitoria (kă-lĭf′ĕr-ă) The common blowfly, whose larvae sometimes infest human wounds, a condition known as myiasis.

callomania (kăl″ō-mā′nē-ă) [Gr. *kalos,* beautiful, + *mania,* madness] **1.** A delusional belief in one's own beauty as a manifestation of mental illness or psychosis. **2.** Unrealistic attraction to something only because of its beauty.

callosal (kă-lō′săl) [L. *callus,* hardened skin] Pert. to the corpus callosum.

callosity, callositas (kă-lŏs′ĭ-tē, -ĭ-tăs) [L. *callosus,* hard] A circumscribed thickening and hypertrophy of the horny layer of the skin. It may be oval or elongated, gray or brown, slightly elevated, with a smooth burnished surface. It appears on the flexor surfaces of hands and feet and is caused by friction, pressure, or other irritation.

TREATMENT: Salicylic acid or careful shaving will remove the callosity temporarily. Removal is made permanent only by elimination of the cause. SYN: *callus.*

callosomarginal (kă-lō″sō-măr′jĭ-năl) [L. *callus,* hardened skin, + *margo,* margin] Pert. to the corpus callosum and marginal gyrus; marking the sulcus between them.

callosum (kă-lō′sŭm) [L. *callosus,* hard] Corpus callosum.

callous (kăl′ŭs) Hard; like a callus.

callus (kăl′ŭs) [L., hardened skin] **1.** Callosity. **2.** The osseous material woven between the ends of a fractured bone that is ultimately replaced by true bone in the healing process. SEE: *porosis.*

definitive c. The exudate, found between two ends of a fractured bone, that develops into true bone.

provisional c. A temporary deposit between the ends of a fractured bone that is reabsorbed when true bone develops.

calmative (kăl′mă-tĭv) **1.** Sedative; soothing. **2.** An agent that acts as a sedative.

calmodulins Intracellular proteins that combine with calcium ions to activate the contraction of smooth muscle and other processes.

calomel (kăl′ŏ-mĕl) [Gr. *kalos,* beautiful, + *melas,* black] Mercurous chloride.

calor (kā′lor) [L., heat] **1.** Heat. **2.** The heat of fever. It is one of the five classic signs of inflammation, the others being redness (rubor), swelling (tumor), pain (dolor), and loss of function (functio laesa).

Calori's bursa (kăl-ō′rēz) [Luigi Calori, It. anatomist, 1807–1896] The bursa found between the arch of the aorta and the trachea.

caloric (kă-lor′ĭk) [L. *calor,* heat] Relating to heat or to a calorie.

caloric test A procedure used to assess vestibular function in patients who complain of dizziness or exhibit standing balance disturbances or unexplained sensorineural hearing loss. With the patient supine, each ear canal is irrigated with warm (44°C) water for 30 sec, followed by irrigation with cold (30°C) water. Warm water elicits rotatory nystagmus to the side being irrigated; cold water produces the opposite reaction (i.e., nystagmus to the opposite side). SYN: *oculovestibular test; Bárány's caloric test.*

calorie (kăl′ŏ-rē) [L. *calor,* heat] A unit of heat. A calorie may be equated to work or to other units of heat measurement. Small calories are converted to joules by multiplying by 4.1855.

gram c. Small c.

kilogram c. Large calorie; one thousand calories.

large c. ABBR: C, Cal, or kcal. The amount of heat needed to change the temperature of 1 kg of water from 14.5°C to 15.5°C. It is commonly used in metabolic studies and in reference to human nutrition. It is always capitalized to distinguish it from a small calorie. SYN: *kilogram c.; kilocalorie.*

small c. ABBR: c, cal. The amount of heat needed to change the temperature of 1 g of water 1°C. SYN: *gram c.*

calorifacient (kă-lor″ĭ-fā′shĕnt) [L. *calor,* heat, + *faciens,* making] Producing heat.

calorific (kăl″ō-rĭf′ĭk) Producing heat.

calorigenic (kă-lor″ĭ-jĕn′ĭk) [″ + Gr. *gennan,* to produce] Pert. to the production of heat or energy.

calorimeter (kăl″ō-rĭm′ĕ-tĕr) [″ + Gr. *metron,* measure] An instrument for determining the amount of heat exchanged in a chemical reaction or by the animal body under specific conditions.

bomb c. An apparatus for determining potential food energy. Heat produced in combustion is measured by the amount of heat absorbed by a known quantity of water in which the calorimeter is immersed.

respiration c. An apparatus for measuring heat produced from exchange of respiratory gases.

calorimetry (kăl″ō-rĭm′ĕ-trē) The determination of heat loss or gain.

calsequestrin (kăl-sĕ-kwĕs′trĭn) A protein in the sarcoplasmic reticulum of muscle cells that regulates the concentration of calcium ions.

calvaria (kăl-vā′rē-ă) [L., skull] The domelike superior portion of the cranium, composed of the superior portions of the frontal, parietal, and occipital bones. SYN: *skullcap*.

Calvé-Perthes disease (kăl-vā′pĕr′tās) [Jacques Calvé, Fr. orthopedist, 1875–1954; Georg C. Perthes, Ger. surgeon, 1869–1927] A disorder marked by aseptic necrosis of the epiphysis of the head of the femur.

calx (kălks) [L.] **1.** Lime. **2.** Heel.

c. chlorinata Chlorinated lime. It is used as a deodorant and disinfectant.

calyces Pl. of calyx.

calyciform (kă-lĭs′ĭ-form) [Gr. *kalyx,* cup of a flower, + L. *forma,* shape] Cup-shaped.

Calymmatobacterium granulomatis (kă-lĭm″mă-tō-băk-tē′rē-ŭm) The gram-negative bacillus that causes granuloma inguinale. The presence of Donovan bodies in lesions is diagnostic.

calyx (kā′lĭx) *pl.* **calyces** [Gr. *kalyx,* cup of a flower] **1.** Any cuplike organ or cavity. **2.** A cuplike extension of the renal pelvis that encloses the papilla of a renal pyramid; urine from the papillary duct is emptied into it.

CAM *complementary and alternative medicine.*

camera (kăm′ĕr-ă) [Gr. *kamara,* vault] In anatomy, a chamber or cavity.

c. anterior bulbi The anterior chamber of the eye between the cornea and the iris.

c. posterior bulbi The posterior chamber of the eye between the iris and the lens.

camomile The flowering heads of the plant *Anthemis nobilis.* They are used in bitters to improve appetite and digestion and in alternative medicine as a tea. Hypersensitivity reactions to camomile may produce dermatitis, asthma, or anaphylaxis. SYN: *chamomile*.

cAMP *cyclic adenosine monophosphate.*

camphor (kăm′for) [Malay, *kapur,* chalk] A gum obtained from an evergreen tree native to China and Japan. Topically, as a 0.1% preparation, it is used as an antipruritic.

camphorated Combined with or containing camphor.

camphorated oil Liniment containing camphor.

camphor poisoning SEE: *Poisons and Poisoning Appendix.*

campimeter (kămp-ĭm′ĕ-tĕr) [L. *campus,* field, + Gr. *metron,* measure] A device for measuring the field of vision.

campimetry (kămp-ĭm′ĕ-trē) Perimetry (2).

campospasm Camptocormia.

camptocormia (kămp″tō-kor′mē-ă) [Gr. *kamptos,* bent, + *kormos,* trunk] A deformity marked by habitual forward flexion of the trunk when the individual is erect. SYN: *camptospasm*.

camptodactylia (kămp″tō-dăk-tĭl′ē-ă) [″ + *dactylos,* finger] Permanent flexion of the fingers or toes.

camptomelic dwarfism A condition in which infants have craniofacial anomalies, defects of the ribs, and scapular hypoplasia. The cause is unknown, and death usually occurs in the neonatal period.

camptothecin (kămp″tō-thē′sĭn) ABBR: CPT. An inhibitor of the enzyme topoisomerase I. Medications derived from this agent (including irinotecan and topotecan) are used to treat a variety of cancers.

camptospasm (kămp′tō-spăzm) [″ + *spasmos,* spasm] Camptocormia.

Campylobacter (kăm′pĭ-lō-băk′tĕr) [Gr. *kampylos,* curved, + *bakterion,* little rod] A genus of gram-negative, spirally curved, rod-shaped bacteria of the family Spirillaceae that are motile and non–spore-forming. One or both ends of the cell have a single polar flagellum.

C. fetus A species with several subspecies that can cause disease in both humans and animals.

C. jejuni A subspecies of *C. fetus* formerly called *Vibrio fetus.* It is the most frequent bacterial cause of gastroenteritis in the U.S. The disease is usually self-limiting. Treatment consists of fluid and electrolyte replacement and administration of the antibiotic to which the organism is sensitive. Infection with *Campylobacter jejuni* is strongly associated with Guillain-Barré syndrome.

Canadian Nurses' Association ABBR: CNA. The official national organization for professional nurses from the 10 provinces of Canada and the Northwest Territories. All services provided by the organization are offered in English and French.

Canadian Nurses' Association Testing Service ABBR: CNATS. An organization affiliated with the Canadian Nurses' Association that is responsible for administering the nursing licensure examination to graduates of approved nursing schools. Successful completion of the examination qualifies the candidate as a registered nurse. The examination is analogous to the National Council Licensure Examination (NCLEX) in the U.S.

Canadian Occupational Performance Measure ABBR: COPM. An outcome measure designed for use by occupational therapists to assess self-care, productivity, and leisure. The patient iden-

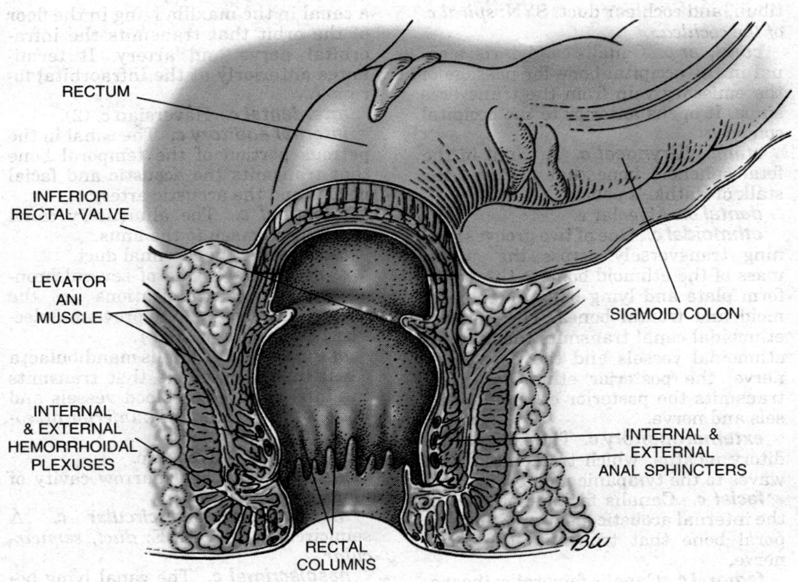

ANAL CANAL

tifies problems in daily function that are then measured on the basis of performance and client satisfaction.

canal (kă-năl′) [L. *canalis,* channel] A narrow tube, channel, or passageway. SEE: *duct; foramen; groove; space.*

adductor c. A triangular space lying beneath the sartorius muscle and between the adductor longus and vastus medialis muscles. It extends from the apex of the femoral triangle to the popliteal space and transmits the femoral vessels and the saphenous nerve. Also called *Hunter's canal.*

Alcock's c. Pudendal c.

alimentary c. The digestive tract from the mouth through the anus.

alveolar c. Canalis alveolaris; one of several canals in the maxilla that transmit the posterior superior alveolar blood vessels and nerves to the upper teeth. SYN: *dental c.; maxillary c.*

anal c. The terminal portion of the large intestine, its external aperture being the anus. This includes the internal and external sphincter muscles of the anus. The canal remains closed except during defecation and passage of flatus. It is about 1½ in. (3.8 cm) long. SEE: illus.

auditory c. One of the two canals associated with the structures of each ear. They are the external auditory canal, leading from the external auditory meatus to the tympanic membrane, length less than 1 in. (2.5 cm); and the internal auditory canal, leading from the structures of the inner ear to the internal auditory meatus and the cranial cavity. Both internal auditory canals transmit the nerves of hearing and equilibrium. SEE: *external auditory c.; internal auditory c.*

birth c. The passageway through which the fetus passes during delivery; specifically, the cervix, vagina, and vulva.

bony semicircular c. One of several canals located in the bony labyrinth of the internal ear and enclosing the three semicircular ducts (superior, posterior, and lateral) that open into the vestibule. They are enclosed within the petrous portion of the temporal bone.

carotid c. Canalis caroticus; a canal in the petrous portion of the temporal bone that transmits the internal carotid artery and the interior carotid plexus of sympathetic nerves.

central c. of bone The haversian canal of an osteon in bone.

central c. of spinal cord Canalis centralis; a small canal in the center of the spinal cord extending from the fourth ventricle to the conus medullaris. It contains cerebrospinal fluid.

cervical c. The anatomic portion of the uterus between the internal and the external os. SYN: *cervix uteri.*

cochlear spiral c. Canalis spiralis cochleae; a part of the bony labyrinth of the ear. A spiral tube about 30 mm long makes two and three quarters turns about a central bony axis, the modiolus. It contains the scala tympani, scala vestibuli, and cochlear duct. SYN: *spiral c. of the cochlea.*

condylar c. Canalis condylaris; a canal in the occipital bone for passage of the emissary vein from the transverse sinus. It opens anterior to the occipital condyle.

craniopharyngeal c. A canal in the fetal sphenoid bone that contains the stalk of Rathke's pouch.

dental c. Alveolar c.

ethmoidal c. One of two grooves running transversely across the lateral mass of the ethmoid bone to the cribriform plate and lying between the ethmoid and frontal bones. The anterior ethmoidal canal transmits the anterior ethmoidal vessels and the nasociliary nerve; the posterior ethmoidal canal transmits the posterior ethmoidal vessels and nerve.

external auditory c. The external auditory meatus, which transmits sound waves to the tympanic membrane.

facial c. Canalis facialis; a canal in the internal acoustic meatus of the temporal bone that transmits the facial nerve.

femoral c. Canalis femoralis; the medial division of the femoral sheath. It is a short compartment about 1.5 cm long, lying behind the inguinal ligament. It contains some lymphatic vessels and a lymph node.

gastric c. A longitudinal groove on the inner surface of the stomach following the lesser curvature. It extends from the esophagus to the pylorus.

haversian c. **1.** One of many minute canals found in compact bone that contain blood and lymph vessels, nerves, and sometimes marrow, each surrounded by lamellae of bone constituting a haversian system. SEE: *bone.* **2.** A canal in osseous tissue that carries a neurovascular bundle to the teeth, seen most often in periapical radiographs of the mandible. SYN: *interdental c.*

hyaloid c. Canalis hyaloideus; a canal in the vitreous body of the eye extending from the optic papilla to the central posterior surface of the lens. It serves as a lymph channel. In the fetus the canal contains the hyaloid artery. This normally disappears 6 weeks before birth.

hypoglossal c. Canalis hypoglossi; a canal in the occipital bone that transmits the hypoglossal nerve and a branch of the posterior meningeal artery.

incisive c. Canalis incisivus; a short canal in the maxillary bone leading from the incisive fossa in the roof of the mouth to the floor of the nasal cavity. It transmits the nasopalatine nerve and the branches of the greater palatine arteries to the nasal fossa.

inferior alveolar c. Mandibular c.

infraorbital c. Canalis infraorbitalis; a canal in the maxilla lying in the floor of the orbit that transmits the infraorbital nerve and artery. It terminates anteriorly at the infraorbital foramen.

interdental c. Haversian c. (2).

internal auditory c. The canal in the petrous portion of the temporal bone that transmits the acoustic and facial nerves and the acoustic artery.

intestinal c. The alimentary canal from the stomach to the anus.

lacrimal c. The lacrimal duct.

c. of Lambert One of several bronchoalveolar communications in the lung. These may help to prevent atelectasis. SEE: *pores of Kohn.*

mandibular c. Canalis mandibulae; a canal in the mandible that transmits the inferior alveolar blood vessels and nerve to the teeth. SYN: *inferior alveolar c.*

maxillary c. Alveolar c.

medullary c. The marrow cavity of long bones.

membranous semicircular c. A semicircular duct. SEE: *duct, semicircular.*

nasolacrimal c. The canal lying between the lacrimal bone and the inferior nasal conchae. It contains the nasolacrimal duct.

nutrient c. An opening on the surface of compact bone through which blood vessels gain access to the osteons (haversian systems) and the marrow cavity of long bones.

obturator c. An opening in the obturator membrane of the hip bone that transmits the obturator vessels and nerve.

optic c. The foramen through which the optic nerve passes.

pharyngeal c. A canal between the sphenoid and palatine bones that transmits branches of the sphenopalatine vessels.

portal c. The connective tissue (a continuation of Glisson's capsule) and its contained vessels (interlobular branches of the hepatic artery, portal vein, and bile duct and lymphatic vessel) located between adjoining liver lobules.

pterygoid c. Canalis pterygoideus; a canal of the sphenoid bone transmitting the pterygoid vessels, artery, and nerve.

pterygopalatine c. Canalis palatinus major, a canal between the maxillary and palatine bones that transmits the descending palatine nerves and artery.

pudendal c. A canal on the pelvic surface of the obturator internus muscle formed by the obturator fascia. It transmits the pudendal vessels and nerve. SYN: *Alcock's c.*

pulp c. The part of the tooth that extends from the pulp chamber to the apical foramen. It contains arteries, veins, lymphatic vessels, and sensory nerve endings.

root c. **1.** The passageway in the root of a tooth through which the nerve and blood vessels pass. **2.** Colloquially, the procedure for preserving a tooth by removing its diseased pulp cavity.

sacral c. Canalis sacralis; a cavity within the sacrum. It is a continuation of the vertebral canal.

Schlemm's c. The space or series of spaces at the junction of the iris and the cornea of the eye into which aqueous humor is drained from the anterior chamber through the pectinate villi.

semicircular c. SEE: *bony semicircular c.; membranous semicircular c.*

spinal c. Vertebral c.

spiral c. of the cochlea Cochlear spiral c.

spiral c. of the modiolus Canalis spiralis modioli; a series of irregular spaces that follow the course of the attached margin of the osseous spiral lamina to the modiolus. They transmit filaments of the cochlear nerve and blood vessels. The spiral ganglion lies in the spiral canal.

uterine c. The cavity of the uterus.

uterocervical c. The cavity of the cervix of the uterus.

uterovaginal c. The combined cavities of the uterus and vagina.

vaginal c. The cavity of the vagina. The vaginal walls can expand but are normally in contact with each other; thus, the cavity is a potential space.

vertebral c. Canalis vertebralis, the cavity formed by the foramina of the vertebral column. It contains the spinal cord and its meninges.

Volkmann's c. Small canals found in bone through which blood vessels pass from the periosteum. They connect with the blood vessels of haversian canals or the marrow cavity.

canaliculus (kăn″ă-lĭk′ū-lŭs) *pl.* **canaliculi** [L. *canalicularis*] A small channel or canal. In bone or cementum, radiating out from lacunae and anastomosing with canaliculi of neighboring lacunae. **canalicular** (-lĭk′ū-lăr), *adj.*

canalis (kă-nā′lĭs) *pl.* **canales** [L., channel] Canal.

canalization (kăn″ăl-ī-zā′shŭn) Formation of channels in tissue.

canavanine (kă-năv′ă-nĭn) An amino acid originally isolated from soybean meal. It prevents growth of some bacteria.

Canavan's disease An autosomal recessive disorder of infants, marked by spongy white matter with Alzheimer's type II cells. Also called *Canavan–van Bogaert–Bertrand disease.*

cancellated (kăn′sĕ-lāt″ĕd) [L. *cancellus,* lattice] Reticulated; said of a lattice-like structure.

cancelli (kăn-sĕl′ī) Pl. of cancellus.

cancellous (kăn′sĕl-ŭs) Having a reticular or latticework structure, as the spongy tissue of bone.

cancellus (kăn-sĕl′ŭs) *pl.* **cancelli** [L.] An osseous plate composing cancellous bone; any structure arranged as a lattice.

cancer (kăn′sĕr) [G. *karkinos,* crab] Malignant neoplasia marked by the uncontrolled growth of cells, often with invasion of healthy tissues locally or throughout the body. Cancer is the second leading cause of death in the U.S., after the cardiovascular diseases. More than 500,000 Americans die of cancer each year, and twice that number are newly diagnosed with cancer annually. The most common cancers in the U.S. are lung, breast, colon, prostate, and skin. Because most cancers occur in patients who are age 65 or older, the incidence of cancer is expected to increase as the population ages. More than 200 kinds of cancer have been identified. Cancers that arise from epithelial tissues are called *carcinomas;* from mesenchymal tissues, *sarcomas;* from lymphatic cells, *lymphomas;* from blood-forming cells, *leukemias.* SYN: *malignancy* (2). SEE: *carcinoma; leukemia; lymphoma; oncogene; sarcoma.*

Cancer cells have several reproductive advantages over normal cells. They can make proteins that stimulate their own growth or that stimulate new blood vessels to bring them nourishment. They can produce enzymes that prevent their chromosomes from aging. They can invade the bloodstream and find places to grow in new tissues.

Usually, as cancer cells proliferate, they become increasingly abnormal and require more of the body's metabolic output for their growth and development. Damage caused by their invasion of healthy tissues results in organ malfunction, pain, and, often, death. SEE: illus. (Cancer Statistics).

ETIOLOGY: Ionizing radiation, ultraviolet light, some viruses, and drugs that damage nucleic acids may initiate the genetic lesions that result in cancers. The best-known and most widespread type of carcinogen exposure, however, results from the consumption of tobacco. The American Cancer Society estimates that one-third of the cancer deaths that occur annually in the U.S. are related to nutrition and other lifestyle factors. Some cancers are familial (i.e., caused by genetic injuries that are transmitted from parents to offspring); others result from occupational exposures to cancer-causing agents. Ironically, cytotoxic drugs used to treat some cancers may damage chromosomes and occasionally cause secondary malignancies.

SYMPTOMS: Symptoms of widespread cancer include pain, malnutrition, weakness, fatigue, bone fractures, stroke-like syndromes, and many others. Early warning signs of cancer may

Leading Sites of New Cancer Cases and Deaths — 2000 Estimates

CANCER CASES BY SITE AND SEX

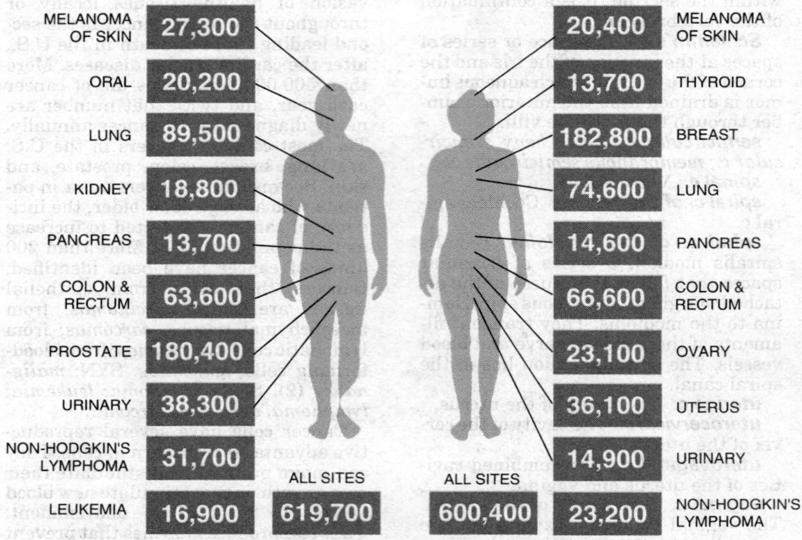

Excluding basal and squamous cell skin cancers and in situ carcinoma except bladder.

CANCER DEATHS BY SITE AND SEX

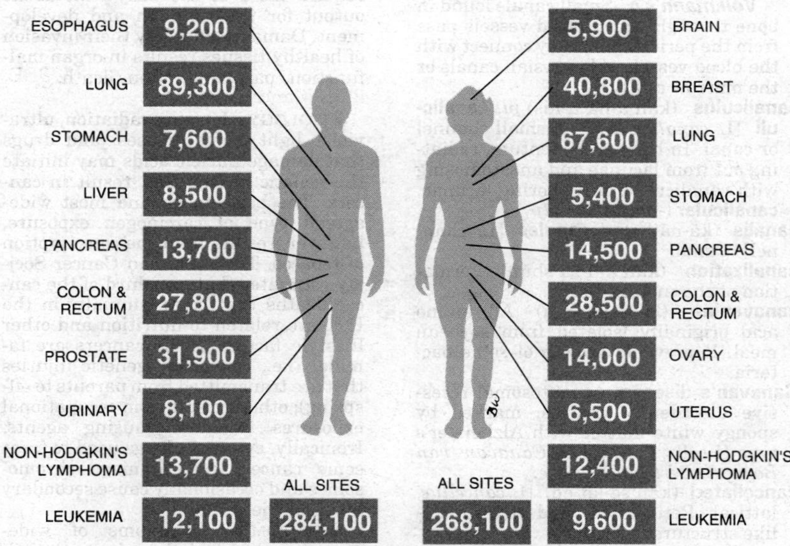

Source: Cancer Facts and Figures 2000, American Cancer Society.

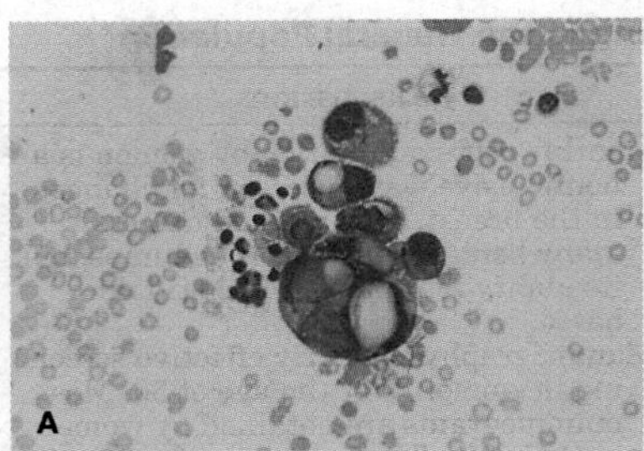

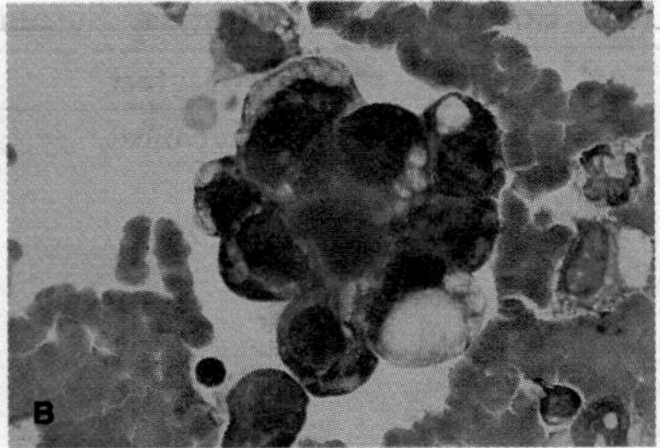

CANCER

Colon (A) and ovarian (B) cancer cells in peritoneal fluid (orig. mag. ×500)

be remembered by the mnemonic. CAUTION. *C*hange in bowel or bladder habit; *A* sore that does not heal; *U*nusual bleeding or discharge; *T*hickening or mass in the breast or other body parts; *I*ndigestion or difficulty in swallowing; *O*bvious change in a wart or a mole; *N*agging cough or hoarseness. Individuals should seek prompt medical attention if they observe any of these signs.

DIAGNOSIS: The location of a suspected lesion often dictates the modality used for cancer diagnosis. Endoscopy and radiography (such as x-ray studies, computed tomography, magnetic resonance imaging, ultrasonography, and mammography) typically are used to locate and assess the extent of the disease, but definitive diagnosis still rests on the examination of cytological specimens (e.g., Papanicolaou test) or the pathological review of biopsy specimens. SEE: illus. (Cancer); table.

Screening for cancers can identify some malignancies before they have invaded neighboring tissues or become widespread. The most widely used screening tests include the Papanicolaou test for cervical cancer, mammography for breast cancer, prostate specific antigen tests for prostate carcinoma, and occult blood tests for intestinal cancers.

TREATMENT: Surgery, chemotherapy, hormone therapy, radiation therapy, and combined-modality therapies often are effective methods for treating patients with cancer. The specific treatment used depends on the cancer's cell type, stage, and location, and the patient's general health.

The pain associated with cancer often is severe. Cancer patients also may suffer depression and significant anxiety, and have nutritional deficits. Guidelines for addressing these critical issues have been published widely, for example, by the U.S. Department of Health and Human Services' Agency for Health Care Policy and Research. Publications may be obtained by calling 1-800-4-CANCER or by accessing websites such as that of the American Cancer Society (www.cancer.org).

PATIENT CARE: Collaborative efforts of the entire health-care team must be coordinated, and participation of the patient and family in care must be encouraged. The patient's knowledge of the disease process is determined, misinformation corrected, and verbal and written information supplied about the disease, its progression, its treatment, and expected outcomes. The patient's and family's positive coping mechanisms are identified and supported, and verbalization of feelings and fears, particularly with regard to changes in body image, pain and suffering, and dying and death, is encouraged.

Assistance is provided with personal hygiene and physical care. Physical care is directed at the maintenance of fluid and electrolyte balance and proper nutrition. Nutrition is a special concern because tumors compete with normal tissues for nutrients and grow at their expense and because the disease or treatments can cause anorexia, altered taste sensations, mouth ulcerations, vomiting, diarrhea, and draining fistulas. Nutritional support includes assessing the patient's status and problems, experimenting to find foods that the patient can tolerate, avoiding highly aromatic foods, and offering frequent small meals of high-calorie, high-nutrient soft foods along with fluids to limit fatigue and to encourge overall intake. Elimination is maintained by administering stool softeners as necessary if analgesic drugs result in constipation.

Using careful, gentle handling techniques, the health care professional assists with range-of-motion exercises, encourages ambulation when possible, and turns and repositions the patient frequently to decrease the deleterious multisystemic effects of immobilization. Comfort is achieved through correct body alignment, noninvasive measures

Controversies in Cancer Screening in the General Population*

Test	To Detect	Discussion
Breast self-examination	Breast cancer	Monthly self-examination by women is a noninvasive way to screen for changes in the breast. This method detects many benign and cancerous lumps, but its ability to prolong life is still debated.
Mammography	Breast cancer	Mammography is clearly effective screening in women over the age of 50. Most mammograms are obtained by women in their 40s. The incidence of cancer is higher in later life, when mammography use tends to decline.
Digital rectal examination (DRE)	Colorectal cancer, prostate cancer	DRE is easy to perform and inexpensive, but its cancer screening value is small, and when it detects cancers, there is no proof the test results in better patient outcomes.
Fecal occult blood test	Colorectal cancer	Testing stool specimens for hidden bleeding detects many cancers, but whether it prolongs life is unproven. Its usefulness when contrasted with colonoscopy and sigmoidoscopy is debated.
Chest x-ray, sputum cytology	Lung cancer	Prospective studies have not demonstrated any value to screening for lung cancers with these tests, even among smokers. It is not known if other tests might be more effective screening tools.
Prostate specific result antigen (PSA)	Prostate cancer	PSA testing detects many previously undetected prostate cancers, but may result in increased death and disease due to complications from subsequent surgery. Refinements in its application may improve its usefulness as a screening tool.
Genetic testing	For predisposition to a variety of cancers	The predictive value of genetic testing for cancer is very small. Experts are debating the emotional and ethical consequences of genetic cancer screening tests.

* Note: Cancer screening tests are most likely to be useful when (1) the cancer is common and deadly; (2) the test reliably distinguishes between healthy and diseased people; (3) early detection of the disease leads to improved treatments; (4) treatments are safe and well-tolerated; (5) the psychological effects of test results are addressed sensitively and carefully; (6) the tests are applied to people who will truly benefit from them.

such as guided imagery and cutaneous stimulation, and prescribed pharmacological measures, preferably administered on a regular schedule to prevent pain, with additional dosing to relieve breakthrough pain. Emotional assistance includes decreasing the patient's fears of helplessness and loss of control; providing hope for remission or long-term survival, but avoiding giving false hope; and providing the patient with realistic reassurance about pain control, comfort, and rest.

Hospice care if needed is discussed with the patient and family. Family members are encouraged to assume an active role in the patient's care. Communication is fostered between patient and family and other health-care providers, and the patient is assisted to maintain control and to carry out realistic decision making about issues affecting life and death.

To provide effective emotional support to the patient and family, health care professionals must understand and cope with personal feelings about terminal illness and death and seek assistance with grieving and in developing a personal philosophy about dying and death. They will then be better able to listen sensitively to patients' concerns, to offer genuine understanding and comfort, and to help patients and family work through their grief. SEE: *Nursing Diagnoses Appendix.*

bone c. Any malignancy of bone tissue. Primary bone tumors (such as osteosarcomas) are rare in adults; they are seen more often in children and adolescents. Secondary or metastatic bone tumors are far more common. Tumors arising in other areas of the body that metastasize to the bones most often spread from organs such as prostate or breast.

cervical c. A malignant neoplasm of the cervix of the uterus (cervix uteri). With an incidence of 15:100,000, it is the third most common cancer of the female reproductive tract, and causes 5% of all cancer deaths among women. Although it may occur in younger women, the average age at diagnosis is 54. The disease is insidious, asymptomatic in the early stages, and best treated when recognized at an early stage.

ETIOLOGY: Some strains of the human papillomavirus (HPV), a common sexually transmitted infection, are carcinogenic to cervical epithelium. Along with other risk factors (such as tobacco smoking, early age at first intercourse, and having multiple sex partners), HPV plays a role in the development of cervical cancer.

DIAGNOSIS: Periodic Papanicolaou tests are recommended for all sexually active women. The tests identify cellular changes with 95% accuracy. Dilatation and curettage, punch biopsy, and colposcopy may be done if Pap test findings raise the suspicion of cancer. SEE: *Bethesda System, The; cervical intraepithelial neoplasia; colposcopy; cryosurgery; loop electrode excision procedure; Papanicolaou test.*

TREATMENT: Management varies from cryotherapy or laser therapy for low-grade squamous intraepithelial lesions, conization for carcinoma in situ, to hysterectomy for preinvasive cervical cancer in women who are not planning to have children. Stage-related management of invasive cervical carcinoma includes radiation and/or hysterectomy.

chimney sweeps' c. Cancer of the skin of the scrotum due to chronic irritation by coal soot.

colorectal c. Colorectal carcinoma.

hard c. A cylindrical cancer composed of fibrous tissue. SYN: *scirrhous c.*

head and neck c. Squamous cell carcinoma usually arising in the pharynx, oral cavity, or larynx.

lip c. A squamous cell carcinoma of the lower lip usually seen in men or smokers.

lung c. The deadliest form of cancer in the U.S., responsible for about 160,000 deaths annually. The term includes four cell types: squamous cell carcinoma, adenocarcinoma, large cell cancer, and small cell cancer. The vast majority are caused by carcinogens in tobacco smoke. Survival after diagnosis is poor—only one of seven affected persons lives for 5 years. Treatments include lung surgery, radiation therapy, and chemotherapy. SYN: *bronchogenic carcinoma.*

oral cavity c. Squamous cell carcinoma of the mouth or tongue. Oral cavity cancers are only rarely caused by salivary gland tumors or sarcomas.

ETIOLOGY: In patients over the age of 40, the disease usually results from exposure to tobacco smoke, chewing tobacco, and/or alcohol.

ovarian c. Any malignant growth in an ovary. About 85% to 90% of ovarian cancers arise from the surface epithelium of the ovary. In the U.S. about 25,000 new cases of ovarian cancer are diagnosed each year, most when the disease is already at an advanced stage because early detection of the disease is still unsatisfactory. Currently, more women die of epithelial ovarian cancer than of all other gynecological cancers combined. SEE: *inhibin.*

primary c. The original cell or tissue type from which a metastatic cancer arises.

scirrhous c. Hard c.

c. of unknown primary site Disseminated cancer in which the original tissue type is uncertain. Cancer of unknown primary site generally has a poor prognosis.

ETIOLOGY: Patients with cancer of unknown cell type are usually evaluated for tumors that might respond well to therapy, such as a lymphoma, a thyroid cancer, a germ cell tumor, or neoplasms of the breast or prostate.

vulvar c. Any malignant neoplasm of the vulva. Of these, 90% are squamous cell carcinomas and the remainder are caused by adenocarcinomas, sarcomas, or Paget's disease.

Vulvar cancer accounts for 4% of all gynecological malignancies. More than 50% of cases occur in postmenopausal women between 65 and 70 years of age. Generally, vulvar cancers are localized, slow-growing, and marked by late metastasis to the regional lymph nodes. Treatment may include surgery and/or radiation therapy. SEE: *vulvectomy.*

cancer cell A cell present in a neoplasm and differentiated from normal tissue cells because of its degree of anaplasia, irregularity of shape, indistinct outline, nuclear size, changes in the structure of the nucleus and cytoplasm, increased number of mitoses, and ability to metastasize.

cancer, chemoprevention of The use of certain foods and drugs to prevent the progression of preneoplastic and some neoplastic conditions. This topic is the object of extensive investigation.

cancer cluster The occurrence of a rare

type of cancer in a small geographical area (or a defined population) in much greater numbers than would be expected through chance alone.

cancer grading and staging The standardized procedure for expressing cancer cell differentiation, called grading, and the extent of dissemination of the cancer, called staging. This procedure is very helpful in comparing the results of various forms of therapy. Cancer is graded on the differentiation of the tumor cells and the number of mitoses present. These are thought to be correlated with the ability of the tumor to grow and spread. Some cancers are graded I to IV, the latter being the most anaplastic and having the least resemblance to normal tissue.

Cancers are staged according to size, amount of local spread (metastases), and whether blood-borne metastasis has occurred. There are two major staging systems. The TNM judges the size of primary tumor (T), evidence of regional extension or nodes (N), and evidence of metastases (M). Another system classifies cancers as Stage 0 to IV according to the size of the tumor and its spread.

It is not possible to determine the site of the primary malignancy for some metastatic cancers. The most frequent cell types are adenocarcinoma, melanoma, lymphoma, sarcoma, and squamous cell carcinoma. Even though the prognosis is poor for affected patients, their response may be improved if the cell type is specifically identified.

cancericidal (kăn″sĕr-ĭ-sī′dăl) [L. *cancer,* crab, + *cidus,* killing] Lethal to malignant cells.

cancerigenic (kăn″sĕr-ĭ-jĕn′ĭk) [″ + Gr. *gennan,* to produce] Carcinogenic.

Cancer Information Service A program sponsored by the National Cancer Institute that provides cancer information to patients and their families, health professionals, and the general public. Information may be obtained by calling the toll-free number 1-800-4-CANCER.

cancerogenic (kăn″sĕr-ō-jĕn′ĭk) [″ + Gr. *gennan,* to produce] Carcinogenic.

cancerophobia [″ + Gr. *phobos,* fear] Unreasonable fear of cancer.

cancerous (kăn′sĕr-ŭs) Pert. to malignant growth.

cancer screening A program to detect cancer before it causes symptoms or signs, esp. before it metastasizes and threatens life or health.

cancra (kăng′kră) Pl. of cancrum.

cancroid (kăng′kroyd) [″ + Gr. *eidos,* form, shape] **1.** Like a cancer. **2.** A type of keloid. **3.** Epithelioma.

cancrum (kăng′krŭm) *pl.* **cancra** [L. *cancer,* crab, creeping ulcer] A rapidly spreading ulcer.

c. nasi A gangrenous inflammation of the nasal membranes.

c. oris Gangrenous destruction of oral and facial tissues occurring as a consequence of an infection of the gums (necrotizing ulcerative gingivitis), usually with anaerobic bacteria or herpes viruses. The disease is most commonly found in children who live in extremely impoverished circumstances, are severely malnourished, have poor oral hygiene, or a recent measles infection. It is usually found in children from underdeveloped nations. SYN: *noma.*

c. pudendi Ulceration of the vulva.

candela (kăn-dĕl′ă) [L. *candela,* candle] SYMB: cd. The SI base unit of the intensity of light.

candicidin (kăn″dĭ-sī′dĭn) An antibiotic produced by certain species of *Streptomyces.*

Candida (kăn′dĭ-dă) [L. *candidus,* glowing white] A genus of yeasts that develop a pseudomycelium and reproduce by budding. *Candida* (formerly *Monilia*) species are part of the normal flora of the mouth, skin, intestinal tract, and vagina. SEE: illus.

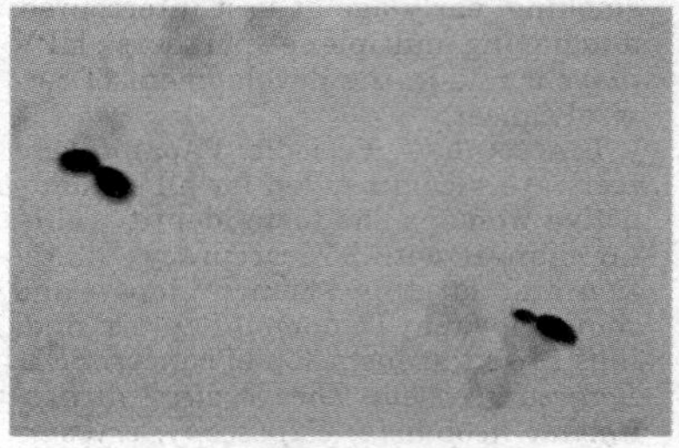

CANDIDA

Gram stain of *Candida* vaginitis

C. albicans A small, oval budding fungus that is the primary etiological organism of moniliasis (candidiasis). It was formerly called *Monilia albicans.* SEE: illus.

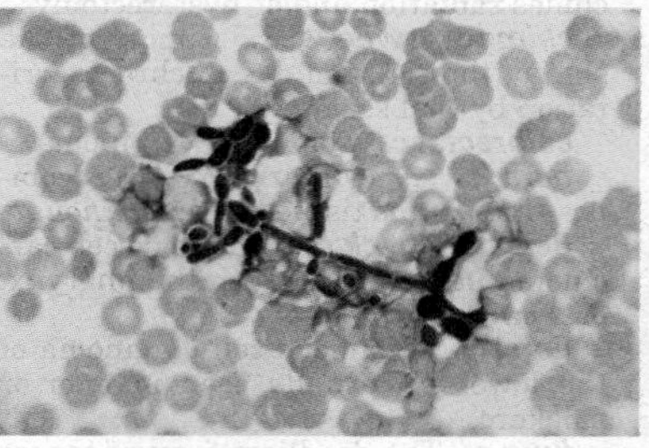

CANDIDA ALBICANS

C. albicans (purple) in blood (×640)

candidemia The presence of yeast from the genus *Candida* in the blood.

candidiasis (kăn″dĭ-dī′ă-sĭs) Infection of the skin or mucous membrane with any species of *Candida,* but chiefly *Candida albicans*. *Candida* species are part of the body's normal flora. *Candida* grows in warm, moist areas, causing superficial infections of the mouth, vagina, nails, and skinfolds in healthy persons. In patients with immunodeficiencies, central venous lines, and burns, or those receiving peritoneal dialysis, it can invade the bloodstream, causing disseminated infections. SEE: illus.; *normal flora*; *thrush*.

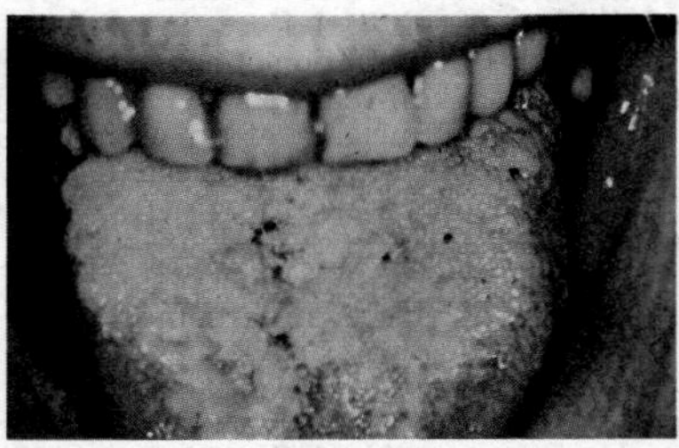

CANDIDIASIS

ETIOLOGY: *Candida* infections are due to a disruption in the composition of normal flora or a change in host defenses. Antibiotic therapy, which destroys the bacteria in normal flora, and inhaled or systemic corticosteroid therapy, which decreases white blood cell activity, are common treatments that may cause candidiasis. Vulvovaginal candidiasis is common during pregnancy, possibly as the result of increased estrogen levels. Infections of the nailbeds (paronychia) can occur in people whose hands are frequently in water or who wear occlusive gloves. Chronic mucocutaneous candidiasis is common in people with AIDS. In AIDS patients, systemic fungal infections may be present in any organ, including the brain, heart, kidneys, and eyes.

SYMPTOMS: Oral lesions (thrush) are raised, white patches on the mucosa and tongue that can be easily scraped off, revealing an underlying red, irritated surface. Skin lesions are red and macerated, and are usually located in skinfolds of the groin or abdomen and under pendulous breasts. Vaginal infections are characterized by a thick, cheesy discharge and itching. The symptoms produced in systemic infections depend on the extent of the infection and the organs affected.

TREATMENT: Oral candidiasis is treated with a single dose of fluconazole or with clotrimazole lozenges or nystatin oral solution (which must be held in the mouth for several minutes before swallowing) for 14 days. Topical forms of amphotericin B, clotrimazole, econazole, nystatin, or miconazole are effective for skin infections. Fluconazole is used for oral or vaginal infections in patients with AIDS. Amphotericin B is the drug of choice in treating patients with systemic infections unless they are neutropenic, in which case fluconazole is used. Some strains of *Candida albicans* are resistant to fluconazole. Pregnant women should consult their health care providers before taking or applying these drugs.

PATIENT CARE: Patients with thrush need clear explanations about the need to swish nystatin solution in their mouths for several minutes before swallowing to obtain maximum benefit. A nonirritating mouthwash and a soft toothbrush or sponge toothette are provided to loosen tenacious secretions without causing irritation. A topical anesthetic will help relieve mouth discomfort, and a soft diet may be helpful. The patient's intake should be monitored: mouth pain may interfere with nutritional intake, esp. in those recovering from surgery, trauma, or severe infection. The patient is weighed twice a week to assess nutritional status.

Patients who are obese or incontinent of urine are at special risk for *Candida* infection, esp. if they are receiving antibiotics. Skin folds should be carefully washed and dried, and antifungal cream or powder should be applied, usually 3–4 times a day. When possible, the affected area should be exposed to the air.

Patients with vulvovaginal candidiasis should be reminded not to wear constricting clothing such as pantyhose. If dyspareunia occurs, the patient is counseled that sexual impairment should resolve as the infection subsides, and to complete the full course of medication as prescribed. Although the sexual partners of infected patients usually will not need treatment, partners of patients with recurrent vaginal infections should be examined and treated if indicated to prevent ongoing reinfections.

Vital signs are monitored because of the risk of septic shock. Supportive care includes premedication with antipyretics, antihistamines, or corticosteroids to minimize hypersensitivity reactions if the patient is receiving intravenous amphotericin B.

candle (kăn′dl) [L. *candela*] A solid mass of combustible material such as tallow or wax in which a wick is embedded. When the wick is lighted, the wax burns slowly to produce heat and light. Candles can be used in bacteriology, where they are placed lighted in an airtight jar and allowed to extinguish themselves. This process produces an atmosphere containing approx. 10%

carbon dioxide. This carbon dioxide concentration is required for culturing certain organisms, particularly *Neisseria gonorrhoeae*.

cane (kān) An assistive device prescribed to provide support during ambulation and transfers for individuals with weakness, instability, pain, or balance loss. It also may be used to unload a lower extremity joint or to partially eliminate weight-bearing. Standard (conventional) canes are made from wood or aluminum and have a variety of hand grip styles. Other styles include tripod canes, quadruped (quad) canes, and walk ("hemi") canes.

canine (kā′nīn) [L. *caninus,* dog] **1.** Pert. to a dog. **2.** A canine tooth; any of the four teeth, also known as the eyeteeth (upper and lower), between the incisors and molars. SEE: *dentition* for illus.

canities (kăn-ĭsh′ē-ēz) [L., gray hair] Congenital (rare) or acquired whiteness of the hair. The acquired form may develop rapidly or slowly and be partial or complete.

c. unguium Gray or white streaks in the nails. SYN: *leukonychia*.

cannabis sativa (kăn′ă-bĭs) [Gr. *kannabis,* hemp] Marijuana.

cannibalism The human consumption of human flesh. SEE: *kuru*.

cannula (kăn′ū-lă) [L., a small reed] A tube or sheath enclosing a trocar; the tube allowing the escape of fluid after withdrawal of the trocar from the body.

nasal c. Tubing used to deliver oxygen at levels from 1 to 6 L/min. The nasal prongs of the cannula extend approx. 1 cm into each naris and are connected to a common tube, which is then connected to the oxygen source. It is used in situations such as cardiac disease, in which a low-flow, small-percentage oxygen therapy is desirable. The exact percentage of oxygen delivered to the patient varies with respiratory rate and other factors.

cannulate (kăn′ū-lāt) To introduce a cannula through a passageway.

cannulation of large veins, venous cannulation Gaining access to venous circulation by placing a flexible catheter into one of the large veins, usually the femoral, subclavian, or jugular vein. The cannula may be used to provide hyperalimentation; to administer drugs; or to replace fluids, among other uses.

CAUTION: Potential complications of venous cannulation include bleeding, infection, pneumothorax, arterial puncture, and injury to internal organs, among others.

cantharides (kăn-thăr′ĭ-dēz) *sing.,* **cantharis** [Gr. *kantharis,* beetle, + *eidos,* form, shape] Dried insects of the species *Cantharis vesicatoria;* poisonous if taken internally in large doses. It was formerly used externally as a counterirritant and vesicant, and internally for its supposed aphrodisiac effect. It is no longer used. SYN: *Spanish fly*. **cantharidal** (-thăr′ĭ-dăl), *adj.*

Cantharis (kăn′thă-rĭs) A genus of beetles, *C. vesicatoria,* known as Spanish fly. SEE: *cantharides*.

canthectomy (kăn-thĕk′tō-mē) [Gr. *kanthos,* angle, + *ektome,* excision] Excision of a canthus.

canthi (kăn′thī) Pl. of canthus.

canthitis (kăn-thī′tĭs) [″ + *itis,* inflammation] Inflammation of a canthus.

cantholysis (kăn-thŏl′ĭ-sĭs) [″ + *lysis,* dissolution] Incision of an optic canthus of an eye to widen the palpebral slit.

canthoplasty (kăn′thō-plăs″tē) [″ + *plassein,* to form] **1.** Plastic surgery of an optic canthus. **2.** Enlargement of the palpebral fissure by division of the external canthus.

canthorrhaphy (kăn-thor′ă-fē) [″ + *rhaphe,* seam, ridge] Suturing of a canthus.

canthotomy (kăn-thŏt′ō-mē) [″ + *tome,* incision] Surgical division of a canthus.

canthus (kăn′thŭs) *pl.* **canthi** [Gr. *kanthos,* angle] The angle at either end of the slit between the eyelids; the external canthus (commissura palpebrarum lateralis) and the internal canthus (commissura palpebrarum medialis). **canthal** (-thăl), *adj.*

CaO Calcium oxide.

CaO_2 The content of oxygen in arterial blood.

$Ca(OH)_2$ Calcium hydroxide.

C.A.O.T. *Canadian Association of Occupational Therapists.*

cap (kăp) [LL. *cappa,* hood] **1.** A covering. SYN: *tegmentum*. **2.** The first part of the duodenum. SYN: *pyloric cap*. **3.** The protective covering of a developing tooth. **4.** The artificial covering of a tooth, used for cosmetic reasons. SEE: *enamel organ*.

cradle c. Seborrheic dermatitis of the newborn, usually appearing on the scalp, face, and head. Thick, yellowish, crusted lesions develop on the scalp, and scaling, papules, or fissuring appears behind the ears and on the face. SEE: *seborrhea*.

TREATMENT: The head is cleansed with a mild shampoo daily. Corticosteroid cream is applied to the affected area twice daily.

knee c. Patella.

cap [L.] *capiat,* let (the patient) take.

CAP *College of American Pathologists.*

capacitance (kă-păs′ĭ-tăns) [L. *capacitas,* holding] **1.** The ability to store an electrical charge. **2.** The ratio of the charge transferred between a pair of conductors to the potential difference between the conductors.

capacitation (kă-păs″ĭ-tā′shŭn) A natural process that helps sperm cells to fertilize ova. As they travel through the female reproductive tract, the plasma membranes of sperm cells break down, exposing the acrosomes to the acidic environment surrounding the corona radiata of the ovum. This attracts the sperm to the ovum and releases spermatic enzymes responsible for penetration. The process requires about 7 hr.

capacitor (kă-păs′ĭ-tor) An electronic device for storing electric charges.

capacity **1.** The potential ability to contain; the potential power to do something. **2.** Cubic content. **3.** The ability to perform mentally. **4.** The measure of the electrical output of a generator.

forced vital c. ABBR: FVC. The volume of gas exhaled from the completely inflated lungs during a maximal expiratory effort.

PATIENT CARE: Patients with a significantly reduced vital capacity are prone to respiratory failure, esp. during the immediate postoperative period.

maximum aerobic c. ABBR: $VO_{2\ max}$ BP. The maximum amount of physiological work that an individual can do, as measured by oxygen consumption. $VO_{2\ max}$ is determined by the combination of aging and cardiovascular conditioning and is associated with the efficiency of oxygen extraction in the tissues.

timed vital c. A test of vital capacity of the lungs expressed with respect to the volume of air that can be quickly and forcibly breathed out in a certain amount of time. SEE: FEV_1.

total lung c. ABBR: TLC. The volume of air in the lungs after a maximal inspiration. This amount is important in evaluating the ability of the lung to exchange oxygen and carbon dioxide. SEE: *pulmonary function test; vital c.; volume, residual*.

vital c. The volume of air that can be exhaled from the lungs after a maximal inspiration. This amount is important in evaluating the ability of the lung to exchange oxygen and carbon dioxide. SEE: *pulmonary function test; total lung c.; volume, residual*.

CAPD *continuous ambulatory peritoneal dialysis*.

Capdepont-Hodge syndrome Dentinogenesis imperfecta.

capeline (kăp′ĕ-lĭn) [Fr., a hat] A bandage used for the head or for the stump of an amputated limb.

Capgras' syndrome [Jean Marie Joseph Capgras, Fr. psychiatrist, 1873–1950] The patient's delusion that a close relative or friend has been replaced by an impostor.

capillarectasia (kăp″ĭ-lăr″ĕk-tā′sē-ă) [L. *capillaris,* hairlike, + Gr. *ektasis,* dilatation] Distention of capillary vessels.

Capillaria (kăp″ĭ-lăr′ē-ă) A genus of parasitic nematodes.

C. philippinensis A species of roundworm discovered in the Philippines. It causes severe diarrhea, malabsorption, and enteric protein loss in humans; mortality is high.

capillariasis (kăp″ĭ-lă-rī′ă-sĭs) [*Capillaria* + Gr. *-iasis,* condition] A disease, first described in 1968, caused by infestation of the small bowel with the roundworm *Capillaria*. Treatment is with thiabendazole or albendazole.

capillaritis (kăp″ĭ-lăr-ī′tĭs) [″ + Gr. *itis,* inflammation] Telangiitis.

capillarity (kăp″ĭ-lăr′ĭ-tē) Capillary action.

capillaropathy (kăp″ĭ-lăr-ŏp′ă-thē) [″ + Gr. *pathos,* disease] A capillary disorder or disease.

capillaroscopy (kăp″ĭ-lăr-ŏs′kō-pē) [″ + Gr. *skopein,* to examine] Examination of capillaries for diagnostic purposes.

capillary (kăp′ĭ-lăr″ē) *pl.* **capillaries** [L. *capillaris,* hairlike] **1.** Any of the minute blood vessels, averaging 0.008 mm in diameter, that connect the ends of the smallest arteries (arterioles) with the beginnings of the smallest veins (venules). **2.** Pert. to a hair; hairlike.

arterial c. One of the very small vessels that are the terminal branches of the arterioles or metarterioles.

bile c. One of the intercellular biliary passageways that convey bile from liver cells to the interlobular bile ducts. Also called *bile canaliculus*.

blood c. One of the minute blood vessels that convey blood from the arterioles to the venules and form an anastomosing network that brings the blood into intimate relationship with the tissue cells. Its wall consists of a single layer of squamous cells (endothelium) through which oxygen diffuses to the tissue and products of metabolic activity enter the bloodstream. Blood capillaries average about 8 μm in diameter.

venous c. One of the minute vessels that convey blood from a capillary network into the small veins (venules).

capillary attraction Capillary action.

capillary nail refill test Blanch test.

capillus (kă-pĭl′ŭs) *pl.* **capilli** [L., a hair] **1.** A hair, esp. of the head. **2.** A filament. **3.** A hair's breadth.

capital (căp′ĭ-tăl) [L. *capitalis*] Pert. to the head.

capital punishment Sentencing a criminal to death and carrying out the sentence via a legal method such as hanging, electrocution, or lethal injection.

capitate (kăp′ĭ-tāt) [L. *caput,* head] Head-shaped; having a rounded extremity.

capitation (kăp″ĭ-tā′shŭn) A form of reimbursement for health care services in which the health insurer assigns a finite number of patients to the care of a subcontracting provider. The health care provider is paid a predetermined amount for each patient enrolled in his or her care. This arrangement provides incentives to the provider to limit health care costs, by placing the provider at financial risk if the cost of care provided exceeds the payment received.

capitation fee (kăp″ĭ-tā′shŭn) The amount paid a physician annually from each patient in a medical group plan.

capitatum (kăp″ĭ-tā′tŭm) Os capitatum; the third bone in the distal row of the carpus (i.e., the wrist). SYN: *os magnum*.

capitellum (kăp″ĭ-tĕl′ŭm) [L., small head] The round eminence at the lower end of the humerus articulating with the radius; the radial head of the humerus. SYN: *capitulum humeri*.

capitular (kă-pĭt′ū-lăr) Pert. to a capitulum.

capitulum (kă-pĭt′ū-lŭm, -pĭch′ŭ-lŭm) *pl.* **capitula** [L., small head] A small, rounded articular end of a bone.

c. fibulae The proximal extremity or head of the fibula. It articulates with the tibia.

c. humeri Capitellum.

c. mallei In the middle ear, the head (the large rounded extremity) of the malleus. It carries the facet for the incus.

c. stapedis The head of the stapes. It articulates with the lenticular process of the incus of the middle ear.

Caplan's syndrome [Anthony Caplan, Brit. physician, 1907–1976] Rheumatoid arthritis and pneumoconiosis with progressive massive fibrosis of the lung in coal workers. SYN: *pneumoconiosis*.

Capnocytophaga A genus of gram-negative, facultative, anaerobic bacteria that may be isolated from the oral cavity of humans and canines and are associated with serious systemic infections, esp. in asplenic patients.

C. canimorsus A species associated with infections from dog bites. The resulting illness may be mild or life threatening. Alcoholics, splenectomized individuals, and those taking corticosteroids are esp. susceptible, but the illness can be fatal even in previously healthy people. Treatment consists of penicillin; it may be given prophylactically to asplenic patients following a dog bite.

capnography Continuous recording of the carbon dioxide level in expired air in mechanically ventilated patients.

capnometry (kăp-nŏm′ĕ-trē) The measurement of the concentration of carbon dioxide in the exhaled breath of a critically ill person, typically a victim of cardiac or respiratory arrest or a patient receiving mechanical ventilation.

capnophilic (kăp-nō-fĭl′ĭk) [Gr. *kapnos*, smoke, + *philein*, to love] Pert. to bacteria that grow best in an atmosphere containing carbon dioxide.

capotement (kă-pōt-mŏn′) [Fr.] A splashing sound that may be heard when the dilated stomach contains air and fluid.

capping (kăp′ĭng) **1.** Pulp capping. **2.** Placing an artificial crown on a tooth for cosmetic purposes. **3.** In immunology, the aggregation of living B lymphocytes that have reacted with fluorescein-labeled anti-immune globulin cells to form a polar cap.

capsicum (kăp′sĭ-kŭm) The fruit of pepper plants, of which there are more than 200 varieties, including jalapeno and tabasco. It is used topically as an analgesic.

capsid (kăp′sĭd) The protein covering around the central core of a virus. The capsid, which develops from protein units called protomers, protects the nucleic acid in the core of the virus from the destructive enzymes in biological fluids and promotes attachment of the virus to susceptible cells.

capsitis (kăp-sī′tĭs) [L. *capsa*, box, + Gr. *itis*, inflammation] Capsulitis of the crystalline lens of the eye.

capsomer (kăp′sō-mĕr) [″ + Gr. *meros*, part] Short ribbons of protein that make up a portion of the capsid of a virus.

capsula [L., little box] *pl.* **capsulae** A sheath or continuous enclosure around an organ or structure.

c. articularis The capsule of a joint.

c. bulbi Tenon's capsule.

c. fibrosa perivascularis Glisson's capsule.

c. glomeruli Bowman's capsule.

c. lentis The crystalline lens capsule of the eye.

capsular Pert. to a capsule.

capsulation Enclosure in a capsule.

capsule [L. *capsula*, little box] **1.** A sheath or continuous enclosure around an organ or structure. **2.** A special container made of gelatin, sized for a single dose of a drug. The enclosure prevents the patient from tasting the drug.

articular c. Joint c.

auditory c. The embryonic cartilaginous capsule that encloses the developing ear.

bacterial c. The polysaccharide or polypeptide layer that surrounds the cell wall of some bacteria; it provides resistance to phagocytosis. Capsules are antigenic, yet nontoxic, and are used in some vaccines.

Bowman's c. The glomerular capsule of the kidneys. SYN: *glomerular c.*

cartilage c. The layer of matrix that forms the innermost portion of the wall of a lacuna enclosing a single cell or a group of cartilage cells. It is basophilic.

Glisson's c. An outer capsule of fibrous tissue that covers the liver, its ducts, and its vessels. SYN: *capsula fibrosa perivascularis*.

glomerular c. Bowman's capsule.

joint c. The sleevelike membrane that encloses the ends of bones in a diarthrodial joint. It consists of an outer fibrous layer and an inner synovial layer and contains synovial fluid. SYN: *articular c.*

c. of the kidney Renal c.

lens c. A transparent, connective tissue membrane that surrounds and encloses the lens of the eye.

nasal c. The cartilaginous capsule that develops in the embryonic skull to enclose the nasal cavity.

optic c. The cartilaginous capsule that develops in the embryonic skull to enclose the eye.

otic c. The cartilaginous capsule that develops in the embryonic skull to enclose the ear.

c. of Tenon The thin fibrous sac enveloping the eyeball, forming a socket in which it rotates.

renal c. The fibrous membrane on the outer surface of a kidney, which is in turn enclosed by adipose tissue that cushions the kidney. SYN: *c. of the kidney.*

suprarenal c. A tough connective tissue capsule that encloses the adrenal gland.

temporomandibular joint c. The fibrous covering of the synovial joint between the skull and mandible on each side of the head.

capsulectomy (kăp″sū-lĕk′tō-mē) [L. *capsula,* little box, + Gr. *ektome,* excision] Surgical removal of a capsule.

capsulitis (kăp″sū-lī′tĭs) [″ + Gr. *itis,* inflammation] Inflammation of a capsule.

capsulociliary (kăp″sū-lō-sĭl′ē-ĕr-ē) [″ + *ciliaris,* pert. to the eyelashes] Pert. to the lens capsule and the ciliary structures of the eye.

capsulolenticular (kăp″sū-lō-lĕn-tĭk′ū-lăr) [″ + *lenticularis,* pert. to a lens] Pert. to the capsule of the eye and the lens.

capsuloplasty (kăp′sū-lō-plăs″tē) [″ + Gr. *plassein,* to mold] Plastic surgery of a capsule, esp. a joint capsule.

capsulorhexis (kăp″sū-lor-ĕk′sĭs) A common method of cataract extraction in which a circular incision is made in the anterior capsule to permit lens extraction.

capsulorrhaphy (kăp″sū-lor′ă-fē) [″ + Gr. *rhaphe,* seam, ridge] Suture of a joint capsule or of a tear in a capsule.

capsulotome (kăp′sū-lō-tōm″) [″ + Gr. *tome,* incision] An instrument for incising the capsule of the crystalline lens.

capsulotomy (kăp″sū-lŏt′ō-mē) Cutting of a capsule of the lens or a joint.

laser c. The use of a laser to make a hole in the capsule surrounding the lens of the eye to let light pass. Extracapsular removal of a cataract allows the capsule surrounding the lens to remain in the eye; however, if the capsule becomes cloudy, laser capsulotomy is used to restore vision.

captioning The display of spoken words as text on a television or a movie screen, to improve the comprehension of dialogue by hearing-impaired individuals.

captopril A drug that blocks the conversion of angiotensin I to angiotensin II. It is used primarily to treat high blood pressure and congestive heart failure. It also can be used in the diagnosis of renovascular hypertension and in the management of the renal crises that occur in systemic sclerosis (scleroderma). Important side effects of the medication are cough, angioedema, and hypotension.

capture In atomic physics, the joining of an elementary particle such as an electron or neutron with the atomic nucleus.

ventricular c. The normal response of the ventricle of the heart to the electrical impulse from the electrical conducting system.

caput (kā′pŭt, kăp′ŭt) *pl.* **capita** [L.] **1.** The head. **2.** The chief extremity of an organ.

c. medusae A plexus of dilated veins around the umbilicus, seen in patients with portal hypertension (usually as a result of cirrhosis of the liver). It may be seen in newborns.

c. succedaneum Diffuse edema of the fetal scalp that crosses the suture lines. Head compression against the cervix impedes venous return, forcing serum into the interstitial tissues. The swelling reabsorbs within 1 to 3 days.

carbacephem (kăr-bă-sĕph′ĕm) A class of broad-spectrum antibiotic drugs, derived from cephalosporins, that resist degradation by bacterial beta-lactamases. One drug in this class is loracarbef.

carbachol (kăr′bă-kŏl) A drug with action similar to that of acetylcholine. It is used intraocularly to produce miosis during eye surgery and topically to lower intraocular pressure in glaucoma.

carbamazepine (kăr-bă-măz′ĕ-pēn) A drug used to treat trigeminal neuralgia, temporal lobe epilepsy, bipolar disorder, and chronic pain. Trade name is Tegretol.

carbamide (kăr′bă-mīd, kăr-băm′īd) $CO(NH)_2$; urea in an anhydrous, sterile powder form.

carbaminohemoglobin (kăr-băm″ĭ-nō-hē″mō-glō′bĭn) A chemical combination of carbon dioxide and hemoglobin.

carbapenem A class of antibiotics with a broad spectrum of action against gram-positive, gram-negative, and anaerobic germs. The carbapenems include imipenem and meropenem.

carbenicillin indanyl sodium (kăr″bĕn-ĭ-sĭl′ĭn) An antibiotic derived from penicillin that can be used to treat infections with *Pseudomonas aeruginosa.* Trade name is Geocillin.

carbidopa (kăr″bĭ-dō′pă) A drug used with levodopa to treat parkinsonism.

carbohydrase (kăr″bō-hī′drās) One of a group of enzymes (such as amylase and lactase) that hydrolyze carbohydrates.

carbohydrate (kăr″bō-hī′drāt) [L. *carbo,* carbon, + Gr. *hydor,* water] One of a group of chemical substances, including sugars, glycogen, starches, dextrins, and celluloses, that contain only carbon, oxygen, and hydrogen. Usually the ratio of hydrogen to oxygen is 2 to 1. Glucose and its polymers (including starch and cellulose) are estimated to be the most abundant organic chemical compounds on earth, surpassing in quantity even the great stores of fuel hydrocarbons beneath the earth's crust. Carbohydrates are one of the six classes of nutrients needed by the body (the others are proteins, fats, minerals, vitamins, and water).

Green plants use the sun's energy to combine carbon dioxide and water to form carbohydrates. Most plant carbohydrates (celluloses) are unavailable for direct metabolism by vertebrates. However, the bacteria present in the intestinal tracts of some vertebrates break down cellulose to molecules that can be absorbed. The human intestinal tract lacks the enzyme that splits cellulose into sugar molecules, but humans do split starch into maltose by means of their salivary and pancreatic amylases.

CLASSIFICATION: Carbohydrates are grouped according to the number of carbon atoms they contain and how many of the basic types are combined into larger molecules. The most common simple sugars, monosaccharides, contain five or six carbon atoms and are called pentoses and hexoses, respectively. Two monosaccharides linked together are called a disaccharide. A series (chain) of monosaccharides or disaccharides is called a polysaccharide. Ribose and deoxyribose are the most important pentoses; glucose, fructose, and galactose are the most important hexoses in human metabolism. The disaccharide sugars in the diet are maltose (2 D-glucose molecules), sucrose or cane sugar (glucose and fructose), and lactose or milk sugar (D-glucose and D-galactose). These sugars are split and eventually converted to glucose by enzyme action. The two important polysaccharides are starch and glycogen; the latter is called animal starch. The basic monosaccharide building block for both of these large polymers is glucose. Dietary starch and glycogen are metabolized first to glucose and then to carbon dioxide and water in humans. SEE: table (Classification of Important Carbohydrates).

FUNCTION: Carbohydrates are a basic source of energy. They are stored in the body as glycogen in virtually all tissues, but principally in the liver and muscles. Carbohydrates can be mobilized from those sites, making these stores an important source of reserve energy.

DIGESTION AND ABSORPTION: Cooked but not raw starch is broken down to disaccharide by salivary amylase. Both cooked and raw starches are split in the small intestine by pancreatic amylase. Disaccharides cannot be absorbed until they have been split into monosaccharides by the enzymes present in the brush border of cells lining the intestinal tract. Glucose and galactose are the actively absorbed sugars. Fructose is absorbed by diffusion. SEE: table (Digestion of Carbohydrates).

METABOLISM: Although very complex at the molecular level, carbohydrate metabolism can be explained as follows. Carbohydrates are absorbed as glucose, galactose, or fructose. Fructose and galactose are converted to glucose by the liver and are then available for energy production, or they may be stored after conversion to glycogen. The glycogen is available for metabolism to

Classification of Important Carbohydrates

Classification	Examples	Some Properties
Monosaccharides $C_6H_{12}O_6$	Glucose	Crystalline, sweet, very soluble, readily absorbed
Pentoses $C_5H_{10}O_5$ or $C_5H_{10}O_4$	Ribose Deoxyribose	Part of nucleic acid, RNA Part of nucleic acid, DNA
Disaccharides $(C_6H_{10}O_5)_2 \cdot H_2O$ or $C_{12}H_{22}O_{11}$ hydrolyzed to simple sugars	Sucrose Lactose Maltose	Crystalline, sweet, soluble, digestible Present in milk
Polysaccharides $(C_6H_{10}O_5)_n$ composed of many molecules of simple sugars. (Since polysaccharides can be composed of various numbers of monosaccharides and disaccharides, n refers to an unknown number of these groups.)	Starch Dextrin Cellulose Glycogen	Amorphous, little or no flavor, less soluble. Vary in solubility and digestibility.

Digestion of Carbohydrates

Enzyme	Produced in	Carbohydrates Digested	End Product
Sucrase (invertase)	Small intestine	Sucrose	Glucose and fructose
Maltases	Small intestine and mucosal cells of small intestine	Maltose	Two D-glucose
Lactase	Small intestine	Lactose	D-glucose and D-galactose
Salivary amylase	Saliva (mouth)	Cooked starch, glycogen, and dextrins	Maltose
Pancreatic amylase	Pancreas	Raw and cooked starch and glycogen	Maltose

glucose whenever reserve energy is needed. SEE: *muscle metabolism*.

SOURCES: Carbohydrates are present in food in digestible and indigestible forms. The digestible type are an important source of energy. Those that cannot be used, usually some form of cellulose, are beneficial in adding bulk to the diet. Whole grains, vegetables, legumes (peas and beans), tubers (potatoes), fruits, honey, and refined sugar are excellent sources of carbohydrate. Calories derived from sugar and candy have been termed "empty" calories because these foods lack essential amino acids, vitamins, and minerals. SEE: *fiber, dietary*.

NUTRITION: Carbohydrates contain 4.1 kcal/g and are esp. useful as a quick source of energy as they are readily digested.

carbohydrate loading Dietary manipulation to enhance the amount of glycogen stored in muscle tissue. This technique is used by athletes before high-intensity endurance events such as a marathon foot race. Phase I is begun 7 days before competition. It depletes glycogen from specific muscles used in the event by exercise to exhaustion in the sport for which the athlete is preparing. The glycogen exhaustion is maintained by a high-fat, high-protein diet for 3 days. It is important to include 100 g of carbohydrate to prevent ketosis. Phase II consists of a high-carbohydrate diet of at least 1000 to 2000 kcal for 3 days. This is called the supersaturation phase because the goal is to enhance glycogen storage. Glycogen synthesis is facilitated by the extended period of depletion in phase I. Carbohydrates used should be complex ones (as in grain-derived foods such as bread and pasta) rather than simple carbohydrates (as in candy and soft drinks). Phase III begins on the day of the event. Any type of food may be eaten up to 4 to 6 hr before competition. Food eaten from that time up to the time of competition is a matter of individual preference.

carbolize (kăr′bŏl-īz) To mix with or add carbolic acid.

carbon [L. *carbo*, carbon] SYMB: C. The nonmetallic element that is the characteristic constituent of organic compounds; average atomic mass 12.0111, atomic number 6.

Carbon occurs in two pure forms, diamond and graphite, and in impure form in charcoal, coke, and soot. Its compounds are constituents of all living tissue. Carbon combines with hydrogen, nitrogen, and oxygen to form the basis of all organic matter. Organic carbon compounds provide energy in foods.

impregnated c. An electrode having a carbon shell with a core of various metals or salts of metals for use in a carbon arc lamp.

carbon-14 SYMB: ^{14}C. A radioactive isotope of carbon with a half-life of 5600 years. It is used as a tracer in metabolic studies and in archaeology to date materials containing carbon.

carbonate (kăr′bŏn-āt) [L. *carbo*, carbon] Any salt of carbonic acid.

c. of soda Sodium carbonate used commercially in crude form, such as washing soda. The free alkali present is irritating and in strong concentrations has the effect of sodium hydroxide.

carbon dioxide SYMB: CO_2. A colorless gas that is heavier than air and is produced in the combustion or decomposition of carbon or its compounds. It is the final metabolic product of carbon compounds present in food. The body eliminates CO_2 through the lungs, in urine, and in perspiration. It is also given off by decomposition of vegetable and animal matter and is formed by alcoholic fermentation as in rising bread. Green plants absorb it directly from the air and use it in photosynthesis. Approx. 1 sq m of leaf surface can absorb the CO_2 from 2500 L of air in 1 hr. An acre of trees uses an estimated 4½ tons (4082 kg) of CO_2 a year. Commercially, CO_2 gas is used in carbonated drinks and the solid form is used to make dry ice.

c.d. combining power The amount of carbon dioxide that the blood can hold in chemical combination. CO_2 in aqueous solution forms carbonic acid; the amount of this acid that the blood serum can take up is a measure of its reserve power to prevent acidosis. The normal amount is 50 to 70 ml/dl of blood (usually expressed as 50 to 70 vol%). Values below 50 indicate acidosis; above 70, alkalosis.

c.d. inhalation Providing the patient with a mixture of oxygen and carbon dioxide. It can be used as an accessory to artificial respiration when resuscitation equipment, such as a bag-valve-mask, is not available. In the past, it also was used to stimulate breathing and to treat persistent hiccups.

c.d. poisoning Toxicity from carbon dioxide inhalation. In small quantities (up to about 5%) in inspired air, CO_2 stimulates respiration in humans; in greater quantities it produces an uncomfortable degree of mental activity with confusion. Although not toxic in low concentrations, CO_2 can cause death by suffocation. Poisoning is rarely fatal unless exposure occurs in a closed space.

SYMPTOMS: Symptoms include a sensation of pressure in the head, ringing in the ears, an acid taste in the mouth, and a slight burning in the nose. With massive exposures to very concentrated carbon dioxide, respiratory depression and coma may occur.

TREATMENT: The patient should be removed to fresh air and given oxygen and, if needed, ventilatory assistance.

c.d. solid therapy Solid carbon dioxide (CO_2 snow) used for therapeutic refrigeration. Solid CO_2 has a temperature of 80°C below zero. Its application to the skin for 1 to 2 sec causes superficial frostbite; 4 to 5 sec, a blister; 10 to 15 sec, superficial necrosis; and 15 to 45 sec, ulceration. It is used mostly for removal of certain nevi and warts, occasionally for telangiectasia.

carbonemia (kăr″bō-nē′mē-ă) [L. *carbo,* carbon, + Gr. *haima,* blood] An excess accumulation of carbonic acid in the blood.

carbonic Pert. to carbon.

c. anhydrase An enzyme that catalyzes union of water and carbon dioxide to form carbonic acid, or performs the reverse action. It is present in red blood cells.

carbonize (kăr′bŏn-īz) To char or convert into charcoal.

carbon monoxide SYMB: CO. A poisonous gas resulting from the inefficient and incomplete combustion of organic fuels. Colorless, tasteless, and odorless, it cannot be detected by the senses. Carbon monoxide is distributed widely because of imperfect combustion and oxidation and is found, for example, in the exhaust gas from the internal combustion engines in most motor-powered vehicles, and in sewers, cellars, and mines.

c.m. poisoning Toxicity that results from inhalation of small amounts of carbon monoxide (CO) over a long period or from large amounts inhaled for a short time. In the U.S., where exposure to smoke, car exhaust, and other sources of combustion is common (esp. during the winter months), CO poisoning is one of the most frequent, and potentially deadliest, intoxications. CO poisoning results from the avid chemical combination of the gas with hemoglobin, forming carboxyhemoglobin (COHb), a long-lasting substance that inhibits the binding of oxygen to hemoglobin and prevents oxygenation of tissues. SEE: *Poisons and Poisoning Appendix.*

CAUTION: Health care professionals should not rely on a "cherry red" appearance of the mucous membranes or skin to diagnose severe CO intoxications, as this physical finding rarely is present. It is advisable in any case of suspected CO exposure to check the COHb level.

SYMPTOMS: The symptoms of CO poisoning vary with the level of exposure and the concentration of COHb in the bloodstream. At levels of less than 10%, patients may be symptom-free or may complain only of headache. (Heavy cigarette smoking may produce levels as high as 7% to 9%.) COHb levels of 30% produce mild neurological impairment (dizziness, fatigue, difficulty concentrating), and levels of 50% may cause seizures or coma. Death is likely when COHb levels exceed 70%.

TREATMENT: The affected person should be removed immediately from exposure to CO. Individuals with a COHb level greater than 25% are admitted to the hospital. Using a tight-fitting mask, 100% oxygen is given, under pressure (hyperbaric) if possible. Artificial respiration should be used if indicated. The patient should be kept at bedrest to reduce the body's oxygen requirements.

COMPLICATIONS: When exposed patients recover, they often have some central nervous system complications, such as memory disturbances, difficulty concentrating, or tremor, among others. These complications usually disappear over time, but occasionally permanent neurological dysfunction follows CO intoxication.

PREVENTION: Combustible products and internal combustion engines should not be used in closed spaces, such as ga-

Toxic Symptoms of Carbon Monoxide

Carbon Monoxide Concentration		Response
Percent in Air	**Parts per Million**	
0.005	50	No apparent toxic symptoms.
0.01	100	Can be tolerated for several hr without symptoms.
0.02	200	Possible mild frontal headache in 2–3 hr.
0.08	800	Headache, dizziness, and nausea in 45 min; collapse and possible unconsciousness in 2 hr.
0.16	1600	Headache, dizziness, and nausea in 20 min; collapse and possible death in 2 hr.
0.32	3200	Headache and dizziness in 5–10 min; unconsciousness and possible death in 10–15 min.
0.64	6400	Headache and dizziness in 1–2 min; possible death in 10–15 min.
1.28	12,800	Immediate unconsciousness; possible death in 1–3 min.

SOURCE: Adapted from Hamilton, A, and Hardy, H: Industrial Toxicology, ed 3. Publishing Sciences Group, Littleton, MA, 1974.

rages, homes, auditoriums, or sports facilities. Many CO exposures are preventable. SEE: table.

carbon tetrachloride (tĕt″ră-klō′rīd) SYMB: CCl_4. A clear, colorless liquid, not flammable, with an odor like that of chloroform. Although having narcotic and anesthetic properties resembling chloroform, it is too toxic to be suitable as an anesthetic or for any medical use. Inhalation of a small quantity can produce death due to the toxic damage to the liver and kidney.

c.t. poisoning Toxic effects due to prolonged inhalation of carbon tetrachloride. Consequences include irritation of the eyes, nose, and throat, headache, confusion, central nervous system depression, visual disturbances, nausea, anorexia, hepatitis, nephropathy, and cardiac arrhythmias.

TREATMENT: Clothes contaminated with carbon tetrachloride are removed. Oxygen, artificial respiration, gastric decontamination, and management of cardiac rhythms are often needed. SEE: *Poisons and Poisoning Appendix.*

carbonuria (kăr″bō-nū′rē-ă) [L. *carbo,* carbon, + Gr. *ouron,* urine] The presence or excretion of carbon compounds in the urine.

carbonyl (kăr′bŏn-ĭl) [″ + Gr. *hyle,* matter] The divalent radical carbon monoxide, characteristic of aldehydes and ketones.

carboplatin A cytotoxic, platinum-containing drug used to treat ovarian cancer. SEE: *cisplatin.*

carboxyhemoglobin (kăr-bŏk″sē-hē″mō-glō′bĭn) [″ + Gr. *oxys,* acid, + *haima,* blood, + L. *globus,* sphere] A compound formed by carbon monoxide and hemoglobin in carbon monoxide poisoning.

carboxyhemoglobinemia The presence of carboxyhemoglobin in the blood. SEE: *carbon monoxide poisoning.*

carboxyl (kăr-bŏk′sĭl) The characteristic group (—COOH) of organic carboxylic acids, such as formic acid (HCOOH) and acetic acid (CH_2COOH).

carboxylase (kăr-bŏk′sĭ-lās) An enzyme that catalyzes the removal of the carboxyl group (COOH) from amino acids. Found in brewer's yeast, it catalyzes the decarboxylation of pyruvic acid by producing acetaldehyde and carbon dioxide. In the body, this process requires the presence of vitamin B_1 (thiamine), which acts as a coenzyme.

carboxylation In chemistry, the replacement of hydrogen by a carboxyl (—COOH) group.

carbuncle, carbunculus (kăr′bŭng″k′l, kăr-bŭng′kū-lŭs) [L. *carbunculus,* small glowing ember] An abscess of the skin, formed by the merger of two or more boils (furuncles). **carbuncular** (-bŭng′kū-lăr), *adj.* SEE: *boil.*

ETIOLOGY: Staphylococci are the usual cause. They may be introduced into the skin by chafing, pressure, shaving, or by pits or cracks that result from dermatitis.

SYMPTOMS: The lesions are often tender, red, warm, and swollen.

TREATMENT: Warm compresses, incision and drainage, and/or antibiotics (such as first-generation cephalosporins) are usually effective.

PATIENT CARE: Patients or caregivers are taught to change the dressings at least twice a day to remove infected material, and to prevent the spread of infection in the home by avoiding contact with wound drainage, disposing of dressings in sealed bags, and washing contaminated linens separately in very hot water. SEE: *Standard and Universal Precautions Appendix.*

carbunculosis (kăr-bŭng″kū-lō′sĭs) [″ + Gr. *osis,* condition] The appearance of several carbuncles in succession.

carcass (kăr′kăs) A dead body; usually applied to nonhuman bodies.

carcin- SEE: *carcino-*.

carcino-, carcin- [Gr. *karkinos,* cancer] Combining form meaning *cancer*.

carcinogen (kăr′sĭn-, kăr-sĭn′ō-jĕn) Any substance or agent that produces cancer or increases the risk of developing cancer in humans or animals.

chemical c. Any chemical substance capable of causing cancer.

carcinogenesis (kăr″sĭ-nō-jĕn′ĕ-sĭs) [Gr. *karkinos,* crab, + *genesis,* generation, birth] The transformation of normal cells into cancer cells, often as a result of chemical, viral, or radioactive damage to genes.

carcinogenic (kăr″sĭ-nō-jĕn′ĭk) Producing cancer.

carcinoid (kăr′sĭ-noid) [″ + *eidos,* form, shape] A tumor derived from the neuroendocrine cells in the intestinal tract, bile ducts, pancreas, bronchus, or ovary. It secretes serotonin (5-hydroxytryptamine) and other vasoactive substances.

carcinoid syndrome A group of symptoms produced by carcinoid tumors that secrete excessive amounts of serotonin, bradykinin, and other powerful vasoactive chemicals.

SYMPTOMS: One or more of the following may occur: brief episodes of flushing, esp. of the face and neck, tachycardia, facial and periorbital edema, hypotension, intermittent abdominal pain with diarrhea, valvular heart lesions, weight loss, hypoproteinemia, and ascites. When carcinoid tumors are found in the bronchi, intermittent bronchospasm may be the presenting symptom. Endocardial fibrosis and symptoms of pellagra may occasionally occur.

DIAGNOSIS: The diagnosis is based on clinical presentation, greatly increased excretion of 5-HIAA in urine, and uptake by tumors of specific radioisotopes, such as MIBG or pentreotide.

TREATMENT: Isolated tumors can be surgically removed. Multiple metastatic tumors can be treated with arterial embolization and with variable success with chemotherapy.

carcinolysis (kăr″sĭ-nŏl′ĭ-sĭs) [Gr. *karkinos,* crab, + *lysis,* dissolution] Destruction of carcinoma cells. **carcinolytic** (-nō-lĭt′ĭk), *adj.*

carcinoma (kăr″sĭ-nō′mă) [″ + *oma,* tumor] A new growth or malignant tumor that occurs in epithelial tissue and may infiltrate local tissues or produce metastases. It may affect almost any organ or part of the body and spread by direct extension, through lymphatics, or through the bloodstream. The causes vary with tumor type.

alveolar cell c. A type of lung carcinoma.

basal cell c. A skin malignancy that rarely metastasizes but may be locally invasive. Typically it begins as a small, shiny papule. The lesion enlarges to form a whitish border around a central depression or ulcer that may bleed. When the lesion reaches this stage, it is often called a rodent ulcer. After biopsy, the removal method used is determined by the size, location, and appearance of the lesion. SYN: *basal cell epithelioma.* SEE: illus.

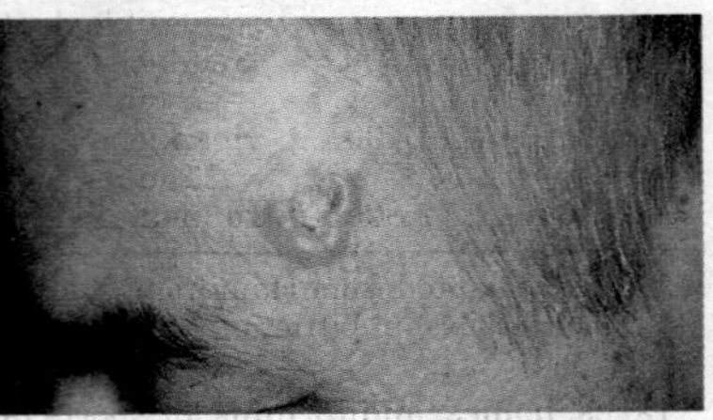

BASAL CELL CARCINOMA

bronchogenic c. Lung cancer.

chorionic c. Choriocarcinoma.

colorectal c. A malignant neoplasm of the colon or rectum, responsible for an estimated annual mortality of 57,000 people in the U.S. It is the third most common cause of cancer death in the U.S. SYN: *colorectal cancer; carcinoma of the colon.*

SYMPTOMS: Symptoms are variable and include change in the usual pattern of bowel habits, esp. in patients over 40 years of age; recent onset of constipation, diarrhea, or tenesmus in an older patient; bright red or dark blood in the stool. Laboratory findings may include iron-deficiency anemia or positive fecal occult blood tests.

DIAGNOSIS: Diagnosis is based on findings from the digital rectal examination, anoscopy, proctosigmoidoscopy, colonoscopy, barium enema examination, and biopsy of suspicious lesions and polyps.

TREATMENT: Surgery is the primary form of treatment. Radiation therapy alone, or in combination with surgery and chemotherapy, can be used as adjuvant therapy.

embryonal c. A malignant, aggressive germ cell tumor that may metastasize widely. It can occur in young adults of either sex.

epidermoid c. Squamous cell c.

giant cell c. Carcinoma marked by the presence of unusually large cells.

glandular c. Adenocarcinoma.

c. in situ ABBR: CIS. Malignant cell changes in the epithelial tissue that do not extend beyond the basement membrane.

medullary c. Carcinoma in which

there is a predominance of cells and little fibrous tissue.

melanotic c. Carcinoma containing melanin.

mucinous c. Carcinoma in which the glandular tissue secretes mucin.

oat cell c. A poorly differentiated tumor of the bronchus that contains small oat-shaped cells. SYN: *small cell c.*

scirrhous c. Hard cancer.

small cell c. Oat cell c.

squamous cell c. Carcinoma that develops primarily from squamous cells, e.g., on the skin or in the mouth, lungs, bronchi, esophagus, or cervix. SEE: illus.

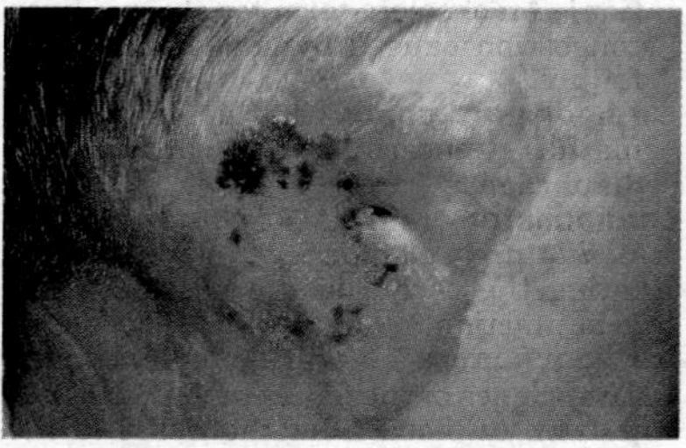

SQUAMOUS CELL CARCINOMA

carcinomatophobia (kăr″sĭ-nō″mă-tō-fō′bē-ă) [Gr. *karkinos,* crab, + *oma,* tumor, + *phobos,* fear] Morbid fear of cancer.

carcinomatosis (kăr″sĭ-nō″mă-tō′sĭs) [″ + ″ + *osis,* condition] Widespread dissemination of carcinoma in the body. SYN: *carcinosis.*

carcinophilia (kăr″sĭ-nō-fĭl′ē-ă) [″ + *philos,* love] An affinity for cancer cells.

carcinosarcoma (kăr″sĭ-nō-săr-kō′mă) [″ + *sarx,* flesh, + *oma,* tumor] A malignant tumor containing the elements of both carcinoma and sarcoma.

embryonal c. A malignant germ-cell tumor derived from embryonic cells.

carcinosis (kăr″sĭ-nō′sĭs) [″ + *osis,* condition] Carcinomatosis.

cardamom, cardamon [Gr. *kardamomon*] The dried ripe fruit of an herb, *Elettaria repens* or *E. cardamomum.* It is used as an aromatic and carminative.

Cardarelli's sign (kăr″dă-rĕl′lēz) [Antonio Cardarelli, It. physician, 1831–1926] Pulsating movement of the trachea to one side. It may be present with aortic aneurysm.

cardi- SEE: *cardio-.*

cardia (kăr′dē-ă) [Gr. *kardia,* heart] The upper orifice of the stomach connecting with the esophagus.

cardiac (kăr′dē-ăk) [L. *cardiacus*] **1.** Pert. to the heart. **2.** Pert. to the cardia.

cardiac arrest Sudden cessation of functional circulation. In the U.S., about 1000 people die daily as a result of cardiac arrest. SEE: *arrhythmia; myocardial infarction.*

ETIOLOGY: Coronary artery disease is present in the majority of victims, and cardiac arrest usually is caused by myocardial infarction or ventricular arrhythmias. Other contributors include cardiomyopathies, valvular heart disease, diseases of the electrical conducting system of the heart (such as the long QT syndrome or the Wolff-Parkinson-White syndrome), myocarditis, chest trauma, severe electrolyte disturbances, and intoxications with drugs of abuse or prescribed agents (e.g., digitalis). Physical exertion or extreme emotional stress sometimes precipitates cardiac arrest.

SYMPTOMS: Abrupt loss of consciousness, followed by death occurring within an hour of the onset of the illness (i.e., sudden death) is the typical presentation of cardiac arrest.

TREATMENT: Opening the airway, establishing effective respirations, and restoring circulation (with early defibrillation) are the keys to treating cardiac arrest. The effectiveness of treatment depends on the speed with which resuscitation begins and the patient's underlying condition. Because most episodes of sudden cardiac arrest are unwitnessed, no intervention usually is given. Spontaneous recovery from cardiac arrest is rare. For resuscitated patients, therapies may include implantable defibrillators, beta blockers, antiarrhythmic drugs, and in patients with coronary artery disease, modification of risk factors (i.e., treatment of hypertension, smoking cessation, and lipid-lowering diets and drugs). SEE: *advanced cardiac life support.*

sudden c.a. ABBR: SCA. Cardiac arrest.

cardiac compensation The ability of the heart to compensate for impaired functioning through muscle hypertrophy or other means.

cardiac failure A condition resulting from the heart's inability to pump sufficient blood to meet the body's needs. SEE: *heart failure.*

cardiac hypertrophy Enlargement of the heart's muscles or chambers.

cardiac output, decreased A state in which the blood pumped by the heart is inadequate to meet the metabolic demands of the body. (NOTE: In a hypermetabolic state, although cardiac output may be within normal range, it may still be inadequate to meet the needs of the body's tissues. Cardiac output and tissue perfusion are interrelated. When cardiac output is decreased, tissue perfusion problems will develop. Tissue perfusion also can be impaired when there is normal or high cardiac output, for example, in septic shock.) SEE: *Nursing Diagnoses Appendix.*

cardiac plexus Plexus cardiacus; the nerve plexus at the base of the heart made up of branches of the vagus nerves and sympathetic trunks. Afferent nerves from this plexus provide the nerve supply to the heart.

cardiac reflex An involuntary response consisting of a change in cardiac rate. Stimulation of sensory nerve endings in the wall of the carotid sinus by increased arterial blood pressure reflexively slows the heart (Marey's law). Stimulation of vagus fibers in the right side of the heart by increased venous return reflexively increases the heart rate (Bainbridge's reflex).

cardiac silhouette The shadow on the chest radiograph created by the heart. A large cardiac silhouette is consistent with congestive heart failure.

cardiac surgery Any operation on the heart and/or the proximal great vessels. SEE: *Nursing Diagnoses Appendix.*

cardialgia (kăr″dē-ăl′jē-ă) [Gr. *kardia,* heart, + *algos,* pain] Pain at the pit of the stomach or region of the heart, usually occurring in paroxysms.

cardiaortic (kăr″dē-ā-or′tĭk) [″ + *aorte,* aorta] Pert. to the heart and aorta.

cardiasthenia (kăr″dē-ăs-thē′nē-ă) [″ + *astheneia,* weakness] An obsolete term for a somatization disorder with prominent cardiac symptoms.

cardiasthma (kăr″dē-ăz′mă) [″ + *asthma,* panting] Dyspnea due to heart disease.

cardiectasia, cardiectasis (kăr″dē-ĕk-tā′sē-ă, -ĕk′tă-sĭs) [″ + *ektasis,* dilatation] Dilatation of the heart.

cardiectomy (kăr″dē-ĕk′tō-mē) [″ + *ektome,* excision] **1.** Excision of the gastric cardia. **2.** Harvesting of the heart and adjacent great vessels for transplantation.

Cardiff Count-to-Ten chart A way to assess intrauterine well-being in which the expectant woman records fetal movement during her usual activities. There should be at least 10 movements within a 12-hour period; if fewer than 10 movements are perceived, further medical evaluation is needed.

cardinal [LL. *cardinalis,* important] Of primary importance, as in the cardinal signs: temperature, pulse, respiration, and blood pressure.

cardio-, cardi- [Gr. *kardia,* heart] Combining form meaning *heart.*

cardioaccelerator (kăr″dē-ō-ăk-sĕl′ĕr-ā-tor) [″ + L. *accelerare,* to hasten] Something that increases the rate of the heartbeat.

cardioactive (kăr″dē-ō-ăk′tĭv) [″ + L. *activus,* acting] Acting on the heart.

cardioangiography (kăr″dē-ō-ăn″jē-ŏg′ră-fē) [″ + *angeion,* vessel, + *graphein,* to write] Angiocardiography.

cardioangiology (kăr″dē-ō-ăn″jē-ŏl′ō-jē) [″ + ″ + *logos,* word, reason] The science of the heart and blood vessels.

cardioaortic (kăr″dē-ō-ā-or′tĭk) [″ + *aorte,* aorta] Pert. to the heart and the aorta.

cardiocele (kăr′dē-ō-sēl) [″ + *kele,* tumor, swelling] A herniation or protrusion of the heart through an opening in the diaphragm or through a wound.

cardiocentesis Cardiopuncture.

cardiochalasia (kăr″dē-ō-kă-lā′zē-ă) [″ + *chalasis,* relaxation] Relaxation of the muscles of the cardiac sphincter of the stomach.

cardiocirrhosis (kăr″dē-ō-sĭr-rō′sĭs) [″ + *kirrhos,* orange-yellow, + *osis,* condition] An obsolete term for chronic liver congestion caused by congestive heart failure.

cardiodiaphragmatic (kăr″dē-ō-dī″ă-frăg-măt′ĭk) Concerning the heart and the diaphragm.

cardiodilator (kăr″dē-ō-dī′lā-tor) [″ + L. *dilatare,* to enlarge] A device for dilating the cardia of the gastroesophageal junction.

cardiodynamics (kăr″dē-ō-dī-năm′ĭks) The science of the forces involved in propulsion of blood from the heart to the tissues and back to the heart.

cardiodynia (kăr″dē-ō-dĭn′ē-ă) [Gr. *kardia,* heart, + *odyne,* pain] Pain in the region of the heart.

cardioesophageal Pert. to the junction of the esophagus and the stomach.

cardioesophageal reflux SEE: *gastroesophageal reflux.*

cardiogenesis (kăr″dē-ō-jĕn′ĕ-sĭs) [″ + *genesis,* generation, birth] Formation and growth of the embryonic heart.

cardiogenic (kăr″dē-ō-jĕn′ĭk) [″ + *gennan,* to produce] Originating in the heart.

cardiogram (kăr′dē-ō-grăm″) [″ + *gramma,* something written] A graph of the electrical activity of the heart muscle, made with an electrocardiograph machine. SYN: *electrocardiogram.*

cardiograph (kăr′dē-ō-grăf″) [″ + *graphein,* to write] A device for registering the electrical activity of the heart muscle.

cardiography (kăr″dē-ŏg′ră-fē) The recording and study of the electrical activity of the heart. **cardiographic** (-ō-grăf′ĭk), *adj.*

cardiohepatic (kăr″dē-ō-hĕ-păt′ĭk) [″ + *hepatos,* liver] Pert. to the heart and liver.

cardiohepatomegaly (kăr″dē-ō-hĕp″ă-tō-mĕg′ă-lē) [″ + ″+ *megas,* large] Enlargement of the heart and liver.

cardioinhibitory (kăr″dē-ō-ĭn-hĭb′ĭ-tō-rē) [″ + L. *inhibere,* to check] Inhibiting the action of the heart.

cardiokinetic (kăr″dē-ō-kĭ-nĕt′ĭk) [″ + *kinesis,* movement] Pert. to the action of the heart.

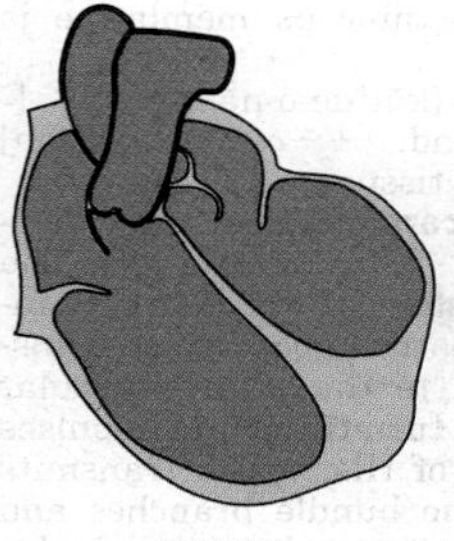

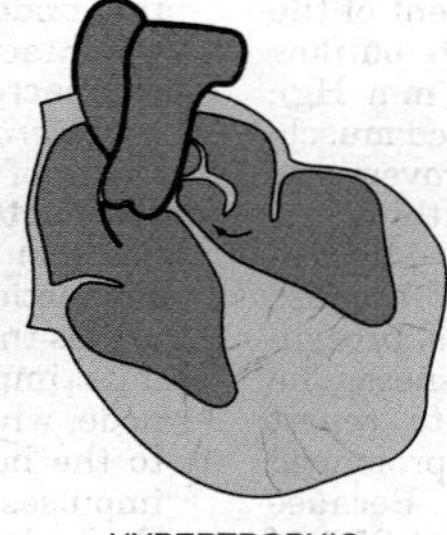

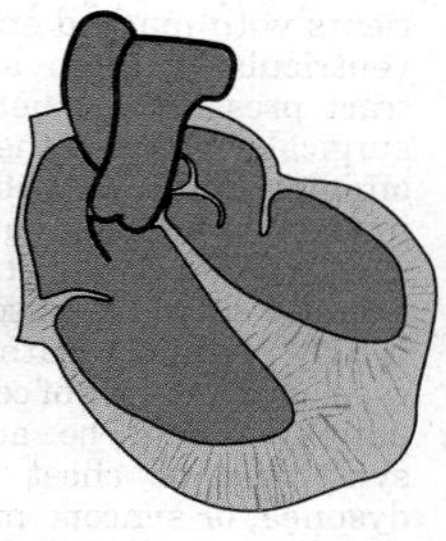

CARDIOMYOPATHIES

cardiokymography ABBR: CKG. An obsolete radiographic method of recording the outline of the heart as it beats. Its usefulness in clinical medicine has not been shown.

cardiolipin (kăr″dē-ō-lĭp′ĭn) [″ + *lipos,* fat] Previously used term for diphosphatidylglycerol.

cardiolith (kăr′dē-ō-lĭth″) [″ + *lithos,* stone] A concretion or calculus in the heart.

cardiologist (kăr-dē-ŏl′ō-jĭst) [″ + *logos,* word, reason] A physician specializing in treatment of heart disease.

cardiology (kăr-dē-ŏl′ō-jē) The study of the physiology and pathology of the heart.

nuclear c. A noninvasive method for studying cardiovascular disease by use of nuclear imaging techniques. These tests are usually done while the individual is exercising. Coronary artery disease can be investigated as can damage to the myocardium following coronary infarction. The size and function of the ventricles can be evaluated using these techniques.

cardiolysin (kăr″dē-ŏl′ĭ-sĭn) [″ + *lysis,* dissolution] An antibody acting destructively on the heart muscle.

cardiolysis (kăr-dē-ŏl′ĭ-sĭs) An operation that separates adhesions constricting the heart in adhesive mediastinopericarditis. It involves resection of the ribs and sternum over the pericardium.

cardiomalacia (kăr″dē-ō-mă-lā′shē-ă) [Gr. *kardia,* heart, + *malakia,* softening] Softening of the heart muscle.

cardiomegaly (kăr″dē-ō-mĕg′ă-lē) [″ + *megas,* large] Enlargement of the heart.

cardiomotility (kăr″dē-ō-mō-tĭl′ĭ-tē) [″ + L. *motilis,* moving] The ability of the heart to move.

cardiomyoliposis (kăr″dē-ō-mī″ō-lĭp-ō′sĭs) [″ + *mys,* muscle, + *lipos,* fat, + *osis,* condition] Fatty degeneration of the heart.

cardiomyopathy (kăr″dē-ō-mī-ŏp′ă-thē) [″ + ″ + *pathos,* disease, suffering] ABBR: CMP. Any disease that affects the heart muscle, diminishing cardiac performance. SEE: *myocarditis.*

alcoholic c. Heart muscle damage caused by years of heavy alcohol usage. Affected patients have enlarged (dilated) hearts and left ventricular failure. Abstinence from alcohol may halt or reverse the course of the illness in some individuals.

congestive c. Myocardial disease associated with enlargement of the left ventricle of the heart and congestive heart failure.

constrictive c. Restrictive c.

hypertrophic c. ABBR: HCM. A heart muscle disease of uncertain cause, marked by excessive and disorganized growth of myofibrils, impaired filling of the heart (diastolic dysfunction), a reduction in the size of ventricular cavities, and often, ventricular arrhythmias and sudden death. Examination of the heart by echocardiography or other modalities may show the heart's enlargement to be most pronounced in the interventricular septum. Hypertrophy in that location may limit the flow of blood (and increase pressure gradients) from the left ventricle to the aorta. Abnormal anterior motion of the mitral valve during systole also may be found. These two findings are often designated on echocardiographic reports of patients with HCM by the following abbreviation: ASH-SAM ("asymmetric septal hypertrophy–systolic anterior motion" of the mitral valve). SEE: illus.

SYMPTOMS: Although they may be asymptomatic for many years, patients commonly report shortness of breath, fatigue, chest pain, orthopnea, and other symptoms of congestive heart failure after the heart muscle markedly enlarges. Ventricular arrhythmias are common; they may result in palpitations, syncope, or sudden death.

TREATMENT: Drug therapies include beta blocking and calcium channel blocking drugs (such as verapamil). Anticoagulants and antiarrhythmic agents are used occasionally as well. For patients with marked enlargement of the ventricular septum and high outflow tract pressure gradients (50 mm Hg), surgical removal of the enlarged muscle often produces favorable improvements in exercise tolerance and breathing.

PATIENT CARE: Strenuous physical exercise should be discouraged because it may produce breathlessness, presyncope, or frank loss of consciousness. The patient should be advised to report symptoms of chest pain, prolonged dyspnea, or syncope promptly. Because HCM may be familial in about 25% of patients, first-degree relatives of affected persons should be referred for evaluation.

idiopathic dilated c. ABBR: IDC. Heart muscle weakness of occult or uncertain cause, possibly due to viral infections, unrecognized toxic exposures, or a genetic predisposition, but not to ischemia, hypothyroidism, hypertension, valvular disease, or alcohol abuse. SEE: illus.

TREATMENT: General supportive therapy includes rest, weight control, abstinence from tobacco, and moderate exercise at a level that does not cause symptoms. A salt-restricted diet is recommended. Therapy includes the use of vasodilators, such as ACE inhibitors and diuretics like furosemide. Anticoagulants are important to prevent thrombus formation. IDC is a principal indication for cardiac transplant.

c. of overload Enlargement of heart muscle, as a result of long-standing or severe hypertension or aortic stenosis. Like all other forms of cardiomyopathy, the end result is heart failure.

primary c. Cardiomyopathy in which the origin (i.e., cause) is unknown.

restrictive c. A disease of the heart muscle associated with lack of flexibility of the ventricular walls. Common causes include hemochromatosis, amyloidosis, and other diseases in which the heart is infiltrated by foreign material, or scarred. SEE: illus.

secondary c. Any cardiomyopathy in which the cause is either known or associated with a well-defined systemic disease. Included are cardiomyopathies associated with inflammation, toxic chemicals, metabolic abnormalities, and inherited muscle disorders.

cardiomyopexy (kăr′dē-ō-mī′ō-pĕk″sē) [″ + ″ + *pexis,* fixation] Surgical fixation of a vascular tissue such as pectoral muscle to the cardiac muscle and pericardium to improve blood supply to the myocardium.

cardiomyoplasty Surgical implantation of skeletal muscle to either supplement or replace myocardial muscle.

cardiomyotomy Surgical therapy for achalasia. The muscles surrounding the cardioesophageal junction are cut, while the underlying mucous membrane is left intact.

cardionecrosis (kăr″dē-ō-nĕ-krō′sĭs) [″ + *nekros,* dead, + *osis,* condition] Death of heart tissue.

cardionecteur, cardionector (kăr″dē-ō-nĕk′tĕr) [″ + L. *nektor,* joiner] The conduction system of the heart. It includes the sinoatrial node, which transmits impulses to the atrioventricular node, which in turn transmits impulses to the bundle of His, which transmits impulses to the bundle branches and Purkinje fibers to produce ventricular contraction.

cardionephric (kăr″dē-ō-nĕf′rĭk) [″ + *nephros,* kidney] Pert. to the heart and kidney.

cardioneural (kăr″dē-ō-nū′răl) [″ + *neuron,* nerve] Pert. to nervous control of the heart.

cardioneurosis (kăr″dē-ō-nū-rō′sĭs) [″ + ″ + *osis,* condition] Functional neurosis with cardiac symptoms.

cardiopathy (kăr″dē-ŏp′ă-thē) [″ + *pathos,* disease, suffering] Any disease of the heart.

cardiopericarditis (kăr″dē-ō-pĕr″ĭ-kăr-dī′tĭs) [″ + *peri,* around, + *kardia,* heart, + *itis,* inflammation] Inflammation of the myocardium and pericardium.

cardiophobia (kăr″dē-ō-fō′bē-ă) [″ + *phobos,* fear] Morbid fear of heart disease.

cardioplasty (kăr″dē-ō-plăs′tē) [″ + *plassein,* to form] An operation on the cardiac sphincter of the stomach to relieve cardiospasm.

cardioplegia (kăr″dē-ō-plē′jē-ă) [″ + *plege,* stroke] Intentional, temporary arrest of cardiac function by means of hypothermia, medication, or electrical stimuli to reduce the need of the myocardium for oxygen. This is done during surgery requiring cardiopulmonary bypass.

cardiopneumograph (kăr″dē-ō-nū′mō-grăf) [″ + ″ + *graphein,* to write] A device for recording the motion of the heart and lungs.

cardioptosis (kăr″dē-ŏp-tō′sĭs) [″ + *ptosis,* a dropping] Prolapse of the heart.

cardiopulmonary (kăr″dē-ō-pŭl′mō-nĕr-ē) [″ + L. *pulmo,* lung] Pert. to the heart and lungs.

cardiopulmonary arrest Cardiac arrest.

cardiopuncture [″ + L. *punctura,* piercing] Surgical incision or puncture of the heart. SYN: *cardiocentesis*.

cardiopyloric (kăr″dē-ō-pī-lor′ĭk) [″ + *pyloros,* gatekeeper] Pert. to the cardiac and pyloric ends of the stomach.

cardiorenal (kăr″dē-ō-rē′năl) [Gr. *kardia,* heart, + L. *renalis,* pert. to kidney] Pert. to both the heart and the kidneys.

cardiorrhaphy (kăr″dē-or′ă-fē) [″ +

rhaphe, seam, ridge] Suturing of the heart muscle.

cardiorrhexis (kăr″dē-ō-rĕk′sĭs) [″ + *rhexis,* rupture] Rupture of the heart.

cardiosclerosis (kăr″dē-ō-sklĕ-rō′sĭs) [″ + *sklerosis,* hardening] Hardening of the cardiac tissues and arteries.

cardiospasm (kăr′dē-ō-spăzm) [″ + *spasmos,* a convulsion] Achalasia of the esophagus. SYN: *achalasia of the cardia.*

cardiotachometer (kăr″dē-ō-tăk-ŏm′ĕ-tĕr) [Gr. *kardia,* heart, + *tachos,* speed, + *metron,* measure] An instrument for measuring the heart rate over a long period.

cardiotherapy (kăr″dē-ō-thĕr′ă-pē) [″ + *therapeia,* treatment] The treatment of cardiac diseases.

cardiothyrotoxicosis (kăr″dē-ō-thī″rō-tŏk″sĭ-kō′sĭs) [″ + *thyreos,* shield, + *toxikon,* poison, + *osis,* condition] Heart disease due to hyperthyroidism.

cardiotomy (kăr″dē-ŏt′ō-mē) [″ + *tome,* incision] Incision of the heart.

cardiotonic (kăr″dē-ō-tŏn′ĭk) [″ + *tonos,* tone] Increasing the tonicity of the heart. Various drugs, including digitalis, are cardiotonic. SEE: *inotropic.*

cardiotoxic (kăr″dē-ō-tŏk′sĭk) [″ + *toxikon,* poisoning] Poisonous to the heart.

cardiovalvulitis (kăr″dē-ō-văl″vū-lī′tĭs) [″ + L. *valvula,* valve, + Gr. *itis,* inflammation] Inflammation of the heart valves.

cardiovalvulotome (kăr″dē-ō-văl′vū-lō-tōm″) [″ + ″ + Gr. *tome,* incision] An instrument for excising part of a valve, esp. the mitral valve.

cardiovascular (kăr″dē-ō-văs′kū-lăr) [″ + L. *vasculum,* small vessel] Pert. to the heart and blood vessels.

cardiovascular collapse Sudden loss of effective blood flow to the tissues, which may be caused by such conditions as cardiogenic shock, vasovagal syncope, or postural hypotension. SEE: *cardiac arrest.*

cardiovascular reflex **1.** A sympathetic increase in heart rate when increased pressure in, or distention of, great veins occurs. **2.** Reflex vasoconstriction resulting from reduced venous pressure.

cardioversion (kăr′dē-ō-vĕr″zhŭn) [″ + L. *versio,* a turning] The restoration of normal sinus rhythm by chemical or electrical means. When performed medicinally, the procedure relies on the oral or intravenous administration of antiarrhythmic drugs. Electrical cardioversion relies instead on the delivery of synchronized shock of direct electrical current across the chest wall. It is used to terminate arrhythmias such as atrial fibrillation, atrial flutter, supraventricular tachycardia, and well-tolerated ventricular tachycardia. Unlike defibrillation, which is an unsynchronized shock applied during dire emergencies, electrical cardioversion is timed to avoid the T wave of cardiac repolarization to avoid triggering malignant arrhythmias. A patient will almost always require sedation and analgesia before the procedure.

CAUTION: Electrical cardioversion should not be used in patients who have recently eaten (because of the risk of regurgitation of stomach contents), in patients with severe electrolyte abnormalities, in patients with some drug overdoses, or in patients unable or unwilling to give informed consent. Patients need to be advised of the risks of cardioversion, including the rare precipitation of ventricular fibrillation and ventricular tachycardia, the development of bradyarrhythmias or heart blocks, and the possibility of embolic stroke.

PATIENT CARE: The procedure, expected sensations, complications, and risks are explained to and clarified for the patient. Emotional support is provided throughout the procedure and at its conclusion. The patient's medication history is reviewed, and cardiac glycoside use is reported to the health care provider, along with the patient's electrolyte levels. Emergency equipment (including ACLS drugs, a bag-valve-mask resuscitator, supplemental oxygen, suction, laryngoscope and appropriate size ET tube, defibrillator, and supplies for intravenous injection) are assembled at the bedside. In the hospital setting, emergency personnel (respiratory technicians, anesthesiologists, nurses, and paramedics) may assist the attending physician. The patient's vital signs are checked, an intravenous infusion is started, and the patient is connected to a continuous ECG monitor. Dentures are removed from the mouth, and necklaces or pendants, as well as nitroglycerin patches, are removed from the chest and neck. Chest electrodes are placed to facilitate recording of tall R waves without interfering with paddle placement. A 12-lead ECG is obtained and the patient is given enriched oxygen to breathe. The patient is placed in a supine position, and adequate ventilation and oxygenation are ensured by observation and oximetry. A sedative, such as diazepam, is provided as prescribed unless the patient is profoundly hypotensive. The defibrillator leads are attached to the patient. The cardioverter/defibrillator is set to synchronize with the patient's QRS complex, and the recording is checked to ensure that each R wave is marked. The control is set to the energy level prescribed by the health care provider or by protocol. The defibrillation pads for hands-free operation (or manual paddles) are placed in prescribed positions on the chest wall. All personnel in attendance are cleared from direct contact with the patient or his or her bed. After this is carefully verified, the electrical current is discharged. The monitor is immediately analyzed to ensure that the dysrhythmia has resolved. If it has not, the procedure is repeated, usually with a higher energy setting. After successful cardioversion, health care personnel monitor the posttreatment rhythm and vital signs until the patient's stability is assured. The patient's skin is inspected for burns. SEE: *defibrillation*.

cardioverter (kăr′dē-ō-vĕr″tĕr) A device used to administer electrical shocks to the heart through electrodes placed on the chest wall or on the surface of the heart itself. It is used in the emergency management of cardiac dysrhythmias such as ventricular or supraventricular tachycardias. Changing the dysrhythmia to normal sinus rhythm is called cardioversion. SEE: *defibrillator*.

automatic implantable c. An implantable device for detecting and terminating ventricular tachycardia or fibrillation.

carditis (kăr-dī′tĭs) [″ + *itis*, inflammation] Inflammation of the layers of the heart. It usually involves two of the following: pericardium, myocardium, or endocardium.

Coxsackie c. Carditis or pericarditis that may occur in infections with enteroviruses of the Coxsackie groups, and also with echovirus groups.

rheumatic c. Inflammation of cardiac tissue as a result of acute rheumatic fever. Mitral insufficiency is a prominent feature, and aortic insufficiency is sometimes present as well.

care, cluster A system of home care for the elderly that allows the needs of many clients who live in proximity to be met by a team of workers.

care, culturally competent The provision of health care with professional tolerance and respect for individuals of all ages, nationalities, races, genders, beliefs, and behaviors.

care, day The supervision of dependents during working hours. The goals of day care are to provide adequate, affordable care for young children or dependent adults, esp. while employed caregivers are at work.

c., adult day ABBR: ADC. A licensed agency where chronically ill, disabled, or cognitively impaired persons can stay during the day under health care supervision. Most people who attend adult day care are elderly and need some assistance with care. They are able to participate in structured activities programs and to ambulate with or without an assistive device. Most day care centers operate 5 days a week for 8 to 12 hr a day.

care, end-of-life Supportive care for dying patients. Such care can include invasive interventions like advanced cardiac life support, or supportive interventions, like educational, emotional, or social assistance to patients with terminal illnesses.

care, family-centered The integration and collaboration of family members in the patient care team, esp. in the care of dependent infants, children, or adults with complex or ongoing health care needs.

care, home health The provision of equipment and services to patients in their homes to restore and maintain the individual's maximal levels of comfort, function, and health.

care, intensive Care of critically ill patients.

care, long-term ABBR: LTC. **1.** A range of continuous health care or social services for individuals with chronic physical or mental impairments, or both. LTC provides for basic needs and promotes optimal functioning. SEE: *Nursing Diagnoses Appendix*. **2.** Used interchangeably with nursing home care.

care, medical The use of medical skill to benefit a patient.

care, mouth Personal and bedside care of the oral cavity including the gingivae, teeth, lips, epithelial covering of the mucosa, pharynx, and tongue. When ill, persons who would normally be able to provide their own oral hygiene may require assistance in maintaining a healthy oral environment. The intensity and frequency of care is dictated by patient comfort; the severity of the illness; potential or existing irritation or inflammation secondary to trauma or therapy; and the patient's state of consciousness, level of cooperation, and ability to provide self-care. SEE: *stomatitis*.

care, personal Self-care (2).

care, primary Integrated, accessible health care, provided where the patient first seeks medical assistance, by clinicians who are responsible for most of a patient's personal health care, including health maintenance, therapy during illnesses, and consultation with specialists.

care, respiratory The evaluation, treatment, and rehabilitation of patients with cardiopulmonary disease by respiratory therapy professionals working under a physician's supervision.

care, respite Provision of short-term care to older or disabled persons in the community to allow caregivers a temporary relief from their responsibilities. Respite care is similar to adult day care, but organized activities or services are not available. The care may be provided either in the patient's home, church, community center, nursing home, or caregiver's home.

care, secondary medical Medical care of a patient by a physician acting as a consultant. The provider of primary medical care usually refers the patient for expert or specialty consultation, or a second opinion.

care, skilled Medical care provided by licensed professionals working under the direction of a physician.

care, tertiary medical Medical care of a patient in a facility staffed and equipped to administer comprehensive care. In the usual situation, this level of care is provided in a large hospital to which the patient has been referred or transferred.

care, transitional Health care services provided to patients after hospitalization in an acute care facility, before they are ready to return to their homes. Transitional care shortens acute hospital stays, decreases health care costs, and provides a period for recuperation for patients who are still unable to thrive independently. Facilities used in transitional care include rehabilitation units, long-term care hospitals, subacute care facilities, hospice services, and some home care services.

caregiver One who provides care to a dependent or partially dependent patient. In an acute care setting, the caregiver is most often a professional; however, in the home care situation, this person is often a family member. Care of caregivers is a focus of nurses, social workers, and other health care providers who manage chronically ill patients. Generally, caregivers need emotional support and comfort owing to the extreme stress of their lives. SEE: *caregiver burden*.

caregiver burden The perception of stress and fatigue caused by the sustained effort required in caring for persons with chronic illness or other conditions with special needs for care.

caregiver role strain A caregiver's felt or exhibited difficulty in performing the family caregiver role. SEE: *Nursing Diagnoses Appendix*.

caregiver role strain, risk for The vulnerability of the caregiver for felt difficulty in performing the family caregiver role. SEE: *Nursing Diagnoses Appendix*.

Caregiver Stress Inventory ABBR: CSI. A 50-item scale specific to professionals caring for dependent patients. It is divided into three subscales measuring stress related to the patient's verbal and physical behavior, the patient's mental, emotional, and social behavior, and the resources, knowledge, and abilities of the staff.

C.A.R.F. *Commission on Accreditation of Rehabilitation Facilities.*

caries (kār′ēz, kār′ĭ-ēz) [L., rottenness] Gradual decay and disintegration of soft or bony tissue or of a tooth. If the decay progresses, the surrounding tissue becomes inflamed and an abscess forms (e.g., chronic abscess, tuberculosis, and bacterial invasion of teeth). In caries, the bone disintegrates by pieces, whereas in necrosis, large masses of bone are involved. SYN: *dental cavity*. **carious** (-rē-ŭs), *adj.*

arrested c. Apparent lack of progress in a carious lesion between dental examinations.

bottle mouth c. Extensive caries and discoloration of the teeth observed in children from 19 months to 4 years of age who have had prolonged bottle feedings.

cervical c. Caries involving the neck of the tooth, slightly above or below the junction between the root cementum and the enamel crown.

classification of c. G. V. Black's classification of dental caries according to the part of the tooth involved: class I, occlusal; class II, interproximal, commonly at the dentinoenamel junction of bicuspids and molars; class III, interproximal surfaces not involving incisal surfaces; class IV, interproximal but involving an incisal surface; class V, the faciocervical area.

dental c. Tooth decay; progressive decalcification of the enamel and dentin of a tooth. The causes are not fully known, but minimizing intake of dietary refined carbohydrates and good dental hygiene prevent growth of bacteria that contribute to the development of caries. Proper brushing of the teeth is effective in preventing and removing dental plaque in all areas except those between the teeth and deep fissures. Use of dental floss or tape removes plaque from between adjacent tooth surfaces; deep pits and fissures may be sealed by the application of resins. The sealant may need to be replaced periodically. Early detection and dental restorations offer the best form of control once caries has formed. Topical application of fluoride promotes resistance to dental caries. Dental caries is less likely to develop if appropriate amounts of fluoride are ingested while the teeth are developing. It is important that excess fluoride not be ingested because greater amounts than required (about 1 mg/day) cause mottling of the teeth. Fluoride in the diet does not obviate the need for topical application of fluoride to the teeth. SYN: *dental cavity*. SEE: illus.; *dental plaque*.

incipient c. One of the two distinct stages in the development of a carious dental lesion. The first stage is the incipient lesion, marked by the appearance of a white spot. Microscopic pores course through the enamel to the subsurface demineralization, where the main body of the lesion is located.

necrotic c. A disease in which

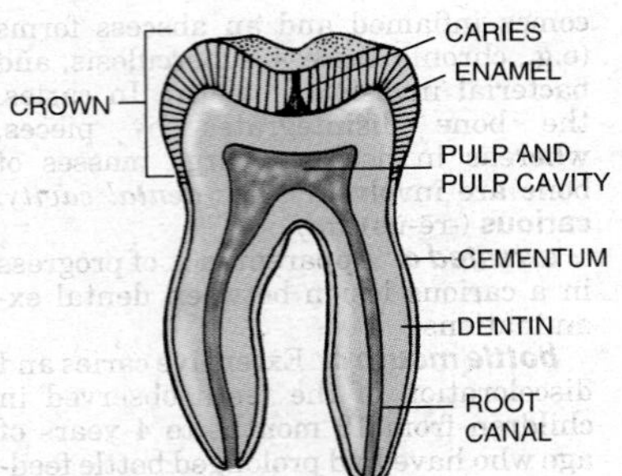

ACID BREAKS DOWN THE ENAMEL THAT COVERS THE CROWN OF THE TOOTH

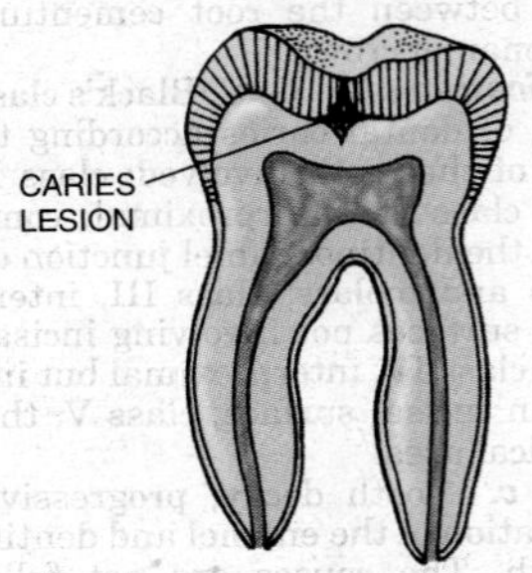

DECAY PENETRATES THE DENTIN, THE LAYER UNDER THE ENAMEL

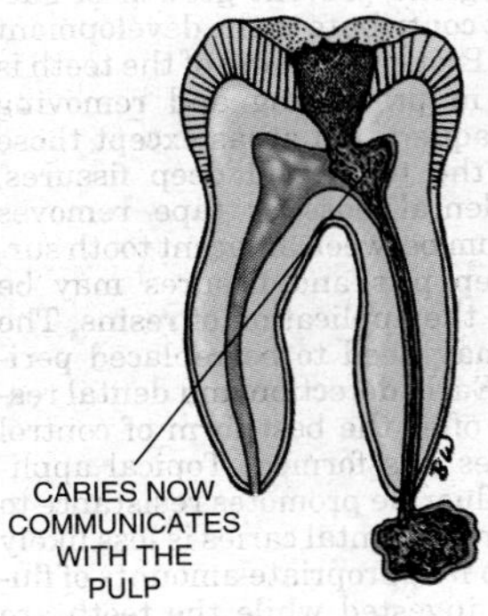

THE CAVITY, IF NOT REPAIRED, SPREADS INTO THE PULP OF THE TOOTH. THIS MAY CAUSE INFLAMMATION AND AN ABSCESS. THEN THE TOOTH MAY HAVE TO BE EXTRACTED.

DENTAL CARIES

masses of bone lie in a suppurating cavity.

pit and fissure c. Caries in the pits and fissures of tooth enamel.

radiation c. Dental caries that develops as a side effect of treatment of malignancies of the oral cavity with ionizing radiation. The etiology is, in part, due to the dysfunction of the salivary glands.

rampant c. A sudden onset of widespread caries that affects most of the teeth and penetrates quickly to the dental pulp.

recurrent c. Dental caries that develops at the small imperfections between the tooth surface and a restoration, caused by plaque at the imperfections. SYN: *secondary c.*

root c. Caries on the root of a tooth. The root is more susceptible to decay than the rest of the tooth due to the lack of an enamel covering, difficulty in maintaining a clean root surface, and the lack of effective preventive therapies.

secondary c. Recurrent c.

c. sicca Bony destruction such as that caused by infection with syphilis.

spinal c. Pott's disease.

carina (kă-rī′nă) *pl.* **carinae** [L., keel of a boat] A structure with a projecting central ridge.

c. nasi The olfactory nasal sulcus.

c. tracheae The ridge at the lower end of the trachea separating the openings of the two primary bronchi.

c. urethralis The ridge extending posteriorly from the urethral orifice and continuous with the anterior column of the vagina.

carinate (kăr′ĭ-nāt) [L. *carina,* keel of a boat] Keel-shaped; having a conspicuous central ridge.

caring behaviors The actions or responses of providing patient services.

PATIENT CARE: The following are the 10 highest-ranked caring behaviors, derived from nursing literature, then selected by nurses as evident in caring situations with patients: attentive listening, comforting, honesty, patience, responsibility, providing information so the patient can make an informed decision, touch, sensitivity, respect, addressing the patient by name.

carioca (kăr-ē-ō-kăh) A bean (legume) that is a good source of vegetable protein and fiber.

cariogenesis (kār″ē-ō-jĕn′ĕ-sĭs) [L. *caries,* rottenness, + Gr. *genesis,* generation, birth] The formation of caries. SEE: *dental caries.*

cariogenic (kā″rē-ō-jĕn′ĭk) [″ + Gr. *gennan,* to produce] Conducive to caries formation.

cariostatic (kā″rē-ō-stăt′ĭk) Able to prevent the formation of dental caries.

carious (kā′rē-ŭs) **1.** Affected with or pert. to caries. **2.** Having pits or perforations.

carisoprodol (kăr″ī-sō-prō′dŏl) A drug that relaxes muscles by acting on the central nervous system. Toxic levels of the drug may accumulate after prolonged use.

carminative (kăr-mĭn′ă-tĭv) [L. *carmin-*

ativus, cleanse] An agent that helps to prevent gas formation in the gastrointestinal tract.

carmustine (BCNU) An antineoplastic drug. Trade name is BiCNU.

carnal (kăr′năl) [L. *carnalis,* flesh] Pert. to the desires and appetites of the flesh; sensual.

carneous (kăr′nē-ŭs) [L. *carneus,* fleshy] Fleshy.

Carnett's sign (kăr′nĕtz) [J. B. Carnett, American physician] In evaluating a surgical abdomen, decreased abdominal tenderness to palpation after the supine patient elevates his or her head from the bed. The sign indicates that acute abdominal pain originates in the rectus muscle sheath rather than the peritoneum.

carnitine (kăr′nĭ-tĭn) A chemical, γ-trimethylamine-β-hydroxybutyrate, important in metabolizing palmitic and stearic acids. It has been used therapeutically in treating myopathy due to carnitine deficiency.

carnivore (kăr′nĭ-vor) An animal that eats primarily meat, particularly an animal of the order Carnivora, which includes cats, dogs, and bears.

carnivorous (kăr-nĭv′ō-rŭs) [L. *carnivorus*] Flesh-eating.

carnophobia (kăr″nō-fō′bē-ă) [″ + Gr. *phobos,* fear] An abnormal aversion to meat.

carnose (kăr′nōs) Having the consistency of or resembling flesh.

carnosine (kăr′nō-sĭn) $C_9H_{14}N_4O_3$; a chemical, β-alanylhistidine, present in brain and muscle. Its function is unknown.

carnosity (kăr-nŏs′ĭ-tē) [L. *carnositas,* fleshiness] An excrescence resembling flesh; a fleshy growth.

carotenase (kăr-ŏt′ĕ-nās) [Gr. *karoton,* carrot] An enzyme that converts carotene into vitamin A. SYN: *carotinase.*

carotene (kăr′ō-tēn) [Gr. *karoton*] One of several yellow to red antioxidant compounds that are biochemical precursors to vitamin A. Many fresh fruits and vegetables (including carrots, squash, sweet potatoes, corn, apricots, and oranges) are richly endowed with these chemicals. They may play a part in preventing atherosclerosis, neurodegenerative diseases, cancers, and retinal degeneration.

Retinol is the form of vitamin A found in mammals. One retinol equivalent is equal to 6 μg of beta-carotene. Beta-carotene is a safer food supplement than vitamin A because the latter has much greater toxic potential in large doses.

carotenemia (kăr″ō-tĕ-nē′mē-ă) [″ + *haima,* blood] Carotene in the blood, marked by yellowing of the skin (pseudojaundice). It can be distinguished from true jaundice by the lack of yellow discoloration of the conjunctivae in carotenemia.

carotenoid (kă-rŏt′ĕ-noyd) [″ + *eidos,* form, shape] **1.** One of a group of more than 500 yellow, orange, or red fat-soluble pigments found naturally in fruits and vegetables and acting as antioxidants in the body. About 50 carotenoids are precursors of vitamin A. Beta-carotene, the most abundant carotenoid, has the most provitamin A activity. **2.** Resembling carotene.

carotic (kă-rŏt′ĭk) [Gr. *karos,* deep sleep] **1.** Carotid. **2.** Resembling stupor; stupefying.

caroticotympanic (kă-rŏt″ĭ-kō-tĭm-păn′ĭk) Pert. to the carotid canal and the tympanic cavity (the middle ear).

carotid (kă-rŏt′ĭd) [Gr. *karos,* deep sleep] **1.** Pert. to the right and left common carotid arteries, which form the principal blood supply to the head and neck. The left arises directly from the aortic arch and the right from the brachiocephalic artery. Each of these two arteries divides to form external and internal carotid arteries. **2.** Pert. to any carotid part, such as the carotid sinus.

carotid siphon The S-shaped terminal portion of the internal carotid artery. It is the origin of most of the arteries to the brain.

carotidynia, carotodynia (kăr-ŏt″ĭ-dĭn′ē-ă) [″ + *odyne,* pain] Pain in the face, neck, or jaw. It may be produced in persons with atypical facial neuralgia by pressure on the common carotid artery. The pain is dull and referred to the same side to which pressure was applied. Treatment is with analgesics.

carotinase Carotenase.

carotinemia Carotenemia.

carpal (kăr′păl) [Gr. *karpalis*] Pert. to the carpus or wrist.

carpal boss A bony growth on the dorsal surface of the third metacarpocarpal joint.

carpale (kăr-pā′lē) [Gr. *karpos*] Any wrist bone.

carpal spasm Involuntary contraction of the muscles of the hand. SEE: *tetany.*

carpal tunnel syndrome Pain or numbness that affects some part of the median nerve distribution of the hand (the palmar side of the thumb, the index finger, the radial half of the ring finger, and the radial half of the palm) and may radiate into the arm. Patients may have a history of cumulative trauma to the wrist, for example, in carpenters, rowers, typists, computer users, or those who regularly use vibrating tools or machinery. In addition, the condition may occur after wrist fracture, in pregnancy, or as a consequence of systemic or metabolic disorders such as diabetes mellitus, hypothyroidism, acromegaly, and amyloidosis. SEE: *repetitive motion injury.*

TREATMENT: The patient should rest the extremity, avoiding anything that aggravates the symptoms. This may require splinting of the wrist for several weeks to relieve tension on the median nerve. The patient's job requirements should be analyzed and recommendations provided for modified tools or a change in job assignment. The patient is taught how to avoid tension on the median nerve. Other treatments may include yoga, corticosteroid injections, or surgery.

PATIENT CARE: The patient is evaluated for symptoms, degree of immobility, and changes that may have occurred over time. The patient's ability to make a fist is assessed, and the fingernails are inspected for atrophy and for surrounding dry, shiny skin. The transverse carpal ligament over the median nerve is lightly percussed to elicit pain, burning, numbness, or tingling in the hands and fingers (Tinel's sign). The patient is instructed to flex the wrists for 30 sec, and the hands and fingers are assessed for pain and numbness. The prescribed analgesic drug is administered, the patient's response evaluated, and the patient instructed in the drug's use, including the need to take it with food or antacids if stomach upset or irritation occurs. The patient should use the hands for self-care as much as immobility and pain allow. If a splint is prescribed to relieve symptoms, the patient is taught how to apply it without making it too tight, and how to remove it and perform gentle range-of-motion exercises daily.

Lifestyle changes needed to help minimize symptoms are demonstrated and explained to the patient. Occupational counseling is suggested if the syndrome necessitates a change in jobs.

The need for diagnostic studies, such as nerve conduction tests or electromyography, and expected sensations are explained. If surgery (carpal tunnel release) is required, the patient is prepared by explaining the procedure and expected sensations. Postoperatively, neurovascular status in the affected extremity is carefully assessed, and the patient is encouraged to keep the hand elevated to reduce swelling and discomfort. The patient should perform prescribed wrist and finger exercises daily to improve circulation and to enhance muscle tone; he or she can perform these exercises in warm water if they are painful (wearing a surgical glove if dressings are still in place). He or she should avoid lifting anything weighing more than a few ounces. The patient should report severe, persistent pain or tenderness, which may point to tenosynovitis or hematoma formation. The incision should be kept clean and dry, and dressings changed daily until the incision has healed completely. Dressings should also be checked for bleeding; any unusual bleeding or drainage should be reported. The patient is encouraged to express any concerns, and support is offered. SEE: *Nursing Diagnoses Appendix*.

carpectomy (kăr-pĕk′tō-mē) [″ + *ektome,* excision] Excision of the carpus or a portion of it.

carphology, carphologia (kăr-fō-lō′jē-ă, -fŏl′ō-jē) [Gr. *karphos,* dry twig, + *legein,* to pluck] Involuntary picking at bedclothes, seen esp. in febrile delirium. SYN: *floccillation*.

carpo- [Gr. *karpos*] Combining form for carpus.

carpometacarpal [″ + *meta,* beyond, + *karpos,* wrist] Pert. to both the carpus and the metacarpus.

carpopedal (kăr″pō-pĕd′ăl) [″ + L. *ped,* foot] Pert. to both the wrist and the foot.

carpoptosis (kăr″pŏp-tō′sĭs) [″ + *ptosis,* a falling] Wrist drop.

carpus (kăr′pŭs) [L.] The eight bones of the wrist joint. SEE: *skeleton; wrist drop*.

carrageen, carragheen (kăr′ă-gēn) Irish moss; dried red alga, *Chondrus crispus,* from which the substance carrageenan, or carragheenan, is obtained. It is used as a demulcent and thickening agent in medicines and foods. SYN: *Irish moss*.

Carrel-Dakin treatment (kăr-ĕl′dā′kĭn) [Alexis Carrel, Fr.-U.S. surgeon, 1873–1944; Henry D. Dakin, U.S. chemist, 1880–1952] A method of wound irrigation first used in 1915. The wound is intermittently irrigated with Dakin's solution.

carrier [O. Fr. *carier,* to bear] **1.** A person who harbors a specific pathogenic organism, has no discernible symptoms or signs of the disease, and is potentially capable of spreading the organism to others. **2.** An animal, insect, or substance (e.g., food, water, feces) that can transmit infectious organisms. SYN: *vector*. SEE: *fomes; isolation; microorganism; Standard and Universal Precautions Appendix; communicable disease* for table. **3.** A molecule that when combined with another substance can pass through a cell membrane, as occurs in facilitated diffusion or some active transport mechanisms. **4.** A heterozygote; one who carries a recessive gene together with its normal allele. **5.** An instrument or apparatus for transporting something; in dentistry, for example, an amalgam carrier.

active c. One who harbors a pathogenic organism for a considerable period after recovery from disease caused by it.

convalescent c. One who harbors an infective organism during recovery from the disease caused by the organism.

genetic c. One whose chromosomes contain a pathological mutant gene that may be transmitted to offspring. In some cases, such as Tay-Sachs disease, this can be detected prenatally by a laboratory test done on amniotic fluid.

incubatory c. One who harbors and spreads an infectious organism during the incubation period of a disease.

intermittent c. One who is capable of spreading infectious organisms at intervals.

carrier-free (kăr′ē-ĕr-frē) Not attached to a carrier; said of radioactive isotopes.

Carrion's disease (kăr-ē-ōnz′) [Daniel A. Carrion, 1850–1885, a Peruvian student who died after voluntarily injecting himself with a disease] Bartonellosis.

carry-over The portion of analyte brought from one reaction segment to the next. The accuracy of laboratory test results may be altered by contaminants that are transferred from one reaction to the following one.

cartilage (kăr′tĭ-lĭj) [L. *cartilago,* gristle] A specialized type of dense connective tissue consisting of cells embedded in a ground substance or matrix. The matrix is firm and compact and can withstand considerable pressure or tension. Cartilage is bluish-white or gray and is semiopaque; it has no nerve or blood supply of its own. The cells lie in cavities called lacunae. They may be single or in groups of two, three, or four.

Cartilage forms parts of joints in the adult skeleton, such as between vertebral bodies and on the articular surfaces of bones. It also occurs in the costal cartilages of the ribs, in the nasal septum, in the external ear and lining of the eustachian tube, in the wall of the larynx, and in the trachea and bronchi. It forms the major portion of the embryonic skeleton, providing a model in which most bones develop.

articular c. The thin layer of smooth, hyaline cartilage located on the joint surfaces of a bone, as in a synovial joint.

costal c. A cartilage that connects the end of a true rib with the sternum or the end of a false rib with the costal cartilage above.

cricoid c. The lowermost cartilage of the larynx; shaped like a signet ring, the broad portion or lamina being posterior, the anterior portion forming the arch. SEE: *larynx* for illus.

cuneiform c. One of two small pieces of elastic cartilage that lie in the aryepiglottic fold of the larynx immediately anterior to the arytenoid cartilage.

elastic c. Cartilage that contains elastin fibers in the matrix. Found in the epiglottis, external ear, and auditory tube, it strengthens these and maintains their shape. SYN: *yellow c.*

fibrous c. Fibrocartilage.

hyaline c. A bluish-white, glassy, translucent cartilage. The matrix appears homogeneous although it contains collagenous fibers forming a fine network. The walls of the lacunae stain intensely with basic dyes. Hyaline cartilage is flexible and slightly elastic. Its surface is covered by the perichondrium except on articular surfaces. It is found in articular cartilage, costal cartilages, the nasal septum, the larynx, and the trachea.

repair of c. defects The experimental treatment of full-thickness knee cartilage defects by culturing cartilage cells from the patient and then implanting them in cartilage tears. The cells are covered with a thin patch of bone tissue.

semilunar c. One of two crescentic cartilages (medial and lateral) of the knee joint between the femur and tibia.

shark c. An alternative medical therapy for cancer. Its efficacy is unproven.

thyroid c. The largest cartilage of the larynx, a shield-shaped cartilage that forms the prominence known as the Adam's apple.

yellow c. Elastic c.

cartilaginification (kăr″tĭ-lă-jĭn″ĭ-fĭ-kā′shŭn) [″ + *facere,* to make] Cartilage formation or chondrification; the development of cartilage from undifferentiated tissue.

cartilaginoid (kăr″tĭ-lăj′ĭ-noyd) [″ + Gr. *eidos,* form, shape] Resembling cartilage.

cartilaginous (kăr″tĭ-lăj′ĭ-nŭs) Pert. to or consisting of cartilage.

cartilago (kăr″tĭ-lă′gō) *pl.* **cartilagines** [L.] Cartilage.

caruncle (kăr′ŭng-kl) [L. *caruncula,* small flesh] A small fleshy growth.

lacrimal c. A small reddish elevation found on the conjunctiva near the inner canthus, at the medial angle of the eye.

sublingual c. A protuberance on each side of the frenulum of the tongue, containing the openings of the ducts from the submandibular and sublingual salivary glands.

urethral c. A small, red, papillary growth that is highly vascular and is sometimes found in the urinary meatus in females. It is characterized by pain on urination and is very sensitive to friction.

caruncula (kăr-ŭng′kū-lă) *pl.* **carunculae** [L.] Caruncle.

c. hymenales Small irregular nodules representing remains of the hymen.

Carvallo's sign [J. M. Rivero-Carvallo, contemporary Mexican physician] An increase in intensity of the presystolic murmur heard in patients with tricuspid stenosis during inspiration, and its decrease during expiration. This is best demonstrated with the patient in an erect position.

carvedilol (kăr-vē′dĭ-lōl) A beta- and alpha-blocking drug that can be used to treat high blood pressure and congestive heart failure. Trade name is Coreg.

carve-out In managed care, a service or benefit for a specific disease, condition, or population that is contracted for separately from the rest of a health insurance plan. Carve-outs typically are used in managed care contracts to identify the costs associated with esp. expensive forms of care, such as mental health or substance abuse services.

carver A knife or other instrument used to fashion or shape an object. In dentistry, it is used with artificial teeth or dental restorations.

amalgam c. A small, sharp instrument of varying shape used to carve or contour amalgam for interdental occlusion.

wax c. A blunt instrument of varying shape to heat and carve or shape wax patterns.

cary-, caryo- [Gr. *karyon,* nucleus] Combining form meaning *nucleus.*

CAS *Coronary artery scan.*

Casal necklace [Gaspar Casal, Sp. physician, 1691–1759] Bilaterally symmetrical lesions of the neck that represent a portion of the skin's involvement in pellagra. The lesions begin as erythemas and progress to vesiculation and crusting.

cascade (kăs-kād′) The continuation of a process through a series of steps, each step initiating the next, until the final step is reached. The action may or may not become amplified as each step progresses.

perineal c. cleansing douche.

cascara sagrada (kăs-kăr′ă să-gră′dă) The dried bark of *Rhamnus purshiana,* a small tree grown on the western U.S. coast and in parts of South America. It is the main ingredient in aromatic cascara sagrada fluid extract, a cathartic.

case [L. *casus,* happening] **1.** An occurrence of disease; incorrectly used to refer to a patient. **2.** An enclosing structure.

index c. The initial individual whose condition leads to the investigation of a hereditary or infectious disorder.

caseate (kā′sē-āt) [L. *caseus,* cheese] To undergo cheesy degeneration, as in certain necroses.

caseation (kā″sē-ā′shŭn) **1.** The process in which necrotic tissue is converted into a granular amorphous mass resembling cheese. **2.** The precipitation of casein during coagulation of milk.

case control In epidemiology, a study in which index cases are matched with comparison cases to discover risk factors or exposure.

casefinding An active attempt to identify persons who have a certain disease. SEE: *epidemiology.*

case history The complete medical, family, social, and psychiatric history of a patient up to the time of admission for the present illness.

casein (kā′sē-ĭn) [L. *caseus,* cheese] The principal protein in milk, which forms curds at acid pH. When coagulated by rennin or acid, it becomes one of the principal ingredients of cheese.

case law Opinions or decisions made by the courts.

case management An individualized approach to coordinating patient care services, esp. when clients with complex needs or chronic medical problems require multifaceted or interdisciplinary care. Case management is a particularly valuable approach to meeting the service needs of impaired elderly persons and others with chronic medical disabilities.

hospital c.m. A system of patient care delivery in which a case manager, typically a registered nurse, coordinates interdisciplinary care for a group of patients. The advantages of hospital case management are improved quality, continuity of care, and decreased hospital costs.

caseous (kā′sē-ŭs) **1.** Resembling cheese. **2.** Pert. to transformation of tissues into a cheesy mass.

$CaSO_4$ Calcium sulfate.

caspase A protein that regulates programmed cellular death (apoptosis).

cassava A group of perennial herbs of the genus *Manihot.* The plant is one of the most efficient converters of solar energy to carbohydrate. The root of *M. esculenta* provides an excellent source of starch and can thrive in poor, dry, acid soils. To be suitable for eating, the root is processed by one of several methods to remove or control the amount of cyanide present. Tapioca is made from cassava.

cassette (kă-sĕt′) [Fr., little box] **1.** A flat, lightproof box with an intensifying screen, for holding x-ray film. SEE: il-

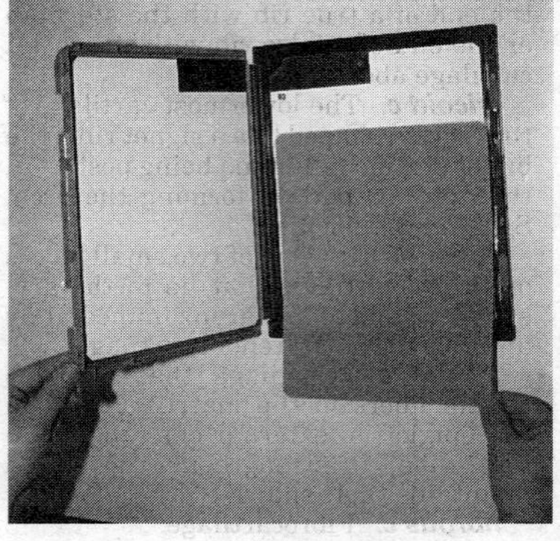

CASSETTE AND FILM

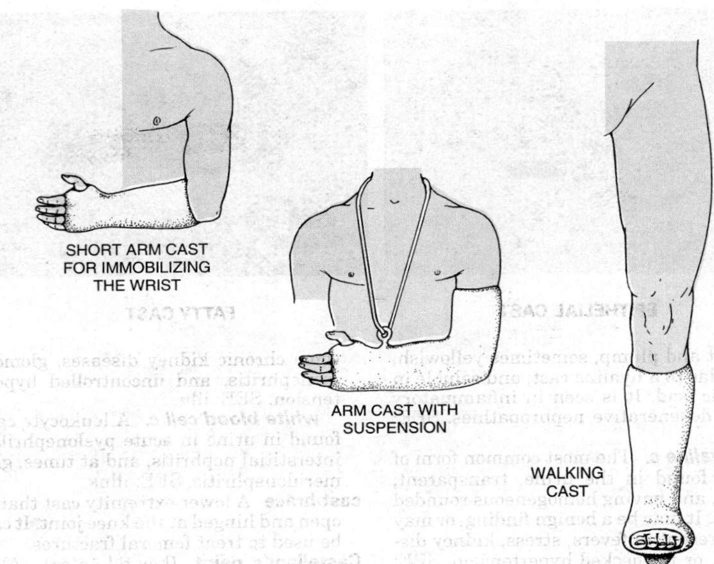

CASTS

lus. **2.** A case used for film or magnetic tape.

cassette, screen-type A light-tight film holder.

cast [ME. *casten,* to carry] **1.** In dentistry, a positive copy of jaw tissues over which denture bases may be made. **2.** To make an accurate metallic reproduction of a wax pattern of a dental appliance, tooth crown, or inlay cavity preparation. **3.** Pliable or fibrous material shed in various pathological conditions; the product of effusion. It is molded to the shape of the part in which it has been accumulated. Casts are classified as bronchial, intestinal, nasal, esophageal, renal, tracheal, urethral, and vaginal; constituents are classified as bloody, fatty, fibrinous, granular, hyaline, mucous, and waxy. **4.** A solid mold of a part, usually applied in situ for immobilization as in fractures, dislocations, and other severe injuries. It is usually made of plaster of Paris, sodium silicate, starch, or dextrin that is rubbed into crinoline, then soaked in water, carefully applied to the immobilized part, and allowed to harden. Synthetic materials, such as fiberglass, are also used, esp. for non–weight-bearing parts of the body. SEE: illus.

PATIENT CARE: Neurovascular status distal to the cast is monitored; and any deterioration in circulation and in sensory or motor abilities, such as paresthesias, paralysis, diminished pulses, pallor, coldness, or pain, is documented and reported. Pain or burning under the cast, including the region involved, is also documented and reported. The cast is bivalved or removed to relieve pressure. Objects should not be placed inside a cast to relieve itching, but relief often can be obtained by applying cold (a well-sealed ice bag) to the cast over the area that itches, or by scratching the opposite extremity in the same area. The patient is instructed in cast care and ways to protect the cast from damage; prescribed exercises or activity limitations; and use of any assistive devices such as slings, crutches, or walker. SEE: *Nursing Diagnoses Appendix.*

body c. A cast used to immobilize the spine. It may extend from the thorax to the groin.

bronchial c. A cast seen in the sputum of patients with asthma and some patients with bronchitis.

broomstick c. A type of cast used following skin traction for Legg's disease (Legg-Calvé-Perthes disease). A bar is used between upper femoral casts to maintain abduction. SEE: *Legg's disease.*

epithelial c. Tubular epithelial cells in the urine, a finding in some cases of glomerulonephritis. SEE: illus.

fatty c. A urinary cast, consisting of a mass of fatty globules, seen in the examination of patients with nephrosis. SEE: illus.

fibrinous c. A yellow-brown cast sometimes seen in glomerulonephritis.

granular c. A coarse or fine granule,

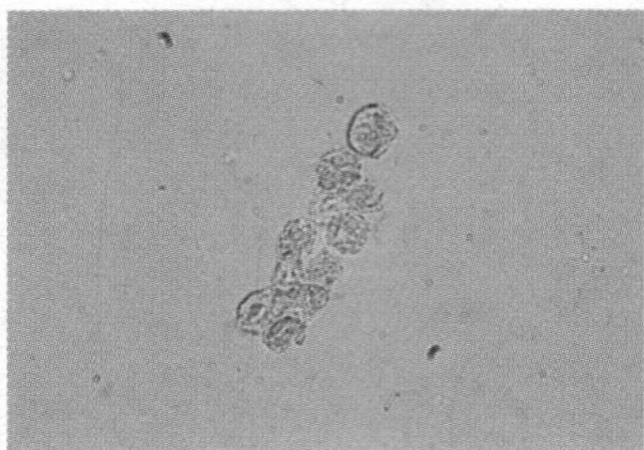
EPITHELIAL CAST

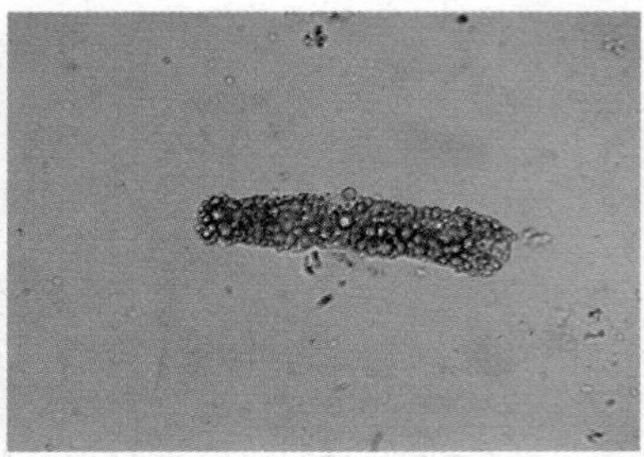
FATTY CAST

short and plump, sometimes yellowish, similar to a hyaline cast, and soluble in acetic acid. It is seen in inflammatory and degenerative nephropathies. SEE: *cast*.

hyaline c. The most common form of cast found in the urine, transparent, pale, and having homogeneous rounded ends. It may be a benign finding, or may be present in fevers, stress, kidney disease, or unchecked hypertension. SEE: illus.

light c. A cast used in orthopedics, made of a lightweight material that is usually applied and then hardened by treating with the heat from a light.

minerva c. A body cast that extends from the top of the head to the iliac crests, leaving the facial features exposed, but supporting the chin and neck. It is used to treat odontoid fractures in children.

red blood cell c. A urinary cast composed principally of red blood cells strongly suggestive of glomerulonephritis. SEE: illus.

urinary c. A cylindrical clump of cells and proteins found in the urine in a wide variety of diseases and conditions. SEE: *Tamm-Horsfall mucoprotein*.

uterine c. A cast from the uterus passed in exfoliative endometritis or membranous dysmenorrhea.

waxy c. A light yellowish, well-defined urinary cast probably made up of disintegrating kidney cells, found in some chronic kidney diseases, glomerulonephritis, and uncontrolled hypertension. SEE: illus.

white blood cell c. A leukocyte cast found in urine in acute pyelonephritis, interstitial nephritis, and at times, glomerulonephritis. SEE: illus.

cast-brace A lower extremity cast that is open and hinged at the knee joint. It can be used to treat femoral fractures.

Castellani's paint (kăs-tĕl-ăn′ēz) [Aldo Castellani, It. physician, 1878–1971] Paint used to disinfect skin and to treat fungus infections of the skin. Its components are phenol, resorcinol, basic fuchsin, boric acid, and acetone.

casting The forming of an object in a mold.

Castleman's disease (kăs′l-mănz) [Benjamin Castleman, U.S. pathologist, 1906–1982] An occasionally aggressive illness marked by excessive growth of lymphoid tissue either localized in a single lymph node group or in multiple regions of the body. Although the cause is not precisely known, its associations with acquired immunodeficiency syndrome, Kaposi's sarcoma, and human herpes virus 8 infection have led some experts to propose that it has an infectious basis. Localized disease responds well to surgical resection. Widespread disease can sometimes be treated effectively with chemotherapy.

Castle's intrinsic factor Intrinsic factor.

castor oil A fixed oil expressed from the

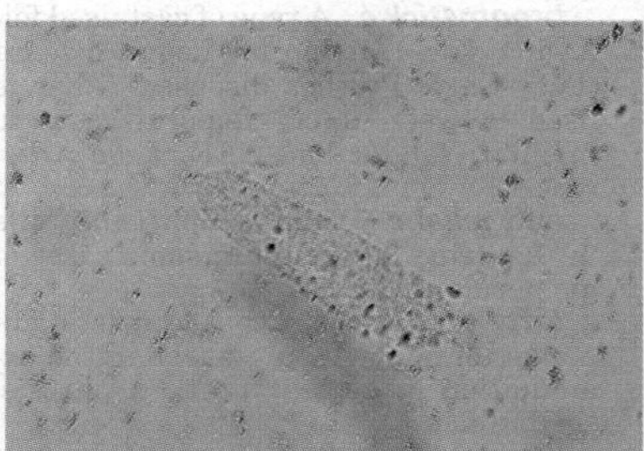
HYALINE CAST

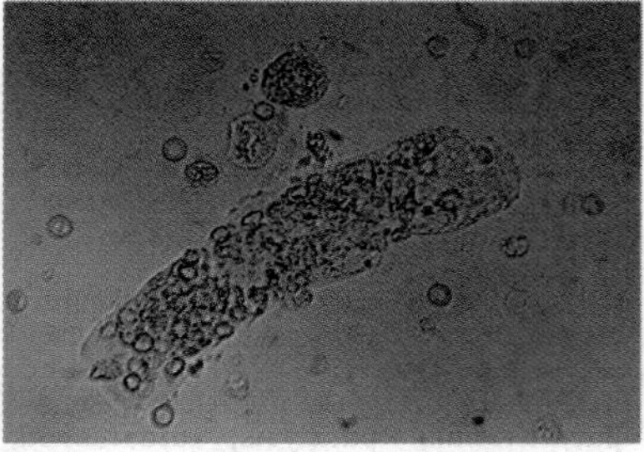
RED BLOOD CELL CAST

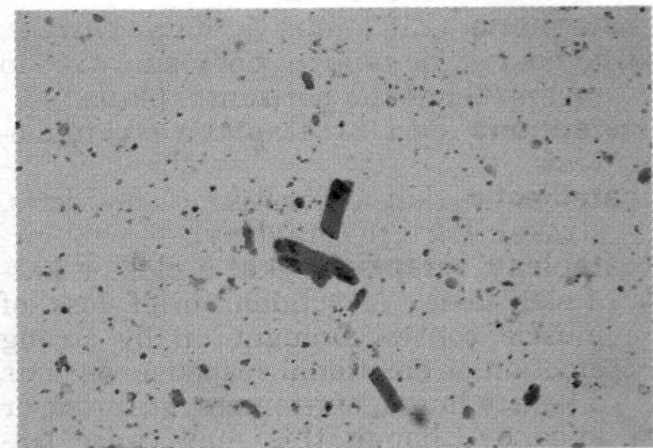

WAXY CAST

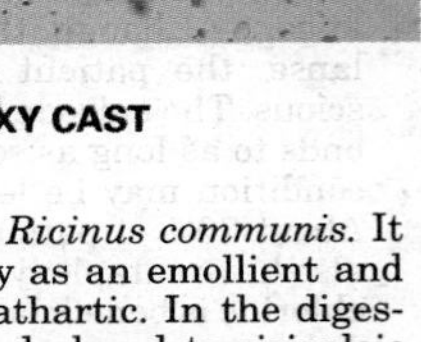

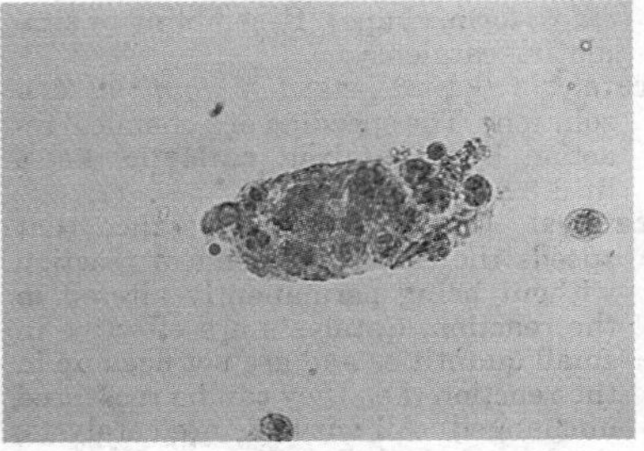

WHITE BLOOD CELL CAST

seed of the plant *Ricinus communis.* It is used externally as an emollient and internally as a cathartic. In the digestive tract it is hydrolyzed to ricinoleic acid, which acts as an irritant type of laxative.

castrate (kăs′trāt) [L. *castrare,* to prune] **1.** To remove the testicles or ovaries. SEE: *spay*. **2.** To render an individual incapable of reproduction. **3.** To spay or neuter. **4.** To deprive an individual of sex hormones by medical means, esp. in the treatment of hormone-sensitive illnesses. **5.** One who has been rendered incapable of reproduction.

castrated Rendered incapable of reproduction by removal of the testicles or ovaries.

castration (kăs-trā′shŭn) **1.** Excision of the testicles or ovaries. **2.** Destruction or inactivation of the gonads.

female c. Removal of the ovaries. SYN: *oophorectomy; spaying*.

male c. Removal of the testes. SYN: *orchiectomy*.

parasitic c. Destruction of the gonads by parasitic organisms early in life. It may result from direct infestation of the gonad or indirectly from effects of infestation in other parts of the body.

castration anxiety, castration complex Anxiety about the possibility of injury to or loss of the testicles or ovaries.

casualty (kăz′ū-ăl-tē) [L. *casualis,* accidental] **1.** An accident causing injury or death. **2.** A person injured or killed in an accident or preventable traumatic event. **3.** A military person captured, missing, injured, or killed.

casuistics (kăz-ū-ĭs′tĭks) [L. *casus,* chance] **1.** Analysis of clinical case records to establish the general characteristics of a disease. **2.** In moral questions, the determination of right and wrong by application of ethical principles to a particular case.

cata- [Gr. *kata,* down] Prefix indicating *down, downward, destructive,* or *against.*

catabasis (kă-tăb′ă-sĭs) [Gr. *kata,* down, + *basis,* going] The decline of a disease.

catabatic (kăt-ă-băt′ĭk) Pert. to catabasis.

catabolin (kă-tăb′ō-lĭn) Catabolite.

catabolism (kă-tăb′ō-lĭzm) [Gr. *katabole,* a casting down, + *-ismos,* condition] The destructive phase of metabolism; the opposite of anabolism. Catabolism includes all the processes in which complex substances are converted into simpler ones, usually with the release of energy. SEE: *anabolism; metabolism.* **catabolic** (kăt″ă-bŏl′ĭk), *adj.*

catabolite (kă-tăb′ō-līt) Any product of catabolism. SYN: *catabolin.*

catacrotic (kăt″ă-krŏt′ĭk) [″ + *krotos,* beat] Indicating the downstroke of pulse tracing interrupted by an upstroke.

catacrotism (kă-tăk′rō-tĭzm) [″ + ″ + *-ismos,* condition] A pulse with one or more secondary expansions of the artery following the main beat.

catadicrotic (kăt″ă-dī-krŏt′ĭk) [″ + *dis,* twice, + *krotos,* beat] Manifesting one or more secondary expansions of a pulse on the descending limb of the tracing.

catadicrotism (kăt″ă-dī′krō-tĭzm) [″ + ″ + ″ + *-ismos,* condition] Two minor expansions following the main beat of an artery.

catagen (kăt′ă-jĕn) [″ + *gennan,* to produce] The intermediate phase of the hair-growth cycle, between the growth or anagen stage and the resting or telogen phase.

catagenesis (kăt″ă-jĕn′ĕ-sĭs) [″ + *genesis,* generation, birth] Retrogression or involution.

catalase (kăt′ă-lās) An enzyme present in almost all cells that catalyzes the decomposition of hydrogen peroxide to water and oxygen.

catalepsy (kăt′ă-lĕp″sē) [Gr. *kata,* down, + *lepsis,* seizure] A condition seen in some patients after parietal lobe strokes and some psychotic patients in which patients may appear to be in a trance or may assume rigidly held body postures. **cataleptic** (kăt″ă-lĕp′tĭk), *adj.*

cataleptoid (kăt″ă-lĕp′toyd) [″ + ″ +

eidos, form, shape] Resembling or simulating catalepsy.

catalysis (kă-tăl'ĭ-sĭs) [Gr. *katalysis,* dissolution] The speeding of a chemical reaction by a catalyst. **catalytic** (kăt-ă lĭt'ĭk), *adj.*

catalyst (kăt'ă-lĭst) A substance that speeds the rate of a chemical reaction without being permanently altered in the reaction. Catalysts are effective in small quantities and are not used up in the reaction (i.e., they can be recovered unchanged). All enzymes are catalysts; the human body has thousands of enzymes, each specific for a particular reaction. For example, pepsin catalyzes the hydrolysis of protein; amylase catalyzes the hydrolysis of starch; transaminases catalyze the transfer of an amino group from one molecule to another. SYN: *catalyzer.*

catalyze (kăt'ă-līz) [Gr. *katalysis,* dissolution] To cause catalysis.

catalyzer (kăt'ă-lī-zĕr) A catalyst.

catamenia (kăt-ă-mē'nē-ă) [Gr. *kata,* according to, + *men,* month] Menstruation. **catamenial** (-ăl), *adj.*

catamnesis (kăt-ăm-nē'sĭs) [Gr. *kata,* down, + *mneme,* memory] A patient's medical history after treatment; the follow-up history. SEE: *anamnesis.*

cataphasia (kăt-ă-fā'zē-ă) [" + *phasis,* speech] A speech disorder causing an involuntary repetition of the same word.

cataphoresis (kăt"ă-fō-rē'sĭs) [Gr. *kata,* down, + *phoresis,* being carried] Transmission of electronegative ions or drugs into the body tissues or through a membrane by use of an electric current.

cataphoria (kăt"ă-fō'rē-ă) [" + *pherein,* to bear] The tendency of visual axes to incline below the horizontal plane.

cataphoric Pert. to cataphora or cataphoresis.

cataplectic (kăt-ă-plĕk'tĭk) [" + *plexis,* stroke] Pert. to cataplexy.

cataplexy, cataplexia (kăt'ă-plĕks-ē, kăt-ă-plĕk'sē-ă) A sudden, brief loss of muscle control brought on by strong emotion or emotional response, such as a hearty laugh, excitement, surprise, or anger. Although this may cause collapse, the patient remains fully conscious. The episode lasts from a few seconds to as long as several minutes. The condition may be less severe with age. About 70% of patients with narcolepsy also have cataplexy. Imipramine hydrochloride is beneficial in treating this disorder.

cataract (kăt'ă-răkt) [L. *cataracta,* waterfall] An opacity of the lens of the eye, usually occurring as a result of aging, trauma, endocrine or metabolic disease, intraocular disease, or as a side effect of the use of tobacco or certain medications (such as steroids). Cataracts are the most common cause of blindness in adults. SEE: illus; *visual field* for illus.

Symptoms: At first, vision is distorted, particularly during night driving or in very bright light, due to light sensitivity (photophobia). As the cataract progresses, severe visual impairment develops.

Prevalence: After the age of 65, 90% of all adults have cataracts.

Treatment: Surgical removal of the

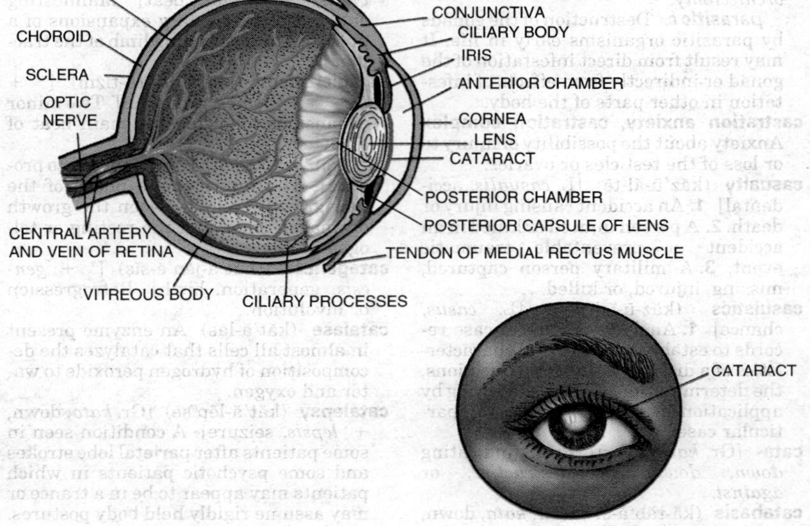

CATARACT

lens is the only effective treatment. In the U.S. about a million cataract surgeries are performed annually. Typically, the lens and its anterior capsule are removed, leaving the posterior capsule of the lens in place. Ultrasound may be used to fragment the cataract (a process called "phacoemulsification") so that the particles of the lens may be removed through a tiny incision. SEE: *intraocular lens; phacoemulsification*.

PATIENT CARE: *Preoperative:* The procedure is explained to the patient. An antiseptic facial scrub is performed. Mydriatic and cycloplegic eye drops are instilled to dilate the pupil, and osmotic diuretics are given to reduce intraocular pressure. Antibiotics, a sedative, and a local anesthetic are provided.

Postoperative: The nurse orients the patient to the surroundings and speaks with him or her at frequent intervals to decrease the effects of sensory deprivation. Any severe pain, which may signify an increase in intraocular pressure or hemorrhage; increased drainage; bleeding; or fever, are assessed, documented, and reported. Prescribed antiemetics are administered, and the patient is instructed about use of prescribed analgesics. An eye patch and shield are required temporarily to prevent injury and infection; these coverings will result in temporary loss of peripheral vision on the operative side. The patient will need help when getting up from bed and should sleep on the unaffected side to reduce intraocular pressure. Safety measures, such as using up-and-down head movements to judge distance and turning the head fully toward the operative side to view objects in that area, help to protect the patient from injury due to decreased peripheral vision. Both patient and family are taught how to change an eye patch, to inspect the eye for redness or watering and to report these conditions as well as any photophobia or sudden visual changes, to instill eye drops as prescribed, and to maintain the eye patch and shield as directed (usually for several weeks, esp. during sleep).

Activities that raise intraocular pressure, including heavy lifting, bending from the waist, straining during defecation, or vigorous coughing and sneezing, should be avoided. Strenuous activity should also be avoided for 6 to 10 weeks or as directed by the ophthalmologist. Keeping follow-up appointments is important. Dark glasses should be worn to counteract glare. If the patient will be wearing contact lenses, proper insertion, removal, and care are explained, as is the need to visit the ophthalmologist routinely for removal, cleaning, and reinsertion of extended-wear lenses. SEE: *Nursing Diagnoses Appendix*.

capsular c. A cataract occurring in the capsule.

hypermature c. Overripe c.

immature c. An early cataract, too poorly developed to require therapy.

lenticular c. A cataract occurring in the lens.

mature c. Sufficiently dense changes in the anterior cortex of the lens to prevent the examiner from viewing the posterior portion of the lens and the posterior portion of the eye; that is, the entire lens is opaque and ophthalmoscopic examination of the eye past the lens is not possible. SYN: *ripe c.*

morgagnian c. SEE: *Morgagni's cataract*.

nuclear c. A cataract in which the central portion of the lens is opacified.

overripe c. A cataract in which the lens solidifies and shrinks. This stage follows the mature stage. SYN: *hypermature c.*

radiation c. A cataract caused by exposure to radiation, esp. from sunlight.

ripe c. Mature c.

senile c. A cataract occurring in an elderly person.

cataractogenic (kăt″ă-răk″tō-jĕn′ĭk) [L. *cataracta,* waterfall, + Gr. *gennan,* to produce] Causing or forming cataracts.

catarrh (kă-tăr′) [Gr. *katarrhein,* to flow down] Term formerly applied to inflammation of mucous membranes, esp. of the head and throat. **catarrhal** (-ăl), *adj.*

dry c. An obsolete term for a nonproductive cough.

vernal c. Allergic conjunctivitis.

catastrophizing (kă-tăs′trō-fī-zĭng) Exaggerated focus on perceived failures in one's past, present, or future; associated with mood disorders, especially depression, and chronic pain.

catatonia (kăt-ă-tō′nē-ă) [″ + *tonos,* tension] **1.** A phase of schizophrenia in which the patient is unresponsive, marked by the tendency to assume and remain in a fixed posture and the inability to move or talk. **2.** Stupor. **catatonic** (-tŏn′ĭk), *adj.*

catatricrotic (kăt″ă-trī-krŏt′ĭk) [″ + *treis,* three, + *krotos,* beat] Manifesting a third impulse in the descending stroke of the sphygmogram of the pulse.

catatricrotism (kăt″ă-trī′krō-tĭzm) A condition in which the pulse shows a third impulse in the descending stroke of a pulse tracing.

catatropia (kăt″ă-trō′pē-ă) [″ + *tropos,* turning] A condition in which both eyes are turned downward.

cat-cry syndrome SEE: *syndrome, cri du chat*.

catecholamine (kăt″ĕ-kōl′ă-mēn) One of many biologically active amines, including metanephrine, dopamine, epinephrine and norepinephrine, derived from the amino acid tyrosine. They have a marked effect on the nervous and cardiovascular systems, metabolic rate, temperature, and smooth muscle.

catelectrotonus (kăt″ē-lĕk-trŏt′ō-nŭs) [″ + *elektron,* amber, + *tonos,* tension] The increased excitability produced in a nerve or muscle in the region near the cathode during the passage of an electric current.

catenating (kăt′ĕn-āt″ĭng) [L. *catena,* chain] **1.** Pert. to a disease that is linked with another. **2.** Forming a series of symptoms.

catenation Concatenation.

catenoid (kăt′ĕ-noyd) [″ + Gr. *eidos,* form, shape] Chainlike; pert. to protozoan colonies whose individuals are joined end to end.

catgut Sheep intestine twisted for use as an absorbable ligature.

chromic c. Catgut treated with chromium trioxide. This enhances the strength of the suture material and delays its absorption.

catharsis (kă-thăr′sĭs) [Gr. *katharsis,* purification] **1.** Purgative action of the bowels. **2.** The Freudian method of freeing the mind by recalling from the patient's memory the events or experiences that were the original causes of a psychoneurosis. SEE: *abreaction.*

cathartic (kă-thăr′tĭk) [Gr. *kathartikos,* purging] An active purgative, producing bowel movements (e.g., cascara sagrada, castor oil). SEE: *purgative.*

cathepsins (kă-thĕp′sĭns) A group of protein-destroying, lysosomal enzymes found in nearly every cell in the body. Many of these enzymes are released by cancer cells in excessive amounts, a factor that contributes to the invasiveness of tumors into neighboring tissues. The detection of cathepsins in tumors is strongly correlated with metastasis.

catheter (kăth′ĕ-tĕr) [Gr. *katheter,* something inserted] A tube passed through the body for evacuating fluids or injecting them into body cavities. It may be made of elastic, elastic web, rubber, glass, metal, or plastic. SEE: illus.

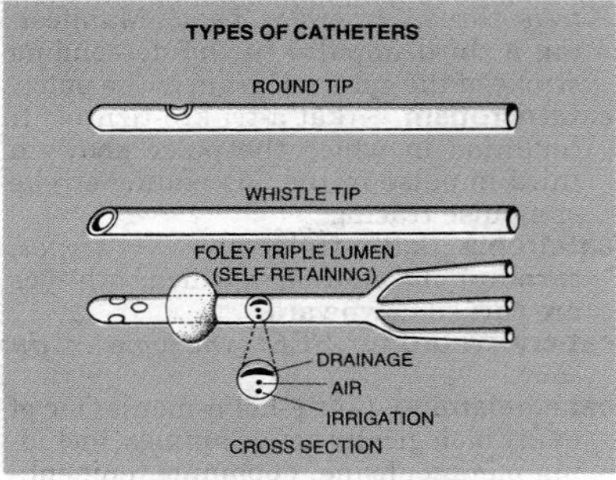

antimicrobial-impregnated central c. An intravenous tube saturated with antibiotics; designed to decrease the likelihood of colonization or infection of indwelling infusion lines.

arterial c. A catheter inserted into an artery to measure pressure, remove blood, inject medication or radiographic contrast media, or perform an interventional radiological procedure.

balloon c. A double-lumened catheter surrounded by a balloon. The balloon may be expanded by injecting air, saline, or contrast medium.

cardiac c. A long, fine catheter specially designed for passage through the lumen of a blood vessel into the arteries or chambers of the heart. SEE: *cardiac catheterization.*

central c. A catheter inserted into a central vein or artery for diagnostic or therapeutic purposes or both.

central venous c. A catheter inserted into the superior vena cava to permit intermittent or continuous monitoring of central venous pressure, to administer medications or nutrition, or to facilitate obtaining blood samples for chemical analysis. SEE: illus.

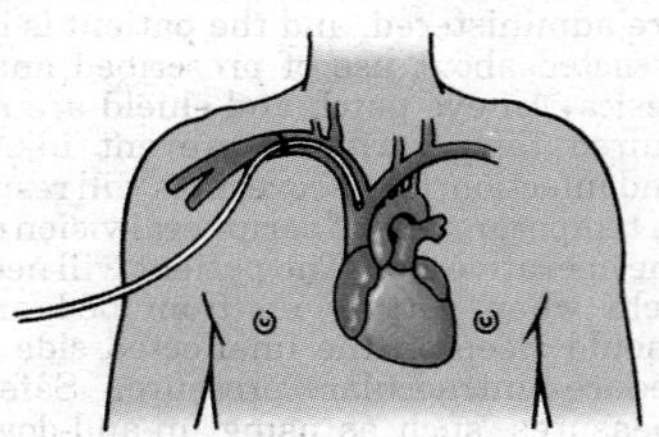

CATHETER (LINE) ENTERING VEIN

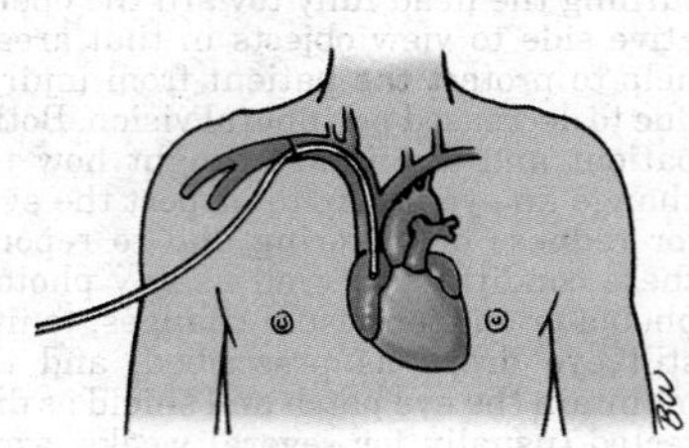

CATHETER TIP IN PLACE IN RIGHT ATRIUM

CENTRAL VENOUS CATHETER (SUBCLAVIAN)

condom c. A specially designed condom that includes a catheter attached to the end. The catheter carries urine to a collecting bag. Its use prevents men with urinary incontinence from soiling clothes or bed linens.

CAUTION: Continual use of this device may excoriate the skin of the penis.

double-channel c. A catheter providing for inflow and outflow.

elbowed c. Prostatic c.

eustachian c. A catheter passed into the eustachian tube through the nasal passages to ventilate the middle ear.

female c. A catheter about 5 in. (12.7 cm) long, used to pass into a woman's bladder.

Foley c. SEE: *Foley catheter*.

heparin-bonded c. A pulmonary artery catheter with a heparin coating to reduce the risk of thrombus formation.

impregnated c. A catheter that is coated with a medication designed to prevent complications of prolonged insertion in the body. Commonly used coatings include antibiotics and antiseptics.

indwelling c. Any catheter that is allowed to remain in place in a vein, artery, or body cavity.

intra-aortic c. SEE: *intra-aortic balloon counterpulsation*.

intravenous c. A catheter inserted into a vein to administer fluids or medications or to measure pressure.

Karman c. SEE: *Karman catheter*.

male c. A catheter 12 to 13 in. (30.5 to 33 cm) long, used to pass into a man's bladder.

pacing c. A catheter inserted most commonly into the right side of the heart via the brachial, femoral, internal jugular, or subclavian vein for temporary pacing of the heart. The pacing wires or leads provide the electrical stimulus from an external source (called a "pulse generator").

peripherally inserted central c. ABBR: PICC. A soft, flexible central venous catheter, inserted in a vein in the arm and advanced until the tip is positioned in the axillary, subclavian, or bracheocephalic vein. It may also be advanced into the superior vena cava. A PICC is commonly used for prolonged antibiotic therapy, total parenteral nutrition, or continuous opioid infusion.

pharyngeal suction c. A rigid tube used to suction the pharynx during direct visualization. SYN: *Yankauer suction c.*

presternal c. A catheter used for peritoneal dialysis that exits the chest instead of the lower abdomen. It is made of two silicone rubber tubes joined at the implantation site by a titanium connector that links its abdominal and presternal parts.

prostatic c. A catheter, 15 to 16 in. (38 to 40.6 cm) long, with a short elbowed tip designed to pass prostatic obstruction. SYN: *elbowed c.*

pulmonary artery c. A catheter inserted into the pulmonary artery to measure pulmonary artery pressures, pulmonary capillary wedge pressure, and cardiac output.

self-retaining c. A bladder catheter designed to remain in place (e.g., a Foley catheter).

suprapubic c. A urinary catheter used for closed drainage. It is inserted through the skin, about 2.5 cm above the symphysis pubis, into the distended bladder. This is usually done under general anesthesia. If it is to remain in place, it is sutured to the abdominal skin.

Swan-Ganz c. SEE: *Swan-Ganz catheter*.

Tenckhoff peritoneal c. SEE: *Tenckhoff peritoneal catheter*.

triple-lumen c. A central catheter containing three separate channels or passageways.

tunneled central venous c. An intravenous catheter inserted into the subclavian or internal jugular vein and then advanced into the right atrium or superior vena cava. The proximal end is tunneled subcutaneously from the insertion site and brought out through the skin at an exit site below the nipple line. Commonly used tunneled catheters include the Hickman and Broviac catheters.

vertebrated c. A catheter in sections to be fitted together so that it is flexible.

winged c. A catheter with little flaps at each side of the beak to help retain it in the bladder.

Yankauer suction c. SEE: *Yankauer suction catheter*.

catheterization (kăth″ĕ-tĕr-ĭ-zā′shŭn) [Gr. *katheterismos*] Use or passage of a catheter.

cardiac c. Percutaneous intravascular insertion of a catheter into any chamber of the heart or great vessels for diagnosis, assessment of abnormalities, interventional treatment, and evaluation of the effects of pathology on the heart and great vessels. Diagnostic tests that can be performed with cardiac catheterization include the following:

1. Assessments of coronary artery anatomy and patency
2. Estimates of cardiac ejection fraction and wall motion
3. Evaluations of the cardiac valves
4. Measurements of intracardiac pressures
5. Biopsies of the endomyocardium

Patient Care: *Precatheterization:* The nurse prepares the patient physically and emotionally by explaining the procedure and expected sensations. The patient's vital signs, including the presence and intensity of peripheral pulses, are assessed to establish a baseline measure. Anxiety and activity levels are documented, as well as the presence and pattern of any chest pain. Any known allergies, particularly to shellfish or iodine (suggestive of sensitivity to radiopaque dye), are also documented, and the cardiologist is alerted to these allergies or any changes in the patient's condition. The groin is shaved and cleansed, and the patient is informed that an oral or intravenous mild sedative (rather than general anesthesia) will probably be given before or during the procedure, so that he or she is able to cough and breathe deeply as instructed during testing. A radiopaque contrast medium is injected into the arteries and nitroglycerin may be administered to aid visualization. After the injection, the patient may feel lightheaded, warm, or nauseated for a few moments. The patient will have to lie on the back for several hours after the procedure and should report chest pain immediately both during and after the procedure.

During catheterization: Support personnel assist with the procedure according to protocol by monitoring cardiac pressures and rhythm and the results of hemodynamic studies. Patient comfort and safety are assured; and changes in emotional status, level of consciousness, and verbal and nonverbal responses are assessed to determine the patient's response to the procedure and need for reassurance or medication to prevent vasovagal reactions or coronary artery spasm. Any complications, such as cardiac dysrhythmias or allergic reaction to the contrast medium, are also evaluated and reported.

Postcatheterization: The nurse provides emotional support to the patient and answers questions. Cardiac rhythm and vital signs (including apical pulse and temperature) are monitored until stable according to protocol (usually every 15 min for the first 1 to 2 hr) or more frequently as the patient's condition requires. The blood pressure should not be checked in any limb used for catheter insertion. The dressing is inspected frequently for signs of bleeding, and the patient is instructed to report any increase in dressing tightness (which may indicate hematoma formation). Pressure is applied over the entry site and the extremity is maintained in extension according to protocol. The patient is cautioned to avoid flexion or hyperextension of the affected limb for 12 to 24 hr depending on protocol.

Neurovascular status of the involved extremity distal to the insertion site is monitored for changes, which may indicate arterial thrombosis (the most frequent complication), embolus, or another complication requiring immediate attention. The head of the bed is elevated no more than 30 degrees, and the patient is confined to bedrest. The patient may complain of urinary urgency immediately after the procedure. Fluids are given to flush out the dense radiopaque contrast medium, and urine output is monitored, esp. in patients with impaired renal function. The patient is assessed for complications such as pericardial tamponade, myocardial infarction, pulmonary embolism, stroke, congestive heart failure, cardiac dysrhythmia, infection, and thrombophlebitis. The patient's preoperative medication regimen is resumed as prescribed (or revised).

The patient will need to be driven home, and a responsible adult should be in attendance until the next morning. Both patient and family are provided with written discharge instructions explaining the need to report any of the following symptoms to the physician: bleeding or swelling at the entry site; increased tenderness; redness; drainage or pain at the entry site; fever; and any changes in color, temperature, or sensation in the involved extremity. The patient may take acetaminophen or other nonaspirin analgesic every 3 to 4 hr as needed for pain. The entry site should be covered with an adhesive bandage for 24 hr or until stitches, if present, are removed (usually within 6 days). The patient usually is permitted to shower the day after the procedure and to take a tub bath 48 hr after the procedure (if no sutures are present). Strenuous activity should be avoided for 24 hr after the procedure.

urinary bladder c. Introduction of a drainage tube through the urethra into the bladder to withdraw urine. Catheterization of the bladder may be performed when sterile urinary specimens are needed for laboratory analysis, when precise monitoring of urinary output is required (e.g., in the critical care unit), or when patients have chronic voiding difficulties.

Patients with chronic difficulty urinating sometimes are given indwelling urinary catheters; as an alternative, they may be instructed in the technique of clean, intermittent self-catheterization. To do this, they need to learn about their urethral anatomy and about methods they can use to avoid introducing germs into the urinary bladder (handwashing, periurethral and catheter cleansing, and catheter storage). Most patients need to catheterize themselves four or five times daily. Carefully performed intermittent catheterization is less likely to cause urinary tract infection than is chronic indwelling urinary catheterization. SEE: illus.

PATIENT CARE: After the procedure is explained to the patient, the proper equipment is assembled, and the catheter is connected to a closed drainage bag, if necessary. The balloon at the tip of the catheter is inflated (and deflated) before its insertion to make sure that it

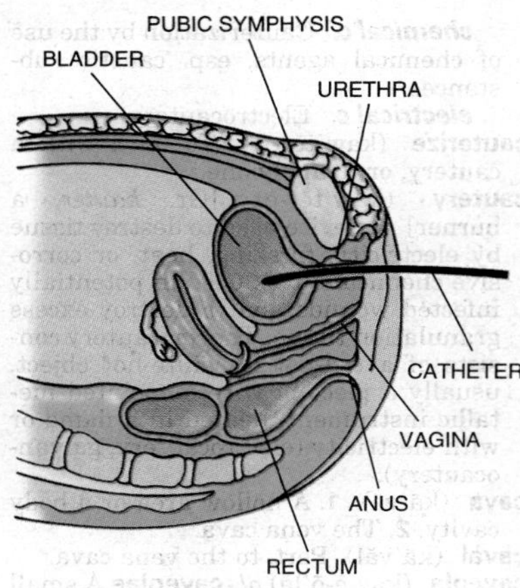

FEMALE

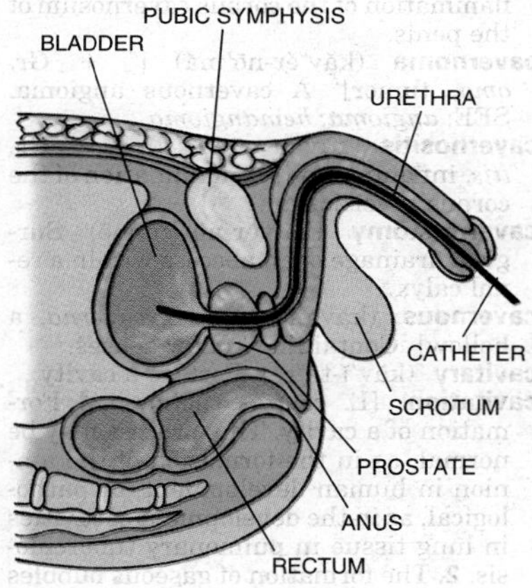

MALE

CATHETERIZATION OF URINARY BLADDER

will stay in place after entering the bladder. The patient is properly positioned and draped (see instructions for female and male patients); the site is prepared with antiseptic solution and the catheter is gently inserted. Sterile technique is maintained throughout these procedures, and the indwelling catheter is connected to a closed drainage system prior to insertion. The tube is secured to the patient's leg, the drainage tubing is looped on the bed, and the tubing leading to the collection bag is straightened to facilitate gravity drainage. The collection bag is suspended above the floor. The drainage tube is prevented from touching a surface when the collection bag is emptied; the spout is wiped with an alcohol swab before being refastened to the bag. The meatal area should be cleansed daily. The patient's ability to void and remain continent is periodically evaluated and catheterization is discontinued when possible. Results of the procedure, including the character and volume of urine drained and the patient's response, are observed and documented.

Female: The patient should be in the dorsal recumbent position on a firm mattress or examining table to enhance visualization of the urinary meatus. Alternately, the lithotomy position, with buttocks at the edge of the examining table and feet in stirrups, may be used. For female patients with difficulties involving hip and knee movements, the Sims' or left lateral position may be more comfortable and allow for better visualization. Pillows may be placed under the head and shoulders to relax the abdominal muscles.

Male: The patient should be in a supine position with legs extended. Lubricant is instilled directly into the urethra with a prefilled syringe to facilitate passage of the tube. After the procedure, care should be taken to return the prepuce to its normal position to prevent any subsequent swelling.

catheterize (kăth′ĕ-tĕr-īz) To pass or introduce a catheter into a part; usually referring to bladder catheterization.

cathexis [Gr. *kathexis,* retention] The emotional or mental energy used in concentrating on an object or idea.

cathode ABBR: ca. **1.** The negative electrode from which electrons are emitted; the opposite of the anode or positive pole. **2.** In a vacuum tube, the electrode that serves as the source of the electron stream.

cathodic (kă-thŏd′ĭk) **1.** Pert. to a cathode. **2.** Proceeding outwardly or efferently as applied to a nerve impulse.

cation (kăt′ī-ŏn) [Gr. *kation,* descending] An ion with a positive electric charge; opposite of anion. It is attracted by the cathode (negative pole).

catoptrophobia A morbid fear of mirrors or of breaking them.

CAT scan Computed axial tomography scan. Modern computerized tomography units are capable of a multitude of image reconstructions in addition to simple axial imaging. The proper term is “computed tomography” or “CT.”

Caucasian Pert. unscientifically to individuals of European or Northern African descent. **caucasoid,** *adj.*

cauda (kaw′dă) *pl.* **caudae** [L.] A tail or taillike structure.

c. epididymidis The inferior portion of the epididymis that is continuous with the ductus deferens.

c. equina The terminal portion of the spinal cord and the spinal nerves below the first lumbar nerve.

c. helicis A pointed process extending inferiorly from the helix of the auricular cartilage of the ear.

c. pancreatis The tail of the pancreas.

c. striati A tail-like posterior extremity of the corpus striatum.

caudad (kaw′dăd) [L. *cauda,* tail, + *ad,* toward] Toward the tail; in a posterior direction.

caudal (kawd′ăl) [L. *caudalis*] **1.** Pert. to any tail-like structure. **2.** Inferior in position.

caudate (kaw′dāt) [L. *caudatus*] Possessing a tail.

caudocephalad (kaw-dō-sĕf′ă-lăd) [L. *cauda,* tail, + Gr. *kephale,* head, + L. *ad,* toward] Moving from the tail end toward the head.

caul (kawl) [O.Fr. *cale,* a small cap] Membranes or portions of the amnion covering the head of the fetus at birth.

causalgia (kaw-săl′jē-ă) [″ + *algos,* pain] Intense burning pain accompanied by trophic skin changes, due to injury of nerve fibers.

cause [L. *causa*] Something that brings about a particular condition, result, or effect.

antecedent c. An event or condition that predisposes to a disease or condition.

determining c. The final event or condition that brings about a disease or condition.

necessary and sufficient c. In logic, an antecedent condition that is wholly and solely capable of producing an effect.

predisposing c. Something that favors the development of a disease or condition.

proximate c. An event or condition that immediately precedes and causes a disease or condition.

remote c. An event or condition that is not immediate in its effect but predisposes to the development of a disease or condition.

ultimate c. The remote event or condition that initiated a train of events resulting in the development of a disease or condition.

caustic (kaw′stĭk) [Gr. *kaustikos,* capable of burning] **1.** Corrosive and burning; destructive to living tissue. **2.** An agent, particularly an alkali, that destroys living tissue (e.g., silver nitrate, potassium hydroxide, nitric acid). SEE: *poisoning; Poisons and Poisoning Appendix.*

cauterant (kaw′tĕr-ănt) [Gr. *kauter,* a burner] **1.** Cauterizing. **2.** A cauterizing agent.

cauterization (kaw″tĕr-ī-zā′shŭn) [Gr. *kauteriazein,* to burn] Destruction of tissue with a caustic, an electric current, a hot iron, or by freezing.

chemical c. Cauterization by the use of chemical agents, esp. caustic substances.

electrical c. Electrocautery.

cauterize (kaw′tĕr-īz) To burn with a cautery, or to apply one.

cautery (kaw′tĕr-ē) [Gr. *kauter,* a burner] A device used to destroy tissue by electricity, freezing, heat, or corrosive chemicals. It is used in potentially infected wounds and to destroy excess granulation tissue. Thermocautery consists of a red-hot or white-hot object, usually a piece of wire or pointed metallic instrument, heated in a flame or with electricity (electrocautery, galvanocautery).

cava (kā′vă) **1.** A hollow area or a body cavity. **2.** The vena cava.

caval (kā′văl) Pert. to the vena cava.

caveola (kăv-ē-ō′lă) *pl.* **caveolae** A small pit or depression formed on the cell surface during pinocytosis.

cavernitis (kăv″ĕr-nī′tĭs) [L. *caverna,* hollow, + Gr. *itis,* inflammation] Inflammation of the corpus cavernosum of the penis.

cavernoma (kăv″ĕr-nō′mă) [″ + Gr. *oma,* tumor] A cavernous angioma. SEE: *angioma; hemangioma.*

cavernositis (kăv″ĕr-nō-sī′tĭs) [″ + Gr. *itis,* inflammation] Inflammation of the corpus cavernosum.

cavernostomy (kă-vĕr-nŏs′tō-mē) Surgical drainage of an abscess within a renal calyx.

cavernous (kăv′ĕr-nŭs) [L. *caverna,* a hollow] Containing hollow spaces.

cavitary (kăv′ĭ-tā″rē) Pert. to a cavity.

cavitation [L. *cavitas,* hollow] **1.** Formation of a cavity. This process may be normal, as in the formation of the amnion in human development, or pathological, as in the development of cavities in lung tissue in pulmonary tuberculosis. **2.** The formation of gaseous bubbles in body fluids during exposure to ultrasonic energy; known as acoustic cavitation.

cavitis (kā-vī′tĭs) [″ + Gr. *itis,* inflammation] Inflammation of a vena cava.

cavity (kăv′ĭ-tē) [L. *cavitas,* hollow] A hollow space, such as a body organ or the hole in a tooth produced by caries.

abdominal c. The ventral cavity between the diaphragm and pelvis, containing the abdominal organs. It is lined with a serous membrane, the peritoneum, and contains the following organs: stomach with the lower portion of the esophagus, small and large intestines (except sigmoid colon and rectum), liver, gallbladder, spleen, pancreas, adrenal glands, kidneys, and ureters. It is continuous with the pelvic cavity; the two constitute the abdominopelvic cavity. SEE: *abdomen; abdominal quadrants* for illus.

alveolar c. A tooth socket.

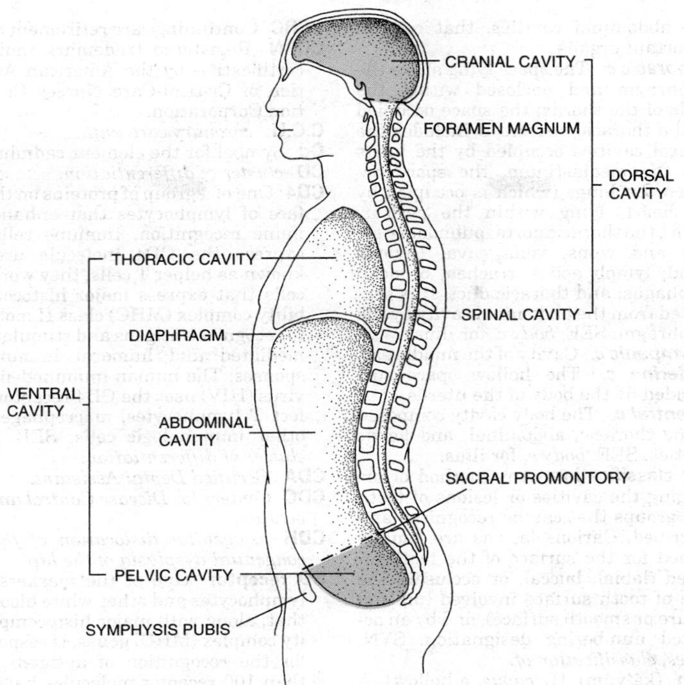

CAVITIES OF THE BODY

articular c. The synovial cavity of a joint.

body c. Either of the two major body cavities, one containing the viscera of the thorax, abdomen, and pelvic areas (ventral), and the other composed of the cranial and spinal cavities (dorsal). SYN: *coelom*. SEE: illus.

buccal c. Oral c.

cotyloid c. Acetabulum.

cranial c. The cavity of the skull, which contains the brain.

dental c. Caries.

dorsal c. The body cavity composed of the cranial and spinal cavities. SEE: *body c.* for illus.

glenoid c. A shallow concavity on the lateral surface of the head of the scapula that receives the head of the humerus.

joint c. The articular cavity or space enclosed by the synovial membrane and articular cartilages. It contains synovial fluid.

lesser peritoneal c. Omental bursa.

oral c. The cavity of the mouth. It includes the vestibule and oral cavity proper. SYN: *buccal c.*

pelvic c. The bony hollow formed by the innominate bones, the sacrum, and the coccyx. The major pelvic cavity lies between the iliac fossae and above the iliopectineal lines. The minor pelvic cavity lies below the iliopectineal lines. SEE: *pelvis*.

pericardial c. The potential space between the epicardium (visceral pericardium) and the parietal pericardium. SEE: *friction rub, pericardial; pericarditis*.

peritoneal c. The potential space between the parietal peritoneum, which lines the abdominal wall, and the visceral peritoneum, which forms the surface layer of the visceral organs. It contains serous fluid.

pleural c. The potential space between the parietal pleura that lines the thoracic cavity and the visceral pleura that covers the lungs. It contains serous fluid that prevents friction.

pulp c. The cavity in a tooth containing the dental pulp and nerve termination.

Rosenmüller's c. The cavity on either side of the openings of the eustachian tube.

serous c. The space between two layers of serous membrane (e.g., the pleural, pericardial, and peritoneal cavities).

spinal c. The cavity that contains the spinal cord. SEE: *body c.* for illus.

splanchnic c. One of the cavities of the body, such as the cranial, thoracic, and abdominal cavities, that contain important organs.

thoracic c. The space lying above the diaphragm and enclosed within the walls of the thorax; the space occupied by the thoracic viscera. It includes the pleural cavities occupied by the lungs and the mediastinum, the space between the lungs (which is occupied by the heart, lying within the pericardium), the thoracic aorta, pulmonary artery and veins, vena cava, thymus gland, lymph nodes, trachea, bronchi, esophagus, and thoracic duct. It is separated from the abdominal cavity by the diaphragm. SEE: *body c.* for illus.

tympanic c. Cavity of the middle ear.

uterine c. The hollow space surrounded by the body of the uterus.

ventral c. The body cavity composed of the thoracic, abdominal, and pelvic cavities. SEE: *body c.* for illus.

cavity classification Any method of arranging the cavities or lesions of teeth into groups that can be recognized and described. Carious lesions are usually named for the surface of the tooth affected (labial, buccal, or occlusal), the type of tooth surface involved (pit and fissure or smooth surface), and by an accepted numbering designation. SYN: *caries, classification of.*

cavum (kā′vŭm) [L. *cavus,* a hollow] A cavity or space.

c. abdominis Abdominal cavity.

c. conchae The inferior portion of the cavity of the auricle of the ear. It leads to the external acoustic meatus.

c. mediastinale Mediastinum (2).

c. medullare The medullary cavity of a long bone.

c. oris Oral cavity.

c. pelvis Pelvic cavity.

c. septi pellucidi The cavity of the septum pellucidum of the brain.

c. trigeminale The space between the two layers of the dura mater of the brain in which the trigeminal ganglion is located. SYN: *Meckel's space.*

c. tympani The cavity of the middle ear.

c. uteri The cavity of the uterus.

cavus (kā′vŭs) [L., hollow] Talipes arcuatus.

cayenne pepper (kī-ĕn′, kā-ĕn′) Capsicum.

C bar The curved part of a hand splint that maintains the thumb web space.

CBC *complete blood count.*

C.C. *chief complaint; Commission Certified.*

cc *cubic centimeter.*

$CCl_3 \cdot CHO$ Chloral.

CCl_4 Carbon tetrachloride.

CCPD *continuous cycling peritoneal dialysis.*

CCR5 coreceptor A cell surface receptor found on macrophages that facilitates entry of HIV-1 into these cells.

CCRC Continuing care retirement center.

CCRN Registered trademark indicating certification by the American Association of Critical-Care Nurses Certification Corporation.

C.C.U. *coronary care unit.*

Cd Symbol for the element cadmium.

CD *cluster of differentiation.*

CD4 One of a group of proteins on the surface of lymphocytes that enhance immune recognition. Immune cells that express the CD4 molecule are also known as helper T cells; they work with cells that express major histocompatibility complex (MHC) class II molecules to recognize antigens and stimulate cell-mediated and humoral immune responses. The human immunodeficiency virus (HIV) uses the CD4 receptor to infect T lymphocytes, macrophages, and other immunologic cells. SEE: *AIDS; cluster of differentiation.*

CDA *Certified Dental Assistant.*

CDC *Centers for Disease Control and Prevention.*

CDH *congenital dislocation of the hip; congenital dysplasia of the hip*

CD receptor One of the markers on T lymphocytes and other white blood cells that, along with major histocompatibility complex (MHC) genes, is responsible for the recognition of antigens. More than 100 receptor molecules have been identified. CD4 receptors on T4 lymphocytes are the sites to which human immunodeficiency virus (HIV) binds, producing infection. SEE: *AIDS; cluster of differentiation.*

Ce Symbol for the element cerium.

CEA Carcinoembryonic antigen.

cebocephalus (sē″bō-sĕf′ă-lŭs) [Gr. *kebos,* monkey, + *kephale,* head] A fetus with a monkey-like head.

cecal (sē′kăl) [L. *caecalis,* pert. to blindness] **1.** Pert. to the cecum. **2.** Blind, terminating in a closed extremity.

cecectomy (sē-sĕk′tō-mē) [L. *caecum,* blindness, + Gr. *ektome,* excision] Surgical removal of the cecum.

cecitis (sē-sī′tĭs) [″ + Gr. *itis,* inflammation] Inflammation of the cecum.

cecocolopexy (sē″kō-kō′lō-pĕk″sē) [″ + Gr. *kolon,* colon, + *pexis,* fixation] Surgical fixation of the colon and the cecum.

cecocolostomy (sē″kō-kō-lŏs′tō-mē) [″ + ″ + *stoma,* mouth] A colostomy joining the cecum to the colon.

cecoileostomy (sē″kō-ĭl″ē-ŏs′tō-mē) [″ + *ileum,* ileum, + Gr. *stoma,* mouth] Surgical formation of an anastomosis between the cecum and the ileum.

cecopexy (sē′kō-pĕk″sē) [″ + Gr. *pexis,* fixation] Surgical fixation of the cecum to the abdominal wall.

cecoplication (sē″kō-plĭ-kā′shŭn) [″ + *plica,* fold] The reduction of a dilated cecum by making a fold in its wall.

cecoptosis (sē″kŏp-tō′sĭs) [″ + Gr. *pto-*

sis, a dropping] Falling displacement of the cecum.

cecosigmoidostomy (sē″kō-sĭg″moy-dŏs′tō-mē) [″ + Gr. *sigmoeides,* shaped like Gr. letter Σ (sigma), + *stoma,* mouth] A surgical connection between the cecum and the sigmoid.

cecostomy (sē-kŏs′tō-mē) [″ + Gr. *stoma,* mouth] Surgical formation of an artificial opening into the cecum.

cecotomy (sē-kŏt′ō-mē) [″ + Gr. *tome,* incision] An incision into the cecum.

cecum, caecum (sē′kŭm) [L. *caecum,* blindness] A blind pouch or cul-de-sac that forms the first portion of the large intestine, located below the entrance of the ileum at the ileocecal valve. It averages about 6 cm in length and 7.5 cm in width. At its lower end is the vermiform appendix. SEE: *colon*.

cefamandole nafate An antibacterial drug. It is a second-generation cephalosporin. Trade name is Mandol.

cefoxitin sodium An antibacterial drug with a spectrum of action that includes some gram-positive, gram-negative, and anaerobic germs. This second-generation cephalosporin is often used to treat pelvic and intra-abdominal infections, among others.

ceftriaxone (sĕf-trī′-ăx-ōn) An injectable, third-generation cephalosporin with a long half-life that can be given once daily. It is used to treat a wide spectrum of respiratory, gastrointestinal, and urinary infections. Trade name is Rocephin.

cel- SEE: *celo-*.

-cele [Gr. *kele,* tumor, swelling; *koilia,* cavity] Suffix indicating *swelling, hernia,* or *tumor*.

celecoxib (sĕl-ĕ-cŏk′sĭb) A nonsteroidal anti-inflammatory drug approved for the treatment of osteoarthritis and rheumatoid arthritis.

celiac (sē′lē-ăk) [Gr. *koilia,* belly] Pert. to the abdominal cavity.

celiectomy (sē″lē-ĕk′tō-mē) [″ + *ektome,* excision] **1.** Surgical removal of an abdominal organ. **2.** Excision of the celiac branches of the vagus nerve.

celiocentesis (sē″lē-ō-sĕn-tē′sĭs) [″ + *kentesis,* puncture] Puncture of the abdomen.

celiocolpotomy (sē″lē-ō-kōl-pŏt′ō-mē) [″ + *kolpos,* vagina, + *tome,* incision] A surgical incision of the vagina through the abdominal wall.

celioenterotomy (sē″lē-ō-ĕn″tĕr-ŏt′ō-mē) [″ + *enteron,* intestine, + *tome,* incision] An incision in the abdominal wall to gain access to the intestines.

celiogastrostomy (sē″lē-ō-găs-trŏs′tō-mē) [″ + *gaster,* stomach, + *stoma,* mouth] Laparogastrostomy.

celiogastrotomy (sē″lē-ō-găs-trŏt′ō-mē) [Gr. *koilia,* belly, + *gaster,* stomach, + *tome,* incision] Laparogastrotomy.

celiohysterectomy (sē″lē-ō-hĭs-tĕr-ĕk′tō-mē) [″ + *hystera,* uterus, + *ektome,* excision] Removal of the uterus through the abdomen.

celiohysterotomy (sē″lē-ō-hĭs″tĕr-ŏt′ō-mē) [″ + ″ + *tome,* incision] An incision into the uterus through the abdominal wall.

celioma (sē-lē-ō′mă) [″ + *oma,* tumor] An abdominal tumor.

celiomyomectomy (sē″lē-ō-mī″ō-mĕk′tō-mē) [″ + ″ + *oma,* tumor, + *ektome,* excision] Cutting of muscular tissue via an abdominal incision.

celiomyomotomy (sē″lē-ō-mī″ō-mŏt′ō-mē) [″ + ″ + ″ + *tome,* incision] Incision of the abdominal muscles.

celiomyositis (sē″lē-ō-mī″ō-sī′tĭs) [″ + ″ + *itis,* inflammation] Inflammation of the abdominal muscles.

celioparacentesis (sē″lē-ō-păr″ă-sĕn-tē′sĭs) [″ + *para,* beside, + *kentesis,* puncture] Needle puncture of the abdomen for tapping or drainage.

celiopathy (sē″lē-ŏp′ă-thē) [″ + *pathos,* disease, suffering] Any disease of the abdomen.

celiorrhaphy (sē″lē-or′ă-fē) [″ + *rhaphe,* seam, ridge] Laparorrhaphy.

celiosalpingectomy (sē″lē-ō-săl″pĭn-jĕk′tō-mē) [″ + *salpinx,* tube, + *ektome,* excision] Removal of the fallopian tubes through an abdominal incision.

celioscope (sē′lē-ō-skōp) [″ + *skopein,* to examine] An endoscope for visual examination of a body cavity.

celioscopy (sē″lē-ŏs′kō-pē) Examination of a body cavity through a celioscope.

celiotomy (sē″lē-ŏt′ō-mē) [″ + *tome,* incision] Surgical incision into the abdominal cavity.

vaginal c. Incision into the abdomen through the vagina.

cell [L. *cella,* a chamber] A mass of protoplasm containing a nucleus or nuclear material; the structural unit of all animals and plants. Cells and cell products form all the body tissues; their structures are correlated with the functions of the organs of which these tissues are a part. Cells arise only from pre-existing cells, through cell division. Growth and development result from the increase in numbers of cells and their differentiation into different types of tissues. Specialized germ cells, the spermatozoa and ova, contain the genes to be passed to offspring.

STRUCTURE: A typical cell has a nucleus surrounded by cytoplasm. The nucleus is bounded by a double-layered nuclear membrane and contains the chromosomes, which are made of DNA and protein. One or more nucleoli, made of protein, RNA, and DNA, may be present; these are sites of ribosome formation. The cell membrane is made of phospholipids, protein, and cholesterol; it forms the outer boundary of the cells

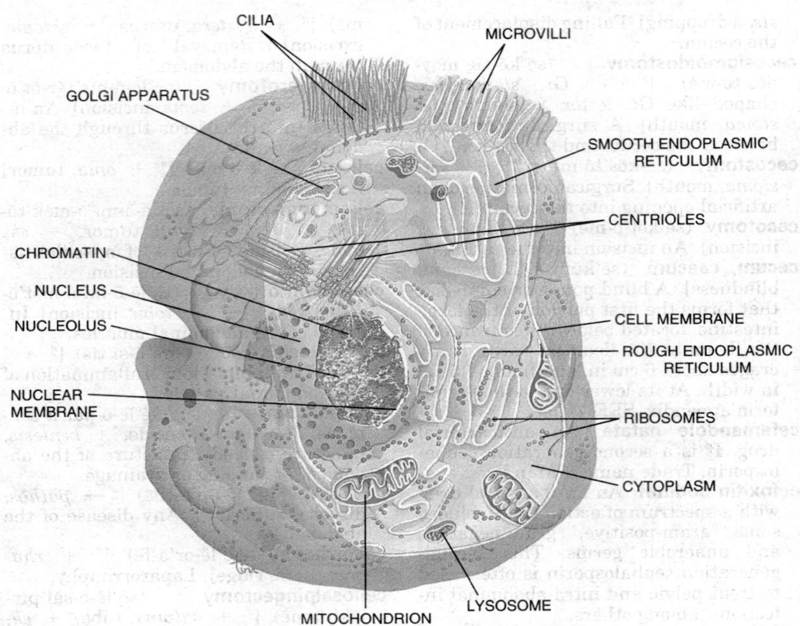

GENERALIZED HUMAN CELL AND ORGANELLES

and selectively allows substances to enter or leave the cell. Within the cell are cell organelles, including ribosomes, endoplasmic reticulum, mitochondria, Golgi apparatus, centrioles, and lysosomes; each has a specific function. SEE: illus.

CELL DIVISION: *Meiosis* is the type of cell division in which two successive divisions of the germ cell nuclei produce cells that contain half the number of chromosomes present in somatic cells. In *mitosis,* the other type of cell division, each daughter cell contains the same number of chromosomes as the parent cell. SEE: *meiosis* and *mitosis* for illus.

accessory c. A monocyte or macrophage; refers to the immune response. SEE: *antigen-presenting cell; macrophage.*

acidophil c. A cell with an affinity for staining with acid dyes.

acinar c. A cell present in the acinus of an acinous gland (e.g., of the pancreas).

adipose c. Fat c.

adventitial c. A macrophage along a blood vessel, together with perivascular undifferentiated cells associated with it.

alpha c. A cell of the anterior lobe of the pituitary and the pancreas. In the latter, these cells are the source of glucagon.

alveolar c., type I One of the thin, flat cells that form the epithelium of the alveoli.

alveolar c., type II An epithelial cell of the alveoli of the lungs that secretes pulmonary surfactant.

ameloblast c. The type of cell that produces the enamel rods of the tooth crown.

argentaffin c. A cell in the epithelium of the stomach, intestines, and appendix that secretes serotonin.

B c. A lymphocyte that matures in the bone marrow and then migrates to lymphoid tissues, where a foreign antigen stimulates it to produce antibodies. All B cells are antigen specific and respond to only one foreign protein. The spleen and lymph nodes contain many B cells that, because of the large amount of blood passing through these organs, become exposed to new antigens. After a B cell comes in contact with an antigen, it differentiates into either a plasma cell or a memory cell, and then proliferates. Plasma cells produce antigen-specific antibodies. Memory cells are available to produce antibodies quickly if the same antigen reappears. The antigen-antibody reaction is part of the humoral immune response. It is the basis for vaccination and plays a major role in defense against infection from common organisms. SYN: *B lymphocyte.* SEE: *plasma c.; T c. antibody; antigen; cytokine; immunoglobulin; vaccination.*

band c. The developing leukocyte at a stage at which the nucleus is not segmented.

basal c. A type of cell in the deepest layer of the epidermis.

basket c. **1.** A branching basal or myoepithelial cell of the salivary and other glands. **2.** A type of cell in the cer ebellar cortex in which Purkinje cells rest.

basophil c. A cell with an affinity for staining with basic dyes.

beta c. **1.** One of the insulin-secreting cells of the pancreas that constitute the bulk of the islets of Langerhans. **2.** A basophil cell of the anterior lobe of the pituitary.

Betz c. SEE: *Betz cell.*

bipolar c. A neuron with two processes, an axon and a dendrite. It is found in the retina of the eye and in the cochlear and vestibular ganglia of the acoustic nerve.

blast c. **1.** A newly formed cell of any type. Large numbers of blast cells in the peripheral blood indicate that the bone marrow is producing a high level of the particular cell (e.g., lymphoblast [lymphocyte], monoblast [monocyte]). **2.** A cell that produces something, such as an osteoblast that produces bone matrix.

blood c. Any type of nucleated or non-nucleated cell normally found in the blood or blood-forming tissues. SEE: *blood* for illus.

burr c. An erythrocyte with 10 to 30 spicules distributed over the surface of the cell, as seen in heart disease, stomach cancer, kidney disease, and dehydration. SEE: illus.

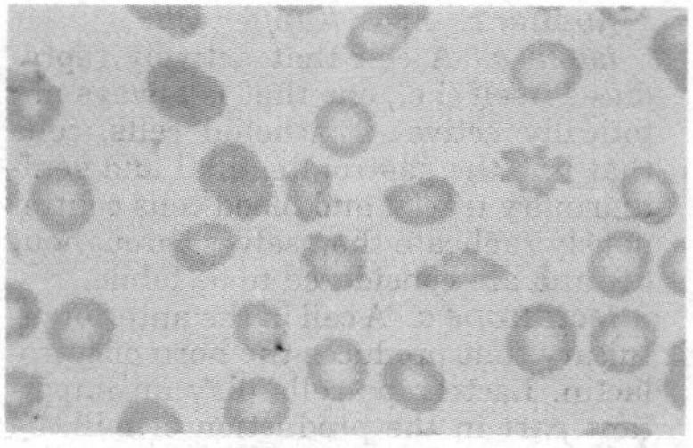

BURR CELLS

capsule c. Satellite c.

castration c. An enlarged and vacuolated basophil cell seen in the pituitary in gonadal insufficiency or following castration.

cementoblast c. One of the cells that produce the cementum layer, which covers the tooth root and provides attachment for the supporting periodontal ligament.

cementocyte c. One of the cells trapped within cementum that maintain cementum as a living calcified tissue by their metabolic activity.

centroacinar c. A duct cell of the pancreas more or less invaginated into the lumen of an acinus.

chalice c. Goblet c.

chief c. **1.** One of the cells of the parathyroid gland that secrete the parathyroid hormone. **2.** One of the secretory cells that line the gastric glands and secrete pepsin or its precursor. **3.** A chromophobe cell of the pituitary.

chromaffin c. An epinephrine-containing cell of the adrenal medulla whose granules stain brown when cells are stained with a fluid containing potassium bichromate.

cleavage c. A cell that results from mitosis or splitting of the fertilized ovum; a blastomere.

clue c. A vaginal epithelial cell, thickly coated with coccobacillary organisms; a hallmark of bacterial vaginosis. SEE: illus; *Gardnerella vaginalis.*

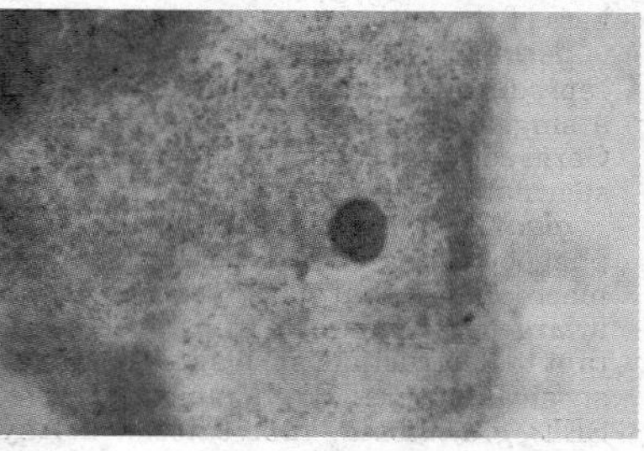

CLUE CELL

columnar c. An epithelial cell with height greater than its width.

cone c. A cell in the retina whose scleral end forms a cone that serves as a light receptor. Vision in bright light, color vision, and acute vision depend on the function of the cones. SEE: *rod c.*

cuboid c. A cell with height about equal to width and depth.

cytotoxic T c. A CD8 + T lymphocyte that can destroy microorganisms directly. SEE: *T c.*

daughter c. Any cell formed from the division of a mother cell.

delta c. A cell of the islets of Langerhans of the pancreas that secretes somatostatin.

dendritic c. One type of antigen-presenting cell that helps T cells respond to foreign antigens. They are found in epithelial tissues and include the Langerhans' cells of the skin and interdigitating cells in lymph nodes; they also circulate in the blood.

endothelial c. One of the flat cells that form the lining of the blood and lymph vessels.

ependymal c. One of the cells of the developing neural tube that give rise to the ependyma. They originate from spongioblasts derived from the neural epithelium.

epithelial c. One of the cells forming

the epithelial surfaces of membranes and skin. SEE: *epithelial tissue*.

ethmoidal c. One of several cavities that honeycomb the lateral masses of the ethmoid bone, forming a part of the paranasal air sinuses. SYN: *ethmoid sinus*.

fat c. A cell that stores fat. SYN: *adipose c.; adipocyte; lipocyte*.

flame c. A bone marrow cell with a bright-red cytoplasm, occasionally found in the marrow of patients with multiple myeloma.

foam c. A cell that contains vacuoles; a lipid-filled macrophage.

ganglion c. **1.** Any neuron whose cell body is located within a ganglion. **2.** A neuron of the retina of the eye whose cell body lies in the ganglion cell layer. The axons of ganglion cells form the fibers of the optic nerve.

germ c. A cell whose function is to reproduce the organism. It usually has a single set of chromosomes (haploid). Germ cells are called ova in females and spermatozoa in males.

giant c. **1.** An active, multinucleated phagocyte created by several individual macrophages that have merged around a large pathogen or a substance resistant to destruction, such as a splinter or surgical suture. SYN: *megakaryocyte*. SEE: *granuloma; tuberculosis*. **2.** Any large cell, containing one or multiple nuclei.

glia c. Neuroglia c.

goblet c. An epithelial cell, containing a large globule of mucin, giving it the appearance of a goblet. SYN: *chalice c.*

Golgi c. SEE: *Golgi cell*.

granule c. A small neuron of the cerebrum or the cerebellum that contains granules.

gustatory c. A neuroepithelial cell or taste cell of a taste bud.

hair c. An epithelial cell possessing fine nonmotile cilia found in the maculae and the organ of Corti of the membranous labyrinth of the inner ear. These cells are receptors for the senses of position and hearing.

HeLa c. An immortal cancer cell that has been maintained in continuous tissue cultures for decades from a patient with carcinoma of the cervix. It is named for the first two letters of the patient's first and last names, Henrietta Lacks. HeLa cells have been used in thousands of experiments on cell growth, differentiation, and cancer, and in virology, pharmacology, and other fields.

helper T c. A type of T lymphocyte, whose surface is marked by CD4 receptors, that is involved in both cell-mediated and antibody-mediated immune responses. It secretes cytokines (chemical messengers) that stimulate the activity of B cells and other T cells and binds with class II histocompatibility antigens, which are processed by macrophages and other antigen-presenting cells. SEE: *antigen processing; T c.; cell-mediated immunity*.

horizontal c. A neuron of the inner nuclear layer of the retina. The axons of these cells run horizontally and connect various parts of the retina.

Hürthle c. SEE: *Hürthle cell*.

hybridoma c. SEE: *hybridoma*.

hyperchromatic c. All or part of a cell that contains more than the normal number of chromosomes and hence stains more densely.

interstitial c. One of the many cells found in connective tissue of the ovary, in the seminiferous tubules of the testes, and in the medulla and cortex of the kidney. The cells in the testes and ovaries produce hormones such as testosterone and estrogen.

islet c. A cell of the islets of Langerhans of the pancreas.

juvenile c. The early developmental form of a white blood cell.

juxtaglomerular c. A modified smooth muscle cell in the wall of the afferent arteriole leading to a glomerulus of the kidney. This type of cell secretes renin when blood pressure decreases to activate the renin-angiotensin mechanism, which elevates blood pressure and increases sodium retention.

killer c. Natural killer c.

killer T c. SEE: *cytotoxic T c.*

Kupffer c. SEE: *Kupffer cell*.

labile c. A cell that actively reproduces itself (i.e., one that is always mitotically active). Epithelial cells, cells that line the gastrointestinal and genitourinary tracts, and blood cells continuously replicate themselves throughout life and are considered to be labile.

lactotrope c. A cell in the anterior pituitary that produces the hormone prolactin. Lactotrope cells play an important part in the production of milk by the mammary glands, both in postpartum women and in patients with prolactinomas.

L.E. c. SEE: *L.E. cell*.

Leydig's c. SEE: *Leydig's cell*.

littoral c. A macrophage found in the sinuses of lymphatic tissue.

lutein c. A cell of the corpus luteum of the ovary that contains fatty yellowish granules. Granulose lutein cells are hypertrophied follicle cells; these lutein (paralutein) cells develop from the theca interna.

lymph c. A term formerly used to describe a lymphocyte.

lymphokine-activated killer c. ABBR: LAK cell. Natural killer cells, obtained from the patient's blood, that have been activated in a culture with interleukin-2. LAK cells are used, with some success, to treat patients with solid malignant tumors.

mast c. A cell found in connective tissue of vertebrates that contains heparin and histamine.

mastoid c. An old term for one of the mastoid sinuses of the temporal bone.

memory c. A cell derived from B or T lymphocytes that can quickly recognize a foreign antigen to which the body has been previously exposed. Memory T cells stimulate T helper lymphocytes and cytotoxic T cells; memory B cells stimulate the production of antigen-specific antibodies by B plasma cells. Both types of memory cells survive for years, providing a durable immune response against foreign antigens. SEE: *B c.; lymphocyte.*

microglia c. A neuroglial cell of mesodermal origin present in the brain and spinal cord and capable of phagocytosis.

mossy c. A protoplasmic astrocyte; one of two types of neuroglial cell, containing many branching processes. SEE: *neuroglia.*

mother c. A cell that gives rise to similar cells through fission or budding. SYN: *parent c.*

mucous c. A cell that secretes mucus; found in mucus-secreting glands.

myeloma c. A cell present in the bone marrow of patients with multiple myeloma.

myoepithelial c. A spindle-shaped or branched contractile epithelial cell found between glandular cells and basement membrane of sweat, mammary, and salivary glands.

natural killer c. ABBR: NK cell. A large granular lymphocyte that bonds to cells and lyses them by releasing cytotoxins. Unlike other lymphocytes, these cells do not have B cell or T cell surface markers, and they can be activated without previous antigen exposure. NK cells destroy cells infected with viruses and some types of tumor cells in cultures. They also secrete gamma interferon (INFγ), tumor necrosis factor alpha (TNFα), and granulocyte-macrophage colony-stimulating factor (GMCSF), enhancing the effect of T lymphocytes.

nerve c. A neuron, a cell of nerves that has processes extending from the cell body. One process, the axon, transmits nerve impulses away from the body; the other, the dendrite, receives impulses and transmits them to the cell body.

neuroglia c. A non-nerve cell of the supporting tissue of the central nervous system and the retina of the eye. This type includes astrocytes, oligodendrocytes, and microglia. SYN: *glia c.*

Niemann-Pick c. SEE: *Niemann-Pick cell.*

null c. A white blood cell that is a lymphocyte but does not have the characteristics of either a T cell or a B cell.

odontoblast c. A cell that produces dentin and is responsible for the sensitivity of and metabolism of dentin in the tooth.

olfactory c. A special cell of the olfactory mucosa that has a combined neuroepithelial function.

osteoblast c. A mesodermal cell that produces the bone matrix and forms bone layer by layer on its surface.

osteocyte c. A type of cell trapped within bone matrix that maintains bone as a living tissue by its metabolic activity.

oxyntic c. A parietal cell of the stomach. In humans, hydrochloric acid is formed in these cells.

parent c. Mother c.

phalangeal c. One of the cells supporting the hair cells of the organ of Corti. These cells form several rows of outer phalangeal cells (Deiters' cells) and a single row of inner phalangeal cells.

pigment c. Any cell that normally contains pigment granules.

plasma c. A cell derived from B lymphocytes that has been sensitized to a specific foreign antigen and produces antibodies to that particular antigen. It may be found in the blood or in tissue fluid. SYN: *plasmacyte.*

prickle c. A cell possessing spinelike protoplasmic processes that connect with similar processes of adjoining cells. These are found in the stratum spinosum (Malphighian layer) of the epidermis of keratinized epithelium.

primordial c. One of the original germ cells that in the embryo migrate to the gonadal ridge, where they form all of the germ cells.

Purkinje c. SEE: *Purkinje cell.*

pus c. A leukocyte present in pus. Cells of this type are often degenerated or necrotic.

pyramidal c. A nerve cell of the cerebral cortex.

red c. The erythrocyte of the blood. Its principal purpose is to transport oxygen to the cells of the body. The hemoglobin that the red cell contains is oxygenated in the lungs, and the oxygen contained in the arterial system is released to the tissues from capillaries.

Renshaw c. SEE: *Renshaw cell.*

reticular c. **1.** An undifferentiated cell of the spleen, bone marrow, or lymphatic tissue that can develop into one of several types of connective tissue cells or into a macrophage. **2.** A cell of reticular connective tissue. SEE: *reticular tissue.*

reticuloendothelial c. An out-of-date term for a cell of the mononuclear phagocytic system.

Rieder c. SEE: *Rieder cell.*

rod c. A cell in the retina of the eye whose scleral end is long and narrow, forming a rod that acts as a sensory element. Rods are stimulated by dim light. SEE: *cone c.*

rosette c. A rose-shaped cluster of phagocytes surrounding lysed nuclear material or red blood cells. Rosette cells occur frequently in blood in which L.E. cells are present. Rosette cells are not diagnostic of lupus erythematosus. SEE: *L.E. cell.*

Rouget c. SEE: *Rouget cell.*

satellite c. **1.** A stem cell associated with skeletal muscle that may form a limited number of new muscle cells after injury. **2.** One of the neuroglia cells enclosing the cell bodies of sensory neurons in spinal ganglia. SYN: *capsule c.*

segmented c. A segmented neutrophil (i.e., one with a nucleus of two or more lobes connected by slender filaments).

sensory c. A cell that when stimulated gives rise to nerve impulses that are conveyed to the central nervous system.

septal c. A type II alveolar cell that secretes pulmonary surfactant; it is attached to or in the septa of the lungs.

Sertoli c. SEE: *Sertoli cell.*

sickle c. An abnormal erythrocyte shaped like a sickle. SEE: *anemia, sickle cell.*

signet-ring c. A vacuolated cell with the nucleus off center. Mucus-secreting adenocarcinomas usually contain these cells.

somatic c. A cell that is not a germ cell. Somatic cells have two sets of chromosomes (diploid) and include cells of many different shapes and functions.

spider c. Astrocyte.

squamous c. A flat, scaly, epithelial cell.

stellate c. A star-shaped cell with processes extending from it (e.g., astrocytes and Kupffer's cells).

stellate reticuloendothelial c. Old name for Kupffer cells, the macrophages that line the sinusoids of the liver. SYN: *Kupffer cell.*

stem c. **1.** Any cell that can give rise to more specifically differentiated daughter cells. Stem cells can be harvested from bone marrow or the peripheral blood and used in hematological transplants. **2.** In transplantation, a hematopoietic cell in bone marrow, umbilical cord blood, and peripheral blood, capable of reconstituting bone marrow (i.e., after myeloablative conditioning chemoradiotherapy) to restore lymphohematopoietic function.

stem c. rescue In patients being treated with high doses of chemotherapy or radiation therapy, the removal of stem cells (the precursors to red and white blood cells and platelets) from the patient's blood before treatment and their reinfusion after treatment. Granulocyte colony stimulating factor, erythropoietin, and other growth factors are administered to stimulate proliferation of the stem cells after reinfusion. Until adequate numbers of cells repopulate the patient's marrow and bloodstream, the patient is at high risk for infection and bleeding.

Stem cell rescue is used in patients with solid tumors not involving bone marrow who require treatments that would destroy the blood-forming (hematopoietic) cells. The process is immunologically advantageous because the cells infused are the patient's own cells, and thus do not have foreign antigens.

Sternberg-Reed c. SEE: *Reed-Sternberg cell.*

stipple c. A red blood cell that contains small basophilic-staining dots. It is seen in lead poisoning, malaria, severe anemia, and leukemia.

suppressor T c. A previously used term for a type of lymphocyte that inhibits CD4+ and B cell activity. Because no specific CD markers have been identified for these cells, it is unclear whether they exist as a separate group.

sympathicotrophic c. One of the large epithelial cells that occur in groups in the hilus of the ovary. They are thought to be chromaffin cells.

sympathochromaffin c. A chromaffin cell of ectodermal origin present in the fetal adrenal gland. Sympathetic and medullary cells originate from these cells.

T c. A lymphoid cell from the bone marrow that migrates to the thymus gland, where it develops into a mature differentiated lymphocyte that circulates between blood and lymph, serving as one of the primary cells of the immune response. Immature T cells are called thymocytes. Mature T cells are "antigen specific": T cell receptor (TCR) proteins on the surface of each T cell detect only one antigen. T cells are identified by surface protein markers called clusters of differentiation (CDs). All T cells have the CD3 marker; additional markers differentiate T subsets. CD4 T helper cells serve primarily as regulators, secreting cytokines that stimulate the activities of other white blood cells. CD8 T cells (cytotoxic T cells), effector cells that directly lyse (kill) organisms, are an important defense against viruses. Most CD8 T cells also produce gamma interferon (INFγ), one of the strongest stimulators of macrophage activity. Natural killer cells, originally believed to be a subset of T cells, are now recognized as being a third type of lymphocyte. SYN: *T lymphocyte.* SEE: *immune response; lymphocyte; immunological surveillance; T-cell receptor.*

T cells cannot recognize foreign antigens without the help of macrophages and other antigen-presenting cells (APCs), which change antigenic proteins into peptides that bind with major histocompatibility complex molecules. However, once the macrophage has helped them identify an antigen as "nonself," T cells dominate the specific immune response, directing macrophages, B cells, and other T cells in the body's defense. T cells also play a major role in graft rejection and other type IV hypersensitivity reactions, as well as in tumor cell recognition and destruction, because of the unique antigens these cells carry. SEE: *cytokine; cell-mediated immunity*.

target c. An erythrocyte with a rounded central area surrounded by a lightly stained clear ring, which in turn is surrounded by a dense ring of peripheral cytoplasm. It is present in certain blood disorders, such as thalassemia, and in patients who have no spleen.

tart c. A phagocyte that has ingested the unaltered nuclei of cells. These nuclei can be observed unchanged within the phagocytic cell.

taste c. A cell of a taste bud.

totipotent c. An undifferentiated embryonic cell that has the potential to develop into any type of cell.

Touton giant c. SEE: *Touton cell*.

Türk's irritation c. SEE: *Türk's irritation cell*.

Tzanck c. SEE: *Tzanck cell*.

undifferentiated c. A cell resembling an embryonic cell in that it has not demonstrated a change into a mature cell of any type.

visual c. A rod cell or cone cell of the retina.

wandering c. A rarely used term for a cell (such as a macrophage) that moves like an amoeba.

white c. Any of the leukocytes of the blood.

zymogenic c. Any of the chief cells or enzyme-producing cells of the gastric glands.

cell bank A facility for keeping cells frozen at extremely low temperatures. These cells are used for investigating hereditary diseases, human aging, and cancer. Collections of banked cells are kept by the National Institutes of Health (the Human Genetic Mutant Cell Repository and the Aging Cell Repository) and at the Cornell Institute for Medical Research.

cell counter, electronic An electronic instrument used to count blood cells, employing either an electrical resistance or an optical gating technique. SEE: *flow cytometry*.

cell cycle The series of events that occur during the growth and development of a cell. SEE: *meiosis* and *mitosis* for illus.

cell division The fission of a cell. SEE: *meiosis* and *mitosis* for illus.

cell-free Pertaining to fluids or tissues that contain no cells or in which all the cells have been disintegrated by laboratory treatment.

cell growth cycle The order of physical and biochemical events that occur during the growth of cells. In tissue culture studies, the cyclic changes are divided into specific periods or phases: the DNA synthesis or S period, the G_2 period or gap, the M or mitotic period, and the G_1 period.

cell kill In antineoplastic therapy, the number of malignant tumor cells destroyed by a treatment.

cell kinetics The study of cells and their growth and division. Study of these factors has led to understanding of cancer cells and has been useful in developing chemotherapeutic methods.

cell mass In embryology, the mass of cells that develops into an organ or structure.

cellobiose (sĕl″ō-bī′ōs) A disaccharide resulting from the hydrolysis of cellulose.

cellophane (sĕl′ō-fān) A thin, transparent, waterproof sheet of cellulose acetate. It is used as a dialysis membrane.

cell organelle Any of the structures in the cytoplasm of a cell. These include mitochondria, endoplasmic reticulum, Golgi complex, ribosomes, lysosomes, and centriole. SEE: *cell* for illus.

cell saver An apparatus that aspirates extravasated blood in an operative field; after appropriate filtration the blood may be returned to the patient. This device cannot be used when the blood returned to the patient may be infected or contaminated (e.g., in perforated diverticulitis). SEE: *blood salvage*.

cell sorting The separation of cells from one another, based on physical or chemical properties. Cell-separation techniques are used to collect uniform populations of cells from tissues or fluids in which many different cell types are present. The collected cells can then be used for transplantation or scientific study. Common methods of separating cells include cloning, centrifugation, electrophoresis, magnetism, and antibody- or fluorescent-binding. SEE: *flow cytometry*.

fluorescence-activated c. s. ABBR: FACS. A method of separating cells by selectively tagging them with colored fluorescent dyes bound to specific cellular structures or molecules.

cellucidal (sĕl″ū-sī′dăl) [L. *cella,* a chamber, + *caedere,* to kill] Destructive to cells.

cellula (sĕl′ū-lă) *pl.* **cellulae** [L., little cell] **1.** A minute cell. **2.** A small compartment.

cellular (sĕl′ū-lăr) Pertaining to, composed of, or derived from cells.

cellular immunity T-cell–mediated immune functions requiring cell interactions (e.g., graft rejection, or destruction of infected cells).

cellulase (sĕl′ū-lās) An enzyme that converts cellulose to cellobiose. It is present in some microorganisms and marine life.

cellulifugal (sĕl″ū-lĭf′ū-găl) [″ + *fugere*, to flee] Extending or moving away from a cell.

cellulipetal (sĕl″ū-lĭp′ĭ-tăl) [″ + *petere*, to seek] Extending or moving toward a cell.

cellulite A nontechnical term for subcutaneous deposits of fat, especially in the buttocks, legs, and thighs.

cellulitis (sĕl-ū-lī′tĭs) [″ + Gr. *itis*, inflammation] A spreading bacterial infection of the skin, usually caused by streptococcal or staphylococcal infections, that results in severe inflammation with erythema, warmth, and localized edema. The extremities, esp. the lower legs, are the most common sites. Adjacent soft tissue may be involved, esp. in patients with diabetes mellitus. Cellulitis involving the face is called erysipelas. When it affects the lower extremities, cellulitis must be differentiated from stasis dermatitis, which is associated most commonly with bilateral, chronic dependent edema, and occasionally with deep venous thrombosis. Patients with diabetes mellitus are at increased risk for cellulitis because of the peripheral vascular disease, neuropathy, and decreased immune function associated with diabetes. SEE: illus.; *necrotizing fasciitis*.

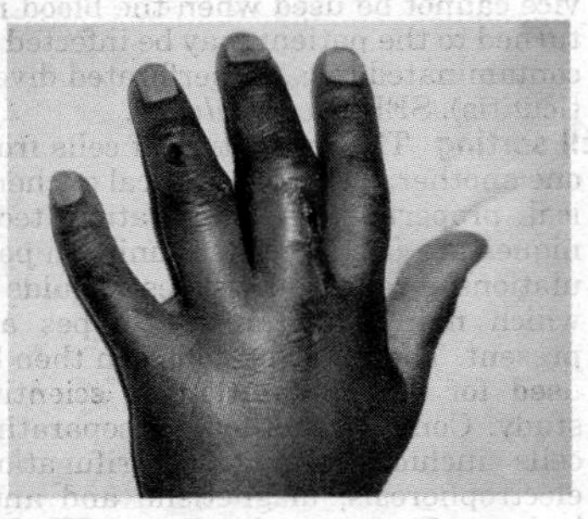

CELLULITIS

ETIOLOGY: Bacteria gain access through breaks in the skin and spread rapidly; lesions between the toes from athlete's foot are common entry sites.

TREATMENT: For mild cases of cellulitis, oral dicloxacillin or cefazolin is effective. For severe cases, intravenous penicillinase-resistant penicillins are used; imipenem and surgical débridement to obtain cultures and to rule out fasciitis are recommended for patients with diabetes.

CAUTION: Rarely, group A streptococcal cellulitis may be complicated by exfoliative dermatitis or infection of the subcutaneous fat and fascia, causing necrosis (necrotizing fasciitis), a condition popularly ascribed to the action of "flesh-eating bacteria."

pelvic c. Parametritis.

postseptal c. Facial infection invading the orbit.

preseptal c. Soft tissue infection limited to the tissues that are anterior to the orbital septum.

cellulofibrous (sĕl″ū-lō-fī′brŭs) [″ + *fibra*, fiber] Both cellular and fibrous.

cellulose (sĕl′ū-lōs) [L. *cellula*, little cell] A polysaccharide that forms plant fiber; a fibrous form of carbohydrate, $(C_6H_{10}O_5)_n$, constituting the supporting framework of most plants. It is composed of many glucose units. When ingested, it stimulates peristalsis and promotes intestinal elimination. When ingested by humans, cellulose provides no nutrient value because it is not chemically changed or absorbed in digestion; it remains a polysaccharide.

Some foods that contain cellulose are apples, apricots, asparagus, beans, beets, bran flakes, broccoli, cabbage, celery, mushrooms, oatmeal, onions, oranges, parsnips, prunes, spinach, turnips, wheat flakes, whole grains, and whole wheat bread. SEE: *fiber, dietary*.

c. acetate **1.** A support medium commonly used in electrophoresis. **2.** A semi-synthetic dialysis membrane. Normally it is white. When treated with a clearing agent of methanol and acetic acid, it becomes transparent. allowing the sample bands to be visualized.

carboxymethyl sodium c. ABBR: CMC. Carboxymethyl cellulose sodium.

oxidized c. Cellulose that has been oxidized and is made to resemble cotton or gauze. It is used to arrest bleeding by direct application to the site of hemorrhage.

cellulose triacetate c. A semi-synthetic dialysis membrane with excellent biocompatibility that can be used in high-flux dialyzers.

cellulotoxic (sĕl″ū-lō-tŏk′sĭk) [″ + Gr. *toxikon*, poison] **1.** Poisonous to cells. **2.** Caused by cell toxins.

cell wall A wall made of cellulose and other materials that encloses a plant cell in a rigid framework. Plant cells have both cell membranes and cell walls. Plant cell walls cannot be digested by humans. SEE: *cellulose*.

celo-, cel- [Gr. *kele*, tumor, swelling] Combining form meaning *tumor* or *hernia*.

celo-, cel- [Gr. *koilia*, cavity] Combining form meaning *cavity*.

celom, celoma (sē′lŏm, sē-lō′mă) [Gr. *koiloma,* a hollow] The coelom.

celoschisis (sē-lŏs′kĭ-sĭs) [Gr. *koilia,* cavity, + *schisis,* fissure] A congenital fissure of the abdominal wall.

celoscope (sē′lō-skōp) [″ + *skopein,* to examine] A device for visual examination of a body cavity.

celosomia (sē-lō-sō′mē-ă) [″ + *soma,* body] A congenital fissure of the sternum with herniation of the fetal viscera.

Celsius scale (sĕl′sē-ŭs) [Anders Celsius, Swedish astronomer, 1701–1744] A temperature scale on which the boiling point of water is 100° and the freezing point is 0°. This is the official scientific name of the temperature scale, also called the centigrade scale. SEE: *Fahrenheit scale* for table; *Celsius thermometer* for table; *Conversion Factors Appendix.*

cement (sē-mĕnt′) **1.** Any material that hardens into a firm mass when prepared appropriately. **2.** To cause two objects to stick together, as in using an adhesive to join a gold inlay to the cavity of a tooth and to insulate the pulp from metallic fillings. **3.** The material used to make one substance adhere to another.

glass ionomer c. A dental adhesive made from powdered aluminosilicate glass and liquid polyacrylic acid, used as a lining for dental cavities; as a permanent dental restorative material; and, as a result of leakage, as a source of fluoride. The cement is not recommended for Class II or IV restorations.

silicate c. A hard, translucent, tooth-colored restorative material. Silicate cement is produced by mixing aluminosilicate (an acid-based powdered glass) with liquid phosphoric acid. Because the cement is damaging to pulp of the tooth, pulp protection is required. Leakage often occurs at the margins of a silicate cement, but the fluoride released prevents caries.

CAUTION: Pulp protection is required.

zinc phosphate c. The oldest of the dental cements, composed of a powder (zinc oxide and magnesium oxide) and a liquid (phosphoric acid and water). An acid-base reaction occurs when the powder and liquid are mixed. The set cement is unreacted zinc oxide particles suspended within a matrix of zinc aluminophosphate. The cement is used for inlays, crowns, bridges, and orthodontic appliances.

zinc polycarboxylate c. Dental cement that can be used to attach cast restorations and orthodontic appliances and as a thermal insulating base. It forms an adhesive bond with enamel. It is produced by mixing a powder containing zinc oxide and magnesium oxide with a liquid solution of polyacrylic acid.

cementation The use of a plastic or moldable substance to seal joints and cement or join substances together. SYN: *luting.*

cementicle (sē-mĕn′tĭ-kl) The small calcified area in the periodontal membrane of the root of a tooth.

cementitis (sē″mĕn-tī′tĭs) [L. *cementum,* cement, + Gr. *itis,* inflammation] Inflammation of the dental cementum.

cementoblast (sē-mĕn′tō-blăst) [″ + Gr. *blastos,* germ] A cell of the inner layer of the dental sac of a developing tooth. It deposits cementum on the dentin of the root.

cementoclasia (sē-mĕn″tō-klā′sē-ă) [″ + Gr. *klasis,* breaking] Decay of the cementum of a tooth root.

cementoclast (sē-mĕn′tō-klăst) A very large multinucleated cell associated with the removal of cementum during root resorption, more correctly called an odontoclast.

cementogenesis (sē-mĕn″tō-jĕn′ĕ-sĭs) [″ + Gr. *genesis,* generation] The development of cementum on the root dentin of a tooth.

cementoid (sē″mĕn′toyd) [″ + Gr. *eidos,* form, shape] The noncalcified matrix of cementum.

cementoma (sē″mĕn-tō′mă) [″ + Gr. *oma,* tumor] A benign fibrous connective tissue growth containing small masses of cementum, usually found in the periodontal ligament near the apex of the tooth.

cementum (sē-mĕn′tŭm) [L.] The thin layer of calcified tissue formed by cementoblasts which covers the tooth root. In it are embedded the collagenous fibers of the periodontal ligament, which are also attached to the surrounding alveolar bone proper, thereby supporting the tooth. Also called *substantia ossea dentis.*

CEN *certified emergency nurse.*

cenosite (sĕn′ō-, sē′nō-sīt) [Gr. *koinos,* common, + *sitos,* food] A parasitic microorganism that can live without a host.

cenotophobia (sĕn″ō-, sē″nō-tō-fō′bē-ă) [Gr. *kainotes,* novelty, + *phobos,* fear] Pathological aversion to new things and new ideas. SYN: *cainotophobia.*

cenotype (sē′nō-, sĕn′ō-tīp) [″ + *typos,* a type] An original type; term used in ontogeny and cytology.

censor (sĕn′sĕr) [L. *censor,* judge] In psychoanalysis, a psychic inhibition that prevents abhorrent unconscious thoughts or impulses from being expressed objectively in any form recognized at the conscious level.

census In hospital management, the number of patients in the hospital.

centenarian A person over the age of 100.

center (sĕn′tĕr) [L. *centrum,* center] **1.** The middle point of a body. **2.** A group of nerve cells within the central nervous system that controls a specific activity or function. **3.** A facility specializing in a particular service.

apneustic c. A cluster of brainstem neurons that regulate breathing.

auditory c. The center for hearing in the anterior gyri of the transverse temporal gyri. SEE: *area, auditory.*

autonomic c. The center in the brain or spinal cord that regulates any of the activities under the control of the autonomic nervous system. Most centers are located in the hypothalamus, medulla oblongata, and spinal cord.

Broca's c. SEE: *Broca's area.*

burn c. A hospital-based health care facility staffed with specialists essential to the comprehensive care of burn patients.

cardioaccelerator c. The center in the medulla oblongata that gives rise to impulses that speed up the heart rate. Impulses reach the heart by way of sympathetic fibers.

cardioinhibitory c. The center in the medulla oblongata containing neurons whose axons, parasympathetic fibers, pass by way of the vagus nerves to the heart. Impulses from this center cause the heart rate to slow down.

chondrification c. The center of cartilage formation.

ciliospinal c. The center in the spinal cord that transmits sympathetic impulses that dilate the pupils of the eyes.

community health c. A health care facility for treatment of ambulatory patients. SYN: *neighborhood health c.*

defecation c. Either of two centers, a medullary center located in the medulla oblongata and a spinal center located in the second to fourth sacral segments of the spinal cord. The anospinal centers control the sphincter reflexes for defecation.

deglutition c. The center in the medulla oblongata on the floor of the fourth ventricle that controls swallowing.

epiotic c. The ossification center of the temporal bone, forming the upper and posterior part of the auditory capsule.

feeding c. An area in the ventrolateral nucleus of the hypothalamus that originates signals to the cerebral cortex that stimulate eating. SEE: *satiety c.; set point weight.*

germinal c. A collection of B cells undergoing proliferation within the follicle of a lymph node or other lymphoid tissue after antigen stimulation.

gustatory c. The cerebral center that controls taste. SYN: *taste c.; taste area.*

heat-regulating c. One of two centers, a heat loss and a heat production center, located in the hypothalamus. They regulate body temperature.

higher c. **1.** The center in the cerebrum from which impulses based on conscious sensations, wishes, or desires are initiated. **2.** A center in any portion of the brain, in contrast to one in the spinal cord.

independent living c. A facility in the community that coordinates services for the disabled, including counseling, training, rehabilitation, assistance with devices, and respite care.

inspiratory c. The respiratory center in the medulla that generates impulses that cause contraction of the diaphragm and external intercostal muscles.

lower c. A center in the brainstem or spinal cord.

micturition c. A center that controls the reflexes of the urinary bladder. These are located in the second to fourth and fourth to sixth sacral segments of the cord. Higher centers are present in the medulla oblongata, hypothalamus, and cerebrum.

motor cortical c. An area in the frontal lobe in which impulses for voluntary movements originate.

neighborhood health c. Community health c.

nerve c. An area in the central nervous system or in a ganglion that is responsible for certain functions; examples include the motor areas in the frontal lobes of the cerebrum.

ossification c. The spot in bones where ossification begins.

pneumotaxic c. The center in the pons that rhythmically inhibits inspiration.

psychocortical c. One of the centers of the cerebral cortex concerned with voluntary muscular contractions.

reflex c. A region within the brain or spinal cord where connections (synapses) are made between afferent and efferent neurons of a reflex arc.

respiratory c. One of four centers in the medulla oblongata or pons that helps regulate breathing. The medulla contains the inspiration center and the expiration center; the pons contains the apneustic center and the pneumotaxic center.

satiety c. An area in the ventromedial hypothalamus that modulates the stimulus to eat by sending inhibitory impulses, following a meal, to the feeding center, also located in the hypothalamus. Blood glucose and insulin level influence its activity.

senior c. A community building or meeting room where elderly persons congregate for services and activities that reflect their interests, enhance their dignity, support their independence, and encourage their involvement with the community.

speech c. Broca's area.

suicide prevention c. A health care facility dedicated to preventing suicide by counseling and crisis intervention.

taste c. Gustatory c.

temperature c. Thermoregulatory c.

thermoregulatory c. One of the temperature-regulating centers in the hypothalamus. SYN: *temperature c.*

vasoconstrictor c. The center in the medulla oblongata that brings about the constriction of blood vessels.

vasodilator c. The center in the medulla oblongata that brings about the dilation of blood vessels.

vasomotor c. The center that controls the diameter of blood vessels; the vasoconstrictor and vasodilator centers.

visual c. A center in the occipital lobes of the cerebrum that receives visual information transmitted from the retina.

word c. The area in the dominant hemisphere of the brain that recognizes and perceives spoken or written words.

centering In complementary medicine and meditation, an attempt to attain a state of self-awareness, relaxation, and psychological balance.

Centers for Disease Control and Prevention ABBR: CDC. A division of the U.S. Public Health Service in Atlanta, Georgia, that investigates and controls various diseases, especially those that have epidemic potential. The agency is also responsible for national programs to improve laboratory conditions and encourage health and safety in the workplace.

Centers for Education and Research on Therapeutics ABBR: CERT. A division of the Agency for Healthcare Research and Quality that directs efforts toward improving patient outcomes by reducing the incidence of medical errors. The program focuses on supporting research and disseminating current information about the appropriate use of therapeutic agents.

centesis (sěn-tē′sĭs) [Gr. *kentesis,* puncture] Puncture of a cavity.

centigrade (sěn′tĭ-grād) [L. *centum,* a hundred, + *gradus,* a step] ABBR: C. **1.** Having 100 degrees. **2.** Pertaining to a thermometer divided into 100°. The boiling point of water is 100° and the freezing point is 0°.

centigram (sěn′tĭ-grăm) [″ + Gr. *gramma,* a small weight] One hundredth of a gram.

centiliter (sěn′tĭ-lē-tĕr) [″ + Gr. *litra,* measure of wt.] One hundredth of a liter. SEE: *metric system.*

centimeter (sěn′tĭ-mē-tĕr) [″ + Gr. *metron,* measure] ABBR: cm. One hundredth of a meter. SEE: *metric system.*

centimorgan ABBR: cM. One hundredth of a morgan; a measure of genetic distance that indicates the likelihood of crossover of two loci on a gene.

centinormal (sěn″tĭ-nor′măl) [″ + *norma,* rule] One hundredth of the normal, as the strength of a solution.

centipede (sěn′tĭ-pēd″) [″ + *pes,* foot] An arthropod of the subclass Chilopoda distinguished by an elongated flattened body of many segments, each with a pair of jointed legs. The first pair of appendages are hooklike claws bearing openings of ducts from poison glands. The bites of large tropical centipedes may cause severe local and sometimes general symptoms, but they are rarely fatal.

centipoise (sěn′tĭ-poyz) A unit of viscosity, one hundredth of a poise. SEE: *poise.*

centrad (sěn′trăd) [Gr. *kentron,* center, + L. *ad,* toward] Toward the center.

central (sěn′trăl) **1.** Situated at or pertaining to a center. **2.** Principal or controlling.

central core disease A rare autosomal dominant polymyopathy marked by hypotonia, delay in walking, a propensity for malignant hyperthermia, and muscle weakness. When muscle fibers from the affected person are stained in certain ways and studied microscopically, a central area does not stain. The disease is caused by a defect in the calcium release channel of the sarcoplasmic reticulum of skeletal muscle.

central intravenous line SEE: *catheter, central venous; central line.*

central line A venous access device inserted into and kept in the vena cava, innominate, or subclavian veins. It is used to infuse fluids and medicines, or for gaining access to the heart to measure pressures in the venous circulation. Keeping the line open permits later venous access when the veins might be collapsed and difficult to enter. SEE: *catheter, central venous.*

centration The ability of the preschool child to focus or center attention on only one aspect or characteristic of a situation at a time. It was first described by Piaget.

centre Center.

centriciput (sěn-trĭs′ĭ-pŭt) [″ + L. *caput,* head] The central part of the upper surface of the skull between the occiput and sinciput.

centrifugal (sěn-trĭf′ū-găl) [″ + L. *fugere,* to flee] Receding from the center. SYN: *axifugal.* SEE: *centrifuge.*

centrifuge (sěn′trĭ-fūj) A device that spins test tubes at high speeds. Centrifugal force causes the heavy particles in the liquid to settle to the bottom of the tubes and the lighter liquid to go to the top. When unclotted blood is centrifuged, the plasma goes to the top and the heavy red cells go to the bottom of the tube. The white blood cells are heavier than the plasma but lighter than the red blood cells. Therefore they form a thin layer between the red blood cells and the plasma. SEE: *buffy coat.*

human c. A device that accommodates a human subject being rotated while suspended from a long arm. It is used to investigate the ability of subjects to withstand positive gravitational forces.

centrilobular (sĕn″trĭ-lŏb′ū-lăr) Pertaining to the center of a lobule.

centriole (sĕn′trē-ōl) A minute organelle consisting of a hollow cylinder closed at one end and open at the other, found in the cell center or attraction sphere of a cell. Before mitosis it divides, forming two daughter centrioles (diplosomes). During mitosis the centrioles migrate to opposite poles of the cell, and each forms the center of the aster to which the spindle fibers are attached. SEE: *mitosis.*

centripetal (sĕn-trĭp′ĕ-tăl) [″ + L. *petere,* to seek] Directed toward the axis. SYN: *axipetal.*

centrocyte (sĕn′trō-sīt) [″ + *kytos,* cell] A cell with single and double hematoxylin-stainable granules of varying size in its protoplasm.

centrodesmus (sĕn-trō-dĕz′mŭs) [Gr. *kentron,* center, + *desmos,* a band] The matter connecting the two centrosomes in a nucleus during mitosis.

centrolecithal (sĕn″trō-lĕs′ĭ-thăl) [″ + *lekithos,* yoke] Pertaining to an egg, especially an ovum, with the yolk centrally located.

centromere (sĕn′trō-mēr) [″ + *meros,* part] A constricted region of a chromosome, a specific sequence of about 200 nucleotides that connects the chromatids during cell division. Attached to this DNA is a protein disk called a kinetochore, which attaches the pair of chromatids to a spindle fiber.

centrosclerosis (sĕn″trō-sklĕ-rō′sĭs) [″ + *sklerosis,* a hardening] Filling of the bone marrow space with bone tissue.

centrosome (sĕn′trō-sōm) [″ + *soma,* body] A region of the cytoplasm of a cell usually lying near the nucleus, containing in its center one or two centrioles, the diplosomes. SEE: *mitosis.*

centrosphere (sĕn′trō-sfēr) [″ + *sphaira,* sphere] The cytoplasm of the centrosome.

centrostaltic (sĕn″trō-stăl′tĭk) [″ + *stellein,* send forth] Pert. to a center of motion.

centrum (sĕn′trŭm) *pl.* **centra** [L.] **1.** Any center, esp. an anatomical one. **2.** The body of a vertebra.

c. semiovale The mass of white matter at the center of each cerebral hemisphere.

c. tendineum The central tendon of the diaphragm.

cepacia SEE: *Pseudomonas cepacia.*

cephalad (sĕf′ă-lăd) [Gr. *kephale,* head, + L. *ad,* toward] Toward the head.

cephalalgia (sĕf-ă-lăl′jē-ă) [″ + *algos,* pain] Headache. SYN: *cephalodynia.*

cephalalgic (-jĭk), *adj.*

cephalea (sĕf-ă-lē′ă) [Gr. *kephale,* head] Cephalalgia.

cephaledema (sĕf″ăl-ĕ-dē′mă) [″ + *oidema,* swelling] Edema of the head, esp. of the brain.

cephalexin (sĕf″ă-lĕk′sĭn) A first-generation cephalosporin antibiotic. It treats gram-positive and some gram-negative bacteria.

cephalhematocele (sĕf″ăl-hē-măt′ō-sēl) [″ + *haima,* blood, + *kele,* tumor] A bloody tumor communicating with the dural sinuses.

cephalic (sĕ-făl′ĭk) [L. *cephalicus*] **1.** Cranial. **2.** Superior in position.

cephalohematoma (sĕf″ăl-hē″mă-tō′mă) [″ + ″ + *oma,* tumor] A mass composed of clotted blood, located between the periosteum and the skull of a newborn. It is confined between suture lines and usually is unilateral. The cause is rupture of periosteal bridging veins due to pressure and friction during labor and delivery. The blood reabsorbs gradually within a few weeks of birth.

cephalocele (sĕf′ă-lō-sēl) [″ + *kele,* hernia] Protrusion of the brain from the cranial cavity.

cephalocentesis (sĕf″ă-lō-sĕn-tē′sĭs) [″ + *kentesis,* puncture] Surgical puncture of the cranium.

cephalodynia (sĕf″ă-lō-dĭn′ē-ă) [″ + *odyne,* pain] Headache.

cephalogyric (sĕf″ă-lō-jī′rĭk) [″ + *gyros,* a turn] Pert. to rotation of the head.

cephalohemometer (sĕf″ă-lō-hē-mŏm′ĕ-tĕr) [″ + *haima,* blood, + *metron,* measure] An instrument for determining changes in intracranial blood pressure.

cephalomenia (sĕf″ă-lō-mē′nē-ă) [″ + *men,* month] Vicarious menstruation from the nose or head.

cephalomeningitis (sĕf″ă-lō-mĕn″ĭn-jī′tĭs) [″ + *meninx,* membrane, + *itis,* inflammation] Inflammation of the cerebral meninges.

cephalometer (sĕf-ă-lŏm′ĕ-tĕr) [″ + *metron,* measure] **1.** A device for measuring the head. **2.** In radiology, a device that maintains the head in a certain position for radiographic examination and measurement.

cephalometry (sĕf″ă-lŏm′ĕ-trē) Measurement of the head of a living person by using certain bony points directly, or by tracing radiographs made using well-established planes for linear and angular measurements. This technique is used in dentistry to assess growth and to determine orthodontic or prosthetic treatment plans.

cephalomotor (sĕf″ă-lō-mō′tor) [Gr. *kephale,* head, + L. *motus,* motion] Pert. to movements of the head.

cephalonia (sĕf″ă-lō′nē-ă) A condition

marked by mental retardation and enlargement of the head.

cephalopathy (sĕf″ă-lŏp′ă-thē) [″ + *pathos,* disease, suffering] Any disease of the head or brain.

cephalopelvic (sĕf″ă-lō-pĕl′vĭk) Pert. to the relationship between the measurements of the fetal head and the diameters of the maternal pelvis, esp. to the size of the pelvic outlet through which the fetal head will pass during delivery.

cephaloplegia (sĕf″ă-lō-plē′jē-ă) [″ + *plege,* stroke] Paralysis of head or neck muscles or both.

cephalorhachidian (sĕf″ă-lō-ră-kĭd′ē-ăn) [″ + *rhachis,* spine] Pert. to the head and spine.

cephaloridine (sĕf″ă-lor′ĭ-dēn) An analogue of the antibiotic cephalosporin C.

cephalosporin (sĕf″ă-lō-spor′ĭn) General term for a group of antibiotic derivatives of cephalosporin C, which is obtained from the fungus *Cephalosporium.*

first-generation c. Group of cephalosporin antibiotics capable of killing gram-positive cocci such as *Staphylococcus aureus,* streptococci, and some aerobic gram-negative rods. These agents are commonly used to treat skin and soft tissue infections, uncomplicated respiratory tract infections, and urinary tract infections. Examples of first generation cephalosporins are cephalothin, cephaloridine, cephapirin, cefazolin, cephradine, cephalexin, and cefadroxil.

second-generation c. Group of cephalosporin antibiotics possessing some ability to kill gram-positive cocci such as staphylococci and streptococci, as well as aerobic gram-negative rods. Some agents, namely cefotetan, cefoxitin, and cefmetazole, can be used to treat anaerobic infections. Examples of second-generation cephalosporins are cefamandole, cefuroxime, cefonicid, ceforanide, cefixime, cefaclor, cefoxitin, cefotetan, and cefmetazole.

third-generation c. Group of cephalosporin antibiotics capable of killing aerobic gram-negative rods. These agents are commonly used for treatment of pneumonia and meningitis. Some agents, namely ceftazidime and cefoperazone, have excellent activity against *Pseudomonas aeruginosa*. Examples of third-generation cephalosporins are cefsulodin, cefotaxime, ceftizoxime, ceftriaxone, cefoperazone, moxalactam, and ceftazidime.

Cephalosporium A genus of imperfect fungi that inhabit soil. Cephalosporins are derived from them.

cephalothin sodium (sĕf′ă-lō-thĭn″) A first-generation cephalosporin antibiotic that treats infections caused by gram-positive and a small number of gram-negative bacteria. Trade name is Keflin.

cephalothoracic (sĕf″ă-lō-thō-răs′ĭk) [″ + *thorakos,* chest] Pert. to the head and thorax.

cephalothoracopagus (sĕf″ă-lō-thō″ră-kŏp′ă-gŭs) [″ + ″ + *pagos,* thing fixed] A double fetus joined at the head and thorax.

cephalotome (sĕf′ă-lō-tōm) [″ + *tome,* incision] An instrument for cutting the head of the fetus to facilitate delivery.

cephalotomy (sĕf-ă-lŏt′ō-mē) Cutting the fetal head to facilitate delivery.

cephapirin sodium (sĕf-ă-pī′rĭn) A first-generation cephalosporin. Trade name is Cefadyl.

ceptor (sĕp′tor) [L. *receptor,* receiver] Receptor (2).

chemical c. A ceptor that detects chemical changes in the body.

contact c. A ceptor that receives stimuli contributed by direct physical contact.

distance c. A ceptor that perceives stimuli remote from the immediate environment.

cera (sē′ră) [L.] Wax (1).

c. alba White wax.

c. flava Yellow wax.

ceramics, dental [Gr. *keramos,* potter's clay] The use of porcelain or porcelain-type materials in dental work.

ceramide (sĕr′ă-mīd) A class of lipids that do not contain glycerol. They are derived from a sphingosine. Glycosphingolipids and sphingomyelins are derived from ceramides.

c. oligosaccharides A class of glycosphingolipids.

ceramodontia (sē-răm″ō-dŏn′sheē-ă) [Gr. *keramos,* potter's clay, + *odous,* tooth] SEE: *ceramics, dental.*

cerate ceratum (sē′rāt) [L. *ceratum*] A medicinal formulation for topical use containing wax. It can be spread easily with a spatula on muslin or similar material at ordinary temperature, but is not soft enough to liquefy and run when applied to the skin. It is rarely prescribed.

ceratocele (sĕr′ă-tō-sēl) [Gr. *keras,* horn, + *kele,* hernia] Keratocele.

ceratotome (sē-răt′ō-tōm) [″ + *tome,* incision] A knife for division of the cornea.

cercaria (sĕr-kā′rē-ă) *pl.* **cercariae** [Gr. *kerkos,* tail] A free-swimming stage in the development of a fluke or trematode. Cercariae develop within sporocysts or rediae that parasitize snails or bivalve mollusks. They emerge from the mollusk and either enter their final host directly or encyst in an intermediate host that is ingested by the final host. In the latter case, the encysted tailless form is known as a metacercaria. SEE: *fluke; trematode.*

cercaricide An agent that is lethal to cercaria.

cerclage (sār-klŏzh′) [Fr., hooping] Encircling tissues with a ligature, wire, or loop.

cervical c. The use of ligatures around the cervix uteri to treat cervical incompetence during pregnancy. This has been used to prevent spontaneous abortion, although its efficacy is uncertain. SEE: *Shirodkar operation.*

Cercomonas (sĕr-kŏm′ō-năs) [Gr. *kerkos,* tail, + *monas,* unit] A genus of free-living flagellate protozoa. It may be present in stale specimens of feces or urine. It is not pathogenic.

cercomoniasis (sĕr″kō-mō-nī′ă-sĭs) Infestation with *Cercomonas intestinalis.*

Cercopithecine herpesvirus 1 A virus that is prevalent in macaques but not other primates; humans who handle macaques may be infected by bites or exposure to animal blood or body fluids. Although in macaques the virus causes a herpetic rash, in humans it often produces deadly infections of the brain and meninges.

cercus (sĕr′kŭs) *pl.* **cerci** [L., tail] A hairlike structure.

cerea flexibilitas (sē′rē-ă flĕk″sĭ-bĭl′ĭ-tăs) [L. *cera,* wax, + *flexibilitas,* flexibility] A cataleptic state in which limbs retain any position in which they are placed. It is characteristic of catatonic patients. SEE: *catalepsy.*

cereal [L. *cerealis,* of grain] An edible seed or grain. All cereals are similar in composition. Carbohydrates are the principal nutrient present and protein is next. Cereals contain 70% to 80% carbohydrate in the form of starch, and 8% to 15% protein. Many cereals are high in fiber. Vitamin B complex is abundant in wheat germ.

cerebellifugal (sĕr″ĕ-bĕl-ĭ-fū′găl) [L. *cerebellum,* little brain, + *fugere,* to flee] Extending or proceeding from the cerebellum.

cerebellipetal (sĕr″ĕ-bĕl-lĭp′ĭ-tăl) [″ + *petere,* to seek] Extending toward the cerebellum.

cerebellitis (sĕr″ĕ-bĕl-ī′tĭs) [″ + Gr. *itis,* inflammation] Inflammation of the cerebellum.

cerebellospinal (sĕr″ĕ-bĕl-ō-spī′năl) [″ + *spina,* thorn] Pert. to the cerebellum and spinal cord.

cerebellum (sĕr-ĕ-bĕl′ŭm) [L., little brain] The portion of the brain forming the largest segment of the rhombencephalon. It lies dorsal to the pons and medulla oblongata, overhanging the latter. It consists of two lateral cerebellar hemispheres and a narrow medial portion, the vermis. It is connected to the brainstem by three pairs of fiber bundles, the inferior, middle, and superior peduncles. The cerebellum is involved in synergic control of skeletal muscles and plays an important role in the coordination of voluntary movements. It receives afferent impulses and discharges efferent impulses but is not a reflex center in the usual sense; however, it may reinforce some reflexes and inhibit others. SEE: illus.

Although the cerebellum does not initiate movements, it interrelates with many brainstem structures in executing various movements, including maintaining proper posture and balance; walking and running; fine voluntary movements as required in writing, dressing, eating, and playing musical instruments; and smooth tracking movements of the eyes. The cerebellum controls the property of movements, such as speed, acceleration, and trajectory. **cerebellar** (-ăr), *adj.*

cerebral dominance The control of speech and handedness by one hemisphere of the brain. In 90% to 95% of human beings the left cerebral hemisphere is functionally dominant, and those persons are right-handed. A lesion to the left cerebral hemisphere of such persons (e.g., a stroke or tumor) will produce aphasia and right-sided paralysis. Aphasia rarely occurs in right-handed persons as a result of a right cerebral lesion. In 60% of left-handed individuals with aphasia owing to a cerebral lesion, the left side is affected. In some left-handed patients, it is possible that language function is controlled partially by both the left and right cerebal hemispheres. SEE: *stroke.*

cerebration (sĕr″ĕ-brā′shŭn) [L. *cerebratio,* brain activity] Mental activity; thinking.

cerebrifugal (sĕr″ĕ-brĭf′ū-găl) [L. *cerebrum,* brain, + *fugere,* to flee] Away from the brain; pert. to efferent nerve fibers.

cerebripetal (sĕr″ĕ-brĭp′ĕ-tăl) [″ + *petere,* to seek] Proceeding toward the cerebrum; pert. to afferent nerve fibers or impulses.

cerebroid (sĕr′ē-broyd) [″ + Gr. *eidos,* form, shape] Resembling brain tissue.

cerebromeningitis (sĕr″ĕ-brō-mĕn″ĭn-jī′tĭs) [″ + Gr. *meninx,* membrane, + *itis,* inflammation] Inflammation of the cerebrum and its membranes.

cerebropathy (sĕr-ĕ-brŏp′ă-thē) [″ + *pathos,* disease, suffering] Any disease of the brain, esp. the cerebrum.

cerebrophysiology (sĕr″ĕ-brō-fĭz-ē-ŏl′ō-jē) [″ + Gr. *physis,* nature, + *logos,* word, reason] The physiology of the brain.

cerebropontile (sĕr″ĕ-brō-pŏn′tĭl) [″ + *pons,* bridge] Pert. to the cerebrum and pons varolii.

cerebrosclerosis (sĕr″ĕ-brō″sklĕ-rō′sĭs) [″ + Gr. *sklerosis,* hardening] Hardening of the brain, esp. of the cerebrum.

cerebroside (sĕr′ĕ-brō-sīd″) A lipid or fatty substance present in nerve and other tissues.

cerebrosidosis (sĕr″ĕ-brō″sī-dō′sĭs) A form of lipoidosis with kerasin in the fatty cells. SEE: *Gaucher's disease.*

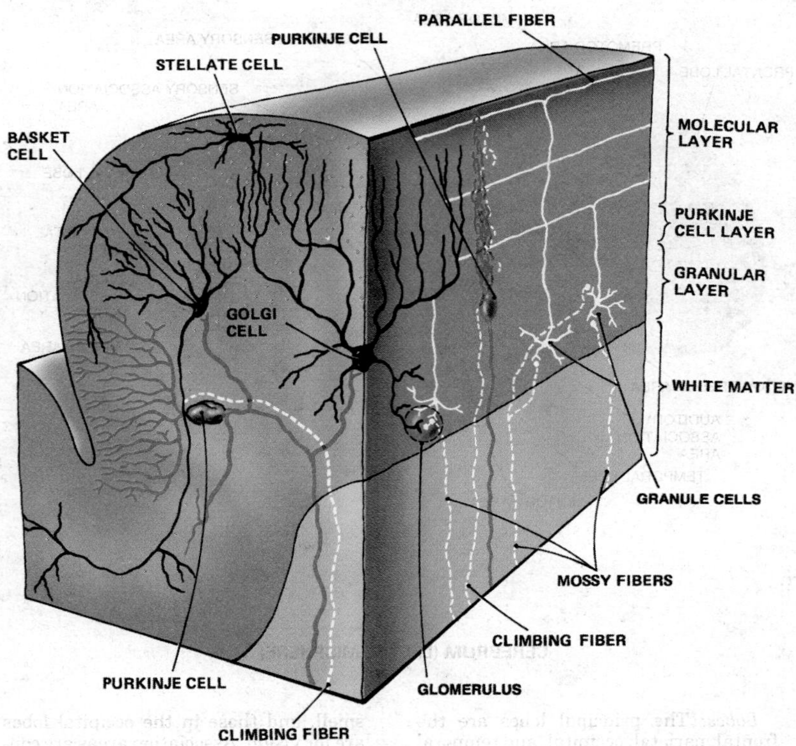

CEREBELLUM

Layers of the cerebellar cortex

cerebrospinal (sĕr″ĕ-brō-spī′năl) [″ + *spina,* thorn] Pert. to the brain and spinal cord, as the cerebrospinal axis.

cerebrospinal axis The central nervous system.

cerebrospinal puncture A puncture for the collection of cerebrospinal fluid or the injection of contrast media or medications. Puncture sites include the spaces around the spinal cord (lumbar puncture), the cisterna magna (cisternal puncture), or open fontanelles in infants (ventricular puncture).

cerebrotomy (sĕr″ĕ-brŏt′ō-mē) [L. *cerebrum,* brain, + Gr. *tome,* incision] **1.** Incision of the brain to evacuate an abscess. **2.** Dissection of the brain.

cerebrovascular (sĕr″ĕ-brō-văs′kū-lăr) [″ + *vasculum,* vessel] Pert. to the blood vessels of the brain, esp. to pathological changes.

cerebrum (sĕr′ĕ-brŭm, sĕr-ē′brŭm) [L.] The largest part of the brain, consisting of two hemispheres separated by a deep longitudinal fissure. The hemispheres are united by three commissures—the corpus callosum and the anterior and posterior hippocampal commissures. The surface of each hemisphere is thrown into numerous folds or convolutions called gyri, which are separated by furrows called fissures or sulci.

EMBRYOLOGY: The cerebrum develops from the telencephalon, the most anterior portion of the prosencephalon or forebrain.

ANATOMY: Each cerebral hemisphere consists of three primary portions—the rhinencephalon or olfactory lobe, the corpus striatum, and the pallium or cerebral cortex. The cortex is a layer of gray matter that forms the surface of each hemisphere. The part in the rhinencephalon (phylogenetically the oldest) is called the archipallium; the larger nonolfactory cortex is called the neopallium. The cerebrum contains two cavities, the lateral ventricles (right and left) and the rostral portion of the third ventricle. The white matter of each hemisphere consists of three kinds of myelinated fibers: commissural fibers, which pass from one hemisphere to the other; projection fibers, which convey impulses to and from the cortex; and association fibers, which connect various parts of the cortex within one hemisphere.

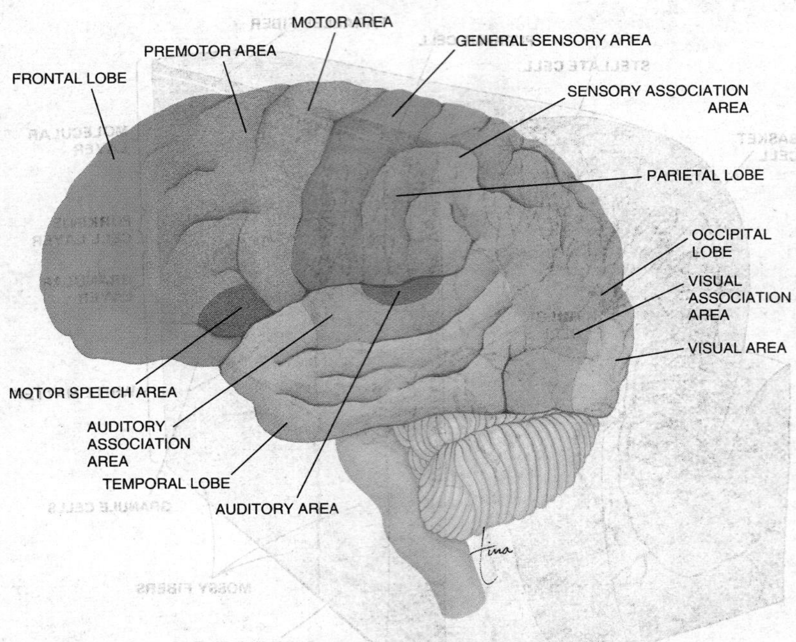

CEREBRUM (LEFT HEMISPHERE)

Lobes: The principal lobes are the frontal, parietal, occipital, and temporal lobes and the central (the insula or island of Reil). *Basal ganglia:* Masses of gray matter are deeply embedded within each hemisphere. They are the caudate, lentiform, and amygdaloid nuclei and the claustrum. *Fissures and sulci:* These include the lateral cerebral fissure (of Sylvius), the central sulcus (of Rolando), the parieto-occipital fissure, the calcarine fissure, the cingulate sulcus, the collateral fissure, the sulcus circularis, and the longitudinal cerebral fissure. *Gyri:* These include the superior, middle, and inferior frontal gyri, the anterior and posterior central gyri, the superior, middle, and inferior temporal gyri, and the cingulate, lingual, fusiform, and hippocampal gyri.

PHYSIOLOGY: The cerebrum is concerned with sensations (the interpretation of sensory impulses) and all voluntary muscular activities. It is the seat of consciousness and the center of the higher mental faculties such as memory, learning, reasoning, judgment, intelligence, and the emotions. SEE: illus.

On the basis of function, several areas have been identified and located. Motor areas in the frontal lobes initiate all voluntary movement of skeletal muscles. Sensory areas in the parietal lobes are for taste and cutaneous senses, those in the temporal lobes are for hearing and smell, and those in the occipital lobes are for vision. Association areas are concerned with integration, analysis, learning, and memory.

cerium (sē′rē-ŭm) [L.] SYMB: Ce. A metallic element obtained from the rare earths; atomic weight 140.12, atomic number 58.

ceroid (sē′royd) A fatty pigment present in various tissues.

ceroma (sē-rō′mă) [L. *cera,* wax, + Gr. *oma,* tumor] A waxy tumor that has undergone amyloid degeneration.

ceroplasty (sē′rō-plăs″tē) [″ + Gr. *plassein,* to mold] The manufacture of anatomical models and pathological specimens in wax.

CERT *Centers for Education and Research on Therapeutics.*

certifiable (sĕr″tĭ-fī′ă-b'l) **1.** Pert. to infectious diseases that must be reported or registered with the health authorities. **2.** In forensic medicine, a term applied to a mentally incompetent individual who requires the care of a guardian or institution.

certification (sĕr″tĭ-fĭ-kā′shŭn) **1.** A legal document prepared by an official body that indicates a person or institution has met certain standards, or that a person has completed a prescribed course of instruction or training. **2.** The completion of a form indicating the cause of death. **3.** The legal process of declaring a person insane or mentally incompetent on the basis of medical evidence.

certified emergency nurse ABBR: CEN. A nurse who has passed the examination administered by the Board of Certification of Emergency Nursing. To maintain certification as a CEN, a nurse must recertify every 4 years; a formal examination is required every 8 years, and continuing education credits can be submitted as proof of professional competence during alternate 4-year cycles.

certify [L. *certus,* certain, + *facio,* to make] **1.** To confirm or verify. **2.** To make a declaration concerning the sanity of an individual. **3.** To report certain specified diseases to public health authorities.

ceruloplasmin (sĕ-roo″lō-plăz′mĭn) A blue glycoprotein to which most of the copper in the blood is attached. It is decreased in Wilson's disease.

cerumen (sĕ-roo′mĕn) [L. *cera,* wax] A substance secreted by glands at the outer third of the ear canal. Usually cerumen does not accumulate in the ear canal, but it may clog the channel in some persons; the cerumen may become impacted and must be physically removed, not by irrigation of the canal but by use of a curette. Soft cerumen is easily removed by gentle syringe instillation of water in the canal. **ceruminal, ceruminous** (-mĭ-năl, -mĭ-nŭs), *adj.*

ceruminolysis (sĕ-roo″mĭ-nŏl′ĭ-sĭs) The dissolution or disintegration of cerumen in the external ear canal.

ceruminolytic agent (sĕ-roo″mĭ-nō-lĭt′ĭk) An agent that dissolves cerumen in the external ear canal. Obstruction of the ear canal with cerumen can cause itching, pain, and temporary conductive hearing loss. The first approach to treatment should be removal of the obstruction manually with a blunt curette or loop or by irrigation. Cerumen solvents are not always recommended because they often do not eliminate the problem and frequently cause maceration of skin of the canal and allergic reactions.

ceruminosis (sĕ-roo″mĭ-nō′sĭs) [″ + Gr. *osis,* condition] Excessive secretion of cerumen.

ceruminous gland One of the modified sweat glands in the skin lining the external auditory canal that secrete cerumen.

cervic- SEE: *cervico-*.

cervical (sĕr′vĭ-kăl) [L. *cervicalis*] **1.** Pert. to or in the region of the neck. **2.** Pert. to the cervix of an organ, as the cervix uteri.

cervical cap A contraceptive device made of a flexible material that is shaped to provide a covering for the uterine cervix.

cervical intraepithelial neoplasia ABBR: CIN. Dysplasia of the basal layers of the squamous epithelium of the uterine cervix. This may progress to involve deeper layers of the epithelium. Grades 1, 2, and 3 represent increasing progression of the pathological process. Grade 3 (CIN 3) represents carcinoma in situ. CIN 3 is also classed stage 0 of cancer of the cervix. SEE: *Bethesda System, The; cervix, cancer of*.

cervical nerve A nerve in the first eight pairs of spinal nerves. SEE: *skeleton; spinal nerve*.

cervical plexus A network formed by the first four cervical spinal nerves. It innervates parts of the face, neck, shoulder, and chest, and gives rise to the phrenic nerve to the diaphragm.

cervical rib syndrome Pain and paresthesias in the the hand, neck, shoulder, or arms, usually due to compression of the brachial plexus of nerves by an accessory cervical rib. SEE: *scalenus syndrome*.

cervical ripening The biochemical changes in the cervix that take place gradually over the last few weeks of gestation in preparation for childbirth. The cervix softens, and its potential for stretching increases. Normally this occurs naturally, but in postterm pregnancies it may be necessary to use mechanical dilators or drugs. Placement of *Laminaria digitata* or prostaglandin E analogs (e.g., misoprostol) in the vagina or cervical canal promotes cervical ripening and onset of labor but does not reduce the rate of cesarean deliveries.

PATIENT CARE: Fetal status is assessed by monitoring the heart rate for 30 min before gel insertion and for approx. 1 hr after the procedure. The woman is assessed for uterine contractions and signs of hyperstimulation, nausea, or vomiting. If hyperstimulation occurs, the gel is removed, and the primary health care provider is notified.

cervicectomy (sĕr″vĭ-sĕk′tō-mē) [L. *cervix,* neck, + Gr. *ektome,* excision] Surgical removal of the cervix uteri.

cervices Pl. of cervix.

cervicitis (sĕr-vĭ-sī′tĭs) [″ + Gr. *itis,* inflammation] Inflammation of the cervix uteri.

cervico-, cervic- (sĕr′vĭ-kō) [L. *cervix*] Combining form pert. to the neck or to the neck of an organ.

cervicobrachial (sĕr″vĭ-kō-brā′kē-ăl) [″ + Gr. *brachion,* arm] Pert. to the neck and arm.

cervicocolpitis (sĕr″vĭ-kō-kŏl-pī′tĭs) [″ + Gr. *kolpos,* vagina, + *itis,* inflammation] Inflammation of the cervix uteri and vagina.

cervicodynia (sĕr″vĭ-kō-dĭn′ē-ă) [″ + Gr. *odyne,* pain] A pain or cramp of the neck; cervical neuralgia.

cervicofacial (sĕr″vĭ-kō-fā′shē-ăl) [″ + *facies,* face] Pert. to the neck and face.

cervicogenic (sĕr″vĭ-kō-jĕn′ĭk) Relating to, or beginning in, the upper segments of the cervical spine or neighboring soft tissues.

cervicography Photographic study of the uterine cervix.

cervicovaginitis (sĕr″vĭ-kō-văj″ĭ-nī′tĭs) [″ + *vagina,* sheath, + Gr. *itis,* inflammation] Inflammation of the cervix uteri and the vagina.

cervicovesical (sĕr″vĭ-kō-vĕs′ĭ-kăl) [″ + *vesica,* bladder] Pert. to the cervix uteri and bladder.

cervix (sĕr′vĭks) *pl.* **cervices** [L.] The neck or a part of an organ resembling a neck.

c. uteri The neck of the uterus; the lower part from the internal os outward to the external os. It is rounded and conical, and a portion protrudes into the vagina. It is about 1 in. (2.5 cm) long and is penetrated by the cervical canal, through which the fetus and menstrual flow escape. It may be torn in childbirth, esp. in a primigravida.

Deeper tears may occur in manual dilatation and use of forceps; breech presentation also may be a cause. Laceration may be single, bilateral, stellate, or incomplete. Tears are repaired by suturing to prevent hemorrhage and later complications. SYN: *cervical canal.*

c. vesicae Neck of the bladder.

c.e.s. *central excitatory state.*

cesarean birth Cesarean section.

cesarean-obtained barrier-sustained ABBR: COBS. Used in reference to animals delivered sterilely by cesarean section and maintained in a germ-free environment.

cesarean section Delivery of the fetus by means of incision into the uterus. Operative approaches and techniques vary. A horizontal incision through the lower uterine segment is most common; the classic vertical midline incision may be used in times of profound fetal distress. Elective cesarean section is indicated for known cephalopelvic disproportion, malpresentations, and active herpes infection. The most common reason for emergency cesarean delivery is fetal distress. Many women can experience successful vaginal birth with a later pregnancy.

PATIENT CARE: *Preoperative:* The procedure is explained to the patient and her partner. The partner should be included in the experience if possible. Baseline measures of maternal vital signs and fetal heart rate are obtained; maternal and fetal status are monitored until delivery according to protocol. Laboratory data, ultrasound results, or the results of other studies are available to the obstetrical team. The operative area is prepared according to the surgeon's preference, and an indwelling urinary catheter is inserted as prescribed. An intravenous infusion with a large-bore catheter is started, and oral food and fluid are restricted as time permits. Blood replacement is prepared only as the surgeon requests. The patient is premedicated to reduce anxiety and discomfort.

Postoperative: On recovery from general anesthesia, or as soon as possible thereafter, the mother is allowed to see, hold, and touch her newborn. The pediatrician or nurse midwife assesses the newborn's status. Vital signs are monitored for mother and baby. The dressing and perineal pad are assessed for bleeding. The fundus is gently palpated for firmness (avoiding the incision), and intravenous oxytocin is administered as prescribed. If general anesthesia is used, routine postoperative care and positioning are provided; if regional anesthesia is used, the anesthesia level is assessed until sensation has completely returned. Intake and output are monitored, and any evidence of blood-tinged urine is documented and reported. Cold is applied to the incision to control pain and swelling if prescribed, analgesics are administered, and noninvasive pain-relief measures are instituted. The mother is assisted to turn from side to side and is encouraged to breathe deeply, cough, and use incentive spirometry to improve ventilation and to mobilize secretions. When bowel sounds have returned, oral fluids and food are encouraged and bowel and bladder activity are monitored.

The patient is assisted with early ambulation and urged to visit her newborn in the nursery if the neonate is not healthy enough to be brought to her bedside. Usual postpartal instruction is provided regarding fundus, lochia, and perineal care; breast and nipple care; and infant care. Instruction is also given on incision care and the need to report any hemorrhage, chest or leg pain (possible thrombosis), dyspnea, separation of the wound's edges, or signs of infection, such as fever, difficult urination, or flank pain. Any activity restrictions after discharge are discussed with both the woman and her partner. SEE: *Nursing Diagnoses Appendix.*

cervical c.s. Surgical removal of the fetus, placenta, and membranes through an incision in the portion of the uterus just above the cervix.

classic c.s. Surgical removal of the fetus, placenta, and membranes through an incision in the abdominal and uterine walls.

extraperitoneal c.s. Surgical removal of the fetus, placenta, and membranes through an incision into the lowest portion of the anterior aspect of the uterus. This approach does not entail entering the peritoneal cavity.

low transverse c.s. Surgical removal of the fetus, placenta, and membranes through a transverse incision into the lower uterine segment. Use of this incision is associated with a decreased incidence of maternal and fetal mortality and morbidity in future pregnancies.

postmortem c.s. Surgical removal of the fetus from the uterus immediately after maternal death.

cesium (sē′zē-ŭm) [L. *caesius,* sky blue] SYMB: Cs. A metallic element; atomic weight 132.905, atomic number 55. It has several isotopes. The radioactive isotope ^{137}Cs, which has a half-life of 30 years, is used therapeutically for irradiation of cancerous tissue.

cesspool Colloquial term for *septic tank.*

Cestan-Chenais syndrome (sĕs-tăn′shĕn-ā′) [Raymond Cestan, Fr. neurologist, 1872–1934; Louis J. Chenais, Fr. physician, 1872–1950] A neurological disorder produced by a lesion of the pontobulbar area of the brain.

Cestoda (sĕs-tōd′ă) [Gr. *kestos,* girdle] A subclass of the class Cestoidea, phylum Platyhelminthes, which includes the tapeworms, having a scolex and a chain of segments (proglottids) (e.g., *Taenia,* intestinal parasites of humans and other vertebrates).

cestode (sĕs′tōd) [″ + *eidos,* form, shape] A tapeworm; a member of the Cestoda family. **cestoid** (-toyd), *adj.*

cestodiasis (sĕs″tō-dī′ă-sĭs) [″ + ″ + *-iasis,* condition] Infestation with tapeworms. SEE: *Cestoda.*

Cestoidea (sĕs-toy′dē-ă) A class of flatworms of the phylum Platyhelminthes; it includes the tapeworms.

cetylpyridinium chloride An anti-infective agent used topically and as a preservative in the manufacture of drugs.

CF *Christmas factor; citrovorum factor.*

Cf Symbol for the element californium.

C.F.T. *complement fixation test.*

CGD *Chronic granulomatous disease.*

cGMP *cyclic guanosine monophosphate.*

C.G.S. *centimeter-gram-second,* a name given to a system of units for length, weight, and time.

CH_4 Methane.

C_2H_2 Acetylene.

C_2H_4 Ethylene.

C_6H_6 Benzene.

Chaddock's reflex (chăd′ŏks) [Charles G. Chaddock, U.S. neurologist, 1861–1936] **1.** Extension of the great toe when the outer edge of the dorsum of the foot is stroked. It is present in disease of the corticospinal tract. **2.** Flexion of the wrist and fanning of the fingers when the tendon of the palmaris longus muscle is pressed.

Chadwick's sign [James R. Chadwick, U.S. gynecologist, 1844–1905] A deep blue-violet color of the cervix and vagina caused by increased vascularity; a probable sign of pregnancy that becomes evident around the fourth week of gestation.

chafe (chāf) [O.Fr. *chaufer,* to warm] To injure by rubbing or friction.

chafing (chāf′ĭng) A superficial inflammation that develops when skin is subjected to friction from clothing or adjacent skin. This may occur at the axilla, groin, or anal region, between digits of hands and feet, or at the neck or wrists. Erythema, maceration, and sometimes fissuring occur. Bacterial or fungal infection may result secondarily.

Chagas' disease (chăg′ăs) [Carlos Chagas, Braz. physician, 1879–1934] American trypanosomiasis.

chagoma An erythematous swelling following the bite of the parasite that transmits trypanosomiasis. SEE: *trypanosomiasis, South American.*

chain (chān) [O.Fr. *chaine,* chain] **1.** A related series of events or things. **2.** In bacteriology, bacterial organisms strung together. **3.** In chemistry, the linkage of atoms in a straight line or in a circle or ring. The ring or straight-line structures may have side chains branching off from the main compound.

electron transport c. SEE: *cytochrome transport system.*

food c. The sequential transfer of food energy from green plants to animals that eat plants, then to animals that eat the plant-eating animals. For example, cows eat plants; other animals including humans eat the meat of cows. Interruption of the chain at any point may produce ecological disruptions.

heavy c. The large polypeptide chains of antibodies. SEE: *heavy chain disease.*

J c. The joining portion of a polymeric immunoglobulin, found in dimeric and polymeric IgA and pentameric IgM.

kinematic c. A series of bones connected by joints. Movement of one segment influences other parts of the chain.

light c. The small polypeptide chains of antibodies.

chaining (chān′ĭng) A behavioral therapy process whereby reinforcement is given for behaviors related to established behavior. Also called *chained reinforcement.*

chain of custody In legal medicine, the procedure for ensuring that material obtained for diagnosis has been taken from the named patient, is properly labeled, and has not been tampered with en route to the laboratory. SEE: *rape.*

chain of survival In emergency cardiac care, the idea that the survival of patients in cardiac arrest depends on the linkage of the following: 1. early access, 2. early CPR, 3. early defibrillation, 4. early advanced life support. If for any reason any one of these links is missing or delayed, the chance of survival decreases considerably. SEE: *cardiopulmonary resuscitatio.*

chair, birthing SEE: *birthing chair.*

chakra (chah′kruh, shah′kruh) In yoga philosophy any of the seven energy centers that run parallel to the spine in the human body.

chalasia (kă-lā′zē-ă) [Gr. *chalasis,* relaxation] Relaxation of sphincters.

chalazion (kă-lā′zē-ōn) *pl.* **chalazia, chalazions** [Gr. *khalaza,* hailstone] A small, hard benign tumor analogous to a sebaceous cyst developing on the eyelids, formed by distention of a meibomian gland with secretion. SYN: *meibomian cyst.* SEE: *steatoma.*

chalicosis (kăl-ĭ-kō′sĭs) [Gr. *chalix,* limestone, + *osis,* condition] Pneumonoconiosis associated with the inhalation of dust produced by stone cutting.

chalinoplasty (kăl′ĭ-nō-plăs″tē) [Gr. *chalinos,* corner of mouth, + *plassein,* to mold] An obsolete term for plastic surgery of the mouth and lips, esp. of the corners of the mouth.

challenge (chăl′ĕnj) In immunology, administration of a specific antigen to an individual known to be sensitive to that antigen in order to produce an immune response.

food c. Exposing a patient to a substance to which the patient is thought to react adversely. Ethically, the test cannot be performed without the patient's permission, but for accuracy the test foods should be disguised during the test. Typically, food challenges are performed after the patient has eliminated the suspected food from his or her diet for 1 or 2 weeks. To eliminate bias, the patient should agree to ingest several disguised foods that he or she is known to tolerate, in addition to the suspected food. SEE: *elimination d.*

peremptory c. A challenge to remove a juror from a prospective jury without cause.

challenge for cause A request that a prospective juror not be allowed to serve for specific reasons or causes (e.g., concerns about potential bias or prejudice).

chalone (kăl′ōn) [Gr. *chalan,* to relax] A protein that inhibits mitosis in the tissue in which it is produced.

chamber (chām′bĕr) [Gr. *kamara,* vault] A compartment or closed space.

altitude c. Low-pressure c.

anterior c. The space between the cornea and iris of the eye. SEE: *posterior c.*

aqueous c. The anterior and posterior chambers of the eye, containing the aqueous humor.

hyperbaric c. An airtight enclosure strong enough to withstand high internal pressure. It is used to expose animals, humans, or an entire surgical team to increased air pressure. SYN: *pressure c.* SEE: *oxygenation, hyperbaric.*

ionization c. A device used to measure radiation by equating ion production in a gas chamber with the intensity of an electrical charge.

low-pressure c. An enclosure designed to simulate high altitudes by exposing humans or animals to low atmospheric pressure. Such studies are essential for simulated flights into the atmosphere and space. SYN: *altitude c.*

posterior c. In the eye, the space behind the iris and in front of the vitreous body. It is occupied by the lens, its zonules, and the aqueous humor. SEE: *anterior c.; eye* for illus.

pressure c. Hyperbaric c.

pulp c. The central cavity of a tooth. The pulp canal contains arteries, veins, lymphatic vessels, and sensory nerve endings. Anatomically, the pulp chamber can be divided into the body and the pulp horns. Pulp horns correspond to the cusps of the teeth. SEE: *pulp canal; pulp cavity.*

vitreous c. The cavity behind the lens in the eye that contains the vitreous humor.

chamomile (kăm′ĕ-mīl) [Gr. *khamaemelon,* earth apple] The flowers of the genus *Anthemis;* they yield a bluish volatile oil and a bitter infusion.

chance **1.** That which occurs randomly. **2.** An accident.

chancre (shăng′kĕr) [Fr., ulcer] A hard, syphilitic primary ulcer, the first sign of syphilis, appearing approx. 2 to 3 weeks after infection. SEE: illus.; *syphilis.* **chancrous** (-krŭs), *adj.*

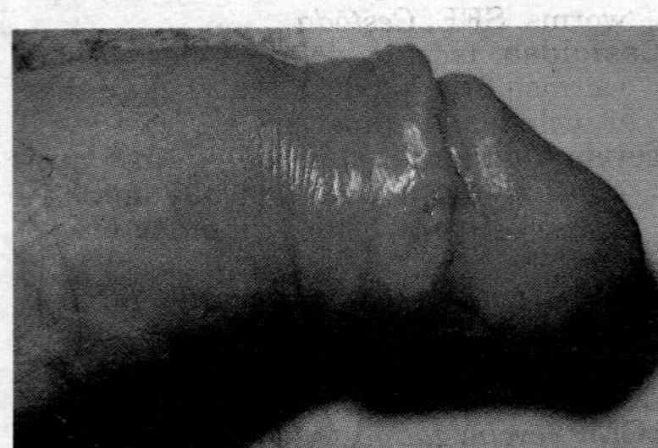

TYPICAL CHANCRE OF PRIMARY SYPHILIS

SYMPTOMS: The ulcer begins as a painless erosion or papule that ulcerates superficially. It generally occurs alone. It has a scooped-out appearance due to level or sloping edges that are adherent, and a shining red or raw floor. The ulcer heals without leaving a scar. It may appear at almost any site including the mouth, penis, urethra, hand, toe, eyelid, conjunctiva, vagina, or cervix. Discovery of these organisms in the chancre is the basis for the positive dark-field test for syphilis. SYN: *hard c.; hunterian c.; true c.*

CAUTION: During the chancre stage, syphilis is highly contagious. The chancre contains many spirochetes.

hard c. Chancre.
hunterian c. Chancre.
simple c. Chancroid.
soft c. Chancroid.
true c. Chancre.

chancroid (shăng′kroyd) [″ + Gr. *eidos,* form, shape] A sexually transmitted infection, caused by the *Haemophilus ducreyi* (a gram-negative bacillus). Its hallmark is the appearance on the genitals of one or more painful ulcers. The incubation period is typically 2 to 5 days, although longer incubations have been reported. The genital chancre of syphilis is clinically distinguished from that of chancroid in that the syphilitic ulcer is painless. Cultures on chocolate agar are used to confirm the diagnosis. Ceftriaxone and macrolide antibiotics (such as erythromycin or azithromycin) treat the infection. SEE: illus.

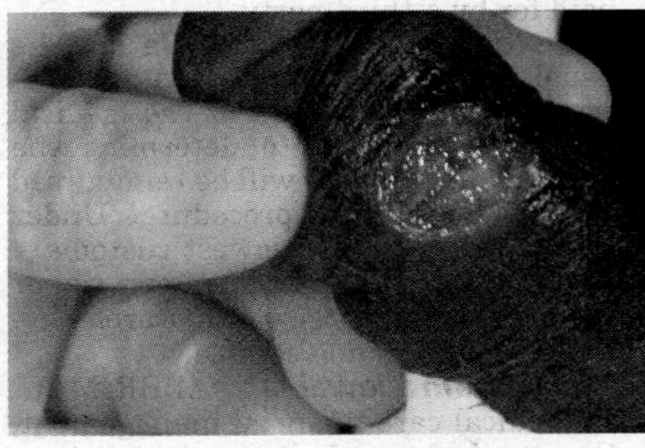

CHANCROID

SYMPTOMS: A chancroid begins with multiple pustules or ulcers having abrupt edges, a rough floor, yellow exudate, and purulent secretion. It is sensitive and inflamed. It heals rapidly, leaving a scar. Chancroids may affect the penis, urethra, vulva, or anus. Multiple lesions may develop by autoinoculation. Types include transient, phagedenic, giant, and serpiginous.

change, fatty Any abnormal accumulation of fat within parenchymal cells. It may occur in the heart or other organs. When seen in the liver, it often is a result of excessive and prolonged alcohol intake or obesity.

change of life Menopause.

channel [L. *canalis,* a waterpipe] **1.** A conduit, groove, or passageway through which various materials may flow. **2.** In cell biology, a passageway in the cell membrane through which materials may pass.

gated c. An ion channel in a cell membrane that opens or closes in response to a stimulus such as a neurotransmitter or to a change in pressure, voltage, or light.

ion c. A protein that spans the lipid bilayer of the cell membrane and regulates the movement of charged particles (e.g., electrolytes) into and out of cells.

leakage c. An ion channel in a cell membrane that is always open, making the membrane permeable to ions.

nongated c. Leakage c.

receptor-operated c. A conduit in a cell membrane through which ions pass when a neurotransmitter binds to its receptor site.

voltage c. A glycosylated protein in a cell membrane through which ions pass when the electrical potential of the membrane shifts.

voltage-gated c. A gated ion channel that opens in response to a change in the membrane potential of a cell membrane; such channels give muscle fibers and neurons their ability to generate and propagate impulses.

voltage-regulated c. Voltage-gated c.

chaperone (shăp-ĕr-ōn′) **1.** An individual who accompanies a health care provider during the examination of a disrobed patient to ensure that sexual boundary violations do not occur. **2.** Molecular chaperone.

molecular c. A protein that shapes other protein molecules so they can work optimally as receptors or can be secreted or cleared from cells.

chapped (chăpt) [ME. *chappen*] Inflamed, roughened, fissured, as from exposure to cold.

character (kăr′ăk-tĕr) **1.** A person's pattern of thought and action, esp. regarding moral choices. Character differs from personality, although in psychiatry the terms are often used interchangeably. **2.** The feature of an organism or individual that results from the expression of genetic information inherited from the parents.

characteristic (kăr″ăk-tĕr-ĭs′tĭk) **1.** A trait or character that is typical of an organism or individual. **2.** In logarithmic expressions, the number to the left of the decimal point, as distinguished from the mantissa, which is the number to the right of the decimal point.

acquired c. A trait or quality that was not inherited but is the result of environmental influence.

anal c. A term sometimes used to describe an individual with obsessive-compulsive personality disorder.

dominant c. In genetics, a trait that is expressed although it is present in only one gene.

primary sex c. An inherited trait directly concerned with the reproductive tract.

recessive c. In genetics, a trait that is not expressed unless it is present in the genes received from both parents.

secondary sex c. A gender-related physical attribute that normally develops under the influence of sex hormones at puberty. Voice quality, facial hair, and body fat distribution are examples.

sex-conditioned c. A genetic trait carried by both sexes but expressed or inhibited by the sex of the individual.

sex-limited c. A trait present in only one sex even though the gene responsible is present in both sexes.

sex-linked c. A trait for which the gene is present on one of the sex chromosomes.

characterize To mark, identify, or describe the attributes of something. This helps to distinguish an individual or material from other examples of similar individuals or materials.

charcoal (chăr'kōl) [ME. *charcole*] A black granular mass or fine powder prepared from soft charred wood.

ACTION/USES: In treating persons who have ingested organic poisons, activated charcoal is given orally as a suspension in water, using 8 ml of diluent per gram of charcoal. This may be given to infants by using a nippled bottle. The dose is 1 to 2 g/kg of body weight. Superactivated charcoal is two to three times more effective than activated charcoal. Charcoal should be administered as soon as possible after intake of the toxin. It is contraindicated in patients who have ingested corrosive chemicals. Ionized chemicals such as acids, alkalis, and salts of cyanide, iron, and lithium are not well absorbed by charcoal.

superactivated c. A type of charcoal used in treating poisoning. It is several more times as effective as activated charcoal. Trade name is SuperChar.

Charcot's joint (shăr-kōz') [Jean M. Charcot, Fr. neurologist, 1825–1893] A type of diseased joint, marked by hypermobility, associated with tabes dorsalis, syringomyelia, or other conditions involving spinal cord disease or injury. Bone decalcification occurs on the joint surfaces, accompanied by bony overgrowth about the margins. Pain is usually absent, although there are exceptions. Deformity and instability of the joint are characteristic.

Charcot-Bouchard aneurysm [Charcot; Charles Jacques Bouchard, Fr. physician, 1837–1886] A microaneurysm in a small artery of the brain thought, in the past, to be a cause of intracranial hemorrhage.

Charcot-Leyden crystal (shăr-kō'lī'dĕn) [Charcot; Ernest V. von Leyden, Ger. physician, 1832–1910] A type of colorless, hexagonal, double-pointed, often needle-like crystal found in the sputum in asthma and bronchial bronchitis or in the feces in ulceration of the intestine, esp. amebiasis.

Charcot-Marie-Tooth disease [Charcot; Pierre Marie, Fr. neurologist, 1853–1940; Howard Henry Tooth, Brit. physician, 1856–1925] A form of progressive neural atrophy of muscles supplied by the peroneal nerves. There are numerous variants of the disease: some are transmitted on the X chromosome and some are autosomal recessive. In all versions, there is a defect in the myelination of peripheral nerves, causing motor deficits (such as footdrop) and loss of sensation. SYN: *peroneal muscular atrophy*.

Charcot's triad **1.** The combination of nystagmus, intention tremor, and scanning speech. It is frequently associated with multiple sclerosis. **2.** The combination of right upper quadrant abdominal pain, fever, and jaundice—a marker of cholangitis.

charge **1.** In electricity, the amount of electrical force present. **2.** To add electrical energy to a battery. **3.** The cost to the patient and/or the third-party payer for a medical service or hospitalization.

covered c. Medical services that are paid for by a third-party.

customary and reasonable c. The usual cost of a specific service to a patient. The term is used in the medical insurance industry to determine the amount the provider will be reimbursed for the service or procedure. Under Medicare, this is the lowest customary charge by a physician for a service, or the prevailing charge of other area physicians for the same service.

maximum allowable c. ABBR: MAC. In medical care financial management, the maximum reimbursement rate a health plan will allow for the cost of services such as prescribed medicines or professional fees.

charlatan (shăr'lă-tăn) [It. *ciarlatano*] A pretender to special knowledge or ability, as in medicine. SYN: *quack*.

charlatanry (shăr'lă-tăn-rē) Undue pretension to knowledge or skill that is not possessed.

Charles' law (shărl) [Jacques A. C. Charles, Fr. physicist, 1746–1823] At constant pressure, a given amount of gas expands its volume in direct proportion to the absolute temperature. SYN: *Gay-Lussac's law*. SEE: *Boyle's law*.

charleyhorse A colloquial term for pain and tenderness in the fibromuscular tissue of the thighs, usually caused by muscle strain or tear. The condition is marked by sudden onset and aggravation on movement. Relief can be obtained from rest, local applications of cold, gentle massage, and nonsteroidal anti-inflammatory drugs.

chart [L. *charta,* paper] **1.** A form or sheet of paper used to record the course of a patient's illness. It includes records of temperature, pulse, respiratory rate, blood pressure, urinary and fecal output, and doctors' and nurses' notes. **2.** To record on a graph the sequence of events such as vital signs. SEE: *charting*. **3.** The complete clinical record of a

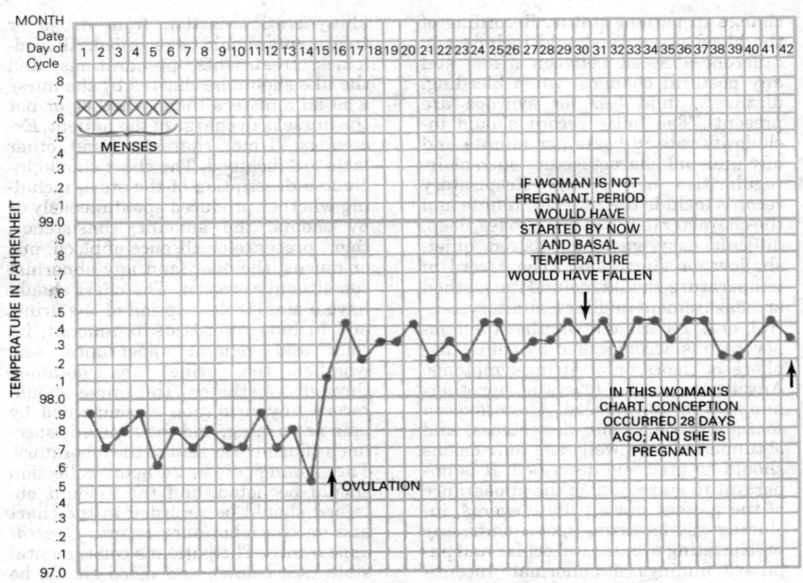

BASAL BODY TEMPERATURE CHART

patient, including physical and psychosocial state of health as well as results of diagnostic tests. Plans for meeting the needs of the patient are also included. SEE: *problem-oriented medical record*. **4.** To record the clinical, radiographic, and forensic findings of the teeth and surrounding tissues.

basal temperature c. A daily chart of temperature (usually taken rectally) obtained upon awakening. Some women are able to predict the time of ovulation by carefully analyzing the character and rhythm of the temperature chart. This information and other data can be used to establish that the woman is ovulating. Use of this method to control conception by predicting time of ovulation is unreliable in most cases. SEE: illus.; *conception; luteal phase defect*.

dental c. A diagram of the teeth on which clinical and radiographic findings can be recorded. These often include existing restorations, decayed surfaces, missing teeth, and periodontal conditions.

charta (kăr′tă) [L.] A preparation intended principally for external application, made either by saturating paper with medicinal substances or by applying the latter to the surface of the paper by adding adhesive liquid.

charting The process of making a tabulated record of a patient's progress and treatment during an illness, outpatient procedure, office visit, or hospitalization. The physician and other health care providers need detailed information about the patient that the nurse or other members of the health care team may contribute through observation and contact. These notes and flow sheet entries contain details used in planning, implementing, and evaluating patient care. SEE: *nursing process; problem-oriented medical record*.

CAUTION: Verbal reports are not sufficient; they may be misunderstood or forgotten.

Written documentation is considered legal evidence. It must be recorded promptly and be dated and timed, and be clear, concise, and legible. Mistakes should be corrected by noting the mistaken entry and correction, or by placing a single line through the mistaken entry and writing the correction immediately after. If an entry is made late, it should follow the most recent entry in the chart and include the date and time when it was made. Slang should not be used. Since charting procedures may differ among health care institutions, it is crucial to learn to use the system specified in one's own facility.

The following subheadings exemplify those aspects of patient care found in complete nursing records: *Vital signs*: including blood pressure, pulse, respiration, and temperature. They are recorded on admission and before the patient goes for procedures, to the operating room, or with any significant change in patient status. Recording of the blood pressure should include any differences noted between arms, and any postural changes (when bleeding, dizziness, fluid loss, or syncope are present). The pulse record should include its rate in beats per minute and any unusual characteristics such as irregularities of rhythm. Respiratory records include the rate per minute and the character (e.g. Cheyne-Stokes, deep, difficult, easy, gasping, labored, quiet, shallow, or stertorous). The record of temperature should include the method of measurement (axillary, auditory, central, oral, rectal) and whether the temperature is accompanied by chills, diaphoresis, rigors, or localizing symptoms. Any treatment for fevers of hypothermia should be recorded. *Alterations in consciousness*: Coma, drowsiness, and obtundation as well as convulsions should be precisely described. It is important to make note of the appearance of the patient during these events, including any localizing movements, any precipitating events, and ocular and pupillary findings if abnormal. Incontinence of bowel or bladder, and unintentional injury to self during changes in consciousness should be noted, as well as any delay in recovery to normal awareness. *Diet*: The percentage of intake for each meal and type of meals consumed are recorded. If a calorie count is needed, the type and amount of each food and liquid taken are recorded. If the patient is being monitored for intake and output, the amount of each liquid consumed is documented. The following should be included in dietary records: amount of liquids taken; hours of giving; type of diet (full, light, soft, liquid, special); and appetite. The description of appetite may include remarks about special likes or dislikes, difficulties with ingestion, or alterations in digestion. *Discharge or death*: The date and hour of discharge or death and the name of the person who ordered the discharge or pronounced the death should be given. *Dressings*: This chart should include the changes of dressings on wounds and the amount and character of drainage (including the phrase "Specimen Saved," if this was done). In addition, the hour, the person who changed the dressing, the removal of stitches or drains, and the patient's reaction to the dressing change should be recorded. *Drugs*: The name of each medicine, the dosage, the route of administration, the time of administration, and the frequency should be confined to the prescribed column of the medical record. When preparations are dispensed in liquid form, the actual dose given should be recorded rather than the amount of solution. Any unfavorable, unusual, or idiosyncratic reaction from drugs or treatments should be recorded. All medicines, treatments, preparations, and the like should be charted by the nurse who administers them whether or not the nurse is in charge of the patient. *Excretions*: Time, character, and other facts are included. The chart should include a description of the stool, including whether produced spontaneously or by enema, the amount, consistency, color, presence or absence of blood, pus or mucus, the odor, and any abnormal constituents present. The chart should have a similar description of the urine, and include records of its amount, its color and general appearance, and whether the urine was obtained through a catheter. The nurse should record any urination accompanied by pain or burning, and the time any specimen of urine was sent to the laboratory. The timing of a 24-hour collection should be noted, and the amount obtained should be recorded in the chart and on the laboratory record. *General appearance*: The patient's color, mental state (see below), and mood should be documented. *Hemorrhages and discharges*: These should be described, and any unusual specimens saved for examination. *Infant feeding*: Breast versus bottle feeding are noted, and any maternal education is given. Any formula given should be recorded the first time; afterward, the amount given suffices. If infants regurgitate, the approximate amount is recorded. *Laboratory*: The date and time, type of specimen, ordering physician, method of transport, and courier are all noted. SEE: *chain of custody*. *Mental state*: The record should document the patient's alertness and awareness, cooperativeness, delirium or delusion, depression, hallucinosis, psychotic symptoms, and teaching and learning ability. Reactions to visitors and mood change after visitors depart should be reported. This is esp. important in psychiatric patients. *Nausea*: The chart should record whether nausea was accompanied by vomiting, and whether it followed certain foods, drugs, interventions, or treatments. *Nerves*: All symptoms of nervousness or excitability should be noted. *Nursing care*: The nurse should chart and date all activities, ambulation, assessments, independent interventions, medications given, and special treatments. *Pain*: The record should include the character (e.g., sharp, dull, burning, grinding, throbbing), onset, location, duration, and any factors that exacerbate the pain or facilitate its remission. *Personal care*: Baths, personal hygiene, and the patient's reactions to these should be recorded. For women, this includes menstruation and the type of menstrual protection used. *Physician*: The physician's visit is recorded as are any verbal or telephone orders and the time they are expressed or written, and carried out. *Physical therapy*: The hour of going for treatment, the hour of return, and the condition of the patient should be charted. *Sleep*: Hours of sleep during both day and night are charted. If an accurate estimate is impossible, an approximation is made and noted as such. Abnormalities of sleep, such as apneic periods, bruxism, nightmares, and sleepwalking are recorded. *Surgery*: Documentation includes the procedure, preparation (including medications), the time, the admission and discharge from the postanesthesia care unit (PACU) or critical care unit; the transfer to the patient's room, the condition, lines, monitors, tubes, and assessment on return to the room; and the results of assessments during the first few hours after surgery. PACU and critical care nurses record treatment and condition while the patient is under their care. *Symptoms*: An accurate description of all symptoms should be given. The remarks should include both subjective and objective findings. *Time*: Everything relating to the patient's progress should be charted as it occurs. *Treatments*: The hour of treatment, the nature of the treatment, the provider of the treatment, and the patient's reaction are recorded. *Radiographic studies*: The type of study, its hour of initiation, the location of the study, the transportation involved, the practitioners, and the patient's subsequent condition are all recorded. *Visits of family or clergy*: The hour, the name of the visitor, and the rite performed are charted, as well as the patient's response. *Miscellaneous*: Any sudden or marked change in the patient's condition is charted, as well as any subsequent notification of the patient's relatives, physician, or clergy.

dental c. Recording on a chart the clinical findings in the mouth. Each tooth is examined and the gingival sulcus probed. Restorations and missing teeth are noted, as are periodontal pocket depth and the conditions of all soft tissues.

chartula (kăr'tū-lă) [L., small piece of paper] A paper folded to form a receptacle containing a dose of medicine.

chasma (kăz'mă) [Gr., a cleft] An opening, gap, or wide cleft.

chaude-pisse (shōd-pēs') [Fr.] A burning sensation during urination, esp. in acute gonorrhea.

chaulmoogra oil (chŏl-moo'gră, chŏl-mŏ'gră) [Bengali *caulmugra*] A vegetable oil used to treat leprosy and some dermatoses. Although generally replaced by sulfones in treatment of leprosy, chaulmoogra oil is still used in endemic areas because of its availability and low cost. Also spelled *chaulmugra* or *chaulmaugra*.

Chaussier's areola (shō-sē-āz') [François Chaussier, Fr. physician, 1746–1828] Indurated tissue around the lesion of a malignant pustule.

CHB *complete heart block*.

Ch.B. *Bachelor of Surgery;* used mostly in the United Kingdom.

CHD *congenital hip dislocation; congenital heart disease; coronary heart disease.*

check [O.Fr. *eschec*] **1.** To slow down or arrest the course of a condition. **2.** To verify.

check bite A sheet of hard wax used to make an impression of teeth to check articulation.

check-up General term for a visit to a health care provider for a history and physical examination.

Chédiak-Higashi syndrome (shē'dē-ăk-hē-gă'shē) [M. Chédiak and O. Higashi, contemporary French and Japanese physicians, respectively] A lethal metabolic disorder, inherited as an autosomal recessive trait, in which neutrophils contain peroxidase-positive inclusion bodies. Partial albinism, photophobia, and pale optic fundi are clinical features. Children usually die by 5 to 10 years of age of a lymphoma-like disease.

cheek [AS. *ceace*] **1.** The side of the face forming the lateral wall of the mouth below the eye. SYN: *bucca*. **2.** The buttock.

cheekbone The malar bone. SEE: *zygomatic bone*.

cheek retractor A device that encloses the cheek at the angle of the mouth for proper exposure of the operating field.

cheil- SEE: *cheilo-*.

cheilectomy (kī-lĕk'tō-mē) [Gr. *cheilos,* lip, + *ektome,* excision] **1.** Surgical removal of abnormal bone around a joint to facilitate joint mobility. **2.** Surgical removal of a lip.

cheilectropion (kī''lĕk-trō'pē-ŏn) [" + *ektrope,* a turning aside] Eversion of the lip.

cheilitis (kī-lī'tĭs) [" + *itis,* inflammation] Inflammation of the lip.

angular c. An inflammation of the corners of the mouth. The cause is bacterial infection of the skin. Erythema and painful fissures are present. This condition usually occurs in edentulous patients. SYN: *perlèche*.

solar c. Skin changes including papules and plaques that occur on sun-exposed areas of the lips.

c. venenata Dermatitis of the lips resulting from chemical irritants in lipsticks, lip cream, and various other materials.

cheilo-, cheil- Combining form meaning *lip*. SEE: *chilo-*.

cheilognathopalatoschisis (kī''lō-nă''thō-păl-ă-tŏs′kĭ-sĭs) [″ + *gnathos,* jaw, + L. *palatum,* palate, + Gr. *schisis,* a splitting] A developmental anomaly in which there is a cleft in the hard and soft palates, upper jaw, and lip.

cheilophagia (kī″lō-fā′jē-ă) [″ + *phagein,* to eat] The habit of biting one's own lip.

cheiloplasty (kī′lō-plăs″tē) [″ + *plassein,* to form] Plastic surgery on the lips.

cheilorrhaphy (kī-lor′ă-fē) [″ + *rhaphe,* seam, ridge] Surgical repair of a cleft lip.

cheiloschisis (kī-lŏs′kĭ-sĭs) [″ + *schisis,* a splitting] Cleft lip.

cheilosis (kī-lō′sĭs) [″ + *osis,* condition] A morbid condition in which the lips become reddened and develop fissures at the angles. It is seen frequently in vitamin B complex deficiencies, esp. riboflavin.

cheilostomatoplasty (kī″lō-stō-măt′ō-plăs″tē) [″ + *stoma,* mouth, + *plassein,* to form] Plastic surgery and restoration of the mouth.

cheilotomy, chilotomy (kī-lŏt′ō-mē) [″ + *tome,* incision] Excision of part of the lip.

cheirognostic, chirognostic (kī″rŏg-nŏs′tĭk) [Gr. *cheir,* hand, + *gnostikos,* knowing] Able to distinguish the left from the right side of the body; able to perceive which side of the body is being stimulated.

cheirology (kī-rŏl′ō-jē) [″ + *logos,* word, reason] Representing words by signs made with the fingers.

cheirospasm (kī′rō-spăsm) [″ + Gr. *spasmos,* a convulsion] Writer's cramp; a spasm of the muscles of the hand.

chelate (kē′lāt) [Gr. *chele,* claw] **1.** In chemistry, to grasp a metallic ion in a ring-shaped molecule. **2.** In toxicology, to use a compound to enclose or sequester a toxic substance, rendering it inactive or less injurious. SEE: *poisoning; Poisons and Poisoning Appendix.*

chelation (kē-lā′shŭn) [Gr. *chele,* claw] The combining of metallic ions with certain heterocyclic ring structures so that the ion is held by chemical bonds from each participating ring. Clinically, this technique is used in poisonings brought on by exposure to or ingestion of metals such as arsenic, iron, lead, and mercury. SEE: *poisoning; Poisons and Poisoning Appendix.*

cheloid (kē′loyd) [Gr. *kele,* tumor, swelling, + *eidos,* form, shape] Keloid.

chemabrasion (kēm-ă-brā′shŭn) The use of a chemical to destroy superficial layers of skin. This technique may be used to treat scars, tattoos, or abnormal pigmentation. SYN: *chemexfoliation.*

chemexfoliation (kēm′ĕks-fō′lē-ā″shŭn) Chemabrasion.

CHEMFET *chemically sensitive field effect transistor.*

chemical [Gr. *chemeia,* chemistry] Pert. to chemistry.

Chemical Abstract Service ABBR: CAS. A branch of the American Chemical Society that maintains a registry of chemicals, active ingredients used in drugs, and food additives. Each chemical is assigned a permanent CAS number through which current data can be traced.

chemical barriers **1.** The chemical characteristics of certain areas of the body that oppose colonization by microorganisms. Examples are the acidic properties of the stomach mucosa and urinary bladder, which effectively prevent invasion by pathogenic microorganisms. **2.** A contraceptive cream, foam, jelly, or suppository that contains chemical spermicides.

chemical change A process in which molecular bonds break or form between electron-sharing atoms or molecules to create substances with new properties or characteristics. For example, oxygen and hydrogen combine to form water. Sodium (a metal) and chlorine (a gas) combine to form sodium chloride, or common salt. Glucose ($C_6H_{10}O_5$) is metabolized to carbon dioxide (CO_2) and water (H_2O). Oxygen combines with hemoglobin to form oxyhemoglobin when the hemoglobin in the blood comes into contact with the oxygen in the air contained in the alveoli of the lungs. A chemical change is also known as a chemical reaction.

chemical compound **1.** A substance consisting of two or more chemical elements, in specific proportions and in chemical combination, for which a chemical formula can be written. Examples include water (H_2O) and salt (NaCl). **2.** A substance that can be separated chemically into simpler substances.

chemical disaster The accidental release of large amounts of toxins into the environment. The effects suffered by people in the area are determined by the toxicity of the chemical, its speed in spreading, its composition (liquid, solid, or gaseous), and the spill site, esp. its proximity to a water supply or buildings. The major effect may be due to the chemical itself or to a resulting fire or explosion. The catastrophic release of chemicals may overwhelm, at least temporarily, local or regional health care resources. SEE: *chemical warfare.*

chemical element SEE: *element.*

chemically sensitive field effect transistor ABBR: CHEMFET. A specialized chemical sensor found in some clinical laboratory instruments.

chemical reflex Chemoreflex.

chemical warfare The tactics and technique of conducting warfare by using toxic chemical agents. The chemicals include nerve gases; agents that cause temporary blindness, paralysis, hallucinations, or deafness; eye and lung irritants; blistering agents, including mustard gas; defoliants; and herbicides. SEE: *biological warfare*.

chemiluminescence, chemoluminescence (kĕm″ĭ-loo″mĭ-nĕs′ĕns, kĕm″ō-loo″mĭ-nĕs′ĕns) Cold light or light resulting from a chemical reaction and without heat production. Certain bacteria, fungi, and fireflies produce this type of light. SEE: *luciferase*.

chemist (kĕm′ĭst) Someone who is trained in chemistry.

chemistry [Gr. *chemeia,* chemistry] The science dealing with the molecular and atomic structure of matter and the composition of substances—their formation, decomposition, and various transformations.

analytical c. Chemistry concerned with the detection of chemical substances (qualitative analysis) or the determination of the amounts of substances (quantitative analysis) in a compound.

biological c. Biochemistry.

general c. The study of the entire field of chemistry with emphasis on fundamental concepts or laws.

inorganic c. The chemistry of compounds not containing carbon.

nuclear c. Radiochemistry; the study of changes that take place within the nucleus of an atom, esp. when the nucleus is bombarded by electrons, neutrons, or other subatomic particles.

organic c. The branch of chemistry dealing with substances that contain carbon compounds.

pathological c. The study of chemical changes induced by disease processes (e.g., changes in the chemistry of organs and tissues, blood, secretions, or excretions).

pharmaceutical c. The chemistry of medicines, their composition, synthesis, analysis, storage, and actions.

physical c. Theoretical chemistry; the chemistry concerned with fundamental laws underlying chemical changes and the mathematical expression of these laws.

physiological c. The study of the chemistry of living matter and the changes occurring in the metabolic activities of plants and animals.

chemocautery (kĕm″ō-kaw′tĕr-ē) [Gr. *chemeia,* chemistry, + *kauterion,* branding iron] Cauterization by chemical agents.

chemoceptor (kĕm′ō-sĕp-tĕr) Chemoreceptor.

chemocoagulation (kē″mō-kō-ăg″ū-lā′shŭn) [″ + L. *coaglutio,* coagulation] Coagulation caused by chemical agents.

chemodectoma (kē″mō-dĕk-tō′mă) [″ + *dektikos,* receptive, + *oma,* tumor] A tumor of the chemoreceptor system. SEE: *paraganglioma*.

chemokine Any cytokine that causes chemotaxis, attracting neutrophils, monocytes, and T lymphocytes to assist in destroying an invading microorganism. SEE: *cytokine; inflammation*.

chemokinesis The accelerated random locomotion of cells, usually in response to chemical stimuli.

chemoluminescence Chemiluminescence.

chemolysis (kē-mŏl′ĭ-sĭs) [″ + *lysis,* dissolution] Destruction by chemical action.

chemonucleolysis (kēm″ō-nū-klē-ŏl′ĭ-sĭs) A method of dissolving a herniated nucleus pulposus, by injecting the enzyme chymopapain into it. This procedure is controversial and is contraindicated for patients with a herniated lumbar disk in which the nucleus pulposus protrudes through the annulus.

chemopallidectomy (kē″mō-păl″ĭ-dĕk′tō-mē) [″ + L. *pallidum,* globus pallidus, + Gr. *ektome,* excision] Destruction of a portion of the globus pallidus of the brain with drugs or chemicals.

chemoprophylaxis (kē″mō-prō″fĭ-lăk′sĭs) The use of a drug or chemical to prevent a disease (e.g., the taking of an appropriate medicine to prevent malaria).

chemopsychiatry (kē″mō-sī-kī′ă-trē) The use of drugs in treating psychiatric illnesses.

chemoreceptor (kē″mō-rē-sĕp′tor) [″ + L. *recipere,* to receive] A sense organ or sensory nerve ending (as in a taste bud) that is stimulated by and reacts to certain chemical stimuli and that is located outside the central nervous system. Chemoreceptors are found in the large arteries of the thorax and neck (carotid and aortic bodies), the taste buds, and the olfactory cells of the nose. SYN: *chemoceptor*. SEE: *carotid body; taste bud*.

chemoreflex (kē″mō-rē′flĕks) [″ + L. *reflectere,* to bend back] Any involuntary response initiated by a chemical stimulus. SYN: *chemical reflex*.

chemoresistance (kē″mō-rē-zĭs′tăns) The resistance of a cell or microorganism to the expected actions of drugs or chemicals.

chemosensitive (kē″mō-sĕn′sĭ-tĭv) Reacting to the action of a chemical or a change in chemical composition.

chemosensory (kē″mō-sĕn′sō-rē) Pert. to the sensory detection of a chemical, esp. by odor.

chemoserotherapy (kē″mō-sē″rō-thĕr′ă-pē) The combined use of a drug and serum in treating disease.

chemosis (kē-mō′sĭs) [Gr. *cheme,* cockleshell, + *osis,* condition] Edema of the conjunctiva around the cornea. **chemotic** (-mŏt′ĭk), *adj.*

chemosterilant (kē″mō-stĕr′ĭ-lănt) **1.** A chemical that kills microorganisms. **2.** A chemical that causes sterility, usually of the male, in organisms such as insects.

chemosurgery Destruction of tissue by the use of chemical compounds.

chemosynthesis (kē″mō-sĭn′thĕ-sĭs) The formation of a chemical compound from other chemicals or agents. In biological systems, this involves metabolism.

chemotactic (kē″mō-tăk′tĭk) Pert. to chemotaxis.

chemotaxin A substance released by bacteria, injured tissue, and white blood cells that stimulates the movement of neutrophils and other white blood cells to the injured area. Complement factors 3a (C3a) and 5a (C5a), cytokines, leukotrienes, prostaglandins, and fragments of fibrin and collagen are common chemotaxins. SEE: *inflammation.*

chemotaxis (kē″mō-tăk′sĭs) [Gr. *chemeia,* chemistry, + *taxis,* arrangement] The movement of additional white blood cells to an area of inflammation in response to the release of chemical mediators by neutrophils, monocytes, and injured tissue. SYN: *chemotropism.*

chemothalamectomy (kē″mō-thăl-ă-mĕk′tō-mē) Chemical destruction of a part of the thalamus.

chemotherapy (kē″mō-thĕr′ă-pē) [″ + *therapeia,* treatment] Drug therapy used, for example, to treat infections, cancers, and other diseases and conditions. SEE: *Nursing Diagnoses Appendix.*

CAUTION: Chemotherapeutic agents used to treat cancer are poisons and pose risks to those who handle them, primarily pharmacists and nurses. Usually, only oncology practitioners specifically trained in chemotherapy administration should perform this task. The most important factor in reducing exposure is the use of proper protection when preparing and administering these agents. After washing hands, the health care provider dons appropriate protective apparel, including surgical powder-free or hypoallergenic latex-free chemotherapy gloves, a disposable impermeable gown, and goggles or a mask with face and eye shield. He or she then gathers equipment to administer the drugs, including normal saline or D5W solution (the same solution should be used for both priming and mixing), IV tubing, the drugs, alcohol swabs, sterile gauze, all equipment required to start an IV line, and plastic-backed absorbent pads. Eating, drinking, smoking, chewing gum, applying cosmetics, and storing food are prohibited in areas where chemotherapeutic drugs are prepared or administered. The drugs should be administered in a calm environment, and all chemotherapy waste and equipment must be discarded in designated waste containers. Health care providers must follow OSHA guidelines when cleaning up drug spills. Spill kits should be available and used, and spill areas cleaned three times using soap and water (skin) or detergent followed by clean water (other surfaces). Gloves also should be worn when handling the patient's excreta. Exposure poses additional risks to female reproductive health, including ectopic pregnancies, spontaneous abortions, and fetal abnormalities.

PATIENT CARE: Antineoplastic agents kill cancer cells, but also kill or injure normal cells and may consequently compromise patient comfort and safety. Bone marrow suppression is a common and potentially serious adverse reaction. Chemotherapy can decrease the numbers of white blood cells, red blood cells, and platelets in the peripheral bloodstream. Leukopenia increases the patient's risk for infection, especially if the granulocyte count falls below 1,000/mm^3. The patient is given information about personal hygiene and potential sites for infection and is taught to recognize signs and symptoms, such as fever, cough, sore throat, or a burning sensation when urinating. The patient is cautioned to avoid crowds and people with colds or flu. Filgrastim (Neupogen) is administered as prescribed to stimulate proliferation and differentiation of hematopoietic cells, specifically neutrophils. Thrombocytopenia (abnormally low platelet count) increases a patient's risk for bleeding when the platelet count falls below 50,000/mm^3; the risk is highest when the platelet count falls below 20,000/mm^3. The patient is assessed and taught to observe for bleeding gums, increased bruising or petechiae, hypermenorrhea, tarry stools, hematuria, and coffee-ground emesis. He or she is advised to avoid cuts and bruises and to use a soft toothbrush and an electric razor. The patient must report sudden headaches, which could indicate intracranial bleeding. He or she should use a stool softener, as prescribed, to avoid colonic irritation and bleeding. Intramuscular injections are avoided to prevent bleeding. Anemia develops slowly over the course of treatment, so the patient's hemoglobin, hematocrit, and red blood cell counts are monitored. Dehydration can lead to a false-normal hematocrit, which decreases when the patient is rehydrated. The patient is assessed for and taught to report any dizziness, fatigue, pallor, or shortness of breath on minimal exertion. He or she must rest more frequently, increase dietary intake of iron-rich foods, and take a multivitamin with iron, as prescribed. Growth factors or colony-stimulating factors are administered as prescribed, and whole blood or packed cells are transfused as prescribed for a symptomatic patient.

Antineoplastics attack cancer cells because they divide rapidly. For the same reason, they also destroy rapidly dividing normal cells. While epithelial damage can affect any mucous membrane, the oral mucosa is the most common site of destruction. Stomatitis is a temporary but disabling phenomenon that may interfere with eating and drinking. It can range from mild and barely noticeable to severe and debilitating malnutrition. Preventive mouth care is initiated and taught to the patient to provide comfort and decrease the severity of mouth pain. Therapeutic mouth care is also provided, including topical antibiotics, if prescribed. The patient can experience nausea and vomiting from gastric mucosal irritation (oral chemotherapy drugs), chemical irritation of the central nervous system (parenteral chemotherapy), or psychogenic factors activated by sensations, suggestions, or anxiety. Chemotherapy-induced nausea and vomiting is of great concern because it can cause fluid and electrolyte imbalance, noncompliance with the treatment regimen, tears at the esophageal-gastric junction leading to massive bleeding (Mallory-Weiss syndrome), wound dehiscence, and pathological fractures. It also reduces quality of life by interfering with the patient's ability and motivation to take an active role in his or her self-care. Such complications are assessed for and prevented as much as possible. Chemical irritation is controlled by administering prescribed combinations of antiemetics that act by different mechanisms, such as serotonin antagonists, prochlorperazine, diphenhydramine, droperidol, and dronabinol. Signs and symptoms of aspiration are monitored, because most antiemetics are sedating. Psychogenic factors can be relieved by using relaxation techniques to minimize feelings of isolation and anxiety prior to and during each treatment. The patient is encouraged to express feelings of anxiety, and to listen to music, engage in relaxation techniques, meditation, or self-hypnosis to help promote feelings of well being and a sense of control.

Hair loss is a distressing adverse reaction to the patient, especially when the patient's body image or self-esteem is closely linked to his or her grooming or appearance. The patient is informed that hair loss usually is gradual, affects both men and women, and may be partial or complete. He or she is reassured if alopecia is reversible after treatment ends.

Chemotherapy extravasation may lead to tissue necrosis, so the patient is taught to immediately report any pain, stinging, burning, swelling, or redness at the injection site. Extravasation must be distinguished from vessel irritation or flare reaction. Vein irritation is felt as aching or tightness along the blood vessel, and the length of the vein may become reddened or darkened, accompanied by swelling. In flare reaction, itching is the major complaint; redness occurs in blotches along the vessel, may look like hives, and subsides within 30 minutes. Blood return from the IV usually can be obtained with both irritation and flare reaction. To help prevent extravasation, peripheral vesicant drugs are administered in small quantities by IV push through the side port of a flowing main IV infusion. If extravasation is suspected, the infusion is stopped and any drug is aspirated. The extremity is elevated, and cold compresses are applied, except for *Vinca* alkaloids, where heat is recommended. Depending on agency protocol, the oncologist is notified, and if a specific antidote for the drug exists, it is administered as prescribed. The main line IV provides direct access to the patient if an undesired reaction occurs; other drugs can be administered quickly to counteract the adverse reaction.

adjuvant c. The giving of cytotoxic drugs to eradicate malignant cells that may remain in the body after surgery or radiation therapy.

combination c. In antineoplastic drug therapy, the use of two or more drugs to treat disease.

consolidation c. Cycles of therapy with cytotoxic drugs after the initial treatment for a cancer. The object is to sustain a remission that has been achieved during induction.

induction c. The initial treatment of advanced cancers or leukemias with high doses of cytotoxic drugs to try to produce a remission.

peritoneal c. Intraperitoneal injection of antineoplastic drugs.

chemotropism (kē-mŏt′rō-pĭzm) [″ + *tropos,* a turning] The growth or movement of an organism in response to a chemical stimulus, such as the movement of bacteria toward nutrients.

CHEMTREC The Chemical Transportation Emergency Center, which provides a 24-hour hotline with product information and emergency advice to rescue personnel at the scene of a hazardous materials incident.

chenodeoxycholic acid A drug given orally to dissolve cholesterol gallstones. SEE: *gallstone.*

cherophobia (kē″rō-fō′bē-ă) [Gr. *chairein,* to rejoice, + *phobos,* fear] Morbid fear of and aversion to gaiety.

cherubism (chĕr′ū-bĭzm) Cherubic appearance of the face of a child due to infiltration of the jaw, esp. the mandible, with masses of vascular fibrous tissue containing giant cells.

chest [AS. *cest,* a box] The thorax, including all the organs (e.g., heart, great vessels, esophagus, trachea, lungs) and tissues (bone, muscle, fat) that lie between the base of the neck and the diaphragm.

PHYSICAL EXAMINATION: *Inspection*: The practitioner inspects the chest to determine the respiratory rate and whether the right and left sides of the chest move symmetrically during breathing. In pneumonia, pleurisy, or rib fracture, for example, the affected side of the chest may have reduced movement as a result of lung consolidation or pain ("splinting" of the chest). Increased movements may be seen in extensive trauma ("flail" chest). The patient in respiratory distress uses accessory muscles of the chest to breathe; retractions of the spaces between the ribs are also seen when patients labor to breathe.

Percussion: The chest wall is tapped with the fingers (sometimes with a reflex hammer) to determine whether it has a normally hollow, or resonant, sound and feel. Dullness perceived during percussion may indicate a pleural effusion or underlying pneumonia. Abnormal tympany may be present in conditions such as emphysema, cavitary lung diseases, or pneumothorax.

Palpation: By pressing or squeezing the soft tissues of the chest, bony instability (fractures), abnormal masses (lipomas or other tumors), edema, or subcutaneous air may be detected.

Auscultation: Chest sounds are assessed using the stethoscope. Abnormal friction sounds may indicate pleurisy, pericarditis, or pulmonary embolism; crackles may be detected in pulmonary edema, pneumonia, or interstitial fibrosis; and wheezes may be heard in reactive airway disease. Intestinal sounds heard in the chest may point to diaphragmatic hernias. Heart sounds are diminished in obesity and pericardial effusion; they are best heard near the xiphoid process in emphysema. Lung sounds may be decreased in patients with chronic obstructive lung diseases, pleural effusion, and other conditions.

emphysematous c. A misnomer for the barrel-shaped appearance of the chest in chronic bronchitis. The thorax is short and round, the anteroposterior diameter is often as long as the transverse diameter, the ribs are horizontal, and the angle formed by divergence of the costal margin from the sternum is obtuse or obliterated.

flail c. A condition of the chest wall due to two or more fractures on each affected rib resulting in a segment of rib that is not attached on either end; the flail segment moves paradoxically in with inspiration and out during expiration.

flat c. A deformity of the chest in which the anteroposterior diameter is short, the thorax long and flat, and the ribs oblique. The scapula is prominent; the spaces above and below the clavicles are depressed. The angle formed by divergence of the costal margins from the sternum is very acute.

funnel c. Pectus excavatum.

pigeon c. A condition in which the sides of the chest are considerably flattened and the sternum is prominent. The sternal ends of the ribs are enlarged or beaded. Often there is a circular constriction of the thorax at the level of the xiphoid cartilage. The condition is often congenital and present in mucopolysaccharidoses.

chest physical therapy, chest physiotherapy ABBR: CPT, Chest P.T. A type of respiratory care usually incorporating postural drainage, cough facilitation, and breathing exercises used for loosening and removing lung secretions. It may include percussion (clapping) and vibration over the affected areas of the lungs, simultaneous with postural drainage to remove secretions. Auscultation of breath sounds is done before and after the procedure. SYN: *pulmonary rehabilitation.*

chest prominences and depressions An unnatural prominence or depression often observed over the lower part of the sternum and generally congenital. The sternal depression has been called "funnel breast" or "shoemaker's breast" (because it may result from pressure of tools). The correct term is pectus excavatum.

A unilateral or local depression may be caused by consolidation, cavity, or pleurisy with fibrous adhesions.

A unilateral or local prominence may be due to pleurisy with effusion; pneumothorax, hydrothorax, or hemothorax; aneurysm or tumor; compensatory emphysema resulting from impairment of the opposite lung; cardiac enlargement (left side); or enlargement of abdominal organs, esp. the liver and spleen.

chest P.T. *chest physical therapy.*

chest regions The anterior, posterior, and lateral chest areas. Anterior divisions (right and left) are the clavicular, infraclavicular, and supraclavicular, the mammary and inframammary, and the upper and lower sternal. Posterior divisions (right and left) are the scapular, infrascapular, interscapular, and suprascapular. Lateral divisions are the axillary and infra-axillary.

chest thump A sharp blow delivered to the precordial area of the chest in an attempt to terminate a lethal cardiac rhythm, such as ventricular fibrillation or ventricular tachycardia.

Cheyne-Stokes respiration (chān′stōks′) [John Cheyne, Scot. physician, 1777–1836; William Stokes, Irish physician, 1804–1878] A breathing pattern marked by a period of apnea lasting 10 to 60 sec, followed by gradually increasing depth and frequency of respirations (hyperventilation). It occurs in dysfunction or depression of the cerebral hemispheres (e.g., in coma), in basal ganglia disease, and occasionally in patients with congestive heart failure. It often indicates a grave prognosis in adults but may be a normal finding in children. SEE: *Cheyne-Stokes respiration* for illus.

CHF *congestive heart failure.*

ch'i, Qi (chē) **1.** In traditional Chinese medicine, the "vital force" or "energy of life." **2.** In molecular biology and biochemistry, a regulatory sequence of base pairs that participate in the repair or recombination of nucleic acid strands.

Chiari's deformity SEE: *Arnold-Chiari deformity.*

Chiari-Frommel syndrome (kē-ăr′ē-frŏm′mĕl) [Hans Chiari, Austrian pathologist, 1851–1916; Richard Julius Ernst Frommel, Ger. gynecologist, 1854–1912] Persistent lactation and amenorrhea following childbirth, caused by continued prolactin secretion and decreased gonadotropin production. A pituitary adenoma may be present.

chiasm, chiasma (kī′ăzm, kī-ăz′mă) [Gr. *khiasma,* cross] A crossing or decussation.

optic c. An X-shaped crossing of the optic nerve fibers in the brain. Past this point, the fibers travel in optic tracts. Fibers that originate in the outer half of the retina end on the same side of the brain; those from the inner half cross over to the opposite, or *contralateral,* side.

chickenpox Varicella.

chiggers (chĭg′ĕrs) The harvest mite; also known as "mower's mite," trombiculid mite, or red bug. During summer months, hikers, outdoor enthusiasts, and field hands may become infested with these nonscabietic mites, which tend to attach to the skin where clothing fits snugly, causing an intensely itchy rash. The skin irritation results from an allergic reaction to the injected saliva of the insect; unlike some other insects, the mites do not feed on human blood. Occasionally chiggers act as vectors for rickettsial diseases, such as scrub typhus. Infestation can be prevented by applying insect repellents to outdoor clothing. SEE: *Tunga.*

TREATMENT: Proprietary preparations are available to kill chiggers. They are applied topically to affected skin. One of these, Kwell, contains hexachlorohexane. Benzyl benzoate ointment and gamma benzene hexachloride are also effective.

chigoe infestation Infestation of a parasite of dogs, pigs, and barefooted humans by the flea *Tunga penetrans.* In humans the usual sites of invasion are the spaces between the toes, where the burrowing female swells and causes a painful open sore.

TREATMENT: The gravid flea is removed with a sterile needle. The site is treated with tincture of iodine, which is toxic to the remaining fleas and eggs.

chi kung (chē-gŏng) Qi gong.

chil- SEE: *chilo-.*

chilblain (chĭl′blān) [AS. *cele,* cold, + *blegen,* to puff] A mild form of cold injury marked by localized redness, burning, and swelling on exposed body parts, esp. in cool, damp climates. The affected skin sometimes blisters or ulcerates. Insufficient blood flow into small blood vessels in the skin may contribute to the formation of chilblains. SYN: *pernio.*

PREVENTION: Patients with a history of chilblains should wear warm, loose-fitting clothing when outdoors in the cold.

child [AS. *cild,* child] Any human between infancy and puberty. SEE: *pediatrics.*

child abuse Emotional, physical, or sexual injury to a child. It may be seen after instances of severe disruption in the process of parental attachment. It may be due to either a positive action or an omission on the part of those responsible for the care of the child. In domestic situations in which a child is abused, it is important to examine other children and infants living in the same home because about 20% will have signs of physical abuse. That examination should be done without delay to attempt to prevent further child abuse in that home. An infant or child must never be allowed to remain in the hostile environment where the abuse occurred; such a situation might be disastrous for the child. SEE: *battered child syndrome; shaken baby syndrome.*

PATIENT CARE: All health care providers, teachers, and others involved with children are responsible for identifying and reporting abusive situations as early as possible. Risks for abuse may be assessed by identifying predisposing parental, child, and environmental characteristics, but these are not by themselves predictors of actual abuse. A detailed history and thorough physical examination should be carried out. Findings should be assessed not only in comparison to known indicators of maltreatment, but also in light of diseases or cultural practices that can simulate abuse. Nurses play an important role in identifying child abuse, since they often are the first health care contacts for child and family (e.g., in the emergency department, physician's office, clinic, or school). They look for a pattern or combination of physical and behavioral signs indicating mistreatment.

Physical neglect may be evidenced by failure to thrive, signs of malnutrition, poor personal hygiene, dental neglect, unclean or inappropriate dress, and frequent injuries from lack of supervision. Behavioral indicators of neglect include dullness and inactivity, excessive passivity or sleepiness, self-stimulating behavior (rocking, finger sucking), and, in the older child, begging or stealing food, frequent school absences, vandalism, shoplifting, or substance abuse.

Emotional abuse and neglect may be suspected, but are difficult to substantiate. Physical indicators include failure to thrive, feeding disorders, enuresis, and sleep disorders. Behavioral indicators include self-stimulating behaviors; lack of social smile and stranger anxiety during infancy; withdrawal; unusual fearfulness; antisocial behavior (destructiveness, cruelty, stealing); being overly compliant, passive, aggressive, or demanding; emotional, language, and intellectual developmental lags; and suicide attempts.

Physical abuse is not always obvious, and may be unusual and perplexing. It requires careful documentation on the part of the health care team in order to protect the child from unnecessary and uncomfortable diagnostic and treatment procedures. Physical indicators include bruises and welts, burns, fractures and dislocations, abrasions and lacerations, and chemical poisonings and illnesses. Behavioral indicators include wariness of physical contact with adults; apparent fear of parents or others in the home; inappropriate affective responses toward the parents or others in the household; clinging behaviors; lying very still while watching the environment; reacting inappropriately to injury; becoming apprehensive when hearing other children cry; being indiscriminately friendly or displaying unexpected affection; developing only superficial relationships; acting out to seek attention; and withdrawal.

When sexual abuse is suspected, a very thorough but gentle and reassuring physical examination must be conducted. Physical indicators may include any injury to the external genitalia, anus, mouth, and throat; torn, stained, or bloody undergarments; pain on urination or recurrent urinary tract infections; pain, swelling, unusual odor, and itching of the genitalia; vaginal or penile discharge, vaginitis, venereal warts, or sexually transmitted diseases; difficulty walking or sitting; or pregnancy in the young adolescent. Behavioral manifestations are numerous, but none are specific. Some indicators include withdrawal and excessive daydreaming; preoccupation with fantasies; poor peer relationships; sudden changes in behavior (anxiety, clinging, weight loss or gain); excessive anger at mother (in incestuous relationships); regressive behavior (thumb-sucking, bed-wetting); sudden onset of fears or phobias (e.g., the dark, men, strangers, particular situations); running away from home; sudden emergence of sexually related problems (public masturbation, age-inappropriate sexual play, promiscuity, overtly seductive behavior); substance abuse; profound personality changes (extreme depression, hostility, aggression, social withdrawal); rapidly declining school performance; and suicide ideation or attempts.

Abuse should be suspected in the presence of physical evidence, including old injuries; conflicting stories about an accident or injury from parents or others; injury blamed on siblings or another party; injury inconsistent with the history given; a history inconsistent with the child's developmental age; a chief complaint that is not associated with physical evidence; inappropriate level of parental concern (absence or an exaggerated response); refusal of parents to sign for needed tests or treatments; excessive delay in seeking treatment; absence of parents for questioning; inappropriate response of the child (little or no response to pain, fear of being touched, excessive or lack of separation anxiety, indiscriminate friendliness to strangers); previous reports of abuse in the family; and/or repeated visits to emergency facilities with injuries (may require checking with other facilities). Often, suspicions may be aroused by a feeling that behaviors are "not right." Examples include parents who have difficulty showing concern or comfort for the child or recognizing his or her physical or emotional feelings; parents who demonstrate anger about the injury, criticize the child, or blame him for the injury; parents who become hostile if questioned about their responsibilities toward the child; and parents who are preoccupied with own needs and how the accident affects them (not the child).

The first priority of care for the abused child is preventing further injury. This usually involves removing the child from the abusive situation by reporting the situation to local authorities. All U.S. states and Canadian provinces have laws for mandatory reporting of such mistreatment. If evidence of abuse is supported, further action is taken. If the child is hospitalized because of injuries, his prescribed treatment regimen is managed. Care consistent with that for a rape victim is provided when sexual abuse is present. All the developmental and other needs of the child are considered and addressed as they would be for any other child-patient. Caregivers act as role-models for parents, helping them to relate positively and constructively to their child and fostering a therapeutic environment. In such an environment, there is no accusation or punishment, only genuine concern and treatment to help parents recognize and change abusive behaviors. Referral to self-help groups, resources for financial aid, improved housing, and child care are important in helping families deal with overwhelming stress.

Education programs in the prenatal period, infancy home visits, and outpatient parent groups provide opportunities for health care providers to give families information about normal growth and development and routine health care. In such cases, families also can share their feelings and concerns, gain support from others, and obtain referrals to appropriate services when needs are identified. Prevention of sexual abuse focuses on teaching children about their bodies, their right to privacy, and their right to say no. Parents and school nurses can discuss such topics with children, using "what if" questions to explore potentially dangerous situations. All need to know that "nice" people can be sexual abusers, and that a change in a child's behavior toward an individual requires investigation. The child always must be reassured that whatever occurred was not his or her fault. Prevention of false accusations also is important, and caregivers play an important role when they carefully document all evidence of abuse, recording exactly what they observed on examination and what behaviors occurred, without interpreting their meaning.

childbearing The act of carrying and being delivered of a child.

delayed c. SEE: *elderly primigravida.*

childbed Historically, the period of parturition during which women remained in bed for labor, delivery, and the traditional 6 weeks' recovery time after childbirth. SYN: *puerperium*. SEE: *childbed fever*.

childbirth The process of giving birth to a child. SYN: *parturition*. SEE: *delivery; labor.*

natural c. The delivery of a fetus without the use of analgesics, sedatives, or anesthesia and less reliance on technology (and more reliance on emotional support during labor and delivery) than may be practical during standard obstetrical care. The woman, and often her partner, go through a training period beginning months before the actual delivery. This training is called psychoprophylactic preparation for childbirth. SEE: *Lamaze technique; psychoprophylactic preparation for childbirth.*

prepared c. Childbirth in which the mother, and often also the father, of the baby has been educated about childbirth, anesthesia, and analgesia during labor. The mother may choose to have natural childbirth or to receive medications or regional anesthesia. SEE: *natural c.*; *Lamaze technique; psychoprophylactic preparation for childbirth.*

child neglect Failure by those responsible for caring for a child to provide for the child's nutritional, emotional, and physical needs.

childproof Designed to be harmless to children; used esp. of medicine containers that children cannot open.

chilectropion Cheilectropion.

chilitis Cheilitis.

chill (chĭl) [AS. *cele,* cold] Involuntary, rapid contraction of muscle groups (shivering) accompanied by the sensation of cold, or the sensation of being cold without shivering. It may be caused by a rising fever associated with an infection, a hypersensitivity reaction to drugs or blood transfusions, exposure to cold temperatures, or a neuroendocrine disturbance in the temperature-regulating centers of the hypothalamus. Severe chills accompanied by violent shaking of the body are called rigors.

chilo-, chil- [Gr. *cheilos,* lip] Combining form meaning *lip.*

Chilomastix mesnili (kī″lō-măs′tĭks mĕs-nĭl′ē) A species of Mastigophora, a protozoon that may cause diarrhea in humans. SEE: illus.

chimera (kī-mē′ră) **1.** A tissue in which two distinct forms of DNA are present. **2.** The conjugation of two different drugs, cells, proteins, or organisms. **3.** A double-egg twin whose blood and blast cells have been mixed in embryo with those of the other twin. Therefore, although each twin originally had a different blood group, each now has a mixed group.

chimpanzee (chĭm-păn′zē) An intelligent ape native to parts of Africa. It is used in experimental medicine because of its similarity to humans.

chin [AS. *cin,* chin] The point of the lower jaw; the region below the lower lip. SYN: *mentum*.

China clay Kaolin.

Chinese restaurant syndrome A group of transient symptoms that some persons report after eating at restaurants that

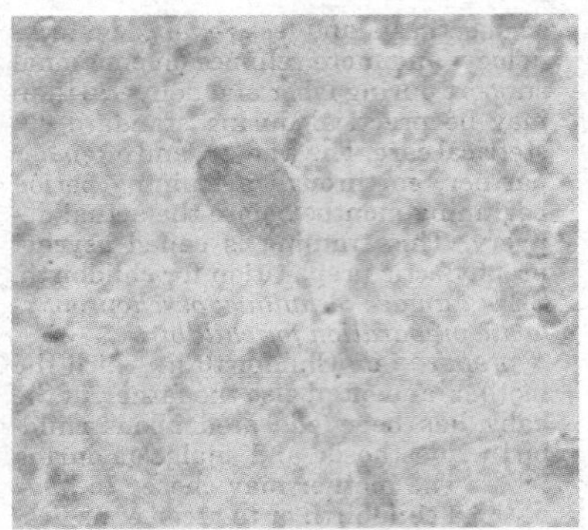

CHILOMASTIX MESNILI

(Orig. mag. ×1000)

add monosodium glutamate (MSG) to some of their recipes. The syndrome may be a valid clinical condition, but it has not been proven that MSG is the cause and its linkage to Chinese ethnicity is pejorative and offensive.

chin jerk Chin reflex.

chin-lift airway technique, head-tilt A method of opening the airway of an unconscious patient by elevating the chin and tilting the head. This provides the maximum opening, esp. in an unconscious patient whose tongue is blocking the airway. SEE: *airway; bag-valve-mask resuscitator; cardiopulmonary resuscitation; Standard and Universal Precautions Appendix.*

CAUTION: This technique is not to be used in patients with potential neck or spinal injuries.

The fingertips are used to bring the patient's chin forward and support the lower jaw, while the neck is extended slightly, by applying gentle pressure to the patient's forehead with the other hand. The patient's mouth must be kept open; however, the thumb must not be used for this purpose to avoid injury to the rescuer.

chiragra (kī-răg′ră) [Gr. *cheir,* hand, + *agra,* seizure] Pain in the hand.

chiralgia (kī-răl′jē-ă) [″ + *algos,* pain] Nontraumatic or neuralgic pain in the hand.

c. paresthetica Numbness and pain in the hand, esp. in the region supplied by the radial nerve.

chirokinesthesia (kī″rō-kĭn″ĕs-thē′zē-ă) [″ + *kinesis,* movement, + *aisthesis,* sensation] A subjective sensation of hand motions.

chiromegaly (kī″rō-mĕg′ă-lē) [″ + *megas,* large] Enlargement of the hands, wrists, or ankles.

chiroplasty (kī′rō-plăs″tē) [″ + *plassein,* to form] Plastic surgery on the hand.

chiropodist (kī-rŏp′ō-dĭst, kĭ-) [″ + *pous,* foot] An obsolete term for podiatrist. SEE: *podiatrist.*

chiropody (kĭ-rŏp′ō-dē) Obsolete term for treatment of foot disorders. SEE: *podiatry.*

chiropractic (kī″rō-prăk′tĭk) [Gr. *cheir,* hand, + *prattein,* to do] A system of health care in which diseases are treated predominantly with manipulation or massage of spinal and musculoskeletal structures, nutritional therapies, and emotional support. Prescription drugs and surgeries are not used. Chiropractic was founded in the U.S. in 1895 by Daniel D. Palmer.

chiropractor A person certified and licensed to provide chiropractic care.

chirospasm (kī′rō-spăzm) [″ + *spasmos,* spasm] A spasm of the hand muscles; writer's cramp.

chisel (chĭs′l) A beveled-edge steel cutting instrument used in dentistry and orthopedics.

chi-square (kī-skwār) A statistical test to determine the correlation between the number of actual occurrences and the expected occurrences. The symbol for chi-square is χ^2.

chitin (kī′tĭn) [Gr. *chiton,* tunic] A polysaccharide that forms the hard exoskeleton of arthropods such as insects and crustaceans. It is also present in the cell walls of some fungi. **chitinous** (-nŭs), *adj.*

chitosan (kī′tō-săn) A polysaccharide made of glucosamine, naturally present in the exoskeleton of crustaceans. It resists digestion in the stomach but degrades in the colon. It is used to protect drugs and oral vaccines for controlled release into the gastrointestinal tract.

Chlamydia (klă-mĭd′ē-ă) [Gr. *chlamys,* cloak] A single genus of intracellular parasites with three recognized species: *C. psittaci, C. trachomatis,* and *C. pneumoniae.* The organisms are characterized as bacteria because of the composition of their cell walls and their growth by binary division; but they grow only intracellularly. These species cause a variety of diseases.

C. pneumoniae A species of *Chlamydia* that is an important cause of pneumonia, bronchitis, and sinusitis. It is believed to be transmitted from person to person by respiratory tract secretions, such as droplets suspended in air. In closed populations, it is spread slowly. Most cases of respiratory infection are mild and rarely require hospitalization. It is possible that this organism is a factor in the development of coronary artery disease. Treatment consists of a daily tetracycline, macrolide, or fluoroquinolone for 14 to 21 days.

C. psittaci A species of *Chlamydia* that is common in birds and animals, thus pet owners, pet shop employees, poultry farmers, and workers in meat processing plants are frequently exposed. After an incubation period of 5 to 15 days, nonspecific symptoms similar to a viral illness with malaise and fever may develop. Alternately the illness may resemble infectious mononucleosis with fever, pharyngitis, hepatosplenomegaly, and adenopathy. The severity may vary from mild or inapparent to a fatal systemic disease. In patients who are untreated, the fatality rate is approximately 20%. Treatment consists of administration of tetracycline or doxycycline for 10 to 21 days. SEE: *ornithosis*.

C. trachomatis A species of *Chlamydia* that causes a great variety of diseases, including genital infections in men and women. The diseases caused by *C. trachomatis* include nonspecific urethritis, neonatal inclusion conjunctivitis, lymphogranuloma venereum, pneumonia, and trachoma.

In industrialized nations *C. trachomatis* is the most common sexually transmitted pathogen (causing an estimated 4 million new infections annually in the U.S.). Men with chlamydial infection experience penile discharge and discomfort while urinating. Women may be asymptomatic or may experience urethral or vaginal discharge, painful or frequent urination, lower abdominal pain, or acute pelvic inflammatory disease, which may result in infertility.

Transmission of the disease can be prevented by avoiding contact with infected persons and by using condoms during intimate sexual activity. A pregnant woman with a chlamydial infection can transmit the disease to her newborn during birth. In newborns, ophthalmic antibiotic solution should be instilled in the conjunctival sac of each eye to prevent neonatal conjunctivitis and blindness caused by *Chlamydia*.

DIAGNOSIS: Several tests are available, including cultures, antigen detection assays, ligase chain reactions, polymerase chain reactions, and enzyme-linked immunoassays.

TREATMENT: Erythromycin, azithromycin, or tetracycline is effective.

CAUTION: Tetracyclines are generally not recommended for pregnant women or children under 8 yr old.

---

chloasma (klō-ăz′mă) [Gr. *chloazein,* to be green] Tan to brown, sharply defined patches of skin pigment, usually found symmetrically on the forehead, temples, cheeks, or upper lip. The excess pigmentation often occurs in pregnant women, in women using oral contraceptives, or in patients with underlying liver disease. Women are affected more often than men. Sun exposure tends to worsen the condition. SYN: *melasma*.

c. gravidarum Brownish pigmentation of the face, often occurring in pregnancy. It usually disappears after delivery. It is also seen in some women who take progestational oral contraceptives. SYN: *mask of pregnancy*. SEE: illus.

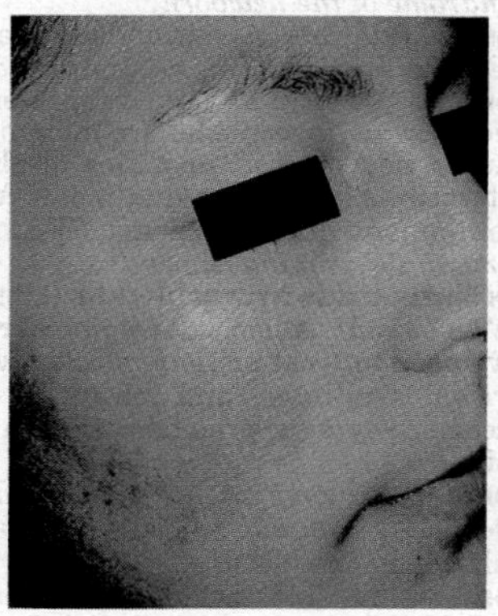

CHLOASMA GRAVIDARUM

c. hepaticum Liver spot.

idiopathic c. Chloasma caused by external agents such as sun, heat, mechanical means, and x-rays.

c. traumaticum Skin discoloration following trauma.

chloracne (klor-ăk′nē) Generalized acne that usually occurs after industrial exposure to chemicals such as polychlorinated biphenyls (PCBs) or dioxin.

chloral (klō′răl) [Gr. *chloras,* green] **1.** An oily liquid having a bitter taste. **2.** Chloral hydrate.

chloral hydrate A drug occasionally used as a sedative and hypnotic. Benzodiazepines (such as temazepam) have largely replaced chloral hydrate.

chloral hydrate poisoning Toxicity caused by excessive ingestion of chloral hydrate. The drug depresses and eventually paralyzes the central nervous system and may cause liver toxicity. There may be nausea and vomiting due to gastric irritation.

TREATMENT: An airway must be maintained and a cuffed endotracheal tube used if necessary. Mechanical ventilation may be required. A slurry of activated charcoal is administered. Beta blockers, such as propranolol, are used to manage arrhythmias. SEE: *Poisons and Poisoning Appendix*.

chlorambucil (klō-răm′bū-sĭl) A cytotoxic agent used in treating chronic lymphocytic leukemia, Hodgkin's disease, and certain lymphomas. Trade name is Leukeran.

chloramphenicol (klō″răm-fĕn′ĭ-kŏl) A broad-spectrum antibiotic employed internationally for the treatment of salmonellosis, ricksettsial diseases, and meningitis. It is taken up readily in the central nervous system. Because it has caused aplastic anemia, which is often fatal, its use in the U.S. is restricted to life-threatening infections that cannot be treated with safer drugs. SEE: *gray syndrome of the newborn*.

chlorate (klō′rāt) A salt of chloric acid. SEE: *Poisons and Poisoning Appendix*.

chlordane (klor′dān) A organochlorine used as an insecticide. In humans it causes neurological toxicities (such as alterations in memory and motor function) among other problems. SEE: *Poisons and Poisoning Appendix*.

chlordiazepoxide hydrochloride (klor″dī-ăz″ĕ-pŏk′sīd) A benzodiazepine derivative used to treat anxiety, alcohol withdrawal syndrome, and insomnia, and occasionally as a premedication in anesthesia.

chloremia (klō-rē′mē-ă) [Gr. *chloros*, green, + *haima*, blood] Increased chloride in the blood.

chlorhexidine (klor-hĕk′sĭ-dēn) A bisbiguanide used as a topical disinfectant and as an oral treatment for plaque and gingivitis. Oral rinses have side effects that include staining, bitter taste, transient loss of taste, and soft tissue ulceration. Rarely, systemic anaphylaxis can occur after exposure of the skin to this agent. The trade name for chlorhexidine is Peridex.

PATIENT CARE: Chlorhexidine rinses should be performed after meals to minimize taste alteration. Patients should not rinse with water following a chlorhexidine rinse.

chlorhexidine gluconate A topical disinfectant. Trade name is Hibiclens.

chlorhydria (klor-hī′drē-ă) [″ + *hydor*, water] An excess of hydrochloric acid in the stomach.

chloride (klō′rīd) [Gr. *chloros*, green] A binary compound of chlorine; a salt of hydrochloric acid. In health, blood serum contains 100 to 110 mmol/L of chloride ions.

FUNCTION: Chloride is the major extracellular anion and contributes to many body functions including the maintenance of osmotic pressure, acid-base balance, muscular activity, and the movement of water between fluid compartments. It is associated with sodium in the blood and was the first electrolyte to be routinely measured in the blood. Chloride ion is secreted in the gastric juice as hydrochloric acid.

chloridemia (klō″rĭ-dē′mē-ă) [″ + *haima*, blood] Chlorides in the blood.

chloride poisoning SEE: *barium salts, absorbable, in Poisons and Poisoning Appendix*.

chloridimeter (klor-ĭ-dim′ĕ-tur) An instrument for determining the amount of chloride in a body fluid.

chloriduria (klō″rĭ-dū′rē-ă) [″ + *ouron*, urine] Excess of chlorides in the urine.

chlorinated (klō′rĭn-ā-tĕd) Impregnated or treated with chlorine.

chlorination (klō″rĭ-nā′shŭn) The addition of chlorine or one of its derivatives to water, to kill microorganisms. For effective disinfection, a concentration of 0.5 to 1 part chlorine per million parts water is necessary. Some studies have suggested an association (but not a causal link) between the chlorination of drinking water and the incidence of cancers and birth defects.

chlorine (klō′rēn) [Gr. *chloros*, green] SYMB: Cl. A highly irritating, very poisonous gas; atomic weight 35.453, atomic number 17. It is destructive to the mucous membranes of the respiratory passages, and excessive inhalation may cause death. Chlorine is an active bleaching agent and germicide, owing to its oxidizing powers. It is used extensively to disinfect water supplies and treat sewage.

chlorite (klō′rīt) A salt of chlorous acid; used as a disinfectant and bleaching agent.

chlorobutanol (klō-rō-bū′tă-nŏl) Colorless crystals with camphor odor and taste. It is used as an antiseptic and local anesthetic in dentistry, and as a preservative in many pharmaceuticals.

INCOMPATIBILITY: Chlorobutanol is decomposed by alkalies and should not be mixed with borax or carbonates. It is soluble in ether, chloroform, and volatile oils.

chloroform (klō′rō-form) [Gr. *chloros*, green, + L. *forma*, form] $CHCl_3$; a heavy, clear, colorless liquid with a strong ether-like odor, formed by the action of chlorinated lime on methyl alcohol. At one time chloroform was administered by inhalation to produce anesthesia, but this use is obsolete.

chloroformism (klō′rō-form″ĭzm) The habit of inhaling chloroform for pleasure.

chloroleukemia (klō″rō-loo-kē′mē-ă) [″ + *leukos*, white, + *haima*, blood] Leukemia with chlorosis.

chloroma (klō-rō′mă) [″ + *oma*, growth] A tumor composed of leukemic cells that may metastasize to the brain, bones, skin, or other locations. Chloromas often have a green appearance due to an abundance of the fluorescent chemical myeloperoxidase.

chloropenia (klō″rō-pē′nē-ă) Hypochloremia. **chloropenic** (-nĭk), *adj*.

chlorophane (klō′rō-fān) [″ + *phainein,* to show] A green-yellow pigment in the retina.

chlorophenothane (klō″rō-fĕn′ō-thān) An insecticide, better known as DDT, not used in the U.S. since the 1970s because of its toxic effects on animals and the environment.

chlorophyll, chlorophyl (klō′rō-fĭl) [″ + *phyllon,* leaf] The green pigment in plants that accomplishes photosynthesis. In this process, carbon dioxide and water are combined to form glucose and oxygen according to the following equation: $6\ CO_2 + 6\ H_2O + \text{light} \rightarrow C_6H_{12}O_6 + 6\ O_2$. The primary energy source for our planet is the sunlight absorbed by chlorophyll. Four forms of chlorophyll (a, b, c, and d) occur in nature. Magnesium is an important component of chlorophyll, and green vegetables are an important dietary source of this mineral.

chloropia, chloropsia (klō-rō′pē-ă, klō-rŏp′sē-ă) [″ + *opsis,* vision] A sign of digitalis toxicity in which viewed objects appear green.

chloroplast, chloroplastid (klō′rō-plăst, klō″rō-plăs′tĭd) [″ + *plastos,* formed] A small green cell organelle found in the leaves and some stems of plants. Chloroplasts are the sites of photosynthesis. They possess a stroma and contain four pigments: chlorophyll a, chlorophyll b, carotene, and xanthophyll.

chloroprivic (klō″rō-prĭv′ĭk) [″ + L. *privare,* to deprive of] Lacking in or caused by loss of chlorides.

chloroprocaine hydrochloride (klō″rō-prō′kān) A local anesthetic.

chloroquine hydrochloride (klō′rō-kwĭn) A white crystalline powder used to treat both malaria and amebic dysentery. SEE: *malaria.*

chlorosis (klō-rō′sĭs) [″ + *osis,* condition] A form of iron-deficiency anemia. SEE: *anemia, iron-deficiency.* **chlorotic** (-rŏt′ĭk), *adj.*

chlorothiazide sodium (klō″rō-thī′ă-zīd) A thiazide diuretic.

chlorpheniramine maleate (klor″fĕn-ĭr′ă-mēn) An antihistamine that may be used orally or by injection. It is available under several trade names, including Chlor-Trimeton and Teldrin.

chlorpromazine (klor-prō′mă-zēn) A tranquilizing agent used primarily in its hydrochloride form to treat schizophrenia. Its side effects may include sedation, slurred speech, and tardive dyskinesia. Trade name is Thorazine.

chlorpromazine poisoning SEE: *Poisons and Poisoning Appendix.*

chlorpropamide (klor-prō′pă-mīd) An oral hypoglycemic agent of the sulfonylurea class. Trade name is Diabinese.

CAUTION: Because of its long duration of action, chlorpropamide causes more prolonged hypoglycemic reactions than other oral drugs for diabetes mellitus.

chlorprothixene (klor-prō-thĭks′ēn) A major tranquilizer used to treat schizophrenia. Its side effects include sedation, slurred speech, and tardive dyskinesia. Trade name is Taractan.

chlortetracycline hydrochloride (klor″tĕt-ră-sī′klēn) A golden-colored, broad-spectrum antibiotic isolated from a strain of *Streptomyces aureofaciens.* It inhibits growth of or destroys some strains of streptococci, staphylococci, pneumococci, rickettsiae. Trade name is Aureomycin.

chlorthalidone (klor-thăl′ĭ-dōn) A mild diuretic with a potency similar to those of the thiazides. Trade name is Hygroton.

chlorzoxazone (klor-zŏk′să-zōn) A muscle relaxant.

Ch.M. *chirurgiae magister,* Master of Surgery.

choana (kō′ă-nă) *pl.* **choanae** [Gr. *choane,* funnel] A funnel-shaped opening, esp. of the posterior nares; one of the communicating passageways between the nasal fossae and the pharynx.

choanoid (kō′ăn-oyd) [″ + *eidos,* form, shape] Shaped like a funnel.

choke [ME. *choken*] To prevent respiration by compressing or obstructing the larynx or trachea.

chokes Respiratory symptoms such as substernal distress, paroxysmal cough, tachypnea, or asphyxia. These may occur in decompression illness, esp. in cases of aeroembolism resulting from exposure to pressure lower than atmospheric.

choke-saver The name of any device designed to clear an obstructed airway. These devices are rarely used because of the ready availability of intubation equipment (e.g., laryngoscopes and McGill forceps). SEE: *Heimlich maneuver.*

choking [ME. *choken,* to suffocate] Upper airway obstruction caused, for example, by a foreign body in the trachea or oropharynx, laryngeal edema or spasm, or external compression of the neck. The choking patient may have gasping or stridorous respirations, repetitive ineffective coughing, an inability to speak, or hypersalivation. Intense agitation may be present. If the airway is not rapidly cleared, asphyxia and hypoxia may produce loss of consciousness or death. SEE: *Heimlich maneuver.*

chol- SEE: *chole-.*

cholagogue (kō′lă-gŏg) [Gr. *chole,* bile, + *agein,* to lead forth] An agent that increases the flow of bile into the intestine (i.e., a choleretic or cholecystagogue).

cholangi- SEE: *cholangio-.*

cholangiectasis (kō-lăn″jē-ĕk′tă-sĭs) [″ + *angeion,* vessel, + *ektasis,* dilatation] Dilation of the bile ducts.

cholangio-, cholangi- [chole + Gr. *angeion,* vessel] Combining form meaning *bile vessel.*

cholangiocarcinoma (kō-lăn″jē-ō-kăr″sĭ-nō′mă) [″ + ″ + *karkinos,* crab, + *oma,* tumor] Carcinoma of the bile ducts.

cholangioenterostomy (kō-lăn″jē-ō-ĕn″tĕr-ŏs′tō-mē) [″ + ″ + *enteron,* intestine, + *stoma,* mouth] Surgical formation of a passage between a bile duct and the intestine.

cholangiogastrostomy (kō-lăn″jē-ō-găs-trŏs′tō-mē) [″ + ″ + *gaster,* stomach, + *stoma,* mouth] Surgical formation of a passage between a bile duct and the stomach.

cholangiography (kō-lăn″jē-ŏg′ră-fē) [″ + ″ + *graphein,* to write] Radiography of the bile ducts, a procedure replaced by ultrasonography.

percutaneous transhepatic c. ABBR: PTC. Direct percutaneous puncture of an intrahepatic duct by a needle inserted through the eighth or ninth intercostal space into the center of the liver. Radiopaque material is injected into the dilated intrahepatic biliary tree. The procedure is useful in determining the cause of obstructive jaundice. SEE: *endoscopic retrograde cholangiopancreatography; jaundice.*

cholangiole (kō-lăn′jē-ōl) [″ + ″ + *ole,* dim. suffix] The small terminal portion of the bile duct.

cholangiolitis (kō-lăn″jē-ō-lī′tĭs) [″ + ″ + ″+ Gr. *itis,* inflammation] Inflammation of the bile ducts, occurring in various forms of hepatitis.

cholangioma (kō-lăn-jē-ō′mă) [″ + *angeion,* vessel, + *oma,* tumor] A tumor of the bile ducts.

cholangiostomy (kō″lăn-jē-ŏs′tō-mē) [″ + ″ + *stoma,* mouth] Surgical formation of a fistula into the bile duct.

cholangiotomy (kō″lăn-jē-ŏt′ō-mē) [″ + ″ + *tome,* incision] Incision of an intrahepatic or extrahepatic bile duct for removal of gallstones.

cholangitis (kō″lăn-jī′tĭs) [″ + *angeion,* vessel, + *itis,* inflammation] Inflammation of the bile ducts.

primary sclerosing c. A chronic liver disease of unknown origin marked by inflammation and obliteration of the intrahepatic and extrahepatic bile ducts. The disease progresses silently and steadily and in most patients leads to cirrhosis, portal hypertension, and liver failure. Seventy percent of patients are men and the mean age at diagnosis is 39. Liver transplantation can be used to treat patients who develop cirrhosis from this disease.

cholanopoiesis (kō″lă-nō-poy-ē′sĭs) [Gr. *chole,* bile, + *ano,* upward, + *poiesis,* making] Synthesis of cholic acid in the liver.

cholate (kō′lāt) Any salt or ester of cholic acid.

chole-, chol- [Gr. *chole,* bile] Combining form meaning *bile* or *gall.*

cholecalciferol (ko″lē-kăl-sĭf′ĕr-ŏl) Vitamin D_3; an antirachitic, oil-soluble vitamin occurring as white, odorless crystals.

cholecyst- SEE: *cholecysto-.*

cholecystagogue (kō″lē-sĭs′tă-gŏg) [″ + ″ + *agogos,* leader] A drug or action that empties the gallbladder.

cholecystalgia (kō″lē-sĭs-tăl′jē-ă) [″ + ″ + *algos,* pain] Biliary colic.

cholecystangiography (kō″lē-sĭs″tăn-jē-ŏg′ră-fē) [″ + ″ + *angeion,* vessel, + *graphein,* to write] Radiographic examination of the gallbladder and bile ducts after injection of a contrast medium, a procedure replaced by ultrasonography.

cholecystectasia (kō″lē-sĭs-tĕk-tā′zē-ă) [″ + ″ + *ektasis,* dilatation] Dilatation of the gallbladder.

cholecystectomy (kō″lē-sĭs-tĕk′tō-mē) [″ + ″ + *ektome,* excision] Removal of the gallbladder by laparoscopic or open surgery. The procedure is performed for symptomatic gallstone disease. In the U.S. alone, more than half a million operations are performed annually, but some hospitals have reported a 20% increase in this number since the introduction of laparoscopic surgery. Surgical complications, including wound infections, adverse reactions to anesthetics, and injury to the liver, gallbladder, or neighboring organs, occur about 5% of the time.

Acute, chronic, or acalculous cholecystitis (i.e., biliary inflammation that is not caused by gallstones), repeated episodes of biliary colic, biliary dyskinesia, gallstone pancreatitis, and occasionally cholangitis are indications for the procedure. The gallbladder does not usually need to be removed for asymptomatic gallstone disease.

PATIENT CARE: *Preoperative:* The patient is informed about the procedure, including the need for drains, catheter, nasogastric tubes, etc.

Postoperative: Vital signs are monitored and dressings are inspected. The patient is assessed for pain and for gastrointestinal and urinary function; analgesics and antiemetics are provided as needed. Fluid and electrolyte balance is monitored, and prescribed replacement therapy is administered. Respiratory status is assessed, and the patient is encouraged to breathe deeply and to perform incentive spirometry as prescribed. The patient is assisted with early ambulation and to splint the abdomen for coughing. Peripheral circulation is evaluated, and venous return is promoted with leg exercises and elastic stockings or pneumatic hose as prescribed.

If a laparoscopic approach is used, the

patient may be discharged the day of or the day after surgery. Clear liquids are offered after recovery from general anesthesia, and the patient resumes a normal diet within a few days. If an open incision is used, the patient is placed in a position of comfort; an NG tube, if used, is attached to low intermittent suction; and the volume and characteristics of drainage from the NG tube and any abdominal drains or T tube are documented. Skin care and appropriate dressings are provided around any drain site.

When peristalsis returns, the NG tube, if used, is removed as directed. Oral intake, beginning with clear liquids, is initiated. A T-tube may be clamped before and after each meal to allow additional bile to enter the intestine. Signs and symptoms of postcholecystectomy syndrome (i.e., fever, abdominal pain, and jaundice) and other complications involving obstructed bile drainage are reported; urine and stool samples are collected for analysis of bile content should any such complications occur.

Discharge teaching for the patient and family includes wound care and T-tube care if appropriate (the T-tube may remain in place up to 2 weeks); the need to report any signs of biliary obstruction (i.e., fever, jaundice, pruritus, pain, dark urine, and clay-colored stools); the importance of daily exercise such as walking; avoidance of heavy lifting or straining for the prescribed period; and any restrictions on motor vehicle operation. Although diet is not restricted, the patient may be more comfortable avoiding excessive intake of fats and gas-forming foods for 4 to 6 weeks. Arrangements for home health care may be necessary. SEE: *Nursing Diagnoses Appendix.*

laparoscopic laser c. Removal of the gallbladder using the laser technique. This procedure may be inappropriate for patients with severe acute cholecystitis, a palpable gallbladder, or evidence of a stone in the common bile duct. The procedure may also be referred to as endoscopic laser cholecystectomy.

PATIENT CARE: The nurse or surgeon explains to the patient that this type of surgery will not be used if the patient is pregnant or has had extensive abdominal surgery (because of concern for adhesions), severe acute cholecystitis, a palpable gallbladder, evidence of a stone in the common bile duct, or a bleeding problem. The patient also is told that, using the videolaserscopy technique, the surgeon will be able to remove the gallbladder without unsightly scarring, as there will be only four small punctures, reducing the risk for wound complications (e.g., infection, hematoma, separation). Risks for other complications such as pneumonia, thrombophlebitis, urinary retention, and paralytic ileus also are decreased, because the procedure enables early mobility and avoids use of parenteral analgesia. Patients usually are happy to hear that they will experience less pain and immobility, require less narcotic analgesia, be discharged the same or the following day, and be able to return to their usual activities (including work) within 3 to 7 days. Preoperative preparation, which usually is similar to that for any other abdominal surgery, is explained.

Postoperatively, the patient is stabilized during a brief stay in postanesthesia, then is transported to a surgical observation unit. The patient is offered clear liquids; carbonated beverages are avoided because they may cause distension and abdominal pressure. If the patient tolerates liquids, the IV is removed, and the patient is offered a regular diet. Analgesics are administered as prescribed as soon as the patient can take liquids. A parenteral narcotic (which may result in drowsiness, reduced intestinal motility, and/or vomiting) is given only if the patient continues to experience pain after taking an analgesic. Once the patient is comfortable, he or she is assisted to walk, as early ambulation speeds recovery. Usually, the patient is fully awake and walking within 3 to 4 hours of arrival on the unit. If he or she experiences shoulder pain, a heating pad may be applied to the area; however, the surgeon usually removes the carbon dioxide at the end of the procedure to prevent this problem. The nurse evaluates readiness for discharge, which usually can occur if the patient is afebrile, walking, eating, and voiding, and has stable vital signs with no evidence of bleeding or bile leakage. To assess for the latter risks, the patient is observed for severe pain and tenderness in the right upper quadrant, an increase in abdominal girth, leakage of bile-colored drainage from the puncture site, a fall in blood pressure, and increased heart rate.

The patient is taught to keep the adhesive bandages covering the puncture site clean and dry. He or she may remove them the next day and bathe or shower as usual. The patient most likely will require little analgesia, but is given a prescription for use as needed. He or she is reminded to pace activity according to energy level. While no special diet is required, the patient may wish to avoid excessive fat intake and gas-forming foods for 4 to 6 weeks. He or she should return to the surgeon for follow-up evaluation as directed, and report any vomiting, abdominal distention, signs of infection, and new or worsening pain.

If the patient requires an abdominal approach, a nasogastric (NG) tube may be placed after surgery to drain the stomach and prevent abdominal distension. A T-tube drain may be in place through an abdominal insertion site. The T-tube's drainage bag will be maintained level with the patient's abdomen to prevent excessive drainage. Once bowel sounds are present (2–3 days), the NG tube is removed, and a clear liquid diet is initiated. The diet is advanced slowly as tolerated, and the T-tube is clamped for an hour before and after each meal as prescribed to allow bile to aid digestion. The T-tube's position and patency are assessed to prevent obstructed bile drainage. Signs of postcholecystectomy syndrome (fever, abdominal pain, and jaundice) are monitored. The patient receives medication for pain as prescribed. The nurse and respiratory therapist support the incision and the patient to enable deep breathing, coughing, and use of incentive spirometry every 3 to 4 hours. If the patient is discharged with the T-tube in place, he or she is taught how to care for the equipment and the wound, and is reminded to return to the surgeon as instructed. The patient is warned to report immediately any signs of biliary obstruction such as fever, jaundice, pruritus, increased pain, dark urine, and clay-colored stools.

cholecystenterorrhaphy (kō″lē-sĭs-tĕn″tĕr-or′ă-fē) [″ + ″ + *enteron,* intestine, + *rhaphe,* seam, ridge] Suture of the gallbladder to the intestinal wall.

cholecystenterostomy (kō″lē-sĭs-tĕn″tĕr-ŏs′tō-mē) [″ + ″ + *enteron,* intestine, + *stoma,* mouth] Surgical formation of a passage between the gallbladder and the small intestine.

cholecystic (kō″lē-sĭs′tĭk) Pert. to the gallbladder.

cholecystitis (kō″lē-sĭs-tī′tĭs) [Gr. *chole,* bile, + *kystis,* bladder, + *itis,* inflammation] Inflammation of the gallbladder, usually caused by obstruction of the biliary ducts by gallstones. Cholecystitis caused by gallstones occurs commonly, esp. in women, patients who are obese, and those who have been dieting. The disease is marked by colicky pain in the right upper quadrant of the abdomen that develops shortly after a meal.

Acalculous cholecystitis, that is, biliary inflammation that is not caused by gallstones, is a disease of the critically ill. It is associated with a high likelihood of abscess formation, gallbladder perforation, gangrene, and death.

ETIOLOGY: Acute cholecystitis is usually caused by obstruction of the biliary ducts, with chemical irritation and often infection of the gallbladder.

SYMPTOMS: Cholecystitis due to gallstones causes right upper quadrant pain that occurs after a fatty meal, as well as fever, chills, nausea, and vomiting. The pain of cholecystitis often radiates into the right shoulder or right side of the back. Jaundice is present in about 20% of patients. In patients in intensive care units, acalculous cholecystitis may present with fever and few other easily identified symptoms.

DIAGNOSIS: Ultrasonography of the right upper quadrant, the diagnostic procedure of choice, reveals cholecystitis in about 90% of patients. Oral cholecystograms, computed tomography of the abdomen, and other diagnostic tests are sometimes used when the disease is suspected clinically but ultrasonography is not diagnostic.

TREATMENT: Cholecystectomy is the usual treatment. Gallbladder drainage (cholecystostomy) is sometimes used as a temporizing procedure in unstable patients. Gallstones lodged in the ampulla of Vater can sometimes be removed with endoscopic retrograde cholangiopancreatography.

PATIENT CARE: During an acute attack, the patient's vital signs and fluid balance are monitored, oral intake is withheld, prescribed antiemetics are administered as necessary, and intravenous fluid and electrolyte therapy is maintained as prescribed. A nasogastric tube may be employed. The patient's comfort is ensured, and prescribed narcotic analgesics and anticholinergics are administered to relieve pain.

Diagnostic tests including pretest instructions and aftercare are explained; the surgeon's explanation of any prescribed surgical interventions, including possible complications, is reinforced; and the patient is prepared physically and emotionally for such procedures.

cholecystnephrostomy (kō″lē-sĭst″nē-frŏs′tō-mē) [″ + *kystis,* bladder, + *nephros,* kidney, + *stoma,* mouth] Surgical formation of a passage between the gallbladder and the renal pelvis.

cholecysto-, cholecyst- [chole + Gr. *kystis,* bladder] Combining form meaning *gallbladder*.

cholecystocolostomy (kō″lē-sĭs″tō-kō-lŏs′tō-mē) [″ + ″ + *kolon,* colon, + *stoma,* mouth] Surgical formation of a passage between the gallbladder and the colon.

cholecystocolotomy (kō″lē-sĭs″tō-kō-lŏt′ō-mē) [″ + ″ + ″ + *tome,* incision] A surgical incision into the gallbladder and colon.

cholecystoduodenostomy (kō″lē-sĭs″tō-dū″ō-dē-nŏs′tō-mē) [″ + ″ + L. *duodeni,* twelve, + Gr. *stoma,* mouth] Surgical formation of a passage between the gallbladder and the duodenum.

cholecystogastrostomy (kō″lē-sĭs″tō-găs-trŏs′tō-mē) [″ + ″ + *gaster,* belly, + *stoma,* mouth] Surgical formation of a passage between the gallbladder and the stomach.

cholecystogram (kō″lē-sĭs′tō-grăm) [″ + ″ + *gramma,* something written] A radiograph of the gallbladder.

cholecystography (kō″lē-sĭs-tŏg′ră-fē) [″ + ″ + *graphein,* to write] Radiography of the gallbladder, a procedure replaced by ultrasonography.

cholecystoileostomy (kō″lē-sĭs″tō-ĭl-ē-ŏs′tō-mē) [″ + *kystis,* bladder, + L. *ileum,* + Gr. *stoma,* mouth] Surgical formation of a passage between the gallbladder and the ileum.

cholecystojejunostomy (kō″lē-sĭs″tō-jĕ-jū-nŏs′tō-mē) [″ + ″ + L. *jejunum,* empty, + Gr. *stoma,* mouth] Surgical formation of a passage between the gallbladder and the jejunum.

cholecystokinin ABBR: CCK. A hormone secreted into the blood by the mucosa of the upper small intestine. It stimulates contraction of the gallbladder and pancreatic secretion.

cholecystolithiasis (kō″lē-sĭs″tō-lĭ-thī′ă-sĭs) [″ + ″ + *lithos,* stone, + *-iasis,* condition] Gallstones in the gallbladder.

cholecystolithotripsy (kō″lē-sĭs″tō-lĭth′ō-trĭp″sē) [″ + ″ + ″ + *tripsis,* a rubbing] Crushing of a gallstone in the unopened gallbladder with an extracorporeal shock-wave lithotriptor; its use is primarily investigational.

cholecystomy (kō″lē-sĭs′tō-mē) [Gr. *chole,* bile, + *kystis,* bladder, + *tome,* incision] Cholecystotomy.

cholecystopathy (kō″lē-sĭs-tŏp′ă-thē) [″ + ″ + *pathos,* disease, suffering] Any gallbladder disorder.

cholecystopexy (kō″lē-sĭs′tō-pĕk″sē) [″ + ″ + *pexis,* fixation] Suturing of the gallbladder to the abdominal wall, in conjunction with cholecystostomy.

cholecystoptosis (kō″lē-sĭs-tŏp-tō′sĭs) [″ + ″ + *ptosis,* a dropping] Downward displacement of the gallbladder.

cholecystorrhaphy (kō″lē-sĭs-tor′ă-fē) [″ + *kystis,* bladder, + *rhaphe,* seam, ridge] Suturing of the gallbladder.

cholecystostomy (kō″lē-sĭs-tŏs′tō-mē) [″ + ″ + *stoma,* mouth] Surgical formation of an opening into the gallbladder through the abdominal wall.

cholecystotomy (kō″lē-sĭs-tŏt′ō-mē) [″ + ″ + *tome,* incision] Incision of the gallbladder through the abdominal wall for removal of gallstones.

choledoch- SEE: *choledocho-*.

choledochal (kō-lē-dŏk′ăl) [″ + *dochos,* receptacle] Pert. to the common bile duct.

choledochectasia (kō-lĕd″ō-kĕk-tā′zē-ă) [″ + ″ + *ektasis,* distention] Distention of the common bile duct.

choledochectomy (kō-lĕd″ō-kĕk′tō-mē) [″ + ″ + *ektome,* excision] Excision of a portion of the common bile duct.

choledochitis (kō″lē-dō-kī′tĭs) [″ + ″ + *itis,* inflammation] Inflammation of the common bile duct.

choledocho-, choledoch- [Gr. *choledochos,* containing bile fr. *chole,* bile + *dechomai,* receptable, to receive] Meaning *bile duct.*

choledochoduodenostomy (kō-lĕd″ō-kō-dū-ō-dē-nŏs′tō-mē) [″ + ″ + L. *duodeni,* twelve, + Gr. *stoma,* mouth] Surgical formation of a passage between the common bile duct and the duodenum.

choledochoenterostomy (kō-lĕd″ŏ-kō-ĕn-tĕr-ŏs′tō-mē) [″ + ″ + *enteron,* intestine, + *stoma,* mouth] Surgical formation of a passage between the common bile duct and the intestine.

choledochography (kō-lĕd″ō-kŏg′ră-fē) [″ + *dochos,* receptacle, + *graphein,* to write] Radiography of the bile duct following administration of a radiopaque contrast medium, a procedure replaced by ultrasonography.

choledochojejunostomy (kō-lĕd″ō-kō-jĕ-jū-nŏs′tō-mē) [″ + ″ + L. *jejunum,* empty, + Gr. *stoma,* mouth] Surgical joining of the common bile duct to the jejunum of the small intestine.

choledocholith (kō-lĕd′ō-kō-lĭth″) [″ + ″ + *lithos,* stone] A calculus, or stone, in the common bile duct.

choledocholithiasis (kō-lĕd″ō-kō-lĭ-thī′ă-sĭs) [″ + ″ + *lithos,* stone, + *-iasis,* condition] Calculi in the common bile duct.

choledocholithotomy (kō-lĕd″ō-kō-lĭth-ŏt′ō-mē) [″ + ″ + ″ + *tome,* incision] Removal of a gallstone through an incision of the bile duct.

choledocholithotripsy (kō-lĕd′ō-kō-lĭth″ō-trĭp-sē) [″ + ″ + ″ + *tripsis,* a crushing] Crushing of a gallstone in the common bile duct.

choledochoplasty (kō-lĕd′ō-kō-plăs″tē) [Gr. *chole,* bile, + *dochos,* receptacle, + *plassein,* to form] Surgical repair of the common bile duct.

choledochorrhaphy (kō-lĕd″ō-kor′ă-fē) [″ + ″ + *rhaphe,* seam, ridge] Suturing of the severed ends of the common bile duct.

choledochostomy (kō-lĕd″ō-kŏs′tō-mē) [″ + ″ + *stoma,* mouth] Surgical formation of a passage into the common bile duct through the abdominal wall.

choledochotomy (kō″lĕd-ō-kŏt′ō-mē) [″ + ″ + *tome,* incision] Surgical incision of the common bile duct.

cholelith Gallstone.

cholelithiasis (kō″lē-lĭ-thī′ă-sĭs) [″ + ″ + *-iasis,* condition] The presence or formation of gallstones. SEE: *cholecystectomy; cholecystitis; colic* (1); *gallstone; lithotripsy.*

cholelithic (kō″lē-lĭth′ĭk) Pert. to or caused by biliary calculus.

cholelithotomy (kō″lē-lĭ-thŏt′ō-mē) [″ + *lithos,* stone, + *tome,* incision] Removal of gallstones through a surgical incision.

cholelithotripsy, cholelithotrity (kō″lē-lĭth′ō-trĭp-sē, kō″lē-lĭ-thŏt′rĭ-tē) [″ + ″ + *tripsis,* a crushing] Crushing of a biliary calculus.

cholemesis (kō-lĕm′ĕ-sĭs) [″ + *emein,* to vomit] Bile in the vomitus.

choleperitoneum (kō″lē-pĕr″ĭ-tō-nē′ŭm) [″ + *peri,* around, + *teinein,* to stretch] Bile in the peritoneum.

cholera (kŏl′ĕr-ă) [L. *cholera,* bilious diarrhea] An acute infection involving the entire small intestine, marked by profuse, watery, secretory diarrhea. Without treatment, the severe loss of fluids and electrolytes can cause dehydration and vascular collapse. The incubation period is from a few hours to 4 or 5 days. Cholera is endemic in India, parts of Asia, and sub-Saharan Africa. SYN: *Asiatic cholera.*

ETIOLOGY: The causative organism, *Vibrio cholerae,* is a short, curved, motile gram-negative rod. Two serotypes have been identified, 01 and 0139 (Bengal). The bacteria do not invade the bowel wall, but produce a potent enterotoxin that causes increased secretion of chloride, bicarbonate, and water into the small intestine, which overwhelms the large intestine's ability to reabsorb. Transmission is through water and food contaminated with excreta of infected persons.

SYMPTOMS: Approximately 80% of patients have mild disease marked by diarrhea and malaise. Severe attacks are characterized by periodic voluminous "rice water" diarrhea, vomiting, and muscle cramps. Without treatment, severe dehydration develops, characterized by loss of skin turgor, dizziness, increased heart rate and respirations, decreased urinary output, and, ultimately, circulatory collapse and hypovolemic shock. Hypoglycemia may be a problem in very young children.

TREATMENT: The use of oral solutions to replace the lost water, sodium, chloride, and bicarbonate has decreased the death rate from cholera by preventing death due to dehydration. A commercial or over-the-counter oral rehydration solution can be used or a solution made by adding 1 level tsp of salt and 1 heaping tsp of sugar to 1 L of water; patients should replace 5% to 7% of body weight (e.g., a 20-kg child would receive 1 to 1.4 L of fluid per day). Hospitalization and intravenous fluid replacement are required if the patient is already dehydrated. Quinolone antibiotics decrease the duration and severity of the disease.

PREVENTION: Cholera vaccine is relatively ineffective. Travelers to developing countries should not drink unboiled water or add ice to beverages, and should not eat raw or partially cooked shellfish, uncooked vegetables or salads, or fruits they have not peeled themselves. They should not assume bottled water is safe, and should swim only in chlorinated swimming pools. They should seek medical attention immediately if diarrhea or a febrile illness develops.

c. sicca A dated term for a fulminating variety of cholera that occurs without vomiting or diarrhea.

choleresis (kŏl-ĕr-ē′sĭs, kō-lĕr′ĕ-sĭs) [Gr. *chole,* bile, + *hairesis,* removal] The secretion of bile by the liver.

choleretic (kŏl-ĕr-ĕt′ĭk) **1.** Stimulating excretion of bile by the liver. **2.** Any agent that increases excretion of bile by the liver.

choleric (kŏl′ĕr-ĭk) Irritable; quick-tempered without apparent cause.

choleriform (kŏl-ĕr′ĭ-form) [L. *cholera,* + *forma,* shape] Resembling cholera.

choleroid (kŏl′ĕr-oyd) [″ + Gr. *eidos,* form, shape] Resembling cholera.

cholerophobia (kŏl″ĕr-ō-fō′bē-ă) [″ + Gr. *phobos,* fear] A morbid fear of acquiring cholera.

cholestasia (kō″lē-stā′zē-ă) [Gr. *chole,* bile, + *stasis,* stoppage] Cholestasis. **cholestatic** (-stăt′ĭk), *adj.*

cholestasis Arrest of the flow of bile. This may be due to intrahepatic causes, obstruction of the bile duct by gallstones, or any process that blocks the bile duct (e.g., cancer). SYN: *cholestasia.*

cholesteatoma (kō″lē-stē″ă-tō′mă) [″ + *steatos,* fat, + *oma,* tumor] An epithelial pocket or cystlike sac filled with keratin debris. It can occur in the meninges, central nervous system, and skull bones, but is most common in the middle ear and mastoid area. The cyst, which is filled with a combination of epithelial cells and cholesterol, most commonly enlarges to occlude the middle ear. Enzymes formed within the sac cause erosion of adjacent bones, including the ossicles, and destroy them. Cholesteatomas are classified as congenital, primary acquired, and secondary acquired.

cholesteremia, cholesterolemia (kō-lĕs″tē-rē′mē-ă, kō-lĕs″tĕr-ŏl-ē′mē-ă) [″ + *stereos,* solid, + *haima,* blood] Hypercholesterolemia.

cholesterol (kō-lĕs′tĕr-ŏl) [″ + *stereos,* solid] $C_{27}H_{45}OH$, a monohydric alcohol; a sterol widely distributed in animal tissues and occurring in egg yolks, various oils, fats, myelin in brain, spinal cord and axons, liver, kidneys, and adrenal glands. It is synthesized in the liver and is a normal constituent of bile. It is the principal constituent of most gallstones and of atherosclerotic plaques found in arteries. It is important in metabolism, serving as a precursor to various steroid hormones (e.g., sex hormones, adrenal corticoids). SEE: illus.

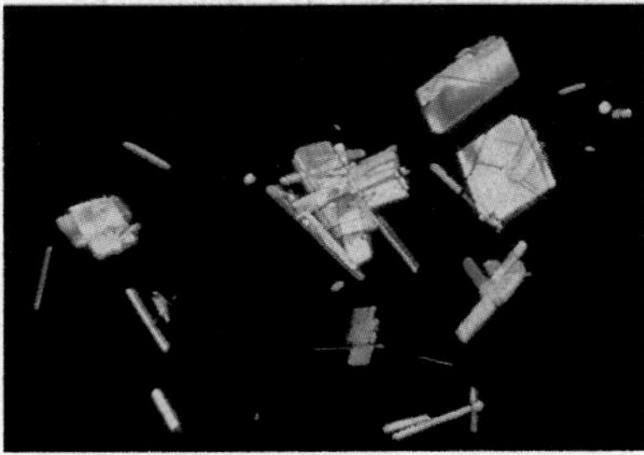

CHOLESTEROL CRYSTALS, POLARIZED

(Orig. mag. ×400)

An elevated blood level of cholesterol increases a person's risks of developing coronary heart disease (CHD). Lowering elevated total blood cholesterol levels, and the levels of low-density lipoprotein cholesterol, reduces the risk of heart attacks both in persons with a prior history of coronary disease and in asymptomatic individuals. Risk categories and recommended actions are included in the accompanying table. SEE: table.

Cholesterol levels may be decreased by eating a diet that is low in cholesterol and fat and high in fiber; exercising regularly; and taking medications. Drugs used to control cholesterol levels include lovastatin (and other "statin" drugs); niacin; bile-acid resins (e.g., cholestyramine); and others.

high-density lipoprotein c. SEE: under *lipoprotein*.

low-density lipoprotein c. SEE: under *lipoprotein*.

total c. The sum of low- and high-density lipoproteins.

cholesterolosis The abnormal accumulation of cholesterol in tissues.

cholestyramine resin (kō″lĕ-stī′ră-mĭn) An ion-exchange resin used to treat itching associated with jaundice and elevated serum lipid levels. Side effects may include bloating and abdominal discomfort. Trade name is Questran.

choleverdin SEE: *biliverdin*.

choline (kō′lĭn, -lēn) [Gr. *chole,* bile] An amine, $C_5H_{15}NO_2$, widely distributed in plant and animal tissues. It is a constituent of lecithin and other phospholipids. It is essential in normal fat and carbohydrate metabolism. A deficiency leads to fatty liver. Choline is also involved in protein metabolism, serving as a methylating agent, and is a precursor of acetylcholine.

cholinergic (kō″lĭn-ĕr′jĭk) [″ + *ergon,* work] **1.** Liberating acetylcholine; used of nerve endings. **2.** An agent that produces the effect of acetylcholine.

cholinergic blocking agent Anticholinergic (2).

cholinesterase (kō″lĭn-ĕs′tĕr-ās) Any enzyme that catalyzes the hydrolysis of choline esters, such as acetylcholinesterase, which catalyzes the breakdown of acetylcholine to acetic acid and choline. Cholinesterases are inhibited by physostigmine (eserine).

cholinoceptive (kō″lĭn-ō-sĕp′tĭv) [″ + L. *receptor,* receiver] Pert. to sites on cells that are acted on by cholinergic transmitters.

cholinolytic (kō″lĭn-ō-lĭt′ĭk) [″ + *lysis,* dissolution] Anticholinergic (2).

cholinomimetic (kō″lĭ-nō-mī-mĕt′ĭk) [″ + *mimetikos,* imitating] Acting in the same way as acetylcholine.

chologenic (kō″lō-jĕn′ĭk) [″ + *gennan,* to produce] Promoting or stimulating bile production.

chololith (kŏl′ō-lĭth) [″ + *lithos,* stone] Obsolete term for gallstone. SEE: *cholelith*.

chololithiasis (kŏl″ō-lĭth-ī′ăs-ĭs) [″ + ″ + *-iasis,* state] Cholelithiasis.

cholorrhea (kŏl″ō-rē′ă) [″ + *rhoia,* flow] Excessive secretion of bile.

chondr- SEE: *chondro-*.

chondral (kŏn′drăl) [Gr. *chondros,* cartilage] Pert. to cartilage.

chondralgia (kŏn-drăl′jē-ă) [″ + *algos,* pain] Pain in or around a cartilage.

chondralloplasia (kŏn″drăl-ō-plā′zē-ă) [″ + *allos,* other, + *plassein,* to form] Cartilage in abnormal places.

chondrectomy (kŏn-drĕk′tō-mē) [″ + *ektome,* excision] Surgical excision of a cartilage.

chondric (kŏn′drĭk) [Gr. *chondros,* cartilage] Pert. to cartilage.

chondrification (kŏn-drĭ-fĭ-kā′shŭn) [″ + L. *facere,* to make] Conversion into cartilage.

chondrigen, chondrogen (kŏn′drĭ-jĕn) [″ + *gennan,* to produce] Previously used term for the basal substance of cartilage and corneal tissue, which turns into chondrin on boiling.

chondrin (kŏn′drĭn) [Gr. *chondros,* cartilage] Gelatin-like matter obtained by boiling cartilage.

chondritis (kŏn-drī′tĭs) [″ + *itis,* inflammation] Inflammation of cartilage.

chondro-, chondr- [Gr. *chondros,* cartilage] meaning *cartilage*.

chondroadenoma (kŏn″drō-ăd-ē-nō′mă) [″ + *aden,* gland, + *oma,* tumor] Cartilaginous tissue in an adenoma.

chondroangioma (kŏn″drō-ăn-jē-ō′ma) [″ + *angeion,* vessel, + *oma,* tumor] Cartilaginous elements in an angioma.

chondroblast (kŏn′drō-blăst) [″ + *blastos,* germ] A cell that forms cartilage. SYN: *chondroplast*.

chondroblastoma (kŏn″drō-blăs-tō′mă) [″ + ″ + *oma,* tumor] A benign neo-

Lipids

Suggested Management of Patients with Raised Lipid Levels

- LDL cholesterol is the primary key to treatment. Diet is first-line therapy and drug intervention is reserved for patients considered to be at a higher risk. Continue diet for at least 6 months before initiating drug therapy; use drug therapy in conjunction with diet, not in place of diet. The greater the risk the more aggressive the intervention.
- If there is evidence of coronary heart disease (CHD), do lipoprotein analysis.
- Initially measure total cholesterol and HDL cholesterol levels; based on these results and the presence or absence of other risk factors, determine course of action or proceed to lipoprotein analysis.
- See American Heart Association (AHA) diet, Step I, and AHA diet, Step II
- Risk factors for atherosclerosis: advanced age, diabetes mellitus, family history, hypertension, male gender, obesity, sedentary lifestyle, tobacco use.

TOTAL AND HDL CHOLESTEROL

Status and Total Cholesterol	HDL Cholesterol	≥2 Positive Risk Factors	Recommendations
Desirable (<200 mg/dL)	≥35 mg/dL	N/A*	• Reassess total and HDL levels in 5 yr. • Provide information on diet, physical activity, and risk factor reduction.
	≤35 mg/dL	N/A	• Do lipoprotein analysis (see below).
Borderline high (200–239 mg/dL)	≥35 mg/dL	No	• Reassess total and HDL levels in 1–2 yr. • Reinforce diet, physical activity, and other risk factor reduction activities.
	≤35 mg/dL	Yes	• Do lipoprotein analysis (see below).
High (≥240 mg/dL)			• Do lipoprotein analysis (see below).

LIPOPROTEIN ANALYSIS

LDL cholesterol = (total cholesterol − HDL) − (triglycerides ÷ 5)

Status and LDL Cholesterol	≥2 Positive Risk Factors	Recommendations
Desirable (<130 mg/dL)	N/A	• Reassess total and HDL in 5 yr. • Provide information on diet, physical activity, and risk factor reduction.
Borderline high-risk (130–159 mg/dL)	No	• Reassess total, HDL, and LDL annually. • Provide information on Step I diet and physical activity.
High-risk (≥160 mg/dL)	Yes	• Clinical workup (history, physical exam, and lab tests) to check for secondary causes or familial disorders. • Consider risk factors that can be changed. • Initiate Step I diet; if diet fails, proceed to Step II diet. • Consider drug therapy if diet fails to obtain desired levels. • **Goal** for borderline high-risk patients with ≥2 negative risk factors is LDL <130 mg/dL. • **Goal** for high-risk patients with no other risk factors is LDL <160 mg/dL.

Table continued on following page

Lipids *(Continued)*

- **When there is evidence of CHD,** the **goal** of therapy is to reduce LDL to ≤100 mg/dL.
  - LDL >100—Do clinical workup and initiate diet or drug therapy.
  - LDL ≤100—Individualize instruction on diet and physical activity and repeat lipoprotein analysis annually.

*N/A = not applicable.
SOURCE: From the Second Report of the Expert Panel on Detection, Evaluation and Treatment of High Blood Cholesterol in Adults, National Heart, Lung, and Blood Institute, National Institutes of Health, NIH Pub. No. 93-3095, September 1993.

plasm in which the cells resemble cartilage cells and the tumor appears to be cartilaginous.

chondrocalcinosis (kŏn″drō-kăl″sĭn-ō′sĭs) [″ + L. *calx,* lime, + Gr. *osis,* condition] Pseudogout; chronic recurrent arthritis clinically similar to gout. The crystals found in the synovial fluid are calcium pyrophosphate dihydrate and not urate crystals. The most commonly involved joint is the knee.

chondroclast (kŏn′drō-klăst) [″ + *klastos,* broken into bits] A giant cell involved in the absorption of cartilage.

chondrocostal (kŏn″drō-kŏs′tăl) [″ + L. *costa,* rib] Pert. to the ribs and costal cartilages.

chondrocranium (kŏn-drō-krā′nē-ŭm) [″ + *kranion,* head] The cartilaginous embryonic cranium before ossification.

chondrocyte (kŏn′drō-sīt) [″ + *kytos,* cell] A cartilage cell.

chondrodermatitis nodularis chronica helicis Growth of nodules on the helix of the ear.

chondrodynia (kŏn″drō-dĭn′ē-ă) [″ + *odyne,* pain] Pain in or about a cartilage.

chondrodysplasia (kŏn″drō-dĭs-plā′zē-ă) [″ + Gr. *dys,* bad, + *plasis,* a molding] A disease, usually hereditary, resulting in disordered growth. It is marked by multiple exostoses of the epiphyses, esp. of the long bones, metacarpals, and phalanges. SYN: *dyschondroplasia.*

chondrodystrophy (kŏn″drō-dĭs′trō-fē) [″ + ″ + *trophe,* nourishment] Achondroplasia.

chondroendothelioma (kŏn″drō-ĕn″dō-thē″lē-ō′mă) [″ + *endon,* within, + *thele,* nipple, + *oma,* tumor] An endothelioma that contains cartilage.

chondroepiphysitis (kŏn″drō-ĕp″ĭ-fĭz-ī′tĭs) [″ + *epiphysis,* a growing on, + *itis,* inflammation] Inflammation of the epiphyseal portion of the bone and the attached cartilage.

chondrofibroma (kŏn″drō-fī-brō′mă) [″ + L. *fibra,* fiber, + Gr. *oma,* tumor] A mixed tumor with elements of chondroma and fibroma.

chondrogenesis (kŏn″drō-jĕn′ĕ-sĭs) [″ + *genesis,* generation, birth] Formation of cartilage. **chondrogenic** (-jĕn′ĭk), *adj.*

chondroid (kŏn′droyd) [″ + *eidos,* form, shape] Resembling cartilage; cartilaginous.

chondroitin (kŏn-drō′ĭ-tĭn) A glycosaminoglycan (complex polysaccharide) present in connective tissue, including the cornea and cartilage. It is promoted as a dietary supplement for use in the treatment of joint pain, usually with glucosamine.

chondrolipoma (kŏn-drō-lĭp-ō′mă) [″ + *lipos,* fat, + *oma,* tumor] A tumor made of cartilaginous and fatty tissue.

chondrology (kŏn-drŏl′ō-jē) [″ + *logos,* word, reason] The scientific study of cartilage.

chondrolysis (kŏn-drŏl′ĭ-sĭs) [″ + *lysis,* dissolution] The breaking down and absorption of cartilage.

chondroma (kŏn-drō′mă) [″ + *oma,* tumor] A slow-growing, painless cartilaginous tumor. It may occur wherever there is cartilage. **chondromatous** (-ă-tŭs), *adj.*

chondromalacia (kŏn-drō-măl-ā′shē-ă) [″ + *malakia,* softness] Softening of the articular cartilage, usually involving the patella.

chondromatosis (kŏn″drō-mă-tō′sĭs) [″ + *oma,* tumor, + *osis,* condition] Formation of multiple chondromas of the hands and feet; often occurs in joint spaces.

chondromucin (kŏn″drō-mū′sĭn) Chondromucoid.

chondromucoid (kŏn″drō-mū′koyd) [″ + L. *mucus,* mucus, + Gr. *eidos,* form, shape] A basophilic glycoprotein present in the interstitial substance of cartilage. SYN: *chondromucin.*

chondromucoprotein (kŏn″drō-mū″kō-prō′tē-ĭn) [″ + ″ + *protos,* first] The ground substance (the fluid or solid material) that occupies the space between the cells and fibers of cartilage.

chondromyoma (kŏn″drō-mī-ō′mă) [″ + *mys,* muscle, + *oma,* tumor] A combined myoma and cartilaginous neoplasm.

chondromyxoma (kŏn″drō-mĭks-ō′mă) [″ + *myxa,* mucus, + *oma,* tumor] A chondroma with myxomatous elements.

chondromyxosarcoma (kŏn-drō-mĭk″sō-săr-kō′mă) [″ + ″ + *sarx,* flesh, + *oma,* tumor] A cartilaginous and sarcomatous tumor.

chondro-osseus (kŏn″drō-ŏs′ē-ŭs) [″ + L. *osseus,* bony] Composed of cartilage and bone.

chondro-osteodystrophy (kŏn″drō-ŏs″tē-ō-dĭs′trō-fē) [″ + *osteon,* bone, + *dys,* bad, + *trophe,* nourishment] Mucopolysaccharidosis IV.

chondropathology (kŏn″drō-pă-thŏl′ō-jē) [Gr. *chondros,* cartilage, + *pathos,* disease, + *logos,* word, reason] The pathology of cartilage disease.

chondropathy (kŏn-drŏp′ă-thē) Any disease of cartilage.

chondroplasia (kŏn″drō-plā′zē-ă) [″ + *plassein,* to mold] The formation of cartilage.

chondroplast (kŏn′drō-plăst) Chondroblast.

chondroplasty (kŏn′drō-plăs″tē) [″ + *plassein,* to mold] Plastic or reparative surgery on cartilage.

chondroporosis (kŏn″drō-pō-rō′sĭs) [″ + *poros,* passage] The porous condition of pathological or normal cartilage during ossification.

chondroprotection (kŏn-drō-prō-tĕk′shŭn) **1.** Cartilage preservation. **2.** The potential of some drugs or nutrients to prevent the degradation of cartilage that occurs with various forms of arthritis.

chondroprotein (kŏn-drō-prō′tē-ĭn) [″ + *protos,* first] Any of a group of glucoproteins found in cartilage, tendons, and connective tissue.

chondrosarcoma (kŏn-drō-săr-kō′mă) [″ + *sarx,* flesh, + *oma,* tumor] A cartilaginous sarcoma.

chondrosin (kŏn′drō-sĭn) Previously used term for material produced when chondroitin sulfate is hydrolyzed.

chondrosis (kŏn-drō′sĭs) [″ + *osis,* condition] The development of cartilage.

chondrosternal (kŏn″drō-stĕr′năl) [″ + *sternon,* chest] Pert. to sternal cartilage.

chondrosternoplasty (kŏn″drō-stĕr′nō-plăs″tē) [″ + ″ + *plassein,* to mold] Surgical correction of a deformed sternum.

chondrotome (kŏn′drō-tōm) [″ + *tome,* incision] A device for cutting cartilage.

chondrotomy (kŏn-drŏt′ō-mē) Dissection or surgical division of cartilage.

chondroxiphoid (kŏn″drō-zī′foyd) [″ + *xiphos,* sword, + *eidos,* form, shape] Pert. to the sternum and the xiphoid process.

Chondrus [L., cartilage] A genus of red algae that includes *Chondrus crispus,* the source of carrageenan, a mucilaginous substance used as an emulsifying agent. *Chondrus* is commonly called Irish moss or carrageen.

choosing death Deciding to die. In particular, an individual may choose to withdraw from chronic kidney dialysis with no medical reason for withdrawing. In one study, stopping dialysis in this situation was three times more common in patients treated at home than in those treated at dialysis centers. SEE: *death; death with dignity; do not attempt resuscitation; suicide.*

Chopart's amputation (shō-părz′) [François Chopart, Fr. surgeon, 1743–1795] Disarticulation at the midtarsal joint.

chorda (kor′dă) *pl.* **chordae** [Gr. *chorde,* cord] A cord or tendon.

c. dorsalis Notochord.

c. gubernaculum An embryonic structure forming a part of the gubernaculum testis in males and the round ligament in females.

c. obliqua The oblique ligament, an oblique cord that connects the shafts of the radius and ulna. It extends from the lateral side of the tubercle of the ulna to a point just below the radial tuberosity.

c. tendinea One of several small tendinous cords that connect the free edges of the atrioventricular valves to the papillary muscles and prevent inversion of these valves during ventricular systole.

c. tympani A branch of the facial nerve that leaves the cranium through the stylomastoid foramen, traverses the tympanic cavity, and joins a branch of the lingual nerve. Efferent fibers innervate the submandibular and sublingual glands; afferent fibers convey taste impulses from the anterior two thirds of the tongue.

c. umbilicalis The umbilical cord connecting the fetus and placenta.

c. vocalis The vocal folds of the larynx.

c. willisii One of several fibrous cords across the superior longitudinal sinus of the brain.

chordal (kor′dăl) Pert. to a chorda, esp. the notochord.

Chordata (kor-dā′tă) [LL., notochord] A phylum of the animal kingdom including all animals that have a notochord during their development (i.e., all vertebrates).

chordee (kor-dē′) [Fr., corded] Painful downward curvature of the penis during erection. It occurs in congenital anomaly (hypospadia) or in urethral infection such as gonorrhea. SEE: *Peyronie's disease.*

chorditis (kor-dī′tĭs) [Gr. *chorde,* cord, + *itis,* inflammation] Inflammation of the spermatic or vocal cord.

c. nodosa Singer's node.

chordoma (kor-dō′mă) [″ + *oma,* tumor] A rare type of tumor that occurs at any place along the vertebral column. It is composed of embryonic nerve tissue and vacuolated physaliform cells. The neoplasm may cause death because of its surgical inaccessibility and the damage caused by the expanding tissue.

chordotomy (kor-dŏt′ō-mē) Cordotomy.

chorea (kō-rē′ă) [Gr. *choreia,* dance] Involuntary dancing or writhing of the limbs or facial muscles. **choreal** (kō-rē'al, kō'rē-ăl), *adj.*

acute c. Sydenham's chorea.

Bergeron's c. Electric c.

chronic c. Huntington's c.

electric c. A rare form of chorea marked by sudden involuntary contraction of a muscle group. This causes violent movements as if the patient had been stimulated by an electric current. SYN: *Bergeron's c.; Dubini's disease.*

epidemic c. Dancing mania; uncontrolled dancing. It was manifested in the 14th century in Europe. SYN: *dancing mania.*

c. gravidarum A form of Sydenham's chorea seen in some pregnant women, usually in those who have had chorea before, esp. in their first pregnancy. SEE: *Sydenham's chorea.*

Henoch's c. A form of progressive electric chorea.

hereditary c. Huntington's chorea.

Huntington's c. SEE: *Huntington's chorea.*

hyoscine c. Movements simulating chorea and sometimes accompanied by delirium, seen in acute scopolamine intoxication.

hysteric c. A form of hysteria with choreiform movements.

mimetic c. Chorea caused by imitative movements.

c. minor Sydenham's chorea.

posthemiplegic c. Chorea affecting partially paralyzed muscles subsequent to a hemiplegic attack.

sporadic c. of the elderly A mild, usually benign disorder of adults marked by chorea-like movements and mild cognitive deficits. It may be related to Huntington's chorea. SEE: *Huntington's chorea.*

choreiform (kō-rē'ĭ-form) [Gr. *choreia,* dance, + L. *forma,* form] Of the nature of chorea.

choreoathetoid (kō″rē-ō-ăth'ĕ-toyd) [″ + *athetos,* not fixed, + *eidos,* form, shape] Pert. to choreoathetosis.

choreoathetosis (kō″rē-ō-ăth″ĕ-tō'sĭs) [″ + ″ + *osis,* condition] A type of athetosis frequently seen in cerebral palsy, marked by extreme range of motion, jerky involuntary movements that are more proximal than distal, and muscle tone fluctuating from hypotonia to hypertonia.

chorioadenoma (kō″rē-ō-ăd″ĕn-ō'mă) [Gr. *chorion,* outer membrane enclosing an embryo, + *aden,* gland, + *oma,* tumor] A rare glandular tumor of the outermost embryonic membrane.

c. destruens A type of hydatidiform mole in which the chorionic villi penetrate the myometrium.

chorioallantois (kō″rē-ō-ă-lăn'tō-ĭs) In embryology, the membrane formed by the union of the chorion and allantois. In the human embryo, this develops into the placenta.

chorioamnionitis (kō″rē-ō-ăm″nē-ō-nī'tĭs) [″ + *amnion,* lamb, + *itis,* inflammation] Inflammation of the amnion, usually secondary to bacterial infection. This condition is an obstetric emergency that may cause conditions such as pneumonia, meningitis, or sepsis in the neonate, and bacteremia or sepsis in the mother.

ETIOLOGY: The most common infectious agents are *Bacteroides* species, *Escherichia coli,* streptococci, and *Prevotella* species.

TREATMENT: Intravenous antibiotics active against the most commonly implicated organisms are given. Typically, these include ampicillin and gentamicin, vancomycin, clindamycin, or metronidazole. SYN: *amnionitis.*

chorioangioma (kō″rē-ō-ăn-jē-ō'mă) [″ + *angeion,* vessel, + *oma,* tumor] A vascular tumor of the chorion.

choriocapillaris (kō″rē-ō-kăp-ĭl-lā'rĭs) [Gr. *choroeides,* resembling a membrane, + L. *capillaris,* hairlike] The capillary layer of choroid.

choriocarcinoma (kō″rē-ō-kăr″sĭ-nō'mă) [Gr. *chorion,* + *karkinoma,* cancer] An extremely rare, very malignant neoplasm, usually of the uterus but sometimes at the site of an ectopic pregnancy. Although the actual cause is unknown, it may occur following a hydatid mole, a normal pregnancy, or an abortion. This cancer may respond dramatically to combined modality therapy using surgery and chemotherapy. SYN: *chorioepithelioma; gestational trophoblastic disease.*

choriocele (kō'rē-ō-sēl) [Gr. *choroeides,* resembling a membrane, + *kele,* tumor, swelling] A protrusion of the choroid coat of the eye through a defective sclera.

chorioepithelioma (kō″rē-ō-ĕp″ĭ-thē″lē-ō'mă) Choriocarcinoma.

choriogenesis (kō″rē-ō-jĕn'ĕ-sĭs) [Gr. *chorion,* chorion, + *genesis,* generation, birth] Formation of the chorion.

chorioid (kō'rē-oyd) Choroid.

choriomeningitis (kō″rē-ō-mĕn″ĭn-jī'tĭs) [″ + *meninx,* membrane, + *itis,* inflammation] Inflammation of the brain, meninges, and often the choroid plexuses.

lymphocytic c. An acute viral infection of the central nervous system marked by flulike symptoms (fever, malaise, headache). The disease is transmitted to humans from house mice.

chorion (kō'rē-ŏn) [Gr.] An extraembryonic membrane that, in early development, forms the outer wall of the blastocyst. It is formed from the trophoblast and its inner lining of mesoderm. From it develop the chorionic villi, which establish an intimate connection with the endometrium, giving rise to the placenta. SEE: *embryo*, *placenta*, and *umbilical cord* for illus.; *trophoblast*. **chorionic** (kō-rē-ŏn′ĭk), *adj.*

c. frondosum The outer surface of the chorion. Its villi contact the decidua basalis. This is the placental portion of the chorion.

c. laeve The smooth, nonvillous portion of the chorion.

chorionepithelioma (kō″rē-ŏn-ĕp″ĭ-thē″lē-ō′mă) [″ + *epi,* on, + *thele,* nipple, + *oma,* tumor] Choriocarcinoma.

chorionic plate In the placenta, the portion of the chorion attached to the uterus.

chorionic villi The vascular projections from the chorion, which will form the fetal portion of the placenta. SEE: *embryo* for illus.

chorionic villus sampling ABBR: CVS. A procedure for obtaining a sample of the chorionic villi. In one method, a catheter is inserted into the cervix and the outer portion of the membranes surrounding the fetus. Microscopic and chemical examination of the sample is useful in prenatal evaluation of the chromosomal, enzymatic, and DNA status of the fetus. CVS may be performed between gestational weeks 8 and 12 in women who are at high-risk for serious fetal chromosomal abnormalities.

chorionitis (kō″rē-ŏn-ī′tĭs) [″ + *itis,* inflammation] Inflammation of the chorion. SYN: *choroidoretinitis; retinochoroiditis.*

chorioretinal (kō″rē-ō-rĕt′ĭ-năl) Pert. to the choroid and retina. SYN: *retinochoroid.*

chorioretinitis (kō″rē-ō-rĕt″ĭn-ī′tĭs) [Gr. *chorioeides,* skinlike, + L. *rete,* network, + Gr. *itis,* inflammation] Inflammation of the choroid and retina, often caused by infections (such as toxoplasmosis, cytomegalovirus, or tuberculosis) or by multisystem diseases (such as sarcidosis). SYN: *choroidoretinitis.*

chorista (kō-rĭs′tă) [Gr. *choristos,* separated] An error of development in which tissues grow in a displaced position. These tissues are histologically normal.

choristoma (kō-rĭs-tō′mă) [″ + *oma,* tumor] A neoplasm in which embryonic cells grow in parts of the body where they do not belong normally.

choroid (kō′royd) [Gr. *chorioeides,* skinlike] The dark blue vascular layer of the eye between the sclera and retina, extending from the ora serrata to the optic nerve. It consists of blood vessels united by connective tissue containing pigmented cells and contains five layers: the suprachoroid, the layer of large vessels, the layer of medium-sized vessels, the layer of capillaries, and the lamina vitrea (a homogeneous membrane next to the pigmentary layer of the retina). It is a part of the uvea or vascular tunic of the eye. SYN: *chorioid.*

choroideremia (kō-roy-dĕr-ē′mē-ă) [″ + *eremia,* destitution] A hereditary primary choroidal degeneration transmitted as an X-linked trait. In males, the earliest symptom is night blindness followed by constricted visual field and eventual blindness. In females, the condition is nonprogressive and vision is usually normal.

choroiditis (kō″royd-ī′tĭs) [″ + *itis,* inflammation] Inflammation of the choroid.

anterior c. Choroiditis in which outlets of exudation are at the choroidal periphery.

areolar c. Choroiditis in which inflammation spreads from around the macula lutea.

central c. Choroiditis in which exudation is limited to the macula.

diffuse c. Choroiditis in which the fundus is covered with spots.

exudative c. Choroiditis in which the choroid is covered with patches of inflammation.

metastatic c. Choroiditis due to embolism.

suppurative c. Choroiditis in which suppuration occurs.

Tay's c. A familial condition marked by degeneration of the choroid, esp. in the region about the macula lutea. It occurs in aged persons.

choroidocyclitis (kō-roy″dō-sĭk-lī′tĭs) [Gr. *chorioeides,* skinlike, + *kyklos,* a circle, + *itis,* inflammation] Inflammation of the choroid coat and ciliary processes.

choroidoiritis (kō-royd″ō-ī-rī′tĭs) [″+ *iris,* iris, + *itis,* inflammation] Inflammation of the choroid coat and iris.

choroidopathy (kō″roy-dŏp′ă-thē) [″+ *pathos,* disease, suffering] Any disease of the choroid.

choroidoretinitis (kō-royd″ō-rĕt″ĭn-ī′tĭs) [″ + L. *rete,* network, + Gr. *itis,* inflammation] Chorioretinitis.

Christian Science A system of religious teaching based on Christian Scientists' interpretation of Scripture, founded in 1866 by Mary Baker Eddy. The system emphasizes healing of disease by mental and spiritual means.

Christian-Weber disease SEE: *Weber-Christian disease.*

Christmas disease [*Christmas,* family name of the first patient with the disease who was studied] A form of hemophilia in males resulting from Factor IX deficiency. It is transmitted as an X-linked trait. SYN: *hemophilia B.*

Christmas factor ABBR: CF. An obsolete term for coagulation factor IX.

chromaffin (krō-măf′ĭn) [Gr. *chroma,* color, + L. *affinis,* having affinity for] **1.** Staining readily with chromium salts. **2.** Denoting the pigmented cells forming the medulla of the adrenal glands and the paraganglia. SYN: *chromaphil.*

chromaffinoma (krō″măf-ĭ-nō′mă) [″ + ″ + Gr. *oma,* tumor] A chromaffin cell tumor. SYN: *paraganglioma.*

chromaffinopathy (krō″măf-ĭn-ŏp′ă-thē) [″ + ″ + Gr. *pathos,* disease] Any disease of chromaffin tissue.

chromaffin reaction Histological demonstration of cytoplasmic granules containing epinephrine when subjected to stains containing chromium salts. Such granules stain green with ferric chloride, yellow with iodine, and brown with osmic acid.

chromaphil (krō′mă-fĭl) [″ + *philein,* to love] Chromaffin.

chromate (krō′māt) [Gr. *chromatos,* color] A salt of chromic acid. SEE: *potassium chromate.*

chromatic (krō-măt′ĭk) Pert. to color.

chromatid (krō′mă-tĭd) One of the two potential chromosomes formed by DNA replication of each chromosome before mitosis and meiosis. They are joined together at the centromere and separate at the end of metaphase; then the new chromosomes migrate to opposite poles of the cell at anaphase.

chromatin (krō′mă-tĭn) [Gr. *chroma,* color] The deeply staining genetic material present in the nucleus of a cell that is not dividing. It is the largely uncoiled chromosomes, made of DNA and protein.

sex c. SEE: *Barr body.*

chromatin-negative Lacking visible chromatin. It is characteristic of cell nuclei of normal human males. SEE: *Barr body.*

chromatinolysis (krō″mă-tĭn-ŏl′ĭ-sĭs) [″ + *lysis,* dissolution] **1.** Destruction of chromatin. **2.** The emptying of a cell, bacterial or other, by lysis.

chromatinorrhexis (krō″mă-tĭn-or-rĕk′sĭs) [″ + *rhexis,* rupture] Splitting of chromatin.

chromatin-positive Having the sex chromatin (the Barr body); characteristic of nuclei in cells of normal females.

chromatism (krō′mă-tĭzm) [″ + *-ismos,* condition] **1.** Unnatural pigmentation. **2.** A chromatic aberration.

chromatogenous (krō″mă-tŏj′ĕn-ŭs) [″ + *gennan,* to produce] Causing pigmentation or color.

chromatogram (krō-măt′ō-grăm) [″+ *gramma,* something written] A record produced by chromatography.

chromatography (krō″mă-tŏg′ră-fē) [″ + *graphein,* to write] The separation of two or more chemical compounds in a liquid or gaseous mixture by their removal at different rates based on differential solubility and absorption/adsorption. This separation is often accomplished by letting the chemicals percolate through a column of a powdered absorbent or by passing them across the surface of an absorbent paper, among other techniques.

adsorption c. Chromatography accomplished by applying the test material to one end of a sheet or column containing a solid. As the material moves, the various constituents adhere to the surface of the particles of the solid at different distances from the starting point according to their chemical characteristics.

column c. A form of adsorption chromatography in which the adsorptive material is packed into a column.

gas c. An analytical technique in which a sample is separated into its component parts between a gaseous mobile phase and a chemically active stationary phase.

gas-liquid c. ABBR: GLC. Chromatography in which a gas moves over a liquid, and chemical substances are separated on the liquid by their different adsorption rates.

high-performance liquid c. ABBR: HPLC. Application of high pressure to liquid chromatography technique to increase separation speed and enhance resolution. SYN: *high pressure liquid chromatography.*

high pressure liquid c. High-performance liquid c.

paper c. Chromatography in which paper strips are used as the porous solid medium.

partition c. Chromatography in which substances in solution are separated by being exposed to two immiscible solvents. The immobile solvent is located between the spaces of an inert material such as starch, cellulose, or silica. The substances move with the mobile solvent as it passes down the column at a rate governed by their partition coefficient.

thin layer c. ABBR: TLC. Chromatography involving the differential adsorption of substances as they pass through a thin layer or sheet of cellulose or some other inert compound.

chromatoid (krō′mă-toyd) [Gr. *chroma,* color, + *eidos,* form, shape] Staining in the same manner as chromatin.

chromatokinesis (krō″mă-tō-kī-nē′sĭs) [″ + *kinesis,* movement] The movement of chromatin during the division of a cell.

chromatolysis (krō″mă-tŏl′ĭ-sĭs) [″ + *lysis,* dissolution] The dissolution of chromophil substance (Nissl bodies) in neurons in certain pathological conditions, or following injury to the cell body or axon. SYN: *chromolysis; karyolysis.*

chromatometer (krō-mă-tŏm′ĕt-ĕr) [″

+ *metron,* measure] A scale of colors for testing color perception.

chromatophil, chromatophilic (krō′mă-tō-fĭl″, krō″mă-tō-fĭl′ĭk) [″ + *philein,* to love] Staining easily.

chromatophore (krō-măt′ō-for) [″ + *phoros,* bearing] A pigment-bearing cell.

chromatopsia (krō″mă-tŏp′sē-ă) [″ + *opsis,* vision] Abnormally colored vision.

chromatoptometry (krō″măt-ŏp-tŏm′ĕ-trē) [″ + *optos,* visible, + *metron,* measure] Measurement of color perception.

chromatosis (krō″mă-tō′sĭs) [″ + *osis,* condition] **1.** Pigmentation. **2.** The pathological deposition of pigment in any part of the body where it is not normally present, or excessive deposition where it is normally present.

chromaturia (krō-mă-tū′rē-ă) [″ + *ouron,* urine] Abnormal color of the urine.

chromesthesia (krō″mĕs-thē′zē-ă) [″ + *aisthesis,* sensation] The association of color sensations with words, taste, smell, or sounds.

chromidrosis, chromhidrosis (krō″mĭd-rō′sĭs) [″ + *hidros,* sweat] Excretion of colored sweat. Red sweat may be caused by an exudation of blood into the sweat glands or by color-producing microorganisms in those glands. This disorder is treated by relief of the underlying condition.

ETIOLOGY: Colored sweat may be due to ingestion or absorption of certain substances, such as pigment-producing bacteria. It may also be caused by certain metabolic disorders.

SYMPTOMS: Colored sweat may be localized in the eyelids, breasts, axillae, and genitocrural regions, and occasionally on the hands and limbs. It may be grayish, bluish, violaceous, brownish, or reddish; it collects on skin, giving a greasy, powdery appearance to parts.

chromium (krō′mē-ŭm) [L., color] SYMB: Cr. A very hard, metallic element; atomic weight 51.996, atomic number 24. It is an essential trace element required for normal uptake.

chromium-51 A radioactive isotope of chromium. The half-life is 27.7 days. Red blood cells are labeled with this isotope in order to study their length of life in the body.

chromium poisoning Toxicity caused by excess chromium (e.g., in mining, welding, or pigment manufacturing). It may cause contact dermatitis, skin burns, or lung, liver, or kidney damage. Treatment after ingestion consists of gastrointestinal irrigation followed by forced diuresis and alkalinization of urine.

chromoblast (krō′mō-blăst) [Gr. *chroma,* color, + *blastos,* germ] An embryonic cell that becomes a pigment cell.

chromocenter (krō′mō-sĕn″tĕr) [″ + *kentros,* middle] Karyosome.

chromocyte (krō′mō-sīt) [″ + *kytos,* cell] Any colored cell.

chromodacryorrhea (krō″mō-dăk″rē-ō-rē′ă) [″ + *dacryon,* tear, + *rhoia,* flow] A flow of blood-stained tears.

chromogen (krō′mō-jĕn) [″ + *gennan,* to produce] Any chemical that may be changed into a colored material.

chromogenesis (krō″mō-jĕn′ĕ-sĭs) [″ + *genesis,* generation, birth] Production of pigment.

chromolipoid (krō″mō-lĭp′oyd) [″ + *lipos,* fat, + *eidos,* form, shape] Lipochrome.

chromolysis (krō-mŏl′ĭ-sĭs) Chromatolysis.

chromomere (krō′mō-mēr) [Gr. *chroma,* color, + *meros,* part] One of a series of chromatin granules found in a chromosome.

chromomycosis (krō″mō-mī-kō′sĭs) [″ + *myxa,* mucus, + *osis,* condition] A chronic fungal skin infection marked by itching and warty plaques on the skin and subcutaneous swellings of the feet, legs, and other exposed areas. Various fungi have been implicated, including *Phialophora verrucosa, P. pedrosoi, P. compacta,* and *Cladosporium carrionii.* Some of these are also called *Fonsecaea pedrosoi* and *F. compacta.*

chromopexic, chromopectic (krō″mō-pĕk′sĭk, -pĕk′tĭk) [″ + *pexis,* fixation] Pert. to fixation of coloring matter, as the liver function in forming bilirubin.

chromophane (krō′mō-făn) [″ + *phainein,* to show] Retinal pigment of some animal species.

chromophil(e) (krō′mō-fĭl, -fīl) [″ + *philein,* to love] **1.** Any structure that stains easily. **2.** One of two types of cells present in the pars distalis of the pituitary gland. It is considered a secretory cell.

chromophilic, chromophilous (krō-mō-fĭl′ĭk, krō-mŏf′ĭl-ŭs) Staining readily.

chromophobe (krō′mō-fōb) [″ + *phobos,* fear] Any cell or tissue that stains either poorly or not at all. A type of cell found in the pars distalis of the pituitary gland.

chromophobia (krō″mō-fō′bē-ă) The condition of staining poorly. **chromophobic** (-bĭk), *adj.*

chromophore (krō′mō-for) [″ + *pherein,* to bear] Any chemical that displays color when present in a cell that has been prepared properly. **chromophoric** (-for′ĭk), *adj.*

chromophose (krō′mō-fōz) [″ + *phos,* light] A subjective sensation of a spot of color in the eye.

chromoprotein (krō″mō-prō′tē-ĭn) [″ + *protos,* first] One of a group of conjugated proteins consisting of a protein combined with hematin or another colored, metal-containing, prosthetic

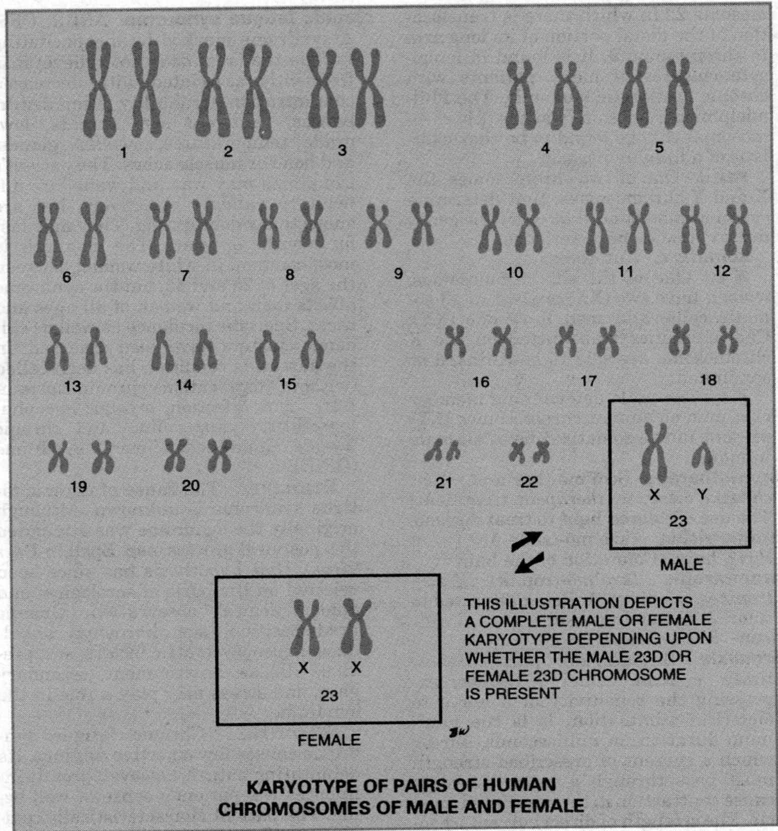

KARYOTYPE OF PAIRS OF HUMAN CHROMOSOMES OF MALE AND FEMALE

group (e.g., hemoglobin, hemocyanin, chlorophyll, flavoproteins, cytochromes).

chromosomal map SEE: *gene mapping*.

chromosome (krō′mō-sōm) [Gr. *chroma*, color, + *soma*, body] A linear strand made of DNA (and associated proteins in eukaryotic cells) that carries genetic information. Chromosomes stain deeply with basic dyes and are especially conspicuous during mitosis. The normal diploid number of chromosomes is constant for each species. For humans, the diploid number is 46 (23 pairs in all somatic cells). In the formation of gametes (ovum and spermatozoon), the number is reduced to one half (haploid number); that is, the ovum and sperm each contain 23 chromosomes. Of these, 22 are autosomes and one is the sex chromosome (X or Y). At fertilization, the chromosomes from the sperm unite with the chromosomes from the ovum. This random union determines the sex of the embryo. The female sex chromosome from the ovum always contributes an X to the embryo. The male sex chromosome may contribute an X or a Y to join with the chromosome derived from the ovum. Thus the embryo may have an XX pair of sex chromosomes, which will produce a girl, or an XY pair, which will produce a boy. SEE: illus; *Barr body; centromere; chromatid; cytogenetics; dominant; gene; heredity; karyotype; mutation; recessive; telomere*.

accessory c. An unpaired sex chromosome. SEE: *sex chromosome*.

banded c. A chromosome specially stained to delineate bands of various width on its regions or loci. This facilitates analysis and investigation of genes and gene-related illnesses.

bivalent c. A double chromosome resulting from the conjugation of two homologous chromosomes in synapsis, which occurs during the first meiotic division.

homologous c. One of a pair of chromosomes that contain genes for the same traits; one is maternal in origin, the other paternal.

Philadelphia c. An abnormal chromosome 22 in which there is translocation of the distal portion of its long arm to chromosome 9. It is found in leukocyte cultures of many patients with chronic myelocytic leukemia. The Philadelphia chromosome was the first chromosomal change found to be characteristic of a human disease.

sex c. One of two chromosomes, the X and Y chromosomes, that determine sex in humans and that carry the genes for sex-linked characteristics.

somatic c. Autosome.

X c. One of the sex chromosomes; women have two (XX) present in all somatic cells, and men have one (XY). Characteristics transmitted on the X chromosome are said to be X-linked or sex-linked.

Y c. The male-determining member of a pair of human chromosomes (XY) present in the somatic cells of all male humans.

chromotherapy (krō″mō-thĕr′ă-pē) [Gr. *chroma,* color, + *therapeia,* treatment] The use of colored light to treat disease.

chromotrichia (krō″mō-trĭk′ē-ă) [″ + *thrix,* hair] Coloration of the hair.

chromotropic (krō″mō-trŏp′ĭk) [″ + *tropikos,* turning] **1.** Being attracted to color. **2.** Attracting color.

chron- SEE: *chrono-*.

chronaxie (krō′năk-sē) [Gr. *chronos,* time, + *axia,* value] A number expressing the sensitivity of a nerve to electrical stimulation. It is the minimum duration, in milliseconds, during which a current of prescribed strength must pass through a motor nerve to cause contraction in the associated muscle. The strength of direct current (rheobasic voltage) that will just suffice if given an indefinite time is first determined, and exactly double this strength is used for the final determinations.

chronic [Gr. *chronos,* time] **1.** Of long duration. **2.** Denoting a disease showing little change or of slow progression; the opposite of acute.

chronic airflow limitation ABBR: CAL. SEE: *chronic obstructive pulmonary disease.*

chronically neurologically impaired ABBR: CNI. Having a general level of intellectual function that is significantly below average and that exists concurrently with deficits in adaptive behavior. These behavioral changes may first appear in childhood or may develop after head trauma or stroke. This condition is sometimes called "organic brain syndrome" in adults or "mental retardation" in children. Chronically neurologically impaired children are often grouped epidemiologically with persons who have other developmental disabilities including chronic epilepsy, autism, and cerebral palsy.

chronic desquamating eosinophilic bronchitis Asthma.

chronic fatigue syndrome ABBR: CFS. A syndrome marked by incapacitating fatigue that rest does not relieve; it is frequently associated with decreased concentration, irritability, sleep disturbances, recurrent sore throats, low-grade temperatures, swollen glands, and bone or muscle aches. The patient's symptoms may wax and wane, are difficult to validate objectively, but are subjectively debilitating. They may last for months or years. The diagnosis is most common in white women between the ages of 25 and 45, but the syndrome affects men and women of all ages and races. Sporadic incidence as well as epidemic clusters have been observed. In the past, this condition has been called (without justification) chronic Epstein-Barr virus infection, myalgic encephalomyelitis, "yuppie flu," and chronic fatigue immunodeficiency syndrome (CFIDS).

ETIOLOGY: The cause of chronic fatigue syndrome is unknown. Although originally the syndrome was attributed to a postviral process (esp. Epstein-Barr virus), that hypothesis has since been rejected on the basis of serological and epidemiological observation. Genetic predisposition, age, hormonal imbalance, neuropsychiatric factors, sex, previous illness, environment, secondary gain, and stress may play a role in the syndrome.

SYMPTOMS: Chronic fatigue syndrome causes few objective findings. Its debilitating nature, however, greatly influences the patient's sense of well-being. The patient characteristically complains of prolonged, overwhelming fatigue, along with sore throat, myalgia, and cognitive dysfunction. No definitive test exists for this disorder. Diagnostic studies should include tests to rule out other similar clinical illnesses.

TREATMENT: Because there is no known cause, treatment focuses on supportive care. Nonsteroidal anti-inflammatory drugs (NSAIDs) may be useful for myalgia or arthralgias; low doses of tricyclic antidepressants sometimes enhance pain control and also may be useful for patients having trouble sleeping. Complex immunological or metabolic therapies have not proven effective.

PATIENT CARE: Activity level and degree of fatigue during activities of daily living are assessed. The patient's emotional response to the illness and coping abilities are evaluated. Emotional support is provided through the long period of diagnostic testing and the protracted, sometimes discouraging course of the illness. Patients are referred for mental health or career counseling as needed or to a local support group if available to help the patient lead as normal a life as possible. Activities should be reduced when fatigue is greatest, but bedrest other than that required for sleep should be avoided because it does not relieve disability. The patient should participate in a graded exercise program, which may be difficult to initiate and maintain but may help him or her feel better. Exercise should be carried out for short periods and slowly increased, to avoid increasing fatigue.

chronicity (krŏn-ĭs′ĭt-ē) The condition of being long lasting or of showing little or slow progress.

chronic sorrow A cyclical, recurring, and potentially progressive pattern of pervasive sadness that is experienced by a parent or caregiver, or individual with chronic illness or disability in response to continual loss, throughout the trajectory of an illness or disability. SEE: *Nursing Diagnoses Appendix.*

This diagnosis was accepted at the NANDA 13th Conference, 1998.

chrono- [Gr. *chronos,* time] Combining form meaning *time* or *timing.*

chronobiology (krŏn″ō-bī-ŏl′ō-jē) [Gr. *chronos,* time, + *bios,* life, + *logos,* word, reason] The study of the effects of time on biochemistry, the release of hormones, sleeping and waking cycles, and related aspects of plant and animal life. SEE: *circadian; clock, biological.*

chronognosis (krŏn″ŏg-nō′sĭs) [″ + *gnosis,* knowledge] The subjective realization of the passage of time.

chronograph (krŏn′ō-grăf) [″ + *graphein,* to write] A device for recording intervals of time.

chronological (krŏn″ō-lŏj′ĭ-kăl) [″ + *logos,* word, reason] Occurring in natural sequence according to time.

chronopharmacology A method used in pharmacokinetics to describe the diurnal changes in plasma drug concentrations.

chronophobia Fear of time or its perceived duration, esp. in prisoners.

chronotaraxis (krō-nō-tăr-ăk′sĭs) [″ + *taraxis,* without order] Being unable to orient oneself with respect to time.

chronotropic (krŏn″ō-trŏp′ĭk) [″ + *tropikos,* turning] Influencing the rate of occurrence of an event, such as the heartbeat. SEE: *inotropic.*

chronotropism [″ + ″ + *-ismos,* condition] Interference with periodic events such as the heartbeat.

negative c. Deceleration of the rate of an event such as the heartbeat.

positive c. Acceleration of the rate of an event such as the heartbeat.

chrysarobin (krĭs″ă-rō′bĭn) [Gr. *chrysos,* gold, + Brazilian *araraba,* bark] A mixture of neutral principles obtained from goa powder, which is deposited in the wood of Araroba, a leguminous tree of South America. It is used topically as an ointment for treatment of certain skin disorders. It promotes the growth of skin tumors in laboratory animals.

chrysiasis (krĭ-sī′ă-sĭs) **1.** Gray patches of skin discoloration after therapeutic administration of gold. **2.** Deposition of gold in tissues. SYN: *auriasis.*

chrysoderma (krĭs″ō-dĕr′mă) [″ + *derma,* skin] Discoloration of the skin due to deposition of gold.

chrysotherapy (krĭs″ō-thĕr′ă-pē) [″ + *therapeia,* treatment] The medical use of gold compounds, e.g., in rheumatoid arthritis.

chunking (chŭn′kĭng) A strategy for improving memory and learning, in which information is arranged into manageable clusters ("chunks") of data. SYN: *grouping.*

Churg-Strauss syndrome (chŭrg-strŏws) [Jacob Churg, U.S. pathologist, b. 1910; Lotte Strauss, U.S. pathologist, b. 1913] A rare systemic vasculitis affecting the respiratory, musculoskeletal, cardiac, and peripheral nervous systems. It typically develops in patients with a history of asthma or allergy and is marked by hypereosinophilia.

Chvostek's sign (vōs′tĕks) [Franz Chvostek, Austrian surgeon, 1835–1884] A spasm of the facial muscles following a tap on the facial nerve; seen in hypocalcemic tetany.

chylangioma (kī″lăn-jē-ō′mă) [Gr. *chylos,* juice, + *angeion,* vessel, + *oma,* tumor] A tumor of the intestinal lymph vessels containing chyle.

chyle (kīl) [Gr. *chylos,* juice] The milk-like, alkaline contents of the lacteals and lymphatic vessels of the intestine, consisting of digestive products and principally absorbed fats. It is carried by the lymphatic vessels to the cisterna chyli, then through the thoracic duct to the left subclavian vein, where it enters the bloodstream. A large amount forms in 24 hr.

chylemia (kī-lē′mē-ă) [″ + *haima,* blood] Chyle in the peripheral circulation.

chylifacient, chylifactive (kī″lĭ-fā′shĕnt, kī-lĭ-făk′tĭv) [″ + L. *facere,* to make] Forming chyle.

chylifaction, chylification (kī-lĭ-făk′shŭn, kī-lĭ-fĭ-kā′shŭn) Chylopoiesis.

chyliferous (kī-lĭf′ĕr-ŭs) [″ + L. *ferre,* to carry] Carrying chyle.

chyliform (kī′lĭ-form) [″ + L. *forma,* shape] Resembling chyle.

chylocele (kī′lō-sēl) [″ + *kele,* tumor, swelling] Distention of the tunica vaginalis testis with chyle.

chyloderma (kī″lō-dĕr′mă) [″ + *derma,* skin] Lymph accumulated in the enlarged lymphatic vessels and thickened skin of the scrotum. SYN: *elephantiasis, scrotal.*

chylomediastinum (kī″lō-mē″dē-ăs-tī′nŭm) [″ + L. *mediastinum,* median] Chyle in the mediastinum.

chylomicron (kī″lō-mī′krŏn) [″ + *mikros,* small] A lipoprotein molecule formed in the small intestine from digested fats for transport of fats to other tissues.

chylopericardium (kī″lō-pĕr″ĭ-kăr′dē-ŭm) [″ + L. *peri,* around, + Gr. *kardia,* heart] Chyle in the pericardium.

chyloperitoneum (kī″lō-pĕr″ĭ-tō-nē′ŭm) [″ + *peritonaion,* peritoneum] Chyle in the peritoneal cavity.

chylopneumothorax (kī″lō-nū″mō-thō′răks) [″ + *pneumon,* air, + *thorax,* chest] Chyle and air in the pleural space.

chylopoiesis (kī″lō-poy-ē′sĭs) [″ + *poiesis,* production] Formation of chyle and its absorption by lacteals in the intestines. SYN: *chylifaction; chylification.*

chylorrhea (kī″lō-rē′ă) [Gr. *chylos,* juice, + *rhoia,* flow] Escape of chyle resulting from rupture of the thoracic duct.

chylothorax [″ + *thorax,* chest] Chyle in the pleural cavities.

chylous (kī′lŭs) Pert. to or of the nature of chyle.

chyluria (kī-lū′rē-ă) [″ + *ouron,* urine] The presence of chyle in the urine, giving it a milky appearance. SYN: *galacturia.*

chymase (kī′mās) An enzyme in gastric juice that accelerates the action of the pancreatic enzymes.

chyme (kīm) [Gr. *chymos,* juice] The mixture of partly digested food and digestive secretions found in the stomach and small intestine during digestion of a meal. It is a varicolored, thick, nearly liquid mass.

chymopapain (kī-mō-pă′pā-ĭn) An enzyme related to papain.

chymosin (kī′mō-sĭn) [Gr. *chymos,* juice] An enzyme that curdles milk; present in the gastric juice of young ruminants. It is the preferred term for rennin because of possible confusion with the term renin.

chymotrypsin (kī″mō-trĭp′sĭn) [″ + *tryein,* to rub, + *pepsis,* digestion] A digestive enzyme produced by the pancreas and functioning in the small intestine that, with trypsin, hydrolyzes proteins to peptones or amino acids. It can be synthesized and given orally to patients with pancreatic insufficiency.

C.I. *chemotherapeutic index* (parasitology); *color index.*

Ci *curie.*

cib Abbreviation for L. *cibus,* food.

cibophobia (sī″bō-fō′bē-ă) [L. *cibus,* food, + Gr. *phobos,* fear] A morbid aversion to or fear of food.

cicatricotomy (sĭk″ă-trĭk-ŏt′ō-mē) [″ + Gr. *tome,* incision] Incision of a cicatrix or scar.

cicatrix (sĭk′ă-trĭks, sĭk-ā′trĭks) [L.] A scar left by a healed wound. Lack of color is due to an absence of pigmentation. Cicatricial tissue is less elastic than normal tissue, so it usually appears contracted. SEE: *keloid.* **cicatricial** (-trĭsh′ăl), *adj.*

cicatrizant (sĭk-ăt′rĭ-zănt) [L. *cicatrix,* scar] Favoring or causing cicatrization; an agent that aids in scar formation.

cicatrization (sĭk″ă-trĭ-zā′shŭn) Healing by scar formation.

cicatrize (sĭk′ă-trīz) To heal by scar tissue.

cicutism (sĭk′ū-tĭzm) Poisoning resulting from ingestion of *Cicuta maculata* or *C. virosa,* water hemlock.

CID *cervical immobilization device.*

Cieszynski's rule A geometric theorem stating that two triangles are equal if they share one complete side and have two equal angles. In dental radiography, the theorem is applied in the bisecting angle technique to guide film placement and angulation of the central beam of the x-ray. The resulting image on the radiograph is the same length as the projected object. SEE: *technique, bisecting angle.*

ciguatera poisoning (sē″gwă-tā′ră) [Sp. Amer. from W. Indies *cigua,* sea snail] A form of fish poisoning caused by eating fish normally considered safe to eat, such as sea bass, grouper, or snapper. The fish become toxic after ingesting certain dinoflagellates, marine plankton that are the source of toxin. Clinically there is tingling of the lips, tongue, and throat with nausea, vomiting, diarrhea, paralysis, and numbness. There is no specific therapy but treatment of respiratory paralysis may be required.

ciguatoxin (sē″gwă-tŏk′sĭn) The toxic substance (acyclic polyther) that causes ciguatera poisoning. The toxin interferes with nerve impulse transmission by altering cell membrane sodium channel polarization.

cilia (sĭl′ē-ă) *sing.,* **cilium** [L. eyelid] **1.** Eyelashes. **2.** Threadlike projections from the free surface of certain epithelial cells such as those lining the trachea, bronchi, and some reproductive ducts (e.g., the fallopian tubes). They propel or sweep materials, such as mucus or dust, across a surface, such as the respiratory tract. SEE: illus.

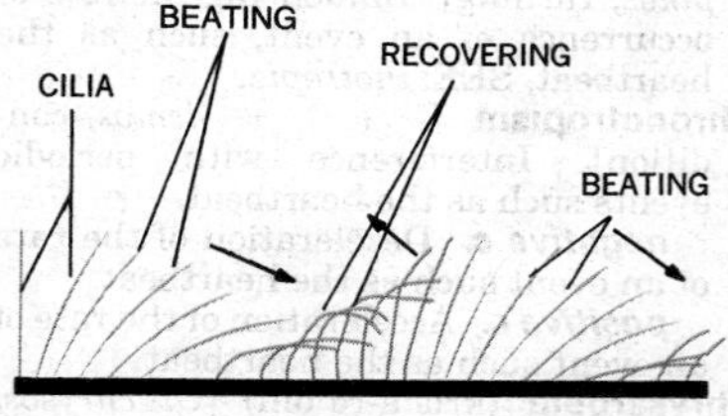

ACTION OF CILIA

immotile c. syndrome A group of inherited conditions characterized by severely impaired movement of the cilia or flagella of the respiratory tract epithelium, sperm, and other cells. Sperm flagella and respiratory tract cilia lack the protein dynein, essential to ciliary movement. SYN: *Kartagener's syndrome*.

ciliariscope (sĭl″ē-ă′rĭ-skōp) [L. *ciliaris,* pert. to eyelid, + Gr. *skopein,* to examine] An instrument for examining the ciliary region of the eye.

ciliarotomy (sĭl″ē-ă-rŏt′ō-mē) [″ + Gr. *tome,* incision] Surgical section of the ciliary zone in glaucoma.

ciliary (sĭl′ē-ĕr″ē) [L. *ciliaris,* pert. to eyelid] Pertaining to any hairlike processes, esp. the eyelashes, and to eye structures such as the ciliary body.

ciliary apparatus Ciliary body.

ciliary artery Any of the branches of the ophthalmic artery that supply the choroid layer.

ciliary muscle The smooth muscle forming a part of the ciliary body of the eye. Contraction pulls the choroid forward, lessening tension on the fibers of the zonula (suspensory ligament) and allowing the lens, which is elastic, to become more spherical. Accommodation for near vision is accomplished by this process.

ciliary nerve, long One of the two or three branches of the nasal nerves supplying the ciliary muscle, iris, and cornea.

ciliary nerve, short One of the several branches of the ciliary ganglion supplying the ciliary muscle, iris, and tunics of the eyeball.

Ciliata (sĭl″ē-ă′tă) Formerly a class of protozoa characterized by locomotion by cilia. Now called Ciliophora, a phylum of the kingdom Protista.

ciliate (sĭl′ē-āt) [L. *cilia,* eyelids] Ciliated.

ciliated (sĭl′ē-ā-tĕd) Possessing cilia.

ciliectomy (sĭl″ē-ĕk′tō-mē) [″ + Gr. *ektome,* excision] Excision of a portion of the ciliary body or ciliary border of the eyelid.

ciliogenesis (sĭl″ē-ō-jĕn′ĕ-sĭs) Formation of cilia.

Ciliophora A phylum of the kingdom Protista that includes unicellular and colonial forms possessing cilia for locomotion. Some are free living and others are parasitic species such as *Balantidium coli*.

ciliospinal (sĭl″ē-ō-spī′năl) [″ + *spinalis,* pert. to a spine] Pert. to the ciliary body and spinal cord.

ciliostatic (sĭl″ē-ō-stăt′ĭk) [″ + Gr. *statos,* placed] Interfering with or preventing movement of the cilia.

ciliotomy (sĭl″ē-ŏt′ō-mē) [″ + Gr. *tome,* incision] Surgical cutting of the ciliary nerve.

ciliotoxicity The action of anything that interferes with ciliary motion.

cilium (sĭl′ē-ŭm) [L.] Sing. of cilia.

cillosis (sĭl-ō′sĭs) [L.] Spasmodic twitching of the eyelid.

cimbia (sĭm′bē-ă) [L.] A slender band of white fibers crossing the ventral surface of a cerebral peduncle.

cimetidine An H_2-receptor antagonist that inhibits the secretion of stomach acid. It is primarily used to treat peptic ulcers and gastroesophageal reflux disease. Trade name is Tagamet. SEE: *peptic ulcer*.

Cimex lectularius (sī′mĕks lĕk-tū-lā′rē-ŭs) The bedbug. An insect belonging to the order Hemiptera. SYN: *Acanthia lectularia*. SEE: *bedbug*.

cimicosis (sĭm″ĭ-kō′sĭs) Itching due to the bite of a bedbug.

CIN *cervical intraepithelial neoplasia.*

CINAHL *Cumulative Index to Nursing and Allied Health Literature,* an index of literature related to nursing and allied health. The index is available in electronic form from 1982 on.

CINAHL-CD A computer-accessible index to nursing and allied health literature. SEE: *CINAHL*.

cinchona (sĭn-kō′nă, -chō′nă) [Sp. *cinchon,* Countess of Cinchon] The dried bark of the tree from which the antimalarial quinine is derived. SEE: *quinine*.

cinchonism (sĭn′kŏn-ĭzm) [″ + Gr. *-ismos,* condition] Poisoning from cinchona or its alkaloids. SYN: *quininism*.

cinclisis (sĭn′klĭ-sĭs) [Gr. *kinklisis,* a wagging] Swift spasmodic movement of any part of the body.

cine- [Gr. *kinesis,* movement] Combining form indicating a relationship to movement.

cineangiocardiography (sĭn″ē-ăn″jē-ō-kăr″dē-ŏg′ră-fē) [Gr. *kinesis,* movement, + *angeion,* vessel, + *kardia,* heart, + *graphein,* to write] Cinefluorographic imaging of the heart chambers or coronary vessels after injection of a radiopaque contrast medium. SEE: *cardiac catheterization*.

radionuclide c. The use of a scintillation camera to record and project the image of a radioisotope as it travels through the heart and great vessels.

cinefluorography (sĭn″ē-floo″or-ŏg′ră-fē) The production of moving images during image-intensified fluoroscopy.

cinematics (sĭn″ĕ-măt′ĭks) [Gr. *kinema,* motion] The science of motion; kinematics.

cinematoradiography (sĭn″ĕ-măt-ō-rā″dē-ŏg′ră-fē) [″ + L. *radius,* ray, + Gr. *graphein,* to write] Radiography of an organ in motion.

cinemicrography (sĭn″ĕ-mī-krŏg′ră-fē) [Gr. *kinesis,* movement, + *mikros,* small, + *graphein,* to write] A motion picture record of an object seen through a microscope.

cineplastics (sĭn″ĕ-plăs′tĭks) [″ + *plassein,* to form] The arrangement of muscles and tendons in a stump after amputation so that it is possible to impart motion and direction to an artificial limb.

cineradiography (sĭn″ĕ-rā″dē-ŏg′ră-fē) [″+ L. *radius,* ray, + Gr. *graphein,* to write] A motion picture record of images produced during fluoroscopic examination.

cinerea (sĭn-ē′rē-ă) [L. *cinereus,* ashen-hued] Gray matter of the brain or spinal cord. **cinereal** (-ăl), *adj.*

cineurography (sĭn″ĕ-ū-rŏg′ră-fē) [″+ *ouron,* urine, + *graphein,* to write] The use of cineradiography to obtain motion pictures of the urinary tract.

cingulotomy (sĭn′gū-lŏt″ō-mē) [L. *cingulum,* girdle, + Gr. *tome,* incision] Surgical excision of the anterior half of the cingulate gyrus of the brain. It may be done to alleviate intractable pain.

cingulum (sĭn′gū-lŭm) *pl.* **cingula** [L., girdle] **1.** A band of association fibers in the cingulate gyrus extending from the anterior perforated substance posteriorly to the hippocampal gyrus. **2.** A convexity on the cervical third of the lingual aspect of incisors and canines. SYN: *basal ridge.*

cinnamic acid A white insoluble powder derived from cinnamon. It is used as a flavoring agent in cooking and in the preparation of perfumes and medicines.

cinnamon A volatile oil derived from the bark of *Cinnamomum zeylanicum.* It is used as a flavoring agent in cooking and in preparing pharmaceutical products.

ciprofloxacin (sĭp-rō-flŏcks′ă-sĭn) A fluoroquinolone antibiotic with a broad spectrum of action; it may be used to treat susceptible genitourinary, intestinal, respiratory, dermatological, and orthopedic infections. Trade name is Cipro.

CAUTION: Its use is contraindicated in pregnant and nursing women.

---

circa (sĭr′kă) [L.] ABBR: c. About; used before dates or figures that are approximate.

circadian (sĭr″kă-dē′ăn, sĭr-kā′dē-ăn) [L. *circa,* about, + *dies,* day] Pert. to events that occur at approx. 24-hr intervals, such as certain physiological phenomena. SEE: *biological clock; desynchronosis; night work, maladaption to.*

circinate (sĕr′sĭ-nāt) [L. *circinatus,* made round] Circular.

circle [L. *circulus,* a little ring] Any ring-shaped structure.

c. of diffusion One or more circles on the projection plane of an image not in focus of the lens of the eye.

c. of Willis SEE: *Willis, circle of.*

Circ-O-Lectric bed A bed that allows the patient's position to be changed from supine to prone because it rotates electromechanically through 180° along its long axis.

circuit (sĕr′kĭt) [L. *circuire,* to go around] **1.** The course or path of an electric current. **2.** The path followed by a fluid circulating in a system of tubes or cavities. **3.** The path followed by nerve impulses in a reflex arc from sensory receptor to effector organ.

ventilator c. The external or internal pneumatic delivery component of a mechanical ventilator.

circular [L. *circularis*] **1.** Shaped like a circle. **2.** Recurrent.

circulation [L. *circulatio*] Movement in a regular or circular course.

bile salt c. Secretion and reuptake of the sodium glycocholate and taurocholate found in hepatic bile. Bile salts enter the duodenum and emulsify fats in the small intestine. They are resorbed in the terminal ileum and returned to the liver in portal blood.

blood c. The movement of blood through the circulatory system. SEE: *artery; heart; circulatory system; vein.*

collateral c. Circulation established through an anastomosis between two vessels supplying or draining two adjacent vascular areas. This enables blood to bypass an obstruction in the larger vessel that supplies or drains both areas, or enables blood to flow to or from a tissue when the principal vessel involved is obstructed.

coronary c. Movement of blood through the vessels of the heart, specifically from the ascending aorta to the epicardial coronary arteries to the penetrating arteries of the myocardium, the coronary arterioles, capillaries, veins, coronary sinus, and into the right atrium. A few of the small veins open directly into the atria and ventricles. SEE: illus.

enterohepatic c. Circulation in which substances secreted by the liver pass into the intestines where some are absorbed into the bloodstream and returned to the liver and re-secreted. Bile and bile salts follow this pathway.

extracorporeal c. Circulation of blood outside the body. This may be through an artificial kidney or a heart-lung device.

fetal c. The course of the flow of blood in a fetus. Oxygenated in the placenta, blood passes through the umbilical vein and ductus venosus to the inferior vena cava and from there to the right atrium. It then follows one of two courses: through the foramen ovale to the left atrium and thence through the aorta to the tissues, or through the right ventricle, pulmonary artery, and ductus arteriosus to the aorta and thence to the tissues. In either case the blood bypasses the lungs, which do not function before birth. Blood returns to the placenta through the umbilical arteries, which are continuations of the hypogastric ar-

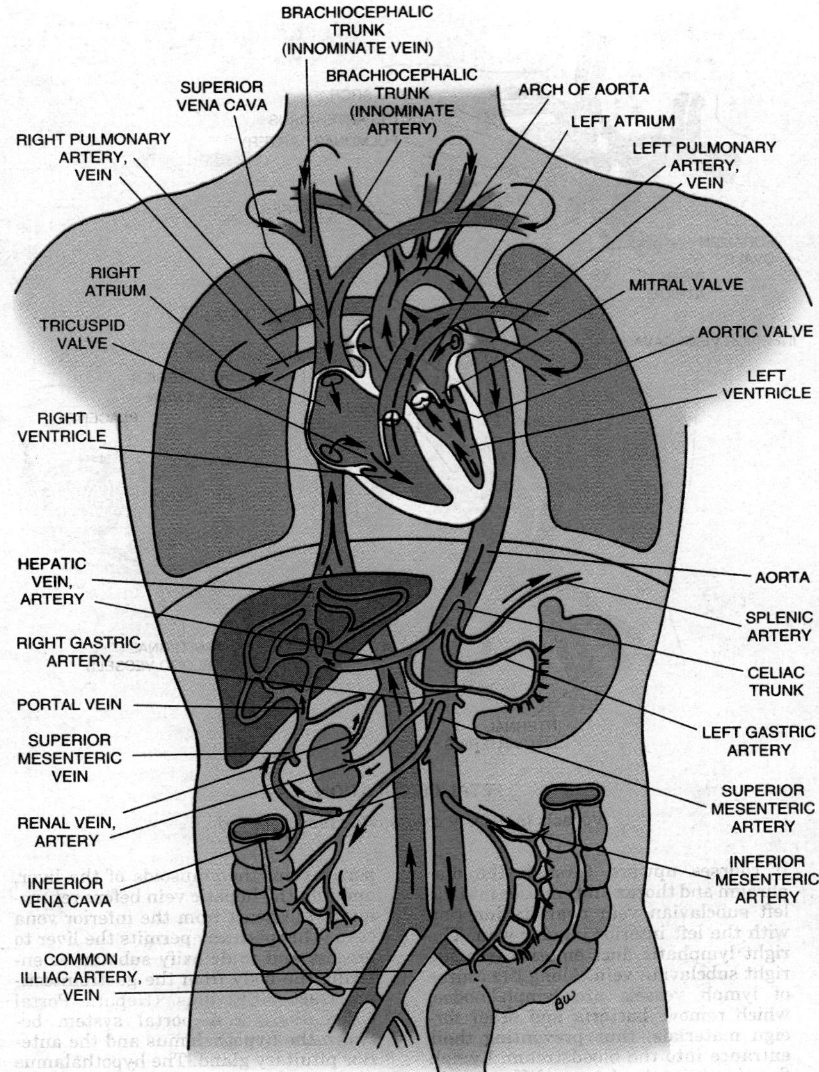

CIRCULATION OF BLOOD THROUGH HEART AND MAJOR VESSELS

teries. At birth or shortly after, the ductus arteriosus and the foramen ovale close, establishing the postpartum circulation. If either fails to close, the baby may be hypoxemic. SEE: illus.; *patent ductus arteriosus*.

lymph c. The flow of lymph from the tissues into the lymphatic collecting system. Lymph is formed from the tissue fluid that fills the interstitial spaces of the body. It is collected into lymph capillaries, which carry the lymph to the larger lymph vessels. These converge to form one of two main trunks, the right lymphatic duct and the thoracic duct. The right lymphatic duct drains the right side of the head, neck, and trunk and the right upper extremity; the thoracic duct drains the rest of the body. The thoracic duct originates at the cisterna chyli, which receives the lymphatics from the abdominal organs and legs.

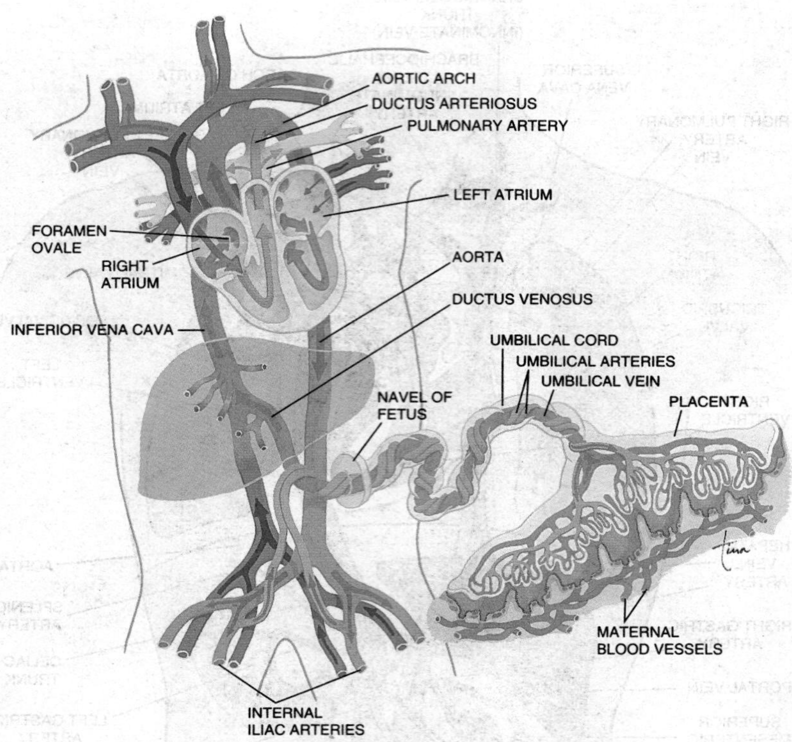

FETAL CIRCULATION

Vessels that carry oxygenated blood are red

It courses upward through the diaphragm and thorax and empties into the left subclavian vein near its junction with the left interior jugular vein. The right lymphatic duct empties into the right subclavian vein. Along the course of lymph vessels are lymph nodes, which remove bacteria and other foreign materials, thus preventing their entrance into the bloodstream. Lymph flow is maintained by a difference in pressure at the two ends of the system. Important accessory factors aiding lymph flow are breathing movements and muscular activity.

persistent fetal c. ABBR: PFC. A condition of newborns in which unoxygenated blood is shunted from the right to the left side of the heart through the ductus arteriosus and the foramen ovale, resulting in hypoxemia. It is caused by pulmonary hypertension and occurs most frequently in small-for-gestational-age infants and infants of diabetic mothers.

portal c. **1.** Blood flow from the abdominal organs that passes through the portal vein, the sinusoids of the liver, and into the hepatic vein before returning to the heart from the inferior vena cava. This pathway permits the liver to process and to detoxify substances entering the body from the gastrointestinal tract. SEE: illus. (Hepatic Portal Circulation). **2.** A portal system between the hypothalamus and the anterior pituitary gland. The hypothalamus secretes releasing or inhibiting hormones into the blood; they are carried directly to the anterior pituitary and stimulate or inhibit secretion of specific hormones. SEE: illus. (Portal Circulation of Hypothalamus-Pituitary).

pulmonary c. The flow of blood from the right ventricle of the heart to the lungs for exchange of oxygen and carbon dioxide in the pulmonary capillaries, then through the pulmonary veins to the left atrium.

systemic c. The general circulation of blood from the left ventricle to the right atrium of the heart.

venous c. Circulation via the veins.

circulation rate The minute volume or

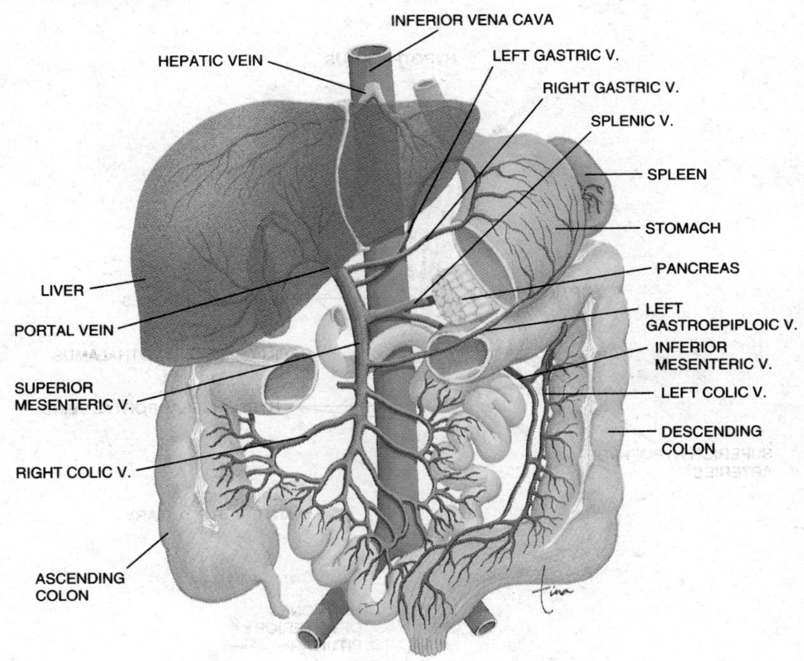

HEPATIC PORTAL CIRCULATION

output of the heart per minute. In an average-sized adult with a pulse rate of 70, the amount is about 3 L/sq m of body surface each minute.

circulation time The time required for a drop of blood to make the complete circuit of both the systemic and pulmonary systems. Circulation time is determined by injecting a substance into a vein and timing its reappearance in arteries at the injection point. The blood with the contained substance must pass through veins to the heart and through the right atrium and ventricle, through the pulmonary circuit to the lungs, and back through the left atrium and ventricle, and then out through the aorta and arteries to the place of detection. Dyes such as fluorescein and methylene blue and substances such as potassium ferrocyanide and histamine have been used as tracers. Average circulation time is 18 to 24 sec.

Circulation time is reduced in anemia and hyperthyroidism and is increased in hypertension, myxedema, and cardiac failure. Circulation time may also be measured by injecting into a vein a substance that can be tasted when it is transported to the tongue. The normal circulation time from an arm vein to the tongue is 10 to 16 sec. In the aorta, the blood flows at a speed of approx. 30 cm/sec.

circulatory Pert. to circulation.

circulatory failure Failure of the cardiovascular system to provide body tissues with enough blood for proper functioning. It may be caused by cardiac failure or peripheral circulatory failure, as occurs in shock, in which there is general peripheral vasodilation with "pooling" of blood in the expanded vascular space, resulting in decreased venous return.

circulatory overload Increased blood volume, usually caused by transfusions or excessive fluid infusions that increase the venous pressure, esp. in patients with heart disease. This can result in heart failure, pulmonary edema, and cyanosis.

circulus (sĕr′kū-lŭs) [L.] Circle.

circum- [L.] Prefix meaning *around.*

circumanal Around the anus.

circumarticular (sĕr″kŭm-ăr-tĭk′ū-lăr) [L. *circum,* around, + *articulus,* small joint] Surrounding a joint. SYN: *periarthric; periarticular.*

circumcision (sĕr″kŭm-sĭ′zhŭn) [L. *circumcisio,* a cutting around] Surgical removal of the end of the foreskin of the penis. Circumcision usually is performed at the request of the parents, in some cases for religious reasons. Considerable controversy exists over whether the procedure has medical benefits: some authorities suggest that circumcision is associated with a reduced risk of human immunodeficiency virus

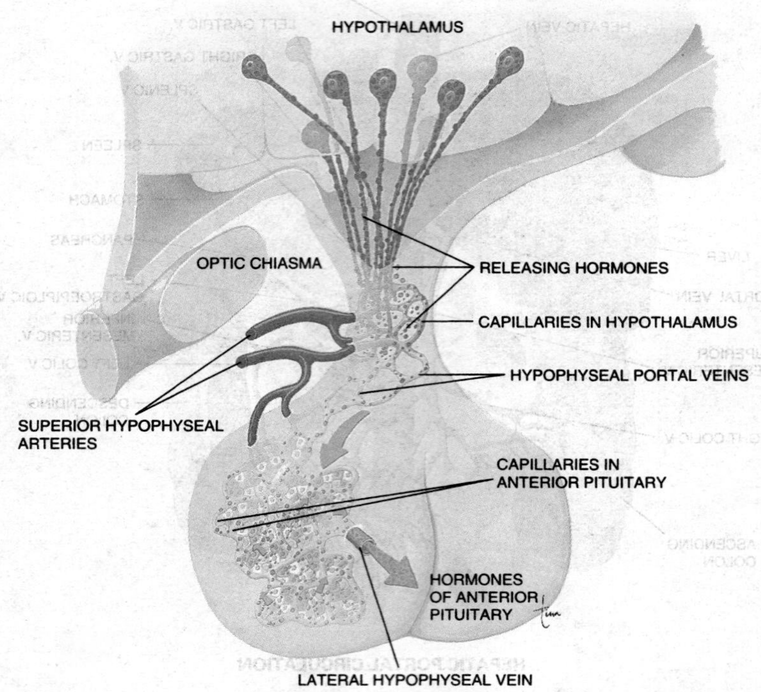

PORTAL CIRCULATION OF HYPOTHALAMUS-PITUITARY

infection, urinary tract infections, sexually transmitted diseases, and penile carcinoma. Other authorities dispute these findings, suggesting that the procedure may have adverse effects on sexual, emotional, or psychological health. If the procedure is performed, anesthesia should always be used.

PATIENT CARE: *Preoperative:* The procedure and expected sensations are explained to the patient or his parents. Adult patients should be reassured that the procedure will not interfere with urinary, sexual, or reproductive function. Necessary equipment, including a restraining board for the newborn, and appropriate anesthetics are assembled. The newborn should not receive food within 1 hr before the procedure.

Postoperative: Vital signs are monitored, and the incision is inspected for bleeding every 15 min for the first hour, then hourly for 12 to 24 hr, as protocol directs. Bleeding is controlled by applying gentle pressure with sterile gauze sponges; any heavy or persistent bleeding should be reported, and preparations made for blood vessel ligation. A sterile petroleum gauze dressing is applied after circumcision, remains in place for 24 hr, and is replaced if it becomes dislodged during that period. The penis is gently washed at diaper change, and fresh sterile petroleum gauze is reapplied. The dressing, glans penis, and sutures, if present, are periodically examined for swelling, redness, or purulent exudate; any signs of infection are reported, and a specimen of the exudate is obtained. A plastic bell instead of petroleum gauze may be used to cover the glans and to prevent hemorrhage and contamination. The newborn is diapered loosely to avoid irritation and should not be positioned on the abdomen for the first few hours after the procedure.

For the adult patient, analgesics are provided, and a topical anesthetic ointment or spray is applied as needed. If prescribed, a sedative is given to help prevent nocturnal penile tumescence and resulting pressure on the suture line. The patient is encouraged to void within 6 hr after the procedure. Either the patient or his family is instructed how to keep the area clean and how to change and apply dressings. They are also instructed to watch for and report renewed bleeding or signs of infection. Adult patients can resume normal sexual activity as soon as healing is complete, usually within a week or so. Use of prescribed analgesics is recommended to relieve discomfort during intercourse.

female c. Partial or complete surgical removal of the clitoris, usually performed before puberty, a procedure widespread in Africa and in certain groups in the Middle East and Far East. The untoward results include infection, loss of pleasure during sexual intercourse, scarring that may prevent sexual intercourse, and death from excessive bleeding or postoperative shock resulting from improper medical care. SYN: *female genital mutilation; genital cutting*. SEE: *infibulation*.

ritual c. The religious rite performed by the Jews and Muslims at the time of removal of the prepuce.

circumclusion (sĕr″kŭm-klū′zhŭn) [L. *circumcludere,* to shut in] Occlusion by use of a pin under an artery and a wire loop over it attached to each end of the pin.

circumcorneal (sĕr″kŭm-kor′nē-ăl) [L. *circum,* around, + *corneus,* horny] Around the cornea.

circumduction (sĕr″kŭm-dŭk′shŭn) [″ + *ducere,* to lead] To revolve around an axis in such a way that the proximal end of a limb or organ is fixed, and the distal end traces a circle.

circumference (sĕr-kŭm′fĕr-ĕns) [″ + *ferre,* to bear] The perimeter of an object or body.

circumferential (sĕr″kŭm-fĕr-ĕn′shăl) **1.** Encircling. **2.** Pert. to the periphery or circumference of an object or body.

circumflex (sĕr′kŭm-flĕks) [″ + *flectere,* to bend] Winding around, as a vessel.

circuminsular (sĕr″kŭm-ĭn′sū-lăr) [″ + *insula,* island] Surrounding the island of Reil in the cerebral cortex.

circumlental (sĕr″kŭm-lĕn′tăl) [″ + *lens,* lens] Surrounding the lens of the eye.

circumnuclear (sĕr″kŭm-nū′klē-ăr) [″ + *nucleus,* kernel] Surrounding the nucleus.

circumocular (sĕr″kŭm-ŏk′ū-lăr) [″ + *oculus,* eye] Surrounding the eye.

circumoral (sĕr″kŭm-ō′răl) [L. *circum,* around, + *os,* mouth] Encircling the mouth.

circumoral pallor A white area around the mouth, contrasting vividly with the color of the face, seen in scarlet fever and many other diseases.

circumorbital (sĕr″kŭm-or′bĭt-ăl) [″ + *orbita,* orbit] Around an orbit.

circumpolarization (sĕr″kŭm-pō″lăr-ĭ-ză′shŭn) [″ + *polaris,* polar] The rotation of a ray of polarized light.

circumrenal (sĕr″kŭm-rē′năl) [″ + *renalis,* pert. to kidney] Surrounding or partly surrounding the kidney.

circumscribed (sĕr′kŭm-skrībd) [″ + *scribere,* to write] Limited in space by something drawn around or confining an area.

circumstantiality (sĕr″kŭm-stăn″shē-ăl′ĭ-tē) [L. *circum,* around, + *stare,* to stand] Disturbance of the associative thought and speech processes in which the patient digresses into unnecessary details and inappropriate thoughts before communicating the central idea. It is observed in schizophrenia, obsessional disturbances, and certain cases of dementia.

circumvallate (sĕr″kŭm-văl′āt) [″ + *vallare,* to wall] Surrounded by a wall or raised structure.

circumvascular (sĕr″kŭm-văs′kū-lăr) [″ + *vasculum,* vessel] Perivascular; around a blood vessel.

cirrhosis (sĭ-rō′sĭs) [Gr. *kirrhos,* orange yellow, + *osis,* condition] A chronic liver disease characterized pathologically by liver scarring with loss of normal hepatic architecture and areas of ineffective regeneration. Clinical symptoms of the disease result from loss of functioning liver cells and increased resistance to blood flow through the liver (portal hypertension). SEE: *alcoholism; encephalopathy; hepatic; esophageal varix; liver*.

ETIOLOGY: In the U.S., alcoholism and chronic viral hepatitis are the most common causes of the illness. Other causes are autoimmune (primary biliary cirrhosis), biliary (sclerosing cholangitis), cardiac (due to right-sided heart failure), nutritional (e.g., fatty liver), genetic (alpha-1-antitrypsin deficiency, hemochromatosis, Wilson's disease) or toxic (exposure to drugs or agents in excess such as vitamin A, carbon tetrachloride, and methotrexate).

SYMPTOMS: Fatigue and malaise are common but nonspecific symptoms of the illness. Anorexia, early satiety, dyspepsia, altered bowel habits, and easy bruising and bleeding also are reported often. Alterations in mental status, personality, or behavior ("hepatic encephalopathy") are common but vary in severity and may not be noticed initially. Pruritus is reported when significant jaundice is present. Signs of the illness may include ascites; asterixis; bleeding from gums, nose, or gastroesophageal varices; "mousy" breath odor; edema; jaundice; and an irregular liver edge with hepatic enlargement (the liver may shrink when complete loss of function is present). Multiple skin findings may include abnormal pigmentation, palmar erythema, spider angiomas, ecchymoses, and dilated abdominal veins. Limited thoracic expansion due to hepatomegaly or ascites and endocrine changes such as menstrual irregularities, testicular atrophy, gynecomastia, and loss of chest and axillary hair may also be present.

TREATMENT: Liver transplantation may be curative, but its use is limited by the number of donor organs available. Shunting procedures to divert blood flow from the hepatic to the systemic circulation may improve portal hypertension and its consequences.

PATIENT CARE: Daily weights are obtained, fluid and electrolyte balance is monitored, and abdominal girth is measured. The ankles, sacrum, and scrotum are also assessed for dependent edema. The stools are inspected for color, amount, and consistency. Stools and vomitus are tested for occult blood. Surface bleeding sites are monitored frequently, and direct pressure is applied to the site if bleeding occurs. The patient is observed for indications of internal bleeding, such as anxiety, epigastric fullness, weakness, and restlessness; and vital signs are monitored as appropriate. Dependent areas are exercised and elevated, and skin breakdown is prevented by eliminating soaps and by using lubricating oils and lotions for bathing. The patient is frequently repositioned. The patient should avoid straining at stool and should use stool softeners as necessary and prescribed. Violent sneezing and nose blowing should also be avoided. A soft toothbrush or sponge stick and an electric razor are used. Aspirin, acetaminophen, or other over-the-counter medication should not be taken without the physician's knowledge. Alcohol or products containing alcohol are prohibited.

Both patient and family may require referral to alcohol cessation and related support groups. Prescribed therapies, including sodium and fluid restriction, dietary modifications, supplemental vitamin therapy, antiemetics, and diuretics, are administered. The patient's response to prescribed therapies is assessed, and the patient is instructed in their use and any adverse reactions. A regimen of moderate exercise alternating with periods of rest is prescribed; energy conservation measures are explained; small, frequent, nutritious meals are recommended; and exposure to infections should be avoided. Appropriate safety measures are instituted, esp. if the patient demonstrates hepatic encephalopathy, and the patient is frequently reoriented to time and place. Albumin is administered and paracentesis performed, if prescribed, to control ascites, and the patient is physically and psychologically prepared for required medical and surgical procedures. SEE: *Nursing Diagnoses Appendix.*

alcoholic c. Cirrhosis resulting from chronic liver damage by alcoholism. Approx. 20% of chronic alcoholics develop cirrhosis.

atrophic c. Cirrhosis in which the liver is decreased in size.

biliary c. Cirrhosis marked by prolonged jaundice due to chronic retention of bile and inflammation of bile ducts. SEE: *obstructive biliary c.; primary biliary c.*

cardiac c. Passive congestion of the liver due to congestive heart failure.

fatty c. Fatty liver.

hypertrophic c. Cirrhosis in which connective tissue hyperplasia causes the liver to be greatly enlarged.

infantile c. Cirrhosis occurring in childhood as a result of protein malnutrition. SEE: *kwashiorkor.*

metabolic c. Cirrhosis resulting from metabolic disease such as hemochromatosis, glycogen storage disease, or Wilson's disease.

obstructive biliary c. Cirrhosis resulting from obstruction of the common duct by a stone or tumor.

primary biliary c. A rare, progressive form of cirrhosis usually occurring in middle-aged women, marked by jaundice, pruritus, fatigue, and autoimmune destruction of the small bile ducts.

syphilitic c. Cirrhosis occurring in tertiary syphilis, in which gummas form in the liver and cause coarse lobulation on healing.

toxic c. An obsolete term for drug-induced hepatitis.

zooparasitic c. Cirrhosis resulting from infestation with animal parasites, esp. blood flukes of the genus *Schistosoma* or liver flukes, *Clonorchis sinensis.*

cirrhotic (sĭ-rŏt′ĭk) Pert. to or affected with cirrhosis.

cirsectomy (sĕr-sĕk′tō-mē) [Gr. *kirsos,* varix, + *ektome,* excision] Excision of a portion of a varicose vein.

cirsoid (sĕr′soyd) Varicose.

cirsomphalos (sĕr-sŏm′fă-lŏs) [″ + *omphalos,* navel] Varicose veins around the navel.

cirsotome (sĕr′sō-tōm) [″ + *tome,* incision] An instrument for cutting varicose veins.

cirsotomy (sĕr-sŏt′ō-mē) Incision of a varicose vein.

C.I.S. *central inhibitory state.*

cis (sĭs) [L., on the same side] In organic chemistry, a form of isomerism in which similar atoms or radicals are on the same side. In genetics, a prefix meaning the location of two or more genes on the same chromosome of a homologous pair.

cisapride (sĭs-ă′prīd) A medication that promotes motor activity throughout the gastrointestinal tract. It is used to treat gastroparesis, ileus, chronic constipation, and gastroesophageal reflux disease. When given with erythromycin or related drugs that prevent its metabolism, it may cause lethal cardiac rhythms. Trade name is Propulsid.

CISD *Critical incident stress debriefing; critical incident stress defusing.*

cisplatin, cis-platinum (sĭs′plă-tĭn) A drug used to treat cancers, especially solid tumors such as testicular and ovarian carcinoma. Common side effects of this drug include severe nausea and vomiting and renal failure.

cis-retinal The form of retinal combined with a glycoprotein opsin (rhodopsin in rods) during darkness. Light striking the retina changes it to *trans*-retinal and begins the generation of a nerve impulse.

cistern (sĭs′tĕrn) A reservoir for storing fluid.

cisterna [L.] A reservoir or cavity.

c. chyli A dilated sac; the origin of the thoracic duct. Into it empty the intestinal, two lumbar, and two descending lymphatic trunks.

c. magna The cranial subarachnoid space between the medulla and the cerebellum; the foramina of the fourth ventricle open into it. Cerebrospinal fluid flows from it into the spinal subarachnoid space.

c. subarachnoidalis A wide space in the cranial cavity between the arachnoid and the pia mater. It contains cerebrospinal fluid.

cisternal (sĭs-tĕr′năl) Concerning a cavity filled with fluid.

cisternography Radiography of the basal cistern of the brain after the injection of a contrast medium into the subarachnoid space, a procedure replaced by computed tomography.

cisvestitism (sĭs-vĕs′tĭ-tĭzm) [L. *cis,* on the same side, + *vestitus,* dressed, + Gr. *-ismos,* condition] Wearing of clothes appropriate to one's sex but suitable for a calling or profession other than one's own. An example would be a civilian who dresses in a uniform of the armed services.

Citelli's syndrome (chē-tĕl′ēz) [Salvatore Citelli, It. laryngologist, 1875–1947] Insomnia or drowsiness and lack of concentration associated with intelligence disorders, seen in children with infected adenoids or sphenoid sinusitis.

citrate (sĭt′rāt, sī′trāt) A compound of citric acid and a base.

sildenafil c. Viagra.

citrated (sĭt′rāt-ĕd) Combined or mixed with citric acid or a citrate.

citrate solution A solution used to prevent clotting of the blood. Its use permits whole blood to be stored in a refrigerator until it is needed for transfusion.

citric acid cycle Krebs cycle.

citronella (sĭt″rŏn-ĕl′ă) A volatile oil obtained from *Cymbopogon citratus,* or lemongrass, that contains geraniol and citronellal. It is used in perfumes and as an insect repellent.

citrulline (sĭt-rŭl′lĭn) An amino acid, $C_6H_{13}N_3O_3$, formed from ornithine. It is sometimes used to treat patients with urea cycle defects because citrulline is not taken up by the liver but is converted to arginine in the kidney.

citrullinemia (sĭt-rŭl″lĭ-nē′mē-ă) A type of aminoaciduria accompanied by increased amounts of citrulline in the blood, urine, and spinal fluid. Clinical findings include ammonia intoxication, liver disease, vomiting, mental retardation, convulsions, and failure to thrive.

Cl **1.** Symbol for the element chlorine. **2.** *chloride; clavicle; Clostridium.*

cladosporiosis (klăd″ō-spō-rē-ō′sĭs) [Gr. *klados,* branch, + *sporos,* seed, + *osis,* condition] A general term for an infection, usually of the central nervous system, caused by the fungus *Cladosporium.*

Cladosporium A genus of fungi. The condition tinea nigra is caused by either *C. werneckii* or *C. mansonii.* SEE: illus.

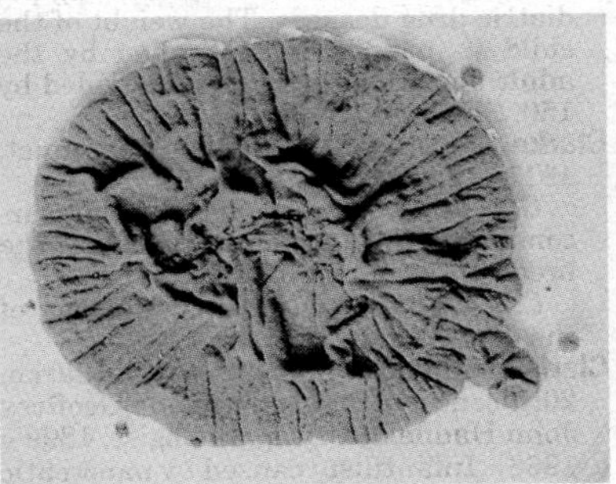

CLADOSPORIUM IN CULTURE

claim (klām) **1.** An assertion of fact. **2.** A request or demand for reimbursement of medical care costs.

clairvoyance (klār-voy′ăns) [Fr.] The alleged ability to be aware of events that occur at a distance without receiving any sensory information concerning those events.

clamp (klămp) [MD. *klampe,* metal clasp] A device used in surgery to grasp, join, compress, or support an organ, tissue, or vessel.

rubber dam c. An attachment that fits on the cervical part of the tooth for retention of a rubber dam.

CLAMS *Clinical Linguistic and Auditory Milestone Scale.*

clang [L. *clangere,* to peal] A loud, metallic sound.

clang association A speech disorder marked by the use of words grouped by their sound or rhyme, rather than their meaning.

clap A colloquial term for gonorrhea.

clapotage, clapotement (klă″pō-tăzh′, klă-pŏt-maw′) [Fr.] Any splashing sound in succussion of a dilated stomach.

clapping (klăp′ĭng) Percussion of the chest to loosen secretions. Also called *cupping* or *tapotement*. The hand is held in a cupped position.

Clapton's lines Green lines on the dental margin of the gums in copper poisoning.

Clara cell [Max Clara, Austrian anatomist, b. 1899] One of the secreting cells in the surface epithelium of the bronchioles. These cells, along with goblet cells, provide secretions for the respiratory tract. The secretion is a mucus-poor protein that coats the epithelium.

clarificant (klăr-ĭf′ĭk-ănt) [L. *clarus,* clear, + *facere,* to make] Any agent that clears turbidity from a liquid.

clarification (klăr″ĭ-fĭ-kā′shŭn) **1.** The removal of turbidity from a solution. **2.** In psychiatry, a technique used to help a patient recognize inconsistencies in his or her statements.

Clark electrode Oxygen electrode.

Clark's rule A method of calculating pediatric drug dosages. The weight of the child in pounds is multiplied by the adult dose and the result is divided by 150. SEE: *dosage*.

Clarke, Jacob A. L. British anatomist, 1817–1880.

C.'s body One of the alveolar sarcomatous intranuclear bodies of the breast.

C.'s column The dorsal nucleus of the spinal cord.

Clarke-Hadfield syndrome [Cecil Clarke, 20th-century Brit. physician; Geoffrey John Hadfield, Brit. pathologist, 1899–1968] Infantilism caused by pancreatic insufficiency. A child suffering from this syndrome is underweight and fails to grow.

clasmatodendrosis (klăz-măt″ō-dĕn-drō′sĭs) [Gr. *klasma,* fragment, + *dendron,* tree, + *osis,* condition] Breaking up of astrocytic protoplasmic expansions.

clasmatosis (klăz″mă-tō′sĭs) [″ + *osis,* condition] Crumbling into small bits; fragmentation, as of cells.

clasp (klăsp) A device for holding objects or tissues together. In dentistry, a type of wire or metal retainer or attachment used to stabilize dentures or prosthetic devices in the mouth.

clasp-knife phenomenon Increased muscle resistance to passive movement of a joint followed by a sudden release of the muscle; commonly seen in patients with spasticity.

class [L. *classis,* division] **1.** In biology, a taxonomic group of clearly defined organisms classified below a phylum and above an order. **2.** In statistics, a group of variables that fall within certain value limits.

classification (klăs″sĭ-fĭ-kā′shŭn) The orderly grouping of similar organisms, animals, individuals, diseases, or pathological findings according to traits or characteristics common to each group.

Dukes c. A system of classifying the extent of spread of adenocarcinoma of the colon or rectum.

classification of living organisms A systematic method of assigning organisms to various groups. Living organisms are classified into five kingdoms: Monera (Prokaryota), Protista, Fungi, Plantae, and Animalia. Within a kingdom, the subdivisions usually are phylum, class, order, family, genus, and species. The genus and species names are referred to as binomial nomenclature, with the larger (genus) category first and the precise species name second. SEE: *taxonomy*.

class restriction The requirement of certain T lymphocytes for the presence of either class I or class II major histocompatibility complex markers on antigen-presenting cells. These markers enable the T cells to recognize and respond to foreign antigens. CD4+ T cells require class II antigens and CD8+ T cells require class I antigens. Class restriction is a type of clonal restriction. SEE: *antigen-presenting cell; clonal restriction*.

clastic (klăs′tĭk) [Gr. *klastos,* broken] Causing division into parts.

clastogenic (klăs′tō-jĕn″ĭc) [″ + *gennan,* to produce] Capable of breaking chromosomes (e.g., able to cause chromosomal abnormalities).

clastothrix (klăs′tō-thrĭks) [″ + *thrix,* hair] Trichoclasia.

Claude's syndrome (klawdz) [Henri Claude, Fr. psychiatrist, 1869–1945] Paralysis of the third cranial nerve, contralateral ataxia, and tremor; caused by a lesion in the red nucleus of the brain.

claudication (klaw-dĭ-kā′shŭn) [L. *claudicare,* to limp] Lameness.

intermittent c. Cramping or pain in leg muscles brought on by a predictable amount of walking (or other form of exercise) and relieved by rest. This symptom is a marker of peripheral vascular disease of the aortoiliac, femoral, or popliteal arteries. It may be present in patients with diffuse atherosclerosis, for example, with arterial insufficiency in the coronary or carotid circulations as well as the limbs. SEE: *peripheral vascular disease*.

PHYSICAL EXAMINATION: The patient often has thin or shiny skin over the parts of the limb with decreased blood flow. Diminished pulses and bruits (audible blood flow through partially blocked arteries) may also be present.

DIAGNOSIS: In patients with a suggestive history, the blood pressure (BP) is measured in the affected limb and divided by the BP in the arm on the same side of the body. This ratio is called the ankle-brachial index (ABI); patients with significant peripheral vascular disease have an ABI of less than 85%. If surgery is contemplated for the patient, angiography may be used to define anatomical obstructions more precisely.

TREATMENT: Affected patients are encouraged to begin a program of regular exercise, to try to maximize collateral blood flow to the legs. Oral pentoxifylline improves the distance patients can walk without pain. For severely limiting claudication, patients may require angioplasty or arterial bypass surgery to respectively open or bypass obstructed arteries.

jaw c. Fatigue or cramping pain felt in the jaw, esp. while eating meats or other tough foods. About half of all patients with giant cell arteritis report this symptom.

venous c. Claudication resulting from inadequate venous drainage.

Claudius' cell (klaw'dē-ŭs) [Friedrich Claudius, Austrian anatomist, 1822–1869] One of the large columnar cells external to the organ of Corti.

Claudius' fossa A small depression on either side of the posterior part of the pelvis; each contains an ovary.

claustrophilia (klaws-trō-fĭl'ē-ă) [L. *claustrum,* a barrier, + Gr. *philein,* to love] Dread of being in an open space; a morbid desire to be shut in with doors and windows closed.

claustrophobia (klaws-trō-fō'bē-ă) [" + Gr. *phobos,* fear] Fear of being confined in any space, as in a locked room.

claustrum (klŏs'trŭm) [L.] **1.** Barrier. **2.** The thin layer of gray matter separating the external capsule of the brain from the island of Reil.

clava (klā'vă) *pl.* **clavae** [L., club] An elevation on the dorsal surface of the medulla oblongata caused by the underlying nucleus gracilis, the superior extremity of the fasciculus gracilis.

clavate (klā'vāt) Club-shaped.

clavicle (klăv'ĭ-k'l) [L. *clavicula,* little key] A bone curved like the letter *f* that articulates with the sternum and the scapula. SYN: *collar bone*.

dislocation of c. Traumatic displacement of either end of the clavicle.

TREATMENT: Open or closed reduction is the treatment.

fracture of c. Physical injury of the clavicle sufficient to fracture it, often as a result of a fall (e.g., from a ladder or bicycle).

SYMPTOMS: Symptoms include swelling, pain, and protuberance with a sharp depression over the injured bone. Palpable deformity and crepitus are commonly present.

TREATMENT: If indicated, an emergency care physician or an orthopedist will reduce the fracture. This usually is done by elevating the arm and lateral fragment so they line up with the medial fragment. The position is maintained by a clavicle strap, spica cast, immobilizing sling, or figure-of-eight wrap between the shoulders and over the back. Healing concludes in about 6 to 8 weeks.

FIRST AID: A ball of cloth or one or two handkerchiefs are tightly rolled and placed under the armpit. An arm sling is applied and the elbow bandaged to the side, with the hand and forearm extending across the chest. Alternatively, the patient may lie on his or her back on the floor with a rolled-up blanket under the shoulders until medical aid arrives. This position keeps the shoulders back and prevents the broken ends of the bone from rubbing.

clavicotomy (klăv"ĭ-kŏt'ō-mē) [" + Gr. *tome,* incision] Surgical division of the clavicle.

clavicular (klă-vĭk'ū-lăr) Pert. to the clavicle.

clavus (klā'vŭs) [L., nail] A corn or callosity.

c. hystericus A sharp pain in the head described as feeling like a nail being driven into the head.

clawfoot A deformity of the foot marked by an excessively high longitudinal arch, usually accompanied by dorsal contracture of the toes.

clawhand A hand marked by hyperextension of the proximal phalanges of the digits and extreme flexion of the middle and distal phalanges. Usually it is caused by injury to the ulnar and median nerves. SYN: *main en griffe*.

claw toe Hammertoe.

Clayton gas Sulfur dioxide; used to fumigate ships.

Clean Air Act A federal law, enacted in 1956 and amended many times since then, that empowers the administration to protect the public health and welfare by defining and attempting to control atmospheric pollutants, including automotive and factory exhausts such as sulfur dioxide, nitrogen dioxide, carbon monoxide, particulates, and lead.

clean-catch method A procedure for obtaining a urine specimen that exposes the culture sample to minimal contamination. For females, the labia are held apart and the periurethral area is cleaned with a mild soap or antibacterial solution, rinsed with copious amounts of plain water, and dried from front to back with a dry gauze pad. The urine is then passed and the specimen collected in a sterile container. It is important that the labia be held apart and that the urine flow directly into the container without touching the skin. If possible, the sample should be obtained after the urine flow is well established (i.e., a midstream specimen). For males, the urethral meatus is cleaned and the midstream specimen is collected in a sterile container. If the male is uncircumcised, the foreskin is retracted before the penis is cleaned.

cleaning, ultrasonic The use of high-frequency vibrations to clean instruments.

Clean Water Act An act originally passed by the federal government in 1972, and since amended several times, that gives the Environmental Protection Agency (EPA) responsibility for developing criteria for water-quality standards and controlling and regulating pollutants discharged into water sources.

clearance The elimination of a substance from the blood plasma by the kidneys. SEE: *renal clearance test*.

estimated creatinine c. ABBR: Calc CrCl. The rate of the removal of creatinine from the serum by the kidney. SEE: *creatinine clearance test*.

clearing agent **1.** A substance that increases the transparency of tissues prepared for microscopic examination. **2.** In radiographic film processing, the active agent in the fixer that clears undeveloped silver bromide crystals from the film. The most common agent is ammonium thiosulfate. SYN: *fixing agent*.

cleavage (klē′vĕj) [AS. *cleofian,* to cleave] **1.** Splitting a complex molecule into two or more simpler ones. **2.** Division of a fertilized egg into many smaller cells or blastomeres. SYN: *segmentation*. SEE: *blastomere; embryo*.

cleft (klĕft) [ME. *clift,* crevice] **1.** A fissure or elongated opening. **2.** Divided or split.

alveolar c. An anomaly resulting from lack of fusion between the medial nasal process and the maxillary process. A cleft maxillary alveolar process is usually associated with a cleft lip or palate or both.

branchial c. An opening between the branchial arches of an embryo. In lower vertebrates it becomes a gill cleft.

facial c. An anomaly resulting from failure of the facial processes of the embryo to fuse. Common types are oblique facial cleft, an open nasolacrimal furrow extending from the eye to the lower portion of the nose that is sometimes continuous with a cleft in the upper lip, and transverse facial cleft, which extends laterally from the angle of the mouth.

synaptic c. The synapse of a neuromuscular junction (between the axon terminal of a motor neuron and the sarcolemma of a muscle fiber). Impulse transmission is accomplished by a neurotransmitter.

cleft cheek Transverse facial cleft.

cleido-, cleid- (klī′dō) [L. *clavis,* key] Combining form pert. to the clavicle.

cleidocostal (klī″dō-kŏs′tăl) [″ + *costa,* rib] Pertaining to the clavicle and ribs.

cleidorrhexis (klī″dō-rĕk′sĭs) [″ + Gr. *rhexis,* rupture] Fracture or folding of the fetal clavicles to facilitate delivery.

cleidotomy (klī-dŏt′ō-mē) [″ + Gr. *tome,* incision] Division of a fetal clavicle to facilitate delivery.

clemastine fumarate (klĕm′ăs-tēn) An antihistamine drug.

clenching (klĕnch′ĭng) **1.** Forcible, repeated contraction of the jaw muscles with the teeth in contact. This causes pulsating, bilateral contractions of the temporalis and pterygomasseteric muscles. It may be done consciously, subconsciously while awake, or during sleep. SEE: *bruxism*. **2.** Tightly closing the fist.

cleptomania (klĕp″tō-mā′nē-ă) Kleptomania.

click (klĭk) **1.** An abrupt, brief sound heard in listening to the heart sounds. **2.** Any brief sound but esp. one heard during a joint movement. **3.** In dentistry, a noise associated with temporomandibular joint movement, sometimes accompanied by pain or joint dysfunction.

client The patient of a health care professional.

climacteric (klī-măk′tĕr-ĭk, klī-măk-tĕr′ĭk) [Gr. *klimakter,* a rung of a ladder] The menopause (i.e., the period that marks cessation of a woman's reproductive ability) in women; the corresponding period of diminished sexual arousal and activity in males. SEE: *menopause*.

climatology, medical [Gr. *klima,* sloping surface of the earth, + *logos,* word, reason] The branch of meteorology that includes the study of climate and its relationship to disease. SEE: *bioclimatology*.

climatotherapy (klī″măt-ō-thĕr′ăp-ē) [″ + *therapeia,* treatment] Treatment of disease by having the patient move to a specialized climate; historically used in the treatment of diseases like tuberculosis (cold, wintry air was thought to contribute to cure).

climax (klī′măks) [Gr. *klimax,* ladder] **1.** The period of greatest intensity. **2.** The sexual orgasm.

clindamycin hydrochloride (klĭn″dă-mī′sĭn) An antibiotic drug that treats infections with gram-positive and anaerobic organisms. Like other antibiotics, it may alter the flora of the gastrointestinal tract, leading to pseudomembranous colitis caused by overgrowth of *Clostridium difficile*.

clinic (klĭn′ĭk) [Gr. *klinikos,* pert. to a bed] **1.** Medical and dental instruction in which patients are observed directly, symptoms noted, and treatments discussed. **2.** A center for physical examination and treatment of ambulatory patients. **3.** A center where preliminary diagnosis is made and treatment given, as an x-ray clinic, a dental clinic, or a child-guidance clinic.

walk-in c. A general medical care clinic that is open to people who do not have an appointment.

clinical **1.** Founded on actual observation

and treatment of patients as distinguished from data or facts obtained from other sources. **2.** Pert. to a clinic.

clinical ecology A form of medical practice based on two concepts: that a broad range of environmental chemicals and foods can cause symptoms of illness (such as malaise, fatigue, dizziness, joint discomfort) and that the immune system is functionally depressed by exposure to many synthetic chemicals in the work place, the home or contemporary agricultural products. The premise of clinical ecology is that these exposures are toxic or that they trigger hypersensitivity reactions, or environmental illness.

clinical judgment The exercise of the clinician's experience and knowledge in diagnosing and treating illness and disease. SEE: *decision analysis*.

Clinical Linguistic and Auditory Milestone Scale ABBR: CLAMS. An office test used to evaluate language development in children from birth to age 3. SEE: *Denver Developmental Screening Test*.

clinical trial A carefully designed and executed investigation of the effects of a drug administered to human subjects. The goal is to define the clinical efficacy and pharmacological effects (toxicity, side effects, incompatibilities, or interactions). The U.S. government requires strict testing of all new drugs before their approval for use as therapeutic agents. SEE: *randomization*.

clinician (klĭn-ĭsh'ăn) [Gr. *klinikos*, pert. to a bed] A health professional with expertise in patient care rather than research or administration.

clinicopathological (klĭn"ĭ-kō-pă"thō-lŏj'ĭk-ăl) Concerning clinical and pathological disease manifestations.

clinicopathological conference ABBR: CPC. A teaching conference in which clinical findings are presented to a physician previously unfamiliar with a case, who then attempts to diagnose the disease that would explain the clinical findings. The exact diagnosis is then presented by the pathologist, who has either examined the tissue removed at surgery or has performed the autopsy.

clinocephaly (klī"nō-sĕf'ă-lē) [Gr. *klinein*, to bend, + *kephale*, head] Congenital flatness or saddle shape of the top of the head, caused by bilateral premature closure of the sphenoparietal sutures.

clinodactyly (klī"nō-dăk'tĭ-lē) [" + *daktylos*, finger] Hypoplasia of the middle phalanx of one or more of the fingers resulting in inward curving of these fingers in patients with Down syndrome.

clinoid (klī'noyd) [Gr. *kline*, bed, + *eidos*, form, shape] Shaped like a bed.

clinometer (klī-nŏm'ĕ-tĕr) [Gr. *klinein*, to slope, + *metron*, measure] An instrument formerly used for estimating torsional deviation of the eyes; used to measure ocular muscle paralysis.

clinoscope (klī'nō-skōp) Clinometer.

clip A device for holding or compressing tissues or other material together (e.g., after surgery; available in a variety of metals and slowly absorbed materials (e.g., polyglycolic acid).

vascular c. Small titanium or polyglycolic acid vessel clamp used to occlude blood vessels or to perform vascular anastomoses. In the anastomotic application, the clips are used in place of sutures. Advocates believe that this everting technique allows for less endothelial trauma and improved bonding of collagen molecules.

clithrophobia (klĭth"rō-fō'bē-ă) [Gr. *kleithria*, keyhole, + *phobos*, fear] A morbid fear of being locked in.

clition (klĭt'ē-ōn) [Gr. *kleitys*, slope] A craniometric point in the center of the highest part of the clivus on the sphenoid bone.

clitoridectomy (klī"tō-rĭd-ĕk'tō-mē) [Gr. *kleitoris*, clitoris, + *ektome*, excision] Excision of the clitoris.

clitoriditis (klī"tō-rĭd-ī'tĭs) Clitoritis.

clitoridotomy (klī"tō-rĭd-ŏt'ō-mē) [" + *tome*, incision] Incision of the clitoris; female circumcision.

clitoris (klī'tō-rĭs, klĭt'ō-rĭs) [Gr. *kleitoris*] One of the structures of the female genitalia; a small erectile body located beneath the anterior labial commissure and partially hidden by the anterior portion of the labia minora.

STRUCTURE: It consists of three parts: a body, two crura, and a glans. The body, about 1 in. (2.5 cm) long, consists of two fused corpora cavernosa. It extends from the pubic arch above to the glans below. The two crura are continuations of the corpora cavernosa and attach them to the inferior rami of the pubic bones. They are covered by the ischiocavernosus muscles. The glans, which forms the free distal end, is a small rounded tubercle composed of erectile tissue. It is highly sensitive. The glans is usually covered by a hoodlike prepuce, and its ventral surface is attached to the frenulum of the labia.

clitorism (klī'tō-rĭzm) **1.** The counterpart of priapism; a long-continued, painful condition with recurring erection of the clitoris. **2.** Clitoral enlargement.

clitoritis (klī"tō-rī'tĭs) Inflammation of the clitoris. SYN: *clitoriditis*.

clitoromegaly (klī"tō-rō-mĕg'ă-lē) [" + *megas*, large] Clitoral enlargement. This may be caused by an endocrine disease or by use of anabolic steroids.

clivus (klī'vŭs) [L., a slope] A surface that slopes, as the sphenoid bone.

c. blumenbachii The slope at the base of the skull.

clo A unit for thermal insulation of clothing; the amount of insulation necessary to maintain comfort in a sitting-resting subject in a normally ventilated room (air movement at the rate of 10 cm/sec) at a temperature of 70°F (21°C) with relative humidity of less than 50%.

cloaca (klō-ā′kă) [L. *cloaca,* a sewer] **1.** A cavity lined with endoderm at the posterior end of the body that serves as a common passageway for urinary, digestive, and reproductive ducts. It exists in adult birds, reptiles, and amphibia, and in the embryos of all vertebrates. **2.** An opening in the sheath covering necrosed bone.

clobetasol propionate A high-potency topical corticosteroid; used for short-term treatment to cortisone-responsive dermatoses.

clock A device for measuring time.

biological c. An internal system in organisms that influences behavior in a rhythmic manner. Functions such as growth, feeding, secretion of hormones, the rate of drug action, the wake-sleep cycle, the menstrual cycle, and reproduction coincide with certain external events such as day and night, the tides, and the seasons. Biological clocks appear to be set by environmental conditions in some animals, but if these animals are isolated from their environment they continue to function according to the usual rhythm. A gradual change in environment does produce a gradual change in the timing of the biological clock. SEE: *circadian; maladaptation to night work; zeitgeber*.

clofazimine (klō-fă′zĭ-mēn) An antimicrobial drug used to treat patients with leprosy or disseminated *Mycobacterium avium-intracellulare* infection. Trade name is Lamprene.

clofibrate (klō-fī′brāt) A drug used to reduce plasma concentration of lipids; used in treating hyperlipoproteinemias III, IV, and V. Trade name is Atromid-S.

clomiphene citrate (klō′mĭ-fēn) A nonsteroidal agent used to stimulate ovulation in women who have potentially functioning pituitary and ovarian systems. Women treated with this medicine who become pregnant have an increased incidence of multiple births. Trade name is Clomid.

clonal (klōn′ăl) Pert. to a clone.

clonal restriction The occurrence of the same characteristics as the parent cell in all clones (offspring) of one B or T lymphocyte. For example, surface receptors are identical, so clones react to the same group of specific antigens as the parent cell does.

clonazepam (klō-năz′ĕ-păm) A benzodiazepine used to treat anxiety, panic, and seizure disorders.

clone (klōn) [Gr. *klon,* a cutting used for propagation] **1.** In microbiology, the asexual progeny of a single cell. **2.** A group of plants propagated from one seedling or stock. Members of the group are identical but do not reproduce from seed. **3.** In tissue cultures or in the body, a group of cells descended from a single cell. The term commonly refers to the multiple offspring of single T or B lymphocytes that have identical surface receptors or immunoglobulins, and to the offspring of malignant cells. **4.** In immunology, a group of lymphocytes that develop from a sensitized lymphocyte; they are all capable of responding to a specific foreign antigen. **5.** In biology, the creation of an embryo from an unfertilized egg and the diploid nucleus of a somatic cell. With the full diploid number of chromosomes, the egg cell begins dividing as if fertilization had taken place. Clones of sheep and cows have been successfully produced.

clonic (klŏn′ĭk) [Gr. *klonos,* turmoil] Pert. to clonus; alternately contracting and relaxing the muscles.

clonicity (klŏn-ĭs′ĭ-tē) The condition of being clonic.

clonicotonic (klŏn″ĭ-kō-tŏn′ĭk) [Gr. *klonos,* turmoil, + *tonikos,* tonic] Both clonic and tonic, as some forms of muscular spasm.

clonidine hydrochloride (klō′nĭ-dēn) A centrally acting alpha-agonist drug used to treat hypertension and opiate withdrawal. Trade name is Catapres.

clonorchiasis (klō″nor-kī′ă-sĭs) A disease caused by the Chinese liver fluke, *Clonorchis sinensis,* which infects the bile ducts of humans. Infection is caused by eating uncooked freshwater fish containing encysted larvae. Early symptoms are loss of appetite and diarrhea; later there may be signs of cirrhosis of the liver. The disease may be prevented by cooking fish thoroughly, or by freezing it at −10°C (14°F) for a minimum of 5 days. The disease rarely causes death. Treatment with Praziquantel is effective.

Clonorchis sinensis (klō-nor′kĭs sī-nĕn′sĭs) The trematode fluke, Chinese liver fluke. It is an important cause of biliary disease, esp. in Asia. SEE: illus.; *clonorchiasis*.

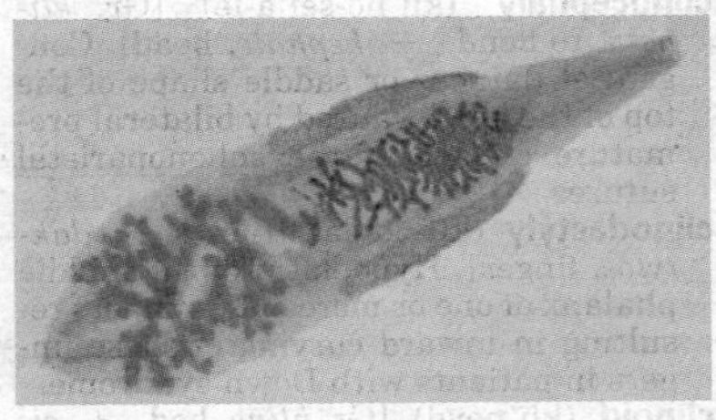

CLONORCHIS SINENSIS

(Orig. mag. ×4)

clonospasm (klŏn′ō-spăzm) [″ + *spasmos,* spasm] Clonic spasm.

clonus (klō′nŭs) Spasmodic alternation of muscular contractions between antagonistic muscle groups caused by a hyperactive stretch reflex from an upper motor neuron lesion. Usually, sustained pressure or stretch of one of the muscles inhibits the reflex.

Cloquet's canal (klō-kāz′) [Jules Germain Cloquet, Fr. surgeon, 1790–1883] An irregular passage (hyaloid) through the center of the vitreous body in the fetus.

closed-packed position The joint position in which there is maximum congruency of the articular surfaces and joint stability is derived from the alignment of bones. This is the opposite of the maximum loose-packed position.

Clostridium (klō-strĭd′ē-ŭm) [Gr. *kloster,* spindle] A genus of bacteria belonging to the family Bacillaceae. These anaerobic, spore-forming rods are widely distributed in nature, with more than 250 species recognized. They are common in the soil and in the intestinal tract of humans and animals and are frequently found in wound infections. In humans several species are pathogenic, being the primary causative agents of gas gangrene.

C. botulinum A species of soil bacteria that may grow in improperly processed food or in wounds under anaerobic conditions; it produces the neurotoxin that causes botulism.

C. chauvoei The organism causing blackleg or symptomatic anthrax in cattle.

C. difficile A species that causes pseudomembranous colitis. Any antibiotic that diminishes the normal colon flora may permit this species to overgrow and release toxins injuring the intestinal mucosa. The infection is treated with oral metronidazole or vancomycin. SEE: *pseudomembranous colitis*.

C. histolyticum A proteolytic organism found in feces and soil, isolated from necrotic war wounds and found in some cases of gas gangrene.

C. novyi A species found in many cases of gas gangrene.

C. perfringens The most common causative agent of gas gangrene. SYN: *C. welchii; gas bacillus*.

C. septicum A species found in cases of gangrene in humans, as well as in cattle, hogs, and other domestic animals.

C. sporogenes A species frequently associated with other organisms in mixed gangrenous infections.

C. tetani The causative organism of tetanus or lockjaw. It produces a powerful exotoxin, one portion of which affects nerve tissue and the other of which is hemolytic. SEE: *tetanus*.

C. welchii C. perfringens.

closure (klō′shŭr) **1.** Shutting or bringing together as in suturing together the edges of a laceration wound. **2.** In psychotherapy, the resolution of an issue that was a topic in therapy and a cause of distress for the patient.

clot (klŏt) [AS. *clott,* lump] **1.** Thrombus. **2.** To coagulate.

agonal c. A clot formed in the heart when death follows prolonged heart failure.

antemortem c. A clot formed in the heart or its cavities before death.

blood c. A coagulated mass of blood. SEE: *blood coagulation*.

chicken fat c. A yellow blood clot appearing to contain no erythrocytes.

currant jelly c. A soft red postmortem blood clot found in the heart and vessels.

distal c. A clot formed in a vessel on the distal side of a ligature.

external c. A clot formed outside a blood vessel.

internal c. A clot formed by coagulation of blood within a vessel.

laminated c. A clot formed in a succession of layers filling an aneurysm.

muscle c. A clot formed in muscle tissue.

passive c. A clot formed in the sac of an aneurysm.

plastic c. A clot formed from the intima of an artery at the point of ligation.

postmortem c. A clot formed in the heart or in a blood vessel after death.

proximal c. A clot formed on the proximal side of a ligature.

stratified c. A clot consisting of layers of different colors. SEE: *coagulation, blood; coagulation factor; thrombosis*.

clothes louse SEE: *Pediculus humanus corporis*.

clothing [AS. *clath,* cloth] Wearing apparel; used both functionally and decoratively. From the medical standpoint, clothes conserve heat or protect the body (e.g., gloves, sunhelmets, and shoes). Air spaces in a fabric and its texture, rather than the material alone, conserve heat. In matted woolen fabrics, the air spaces are destroyed and insulation is lost. Wool and silk absorb more moisture than other fabrics, but silk loses it more readily. Cotton and linen come next, but linen loses moisture more quickly than cotton. Knitted fabrics absorb and dry more readily than woven fabrics of the same material. The temperature inside an individual's hat may vary from 13° to 20°F (7° to 11°C) warmer than the outside temperature. SEE: *clo; hypothermia*.

clotrimazole (klō-trĭm′ă-zōl) An over-the-counter antifungal drug used to treat athlete's foot and other fungal skin infections, including vulvovaginal candidiasis. Intravaginal use occasionally causes burning, redness, and itching in the patient, her sex partner, or both. Trade names are Lotrimin, Gyne-Lotrimin, and Mycelex G.

clotting The formation of a jelly-like coagulum from blood shed at the site of an injury to a blood vessel. This action usually halts blood flow from the wound. SEE: *coagulation, blood*.

cloven spine Congenital defect of spinal canal walls caused by lack of union between laminae of the vertebrae. SYN: *spina bifida cystica*.

clove oil [L. *clavus,* a nail or spike] A volatile oil distilled from the dried flower buds of the clove tree, *Eugenia caryophyllus*. It is used as an antiseptic and an aromatic and is applied directly to relieve pain in teeth.

cloxacillin sodium (klŏks″ă-sĭl′ĭn) A penicillinase-resistant antibiotic used primarily to treat streptococcal and staphylococcal infections.

clozapine A dopamine receptor–blocking drug used to treat psychosis. Trade name is Clozaril.

clubbing (klŭb′ĭng) An enlarged terminal phalanx of the finger. This may be present in chronic obstructive pulmonary disease, interstitial fibrosis of the lungs, cyanotic congenital heart disease, carcinoma of the lung, bacterial endocarditis, and many other illnesses. SYN: *clubbed finger; hippocratic finger*. SEE: illus.

CLUBBING

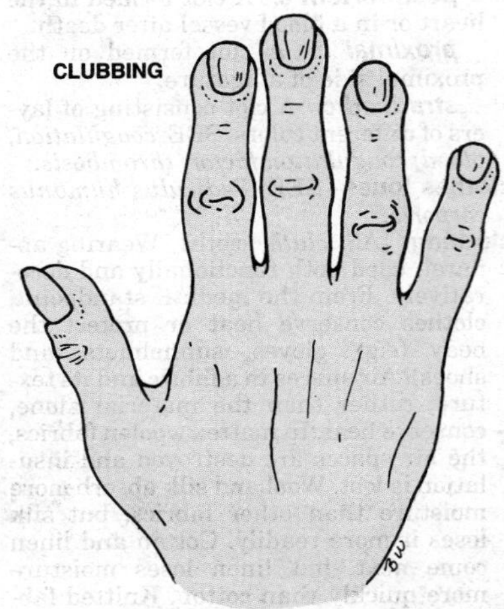

ADVANCED CLUBBING

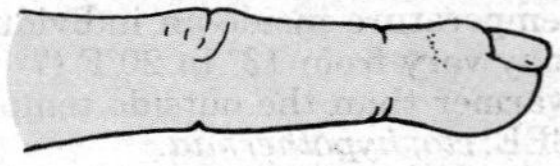

CLUBBING

clubfoot Talipes equinovarus.

clubhand Talipomanus.

clump (klŭmp) [AS. *clympre,* a lump] **1.** A mass of bacteria in solution; may be caused by an agglutination reaction. **2.** To gather together.

clumping Agglutination.

cluster A closely grouped series of events (e.g., cases of a disease) with well-defined distribution patterns in relation to time, place, or risk factor exposure.

c. of differentiation ABBR: CD. A group of protein markers on the surface of a white blood cell. These markers are used to classify immune cell types and establish international nomenclature standards. Although found on many blood cells and some nonblood cells, they are used most often to refer to lymphocytes. Markers for CD3 are found on all mature T cells in association with T-cell antigen receptors; CD2 and CD7 markers are found on immature T cells. Markers for CD4 are found on all T helper cells, macrophages, and some B cells. Markers for CD8 identify cytotoxic T cells, which are essential to the defense against viral infections. Each marker has a specific function in the cell, such as passing a signal from the T-cell receptor to the cytoplasm. SEE: *cell, T*.

cluttering (klŭt′ĕr-ĭng) A form of speech difficulty marked by excessive speed and irregular rhythm, often with condensation of sounds and collapsing of words. It may range in severity from an annoying but generally intelligible speech difficulty to a severe disability with virtually unintelligible speech.

Clutton's joint [Henry Hugh Clutton, Brit. surgeon, 1850–1909] Hydroarthrosis of the knee joint often associated with interstitial keratitis, seen in congenital syphilis.

clysis (klī′sĭs) *pl.* **clyses** [Gr. *klyzein,* to cleanse] Injection of fluid into the body other than orally. Fluid may be injected into tissue spaces, the rectum, or the abdominal cavity. This technique is used to inject fluids parenterally when venipuncture is not possible. SEE: *enteroclysis*.

C.M. *chirurgiae magister,* Master in Surgery.

Cm Symbol for the element curium.

cm *centimeter*.

c/m *counts per minute*.

cm² *square centimeter*.

cm³ *cubic centimeter*.

C.M.A. *Canadian Medical Association*.

C_{max} Maximum concentration of a drug achieved after dosing. SEE: illus.

CMI *cell-mediated immunity*.

c/min *counts per minute*.

c.mm. *cubic millimeter*. This symbol is no longer recommended for use.

CMRR *common mode rejection ratio*.

CMT *certified medical transcriptionist*. SEE: *medical transcriptionist*.

CMV *continuous mandatory ventilation*.

CN *cyanogen*.

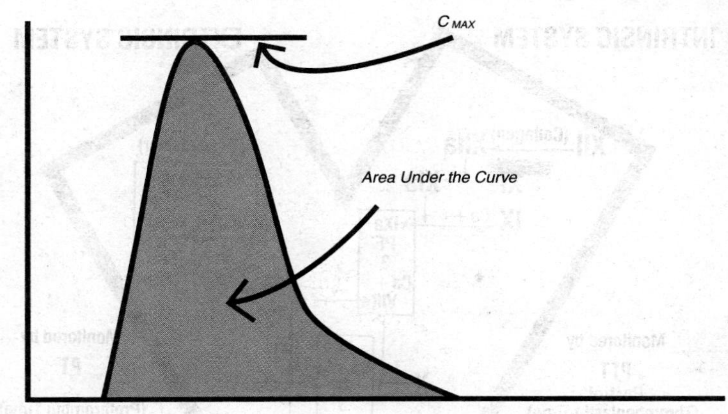

C MAX

C.N.A. *Canadian Nurses' Association.*

C.N.M. *certified nurse-midwife.*

CNS *central nervous system; clinical nurse specialist; coagulase-negative staphylococcus.*

CO Formula for carbon monoxide; *cardiac output*.

CO_2 Formula for carbon dioxide.

CO_2 therapy **1.** Therapeutic application of low temperatures with solid carbon dioxide. SEE: *cryotherapy; hypothermia* (2). **2.** Inhalation of carbon dioxide to stimulate breathing.

Co Symbol for the element cobalt.

Co1 *coccygeal spinal nerve*.

CoA Coenzyme A.

coacervate (kō-ăs′ĕr-vāt) [L. *coacervatus,* heaped up] The formation of an aggregate in a solution that is about to emulsify or in an emulsion that is demulsifying.

coadaptation (kō″ăd-ăp-tā′shŭn) Mutual adaptation of two independent organisms, organs, or persons.

coadministration (cō″ăd-mĭn-ĭ-strā′shŭn) The giving of two or more therapeutic agents at the same time.

coagglutination (kō″ă-gloo″tĭn-ā′shŭn) [L. *coagulare,* to curdle] Use of latex or other inert particles to which an antibody will bind in laboratory tests of agglutination.

coagula (kō-ăg′ū-lă) [L.] Pl. of coagulum.

coagulability (kō-ăg″ū-lă-bĭl′ĭ-tē) The capacity to form clots, esp. blood clots.

coagulable (kō-ăg′ū-lă-b′l) Capable of clotting; likely to clot.

coagulant (kō-ăg′ū-lănt) [L. *coagulans,* congealing] **1.** Something that causes a fluid to coagulate. **2.** Causing coagulation.

coagulase (kō-ăg′ū-lāz) [L. *coagulum,* blood clot] Any enzyme, such as thrombin, that causes coagulation.

coagulate (kō-ăg′ū-lāt) [L. *coagulare,* to congeal] To solidify; to change from a fluid state to a semisolid mass.

coagulated Clotted or curdled.

coagulator (kō-ăg′ū-lāt″ŏr) **1.** A surgical device that utilizes electrical current, light energy, ultrasound, etc., to stop bleeding. **2.** A pharmacological substance used to induce hemostasis or solidification of proteinaceous fluids.

argon beam c. A surgical instrument used to cut or cauterize tissues, which relies on a jet of argon gas to carry electrons into the operative field.

infrared c. A surgical instrument that focuses infrared light energy to cut or damage tissues or to stop bleeding. The device has been used in skin surgery, hair transplantation, ablation of abnormal cardiac conduction pathways, and treatment of internal hemorrhoids, among other applications.

microwave c. A surgical instrument that focuses microwave energy through an antenna to cut or cauterize tissue. The device can be used in open or laparoscopic surgeries.

coagulation, blood (kō-ăg″ū-lā′shŭn) [L. *coagulatio,* clotting] The process of clumping together of blood cells to form a clot. This may occur in vitro, intravascularly, or when a laceration of the skin allows the escape of blood from an artery, vein, or capillary. Coagulation of blood may occur in two pathways, depending on the beginning of the process.

Extrinsic: The extrinsic pathway (in an abbreviated outline form) requires the blood to be exposed to a subendothelial tissue factor originating outside the blood. This factor begins a complex series of chemical reactions involving thromboplastin, factor VII, and calcium;

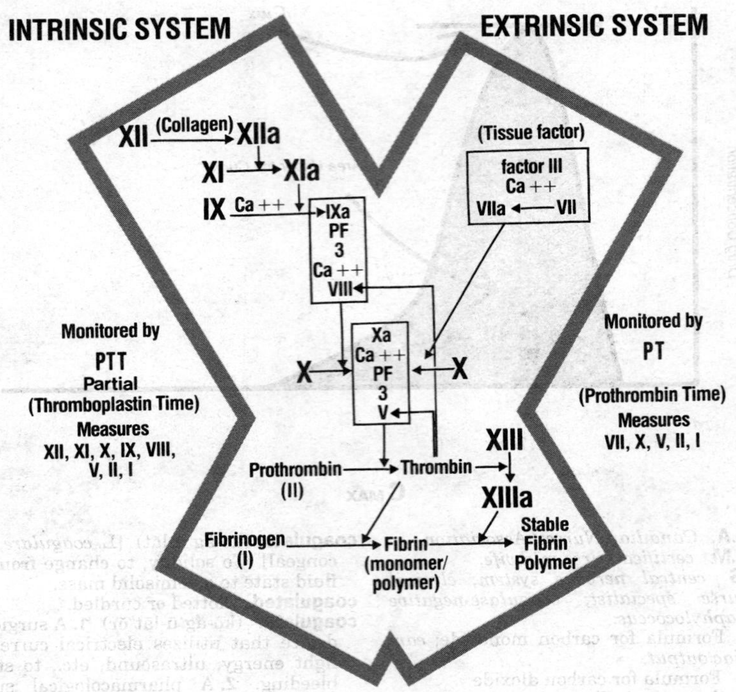

COAGULATION CASCADE

binding to factor X, causing its conversion to factor Xa; and the resulting conversion of prothrombin to thrombin to fibrinogen and eventually fibrin.

Intrinsic: The intrinsic pathway (in abbreviated outline form) occurs when blood is drawn without contamination by tissue factor. This clotting pathway does not require an additive. It is triggered when the blood is exposed to a foreign surface and factor XII is activated. Factor XII may also be activated through limited cleavage by kallikrein. This process is accelerated by high-molecular-weight kininogen (HMWK). This leads to formation of factor XII, a process that produces more HMWK to accelerate kallikrein production. The process continues and factors XI and IX, and HMWK, in concert with calcium, generate factor Xa. The clotting cascade then continues as in the extrinsic pathway, and prothrombin is converted to thrombin, which acts on fibrinogen to produce fibrin. SEE: illus.

coagulopathy (kō-ăg″ū-lŏp′ă-thē) [″ + Gr. *pathos,* disease, suffering] A defect in blood-clotting mechanisms. SEE: *coagulation, blood.*

consumption c. Disseminated intravascular coagulation.

coalesce (kō-ăl-ĕs′) [L. *coalescere*] To fuse; to run or grow together.

coalescence (kō-ă-lĕs′ĕns) The fusion or growing together of two or more body parts.

coal worker's pneumoconiosis ABBR: CWP. A form of pneumoconiosis in which carbon and silica accumulate in the lungs as a result of breathing coal dust. SYN: *black lung.*

coapt (kō′ăpt) [L. *coaptare,* to fit together] To bring together, as in suturing a laceration.

coaptation (kō″ăp-tā′shŭn) [L. *coaptare,* to fit together] The adjustment of separate parts to each other, as the edges of fractures.

coarctate (kō-ărk′tāt) [L. *coarctare,* to tighten] To press together; pressed together.

coarctation (kō″ărk-tā′shŭn) **1.** Compression of the walls of a vessel. **2.** Shriveling. **3.** A stricture.

c. of the aorta A localized congenital malformation resulting in narrowing of the aorta, often resulting in hypertension. Surgical correction of the obstruction may cure high blood pressure in affected patients.

coarctotomy (kō″ărk-tŏt′ō-mē) [″ + Gr. *tome,* incision] Cutting or dividing of a stricture.

coat [L. *cotta,* a tunic] A covering or a layer in the wall of a tubular structure, as the inner coat (tunica intima), middle coat (tunica media), or outer coat (tunica adventitia) of an artery.

Coats' disease [George Coats, Brit. ophthalmologist, 1876–1915] The development of large white masses deep in the blood vessels of the retina. This term is now used to describe at least six separate retinal disorders.

cobalamin (kō-băl′ă-mĭn) Another name for vitamin B_{12}, a complex molecule containing one atom of cobalt. SEE: *cyanocobalamin*.

cobalt (kō′bălt) SYMB: Co. A gray, hard, ductile metal; atomic weight 59.933, atomic number 27, specific gravity 8.9. Cobalt deficiency causes anemia in ruminants, but this has not been demonstrated in humans. Cobalt is an essential element in vitamin B_{12}. Cobalt stimulates production of red blood cells, but its use as a therapeutic agent is not advised. In children, cobalt overdose may cause death. In adults, it may cause anorexia, nausea, vomiting, deafness, and thyroid hyperplasia with resultant compression of the trachea.

cobalt-57 A radioactive isotope of cobalt with a half-life of 272 days.

cobalt-60 A radioactive isotope of cobalt, used as a source of beta and gamma rays in treating malignancies. It has a half-life of 5.27 years.

Coban Trade name for a self-adherent compression bandage used for protection and edema control. Also called *Coban wrap*.

cobra (kō′bră) Any one of a group of poisonous snakes native to parts of Africa and Asia. They all have the ability to expand the neck into a flattened hood.

cobra venom solution Minute quantities of cobra venom in sterile physiological salt solution.

COBS *cesarean-obtained barrier-sustained.*

coca (kō′kă) Dried leaves of the shrub *Erythroxylum coca,* from which several alkaloids including cocaine are obtained.

cocaine Cocaine hydrochloride.

cocaine baby An infant exposed to cocaine in utero through maternal use of the drug. Cocaine crosses the placenta and enters the fetal circulation.

CONSEQUENCES: Cocaine abuse during pregnancy has been correlated with birth defects, intrauterine growth retardation, and perinatal death related to premature separation of the placenta, preterm labor and delivery, low birth weight, and sudden infant death syndrome. Newborns may exhibit signs of drug withdrawal, tachycardia, hyperirritability, muscle rigidity, seizures, and feeding problems. Children who were cocaine babies have short attention spans and learning disorders.

In addition, cocaine use by the father at the time of conception may have a negative effect on sperm quality.

PATIENT CARE: Since cocaine-dependent newborns often experience a significant and agonizing withdrawal syndrome that can last 2 to 3 weeks, they require continual assessment and evaluation. During the withdrawal period, patient care measures are instituted to effect the following outcomes: the infant maintains a patent airway and breathes easily, maintaining adequate oxygen intake, independent respiratory effort, and adequate tissue perfusion; the infant relaxes and sleeps; crying diminishes; the infant is able to remain asleep for 3- to 4-hour periods; the infant recovers from seizures with minimal or no sequelae; the infant ingests and retains sufficient fluids for hydration and nutrients for growth; and the infant's skin remains intact and free from infection.

The parents and significant others are an important part of the care plan. The mother requires considerable support, as her need for and abuse of drugs result in decreased coping abilities. The newborn's withdrawal symptoms, decreased consolability, and poor interactive behaviors stress her coping abilities even further. Home health care, treatment for addiction, and education are important considerations. Health care providers explore with the mother options for infant care, for care of herself, and for future fertility management, employing a sensitive approach that communicates respect for the patient and her ability to make responsible decisions. Depending on the scope of the patient's drug abuse problem, total prevention may be unrealistic; however, the parent is referred for education and social supports to provide opportunities for detoxification and abstinence. Because the newborn's dependence is physiologic, not psychologic, no predisposition to later dependence is thought to be present. The psychosocial environment in which the infant is raised, however, may predispose the baby to addiction. The infant must be referred for child welfare follow-up assessment, evaluation, and action, which may include removing the infant from the birth mother's care temporarily or permanently. SEE: *infant of substance-abusing mother*.

cocaine hydrochloride (kō-kān′, kō′kān) The hydrochloride of an alkaloid obtained from the shrub *Erythroxylum coca,* native to Bolivia and Peru and cultivated extensively in South America. Cocaine is classed as a drug of abuse when used for nonmedical purposes. "Street" names for cocaine include snow, coke, crack, lady, flake, gold dust, green gold, blow, and toot. Medically it is used as a topical anesthetic applied to mucous membranes. SYN: *cocaine*. SEE: *crack; free base; freebasing*.

cocaine hydrochloride poisoning, acute The acute, toxic, systemic reaction to an overdose of cocaine that has been eaten, smoked, inhaled, or injected. SEE: *Nursing Diagnoses Appendix*.

SYMPTOMS: An overdose of cocaine (cocaine toxicity) is an accelerated version of the classic physiological and psychological responses to cocaine use. Initial euphoria gives way to excitability, delirium, tremors, convulsions, tachycardia, and angina pectoris—all signs of overwhelming sympathetic stimulation of the central nervous, cardiovascular, and pulmonary systems. Death usually is due to a cardiovascular event or to respiratory failure. Plasma and liver pseudocholinesterase detoxify cocaine into water-soluble metabolites that are excreted in urine. Anyone with low plasma cholinesterase activity (e.g., fetus, infant, pregnant woman, or individual with liver disease) is especially prone to cocaine toxicity. Persons who congenitally lack pseudocholinesterase are highly sensitive to the effects of any dose of cocaine.

Many chronic cocaine users overdose while taking no more than their usual amount of the drug, when, for example, the purity (pharmacological strength) of an ingested dose is greater than usual. The lethal event is typically a myocardial infarction or ventricular dysrhythmia, such as ventricular fibrillation. Some cocaine users may die instead of intracerebral hemorrhage, that is, bleeding into the brain due to the rupture of an intracranial blood vessel. The presenting findings may include seizures, hemiplegia, aphasia, or coma. Patients admitted for trauma also may be cocaine intoxicated (2/3 of cocaine-related deaths result from traumatic injuries, not drug overdose). Because many signs and symptoms that cocaine produces resemble those that result from injuries, and because cocaine poisoning is life-threatening, emergency department care providers need to quickly distinguish drug-related problems from traumatic injury problems.

TREATMENT: Overdose requires prompt treatment aimed at reducing stimulation of the central nervous system (CNS) and supporting all systems. Hypertension and tachyarrhythmias may respond to diltiazem; naloxone may help reverse the effects of other drugs the patient may have taken, but no drug can reverse a cocaine overdose. To determine what drugs the patient has taken, emergency department personnel obtain blood and urine specimens as quickly as possible, as drug screens may take anywhere from one to 24 hours. The alert patient will often accurately describe the drugs that he or she has taken, including crack cocaine or cocaine in powdered form, taken by snorting or injection.

PATIENT CARE: Vital signs are checked frequently, the patient is attached to a cardiac monitor, and an intravenous line is initiated. Large volumes of fluids are infused to help remove protein breakdown products for the body, a result of rhabdomyolysis. Bilateral lung sounds are auscultated frequently during fluid resuscitation, as aggressive fluid therapy worsens heart failure. Care providers try to control patients physically to prevent them from injuring themselves; if patients demonstrate violent or aggressive behavior, chemical or physical restraints may be required. Calcium channel blockers or a benzodiazepine is administered as prescribed to reduce the patient's blood pressure and heart rate. Seizures, which occur because the brain's seizure threshold is lowered, are treated with diazepam. Because the drug causes hypothalamic thermal regulatory dysfunction, core body temperature is monitored closely. The high ambient temperature associated with hot days seems to exacerbate hyperthermia induced by cocaine poisoning. Elevated temperature is treated with acetaminophen and cooling blankets, cool-air ventilation, and cool saline gastric lavage. CNS stimulation may be followed by CNS depression, characterized by flaccid paralysis, coma, fixed and dilated pupils, respiratory failure, and cardiovascular collapse.

Cocaine smuggling often involves "body packing" (swallowing balloons, condoms, or other objects filled with cocaine). If these items leak, the patient becomes intoxicated, and is at high risk for death. Syncope or seizures are treated symptomatically. If such a patient arrives in the emergency department with cardiac or respiratory arrest, however, he or she usually will die.

If the patient survives the acute poisoning episode, treatment is directed toward helping the patient abstain from drugs and preventing relapses. The patient benefits from consultation with an addictions specialist or mental health nurse practitioner. Studies support the effectiveness of a 12-step program, such as Cocaine Anonymous, to help build a solid recovery program. Other community resources also can be accessed to provide various types of support and to help the patient identify and manage relapse triggers.

cocainism (kō′kān-ĭzm) The habitual use of cocaine. SEE: *cocaine hydrochloride poisoning, acute*.

cocainization (kō″kān-ĭ-zā′shŭn) The use of cocaine to induce analgesia.

cocainomania (kō″kān-ō-mā′nē-ă) An intense desire for cocaine and its effects.

cocarboxylase (kō″kăr-bŏk′sĭ-lās) Thiamine pyrophosphate.

cocarcinogen (kō-kăr′sĭ-nō-jĕn″) A chemical or environmental factor that enhances the action of a carcinogen, the end result being the development of a malignancy.

coccal (kŏk′ăl) Pert. to or caused by cocci.

cocci (kŏk′sī) Pl. of coccus.

Coccidia (kŏk-sĭd′ē-ă) [Gr. *kokkos,* berry] A subclass of the phylum Apicomplexa (apical microtubule complex) of the kingdom Protista. All are intracellular parasites usually infecting epithelial cells of the intestine and associated glands.

coccidian (kŏk-sĭd′ē-ăn) **1.** Pert. to Coccidia. **2.** Any member of the order Coccidia.

Coccidioides A genus of fungi with only one species, *Coccidioides immitis,* that is pathogenic for humans. SEE: illus.; *coccidioidomycosis*.

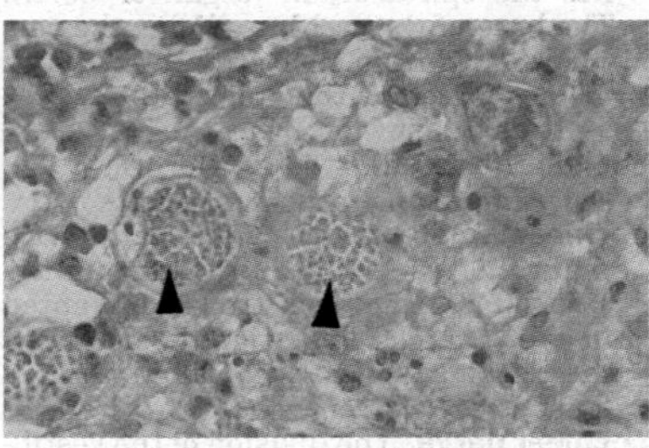

COCCIDIOIDES IMMITIS SPHERULES

(Orig. mag. ×450)

coccidioidin (kŏk″sĭd-ē-oy′dĭn) An antigenic substance prepared from *Coccidioides immitis.* It is used as a skin test in diagnosing coccidioidomycosis.

coccidioidomycosis (kŏk-sĭd″ĭ-oyd-ō-mī-kō′sĭs) [″ + *eidos,* form, shape, + *mykes,* fungus, + *osis,* condition] Infection with the pathogenic fungus, *Coccidioides immitis,* a spore-forming pathogen found in soil. Spores from the fungus (called arthroconidia) circulate in the air when the soil is disturbed, for example, during construction, dust storms, or earthquakes. Persons who inhale the spores may develop active or subclinical infection. SYN: *San Joaquin valley fever*. SEE: *granuloma; Nursing Diagnoses Appendix.*

Approx. 80% of persons in the southwest and western states have positive skin test reactions, which identify those infected. Usually these infections are asymptomatic and require no treatment. In approx. 10% of patients, fever, cough, pleurisy, or rashes such as erythema multiforme occur. Granulomas may be seen on the chest x-ray of patients with fungal pneumonia. Systemic infection involving the skin and meninges of the brain occurs in fewer than 1% of patients but is often fatal. Affected patients are treated with long-term fluconazole or with amphotericin B; these drugs have a 50% to 70% success rate.

DIAGNOSIS: Diagnostic testing for the disease includes collecting blood, sputum, pus from lesions, and tissue for biopsy, using strict secretion precautions. An initial skin test also is administered, as both the primary and disseminated forms produce a positive coccidioidin skin test. A rising serum or body fluid antibody titer indicates dissemination. Additional testing may involve pleural, spinal, and joint fluid for the presence of antibodies. After diagnosis, serial skin testing, blood cultures, and serologic testing are performed to help document the effectiveness of therapy. The patient is cautioned not to wash off the circle marked on the skin for serial testing, as it aids in reading test results.

TREATMENT: Most patients with primary infection recover without therapy. Patients with disseminated disease require prolonged chemotherapy. Amphotericin B is administered for 1 to 3 months. Meningitis due to *Coccidioides immitis* is treated with amphotericin B injected directly into the cerebrospinal fluid.

PROGNOSIS: For primary infection, the prognosis is favorable. Disseminated disease is often fatal.

PATIENT CARE: In mild primary disease, bedrest and adequate fluid intake are encouraged. The amount and color of sputum are recorded, and the patient is monitored for shortness of breath, an indicator of pleural effusion. If arthralgia is present, prescribed analgesics are administered. If the patient has draining lesions, the patient and family are taught about strict secretion precautions, including the "no touch" dressing technique and careful hand washing. In central nervous system (CNS) dissemination, the patient is monitored closely for decreased level of consciousness or change in mood or affect.

Before intrathecal administration of amphotericin B, the procedure is explained to the patient, who is reassured that he or she will receive a local anesthetic prior to lumbar puncture. If the patient is prescribed amphotericin B intravenously, a test dose is administered as prescribed; if tolerated, the treatment dose is infused slowly (rapid infusion may result in circulatory collapse). The dosage (but not the rate) is increased gradually as prescribed. During the infusion, the patient's vital signs are monitored. Temperature may rise and the patient may experience shaking chills and hypotension 1 to 2 hours after the infusion is initiated, but these should subside within 4 hours after the infusion is completed. Fluid intake and output are assessed, with any oliguria and anuria noted. Laboratory results are evaluated for elevated blood urea nitrogen and creatinine levels and hypokalemia. To ease adverse reactions to amphotericin B, antiemetics, antihistamines, and antipyretics or small doses of corticosteroids are administered as prescribed. The patient is warned to report immediately any hearing loss, tinnitus, dizziness, headache, blurred vision, diplopia, and breathing difficulty. Laboratory findings are also monitored for blood dyscrasias and liver failure. The patient is monitored for any seizures, cardiac arrhythmias, respiratory distress, hemorrhagic gastroenteritis, drug extravasation, and anaphylactoid reactions. The patient is informed that therapy may take several months, and the importance of cooperating with the treatment regimen and recommended follow-up studies is emphasized.

coccidiosis (kŏk-sĭd-ē-ō′sĭs) [″ + *osis,* condition] A pathogenic condition resulting from infestation with coccidia. SEE: *Coccidia*.

coccobacilli (kŏk″ō-bă-sĭl′ī) Bacilli that are short, thick, and somewhat ovoid. SEE: *bacterium* for illus.

coccobacteria (kŏk″ō-băk-tē′rē-ă) **1.** Spherical-shaped bacteria. **2.** Any kind of cocci.

coccogenous (kŏk-ŏj′ĕn-ŭs) [Gr. *kokkos,* berry, + *gennan,* to produce] Produced by cocci.

coccoid (kŏk′oyd) [″ + *eidos,* form, shape] Resembling a micrococcus.

coccus (kŏk′ŭs) *pl.* **cocci** [Gr. *kokkos,* berry] A bacterial type that is spherical or ovoid. When cocci appear singly, they are designated micrococci; in pairs, diplococci; in clusters like bunches of grapes, staphylococci; in chains, streptococci; in cubical packets of eight, sarcinae. Many are pathogenic, causing such diseases as strep throat, erysipelas, scarlet fever, rheumatic fever, pneumonia, gonorrhea, meningitis, and puerperal fever. SEE: *bacterium*.

coccyalgia, coccydynia (kŏk″sē-ăl′jē-ă, kŏk″sē-dĭn′ē-ă) [Gr. *kokkyx,* coccyx, + *algos,* pain, + *odyne,* pain] Pain in the coccyx. SYN: *coccygodynia*.

coccygeal (kŏk-sĭj′ē-ăl) Pert. to or in the region of the coccyx.

coccygeal nerve The lowest of the spinal nerves; one of the pair of nerves arising from the coccygeal section of the spinal cord and entering the pudendal plexus.

coccygectomy (kŏk″sĭ-jĕk′tō-mē) [″ + *ektome,* excision] Excision of the coccyx.

coccygeus (kŏk-sĭj′ē-ŭs) Pert. to the coccyx.

coccygodynia (kŏk-sĭ-gō-dĭn′ē-ă) [″ + *odyne,* pain] Coccyalgia.

coccyx (kŏk′sĭks) [Gr. *kokkyx,* coccyx] A small bone at the base of the spinal column in humans, formed by four fused rudimentary vertebrae. It is usually ankylosed and articulated with the sacrum above.

cochineal (kŏch′ĭn-ēl) [L. *coccinus,* scarlet] A dried female insect, *Coccus cacti,* previously used as a dye.

cochlea (kŏk′lē-ă) [Gr. *kokhlos,* land snail] A winding cone-shaped tube forming a portion of the inner ear. It contains the organ of Corti, the receptor for hearing.

The cochlea is coiled, resembling a snail shell, winding two and three quarters turns about a central bony axis, the modiolus. Projecting outward from the modiolus, a thin bony plate, the spiral lamina, partially divides the cochlear canal into an upper passageway, the scala vestibuli, and a lower one, the scala tympani. Between the two scalae is the cochlear duct, in the floor of which lies the spiral organ (organ of Corti). The base of the cochlea adjoins the vestibule. At the cupola or tip, the two scalae are joined at the helicotrema. SEE: illus. **cochlear** (-ăr), *adj.*

cochleariform (kŏk″lē-ăr′ĭ-form) [″ + L. *forma,* shape] Spoon-shaped.

cochlear implant An electrical device that receives sound and transmits the resulting signal to electrodes implanted in the cochlea. That signal stimulates the cochlea so that hearing-impaired persons can perceive sound.

cochlear nerve The division of the vestibulocochlear nerve (eighth cranial nerve) that supplies the cochlea. SEE: *vestibulocochlear nerve*.

cochleitis (kŏk″lē-ī′tĭs) [Gr. *kokhlos,* land snail, + *itis,* inflammation] Inflammation of the cochlea.

cochleo-orbicular reflex SEE: *cochleopalpebral reflex*.

cochleopalpebral reflex (kŏk″lē-ō-păl′pĕ-brăl) Contraction of the orbicularis palpebrarum muscle resulting from a sudden noise produced near the ear. SYN: *cochleo-orbicular reflex*.

cochleovestibular (kŏk″lē-ō-vĕs-tĭb′ū-lăr) [″ + L. *vestibulum,* vestibule] Pert. to the cochlea and vestibule of the ear.

cockroach [Sp. *cucaracha*] *Blatta orientalis,* a common insect of the order Orthoptera that infests homes and food handling and food storage places. They may transmit bacteria, protozoan cysts, and helminth ova to human food and are a common cause of household allergies and asthma.

cocktail (kŏk′tāl) Any beverage containing several ingredients, or any combination of drugs used to treat a disease that would not respond adequately to any of them given alone.

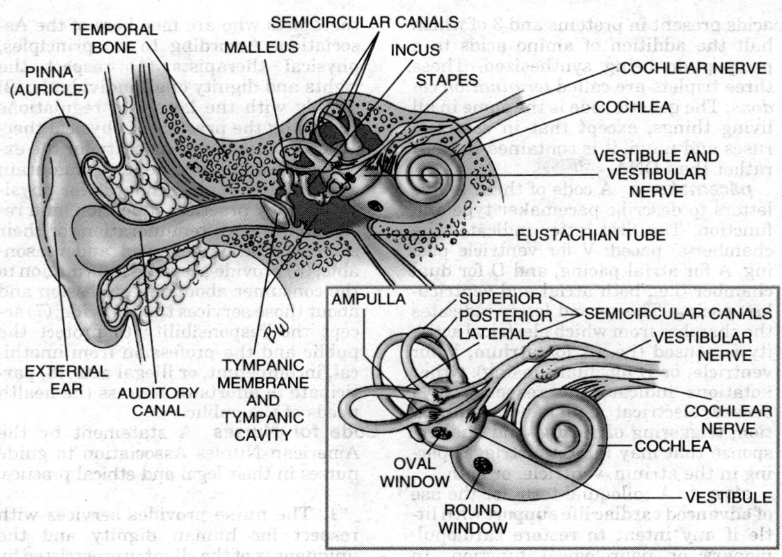

COCHLEA
(In relation to the inner ear and outer auditory apparatus)

GI c. A mixture of a topical anesthetic and antacid sometimes given to patients suspected of having noncardiac chest pain. Its use is controversial because patients having coronary chest pain may also suffer from gastrointestinal lesions that will respond to this therapy, confusing the diagnosis.

lytic c. A mixture of analgesic and phenothiazine derivatives used in anesthesia as a premedication.

cock-up splint A static splint designed to maintain the wrist in either extension or dorsal flexion.

cock-up toe A toe deformity with dorsiflexion of the metatarsophalangeal joint and flexion of the interphalangeal and distal interphalangeal joints. SEE: *hammertoe*.

cocoa butter Theobroma oil; the fat obtained from the roasted seed of *Theobroma cacao.* It is used as a base in suppositories and as a topical skin lubricant.

coconsciousness (kō-kŏn′shŭs-nĕs) Awareness of objects, ideas, or thoughts at the fringe of consciousness.

cocontraction (kō″kŏn-trăk′shŭn) A condition in which muscles around a joint or the spinal column contract simultaneously to provide stability.

coconut "water" [Sp. and Port. *coco,* coconut, + Eng. *nut*] The liquid obtained from an unripe coconut. The composition of the "water" varies with the species of coconut, maturation of the fruit, and location in which it was grown. It is not the treatment of choice for use in treating acute diarrhea because it is poor in sodium, chloride, and bicarbonate while rich in potassium, calcium, and magnesium.

code (kōd) **1.** A collection of rules and regulations or specifications. **2.** A set of symbols that communicate information or conceal it from people not familiar with the true meaning of the symbols. **3.** A form of message used in transmitting information in a hospital, esp. when the information is broadcast over a public address system (e.g., "code blue" or "code 9" could indicate a particular type of emergency to an emergency care team). SEE: *code cart; code drug*. **4.** A system of symbols that represents information contained in a computer data bank.

civil c. Comprehensive written organization of general rules and regulations authorized by the legislature, based on Roman, Spanish, and French civil law. In the U.S., the judicial system that presides over health care issues and lawsuits is governed by the civil code in some states and by common law in other states.

c. of ethics A summary (sometimes in written form) of a profession's values and standards of conduct.

genetic c. The sequence of bases in the DNA of living cells that provides the instructions for the synthesis of polypeptides (proteins) from amino acids. These instructions are contained in 64 nucleotide triplet sequences, called codons, 61 of which specify the 20 amino acids present in proteins and 3 of which halt the addition of amino acids to a polypeptide being synthesized. These three triplets are called *termination codons*. The genetic code is the same in all living things, except that in some viruses and fungi, it is contained in RNA rather than DNA.

pacemaker c. A code of three to five letters to describe pacemaker type and function. The first letter indicates the chamber(s) paced: V for ventricle pacing, A for atrial pacing, and D for dual chamber (i.e., both atrial and ventricular) pacing. The second letter indicates the chamber from which electrical activity is sensed (i.e., A for atrium, V for ventricle, or D for dual sensing). Other notations indicate the response to a sensed electrical signal: none, inhibition, triggering of pacing, and dual response that may inhibit or trigger pacing in the atrium, ventricle, or both.

slow c. A colloquial term for the use of advanced cardiac life support with little if any intent to restore cardiopulmonary or neurological function. In some instances, slow resuscitative efforts are made when professional staff and moribund patients differ with respect to their interpretation of the appropriateness of end of life care. The practice, at best, rests on dubious moral and legal grounds. An alternate term, the "Hollywood Code," implies that the rescue attempt is made as a pretense.

triplet c. In DNA or mRNA, the sequence of three nucleotides that is the code for a particular amino acid. The triplet sequence controls the amino acid sequence during protein synthesis.

code cart A container or cart that can easily and quickly be moved to a patient who has suddenly developed a life-threatening emergency. Supplies should always be replenished and arranged so that the most frequently used first-line drugs and equipment are readily available. Powered equipment, such as a defibrillator, is tested regularly to be certain it is functioning properly. SEE: *basic life support; code* (3).

code drug A medication used to treat acute life-threatening emergencies, such as arrhythmias, cardiac arrest, pulmonary edema, and shock. Included are drugs and equipment required for treating shock, cardiac arrhythmias, and heart block. SEE: *basic life support; code* (3); *code cart*.

Code of Ethics for Physical Therapists A code of ethics that sets forth ethical principles for the physical therapy profession. According to its preamble, members of this profession are responsible for maintaining and promoting ethical practice. This code of ethics, adopted by the American Physical Therapy Association, is binding on physical therapists who are members of the Association. According to its principles, physical therapists (1) respect the rights and dignity of all individuals; (2) comply with the laws and regulations governing the practice of physical therapy; (3) accept responsibility for the exercise of sound judgment; (4) maintain and promote high standards for physical therapy practice, education, and research; (5) seek remuneration for their services that is deserved and reasonable; (6) provide accurate information to the consumer about the profession and about those services they provide; (7) accept the responsibility to protect the public and the profession from unethical, incompetent, or illegal acts; (8) participate in efforts to address the health needs of the public.

Code for Nurses A statement by the American Nurses Association to guide nurses in their legal and ethical practice.

1. The nurse provides services with respect for human dignity and the uniqueness of the client, unrestricted by considerations of social or economic status, personal attributes, or the nature of health problems.
2. The nurse safeguards the client's right to privacy by judiciously protecting information of a confidential nature.
3. The nurse acts to safeguard the client and the public when health care and safety are affected by the incompetent, unethical, or illegal practice of any person.
4. The nurse assumes responsibility and accountability for individual nursing judgments and actions.
5. The nurse maintains competence in nursing.
6. The nurse exercises informed judgment and uses individual competence and qualifications as criteria in seeking consultation, accepting responsibilities, and delegating nursing activities to others.
7. The nurse participates in activities that contribute to the ongoing development of the profession's body of knowledge.
8. The nurse participates in the profession's efforts to implement and improve standards of nursing.
9. The nurse participates in the profession's efforts to establish and maintain conditions of employment conducive to high quality nursing care.
10. The nurse participates in the profession's effort to protect the public from misinformation and misrepresentation and to maintain the integrity of nursing.
11. The nurse collaborates with members of the health professions and other citizens in promoting community and national efforts to meet the health needs of the public.

[From Code for Nurses with Interpretive Statements, Kansas City, MO, American Nurses' Association, 1985]

codeine An alkaloid obtained from opium, or synthetically from morphine as methylmorphine. It is used as an analgesic, a cough suppressant, or a sedative/hypnotic drug. Common side effects include nausea, constipation, itching, or confusion. Tolerance of or dependence on codeine may develop with regular use.

c. phosphate The phosphate of the alkaloid codeine; used because of its free solubility in water.

c. sulfate The sulfate of the alkaloid codeine. It has the same uses as codeine.

codeine poisoning SEE: *opiate poisoning; Poisons and Poisoning Appendix.*

codependency **1.** In psychology, unintentional or conscious reinforcement of another person's addictive or self-destructive behaviors. **2.** In biology, symbiosis.

coding In billing for medical services, the grouping of medical diagnoses within an established category, usually with standard symbols such as those in the International Classification of Diseases.

cod liver oil An oil obtained from codfish liver, which is rich in vitamins A and D.

ACTION/USES: Cod liver oil was widely used in cases of nutritional deficiency to supply vitamins A and D, esp. for prophylaxis of rickets in infants. It is rarely used now because more efficient and more palatable agents are available.

codon (kō′dŏn) A sequence of three bases in a strand of DNA or mRNA (messenger RNA) that is the genetic code for a specific amino acid.

coefficient (kō″ĕ-fĭsh′ĕnt) **1.** In chemistry, a numeral put before a chemical formula or compound to indicate the number of molecules of that substance taking part in the chemical reaction. **2.** An expression of the ratio between two different quantities, or the effect produced by varying certain factors.

activity c. **1.** A factor used in potentiometry to describe the activity of free ions in solution. **2.** A vitamin deficiency factor that describes the enhancement of enzyme activity after saturation with a vitamin.

attenuation c. The calculated remainder of the x-ray beam that is received by the detectors in a computed tomography unit. This value is used to determine the CT (Hounsfield) number.

diffusion c. The number of milliliters of gas at 1 atmosphere of pressure that will diffuse a distance of 1 μm over 1 sq cm/min.

c. of absorption The volume of gas absorbed by a unit volume of a liquid at 0°C and a pressure of 760 mm Hg.

c. of elastic expansion The volumetric expression in cubic centimeters of a compressed gas cylinder under hydrostatic test conditions.

c. of thermal expansion The change in the dimensions of a material when its temperature is raised 1°C. In dentistry, if the relative expansion and contraction of restorative materials, casts, or appliances are not accounted for, the patient may have problems with improper fitting, microleakage, or adhesive debonding.

c. of variation Analytical variability expressed as the standard deviation's percentage of the mean. This mode of expressing the analytical variability enables one to determine if the variability proportion changes with the actual value. It is typically a useful tool when there is a relatively large dynamic range for the quantity being measured. It is subject to misinterpretation if applied to numbers that have already been mathematically manipulated, such as logarithms.

Coelenterata (sē-lĕn″tĕr-ā′tă) A phylum of invertebrates that includes corals, hydras, jellyfish, and sea anemones. Contact with some species can result in sting injuries. SEE: *bite; sting.*

coelom (sē′lŏm) [Gr. *koiloma,* a cavity] The cavity in an embryo between the split layers of lateral mesoderm. In mammals it develops into the pleural, peritoneal, and pericardial cavities. SYN: *body cavity.*

extraembryonic c. In humans, the cavity in the developing blastocyst that lies between the mesoderm of the chorion and the mesoderm covering the amniotic cavity and yolk sac.

coenocyte (sē′nō-sīt, sĕn′ō-sīt) [Gr. *koinos,* common, + *kytos,* cell] A multinucleated mass of protoplasm; a mass of protoplasm in which there are no cell membranes between the nuclei. SYN: *syncytium.*

coenzyme (kō-ĕn′zīm) [L. *co-,* together, + Gr. *en,* in, + *zyme,* leaven] An enzyme activator; a diffusible, heat-stable substance of low molecular weight that, when combined with an inactive protein called apoenzyme, forms an active compound or a complete enzyme called a holoenzyme (e.g., adenylic acid, riboflavin, and coenzymes I and II).

coenzyme A A derivative of pantothenic acid, important as a carrier molecule for acetyl groups in many reactions including the Krebs cycle and the oxidation of fatty acids.

coenzyme Q A dietary supplement promoted by alternative medicine practitioners as an antioxidant.

coenzyme Q10 ABBR: CoQ10. A vitamin-like substance which can be synthesized from tyrosine in a multistep process. It is a coenzyme for several mitochondrial enzymes involved in ATP production. Its reduced form is a potent antioxidant. Coenzyme Q10 is also known as ubiquinone.

coetaneous (kō″ē-tā′nē-ŭs) [″ + *aetas,* age] Having the same age or date.

coexcitation (kō-ĕk-sī-tā′shŭn) [″ + *excitare,* to arouse] Simultaneous excitation of two parts or bodies.

cofactor (kō′făk-tor) **1.** A biochemical or physiological agent that produces an effect in conjunction with other agents. **2.** One of several agents in the development of an illness or epidemic.

coffee The beverage made from the seed of trees of the genus *Coffea,* called coffee beans. Coffee has a 2500-year history of use. Its use is associated with a decreased risk of depression. The possibility that its use causes harm is complicated by the fact that roasted coffee contains more than 700 volatile and nonvolatile compounds. The investigations have not produced evidence that normal consumption of caffeine is a risk factor for cardiovascular disease, birth defects, breast disease, or cancer. SEE: *caffeine; caffeine withdrawal; tea.*

Cogan's syndrome (kō′găns) [David G. Cogan, U.S. ophthalmologist, b. 1908] Interstitial keratitis associated with tinnitus, vertigo, and usually deafness.

cognition (kŏg-nĭsh′ŭn) [L. *cognoscere,* to know] Thinking skills that include language use, calculation, perception, memory, awareness, reasoning, judgment, learning, intellect, social skills, and imagination. **cognitive** (kŏg′nĭ-tĭv), *adj.*

coherent (kō-hēr′ĕnt) [L. *cohaerere,* to stick together] **1.** Sticking together, as parts of bodies or fluids. **2.** Consistent; making a logical whole.

cohesion (kō-hē′zhŭn) The property of adhering.

cohesive (kō-hē′sĭv) Adhesive; sticky.

Cohnheim's areas (kōn′hīmz) [Julius Friedrich Cohnheim, Ger. pathologist, 1839–1884] One of the irregular groups of fibrils seen in a cross section of a striated muscle fiber.

Cohnheim's theory The obsolete theory that tumors result from embryonal cells not used for fetal development.

cohort A selected group of people born during a particular period and traced through life during successive time and age periods. SEE: *analysis, cohort.*

cohort study In epidemiology, a method of investigation using a cohort studied prospectively or retrospectively.

coil (koyl) A continuous material such as tubing, rope, or a spring arranged in a spiral, loop, or circle.

coilonychia (koy″lō-nĭk′ē-ă) [Gr. *koilos,* hollow, + *onyx,* nail] Dystrophy of the fingernails in which they are thin and concave with raised edges. This condition is sometimes associated with iron-deficiency anemia. SEE: *koilonychia* for illus.

coin counting A sliding movement of the tips of the thumb and index finger over each other. This may occur in Parkinson's disease. Also called *pill rolling.*

coinfection The simultaneous infection of an organism or individual cells by two different pathological microorganisms.

coining (koy′nĭng) **1.** A traditional health practice in some Asian subcultures in which a heated coin is placed on the skin to treat certain conditions (such as asthma). A health care provider who is unaware of this practice could, erroneously, attribute the lesion to physical abuse. **2.** In biomedical engineering, a cold-working process used to improve the strength of metals used for biological purposes (e.g., nails used in orthopedic surgeries).

coitarche Age at first sexual intercourse.

coition (kō-ĭsh′ŭn) [L. *coire,* to come together] Coitus.

coitophobia (kō″ĭ-tō-fō′bē-ă) [″ + Gr. *phobos,* fear] Morbid fear of sexual intercourse.

coitus (kō′ĭ-tŭs) Sexual intercourse between a man and a woman by insertion of the penis into the vagina. SYN: *coition; copulation; sexual intercourse.* **coital** (-tăl), *adj.*

c. à la vache Coitus from behind with the woman in the knee-chest position.

c. interruptus Coitus with withdrawal of the penis from the vagina before seminal emission occurs. This is not an effective method of contraception.

c. reservatus Coitus with intentional suppression of ejaculation.

c. Saxonius Coitus with manual pressure of the urethra at the underside of the penis or in the perineum to block the emission of semen at ejaculation; also called the squeeze technique. The woman may do this to prevent her partner's premature ejaculation.

col (kŏl) The nonkeratinized, depressed gingival tissue that lies between adjacent teeth; it extends labiolingually between the interdental papillae below the interproximal contact of the teeth.

Cola (kō′lă) [W. African *kola*] A genus of tropical trees that produce the kola nut. A kola nut extract is used in pharmaceutical preparations and as a main ingredient in some carbonated beverages.

colation (kō-lā′shŭn) [L. *colare,* to strain] Straining, filtering.

colchicine (kŏl′chĭ-sĭn) A medicine used principally to treat and prevent gout. One common side effect of the drug is diarrhea.

COLD *chronic obstructive lung disease.* SEE: *chronic obstructive pulmonary disease.*

cold [AS. *ceald,* cold] **1.** A general term for coryza or inflammation of the respiratory mucous membranes known as the common cold. **2.** Lacking heat or warmth; having a low temperature; the opposite of heat.

chest c. Acute bronchitis

common c. An acute infection of any or all parts of the respiratory tract from the nasal mucosa to the nasal sinuses, throat, larynx, trachea, and bronchi. Common colds occur in most people, usually at least once a year. They are more common in smokers and in children than in healthy adults. The common cold causes more loss of work and school time than any other ailment.

The contagious period begins before the onset of symptoms. Causative viruses are distributed to others by sneezing (aerosolization) and by direct contact with nasal secretions. The incubation period is typically from 12 to 72 hr.

ETIOLOGY: Most colds are caused by rhinoviruses, adenoviruses, coronaviruses, coxsackieviruses, influenza viruses, parainfluenza viruses, or respiratory syncytial viruses.

SYMPTOMS: The common cold is marked by swelling of the nasal mucosa with increased mucus production that may occlude the nasal passages. Sneezing, lacrimation, a sore or scratchy throat, hoarseness, cough, colorful sputum, headache, chills, and malaise are also common. Symptoms usually resolve within 2 days to 2 weeks. If a cold lasts longer than 10 days, or is accompanied by fever or systemic symptoms, it is advisable to consult a health care provider. Persons with chronic diseases, such as diabetes or heart or lung disease, should consult a health care provider if a cold is severe, is accompanied by fever, or lasts more than 10 days.

CONTAGIOUSNESS: The virus may be present in the nasal secretions for a week or longer after the onset of symptoms.

cold agglutinin disease A group of disorders marked by hemolytic anemia, obstruction of the microcirculation, or both. It is caused by agglutination of red blood cells by cold agglutinin. In some people this is caused by a transient infectious disease; in others, the cause is idiopathic. The latter occurs mostly in women over 50 years of age.

cold cream A water-in-oil emulsion ointment base used on the skin.

cold-damp Foggy vapor in a mine charged with carbon dioxide.

cold pressor test A test that measures blood pressure response to the immersion of one hand in ice water. An excessive increase in pressure was once thought to indicate a latent hypertensive state.

coldspray An aerosol coolant used to lower the temperature quickly and thus harden thermoplastic splinting material during fitting or molding.

cold stress SEE: *hypothermia*.

colectomy (kō-lĕk′tō-mē) [Gr. *kolon,* colon, + *ektome,* excision] Excision of part or all of the colon.

coleocystitis (kō″lē-ō-sĭs-tī′tĭs) Colpocystitis.

coleoptosis (kō″lē-ŏp-tō′sĭs) [″ + *ptosis,* a dropping] Prolapse of the wall of the vagina.

coleotomy (kō″lē-ŏt′ō-mē) Colpotomy.

colestipol hydrochloride (kō-lĕs′tĭ-pōl) An anion-exchange resin used to treat hypercholesterolemia. Common side effects include constipation, bloating, and abdominal discomfort.

colibacillemia (kō″lĭ-băs-ĭl-lē′mē-ă) [Gr. *kolon,* colon, + L. *bacillus,* little rod, + Gr. *haima,* blood] *Escherichia coli* in the blood.

colibacillosis (kō″lĭ-băs-ĭ-lō′sĭs) [″ + ″ + Gr. *osis,* condition] Infection with *Escherichia coli.*

colibacilluria (kō-lĭ-băs-ĭl-ū′rē-ă) [″ + ″ + Gr. *ouron,* urine] Presence of *Escherichia coli* in the urine.

colibacillus (kō″lĭ-bă-sĭl′ŭs) [″ + L. *bacillus,* little rod] The colon bacillus, *Escherichia coli.*

colic (kŏl′ĭk) [Gr. *kolikos,* pert. to the colon] **1.** Spasm in any hollow or tubular soft organ accompanied by pain. **2.** Pert. to the colon. SEE: *cholecystalgia; tormina.*

biliary c. Right upper quadrant pain resulting from obstruction of a bile duct by a gallstone.

infantile c. Colic occurring in infants, principally during the first few months. It may respond to substitution of a hypoallergenic formula for that containing cow's milk, or to decreased stimulation of the infant.

intestinal c. Abdominal colic, typically associated with intestinal obstruction or ileus.

lead c. Severe abdominal colic associated with lead poisoning.

menstrual c. Dysmenorrhea.

renal c. Pain in the region of one of the flanks that radiates inferiorly, toward the lower abdomen, groin, scrotum, labia, or thigh. This condition may be associated with the passage of kidney stones.

uterine c. Severe abdominal pain arising in the uterus, usually during the menstrual period. SEE: *dysmenorrhea.*

colica (kŏl′ĭ-kă) [L.] Colic.

colicin (kŏl′ĭ-sĭn) A bacteriocin produced by some strains of *Escherichia coli* that is lethal to other *E. coli.* Since its discovery in 1925, approx. 20 colicins have been described, some produced by bacteria other than *E. coli.* All colicins are now called bacteriocins.

colicky (kŏl′ĭk-ē) Concerning colic or affected by it.

colicolitis (kō″lĭ-kō-lī′tĭs) [Gr. *kolon,* colon, + *kolon,* colon, + *itis,* inflammation] Colitis due to *Escherichia coli.*

colicoplegia (kō″lĭ-kō-plē′jē-ă) [″ + *plege,* stroke] Colic and paralysis due to lead poisoning.

colicystitis (kō″lĭ-sĭs-tī′tĭs) [″ + *kystis,* bladder, + *itis,* inflammation] Inflammation of the bladder resulting from *Escherichia coli* infection.

colicystopyelitis (kō-lĭ-sĭs″tō-pī″ĕ-lī′tĭs) [″ + ″+ *pyelos,* pelvis, + *itis,* inflammation] *Escherichia coli* inflammation of the bladder and renal pelvis.

coliform (kō′lĭ-form) [″ + L. *forma,* form] **1.** Sieve form; cribriform. **2.** A general term applied to some species of the family Enterobacteriaceae, including *Escherichia coli, Enterobacter,* and *Klebsiella* species. Their presence in water, esp. that of *E. coli,* is presumptive evidence of fecal contamination.

colinephritis (kō″lĭ-nē-frī′tĭs) [″ + *nephros,* kidney, + *itis,* inflammation] Nephritis caused by *Escherichia coli.*

coliplication (kō″lĭ-plĭ-kā′shŭn) [″ + L. *plica,* fold] Operation for correcting a dilated colon.

colipuncture (kō′lĭ-pŭnk″chūr) Colocentesis.

colisepsis [″ + *sepsis,* putrefaction] Infection caused by *Escherichia coli.*

colistimethate sodium, sterile (kō-lĭs″tĭ-mĕth′āt) A form of colistin, suitable for use intramuscularly or intravenously.

colistin sulfate (kō-lĭs′tĭn) Polymyxin E; an antibiotic effective against some gram-negative bacteria, esp. *Pseudomonas* organisms, that are resistant to other antibiotics. Trade name is Coly-Mycin S.

colitis (kō-lī′tĭs) [″ + *itis,* inflammation] Inflammation of the colon. SEE: *dysentery; gay bowel syndrome; regional ileitis.*

amebic c. Amebiasis.

antibiotic-associated c. Antibiotic-induced diarrhea. SEE: *pseudomembranous c.*

pseudomembranous c. Colitis associated with antibiotic therapy and, less commonly, with chronic debilitating illnesses in adult patients in the community. It is caused by one of two exotoxins produced by *Clostridium difficile,* which is part of the normal intestinal flora. Broad-spectrum antibiotics disrupt the normal balance of the intestinal flora and allow an overgrowth of strains that produce toxins. The exotoxins damage the mucosa of the colon and produce a pseudomembrane composed of inflammatory exudate. The symptoms—foul-smelling diarrhea with gross blood and mucus, abdominal cramps, fever, and leukocytosis—usually begin 4 to 10 days after the start of antibiotic therapy. The disease is treated by discontinuing previously prescribed antibiotics and beginning therapy with oral metronidazole; use of vancomycin should be limited to patients who do not respond to metronidazole. Diarrhea may reappear in approx. 20% of patients after treatment, necessitating a second course of therapy.

radiation c. Colitis due to damage of the bowel by radiation therapy. The symptoms are those of an inflamed bowel: pain, cramps, diarrhea, and rectal bleeding. Malabsorption may develop as a result of permanent injury to the mucosa.

ulcerative c. An inflammatory bowel disease marked pathologically by continuous inflammation of the intestinal mucosa, which typically involves the anus, rectum, and distal colon, and sometimes affects the entire large intestine. It occurs most often in patients during the second or third decade of life, although a second cluster of cases occurs in patients in their sixties. The disease is associated with an increased incidence of cancer of the colon. SEE: *Crohn's disease; inflammatory bowel disease; Nursing Diagnoses Appendix.*

SYMPTOMS: Bloody diarrhea and pain with the passage of stools are characteristic. In severe cases, patients may have more than 6 bloody bowel movements in a day. Iron deficiency anemia often develops as a result.

TREATMENT: Aminosalicylate drugs and corticosteroids decrease symptoms and improve inflammation. Patients with refractory disease may require colectomy.

PATIENT CARE: The patient is prepared for diagnostic studies and is told that they can be uncomfortable and fatiguing. He or she is assisted to understand and participate in treatment goals: controlling inflammation, maintaining or restoring fluid and electrolyte balance, receiving adequate nutrition and replacing nutritional losses, and preventing complications. The nurse or dietitian teaches the patient about dietary intake, which should be high-caloric, non-spicy, caffeine-free, and low in high residue foods and milk products. Actual dietary and caloric intake must be documented. If the patient is unable to take fluids by mouth, intravenous (IV) fluid and electrolyte replacement are instituted as prescribed. Fluid intake and output are monitored, particularly for frequency, volume, and characteristics of diarrhea. The patient is monitored for dehydration and electrolyte imbalances, particularly hypokalemia, hypernatremia, and anemia.

Prescribed drug therapy is administered; the patient is evaluated for desired and adverse effects and is taught about the particulars of his or her regimen, which usually includes sulfasalazine (5-ASA), prescribed for its antibiotic and anti-inflammatory effects. Studies have shown that, in high-risk patients, 5-ASA given both orally and by enema appears to sustain remission better than oral therapy alone. Since 5-ASA interferes with folate metabolism, use of a folate supplement is encouraged. Corticosteroids such as prednisone often are prescribed to reduce inflammation. The patient is taught that once clinical remission is achieved, steroid therapy can be tapered gradually and discontinued, but should never be summarily stopped. If the patient requires prolonged steroid therapy, he or she must report gastric irritation, edema, personality changes, moon face, and hirsutism. Corticosteroids given chronically may produce many side effects, including bone loss, diabetes mellitus, and cataract, among others. Antispasmodic and antidiarrheal agents (tincture of belladonna, diphenoxylate, loperamide) are used rarely and with great caution because they can precipitate colonic dilation (toxic megacolon). Measures to prevent perianal skin breakdown are reviewed (e.g., cleaning the rectal area thoroughly but gently following each bowel movement, applying a moisture barrier such as petroleum jelly, and changing position frequently).

colla (kŏl′lă) Pl. of collum.

collagen (kŏl′ă-jĕn) [Gr. *kolla,* glue, + *gennan,* to produce] A strong, fibrous insoluble protein found in connective tissue, including the dermis, tendons, ligaments, deep fascia, bone, and cartilage. Collagen is the protein typical of dental tissues (except enamel), forming the matrix of dentin, cementum, and alveolar bone proper. Collagen fibers also form the periodontal ligament, which attaches the teeth to their bony sockets.

collagenase (kŏl-lăj′ĕ-nās) [″ + ″ + *-ase,* enzyme] A member of the metalloproteinase family of enzymes that degrades collagen.

collagenic (kŏl″ă-jĕn′ĭk) Producing or containing collagen.

collagenoblast (kŏl-lăj′ĕ-nō-blăst) [″ + ″ + *blastos,* germ] A fibroblast-derived cell that produces collagen when mature.

collagenolysis (kŏl″ă-jĕn-ŏl′ĭ-sĭs) [″ + ″ + *lysis,* dissolution] The degradation or destruction of collagen.

collagenosis (kŏl-lăj″ĕ-nō′sĭs) [″ + ″ + *osis,* condition] A connective tissue disease.

collapse [L. *collapsus,* fallen to pieces] **1.** A sudden exhaustion, prostration, or weakness due to decreased circulation of the blood. **2.** An abnormal retraction of the walls of an organ.

SYMPTOMS: The symptoms include thirst, dizziness on arising, apathy, lethargy, delirium, frank loss of consciousness, or convulsions. Physical findings include pallor, cold clammy skin, gooseflesh, a thin or thready pulse, an increased respiratory rate, tachycardia, and hypotension.

PATIENT CARE: A patent airway is maintained, the patient's head is lowered, and the lower extremities are elevated slightly in the Trendelenburg position to enhance venous return to the heart. Vital signs and level of consciousness are assessed for signs of shock or aspiration of vomitus. High concentration oxygen by a nonrebreather mask should be administered and oxygen saturation and ventilation evaluated. The patient should be kept warm but not hot. The patient's ECG should be monitored for arrhythmias, and an IV line should be established. If the patient is hypotensive, a rapid infusion of normal saline or lactated Ringer's should be considered. The health care provider remains with the patient, briefly and calmly orienting him or her to surroundings and explaining procedures to provide reassurance of appropriate care.

circulatory c. Shock.

c. of lung An airless state of all or part of a lung. This is normal in the fetus. It is artificially induced by pneumothorax, thoracoplasty, or avulsion of the phrenic nerve. It may occur spontaneously owing to rupture of a bleb on the pleural surface of the lung.

collapsing **1.** Falling into extreme and sudden prostration resembling shock. **2.** Shrinking; disintegrating. **3.** Condensing.

collapsotherapy (kŏ-lăp″sō-thĕr′ă-pē) [L. *collapsus,* fallen to pieces, + Gr. *therapeia,* treatment] Treatment of pulmonary disorders by unilateral pneumothorax and immobilization of the affected lung.

collar (kŏl′ăr) [L. *collum,* neck] **1.** Band worn around the neck. **2.** A structure or marking formed like a neckband. **3.** A device designed to limit movement of the neck.

cervical c. A soft or rigid band of plastic or padded foam that is designed to limit extension, flexion, and lateral movement of the neck. Soft collars usually are reserved for confirmed strains of the neck. SEE: *extrication c.; cervical immobilization device; orthosis; Philadelphia collar.*

extrication c. Rigid cervical c.

c. of Venus Syphilitic leukoderma.

rigid cervical c. A firm plastic collar applied to the neck of a patient whose mechanism of injury may lead to a neck injury. It is designed to limit flexion, extension, and lateral movement of the neck. Because no collar eliminates all movement, patients who have not yet had a fracture ruled out by x-ray examination should remain immobilized to a backboard. SYN: *extrication c.* SEE: *cervical immobilization device.*

collar bone Clavicle.

collateral (kŏ-lăt′ĕr-ăl) [L. *con,* together, + *lateralis,* pert. to a side] **1.** Accom-

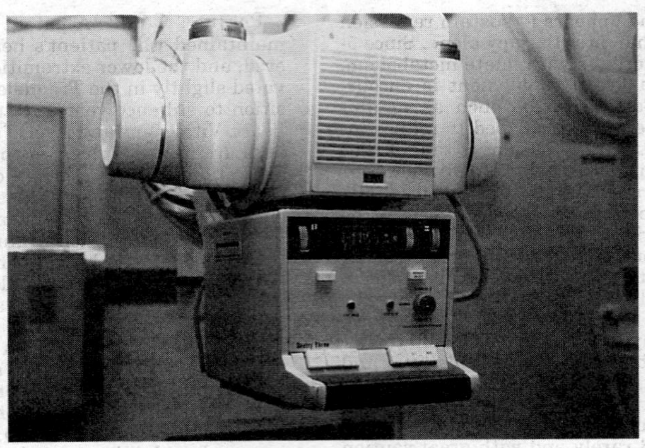

COLLIMATOR BELOW X-RAY TUBE

panying, side by side, as in a small side branch of a blood vessel or nerve. **2.** Subordinate or accessory.

collateral trigone The angle between the diverging inferior and posterior horns of the lateral ventricle.

collectin (kŏl-lĕk′tĭn) A plasma protein that binds carbohydrate molecules in the cell walls of microorganisms and facilitates phagocytosis. SEE: *phagocytosis.*

Colles, Abraham Irish surgeon, 1773–1843.

C.'s fascia The inner layer of the superficial fascia of the perineum.

C.'s fracture A transverse fracture of the distal end of the radius (just above the wrist) with displacement of the hand backward and outward.

PATIENT CARE: A history of the injury is obtained, and the patient is assessed for pain, swelling, mobility, and any deformity of the distal forearm. The areas above and below the fracture site are inspected for color changes and palpated for pulses, temperature, and the presence of sensation. The extremity is temporarily immobilized with a splint, and cold is applied according to protocol to reduce pain and limit swelling. The patient is scheduled for radiography, all procedures are explained, and noninvasive pain relief measures are instituted to reduce discomfort. The nurse or orthopedic technician assists with closed reduction and casting if carried out in the emergency department or refers the patient to an orthopedic surgeon for treatment and follow-up care.

colliculectomy (kŏl-lĭk″ū-lĕk′tō-mē) [L. *colliculus,* mound, + Gr. *ektome,* excision] Removal of the colliculus seminalis.

colliculitis (kŏl-lĭk″ū-lī′tĭs) [″ + Gr. *itis,* inflammation] Inflammation of the colliculus seminalis.

colliculus (kŏl-lĭk′ū-lŭs) *pl.* **colliculi** [L.] A little eminence.

c. bulbi Erectile tissue encircling the male urethra at the entrance to the bulb.

c. cervicalis The crest on the posterior wall of the female urethra.

c. inferior One of two elevations forming the lower portion of the corpora quadrigemina of the midbrain.

c. seminalis An oval enlargement on the crista urethralis, an elevation in the floor of the prostatic portion of the urethra. On its sides are the openings of the ejaculatory ducts and numerous ducts of the prostate gland. SYN: *c. urethralis.*

c. superior One of two elevations forming the upper portion of the corpora quadrigemina of the midbrain.

c. urethralis C. seminalis.

collimation (kŏl″ĭ-mā′shŭn) [L. *collineare,* to align] **1.** The process of making parallel. **2.** In radiography, the process of limiting the scatter and extent of the x-ray beam to the part being radiographed.

collimator (kŏl′ĭ-mā″tur) [L. *collineare,* to align, direct, aim] A radiographic device used to limit the scatter and extent of the x-ray beam. SEE: illus.

colliquation (kŏl″ĭ-kwā′shŭn) [L. *con,* together, + *liquare,* to melt] **1.** Abnormal discharge of a body fluid. **2.** Softening of tissues to liquefaction. **3.** Wasting.

colliquative (kŏ-lĭk′wă-tĭv) Pert. to a liquid and excessive discharge, as a colliquative diarrhea.

collodion (kō-lō′dē-ŏn) [Gr. *kollodes,* resembling glue] A thick fluid coating, made of dissolved pyroxylin, that is used to dress wounds or to supply medications to the skin. When applied, it dries to form a transparent film.

flexible c. A collodion preparation

containing camphor and castor oil. It is more elastic than collodion.

salicylic acid c. A flexible film used to remove accumulated layers of dead skin and scale (e.g., to treat psoriasis, warts, corns, or calluses).

colloid (kŏl′oyd) [Gr. *kollodes,* glutinous] **1.** A gluelike substance, such as a protein or starch, whose particles (molecules or aggregates of molecules), when dispersed as much as possible in a solvent, remain uniformly distributed and do not form a true solution. **2.** The size of a microscopic colloid; particles ranging from 10^{-9} to 10^{-11} meters (1 to 100 nm). **3.** A homogeneous gel found within the follicles of the thyroid gland and containing the thyroid hormones. **4.** A substance used as a plasma expander in place of blood. **colloidal** (-loyd′ăl), *adj.*

thyroid c. A semifluid, jelly-like substance filling the follicles of the thyroid gland. It contains the thyroid hormones.

colloid chemistry The application of chemistry to systems and substances, and the problems of emulsions, mists, foams, and suspensions.

colloidin (kŏl-loy′dĭn) A jelly-like substance seen in colloid degeneration.

colloidoclasia (kŏl-oyd″ō-klā′sē-ă) [″ + *klasis,* fracture] An obsolete term for an alteration in the equilibrium of body colloids, thought to be responsible for anaphylaxis.

colloidopexy (kŏl-oyd′ō-pĕk″sē) [″ + *pexis,* fixation] Fixation of colloids during metabolism.

colloma (kŏ-lō′mă) [Gr. *kolla,* glue, + *oma,* tumor] A colloid degeneration of a cancer.

collopexia (kŏl″ō-pĕk′sē-ă) [L. *collum,* neck, + Gr. *pexis,* fixation] Fixation of the cervix uteri.

collum (kŏl′lŭm) *pl.* **colla** [L.] **1.** The necklike part of an organ. **2.** The neck.

collyrium (kō-lĭr′ē-ŭm) [Gr. *kollyrion,* eye salve] An eyewash or lotion for the eye.

coloboma (kŏl″ō-bō′mă) [Gr. *koloboma,* a mutilation] A lesion or defect of the eye, usually a fissure or cleft of the iris, ciliary body, or choroid. It may be congenital, pathological, or surgical. Sometimes the eyelid is involved.

colocecostomy (kō″lō-sē-kŏs′tō-mē) [Gr. *kolon,* colon, + L. *caecum,* blindness, + Gr. *stoma,* mouth] Surgical joining of the colon to the cecum of the small intestine.

colocentesis (kō″lō-sĕn-tē′sĭs) [″ + *kentesis,* puncture] Surgical puncture of the colon to relieve distention. SYN: *colipuncture; colopuncture.*

colocolostomy (kō″lō-kō-lŏs′tō-mē) [″ + *kolon,* colon, + *stoma,* mouth] The surgical formation of a passage between two portions of the colon.

colocutaneous (kō″lō-kū-tā′nē-ŭs) [″ + L. *cutis,* skin] **1.** Pert. to the colon and the skin. **2.** Pert. to a pathological or surgical connection between the colon and the skin. SEE: *colostomy.*

coloenteritis (kō″lō-ĕn″tĕr-ī′tĭs) [Gr. *kolon,* colon, + *enteron,* intestine, + *itis,* inflammation] Inflammation of the mucous membrane of the small and large intestines.

colofixation (kō″lō-fĭk-sā′shŭn) Suspension of the colon.

colon [L.; Gr. *kolon*] The large intestine from the end of the ileum to the anal canal that surrounds the anus, about 59 in. (1.5 m) long; divided into the ascending, the transverse, the descending, and the sigmoid or pelvic colon. Beginning at the cecum, the first part of the large intestine (ascending colon) passes upward to the right colic or hepatic flexure, where it turns as the transverse colon passing ventral to the liver and stomach. On reaching the spleen, it turns downward (left colic or splenic flexure) and continues as the descending colon to the brim of the pelvis, where it is continuous with the sigmoid colon and extends to the rectum. SEE: illus.

FUNCTION: *Mechanical:* The colon mixes the intestinal contents. *Chemical:* The colon does not secrete digestive enzymes. The products of bacterial action that are absorbed into the bloodstream are carried by the portal circulation to the liver before they enter the general circulation. More water is absorbed in the colon than in the small intestine. In this way, body fluids are conserved, and despite the large volumes of secretions added to the food during its progress through the alimentary canal, the contents of the colon are gradually dehydrated until they assume the consistency of normal feces or even become quite hard. SEE: *absorption, colon; defecation.* **colonic** (kō-lŏn′ĭk), *adj.*

bacteria of the c. The normal microbial flora in the colon, some of which may produce vitamins, esp. vitamin K; metabolize proteins and sugars; produce organic acids and ammonia; and deconjugate bile acids. Several conditions, such as use of antibiotics, corticosteroids, or dieting, may alter the normal flora. Although *Escherichia coli* is the most widely known bacterium that inhabits the colon, it is not the most common, being outnumbered by anaerobic *Bacteroides* species by a very wide margin. SEE: *intestinal flora.*

carcinoma of the c. Colorectal carcinoma.

irritable c. irritable bowel syndrome.

polyp of c. SEE: *polyp, colonic.*

toxic dilatation of c. toxic megacolon.

colonalgia (kō″lŏn-ăl′jē-ă) [Gr. *kolon,* colon, + *algos,* pain] Pain in the colon.

colonitis (kō-lŏn-ī′tĭs) [″ + *itis,* inflammation] Colitis.

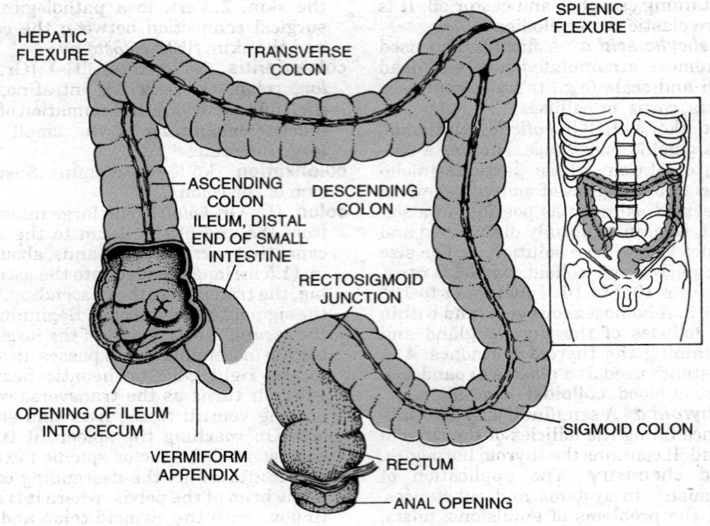

COLON AND RECTUM

colonization (kŏl″ŏ-nĭ-zā′shŭn) **1.** The growth of microorganisms, esp. bacteria, in a particular body site. **2.** Innidiation.

colonopathy (kō″lō-nŏp′ă-thē) [Gr. *kolon,* colon, + *pathos,* disease] Any disease of the colon.

colonopexy (kō-lŏn′ō-pĕk″sē) [″ + *pexis,* fixation] Surgical attachment of part of the colon to the abdominal wall.

colonorrhagia (kō″lŏn-ō-rā′jē-ă) [″ + *rhegnynai,* to burst forth] Hemorrhage from the colon.

colonorrhea (kō″lŏn-ō-rē′ă) [″ + *rhoia,* flow] **1.** Colitis. **2.** Discharge of watery fluid from the colon.

colonoscope (kō-lŏn′ō-skōp) [″ + *skopein,* to examine] An instrument for examining the colon. SEE: *sigmoidoscope*.

colonoscopy (kō″lŏn-ŏs′kō-pē) Visualization of the lower gastrointestinal tract; most often refers to insertion of a flexible endoscope through the anus to inspect the entire colon and terminal ileum. SYN: *coloscopy*.

colony (kŏl′ō-nē) [L. *colonia*] A growth of microorganisms in a culture; usually considered to have grown from a single organism.

colony-stimulating factor-1 ABBR: CSF-1. A protein in human serum that promotes monocyte differentiation. SEE: *granulocyte-macrophage colony-stimulating factor*.

colopexostomy (kō″lō-pĕks-ŏs′tō-mē) [Gr. *kolon,* colon, + *pexis,* fixation, + *stoma,* mouth] A procedure formerly used to make an artificial anus by resecting the colon and fixing it to the abdominal wall.

colopexotomy (kō″lō-pĕks-ŏt′ō-mē) [″ + ″ + *tome,* incision] Incision and fixation of the colon.

colopexy, colopexia (kō′lō-pĕk″sē, -pĕks′ē-ă) Fixation of the sigmoid colon or cecum to the abdominal wall by suture.

coloplication (kō″lō-plĭ-kā′shŭn) [″ + L. *plica,* fold] An obsolete technique of surgically folding the colon to reduce its lumen.

coloproctectomy (kō″lō-prŏk-tĕk′tō-mē) [″ + *proktos,* anus, + *ektome,* excision] Surgical removal of the rectum and colon.

coloproctitis [″ + ″ + *itis,* inflammation] Colonic and rectal inflammation. SYN: *colorectitis*.

coloproctostomy (kō″lō-prŏk-tŏs′tō-mē) [″ + ″ + *stoma,* mouth] Surgical creation of a passage between a segment of the colon and the rectum.

coloptosis (kō-lŏp-tō′sĭs) A downward displacement of the colon.

colopuncture (kō′lō-pŭnk-chūr) [″ + L. *punctura,* piercing] Colocentesis.

color [L.] A visible quality, distinct from form, light, texture, size, brightness, and shade, that distinguishes some objects from others.

complemental c. One of two spectral colors that produce white light when blended.

primary c. Any of the three colors of light—red, green, and violet—that can be mixed to produce all the colors perceived by the human eye. Pigments that can be so mixed are red, yellow, and blue.

color additive Any dye, pigment, or substance that can impart color when added or applied to a food, drug, or cosmetic. Use of color additives in the U.S. is regulated by the Food and Drug Administration (FDA). Food Drug and Cosmetic (FD&C) colors certified for food use are FD&C Blue No. 1, No. 2, and No. 3; Green No. 3; Red No. 3 and No. 40; and Yellow No. 5 and No. 6.

color blindness A genetic or acquired abnormality of color perception. Complete color blindness, a rare disease, is called achromatopsia. Red-green color blindness, which affects about 8% of the male population, is an X-linked trait. Although the term "color blindness" is used frequently, it is inaccurate. "Color deficiency" is a more accurate description. SEE: illus.

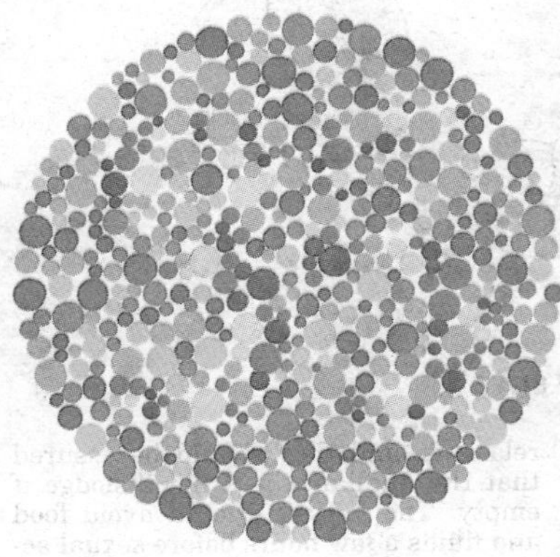

TEST FOR COLOR BLINDNESS

color deficiency A preferred term for color blindness, the inability to identify one or more of the primary colors.

colorectal carcinoma A malignant neoplasm of the colon or rectum, of which an estimated 55,000 persons in the U.S. die annually. It is the second most common cause of death from cancer in the U.S. SYN: *carcinoma of the colon.*

SYMPTOMS: Initial symptoms are nonspecific and include change in the usual pattern of bowel habits, esp. in patients over 40 years of age; recent onset of constipation, diarrhea, or tenesmus in an older patient; bright red or dark blood in the stool. Laboratory findings may reveal a hypochromic microcytic anemia.

DIAGNOSIS: Diagnosis is based on findings from the digital rectal examination, anoscopy, proctosigmoidoscopy, colonoscopy, barium enema examination, and biopsy of suspicious lesions and polyps.

TREATMENT: Surgical resection is the treatment for this disease. Chemotherapy (e.g., with levamisole hydrochloride and fluorouracil or local radiation therapy) is given if the cancer has metastasized to regional lymph nodes.

colorectitis (kō″lō-rĕk-tī′tĭs) Coloproctitis.

colorectostomy (kō″lō-rĕk-tŏs′tō-mē) [″ + ″ + Gr. *stoma,* mouth] Surgical formation of a passage between the colon and rectum.

colorectum (kōl″ō-rĕk′tŭm) The colon and rectum.

color gustation A sense of color aroused by stimulation of taste receptors.

color hearing A sense of color caused by a sound.

colorimeter (kŭl″or-ĭm′ĕ-tĕr) [L. *color,* color, + Gr. *metron,* measure] An instrument for measuring the intensity of color in a substance or fluid, esp. one for determining the amount of hemoglobin in the blood.

colorimetry A photometric technique that measures the absorption of light by colors in a test solution, as compared with that in a standard solution.

color index An outmoded method of expressing the amount of hemoglobin present in each red cell.

colorrhaphy (kō-lor′ă-fē) [Gr. *kolon,* colon, + *rhaphe,* seam, ridge] Suture of the colon.

coloscopy (kō-lŏs′kō-pē) Visual examination of the colon through a sigmoidoscope or colonoscope. SEE: *colonoscope.*

colosigmoidostomy (kō″lō-sĭg″moy-dŏs′tō-mē) [″ + *sigmoeides,* shaped like Gr. Σ, + *stoma,* mouth] Surgical joining of the descending colon to the sigmoid colon.

colostomy (kō-lŏs′tō-mē) [Gr. *kolon,* colon, + *stoma,* mouth] The opening of a portion of the colon through the abdominal wall to its skin surface. A colostomy is established in cases of distal obstruction, inflammatory process, including perforation, and when the distal colon or rectum is surgically resected. A temporary colostomy is performed to divert the fecal stream from an inflamed or operative site. SEE: illus.; *ostomy* for colostomy care.

PATIENT CARE: *Preoperative:* When the possibility exists that a patient will need to have a colostomy created (even when surgery is performed in an emergency), the patient and family are advised about the nature of the colostomy, including temporary versus permanent stoma and general principles of aftercare. The patient is assured that he or she will be able to resume a normal lifestyle with a stoma. Except in an extreme emergency (e.g., perforation, penetrating trauma, etc.), preparation for colon surgery with laxatives, enemas, and antibacterial agents is coordinated with the surgery's starting time. Intravenous hydration is instituted.

Postoperative: Routine care, including the use of various monitors, pneumatic hose, and pulmonary toilet measures, along with special attention given to in-

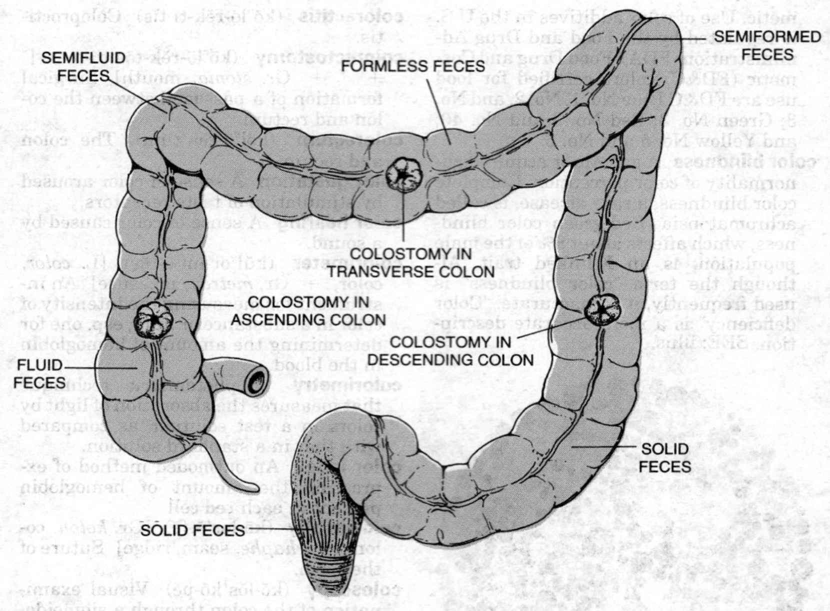

COLOSTOMY SITES

specting the stoma for viability and the surrounding skin for irritation and excoriation. The stoma should be smooth, cherry red, and slightly edematous. Any discoloration or excessive swelling is documented and reported. The stoma and surrounding skin are gently cleansed and dried thoroughly. A drainage bag is applied by fitting a karaya adhesive ring (or other appliance) before the patient leaves the operating room to ensure a firm seal and to prevent leakage without constricting the stoma. Nonirritating skin barriers are used as appropriate.

Avoidance of dehydration and maintenance of electrolyte balance are emphasized until the patient is able to eat a normal diet. Stool consistency is observed. If colostomy irrigations are prescribed, the patient is advised that the procedure is similar to an enema. The patient is advised to return to a normal diet judiciously, adding new foods gradually while observing their effect. He or she should avoid gas-forming, odoriferous, spicy, and irritating foods. Colostomy requires a difficult adjustment by both patient and family; they are encouraged to verbalize their fears and concerns, and support is offered. The patient is reassured of the ability to regain continence with dietary control and bowel retraining. Both patient and partner are encouraged to discuss their feelings and concerns about body image changes and about resumption of sexual relations, and they should be assured that the appliance will not dislodge if empty. The patient should avoid food and fluids a few hours before sexual activity. Depression is not uncommon after ostomy surgery, and psychological counseling is recommended if depression persists. SEE: *Nursing Diagnoses Appendix.*

double-barrel c. A temporary colostomy with two openings into the colon: one distal and one proximal. Elimination occurs through the proximal stoma, allowing the distal length of the colon to rest and heal. When healing is complete, the two ends are rejoined and returned to the peritoneal cavity, and normal function resumes. In colitis, resection rather than reanastomosis is performed.

terminal c. A colostomy in which the proximal cut end of the colon is formed into a stoma and the distal colon is either resected or closed.

wet c. **1.** A colostomy in the right side of the colon or in the ileum. The drainage from this type of colostomy is liquid. **2.** A colostomy in the left side of the colon distal to the point where the ureters have been anastomosed to it. Thus the urine and fecal material are excreted through the same stoma.

colostrorrhea (kō-lŏs″trō-rē′ă) [L. *colostrum,* + Gr. *rhoia,* flow] Abnormal secretion of colostrum.

colostrum [L.] Breast fluid that may be secreted from the second trimester of pregnancy onward but that is most evident in the first 2 to 3 days after birth and before the onset of true lactation. This thin yellowish fluid contains a great number of proteins and calories in addition to immune globulins.

colotomy (kō-lŏt′ō-mē) [Gr. *kolon*, colon, + *tome*, incision] Incision of the colon.

colovaginal (kō″lō-văj′ĭ-năl) Concerning the colon and vagina or communication between the two.

colovesical (kō″lō-vĕs′ĭ-kăl) Concerning the colon and the urinary bladder or communication between the two.

colp- SEE: *colpo-*.

colpalgia (kŏl-păl′jē-ă) [Gr. *kolpos*, vagina, + *algos*, pain] Vaginal pain.

colpectomy (kŏl-pĕk′tō-mē) [″ + *ektome*, excision] Surgical removal of the vagina.

colpeurysis (kŏl-pū′rĭs-ĭs) Surgical dilatation of the vagina.

colpitis (kŏl-pīt′ĭs) Vaginitis (2).

c. macularis Small erythematous lesions on the squamous epithelium of the upper vagina and cervix. The lesions are seen best by use of colposcopy, and have the appearance of "strawberry spots." These spots have a high positive predictive value for women with trichomoniasis. SEE: *Trichomonas vaginalis*.

colpo-, colp-, kolpo-, kolp- [Gr. *kolpos*, vagina] combining form meaning *vagina*.

colpocele (kŏl′pō-sēl) [″ + *kele*, tumor, swelling] A hernia into the vagina.

colpoceliotomy (kŏl″pō-sē″lē-ŏt′ō-mē) [″ + *koilia*, belly, + *tome*, incision] An incision into the abdomen through the vagina. SEE: *culdoscopy*.

colpocleisis (kŏl″pō-klī′sĭs) [″ + *kleisis*, a closure] Surgical occlusion of the vagina.

colpocystitis (kŏl″pō-sĭs-tī′tĭs) [″ + *kystis*, bladder, + *itis*, inflammation] Inflammation of the vagina and bladder. SYN: *coleocystitis*.

colpocystocele (kŏl″-pō-sĭs′tō-sēl) [″ + *kystis*, bladder, + *kele*, tumor, swelling] Prolapse of the bladder into the vagina.

colpocystoplasty (kŏl″pō-sĭs′tō-plăs″tē) [″ + ″ + *plassein*, to form] Surgical repair of a vesicovaginal fistula.

colpocystotomy (kŏl″pō-sĭs-tŏt′ō-mē) [″ + ″ + *tome*, incision] An incision into the bladder through the vagina. This procedure is no longer used, as better surgical approaches to the bladder are available.

colpocystourethropexy (kŏl″pō-sĭs-tō-ū-rē′thrō-pĕks-ē) The transvaginal surgical suspension of the urethra and bladder—used to treat urinary incontinence in women. The surgery restores the proper cystourethral angle for normal urinary continence.

Patient Care: Vital signs are recorded postoperatively. The drainage catheter is checked. The patient is encouraged to maintain a high intake of fluids to help prevent infection. Intake and output measurements must be recorded.

colpohyperplasia (kŏl″pō-hī-pĕr-plā′zē-ă) [″ + *hyper*, over, + *plasis*, a forming] Excessive growth of the mucous membrane of the vagina.

c. cystica Infectious inflammation of the vaginal walls marked by the production of small blebs.

colpomicroscope (kŏl″pō-mī′krō-skōp) [″ + *mikros*, small, + *skopein*, to view] colposcope.

colpomyomectomy (kŏl″pō-mī″ō-mĕk′tō-mē) [″ + *mys*, muscle, + *oma*, tumor, + *ektome*, excision] Removal of a fibroid tumor of the uterus through the vagina.

colpomyomotomy (kŏl″pō-mī″ō-mŏt′ō-mē) [″ + ″ + ″ + *tome*, incision] Incision of the uterus through the vagina for removal of a tumor.

colpoperineoplasty (kŏl″pō-pĕr″ĭn-ē′ō-plăs″tē) [″ + *perinaion*, perineum, + *plassein*, to form] Plastic surgery on the vagina and perineum.

colpoperineorrhaphy (kŏl″pō-pĕr″ĭn-ē-or′ră-fē) [″ + ″ + *rhaphe*, seam, ridge] Surgical repair of perineal tears in the vagina.

colpopexy (kŏl′pō-pĕk″sē) [″ + *pexis*, fixation] Suture of a relaxed and prolapsed vagina to the abdominal wall.

colpoplasty (kŏl′pō-plăs″tē) [″ + *plassein*, to form] Plastic surgery of the vagina.

colpoptosis (kŏl″pŏp-tō′sĭs) [″ + *ptosis*, a dropping] Prolapse of the vagina.

colporrhaphy (kŏl-por′ă-fē) [″ + *rhaphe*, seam, ridge] Suture of the vagina.

colporrhexis (kŏl″pō-rĕk′sĭs) [″ + *rhexis*, rupture] Laceration or rupture of the vaginal walls.

colposcope (kŏl′pō-skōp) [″ + *skopein*, to examine] An instrument used to examine the tissues of the vagina and cervix through a magnifying lens. SYN: *colpomicroscope*.

colposcopy (kŏl-pŏs′kō-pē) The examination of vaginal and cervical tissues by means of a colposcope. Colposcopy is used to select sites of abnormal epithelium for biopsy in patients with abnormal Pap smears. It is helpful in defining tumor extension, for evaluating benign lesions, and in postpubertal vaginal examination of diethylstilbestrol-exposed daughters.

colpostat (kŏl′pō-stăt) [″ + *statikos*, standing] A device for holding an instrument, such as a radium applicator, in place in the vagina.

colpostenosis (kŏl″pō-stĕn-ō′sĭs) [″ + *stenosis*, narrowing] Stenosis or narrowing of the vagina.

colposuspension (kŏl″pō-sŭs-pĕn′shŭn) colpocystourethropexy.

colpotomy (kŏl-pŏt′ō-mē) [″ + *tome*,

incision] An incision into the wall of the vagina. SYN: *coleotomy*.

colpoureterotomy (kŏl″pō-ū-rē″tĕr-ŏt′ō-mē) [″ + ″ + *tome*, incision] Incision of the ureter through the vagina.

columbium Former name for the element niobium.

columella (kŏl″ū-mĕl′lă) [L., small column] **1.** A little column. **2.** In microbiology or mycology, the portion of the sporangiophore on which the spores are borne.

c. cochleae The modiolus of the cochlea.

c. nasi The anterior part of the septum of the nose.

column (kŏl′ŭm) [L. *columna*, pillar] A cylindrical supporting structure.

anal c. Vertical folds in the anal canal. SYN: *rectal c.*

anterior c. The anterior portion of the gray matter on each side of the spinal cord; in reference to white matter, the anterior funiculus.

c. of Burdach Fasciculus cuneatus.

Clarke's c. A group of large cells in the medial portion of the base of the posterior gray column of the spinal cord.

fornix c. A column of the fornix; two arched bands of fibers that form its anterior portion. The fibers lead to the mammillary body.

gray c. Gray matter in the anterior and posterior horns of the spinal cord.

lateral c. **1.** A column in the lateral portion of the gray matter of the spinal cord. It contains cell bodies of preganglionic neurons of the sympathetic nervous system. **2.** The lateral funiculus or the white matter between roots of spinal nerves.

c. of Goll Fasciculus gracilis.

c. of Gowers The tract of ascending fibers anterior to the direct cerebellar column and on the lateral surface of the spinal cord.

c. of Morgagni One of several vertical ridges in the mucous membrane at the junction of the anus and rectum.

posterior c. **1.** The posterior horn of the gray matter of the spinal cord. It consists of an expanded portion or caput connected by a narrower cervix to the main portion of the gray matter. **2.** The posterior funiculus of the white matter.

rectal c. Anal c.

renal c. A column of Bertin, cortical material of the kidney that extends centrally, separating the pyramids.

spinal c. Vertebral c. SEE: illus.

vertebral c. The portion of the axial skeleton consisting of vertebrae (7 cervical, 12 thoracic, 5 lumbar, the sacrum, and the coccyx) joined together by intervertebral disks and fibrous tissue. It forms the main supporting axis of the body, encloses and protects the spinal cord, and attaches the appendicular skeleton and muscles for moving the various body parts. SYN: *spinal c.*

columna (kō-lŭm′nă) *pl.* **columnae** [L.] A column or pillar.

c. carnea Trabecula carnea cordis.

c. nasi The nasal septum.

c. rugarum vaginae The folds of mucous membrane of the vagina that are arranged in a columnar fashion.

coma (kō′mă) [Gr. *koma*, a deep sleep] A state of unconsciousness from which one cannot be aroused. Coma is the most severe of the alterations of consciousness. It differs from sleep in that comatose patients will not awaken with stimulation; it differs from lethargy, drowsiness, or stupor (states in which patients are slow to respond) in that comatose patients are completely unresponsive. Finally, it differs from delirium, confusion, or hallucinosis (states in which patients' sense of reality is distorted and expressions are bizarre) in that comatose patients cannot express themselves at all. SEE: *Glasgow Coma Scale*.

ETIOLOGY: Two thirds of the time, coma results from diffuse brain injury or intoxication, such as may be caused by drug overdose, poisoning, hypoglycemia, uremia, liver failure, infection, or closed-head trauma. In about one third of cases, coma results from intracranial lesions, such as massive strokes, brain tumors, or abscesses. For these focal injuries to depress consciousness, the lesion must result in compression or injury to the brain's reticular activating system (the network of cells responsible for arousal). Rarely, coma is feigned by patients with psychiatric illnesses.

TREATMENT: The airway, breathing, and circulation are supported. The cervical spine is protected if there is any question of traumatic injury to the head and neck. A rapid physical examination is performed to determine whether the patient has focal neurological deficits. Simultaneously, intravenous dextrose, naloxone, and thiamine are given (to try to reverse narcotic overdose or diabetic coma). If the examination reveals focal findings, an intracranial lesion may be present and should be quickly diagnosed (with brain scans) and treated (e.g., with neurosurgery if appropriate). If the patient is neurologically nonfocal, treatment focuses on metabolic support, the administration of antidotes for any proven intoxications, and treatment for infections.

FIRST AID: If neck trauma is suspected, the patient should not be moved except in-line traction to position the head to help clear the airway. Sudden movement of the patient by unskilled persons may be dangerous.

CAUTION: If there is a question of whether the coma is due to an overdose of insulin or to hypoglycemia, it is crucial to

mary care provider (blood glucose above 200 mg/dl, inability to eat, or vomiting). The patient also is referred to a home care nurse for further monitoring as necessary, and to a community-based diabetic education course for better understanding and control of diabetes.

hepatic c. Coma resulting from portal-systemic encephalopathy.

hyperosmolar nonketotic c. ABBR: HNC. A coma in which the patient has a relative insulin deficiency and resulting hyperglycemia, but enough insulin to prevent fatty acid breakdown. The condition occurs most often in patients with type 2 diabetes and involves hyperosmolarity of extracellular fluids and subsequent intracellular dehydration. It often is precipitated by severe physical stress or by extreme or prolonged dehydration.

hypoglycemic c. Unconsciousness caused by very low blood sugars, usually less than 40 mg/dl. The most common cause is a reaction to insulin or an oral hypoglycemic agent. The patient typically will recognize, after reviving, that coma was preceded by heavy exercise, limited caloric intake, or a recent increase in the dose of diabetic medications. Occasionally alcoholic patients, patients with salicylate overdoses, or severely malnourished patients will present with coma and low blood sugar. Very rarely, the hypoglycemic patient will be found to have an insulin-secreting tumor of the pancreas.

irreversible c. A coma from which the patient cannot recover.

Kussmaul's c. The coma, acidosis, and deep breathing in diabetic coma.

myxedema c. Unresponsiveness or lethargy that results from severe or neglected hypothyroidism. It is marked by neurological dysfunction, by respiratory depression, and by lowered body temperature, blood pressure, blood sugar, and serum sodium. The condition is an endocrinological crisis that requires treatment with thyroid and adrenocortical hormones, fluids, and glucose; gradual rewarming; ventilatory support; and intensive monitoring.

uremic c. Loss of consciousness caused by the toxic effects of the nitrogen-containing wastes and inorganic acids that accumulate in the bloodstream of patients in renal failure. Coma in renal failure usually occurs after other uremic symptoms, such as loss of appetite, confusion, lethargy, or seizures.

vigil c. Akinetic mutism.

comatose (kō′mă-tōs) In a coma.

combitube, airway combitube A multilumen airway that consists of an endotracheal and pharyngeal tube molded into a single unit. It is used to intubate adult patients when traditional airways are unavailable or unsuccessful.

combustion (kŏm-bŭst′yŭn) **1.** Burning. **2.** In metabolism, the oxidation of food with production of heat.

comedo (kŏm′ē-dō) *pl.* **comedones, comedos** [L. *comedere,* to eat up] The typical small skin lesion of acne vulgaris and seborrheic dermatitis. The closed form is called a whitehead. It consists of a papule from which the contents are not easily expressed. When inflamed these lesions form pustules and nodules. The open form of comedo, called a blackhead, is rarely inflamed. It has a dilated opening from which the oily debris is easily expressed. Both forms are usually located on the face, but the chest and back may be involved. SEE: illus.

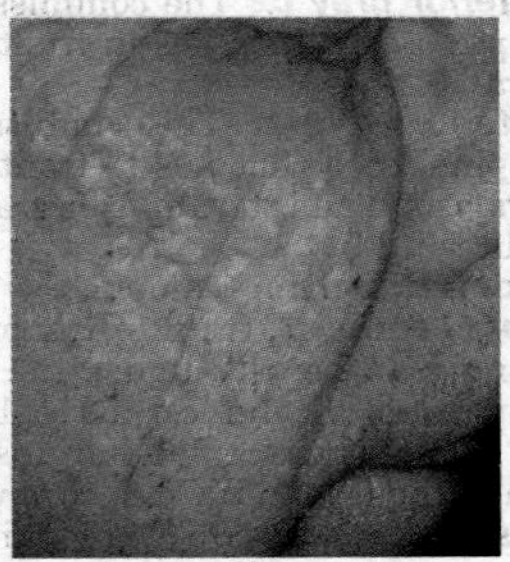

COMEDONES

comes (kō′mēz) *pl.* **comites** [L., companion] A blood vessel that accompanies a nerve or another blood vessel.

comfrey (cŭm′frē) A hardy perennial, *Symphytum officinale,* whose oil from the leaves and roots has been used in ointments to promote wound healing. Because it contains known liver toxins, comfrey is not recommended for use in tea and should not be taken internally.

comity (kŏ′mĭ-tē) In interpersonal relations or social interactions, the condition of politeness, courtesy, and respect.

comma tract of Schultze The fasciculus interfascicularis, a tract of descending fibers located between the fasciculus cuneatus and fasciculus gracilis in the posterior funiculus of the spinal cord.

commensal (kŏ-mĕn′săl) [L. *com-,* together, + *mensa,* table] Either of the two organisms of different species that live in a close but nonparasitic relationship. SEE: *commensalism; symbiosis.*

commensalism (kŏ-mĕn′săl-ĭzm″) The symbiotic relationship of two organisms of different species in which neither is harmful to the other and one gains some benefit such as protection or nourishment (e.g., nonpathogenic bacteria in the human intestine).

comminute (kŏm′ĭ-nūt) [L. *com-,* together, + *minuere,* to crumble] To break into pieces.

comminution (kŏm″ĭ-nū′shŭn) [L. *comminutio,* crumbling] The reduction of a solid body to varying sizes by grating, pulverizing, slicing, granulating, and other processes.

commissura (kŏm″mĭ-sū′ră) *pl.* **commissurae** [L.] Commissure.

commissure (kŏm′ĭ-shūr) [L. *commissura,* a joining together] **1.** A transverse band of nerve fibers passing over the midline in the central nervous system. **2.** The meeting of two structures, as the lips, eyelids, or labia, across the midline or dividing space. **commissural** (kŏm-mĭs′ū-răl), *adj.*

anterior cerebral c. The band of white fibers that passes through the lamina terminalis, connecting the two cerebral hemispheres.

anterior gray c. The commissure in the spinal cord that lies in front of the central canal.

anterior white c. The commissure in the spinal cord that lies in front of the central canal and the anterior gray commissure.

c. of fornix Hippocampal c.

hippocampal c. A thin sheet of fibers passing transversely under the posterior portion of the corpus callosum. They connect the medial margins of the crura of the fornix. SYN: *c. of fornix.*

posterior c. of brain The commissure just above the midbrain containing fibers that connect the superior colliculi.

posterior c. of spinal cord The gray commissure connecting the halves of the spinal cord, lying behind the central canal.

commissurorrhaphy (kŏm″ĭ-shūr-or′ă-fē) [″ + Gr. *rhaphe,* seam, ridge] The surgical joining of the parts of a commissure to decrease the size of the opening.

commissurotomy (kŏm″ĭ-shūr-ŏt′ō-mē) [″ + Gr. *tome,* incision] Surgical incision of any commissure; used in treating mitral stenosis to increase the size of the mitral orifice. This is done by incising the adhesions that cause the leaves of the valve to stick together. Commissurotomy may also be used in treating certain psychiatric conditions by incising the anterior commissure of the brain.

commitment (kŏ-mĭt′mĕnt) The legal procedure for hospitalization of a patient who may not be competent to choose to be hospitalized. Confining a patient without his or her consent may be necessary, for example, to care for suicidal patients, patients with altered mental status, or persons with certain contagious diseases. SEE: *certification.*

committee, patient care advisory A multidisciplinary group of individuals who advise health-care agencies facing ethical dilemmas. This committee usually comprises health-care professionals, clergy, legal counsel, and administrative personnel. Also called *institutional ethics committee.* SEE: *institutional review board.*

commode A receptacle suitable for use as a toilet.

bedside c. A portable toilet that enables a patient to sit comfortably while using it. For many patients using a bedside commode is less stressful than using a bedpan.

commotio cordis (kō-mō′shē-ō kŏr′dĭs) Sudden death following blunt chest trauma. At autopsy, no pathological findings are demonstrated. The syndrome is believed to be caused by ventricular fibrillation.

communicans (kŏ-mū′nĕ-kănz) [L. *communicare,* to connect with] One of several communicating nerves or arteries.

communication, augmentative Any method or device that improves a person's ability to share information with, or receive information from others. The term is used esp. with respect to techniques that promote the exchange of language and symbols with speech- and hearing-impaired individuals. Technologies that assist communication include hearing aids, communication boards, and portable electronic devices that display, print out, or synthesize speech. SEE: *communication board.*

communication board Any device with letters, pictures, or words that lets patients with impaired physical and verbal ability express themselves.

communication, impaired verbal The state in which an individual experiences a decreased, delayed, or absent ability to receive, process, transmit, and use a system of symbols or anything that has meaning, i.e., transmits meaning. SEE: *Nursing Diagnoses Appendix.*

communication, nonverbal In interpersonal relationships, the use of communication techniques that do not involve words. A grimace, shrug, silence, smile, wink, raised eyebrows, avoidance, turning away, or even fighting are examples of nonverbal communication.

communicator An electronic device that permits persons with impaired verbal and physical ability to communicate through graphic or symbolic light-emitting diode (LED) displays, printed messages, or synthetic speech.

community coping, enhanced, potential for A pattern of community activities for adaptation and problem solving that is satisfactory for meeting the demands or needs of the community but can be improved for management of current and future problems/stressors. SEE: *Nursing Diagnoses Appendix.*

community coping, ineffective A pattern of community activities for adaptation and problem solving that is unsatisfactory for meeting the demands or needs of the community. SEE: *Nursing Diagnoses Appendix.*

Comolli's sign (kō-mōl'lēz) [Antonio Comolli, It. pathologist, b. 1879] A triangular swelling corresponding to the outline of the fractured scapula.

comorbid disease A disease that worsens or impacts a primary disease (e.g., the primary disease could be cancer and the comorbid disease emphysema).

compact Closely and tightly packed together; solid.

compaction (kŏm-păk'shŭn) **1.** Simultaneous engagement of the presenting parts of twins in the pelvis so that labor cannot progress. **2.** In dentistry, the act or process of joining or packing together powdered gold, mat gold, or gold foil in a prepared cavity in a tooth.

comparative negligence In forensic medicine, negligence of the plaintiff and defendant measured in terms of percentages. Damages awarded are decreased in proportion to the plaintiff's amount of negligence provided it is less than that of the defendant.

compartment syndrome Elevation of tissue pressure within a closed fascial compartment, causing a decreased arteriovenous pressure and decreased muscular perfusion. Acutely, compartment syndromes are caused by hemorrhage and/or edema within a closed space, or external compression or arterial occlusion that induces postischemic reperfusion. Chronic compartment syndromes (also known as exertional or recurrent compartment syndromes) may result from muscular expansion during exercise or decreased size of the anatomical compartment.

SYMPTOMS: Both types of compartment syndrome are marked by limb redness, swelling, and pain. The overlying skin may feel hard. As intracompartmental pressure increases, distal neurovascular function may become compromised. Chronic compartment syndrome is definitively diagnosed by measuring the intramuscular pressure while the patient is at rest and during exertion.

TREATMENT: Acute compartment syndromes should be managed with topically applied ice and elevation of the limb. External compression should be avoided because of the risk of increasing intracompartmental pressure. Absent or diminished distal pulses require prompt surgical consultation.

PATIENT CARE: The patient with acute compartment syndrome may need a fasciotomy if symptoms are not resolved in 30 min. Fasciotomy may also be required to relieve the symptoms of chronic compartment syndrome.

chronic c. s. An increase in intracompartmental pressure that may occur during exercise or other forms of exertional activity. The increased intracompartmental pressure decreases blood flow to the distal extremity and impairs nerve function.

ETIOLOGY: Individuals who have herniated muscles that occlude the neurovascular network, unyielding fascia in a closed compartment or excessive hypertrophy of muscles during exercise are predisposed to chronic compartment syndrome, as are athletes who use anabolic steroids.

SYMPTOMS: The patient will complain of pain, numbness, and weakness in the involved extremity during exercise. Inspection may also reveal cyanosis and swelling in the distal portion of the involved limb. Symptoms may subside following activity or may lead to muscle necrosis, requiring fasciotomy.

exertional c. s. Chronic c. s.

recurrent anterior c. s. Chronic c. s.

recurrent c. s. Chronic c. s.

compassion Deep awareness of the pain and suffering of others; empathy.

compassionate use The administration of investigational drugs to a patient in a special circumstance in which it is felt that the drug may be lifesaving or effective when no other therapy would be. The procedure requires the treating physician to contact either the Food and Drug Administration or the drug manufacturer to obtain permission.

compatibility **1.** The suitability to be mixed or taken together without unfavorable results, as drugs. **2.** The ability of two individuals or groups to interact without undue strife or tension.

compatible In pharmacology, pert. to the ability to combine two medicines without interfering with their action.

compensating Making up for a deficiency.

compensation **1.** Making up for a defect, as cardiac circulation competent to meet demands regardless of valvular defect. **2.** In psychoanalysis, a psychic mechanism in which an individual who feels himself or herself to be inadequate (e.g., because of neuroses, character defects, or a physical disability) makes up for this perception by stressing or using other personal strengths and assets. Sublimation is often similar, but varies by substituting a higher social goal to gratify the infrasocial drive by replacement rather than mere camouflaging. **3.** Restitution by payment to a person injured, esp. in the workplace.

failure of c. The inability of the heart muscle or other diseased organs to meet the body's needs. In cardiac failure, this results in pulmonary congestion, difficulty breathing, and sometimes hypotension or lower extremity swelling. Causes of cardiac compensatory failure may include heart disease, valvular heart disease, or cardiomyopathies.

competence (kŏm'pĕ-tĕns) **1.** In psychiatry, being able to manage one's affairs, and by inference, being sane; usually stated as mental competence. **2.** Performance in a manner that satisfies the demands of a situation; interaction effectively with the environment.

competition (kŏm″pĕ-tĭsh′ŭn) The simultaneous attempt of similar substances to attach to a receptor site of a cell membrane.

complaint (kŏm-plānt′) **1.** Verbal or other communication of the principal reason the patient is seeking medical assistance. **2.** The initial pleading or document that commences a legal action, states grounds for such an action, names the parties to the lawsuit, and demands for relief. SYN: *petition*.

chief c. The symptom or group of symptoms that represents the primary reason for a patient's seeking health care.

complement (kŏm′plĕ-mĕnt) [L. *complere,* to complete] A group of proteins in the blood that play a vital role in the body's immune defenses through a cascade of interactions. Components of complement are labeled C1 through C9. Complement acts by directly lysing (killing) organisms; by opsonizing an antigen, thus stimulating phagocytosis; and by stimulating inflammation and the B-cell–mediated immune response. All complement proteins lie inactive in the blood until activated by either the classic or the alternative pathways.

The lack of C3 increases susceptibility to common bacterial infections, whereas deficits in C5 through C9 are usually associated with increased incidence of autoimmune diseases, particularly systemic lupus erythematosus and glomerulonephritis. Lack of C1 causes hereditary angioedema of the extremities and gastrointestinal tract. The lack of any of the more than 25 proteins involved in the complement system may affect the body's defenses adversely.

complemental, complementary Supplying something that is lacking in another system or entity.

complementarity In individual and group interactions, the extent to which emotional requirements are met.

complement fixation A common blood assay used to determine if antigen-antibody reactions have occurred. Complement that combines with the antigen-antibody complex becomes inactive and is unable to lyse (kill) red blood cells in vitro. The degree of complement fixation is determined by the number of red blood cells destroyed, which indicates the amount of free complement not bound to the antigen-antibody complexes. Complement fixation can measure the severity of an infection because it helps indicate the extent and effectiveness of antigen-antibody reactions occurring in the body.

complex [L. *complexus,* woven together] **1.** All the ideas, feelings, and sensations connected with a subject. **2.** Intricate. **3.** An atrial or ventricular systole as it appears on an electrocardiograph tracing. **4.** A subconscious idea (or group of ideas) that has become associated with a repressed wish or emotional experience and that may influence behavior, although the person may not realize the connection with the repressed thoughts or actions. **5.** In Freudian theory, a grouping of ideas with an emotional background. These may be harmless, and the individual may be fully aware of them (e.g., an artist sees every object with a view to a possible picture and is said to have established a complex for art). Often, however, the complex is aroused by some painful emotional reaction such as fright or excessive grief that, instead of being allowed a natural outlet, becomes unconsciously repressed and later manifests itself in some abnormality of mind or behavior. According to Freud, the best method of determining the complex is through psychoanalysis. SEE: *Electra complex; Jocasta complex; Oedipus complex*.

castration c. A morbid fear of being castrated.

Ghon c. The primary lesion in tuberculosis, consisting of the affected area of the lung and a corresponding lymph node. These usually heal and become calcified. If the calcium surrounding the lesion is later dissolved, the contained tubercle bacilli are free to spread throughout the body. SEE: *miliary tuberculosis*.

Golgi c. Golgi apparatus.

inferiority c. The condition of having low self-esteem; a 20th-century term stemming from Adlerian therapy.

membrane attack c. The combination of complement factors C5 through C9 that directly attack and kill the cell membranes of microorganisms during the terminal attack phase of the complement cascade. SEE: *complement; inflammation*.

nodal premature c. ABBR: NPC. Ectopic cardiac beat originating in the atrioventricular node.

superiority c. Exaggerated conviction of one's own superiority; the pretense of being superior to compensate for a real or imagined inferiority.

complexion (kŏm-plĕk′shŭn) The color and appearance of the facial skin.

complexus (kŏm-plĕk′sŭs) [L.] Semispinalis capitis muscle. SEE: *muscle*.

compliance (kŏm-plī′ăns) **1.** The property of altering size and shape in response to application of force, weight, or release from force. The lung and thoracic cage of a child may have a high degree of compliance as compared with that of an elderly person. SEE: *elastance*. **2.** The extent to which a patient's behavior coincides with medical advice. Compliance may be estimated by carefully questioning the patient and family members, evaluating the degree of clinical response to therapy, the presence or absence of side effects from drugs, measuring serum drug levels or testing for excretion of the drug in the urine, and counting remaining pills.

dynamic c. A measure of the ease of lung inflation with positive pressure.

effective c. Patient compliance during positive-pressure breathing using a tidal volume corrected for compressed volume divided by static pressure.

frequency-dependent c. A condition in which pulmonary compliance decreases with rapid breathing; used to identify small airway disease.

pulmonary c. A measure of the force required to distend the lungs.

static c. A volume-to-pressure measurement of lung distensibility with exhalation against a closed system, taken under conditions of no airflow.

tubing c. The ability of ventilator tubing to expand when pressurized. It is calculated by closing the ventilator circuit and measuring the volume under pressurization.

complication [L. *cum,* with, + *plicare,* to fold] An added difficulty; a complex state; a disease or accident superimposed on another without being specifically related, yet affecting or modifying the prognosis of the original disease (e.g., pneumonia is a complication of measles and is the cause of many deaths from that disease).

component A constituent part.

component blood therapy SEE: *blood component therapy*.

compos mentis (kŏm″pŭs mĕn′tĭs) [L.] Of sound mind; sane. SEE: *non compos mentis*.

compound [L. *componere,* to place together] **1.** A substance composed of two or more units or parts combined in definite proportions by weight and having specific properties of its own. Compounds are formed by all living organisms and are of two types, organic and inorganic. **2.** Made up of more than one part.

impression c. A nonelastic molding used in dentistry to make imprints of teeth and other oral tissues. Impression compound is a thermoplastic material (i.e., it softens when heated and solidifies without chemical change when cooled).

inorganic c. One of many compounds that, in general, contain no carbon.

organic c. A compound containing carbon. Such compounds include carbohydrates, proteins, and fats.

sulfonylurea c. An oral hypoglycemic agent, helpful in the treatment of type 2 diabetes mellitus.

comprehend To understand something.

compress (kŏm′prĕs) A cloth, wet or dry, folded and applied firmly to a body part.

cold c. A soft, absorbent cloth, several layers thick, dipped in cold water, slightly wrung out, and applied to the part being treated. To maintain constant temperature, the compress is frequently renewed, or an ice bag or rubber coil through which ice water is circulating is placed on it. The duration of the application is usually 10 to 20 min.

hot c. A soft, absorbent cloth folded into several layers, dipped in hot water 107° to 115°F (41.7° to 46.1°C), barely wrung out, and placed on the part to be treated. It is covered with a piece of cloth. The temperature is maintained at a constant level by renewing the compress or by applying a rubber coil through which hot water 107° to 115°F (41.7° to 46.1°C) is circulated.

wet c. Two or more folds of soft cloth wrung out of water at prescribed temperatures and covered with fabric.

compress (kŏm-prĕs′) [L. *compressus,* squeezed together] **1.** To press together into a smaller space. **2.** To close by squeezing together, as a wound.

compression (kŏm-prĕsh′ŭn) [L. *compressio,* a compression] A squeezing together; the condition of being pressed together.

cerebral c. Potentially life-threatening pressure on the brain produced by increased intracranial fluids, embolism, thrombosis, tumors, skull fractures, or aneurysms.

SYMPTOMS: The condition is marked by alterations of consciousness, nausea and vomiting, limb paralysis, and cranial nerve deficits. It may present as, or progress to, brain death. SEE: *Glasgow Coma Scale*.

PATIENT CARE: The patient is closely assessed for signs and symptoms of increased intracranial pressure, respiratory distress, convulsions, bleeding from the ears or nose, or drainage of cerebrospinal fluid from the ears or nose (which most probably indicates a fracture). Neurological status is monitored for any alterations in level of consciousness, pupillary signs, ocular movements, verbal response, sensory and motor function (including voluntary and involuntary movements), or behavioral and mental capabilities; and vital signs are assessed, esp. respiratory patterns. Any signs of deterioration are documented and reported. Seizure precautions are maintained.

digital c. Compression of blood vessels with the fingers to stop hemorrhage.

myelitis c. Compression due to pressure on the spinal cord, often caused by a tumor.

compression glove Any type of glove made of stretch material so that pressure is maintained against the fingers and hands. This helps to reduce edema.

compressor **1.** An instrument or device that applies a compressive force, as in compaction of gold. **2.** A muscle that compresses a part, as the compressor hemispherium bulbi, which compresses the bulb of the urethra.

air c. A machine that compresses air into storage tanks for use in air syringes, air turbine handpieces, and other air-driven tools.

compromised host A person who lacks resistance to infection owing to a deficiency in any of the host defenses. SEE: *AIDS; host defense mechanisms; immunocompromised.*

Compton scattering An interaction between x-rays and matter in which the incoming photon ejects a loosely bound outer-shell electron. The resulting change in the direction of the x-ray photon causes scatter, increasing the dose and degrading the radiographic image. Most interactions between x-rays and matter are of this type, esp. at high energies.

compulsion (kŏm-pŭl′shŭn) [L. *compulsio,* compulsion] A repetitive stereotyped act performed to relieve fear connected with obsession. It is dictated by the subconscious against the person's wishes and, if denied, causes uneasiness. **compulsive** (-sĭv), *adj.*

compulsory (kŏm-pŭl′sor-ē) Compelling action against one's will.

CON *certificate of need.*

con- [L.] Prefix meaning *together* or *with.* SEE: *syn-.*

con-A *concanavalin-A.*

conarium (kō-nā′rē-ŭm) [L.] The pineal body of the brain.

conation (kō-nā′shŭn) [L. *conatio,* an attempt] The initiative, impulse, and drive to act. All of these may be diminished in cerebral diseases, esp. those involving the medial orbital parts of the frontal lobes. SEE: *abulia.*

concanavalin-A (kŏn″kā-năv′ĭ-lĭn) ABBR: con-A. A protein derived from the jack bean used to stimulate proliferation of T lymphocytes. SEE: *mitogen.*

concatenation (kŏn-kăt″ĭ-nā′shŭn) [L. *con,* together, + *catena,* chain] A group of events or effects acting in concert or occurring at the same time.

Concato's disease (kŏn-kŏ′tōs) [Luigi M. Concato, It. physician, 1825–1882] Polyserositis.

concave (kŏn′kāv, kŏn-kāv′) [″ + *cavus,* hollow] Having a spherically depressed or hollow surface.

concavity (kŏn-kăv′ĭ-tē) A surface with curved, bowl-like sides.

concavoconcave (kŏn-kā″vō-kŏn′kāv) [″ + *cavus,* hollow, + *con,* with, + *cavus,* hollow] Concave on opposing sides.

concavoconvex (kŏn-kā″vō-kŏn′věks) [″ + ″ + *convexus,* vaulted] Concave on one side and convex on the opposite surface. SEE: *convex.*

concealment (kŏn-sēl′měnt) **1.** In medicolegal affairs, failure to provide information or evidence. **2.** In research, techniques used to guarantee blinding of subjects and investigators. **3.** In patient care, shielding a patient from his or her diagnosis. **4.** In plastic surgery, the hiding of a structure with an undesirable appearance. **5.** In electrocardiography, the invisibility of a rhythm or conduction disturbance.

conceive (kŏn-sēv′) [L. *concipere,* to take to oneself] **1.** To become pregnant. **2.** To form a mental image or to bring into mind; to form an idea.

concentration (kŏn-sěn-trā′shŭn) [L. *con,* together with, + *centrum,* center] **1.** Fixation of the mind on one subject to the exclusion of all other thoughts. **2.** An increase in the strength of a fluid by evaporation. **3.** The amount of a substance in a mixture or solution expressed as weight or mass per unit volume.

airborne c. The mass of particulate substances or fibers, or the vapor percentage of dissolved pollutants in a specific volume of air. The heavier the concentration, the greater the risk of diseases caused by inhalation.

hydrogen ion c. [H^+], the relative proportion of hydrogen ions in a solution, the factor responsible for the acidic properties of a solution. SEE: *pH.*

mass c. SYMB: ρ. The amount of matter of any substance divided by its volume. In the metric system, ρ is defined in kilograms per liter (kg/L). SEE: *substance c.*

mean corpuscular hemoglobin c. ABBR: MCHC. The average concentration of hemoglobin in a given volume (usually 100 ml) of packed red blood cells, obtained by multiplying the number of grams of hemoglobin in the unit volume by 100 and dividing by the hematocrit.

minimum bactericidal c. Minimum lethal c.

minimum inhibitory c. ABBR: MIC. The lowest concentration of an antimicrobial drug that prevents visible bacterial growth in a defined growth medium.

minimum lethal c. ABBR: MLC. The lowest concentration of an antimicrobial that kills a defined fraction of bacteria or fungi. SYN: *minimum bactericidal c.*

substance c. SYMB: *c.* The amount of a specified material in the total volume of a system. SEE: *mass c.*

concentric (kŏn-sěn′trĭk) [″ + *centrum,* center] Having a common center.

concept (kŏn′sěpt) [L. *conceptum,* something understood] An idea.

conception (kŏn-sěp′shŭn) **1.** The mental process of forming an idea. **2.** The onset of pregnancy marked by implantation of a fertilized ovum in the uterine wall. SEE: *contraception; fertilization; implantation.*

conceptual models in nursing A set of abstract and general concepts and propositions that provide a distinctive frame of reference for viewing the person, environment, health, and nursing actions; used to guide nursing practice, research, education, and administration. SEE: Nursing Theory Appendix.

conceptus (kŏn-sĕp′tŭs) The products of conception.

concha (kŏng′kă) *pl.* **conchae** [Gr. *konche,* shell] **1.** The outer ear or the pinna. **2.** One of the three nasal conchae. SEE: *nasal concha.*

c. auriculae A concavity on the median surface of the auricle of the ear, divided by a ridge into the upper cymba conchae and a lower cavum conchae. The latter leads to the external auditory meatus.

c. bullosa A distention of the turbinate bone due to cyst formation.

nasal c. One of the three scroll-like bones that project medially from the lateral wall of the nasal cavity; a turbinate bone. The superior and middle conchae are processes of the lateral mass of the ethmoid bone; the inferior concha is a facial bone. Each overlies a meatus.

c. sphenoidalis In a fetal skull, one of the two curved plates located on the anterior portion of the body of the sphenoid bone and forming part of the roof of the nasal cavity.

conchoidal (kŏng-koy′dăl) [″ + *eidos,* form, shape] Shell-shaped.

conchoscope (kŏng′kō-skōp) [″ + *skopein,* to examine] An instrument for examining the nasal cavity.

conchotome (kŏng′kō-tōm) [″ + *tome,* incision] A device for excising the middle turbinate bone.

concoction (kŏn-kŏk′shŭn) [L. *con,* with, + *coquere,* to cook] A mixture of two medicinal substances, usually done with the aid of heat.

concomitant (kŏn-kŏm′ĭ-tănt) [″ + *comes,* companion] Accessory; taking place at the same time.

concordance (kŏn-kor′dăns) In twins, the equal representation of a genetic trait in each.

concrement (kŏn′krē-mĕnt) [L. *concrementum*] A concretion as of protein and other substances. If infiltrated with calcium salts, it is termed a calculus.

concrescence (kŏn-krĕs′ĕns) [L. *con,* with, + *crescere,* to grow] The union of separate parts; coalescence, esp. the attachment of a tooth to an adjacent one by deposition of cementum to the roots.

concrete (kŏn′krēt, kŏn-krēt′) [L. *concretus,* solid] Condensed, hardened, or solidified.

concretio cordis (kŏn-krē′shē-ō kor′dĭs) Obliteration of the pericardial space caused by chronic constrictive pericarditis.

concretion (kŏn-krē′shŭn) [″ + *crescere,* to grow] Calculus.

concussion (kŏn-kŭsh′ŭn) [L. *concussus,* shaken violently] **1.** An injury resulting from impact with an object. **2.** Partial or complete loss of function, as that resulting from a blow or fall.

c. of brain An imprecise term for a traumatic brain injury.

c. of labyrinth Deafness resulting from a blow to the head or ear.

spinal c. Loss of function in the spinal cord resulting from a blow or severe jarring.

condensation (kŏn″dĕn-sā′shŭn) [L, *con,* with, + *densare,* to make thick] **1.** Making more dense or compact. **2.** Changing of a liquid to a solid or a gas to a liquid. **3.** In psychoanalysis, the union of ideas to form a new mental pattern. **4.** In chemistry, a type of reaction in which two or more molecules of the same substance react with each other and form a new and heavier substance with different chemical properties. **5.** A mechanical process used in dentistry to pack amalgam into a cavity preparation. The goal of condensation is to produce a homogeneous restorative material with an absence of voids. Condensation is also a method of placing a direct gold restoration, improving the physical properties of the gold foil used and forcing the foil to adapt to the cavity preparation.

condenser (kŏn-dĕn′sĕr) **1.** A device for solidifying vapors and liquids. **2.** An instrument or tool used to compact and condense restorative materials in dental cavity preparations; also called a plugger.

electrical c. A device for storing electricity by using two conducting surfaces and a nonconductor.

substage c. The part of the lens system of a microscope that supplies the illumination critical to the resolving power of the instrument; also called an Abbé condenser.

condiment (kŏn′dĭ-mĕnt) [L. *condire,* to pickle] An appetizing ingredient added to food.

CLASSIFICATION: *Aromatic*: vanilla, cinnamon, cloves, chervil, parsley, bay leaf. *Acrid or peppery*: pepper, ginger, tabasco, all-spice. *Alliaceous or allylic*: onion, mustard, horseradish. *Acid*: vinegar, capers, gherkins, citron. *Animal origin*: caviar, anchovies. *Miscellaneous*: salt, sugar, truffles.

In general, with the exception of sugar, condiments have little nutritional value. They are appetizers, stimulating the secretion of saliva and intestinal juices.

condition **1.** A state of health; physical, esp. athletic, fitness. **2.** To train a person or animal to respond in a predictable way to a stimulus.

conditioning (kŏn-dĭsh′ŭn-ĭng) **1.** Improving the physical capability of a person by an exercise program. **2.** In psychology, the use of a special and different stimulus in conjunction with a familiar one. After a sufficient period in which the two stimuli have been presented simultaneously, the special stimulus alone will cause the response that could originally be produced only by the familiar stimulus. The late Russian physiologist Ivan Pavlov used dogs to demonstrate that the strange stimulus, ringing of a bell, could cause the animal to salivate if the test was done after a period of *conditioning* during which the bell and the familiar stimulus, food, were presented simultaneously. Also called *classical conditioning*.

aversive c. SEE: *aversion therapy*.

operant c. The learning of a particular action or type of behavior followed by a reward. This technique was publicized by the Harvard psychologist B. F. Skinner, who trained animals to activate (by pecking, in the case of a pigeon, or pressing a bar, in the case of a rat) an apparatus that released a pellet of food.

condom (kŏn′dŭm) [L. *condus*, a receptacle] A thin, flexible penile sheath made of synthetic or natural materials. Condoms are used commonly during sexual intercourse to prevent conception by capturing ejaculated semen. Latex condoms also shield against sexually transmitted infections. Their effectiveness is affected by careful handling (to avoid punctures, tears, or slippage), usage before sexual contact (to prevent inadvertent transmission of sperm or germs), and allowing sufficient space for ejaculation (to prevent condom rupture). To avoid damage to condoms, only water-soluble lubricants should be used to facilitate vaginal entry. Condoms should not be reused. SEE: *contraception; sexually transmitted disease*.

CAUTION: Only a water-based lubricant such as K-Y Jelly should be used with a condom. Oil-based products begin to deteriorate latex in less than 1 min.

female c. An intravaginal device, similar to the male condom, that is designed to prevent unwanted pregnancy and sexually transmitted diseases. It consists of a soft loose-fitting polyurethane sheath closed at one end. A flexible polyurethane ring is inside the closed end and another is at the open end. The inner ring is used for insertion, covering the cervix the way a contraceptive diaphragm does and also anchoring and positioning the condom well inside the vagina. During use the external ring remains outside the vagina and covers the area around the vaginal opening. This prevents contact between the labia and the base of the penis. The female condom is prelubricated and additional lubrication is provided in the package. It is designed for one-time use. As a contraceptive, it is as effective as other barrier methods.

conductance (kŏn-dŭk′tăns) [L. *conducere*, to lead] The conducting ability of a body or a circuit for electricity. The best conductor is one that offers the least resistance such as gold, silver, or copper. When expressed as a numerical value, conductance is the reciprocal of resistance. The unit is the ohm.

airway c. ABBR: G. The amount of airflow divided by the amount of pressure that produces it; a measure of the ability of the respiratory airways to maintain airflow.

conduction (kŏn-dŭk′shŭn) **1.** The process whereby a state of excitation affects adjacent portions of a tissue or cell, so that the disturbance is transmitted to remote points. Conduction occurs not only in the fibers of the nervous system but also in muscle fibers. **2.** The transfer of electrons, ions, heat, or sound waves through a conductor or conducting medium.

bone c. Sound conduction through the cranial bones.

conductivity (kŏn″dŭk-tĭv′ĭ-tē) The specific electric conducting ability of a substance. Conductivity is the reciprocal of unit resistance or resistivity. The unit is the ohm/cm. Specific conductivity is sometimes expressed as a percentage. In such cases, it is given as a percentage of the conductivity of pure copper under certain standard conditions.

conductor (kŏn-dŭk′tor) **1.** A medium that transmits a force, a signal, or electricity. **2.** A guide directing a surgical knife or probe.

conduit (kŏn′doo-ĭt) A channel, esp. one constructed surgically.

ileal c. A method of diverting the urinary flow by transplanting the ureters into a prepared and isolated segment of the ileum, which is sutured closed on one end. The other end is connected to an opening in the abdominal wall. Urine is collected there in a special receptacle.

condylar (kŏn′dĭ-lăr) [Gr. *kondylos*, knuckle] Pert. to a condyle.

condylarthrosis (kŏn″dĭl-ăr-thrō′sĭs) [″ + *arthrosis*, a joint] A form of diarthrosis; an ovoid head in an elliptical cavity.

condyle (kŏn′dīl) *pl.* **condyles** [Gr. *kondylos*, knuckle] A rounded protuberance at the end of a bone forming an articulation.

condylectomy (kŏn″dĭ-lĕk′tō-mē) [″ + *ektome*, excision] Excision of a condyle.

condylion (kŏn-dĭl′ē-ŏn) [Gr. *kondylion*, knob] A point on the lateral or medial surface of the mandibular condyle.

condyloid (kŏn′dĭ-loyd) [Gr. *kondylos,* knuckle, + *eidos,* form, shape] Pert. to or resembling a condyle.

condyloma (kŏn″dĭ-lō′mă) *pl.* **condylomata** [Gr. *kondyloma,* wart] A wart, found on the genitals or near the anus, with a textured surface that may resemble coral, cauliflower, or cobblestone.

c. acuminatum A genital wart caused by human papilloma virus infection, typically transmitted by sexual contact. It is caused by various types of human papilloma virus and may be spread by physical contact with an area containing a wart. The spread of a wart from one labium to the other by autoinoculation is possible. The virus that causes the wart is usually transmitted sexually. SYN: *genital wart.* SEE: illus.

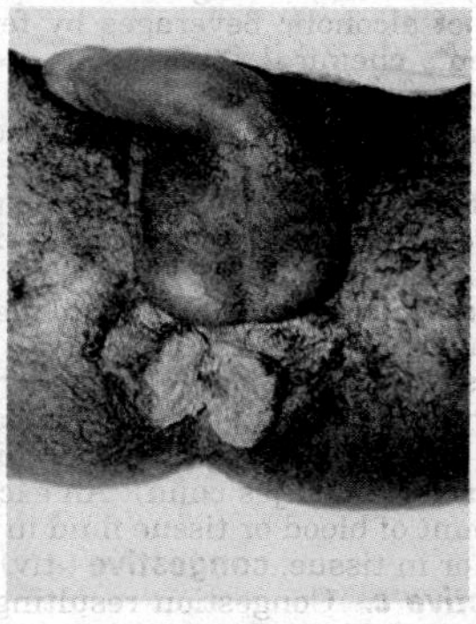

CONDYLOMA (PERIANAL WARTS)

TREATMENT: Topically applied liquid nitrogen, imiquimod cream, fluorouracil, or podophyllin may prove effective; multiple treatments are usually needed.

c. latum A mucous patch, characteristic of syphilis, on the vulva or anus. It is flat, coated with gray exudate and has a delimited area. SYN: *moist papule.*

condylomatous (kŏn″dĭ-lō′mă-tŭs) Pert. to a condyloma.

condylotomy (kŏn″dĭ-lŏt′ō-mē) [Gr. *kondylos,* knuckle, + *tome,* incision] Division of a condyle without its removal.

condylus (kŏn′dĭ-lŭs) *pl.* **condyli** Condyle.

cone (kōn) [Gr. *konos,* cone] **1.** A solid or hollow three-dimensional figure with a circular base and sides sloping up to a point. **2.** In the outer layer of the retina (the layer adjacent to the choroid), one of the flask-shaped cells that are stimulated by the wavelengths of light of different colors. The cones are essential for color discrimination. SYN: *retinal c.; cone cell.* SEE: *retina* for illus.; *rod; rod cell.* **3.** A hollow, tapered, cylindrical device used in upper-extremity exercise to improve grasp, coordination, and range of motion. **4.** A device on a dental radiography machine that indicates the direction of the central beam and helps to establish the desired source-to-film distance.

c. of light One of the triangular areas of reflected light on the membrana tympani extending downward from the umbo.

ocular c. A cone of light in the eye with the point on the retina.

retinal c. One of the specialized cone-shaped cells of the retina. These cells, along with the retinal rods, are light sensitive. The cones receive color stimuli. SYN: *cone* (2).

cone cutting Failure to cover or expose the whole area of a radiograph with the useful beam. The film is only partially exposed.

cone shell poisoning A toxic reaction to the neurotoxin delivered by the pointed, hollow teeth of the marine animal contained in the cone shell. Intense local pain, swelling, and numbness may last several days. In severe poisoning, muscular incoordination and weakness can progress to respiratory paralysis. Although death can occur, recovery within 24 hr is the usual outcome. There is no specific therapy, but supportive measures including artificial respiration and supplemental oxygen may be needed.

conexus (kŏ-nĕk′sŭs) [L.] A connecting structure.

confabulation (kŏn-făb″ū-lā′shŭn) [L. *confabulari,* to talk together] A behavioral reaction to memory loss in which the patient fills in memory gaps with inappropriate words or fabricated ideas, often in great detail. Confabulation is a common finding in patients with Korsakoff's syndrome.

confectio, confection (kŏn-fĕk′shē-ō, -shŭn) [L. *conficere,* to prepare] A sugar-like soft solid in which one or more medicinal substances are incorporated so that they can be administered agreeably and preserved conveniently. The use of confections is rare in contemporary medicine.

confidence level The probability associated with a confidence interval, and stated as a part of that interval.

confidentiality The maintenance of privacy, by not sharing or divulging to a third party privileged or entrusted information. Patients' knowledge that they may safely discuss sensitive matters with their health care providers is necessary for successful, caring, and effective diagnosis and treatment. Matters discussed in confidence are held in secret, except in the rare instances when the information presents a clear threat to the health and well-being of another person, or in cases in which public health may be compromised by not revealing the information. In these instances, it is unethical and illegal not to disclose the information. SEE: *forensic medicine; privileged communication.*

configuration (kŏn-fĭg″ū-rā′shŭn) **1.** The shape and appearance of something. **2.** In chemistry, the position of atoms in a molecule.

activity c. An assessment approach used by occupational therapists to determine an individual's usual use of time during a typical week. The technique is designed to elicit the person's perceptions of the nature of daily activities and satisfaction with them.

confinement (kŏn-fīn′mĕnt) [O.Fr. *confiner,* to restrain in a place] **1.** Historically, the 6-week period between the day of parturition and the end of the puerperium when women were expected to absent themselves from society, remain at home to recover, and be cared for by their family members. **2.** Hospitalization, esp. for labor and delivery. **3.** The experience of being restrained to a physical space in order to limit activity.

conflict (kŏn′flĭkt) [L. *confligere,* to contend] **1.** The opposing action of incompatible substances. **2.** In psychiatry, the conscious or unconscious struggle between two opposing desires or courses of action; applied to a state in which social goals dictate behavior contrary to more primitive (often subconscious) desires.

conflict of interest Prejudice or bias that may occur when one's impartiality is compromised by opportunities for personal gain or occupational advancement, or by the chance that one's work may support a favored point of view or social agenda.

confluence of sinuses The union of the sagittal and transverse sinuses.

confluent (kŏn′floo-ĕnt) [L. *confluere,* to run together] Running together, as when pustules merge.

conformation (kŏn″for-mā′shŭn) The form or shape of a part, body, material, or molecule.

confrontation (kŏn″frŭn-tā′shŭn) [L. *con,* together with, + *frons,* face] **1.** The examination of two patients together, one with a disease and the other from whom the disease was supposedly contracted. **2.** A method of determining the extent of visual fields in which that of the patient is compared with that of the examiner. **3.** In psychiatry, a feedback procedure in which a patient's behavior and apparent feelings are presented to facilitate better understanding of his or her actions.

confusion (kŏn-fū′zhŭn) Not being aware of or oriented to time, place, or self.

acute c. The abrupt onset of a cluster of global, transient changes and disturbances in attention, cognition, psychomotor activity, level of consciousness, and/or sleep-wake cycle. SYN: *acute confusional state.* SEE: *delirium; Nursing Diagnoses Appendix.*

chronic c. An irreversible, long-standing, and/or progressive deterioration of intellect and personality characterized by decreased ability to interpret environmental stimuli, decreased capacity for intellectual thought processes, and disturbances of memory, orientation, and behavior. SEE: *dementia; Nursing Diagnoses Appendix.*

mental c. An abnormal mental state in which the individual experiences reduced mental functions, attentiveness, alertness, and ability to comprehend the environment.

confusional state, acute SEE: *acute c.*

congener (kŏn′jĕn-ĕr) [L. *con,* together, + *genus,* race] **1.** Two or more muscles with the same function. **2.** Something that resembles something else in structure, function, or origin. In the production of alcoholic beverages by fermentation, chemical substances termed congeners are also produced. These chemicals, more than 100 of which are known, impart aroma and flavor to the alcoholic compound. The precise role of these congeners in producing toxic effects is unknown.

congenital (kŏn-jĕn′ĭ-tăl) [L. *congenitus,* born together] Present at birth.

congested (kŏn-jĕs′tĕd) [L. *congerere,* to heap together] Containing an abnormal amount of blood or tissue fluid.

congestion (kŏn-jĕs′chŭn) An excessive amount of blood or tissue fluid in an organ or in tissue. **congestive** (-tĭv), *adj.*

active c. Congestion resulting from increased blood flow to a part or from dilatation of blood vessels.

passive c. Hyperemia of an organ resulting from interference with blood flow from capillaries into venules, for example, in congestive heart failure.

pulmonary c. The accumulation of an abnormal amount of blood in the pulmonary vascular bed. It usually occurs in association with heart failure.

conglobate (kŏn′glō-bāt) [L. *con,* together, + *globare,* to make round] In one mass, as lymph glands.

conglobation (kŏn″glō-bā′shŭn) An aggregation of particles in a rounded mass.

conglomerate (kŏn-glŏm′ĕr-āt) [″ + *glomerare,* to heap] **1.** An aggregation in one mass. **2.** Clustered; heaped together.

conglutinant (kŏn-gloo′tĭ-nănt) Promoting adhesion, as of the edges of a wound.

congregate housing A group residence, usually for elderly persons, which encourages independence and community living. The tenants may need some medical or social assistance, but not enough to require hospitalization or nursing home care. Congregate housing can also be used by head-injured patients, spinal cord-injured patients, recovering alcoholics, and others. SEE: *assisted living.*

coniasis (kō-nī′ă-sĭs) [Gr. *konis,* dust, + *-iasis,* condition] Dustlike calculi in gallbladder and bile ducts.

conidia (kō-nĭd′ē-ă) *sing.,* **conidium** Asexual spores of fungi.

conidiophore (kŏn-ĭd′ē-ō-for) [″ + *phoros,* bearing] The stalk supporting conidia.

coniofibrosis (kō″nē-ō-fī-brō′sĭs) [Gr. *konis,* dust, + L. *fibra,* fiber, + Gr. *osis,* condition] Pneumoconiosis produced by dust such as that from asbestos or silica. This causes fibrosis to develop in the lung.

coniology (kō-nē-ŏl′ŏ-jē) [″ + *logos,* study of] The study of dust and its effects.

coniosis (kō″nē-ō′sĭs) [″ + *osis,* condition] Any condition caused by inhalation of dust.

coniosporosis (kō″nē-ō-spō-rō′sĭs) [″ + *sporos,* seed, + *osis,* condition] A hypersensitivity reaction consisting of asthma and pneumonitis caused by breathing the spores of *Cryptostroma corticale* or *Coniosporium corticale.* These fungi grow under the bark of some types of trees. Workers who strip the bark from these trees may develop this condition.

coniotomy (kō″nē-ŏt′ō-mē) [Gr. *konos,* cone, + *tome,* incision] Cricothyrotomy.

conization (kŏn″ĭ-zā′shŭn) [Gr. *konos,* cone] SYN: *cone biopsy.*

conjugata (kŏn″jū-gā′tă) Conjugate (2).

c. diagonalis Diagonal conjugate.

c. vera True conjugate.

conjugate (kŏn′jū-gāt) **1.** Paired or joined. **2.** An important diameter of the pelvis, measured from the center of the promontory of the sacrum to the back of the symphysis pubis. In obstetrics, the diagonal conjugate is measured and the true conjugate is estimated. SYN: *conjugata.* SEE: *diagonal c.*

diagonal c. The distance between the sacral promontory and the lower inner surface of the symphysis pubis, usually more than 4.52 in. (11.5 cm). SYN: *conjugata diagonalis.*

c. diameter Conjugate (2).

external c. The diameter measured (with calipers) from the spine of the last lumbar vertebra to the front of the pubes; it is normally about 8 in. (20.3 cm).

obstetrical c. The distance between the sacral promontory and a point slightly below the upper inner margin of the symphysis pubis; the shortest diameter to which the fetal head must accommodate to descend successfully through the pelvic inlet.

true c. In obstetrics, the distance between the midline superior point of the sacrum and the upper margin of the symphysis pubis. It is the anteroposterior diameter of the pelvic inlet, estimated by subtracting 1.5 to 2 cm from the measurement of the diagonal conjugate. SYN: *conjugata vera.*

conjugation (kŏn″jū-gā′shŭn) **1.** A coupling. **2.** In biology, the union of two unicellular organisms accompanied by an interchange of nuclear material as in *Paramecium.*

conjunctiva (kŏn″jŭnk-tī′vă, kŏn-jŭnk′tĭ-vă) [L. *conjungere,* to join together] The mucous membrane that lines the eyelids and is reflected onto the eyeball.

DIVISIONS: The palpebral conjunctiva covers the undersurface of the eyelids. The bulbar conjunctiva coats the anterior portion of the eyeball. The fornix conjunctiva is the transition portion forming a fold between the lid and the globe.

INSPECTION: The palpebral and ocular portions should be examined. Color, degree of moisture, presence of foreign bodies or petechial hemorrhages, and inflammation should be observed.

PATHOLOGY: Conjunctival pathology includes trachoma, pannus, and discoloration. Yellowish discoloration is seen in jaundice and pale conjunctivae are seen in anemias. Note: The skin of a person with hypercarotinemia is yellow, but the conjunctivae are not.

conjunctivitis (kŏn-jŭnk″tĭ-vī′tĭs) [″ + Gr. *itis,* inflammation] Inflammation of the conjunctiva. Treatment is directed against the specific cause.

actinic c. Conjunctivitis resulting from exposure to ultraviolet (actinic) radiation.

acute contagious c. Pinkeye.

acute hemorrhagic c. A contagious viral eye infection marked by rapid onset of pain. It causes swollen eyelids, hyperemia of the conjunctiva, and later subconjunctival hemorrhage. The disease, which is self-limited and for which there is no specific therapy, usually affects both eyes. Several viral agents can cause this disease, including enterovirus 70, echovirus 7, and a variant of coxsackievirus A24.

angular c. of Morax-Axenfeld Conjunctivitis affecting the inner angle of the conjunctivae.

catarrhal c. Conjunctivitis due to causes such as foreign bodies, bacteria, or irritation from heat, cold, or chemicals.

chlamydial c. Conjunctivitis caused by *Chlamydia trachomatis.* In newborns this type of conjunctivitis is encountered more frequently than ophthalmia neonatorum caused by gonococci. Prophylaxis for chlamydial conjunctivitis is 1% silver nitrate. If the disease develops, drugs such as azithromycin, quinolones, or sulfa-based antibiotics are used.

follicular c. A type of conjunctivitis characterized by pinkish round bodies in the retrotarsal fold.

gonorrheal c. A severe, acute form of purulent conjunctivitis caused by *Neis-*

seria gonorrhoeae. SEE: *ophthalmia neonatorum.*

granular c. Acute contagious inflammatory conjunctivitis with granular elevations on the lids that ulcerate and scar.

inclusion c. An acute purulent inflammation of the conjunctivae caused by *Chlamydia trachomatis.* The newborn is infected as it passes through the mother's genital tract. Adults may be infected by a sex partner.

ligneous c. A rare eye disease in which fibrin deposits create woody plaques on the conjunctiva. Similar plaques may develop in the airways and genitalia. The disease often is found in patients with a deficiency in plasminogen levels.

membranous c. Acute conjunctivitis marked by a false membrane with or without infiltration.

c. of newborn Ophthalmia neonatorum.

phlyctenular c. An allergenic form of conjunctivitis common in children and marked by nodules that may ulcerate.

purulent c. A form of conjunctivitis caused by organisms producing pus, esp. gonococci.

seasonal c. Allergic inflammation of the conjunctiva that occurs because of exposure to pollens, grasses, and other antigens.

vernal c. Conjunctivitis beginning in the spring; due to allergy.

conjunctivoma (kŏn-jŭnk″tĭ-vō′mă) [L. *conjungere,* to join together, + Gr. *oma,* tumor] A tumor of the conjunctiva.

conjunctivoplasty (kŏn″jŭnk-tī′vō-plăs″tē) [″ + Gr. *plassein,* to form] Removal of part of the cornea and replacement with flaps from the conjunctiva.

connective [L. *connectere,* to bind together] Connecting or binding together.

connexon (kŏn-ĕks′ŭn) A protein that forms tunnels across gap junctions, enabling ions or small molecules, such as glucose, to pass from one cell to another.

Conn's syndrome [J. W. Conn, U.S. physician, b. 1907] Primary hyperaldosteronism. Clinical findings include muscle weakness, polyuria, hypertension, hypokalemia, and alkalosis associated with an abnormally high rate of aldosterone secretion by the adrenal cortex. SEE: *Nursing Diagnoses Appendix.*

conoid (kō′noyd) [Gr. *konos,* cone, + *eidos,* form, shape] Resembling a cone; conical.

conoid tubercle An eminence on the inferior surface of the clavicle to which the conoid ligament is attached.

consanguinity (kŏn″săn-gwĭn′ĭ-tē) [L. *consanguinitas,* kinship] Relationship by blood (i.e., descent from a common ancestor).

conscience (kon′shŭntz) One's inner sense of what is right, wrong, or fair, esp. regarding relations with people or society. This sense can inhibit or reinforce the individual's actions and thoughts. SEE: *superego.*

conscious (kŏn′shŭs) [L. *conscius,* aware] Being aware and having perception; awake. SEE: *coma.*

consciousness Arousal accompanied by awareness of one's environment. In practice, consciousness is said to be present when a person is awake, alert, and oriented to his or her surroundings (i.e., where one is, who one is, what the date is).

Alterations of consciousness are common. Sleep is an altered state of consciousness from which one can be easily aroused. Stupor and lethargy are conditions in which one's level of arousal is diminished. In coma, one cannot be aroused. Other alterations in consciousness occur in delirium, dementia, hallucinosis, or intoxication, when persons may be fully aroused but have impaired perceptions of themselves and their environment.

clouding of c. In delirium, a state in which awareness of the environment is impaired.

cost c. Awareness of economic limits in the practice of medicine.

disintegration of c. In classic psychoanalysis, disorganization of the personality. It is produced by the contents of the unconscious gradually disrupting the conscious.

levels of c. States of arousal and awareness, ranging from fully awake and oriented to one's environment to comatose. It is important to use a standardized system of description rather than vague terms such as semiconscious, semicomatose, or semistuporous.

Alert wakefulness: The patient perceives the environment clearly and responds quickly and appropriately to visual, auditory, and other sensory stimuli.

Drowsiness: The patient does not perceive the environment fully and responds to stimuli appropriately but slowly or with delay. He or she may be roused by verbal stimuli but may ignore some of them. The patient is capable of verbal response unless aphasia, aphonia, or anarthria is present. Lethargy and obtundation also describe the drowsy state.

Stupor: The patient is aroused by intense stimuli only. Loud noise may elicit a nonspecific reaction. Motor response and reflex reactions are usually preserved unless the patient is paralyzed.

Coma: The patient does not perceive the environment and intense stimuli produce a rudimentary response if any.

The presence of reflex reactions depends on the location of the lesion(s) in the nervous system.

consensual (kŏn-sĕn′shū-ăl) [L. *consensus,* agreement] **1.** Pert. to reflex stimulation of one part or side produced by excitation of another part or the opposite side. **2.** Mutually agreeable. **3.** Consenting.

consensual light reflex The reaction of both pupils that occurs when one eye is exposed to a greater intensity of light than the other. SEE: *reflex, pupillary.*

consent The granting of permission by the patient for another person to perform an act (e.g., permission for a surgical or therapeutic procedure or experiment to be performed by a physician, dentist, or other health-care professional).

implied c. Nonverbal consent suggested by the actions by the patient, as when he or she enters the dental office and sits in a dental chair. This suggests that the patient seeks examination, diagnosis, and consultation.

informed c. A voluntary agreement made by a well-advised and mentally competent patient to be treated or randomized into a research study. The health care provider should provide full disclosure of information regarding the material risks, benefits of the proposed treatment, alternatives, and consequences of no treatment, so that the patient can make an intelligent, or informed, choice.

consenting adult A mature individual who agrees to participate in social or sexual activity by virtue of his or her own desire or free will.

consequence (kŏn′sē-kwĕns) **1.** Any result, conclusion, or effect. **2.** In psychology, the end result of a behavior, which may be positive, negative, or neutral.

conservative (kŏn-sĕr′vă-tĭv) [L. *conservare,* to preserve] Pert. to the use of a simple rather than a radical method of medical or surgical therapy.

conservation A cognitive principle, first described by Piaget, indicating that a certain quantity remains constant despite the transformation of shape. Children develop conservation ability for number, length, liquid amount, solid amount, space, weight, and volume.

conservation model A conceptual model of nursing developed by Myra Levine. The person is viewed as a holistic being who adapts to environmental challenges. In this model the goal of nursing is to promote wholeness through conservation of energy, structural integrity, personal integrity, and social integrity. SEE: *Nursing Theory Appendix.*

conservator (kŏn-sĕr′vă-tŏr) A person appointed by the courts to manage the affairs of another person (called the conservatee), esp. if there is strong evidence that the conservatee is incapable of managing his or her own affairs. SEE: *guardianship.*

conservatorship The preservation and protection of a dependent person's self and property by another individual. The term does not refer to imprisonment or confinement in a psychiatric facility. This is called *guardianship* in some states.

consolidation (kŏn-sŏl-ĭ-dā′shŭn) [L. *consolidare,* to make firm] The process of becoming solid, esp. in connection with the lungs. Solidification of the lungs is caused by pathological engorgement of the lung tissues as occurs in acute pneumonia.

constant (kŏn′stănt) [L. *constans,* standing together] **1.** Unchanging. **2.** A condition, fact, or situation that does not change.

constellation (kŏn″stĕl-lā′shŭn) [L. *con,* together, + *stella,* star] A group, set, or configuration of objects, individuals, or conditions.

constipation (kŏn″stĭ-pā′shŭn) [L. *constipare,* to press together] A decrease in a person's normal frequency of defecation accompanied by difficult or incomplete passage of stool and/or passage of excessively hard, dry stool. SEE: *Nursing Diagnoses Appendix.*

ETIOLOGY: Predisposing factors in healthy individuals include a diet that lacks fiber, inadequate consumption of fluids, a sedentary lifestyle, and advancing age. Many drugs, including opiates, antidepressants, calcium channel blockers, antiemetics, and anticholinergics (among others) cause constipation as well. Among metabolic illnesses, hypothyroidism and disorders of calcium metabolism occasionally contribute to difficulty with the passage of stools. Pathological lesions of the bowel, such as diverticular disease, anorectal gonorrhea, hemorrhoids, or obstructions due to tumors, adhesions, or incarcerated hernias, may also be responsible.

NOTE: Normal bowel frequency varies from person to person. Some individuals normally have three bowel movements daily, while others have a normal pattern of one or two bowel movements a week.

CAUTION: A change in frequency of bowel movements may be a sign of serious intestinal or colonic disease (e.g., a malignancy). A change in bowel habits should be discussed with a physician.

TREATMENT: Consumption of fresh vegetables, fruits, and grains helps prevent constipation. Medications to alleviate constipation include docusate, bulk-forming laxatives (such as psyllium), magnesium-containing compounds, lactulose, and a variety of enemas.

atonic c. Constipation due to weakness or paralysis of the muscles of the colon and rectum.

colonic c. The state in which an individual's pattern of elimination is characterized by hard, dry stools which results from a delay in passage of food residue.

obstructive c. Constipation due to a mechanical obstruction of the intestines, e.g., by hernias, adhesions, or tumors.

perceived c. The state in which an individual makes a self-diagnosis of constipation and ensures a daily bowel movement through use of laxatives, enemas, and suppositories. SEE: *Nursing Diagnoses Appendix.*

risk for c. A nursing diagnosis approved at the 13th NANDA Conference (1998); at risk for a decrease in a person's normal frequency of defecation accompanied by difficult or incomplete passage of stool and/or passage of excessively hard, dry stool. SEE: *Nursing Diagnoses Appendix.*

spastic c. Constipation due to excessive tonicity of the intestinal wall, esp. the colon.

constitution (kŏn-stĭ-tū′shŭn) [L. *constituere,* to establish] The physical makeup and functional habits of the body. **constitutional** (-ăl), *adj.*

constriction [L. *con,* together, + *stringere,* to draw] **1.** The binding or squeezing of a part. **2.** The narrowing of a vessel or opening (e.g., blood vessels or the pupil of the eye).

constrictor **1.** Something that binds or restricts a part. **2.** A muscle that constricts a vessel, opening, or passageway, as the constrictors of the faucial isthmus and pharynx and the circular fibers of the iris, intestine, and blood vessels.

consultant [L. *consultare,* to counsel] A health care worker, such as a nurse, physician, dentist, pharmacist, or psychologist, who acts in an advisory capacity.

consultation For a specific patient, diagnosis and proposed treatment by two or more health care workers at one time, one of whom usually is specially trained in the problem confronting the patient.

consummation The first act of sexual intercourse after marriage.

consumption (kŏn-sŭmp′shŭn) [L. *consumere,* to waste away] **1.** Tuberculosis. **2.** Wasting. **3.** The using up of anything.

consumption-coagulopathy Disseminated intravascular coagulation.

consumptive Pert. to or afflicted with tuberculosis.

contact [L. *con,* with, + *tangere,* to touch] **1.** Mutual touching or apposition of two bodies. **2.** One who has been recently exposed to a contagious disease.

complete c. The contact that occurs when the entire proximal surface of a tooth touches the entire surface of an adjoining tooth, proximally.

defective occlusal c. Interceptive occlusal c.

direct c. Transmission of a communicable disease from the host to a healthy person by way of body fluids, such as respiratory droplets, blood, and semen; cutaneous contact; or placental transmission.

indirect c. Transmission of a communicable disease by any medium between the host and the susceptible person. The medium may be, for example, contaminated food or water; medical supplies; the hands of a health care worker; clothing; or an arthropod vector. SEE: *fomes.*

interceptive occlusal c. Tooth contact that can divert the mandible from a normal to an abnormal path of motion. SYN: *defective occlusal c.*

intercuspal c. Contact between the cusps of opening teeth.

occlusal c. The normal contact between teeth when the maxilla and mandible are brought together in habitual or centric occlusion.

proximal c. Touching of teeth on their adjacent surfaces.

contactant (kŏn-tăk′tănt) A substance that produces an allergic or sensitivity response when it contacts the skin directly.

contact lens SEE: under *lens.*

contact surface A proximal tooth surface.

contagion (kŏn-tā′jŭn) [L. *contingere,* to touch] **1.** A transmissible infectious disease. **2.** Any virus or other microorganism that causes a contagious disease. SEE: *virulent; virus.*

contagious (kŏn-tā′jŭs) Capable of being transmitted from one individual to another. SEE: *infectious.*

contagious pustular dermatitis A cutaneous disease of sheep and goats transmitted to humans by direct contact. The lesion on humans is usually solitary and on the hands, arms, or face. This maculopapular area may progress to a pustule up to 3 cm in diameter and may last 3 to 6 weeks. The etiological agent is *Parapoxvirus,* which is a genus of poxvirus. There is no specific treatment. SYN: *orf.*

contagium (kŏn-tā′jē-ŭm) [L.] The agent causing infection.

container (kŏn-tā′nĕr) A receptacle for storing a medical specimen or supplies. Use of sterile disposable containers for collecting specimens is recommended, since contamination of the container may alter the results of the specimen analysis and therefore interfere with the diagnosis. SEE: *Standard and Universal Precautions Appendix.*

containment (kŏn-tān′mĕnt) **1.** In public health, the control or eradication of infectious diseases. **2.** In environmental health, the prevention of spread of toxic substances into the environment. **3.** In health care delivery, the restricting and controlling of excess spending on health care. SYN: *cost c.*

cost c. The management and control of health care expenditures.

contaminant (kŏn-tăm′ĭ-nănt) A substance or organism that soils, stains, pollutes, or renders something unfit for use.

contaminate (kŏn-tăm′ĭ-nāt) [L. *contaminare,* to render impure] **1.** To soil, stain, or pollute. **2.** To render unfit for use through introduction of a harmful or injurious substance. **3.** To make impure or unclean. **4.** To deposit a radioactive substance in any place where it is not supposed to be.

contamination **1.** The act of contaminating, esp. the introduction of pathogens or infectious material into or on normally clean or sterile objects, spaces, or surfaces. **2.** In psychiatry, the fusion and condensation of words so that they run together when spoken.

radiation c. Radiation in or on a place where it is not wanted.

contiguity (kŏn″tĭ-gū′ĭ-tē) [L. *contiguus,* touching] Contact or close association.

law of c. The law stating that if two ideas occur in association, they are likely to be repeated.

solution of c. The dislocation or displacement of two normally contiguous parts.

continence (kŏn′tĭ-nĕns) [L. *continere,* to hold together] Self-restraint, used esp. in reference to refraining from sexual intercourse, and to the ability to control urination and defecation. SEE: *incontinence.*

continent (kŏn′tĭ-nĕnt) **1.** Able to control urination and defecation. **2.** Not engaging in sexual intercourse. SEE: *continence.*

continuing care community A type of managed care that combines health insurance, housing, and social care, usually for the elderly. The participant enters a contractual arrangement, in which he or she receives a residence and long-term care on an as-needed basis in exchange for an agreed-upon fee.

continuing education, continuing medical education ABBR: CE; CME. Postgraduate education in the health professions; the enhancement or expansion of an individual's knowledge or skills through coursework; home study; live, audio, or video conferences; electronic media; or clinical practice. Postgraduate courses may be required for continued certification or licensure requirements in a practice such as medicine, nursing, physical therapy, respiratory therapy, and social work.

continuity (kŏn″tĭ-nū′ĭ-tē) [L. *continuus,* continued] The condition of being unbroken, uninterrupted, or intimately united.

continuous spectrum **1.** An unbroken series of wavelengths, either visible or invisible. **2.** An unbroken range of radiations of different wavelengths in any portion of the invisible spectrum.

continuous subcutaneous insulin infusion ABBR: CSII. SEE: *insulin pump.*

continuum of care The range of services required by chronically ill, impaired, or elderly persons. Services include preventive measures, acute medical treatment, rehabilitative and supportive care, and social services, to meet the needs of clients in the community or institutional settings. These take place in the community and in many institutional settings.

contour (kŏn′toor) [It. *contornare,* to go around] **1.** The outline or surface configuration of a part. **2.** To shape or form a surface, as in carving dental restorations to approximate the conditions of the original tooth surface.

gingival c. The normal arching appearance of the gingiva along the cervical part of the teeth and rounding off toward the attached gingiva.

gingival denture c. The form of the denture base or other materials around the cervical parts of artificial teeth.

contoured (kŏn′toord) Having an irregular, undulating surface resembling a relief map; said of bacterial colonies.

contra- [L.] Prefix indicating *opposite* or *against.*

contra-aperture [L. *contra,* against, + *apertura,* opening] A second opening made in an abscess.

contraception (kŏn″tră-sĕp′shŭn) [″ + *conceptio,* a conceiving] The prevention of conception.

emergency c. Postcoital contraception.

postcoital c. ABBR: PCC. The prevention of conception in the immediate postcoital period. These methods include insertion of an intrauterine device within 5 days of unprotected coitus and administering diethylstilbestrol, mifepristone (RU 486), or levonorgestrel. Of the various methods available for this purpose, only the use of combined oral contraceptive pills has been approved by the U.S. Food and Drug Administration.

contraceptive (kŏn″tră-sĕp′tĭv) Any process, device, or method that prevents conception. Categories of contraceptives include steroids; chemical; physical or barrier; combinations of physical or barrier and chemical; "natural"; abstinence; and permanent surgical procedures. SEE: table; *abortion.*

Contraceptive Use by Women, 15 to 44 Years Old: 1995 (Based on Samples of the Female Population of the United States)

Contraceptive Status and Method	All Women[1]	Age 15–24 Years	25–34 Years	35–44 Years	Race White	Black	Hispanic
All women (1,000)	58,381	17,637	21,728	19,016	42,968	7,510	5,500
Percent Distribution							
Sterile	32.1	3.8	26.4	64.6	32.9	34.0	27.5
Surgically sterile	30.2	3.1	24.8	61.1	31.2	31.4	23.9
Noncontraceptively sterile[2]	5.2	0.3	2.7	12.5	5.4	6.5	3.2
Contraceptively sterile[3]	25.0	2.8	22.1	48.6	25.8	24.9	20.7
Nonsurgically sterile[4]	1.9	0.7	1.6	3.5	1.7	2.6	3.6
Pregnant, postpartum	5.4	7.0	7.9	1.2	5.2	5.5	7.7
Seeking pregnancy	4.0	1.8	7.6	2.0	3.7	4.7	5.1
Other nonusers	24.2	46.4	17.1	12.0	23.6	22.1	28.3
Never had intercourse	9.4	26.4	2.8	1.3	8.7	7.0	16.4
No intercourse in last month	7.0	7.7	7.1	6.4	7.2	7.5	5.1
Had intercourse in last month	7.8	12.3	7.2	4.3	7.7	7.6	6.8
Nonsurgical contraceptors	34.3	41.2	41.3	20.1	34.6	33.8	31.7
Pill	16.9	23.9	22.0	4.7	17.3	16.7	16.4
IUD	0.8	0.2	0.4	1.8	0.8	0.8	1.0
Diaphragm	1.7	0.2	2.3	2.4	1.8	1.0	0.8
Condom	10.5	13.9	11.0	6.7	10.3	11.4	8.9
Periodic abstinence	1.6	1.0	2.0	1.6	1.6	0.7	1.9
Natural family planning	0.2	0.1	0.4	0.2	0.2	—	—
Withdrawal	0.6	0.6	0.6	0.5	0.6	0.4	0.4
Other methods[5]	2.3	1.4	3.0	2.4	2.2	2.8	2.3

SOURCE: Adapted from U.S. National Center for Health Statistics. *Advance Data from Vital and Health Statistics.*

—Represents or rounds to zero.

[1] Includes other races, not shown separately.

[2] Persons who had sterilizing operation and who gave as one reason that they had medical problems with their reproductive organs.

[3] Includes all other sterilization operations, and sterilization of the husband or current partner.

[4] Persons sterile from illness, accident, or congenital conditions.

[5] Douche, suppository, and less frequently used methods.

STEROIDS: Oral contraceptives, colloquially termed “the pill,” consist of chemicals that are quite similar to natural hormones (estrogen or progesterone). They act by preventing ovulation. When taken according to instructions, these pills are almost 100% effective. Long-acting contraceptives including the implanted levonorgestrel are available. Diethylstilbestrol is used as a “morning-after” contraceptive, esp. in cases of rape or incest.

CHEMICAL: Spermicides in the form of foam, cream, jelly, spermicide-impregnated sponge, or suppositories are placed in the vagina before intercourse. They may be used alone or in combination with a barrier contraceptive. They act by killing the sperm. Douching after intercourse is not effective enough to be considered a method of contraception.

PHYSICAL OR BARRIER: Intrauterine contraceptive devices (IUDs) are plastic or metal objects placed inside the uterus. They are thought to prevent the fertilized egg from attaching itself to the lining of the uterus. Their effectiveness is only slightly lower than that of oral contraceptives. Diaphragms are made of a dome-shaped piece of rubber with a flexible spring circling the edge. They are available in various sizes and are inserted into the vagina so as to cover the cervix. A diaphragm must be used in conjunction with a chemical spermicide, which is used before positioning the diaphragm. A specially fitted cervical cap is also available as a barrier-type contraceptive. A sponge impregnated with a contraceptive cream or jelly is available. It is placed in the vagina up to several hours prior to intercourse. The male partner can use a condom, a flexible tube-shaped barrier placed over the erect penis so that the ejaculate is contained in the tube and is not deposited in the vagina. Made of rubber or animal membranes, condoms are available in both dry and wet-lubricated forms and in various colors. Used properly, the condom is a reliable means of contraception. It is more effective if combined with a chemical spermicide. Condoms also help prevent transmission of diseases by sexual intercourse by providing a physical barrier. SEE: *condom*.

NATURAL: These methods involve abstaining from intercourse for a specified number of days before, during, and after ovulation. The rhythm method is based on calculating the fertile period by the use of a calendar, on which the supposed infertile days are marked. In practice, this method has a high rate of failure. Other methods include determining ovulation by keeping a basal temperature chart and judging the time of ovulation by observing cyclical changes in the cervical mucus. SEE: *basal temperature chart*.

Sophisticated home-diagnostic tests for the hormonal changes present at ovulation are available. Withdrawal, the removal of the penis from the vagina just before ejaculation, is subject to a high failure rate because sperm may be contained in the pre-ejaculatory fluid from the penis.

PERMANENT: *For women:* Tubal ligation involves surgical division of the fallopian tubes and ligation of the cut ends. This procedure does not interfere with the subsequent enjoyment of sexual intercourse. This form of sterilization is effective but virtually irreversible. *For men:* Vasectomy consists of cutting the vas deferens and ligating each end so that the sperm can no longer travel from the testicle to the urethra. The procedure must be done bilaterally and the ejaculate tested for several months postoperatively to make certain sperm are not present. Until two successive tests reveal absence of sperm, the method should not be regarded as having succeeded. Attempts to reverse this surgical procedure have succeeded in only a small percentage of cases. Vasectomy does not interfere with the normal enjoyment of sexual intercourse.

contract (kŏn-trăkt′) [L. *contrahere,* to draw together] **1.** To draw together, reduce in size, or shorten. **2.** To acquire through infection, as to contract a disease. **3.** In psychology or psychiatry, the patient's commitment to attempt to alter behavior or to take a specific course of action. **4.** An agreement consisting of one or more legally enforceable promises among two or more parties such as people, corporations, and partnerships. Four elements are in a contractual relationship: offer, acceptance, consideration, and breach. In health care, contracts are used to govern relationships, for example, between employees and employers, insurers and the insured, or health care providers and patients.

contractile (kŏn-trăk′tĭl) Able to contract or shorten.

contractility (kŏn-trăk-tĭl′ĭ-tē) **1.** Having the ability to contract or shorten. **2.** In cardiac physiology, the force with which left ventricular ejection occurs. It is independent of the effects of preload or afterload.

contraction (kŏn-trăk′shŭn) A shortening or tightening, as of a muscle; a shrinking or a reduction in size.

Braxton Hicks c. SEE: *Braxton Hicks contractions*.

carpopedal c. A contraction of the flexor muscles of the hands and feet due to tetany, hypocalcemia, or hyperventilation.

hourglass c. An excessive, irregular contraction of an organ at its center. SEE: *ectasia*.

idiomuscular c. Motion produced by degenerated muscles without nerve stimulus.

isoinertial muscle c. Shortening and increased tension in a muscle against a constant load or resistance.

isometric c. A muscular contraction in which the muscle increases tension but does not change its length; also called a *static muscle contraction*.

isotonic c. A muscular contraction in which the muscle maintains constant tension by changing its length during the action.

tetanic c. **1.** Continuous muscular contraction. **2.** A sudden, strong, sustained uterine contraction that jeopardizes maternal and fetal status. It may occur during oxytocin induction or stimulation of labor and can cause profound fetal distress, premature placental separation, or uterine rupture.

tonic c. Spasmodic contraction of a muscle for an extended period.

contraction stress test ABBR: CST. A procedure used to evaluate placental sufficiency by assessing fetal response to the physiological stress of artificially induced uterine contractions. Contractions may be generated by breast stimulation or by the oxytocin challenge test. SEE: *oxytocin challenge test*.

contracture (kŏn-trăk′chūr) [L. *contractura*] Fibrosis of connective tissue in skin, fascia, muscle, or a joint capsule that prevents normal mobility of the related tissue or joint.

Dupuytren's c. SEE: *Dupuytren's contracture*.

fibrotic c. Contraction of a muscle in which the muscle tissue has been replaced by fibrous tissue because of injury.

functional c. Contraction of a muscle that decreases during anesthesia or sleep.

myostatic c. Adaptive shortening of muscle, usually caused by immobilization and without tissue pathology.

physiological c. A temporary condition in which tension and shortening of a muscle are maintained for a considerable time although there is no tetanus. It may be induced by heat, illness, drug action, or acids.

pseudomyostatic c. Apparent permanent contraction of a muscle due to a central nervous system lesion, resulting in loss of range of motion and resistance of the muscle to stretch.

Volkmann's c. Pronation and flexion of the hand, with atrophy of the forearm muscles, resulting from circulatory impairment due to pressure from a cast, constricting dressings, or injury to the radial artery. This can be prevented by alertness to signs of cold, pallor, cyanosis, pain, and swelling of the part below the injury or constriction and removal of the cause.

contrafissura (kŏn″tră-fĭ-shū′ră) [L. *contra,* against, + *fissura,* fissure] A skull fracture at a point opposite where the blow was received. SEE: *contrecoup*.

contraindication (kŏn″tră-ĭn-dĭ-kā′shŭn) [″ + *indicare,* to point out] Any symptom or circumstance that makes treatment with a drug or device unsafe or inappropriate.

contralateral (kŏn″tră-lăt′ĕr-ăl) [″ + *latus,* side] Originating in or affecting the opposite side of the body, as opposed to homolateral and ipsilateral.

contralateral reflex **1.** Passive flexion of one part following flexion of another. **2.** Passive flexion of one leg, causing similar movement of the opposite leg.

contrast (kŏn′trăst) In radiology, The difference between adjacent densities in an image. This is controlled by the energy of the beam and influenced by the characteristics of the part radiographed, production of scatter radiation, type of film and screen combination, and processing.

contrast medium In radiology, a substance used to fill hollow organs or blood vessels to highlight their internal structure or distinguish them from neighboring anatomical features. The substance can be radiopaque and positive (e.g., barium sulfate, tri-iodinated media) or radiolucent and negative (e.g., air). Barium sulfate is a commonly used contrast agent for the gastrointestinal tract; it may be swallowed (for upper GI studies) or given as an enema (to visualize the colon).

high-osmolarity c.m. ABBR: HOCM. A water-soluble contrast medium with high osmolarity. These agents increase the probability of an adverse reaction and are generally ionic.

low-osmolarity c.m. ABBR: LOCM. A water-soluble contrast medium with low osmolarity. These agents produce fewer undesired effects after intravascular administration than do high-osmolarity contrast media. They are generally nonionic, with the exception of Hexabrix (an ionic dimer).

nonionic c.m. A water-soluble contrast medium whose molecules do not dissociate into cations and anions in solution. These agents tend to have low osmolarity. They decrease the risk of adverse reactions, but are costly.

tri-iodinated c.m. A derivative of tri-iodobenzoic acid that is the base for water-soluble contrast media. It contains three atoms of iodine per molecule.

contrast bath A method of stimulating blood circulation by having the patient sit on the side of a bathtub and spraying the feet and legs with warm water for 1 min and cold water for 1 min.

contravolitional (kŏn″tră-vō-lĭ′shŭn-ăl) [L. *contra,* against, + *velle,* to wish] In opposition to or without the will; involuntary.

contrecoup (kŏn-tr-koo′) An injury to parts of the brain located on the side opposite that of the primary injury, as when a blow to the back of the head forces the frontal and temporal lobes against the irregular bones of the anterior portion of the cranial vault.

contributory negligence In forensic medicine, the concept that the plaintiff's negligence in combination with the defendant's negligence is the cause of the plaintiff's injuries or damages.

control (kŏn-trōl′) [L. *contra,* against, + *rotulus,* little wheel] **1.** To regulate or maintain. **2.** A standard against which observations or conclusions may be checked to establish their validity, as a control animal (e.g., one that has not been exposed to the treatment or condition being studied in the other animals). **3.** In clinical investigations, a research subject whose age, sex, race, behavior, weight, or health matches as many features of the population being studied as is possible or appropriate. When cases and controls are closely matched, the validity of results increases.

automatic exposure c. ABBR: AEC. In radiology, an ionization chamber or solid-state device that terminates the radiation exposure at a preset level. SYN: *phototimer*.

infection c. In medical care, institutional procedures and policies for monitoring and attempting to control the transmission of communicable diseases. This includes establishing sanitation, sterilization, and isolation procedures.

motor c. The neural and biomechanical basis of planned, coordinated movement. SEE: *motor learning*.

controlled substance act The Comprehensive Drug Abuse Prevention and Control Act; a law enacted in 1971 to control the distribution and use of all depressant and stimulant drugs and other drugs of abuse or potential abuse as may be designated by the Drug Enforcement Administration of the Department of Justice.

The act specifies record keeping by the pharmacist, the format for prescription writing, and the limit on the amount of a drug that can be legally dispensed. This limit and whether refills are allowed varies with the nature of the drug. Centrally acting drugs such as narcotics, stimulants, and certain sedatives are divided into five classes called schedules I through V. Schedule I drugs are experimental. Prescriptions for schedule II drugs may not be refilled. Prescriptions for schedule III and IV drugs may be refilled up to five times within 6 months of the time the initial prescription was written. Schedule V drugs are restricted only to the extent that all nonscheduled prescription drugs are regulated.

Controlled substances are labeled with a large "C" followed by the Roman numeral designation. Alternatively the Roman numeral is within the large "C."

contuse (kŏn-tooz′) [L. *contundere,* to bruise] To bruise.

contusion (kŏn-too′zhŭn) Bruise.

conus (kō′nŭs) [Gr. *konos*] **1.** A cone. **2.** A posterior staphyloma of a myopic eye.

c. arteriosus The upper rounded anterior angle of the right cardiac ventricle, where the pulmonary artery arises.

c. medullaris The conical portion of the lower spinal cord.

convalescence (kŏn″văl-ĕs′ĕns) [L. *convalescere,* to become strong] The period of recovery after a disease or an operation.

convalescent **1.** Getting well. **2.** One who is recovering from a disease or operation.

convalescent diet A diet suitable for the condition from which the patient is recovering.

convection (kŏn-vĕk′shŭn) [L. *convehere,* to convey] **1.** Heat transference by means of currents in liquids or gases. **2.** Loss of body heat by means of transfer to the surrounding cooler air.

convergence (kŏn-vĕr′jĕns) [L. *con,* with, + *vergere,* to incline] **1.** The moving of two or more objects toward the same point. **2.** In reflex activity, the coming together of several axons or afferent fibers on one or a few motor neurons; the condition in which impulses from several sensory receptors converge on the same motor center, resulting in a limited and specific response. **3.** The directing of visual lines to a nearby point.

convergent (kŏn-vĕr′jĕnt) Tending toward a common point.

conversion (kŏn-vĕr′zhŭn) [L. *convertere,* to turn round] **1.** The change from one condition to another. For example, a patient with an arrhythmia may convert from atrial fibrillation to sinus rhythm, or a patient with no evidence of tuberculosis may convert to a positive purified protein derivative status. **2.** In obstetrics, a change in position of a fetus in the uterus by the physician to facilitate delivery. SEE: *version*.

conversion disorder A psychological disorder marked by symptoms or deficits affecting motor or sensory function that mimic a neurological or general medical disease. Psychological factors are associated with and precede the condition. Symptoms may include loss of sense of touch, double vision, blindness, deafness, paralysis, and hallucinations. Individuals with conversion symptoms show "la belle indifference" or relative lack of concern. The symptoms are not intentionally produced or feigned. The diagnosis cannot be established if the condition can be explained by the effects of medication or a neurological or other general medical condition. SYN: *somatoform disorder*.

conversion symptom SEE: *somatoform disorder*.

convex (kŏn′vĕks, kŏn-vĕks′) [L. *convexus,* vaulted, arched] Curved evenly; resembling the segment of a sphere.

convexoconcave (kŏn-vĕk″sō-kŏn′kāv, -kŏn-kāv′) Concavoconvex.

convexoconvex [″ + *convexus,* arched] Convex on two opposite faces.

convolute, convoluted (kŏn′vō-loot; -loot′ĕd) [L. *convolvere,* to roll together] Rolled, as a scroll.

convolution (kŏn″vō-loo′shŭn) [L. *convolvere,* to roll together] **1.** A turn, fold, or coil of anything that is convoluted. **2.** In anatomy, a gyrus, one of the many folds on the surface of the cerebral hemispheres. They are separated by grooves (sulci or fissures). SEE: *gyrus.*

angular c. A gyrus forming the posterior portion of the inferior parietal lobule.

annectant c. One of the four gyri connecting the convolutions on the upper surface of the occipital lobe with the parietal and temporosphenoidal lobes.

anterior choroid c. Gyrus choroides.

anterior orbital c. The convolution that lies in front of the orbital sulcus.

Arnold's c. One of the gyri posteriores inferiores.

ascending frontal c. The convolution forming the anterior boundary of Rolando's fissure.

ascending parietal c. The convolution parallel to the ascending frontal convolution, separated from it by Rolando's fissure, except at the extremities, where they are generally united.

Broca's c. Broca's area.

callosal c. Cingulate gyrus.

cerebral c. One of the convolutions of the cerebrum.

c. of corpus callosum Gyrus fornicatus.

cuneate c. Gyral isthmus.

dentate c. A small, notched gyrus, rudimentary in humans, situated in the dentate fissure.

exterior olfactory c. One of the small projections forming the outer boundary of the olfactory grooves.

hippocampal c. Uncinate gyrus.

inferior frontal c. The lower and outer part of the frontal lobe.

inferior occipital c. A small convolution lying between the middle and inferior occipital fissures.

insular c. One of a group of small convolutions forming the island of Reil, entirely concealed by the operculum.

intestinal c. A coil of the intestines.

marginal c. The convolution beginning in front of the locus perforatus anterior and bounding the longitudinal fissure on the mesial aspect of the hemisphere.

middle frontal c. Second frontal c.

middle occipital c. The convolution between the first and third occipital convolutions.

middle temporosphenoidal c. A small gyrus continuous with the middle occipital or angular gyrus.

occipitotemporal c. One of two small convolutions on the lower surface of the temporosphenoidal lobe.

olfactory c. Olfactory lobe.

orbital c. One of the small gyri on the orbital surface of the frontal lobe.

parietal c. The ascending parietal or the superior parietal convolution.

posterior orbital c. A small convolution on the posterior and outer side of the orbital sulcus, and continuous with the inferior frontal convolution.

second frontal c. A convolution on the frontal lobes, lying posteriorly between the superior and inferior frontal sulci. SYN: *middle frontal c.*

superior frontal c. A convolution that bounds the great longitudinal fissure, originating behind the upper end of the ascending frontal convolution.

superior occipital c. The uppermost of the three convolutions on the superior surface of the occipital lobe.

superior parietal c. The portion of the parietal lobe limited anteriorly by the upper part of Rolando's fissure, posteriorly by the exterior parieto-occipital fissure, and inferiorly by the intraparietal sulcus.

superior temporosphenoidal c. The uppermost of three convolutions forming the temporosphenoidal lobe. It is just below and parallel to the sylvian fissure.

supramarginal c. The anterior portion of the interior parietal lobule behind the inferior extremity of the intraparietal sulcus, below which it joins the ascending parietal convolution.

c. of the sylvian fissure The convolution that bounds the fissure of Sylvius.

transverse orbital c. The gyrus occupying the posterior portion of the inferior surface of the frontal lobe, at the anterior extremity of the fissure of Sylvius.

uncinate c. The convolution extending from near the posterior extremity of the occipital lobe to the apex of the temporosphenoidal lobe.

convulsant (kŏn-vŭl′sănt) [L. *convellere,* to pull together] **1.** An agent that produces a convulsion. **2.** Causing the onset of a convulsion.

convulsion (kŏn-vŭl′shŭn) Paroxysms of involuntary muscular contractions and relaxations.

NOTE: It is important for the person who observes the convulsion to record on the chart the following: time of onset, duration, whether the convulsion started in a certain area of the body or became generalized from the start, type of contractions, whether the patient became incontinent, and whether the convulsion caused the patient to be injured or strike the head. This information, in addition to its medicolegal importance, is valuable in diagnosis and in caring for the patient.

ETIOLOGY: Common causes are epilepsy, eclampsia, meningitis, heat cramps, brain lesions, tetanus, uremia, hypoxemia, hypotension, and many poisonings. In children, the cause is often fever.

TREATMENT: Febrile convulsions in children are usually controlled by suppressing fever with acetaminophen. In adults a specific diagnosis should be made. Diagnostic testing may include assessments of serum chemistries, oxygenation, alcohol levels, brain scanning, or lumbar puncture. The patient should be prevented from self-injury and from the aspiration of oral or gastrointestinal contents. If fever is present, antipyretic drugs may be helpful. Sedatives or anesthesia may be ordered by the physician. Aftercare includes rest in bed. SEE: *febrile convulsion.*

clonic c. A convulsion with intermittent contractions, the muscles being alternately contracted and relaxed.

febrile c. A tonic-clonic seizure occurring in children between ages 6 months and 5 years who have no other signs of CNS infection or CNS abnormalities. About 3% to 5% of kids will have this type of seizure, thought to be caused by a rapid rise in body temperature to 102.5°F or higher. Boys are more susceptible than girls. The seizure rarely lasts more than 10 minutes, and repeat seizures during the same febrile episode are uncommon. The risk for a seizure during the next febrile illness is 30%, and for the episode after that 17%. A complete history and physical examination should include neurological appraisal to rule out other causes, such as epilepsy; acute lead encephalopathy; cerebral concussion, hemorrhage, or tumor; hypoglycemia; or poisoning with a convulsant drug. SEE: *epilepsy.*

TREATMENT: Appropriate therapy, such as acetaminophen or ibuprofen, should be instituted to reduce the fever. Oral diazepam (Valium) may be administered while fever is present to prevent seizure recurrence, though in many children the seizure is the first indication of fever. The measures to reduce the temperature must not be so vigorous as to cause hypothermia. Ice water baths and vigorous fanning with application of alcohol should not be used. The application of cool compresses with a gentle flow of air over the body is sufficient. A hypothermia blanket is also suitable. The efficacy and advisability of daily anticonvulsant drug therapy for children with recurrent febrile seizures have not been proven.

CAUTION: 1. If the fever is due to influenza or varicella, salicylates should not be administered; their use could increase the risk for developing Reye's syndrome. 2. Prolonged treatment with phenobarbital depresses cognitive function in children and produces marked personality changes in about 15% of them.

---

hysterical c. An old term for a pseudoseizure.

mimetic c. A facial muscle spasm.

puerperal c. Spontaneous paroxysmal muscular contractions and relaxation in the postpartum woman.

salaam c. Nodding spasm.

tonic c. Convulsion in which the contractions are maintained for a time, as in tetany.

toxic c. Convulsion caused by the action of a toxin on the nervous system.

uremic c. Seizures caused by the toxic effects of accumulated waste products and inorganic acids in renal failure.

convulsive (kŏn-vŭl′sĭv) Pert. to convulsions.

cooking [L. *coquere,* to cook] The process of heating foods to prepare them for eating. Cooking makes most foods more palatable and easier to chew, improves their digestibility, and destroys or inactivates harmful organisms or toxins that may be present. Cooking releases the aromatic substances and extractives that contribute odors and taste to foods. These odors help to stimulate the appetite.

CAUTION: Not all toxic substances are inactivated by heat. Most microorganisms and parasites are destroyed in the ordinary process of cooking, but some require a higher degree of heat and longer cooking to effect this result. Pork must be cooked completely throughout to kill the encysted larvae of *Trichinella.*

ACTION: *Protein:* Soluble proteins become coagulated. *Soluble substances:* These, including heat-labile vitamins, are often inactivated by boiling, and even mineral substances and starches, although insoluble to a certain extent, may be altered in this process. *Starch:* The starch granules swell and are changed from insoluble (raw) starch to soluble starch capable of being converted into sugar during digestion and of being assimilated in the system.

Cooley's anemia [Thomas Cooley, U.S. pediatrician, 1871–1945] Thalassemia major.

Coombs' test [R. R. A. Coombs, Brit. immunologist, b. 1921] A laboratory test for the presence of antibodies, usually blood type antibodies, in serum. The patient's serum is incubated with red blood cells (RBCs) with known antigenic markers; if antibodies to the antigen are present in the serum, they bind with the RBCs. When antihuman globulin is added, RBC clumping (agglutination) occurs. The test is used for crossmatching blood before transfusions to ensure that no antigen-antibody reactions will occur and to test for the presence of specific antibodies to RBCs.

Cooper's ligaments [Sir Astley Paston Cooper, Eng. surgeon, 1768–1841] Supportive fibrous structures throughout the breast that partially sheathe the lobes shaping the breast. These ligaments affect the image of the glandular tissue on a mammogram.

coordination (kō-or″dĭn-ā′shŭn) [L. *co-*, same, + *ordinare,* to arrange] **1.** The working together of various muscles to produce certain movements. The ability to produce coordinated movement is necessary to execute fine motor skills, manipulate objects, and perform gross motor tasks. Coordinated movement requires sequencing of muscle activity and stability of proximal musculature. **2.** The working together of different body systems in a given process, as the conjoint action of glandular secretion and involuntary muscles in digestion.

copayment (kō′pā-mĕnt) The fee insured persons must pay, in addition to their health insurance premiums and deductibles, for specific medical services such as emergency department visits, appointments with primary care providers, laboratory studies, prescriptions, or x-ray examination.

COPD *chronic obstructive pulmonary disease.*

cope (kōp) [ME. *caupen,* to contend with] **1.** To deal effectively with and handle stresses. **2.** The upper half of a flask used in casting. **3.** In dentistry, the cavity side of a denture flask.

coping Adapting to and managing change, stress, or opportunity, such as those associated with acute or chronic illness, disability, pain, death, relocation, work, changes in family structure, new relationships, or new ideas—that is, the unexpected.

defensive c. The state in which an individual repeatedly projects falsely positive self-evaluation based on a self-protective pattern which defends against underlying perceived threats to positive self-regard. SEE: *Nursing Diagnoses Appendix.*

ineffective individual c. Inadequate adaptive behaviors and abilities of a person in meeting life's demands and roles. SEE: *Nursing Diagnoses Appendix.*

c. mechanism A conscious or physical effort to manage anxiety or a stressful situation.

c. skills The characteristics or behavior patterns of a person that enhance adaptation. Coping skills include a stable value or religious belief system, problem solving, social skills, health-energy, and commitment to a social network.

copolymer (kō-pŏl′ĭ-mĕr) A polymer composed of two kinds of monomers.

copper [L. *cuprum*] SYMB: Cu. A metal, small quantities of which are used by the body, with atomic weight 63.54, atomic number 29, and specific gravity 8.96. Its salts are irritant poisons. Symptoms of deficiency include anemia, weakness, impaired respiration and growth, and poor use of iron. SEE: *Wilson's disease; Poisons and Poisoning Appendix.*

FUNCTION: The total body content of copper is 100 to 150 mg; the amount normally ingested each day is less than 2 mg. It is found in many vegetable and animal tissues. Copper is an essential component of several enzymes, including those for hemoglobin synthesis and cell respiration. It is stored in the liver, and excess is excreted in bile or by the kidneys.

copperas (kŏp′ĕr-ăs) An impure form of ferrous sulfate that is used as a disinfectant and deodorizer. SEE: *ferrous sulfate.*

copperhead A poisonous snake, *Agkistrodon contortrix,* common in the southern, eastern, and central U.S. SEE: *snake bite.*

copper sulfate $CuSO_4 \cdot 5H_2O$; deep-blue shiny crystals or granular powder. It is used as an astringent in proper dilution and also as an algicide.

copper sulfate poisoning The systemic response to ingestion of toxic amounts of copper sulfate, a pesticide. Large ingestions may cause liver failure, acute renal failure, and shock.

TREATMENT: Penicillamine or dimercaprol should be given. The caregiver should monitor vital signs, treat shock, administer oxygen if needed, control convulsions, and maintain electrolyte balance. SEE: *Poisons and Poisoning Appendix.*

copremesis (kŏp-rĕm′ĕ-sĭs) [Gr. *kopros,* dung, + *emesis,* vomiting] The vomiting of fecal material.

coproantibody (kŏp″rō-ăn′tĭ-bŏd″ē) Any one of a group of antibodies to various bacteria in the feces. They are of the IgA type. Their ability to protect the host has not been shown.

coprolagnia (kŏp″rō-lăg′nē-ă) [″ + *lagneia,* lust] An erotic satisfaction at the sight or odor of excreta.

coprolalia (kŏp″rō-lā′lē-ă) [″ + *lalia,* babble] The use of vulgar, obscene, or sacrilegious language, seen in schizophrenia and Tourette's syndrome.

coprolith (kŏp′rō-lĭth) [″ + *lithos,* stone] Hard, inspissated feces.

coprology (kŏp-rŏl′ō-jē) [″ + *logos,* word, reason] Scientific study of the feces. SYN: *scatology* (1).

coprophagy (kŏp-rŏf′ă-jē) [″ + *phagein,* to eat] The eating of excrement. SYN: *scatophagy.*

coprophilia (kŏp″rŏ-fĭl′ē-ă) [″ + *philein,* to love] Abnormal interest in feces; a perversion in adults.

coprophilic A term applied to organisms that normally live in fecal material.

coprophobia (kŏp″rŏ-fō′bē-ă) [″ + *phobos,* fear] Abnormal fear of defecation and feces.

coproporphyria (kŏp″rō-por-fĭr′ē-ă) [″ + *porphyra,* purple] An inherited form of porphyria in which an excess amount of coproporphyrin is excreted in the feces.

coproporphyrin (kŏp″rō-por′fĭr-ĭn) A porphyrin present in urine and feces. Coproporphyrins I and II are normally present in minute and equal amounts, but quantities are altered in certain diseases such as poliomyelitis and in infectious hepatitis and lead poisoning.

coproporphyrinuria (kŏp″rō-por″fĭr-ĭn-ū′rē-ă) Excess coproporphyrin in the urine.

coprozoa (kŏp″rō-zō′ă) [″ + *zoon,* animal] Protozoa in the fecal matter outside of the intestine.

copula (kŏp′ū-lă) [L., link] **1.** Any connecting part. **2.** A median elevation on the floor of the embryonic pharynx that is the future root of the tongue; copula linguae.

copulation (kŏp″ū-lā′shŭn) [L. *copulatio*] The act of uniting in sexual intercourse. SYN: *coition; coitus*.

cor (kor) [L.] Heart.

coracoacromial (kor″ă-kō-ă-krō′mē-ăl) [Gr. *korax,* raven, + *akron,* point, + *omos,* shoulder] Pert. to the acromial and coracoid processes.

coracoid (kor′ă-koyd) [″ + *eidos,* form, shape] Shaped like a crow's beak.

cord [Gr. *khorde*] **1.** A stringlike structure. **2.** The umbilical cord. **3.** A firm elongated structure consistent with a thrombosed vein, esp. in the extremities, where it may be felt on palpation.

nuchal c. The condition in which the umbilical cord is found wrapped around the neck of the fetus during delivery. If the cord cannot be unwrapped easily, or if there is more than one loop, the cord should be clamped and cut before delivery continues.

spermatic c. The cord by which the testis is connected to the abdominal inguinal ring. It surrounds the ductus deferens, blood vessels, lymphatics, and nerves supplying the testis and epididymis. These are enclosed in the cremasteric fascia, which forms an investing sheath.

spinal c. The portion of the central nervous system contained in the spinal canal. The center of the cord is gray matter in the shape of the letter H; it consists of the cell bodies and dendrites of motor neurons and interneurons. The white matter is arranged in tracts outside the gray matter. It consists of myelinated axons that transmit impulses to and from the brain, or between levels of the gray matter of the spinal cord, or that will leave the cord and become peripheral nerves. The cord is the pathway for sensory impulses to the brain and motor impulses from the brain. It also serves as a reflex center for many reflex acts.

umbilical c. The cord that connects the circulatory system of the fetus to the placenta.

vocal c. One of two thin, reedlike folds of tissue within the larynx that vibrate with the passage of air between them, producing sounds that are the basis of speech. SEE: illus.

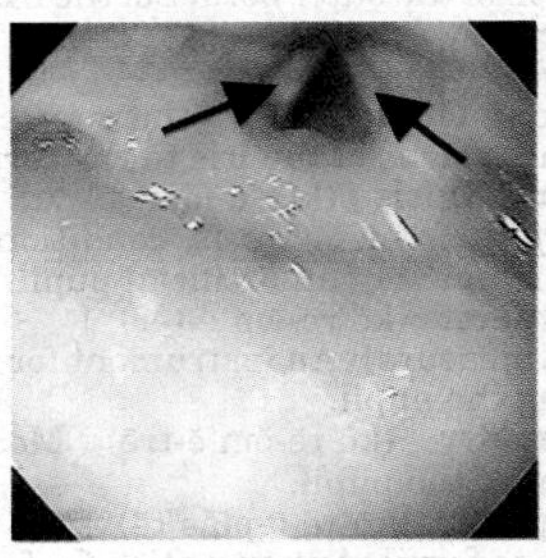

VOCAL CORDS

cordal (kor′dăl) Pert. to a cord (e.g., a spinal or vocal cord).

cordate (kor′dāt) [L. *cor,* heart] Shaped like a heart.

cord bladder Distention of the bladder without discomfort. Symptoms include a tendency to void frequently and dribbling after urination. The condition is caused by a lesion affecting the posterior roots of the spinal column at the level of bladder innervation above the sacrum.

cordectomy (kor-dĕk′tō-mē) [Gr. *khorde,* cord, + *ektome,* excision] Surgical removal of a cord.

cordiform (kor′dĭ-form) [L. *cor,* heart, + *forma,* shape] Shaped like a heart.

corditis (kor-dī′tĭs) Funiculitis.

cordocentesis Withdrawal of a sample of fetal blood from the umbilical cord with a needle inserted into the abdomen. Ultrasonic guidance is used to select a puncture site near the insertion of the placenta.

cordopexy (kor′dō-pĕk″sē) [″ + *pexis,* fixation] Surgical fixation of anatomical cords, esp. the vocal cords.

cordotomy (kor-dŏt′ō-mē) [″ + *tome,* incision] Spinal cord section of lateral pathways to relieve pain.

core (kor) The center of a structure.

coreceptor (kō-rē-sĕp′tŏr) A structure on a cell membrane that enhances the action of the cell receptor.

CXCR4 c. A cell surface receptor found on T cells that facilitates entry of HIV-1 to these cells.

coreclisis (kor″ē-klī′sĭs) [Gr. *kore,* pupil of the eye, + *kleisis,* closure] Occlusion of the pupil.

corectasia, corectasis (kor-ĕk-tā′zē-ă, -ĕk′tă-sĭs) [″ + *ektasis,* dilatation]

Dilatation of the pupil of the eye resulting from disease.

corectome (kō-rĕk′tōm) Iridectome.

corectomy (kō-rĕk′tō-mē) Iridectomy.

corectopia (kor-ĕk-tō′pē-ă) [″ + *ek,* out of, + *topos,* place] A condition in which the pupil is to one side of the center of the iris.

coredialysis (kō″rē-dī-ăl′ĭ-sĭs) [″ + *dia,* through, + *lysis,* dissolution] Separation of the outer border of the iris from its ciliary attachment.

corelysis (kor-ĕl′ĭ-sĭs) [″ + *lysis,* dissolution] Obliteration of the pupil caused by adhesions of the iris to the cornea.

coremorphosis (kor″ē-mor-fō′sĭs) [″ + *morphe,* form, + *osis,* condition] Establishment of an artificial pupil.

coreometer (kō″rē-ŏm′ĕ-tĕr) [″ + *metron,* measure] An instrument for measuring the pupil.

coreometry (kō″rē-ŏm′ĕ-trē) Measurement of the pupil.

coreoplasty (kō′rē-ō-plăs″tē) [″ + *plassein,* to form] Any operation for forming an artificial pupil.

corepressor (kō″rē-prĕs′sor) The substance capable of activating the repressor produced by a regulator gene.

corestenoma (kor″ē-stĕn-ō′mă) [″ + *stenoma,* contraction] Narrowing of the pupil.

c. congenitum Partial congenital obliteration of the pupil by outgrowths from the iris that form a partial gridlike covering over the pupil.

coretomedialysis (kor″ĕt-ō-mē-dē-ăl′ĭ-sĭs) [″ + *tome,* incision, + *dialysis, dia,* through, + *lysis,* dissolution] Making of an artificial pupil through the iris.

coretomy (kō-rĕt′ō-mē) Iridotomy.

CORF Comprehensive outpatient rehabilitation facility.

Cori cycle (kō′rē) [Carl Ferdinand Cori, Czech.-born U.S. physician and biochemist, 1896–1984; Gerty T. Cori, Czech.-born U.S. biochemist, 1896–1957] The cycle in carbohydrate metabolism in which muscle glycogen breaks down, forms lactic acid, which enters the bloodstream, and is converted to liver glycogen. Liver glycogen then breaks down into glucose, which is carried to muscles, where it is reconverted to muscle glycogen.

corium (kō′rē-ŭm) *pl.* **coria** [L., skin] Dermis. SYN: *cutis vera.* SEE: *skin* for illus.

corm (korm) [Gr. *kormos,* a trimmed tree trunk] A short, bulb-shaped underground stem of a plant such as the autumn crocus, a source of colchicine.

corn [L. *cornu,* horn] A horny induration and thickening of the skin that may be hard or soft according to location. Pressure, friction, or both cause this condition. SYN: *clavus; heloma.*

SYMPTOMS: Hard corns on exposed surfaces have a horny, conical core extending down into the derma, causing pain and irritation. Soft corns that occur between the toes are kept soft by moisture and maceration. This may lead to inflammation or infection beneath the corn. Infection with pyogenic organisms results in suppuration.

TREATMENT: Properly fitting shoes of soft leather and proper shape should be worn. Spongelike materials that absorb energy and thus prevent friction are available for lining shoes or bandaging the area of the foot being abraded. Local application of a keratolytic agent is effective for removal of the corn. Corn pads are used to relieve pressure. A podiatrist may remove corns with a scalpel. Patients with diabetes or a circulatory condition who have corns need special care to prevent foot infections.

cornea (kor′nē-ă) [L. *corneus,* horny] The transparent anterior portion of the sclera (the fibrous outer layer of the eyeball), about one sixth of its surface. Beyond the edge of the cornea is the sclera, or "white" of the eye. The curvature of the cornea is greater than that of the remainder of the sclera; the cornea is the first part of the eye that refracts light. It is composed of five layers: an epithelial layer, Bowman's membrane (anterior limiting membrane), the substantia propria corneae, vitreous membrane, and a layer of endothelium. **corneal** (-ăl), *adj.*

corneal impression test In diagnosing rabies, the immunofluorescent staining of material obtained from the corneas of patients suspected of having the disease. The rabies virus may be seen in the stained material.

corneal transplant The implantation of a cornea from a healthy donor eye. This is the most common organ transplantation procedure in the U.S. There are two major types of procedures. Lamellar keratoplasty, or split-thickness technique, involves removing a portion of the anterior host cornea and attaching a partial thickness of the donor cornea. Penetrating keratoplasty, or full-thickness transplantation, involves complete removal of the patient's cornea and replacement with the donor cornea.

Transmission of donor disease to the recipient is rare, but rabies, Creutzfeldt-Jakob disease, and hepatitis B have been acquired by graft recipients. The technique is more likely to be successful when histocompatibility matching of donor and recipient is as close as possible. The success rate is more than 90% at 1 year. SEE: *keratoplasty.*

PATIENT CARE: *Preoperative:* The surgical transplant procedure is explained, including duration (1 hr), the need to remain still throughout the procedure, and expected sensations. A preoperative sedative is given.

Postoperative: Evidence of any sudden, sharp, or excessive pain; bloody, purulent, or clear viscous drainage; or fever is reported immediately. Prescribed corticosteroid eye drops or topical antibiotics are administered to prevent inflammation and graft rejection, and prescribed analgesics are provided as necessary. A calm, restful environment is provided, and the patient is instructed to lie on the back or on the unaffected side, with the head of the bed flat or slightly elevated according to protocol. Rapid head movements, hard coughing or sneezing, or any other activities that could increase intraocular pressure should be avoided, and the patient should not squint or rub the eyes. Assistance is provided with standing or walking until the patient adjusts to vision changes, and personal items should be within the patient's field of vision.

Both patient and family are taught to recognize signs of graft rejection such as inflammation, cloudiness, drainage, and pain at the graft site and to report such signs immediately. Graft rejection may occur years after surgery; consequently, the graft must be assessed daily for the rest of the patient's life. The patient is encouraged to verbalize feelings of anxiety and concerns about graft rejection, and is helped to develop effective coping behaviors to deal with these feelings and concerns. Photophobia is a common adverse reaction, but it will gradually decrease as healing progresses; patients are advised to wear dark glasses in bright light. The patient is taught how to correctly instill prescribed eye drops and should wear an eye shield when sleeping.

corneitis (kor″nē-ī′tĭs) [L. *corneus,* horny, + Gr. *itis,* inflammation] Keratitis.

Cornelia de Lange's syndrome De Lange's syndrome.

Cornell Medical Index A lengthy, all-inclusive, self-administered medical and health history form developed at Cornell University Medical School.

corneoblepharon (kor″nē-ō-blĕf′ă-rŏn) [″ + Gr. *blepharon,* eyelid] Adhesion of the eyelid to the cornea.

corneomandibular reflex (kor″nē-ō-măn-dĭb′ū-lăr) Deflexion of the mandible toward the opposite side when the cornea is irritated while the mouth is open and relaxed.

corneosclera (kor″nē-ō-sklē′ră) [L. *corneus,* horny, + *skleros,* hard] The cornea and sclera, constituting the tunica fibrosa or fibrous coat of the eye.

corneous (kor′nē-ŭs) [L. *corneus*] Horny; hornlike.

corneum (kor′nē-ŭm) [L., horny] Stratum corneum.

corniculate (kor-nĭk′ū-lāt) Containing small horn-shaped projections.

corniculum (kor-nĭk′ū-lŭm) [L., little horn] A small hornlike process.

cornification (kor″nĭ-fĭ-kā′shŭn) Keratinization.

cornified (kor′nĭ-fīd) Changed into horny tissue.

cornu (kor′nū) *pl.* **cornua** [L., horn] Any projection like a horn. **cornual** (-ăl), *adj.*

c. ammonis The hippocampus major of the brain.

c. anterius The anterior horn of the lateral ventricle.

c. coccygeum One of the two upward-projecting processes that articulate with the sacrum.

c. cutaneum A hornlike excrescence on the skin.

c. of the hyoid The greater or the lesser horn of the hyoid bone.

c. inferius The inferior horn of the lateral ventricle of the brain.

c. posterius The posterior horn of the lateral ventricle.

c. of the sacrum The two small processes projecting inferiorly on either side of the sacral hiatus leading into the sacral canal.

c. of the uterus The entry point of the fallopian tube into the uterine cavity.

corona (kŏ-rō′nă) [Gr. *korone,* crown] Any structure resembling a crown. **coronal** (-năl), *adj.*

c. capitis The crown of the head.

c. ciliaris The circular figure on the inner surface of the ciliary body.

c. dentis The crown of a tooth.

c. glandis The posterior border of the glans penis.

c. radiata **1.** The ascending and descending fibers of the internal capsule of the brain that extend in all directions to the cerebral cortex above the corpus callosum. Many of the fibers arise in the thalamus. **2.** A thin mass of follicle cells that adhere firmly to the zona pellucida of the human ovum after ovulation.

c. veneris Syphilitic blotches on the forehead that parallel the hairline.

coronary (kor′ō-nă-rē) [L. *coronarius,* pert. to a crown or circle] Encircling, as the blood vessels that supply blood directly to the heart muscle; loosely used to refer to the heart and to coronary artery disease. *Coronary pain* is usually dull and heavy and may radiate to the arm, jaw, shoulders, or back. Typically, the patient describes the pain as being viselike or producing a feeling of compression or squeezing of the chest.

café c. Chest pain, cyanosis, and collapse (or sudden death) during a meal, caused by aspiration of a bolus of food into the trachea. The Heimlich maneuver may be used to clear the obstructed airway.

coronary artery **1.** One of a pair of arteries that supply blood to the myocardium of the heart. They arise within the

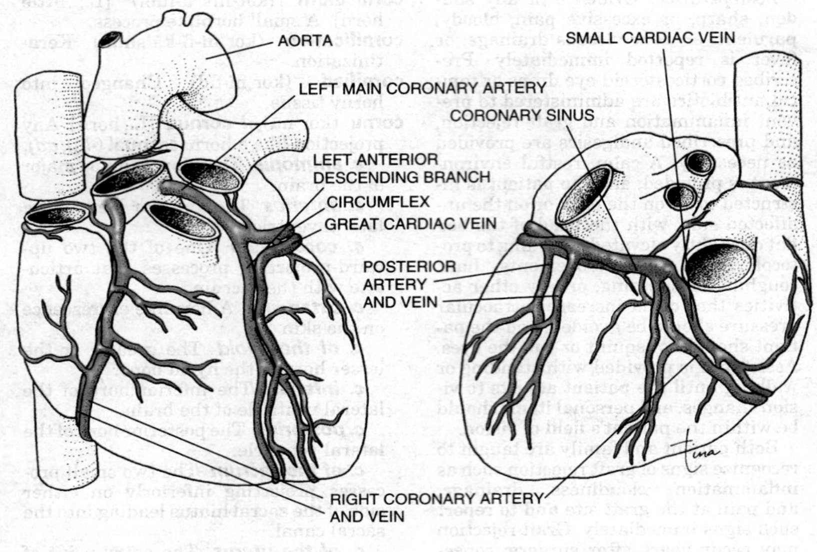

CORONARY ARTERIES

(A) anterior, (B) posterior

right and left aortic sinuses at the base of the aorta. Decreased flow of blood through these arteries induces attacks of angina pectoris. SEE: illus. **2.** The cervical branch of the uterine artery.

coronary artery bypass surgery Surgical establishment of a shunt that permits blood to travel from the aorta or internal mammary artery to a branch of the coronary artery at a point past an obstruction. It is used in treating coronary artery disease.

PATIENT CARE: *Preoperative:* The surgical procedure and the equipment and procedures used in the postanesthesia and intensive care units are explained. If possible, a tour of the facilities is arranged for the patient. The nurse assists with insertion of arterial and central lines and initiates cardiac monitoring when the patient enters the operating room.

Postoperative: Initially after surgery, the patient will have an endotracheal tube; will be mechanically ventilated and connected to a cardiac monitor; and will have a nasogastric tube, a chest tube and drainage system, an indwelling urinary catheter, arterial and venous lines, epicardial pacing wires, and a pulmonary artery catheter.

Signs of hemodynamic compromise, such as severe hypotension, decreased cardiac output, and shock, are monitored, and vital signs are obtained and documented according to protocol until the patient's condition stabilizes. Disturbances in heart rate or rhythm are monitored, and any abnormalities are documented and reported. Preparations are made to initiate or assist with epicardial pacing, cardioversion, or defibrillation as necessary. Pulmonary artery, central venous, and left arterial pressures are monitored, and arterial pressure is maintained within prescribed guidelines (usually between 110 and 70 mm Hg). Peripheral pulses, capillary refill time, and skin temperature and color are assessed frequently, and the chest is auscultated for changes in heart sounds or pulmonary congestion. Any abnormalities are documented and reported to the surgeon. Tissue oxygenation is monitored by assessing breath sounds, chest excursion, symmetry of chest expansion, pulse oximeter, and arterial blood gas (ABG) values. Ventilator settings are adjusted as needed. Fluid intake and output and electrolyte levels are assessed for imbalances. Chest tube drainage is maintained at the prescribed negative pressure (usually −10 to −40 cm H_2O), and chest tubes are inspected for patency. The patient is assessed for hemorrhage, excessive drainage (200 ml/hr), and sudden decrease or cessation of drainage. Prescribed analgesics and other medications are administered.

Throughout the recovery period, the patient is evaluated for indications of cerebrovascular accident, pulmonary embolism, and impaired renal perfusion. After the patient is weaned from the ventilator and extubated, chest physiotherapy and incentive spirometry are instituted, and the patient is encouraged to breathe deeply and cough and assisted to change position frequently. Assistance is also provided with range-of-motion exercises and with active leg movement and gluteal and quadriceps setting exercises.

Before discharge, the patient is instructed to report any signs of infection (i.e., fever; sore throat; redness, swelling, or drainage from the leg or chest incisions) or cardiac complications (i.e., angina, dizziness, rapid or irregular pulse, or increasing fatigue or prolonged recovery time following activity or exercise). Postcardiotomy syndrome, characterized by fever, muscle and joint pain, weakness, or chest discomfort, often develops after open heart surgery. Postoperative depression may also develop weeks after discharge; both patient and family are reassured that this is normal and usually passes quickly. The patient is advised to observe any tobacco, sodium, cholesterol, fat, and calorie restrictions, which may help reduce the risk of recurrent arterial occlusion. The patient needs to maintain a balance between activity and rest and should schedule a short afternoon rest period and plan to get 8 hours' sleep nightly. Frequent rest should also follow any tiring activity. Participation in the prescribed cardiac rehabilitative exercise program is recommended, and any activity restrictions (avoiding lifting heavy objects, driving a car, or doing strenuous work until specific permission is granted) are reinforced. Appropriate reassurance is offered that the patient can climb stairs, engage in sexual activity, take baths or shower, and do light chores. The patient is referred to local information and support groups or organizations, such as the American Heart Association. SEE: *Nursing Diagnoses Appendix.*

coronary artery disease ABBR: CAD. Narrowing of the coronary arteries, usually as a result of atherosclerosis. It is the single most common cause of death in industrialized nations. SEE: illus.; *angina pectoris; cholesterol; ischemic heart disease; lipoprotein; percutaneous transluminal coronary angioplasty; coronary thrombosis.*

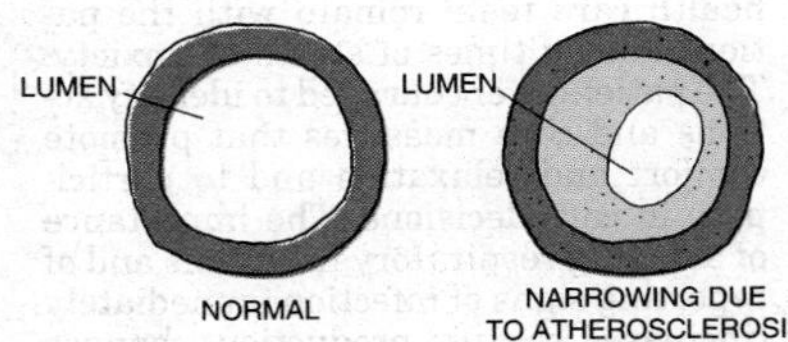

NORMAL AND DISEASED CORONARY ARTERIES

Stenoses within the coronary circulation most commonly occur in people who smoke or who have diabetes mellitus, hypertension, adverse lipid profiles, or a familial predisposition to coronary heart disease. CAD tends to worsen as people age and is more common in men than in women. If blockages within the coronary arteries limit the flow of oxygenated blood to the myocardium, ischemia or infarction of the heart muscle may occur.

SYMPTOMS: Typically, patients who experience symptoms due to CAD report pain, burning, or pressure in the chest (angina pectoris) that begins or worsens with exertion, emotion, exposure to cold air, or the eating of a large meal. The pain may be described as a suffocating feeling or may be experienced as shortness of breath. It is often located beneath the sternum and can radiate to the upper chest, neck, jaw, shoulders, back, or arms. It may cause bloating, nausea, vomiting, or perspiration. However, many patients may not recognize the symptoms of coronary artery disease, a condition called "silent ischemia," or they may attribute their symptoms to another cause (e.g., indigestion).

TREATMENT: A low-fat, low-cholesterol diet, a regular program of sustained exercise, and smoking cessation all help patients to limit CAD. Medications to control hypertension, lipids, and ischemia (such as beta blockers, statins, and nitrates) also alleviate symptoms. Invasive approaches to reopen narrowed arteries are helpful in some patients. These include coronary angioplasty, stent placement, atherectomy, and coronary artery bypass surgery.

coronary artery scan ABBR: CAS. A noninvasive diagnostic computed tomography scan that may identify patients at risk for atherosclerosis and coronary disease episodes by measuring calcium in the coronary arteries.

coronary artery spasm Intermittent constriction of the large coronary arteries. This may lead to angina pectoris in various conditions and is not necessarily associated with exertion. SEE: *Prinzmetal's angina.*

coronary atherectomy A technique of removing obstructions from the coronary artery with a cutting instrument inserted through a cardiac catheter.

coronary blood flow The amount of blood flowing to the coronary arteries. This may be measured by one of several techniques including indicator dilution or use of radioisotopes.

coronary care unit A specially equipped

area of a hospital providing intensive nursing and medical care for patients who have acute coronary thrombosis.

coronary plexus A network of autonomic nerve fibers that lies close to the base of the heart.

coronary sinus The vessel or passage that receives the cardiac veins from the heart. It opens into the right atrium. SEE: *coronary artery* for illus.

coronavirus (kor″ō-nă-vī′rŭs-ĕs) [L. *corona,* crown, + *virus,* poison] One of a group of viruses, morphologically similar, ether sensitive, and containing RNA, that are responsible for some common colds. They are so named because their microscopic appearance is that of a virus particle surrounded by a crown.

coroner (kor′ŏ-nĕr) [L. *corona,* crown] An official (originally, English crown officer) who investigates and holds inquests concerning people dead from unknown or violent causes. The coroner may or may not be a physician, depending on the law in each state.

coronoid (kor′ō-noyd) [Gr. *korone,* something curved, kind of crown, + *eidos,* form, shape] Shaped like a crown.

coronoidectomy (kor″ō-noy-dĕk′tō-mē) [″ + ″ + *ektome,* excision] Excision of the coronoid process of the mandible.

coroparelcysis (kor″ō-păr-ĕl′sĭ-sĭs) [Gr. *kore,* pupil, + *parelkein,* to draw aside] Surgical moving of the pupil to one side so that it no longer lies under a scar but under a transparent area.

coroscopy (kō-rŏs′kō-pē) [″ + *skopein,* to examine] Shadow test to determine refractive error of an eye. SYN: *retinoscopy; skiascopy.*

corotomy (kō-rŏt′ō-mē) Iridotomy.

corpora (kor′pō-ră) Pl. of corpus.

c. arantii Tubercles found in the center of the semilunar valves of the heart.

c. arenacea Psammoma bodies found in the pineal body. SYN: *brain sand.*

c. olivaria Two oval masses behind the pyramids of the medulla oblongata.

c. para-aortica Aortic bodies.

c. quadrigemina The superior portion of the midbrain consisting of two pairs of rounded bodies, the superior and inferior colliculi.

corporeal (kor-pō′rē-ăl) Having a physical body.

corpse (korps) [L. *corpus,* body] The dead human body.

corpsman (kor′măn) An enlisted person in the U.S. Armed Forces who works as a member of the medical team. During duty in the armed forces he or she receives training and experience in one or more health-related fields. In wartime, a corpsman may be assigned as the only medically trained person to a field unit or a small ship. SYN: *medic; medical corpsman.*

corpulence (kor′pū-lĕns) [L. *corpulentia*] Obesity. **corpulent** (-lĕnt), *adj.*

cor pulmonale Hypertrophy or failure of the right ventricle resulting from disorders of the lungs, pulmonary vessels, or chest wall. Living for an extended period at a high altitude also may cause this condition.

SYMPTOMS: Symptoms include chronic productive cough, exertional dyspnea, wheezing, fatigue, weakness, drowsiness, and alterations in level of consciousness. On physical examination, dependent edema is present, and the neck veins are distended. The pulse is weak. A gallop rhythm, tricuspid insufficiency, or a right ventricular heave may be present. Sometimes an early right ventricular murmur or a systolic pulmonary ejection sound may be heard. The liver is enlarged and tender, and hepatojugular reflux is present.

PATIENT CARE: Serum potassium levels are monitored closely if diuretics are prescribed, signs of digitalis toxicity (anorexia, nausea, vomiting) are noted, and cardiac arrhythmias are monitored. Periodically, arterial blood gas levels are measured, and signs of respiratory failure are noted. Prescribed medications are administered and evaluated for desired effects, such as improvements in oxygenation, ventilation, or edema, and any adverse reactions, such as cardiac decompensation. A nutritious diet (limiting carbohydrates if the patient is a carbon dioxide retainer) is provided in frequent small meals to limit fatigue. Fluid retention is prevented by limiting the patient's intake as prescribed (usually 1 to 2 L daily) and by providing a low-sodium diet. The rationale for fluid restriction is explained, because those patients with chronic obstructive pulmonary disease would previously have been encouraged to increase fluid intake to help loosen and thin secretions. Frequent position changes are encouraged and meticulous respiratory care is provided, including prescribed oxygen therapy and breathing exercises or chest physiotherapy. Assistance is provided to help the patient rinse the mouth after respiratory therapies.

Care activities are paced and rest periods provided. The patient is encouraged to verbalize fears and concerns about the illness, and members of the health care team remain with the patient during times of stress or anxiety. The patient is encouraged to identify actions and care measures that promote comfort and relaxation and to participate in care decisions. The importance of avoiding respiratory infections and of reporting signs of infection immediately (increased sputum production, changes in sputum color, increased coughing or wheezing, fever, chest pain, and tightness in the chest) is stressed. Immunizations against influenza and pneumococcal pneumonia are recommended. Use of over-the-counter medications should be avoided unless the health care provider is consulted first. If the patient needs supplemental oxygen or suctioning at home, referral is made to a social service agency for assistance in obtaining the necessary equipment, and correct procedures are taught for equipment use. As appropriate, the patient is referred to smoking cessation programs, nicotine patch therapy, and local support groups.

corpus (kor′pŭs) *pl.* **corpora** [L., body] The principal part of any organ; any mass or body.

c. albicans A mass of fibrous tissue that replaces the regressing corpus luteum following rupture of the graafian follicle. It forms a white scar that gradually decreases and eventually disappears.

c. amygdaloideum Almond-shaped gray matter in the lateral wall and roof of the third ventricle of the brain.

c. amylaceum A mass having an irregular laminated structure like a starch grain; found in the prostate, meninges, lungs, and other organs in various pathologies. SYN: *colloid corpuscle*.

c. annulare Pons varolii.

c. callosum The great commissure of the brain that connects the cerebral hemispheres. SYN: *callosum*.

c. cavernosum Any erectile tissue, esp. the erectile bodies of the penis, clitoris, male or female urethra, bulb of the vestibule, or nasal conchae.

c. cavernosum penis One of the two columns of erectile tissue on the dorsum of the penis.

c. cerebellum One of the two lateral portions of the cerebellum exclusive of the central flocculonodular node.

c. ciliare Ciliary body.

c. dentatum The gray layer in the white matter of the cerebellum. SYN: *c. rhomboidale*.

c. fimbriatum The white matter edging the lower cornu of the lateral ventricle.

c. fornicis The body of the fornix.

c. geniculatum The medial or lateral geniculate body; a mass of gray matter lying in the thalamus.

c. hemorrhagicum A blood clot formed in the cavity left by rupture of the graafian follicle.

c. highmorianum Mediastinum testis.

c. interpedunculare The gray matter between the peduncles in front of the pons varolii.

c. luteum The small yellow endocrine structure that develops within a ruptured ovarian follicle and secretes progesterone and estrogen. SEE: *fertilization* for illus.

c. Luysii C. subthalamicum.

c. mammillare Mamillary body.

c. restiforme Restiform body.

c. rhomboidale C. dentatum.

c. spongiosum Erectile tissue surrounding the male urethra.

c. striatum A structure in the cerebral hemispheres consisting of two basal ganglia (the caudate and lentiform nuclei) and the fibers of the internal capsule that separate them.

c. subthalamicum The subthalamic nucleus, lying in the ventral thalamus. SYN: *c.Luysii*.

c. trapezoideum Trapezoid body.

c. uteri The main body of the uterus, located above the cervix.

c. vitreum The vitreous part of the eye.

c. wolffianum Wolffian body.

corpuscle (kor′pŭs-ĕl) [L. *corpusculum*, little body] **1.** Any small rounded body. **2.** An encapsulated sensory nerve ending. **3.** Old term for a blood cell. SEE: *erythrocyte; leukocyte*. **corpuscular** (kor-pŭs′kū-lăr), *adj.*

axis c. The center of a tactile corpuscle.

blood c. An erythrocyte or leukocyte.

bone c. Bone cell.

cancroid c. The characteristic nodule in cutaneous epithelioma.

cartilage c. A cell characteristic of cartilage.

chromophil c. Nissl body.

chyle c. A corpuscle seen in chyle.

colloid c. Corpus amylaceum.

colostrum c. A cell containing phagocytosed fat globules, present in milk secreted the first few days after parturition; also called *colostrum body*.

corneal c. A type of connective tissue cell found in the fibrous tissue of the cornea.

Drysdale's c. SEE: *Drysdale's corpuscle*.

genital c. An encapsulated sensory nerve ending resembling a pacinian corpuscle that is found in the skin of the external genitalia and nipple.

ghost c. Achromatocyte.

Gierke's c. Hassall's c.

Golgi-Mazzoni c. A tactile corpuscle in the skin of the fingertips.

Hassall's c. A corpuscle in the thymus gland. SYN: *Gierke's c.*

Krause's c. One of the sensory encapsulated nerve endings in the mucosa of the genitalia, mouth, nose, and eyes.

lymph c. Lymphocyte.

malpighian c. **1.** Renal c. **2.** A malpighian body of the spleen.

Mazzoni's c. A nerve ending resembling a Krause corpuscle.

Meissner's c. SEE: *Meissner's corpuscle*.

milk c. A fat-filled globule present in milk. It represents the distal end of a mammary gland cell broken off in apocrine secretion.

pacinian c. A large, ovoid, sensory end organ consisting of concentric layers or lamellae of connective tissue surrounding a nerve ending. Pacinian corpuscles are present in the dermis, tendons, intermuscular septa, connective tissue membranes, and sometimes internal organs, and function as proprioceptive and deep pressure receptors.

phantom c. Achromatocyte.

Purkinje's c. SEE: *Purkinje cell.*

red c. Erythrocyte.

renal c. A glomerulus and the capsule (Bowman's capsule) that surrounds it. It is located at the proximal end of a renal tubule. SYN: *malpighian c.* (1).

reticulated c. Reticulocyte.

splenic c. A nodule of lymphatic tissue in the spleen.

tactile c. A sensory end organ that responds to touch, as Meissner's corpuscle. Tactile corpuscles are located in the dermal papillae just beneath the epidermis and are most numerous on the fingertips, toes, soles, palms, lips, nipples, and tip of the tongue.

terminal c. A nerve ending.

white c. Leukocyte.

corpuscular (kor-pŭs'kū-lăr) Pert. to corpuscles.

correction The altering of a condition that is abnormal or malfunctioning.

corrective (kŏ-rĕk'tĭv) [L. *corrigere,* to correct] **1.** A drug that modifies the action of another. **2.** Pert. to such a drug.

correlation (kor"ĕ-lā'shŭn) [L. *com-,* together, + *relatio,* relation] **1.** In statistics, the degree to which one variable increases or decreases with respect to another variable. A variable can have a positive or negative correlation with another variable. The positive correlation exists when the coefficient of correlation is +1 or greater; the negative correlation exists when the coefficient is −1 or less; the correlation is considered to be nonexistent when the value is zero. **2.** The processes by which the various activities of the body, esp. nervous impulses, occur in relation to each other.

correspondence The act or condition of corresponding (i.e., occurring in proper relationship to other phenomena).

retinal c. A condition occurring in normal vision in which the images formed on the maculae or other points of both retinas are mentally blended and seen as a single image.

corresponding Agreeing with, matching, or fitting.

Corrigan's pulse (kor'ĭ-găns) [Sir Dominic J. Corrigan, Ir. physician, 1802–1880] Waterhammer pulse.

corroborating (kŏr-ŏb'ō-rā-tĭng) Confirming or supporting with evidence.

corrosion (kŏ-rō'zhŭn) [L *corrodere,* to corrode] The slow disintegration or wearing away of something by a destructive agent.

corrosive (kŏ-rō'sĭv) Producing corrosion.

corrugator (kor'ū-gā"tor) [L. *con,* together, + *rugare,* to wrinkle] A muscle that lies above the orbit, arises medially from the frontal bone, and has its insertion on the skin of the medial half of the eyebrows. It draws the brow medially and inferiorly.

cortex (kor'tĕks) *pl.* **cortices** [L., rind] **1.** The outer layer of an organ as distinguished from the inner medulla, as in the adrenal gland, kidney, ovary, lymph node, thymus, and cerebrum and cerebellum. **2.** The outer layer of a structure, as a hair or the lens of the eye. **3.** The outer superficial portion of the stem or root of a plant.

adrenal c. The outer layer of the adrenal gland, which secretes mineralocorticoids, androgens, and glucocorticoids.

cerebellar c. The surface layer of the cerebellum consisting of three layers: the outer or molecular, the middle, and the inner or granular. Purkinje's cells are present in the middle layer.

cerebral c. The thin, convoluted surface layer of gray matter of the cerebral hemispheres, consisting principally of cell bodies of neurons arranged in five layers. There are also numerous fibers.

interpretive c. The temporal cortex, where memories of the past may be evoked by electrical stimulation.

olfactory c. The portion of the cerebral cortex concerned with the sense of smell. It includes the pyriform lobe and the hippocampal formation.

renal c. SEE: *kidney.*

Corti, Alfonso Giacomo Gaspare (kor'tē) Italian anatomist, 1822–1876.

canal of C. A triangular-shaped canal extending the entire length of the organ of Corti. Its walls are formed by the external and internal pillar cells.

C.'s membrane A delicate gelatinous film that covers the cochlear duct of the inner ear. SEE: *organ of C.*

organ of C. An elongated spiral structure running the entire length of the cochlea in the floor of the cochlear duct and resting on the basilar membrane. It is the end organ of hearing and contains hair cells, supporting cells, and neuroepithelial receptors stimulated by sound waves. SYN: *organum spirale; spiral organ.* SEE: illus.; *C. membrane; Claudius' cell; ear.*

cortical (kor'tĭ-kăl) Pert. to a cortex.

corticate (kor'tĭ-kāt) Possessing a cortex or bark.

corticectomy (kor"tĭ-sĕk'tō-mē) [" + Gr. *ektome,* excision] Surgical removal of a portion of the cerebral cortex.

cortices (kor'tĭ-sēz) Pl. of cortex.

corticifugal (kor"tĭ-sĭf'ū-găl) [L. *cortex,* rind, + *fugere,* to flee] Conducting impulses away from the outer surface, or cortex; particularly denoting axons of

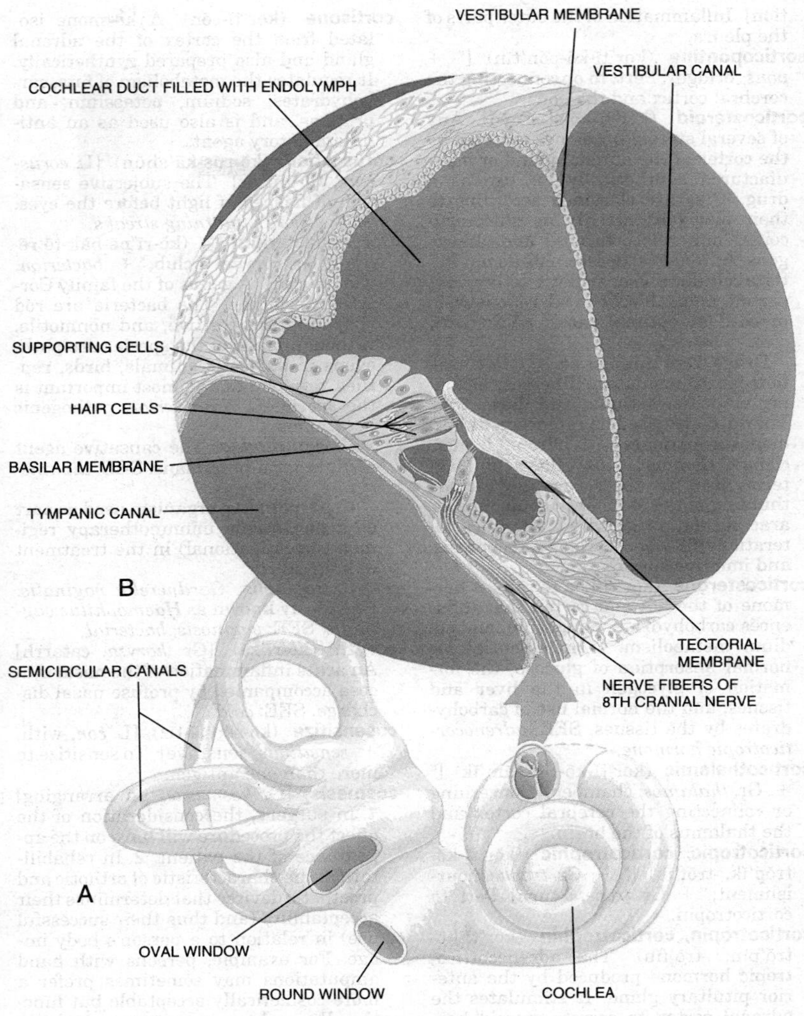

ORGAN OF CORTI

(A) inner ear structure, (B) organ of Corti within the cochlea

the pyramidal cells of the cerebral cortex. SYN: *corticoefferent*.

corticipetal (kor″tĭ-sĭp′ĕ-tăl) [″ + *petere,* to seek] Conducting impulses toward the outer surface, or cortex; particularly denoting thalamic radiation fibers conveying impulses to sensory areas of the cerebral cortex. SYN: *corticoafferent*.

corticoadrenal (kor″tĭ-kō-ăd-rē′năl) [″ + *ad,* toward, + *ren,* kidney] Pert. to the cortex of the adrenal gland.

corticoafferent (kor″tĭ-kō-ăf′fĕr-ĕnt) [″ + *adferre,* to bear to] Corticipetal.

corticobulbar (kor″tĭ-kō-bŭl′băr) [″ + *bulbus,* bulb] Pert. to the cerebral cortex and upper portion of the brainstem, as the corticobulbar tract.

corticoefferent (kor″tĭ-kō-ĕf′ĕr-ĕnt) [″ + *effere,* to bring out of] Corticifugal.

corticoid (kor′tĭ-koyd) [″ + Gr. *eidos,* form, shape] Corticosteroid.

corticopeduncular (kor″tĭ-kō-pē-dŭng′kū-lăr) [″ + *pedunculus,* little foot] Pert. to the cerebral cortex and cerebral peduncles.

corticopleuritis (kor″tĭ-kō-ploo-rī′tĭs) [″ + Gr. *pleura,* rib, + *itis,* inflammation] Inflammation of the outer parts of the pleura.

corticopontine (kor″tĭ-kō-pŏn′tīn) [″ + *pons*, bridge] Pert. to or connecting the cerebral cortex and the pons.

corticosteroid (kor″tĭ-kō-stēr′oyd) Any of several steroid hormones secreted by the cortex of the adrenal gland or manufactured synthetically for use as a drug. They are classified according to their biological activity as glucocorticoids, mineralocorticoids, and androgens. Adrenal corticosteroids do not initiate cellular and enzymatic activity but permit many biochemical reactions to proceed at optimal rates. SYN: *corticoid*.

Drugs from this class are widely used to treat inflammatory illnesses, including arthritis, asthma, and dermatitis. They are also used as replacement hormones in patients with adrenal insufficiency. Common side effects of long-term use of these agents include thinning of the skin, easy bruising, cataract formation, glucose intolerance, alterations in sleep cycles, osteoporosis, and immune suppression.

corticosterone (kor″tĭ-kŏs′tĕ-rōn) A hormone of the adrenal cortex that influences carbohydrate, potassium, and sodium metabolism. It is essential for normal absorption of glucose, the formation of glycogen in the liver and tissues, and the normal use of carbohydrates by the tissues. SEE: *adrenocorticotropic hormone*.

corticothalamic (kor″tĭ-kō-thă-lăm′ĭk) [″ + Gr. *thalamos*, chamber] Concerning or connecting the cerebral cortex and the thalamus of the brain.

corticotropic, corticotrophic (kor″tĭ-kō-trŏp′ĭk, -trŏf′ĭk) [″ + Gr. *trophe*, nourishment; ″ + Gr. *trope*, a turn] Pert. to corticotropin.

corticotropin, corticotrophin (kor″tĭ-kō-trō′pĭn, -trō′fĭn) The adrenocorticotropic hormone produced by the anterior pituitary gland. It stimulates the adrenal cortex to secrete steroid hormones. SYN: *adrenocorticotropic hormone*.

corticotropin production, ectopic The production of corticotropin by nonendocrine tissue. This is usually but not always associated with a cancer such as a small-cell cancer of the lung. In some cases, the production site may not be found. SEE: *dexamethasone suppression test*.

cortin (kor′tĭn) [L. *cortex*, rind] An extract of the cortex of the adrenal gland; contains a mixture of the active steroid agents such as corticosterone.

cortisol (kor′tĭ-sŏl) A glucocortical hormone of the adrenal cortex, usually referred to pharmaceutically as hydrocortisone. It is closely related to cortisone in its physiological effects.

cortisone (kor′tĭ-sōn) A hormone isolated from the cortex of the adrenal gland and also prepared synthetically. It regulates the metabolism of fats, carbohydrates, sodium, potassium, and proteins, and is also used as an anti-inflammatory agent.

coruscation (kŏ-rŭs-kā′shŭn) [L. *coruscare*, to glitter] The subjective sensation of flashes of light before the eyes. SEE: *Moore's lightning streaks*.

Corynebacterium (kō-rī″nē-băk-tē′rē-ŭm) [Gr. *coryne*, a club, + *bacterion*, a small rod] A genus of the family Corynebacteriaceae. The bacteria are rod shaped, gram positive, and nonmotile. Although many of the species are pathogens in domestic animals, birds, reptiles, and plants, the most important is the species *C. diphtheriae*, pathogenic in humans.

C. diphtheriae The causative agent of diphtheria in humans. SEE: *diphtheria*.

C. parvum An organism used as part of a nonspecific immunotherapy regimen (investigational) in the treatment of lung cancer.

C. vaginalis *Gardnerella vaginalis*. Previously known as *Haemophilus vaginalis*. SEE: *vaginosis, bacterial*.

coryza (kŏ-rī′ză) [Gr. *koryza*, catarrh] An acute inflammation of the nasal mucosa accompanied by profuse nasal discharge. SEE: *cold*.

cosensitize (kō-sĕn′sĭ-tīz) [L. *con*, with, + *sensitivus*, sensitive] To sensitize to more than one antigen.

cosmesis [G. *kosmesus*, an arranging] **1.** In surgery, the consideration of the effect the procedure will have on the appearance of the patient. **2.** In rehabilitation, the characteristic of orthotic and prosthetic devices that determines their acceptability (and thus their successful use) in relation to a person's body image. For example, persons with hand amputations may sometimes prefer a more cosmetically acceptable but functionally useless glove over a less appealing but highly functional artificial limb with a stainless steel terminal device.

cosmetic (kŏz-mĕt′ĭk) **1.** A preparation such as powder or cream for improving appearance. **2.** Serving to preserve or promote appearance.

costa (kŏs′tă) *pl.* **costae** [L.] Rib.

c. fluctuans Floating rib.

c. spuria False rib.

c. vera True rib.

costal (kŏs′tăl) Pert. to a rib.

costalgia (kŏs-tăl′jē-ă) [L. *costa*, rib, + Gr. *algos*, pain] Pain in a rib or the intercostal spaces (e.g., intercostal neuralgia).

cost awareness In the economics of medical care, knowledge and consideration of the comparative costs of preventive actions versus the treatment of avoidable illness and disability.

cost-effectiveness An assessment or determination of the most efficient and least expensive approaches to providing health care and preventive medicine services. One component, health education, focuses on helping people to assume some responsibility for their own health maintenance and avoid preventable illness and disability. Accident prevention programs, immunization drives, and "safe sex" campaigns are designed to reduce the number of patients who will suffer preventable illnesses. To control costs, health care providers also must understand the comparative value of procedures and medicines. SEE: *preventive medicine; preventive nursing.* **cost-effective,** *adj.*

costectomy (kŏs-tĕk′tō-mē) [″ + Gr. *ektome,* excision] Surgical excision or resection of a rib.

Costen's syndrome [James B. Costen, U.S. otolaryngologist, 1895–1961] Temporomandibular joint syndrome.

costocervical (kŏs″tō-sĕr′vĭ-kăl) Concerning the ribs and neck.

costochondral (kŏs″tō-kŏn′drăl) [L. *costa,* rib, + Gr. *chondros,* cartilage] Pert. to a rib and its cartilage.

costochondritis (kŏs″tō-kŏn drī′tĭs) [L. *costa,* rib, + Gr. *chondros,* cartilage, + Gr. *itis,* inflammation of] Inflammation of the costochondral joints of the chest, which can cause chest pain. The pain of costochondritis can sometimes be distinguished from other, more serious forms of chest pain by its reproducibility on palpation of the involved joints and the absence of abnormalities on chest x-ray examinations, electrocardiograms, and blood tests. SEE: *arthritis; costochondral.*

SYMPTOMS: Symptoms include pain and tenderness over the joints lateral to the sternum.

TREATMENT: Use of a nonsteroidal anti-inflammatory agent often helps reduce the discomfort, which normally resolves spontaneously over time.

costoclavicular (kŏs″tō-klă-vĭk′ū-lăr) [″ + *clavicula,* a little key] Pert. to the ribs and clavicle.

costocoracoid (kŏs″tō-kor′ă-koyd) [″ + Gr. *korax,* crow, + *eidos,* form, shape] Pert. to the ribs and coracoid process of the scapula.

costophrenic [″ + Gr. *phren,* diaphragm] Pert. to the ribs and diaphragm.

costopneumopexy (kŏs″tō-nū′mō-pĕk″sē) [″ + Gr. *pneumon,* lung, + *pexis,* fixation] Anchoring a lung to a rib.

costosternal (kŏs″tō-stĕr′năl) [″ + Gr. *sternon,* chest] Pert. to a rib and the sternum.

costosternoplasty (kŏs″tō-stĕr′nō-plăs″tē) [″ + ″ + *plassein,* to form] Surgical repair of funnel chest. A portion of a rib is used to support the sternum.

costotome (kŏs′tō-tōm) [″ + Gr. *tome,* incision] Knife or shears for cutting through a rib or cartilage.

costotomy (kŏs-tŏt′ō-mē) **1.** Incision or division of a rib or part of one. **2.** Excision of a rib. SYN: *costectomy.*

costotransverse (kŏs″tō-trăns-vĕrs′) [″ + *transvertere,* to turn across] Pert. to the ribs and transverse processes of articulating vertebrae.

costovertebral (kŏs″tō-vĕr′tĕ-brăl) [″ + *vertebra,* joint] Pert. to a rib and a vertebra.

costoxiphoid (kŏs″tō-zī′foyd) [″ + Gr. *xiphos,* sword, + *eidos,* form, shape] Concerning or connecting the ribs and the xiphoid process of the sternum.

cosyntropin (kō-sĭn-trō′pĭn) Synthetic adrenocorticotropic hormone (ACTH). It is used to test for adrenal insufficiency by giving the medication parenterally and checking plasma cortisol levels at timed intervals. If the levels fail to rise appropriately, adrenal insufficiency is present.

C.O.T.A. *certified occupational therapy assistant.*

cotinine The principal metabolite of nicotine; excreted in the urine. Its detection indicates that the individual has recently smoked cigarettes or inhaled second-hand smoke. SEE: *tobacco.*

cotton [ME. *cotoun,* from Arabic *qutn,* cotton] A soft, white, fibrous material obtained from the fibers enclosing the seeds of various plants of the Malvaceae, esp. those of the genus *Gossypium.*

purified c. Cotton fibers from which the oil has been completely removed. This enhances the ability to absorb liquids.

styptic c. Cotton impregnated with an astringent.

cotton-wool spot A tiny infarct in the retina, present in hypertension, diabetes mellitus, bacterial endocarditis, and other diseases.

co-twin (kō-twĭn) Either one of twins.

cotyledon (kŏt″ĭ-lē′dŏn) [Gr. *kotyledon,* hollow of a cup] **1.** A mass of villi on the chorionic surface of the placenta. **2.** Any of the rounded portions into which the placenta's uterine surface is divided. **3.** The seed leaf of a plant embryo.

cotyloid (kŏt′ĭ-loyd) [Gr. *kotyloeides,* cup-shaped] Shaped like a cup.

cough (kawf) [ME. *coughen*] A forceful and sometimes violent expiratory effort preceded by a preliminary inspiration. The glottis is partially closed, the accessory muscles of expiration are brought into action, and the air is noisily expelled.

There is no one course of therapy for a cough, as it may be due to a variety of conditions. Each disease is evaluated and treated accordingly. It is usually inadvisable to suppress completely coughs due to inflammation of the respiratory tract. This is particularly true if sputum is produced as a result of coughing. SEE: *expectoration*.

aneurysmal c. A cough that is brassy and clanging, sometimes heard in patients who have an aortic aneurysm.

brassy c. A cough heard in patients who have pressure on the left recurrent laryngeal nerve, as in aortic aneurysm or in those with laryngeal inflammation.

bronchial c. A cough heard in patients with bronchiectasis or bronchitis. It may be provoked by a change of posture, as when getting up in the morning, and produces frothy mucus that is copious, dirty gray, and has a fetid odor. The cough is hacking and irritating in the earlier stages; in later stages it is looser and easier.

diphtherial c. A cough heard in laryngeal diphtheria. It is noisy and brassy, and breathing is stridulous.

dry c. A cough unaccompanied by sputum production.

ear c. A reflex cough induced by irritation in the ear that stimulates Arnold's nerve (ramus auricularis nervi vagi).

hacking c. A series of repeated efforts, as in many respiratory infections.

harsh c. A metallic cough occurring in laryngitis.

moist c. A loose cough accompanied by production of mucus or exudate.

paroxysmal c. A cough occurring in whooping cough and bronchiectasis.

productive c. A cough in which mucus or an exudate is expectorated.

pulmonary c. A cough that is deep and pleuritic, seen in pneumonia. It may be hacking and irritating in the early stages of lung infection; in later stages, it is frequent, paroxysmal, and productive. SEE: *sputum*.

reflex c. A cough due to irritation from the middle ear, pharynx, stomach, or intestine. It may occur singly or coupled, or may be hacking. Stimulation of Arnold's nerve of the ear can cause this type of cough.

whooping c. **1.** Pertussis. **2.** The paroxysmal cough ending in a whooping inspiration that occurs in pertussis.

coulomb (koo′lŏm, -lōm) [Charles A. de Coulomb, Fr. physicist, 1736–1806] ABBR: C. A unit of electrical quantity; the quantity of electricity that flows across a surface when a steady current of 1 ampere flows for 1 sec.

coumarin anticoagulant One of a group of natural and synthetic compounds that inhibit blood clotting by antagonizing the biosynthesis of vitamin K–dependent coagulation factors in the liver. SEE: *dicumarol; warfarin sodium*.

counseling The providing of advice and guidance to a patient by a health professional.

count **1.** The number of units in a sample or object. **2.** To enumerate.

absolute neutrophil c. ABBR: ANC. The actual number of neutrophils in a cubic millimeter of blood. The approximate normal range is 3000 to 6000 cells/mm^3. This figure is measured before and after drugs are given that may lower neutrophil counts, such as those used in cancer chemotherapy. Generally, chemotherapy is not given unless the patient's ANC is greater than 1000. Patients with an ANC of less than 500 cells/mm^3 are at high risk for infection. SEE: *neutrophil*.

CAUTION: The development of fever in a patient with neutropenia secondary to chemotherapy is an indication for urgent medical evaluation and prompt institution of antibiotics with activity against gram-negative organisms.

---

absolute phagocyte c. ABBR: APC. The number of phagocytes (neutrophils and monocytes-macrophages) in a cubic millimeter of blood. The APC is the sum of the neutrophils ("segs" and "bands"), monocytes, and macrophages times one hundredth of the white blood cell count. This figure is used to measure bone marrow production of these cells before and after cancer chemotherapy. SEE: *absolute neutrophil c.; blood count*.

counter (kown′tĕr) A device for counting anything.

colony c. An apparatus for counting bacterial colonies in a culture plate.

Coulter c. An automated device that counts blood cells.

impedance c. A blood cell counter that uses cell membrane electrical impedance to determine the volume of cells in a solution.

particle c. An electronic device for counting and differentiating cells, platelets, and small particles according to their volume.

scintillation c. A device for detecting and counting radiation. Flashes of light are produced when radiation is detected.

counteract (kown″tĕr-ăkt′) To act against or in opposition to.

counteraction (kown″tĕr-ăk′shŭn) The action of a drug or chemical agent having an action opposing that of another agent.

countercurrent exchanger The exchange of chemicals between two streams of fluid flowing in opposite directions on either side of a permeable membrane. This permits the fluid leaving one side of the membrane to be similar to the composition of the fluid entering the other end of the other stream.

counterextension (kown″tĕr-ĕks-tĕn′shŭn) [L. *contra,* against, + *extendere,* to extend] Back pull or resistance to extension on a limb.

counterimmunoelectrophoresis (kown″tĕr-ĭm″ū-nō-ē-lĕk″trō-fō-rē′sĭs) [″ + *immunis,* safe, + Gr. *elektron,* amber, + *phoresis,* bearing] The process in which antigens and antibodies are placed in separate wells and an electric current is passed through the diffusion medium. Antigens migrate to the anode and antibodies to the cathode. If the antigen and antibody correspond to each other, they will precipitate and form a precipitin band or line upon meeting in the diffusion medium.

counterincision (kown″tĕr-ĭn-sĭzh′ŭn) [″ + *incisio,* incision] A second incision made to promote drainage or relieve the stress on a wound as it is sutured.

counterirritant (kown″tĕr-ĭr′ĭ-tănt) [″ + *irritare,* to excite] An agent such as mustard plaster that is applied locally to produce inflammatory reaction for the purpose of affecting some other part, usually adjacent to or underlying the surface irritated. Three degrees of irritation are produced by the following classes of agents: 1. rubefacients, which redden the skin; 2. vesicants, which produce a blister or vesicle; and 3. escharotics, which form an eschar or slough or cause death of tissue. SEE: *acupuncture; escharotic; moxibustion; plaster, mustard.*

counterirritation (kown″tĕr-ĭr″ĭ-tā′shŭn) Superficial irritation that relieves some other irritation of deeper structures.

counteropening (kown″tĕr-ō′pĕn-ĭng) [L. *contra,* against, + AS. *open,* open] A second opening, as in an abscess that is not draining satisfactorily from the first incision.

counterpressure instrument An instrument that provides counterretraction to offset that exerted by the exit of a needle.

counterpulsation, intra-aortic balloon, intra-aortic balloon pump ABBR: IABC. The treatment of medically unmanageable cardiogenic shock with a balloon attached to a catheter inserted through the femoral artery into the descending thoracic aorta. The balloon is inflated in diastole to increase coronary blood flow, and deflated during systole to lower systemic resistance and improve tissue perfusion.

counterresistance A term rooted in Freudian psychoanalysis that refers to resistance by a psychotherapist that corresponds to the patient's resistance to closeness and change of life patterns. Examples include coming late to sessions, avoiding certain subjects, and fascination with the patient. Three types are countertransferance, characterological resistance, and cultural resistance.

countershock The application of electric current to the heart, by internal paddles, external paddles, or electrodes. SEE: *cardioversion; defibrillation.*

counterstain (kown′tĕr-stān) Application of a different stain to tissues that have already been prepared for microscopic examination by having been stained. The added stain helps to contrast the tissues originally stained.

countertraction (kown″tĕr-trăk′shŭn) The application of traction so the force opposes the traction already established; used in reducing fractures and assisting with surgical dissection.

countertransference (kown″tĕr-trăns-fĕr′ĕns) In psychoanalytic theory, the development by the analyst of an emotional (i.e., transference) relationship with the patient. In this situation, the therapist may lose objectivity.

coup SEE: *contrecoup.*

couple **1.** To join together. **2.** To have sexual intercourse.

coupling (kŭp′lĭng) In cardiology, the regular occurrence of a premature beat just after a normal heart beat.

Courvoisier, Ludwig Georg (koor-vwă′zē-ā) Swiss surgeon, 1843–1918.

C. law Law that states that disease processes associated with prior inflammation of the gallbladder (e.g., gallstones) produce scarring, which prevents enlargement of the gland. When the common bile duct is obstructed by cancer, the gallbladder becomes palpably dilated. SEE: *C. sign.*

C. sign Painless enlargement of the gallbladder in a jaundiced patient. The sign suggests a cancer obstructing the biliary tree.

couvade (koo-văd′) The custom in some primitive cultures of the father remaining in bed as if ill during the time the mother is confined for childbirth. In other cultures, expectant fathers may experience psychosomatic pregnancy-simulating symptoms of nausea, fatigue, and backache.

Couvelaire uterus [Alexandre Couvelaire, French obstetrician, 1873–1948] The condition in which blood escaping from an abruptio placentae centralis is extravasated into the uterine musculature. This acute condition may be associated with disseminated intravascular coagulation, and hysterectomy may be required.

covalence (kō-văl′ĕns) The sharing of electrons between two atoms, which bonds the atoms. **covalent** (-ĕnt), *adj.*

covariance (kō-vā′rē-ăns) In statistics, the expected value of the product of the deviations of corresponding values of two variables from their respective means.

covariant (kō-vā′rē-ănt) In mathematics, pert. to variation of one variable with another so that a specified relationship is unchanged.

cover **1.** To provide protection from potential illnesses with drugs, e.g. to cover a patient with a fever with antibiotics pending results of cultures. **2.** Concealment or protection from projectiles such as bullets, used by emergency medical providers when rescuing patients from violent settings. Examples would include engine blocks or brick walls. **3.** A blanket or other garment to warm or reassure a patient.

cover glass, cover slip A thin glass disk to cover a tissue or bacterial specimen to be examined microscopically.

Cowden's disease, Cowden's syndrome [Cowden, family name of first patient described] Multiple hamartoma.

Cowling's rule A method for calculation of pediatric drug dosages in which the age of the child at the next birthday is divided by 24. However, the most safe and accurate methods of pediatric dosage calculation include the weight and body surface area or both of the patient. SEE: *Clark's rule.*

Cowper's glands [William Cowper, Brit. anatomist, 1666–1709] Bulbourethral glands.

cowperitis (kow″pĕr-ī′tĭs) [*Cowper* + Gr. *itis,* inflammation] Inflammation of Cowper's glands.

cowpox (kow′poks) Vaccinia.

coxa (kŏk′să) *pl.* **coxae** [L.] **1.** Hip. **2.** Hip joint.

c. plana Legg's disease.

c. valga A deformity produced when the angle of the head of the femur with the shaft is increased above 120°, as opposed to coxa vara.

c. vara A deformity produced when the angle made by the head of the femur with the shaft is decreased below 120°. In coxa vara it may be 80° to 90°. Coxa vara may occur in rickets, bone injury, or congenitally.

coxalgia (kŏk-săl′jē-ă) [L. *coxa,* hip, + Gr. *algos,* pain] Pain in the hip.

coxarthrosis (kŏks″ărth-rō′sĭs) [″ + Gr. *arthron,* joint, + *osis,* condition] Arthrosis of the hip joint.

Coxiella (kŏk″sē-ĕl′lă) [Harold Rae Cox, U.S. bacteriologist, b. 1907] A genus of bacteria of the order Rickettsiales.

C. burnetii Causative organism of Q fever.

coxitis (kŏk-sī′tĭs) [L. *coxa,* hip, + Gr. *itis,* inflammation] Inflammation of the hip joint.

coxodynia (kŏk″sō-dĭn′ē-ă) [″ + Gr. *odyne,* pain] Pain in the hip joint.

coxofemoral (kŏk″sō-fĕm′ŏ-răl) [″ + *femur,* thigh] Pert. to the hip and femur.

coxotuberculosis (kŏk″sō-tū-bĕr″kū-lō′sĭs) [″ + *tuberculum,* a little swelling, + *osis,* diseased condition] Tuberculosis of the hip joint.

coxsackievirus (kŏk-săk′ē-vī″rŭs) Any of a group of viruses, the first of which was isolated in 1948 from two children in Coxsackie, New York. There are 23 group A and 6 group B coxsackieviruses. Most coxsackievirus infections in humans are mild, but the viruses produce a variety of important illnesses including aseptic meningitis, herpangina, epidemic pleurodynia, epidemic hemorrhagic conjunctivitis, acute upper respiratory infection, and myocarditis. SEE: *picornavirus.*

cozymase (kō-zī′mās) ABBR: NAD. Nicotinamide-adenine dinucleotide.

C.P. *candle power; cerebral palsy; chemically pure.*

C.P.A. *Canadian Physiotherapy Association.*

CPAP *continuous positive air pressure.*

C. Ped. *certified pedorthist.*

CPFT *Certified Pulmonary Function Technician.*

CPK *creatine phosphokinase.*

c.p.m. *counts per minute.*

CPPV *continuous positive pressure ventilation.*

CPR *cardiopulmonary resuscitation.*

C. bystander A lay person who provides CPR and who is not part of the organized emergency response system in a community.

C.P.S. *cycles per second.*

CPT *chest physical therapy.*

CR *conditioned reflex; complement receptor.*

C.R. *crown-rump; central ray.*

Cr Symbol for the element chromium.

crack Street name for a form of cocaine prepared from an aqueous solution of cocaine hydrochloride to which ammonia (with or without baking soda) has been added. This causes the alkaloidal form of cocaine to be precipitated. Because crack is not destroyed by heating, it may be smoked. The neuropsychiatric effects of crack are very brief compared with those of ingested or injected cocaine, but more intense. Adverse physiological effects of the drug include changes in behavior, compulsive use (addiction), cardiac dysrhythmias, coronary ischemia, stroke, and damage to the fetus during pregnancy, among others. SEE: *cocaine hydrochloride poisoning, acute.*

crack baby An infant exposed to crack cocaine in utero owing to the mother's use of the drug during pregnancy. SEE: *cocaine baby.*

cracking joint The sound produced by forcible movement of a joint by contracting the muscles that contract or extend a joint, esp. the metacarpophalangeal joints. The cause is not known. SEE: *crepitation.*

crackle An adventitious lung sound heard on auscultation of the chest, produced by air passing over retained airway secretions or the sudden opening of collapsed airways. It may be heard on inspiration or expiration. A crackle is a discontinuous adventitious lung sound as opposed to a wheeze, which is continuous. Crackles are described as fine or coarse. SYN: *rale.* SEE: *sounds, adventitious lung.*

coarse c. Louder, rather long, low-pitched lung sounds. Coarse inspiratory and expiratory crackles indicate excessive airway secretion.

fine c. Soft, very short, high-pitched lung sounds. Fine, late-inspiratory crackles are often heard in pulmonary fibrosis and acute pulmonary edema.

late-inspiratory c. A discontinuous adventitious lung sound that is present in the latter half of inhalation.

PATIENT CARE: The presence of late-inspiratory crackles is indicative of restrictive lung disorders such as atelectasis or pulmonary fibrosis.

cradle [AS. *cradel*] A lightweight frame placed over part of the bed and patient to provide protection of an injured or burned part or to contain either heat or cold.

cramp [ME. *crampe*] **1.** A pain, usually sudden and intermittent, of almost any area of the body, esp. abdominal and pelvic viscera. SEE: *dysmenorrhea.* **2.** A painful, involuntary skeletal muscle contraction. SEE: *heat c.; muscle c.; writer's c.; systremma.*

TREATMENT: Therapy depends on the cramp's cause and location. In muscular cramps, the muscle is extended and compressed, and heat and massage are applied.

heat c. Skeletal muscle spasm caused by the excess fluid and/or electrolyte loss that occurs with profuse sweating. The usual muscles affected are those used during work (i.e., the hand, arm, or leg muscles). The cramps may come on during work or up to 18 hr after completing a work shift.

TREATMENT: The patient should be rehydrated by drinking cool water or an electrolyte-containing drink, such as diluted juice or a commercially marketed sports drink. The severity of the cramp can be decreased through passive stretching and/or massage of the muscle. Severe heat cramps may require the use of an intravenous electrolyte solution, such as normal saline or Ringer's solution.

PREVENTION: Heat cramps may be prevented by maintaining proper hydration by drinking water or commercial electrolyte drinks before and during exposure to hot, humid environments. Normal dietary amounts of electrolytes and salt should be encouraged during meals.

menstrual c. An abdominal cramp associated with menstruation. SEE: *dysmenorrhea.*

muscle c. A painful, involuntary skeletal muscle contraction. This may occur at rest or during exercise, is asymmetrical, and usually affects the gastrocnemius muscle and small muscles of the foot. Ordinary muscle cramps are not due to fluid or electrolyte abnormality. These cramps begin when a muscle already in its most shortened position involuntarily contracts.

TREATMENT: Passive stretching of the involved muscle and active contraction of the antagonists will relieve an established cramp. Quinine, methocarbamol, chloroquine, and other drugs may help to relieve muscle cramps.

occupational c. A form of focal dystonia in which agonist and antagonist muscles contract at the same time. This can occur in writers, pianists, typists, and almost any occupation; they are not considered to have an emotional basis.

TREATMENT: Rest from the specific task and administration of anticholinergics and benzodiazepine may provide temporary relief.

pianists' c. Spasm, or occupational neurosis, of muscles of fingers and forearms from piano playing.

writer's c. A cramp affecting muscles of the thumb and two adjacent fingers after prolonged writing.

cranberry (krăn'bĕr-ē) A tart red fruit produced by plants of the genus *Vaccinium* and used in the treatment and prevention of urinary tract infections (UTIs). Scientific evidence of its effectiveness in treating UTIs is not definitive.

crani- SEE: *cranio-.*

cranial (krā'nē-ăl) [L. *cranialis*] Pert. to the cranium.

craniectomy (krā-nē-ĕk'tŏ-mē) [Gr. *kranion,* skull, + *ektome,* excision] Opening of the skull and removal of a portion of it.

cranio-, crani- [Gr. *kranion,* L. *cranium,* skull] Combining form meaning *skull.*

cranioacromial (krā"nē-ō-ă-krō'mē-ăl) [Gr. *kranion,* skull, + *akron,* extremity] Relating to the cranium and the acromion.

craniocaudal (krā"nē-ō-kawd'ăl) [" + L. *cauda,* tail] Direction from head to foot.

craniocele (krā'nē-ō-sēl) [" + *kele,* tumor, swelling] Protrusion of the brain from the skull. SEE: *encephalocele.*

craniocerebral (krā"nē-ō-sĕr-ē'brăl) [" + L. *cerebrum,* brain] Relating to the skull and brain.

cranioclasis (krā"nē-ŏk'lă-sĭs) [" + *klasis,* fracture] Crushing of the fetal head to permit delivery.

cranioclast (krā'nē-ō-klăst) [" + *klastos,* broken] An instrument for crushing the fetal skull to facilitate delivery.

cranioclasty (krā'nē-ō-klăs"tē) Crushing the skull of a dead fetus to enable vaginal delivery when the disparity between the diameters of the fetal head and maternal pelvis prohibit descent.

craniocleidodysostosis (krā″nē-ō-klī″dō-dĭs-ŏs-tō′sĭs) [″ + *kleis,* clavicle, + *dys,* bad, + *osteon,* bone, + *osis,* condition] A congenital condition that involves defective ossification of the bones of the head and face, and of the clavicles.

craniodidymus (krā″nē-ō-dĭd′ĭ-mŭs) [″ + *didymos,* twin] A congenitally deformed fetus with two heads.

craniofacial (krā″nē-ō-fā′shăl) Concerning the head and face.

craniograph (krā′nē-ō-grăf) [″ + *graphein,* to write] A device for making graphs of the skull.

craniology (krā″nē-ŏl′ō-jē) [″ + *logos,* word, reason] The study of the skull.

craniomalacia (krā-nē-ō-mă-lā′shē-ă) [″ + *malakia,* softening] Softening of the skull bones.

craniometer (krā-nē-ŏm′ĕ-tĕr) [″ + *metron,* measure] Instrument for making cranial measurements.

craniometry (krā-nē-ŏm′ĕ-trē) [″ + *metron,* measure] Study of the skull and measurement of its bones.

craniopagus (krā-nē-ŏp′ă-gŭs) [″ + *pagos,* a fixed or solid thing] Twins joined at the skulls.

craniopharyngeal (krā″nē-ō-făr-ĭn′jē-ăl) [″ + *pharynx,* throat] Pert. to the cranium and pharynx.

craniopharyngioma (krā″nē-ō-făr-ĭn-jē-ō′mă) [″ + ″ + *oma,* tumor] A tumor of a portion of the pituitary gland that often causes hormone deficiencies.

cranioplasty (krā′nē-ō-plăs-tē) [″ + *plassein,* to form] Surgical correction of defects of the skull.

craniopuncture (krā′nē-ō-pŭnk″chūr) [″ + L. *punctura,* puncture] Puncture of the skull.

craniorhachischisis (krā″nē-ō-ră-kĭs′kĭ-sĭs) [″ + *rhachis,* spine, + *schizein,* to split] A congenital fissure of the skull and spine.

craniosacral (krā″nē-ō-sā′krăl) Concerning the skull and sacrum.

cranioschisis (krā″nē-ŏs′kĭ-sĭs) [″ + *schizein,* to split] A congenital fissure of the skull.

craniosclerosis (krā″nē-ō-sklē-rō′sĭs) [″ + *skleros,* hard, + *osis,* condition] An abnormal thickening of the skull bones; usually associated with rickets.

cranioscopy (krā″nē-ŏs′kō-pē) [″ + *skopein,* to examine] Endoscopic examination of intracranial structures.

craniospinal (krā′nē-ō-spī′năl) Concerning the skull and spine.

craniostenosis (krā″nē-ō-stē-nō′sĭs) [″ + *stenosis,* act of narrowing] A contracted skull caused by premature closure of the cranial sutures.

craniostosis (krā-nē-ŏs-tō′sĭs) [″ + *osteon,* bone, + *osis,* condition] Congenital ossification of the cranial sutures.

craniosynostosis (krā″nē-ō-sĭn″ŏs-tō′sĭs) [″ + *syn,* together, + *osteon,* bone, + *osis,* condition] Premature closure of the skull sutures.

craniotabes (krā″nē-ō-tā′bēz) [″ + L. *tabes,* a wasting] In infancy, an abnormal softening of the skull bones. Those in the occipital region become almost paper thin. This condition may be the result of marasmus, rickets, or syphilis.

craniotome (krā′nē-ō-tōm) [″ + *tome,* incision] A device for forcibly perforating and dividing a fetal skull in labor in order to allow labor to continue. This is done when the fetus has died in utero.

craniotomy (krā-nē-ŏt′ō-mē) **1.** Incision through the cranium. This is done to gain access to the brain during neurosurgical procedures. SYN: *cranioclasty.*

PATIENT CARE: *Preoperative:* Procedures are explained, including antiseptic shampooing of the hair and scalp, shaving of the head, insertion of peripheral arterial and venous lines and indwelling urinary catheter, and application of pneumatic compression dressings. The patient is prepared for postoperative recovery in the neurological intensive care unit: the presence of a large bulky head dressing, possibly with drains; use of corticosteroids, antibiotics, and analgesics; use of monitoring equipment; postoperative positioning and exercise regimens; and other specific care measures.

Postoperative: Neurological status is assessed according to protocol (every 15 to 30 min for the first 12 hr, then every hour for the next 12 hr, then every 4 hr or more frequently, depending on the patient's stability). Patterns indicating deterioration are immediately reported. Serum electrolyte values are evaluated daily because decreased sodium, chloride, or potassium can alter neurological status, necessitating a change in treatment. Measures are taken to prevent increased intracranial pressure (ICP), and if level of consciousness is decreased, the airway is protected by positioning the patient on the side. The patient's head is elevated 15° to 30° to increase venous return and to aid ventilatory effort.

The patient is gently repositioned every 2 hr and is encouraged to breathe deeply and cough without straining; the airway is gently suctioned if necessary. Fluid is restricted as prescribed or according to protocol, to minimize cerebral edema and prevent increased ICP and seizures. Wound care is provided as appropriate; dressings are assessed for increased tightness (indicative of swelling); and closed drainage systems are checked for patency and for volume and characteristics of any drainage. Excessive bloody drainage, possibly indicating cerebral hemorrhage, and any clear or yellow drainage, indicating a cerebrospinal fluid leak, is reported to the surgeon. The patient is observed for signs of wound infection.

Prescribed stool softeners are also administered to prevent increased ICP from straining during defecation. Before discharge, the patient and family are taught to perform wound care; to assess the incision regularly for redness, warmth, or tenderness; and to report such findings to the neurosurgeon. If self-conscious about appearance, the patient can wear a wig, hat, or scarf until the hair grows back and can apply a lanolin-based lotion to the scalp (but not to the incision line) to keep it supple and to decrease itching as the hair grows. Prescribed medications, such as anticonvulsants, may be continued after discharge.

2. After the death of a fetus, the breaking up of the fetal skull to facilitate delivery in difficult parturition.

craniotonoscopy (krā″nē-ō-tō-nŏs′kō-pē) [″ + *tonos,* tone, + *skopein,* to examine] Auscultatory percussion of the cranium.

craniotrypesis (krā″nē-ō-trĭ-pē′sis) [″ + Gr. *trypesis,* a boring] The introduction of trephine or burr holes into the cranial bones.

craniotympanic (krā″nē-ō-tĭm-păn′ĭk) [″ + *tympanon,* kettle-drum] Pert. to the skull and middle ear.

cranium (krā′nē-ŭm) *pl.* **crania** [L.] The portion of the skull that encloses the brain, consisting of single frontal, occipital, sphenoid, and ethmoid bones and the paired temporal and parietal bones. SEE: *skeleton.*

crank (krănk) A slang term for methamphetamine hydrochloride.

crapulous [L. *crapula,* excessive drinking] Relating to the effects of excessive drinking and eating; relating to intoxication.

crash cart A mobile medicine chest for storing and transporting the equipment, medications, and supplies needed to manage life-threatening emergencies (e.g., anaphylaxis, cardiac arrest or dysrhythmias, pulmonary edema, shock, or major trauma).

crater (krā′tĕr) A circular depression with an elevated area at the periphery.

crateriform (krā-tĕr′ĭ-form) [Gr. *krater,* bowl, + L. *forma,* shape] In bacteriology, relating to colonies that are saucer shaped, crater-like, or goblet shaped.

Crawford Small Parts Dexterity Test A performance test that uses the manipulation of small tools under standardized conditions to measure fine motor skills and eye-hand coordination.

crazing Minute fissures on the surface of natural or artificial teeth.

cream The fat portion of milk. When untreated milk is allowed to stand undisturbed, the cream rises to the top of the container. Approx. 90% of the calories in cream come from fat.

crease (krēs) [ME. *crest,* crest] A line produced by a fold.

gluteofemoral c. The crease that bounds the inferior border of the buttocks.

inframammary c. The attachment of the inferior breast to the chest wall; the location of the film during craniocaudal filming of the breast.

creatinase (krē-ăt′ĭn-ās) [Gr. *kreas,* flesh, + *-ase,* enzyme] An enzyme that decomposes creatinine.

creatine (krē′ă-tĭn) [Gr. *kreas,* flesh] $C_4H_9O_2N_3$; a colorless, crystalline substance that can be isolated from various animal organs and body fluids. It combines readily with phosphate to form phosphocreatine (creatine phosphate), which serves as a source of high-energy phosphate released in the anaerobic phase of muscle contraction. Creatine may be present in a greater quantity in the urine of women than in that of men. Creatine excretion is increased in pregnancy and decreased in hypothyroidism.

creatine kinase An enzyme that catalyzes the reversible transfer of high-energy phosphate between creatine and phosphocreatine and between adenosine diphosphate (ADP) and adenosine triphosphate (ATP). Different isoforms predominate in different tissues (skeletal muscle [CK-MM], cardiac muscle [CK-MB], and the brain [CK-BB]), aiding in differential diagnosis of conditions in which this enzyme is present in the bloodstream.

The serum level of CK-MB may be increased 10 to 25 times the normal level in the first 10 to 14 hr after myocardial infarction and return to normal within 2 to 4 days, provided that no further heart muscle necrosis occurs. Serum levels of CK-MB are also increased in progressive muscular dystrophy, in myocarditis, and following trauma to skeletal muscle. Serum CK-MB levels are not elevated in liver disease or pulmonary infarction.

creatinemia (krē″ă-tĭn-ē′mē-ă) [″ + *haima,* blood] An excess of creatine in circulating blood.

creatinine (krē-ăt′ĭn-ĭn) [Gr. *kreas,* flesh] $C_4H_7ON_3$; the decomposition product of the metabolism of phosphocreatine, a source of energy for muscle contraction. Increased quantities of it are found in advanced stages of renal disease. It is a normal, alkaline constituent of urine and blood. The average normal serum creatinine value is less than 1.2 mg/dL. About 0.02 g/kg of body weight is excreted by the kidneys per day. SEE: *blood urea nitrogen.*

creatinuria (krē-ă″tĭn-ū′rē-ă) [″ + *ouron,* urine] Excess concentration of creatinine in urine.

creatorrhea (krē″ă-tō-rē′ă) [″ + *rhoia,*

flow] The presence of undigested muscle fibers in the feces, seen in some cases of pancreatic disease.

credentialing (krē-dĕn′shăl-ĭng) Recognition by licensure, certification, proof of professional competence, or award of a degree in the field in which an individual has met certain educational or occupational standards.

Credé's method (krā-dāz′) [Karl S. F. Credé, Ger. gynecologist, 1819–1892] **1.** The means whereby the placenta is expelled by downward pressure on the uterus through the abdominal wall with the thumb on the posterior surface of the fundus uteri and the flat of the hand on the anterior surface, the pressure being applied in the direction of the birth canal. This may cause inversion of the uterus if done improperly. **2.** For treatment of the eyes of the newborn, the use of 1% silver nitrate solution instilled into the eyes immediately after birth for the prevention of ophthalmia neonatorum (gonorrheal ophthalmia). **3.** For emptying a flaccid bladder, the method of applying pressure over the symphysis pubis to expel the urine periodically. This technique is sometimes used therapeutically to initiate voiding in bladder retention for persons with paralysis following spinal cord injury (neurogenic bladder).

creep (krēp) [AS.] The time-dependent plastic deformation of a material under a static load or constant stress. Creep may be destructive to a dental amalgam restoration.

cremains [contraction of *cre*mated re*mains*] That which remains after the body has been prepared for burial by cremation.

cremaster (krē-măs′tĕr) [L., to suspend] One of the fascia-like muscles suspending and enveloping the testicles and spermatic cord. **cremasteric** (-ĭk), *adj.*

cremate (krē′māt) [L. *crematio,* a burning] To dispose of the body of a dead person by burning. The ashes may or may not be buried.

crematorium (krē″mă-tō′rē-ŭm) [L.] A place for the burning of corpses.

crenate (krē′nāt) [L. *crenatus*] Notched or scalloped, as crenated condition of blood corpuscles.

crenation (krē-nā′shŭn) The conversion of normally round red corpuscles into shrunken, knobbed, starry forms, as when blood is mixed with salt solution of 5% strength. SEE: *plasmolysis.*

crenocyte (krē′nō-sīt) Crenated red blood cell.

creosote (krē′ō-sōt) [Gr. *kreas,* flesh, + *sozein,* to preserve] A mixture of phenols obtained from the destructive distillation of coal or wood. This toxic substance has been used as a disinfectant and as a preserver of wood. Because creosote is a potent carcinogen, contact with it should be avoided by wearing protective garments, gloves, and masks.

crepitant (krĕp′ĭ-tănt) [L. *crepitare*] Crackling; having or making a crackling sound.

crepitation (krĕp-ĭ-tā′shŭn) **1.** A crackling sound heard in certain diseases, as the crackle heard in pneumonia. **2.** A grating sound heard on movement of ends of a broken bone. **3.** A clicking or crackling sound often heard in movements of joints, such as the temporomandibular, elbow, or patellofemoral joints, due to roughness and irregularities in the articulating surfaces. SEE: *temporomandibular joint syndrome.*

crepuscular (krē-pŭs′kū-lăr) [L. *crepusculum,* twilight] Pert. to twilight; used to describe twilight mental state.

crescent (krĕs′ĕnt) [L. *crescens*] Shaped like a sickle or the new moon.

articular c. A crescent-shaped cartilage present in certain joints, as the menisci of the knee joint.

c. body Achromocyte.

myopic c. A grayish patch in the fundus of the eye caused by atrophy of the choroid.

c. of Giannuzzi A crescent-shaped group of serous cells lying at the base of or along the side of a mucous alveolus of a salivary gland.

crescentic (krĕs-ĕn′tĭk) Sickle-shaped.

cresol (krē′sŏl) Yellow-brown liquid obtained from coal tar and containing not more than 5% of phenol, used as a disinfectant in a 1% to 5% solution for articles or areas that do not come in direct contact with food.

cresomania, croesomania (krē″sō-mā′nē-ă) [Croesus, wealthy king of Lydia, 6th century B.C.] Delusion of possessing great wealth.

crest [L. *crista,* crest] A ridge or an elongated prominence, esp. one on a bone.

alveolar c. The most coronal portion of the bone surrounding the tooth; the continuous upper ridge of bone of the alveolar process, which is usually the first bone lost as a result of periodontal disease.

iliac c. The anatomical landmark for the superior margin of the pelvis, located between the anterior superior and posterior superior iliac spines.

intertrochanteric c. On the posterior femoral shaft, the ridge of bone extending from the greater to the lesser trochanter. SYN: *intertrochanteric line.*

CREST syndrome The presence of calcinosis, *R*aynaud's phenomenon, *e*sophageal dysfunction, *s*clerodactyly, and *t*elangiectasia, a variant of progressive systemic sclerosis.

cretin (krē′tĭn) [Fr.] A person afflicted with congenital hypothyroidism. SEE: *cretinism.* **cretinous** (-ŭs), *adj.*

cretinism (krē′tĭn-ĭzm) [″ + Gr. *-ismos,* condition] A congenital condition caused by a lack of thyroid hormones, characterized by arrested physical and mental development, myxedema, dystrophy of the bones and soft tissues, and lowered basal metabolism. The treatment consists of administration of synthetic thyroid hormones. The acquired form of severe hypothyroidism is referred to as myxedema.

cretinoid (krē'tĭ-noyd) [" + Gr. *eidos,* form, shape] Having the symptoms of cretinism, or resembling a cretin, owing to a congenital condition.

Creutzfeldt-Jakob disease [Hans Gerhard Creutzfeldt, 1885–1964; Alfons Maria Jakob, 1884–1931, German psychiatrists] ABBR: CJD. A central nervous system disease that causes rapidly progressive dementia usually accompanied by muscle jerking, difficulty walking, and aphasia. The causative agent is assumed to be a prion, and may be related to the agent that causes bovine spongiform encephalopathy ("mad cow disease"). Creutzfeldt-Jakob disease has developed in the recipient of a cornea from a donor with the disease, and in a few recipients of human growth hormone. There is no treatment, and the disease is fatal.

CAUTION: The causative agent of CJD is extremely resistant to most sterilization procedures. SEE: *Standard and Universal Precautions Appendix.*

---

crevice (krĕv'ĭs) [Fr. *crever,* to break] A small fissure or crack.

gingival c. The fissure produced by the marginal gingiva with the tooth surface. SYN: *gingival pocket; periodontal pocket; sulcus.*

crevicular (krĕv-ĭk'ū-lăr) Pert. to the gingival crevice or sulcus. SYN: *sulcus; gingival pocket; periodontal pocket.*

CRF *corticotropin-releasing factor.*

crib (krĭb) [AS. *cribbe,* manger] **1.** A framework around a denture or a natural tooth to serve as a brace or supporting structure. **2.** A small bed with long legs and high sides for an infant or young child.

cribrate (krĭb'rāt) [L. *cribratus*] Profusely pitted or perforated like a sieve.

cribration (krĭb-rā'shŭn) The state of being perforated.

cribriform (krĭb'rĭ-form) [L. *cribrum,* a sieve, + *forma,* form] Sievelike.

crick A muscle spasm or cramp, esp. in the neck.

cricoarytenoid (krī"kō-ă-rĭt'ĕn-oyd) [Gr. *krikos,* ring, + *arytaina,* pitcher, + *eidos,* form, shape] Extending between the cricoid and arytenoid cartilages.

cricoid (krī'koyd) [" + *eidos,* form, shape] Shaped like a signet ring.

cricoidectomy (krī"koyd-ĕk'tō-mē) [" + " + *ektome,* excision] Excision of the cricoid cartilage.

cricoidynia (krī-koy-dĭn'ē-ă) [" + " + *odyne,* pain] Pain in the cricoid cartilage.

cricopharyngeal (krī"kō-făr-ĭn'jē-ăl) [" + *pharynx,* throat] Pert. to the cricoid cartilage and pharynx.

cricothyroid (krī-kō-thī'royd) [" + *thyreos,* shield, + *eidos,* form, shape] Pert. to the thyroid and cricoid cartilages.

cricothyrotomy (krī"kō-thī-rŏt'ō-mē) [" + " + *tome,* incision] Division of the cricoid and thyroid cartilages. SYN: *coniotomy.*

cricotomy (krī-kŏt'ō-mē) [" + *tome,* incision] Division of the cricoid cartilage.

cricotracheotomy (krī"kō-trā"kē-ŏt'ō-mē) [" + *tracheia,* windpipe, + *tome,* incision] Division of the cricoid cartilage and upper trachea in closure of the glottis.

Crigler-Najjar syndrome (krēg'lĕr-nă'hār) [John Fielding Crigler, U.S. physician, b. 1919; Victor A. Najjar, U.S. physician, b. 1914] One of two familial forms of congenital hyperbilirubinemia associated with brain damage as a result of bilirubin deposition in the brain (kernicterus). The syndrome is caused by an enzyme deficiency in the liver that causes faulty bilirubin conjugation. It is transmitted as an autosomal recessive trait; death may occur within 15 months after birth in the more severe form.

crinogenic (krĭn"ō-jĕn'ĭk) [Gr. *krinein,* to secrete, + *gennan,* to produce] Producing or stimulating secretion.

crisis (krī'sĭs) *pl.* **crises** [Gr. *krisis,* turning point] **1.** The turning point of a disease; a very critical period often marked by a long sleep and profuse perspiration. **2.** The term used for the sudden descent of a high temperature to normal or below; generally occurs within 24 hr. **3.** Sharp paroxysms of pain occurring over the course of a few days in certain diseases. **4.** In counseling, an unstable period in a person's life characterized by inability to adapt to a change resulting from a precipitating event. SEE: *crisis intervention.*

abdominal c. Severe pain in the abdomen caused by biliary or renal colic, testicular or ovarian torsion, sickle cell anemia, bowel obstruction, or related illnesses.

addisonian c. Acute adrenal insufficiency.

celiac c. The rapid onset of malnutrition in celiac disease with severe watery diarrhea, vomiting, dehydration, and acidosis. Vigorous antibiotic and nutritional therapy is required.

Dietl's c. A sudden, severe attack of gastric pain, chills, fever, nausea, and collapse. In cases of floating kidney, the ureter becomes kinked and urine is obstructed, producing symptoms of renal colic.

salt-losing c. Acute vomiting, dehydration, hypotension, and sudden death as a result of acute loss of sodium; may be caused by adrenal hyperplasia, salt-losing nephritis, or gastrointestinal disease.

sickle cell c. Vaso-occlusive c. (in sickle cell disease).

tabetic c. Abdominal pain due to tabes dorsalis in patients with syphilis.

thyroid c. Thyroid storm.

true c. Temperature drop accompanied by a fall in the pulse rate.

vaso-occlusive c. (in sickle cell disease) Painful occlusions of blood vessels in bones, the chest, the lungs, or the abdomen, in patients with sickle cell anemia. The syndrome is caused by sickling of blood cells in small blood vessels, with resulting infarction and tissue death. SYN: *sickle cell crisis.*

crisis intervention Problem-solving activity intended to correct or prevent the continuation of a crisis, as in poison control centers or suicide prevention services. Usually these activities are mediated through telephone services or clinics operated by professional or paraprofessional workers in the medical and social fields.

crista (krĭs′tă) *pl.* **cristae** [L.] **1.** A crest or ridge. **2.** A projection, sometimes branched, of the inner wall of a mitochondrion into its fluid-filled cavity.

c. ampullaris A localized thickening of the membrane lining the ampullae of the semicircular canals; it is covered with neuroepithelium containing hair cells that are stimulated by movement of the head.

c. galli A ridge on the ethmoid bone to which the falx cerebri is attached.

c. lacrimalis posterior A vertical ridge on the lateral surface of the lacrimal bone.

c. spiralis A ridge on the spiral lamina of the cochlea.

criterion (krī-tē′rē-ŏn) *pl.* **criteria** [Gr. *kriterion,* a means for judging] A standard or attribute for judging a condition or establishing a diagnosis.

critical (krĭt′ĭ-kăl) [Gr. *kritikos,* critical] **1.** Pert. to a crisis. **2.** Dangerous. **3.** Extremely ill.

critical care unit SEE: *intensive care unit.*

critical incident stress debriefing, critical incident stress defusing ABBR: CISD. A group session conducted by mental health professionals and emergency medical service peers for rescuers after a tragic incident, such as the death of a partner, serious injuries to children, a mass casualty incident, or other disaster. A CISD is not a critique but rather an open discussion about rescuers' thoughts about an incident, combined with some teaching about the effects of stress that can be expected over the next few days to weeks.

CRM *Certified Reference Material.*

CRNA *certified registered nurse anesthetist.*

Crohn's disease (krōnz) [Burrill B. Crohn, U.S. gastroenterologist, 1884–1983] An inflammatory bowel disease marked by patchy areas of full-thickness inflammation anywhere in the gastrointestinal tract, from the mouth to the anus. It frequently involves the terminal ileum of the small intestine or the proximal large intestine, and may be responsible for abdominal pain, diarrhea, malabsorption, fistula formation between the intestines and other organs, and bloody stools. Like ulcerative colitis, it is most common in the second and third decades of life. SEE: *inflammatory bowel disease; Nursing Diagnoses Appendix.*

TREATMENT: Medical therapies include anti-inflammatory drugs, such as corticosteroids, aminosalicylates, such as mesalamine, and antibodies to tumor necrosis factor. Nutritional support of the patient may be needed during flares of the disease. Surgical removal of diseased bowel segments often is followed by relapse and may result in malnutrition.

cromolyn sodium (krō′mŏ-lĭn) A prophylactic mast cell stabilizer used to prevent asthma, allergies, rhinitis, and conjunctivitis.

Crookes' dark space [Sir William Crookes, Brit. physicist, 1832–1919] The nonluminous region enveloping the outline of the cathode in a discharge tube. SEE: *cathode.*

Crookes' tube An early form of vacuum discharge tube used for the study of cathode rays.

Crosby capsule [William Holmes Crosby, Jr., U.S. physician, b. 1914] A device attached to a flexible tube that is introduced into the gastrointestinal tract per os. It is designed so that a sample of tissue may be obtained from the mucosal surface with which it is in contact. The capsule is then removed and the tissue examined for evidence of pathological changes.

cross [L. *crux*] **1.** Any structure or figure in the shape of a cross. **2.** In genetics, the mating or the offspring of the mating of two individuals of different strains, varieties, or species.

crossbirth Presentation of the fetus in which the long axis of the fetus is at right angles to that of the mother and requires version or cesarean delivery. Also called *transverse lie.*

cross bite A form of dental malocclusion in the buccolingual direction.

crossbreeding Mating of individuals of different breeds or strains.

cross-bridge In the sarcomere of a muscle cell, the portion of the myosin filaments that pulls the actin filaments toward the center of a sarcomere during contraction.

cross-cultural Concerning the physiological and social differences and similarities of two or more cultures.

cross-dress To dress in clothing appropriate for one of the opposite sex.

crossed Passing from one side to the other, as the crossed corticospinal tract, in which nerve fibers cross from one side of the medulla to the other.

crossed finger technique A hazardous method of opening an unconscious patient's mouth by placing the thumb and index finger of a gloved hand on opposite rows of teeth and spreading the jaw open.

cross education Contralateral facilitation or changes resulting from exercise.

cross-eye Manifest inward deviation of the visual axis of one eye toward that of the other eye when looking at an object. SYN: *esotropia*. SEE: *squint; strabismus*.

cross-fertilization Fusion of male and female gametes from different individuals.

crossing over In genetics, the mutual interchange of blocks of genes between two homologous chromosomes. It occurs during synapsis in meiosis. In this process, there is no gain or loss of genetic material, but a recombination does occur.

crossmatching A test to establish blood compatibility before transfusion. SEE: *blood group*.

crossover The result of the reciprocal exchange of genetic material between chromosomes.

cross-training **1.** A cost-containment measure whereby instruction and experience are provided to enable health care workers to perform procedures and provide services previously limited to other members of the health team. **2.** In physical fitness training, the use of one or more sports to train for another. For example, training in both cycling and running strengthens all of the leg muscle groups and makes them less vulnerable to injury.

Crotalus (krŏt′ă-lŭs) [Gr. *krotalon,* rattle] A genus of snakes that includes most rattlesnakes; all are highly poisonous.

crotamiton (krō″tă-mī′tŏn) A scabicide. Trade name for a preparation of which crotamiton is a component is Eurax.

crotaphion (krō-tăf′ē-ŏn) [Gr. *krotaphos,* the temple] The tip of the greater wing of the sphenoid bone.

crotonism (krō′tŏn-ĭzm) Poisoning from croton oil.

croton oil (krō′tŏn) [Gr. *kroton,* castor oil plant seed] Oleum tiglii; a fixed oil expressed from the seed of the croton plant, *Croton tiglium.* It is toxic to skin, heart, muscle, and the gastrointestinal tract.

croup (croop) An acute viral disease of early childhood, usually occurring from age 6 months to 3 years, marked by a resonant barking cough (described as sounding "seallike") and varying degrees of respiratory distress. Inflammation and spasm of the larynx, trachea, and bronchi account for most of the symptoms. With increasing respiratory distress, the child becomes more hypoxic and hypercapnic.

ETIOLOGY: With the control of the bacterial agent *Haemophilus influenzae* type b through immunizations (the HIB shot), croup is now caused almost exclusively by viruses, especially parainfluenza, respiratory syncytial, and influenza viruses.

DIAGNOSIS: Diagnosis is based on characteristic clinical findings and x-ray examination of the neck, which may show subglottic narrowing of air within the trachea.

TREATMENT: Supportive measures include rest, supervised hydration, and inhalation of cool mist (e.g., in an oxygen tent) to reduce the viscosity of respiratory secretions. Oral corticosteroids are routinely prescribed. Hospitalization may be needed for more severe cases; nebulized racemic epinephrine and oxygen therapy may be needed. Intubation is rarely required unless the patient shows evidence of respiratory fatigue or hypoxia. Antibiotics are seldom needed because the viruses involved do not predispose to secondary bacterial infections. The vast majority of children, even those hospitalized, recover without complications. SEE: *racemic epinephrine*.

PATIENT CARE: A quiet, calm environment is maintained, all procedures are explained to the family, and support and reassurance are provided to the child and family to reduce fear and anxiety. Ventilation and heart rate are monitored, and a high-humidity atmosphere is provided, with cool moisture to help control fever, if present, but the child is kept dry to prevent chilling. Antipyretics are provided for fever. If the child becomes dehydrated, oral or intravenous rehydration is administered. Sore throat is relieved with water-based ices (fruit sherbets, iced Popsicles), and thicker fluids are avoided if the child is producing thick mucus or has difficulty swallowing. Humidified air is provided at home by a cool mist humidifier or by running hot water in the shower or sink in a closed bathroom. SEE: *Nursing Diagnoses Appendix*.

diphtheritic c. Laryngeal diphtheria.

membranous c. Inflammation of the larynx with exudation forming a false membrane. SYN: *croupous laryngitis*. SEE: *Nursing Diagnoses Appendix*.

SYMPTOMS: Symptoms include those of laryngitis; loss of voice; noisy, difficult, and stridulous breathing; weak, rapid pulse; livid skin; and moderate fever.

ETIOLOGY: Several viruses may cause this disease. These include parainfluenza, respiratory syncytial virus, and various influenza viruses.

TREATMENT: The air should be humidified by whatever means is available such as vaporizers or steam. Antibiotics are indicated only if there is secondary bacterial infection; corticosteroids are of no benefit. If hypoxia is present, inhalation of 40% concentration of well-humidified oxygen is indicated. This is best accomplished by use of a face mask. SEE: *steam tent.*

spasmodic c. A form of childhood croup that typically occurs in the middle of the night. The characteristic barky cough is present, but there are no other signs of viral illness. The child is perfectly fine the next morning, only to have a repeat of symptoms the next 2 or 3 nights. Hospitalization is rarely required. An allergic etiology is suspected. Antihistamines occasionally provide effective treatment.

croupous (kroo′pŭs) Pert. to croup or having a fibrinous exudation.

Crouzon's disease (kroo-zŏnz′) [Octave Crouzon, Fr. neurologist, 1874–1938] A congenital disease characterized by hypertelorism (widely spaced eyes), craniofacial dysostosis, exophthalmos, optic atrophy, and divergent squint.

crowing (krō′ĭng) A noisy, harsh sound on inspiration.

crown [L. *corona,* wreath] The top or highest part of an organ, tooth, or other structure, as the top of the head; the corona.

anatomical c. The part of a tooth extending from the cementoenamel junction to the occlusal surface or the incisal edge.

clinical c. The portion of the natural tooth that is exposed in the mouth, from the gingiva to the occlusal plane or the incisal edge.

dental c. SEE: *crownwork.*

crowning [L. *corona,* wreath] Visible presentation of the fetal head at the vaginal introitus. It occurs when the largest diameter of the infant's head comes through the vulvar opening.

crown-rump ABBR: CR. The axis for measurement of a fetus.

crownwork An artificial surface for a tooth.

CRP *C-reactive protein.*

CRT *cathode ray tube.*

CRTT *certified respiratory therapy technician.*

crucial (kroo′shăl) [L. *crucialis*] **1.** Cross-shaped. **2.** Decisive; of supreme importance; critical.

cruciate (kroo′shē-āt) Cross-shaped, as in the cruciate ligaments of the knee.

crucible (kroo′sĭ-b′l) [L. *crucibulum*] A dish or container for substances that are being melted, burned, or dehydrated while exposed to high temperatures.

cruciform (kroo′sĭ-form) [L. *crux,* cross, + *forma,* shape] Shaped like a cross.

crude (krood) [L. *crudus,* raw] Raw, unrefined, or in a natural state.

crura (kroo′ră) *sing.,* **crus** [L., legs] A pair of elongated masses or diverging bands, resembling legs.

c. cerebelli Cerebellar peduncles.

c. cerebri A pair of bands joining the cerebrum to the medulla and pons.

c. of diaphragm Two pillars connecting the spinal column and diaphragm.

c. of the fornix Arches made by division of the fornicate extremities.

crural (kroo′răl) [L. *cruralis*] Pert. to the leg or thigh; femoral.

c. nerve Femoral nerve.

c. palsy Paralysis of the nerves of the legs (e.g., 12th thoracic, first to fifth lumbar, and first to third sacral spinal nerves).

crus (krŭs) *pl.* **crura** [L.] **1.** Leg. **2.** Any structure resembling the leg.

c. cerebri Either of the two peduncles connecting the cerebrum with the pons.

crush syndrome The tissue damage and systemic effects of prolonged traumatic muscle compression. Crushing injuries may cause compartment syndromes, muscle necrosis, and leakage of muscle cell contents into the systemic circulation, especially after blood flow is restored to damaged tissues. Kidney failure may occur when myoglobin released from injured muscles blocks renal tubules. Electrolyte and acid base disturbances are common. Treatment may include local surgical care, metabolic support, hydration, and alkalinization of the urine. SEE: *renal failure, acute; reperfusion; rhabdomyolysis.*

crust, crusta [L. *crusta*] **1.** Dried serum, pus, or blood on the skin surface. Crusts are seen in diseases in which the skin weeps, such as eczema, impetigo, and seborrhea. They are often yellow-brown, dirty cream-colored, or honey-colored. **2.** An outer covering or coat.

crutch [AS. *crycc*] An assistive device prescribed to provide support during ambulation and transfers for individuals with paralysis, weakness, or injury. It also may be used to provide support for balance loss or to minimize or eliminate weight bearing on lower extremities. A variety of crutches that serve this purpose are available. The most common is the axillary crutch, which generally is constructed of wood or aluminum. This type of crutch consists of a curved surface that fits directly under the axilla, and double uprights connected by a hand grip that converge into a single contact point at the distal end. A rubber suction tip generally is fitted to this distal end for safety. The axillary crutch can be adjusted to suit the user's height. Other variations include the forearm crutch or lofstrand crutch. This aluminum crutch consists of a single metal tube, a hand grip, and a metal cuff that surrounds the proximal forearm. Platform adaptations for forearm crutches, which allow individuals to bear weight through the forearm, are available.

PATIENT CARE: Depending on activity restrictions, the patient is taught an appropriate gait pattern for crutch walking, including negotiating stairs and moving safely through doorways. The patient should not lean on the crutches during ambulation or when transferring from a standing to sitting position. Prolonged or excessive pressure in the axilla can lead to axillary nerve damage. The patient's safety and dexterity while on crutches are evaluated, and use of a walker may be recommended if safety is a concern.

Crutchfield tongs [William Gayle Crutchfield, U.S. surgeon, 1900–1972] A traction device whose pins are inserted into the skull to distract and/or immobilize the neck. Crutchfield tongs are used to stabilize fractures of the cervical spine.

Cruveilhier-Baumgarten syndrome (kroo-vāl-yā'bŏm'găr-tĕn) [Jean Cruveilhier, Fr. pathologist, 1791–1874; Paul Clemens von Baumgarten, Ger. pathologist, 1848–1928] Cirrhosis of the liver caused by patency of the umbilical or paraumbilical veins and the resultant collateral circulation. It is associated with prominent periumbilical veins, portal hypertension, liver atrophy, and splenomegaly.

cry- SEE: *cryo-*.

cry (krī) The production of inarticulate sounds, with or without weeping, which may be sudden, loud, or quiet as in a sob. These sounds are made in response to a variety of stimuli: fright, fear, pain, apprehension, sadness, glee, or joy. They may occur during nightmares. SEE: *cry reflex*.

cephalic c. A sudden shrill cry by an infant that may be indicative of cerebral disease.

epileptic c. A sudden, loud cry that may accompany the onset of an epileptic seizure.

hydrocephalic c. An involuntary night cry by a child with acute tuberculous meningitis or acute-onset hydrocephalus.

cryalgesia (krī-ăl-jē'zē-ă) [Gr. *kryos*, cold, + *algos*, pain] Pain from the application of cold.

cryanesthesia (krī-ăn-ĕs-thē'zē-ă) [" + *an-*, not, + *aisthesis*, sensation] Loss of sense of cold.

cryesthesia (krī-ĕs-thē'zē-ă) [" + *aisthesis*, sensation] Sensitivity to the cold.

cry for help An action by an individual who is potentially suicidal or severely depressed to inform others of his or her distress. This may be done by leaving obvious or cryptic messages or making telephone calls that are later interpreted to mean that the individual was asking for help more or less covertly.

crymodynia (krī"mō-dĭn'ē-ă) [Gr. *krymos*, frost, + *odyne*, pain] Pain from cold, esp. rheumatic pain aggravated by cold or damp weather.

crymophilic (krī"mō-fĭl'ĭk) [" + *philein*, to love] Cryophilic.

crymotherapy (krī"mō-thĕr'ă-pē) [" + *therapeia*, treatment] Cryotherapy.

cryo-, cry- [Gr. *krymos*, cold] Combining form concerning cold. SEE: *psychro-*.

cryoanesthesia SEE: *anesthesia, refrigeration*.

cryobank (krī'ō-bănk) A facility for storage of biological tissues at very low temperatures.

cryobiology (krī"ō-bī-ŏl'ō-jē) [" + *bios*, life, + *logos*, word, reason] The study of the effect of cold on biological systems.

cryocautery (krī"ō-kaw'tĕr-ē) [" + *kauter*, a burner] A device for application of cold sufficient to kill tissue.

cryocrit (krī'ō-krĭt) [" + *krinein*, to separate] The proportion of cold-precipitable protein in a serum sample. The cryocrit is used as a measure of immune complex formed in response to various agents, such as viruses.

cryoextraction (krī"ō-ĕks-trăk'shŭn) The use of a cooling probe introduced into the lens of the eye to produce an ice ball limited to the lens. The ice ball, which includes the lens, is then removed. This can be used to treat ophthalmic conditions, such as hemangiomas or cataracts.

cryofibrinogen (krī"ō-fī-brĭn'ō-jĕn) An abnormal fibrinogen that precipitates when cooled and dissolves when reheated to body temperature.

cryogen (krī'ō-jĕn) [" + *gennan*, to produce] A substance that produces low temperatures.

cryogenic (krī"ō-jĕn'ĭk) Producing or pert. to low temperatures.

cryoglobulin (krī"ō-glŏb'ū-lĭn) [" + L. *globulus*, globule] An abnormal globulin that precipitates when cooled and dissolves when reheated to body temperature.

cryoglobulinemia (krī"ō-glŏb"ū-lĭn-ē'mē-ă) [" + " + Gr. *haima*, blood] The presence in the blood of an abnormal protein that forms gels at low temperatures. It is found in association with pathological conditions such as hepatitis C viral infection, multiple myeloma, leukemia, and certain forms of pneumonia.

cryohypophysectomy (krī"ō-hī"pō-fĭz-ĕk'tō-mē) [Gr. *kryos*, cold, + *hypo*, under, + *physis*, growth, + *ektome*, excision] Destruction of the hypophysis by the use of cold.

cryokinetics (krī"ō-kĭ-nĕt'ĭks) [" + *kinesis*, motion] The therapeutic use of

General Indications and Contraindications for Cryotherapy

Indications	Contraindications
Acute or chronic muscle spasm	Advanced diabetes mellitus
Acute or chronic pain; neuralgia	Anesthetic skin
Acute injury or inflammation	Cardiac or respiratory involvement
Small, superficial, first-degree burns	Circulatory insufficiency
Postsurgical pain and edema	Cold allergy
In conjunction with rehabilitation exercises	Raynaud's phenomenon (advanced)
Spasticity accompanying central nervous system disorders	Second- or third-degree burns
	Uncovered open wounds

SOURCE: Adapted from Starkey, C: Therapeutic Modalities, ed 2., F. A. Davis Co., Philadelphia, 1999, p. 113.

cold (such as ice packs or ice immersion) before active exercise. The application of cold increases the amount of motion that is available to a joint by decreasing pain. Active exercise increases range of motion, improves tissue tensile strength, and enhances healing. SEE: *cryotherapy*.

TREATMENT: Cold therapy is administered to the patient until skin numbness is reported. Non-weight-bearing or weight-bearing exercises are then implemented without causing pain.

CAUTION: This technique should not be used in patients for whom cold application cryotherapy or active exercise is contraindicated.

cryolesion **1.** The cooling of an area in order to injure or destroy it. SYN: *cryotherapy*. **2.** A lesion produced by exposure to cold (e.g., frostbite).

cryophilic (krī″ō-fĭl′ĭk) [″ + *philein*, to love] Showing preference for cold, as in psychrophilic bacteria. SYN: *crymophilic; psychrophilic*.

cryoprecipitate (krī″ō-prē-sĭp′ĭ-tāt) **1.** The precipitate formed when serum from patients with rheumatoid arthritis, glomerulonephritis, systemic lupus erythematosus, and other chronic diseases in which immune complexes are found is stored at 4°C. **2.** A derivative of plasma that contains fibrinogen, clotting factor VIII, and fibronectin. It is used for bleeding disorders.

cryopreservation The preservation at very low temperatures of biological materials such as blood or plasma, embryos or sperm, or other tissues. After thawing, the preserved material can be used for its original biological purpose.

cryoprobe (krī′ō-prōb) A device for applying cold to a tissue. Liquid nitrogen is the coolant frequently used. SEE: *cryoextraction*.

cryoprotectant A drug that permits cells to survive freezing and thawing.

cryoprotective (krī″ō-prō-tĕk′tĭv) Pert. to a chemical that protects cells from the effect of cold.

cryoprotein (krī″ō-prō′tē-ĭn) Any protein that precipitates when cooled below body temperature. SEE: *cryofibrinogen; cryoglobulin*.

cryostat (krī′ō-stăt) A device for maintaining very low temperatures.

cryostretch (krī′ō-strĕch) [″ + AS. *streccan*, extend] A technique used to reduce muscle spasm by combining cold applications to produce numbness with proprioceptive neuromuscular facilitation. The body part is numbed using an ice pack and then exercised using proprioceptive neuromuscular facilitation. The ice application and exercise are repeated, to stretch and fatigue the involved muscle group.

cryosurgery (krī″ō-sĕr′jĕr-ē) [″ + ME. *surgerie*, surgery] The use of extremely cold probes to destroy unwanted, cancerous, or infected tissues. Cryosurgery has been used to treat a variety of lesions, including metastatic liver cancer, prostate cancer, sun-induced skin cancers, warts, cutaneous leishmaniasis, and even abnormal conduction pathways in the heart or nervous system. Liquid nitrogen is often used.

cryothalamotomy (krī″ō-thăl″ă-mŏt′ō-mē) [″ + L. *thalamus*, inner chamber, + Gr. *tome*, incision] The destruction of a portion of the brain by cooling the end of a slender probe placed in the thalamus, usually done by circulating liquid nitrogen through the hollow stylus. This is rarely used to treat parkinsonism.

cryotherapy (krī-ō-thĕr′ă-pē) [″ + *therapeia*, treatment] The removal of heat from a body part to decrease cellular metabolism, improve cellular survival, decrease inflammation, decrease pain and spasm, and promote vasoconstriction. SEE: table.

cryotolerant (krī″ō-tŏl′ĕr-ănt) [″ + L. *tolerare*, to bear] Able to tolerate very low temperatures.

crypt (krĭpt) [Gr. *kryptos*, hidden] **1.** A small sac or cavity extending into an epithelial surface. **2.** A tubular gland, esp. one of the intestine.

anal c. One of a number of small indentations lying immediately behind the junction of the anal skin and rectal mucosa.

dental c. A space in the bony jaw occupied by a developing tooth.

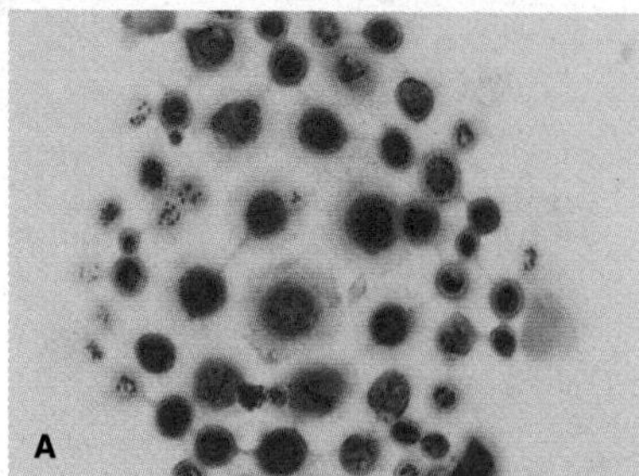

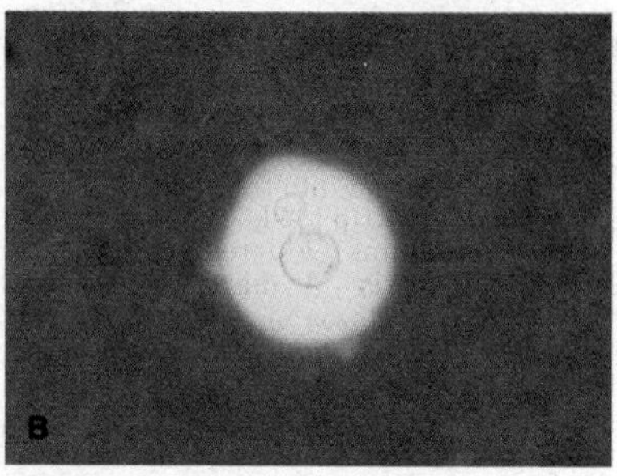

CRYPTOCOCCUS NEOFORMANS

(A) cerebrospinal fluid (orig. mag. ×1000), (B) India ink preparation showing large capsule (orig. mag. ×400)

c. of iris An irregular excavation on the anterior surface of the iris near the pupillary and ciliary margins.

c. of Lieberkühn A tubular intestinal gland that secretes fluids and digestive enzymes. Its wall is composed of columnar epithelium containing argentaffin cells and, at the base of the gland, cells of Paneth. They open between bases of the villi.

synoviparous c. A saclike extension of the synovial cavity into the capsule of a joint. Sometimes these crypts become blind sacs.

tonsillar c. A deep invagination of the stratified epithelium into the lymphatic tissue of the lingual or palatine tonsils. It may be branched.

cryptanamnesia (krĭpt″ăn-ăm-nē′zē-ă) [″ + *an-*, not, + *amnesia,* forgetfulness] Cryptomnesia.

cryptectomy (krĭp-tĕk′tō-mē) [″ + *ektome,* excision] Excision of a crypt.

cryptesthesia (krĭp-tĕs-thē′zē-ă) [″ + *aisthesis,* sensation] Subconscious awareness of facts or occurrences other than through the senses or rational thinking, such as through intuition or alleged clairvoyance.

cryptic (krĭp′tĭk) [Gr. *kryptikos,* hidden] **1.** Having a hidden meaning; occult. **2.** Tending to hide or disguise.

cryptitis (krĭp-tī′tĭs) [Gr. *kryptos,* hidden, + *itis,* inflammation] Inflammation of a crypt or follicle, esp. an anal crypt.

cryptocephalus (krĭp″tō-sĕf′ă-lŭs) [″ + *kephale,* head] A congenital deformity in which the head is inapparent.

cryptococcosis (krĭp″tō-kŏk-ō′sĭs) [″ + *kokkos,* berry, + *osis,* condition] Infection with the opportunistic fungus *Cryptococcus neoformans,* a spore-forming yeast present worldwide in the soil and in bird droppings. Humans contract the disease by inhalation. It may occur in healthy persons but is most common in immunosuppressed patients such as those with AIDS, leukemia, or organ transplants. Infection typically involves the brain and meninges but may affect the lungs, skin, liver, or bone. Immune competent persons respond to short-term treatment with amphotericin B and fluconazole, but many months of suppressive therapy with these drugs are needed in patients with AIDS. SYN: *torulosis*. SEE: *acquired immunodeficiency syndrome; amphotericin B*.

Cryptococcus (krĭp″tō-kŏk′ŭs) A genus of pathogenic yeastlike fungi. The former term was *Torula.*

C. neoformans A species that is the causative agent of cryptococcosis. SEE: illus.

cryptodidymus (krĭp-tō-dĭd′ĭ-mŭs) [″ + *didymos,* twin] A congenital anomaly in which one fetus is concealed within another.

cryptogenic (krĭp″tō-jĕn′ĭk) [″ + *gennan,* to produce] Of unknown or indeterminate origin.

cryptolith (krĭp′tō-lĭth) [″ + *lithos,* stone] A concretion in a glandular follicle.

cryptomenorrhea (krĭp″tō-mĕn″ō-rē′ă) [″ + *men,* month, + *rhoia,* flow] Monthly subjective symptoms of menses without flow of blood; may be caused by an imperforate hymen.

cryptomerorachischisis (krĭp″tō-mē″rō-ră-kĭs′kĭ-sĭs) [″ + *meros,* part, + *rhachis,* spine, + *schisis,* a splitting] Spina bifida occulta without a tumor but with bony deficiency.

cryptomnesia (krĭp-tŏm-nē′zē-ă) [″ + *mnesis,* memory] Subconscious memory. SYN: *cryptanamnesia*.

cryptophthalmus (krĭp″tŏf-thăl′mŭs) [″ + *ophthalmos,* eye] Complete congenital adhesion of the eyelid to the globe of the eye.

cryptoplasmic (krĭp″tō-plăz′mĭk) [″ + LL. *plasma,* form, mold] Having existence in a concealed form.

cryptorchid, cryptorchis (krĭpt-or′kĭd, -or′kĭs) [″+ *orchis,* testis] An individual in whom either or both testicles have not descended into the scrotum. SEE: *monorchid*.

cryptorchidectomy (krĭpt″or-kĭ-dĕk′tō-mē) [″ + ″ + *ektome,* excision] Operation for correction of an undescended testicle.

cryptorchidism, cryptorchism (krĭpt-or′kĭd-ĭzm, -kĭzm) [″ + *orchis,* testis, + *-ismos,* condition] Failure of the testicles to descend into the scrotum.

cryptoscope (krĭp′tō-skōp) [″ + *skopein,* to examine] Fluoroscope.

cryptosporidiosis A diarrheal disease caused by protozoa of the genus *Cryptosporidium* and often transmitted to humans after exposure to water or food that has been contaminated with cysts found in animal waste. *C. parvum* is the most common species associated with human infections. The typical infection in immunocompetent individuals causes explosive diarrhea and abdominal cramps following an incubation period of 4 to 14 days. Symptoms usually last 5 to 11 days but may continue for a month. In immunocompromised patients cryptosporidiosis often causes dehydration or death. This disease is commonly seen in patients with AIDS and in immunocompromised cancer and organ transplant patients. In immunocompetent patients, no effective specific therapy exists, and the disease is self-limiting. In the immunocompromised patient, the only effective therapy is reversal of the immunological defect.

When the organism contaminates public water supplies, hundreds of thousands of those drinking that water may develop diarrhea. A water-borne infection with *Cryptosporidium* caused an estimated 400,000 cases of diarrhea in Milwaukee in the 1990s. This outbreak was attributed to contamination of the municipal water supply by grazing livestock. Resistant to chlorine, cryptosporidial cysts are incompletely removed by standard water-filtration systems. The least expensive method of killing the organism in water is to boil the water. Some types of bottled water that come from above-ground sources may contain cryptosporidia. Water filters effective against the organism are labeled “absolute 1 micron” or “National Sanitation Foundation (NSF) certified for Standard 53 cyst removal.”

CAUTION: Stools from affected patients are highly infectious. Standard techniques must be used in handling and disposing of them. SEE: *Standard and Universal Precautions Appendix.*

Cryptosporidium A genus of protozoa in the kingdom Protista classed as a coccidian parasite. It is an important cause of diarrhea, esp. in immunocompromised patients, but may cause large outbreaks in the general population when it contaminates supplies of drinking water. SEE: illus.; *cryptosporidiosis.*

cryptoxanthin (krĭp″tō-zăn′thĭn) A sub-

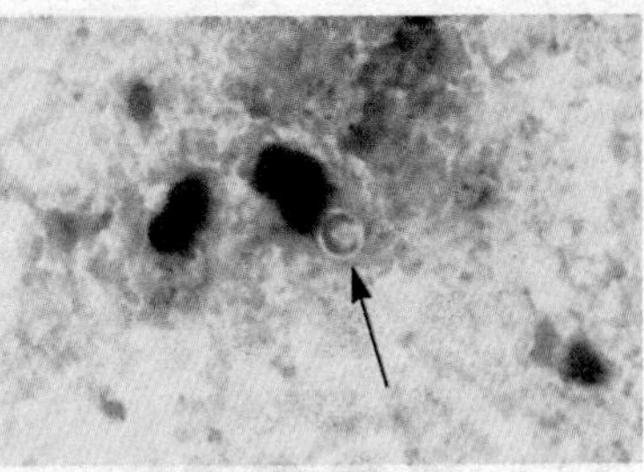

CRYPTOSPORIDIUM IN STOOL SPECIMEN

(Orig. mag. ×500)

stance present in a variety of foods (e.g., eggs and corn) that can be converted to vitamin A in the body.

cry reflex **1.** The normal ability of an infant to cry; not usually present in premature infants. **2.** The spontaneous crying by infants during sleep. It may be caused by a painful joint disease.

crystal (krĭs′tăl) [Gr. *krystallos,* ice] A solid in which atoms are arranged in a specific symmetrical pattern, forming distinct lattices, with definable fixed angles, faces, walls, and interatomic relationships. Examples include ice and many salts.

apatite c. In dentistry, the hydroxyapatite crystal typical of calcified tissues; a complex of calcium phosphate and other elements, present in bone and in the cementum, dentin, and enamel layers of teeth. The most dense crystalline pattern is found in enamel, the hardest tissue of the body.

Charcot-Leyden c. A protein-containing crystal found in diseased tissues wherein eosinophils are being destroyed. It is present in sputum from asthma patients, leukemic blood, and pleural effusions containing large numbers of eosinophils.

Charcot-Neumann c. A spermin crystal found in semen and some animal tissues.

Charcot-Robin c. A type of crystal formed in the blood in leukemia.

c. of hemin Hemin.

liquid c. A substance that alters its color or changes from opaque to transparent when subjected to changes in temperature, electric current, pressure, or electromagnetic waves, or when impurities are present. Liquid crystals have been used to detect temperature fluctuation in infants, and may be divided into two general classes: cholestric, which change color, and nematic, which can change back and forth from transparent to opaque.

spermin c. A crystal composed of spermine phosphate and seen in prostatic fluid on addition of a drop of ammonium phosphate solution.

crystallin (krĭs′tăl-ĭn) Globulin of the crystalline lens.

crystalline (krĭs′tă-līn) Resembling crystal.

c. deposits An acid group including the urates, oxalates, carbonates, and sulfates. The alkaline group includes the phosphates and cholesterin ammonium urate.

crystallization (krĭs″tă-lī-zā′shŭn) [Gr. *krystallos,* ice] The formation of crystals.

crystallography (krĭs″tă-lŏg′ră-fē) [″ + *graphein,* to write] The study of crystals; useful in investigating renal calculi.

crystalloid [″ + *eidos,* form, shape] **1.** Like a crystal. **2.** A substance capable of crystallization, which in solution can be diffused through animal membranes; the opposite of colloid.

crystalloiditis (krĭs″tăl-oyd-ī′tĭs) [″ + ″ + *itis,* inflammation] Inflammation of the crystalline lens.

crystallophobia [Gr. *krystallos,* ice, + *phobos,* fear] An abnormal fear of glass or objects made of glass.

crystalluria (krĭs-tă-lū′rē-ă) [″ + *ouron,* urine] The appearance of crystals in the urine. It may occur following the administration of many drugs, including sulfonamides. It can be prevented by adequate hydration.

CS *cesarean section.*

Cs Symbol for the element cesium.

c-section ABBR: CS. Operative delivery of the fetus. SYN: *cesarean section.*

CSF *cerebrospinal fluid.*

CST *Certified Surgical Technologist.*

C substance A complex carbohydrate present in the cell wall of pneumococcal cells. SEE: *C-reactive protein.*

CT *computed tomography.*

C.T.D. *connective tissue disease.*

Ctenocephalides (tĕn-ō-sĕf-ăl′ĭ-dēz) [Gr. *ktenodes,* like a cockle, + *kephale,* head] A genus of fleas belonging to the order Siphonaptera. Common species are *C. canis* and *C. felis,* the dog flea and cat flea, respectively. The adults feed on their hosts, whereas the larvae live on dried blood and feces of adult fleas. Adults may attack humans and other animals. They serve as intermediate hosts of the dog tapeworm, *Dipylidium caninum,* and may transmit other helminth and protozoan infections.

C-terminal In chemical nomenclature, the alpha carboxyl group of the last amino acid of a molecule.

CTZ *chemoreceptor trigger zone.*

Cu [L. *cuprum*] Symbol for the element copper.

cubic measure A unit or a system of units used to measure volume or capacity as distinguished from liquid measure. SEE: *Weights and Measures Appendix.*

cubital (kū′bĭ-tăl) [L. *cubitum,* elbow] Pert. to the ulna or to the forearm.

cubital fossa Antecubital fossa.

cubitus (kū′bĭ-tŭs) [L] Elbow; forearm; ulna.

c. valgus A deformity of the arm in which the forearm deviates laterally; may be congenital or caused by injury or disease. In women, slight cubitus valgus is normal and is one of the secondary sex characteristics.

c. varus A deformity of the arm in which the forearm deviates medially.

cuboid (kū′boyd) [Gr. *kubos,* cube, + *eidos,* form, shape] Like a cube.

cu cm *cubic centimeter.*

cucurbit (kū-kĕr′bĭt) [L. *cucurbita,* gourd] Cupping glass. SEE: *cupping.*

cue In psychology, a stimulus or set of stimuli that results in action or attempted action.

cuff (kŭf) [ME. *cuffe,* glove] An anatomical structure encircling a part.

attached gingival c. Attachment or junctional epithelium attached to the calcified root of the tooth apical to the gingival sulcus.

gingival c. The most coronal portion of the gingiva around the tooth.

rotator c. A musculotendinous structure consisting of supraspinatus, infraspinatus, teres minor, and subscapularis tendons blending with the shoulder joint capsule. The muscles, which surround the glenohumeral joint below the superficial musculature, stabilize and control the head of the humerus in all arm motions, function with the deltoid to abduct the arm, and rotate the humerus. Weakness in the cuff muscles may lead to impingement syndromes and tendinitis; tears in the cuff may lead to subluxations; and calcification may lead to immobilization of the shoulder.

cuffing (kŭf′ĭng) A collection of inflammatory cells in the shape of a ring around small blood vessels.

cuirass (kwē-răs′) [Fr. *cuirasse,* breastplate] A firm bandage around the chest.

cul-de-sac (kŭl″dĭ-săk′) [Fr., bottom of the sack] **1.** A blind pouch or cavity. **2.** The rectouterine pouch or pouch of Douglas, an extension of the peritoneal cavity, which lies between the rectum and posterior wall of the uterus.

culdocentesis (kŭl″dō-sĕn-tē′sĭs) [″ + Gr. *kentesis,* puncture] The procedure for obtaining specimens from the posterior vaginal cul-de-sac by aspiration or surgical incision through the vaginal wall, performed for therapeutic or diagnostic reasons.

culdoscope (kŭl′dō-skōp) An endoscope used in performing a culdoscopic examination.

culdoscopy (kŭl-dŏs′kō-pē) Examination of the viscera of the female pelvic cavity after introduction of an endoscope through the wall of the posterior fornix of the vagina.

-cule, -cle [L.] Suffix indicating little, as molecule, corpuscle.

Culex (kū'lĕks) [L., gnat] A genus of small to medium-sized mosquitoes of cosmopolitan distribution. Some species are vectors of disease organisms.

C. pipiens The common house mosquito; serves as a vector of *Wuchereria bancrofti,* the causative agent of filariasis.

C. quinquefasciatus Mosquito common in the tropics and subtropics; the most important intermediate host of *Wuchereria bancrofti.*

Culicidae (kū-lĭs'ĭ-dē) A family of insects belonging to the order Diptera; includes the mosquitoes.

culicide (kū'lĭ-sīd) [L. *culex,* gnat, + *caedere,* to kill] An agent that destroys gnats and mosquitoes.

Cullen's sign (kŭl'ĕnz) [Thomas Stephen Cullen, U.S. gynecologist, 1868–1953] Bluish discoloration of the periumbilical skin caused by intraperitoneal hemorrhage. This may be caused by ruptured ectopic pregnancy or acute pancreatitis.

culling The process of removal of abnormal or damaged blood cells from the circulation by the spleen. SEE: *pitting; spleen.*

culmen (kŭl'mĕn) *pl.* **culmina** [L., summit] **1.** The top or summit of a thing. **2.** The most prominent part of the vermis superior of the cerebellum, located near its anterior extremity.

cult [L. *cultus,* care] A group of people with an obsessive commitment to an ideal or principle or to an individual personifying that ideal.

cultivation (kŭl"tĭ-vā'shŭn) [L. *cultivare,* to cultivate] The propagation of living organisms, esp. growing microorganisms in an artificial medium.

cultural (kŭl'tū-răl) [L. *cultura,* tillage] Pert. to cultures of microorganisms.

cultural formulation A systematic review of a person's cultural background and the role of culture in the manifestation of symptoms and dysfunction. It includes the cultural identity of the individual, cultural explanations of the illness, cultural factors related to the environment and individual functioning, cultural elements of the clinician-patient relationship, and a general discussion of how cultural considerations may influence the diagnosis and treatment of a psychiatric illness.

culture (kŭl'tūr) **1.** The propagation of microorganisms or of living tissue cells in special media that are conducive to their growth. **2.** Shared human artifacts, attitudes, beliefs, customs, entertainment, ideas, language, laws, learning, and moral conduct.

blood c. A culture used to identify bacteria, fungi, or viruses in the blood. This test consists of withdrawing blood from a vein under sterile precautions, placing it in or on suitable culture media, and determining whether or not microbes grow in the media. If organisms do grow, they are identified by bacteriological methods. Multiple blood cultures may be needed to isolate an organism.

cell c. The growth of cells in vitro for experimental purposes. The cells proliferate but do not organize into tissue.

contaminated c. Culture in which bacteria from a foreign source have infiltrated the growth medium.

continuous flow c. A bacterial culture in which a fresh flow of culture medium is maintained. This allows the bacteria to maintain their growth rate.

corporate c. Institutional values, for example, of a corporation, hospital, professional association, or other health care entity.

gelatin c. A culture of bacteria on a gelatin medium.

hanging block c. A thin slice of agar seeded on its surface with bacteria and then inverted on a cover slip and sealed in the concavity of a hollow glass slide.

hanging drop c. A culture accomplished by inoculating the bacterium into a drop of culture medium on a cover glass and mounting it upside down over the depression on a concave slide.

negative c. A culture made from suspected matter that fails to reveal the suspected organism.

positive c. A culture that reveals the suspected organism.

pure c. A culture of a single form of microorganism uncontaminated by other organisms.

c. shock The emotional trauma of being exposed to the culture, mores, and customs of a culture that is vastly different from the one to which one has been accustomed.

slant c. A culture in which the medium is placed in a tube that is slanted to allow greater surface for growth of the inoculum of bacteria.

stab c. A bacterial culture made by thrusting into the culture medium a point inoculated with the matter under examination.

stock c. A permanent culture from which transfers may be made.

streak c. The spreading of the bacteria inoculum by drawing a wire containing the inoculum across the surface of the medium.

tissue c. A culture in which tissue cells are grown in artificial nutrient media.

type c. A culture of standard strains of bacteria that are maintained in a suitable storage area. These permit bacteriologists to compare known strains with unknown or partially identified strains.

cu mm *cubic millimeter.*

cumulative (kū'mū-lă-tĭv) [L. *cumulus,* a heap] Increasing in effect by successive additions.

cumulative drug action The action of repeated doses of drugs that are not immediately eliminated from the body. For example, preparations containing lead, silver, and mercury tend to accumulate in the system and can produce symptoms of poisoning.

Cumulative Index to Nursing and Allied Health Literature SEE: *CINAHL*.

cumulus (kū'mū-lŭs) [L., a little mound] A small elevation; a heap of cells.

c. oophorus A solid mass of follicular cells that surrounds the developing ovarian follicle. It projects into the antrum of the graafian follicle. SYN: *discus proligerus*.

cuneate (kū'nē-āt) [L. *cuneus,* wedge] Wedge-shaped.

cuneiform (kū-nē'ĭ-form) [" + *forma,* shape] Wedge-shaped.

cuneo- (kū'nē-ō) [L. *cuneus,* wedge] Combining form rel. to a wedge.

cuneocuboid (kū"nē-ō-kū'boyd) [" + Gr. *kubos,* cube, + *eidos,* form, shape] Pert. to cuboid and cuneiform bones.

cuneus (kū'nē-ŭs) *pl.* **cunei** [L., wedge] A wedge-shaped lobule of the brain on the mesial surface of the occipital lobe.

cuniculus (kū-nĭk'ū-lŭs) *pl.* **cuniculi** [L., an underground passage] A burrow in the epidermis made by scabies.

cunnilinguist (kŭn-ĭ-lĭn'gwĭst) [L. *cunnus,* pudenda, + *lingua,* tongue] One who practices cunnilingus.

cunnilingus (kŭn-ĭ-lĭn'gŭs) Sexual activity in which the mouth and tongue are used to stimulate the female genitalia. SEE: *fellatio*.

cunnus (kŭn'ŭs) [L.] The vulva; pudenda.

cup [LL. *cuppa,* drinking vessel] **1.** Small drinking vessel. **2.** A cupping glass. SEE: *cupping*. **3.** An athletic supporter (jock strap) reinforced with a piece of firm material to cover the male genitalia; worn to protect the penis and testicles during vigorous and contact sports. **4.** Either of the two cup-shaped halves of a brassiere that fit over a breast. **5.** A method of producing counterirritation. SEE: *cupping*.

favus c. A cup-shaped crust that develops in certain fungal infections. SEE: *favus*.

glaucomatous c. A depression in the optic disk occurring in late stages of glaucoma.

optic c. In the embryo, a double-layered cuplike structure connected to the diencephalon by a tubular optic stalk. It gives rise to the sensory and pigmented layers of the retina.

physiological c. A slight concavity in the center of the optic disk.

cup arthroplasty of hip Surgical technique for remodeling the femoral head and acetabulum and then covering the head with a metal cup. It is rarely used in treating arthritis of the hip. Total hip replacement is usually the procedure of choice in the elderly as well as in young adults on a selective basis.

cupola, cupula (kū'pō-lă, -pū-lă) [L. *cupula,* little tub] **1.** The little dome at the apex of the cochlea and spiral canal of the ear. **2.** The portion of costal pleura that extends superiorly into the root of the neck. It is dome shaped and accommodates the apex of the lung.

cupping Application to the skin of a glass vessel, from which air has been exhausted by heat, or of a special suction apparatus in order to draw blood to the surface. This is done to produce counterirritation. SEE: *leech; moxibustion*.

cupric (kū'prĭk) Concerning divalent copper, Cu^{++}, in solution.

c.sulfate The pentahydrate salt of copper, $CuSO_4 \cdot 5H_2O$, used as an antidote in treating phosphorus poisoning.

cuprous (kū'prŭs) Concerning monovalent copper, Cu^+, in a compound.

cuprum (kū'prŭm) [L.] ABBR: Cu. Copper.

cupruresis (kū"proo-rē'sĭs) [L. *cuprum,* copper, + Gr. *ouresis,* to void urine] Excretion of copper in the urine.

CUPS *Critical, unstable, potentially unstable, and stable;* patient priority classifications used during the initial assessment of a patient.

cupulolithiasis (kū"pū-lō-lĭth-ī'ă-sis) [L. dim. of *cupa,* a tub, + Gr. *lithos,* stone, + *iasis,* state or condition of] A disease of calculi in the cupula of the posterior semicircular canal of the middle ear. The condition may be associated with positional vertigo.

curanderismo (kū-răn-dăr-ēs'mō) A traditional Mexican-American folk medicine based on a belief that magic and ritual can be used to treat a broad spectrum of illnesses. Practitioners are known as curanderas (females) and curanderos (males).

curare (kū-, koo-răr'ē) [phonetic equivalent of a South American Indian name for extracts of plants used as arrow poisons] A paralytic drug, derived from natural plant resins, that is used by indigenous South American hunters to immobilize prey. Synthetic derivatives of this agent are used medicinally to relax skeletal muscles during anesthesia and critical care. SEE: *tubocurarine chloride*.

curarization (kū"răr-ī-zā'shŭn) Paralysis induced by curare or by a drug like curare (e.g., pancuronium or vecuronium).

curative (kū'ră-tĭv) [L. *curare,* to take care of] Having healing or remedial properties.

curb cut An area in which a sidewalk has been modified or designed to eliminate the vertical curb. By providing a gradual slope to the street at this point, an environmental obstacle has been removed, thus improving access for persons with wheelchairs, who have difficulty walking, or for persons pushing wheeled vehicles.

curd [ME] Milk coagulum, composed mainly of casein.

cure [L. *cura,* care] **1.** Course of treatment to restore health. **2.** Restoration to health.

curet, curette (kū-rĕt′) [Fr. *curette,* a cleanser] **1.** A spoon-shaped scraping instrument for removing foreign tissue matter from a cavity. **2.** In dentistry, one of a variety of sharp instruments used to remove calculus and to smooth tooth roots or to remove soft tissues from a periodontal pocket or extraction site.

curettage (kū″rĕ-tăzh′) [Fr.] **1.** Scraping of a cavity. SYN: *curettement.* **2.** The use of a curet in removal of necrotic tissue from around the tooth, dental granulomata, or cysts and tissue fragments or debris from the bony socket after tooth extraction; also called débridement.

periapical c. Use of a curet to remove pathological tissues from around the apex of the tooth root.

suction c. Vacuum aspiration.

uterine c. Scraping to remove the contents of the lining of the uterus. This procedure is used to evacuate the uterus following inevitable or incomplete abortion, to produce abortion, to obtain specimens for use in diagnosis, and to remove growths, such as polyps.

PATIENT CARE: *Preoperative:* The health care provider explains and clarifies the procedure, answers any questions, and describes expected sensations. Physical preparation of the patient is completed according to protocol, and the patient is placed in the lithotomy position. Asepsis is maintained throughout the procedure.

Postoperative: Vital signs are monitored until they are stable, and the patient is monitored until she is able to tolerate liquids by mouth and to urinate without difficulty. A perineal pad count is performed to determine the extent of uterine bleeding, and excessive bleeding is documented and reported to the health care provider. Prescribed analgesics are administered to relieve pain and discomfort. Before discharge, the patient is instructed to report profuse bleeding immediately; to report any bleeding lasting longer than 10 days; to avoid use of tampons, diaphragms, and douches; and to report signs of infections such as fever or foul-smelling vaginal discharge. Gradual resumption of usual activities is encouraged as long as they do not result in vaginal bleeding. During discharge teaching, the importance of reporting any of the following promptly is emphasized: heavy bleeding, bleeding that persists for more than 10 days, severe pain, and any signs of infection, such as fever or foul-smelling discharge. The woman is counseled to avoid the use of tampons or douches, and to abstain from intercourse for 2 weeks or until after the follow-up examination.

curettement (kū-rĕt′mĕnt) [Fr.] Curettage.

Curie (kūr′ē, kū-rē′) **1.** Marie, the Polish-born Fr. chemist, 1867–1934, who discovered the radioactivity of thorium, who discovered polonium and radium, and who isolated radium from pitchblende. She was awarded the Nobel Prize in physics in 1903 with her husband, and in chemistry in 1911. **2.** Pierre, Fr. chemist, 1859–1906, who, with his wife, was awarded the Nobel Prize in 1903.

curie [Marie Curie] ABBR: Ci. The quantity of a radioactive substance which has 3.7×10^{10} transitions, or disintegrations, per second. One gram of radium has almost exactly 3.7×10^{10} transitions per second. Thus 1 Ci of radium has a mass of almost exactly 1 g. SEE: *becquerel.*

curietherapy (kū″rē-thĕr′ă-pē) [″ + Gr. *therapeia,* treatment] Radium therapy.

curium (kū′rē-ŭm) [Pierre and Marie Curie] SYMB: Cm. An artificially made element of the actinide series; atomic weight of the longest-lived isotope, 247, atomic number 96. The half-life of the most stable isotope is 16 million years.

Curling's ulcer (kŭr′lĭngz) [Thomas Curling, Brit. physician, 1811–1888] An acute peptic ulcer that sometimes follows acute stress (e.g., a severe burn); a form of stress ulcer.

current [L. *currere,* to run] A flow, as of water or the transference of electrical impulses.

alternating c. ABBR: ac; AC. A current that periodically flows in opposite directions; may be either sinusoidal or nonsinusoidal. The alternating current wave usually used therapeutically is the sinusoidal.

direct c. ABBR: dc; DC. A current that flows in one direction only, used medically for cardioversion and defibrillation of dysrhythmias.

curriculum (kŭ-rĭk′ū-lŭm) [L.] **1.** A course of study. **2.** An outline or summary of available courses of study in an academic discipline or educational institution.

Curschmann's spirals (koorsh′mănz) [Heinrich Curschmann, Ger. physician, 1846–1910] Coiled spirals of mucus occasionally seen in sputum of asthma patients. SEE: *sputum.*

curse (kĕrs) **1.** To attempt to inflict injury by appeal to a malevolent supernatural power. **2.** Injury assumed to have been inflicted by a malevolent supernatural power. **3.** To use foul, offensive language.

curvature [L. *curvatura,* a slope] A normal or abnormal bending or sloping away; a curve.

angular c. A sharp bending of the vertebral column.

c. of spine One of four normal curves or flexures of the vertebral column as seen in profile: cervical, thoracic, lumbar, and sacral. Abnormal curvatures may occur as a result of maldevelopment or disease processes. SEE: *kyphosis; lordosis; scoliosis*.

curve [L. *curvus*] A bend, chart or graph.

characteristic c. Sensitometric c.

D log E c. Sensitometric c.

dye-dilution c. A graph of the disappearance rate of a known amount of injected dye from the circulation; used to measure cardiac function.

epidemic c. A chart or graph in which the number of new cases of an illness is plotted over time.

Hurter and Driffield c. ABBR: H and D curve. Sensitometric c.

learning c. A graph of the effect of learning or practice on the performance of an intellectual or physical task.

normal c. In statistics, the theoretical frequency of a set of data. It is usually a bell-shaped curve. SYN: *normal distribution*.

c. of Carus An arc corresponding to the pelvic axis. At the end of the second stage of labor, when the fetal head reaches the curve of Carus, it is directed upward toward the vaginal introitus and forced into extension by the resistance of the pelvic floor.

sensitometric c. In radiographic film analysis, the curve derived by graphing the exposure to the film versus the film density. Analysis yields information about the contrast, speed, latitude, and maximum and minimum densities of the film or film-screen system. SYN: *characteristic c.; D log E c.; Hurter and Driffield c.*

c. of Spee A curve established by viewing the occlusal alignment of teeth, beginning with the tip of the lower canine and extending back along the buccal cusps of the natural premolar and molar teeth to the ramus of the mandible.

time-temperature cooling c. The mathematical relation that plots the physical and chemical behaviors of dental (and other) materials as their temperature decreases over time.

curvilinear Concerning or pert. to a curved line.

Cushing, Harvey (koosh'ĭng) U.S. surgeon, 1869–1939.

C.'s disease Cushing's syndrome caused by excessive production of adrenocorticotropic hormone in the body.

C.'s syndrome The signs and symptoms that result from prolonged exposure to excessive glucocorticoid hormones. Glucocorticoids are naturally excreted by the adrenal glands; however, Cushing's syndrome is a side effect of the pharmacological use of steroids in the management of inflammatory illnesses, such as reactive airways disease or arthritis. Glucocorticoid excess that results from pituitary or adrenal adenomas, or from the production of excess levels of adrenocorticotropic hormone, is exceptionally rare (it is called Cushing's disease).

SYMPTOMS: The affected patient may complain of muscular weakness, thinning of the skin, easy bruising, weight gain, rounding of facial features ("moon-like" facies), or psychological depression. Symptoms of diabetes mellitus such as thirst, polyuria, and polyphagia may be present because glucocorticoid hormones oppose the action of insulin. On physical examination patients may have obesity that affects the face, upper back and trunk, but spares the limbs. The abdominal skin may be marked by purplish lines called striae. Hypertension is often present.

TREATMENT: Cushing's syndrome caused by the chronic use of steroid hormones may improve if steroids can be given every other day, or if high doses of these medications can be gradually tapered. When Cushing's disease is present, surgery to remove the responsible adenoma is usually needed.

PATIENT CARE: When prolonged administration of therapeutic, as opposed to replacement, doses of adrenocortical hormones is required, the patient is monitored for development of adverse reactions. A diet high in protein and potassium but low in calories, carbohydrates, and sodium is provided. The patient is assisted to adjust to changes in body image and strength. Realistic reassurance and emotional support are provided, and the patient is encouraged to verbalize feelings about losses and to develop positive coping strategies. Intermittent rest periods are recommended, and assistance is provided with mobility, esp. with movements requiring arm-shoulder strength. Safety measures are instituted to prevent falls. Patient teaching should include information about the risk for the development of diabetes mellitus, cataracts, easy bruising, and infections. SEE: *Nursing Diagnoses Appendix*.

C.'s ulcer A stress-related ulcer that occurs in some patients after head injury as a result of the hypersecretion of gastric acid. SEE: *stress ulcer*.

Cushing response A reflex due to cerebral ischemia that causes an increase in systemic blood pressure. This maintains cerebral perfusion during increased intracranial pressure.

cushingoid (koosh'ĭng-oyd) Having physical characteristics that result from excess exposure to corticosteroids, such as a rounded face, weight gain, or thin, easily bruised skin.

cushion In anatomy, a mass of connective tissue, usually adipose, that acts to prevent undue pressure on underlying tissues or structures.

wheelchair c. A padded surface for wheelchair seats designed to prevent pressure sores. There are several static varieties, including air-filled, polyurethane foam, and flotation, the latter filled with water or gel. Dynamic surfaces, which require an external power source, protect pressure points by alternating high and low air pressures through a system of valves and pumps. SYN: *pressure relief device.*

cusp (kŭsp) [L. *cuspis,* point] **1.** A rounded or cone-shaped point on the crown of a tooth. **2.** One of the leaflike divisions or parts of the valves of the heart. SEE: *bicuspid valve; semilunar cusp; tricuspid valve.*

Carabelli's c. An accessory cusp found on the upper first molar.

plunger c. A cusp of a tooth that tends to forcibly wedge food into interproximal areas, causing an impaction. Cusp points should be rounded, shortened, or reduced with a dental drill.

cuspid (kŭs′pĭd) The canine teeth. SEE: *dentition* for illus.

cuspidate (kŭs′pĭ-dāt) [L. *cuspidatus*] Having cusps.

custom A generally accepted practice or behavior by a particular group of people or a social group.

cut 1. Separating or dividing of tissues by use of a sharp surgical instrument such as a scalpel. **2.** To dilute a substance in order to decrease the concentration of the active ingredient.

cutaneous (kū-tā′nē-ŭs) [L. *cutis,* skin] Pert. to the skin. SYN: *integumentary.*

cutaneous nerves Nerves that provide sensory pathways for stimuli to the skin. SEE: *Nerves Appendix.*

cutaneous respiration The transpiration of gases through the skin.

cutdown (kŭt′down) A surgical procedure for locating a vein or artery to permit intravenous or intra-arterial administration of fluids or drugs; required in patients with vascular collapse caused by shock or other conditions.

cuticle (kū′tĭ-k′l) [L. *cuticula,* little skin] A layer of solid or semisolid tissue that covers the free surface of a layer of epithelial cells. It may be horny or chitinous, and sometimes is calcified. Examples include the enamel cuticle of a tooth and the capsule of the lens of the eye.

acquired c. A layer of salivary products, bacteria, and food debris on the surface of the teeth; not a true cuticle. SYN: *pellicle.*

attachment c. Dental c.

dental c. The glycosaminoglycans layer produced by attachment epithelium on the cementum of the tooth root. It is continuous with and identical in origin and function to enamel cuticle, which is present on the enamel crown. SYN: *attachment c.*

enamel c. The thin, calcified layer that covers the enamel crown of the tooth prior to eruption. Remnants that persist after decalcification of the tooth for microscopy are called Nasmyth's membrane. SYN: *cuticula dentis.*

cuticula (kū-tĭk′ū-lă) [L.] Cuticle.

c. dentis A skinlike membrane that may cover the teeth after they have erupted and usually is lost in ordinary mastication of food. The membrane is easily removed by a dentist. SYN: *enamel cuticle; Nasmyth's membrane.*

cuticularization (kū-tĭk″ū-lăr-ī-zā′shŭn) Growth of skin over a sore or wound.

cutin (kū′tĭn) [L. *cutis,* skin] A wax that combines with cellulose to form the cuticle of plants.

cutireaction (kū″tē-rē-ăk′shŭn) An inflammatory or irritative reaction appearing on the skin; skin reaction.

von Pirquet's c. The reaction of the skin after inoculation with tuberculosis toxins.

cutis (kū′tĭs) [L.] The skin; consisting of the epidermis and the corium (dermis), and resting on the subcutaneous tissue.

c. anserina Piloerection.

c. aurantiasis Yellow discoloration of the skin resulting from ingesting excessive quantities of vegetables, such as carrots, containing carotenoid pigments. SEE: *carotenemia.*

c. hyperelastica Ehlers-Danlos syndrome.

c. laxa A rare inherited condition in which there is loss of elastic fibers of the skin. The skin becomes so loose it hangs and sags. Pulmonary emphysema, intestinal diverticula, and hernias also may be present. There are at least three inheritable patterns of this disease. There is no known treatment. SYN: *c. pendula.*

c. marmorata Transient mottling of the skin caused by exposure to decreased temperature. SYN: *mottling.*

c. pendula C. laxa.

c. vera Dermis.

c. verticis gyrata Convoluted scalp folds 1 to 2 cm thick. It may develop any time from birth to adolescence and is more common in males. The skin cannot be flattened by traction.

cutization (kū-tĭ-zā′shŭn) Skinlike changes in a mucous membrane as a result of continued inflammation.

cut throat Laceration of the throat. The seriousness of the injury depends on the angle of thrust of the cutting object, the location of the injury, and the amount of tissue damage.

FIRST AID: The patient should be transported to the nearest appropriate facility for evaluation. (If there is bleeding into the airway, the patient should be positioned so blood flows away from the pharynx. This may require a head-low position.) If the trachea is severed, it should be kept open and free of clots. Bleeding points should be compressed with sterile cloths. Vital signs should be monitored closely. Artificial respiration should be given if necessary.

cuvette (kŭv-ĕt′) [Fr. *cuve,* a tub] A small transparent glass or plastic container, esp. one used to hold liquids to be examined photometrically.

CV *coefficient of variation.*

CVA *cerebrovascular accident.*

CVD *cardiovascular disease.*

CVP *central venous pressure.*

cyan- SEE: *cyano-.*

cyanephidrosis (sī″ăn-ĕf″ĭ-drō′sĭs) [Gr. *kyanos,* dark blue, + *ephidrosis,* sweating] Bluish sweat.

cyanhemoglobin (sī″ăn-hē″mō-glō′bĭn) Hemoglobin combined with cyanide.

cyanhidrosis (sī-ăn-hī-drō′sĭs) [″ + *hidrosis,* sweat] Exuding bluish sweat.

cyanide (sī′ă-nīd″) A compound containing the radical —CN, as potassium cyanide (KCN), sodium cyanide (NaCN).

cyanide poisoning Intoxication with any of several cyanide-containing compounds, which are among the most potent blockers of cellular oxygenation. They inhibit respiration by blocking oxidative phosphorylation at the cellular level. SEE: *Poisons and Poisoning Appendix.*

The most common patients are jewelers, metal platers, persons who handle rodenticides, victims of smoke inhalation, and patients treated with very high doses of sodium nitroprusside. Rarely, cyanide poisoning results from the ingestion of certain fruits, such as the bitter cassava and some stone fruits.

SYMPTOMS: Palpitations, disorientation, and confusion may be rapidly followed by respiratory failure, seizures, coma, and death in patients who suffer large exposures. Smaller exposures may produce anxiety, dizziness, headache, and shortness of breath. Patients may report that they have detected an odor of bitter almonds at the time of exposure to cyanide.

TREATMENT: The patient is immediately treated with gastric lavage, and activated charcoal is given to adsorb to whatever toxin may remain in the gastrointestinal tract. Emesis is contraindicated. Oxygen is immediately provided; intubation and mechanical ventilation may be needed when the patient has suffered respiratory failure. Antidotes to cyanide poisoning include amyl nitrate, sodium nitrite, and sodium thiosulfate.

cyanmethemoglobin (sī″ăn-mĕt″hē-mō-glō′bĭn) Combination of cyanide and methemoglobin.

cyano-, cyan- [Gr. *kyanos,* dark blue] Combining form meaning *blue.*

cyanoacrylate adhesives Monomers of *N*-alkyl cyanoacrylate that have been used as a tissue adhesive in the repair of simple lacerations (e.g., of the arms or legs). Commercially available versions are called "superglue."

CAUTION: "Superglues" can cause tissues to adhere firmly to each other. They should not be used near the eyes or mouth, or on the hands, to avoid bonding these tissues together.

cyanocobalamin (sī″ăn-ō-kō-băl′ă-mĭn) Vitamin B_{12}, essential for DNA synthesis, esp. in red blood cell formation. It is used in treating pernicious anemia.

cyanoderma (sī″ă-nō-dĕr′mă) [″ + *derma,* skin] Cyanosis.

cyanogen (sī-ăn′ō-jĕn) [″ + *gennan,* to produce] **1.** The radical CN. **2.** A poisonous gas, CN—CN.

cyanomycosis (sī″ăn-ō-mī-kō′sĭs) [″ + *mykes,* fungus, + *osis,* condition] The development of blue pus due to *Micrococcus pyocyaneus.*

cyanophilous (sī-ăn-ŏf′ĭl-ŭs) Having an affinity for a blue dye or stain.

cyanopia, cyanopsia (sī-ăn-ō′pē-ă, -ŏp′sē-ă) [″ + *opsis,* vision] Vision in which all objects appear to be blue.

cyanosed Affected with cyanosis.

cyanosis (sī-ă-nō′sĭs) [″ + *osis,* condition] A blue, gray, slate, or dark purple discoloration of the skin or mucous membranes caused by deoxygenated or reduced hemoglobin in the blood. Cyanosis is found most often in hypoxemic patients and rarely in patients with methemoglobinemias. Occasionally, a bluish skin tint that superficially resembles cyanosis results from exposure to the cold. In the very young patient, cyanosis may point to a congenital heart defect.

ETIOLOGY: This condition usually is caused by inadequate oxygenation of the bloodstream.

TREATMENT: Supplemental oxygenation is supplied to cyanotic patients who are proven to be hypoxemic. SEE: *asphyxia.*

CAUTION: Oximetry or arterial blood gas analysis should be used to determine whether a patient is adequately oxygenated. Relying only on the appearance of the skin or mucous membranes to determine hypoxemia may result in misdiagnosis.

central c. A bluish discoloration of the mucous membranes in the mouth, indicating hypoxemia and respiratory failure.

TREATMENT: If hypoxemia is confirmed by oximetry or blood gas analysis, supplemental oxygen is provided.

PATIENT CARE: The patient's vital

signs, blood gases, and sensorium should be monitored closely, as this sign may indicate hypoxemia accompanying impending respiratory failure. SYN: *circumoral c.*

circumoral c. Central c.

congenital c. Cyanosis usually associated with stenosis of the pulmonary artery orifice, an imperforate ventricular septum, or a patent foramen ovale or ductus arteriosus. SEE: *tetralogy of Fallot.*

delayed c. Tardive c.

enterogenous c. Cyanosis induced by intestinal absorption of toxins or by certain drugs. SEE: *methemoglobinemia.*

peripheral c. A bluish discoloration of the digits.

PATIENT CARE: The patient's vital signs, oxygen saturation, blood gases, and mental status should be monitored closely.

c. retinae Bluish appearance of the retina seen in congenital heart disease, polycythemia, and in certain poisonings, such as dinitrobenzol.

tardive c. Cyanosis caused by congenital heart disease and appearing only after cardiac failure. SYN: *delayed c.*

cyanotic (sī-ăn-ŏt′ĭk) Of the nature of, affected with, or pert. to cyanosis.

cyanuria (sī″ă-nū′rē-ă) The voiding of blue urine.

cybernetics (sī″bĕr-nĕt′ĭks) [Gr. *kybernetes,* helmsman] The science of control and communication in biological, electronic, and mechanical systems. This includes analysis of feedback mechanisms that serve to govern or modify the actions of various systems.

cyberphilia (sī″bĕr-fĭl′ē-ă) [″ + *philein,* to love] Fascination with the use of machines, esp. computers, their use, and their programming.

cyberphobia (sī″bĕr-fō′bē-ă) [″ + *phobos,* fear] Tension, anxiety, and stress in persons required to work with a computer.

cycad (sī′kăd) A variety of plants including *Cycas revoluta* and *C. circinalis,* from which cycasin has been isolated.

cycasin (sī′kă-sĭn) A carcinogenic substance present in cycad plants.

cycl- SEE: *cyclo-.*

cyclamate (sī′klă-māt) A salt of cyclamic acid that is used as a nonnutritive artificial sweetener. It is about 30 times as sweet as sugar. Its use is banned in the U.S., but it is widely used in Canada and Europe.

cyclarthrosis (sī-klăr-thrō′sĭs) [Gr. *kyklos,* circle, + *arthron,* joint, + *osis,* condition] A lateral ginglymus or pivot joint, which makes rotation possible.

cycle (sī′kl) [Gr. *kyklos,* circle] A series of movements or events; a sequence usually recurring at regular intervals.

cardiac c. The period from the beginning of one heartbeat to the beginning of the succeeding beat, including *systole,* the contraction of the atria and ventricles that propels the blood, and *diastole,* the period during which the cavities are being refilled with blood. Normally, the atria contract immediately before the ventricles. The ordinary cycle lasts 0.8 sec with the heart beating approx. 60 to 85 times a minute in the adult at rest. Atrial systole lasts 0.1 sec; ventricular systole 0.3 sec, and diastole 0.4 sec; although the heart seems to be working continuously, it actually rests for a good portion of each cardiac cycle. SEE: illus.

gastric c. The progression of peristaltic waves over the stomach wall.

genesial c. **1.** The period from puberty to menopause. **2.** The period of sexual maturity.

glycolytic c. The successive steps by which glucose is broken down in living tissue.

life c. All of the developmental history of an organism whether in a free-living condition or in a host (e.g., as a parasite that experiences part of its cycle inside another organism).

menstrual c. A series of periodically recurring changes in the hormonal status of women and in the endometrium of the uterus, culminating in menstruation. SEE: *menstruation.*

stimulated c. An assisted reproductive technology cycle in which a woman receives drugs to stimulate her ovaries to produce additional follicles. SEE: *unstimulated c.*

stretch-shortening c. An eccentric muscle contraction followed immediately by a concentric contraction. The elastic potentiation that occurs during the eccentric phase increases the force of output of the concentric contraction. Exercises incorporating this phenomenon are called plyometrics. SEE: *plyometrics.*

unstimulated c. An assisted reproductive technology cycle in which a woman does not receive drugs to stimulate her ovaries to produce additional follicles. SEE: *stimulated c.*

cyclectomy (sī-klĕk′tō-mē) [Gr. *kyklos,* circle, + *ektome,* excision] **1.** Excision of part of the ciliary body or muscle. **2.** Excision of the ciliary border of the eyelids.

cycles per second ABBR: cps. SEE: *hertz.*

cyclic (sī′klĭk) **1.** Periodic. **2.** Having a ring-shaped structure.

cyclic AMP Adenosine 3′,5′-cyclic monophosphate.

cyclic AMP synthetase Adenylate cyclase.

cyclicotomy (sĭk″lĭ-kŏt′ō-mē) [″ + *tome,* incision] Cutting of the ciliary muscle.

cyclins A group of proteins important in regulating mitosis.

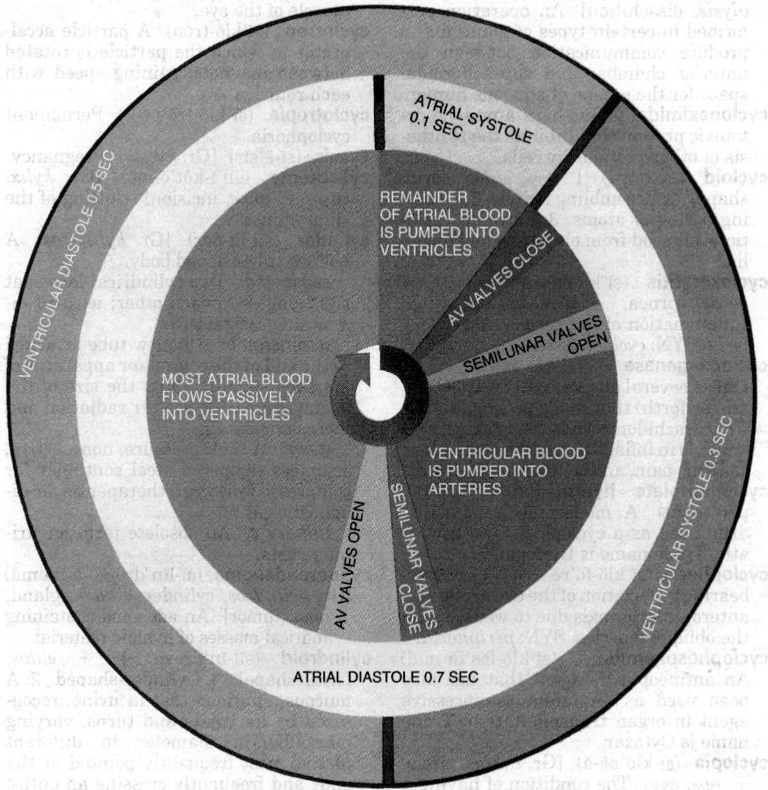

CARDIAC CYCLE (ONE HEARTBEAT, PULSE 75)

The outer circle represents the ventricles, the middle circle the atria, and the inner circle the movement of blood and its effect on the heart valves

cyclitis (sĭk-lī′tĭs) [″ + *itis,* inflammation] An inflammation of the ciliary body of the eye.

SYMPTOMS: The patient exhibits tenderness in the ciliary region, swelling of the upper lid, circumcorneal injection, deposits on Descemet's membrane, reduced or hazy vision, and increased or decreased intraocular tension. Pain in or about the eye is present, which is worse at night and on pressure. Its course is rapid and progressively unfavorable. Complications include iritis, choroiditis, scleritis, and glaucoma.

TREATMENT: Anti-inflammatory drugs such as corticosteroids are used. Cataract surgery is helpful in some cases.

plastic c. Ciliary body inflammation accompanied by inflammation of the entire uveal tract, giving rise to a fibrinous exudate in the anterior chamber and vitreous.

purulent c. Suppurative inflammation of the ciliary body and iris.

serous c. Simple inflammation of the ciliary body without iritis.

cyclizine hydrochloride An antihistamine used in treating and preventing motion sickness. Trade name is Marezine.

cyclo-, cycl- [Gr. *kyklos,* circle] **1.** Combining form meaning *circular* or pert. to a cycle. **2.** Combining form meaning pert. to the ciliary body of the eye.

cycloceratitis (sī″klō-sĕr″ă-tī′tĭs) Cyclokeratitis.

cyclochoroiditis (sī″klō-kō″royd-ī′tĭs) [″ + *chorioeides,* skinlike, + *itis,* inflammation] Inflammation of the ciliary body and choroid coat of the eye.

cyclodextrin (sī-klō-dĕks′trĭn) A molecule made of linked dextrose subunits that can be used in drug delivery in the body. Cyclodextrins have lipid centers surrounded by water-soluble exteriors. This combination allows fat-soluble medicines to be carried through the bloodstream to lipid-rich organs like the brain.

cyclodialysis (sī″klō-dī-ăl′ĭ-sĭs) [″ + *dialysis,* dissolution] An operation performed in certain types of glaucoma to produce communication between the anterior chamber and suprachoroidal space for the escape of aqueous humor.

cycloheximide (sī″klō-hĕks′ă-mīd) A cytotoxic protein that inhibits the synthesis of other proteins by cells.

cycloid (sī′kloyd) [″ + *eidos,* form, shape] **1.** Resembling a circle. **2.** Denoting a ring of atoms. **3.** Extreme variations of mood from elation to melancholia.

cyclokeratitis (sī″klō-kĕr-ă-tī′tĭs) [″ + *keras,* cornea, + *itis,* inflammation] Inflammation of the cornea and ciliary body. SYN: *cycloceratitis.*

cyclooxygenase (sī′klō-ŏks-sī″gĕn-āz) One of several enzymes (COX-1, COX-2, and so forth) that make prostaglandins from arachidonic acids. They play a central role in inflammatory diseases, blood clotting, pain, and cellular proliferation.

cyclopentolate hydrochloride (sī″klō-pĕn′tō-lāt) A moderately long-acting drug used as a cycloplegic and mydriatic. Trade name is Cyclogyl.

cyclophoria (sī″klō-fō′rē-ă) [″ + *phoros,* bearing] Deviation of the eye around its anteroposterior axis due to weakness of the oblique muscles. SYN: *periphoria.*

cyclophosphamide (sī″klō-fŏs′fă-mīd) An antineoplastic agent that has also been used as an immunosuppressive agent in organ transplantation. Trade name is Cytoxan.

cyclopia (sī-klō′pē-ă) [Gr. *kyklos,* circle, + *ops,* eye] The condition of having a single eye.

cycloplegia (sī″klō-plē′jē-ă) [″ + *plege,* a stroke] Paralysis of the ciliary muscle. This can be an anticholinergic side effect of antipsychotic or antidepressant medications.

cycloplegic (sī″klō-plē′jĭk) Producing cycloplegia.

cyclopropane (sī″klō-prō′pān) C_3H_6; a flammable anesthetic agent rarely used since the 1960s because of its potential to ignite and its adverse effects on ventilation.

cyclops (sī′klŏps) A fetal malformation in which there is only one eye. SYN: *monoculus* (2).

cycloserine (sī″klō-sĕr′ĕn) A broad-spectrum antibiotic that has been used in combination with other drugs to treat tuberculosis. It is contraindicated in patients with epilepsy and in those with depression or anxiety.

cyclosis (sī-klō′sĭs) [Gr. *kyklosis,* circulation] A streaming movement of protoplasm, as is seen in certain plant and animal cells.

cyclosporine (sī′klō-spor-een) An immunosuppressive drug useful in suppressing rejection phenomena in organ transplant recipients.

cyclotomy (sī-klŏt′ō-mē) [″ + *tome,* incision] Surgical incision of the ciliary muscle of the eye.

cyclotron (sī′klō-trŏn) A particle accelerator in which the particle is rotated between magnets, gaining speed with each rotation.

cyclotropia (sī″klō-trō′pē-ă) Permanent cyclophoria.

cyesis (sī-ē′sĭs) [Gr. *kyesis*] Pregnancy.

cylicotomy (sĭl″ĭ-kŏt′ō-mē) [Gr. *kylix,* cup, + *tome,* incision] Cutting of the ciliary muscle.

cylinder (sĭl′ĭn-dĕr) [Gr. *kylindros*] A hollow, tube-shaped body.

crossed c. Two cylindrical lenses at right angles to each other; used in diagnosing astigmatism.

extension c. A hollow tube attached to the end of the collimator apparatus of an x-ray tube. It limits the size of the beam, decreasing scatter radiation and increasing detail.

gas c. A high-pressure, nonreactive, seamless tempered steel container for compressed medical, therapeutic, or diagnostic gas.

urinary c. An obsolete term for urinary casts.

cylindroadenoma (sĭ-lĭn″drō-ăd″ē-nō′mă) [Gr. *kylindros,* cylinder,+ *aden,* gland, + *oma,* tumor] An adenoma containing cylindrical masses of hyaline material.

cylindroid (sĭl-ĭn′droyd) [″ + *eidos,* form, shape] **1.** Cylinder-shaped. **2.** A mucous, spurious cast in urine; recognized by its twists and turns, varying markedly in diameter in different places, most frequently pointed at the ends and frequently crossing an entire field. It does not usually have cellular intrusions.

cylindroma (sĭl″ĭn-drō′mă) [″ + *oma,* tumor] A skin tumor of apocrine origin usually found on the face or forehead containing a collection of cells forming cylinders.

cylindruria (sĭl″ĭn-drū′rē-ă) [″ + *ouron,* urine] The presence of cylindroids in the urine.

cymbocephalic (sĭm″bō-sĕ-făl′ĭk) [Gr. *kymbe,* boat, + *kephale,* head] Having a boat-shaped head.

cynanthropy (sĭn-ăn′thrō-pē) [Gr. *kyon,* dog, + *anthropos,* man] Insanity in which the patient behaves like a dog.

cynic spasm [Gr. *kynikos,* doglike] Spasm of the facial muscles causing a grin or snarl like a dog. SYN: *risus sardonicus.*

cynophobia (sī″nō-fō′bē-ă) [″ + *phobos,* fear] **1.** Unreasonable fear of dogs. **2.** Morbid fear of rabies. SYN: *lyssophobia* (2).

CYP3A4 One isoenzyme form of the cytochrome p450 system involved in the metabolism of many drugs. Drugs that alter this enzyme system can influence the metabolism of other agents taken by patients and cause unanticipated toxic effects.

cypridophobia (sĭp″rĭ-dō-fō′bē-ă) [Gr. *Kypris,* Venus, + *phobos,* fear] **1.** Morbid fear of sexually transmitted diseases. **2.** Abnormal fear of the sexual act. **3.** False belief of having a sexually transmitted disease.

cypriphobia (sĭp-rĭ-fō′bē-ă) Morbid aversion to and fear of coitus.

cyproheptadine hydrochloride (sī″prō-hĕp′tă-dēn) An antihistamine that can also be used to prevent headache pain. A common side effect of regular use is weight gain.

cyrtosis (sĭr-tō′sĭs) [″ + *osis,* condition] Any abnormal curvature of the spine. SEE: *kyphosis*.

cyst- SEE: *cysto-*.

cyst (sĭst) [Gr. *kystis,* bladder, sac] **1.** A closed sac or pouch, with a definite wall, that contains fluid, semifluid, or solid material. It is usually an abnormal structure resulting from developmental anomalies, obstruction of ducts, or parasitic infection. **2.** In biology, a structure formed by and enclosing certain organisms, in which they become inactive, as the cyst of certain protozoans or of the metacercariae of flukes.

adventitious c. A cyst formed around a foreign body.

alveolar c. Dilation and rupture of pulmonary alveoli to form air cysts.

apical c. A cyst near the apex of the tooth root.

blood c. Hematoma.

blue dome c. A cyst close to the surface of the breast. The blue color is caused by bleeding into the cyst.

branchial c. Cervical c.

cervical c. A closed epithelial sac derived from a branchial groove of its corresponding pharyngeal pouch. SYN: *branchial c.*

chocolate c. An ovarian cyst with darkly pigmented gelatinous contents.

colloid c. A cyst with gelatinous contents.

congenital c. A cyst present at birth resulting from abnormal development, as a dermoid cyst, imperfect closure of a structure as in spina bifida cystica, or nonclosure of embryonic clefts, ducts, or tubules, such as cervical cysts.

daughter c. A cyst growing out of the walls of another cyst.

dental c. A cyst that forms from any of the odontogenic tissues.

dentigerous c. A fluid-filled cyst usually surrounding the crown of an unerupted tooth; often involves incomplete enamel formation. SYN: *eruption c.; follicular c.; follicular odontoma*. SEE: *dermoid c.*

dermoid c. **1.** An ovarian teratoma. **2.** A nonmalignant cystic tumor containing elements derived from the ectoderm, such as hair, teeth, or skin. These tumors occur frequently in the ovary but may develop in other organs such as the lungs.

distention c. A cyst formed in a natural enclosed cavity, as a follicular cyst of the ovary.

echinococcus c. Hydatid c.

epidermoid c. A cyst filled with keratin, sebum, and skin debris that may form on the scalp, the back of the neck, or the axilla. It is benign, but can be removed surgically. SYN: *sebaceous c.*

eruption c. Dentigerous c.

extravasation c. A cyst arising from hemorrhage or escape of other body fluids into tissues.

exudation c. A cyst caused by trapping of an exudate in a closed area.

follicular c. A cyst arising from a follicle, as a follicular cyst of the thyroid gland, the ovary, or a forming tooth. SYN: *dentigerous c.*

Gartner's c. A cyst developing from a vestigial mesonephric duct (Gartner's duct) in a female.

hydatid c. A cyst formed by the growth of the larval form of *Echinococcus granulosus,* usually in the liver. SYN: *echinococcus c.*

implantation c. A cyst resulting from displacement of portions of the epidermis as may occur in injuries.

intraligamentary c. A cystic formation between the layers of the broad ligament.

involutional c. A cyst occurring in the normal involution of an organ or structure, as in the mammary gland.

keratin c. A cyst containing keratin.

meibomian c. Chalazion.

meniscus c. A fluid-filled cyst often associated with a degenerative horizontal meniscal tear, more frequently seen in the lateral meniscus of the knee. This ganglion-like cyst is a palpable mass at the joint line of the knee and can be visualized by arthrography and magnetic resonance imaging.

morgagnian c. A cystlike remnant of the müllerian duct that is attached to the fallopian tube.

mother c. A hydatid cyst enveloping smaller ones.

mucous c. A retention cyst composed of mucus.

nabothian c. SEE: *nabothian cyst.*

odontogenic c. A cyst associated with the teeth, such as a dentigerous or radicular cyst.

ovarian c. A cyst in the ovary. SEE: *ovary*.

parasitic c. A cyst enclosing the larval form of certain parasites, as the cysticercus or hydatid of tapeworms or the larva of certain nematodes (i.e., *Trichinella*).

parovarian c. A cyst of the parovarium.

pilar c. An epithelial cyst with a wall that resembles the follicular epithelium. It is filled with a homogeneous mixture of keratin and lipid. SYN: *trichilemma c.*

pilonidal c. A cyst in the sacrococcygeal region, usually at the upper end of the intergluteal cleft. It is due to a developmental defect that permits epithelial tissue to be trapped below the skin. This type of cyst may become symptomatic in early adulthood when an infected draining sinus forms. SYN: *pilonidal fistula.*

popliteal c. Baker's cyst.

porencephalic c. An anomalous cavity of the brain that communicates with the ventricular system.

proliferative c. A cyst lined with epithelium that proliferates, forming projections that extend into the cavity of the cyst.

radicular c. A granulomatous cyst located alongside the root of a tooth.

retention c. A cyst retaining the secretion of a gland, as in a mucous or sebaceous cyst.

sebaceous c. Epidermoid c.

seminal c. A cyst of the epididymis, ductus deferens, or other sperm-carrying ducts that contain semen.

suprasellar c. A cyst of the hypophyseal stalk just above the floor of the sella turcica. Its wall is frequently calcified or ossified.

trichilemma c. Pilar c.

tubo-ovarian c. An ovarian cyst that ruptures into the lumen of an adherent uterine tube.

unilocular c. A cyst containing only one cavity.

vaginal c. A cyst in the vagina.

vitelline c. A congenital cyst of the gastrointestinal canal. Lined with ciliated epithelium, it is the remains of the omphalomesenteric duct.

cystadenocarcinoma (sĭs-tăd″ē-nō-kăr″sĭ-nō′mă) [Gr. *kystis,* bladder, + *aden,* gland, + *karkinos,* crab, + *oma,* tumor] A glandular malignancy that forms cysts as it grows.

cystadenoma (sĭst″ăd-ĕn-ō′mă) [″ + ″ + *oma,* tumor] An adenoma containing cysts; cystoma blended with adenoma.

pseudomucinous c. A cyst filled with a thick, viscid fluid and lined with tall epithelial cells.

serous c. A cyst filled with a clear serous fluid and lined with cuboidal epithelial cells.

cystalgia (sĭs-tăl′jē-ă) [″ + *algos,* pain] Pain in the bladder. SYN: *cystodynia.*

cystathionine (sĭs″tă-thī′ō-nĭn) $C_7H_{14}N_2O_4S$; an intermediate compound in the metabolism of methionine to cysteine.

cystathioninuria (sĭs″tă-thī″ō-nĭ-nū′rē-ă) A hereditary disease caused by a deficiency of the enzyme important in metabolizing cystathionine, resulting in mental retardation, thrombocytopenia, and acidosis.

cystectasy (sĭs-tĕk′tă-sē) [″ + *ektasis,* dilatation] **1.** An operation for extracting a stone from the bladder by dividing the membranous portion of the urethra and then dilating the neck of the bladder. **2.** Dilatation of the bladder.

cystectomy (sĭs-tĕk′tō-mē) [″ + *ektome,* excision] **1.** Removal of a cyst. **2.** Excision of the cystic duct and the gallbladder, or just the cystic duct. **3.** Excision of the urinary bladder or a part of it.

cysteic acid $C_3H_7NO_5S$; acid produced by the oxidation of cysteine. Further oxidation produces taurine.

cysteine hydrochloride (sĭs′tē-ĭn, sĭs-tē′ĭn) An amino acid, $C_3H_7NO_2S \cdot HCl \cdot H_2O$, containing sulfur and found in many proteins. It is valuable as a source of sulfur in metabolism.

cystelcosis (sĭs″tĕl-kō′sĭs) [″ + *helkosis,* ulceration] Ulceration of the urinary bladder.

cystic (sĭs′tĭk) [Gr. *kystis,* bladder] **1.** Of or pert. to a cyst. **2.** Pert. to the gallbladder. **3.** Pert. to the urinary bladder.

cysticercoid (sĭs″tĭ-sĕr′koyd) [″ + *kerkos,* tail, + *eidos,* form, shape] The larval encysted form of a tapeworm. It differs from a cysticercus in having a much reduced bladder.

cysticercosis (sĭs″tĭ-sĕr-kō′sĭs) [″ + ″ + *osis,* condition] Infestation with the larvae of the pork tapeworm. It occurs when ingested *Taenia solium* larvae from uncooked pork burrow through the intestinal wall and are carried to other tissues through the blood. They may encyst in the heart, eye, muscles, or brain. In the brain, they may cause a wide variety of neurological symptoms, including seizures. A patient history of eating undercooked pork or other meats may be helpful in establishing the diagnosis, esp. in adults with new-onset seizures who are found to have multiple cystic lesions in the brain.

TREATMENT: Anticonvulsants are used to control seizures. Antiparasitic drugs such as praziquantel or albendazole are effective.

cysticercus (sĭs″tĭ-sĕr′kŭs) *pl.* **cysticerci** The encysted larval form of a tapeworm, consisting of a rounded cyst or bladder into which the scolex is invaginated. SYN: *bladder worm.*

c. cellulosae The bladder worm that is the larva of the pork tapeworm, *Taenia solium.*

cystic fibrosis ABBR: CF. A potentially fatal autosomal recessive disease that manifests itself in multiple body systems including the lungs, the pancreas, the urogenital system, the skeleton, and the skin; it causes chronic obstructive pulmonary disease, frequent lung infections, deficient elaboration of pancreatic enzymes, osteoporosis, and an abnormally high electrolyte concentration in the sweat. The name is derived from the characteristic histologic changes in the pancreas. CF usually begins in infancy and is the major cause of severe chronic lung disease in children. In the U.S., CF occurs in 1 in 2500 white live births and 1 in 17,000 black live births. Also called *fibrocystic disease of pancreas*. SYN: *mucoviscidosis*.

SYMPTOMS: A great variety of clinical manifestations may be present, including nasal polyposis; bronchiectasis; bronchitis; pneumonia; respiratory failure; gallbladder diseases; intussusception; meconium ileus; salt depletion; pancreatic exocrine deficiency causing intestinal malabsorption of fats, proteins, and, to a lesser extent, carbohydrates; pancreatitis; peptic ulcer; rectal prolapse; diabetes; nutritional deficiencies; arthritis; absent vas deferens with consequent aspermia and absence of fructose in the ejaculate; failure to thrive; and delayed puberty.

TREATMENT: Therapy must be individualized, carefully monitored, and continued throughout life. Pulmonary infection is controlled with antibiotics. It is essential that secretions be cleared from the airway by intermittent aerosol therapy. A mucolytic agent such as *N*-acetylcysteine may be helpful, as well as postural drainage, mist inhalation, and bronchodilator therapy. Bronchoalveolar lavage has been of use in some patients. In addition, bronchial drainage may be improved by use of aerosolized recombinant human DNase (rhDNase). Use of a Flutter device for airway mucus clearance is considerably more effective in increasing sputum expectoration than traditional postural drainage and clapping the chest. Lung transplantation may also be used to treat CF. High doses of ibuprofen taken consistently for years may slow progression of the disease, by limiting airway inflammation. SEE: *bronchoalveolar lavage; Flutter device*.

PROGNOSIS: Median cumulative survival is approximately 30 years, with males surviving much longer than females for unknown reasons.

PATIENT CARE: Both patient and family are taught to perform pulmonary chest physiotherapy followed by deep breathing and coughing to help mobilize secretions. Fluid intake is encouraged to thin inspissated secretions. Humidified air, with intermittent positive-pressure breathing therapy if prescribed, is provided; and prescribed pancreatic enzyme replacement is administered with meals and snacks. Dornase alpha is also administered by nebulizer as prescribed. A DNA enzyme produced by recombinant gene therapy, the drug is used to reduce the frequency of respiratory infections, to decrease sputum thickness (viscosity), and to improve pulmonary functioning in patients with cystic fibrosis.

The patient should take precautions (e.g., annual influenza immunization and at least one pneumococcal vaccination) to prevent respiratory infections, and should learn to recognize and report signs and symptoms and to initiate prescribed antibiotic prophylaxis promptly. A well-balanced high-calorie, high-protein diet is recommended, including replacement of fat-soluble vitamins if laboratory analysis indicates any deficiencies. Aerobic exercise and physical activity within permitted limits are encouraged; breathing exercises should be performed during activity to improve ventilatory capacity and activity tolerance. The child is encouraged in age-appropriate developmental tasks, and acceptable activities are substituted for those in which the child is unable to participate.

Caregivers involve the child in care by offering valid choices and encouraging decision making. The family is encouraged to discuss their feelings and concerns. Genetic testing is explained. Realistic reassurance is offered regarding expectations after an exacerbation, and emotional support is provided to help both patient and family work through feelings of anticipatory grief. Referral is made to available local chapters of support groups such as the Cystic Fibrosis Foundation. SEE: *Nursing Diagnoses Appendix*.

cysticotomy (sĭs″tĭ-kŏt′ō-mē) [″ + *tome,* incision] Incision of cystic bile duct. SYN: *choledochotomy*.

cystiform (sĭs′tĭ-form) [″ + L. *forma,* form] Having the form of a cyst.

cystigerous (sĭs-tĭj′ĕr-ŭs) [″ + L. *gerere,* to bear] Containing cysts.

cystine (sĭs′tēn) [Gr. *kystis,* bladder] $C_6H_{12}N_2S_2O_4$; a sulfur-containing amino acid, produced by the action of acids on proteins that contain this compound. It is an important source of sulfur in metabolism.

cystinemia (sĭs″tĭ-nē′mē-ă) [*cystine* + Gr. *haima,* blood] The presence of cystine in the blood.

cystinosis (sĭs′tĭ-nō′sĭs) [″ + Gr. *osis,* condition] An inherited disease of cystine metabolism resulting in abnormal deposition of cystine in body tissues. The cause is disordered proximal renal tubular function. Clinically, failure to grow is accompanied by the development of rickets, corneal opacities, acidosis, and deposition of cystine in tissues. SYN: *cystine storage disease*.

cystinuria (sĭs″tĭ-nū′rē-ă) [″ + *ouron,* urine] **1.** The presence of cystine in the urine. **2.** A hereditary metabolic disorder characterized by excretion of large amounts of cystine, lysine, arginine, and ornithine in the urine. It results in the development of recurrent urinary calculi.

cystitis (sĭs-tī′tĭs) [Gr. *kystis,* bladder, + *itis,* inflammation] Bladder inflammation usually occurring as a result of a urinary tract infection. Associated organs (kidney, prostate, urethra) may be involved. This condition may be acute or chronic. SEE: *Nursing Diagnoses Appendix.*

SYMPTOMS: Cystitis is marked by urinary urgency, frequency, and pain. Bladder spasms and perineal aching or fullness are also reported.

TREATMENT: Antibiotics are useful in treating the infection, but more definitive therapy is required if the basic cause is a kidney stone or a structural defect in the urinary tract such as obstruction.

PATIENT CARE: The patient is assessed for pain, burning, urinary frequency, bladder spasms, chills, and fever. The urinary bladder is palpated and percussed for distention. Volume and frequency of urinary output are monitored, and urine is inspected for cloudiness and gross hematuria. A clean-catch or catheterized specimen is sent to the laboratory for urinalysis and culture and sensitivity tests. Oral fluid intake is encouraged to dilute urine and to decrease pain on voiding. Heat is applied to the lower abdomen to decrease bladder spasms. Urinary antiseptics, analgesics, and antibiotics are administered and evaluated for therapeutic effectiveness and any adverse reactions. The patient is warned that urinary antiseptics such as phenazopyridine hydrochloride (Pyridium) will color the urine reddish orange and may stain fabric. The importance of follow-up urinalysis and culture testing to ensure that the cause of cystitis has been eliminated is emphasized.

interstitial c. A chronically painful inflammatory bladder condition, the etiology of which is often undetermined. It sometimes occurs as a result of exposure to drugs such as cyclophosphamide or ciprofloxacin but more often is idiopathic.

Most commonly, the disease is seen in women 30 to 70 years of age. The disease is not life-threatening, but the pain can make a patient's life intolerable. The most common symptoms are urinary frequency, nocturia, and suprapubic pain on bladder filling. There is no curative medical therapy, but hydraulic distention of the bladder, intravesical instillations, transcutaneous electrical nerve stimulation, and antidepressants, as well as a variety of alternative medicines, have been tried, with variable success. Some patients are treated with urinary diversion procedures or cystectomy. If these fail, the tricyclic antidepressant amitriptyline has been beneficial. Transcutaneous electrical nerve stimulation and intravesical heparin instillation have also been used.

cystitome (sĭs′tĭ-tōm) [″ + *tome,* incision] Instrument for incision into the sac of the crystalline lens.

cystitomy (sĭs-tĭt′ō-mē) **1.** Surgical incision of a cavity. **2.** Incision of the capsule of the crystalline lens. **3.** Incision into the gallbladder. SYN: *cholecystotomy.*

cysto-, cyst- [Gr. *kystis,* bladder] Combining form denoting a relationship to the urinary bladder or a cyst.

cystoadenoma (sĭs″tō-ăd″ĕ-nō′mă) [″ + *aden,* gland, + *oma,* tumor] A tumor containing cystic and adenomatous elements.

cystocele (sĭs′tō-sēl) [″ + *kele,* tumor, swelling] A bladder hernia that protrudes into the vagina. Injury to the vesicovaginal fascia during delivery may allow the bladder to pouch into the vagina, causing a cystocele. It may cause urinary frequency, urgency, and dysuria. SYN: *vesicocele.*

cystocolostomy (sĭs″tō-kō-lŏs′tō-mē) [″ + *kolon,* colon, + *stoma,* mouth] Formation of communication between the gallbladder and colon.

cystodiaphanoscopy (sĭs″tō-dī″ă-făn-ŏs′kō-pē) [″ + *dia,* through, + *phanein,* to shine, + *skopein,* to examine] Transillumination of the abdomen by an electric light in the bladder.

cystodynia (sĭs″tō-dĭn′ē-ă) [″ + *odyne,* pain] Cystalgia.

cystoelytroplasty (sĭs″tō-ē-lĭt′rō-plăs-tē) [″ + *elytron,* sheath, + *plassein,* to form] Repair of a vesicovaginal fistula.

cystoepiplocele (sĭs″tō-ē-pĭp′lō-sēl) [″ + *epiploon,* omentum, + *kele,* tumor, swelling] Herniation of a portion of the bladder and the omentum.

cystoepithelioma (sĭs″tō-ĕp″ĭ-thē″lē-ō′mă) [″ + *epi,* upon, + *thele,* nipple, + *oma,* tumor] Epithelioma in the stage of cystic degeneration.

cystofibroma (sĭs″tō-fī-brō′mă) [″ + L. *fibra,* fiber, + Gr. *oma,* tumor] Fibrous tumor containing cysts.

cystogastrostomy (sĭs″tō-găs-trŏs′tō-mē) [″ + *gaster,* stomach, + *stoma,* mouth] Joining an adjacent cyst, usually of the pancreas, to the stomach.

cystogram (sĭs′tō-grăm) [″ + *gramma,* something written] A radiograph of the bladder.

cystography (sĭs-tŏg′ră-fē) [″ + *graphein,* to write] Radiography of any cyst into which a contrast medium has been instilled, esp. the bladder.

cystoid (sĭs′toyd) [″ + *eidos,* form, shape] Resembling a cyst.

cystojejunostomy (sĭs″tō-jē-jū-nŏs′tō-mē) [″ + L. *jejunum,* empty, + Gr. *stoma,* mouth] Joining of an adjacent cyst to the jejunum.

cystolith (sĭs′tō-lĭth) [″ + *lithos,* stone] Vesical calculus.

cystolithectomy (sĭs-tō-lĭ-thĕk′tō-mē) [″ + *lithos,* stone, + *ektome,* excision] Excision of a stone from the bladder.

cystolithiasis (sĭs-tō-lĭ-thī′ă-sĭs) [Gr.

kystis, bladder, + *lithos,* stone, + *-iasis,* condition] Formation of stones in the bladder.

cystolithic (sĭs″tō-lĭth′ĭk) Pert. to a bladder stone.

cystolitholapaxy (sĭs′tō-lĭth-ăl-ō-pĕk-sē) The removal of a kidney stone from the bladder by crushing the particles and extracting them by irrigation.

cystolutein (sĭs″tō-loo′tē-ĭn) [″ + L. *luteus,* yellow] Yellow pigment found in some ovarian cysts.

cystoma (sĭs-tō′mă) *pl.* **cystomata, cystomas** [″ + *oma,* tumor] A cystic tumor; a growth containing cysts.

cystometer (sĭs-tŏm′ĕ-tĕr) [″ + *metron,* measure] A device for estimating the capacity of the bladder and pressure changes in it during micturition.

cystometrography (sĭs″tō-mĕ-trŏg′ră-fē) [″ + ″ + *graphein,* to write] A graphic record of the pressure in the bladder at varying stages of filling.

cystomorphous (sĭs″tō-mor′fŭs) [″ + *morphe,* form] Cystlike; cystoid.

cystopexy (sĭs′tō-pĕk″sē) [″ + *pexis,* fixation] Surgical fixation of the bladder to the wall of the abdomen.

cystoplasty (sĭs′tō-plăs″tē) [″ + *plassein,* to form] Plastic operation on the bladder.

cystoplegia (sĭs″tō-plē′jē-ă) [″ + *plege,* stroke] Paralysis of the bladder.

cystoproctostomy (sĭs″tō-prŏk-tŏs′tō-mē) [″ + *proktos,* rectum, + *stoma,* mouth] Surgical formation of a connection between the urinary bladder and the rectum.

cystoptosia, cystoptosis (sĭs″tŏp-tō′sē-ă, -sĭs) [″ + *ptosis,* a dropping] Prolapse into the urethra of the vesical mucous membrane.

cystoradiography (sĭs″tō-rā″dē-ŏg′ră-fē) [″ + L. *radius,* ray, + Gr. *graphein,* to write] Radiography of the gallbladder or urinary bladder.

cystorrhaphy (sĭst-or′ă-fē) [″ + *rhaphe,* seam, ridge] Surgical suture of the bladder.

cystorrhea (sĭs″tō-rē′ă) [″ + *rhoia,* flow] A discharge of mucus from the urinary bladder.

cystorrhexis [″ + *rhexis,* rupture] Rupture of the bladder.

cystosarcoma (sĭs″tō-săr-kō′mă) [″ + *sarx,* flesh, + *oma,* tumor] A sarcoma containing cysts or cystic formations.

cystoscope (sĭst′ō-skōp) [″ + *skopein,* to examine] An instrument for interior examination of bladder and ureter. It is introduced through the urethra into the bladder.

cystoscopy (sĭs-tŏs′kō-pē) [″ + *skopein,* to examine] Examination of the bladder with a cystoscope.

cystospasm (sĭs′tō-spăzm) [Gr. *kystis,* bladder, + *spasmos,* a convulsion] A spasmodic contraction of the urinary bladder.

cystostomy (sĭs-tŏs′tō-mē) [″ + *stoma,* mouth] Surgical incision into the bladder.

cystotome (sĭs′tō-tōm) [″ + *tome,* incision] An instrument for incision of the bladder.

cystotomy (sĭs-tŏt′ō-mē) [″ + *tome,* incision] Incision of the bladder.

suprapubic c. Surgical opening of the bladder from just above the symphysis pubis.

cystotrachelotomy (sĭs″tō-trā″kē-lŏt′ō-mē) [″ + *trachelos,* neck, + *tome,* incision] Incision into the neck of the bladder.

cystoureteritis (sĭs″tō-ū-rē″tĕr-ī′tĭs) [″ + *oureter,* ureter, + *itis,* inflammation] Inflammation of the ureter and urinary bladder.

cystoureterogram (sĭs″tō-ū-rē′tĕr-ō-grăm) [″ + ″ + *gramma,* something written] A radiograph of the bladder and ureter obtained after instillation of a contrast medium.

cystourethritis (sĭs″tō-ū″rē-thrī′tĭs) [″ + *ourethra,* urethra, + *itis,* inflammation] Inflammation of the urinary bladder and urethra.

cystourethrocele (sĭs″tō-ū-rē′thrō-sēl) [″ + ″ + *kele,* tumor, swelling] Prolapse of the bladder and urethra of the female.

cystourethrography (sĭs″tō-ū-rē-thrŏg′ră-fē) [″ + ″ + *graphein,* to write] Radiography of the bladder and urethra by use of a radiopaque contrast medium.

chain c. Radiography in which a sterile beaded radiopaque chain is introduced into the bladder by means of a special catheter so that one end of the chain is in the bladder and the other extends outside via the urethra. This examination is useful in demonstrating anatomical relationships, esp. in women with persistent urinary incontinence.

voiding c. Cystourethrography done before, during, and after voiding.

cystourethropexy, retropubic A general term for a surgical procedure for correction of stress urinary incontinence.

cystourethroscope (sĭs″tō-ū-rē′thrō-skōp) [″ + *ourethra,* urethra, + *skopein,* to examine] A device for examining the posterior urethra and urinary bladder.

cystovesiculography (sĭs″tō-vĕ-sĭk-ū-lŏg′ră-fē) Radiography of the bladder and seminal vesicles after instillation of a contrast medium.

cyt- SEE: *cyto-.*

cytarabine (sī-tăr′ă-bēn) A drug originally developed as an antileukemic agent, also used in treating herpesvirus hominis infections that cause either keratitis or encephalitis. SYN: *cytosine arabinoside; ara-C.* SEE: *ara-A.*

-cyte (sīt) [Gr. *kytos,* cell] Suffix denoting cell.

cytidine (sī′tĭ-dĭn) A nucleoside that is one of the four main riboside components of ribonucleic acid. It consists of a cytosine and D-ribose.

cyto-, cyt- [Gr. *kytos,* cell] Combining form meaning *cell.*

cytoanalyzer (sī″tō-ăn″ă-lī′zĕr) An automated device for detecting malignant cells in microscopic preparations or in fluids. It is used in conjunction with professional analysis.

cytoarchitectonic (sī″tō-ărk″ĭ-tĕk-tŏn′ĭk) [″ + *architektonike,* architecture] Pert. to structure and arrangement of cells.

cytobiology (sī″tō-bī-ŏl′ō-jē) [″ + *bios,* life, + *logos,* word, reason] Biology of cells.

cytobiotaxis (sī″tō-bī-ō-tăk′sĭs) [″ + ″ + *taxis,* arrangement] The influence of living cells on other living cells. SYN: *cytoclesis*.

cytoblast (sī′tō-blăst) [″ + *blastos,* germ] A cell nucleus. SEE: *cyton*.

cytocentrum (sī″tō-sĕn′trŭm) [″ + *kentron,* center] A minute body in the cytoplasm of a cell close to the nucleus. SYN: *centrosome*. SEE: *sphere, attraction*.

cytochalasin B (sī″tō-kăl′ă-sĭn) A chemical that destroys the contractile microfilaments in cells. This fragments cells and permits the fragments to be investigated.

cytochemistry (sī″tō-kĕm′ĭs-trē) The chemistry of the living cell.

cytochrome (sī′tō-krōm) [″ + *chroma,* color] An iron-containing protein found in the mitochondria of eukaryotic cells; each is given a letter name (a, b, c). The cytochrome transport system (electron transport chain) is the last stage in aerobic cell respiration. SEE: *c. oxidase; c. P450; cytochrome transport system*.

c. P450 A group of enzymes present in every type of cell in the body except red blood cells and skeletal muscle cells. They are important in metabolizing substances normally present in the body such as steroids, fat-soluble vitamins, fatty acids, prostaglandins, and alkaloids. The P450 enzymes also detoxify drugs and a great number of environmental pollutants, such as carcinogens present in tobacco smoke and charcoal-broiled meat, polychlorinated biphenyls, and dioxin. Specialized types of cytochrome P450 are involved in the synthesis of nitric oxide.

cytochylema (sī″tō-kī-lē′mă) [Gr. *kytos,* cell, + *chylos,* juice] Hyaloplasm.

cytocidal (sī″tō-sī′dăl) [″ + L. *caedere,* to kill] Lethal to cells.

cytocide (sī′tō-sīd) An agent that kills cells.

cytoclasis (sī″tŏk′lă-sĭs) [″ + *klasis,* destruction] Destruction of cells.

cytoclastic [″ + *klasis,* destruction] Destructive to cells.

cytoclesis (sī″tō-klē′sĭs) [″ + *klesis,* a call] Cytobiotaxis.

cytodendrite (sī″tō-dĕn′drīt) [″ + *dendron,* tree] An obsolete term for dendrite.

cytodiagnosis (sī″tō-dī″ăg-nō′sĭs) [″ + *dia,* through, + *gignoskein,* to know] Diagnosis of pathogenic conditions by the study of cells present in exudates, fluids, and so forth.

cytodieresis (sī″tō-dī-ĕr′ē-sĭs) [″ + *diairesis,* division] Cytokinesis.

cytodistal (sī″tō-dĭs′tăl) [″ + *distare,* to be distant] Pert. to a neoplasm remote from the cell of origin.

cytogenesis (sī″tō-jĕn′ĕs-ĭs) [″ + *genesis,* generation, birth] Origin and development of the cell.

cytogenetics (sī″tō-jĕ-nĕt′ĭks) The study of the structure and function of chromosomes. Clinically, the science of cytogenetics has been applied to the diagnosis and management of congenital disorders. The diagnosis of some fetal abnormalities can be made by chromosomal analysis of chorionic villus samples as early as 8 to 14 weeks' gestation. SEE: *amniocentesis; chorionic villus sampling*.

cytogenic (sī-tō-jĕn′ĭk) [″ + *gennan,* to produce] Producing cells or promoting the production of cells.

cytogenous (si-tŏj′ĕn-ŭs) [″ + *gennan,* to produce] Producing cells.

cytogeny (sī-tŏj′ĕ-nē) [″ + *genesis,* generation, birth] The formation and development of the cell.

cytogerontology The study of cell aging developed by Leonard Hayflick.

cytoglycopenia (sī″tō-glī-kō-pē′nē-ă) [″ + *glykys,* sweet, + *penia,* poverty] Deficient glucose of blood cells; also called cytoglucopenia.

cytohistogenesis (sī″tō-hĭs″tō-jĕn′ĕ-sĭs) [″ + *histos,* web, + *genesis,* generation, birth] The structural development of cells.

cytohyaloplasm (sī″tō-hī′ăl-ō-plăzm) [″ + *hyalos,* glass, + LL. *plasma,* form, mold] Cytoplasm.

cytoid (sī′toyd) [″ + *eidos,* form, shape] Resembling a cell.

cytoinhibition (sī″tō-ĭn″hĭ-bĭsh′ŭn) [″ + L. *inhibere,* to restrain] Phagocytic cell action that prevents the destruction of ingested bacteria by the cell.

cytokine One of more than 100 distinct proteins produced primarily by white blood cells. They provide signals to regulate immunological aspects of cell growth and function during both inflammation and specific immune response. Each cytokine is secreted by a specific cell in response to a specific stimulus. Cytokines produced by monocytes or macrophages and lymphocytes are called monokines and lymphokines, respectively. Cytokines include the interleukins, interferons, tumor necrosis factors, erythropoietin, and colony-stimulating factors. They act by changing the cells that produce them (autocrine effect) and altering other cells close to them (paracrine effect); a few affect cells systemically (endocrine effect).

SEE: *granulocyte-macrophage colony-stimulating factor; immune response; inflammation; interferon; interleukin; macrophage; tumor necrosis factor.*

cytokinesis (sī″tō-kĭ-nē′sĭs) [″ + *kinesis,* movement] The separation of the cytoplasm into two parts, which occurs in the latter stages of mitosis or cell division. SYN: *cytodieresis.*

cytologist A person trained in cytology.

cytology (sī-tŏl′ō-jē) [″ + *logos,* word, reason] The science that deals with the formation, structure, and function of cells.

cytolymph (sī′tō-lĭmf) [″ + L. *lympha,* lymph] Hyaloplasm.

cytolysin (sī-tŏl′ĭ-sĭn) [″ + *lysis,* dissolution] An antibody that causes disintegration of cells.

cytolysis (sī-tŏl′ĭ-sĭs) Dissolution or destruction of living cells.

cytomegalovirus (sī″tō-mĕg″ă-lō-vī′rŭs) A widely distributed species-specific herpesvirus; in humans, it inhabits many different tissues and causes cytomegalic inclusion disease. A mother with a latent infection may transmit the virus to her fetus either transplacentally or at the time of birth. The virus may also be transmitted by blood transfusion. Although it is usually not harmful to those with functional immune systems, it may cause a fatal pneumonia in immunocompromised patients. Cytomegalovirus may infect the retina and cause blindness in AIDS patients.

cytomegalovirus infection ABBR: CMV infection. A persistent, latent infection of white blood cells caused by cytomegalovirus (CMV), a beta-group herpesvirus. Approx. 60% of persons over age 35 have been infected with CMV, usually during childhood or early adulthood; the incidence appears to be higher in persons with low socioeconomic status. Primary infection is usually mild in persons with normal immune function, but CMV can be reactivated and cause overt disease in pregnant women, persons with AIDS, or those receiving immunosuppressive therapy following organ transplantation. SEE: *Nursing Diagnoses Appendix.*

During pregnancy, the woman can transmit the virus to the fetus, with devastating results. Approx 10% of infected infants develop CMV inclusion disease, marked by anemia, thrombocytopenia, purpura, hepatosplenomegaly, microcephaly, and abnormal mental or motor development; more than 50% of these infants die. Most fetal infections occur when the mother is infected with CMV for the first time during this pregnancy, but they may also occur following reinfection or reactivation of the virus. Patients with AIDS or organ transplants may develop disseminated infection that causes retinitis, esophagitis, colitis, meningoencephalitis, pneumonitis, and inflammation of the renal tubules.

ETIOLOGY: CMV is transmitted from person to person by sexual activity, during pregnancy or delivery, during organ transplantation, or by contaminated secretions; rarely (<5%) blood transfusions contain latent CMV. Health care workers caring for infected newborns or immunosuppressed patients are at no greater risk for acquiring CMV infection than are those who care for other groups of patients (approx. 3%). Pregnant women and all health care workers should strictly adhere to standard infection control precautions.

SYMPTOMS: Primary infection in healthy persons is usually asymptomatic, but some persons develop mononucleosis-type symptoms (fever, sore throat, swollen glands). Symptoms in immunosuppressed patients are related to the organ system infected by CMV and include blurred vision progressing to blindness; severe diarrhea; and cough, dyspnea, and hypoxemia. Antibodies seen in the blood identify infection but do not protect against reactivation of the virus.

TREATMENT: Antiviral agents such as ganciclovir and foscarnet are used to treat retinitis, colitis, and pneumonitis in immunosuppressed patients; chronic antiviral therapy has been used to suppress CMV, but this protocol has not been effective in preventing recurrence of CMV or development of meningoencephalitis. Ganciclovir has limited effect in congenital CMV. No vaccine is available.

cytometaplasia (sī″tō-mĕt″ă-plā′zē-ă) [Gr. *kytos,* cell, + *metaplasis,* change] Change in form or function of cells.

cytometer (sī-tŏm′ĕ-ter) [″ + *metron,* measure] An instrument for counting and measuring cells.

flow c. A device for measuring thousands of cells as they are forced one at a time through a focused light beam, usually a laser. Cells studied by this device need to be in an evenly dispersed suspension.

cytometry (sī-tŏm′ĕ-trē) The counting and measuring of cells.

flow c. A technique for analyzing individual cells passing through a detector system. In one method, the cells are tagged with a monoclonal antibody carrying a fluorescent label. They pass through the detector at about 10,000 cells per second. Flow cytometry has many clinical and research applications. These include analysis of cell size, structure, and viability; examination of DNA and RNA in the cells; determination of pH in the cells; and chromosome analysis. Flow cytometry is also used to determine the percentages of cells in various stages of development in a population, making it possible to estimate

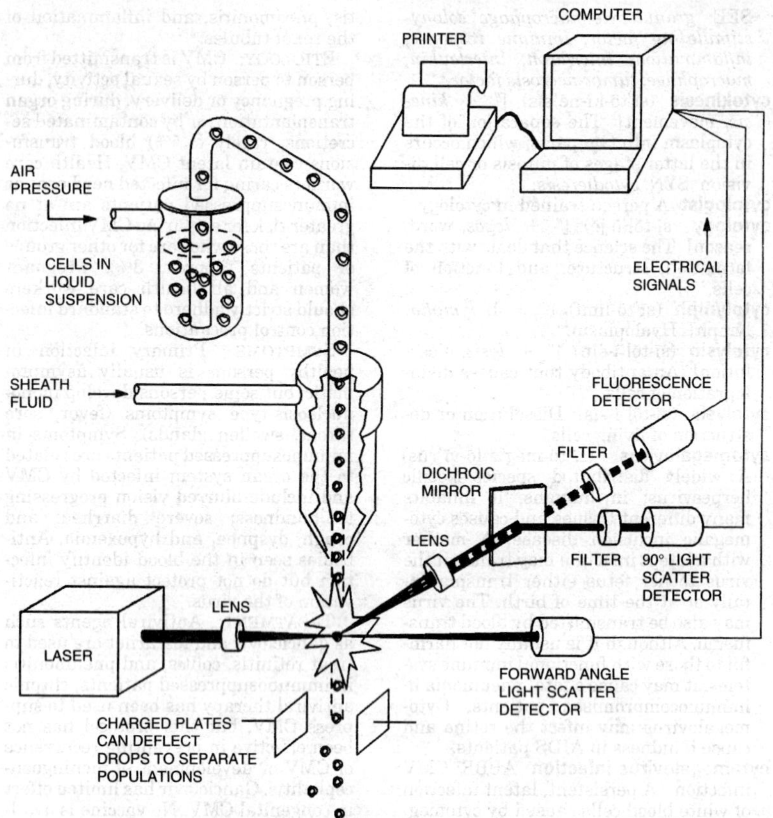

FLOW CYTOMETRY

Components of a laser-based flow cytometer

the extent or controllability of a malignant tumor. Monitoring the number of populations of T cells, B cells, and T helper and suppressor cells, and using that information to calculate the helper : suppressor ratio, assists in determining the patient's immune status. Flow cytometry has been used in monitoring survival of transplanted organs and tissues such as bone marrow. SEE: illus.; *cell sorting*.

cytomicrosome (sī-tō-mī′krō-sōm) [″ + *mikros,* small, + *soma,* body] One of the minute granules in the protoplasm (cytoplasm) of the cell.

cytomitome (sī″tō-mī′tōm) [″ + *mitos,* thread] Any part of the network of the cytoplasm.

cytomorphology (sī″tō-mor-fŏl′ō-jē) [″ + *morphe,* form, + *logos,* word, reason] The study of the structure of cells.

cytomorphosis (sī″tō-mor-fō′sĭs) [″ + ″ + *osis,* condition] The cellular transformations that a cell undergoes during its life.

cyton (sī′tŏn) [Gr. *kytos,* cell] **1.** A cell. **2.** The cell body of a neuron. SYN: *perikaryon*.

cytopathic (sī″tō-păth′ĭk) [″ + *pathos,* disease] Concerning pathological changes in cells, esp. those injured or destroyed by viruses or other microorganisms. SYN: *cytopathogenic*.

cytopathogenic (sī″tō-păth″ō-jĕn′ĭk) [″ + *pathos,* disease, + *gennan,* to produce] Cytopathic.

cytopathology (sī″tō-păth-ŏl′ō-jē) [″ + ″ + *logos,* word, reason] The study of the cellular changes in disease.

cytopenia [″ + *penia,* lack] Diminution of cellular elements in blood or other tissues.

cytophagocytosis (sī″tō-făg″ō-sī-tō′sĭs) [″ + *phagein,* to eat, + *kytos,* cell, + *osis,* condition] Cytophagy.

cytophagy (sī-tŏf′ă-jē) The destruction of other cells by phagocytes. SYN: *cytophagocytosis*.

cytophotometry SEE: *flow cytometry*.

cytophylaxis (sī″tō-fī-lăk′sĭs) [″ + *phylaxis,* protection] The protection of cells against lysis.

cytophyletic (sī″tō-fī-lĕt′ĭk) [″ + *phyle,* tribe] Pert. to the genealogy of cells.
cytophysics (sī″tō-fĭz′ĭks) [″ + *physike,* (study of) nature] The physics of cellular activity.
cytophysiology (sī″tō-fĭz-ē-ŏl′ō-jē) [″ + *physis,* nature, + *logos,* word, reason] Physiology of the cell.
cytoplasm (sī′tō-plăzm) [″ + LL. *plasma,* form, mold, from Gr. *plassein,* to mold, spread out] The protoplasm of a cell outside the nucleus. SEE: *cell.*
cytoplast (sī′tō-plăst) The cytoplasm of a cell as distinguished from the contents of the nucleus.
cytoproximal (sī″tō-prŏk′sĭ-măl) [″ + L. *proximus,* nearest] Pert. to the portion of an axon nearest to the cell body from which it originates.
cytoreduction Cellular killing, usually of cancerous cell clones, with chemotherapy.
cytoreticulum (sī″tō-rĕ-tĭk′ū-lŭm) [″ + L. *reticulum,* network] The fibrillar network supporting fluid of protoplasm.
cytorrhyctes (sī″tō-rĭk′tēz) [″ + *oryssein,* to dig] Inclusion bodies in cells. Composed of virus elementary bodies, they were once thought to be of protozoal origin.
cytoscopy (sī-tŏs′kō-pē) [″ + *skopein,* to examine] Microscopic examination of cells for diagnostic purposes.
cytosine (sī′tō-sĭn) $C_4H_5N_3O$; a pyrimidine base that is part of DNA and RNA. In DNA it is paired with guanine.
 c. arabinoside Cytarabine.
cytoskeleton (sī″tō-skĕl′ĕ-tŏn) The internal structural framework of a cell consisting of three types of filaments: microfilaments, microtubules, and intermediate filaments. These form a dynamic framework for maintaining cell shape and allowing rapid changes in the three-dimensional structure of the cell.
cytosol (sī′tō-sŏl) The fluid of cytoplasm; it contains water, dissolved ions and nutrients, and enzymes. SYN: *hyaloplasm.*
cytosome (sī′tō-sōm) [″ + *soma,* body] The portion of a cell exclusive of the nucleus.
cytostasis (sī-tŏs′tă-sĭs) [Gr. *kytos,* cell, + *stasis,* standing still] Stasis of white blood cells, as in the early stage of inflammation.
cytostatic (sī″tŏ-stăt′ĭk) [″ + *stasis,* standing still] Preventing the growth and proliferation of cells.
cytotactic (sī″tō-tăk′tĭk) Pert. to cytotaxia.
cytotaxia, cytotaxis (sī-tō-tăk′sē-ă, -sĭs) [″ + *taxis,* arrangement] Attraction or repulsion of cells for each other.
cytotechnologist A medical laboratory technologist who works under the supervision of a pathologist to examine cells in order to diagnose cancer or other diseases.
cytotechnology Microscopic examination of cells to identify abnormalities.
cytotherapy [″ + *therapeia,* treatment] **1.** Treatment by use of glandular extracts; organotherapy. **2.** Use of cytotoxic or cytolytic substances or serums to treat disease.
cytothesis (sī-tŏth′ĕ-sĭs) [″ + *thesis,* a placing] Restoration or repair of injured cells.
cytotoxic (sī″tō-tŏks′ĭk) Destructive to cells.
cytotoxic agent Any drug that destroys cells or prevents them from multiplying. Cytotoxic agents are used for the treatment of cancers and severe immunological disorders (such as vasculitis or some forms of glomerulonephritis). An ideal agent (which has not yet been made) would destroy proliferating cells without injuring the normal cells of the body.
cytotoxin (sī″tō-tŏk′sĭn) [″ + *toxikon,* poison] An antibody or toxin that attacks the cells of particular organs. SEE: *endotoxin; erythrotoxin; exotoxin; leukocidin; lysis; neurotoxin.*
cytotrophoblast (sī″tō-trō′fō-blăst) [″ + *trophe,* nourishment, + *blastos,* germ] The thin inner layer of the trophoblast composed of cuboidal cells, the outer layer being the syntrophoblast. SYN: *Langhans' layer.*
cytotropic (sī″tō-trŏp′ĭk, -trōp′ĭk) [″ + *trope,* a turn] Having an affinity for cells.
cytotropism (sī-tŏt′rō-pĭzm) [″ + *trope,* a turn, + *-ismos,* condition] The movement of cells toward or away from a stimulus such as drugs, viruses, bacteria, or physical conditions such as heat or cold.
cytozoic (sī″tō-zō′ĭk) [″ + *zoon,* animal] Living within or attached to a cell, as certain protozoa.
cytozoon (sī-tō-zō′ŏn) A protozoon that lives as an intracellular parasite.
cyturia (sĭ-tū′rē-ă) [Gr. *kytos,* cell, + *ouron,* urine] The presence of any kind of cells in the urine.
Czermak's spaces (chār′măks) [Johann Czermak, Ger. physiologist, 1828–1873] The interglobular spaces in dentin caused by failure of calcification. SYN: *interglobular spaces.*

D

Δ, δ Upper- and lower-case delta, respectively; the fourth letter of the Greek alphabet.

D **1.** L. *da,* give; *date; daughter; deciduous;* L. *detur,* let it be given; *died; diopter; divorced; doctor.* **2.** Symbol for the element deuterium.

D- In biochemistry, a prefix indicating the structure of certain organic compounds with asymmetric carbon atoms. If a carbon atom is attached to four different substituent groups that can be arranged in two ways and represent nonsuperimposable mirror images, it is classed as asymmetrical. The name of such a compound is preceded by D. When there are only three dissimilar groups around the carbon atom, only one configuration in space is possible. The carbon atom is classed as symmetrical (or chiral), and the name is preceded by L.

In other chemical nomenclature, a lower-case *d-* or *l-* indicates the rotational direction of a polarized light shined through a solution of the compound. When the plane of the light is rotated to the right (i.e., is dextrorotatory), the compound's name is preceded by *d-*. When the light is rotated to the left (i.e., is levorotatory), the name is preceded by *l-*.

If a D compound that has an asymmetrical carbon can also rotate light and is dextrorotatory, its name is preceded by D(+); if levorotatory, D(−). If the asymmetrical carbon is of the L form and is dextrorotatory, its name is prefixed by L(+); if it is levorotatory, the name is preceded by L(−).

d *density;* L. *dexter* or *dextro,* right; L. *dies,* day; *distal; dorsal; duration.*

2,4-D Herbicide, 2,4-dichlorophenoxyacetic acid, that acts by stimulating broad-leaf plants to grow. It is toxic to humans and animals.

D/A *digital to analog.*

Da Symbol for dalton.

daboia, daboya (dă-boy′ă) Russell's viper, a large poisonous snake of India, Burma, and Thailand. Its venom is used to enhance the action of certain blood coagulation factors.

dacarbazine (dă-kăr′bă-zēn) An alkylating agent used in treating neoplasms including malignant melanoma and Hodgkin's disease.

dacryadenalgia (dăk″rē-ăd-ĕn-ăl′jē-ă) [Gr. *dakryon,* tear, + *aden,* gland, + *algos,* pain] Pain in a lacrimal gland. SYN: *dacryoadenalgia.*

dacryadenitis (dăk″rē-ăd-ĕ-nī′tĭs) [″ + ″ + *itis,* inflammation] Inflammation of a lacrimal gland.

dacryadenoscirrhus (dăk″rē-ăd″ĕn-ō-skĭr′us) [″ + ″ + *skirrhos,* hardening] Induration of a lacrimal gland.

dacryagogatresia (dăk″rē-ă-gŏg″ă-trē′sē-ă) [Gr. *dakryon,* tear, + *agogos,* leading, + *a-,* not, + *tresis,* perforate] Occlusion of a tear duct.

dacryagogue (dăk′rē-ă-gŏg) An agent that stimulates the secretion of tears.

dacrycystalgia (dăk″rē-sĭs-tăl′jē-ă) [″ + *kystis,* cyst, + *algos,* pain] Pain in a lacrimal sac. SYN: *dacryocystalgia.*

dacryelcosis (dăk″rē-ĕl-kō′sĭs) [″ + *helkosis,* ulceration] Ulceration of the lacrimal apparatus.

dacryoadenalgia (dăk″rē-ō-ăd″ĕn-ăl′jē-ă) [″ + *aden,* gland, + *algos,* pain] Pain in a lacrimal gland. SYN: *dacryadenalgia.*

dacryoadenectomy (dăk″rē-ō-ăd″ĕ-nĕk′tō-mē) [″ + ″ + *ektome,* excision] Surgical removal of a lacrimal gland.

dacryoadenitis (dăk″rē-ō-ăd″ĕn-ī′tĭs) [″ + ″ + *itis,* inflammation] Inflammation of a lacrimal gland. It is rare, seen as a complication in epidemic parotitis (mumps involving the lacrimal gland), and present in Mikulicz's disease. It may be acute or chronic.

dacryoblennorrhea (dăk″rē-ō-blĕn″ō-rē′ă) [″ + *blenna,* mucus, + *rhoia,* flow] Discharge of mucus from a lacrimal sac, and chronic inflammation of the sac.

dacryocele (dăk′rē-ō-sēl) [″ + *kele,* tumor, swelling] Protrusion of a lacrimal sac.

dacryocyst (dăk′rē-ō-sĭst) [″ + *kystis,* cyst] Lacrimal sac.

dacryocystalgia (dăk″rē-ō-sĭs-tăl′jē-ă) [″ + ″ + *algos,* pain] Pain in a lacrimal sac. SYN: *dacrycystalgia.*

dacryocystectomy (dăk″rē-ō-sĭs-tĕk′tō-mē) [″ + *kystis,* cyst, + *ektome,* excision] Excision of membranes of the lacrimal sac.

dacryocystitis (dăk″rē-ō-sĭs-tī′tĭs) [″ + ″ + *itis,* inflammation] Inflammation of a lacrimal sac, including the mucous membrane of the sac and submucous membrane. It may occasionally extend the surrounding connective tissue and cause periorbital cellulitis. It is usually secondary to prolonged obstruction of a nasolacrimal duct.

SYMPTOMS: The symptoms are profuse tearing (epiphora); redness and swelling in the lacrimal sac, which may also extend to the lids and conjunctiva; pain, esp. on pressure over the sac.

TREATMENT: Hot compresses should

be applied to the area. Appropriate topical and systemic antibiotic therapy depend on the organisms isolated from the inflamed area. The physician should incise and drain the sac if it is fluctuant; attempt to restore permeability of the duct with a probe when acute symptoms have subsided; and in chronic cases, extirpate the sac or perform an intranasal operation (dacryocystorhinostomy).

dacryocystoblennorrhea (dăk″rē-ō-sĭs″tō-blĕn-ō-rē′ă) [″ + ″ + *blenna,* mucus, + *rhoia,* flow] Chronic inflammation of and discharge from a lacrimal sac.

dacryocystocele (dăk″rē-ō-sĭs′tō-sēl) [Gr. *dakryon,* tear, + *kystis,* cyst, + *kele,* tumor, swelling] A herniated protrusion of a lacrimal sac.

dacryocystography (dăk″rē-ō-sĭs-tŏg′ră-fē) [″ + ″ + *graphein,* to write] Radiographic examination of the nasolacrimal drainage system after introduction of a contrast agent.

dacryocystoptosis (dăk″rē-ō-sĭs-tŏp-tō′sĭs) [″ + ″ + *ptosis,* a dropping] Prolapse of a lacrimal sac.

dacryocystorhinostenosis (dăk″rē-ō-sĭs″tō-rī-nō-stĕ-nō′sĭs) [″ + ″ + *rhis,* nose, + *stenosis,* act of narrowing] Narrowing or obliteration of the canal connecting a lacrimal sac with the nasal cavity. Patency is tested by placing a weak sugar solution in the conjunctival space. If the duct is patent, the patient will report a sweet taste in the mouth.

dacryocystorhinostomy (dăk″rē-ō-sĭs″tō-rī-nŏs′tō-mē) [″ + ″ + ″ + *stoma,* mouth] Surgical connecting of the lumen of a lacrimal sac with the nasal cavity.

dacryocystorhinotomy (dăk″rē-ō-sĭs″tō-rī-nŏt′ō-mē) [″ + ″ + ″ + *tome,* incision] Surgical probing of the duct leading from a lacrimal sac into the nose.

dacryocystosyringotomy (dăk″rē-ō-sĭs″tō-sĭr″ĭn-gŏt′ō-mē) [″ + *kystis,* cyst, + *syrinx,* tube, + *tome,* incision] A surgically created opening between a lacrimal sac and the nasal cavity.

dacryocystotome (dăk″rē-ō-sĭs′tō-tōm) [″ + ″ + *tome,* incision] A device for incision of a lacrimal sac.

dacryocystotomy (dăk″rē-ō-sĭs-tŏt′ō-mē) Incision of a lacrimal sac.

dacryogenic Promoting the shedding of tears.

dacryohelcosis (dăk″rē-ō-hĕl-kō′sĭs) [″ + *helcosis,* ulceration] Ulceration of a lacrimal sac or duct.

dacryohemorrhea (dăk″rē-ō-hĕm″ō-rē′ă) [″ + *haima,* blood, + *rhoia,* flow] Discharge of bloody tears.

dacryolithiasis (dăk″rē-ō-lĭ-thī′ă-sĭs) [″ + *lithiasis,* formation of stones] Presence of stones or calculi in the lacrimal apparatus.

dacryoma (dăk″rē-ō′mă) [″ + *oma,* tumor] **1.** A lacrimal tumor. **2.** A tumor-like swelling due to obstruction of the lacrimal duct.

dacryon (dăk′rē-ŏn) [Gr. *dakryon*] The lacrimal juncture point of the lacrimal, frontal, and upper maxillary bones.

dacryopyorrhea (dăk″rē-ō-pī″ō-rē′ă) [″ + *pyon,* pus, + *rhoia,* discharge] Discharge of pus from a lacrimal duct.

dacryopyosis [″ + *pyosis,* suppuration] Suppuration in a lacrimal sac or duct.

dacryorrhea (dăk″rē-ō-rē′ă) [″ + *rhoia,* flow] Excessive flow of tears.

dacryosolenitis (dăk″rē-ō-sō-lĕn-ī′tĭs) [″ + *solen,* duct, + *itis,* inflammation] Inflammation of a lacrimal or nasal duct.

dacryostenosis (dăk″rē-ō-stĕn-ō′sĭs) [″ + *stenosis,* act of narrowing] Obstruction or narrowing of a lacrimal or nasal duct.

dacryosyrinx (dăk″rē-ō-sī′rĭnks) [″ + *syrinx,* tube] A lacrimal fistula.

dactinomycin An antibiotic used in cancer chemotherapy, esp. in the treatment of Wilms' tumor.

dactyl (dăk′tĭl) [Gr. *daktylos,* finger] A finger or toe; a digit of the hand or foot.

dactyl- SEE: *dactylo-*.

dactyledema (dăk″tĭl-ĕ-dē′mă) [″ + *oidema,* swelling] Edema of the fingers or toes.

dactylion Adhesions between or union of fingers or toes.

dactylitis [″ + *itis,* inflammation] Chronic inflammation of finger and toe bones in very young children, usually of tuberculous or syphilitic origin.

sickle cell d. Painful swelling of the feet and hands during the first several years of life in children with sickle cell anemia.

dactylo-, dactyl- [Gr. *dactylosdaktylos,* finger, toe] Combining form meaning *finger or toe.*

dactylogryposis (dăk″tĭ-lō-grĭ-pō′sĭs) [″ + *gryposis,* curve] Permanent contraction of the fingers.

dactylolysis (dăk″tĭ-lŏl′ĭ-sĭs) [″ + *lysis,* dissolution] Spontaneous dropping off of fingers or toes, seen in leprosy and ainhum and sometimes produced in utero when a hair firmly wrapped around a digit causes amputation.

dactylomegaly (dăk″tĭ-lō-mĕg′ă-lē) [″ + *megas,* large] Abnormally large size of fingers and toes. SEE: *acromegaly.*

dactylospasm (dăk′tĭ-lō-spăzm) [″ + *spasmos,* a convulsion] Cramp of a finger or toe.

dactylus (dăk′tĭ-lŭs) [Gr. *daktylos*] Digit.

dairy food substitute A food resembling an existing dairy food in taste and appearance but differing in composition from the dairy food for which it is substituted.

Dakin's solution (dā′kĭns) [Henry D. Dakin, U.S. chemist, 1880–1952] A dilute, neutral solution of sodium hypochlorite and boric acid. It was developed during World War I and is still used for cleansing wounds.

Dale reaction [Sir Henry H. Dale, 1875–1968, Brit. scientist and Nobel Prize winner in 1936] An old test used to demonstrate the ability of muscle tissues from an anaphylactic organism to contract on re-exposure to the antigen. Either guinea pig uterine muscle or intestine is used. The test is very specific, as unrelated antigens will not cause the sensitized muscle to contract. SYN: *Schultz reaction*.

dalton (dawl'tŏn) ABBR: Da. An arbitrary unit of mass equal to 1⁄12 the mass of carbon 12, or 1.657×-10^{-24} g; also called atomic mass unit.

Dalton's law [John Dalton, Brit. chemist, 1766–1844] A law that states that, in a mixture of gases, the total pressure is equal to the sum of the partial pressures of each gas.

dam A thin sheet of rubber used in dentistry and surgery to isolate a part from the surrounding tissues and fluids.

damages The compensation or payment awarded by the courts to an injured party.

compensatory d. In a lawsuit, money awarded to an injured individual to repay that person for the actual costs that have resulted from the injury. The damages should restore the injured party to his or her pre-injury status.

punitive d. In lawsuits, the money awarded to the victorious party to punish the losing party for acts of misconduct.

damp 1. Moist, humid. **2.** A noxious gas in a mine.

damping Steady diminution of the amplitude of successive vibrations, as of an electric wave or current.

danazol (dă'nă-zōl) A drug that suppresses the action of the anterior pituitary; used to treat endometriosis, fibrocystic breast disease, and angioedema.

dancing disease In Europe during the Middle Ages, an epidemic chorea supposed to have been caused by the bite of the tarantula. SEE: *tarantism*.

dancing mania Epidemic chorea.

D and C *dilation and curettage*.

D and E *dilation and evacuation* of the uterus. SEE: *dilation and curettage*.

dander (dăn'dĕr) Small scales from the skin, hair, or feathers of animals, which may provoke allergic reactions in sensitized individuals.

dandruff Scale that exfoliates from the outer layer of the skin, esp. from the scalp.

TREATMENT: Several over-the-counter products, including salicylic acid, pyrithione zinc, and selenium sulfide, provide effective treatment.

dandy fever Dengue; an acute, epidemic, febrile disease occurring in tropical areas.

Dandy-Walker syndrome (dăn'dē-wawk'ĕr) [Walter E. Dandy, U.S. neurosurgeon, 1886–1946; Arthur E. Walker, U.S. surgeon, b. 1907] Congenital hydrocephalus caused by blockage of the foramina of Magendie and Luschka, through which the cerebrospinal fluid passes.

Dane particle [David S. Dane, contemporary Brit. virologist] A viral particle present in the serum of patients with hepatitis B. Dane particles contain DNA and are infectious.

dantrolene sodium (dăn'trō-lēn) A muscle relaxant used to relieve spasticity.

Danysz phenomenon [Jean Danysz, Polish-born pathologist in France, 1860–1928] A phenomenon that illustrates the reversibility of precipitation of antibody and antigen complexes. When a specified amount of diphtheria toxin is added all at once to an antitoxin serum, the mixture is nontoxic; but when the same quantity of toxin is added in portions at about 30-min intervals, the mixture is toxic.

dapsone (dăp'sōn) An antibacterial sulfone that was once the drug of choice for treating leprosy; also used to treat patients with dermatitis herpetiformis and some who have malaria or *Pneumocystis carinii* pneumonia. Frequent blood studies must be performed on patients receiving this drug for prolonged periods, as hemolysis, leukopenia, and methemoglobinemia can occur.

Darier, Ferdinand Jean (dăr-ē-ā') French dermatologist, 1856–1938.

D.'s disease A rare autosomal dominant skin disease in which the patient is marked by numerous warty papules that merge into large plaques. The lesions often become infected and may have an offensive odor. SYN: *keratosis follicularis*.

D.'s sign The skin change produced when the skin lesion in urticaria pigmentosa is rubbed briskly. The area usually begins to itch and becomes raised and surrounded by erythema. SEE: illus.; *mastocytosis; urticaria pigmentosa*.

darkroom A room designed to be devoid of light. The darkroom is necessary for the development of radiographic film.

Darling's disease (dăr'lĭngz) [Samuel Taylor Darling, U.S. pathologist, 1872–1925] Histoplasmosis.

dartoid (dăr'toyd) [Gr. *dartos*, skinned, + *eidos*, form, shape] Resembling the tunica dartos in its slow, involuntary contractions.

dartos [Gr.] The muscular, contractile tissue beneath the skin of the scrotum. SYN: *tunica dartos*.

dartos muliebris A veil-like smooth mus-

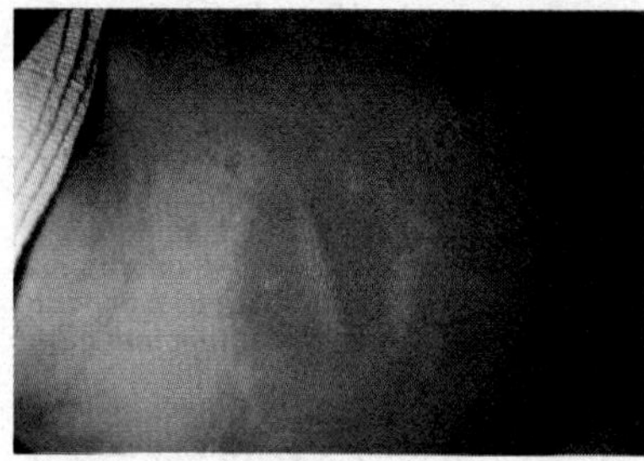

DARIER'S SIGN

cle just under the skin of the labia majora.

dartos muscle reflex Wormlike contraction of the dartos muscle following sudden cold application to the perineum.

dartrous [Gr. *dartos,* skinned] Of the nature of herpes; herpetic.

darwinian ear [Charles Robert Darwin, Brit. naturalist, 1809–1882] An exaggeration of the darwinian tubercle.

darwinian tubercle [Charles Robert Darwin, Brit. naturalist, 1809–1882] A blunt point projecting from the upper part of the helix of the ear.

darwinism (dăr′wĭ-nĭzm) The theory of biological evolution through natural selection.

Datura (dā-tū′ră) A genus of plants, one member of which, *Datura stramonium,* contains constituents of hyoscyamine and scopolamine, which have anticholinergic properties.

daughter (daw′tĕr) **1.** The product of the decay of a radioactive element. **2.** A product of cell division, as a daughter cell or daughter nucleus. **3.** One's female child.

daughter, DES The daughter of a mother who received diethylstilbestrol (DES) during pregnancy. SEE: *DES syndrome; diethylstilbestrol.*

daunorubicin hydrochloride An antineoplastic drug of the anthracine drug class used in leukemia and solid tumors.

Davidsohn's sign [Hermann Davidsohn, Ger. physician, 1842–1911] Lessening or absence of the pupillary light reflex when an electric light is held in the closed mouth. It indicates the presence of a tumor or fluid in the maxillary sinus.

DAWN *Drug Abuse Warning Network.*

dawn phenomenon A marked increase in insulin requirements between 6 A.M. and 9 A.M. as compared with the midnight to 6 A.M. period. The increased dose of insulin required during this period is in contrast to the Somogyi phenomenon, which is managed by decreasing insulin during the critical period. Dawn phenomenon may occur in persons with diabetes mellitus of either type and in some normal persons. SEE: *diabetes mellitus.*

day care center A place for the care of preschool children whose parents are for any reason unable to care for their children during normal working hours.

adult d.c.c. A center for daytime supervision of adult patients. These centers provide supervised social, recreational, and health-related activities, usually in a group setting. The centers permit caregivers a respite and free them for other activities (work, play, appointments, socialization) during the day.

daydream Mental musing or fantasy while awake.

dazzle Dimming of vision due to intense stimulus of very bright light. SEE: *glare.*

dB, db *decibel.*

D.C. *Doctor of Chiropractic; direct current.*

d/c *discontinue.*

DCAP-BTLS An acronym that stands for deformities, contusions, abrasions, penetrations or perforations, burns, tenderness, lacerations, and swelling; to remember what is observed for when looking at soft tissue during the assessment of a patient.

DCIS *ductal carcinoma in situ.*

ddc Zalcitabine.

DDD pacing SEE: *pacemaker, artificial cardiac.*

ddi Didanosine.

d-dimer A byproduct of the degradation of blood clots, specifically, of the fibrin within a thrombus. The detection of this substance aids in the diagnosis of deep venous thrombosis and pulmonary embolism.

D.D.S. *Doctor of Dental Surgery.* SEE: *D.M.D.*

DDT Dichlorodiphenyltrichloroethane, now called chlorophenothane; a powerful insecticide effective against a wide variety of insects, esp. the flea, fly, louse, mosquito, bedbug, cockroach, Japanese beetle, and European corn borer. However, many species develop resistant populations, and birds and fish that feed on affected insects suffer toxic effects. In 1972, the U.S. banned DDT except for essential public health use and a few minor uses to protect crops for which there were no effective alternatives.

When ingested orally, it may cause acute poisoning. Symptoms are vomiting, numbness and partial paralysis of limbs, anorexia, tremors, and depression, resulting in death. SEE: *Poisons and Poisoning Appendix.*

de- [L. *de,* from] Prefix indicating *down* or *from.*

deacidification [″ + *acidus,* sour, + *facere,* to make] Neutralization of acidity.

deactivation [″ + *activus,* acting] The process of becoming or making inactive.

dead [AS. *dead*] Without life or life processes. SEE: *death*.

deadman switch A switch or control that requires continuous pressure by the operator.

deadspace The portion of the tidal volume not participating in gas exchange.

alveolar d. The volume of gas in alveoli that are ventilated but not perfused with capillary blood.

anatomical d. In pulmonary physiology, the air in the mouth, nose, pharynx, larynx, trachea, and bronchial tree at the end of inhalation. This is termed dead space because the air does not reach the alveoli and is not involved in gas exchange. One purpose of this space is to permit warming of very cold inhaled air before it comes in contact with the alveoli.

mechanical d. The volume of gas exhaled into a tubing system and rebreathed on the subsequent breath.

physiological d. The sum of anatomical and alveolar deadspace.

dead tooth A nonvital tooth by clinical standards, having had the pulp removed by endodontic treatment. The term is a poor choice because, if the periodontal tissues are healthy, the tooth will continue to function without symptoms.

deaf [AS. *deaf*] **1.** Partially or completely lacking the sense of hearing. **2.** Unwilling to listen; heedless.

deafferentation (dē-ăf″ĕr-ĕn-tā′shŭn) Cutting off of the afferent nerve supply. SEE: *denervation*.

deaf-mute A person who is unable to hear or speak.

deaf-mutism The state of being both deaf and unable to speak.

deafness [AS.] Complete or partial loss of the ability to hear. The deficit may be temporary or permanent. More than 20 million Americans have hearing impairment; most of them are older than age 65, although about 5% are children. Hereditary forms of hearing impairment affect about 1 newborn out of 2000. In this population, hearing deficits may impair language acquisition and speech. Acquired hearing loss impacts the lives of nearly half of all individuals over the age of 80, in whom it may be a prominent cause of social isolation or depression. SYN: *hearing loss*.

ETIOLOGY: Hearing impairment has multiple causes. Congenital deafness occurs in such syndromes as neurofibromatosis or Usher's syndrome. Toxic deafness may result from exposure to agents like salicylates, diuretics, or aminoglycoside antibiotics or infections of the central nervous system (meningococcal meningitis, syphilis) or of the eighth cranial nerve. Many viruses may contribute to loss of hearing as may prolonged or repetitive exposures to environmental noise. Otosclerosis is an example of bilateral hearing loss due to progressive ossification of the annular ligaments of the ear. Sudden hearing loss may result from ear trauma, fistulae, stroke, drug exposures, cancer, multiple sclerosis, vasculitis, Ménière's disease, and numerous other conditions. Not infrequently, adult patients with unilateral conductive hearing loss have a cerumen impaction.

DIAGNOSIS: Simple bedside tests, such as assessing a patient's ability to hear a whispered phrase or the sound of fingers, may suggest hearing impairment. Tuning fork tests that compare air and bone conduction of sound help clinicians identify whether hearing loss is due to conductive or sensorineural causes. Audiometry provides definitive diagnosis.

TREATMENT: Therapy depends on the underlying condition. Cerumen impaction, for example, responds to irrigation of the external auditory canal, while otosclerosis may respond to the intra-aural placement of prostheses. Other forms of therapy include the use of hearing amplifiers or cochlear implants, or education in lip reading or sign language.

PATIENT CARE: Patients can prevent damage to hearing from excessively loud noises by wearing sound-muffling ear plugs or muffs when exposed to loud noise from any source, esp. industrial noise, and by recognizing that loud music can be as detrimental to hearing as the noise of a jackhammer. Patients should avoid cleaning inside the ears or putting sharp objects in them. Many antibiotics and chemotherapeutic drugs are ototoxic, and hearing should be evaluated continually when such drugs are used.

When interacting with a person with a hearing deficit, the health care professional should make his or her presence known to the patient by sight or gentle touch before beginning to speak. If possible, background noise should be decreased or the patient removed from a noisy area before the other person speaks. The health care professional's face should be illuminated to facilitate the patient's visualization of the lips and expressions. The health care professional faces directly to the patient's face or toward the ear with the best hearing and does not turn away while speaking. To facilitate lip reading, short words and simple sentences should be used and spoken clearly and distinctly in a normal tone and speed. Exaggerated mouthing of words or loud tones should be avoided. Placing a stethoscope in the patient's ears and speaking into the bell helps to cut out extraneous sounds and to direct words into the patient's ears. If the patient is literate, sign language or finger spelling may be used to communicate. Written information should be presented clearly and in large letters, esp. if the patient has poor visual acuity.

acoustic trauma d. Impaired hearing due to repeated exposure to loud noise.

acquired d. Loss of hearing that is not present at birth but develops later in life.

aviator's d. A temporary or permanent nerve deafness found in some aviators. It is caused by prolonged exposure to loud noise.

bass d. Inability to hear low-frequency tones.

central d. Deafness resulting from lesions of the auditory tracts of the brain or the auditory centers of the cerebral cortex.

cerebral d. Cortical d.

ceruminous d. Deafness due to plugs of cerumen (ear wax) blocking the ear canal.

conduction d. Deafness resulting from any condition that prevents sound waves from being transmitted to the auditory receptors. It may result from wax obstructing the external auditory meatus, inflammation of the middle ear, ankylosis of the ear bones, or fixation of the footplate of the stirrup. SEE: *otosclerosis; Rinne test; Weber test.*

cortical d. Deafness due to disease of the cortical centers without a lesion. SYN: *cerebral d.*

hereditary d. Hearing loss passed down through generations of a family.

high-frequency d. Inability to hear high-frequency sounds.

hysterical d. An out-of-date term for functional deafness.

nerve d. Deafness due to a lesion of the auditory nerve or central neural pathways.

nonsyndromic d. Any form of hereditary hearing impairment caused by one of dozens of genetic mutations (e.g., in somatic, mitochondrial, or X-linked genes).

occupational d. Deafness caused by working in places where noise levels are quite high. Persons working in such an environment should wear protective devices.

ototoxic d. Hearing loss due to the toxic effect of certain chemicals or medicines on the eighth cranial nerve. Aminoglycosides are responsible occasionally.

perceptive d. Deafness resulting from lesions involving sensory receptors of the cochlea or fibers of the acoustic nerve, or a combination of these.

postlingual d. Hearing impairment that develops after a patient has learned language.

prelingual d. Hearing impairment that is present in infancy and childhood, before language skills are acquired.

psychic d. A condition in which auditory sensations are perceived but not comprehended.

pure word d. A form of aphasia in which sounds and words are heard but linguistic comprehension is absent.

sensorineural d. Deafness due to defective function of the cochlea or acoustic nerve.

tone d. Inability to distinguish musical sounds.

deamidase (dē-ăm′ĭ-dās) An enzyme that splits amides to form carboxylic acid and ammonia.

deamidization (dē-ăm″ĭ-dĭ-zā′shŭn) The removal of an amide group by hydrolysis.

deaminase An enzyme that causes the removal of an amino group from organic compounds.

deamination Deaminization.

deaminization Loss of the NH_2 radical from amino compounds. Alanine can be deaminized to give ammonia and pyruvic acid: $CH_3CH(NH_2)COOH + O{=}CH^3CO \cdot COOH + NH^3$. Deaminization may be simple, oxidative, or hydrolytic. Oxidizing enzymes are called deamination enzymes when the oxidation is accompanied by splitting off of amino groups. Deaminization is the first step in the use of amino acids in cell respiration; the NH_2 is converted to urea. SYN: *deamination.*

dearterialization (dē″ăr′tēr″ē-ăl-ī-zā′shŭn) [L. *de,* from, + Gr. *arteria,* artery] Changing of arterial into venous blood; deoxygenation.

dearticulation (dē″ăr-tĭk″ū-lā′shŭn) Dislocation of a joint.

death [AS. *death*] Permanent cessation of all vital functions, including those of the heart, lungs, and brain. SEE: table; *brain d.; euthanasia; life.*

Signs: The principal clinical signs of death are apnea (the absence of respirations) and asystole (the absence of heartbeat). Other indications may need to be relied on in individuals who are receiving mechanical life support. These include the loss of cranial nerve reflexes and the cessation of the electrical activity of the brain.

Patient Care: Legal procedures and institutional protocols should be followed in the determination of death. The times of cessation of breathing and heartbeat are documented, and the physician or other legally authorized health care professional is notified and requested to certify death. The family is notified according to institutional policy, and emotional support is provided. Auxiliary equipment is removed, but the hospital identification bracelet is left in place. The body is cleansed, clean dressings are applied as necessary, and

Ten Leading Causes of Death and Disability in the World (1990)

Deaths	(in millions)	Disability	YLD's* (in thousands)
Ischemic heart disease	6.3	Unipolar major depression	50.8
Cerebrovascular disease	4.4	Iron-deficiency anemia	22
Lower respiratory infections	4.3	Falls	22
Diarrheal diseases	2.9	Alcohol use	15.8
Perinatal conditions	2.4	Chronic obstructive pulmonary disease	14.7
Chronic obstructive pulmonary disease	2.2	Bipolar disorder	14.1
Tuberculosis	2.0	Congenital anomalies	13.5
Measles	1.1	Osteoarthritis	13.3
Road traffic accidents	1.0	Schizophrenia	12.1
Trachea, bronchus, and lung cancers	0.9	Obsessive-compulsive disorders	10.2

*Years of life lived with disability

SOURCE: From Murray, Christopher J. L. and Lopez, Alan D.: The Global Burden of Disease, Harvard School of Public Health, Cambridge, MA 1996, p179 and p236.

the rectum is packed with absorbent material to prevent drainage. The patient is placed in a supine position with the limbs extended and the head slightly elevated. Dentures are inserted, if appropriate; the mouth and eyes are closed; and the body is covered to the chin with a sheet.

The patient's belongings are collected and documented. Witnesses should be present, esp. if personal items have great sentimental or monetary value. The family is encouraged to visit, touch, and hold the patient's body as desired. In some situations (e.g., neonatal death, accidental death) and according to protocol, a photograph of the deceased is obtained to assist the family in grieving and remembering their loved one. A health care professional and a family member sign for and remove the patient's belongings.

After the family has gone, the body is prepared for the morgue. Body tags, imprinted with the patient's identification plate or card information (name, identification number, room and bed number, attending physician), along with the date and time of death, are tied to the patient's foot or wrist as well as to the outside of the shroud. The body is then transported to the morgue and placed in a refrigerated unit according to protocol.

biological d. Death due directly to natural causes.

black d. Former name for bubonic plague.

brain d. The cessation of brain function. The criteria for concluding that the brain has died include lack of response to stimuli, lack of all reflexes, absent respirations, and an isoelectric electroencephalogram that for at least 30 min will not change in response to sound or pain stimuli. Other criteria that are sometimes used include loss of afferent cerebral evoked potentials, loss of isotope uptake during brain scans, or absence of cerebral perfusion on Doppler sonography. Before making this diagnosis, two physicians, including one experienced in caring for severely brain-damaged patients, should review the medical records. It is inadvisable for physicians associated with transplantion procedures to participate in the review. The patient's body may be kept "alive" briefly by life-support devices if the patient is an organ donor.

CAUTION: Some drugs (e.g., barbiturates, methaqualone, diazepam, mecloqualone, meprobamate, trichloroethylene) can produce short isoelectric periods on encephalograms. Hypothermia must also be excluded as the cause of apparent brain death.

crib d. Sudden infant death syndrome.

fetal d. Spontaneous demise of the fetus occurring after the 20th week of gestation. The cause is often unknown; however, fetal death often is associated with maternal infection, diabetes mellitus, fetal and placental abnormalities, and pre-eclampsia.

functional d. Central nervous system death with vital functions being artificially supported.

good d. Death in which the rights of the individual have been respected, and during which the dying person was made as comfortable as possible and was in the company of persons he or she knew and loved. SEE: *living will*.

local d. Gangrene or necrosis of a part.

man-made d. Death due to something other than natural causes (e.g., murder, war, political violence).

molecular d. Death of cell life.

neocortical d. Persistent vegetative state.

sudden d. Death occurring unexpectedly and instantaneously or within 1 hr of the onset of symptoms in a patient with or without known preexisting heart disease. Sudden death due to cardiac conditions occurs in the U.S. at the rate of one a minute. It may be caused by cardiovascular conditions, including ischemic heart disease, aortic stenosis, coronary embolism, myocarditis, ruptured or dissecting aortic aneurysm, Stokes-Adams syndrome, stroke, pulmonary thromboembolism, and other, noncardiovascular-related disorders, such as electrolyte imbalance and drug toxicity.

wrongful d. Loss of life caused by negligent, illegitimate, or illegal acts.

deathbed statement A declaration made at the time immediately preceding death. Such a statement, if made with the consciousness and belief that death is impending and in the presence of a witness, is legally considered as binding as a statement made under oath. SYN: *antemortem statement.*

death investigation The customary investigation of a violent, suspicious, or unexpected death, or of a death unattended by a physician. The investigation is, by law, done by an officially appointed person. The investigation system includes medical examiners, coroners, or both a combined medical examiner and coroner. The system used varies from state to state. SEE: *coroner.*

death with dignity Death that is allowed to occur in accordance with the wishes of a patient. An individual may choose to withdraw from chronic medical therapies (e.g., when there is little expectation of cure). Patients who choose death rather than active treatment often have advanced malignancies, poor performance status, major depression, poor social supports, or a desire for a palliative approach to end-of-life care.

debilitant [L. *debilis,* weak] **1.** A remedy used to reduce excitement. **2.** Something that weakens.

debilitate To produce weakness or debility.

debility Weakness or lack of strength.

débouchement (dā-boosh-mŏn′) [Fr.] An opening or emptying into another part.

Debove's membrane (dĕ-bōvz′) [Georges Maurice Debove, Fr. physician, 1845–1920] A layer of connective tissue cells between the epithelium and basement tissue of respiratory and intestinal epithelia.

débride (dā-brēd′) [Fr.] To perform the action of débridement.

débridement (dā-brēd-mŏn′) [Fr.] The removal of foreign material and dead or damaged tissue, esp. in a wound.

canal d. The removal of organic and inorganic debris from a dental root canal by mechanical or chemical methods. This procedure is done in preparation for sealing the canal to prevent further decay of the tooth.

enzymatic d. Use of proteolytic enzymes to remove dead tissue from a wound. The enzymes do not attack viable tissues.

epithelial d. The removal of the entire epithelial lining or attachment epithelium from a periodontal pocket.

debris (dĕ-brē′) [Fr., remains] The remains of broken-down or damaged cells or tissue.

debt (dĕt) Deficit.

oxygen d. After strenuous (i.e., anaerobic) physical activity, the oxygen required (in addition to that required in the resting, or recovery, period) to oxidize the excess lactic acid produced and to replenish the depleted stores of adenosine triphosphate and phosphocreatine.

debulking Surgery to remove a large portion of a tumor when complete excision is not possible.

deca-, dec- [Gr. *deka*] Prefix indicating *ten.*

decagram (dĕk′ă″grăm) [Gr. *deka,* ten, + *gramma,* small weight] A mass equal to 10 g.

decalcification (dē″kăl-sĭ-fĭ-kā′shŭn) [L. *de,* from, + *calx,* lime, + *facere,* to make] The removal or withdrawal of calcium salts from bone or teeth.

decalcify **1.** To soften bone through removal of calcium or its salts by acids. **2.** To remove the mineral content from bones or teeth so that sections can be cut and stained for microscopic examination.

decaliter (dĕk′ă-lē″tĕr) [Gr. *deka,* ten, + Fr. *litre,* liter] A measure of 10 L, equivalent to 10,000 ml, or about 10.57 qt. SEE: *deciliter.*

decameter (dĕk′ă-mē-tĕr) [Gr. *deka,* ten, + *metron,* measure] A measure of 10 m; 393.71 in.

decannulation (dē-kăn″nū-lā′shŭn) The removal of a cannula.

decanormal (dĕk″ă-nor′măl) [″ + L. *norma,* rule] Pert. to a solution 10 times as strong as one normal solution. It contains 10 gram-equivalent weights of the substance per liter. SEE: *normal.*

decant (dē-kănt′) [L. *de,* from, + *canthus,* rim of a vessel] To pour off liquid so the sediment remains in the bottom of the container.

decantation Gentle pouring off of a liquid so the sediment remains.

decapitation (dē-kăp″ĭ-tā′shŭn) [″ +

caput, head] **1.** Separation of the head from the body; beheading. **2.** Separation of the head from the shaft of a bone.

decapsulation [" + *capsula,* little box] Removal of a capsule of an organ.

decarboxylase (dē"kăr-bŏk'sĭ-lās) An enzyme that catalyzes the release of carbon dioxide from compounds such as amino acids.

decarboxylation (dē"kăr-bŏks-ĭ-lā'shŭn) A chemical reaction whereby the carboxyl group, —COOH, is removed from an organic compound.

decarboxylization (dē"kăr-bŏks-ĭ-lĭ-zā'shŭn) Decarboxylation.

decay (dē-kā') [" + *cadere,* to fall, die] **1.** Gradual loss of vigor with physical and mental deterioration as may occur in aging. **2.** To waste away. **3.** Decomposition of organic matter by the action of microorganisms. SEE: *caries*; *cementoclasia*. **4.** Disintegration of radioactive substances.

radioactive d. The continual loss of energy by radioactive substances. Disintegration of the nucleus by the emission of alpha, beta, or gamma rays eventually results in the complete loss of radioactivity. The time required for some materials to become stable may be minutes and, for others, thousands of years. SEE: *half-life*.

tooth d. Caries.

deceleration (dē-sĕl"ĕ-rā'shŭn) **1.** A rapid decrease in velocity. **2.** A fall in the baseline fetal heart rate as recorded by the fetal monitor.

Early deceleration coincides with uterine contractions and reflects the fetal vagal response to head compression during these contractions. Normal baseline variability is evident throughout the interval between uterine contractions. *Late deceleration* occurs after contraction and reflects insufficient blood flow through the intervillous spaces of the placenta. *Variable deceleration* does not occur at any consistent point during contractions. The monitor record also exhibits different degrees and shapes. Variable deceleration indicates interference with blood flow through the umbilical vessels caused by cord compression. SEE: *fetal distress*.

deceleration injury An injury in which a moving body hits a stationary object, for example, when a falling patient lands improperly on the ground.

decerebrate (dē-sĕr'ĕ-brāt) [" + *cerebrum,* brain] **1.** To eliminate cerebral function by decerebration. **2.** A person or animal who has been subjected to decerebration.

decerebrate posture The rigid body position assumed by a patient who has lost cerebral control of spinal reflexes, usually as a result of an intracranial catastrophe. The patient's arms are stiff and extended, the forearms are pronated, and the deep tendon reflexes exaggerated.

decerebration (dē-sĕr-ĕ-brā'shŭn) Removal of the brain or cutting of the spinal cord at the level of the brainstem. SEE: *pithing*.

dechlorination, dechloridation [" + Gr. *chloros,* green] Reduction in the amount of chlorides in the body by reduction of or withdrawal of salt in the diet.

deci- [L. *decimus,* tenth] Prefix indicating *one tenth.*

decibel (dĕs'ĭ-bĕl) [L. *decimus,* tenth, + *bel,* unit of sound] The unit for expressing logarithmically the pressure or power (and thus degree of intensity or loudness) of sound.

decidophobia [*decide* + Gr. *phobos,* fear] Fear of making a decision; a slang term.

decidua (dē-sĭd'ū-ă) [L. *deciduus,* falling off] The endometrium or lining of the uterus during pregnancy, and the tissue around the ectopically located fertilized ovum, e.g., in the fallopian tube or peritoneal cavity. The gland structures of the endometrium and the interstitial cells undergo marked hypertrophy. The decidua divides itself into an outer compact layer and an inner spongy layer. **decidual** (-ăl), *adj.*

d. basalis The part of the decidua that unites with the chorion to form the placenta. SYN: *d. serotina*.

d. capsularis The part of the decidua that surrounds the chorionic sac.

d. menstrualis The layer of the uterine endometrium that is shed during menstruation.

d. parietalis The endometrium during pregnancy except at the site of the implanted blastocyst.

d. serotina D. basalis.

deciduation (dē-sĭd"ū-ā'shŭn) The loss of the decidua during menstruation.

deciduitis (dē-sĭd"ū-ī'tĭs) [" + Gr. *itis,* inflammation] Inflammation of the decidua.

deciduoma (dē-sĭd"ū-ō'mă) [" + Gr. *oma,* tumor] A uterine tumor containing decidual tissue, thought to arise from portions of decidua retained within the uterus following an abortion.

benign d. During pregnancy, the normal invasion of the uterine musculature by the syncytium, which disappears after the gestation is completed.

Loeb's d. Decidual tissue produced within the uteri of experimental animals as a result of mechanical or hormonal stimulation.

malignant d. A uterine tumor consisting of syncytial and Langhans cells, which tend to spread systemically (metastasize) by way of the bloodstream. Specific therapy with methotrexate may cause a complete remission. SYN: *choriocarcinoma; chorioepithelioma*.

ETIOLOGY: This tumor may arise following a full-term pregnancy, an ectopic pregnancy, an abortion, a miscarriage, or a molar pregnancy.

DIAGNOSIS: The diagnosis may be made by histological study, aided by the symptoms and the pregnancy test, the results of which remain strongly positive during the presence of this type of tumor.

TREATMENT: Chemotherapy with dactinomycin or the folic acid antagonist methotrexate should be administered.

deciduosarcoma [″ + Gr. *sarx,* flesh, + *oma,* tumor] A tumor of the chorion. SYN: *choriocarcinoma; chorioepithelioma.*

deciduous (dē-sĭd′ū-ŭs) [L. *deciduus*] Falling off; subject to being shed.

decigram (dĕs′ĭ-grăm) [L. *decimus,* tenth, + Gr. *gramma,* small weight] One tenth of a gram.

deciliter (dĕs′ĭ-lē-tĕr) [″ + Fr. *litre*] ABBR: dL. A unit of volume in the SI system of measurement that is equal to 0.1 L or 100 ml.

decimeter (dĕs′ĭ-mē″tĕr) [″ + Gr. *metron,* measure] One tenth of a meter.

decinormal (dĕs″ĭ-nor′măl) [″ + *norma,* rule] Having one tenth the strength of a normal solution. SEE: *normal.*

decipara (dē-sĭp′ă-ră) [″ + *parere,* to bring forth, to bear] A woman who has given birth for the tenth time to an infant or infants, alive or dead, weighing 500 g or more.

decisional conflict The state of uncertainty about the course of action to be taken when choice among competing actions involves risk, loss, or challenge to personal life values. SEE: *Nursing Diagnoses Appendix.*

decision analysis A logically consistent approach to making a medical decision when its consequences cannot be foretold with certainty. Uncertainties in medical practice are due to many factors including biological variation and limitations in the clinical data available for an individual patient. There are three steps in this process: the outcome, or consequences, of each option is described schematically by the use of a decision tree; probability is used to quantify the uncertainties inherent in each option; and each possible outcome is designated by a number that measures the patient's preference for that outcome as compared with the others. After the last step is completed, each outcome is assigned a "utility" value in which 1.0 indicates a perfect outcome and 0 is the worst possibility. Decision analysis may someday achieve widespread clinical usage in helping members of the health care team and the patient make logical choices concerning management of illness.

decision making The process of using all of the available information about a patient and arriving at a decision concerning the therapeutic plan.

decision tree A graphical analysis of the decisions or choices available to the physician in deciding a course of treatment. Included in the graph are the probabilities of all of the events that may result from each decision. SEE: *decision analysis.*

Declaration of Geneva A statement adopted in 1948 by the Second General Assembly of the World Medical Association. Some medical schools use it at graduation exercises.

"At the time of being admitted as Member of the Medical Profession I solemnly pledge myself to consecrate my life to the service of humanity. I will give to my teachers the respect and gratitude which is their due; I will practice my profession with conscience and dignity. The health of my patient will be my first consideration; I will respect the secrets which are confided in me; I will maintain by all the means in my power, the honor and the noble traditions of the medical profession; my colleagues will be my brothers; I will not permit considerations of religion, nationality, race, party politics or social standing to intervene between my duty and my patient; I will maintain the utmost respect for human life, from the time of conception; even under threat, I will not use my medical knowledge contrary to the laws of humanity. I make these promises solemnly, freely and upon my honor." SEE: *Hippocratic oath; Nightingale Pledge; Prayer of Maimonides.*

Declaration of Hawaii Ethical and practice guidelines developed by the World Psychiatric Association for the worldwide practice of psychiatry. It defines psychiatry as medical treatment of psychiatric disorders, requires maintenance and use of current clinical knowledge, describes the parameters of the therapist–patient relationship, and the need to safeguard an incapacitated or judgment-impaired individual's rights. Assessments are to be performed with full knowledge by the person being assessed and confidentiality is protected in the course of the therapeutic intervention. Research is to be undertaken with the supervision of an ethical committee, and established rules are followed for research by individuals properly trained for research.

declination (dĕk″lĭ-nā′shŭn) Cyclophoria.

declinator (dĕk′lĭn-ā″tor) [L. *declinare,* to turn aside] An instrument used during trephining for holding apart the dura mater.

decline (dē-klīn′) **1.** Progressive decrease. **2.** The declining period of a disease.

functional d. The loss of independent function that often accompanies an acute illness, a restriction in one's activities, or a change in one's diet, esp. in elderly persons.

declivis cerebelli (dē-klīv'ĭs sĕr-ĕ-bĕl'ī) [L.] The sloping posterior portion of the monticulus of the superior vermis of the cerebellum.

decoction (dē-kŏk'shŭn) [L. *de,* down, + *coquere,* to boil] A liquid medicinal preparation made by boiling vegetable substances with water. Although liquid extracts such as these are no longer used in western medicine, they are actively employed by herbalists and practitioners of traditional Chinese medicine.

decoloration (dē-kŭl"or-ā'shŭn) Loss or removal of color or pigment.

decompensation [L. *de,* from, + *compensare,* to make good again] **1.** Failure of the heart to maintain adequate circulation, or failure of other organs to work properly during stress or illness. **2.** In psychology, failure of defense mechanisms such as occurs in initial and subsequent episodes of acute mental illness.

decomposition (dē-kŏm-pō-zĭsh'ŭn) [" + *componere,* to put together] **1.** The putrefactive process; decay. **2.** Reducing a compound body to its simpler constituents. SEE: *biodegradation; fermentation; resolution.*

double d. A chemical change in which the molecules of two interacting compounds exchange a portion of their constituents.

hydrolytic d. A chemical change in substances due to addition of a molecule of water.

simple d. A chemical change by which a molecule of a single compound breaks into its simpler constituents or substitutes the entire molecule of another body for one of these constituents.

decompress (dē'kŏm-prĕs) **1.** To pass from a state of stress to tranquillity. **2.** To relieve pressure, esp. that produced by air or gas.

decompression [" + *compressio,* a squeezing together] **1.** The removal of pressure, as from gas in the intestinal tract. SEE: *Wangensteen tube.* **2.** The slow reduction or removal of pressure on deep-sea divers and caisson workers to prevent development of nitrogen bubbles in the tissue spaces.

explosive d. In aviators or divers, decompression resulting from an extremely rapid rate of change to a much lesser pressure. This may occur if a high-altitude aircraft suddenly loses its cabin pressure or if a diver ascends rapidly. Either of these causes violent expansion of body gases. SEE: *decompression illness.*

decompression illness A condition that develops when gas bubbles expand in tissues. Body fluids and tissues normally contain some dissolved gases. During activities performed at high atmospheric pressures, for example deep underwater diving, the body may become supersaturated with gases, which may rise out of solution on rapid return to atmospheric pressures. Gas bubbles that enter joints can cause musculoskeletal pain, free gases in the skin can cause itching and rash, and gas in the lungs and brain can cause chest pain, choking, or neurological dysfunction.

TREATMENT: Affected patients should be transported to specialized treatment centers where recompression or hyperbaric chambers are available.

deconditioning A loss of physical fitness due to failure to maintain an optimal level of physical activity or training. Inactivity for any reason may lead to deconditioning. For example, individuals placed on prolonged bedrest may experience overall deconditioning of the musculoskeletal and cardiopulmonary systems.

decongestant **1.** Reducing congestion or swelling. **2.** An agent that reduces congestion, esp. nasal.

decontamination The use of physical, chemical, or other means to remove, inactivate, or destroy harmful microorganisms or poisonous or radioactive chemicals from persons, spaces, surfaces, or objects. Decontamination of people exposed to hazardous materials should be performed in an orderly fashion. Tools and outer gloves should be removed first; surface contaminants should next be blown or washed away; any breathing apparatus, protective equipment, and clothing should then be removed, followed by careful washing and drying of the skin. Finally, the exposed person should be medically monitored until he or she is judged to be safe from the toxic effects of the exposure.

gastrointestinal d. Cleansing of the gastrointestinal tract to remove toxic substances, pills taken in overdose, or microorganisms. Activated charcoal or polyethylene glycol solutions (e.g., Golytely) given orally reduce the uptake of many drugs from the gastrointestinal tract. Before bowel surgery, oral antibiotics (e.g., neomycin) may be given to reduce the number of bacteria within the intestines.

decorticate posture The characteristic posture of a patient with a lesion at or above the upper brainstem. The patient is rigidly still with arms flexed, fists clenched, and legs extended.

decortication [" + *cortex,* bark] Removal of the surface layer of an organ or structure, as removal of a portion of the cortex of the brain from the underlying white matter.

pulmonary d. Removal of the pleura of the lung or a portion of the surface lung tissue.

renal d. Removal of the capsule of the kidney.

decrement (dĕk′rĕ-mĕnt) [L. *decrementum,* decrease] **1.** The period in the course of a febrile disease when the fever subsides. **2.** A reduction in the response of the nervous system to repeated stimulation. **3.** A decrease in the quantity or force of an entity. **4.** The portion of each uterine contraction between acme and baseline. The downslope is recorded by the fetal monitor.

decrepitate (dē-krĕp′ĭ-tāt) [L. *decrepitare,* to crackle] To cause decrepitation.

decrepitation A crackling noise.

decrepitude (dē-krĕp′ĭ-tūd) A state of general feebleness and decline that sometimes accompanies old age; weakness; infirmity.

decrudescence (dē-kroo-dĕs′ĕns) A decrease in the severity of disease symptoms.

decubation (dē-kū-bā′shŭn) [L. *de,* down, + *cumbere,* to lie] **1.** The act of lying down. **2.** The recovery stage of an infectious disease.

decubitus (dē-kū′bĭ-tŭs) [L., a lying down] A patient's position in bed. **decubital** (-tăl), *adj.*

Andral's d. Lying on the sound side during the early stages of pleurisy.

dorsal d. Lying on the back.

lateral d. Lying on the side.

ventral d. Lying on the stomach.

decubitus Pressure sore.

acute d. A bedsore that develops rapidly (e.g., after a stroke or paralytic illness).

decubitus projection A radiographic procedure, using the decubitus positions and the central ray of the x-ray beam placed horizontally, that aids in the demonstration of air-fluid levels.

decubitus ulcer Pressure sore.

decussate (dē-kŭs′āt) [L. *decussare,* to make an X] **1.** To cross, or crossed, as in the form of an X. **2.** Interlacing or crossing of parts.

decussation **1.** A crossing of structures in form of an X. **2.** A place of crossing. SYN: *chiasma.*

d. of pyramids Crossing of fibers of pyramids of the medulla oblongata from one pyramid to the other.

optic d. Crossing of fibers of the optic nerves; the optic chiasma.

dedifferentiation **1.** The return of parts to a homogeneous state. **2.** The process by which mature differentiated cells or tissues become sites of origin for immature elements of the same type, as in some cancers.

deductible An expense borne by an insured party before any obligated payments are made by the insurer.

deduction (dē-dŭk′shŭn) Reasoning from the general to the particular.

de-efferented state Locked-in syndrome.

deep [AS. *deop*] Below the surface.

deer fly A biting fly, *Chrysops discalis,* that transmits the causative organism of deer fly fever, a form of tularemia.

deer fly fever Tularemia.

DEET *N, N*-diethyl-3-methylbenzamide, a potent, broad-spectrum insect repellent.

DEF *decayed, extracted, filled.*

defamation In law, an intentional wrong that occurs when a person communicates to a third party false information that injures or harms an individual. Oral defamation is slander. Written defamation is libel.

defatted [L. *de,* from, + AS. *faelt,* to fatten] Freed from or deprived of fat.

defecalgesiophobia (dĕf″ĕ-kăl″jē-sē-ō-fō′bē-ă) [L. *defaecare,* to remove dregs, + Gr. *algesis,* sense of pain, + *phobos,* fear] Fear of defecating because of pain.

defecation (dĕf-ĕ-kā′shŭn) [L. *defaecare,* to remove dregs] Evacuation of the bowels. The bulk of the feces depends on the amount and composition of food ingested. One does not, however, have to eat to have bowel movements. A large quantity of cellular material is desquamated from the epithelial lining of the intestinal tract each day. The food residues, reaching the rectum, cause the urge to defecate. The sensation is related to periodic increase of pressure within the rectum and contracture of its musculature. The expulsion of a fecal mass is accompanied by coordinated action of the following mechanisms: involuntary contraction of the circular muscle of the rectum behind the bowel mass followed by contraction of the longitudinal muscle; relaxation of the internal (involuntary) and external (voluntary) sphincter ani; voluntary closure of the glottis, fixation of the chest, and contraction of the abdominal muscles, causing an increase in intra-abdominal pressure. SEE: *constipation; feces; stool.*

defecography (dĕ″fē-kŏ′grăfē) Radiography of the anorectal region after instillation of a barium paste into the rectum. The defecation process is imaged by direct filming or video recording.

defect (dē′fĕkt) A flaw or imperfection.

alcohol-related birth d. A congenital abnormality that reflects the teratogenic effects of maternal alcohol use on developing fetal structures. The most common abnormalities involve the heart, eyes, kidneys, and skeleton. SEE: *effects, fetal alcohol; fetal alcohol syndrome.*

congenital d. An imperfection present at birth.

congenital heart d. A structural abnormality of the heart and great blood vessels that occurs during intrauterine development. Abnormalities are commonly classified by the presence or absence of cyanosis. Acyanotic abnormalities include atrial and ventricular septal defects, coarctation of the aorta, and patent ductus arteriosus. Cyanotic defects include tetralogy of Fallot, transposition of the great vessels, and hypoplastic left heart syndrome.

filling d. An interruption of the contour of a body structure revealed by radiographic contrast material. It may be due to an obstruction caused by blood clots, emboli, malignancies, or extrinsic compression.

intraventricular conduction d. ABBR: IVCD. In electrocardiography, abnormally slow conduction through the ventricles that is greater than 0.12 seconds but less than 0.16 seconds. It is sometimes referred to as incomplete bundle branch block.

luteal phase d. A deficiency in either the amount or the duration of postovulatory progesterone secretion by the corpus luteum. Insufficient hormonal stimulation results in inadequate preparation of the endometrium for successful implantation and support of the growing embryo. This rare condition is associated with infertility or habitual spontaneous first-trimester abortion. SEE: *menstrual cycle.*

septal d. A defect in one or more of the septa between the heart chambers.

defective [L. *defectus,* a failure] **1.** Not perfect. **2.** A person deficient in one or more physical, mental, or moral powers.

defendant In law, the person, entity, or party charged or sued in a legal action that seeks damages or other legal relief. SEE: *plaintiff.*

defense [L. *defendere,* to repel] **1.** Resistance to disease. **2.** Protective action against harm or injury.

defense reflex Retraction or tension in defense against an action or threatened action.

defensin [term coined by Robert I. Lehrer, U.S. physician, b. 1938] Destructive peptides (groups of amino acids) found in the granules of neutrophils and other phagocytic cells that kill bacteria and fungi by destroying their membranes. Defensins are active against bacteria, fungi, and enveloped viruses in vitro. They may contribute to host defenses against susceptible organisms.

defensive Defending; protecting from injury.

defensive medicine The use of excessive health care resources to prevent malpractice litigation.

deferens (dĕf′ĕr-ĕnz) [L. *deferens,* carrying away] Deferent.

deferent (dĕf′ĕr-ĕnt) Conveying something away from or downward. SEE: *afferent; efferent.*

deferentectomy (dĕf-ĕr-ĕn-tĕk′tō-mē) [″ + Gr. *ektome,* excision] Cutting of a ductus deferens.

deferential (dĕf-ĕr-ĕn′shăl) [L. *deferre,* to bring to] Pert. to or accompanying the ductus deferens.

deferentitis (dĕf″ĕr-ĕn-tī′tĭs) [″ + Gr. *itis,* inflammation] Inflammation of the ductus deferens.

deferoxamine mesylate (dĕ-fĕr-ŏks′ă-mēn) A drug with a very high affinity for iron. It is used parenterally to reduce the iron overload in patients with hemochromatosis, acute iron poisoning, or multiple blood transfusions.

defervescence [L. *defervescere,* to become calm] The period that marks the subsidence of fever to normal temperature.

defibrillation 1. Termination of ventricular fibrillation (vfib) with electrical countershock(s). This is the single most important intervention a rescuer can take in patients who have suffered cardiac arrest due to vfib or pulseless ventricular tachycardia. **2.** A term formerly used to signify termination of atrial fibrillation. The contemporary terms are conversion or cardioversion.

defibrillator (dē-fĭb″rĭ-lā′tor) An electric device that produces defibrillation of the heart. It may be used externally or in the form of an automatic implanted cardioverter defibrillator. The latter is used in patients who have had a life-threatening ventricular tachyarrhythmia or cardiac arrest and in whom drug therapy to prevent ventricular fibrillation is ineffective or poorly tolerated. SEE: *cardioversion.*

automatic external d. Fully automatic defibrillator.

automatic implanted cardioverter d. ABBR: AICD. A defibrillator surgically implanted in patients at high risk for sudden cardiac (arrhythmia-induced) death. The device automatically detects and treats life-threatening arrhythmias.

fully automatic d. A defibrillator that performs all functions by computer (analyzes rhythm, selects an energy level, charges the machine, and shocks the patient). The operator applies adhesive paddles and turns the machine on, then makes certain that no one is in contact with the patient.

manual d. A defibrillator that requires the operator to assess the need for defibrillation (by reviewing monitor data and the patient's clinical condition), select an energy level, charge the machine, and deliver shock.

semi-automatic d. A defibrillator that assesses rhythm and gives voice prompts to the operator concerning the patient's condition, the energy level, charging, and shocking the patient.

defibrination, defibrinization [L. *de,* from, + *fibra,* fiber] The process of removing fibrin, usually from blood. SEE: *coagulation, blood.*

deficiency (dē-fĭsh′ĕn-sē) [L. *deficere,* to

lack] A lack; less than the normal amount.

branching enzyme d. Type IV glycogen storage disease.

deficit (dĕf′ĭ-sĭt) A deficiency (e.g., a loss of neurological function after a stroke).

isomolar volume d. An equal proportion of loss of water and electrolytes from the body.

reversible ischemic neurological d. ABBR: RIND. A transient stroke resulting from a decrease in cerebral blood flow. Symptoms typically last longer than 24 hr but less than 1 week.

defined medium SEE: *defined medium*.

definition [L. *definire,* to limit] **1.** The precise determination of limits, esp. of a disease process. **2.** The detail with which images are recorded on radiographic film or screens.

definitive Clear and final; without question.

deflection (dē-flĕk′shŭn) A turning away from a previous or usual course.

defloration (dĕf″lō-rā′shŭn) [L. *de,* from, + *flos, flor-,* flower] Rupture of the hymen during coitus, by accident, surgically, or through vaginal examination. Not many women have a hymen that is of such size or consistency as to require its surgical rupture. SEE: *hymen; virginity*.

deflorescence Disappearance of an eruption of the skin.

defluvium (dē-floo′vē-ŭm) [L.] The process of falling out.

deformability (dē-form″ă-bĭl′ĭ-tē) Capability of being deformed.

deformation [L. *de,* from, + *forma,* form] **1.** The act of deforming. **2.** A disfiguration.

deformity Alteration in the natural form of a part or organ; distortion of any part or general disfigurement of the body. It may be acquired or congenital. If present after injury, deformity usually implies the presence of fracture, dislocation, or both. It may be due to extensive swelling, extravasation of blood, or rupture of muscles.

anterior d. Abnormal anterior convexity of the spine. SYN: *lordosis*.

gunstock d. A deformity in which the forearm, when extended, makes an angle with the arm because of displacement of the axis of the extended arm. It is caused by a condylar fracture at the elbow.

habit-tic d. Horizontal sharp grooving in a band across the tip of the nailbed. This is caused by biting or picking the proximal nail fold of the thumb with the index fingernail.

Madelung's d. SEE: *Madelung's deformity*.

seal fin d. Obsolete term for ulnar deviation of the fingers in rheumatoid arthritis.

silverfork d. The peculiar deformity seen in Colles' fracture of the forearm. SYN: *Velpeau's d.* SEE: *Colles' fracture*.

Sprengel's d. Congenital upward displacement of the scapula.

Velpeau's d. Silverfork d.

Volkmann's d. Congenital tibiotarsal dislocation.

defurfuration (dē″fĕr-fū-rā′shŭn) [″ + *furfur,* bran] Shedding of epidermis in scales; branny desquamation. It may occur in various skin conditions, including seborrheic dermatitis (dandruff), psoriasis, ichthyosis, and eczema.

deg *degeneration; degree.*

deganglionate (dē-găn′glē-ŏn-āt″) [″ + Gr. *ganglion,* knot] To deprive of ganglia.

degenerate [L. *degenerare,* to fall from one's ancestral quality] **1.** To deteriorate. **2.** Characterized by deterioration.

degeneration [L. *degeneratio*] Deterioration or impairment of an organ or part in the structure of cells and the substances of which they are a component; opposed to regeneration. **degenerative,** *adj.*

age-related macular d. SEE: *macular degeneration*.

ascending d. Nerve fiber degeneration progressing to the center from the periphery.

calcareous d. Infiltration of inorganic calcium into tissues.

caseous d. Cheesy alteration of tissues as seen in tuberculosis.

cloudy swelling d. A condition in which protein in cells forms minute visible droplets that give the cells a cloudy appearance. It may occur in any inflamed tissue.

colloid d. Mucoid degeneration seen in the protoplasm of epithelial cells.

congenital macular d. Congenital degeneration of the macula of the eye.

cystic d. Cyst formation accompanying degeneration.

descending d. Nerve fiber degeneration progressing toward the periphery from the original lesion.

fatty d. Deposition of abnormal amounts of fat in the cytoplasm of cells, or replacement or infiltration of tissues by fat cells.

fibroid d. Change of membranous tissue into fibrous tissue.

granulovacuolar d. A pathological finding in the brain cells of some patients with Alzheimer's dementia, in which the neuronal cytoplasm is partly replaced by cavities that contain particles resembling grit or sand.

gray d. Degeneration in myelinated nerve tissue due to chronic inflammation, causing it to turn gray.

hepatocerebral d. Loss of nerve and supporting cells of the brain as a result of multiple episodes of hepatic encephalopathy or coma. This condition may be caused by Wilson's disease or other insults to the liver, such as may occur in hepatic coma produced by alcoholic, drug-induced, or viral hepatitis.

hepatolenticular d. Wilson's disease.

hyaline d. A form of degeneration in which the tissues assume a homogeneous and glassy appearance. It is caused by hyaline deposits replacing musculoelastic elements of blood vessels with a firm, transparent substance that causes loss of elasticity. It is responsible for hardening of the arteries and is often followed by calcification or deposit of lime salts in dead tissue. Calcification also may result in concretions. SYN: *vitreous d.; Zenker's d.*

hydropic d. Pathological change in cells marked by the appearance of water droplets in the cytoplasm.

lipoidal d. Deposition of fat droplets in cells.

mucoid d. Deposition of mucus in the connective tissues. SYN: *myxomatous d.*

mucous d. Deposition of mucus or mucoid substance in the connective tissue of organs or in epithelial cells.

myxomatous d. Mucoid d.

Nissl d. Nerve cell degeneration after division of the axon.

pigmentary d. Degeneration in which affected cells develop an abnormal color.

polypoid d. Formation of polyp-like growths on mucous membranes.

secondary d. Wallerian d.

senile d. The bodily and mental changes that occur during pathological aging.

senile macular d. ABBR: SMD. Degeneration of the retina that may begin and increase as a person ages.

spongy d. Familial demyelination of the deep layers of the cerebral cortex. The affected area has a spongy appearance. Symptoms include mental retardation, enlarged head, muscular flaccidity, and blindness. Death usually occurs before 18 months of age.

subacute combined d. of spinal cord Degeneration of the posterior and lateral columns of the spinal column. Clinically, paresthesia, sensory ataxia, and sometimes spastic paraplegia are present. The disease is the result of pernicious anemia.

vitreous d. Hyaline d.

wallerian d. Nerve fiber degeneration after separation from its nutritive center. SYN: *secondary d.*

Zenker's d. Hyaline d.

deglutition (dē″gloo-tĭsh′ŭn) The act of swallowing.

deglutitive Pert. to deglutition.

degradation (dĕg″rĕ-dā′shŭn) [LL. *degradare,* to go down a step] Physical, metabolic, or chemical change to a less complex form. Foods are physically degraded during chewing, and then chemically degraded from complete compounds, such as proteins and starches, to amino acids and sugars, respectively. SEE: *biodegradation.*

degranulation The release of chemical mediators from preformed storage depots in cells, esp. hematological cells such as neutrophils, mast cells, basophils, macrophages, and platelets.

degree (dĕ-grē′) **1.** A unit of measurement on a scale. **2.** A unit of angular measure. **3.** A stage of severity of a disease or injury (e.g., second-degree burn). **4.** Evidence of academic attainment granted by the institution in which the individual studied.

degrees of freedom ABBR: d.f. In defining the properties of a statistical sample, the number of independent observations in a quantity. For example, if a sample contains a total of 10 children who are being classified by hair color (brown, black, or blond) and it is known that four of the children have blond hair, then there are two degrees of freedom. If, at the beginning of the investigation, the hair color of all the subjects is unknown, there are three degrees of freedom.

degustation (dē″gŭs-tā′shŭn) [L. *degustatio*] The sense of taste; the function or act of tasting.

dehiscence (dē-hĭs′ĕns) [L. *dehiscere,* to gape] **1.** A bursting open, as of a graafian follicle or a wound, esp. a surgical abdominal wound. **2.** In dentistry, an isolated area in which the tooth root is denuded of bone from the margin nearly to the apex. It occurs more often in anterior than posterior teeth, and more on the vestibular than the oral surface.

PATIENT CARE: Dehiscence can be lessened by assessing nutritional status and risk factors such as obesity or malnourishment before surgery; by ensuring proper nutrition as time permits; and by providing support for the wound during coughing and movements that strain the incision. Surgically, stay sutures, wound bridges, etc., may minimize cases at risk. If dehiscence occurs, the surgeon is notified immediately, and the wound is covered with a sterile dressing or towel moistened with warm sterile physiological saline solution. The covering may need to be held in place by hand to keep abdominal tissues from "spilling" into the bed until a restraining bandage can be applied. The patient should flex the knees slightly to decrease tension on the abdominal muscles. The patient is kept calm and quiet, is reassured that measures are being taken to care for the wound, and is prepared physically and emotionally for surgery to close the wound. SEE: *Nursing Diagnoses Appendix.*

dehumanization (dē-hū″măn-ī-zā′shŭn) [L. *de,* from, + *humanus,* human] Loss of human qualities, as occurs in persons who are psychotic or in previously normal individuals subjected to torture or mental stress imposed by others, as could occur in prisoners.

dehumidifier (dē″hū-mĭd′ĭ-fī″ĕr) A device for removing moisture from the air.

dehydrate [L. *de,* from, + Gr. *hydor,* water] **1.** In chemistry, to deprive of, lose, or become free of water. **2.** To lose or be deprived of water from the body or tissues. **3.** To become dry.

dehydration (dē″hī-drā′shŭn) **1.** Removal of water from a substance. **2.** The clinical consequences of negative fluid balance (i.e., of fluid intakes that fail to match fluid losses). Dehydration is marked by thirst, orthostatic hypotension, tachycardia, elevated plasma sodium levels, hyperosmolality, and in severe instances, cellular disruption, renal failure, or death. SEE: *Nursing Diagnoses Appendix.*

ETIOLOGY: Worldwide, the most common cause of dehydration is diarrhea. In industrialized nations, dehydration also is caused by vomiting, fevers, heat-related illnesses, diabetes mellitus, diuretic use, thyrotoxicosis, hypercalcemia, and other illnesses. Patients at risk for dehydration include those with an impaired level of consciousness and/or an inability to ingest oral fluids, patients receiving only high-protein enteral feedings, older adults who don't drink enough water, and patients (especially infants and children) with watery diarrhea. Clinical states that can produce hypertonicity and dehydration include a deficiency in synthesis or release of antidiuretic hormone (ADH) from the posterior pituitary gland (diabetes insipidus); a decrease in renal responsiveness to ADH; osmotic diuresis (hyperglycemic states, administration of osmotic diuretics); excessive pulmonary water loss in high fever states (especially in children); and excessive sweating without water replacement.

CAUTION: Dehydration should not be confused with fluid volume deficit. In the latter condition, water and electrolytes are lost in the same proportion as they exist in normal body fluids; thus, the electrolyte to water ratio remains unchanged. In dehydration, water is the primary deficiency, resulting in increased levels of electrolytes or hypertonicity.

PATIENT CARE: The goal of treatment in dehydration is to determine and treat the underlying cause. The patient is assessed for decreased skin turgor; dry, sticky mucous membranes; rough, dry tongue; weight loss; fever; restlessness; agitation; and weakness. Cardiovascular findings include orthostatic hypotension, decreased cardiovascular pressure, and a rapid weak pulse. Hard stools result if the patient's problem is not primarily watery diarrhea. Urinary findings include a decrease in urine volume (oliguria), specific gravity greater than 1.030, and an increase in urine osmolality. Blood serum studies reveal increased sodium, protein, hematocrit, and serum osmolality.

Continued water loss is prevented, and water replacement is provided as prescribed, usually beginning with 5% dextrose in water solution intravenously, if the patient cannot ingest oral fluids. Once adequate renal function is present, electrolytes can be added to the infusion based upon periodic evaluation of serum electrolyte levels.

dehydroandrosterone (dē-hī″drō-ăn-drō-stēr′ōn, -drŏs′tĕr-ōn) A previously used name for dehydroepiandrosterone.

dehydrocholesterol (dē-hī″drō-kō-lĕs′tĕr-ŏl) A sterol found in the skin and other tissues that forms vitamin D after activation by irradiation.

dehydrocholic acid A bile salt that stimulates production of bile from the liver.

dehydrocorticosterone (dē-hī″drō-kor-tĭ-kōs′tĕr-ōn) A physiologically active steroid, $C_{21}H_{28}O_4$, isolated from the adrenal cortex. It is important in water and salt metabolism. Also called 11-dehydrocorticosterone (formerly: Kendall's compound A). SEE: *adrenal gland.*

dehydroepiandrosterone (dē-hī″drō-ĕp″ē-ăn-drŏs′tĕr-ōn) An androgenic substance, $C_{19}H_{28}O_2$, present in urine. It has about one fifth the potency of androsterone. The level of this hormone in plasma decreases with age. It is promoted as an antiaging, anticancer, and antiatherosclerosis agent by alternative medicine practitioners.

dehydrogenase (dē-hī-drŏj′ĕ-nās) An enzyme that catalyzes the oxidation of a specific substance, causing it to give up its hydrogen.

alcohol d. An enzyme that catabolizes ethyl alcohol (ethanol) in the liver. When ethanol is consumed in relatively large amounts, it is instead catabolized by the microsomal ethanol oxidizing system, also in the liver. SEE: *system, microsomal ethanol oxidizing.*

dehydrogenate (dē-hī″drŏj′ĕn-āt) To remove hydrogen from a chemical compound.

dehydroisoandrosterone (dĕ-hī″drō-ī″sō-ăn-drŏs′tĕr-ōn) A 17-ketosteroid excreted in normal male urine. It possesses androgenic activity.

deinstitutionalization The placement of hospitalized psychiatric patients in the community in halfway houses, community mental health centers, residential hotels, group homes, or boarding houses.

deionization (dē-ī″ŏn-ī-zā′shŭn) Removal of ions from a substance, producing a substance free of minerals.

Deiters' cells (dī′tĕrz) [Otto F. C. Deiters, Ger. anatomist, 1834–1863] **1.** Supporting cells in the organ of Corti. **2.** Neuroglia cell.

Deiters' nucleus Collection of cells behind the acoustic nucleus.

déjà entendu (dā′zhă ŏn-tŏn-doo′) [Fr., already heard] **1.** Recognition of something previously understood. **2.** The illusion that what one is hearing was heard previously.

déjà vu (dā′zhă voo) [Fr., already seen] The illusion that something seen or some situation being experienced for the first time has been previously seen or experienced.

dejecta (dē-jĕk′tă) [L. *dejectio,* injection] Feces; intestinal waste.

dejection, dejecture (dē-jĕk′shŭn, -tūr) **1.** A cast-down feeling or mental depression. **2.** Defecation or act of defecation.

Déjérine, Joseph Jules (dā″zhĕr-ēn′) French neurologist, 1849–1917.

D.'s disease Interstitial neuritis of infants.

D.'s syndrome A condition in which deep sensation is depressed but tactile sense is normal, caused by a lesion of the long root fibers of the posterior spinal column.

Déjérine-Sottas disease Progressive and hypertrophic interstitial neuritis of infants. It progresses slowly; the life span may be normal.

dekaliter A unit of volume in the SI system of measurement that is equal to 10 L. SEE: *decaliter; deciliter.*

delacrimation (dē-lăk″rĭ-mā′shŭn) [L. *de,* from, + *lacrima,* tear] Excessive flow of tears. SEE: *epiphora.*

delamination (dē-lăm″ĭn-ā′shŭn) [″ + *lamina,* plate] Division into layers, esp. that of a blastoderm into two layers—epiblast and hypoblast.

de Lange's syndrome [Cornelia de Lange, Dutch pediatrician, 1871–1950] A congenital disorder marked by mental retardation, a small round head, thin lips, downward curve of the mouth, small feet, short stature, failure to thrive, and generalized hirsutism. Mental retardation is present and autism may develop. The cause is unknown. SYN: *Cornelia de Lange's syndrome.*

delead (dē-lĕd) To remove lead from the body or a tissue. SEE: *chelate.*

deleterious (dĕl″ĕ-tē′rē-ŭs) [Gr. *deleterios*] Harmful.

deletion (dē-lē′shŭn) In cytogenetics, the loss of a portion of a chromosome.

Delhi boil Aleppo boil.

delicate Having a fine, fragile structure.

delimitation [L. *de,* from, + *limitare,* to limit] Determination of limits of an area or organ in diagnosis.

delinquent (dē-lĭn′kwĕnt) **1.** Someone, esp. a juvenile, whose behavior is criminal or antisocial. **2.** Of a criminal or antisocial nature.

deliquescence (dĕl″ĭ-kwĕs′ĕns) The process of becoming liquefied or moist by absorbing of water from the air. Ordinary table salt has this property. **deliquescent,** *adj.*

délire de toucher (dā-lĕr′ dŭ too-shā′) [Fr.] An abnormal desire to touch or feel things.

deliriant, delirifacient (dē-lĭr′ē-ănt, dē-lĭr″ĭ-fā′shĭ-ĕnt) [L. *delirare,* to be deranged] An agent that produces delirium (e.g., atropine or hyoscine).

delirium (dē-lĭr′ē-ŭm) [L.] An acute, reversible state of agitated confusion. Delirium is marked by disorientation without drowsiness; hallucinations or delusions; difficulty in focusing attention; inability to rest or sleep; and emotional, physical, and autonomic overactivity.

ETIOLOGY: Common causes include drug and alcohol withdrawal; medication side effects; infections (esp. sepsis); pain; surgery or trauma; hypoxia; electrolyte and acid-base imbalances; sensory deprivation and sensory overload.

TREATMENT: Treatment involves determining the cause of the delirium and removing or resolving it if possible.

PATIENT CARE: The caregiver calmly assesses the patient for changes in behavior and meets the patient's needs for comfort. The patient benefits from reality orientation and reorientation. Large clocks and calendars help to keep the patient oriented to date and time. Conversation, distraction, games, and shared activities are preferable to physical restraints because restraints may increase fear and agitation and injure confused patients.

acute d. Delirium developing suddenly.

alcoholic d. D. tremens.

d. cordis Atrial fibrillation.

d. epilepticum Delirium following an epileptic attack or appearing instead of an attack.

febrile d. Delirium occurring with fever.

d. of negation Delirium in which the patient thinks body parts are missing.

d. of persecution Delirium in which the patient feels persecuted by surrounding persons.

partial d. Delirium acting on only a portion of the mental faculties, causing only some of the patient's actions to be unreasonable.

senile d. An intermittent or permanent state of disorientation, hallucinations, confusion, and wandering that may come on abruptly in old age or may be associated with senile dementia.

toxic d. Delirium produced by a toxin.

traumatic d. Delirium following injury or shock.

d. tremens ABBR: DT. The most severe expression of alcohol withdrawal syndrome, marked by visual, auditory, or tactile hallucinations, extreme disorientation, restlessness, and hyperactivity of the autonomic nervous system (evidenced by such findings as pupillary dilation, fever, tachycardia, hypertension, and profuse sweating). About 15% of affected patients may die, usually as a result of co-morbid illnesses. In most affected patients, recovery occurs within 3 to 5 days. SYN: *alcoholic d.* SEE: *alcoholism; alcohol withdrawal syndrome.*

TREATMENT: Sedation with benzodiazepines is the cornerstone of therapy. Other principles of general supportive care include airway protection (and intubation, when indicated); fluid and electrolyte resuscitation; hemodynamic support; protection of the patient from injury; and seizure precautions. Co-morbid conditions resulting from chronic alcoholism, such as pancreatitis, esophagitis, hepatitis, or malnutrition, may complicate therapy.

PATIENT CARE: The patient and those around him or her are protected from harm while prescribed treatment is carried out to relieve withdrawal symptoms. The patient's mental status, cardiopulmonary and hepatic function, and vital signs, including body temperature, are monitored in anticipation of complicating hyperthermia or circulatory collapse. Prescribed drug and fluid therapy, titrated to the patient's symptoms and blood pressure response, are administered; and the patient's need for anticonvulsant drugs is evaluated, and such drugs given as prescribed. A calm, nonstressful, evenly illuminated environment is provided to reduce visual hallucinations. The patient is called by name, surroundings are validated frequently to orient the patient to reality, and all procedures are explained. The patient is observed closely and left alone as little as possible. Physical restraints should be reserved for patients who are combative or who have attempted to injure themselves. Patience, tact, understanding, and support are imperative throughout the acute withdrawal period. Once the acute withdrawal has subsided, the patient is advised of the need for further treatment and supportive counseling. SEE: *Nursing Diagnoses Appendix.*

CAUTION: It is crucial to distinguish the signs and symptoms of alcoholic delirium from those caused by intracerebral hemorrhage, meningitis, or intoxications with substances other than alcohol. Evaluation of the patient suspected of having DTs may therefore require neuroimaging, lumbar puncture, or drug screening.

---

deliver [L. *deliberare,* to free completely] **1.** To aid in childbirth. **2.** To remove or extract, as a tumor from a cystic enclosure or a cataract.

delivery Giving birth to a child, together with the placenta and membranes, by a parturient woman. SEE: *labor.*

abdominal d. Delivery of a child by cesarean section.

breech d. Delivery of the fetus that presents in the breech position (i.e., the buttocks are the first part of the body to be delivered). Also called *breech extraction.* SEE: *breech presentation.*

forceps d. Delivery of a child by application of forceps to the fetal head. These may be applied prior to head engagement. This method is called *high forceps delivery;* if the forceps are applied after the head is visible, *low forceps delivery;* or, if they are applied after engagement but prior to the head becoming visible, *midforceps delivery.*

postmortem d. Delivery of the child by either the abdominal or vaginal route after death of the mother.

precipitous d. An unexpected birth caused by swift progression through the second stage of labor with rapid fetal descent and expulsion. SEE: *precipitate labor.*

PATIENT CARE: Although primiparas may experience unduly rapid labor and delivery, the event is more common among multiparas. Signs to be particularly alert for are an accelerating second stage, such as the abrupt onset of strong contractions, an intense urge to bear down, or the patient's conviction that delivery is imminent. To diminish the urge to push, the woman should be encouraged to pant.

Emergency delivery by health care professionals. If time permits, the health care provider opens the emergency delivery pack, scrubs, and gloves, and places a sterile drape under the patient's buttocks. As crowning occurs, the health care provider uses the dominant hand to gently support the oncoming fetal head and the other hand to support the woman's perineum. If the amniotic sac is intact, the membranes are broken. The head should be born between contractions and supported as it emerges. The health care provider immediately feels for a nuchal cord. If the cord loosely encircles the infant's neck, it should be slipped over the infant's head. If it is tightly looped, two clamps are used to occlude the cord, and cut it between them. The clamp is left in place. The health care provider unwinds the cord and suctions the infant's nose and mouth. He or she places one hand on either side of the infant's head and gently exerts downward traction to deliver the anterior shoulder. Gentle upward traction assists delivery of the posterior shoulder, and the body emerges as the mother gently pushes. Standard birthing protocols are then followed, such as using a bulb syringe to suction the newborn as needed, drying the infant, and placing the newborn on the mother's abdomen in a head-dependent position to facilitate drainage of mucus and fluid. The patient is assessed for signs of placental separation (small gush of blood, more cord protruding from the vagina, fundal rebound). Traction on the cord to hasten placental separation is contraindicated. The postdelivery status of the mother and newborn is assessed and recorded.

premature d. Preterm d.

preterm d. Childbirth that occurs between the date of fetal viability and the end of the 37th week of gestation. SYN: *premature d.* SEE: *preterm labor*.

spontaneous d. Delivery of an infant without external aid.

vaginal d. Expulsion of a child, placenta, and membranes through the birth canal.

dellen (dĕl′ĕn) A depression or thinning in the corneal surface of the eye. It may be due to swelling of adjacent tissue from wearing contact lenses or degenerative changes.

delomorphous cell A granular cell that stains easily. It is found next to the basement membrane in the stomach and the glands in the cardiac region.

delousing (dē-lows′ĭng) [L. *de,* from, + AS. *lus,* louse] Ridding the body of lice. SEE: *louse*.

delta 1. Δ or δ, respectively, the uppercase and lowercase symbols for the fourth letter of the Greek alphabet. **2.** A triangular space. **3.** Change in value or amount of something being measured or monitored.

deltacortisone (dĕl″tă-kor′tĭ-sōn) Prednisone, a steroid hormone with glucocorticoid activity.

delta fornicis (dĕl′tă for′nĭ-sĭs) [L.] A triangular surface on the lower side of the fornix.

delta hepatitis virus ABBR: HDV. SEE: *hepatitis D*.

deltoid [Gr. *delta,* letter d, + *eidos,* form, shape] Shaped like the uppercase form of the Greek letter delta (Δ); triangular.

deltoid muscle The large triangular muscle that covers the shoulder joint.

deltoid ridge The ridge on the humerus where the deltoid muscle is attached.

delusion (dē-loo′zhŭn) [L. *deludere,* to cheat] A false belief brought about without appropriate external stimulation and inconsistent with the individual's own knowledge and experience. It is seen most often in psychoses, in which patients cannot separate delusion from reality. It differs from hallucination, in that the latter involves the false excitation of one or more senses. The most serious delusions are those that cause patients to harm others or themselves (e.g., fear of being poisoned may cause the patient to refuse food). Delusions may lead to suicide or self-injury. False beliefs might include being persecuted or being guilty of an unpardonable sin.

d. of control A delusion that one's thoughts and actions are under the control of an external force.

depressive d. A delusion causing a saddened state.

expansive d. An unreasonable conviction of one's own power, importance, or wealth, accompanied by a feeling of well-being, seen in manic patients. These beliefs are not consistent with reality. SEE: *megalomania*.

fixed d. A delusion that remains unaltered.

d. of grandeur A false sense of possessing wealth or power. SYN: *megalomania*.

d. of negation Nihilistic d.

nihilistic d. A delusion that everything has ceased to exist. SYN: *d. of negation*.

d. of persecution A delusion in which patients believe people or agencies are seeking to injure or harass them.

reference d. A delusion that causes the patient to read an unintended meaning into the acts or words of others; often the interpretation is of slight or ridicule.

systematized d. A logical correlation with false reasoning and deduction.

unsystematized d. A delusion with no correlation between ideas and actual circumstances.

delusional Pert. to a delusion.

demand 1. A need for something. **2.** A legal obligation asserted in courts, such as a payment of a debt or monetary award for injuries suffered by the plaintiff and allegedly caused by the defendant. **3.** In health care delivery, the amount of care a population seeks to use.

biological oxygen d. The amount of oxygen required for a biological reaction, esp. the oxygen required to oxidize materials in natural water supplies, such as rivers or lakes. SEE: *eutrophication*.

specific adaptations to imposed d. ABBR: SAID. A principle in exercise prescription that any tissue will alter its structure to accommodate the stresses placed on it. The intensity and direction of force, type and speed of muscle contraction, frequency and duration of exercise, range of motion, and external environment each influence tissue adaptation. In physical therapy, this principle is used to prescribe the best exercises to regain function in work, sports, or other activities.

demand valve manually cycled resuscitator A multifunction resuscitator that uses high-flow oxygen. This device often can be triggered by negative pressure caused by an inhaling patient, as well as operated by a button while the operator watches the patient's chest rise. During resuscitation, it is necessary to use the positive pressure aspect of this device and manually trigger or compress the button, as the patient is not able to open up the valve by inhaling. These devices should be fitted with an overinflation high-pressure alarm to avoid gastric distention and/or barotrauma.

demarcation (dē″măr-kā′shŭn) [L. *demarcare,* to limit] A limit or boundary.

demasculinization Loss of male sexual characteristics. This may be caused by lack of the male hormone or by the action of certain drugs.

demecarium bromide (dĕm″ē-kā′rē-ŭm) An anticholinesterase agent used in treating glaucoma.

demeclocycline hydrochloride (dĕm″ĕ-klō-sī′klēn) A tetracycline-type antibiotic, used primarily to treat the syndrome of inappropriate secretion of antidiuretic hormone. The drug interferes with the action of antidiuretic hormone at the renal collecting ducts.

demented Chronically cognitively impaired. SEE: *dementia.*

dementia (dē-mĕn′shē-ă) [L. *dementare,* to make insane] A progressive, irreversible decline in mental function, marked by memory impairment and, often, deficits in reasoning, judgment, abstract thought, registration, comprehension, learning, task execution, and use of language. The cognitive impairments diminish a person's social, occupational, and intellectual abilities. Dementia is largely, although by no means exclusively, a disease of the aged. In the U.S., 20% to 40% of individuals over age 85 suffer dementia. The condition is somewhat more common in women than in men. It must be distinguished by careful clinical examination from delirium, psychosis, depression, and the effects of medications. SEE: *Alzheimer's disease; Huntington's chorea; Parkinson's disease.*

SYMPTOMS: The onset of primary dementia may be slow, over months or years. Memory deficits, impaired abstract thinking, poor judgment, and clouding of consciousness and orientation are not present until the terminal stages; depression, agitation, sleeplessness, and paranoid ideation may be present. Patients become dependent for activities of daily living and typically die from complications of immobility in the terminal stage.

ETIOLOGY: Dementia may result from many illnesses, including AIDS, chronic alcoholism, Alzheimer's disease, vitamin B_{12} deficiency, carbon monoxide poisoning, cerebral anoxia, hypothyroidism, subdural hematoma, multiple brain infarcts, and others.

TREATMENT: A limited benefit is obtained in some patients treated with donepezil, tacrine, or gingko biloba.

alcoholic d. Dementia in the terminal portion of the chronic alcoholic state.

apoplectic d. Dementia due to cerebral hemorrhage or tumor.

dialysis d. A neurological disturbance seen in patients who have been on dialysis for several years. There are speech difficulties, myoclonus, dementia, seizures, and eventually death. The causative agent is presumed to be aluminum in the dialysate.

epileptic d. Dementia seen in some cases of long-term epilepsy.

multi-infarct d. Dementia resulting from multiple small strokes. After Alzheimer's disease, it is the most common form of dementia in the U.S. It has a distinctive natural history, unlike Alzheimer's disease, which develops insidiously. The cognitive deficits of multi-infarct dementia appear suddenly, in "step-wise" fashion. The disease is rare before middle age, and is most common in patients with hypertension, diabetes mellitus, or other risk factors for generalized atherosclerosis. Brain imaging in patients with this form of dementia shows multiple lacunar infarctions. SYN: *vascular d.*

d. paralytica A form of neurosyphilis marked by a sudden onset with irritability and deterioration of memory and concentration. Behavior deteriorates and emotional instability develops. Neurasthenia, depression, and delusions of grandeur with lack of insight may be present.

postfebrile d. Dementia following a severe febrile illness.

presenile d. Dementia beginning in middle age, usually resulting from cerebral arteriosclerosis or Alzheimer's disease. The symptoms are apathy, loss of memory, and disturbances of speech and gait. SEE: *Nursing Diagnoses Appendix.*

primary d. Dementia associated with Alzheimer's disease.

d. pugilistica Traumatic dementia; that is, dementia caused by physical injury to the brain. It is sometimes referred to colloquially as "boxer's brain."

senile d. of the Alzheimer's type ABBR: SDAT. Alzheimer's disease.

syphilitic d. Dementia caused by a lesion of syphilis.

toxic d. Dementia due to excessive use of a drug or drugs toxic to the central nervous system.

vascular d. Multi-infarct d.

demi- [L. *dimidius,* half] Prefix indicating *half.*

demibain (dĕm′ĭ-băn) [Fr., half bath] Half a bath. A sitz bath.

demifacet In the thoracic spine, T1 through T9, a notch on the superior and inferior aspects of the posterior vertebral bodies that articulates with the head of the rib.

demilune (dĕm′ĭ-loon) [L. *dimidius,* half, + *luna,* moon] A crescent-shaped group of serous cells that form a caplike structure over a mucous alveolus. They are present in mixed glands, esp. the submandibular gland.

demineralization [L. *de,* from, + *minare,* to mine] Loss of mineral salts, esp. from the bones. It occurs commonly in juxta-articular or peri-articular locations in patients with rheumatoid arthritis. SEE: *decalcification.*

demise (dĕ-mīz′) [L. *dimittere,* to dismiss] Death.

demodectic (dĕm-ō-dĕk′tĭk) Concerning or caused by the mite *Demodex.*

Demodex [Gr. *demos,* fat, + *dex,* worm] A genus of mites and ticks of the class Arachnida and order Acarina.

D. folliculorum The hair follicle or face mite; an almost microscopic elongated wormlike organism that infests hair follicles and sebaceous glands of various mammals, including humans.

demography (dē-mŏg′ră-fē) [Gr. *demos,* people, + *graphein,* to write] The study of measurable characteristics of human populations such as their size, growth, density, age, race and sex distribution, or marital status. This information may be used to forecast health needs and the use of health services.

demoniac 1. Concerning or resembling a demon. **2.** Frenzied, as if possessed by demons or evil spirits.

demorphinization (dē-mor″fĭn-ī-zā′shŭn) Gradual decrease in the dose of morphine being used by one addicted to that drug.

demotivate To cause loss of incentive or motivation.

Demours′ membrane (dē-mūr′) [Pierre Demours, Fr. ophthalmologist, 1702–1795] A fine membrane between the endothelial layer of the cornea and the substantia propria. SYN: *Descemet's membrane.*

demucosation (dē″mū-kō-sā′shŭn) [L. *demucosatio*] Removal of mucosa from any part of body.

demulcent [L. *demulcens,* stroking softly] An oily or mucilaginous agent used to soothe or soften an irritated surface, esp. mucous membranes. SEE: *emollient.*

de Musset's sign SEE: *Musset's sign.*

demyelinate (dē-mī′ĕ-lĭ-nāt) [″ + Gr. *myelos,* marrow] To remove the myelin sheath of nerve tissue.

demyelinating An inflammatory process of nerves that destroys normal, healthy myelin.

demyelination Destruction or removal of the myelin sheath of nerve tissue, seen in Guillain-Barré syndrome, multiple sclerosis, and many other neurological diseases.

denaturation (dē-nā″chŭr-ā′shŭn) **1.** Addition of a substance to alcohol that makes it toxic and unfit for human consumption but usually does not interfere with its use for other purposes. **2.** A change in conditions (temperature, addition of a substance) that causes an irreversible change in a protein's structure, usually resulting in precipitation of the protein.

denatured [″ + *natura,* nature] **1.** A change in the usual character of a substance, as when the addition of methanol to alcohol renders it unfit for consumption. **2.** Structurally altered.

dendraxon (dĕn-drăk′sŏn) [Gr. *dendron,* tree, + *axon,* axle] A term formerly used to indicate the terminal filaments of an axon.

dendric (dĕn′drĭk) Pert. to or possessing a dendron.

dendriform (dĕn′drĭ-form) [″ + L. *forma,* shape] Branching or treelike.

dendrite (dĕn′drīt) [Gr. *dendrites,* pert. to a tree] A branched cytoplasmic process of a neuron that conducts impulses to the cell body. There are usually several to a cell. They form synaptic connections with other neurons. SYN: *dendron; neurodendrite.* SEE: illus.

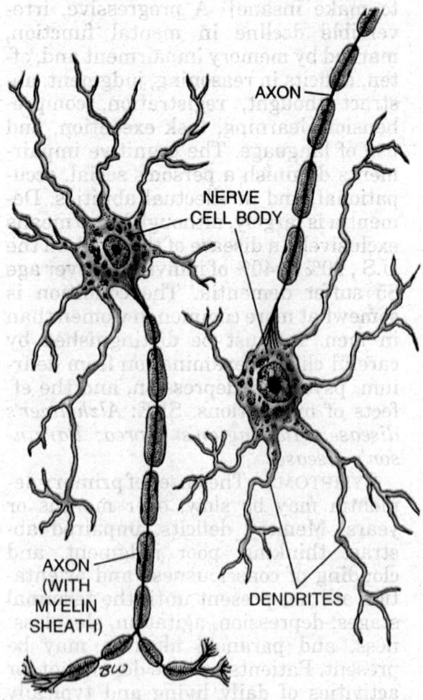

DENDRITES

extracapsular d. A dendrite of a neuron of autonomic ganglia that pierces the capsule surrounding the cell and extends for a considerable distance from the cell body.

intracapsular d. A dendrite of a neuron of autonomic ganglia that branches beneath the capsule, forming a network about the cell body.

dendritic Treelike.

dendritic calculus A renal stone molded in the form of the pelvis and calyces.

dendroid (dĕn′droyd) [″ + *eidos,* form, shape] **1.** Dendriform; dendritic; pert. to dendrites. **2.** Arborescent; treelike.

dendron (dĕn′drŏn) [Gr., tree] A dendrite; a cytoplasmic branch from a nerve cell. SYN: *neurodendrite.*

dendrophagocytosis (dĕn″drō-făg-ō-sī-tō′sĭs) [Gr. *dendron,* tree, + *phagein,* to eat, + *kytos,* cell, + *osis,* condition] Absorption of portions of astrocytes by microglia cells.

denervation [L. *de,* from, + Gr. *neuron,* nerve] **1.** Excision, incision, or blocking of a nerve supply. **2.** A condition in which the afferent and efferent nerves are cut. SEE: *deafferentation.*

dengue (dāng′gā, -gĕ) [Sp.] An acute febrile illness, often presenting with severe musculoskeletal pain, caused by one of four serotypes of flavivirus. The disease is transmitted to humans by the bite of the *Aedes aegypti* mosquito. It is endemic in tropical regions of the world and a major health problem in Southeast Asia, Mexico, and Central America, where it causes periodic epidemic disease. Worldwide, tens of millions of people have been infected. Outbreaks occur sporadically in southern Texas and the southeastern U.S. (approx. 200 confirmed cases in 1997). SYN: *breakbone fever; dengue fever.*

SYMPTOMS: The incubation period of 5 to 7 days precedes sudden onset of fever, myalgia, arthralgias, headache, and abdominal pain; a rash may develop 3 days later. Most patients recover without a problem. About 5% of patients develop bleeding into the brain and lungs, with severe neutropenia and thrombocytopenia (dengue hemorrhagic fever). This illness often affects children and is frequently fatal.

ETIOLOGY: Dengue is caused by the Group B arbovirus transmitted by mosquitoes. The incubation period is 3 to 15 days, usually 5 to 6 days.

TREATMENT: Dengue is treated with antipyretics and analgesics. No drugs are effective against the virus. Candidate vaccines are being tested for disease prevention.

denial (dĕ-nī′ăl) **1.** Refusal to admit the reality, or to acknowledge the presence or existence, of something; keeping of anxiety-producing realities from conscious awareness. This is a defense mechanism. **2.** In medical care reimbursement, the decision by the patient's insurer that part or all of the medical care administered was not justified. The result of the denial is that the insurer refuses to pay for all or a portion of the medical costs incurred.

ineffective d. The state of a conscious or unconscious attempt to disavow the knowledge or meaning of an event to reduce anxiety/fear to the detriment of health. SEE: *Nursing Diagnoses Appendix.*

denial and isolation According to Elisabeth Kübler-Ross, the initial emotional reactions to being told of impending death. Individuals refuse to accept the diagnosis and seek additional professional opinions in the hope that the predicted outcome is erroneous. When these efforts are in vain, the patient feels isolated and abandoned. SEE: *acceptance.*

denitrify To remove nitrogen from something.

denitrogenation In aerospace medicine, the removal of nitrogen from the body of a person preparing to fly in an environment in which the barometric pressure will be much lower than at sea level. Prior to the flight, the person breathes 100% oxygen for a variable length of time, depending on the anticipated degree of reduced barometric pressure. SYN: *preoxygenation.* SEE: *decompression illness.*

Dennie's line [Charles Clayton Dennie, U.S. dermatologist, 1883–1971] An extra fold of skin below the lower eyelid. It may be present in patients with atopic dermatitis.

dens (dĕnz) *pl.* **dentes** [L.] **1.** A tooth. SEE: *dentition* for illus. **2.** The odontoid process of the axis, which serves as a pivot for the rotation of the atlas.

d. bicuspidus D. premolaris.

d. caninus A canine tooth.

d. deciduus A milk tooth, or first tooth.

d. incisivus An incisor tooth.

d. in dente A dental anomaly in which the radiograph of a tooth shows the outline of a second dental structure inside it. Outwardly, on inspection, the visible tooth is normal. SYN: *d. invaginatus.*

d. invaginatus D. in dente.

d. molaris A molar tooth, or grinder.

d. permanens One of the 32 permanent teeth. SYN: *permanent dentition.*

d. premolaris A premolar tooth. SYN: *d. bicuspidus.*

d. serotinus A wisdom tooth (third molar).

densitometer (dĕn″sĭ-tŏm′ĕ-tĕr) **1.** An instrument that measures bacterial growth and the effect on it of antiseptics and bacteriophages. **2.** In radiology, an instrument that measures the optical density of a radiograph. SEE: illus.

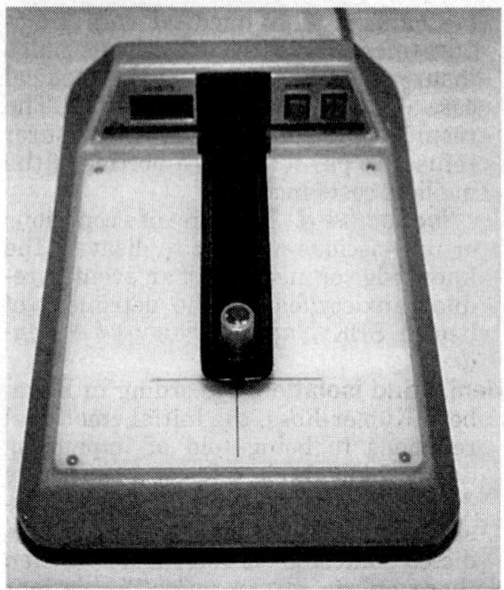

DENSITOMETER

densitometry (děn″sĭ-tŏm′ĕ-trē) **1.** The determination of the density of a substance (e.g., bone). **2.** The determination of the amount of ionizing radiation to which a person has been exposed.

density [L. *densitas,* thickness] **1.** The relative weight of a substance compared with a reference standard. SEE: *specific gravity.* **2.** The quality of being dense. **3.** The degree of blackness on a radiograph or the relationship between the light given and the light passing through a radiograph.

bone mass d. ABBR: BMD. The heft of the skeleton. BMD is reduced in osteoporosis, and the reduction in skeletal mass predisposes patients to fractures. BMD can be measured by dual x-ray absorptiometry (DEXA) and several other techniques. All women over age 65 should have some form of BMD measurement, so that fracture-preventing treatments can be started if osteopenia is found. Any woman with an osteoporotic fracture or multiple risk factors for osteoporosis, regardless of age, should also have her BMD measured.

caloric d. Calories per gram of food. The number of calories in a given mass of food influences hunger and feeding behaviors in animals and humans. When a limited amount of food is available, foods of higher caloric density are more likely to satisfy hunger than equivalent amounts of food with fewer calories. Calorically dense foods that provide little in the way of micronutrients are often termed empty calories. SEE: *satiety.*

nutrient d. The ratio of the nutrients present in a food, relative to its caloric value.

dent- SEE: *dento-.*

dental Pert. to the teeth.

dental chart A diagram of the mouth on which clinical and radiographic findings can be recorded. It often includes restorations, decayed surfaces, missing teeth, and periodontal conditions.

dental consonant A consonant pronounced with the tongue at or near the front upper teeth. The term is used in speech therapy.

dental curve The curve or bow of the line of the teeth. Its different portions are described as follows: *alignment curve,* the line passing through the center of the teeth from the middle line through the last molar; *buccal curve,* the curve extending from the cuspid to the third molar; *compensating curve,* the occlusal line of the bicuspids and molars; *labial curve,* the curve extending from cuspid to cuspid.

dental dysfunction Malfunctioning of the parts of the dental structure.

dental emergency An acute condition affecting the teeth, such as inflammation of the soft tissues surrounding teeth or posttreatment complications of dental surgery. It is best treated by a dentist. Nevertheless, the primary care physician and other health care professionals must be familiar with these emergency conditions and their management. SEE: table.

dental engineering Use of the principles of engineering in dentistry.

dental geriatrics The scientific study and treatment of dental conditions of the aged.

dentalgia (děn-tăl′jē-ă) [L. *dens,* tooth, + Gr. *algos,* pain] Toothache.

dental handpiece An instrument designed to hold the rotary instruments used in dentistry to remove tooth structure or to smooth and polish restorative materials; it may be powered by electric motor or air turbines.

dental index A system of numbers for indicating comparative size of the teeth.

dental material Any of several types of colloids, plastics, resins, and metal alloys used in dentistry to take impressions, restore teeth, or duplicate dentition.

dental tape Waxed or unwaxed thin tape used for cleaning and removing plaque from between the teeth.

dental trephination Surgical creation of a drainage tract, with a bur or sharp instrument, in the soft tissue or bone overlying a tooth root apex. This is usually done to permit drainage of an apical abscess. SYN: *apicostomy.*

dentate (děn′tāt) [L. *dentatus,* toothed] Notched; having short triangular divisions at the margin; toothed.

dentes *sing.,* **dens** [L.] Teeth.

denti- SEE: *dento-.*

dentia (děn′shē-ă) [L.] Eruption of teeth.

d. praecox Premature eruption of teeth.

Signs and Symptoms and Recommended Emergency Management of Odontogenic Problems

Condition	Signs and Symptoms	Management
Periodontal disease		
Periodontal abscess	Localized pain Swelling of gingivae Possible sinus tract Lack of response to percussion Periodontal pocketing	Curettage to establish drainage Antibiotics Warm saline rinses Soft diet Referral to dentist
Pericoronitis	Pain and generalized soreness Inflamed operculum over partially erupted tooth	Irrigation Warm saline rinses Gentle massage with toothbrush Antibiotics for fever and lymphadenopathy Referral to dentist for possible tissue excision or tooth removal
Necrotizing ulcerative gingivitis	Generalized pain Bleeding gums Fetid odor Generalized gingival inflammation Necrotic tissue Loss of interdental papillae Fever	Brushing, flossing, general débridement Daily saline rinses Hydration Referral to dentist Antibiotics if necessary Dietary recommendations Rinse twice daily with 1.2% chlorhexidine rinse
Primary herpetic gingivostomatitis (highly infectious)	Gingival ulceration Fever Punctate lesions of gingivae and possibly dorsum of tongue, buccal mucosa, floor of mouth, lips Malaise Headache Irritability Lymphadenopathy	Rest Diluted mouthwashes Increased fluid intake Soft diet Topical analgesics Referral to dentist
Pulpitis and periapical problems		
Reversible pulpitis	Sharp, transient pain response to cold stimuli Recent dental restoration	Analgesics Avoidance of thermal stimuli Referral to dentist
Irreversible pulpitis	Spontaneous pain Persistent pain response to thermal stimuli	Referral to dentist for removal of pulp or extraction of tooth
Periapical inflammation	Acute pain on percussion	Examination for lymph node involvement, intraoral and extraoral swelling, fever Analgesics Referral to dentist
Periapical abscess	Tooth sensitive to touch Tooth mobile Fever Swelling	Thorough systemic examination Incision and drainage Antibiotics Analgesics Warm water rinses Referral to dentist

Table continued on following page

Signs and Symptoms and Recommended Emergency Management of Odontogenic Problems (Continued)

Condition	Signs and Symptoms	Management
Posttreatment complications		
Alveolar osteitis (dry socket)	Throbbing pain 2–4 days after extraction	Irrigation of extraction site Sedative dressing (eugenol) Analgesics Gauze packs, bone wax, or gelatin sponge to control hemorrhage Referral to dentist
Tooth sensitivity	Imbalance when teeth contact Thermal sensitivity Pain on closing mouth	Referral to dentist

SOURCE: Adapted from Comer, RW, et al: Dental emergencies. Postgrad Med 85(3):63, Feb. 1989.

d. tarda Delayed eruption of teeth.

dentibuccal (dĕn-tĭ-bŭk'l) [L. *dens,* tooth, + *bucca,* cheek] Pert. to both the cheek and the teeth.

denticle (dĕn'tĭ-kl) [L. *denticulus,* little tooth] **1.** A small toothlike projection. **2.** A calcified structure within the pulp of the tooth. SYN: *pulp stone*.

denticulate [L. *denticulatus,* small-toothed] Finely toothed or serrated.

denticulate body The corpus dentatum of the cerebellum.

dentification [L. *dens,* tooth, + *facere,* to make] Conversion into dental structure.

dentiform [" + *forma,* shape] Toothlike.

dentifrice (dĕn'tĭ-frĭs) [" + *fricare,* to rub] A paste, liquid, gel, or powder for cleaning teeth. A dentifrice may be cosmetic or therapeutic. Cosmetic dentifrices must clean and polish; therapeutic dentifrices must reduce some disease process in the oral cavity. Each dentifrice generally contains an abrasive, water, humectants, a foaming agent, a binder, a flavoring agent, a sweetener, a therapeutic agent, a coloring material, and a preservative.

dentigerous (dĕn-tĭj'ĕr-ŭs) [" + *gerere,* to bear] Having or containing teeth.

dentilabial (dĕn-tĭ-lā'bē-ăl) [" + *labium,* lip] Pert. to both the teeth and the lips.

dentilingual (dĕn-tĭ-lĭn'gwăl) [" + *lingua,* tongue] Pert. to both the teeth and the tongue.

dentin (dĕn'tĭn) [L. *dens,* tooth] The calcified part of the tooth surrounding the pulp chamber, covered by enamel in the crown and cementum in the root area. Dentin is called primary, secondary, or reparative according to its location inside the tooth and its relative sensitivity.

interglobular d. Dentin that contains spaces or hypomineralized areas between mineralized globules or calcospherites.

dentinal Pert. to dentin.

dentinoclast (dĕn'tĭn-ō-clăst) [" + Gr. *clastos,* broken] A multinucleate cell indistinguishable from an osteoclast. It is involved with resorption of dentin. The same cells probably resorbed cementum before contacting dentin and would be better called odontoclasts. SEE: *osteoclast*.

dentinogenesis (dĕn"tĭn-ō-jĕn'ĕ-sĭs) [" + *genesis,* generation, birth] Formation of dentin in the development of a tooth.

d. imperfecta Hereditary aplasia or hypoplasia of the enamel and dentin of a tooth, resulting in misshapen blue or brown teeth.

dentinoid [" + Gr. *eidos,* form, shape] **1.** Resembling dentin. **2.** The noncalcified matrix of dentin, similar to the noncalcified matrix of bone, which is called osteoid. SYN: *dentoidin; predentin*.

dentinoma [" + Gr. *oma,* tumor] A tumor composed of tissues from which the teeth originate, consisting mainly of dentin.

dentinosteoid (dĕn"tĭn-ŏs'tē-oyd) [" + Gr. *osteon,* bone, + *eidos,* form, shape] A tumor composed of dentin and bone.

dentist [L. *dens,* tooth] ABBR: D.D.S., D.M.D. One who has been professionally trained and licensed to practice dentistry.

dentistry **1.** The branch of medicine dealing with the care of the teeth and associated structures of the oral cavity. It is concerned with the prevention, diagnosis, and treatment of diseases of the teeth and gums. **2.** The art or profession of a dentist.

esthetic d. Repair and restoration or replacement of carious or broken teeth.

forensic d. The area of dentistry particularly related to jurisprudence; usually, the identification of unknown persons by the details of their dentition and tooth restorations.

Whereas forensic medicine often is used to establish the time and cause of death, forensic dentistry may be used to establish identity on the basis of dental records only.

four-handed d. Extensive use of a chairside dental assistant to facilitate and enhance the productivity of the dentist.

geriatric d. Dental geriatrics.

hospital d. The practice of dentistry in a hospital where the dentist is an integral part of the comprehensive health care team.

operative d. The branch of dentistry dealing with restorative dental surgery.

preventive d. That phase of dentistry concerned with the maintenance of the normal masticatory apparatus by teaching good oral hygiene and dietary practice, and preserving dental health by early restorative procedures.

prosthodontic d. The replacement of defective or missing teeth with artificial appliances such as bridges, crowns, and dentures.

public health d. The area of dentistry that seeks to improve the dental health of communities by epidemiological studies, research in preventive methods, and better distribution, management, and use of dental skills.

dentition [L. *dentitio*] The type, number, and arrangement of teeth in the dental arch. SEE: illus.; *teeth* for illus.

altered d. A nursing diagnosis accepted at the NANDA 13th conference (1998); disruption in tooth development/eruption patterns or structural integrity of individual teeth. SEE: *Nursing Diagnoses Appendix.*

diphyodont d. Two sets of teeth (i.e., primary and permanent, as in many mammals and humans).

heterodont d. A set of teeth of various shapes which may serve different functions (e.g., incisors, canines, and molars).

mixed d. A set of both primary and permanent teeth, as in humans between 6 and 13 years of age.

monophyodont d. A single set of teeth.

permanent d. The 32 permanent teeth, which begin to erupt at about 6 years of age in humans. These are completed by the 16th year with the exception of third molars, which appear between the 18th and 25th years. The incisors are followed by the bicuspids (premolars) and the canines; then the second molars are followed by the third molars. In some individuals the third molars, although present beneath the

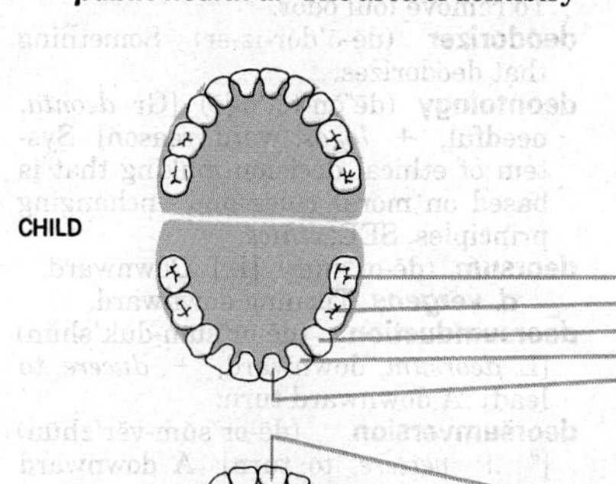

ERUPTION OF DECIDUOUS (MILK) TEETH

UPPER	ERUPTION
CENTRAL INCISOR	5–7 MO
LATERAL INCISOR	7–10 MO
(CUSPID) CANINE	16–20 MO
FIRST MOLAR	10–16 MO
SECOND MOLAR	20–30 MO
LOWER	
SECOND MOLAR	20–30 MO
FIRST MOLAR	10–16 MO
(CUSPID) CANINE	16–20 MO
LATERAL INCISOR	8–11 MO
CENTRAL INCISOR	6–8 MO

ERUPTION OF PERMANENT TEETH

UPPER	COMPLETED BY
CENTRAL INCISOR	9–10 YR
LATERAL INCISOR	10–11 YR
(CUSPID) CANINE	12–15 YR
FIRST PREMOLAR (BICUSPID)	12–13 YR
SECOND PREMOLAR (BICUSPID)	12–14 YR
FIRST MOLAR	6–7 YR
SECOND MOLAR	14–16 YR
THIRD MOLAR	18–25 YR
LOWER	
THIRD MOLAR	18–25 YR
SECOND MOLAR	13–16 YR
SECOND PREMOLAR (BICUSPID)	13–14 YR
FIRST PREMOLAR (BICUSPID)	12–15 YR
FIRST MOLAR	6–7 YR
(CUSPID) CANINE	10–13 YR
LATERAL INCISOR	9–10 YR
CENTRAL INCISOR	8–9 YR

DENTITION

gingiva, do not erupt. The appearance of the first molars is highly variable, but in some instances they may be the first permanent teeth to appear. SYN: *dens permanens*. SEE: *teeth*.

polyphyodont d. Several successive sets of teeth developing during a lifetime.

primary d. The 20 primary or deciduous teeth in humans. In general, the order of eruption is two lower central incisors, 6 to 8 months; two upper central incisors, 5 to 7 months; two lower lateral incisors, 8 to 11 months; two upper lateral incisors, 7 to 10 months; four canines (cuspids), lower and upper, 16 to 20 months; four first molars, lower and upper, 10 to 16 months; four second molars, upper and lower, 20 to 30 months.

dento-, denti-, dent- Combining form concerning teeth.

dentoalveolar (dĕn″tō-ăl-vē′ō-lăr) [L. *dens,* tooth, + *alveolus,* small hollow] Pert. to the alveolus of a tooth and the tooth itself.

dentoalveolitis (dĕn″to-ăl″vē-ō-lī′tĭs) [″ + ″ + Gr. *itis,* inflammation] A purulent inflammation of the tooth socket linings characterized by loose teeth and shrinkage of the gum.

dentofacial (dĕn″tō-fā′shăl) Concerning the teeth and face.

dentoid [″ + Gr. *eidos,* form, shape] Dentiform; odontoid; tooth-shaped.

dentoidin The organic ground substance of dentin. SYN: *dentinoid; predentin*.

dentolegal Concerning dentistry and legal matters.

dentulous (dĕn′tū-lŭs) Having one's natural teeth. SEE: *edentulous*.

denture (dĕn′chūr) A partial or complete set of artificial teeth set in appropriate plastic materials to substitute for the natural dentition and related tissues. SYN: *dental prosthesis*.

PATIENT CARE: Proper denture care involves cleansing the dentures after each meal by gently brushing them with warm water and by scrubbing them with only moderate pressure. Cleansing solutions and mixtures accepted by the American Dental Association are ammonia water 28% (2 ml in 30 ml water); trisodium phosphate (0.6 g in 30 ml water); sodium hypochlorite, or bleach (2 ml in 120 ml water). Dentures should be properly fitted in the patient's mouth; when stored outside the mouth, they should be placed in a well-identified, opaque, closed container. Dentures are stored wet or dry according to their particular composition and according to instructions by the dentist. Dentures are removed from comatose or moribund patients as well as from patients undergoing surgery.

fixed partial d. A dental restoration of one or more missing teeth that is cemented to prepared natural teeth.

full d. A dental appliance that replaces all of the teeth in both jaws.

immediate d. A complete set of artificial teeth inserted immediately after removal (extraction) of natural teeth.

implant d. An artificial denture placed in and supported by bone. The denture may be implanted at the site of a previously removed natural tooth. SEE: *implant, dental* for illus.

partial d. A dental appliance replacing less than the full number of teeth in either jaw.

denturist A person licensed in some states to fabricate and fit dentures. This person is not a dentist or a dental technician.

denucleated (dē-nū′klē-āt″ĕd) [L. *de,* from, + *nucleus,* kernel] Deprived of a nucleus.

denudation [L. *denudare,* to lay bare] Removal of a protecting layer or covering through surgery, pathological change, or trauma.

Denver classification A system for classifying chromosomes based on the size and position of the centromere. SEE: *chromosome*.

Denver Developmental Screening Test ABBR: DDST. A widely used screening test to detect problems in the development of very young children.

deodorant (dē-ō′dor-ănt) [″ + *odorare,* to perfume] An agent that masks or absorbs foul odors. SEE: *odor*.

deodorize (dē-ō′dor-īz) [″ + *odor,* odor] To remove foul odor.

deodorizer (dē-ō′dor-īz-ĕr) Something that deodorizes.

deontology (dē″ŏn-tŏl′ō-jē) [Gr. *deonta,* needful, + *logos,* word, reason] System of ethical decision making that is based on moral rules and unchanging principles. SEE: *ethics*.

deorsum (dē-or′sŭm) [L.] Downward.

d. vergens Turning downward.

deorsumduction (dē-or″sŭm-dŭk′shŭn) [L. *deorsum,* downward, + *ducere,* to lead] A downward turn.

deorsumversion (dē-or″sŭm-vĕr′zhŭn) [″ + *vertere,* to turn] A downward turning or movement of the eyes.

deossification (dē-ŏs″ĭ-fĭ-kā′shŭn) [L. *de,* from, + *os,* bone, + *facere,* to make] Loss or removal of mineral matter from bone or osseous tissue.

deoxidation The process of depriving a chemical compound of oxygen.

deoxidizer (dē-ŏk′sĭ-dī-zĕr) An agent that removes oxygen.

deoxycholic acid (dē-ŏk″sē-kō′lĭk) $C_{24}H_{40}O_4$. A crystalline acid found in bile.

deoxycorticosterone (dē-ŏk″sē-kor″tē-kŏs′tĕr-ōn) A hormone from the adrenal gland. It acts principally on salt and water metabolism.

deoxygenation (dē-ŏk″sĭ-jĕn-ā′shŭn)

Removal of oxygen from a chemical compound or tissue.

deoxyhemoglobin Chemically reduced (deoxygenated) hemoglobin.

deoxyribonuclease (dē-ŏk″sē-rī″bō-nū′klē-ās) ABBR: DNase. An enzyme that hydrolyzes and thus depolymerizes deoxyribonucleic acid (DNA).

deoxyribonucleoprotein (dē-ŏk″sē-rī″bō-nū″klē-ō-prō′tē-ĭn) One of a class of conjugated proteins that contain deoxyribonucleic acid.

deoxyribonucleoside (dē-ŏk″sē-rī″bō-nū′klē-ō-sīd) One of a class of nucleotides in which the pentose is 2-deoxyribose.

deoxyribose (dē-ŏk″sē-rī′bōs) A pentose sugar that is part of DNA.

Department of Health and Human Services ABBR: DHHS. The U.S. Government agency that administers federal health programs, including the Federal Drug Administration and the Centers for Disease Control and Prevention. Its previous name was Department of Health, Education and Welfare.

dependence (dē-pĕn′dĕns) [L. *dependere,* to hang down] **1.** A form of behavior that suggests inability to make decisions. **2.** A psychic craving for a drug that may or may not be accompanied by physiological dependency. **3.** A state of reliance on another. SEE: *habituation; withdrawal.*

dependent care The support and nurturing of persons who cannot meet their own needs, such as the frail elderly, children, or functionally impaired adults.

depersonalization disorder The belief that one's own reality is temporarily lost or altered. The patient feels estranged or unreal and may feel that the extremities have changed size. A feeling of being automated or as if in a dream may be present. The onset is usually rapid, and it usually occurs in adolescence or under extreme stress, fatigue, or anxiety.

depersonalize To make impersonal; to deprive of personality or individuality.

dephosphorylation (dē-fŏs″for-ĭ-lā′shŭn) [L. *de,* from, + *phosphorylation*] Removal of a phosphate group from a compound.

depigmentation (dē″pĭg-mĕn-tā′shŭn) **1.** The pathological loss of normal pigment as in vitiligo. **2.** Removal of pigment, esp. from the skin, by chemical or physical means.

depilate (dĕp′ĭl-āt) [L. *depilare,* to deprive of hair] To remove hair.

depilation (dĕp″ĭl-ā′shŭn) Hair removal. SEE: *epilation.*

depilatory An agent used to remove hair.

depilatory technique One of several temporary procedures to remove hair from the body, including shaving the area, plucking a few unwanted hairs, chemical means, or wax treatment. If chemical depilation is used, care must be taken to avoid skin irritation. The wax treatment involves application of molten wax, which is allowed to cool; then, when the wax is pulled away, the hair comes with it. Permanent depilation is accomplished by electrolysis of each hair follicle. This time-consuming process is done by an electrologist trained in the technique. SEE: *electrolysis; hirsutism.*

deplete (dē-plēt′) [L. *depletus,* emptied] To empty; to produce depletion.

depletion (dē-plē′shŭn) Removal of substances such as blood, fluids, iron, fat, or protein from the body.

depolarization (dē-pō″lăr-ĭ-zā′shŭn) [″ + *polus,* pole] A reversal of charges at a cell membrane; an electrical change in an excitable cell in which the inside of the cell becomes positive (less negative) in relation to the outside. This is the opposite of polarization and is caused by a rapid inflow of sodium ions. SEE: illus.

depolymerization (dē-pŏl″ĭ-mĕr-ĭ-zā′shŭn) The breakdown or splitting of polymers into their basic building blocks or monomers. The glucose monomer may be polymerized to form the large glycogen polymer and then broken down (i.e., depolymerized) to form glucose.

deponent (dē-pō′nĕnt) One who testifies under oath about the facts at issue in litigation; the testimony is transcribed to become part of the legal record.

deposit (dē-pŏz′ĭt) [L. *depositus,* having put aside] **1.** Sediment. **2.** Matter collected in any part of an organism.

calcareous d. A deposit of calcified material, as in calculus on teeth.

tooth d. Soft or hard material deposited on the surface of a tooth. Also called *plaque* or *calculus.*

deposition **1.** Pretrial discovery device in which the person being questioned (the deponent) is placed under oath and asked to testify about issues on the subject of litigation, which is then transcribed. **2.** The sedimentation of particles previously suspended or circulating in solution.

diffusion d. The accumulation of aerosol particles on a surface due to their random bombardment by gas molecules.

depot (dē′pō, dĕp′ō) [Fr. *depot,* fr. L. *depositum*] A place of storage, esp. in the body, such as a fat depot or a drug depot. Drugs that remain in long-term storage in the body after injection include hormonal agents (such as progesterone, testosterone, insulin, and leuprolide) and antipsychotic agents (such as haloperidol and risperidone), among others.

depravation (dĕp″ră-vā′shŭn) [L. *depravare,* completely destroyed] A patholog-

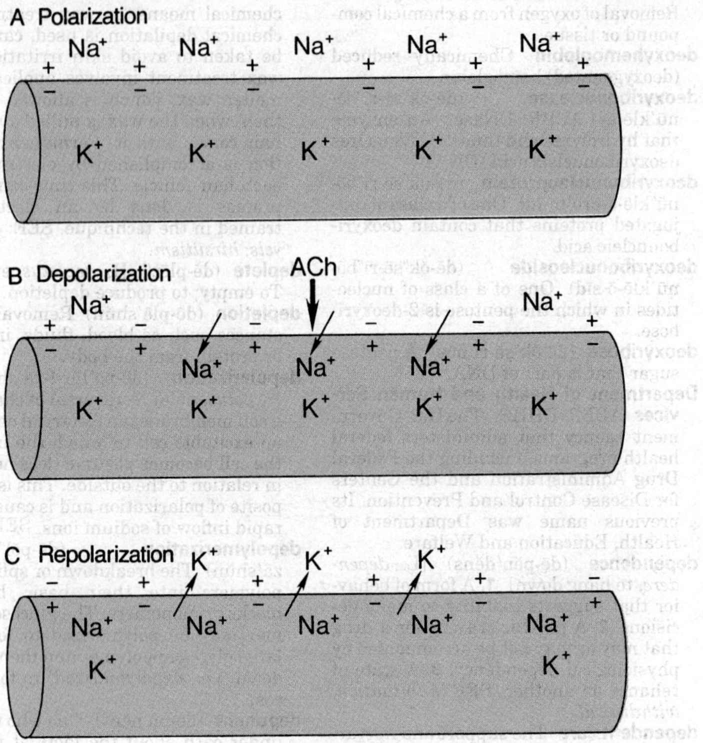

A Polarization

B Depolarization

C Repolarization

DEPOLARIZATION

Electrical charges and ion concentrations at the cell membrane; (A) polarization, (B) depolarization, (C) repolarization

ical deterioration of function or secretion.

depressant [L. *depressus*, pressed down] An agent that decreases the level of a body function or nerve activity (e.g., a sedative medicine).

cardiac d. An agent that decreases heart rate and contractility.

cerebral d. An agent that sedates or tranquilizes.

motor d. An agent that lessens contractions of involuntary muscles.

respiratory d. An agent that lessens frequency and depth of breathing.

depressed (dĕ-prĕst′) **1.** Below the normal level, as when fragments of bone are forced below their normal level and that of surrounding portions of bone. **2.** Low in spirits; dejected. **3.** Having a decreased level of function. SEE: *depression*.

depression (dē-prĕsh′ŭn) [L. *depressio*, a pressing down] **1.** A hollow or lowered region. **2.** The lowering of a part, such as the mandible. **3.** The decrease of a vital function such as respiration. **4.** One of several mood disorders marked by loss of interest or pleasure in living. Disorders linked to depression include dysthymia, major depressive disorder, schizoaffective disorders, bipolar disorders, seasonal affective disorders, and mood disorders caused by substance abuse or other medical conditions.

The depressive disorders are common: for example, about one in five women may suffer major depression at some point during her lifetime; the prevalence of major depression in men is about 1 in 10. Worldwide, depression is considered to be the fourth most serious illness as far as the overall burden it imposes on people's health. Depressed patients have more medical illnesses and a higher risk of self-injury and suicide than patients without mood disorders.

SYMPTOMS: Characteristic symptoms of the depressive disorders include persistent sadness, hopelessness, or tearfulness; loss of energy (or persistent fatigue); persistent feelings of guilt or self-criticism; a sense of worthlessness; irritability; an inability to concentrate; decreased interest in daily activities; changes in appetite or body weight; insomnia or excessive sleep; and recurrent thoughts of death or suicide. These symptoms cause pervasive deficits in social functioning.

TREATMENT: Psychotherapies, behavioral therapies, electroconvulsive ("shock") therapies, and psychoactive drugs are effective in the treatment of depressive disorders.

CAUTION: Depressed persons who express suicidal thoughts should not be left alone, esp. if hospitalized.

PATIENT CARE: The patient is assessed for feelings of worthlessness or self-reproach, inappropriate guilt, concern with death, and attempts at self-injury. Level of activity and socialization are evaluated. Adequate nutrition and fluids are provided. Dietary interventions and increased physical activity are recommended to manage drug-induced constipation; assistance with grooming and other activities of daily living may be required. A structured routine, including noncompetitive activities, is provided to build the patient's self-confidence and to encourage interaction. Health care professionals should express warmth and interest in the patient, and be optimistic while guarding against excessive cheerfulness. Support is gradually reduced as the patient demonstrates an increasing ability to resume self-care. Drug therapies are administered and evaluated.

If electroconvulsive therapy (ECT) is required, the patient is informed that a series of treatments may be needed. Before each ECT session, the prescribed sedative is administered, and a nasal or oral airway inserted. Vital signs are monitored, and support is offered by talking calmly or by gentle touch. After ECT, mental status and response to therapy are evaluated. The patient may be drowsy and experience transient amnesia but should become alert and oriented within 30 min. The period of disorientation lengthens after subsequent treatments. SEE: *Nursing Diagnoses Appendix.*

anaclitic d. Depression in infants suddenly separated from their mothers between the first months and 1 year of age. The loss of the love, affection, and nurturing usually present in the mother–child relationship may cause severe disturbances in health and in motor, language, and social development, or may occasionally lead to death. Symptoms first found in affected infants include crying, panic behavior, and increased motor activity. Later, psychologically abandoned or neglected infants manifest dejection, apathy, staring into space, and silent crying. Recovery is possible if the actual mother or a surrogate is available to meet the infant's needs for parental support.

bipolar d. SEE: *bipolar disorder.*

endogenous d. Melancholia.

postpartum d. Depression in a new mother in which the signs and symptoms do not dissipate within several weeks following delivery, or strong feelings of dejection and anger beginning 1 to 2 months after childbirth. The symptoms are tearfulness, despondency, a feeling of hopelessness, inadequacy, inability to cope with infant care, mood swings, extreme anxiety over the infant, guilt of not loving the infant enough, irritability, fatigue, loss of normal interests, and insomnia. This depression occurs in about 3% of women and may occur in other family members, including the father. SEE: *postpartum blues.*

post-stroke d. A dysphoric mood disorder that follows a cerebral infarction, found in about a quarter of all patients who suffer a stroke. Although for many years depression after strokes was thought to occur mainly in patients who had injured the nondominant hemisphere of the brain, research has shown that this phenomenon is most common in female patients and patients who have had higher education.

reactive d. Depression that is usually self-limiting, following a serious event such as a death in the family, the loss of a job, or a personal financial catastrophe. The disorder is longer lasting and more marked than the normal reaction.

unipolar d. Depression.

depressive disorder Depression. SEE: *Nursing Diagnoses Appendix.*

depressomotor (dē-prĕs′ō-mō″tor) [″ + *motor,* mover] Having the ability to diminish muscular movements by lessening the impulses for motion sent from the brain or spinal cord; said of drugs.

depressor [L.] An instrument for drawing down a body part.

tongue d. A device used to draw down and displace the tongue to facilitate visual examination of the throat.

depressor fiber A nerve that decreases arterial muscle tone and, as a result, lowers blood pressure.

depressor reflex A reflex that results in slowed muscle activity, as in the heart rate.

deprivation (dĕp″rĭ-vā′shŭn) [L. *de,* from, + *privare,* to remove] Loss or absence of a necessary part or function.

androgen d. The chemical suppression of male sex hormones to prevent their stimulatory effects on various hormone-sensitive illnesses, including prostate cancer and predatory sexual behavior. SYN: *androgen suppression.*

emotional d. Isolation of an individual, esp. an infant, from normal emotional stimuli. In infants, this produces impairment of mental and physical development.

sensory d. The absence of usual and accustomed visual, auditory, tactile, or other stimuli (e.g., in patients whose eyes are bandaged for extended periods following eye surgery, patients on respirators, astronauts, or persons imprisoned in dark, soundproof cells). The long-lasting absence of normal stimuli eventually produces psychological and neurological symptoms, including auditory and visual hallucinations, anxiety, depression, and delusions.

In psychological experimentation, sensory deprivation may be achieved by confining a volunteer wearing gloves, an eye mask, and ear muffs in a small soundproof room or by immersing an individual equipped for underwater breathing in a tank of water that is devoid of stimuli except for the sound of breathing.

PATIENT CARE: The patient's usual response to prolonged quiet or isolation is assessed. Patients who require more environmental stimuli (radio, TV noise, social contact) suffer more (and more quickly) than do those who prefer quiet. Stimulation is provided to replace those stimuli which the patient is deprived of. Caregivers tell those patients who cannot see or whose visual field is limited by position or equipment about weather, time of day, and surrounding colors. They also describe equipment, locations, food, and other features of the environment that the patient wants to experience, but cannot see, allowing touch to help replace vision. For the patient whose hearing is reduced by location or equipment (or by effects of drug therapy), devices are used that assist hearing-impaired persons to understand speech. Sensory-deprived patients are encouraged to use radio or TV as desired, and the health care professional makes frequent visits to prevent these patients from feeling abandoned. Therapies are related to time of day (before breakfast, after dinner, at bedtime, etc.), and a clock and calendar are provided to assist with time orientation. Reported auditory or visual hallucinations should be investigated thoroughly and a source sought that could simulate the sound or sight reported by the patient (e.g., linen cart may sound like truck going by, curtain moving may look like ghost). Caregivers validate reality for the patient by changing lighting or altering external noises to eliminate confusion.

sleep d., effects of SEE: *sleep*.

deprogram To free an individual from some mentally harmful cult, religion, or political brainwashing program.

depth [ME. *depthe*] **1.** The distance between an elevated and a depressed point; a measure of height. **2.** Richness; intensity; the quality of being deep.

depth dose The actual amount of radiation exposure at a specific point below the surface of the body.

depth psychology The psychology of unconscious behavior, as opposed to psychology of conscious behavior.

depulization (dē-pūl″ĭ-zā′shŭn) [L. *de,* from, + *pulex,* flea] Destruction of fleas, including those that carry plague.

depurant (dĕp′ū-rănt) [L. *depurare,* to purify] **1.** A medicine that helps to purify by promoting the removal of waste material from the body. **2.** Any agent that removes waste material.

depuration The process of freeing from impurities. **depurative,** *adj.*

depurator An agent that purifies.

de Quervain's tenosynovitis (kār′vañz) [Fritz de Quervain, Swiss surgeon, 1868–1940] Chronic tenosynovitis of the abductor pollicis longus and extensor pollicis brevis muscles. Also called Quervain's disease.

deradelphus (dĕr-ă-dĕl′fŭs) [Gr. *dere,* neck, + *adelphos,* brother] A pair of malformed twins, fused above the thorax and having one head, but separated below the chest as two bodies.

derangement (dē-rānj′mĕnt) [Fr. *deranger,* unbalance] **1.** Lack of order or organization, esp. as compared with the previous condition; confusion. **2.** A defect in the annulus fibrosus of the intervertebral disk allowing the nucleus pulposus to herniate.

Dercum's disease (dĕr′kŭms) [Francis X. Dercum, U.S. neurologist, 1856–1931] The appearance of multiple painful fatty nodules (lipomas) in the skin of adults, esp. overweight or postmenopausal women. SYN: *adiposis dolorosa.*

derealization A sense that reality has changed; a sense of detachment from one's surroundings.

dereism (dē′rē-ĭzm) [L. *de,* from, + *res,* thing] In psychiatry, activity and thought based on fantasy and wishes rather than logic or reason; overexercise of the imagination to the extent of ignoring reality, as seen in daydreaming. SEE: *autism*. **dereistic** (dē-rē-ĭst′ik), *adj.*

derencephalus (dĕr″ĕn-sĕf′ă-lŭs) [Gr. *dere,* neck, + *enkephalos,* brain] A congenitally deformed fetus with a rudimentary skull and bifid cervical vertebrae.

derivation (dĕr″ĭ-vā′shŭn) [L. *derivare,* to draw off] The source or origin of a substance or idea.

derivative (dĕ-rĭv′ă-tĭv) **1.** Something that is not original or fundamental. **2.** Something derived from another body or substance. **3.** Something that produces derivation. **4.** In embryology, anything that develops from a preceding structure, as the derivatives of the germ layers.

derm- SEE: *dermato-*.

derm, derma [Gr. *derma,* skin] True skin. **dermal,** *adj.*

dermabrasion (dĕrm′ă-brā″zhŭn) [″ + L. *abrasio,* wearing away] A surgical procedure used to resurface the skin. It may remove acne scars, nevi, tattoos, or fine wrinkles on the skin. Complications of the procedure include infection, skin pigment changes, or scarring. SEE: *skin, chemical peel of; planing.*

Dermacentor (dĕr″mă-sĕn′tor) A genus of ticks belonging to the order Acarina, family Ixodidae.

D. andersoni The wood tick, a species of ticks that is parasitic on humans or other mammals during some part of its life cycle. It may cause tick paralysis, and is a vector of Rocky Mountain spotted fever, scrub typhus, tularemia, brucellosis, Q fever, and several forms of viral encephalomyelitis.

D. variabilis A species of ticks similar to *D. andersoni.* In the central and eastern U.S., it is the main vector for Rocky Mountain spotted fever. It is parasitic to dogs, horses, cattle, rabbits, and humans.

dermad [Gr. *derma,* skin, + L. *ad,* toward] Toward the skin; externally.

dermalgia (dĕr-măl′jē-ă) [″ + *algos,* pain] Pain localized in the skin.

dermamyiasis (dĕr-mă-mī-ī′ă-sĭs) [″ + *myia,* fly, + *-iasis,* condition] A skin disease caused by infestation by the larvae of dipterous insects. SEE: *myiasis.*

dermat- SEE: *dermato-*.

dermatalgia (dĕr″mă-tăl′jē-ă) [Gr. *dermatos,* skin, + *algos,* pain] A paresthesia with localized pain in the skin. SYN: *dermalgia.*

dermatatrophia (dĕrm″ăt-ă-trō′fē-ă) [″ + *atrophia,* atrophy] Atrophy of the skin.

dermatitis (dĕr″mă-tī′tĭs) *pl.* **dermatitides** [Gr. *dermatos,* skin, + *itis,* inflammation] An inflammatory rash marked by itching and redness. SEE: *eczema.*

ETIOLOGY: Inflammation of the skin may be caused by numerous conditions, including contact with skin irritants, such as the oil that causes poison ivy or oak; venous stasis, with edema and vesicle formation near the ankles; habitual scratching, as is found in neurodermatitis; dry skin, such as in winter itch; ultraviolet light, as in photosensitivity reactions; and many others.

TREATMENT: When a source of dermatitis is identifiable (e.g., in contact dermatitis due to a detergent or topical cosmetic), the best treatment is to avoid the irritating substance and to cleanse any affected area immediately with mild soap and water. Once skin inflammation is established, topical corticosteroid ointments or systemic steroids and antihistamines may be used.

PATIENT CARE: The patient should avoid known skin irritants. Tepid baths, cool compresses, and astringents sometimes help relieve inflammation and itch. Drug therapy is administered and evaluated for desired effects and adverse reactions. The patient is taught how to apply topical medications and is educated about specific side effects of oral medications. Scratching is discouraged since it worsens dermatitis. The patient is encouraged to express feelings about the condition.

actinic d. A chronic red or eczematous rash, usually on the face or exposed skin surfaces, that typically results from exposure and sensitization to ultraviolet rays. Adults over age 50 may be affected. SYN: *photosensitivity d.*

allergic contact d. Contact d.

atopic d. Chronic dermatitis of unknown etiology found in patients with a history of allergy. The disease usually begins after the first 2 months of life, and affected individuals may experience exacerbations and remissions throughout childhood and adulthood. In many cases, the family has a history of allergy or atopy; if both parents have atopic dermatitis, the chances are nearly 80% that their children will have it as well. The skin lesions consist of reddened, cracked, and thickened skin that can become exudative and crusty from scratching. Scarring or secondary infection may occur. Most patients have an elevated level of immunoglobulin E in their serum. SEE: illus.

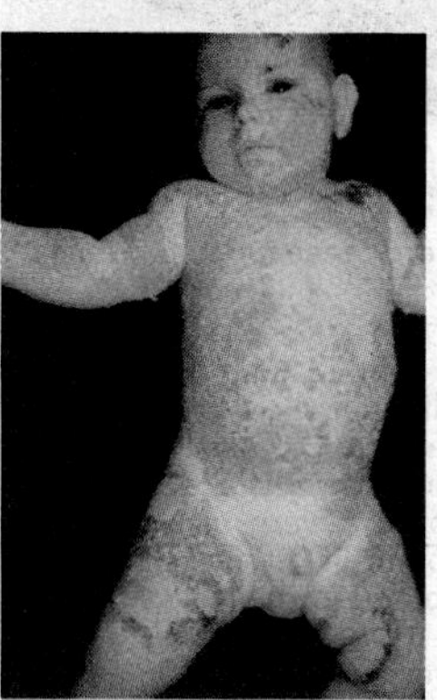

ATOPIC DERMATITIS

TREATMENT: The patient should avoid soaps and ointments. Bathing is kept to a minimum, but bath oils may help to prevent drying of the skin. Clothing should be soft textured and should not contain wool. Fingernails should be kept short to decrease damage from scratching. Antihistamines may help to reduce itching at night. Heavy exercise should be avoided because it induces perspiration. A nonlipid softening lotion followed by a corticosteroid in a propylene glycol base may effectively treat acute exacerbations; when large areas of the body are involved, oral steroids may be needed. Antistaphylococcal antibiotics may be needed to control secondary infection.

berloque d. A type of phytophotodermatitis with postinflammatory hyperpigmentation at the site of application of perfumes or colognes containing oil of bergamot.

d. calorica Inflammation due to heat, as in sunburn, or cold.

cercarial d. Swimmer's itch.

contact d. Inflammation and irritation of the skin due to contact with allergens or an irritating substance. Allergic contact dermatitis is caused by a T-cell–mediated hypersensitivity reaction to environmental allergens, either natural or synthetic. Nonallergic contact dermatitis is usually due to exposure to a harsh or highly concentrated acid, base, or soap. SYN: *d. venenata* (1). SEE: illus.

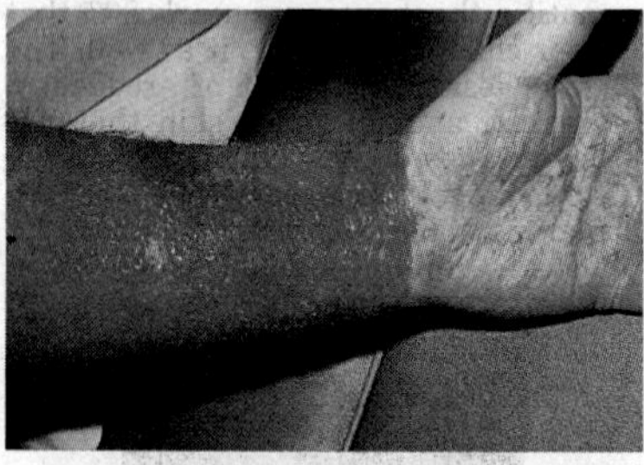

CONTACT DERMATITIS

Allergic reaction to topical anesthetic

SYMPTOMS: Skin changes, which appear 4 to 48 hours after exposure, depending on the degree of sensitivity to the allergen, consist of erythema, local edema, and blisters. The blisters may weep in severe cases. Most patients complain of intense itching. Signs and symptoms of the disease usually last 10 to 14 days. Re-exposure to the cause will trigger a relapse.

TREATMENT: Tepid baths, cool compresses, topical astringents (such as solutions of aluminum acetate), antihistamines, and corticosteroids all provide some relief.

diaper d. Diaper rash.

exfoliative d. Generalized reddening and inflammation of the skin surface, often followed by scaling. The condition may be caused by leukemias or lymphomas that infiltrate the skin; extensive psoriasis; drug reactions (e.g., vancomycin); allergies, seborrhea, or atopy. The condition is often associated with systemic findings, including lymphadenopathy, hepatic and splenic enlargement, fever, anemia, eosinophilia, and decreases in serum albumin.

When the skin involvement is extensive the patient may become depressed because of the cosmetic changes.

TREATMENT: Therapy is directed at treating the underlying cause.

factitial d. A skin irritation or injury that is self-inflicted.

d. herpetiformis A chronic inflammatory disease characterized by erythematous, papular, vesicular, bullous, or pustular lesions with a tendency to grouping and with intense itching and burning.

ETIOLOGY: The direct cause is unknown. The condition occurs mostly in men; no age is exempt. Some patients have associated asymptomatic gluten-sensitive enteropathy. In those persons the HLA-B8 antigen may be present.

SYMPTOMS: The lesions develop suddenly and spread peripherally. The disease is variable and erratic, and an attack may be prolonged for weeks or months. Secondary infection may follow trauma to the inflamed areas.

TREATMENT: Oral dapsone provides substantial relief of symptoms in a few days. Sulfapyridine also may be used.

d. hiemalis Winter itch.

d. infectiosa eczematoides A pustular eruption during or following a pyogenic disease.

meadow d. A blistering but not itchy rash that appears on the exposed skin of hikers, florists, gardeners, and individuals who work outdoors in sunny climates. It is a phototoxic reaction caused by exposure to light-sensitizing chemicals in some plants (such as parsley, rue, bergamot, and fig).

d. medicamentosa Drug rash.

d. multiformis A form of dermatitis with pustular lesions.

d. papillaris capillitii Formation on the scalp and neck of papules interspersed with pustules. The rash ultimately produces scarlike elevations resembling keloids.

photoallergic contact d. Photoallergy.

photosensitivity d. Actinic d.

poison ivy d. Dermatitis resulting from irritation or sensitization of the skin by urushiol, the toxic resin of the poison ivy plant. There is no absolute immunity, although susceptibility varies greatly, even in the same individual.

Persons sensitive to poison ivy may also react to contact with other plants such as the mango rind and cashew oil. These plants contain chemicals that cross-react with the sap present in poison ivy, poison oak, and poison sumac.

SYMPTOMS: An interval of time elapses between skin contact with the poison and first appearance of symptoms, varying from a few hours to several days and depending on the sensitivity of the patient and the condition of the skin. Moderate itching or a burning sensation is soon followed by small blisters; later manifestations vary. Blisters usually rupture and are followed by oozing of serum and subsequent crusting.

PREVENTION: Certain substances, including organoclay compounds, have been useful in preventing poison ivy dermatitis. They are sprayed on the skin, where they serve as a barrier to prevent the irritating agent, urushiol, from bonding with the skin. Organoclay compounds are present in some antiperspirants. Shoes and clothes as well as the hair of cats and dogs can carry the toxic resin to those who handle them.

TREATMENT: In mild dermatitis, a lotion to relieve itching is usually sufficient. In severe dermatitis, cool, wet dressings or compresses, potassium permanganate baths, and perhaps a course of intramuscular or oral corticosteroid therapy will be required. Sedation is also necessary in some cases.

Application of moderately hot water to nonblistered areas for 2 or 3 min may provide symptomatic relief from itching and burning. The comfort produced is dramatic and may last several hours.

PATIENT CARE: Prevention is important in both persons with known sensitivity and those with no previous contact with or reaction to the plant. Patient teaching focuses on helping the patient to recognize the plant, to avoid contact with it, and to wear long-sleeved shirts and long pants in wooded areas. If contact occurs, the patient should wash with soap and water immediately to remove the toxic oil.

primary d. Dermatitis that is a direct rather than an allergic response.

radiation d. Dermatitis due to radiation exposure.

rhus d. Contact dermatitis caused by the toxic resin in poison ivy or oak. SEE: *poison ivy dermatitis; Toxicodendron.*

schistosome d. Swimmer's itch.

d. seborrheica An acute or subacute inflammatory skin disease of unknown cause, beginning on the scalp and characterized by rounded, irregular, or circinate lesions covered with yellow or brown-gray greasy scales. SYN: *pityriasis capitis; seborrhea corporis; seborrhea sicca.* SEE: *Nursing Diagnoses Appendix.*

SYMPTOMS: On the scalp, it may be dry with abundant grayish branny scales, or oozing and crusted, constituting eczema capitis, and may spread to the forehead and postauricular regions. The forehead shows scaly and infiltrated lesions with dark red bases, some itching, and localized loss of hair. The eyebrows and eyelashes show dry, dirty white scales with itching. On nasolabial folds or the vermilion border of the lips, there is inflammation with itching. On the sternal region, the lesions are greasy to the touch. Eruptions may appear in interscapular, axillary, and genitocrural regions also.

TREATMENT: Because there is no known cure for this condition, therapeutic objectives are to control the disorder and allow the skin to repair itself. When the condition is limited to the scalp, frequent shampooing and use of mild keratolytic agents is indicated. Selenium-containing shampoos have been helpful. Generalized seborrheic dermatitis requires careful attention including scrupulous skin hygiene, keeping the skin as dry as possible, and using dusting powders. Topical and systemic cortisone preparations may be required.

PATIENT CARE: The nurse or primary care provider explains to the patient that the condition has remissions and exacerbations; also, that hormone imbalances, nutritional status, infection, and emotional stress influence its course. The patient is taught topical application of prescribed corticosteroid cream to the body and face, used to allay secondary inflammation. He or she is warned to use this medication with caution near the eyelids, because it can lead to glaucoma in at risk patients. To avoid developing a secondary *Candida* yeast infection in body creases or folds, the patient is advised to carefully cleanse these areas, to dry gently but thoroughly, and to ensure that the skin is well aerated. He or she is taught to treat seborrheic scalp conditions (dandruff) with proper and frequent shampooing, alternating two or three different types of shampoo to prevent the development of resistance to a particular product. He or she also should remove external irritants and avoid excessive heat and perspiration. Rubbing and scratching the skin are discouraged, as they prolong exacerbations and increase the risk for secondary infection and excoriation, especially since scaly, pruritic lesions present in skin areas with high bacteria counts. Oral antibiotics (e.g., tetracycline) may be prescribed (as in acne vulgaris) in small doses over a prolonged period to reduce bacterial colonization. The patient is advised to take tetracycline at least 1 hour before or 2 hours after meals, since the drug is poorly absorbed with food. The patient also is taught about the drug's adverse effects (photosensitivity, birth defects, nausea, vomiting, and candidal vaginitis) and their management. The patient is encouraged to adhere to the treatment regimen, to deal with increasing frustration, and to handle body image problems.

stasis d. Eczema of the legs with edema, pigmentation, and sometimes chronic inflammation. It is usually due to impaired return of blood from the legs. Compression stockings help the rash to resolve gradually. SEE: illus.

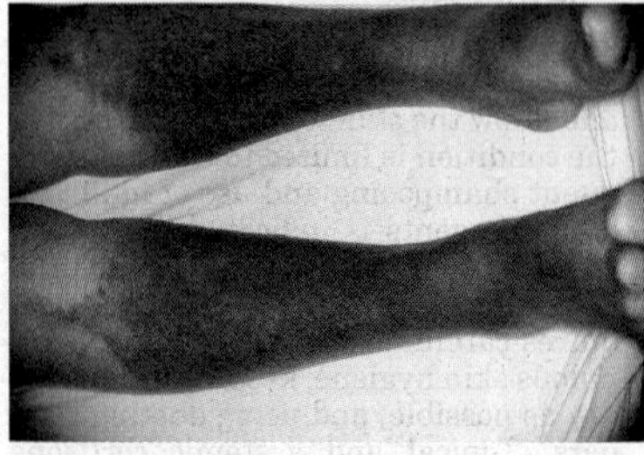

STASIS DERMATITIS

d. venenata **1.** Contact d. **2.** Any inflammation caused by local action of various animal, vegetable, or mineral substances contacting the surface of the skin.

d. verrucosa A chronic fungal infection of the skin characterized by the formation of wartlike nodules. These may enlarge and form papillomatous structures that sometimes ulcerate.

ETIOLOGY: This condition may be due to one of several fungi including *Hormodendrum pedrosoi* or *Phialophora verrucosa.*

x-ray d. Skin inflammation due to effects of x-rays.

dermato-, dermat-, derm- Combining form meaning *skin.*

dermatoautoplasty (dĕr″mă-tō-aw′tō-plăs″tē) [Gr. *dermatos,* skin, + *autos,* self, + *plassein,* to form] Grafting of skin taken from some portion of the patient's own body.

Dermatobia (dĕr″mă-tō′bē-ă) [″ + *bios,* life] A genus of botflies belonging to the order Diptera of the family Oestridae.

D. hominis A species of botflies, found in parts of tropical America, whose larvae infest humans and cattle. The eggs are transported by mosquitoes.

dermatobiasis (dĕr″mă-tō-bī′ă-sĭs) Infestation by the larvae of *Dermatobia hominis,* the eggs of which are carried to the skin by mosquitoes. The larvae then hatch and bore into the skin while the mosquito feeds. Marblelike boils form at the site of infestation.

dermatocele (dĕr′mă-tō-sēl″) [″ + *kele,* tumor, swelling] A tendency of hypertrophied skin and subcutaneous tissue to hang loosely in folds. SYN: *dermatolysis.*

d. lipomatosa A pedunculated lipoma with cystic degeneration.

dermatocelidosis (dĕr″mă-tō-sĕl″ĭ-dō′sĭs) [″ + *kelis,* spot, + *osis,* condition] A macular eruption; a freckle. SYN: *dermatokelidosis.*

dermatocellulitis (dĕr″mă-tō-sĕl″ū-lī′tĭs) [″ + L. *cellula,* little cell, + Gr. *itis,* inflammation] Inflammation of subcutaneous connective tissue.

dermatoconiosis (dĕr″mă-tō-kō″nē-ō′sĭs) [″ + *konia,* dust] Any irritation of the skin caused by dust, esp. one due to occupational exposure.

dermatocyst (dĕr′mă-tō-sĭst) [″ + *kystis,* cyst] A skin cyst.

dermatofibroma [″ + L. *fibra,* fiber, + Gr. *oma,* tumor] A firm but freely movable benign skin nodule, often found on the lower extremities. SEE: illus.; *dimple sign.*

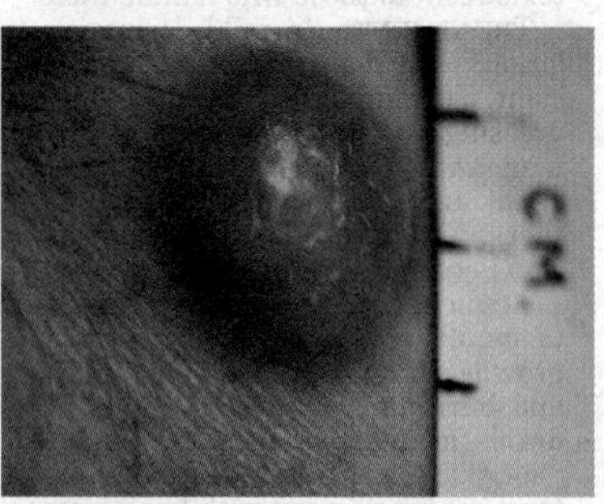

DERMATOFIBROMA

dermatofibrosarcoma (dĕr″mă-tō-fī″brō-săr-kō′mă) [″ + ″ + Gr. *sarx,* flesh, + *oma,* tumor] Fibrosarcoma of the skin.

dermatogen (dĕr-măt′ō-jĕn) [″ + *gennan,* to produce] Antigen from a skin disease.

dermatogenous (dĕr″mă-tŏj′ĕn-ŭs) Producing skin or skin disease.

dermatoglyphics (dĕr″mă-tō-glĭf′ĭks) [″ + *glyphe,* a carving] Study of the surface markings of the skin, esp. those of hands and feet, used in identification and genetic studies. SEE: *fingerprint* for illus.

dermatographism Dermographism.

dermatoheliosis Sun-induced degenerative changes in the skin. Included are wrinkling, atrophy, hypermelanotic and hypomelanotic macules, telangiectasia, yellow papules and plaques, keratoses, and degeneration of elastic tissue. This condition can be prevented by avoiding exposure to the sun or by using topically applied effective sunscreens.

dermatoheteroplasty (dĕr″mă-tō-hĕt′ĕr-ō-plăs″tē) [″ + *heteros,* other, + *plassein,* to mold] Skin grafting from a member of a different species.

dermatokelidosis (dĕr″mă-tō-kĕl″ĭ-dō′sĭs) Dermatocelidosis.

dermatologist (dĕr″mă-tŏl′ō-jĭst) [Gr. *dermatos,* skin, + *logos,* word, reason] A physician who specializes in treating diseases of the skin.

dermatology (dĕr″mă-tŏl′ō-jē) The science of the skin and its diseases.

dermatolysis (dĕr″mă-tŏl′ĭ-sĭs) [″ + *lysis,* dissolution] A tendency of hypertrophied skin and subcutaneous tissue to hang in folds; loose skin. SYN: *cutis laxa; cutis pendula; pachydermatocele* (1).

dermatoma (dĕr″mă-tō′mă) [″ + *oma,* tumor] A circumscribed thickening of skin.

dermatome (dĕr′mă-tōm) [Gr. *derma,* skin, + *tome,* incision] **1.** An instrument for cutting thin slices for skin transplantation. **2.** A band or region of skin supplied by a single sensory nerve. SEE: illus. **3.** The lateral portion of the somite of an embryo, where the dermis of the skin originates; the cutis plate.

dermatomere (dĕr′mă-tō-mēr) [Gr. *dermatos,* skin, + *meros,* part] A segment of embryonic integument.

dermatomucosomyositis (dĕr″mă-tō-mū-kō″sō-mī-ō-sī′tĭs) [″ + L. *mucosa,* mucous membrane, + Gr. *mys,* muscle, + *itis,* inflammation] An inflammation involving the mucosa and muscles.

dermatomycosis (dĕr″mă-tō-mī-kō′sĭs) *pl.* **dermatomycoses** [″ + *mykes,* fungus, + *osis,* condition] A skin infection caused by certain fungi of the genera *Trichophyton, Epidermophyton,* and *Microsporum.* SYN: *tinea.*

dermatomyoma [″ + *mys,* muscle, + *oma,* tumor] Myoma of the skin.

dermatomyositis (dĕr″mă-tō-mī″ō-sī′tĭs) [″ + ″ + *itis,* inflammation] An acute, subacute, or chronic disease of connective tissue, of unknown cause, marked by edema, rash, weakness, pain, and inflammation of the muscles. SEE: illus.

SYMPTOMS: Symptoms include fever, malaise, and weakness, esp. of the pelvic and shoulder girdle muscles; skin and mucosal lesions (e.g., Gottron's papules), and joint discomfort. About one third of patients have dysphagia.

TREATMENT: The treatment is symptomatic and includes bedrest, physical therapy, and steroids. Other anti-inflammatory agents may be helpful, too. Cytotoxic drugs such as azathioprine, cyclophosphamide, and methotrexate are often beneficial in patients who do not respond to adrenocortical steroids.

PATIENT CARE: The patient's level of discomfort, muscle weakness, and joint range of motion are assessed and documented daily. The patient's face, neck, upper back, chest, nailbeds, eyelids, and interphalangeal joints are evaluated for rashes, and any findings are documented. Frequent assistance is provided to help the patient reposition in correct body alignment; appropriate supportive devices and graduated exercises are used to prevent and treat muscle atrophy and joint contractures. Warm baths, moist heat, and massage are provided to relieve stiffness, and prescribed analgesics are administered. Oral lesions are irrigated with warm saline solution as necessary. Tepid sponge baths and compresses are used to relieve pruritus and to prevent scratching; antihistamines are also administered as prescribed. Self-care activities, with assistance if necessary, are encouraged and paced according to the patient's response. Prescribed corticosteroid or cytotoxic drugs are administered, and the patient's response is evaluated.

Both patient and family are educated about the disease process, treatment expectations, and possible adverse reactions to corticosteroid and cytotoxic drugs. Good nutrition and a low-sodium diet are recommended to prevent fluid retention. The patient should be educated about the potential side effects of therapy (e.g., those associated with chronic, high-dose corticosteroids). The patient is encouraged to express feelings, fears, and concerns about the illness; realistic support and encouragement are provided.

dermatopathology [″ + ″ + *logos,* word, reason] The study of skin diseases.

dermatopathy, dermatopathia (dĕr″mă-tŏp′ă-thē) Any skin disease.

dermatophiliasis (dĕr″mă-tō-fĭ-lī′ă-sĭs) **1.** Infestation with *Tunga penetrans,* a pathogenic actinomycete. **2.** Dermatophilosis.

dermatophilosis (dĕr″mă-tō-fĭ-lō′sĭs) An actinomycotic infection that occurs in certain hooved animals and rarely in humans. SYN: *dermatophiliasis.*

dermatophobia [″ + *phobos,* fear] Abnormal fear of having a skin disease.

dermatophyte (dĕr′mă-tō-fīt) [″ + *phyton,* plant] A fungal parasite that grows in or on the skin. Dermatophytes rarely penetrate deeper than the epidermis or its appendages—hair and nails. They cause such skin diseases as favus, tinea, ringworm, and eczema. Important dermatophytes include the genera *Microsporum, Trichophyton,* and *Epidermophyton.*

dermatophytid (dĕr″mă-tŏf′ĭ-tĭd) A toxic rash or eruption occurring in dermatomycosis.

dermatophytosis (dĕr″mă-tō-fī-tō′sĭs) [″ + *phyton,* plant, + *osis,* condition] Athlete's foot.

dermatoplastic [″ + *plassein,* to form] Pert. to skin grafting.

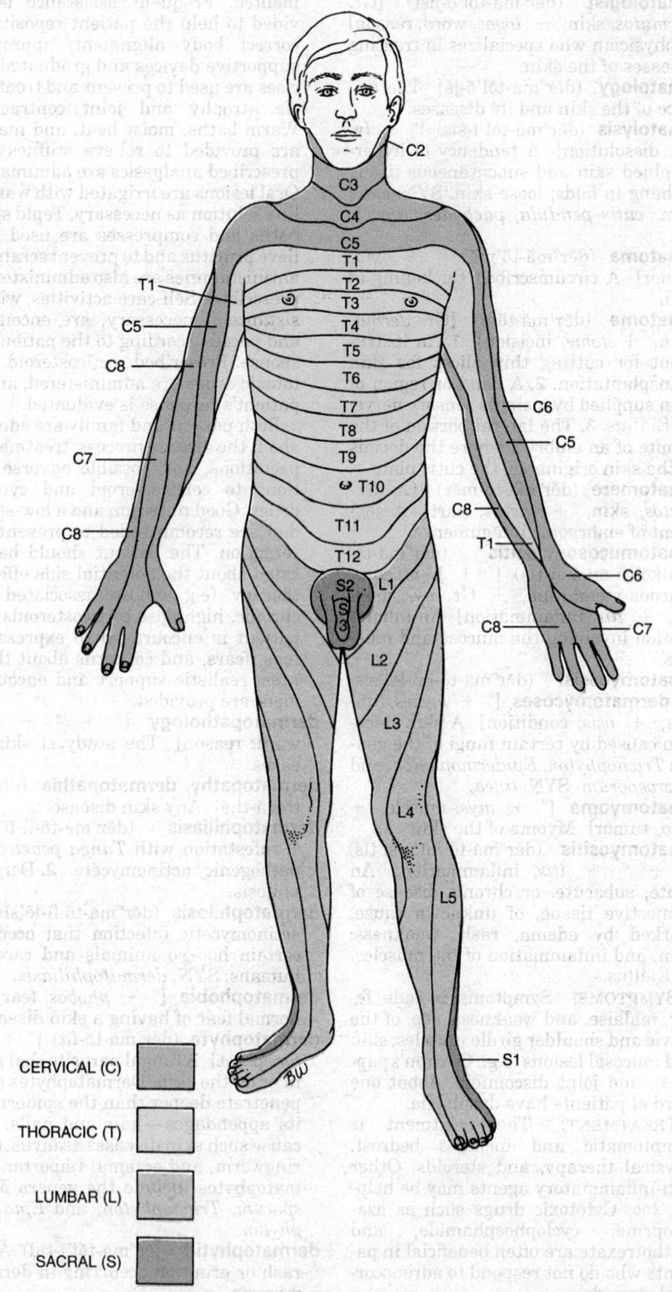
C2
C3
C4
C5
T1
T2
T3
T4
T5
T6
T7
T8
T9
T10
T11
T12
S2
S3
L1
L2
L3
L4
L5
S1
C5
C8
C7
C8
C6
C5
C8
T1
C6
C8
C7
CERVICAL (C)
THORACIC (T)
LUMBAR (L)
SACRAL (S)

DERMATOME

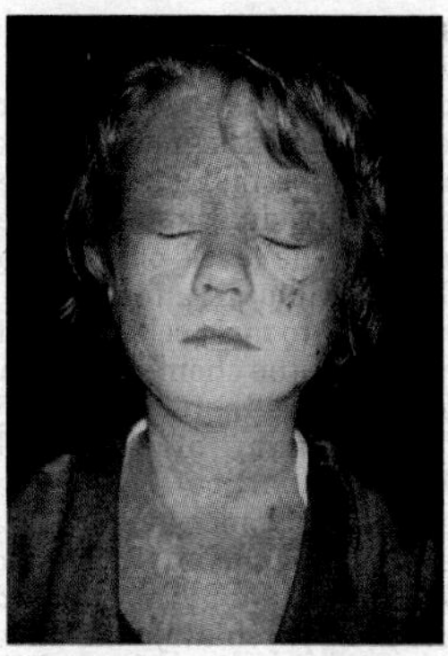

DERMATOMYOSITIS

dermatoplasty (děr′mă-tō-plăs″tē) Transplantion of living skin to cover cutaneous defects caused by injury, operation, or disease.

PATIENT CARE: Techniques are employed during surgery to protect the graft from dislodgement. Postoperative measures include use of splints and dressings, which are employed to minimize trauma, prevent undue motion, prevent infection, and promote healing of the donor site. Signs of infection such as fever and pain are monitored, and assistance is offered to help the patient to cope with altered mobility. Any discomfort is assessed, and pain relief provided as indicated. Nutrition is emphasized to aid healing.

dermatorrhexis [″ + *rhexis,* rupture] Rupture of the skin and capillaries in the skin.

dermatosclerosis (děr″mă-tō-sklěr-ō′sĭs) [″ + *sklerosis,* hardening] Infiltration of the skin with fibrous material.

dermatoscopy Microscopy.

dermatosis (děr″mă-tō′sĭs) *pl.* **dermatoses** [″ + *osis,* condition] Any skin disease, esp. any noninflammatory skin disease. SEE: *dermatitis*.

d. papulosa nigra An eruption consisting of many tiny tumors, or milia, on facial skin. It is more common in blacks than in other ethnic groups.

progressive pigmentary d. A slowly progressive eruption of reddish papules principally on the legs.

dermatosome (děr′mă-tō-sōm) [″ + *soma,* body] A section of the equatorial plate in mitosis.

dermatotherapy [″ + *therapeia,* treatment] Treatment of skin disease.

dermatotome (děr′mă-tō-tōm″) [″ + *tome,* incision] **1.** One of the fetal skin segments. **2.** A knife for incising the skin or small lesions. SYN: *dermatome* (1).

dermatotropic (děr″mă-tō-trŏp′ĭk) [″ + *trope,* a turning] Acting preferentially on the skin.

dermatozoon [″ + *zoon,* animal] An animal parasite of the skin.

dermatozoonosis (děr″mă-tō-zō″ō-nō′sĭs) [″ + ″ + *nosos,* disease] Any skin disease caused by an animal parasite.

dermic (děr′mĭk) [Gr. *derma,* skin] Pert. to the skin.

dermis (děr′mĭs) [L.] The layer of the skin lying immediately under the epidermis; the true skin. It consists of two layers, papillary and reticular. The corium dermis is composed of fibrous connective tissue made of collagen and elastin, and contains numerous capillaries, lymphatics, and nerve endings. In it are hair follicles and their smooth muscle fibers, sebaceous glands and sweat glands, and their ducts. SYN: *corium; cutis vera*.

dermoblast [Gr. *derma,* skin, + *blastos,* germ] Part of the mesoblastic layer, developing into the corium.

dermographia, dermography A form of urticaria due to allergy.

dermographism A form of urticaria (hives) in which a pale raised wheal and red flare are produced on the skin when it is gently stroked or scratched. SYN: *dermatographism*. SEE: illus.

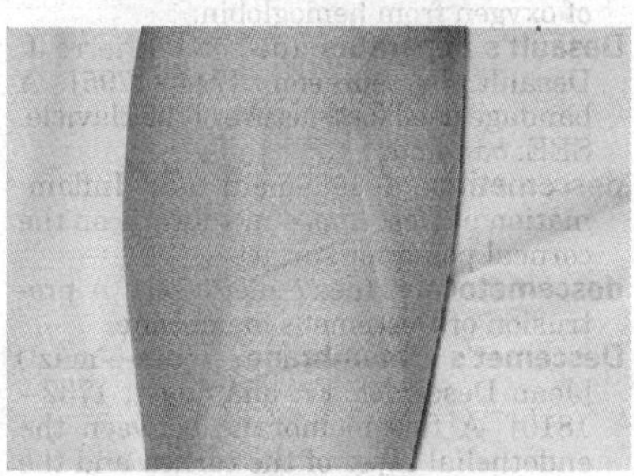

DERMOGRAPHISM

dermoid (děr′moyd) [″ + *eidos,* form, shape] **1.** Resembling the skin. **2.** Dermoid cyst.

dermoidectomy (děr″moyd-ěk′tō-mē) [″ + ″ + *ektome,* excision] Excision of a dermoid cystectomy.

dermolipoma (děr″mō-lī-pō′mă) **1.** A growth of yellow fatty tissue beneath the bulbar conjunctiva. **2.** A lipoma of the skin.

dermomycosis (děr″mō-mī-kō′sĭs) [″ + *mykes,* fungus, + *osis,* condition] A skin disease produced by a fungus; dermatomycosis. SYN: *tinea*.

dermonosology (děr″mō-nō-sŏl′ō-jē) [″ + *nosos,* disease, + *logos,* word, reason] The science of classification of skin diseases.

dermoskeleton [″ + *skeleton*] The apparent external covering of the body;

the hair, nails, and teeth in humans. SYN: *exoskeleton*.

dermosynovitis (dĕr″mō-sĭn-ō-vī′tĭs) [″ + L. *synovia*, joint fluid, + Gr. *itis*, inflammation] Inflammation of the skin overlying an inflamed bursa or tendon.

dermovascular (dĕr″mō-văs′kū-lăr) [″ + *vas*, vessel] Concerning the skin and its blood vessels.

derodidymus (dĕr″ō-dĭd′ĭ-mŭs) [Gr. *dere*, neck, + *didymos*, double] A malformed fetus with two necks and heads but a single body and normal limbs. SYN: *dicephalus*.

DES *diethylstilbestrol*.

desalination Partial or complete removal of salts from a substance, as from seawater or brackish water, so that it is suitable for agricultural or household purposes but not for drinking.

desaturation [L. *de*, from, + *saturare*, to fill] 1. A process whereby a saturated organic compound is converted into an unsaturated one, as when stearic acid, $C_{18}H_{36}O_2$, is changed into oleic acid, $C_{18}H_{34}O_2$. The product has different physical and chemical properties after this transformation. SEE: *saturated hydrocarbon*. **2.** The removal of a component from a chemical solution (e.g., a solute from a solvent). **3.** The dissociation of oxygen from hemoglobin.

Desault's apparatus (dĕ-sōz′) [Pierre J. Desault, Fr. surgeon, 1744–1795] A bandage used for fracture of the clavicle. SEE: *bandage*.

descemetitis (dĕs″ĕ-mĕ-tī′tĭs) Inflammation of Descemet's membrane on the corneal posterior surface.

descemetocele (dĕs″ĕ-mĕt′ō-sēl) A protrusion of Descemet's membrane.

Descemet's membrane (dĕs-ĕ-māz′) [Jean Descemet, Fr. anatomist, 1732–1810] A fine membrane between the endothelial layer of the cornea and the substantia propria. SYN: *vitreous membrane*.

descendens (dē-sĕn′dĕns) [L. *de*, from, + *scendere*, to climb] Descending; a descending structure.

d. hypoglossi A branch of the hypoglossal nerve occurring at the point at which the nerve curves around the occipital artery, which passes down obliquely across (sometimes within) the sheath of the carotid vessels to form a loop just below the middle of the neck with branches of the second and third cervical nerves.

descensus (dē-sĕn′sŭs) [L.] The process of falling; descent.

d. testis The normal passage of the testicle from the abdominal cavity down into the scrotum. This occurs during the last few months of fetal life. SYN: *migration of testicle*.

d. uteri Prolapse of uterus.

d. ventriculi Downward displacement of the stomach. SYN: *gastroptosis*.

desensitization **1.** Treatment of an allergy by repeated injections of a dilute solution containing the allergen. The concentration is designed to be too weak to cause symptoms, but strong enough to promote gradual immune tolerance. It increases the levels of immunoglobulin G, which blocks immunoglobulin E from binding to mast cells and initiating the release of the chemical mediators of inflammation. Although not always successful, densensitization is still commonly used, particularly for patients whose allergic response to an antigen is systemic anaphylaxis. SYN: *hyposensitization*. SEE: *allergy; anaphylaxis; tolerance*. **2.** In psychiatry, the alleviation of an emotionally upsetting life situation.

CAUTION: The patient must be closely monitored for signs of anaphylaxis for at least 20 min after each injection of dilute antigen. Emergency drug therapy is maintained nearby for immediate treatment of anaphylaxis. Prescribed antihistamine therapy is provided to relieve lesser allergic symptoms (urticaria, pruritus, wheezing).

phobic d. A method of treating phobias in which the patient is taught to relax while slowly re-entering the phobic situation, first in imagination and then in real life. Anxiety and fear are kept to a minimum at all times. SEE: *implosion flooding*.

systematic d. A form of behavior therapy, used particularly for phobias, in which the patient is gradually exposed to anxiety-producing stimuli until they no longer produce anxiety. SEE: *implosion flooding*.

desensitize [L. *de*, from, + *sentire*, to perceive] **1.** To deprive of or lessen sensitivity by nerve section or blocking. **2.** To abate anaphylactic sensitivity by administration of the specific antigen in low dosage.

desert fever, desert rheumatism Coccidioidomycosis.

desexualize (dē-sĕks′ū-ăl-īz) [″ + *sexus*, sex] To castrate; to remove sexual traits.

desferrioxamine (dĕs-fĕr′ē-ŏks′ă-mēn) Deferoxamine mesylate.

desiccant (dĕs′ĭ-kănt) Causing desiccation or dryness.

desiccate (dĕs′ĭ-kāt) [L. *desiccare*, to dry up] To dry.

desiccation (dĕs″ĭ-kā′shŭn) The process of drying up. SEE: *electrodesiccation*.

desipramine hydrochloride (dĕs-ĭp′ră-mēn) A tricyclic antidepressant.

deslanoside (dĕs-lăn′ō-sīd) A cardiac glycoside, obtained from digitalis leaf, that slows the heart rate and increases the strength of cardiac muscles.

desmepithelium (dĕs-mĕp-ĭ-thē′lē-ŭm) [″ + *epi,* upon, + *thele,* nipple] The epithelial lining of vessels and synovial cavities.

desmitis (dĕs-mī′tĭs) [″ + *itis,* inflammation] Inflammation of a ligament.

desmo- [Gr. *desmos,* band] Combining form indicating a band or ligament.

desmocranium (dĕs″mō-krā′nē-ŭm) [″ + L. *cranium*] In the embryo, the earliest form of the skull.

desmocyte (dĕs′mō-sīt) [″ + *kytos,* cell] A connective tissue cell. SYN: *fibroblast; fibrocyte.*

desmocytoma (dĕs″mō-sī-tō′mă) [″ + ″ + *oma,* tumor] A tumor formed of desmocytes. A sarcoma.

desmogenous (dĕs-mŏj′ĕ-nŭs) [″ + *gennan,* to produce] Originating in connective tissue.

desmoid (dĕs′moyd) [″ + *eidos,* form, shape] **1.** Tendonlike. SYN: *fibroid* (1). **2.** A very tough and firm fibroma.

desmology (dĕs-mŏl′ō-jē) [″ + *logos,* word, reason] The science of tendons and ligaments.

desmoma [″ + *oma,* tumor] A tumor of the connective tissue.

desmoneoplasm (dĕs″mō-nē′ō-plăzm) [″ + *neos,* new, + LL. *plasma,* form, mold] A newly developed connective tissue tumor.

desmopathy (dĕs-mŏp′ă-thē) [″ + *pathos,* disease, suffering] Any disease affecting ligaments.

desmoplasia (dĕs-mō-plā′zē-ă) [″ + Gr. *plassein,* to form] An abnormal tendency to form fibrous tissue or adhesive bands.

desmoplastic [″ + *plassein,* to form] Causing or forming adhesions.

desmopressin acetate A synthetic antidiuretic, a vasopressin analogue, with greater antidiuretic activity but less pressor activity than vasopressin. Desmopressin is used to treat central diabetes insipidus, primary nocturnal enuresis (bedwetting), and bleeding caused by mild forms of hemophilia A or von Willebrand's disease.

desmopyknosis (dĕs″mō-pĭk-nō′sĭs) [″ + *pyknosis,* condensation] A surgical procedure for shortening round ligaments by attaching them by loops to the anterior uterine wall.

desmorrhexis (dĕs-mō-rĕk′sĭs) [″ + *rhexis,* rupture] Rupture of a ligament.

desmosis (dĕs-mō′sĭs) [″ + *osis,* condition] Any disease of the connective tissue.

desmosome (dĕs′mō-sōm) [″ + *soma,* body] A structure binding adjacent epithelial cells.

desmotomy (dĕs-mŏt′ō-mē) [″ + *tome,* incision] Dissection of a ligament.

desoximetasone (dĕs-ŏk″sē-mĕt′ă-sōn) A corticosteroid used topically.

desoxy- Prefix meaning deoxidized or a reduced form of.

desoxycorticosterone (dĕs-ŏk″sē-kor-tĭ-kŏs′tĕr-ōn) An active steroid hormone produced by the adrenal cortex. It plays an important role in the regulation of water and salt metabolism.

d. acetate An acetate ester of desoxycorticosterone and the form in which the hormone is usually administered in its therapeutic use. It may be injected intramuscularly or used buccally.

despair The eighth stage in Erikson's developmental theory; the opposite of ego integrity. The individual experiences sorrow over past life events and dismay over a foreshortened life.

desquamate (dĕs′kwă-māt) [L. *desquamare,* to remove scales] To shed or scale off the surface epithelium.

desquamation (dĕs″kwă-mā′shŭn) **1.** Shedding of the epidermis. **2.** The peeling skin characteristic of postmature infants.

furfuraceous d. Shedding of branlike scales.

desquamative (dĕs-kwŏm′ă-tĭv) Of the nature of desquamation, or pert. to or causing it. SYN: *keratolytic.*

DES syndrome The occurrence of neoplasms and malformation of the vagina in young women whose mothers received diethylstilbestrol early in their pregnancy. SEE: *DES daughter.*

destructive [L. *destructus,* destroyed] Causing ruin or destruction; the opposite of constructive.

destructive lesion A pathological change such as an infection, tumor, or injury that causes the death of tissue or an organ.

desulfhydrase (dē″sŭlf-hī′drās) An enzyme that cleaves cysteine into hydrogen sulfide, ammonia, and pyruvic acid.

desynchronosis (dē-sĭn″krō-nō′sĭs) [″ + Gr. *synkhronos,* same time] An upset of a person's internal biological clock, caused by the difference between the time at a person's present location and the time to which the person is accustomed. This condition occurs in persons traveling across several time zones in a short period. The lay term for this condition is "jet lag."

DET *diethyltryptamine.*

det L. *detur,* let it be given.

detachment [O.Fr. *destachier,* to unfasten] The process of separation.

detail In radiology, the sharpness with which an image is presented on a radiograph.

detector [L. *detectus,* uncovered] A device for determining the presence of something.

flame ionization d. ABBR: FID. A device used in gas chromatography in which a sample burned in a flame changes the conductivity between two electrodes.

lie d. Polygraph.

optical d. The sensor in a typical colorimeter or photometer that senses the light transmitted by the sample.

radiation d. An instrument used to detect the presence of radiation. SEE: *dosimeter*.

detergent [L. *detergere,* to cleanse] **1.** Something that purges or cleanses; cleansing. **2.** A cleaning or wetting agent prepared synthetically from any of several chemicals. These are classed as anionic if they have a negative electric charge or cationic if they have a positive charge. SEE: *soap*.

deterioration [L. *deteriorare,* to deteriorate] Retrogression; said of impairment of mental or physical functions.

determinant (dē-tĕr′mĭ-nănt) [L. *determinare,* to limit] That which determines the character of something.

determination [L. *determinatus,* limiting] The establishing of the nature or precise identity of a substance, organism, or event.

determinism (dē-tĕr′mĭn-ĭzm) [″ + Gr. *-ismos,* condition] The theory that all human action is the result of predetermined and inevitable physical, psychological, or environmental conditions that are uninfluenced by the will of the individual.

detersive [L. *detergere,* to cleanse] Detergent (1).

detortion, detorsion (dē-tor′shŭn) **1.** Surgical therapy for torsion of a testicle, ureter, or volvulus of the bowel. **2.** Correction of any bodily curvature or deformity.

detoxification [″ + ″ + L. *facere,* to make] **1.** Reduction of the toxic properties of a poisonous substance. SEE: *biotransformation*. **2.** The process of removing the physiological effects of a drug or substance from an addicted individual.

detoxify (dē-tŏk′sĭ-fī) **1.** To remove the toxic quality of a substance. **2.** To treat a toxic overdose of any medicine, but esp. of the toxic state produced by drug abuse or acute alcoholism.

detrition (dē-trĭsh′ŭn) [L. *detritus,* to rub away] The wearing away of a part, esp. through friction, as of the teeth. SEE: *bruxism*.

detritus (dĭ-trī′tŭs) [L., to rub away] Any broken-down, degenerative, or carious matter produced by disintegration.

detrusor hyperactivity with impaired contractility ABBR: DHIC. A condition in which urinary incontinence is produced by an overactive detrusor muscle coexisting with a weak bladder. This is a common urologic abnormality in the elderly.

detrusor instability Contractions of the muscles of the urinary bladder during the filling phase of a urodynamic study, or during coughing, sneezing, or other activities that raise intra-abdominal pressures. It is a cause of urinary incontinence, esp. in women. Some experts believe detrusor overactivity to be the most common cause of urinary incontinence in the elderly. Causes include urethral obstruction, cystitis, bladder carcinoma, stroke, Parkinson's disease, and multiple sclerosis. SYN: *detrusor overactivity*.

detrusor overactivity Detrusor instability.

detrusor urinae (dē-trū′sor ū-rĭ′nē) [L.] The external longitudinal layer of the muscular coat of the bladder.

detumescence (dē″tū-mĕs′ĕns) [L. *de,* down, + *tumescere,* to swell] **1.** Subsidence of a swelling. **2.** Subsidence of the swelling of erectile tissue of the genital organs (penis or clitoris) following erection.

deuter- SEE: *deutero-*.

deuteranomalopia (doo″tĕr-ă-nŏm″ă-lō′pē-ă) [″ + *anomalos,* irregular, + *ops,* eye] Partial color blindness in which the primary colors are perceived but green is poorly appreciated.

deuteranopia, deuteranopsia (dū″tĕr-ăn-ō′pē-ă, -ŏp′sē-ă) [″ + *anopia,* blindness] Green blindness; color blindness in which there is a defect in the perception of green. SEE: *color blindness*.

deuterate (dū′tĕr-āt) To combine with deuterium.

deuterium (dū-tē′rē-ŭm) [Gr. *deuteros,* second] SYMB: H^2 or D. The isotope of hydrogen, whose mass is 2, sometimes called heavy hydrogen.

d. oxide An isotope of water in which hydrogen has been displaced by its isotope, deuterium. Its properties differ from ordinary water in that it has higher freezing and boiling points and is incapable of supporting life. SYN: *heavy water*.

deutero-, deuter-, deuto- [Gr. *deuteros,* second] Prefix indicating *second* or *secondary*.

deuteron (dū′tĕr-ŏn) SYMB: d. The nucleus of deuterium or heavy hydrogen.

deuteroplasm [″ + LL. *plasma,* form, mold] The reserve food supply in the yolk or ovum.

deuto- SEE: *deutero-*.

deutoscolex (dū″tō-skō′lĕks) [″ + *skolex,* worm] A secondary daughter cyst that develops on the inner wall of a hydatid cyst.

devascularization (dē-văs″kū-lăr-ĭ-zā′shŭn) [″ + *vascularis,* pert. to a vessel] A decrease in the blood supply to a body part by pathologic or surgical process.

developer In radiology and photography, the solution used to make the latent image visible on the radiographic film.

development [O.Fr. *desveloper,* to unwrap] Growth to full size or maturity, as in the progress of an egg to the adult state. SEE: *growth*.

cognitive d. The sequential acquisition of the ability to learn, reason, and analyze that begins in infancy and progresses as the individual matures.

psychomotor and physical d. of infant SEE: *psychomotor and physical development of infant.*

risk for altered d. A nursing diagnosis approved at the 13th NANDA Conference (1998); at risk for delay of 25% or more in one or more of the areas of social or self-regulatory behavior, or cognitive, language, gross, or fine motor skills. SEE: *Nursing Diagnoses Appendix.*

developmental Pert. to development.

developmental delay An impairment in the performance of tasks or the meeting of milestones that a child should achieve by a specific chronological age. The diagnosis of a developmental delay is made with diagnostic testing that assesses cognitive, physical, social, and emotional development, as well as communication and adaptive skills.

developmental milestone A skill regarded as having special importance in the development of infants and toddlers and usually associated with a particular age range (e.g., sitting, crawling, walking).

deviance [L. *deviare,* to turn aside] A variation from the accepted norm.

deviant Something (or someone) that is variant when compared with the norm or an accepted standard.

sex d. One whose sexual behavior is considered to be abnormal or socially unacceptable. SEE: *paraphilia.*

deviant behavior Any action considered to be abnormal.

deviate (dē′vē-āt″) [L. *deviare,* to turn aside] **1.** To move steadily away from a designated norm. **2.** An individual whose behavior, esp. sexual behavior, is so far removed from societal norms that it is classed as socially, morally, or legally unacceptable.

deviation (dē-vē-ā′shŭn) **1.** A departure from the normal. **2.** To alter course or direction.

axis d. A change in the direction of the major electrical axis of the heart as determined by the electrocardiogram.

conjugate d. Deviation of the eyes to the same side.

minimum d. The smallest deviation that a prism can produce.

standard d. ABBR: SD. In statistics, the measure of variability from the central tendency of any frequency curve. It is the square root of the variance.

device (dĭ-vīs′) [O.Fr. *devis,* contrivance] An apparatus, machine, or shaped object constructed to perform a specific function.

abduction d. A trapezoid-shaped pillow, wedge, or splint placed between the legs to prevent adduction. It is commonly used postoperatively for patients having total hip replacement or open reduction or internal fixation of the hip.

adapted seating d. ABBR: ASD. A device that provides proper positioning for persons with limited motor control. These include seating inserts, wheelchairs, and postural support systems designed to prevent deformities and enhance function. SYN: *seating system.*

adaptive d. Assistive technology.

assistive d. Assistive technology.

augmentative d. A tool that helps individuals with limited or absent speech to communicate. Examples include communication boards, pictographs (symbols that look like the things they represent), or ideographs (symbols representing ideas).

belay d. A mechanism designed to use friction to brake or slow the movement of a rope, to protect a patient, basket, climber, or other rescuer.

cervical immobilization d. ABBR: CID. Any stiff neck brace or collar used to prevent movement of the cervical spine.

esophageal intubation detector d. A syringe that is attached to the endotracheal tube immediately after an intubation attempt. If aspiration is difficult or stomach contents are withdrawn, or both, the endotracheal (ET) tube may have been placed in the esophagus and needs to be removed and reinserted. If aspiration is easy and free of stomach contents there is a good chance that the ET tube is located in the trachea; the rescuer should then confirm tube placement by other techniques (e.g., a combination of auscultation, x-ray, and pulse oximetry).

flow-restricted oxygen-powered ventilation d. ABBR: FROPVD. A ventilation device that provides a peak flow rate of 100% oxygen at up to 40 L/min.

head immobilization d. A device that attaches to a long back board and holds the patient's head in neutral alignment. Also called *cervical immobilization device.* SEE: *back board, long.*

input d. In assistive technology, the apparatus that activates an electronic device. This can be a manual switch, a remote control, or a joystick. SEE: *switch.*

Kendrick extrication d. SEE: *Kendrick extrication device.*

listening d. A speech amplifier that aids hearing-impaired individuals in direct person-to-person communication or telephone conversation. Such devices differ from conventional hearing aids in that they reduce interference from background noises.

needleless d. A device used to inject drugs and fluids that has no exposed sharp surface. It is designed to decrease the risk of needle-stick injuries by health care professionals.

personal flotation d. ABBR: PFD. A life vest used to prevent drowning and near drowning. People engaged in water sports, such as boating or water skiing, or rescuers working on or near the water should wear PFDs at all times. The U.S. Coast Guard sets standards and establishes specifications for the manufacture and use of PFDs.

pointing d. A type of input device for sending commands to a computer. Moving the device results in movement of a cursor on the monitor or computer screen. Pointing devices range from the conventional desktop mouse, trackball, and touch-sensitive screens to infrared and ultrasound pointers mounted on the head. SEE: *pointer, light; switch.*

position-indicating d. ABBR: PID. A device used to guide the direction of the x-ray beam during the exposure of dental radiographs. These devices improve and standardize dental radiographic imaging and reduce the patient's risk of radiation exposure.

positive beam limiting d. A collimator that automatically adjusts the size of the radiation field to match the size of the imaging device. Also called *automatic collimator.*

pressure relief d. Wheelchair cushion.

protective d. An external support applied to vulnerable joints or other body parts to guard against injury. Protective devices include helmets, braces, tape or wrapping, and padding.

sequential compression d. An air-filled sleeve wrapped around the leg to prevent deep venous thrombosis. The sleeve is attached to a pneumatic pump that alternately inflates and deflates it.

telecommunication d. for the deaf A device that allows hearing-impaired people to use the telephone even if they cannot comprehend speech. A keyboard and display screen are used.

devil's grip Epidemic pleurodynia.

deviometer (dē″vē-ŏm′ĕ-tĕr) [L. *de,* from, + *via,* way, + Gr. *metron,* measure] A machine for estimating degrees of strabismus.

devitalization [″ + *vita,* life] **1.** Destruction or loss of vitality. **2.** Anesthetizing of the sensitive pulp of a tooth; known as killing the nerve.

dexamethasone (dĕk″să-mĕth′ă-sōn) A synthetic glucocorticoid drug.

dexamethasone suppression test A test performed by administering dexamethasone to determine the effect on cortisol production. This is done as part of the diagnostic investigation for Cushing's syndrome. Normally this test causes a decrease in cortisol production, but in a patient with Cushing's syndrome, suppression is minimal. The test may be positive in patients with ectopic corticotropin production. SEE: *corticotropin production, ectopic; Cushing's syndrome.*

dexbrompheniramine maleate (dĕks″ brŏm-fĕn-ĭr′ă-mēn) An antihistamine.

dexchlorpheniramine maleate (dĕks″ klor-fĕn-ĭr′ă-mēn) An antihistamine.

dexter (dĕks′tĕr) [L.] On the right side. SEE: *sinister.*

dexterity Skill in using the hands, usually requiring both fine and gross motor coordination.

dextrad (dĕks′trăd) [L. *dexter,* right, + *ad,* toward] **1.** Toward the right side. **2.** A right-handed person.

dextral (dĕks′trăl) Pert. to the right side.

dextrality (dĕks-trăl′ĭ-tē) Right-handedness. SEE: *sinistrality.*

dextran (dĕks′trăn) [L. *dexter,* right] A polysaccharide produced by the action of *Leuconostoc mesenteroides* on sucrose. It is available in various molecular weights and is used as a plasma volume expander.

dextranomer beads A cross-linked network of dextran prepared in the form of beads. Because this compound has great ability to absorb moisture, it has been used in helping to débride wounds. SEE: *decubitus ulcer.*

dextrase (dĕks′trās) An enzyme that splits dextrose and converts it into lactic acid.

dextraural (dĕks-traw′răl) [L. *dexter,* right, + *auris,* ear] Hearing better with the right ear.

dextrin (dĕks′trĭn) [L. *dexter,* right] A yellow-white powder that forms mucilaginous solutions in water and can be prepared by the action of heat or acid on starch. It is a carbohydrate of the formula $(C_6H_{10}O_5)_{11}$. In digestion, it is a soluble or gummy matter into which starch is converted by diastase; it is the result of the first chemical change in the digestion of starch.

dextro- [L. *dexter,* right] Combining form meaning *to the right.*

dextroamphetamine sulfate (dĕks″trō-ăm-fĕt′ă-mēn sŭl′fāt) A compound related to amphetamine sulfate (i.e., an isomer of amphetamine); sometimes written D-amphetamine sulfate or dextroamphetamine sulfate. It is used as a central nervous system stimulant in attention deficit hyperactivity disorder and occasionally as a treatment for depression in patients with terminal illnesses. Prolonged use can cause psychological dependence. The "street" name is "speed."

dextrocardia (dĕks″trō-kăr′dē-ă) [″ + Gr. *kardia,* heart] The condition of having the heart on the right side of the body.

dextrocular (dĕks-trŏk′ū-lăr) [″ + *oculus,* eye] Having a stronger right eye than left.

dextrocularity (dĕks″trŏk-ū-lăr′ĭ-tē) The condition of having the right eye stronger than the left.

dextroduction [″ + *ducere,* to lead] Movement of the visual axis to the right.

dextrogastria [″ + Gr. *gaster,* belly] The condition of having the stomach on the right side of the body.

dextromanual [″ + *manus,* hand] Right-handed.

dextromethorphan (dĕk″strō-mĕth′or-făn) A cough suppressant. A great number of cough medicines include this drug in their formula.

dextropedal (dĕks-trŏp′ĕ-dăl) [″ + *pes, ped-,* foot] Having greater dexterity in using the right leg than the left.

dextrophobia [″ + Gr. *phobos,* fear] Abnormal aversion to objects on the right side of the body.

dextroposition (dĕks″trō-pō-zĭsh′ŭn) Displacement to the right.

dextroposition of the great vessels Transposition of the great vessels.

dextropropoxyphene (dĕk″strō-prō-pŏk′sē-fēn) Propoxyphene, a mild narcotic analgesic that can cause addiction and may be fatal in an overdose.

dextrorotatory (dĕks″trō-rō′tă-tor-ē) [″ + *rotare,* to turn] Causing to turn to the right, applied esp. to substances that turn polarized rays of light to the right.

dextrose (dĕks′trōs) Glucose.

dextrose and sodium chloride injection A sterile solution of dextrose, salt, and water for use intravenously. It contains no antimicrobial agents.

dextrosinistral (dĕks″trō-sĭn′ĭs-trăl) [L. *dexter,* right, + *sinister,* left] From right to left.

dextrosuria (dĕks-trō-sū′rē-ă) Dextrose in the urine.

dextrotropic, dextrotropous (dĕks″trō-trŏp′ĭk, -trō′pŭs) [″ + Gr. *tropos,* a turning] Turning to the right.

dextroversion [″ + *vertere,* to turn] Turned or located toward the right.

DFP *di-isopropyl fluorophosphate.* SEE: *isoflurophate.*

dg *decigram.*

DHEA *Dehydroepiandrosterone.*

di- [Gr. *dis,* twice] Prefix indicating *twice, double,* or *two.*

diabetes (dī″ă-bē′tēz) [Gr. *diabetes,* passing through] A general term for diseases marked by excessive urination; usually refers to diabetes mellitus. SEE: *Nursing Diagnoses Appendix.*

brittle d. Diabetes mellitus that is exceptionally difficult to control. The disease is marked by alternating episodes of hypoglycemia and hyperglycemia. Frequent adjustments of dietary intake and insulin dosage are required.

ETIOLOGY: Diabetes may be brittle when 1. insulin is not well-absorbed; 2. insulin requirements vary rapidly; 3. insulin is improperly prepared or administered; 4. the Somogyi phenomenon is present; 5. the patient has coexisting anorexia or bulimia; 6. the patient's daily exercise routine, diet, or medication schedule varies; or 7. physiological or psychological stress is persistent.

bronze d. Hemochromatosis.

chemical d. **1.** Asymptomatic diabetes mellitus; that is, a stage of diabetes mellitus (DM) in which no obvious clinical signs and symptoms of the disease are present, but blood sugar measurements are abnormal. **2.** Type 2 DM occurring in an obese child or adolescent. The syndrome is sometimes referred to as "mature onset diabetes of youth" (MODY).

endocrine d. Diabetes mellitus that results from diseases of the pituitary, thyroid, or adrenal glands or from the ovaries.

gestational d. Diabetes mellitus that begins during pregnancy, typically in the second or third trimester. It occurs in 1% to 4% of pregnancies and requires careful treatment to prevent fetal anomalies (e.g., macrosomia) and maternal complications (e.g., pregnancy-induced hypertension, eclampsia, and the need for cesarean delivery).

Although gestational diabetes usually subsides after delivery, more than one third of women with gestational diabetes will eventually develop type 2 diabetes mellitus during their lifetimes.

iatrogenic d. Diabetes mellitus brought on by administration of drugs such as corticosteroids, certain diuretics, or birth control pills.

immune-mediated d. mellitus Type 1 diabetes.

d. insipidus ABBR: DI. Excessive urination caused either by inadequate amounts of antidiuretic hormone in the body (hypothalamic DI) or by failure of the kidney to respond to antidiuretic hormone (nephrogenic DI). Urinary output is often massive (e.g., 5 to 10 L/day), which may result in dehydration, esp. in patients who cannot drink enough liquid to replace urinary losses (e.g., those with impaired consciousness). The urine is dilute (specific gravity is often below 1.005), and typically the patient's serum sodium level and osmolality rise as free water is dumped into the urine. If water deficits are not matched or the urinary losses are not prevented, death will result from dehydration.

ETIOLOGY: DI usually results from hypothalamic injury (e.g., brain trauma or neurosurgery) or from the effects of certain drugs (e.g., lithium or demeclocycline) on the renal resorption of water. Other representative causes include sickle cell anemia (in which renal infarcts damage the kidney's ability to retain water), hypothyroidism, adrenal insufficiency, inherited disorders of antidiuretic hormone production, and sarcoidosis.

SYMPTOMS: The primary symptoms

are urinary frequency, thirst, and dehydration.

TREATMENT: When DI is a side effect of drug therapy, the offending drug is withheld. DI caused by failure of the hypothalamus to secrete antidiuretic hormone is treated with synthetic vasopressin.

PROGNOSIS: The prognosis is usually good when the disease is recognized and appropriately managed.

PATIENT CARE: Fluid balance is monitored. Fluid intake and output, urine specific gravity, and weight are assessed for evidence of dehydration and hypovolemic hypotension. Serum electrolyte and blood urea nitrogen levels are monitored.

The patient is instructed in nasal insufflation of vasopressin or administration of subcutaneous or intramuscular hormones. The length of the therapy and the importance of taking medications as prescribed and not discontinuing them abruptly are stressed. Meticulous skin and oral care are provided; use of a soft toothbrush is recommended, and petroleum jelly is applied to the lips and an emollient lotion to the skin to reduce dryness. Adequate fluid intake should be maintained.

Both the patient and family are taught to identify signs of dehydration and to report signs of severe dehydration and impending hypovolemia. The patient is taught to measure intake and output, to monitor weight daily, and to use a hydrometer to measure urine specific gravity. The patient should wear or carry a medical identification tag and keep a supply of medication with him or her at all times.

insulin-dependent d. mellitus ABBR: IDDM. Type 1 diabetes.

juvenile-onset d. Type 1 diabetes.

latent d. Diabetes mellitus that manifests itself during times of stress such as pregnancy, infectious disease, weight gain, or trauma. Previous to the stress, no clinical or laboratory findings of diabetes are present. There is a very strong chance that such individuals will eventually develop overt type 2 diabetes mellitus.

mature-onset d. of youth ABBR: MODY. Type 2 DM that presents during childhood or adolescence, typically as an autosomal dominant trait in which there is diminished, but not absent, insulin production by the pancreas. Children with this form of diabetes mellitus are not prone to diabetic ketoacidosis.

d. mellitus A chronic metabolic disorder marked by hyperglycemia. Diabetes mellitus (DM) results either from failure of the pancreas to produce insulin (type 1 DM) or from insulin resistance, with inadequate insulin secretion to sustain normal metabolism (type 2 DM). Either type of DM may damage blood vessels, nerves, kidneys, the retina, and in pregnancy, the developing fetus. Type 1, or insulin-dependent, DM has a prevalence of just 0.3% to 0.4%. Type 2 DM (previously known as "adult-onset" DM) has a prevalence in the general population of 6.6%. In some populations (e.g., elderly persons, Native Americans, blacks, Pacific Islanders, Mexican Americans), it is present in nearly 20% of adults. Type 2 DM primarily affects obese middle-aged people with sedentary lifestyles, whereas type 1 DM (formerly called "juvenile-onset" DM) occurs usually in children, most of whom are active and thin. SEE: table; *dawn phenomenon; insulin; insulin pump; insulin resistance; diabetic polyneuropathy; Somogyi phenomenon.*

Type 1 DM usually presents as an acute illness with dehydration and often diabetic ketoacidosis. Type 2 DM is often asymptomatic in its early years and therefore occult. The American Diabetes Association (1-800-DIABETES) estimates that more than 5 million Americans have type 2 DM without knowing it. Diagnosis is based on a fasting plasma glucose level greater than 126 mg/dl on more than one occasion or a glucose level exceeding 200 mg/dl in a patient with excessive urinary volume (polyuria), excessive thirst (polydipsia), and weight loss.

ETIOLOGY: Type 1 DM is caused by autoimmune destruction of the insulin-secreting beta cells of the pancreas. The loss of these cells results in nearly complete insulin deficiency; without exogenous insulin, type 1 DM is rapidly fatal. Type 2 DM results partly from a decreased sensitivity of muscle cells to insulin-mediated glucose uptake and partly from a relative decrease in pancreatic insulin secretion.

SYMPTOMS: Classic symptoms of DM are polyuria, polydipsia, and weight loss. In addition, patients with hyperglycemia often have blurred vision, increased food consumption (polyphagia), and generalized weakness. When a patient with type 1 DM loses metabolic control (e.g., during infections or periods of noncompliance with therapy), symptoms of diabetic ketoacidosis occur. These may include nausea, vomiting, dizziness on arising, intoxication, delirium, coma, or death. Chronic complications of hyperglycemia include retinopathy and blindness, peripheral and autonomic neuropathies, glomerulosclerosis of the kidneys (with proteinuria, nephrotic syndrome, or end-stage renal failure), coronary and peripheral vascular disease, and reduced resistance to infections. Patients with DM often also sustain ulcerations of the feet, which

Comparison of Diabetic Ketoacidosis and Hypoglycemia

	Diabetic Ketoacidosis	Hypoglycemia
Onset	Gradual	Often sudden
History	Often acute infection in a diabetic or insufficient insulin intake Previous history of diabetes may be absent	Recent insulin injection, inadequate meal, or excessive exercise after insulin
Musculoskeletal	Muscle wasting or weight loss	Weakness Tremor Muscle twitching
Gastrointestinal	Abdominal pains or cramps, sometimes acute Nausea and vomiting	Nausea and vomiting
Central nervous system	Headache Double or blurred vision Irritability	Confusion, delirium, or seizures
Cardiovascular	Tachycardia Orthostatic hypotension	Variable
Skin	Flushed, dry	Diaphoretic, pale
Respiratory	Air hunger Acetone odor of breath Dyspnea	Variable Increased respiratory rate
Laboratory values	Elevated blood glucose (200 mg/dl) Glucose and ketones in blood and urine	Subnormal blood glucose (0–50 mg/dl) Absence of glucose and ketones in urine unless bladder is full

may result in osteomyelitis and the need for amputation.

TREATMENT: DM types 1 and 2 are both treated with specialized diets, regular exercise, intensive foot and eye care, and medications.

Patients with type 1 DM, unless they have had a pancreatic transplant, require insulin to live; intensive therapy with insulin to limit hyperglycemia ("tight control") is more effective than conventional therapy in preventing the progression of serious microvascular complications such as kidney and retinal diseases. Intensive therapy consists of three or more doses of insulin injected or administered by infusion pump daily, with frequent self-monitoring of blood glucose levels as well as frequent changes in therapy as a result of contacts with health care professionals. Some negative aspects of intensive therapy include a three times more frequent occurrence of severe hypoglycemia, weight gain, and an adverse effect on serum lipid levels (i.e., a rise in total cholesterol, LDL cholesterol, and triglycerides, and a fall in HDL cholesterol). Participation in an intensive therapy program requires a motivated patient.

Some patients with type 2 DM can control their disease with a calorically restricted diet (e.g., 1600 to 1800 cal/day) and regular aerobic exercise. Most patients, however, require the addition of some form of oral hypoglycemic drug or insulin. Oral agents to control DM include sulfonylurea drugs (e.g., tolazamide, tolbutamide, glyburide, or glipizide), which typically increase pancreatic secretion of insulin; biguanides or thiazolidinediones (e.g., metformin or troglitazone), which increase cellular sensitivity to insulin; or α-glucosidase inhibitors (e.g., acarbose), which decrease the absorption of carbohydrates from the gastrointestinal tract. When combinations of these agents fail to normalize blood sugar levels, insulin injections are added.

PREVENTION OF COMPLICATIONS: Patients with DM should avoid using tobacco products, actively manage their serum lipid levels, and keep hypertension under optimal control because failure to do so may result in a risk of atherosclerosis much higher than that of the general public. Other elements in good diabetic care include receiving regular vaccinations (e.g., to prevent influenza and pneumococcal pneumonia).

PROGNOSIS: Diabetes is a chronic, incurable disease, but symptoms can be ameliorated and life prolonged by proper therapy. The isolation and eventual production of insulin in 1922 by Canadian physicians Banting and Best made it possible to allow persons with the disease to lead a normal life.

PATIENT CARE: The diabetic patient should learn to recognize symptoms of low blood sugar (such as confusion, sweats, and palpitations) as well as those of high blood sugar, such as polyuria and polydipsia. When either condition results in hospitalization, vital signs, weight, fluid intake, urine output, and caloric intake are accurately documented. Serum glucose and ketone levels are evaluated. The effects of diabetes on other body systems, such as cerebrovascular, coronary artery, and peripheral vascular impairment; visual impairment; and peripheral and autonomic nervous system impairment are assessed. The patient is observed for signs and symptoms of diabetic neuropathy, such as numbness or pain in the hands and feet, decreased vibratory sense, footdrop, and neurogenic bladder. The urine is checked for microalbumin or overt protein losses, an early indication of nephropathy.

Insulin or oral hypoglycemic agents are administered as prescribed and their action and use explained. With help from a dietitian, a diet is planned based on the recommended amount of calories, protein, carbohydrates, and fats. The patient learns how to choose food exchanges and how to read food container labels. A steady, consistent level of daily exercise is prescribed, and participation in a supervised exercise program is recommended.

Hypoglycemic reactions are promptly treated by giving carbohydrates (oral orange juice, hard candy, honey, or any sugar-containing food); as necessary, SC or IM glucagon or IV dextrose (if the patient is not conscious) is administered. Hyperglycemic crises are treated initially with prescribed intravenous fluids and insulin, and later, with potassium replacement based on laboratory values.

Skin care, esp. to the feet and legs, is provided, and the patient is instructed in these techniques. All injuries, cuts, and blisters should be treated promptly. The patient should avoid constricting hose, slippers, shoes, bed linens, and walking barefoot. The patient is referred to a podiatrist for ongoing foot care and is warned that decreased sensation can mask injuries. Regular ophthalmological examinations are recommended for early detection of diabetic retinopathy.

The patient is educated about diabetes, its possible complications and their management, and the importance of strict adherence to the prescribed therapy. Emotional support and a realistic assessment of the patient's condition are offered; this assessment should stress that, with proper treatment, the patient can have a near-normal lifestyle and life expectancy. Assistance is offered to help the patient to develop positive coping strategies. The patient and family may be referred for counseling and to local and national support and information groups. SEE: *Nursing Diagnoses Appendix.*

non-insulin-dependent d. mellitus ABBR: NIDDM. Type 2 d. SEE: *type 1 d.* for table.

pancreatic d. Diabetes associated with disease of the pancreas, such as chronic or recurrent pancreatitis.

phlorhizin d. Glycosuria caused by administration of phlorhizin.

renal d. Renal glycosuria; this condition is marked by a low renal threshold for glucose. Glucose tolerance is normal and diabetic symptoms are lacking.

secondary d. mellitus DM that results from damage to the pancreas (e.g., after frequent episodes of pancreatitis), or from drugs such as corticosteroids (which increase resistance to the effects of insulin).

strict control of d. Regulation of blood sugars to normal, or nearly normal levels, both before and after meals. Tight control has been shown to prevent microvascular complications of diabetes mellitus (DM), such as blindness, nerve damage, and kidney failure.

Patients with meticulously controlled DM typically have a hemoglobin A1c level of about 7%; fasting blood sugars that are less than 110 mg/dl; and postprandial blood sugars that are less than 180 mg/dl. Strategies to attain these levels including paying careful attention to dietary regimens, exercising regularly, and monitoring blood sugars, oral medications, and insulin doses frequently throughout the day. SYN: *tight control of d.*

tight control of d. Strict control of d.

true d. D. mellitus.

type 1 d. Diabetes mellitus that usually has its onset before the age of 25 years, in which the essential abnormality is related to absolute insulin deficiency. SYN: *juvenile-onset d.* SEE: table.

type 2 d. A group of forms of diabetes mellitus that occur predominantly in adults. The insulin produced is sufficient to prevent ketoacidosis but insufficient to meet the total needs of the body. This form of diabetes in nonobese patients can usually be controlled by diet and oral hypoglycemic agents, such as sulfonylurea drugs or metformin, a nonsulfonylurea drug. Occasionally insulin therapy is required. In some patients the condition can be controlled

Comparison of Type 1 Insulin-Dependent Diabetes Mellitus and Type 2 Non–Insulin-Dependent Diabetes Mellitus

	Type 1	Type 2
Age at onset	Usually under 30	Usually over 40
Symptom onset	Abrupt	Gradual
Body weight	Normal	Obese—80%
HLA association	Positive	Negative
Family history	Common	Nearly universal
Insulin in blood	Little to none	Some usually present
Islet cell antibodies	Present at onset	Absent
Prevalence	0.2%–0.3%	6%
Symptoms	Polyuria, polydipsia, polyphagia, weight loss, ketoacidosis	Polyuria, polydipsia, peripheral neuropathy
Control	Insulin, diet, and exercise	Diet, exercise, and often oral hypoglycemic drugs or insulin
Vascular and neural changes	Eventually develop	Will usually develop
Stability of condition	Fluctuates, may be difficult to control	May be difficult to control in poorly motivated patients

by careful diet and regular exercise. SYN: *non–insulin-dependent d. mellitus*. SEE: *type 1 diabetes* for table.

diabetic (dī-ă-bĕt′ĭk) Pert. to diabetes.

diabetic center An area in the floor of the fourth ventricle of the brain.

diabetic ear "Malignant" otitis media often caused by infection with *Pseudomonas aeruginosa*. SEE: *otitis media*.

diabetic ketoacidosis Acidosis caused by an accumulation of ketone bodies, in advanced stages of uncontrolled diabetes mellitus. SEE: *diabetic coma; Nursing Diagnoses Appendix*.

diabetogenic (dī″ă-bĕt″ō-jĕn′ĭk) [″ + *gennan*, to produce] Causing diabetes.

diabetogenous (dī″ă-bē-tŏj′ĕn-ŭs) Caused by diabetes.

diacele (dī′ă-sēl) [Gr. *dia*, between, + *koilia*, a hollow] The third ventricle of the brain.

diacetate (dī-ăs′ĕ-tāt) A salt of diacetic acid.

diacetemia (dī-ăs″ĕ-tē′mē-ă) The presence of diacetic acid in the blood.

diacetic acid (dī″ă-sĕt′ĭk) Acetoacetic acid, found in acidosis and in the urine of diabetic persons. Like acetone, it is found in uncontrolled diabetes and in any condition that produces starvation and excessive fat metabolism, such as persistent vomiting.

diacetonuria, diaceturia (dī-ăs″ĕ-tō-nū′rē-ă, dī-ăs″ĕ-tū′rē-ă) Diacetic acid in urine.

diacetylmorphine (dī″ă-sē″tĭl-mor′fēn) Heroin.

diacidic (dī-ăs′ĭd-ĭk) [Gr. *dis*, twice, + L. *acidus*, soured] Containing two acidic hydrogen ions.

diaclasis (dī-ă-klā′sĭs) [Gr. *dia*, through, + *klan*, to break] A surgical procedure in which a bone is intentionally fractured. SYN: *osteoclasia*.

diaclast (dī′ă-klăst) [″ + *klan*, to break] A device for perforating the fetal skull.

diacrinous (dī-ăk′rĭn-ŭs) [Gr. *diakrinein*, to separate] Pert. to cells that secrete into ducts rather than into the vascular system. SYN: *exocrine*.

diaderm [Gr. *dia*, through, + *derma*, skin] A blastoderm composed of ectoderm and endoderm, and containing between them the segmentation cavity.

diadochokinesia (dī-ăd″ō-kō-kĭn-ē′zē-ă) [Gr. *diadokos*, succeeding, + *kinesis*, movement] The ability to make antagonistic movements, such as pronation and supination of the hands in quick succession. SEE: *disdiadochokinesia*.

diagnose (dī′ăg-nōs) [Gr. *diagignoskein*, to discern] To determine the cause and nature of a pathological condition; to recognize a disease.

diagnosis (dī″ăg-nō′sĭs) *pl.* **diagnoses** **1.** The term denoting the disease or syndrome a person has or is believed to have. **2.** The use of scientific or clinical methods to establish the cause and nature of a person's illness. This is done by evaluating the history of the disease process, the signs and symptoms, the laboratory data, and special tests such as radiography and electrocardiography. The value of establishing a diagnosis is to provide a logical basis for treatment and prognosis.

antenatal d. Prenatal d.

clinical d. Identification of a disease by history, physical examination, laboratory studies, and radiological studies.

cytological d. Identification of a disease based on cells present in body tissues or exudates.

differential d. Identification of a disease by comparison of illnesses that share features of the presenting illness, but differ in some critical ways.

dual d. The presence of mental illness in a patient with a history of concurrent substance abuse.

d. by exclusion Identification of a disease by eliminating other implausible diagnoses.

medical d. The identification of the cause of the patient's illness or discomfort. SYN: *clinical d.*

nursing d. SEE: *nursing diagnosis.*

oral d. The procedure or special area of dentistry devoted to the compilation and study of the patient's dental history, and a detailed clinical examination of the oral tissues and radiographs to assess the level of oral health, with the object of developing a treatment plan to restore tooth structure and proper occlusion and to promote healing and better oral health.

pathological d. Determining the cause(s) of an illness or disease by examining fluids and tissues from the patient before or after death. The examination may be performed on blood, plasma, microscopic tissue samples, or gross specimens. SEE: *autopsy; pathology.*

physical d. Identification of an illness or abnormality by looking at, listening to, percussing, or palpating the patient. In contemporary health care, diagnostic imaging (e.g., ultrasound, nuclear medicine, CT and MRI scans) has replaced, amid much controversy, many traditional physical diagnostic skills.

physical therapist d. **1.** The clinical classification by a physical therapist of a patient's impairments, functional limitations, and disabilities. **2.** The use of data obtained by physical therapy examination and other relevant information to determine the cause and nature of a patient's impairments, functional limitations, and disabilities.

prenatal d. Identification of disease or congenital defects of the fetus during gestation. A growing number of pathologic conditions can be diagnosed by analyses of maternal blood and such tests as chorionic villi sampling, ultrasound, embryoscopy, amniocentesis, and fetoscopy. Thus, the gender, inherited characteristics, and current status of the fetus can be identified as early as the first trimester, helping parents in their decision-making if findings indicate an incurable disorder. Midtrimester and last trimester tests provide information regarding the physical characteristics of the fetus and placenta, and analysis of amniotic fluid allows estimation of fetal age and maturity, and may improve intrauterine management of treatable disorders. SEE: *prenatal surgery.*

primary d. Diagnosis of the most important disease process or the underlying disease process afflicting a patient.

radiographic d. Identification of an illness by the interpretation of radiographic findings.

serological d. Identification of an illness through a serological test such as that for syphilis or typhoid.

tongue d. In traditional Chinese medicine, the methodical evaluation of the appearance of the tongue to determine the cause of a complaint or syndrome.

diagnosis-related group ABBR: DRG. An indexing or classification system designed to standardize prospective payment for medical care. Diseases and conditions are assigned to a single DRG when they are felt to share similar clinical and health care utilization features. The reimbursement for treating all individuals within the same DRG is the same, regardless of actual cost to the health care facility.

diagnostic Pert. to a diagnosis.

in vitro d. ABBR: IVD. Any device, reagent, material, or system designed for use in the laboratory diagnosis of disease or health status. The term also refers to a general category of entities that are highly and specifically regulated by the U.S. Food and Drug Administration and other regulatory bodies.

Diagnostic and Statistical Manual of Mental Disorders (Fourth Edition) ABBR: DSM-IV. The standard nomenclature of emotional illness used by all health care practitioners. DSM-IV, published by the American Psychiatric Association, was introduced in 1994.

diagnostician (dī″ăg-nŏs-tĭsh′ŭn) [Gr. *diagignoskein,* to discern] One skilled in diagnosis.

diakinesis (dī″ă-kĭ-nē′sĭs) [Gr. *dia,* through, + *kinesis,* motion] In cell division, the final stage in the prophase of meiosis. During this stage of cell division, the homologous chromosomes shorten and thicken.

dial (dī′ăl) [L. *dialis,* daily, fr. *dies,* day] A graduated circular face, similar to a clock face, on which some measurement is indicated by a pointer that moves as the entity being measured (pressure, temperature, or heat) changes.

astigmatic d. A circular dial with black lines of uniform width drawn as if they were connecting opposing numbers on the face of a clock. It is used in testing for astigmatism.

dialy- [Gr. *dia,* through, + *lysis,* dissolution] Prefix denoting *separation.*

dialysance (dī″ă-lī′săns) In renal dialysis, the minute rate of net exchange of a substance between blood and dialysis fluid per unit of blood-bath concentration gradient.

dialysate (dī-ăl′ĭ-sāt) **1.** A liquid that has been dialyzed. **2.** In renal failure, the fluid used to remove or deliver compounds or electrolytes that the failing kidney cannot excrete or retain in the proper concentrations.

dialysis (dī-ăl′ĭ-sĭs) [Gr. *dia,* through, + *lysis,* dissolution] **1.** The passage of a solute through a membrane. **2.** The process of diffusing blood across a semipermeable membrane to remove toxic materials and to maintain fluid, electrolyte, and acid-base balance in cases of impaired kidney function or absence of the kidneys. SEE: *hemodialysis; Nursing Diagnoses Appendix.*

chronic ambulatory peritoneal d. Continuous ambulatory peritoneal d.

continuous ambulatory peritoneal d. ABBR: CAPD. Dialysis in which fluid is infused into the peritoneum through an implanted catheter and then drained from the body after absorbing metabolic toxins. The peritoneal lining serves as the dialytic membrane. CAPD is an alternative to hemodialysis for patients with end-stage renal disease. It removes fluids, electrolytes, and nitrogen-containing wastes from the body by osmosis, but does so somewhat less efficiently than hemodialysis. Scrupulous antiseptic technique is needed to avoid introducing infectious microorganisms into the dialysate and peritoneum. Nonetheless, the technique has several benefits. It can be performed at home by patients (increasing their autonomy); it avoids the hypotension sometimes associated with hemodialysis; and it is better tolerated than hemodialysis, because it is less likely to produce rapid shifts in the concentration of urea, electrolytes, and other solutes in the bloodstream. SYN: *chronic ambulatory peritoneal d.* SEE: *peritoneal dialysis.*

continuous cyclic peritoneal d. ABBR: CCPD. Dialysis performed every night with fluid remaining in the peritoneal cavity until the next night.

intermittent peritoneal d. ABBR: IPD. Dialysis using automated equipment, often performed overnight. The fluid is drained from the peritoneal cavity at the end of the treatment.

peritoneal d. Dialysis in which the lining of the peritoneal cavity is used as the dialyzing membrane. Dialyzing fluid introduced into the peritoneal cavity is left there for 1 or 2 hr and is then removed.

This technique is used to remove toxic substances from the body by perfusing specific warm sterile chemical solutions through the peritoneal cavity. It is used in treating renal failure and in certain types of poisoning. Some of the drugs and chemicals that may be so removed are salicylates, barbiturates, meprobamate, amphetamines, bromide, methanol, boric acid, sulfonamide, and various antibiotics.

This technique, using chilled, sterile isotonic saline, has been used in treating heatstroke. SEE: *Nursing Diagnoses Appendix.*

CAUTION: Although peritoneal dialysis may be performed at home, regular follow-up with health care professionals is needed to optimize its safety and effectiveness.

PATIENT CARE: Strict aseptic technique is maintained throughout the procedure. The patient is observed for signs of peritonitis, pain, respiratory difficulty, and low blood pressure. Many persons can ably perform the procedure using equipment designed for home use. The patient's understanding of the procedure and its rationale, care of the peritoneal catheter, and symptoms of infection is verified. Medication schedule can be changed before and after dialysis. The patient's ability to adjust his or her lifestyle to provide a balance of adequate rest and activity is evaluated.

renal d. Hemodialysis.

dialysis acidosis Metabolic acidosis due to prolonged hemodialysis in which the pH of the dialysis bath has been inadvertently reduced by the action of contaminating bacteria.

dialysis disequilibrium A disturbance in which nausea, vomiting, drowsiness, headache, and seizures occur shortly after the patient begins hemodialysis or peritoneal dialysis. The cause is related to the rapid correction of metabolic abnormalities in the uremic patient. SYN: *disequilibrium syndrome.*

dialyze (dī′ă-līz) To perform a dialysis or to undergo one.

dialytic Belonging to or resembling the process of dialysis.

dialyzable (dī-ă-līz′ă-b′l) Capable of receiving dialysis.

dialyzer (dī′ă-līz″ĕr) [Gr. *dia,* through, + *lysis,* dissolution] The apparatus used in performing dialysis.

diameter (dī-ăm′ĕ-tĕr) [″ + *metron,* a measure] The distance from any point on the periphery of a surface, body, or space to the opposite point.

anteroposterior d. of pelvic cavity The distance between the middle of the symphysis pubis and the upper border of the third sacral vertebra (about 13.5 cm in women).

anteroposterior d. of pelvic inlet

The distance from the posterior surface of the symphysis pubis to the promontory of the sacrum (about 11 cm in women). SYN: *conjugata vera; true conjugate d. of pelvic inlet.*

anteroposterior d. of pelvic outlet The distance between the tip of the coccyx and the lower edge of the symphysis pubis.

bigonial d. The distance between the two gonia. The gonion is the anthropometric point at the most inferior, posterior, and lateral points on the angle of the mandible.

biparietal d. The transverse distance between the parietal eminences on each side of the head (about 9.25 cm).

bitemporal d. The distance between the temporal bones (about 8 cm).

bitrochanteric d. The distance between the highest points of the greater trochanters.

bizygomatic d. The greatest transverse distance between the most prominent points of the zygomatic arches.

buccolingual d. The measurement of a tooth from the buccal to the lingual surface.

cervicobregmatic d. The distance between the anterior fontanel and the junction of the neck with the floor of the mouth.

diagonal conjugate d. of pelvis The distance from the upper part of the symphysis pubis to the most distant part of the brim of the pelvis.

external conjugate d. The anteroposterior diameter of the pelvic inlet measured externally; the distance from the skin over the upper part of the symphysis pubis to the skin over a point corresponding to the sacral promontory. SYN: *Baudelocque's diameter.*

frontomental d. The distance from the top of the forehead to the point of the chin.

interspinous d. The distance between the two anterior superior spines of the ilia.

intertuberous d. The distance between the ischial tuberosities. Most commonly, this measure of the female pelvic outlet is greater than 9 cm, allowing the exit of an average-sized term fetus.

labiolingual d. The measurement of an anterior tooth from the labial to the lingual surface.

mentobregmatic d. The distance from the chin to the middle of the anterior fontanel.

mesiodistal d. The measurement of a tooth from the ventral or mesial surface to the distal or dorsal surface.

obstetrical d. of pelvic inlet The shortest distance between the sacrum and the symphysis pubis. This diameter is shorter than the true conjugate. SYN: *obstetrical conjugate.*

occipitofrontal d. The distance from the posterior fontanel to the root of the nose.

occipitomental d. The greatest distance between the most prominent portion of the occiput and the point of the chin (about 13.5 cm).

d. of pelvis Any diameter of the pelvis found by measuring a straight line between any two points. *Anteroposterior:* the distance between the sacrovertebral angle and the symphysis pubis. *Bi-ischial:* the distance between the ischial spines. *Conjugata diagonalis:* the distance between the sacrovertebral angle and the symphysis pubis. *Conjugata vera:* the true conjugate between the sacrovertebral angle and the middle of the posterior aspect of the symphysis pubis (about 1.5 cm less than the diagonal conjugate). *Intercristal:* the distance between the crests of the ilia. *Interspinous:* the distance between the spines of the ilium. *Intertrochanteric:* the distance between the greater trochanters when the hips are extended and the legs are held together. *Obstetrical conjugate:* the distance between the promontory of the sacrum and the upper edge of the symphysis pubis. SEE: *pelvis.*

true conjugate d. of pelvic inlet Anteroposterior d. of pelvic inlet.

diamid(e) (dī-ăm′ĭd, -īd) [L. *di,* two, + *amide*] A compound that contains two amine groups. The term is sometimes used incorrectly to indicate a diamine or hydrazine.

diamidine (dī-ăm′ĭ-dēn) Any chemical compound that contains two amidine, $C(NH)NH_2$, groups.

diamine (dī-ăm′ĭn, -ēn) A chemical compound with two amino, $—NH_2$, groups.

diaminuria (dī-ăm″ĭ-nū′rē-ă) Presence of diamines in the urine.

diapause (dī′ă-pawz) [Gr. *dia,* through, + *pausis,* pause] The state of metabolic inactivity that some plants, seeds, eggs, and insect forms assume to survive adverse conditions such as winter.

diapedesis (dī″ă-pĕd-ē′sĭs) [″ + *pedan,* to leap] The movement of white blood cells and other cells out of small arterioles, venules, and capillaries as part of the inflammatory response. The cells move through gaps between cells in the vessel walls. SEE: *inflammation.*

diaphane (dī′ă-fān) [Gr. *dia,* through, + *phainein,* to appear] A very small electric light used in transillumination.

diaphanography Transillumination of the breast.

diaphanometer (dī″ă-făn-ŏm′ĕ-tĕr) [″ + ″ + *metron,* measure] A device for estimating the amount of solids in a fluid by its transparency.

diaphanometry (dī″ă-făn-ŏm′ĕ-trē) Determination of the translucency of a fluid (e.g., urine).

diaphanoscope (dī-ă-făn′ō-skōp) [″ +

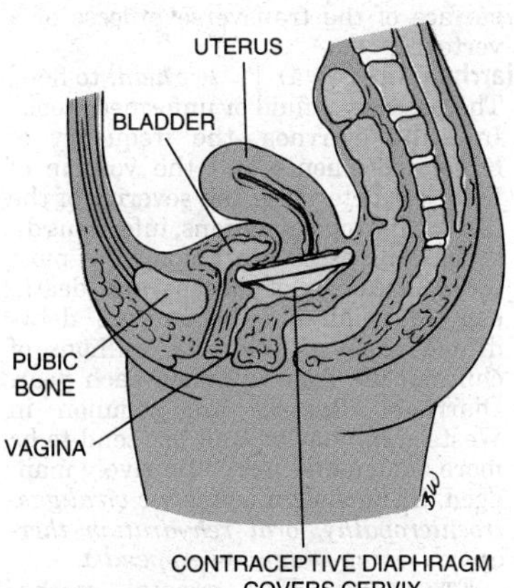

CONTRACEPTIVE DIAPHRAGM

phainein, to appear, + *skopein,* to examine] A device for transillumination of body cavities.

diaphanoscopy (dī″ă-făn-ŏs′kō-pē) Examination using the diaphanoscope; transillumination.

diaphemetric (dī″ă-fē-mĕt′rĭk) [″ + *haphe,* touch, + *metron,* measure] Pert. to the degree of tactile sensibility.

diaphorase (dī-ăf′ō-rās) The flavoprotein catalyst of the reoxidation of nicotinamide-adenine dinucleotide (NAD) or nicotinamide-adenine dinucleotide phosphate (NADP) by the mitochondrial electron transport chain.

diaphoresis (dī″ă-fō-rē′sĭs) [″ + *pherein,* to carry] Profuse sweating.

diaphoretic (dī″ă-fō-rĕt′ĭk) [″ + *pherein,* to carry] **1.** A sudorific, or an agent that increases perspiration. **2.** Covered by sweat.

diaphragm (dī′ă-frăm) [Gr. *diaphragma,* a partition] **1.** A thin membrane such as one used for dialysis. **2.** In microscopy, an apparatus located beneath the opening in the stage and permitting regulation of the amount of light passing through the object. **3.** A rubber or plastic cup that fits over the cervix uteri, used for contraceptive purposes. SEE: illus (Contraceptive Diaphragm). **4.** The dome-shaped skeletal muscle that separates the abdomen from the thoracic cavity with its convexity upward. It contracts with each inspiration, flattening downward, permitting the bases of the lungs to descend. It relaxes with each expiration, and then returns to its resting dome-shaped position because of the elastic recoil of the lung. The deeper the inspiration, the lower the diaphragm descends; the greater the expiration, the higher it rises.

Its origin is at a level with the sixth ribs or intercostal spaces anteriorly and the 11th or 12th ribs posteriorly. The right half rests higher than the left. The lower surface is in relation to the suprarenal bodies of the kidney, the liver, the spleen, and the cardiac end of the stomach. It aids in defecation and parturition by its ability to increase intra-abdominal pressure while the person attempts to exhale with the glottis closed. It becomes spasmodic during hiccups and sneezing. SEE: illus. (Movement of Rib Cage and Diaphragm During Respiration); *Boerhaave syndrome.*

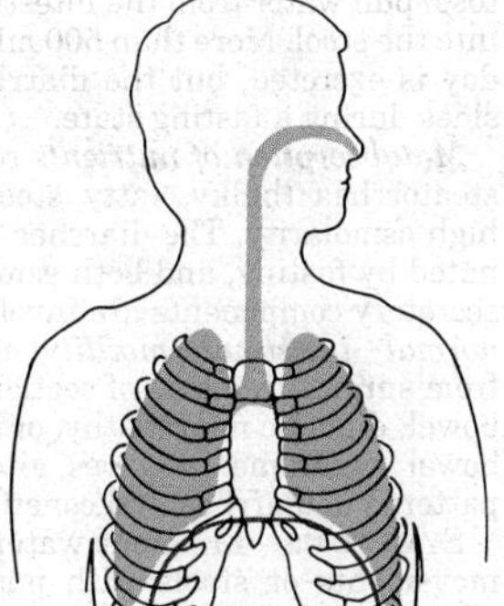

INHALATION
THE DIAPHRAGM HAS CONTRACTED
AND DESCENDED AND THE RIB CAGE
HAS BEEN PULLED UP AND OUT TO
EXPAND THE LUNGS

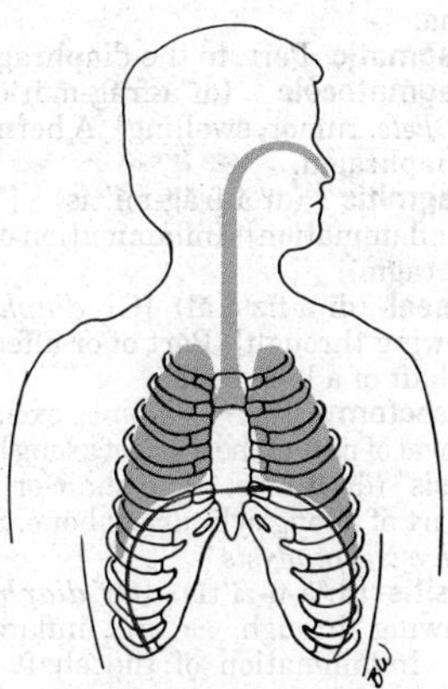

MOVEMENT OF RIB CAGE AND DIAPHRAGM DURING RESPIRATION

Bucky d. A grid suspended immediately beneath the radiography table and above the film tray, constructed to increase image contrast by eliminating the effects of backscatter and secondary radiation when radiographs of dense structures are taken. It is also called the Potter-Bucky diaphragm.

hernia of d. A congenital or traumatic protrusion of abdominal contents through the diaphragm.

pelvic d. The musculofascial layer forming the lower boundary of the abdominopelvic cavity. It is funnel shaped and is pierced in the midline by the urethra, vagina, and rectum. It consists of a muscular layer made up of the paired levator ani and coccygeus muscles. The fascial layer consists of two portions, the parietal and visceral layers. The parietal layer comprises the peritoneum continuous with the connective tissue sheaths of the psoas and iliac muscles. The visceral layer is split from the parietal layer at the white line passing downward and inward to form the upper sheath of the levator ani muscles; the anterior part of this layer unites the bladder with the posterior wall of the pubes. The middle portion splits into three parts: the vesical layer, investing the bladder and urethra; the rectovaginal layer, forming the rectovaginal septum; and the rectal layer, investing the rectum. The posterior part is the base of the broad ligament, where it sheaths the uterine arteries and supports the cervix.

urogenital d. The urogenital trigone, or triangular ligament. A musculofascial sheath that lies between the ischiopubic rami, it is superficial to the pelvic diaphragm. In males it surrounds the membranous urethra; in females, the vagina.

diaphragmatic Pert. to the diaphragm.

diaphragmatocele (dī″ă-frăg-măt′ō-sēl) [″ + *kele,* tumor, swelling] A hernia of the diaphragm.

diaphragmitis (dī″ă-frăg-mī′tĭs) [″ + *itis,* inflammation] Inflammation of the diaphragm.

diaphyseal (dī″ă-fĭz′ē-ăl) [Gr. *diaphysis,* a growing through] Part of or affecting the shaft of a long bone.

diaphysectomy [″ + *ektome,* excision] Removal of part of the shaft of a long bone.

diaphysis (dī-ăf′ĭ-sĭs) The shaft or middle part of a long cylindrical bone. SEE: *apophysis; epiphysis.*

diaphysitis (dī″ă-fĭ-zī′tĭs) [Gr. *diaphysis,* a growing through, + *itis,* inflammation] Inflammation of the shaft of a long bone.

diaplexus [Gr. *dia,* through, + L. *plexus,* braid] The choroid plexus of the third ventricle.

diapophysis (dī-ă-pŏf′ĭ-sĭs) [″ + *apophysis,* outgrowth] The upper articular surface of the transverse process of a vertebra.

diarrhea (dī-ă-rē′ă) [″ + *rhein,* to flow] The passage of fluid or unformed stools. In acute diarrhea, the frequency of bowel movements and the volume of fluid lost determine the severity of the illness. In tropical nations, infectious diarrheal illnesses are among the most common causes of disease and death, esp. in children, who become dehydrated easily. Worldwide, millions of children die from diarrhea each year. Diarrheal illnesses are common in Western nations as well but tend to be more benign and more effectively managed. SEE: *cholera; epidemic viral gastroenteropathy; oral rehydration therapy; Nursing Diagnoses Appendix.*

ETIOLOGY: Five general mechanisms may cause diarrhea. *Excessive secretion,* or secretory diarrhea, is usually caused by infectious organisms (e.g., rotavirus) or enterotoxins (e.g., *Escherichia coli, Campylobacter difficile*), which produce excessive secretion of electrolytes and water. More than 500 ml of stool/day is excreted even during fasting. In *inflammatory or exudative disorders,* infectious organisms (e.g., *Salmonella, Shigella*) damage the intestinal mucosa; the stools often contain blood or pus and can be of small volume (dysentery) or large. The diarrhea continues during fasting. Transmission of infectious organisms is most commonly person-to-person or through contaminated water or food. The incubation period and duration of illness vary, depending on the organism involved. The diarrhea may be bloody.

Osmotic diarrhea occurs when highly concentrated substances that cannot be absorbed (e.g., antacids, lactulose, lactose) pull water from the intestinal wall into the stool. More than 500 ml of stool/day is excreted, but the diarrhea subsides during a fasting state.

Malabsorption of nutrients results in steatorrhea (bulky, fatty stools) with high osmolarity. The diarrhea is eliminated by fasting, and both osmotic and secretory components are involved. *Abnormal intestinal motility* resulting from surgical removal of sections of the bowel, diabetic neuropathy, or irritable bowel syndrome produces alternating patterns of diarrhea and constipation.

SYMPTOMS: Frequent watery bowel movements or stools with pus, blood, oils, or mucus are characteristic of diarrhea, as are abdominal cramping, bloating, or rectal discomfort. When volume losses from diarrhea are large, symptoms of dehydration or electrolyte imbalance, such as dizziness, thirst, and prostration, are common.

TREATMENT: Fluid replacement is the key to successful management of acute diarrhea and the prevention of its complications. Oral rehydration solutions are inexpensive and effective tools for volume repletion. Intravenous fluids are more costly. Infectious causes of diarrhea are often managed with antibiotics (such as sulfa drugs or quinolones). Antidiarrheal agents include kaolin derivatives, loperamide, and paregorics. Alternative medicine practitioners advocate herbal remedies such as arrowroot. The management of chronic diarrhea depends on the underlying cause.

PATIENT CARE: The patient is assessed for signs and symptoms of dehydration and of metabolic disarray or renal failure, such as headache, lethargy, decreasing level of consciousness, and compensatory hyperventilation. The frequency, consistency, color, and volume of stools are monitored, and bowel sounds auscultated for changes from normal patterns. Fluid balance, intake and output, and daily weights are also monitored. Prescribed oral or intravenous fluid and electrolyte and nutrient replacements are administered, and the patient's response is evaluated. The anal area is assessed for skin excoriation and gently but thoroughly washed and rinsed after each bowel movement, and protective ointment is applied. Universal precautions are observed for these interventions. Antidiarrheal medications are administered as prescribed.

The spread of infectious diarrhea is prevented by practicing and teaching thorough handwashing and hygiene measures, by correctly handling and refrigerating foods at risk for bacterial contamination, and by reporting diarrheal pathogens to appropriate public health authorities.

acute d. Diarrhea marked by sudden onset.

antibiotic-associated d. Mild to moderate diarrhea in individuals taking oral antibiotics. The antibiotics destroy the normal flora in the gastrointestinal tract. SEE: *pseudomembranous colitis.*

dysenteric d. Dysentery.

emotional d. Diarrhea caused by emotional stress.

epidemic d. in the newborn Contagious diarrhea in a newborn caused by pathogenic strains of *Escherichia coli,* occurring in epidemics in hospitals.

factitious d. Self-induced diarrhea. This can be accomplished, for example, by self-medication with laxatives. SEE: *Munchausen syndrome.*

fatty d. Steatorrhea.

infantile d. Diarrhea in children under 2 years of age. Most commonly, it is caused by infectious enterocolitis due to rotavirus, Norwalk virus, and *Escherichia coli.* SEE: *enterocolitis.*

SYMPTOMS: Frequent watery stools, occasionally accompanied by evidence of dehydration, are the primary findings.

TREATMENT: Each year the deaths of thousands of children with diarrhea are prevented by the use of oral rehydration solutions consisting of clean (i.e., potable) water, salt, potassium, bicarbonate, and glucose. SEE: *oral rehydration solution.*

lienteric d. Watery stools with undigested food particles.

membranous d. Diarrhea with pieces of intestinal mucosa.

mucous d. Diarrhea with mucus.

osmotic d. Diarrhea caused by the retention of osmotically active solutes in the small intestine. This causes fluid to be drawn into the intestinal lumen. The retained fluid is more than the colon can resorb. The solute may be the result of maldigestion, malabsorbed nutrient, or drugs.

purulent d. Diarrhea with pus, a result of intestinal ulceration.

secretory d. Diarrhea in which there is a large volume of fecal output caused by abnormalities of the movement of fluid and electrolytes into the intestinal lumen. This can be caused by hormonal abnormalities present in disorders such as carcinoid syndrome, Zollinger-Ellison syndrome, certain types of pancreatic adenomas, and medullary carcinomas of the thyroid.

simple d. Diarrhea in which stools contain only normal excreta.

summer d. Diarrhea occurring in children during months when rotavirus is not prevalent. *Shigella, Campylobacter jejuni,* and cryptosporidia are among the most common causes.

travelers' d. ABBR: TD. Diarrhea experienced by travelers, esp. those who go to tropical countries. The most common causes are enterotoxigenic *Escherichia coli,* amebas, *Giardia, Cyclospora, Cryptosporidium, Shigella, Salmonella,* and *Campylobacter*. The disease is common, affecting as many as 40% of travelers to underdeveloped nations. There is no completely effective method of prevention, but avoidance of tap water, fresh fruits and vegetables, iced drinks, or inadequately cooked foods is helpful. Fish and shellfish may contain biotoxins even when well cooked; local residents can provide valuable advice concerning which fish to avoid. Loperamide with a quinolone antibiotic (e.g., ciprofloxacin) used after the passage of the first loose stool frequently aborts the illness, but children and pregnant women should not take quinolones. As with other forms of diarrhea, rehydration is crucial. Antidiarrheals are used for comfort.

diarthric (dī-ăr′thrĭk) [Gr. *dis,* two, + *arthron,* joint] Pert. to two or more joints.

diarthrosis [Gr., a movable articulation] An articulation in which opposing bones move freely (e.g., a hinge joint or a pivot joint).

diarticular [Gr. *dis,* two, + L. *articulus,* joint] Pert. to two joints; specifically, the temporomandibular joints, where the mandible articulates in two places with the skull.

diaschisis (dī-ăs-kī′sĭs) In a person with a focal brain injury, a reduction in synaptic activity (and often, cerebral blood flow and metabolism) in a part of the brain that is remote from the injury. Brain functions that are lost as a result of diaschisis often are restored with rehabilitation or the return of blood flow.

diascope (dī′ă-skōp) [Gr. *dia,* through, + *skopein,* to examine] A glass plate held against the skin for examining superficial lesions. Erythematous lesions will show the compressed capillary bed, but a hemorrhagic area will not blanch when the glass is pressed against the skin.

diascopy (dī-ă′skō-pē) Examination of skin lesions by means of a diascope. SEE: illus.

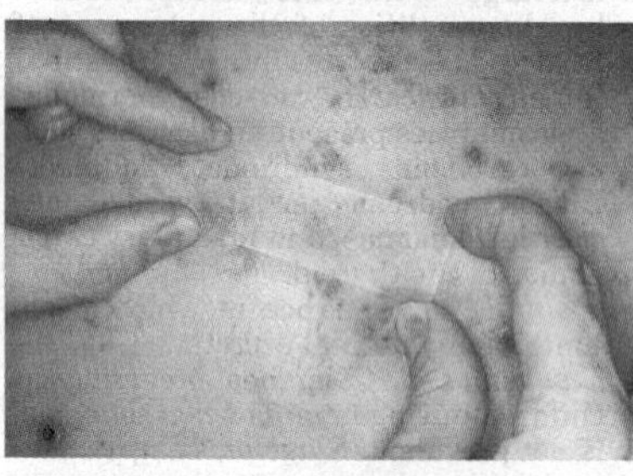

DIASCOPY

diastalsis (dī-ă-stăl′sĭs) [″ + *stalsis,* contraction] A wave of inhibition before a forward contraction in the intestine. The process is similar to peristalsis.

diastaltic **1.** Pert. to diastalsis. **2.** Denoting reflex action.

diastase (dī′ăs-tās) [Gr. *diastasis,* a separation] A specific enzyme in plant cells, such as sprouting grains and malt, that converts starch into sugar.

diastasis (dī-ăs′tă-sĭs) [Gr.] **1.** In surgery, injury to a bone involving separation of an epiphysis. **2.** In cardiac physiology, the last part of diastole. It follows the period of most rapid diastolic filling of the ventricles, consists of a period of retarded inflow of blood from atria into ventricles, lasts (in humans under average conditions) about 0.2 sec, and is immediately followed by atrial systole.

d. recti A separation of the two halves of the rectus abdominis muscles in the midline at the linea alba. This condition is benign when it occurs in pregnant women.

diastema (dī″ă-stē′mă) *pl.* **diastemata** [Gr. *diastema,* an interval or space] **1.** A fissure. **2.** A space between two adjacent teeth.

diastematocrania (dī″ă-stĕm″ă-tō-krā′nē-ă) [″ + *kranion,* cranium] A congenital sagittal fissure of the skull.

diastematomyelia (dī″ă-stĕm″ă-tō-mī-ē′lē-ă) [″ + *myelos,* marrow] A congenital fissure of the spinal cord, frequently associated with spina bifida cystica.

diastematopyelia (dī″ă-stĕm″ă-tō-pī-ē′lē-ă) [″ + *pyelos,* pelvis] A congenital median slit of the pelvis.

diaster [Gr. *dis,* two, + *aster,* star] A double star figure formed during mitosis. SYN: *amphiaster.*

diastole (dī-ăs′tō-lē) [Gr. *diastellein,* to expand] **1.** The normal period in the heart cycle during which the muscle fibers lengthen, the heart dilates, and the cavities fill with blood; diastole of the atria occurs before that of the ventricles. **2.** The period of cardiac muscle relaxation alternating with systole or contraction. SEE: *blood pressure; heart; murmur; pulse; systole.*

diastolic (dī-ăs-tŏl′ĭk) Pert. to diastole.

diataxia [Gr. *dis,* two, + *ataxia,* lack of order] Bilateral ataxia.

diatela, diatele (dī-ă-tē′lă, -tēl′) [Gr. *dia,* between, + L. *tela,* web] The membranous roof of the third ventricle.

diaterma [″ + *terma,* end] A portion of the floor of the third ventricle.

diathermal (dī″ă-thĕr′măl) [Gr. *dia,* through, + *therme,* heat] Able to absorb heat rays.

diathermic Of the nature of diathermy or of its results.

diathermy (dī′ă-thĕr″mē) [Gr. *dia,* through, + *therme,* heat] The therapeutic use of a high-frequency current to generate heat within some part of the body. The frequency is greater than the maximum frequency for neuromuscular response and ranges from several hundred thousand to millions of cycles per second. It is used to increase blood flow to specific areas. It should not be used in the acute stage of recovery from trauma.

medical d. The generation of heat within the body by the application of high-frequency oscillatory current for warming, but not damaging, tissues.

short-wave d. Diathermy using wavelengths of 3 to 30 m.

surgical d. Diathermy of high frequency for electrocoagulation or cauterization.

diathesis (dī-ăth′ĕ-sĭs) [Gr. *diatithenai,* to dispose] A constitutional predisposition to certain diseases or conditions.

diathetic Pert. to diathesis.

diatom (dī′ă-tŏm) [Gr. *diatemnein,* to cut through] One of a group of unicellular, microscopic algae, numerous in freshwater and saltwater. Its cell walls are made of silica.

diatomic **1.** Containing two atoms; said of molecules. **2.** Bivalent.

diatrizoate meglumine (dī″ă-trī-zō′āt) A

high-osmolarity, water-soluble ionic contrast medium with the cation consisting of meglumine during ionic dissociation. It is used intra-arterially to visualize the arteries and veins of the heart and brain, great vessels such as the aorta, and the kidneys and bladder.

diatrizoate sodium A high-osmolarity, water-soluble contrast medium with the cation consisting of sodium during ionic dissociation. It is used to visualize various hollow body organs such as the kidney, bladder, uterus, and fallopian tubes.

diaxon, diaxone [Gr. *dis,* two, + *axon,* axis] A neuron having two axons.

diazepam (dī-ăz′ĕ-păm) An antianxiety and sedative drug used extensively in the U.S. It is used to treat status epilepticus, acute cocaine poisoning, and a variety of anxiety disorders. Prolonged use may cause dependence or tolerance.

diazo- A prefix used in chemistry to indicate that a compound contains the —N=N— group.

diazo reaction A deep red color in urine, produced by the action of *p*-diazobenzene-sulfonic acid and ammonia on aromatic substances found in the urine in certain conditions.

diazotize (dī-ăz′ō-tīz) In chemistry, to convert NH_2 groups into diazo, —N=N—, groups.

diazoxide (dī-ăz-ŏk′sīd) A drug used to lower blood pressure in acute hypertension emergencies, and to treat hypoglycemia due to hyperinsulinism.

dibasic (dī-bā′sĭk) [″ + *basis,* base] Capable of neutralizing or accepting two hydrogen ions.

diblastula (dī-blăs′tū-lă) [″ + *blastos,* sprout] A blastula containing the ectoderm and endoderm.

Dibothriocephalus (dī-bŏth″rē-ō-sĕf′ăl-ŭs) Former name for the genus *Diphyllobothrium.*

dibucaine hydrochloride A local anesthetic similar to cocaine in action when applied topically and similar to procaine and cocaine when injected.

DIC *disseminated intravascular coagulation.*

dicalcic, dicalcium (dī-kăl′sĭk) [″ + L. *calx,* lime] Containing two atoms of calcium.

dicalcium phosphate (dī-kăl′sē-ŭm fŏs′fāt) Dibasic calcium phosphate. It is used as a source of calcium to supplement the diet.

dicentric (dī-sĕn′trĭk) Having two centers or two centromeres.

dicephalus (dī-sĕf′ă-lŭs) [″ + *kephale,* head] A congenitally deformed fetus with two heads.

2,4-dichlorophenoxyacetic acid ABBR: 2,4-D. A toxic substance previously used as a weed killer. SEE: *Poisons and Poisoning Appendix.*

dichlorphenamide (dī″klor-fĕn′ă-mīd) A carbonic anhydrase inhibitor used in treating glaucoma.

dichorionic (dī″kō-rē-ŏn′ĭk) Having two chorions. This may occur in two-egg (dizygotic) twins.

dichotomy, dichotomization (dī-kŏt′ō-mē, dī-kŏt″ō-mī-zā′shŭn) [Gr. *dicha,* twofold, + *tome,* incision] **1.** Bifurcation of a vein. **2.** Cutting or dividing into two parts.

dichroic (dī-krō′ĭk) Pert. to dichroism.

dichroic mirror An optical device used in some spectrophotometers to split a beam of light into reference and sample beams.

dichroism (dī′krō-ĭzm) [Gr. *dis,* two, + *chroa,* color] The property of appearing to be one color by direct light and another by transmitted light.

dichromate (dī-krō′māt) A chemical that contains the Cr_2O_7 group.

dichromatic Able to see only two colors.

dichromatism (dī-krō′mă-tĭzm) The ability to distinguish only two primary colors. SYN: *dichromatopsia.*

dichromatopsia (dī″krō-mă-tŏp′sē-ă) [″ + *chroma,* color, + *opsis,* sight] Dichromatism.

dichromic **1.** Containing two atoms of chromium. **2.** Seeing only two colors.

dichromophil [″ + *chroma,* color, + *philein,* to love] Double staining with both acid and basic dyes.

dichromophilism (dī″krō-mŏf′ĭl-ĭzm) [″ + ″ + ″ + *-ismos,* condition] The capacity for double staining.

Dick method [George F. Dick, 1881–1967, and Gladys H. Dick, 1881–1963, U.S. bacteriologists] A toxin-antitoxin injection formerly used to prevent scarlet fever.

Dick test A test formerly used to assess susceptibility to scarlet fever, in which the erythrogenic toxin from Streptococcus was injected subcutaneously, and the injection site was checked for inflammatory changes in 12 to 24 hr. SEE: *Schick test.*

dicloxacillin sodium (dī-klŏks″ă-sĭl′ĭn) A semisynthetic penicillin useful in treating penicillinase-resistant staphylococci.

dicoelous (dī-sē′lŭs) [″ + *koilos,* hollow] **1.** Concave or hollowed out on two sides. **2.** Containing two cavities.

dicophane (dī′kō-fān) A powerful insecticide now rarely used because of its toxicity. SYN: *chlorophenothane; DDT.*

dicoria (dī-kō′rē-ă) [″ + *kore,* pupil] A double pupil in each eye.

dicoumarol (dī-koo′mă-rŏl) Dicumarol.

dicrotic (dī-krŏt′ĭk) [Gr. *dikrotos,* beating double] Having one heartbeat for two arterial pulsations; relating to a double pulse.

dicrotic notch In a pulse tracing, a notch on the descending limb.

dicrotic wave A positive wave following the dicrotic notch.

dicrotism (dī′krŏt-ĭzm) [″ + *-ismos,* condition] The state of being dicrotic.

dictyoma, diktyoma (dĭk″tē-ō′mă) [Gr.

diktyon, net, + *oma,* tumor] A tumor of the ciliary epithelium.

dictyosome (dĭk′tē-ō-sōm) [″ + *soma,* body] A cytoplasmic body similar to the Golgi apparatus. It is thought to be a dispersed piece of the Golgi apparatus.

dicumarol (dī-koo′mă-rŏl) An anticoagulant drug. SEE: *warfarin sodium.*

dicyclic (dī-sī′klĭk) **1.** Having or concerning two cycles. **2.** In chemistry, containing two cyclic ring structures.

dicyclomine hydrochloride (dī-sī′klō-mēn) An anticholinergic drug used as an antispasmodic.

didactic (dī-dăk′tĭk) [Gr. *didaktikos*] Concerning instruction by lectures and use of texts as opposed to clinical or bedside teaching.

didactylism (dī-dăk′tĭ-lĭzm) [Gr. *dis,* two, + *daktylos,* finger] The congenital condition of having only two digits on a hand or foot.

didanosine ABBR: ddI. A reverse transcriptase inhibitor drug used, usually in combination with other agents, to treat infections with the human immunodeficiency virus. Trade name is Videx.

didelphic (dī-dĕl′fĭk) [″ + *delphys,* uterus] Having or pert. to a double uterus.

didymalgia, didymodynia (dĭd-ĭ-măl′jē-ă, dĭd″ĭ-mō-dĭn′ē-ă) [Gr. *didymos,* twin, + *algos,* pain] Pain in a testicle.

didymitis (dĭd-ĭ-mī′tĭs) [″ + *itis,* inflammation] Inflammation of a testicle. SYN: *orchitis.*

didymus (dĭd′ĭ-mŭs) [Gr. *didymos,* twin] **1.** Twin. **2.** A congenital abnormality involving joined twins. **3.** Testis.

die **1.** To cease living. **2.** In dentistry, a positive duplicate made from an impression of a tooth.

dieldrin (dī-ĕl′drĭn) A chlorinated hydrocarbon used as an insecticide. It is toxic to humans and marine and terrestrial animals. SEE: *Poisons and Poisoning Appendix.*

dielectric [Gr. *dia,* through, + *elektron,* amber] Insulating by offering great resistance to the passage of electricity by conduction.

diencephalon (dī″ĕn-sĕf′ă-lŏn) [Gr. *dis,* two, + *enkephalos,* brain] The second portion of the brain, or that lying between the telencephalon and mesencephalon. It includes the epithalamus, thalamus, metathalamus, and hypothalamus. SYN: *interbrain; thalamencephalon.*

dienestrol (dī″ēn-ĕs′trŏl) A nonsteroid, synthetic estrogen used for estrogen therapy.

Dientamoeba (dī″ĕn-tă-mē′bă) A genus of parasitic protozoa marked by possession of two similar nuclei.

D. fragilis A species of parasitic ameba inhabiting the intestine of humans. Persons infected may have diarrhea with blood or mucus, abdominal pain, and anal pruritus. This organism has been found inside the eggs of pinworms, and the eggs are thought to serve as the vector.

dieresis (dī-ĕr′ĕ-sĭs) [Gr. *diairesis,* a division] **1.** Breaking up or dispersion of things normally joined, as by an ulcer. **2.** Mechanical separation of parts by surgical means.

dieretic Pert. to dieresis; dissolvable or separable.

diet [Gr. *diaita,* way of living] **1.** Liquid and solid food substances regularly consumed in the course of normal living. **2.** A prescribed allowance of food adapted for a particular state of health or disease, as a diet prescribed for use by a diabetic. SEE: table. **3.** To eat or drink sparingly in accordance with prescribed rules. SEE: *energy expenditure, basal.*

acid-ash d. A diet designed to acidify the urine. It contains acidic foods such as meat, fish, eggs, and cereals and is lacking in fruits, vegetables, cheese, and milk.

alkali-ash d. A diet designed to produce an alkaline urine. It contains foods such as fruits, vegetables, and milk and is lacking in meat, fish, eggs, and cereals.

American Heart Association d., Step I A meal plan in which no more than 30% of consumed calories come from fats (10% as saturated fat), and in which cholesterol intake is less than 300 mg/day.

American Heart Association d., Step II A meal plan in which less than 30% of total calories are consumed as fat, (7% as saturated fat) and cholesterol intake is limited to less than 200 mg/day. This diet is recommended esp. for patients with abnormal serum lipid levels who have known coronary artery disease.

balanced d. A diet adequate in energy-providing substances (carbohydrates and fats), tissue-building compounds (proteins), inorganic chemicals (water and mineral salts), agents that regulate or catalyze metabolic processes (vitamins), and substances for certain physiological processes, such as bulk for promoting peristaltic movements of the digestive tract.

DASH d. *Dietary Approaches to Stop Hypertension diet.*

Dietary Approaches to Stop Hypertension d. ABBR: DASH diet. A specific diet proven to treat stage I hypertension, consisting of generous amounts of cereals, fruits, and vegetables (for fiber, vitamins, and minerals), and low-fat dairy products and lean meats (to maximize protein intake without too much saturated fat and cholesterol). Guidelines for a diet of 2000 calories daily include seven to eight servings of grains and grain products; four to five servings of vegetables; four to five servings of fruits; two to three servings of

The DASH Diet

Food Group	Daily Servings	Serving Sizes	Examples and Notes	Significance of Each Food Group to the DASH Diet Pattern
Grains and grain products	7–8	1 slice bread; 1/2 C dry cereal; 1/2 C cooked rice, pasta, or cereal	whole wheat bread, English muffin, pita bread, bagel, cereals, grits, oatmeal	major sources of energy and fiber
Vegetables	4–5	1 C raw leafy vegetable, 1/2 C cooked vegetable; 6 oz vegetable juice	tomatoes, potatoes, carrots, peas, squash, broccoli, turnip greens, collards, kale, spinach, artichokes, sweet potatoes, beans	rich sources of potassium, magnesium, and fiber
Fruits	4–5	6 oz fruit juice; 1 medium fruit; 1/4 C dried fruit; 1/2 C fresh, frozen, or canned fruit	apricots, bananas, dates, oranges, orange juice, grapefruit, grapefruit juice, mangoes, melons, peaches, pineapples, prunes, raisins, strawberries, tangerines	important sources of potassium, magnesium, and fiber
Low fat or nonfat dairy foods	2–3	8 oz milk, 1 C yogurt, 1.5 oz cheese	skim or 1% milk, skim or low fat buttermilk, nonfat or lowfat yogurt, part skim mozzarella cheese, nonfat cheese	major sources of calcium and protein
Meats, poultry, and fish	2 or less	3 oz cooked meats, poultry, or fish	select only lean; trim away visible fats; broil, roast, or boil, instead of frying; remove skin from poultry	rich sources of protein and magnesium
Nuts, seeds, and legumes	4–5 per week	1.5 oz or 1/3 C nuts, 1/2 oz or 2 Tbsp seeds, 1/2 C cooked legumes	almonds, filberts, mixed nuts, peanuts, walnuts, sunflower seeds, kidney beans, lentils	rich sources of energy, magnesium, potassium, protein, and fiber

SOURCE: National Institutes of Health. September 1998. Facts about the DASH diet. Available from World Wide Web: ⟨http://www.nih.gov/health/public/heart/hbp/dash/dashdiet.pdf⟩.

low-fat or nonfat dairy products; two or fewer servings of lean meats, proteins, and fish. The plan also permits four to five weekly servings of nuts, seeds, and legumes per week. It is recommended that sodium intake be less than 3 g/day. Compared with the diet recommended in the Food Guide Pyramid, this diet contains more fruits and vegetables but less fat. SEE: table.

elimination d. A method for assessing allergic responses to foods. To this, foods that are suspected of causing problems are added one at a time to determine whether any of them cause an adverse reaction.

gluten-free d. Elimination of gluten from the diet by avoiding all products containing wheat, buckwheat, rye, oats, or barley. Because gluten is present in many foods containing thickened sauces, the diet must be discussed with a dietitian. It is the basis of management for celiac disease. SEE: *celiac sprue; sprue.*

high-calorie d. A diet that contains more calories than normally required for an individual's metabolic and energy needs and therefore places the individual in positive energy balance. The diet should include three meals plus between-meal feedings, avoiding fermentable and bulky foods. A high-calorie diet may be used to prevent weight loss in wasting diseases, in high basal metabolism, and after a long illness; in deficiency caused by anorexia, poverty, and poor dietary habits; and during lactation (when an extra 1000 and 1200 kcal each day are indicated).

high-carbohydrate d. A meal plan in which more than 45% of total calories are consumed as carbohydrates. Some endurance athletes (e.g., marathon runners) favor this type of eating.

high-cellulose d. High-residue d.

high-residue d. A diet that contains considerable amounts of substances such as fiber or cellulose, which the human body is unable to metabolize and absorb. This diet is particularly useful in treating constipation and may be beneficial also in preventing certain diseases of the gastrointestinal tract. Lay persons may refer to a high-residue diet as one containing a lot of roughage. SYN: *high-cellulose d.* SEE: *fiber.*

ketogenic d. A diet that produces acetone or ketone bodies, or mild acidosis. It can cause severe ion imbalance and can result in coma or death.

light d. A diet consisting of all foods allowed in a soft diet, plus whole-grain cereals, easily digested raw fruits, and vegetables. Foods are not pureed or ground. This diet is used as an intermediate regimen for patients who do not require a soft diet but are not yet able to resume a full diet.

liquid d. A diet for persons unable to tolerate solid food or for patients whose gastrointestinal tract must be free of solid matter. This type of diet may contain coffee with hot milk, tea, water, milk in all forms, milk and cream mixtures, cocoa, strained cream soups, fruit juices, meat juices, beef tea, clear broths, gruels, strained meat soups, and eggnogs.

liquid protein d. A severely calorically restricted diet, lacking carbohydrates, fats, and many minerals and vitamins. Its use has been associated on occasion with cardiac rhythm disturbances and sudden cardiac death.

low carbohydrate, hypocaloric d. A meal regimen that limits total calories, usually to about 1200 calories per day, and total carbohydrates to no more than about 25% of total calories. Although this form of dietary restriction does not create more weight loss than calorically restricted high-carbohydrate diets, it does reduce fasting levels of insulin and triglycerides, and may be preferable for inactive or obese patients with type 2 diabetes mellitus or impaired glucose tolerance.

low-protein d. A diet that contains a limited amount of protein. The principal sources of food energy are fats and carbohydrates. This diet is used to treat end-stage renal and hepatic disease.

low-salt d. A diet in which no salt is allowed on the patient's tray and no salty foods are served. This diet is used in treating hypertension and congestive heart failure.

macrobiotic d. A diet consisting of unprocessed foods, vegetables, beans, whole grains, and some fish and fruits.

Mediterranean d. A well-tolerated and palatable diet that mimics the traditional cuisine of Italy, Greece, and the islands of the Mediterranean Sea. It includes fish and other seafood, wine, and olive oil, and derives about 25% to 35% of its calories from fat, but the primary fat is olive oil, a monounsaturated fat.

minimum residue d. A diet used for short periods to ensure a minimum of solid material in the intestinal tract. Foods allowed include one glass of milk per day, clear fluids and juices, lean meat, noodles, and refined cereals.

National Cholesterol Education Program d. A two-step approach designed to lower blood cholesterol in adults, children, and adolescents. It is similar to the Step I and Step II diets designed by the American Heart Association.

National Renal d. A diet designed by the American Dietetic Association (ADA) and the National Kidney Foundation for the treatment of kidney disease. It consists of six food planning systems based on the ADA Exchange Lists. The presence of diabetes and the use of peritoneal dialysis and hemodialysis are considered.

Paleolithic d. A meal regimen that mimics the food choices of modern hunter-gatherer societies or primitive human cultures. It includes nuts, fruits, vegetables, wild game, and fish and typically derives about 21% of its calories from fat.

"Prudent d." A diet designed by the American Heart Association for protection against and treatment of cardiovascular disease. A multistep approach decreases fat, cholesterol, and protein.

purine-restricted d. A diet that limits purine and fats and encourages fluid intake; used to control the excessive levels of uric acid caused by gout.

reducing d. A diet designed to help people lose weight (i.e., a diet with a restricted number of calories and a carefully crafted balance of other nutrients.

Diseases in Which Diet Plays an Important Role

Condition	Consensus Recommendations
Celiac sprue	Avoid glutens
Cholelithiasis	Avoid fatty foods
Cirrhosis	Limit sodium; limit protein intake
Coronary artery disease	American Heart Association diets
Congestive heart failure	Limit sodium
Diabetes mellitus	American Diabetic Association Diet, calorie limited; exercise
Diverticulosis	Low-residue diet
Dysphagia	Special consistency diets as indicated by testing/tolerance
Esophagitis	Avoid alcohol, nonsteroidal drugs, tobacco; consume thick liquids
Gastroesophageal reflux	Avoid caffeine, chocolates, mints, or late meals
Gout	Limit alcohol and purine intake
Hyperhomocysteinemia	Increase consumption of folates, vitamin B_{12}
Hyperlipidemias	National Cholesterol Education Program Diet with limited fat and cholesterol, and increased fiber
Iron deficiency anemia	Iron supplements with vitamin C
Irritable bowel syndrome	Increase fiber content of meals, limit dairy products
Kidney stone formers	Liberal fluid intake
Nephrotic syndrome	Limit sodium intake
Obesity	Caloric restriction, accompanied by increased exercise
Osteoporosis	Supplement calcium and vitamin D; limit alcohol and tobacco
Pernicious anemia	Supplement cyanocobalamin (vitamin B_{12})
Renal failure	Limit sodium, potassium, protein, and fluids
Women and men, over 25 yr of age	Supplement calcium

soft d. A diet consisting of nothing but soft or semisolid foods or liquids, including fish, eggs, cheese, chicken, cereals, bread, toast, and butter. Excluded are red meats, vegetables or fruits having seeds or thick skins, cellulose, raw fruits, and salads. SYN: *convalescent diet*.

very low calorie d. A commercially available diet in which caloric intake may be from 400 to 800 kcal/day. The very low calorie diet is usually in the form of a powdered supplement that is taken 3 to 5 times a day with large amounts of water. This type of diet can be effective, but the long-range efficacy in maintaining the weight loss may be discouraging.

weight reduction d. A diet that reduces the caloric content sufficiently to cause weight loss. Normal metabolism must be preserved, and bulk, mineral, protein, vitamin, and water requirements must be met. During weight loss, intake should be 600 to 1500 kcal below maintenance levels for the individual's weight.

Western d. A diet with inadequate fiber and excessive quantities of refined carbohydrates. The Western diet has been implicated in many diseases in industrialized nations, including diabetes, atherosclerosis, and obesity.

yo-yo d. A popular term to describe a dietary practice resulting in alternating cycles of losing and regaining weight. The demonstration of successful weight loss should be emphasized to motivate the patient to commit to lifelong changes in behaviors related to diet and physical activity. SYN: *weight cycling*.

dietary (dī′ĕ-tā″rē) **1.** Pert. to diet. **2.** A system of dieting. **3.** A regulated food allowance.

Dietary Guidelines for Americans Recommendations issued in 2000 from the Center for Nutrition Policy and Promotion at the U.S. Department of Agriculture for planning and eating a healthy diet. SEE: table; *Food Guide Pyramid*.

Dietary Reference Intakes ABBR: DRI. In the U.S., federally recommended dietary allowances, adequate intakes, tolerable upper intake levels, and estimated average requirements for essential nutrients and other food components in the diet.

dietetic (dī″ĕ-tĕt′ĭk) **1.** Pert. to diet or its regulation. **2.** Food specially prepared for restrictive diets.

dietetics [Gr. *diaitetikos*] The science of applying nutritional data to the regulation of the diet of healthy and sick individuals. Some fundamental principles and facts of this science are summarized here.

Dietary Guidelines for Americans

Aim for a healthy weight.
Be physically active each day.
Choose a variety of grains daily, especially whole grains.
Choose a variety of fruits and vegetables daily.
Keep food safe to eat.
Choose a diet low in saturated fat and cholesterol and moderate in total fat.
Choose beverages and foods that limit your intake of sugars.
Choose and prepare foods with less salt.
If you drink alcoholic beverages, do so in moderation.

SOURCE: U.S. Department of Agriculture

CONSERVATION OF ENERGY: To produce metabolic balance, the number of calories consumed must equal the energy required for basic metabolic needs plus additional energy output resulting from muscular work and added heat losses. Thus a person whose basal rate is 1000 kcal per 24 hr may do work and lose heat during the day, adding about 1500 kcal to the energy output; he or she must, therefore, obtain 2500 kcal per day.

One g of fat yields approx. 9 kcal. One g of carbohydrate or protein yields about 4 kcal.

NOTE: To convert kilocalories to kilojoules, multiply them by 4.1855.

CONSERVATION OF MATTER: Everything that leaves the body, whether exhaled as carbon dioxide and water or excreted as urea and minerals, must be replaced by food. Thus, a person excreting 10 g of nitrogen daily must receive the same in his or her diet, for the element can be neither created nor destroyed. This metabolic balance may be monitored by careful chemical analysis of all that is eaten and excreted.

diethylcarbamazine citrate (dī-ĕth″ĭl-kăr-băm′ă-zēn) A medicine used in treating filarial infections.

di-2-ethylhexyl phthalate (dī-2-ĕth″ĭl-hĕks-ĭl fthăl′āt) ABBR: DHEP. A plastic form of polyvinyl chloride used to manufacture intravenous (IV) tubing and containers. It may leach into IV solutions during the administration of fluids and blood products, producing toxic effects.

diethylpropion hydrochloride (dī-ĕth″ĭl-prō′pē-ŏn) An adrenergic drug with actions similar to those of the amphetamines.

diethylstilbestrol (dī-ĕth″ĭl-stĭl″bĕs′trŏl) ABBR: DES. A synthetic preparation possessing estrogenic properties. It is several times more potent than natural estrogens and may be given orally. It is used therapeutically in the treatment of menopausal disturbances and other disorders due to estrogen deficiencies. SEE: *DES daughter; DES syndrome.*

CAUTION: Diethylstilbestrol should not be administered during pregnancy. Such use has been found to be related to subsequent vaginal malignancies in the daughters of mothers who were given it.

This drug was once used extensively during pregnancy to treat threatened and habitual abortion. An estimated 5 million to 10 million Americans received DES during pregnancy or were exposed to the drug in utero. Those who were exposed to DES in utero were found to be at risk of developing reproductive tract abnormalities such as clear-cell cervicovaginal cancer in women and reproductive tract abnormalities in men. These findings were reported in 1970; the use of the drug during pregnancy was subsequently banned in the U.S. in 1971 and in Europe in 1978. Women who took the drug are now known as DES mothers and their daughters and sons are known as DES daughters and DES sons, respectively.

diethyltoluamide (dī-ĕth″ĭl-tŏl-ū′ă-mīd) ABBR: DEET. An effective insect repellent, esp. for repelling arthropods such as ticks and mosquitoes and flies.

diethyltryptamine (dī-ĕth″ĭl-trĭp′tă-mĭn) A hallucinogenic agent that at low doses has effects similar to those of LSD.

dietitian, dietician (dī-ĕ-tĭsh′ăn) [Gr. *diaita,* way of living] An individual whose training and experience are in the area of nutrition, and who has the ability to apply that information to the dietary needs of the healthy and sick.

registered d. ABBR: RD. A specialist in dietetics who has met the requirements for certification stipulated by the American Dietetic Association.

dietotherapy (dī″ĕ-tō-thĕr′ă-pē) Use of the sciences of dietetics and nutrition in treating disease.

Dieulafoy's triad (dyū-lă-fwăhz′) [Georges Dieulafoy, Fr. physician, 1839–1911] Tenderness, muscular contraction, and skin hyperesthesia at McBurney's point in acute appendicitis.

differential (dĭf″ĕr-ĕn′shăl) [L. *differre,* to carry apart] Marked by or relating to differences.

differential amplifier An amplifier used to increase the difference between two signals, one of which is usually a reference.

differentiation **1.** In embryology, the acquiring of individual characteristics. This occurs in progressive diversification of cells of the developing pre-embryo and embryo. **2.** The distinguishing of one disease from another. **3.** In psychiatry, the integration of emotional and intellectual functions in an individual.

lymphocyte d. The process by which immature lymphocytes are stimulated to become functional T and B cells able to recognize and respond to antigens.

diffraction (dĭ-frăk′shŭn) [L. *diffringere,* to break to pieces] The change occurring in light when it passes through crystals, prisms, or parallel bars in a grating, in which the rays are deflected and thus appear to be turned aside. This produces dark or colored bands or lines. The term is also applied to similar phenomena in sound.

diffraction grating The device in a spectrophotometer that disperses white light into the colors (wavelengths) of the electromagnetic spectrum, using multiple lines precisely etched into an optically aligned material such as a specialized mirror or metal plate.

diffusate (dĭf′ū-sāt) [L. *dis,* apart, + *fundere,* to pour] In dialysis, the portion of a liquid that passes through a membrane and that contains crystalloid matter in solution. SYN: *dialysate.*

diffuse (dĭ-fūs′) Spreading, scattered, spread.

diffusible (dĭ-fūz′ĭ-bl) Capable of being diffused.

diffusing capacity The ability of gas to cross the alveolar-capillary membrane in the lung. This may be measured by using the rate of movement of a single breath of inhaled 0.3% carbon monoxide across the alveolar-capillary membrane.

diffusion (dĭ-fū′zhŭn) [″ + *fundere,* to pour] **1.** The tendency of molecules of a substance (gaseous, liquid, or solid) to move from a region of high concentration to one of lower concentration. **2.** Absorption of a liquid, such as the absorption by cells of water from lymph when the percentage of salt is less in the lymph than in the cells. When the percentage is greater in the lymph, water is withdrawn from the cells. SEE: *osmosis.* **3.** A process whereby various gases interpenetrate and become mixed through the incessant motion of their molecules. Similarly, if aqueous solutions of different materials stand in contact, mixing occurs on standing even if the solutions are separated by thin membranes. SEE: illus.

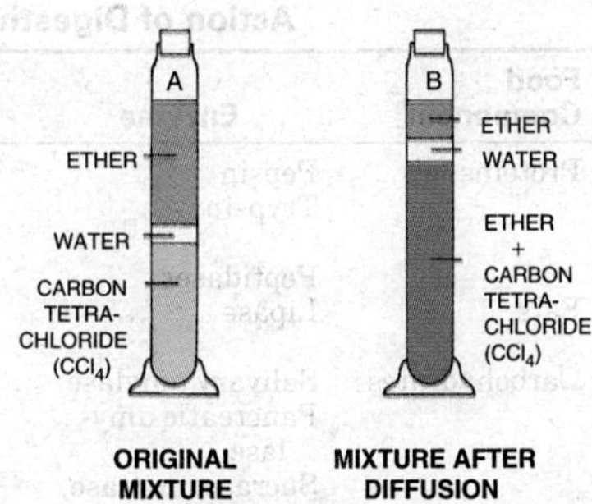

DIFFUSION

facilitated d. The movement of a substance (such as glucose) through a cell membrane with the help of membrane proteins acting as carrier molecules.

digastric (dī-găs′trĭk) [Gr. *dis,* twice, + *gaster,* belly] Having two bellies; said of certain muscles.

Digenetica (dī-jĕ-nĕt′ĭ-kă) An order of parasitic flatworms belonging to the class Trematoda. It reproduces asexually, lives usually in molluscs, and alternates with a sexual generation living in vertebrates as their final host. It includes all four groups of flukes parasitic in humans. SEE: *fluke.*

digest [L. *dis,* apart, + *gerere,* to carry] **1.** To undergo the process involved in changing food from a solid physical form to a soft, moisturized mass broken down in the intestinal tract by chemicals, bacteria, and enzymes. SEE: *metabolism.* **2.** To make a condensation of a subject.

digestant **1.** An agent that digests food or aids in digestion, such as pepsin or pancreatin. **2.** A preparation made from the digestive glands or lining membrane of the stomach, classified according to the foods it digests, such as carbohydrate or protein.

digestible Capable of being digested.

digestion [L. *digestio,* a taking apart] The process by which food is broken down mechanically and chemically in the gastrointestinal tract and converted into absorbable forms. Salts (minerals), water, and monosaccharides can be absorbed unchanged, but starches, fats, and proteins must be broken down into smaller molecules. This is brought about by enzymes, each of which acts on a specific type of food and requires a specific pH to be effective. SEE: tables.

Hormones released by the gastrointestinal mucosa stimulate the secretion of digestive enzymes and bile and influence the motility (peristalsis) of the stomach and intestines. Starches and disaccharides are digested to monosaccharides; fats are digested to fatty acids and glycerol; proteins are digested to amino acids. During digestion, vitamins and minerals are liberated from these large organic molecules. SEE: *intestinal hormone.*

artificial d. Digestion outside the living organism by an enzyme.

chemical d. The conversion of complex food molecules into simpler molecules by the action of digestive enzymes. SEE: tables.

duodenal d. The part of digestion

Action of Digestive Enzymes on Food

Food Component	Enzyme	Secretion	Site of Action
Proteins	Pepsin	Gastric juice, acid	Stomach
	Trypsin	Pancreatic juice, alkaline	Small intestine
	Peptidases	Intestinal juice	Small intestine
Fats	Lipase	Gastric juice	Stomach
		Pancreatic juice	Small intestine
Carbohydrates	Salivary amylase	Saliva, alkaline	Mouth
	Pancreatic amylase	Pancreatic juice	Small intestine
	Sucrase, maltase, lactase	Intestinal juice	Small intestine

that occurs in the duodenum where stomach contents mix with biliary and pancreatic secretions. SEE: *duodenum*.

extracellular d. Digestion occurring outside a cell, such as the digestion of tissue by bacterial enzymes (toxins).

gastric d. The phase of digestion that occurs in the stomach while food is being temporarily stored and mixed in it. The semisolid mass of food known as chyme is mixed with saliva and the gastric juices, which include hydrochloric acid, mucus, pepsin, intrinsic factor, salts, and some lipase. The general result of gastric digestion is the reduction of the ingested mass to a gray mixture called acid chyme.

CHEMICAL ASPECTS: During a meal, stimuli from the brain are carried to the stomach by way of the vagal nerves. These stimuli are produced by the sensations of sight, smell, and taste. In addition, the stretching of the stomach wall stimulates the gastric glands, causing the hormone gastrin to be discharged from the pyloric region into the blood. The circulating gastrin reaches the gastric glands and causes them to secrete.

The food undergoes certain changes while in the stomach. Pepsin acts on high molecular weight proteins, hydrolyzing them to peptones, and also coagulates milk. Hydrochloric acid is essential for the activity of pepsin and is responsible for the antiseptic action of the gastric juice. SEE: *digestion*.

MOTOR ASPECTS: When food first enters the stomach, the stomach is relaxed; then it increases its pressure on the contents. The cardiac sphincter closes firmly to prevent regurgitation into the esophagus. Contractions of the pyloric region of the stomach become more forceful. At first the pyloric sphincter is closed; the result is physical mixing of the food and the beginning of chemical digestion. Then, at intervals, the pyloric sphincter relaxes to permit acid chyme to gradually enter the duodenum. How quickly the chyme leaves the stomach is influenced by the amount of the feeding, its osmotic character, and the amount of fat present. In general, a

Action of Digestive Secretions on Proteins, Fats, and Carbohydrates

Secretion	Proteins	Fats	Carbohydrates
Saliva			Cooked starch into maltose
Gastric juice	Curdles milk Proteins into polypeptides		
Pancreatic enzymes	Polypeptides to peptides	Fats to fatty acids and glycerol	Raw and cooked starch into maltose
Bile		Emulsifies fats	
Intestinal juice	Completes the metabolism of peptides into amino acids		Completes the conversion of all sugars into the simplest form NOTE: Disaccharides are hydrolyzed to monosaccharides in the mucosal cells lining the small intestine.

high-fat meal leaves the stomach more slowly than a low-fat meal. SEE: *digestion, duodenal*.

intestinal d. The part of digestion that occurs in the intestine. SEE: *absorption; large intestine; small intestine*.

intracellular d. The consumption and chemical degradation of materials ingested by cells (such as bacteria, viruses, or large molecules) within vacuoles in the cytoplasm.

mechanical d. The conversion of food into small pieces by chewing, churning of the stomach, or emulsifying action of bile salts, thereby exposing more surface area to digestive enzymes.

oral d. The portion of the digestive process taking place in the mouth. It includes the physical process of chewing food and the chemical process of starch splitting by the enzyme amylase, present in the saliva.

pancreatic d. The digestion of proteins and fats by pancreatic enzymes that are released into the intestine.

salivary d. Digestion of starches by salivary amylase.

digestive (dī-jĕs′tĭv) Pert. to digestion.

digestive juice One of several secretions that aid in processes of digestion.

digit (dĭj′ĭt) *pl.* **digits** [L. *digitus,* finger] A finger or toe. **digital** (-ĭ-tăl), *adj.*

digital amniotome A small apparatus that fits over the tip of the index finger. A small knifelike projection at the end of the device is used to puncture the bag of waters before delivery of the fetus. This usually expedites progression of labor.

digitalis (dĭj″ĭ-tăl′ĭs) [L. *digitus,* finger] An antiarrhythmic and cardiotonic drug, derived from the dried leaves of *Digitalis purpurea,* the common foxglove. It is also found in smaller quantities in the leaves of other plants, such as rhododendrons. SEE: *digitalis poisoning; Poisons and Poisoning Appendix.*

ACTION/USES: Digitalis glycosides increase the force of myocardial contraction, increase the refractory period of the atrioventricular node, and to a lesser degree affect the sinoatrial node. Digitalis increases cardiac output by increasing the contractility of cardiac muscle. Digitalis is used to treat patients with congestive heart failure; it contributes to an improvement in exercise tolerance in these patients. Digitalis glycosides can also be used to control heart rate in patients with atrial fibrillation, atrial flutter, and supraventricular tachycardias.

PRECAUTIONS: Potassium depletion, which may accompany diuresis, sensitizes the myocardium to digitalis and may permit toxicity to develop with what would otherwise be the usual dose. Patients with acute myocardial infarction, severe pulmonary disease, or far-advanced heart failure may be more sensitive to digitalis and thus prone to develop arrhythmia. Calcium affects the heart in a manner similar to that of digitalis; its use in a digitalized patient may produce serious arrhythmias. In myxedema, digitalis requirements are decreased because the excretion rate of the drug is decreased. Patients with incomplete atrioventricular block, esp. those with Stokes-Adams attacks, may develop complete heart block if given digitalis. Because renal insufficiency delays the excretion of digitalis, the dose of the drug must be decreased in patients with this problem. Digitalis glycosides interact with many other drugs used to treat patients with heart failure, such as warfarin and amiodarone. Patients taking agents that alter drug levels of digitalis may need frequent clinical assessment to prevent digitalis toxicity. Elderly patients, in whom the drug is most often used, are at greatest risk for digitalis toxicity.

digitalis poisoning Toxicity that may develop acutely or chronically from the cumulative effect of digitalis. Its most common adverse effects include anorexia, nausea, vomiting, atrial tachycardia and other dysrhythmias, atrioventricular heart blocks, confusion, dizziness, or neurological depression. Digitalis toxicity is a potentially life-threatening, and frequently a drug-related, complication. SEE: *Nursing Diagnoses Appendix.*

SYMPTOMS: Extracardiac signs develop initially in most patients, the first of which is almost always anorexia. Nausea and vomiting, sometimes with abdominal pain and increased salivation, usually appear 1 to 2 days later. Other symptoms include fatigue, drowsiness, general muscle weakness, and visual disturbances such as blurring of vision, yellow-green or white halos around visual images, light flashes, photophobia, and diplopia. Mental disturbances, such as agitation, hallucinations, and disorientation, are especially common in elderly atherosclerotic patients. If the early signs are unheeded, 80% of patients eventually will show more serious cardiac signs. Toxic concentrations of digitalis can cause nearly every known arrhythmia. They can decrease heart rate by slowing conduction and increasing the refractory period at the AV node, or they can increase the rate by creating abnormal pacemaker activity in the conductive tissue. SEE: illus.

PATIENT CARE: Because a fine line separates therapeutic and toxic levels, health care providers must be alert to signs of digitalis poisoning in patients. Elderly patients and those with liver or

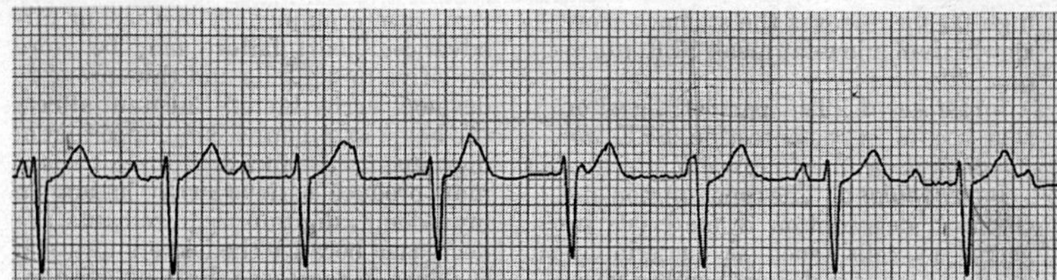

DIGITALIS POISONING

Atrial and junctional tachycardia caused by digitalis toxicity

kidney disease are at especially high risk because their absorption, metabolism, and excretion rates are unpredictable. Health care providers also must watch for changes in physical condition that can alter a patient's response to digitalis, including vomiting, diarrhea, or other gastrointestinal upset; acid-base or electrolyte disturbances (e.g., hypokalemia, hypomagnesemia, or hypercalcemia), which change the heart's sensitivity to digitalis; hypothyroidism, which disrupts the patient's ability to metabolize digitalis; and liver or kidney disease, which alters metabolism and excretion. Changes in a treatment regimen also can predispose the patient to toxicity, especially the addition of or increase in dosages of drugs such as antiarrhythmics, calcium channel blockers, or potassium-wasting diuretics. Assessment for digitalis toxicity is necessary if electrical cardioversion is used to restore a patient to sinus rhythm, as this procedure increases the heart's sensitivity to digitalis.

Because digitalis toxicity develops quickly and insidiously, the patient is taught early symptoms to report. Extracardiac signs can be missed or mistaken for complications of another condition being treated (e.g., pneumonia). Health care providers need to compare the patient's current appetite and activity to previous reports, and watch the patient's laboratory reports for electrolyte imbalances. Heart rate is auscultated, and the patient is taught to count his or her pulse for a full minute prior to dosing or when suspicious of toxicity. Significant decreases or increases in rate, skipped beats, or new irregularities must be reported, since toxic concentrations can lead to ventricular fibrillation and death. If toxicity is suspected, an ECG is performed; signs of digitalis toxicity include first degree AV block with depressed ST segments, shortened QT intervals, and flattened T waves. In the presence of such changes, the primary care provider should order a serum digoxin level to confirm toxicity, as well as serum electrolyte levels. Cardiac monitoring for rate and rhythm should continue. Since hypokalemia is a major cause of digitalis toxicity, adequate potassium intake is essential. The patient is advised about potassium-rich foods and prescribed potassium supplements, available in various forms. The patient learns how to take the prescribed form while preventing gastric complications. He or she is warned that being under stress and having diarrhea both result in excessive potassium losses and should be reported. The patient is advised not to take OTC medications without notifying his primary care provider, as these may alter his or her sensitivity to digitalis. The patient also is taught not to substitute one brand of prescribed drug for another, as bioavailability may differ.

Digitalis poisoning also can occur because of accidental or purposeful overdose. Emergency department personnel remove the drug from the stomach by emesis or lavage, wash out the absorbed drug with intravenous fluids, provide potassium as prescribed, monitor cardiac status, and treat cardiac arrhythmias as they arise. They also administer digoxin immune FAB (ovine) if prescribed, to bind molecules of unbound digoxin and especially longer-acting digitoxin, making them unavailable for binding at cell action sites.

digitalization (dĭj″ĭ-tăl-ĭ-zā′shŭn) **1.** Subjection of an organism to the action of digitalis. **2.** Providing a loading dose of digoxin to a patient, to reach a therapeutic drug level rapidly.

digital radiography Radiography using computerized imaging instead of conventional film or screen imaging.

digitate [L. *digitus,* finger] Having finger-like impressions or processes.

digitation (dĭj-ĭ-tā′shŭn) A finger-like process.

digiti (dĭj′ĭ-tī) Pl. of digitus.

digitiform (dĭj′ĭ-tĭ-form) Similar to a finger.

digitoxin (dĭj-ĭ-tŏk′sĭn) A cardiotoxic glycoside obtained from various species of foxglove, used infrequently to treat heart failure and atrial arrhythmias. SEE: *digitalis.*

digit span test A test of immediate memory. The patient is asked to repeat a string of numerals spoken by the examiner. The string is made progressively longer in order to determine the numerals that can be recalled. Normally six or seven numbers can be repeated. SEE: *memory; object span test; temporal-sequential organization.*

digitus [L] A finger or toe.

diglossia (dī-glŏs′ē-ă) [Gr. *dis,* double, + *glossa,* tongue] The condition of having a double tongue.

diglyceride (dī-glĭs′ĕr-īd) A glyceride combined with two fatty acid molecules. SEE: *triglycerides.*

dignathus (dĭg-nā′thŭs) [″ + *gnathos,* jaw] Having two jaws due to a congenital deformity.

digoxin (dĭ-jŏk′sĭn) The most frequently prescribed digitalis glycoside. It may be used orally or intravenously to treat patients with congestive heart failure, atrial fibrillation, atrial flutter, and supraventricular tachycardias.

digoxin immune Fab (ovine) for injection A monoclonal antibody for use in treating life-threatening overdose of digoxin or digitoxin. This fragment antigen binding (Fab) substance combines with molecules of digoxin or digitoxin, which are then excreted by the kidneys.

dihydric (dī-hī′drĭk) A compound containing two hydrogen atoms.

dihydrocodeinone bitartrate (dī-hī″drō-kō′dē-ĭ-nōn) An opioid analgesic used to treat pain, often in combination with acetaminophen.

dihydroergotamine mesylate (dī-hī″drō-ĕr-gŏt′ă-mēn) A vasoconstrictor used in treating migraine.

dihydrosphingosine $CH_3—[CH_2]_{14}—CHOH—CH(NH_2)—CH_2OH$; a long-chain amino alcohol present in sphingolipids, also known as sphinganine. SEE: *sphingolipid; sphingosine.*

dihydrotachysterol (dī-hī″drō-tăk-ĭs′tĕr-ŏl) A hydrogenated tachysterol; a steroid obtained by irradiation of ergosterol. It aids the absorption of calcium from the digestive tract in hypoparathyroidism.

dihydroxyaluminum aminoacetate (dī″hī-drŏk″sē-ă-lū′mĭ-nŭm) An antacid used in treating gastric hyperacidity.

dihydroxyaluminum sodium carbonate A gastric antacid preparation.

dihydroxycholecalciferol (dī″hī-drŏk″sē-kō″lē-kăl-sĭf′ĕ-rŏl) One of the vitamin D analogues and metabolites that influence the body's absorption and use of calcium and phosphorus. Vitamin D and its analogues prevent and are used to treat rickets, osteodystrophy, hypocalcemia, and hypophosphatemia. SEE: *Vitamins Appendix.*

3,4-dihydroxyphenylalanine (dī-hī-drŏk″sē-fĕn″ĭl-ăl′ă-nēn) Dopa.

di-iodohydroxyquin (dī″ī-ō″dō-hī-drŏk′sē-kwĭn) The previously used name for iodoquinol.

diktyoma Dictyoma.

dilaceration (dī″lăs-ĕr-ā′shŭn) [L. *dilacerare,* to tear apart] **1.** A tearing apart, as of a cataract. SEE: *discission.* **2.** Bending of the root of a tooth due to injury during development.

dilatant (dī-lā′tănt) [L. *dilatare,* to enlarge] Anything that causes dilation.

dilatation (dĭl-ă-tā′shŭn) **1.** Expansion of an organ or vessel. **2.** Expansion of an orifice with a dilator.

cervical d. The gradual opening of the cervical os during labor to allow the fetus to leave the uterus.

digital d. Dilatation of an opening or a cavity by use of the fingers.

heart d. Abnormal increase in the size of the cavities of the heart, a common result of valvular disease or hypertension.

stomach d. Distention of the stomach caused by food or gas. Acute dilatation of the stomach or acute gastromesenteric ileus may occur as a postoperative or postpartum condition and usually results from obstruction of the duodenum or pylorus.

dilation **1.** Expansion of an orifice with a dilator. **2.** Expansion of an organ, orifice, or vessel. SYN: *dilatation.*

dilation and curettage ABBR: D and C. A surgical procedure that expands the cervical canal of the uterus (dilation) so that the surface lining of the uterine wall can be scraped (curettage).

PATIENT CARE: Preoperatively, the patient's understanding of the procedure is ascertained, with any misconceptions clarified. She is told what she will experience, and what to expect after the procedure. The patient usually will be allowed nothing to eat or drink after midnight. Perineal shave, enema, and vaginal douche usually are not performed, unless they are the preference of the gynecologic-surgeon.

Postoperatively, the patient's vital signs are assessed frequently until stable, and the amount and type of vaginal bleeding are monitored, with a pad count kept. Once the patient has voided and is tolerating oral intake, she is discharged.

Post-discharge care is reviewed with the patient, including concerns to report. The patient should not need to change pads more than hourly and should keep a pad count, noticing if the pads are soaked through. She may pass a few small clots, but should report bleeding that exceeds saturating one pad per hour for a total of 8 over the first 8 hours. The patient then should experience only spotting, which may last a few weeks. Usually, she should not use tampons for at least 1 week after surgery. Abdominal cramping is not unusual for the first few days; it usually can be relieved by taking a mild analgesic (e.g., acetaminophen, aspirin) or placing a heating pad or hot water bottle on the lower abdomen. The patient should check her temperature every 4 hours for 2 days and notify the gynecologist of any elevation over 100°F. Usually, the patient is told to refrain from intercourse for 2 weeks or until her postoperative visit, scheduled according to the gynecologic-surgeon's wishes. SEE: *Nursing Diagnoses Appendix.*

dilation and evacuation ABBR: D and E. During the second trimester, removal of the products of conception by suction curettage and use of forceps.

dilator (dī-lā′tor) [L. *dilatare,* to expand] An instrument for dilating muscles or for stretching cavities or openings.

Barnes' d. A rubber bag filled with fluid for dilation of the cervix uteri.

Bossi's d. A multiple-pronged instrument that dilates by separation of its prongs. It is used for dilation of the cervix uteri.

Goodell's d. An instrument similar to the Bossi dilator except that it has three prongs.

gynecological d. An instrument for dilating the cervix uteri.

Hegar's d. Graduated metal sounds that are inserted into the cervical canal and cause a graded dilation.

tent d. A small cone made of seaweed, sponge, or tree roots, which is inserted into the uterine canal dry and, on absorbing moisture, expands to cause a slow dilation. SEE: *Laminaria digitata.*

vaginal d. A glass, plastic, or metal device for dilating the vagina.

dildo, dildoe An artificial penis-shaped device used intravaginally to simulate sexual intercourse.

dill (dĭl) A hardy annual, Anethum graveolens, whose leaves and seeds are used primarily to flavor foods. It is also used as an antiflatulent and antispasmodic, but scientific evidence of its effectiveness is lacking.

diluent (dĭl′ū-ĕnt) [L. *diluere,* to wash away] An agent that dilutes the substance or solution to which it is added.

dilution (dī-loo′shŭn) **1.** The process of attenuating or weakening a substance. **2.** A diluted substance.

dimenhydrinate (dī″mĕn-hī′drĭn-āt) A drug used to prevent or treat motion sickness and to control nausea, vomiting, and dizziness in other conditions.

dimension, vertical A vertical measurement of the face; used in dentistry for growth studies and for reference in denture placement.

dimer (dī′mĕr) **1.** In chemistry, esp. polymer chemistry, a combination of two identical molecules to form a single compound. **2.** In virology, a capsomer containing two subunits.

dimercaprol (dī-mĕr-kăp′rōl) $C_3H_8OS_2$; a compound, 2,3-dimercaptopropanol, used as an antidote in poisoning from heavy metals such as arsenic, gold, and mercury. It is a colorless liquid with a disagreeable odor. Mixed with benzyl benzoate and oil, it is administered intramuscularly.

dimethicone (dī-mĕth′ĭ-kōn) A silicone oil used to protect the skin against water-soluble irritants.

dimethylamine (dī-mĕth″ĭl-ăm′ĭn) $(CH_3)_2NH$; a malodorous product of decay of materials that contain proteins.

p-dimethylaminoazobenzene (dī-mĕth″ĭl-ăm″ĭ-nō-ăz″ō-bĕn′zēn) A carcinogenic dye, butter yellow.

dimethylmercury (dī-mĕth-ĭl-mĕr′kū-rē) An exceptionally toxic form of mercury that may cause disease and death even after minute exposures. It is readily absorbed through the skin and respiratory tract. SEE: *mercury poisoning.*

dimethyl phthalate (dī-mĕth″ĭl thăl′āt) An insect repellent.

dimethyl sulfoxide (dī-mĕth′ĭl sŭlf-ŏks′īd) ABBR: DMSO. A solvent used to treat interstitial cystitis. The drug was previously believed to improve the absorption of medications from the skin, and it was used to treat rheumatic diseases. There is no objective evidence that DMSO is effective for either use.

dimethyltryptamine (dī-mĕth″ĭl-trĭp′tă-mēn) An agent that in low doses has hallucinogenic action like that of LSD.

dimetria (dī-mē′trē-ă) [Gr. *dis,* double, + *metra,* uterus] Double uterus.

dimorphous (dī-mor′fŭs) [″ + *morphe,* form] Occurring in two different forms.

dimple A small depression in the skin, esp. of the cheek or chin.

dimple sign A sign used to differentiate a benign lesion, dermatofibroma, from nodular melanoma, which it may mimic. On application of lateral pressure with the thumb and index finger, the dermatofibroma dimples or becomes indented; melanomas, melanocytic nevi, and normal skin protrude above the initial plane.

dimpling The formation of slight depressions in the flesh due to retraction of the subcutaneous tissue. It occurs in certain carcinomas, such as cancer of the breast. SEE: *peau d'orange.*

2,4-dinitrophenol (dī-nī″trō-fē′nŏl) $C_6H_4N_2O_5$; a toxic compound formerly used to make dyes. SEE: *Poisons and Poisoning Appendix.*

Dinoflagellata (dī″nō-flăj″ĕ-lā′tă) [″ + *flagellum,* whip] A phylum of the kingdom Protista; photosynthetic unicellular organisms that are part of the phytoplankton in fresh and ocean water. Some marine species bloom explosively in what are called "red tides"; shellfish that feed on the dinoflagellates are toxic to humans (paralytic shellfish poisoning). Another species produces ciguatera toxin, which is poisonous to fish and to humans who consume such fish.

dinoprostone (dī'nō-prŏs-tōn) A form of prostaglandin E_2. The gel form is used to produce cervical ripening and to stimulate myometrial contractions, thus reducing oxytocin requirements to induce and shorten labor. Vaginal suppositories containing dinoprostone may be used to induce midtrimester abortion, to engender expulsion of a retained dead fetus (missed abortion), and to treat benign hydatidiform mole. SEE: *prostaglandin.*

dinucleotide (dī-nū'klē-ō-tīd) The product of cleaving a polynucleotide.

Dioctophyma (dī-ŏk"tō-fī'mă) A genus of roundworms found in dogs but rarely in humans.

dioctyl calcium sulfosuccinate (dī-ŏk'tĭl) A stool softener. The name was previously used for docusate calcium.

dioctyl sodium sulfosuccinate Previously used name for docusate sodium.

Diogenes syndrome [Diogenes, Gr. philosopher, 4th century B.C.] A lack of interest in personal cleanliness or cleanliness of the home, usually occurring in elderly individuals who live alone. Affected persons usually are undernourished, but not necessarily from poverty; this condition occurs in all socioeconomic circumstances.

diopter (dī-ŏp'tĕr, dī'ŏp-) [Gr. *dia,* through, + *optos,* visible] The refractive power of a lens; the reciprocal of the focal length expressed in meters. It is used as a unit of measurement in refraction. **dioptric** (-ŏp'trĭk), *adj.*

dioptometer (dī"ŏp-tŏm'ĕ-tĕr) [" + " + *metron,* measure] A device for measuring ocular refraction.

dioptometry (dī"ŏp-tŏm'ĕ-trē) The determination of refraction and accommodation of the eye.

dioptrics (dī-ŏp'trĭks) The science of light refraction.

diovulatory (dī-ŏv'ū-lă-tō"rē) Producing two ova in the same ovarian cycle.

dioxide (dī-ŏk'sīd) [Gr. *dis,* two, + *oxys,* sharp] A compound having two oxygen atoms per molecule.

dioxin 2,3,7,8-tetrachlorodibenzo-*p*-dioxin (TCDD); a toxic, cancer-causing chemical. Initial exposure to this agent can produce chloracne, liver injury, and peripheral neuropathy. It has been used as a herbicide (e.g., during the Vietnam War, when it was called "agent orange") and is an unwanted pollutant released by some industrial and agricultural processes. Dioxin-like compounds are also released by the degradation of some other organic molecules. SEE: *Agent Orange; pentachlorophenol; polychlorinated biphenyls; 2,4,5-trichlorophenoxyacetic acid.*

dioxybenzone (dī-ŏks"ĭ-bĕn'zōn) A topical sunscreen that blocks ultraviolet A and B.

dipalmityl lecithin ABBR: DPL. A major constituent of pulmonary surfactant.

dipeptid(e) (dī-pĕp'tĭd, -tīd) [" + *peptein,* to digest] A derived protein obtained by hydrolysis of proteins or condensation of amino acids.

dipeptidase (dī-pĕp'tĭ-dās) An enzyme that catalyzes the hydrolysis of dipeptides to amino acids.

Dipetalonema perstans (dī-pĕt"ă-lō-nē'mă) A species of filariae that infests wild or domestic animals and occasionally humans. In humans, the adult worm migrates to the subcutaneous tissue and produces a nodule. Rarely, the adult worm may be seen beneath the conjunctiva.

diphallus (dī-făl'ŭs) [" + *phallos,* penis] A condition in which there is either complete or incomplete doubling of the penis or clitoris.

diphasic (dī-fā'zĭk) [" + *phasis,* a phase] Having two phases.

diphenhydramine hydrochloride (dī"fĕn-hī'dră-mēn hī-drō-klō'rīd) An antihistamine. Tradename is Benadryl.

diphenoxylate hydrochloride (dī"fĕn-ŏk'sĭ-lāt) A smooth muscle relaxant used in combination with atropine in treating diarrhea.

diphenylhydantoin sodium (dī-fĕn"ĭl-hī-dăn'tō-ĭn) An anticonvulsant, also known as phenytoin, used to treat grand mal, partial complex, and simple seizures. Its official name is phenytoin. Trade name is Dilantin.

diphonia (dī-fō'nē-ă) [Gr. *dis,* two, + *phone,* voice] Simultaneous production of two different voice tones. SYN: *diplophonia.*

diphosphatidylglycerol An extract of beef hearts that contains phosphorylated polysaccharide esters of fatty acids. It is used in certain tests for syphilis.

2,3-diphosphoglycerate ABBR: 2,3-DPG. An organic phosphate in red blood cells that alters the affinity of hemoglobin for oxygen. Blood cells stored in a blood bank lose 2,3-diphosphoglycerate, but once they are infused, the substance is resynthesized or reactivated.

diphtheria (dĭf-thē'rē-ă) [Gr. *diphthera,* membrane] A rare bacterial infectious disease marked by the formation of a membrane over the tonsils, uvula, soft palate, and posterior pharynx and occasionally on the skin. The membrane is created by a thick, inflammatory exudate. SEE: *antitoxin; exotoxin; sepsis; diphtheria toxoid.* **diphtherial** (-thē'rē-ăl), *adj.*

ETIOLOGY: The causative organism is *Corynebacterium diphtheriae,* a gram-positive nonmotile, non-spore-forming, club-shaped bacillus. Airborne droplets transmit the organism from person to person. An effective vaccination program has made the incidence of the disease rare in the U.S., except among groups of people who do not receive immunizations because of religious or other reasons. The lack of virulent strains to reinforce immunity, however, has resulted in loss of immunity in some older adults. The incubation period is 2 to 5 days, and occasionally longer.

IMMUNIZATION: Immunization is accomplished by the administration of three doses at least 4 weeks apart, beginning at 2 months of age. Diphtheria toxoid (inactivated exotoxin capable of producing antibodies) is given, in combination with pertussis vaccine and tetanus toxoid; a fourth dose is given 1 year later. Booster doses are administered if a child under 6 years old is exposed to diphtheria. Adults may receive a booster of diphtheria toxoid when tetanus toxoid boosters are given every 10 years. Immunity to diphtheria is assessed by measuring antibody levels in the blood or, rarely, by the Schick test, in which small doses of inactivated toxin are administered intradermally; the presence of necrosis at the site indicates that protective antibodies are not present.

SYMPTOMS: Patients present with fever, malaise, cervical lymphadenopathy, and sore throat. A tough yellow-white or gray pseudomembrane forms in the throat, as the result of an inflammatory process. It contains cell debris and fibrin and, unlike the exudate caused by streptococci, is difficult to remove and can obstruct air flow. As the bacteria multiply, they produce a potent exotoxin that prevents protein synthesis in cells. Once the exotoxin has spread to the bloodstream, signs of sepsis develop. The toxin can cause peripheral nerve paralysis and myocarditis, resulting in death.

DIFFERENTIAL DIAGNOSIS: Similar symptoms may be due to tonsillitis, scarlet fever, acute pharyngitis, streptococcus sore throat, peritonsillar abscess, infectious mononucleosis, Vincent's angina, acute moniliasis, primary HIV retroviral syndrome, and staphylococcus infections in the respiratory tract following chemotherapy. Examination of a smear from the infected area is advisable; cultures should be obtained in every instance to confirm the diagnosis. In the laryngeal type of diphtheria, edema of the glottis, foreign bodies, and retropharyngeal abscess must be considered.

TREATMENT: If an adult or nonimmunized child shows signs of infection, diphtheria antitoxin, containing preformed antibodies, is administered immediately, without waiting for laboratory confirmation of the diagnosis. Because antitoxin is made from animal serum, hypersensitivity must be assessed first using an intradermal injection of 1:10 dilute antitoxin. Intravenous erythromycin administered for 7 to 14 days may decrease exotoxin production by the *C. diphtheriae* and limit spread of the disease. Patients should be hospitalized in an intensive care unit without delay and diphtheria antitoxin administered intravenously even before culture results are known.

CAUTION: A skin test for type III hypersensitivity must precede administration of the antitoxin.

PATIENT CARE: The patient is monitored for respiratory distress, sepsis, and myocardial or neural involvement. Humidified oxygen is administered to maintain saturated hemoglobin (SaO_2) above 92%, and the patient is assessed for increased ventilatory effort, use of accessory muscles, nasal flaring, stridor, cyanosis, and agitation or decreased level of consciousness. Hypotension, tachycardia, and rales on auscultation may indicate heart failure. Sepsis may produce fever, tachycardia, and hypotension. Neuromuscular involvement is assessed through weakness, paralysis, or sensory changes. All data are clearly documented. Patients who receive antitoxin are closely observed for local or systemic anaphylaxis.

Strict isolation is maintained until two consecutive negative nasopharyngeal cultures have been obtained at least 1 week after drug therapy ceases. Nonimmunized members of the patient's household are advised to receive diphtheria toxoid appropriate to age and to complete the proper series of diphtheria immunizations. All cases of diphtheria must be reported to local public health authorities. Families are prepared for a prolonged convalescence, esp. if the patient has neuromuscular involvement.

cutaneous d. A skin infection, usually at the site of a wound, caused by *C. diphtheriae,* usually occurring in humid, tropical regions with poor sanitation. It is characterized by slow healing, shallow ulcers containing a tough grayish membrane. It is treated with diphtheria antitoxin and penicillin or erythromycin.

laryngeal d. A complication of diphtheria caused by extension of the membrane from the pharynx with gradual occlusion of the airway. The signs are restlessness, use of accessory respiration muscles, and development of cyanosis. If this condition is not remedied effectively, death results.

surgical d. Diphtheritic membrane formation on wounds.

diphtheria antitoxin **1.** The protective antibody formed after exposure to *Cor-*

ynebacterium diphtheriae or its toxoid. The object of immunization with diphtheria toxoid is to develop high enough titers of this antibody to prevent diphtheria on subsequent exposures. **2.** Solution containing preformed antibodies to *C. diphtheriae,* used to treat diphtheria. Skin tests to assess for type III hypersensitivity are necessary before administration because the solution is obtained from animal serum.

diphtheria toxin for Schick test The toxin used for determining immunity to diphtheria. SEE: *Schick test.*

diphtheroid (dĭf′thĕ-royd) [″ + *eidos,* form, shape] **1.** Resembling diphtheria or the bacteria that cause diphtheria. **2.** A false membrane or pseudomembrane not due to *Corynebacterium diphtheriae.*

diphthongia (dĭf-thŏn′jē-ă) [Gr. *dis,* two, + *phtongos,* voice] The simultaneous utterance of two vocal sounds of different pitch in pathological conditions of the larynx.

Diphyllobothrium (dī-fĭl″ō-bŏth′rē-ŭm) [″ + *phyllon,* leaf, + *bothrion,* pit] A genus of tapeworm belonging to the order Pseudophyllidea and marked by possession of a scolex with two slitlike grooves or bothria. Formerly called *Dibothriocephalus.*

D. cordatum The heart-shaped tapeworm, a small species infesting dogs and seals in Greenland, formerly known as *D. mansoni.* The plerocercoids are occasionally found in humans.

D. erinacei A species infesting dogs, cats, and other carnivores. Larval stages are occasionally found in humans.

D. latum The broad or fish tapeworm. The adult lives in the intestine of fish-eating mammals, including humans. The largest tapeworm infesting humans, it may reach a length of 50 to 60 ft or 15.2 to 18.3 m (average 20 ft or 6.1 m). The eggs develop into ciliated larvae that are eaten by small crustaceans called copepods. The larvae pass through several stages in the copepods, and develop further after the copepods are eaten by fish, finally encysting in fish muscle. People acquire infection by eating raw or poorly cooked fish that contains cysts. Infection can be prevented by thoroughly cooking all freshwater fish, or by keeping the fish frozen at −10°C (14°F) for 48 hr before eating. SEE: illus.

SYMPTOMS: Patients often report abdominal pain, loss of weight, digestive disorders, progressive weakness, and symptoms of pernicious anemia because the worm absorbs ingested vitamin B_{12} from the gastrointestinal tract.

TREATMENT: Praziquantel is used to treat the infestation.

diphyodont (dĭf′ē-ō-dŏnt) [″ + *phyein,* to produce, + *odous,* tooth] Having two sets of teeth, a primary and a permanent set, as in humans.

diplacusis (dĭp″lă-kū′sĭs) [″ + *akousis,* hearing] A disturbed perception of pitch in which two tones are heard for every sound produced.

diplegia (dī-plē′jē-ă) [Gr. *dis,* twice, + *plege,* a stroke] **1.** Paralysis of similar parts on both sides of the body. **2.** In cerebral palsy, excessive stiffness usually in all limbs, but greater stiffness in the legs than in the arms. **diplegic** (-jĭk), *adj.*

infantile d. Birth palsy.

spastic d. Congenital spastic stiffness of the limbs.

diplo- Combining form meaning *double* or *twin.*

diploalbuminuria (dĭp″lō-ăl-bū″mĭn-ū′rē-ă) [Gr. *diplous,* double, + L. *albumen,* white of egg, + Gr. *ouron,* urine] The coexistence of physiological and pathological albuminuria.

diplobacillus [″ + L. *bacillus,* a little stick] A double bacillus, the two being linked end to end.

diplobacterium [″ + *bakterion,* little rod] An organism made up of two adherent bacteria.

diploblastic (dĭp″lō-blăs′tĭk) [″ + *blastos,* germ] Having two germ layers, used of the ectoderm and endoderm.

diplocardia [″ + *kardia,* heart] A condition in which the two lateral halves of the heart are partially separated by a groove.

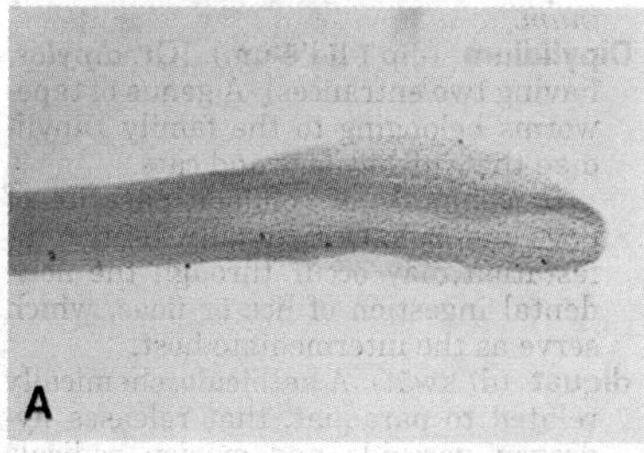

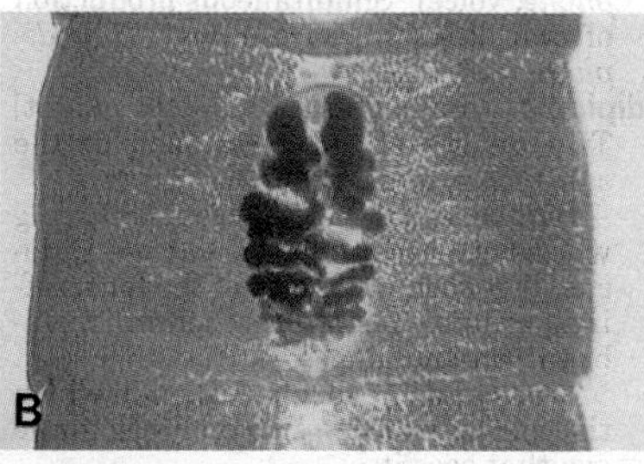

DIPHYLLOBOTHRIUM LATUM

(A) Scolex with grooved suckers (orig. mag. ×5), (B) proglottid (orig. mag. ×10)

diplocephaly (dĭp″lō-sĕf′ă-lē) [″ + *kephale,* head] The condition of having two heads.

diplococcemia (dĭp″lō-kŏk-sē′mē-ă) [″ + *kokkos,* berry, + *haima,* blood] The presence of diplococci in the blood.

Diplococcus (dĭp-lō-kŏk′ŭs) [″ + *kokkus,* berry] A genus of bacteria belonging to the family Lactobacillaceae. They are gram-positive organisms occurring in pairs.

D. pneumoniae SEE: *Streptococcus pneumoniae.*

diplococcus (dĭp″lō-kŏk′ŭs) *pl.* **diplococci** Any of various spherical bacteria appearing in pairs. SEE: *bacterium* for illus; *Neisseria gonorrhoeae* for illus.

diplocoria (dĭp″lō-kō′rē-ă) [″ + *kore,* pupil] A double pupil in the eye.

diploë (dĭp′lō-ē) [Gr. *diploē,* fold] Spongy bone containing red bone marrow between the two layers of compact bone of the skull bones. **diploetic** (-lō-e′tĭc), *adj.*

diplogenesis [Gr. *diplous,* double, + *genesis,* generation, birth] The condition of having two parts or producing two substances; the production of a double fetus or the doubling of some fetal parts.

diploid (dĭp′loyd) [″ + *eidos,* form, shape] Having two sets of chromosomes; said of somatic cells, which contain twice the number of chromosomes present in the egg or sperm. SEE: *chromosome; meiosis; mitosis.*

diplokaryon (dĭp″lō-kăr′ē-ŏn) [″ + *karyon,* nucleus] A nucleus containing twice the diploid number of chromosomes.

diplomyelia (dĭp″lō-mī-ē′lē-ă) [″ + *myelos,* marrow] A condition in certain types of spina bifida in which the spinal cord appears to be doubled due to a lengthwise fissure.

diploneural [″ + *neuron,* nerve] Having two nerves from different origins, as certain muscles.

diplopagus (dĭp-lŏp′ă-gŭs) [″+ *pagos,* a thing fixed] Conjoined and sharing some organs, said of twins with this condition.

diplophonia (dĭp-lō-fō′nē-ă) [″ + *phone,* voice] Simultaneous production of two different voice tones. SYN: *diphonia.*

diplopia (dĭp-lō′pē-ă) [″ + *ope,* sight] Two images of an object seen at the same time. SYN: *doublev.*

binocular d. Double vision occurring when both eyes are used but not in focus. It is seen in disease of the lens, retina, cranial nerve, cerebellum, cerebrum, and meninges.

crossed d. Binocular vision in which the image is on the side opposite to the eye that sees it.

homonymous d. Uncrossed d.

monocular d. Double vision with one eye.

uncrossed d. Double vision in which the image appears on the same side as the eye that sees it. SYN: *homonymous d.* SEE: *crossed d.*

vertical d. Double vision with one of two images higher than the other.

diploscope [″ + *skopein,* to examine] A device for studying binocular vision.

diplosomatia, diplosomia (dĭp″lō-sō-mā′shē-ă, dip″lō-sō′mē-ă) [″ + *soma,* body] A condition in which twins are joined at one or more points.

diplotene (dĭp′lō-tēn) In cell division, the stage of the first meiotic prophase, when the homologous pairs of chromatids begin to separate.

dipole (dī′pōl) A molecule in which each end has an equal but opposite charge. The intensity of the charge is given by its dielectric moment or constant.

dipping 1. Palpation of the liver by a quick depressive movement of the fingers while the hand is held flat on the abdomen. **2.** Immersion of an object in a solution, esp. applied to the dipping of cattle or dogs for tick control.

diprosopus (dĭp-rō-sōp′ŭs) [Gr. *dis,* twice, + *prosopon,* face] A malformed fetus with a double face.

dipsophobia (dĭp-sō-fō′bē-ă) [″ + *phobos,* fear] Morbid fear of drinking.

dipsosis (dĭp-sō′sĭs) [″ + *osis,* condition] Abnormal thirst.

dipstick (dĭp′stĭk) A chemical-impregnated paper strip used for analysis of body fluids, principally urine.

Diptera (dĭp′tĕr-ă) [Gr. *dipteros,* having two wings] An order of insects characterized by sucking or piercing mouth parts, one pair of wings, and complete metamorphosis. It includes the flies, gnats, midges, and mosquitoes. It contains many species involved in the transmission of pathogenic organisms, such as malaria.

dipterous (dĭp′tĕr-ŭs) Having two wings; characteristic of the order Diptera.

dipygus (dī-pī′gŭs) [Gr. *dis,* two, + *pyge,* rump] Having a double pelvis; said of a congenitally deformed fetus.

dipylidiasis (dĭp″ĭ-lĭ-dī′ă-sĭs) Infestation with the tapeworm *Dipylidium caninum.*

Dipylidium (dĭp″ĭ-lĭd′ē-ŭm) [Gr. *dipylos,* having two entrances] A genus of tapeworms belonging to the family Dipylidiae that infests dogs and cats.

D. caninum A common parasite of dogs and cats. Occasionally, human infestation may occur through the accidental ingestion of lice or fleas, which serve as the intermediate host.

diquat (dī′kwăt) A herbicide, chemically related to paraquat, that releases hydrogen peroxide and oxygen radicals when consumed. It can cause nausea, vomiting, renal failure, altered mental status, and cardiac arrhythmias.

directionality The ability to perceive one's position in relation to the environment; the sense of direction. Problems with directionality are frequently found in children with learning disabilities or suspected minimal brain dysfunction.

direction, direct medical Giving a physician's medical orders, on-line, on the radio, or on the telephone, to the EMS providers at the scene of an emergency.

direct light reflex Prompt contraction of the sphincter of the iris when light entering through the pupil strikes the retina.

directly observed therapy ABBR: DOT. Oral administration of a drug(s) to a patient and observing to ensure the drug is swallowed. DOT is especially important in treating patients with infectious diseases (such as tuberculosis) in which development of drug-resistant microorganisms is likely to threaten public health if the drug is not taken exactly as prescribed.

director A grooved device for guiding a knife in surgery.

direct reflex A reflex in which response occurs on the same side as the stimulus.

dirigomotor (dĭr″i-gō-mō′tor) [L. *dirigere,* to direct, + *motor,* mover] Controlling or directing muscular activity.

Dirofilaria (dī″rō-fĭ-lā′rē-ă) A genus of filariae.

D. immitis Heartworm, a species of filariae that occurs in dogs, but may infest humans.

dis- [L. *dis,* apart] Prefix indicating *free of, undone from.*

dis- [Gr. *dis,* twice] Prefix meaning *double* or *twice.*

disability (dĭs″ă-bĭl′ĭ-tē) Any physical, mental, or functional impairment that limits a major activity. It may be partial or complete. The definition of disability is controversial. To some experts it refers to any restriction or inability to perform socially defined roles or tasks that are expected of an individual in specific social contexts. Another concept of disability is that it is any restriction or lack of ability to perform tasks or roles in the manner previously considered normal for an individual. SYN: *activity limitation; functional limitation.* SEE: *death* for table; *handicap.*

developmental d. A condition due to congenital abnormality, trauma, deprivation, or disease that interrupts or delays the sequence and rate of normal growth, development, and maturation.

excess d. The discrepancy that exists when a person's functional limitations are greater than those warranted by the objective degree of impairment. Often excess disability is created by attitudes and policies that create barriers to a disabled person's full participation.

learning d. Learning disorder.

disability analysis The attempt to determine the relative importance of life events that contribute to functional impairments. Determining the relationship between occupational or other exposures and the development of chronic illness is often a complex task. For example, chronic obstructive lung diseases may result from non-occupational factors such as tobacco abuse or genetic illnesses such as alpha-1 antitrypsin disease, or they may result from job-related exposures to chemicals, dusts, or asbestos. Similarly, hearing loss may occur as a natural consequence of aging or as a result of exposures to high levels of noise at work (e.g., with heavy machinery) or during recreation (pursuits such as motorcycle riding or snowmobiling).

disaccharidase (dī-săk′ă-rĭ-dās) A group of enzymes that split disaccharides into monosaccharides.

disaccharide (dī-săk′ĭ-rĭd) [Gr. *dis,* twice, + *sakkharon,* sugar] A carbohydrate composed of two monosaccharides. SEE: *carbohydrate.*

disarticulation [L. *dis,* apart, + *articulus,* joint] Amputation through a joint.

disassimilation [″ + *ad,* to, + *similare,* to make like] The conversion of assimilated material into less complex compounds for energy production.

disaster [″ + L. *astrum,* star, ill-starred] A natural or man-made occurrence such as a flood, tornado, earthquake, forest fire, bridge or building collapse, nuclear reactor accident, war, explosion, terrorist attack or bombing, or train wreck. The need for emergency evacuation and medical services is increased during and following a disaster. It is essential that hospitals and community services have a plan for the expeditious mobilization and use of their services at such times.

disaster medical assistance team ABBR: DMAT. A group of specially trained and readily mobilized medical and rescue workers available to respond to a mass casualty incident on short notice. Team members include physicians, nurses, paramedics, firefighters, and other support personnel.

disaster planning A procedure for coping with mass casualties or massive disruptions of normal health care services as a result of human or natural catastrophes. In the U.S., the Joint Commission on the Accreditation of Health Organizations (JCAHO) requires that all hospitals have a written plan in place, and that drills be performed twice a year to assess the plan's usefulness. The plan should address major problems such as airplane crashes, contamination of the water supply, earthquakes, electrical power failures, explosions, famine, fire, flood, or terrorist attacks. The plan may be for a local community, region or state, and should link health care resources with other public services and the media.

disc SEE: *disk*.

discharge (dĭs-chărj′, dĭs′chărj) [ME. *dischargen,* to discharge] **1.** To release from care; done by a physician, other medical care worker, or a medical care facility. **2.** The escape (esp. by violence) of pent-up or accumulated energy or of explosive material. **3.** The flowing away of a secretion or excretion of pus, feces, urine, and so forth. **4.** The material thus ejected.

cerebrocortical d. The electrical activity of an injured or malfunctioning portion of the cerebral cortex that gives rise to a seizure.

convective d. The discharge from a high-potential source in the form of electrical energy passing through the air to the patient.

disruptive d. The passage of current through an insulating medium due to the breakdown of the medium under electrostatic stress.

lochial d. Uterine excretion following childbirth. SEE: *lochia*.

discharge summary A summary of the hospital or clinic record of a patient, prepared when the patient is released from the medical care facility.

discharging The emission of or the flowing out of material, as the discharge of pus from a lesion; excretion.

discharging lesion A lesion of a nerve center in the brain that suddenly discharges motor impulses.

discipline A branch or domain of knowledge, instruction, or learning. Nursing, medicine, physical therapy, and social work are examples of health-related or professional disciplines. History, sociology, psychology, chemistry, and physics are examples of academic disciplines.

discission (dĭs-sĭzh′ŭn) [L. *dis,* apart, + *scindere,* to cut] Rupture of the capsule of the crystalline lens in cataract surgery.

disclosing agent A diagnostic aid used in dentistry to stain areas of the teeth that are not being cleaned adequately. Typically, a dye such as erythrosine sodium is used to color dental plaque, so that inadequately brushed surfaces can be demonstrated to patients.

discoblastic [″ + *blastos,* germ] Meroblastic.

discoblastula (dĭs″kō-blăs′tū-lă) A modified blastula found in highly telolecithal eggs, as in birds in which the blastomeres form a cellular cap (germinal disk or blastoderm) that is separated from the yolk by a space, the blastocele.

discogenic (dĭs″kō-jĕn′ĭk) [″ + *gennan,* to produce] Caused by an intervertebral disk.

discography (dĭs-kŏg′ră-fē) Use of a contrast medium injected into the intervertebral disk so that it can be examined radiographically.

discoid Like a disk.

disconnection syndrome Disturbance of the visual and language functions of the central nervous system due to interruption of the connections between two cerebral hemispheres in the corpus callosum, occlusion of the anterior cerebral artery, or interruption of the connections between different parts of one hemisphere. These disorders also may be produced by tumors or hypoxia. They can manifest in several ways including the inability, when blindfolded, to match an object held in one hand with that in the other; the inability to execute a command with the right hand but not the left; if blindfolded, the ability to correctly name objects held in the right hand but not those in the left; and the inability to understand spoken language while being able to speak normally. SEE: *inattention, unilateral*.

discoplacenta [Gr. *diskos,* quoit, + *plakous,* a flat cake] A disklike placenta.

discordance (dĭs-kor′dăns) In genetics, the expression of a trait in only one of a twin pair. SEE: *concordance*.

discordant (dĭs-kor′dănt) Resulting from or producing conflict with one's self image.

discovery Pretrial device used to obtain or discover all information, facts, and circumstances surrounding the allegations at issue in the lawsuit so that parties can better prepare for trial. Techniques include interrogatories, requests for production of documents and things, admissions of facts, physical and mental examinations, and depositions.

discrete (dĭs-krēt′) [L. *discretus,* separated] Separate; said of certain eruptions on the skin. SEE: *confluent*.

discrimination [L. *discriminare,* to divide] **1.** The process of distinguishing or differentiating. **2.** Unequal and unfair treatment or denial of privileges without reasonable cause. Federal statutes prohibit discrimination based on age, sex, sexual preference, religion, race, national origin, and disability.

figure-ground d. The ability to see the outline of an object as distinct from visually competing background stimuli. This ability is often impaired following central nervous system damage.

one-point d. The ability to locate specifically a point of pressure on the surface of the skin.

tonal d. The ability to distinguish one tone from another. This is dependent on the integrity of the transverse fibers of the basilar membrane of the organ of Corti.

two-point d. The ability to localize two points of pressure on the surface of the skin and to identify them as discrete sensations. SYN: *tactile discrimination.* SEE: *two-point discrimination test.*

discus [Gr. *diskos,* quoit] Disk.

d. articularis Articular disk.

d. proligerus Cumulus oophorus.

disdiaclast (dĭs-dī′ă-klăst) [Gr. *dis,* twice, + *diaklan,* to break through] A doubly refracting area in the tissues of striated muscles.

disdiadochokinesia (dĭs-dī″ă-dō″kō-kĭ-nē′zē-ă) [L. *dis,* apart, + Gr. *diadochos,* succeeding, + *kinesis,* movement] The inability to make finely coordinated antagonistic movements, as when quickly supinating and pronating the hand. SEE: *diadochokinesia.*

disease (dĭ-zēz′) [Fr. *des,* from, + *aise,* ease] A condition marked by subjective complaints, a specific history, and clinical signs, symptoms, and laboratory or radiographic findings. The concepts of disease and illness differ in that disease is usually tangible or measurable, whereas illness (and associated pain, suffering, or distress) is highly individual and personal. Thus, a person may have a serious but symptom-free disease (e.g., hypertension) without any illness. Conversely, a person may be extremely ill (e.g., with posttraumatic stress disorder) but have no obvious evidence of disease.

acute d. A disease having a rapid onset and relatively short duration.

anticipated d. A disease that may be predicted to occur in individuals with a certain genetic, physical, or environmental predisposition.

aortic branch d. Takayasu's arteritis.

autoimmune d. A disease produced when the body's normal tolerance of the antigens on its own cells (i.e., self-antigens or autoantigens [AAg]) is disrupted. Current theories are that the loss of self-tolerance is the result of damage to AAgs by microorganisms, a strong similarity in appearance between the AAg and a foreign antigen, or a foreign antigen linking with an AAg. Autoantibodies (AAbs) produced either by B lymphocytes or self-reacting T lymphocytes attack normal cells whose surface contains a "self" antigen, or autoantigen, destroying the tissue. Both inherited risk factors and environmental factors are considered significant in the development of autoimmune disease. Researchers have found links between AAb production and the inheritance of certain histocompatibility antigens, indicating that genetic susceptibility is probably a component in autoimmune diseases. Other unknown factors within the immune system may prevent it from stopping the abnormal inflammatory process once it has begun.

Many diseases are based on AAb-AAg reactions. Systemic lupus erythematosus and rheumatoid arthritis are autoimmune diseases in which multiple tissues are affected. Some autoimmune disorders manifest themselves primarily in only one or two tissues (even though they too are systemic). The damage to cardiac valves in rheumatic fever occurs because AAgs on the valves are similar in structure to antigens on Group A beta-hemolytic streptococci. Insulin-dependent diabetes mellitus is caused by AAb destruction of the islets of Langerhans, and multiple sclerosis is caused by AAb destruction of the myelin sheath covering nerves. Hemolytic anemia, some forms of glomerulonephritis, myasthenia gravis, chronic thyroiditis, Reiter's syndrome, and Graves' disease are additional examples of autoimmune diseases. SEE: *antigen; autoantibody; autoantigen; autoimmunity; histocompatability locus antigen; inflammation.*

Blount's d. SEE: *Blount's disease.*

cardiovascular d. ABBR: CVD. Any disease of the heart or blood vessels, including atherosclerosis, cardiomyopathy, coronary artery disease, peripheral vascular disease, and others.

cat scratch d. A febrile disease characterized by lymphadenitis, and in some cases conjunctivitis, uveitis, endocarditis, osteomyelitis, or central nervous system infections, transmitted to people by cats, esp. kittens. Fever, malaise, headache, and anorexia accompany the lymphadenopathy. The causative organism is *Bartonella henselae* (formerly *Rochalimaea*), a gram-negative rod that in cats usually produces asymptomatic infection. Diagnosis is based on clinical findings combined with the history of cat contact and positive results from a cat scratch antigen skin test. Antibiotics are not recommended in mild disease but aminoglycosides, quinolones, or macrolides may be indicated for severe, disseminated disease. SEE: *bacillary angiomatosis; Bartonella; Nursing Diagnoses Appendix.*

PATIENT CARE: The patient is assessed for related symptoms and a history of cat contact. Prescribed cat scratch antigen skin testing is explained and administered. The patient is taught how to use hot compresses, and how to handle and dispose of contaminated dressings. He or she also is advised to report headache, sore throat, stiff neck, and ongoing fever (especially if accompanied by chills or night sweats), as these may be indicators of rare complications. The patient is referred for further immune system evaluation if immunodeficiency is suspected.

celiac d. SEE: *celiac sprue.*

chronic d. A disease having a slow onset and lasting for a long period of time.

chronic granulomatous d. ABBR: CGD. A rare, congenital, and often fatal immunodeficiency marked by recurrent infections caused by a defect in white blood cells. The polymorphonuclear leukocytes of affected children are able to ingest but not kill certain bacteria. Chronic granulomatous disease occurs mostly in boys with X-linked (i.e., sex-linked) inheritance, although an autosomal recessive variant of the disease is also known. Twenty percent of reported cases occur in girls. Manifestations of this disease include widespread granulomatous lesions of the skin, lungs, and lymph nodes. Also present are hypergammaglobulinemia, anemia, and leukocytosis.

SCREENING: The nitroblue tetrazolium test is used for screening high-risk persons (e.g., family members).

SYMPTOMS: Symptoms include chronic and acute infections of the skin, liver, lymph nodes, intestinal tract, and bone, often involving bacteria or other microorganisms that usually do not cause infections in patients with normal immune function. SEE: *phagocytosis*.

TREATMENT: The course of the disease has improved owing to continual or intermittent antibiotic use and the advent of bone marrow transplantation. Interferon therapy and gene therapy are being investigated as possible cures.

chronic obstructive lung d. ABBR: COLD. Chronic obstructive pulmonary d.

chronic obstructive pulmonary d. ABBR: COPD. A group of debilitating, progressive and potentially fatal lung diseases that have in common increased resistance to air movement, prolongation of the expiratory phase of respiration, and loss of the normal elasticity of the lung. The chronic obstructive lung diseases include emphysema, chronic obstructive bronchitis, chronic bronchitis, and asthmatic bronchitis. Taken together they make up the fourth most common cause of death in the U.S. SYN: *chronic obstructive lung d.*

ETIOLOGY: Most patients with chronic airflow limitations are now or once were smokers, and their lung disease is a direct consequence of the toxic effects of tobacco smoke on the lung. A smaller number have been exposed to environmental tobacco smoke or to dusts or smoke at work. Individuals who are genetically lacking the enzyme α-1 antitrypsin also develop COPD, typically at an earlier age than smokers (in their 40s instead of their 50s or 60s); this disease affects approximately 1 person in 2000 in the U.S.

SYMPTOMS: All of the diseases in this group are marked by difficulty breathing during exertion, as well as chronic cough and sputum production.

TREATMENT: Quitting smoking is the cornerstone of disease management because it slows the deterioration of lung function in COPD. Additional preventive therapies include influenza and pneumococcal vaccinations. Drugs for COPD have variable effectiveness, and only a few are benign. Most patients will be treated with an inhaled anticholinergic drug (ipratropium). Supplemental oxygen decreases mortality and improves the quality of life in patients with severe COPD. The beta-agonist drugs (e.g., albuterol) are much less useful in COPD than in asthma, and may be completely ineffective. Theophylline can be used, but careful management of drug levels is needed to avoid toxicity and drug interactions. Inhaled or oral steroid therapy helps with any inflammatory component of the illness, but long-term use of steroids can cause side effects such as diabetes, psychological disturbances, osteoporosis, thinning of the skin, and cataracts. Pulmonary rehabilitation programs are helpful.

When patients have acute worsening of their breathing difficulties ("exacerbations") high-dose corticosteroids and antibiotics are frequently beneficial.

PATIENT CARE: The respiratory therapist teaches breathing and coughing exercises and postural drainage to strengthen respiratory muscles and to mobilize secretions. The patient is encouraged to participate in a pulmonary rehabilitation program, as well as to stop smoking and avoid other respiratory irritants. Patients are instructed to avoid contact with other persons with respiratory infections and taught the use of prescribed prophylactic antibiotics and bronchodilator therapy. Frequent small meals and adequate fluid intake are encouraged. The patient's schedule alternates periods of activity with rest. The patient and family are assisted with disease-related lifestyle changes and are encouraged to express their feelings and concerns about the illness and its treatment.

The respiratory therapist monitors arterial blood gases and pulmonary function studies to determine the extent of the disease and proper treatment in consultation with the attending physician. Acute exacerbation occurs when the patient acquires a respiratory infection or other complication and must be recognized and treated promptly. Aerosol and humidity therapy is useful to thin thick sputum and promote bronchial hygiene. Low-concentration oxygen therapy is applied as needed to keep the PAO_2 between 60 and 80 mm Hg. Aerosolized bronchodilators are used to reduce dyspnea and promote improved cough. Mechanical ventilation is reserved for the patient in acute respiratory failure due to a superimposed condition that is reversible and not responding to initial therapy.

CAUTION: 1. In hypoxic patients, oxygen therapy must be adjusted carefully to optimize arterial oxygen saturation. 2. Before traveling on airplanes, patients with COPD should consult their health care providers about special oxygen needs.

communicable d. A disease that may be transmitted directly or indirectly from one individual to another. SEE: table; *Standard and Universal Precautions Appendix.*

complicating d. A disease that occurs during the course of another disease.

congenital d. A disease that is present at birth. It may be due to hereditary factors, prenatal infection, injury, or the effect of a drug the mother took during pregnancy.

connective tissue d. ABBR: CTD. A group of diseases that affect connective tissue, including muscle, cartilage, tendons, vessels, skin, and ligaments. CTDs may be acute but are usually chronic. They may be localized or systemic and are marked by inflammatory or autoimmune injury. Examples of such diseases include systemic lupus erythematosus, rheumatoid arthritis, systemic sclerosis, and the vasculitides.

contagious d. Any disease (usually an infectious disease) readily transmitted from one person to another.

cystine storage d. An inherited disease of cystine metabolism resulting in abnormal deposition of cystine in body tissues. The cause is disordered proximal renal tubular function. Clinically, the child fails to grow and develops rickets, corneal opacities, and acidosis.

deficiency d. A condition due to lack of a substance essential in body metabolism. The deficiency may be due to inadequate intake, digestion, absorption, or use of foods, minerals, water, or vitamins. It may also be due to excess loss through excretion or to an intestinal parasite such as hookworm or tapeworm. Deficiency diseases include night blindness and keratomalacia (caused by lack of vitamin A); beriberi and polyneuritis (lack of thiamine); pellagra (lack of niacin); scurvy (lack of vitamin C); rickets and osteomalacia (lack of vitamin D); pernicious anemia (lack of gastric intrinsic factor and vitamin B_{12}).

degenerative d. An illness resulting from the deterioration of tissues and organs, characteristic of aging or repetitive injury.

degenerative joint d. Osteoarthritis.

demyelinating d. A disturbance of nerve cells due to destruction of their myelin sheaths.

de Quervain's d. de Quervain's tenosynovitis.

endemic d. A disease that is present more or less continuously, or recurs frequently, in a community.

epidemic d. A disease that attacks a large number of individuals in a community at the same time.

epizootic d. An epidemic that affects animals of a particular area, usually in a short period of time.

extrapyramidal d. Any of several degenerative diseases of the nervous system that involve the extrapyramidal system and the basal ganglion of the brain. Symptoms include tremors, chorea, athetosis, and dystonia. Parkinsonism is a form of extrapyramidal disease.

familial d. A disease that occurs in several members of the same family.

fibrocystic d. of the breast A nonspecific diagnosis for a condition marked by palpable lumps in the breasts, usually associated with pain and tenderness, that fluctuate with the menstrual cycle. At least 50% of women of reproductive age have palpably irregular breasts caused by this condition. SYN: *cystic mastitis.* SEE: *breast self-examination.*

Women with fibrocystic breast disease have a two to five times greater risk of developing breast cancer. Some women with this disease have atypical hyperplasia in the lesion. If these patients also have a family history of breast cancer, their risk of developing breast cancer is greatly increased. They should have a breast examination every 6 months and mammography once a year.

TREATMENT: Fine-needle aspiration or another tissue sampling technique may be used to establish the diagnosis. Severe discomfort may be reduced by prescribing a mild daily diuretic to be taken 7 to 10 days before each menses. Androgenic hormone therapy (Danazol) may relieve pain and reduce nodularity. Pain and tenderness subside within a month of starting therapy, but nodule elimination may require up to 6 months. Symptoms return on Danazol cessation.

PATIENT CARE: Emotional support is provided for women who have a heightened awareness and fear of developing breast cancer. Patient teaching includes discussing and demonstrating breast self-examination, with emphasis placed on the importance of monthly self-exams, periodic mammography, and annual examinations by a health care professional. The accuracy of the patient's self-exam is evaluated by asking her to locate any currently palpable lumps and to describe the present contour and texture (feel) of her breasts. Self-care techniques include limiting intake of caffeine and foods containing

Method of Transmission of Some Common Communicable Diseases

Disease	How Agent Leaves the Body	How Organisms May Be Transmitted	Method of Entry into the Body
Acquired immunodeficiency syndrome (AIDS)	Blood, semen, or other body fluids, including breast milk	Sexual contact Contact with blood or mucous membranes or by way of contaminated syringes Placental transmission	Reproductive tract Contact with blood Placental transmission Breastfeeding
Cholera	Feces	Water or food contaminated with feces	Mouth to intestine
Diphtheria	Sputum and discharges from nose and throat Skin lesions (rare)	Droplet infection from patient coughing	Through mouth or nose to throat
Gonococcal disease	Discharges from infected mucous membranes	Sexual activity	Reproductive tract or any mucous membrane
Hepatitis A, viral	Feces	Food or water contaminated with feces	Mouth to intestine
Hepatitis B, viral and delta hepatitis	Blood and serum-derived fluids, including semen and vaginal fluids	Contact with blood and body fluids	Exposure to body fluids including during sexual activity, injection drug abuse, or surgery Contact with blood
Hepatitis C	Blood and other body fluids	Parenteral drug use Laboratory exposure to blood Health care workers exposed to blood (i.e., dentists and their assistants, and clinical and laboratory staff)	Infected blood Contaminated needles Cuts; mucosal exposures
Hookworm	Feces	Cutaneous contact with soil polluted with feces Eggs in feces hatch in sandy soil	Larvae enter through skin (esp. of feet), migrate through the body, and settle in small intestine
Influenza	As in pneumonia	Respiratory droplets or objects contaminated with discharges	As in pneumonia
Leprosy	Cutaneous or mucosal lesions that contain bacilli Respiratory droplets	Cutaneous contact or nasal discharges of untreated patients	Nose or broken skin

Method of Transmission of Some Common Communicable Diseases

Disease	How Agent Leaves the Body	How Organisms May Be Transmitted	Method of Entry into the Body
Measles (rubeola)	As in streptococcal pharyngitis	As in streptococcal pharyngitis	As in streptococcal pharyngitis
Meningitis, meningococcal	Discharges from nose and throat	Respiratory droplets	Mouth and nose
Mumps	Discharges from infected glands and mouth	Respiratory droplets and saliva	Mouth and nose
Ophthalmia neonatorum (gonococcal infection of eyes of newborn)	Vaginal secretions of infected mother	Contact with infected areas of vagina of infected mother during birth	Directly on conjunctiva
Pertussis	Discharges from respiratory tract	Respiratory droplets	Mouth and nose
Pneumonia	Sputum and discharges from nose and throat	Respiratory droplets	Through mouth and nose to lungs
Poliomyelitis	Discharges from nose and throat, and via feces	Respiratory droplets Contaminated water	Through mouth and nose
Rubella	As in streptococcal pharyngitis	As in streptococcal pharyngitis	As in streptococcal pharyngitis
Streptococcal pharyngitis	Discharges from nose and throat	Respiratory droplets	Through mouth and nose
Syphilis	Lesions	Sexual intercourse; contact with skin or mucous membrane lesions	Directly into blood and tissues through breaks in skin or membrane
	Blood	Contaminated needles and syringes	Contaminated needles and syringes
	Transfer through placenta to fetus		
Trachoma	Discharges from infected eyes	Cutaneous contact Hands, towels, handkerchiefs	Directly on conjunctiva
Tuberculosis, bovine		Milk from infected cow	Mouth to intestine
Tuberculosis, human	Sputum	Droplet infection from person coughing with mouth uncovered	Through nose to lungs or intestines
Typhoid fever	Feces and urine	Food or water contaminated with feces, or urine from patients	Through mouth via infected food or water and thence to intestinal tract

methylxanthines, consuming a low-salt premenstrual diet, and taking supplementary vitamin E.

If pain and tenderness are bothersome, suggestions may include using aspirin or other nonsteroidal anti-inflammatory over-the-counter drugs and wearing a well-fitting brassiere day and night. Women for whom Danazol has been prescribed are instructed to take the medication precisely as prescribed, to discontinue the use of oral contraceptives, and to use an alternative technique of birth control. The patient is instructed about signs and symptoms to report promptly to the primary caregiver and about the importance of return visits as scheduled.

fibrocystic d. of the pancreas Cystic fibrosis.

fifth d. Erythema infectiosum.

focal d. A disease located at a specific and distinct area such as the tonsils, adenoids, or a boil.

food-borne d. Illnesses caused by the ingestion of contaminated or toxic nutrients. Among the food-borne diseases are infectious diarrheas (e.g., those caused by *Salmonella, Shigella,* cholera, *Escherichia coli, Campylobacter*); helminth diseases (e.g., those caused by beef, pork, or pike tapeworms); protozoan infections (e.g., giardiasis); food poisoning (toxins produced by *Bacillus cereus, Staphylococcus aureus, Clostridium botulinum,* mushrooms, or ciguatera); and viral illnesses (esp. hepatitis A).

Proper selection, collection, preparation, and serving of food can reduce the risk of food-borne disease, esp. if combined with regular inspections of food-service facilities and periodic evaluations of food-service workers.

foot and mouth d. A viral disease of cattle and horses that is rarely transmitted to humans.

SYMPTOMS: In humans, symptoms include fever, headache, and malaise with dryness and burning sensation of the mouth. Vesicles develop on the lips, tongue, mouth, palms, and soles.

TREATMENT: Therapy is symptomatic. Full recovery occurs in 2 to 3 weeks. A variety of preventive vaccines are available.

functional d. A general term for inorganic disease or a disease in which organic changes are not evident; a disturbance of the function of any organ.

gestational trophoblastic d. ABBR: GTD. Any of several neoplastic diseases of the fetal chorion, including complete and partial hydatidiform mole, chorioadenoma destruens, and choriocarcinoma. Sudden rapid uterine enlargement and early second-trimester vaginal bleeding characterize all forms of GTD. Other common signs include hyperemesis gravidarum, pregnancy-induced hypertension before 24 weeks' gestation, vaginal discharge of hydropic vesicles, and an absence of fetal heart tones.

TREATMENT: Aggressive forms of GTD (e.g., choriocarcinoma), which can metastasize throughout the body, are treated with chemotherapy, radiation therapy, and surgery. Moles and chorioadenoma destruens are treated with prompt evacuation of the uterus.

PATIENT CARE: Close follow-up care of patients with GTD is needed to detect recurrent disease before it has a chance to spread. Quantitative serum hCG levels should be drawn every 2 weeks until normal, then monthly for 1 year. Affected women should avoid pregnancy during the year-long follow-up period. SEE: *choriocarcinoma*.

glucuronidase deficiency d. mucopolysaccharidosis VII.

glycogen storage d. SEE: *glycogen storage disease*.

heavy chain d. A group of diseases involving serum immunoglobulins. The globulins contain heavy chain subunits. If immunoglobulin A is affected, abdominal lymphoma and malabsorption occur. If immunoglobulin D is involved, a clinical picture similar to multiple myeloma is present. If immunoglobulin G is affected, there are lymphadenopathy, weakness, weight loss, and repeated bacterial infections. If immunoglobulin M is involved, the lymphadenopathy affects the abdominal lymph nodes, the liver, and the spleen. Bence Jones proteinuria is present.

hemolytic d. of the newborn Erythroblastosis fetalis.

hemorrhagic d. of the newborn A bleeding tendency in newborns characterized by melena, purpura, and prothrombin deficiency. The disease is self-limiting.

hereditary d. A disease due to genetic factors transmitted from parent to offspring.

hookworm d. Hookworm.

hydatid d. The disease produced by the cysts of the larval stage of the tapeworm *Echinococcus*. SYN: *echinococcosis*. SEE: *hydatid*.

iatrogenic d. A disease caused by or arising as a complication of medical or surgical intervention.

idiopathic d. A disease for which no causative factor can be recognized.

infectious d. Any disease caused by growth of pathogenic microorganisms in the body. SEE: *quarantine; incubation* for table.

inflammatory bowel d. ABBR: IBD. The term for a number of chronic, relapsing inflammatory diseases of the gastrointestinal tract of unknown etiology. The two most common types are ulcerative colitis and Crohn's disease.

PATHOLOGY: Ulcerative colitis is limited to the superficial layers of the wall of the colon, whereas Crohn's disease may involve all layers of the bowel wall, from the oropharynx to the anus. The inflammation of ulcerative colitis is continuous throughout the affected bowel, producing a raw, ulcerated, or effaced lumen. In contrast, Crohn's disease is characterized by patchy areas of granulomatous inflammation, creating a cobblestoned mucosal surface that may develop deep fissures or a thickened, rubbery texture. In Crohn's disease but not ulcerative colitis, fistulas to adjacent sections of the bowel, vagina, and bladder may develop.

DIAGNOSIS: Barium studies of the upper and lower gastrointestinal tract and endoscopic examinations are used to diagnose IBD.

intercurrent d. A disease occurring during the course of another, unrelated disease.

ion channel d. A group of diseases marked clinically by muscular weakness, absent muscle tone, or episodic muscular paralysis. The diseases are caused by congenital defects in the cell membrane proteins that move ions into and out of the cell. These defects alter the cells' resting potential, action potential, or both, and make them "fire" ineffectively.

iron storage d. Hemochromatosis.

kinky hair d. A congenital syndrome caused by an autosomal recessive gene, consisting of short, sparse, often poorly pigmented, kinky hair and physical and mental retardation. The disease is due to a metabolic defect that causes an abnormality in the fatty acid composition of the gray matter of the brain. Death follows progressive severe degenerative changes in the central nervous system.

Lenegre's d. SEE: *Lenegre's disease.*

lysosomal storage d. A disease caused by deficiency of specific lysosomal enzymes that normally degrade glycoproteins, glycolipids, or mucopolysaccharides. Thus, the substances that cannot be catabolized accumulate in lysosomes. Specific enzymes account for specific storage diseases. Included in this group are Gaucher's, Hurler's, Tay-Sachs, Niemann-Pick, Fabry's, Morquio's, Scheie's, and Maroteaux-Lamy diseases.

mad cow d. Bovine spongiform encephalopathy.

malignant d. **1.** Cancer. **2.** A disease, including but not limited to cancer, in which the progress is extremely rapid and generally threatening or resulting in death within a short time.

Mediterranean d. Thalassemia.

metabolic d. A disease due to abnormal biochemistry, usually as a result of an absent or deficient enzyme. Metabolic diseases also are known as inborn errors of metabolism.

mixed connective tissue d. ABBR: MCTD. A rare disease that combines the signs and symptoms of several connective tissue diseases, including systemic lupus erythematosus, scleroderma, rheumatoid arthritis, and/or polymyositis. The cause is unknown.

motor neuron d. One of several diseases of the motor neurons: progressive muscular atrophy, progressive bulbar palsy, and amyotrophic lateral sclerosis. These diseases are marked by degeneration of anterior horn cells of the spinal cord, the motor cranial nerve nuclei, and the corticospinal tracts. They occur principally in men. In the U.S., amyotrophic lateral sclerosis is commonly known as Lou Gehrig's disease, named for a well-known athlete whose baseball career and life ended prematurely as a result of this disease.

notifiable d. In the U.S., a disease or condition that is under surveillance by public health officials (e.g., at the Centers for Disease Control and Prevention or the Council of State and Territorial Epidemiologists) typically because of its widespread effects on public health or its explosive consequences. Regulations require that clinical or laboratory staff report instances of the Hantavirus pulmonary syndrome, meningococcal disease, yellow fever, elevated blood lead levels, silicosis, tobacco use, and many other illnesses to public health authorities. SYN: *reportable d.*

occupational d. A disease resulting from factors associated with the occupation in which the patient is engaged.

organic d. A disease resulting from recognizable anatomical changes in an organ or tissue of the body.

pandemic d. An extremely widespread epidemic disease involving populations in large geographic areas.

parasitic d. A disease resulting from the growth and development of parasitic organisms (plants or animals) in or on the body.

periodontal d. SEE: *periodontitis.*

polycystic kidney d. ABBR: PKD. Any of several hereditary disorders in which cysts form in the kidneys and other organs, eventually destroying kidney tissue and function. The autosomal recessive form usually appears in early childhood; the autosomal dominant form usually develops later in life. Definitive treatments are dialysis and kidney transplant. Because cerebral aneurysms are commonly found in adults with PKD, patients with this disorder are often screened with computed tomography or magnetic resonance imaging studies of the brain.

psychosomatic d. An outdated term for a somatoform disorder, that is, a physical illness caused or exacerbated by psychological factors. Conditions in the general category of psychosomatic disorders are neurodermatitis, mass psychogenic illness and some forms of noncardiac chest pain.

NOTE: It is not possible for a human being to be consciously sick without some interplay between the emotions and the bodily functions.

pulmonary veno-occlusive d. A condition that may complicate organ transplantation rejection. It is marked by extensive occlusion of the small and medium-sized veins of the lung by loose, sparsely cellular, fibrous tissue. Some larger veins may be involved. This disease produces severe pulmonary venous hypertension.

reactive airway d. Any disease in which there is reversible bronchospasm, such as asthma. SEE: *asthma*.

reportable d. Notifiable d.

restrictive lung d. Any chest disease that results in reduced lung volumes.

secondary d. A disease caused by another disease, as when obesity causes diseases of the joints and muscles of the lower limbs due to the increased trauma of transporting and supporting the added weight.

self-limited d. A disease that eventually goes away even if untreated.

storage d. A disorder involving abnormal deposition of a substance in body tissues. SEE: *glycogen storage disease; Wilson's disease.*

subacute d. A disease in which symptoms are less pronounced but more prolonged than in an acute disease; this type is intermediate between acute and chronic disease.

systemic d. A generalized disease rather than a localized or focal one.

thyrotoxic heart d. A disease due to increased activity of the thyroid gland, marked by cardiac enlargement, atrial fibrillation, and high-output heart failure. SEE: *thyrotoxicosis*.

trophoblastic d. ABBR: TD. Any neoplasm of trophoblastic origin. SEE: *chorioadenoma destruens; choriocarcinoma; hydatid mole*.

venereal d. ABBR: VD. Sexually transmitted disease.

disease burden The total effect of a disease or diseases on an individual as well as society. Knowledge concerning this is important, particularly in attempting to plan prevention programs and in evaluating the success or failure of intervention. However, without a rational system for measuring disease burden, the concept is of little value. In 1993 the disease-adjusted life-year (DALY) concept was described in a publication from the World Bank. It is based on the quantitation not only of mortality but also of suffering and loss of health. Data obtained using the DALY concept permit establishing the priority for treating specific diseases and conditions. The goal of global disease assessments is to allot research and treatment resources according to where they would have the best chance to make a difference in alleviating suffering and prevention of death from specific illnesses.

Disease State Management Program ABBR: DSM. A program of health care specific to a designated population (i.e., diabetic patients), offering an organized, systematic pathway to guide clinicians and patients through predetermined steps to measurable outcomes. The program encompasses five elements: clinical guidelines, a coordinated delivery system, health care provider support, patient support and education, and outcomes management.

disengagement [Fr.] **1.** The emergence of the fetal head from within the maternal pelvis. **2.** Any withdrawal from participation in customary social activity. **3.** In psychiatry, autonomous functioning with little or no emotional attachment and a distorted sense of independence.

disentanglement A rescue technique used to free a trapped victim that involves removing the wreckage from around the patient (rather than removing the patient from the wreckage). For example, freeing a person trapped in a crushed car often requires the car to be pried apart with heavy rescue tools capable of cutting through metal.

disequilibrium (dĭs-ē″kwĭ-lĭb′rē-ŭm) [L. *dis,* apart, + *aequus,* equal, + *libra,* balance] An unequal and unstable equilibrium.

disequilibrium syndrome Dialysis disequilibrium.

disharmony Lack of harmony; discord.

disinfect (dĭs-ĭn-fĕkt′) [″ + *inficere,* to corrupt] To free from infection by physical or chemical means.

disinfectant A substance that prevents infection by killing bacteria. Most disinfectants are used on equipment or surfaces rather than in or on the body. Common disinfectants are halogens: chlorine, iodine; salts of heavy metals: mercuric chloride (bichloride of mercury), silver nitrate; boric acid; chloride of lime; organic compounds: formaldehyde, alcohol 70%, iodoform, organic acids, phenol (carbolic acid), cresols, benzoic and salicylic acids and their sodium salts; and miscellaneous substances: thymol, hydrogen peroxide, potassium permanganate, ethylene oxide. The term is usually applied to a chemical or physical agent that kills vegetative forms of microorganisms.

disinfection The application of a disinfectant to materials and surfaces to destroy pathogenic microorganisms.

concurrent d. Prompt disinfection and suitable disposal of infected excreta during the entire course of a disease.

d. of field of operation Disinfection of the area of the body where surgery is to be performed. Universally accepted fields of preparation for most surgical procedures have been widely published. Preparation should extend well beyond the operative site. A variety of disinfection solutions are available, including povidone-iodine, benzalkonium chloride, and chlorhexidine gluconate. These agents may be used in aqueous or soap-based preparations. Mucous membranes may be cleansed by nonirritating agents or not at all.

CAUTION: The mucous membranes are active, absorbing surfaces, and therefore solutions of some potent antiseptics may not be used in these areas. In the past, the use of mercury-based antiseptics in the vagina, uterus, or rectum resulted in serious poisoning and in some instances death.

---

terminal d. Disinfection of the room and infected materials at the end of the infectious stage of a disease.

disinfestation (dĭs″ĭn-fĕs-tā′shŭn) [L. *dis,* apart, + *infestare,* to strike at] The process of killing infesting insects or parasites.

disinhibition (dĭs″ĭn-hĭ-bĭsh′ŭn) **1.** Abolition or countering of inhibition. **2.** In psychiatry, freedom to act in accordance with one's drives with a decrease in social or cultural constraint. **3.** Loss of typical behavioral or social restraints. Unusually outgoing, intrusive, loud, or disruptive behaviors (e.g., in mania or in diseases that affect the frontal lobes of the brain) are exhibited.

disinsertion Detachment of the retina at its periphery. SYN: *retinodialysis.*

disintegration [″ + *integer,* entire] **1.** The product of catabolism; the falling apart of the constituents of a substance. **2.** Disorganization of the psyche.

disjoint To disarticulate or to separate bones from their natural positions in a joint.

disjunction (dĭs-jŭnk′shŭn) Separation of the homologous pairs of chromosomes during anaphase of the first meiotic division.

disk [Gr. *diskos,* a disk] A flat, round, platelike structure. SYN: *disc.*

anisotropic d. SEE: *band, A.*

articular d. The biconcave oval disk of fibrous connective tissue that separates the two joint cavities of the temporomandibular joint on each side.

choked d. A swollen optic disk due to inflammation or edema. SYN: *papilledema.*

dental d. A thin circular paper or other substance carrying polishing or cutting materials; it is driven by a dental engine and used in a variety of procedures with natural or artificial teeth.

embryonic d. An oval disk of cells in the blastocyst of a mammal from which the embryo proper develops. Its lower layer, the endoderm, forms the roof of the yolk sac. Its upper layer, the ectoderm, forms the floor of the amniotic cavity. The primitive streak develops on the upper surface of the disk. SEE: *embryo* for illus.

epiphyseal d. A disk of cartilage at the junction of the diaphysis and epiphyses of growing long bones. Cartilage synthesis provides for growth in length; eventually the cartilage is replaced by bone.

germinal d. A disk of cells on the surface of the yolk of a teloblastic egg from which the embryo develops. SYN: *proligerous d.; blastoderm.*

herniated intervertebral d. A rupture of the nucleus pulposus, causing pain and impingement of spinal nerves. SYN: *slipped d.* SEE: *herniation of nucleus pulposus* for illus.

intercalated d. A modification of the cell membrane of adjacent cardiac muscle cells; it contains intercellular junctions for electrical and mechanical linkage of contiguous cells.

intervertebral d. The fibrocartilaginous tissue between the vertebral bodies. The outer portion is the anulus fibrosus; the inner portion is the nucleus pulposus. The disk is a shock absorber, or cushion, and permits movement.

M d. M line.

Merkel's d. The tiny expanded end of a sensory nerve fiber found in the epidermis and in the epithelial root sheath of a hair. SYN: *tactile d.*

optic d. The area of the retina where the optic nerve enters. SYN: *blind spot* (1).

proligerous d. Germinal d.

slipped d. Lay term for *herniated intervertebral disk.*

tactile d. Merkel's d.

Z d. Z line.

diskectomy (dĭs-kĕk′tō-mē) Surgical removal of a herniated intervertebral disk.

diskiform (dĭs′kĭ-form) Shaped like a dish or disk.

diskitis (dĭsk-ī′tĭs) [Gr. *diskos,* disk, + *itis,* inflammation] Inflammation of a disk, esp. an interarticular cartilage. SYN: *meniscitis.*

dislocation [L. *dis,* apart, + *locare,* to place] The displacement of any part, esp. the temporary displacement of a bone from its normal position in a joint.

closed d. Simple d.

complete d. A dislocation that separates the surfaces of a joint completely.

complicated d. A dislocation associated with other major injuries.

compound d. A dislocation in which the joint communicates with the external air.

condylar d. In the jaw, a displacement of the mandibular condyle in front of the condylar eminence. It is often caused by keeping the mouth wide open for an extended time, as in dental treatment that involves a rubber dam. SEE: *subluxation*.

congenital d. A dislocation existing from or before birth.

consecutive d. A dislocation in which the luxated bone has changed position since its first displacement.

divergent d. A dislocation in which the ulna and radius are displaced separately. It also may involve the tibia and fibula.

habitual d. A dislocation that often recurs after replacement.

incomplete d. A slight displacement. SYN: *Partial d.* SEE: *subluxation* (1).

mandibular d. SEE: *subluxation*.

metacarpophalangeal joint d. The dislocation of the joint between the carpals and the phalanges, usually involving the index finger or small finger of the hand. The dislocation may be simple and respond to closed manipulation or be complex and require surgery.

Monteggia's d. A dislocation of the hip joint in which the head of the femur is near the anterosuperior spine of the ilium.

Nélaton's d. Dislocation of the ankle in which the talus is forced up between the end of the tibia and the fibula.

old d. A dislocation in which no reduction has been accomplished even after many days, weeks, or months.

partial d. Incomplete d.

pathological d. A dislocation resulting from paralysis or disease of the joint or supporting tissues.

primitive d. A dislocation in which the bones remain as originally displaced.

recent d. A dislocation seen shortly after it occurred.

simple d. A dislocation in which the joint is not penetrated by a wound. SYN: *closed d.*

slipped d. SEE: *herniated intervertebral disk*.

subastragalar d. Separation of the calcaneum and the scaphoid from the talus.

traumatic d. Dislocation due to injury or violence.

dismember To remove an extremity or a portion of it.

dismutase (dĭs-mū′tās) An enzyme that acts on two molecules of the same substance. One of these is oxidized and the other reduced; two new compounds are thus produced.

superoxide d. An enzyme present in aerobic but not in strictly anaerobic bacteria. It destroys the poisonous, highly reactive free-radical form of O_2, superoxide (O_2^-), formed by flavoenzymes. Thus, aerobic bacteria are protected from the lethal effect of superoxide by the action of this enzyme.

disocclusion Loss of contact between opposing teeth.

disomus (dī-sō′mŭs) [Gr. *dis*, twice, + *soma*, body] A malformed fetus with a double trunk.

disopyramide phosphate (dī-sō-pēr′ă-mīd) A drug used in treating cardiac arrhythmias. Trade name is Norpace.

disorder A pathologic condition of the mind or body. SEE: *disease*.

acute stress d. A disorder characterized by severe anxiety, dissociative symptoms, and depersonalization. Symptoms occur within 1 month of exposure to an extremely traumatic stressor and persist for at least 2 days.

amnestic d. A group of disorders marked by memory disturbance that is due either to the direct physiological effects of a general medical condition or to the persistent effects of a drug, toxin, or similar substance. Affected patients are unable to recall previously learned information or past events, and social or occupational functioning is significantly impaired.

articulation d. Inability to produce speech sounds (phonemes) correctly because of imprecise placement, timing, pressure, speed, or flow of movement of the lips, tongue, or throat.

balance d. Any condition that affects a person's ability to feel steady while walking, sitting, standing, resting, working, or turning. Some common examples include disease of the labyrinth of the ear, cerebellar strokes, and seasickness.

bipolar d. A psychological disorder marked by manic and depressive episodes. Bipolar disorders are divided into four main categories: bipolar I, bipolar II, cyclothymia, and nonspecified disorders. Mania is the essential feature of bipolar I, whereas recurrent moods of both mania and depression mark bipolar II. SEE: *Nursing Diagnoses Appendix.*

TREATMENT: Often the first-line choice of medication is lithium carbonate. If there are concerns about the side effects of lithium or it is found to be ineffective, valproate and carbamazepine may be tried.

body dysmorphic d. ABBR: BDD. A

preoccupation with one or more imagined defects in appearance.

central auditory processing d. Inability to differentiate, recognize, or understand sounds in individuals with normal hearing and intelligence.

character d. A personality disorder manifested by a chronic, habitual, maladaptive pattern of reaction that is relatively inflexible, limits the optimal use of potentialities, and often provokes the responses from the environment that the individual wants to avoid.

childhood disintegrative d. A personality disorder of children marked by regression in many areas of functioning after at least 2 yr of normal development. Individuals exhibit social, communicative, and behavioral characteristics similar to those of autistic disorder. Also called *Heller's syndrome, dementia infantalis,* or *disintegrative psychosis*.

developmental articulation d. Phonological disorder.

developmental coordination d. Exceptional clumsiness, or an unusual delay in meeting motor milestones of childhood, when such a delay results in functional impairment and cannot be attributed to other medical conditions. SYN: *motor skills d.*

d. of written expression An inability to draft grammatically correct phrases, sentences, or paragraphs, which impairs one's advancement in school or work. This communication disorder is said to be present only when 1) it cannot be attributed to sensory, medical, or neurological deficits (such as hearing impairment); and 2) it is an isolated deficit, out of proportion to one's age and measured intelligence.

disruptive behavior d. attention-deficit hyperactivity disorder. SEE: *Nursing Diagnoses Appendix.*

dissociative identity d. Formerly known as "multiple personality disorder," a rare, but increasingly reported, psychiatric illness in which a person has two (or more) distinct personalities. The patient's personalities may vary broadly with respect to interests, communication styles, aggression, and gender. Amnesia for differing personalities is characteristic.

ETIOLOGY: Patients often report a history of abuse in childhood, but whether this causes the syndrome is unknown.

expressive language d. Failure of a child to learn how to speak, write, or use sign language properly, despite having normal understanding of language and otherwise normal cognitive functions. The impairment in language use is apparent in the child's abnormal composition of sentences, frequent grammatical errors, limited word choices, and difficulty in learning new vocabulary.

factitious d. A disorder that is not real, genuine, or natural. The symptoms, physical and psychological, are produced by the individual and are under voluntary control. These symptoms and the behavior are used to pursue a goal (i.e., to assume the role of patient and to stay in a hospital). This is attained by various means, such as taking anticoagulants or other drugs when they are not needed, or feigning pain with nausea and vomiting, dizziness, fainting, fever of unknown origin, or other illnesses. Mental symptoms may include memory loss, hallucinations, and uncooperativeness. Affected patients have a severe personality disturbance. SEE: *malinger; Munchausen syndrome*.

functional d. SEE: *functional illness*.

gender identity d. A disorder marked by a strong cross-gender identification and a persistent discomfort with the biologically assigned sex. Generally, adults with the disorder are preoccupied with the wish to live as a member of the other sex; this often impairs the social, occupational, or other types of functioning. SEE: *Nursing Diagnoses Appendix.*

habit d. A tension-discharging phenomenon such as head banging, body rocking, thumb sucking, nail biting, hair pulling, tics, or teeth grinding, usually beginning in childhood. The habit's importance depends upon its etiology and persistence. Almost all children will demonstrate one or more of these disorders during their development, but if it does not interfere with function it should be of no concern.

impulse-control d. A disorder marked by failure to resist impulses, drives, or temptations that cause harm. Impulse-control disorders include kleptomania, pyromania, pathological gambling, trichotillomania, and intermittent explosive disorder.

inhalant-induced d. Any disease produced by sniffing or breathing toxic vapors, such as those in petroleum distillates. Abuse may lead to anxiety, psychosis, liver disease, and peripheral or central nervous system damage.

intermittent explosive d. A personality disorder marked by episodes of impulsive aggressiveness that are out of proportion to precipitating events. In contrast to amok, a culture-specific, one-time outburst, intermittent explosive disorder is a pattern of behavior. It may result in serious assaults or destruction of property.

late luteal phase dysphoric d. SEE: *premenstrual dysphoric disorder*.

learning d. One of a variety of disorders characterized by difficulty reading, writing, or using mathematical symbols that is two standard deviations below the norm for one's age and otherwise normal intelligence. The condition may become apparent at an early age but usually is not recognized until the child begins formal education in school. The frequency of this condition in boys is five times that in girls. About 5% of children in school use special educational services because of learning disorders.

mental d. An imprecise term for a clinically significant behavioral or psychological syndrome or pattern typically associated with either a distressing symptom or impaired function. It is important to remember that different individuals described as having the same mental disorder are not alike in the way they react to their illness and how they need to be treated.

motor skills d. Developmental coordination d.

myeloproliferative d. Any of several hematologic malignancies marked by the excessive multiplication of one or more types of blood cells. These disorders include polycythemia rubra vera, essential thrombocytosis, chronic myeloid leukemia, and idiopathic myelofibrosis.

neurogenic communication d. Inability to exchange information with others because of hearing, speech, or language problems caused by impaired functioning of the nervous system.

pain d. A mental disorder in which pain is the predominant symptom, is of such severity to warrant clinical attention, and interferes with function. Psychological factors are important in the onset, severity, exacerbation, or maintenance of the pain. The condition is not intentionally produced or feigned.

phonological d. A disorder in which the individual does not use speech sounds that are appropriate for age and dialect. The disorder may involve production, use, organization, or omission of sounds.

protraction d. Primary dysfunctional labor.

reactive attachment d. A developmental disorder of infancy or early childhood marked either by social isolation and withdrawal or by indiscriminate sociability. The disorder may result from neglect of the child by his or her primary caregiver or from frequent changes in caregivers (esp. in children who have lost their parents or who have been moved frequently from one foster home to another).

relational d. Marked impairments in communication or other aspects of interpersonal interactions among family members, spouses, or coworkers.

sleep-related d. Multiple arousals interfering with restful sleep that occur as a result of airway obstruction, for example, during snoring. Excessive daytime sleepiness is the most common presenting complaint. The person may feel drowsy or fall asleep while talking, eating, or driving. Electrocardiographic abnormalities, elevated pulmonary and systolic arterial pressure, cardiac arrhythmias, and oxyhemoglobin desaturation may be associated laboratory findings. The disorder occurs in both sexes and often has a chronic course.

speech d. Any abnormality that prevents an individual from communicating by means of spoken words. The disorder may develop from such diverse sources as nerve injury to the brain, muscular paralysis of the organs of speech, structural defects of the mouth, teeth, or tongue, somatization disorders, or cognitive deficits.

substance dependence d. An addictive disorder of compulsive drug use. It is marked by a cluster of behavioral and physiological symptoms that indicate continual use of the substance despite significant related problems. The term includes a variety of substances but usually excludes caffeine. Patients develop a tolerance for the substance and require progressively greater amounts to elicit the effects desired. In addition, patients experience physical and psychological signs and symptoms of withdrawal if the agent is not used. SEE: *substance-induced d.; substance-related d.; substance abuse.*

substance-induced d. A disorder related to drug use but excluding drug dependency. Substance-induced disorders include intoxication, withdrawal, and other substance-induced mental disorders such as delirium and psychosis. SEE: *substance dependence d.; substance-related d.; substance abuse.*

substance-related d. Any disorder related to drug abuse or the effects of medication. Substances include alcohol, amphetamines, cannabis, cocaine, hallucinogens, inhalants, nicotine, opioids, phencyclidine (PCP), sedatives, hypnotics, and anxiolytics. SEE: *substance dependence d.; substance-induced d.; substance abuse.*

disorganization [L. *dis,* apart, + Gr. *organon,* a unified organ] Alteration in an organic part, causing it to lose most or all of its distinctive characteristics.

disorganized infant behavior Disintegrated physiological and neurobehavioral responses to the environment. SEE: *Nursing Diagnoses Appendix.*

disorganized infant behavior, risk for Risk for alteration in integration and modulation of the physiological and behavioral systems of functioning (i.e., autonomic, motor, state, organizational, self-regulatory, and attentional-interactional systems). SEE: *Nursing Diagnoses Appendix.*

disorientation (dĭs″ō-rē-ĕn-tā′shŭn) [″ + *oriens,* arising] Inability to estimate direction or location, or to be cognizant of time or of persons.

spatial d. In aerospace medicine, a term used to describe a variety of incidents occurring in flight, when the pilot fails to sense correctly the position, motion, or attitude of the aircraft or himself or herself within the coordinate system provided by the surface of the earth and gravitation.

disparate [L. *disparitas,* unequal] Dissimilar, not equally paired.

dispensary [L. *dispensare,* to give out] **1.** A clinic or similar place for obtaining medical care. **2.** An outpatient pharmacy.

dispensatory (dĭs-pĕn′să-tō-rē) [L. *dispensatorium*] A publication, in book form, of the description and composition of medicines.

dispense (dĭs-pĕns′) To prepare or deliver medicines.

dispersate (dĭs′pŭr-sāt) A suspension of finely divided particles in a liquid.

disperse (dĭs-pĕrs′) [L. *dis,* apart, + *spargere,* to scatter] **1.** To scatter, esp. applied to light rays. **2.** To dissipate or cause to disappear, as a tumor or the particles of a colloidal system.

dispersion (dĭs-pĕr′zhŭn) **1.** The act of dispersing. **2.** That which is dispersed.

coarse d. Suspension (3).

colloidal d. A mixture containing colloid particles that fail to settle out and are held in suspension. They are common in animal and plant tissues; the protoplasm of cells is an example. Particles of colloidal dispersions are too large to pass through cell membranes. Such dispersions usually appear cloudy.

molecular d. A true solution.

QTc d. In electrocardiography, variation in the corrected QT interval in different leads. This has been correlated with an increased incidence of ventricular arrhythmias and sudden death.

dispersoid A colloid with very finely divided particles.

dispersonalization (dĭs-pĕr″sŏn-ăl-ī-zā′shŭn) A mental state in which the individual denies the existence of his or her personality or parts of the body.

displacement [Fr. *deplacer,* to lay aside] **1.** Removal from the normal or usual position or place. **2.** Addition to a fluid of another more dense, causing the first fluid to be dispersed. **3.** Transference of emotion from the original idea with which it was associated to a different idea, thus allowing the patient to avoid acknowledging the original source.

disposition [L. *disponere,* to arrange] **1.** A natural tendency or aptitude exhibited by an individual or group. It may be manifested by acquiring a certain disease, presumably due to hereditary factors. **2.** The sum of a person's behavior as determined by his or her mood. SEE: *diathesis.*

disproportion (dĭs″prō-por′shŭn) A size different from that considered to be normal.

cephalopelvic d. ABBR: CPD. Disparity between the dimensions of the fetal head and those of the maternal pelvis. When the fetal head is larger than the pelvic diameters through which it must pass, or when the head is extended as in a face or brow presentation and cannot rotate to accommodate to the size and shape of the birth canal, fetal descent and delivery are not possible.

dissect (dĭ-sĕkt′, dī-sĕkt′) [L. *dissecare,* to cut up] To separate tissues and parts of a cadaver for anatomical study.

dissection (dĭ-, dī-sĕk′shŭn) In surgical procedures, the separation and delineation of tissues for study.

blunt d. In surgical procedures, separation of tissues by use of a blunt instrument. This provides minimal damage to the part being dissected if anatomical planes are observed. In various pathologic states, sharp dissection may be less traumatic.

carotid artery d. Longitudinal tearing of the carotid artery, a rare cause of stroke, occurring esp. in patients who have suffered trauma or twisting of the head and neck.

SYMPTOMS: Patients may report the sudden onset of unilateral neck pain that radiates toward the head, along with new neurological deficits.

radical neck d. The removal of the sternocleidomastoid muscle, internal jugular vein, spinal accessory nerve, and lymph nodes of the neck. The surgery is used primarily for the treatment of head and neck cancers.

selective neck d. One of several operations used for staging and treatment of neck cancers. In the most commonly used approach, the tissues above the omohyoid, including the submandibular gland and lymphatics, are removed.

sharp d. In surgical procedures, gaining access to tissues by incising them with some sort of sharp instrument such as a scalpel.

dissemble To mislead, to give a false impression, or to conceal the truth.

disseminated [L. *dis,* apart, + *seminare,* to sow] Scattered or distributed over a considerable area, esp. applied to disease organisms; scattered throughout an organ or the body.

disseminated intravascular coagulation ABBR: DIC. A pathological condition in which the coagulation pathways are hyperstimulated, resulting in diffuse rather than localized activation of coagulation factors. Clotting factors are consumed to such an extent that generalized bleeding may occur. This tendency is referred to as consumptive coagulopathy. SEE: *acute respiratory distress syndrome; hypofibrinogenemia; sepsis; serine protease inhibitor; systemic inflammatory response syndrome; Nursing Diagnoses Appendix.*

ETIOLOGY: Various conditions have been associated with DIC, including sepsis; trauma; pancreatitis; acute intravascular hemolysis; acute viral, rickettsial, or protozoal infection; abruptio placentae; septic abortion; surgical procedures; heatstroke; certain poisonous snake bites; severe head injury; malignancy; retained dead fetus; liver disease; and systemic lupus erythematosus.

SYMPTOMS: Symptoms of DIC include bleeding from surgical or invasive procedure sites and bleeding gums, cutaneous oozing, petechiae, ecchymoses, blood vessel clotting (with symptoms of local ischemia), and hematomas. The patient may also experience nausea and vomiting; severe muscle, back, and abdominal pain; chest pain; hemoptysis; epistaxis; seizures; and oliguria. Peripheral pulses and blood pressure may be decreased; the patient may demonstrate confusion or other changes in mental status. SEE: illus.

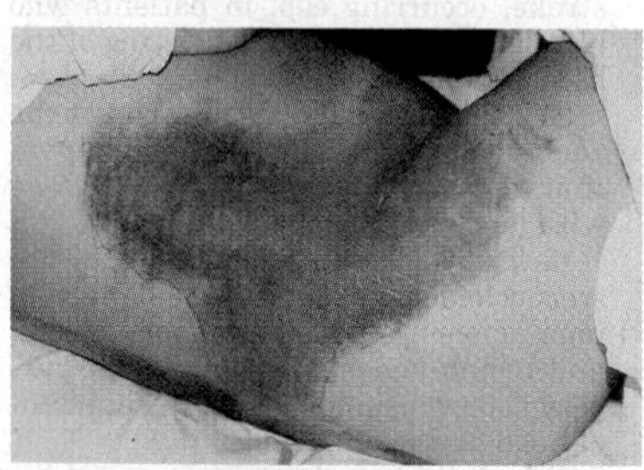

DISSEMINATED INTRAVASCULAR COAGULATION

Bleeding into the skin

TREATMENT: The primary illness must be treated. In some cases, depending on the etiology, heparins or antithrombin III may be administered; patients should receive transfusional support if blood loss is severe.

PATIENT CARE: In acute DIC, intake and output are monitored hourly, esp. when blood products are given, and the patient is observed for transfusion reactions and fluid overload. The blood pressure cuff is used infrequently to avoid triggering subcutaneous bleeding. Any emesis, drainage, urine, or stool should undergo a test for occult blood, and dressings and linens should be weighed to measure the amount of blood lost. Daily weights are obtained, particularly in cases of renal involvement. The patient is observed closely for signs of shock, and the abdominal girth measured every 2 to 4 hr if intra-abdominal bleeding is suspected.

The results of serial blood studies, such as hemoglobin and hematocrit and coagulation studies, are monitored. All venipuncture sites are checked frequently for bleeding. Analgesics are given as prescribed, as well as heparin therapy if prescribed (the latter is controversial). The patient is repositioned every 2 hr, and meticulous skin care is provided. Prescribed oxygen therapy is administered. Areas at risk can be washed gently with hydrogen peroxide and water to remove crusted blood. Pressure, cold compresses, and topical hemostatic agents are applied to control bleeding. Parenteral injections are avoided and venipunctures limited whenever possible; pressure should be applied to an injection site for at least 10 min after removal of a needle or intravenous catheter. The patient is protected from injury by enforcing complete bedrest during bleeding episodes and by padding the bed rails if the patient is at risk for agitation. Frequent rest periods are provided.

The disorder, the patient's progress, and treatment options and posttreatment appearance are explained and the patient and family are encouraged to express their feelings and concerns and are referred for further counseling or support as needed.

dissipation (dĭs-ĭ-pā′shŭn) [L. *dissipare,* to scatter] **1.** Dispersion of matter. **2.** The act of living a wasteful and dissolute life, esp. drinking alcoholic beverages to excess.

dissociation (dĭs-sō″sē-ā′shŭn) [L. *dis,* apart, + *sociatio,* union] **1.** Separation, as the separation by heat of a complex compound into simpler molecules. **2.** The ability to move one body segment independently of another. **3.** In psychiatry, the breaking off of normal thought processes from consciousness, as can occur in amnesia, conversion reaction, or as a result of psychoactive drugs. SEE: *hysteria.*

atrioventricular d. Dissociation that occurs when the independent pacemakers of the atria and ventricles of the heart are not synchronized. This is a hallmark of third-degree heart block.

microbic d. A change in the morphology of a cultured microbial colony due to mutation or selection.

d. of personality A split in consciousness resulting in two different phases of personality, neither being aware of the words, acts, and feelings of the other. SEE: *dissociative identity disorder; multiple personality; vigilambulism; Nursing Diagnoses Appendix.*

psychological d. A disunion of mind of which the person is not aware (e.g., dual personality, fugue, somnambulism, selective amnesia).

dissolution [L. *dissolvere,* to dissolve] **1.** Death. **2.** A pathological resolution or breaking up of the integrity of an anatomical entity.

dissolve (dĭ-zŏlv′) [L. *dissolvere,* to dissolve] To cause absorption of a solid in and by a liquid.

dissonance (dĭs′ō-năns) **1.** Discord or disagreement. **2.** Unpleasant sounds, particularly musical ones.

cognitive d. Incongruity of thought, philosophy, or action.

distad (dĭs′tăd) [L. *distare,* to be distant] Away from the center.

distal (dĭs′tăl) [L. *distare,* to be distant] **1.** Farthest from the center, from a medial line, or from the trunk; opposed to proximal. **2.** In dentistry, the tooth surface farthest from the midline of the arch.

distance The space between two objects.

focal d. The distance from the optical center of a lens to the focal point.

focus-film d. The distance between the focal target of an x-ray and the film.

interocclusal d. The distance between the occlusal surfaces of opposed teeth when the mandible is at rest.

interocular d. The distance between the eyes. SEE: *hypertelorism.*

interpupillary d. The distance between the centers of the pupils of the eyes.

object-film d. ABBR: OFD. In radiography, the distance between the anatomical structure to be imaged and the radiographic film.

source-skin d. In radiography, the distance from a radiation source to a patient's skin.

source-to-image receptor d. ABBR: SID. In radiography, the distance from the x-ray tube to the radiographical film or the image digitizer.

target-skin d. ABBR: TSD. The distance at which it is safe to deliver an appropriately timed exposure of ionizing radiation for treatment or diagnosis.

distemper (dĭs-tĕm′pĕr) In veterinary medicine, one of several virus infections of animals that cause fever, anorexia, and nerve disease.

distend [L. *distendere,* to stretch out] **1.** To stretch out. **2.** To become inflated.

distensibility (dĭs-tĕn″sĭ-bĭl′ĭ-tē) The ability to become distended.

distention The state of being distended.

distichiasis (dĭs″tĭ-kī′ă-sĭs) [Gr. *distichia,* a double row] A condition in which there are two rows of eyelashes, one or both being directed inward toward the eye.

distill (dĭs-tĭl′) [L. *destillare,* to drop from] To vaporize by heat and condense and collect the volatilized products.

distillate (dĭs′tĭl-āt, dĭs-tĭl′āt) That which has been derived from the distillation process.

distillation Condensation of a vapor that has been obtained from a liquid heated to the volatilization point, as the condensation of steam from boiling water. Distillation is used to purify water and for other purposes. Distilled water should be stored in covered containers because it readily takes up impurities from the atmosphere.

destructive d. The process of decomposing complex organic compounds by heat in the absence of air and condensing the vapor of the liquid products.

dry d. Distillation of solids without added liquids.

fractional d. Separation of liquids based on the difference in their boiling points.

distobuccal (dĭs″tō-bŭk′ăl) [L. *distare,* to be distant, + *bucca,* cheek] Pert. to the distal and buccal walls of bicuspid and molar teeth; also pert. to the distal or buccal walls of a cavity preparation.

distoclusion (dĭs″tō-kloo′zhŭn) A condition in which the lower teeth meet the upper teeth behind the normal position.

distogingival (dĭs″tō-jĭn′jĭ-văl) [″ + *gingiva,* gum] Pert. to the distal and gingival walls of a cavity being prepared for restoration.

distolabial (dĭs″tō-lā′bē-ăl) [″ + *labialis,* lips] Pert. to the distal and labial surfaces of a tooth.

distolingual (dĭs″tō-lĭng′gwăl) [″ + *lingua,* tongue] Pert. to the distal and lingual surfaces of a tooth.

distome A fluke with two suckers, an oral and a ventral sucker, or acetabulum.

distomia (dī-stō′mē-ă) [Gr. *dis,* two, + *stoma,* mouth] A congenital deformation producing a fetus with two mouths.

disto-occlusal (dĭs″tō-ŏ-kloo′zăl) Concerning the distal and occlusal surfaces of a tooth or the distal and occlusal walls of a cavity preparation.

distortion [L. *distortio,* twist, writhe] **1.** A twisting or bending out of regular shape. **2.** A writhing or twisting movement as of the muscles of the face. **3.** A deformity in which the part or structure is altered in shape. **4.** In ophthalmology, visual perception of an image that does not provide a true picture, due to astigmatism or to retinal abnormalities. **5.** In psychiatry, the process of modifying unconscious mental elements so that they can enter consciousness without being censored. **6.** In radiology, the difference in size and shape of a radiographic image as compared with the actual part examined. **7.** Variation in the amplitude or frequency of a signal that may be caused by overdriving the amplifier in the circuit.

distractibility Inability to focus one's attention; loss of the ability to concentrate.

distraction (dĭs-trăk′shŭn) [L. *dis,* apart, + *tractio,* a drawing] **1.** A state of mental confusion or derangement. **2.** Separation of joint surfaces by extension without injury or dislocation of the parts. **3.** A joint mobilization technique causing separation of opposing joint surfaces. It is used to inhibit pain, move synovial fluid, or stretch a tight joint capsule.

distraught (dĭs-trawt′) [L. *distrahere,* to perplex] In doubt, deeply troubled, and having conflicting thoughts. The patient may be frantic and may need to be continuously occupied.

distress (dĭs-trĕs′) [L. *distringere,* to draw apart] Physical or mental pain or suffering.

fetal d. A nonspecific clinical diagnosis indicating pathology in the fetus. The distress, which may be due to lack of oxygen, is judged by fetal heart rate or biochemical changes in the amniotic fluid or fetal blood.

distribution [L. *dis,* apart, + *tribuere,* to allot] **1.** The dividing and spreading of anything, esp. blood vessels and nerves, to tissues. **2.** The presence of entities, such as hair, fat, or nutrients, at various sites or in particular patterns throughout the body. **3.** In demography or statistics, the location pattern of particular individuals who are ill, or of events.

frequency d. In statistics, the grouping of data by rate of occurrence at arbitrarily determined values although the variable may vary continuously (e.g., disease occurrences could be grouped by weeks, months, or years rather than by the precise day of occurrence).

gaussian d. Normal d.

normal d. In statistics, the smooth, bell-shaped, hypothetical curve made by a frequency distribution diagram in which the occurrences are plotted on the vertical axis (ordinate), and the values of the variable are plotted on the horizontal axis (abscissa). Also called *bell-shaped curve* or *gaussian curve.* SYN: *gaussian d.*

districhiasis (dĭs-trĭk-ī′ă-sĭs) [Gr. *dis,* double, + *thrix,* hair] A condition in which two hairs grow from the same hair follicle.

disturbance **1.** Interruption of the normal sequence of continuity. **2.** A departure from the considered norm.

emotional d. Mental disorder.

disulfate (dī-sŭl′fāt) A compound containing two sulfate radicals. SEE: *bisulfate.*

disulfiram (dī-sŭl′fĭ-răm) Antabuse.

disulfiram poisoning SEE: *Antabuse in Poisons and Poisoning Appendix.*

disuse syndrome, risk for A state in which an individual is at risk for deterioration of body systems as the result of prescribed or unavoidable musculoskeletal inactivity. SEE: *Nursing Diagnoses Appendix.*

Dittrich's plugs (dĭt′rĭks) [Franz Dittrich, Ger. pathologist, 1815–1859] Small particles in fetid sputum composed of pus, detritus, bacteria, and fat globules.

diurese (dī″ū-rēs′) To cause diuresis.

diuresis (dī″ū-rē′sĭs) [Gr. *diourein,* to urinate] The secretion and passage of large amounts of urine. Diuresis occurs as a complication of metabolic disorders such as diabetes mellitus, diabetes insipidus, and hypercalcemia, among others. It also occurs when obstruction to urinary flow is suddenly relieved ("postobstructive diuresis"), after childbirth, and after supraventricular tachycardias.

Diuretic drugs are used to manage conditions marked by fluid overload, such as congestive heart failure, cirrhosis, and nephrotic syndrome. They are also used to manage cerebral edema, hyperkalemia, and some intoxications. SEE: *diuretic.*

postpartum d. Excessive fluid excretion after childbirth, typically more than 3 L/day.

Patient Care: The nurse should be particularly alert to the potential for rapid bladder distention during the final stage of labor and immediately postpartum. A distended bladder is the most common cause of fundal displacement, loss of uterine tone, a boggy uterus, and excessive bleeding. Despite the marked increase in urine formation related to the rapid postbirth fluid shift, the woman may be unaware of a need to void because of urethral edema, trauma, or the continuing effects of regional anesthesia or analgesia. Spontaneous bladder emptying is encouraged by early ambulation, running water, and warm perineal cascades; catheterization may be necessary if nursing measures are unsuccessful and distention increases.

diuretic (dī″ū-rĕt′ĭk) **1.** Increasing urine secretion. SEE: *diuresis.* **2.** An agent that increases urine output. Diuretics are used to treat hypertension, congestive heart failure, and edema. Common side effects of these agents are potassium depletion, low blood pressure, dehydration, and hyponatremia.

diurnal [L. *dies,* day] **1.** Daily. **2.** Happening in the daytime or pert. to it. SEE: *circadian; clock, biological; desynchronosis; nocturnal.*

divagation (dī-vă-gā′shŭn) [L. *divagatus,* to wander off] **1.** Wandering astray. **2.** Rambling or incoherent speech.

divalent (dī-vā′lĕnt) In a molecule, having an electric charge of two. SYN: *bivalent.*

divergence (dī-vĕr′jĕns) [L. *divergere,* to

turn aside] Separation from a common center, especially that of the eyes.

divergent Radiating in different directions.

diversional activity deficit The state in which an individual experiences a decreased stimulation from or interest or engagement in recreational or leisure activities (because of internal/external factors that may or may not be beyond the individual's control). SEE: *Nursing Diagnoses Appendix.*

diverticulectomy (dī″vĕr-tĭk″ū-lĕk′tō-mē) [″ + Gr. *ektome,* excision] Surgical removal of a diverticulum.

diverticulitis (dī″vĕr-tĭk″ū-lī′tĭs) [″ + Gr. *itis,* inflammation] Inflammation of a diverticulum or diverticula in the intestinal tract, esp. in the colon, causing pain, anorexia, fevers, and occasionally peritonitis. SEE: *Nursing Diagnoses Appendix.*

PATIENT CARE: During an acute episode, prescribed treatment with fluid and electrolyte replacement, antibiotic, antispasmodic, analgesic, and stool softener therapy, and nasogastric suction if required, is initiated. The patient is observed for increasing or decreasing distress and for any adverse reactions to the therapy. Stools are inspected for mucus, blood, and consistency, and the frequency of bowel movements is noted. The patient is assessed for fever, increasing abdominal pain, blood in the stools, and leukocytosis. Rest is prescribed, and the patient is instructed not to lift, strain, bend, cough, or perform other actions that increase intra-abdominal pressure. When the patient resumes a normal diet, stool softeners may be employed.

Patients with chronic diverticulitis are educated about the disease and its symptoms. A well-balanced diet that provides dietary roughage in the form of fruit, vegetable, and cereal fiber, but that is nonirritating to the bowel, is recommended; and fluid intake should be increased to 2 to 3 L daily (unless otherwise restricted). Constipation and straining at stool should be avoided, and the patient is advised to relieve constipation with stool softeners and bulk cathartics, taken with plenty of water. The importance of regular medical evaluation is emphasized.

acute d. Diverticulitis in which the symptoms are similar to those of appendicitis but usually located in the left rather than the right lower quadrant of the abdomen: inflammation of the peritoneum, formation of an abscess, and in untreated patients, intestinal gangrene accompanied by perforation.

chronic d. Diverticulitis marked by worsening constipation, mucus in the stools, and intermittent left lower quadrant abdominal pains. The walls of the bowels may thicken, which may produce stricture formation and chronic intestinal obstruction.

diverticulosis (dī″vĕr-tĭk″ū-lō′sĭs) [″ + Gr. *osis,* condition] Diverticula in the colon without inflammation or symptoms. Only a small percentage of persons with diverticulosis develop diverticulitis.

diverticulum (dī″vĕr-tĭk′ū-lŭm) *pl.* **diverticula** [L. *devertere,* to turn aside] A sac or pouch in the walls of a canal or organ. SEE: illus.

d. of the colon An outpocketing of the colon. These may be asymptomatic until they become inflamed.

d. of the duodenum A diverticulum commonly located near the entrance of the common bile or pancreatic duct.

false d. A diverticulum without a muscular coat in the wall or pouch. This type of diverticulum is acquired.

gastric d. A pulsion-type diverticulum usually on the lesser curvature of the esophagogastric junction.

d. of the jejunum A diverticulum usually marked by severe pain in the upper abdomen, followed occasionally by a massive hemorrhage from the intestine.

Meckel's d. SEE: *Meckel's diverticulum.*

d. of the stomach A diverticulum of the stomach wall.

true d. A diverticulum involving all the coats of muscle in the pouch wall. It is usually congenital.

Zenker's d. SEE: *Zenker's diverticulum.*

divulsion (dĭ-vŭl′shŭn) [L. *dis,* apart, + *vellere,* to pluck] A forcible pulling apart.

divulsor (dĭ-vŭl′sor) [L. *dis,* apart, + *vellere,* to pluck] A device for dilatation of a part, esp. the urethra.

pterygium d. An instrument for separating the corneal portion of the pterygium.

tendon d. A device for separating a tendon from the surrounding tissue.

Dix, Dorothea Lynde A Massachusetts schoolteacher (1802–1887) who crusaded for prison reform and for care of the mentally ill. She was responsible for founding many hospitals in the U.S., Canada, and several other countries. During the Civil War, she organized the nursing service of the Union armies.

dizziness [AS. *dysig,* foolish] **1.** Lightheadedness, unsteadiness, loss of spatial orientation, or loss of balance. **2.** Generalized weakness, faintness, or presyncope. **3.** Mental uncertainty; difficulty concentrating; feeling disconnected from one's normal sense of clarity or focus. SYN: *giddiness.* SEE: *vertigo.*

DJD *degenerative joint disease.*

DKA *diabetic ketoacidosis.*

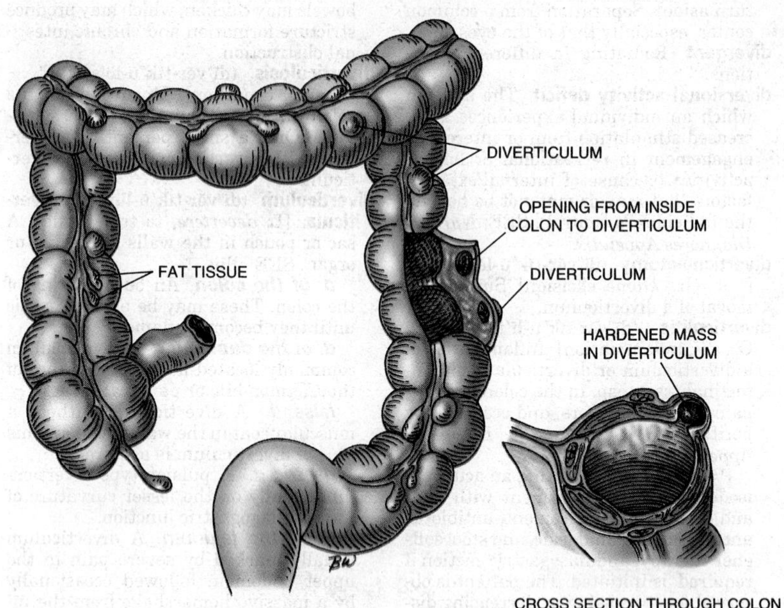

MULTIPLE DIVERTICULA OF THE COLON

dl *deciliter.*

DM *diabetes mellitus.*

DMARD *Disease-modifying antirheumatic drug.*

D.M.D. *Doctor of Dental Medicine.*

DMSO *dimethyl sulfoxide.*

DMT *dimethyltryptamine.*

DNA *deoxyribonucleic acid.*

mitochondrial D. ABBR: mtDNA. Deoxyribonucleic acid (DNA) in the intracellular bodies known as mitochondria. It differs from nuclear DNA in its nucleotide sequences, its size (about 16.5 kb), and its source (it is derived solely from the egg, not the sperm). Alterations in mtDNA caused by reactive oxygen are thought to play an important part in human aging.

DNA fingerprint A distinctive pattern of bands formed by repeating sequences of base pairs of satellite DNA. The identification of the pattern can help establish the origin of tissues and body fluids, and identify bacterial strains in infectious outbreaks.

DNA probe A single-strand DNA fragment used to detect the complementary fragment. DNA probes are used widely in bacteriology. Recombinant DNA techniques are used to isolate, reproduce, and label a portion of the genetic material, DNA, from the nucleus of a microorganism that is specific for it. This fragment can be added to a specimen containing the organisms. The specimen and known DNA are treated so that the DNA strands from the organisms in the specimen are separated into single strands. The DNA from the specimen rejoins (is annealed to) the known labeled DNA and is thereby labeled. This permits the identification of a single pathogenic organism in a specimen that contains many different microorganisms.

DNAR *do not attempt resuscitation.*

DNR *do not resuscitate.*

DNSc, DNS *Doctor of Nursing Science.*

D.O. *Doctor of Osteopathy.*

DOA *dead on arrival* (at a hospital).

Dobell's solution (dō′bĕlz) [Horace B. Dobell, Brit. physician, 1828–1917] Carbolic acid, borax, sodium bicarbonate, glycerine, and water in solution.

Dobie's globule (dō′bēz) [William M. Dobie, Brit. physician, 1828–1915] Z disk.

dobutamine hydrochloride A synthetic beta-agonist whose primary effect is to increase cardiac contractility, with little effect on systemic vascular resistance. It produces less tachycardia than dopamine, and has no effect on renal blood flow. It is of use in congestive heart failure and cardiogenic shock.

doctor [L. *docere*, to teach] **1.** The recipient of an advanced degree, such as doctor of medicine (M.D.), doctor of osteopathy (D.O.), doctor of philosophy (Ph.D.), doctor of science (D.Sc.), doctor of nursing science (DNS), doctor of dental medicine (D.M.D.), doctor of education (Ed.D.), or doctor of divinity (D.D.). **2.** One who, after graduating from a medical, veterinary, or dental school, successfully passes an examination and is licensed by a state government to practice medicine, veterinary medicine, or dentistry. SEE: *optometry; osteopathy*. Because of the great variety of doctoral degrees, the use of the word doctor is sometimes confusing. This may be remedied by using the word physician when writing or speaking of those who possess an M.D. or D.O. (doctor of osteopathy) degree.

barefoot d. A practitioner of traditional or native medicine in the People's Republic of China. These individuals have not attended a medical school.

doctor-patient relationship All the interactions between a patient and a health care professional. These interactions establish the basis for interpersonal communication, trust, compliance, and satisfaction.

doctrine (dŏk'trĭn) A system of principles taught or advocated.

documentation (dŏk″ū-mĕn-tā'shŭn) **1.** Manuals, instruction books, and programs or help menus that provide guidance to a user. **2.** Recording in a medical record pertinent medical information concerning a patient. This may be in the form of written data in the patient's chart or transcribed by electronic means (i.e., storing the information in a computer). SEE: *charting*.

docusate calcium (dŏk'ū-sāt) A stool softener.

docusate sodium A stool softener.

dogmatic Pert. to the expression of opinions in an uncompromising, arrogant manner.

Döhle bodies (dē'lēz) [Paul Döhle, Ger. pathologist, 1855–1928] A leukocyte inclusion in the periphery of a neutrophil. It is composed of liquefied endoplasmic reticulum and is frequently accompanied by toxic granulations. Döhle bodies are present in association with burns, severe or systemic infections, exposure to cytotoxic agents, uncomplicated pregnancy, trauma, and neoplastic diseases. SEE: illus.

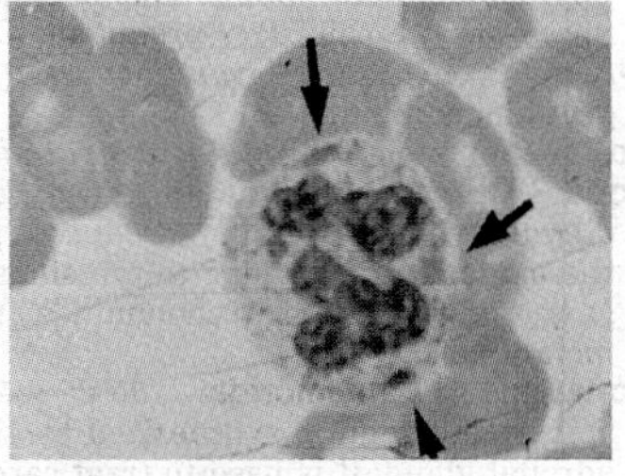

DOHLE BODIES

(Orig. mag. ×1000)

dol Symbol for degree of pain intensity registered on the dolorimeter.

dolichocephalic (dŏl″ĭ-kō-sĭ-făl'ĭk) [Gr. *dolichos,* long, + *kephale,* head] Having a skull with a long anteroposterior diameter.

dolichocolon (dŏl″ĭ-kō-kō'lŏn) [″ + *kolon,* colon] An abnormally long colon.

dolichofacial (dŏl″ĭ-kō-fā'shăl) Having a long face.

dolichohieric (dŏl″ĭ-kō-hī-ĕr'ĭk) [″ + *hieron,* sacred] Having a long, slender sacrum.

dolichomorphic (dŏl″ĭ-kō-mor'fĭk) [″ + *morphe,* form] Pert. to a body type that is long and slender. SEE: *ectomorph*.

dolichopellic, dolichopelvic (dŏl″ĭ-kō-pĕl'ĭk, -pĕl'vĭk) [″ + *pyelos,* an oblong trough] Having an abnormally long or narrow pelvis.

dolichosigmoid (dŏl″ĭ-kō-sĭg'moyd) [″ + *sigmoeides,* sigmoid] Having an abnormally long sigmoid colon.

dolichuranic (dŏl″ĭk-ū-răn'ĭk) [″ + *ouranos,* palate] Having a long alveolar arch of the maxilla.

doll's eye maneuver A test of the oculocephalic reflex that can be used to assess the integrity of the brainstem in neonates and comatose patients. During the evaluation of the comatose patient, with the patient's eyes held open, the head is quickly rotated from one side to the other. Both eyes should deviate to the side opposite the direction of head rotation. If this response is absent, there may be damage to the brainstem or oculomotor nerves. By contrast, in the evaluation of the newborn (whose nervous system is immature), the irises normally remain in midline despite the rotation of the head. SEE: *coma*.

doll's eye movement Oculocephalic reflex.

dolor (dō'lor) *pl.* **dolores** [L.] Pain. This is one of the principal indications of inflammation. The others are rubor (redness), tumor (swelling), functio laesa (loss of function), and calor (heat).

dolorimeter (dō″lor-ĭm'ĭ-tĕr) [″ + Gr. *metron,* measure] A device that applies pressure evenly and reproducibly to a body part; it can be used to measure a patient's pain tolerance (e.g., in arthritis or fibromyalgia).

dolorogenic [″ + Gr. *gennan,* to produce] Causing pain.

domain In immunology, the portion of a protein, such as an immunoglobulin, that has a functional role independent of the remainder of the protein.

domatophobia (dō-măt-ō-fō'bē-ă) [Gr. *doma,* house, + *phobos,* fear] Abnormal aversion to being in a house; a form of claustrophobia.

domiciliary (dŏm″ĭ-sĭl'ē-ār″ē) [L. *domus,* house] Pert. to or carried on in a house.

domiciliary care facility A home providing mainly custodial and personal care for persons who do not require medical or nursing supervision, but may need assistance with activities of daily living because of a physical or mental disability. This may also be referred to as a sheltered living environment. SEE: *adult foster care.*

dominance [L. *dominans,* ruling] **1.** A genetic pattern of inheritance in which one of an allelic pair of genes has the capacity to suppress the expression of the other so that the first prevails in the heterozygote. **2.** Often, the preferred hand or side of the body, as in right-hand dominance. **3.** In psychiatry, the tendency to be commanding or controlling of others.

ocular d. The use of one eye by choice for particular tasks such as aiming a gun. This may or may not be related to right-hand or left-hand dominance.

dominant In genetics, concerning a trait or characteristic that is expressed in the offspring although it is carried on only one of the homologous chromosomes. SEE: *recessive.*

domoic acid A toxin that resembles the brain's main excitatory amino acid (glutamate); when ingested it may cause continuous seizures.

Donath-Landsteiner phenomenon (dō′năth-lănd′stī-nĕr) [Julius Donath, Austrian physician, 1870–1950; Karl L. Landsteiner, Austrian-born U.S. biologist, 1868–1943] A test for paroxysmal hemoglobinuria. Blood from the patient is cooled to 5°C, and a cold hemolysin in the plasma combines with the red blood cells if the patient has the disease. On warming, the sensitized red cells are hemolyzed by the complement normally present.

donation, organ Donation of organs for transplantation in human beings. The success rate of transplantation procedures has led to a great demand for organ donation. Donating an organ does not disfigure the body of the deceased. The family of the donor is not responsible for the expense of providing the organ or tissue. The major religious organizations support organ and tissue donation. SEE: *donor card; transplantation.*

donee (dō-nē′) [L. *donare,* to give] One who receives something, such as a blood transfusion, from a donor.

donepezil hydrochloride A cholinesterase inhibitor that improves cognitive abilities in patients with Alzheimer's dementia. Its most frequent side effects are diarrhea, nausea, and headache. Trade name is Aricept.

Don Juan [After the legendary, promiscuous Spanish nobleman, Don Juan de Tenorio] A man who behaves in a sexually promiscuous manner. Some psychologists suggest this arises from insecurity concerning his masculinity or latent and unconscious homosexual preference.

Donnan's equilibrium (dŏn′ănz) [Frederick G. Donnan, Brit. chemist, 1871–1956] A condition in which an equilibrium is established between two solutions separated by a semipermeable membrane so that the sum of the anions and cations on one side is equal to that on the other side.

Donohue's syndrome SEE: *leprechaunism.*

donor **1.** A person who furnishes blood, tissue, or an organ to be used in another person. **2.** In chemistry, a compound that frees part of itself to unite with another compound called an acceptor.

universal d. A person whose blood is of group O and is therefore usually compatible with most other blood types. In actual practice this compatibility rarely occurs because of the many factors besides the major blood antigens (A, B, AB) that determine compatibility.

donor card A document used by a person who wishes to make an anatomical gift, at the time of his or her death, of an organ or other body part needed for transplantation. SEE: illus; *transplantation.*

do not attempt resuscitation ABBR: DNAR. An order somewhat more precise than "do not resuscitate" (DNR). DNR implies that, if a resuscitation attempt is made, the patient can be revived. DNAR indicates that resuscitation efforts should not be attempted regardless of their expected outcome. SEE: *do not resuscitate.*

do not resuscitate ABBR: DNR. An order stating that a patient should not be revived. It may be written by a physician at the patient's request. If the patient is not competent or is unable to make such a decision, the family, legal guardian, or health care proxy may request and give consent for such an order to be written on the patient's chart and followed by the health care providers. The hospital or physician should have policies regarding time limits and reordering. SEE: *do not attempt resuscitation.*

Donovan body [Charles Donovan, Ir. physician, 1863–1951] The common name for the causative organism, *Calymmatobacterium granulomatis,* of granuloma inguinale.

donovanosis SEE: *granuloma inguinale.*

dopa, DOPA A chemical substance, 3,4-dihydroxyphenylalanine, produced by the oxidation of tyrosine to tyrosinase. It is a precursor of catecholamines and melanin.

dopamine hydrochloride (dō′pă-mēn) **1.** A catecholamine synthesized by the adrenal gland; it is used to treat cardiogenic and septic shock. Its effects on receptors in the kidneys, blood vessels, and heart vary with the dose of the drug

UNIFORM DONOR CARD

OF____

Print or type name of donor

In the hope that I may help others, I hereby make this anatomical gift, if medically acceptable, to take effect upon my death. The words and marks below indicate my desires.

I give: (a) _____ any needed organs or parts

(b) _____ only the following organs or parts

____

Specify the organ(s) or part(s)

for the purposes of transplantation, therapy, medical research or education;

(c) _____ my body for anatomical study if needed.

Limitations or special wishes, if any:____________________________

Signed by the donor and the following two witnesses in the presence of each other:

____________________ ____________________

Signature of Donor — Date of Birth of Donor

____________________ ____________________

Date Signed — City & State

____________________ ____________________

Witness — Witness

This is a legal document under the Uniform Anatomical Gift Act or similar laws.

that is given. At low doses (0.5 to 2.0 μg/kg/min) it increases blood flow to renal, mesenteric, cerebral, and coronary blood vessels. Intermediate doses (about 2.0 to 10.0 μg/kg/min) increase the force of heart muscle contraction, improve cardiac output, and increase heart rate. High doses (more than 10.0 μg/kg/min) elevate blood pressure by causing vasoconstriction. **2.** A catecholamine neurotransmitter, or brain messenger, implicated in some forms of psychosis and abnormal movement disorders.

CAUTION: This drug should not be administered by intravenous push. The intravenous line should be monitored frequently to make certain there is no extravasation. Other drugs should not be administered in the same intravenous line. Use is discontinued gradually. When dopamine is used in life-threatening states of shock, blood pressure and renal function must be monitored carefully.

dopaminergic (dō″pă-mēn-ĕr′jĭk) **1.** Caused by dopamine. **2.** Concerning tissues that are influenced by dopamine.

dopa-oxidase (dō″pă-ŏk′sĭ-dās) An enzyme in some epithelial cells that converts dopa to melanin.

dope A slang term used to describe almost any drug of abuse. SEE: *doping; blood doping*.

doping In athletic medicine, use of a drug or blood product by an athlete to improve performance. The existence of a drug that safely accomplishes this has not been demonstrated. The administration of anabolic hormones to women causes signs of masculinization, including facial hair growth, deepening of the voice, and clitoromegaly.

blood d. The practice by athletes of storing several units of their own blood and having it transfused to themselves a day or two before competition. The safety and effectiveness of this practice is questionable, and it is unapproved by sports governing bodies.

Doppler echocardiography The use of ultrasound technology to determine blood flow velocity in different locations in the heart, but esp. across the heart valves. SEE: *echocardiography*.

Doppler effect (dŏp′lĕr) [Johann Christian Doppler, Austrian scientist, 1803–1853] The variation of the apparent frequency of waves, such as sound waves, with change in distance between the source and the receiver. The frequency seems to increase as the distance decreases and to decrease as the distance increases.

Doppler measurement of blood pressure and fetal heart rate Use of Doppler sound waves to determine systolic blood pressure, as well as to determine the fetal heart rate.

Doppler velocimetry The use of Doppler ultrasound to determine the speed of blood flow through arteries and veins. During pregnancy, for example, Doppler ultrasonography can determine whether blood flow rates are adequate in the uterine artery, placenta, and umbilical cord vessels. SEE: *uteroplacental insufficiency*.

doraphobia (dō″ră-fō′bē-ă) [Gr. *dora,* hide, + *phobos,* fear] Abnormal aversion to touching the hair or fur of animals.

Dorello's canal [Primo Dorello, It. anatomist, 1872–1963] A bony canal in the tip of the temporal bone enclosing the abducens nerve.

Dorendorf's sign [Hans Dorendorf, Ger. physician, b. 1866] A filling or fullness of the supraclavicular groove in an aneurysm of the aortic arch.

dormancy **1.** The condition of greatly reduced metabolic activity that permits long-term survival and possible reactivation. The term refers to bacterial endospores, protozoan cysts, larval stages of some worm parasites, and viruses such as herpesviruses. **2.** The state in which a disease or disease process is no longer active. **dormant,** *adj.*

dornase (dor′nās) Short for deoxyribonuclease.

d. alfa An enzyme that lessens the viscosity of sputum by cleaving DNA deposited in it. It is used to treat patients with cystic fibrosis, who have exceptionally thick pulmonary secretions that are hard to expectorate.

pancreatic d. Dornase prepared from beef pancreas, used to loosen thick pulmonary secretions.

dors- SEE: *dorso-*.

dorsabdominal [L. *dorsum,* back, + *abdomen,* belly] Pert. to the back and abdomen.

dorsad (dōr′săd) [″ + *ad,* toward] Toward the back.

dorsal (dōr′săl) [L. *dorsum,* back] **1.** Pert. to the back. **2.** Indicating a position toward a rear part; opposed to ventral.

dorsal cord stimulation A procedure for relieving pain by electric stimulation of the spinal cord through electrodes sutured to the posterior spinal cord.

dorsalgia (dōr-săl′jē-ă) [″ + Gr. *algos,* pain] Pain in the back. SYN: *notalgia*.

dorsalis (dor-sā′lĭs) [L.] Dorsal (i.e., pert. to the back).

dorsal nerve A branch of spinal nerves that passes dorsally to innervate skin, muscle, and bone near the vertebral column; also called a *dorsal ramus* or *posterior branch*.

dorsal reflex Irritation of the skin over the erector spinae muscles, causing contraction of muscles of the back.

dorsal slit A surgical method of making the foreskin of the penis easily retractable. The foreskin is cut in the dorsal midline but not far enough to extend into the mucous membrane next to the glans.

dorsi- SEE: *dorso-*.

dorsiduct [L. *dorsum,* back, + *ducere,* to lead] To draw toward the back or backward.

dorsiduction Drawing toward the back.

dorsiflect (dor′sĭ-flĕkt) [″ + *flectere,* to bend] To bend backward.

dorsiflexion Movement of a part at a joint to bend the part toward the dorsum, or posterior aspect of the body. Thus, dorsiflexion of the foot indicates movement backward, in which the foot moves toward its top, or dorsum; the opposite of plantar flexion. Dorsiflexion of the toes indicates a movement of the toes away from the sole of the foot. When the hand is extended, or bent backward at the wrist, it is dorsiflexed; this is the opposite of palmar flexion, or volar flexion of the wrist.

dorsimesal (dor″sĭ-mĕs′ăl) In the direction of the dorsimeson.

dorsimeson (dor-sĭ-mĕs′ŏn) [″ + Gr. *meson,* middle] The median plane of the back.

dorsispinal (dor″sĭ-spī′năl) [″ + *spina,* thorn] Pert. to the back and spine.

dorso-, dorsi-, dors- Combining form indicating *back.*

dorsocephalad (dor″sō-sĕf′ă-lăd) [″ + Gr. *kephale,* head, + L. *ad,* toward] Situated toward the back of the head.

dorsodynia (dor″sō-dĭn′ē-ă) [″ + Gr. *odyne,* pain] Pain in the muscles of the upper part of the back.

dorsolateral (dor″sō-lăt′ĕr-ăl) Pert. to the back and side.

dorsolumbar Pert. to the lower thoracic and upper lumbar (loin) area of the back.

dorsoplantar (dor″sō-plăn′tăr) [″ + *planta,* sole of the foot] From the top to the bottom of the foot.

dorsosacral [″ + *sacrum,* sacred bone] Pert. to the lower back.

dorsoventral (dor″sō-vĕn′trăl) Concerning the back and frontal surfaces of the body.

dorsum [L.] The back or posterior surface of a part; in the foot, the top of the foot.

dosage [Gr. *dosis,* a giving] The determination of the amount, frequency, and number of doses of medication or radiation for a patient.

d. calculation for children Specialized determination of dosage allowing for the body mass and metabolic rate of pediatric patients. There is no absolutely reliable formula for calculating the dosage of a medicine an infant or child should receive. Those systems that use body surface area are most accurate. SEE: *body surface area.*

dose (dōs) [Gr. *dosis,* a giving] The amount of medicine or radiation to be administered at one time.

absorbed d. SEE: under *radiation absorbed dose.*

air d. The intensity of radiation measured in air at the target.

bolus d. An amount of medicine given intravenously at a controlled but rapid rate.

booster d. SEE: *booster.*

cumulative d. **1.** The total dose resulting from repeated exposure to radiation, either to one site or to the whole body. **2.** The amount of a drug present in the body after repeated doses.

curative d. The dose required to cure an illness or disease.

divided d. Fractional portions administered at short intervals.

equianalgesic d. A dose of one form of analgesic drug equivalent in pain-relieving potential to another analgesic. In pain control, this equivalence permits substitution of one analgesic to avoid undesired side effects from another.

erythema d. The smallest amount of radiation (e.g., ultraviolet A rays or x-rays) that will redden or burn the skin. SYN: *threshold d.*

fatal d. A dose that kills. SEE: *median lethal d.*

infective d. The amount of an infectious organism, esp. a bacterium or virus, that will cause disease.

maintenance d. The dose required to maintain the desired effect.

maximum d. The largest dose that is safe to administer.

maximum permissible d. ABBR: MPD. The highest dose of radiation allowed to a person exposed over 1 year, an absolute concept replaced by effective dose limits.

mean marrow d. ABBR: MMD. An estimated measure of average exposure to the entire active bone marrow by ionizing radiation. The percentage of active bone marrow in the useful beam is multiplied by the average absorbed dose.

median curative d. A dose that cures half of the persons treated.

median infective d. ABBR: ID_{50}. An infective dose that causes disease in half of the susceptible subjects given that dose.

median lethal d. ABBR: LD_{50}. The amount of a substance, bacterium, or toxin that will kill 50% of the animals exposed to it. SEE: *minimum lethal d.*

minimum d. The smallest effective dose.

minimum lethal d. The smallest amount of a substance capable of producing death. SEE: *median lethal d.*

primary d. The initial, large dose given to provide a high blood level without delay.

skin d. A radiation dose to the skin including secondary radiation from backscatter.

therapeutic d. The dose required to produce the desired effect.

threshold d. Erythema d.

tissue tolerance d. The largest dose, esp. of radiation, that will not harm tissues.

tolerance d. The dose of a drug or physical agent such as radiation that can be received without harm. This dose will vary between individuals.

toxic d. A dose that causes signs and symptoms of drug toxicity.

dose escalation A progressive increase in the strength of any treatment (e.g., a drug or a radiation dose), to improve its tolerability or maximize its effect.

dose response curve A graph that charts the effect of a specific dose of drug, chemical, or ionizing radiation. In radiology, also called *survival curve.*

dosimeter (dō-sĭm′ĭ-tĕr) [″ + *metron,* measure] A device for measuring x-ray output.

dosimetric (dō″sĭ-mĕt′rĭk) Pert. to dosimetry.

dosimetry (dō-sĭm′ĕ-trē) [″ + *metron,* measure] Measurement of doses.

DOT *directly observed therapy.*

dotage [ME. *doten,* to be silly] Cognitive impairment.

double (dŭb′l) [L. *duplus,* twofold] Being twofold; combining two qualities.

double-blind technique A method of scientific investigation in which neither the subject nor the investigator knows what treatment, if any, the subject is receiving. At the completion of the experiment, the treatment protocol is revealed and data are analyzed with respect to the various treatments used. This method attempts to eliminate observer and subject bias. SEE: *open-label study*.

double chin Buccula.

double personality A split in consciousness, neither personality being aware of the actions and words of the other. SEE: *multiple personality*.

double reading Evaluation of the results of a test, especially a mammogram, by two individuals. SEE: *mammography*.

double uterus A congenital anomaly in which abnormalities in the formation of the Mullerian ducts result in a duplication of the uterus, a uterus with a divided cavity, or sometimes, two copies of the cervix or vagina. SYN: *dimetria; uterus didelphys*.

douche (doosh) [Fr.] A current of vapor or a stream of water directed against a body part. A douche may be plain water or a medicated solution. It may be for personal hygiene or treatment of a local condition.

air d. An air current directed onto the body for therapeutic purposes, usually directed to the tympanum for opening the eustachian tube.

astringent d. A douche containing substances such as alum or zinc sulfate for shrinking the mucous membrane.

circular d. A fine spray or application of water to the body through horizontal needle-sized jets. Several small rows of sprays project the water from four directions simultaneously.

cleansing d. An external or perineal douche for cleansing genitalia following defecation or after operations such as hemorrhoidectomy, curettage, rectal surgery, circumcision, or perineorrhaphy. A mild antiseptic or disinfectant solution, 98° to 104°F (36.7° to 40°C), is poured or sprayed over the parts, followed by gentle drying and inspection for cleanliness. SYN: *perineal cascade*.

deodorizing d. An over-the-counter feminine hygiene product. Routine use of such products is unnecessary and may be harmful because it may alter the normal vaginal flora and increase susceptibility to infections.

high d. Vaginal irrigation or instillation in which the bag is at least 4 ft (1.2 m) above the hips of the patient.

jet d. A douche applied to the body in a solid stream from the douche hose.

medicated d. A douche containing a medicinal substance for the treatment of local conditions.

nasal d. An injection of fluid into the nostril with fluid escaping through the nasopharynx out of the mouth. The patient should keep the mouth open and the glottis closed to prevent fluid from entering the throat and bronchus, and should not blow his or her nose during the treatment. The force of the douche must be moderate. The container should not be suspended more than 6 in. (9.2 cm) above the patient. An atomized spray works more quickly.

neutral d. A douche given at the average surface temperature of the body (i.e., 90° to 97°F [32.2° to 36.1°C]).

perineal d. A spray projected upward from a bidet, placed just above the floor; the patient sits on the seat and receives the douche on the perineum.

vaginal d. Gentle, low pressure irrigation of the vagina. Common protocols for antiseptic irrigations require preparing and administering 1000 to 2000 ml of 105° F (40.5° C) povidone-iodine solution while maintaining universal precautions. For hemostasis, solution temperature is increased to 118° F or 120° F (47.8° to 48.9° C). The container should be elevated up to 2 ft (61 cm) above the woman's pelvis to allow slow, low pressure flow of the solution.

NOTE: The vagina, like many other areas of the body, can cleanse itself. Thus there is very little reason for a normal, healthy woman to use a vaginal douche. Douching can upset the balance of the vaginal flora and change the vaginal pH, thus predisposing the woman to vaginitis. There is no evidence that a postcoital vaginal douche is effective as a contraceptive.

In at least one investigation, vaginal douching has been shown to be a risk factor for pelvic inflammatory disease (PID). The more frequently the subjects douched, the more likely they were to have PID.

Douglas bag [Claude G. Douglas, Brit. physiologist, 1882–1963] A container, usually a bag made of flexible material, for collecting expired air. It is used in investigating respiratory function and physiology.

Douglas' cul-de-sac, Douglas' pouch [James Douglas, Scot. anatomist, 1675–1742] The peritoneal space or pouch that lies behind the uterus and in front of the rectum.

Douglas' fold The arcuate line of the sheath of the rectus abdominis muscle.

douglasitis (dŭg-lăs-ī'tĭs) Inflammation of Douglas' cul-de-sac.

doula (doo'lă) **1.** A woman trained to provide emotional support, guidance, and comfort measures during childbirth. **2.** Highest ranking ancient Greek female servant who assisted women during childbirth.

dowager's hump Cervical lordosis with dorsal kyphosis due to slow loss of bone (i.e., osteoporosis). This may occur at any age but is seen most commonly in elderly women.

dowel [ME. *dowle*, peg] A metal pin for fastening an artificial crown to a tooth root.

down **1.** Lanugo, the fine hairs of the

skin of the newborn. **2.** The fine soft feathers of the young of some birds and the small feathers underneath the large feathers of adult birds, particularly waterfowl. It is used in clothing to give protection from the cold.

downregulate To inhibit or suppress the normal response of an organ or system (e.g., the immune system or the central nervous system). SEE: *immunocompromised.*

Down syndrome [J. Langdon Down, Brit. physician, 1828–1896] The clinical consequences of having three copies of chromosome 21. The condition is marked by mild to moderate mental retardation and physical characteristics that include a sloping forehead, low-set ears with small canals, and short broad hands with a single palmar crease ("simian" crease). Cardiac valvular disease and a tendency to develop Alzheimer-like changes in the brain are common consequences of the syndrome. The syndrome is present in about 1 in 700 births in the U.S. and is more common in women over age 40. In women who conceive after age 45, the syndrome affects 1 in 25 births. SYN: *trisomy 21.* SEE: *amniocentesis; chorionic villus sampling; mosaicism; Nursing Diagnoses Appendix.*

Women at high risk of giving birth to a child with Down syndrome are those over 40; those who have had a previous child with the syndrome; and those who themselves have Down syndrome (pregnancy is rare in this condition). In addition, there is a high risk of having a child with Down syndrome when there is parental mosaicism with a 21 trisomic cell population.

ETIOLOGY: Patients with Down syndrome have an extra chromosome, usually number 21 or 22.

DIAGNOSIS: Amniocentesis or chorionic villus sampling can be used to diagnose the syndrome early in pregnancy.

GENETIC MOSAICISM: The possibility of mosaicism should be explored when children who exhibit classic physical characteristics of Down syndrome later demonstrate normal or near-normal developmental cognitive abilities.

PATIENT CARE: The importance of amniocentesis in detecting the syndrome is explained to the at-risk pregnant woman and her partner or support person. Procedural and sensation information to communicate includes that the test can be conducted anytime after the 14th week of pregnancy (when sufficient amniotic fluid is present); only a small amount of fluid will be removed; and the potential for complications to the fetus or woman is less than 1%.

Throughout the procedure, emotional support is provided, and explanations are reinforced. Following the procedure, fetal heart rate is monitored for 30 minutes, and the woman is assessed for uterine contractions. If test results are positive, the patient is referred for genetic counseling. If she elects to have a therapeutic abortion, physical and emotional support are provided throughout and after the procedure, and post-procedure care is explained.

If the pregnancy continues, the patient and her partner must understand the multisystem anomalies that may occur. Postdelivery, the infant is assessed for the major clinical manifestations, including physical characteristics and congenital anomalies. Parental responses, including grief, are anticipated. The family is taught about management of the infant, beginning with possible feeding problems related to poor sucking ability and the risk for upper respiratory infections. A social worker may explore with the family available support systems and social and financial resources, making referrals to community agencies as appropriate.

The child with Down syndrome requires ongoing assessment for mental retardation, social development, sensory problems, physical growth, sexual development, and congenital anomalies. The parents are advised that surgery may be indicated for correction of serious congenital anomalies. The child's participation in self-care, recreational, vocational, educational, and social opportunities to his or her maximum capabilities is encouraged. The family also is encouraged and assisted to investigate opportunities for and with the child, such as Special Olympics, sheltered workshops, and residential care settings, and to use available supportive services to identify and develop realistic goals for the growing child's future.

doxapram hydrochloride (dŏk′să-prăm) A respiratory stimulant.

doxorubicin hydrochloride (dŏk″sō-rū′bĭ-sĭn) A drug used in the treatment of breast cancer, esophageal cancers, sarcomas, and lymphomas. It has many side effects, one of which is cardiac muscle damage.

doxycycline (dŏk″sē-sī′klēn) A broad-spectrum antibiotic of the tetracycline group.

doxylamine succinate (dŏk-sĭl′ă-mēn) An antihistamine.

Doyère's eminence (dwă-yārz′) [Louis Doyère, Fr. physiologist, 1811–1863] An elevation where a nerve fiber enters a muscle.

D.P. *Doctor of Pharmacy.*

2,3-D.P.G. *2,3-diphosphoglycerate.*

D.P.M. *Doctor of Podiatric Medicine.*

DR *reaction of degeneration.*

Dr. *Doctor.*

dr *drachm; dram.*

drachm Dram.

dracontiasis (drăk″ŏn-tī′ă-sĭs) [Gr. *drakontion,* little dragon] Dracunculiasis.

dracunculiasis (dră-kŭng″kū-lī′ă-sĭs) Infestation with the nematode *Dracunculus medinensis.*

dracunculosis (dră-kŭng″kū-lō′sĭs) Dracunculiasis.

Dracunculus (dră-kŭng′kū-lŭs) A genus of parasitic nematodes.

D. medinensis The guinea worm or "fiery serpent." This species of nematode is a common human parasite, esp. in Africa and India. Infection of humans occurs when water containing infected crustacea of the genus *Cyclops* is swallowed. The larvae are liberated in the stomach or duodenum, then migrate through the viscera and become adults. The adult female, after mating, burrows under the skin of the leg. Larvae are discharged into the environment through the ulcer caused by the worm, esp. when the legs are in water. The infection may be prevented by boiling suspect water, treating it with chlorine, or filtering it to remove the infected *Cyclops.*

TREATMENT: The head of the adult worm can be seen in the ulcer. Slow traction on the worm will remove it. This is done by making a small incision, grasping the front end of the worm, and winding it around a small object. The winding is increased each day until the worm is removed. It is important not to break the worm. Use of thiabendazole or metronidazole has no effect on the worms themselves but produces resolution of the skin inflammation in several days. Unerupted worms may be removed surgically under local anesthesia. SEE: illus.

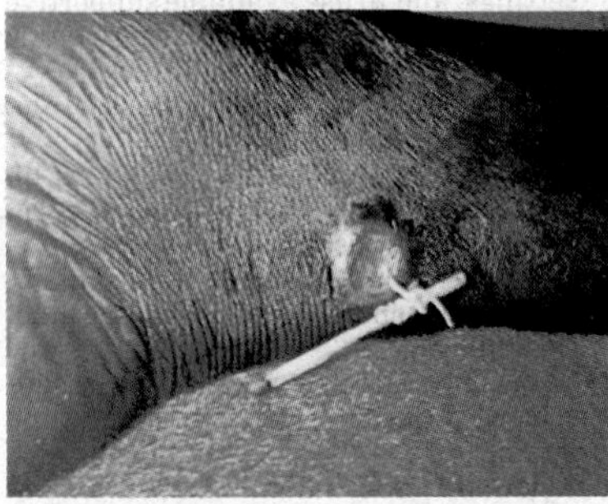

DRACUNCULUS MEDINENSIS

Guinea worm being removed from ulcer

draft, draught A dose of liquid medicine intended to be taken all at once.

drain (drān) [AS. *dreahnian,* to draw off] **1.** An exit or tube for discharge of a morbid matter. **2.** To draw off a fluid.

capillary d. A drawing off by capillary attraction.

cigarette d. A drain made by covering a small strip of gauze with rubber.

Mikulicz's d. SEE: *Mikulicz's drain.*

nonabsorbable d. A drain made from horsehair, gauze, rubber, glass, or metal. Types are abdominal, antral, perineal, and suprapubic.

Penrose d. [Charles B. Penrose, 20th-century American surgeon] A drain made of a piece of small rubber tubing.

drainage (drān′ĭj) The flow or withdrawal of fluids from a wound or cavity, such as pus from a cavity or wound. SEE: *autodrainage; drain.*

capillary d. Drainage by means of capillary attraction.

chest d. Placement of a drainage tube in the chest cavity, usually in the pleural space. The tube is used to drain air, fluid, or blood from the pleural space so the compressed and collapsed lung can expand. The tube is connected to a system that produces suction. This helps to remove the material from the pleural space and also prevents air from being sucked into the space.

closed d. Drainage of a wound or body space so that the air is excluded.

closed sterile d. A sterile tube draining a body site, such as the abdominal cavity or pleural space, that is designed to prevent the entry of air and bacteria into the tubing or the area being drained.

negative pressure d. Drainage in which negative pressure is maintained in the tube. It is used in treating pneumothorax and in certain types of drains or catheters in the intestinal tract, body cavity, or surgical wound. SYN: *suction d.*

open d. Drainage of a wound or body cavity so that air is not excluded from the area of the cavity.

postural d. Positioning a patient so that gravity can be used to assist in the removal of secretions from specific lobes of the lung, bronchi, or lung cavities. The technique can be used in the treatment of pneumonias and other pulmonary infections, bronchiectasis, chronic bronchitis, or any patient having difficulty with retained secretions. SEE: *postural drainage* for illus.

suction d. Negative pressure d.

tidal d. A method, controlled mechanically, of filling the bladder with solution by gravity and periodically emptying the bladder with a catheter. It is usually used when the patient lacks bladder control as in injuries or lesions of the spinal cord.

Wangensteen d. SEE: *Wangensteen tube.*

drained weight The actual weight of food that has been allowed to drain to remove the liquids in which it has been prepared.

dram (drăm) [Gr. *drachme*, a Gr. unit of weight] ABBR: dr. SYMB: ʒ. A unit of weight in the apothecaries' system. SYN: *drachm*.

dramatism [Gr. *drama*, acting, + *-ismos*, condition] Dramatic behavior and lofty speech seen in psychological disturbances.

drapetomania (drăp″ĕt-ō-mā′nē-ă) [Gr. *drapetes*, runaway, + *mania*, madness] An insane impulse to wander from home.

drastic [Gr. *drastikos*, effective] **1.** Acting strongly. **2.** A very active cathartic, usually producing many explosive bowel movements accompanied by pain and tenesmus. The use of this type of cathartic is not advisable.

draught (drăft) [ME. *draught*, a pulling] **1.** A drink. **2.** Liquid drawn into the mouth. **3.** A breeze produced by wind or a fan. **4.** Draft.

Draw-a-Person test A widely used projective assessment that is assumed to reveal information about a patient's body image or self-concept. SYN: *Machover test*.

drawer sign, drawer test Determination of the instability of ligaments by forcibly displacing one bone or structure relative to another.

1. Assessment of the cruciate ligament(s) of the knee. The knee is flexed to 90 degrees, with the foot stabilized on the examination table. The examiner applies an anterior, then a posterior, force against the upper tibia, perpendicular to the long axis of the leg. An increased glide, anterior or posterior, of the tibia is caused by rupture of the anterior or posterior cruciate ligament, respectively.

2. Assessment of the anterior talofibular ligament of the ankle. The foot is placed in its neutral position, the knee is flexed to a minimum of 20 degrees to release the tension of the gastrocnemius muscle, and the tibia is stabilized. The examiner cups the posterior and plantar surface of the calcaneus and draws the foot forward, observing for increased displacement of the lateral foot and talus relative to the opposite extremity. These findings would suggest rupture of the ligament.

DRE *digital rectal examination*.

dream [AS. *dream*, joy] The occurrence of ideas, emotions, visual imagery, and other sensations during sleep. Some dreams may be recalled on awakening; others may not be. SEE: *REM; sleep; sleep disorder; wet dream*.

Interpretation of the meaning of dreams has been of interest to human beings since the dawn of history and to psychoanalysts for the past 100 years. The idea that a dream conceals a meaning buried deep in the subconscious is probably mistaken, and is difficult to confirm scientifically, although it is still accepted by many psychoanalysts. Less controversial are the research results correlating changes in the electroencephalogram and rapid eye movements (REM) during sleep with dream activity. Under experimental conditions, it has been possible to communicate with the person who is dreaming. Some animals (i.e., cats and dogs) are believed to dream. *The Interpretation of Dreams*, a work by Sigmund Freud, was one of the first rigorous attempts to study dreaming.

drench A dose of medicine that is administered to an animal by pouring it into its mouth.

drepanocyte (drĕp′ă-nō-sīt) [Gr. *drepane*, sickle, + *kytos*, cell] Sickle cell.

drepanocytemia (drĕp″ă-nō-sī-tē′mē-ă) [″ + ″ + *haima*, blood] Sickle cell anemia.

drepanocytic (drĕp″ă-nō-sĭt′ĭk) Pert. to or resembling a sickle cell.

dressing [O.Fr. *dresser*, to prepare] A covering, protective or supportive, for diseased or injured parts.

Patient Care: The procedure and expected sensations are explained to the patient. His or her privacy is ensured, and necessary supplies are assembled. Strict aseptic technique is followed during dressing changes, and dressings are properly disposed of in biohazard containers. Personnel must wash their hands before and after the procedure. The wound or incision and dressing are assessed for the presence and character of any drainage, and the findings are documented. The condition of the wound or suture line is also checked, and the presence of erythema or edema is noted. Instruction in wound assessment and dressing change techniques is provided to the patient and his or her family members.

absorbent d. A dressing consisting of gauze, sterilized gauze, or absorbent cotton.

antiseptic d. A dressing consisting of gauze permeated with an antiseptic solution.

clear transparent covering d. Transparent synthetic d.

dry d. A dressing consisting of dry gauze, absorbent cotton, or other dry material.

film d. A transparent wound covering, made of polyurethane, that enables health care providers to visually inspect an injured part as it heals. The dressing allows water vapor to escape from the wound but does not permit liquids or bacteria to enter.

foam d. An opaque polyurethane dressing that is permeable to vapors but partially occlusive to liquids. It is typically used to cover wounds over bony ridges or near inflamed skin.

hydrocolloid d. A flexible dressing made of an adhesive, gumlike (hydrocolloid) material such as karaya or pectin covered with a water-resistant film. The dressing keeps the wound surface moist, but, because it excludes air, it may promote anaerobic bacterial growth. It should not be used on wounds that are, or are suspected to be, infected. The directions that come with the dressing should be followed.

nonadherent d. A dressing that has little or no tendency to stick to dried secretions from the wound.

occlusive d. A dressing that seals a wound completely to prevent infection from outside and to prevent inner moisture from escaping through the dressing.

pressure d. A dressing used to apply pressure to the wound. It may be used following skin grafting.

protective d. A dressing applied for the purpose of preventing injury or infection to the treated part.

self-adhering roller d. A rolled gauze strip made of a material that adheres to one side of the gauze. It comes in various widths.

transparent synthetic d. A dressing usually made of a plastic material with the skin-contact side coated with a hypoallergenic adhesive. SYN: *clear transparent covering d.*

universal d. A large flat bandage that may be folded several times to make a relatively large dressing or folded several more times to make a smaller and thicker dressing. This process can be continued until the unit is suitable for use as a cervical collar. The bandage is easily made and stored. SEE: *cervical collar* for illus.

warm moist d. A dressing that most commonly uses a normal saline solution no hotter than the bare forearm of the nurse can tolerate. The sterile towel is unfolded, and the gauze dressing is dropped into it. Then the center of the towel is immersed in solution and wrung out by turning the dry ends in opposite directions. The dressing is applied with sterile forceps directly to the wound. Sometimes a dry sterile towel is used over it to keep the dressing in place. Heat is best maintained by infrared lamp.

CAUTION: Care must be taken not to burn the patient.

water d. A dressing consisting of gauze, cotton, or similar material that is kept wet by the application of sterilized water.

wet-to-dry d. A dressing consisting of gauze moistened by sterile solution applied directly and conforming to the wound and covered with dry gauze pads and a bandage. Gentle removal of the dressing after it has dried provides some degree of débridement of the wound; the process is then repeated at intervals.

dressing stick An adaptive device de-

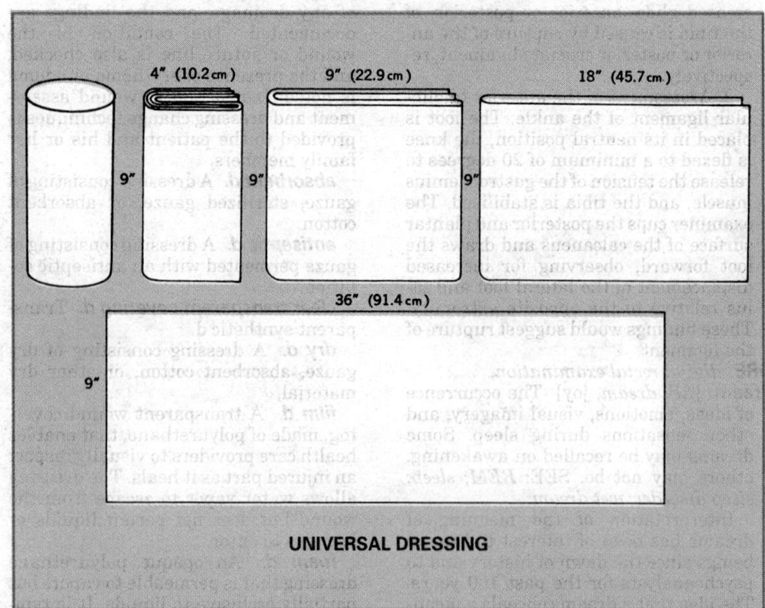

UNIVERSAL DRESSING

signed to permit independent dressing by persons with limited motion. Also called *dressing wand.*

Dressler's syndrome [William Dressler, U.S. physician, 1890–1960] Postmyocardial infarction syndrome, characterized by pleuritic chest pain, pericarditis, fever, and leukocytosis.

DRG *diagnosis-related group.*

drift Movement, often in an aimless fashion.

genetic d. The chance variation of genetic frequency, seen most often in a small population.

mesial d. Movement of teeth in the arch in a mesial or ventral direction due to occlusal forces and interproximal wear of teeth.

drill A device for rotating a sharp and shaped cutting instrument, used for preparing teeth for restoration and in orthopedics. SEE: *bur.*

Drinker respirator [Philip Drinker, U.S. engineer in industrial hygiene, 1894–1972] An obsolete apparatus in which alternating positive and negative air pressure on the patient's thoracic area was used to produce artificial respiration by allowing the air in the otherwise immobile lung to be alternately filled with air and emptied. This device is commonly called an *iron lung.*

drip [ME. *drippen,* to drip] **1.** To fall in drops. **2.** To instill a liquid slowly, drop by drop.

gravity d. Infusion of an intravenous solution by hanging the source of the solution above the patient and controlling the rate of flow with a manually operated clamp.

intravenous d. Slow injection of a solution into a vein a drop at a time.

Murphy d. Slow rectal instillation of a fluid drop by drop.

nasal d. A method of administering fluid slowly to dehydrated babies by means of a catheter with one end placed through the nose into the esophagus.

postnasal d. A condition due to rhinitis or sinusitis in which a discharge flows from the nasopharynx region into the oropharynx.

drive (drīv) [AS. *drifan*] The force or impulse to act.

drive control One of various devices and adapted equipment, including hand or foot controls, for modifying a motor vehicle for use by persons with physical disability.

dromomania (drō″mō-mā′nē-ă) [Gr. *dromos,* a running, + *mania,* madness] An insane impulse to wander.

dromotropic [″ + *tropikos,* a turning] Affecting the conductivity of nerve or muscle fibers. SEE: *inotropic.*

dronabinol The principal psychoactive substance present in Cannabis sativa (marijuana). The trade name is Marinol. SEE: *marijuana.*

drooling Ptyalism.

drop [AS. *dropa*] **1.** A minute spherical mass of liquid. **2.** Failure of a part to maintain its normal position, usually due to paralysis or injury.

culture d. A bacterial culture in a drop of culture medium.

foot d. A condition in which the toes drag and the foot hangs, caused by paralysis of the anterior tibial muscles.

hanging d. Application of a drop of solution to a small glass coverslip. This is then inverted over a glass slide with a depression in it. The contents of the suspended solution can be examined microscopically.

"knock-out" d. A colloquial term for a sedative.

nose d. Medication instilled in or sprayed into the nasal cavity.

wrist d. Paralysis of extensor muscles causing the hand to hang down from the forearm.

drop attack A sudden fall with loss of muscular tone and loss of consciousness. Drop attacks may occur in patients with arrhythmias, autonomic failure, epilepsy, narcolepsy, strokes, and other diseases and conditions. Treatment depends on the underlying cause.

droperidol (drō-pĕr′ĭ-dŏl) A drug used for three purposes: to premedicate patients for surgery; to prevent and treat nausea and vomiting; and to sedate agitated and psychotic patients.

droplet A very small drop.

dropper A tube, usually narrowed at one end, for dispensing drops of liquid. If water is so dispensed, about 20 drops equals 1 ml. SEE: *medicine dropper.*

medicine d. According to *USP XXII,* a tube made of glass or other suitable transparent material that generally is fitted with a collapsible bulb and, while varying in capacity, is constricted at the delivery end to a round opening having an external diameter of 3 mm. When held vertically, it delivers water in drops each weighing between 45 mg and 55 mg.

In using a medicine dropper, one should keep in mind that few medicinal liquids have the same surface and flow characteristics as water, and therefore the size of drops may vary considerably from one preparation to another.

When accurate dosing is important, one should use a dropper that has been calibrated for and supplied with the preparation. The volume error incurred in measuring any liquid by means of a calibrated dropper should not exceed 15% under normal use conditions.

dropsy (drŏp′sē) [Gr. *hydor,* water] An obsolete term for generalized edema.

Drosophila (drō-sŏf′ĭ-lă) A genus of flies belonging to the order Diptera. It includes the common fruit flies.

D. melanogaster A genus of fruit flies used extensively in the study of genetics. The development of the chromosome theory of heredity was largely the outcome of research on this species.

drowning [ME. *dr(o)unen,* to drown] Death resulting from immersion and suffocation in a liquid.

near d. Survival after immersion in water. About 330,000 persons, most of whom are children, adolescents, or young adults, survive an immersion injury in the U.S. each year, and of these, about 10% receive professional attention. Many who suffer near drowning do so because of preventable or avoidable conditions, such as the use of alcohol or drugs in aquatic settings or the inadequate supervision of children by adults. Water sports (e.g., diving, swimming, surfing, or skiing) and boating or fishing accidents also are common causes of near drowning. A small percentage of near drowning episodes occurs when patients with known seizure disorders convulse while swimming or boating.

ETIOLOGY: The injuries suffered result from breath holding ("dry drowning"), the aspiration of water into the lungs ("wet drowning"), and/or hypothermia.

SYMPTOMS: Common symptoms of near drowning result from oxygen deprivation, retention of carbon dioxide, or direct damage to the lungs by water. These include cough, dyspnea, coma, and seizures. Additional complications of prolonged immersion may include aspiration pneumonitis, noncardiogenic pulmonary edema, electrolyte disorders, hemolysis, disseminated intravascular coagulation, and arrhythmias.

TREATMENT: In unconscious patients rescued from water, the airway is secured, ventilation is provided, and cardiopulmonary resuscitation is begun. Oxygen, cardiac, and blood pressure monitoring, rewarming techniques, and other forms of support are provided (e.g., anticonvulsants are given for seizures; electrolyte and acid-base disorders are corrected).

PROGNOSIS: Most patients who are rapidly resuscitated from a dry drowning episode recover fully. The recovery of near drowning victims who have inhaled water into the lungs depends on the underlying health of the victim, the duration of immersion, and the speed and efficiency with which oxygenation, ventilation, and perfusion are restored.

drownproofing A method of staying afloat by using a minimum amount of energy. It may be kept up for hours even by nonswimmers, whereas only the most fit and expert could swim for more than 30 min. Details of the drownproofing technique may be obtained from local chapters of the American Red Cross. SEE: illus.

TECHNIQUE: 1. *Rest:* The person takes a deep breath and sinks vertically beneath the surface, relaxes the arms and legs, keeps the chin down, and allows the fingertips to brush against the knees. The neck is relaxed and the back of the head is above the surface. 2. *Get set:* The arms are raised gently to a crossed position with the back of the wrists touching the forehead. At the same time, the person steps forward with one leg and backward with the other. 3. *Lift head, exhale:* With the arms and legs in the previous position, the head is raised quickly but smoothly to the vertical position and the person exhales through the nose. 4. *Stroke and kick, inhale:* To support the head above the surface while inhaling through the mouth, the arms sweep gently outward and downward and both feet step downward. 5. *Head down, press:* As the person drops beneath the surface, the head goes down and the arms and hands press downward to arrest descent. 6. *Rest:* It is important to relax completely as in the first step for 6 to 10 sec.

drowsiness The state of almost falling asleep.

daytime d. Drowsiness occurring

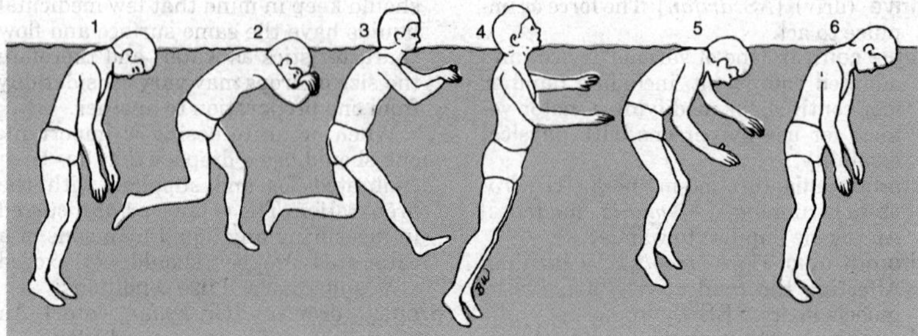

1, Rest. 2, Get set. 3, Lift head, exhale. 4, Stroke and kick, inhale. 5, Head down, press. 6, Rest.

DROWNPROOFING TECHNIQUE

during the day rather than just before normal bedtime. The cause may be inadequate sleep the preceding night; however, it may also be associated with anxiety, ill health, or side effects of either prescribed drugs or drugs of abuse. The condition is not equivalent to narcolepsy.

Dr.P.H. *Doctor of Public Health.*

DRSP *Drug-resistant Streptococcus pneumoniae.*

drug [O.Fr. *drogue,* chemical material] Any substance that, when taken into a living organism, may modify one or more of its functions.

adverse d. reaction An unwanted response to a therapeutic drug. Health professionals are encouraged to report all adverse events related to drugs or medical devices to the manufacturer and the Food and Drug Administration (FDA), to aid in monitoring the safety of marketed medical products. SEE: *MedWatch; post-marketing surveillance.* SYN: *drug reaction.*

brake d. A popular term for a hormonal agent that prevents excessive growth in children.

designer d. A term coined by Gary Henderson, contemporary pharmacologist, meaning an illicitly produced drug of abuse such as methamphetamine, fentanyl and its analogues, and phencyclidine hydrochloride (PCP). In several attempts to produce these drugs, toxic chemicals have been made. Also, the compounds are not standardized with respect to potency, so deaths from overdose may occur.

disease-modifying antirheumatic d. ABBR: DMARD. A drug used to treat rheumatoid arthritis that acts slower than nonsteroidal anti-inflammatory drugs. Included are hydroxychloroquine, intramuscular gold preparations, D-penicillamine, methotrexate, and azathioprine.

generic d. SEE: *generic drug.*

investigational new d. ABBR: IND. A drug available only for experimental purposes because its safety and effectiveness have not been proven; thus, the U.S. Food and Drug Administration has not approved its use except in research.

look-alike d. One of a group of solid dosage forms of drugs that mimic various prescription drugs by size, shape, color, and markings. Some of these may be controlled drugs.

neuromuscular blocking d. A type of drug used during the administration of anesthesia to allow surgical access to body cavities, in particular the abdomen and thorax, by preventing voluntary or reflex muscle movement. These drugs are also used to facilitate compliance in critically ill patients undergoing intensive therapy such as mechanical ventilation.

new d. A drug for which premarketing approval is required by the Food, Drug and Cosmetic Act. For the most part, new prescription drugs have been regulated by new drug application and premarket approval regulations, but most drugs sold over the counter (OTC) and directly to the public (i.e., nonprescription drugs) have not. There has been increased interest in evaluating the safety and efficacy of at least some OTC drugs.

nonprescription d. Over-the-counter medication.

recreational d. A drug used for enjoyment rather than for a medical purpose.

scheduled d. SEE: *controlled substance act.*

street d. A drug obtained illegally. Usually it is a drug of abuse.

drug abuse The use or overuse, usually by self-administration, of any drug in a manner that deviates from the prescribed pattern.

Health care workers, many of whom have easy access to narcotics, are at high risk of abusing analgesics. Increased awareness of this problem has led hospitals to establish special programs for identifying these individuals, esp. physicians, nurses, and pharmacists, in order to provide support and education in an attempt to control the problem and prevent loss of license.

Drug Abuse Warning Network ABBR: DAWN. A system for obtaining statistical data concerning admission to a sample of emergency treatment facilities for drug abuse.

drug addiction A compulsive and maladaptive dependence on a drug that produces adverse psychological, physical, economic, social, or legal ramifications. SEE: *substance abuse; substance dependence.*

drug administration *Acids:* When administered orally, acids should be given well diluted through a glass tube or by stomach tube because they are corrosive to the enamel and dentin of the teeth. They should be given with much water, and the drinking tube should be placed well back in the mouth to prevent the fluid coming in contact with the teeth before passing into the throat. Diluted hydrochloric acid is one preparation that should always be given using this technique.

Habit-forming drugs: These drugs should be given as ordered by the physician.

Horse serum: When injections containing it are administered, information should be obtained as to whether the patient has ever received vaccine containing horse serum and what reaction there was at that time. If the patient is allergic to horse serum, a sensitivity test should always be done by injecting hypodermically a few drops of the greatly diluted material containing horse serum. Reaction occurs within a short time. A small spot appears at the site of the injection if the patient is allergic. The physician will provide instructions for desensitizing a person allergic to horse serum.

Insulin: When insulin is administered, it should be given hypodermically or intravenously according to the instructions of the attending physician. The type of insulin, dosage, and dosing frequency vary greatly with each patient. SEE: *insulin pump.*

Laxatives: These are best given in the evening because they usually take 6 to 8 hr to produce an effect. Saline purgatives are usually given well diluted on an empty stomach in the morning. Other purgatives usually are given as ordered and needed.

Mouthwash: Stock solutions used for mouthwash should be diluted by half or more before being given to the patient. Only enough for the immediate mouth washing should be given to the patient at a particular time.

Oxygen: The most commonly used method for administration of oxygen consists of inserting a cannula into both nostrils. Oxygen may also be given from a tank by means of a mask over the patient's nose and mouth, by an endotracheal tube, or the patient may be placed in an oxygen tent, chamber, or room. The last two methods are not only expensive and less effective than use of a mask or nasal catheters but are also extremely dangerous and must be used cautiously because of the fire hazard. Oxygen given by cannula should be hydrated by bubbling through water before passage into the nose. Dry oxygen in high concentration for a prolonged period will cause irritation of the nasal and lower respiratory mucosa.

Saline purgatives: These should always be given to the patient when the stomach is empty, preferably in the morning.

Sleeping pills: All such preparations should be given from 30 min to 1 hr before sleep is desired. All procedures should be finished before the drug is given so that nothing disturbs the patient after the drug is administered.

Vaccines: The route of administration varies with each specific vaccine; most are given orally or intramuscularly.

drug companion A medication whose efficacy depends on its use with a second agent. The same drug may have little effect when used alone.

drug delivery, new methods of Several methods of drug delivery have been used experimentally. Included are chemical modification of a drug to enable it to penetrate membranes such as the blood-brain barrier; incorporation of microparticles in colloidal carriers made of proteins, carbohydrates, lipids, or synthetic polymers; controlled-release systems that permit a drug to be delivered for very long periods; and transdermal controlled-release systems (e.g., those currently in use for administration of scopolamine or nitroglycerin). In addition to the use of various carriers for drugs, cell transplantation could be used to provide therapeutic agents, and the possibility of inserting genes into cells to produce desired effects is being explored. SEE: *liposome.*

drug dependence A psychic (and sometimes physical) state resulting from interaction of a living organism and a drug. Characteristic behavioral and other responses include a compulsion to take the drug on a continuous or periodic basis to experience its psychic effects or to avoid the discomfort of its absence. Tolerance may be present. A person may become dependent on more than one drug.

Drug Enforcement Agency number ABBR: DEA number. A number assigned by the DEA to health care providers indicating that the person or facility is registered with the DEA to prescribe controlled substances.

drug-fast Drug-resistant.

Drug-Free Workplace Act of 1988 Federal legislation requiring all organizations applying for federal grants to certify that a "good faith" effort will be made to prevent substance abuse in the workplace.

druggist (drŭg′ĭst) Pharmacist.

drug handling It is important to carefully read the label or other printed instruction issued with medications. The ordered doses (quantities) should be measured accurately and never estimated. A measuring glass or spoon marked in milliliters, ounces, or both should be used. In giving a dose of medicine, it is necessary to know to whom it has to be given, what has to be given, when it has to be given, and the prescribed amount. If medicine is to be taken orally, the patient should be observed until he or she has actually swallowed it.

NOTE: The cover must never be left off the container because a necessary property may evaporate, the drug may become dangerously concentrated, or it may absorb moisture from the air and become difficult to handle or dilute. The drug storage compartment must be kept locked.

drug interaction The combined effect of drugs taken concurrently. The result may be antagonism or synergism, and consequently may be lethal in some cases. It is important for the patient, physician, and nurse to be aware of the

Comparison of Toxic and Allergic Drug Reactions

	Toxic	Allergic
Incidence	May occur with any drug	Occurs infrequently
Dosage	Usually high	Therapeutic
Reaction time	May occur with first dose, or may be due to cumulative effect	Usually only upon re-exposure, but some drugs cross-react with chemicals of similar structure
Symptoms	May be similar to pharmacological action of drug	Not related to pharmacological action of drug
Associated disorders	None	Asthma, hay fever

potential interaction of drugs that are prescribed as well as those that the patient may be self-administering.

Many patients, esp. the elderly, may take several medicines each day. The chances of developing an undesired drug interaction increase rapidly with the number of drugs used. It is estimated that if eight or more medications are being used, there is a 100% chance of interaction.

drug overdose The clinical consequence of any excess dose of a drug (e.g., of a self-administered, potentially lethal dose of a drug of abuse, an antidepressant, a non-narcotic pain reliever, or other medication). Drug overdose may be unintentional or deliberate. When such a dose results in coma or death, the person is said to have OD'd (i.e., overdosed).

PATIENT CARE: Emergency department personnel assess the patient's airway, breathing, circulation, level of consciousness, and vital signs, and try to ascertain (from the patient or significant others) what drug was taken, how much, when, and by what route. Blood and urine (and when it becomes available, emesis) are sent to the laboratory for toxicology screening to aid in identifying specific substances.

If the drug was administered by inhalation or parenterally, or if time lapse has allowed for absorption, an intravenous site is established, and fluid is administered as prescribed to help flush out the substance. If the patient is unconscious on admission, he or she will be given a narcotic antagonist, a bolus of 50% dextrose in water, and 50 to 100 mg of thiamine routinely to reverse rapidly the potential effects of opiates or low blood sugar. Depending on the patient's response to the drug's actions (e.g., CNS depression or stimulation, respiratory depression, cardiac arrhythmias, or renal failure), emergency department personnel provide necessary supportive therapies (e.g., airway intubation and ventilation), activated charcoal, or bowel irrigation. Because absorption rates vary and may fluctuate, the patient requires frequent reassessment with immediate intervention as appropriate.

The possibility of attempted suicide should be considered in any case of drug overdose. A psychiatric history is obtained, with any history of depression noted. Suicide precautions are established to protect the patient from further self-injury. SEE: *Nursing Diagnoses Appendix.*

drug product problem reporting program A program managed by the U.S. Pharmacopeial Convention, Inc., that informs the product manufacturer, the labeler, and the Food and Drug Administration (FDA) of potential health hazards and defective drug products. The reports may be submitted by any health professional.

drug reaction Adverse and undesired reaction to a substance taken for its pharmacological effects. An estimated 15% of hospitalized patients develop toxic or allergic drug reactions. SEE: table.

drug-resistant **1.** Unaffected by chemotherapy. **2.** Unable to be killed or eradicated with antibiotics, said of certain bacteria. SYN: *drug-fast*.

drug screen A clinical laboratory procedure that checks a patient's blood or urine sample for presence of certain drugs such as barbiturates, opioids, or amphetamines. Also called a *tox screen*.

drug testing, mandated The enforced testing of individuals for evidence of drug use or abuse. Certain U.S. governmental regulatory agencies have instituted programs for testing employees in industries important to public safety such as ground and air transportation. To date, the programs have not mandated testing for alcohol abuse.

drug user, injection An individual who self-administers drugs, usually to attain a euphoric or altered state of consciousness. The practice is rarely performed aseptically and may result in the spreading of communicable diseases or in self-injury.

drum The membrane of the tympanic

cavity; the tympanum or cavity of the middle ear.

drunkenness [AS. *drinean,* to drink] Alcoholic intoxication. In legal medicine, intoxication or being "under the influence" of alcohol is defined according to the concentration of alcohol in the blood or exhaled air. The precise concentration used to define legal intoxication varies among states. Drivers are considered intoxicated with alcohol (in many states) when the blood level is 0.1% or more. A blood alcohol level over 0.5% is sufficient to cause alcoholic coma in most people.

drusen (droo'zĕn) [Ger. *Duse,* weathered ore] Small, hyaline, globular pathological growths on the optic papilla or on Descemet's membrane.

dry measure A measure of volume for dry commodities. SEE: *Weights and Measures Appendix.*

dry mouth, mouth dryness Decreased production or lack of saliva. This condition may be due to the action of drugs such as diuretics, antihistamines, and anticholinergics; dehydration; anxiety; radiation therapy to the head or neck; or Sjögren's syndrome (an autoimmune disease that affects the salivary glands). SYN: *xerostomia.* SEE: *Sjögren's syndrome; artificial saliva.*

SYMPTOMS: Mouth dryness interferes with speech, swallowing, denture retention, and maintaining oral hygiene.

TREATMENT: The patient should avoid using the drugs mentioned. Careful attention to oral hygiene is necessary. Frequent sips of sugar-free fluids and use of a saliva substitute may provide some relief. Oral fluid intake ameliorates dry mouth due to dehydration. Pilocarpine may increase saliva production.

Drysdale's corpuscle (drīz'dālz) [Thomas M. Drysdale, U.S. gynecologist, 1831–1904] A type of nonnucleated granular cell found in the fluid of certain ovarian cysts.

DSA *digital subtraction angiography.*

DSM-IV *Diagnostic and Statistical Manual of Mental Disorders (Fourth Edition).*

d4t Stavudine, a nucleoside analogue reverse transcriptase inhibitor used in the treatment of HIV-1.

DT *delirium tremens.*

dualism (dū'ă-lĭzm) [L. *duo,* two, + Gr. *-ismos,* condition] **1.** The condition of being double or twofold. **2.** The theory that human beings consist of two entities, mind and matter, that are independent of each other. **3.** The theory that various blood cells arise from two types of stem cells: myeloblasts, giving rise to the myeloid elements, and lymphoblasts, giving rise to the lymphoid elements.

DUB *dysfunctional uterine bleeding.*

Dubini's disease (dū-bē'nēz) [Angelo Dubini, It. physician, 1813–1902] Rapid rhythmic contractions of a group or groups of muscles. SYN: *electric chorea; spasmus Dubini.*

Dubin-Johnson syndrome [Isadore Nathan Dubin, U.S. pathologist, 1913–1980; Frank B. Johnson, U.S. pathologist, b. 1919] An inherited defect of bile metabolism that causes retention of conjugated bilirubin in hepatic cells. The patient is asymptomatic except for mild intermittent jaundice. No treatment is required.

duboisine (dū-bŏy'sēn) An alkaloid derivative of the plant *Duboisia myoporoides.* It is a form of hyoscyamine used as a mydriatic.

Dubowitz tool, Dubowitz score [Lilly and Victor Dubowitz, contemporary South African physicians] A method of estimating the gestational age of an infant based on 21 strictly defined physical and neurological signs. This method provides the correct gestational age ±2 weeks in 95% of infants.

Duchenne, Guillaume B. A. (dū-shĕn') French neurologist, 1806–1875.

D.'s disease Degeneration of the posterior roots and column of the spinal cord and of the brainstem. It is marked by attacks of pain, progressive ataxia, loss of reflexes, functional disorders of the bladder, larynx, and gastrointestinal system, and impotence. This disorder develops in conjunction with syphilis and most frequently affects middle-aged men. SYN: *tabes dorsalis.*

D.'s muscular dystrophy Pseudohypertrophic muscular dystrophy marked by weakness and pseudohypertrophy of the affected muscles. It is caused by mutation of the gene responsible for producing the protein dystrophin. The disease begins in childhood, is progressive, and affects the shoulder and pelvic girdle muscles. The disease, mostly of males, is transmitted as a sex-linked recessive trait. Most patients die before age 20. SEE: *Nursing Diagnoses Appendix.*

D.'s paralysis Bulbar paralysis.

Duchenne-Aran disease (dū-shĕn'ăr-ăn') [Duchenne; Francois Amilcar Aran, Fr. physician, 1817–1861] Spinal muscular atrophy.

Duchenne-Erb paralysis (dū-shĕn'ayrb) [Duchenne; Wilhelm Heinrich Erb, Ger. neurologist, 1840–1921] Erb's paralysis.

duct [L. *ducere,* to lead] **1.** A narrow tubular vessel or channel, esp. one that conveys secretions from a gland. **2.** A narrow enclosed channel containing a fluid (e.g., the semicircular duct of the ear).

accessory pancreatic d. A duct of the pancreas leading into the pancreatic duct or the duodenum near the mouth of the common bile duct. SYN: *d. of Santorini.*

alveolar d. A branch of a respiratory bronchiole that leads to the alveolar sacs of the lungs. SEE: *alveolus* for illus.

Bartholin's d. The major duct of the sublingual gland.

biliary d. A canal that carries bile. The intrahepatic ducts include the bile canaliculi and interlobular ducts; the extrahepatic ducts include the hepatic, cystic, and common bile ducts. Also called *bile duct.*

cochlear d. Canal of the cochlea.

common bile d. The duct that carries bile and pancreatic juice to the duodenum. It is formed by the union of the cystic duct of the gallbladder and the hepatic duct of the liver and is joined by the main pancreatic duct. SYN: *ductus choledochus*. SEE: *biliary tract* for illus.

cystic d. The secretory duct of the gallbladder. It unites with the hepatic duct from the liver to form the common bile duct. SEE: *biliary tract* for illus.

efferent d. One of a group of 12 to 14 small tubes that constitute the efferent ducts of the testis. They lie within the epididymis and connect the rete testis with the ductus epididymidis. Their coiled portions constitute the lobuli epididymidis.

ejaculatory d. The duct that conveys sperm from the vas deferens and secretions from the seminal vesicle to the urethra.

endolymphatic d. In the embryo, a tubular projection of the otocyst ending in a blind extremity, the endolymphatic sac. In the adult, it connects the endolymphatic sac with the utricle and saccule of the inner ear.

d. of the epoophoron Gartner's d.

excretory d. Any duct that conveys a waste product from an organ, such as the collecting duct of the renal tubule.

Gartner's d. The caudal part of the mesonephric duct, extending from the parovarium through the broad ligament into the vagina. SYN: *d. of the epoophoron.*

hepatic d. A duct that receives bile from the right or left lobe of the liver and carries it to the common bile duct. SYN: *ductus hepaticus dexter; ductus hepaticus sinister*.

intercalated d. One of several short, narrow ducts that lie between the secretory ducts and the terminal alveoli in the parotid and submandibular glands and in the pancreas.

interlobular d. A duct passing between lobules within a gland (e.g., one of the ducts carrying bile).

lacrimal d. One of two short ducts, inferior and superior, that convey tears from the lacrimal lake to the lacrimal sac. Their openings are on the margins of the upper and lower eyelids. SYN: *lacrimal canal.*

lactiferous d. One of 15 to 20 ducts that drain the lobes of the mammary gland. Each opens in a slight depression in the tip of the nipple. SYN: *milk d.*

lymphatic d. One of two main ducts conveying lymph to the bloodstream: the left lymphatic (thoracic) and the right lymphatic duct, which drains lymph from the right side of the body above the diaphragm. It discharges into the right subclavian vein. It is smaller than the left lymphatic duct. SEE: *thoracic d.; lymphatic system* for illus.

mesonephric d. Embryonic duct that connects the mesonephros with the cloaca. In males it develops into the reproductive ducts (the duct of the epididymis, deferent duct, seminal vesicle, and ejaculatory duct). In females it develops into the duct of the epoophoron, a rudimentary structure. SYN: *wolffian d.*

milk d. Lactiferous d.

müllerian d. One of the bilateral ducts in the embryo that form the uterus, vagina, and fallopian tubes. SYN: *Müller's duct*.

nasolacrimal d. A duct that conveys tears from the lacrimal sac to the nasal cavity. It opens beneath the inferior nasal concha.

omphalomesenteric d. Vitelline d.

pancreatic d. The duct that conveys pancreatic juice to the common bile duct and duodenum. SYN: *d. of Wirsung*.

papillary d. Any of the large ducts formed by the uniting of the collecting tubules of the kidney.

paramesonephric d. The genital canal in the embryo. In females it develops into the oviducts, uterus, and vagina; in males it degenerates to form the appendix testis.

paraurethral d. Skene's d.

parotid d. A duct through which secretions from the parotid gland enter the oral cavity. The duct is approx. 2 in. (5.1 cm) long. It extends from the anterior border of the parotid gland, crossing the masseter muscle and piercing the buccinator muscle, and then runs between the buccinator muscle and the mucous membrane. It opens into the mouth opposite the second upper molar. The transverse facial artery is above the duct, and the buccal branch of the seventh cranial nerve is below. Stenosis of the duct causes pain and swelling in the parotid gland. SYN: *Stensen's d.*

prostatic d. One of about 20 ducts that discharge prostatic secretion into the urethra. SYN: *ductus prostaticus*.

d. of Rivinus One of 5 to 15 ducts (the minor sublingual ducts) that drain the posterior portion of the sublingual gland.

salivary d. Any of the ducts that drain a salivary gland.

d. of Santorini Accessory pancreatic d.

secretory d. Any of the smaller canals of a gland.

segmental d. One of a pair of embryonic tubes located between the visceral and parietal layers of the mesoblast on each side of the body.

semicircular d. One of three membranous tubes forming a part of the membranous labyrinth of the inner ear. They lie within the semicircular canals and bear corresponding names: anterior, posterior, and lateral.

seminal d. Any of the ducts that convey sperm, specifically the ductus deferens and the ejaculatory duct.

Skene's d. One of the two slender ducts of Skene's glands that open on either side of the urethral orifice in women. SYN: *paraurethral d.*

spermatic d. The secretory duct of the testicle that later joins the duct of the seminal vesicle to become the ejaculatory duct. SYN: *ductus deferens; testicular d.; vas deferens.*

Stensen's d. Parotid d.

striated d. One of a class of ducts contained within the lobules of glands, esp. salivary glands, that contain radially appearing striations within the cells, denoting the presence of mitochondria.

sublingual d. Any of the secretory ducts of the sublingual gland. SEE: *Bartholin's d.*

submandibular d. A duct of the submandibular gland. It opens on a papilla at the side of the frenulum of the tongue. SYN: *Wharton's d.*

tear d. A duct that conveys tears. These include secretory ducts of lacrimal glands, and lacrimal and nasolacrimal ducts.

testicular d. Spermatic d.

thoracic d. The duct that drains lymph from the left side of the body above the diaphragm and all of the body below the diaphragm, and discharges into the left subclavian vein.

umbilical d. Vitelline d.

utriculosaccular d. A narrow tube emanating from the utricle, connecting it to the saccule, and opening into the endolymphatic duct of the inner ear.

vitelline d. The narrow duct that, in the embryo, connects the yolk sac (umbilical vesicle) with the intestine. SYN: *omphalomesenteric d.; umbilical d.; yolk stalk.*

Wharton's d. Submandibular d.

d. of Wirsung Pancreatic d.

wolffian d. Mesonephric d.

duct ectasia An inflammatory condition of the lactiferous ducts of the breast. There is nipple discharge, nipple inversion, and periareolar sepsis. This may occur at any age following menarche. The condition resembles carcinoma of the breast.

ETIOLOGY: The cause is unknown, but in some cases may be associated with hyperprolactinemia due to a pituitary tumor.

TREATMENT: Duct ectasia is treated with surgical drainage of the abscess and antibiotics.

ductal carcinoma in situ of breast SEE: under *breast.*

ductile (dŭk′tĭl) [L. *ductilis,* fr. *ducere,* to lead] Capable of being elongated without breaking.

duction In ophthalmology, the rotation of an eye about an axis. This movement is controlled by the action of the extraocular muscles.

ductless [L. *ducere,* to lead, + AS. *loessa,* less] Having no duct; secreting only into capillaries.

ductogram (dŭk′tō-grăm) Injection of radiographic contrast into a duct of the breast, to determine the cause of nipple discharge.

ductule (dŭk′tūl) A very small duct.

aberrant d. One of a group of small tubules associated with the epididymis. They end blindly, representing the vestigial remains of the caudal group of mesonephric tubules.

ductus (dŭk′tŭs) *pl.* **ductus** Duct.

d. arteriosus A channel of communication between the main pulmonary artery and the aorta of the fetus.

d. choledochus The common bile duct.

d. cochlearis The cochlear duct. SYN: *scala media.*

d. deferens Vas deferens.

d. epoophori longitudinalis Gartner's duct.

d. hemithoracicus The ascending branch of the thoracic duct, opening into either the left lymphatic duct or close to the angle of union of the right subclavian and right internal jugular veins.

d. hepaticus Hepatic duct.

d. hepaticus dexter The duct that originates in the right lobe of the liver and unites with the ductus hepaticus sinister to form the hepatic duct. It drains the right and caudate lobes.

d. hepaticus sinister The duct that originates in the left lobe of the liver and unites with the ductus hepaticus dexter to form the hepatic duct. It drains the left and caudate lobes.

patent d. arteriosus SEE: *patent ductus arteriosus.*

d. prostaticus One of the ducts that carry secretions from the prostate into the urethra.

d. reuniens The endolymph-containing canal of the inner ear that connects the saccule with the cochlear duct. Also called *Hensen's canal.*

d. utriculosaccularis Utriculosaccular duct.

d. venosus The smaller, shorter, and posterior of two branches into which the umbilical vein divides after entering the abdomen of the fetus. It empties into the inferior vena cava.

Duffy system A blood group consisting of two antigens determined by allelic genes. SEE: *blood group*.

Duke method SEE: *bleeding time*.

dull [ME. *dul*] **1.** Not resonant on percussion. **2.** Not mentally alert. **3.** Having a boring personality.

dullness 1. Lack of normal resonance on percussion. **2.** The state of being dull.

shifting d. An area of dullness, found on percussion of the abdominal cavity to shift as body position is changed. This indicates a collection of peritoneal fluid in the cavity.

dumb [AS.] Lacking the power or faculty to speak. SYN: *mute*.

dumbness Muteness.

dumping 1. In medical care, the practice of transferring a patient who is unable to pay for care to a hospital that accepts such patients. **2.** The abandonment of infirm patients in health care facilities.

Duncan's mechanism The progress of placental separation inward from the edges, presenting the maternal surface of the placenta on expulsion. SEE: *Schulze mechanism*.

duoden- SEE: *duodeno-*.

duodenal (dū-ō-dē′năl, dū-ŏd′ĕ-năl) [L. *duodeni*, twelve] Pert. to the duodenum.

duodenal delay Delay in the movement of food through the duodenum due to conditions such as inflammation of the lower portion of the intestine, which reflexly inhibits duodenal movements.

duodenectasis (dū″ō-dĕn-ĕk′tă-sĭs) [″ + Gr. *ektasis*, expansion] Chronic dilatation of the duodenum.

duodenectomy (dū″ō-dĕn-ĕk′tō-mē) [″ + Gr. *ektome*, excision] Excision of part or all of the duodenum.

duodenitis (dū″ŏd-ĕ-nī′tĭs) [″ + Gr. *itis*, inflammation] Inflammation of the duodenum, usually resulting from *Helicobacter pylori* or the use of alcohol, tobacco, or nonsteroidal anti-inflammatory drugs.

duodeno-, duoden- [L. *duodeni*, twelve] Combining form meaning *duodenum* (first part of the small intestine).

duodenocholecystostomy (dū″ō-dē″nō-kō-lĭ-sĭs-tŏs′tō-mē) [″ + Gr. *chole*, bile, + *kystis*, bladder, + *stoma*, mouth] Surgical formation of a passage between the duodenum and the gallbladder. SYN: *duodenocystostomy*.

duodenocholedochotomy (dū″ō-dē″nō-kō-lĕd-ō-kŏt′ō-mē) [″ + Gr. *choledochos*, bile duct, + *tome*, incision] Surgical incision of the duodenum to gain access to the common bile duct.

duodenocystostomy Duodenocholecystostomy.

duodenoenterostomy (dū″ō-dē″nō-ĕn″tĕr-ŏs′tō-mē) [″ + Gr. *enteron*, intestine, + *stoma*, mouth] The formation of a passage between the duodenum and the intestine.

duodenogram (dū-ŏd′ĕ-nō-grăm) [″ + Gr. *gramma*, something written] A radiograph of the duodenum after it has been filled with a contrast medium.

duodenography (dū″ō-dē-nŏg′ră-fē) [″ + Gr. *graphein*, to write] Radiographic examination of the duodenum.

hypotonic d. Radiographic examination of the duodenum after medication has been administered to halt the peristaltic action of the gastrointestinal tract.

duodenohepatic (dū-ŏd″ĕ-nō″hĕ-păt′ĭk) [″ + Gr. *hepatos*, liver] Pert. to the duodenum and liver.

duodenoileostomy (dū″ō-dē″nō-ĭl″ē-ŏs′tō-mē) Surgical formation of a passage between the duodenum and the ileum when the jejunum has been surgically excised.

duodenojejunostomy (dū″ō-dē″nō-jĕ-joo-nŏs′tō-mē) [″ + *jejunum*, empty, + Gr. *stoma*, mouth] Surgical creation of a passage between the duodenum and the jejunum.

duodenorrhaphy (dū″ō-dĕ-nor′ă-fē) [″ + Gr. *rhaphe*, seam, ridge] Suturing of the duodenum.

duodenoscopy (dū″ŏd-ĕ-nŏs′kō-pē) [″ + Gr. *skopein*, to examine] Inspection of the duodenum with an endoscope.

duodenostomy (dū″ŏd-ĕ-nŏs′tō-mē) [″ + Gr. *stoma*, mouth] Surgical creation of a permanent opening into the duodenum through the wall of the abdomen.

duodenotomy (dū″ŏd-ĕ-nŏt′ō-mē) [″ + Gr. *tome*, incision] An incision into the duodenum.

duodenum (dū″ō-dē′nŭm, dū-ŏd′ĕ-nŭm) [L. *duodeni*, twelve] The first part of the small intestine, between the pylorus and the jejunum; it is 8 to 11 in. (20 to 28 cm) long. The duodenum receives hepatic and pancreatic secretions through the common bile duct. SEE: *liver; pancreas; digestive system* for illus.

ANATOMY: The wall of the duodenum contains circular folds (plicae circulares) and villi, both of which increase the surface area. The microvilli of the epithelial cells are called the *brush border*, which also increases surface area for absorption. Intestinal glands (of Lieberkuhn) between the bases of the villi secrete digestive enzymes, and Brunner's glands in the submucosa secrete mucus. The common bile duct opens at the ampulla of Vater. The nerve supply is both sympathetic (the celiac plexus) and parasympathetic (the vagus nerves). Blood is supplied by branches of the hepatic and superior mesenteric arteries. SEE: *digestive system* for illus.

FUNCTION: Acid chyme enters the duodenum from the stomach, as do bile from the liver via the gallbladder and pancreatic juice from the pancreas. Bile salts emulsify fats; bile and pancreatic bicarbonate juice neutralize the acidity of the chyme. Pancreatic enzymes are lipase, which digests emulsified fats to fatty acids and glycerol; amylase, which digests starch to maltose; and trypsin, chymotrypsin, and carboxypeptidase, which continue the protein digestion begun in the stomach by pepsin. Intestinal enzymes are peptidases, which complete protein digestion to amino acids, and sucrase, maltase, and lactase, which digest disaccharides to monosaccharides. Some of these enzymes are in the brush border of the intestinal epithelium and are not secreted into the lumen. Three hormones are secreted by the duodenum when chyme enters. Gastric inhibitory peptide decreases gastric motility and secretions. Secretin stimulates the pancreas to secrete sodium bicarbonate and the liver to produce bile. Cholecystokinin stimulates secretion of enzymes from the pancreas and contraction of the gallbladder to propel bile into the common bile duct.

The end products of digestion (amino acids, monosaccharides, fatty acids, glycerol, vitamins, minerals, and water) are absorbed into the capillaries or lacteals within the villi. Blood from the small intestine passes through the liver by way of the portal vein before returning to the heart.

duplication, duplicature [L. *duplicare,* to double] Doubling or folding of a part or an organ; the state of being folded.

duplicitas (dū-plĭs′ĭ-tăs) A fetal abnormality in which an organ or a part is doubled or apparently doubled.

dupp (dŭp) In cardiac auscultation, the expression for the second heart sound heard over the apex. This sound is shorter and of higher pitch than *lubb,* the first heart sound. SEE: *auscultation; heart.*

Dupuytren, Baron Guillaume (dū-pwē-trăn′) French surgeon, 1777–1835.

D.'s contracture Contracture of palmar fascia usually causing the ring and little fingers to bend into the palm so that they cannot be extended. This condition tends to occur in families, after middle age, and more frequently in men. There is no correlation between occupation and development of this condition. It is associated with liver disease and long-term use of phenytoin. SEE: illus.

ETIOLOGY: The cause is unknown.

TREATMENT: The tissue causing the contracture is removed surgically.

D.'s fracture A fracture dislocation of the ankle. The talus is displaced upward.

dura (dū′ră) [L. *durus,* hard] Dura mater.

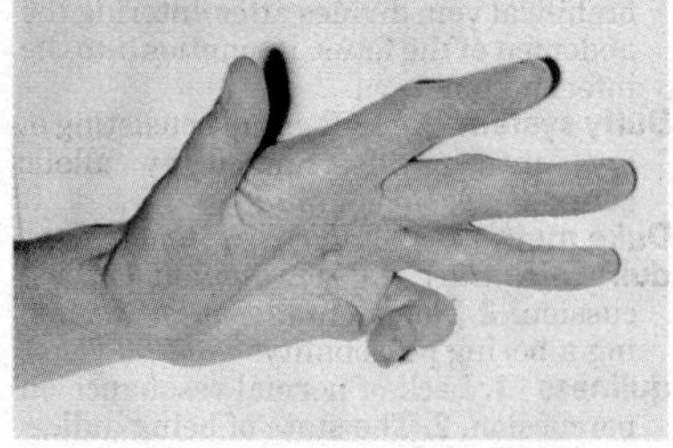

DUPUYTREN'S CONTRACTURE

durable medical equipment ABBR: DME. Assistive devices used by patients at home, such as walkers, electric beds, and bedside commodes.

dural (dū′răl) [L. *durus,* hard] Pert. to the dura.

duramatral An obsolete synonym for dural.

Durand-Nicolas-Favre disease Lymphogranuloma venereum.

duraplasty [″ + Gr. *plassein,* to form] Plastic repair of the dura mater.

duration **1.** The period of time something has been present. **2.** In obstetrics, the time between the beginning and the end of one uterine contraction.

durematoma (dū″rĕm-ă-tō′mă) [″ + Gr. *haima,* blood, + *oma,* tumor] Accumulation of blood between the arachnoid and the dura.

duritis (dū-rī′tĭs) [″ + Gr. *itis,* inflammation] Inflammation of the dura. SYN: *pachymeningitis.*

duroarachnitis (dū″rō-ăr″ăk-nī′tĭs) [″ + Gr. *arachne,* spider, + *itis,* inflammation] Inflammation of the dura and the arachnoid membrane.

Duroziez' murmur (dū-rō″zē-āz′) [Paul Louis Duroziez, Fr. physician, 1826–1897] The systolic and diastolic murmur heard over peripheral arteries in patients with aortic insufficiency. The murmur is audible when pressure is applied to the area just distal to the stethoscope.

dust Minute, fine particles of earth; any powder, esp. something that has settled from the air.

blood d. Hemoconia.

ear d. Fine calcified bodies found in the gelatinous substance of the otolithic membrane of the ear; otoconium or otoliths.

house d. The total of particles present in the air in a house. Materials included are mites, hairs, fibers, pollens, and smoke particles.

dust cell A macrophage in the walls of the alveoli of the lungs that ingests pathogens and particles of air pollution.

dusting powder Any fine powder for dusting on skin.

absorbable d.p. Powder prepared

from cornstarch. It is used as a lubricant for surgical gloves.

duty to warn An obligation to advise a patient about potential risks of a treatment or procedure.

Duverney's fracture (dū-vĕr-nāz′) [Joseph G. Duverney, Fr. anatomist, 1648–1730] A fracture of the ilium.

Duverney's gland Vulvovaginal gland.

D.V.M. *Doctor of Veterinary Medicine.*

dwarf [AS. *dweorg,* dwarf] An abnormally short or undersized person. SEE: *achondroplasia; cretinism; micromelus.*

achondroplastic d. A type of dwarf characterized by a normal trunk but shortened extremities, a large head, and prominent buttocks.

asexual d. A dwarf with deficient sexual development.

hypophyseal d. A dwarf whose condition resulted from hypofunction of the anterior lobe of the hypophysis. SYN: *pituitary d.*

hypopituitary d. Short stature resulting from insufficient production of growth hormone.

infantile d. A dwarf with marked physical, mental, and sexual underdevelopment.

Laron d. A dwarf who has either deficient levels of insulin-like growth factor I or abnormal cellular receptors for this hormone.

micromelic d. A dwarf with very small limbs.

ovarian d. A woman who is undersized due to absence or underdevelopment of the ovaries.

phocomelic d. A dwarf with abnormally short diaphyses of either pair of extremities or of all four.

physiological d. A person normally developed except for unusually short stature.

pituitary d. Hypophyseal d.

primordial d. A dwarf who has a selective deficiency of growth hormone but otherwise normal endocrine function.

rachitic d. A dwarf whose condition is due to rickets.

renal d. A dwarf whose condition is due to renal osteodystrophy.

thanatophoric d. A dwarf whose condition is caused by generalized failure of endochondral bone formation. This condition is characterized by a large head, a prominent forehead, hypertelorism, a saddle nose, and short limbs extending straight out from the trunk. Most affected infants die soon after birth.

dwarfism The condition of being abnormally small. It may be hereditary or a result of endocrine dysfunction, nutritional deficiency, renal insufficiency, diseases of the skeleton, or other causes.

Dwyer instrumentation A surgical procedure for stabilization of scoliosis. The spine is approached from the front and bolts are inserted transversely through each vertebra. A cable attached to the bolts is applied to the convexity of the curve and the vertebrae are pulled together.

Dy Symbol for the element dysprosium.

dyad [Gr. *duas,* pair] **1.** A pair. **2.** A pair of chromosomes formed by the division of a tetrad in meiosis. A dyad is a single chromosome that has already replicated for a subsequent division. **3.** In chemistry, a bivalent element or radical. **4.** In psychiatry, two people in an interactional situation.

dyadic Pert. to the social interaction between two people.

dyclonine hydrochloride (dī′klō-nēn) A topical anesthetic used in otolaryngology.

dye Any substance that is of itself colored or that is used to impart color to another material, such as a thin slice of tissue prepared for microscopic examination. Dyes may also be employed in manufacturing test reagents used in medical laboratories.

dying **1.** The end of life and the transition to death. SEE: *acceptance; advance directive; assisted suicide; death; death with dignity; end-of-life care.* **2.** Degenerating (e.g., "dying back").

dynamic (dī-năm′ĭk) [Gr. *dynamis,* power] Pert. to vital force or inherent power; opposed to static.

dynamics The science of bodies in motion and their forces.

group d. In politics, sociology, and psychology, a study of the forces and conditions that influence the actions of the entire group as well as the relations of the individuals to each other in the group.

population d. SEE: *population dynamics.*

dynamogenic [″ + *gennan,* to produce] Pert. to or caused by an increase of energy.

dynamograph (dī-năm′ō-grăf) [″ + *graphein,* to write] A device for recording muscular strength.

dynamometer (dī″nă-mŏm′ĕ-tĕr) [″ + *metron,* measure] **1.** A device for measuring muscular strength. **2.** A device for determining the magnifying power of a lens.

dynamoscope (dī-năm′ō-skōp) [″ + *skopein,* to examine] An instrument for auscultation of muscles.

dynamoscopy (dī-năm-ŏs′kō-pē) **1.** Auscultation of muscles. **2.** Visual evaluation of the function of an organ or system.

dyne (dīn) [Gr. *dynamis,* power] The force needed for imparting an acceleration of 1 cm per second to a 1-g mass.

dynein A very large protein that has a molecular configuration resembling arms. Contraction of these arms facilitates the movement of cilia and flagella of bacteria. SEE: *immotile cilia syndrome; Kartagener's syndrome.*

-dynia Suffix meaning *pain.* SEE: *-algia.*

dynorphin (dī-nŏr'fĭn) An opiate-like chemical found in the brain, which blocks transmission of pain signals along nerve fibers.

dys- [Gr.] Prefix meaning *bad, difficult, painful.*

dysacousia, dysacusis, dysacousma (dĭs″ă-koo'zē-ă, -koo'sĭs, -kooz'mă) [Gr. *dys,* bad, + *akousis,* hearing] **1.** Discomfort caused by loud noises. **2.** Difficulty in hearing.

dysadrenalism (dĭs″ăd-rē'năl-ĭzm) Disordered function or disease of the adrenal gland.

dysantigraphia (dĭs″ăn-tĭ-grăf'ē-ă) [″ + *anti,* against, + *graphein,* to write] Inability to copy writing or printed letters.

dysaphia (dĭs-ă'fē-ă) [″ + *haphe,* touch] Dullness of the sense of touch.

dysaptation, dysadaptation Impaired ability of the iris of the eye to accommodate to varying intensities of light.

dysarthria (dĭs-ăr'thrē-ă) [″ + *arthroun,* to utter distinctly] Impairments or clumsiness in the uttering of words due to diseases that affect the oral, lingual, or pharyngeal muscles. The patient's speech may be difficult to understand, but there is no evidence of aphasia.

dysarthrosis [″ + *arthrosis,* joint] Joint malformation or deformity.

dysautonomia (dĭs″aw-tō-nō'mē-ă) [″ + *autonomia,* freedom to use one's own laws] A rare hereditary disease involving the autonomic nervous system and characterized by mental retardation, motor incoordination, vomiting, frequent infections, and convulsions. It is seen almost exclusively in Ashkenazi Jews. SEE: *Mecholyl test.*

dysbarism (dĭs'băr-ĭzm) [″ + *barys,* heavy, + *-ismos,* condition] Decompression illness.

dysbasia (dĭs-bā'zē-ă) [″ + *basis,* a step] Difficulty in walking, esp. when due to disease of the brain or spinal cord.

dysboulia (dĭs-bū'lē-ă) [″ + *boulē,* will] **1.** Inability to fix the attention; difficulty experienced in thinking; mind weariness. **2.** Weak and uncertain willpower.

dyscalculia (dĭs″kăl-kū'lē-ă) [″ + L. *calculare,* to compute] An inability to make calculations. It may be found in childhood as a learning disability or may result from a stroke.

dyscephaly (dĭs-sĕf'ă-lē) Malformation of the head and facial bones.

dyschezia (dĭs-kē'zē-ă) [″ + *chezein,* to defecate] Painful or difficult bowel movements.

dyschiria (dĭs-kī'rē-ă) [″ + *cheir,* hand] Inability to tell which side of the body has been touched. If the sensation is referred to the wrong side it is called allochiria, or allesthesia. If referred to both sides it is called synchiria. SYN: *acheiria.*

dyschondroplasia (dĭs″kŏn-drō-plā'zē-ă) Chondrodysplasia.

dyschroa, dyschroia (dĭs-krō'ă, dis-kroy'ă) [″+ *chroia,* complexion] Discolored skin, esp. of the face; poor or bad complexion.

dyschromatopsia (dĭs″krō-mă-tŏp'sē-ă) [″ + *chroma,* color, + *opsis,* vision] Imperfect color vision.

dyschromia Discoloration, as of the skin.

nail d. Discoloration of fingernails and toenails. Pigmented bands in the nails may be related to Addison's disease, Peutz-Jeghers syndrome, pregnancy, use of minocycline, radiotherapy, cytotoxic drugs, antimalarials, and zidovudine therapy in AIDS patients.

dyschronism (dĭs-krō'nĭzm) [″ + *chronos,* time] A disturbed sense of time esp. that occurring after transportation from one time zone to another that is 5 to 10 hr ahead or behind. This leads to disturbances of sleep/wake cycles. SYN: *jet lag.*

dyscoria (dĭs-kō'rē-ă) [″ + *kore,* pupil] Abnormal form or shape of the pupil.

dyscrasia (dĭs-krā'zē-ă) [Gr. *dyskrasia,* bad temperament] An old term meaning abnormal mixture of the four humors. The word is now used as a synonym for disease, esp. hematologic disease.

dysdiadochokinesia (dĭs″dī-ăd″ō-kō-kĭ-nē'sē-ă) [″ + *diadochos,* succeeding, + *kinesis,* movement] An impairment in making smooth and rapid, alternating movements (e.g., turning the palms of the hands rapidly up and down on one's lap). This is one of the impairments brought on by malfunctioning of the cerebellum.

dysembryoplasia (dĭs-ĕm″brē-ō-plā'sē-ă) [″ + *embryon,* embryo, + *plassein,* to form] Fetal malformation occurring during growth of the embryo.

dysenteric (dĭs″ĕn-tĕr'ĭk) Pert. to dysentery.

dysentery (dĭs'ĕn-tĕr″ē) [″ + *enteron,* intestine] Diarrhea containing blood and mucus, resulting from inflammation of the walls of the gastrointestinal tract, esp. the colon. Abdominal pain, rectal urgency, and sometimes fever are present. Dysentery is caused by bacterial, viral, protozoan, or parasitic infections and is most common in places with inadequate sanitation, where food and water become contaminated with pathogens. SEE: *diarrhea; Escherichia coli; Shigella.*

TREATMENT: Prevention of infection is the major emphasis of health care providers, by improving the handling of waste products in the community and teaching proper techniques for handling, cooking, and storing food. Patients, particularly infants, may become severely dehydrated, develop metabolic acidosis, and require rehydration and, on occasion, antibiotic therapy.

PATIENT CARE: The basic principles of food handling should be taught to all those in the home. The need to wash hands frequently, particularly after using the toilet; using a meat thermometer to check that meat and dishes containing eggs are adequately cooked; refrigerating foods (below 40°F) until just before cooking and within 1 hr after cooking (esp. in warm weather); separating raw and cooked food and not using the same utensils or dishes for raw and cooked foods.

amebic d. Amebiasis.

bacillary d. Diarrheal illness caused by bacterial infections of the colon, esp. strains of *Shigella, Salmonella, Campylobacter,* and *Escherichia coli.* It can be relatively mild or severe, endemic or epidemic in presentation. Virulent strains (e.g., *Shigella dysenteriae* and 0157:H7 *E. coli*) release exotoxins that can cause systemic infection and damage to the glomeruli of the kidney (hemolytic-uremic syndrome). SEE: *Campylobacter jejuni; Escherichia coli; hemolytic uremic syndrome; Salmonella; Shigella.*

balantidial d. Dysentery caused by the ciliate protozoan *Balantidium coli.*

malignant d. A form of dysentery in which symptoms are very pronounced and dehydration occurs rapidly, usually terminating fatally.

viral d. Dysentery caused by a virus, esp. rotaviruses, Norwalk-like viruses, coronaviruses, and enteric adenoviruses.

dysesthesia (dĭs″ĕs-thē′zē-ă) [″ + *esthesia,* sensation] Abnormal sensations on the skin, such as a feeling of numbness, tingling, prickling, or a burning or cutting pain. SEE: *paresthesia.*

auditory d. Abnormal discomfort from loud noises. SYN: *dysacousia.*

d. pedis Severe itching and burning of the plantar surface of the feet and toes. This may occur as a result of athlete's foot or as a reaction to heparin therapy.

vulvar d. Generalized constant, severe burning vulvar pain of unknown origin. SYN: *idiopathic vulvodynia.* SEE: *vulvodynia.*

dysfluency (dĭs-flū′ĕn-sē) Hesitant or halting verbal or written language use. This lack of linguistic fluency may be normal during the early phases of language acquisition (e.g., in childhood). SEE: *stuttering.*

dysfunction (dĭs-fŭnk′shŭn) [″+ L. *functio,* a performance] Abnormal, inadequate, or impaired action of an organ or part.

erectile d. ABBR: ED. The inability to achieve or sustain a penile erection for sexual intercourse. The many causes of erectile dysfunction include tension or anxiety, vascular diseases of the pelvis, spinal cord injuries, autonomic nervous system disorders, testosterone deficiencies, and medication side effects. SYN: *impotence.*

dysgammaglobulinemia Disproportion in the concentration of immunoglobulins in the blood. It may be congenital or acquired.

dysgenesis (dĭs-jĕn′ĕ-sĭs) [″ + *genesis,* generation, birth] Defective or abnormal development, particularly in the embryo.

gonadal d. A congenital endocrine disorder caused by failure of the ovaries to respond to pituitary hormone (gonadotropin) stimulation. Clinically there is amenorrhea, failure of sexual maturation, and usually short stature. About one third of these patients have webbing of the neck and may have cubitus valgus. Intelligence may be impaired. SYN: *Turner's syndrome.*

ETIOLOGY: The cause is a defect in or absence of the second sex chromosome.

dysgenic [″ + *gennan,* to produce] Pert. to dysgenesis.

dysgenitalism [″ + L. *genitalia,* organs of reproduction, + Gr. *-ismos,* condition] A condition caused by abnormal genital development.

dysgerminoma (dĭs″jĕr-mĭn-ō′mă) [″ + L. *germen,* a sprout, + Gr. *oma,* tumor] A malignant neoplasm of the ovary.

dysgeusia (dĭs-gū′zē-ă) [″ + *geusis,* taste] Impairment or perversion of the gustatory sense so that normal tastes are interpreted as being unpleasant or completely different from the characteristic taste of a particular food or chemical compound. SEE: *cacogeusia; heterogeusia; hypogeusia, idiopathic; phantogeusia.*

dysglobulinemia (dĭs-glŏb″ū-lĭn-ē′mē-ă) [″ + L. *globulus,* globule, + Gr. *haima,* blood] Abnormality of the amount or quality of blood globulins.

dysgnathia (dĭs-nā′thē-ă) [″ + *gnathos,* jaw] Abnormality of the mandible and maxilla.

dysgonesis (dĭs″gō-nē′sĭs) [Gr. *dys,* bad, + *gone,* seed] **1.** A functional disorder of the genital organs. **2.** Poor growth of bacterial culture.

dysgonic Pert. to a bacterial culture of sparse growth.

dysgraphia (dĭs-grăf′ē-ă) [″ + *graphein,* to write] **1.** Inability to write properly, usually the result of a brain lesion. **2.** Writer's cramp.

dyshemoglobin (dĭs-hĕm″ō-glō′bĭn)

ABBR: dysHb. A hemoglobin derivative that is incapable of reversibly associating with oxygen, and so is unable to carry oxygen from the lungs to the cells. The primary defect in dyshemoglobins is a chemical (or stereochemical) alteration of the heme prosthetic group. Two common dyshemoglobins are carboxyhemoglobin—COHb—in which carbon monoxide is covalently bonded to the hemoglobin molecule, and methemoglobin—metHb—in which the ferrous iron is oxidized to the ferric form. Other, indeterminate dyshemoglobins exist in minute amounts in circulating blood.

dyshidrosis, dyshidria, dysidrosis (dĭs-hī-drō'sĭs) [″ + ″ + *osis,* condition] **1.** A disorder of the sweating apparatus. **2.** A recurrent vesicular eruption on the skin of the hands and feet marked by intense itching. SEE: *pompholyx.*

TREATMENT: The control of sweating or proper absorption of perspiration is beneficial. For the feet, wearing absorbent socks and well-ventilated shoes and applying substances that reduce sweating help to control symptoms. Individuals who do not wear shoes are rarely found to have this disorder. Acute attacks respond to treatment with a corticosteroid in an ointment combined with iodoquinol. This is applied at night with an occlusive dressing.

dyskaryosis (dĭs-kăr″ē-ō'sĭs) Abnormality of the nucleus of a cell.

dyskeratosis (dĭs″kĕr-ă-tō'sĭs) [″ + *keras,* horn, + *osis,* condition] **1.** Epithelial alterations in which certain isolated malpighian cells become differentiated. **2.** Any alteration in the keratinization of the epithelial cells of the epidermis. This is characteristic of many skin disorders.

dyskinesia (dĭs″kĭ-nē'sē-ă) [″ + *kinesis,* movement] A defect in the ability to perform voluntary movement.

biliary d. Symptoms of recurrent biliary colic in patients without gallstones, who nonetheless have an abnormal gallbladder ejection fraction on cholecystokinin-stimulated studies of the gallbladder.

d. intermittens Periodic or intermittent inability to execute voluntary limb movements.

tardive d. A neurological syndrome marked by slow, rhythmical, automatic stereotyped movements, either generalized or in single muscle groups. These occur as an undesired effect of therapy with certain psychotropic drugs, esp. the phenothiazines.

uterine d. Pain in the uterus on movement.

dyskinetic Concerning dyskinesia.

dyslalia (dĭs-lā'lē-ă) [″ + *lalein,* to talk] Impairment of speech due to a defect of the speech organs.

dyslexia (dĭs-lĕk'sē-ă) [″ + *lexis,* diction] Difficulty using and interpreting written forms of communication by an individual whose vision and general intelligence are otherwise unimpaired. The condition is usually noticed in schoolchildren by the third grade. They can see and recognize letters but have difficulty spelling and writing words. They have no difficulty recognizing the meaning of objects and pictures and typically have no other learning disorders. SEE: *learning disorder.*

ETIOLOGY: Although the exact cause is unknown, evidence suggests that dyslexia may be caused by an inability to break words into sounds and assemble word sounds from written language.

dyslogia (dĭs-lō'jē-ă) [″ + *logos,* word, reason] Difficulty in expressing ideas.

dysmasesis (dĭs″mă-sē'sĭs) [″ + *masesis,* mastication] Difficulty in masticating.

dysmaturity A condition in which newborns weigh less than established normal parameters for the estimated gestational age. SEE: *intrauterine growth restriction.*

dysmegalopsia [″ + *megas,* big, + *opsis,* vision] Inability to visualize correctly the size of objects; they appear larger than they really are.

dysmelia (dĭs-mē'lē-ă) [″ + *melos,* limb] Congenital deformity or absence of a portion of one or more limbs.

dysmenorrhea (dĭs″mĕn-ō-rē'ă) [″ + *men,* month, + *rhein,* to flow] Pain in association with menstruation. One of the most frequent gynecological disorders, it is classified as primary or secondary. An estimated 50% of menstruating women experience this disorder, and about 10% of these are incapacitated for several days each period. This disorder is the greatest single cause of absence from school and work among menstrual-age women. In the U.S., this illness causes the loss of an estimated 140,000,000 work hours each year. SEE: *premenstrual tension syndrome; Nursing Diagnoses Appendix.*

PATIENT CARE: Young women experiencing discomfort or pain during menstruation are encouraged to seek medical evaluation to attempt to determine the cause. Support and assistance are offered to help the patient to deal with the problem. Application of mild heat to the abdomen may be helpful. A well-balanced diet and moderate exercise is encouraged. Noninvasive pain relief measures such as relaxation, distraction, and guided imagery are employed, and the patient is referred for biofeedback training to control pain, and to support and self-help groups.

congestive d. A condition caused by excessive fluid in the pelvis.

inflammatory d. A condition caused by pelvic inflammation.

membranous d. A severe spasmodic dysmenorrhea that is accompanied by the passage of a cast or partial cast of the uterine cavity.

primary d. Painful menses.

SYMPTOMS: The pain usually begins just before or at menarche. The pain is spasmodic and located in the lower abdomen, but it may also radiate to the back and thighs. Some individuals also experience nausea, vomiting, diarrhea, low back pain, headache, dizziness, and in severe cases, syncope and collapse. These symptoms may last from a few hours to several days but seldom persist for more than 3 days. They tend to decrease or disappear after the individual has experienced childbirth the first time, and to decrease with age. Primary dysmenorrhea is much more common than secondary dysmenorrhea.

ETIOLOGY: The exact cause is unknown, but uterine ischemia due to increased production of prostaglandins with increased contractility of the muscles of the uterus (i.e., the myometrium) is thought to be the principal mechanism. As in any disease or symptom, the individual's reaction to and tolerance of pain influences the extent of the disability experienced. Primary dysmenorrhea is not a behavioral or psychological disorder.

One study revealed that prevalence and severity of dysmenorrhea might have been reduced in those who used oral contraceptives, and that severity was increased in those who had long duration of menstrual flow, who smoked, and who had had early menarche. Exercise did not influence the prevalence or severity of dysmenorrhea.

DIAGNOSIS: Cramping, labor-like pains that start just before or at onset of menstruation are characteristic of dysmenorrhea.

TREATMENT: Effective drugs are oral contraceptives and nonsteroidal anti-inflammatory drugs including aspirin. These medicines should be taken in the appropriate dose 3 to 4 times a day and with milk to lessen the chance of gastric irritation.

secondary d. Painful menses that manifest some years after menarche. The diagnosis is strongly suggested by a history or finding of use of an intrauterine device; pelvic inflammatory disease; endometriosis; uterine leiomyomas; adenomyosis; fertility problems related to imperforate hymen; cervical stenosis; ovarian cysts; or pronounced uterine retroflexion and/or retroversion.

TREATMENT: Nonsteroidal anti-inflammatory drugs are recommended for pain management. Medical or surgical management is directed toward resolving the underlying problem.

dysmetria (dĭs-mē′trē-ă) [Gr. *dys,* bad, + *metron,* measure] An inability to control the range of movement (e.g., on trying to touch an object with an index finger).

dysmetropsia [″ + ″ + *opsis,* vision] Inability to visualize correctly the size and shape of things.

dysmimia (dĭs-mĭm′ē-ă) [″ + *mimos,* imitation] **1.** Inability to express oneself by gestures or signs. **2.** Inability to imitate.

dysmnesia (dĭs-nē′zē-ă) [″ + *mneme,* memory] Any impairment of memory.

dysmorphic (dĭs-mor′fĭk) Misshapen.

dysmorphophobia (dĭs″mor-fō-fō′bē-ă) [″ + *morphe,* formed, + *phobos,* fear] Irrational fear of being deformed or the illusion that one is deformed.

dysmotility (dĭs′mō-tĭl″ĭ-tī) Any abnormality of smooth muscle function in the gastrointestinal tract, such as gastroparesis, gastric atony, intestinal pseudo-obstruction, or biliary dyskinesia.

dysmyotonia (dĭs″mī-ō-tō′nē-ă) [″ + *mys,* muscle, + *tonos,* tone] Muscle atony; abnormal muscle tonicity.

dysnomia An aphasia in which the patient forgets words or has difficulty finding words for written or oral expression.

dysodontiasis (dĭs″ō-dŏn-tī′ă-sĭs) [″ + *odous,* tooth, + *-iasis,* process] Painful or difficult dentition.

dysomnia (dĭs-ŏm′nē-ă) [″ + L. *somnus,* sleep] Any disturbance involving the amount, quality, or timing of sleep. SEE: *sleep.*

dysontogenesis (dĭs″ŏn-tō-jĕn′ĕ-sĭs) [″ + *ontos,* being, + *gennan,* to produce] Defective development of an organism, esp. of an embryo. **dysontogenetic,** *adj.*

dysopia, dysopsia (dĭs-ō′pē-ă, -ŏp′sē-ă) [″ + *opsis,* vision] Defective vision.

dysosmia (dĭs-ŏz′mē-ă) [″ + *osme,* smell] Distortion of normal smell perception.

dysostosis (dĭs″ŏs-tō′sĭs) [″ + *osteon,* bone, + *osis,* condition] Defective ossification.

cleidocranial d. A congenital ossification of the skull with partial atrophy of the clavicles.

craniocerebral d. A hereditary disease marked by ocular hypertelorism, exophthalmos, strabismus, widening of the skull, high forehead, beaked nose, and hypoplasia of the maxilla.

mandibulofacial d. A condition marked by hypoplasia of the facial bones, downward sloping of the palpebral tissues, defects of the ear, macrostomia, and a fish-faced appearance. It occurs in two forms that are thought to be autosomal dominants.

maxillofacial d. Hypoplasia of the maxillae and nasal bones resulting in a flattened face, elongated nose, and small maxillary arch with crowding or malocclusion of teeth. SYN: *Binder's syndrome; maxillofacial syndrome.*

dysoxia (dĭs-ŏk′sē-ă) [″ + L. *oxidum*] A condition in which tissues cannot make full use of the available oxygen.

dysoxidizable [″ + L. *oxidum,* oxide] Difficult to oxidize.

dyspancreatism [″ + *pankreas,* pancreas, + *-ismos,* condition] Impaired pancreatic function.

dyspareunia (dĭs″pă-rū′nē-ă) [″ + *pareunos,* lying beside] Pain in the labia, vagina, or pelvis during or after sexual intercourse.

ETIOLOGY: Causes are infections in the reproductive tract, inadequate vaginal lubrication, uterine myomata, endometriosis, atrophy of the vaginal mucosa, psychosomatic disorders, and vaginal foreign bodies.

TREATMENT: Specific therapy is for primary disease; counseling is given with respect to appropriate vaginal and vulval lubrication. Vaseline is of no benefit.

dyspepsia (dĭs-pĕp′sē-ă) [″ + *peptein,* to digest] Upper abdominal discomfort, often chronic or persistent, colloquially referred to as "indigestion." It is sometimes related to the ingestion of food, and may be a side effect of many medications. It may include such symptoms as fullness, eructation, bloating, nausea, loss of appetite, or upper abdominal pain. SYN: *indigestion.*

acid d. Dyspepsia due to excessive acidity of the stomach or reflux of acid into the esophagus.

alcoholic d. Dyspepsia caused by excessive use of alcoholic beverages.

biliary d. A form of dyspepsia in which there is insufficient quantity or quality of bile secretion.

cardiac d. Cardiac ischemia that presents with nausea, bloating, indigestion, or other upper abdominal symptoms.

gastric d. Dyspepsia caused by faulty stomach function (e.g., delayed gastric emptying in patients with diabetes mellitus).

gastrointestinal d. Dyspepsia caused by faulty function of the stomach and intestines.

hepatic d. Dyspepsia caused by liver disease.

hysterical d. An obsolete term for functional digestive diseases.

nonulcer d. Upper abdominal discomfort, often chronic, in which endoscopy reveals nondiagnostic, or normal, findings. The role of the bacterium *Helicobacter pylori* in this syndrome is controversial.

dyspeptic (dĭs-pĕp′tĭk) **1.** Affected with or pert. to dyspepsia. **2.** One afflicted with dyspepsia.

dyspermasia [″ + *sperma,* seed] Dyspermia.

dyspermia Difficult or painful emission of sperm during coitus.

dysphagia (dĭs-fā′jē-ă) [″ + *phagein,* to eat] Inability to swallow or difficulty in swallowing. SEE: *achalasia; cardiospasm.*

d. constricta Dysphagia due to narrowing of the pharynx or esophagus.

d. lusoria Dysphagia caused by pressure exerted on the esophagus by an anomaly of the right subclavian artery.

oral phase d. An inability to coordinate chewing and swallowing a bolus of food placed in the mouth.

oropharyngeal d. Difficulty in propelling food or liquid from the oral cavity into the esophagus.

d. paralytica Dysphagia due to paralysis of the muscles of deglutition and of the esophagus.

pharyngeal d. Aspiration of food into the trachea during the act of swallowing.

d. spastica Dysphagia resulting from a spasm of the pharyngeal or esophageal muscles.

dysphasia (dĭs-fā′zē-ă) [″ + *phasis,* speech] Impairment of speech resulting from a brain lesion or neurodevelopmental disorder. SYN: *dysphrasia.*

dysphonia (dĭs-fō′nē-ă) [″ + *phone,* voice] Difficulty in speaking; hoarseness.

d. clericorum Hoarseness due to public speaking; vocal overuse.

d. puberum Change or breaking in the voice in boys during puberty.

spasmodic d. A strained, strangled, or an abnormally breathy voice in a patient with normal laryngeal anatomy. Flexible laryngoscopy reveals laryngeal tremor or spasm during respiration or vocalization. Adductor or abductor muscle spasms may cause the dysfunction. Adductor spasms respond to the injection of botulinum toxin into the thyroarytenoid muscles. Usually, the response lasts several months but provides only partial symptomatic relief.

dysphoria (dĭs-fō′rē-ă) [″ + *pherein,* to bear] A long-lasting mood disorder marked by depression and unrest without apparent cause; a mood of general dissatisfaction, restlessness, anxiety, discomfort, and unhappiness.

dysphrasia (dĭs-frā′zē-ă) [Gr. *dys,* bad, + *phrasis,* speech] Dysphasia.

dysphylaxia (dĭs-fĭ-lăk′sē-ă) [″ + *phylaxis,* protection] Waking too early from sleep.

dyspigmentation (dĭs″pĭg-mĕn-tā′shŭn) Abnormality of the skin or hair pigment.

dyspituitarism (dĭs″pĭ-tū′ĭ-tăr-ĭzm) [″ + L. *pituita,* mucus, + Gr. *-ismos,* condition] Any condition due to a disorder of the pituitary gland.

dysplasia (dĭs-plā′zē-ă) [″ + *plassein,* to form] Abnormal development of tissue. SYN: *alloplasia; heteroplasia.*

anhidrotic d. A congenital condition marked by absent or deficient sweat glands, intolerance of heat, and abnormal development of teeth and nails.

bronchopulmonary d. An iatrogenic chronic lung disease that develops in premature infants after a period of positive pressure ventilation.

cervical d. Abnormal changes in the tissues covering the cervix uteri.

chondroectodermal d. A condition marked by defective development of bones, nails, teeth, and hair and by congenital heart disease. SYN: *Ellis–van Creveld syndrome.*

hereditary ectodermal d. A form of anhidrotic dysplasia marked by few or absent sweat glands and hair follicles, smooth shiny skin, abnormal or absent teeth, nail deformities, cataracts or corneal alterations, absence of mammary glands, a concave face, prominent eyebrows, conjunctivitis, deficient hair growth, and mental retardation.

monostotic fibrous d. Replacement of bone by fibrous tissue, marked by pain usually in the tibia or femur. The cause is unknown.

polyostotic fibrous d. Replacement of bone by a vascular fibrous tissue, marked by difficulty in walking and multiple bone deformities and fractures. It usually commences in childhood. The cause is unknown.

dyspnea (dĭsp-nē′ă, dĭsp′nē-ă) [″ + *pnoē,* breathing] Air hunger resulting in labored or difficult breathing, sometimes accompanied by pain. It is normal when due to vigorous work or athletic activity. SYN: *air hunger; breathlessness.* **dyspneic** (-nē-ĭc), *adj.*

SYMPTOMS: The patient reports that his or her work of breathing is excessive. Signs of dyspnea may include audibly labored breathing, retraction of intercostal spaces, a distressed facial expression, dilated nostrils, paradoxical movements of the chest and abdomen, gasping, and occasionally cyanosis.

PATIENT CARE: The patient is assessed for airway patency, and a complete respiratory assessment is performed to identify additional signs and symptoms of respiratory distress and alleviating and aggravating factors. Arterial blood gas values are obtained if indicated, and oxygen saturation is monitored. The patient is placed in a high Fowler, orthopneic, or other comfortable position. Oxygen and medications are administered as prescribed, and the patient's response is evaluated and documented. The nurse or respiratory therapist remains with the patient until breathing becomes less labored and anxiety has decreased.

cardiac d. Difficulty breathing that results from inadequate cardiac output (i.e., from heart failure).

expiratory d. Difficult breathing associated with obstructive lung diseases such as asthma or chronic bronchitis. Wheezing is often present.

inspiratory d. Difficult breathing due to interference with the passage of air to the lungs. SEE: *stridor.*

paroxysmal-nocturnal d. ABBR: PND. Sudden attacks of shortness of breath that usually occur when patients are asleep in bed. The affected patient awakens gasping for air and tries to sit up (often near a window) to relieve the symptom. PND is one of the classic symptoms of left ventricular failure, although it may also occasionally be caused by sleep apnea or by nocturnal cardiac ischemia.

dyspraxia (dĭs-prăk′sē-ă) [″ + *prassein,* achieve] A disturbance in the programming, control, and execution of volitional movements. It cannot be explained by absence of comprehension, inadequate attention, or lack of cooperation; it is usually associated with a stroke, head injury, or any condition affecting the cerebral hemispheres.

dysprosium (dĭs-prō′sē-ŭm) SYMB: Dy. A metallic element of the yttrium group of rare earths with atomic number 66 and an atomic mass of 162.50.

dysprosody Lack of the normal rhythm, melody, and articulation of speech. This condition may be present in patients with parkinsonism and in other disorders.

dysraphia, dysraphism (dĭs-rā′fē-ă, -fĭzm) [″ + *rhaphe,* seam, ridge] In the embryo, failure of raphe formation or failure of fusion of parts that normally fuse. SEE: *neural tube defect.*

spinal d. A general term applied to failure of fusion of parts along the dorsal midline that may involve any of the following structures: skin, vertebrae, skull, meninges, brain, and spinal cord.

dysreflexia The state in which an individual with a spinal cord injury at T-7 or above experiences a life-threatening uninhibited sympathetic response of the nervous system to a noxious stimulus. SEE: *Nursing Diagnoses Appendix.*

risk for autonomic d. A nursing diagnosis approved at the 13th NANDA Conference in 1998; a lifelong threatening uninhibited response of the sympathetic nervous system for an individual with a spinal cord injury or lesion at T8 or above who has recovered from spinal shock. SEE: *Nursing Diagnoses Appendix.*

dysrhythmia (dĭs-rĭth′mē-ă) [″ + *rhythmos,* rhythm] Abnormal, disordered, or disturbed rhythm.

cardiac d. SEE: *Nursing Diagnoses Appendix.*

dyssomnia Sleep disorders characterized by a disturbance in the amount, quality, or timing of sleep. They include primary insomnia, primary hypersomnia, narcolepsy, breathing-related sleep disorders, altitude insomnia, food allergy insomnia, environmental sleep disorder, and circadian rhythm sleep disorders. SEE: *sleep; sleep disorder*.

dysstasia [" + *stasis,* standing] Difficulty in standing.

dyssynergy (dĭs-sĭn′ĕr-jē) Uncoordinated contractions of heart muscle fibers.

dystaxia (dĭs-tăk′sē-ă) [" + *taxis,* arrangement] Partial ataxia.

dystectia (dĭs-tĕk′shē-ă) [" + L. *tectum,* roof] Failure of the embryonic neural tube to close during development. This is a cause of congenital spina bifida and meningocele.

dysthanasia An undignified and painful death due to inadequate control of symptoms (e.g., pain) at the end of life.

dysthymia (dĭs-thī′mē-ă) [" + *thymos,* mind] Dysthymic disorder. SEE: *Nursing Diagnoses Appendix.*

dysthymic disorder A chronically depressed mood that is present more than 50% of the time for at least 2 years in adults or 1 year for children or adolescents. Affected persons describe themselves as being chronically sad and "down in the dumps." SYN: *dysthymia.*

SYMPTOMS: The symptoms include poor appetite or overeating, insomnia or hypersomnia, low energy or fatigue, low self-esteem, poor concentration or difficulty making decisions, and feelings of hopelessness. The diagnosis of this disorder is not made if the patient has ever had a manic, hypomanic, or mixed manic and hypomanic episode.

TREATMENT: Treatment traditionally has included tricyclic antidepressants, monoamine oxidase inhibitors, or newer second-generation antidepressants such as fluoxetine, bupropion, paroxetine, and sertraline. The latter drugs have the advantage of having no anticholinergic side effects, not causing weight gain, and not altering cardiac condition. They may, however, cause nausea, weight loss, or insomnia.

PATIENT CARE: All professional care providers teach the patient about depression, emphasizing available methods to relieve symptoms. As the patient learns to recognize depressive thought patterns, he or she can begin to consciously substitute self-affirming thoughts. The patient is encouraged to talk about and write down his or her feelings. Health care providers listen attentively and respectfully and share their observations of the patient's behavior, while avoiding feigned cheerfulness and judgmental responses. A structured routine with noncompetitive and group activities may help build the patient's self-confidence and ability to socialize. The patient is assessed for suicidal thoughts and ideation, and suicide precautions are instituted for patients at risk. The patient who is too depressed to care for his or her own needs is assisted with personal hygiene and is encouraged to eat. Increasing high fiber foods and fluids may relieve constipation; warm milk or a backrub at bedtime can improve sleep.

If antidepressant drug therapy has been prescribed, the patient is taught about the medications and is monitored for desired, adverse, and side effects. For drugs that produce anticholinergic effects, sugarless gum or hard candy may relieve dry mouth. For drugs that are sedating, the patient should avoid activities that require alertness. The patient taking a tricyclic antidepressant should avoid alcohol and other central nervous system depressants. The patient taking an monoamine oxidase inhibitor should avoid foods that contain tyramine, since ingestion could result in a hypertensive crisis. The patient is reminded that most antidepressants take several weeks to work.

dysthyreosis (dĭs″thī-rē-ō′sĭs) [" + *thyreos,* shield, + *osis,* condition] Dysthyroidism.

dysthyroid (dĭs′thī-rŏyd) A state of abnormal thyroid functioning.

dysthyroidism (dĭs-thī′roy-dĭzm) [" + " + *eidos,* form, shape, + *-ismos,* condition] Imperfect development and function of the thyroid gland. SYN: *dysthyreosis.*

dystocia (dĭs-tō′sē-ă) [" + *tokos,* birth] Difficult labor. It may be produced by either the size of the fetus or the small size of the pelvic outlet.

FETAL CAUSES: Large fetal size (macrosomia) usually causes this condition. Other factors are malpositions of the fetus (transverse, face, brow, breech, or compound presentation), abnormalities of the fetus (hydrocephalus, tumors of the neck or abdomen, hydrops), and multiple pregnancy (interlocked twins).

MATERNAL CAUSES: *Uterus:* Causes include primary and secondary uterine inertia, congenital anomalies (bicornuate uterus), tumors (fibroids, carcinoma of the cervix), and abnormal fixation of the uterus by previous operation. *Bony pelvis:* Causes include flat or generally contracted pelvis, funnel pelvis, exostoses of the pelvic bones, and tumors of the pelvic bones. *Cervix uteri:* Causes include Bandl's contraction ring, a rigid cervix that will not dilate, and stenosis and stricture preventing dilatation. *Ovary:* Ovarian cysts may block the pelvis. *Vagina and vulva:* Causes include cysts, tumors, atresias, and stenoses.

Pelvic soft tissues: A distended bladder or colon may interfere.

DIAGNOSIS: Dystocia generally can be detected by vaginal examination, ultrasound, and external pelvimetry before the patient goes into labor.

TREATMENT: Treatment varies according to the condition that causes the dystocia. The goal is correction of the abnormality in order to allow the fetus to pass. If this is not possible, operative delivery is necessary. SEE: *cesarean section.*

dystonia (dĭs-tō′nē-ă) [″ + *tonos,* tone] Prolonged muscular contractions that may cause twisting (torsion) of body parts, repetitive movements, and increased muscular tone. These movements may be in the form of rhythmic jerks. The condition may progress in childhood, but progression is rare in adults. In children the legs are usually affected first. **dystonic,** *adj.*

ETIOLOGY: Drugs used to treat psychosis or Parkinson's disease, strokes, brain tumors, toxic levels of manganese or carbon dioxide, viral encephalitis, and other conditions may produce dystonia.

TREATMENT: Offending drugs are withdrawn, and the patient may be treated with diphenhydramine. Focal dystonias, such as blepharospasm or torticollis, may be treated with injected botulinum toxin, which paralyzes hypertonic muscle groups. Physiotherapy may also be helpful.

d. musculum deformans A rare progressive syndrome that usually begins in childhood and in most patients is invariably progressive. It is marked by distorted twisting or movement of a part or all of the body. The posture may be bizarre and the position is sustained. The inherited pattern is seen in families from northern Europe. The patient remains mentally normal. The bizarre posture is abolished in sleep, but eventually it may persist even then. Also called *torsion dystonia of childhood.*

ETIOLOGY: The cause is unknown.

TREATMENT: It is important that the patient not be treated as if the disease were due to hysteria or mental illness. There is no specific therapy but anticholinergics and reserpine may be of benefit. The most effective therapy has involved use of cryothalamectomy to destroy a portion of the ventrolateral nucleus of the thalamus.

dystopia (dĭs-tō′pē-ă) [″ + *topos,* place] Malposition (1); displacement of any organ.

d. canthorum Lateral displacement of the inner canthi of the eyes. **dystopic** (-tŏp′ik), *adj.*

dystrophia (dĭs-trō′fē-ă) Dystrophy.

dystrophin A protein of skeletal and cardiac muscle. Its precise function is unknown, but its production is impaired by the gene for Duchenne's muscular dystrophy.

dystrophoneurosis (dĭs-trŏf″ō-nū-rō′sĭs) [″ + *trephein,* to nourish, + *neuron,* nerve, + *osis,* condition] Defective nutrition caused by disease of the nervous system.

dystrophy (dĭs′trō-fē) [Gr. *dys,* bad, + *trephein,* to nourish] A disorder caused by defective nutrition or metabolism. **dystrophic** (-fĭk), *adj.*

adiposogenital d. A condition marked by obesity and hypogenitalism due to a disturbance in the hypothalamus, which controls food intake, and of the pituitary, which controls gonadal development. SYN: *Fröhlich's syndrome.*

facioscapulohumeral muscular d. Landouzy-Déjérine d.

Landouzy-Déjérine d. A hereditary form of progressive muscular dystrophy with onset in childhood or adolescence. It is marked by atrophic changes in the muscles of the shoulder girdle and face, inability to raise the arms above the head, myopathic facies, eyelids that remain partly open in sleep, and inability to whistle or purse the lips. SYN: *facioscapulohumeral muscular d.; Landouzy-Déjérine atrophy.*

progressive muscular d. Spinal muscular atrophy.

pseudohypertrophic muscular d. A hereditary disease usually beginning in childhood in which muscular ability is lost. At first there is muscular pseudohypertrophy, followed by atrophy.

dysuria (dĭs-ū′rē-ă) [″ + *ouron,* urine] Painful or difficult urination, symptomatic of numerous conditions. Dysuria may indicate cystitis; urethritis; infection anywhere in the urinary tract; urethral stricture; hypertrophied, cancerous, or ulcerated prostate in men; prolapse of the uterus in women; pelvic peritonitis and abscess; metritis; cancer of the cervix; dysmenorrhea; or psychological abnormalities. The condition may also be caused by certain medications, esp. opiates and medicines used to prevent motion sickness. Pain and burning may be caused by concentrated acid urine. SEE: *urinary tract infection.*

dyszoospermia (dĭs″zō-ō-spĕrm′ē-ă) [″ + ″ + *sperma,* seed] Imperfect formation of spermatozoa.

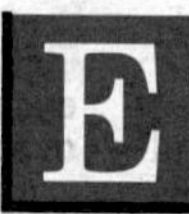

E *emmetropia; energy; Escherichia; eye.*
E_1 *estrone.*
E_2 *estradiol.*
E_3 *estriol.*
e *electric charge; electron;* L. *ex,* from.
ea *each.*
EACA *epsilon-aminocaproic acid.*
ead L. *eadem,* the same.
Eales' disease (ēlz) [Henry Eales, Brit. physician, 1852–1913] Recurrent hemorrhages into the retina and vitreous, most commonly seen in men in the second and third decades of life. The cause is unknown.

ear [AS. *ear*] The organ of hearing and equilibrium. The ear consists of external, internal, and middle portions, and is innervated by the eighth cranial nerve. SEE: illus.

The pathway of hearing is as follows: the auricle funnels sound waves from the environment through the external auditory canal to the tympanic membrane, making this thin epithelial structure vibrate. The vibrations are transmitted to the middle ear ossicles, the malleus, incus, and stapes, then to the perilymph and endolymph in the inner ear labyrinth. The receptors are part of the organ of Corti; they generate impulses transmitted by the cochlear branch of the eighth cranial nerve to the spiral ganglion and auditory tracts of the brain. The auditory areas are in the temporal lobes.

The healthy human ear responds to a variety of sounds, with frequencies ranging from about 20 to 20,000 Hz. It is most sensitive, however, to sounds whose frequencies fall in the 1500- to 3000-Hz range, the frequency range of most human speech. SEE: *hearing*.

The receptors for equilibrium are in the utricle and saccule, and in the semicircular ducts of the inner ear; they are innervated by the vestibular branch of the eighth cranial nerve. Impulses from the utricle and saccule provide information about the position of the head, those from the semicircular ducts about the speed and direction of three-dimensional movement.

Blainville's e. [Henri Marie Ducrotay de Blainville, Fr. scientist, 1777–1850] Congenital asymmetry of the ears.

Cagot e. An ear without a lower lobe.

cauliflower e. A colloquial term for a thickening of the external ear resulting from trauma. It is commonly seen in boxers. Plastic surgery may restore the ear to a normal shape.

external e. The portion of the ear consisting of the auricle and external auditory canal, and separated from the middle ear by the tympanic membrane or eardrum. SYN: *auris externa; outer e.*

foreign bodies in e. Objects that enter the ear accidentally or are inserted deliberately. These are usually insects, pebbles, beans or peas, cotton swabs, or coins.

SYMPTOMS: Foreign objects cause pain, ringing, or buzzing in the ear. A live insect usually causes a noise.

TREATMENT: To remove insects from the ear, a few drops of lidocaine should be instilled. Inorganic foreign bodies can be removed with small forceps by a health care provider.

glue e. The chronic accumulation of a viscous exudate in the middle ear, occurring principally in children who are 5 to 8 years old. It causes deafness, which can be treated by removal of the exudate.

inner e. internal e.

internal e. The portion of the ear consisting of the cochlea, containing the sensory receptors for hearing, the organ of Corti, and the vestibule and semicircular canals, which include the receptors for static and dynamic equilibrium. The receptors are innervated by the vestibulocochlear nerve. SYN: *auris interna; inner e.*

middle e. The tympanic cavity, an irregular air-filled space in the temporal bone. Anteriorly, it communicates with the eustachian tube, which forms an open channel between the middle ear and the cavity of the nasopharynx. Posteriorly, the middle ear opens into the mastoid antrum, which in turn communicates with the mastoid sinuses. Of the three potential openings into the middle ear, two—the tympanic membrane and the round window—are covered. The third one is the eustachian tube. Three ossicles (small bones) joined together, the malleus, incus, and stapes, extend from the tympanic membrane to the oval window of the inner ear. SYN: *auris media*. SEE: *eardrum; tympanum*.

Mozart e. SEE: *Mozart ear*.

nerve supply of e. *External:* The branches of the facial, vagus, and mandibular nerves and the nerves from the cervical plexus. *Middle:* The tympanic plexus and the branches of the mandibular, vagus, and facial nerves. *Internal:* The vestibulocochlear nerve (eighth cranial).

outer e. external e.

pierced e. An ear lobe that has been

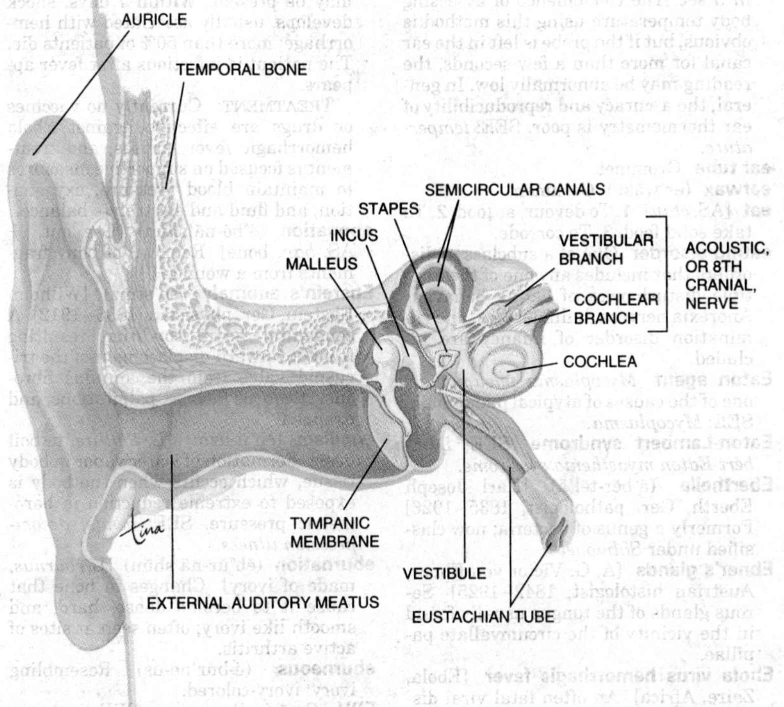

STRUCTURE OF THE EAR

pierced with a needle so that a permanent channel will remain, permitting the wearing of an earring attached to the ear by a connector that passes through the channel.

surfer's e. SEE: *surfer's ear*.

earache Pain in the ear. SYN: *otalgia; otodynia*.

ear bone One of the ossicles of the tympanic cavity: the malleus, incus, and stapes. SEE: *ear* for illus.

eardrops A medication in liquid form for instillation into the external ear canal, usually to treat infections or loosen cerumen.

CAUTION: Eardrops should not be used if the tympanic membrane is damaged or broken.

eardrum (ēr′drŭm) The membrane at the junction of the external auditory canal and the middle ear cavity. SYN: *tympanum*.

ear plug A device for preventing sound from entering the ear by occluding the external auditory canal.

CAUTION: Ear plugs should not be used during swimming, diving, or flying because they may interfere with pressure equalization.

earth 1. The third planet from the sun, located between Venus and Mars. The diameter of the earth at the equator is 7926 miles (12,755 km). It is 92.9 million miles (149.6 million km) from the sun, and it makes one revolution around the sun every 365.26 days. Its only natural satellite is the moon. **2.** The soil on the surface of the planet earth.

alkaline e. A general term for the oxides of calcium, strontium, magnesium, and barium.

diatomaceous e. Silica containing fossilized shells of microscopic algae with a siliceous or calcium-containing cell wall. It is used in insulating material and filters and as an absorbent.

fuller's e. Clay that is similar to kaolin. It is used as an absorbent, as a filler in textiles, and in cosmetics.

earth eating Eating of clay or dirt, sometimes by children as a form of pica.

ear thermometry Determination of the temperature of the tympanic membrane by use of a device for rapidly sensing infrared radiation from the membrane. Commercially available devices do this in 3 sec. The convenience of assessing body temperature using this method is obvious, but if the probe is left in the ear canal for more than a few seconds, the reading may be abnormally low. In general, the accuracy and reproducibility of ear thermometry is poor. SEE: *temperature.*

ear tube Grommet.

earwax (ēr′wăks) Cerumen.

eat [AS. *etan*] **1.** To devour, as food. **2.** To take solid food. **3.** To corrode.

eating disorder One of a subclass of disorders that includes any one of the multiple disturbances of eating behavior. Anorexia nervosa, bulimia, pica, and rumination disorder of infancy are included.

Eaton agent *Mycoplasma pneumoniae,* one of the causes of atypical pneumonia. SEE: *Mycoplasma.*

Eaton-Lambert syndrome SEE: *Lambert-Eaton myasthenia syndrome.*

Eberthella (ā″bĕr-tĕl′ă) [Karl Joseph Eberth, Ger. pathologist, 1835–1926] Formerly a genus of bacteria; now classified under *Salmonella.*

Ebner's glands [A. G. Victor von Ebner, Austrian histologist, 1842–1925] Serous glands of the tongue usually found in the vicinity of the circumvallate papillae.

Ebola virus hemorrhagic fever [Ebola, Zaire, Africa] An often fatal viral disease that has appeared in sporadic outbreaks in Africa. The clinical presentation of widespread bleeding into many organs and fever is similar to that seen in Lassa, Marburg, and Congo-Crimean viral hemorrhagic fevers.

ETIOLOGY: The disease is caused by one of three species of Ebola virus, a Filoviridae virus that is distinguished by long threadlike strands of RNA. The animal host (reservoir) has not been identified, limiting study of the disease. In each outbreak, the first human infection is believed to be caused by a bite from an infected animal. Subsequent cases are the result of contact with blood or body secretions from an infected person, or the reuse of contaminated needles and syringes.

The use of standard barrier precautions prevents transmission, with the addition of leg and shoe covers if large amounts of blood, vomit, or diarrhea are present; negative pressure isolation rooms are used if available. Ebola virus spread between humans by airborne droplets has never been documented, but face masks are recommended if the patient has respiratory symptoms. All equipment must be sterilized before reuse.

SYMPTOMS: The incubation period of 2-3 weeks is followed by sudden onset of high fever, myalgia, diarrhea, headache, fatigue and abdominal pain; a rash, sore throat, and conjunctivitis may be present. Within 7 days, shock develops, usually associated with hemorrhage; more than 50% of patients die. The patient is infectious after fever appears.

TREATMENT: Currently no vaccines or drugs are effective against Ebola hemorrhagic fever viruses, and treatment is focused on supportive measures to maintain blood pressure, oxygenation, and fluid and electrolyte balance.

ebonation (ē″bō-nā′shŭn) [L. *e,* out, + AS. *ban,* bone] Removal of bony fragments from a wound.

Ebstein's anomaly (ĕb′stīnz) [Wilhelm Ebstein, Ger. physician, 1836–1912] A congenital heart condition resulting from downward displacement of the tricuspid valve from the annulus fibrosus. It causes fatigue, palpitations, and dyspnea.

ebullism (ĕb′ū-lĭzm) [L. *ebullire,* to boil over] Formation of water vapor in body tissue, which occurs when the body is exposed to extreme reduction in barometric pressure. SEE: *bends; decompression illness.*

eburnation (ĕb″ŭr-nā′shŭn) [L. *eburnus,* made of ivory] Changes in bone that cause it to become dense, hard, and smooth like ivory; often seen at sites of active arthritis.

eburneous (ĕ-bŭr′nē-ŭs) Resembling ivory; ivory-colored.

EBV *Epstein-Barr virus.* SEE: *mononucleosis, infectious.*

EC *Enzyme Commission; enteric coated.*

ecaudate (ē-kaw′dāt) [L. *e,* without, + *cauda,* tail] Without a tail.

ecbolic (ĕk-bŏl′ĭk) [Gr. *ekbolikos,* throwing out] **1.** Hastening uterine evacuation by causing contractions of the uterine muscles. **2.** Any agent producing or hastening labor or abortion. SYN: *oxytocic.*

ECC *emergency cardiac care; external cardiac compression.*

eccentric (ĕk-sĕn′trĭk) [Gr. *ek,* out, + *kentron,* center] **1.** Proceeding away from a center. **2.** Peripheral. **3.** Departing from the usual, as in dress or conduct.

eccentric muscle contraction SEE: *muscle contraction, eccentric.*

eccentro-osteochondrodysplasia (ĕk-sĕn″trō-ŏs″tē-ō-kŏn″drō-dĭs-plā′zhē-ă) [Gr. *ekkentros,* from the center, + *osteon,* bone, + *chondros,* cartilage, + *dys,* bad, + *plassein,* to form] A pathological condition of bones caused by imperfect bone formation. Ossification occurs in several different centers instead of in one common center.

ecchondroma (ĕk-ŏn-drō′mă) [Gr. *ek,* out, + *chondros,* cartilage, + *oma,* tumor] A chondroma or cartilaginous tumor.

ecchondrotome (ĕk-ŏn′drō-tōm) [″ + ″ + *tome,* incision] A knife for excision of cartilage.

ecchymosis (ĕk-ĭ-mō′sĭs) *pl.* **ecchymoses** [″ + ″ + *osis,* condition] A bruise, that is, superficial bleeding under the skin or a mucous membrane. SEE: illus. **ecchymotic** (-mŏt′ĭk), *adj.*

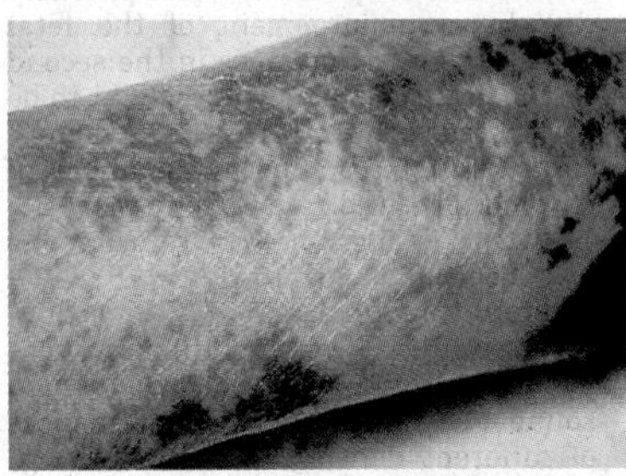

ECCHYMOSIS OF LEG

eccrine (ĕk′rĭn) [Gr. *ekkrinein,* to secrete] Pert. to secretion, esp. of sweat. SEE: *apocrine; endocrine; exocrine.*

eccrine sweat gland One of many glands distributed over the entire skin surface that, because they secrete sweat, are important in regulating body heat. The total number of glands ranges from 2 million to 5 million. There are over 400 per square centimeter on the palms and about 80 per square centimeter on the thighs. SEE: *sweat gland* for illus.

eccritic (ĕk-krĭt′ĭk) [Gr. *ekkritikos*] **1.** Promoting excretion. **2.** An agent that promotes excretion.

ecdysis (ĕk′dĭ-sĭs) *pl.* **ecdyses** [Gr. *ekdysis,* getting out] **1.** The shedding or sloughing off of the epidermis of the skin. SYN: *desquamation.* **2.** The shedding (molting) of the outer covering of the body as occurs in certain animals such as insects, crustaceans, and snakes.

ECF *extracellular fluid.*

ECG, ecg *electrocardiogram.*

echidnase (ĕ-kĭd′nās) [Gr. *echidna,* viper] An enzyme present in the venom of vipers that produces inflammation.

echidnin (ĕ-kĭd′nĭn) The venom of poisonous snakes.

Echidnophaga (ĕk″ĭd-nŏf′ă-gă) A genus of fleas belonging to the family Pulicidae.

E. gallinacea The sticktight flea, an important flea pest of poultry. It collects in clusters on the heads of poultry and in the ears of mammals. It may infest humans, esp. children.

Echinacea purpurea (ĕk-ĭ-nā′sē-ah) A native American herbaceous perennial (purple coneflower) of the family Compositae whose root and leaf extracts are used topically to promote wound healing and internally to improve the immune system. However, no conclusions have been reached yet about its use as a therapeutic agent or about a safe dosage of over-the-counter supplements. SEE: illus.

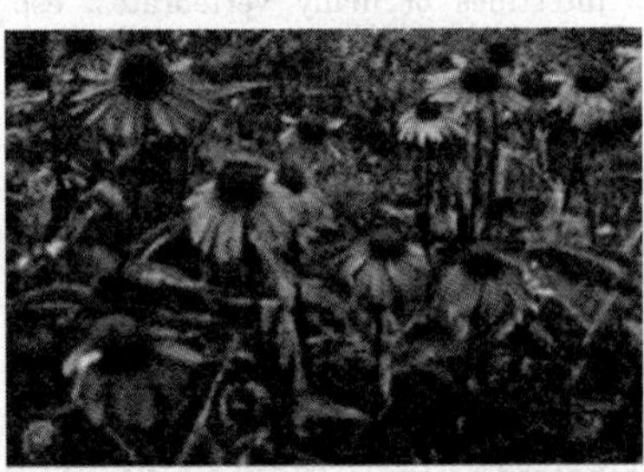

ECHINACEA PURPUREA

echinate (ĕk′ĭ-nāt) [Gr. *echinos,* hedgehog] **1.** Spiny. **2.** In agar streak, a growth with pitted or toothed margins along the inoculation line; in stab cultures, coiled growth with pointed outgrowths. SYN: *echinulate.*

echinococcosis (ĕ-kī″nō-kŏk-ō′sĭs, ĕk″ĭ-nō-kŏk-ō′sĭs) [″ + *kokkos,* berry, + *osis,* condition] Infestation with *Echinococcus.*

echinococcotomy (ĕ-kī″nō-kŏk-ŏt′ō-mē) [″ + ″ + *tome,* incision] An operation for evacuation of an echinococcal cyst.

Echinococcus (ĕ-kī″nō-kŏk′ŭs) *pl.* **Echinococci** A genus of tapeworms. They are minute forms consisting of a scolex and three or four proglottids.

E. granulosus A species of tapeworms that infests dogs and other carnivores. Its larva, called a hydatid, develops in other mammals, including humans, and causes the formation of hydatid cysts in the liver or lungs. SEE: illus.; *hydatid.*

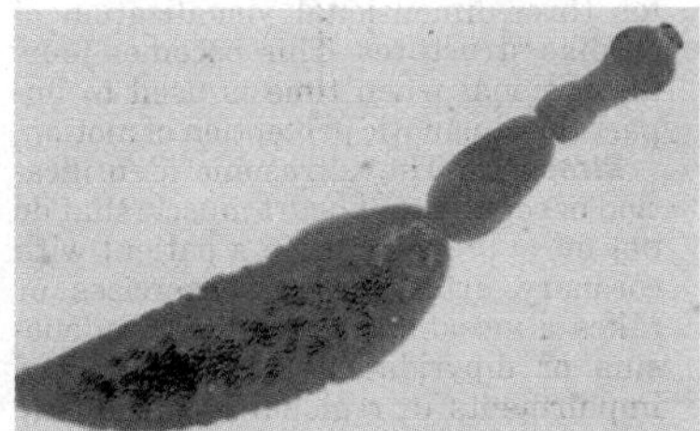

ECHINOCOCCUS GRANULOSUS

(Orig. mag. ×5)

E. hydatidosus A variety of *Echinococcus* characterized by development of daughter cysts from the mother cyst. SEE: *hydatid.*

echinocyte An abnormal erythrocyte with multiple, regular, spiny projections from the surface.

Echinostoma (ĕk″ĭ-nŏs′tō-mă) [″ + *stoma,* mouth] A genus of flukes characterized by a spiny body and the presence of a collar of spines near the anterior end. They are found in the intestines of many vertebrates, esp. aquatic birds. They occasionally occur as accidental parasites in humans.

echinulate (ĕ-kĭn′ū-lāt) A bacterial growth having pointed processes or spines. SYN: *echinate*.

echo (ĕk′ō) [Gr. *ekho*] A reverberating sound produced when sound waves are reflected back to their source.

amphoric e. A sound, sometimes heard in auscultation of the chest, resembling the sound of air blown over the mouth of a bottle. SEE: *chest*.

echocardiogram (ĕk″ō-kăr′dē-ō-grăm″) The graphic record produced by echocardiography.

echocardiography (ĕk″ō-kăr″dē-ŏg′ră-fē) A noninvasive diagnostic method that uses ultrasound to visualize cardiac structures. The heart's valves, walls, and chambers can be evaluated, and intracardiac masses or clots can often be seen.

dobutamine stress e. ABBR: DSE. A noninvasive test for coronary artery disease in which dobutamine is given to patients to increase the workload of the heart, and then the heart is evaluated with ultrasonic imaging. Regions of the heart that do not receive adequate blood flow (ischemic regions) contract poorly during the stress of the test but normally when the patient is at rest. Heart muscle that does not contract normally either at rest or with stimulation has been injured previously by myocardial infarction.

Doppler e. SEE: *Doppler echocardiography*.

multidimensional visualization e. An experimental echocardiographic technique using computer technology for three-dimensional visualization of cardiac structures. This becomes four-dimensional when time is used to impart the cinematic perception of motion.

stress e. The ultrasonic identification of segments of heart muscle that do not move properly when a patient with coronary artery disease exercises or takes a vasodilating drug (e.g., adenosine or dipyridamole). Stress-induced impairments in regional heart muscle activity are used as markers of obstructions in specific coronary arteries.

transesophageal e. ABBR: TEE. An invasive technique for obtaining echocardiographic images in which the ultrasonographic transducer is introduced into the esophagus. TEE is useful in detecting cardiac sources of emboli, prosthetic heart valve malfunction, endocarditis, aortic dissection, cardiac tumors, and valvular and congenital heart disease.

echoencephalogram (ĕk″ō-ĕn-sĕf′ă-lō-grăm″) Recording of the ultrasonic echoes of the brain, a technique that is rarely used since the advent of computed tomography and magnetic resonance imaging.

echogenic bowel A hyperechoic mass that may be seen in the fetal abdomen. If ascites is not present, this is probably due to an enlargement of the fetal bowel. Finding this mass in the second trimester of pregnancy is thought to be associated with an increased and significant risk of an abnormal number of chromosomes (i.e., aneuploidy).

echogram (ĕk′ō-grăm) The record made by echography.

echography (ĕk-ŏg′ră-fē) [″ + *graphein,* to write] The use of ultrasound to photograph the echo produced when sound waves are reflected from tissues of different density. SEE: *ultrasonography*.

echolalia (ĕk-ō-lā′lē-ă) [″ + *lalia,* talk, babble] Involuntary repetition of words spoken by others.

echomimia (ĕk″ō-mĭm′ē-ă) [″ + *mimesis,* imitation] Imitation of the actions of others, as seen in schizophrenia. SYN: *echopraxia*.

echopathy (ĕ-kŏp′ă-thē) [″ + *pathos,* disease, suffering] Pathological repetition of another's actions and words.

echophotony (ĕk″ō-fŏt′ō-nē) [″ + *phos,* light, + *tonos,* tone] Mental association of certain sounds with particular colors.

echopraxia (ĕk″ō-prăk′sē-ă) [″ + *prassein,* to perform] Meaningless imitation of motions made by others. SYN: *echomimia*.

echo sign Repetition of the closing word of a sentence, a sign of epilepsy or other brain conditions.

echothiophate iodide (ĕk″ō-thī′ō-fāt) A cholinergic drug used topically in the eye for treatment of glaucoma.

ECHO virus A virus belonging to the group originally known as *E*nteric *C*ytopathogenic *H*uman *O*rphan group. They are associated with viral meningitis, enteritis, pleurodynia, acute respiratory infection, and myocarditis.

Eck's fistula (ĕks) [N. V. Eck, Russian physiologist, 1847–1908] An artificial communication between the portal vein and the inferior vena cava, used in experimental surgery in animals.

eclampsia (ĕ-klămp′sē-ă) [″ + *lampein,* to shine] A severe hypertensive disorder of pregnancy characterized by convulsions and coma, occurring between 20 weeks' gestation and the end of the first postpartum week. Eclampsia is the most serious complication of pregnancy-induced hypertension. It occurs in 0.5% to 4.0% of all deliveries; roughly 25% of seizures occur within the first 72 hr of delivery. Perinatal mortality is about 20%. SEE: *pregnancy-induced hypertension*.

ETIOLOGY: Although the cause is unknown, risk factors include pre-existing hypertension and glomerulonephritis. SEE: *pre-eclampsia*.

SYMPTOMS: The woman exhibits one or more grand mal seizures. Coma, which follows the convulsive episode, may be short or persist for more than an hour. Without treatment, seizures may recur within minutes. SEE: *epilepsy*.

PATHOLOGY: Organ damage is seen most frequently in the kidney, liver, brain, and placenta. The kidney shows degenerated tubal nephritis; the tubal epithelium shows cloudy swelling, fatty degeneration, and coagulation necrosis. The liver is enlarged and mottled, showing portal vein thrombosis and degeneration of the periphery of the lobules with subcapsular hemorrhages. Edema, hyperemia, thrombosis, and hemorrhages are present in the brain. The placenta shows infarcts, thromboses, and hemorrhages. There is also retinal edema.

TREATMENT: Immediate and effective seizure management is vital. In the attempt to abort subsequent seizure activity, an intravenous bolus and a continuous infusion of magnesium sulfate are administered. An indwelling catheter is inserted and hourly output measured; oliguria is an ominous sign that may indicate renal failure or magnesium toxicity. If applicable, induction of labor or cesarean delivery may be necessary.

CAUTION: The routine use of diuretics in pregnancy is contraindicated because diuretics are of no benefit and may do considerable harm by masking signs and symptoms that would alert the patient and the physician to the onset of eclampsia.

Delivery: Delivery is not indicated until the patient has reached a stable condition, usually within 4 to 6 hr. If she is in active labor, the most conservative methods should be followed. Cesarean section should not be done unless there is some other obstetrical reason. If medical management brings no improvement, however, labor must be instituted by administration of an oxytocic agent. Cesarean section may be required.

PATIENT CARE: Emergency care is provided during convulsions, and prescribed medications are administered as directed. Post seizure, the woman should be positioned on her left side to facilitate increased placental perfusion. Siderails should be elevated to protect the patient from injury during any further seizures. Both fetal and maternal response to magnesium sulfate must be monitored closely because of the risk of toxicity. Signs of maternal magnesium toxicity include absence of patellar reflexes; respiratory rate less than 12 breaths/min; urinary output less than 30 ml/hr; serum magnesium level greater than 8 mg/dl; flushing and muscle flaccidity; fetal bradycardia; or severe maternal hypotension. Calcium gluconate must be immediately available at bedside to counteract the effects of magnesium therapy. The health care provider also must be particularly alert to signs of impending labor and abruptio placentae.

Emotional support and information are given to the woman and her family. Postdelivery assessments vary in frequency depending on the woman's condition, eventually regressing to every 4 hr for 48 hr postpartum. Although infants of eclamptic mothers may be small for gestational age, they sometimes fare better than other premature babies of similar weight because they have developed adaptive ventilatory and other responses to intrauterine stress. Assessments continue every 4 hr for 48 hr after delivery. SEE: *Patient Care* under *pregnancy-induced hypertension*.

eclamptic Rel. to, or of the nature of, eclampsia.

eclamptogenic (ĕk-lămp″tō-jĕn′ĭk) [Gr. *ek*, out, + *lampein*, to shine, + *gennan*, to produce] Causing eclampsia.

eclectic (ĕk-lĕk′tĭk) [Gr. *eklektikos*, selecting] Selecting what elements seem best from various sources.

eclecticism (ĕk-lĕk′tĭ-sĭzm) [″ + *-ismos*, state of] A former system of medicine that treated disease through specific remedies for individual signs or symptoms rather than for distinct diseases. The remedies were principally botanical.

ecmnesia (ĕk-nē′zē-ă) [Gr. *ek*, out, + *mnesis*, memory] A term formerly used to indicate impaired recall of recent events.

ECMO *extracorporeal membrane oxygenator.*

ecocide (ĕk″ō-sīd′) [Gr. *oikos*, house, + L. *caedere*, to kill] Willful destruction of some portion of the environment.

E. coli. Escherichia coli.

ecological fallacy In epidemiology, the erroneous attempt to determine from population studies the risk of a particular individual's developing a disease.

ecological terrorism The threat to use violent acts that would harm the quality of the environment in order to blackmail a group or society.

ecology (ē-kŏl′ō-jē) [Gr. *oikos*, house, + *logos*, word, reason] The science of the relations and interactions of the totality of organisms to their environment, including the relations and interactions of organisms to each other in that environment.

ecomap A family interview and assessment tool that delineates the needs, patterns, and relationships among family members and the environment.

Economo's disease Encephalitis lethargica.

economy of movement [Gr. *oikos,* house, + *nomos,* law] The efficient, energy-sparing motion or activity of the system or body.

écorché (ā″kor-shā′) [Fr.] A representation of an animal or human form without skin so that the muscles are clearly seen.

ecosphere (ĕk′ō-sfēr″) [Gr. *oikos,* house, + L. *sphera,* ball] The portions of the earth habitable by microorganisms, plants, and animals.

ecostate (ē-kŏs′tāt) [L. *e,* without, + *costa,* rib] Without ribs.

ecosystem (ĕk′ō-sĭs″tĕm) The smallest ecological unit; the microorganisms, plants, and animals and their environment in a defined area.

écouvillonage (ā-koo″vē-yŏ-năzh′) [Fr. *ecouvillon,* a stiff brush or swab] The cleansing and application of remedies to a cavity by means of a brush or swab.

écrasement (ā-krăz-mŏn′) [Fr.] Excision by means of an écraseur.

écraseur (ā-kră-zĕr′) [Fr., crusher] A wire loop used for excisions.

EC space *extracellular space.*

ecstasy (ĕk′stă-sē) [Gr. *ekstasis,* a standing out] **1.** An exhilarated, trancelike condition or state of exalted delight. **2.** A so-called designer drug, 3,4-methylenedioxymethamphetamine (MDMA). Use of the drug has been associated with hyperthermia, disseminated intravascular coagulation, liver damage, hallucinations, convulsions, coma, and death.

TREATMENT: The immediate priorities are to control the convulsions, to measure the core temperature, and to reverse the hyperthermia by rapid rehydration and active cooling measures.

ECT *electroconvulsive therapy.*

ectad [Gr. *ektos,* outside, + L. *ad,* toward] Toward the surface; outward; externally.

ectasia, ectasis (ĕk-tā′sē-ă, ĕk′tă-sĭs) [Gr. *ek,* out, + *teinein,* to stretch] Dilatation of any tubular vessel.

hypostatic e. Dilatation of a blood vessel from the pooling of blood in dependent parts, esp. the legs.

e. iridis Small size of the pupil of the eye caused by displacement of the iris.

ectatic Distensible or capable of being stretched.

ectental [Gr. *ektos,* without, + *entos,* within] Pert. to the entoderm and ectoderm.

ectental line The point of the entodermal and ectodermal junction in the gastrula.

ectethmoid (ĕk-tĕth′moyd) [″ + *ethmos,* sieve, + *eidos,* form, shape] The lateral mass of the ethmoid bone.

ecthyma (ĕk-thī′mă) [Gr. *ek,* out, + *thyein,* to rush] A crusting skin infection caused by pyogenic streptococci. It is similar to impetigo but extends more fully into the epidermis. Typically lesions are found on the shins or the dorsum of the feet.

TREATMENT: Topical skin cleansing, mupirocin ointment, and/or oral antibiotics (such as dicloxacillin) are needed to eradicate the infection.

ectiris (ĕk-tī-rĭs) [Gr. *ektos,* outside, + *iris,* iris] The external portion of the iris.

ecto- [Gr. *ektos,* outside] Combining form meaning *outside.*

ectoantigen (ĕk″tō-ăn′tĭ-gĕn) [″ + *anti,* against, + *gennan,* to produce] **1.** An antigen assumed to have its origin in ectoplasm of bacterial cells. **2.** An antigen loosely attached to the surface of bacteria and capable of being separated from the bacterial cell.

ectoblast (ĕk′tō-blăst) [″ + *blastos,* germ] **1.** The ectoderm. **2.** Any outer membrane, such as the ectoderm.

ectocardia (ĕk′tō-kăr′dē-ă) [″ + *kardia,* heart] Displacement of the heart.

ectocervix (ĕk″tō-sĕr′vĭks) The portion of the canal of the uterine cervix that is lined with squamous epithelium. **ectocervical** (-sĕr′vĭ-kăl), *adj.*

ectochoroidea (ĕk″tō-kō-roy′dē-ă) [″ + *khorioeides,* choroid] The outer layer of the choroid coat of the eye.

ectocondyle (ĕk″tō-kŏn′dĭl) [″ + *kondylos,* knuckle] The outer condyle of a bone.

ectocornea (ĕk-tō-kor′nē-ă) [″ + L. *corneus,* horny] The external layer of the cornea.

ectocuneiform (ĕk-tō-kū′nē-ĭ-form) [″ + L. *cuneus,* wedge, + *forma,* form] The lateral cuneiform bone.

ectodactylism (ĕk″tō-dăk′tĭl-ĭzm) [Gr. *ektrosis,* miscarriage, + *daktylos,* finger, + *ismos,* state of] Lack of a digit or digits.

ectoderm (ĕk′tō-dĕrm) [Gr. *ektos,* outside, + *derma,* skin] The outer layer of cells in the developing embryo. It produces skin structures, the teeth and glands of the mouth, the nervous system, organs of special sense, part of the pituitary gland, and the pineal and suprarenal glands. SYN: *epiblast.* SEE: *endoderm; mesoderm.* **ectodermal, ectodermic** (-ăl, -ĭk), *adj.*

ectoentad (ĕk″tō-ĕn′tăd) [″ + *entos,* within] From the outside inward.

ectogenous (ĕk-tŏj′ĕ-nŭs) [″ + *gennan,* to produce] **1.** Originating outside of a body or structure, as infection. **2.** Able to grow outside of the body, as a parasite.

ectoglia (ĕk-tŏg′lē-ă) [″ + *glia,* glue] The superficial embryonic layer in the beginning of the stratification of the medullary tube of the embryo.

ectogony (ĕk-tŏg′ō-nē) [″ + *gone,* seed] Influence of the embryo on the mother.

ectolecithal (ĕk″tō-lĕs′ĭ-thăl) [″ + *lekithos,* yolk] Pert. to an ovum having food yolk placed near the surface.

ectomere (ĕk′tō-mēr) [″ + *meros,* part] One of the blastomeres forming the ectoderm.

ectomesoblast (ĕk″tō-mĕs′ō-blăst) [″ + *mesos,* middle, + *blastos,* germ] A cell from which the ectoblast and mesoblast develop.

ectomorph (ĕk′tō-morf) [″ + *morphe,* form] A person with a body build marked by predominance of tissues derived from the ectoderm. The body is linear with sparse muscular development. SEE: *endomorph; mesomorph; somatotype.*

-ectomy (ĕk′tō-mē) [Gr. *ektome*] Combining form meaning *excision* of any anatomical structure.

ectopagus (ĕk-tŏp′ă-gŭs) [″ + *pagos,* something fixed] An abnormal fetus consisting of twins fused at the thorax.

ectoparasite (ĕk″tō-păr′ă-sīt″) [″ + Gr. *parasitos,* parasite] A parasite that lives on the outer surface of the body, such as fleas, lice, or ticks.

ectoperitonitis (ĕk″tō-pĕr″ĭ-tō-nī′tĭs) [″ + *peritonaion,* peritoneum, + *itis,* inflammation] Inflammation of the parietal layer of the peritoneum (the layer lining the abdominal wall).

ectophyte (ĕk′tō-fīt) [″ + *phyton,* plant] A parasite of vegetable origin growing on the skin.

ectopia (ĕk-tō′pē-ă) [Gr. *ektopos,* displaced] Malposition or displacement, esp. congenital, of an organ or structure.

e. cordis A malposition of the heart in which it lies outside the thoracic cavity.

e. lentis Displacement of the crystalline lens of the eye.

e. pupillae congenita Congenital displacement of the pupil.

e. renis Displacement of the kidney.

e. testis Displacement of the testis.

e. vesicae Displacement, esp. exstrophy, of the bladder.

visceral e. Umbilical hernia.

ectopic (ĕk-tŏp′ik) In an abnormal position. Opposite of entopic.

ectopic beat, complex Any electrical activation of the heart that originates outside the sinoatrial node.

ectopic hormone production The secretion of hormones by nonendocrine tissue. Ectopically produced hormones may arise from both benign and malignant tissues.

ectopic secretion (ĕk-tŏp′ĭk) Ectopic hormone production.

ectoplasm [Gr. *ektos,* outside, + LL. *plasma,* form, mold] The outermost layer of cell protoplasm. **ectoplasmic, ectoplastic,** *adj.*

ectopotomy (ĕk-tō-pŏt′ō-mē) [Gr. *ektopos,* displaced, + *tome,* incision] Removal of the fetus in ectopic pregnancy.

ectopterygoid (ĕk″tō-tĕr′ĭ-goyd) [Gr. *ektos,* outside, + *pteryx,* wing, + *eidos,* form, shape] The external (lateral) pterygoid muscle. It brings the jaw forward.

ectopy (ĕk′tō-pē) [Gr. *ektopos,* displaced] Displacement of an organ or structure. SYN: *ectopia.*

ectoretina (ĕk″tō-rĕt′ĭ-nă) [Gr. *ektos,* outside, + L. *rete,* net] The outer layer of the retina.

ectostosis (ĕk-tŏs-tō′sĭs) [″ + *osteon,* bone, + *osis,* condition] Formation of bone beneath the periosteum.

ectothrix (ĕk′tō-thrĭks) [″ + *thrix,* hair] Any fungus that produces arthrospores on the hair shafts.

Ectotrichophyton (ĕk″ō-trī-kŏf′ĭ-tŏn) [″ + *thrix,* hair, + *phyton,* plant] A former name for *Trichophyton megalosporon ectothrix,* a genus of parasitic fungi causing tinea or ringworm of the hair.

ectozoon (ĕk-tō-zō′ŏn) [″ + *zoon,* animal] A parasitic animal that lives on the outside of another animal.

ectro- [Gr. *ektrosis,* miscarriage] Combining form meaning *congenital absence.*

ectrodactylism (ĕk″trō-dăk′tĭl-ĭzm) [″ + *daktylos,* finger, + *-ismos,* state of] Congenital absence of all or part of a digit.

ectromelia (ĕk″trō-mē′lē-ă) [″ + *melos,* limb] Hypoplasia of the long bones of the limbs.

ectromelus (ĕk-trŏm′ĕ-lŭs) [″ + *melos,* limb] An individual with ectromelia.

ectropic (ĕk-trō′pĭk) [Gr. *ek,* out, + *trope,* turning] Pert. to complete or partial eversion of a part, generally the eyelid.

ectropion (ĕk-trō′pē-ŏn) Eversion of an edge or margin, as the edge of an eyelid.

ETIOLOGY: Causes include aging or loss of tone of the skin, scarring, infection, and palsy of the facial nerve.

ectrosyndactyly (ĕk″trō-sĭn-dăk′tĭ-lē) [″ + *syn,* together, + *dactylos,* finger] Congenital absence of one or more fingers; the remaining fingers are fused together.

eczema (ĕk′zĕ-mă) [Gr. *ekzein,* to boil out] A general term for an itchy red rash that initially weeps or oozes serum and may become crusted, thickened, or scaly. Eczematous rash may result from various causes, including allergies, irritating chemicals, drugs, scratching or rubbing the skin, or sun exposure. It may be acute or chronic. The rash may become secondarily infected. SEE: *dermatitis.*

TREATMENT: Avoiding the cause of the rash (e.g., a sun-sensitizing drug; the leaves of the poison oak plant; an irritating soap or perfume) prevents recurrences and allows the skin to heal. Locally applied astringent solutions (such as Burow's solution), antihistamines, or corticosteroid ointments, tablets, or injections may relieve the inflammation.

PATIENT CARE: Patients are helped to identify and avoid allergens in their diet or environment. Clothing should be soft textured, preferably cotton, and washed in a mild detergent. Fingernails should be kept short to decrease damage from scratching. Antihistamines may help to reduce itching at night. Maintaining a room temperature below 72°F, using humidifiers during the winter, and bathing in tepid water help keep the skin hydrated and decrease itching. SEE: *Nursing Diagnoses Appendix; Standard and Universal Precautions Appendix.*

asteatotic e. SYN: *winter itch.*

dyshidrotic e. Pompholyx.

erythematous e. Dry, pinkish, ill-defined patches with itching and burning; slight swelling with tendency to spread and coalesce; branny scaling; roughness and dryness of skin. This type may become generalized.

e. herpeticum Massive crops of vesicles that become pustular, occurring when herpes simplex virus infection occurs in a person, usually an infant, with pre-existing eczema. SYN: *Kaposi's varicelliform eruption.*

lichenoid e. Eczema with thickening of the skin.

nummular e. Eczema with coin- or oval-shaped lesions. It is often associated with dry skin and worsens in dry weather. SEE: illus.

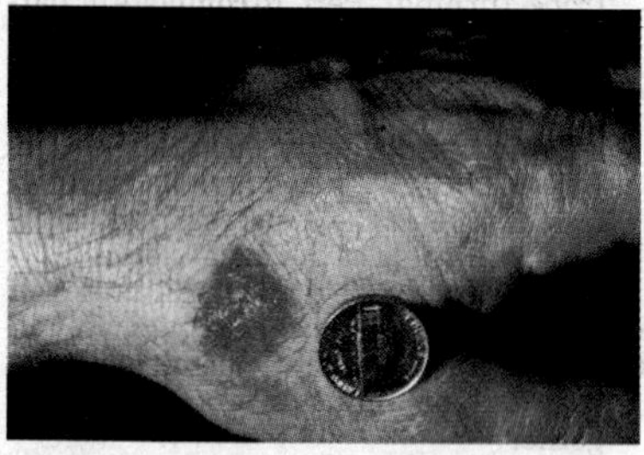

NUMMULAR ECZEMA

pustular e. Follicular, impetiginous, or consecutive eczema including eczema rubrum (red, glazed surface with little oozing), eczema madidans (raw, red, and covered with moisture), eczema fissum (thick, dry, inelastic skin with cracks and fissures), squamous eczema (chronic on soles, legs, scalp; multiple circumscribed, infiltrated patches with thin, dry scales).

seborrheic e. Eczema marked by excessive secretion from the sebaceous glands. SYN: *seborrhea.*

eczematous (ěk-zěm′ă-tŭs) Marked by or resembling eczema.

ED *effective dose; erythema dose.*

E.D. *Emergency Department.*

ED_{50} The median effective dose, producing the desired effect in 50% of subjects tested.

EDC *expected date of confinement.*

EDD *expected date of delivery.*

edema, oedema (ĕ-dē′mă) *pl.* **edemas** or **edemata** [Gr. *oidema,* swelling] A local or generalized condition in which the body tissues contain an excessive amount of tissue fluid. Ascites and hydrothorax are words for excess fluid in the peritoneal and pleural cavities, respectively. Generalized edema was previously termed dropsy. **edematous** (-ăt-ŭs), *adj.*

ETIOLOGY: Edema may result from increased permeability of the capillary walls; increased capillary pressure due to venous obstruction or heart failure; lymphatic obstruction; disturbances in renal function; reduction of plasma proteins; inflammatory conditions; fluid and electrolyte disturbances, particularly those causing sodium retention; malnutrition; starvation; or chemical substances such as bacterial toxins, venoms, caustic substances, and histamine.

TREATMENT: Bedrest helps relieve lower extremity edema. Dietary salt should be restricted to less than 2 g/day. Fluid intake may be restricted to about 1500 ml in 24 hr. This prescription may be relaxed when free diuresis has been attained. Diuretics relieve swelling when renal function is good and when any underlying abnormality of cardiac function, capillary pressure, or salt retention is being corrected simultaneously. One of various effective diuretics may be used. Diuretics are contraindicated in pre-eclampsia and when serum potassium levels are very low (e.g., less than 3.0 mEq/dl. They may be ineffective in cardiac edema associated with advanced renal insufficiency. The diet in edema should be adequate in protein, high in calories, rich in vitamins. Patients with significant edema should weigh themselves daily to gauge fluid loss or retention.

PATIENT CARE: Edema is documented according to type (pitting, nonpitting, or brawny), extent, location, symmetry, and degree of pitting. Areas over bony prominences are palpated for edema by pressing with the fingertip for 5 sec, then releasing. Normally, the tissue should immediately rebound to its original contour, so the depth of indentation is measured and recorded. The patient is questioned about increased tightness of rings, shoes, waistlines of garments, belts, and so forth. Periorbital edema is assessed; abdominal girth and ankle circumference are measured; and the patient's weight and fluid intake and output are monitored.

Fragile edematous tissues are protected from damage by careful handling and positioning and by providing and teaching about special skin care. Edematous extremities are mobilized and elevated to promote venous return, and lung sounds auscultated for evidence of increasing pulmonary congestion. Prescribed therapies, including sodium restriction, diuretics, ACE inhibitors, protein replacement, and elastic stockings or other elastic support garments, are provided, and the patient is instructed in their use.

angioneurotic e. Angioedema.

brain e. Swelling of the brain due to an increase in its water content. It may be caused by a variety of conditions, including increased permeability of brain capillary endothelial cells; swelling of brain cells associated with hypoxia or water intoxication; trauma to the skull; and interstitial edema resulting from obstructive hydrocephalus. SYN: *brain swelling; cerebral e.*

e. bullosum vesicae A form of edema affecting the bladder.

cardiac e. Accumulation of fluid due to congestive heart failure. It is most apparent in the dependent portion of the body and/or the lungs.

cerebral e. Brain e.

dependent e. Edema or swelling of the lower extremities, or if the patient is lying down, of the sacrum.

high-altitude pulmonary e. ABBR: HAPE. Pulmonary edema that may occur in aviators, mountain climbers, or anyone exposed to decreased atmospheric pressure. SEE: *hypoxia*.

inflammatory e. Edema associated with inflammation. The cause is assumed to be damage to the capillary endothelium. It is usually nonpitting and localized, and red, tender, and warm.

laryngeal e. Swelling of the larynx, usually resulting from allergic reaction and causing airway obstruction unless treated. Therapy consists of intravenous or intratracheal epinephrine, emergency tracheostomy, or both.

malignant e. Rapid destruction of tissue by cutaneous or subcutaneous infections, such as anthrax or clostridial species.

e. neonatorum Edema in newborn, esp. premature, infants. This condition is usually transitory, involving the hands, face, feet, and genitalia, and rarely becomes generalized.

pitting e. Edema, usually of the skin of the extremities. When pressed firmly with a finger, the skin maintains the depression produced by the finger.

pulmonary e. A potentially life-threatening accumulation of fluid in the interstitium and alveoli of the lungs. The collected fluid may block the exchange of oxygen and carbon dioxide and produce respiratory failure. SYN: *acute edema of lung*. SEE: *Nursing Diagnoses Appendix.*

ETIOLOGY: Fluid may seep out of the alveolar capillaries if these blood vessels are damaged and become excessively permeable to liquids (noncardiogenic pulmonary edema) or if hydrostatic pressures within blood vessels exceed the strength of the normal alveolar capillary wall (cardiogenic pulmonary edema). Cardiogenic pulmonary edema can result from any condition that causes congestive heart failure, including myocardial infarction, ischemia, or stunning; severe valvular heart disease; arrhythmias; excessive intravenous fluid administration; and diastolic dysfunction, among others.

Noncardiogenic pulmonary edema usually results from blood vessel injury, as occurs in the adult respiratory distress syndrome (sepsis, shock, aspiration pneumonia, airway obstruction). Occasionally, fluid floods the lungs as a result of drug exposure (narcotic overdose), hypoalbuminemia, high-altitude exposure (mountain sickness), and other conditions.

SYMPTOMS: Patients feel as though they are suffocating and often report labored, noisy breathing; cough productive of bloody sputum; air hunger; anxiety; palpitations; and altered mental status. Signs of the condition include a rapid respiratory rate, heaving of the chest and abdomen, intercostal muscle retractions, and cyanosis. To improve the movement of air into and out of the chest, the patient will often sit upright to breathe and resist lying down.

TREATMENT: Oxygen should be administered immediately. Morphine sulfate, nitrates, and loop diuretics are typically given to patients with cardiogenic pulmonary edema. Positive airway pressure ventilation or intubation and ventilator-assisted breathing may be required.

PROGNOSIS: The outlook is good if the condition is stabilized or reversed with treatment.

PATIENT CARE: The patient's head is elevated; respirations and ventilatory effort are assessed. Oxygen is administered as prescribed, with care taken to limit the flow-rate in patients whose respiratory drive is compromised. The lungs are auscultated for adventitious breath sounds, such as crackles, gurgles, and wheezes, and the heart is assessed for apical rate and gallops. The patient is monitored for a cough productive of pink, frothy sputum. His or her skin is checked for diaphoresis and pallor or cyanosis. A medication history is collected, especially for cardiac or respiratory drugs and use of recreational drugs. The patient's cardiac rate and rhythm, blood pressure, and oxygen saturation levels are monitored continuously. An intravenous (IV) line administering normal saline solution (NSS) is inserted at a keep vein open rate to provide access for medication administration. Prescribed first-line drug therapy is administered, and the patient's response to the drugs is evaluated. IV morphine slows respirations and improves hemodynamics and reduces anxiety. It should be administered prior to initiating continuous positive air pressure (CPAP). CPAP, in turn, improves oxygenation and decreases cardiac workload, thus decreasing the need for intubation and ventilation with positive end-expiratory pressure (PEEP). An indwelling urinary catheter is inserted to accurately monitor the patient's fluid status; diuresis should begin within 30 minutes of administration of an IV loop diuretic. Pulmonary edema is a true respiratory emergency that terrifies the patient. All individuals involved with the patient through this crisis must remain as calm and quiet as possible, provide ongoing reassurance, and validate everything occurring through basic and simply understood explanations. Later, health care providers should discuss with the patient his or her feelings about the episode and give more in-depth explanations of what occurred. The at risk patient is taught early warning signs to act on immediately, in an effort to prevent future episodes.

purulent e. Swelling caused by a local collection of pus.

salt-induced e. A form of edema worsened by excess sodium in the diet.

edematogenic (ĕ-dĕm″ă-tō-jĕn′ĭk) Causing edema.

edentia (ē-dĕn′shē-ă) [L. *e,* without, + *dens,* tooth] Absence of teeth.

edentulous (ē-dĕnt′ū-lŭs) Without teeth.

edetate calcium disodium (ĕd′ĕ-tāt) The disodium salt of ethylenediaminetetra-acetic acid. A chelating agent, it is used in diagnosing and treating lead poisoning. Trade names are Calcium Disodium Versenate and Versene CA.

edetate disodium (ĕd′ĕ-tāt dī-sō′dē-ŭm) A chelating agent, disodium dihydrogen ethylenediaminetetra-acetate dihydrate. It is used to treat hypercalcemia.

edge A margin or border.

bevel e. A tooth edge produced by beveling.

cutting e. An angled or sharpened edge for cutting, as an incisor tooth or the blade of a knife.

denture e. The margin or border of a denture.

incisal e. The sharpened edge of a tooth produced by occlusal wear; the labiolingual margin.

edible (ĕd′ĭ-bl) [L. *edere,* to eat] Suitable for food; fit to eat; nonpoisonous.

edrophonium chloride (ĕd″rō-fō′nē-ŭm) A cholinergic drug. Trade name is Tensilon. SEE: *edrophonium test.*

edrophonium test The use of edrophonium chloride to test for the presence of myasthenia gravis. The appropriate dose is injected intravenously; if there is no effect, a larger dose is given within 45 sec. A positive test demonstrates brief improvement in strength unaccompanied by lingual fasciculation. The test may also be used to determine an overdose of a cholinergic drug. An excessive dose of cholinergic drug produces weakness that closely resembles myasthenia. A very small dose of edrophonium chloride given intravenously worsens the weakness if it is due to cholinergic drug overdose and improves it if it is due to myasthenia gravis.

CAUTION: The test should not be performed unless facilities and staff for respiratory resuscitation are immediately available.

EDTA *ethylenediaminetetra-acetic acid.*

education, fieldwork The educational link between the classroom and service delivery settings that takes place in approved facilities under the supervision of a qualified professional.

eduction (ē-dŭk′shŭn) [L. *e,* out, + *ducere,* to lead] Emergence from a particular state or condition (e.g., coming out of the effects of general anesthesia). SEE: *induction* (4).

Edwards' syndrome [James H. Edwards, U.S. geneticist, b. 1928] Trisomy 18.

EE *coefficient of elastic expansion.*

EEE *eastern equine encephalitis.*

EEG *electroencephalogram.*

EENT *eyes, ears, nose, and throat.*

EEOC *Equal Employment Opportunity Commission.*

EFA *essential fatty acid.*

effacement (ĕ-fās′mĕnt) In obstetrics, the thinning of the cervix as the internal os is slowly pulled up into the lower uterine segment.

effect (ĕ-fĕkt′) [L. *effectus,* to accomplish] The result of an action or force.

abstinence e. Withdrawal.

additive e. The therapeutic effect of a combination of two or more drugs that is equal to the sum of the individual drug effects.

Bainbridge e. SEE: *reflex, Bainbridge.*

ceiling e. The optimal potential effect of a medication. Once a therapeutic limit is reached, increases in dose may produce side effects but no further beneficial effects.

cumulative e. A drug effect that is apparent only after several doses have been given. It is caused by excretion or metabolic degradation of only a fraction of each dose given.

fetal alcohol e. fetal alcohol syndrome.

greenhouse e. Planetary warming as a result of the trapping of solar energy beneath atmospheric gases. The composition and concentration of the gases in the atmosphere influence the earth's surface temperature because some gases more effectively retain heat than others. Fossil fuel combustion, which has increased at a rapid rate since the 1950s, has deposited increasing amounts of carbon dioxide in the upper atmosphere. This is thought to be a contributory factor in global warming, a phenomenon suspected of having widespread effects on terrestrial biology. SEE: *global warming; ozone*.

halo e. The giving of an inflated performance appraisal or grade to an employee or student because of the appraiser's tendency to regard all subordinates fondly.

Hawthorne e. [The Hawthorne plant of the Western Electric Company] The tendency of research outcomes to be altered by virtue of their being studied.

mass e. Evidence on a radiological study of the brain that midline structures of the central nervous system have shifted. This finding suggests that pressures within the cranium are abnormally high, that vital anatomic structures may be compressed, and that herniation of the brain and subsequent death may be imminent.

nonstochastic e. A radiation effect whose severity increases in direct proportion to the dose and for which there usually is a threshold. An example is radiation-induced cataracts.

photoelectric e. An interaction between x-rays and matter in which the x-ray photon ejects an inner-shell electron, causing a cascade of outer-shell electrons to fill the hole. The changing of energy shells releases secondary radiation equal to the difference in the binding energies. This absorption reaction increases the patient dose and creates contrast on the radiographic film. It usually occurs at low photon energies.

piezoelectric e. In ultrasound, a change of the mechanical action of the ceramic crystals into an electrical impulse. SEE: *triboluminescence*.

effectiveness (ĕ-fĕk′tĭv-nĕs) The ability to cause the expected or intended effect or result.

effector Any organ stimulated by motor nerve impulses; a muscle that contracts or a gland that secretes. SYN: *effector organ*.

effector cell An active cell of the immune system responsible for destroying or controlling foreign antigens. SEE: *leukocyte*.

effector organ Effector.

effeminate Pert. to a male who has the physical characteristics or mannerisms of a female.

effemination (ĕ-fĕm″ĭ-nā′shŭn) [L. *effeminare,* to make feminine] The production of female physical characteristics in a male. SYN: *feminization*.

efferent [L. *efferens,* to bring out] Carrying away from a central organ or section, as efferent nerves, which conduct impulses from the brain or spinal cord to the periphery; efferent lymph vessels, which convey lymph from lymph nodes; and efferent arterioles, which carry blood from glomeruli of the kidney. Opposite of afferent.

effervesce (ĕf″ĕr-vĕs′) [L. *effervescere,* to boil up] To boil or form bubbles on the surface of a liquid.

effervescence (ĕf-ĕr-vĕs′ĕns) Formation of gas bubbles that rise to the surface of a fluid.

effervescent Bubbling; rising in little bubbles of gas.

efficacy The ability to produce a desired effect.

effleurage (ĕf′lĕ-răzh) A massage technique that employs gentle hand movements along the long axis of limbs or muscles.

abdominal e. Light stroking with the fingertips in a circular pattern from the symphysis pubis to the iliac crests, a Lamaze technique for coping with uterine contractions during the first stage of labor.

efflorescence (ĕf-flor-ĕs′ĕns) [L. *efflorescere,* to bloom] A rash; a redness of the skin. SYN: *exanthem*.

efflorescent Becoming powdery or dry from loss of water in crystallization.

effluent (ĕf′loo-ĕnt) [L. *effluere,* to flow out] **1.** A flowing out. **2.** Fluid material discharged from a sewage treatment or industrial plant.

effluvium (ĕf-loo′vē-ŭm) *pl.* **effluvia** A malodorous outflow of vapor or gas, particularly one that is toxic.

effort Expenditure of physical or mental energy.

effort syndrome A form of anxiety neurosis in which fatigue is the presenting symptom. The fatigue is increased by mild exertion and may be more pronounced in the morning. SEE: *chronic fatigue syndrome*.

effuse (ĕ-fūs′) [L. *effusio,* pour out] Thin, widely spreading; applied to a bacterial growth that forms a very delicate film over a surface.

effusion (ĕ-fū′zhŭn) Escape of fluid into a part, as the pleural cavity, such as pyothorax (pus), hydrothorax (serum), hemothorax (blood), chylothorax (lymph), pneumothorax (air), hydropneumothorax (serum and air), and pyopneumothorax (pus and air).

joint e. Increased fluid within a joint

cavity. There may be increased production of synovial fluid following trauma or with some arthritic disease processes, or blood accumulating in the joint following trauma or surgery or due to hemophilia. Excessive amounts of synovial fluid, pus or blood accumulate in many arthritic diseases (such as gout or rheumatoid arthritis); after trauma; in joint infections; following joint surgery; or in hemophilia.

pericardial e. Fluid in the pericardial cavity, between the visceral and the parietal pericardium. This condition may produce symptoms of cardiac tamponade, such as difficulty breathing.

pleural e. Fluid in the thoracic cavity between the visceral and parietal pleura. It may be seen on a chest radiograph if it exceeds 300 ml.

eflornithine An antineoplastic and antiprotozoal drug. It has been used to treat African sleeping sickness (African trypanosomiasis). Trade name is Ornidyl.

EGCg, EGCG *Epigallocatechin gallate.*

egesta (ē-jĕs′tă) [L. *egere,* to cast forth] Waste matter eliminated from the body, esp. excrement.

egg [AS. *aeg*] **1.** The female sex cell or ovum, applied esp. to a fertilized ovum that is passed from the body and develops outside, as in fowls. **2.** The mammalian ovum.

raw e. An egg in its fresh, uncooked state, esp. one intended for food. Human consumption of raw or inadequately cooked eggs has caused *Salmonella* infections. To kill *Salmonella* organisms, if present, eggs should be boiled for 7 min, fried for 3 min per side, or poached for 5 min. It is unsafe to use sauces or dressings made with raw eggs. Fresh eggs should be stored in the cold; cracked eggs should be discarded. SEE: *salmonellosis.*

eglandulous (ē-glănd′ū-lŭs) [L. *e,* out, + *glandula,* glandule] Without glands.

ego (ē′gō, ĕg′ō) [L. *ego,* I] In psychoanalysis, one of the three major divisions in the model of the psychic apparatus. The others are the id and superego. The ego is involved with consciousness and memory and mediates among primitive instinctual or animal drives (the id), internal social prohibitions (the superego), and reality. The psychoanalytic use of the term should not be confused with its common usage in the sense of self-love or selfishness. SEE: *id; superego.*

egocentric (ē″gō-sĕn′trĭk) [L. *ego,* I, + Gr. *kentron,* center] Pert. to a withdrawal from the external world with concentration on the inner self.

egocentricity The stage of cognitive development in which perception is almost exclusively from the child's own viewpoint and in the child's own way. This stage is characteristic of toddlers and early preschool children.

ego-dystonic (ē″gō-dĭs-tŏn′ĭk) [″ + Gr. *dys,* bad, + *tonos,* tension] Pert. to something repulsive to the individual's self-image.

ego-integrity The eighth stage in Erikson's developmental theory; the opposite of despair. It is the major psychic task of the mature elderly and is marked by a healthy unifying philosophy and the wisdom learned from experience. The individual feels vital, balanced, and whole in relation to the self and the world.

egoism (ē′gō-ĭzm) An inflated estimate of one's value or effectiveness.

egomania (ē″gō-mā′nē-ă) [″ + Gr. *mania,* madness] Abnormal self-esteem and self-interest.

egophony (ē-gŏf′ō-nē) [Gr. *aix,* goat, + *phone,* voice] An abnormal change in tone, somewhat like the bleat of a goat, heard in auscultation of the chest when the subject speaks normally. It is associated with bronchophony and may be heard over the lungs of persons with pleural effusion, or occasionally pneumonia.

ego-syntonic (ē″gō-sĭn-tŏn′ĭk) [″ + Gr. *syn,* together, + *tonos,* tension] Pert. to something that is consistent with the individual's self-image.

egotism (ē′gō-tĭzm) **1.** The tendency to regard oneself more highly than is warranted by the facts, and to boast of one's abilities or achievements. **2.** An inflated sense of self-importance; conceit. SEE: *egoism.*

egotropic (ē″gō-trŏp′ĭk) [L. *ego,* I, + Gr. *tropos,* a turning] Interested chiefly in one's self; self-centered.

EGTA *esophageal gastric tube airway.*

Ehlers-Danlos syndrome (ā′lĕrz-dăn′lŏs) [Edvard Ehlers, Danish dermatologist, 1863–1937; H. A. Danlos, Fr. dermatologist, 1844–1912] An inherited disorder of the elastic connective tissue. The characteristic soft velvety skin is fragile, hyperelastic, and bruises easily. Hyperextensibility of joints, visceral malformations, atrophic scars, pseudotumors, and calcified subcutaneous cysts are present.

Ehrenritter's ganglion (ār′ĕn-rĭt″ĕrs) [Johann Ehrenritter, Austrian anatomist, d. 1790] The superior ganglion of the glossopharyngeal nerve.

ehrlichiosis [Paul Ehrlich, Ger. physician, 1854–1915. Awarded Nobel Prize in medicine in 1908] One of two forms of an infectious disease of monocytes and granulocytes transmitted by tick bites. It was first reported in humans in the U.S. in 1987, and is considered an emerging disease.

ETIOLOGY: Infection is caused by two intracellular bacteria belonging to the Rickettsiaceae family. *Ehrlichia chaffeensis,* carried by the Lone Star tick, causes human monocytic ehrlichiosis (HME); a second species related to *Ehrlichia phagocytophila,* carried by *Ixodes* ticks, causes human granulocytic ehrlichiosis (HGE). Although 30 states have reported cases, HME is found mostly in the southern U.S., while HGE is found in the northern U.S.

SYMPTOMS: Both HME and HGE are marked by nonspecific influenza-like symptoms. A high fever with rigors, headache, malaise, myalgia, leukopenia, and thrombocytopenia are most common; a rash may be present in HME. The symptoms last for approx. 3 weeks; it is unclear if a latent infection remains. Complications of renal failure, cardiomegaly, coagulopathies, or coma occur in 16%, mostly in the elderly. The majority of patients are men over age 40.

TREATMENT: Doxycycline (or other tetracyclines) is the recommended treatment.

DIAGNOSIS: Serological tests are used; a polymerase chain reaction (PCR) applied to whole blood samples can confirm the diagnosis in 24 to 48 hr.

PREVENTION: Ticks should be avoided by avoiding grassy areas where they reside, by wearing long pants and light-colored clothing, and by applying tick repellents to clothing before entering grasslands or woodlands.

After leaving these areas, exposed clothing should be immediately laundered, and the skin bathed and inspected for the presence of adult ticks and tiny nymphs. Any attached ticks should be promptly removed with tweezers, making certain to remove the entire insect.

Ehrlich's side-chain theory (ār′lĭks) [Paul Ehrlich] An outdated hypothesis used early in the 20th century to explain immunological reactions.

eicosa- Combining form used in chemistry to indicate *twenty.*

eicosanoid One of the products of the metabolism of arachidonic acid. Prostaglandins, thromboxanes, and leukotrienes are some of the compounds formed.

EID **1.** *electroimmunodiffusion; electronic infusion device.* **2.** *esophageal intubation detector device.*

eidetic (ī-dĕt′ĭk) [Gr. *eidos,* form, shape] Rel. to or having the ability of total visual recall of anything previously seen.

eighth cranial nerve The acoustic nerve. SYN: *vestibulocochlear nerve.*

Eikenella corrodens (ī″kĕn-ĕl′ă) A gram-negative rod normally present in the mouth.

eikonometer (ī″kō-nŏm′ĕ-tĕr) [Gr. *eikon,* image, + *metron,* measure] An optical instrument used in detecting aniseikonia.

eikonometry Determination of the distance of an object by measuring the image produced by a lens of known focus.

eiloid (ī′loyd) [Gr. *eilein,* to coil, + *eidos,* form, shape] Having a coil-like structure.

Eimeria (ī-mē′rē-ă) A genus of sporozoan parasites belonging to the class Telosporidia, subclass Coccidia. They are intracellular parasites living in the epithelial cells of vertebrates and invertebrates. They rarely are parasitic to humans.

E. hominis A species that has been found in empyema in humans.

einsteinium (īn-stīn′ē-ŭm) [Albert Einstein, German-born U.S. physicist, 1879–1955] A radioactive element with atomic number 99 and an atomic weight of 254.0881. Its symbol is Es.

EIP *end-inspiratory pause.*

Eisenmenger's complex [Victor Eisenmenger, Ger. physician, 1864–1932] A congenital cyanotic heart defect consisting of ventricular septal defect, dextroposition of the aorta, pulmonary hypertension with pulmonary artery enlargement, and hypertrophy of the right ventricle.

Eisenmenger's syndrome [Victor Eisenmenger, Ger. physician, 1864–1932] Pulmonary hypertension that results from any congenital heart defect.

eisodic (ī-sŏd′ĭk) [Gr. *eis,* into, + *hodos,* way] Centripetal or afferent, as nerve fibers of a reflex arc.

ejaculate The semen released during ejaculation.

ejaculatio (ē-jăk″ū-lā′shē-ō) [L.] Sudden expelling; ejaculation.

e. praecox Premature ejaculation.

ejaculation (ē-jăk″ū-lā′shŭn) [L. *ejaculare,* to throw out] Ejection of the seminal fluid from the male urethra.

PHYSIOLOGY: Ejaculation consists of two phases: (1) the passage of semen and the secretions of the accessory organs (bulbourethral and prostate glands and seminal vesicles) into the urethra and (2) the expulsion of the seminal fluid from the urethra. The former is brought about by contraction of the smooth muscle of the ductus deferens and the increased secretory activity of the glands; the latter by the rhythmical contractions of the bulbocavernosus and ischiocavernosus muscles and the levator ani. The prostate discharges its secretions before those of the seminal vesicle. The sensations associated with ejaculation constitute the male orgasm. Ejaculation occurs without ejection of the seminal fluid from the male urethra in patients who have had a prostatectomy. In that case, the ejaculate is in the bladder.

Ejaculation is a reflex phenomenon. Afferent impulses arising principally from stimulation of the glans penis pass to the spinal cord by way of the internal pudendal nerves. Efferent impulses arising from a reflex center located in the upper lumbar region of the cord pass through sympathetic fibers in the hypogastric nerves and plexus to the ductus deferens and seminal vesicles. Other impulses arising from the third and fourth sacral segments pass through the internal pudendal nerves to the ischiocavernosus and bulbocavernosus muscles. Erection of the penis usually precedes ejaculation. Ejaculation occurs normally during copulation, masturbation, or as a nocturnal emission. The seminal fluid normally contains 60 million to 150 million sperm/ml. The volume of the ejaculation is from 2 to 5 ml. SEE: *orgasm; semen.*

premature e. An imprecise term that usually indicates ejaculation occurring very shortly after the onset of sexual excitement, or ejaculation occurring before copulation or before the partner's orgasm. This disorder is usually accompanied by feelings of guilt or relationship difficulties.

retrograde e. Ejaculation in which the seminal fluid is discharged into the bladder rather than through the urethra. Retrograde ejaculation can occur as a consequence of some psychotropic drugs or radical prostatectomy.

ejaculatory Pert. to ejaculation.

ejecta (ē-jĕk'tă) [L. *ejectus,* thrown out, ejected] Material, espcially waste material, excreted by the body. SYN: *dejecta; egesta.*

ejection (ē-jĕk'shŭn) Removal, esp. sudden, of something.

ventricular e. Forceful expulsion of blood from the ventricles of the heart.

ejection fraction In cardiac physiology, the percentage of the blood emptied from the ventricle during systole; the left ventricular ejection fraction averages 60% to 70% in healthy hearts but can be markedly reduced if part of the heart muscle dies (e.g., after myocardial infarction) or in cardiomyopathy or valvular heart disease.

Ekbom's syndrome [Karl A. Ekbom, Swedish neurologist, b. 1907] SEE: *restless legs syndrome.*

EKG Abbreviation for the German *elektrokardiogramm.* SEE: *electrocardiogram.*

ekphorize (ĕk'fō-rīz) [Gr. *ek,* out, + *phorein,* to bear] In psychiatry, to bring back the effect of a psychological experience in an attempt to repeat the experience in memory. SEE: *engram.*

elaboration (ē-lăb″ō-rā'shŭn) In body metabolism, the formation of complex compounds from simpler substances (e.g., formation of proteins from amino acids).

elastance The tendency of a material or body tissue to return to its original form after having been stretched or deformed. SYN: *compliance* (1); *elasticity.*

elastase (ē-lăs'tās) A pancreatic enzyme that cleaves amino acids from proteins in the presence of trypsin.

elastic (ē-lăs'tĭk) [Gr. *elastikos,* driven on, set in motion] Capable of being stretched and then returning to its original state.

intermaxillary e. An elastic band used between the maxillary and mandibular teeth in orthodontic therapy; also called a maxillomandibular elastic.

intramaxillary e. An elastic band used in a horizontal space closure by attachments within the same arch.

vertical e. An elastic applied to arch brackets perpendicularly to the occlusal plane for approximating teeth.

elastic cartilage Yellow cartilage such as is found in the epiglottis, external ears, and auditory tube.

elasticity (ē″lăs-tĭs'ĭ-tē) The quality of returning to original size and shape after compression or stretching.

elastic stocking A stocking worn to apply pressure to the extremity, aiding the return of blood from the extremity to the heart through the deep veins. SEE: *thrombosis, deep venous.*

elastin (ē-lăs'tĭn) An extracellular connective tissue protein that is the principal component of elastic fibers in the middle layer of arteries.

elastinase (ē-lăs'tĭn-ās) An enzyme that dissolves elastin.

elastofibroma (ē-lăs″tō-fī-brō'mă) [″ + L. *fibra,* fiber, + Gr. *oma,* tumor] A benign soft tissue tumor that contains elastic and fibrous elements.

elastoid (ē-lăs'toyd) [″ + *eidos,* form, shape] Pert. to a substance formed by hyaline degeneration.

elastoma (ē″lăs-tō'mă) [″ + *oma,* tumor] A yellow nodular or papular lesion of the skin composed of elastic fibers. Elastomas are seen in the genetic disease pseudoxanthoma elasticum.

elastometer (ē″lăs-tŏm'ĕ-tĕr) [″ + Gr. *metron,* measure] A device for measuring elasticity.

elastometry The measurement of tissue elasticity.

elastorrhexis (ē-lăs″tō-rĕk'sĭs) [″ + *rhexis,* rupture] Rupture of elastic tissue.

elastose (ē-lăs'tōs) A peptone resulting from gastric digestion of elastin.

elation (ē-lā'shŭn) [L. *elatus,* exalted] Joyful emotion. It is pathological when out of accord with the patient's actual circumstances.

elbow (ĕl'bō) [AS. *eln,* forearm, + *boga,* bend] The joint between the arm and forearm. SEE: illus.

golfer's e. Tendonitis occurring at the medial epicondyle. This injury is commonly seen as a result of overuse of the elbow. SYN: *medial humeral epicondylitis.* SEE: *tennis elbow.*

little league e. A form of overuse syndrome marked by inflammation of the medial condyle or fractures of the lateral humeral condyle of the elbow. It is seen in adolescent baseball players, esp. in pitchers. In order to help prevent this condition, Little League Baseball regulations limit the time pitchers may play in any one game.

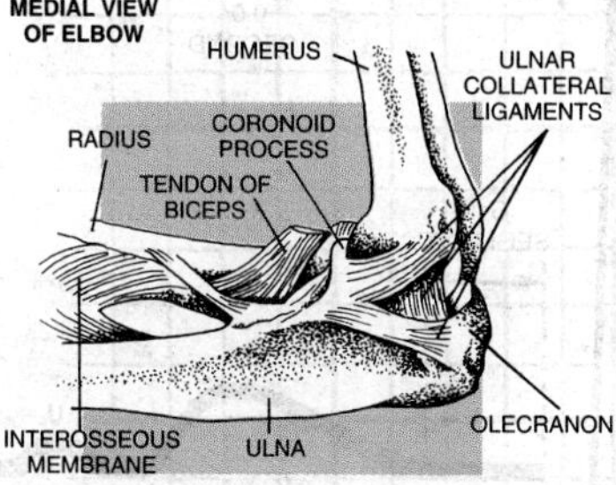

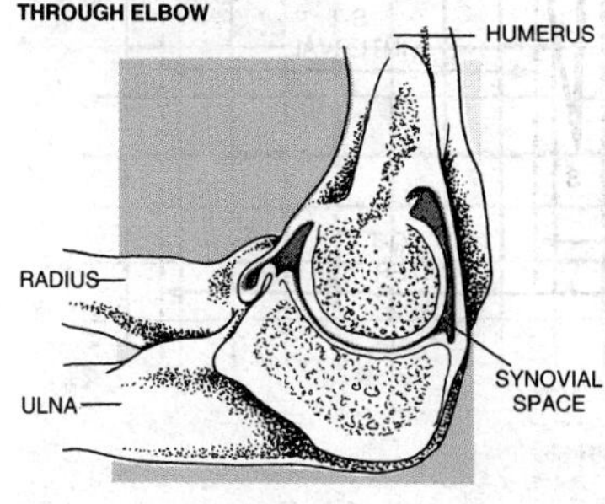

ELBOW JOINT

tennis e. A strain of the lateral forearm muscles near their origin on the lateral epicondyle of the humerus. SYN: *lateral humeral epicondylitis*. SEE: *tennis elbow*.

elbow conformer A splint applied to prevent flexion contractures following burns to the upper extremity. The device is fabricated to conform to the anterior arm. Pressure is applied to the olecranon process by a soft, cupped pad.

elbow unit A component of the upper-extremity prosthesis that permits the arm to bend at the elbow.

elder (ĕl′dĕr) A person over 65 years old.

eldercare Providing health care and assistance with activities of daily living for elderly adults at home. Family members usually provide most of the needed assistance, although friends, professional agencies, or volunteers may participate.

elderly, frail Older persons with functional impairments and poor physiological reserves. Typically, they have difficulty living independently.

elder neglect Elder abuse.

elective therapy A treatment or surgical procedure not requiring immediate attention and therefore planned for the patient's or provider's convenience.

Electra complex [Gr. Elektra, Agamemnon's daughter, who helped assassinate her mother because of love for her father, whom the former had slain] In psychoanalysis, a group of symptoms due to suppressed sexual love of a daughter for her father. SEE: *Jocasta complex; Oedipus complex*.

electric, electrical [Gr. *elektron*, amber] Pert. to, caused by, or resembling electricity.

electrical alternans Beat-to-beat changes in one or more portions of the electrocardiogram.

electrical patch An electrical device for delivering medications transdermally. The slight electric current used in electrical patches allows larger molecules to be transported through the skin. This technique differs from electrophoresis by the electrical current used, which increases the permeability of the skin. SYN: *electroporation*. SEE: *iontophoresis*.

electricity A form of energy that is generated by the interactions of positive and negative charges and that exhibits magnetic, chemical, mechanical, and thermal effects.

frictional e. Static electricity generated by rubbing two objects together.

galvanic e. Electricity generated by chemical action.

induced e. Electricity generated in a body from another body nearby without contact between them.

magnetic e. Electricity induced by a magnetic device.

negative e. An electric charge caused by an excess of negatively charged electrons.

positive e. An electric charge caused by loss of negatively charged electrons.

static e. Electricity generated by friction of certain materials.

electric light baker A device for warming a part, as in arthritis. SEE: *baker*.

electro-, electr- [Gr. *elektron*, amber] Prefix indicating a *relationship to electricity*.

electroanalgesia (ē-lĕk″trō-ăn″ăl-jē′zē-ă) [″ + *analgesia*, want of feeling] Relief from pain by application of low-intensity electric currents locally or through implanted electrodes.

electroanesthesia (ē-lĕk″trō-ăn″ĕs-thē′zē-ă) [″ + *an-*, not, + *aisthesis*, sensation] General anesthesia produced by a device that passes electricity of a certain frequency, amplitude, and wave form through the brain.

electrobiology (ē-lĕk″trō-bī-ŏl′ō-jē) [″ + *bios*, life, + *logos*, word, reason] The science of electrical phenomena in the living body.

electrocardiogram (ē-lĕk″trō-kăr′dē-ō-grăm″) [″ + *kardia*, heart, + *gramma*, something written] ABBR: ECG. A record of the electrical activity of the heart, consisting of waves called P, Q, R, S, T, and sometimes U. The

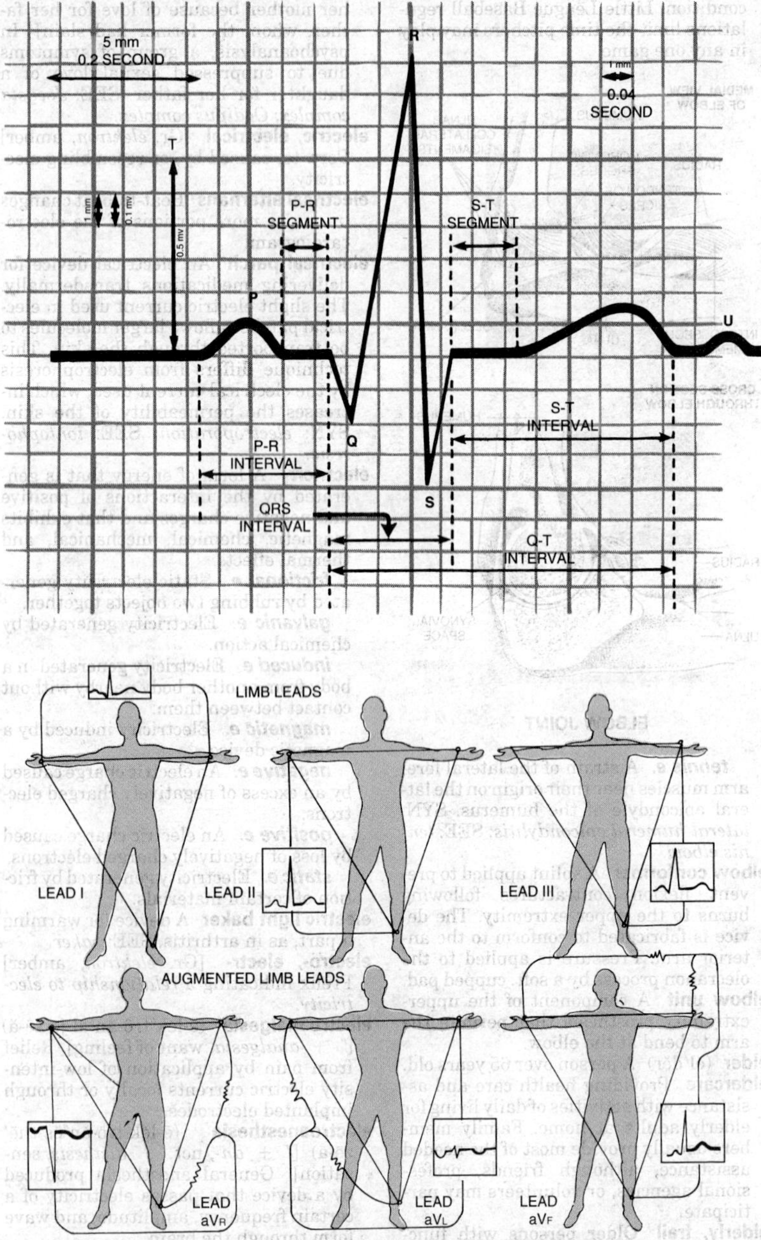

QRST COMPLEX OF ELECTROCARDIOGRAM/ECG LEADS

first, or P, wave is caused by the depolarization of the atria, whose electrical changes in turn cause atrial contraction. The Q, R, and S waves (QRS complex) correspond to depolarization of ventricular muscle. The T wave corresponds to ventricular repolarization. The electrocardiogram gives important information concerning the spread of electricity to the different parts of the heart and is used to diagnose rhythm and conduction disturbances, myocardial infarction or ischemia, chamber enlargement and metabolic disorders, among others. SEE: illus.

signal-averaged e. ABBR: SAECG. An electrocardiographic study, usually performed on patients with unexplained loss of consciousness or suspected dysrhythmias, in which hundreds of QRS complexes are collected, filtered, and analyzed to discover the presence or absence of certain abnormalities in the conducting system of the ventricle. These abnormalities, called late potentials, point to an increased risk of ventricular tachycardia or ventricular fibrillation. The signal-averaging technique allows late potentials to be examined free from random electrical discharges ("noise"), which often are present when only a small number of QRS complexes are evaluated.

electrocardiograph (ē-lĕk″trō-kăr′dē-ō-grăf) [″ + ″ + *graphein,* to write] A device for recording changes in the electrical energy produced by the action of heart muscles.

electrocardiography The creation and study of graphic records (electrocardiograms) produced by electric currents originating in the heart.

electrocardiophonograph (ē-lĕk″trō-kăr″dē-ō-fō′nō-grăf) [Gr. *elektron,* amber, + *kardia,* heart, + *phone,* sound, + *graphein,* to write] A device for recording heart sounds.

electrocautery (ē-lĕk″trō-kaw′tĕr-ē) [″ + *kauterion,* branding iron] Cauterization using a variety of electrical modalities to create thermal energy, including a directly heated metallic applicator, or bipolar or monopolar electrodes.

electrocerebral silence In electroencephalography (EEG), the absence of detectable electrical activity in the cortex of the brain. The EEG tracing shows no deflections from its baseline. This finding is diagnostic of brain death.

electrochemistry [″ + *chemeia,* chemistry] The science of chemical changes produced by electricity.

electrocision (ē-lĕk′trō-sĭ′zhŭn) [″ + L. *caedare,* to cut] Excision by electric current.

electrocoagulation (ē-lĕk″trō-kō-ăg″ū-lā′shŭn) [″ + L. *coagulare,* to thicken] Coagulation of tissue by means of a high-frequency electric current. SEE: *electrocautery*.

electrocochleography (ē-lĕk″trō-kŏk-lē-ŏg′ră-fē) Measurement of electrical activity produced when the cochlea is stimulated. A needle electrode is passed through the eardrum and placed on the cochlea. The electrical activity is then recorded.

electrocontractility (ē-lĕk″trō-kŏn-trăk-tĭl′ĭ-tē) [″ + L. *contrahere,* to contract] Contraction of muscular tissue by electrical stimulation.

electrocorticography (ē-lĕk″trō-kor″tĭ-kŏg′ră-fē) Recording of the electrical impulses from the brain by electrodes placed directly on the cerebral cortex.

electrocution (ē-lĕk″trō-kū′shŭn) [″ + L. *acutus,* sharpened] Destruction of life by means of electric current. SEE: *electric shock; lightning safety rules*.

electrode (ē-lĕk′trōd) [″ + *hodos,* a way] **1.** An electrical terminal or lead. **2.** A conductive medium. **3.** In electrotherapy, an instrument with a point or surface from which to discharge current to a patient's body. **4.** An electrical terminal or lead that is adapted to sense current or voltage in response to specific analytes, for purposes of quantifying the particular analyte.

active e. An electrode that is smaller than a dispersive electrode and produces stimulation in a concentrated area.

calomel e. An electrode that develops a standard electric potential and is used to provide a reference voltage in the circuit for sensing electrodes. It is composed of an amalgam of mercury and mercury chloride. It is used as a standard in determining the pH of fluids.

carbon dioxide e. A blood gas electrode used to measure the carbon dioxide tension (symbolized as P_{CO_2}) in blood. Its operation is based on the diffusion of carbon dioxide from the blood sample through a semipermeable membrane into a buffer solution with a subsequent change in the pH of the buffer. SYN: *Severinghaus electrode*.

coated wire e. ABBR: CWE. A chemical sensor in some clinical laboratory analyzers that functions similarly to a pH electrode. SEE: *hydrogen e.; saturated calomel e.*

depolarizing e. An electrode with greater resistance than the part of the body in the circuit.

dispersive e. An electrode larger than an active electrode. It produces electrical stimulation over a large area. SYN: *indifferent e.*

gas-sensing e. An electrode in which a gas-permeable membrane separates the test solution from an aqueous electrode solution in contact with an ion-selective electrode. Gas permeation of the membrane changes the chemical equilibrium within the electrolyte, and the ion-sensitive electrode detects this change.

glass e. In chemistry, a chemical sensor that uses a glass membrane, as opposed to one that uses an organic or solid state membrane as the sensing surface.

hydrogen e. An electrode that absorbs and measures hydrogen gas; used as the reference for pH measurement in research laboratories.

immobilized enzyme e. A chemical sensor that is highly selective due to a specific enzyme incorporated into its structure.

indifferent e. Dispersive e.

internal reference e. The metal electrode inside all chemical-sensing potentiometric electrodes. The two most commonly used internal reference electrodes are the calomel and the silver/silver chloride.

ion-selective e. A chemical transducer that yields a response to variations in the concentration of a given ion in solution.

liquid membrane e. An electrode in which the sensing membrane is made up of a hydrophobic ion-exchange neutral carrier (ionophore) dissolved in a viscous, water-insoluble solvent. The liquid membrane is physically supported by an inert porous matrix such as cellulose acetate.

multiple point e. Several sets of terminals providing for the use of several electrodes. SEE: *multiterminal*.

negative e. A cathode; the pole by which electric current leaves the generating source.

oxygen e. A blood gas electrode invented by Dr. Leland Clark, used to measure the partial pressure of oxygen (PO_2) in arterial blood. SYN: *Clark electrode; PO_2 e.; polarographic e.*

PO_2 e. Oxygen e.

point e. An electrode with an insulating handle at one end and a small metallic terminal at the other for use in applying static sparks.

polarographic e. Oxygen e.

polymer membrane e. An electrode in which the sensing membrane is an organic polymer containing a hydrophobic ion-exchange neutral carrier (ionophore).

positive e. An anode; the pole opposite a cathode.

reference e. A chemical electrode whose cell potential remains fixed and against which an indicator electrode is compared. The most common reference electrode is the silver/silver chloride (Ag/AgCl) electrode.

saturated calomel e. ABBR: SCE. One of two practical reference electrodes, used with a mercurous chloride (calomel) paste in pH and other potentiometric instruments. The other is the silver/silver chloride electrode. The calomel electrode has been the standard secondary reference electrode used in the laboratory since the introduction of the pH electrode.

solid-state membrane e. An electrode in which the sensing membrane is made of a single crystal or pressed pellet containing the salt of the ion to be sensed.

standard hydrogen e. ABBR: SHE. The standard reference electrode against which all others are measured. Its assigned electrode potential is 0.000 V.

subcutaneous e. An electrode placed beneath the skin.

surface e. An electrode placed on the surface of the skin or exposed organ.

therapeutic e. An electrode used for introduction of medicines through the skin by ionization. SEE: *iontophoresis*.

electrodesiccation (ē-lĕk″trō-dĕs″ĭ-kā′shŭn) [Gr. *elektron*, amber, + L. *desiccare*, to dry up] The destructive drying of cells by application of electrical energy similar to, but to a lesser intensity than electrocoagulation. Electrodesiccation is used for hemostasis of very small capillaries or veins that have been severed during surgery.

electrodiagnosis The use of electrical and electronic devices for diagnostic purposes. This technique is helpful in almost all branches of medicine, but particularly in investigating the function of the heart, nerves, and muscles.

electrodialysis (ē-lĕk″trō-dī-ăl′ĭ-sĭs) *pl.* **electrodialyses** [″ + *dia-*, apart, + *lysis*, dissolution] A method of separating electrolytes from colloids by passing a current through a solution containing both. A semi-permeable membrane is usually used to aid in the separation, with one electrode on each side.

electrodynamometer (ē-lĕk″trō-dī″nă-mŏm′ĕ-tĕr) [″ + *dynamis*, power, + *metron*, measure] An instrument that measures the strength of an electric current.

electroencephalogram (ē-lĕk″trō-ĕn-sĕf′ă-lō-grăm) [″ + *enkephalos*, brain, + *gramma*, something written] ABBR: EEG. A tracing on an electroencephalograph. SEE: illus.; *electroencephalography*.

electroencephalograph (ē-lĕk-trō-ĕn-sĕf′ă-lō-grăf) [″ + ″ + *graphein*, to write] An instrument for recording the electrical activity of the brain. SEE: *electroencephalography*.

electroencephalography Amplification, recording, and analysis of the electrical activity of the brain. The record obtained is called an electroencephalogram (EEG).

Electrodes are placed on the scalp in various locations. The difference between the electric potential of two sites is recorded. The difference between one pair or among many pairs at a time can be obtained. The most frequently seen pattern in the normal adult under resting conditions is the alpha rhythm of 8½ to 12 waves per sec. A characteristic change in the wave occurs during sleep, on opening the eyes, and during periods of concentration. Some persons who have intracranial disease will have a normal EEG and others with no other-

NORMAL AND ABNORMAL ELECTROENCEPHALOGRAM WAVE PATTERNS

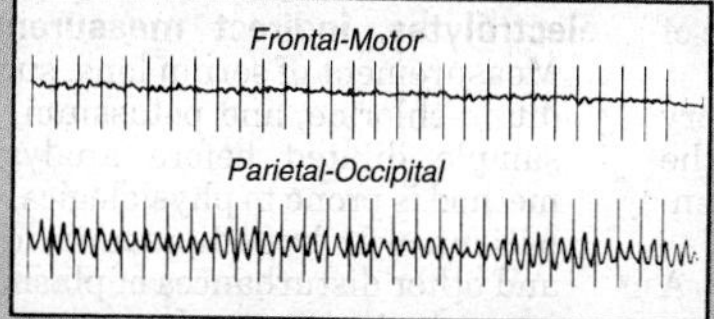

NORMAL ADULT
10/sec. activity in occipital area

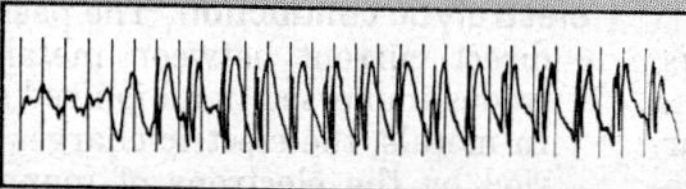

PETIT MAL SEIZURE
Synchronous 3/sec. spikes and waves

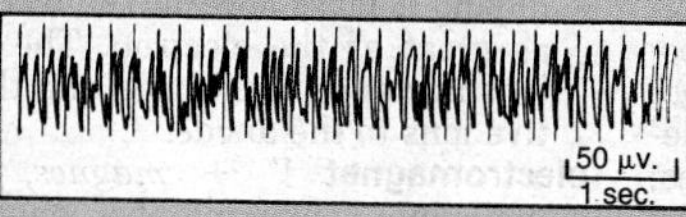

GRAND MAL SEIZURE
High-voltage spikes, generalized

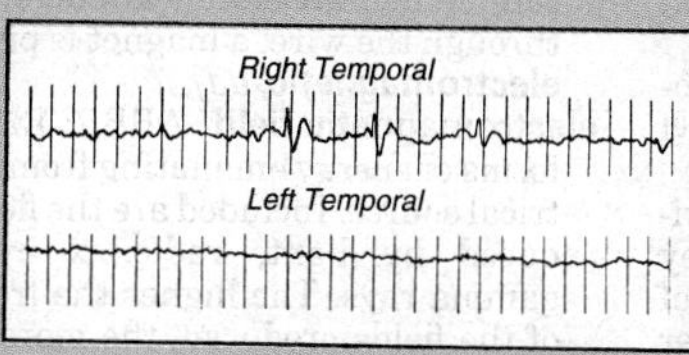

TEMPORAL LOBE EPILEPSY
Right temporal spike focus

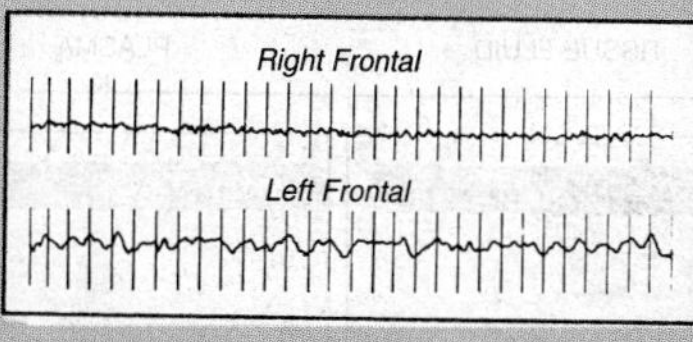

BRAIN TUMOR
Left frontal slow wave focus

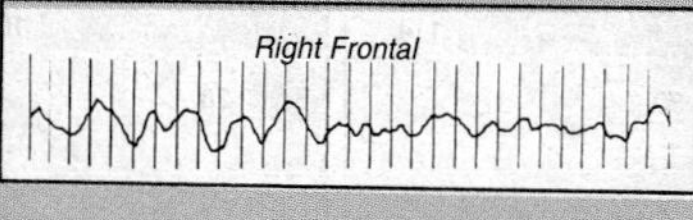

ENCEPHALITIS
Diffuse slowing

SOURCE: Reprinted with permission from The Merck Manual, 13th ed., Merck & Co., Inc., 1977, pp. 1408–1409.

wise demonstrable disease will have an abnormal EEG. Nevertheless, the use of this diagnostic technique has proved to be very helpful in studying epilepsy and convulsive disorders and in localizing lesions in the cerebrum. SEE: *rhythm, alpha; rhythm, beta; wave, theta.*

electrogoniometer (ē-lĕk″trō-gō″nē-ŏm′ĕ-tĕr) An electrical device for measuring angles of joints and their range of motion.

electroimmunodiffusion A laboratory method of identifying antigens in the blood by creating an artificial antigen-antibody reaction.

electrolarynx (ē-lĕk′trō-lăr″ĭnks) A voice-restoring device used by some patients after surgical removal of the larynx. The device works by amplifying breath sounds.

electrolysis (ē″lĕk-trŏl′ĭ-sĭs) [″ + *lysis,* dissolution] The decomposition of a substance by passage of an electric current through it. Hair follicles may be destroyed by this method. SEE: *depilatory technique.*

electrolyte (ē-lĕk′trō-līt) [″ + *lytos,* soluble] **1.** A solution that conducts electricity. **2.** A substance that, in solution, conducts an electric current and is decomposed by its passage. Acids, bases, and salts are common electrolytes. **3.** An ionized salt in blood, tissue fluids, and cells. These salts include sodium, potassium, and chlorine. SEE: illus.

amphoteric e. A solution that produces both hydrogen (H^+) and hydroxyl (OH^-) ions.

fecal e.'s Osmotically and electrically active ions present in stool. They are measured in the evaluation of chronic diarrhea, to determine whether the diarrhea is secretory or osmotic. SEE: *osmotic diarrhea; secretory diarrhea.*

electrolytes, direct measurement of Measurement of serum-plasma ions, such as sodium, chloride, and potassium, without prior dilution of the sample. Direct measurement of electrolytes is considered more physiologically accurate than indirect measurement.

electrolytes, indirect measurement of Measurement of serum ions, such as sodium, chloride, and potassium, using a sample diluted before analysis. The method is prone to physiological error in patients with hyperlipidemia, myeloma, and other disturbances of plasma water concentration.

electrolytic (ē-lĕk″trō-lĭt′ĭk) Caused by or rel. to electrolysis.

electrolytic conduction The passage of a direct current between metallic electrodes immersed in an ionized solution. In metals, the electric charges are carried by the electrons of inappreciable mass. In solutions, the electric charges are carried by electrolytic ions, each having a mass several thousand times as great as the electron. The positive ions move to the cathode and the negative ions to the anode.

electromagnet [″ + *magnes,* magnet] A magnet consisting of a length of insulated wire wound around a soft iron core. When an electrical current flows through the wire, a magnet is produced. **electromagnetic,** *adj.*

electromagnetic field ABBR: EMF. All forms of energy emanating from an electrical source. Included are the fields produced by light, radio, x-rays, and gamma rays. The higher the frequency of the fields produced, the more energy is contained. Thus, the radiated energy

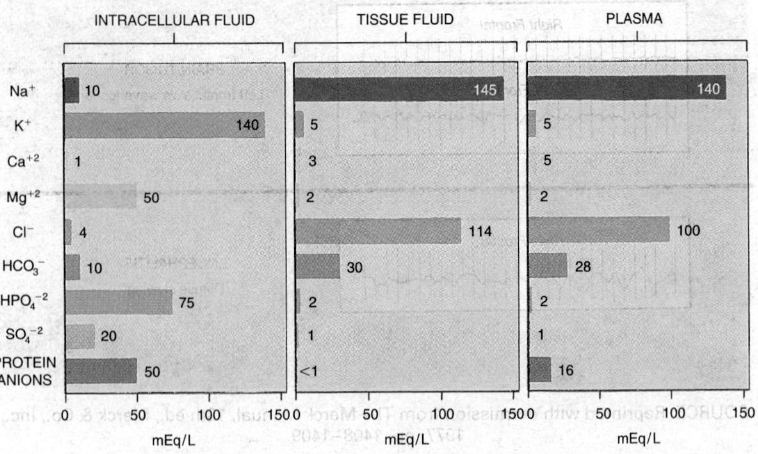

ELECTROLYTE CONCENTRATIONS IN BODY FLUIDS

Electromagnetic Spectrum

Frequency (Hz)	Type of Radiation	Wave-length (cm)
10^{22}		10^{-12}
	Gamma rays	
10^{19}		10^{-9}
	X-rays	
10^{16}		10^{-6}
	Ultraviolet radiation	
10^{15}		10^{-5}
	Visible light	
10^{14}		10^{-4}
	Infrared radiation	
10^{13}		10^{-2}
	Submillimeter waves	
10^{12}		10^{-1}
	Microwaves	
10^{9}		10
	Television and radio waves	
10^{4}		10^{6}

from the 60-cycle frequency of an ordinary household electric line is quite small. The long-range effects of prolonged exposure to EMF are poorly understood.

electromagnetic induction Generation of an electromotive force, in an insulated conductor moving in an electromagnetic field, or in a fixed conductor in a moving magnetic field.

electromagnetic spectrum The complete range of wavelengths of electromagnetic radiation. SEE: table.

electromagnetism Magnetism produced by an electric current.

electromassage [″ + Fr. *masser,* to massage] Massage combined with electrical treatment.

electromotive [″ + L. *motor,* mover] Pert. to the passage of electricity in a current or motion produced by it.

electromyogram (ē-lĕk″trō-mī′ō-grăm) [Gr. *elektron,* amber, + *mys,* muscle, + *gramma,* something written] The graphic record of resting and voluntary muscle activity as a result of electrical stimulation.

electromyography (ē-lĕk″trō-mī-ŏg′ră-fē) [″ + ″ + *graphein,* to write] The preparation, study of, and interpretation of electromyograms.

electron [Gr. *elektron,* amber] An extremely minute particle with a negative electrical charge that revolves about the central core or nucleus of an atom. Its mass is about 1/1840 that of a hydrogen atom, or 9.11 × 10^{-28} g. The negative electrical charge is 1.602 × 10^{-19} coulombs. When emitted from radioactive substances, electrons are known as negative beta particles, or rays.

electronarcosis (ē-lĕk″trō-năr-kō′sĭs) The induction of narcosis or unconsciousness by the application of electricity to the brain.

electron-dense In electron microscopy, having a density that prevents penetration by electrons.

electronegative [″ + L. *negare,* to deny] **1.** The relative attraction of a nucleus for electrons. Using the periodic table, the most electronegative atom is fluorine (upper right), with decreasing electronegativity as one traverses the table down or to the left. **2.** Charged with negative electricity, which results in the attraction of positively charged bodies and the repulsion of negatively charged bodies.

electroneurolysis (ē-lĕk″trō-nū-rŏl′ĭ-sĭs) Destruction of a nerve by use of an electric needle.

electronic Pert. to electrons.

electronic dental anesthesia ABBR: EDA. In dentistry, the use of low levels of electric current to block pain signals en route to the brain. The patient controls the current through a hand-held control. The current creates no discomfort and, unlike local anesthesia, leaves no numbness to wear off once the dental work is completed. SEE: *patient-controlled analgesia.*

electronic fetal monitoring ABBR: EFM. The use of an electronic device to monitor vital signs of the fetus.

electronic infusion device ABBR: EID. A device for monitoring intravenous infusions. The device may have an alarm in case the flow is restricted because of an occlusion of the line. In that case, the alarm will sound when a preset pressure limit is sensed. The device can also signal that an infusion is close to completion. The pressure is regulated by the height at which the container is positioned above the level of the heart when the patient is lying flat. A height of 36 in. (91 cm) provides a pressure of 1.3 lb/sq in. (70 mm Hg). Most EIDs are equipped to stop the flow of the infused liquid if accidental free-flow occurs. SEE: *infusion pump.*

electronics The science of all systems involving the use of electrical devices used for communication, information processing, and control.

electron volt SYMB: eV. The energy acquired by an electron as it passes through a potential of 1 V.

electronystagmography (ē-lĕk″trō-nĭs″tăg-mŏg′ră-fē) [″ + *nystagmos,* drowsiness, + *graphein,* to write] A method of recording the electrical activity of the extraocular muscles. SEE: *nystagmus.*

electro-oculogram (ē-lĕk″trō-ŏk′ū-lō-grăm″) Recording of the electric currents produced by eye movements. SEE: *electroretinogram.*

electropathology (ē-lĕk″trō-pă-thŏl′ō-jē) [″ + *pathos,* disease, suffering, + *logos,* word, reason] Determination of the electrical reaction of muscles and nerves as a means of diagnosis.

electrophobia Irrational fear of electricity.

electrophoresis (ē-lĕk″trō-for-ē′sĭs) [″ + *phoresis,* bearing] The movement of charged colloidal particles through the medium in which they are dispersed as a result of changes in electrical potential. Electrophoretic methods are useful in the analysis of protein mixtures because protein particles move with different velocities depending principally on the number of charges carried by the particle. SEE: *diathermy; iontophoresis; -phoresis.*

electrophrenic (ē-lĕk″trō-frĕn′ĭk) Pert. to stimulation of the phrenic nerve by electricity.

electrophysiology (ē-lĕk″trō-fĭz″ē-ŏl′ō-jē) [″ + *physis,* nature, + *logos,* word, reason] **1.** A field of study that deals with the relationships of body functions to electrical phenomena (e.g., the effects of electrical stimulation on tissues, the production of electric currents by organs and tissues, and the therapeutic use of electric currents). **2.** The study and treatment of cardiac arrhythmias.

electroporation 1. Electrical patch. **2.** The use of electrical current to manipulate cellular metabolism by opening nuclear pores.

electropositive [″ + L. *positivus,* to put, place] Charged with positive electricity, which results in the repulsion of bodies electrified positively and the attraction of bodies electrified negatively.

electroresection (ē-lĕk″trō-rē-sĕk′shŭn) Removal of tissue by use of an electric device such as an electrocautery.

electroretinogram (ē-lĕk″trō-rĕt′ĭ-nō-grăm) ABBR: ERG. A record of the action currents of the retina produced by visual or light stimuli.

electroscission (ē-lĕk″trō-sĭ′zhŭn) [″ + L. *scindere,* to cut] Division of tissues by electrocautery.

electroscope (ē-lĕk′trō-skōp) [″ + *skopein,* to examine] An instrument that detects radiation intensity.

electroshock Shock produced by an electric current, used in psychiatry to treat depression.

electrosleep Sleep produced by the passage of mild electrical impulses through parts of the brain. This technique has been used experimentally in treating insomnia and mental illness.

electrostatic [Gr. *elektron,* amber, + *statikos,* causing to stand] Pert. to static electricity.

electrostimulation, electrical stimulation (ē-lĕk″trō-stĭm″ū-lā′shŭn) ABBR: ES. Use of electric current to affect a tissue, such as nerve, muscle, or bone. In the latter case, the stimulation is used experimentally to facilitate and hasten healing of fractures. SYN: *electrotherapy.* SEE: *bipolar* (2); *monopolar; transcutaneous electrical nerve stimulation.*

electrosynthesis (ē-lĕk″trō-sĭn′thĕ-sĭs) The use of electricity to synthesize chemical compounds.

electrotherapy The use of electricity in treating musculoskeletal dysfunction, pain, or disease. Also called *electrotherapeutics.*

electrotonus (ē-lĕk-trŏt′ō-nŭs) The change in the irritability of a nerve or muscle during the passage of an electric current.

electrovalence (ē-lĕk″trō-vā′lĕns) The ionic linkage between atoms in which each accepts or donates electrons so that each atom ends up with a completed electron shell.

electuary (ē-lĕk′tū-ă-rē) [Gr. *ekleikhein,* to lick up] A medicinal substance mixed with honey or sugar to form a paste suitable for oral consumption.

eleidin (ĕ-lē′ĭ-dĭn) [Gr. *elaion,* oil] A translucent protein present in the stratum lucidum of the epidermis of the palms and soles.

element [L. *elementum,* a rudiment] In chemistry, a substance that cannot be separated into substances different from itself by ordinary chemical processes. Elements exist in free and combined states. There are 109 named elements, plus others yet to be fully characterized and named.

Elements found in the human body include oxygen, aluminum, carbon, cobalt, hydrogen, nitrogen, calcium, phosphorus, potassium, sulfur, sodium, chlorine, magnesium, iron, fluorine, iodine, copper, manganese, and zinc.

trace e. A chemical element present in the body that is consumed as part of the diet in extremely small amounts. These elements, including chromium, manganese, and selenium are involved in metabolism and enzyme activity. Toxic levels for many trace elements may be reached at only several times usual intake.

eleosaccharum (ĕl″ē-ō-săk′ă-rŭm) [″ + *sakcharon,* sugar] A mixture of powdered sugar with a volatile oil.

elephantiasis (ĕl″ĕ-făn-tī′ă-sĭs) [Gr. *elephas,* elephant, + *-iasis,* condition] Massive swelling, esp. of the genitalia and lower extremities, resulting from obstruction of lymphatic vessels, for example by filarial parasites, malignancies, neurofibromatosis, or a familial congenital disease (Milroy's disease). Prolonged swelling can cause an increase in interstitial fibrous tissue and skin puckering or breakdown. In patients with parasitic elephantiasis (i.e., the filarial diseases, which are common in the tropics), single-dose therapy with ivermectin or ivermectin plus albendazole destroys immature but not adult worms. SEE: *lymphedema*.

scrotal e. Swelling of the scrotum, usually as a result of infection of the pelvic lymphatics by filaria. SYN: *chyloderma*.

elephant man disease Colloquial name for Recklinghausen's disease.

elevation (ĕl″ĕ-vā′shŭn) A raised area that protrudes above the surrounding area.

tactile e. A small raised area of the palm and sole that contains a cluster of nerve endings.

elevator [L. *elevare,* to lift up] **1.** A curved retractor for holding the lid away from the globe of the eye. **2.** A retractor for raising depressed bones by levers or screws. **3.** Instrument used for soft tissue; e.g., periosteal elevator. **4.** An instrument of varying design for extracting teeth or removing root or bone fragments.

periosteal e. A surgical instrument for separating the periosteum from the bone.

eleventh cranial nerve The motor nerve, made up of a cranial and a spinal part, that supplies the trapezius and sternomastoid muscles and the pharynx. The accessory portion joins the vagus to supply motor fibers to the pharynx, larynx, and heart. SYN: *accessory nerve; spinal accessory nerve*.

eliminant (ē-lĭm′ĭ-nănt) [L. *e,* out, + *limen,* threshold] **1.** Effecting evacuation. **2.** An agent aiding in elimination.

eliminate (ē-lĭm′ĭ-nāt) To expel; to rid the body of waste material.

elimination **1.** Excretion of waste products by the skin, kidneys, lungs, and intestines. **2.** Leaving out, omitting, removing.

ELISA *enzyme-linked immunosorbent assay*.

elixir (ē-lĭk′sĕr) [L. from Arabic *al-iksir*] A sweetened, aromatic, hydroalcoholic liquid used in the compounding of oral medicines. Elixirs constitute one of the most common types of medicinal preparation taken orally in liquid form.

ellipsis (ē-lĭp′sĭs) [L. *ellīpsis* fr. Gr., a falling short, defective] In psychoanalysis, omission by the patient of important words or ideas during treatment.

ellipsoid (ē-lĭp′soyd) Spindle-shaped.

elliptocyte (ē-lĭp′tō-sīt) An oval-shaped red blood cell. About 11% to 15% of red blood cells are normally oval, but in anemia and hereditary elliptocytosis, the percentage is increased to 25% to 100%. In birds, reptiles, and some other animals, the red cells are normally elliptocytes.

elliptocytosis (ē-lĭp″tō-sī-tō′sĭs) A condition in which the number of elliptocytes is increased. It occurs in some forms of anemia.

hereditary e. An inherited condition in which the red blood cells are oval or elliptical. This anomaly occurs in about 1 in every 2000 births.

Ellis-van Creveld syndrome [Richard W. B. Ellis, Scot. physician, 1902–1966; Simon Creveld, Dutch physician, 1894–1977] A congenital syndrome consisting of polydactyly, chondrodysplasia with acromelic dwarfism, hydrotic ectodermal dysplasia, and congenital heart defects. It is thought to be transmitted as an autosomal trait. SYN: *chondroectodermal dysplasia*.

elongation (ē″lŏng-gā′shŭn) The condition of being extended or lengthened, or the process of extending.

elope To leave a hospital, esp. a psychiatric hospital, without permission.

eluate (ĕl′ū-āt) The material washed out by elution.

eluent (ē-lū′ĕnt) The solvent or dissolving substance used in elution.

elution (ē-lū′shŭn) [L. *e,* out, + *luere,* to wash] In chemistry, separation of one material from another by washing. If a material contains water-soluble and water-insoluble materials, the passage of water (the eluent) through the mixture will remove the portion that is water soluble (the eluate) and leave the water-insoluble residue.

elutriation (ē-lū-trē-ā′shŭn) [L. *elutriare,* to cleanse] The separation of insoluble particles from finer ones by decanting of the fluid.

emaciate (ē-mā′sē-āt) [L. *emaciare,* to make thin] To cause to become excessively lean.

emaciated Excessively thin; wasted.

emaciation The state of being extremely lean. SYN: *wasting*. SEE: *cachexia*.

emailloid (ā-mī′loyd) [Fr. *email,* enamel, + Gr. *eidos,* form, shape] A tumor having its origin in tooth enamel.

emanation [L. *e,* out, + *manare,* to flow] **1.** Something given off; radiation; emission. **2.** A gaseous product of radioactive disintegration.

actinium e. The radioactive gas given off by actinium; a radioactive isotope of actinium. SYN: *actinon*.

radium e. The radioactive gas given off by radium. SYN: *radon*.

thorium e. The radioactive gas given off by thorium. SYN: *thoron*.

emasculation (ē-măs″kū-lā′shŭn) [L. *emasculare,* to castrate] **1.** Castration. **2.** Excision of the entire male genitalia. **3.** Figuratively, the act of making powerless or ineffective.

embalming (ĕm-băm′ĭng) [L. *im-,* on, + *balsamum,* balsam] Preparing a body or part of a body for burial by injecting it with a preservative such as a 4% formaldehyde solution. This is usually done within 48 hr of death. SEE: *Standard and Universal Precautions Appendix.*

embarrass (ĕm-băr′ăs) To interfere with or compromise function.

Embden-Meyerhof pathway [Gustav G. Embden, Ger. biochemist, 1874–1933; Otto Fritz Meyerhof, Ger. biochemist, 1884–1951] A series of metabolic and enzymatic changes that occur in many plants and animals when glucose, glycogen, or starch is metabolized anaerobically to produce acetic acid. The process produces energy in the form of adenosine triphosphate (ATP).

embedding [″ + AS. *bedd,* to bed] In histology, the process by which a piece of tissue is placed in a firm medium such as paraffin to support it and keep it intact during the subsequent cutting into thin sections for microscopic examination.

embolalia, embololalia (ĕm″bō-lā′lē-ă, ĕm″bō-lō-lā′lē-ă) [Gr. *embolos,* thrown in, + *lalia,* babble] The meaningless language of individuals with severe mental illness or organic brain injury. SYN: *embolophrasia.*

embole (ĕm′bō-lē) [Gr. *emballein,* to throw in] **1.** Reduction of a dislocation. **2.** Formation of the gastrula by invagination.

embolectomy (ĕm″bō-lĕk′tō-mē) [″ + *ektome,* excision] Removal of an embolus from a vessel. It may be done surgically or by the use of enzymes that dissolve the clot. The latter method is used in treating acute myocardial infarction and in other areas where blood flow is obstructed by a blood clot. SEE: *tissue plasminogen activator.*

embolic Pert. to or caused by embolism.

emboliform [″ + L. *forma,* form] **1.** Resembling a nucleus. **2.** Wedge-shaped, as the nucleus emboliformis.

embolism (ĕm′bō-lĭzm) [″ + *-ismos,* condition] Sudden obstruction of a blood vessel by debris. Blood clots, cholesterol-containing plaques, masses of bacteria, cancer cells, amniotic fluid, fat from the marrow of broken bones, and injected substances (e.g., air bubbles or particulate matter) all may lodge in blood vessels and obstruct the circulation.

air e. Obstruction of a blood vessel caused by an air bubble.

ETIOLOGY: Air may enter a vessel postoperatively, during change of an intravenous set on a central line or by injection into a central line port or rupture of a central line balloon, during an intravenous injection if the syringe is not properly filled, or from intravenous tubing if fluid is permitted to flow through tubing from which air has not been evacuated. NOTE: A very small amount of air in the tubing or syringe will not cause symptoms.

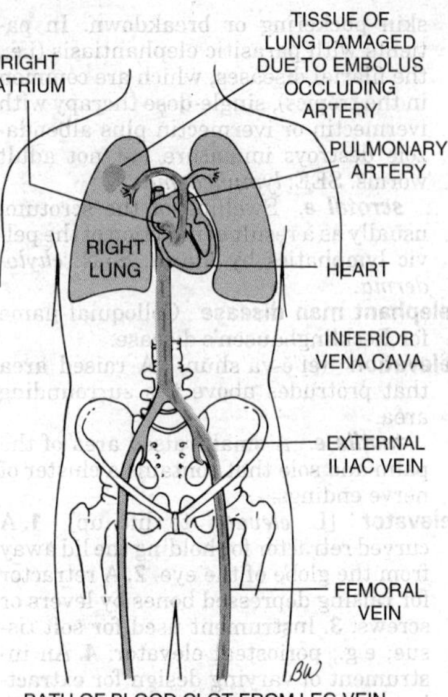

EMBOLISM

SYMPTOMS: Symptoms include sudden onset of dyspnea, unequal breath sounds, hypotension, weak pulse, elevated central venous pressure, cyanosis, sharp chest pains, hemoptysis, a churning murmur over the precordium, and decreasing level of consciousness.

PATIENT CARE: When an air embolism is suspected in the systemic venous circulation (returning to the heart), the patient should immediately be turned on his or her left side with the head down in an attempt to trap air in the right side of the heart. The patient should remain in this position for 20 to 30 min to allow the air to dissolve and disperse through the pulmonary artery. If air is in an IV line, the IV should be stopped and the air evacuated, with a needle and syringe, through the port nearest the patient; otherwise the rate of fluid flow should be slowed to keep the vein open. High concentration oxygen should be administered, with a nonrebreather mask, and the physician should be notified.

Prevention: All air should be purged from the tubing of all IV administration sets before hookup and when solution bags or bottles are changed; air elimination filters should be used close to the patient; infusion devices with air detection capability should be used, as well as locking tubing, locking connection devices, or taped connections. For central lines, to increase peripheral resistance and prevent air from entering the superior vena cava, the patient should be instructed to perform a Valsalva maneuver as the stylet is removed from the catheter, during attachment of the IV tubing, and when adapters or caps are changed on ports.

amniotic fluid e. The entry of amniotic fluid through a tear in the placental membranes into the maternal circulation. The event can occur during labor, delivery, or placental separation. The contents of the fluid (e.g., shed fetal cells, meconium, lanugo, vernix) may produce pulmonary or cerebral emboli, or disseminated intravascular coagulation (DIC).

SYMPTOMS: Chest pain, dyspnea, cyanosis, tachycardia, hemorrhage, hypotension, or shock are potential symptoms. Amniotic fluid embolism is frequently fatal.

drug e. Obstruction of the circulation by injected drugs, debris, or talc, often resulting in pulmonary infarction.

fat e. An embolism caused by globules of fat obstructing blood vessels. It frequently occurs after fracture of long and pelvic bones and may cause disseminated intravascular coagulation.

SYMPTOMS: Findings include agitation, restlessness, delirium, convulsions, coma, tachycardia, tachypnea, dyspnea, wheezing, blood-tinged sputum, copious production of white sputum, and fever, esp. during the first 12 to 24 hr after injury, when fat emboli are most likely to occur. Petechiae may appear on the buccal membranes, conjunctival sacs, and the chest and axillae. Laboratory values may show hypoxemia, decreased hemoglobin level, leukocytosis, thrombocytopenia, increased serum lipase, and fat globules in urine and sputum.

PATIENT CARE: Long bone fractures are immobilized immediately. Patients at risk (i.e., those with fractures of long bones, severe soft tissue bruising, fatty liver injury, or multiple injuries) are assessed for symptoms of fat embolism. Chest radiograph reports are reviewed for evidence of mottled lung fields and right ventricular dilation, and the patient's electrocardiogram is checked for large S waves in lead I, large Q waves in lead III, and right axis deviation.

The patient is placed in the high Fowler's, orthopneic, or other comfortable position to improve ventilation; high concentration oxygen is administered, and endotracheal intubation and mechanical ventilation are initiated as necessary. Prescribed pharmacological agents are administered; these may include steroids, heparin, and diazepam.

paradoxical e. An embolism arising from the venous circulation that enters the arterial circulation by crossing from the right side of the heart to the left side through a patent foramen ovale or septal defect. It may occasionally cause stroke in a patient with a deep venous thrombosis.

pulmonary e. An obstruction of the pulmonary artery or one of its branches, usually caused by an embolus from thrombosis in a lower extremity. Roughly 10% to 15% of patients with the disease will die. Risks for it include genetic predisposition, recent limb or pelvic trauma, surgery, immobilization (especially in hospital), pregnancy, use of hormone replacement, advanced age, cancer, and obesity. Diagnosis is challenging because symptoms are nonspecific and often misinterpreted, and may mimic many other diseases of the limbs or chest. Once the disease is suspected, evaluation may include oximetry, chest x-rays, arterial blood gas analysis, ultrasonography of the limbs, and ventilation/perfusion scanning, among others. Pulmonary angiography is the gold standard test, but is invasive. Treatment includes the administration of anticoagulants such as heparins and warfarin. In critically ill patients intubation and mechanical ventilation may be required. Thrombolytic drugs or thrombolectomy may be attempted. SEE: illus.; *thrombosis, deep venous*.

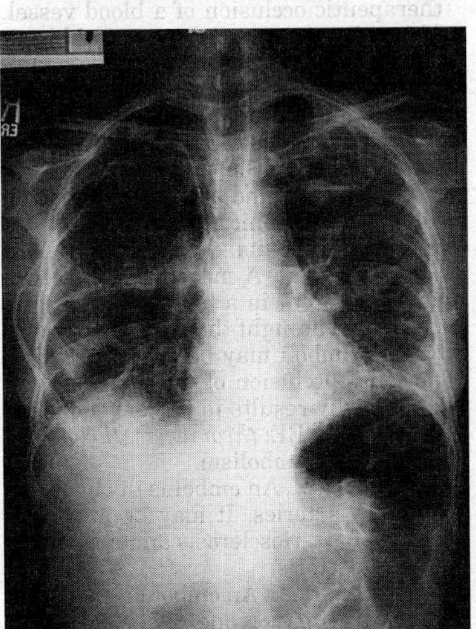

PULMONARY EMBOLISM

Septic pulmonary emboli seen in plain chest x-ray

PATIENT CARE: In the hospitalized patient early mobilization, administration of prophylactic anticoagulants, and compression stockings (elastic or pneumatic) may prevent clot formation. Vital signs, respiratory effort, breath sounds, cardiac rhythm, and urinary output are monitored closely in affected patients. Signs of deterioration are promptly reported. The nurse assists with diagnostic studies and medical treatment, and provides analgesics for pain, prescribed medications, supplemental oxygen, patient education, and emotional support. The respiratory therapist may obtain arterial blood gases to assess oxygenation and administer oxygen as needed. SEE: *Nursing Diagnoses Appendix.*

pyemic e. Septic e.

septic e. An embolism made up of purulent matter that arises from the site of an infection caused by a pyogenic (pus-forming) organism. It can result in the spread of infection to a distant site. SYN: *pyemic e.*

embolization (ĕm-bō-lĭ-zā′shŭn) Obstruction of a blood vessel by intentionally injected material, or by physiologic migration of loosened intravascular plaque, thrombi, etc.

arterial e. Embolotherapy; pathophysiologic migration of an embolus into an artery.

therapeutic e. Embolotherapy.

embolophrasia (ĕm″bŏ-lō-frā′zē-ă) [″ + *phrasis,* utterance] Meaningless speech. SYN: *embolalia.*

embolotherapy The use of any type of embolic material (autologus thrombus, muscle fragment, or foreign body) for therapeutic occlusion of a blood vessel. This technique is used to control bleeding, close fistulae or arteriovenous malformations, devascularize organs, and reduce tumors or varicoceles. Generally a catheter is threaded through the vascular system to the origin of the vessel to be occluded, and an agent is injected under radiographic control.

embolus (ĕm′bō-lŭs) *pl.* **emboli** [Gr. *embolos,* stopper] A mass of undissolved matter present in a blood or lymphatic vessel and brought there by the blood or lymph. Emboli may be solid, liquid, or gaseous. Occlusion of vessels from emboli usually results in the development of infarcts. SEE: *thrombosis; thrombus.*

air e. Air embolism.

coronary e. An embolus in one of the coronary arteries. It may be a complication of arteriosclerosis and may cause angina pectoris.

pulmonary e. An embolus in the pulmonary artery or one of its branches. SEE: *pulmonary embolism.*

embolysis (ĕm-bŏl′ĭ-sĭs) The dissolution of an embolus, esp. one due to a blood clot.

embrasure (ĕm-brā′zhŭr) [Fr., window opening from within] The space formed by the contour and position of adjacent teeth.

buccal e. The embrasure spreading toward the cheek between the molar and premolar teeth.

labial e. The embrasure opening toward the lips between the canine and incisor teeth.

lingual e. The embrasure opening to the lingual sides of the teeth.

occlusal e. The embrasure marked by the marginal ridge on the distal side of one tooth and that on the mesial side of the adjacent tooth, and the contact points.

embryectomy (ĕm″brē-ĕk′tō-mē) [Gr. *embryon,* something that swells in the body, + *ektome,* excision] Removal of an extrauterine embryo.

embryo (ĕm′brē-ō) [Gr. *embryon,* something that swells in the body] **1.** The young of any organism in an early stage of development. **2.** In mammals, the stage of prenatal development between fertilized ovum and fetus. In humans, this stage begins on day 15 after conception and continues through gestational week 8. SEE: illus.

DEVELOPMENT: During this early stage of tissue differentiation and organogenesis, the human embryo is most vulnerable to damage from maternal viral infections such as rubella and from toxic chemicals such as alcohol and tobacco smoke.

Zygote (First week): Following fertilization, cells multiply (cleavage), resulting in the formation of a morula, which in turn develops into a blastocyst consisting of a trophoblast and inner cell mass. The trophoblast gives rise to the fetal membranes and placenta after the blastocyst enters the uterus and begins implantation. *Zygote* (Second week): Two cavities (amniotic cavity and yolk sac) arise within the inner cell mass. These are separated by the embryonic disk, which in the second week consists of an ectoderm and an endoderm layer. *Zygote* (Third week): A mesoderm layer forms between the ectoderm and endoderm layers, and these three germ layers develop into the embryo proper.

Embryo (Second through eighth weeks): The embryo increases in length from about 1.5 mm to 23 mm. The germ layers of the embryonic disk give rise to the principal organ systems, and the embryo begins to show human form. During this period of organogenesis, the embryo is particularly sensitive to the effects of viral infections of the mother (e.g., rubella) and toxic chemicals, including alcohol and tobacco smoke, and is sensitive to hypoxemia.

The epithelium of the alimentary canal, liver, pancreas, and lungs develops from endoderm. Muscle, all connective tissues, blood, lymphatic tissue and the epithelium of blood vessels, body cavities, kidneys, gonads, and suprarenal cortex develop from mesoderm. The epidermis, nervous tissue, hypophysis, and the epithelium of the nasal cavity, mouth, salivary glands, bladder, and urethra develop from ectoderm.

embryocardia (ĕm″brē-ō-kăr′dē-ă) [″ + *kardia,* heart] Heart action in which the first and second sounds are equal

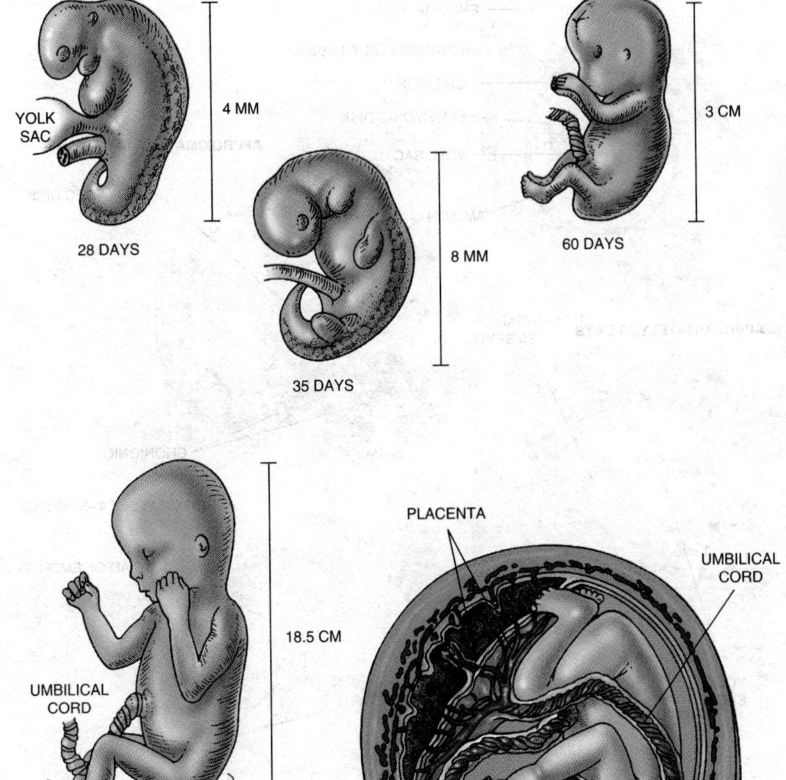

STAGES OF DEVELOPMENT OF HUMAN EMBRYO INCLUDING MATURE FETUS

and resemble the fetal heart sounds; a sign of cardiac distress.

embryocidal (ĕm″brē-ō-sī′dăl) [Gr. *embryon,* something that swells in the body, + L. *cida,* killer] Pert. to anything that kills an embryo.

embryoctony (ĕm″brē-ŏk′tō-nē) [″ + *kteinein,* to kill] Destruction of the fetus in utero, as when delivery is impossible or during abortion. SEE: *craniotomy.*

embryogenetic, embryogenic [″ + *gennan,* to produce] Giving rise to an embryo.

embryogeny (ĕm″brē-ŏj′ĕ-nē) The growth and development of an embryo.

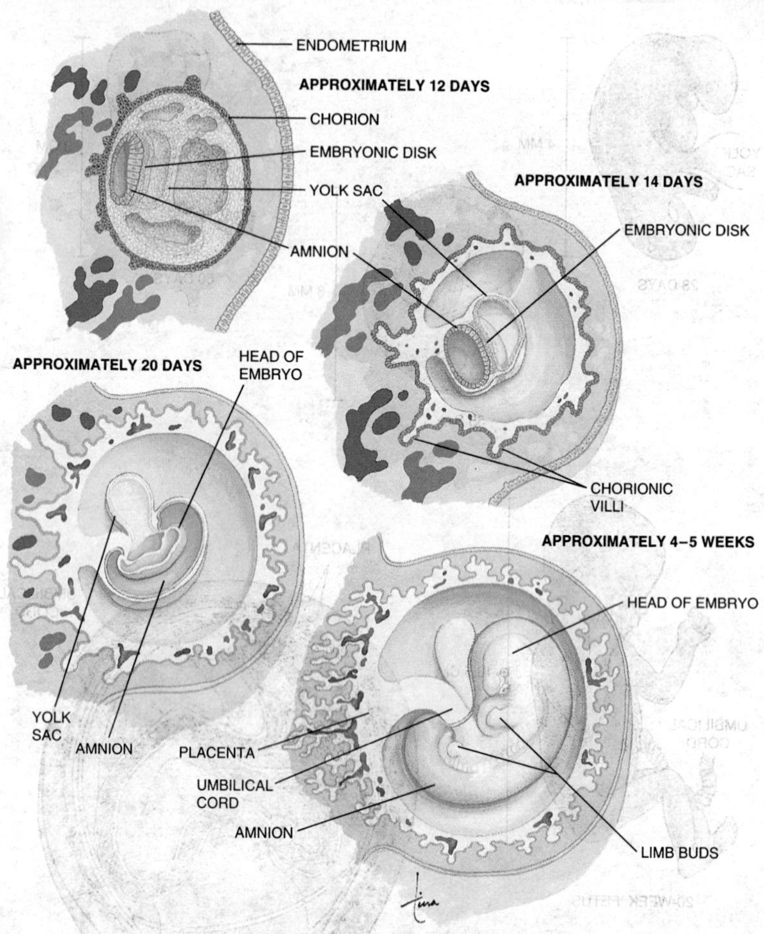

EMBRYONIC DEVELOPMENT

embryography [″ + *graphein,* to write] A treatise on the embryo.

embryology [″ + *logos,* word, reason] The science that deals with the origin and development of an organism in the womb.

embryoma (ĕm-brē-ō′mă) [″ + *oma,* tumor] A tumor, such as Wilms' tumor of the kidney, neuroblastoma, or teratomas, consisting of derivatives of the embryonic germ layers but lacking in organization.

embryonal (ĕm″brē′ō-năl) Pert. to or resembling an embryo.

embryonic (ĕm″brē-ŏn′ĭk) [Gr. *embryon,* something that swells in the body] Pertaining to or in the condition of an embryo.

embryopathy (ĕm″brē-ŏp′ă-thē) [″ + *pathos,* disease, suffering] Any disease of the embryo.

embryoplastic [″ + *plassein,* to form] Having a part in the formation of an embryo; said of cells.

embryoscopy Direct visualization of the fetus or embryo in the uterus by insertion of the light source and image-detecting portion of a fetoscope into the amniotic cavity through a small incision in the abdominal wall. This technique permits visualization and photography, surgical correction of certain types of congenital defects, and collection of amniotic fluid specimens for analysis of chemical and cellular materials. SEE: illus.

embryotomy (ĕm″brē-ŏt′ō-mē) Dissection of a fetus to aid delivery.

embryotoxon (ĕm″brē-ō-tŏks′ŏn) [″ + *toxon,* bow] Congenital marginal opacity of the cornea. SYN: *arcus juvenilis.*

embryo transfer Placement of embryos into the uterus through the cervix after in vitro fertilization (IVF) or, in the

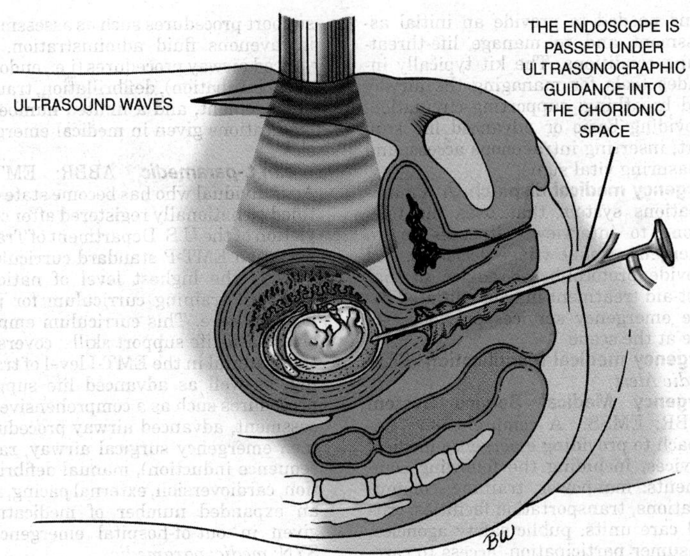
THE ENDOSCOPE IS PASSED UNDER ULTRASONOGRAPHIC GUIDANCE INTO THE CHORIONIC SPACE
ULTRASOUND WAVES
BW
EMBRYOSCOPY

case of gamete intrafallopian transfer (GIFT), into the fallopian tubes. Fertilization is usually done by placing the sperm and ovum in a special culture tube. SEE: *in vitro fertilization; GIFT; surrogate mother*.

embryotroph (ĕm′brē-ō-trōf) [″ + *trophe,* nourishment] A fluid resulting from the enzyme action of the trophoblasts on the neighboring maternal tissue. This fluid nourishes the embryo from the time of implantation into the uterus.

emedullate (ē-mĕd′ū-lāt) [L. *e,* out, + *medulla,* marrow] To remove the marrow from a bone.

emergency [L. *emergere,* to raise up] **1.** Any urgent condition perceived by the patient as requiring immediate medical or surgical evaluation or treatment. **2.** An unexpected serious occurrence that may cause a great number of injuries, which usually require immediate attention. SEE: *disaster planning*.

emergency cardiac care ABBR: ECC. The basic and advanced life support assessment and treatment necessary to manage sudden and often life-threatening events affecting cardiovascular and pulmonary systems. ECC includes identifying the nature of the problem, monitoring the patient closely, providing basic and advanced life support as quickly as possible, preventing complications, reassuring the patient, and transporting the patient to the most appropriate facility for definitive cardiac care. SEE: *advanced cardiac life support; basic life support; cardiopulmonary resuscitation*.

Emergency Department ABBR: E.D. The section of a hospital that treats acute illnesses or injuries.

emergency, fire A situation in which fire may cause death or severe injury. A person whose clothing catches fire should be rolled in a rug or blanket to smother the flames. If an individual is outdoors, rolling in the dirt will smother flames. SEE: *burn; gas; smoke inhalation injury; transportation of the injured*.

If the victim is trapped in a burning building, the occupied room should have the doors and windows closed to prevent cross-breezes from increasing the fire. The window should be opened only if the victim is to be rescued through it. Doors should be opened only a few inches to ascertain the possibility of escape. A burst of flame or hot air can push the door in and asphyxiate anyone in the room. Wet cloths or towels should be held over the mouth and nostrils to keep out smoke and gases.

CAUTION: In attempting to escape from an area filled with smoke or fire, it is important to crawl rather than run. The heat several feet above floor level may be lethal due to superheated gases, but at floor level, it may be cool enough to tolerate. Even when crawling, it is important to proceed as quickly as possible. Carbon monoxide is present in higher concentration at floor level because it is heavier than air.

---

emergency kit A box or bag containing the equipment, supplies, and medications needed to provide an initial assessment and to manage life-threatening conditions. The kit typically includes tools for managing the airway and breathing; supporting circulation; providing basic or advanced life support; inserting intravenous access; and measuring vital signs.

emergency medical dispatch A communications system that uses the telephone to interview witnesses to an emergency, make triage decisions, and provide protocol-based advice so that first-aid treatment may be initiated before emergency services providers arrive at the scene.

emergency medical identification SEE: *Medic Alert.*

Emergency Medical Service System ABBR: EMSS. A comprehensive approach to providing emergency medical services, including the following components: manpower, training, communications, transportation facilities, critical care units, public safety agencies, consumer participation, access to care, patient transfer, coordinated patient record keeping, public information and education, review and evaluation, and disaster planning. SEE: *disaster planning.*

emergency medical services medical direction The physician responsibilities for the patient care and clinical components of an EMS system.

emergency medical technician ABBR: EMT. An individual trained to administer emergency care in a variety of conditions, but esp. to patients who have suffered illnesses such as cardiac arrest, chest pain, stroke, or trauma. EMTs function in an EMS system, are certified by the state after completing instruction, and work under the authority of a supervising medical control physician, using treatment protocols approved by a medical advisory committee. SEE: *Emergency Medical Service System; EMS medical control; EMS treatment protocol; paramedic.*

e.m.t.-basic ABBR: EMT-B. An individual who has become state certified or nationally registered after completion of the U.S. Department of Transportation EMT-B standard curriculum.

e.m.t.-defibrillation ABBR: EMT-D. During the transition from the 1985 to the 1994 U.S. Department of Transportation standard curriculum, the title given in many states to individuals who became certified EMTs in the skill of defibrillation.

e.m.t.-intermediate ABBR: EMT-I. An individual who has become state certified or nationally registered after completion of the U.S. Department of Transportation EMT-I standard curriculum. This curriculum emphasizes basic life support skills as well as advanced life support procedures such as assessment, intravenous fluid administration, advanced airway procedures (i.e., endotracheal intubation), defibrillation, trauma management, and a limited number of medications given in medical emergencies.

e.m.t.-paramedic ABBR: EMT-P. An individual who has become state certified or nationally registered after completion of the U.S. Department of Transportation EMT-P standard curriculum. This is the highest level of national standard training curriculum for prehospital care. This curriculum emphasizes basic life support skills, covers all the material in the EMT-I level of training, as well as advanced life support procedures such as a comprehensive assessment, advanced airway procedures (i.e., emergency surgical airway, rapid sequence induction), manual defibrillation, cardioversion, external pacing, and an expanded number of medications given in out-of-hospital emergencies. SYN: *medic; paramedic.*

Emergency Nurses Association A professional organization representing and certifying nurses who are proficient in emergency care.

emergency readiness Planning in advance for an unexpected crisis, esp. a natural disaster such as a flood or hurricane. The home should be inspected for potential hazards and those discovered should be corrected. Flammable materials such as paints, oils, and fuels should be isolated. Utility shut-off valves should be located and pointed out to all members of the household. It is important to know the location of the nearest public shelter and the time required to go there on foot and by car. Family members should be trained in basic life support techniques. Emergency telephone numbers, including names and telephone numbers of neighbors, should be posted and easily accessible. A first-aid kit should be available and restocked when supplies have been used. Fire extinguishers and flashlights should be in working condition. Supplies of food and water for least 3 days, and protective clothing and blankets, should be available. It is important to provide for the special needs of infants, the elderly, and the ill. Emergency drills should be practiced, including evacuation from the home by various routes in case the usual exits are blocked or surrounded by flames. SEE: *emergency, fire.*

Emergency Room ABBR: E.R. An inaccurate term for Emergency Department.

emergent [L. *emergere,* to raise up] **1.** Growing from a cavity or other part. **2.** Sudden, unforeseen.

emerging infectious disease Any previously unknown communicable illness or any previously controlled contagion whose incidence and prevalence are suddenly rising. In recent years, some emerging (and re-emerging) infections have been bovine spongiform encephalopathy ("mad cow disease"), Ebola hemorrhagic fever, cholera, plague, hemolytic uremic syndrome caused by *Escherichia coli* 0157:H7, drug-resistant strains of enterococcus, and the human immunodeficiency virus, among many others.

emery A granular mineral substance used as an abrasive.

emesis (ĕm′ĕ-sĭs) [Gr. *emein,* to vomit] Vomiting. It may be of gastric, systemic, or neurological origin. SEE: *antiemetic; aspiration; emetic; vomit.*

PATIENT CARE: The relationship of emesis to meals, administered drugs, or other environmental stimuli should be noted. The presence of any aggravating factors (e.g., pain, anxiety, the type of foods eaten, and noxious environmental stimuli), and the type of vomiting, amount, color, and characteristics of the emesis, are documented. Assistance is provided with oral hygiene, and antiemetics are administered, if prescribed, to control vomiting. If vomiting leaves the patient weak, dysphagic, or comatose, safety measures are instituted to prevent aspiration of vomitus into the lungs; these include placing the patient in a side-lying position with the head lowered and having suction and emergency tracheostomy equipment readily available.

chemotherapy-induced e. Vomiting associated with or caused by drug treatments for cancer. Even though this side effect is usually self-limiting and seldom life-threatening, the prospect of it may produce anxiety and depression in many patients. Treatments may include drugs such as dronabinol, granisetron, lorazepam, prochlorperazine, and steroids, among others.

gastric e. Vomiting present in gastric ulcer, gastric carcinoma, acute gastritis, chronic gastritis, hyperacidity and hypersecretion, and pressure on the stomach.

e. gravidarum Vomiting of pregnancy. SEE: *hyperemesis gravidarum.*

irritation e. An old term for vomiting caused by toxins.

nervous e. An old term for emesis resulting from neurological diseases.

reflex e. An old term for gagging.

emetic (ĕ-mĕt′ĭk) [Gr. *emein,* to vomit] An agent that promotes vomiting. An emetic may induce vomiting by irritating the gastrointestinal tract or by stimulating the chemoreceptor trigger zone of the central nervous system. Some drugs, such as narcotic pain relievers and chemotherapeutic agents used to treat cancer, have emetic properties as unwanted side effects of their administration. SEE: *vomiting; vomitus.*

TREATMENT OF DRUG OVERDOSES: Drugs that promote vomiting (such as syrup of ipecac and apomorphine hydrochloride) are given occasionally to treat toxic ingestions. Gastric lavage or the oral administration of activated charcoal usually are preferred for the management of patients who have overdosed on medications, because these methods are generally safer, better tolerated, and more effective than are emetics. Emetics are particularly hazardous in patients with altered mental status or patients who have ingested petroleum distillates, because of the risk of aspiration, and in patients who have ingested corrosive agents, because the emetic drug may worsen the injury to the esophagus and oropharynx. Emetics are also contraindicated in patients with known cardiac or epileptic disorders because they occasionally trigger seizures or arrhythmias. SEE: *Poisons and Poisoning Appendix.*

direct e. An emetic that acts by its presence in the stomach (e.g., mustard).

indirect e. An emetic that acts on the vomiting center of the brain (e.g., apomorphine).

emetine (ĕm′ĕ-tēn) [Gr. *emein,* to vomit] A powdered white alkaloid emetic obtained from ipecac.

bismuth iodide e. A combination of emetine and bismuth containing about 20% emetine and 20% bismuth.

e. hydrochloride The hydrated hydrochloride of an alkaloid obtained from ipecac. It is used for the treatment of both intestinal and extraintestinal amebiasis. It should be used cautiously in elderly or debilitated patients. Children, pregnant women, and patients with serious organic disease should not receive emetine.

emetism [″ + *-ismos,* condition of] Poisoning from an overdose of ipecac.

SYMPTOMS: Symptoms are acute inflammation of the pylorus, hyperemesis, diarrhea, and sometimes aspiration and suffocation.

emetocathartic (ĕm″ĕ-tō-kă-thăr′tĭk) [″ + *katharsis,* a purging] Producing both emesis and catharsis.

emetology (ĕm″ĕ-tŏl′ō-jē) [″ + *logos,* word, reason] The study of the anatomy and physiology of vomiting.

E.M.F. *electromotive force; erythrocyte maturation factor.*

EMG *electromyogram.*

-emia Suffix meaning *blood.* SEE: *hemat-.*

EMIC *emergency maternal and infant care.*

emic (ē′mĭk) In anthropology and transcultural nursing, rel. to a type of disease analysis that focuses on the culture of the patient. The emic perspective emphasizes the subjective experience and cultural beliefs pertinent to the illness experience. For example, in psychiatric settings in the southeastern U.S., many patients believe that their illness is caused by a spell or curse from evil spirits. In these cases, a health care worker using an emic perspective would ask an indigenous health care provider to consult with the patient in addition to providing care within the traditional health care system. SEE: *etic*.

emigration [L. *e,* out, + *migrare,* to move] The passage of white blood cells through the walls of capillaries and into surrounding tissue during inflammation. SEE: *inflammation*.

eminence [" + *minere,* to hang on] A prominence or projection, esp. of a bone.

arcuate e. A rounded eminence on the upper surface of the petrous portion of the temporal bone. SYN: *jugum petrosum*.

articular e. of the temporal bone A rounded eminence forming the anterior boundary of the glenoid fossa.

auditory e. A collection of gray matter on the floor of the fourth ventricle of the brain at its lower part, forming the deep origin of the auditory nerve.

bicipital e. A tuberosity for insertion of the biceps muscle on the radius.

blastodermic e. An elevated mass of cells of a developing ovum forming the blastoderm.

canine e. A vertical ridge on the external surface of the maxilla.

collateral e. An eminence between the middle and posterior horns in the lateral ventricle of the brain.

e. of Doyère A slight elevation of a muscle fiber at the entrance of a nerve fiber into the muscle cell.

frontal e. A rounded prominence on either side of the median line and a little below the center of the frontal bone.

germinal e. The mass of follicle cells that surrounds the ovum. SYN: *cumulus oophorus*.

hypothenar e. An eminence on the ulnar side of the palm, formed by the muscles of the little finger.

iliopectineal e. An eminence on the upper aspect of the pubic bone above the acetabulum, marking the junction of the bone with the ilium.

intercondyloid e. A process on the head of the tibia lying between the two condyles.

mamillary e. A projection of the inner pillars of the fornix. SYN: *corpus mammillare*.

median e. The anterior bodies of the medulla oblongata separated by the anterior median fissure.

nasal e. A prominence on the vertical portion of the frontal bone above the nasal notch and between the two superciliary ridges.

occipital e. A protuberance on the occipital bone.

olivary e. An oval projection at the upper part of the medulla oblongata above the extremity of the lateral column. SYN: *oliva; olivary body*.

parietal e. A marked convexity on the outer surface of the parietal bone.

portal e. One of the small median lobes on the lower surface of the liver.

pyramidal e. An elevation on the mastoid wall of the tympanic cavity. It contains a cavity through which the stapedius muscle passes. SYN: *pyramid of the tympanum*.

thenar e. An eminence formed by muscles on the palm below the thumb.

eminentia (ĕm″ĭn-ĕn′shē-ă) *pl.* **eminentiae** [L.] Eminence.

emiocytosis (ē″mē-ō-sī-tō′sĭs) [L. *emitto,* to send forth, + Gr. *kytos,* cell, + *osis,* condition] The process of movement of intracellular material to the outside. Granules join the cell membrane, which ruptures to allow the substance to be free in the intercellular fluid. SYN: *exocytosis*. SEE: *endocytosis; pinocytosis*.

emissary (ĕm′ĭ-să-rē) [L. *e,* out, + *mittere,* to send] **1.** Providing an outlet. **2.** An outlet.

emissary vein A small vein that pierces the skull and carries blood from the sinuses within the skull to the veins outside it.

emission (ē-mĭsh′ŭn) [L. *e,* out, + *mittere,* to send] An issuance or discharge; the sending forth or discharge of, for example, an atomic particle, an exhalation, or a light or heat wave.

nocturnal e. The involuntary discharge of semen during sleep. SYN: *wet dream*.

thermionic e. The process by which electrons are released from an x-ray filament after a current has been passed through it.

emissivity The ability of a substance or surface to emit radiant energy.

EMIT *Enzyme-multiplied immunoassay technique*.

emit To produce or release something (e.g., light, heat, or sound waves).

EMLA *eutectic mixture of local anesthetics*.

EMLA Cream A topical anesthetic composed of lidocaine and prilocaine. The cream is applied to the skin, covered with an occlusive bandage, and left in place for 1 to 2 hr. This anesthetizes the skin to a depth of about 5 mm so that superficial skin lesions can be removed. Patients will not be aware of a needle piercing the skin; however, they will feel any tissue irritation caused by the fluid injected.

emmenagogue (ĕm-ĕn′ă-gŏg) [Gr. *emmena,* menses, + *agogos,* leading] A substance that promotes or assists the flow of menstrual fluid. SEE: *ecbolic*.

direct e. An agent, such as a hormone, that affects the reproductive tract.

indirect e. An agent that alters menstrual function as a side effect of the treatment of another illness.

emmeniopathy (ĕ-mē″nē-ŏp′ă-thē) [Gr. *emmena,* menses, + *pathos,* disease, suffering] Any disorder of menstruation.

Emmet's operation [Thomas A. Emmet, U.S. gynecologist, 1828–1919] **1.** Uterine trachelorrhaphy (i.e., suturing of a torn uterine cervix). **2.** Suturing of a lacerated perineum. **3.** Conversion of a sessile submucous tumor of the uterus into a pedunculated one.

Additional procedures attributed to Emmet, such as repair of prolapsed uterus and creation of a vesicovaginal fistula, have been superseded by more modern procedures.

emmetrope (ĕm′ĕ-trōp) [Gr. *emmetros,* in measure, + *opsis,* sight] One endowed with normal vision. **emmetropic** (-trŏp′ĭk), *adj.*

emmetropia (ĕm″ĕ-trō′pē-ă) The normal condition of the eye in refraction in which, when the eye is at rest, parallel rays focus exactly on the retina. SEE: illus.; *astigmatism; myopia.*

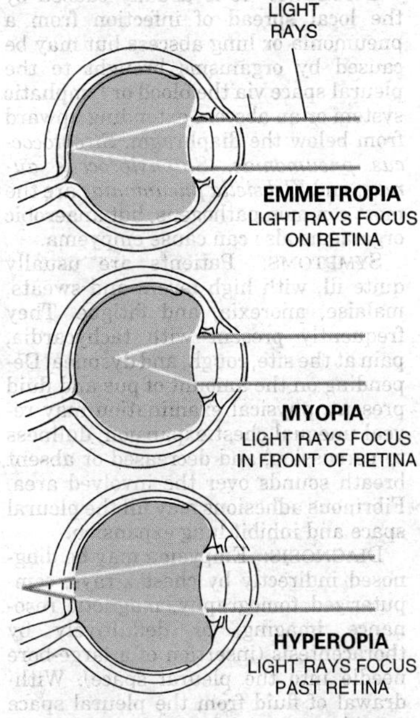

EMMETROPIA, MYOPIA, HYPEROPIA

emollient (ē-mŏl′yĕnt) [L. *e,* out, + *mollire,* to soften] An agent that softens and soothes the surface to which it is applied, usually the skin. SEE: *demulcent.*

emotion (ē-mō′shŭn) [L. *emovere,* to stir up] A mental state or feeling such as fear, hate, love, anger, grief, or joy arising as a subjective experience rather than as a conscious thought. Physiological changes invariably accompany emotions, but such change may not be apparent to either the person experiencing the emotion or an observer. **emotional** (-ăl), *adj.*

DISORDERS: See names of specific mood disorders for more information, e.g. depression, bipolar mood disorders.

emotivity (ē″mō-tĭv′ĭ-tē) One's capability for emotional response.

empathy (ĕm′pă-thē) Awareness of and insight into the feelings, emotions, and behavior of another person and their meaning and significance. It is not the same as sympathy, which is usually nonobjective and noncritical. **empathic** (-pă′thĭk), *adj.*

emperor of pruritus The itching that accompanies poison ivy dermatitis involving the anal area. It is so intense that it is called “the emperor of pruritus.”

emphysema (ĕm″fĭ-sē′mă) [Gr. *emphysan,* to inflate] **1.** Pathological distention of interstitial tissues by gas or air. **2.** A chronic pulmonary disease marked by an abnormal increase in the size of air spaces distal to the terminal bronchiole, with destruction of the alveolar walls. These changes result in a loss of the normal elastic properties of the lungs. **emphysematous** (-ă-tŭs), *adj.*

ETIOLOGY: Tobacco smoking is the most common cause of the tissue destruction found in emphysema. Exposure to environmental dust, smoke, or particulate pollution may also contribute to the disease. A small number of people with emphysema may have developed it as a result of alpha-1-antitrypsin deficiencies, a group of genetic illnesses in which there is inadequate protection against destructive enzyme activity in the lung.

SYMPTOMS: Symptoms include difficulty breathing, esp. during exertion. Weight loss, chronic cough, and wheezing are also characteristic.

TREATMENT: Inhaled bronchodilators, anticholinergics, and anti-inflammatory drugs, such as albuterol, ipratropium, or triamcinolone, may improve respiratory function. Theophylline compounds may help some patients, but they have many drug-drug interactions, and drug toxicity is a frequent problem. Oxygen therapy prevents right heart failure. Lung reduction surgery can eliminate hyperinflated portions of the lungs, allowing the healthier lung tissue that is left behind to expand and contract with improved efficiency. The long-term benefits of this procedure are uncertain.

PATIENT CARE: The patient is protected from environmental bronchial irritants, such as smoke, automobile exhaust, aerosol sprays, and industrial pollutants. The patient's oxygenation, weight, and the results of electrolyte and complete blood count measurements are monitored. The patient is evaluated for infection and other complications, and the effects of the disease on functional capabilities. Prescribed medications are administered by parenteral or oral route or by inhalation.

The patient is encouraged to intersperse normal activities with rest periods. Respiratory infections can be prevented by avoiding contact with infectious persons; by using correct pulmonary hygiene procedures, including thorough hand washing; and by obtaining influenza and pneumococcus immunizations. Frequent small meals of easy-to-chew, easy-to-digest, high-calorie, high-protein foods and food supplements are encouraged. Small meals also reduce intra-abdominal pressure on the diaphragm and reduce dyspnea.

The respiratory therapist and physician monitor the results of arterial blood gases, pulmonary function studies, and breath sounds. Evidence of acute exacerbation is important to detect and presents as heavy use of accessory muscles, a prolonged expiratory time, severe dyspnea, and a decrease in sensorium. The respiratory therapist administers oxygen therapy to maintain adequate oxygenation (PaO_2 60–80 mm Hg) and bronchodilators when needed. Once stable, the patient often benefits from participation in a pulmonary rehabilitation program to promote improved lung function and more efficient breathing techniques. SEE: *Nursing Diagnoses Appendix.*

interlobular e. The presence of air between the lobes of the lung.

subcutaneous e. The presence of air in subcutaneous tissue.

empiric (ĕm-pĭr′ĭk) [Gr. *empeirikos,* skilled, experienced] **1.** Empirical. **2.** A practitioner whose skill or art is based on what has been learned through experience.

empirical (ĕm-pĭr′ĭk-ăl) Based on experience rather than on scientific principles.

empiricism (ĕm-pĭr′ĭs-ĭzm) [Gr. *empeirikos,* skilled, experienced, + *-ismos,* condition of] Experience, not theory, as the basis of medical science.

employment, supported A program of paid work in integrated settings by persons with physical and mental disabilities. Ongoing training is provided by an interdisciplinary team of rehabilitation professionals, employers, and family members.

empowerment **1.** Investing power in another person or group by sharing leadership roles, or helping others to engage fully in a process. **2.** Participating actively and autonomously in policies or events that affect one's health or well-being.

emprosthotonos (ĕm″prŏs-thŏt′ō-nŏs) [Gr. *emprosthen,* forward, + *tonos,* tension] A form of spasm in which the body is flexed forward, sometimes seen in tetanus and strychnine poisoning. Opposite of opisthotonos.

empty follicle syndrome In in vitro fertilization investigations, the absence of oocytes in the stimulated follicle of the ovary. This may be a cause of infertility in some individuals.

empty-sella syndrome A condition, shown by radiography of the skull, in which the sella turcica, which normally contains the pituitary gland, is found to be empty. Clinically, patients may show no endocrine abnormality or may have signs of decreased pituitary function. Hormonal replacement is given to patients with hypopituitarism. In autopsy studies, empty-sella syndrome has been found in about 5% of presumably normal persons. SEE: *pituitary gland.*

empyema (ĕm″pī-ē′mă) [Gr.] A collection of inflamed, infected fluid in a body cavity, typically between the pleura. SEE: *thoracentesis.*

ETIOLOGY: It is usually caused by the local spread of infection from a pneumonia or lung abscess but may be caused by organisms brought to the pleural space via the blood or lymphatic system or an abscess extending upward from below the diaphragm. *Streptococcus pneumoniae, Staphylococcus aureus,* and *Klebsiella pneumoniae* are the most common pathogens, but anaerobic organisms also can cause empyema.

SYMPTOMS: Patients are usually quite ill, with high fevers and sweats, malaise, anorexia, and fatigue. They frequently present with tachycardia, pain at the site, cough, and dyspnea. Depending on the amount of pus and fluid present, physical examination may reveal unequal chest expansion, dullness to percussion, and decreased or absent breath sounds over the involved area. Fibrinous adhesions may fill the pleural space and inhibit lung expansion.

DIAGNOSIS: Empyema may be diagnosed indirectly by chest x-rays, computerized tomography, magnetic resonance imaging, or definitively by thoracentesis (insertion of a large-bore needle into the pleural space). Withdrawal of fluid from the pleural space provides material for a culture and sensitivity test of the organism and helps the infection resolve.

TREATMENT: The purulent exudate and fluid are drained via thoracentesis and underwater-seal chest drainage with suction. Medications such as urokinase may be injected into the pleural space to minimize fibrous adhesions and to help keep the chest tube patent; surgical drainage may be necessary. Intravenous antibiotic therapy is administered based on pathogen sensitivity. The primary infection also is treated.

PATIENT CARE: The patient is monitored for increased respiratory distress and collapse of the portion of the lung (pneumothorax) adjacent to the empyema. Patency of the drainage system is maintained; drainage volume, color, and characteristics are documented; and the patient is protected from accidental dislodgement of the drainage tube. Increased fluid and protein are provided, and breathing exercises and use of incentive spirometry are encouraged. Home health care is arranged as necessary.

interlobular e. A form of empyema with pus between the lobes of the lung.

empyesis (ĕm″pī-ē′sĭs) [Gr., suppuration] **1.** Any skin eruption marked by pustules. **2.** Any accumulation of pus. **3.** Hypopyon, or accumulation of pus in the anterior chamber of the eye.

EMS *emergency medical service.*

EMS communication A communication system that coordinates emergency medical care among ambulances, 911 (telephone) dispatch centers, and hospital emergency departments. Contact includes citizen to EMS, dispatcher to EMS crew, paramedic to doctor, and EMS crew to emergency department, as well as EMS to other public safety organizations (i.e., police, fire, and rescue). SEE: *disaster planning; EMS medical control.*

EMS medical advisory committee Representatives of medical groups that provide medical direction to the EMS system.

EMS medical control Physician direction of life support procedures performed by emergency medical technicians (EMT) and paramedics in prehospital care, including on-line and off-line supervision. *On-line:* The physician provides instruction via radio or telephone to an EMS crew. *Off-line:* The EMS crews receive direction and supervision via treatment protocols, case review, in-service training, and standing orders for treatment.

Medical control is also divided into prospective, immediate, and retrospective forms. *Prospective form:* Treatment protocols for EMTs are developed under a license from the medical director or medical advisory committee. *Immediate form:* Direct medical orders or consultation is given by radio or telephone (defined above as on-line control). *Retrospective form:* Call reports are reviewed to determine whether protocols have been followed.

EMS medical director The physician responsible for ensuring and evaluating the appropriate level of quality of care throughout an EMS system.

EMS standing orders Instructions preapproved by the medical advisory committee directing EMS crews to perform specific advanced life support measures *before* contacting a medical control physician. These orders are implemented in cases in which a delay in treatment could harm the patient (e.g., cardiac arrest).

EMS treatment protocol Written procedures for assessment, treatment, patient transportation, or patient transfer between hospitals. These procedures are part of the official policy of the EMS system and are approved by representatives of the medical advisory committee. The EMS treatment protocols may either be implemented as standing orders or require prior approval of a medical control physician.

EMT *emergency medical technician.*

EMT-B *emergency medical technician-basic.*

EMT-D *emergency medical technician-defibrillation.*

EMT-I *emergency medical technician-intermediate.*

EMT-P *emergency medical technician-paramedic.*

emulsification (ē-mŭl″sĭ-fĭ-kā′shŭn) [L. *emulsio,* emulsion, + *facere,* to make] **1.** The process of making an emulsion, allowing fat and water to mix. **2.** The breaking down of large fat globules in the intestine into smaller, uniformly distributed particles, largely accomplished through the action of bile acids, which lower surface tension.

emulsifier Anything used to make an emulsion.

emulsify (ē-mŭl′sĭ-fī) To form into an emulsion.

emulsion [L. *emulsio*] **1.** A mixture of two liquids not mutually soluble. If they are thoroughly shaken, one divides into globules in what is called the discontinuous or dispersed phase; the other is then the continuous phase. Milk is an emulsion in which butterfat is the discontinuous phase. **2.** In radiology, the part of the radiographic film sensitive to radiation and containing the image after development.

fat e. A combination of liquid, lipid, and an emulsifying system suitable for intravenous use because the lipid has been broken into small droplets that can be suspended in water. Such a solution should not be mixed with other fluids prior to intravenous administration.

emulsoid (ē-mŭl′soyd) [″ + Gr. *eidos,* form, shape] A colloid in an aqueous solution in which the colloid has a marked attraction for water to the extent that the dispersoid contains large quantities of water. Examples are protoplasm, starch, soap, gelatin, and egg white.

E.N.A. *Emergency Nurses Association; extractable nuclear antigen.*

enalapril (ĕn-ăl′-ă-prĭl) An angiotensin-converting enzyme inhibitor used to treat hypertension and congestive heart failure. Trade name is Vasotec.

enamel (ĕn-ăm′ĕl) [O.Fr. *esmail,* enamel] The hard, white, dense, inorganic substance covering the crown of the teeth. Enamel is composed of hydroxyapatite crystal, a calcium-containing salt. The crystals are arranged to form a rod. The enamel rods are organized to form the enamel. Enamel is the hardest substance in the body. Demineralization may result in a carious lesion, or "cavity." SYN: *enamelum.*

aprismatic e. A thin surface layer of the tooth, thought to be solid without individual enamel rods or prisms.

cervical e. Enamel at the neck of the tooth characterized by shorter enamel rods with more prominent incremental lines and perikymata.

gnarled e. Enamel under the cusp of a tooth characterized by twisting, intertwining groups of enamel rods, thought to resist shearing forces.

e. hypoplasia Incomplete development of tooth enamel, usually due to faulty calcium and phosphate metabolism.

mottled e. A condition in which the enamel of the teeth acquires a mottled appearance, often as a result of excessive amounts of fluorides in water or foods. Mottling may also be caused by prolonged administration of tetracyclines to women during the first half of pregnancy, or to children while the teeth are developing. SEE: *fluorosis.*

enamelum Enamel.

enanthem, enanthema (ĕn-ăn′thĕm, -ăn-thē′mă) [Gr. *en,* in, + *anthema,* blossoming] An eruption on a mucous membrane. SEE: *exanthem; Koplik's spots; rash.* **enanthematous** (-thĕm′ă-tŭs), *adj.*

enantio- Combining form meaning *opposite.*

enantiobiosis (ĕn-ăn″tē-ō-bī-ō′sĭs) [Gr. *enantios,* opposite, + *bios,* life] The condition in which associated organisms are antagonistic to each other. SEE: *symbiosis.*

enantiomorph (ĕn-ăn′tē-ō-morf″) One of a pair of isomers, each of which is a mirror image of the other. They may be identical in chemical characteristics, but in solution one rotates a beam of polarized light in one direction and the other in the opposite direction. Isomers are called dextro if they rotate light to the right, and levo if they rotate light to the left.

enarthrosis (ĕn″ăr-thrō′sĭs) *pl.* **enarthroses** [Gr. *en,* in, + *arthron,* joint, + *osis,* condition] Ball-and-socket joint.

en bloc (ĕn blŏk) [Fr., as a whole] As a whole or as en masse; used to refer to surgical excision.

encanthis (ĕn-kăn′thĭs) [Gr. *en,* in, + *kanthos,* angle of the eye] An excrescence or new growth at the inner angle of the eye.

encapsulation [″ + *capsula,* a little box] **1.** Enclosure in a sheath not normal to the part. **2.** Formation of a capsule or a sheath about a structure.

encatarrhaphy (ĕn″kăt-ăr′ă-fē) [Gr. *enkatarrhaptein,* to sew in] Insertion of an organ or tissue into a part where it is not normally found.

encephalalgia (ĕn-sĕf″ăl-ăl′jē-ă) [Gr. *enkephalos,* brain, + *algos,* pain] Deep-seated head pain. SYN: *cephalalgia.*

encephalatrophy (ĕn-sĕf″ă-lăt′rō-fē) [″ + *a-,* not, + *trophe,* nourishment] Cerebral atrophy.

encephalic (ĕn″sĕf-ăl′ĭk) [Gr. *enkephalos,* brain] Pert. to the brain or its cavity.

encephalitis (ĕn-sĕf″ă-lī′tĭs) [″ + *itis,* inflammation] Inflammation of the white and gray matter of the brain. It is almost always associated with inflammation of the meninges (meningoencephalitis) and may involve the spinal cord (encephalomyelitis). In the U.S. about 20,000 cases are reported annually. SEE: *arbovirus; herpesviruses; rabies.*

ETIOLOGY: Viruses (e.g., arbovirus, herpesvirus) are the most common cause of encephalitis. Encephalitis also occurs as a component of rabies and acquired immune deficiency syndrome (AIDS), and as an aftereffect of systemic viral diseases such as influenza, measles, German measles, and chickenpox. CNS involvement occurs in 15% to 20% of patients with AIDS who develop cytomegalovirus infections. Other organisms causing encephalitis in immunosuppressed patients include fungi (e.g., *Candida, Aspergillus,* and *Cryptococcus*) and protozoa (e.g., *Toxoplasma gondii*).

SYMPTOMS: Patients present with a wide variety of neurological signs and symptoms, depending on the infected region of the brain and the type and amount of damage the organism has caused. Seizures, fever, cranial nerve paralysis, abnormal reflexes, and muscle weakness and paralysis are common. Personality changes and confusion usually appear before the patient becomes stuporous or comatose.

DIAGNOSIS: The diagnosis is based on clinical presentation, culture and examination of cerebrospinal fluid, and computerized tomography (CT) scan or magnetic resonance imaging (MRI) results.

TREATMENT: Acyclovir is given for herpes simplex virus infection, the only common viral pathogen for which there is effective treatment. Survival and residual neurological deficits appear to be tied to mental status changes before acyclovir therapy begins. Rabies is treated with rabies immune globulin and vaccine. For other viruses, treatment focuses on supportive care and control of increased intracranial pressure (ICP) using osmotic diuretics (e.g., mannitol), corticosteroids, and drainage.

PATIENT CARE: The acutely ill patient's mental status, level of consciousness, orientation, and motor function are assessed and documented to monitor changes. The head of the bed is raised slightly to promote venous return, and neck flexion is contraindicated. Measures to prevent stimuli that increase ICP are implemented (e.g., preoxygenating with 100% oxygen before suctioning, preventing isometric muscle contraction, using diet and stool softeners to minimize straining at stool, and using turning sheets and head support when turning the patient). Passive and/or active range-of-motion exercises and resistive exercises to prevent contractures, and maintain joint mobility and muscle tone, are used as long as they do not increase ICP.

Normal supportive care is provided in a quiet environment, with lights dimmed without creating shadows, which increase the potential for hallucinations. Rehabilitation programs are usually necessary for the treatment of residual neurological deficits. SEE: *Nursing Diagnoses Appendix.*

acute disseminated e. Postinfectious e.

California (La Crosse) virus e. A viral encephalitis that is the most common mosquito-borne illness in the U.S. It typically affects children in summer or early fall, largely in the Middle Atlantic or midwestern states, causing fever, headache, seizures, and localized muscle paralysis. The primary vector is *Aedes triseriatus*. A full recovery usually follows the illness.

cortical e. Encephalitis of the brain cortex only.

eastern equine e. Encephalitis caused by the eastern equine arbovirus, which is transmitted from horses to humans by mosquitoes; the incubation period is 1 to 2 weeks. Although this is the least common of the arboviruses, mortality is approx. 25%, and those who survive often have neurological problems. In the U.S., it occurs on the East Coast, Gulf Coast, and in the Great Lakes region during the mosquito season from midsummer to early fall.

epidemic e. Any form of encephalitis that occurs as an epidemic.

equine e. Encephalitis caused by either the western or the eastern equine arbovirus, which is carried by mosquitoes from horses. The disease ranges from mild to fatal.

hemorrhagic e. Herpes encephalitis in which there is hemorrhage along with brain inflammation.

herpetic e. Encephalitis caused by infection of the brain with herpes simplex virus-1 (or less often herpes simplex virus-2). This relatively common form of encephalitis typically involves the inferior surfaces of the temporal lobes and may cause hemorrhagic necrosis of brain tissue. It is fatal in at least one third of all cases. Acyclovir (or one of its analogs) is used to treat the infection.

e. hyperplastica Acute encephalitis without suppuration.

infantile e. Encephalitis that occurs in infants. The most common agents are arboviruses and herpes simplex virus.

Japanese (B type) e. Encephalitis caused by the Japanese B type arbovirus, an infection carried by swine. It occurs sporadically in Japan, Taiwan, China, and Korea and is controlled by vaccine.

lead e. Encephalitis due to lead poisoning.

e. lethargica A form of encephalitis that occurred frequently after the influenza pandemic of 1917 and 1918, and rarely since. Its hallmarks include paralysis of oculomotor function and marked sleepiness or coma. Survivors developed a parkinsonism-like illness. SYN: *Economo's disease*.

e. neonatorum A form of encephalitis occurring within the first several weeks of life.

e. periaxialis Inflammation of the white matter of the cerebrum, occurring mainly in the young.

postinfectious e. Encephalitis that follows a systemic viral infection (such as mumps or measles) or a reactivation to varicella-zoster in adults. SYN: *acute disseminated e.*

postvaccinal e. Acute encephalitis following vaccination.

purulent e. Encephalitis characterized by abscesses in the brain.

Russian spring-summer e. Encephalitis due to a tick-borne virus. Humans may also contract it by drinking goat milk.

St. Louis e. Encephalitis caused by the St. Louis arbovirus and carried by mosquitoes. It emerged during an epidemic in the summer of 1933 in and around St. Louis, Missouri. Now endemic in the U.S. (esp. Florida), Trinidad, Jamaica, Panama, and Brazil, it occurs most frequently during summer and early fall.

toxic e. Encephalitis resulting from metal poisonings, such as lead poisoning.

western equine e. A mild type of viral encephalitis that has occurred in the western U.S. and Canada.

Encephalitozoon A genus of the order Microsporidia. SEE: *microsporidiosis*.

encephalocele (ĕn-sĕf′ă-lō-sēl) [Gr. *enkephalos,* brain, + *kele,* hernia] A protrusion of the brain through a cranial fissure. SYN: *hydrencephalocele*.

encephalocystocele (ĕn-sĕf″ă-lō-sĭs′tō-sēl) [″ + *kystis,* sac, + *kele,* tumor, swelling] A hernia of the brain. The hernia sac is filled with cerebrospinal fluid.

encephalogram (ĕn-sĕf′ă-lō-grăm) [″ + *gramma,* something written] A radiograph of the brain, usually performed with air in the ventricles as a contrast medium. This procedure has been replaced by computed tomography and magnetic resonance imaging.

encephalography (ĕn-sĕf″ă-lŏg′ră-fē) [″ + *graphein,* to write] Radiography of the head, esp. examination following the introduction of air into the ventricles through a lumbar or cisternal puncture. This procedure is no longer performed. SEE: *encephalogram*.

encephaloid (ĕn-sĕf′ă-loyd) [″ + *eidos,* form, shape] **1.** Resembling the cerebral substance. **2.** A malignant neoplasm of brainlike texture.

encephalolith (ĕn-sĕf′ă-lō-lĭth) [″ + *lithos,* stone] A calculus of the brain.

encephaloma (ĕn-sĕf″ă-lō-mă) [″ + *oma,* tumor] A tumor of the brain.

encephalomalacia (ĕn-sĕf″ă-lō-mă-lā′sē-ă) [″ + *malakia,* softening] Cerebral softening.

encephalomeningitis (ĕn-sĕf″ă-lō-mĕn″ĭn-jī′tĭs) [″ + *meninx,* membrane, + *itis,* inflammation] Inflammation of the brain and meninges. SYN: *meningoencephalitis*.

encephalomeningocele (ĕn-sĕf″ă-lō-mĕ-nĭng′gō-sēl) [″ + ″ + *kele,* tumor, swelling] A protrusion of membranes and brain substance through the cranium.

encephalomere (ĕn-sĕf′ă-lō-mēr″) [″ + *meros,* part] A primitive segment of the embryonic brain. SYN: *neuromere*.

encephalometer (ĕn-sĕf″ă-lŏm′ĕ-tĕr) [″ + *metron,* measure] An instrument for measuring the cranium and locating brain regions.

encephalomyelitis (ĕn-sĕf″ă-lō-mī-ĕl-ī′tĭs) [″ + *myelos,* marrow, + *itis,* inflammation] Encephalitis that is accompanied by infection and inflammation of the spinal cord. It may follow a viral infection or, in rare instances, a vaccination with a live, weakened virus.

acute disseminated e. An acute disorder of the brain and spinal cord due to causes such as vaccination or acute exanthema. SYN: *postinfectious e*.

benign myalgic e. An epidemic disease of unknown etiology marked by influenza-like symptoms, severe pain, and muscular weakness. SYN: *Iceland disease*.

equine e. A viral disease of horses that may be communicated to humans. It includes eastern and western equine encephalitis.

postinfectious e. Acute disseminated e.

postvaccinal e. Encephalomyelitis following smallpox vaccination.

encephalomyeloneuropathy (ĕn-sĕf″ă-lō-mī″ĕ-lō-nū-rŏp′ă-thē) Any disease involving the brain, spinal cord, and nerves.

encephalomyelopathy (ĕn-sĕf″ă-lō-mī″ĕl-ŏp′ă-thē) [″ + ″ + *pathos,* disease, suffering] Any disease of the brain and spinal cord.

encephalomyeloradiculitis (ĕn-sĕf″ă-lō-mī″ĕ-lō-ră-dĭk″ū-lī′tĭs) Inflammation of the brain, spinal cord, and nerve roots.

encephalomyocarditis (ĕn-sĕf″ă-lō-mī″ō-kăr-dī′tĭs) Any disease involving the brain and cardiac muscle.

encephalon (ĕn-sĕf′ă-lŏn) [Gr. *enkephalos,* brain] The brain, including the cerebrum, cerebellum, medulla oblongata, pons, diencephalon, and midbrain.

encephalopathy (ĕn-sĕf″ă-lŏp′ă-thē) [″ + *pathos,* disease, suffering] Generalized (i.e., not localized) brain dysfunction marked by varying degrees of impairment of speech, cognition, orientation, and arousal. In mild instances, brain dysfunction may be evident only during specialized neuropsychiatric testing; in severe instances (e.g., the last stages of hepatic encephalopathy), the patient may be unresponsive even to unpleasant stimuli.

bovine spongiform e. ABBR: BSE. A progressive neurological disease of cattle, marked by spongelike changes in the brain and spinal cord and associated with rapid and fatal deterioration. SYN: *mad cow disease*. SEE: *Creutzfeldt-Jakob disease; transmissible spongiform e*.

ETIOLOGY: BSE is found in cattle that have been fed offal. An infectious protein (prion) is thought to be the cause.

PREVENTION: Because of the possible link between BSE and rapidly fatal neurological diseases in humans, many countries have banned the use of ruminant proteins in the preparation of cattle feed. This appears to have resulted in a decreasing incidence of BSE.

hepatic e. portal-systemic e.

HIV e. AIDS-dementia complex.

hypertensive e. The abrupt onset of headache and altered mental status (e.g., irritability, confusion, convulsions, and/or coma) that may occur with sudden and extreme elevations in blood pressure (usually diastolic pressures greater than 125 mm Hg). Nausea, vomiting, and visual disturbances are common. The symptoms resolve as the blood pressure is brought under control. Hypertensive encephalopathy is an emergency that requires immediate treatment, usually with intravenous medications.

hypoxic e. The neurological damage that results from depriving the brain of oxygen or blood, or both, for several minutes. The damage may range from a transient loss of short-term memory to persistent vegetative coma. Many conditions can result in an oxygen deficiency in the brain, which is acutely dependent on oxygen, blood, and glucose to work normally. These conditions include carbon monoxide inhalation, cardiac arrest, hypotensive episodes of any kind (e.g., any form of shock), near-drowning, and suffocation. If patients are not rapidly revived and oxygenation restored, the hippocampus, and later the other cerebral structures, may be permanently injured and the patient left with irreversible brain damage.

metabolic e. Any alteration of brain function or consciousness that results from the failure of other internal organs. In the hospital, metabolic encephalopathy is among the most common causes of altered mental status. Renal failure, liver injury, electrolyte or acid-base abnormalities, hypoxia, hypercarbia, or inadequate brain perfusion caused by a failing heart are but a few examples of medical conditions that may produce treatable encephalopathies.

SYMPTOMS: Confusion, irritability, seizures, and coma are common findings.

portal-systemic e. ABBR: PSE. Brain dysfunction present in patients with chronic liver disease and portal hypertension, in which chemicals that the liver normally detoxifies are shunted past it and left to circulate in the blood. Some patients are asymptomatic; others have mild impairments in memory, calculation, speech, affect, or judgment. Severely affected patients may lapse into coma. SYN: *hepatic e.* SEE: *asterixis*.

transmissible spongiform e. Neurological illnesses marked by rapidly developing dementia, or the sudden onset of psychiatric illnesses, often with myoclonus, ataxia, and aphasia. Death may occur within months of onset. These illnesses are believed to be caused by infectious proteins called prions. Examples include kuru, mad cow disease (bovine spongiform encephalopathy), and Creutzfeldt-Jakob disease.

encephalopyosis (ĕn-sĕf″ă-lō-pī-ō′sĭs) [″ + *pyosis,* suppuration] An abscess of the brain.

encephalospinal [″ + L. *spina,* thorn, spine] Pert. to the brain and spinal cord.

encephalotomy (ĕn-sĕf″ă-lŏt′ō-mē) **1.** Brain dissection. **2.** Surgical destruction of the brain of a fetus to facilitate delivery.

enchondroma (ĕn″kŏn-drō′mă) [Gr. *en,* in, + *chondros,* cartilage, + *oma,* tumor] A benign cartilaginous tumor occurring generally where cartilage is absent, or within a bone, where it expands the diaphysis. SYN: *enchondrosis*.

enchondrosarcoma (ĕn-kŏn″drō-săr-kō′mă) [″ + ″ + *sarx,* flesh, + *oma,* tumor] A sarcoma made up of cartilaginous tissue.

enchondrosis (ĕn-kŏn-drō′sĭs) [″ + ″ + *osis,* condition] A benign cartilaginous outgrowth from bone or cartilaginous tissue. SYN: *enchondroma*.

enclave (ĕn′klāv) [Fr. *enclaver,* to enclose] A mass of tissue that becomes enclosed by tissue of another kind.

enclitic (ĕn-klĭt′ĭk) [Gr. *enklinein,* to lean on] Having the planes of the fetal head inclined to those of the maternal pelvis.

encopresis (ĕn-kō-prē′sĭs) [″ + *kopros,* excrement] A condition associated with constipation and fecal retention in which watery colonic contents bypass the hard fecal masses and pass through the rectum. This condition is often confused with diarrhea.

encranial [″ + *kranion,* cranium] Intracranial or within the cranium.

enculturation The process of transmitting to the members of the community the values, beliefs, and customs of the family, the cultural group, and the larger society.

encysted (ĕn-sĭst′ĕd) [″ + *kystis,* bladder, pouch] Surrounded by membrane; encapsulated. SYN: *saccate*.

end [AS. *ende*] A termination; an extremity.

end- SEE: *endo-*.

endadelphos (ĕnd″ă-dĕl′fŏs) [Gr. *endon,* within, + *adelphos,* brother] A congenitally deformed fetus whose twin is enclosed in the body or in a cyst on the fetus.

Endamoeba (ĕn″dă-mē′bă) Entamoeba.

endangiitis, endangeitis (ĕnd″ăn-jē-ī′tĭs) [Gr. *endon,* within, + *angeion,* vessel, + *itis,* inflammation] Inflammation of the endothelium, the innermost layer of a blood vessel. SYN: *endoangiitis; endarteritis; endophlebitis*.

endangium (ĕn-dăn′jē-ŭm) [″ + *angeion,* vessel] The innermost layer, or intima, of a blood vessel.

endaortitis (ĕnd″ā-or-tī′tĭs) [″ + *aorte,* aorta, + *itis,* inflammation] Inflammation of the inner layer of the aorta.

endarterectomy (ĕnd″ăr-tĕr-ĕk′tō-mē) Surgical removal of the lining of an artery. It is performed on almost any major artery that is diseased or blocked, such as the carotid, femoral, or popliteal artery.

carotid e. A surgical technique for removing intra-arterial obstructions of the proximal cervical portion of the internal carotid artery. The technique reduces the risk of stroke when it is performed on a patient with moderate or severe stenoses of the artery, with or without a history of transient ischemic attacks (TIA). SEE: *transient ischemic attack*.

PATIENT CARE: *Preoperative:* To reduce anxiety, the procedure and expected sensations are explained to the patient and family, and their questions answered. The location of the lesion, the atherosclerotic process, and the need to modify risk factors after surgery are discussed. All diagnostic tests used to evaluate carotid disease are explained. If the patient has concurrent coronary artery disease, the electrocardiogram (ECG), coronary angiography, and treadmill exercise stress testing are also explained. Intensive care procedures and equipment (lines, tubes, and machinery) are described to prepare the patient and family for the postoperative course; if possible, a tour of the intensive care unit is arranged. Expected postoperative pain and discomfort are explained, and the patient is instructed in pain assessment and administration of pain relief medications and other noninvasive pain relief measures. The neurological status checks that will be carried out routinely after surgery and normal responses are explained to the patient. An arterial line may be inserted to monitor blood gases and blood pressure, an ECG recorded, a signed consent form obtained before anesthesia, physical preparation of the operative site performed according to protocol or surgeon's preference, and prescribed preoperative sedation administered.

Postoperative: Vital signs (including pupillary changes) are monitored every 15 min for the first hour (or according to protocol) until the patient is stable. (Alteration in blood pressure and heart rate and respirations could indicate cerebral ischemia.) Neurological assessments are performed for the first 24 hr (or according to protocol) to evaluate extremity strength, fine hand movements, speech, level of consciousness, and orientation. Intake and output are monitored hourly for the first 24 hr (or according to protocol). Continuous cardiac and hemodynamic monitoring is performed for the first 24 hr (or according to protocol). Prescribed analgesic medication is administered, and other noninvasive pain relief measures are offered.

Surgical wound care is provided and taught to the patient and family, and the signs and symptoms of infection to be reported to the surgeon (redness, swelling, or drainage from the incision, fever, or sore throat) are reviewed. Patients who smoke cigarettes are encouraged to stop and may be referred to a smoking cessation program or for nicotine patch therapy if appropriate. Modification of risk factors such as high lipid levels or excessive weight is also advised. Prescribed medications are administered, and the patient is instructed in their use and adverse reactions to report to the physician.

The patient who has had a cerebrovascular accident and needs follow-up care is referred to a rehabilitation or home health care agency. Instruction is given in the management of postsurgical neurological, sensory, or motor deficits, and the importance of regular checkups explained. The surgeon or neurologist should be contacted immediately if any new neurological symptoms occur. The patient should wear or carry a medical identification tag to alert others to the condition and treatments in case of an emergency.

endarterial (ĕnd″ăr-tē′rē-ăl) [″ + *arteria,* artery] **1.** Pert. to the inner portion of an artery. **2.** Within an artery.

endarteritis, endoarteritis (ĕnd-ăr-tĕr-ī′tĭs) [″ + ″ + *itis,* inflammation] Infection or inflammation of the lining of a blood vessel.

e. deformans A condition in which the intima is thickened or replaced with atheromatous or calcium-containing deposits.

e. obliterans Chronic progressive thickening of the intima leading to stenosis or obstruction of a lumen.

syphilitic e. Endarteritis caused by syphilis.

endbrain Telencephalon.

end-bud End-bulb.

end-bulb The enlarged tip of the end of an axon.

e. of Krause An encapsulated nerve ending found in the skin and mucous membranes.

endemic [Gr. *en,* in, + *demos,* people] Pert. to a disease that occurs continuously or in expected cycles in a population, with a certain number of cases expected for a given period. Examples include influenza and the common cold. The term is used in contrast to *epidemic*.

endemoepidemic (ĕn-dĕm″ō-ĕp-ĭ-dĕm′ĭk) [″ + ″ + *epi,* on, among, + *demos,* people] Endemic, but becoming epidemic periodically.

endergonic (ĕnd″ĕr-gŏn′ĭk) [Gr. *endon,* within, + *ergon,* work] Pert. to chemical reactions that require energy in order to occur.

end feel In physical therapy and rehabilitation, the feeling experienced by an evaluator when overpressure is applied to tissue at the end of the available range of motion. It is interpreted as abnormal when the quality of the feel is different from normal response at that joint. The feeling may be soft as when two muscle groups are compressed or soft tissues are stretched, firm as when a normal joint or ligament is stretched, or hard as when two bones block motion. Abnormal end feels may include a springy sensation when cartilage is torn within a joint, muscle guarding when a muscle involuntarily responds to acute pain, or muscle spasticity when there is increased tone due to an upper motor neuron lesion or when the feeling is different from that normally experienced for the joint being tested.

end-foot A terminal button; the enlarged end of a nerve fiber that terminates adjacent to the dendrite of another nerve cell.

ending The finish or final portion of a tissue or cell.

endo-, end- Prefix meaning *within*.

endoaneurysmorrhaphy (ĕn″dō-ăn″ū-rĭs-mor′ăf-ē) [Gr. *endon,* within, + *aneurysma,* aneurysm, + *rhaphe,* seam, ridge] Surgical opening of an aneurysmal sac and suturing of its orifice.

endoangiitis (ĕn″dō-ăn-jē-ī′tĭs) [″ + *angeion,* vessel, + *itis,* inflammation] Endangiitis.

endoauscultation (ĕn″dō-ăws″kŭl-tā′shŭn) [″ + L. *auscultare,* to listen to] Auscultation by an esophageal tube passed into the stomach or by a tube passed into the heart.

endobiotic (ĕn″dō-bī-ŏt′ĭk) [″ + *bios,* life] Pert. to an organism living parasitically in the host.

endoblast (ĕn′dō-blăst) [″ + *blastos,* germ] The immature cell that is the precursor of an endodermal cell.

endocardiac, endocardial [″ + *kardia,* heart] Within the heart or arising from the endocardium.

endocarditis (ĕn″dō-kăr-dī′tĭs) [″ + ″ + *itis,* inflammation] Infection or inflammation of the heart valves or of the lining of the heart. In clinical practice, this word is often substituted for infective endocarditis. SEE: *infective e.*

acute bacterial e. ABBR: ABE. Infective endocarditis with a rapid onset, usually a few days to 2 weeks. The infection is typically caused by virulent organisms such as *Staphylococcus aureus,* which may rapidly invade and destroy heart valvular tissue and metastasize to other organs or tissues. SEE: *ulcerative e.*

atypical verrucous e. An infrequently used term for nonbacterial thrombotic endocarditis.

culture-negative e. Infective endocarditis produced by organisms that do not quickly or readily grow in blood cultures, usually because their growth is masked by the previous use of antibiotics or because the germs require special culture media or grow slowly in the laboratory. *Mycoplasma, Ricksettsia,* HACEK organisms, and some fungi produce culture-negative endocarditis. HACEK is an acronym that stands for *Haemophilus, Actinobacillus, Cardiobacterium, Eikenella, Kingella*. SEE: *infective e.*

infective e. ABBR: IE. Endocarditis caused by any microorganism; for example, any species of streptococci or staphylococci; *Haemophilus* spp. or other HACEK bacteria (e.g., *Actinobacillus actinomycetem comitans, Cardiobacterium hominis, Eikenella corrodens,* or *Kingella kingae*); enteric bacteria; ricksettsiae; chlamydiae; or fungi. Traditionally, IE has been categorized as *acute* if the illness has a fulminant onset; *catheter-related* if the causative germ gains access to the heart from an indwelling line; *culture-negative* if echocardiograms reveal vegetations and other criteria for the disease are present, but the causative germs have not been isolated in the laboratory; *left-sided* if it develops on the mitral or aortic valves; *prosthetic* if it occurs on a surgically implanted heart valve; *right-sided* if it develops on the tricuspid or pulmonary valves; and *subacute* if it develops after several weeks or months of anorexia, low-grade fevers, and malaise. In the U.S., most afflicted patients are men. Patients with a history of injection drug abuse, diabetes mellitus, immunosuppressing illnesses, or rheumatic heart disease are more likely than other individuals to become infected.

SYMPTOMS: Patients with *subacute* IE may have vague symptoms, including low-grade fevers, loss of appetite, malaise, and muscle aches. *Acutely* infected patients often present with high fevers; prostration; chills and sweats; stiff joints or back pain; symptoms of heart failure (esp. if the infection has completely disrupted a heart valve or its tethers); heart block (if the infection erodes into the conducting system of the heart); symptoms caused by the spreading of the infection to lungs or meninges (e.g., cough, headache, stiff neck, or confusion); stroke symptoms; symptoms of renal failure; rashes (including petechiae); or other findings. Signs of the illness typically include documented fevers, cardiac murmurs, or nodular eruptions on the hands and feet (Osler's nodes or Janeway lesions). Cottonwool spots may be seen on the retinas of some affected persons.

DIAGNOSIS: Blood cultures, esp. if persistently positive, form the basis for the diagnosis of endocarditis. Contemporary criteria for diagnosis also include visual confirmation of endocardial infection by echocardiography; the presence of several other suggestive anomalies, such as persistent fevers in a patient who is known to inject drugs or a patient with an artificial heart valve; infective emboli in the lungs or other organs; and characteristic skin findings. Occasionally, a patient who dies of a febrile illness may be found to have infective vegetations on the heart valves at autopsy.

TREATMENT: Many patients recover after treatment with prolonged courses of parenteral antibiotics. Some (e.g., those with heart failure or severely injured hearts) may not respond without surgery to replace damaged valves or débride abscesses within the myocardium.

PATIENT CARE: During the acute phase of treatment, patients are monitored for signs of congestive heart failure (e.g., rales, dependent edema, changes in the heart murmur), cerebral emboli (e.g., paralysis, aphasias, changes in mental status), and embolization to the kidney (e.g., decreased urine output, hematuria) or spleen (e.g., upper left quadrant abdominal pain). Blood cultures may be taken periodically to monitor the effectiveness of antibiotic therapy.

Passive and active limb exercises are used to maintain muscle tone until a slow, progressive activity program that limits cardiac workload can be established.

Libman-Sacks e. An eponym for nonbacterial thrombotic endocarditis.

malignant e. **1.** An old term for endocarditis that is rapidly fatal. **2.** Valvular vegetations composed of tumor cells.

mural e. Endocarditis of the lining of the heart chambers but not including the heart valve.

native valve e. Infective endocarditis occurring on a patient's own heart valve(s), rather than on a prosthetic (surgically implanted) valve(s).

nonbacterial thrombotic e. ABBR: NBTE. The presence on the heart valves of vegetations that are produced not by bacteria but by sterile collections of platelets in fibrin. NBTE is characteristically found in severe cases of systemic lupus erythematosus, tuberculosis, or malignancy. The vegetations of NBTE readily embolize, causing infarctions in other organs. SYN: *verrucous e.*

prosthetic valve e. Bacterial infection of a surgically implanted artificial heart valve.

rheumatic e. Valvular inflammation and dysfunction (esp. mitral insufficiency) occurring during acute rheumatic fever.

right-sided e. Endocarditis affecting the tricuspid or pulmonary valve. It is usually the result of a percutaneous infection, and is most often seen in injection drug users.

subacute bacterial e. ABBR: SBE. A heart valve infection that becomes clinically evident after weeks or months. It usually results from infection with streptococcal species that have relatively low virulence (e.g., *Streptococcus viridans*). The infection often develops on a previously abnormal heart valve. SYN: *e. viridans.*

syphilitic e. Endocarditis due to syphilis having extended from the aorta to the aortic valves.

tuberculous e. Endocarditis caused by *Mycobacterium tuberculosis.*

ulcerative e. A rapidly destructive form of acute bacterial endocarditis characterized by necrosis or ulceration of the valves and the growth of bacterial colonies on the valves.

valvular e. Endocarditis affecting the heart valves and not the lining of the heart chambers.

vegetative e. Endocarditis associated with fibrinous clots on ulcerated valvular surfaces.

verrucous e. Nonbacterial thrombotic e.

e. viridans Subacute bacterial e.

endocardium [Gr. *endon,* within, + *kardia,* heart] The endothelial membrane that lines the chambers of the heart and is continuous with the intima (the lining of arteries and veins).

endocervical (ĕn″dō-sĕr′vĭ-kăl) [″ + L. *cervix,* neck] Pert. to the endocervix.

endocervicitis (ĕn″dō-sĕr″vĭ-sī′tĭs) [″ + ″ + Gr. *itis,* inflammation] Inflammation of the mucous lining of the cervix uteri. It is usually chronic, due to infection, and accompanied by cervical erosion.

SYMPTOMS: A white or yellow mucoid discharge is characteristic.

TREATMENT: Depends on the underlying cause.

endocervix (ĕn″dō-sĕr′vĭks) [″ + L. *cervix,* neck] The lining of the canal of the cervix uteri.

endochondral (ĕn″dō-kŏn′drăl) [″ + *chondros,* cartilage] Within a cartilage.

endochondral bone formation One of the two types of bone formation in skeletal development. Each long bone is formed as a cartilage model before bone is laid down, replacing the cartilage.

endochorion (ĕn″dō-kō′rē-ŏn) [″ + *chorion,* chorion] The inner chorion; the vascular layer of the allantois.

endocolitis (ĕn″dō-kō-lī′tĭs) [″ + *kolon,* colon, + *itis,* inflammation] Inflammation of the mucosa of the colon. SEE: *colitis.*

endocorpuscular (ĕn″dō-kor-pŭs′kū-lăr) [″ + L. *corpusculum,* small body (corpuscle)] Within a cell.

endocranial (ĕn″dō-krā′nē-ăl) [″ +

kranion, cranium] **1.** Intracranial or within the cranium. **2.** Pert. to the endocranium.

endocranium (ĕn″dō-krā′nē-ŭm) The dura mater of the brain, which forms the lining membrane of the cranium.

endocrine (ĕn′dō-krīn, -krĭn, -krēn) [″ + *krinein,* to secrete] **1.** An internal secretion. **2.** Pert. to a gland that secretes directly into the bloodstream.

endocrine neoplasm, multiple SEE: *multiple endocrine neoplasia.*

endocrino- [Gr. *endon,* within, + *krinein,* to secrete] Combining form, *endocrine.*

endocrinologist (ĕn″dō-krĭn-ŏl′ō-jĭst) A medical scientist or physician skilled in endocrinology.

endocrinology (ĕn″dō-krĭn-ŏl′ō-jē) [″ + ″ + *logos,* word, reason] The science of the endocrine, or ductless, glands and their functions.

endocrinopathy (ĕn″dō-krĭn-ŏp′ă-thē) [″ + ″ + *pathos,* disease, suffering] Any disease resulting from disorder of an endocrine gland or glands. **endocrinopathic** (-krĭn″-ō-pă′thĭk), *adj.*

endocrinotherapy (ĕn″dō-krĭn″ō-thĕr′ă-pē) [″ + ″ + *therapeia,* treatment] Treatment with endocrine preparations.

endocyst (ĕn′dō-sĭst) [″ + *kystis,* bladder, pouch] The innermost layer of any hydatid cyst.

endocystitis (ĕn′dō-sĭs-tī′tĭs) [″ + ″ + *itis,* inflammation] Inflammation of the mucous membrane of the bladder. SEE: *cystitis.*

endocytosis A method of ingestion of a foreign substance by a cell. The cell membrane invaginates to form a space for the material and then the opening closes to trap the material inside the cell. SEE: *emiocytosis; exocytosis; phagocytosis; pinocytosis.*

endoderm (ĕn′dō-dĕrm) [″ + *derma,* skin] The innermost of the three primary germ layers of a developing embryo. It gives rise to the epithelium of the digestive tract and its associated glands, the respiratory organs, bladder, vagina, and urethra. SYN: *hypoblast.* **endodermal** (-dĕrm′ăl), *adj.*

Endodermophyton (ĕn″dō-dĕr-mŏf′ĭ-tŏn) [″ + *derma,* skin, + *phyton,* a growth] The former name of a genus of parasitic fungi growing in the epidermis. It is now included in the genus *Trichophyton.*

endodontia (ĕn″dō-dŏn′shē-ă) [″ + *odous,* tooth] Endodontics.

endodontics (ĕn″dō-dŏn′tĭks) The branch of dentistry concerned with diagnosis, treatment, and prevention of diseases of the dental pulp and its surrounding tissues.

endodontist A specialist in endodontics.

endodontitis (ĕn″dō-dŏn-tī′tĭs) [″ + *odous,* tooth, + *itis,* inflammation] Inflammation of the dental pulp. SYN: *pulpitis.*

endodontologist Endodontist.

endoectothrix (ĕn″dō-ĕk′tō-thrĭks) [″ + *ektos,* outside, + *thrix,* hair] Any fungus growth on and in the hair.

endogamy (ĕn-dŏg′ă-mē) [″ + *gamos,* marriage] **1.** The custom or tribal restriction of marriage within a tribe or group. **2.** In biology, reproduction by joining together gametes descended from the same ancestral cell.

endogastritis (ĕn″dō-găs-trī′tĭs) [″ + ″ + *itis,* inflammation] Gastritis.

endogenic (ĕn″dō-jĕn′ĭk) [″ + *gennan,* to produce] Endogenous.

endogenous (ĕn-dŏj′ĕ-nŭs) **1.** Produced or originating from within a cell or organism. **2.** Concerning spore formation within the bacterial cell. SYN: *endogenic.*

endogenous opiate-like substance SEE: *endorphin; enkephalin; opiate receptor.*

endoglobar, endoglobular (ĕn″dō-glōb′ăr, ĕn″dō-glŏb′ū-lăr) [Gr. *endon,* within, + L. *globulus,* a globule] Within blood cells.

endognathion (ĕn″dō-năth′ē-ŏn) [Gr. *endon,* within, + *gnathos,* jaw] A point in the inner segment of the intermaxillary bone, or premaxilla.

endointoxication (ĕn″dō-ĭn-tŏk″sĭ-kā′shŭn) [″ + L. *in,* into, + Gr. *toxikon,* poison] Poisoning due to an endogenous toxin, such as hepatoxins, in liver failure, or urea compounds in renal failure.

endolabyrinthitis (ĕn″dō-lăb″ĭ-rĭn-thī′tĭs) [″ + *labyrinthos,* labyrinth, + *itis,* inflammation] Inflammation of the membranous labyrinth.

Endolimax nana (ĕn″dō-lī′măks nă′nă) [″ + *leimax,* meadow] A species of ameba inhabiting the intestines of humans, monkeys, and other mammals. It is usually nonpathogenic in humans and is found in the intestines of healthy persons.

endolumbar [″ + L. *lumbus,* loin] In the lumbar portion of the spinal cord.

endolymph (ĕn′dō-lĭmf) [″ + L. *lympha,* clear fluid] A pale transparent fluid within the membranous labyrinth of the inner ear. **endolymphatic** (-lĭm-făt′ĭk), *adj.*

endolysin (ĕn-dŏl′ĭ-sĭn) [″ + *lysis,* dissolution] A bacterial substance within a leukocyte that destroys bacteria.

endomastoiditis (ĕn″dō-măs″toy-dī′tĭs) [″ + *mastos,* breast, + *eidos,* form, shape, + *itis,* inflammation] Inflammation of the mucosa lining the mastoid cavity and cells.

endometrial (ĕn″dō-mē′trē-ăl) [″ + *metra,* uterus] Pert. to the lining of the uterus.

endometrial cyst An ovarian cyst or tumor lined with endometrial tissue, usually seen in ovarian endometriosis.

endometrial dating Microscopic examination of a suitable, stained specimen from the endometrium to establish the number of days to the next menstrual period. The dating is based on an ideal 28-day cycle. Thus, day 8 indicates menstruation is 20 days away, and day 23 that it is 5 days away. This system was devised by the late Dr. John Rock, a physician at Harvard Medical School, to enable gynecologists to visualize endometria being discussed without having to provide detailed descriptions of the material studied.

endometrial jet washing Collection of fluid that has been used to irrigate the uterine cavity. Cells present in the fluid are examined for evidence of malignancy. This method is used as a screening test for endometrial carcinoma.

endometrioma (ĕn″dō-mē″trē-ō′mă) [Gr. *endon,* within, + *metra,* uterus, + *oma,* tumor] A tumor containing shreds of ectopic endometrium. It is found most frequently in the ovary, the cul-de-sac, the rectovaginal septum, and the peritoneal surface of the posterior portion of the uterus.

endometriosis (ĕn″dō-mē″trē-ō′sĭs) [″ + ″ + *osis,* condition] The presence of functioning ectopic endometrial glands and stroma outside the uterine cavity. Characteristically, the endometrial tissue invades other tissues and spreads by local extension, intraperitoneal seeding, and vascular routes. The endometrial implants may be present in almost any area of the body. In the U.S. this condition is estimated to occur in 10% to 15% of actively menstruating women between the ages of 25 and 44. Estimates are that 25% to 50% of infertile women are affected. The fallopian tubes are common sites of ectopic implantation. Ectopic endometrial cells respond to the same hormonal stimuli as does the uterine endometrium. The cyclic bleeding and local inflammation surrounding the implants may cause fibrosis, adhesions, and tubal occlusion. Infertility may result. SEE: illus.

ETIOLOGY: Although the cause is unknown, hypotheses are that either endometrial cell migration occurs during fetal development, or the cells shed during menstruation are expelled through the fallopian tubes to the peritoneal cavity.

SYMPTOMS: No single symptom is diagnostic. Patients often complain of dysmenorrhea with pelvic pain, premenstrual dyspareunia, sacral backache during menses, and infertility. Dysuria may indicate involvement of the urinary bladder. Cyclic pelvic pain, usually in the lower abdomen, vagina, posterior pelvis, and back, begins 5 to 7 days before menses, reaches a peak, and lasts 2 to 3 days. Premenstrual tenesmus and diarrhea may indicate lower bowel involvement. No correlation exists between the degree of pain and the extent of involvement; many patients are asymptomatic.

DIAGNOSIS: Although history and findings of physical examination may suggest endometriosis, definitive diagnosis of endometriosis can be established only by direct visualization of ectopic lesions or by biopsy.

TREATMENT: Medical and surgical approaches may be used to preserve fer-

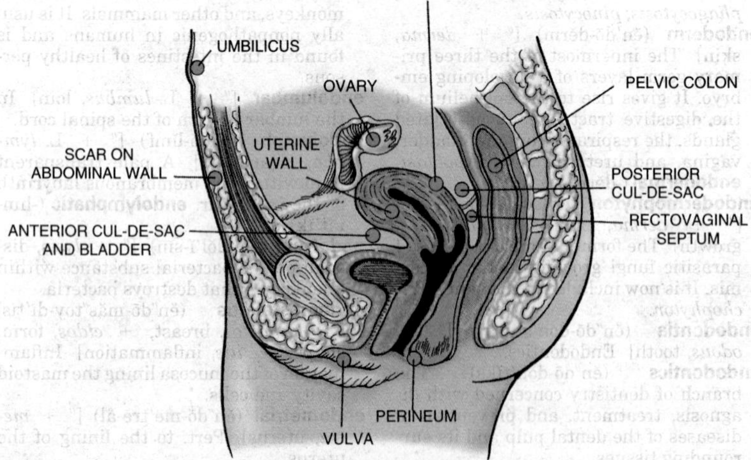

POSSIBLE SITES OF OCCURRENCE OF ENDOMETRIOSIS

tility and to increase the woman's potential for achieving pregnancy. Pharmacological management includes the use of hormonal agents to induce endometrial atrophy by maintaining a chronic state of anovulation. Medroxyprogesterone inhibits ovulation and menstruation by inducing pseudopregnancy. Danazol inhibits pituitary release of gonadotropins. Gonadotropin-releasing hormone (GnRH) analogs inhibit release of follicle-stimulating hormone (FSH) and luteinizing hormone (LH). Methyltestosterone also has been used to cause endometrial atrophy and provide pain relief; however, ovulation and menstruation are not affected, and pregnancy may occur during therapy.

Surgical management includes laparotomy, lysis of adhesions, and removal of aberrant endometrial cysts and implants to encourage fertility. The definitive treatment for endometriosis ends a woman's potential for pregnancy by removal of the uterus, tubes, and ovaries.

PATIENT CARE: Providing emotional support and meeting informational needs are major concerns. The patient is encouraged to verbalize feelings and concerns and to express the effects of the condition on interpersonal relationships. The need for open communication to minimize discomfort and frustration is discussed. The patient is assisted to identify effective coping strategies and to contact counseling and support resources.

Diagnostic and treatment options and procedures are explained. Misconceptions are clarified, and understanding and informed consent are validated. The woman is prepared physically and emotionally for any surgical procedure. Procedures include diagnostic laparoscopy and biopsy; laparoscopy with laser vaporization of implants; laparotomy with excision of ovarian masses, or total hysterectomy with bilateral salpingo-oophorectomy. Prescribed pharmacological treatment and analgesics are administered, and the patient is instructed about the desired effects and potential adverse reactions.

Adolescent girls with a narrow vagina or small vaginal meatus are advised to use sanitary napkins rather than tampons to help prevent retrograde flow. Because infertility is a possible complication, a patient who wants children is advised not to postpone childbearing. An annual pelvic examination and Papanicolaou test is recommended. SEE: *Nursing Diagnoses Appendix.*

peritoneal e. Endometrial tissue found throughout the pelvis.

transplantation e. Endometriosis occurring within an abdominal incision scar following pelvic surgery.

endometritis (ĕn″dō-mē-trī′tĭs) [″ + ″ + *itis,* inflammation] Inflammation of the lining of the uterus. Organisms may migrate through the cervical canal along mucosal surfaces, piggy-back on sperm, or be carried on tampons or intrauterine devices. The inflammation may be acute, subacute, or chronic. The disorder is most common among females of childbearing age. The woman is at highest risk for endometritis during the immediate postpartum period. SEE: *puerperal e.*

ETIOLOGY: Endometritis usually results from an ascending bacterial invasion of the uterine cavity. Common offenders include *Staphylococcus aureus,* a normal commensal resident of human skin; *Escherichia coli,* a common inhabitant of the human bowel; *Chlamydia trachomatis;* and *Neisseria.* SEE: *pelvic inflammatory disease; toxic shock syndrome.*

SYMPTOMS: The woman usually presents with low, cramping abdominal pain, low back pain, dysmenorrhea, dyspareunia, and fever. Depending on the causative organism, a purulent, mucopurulent, or serosanguinous cervical discharge is seen on vaginal examination. Bimanual palpation finds a tender, boggy uterus. SEE: *cervix uteri; endometrium; uterus.*

DIAGNOSIS: Culturing the causative organisms establishes the diagnosis.

TREATMENT: Antibiotics are chosen to cover aerobic and anaerobic bacteria.

PATIENT CARE: The patient should be made aware that the infectious process may move (or have moved) beyond the endometrium, involving fallopian tubes, ovaries, pelvic perineum, pelvic veins, or pelvic connective tissue. This condition is called pelvic inflammatory disease (PID) and may be acute or subacute. The patient is assessed for changes in the amount, color, odor, and consistency of vaginal discharge. Pain also is assessed for and treated as prescribed. The patient is taught about the drug used for treatment, its desired effect, and any adverse effects. In acute cases, the patient may be febrile; fever is treated with antipyretic drugs if it exceeds 101°F and with PO or intravenous (IV) fluids for hydration as required. (The nurse auscultates for bowel sounds, and if they are absent, the patient is kept NPO.) Once culture and sensitivity testing has revealed the bacterial culprit, antibiotic therapy is administered as prescribed, again accompanied by information regarding desired responses and adverse effects. The patient may be placed on bedrest in a semi-Fowler's position to facilitate dependent drainage so that abscesses will not form high in the abdomen. Heat may be applied to the abdomen to improve circulation.

The varied consequences of endometritis are explained. They can include the need for surgery to relieve chronic pain or to manage acute infections that are unresponsive to antibiotic therapy; adhesions; tubal scarring; and infertility. The potential or actual loss of reproductive capabilities can devastate the woman's self-concept. All professional care providers must assist the patient to adjust her self-concept to fit reality and to accept any alterations in a way that promotes future health.

cervical e. Inflammation of the inner portion of the cervix uteri.

decidual e. Inflammation of the mucous membrane of a gravid uterus.

e. dissecans Endometritis accompanied by development of ulcers and shedding of the mucous membrane.

puerperal e. Acute endometritis following childbirth. Risk factors for development of this condition include premature or prolonged rupture of membranes; dystocia with multiple vaginal examinations; poor aseptic technique; trauma related to intrauterine manipulation; and careless perineal care. Constitutional factors that predispose the parturient woman to endometritis include anemia, malnutrition, and hemorrhage. Portals of bacterial entry include the site of previous placental attachment, episiotomy, lacerations, and abrasions.

ETIOLOGY: Aerobic organisms include streptococci, *Gardnerella vaginalis, Escherichia coli, Staphylococcus aureus,* and group A β-hemolytic streptococci. Endometritis that occurs late in the postpartal period is most commonly caused by *Chlamydia trachomatis.*

SYMPTOMS: Abdominal tenderness is common. Severe endometritis may cause fever, chills, tachycardia, extreme uterine tenderness, and subinvolution. Although a moderate-to-profuse foul-smelling vaginal discharge usually is seen, the lochia of women infected by β-hemolytic streptococci is scant, odorless, and serosanguineous to serous.

TREATMENT: Antibiotics that treat aerobic and anaerobic bacteria are administered, usually for a 4- or 5-day course. Supportive therapy includes bedrest, analgesics, and oral and IV fluids.

endometrium (ĕn-dō-mē'trē-ŭm) [Gr. *endon,* within, + *metra,* uterus] The mucous membrane that lines the uterus. It consists of two highly vascular layers of areolar connective tissue; the basilar layer is adjacent to the myometrium, and the functional layer is adjacent to the uterine cavity. Simple columnar epithelium forms the surface of the functional layer and the simple tubular uterine glands. Straight arteries supply blood to the basilar layer; spiral arteries supply the functional layer. Both estrogen and progesterone stimulate the growth of endometrial blood vessels.

Beginning with menarche and ending at menopause, the uterine endometrium passes through cyclical changes that constitute the menstrual cycle. These changes are related to the development and maturation of the graafian follicle in the ovary, the discharge of the ovum, and the subsequent development of the corpus luteum in the ovary.

If the ovum is not fertilized or the zygote not implanted, the functional layer of the endometrium is shed in menstruation.

The cycle then begins again, with the functional layer regenerated by the basilar layer.

Following implantation of the zygote, the endometrium becomes the maternal portion of the placenta; it fuses with the chorion of the embryo. After birth, the uterine lining is shed. SEE: *fertilization* for illus.

proliferative e. Endometrial hypertrophy due to estrogen stimulation during the preovulatory phase of the menstrual cycle. This condition is detected through endometrial biopsy.

secretory e. Histological changes in the endometrium due to the effects of postovulatory progesterone secretion by the corpus luteum. SEE: *luteal phase defect; menstrual cycle.*

endomorph (ĕn"dō-morf') [" + *morphe,* form] A person with a body build marked by predominance of tissues derived from the endoderm. SEE: *ectomorph; mesomorph; somatotype.*

endomyocarditis (ĕn"dō-mī-ō-kăr-dī'tĭs) [" + *mys,* muscle, + *kardia,* heart, + *itis,* inflammation] Inflammation of the endocardium and myocardium.

endomysium (ĕn"dō-mĭs'ē-ŭm) [" + *mys,* muscle] A thin sheath of connective tissue, consisting principally of reticular fibers, that invests each striated muscle fiber and binds the fibers together within a fasciculus.

endoneuritis [" + *neuron,* nerve, + *itis,* inflammation] Inflammation of the endoneurium.

endoneurium (ĕn"dō-nū'rē-ŭm) A delicate connective tissue sheath that surrounds nerve fibers within a fasciculus. SYN: *Henle's sheath.*

endonuclease (ĕn"dō-nū'klē-ās) An enzyme that cleaves the ends of polynucleotides.

restriction e. One of many bacterial enzymes that inactivates foreign DNA but does not interfere with the cell's DNA. This type of enzyme is used to cleave strands of DNA at specific sites.

endoparasite (ĕn"dō-păr'ă-sīt) [" + *para,* beside, + *sitos,* food] Any parasite living within its host.

endopelvic (ĕn"dō-pĕl'vĭk) [" + L. *pelvis,* basin] Within the pelvis.

endopelvic fasciae The downward continuation of the parietal peritoneum of the abdomen to form the pelvic fasciae, which contribute to the support of the pelvic viscera.

endopeptidase (ĕn″dō-pĕp′tĭ-dās) A proteolytic enzyme that cleaves peptides in their centers rather than from their ends.

endopericarditis (ĕn″dō-pĕr″ĭ-kăr-dī′tĭs) [″ + *peri,* around, + *kardia,* heart, + *itis,* inflammation] Endocarditis complicated by pericarditis.

endoperimyocarditis (ĕn″dō-pĕr″ĭ-mī″ō-kăr-dī′tĭs) [″ + ″ + *mys,* muscle, + *kardia,* heart, + *itis,* inflammation] Inflammation of the pericardium, myocardium, and endocardium.

endoperitonitis (ĕn″dō-pĕr″ĭ-tō-nī′tĭs) [″ + *peritonaion,* peritoneum, + *itis,* inflammation] Inflammation of the peritoneum.

endophasia (ĕn″dō-fā′zē-ă) [″ + *phasis,* utterance] Formation of words by the lips without producing sound.

endophasy The silent process of thought and production of unuttered words. This function, called inner speech, is essential to thinking that is done with words. SEE: *exophasy*.

endophlebitis (ĕn″dō-flĕ-bī′tĭs) [″ + *phleps,* vein, + *itis,* inflammation] Inflammation of the inner layer or membrane of a vein. SYN: *endangiitis*.

e. obliterans Endophlebitis causing obliteration of a vein.

e. portalis Inflammation of the portal vein.

endophthalmitis (ĕn″dŏf-thăl-mī′tĭs) [″ + *ophthalmos,* eye, + *itis,* inflammation] Inflammation of the inside of the eye that may or may not be limited to a particular chamber (i.e., anterior or posterior).

endoplasm [″ + LL. *plasma,* form, mold] The central, more fluid portion of the cytoplasm of a cell. Opposed to ectoplasm.

endorphin (ĕn-dor′fĭns, ĕn′dor-fĭns) A polypeptide produced in the brain that acts as an opiate and produces analgesia by binding to opiate receptor sites involved in pain perception. The threshold for pain is therefore increased by this action. The most active of these compounds is beta-endorphin. SYN: *endogenous opiate-like substance*. SEE: *enkephalin; opiate receptor; substance P*.

endorrhachis (ĕn″dō-rā′kĭs) [Gr. *endon,* within, + *rhachis,* spine] The membrane lining the spinal canal. SYN: *dura mater*.

endosalpingitis (ĕn″dō-săl″pĭn-jī′tĭs) [″ + *salpinx,* tube, + *itis,* inflammation] Inflammation of the lining of the fallopian tubes.

endosalpingoma (ĕn″dō-săl″pĭn-gō′mă) An adenomyoma of the uterine tube.

endosalpinx (ĕn″dō-săl′pĭnks) [″ + *salpinx,* tube] The mucous membrane lining the uterine tube.

endoscope (ĕn′dō-skōp) [″ + *skopein,* to examine] A device consisting of a tube and optical system for observing the inside of a hollow organ or cavity. This observation may be done through a natural body opening or a small incision. SYN: *enteroscope*.

endoscopic laser cholecystectomy SEE: *laparoscopic laser cholecystectomy*.

endoscopic mucosectomy Surgical removal of a part of the mucosa of an organ, esp. when cancer is present only in the lining of that organ. Endoscopic mucosectomy sometimes is used to treat superficial cancers of the esophagus.

endoscopic retrograde cholangiopancreatography ABBR: ERCP. Radiography following injection of a radiopaque material into the papilla of Vater. This is done through a fiberoptic endoscope guided by use of fluoroscopy. The procedure is helpful in determining the cause of obstructive jaundice. SEE: *jaundice; percutaneous transhepatic cholangiography*.

endoscopy (ĕn-dŏs′kō-pē) Inspection of body organs or cavities by use of an endoscope.

endoskeleton [″ + *skeleton,* skeleton] The internal bony framework of the body. Opposite of exoskeleton.

endosome (ĕn′dō-sōm) [″ + L. *soma,* body] The vacuole formed when material is absorbed in the cell by endocytosis. The vacuole fuses with lysosomes. SYN: *receptosome*.

endospore [″ + *sporos,* a seed] A thick-walled spore produced by a bacterium to enable it to survive unfavorable environmental conditions.

endostatin (ĕn″dŏ-stăt′ĭn) A protein fragment of collagen that contributes to the regulation of blood vessel growth. It is being investigated for its potential to shrink malignant tumors by decreasing their blood supply.

endosteitis (ĕn″dŏs-tē-ī′tĭs) [″ + *osteon,* bone, + *itis,* inflammation] Inflammation of the endosteum or the medullary cavity of a bone. SYN: *endostitis*.

endosteoma (ĕn-dŏs″tē-ō′mă) [″ + ″ + *oma,* tumor] A tumor in the medullary cavity of a bone.

endosteum (ĕn-dŏs′tē-ŭm) [″ + *osteon,* bone] The membrane lining the marrow cavity of a bone.

endostitis (ĕn″dŏs-tī′tĭs) [″ + ″ + *itis,* inflammation] Endosteitis.

endostoma (ĕn-dŏs-tō′mă) [″ + ″ + *oma,* tumor] An osseous tumor within a bone.

endostosis (ĕn″dŏs-tō′sĭs) [″ + ″ + *osis,* condition] The development of an endostoma.

endotendineum (ĕn″dō-tĕn-dĭn′ē-ŭm) [″ + L. *tendo,* tendon] The connective tissue in tendons between the bundles of fibers.

endothelial (ĕn″dŏ-thē′lē-ăl) [Gr. *endon,* within, + *thele,* nipple] Pert. to or consisting of endothelium.

endothelin A peptide released from the lining of blood vessels that causes blood vessels to constrict and blood pressure to increase. Endothelins are one of several agents involved in raising blood pressure and contributing to congestive heart failure.

endotheliocyte (ĕn″dŏ-thē′lē-ō-sīt″) [″ + ″ + *kytos,* cell] An endothelial cell.

endotheliocytosis (ĕn″dŏ-thē″lē-ō-sī-tō′sĭs) [″ + ″ + ″ + *osis,* condition] An abnormal increase in endothelial cells.

endotheliolysin (ĕn″dŏ-thē-lē-ŏl′ĭ-sĭn) [″ + *thele,* nipple, + *lysis,* dissolution] An antibody found in snake venom that dissolves endothelial cells.

endotheliolytic (ĕn″dŏ-thē-lē-ō-lĭt′ĭk) Capable of destroying endothelial tissue.

endothelioma (ĕn″dŏ-thē-lē-ō′mă) [″ + *thele,* nipple, + *oma,* tumor] A malignant growth of lining cells of the blood vessels.

endotheliomyoma (ĕn″dŏ-thē″lē-ō-mī-ō′mă) [″ + ″ + *mys,* muscle, + *oma,* tumor] A muscular tumor with elements of endothelium.

endotheliomyxoma (ĕn″dŏ-thē″lē-ō-mĭks-ō′mă) [″ + ″ + *myxa,* mucus, + *oma,* tumor] A myxoma with elements of endothelium.

endotheliosis (ĕn″dō-thē″lē-ō′sĭs) Increased growth of endothelium.

endotheliotoxin (ĕn″dō-thē-lē-ō-tŏks′ĭn) [″ + ″ + *toxikon,* poison] A toxin that acts on endothelial capillary cells and causes bleeding.

endothelium (ĕn″dŏ-thē′lē-ŭm) [″ + *thele,* nipple] A form of squamous epithelium consisting of flat cells that line the blood and lymphatic vessels, the heart, and various other body cavities. It is derived from mesoderm. Endothelial cells are metabolically active and produce a number of compounds that affect the vascular lumen and platelets. Included are endothelium-derived relaxing factor (EDRF), prostacyclin, endothelium-derived contracting factors 1 and 2 (EDCF1, EDCF2), endothelium-derived hyperpolarizing factor (EDHF), and thrombomodulin. SEE: *intima.*

endothelium-derived hyperpolarizing factor ABBR: EDHF. A vasodilating substance released by the vascular endothelium. SEE: *endothelium.*

endothelium-derived relaxing factor ABBR: EDRF. An active vasodilator released by the vascular endothelium. It facilitates relaxation of vascular smooth muscle and inhibition of adhesion and aggregation of platelets. When the normal function of the endothelium is disrupted by mechanical trauma, hypertension, hypercholesterolemia, or atherosclerosis, less EDRF is released and the inhibition of platelet aggregation is decreased. In addition, the damaged vessels constrict. This favors the formation of thrombi. SEE: *endothelium.*

endothermal, endothermic [Gr. *endon,* within, + *therme,* heat] **1.** Storing up potential energy or heat. **2.** Absorbing heat. **3.** Pert. to absorption of heat during chemical reactions.

endothermy (ĕn′dō-thĕr″mē) An elevation of the temperature of deep body tissue in response to high-frequency current.

endothrix (ĕn′dō-thrĭks) [″ + *thrix,* hair] Any fungus growing inside the hair shaft.

endotoscope (ĕn-dō′tō-skōp) [″ + *ous,* ear, + *skopein,* to examine] An ear speculum. SYN: *otoscope.*

endotoxemia (ĕn″dō-tŏks-ē′mē-ă) Toxemia due to the presence of endotoxins in the blood.

endotoxicosis (ĕn″dŏ-tŏk″sĭ-kō′sĭs) [Gr. *endon,* within, + *toxikon,* poison, + *osis,* condition] Poisoning due to an endotoxin.

endotoxin A lipopolysaccharide that is part of the cell wall of gram-negative bacteria. It binds with CD14 receptors on leukocytes. The linkage stimulates the release of interleukin-1, tumor necrosis factor and other cytokines, affecting inflammation, the specific immune response, vascular tone, hematopoiesis, and wound healing. When large amounts of lipopolysaccharides are present, the clinical state of sepsis or systemic inflammatory response syndrome occurs. Endotoxins are still active even after bacteria are destroyed; thus, in treating some infections, the positive effects of antibiotics may be delayed or absent. SEE: *bacterium; inflammation; sepsis; systemic inflammatory response syndrome.*

endotracheitis (ĕn″dō-trā-kē-ī′tĭs) [″ + *tracheia,* trachea, + *itis,* inflammation] Inflammation of the tracheal mucosa.

endotrachelitis (ĕn″dō-trā-kĕl-ī′tĭs) [″ + *trachelos,* neck, + *itis,* inflammation] Endocervicitis.

endovasculitis (ĕn″dō-văs″kū-lī′tĭs) [″ + L. *vasculum,* vessel, + Gr. *itis,* inflammation] Endangiitis.

endpoint The final objective, result, or resolution of an illness, treatment, or research protocol.

end product The final material or substance left at the completion of a series of reactions, either chemical or physical.

end-stage The final phase of a disease process.

end-stage renal disease ABBR: ESRD. The stage of chronic renal failure in which the clearance of creatinine has fallen to about 5 ml/min. Renal replacement therapies are required to prevent fatal fluid overload, hyperkalemia, and other uremic complications.

ETIOLOGY: End-stage renal disease may occur as a consequence of many other illnesses, including diabetes mellitus, hypertension, glomerulonephritis, vasculitis, multiple myeloma, analgesic overuse, or any of the causes of acute renal failure (for example, shock, dehydration, post-obstructive nephropathy, or exposure to nephrotoxins such as aminoglycosides, lead, or radiocontrast media).

SYMPTOMS: Patients may complain of fatigue (e.g., as a result of anemia), difficulty concentrating, irritability, personality changes, increased sleepiness, nausea, vomiting, anorexia, edema, breathlessness (if fluid retention results in pulmonary edema) or decreased urination. Some patients who become frankly uremic may become stuporous or comatose; others may develop uremic pericarditis. In general, the early symptoms of renal failure are nonspecific.

TREATMENT: Dialysis (either hemodialysis or peritoneal dialysis) or kidney transplantation are used to restore renal function to patients with end-stage renal disease. Other therapies include the administration of water-soluble vitamins, phosphate-binding medications, erythropoietin, and bicarbonate buffers. Dietary manipulations, typically involving meals with restricted amounts of fluids, sodium, potassium, and protein, prevent complications like fluid retention and hyperkalemia. Tight control of blood pressure and blood sugars in patients with hypertension or diabetes, respectively, will prolong the kidney function and prevent deterioration.

PATIENT CARE: Patients with ESRD should avoid medications that may damage the kidneys (such as nonsteroidal anti-inflammatory drugs) or drugs that may accumulate in toxic concentrations as a result of renal failure (that is, drugs that are normally excreted by the kidneys, such as aspirin, magnesium, or metformin).

endurance The ability to withstand extraordinary mental or physical stress for a prolonged period.

endurance training Physical training for athletic events requiring prolonged effort, such as running a marathon, swimming a long distance, or climbing mountains.

endyma (ĕn′dĭm-ă) [Gr., a garment] Ependyma.

enema (ĕn′ĕ-mă) [Gr.] **1.** The introduction of a solution into the rectum and colon to stimulate bowel activity and cause emptying of the lower intestine, for feeding or therapeutic purposes, to give anesthesia, or to aid in radiographic studies. **2.** A solution introduced into the rectum.

air contrast e. An enema in which two contrast agents, thick barium sulfate and air, are introduced simultaneously under fluoroscopic control followed by multiple radiographs of the colon. This technique produces better visualization of mucosal lining lesions, such as polyps or diverticula, than barium enemas performed without air.

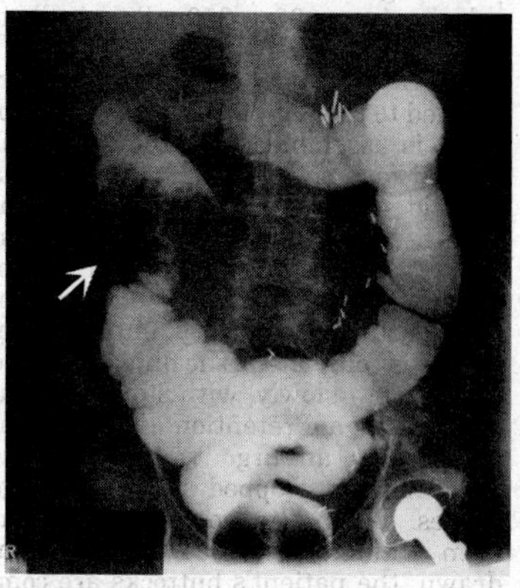

BARIUM ENEMA

Tumor ("apple core" lesion) obstructs flow of barium in ascending colon (Courtesy of Harvey Hatch, MD, Curry General Hospital)

barium e. The use of barium sulfate solution as a contrast agent to facilitate x-ray and fluoroscopic examination of the colon. The examination may be used to screen patients for colon cancer or to identify other colonic lesions, such as diverticula or changes associated with inflammatory bowel disease. Because of the redundancy of the sigmoid colon, barium enema often is used in conjunction with another exam, such as flexible sigmoidoscopy, to improve its sensitivity. Careful preparation of the bowel with laxatives and enemas is critical to eliminate retained feces and improves visualization of the intestinal lumen. SEE: illus.

emollient e. Lubricating e.

high e. An enema designed to reach most of the colon. A rubber tube is inserted into the rectum to carry water as far as possible.

lubricating e. An enema given to soften and ease the passage of feces through the anal canal. SYN: *emollient e.*

medicinal e. Retention e.

nutrient e. An enema containing predigested foods for the purpose of giving sustenance to a patient unable to be fed otherwise. SYN: *nutritive e.*

nutritive e. Nutrient e.

physiological salt solution e. An enema consisting of normal saline solution. It may be used, on rare occasions, to treat dehydration. SYN: *saline e.*

retention e. An enema that may be used to provide nourishment, medication, or anesthetic. It should be made from fluids that will not stimulate peristalsis, such as tap water, soap suds, or physiological saline. A small amount of solution (e.g., 100 to 250 ml) typically is used in adults.

PATIENT CARE: The procedure is explained to the patient. Necessary equipment is assembled, and the patient is draped for privacy and assisted into a left side-lying position with the right knee flexed. The tubing is cleared of air, and the small tube is inserted 3-4 in. into the rectum and is not removed (unless absolutely necessary) until the procedure is completed. The fluid is allowed to flow very slowly, with stops made at intervals to aid retention. If the patient experiences an urge to defecate, the fluid flow is stopped until the urge passes. When the entire volume has been instilled, the tube is quickly withdrawn, the patient's buttocks are compressed together for a few minutes to prevent evacuation, and the patient is encouraged to retain the enema for at least 30 min. The type and amount of fluid instilled, the patient's ability to retain it, and the amount, type, and consistency of the returned fluid and stool are documented. SYN: *medicinal e.*

saline e. Physiological salt solution e.

soapsuds e. An enema consisting of prepared soapsuds or, if liquid soap is used, 30 to 1000 ml of water. Strong soapsuds should not be used because of the danger of injuring intestinal mucosa. Mild white soaps, such as castile, are best.

energetic (ĕn-ĕr-gĕt′ĭk) **1.** Rel. to energy. **2.** Full of energy or vigor.

energetics (ĕn″ĕr-jĕt′ĭks) The study of energy, esp. in relation to human use of energy in the form of food and the expenditure of energy in work or athletic exercise.

energy (ĕn′ĕr-jē) [Gr. *energeia*] The capacity of a system for doing work or its equivalent in the strict physical sense. Energy is manifested in various forms: motion (kinetic energy), position (potential energy), light, heat, ionizing radiation, and sound.

Changes in energy may be physical, chemical, or both. Movement of a part of the body shortens and thickens the muscles involved and changes the position and size of cells temporarily, but intake of oxygen in the blood combined with glucose and fat creates a chemical change and produces heat (energy) and waste products within the cells; fatigue is produced in turn. SEE: *calorie; energy expenditure, basal.*

conservation of e. The principle according to which energy cannot be created or destroyed, but is transformed into other forms.

kinetic e. The energy of motion.

latent e. Energy that exists but is not being used.

potential e. Stored energy.

radiant e. A form of energy transmitted through space. Radio waves, infrared waves, visible rays, ultraviolet waves, x-rays, gamma rays, and cosmic rays are examples of energy in this form. SEE: *electromagnetic spectrum* for table.

energy expenditure, basal ABBR: BEE. The energy used by an individual who is at rest but not asleep. The BEE (expressed as calories) may be calculated by using the Harris-Benedict equations. These account for sex, age, height, and weight. If the individual is sedentary, moderately active, or engaged in strenuous activity, 30%, 40%, or 50%, respectively, are added to the BEE. SEE: *diet; dietetics; food.*

The Harris-Benedict equation involves W (weight in kg), H (height in cm), and A (age in years). The formulae are:

For women: BEE 6.55 + (9.6 × W) + (1.8 × H) – (4.7 × A)

For men: BEE 6.6 + (13.7 × W) + (5 × H) – (6.8 × A)

Hospitalized patients who are nonstressed require 20% more calories than for basal needs.

Energy expended is increased by about 13% over basal needs for each degree centigrade of fever; burn and trauma patients require 40% to 100% more calories than for basal requirements.

energy field disturbance A putative disruption of the flow of energy surrounding a person's being that results in a disharmony of the body, mind, and/or spirit. SEE: *Nursing Diagnoses Appendix.*

enervate (ĕn′ĕr-vāt) To make weak or to lessen the vitality of.

enervation [L. *enervatio*] **1.** Deficiency in nervous strength; weakness. **2.** Resection or removal of a nerve.

ENG *electronystagmography.*

engagement (en-gāj′mĕnt) **1.** In obstetrics, the entry of the largest diameter of the fetal presenting part into the pelvic inlet. SYN: *lightening.* SEE: *labor.* **2.** In the behavioral sciences, a term often used to denote active involvement in everyday activities that have personal meaning.

Engelmann's disk [Theodor W. Engelmann, Ger. physiologist, 1843–1909] H band.

engine A device for converting energy into mechanical motion.

dental e. A machine that rotates dental instruments.

high-speed e. A machine that rotates a dental instrument in excess of 12,000 rpm.

ultraspeed e. A machine that rotates a dental instrument at speeds from 100,000 to 300,000 rpm.

engineering (en-jĭ-nĭr'ĭng) In medical science, the practical application of principles of science and technology to problems posed by health or disease. Branches of this science include human, dental, genetic, and biomechanical, among others.

engorged (ĕn-gorjd') [O. Fr. *engorgier,* to obstruct, to devour] Distended, as with blood or fluids.

engorgement Vascular congestion; distention.

engram (ĕn'grăm) [Gr. *engramm*] A durable protoplasmic mark or trace left by a stimulus in neural tissue.

engrossment An attitude of total focus on something or someone. In obstetrics, the term denotes attachment behavior exhibited by new parents during initial contacts with their newborns.

enhanced organized infant behavior, potential for A pattern of modulation of the physiological and behavioral systems of functioning of an infant (i.e., autonomic, motor, state, organizational, self-regulatory, and attentional-interactional systems) that is satisfactory but that can be improved, resulting in higher levels of integration in response to environmental stimuli. SEE: *Nursing Diagnoses Appendix.*

enhancement (ĕn-hăns'mĕnt) An increase in the effect of ionizing radiation on tissues, produced by the use of oxygen or other chemicals.

enissophobia (ĕn-ĭs"ō-fō'bē-ă) [Gr. *enissein,* to reproach, + *phobos,* fear] Fear of criticism, esp. for having committed a sin.

enkephalin (ĕn-kĕf'ă-lĭn) A pentapeptide produced in the brain. It acts as an opiate and produces analgesia by binding to opiate receptor sites involved in pain perception. The threshold for pain is therefore increased by this action. Enkephalins may have a role in explaining the withdrawal signs of narcotic addiction. SYN: *endogenous opiate-like substance.* SEE: *endorphin; opiate receptor.*

enlargement (ĕn-lărj'mĕnt) An increase in size of anything, esp. of an organ or tissue.

enol (ē'nŏl) A form that a ketone may take by tautomerism. A substance changes from an enol to a ketone by the oscillation of a hydrogen atom from the enol form to the ketone form.

enolase (ē'nō-lās) An enzyme present in muscle tissue that converts phosphoglyceric acid to phosphopyruvic acid.

enology (ē-nŏl'ō-jē) [Gr. *oinos,* wine, + *logos,* word, reason] The science of producing and evaluating wine. Also spelled *oenology.*

enophthalmos (ĕn"ŏf-thăl'mŭs) [Gr. *en,* in, + *ophthalmos,* eye] Recession of the eyeball into the orbit. Opposite of exophthalmos.

enosimania (ĕn"ŏs-ĭ-mā'nē-ă) [Gr. *enosis,* a quaking, + *mania,* madness] A mental state marked by excessive and irrational terror.

enostosis (ĕn"ŏs-tō'sĭs) [Gr. *en,* in, + *osteon,* bone, + *osis,* condition] An osseous tumor within the cavity of a bone.

enriched Having something extra added. For example, vitamins or minerals may be added to a food in order to *enrich* it.

ensiform (ĕn'sĭ-form) [L. *ensis,* sword, + *forma,* form] Xiphoid.

ensisternum (ĕn"sĭs-tĕr'nŭm) [" + Gr. *sternon,* sternum] The lowest portion of the sternum. SYN: *xiphoid process.*

enstrophe (ĕn'strō-fē) [Gr. *en,* in, + *strephein,* to turn] Inversion; a turning inward, esp. of the eyelids.

ENT *ear, nose, and throat.*

ent- SEE: *ento-.*

entad (ĕn'tăd) [" + L. *ad,* toward] Toward the inside; inwardly.

ental (ĕn'tăl) [Gr. *entos,* within] Pert. to the interior; inside; central.

entamebiasis (ĕn"tă-mē-bī'ă-sĭs) [" + *amoibe,* change] Infestation with *Entamoeba.*

Entamoeba (ĕn"tă-mē'bă) A genus of parasitic amebae, several of which are found in the human digestive tract.

E. buccalis E. gingivalis.

E. coli A species of ameba normally found in the human intestinal tract. This species is nonpathogenic to humans.

E. gingivalis A nonpathogenic species of ameba that inhabits the mouth. SYN: *E. buccalis.*

E. histolytica A pathogenic species of ameba, the cause of amebic dysentery and tropical liver abscess. SEE: illus.; *amebiasis.*

enter- SEE: *entero-.*

enteral (ĕn'tĕr-ăl) [Gr. *enteron,* intestine] Within or by way of the intestine.

enteralgia (ĕn"tĕr-ăl'jē-ă) [" + *algos,* pain] Pain in the intestines; intestinal cramps or colic. SYN: *enterodynia.*

enteral tube feeding A means of providing nutrition for a patient unable to consume food normally through the usual route due to a difficulty with chewing or swallowing, or an oral, pharyngeal, or esophageal deformity, a specific blockage or generalized weakness. A patient

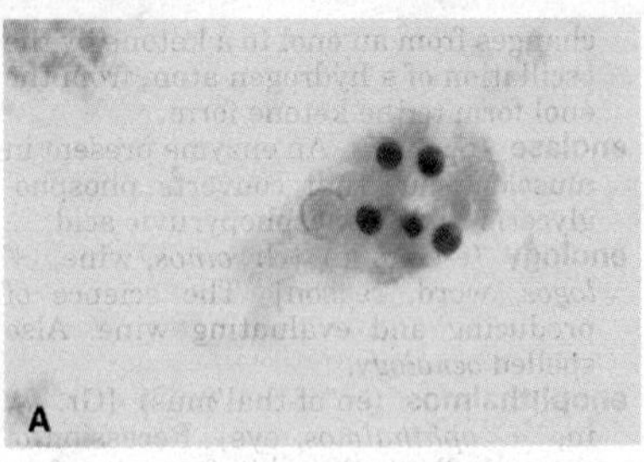

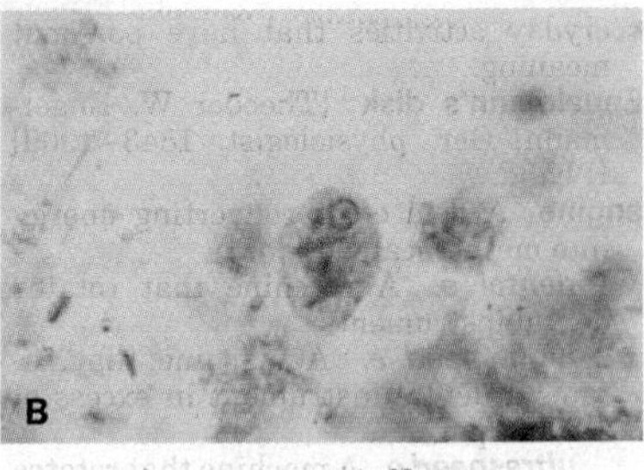

ENTAMOEBA HISTOLYTICA

(A) trophozoite with five ingested red blood cells (orig. mag. ×1000), (B) cyst in fecal debris (orig. mag. ×1000)

is fed an appropriate formula through a tube passed into the stomach or duodenum from the nasal passage (nasogastric or nasoduodenal tube), or by a gastrostomy or jejunostomy tube. SYN: *total enteral n.*

TYPES OF FORMULAS: *Intact nutrient:* These formulas are called "standard." Because the nutrients are "whole," they are appropriate for use whenever normal digestion takes place. They usually provide 1 kcal/ml and can be used orally. *Hydrolyzed nutrient:* In these formulas, the nutrients are "predigested" and are suitable for use whenever malabsorption is present or when the jejunum is the feeding site. These formulas are not appropriate for oral use because of their taste. They are more expensive than intact nutrient formulas. *Elemental (defined):* Because nutrients in these formulas are in the simplest, most basic form, they are rapidly absorbed from the gut. These formulas are not appropriate for oral use. This type of formula is the most expensive. Formulas designed for specific diseases are available. *Modular:* Commercially produced nutritional products may be used as supplements to standard formulas. For example, the addition of a protein module would convert a standard formula to a high-protein formula.

METHODS OF DELIVERY: *Bolus administration:* Formula is delivered in four to six daily feedings by a large syringe attached to the feeding tube in the stomach. This type of delivery is the least well tolerated. *Intermittent infusion:* Formula is delivered four to six times daily over 30 to 60 min per feeding using a pump or gravity. This type of delivery is better tolerated. *Continuous drip:* An infusion pump delivers slow drips 16 to 24 hr/day. This is the best tolerated type of delivery.

enterectomy (ĕn″tĕr-ĕk′tō-mē) [″ + *ektome,* excision] Excision of a portion of the intestines.

enteric (ĕn-tĕr′ĭk) [Gr. *enteron,* intestine] Pert. to the small intestine.

enteric bacilli A broad term for bacilli present in the intestinal tract. Included are gram-negative non–spore-forming facultatively anaerobic bacilli such as *Escherichia, Shigella, Salmonella, Klebsiella,* and *Yersinia.* They may be present in the intestines of vertebrates as normal flora or pathogens.

enteric-coated ABBR: EC. A drug formulation in which tablets or capsules are coated with a compound that does not dissolve until the pill is exposed to the fluids in the small intestine.

enteric fever Typhoid fever.

enteritis (ĕn″tĕr-ī′tĭs) [″ + *itis,* inflammation] Inflammation of the intestines, particularly of the mucosa and submucosa of the small intestine. SEE: *Nursing Diagnoses Appendix.*

regional e. SEE: *ileitis, regional.*

entero-, enter- [Gr. *enteron,* intestine] Combining form meaning *intestines.*

enteroanastomosis (ĕn″tĕr-ō-ăn-ăs″tō-mō′sĭs) [″ + *anastomosis,* opening] An intestinal anastomosis.

enteroantigen (ĕn″tĕr-ō-ăn′tĭ-jĕn) [″ + *anti,* against, + *gennan,* to produce] An antigen derived from the intestines.

Enterobacter A group of enteric gram-negative rods of the family Enterobacteriaceae that occur in soil, dairy products, water, sewage, and the intestinal tracts of humans and animals. Often they are secondary pathogens or produce opportunistic infections. In humans, many of these infections are hospital acquired (nosocomial).

E. aerogenes A species of *Enterobacter* that occurs normally in the intestine of humans and other animals and is found in decayed matter, on grains, and in plants. The organism is important in causing urinary tract infections and intestinal disease when antibiotic therapy causes elimination of other organisms. It was formerly called *Aerobacter aerogenes.*

E. agglomerans A species of *Enterobacter* formerly called *Erwinia*. It has been associated with serious systemic infections, particularly septicemia from contaminated intravenous fluids.

E. cloacae A species of *Enterobacter* that, along with *E. agglomerans*, accounts for most nosocomial infections caused by this genus, esp. those due to intravenous line contamination.

Enterobacteriaceae (ĕn″tĕr-ō-băk-tē″rē-ā′sē-ē) A family of gram-negative, non-spore-forming aerobes. Some are intestinal pathogens, others are usually normal colonizers of the human intestinal tract. Included in the family are *Shigella, Salmonella, Escherichia, Klebsiella, Proteus, Enterobacter,* and *Yersinia.*

enterobiasis (ĕn″tĕr-ō-bī′ă-sĭs) [Gr. *enteron,* intestine, + *bios,* life] Infestation with pinworms *(Enterobius vermicularis).* SYN: *oxyuriasis.*

enterobiliary (ĕn″tĕr-ō-bĭl′ē-ār-ē) [″ + L. *bilis,* bile] Pert. to the intestines and the bile passages.

Enterobius (ĕn″tĕr-ō′bē-ŭs) [″ + *bios,* life] A genus of parasitic nematode worms, formerly *Oxyuris vermicularis.*

E. vermicularis A species of parasitic nematode worms, commonly known as "pinworms," that causes enterobiasis, an infestation of the large intestine. The adult worms live in the cecum and adjacent portions of the colon; the females migrate to the anus and lay their eggs on the perianal skin. Infestations cause irritation of the anal region and allergic reaction of the neighboring skin, accompanied by intense itching, which may result in loss of sleep, excessive irritability, and a secondary infection of the area around the anus as a result of the scratching. Distribution is worldwide. It is estimated that in temperate climates 20% of children have this condition. Female worms average 8 to 13 mm in length and males 2 to 5 mm. SYN: *pinworm.* SEE: illus.

DIAGNOSIS: The presence of adult worms in feces or on the anus confirms the diagnosis. Transparent, pressure-sensitive tape may be applied to the perianal area and then examined microscopically for eggs. This latter test is more likely to be positive in the morning before bathing.

TREATMENT: Pyrantel pamoate, albendazole, or mebendazole is effective. During treatment tight-fitting sleep wear should be used to prevent the eggs from contaminating the bedding. The house, bedding, and night clothes must be thoroughly cleaned daily for several days during treatment. Family recurrences may be prevented if the entire family is treated.

enterocele (ĕn′tĕr-ō-sēl) [″ + *keke,* hernia] **1.** A hernia of the intestine through the vagina. **2.** A posterior vaginal hernia.

enterocentesis (ĕn″tĕr-ō-sĕn-tē′sĭs) [″ + *kentesis,* puncture] Puncture of the intestine to withdraw gas or fluids.

enterocholecystostomy (ĕn″tĕr-ō-kō″lē-sĭs-tŏs′tō-mē) [″ + *chole,* bile, + *kystis,* bladder, + *stoma,* mouth] A surgically created opening between the gallbladder and small intestine. SYN: *cholecystenterostomy.*

enterocholecystotomy (ĕn″tĕr-ō-kō″lē-sĭs-tŏt′ō-mē) [″ + ″ + ″ + *tome,* incision] Incision of both the gallbladder and the intestine.

enteroclysis (ĕn″tĕr-ŏk′lĭ-sĭs) [″ + *klysis,* a washing out] **1.** Injection of a nutrient or medicinal liquid into the bowel. **2.** Irrigation of the colon with a large amount of fluid intended to fill the colon completely and flush it. SEE: *enema.* **3.** Radiography of the small bowel. A tube is advanced into the duodenum under fluoroscopic guidance and barium is given, followed by insufflation of the bowel with air.

Enterococcus (ĕn″tĕr-ō-kŏk′ŭs) A genus of gram-positive bacteria belonging to the family Streptococcaceae, formerly classified as part of the genus *Streptococcus,* but now classified as a separate

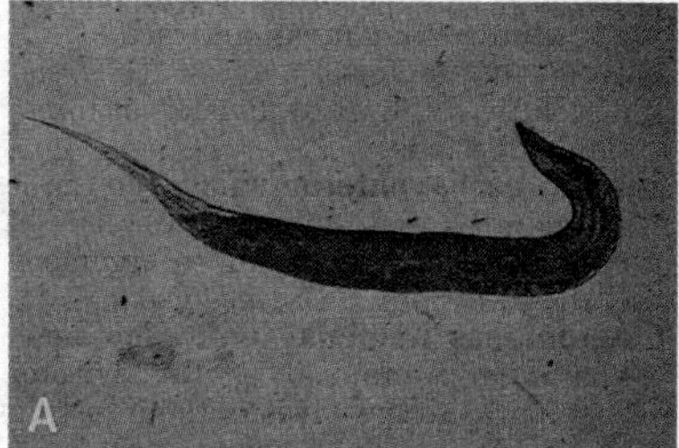

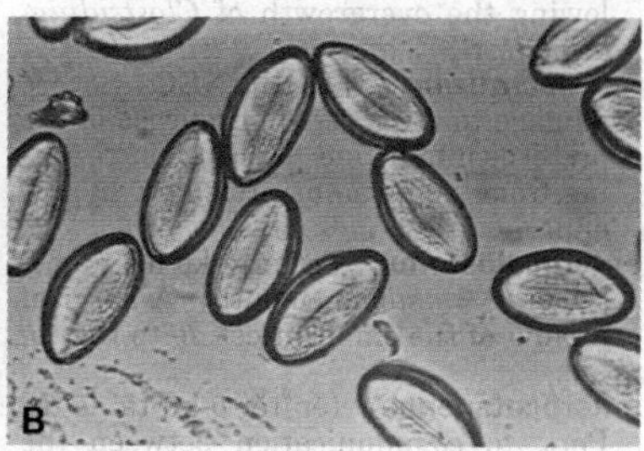

ENTEROBIUS VERMICULARIS

(A) female (orig. mag. ×10), (B) eggs (orig. mag. ×400)

genus. Of the 12 or more species, *E. faecalis* and *E. faecium* are found normally in the human gastrointestinal tract. They may produce urinary tract infections, or other serious infections that are resistant to many antibiotics.

vancomycin-resistant e. ABBR: VRE. A strain of *Enterococcus faecium* resistant to anti-infective agents, including penicillins, aminoglycosides, and vancomycin. Infection with VRE presents a major threat to susceptible patients because no consistently effective antimicrobial drug treatment has been identified and because the resistant genes can be transferred to other gram-positive organisms, such as *Staphylococcus aureus,* making these also more difficult to eradicate.

To prevent the spread of VRE, the organism is identified by culture and sensitivity testing as soon as the infection is recognized. Patients are isolated in private rooms or cohorted with other colonized patients. All persons entering the patient's room don gloves; hands are washed carefully and gloves are removed. Charts and flow sheets should not be taken into the room. Hospitals should heed the guidelines that have been developed for the use of vancomycin, to minimize the spread of vancomycin resistance to other organisms. SEE: *antibiotic resistance; multidrug resistance; Standard and Universal Precautions Appendix.*

enterocolectomy (ĕn″tĕr-ō-kō-lĕk′tō-mē) [″ + *kolon,* colon, + *ektome,* excision] Surgical removal of the terminal ileum, cecum, and ascending colon.

enterocolitis (ĕn″tĕr-ō-kō-lī′tĭs) [″ + ″ + *itis,* inflammation] Inflammation of the small or large bowel, usually as a result of an infectious disease. The most common causative organisms include rotaviruses and other enteric viruses, *Salmonella, Escherichia coli, Shigella, Campylobacter,* and *Yersinia* species. A potentially severe presentation, pseudomembranous enterocolitis, may be induced by prolonged use of antibiotics allowing the overgrowth of *Clostridium difficile*. SEE: *diarrhea; gastroenteritis.*

necrotizing e. ABBR: NEC. Severe damage to the intestinal mucosa of the preterm infant due to ischemia resulting from asphyxia or prolonged hypoxemia.

enterocolostomy (ĕn″tĕr-ō-kō-lŏs′tō-mē) [″ + ″ + *stoma,* mouth] A surgical joining of the small intestine to the colon.

enterocutaneous (ĕn″tĕr-ō-kū-tā′nē-ŭs) Pert. to communication between the skin and intestine.

enterocyst (ĕn′tĕr-ō-sĭst) [Gr. *enteron,* intestine, + *kystis,* bladder] A benign cyst of the intestinal wall.

enterocystocele (ĕn″tĕr-ō-sĭs′tō-sēl) [″ + *kele,* tumor, swelling] A hernia of the bladder wall and intestine.

enterocystoma (ĕn″tĕr-ō-sĭs-tō′mă) [″ + ″ + *oma,* tumor] A cystic tumor of the intestinal wall.

enterocystoplasty (ĕn″tĕr-ō-sĭs′tō-plăs″tē) [″ + ″ + *plastos,* formed] A plastic surgical procedure involving the use of a portion of intestine to enlarge the bladder.

Enterocytozoon A genus of the order Microsporidia. SEE: *microsporidiosis.*

enterodynia (ĕn″tĕr-ō-dĭn′ē-ă) [″ + *odyne,* pain] Enteralgia.

enteroenterostomy (ĕn″tĕr-ō-ĕn″tĕr-ŏs′tō-mē) [″ + *enteron,* intestine, + *stoma,* mouth] Surgical creation of a communication between two intestinal segments.

enteroepiplocele (ĕn″tĕr-ō-ē-pĭp′lō-sēl) [″ + *epiploon,* omentum, + *kele,* tumor, swelling] A hernia of the small intestine and omentum.

enterogastritis (ĕn″tĕr-ō-găs-trī′tĭs) [″ + *gaster,* belly, + *itis,* inflammation] Inflammation of the stomach (gastritis) and the intestines (enteritis).

enterogastrone (ĕn″tĕr-ō-găs′trōn) A hormone such as secretin that is released by the intestinal mucosa and controls the release of food from the stomach into the duodenum by depressing gastric motility and secretion. A fatty meal causes greater secretion of this hormone than a normal meal does.

enterogenous (ĕn″tĕr-ŏj′ĕ-nŭs) [″ + *gennan,* to produce] Originating in the small intestines.

enterohepatic (ĕn″tĕr-ō-hĕ-păt′ĭk) [″ + *hepar,* liver] Pert. to the intestines and liver.

enterohepatitis (ĕn″tĕr-ō-hĕp-ă-tī′tĭs) [″ + ″ + *itis,* inflammation] Inflammation of the intestine and liver.

enterohydrocele (ĕn″tĕr-ō-hī′drō-sēl) [″ + *hydor,* water, + *kele,* tumor, swelling] A hydrocele with a loop of intestine in the sac.

enterokinase (ĕn″tĕr-ō-kī′nās) [″ + *kinesis,* movement] Previous term for enteropeptidase.

enterology [″ + *logos,* word, reason] The study of the intestinal tract.

enterolysis (ĕn″tĕr-ŏl′ĭ-sĭs) [″ + *lysis,* dissolution] Surgical division of intestinal adhesions.

enteromegalia, enteromegaly (ĕn″tĕr-ō-mĕ-gā′lē-ă, ĕn″tĕr-ō-mĕg′ă-lē) [″ + *megas,* large] Abnormal enlargement of the intestines. SYN: *megacolon.*

Enteromonas hominis (ĕn″tĕr-ŏm′ō-năs hŏm′ĭn-ĭs) A minute, flagellated protozoan parasite that lives in the intestine of humans. It is rare and considered nonpathogenic.

enteromycosis (ĕn″tĕr-ō-mī-kō′sĭs) [″ + *mykes,* fungus, + *osis,* diseased condition] A disease of the intestine resulting from bacteria or fungi.

enteromyiasis (ĕn″tĕr-ō-mī-ī′ă-sĭs) [″ + *myia,* fly] A disease caused by the presence of maggots (the larvae of flies) in the intestines.

enteron (ĕn′tĕr-ŏn) [Gr.] Alimentary canal.

enteroneuritis (ĕn″tĕr-ō-nū-rī′tĭs) [″ + *neuron,* nerve, + *itis,* inflammation] Inflammation of the intestinal nerves.

entero-oxyntin A hormone found in animals but not humans believed to be released by the small intestine in response to the presence of chyme. It is thought to cause the parietal cells of the gastric mucosa to release hydrochloric acid. SEE: *gastrin.*

enteroparesis (ĕn″tĕr-ō-păr′ē-sĭs) [″ + *paresis,* relaxation] Reduced peristalsis of the intestines; an old term for ileus.

enteropathogen (ĕn″tĕr-ō-păth′ō-jĕn) [″ + *pathos,* disease, suffering, + *gennan,* to produce] Any microorganism that causes intestinal disease.

enteropathy (ĕn″tĕr-ŏp′ă-thē) [″ + *pathos,* disease, suffering] Any intestinal disease.

gluten-induced e. Celiac sprue.

gluten-sensitive e. Celiac sprue.

radiation e. Damage to the intestines due to radiation.

enteropeptidase (ĕn″tĕr-ō-pĕp′tĭ-dās) An enzyme of the duodenal mucosa that converts pancreatic trypsinogen to active trypsin. Formerly called *enterokinase.*

enteropexy (ĕn′tĕr-ō-pĕks″ē) [″ + *pexis,* fixation] Fixation of the intestine to the abdominal wall or to another portion of the intestine.

enteroplegia (ĕn″tĕr-ō-plē′jē-ă) [″ + *plege,* stroke] Paralysis of the intestines. SEE: *paralytic ileus.*

enteroplex (ĕn′tĕr-ō-plĕks) [″ + *plexis,* a weaving] An instrument for joining cut edges of intestines.

enteroplexy Surgical union of divided parts of the intestine. SYN: *enteroanastomosis.*

enteroptosis (ĕn″tĕr-ŏp-tō′sĭs) [″ + *ptosis,* a falling or dropping] Prolapse of the intestines or abdominal organs.

enterorrhaphy (ĕn″tĕr-or′ă-fē) [″ + *rhaphe,* seam, ridge] Stitching of an intestinal wound, or of the intestines to some other structure.

enterorrhexis (ĕn″tĕr-ō-rĕks′ĭs) [″ + *rhexis,* rupture] Rupture of the intestine.

enteroscope (ĕn′tĕr-ō-skōp″) [″ + *skopein,* to examine] Endoscope

enterosepsis (ĕn″tĕr-ō-sĕp′sĭs) [″ + *sepsis,* decay] A condition in which bacteria in the intestines produce intestinal sepsis. SEE: *enterotoxemia.*

enterospasm (ĕn′tĕr-ō-spăzm) [Gr. *enteron,* intestine, + *spasmos,* spasm] Intermittent painful contractions of the intestines.

enterostasis (ĕn″tĕr-ō-stā′sĭs) [″ + *stasis,* a standing] Cessation of or delay in the passage of food through the intestine; an old term for ileus.

enterostenosis (ĕn″tĕr-ō-stĕ-nō′sĭs) [″ + *stenosis,* a narrowing] Narrowing or stricture of the intestine.

enterostomal therapist ABBR: ET. An individual trained to teach patients proper methods of caring for an ostomy. The certification title is *certified enterostomal therapy nurse* (CETN).

enterostomy (ĕn″tĕr-ŏs′tō-mē) [″ + *stoma,* mouth] A surgically created opening into a portion of the gastrointestinal tract.

enterotoxemia (ĕn″tĕr-ō-tŏk-sē′mē-ă) A condition in which bacterial toxins are absorbed from the intestine and circulate in the blood.

enterotoxigenic (ĕn″tĕr-ō-tŏk″sĭ-jĕn′ĭk) Producing enterotoxins, as in some strains of bacteria.

enterotoxin (ĕn″tĕr-ō-tŏk′sĭn) [″ + *toxikon,* poison] **1.** A toxin produced in or originating in the intestinal contents. **2.** An exotoxin specific for the cells of the intestinal mucosa. **3.** An exotoxin produced by certain species of bacteria that causes various diseases, including food poisoning and toxic shock syndrome.

Enterovirus A group of viruses that originally included poliovirus, coxsackievirus, and ECHO virus, which infected the human gastrointestinal tract. Enteroviruses are now classed as a genus of picornaviruses. SEE: *picornavirus.*

enterozoic (ĕn″tĕr-ō-zō′ĭk) [″ + *zoon,* animal] Pert. to parasites inhabiting the intestines.

enthesitis (ĕn-thē-sī′tĭs) Tenderness to palpation at the site of attachment of bone to a tendon, ligament, or joint capsule. It is usually caused by trauma to the area.

enthlasis (ĕn′thlă-sĭs) [Gr., dent caused by pressure] A depressed fracture of the skull.

entire (ĕn-tīr′) In bacteriology, the smooth, regular border of a bacterial colony.

entitlement **1.** A right or benefit. **2.** A form of compensation granted to an individual because of a special status under the law (e.g., an entitlement to health insurance under the Medicare program).

entity (ĕn′tĭ-tē) [L. *ens,* being] **1.** A thing existing independently, containing in itself all the conditions necessary to individuality. **2.** Something that forms a complete whole, denoting a distinct condition or disease.

ento-, ent- [Gr. *entos,* within] Combining form meaning *within, inside.*

entoblast (ĕn′tō-blăst) [″ + *blastos,* germ] A term formerly used to signify the endoderm.

entocele (ĕn′tō-sēl) [″ + *kele,* tumor, swelling] Internal hernia.

entochondrostosis (ĕn″tō-kŏn″drŏs-tō′sĭs) [″ + *chondros,* cartilage, + *osis,* condition] The development of bone within cartilage.

entochoroidea (ĕn″tō-kō-roy′dē-ă) [″ + *chorioeides,* choroid] The inner layer of the choroid of the eye. SYN: *lamina choriocapillaris.*

entocone (ĕn′tō-kōn) [″ + *konos,* cone] The inner posterior cusp of an upper molar tooth.

entocornea (ĕn″tō-kor′nē-ă) [″ + L. *corneus,* horny] The posterior limiting membrane of the cornea. SYN: *Descemet's membrane.*

entoectad (ĕn″tō-ĕk′tăd) [″ + *ektos,* without, + L. *ad,* toward] Proceeding outward from within.

entome (ĕn′tōm) [Gr. *en,* in, + *tome,* incision] A knife for division of urethral strictures.

entomion (ĕn-tō′mē-ŏn) [Gr. *entome,* notch] The tip of the mastoid angle of the parietal bone.

entomology (ĕn″tō-mŏl′ō-jē) [Gr. *entomon,* insect, + *logos,* word, reason] The study of insects.

medical e. The branch of entomology that deals with insects and their relationship to disease, esp. of humans.

entomophthoramycosis (ĕn-tō-mŏf′thō-ră-mī-kō′sĭs) A disease caused by fungi of the class Zygomycetes, which includes two genera (*Conidiobolus* and *Basidiobolus*) responsible for human disease. *Conidiobolus* causes infections of the heart and face; *Basidiobolus* produces infections in other parts of the body.

SYMPTOMS: Clinically, there is swelling of the nose, perinasal tissues, and mouth. Nodular subcutaneous masses are palpable in the skin.

TREATMENT: Antifungal drugs such as amphotericin B, terbinafine, or ketoconazole are used, often as part of a regimen that includes surgery to remove infected tissues.

entopic [Gr. *en,* in, + *topos,* place] Normally situated; in a normal place. Opposite of ectopic.

entoptic (ĕn-tŏp′tĭk) [Gr. *entos,* within, + *optikos,* seeing] Pert. to the interior of the eye.

entoptic phenomenon A visual phenomenon arising from within the eye, marked by the perception of floating bodies, circles of light, black spots, and transient flashes of light. It may be due to the individual's own blood cells moving through the retinal vessels, or to floaters, which are small specks of tissue floating in the vitreous fluid. SEE: *Moore's lightning streaks; muscae volitantes; photopsia.*

Individuals may see imperfections of their own cornea, lens, and vitreous by looking at a white background through a pinhole held about 17 mm (4.3 in.) from the eye. The person sees a patch of light the size of which varies with the diameter of the pupil. The abnormalities are seen as shadows or bright areas. This method can be used also to see early discrete lens opacities.

entoretina (ĕn″tō-rĕt′ĭ-nă) [″ + L. *rete,* a net] The internal layer of the retina.

entotic (ĕn-tō′tĭk, ĕn-tŏt′ĭk) [″ + *ous,* ear] Pert. to the interior of the ear or to the perception of sound as affected by the condition of the auditory apparatus.

entozoon (ĕn″tō-zō′ŏn) *pl.* **entozoa** [″ + *zoon,* animal] Any animal parasite living within the body of another animal.

entrails The intestines of an animal.

entrain To alter the biological rhythm of an organism so that it assumes a cycle different from a 24-hour one.

entrainment **1.** Gaining control of a heart rhythm (esp. a tachycardic rhythm) with an external stimulus such as a cardiac pacemaker. **2.** The drawing of a second fluid into a stream of gas or fluid by the Bernoulli effect.

entropion (ĕn-trō′pē-ŏn) [Gr. *en,* in, + *trepein,* to turn] An inversion or turning inward of an edge, esp. the margin of the lower eyelid.

cicatricial e. An inversion resulting from scar tissue on the inner surface of the lid.

spastic e. An inversion resulting from a spasm of the orbicularis oculi muscles.

entropionize (ĕn-trō′pē-ō-nīz) To invert or correct by turning in.

entropy (ĕn′trŏ-pē) [Gr. *en,* in, + *trope,* a turning] **1.** The portion of energy within a system that cannot be used for mechanical work but is available for internal use. **2.** The quantity or degree of randomness, disorder, or chaos in a system.

enucleate (ē-nū′klē-āt) [L. *enucleare,* to remove the kernel of] **1.** To remove a part or a mass in its entirety. **2.** To destroy or take out the nucleus of a cell. **3.** To remove the eyeball surgically. **4.** To remove a cataract surgically.

enucleation (ē-nū″klē-ā′shŭn) Removal of an entire mass or part, esp. a tumor or the eyeball, without rupture.

enucleator (ĕ-nū′klē-ā-tor) An instrument for evacuating a tumor mass, such as myoma, intact, e.g., after removal of the ocular globe.

enuresis (ĕn″ū-rē′sĭs) [Gr. *enourein,* to void urine] Involuntary discharge of urine after the age at which bladder control should have been established. In children, voluntary control of urination is usually present by 5 years of age. Nevertheless, nocturnal enuresis is present in about 10% of otherwise healthy 5-year-old children and 1% of normal 15-year-old children. Enuresis is slightly more common in boys than in girls and occurs more frequently in first-born children. This condition has a distinct family tendency. SEE: *nocturnal e.; bladder drill.*

ETIOLOGY: In most instances there is no organic basis for persistent enuresis. These cases are probably due to inadequate or misguided attempts at toilet training. Also, emotional stress, such as the birth of a sibling, a death in the family, or separation from the family, may be associated with the onset of enuresis in a previously continent child. Conditions that may cause enuresis include urinary tract infection, increased fluid intake due to diabetes mellitus, any disease that interferes with the formation of concentrated urine, trauma to or disease of the spinal cord, and epilepsy.

TREATMENT: When no organic disease is present, the use of imipramine as a temporary adjunct may be helpful. This is usually given in a dose of 10 to 50 mg orally at bedtime, but the effectiveness may decrease with continued administration. The bladder may be trained to hold larger amounts of urine. This procedure has decreased the occurrence rate of enuresis. No matter what the cause, the child should not be made to feel guilty or ashamed, and the family and the child should regard enuresis as they would any other condition that lends itself to appropriate therapy. If the child tries too hard to control the condition, it may worsen. Conditioning devices that sound an alarm when bedwetting occurs should not be used unless prescribed by a health care professional familiar with the treatment of enuresis.

CAUTION: Imipramine is not recommended for children under 6 years of age. Blood counts should be taken at least monthly during therapy to detect the possible onset of granulocytosis.

---

diurnal e. Urinary incontinence during the day. Its cause is usually pathological. It may be caused by muscular contractions brought about by laughing, coughing, or crying. SEE: *stress urinary incontinence.*

It often persists for long periods, esp. after protracted illness. It occurs more commonly in women and girls.

nocturnal e. Urinary incontinence during the night, more commonly known as bedwetting. It is irregular and unaccompanied by urgency or frequency. It is more common in boys than in girls.

PATIENT CARE: Fluid should be restricted late in the day and diurnal voidings should be spaced at more than ordinary intervals. The child may be awakened once or twice in the night and, when fully awake, robed and walked to the bathroom. As improvement is noticed, the number of awakenings may be lessened. The foot of the bed may also be elevated. Electronic devices that awaken the child the moment the bed is wet may be helpful. The use of desmopressin acetate nasal spray at bedtime or tricyclic antidepressants, such as imipramine, have been successful in preventing bedwetting. Adults who experience nocturnal enuresis should be evaluated for signs of neurological disorders. SEE: *enuresis.*

primary e. Enuresis in which a child has never been dependably continent.

secondary e. Enuresis in a child with no history of incontinence for a year or more.

envelope (ĕn′vĕ-lōp) A covering or container.

nuclear e. Two parallel membranes containing a narrow perinuclear space and enveloping the nucleus of a cell. Before the advent of electron microscopy, the nucleus was thought to be surrounded by a single, thin membrane. SEE: *nuclear membrane.*

envenomation (ĕn-vĕn″ō-mā′shŭn) The introduction of poisonous venoms into the body by means of a bite or sting.

environment [O. Fr. *en-*, in, + *viron,* circle] The surroundings, conditions, or influences that affect an organism or the cells within it.

neutrothermal e. Thermoneutral e.

thermoneutral e. An environment with an ambient temperature that minimizes the risk of heat loss via conduction, convection, radiation, and evaporation; often used to protect newborns. SYN: *neutrothermal e.*

environmental control unit ABBR: ECU. An electronic device that remotely controls home climate (e.g., heating, air conditioning), security (e.g., lighting, door locks, drapes), and communication devices (telephone, television). ECUs are often, but not exclusively, used by persons with functional limitations.

environmental interpretation syndrome, impaired Consistent lack of orientation to person, place, time, or circumstances over more than 3 to 6 months, necessitating a protective environment. SEE: *Nursing Diagnoses Appendix.*

envy Unhappiness about or the wish to possess qualities, physical attributes, or belongings of someone else.

penis e. SEE: *penis envy.*

enzootic (ĕn″zō-ŏt′ĭk) [Gr. *en,* in, + *zoon,* animal] An endemic disease limited to a small number of animals.

enzygotic (ĕn″zī-gŏt′ĭk) [Gr. *en,* in, + *zygon,* yoke] Developed from the same ovum.

enzyme (ĕn′zīm) [″ + *zyme,* leaven] An organic catalyst produced by living cells but capable of acting outside cells or even in vitro. Enzymes are proteins that change the rate of chemical reactions without needing an external energy source or being changed themselves; an enzyme may catalyze a reaction numerous times. Enzymes are reaction specific in that they act only on certain substances (called substrates). The enzyme and its substrate or substrates form a temporary configuration, called an enzyme-substrate complex, that involves both physical shape and chemical bonding. The enzyme promotes the formation of bonds between separate substrates, or induces the breaking of bonds in a single substrate to form the product or products of the reaction. The human body contains thousands of enzymes, each catalyzing one of the many reactions that take place as part of metabolism.

Each enzyme has an optimum temperature and pH at which it functions most efficiently. For most human enzymes, these would be body temperature and the pH of cells, tissue fluid, or blood. Enzyme activity can be impaired by extremes of temperature or pH, the presence of heavy metals (lead or mercury), dehydration, or ultraviolet radiation. Some enzymes require coenzymes (nonprotein molecules such as vitamins) to function properly; still others require certain minerals (iron, copper, zinc). Certain enzymes are produced in an inactive form (a proenzyme) and must be activated (e.g., inactive pepsinogen is converted to active pepsin by the hydrochloric acid in gastric juice).

ACTION: Of the many human enzymes, the digestive enzymes are probably the most familiar. These are hydrolytic enzymes that catalyze the addition of water molecules to large food molecules to split them into simpler chemicals. Often the name of the enzyme indicates the substrate with the addition of the suffix *-ase*. A lipase splits fats to fatty acids and glycerol; a peptidase splits peptides to amino acids. Some enzymes such as pepsin and trypsin do not end in *-ase;* they were named before this method of nomenclature was instituted.

Enzymes are also needed for synthesis reactions. The synthesis of proteins, nucleic acids, phospholipids for cell membranes, hormones, and glycogen all require one if not many enzymes. DNA polymerase, for example, is needed for DNA replication, which precedes mitosis. Energy production also requires many enzymes. Each step in cell respiration (glycolysis, Krebs cycle, cytochrome transport system) requires a specific enzyme. Deaminases remove the amino groups from excess amino acids so that they may be used for energy. Long-chain fatty acids are split by enzymes into smaller compounds to be used in cell respiration. Blood clotting, the formation of angiotensin II to raise blood pressure, and the transport of carbon dioxide in the blood all require specific enzymes.

activating e. An enzyme that catalyzes the attaching of an amino acid to the appropriate transfer ribonucleic acid.

allosteric e. An enzyme whose activity can change when certain types of effectors, called allosteric effectors, bind to a nonactive site on the enzyme.

amylolytic e. An enzyme that catalyzes the conversion of starch to sugar.

angiotensin-converting e. ABBR: ACE. An enzyme normally found in the capillary endothelium throughout the vascular system. It converts angiotensin I (a part of the renin-angiotensin-aldosterone mechanism of the kidney) to angiotensin II, the final step in the renin-angiotensin mechanism. The latter stimulates aldosterone secretion and therefore sodium retention.

autolytic e. An enzyme that produces autolysis, or cell digestion.

bacterial e. An enzyme produced by bacteria.

branching e. An enzyme, called a glycosyltransferase, that transfers a carbohydrate unit from one molecule to another.

brush border e. An enzyme produced by the cells of the villi and microvilli (brush border) lining the small intestine.

coagulating e. An enzyme that catalyzes the conversion of soluble proteins into insoluble ones. SYN: *coagulase*.

deamidizing e. An enzyme that splits amine off amino acid compounds.

debranching e. An enzyme, dextrin-1-6-glucosidase, that removes a carbohydrate unit from molecules that contain short carbohydrate units attached as side chains.

decarboxylating e. An enzyme, such as carboxylase, that separates carbon dioxide from organic acids.

digestive e. Any enzyme involved in digestive processes in the alimentary canal.

extracellular e. An enzyme that acts outside the cell that produces it.

fermenting e. An enzyme produced by bacteria or yeasts that brings about fermentation, esp. of carbohydrates.

glycolytic e. An enzyme that catalyzes the oxidation of glucose.

hydrolytic e. An enzyme that catalyzes hydrolysis.

inhibitory e. An enzyme that blocks a chemical reaction.

intracellular e. An enzyme that acts within the cell that produces it.

inverting e. An enzyme that catalyzes the hydrolysis of sucrose.

lipolytic e. An enzyme that catalyzes the hydrolysis of fats. SYN: *lipase*.

mucolytic e. An enzyme that depolymerizes mucus by splitting mucoproteins. Examples are lysozyme and hyaluronidase. SYN: *mucinase.*

oxidizing e. An enzyme that catalyzes oxidative reactions. SYN: *oxidase.*

proteolytic e. An enzyme that catalyzes the conversion of proteins into peptides.

redox e. An enzyme that catalyzes oxidation-reduction reactions.

reducing e. An enzyme that removes oxygen. SYN: *reductase.*

respiratory e. An enzyme, such as a cytochrome or a flavoprotein, that acts within tissue cells to catalyze oxidative reactions by releasing energy.

splitting e. An enzyme that facilitates removal of part of a molecule.

transferring e. An enzyme that facilitates the moving of one molecule to another compound. SYN: *transferase.*

uricolytic e. An enzyme that catalyzes the conversion of uric acid into urea.

yellow e. One of a group of flavoproteins involved in cellular oxidations.

Enzyme Commission ABBR: EC. An organization created in 1956 by the International Union of Biochemistry to standardize enzyme nomenclature.

enzyme induction The adaptive increase in the number of molecules of a specific enzyme secondary to either an increase in its synthesis rate or a decrease in its degradation rate.

enzyme-linked immunosorbent assay ABBR: ELISA. A rapid enzyme immunochemical assay method in which either an antibody or an antigen can be coupled to an enzyme. The resulting complex retains both immunological and enzymatic activity. The ELISA method can detect certain bacterial antigens and antibodies as well as hormones; it is one of the primary diagnostic tests for many infectious diseases, including the human immunodeficiency virus (HIV). The sensitivity is enhanced by the addition of an antibody to an enzyme such as alkaline phosphatase. An intense color reaction is produced. These assays are quite sensitive and specific as compared with the radioimmune assay (RIA) tests, and have the advantage of not requiring radioisotopes or the expensive counting apparatus.

enzymology (ĕn″zī-mŏl′ō-jē) The study of enzymes and their actions.

enzymolysis (ĕn-zī-mŏl′ĭ-sĭs) [Gr. *en,* in, + *zyme,* leaven, + *lysis,* dissolution] Chemical change or disintegration due to an enzyme.

enzymopathy (ĕn″zī-mŏp′ă-thē) Any disease involving an enzyme abnormality (can be due to sufficient quantities but defective structure, for example, 2° to mutation).

enzymopenia (ĕn-zī″mō-pē′nē-ă) Deficiency of an enzyme.

enzymuria (ĕn″zī-mū′rē-ă) [″ + ″ + *ouron,* urine] The presence of enzymes in the urine.

EOA *esophageal obturator airway.*

EOM *extraocular muscles.*

eosin (ē′ō-sĭn) [Gr. *eos,* dawn (rose-colored)] Any of several synthetic dyes, including bluish and yellow ones. They are used to stain tissues for microscopic examination.

eosinoblast (ē″ō-sĭn′ō-blăst) [″ + *blastos,* germ] A bone marrow cell that develops into a myelocyte. SYN: *myeloblast.*

eosinopenia (ē″ō-sĭn-ō-pē′nē-ă) [″ + *penia,* poverty] An abnormally small number of eosinophilic cells in the peripheral blood.

eosinophil (ē″ō-sĭn′ō-fĭl) [″ + *philein,* to love] A white blood cell with a polymorphic nucleus and cytoplasmic granules that stain with eosin or other acid stains. Eosinophils are known to destroy parasitic organisms and to play a major role in allergic reactions. They release some of the major chemical mediators that cause bronchoconstriction in asthma. Eosinophils make up 1% to 3% of the white cell count. SEE: *blood* for illus.; *leukocyte.*

eosinophilia (ē″ō-sĭn-ō-fĭl′ē-ă) [Gr. *eos,* dawn, + *philein,* to love] **1.** An unusually large number of eosinophils in the blood. **2.** The characteristic of staining readily with eosin.

urinary e. An abnormal amount of eosinophils in the urine, a finding that sometimes indicates an allergic interstitial nephritis.

eosinophilia-myalgia syndrome, tryptophan-induced Eosinophilia and severe muscle pain and joint stiffness seen in patients with a history of taking oral preparations of the amino acid L-tryptophan.

SYMPTOMS: There is abrupt onset, within a week or so, of pain, edema, and induration of the extremities, esp. the legs. Skin involvement includes alopecia, transient rash, and subjective weakness. The disease is disabling and chronic. To establish the diagnosis, it is necessary to exclude other diseases (e.g., infections or neoplasia) that could cause these findings.

TREATMENT: Treatment is supportive; tryptophan should be discontinued.

eosinophilic (ē″ō-sĭn-ō-fĭl′ĭk) Readily stainable with eosin.

eosinophilous (ē″ō-sĭn-ŏf′ĭ-lŭs) [″ + *philein,* to love] **1.** Easily stainable with eosin. **2.** Having eosinophilia.

eosinotactic (ē″ō-sĭn-ō-tăk′tĭk) [″ + *taktikos,* arranged] Attracting or repulsing eosinophilic cells.

eotaxin (ē-ō-tŏks′ĭn) A chemotactic cytokine produced by epithelial cells that brings eosinophils and T lymphocytes to an area of allergic inflammation. Tumor necrosis factor alpha stimulates its release. SEE: *chemotaxis; cytokine*.

ep- SEE: *epi-*.

EPAP *expiratory positive airway pressure.*

epaxial (ĕp-ăk′sē-ăl) [″ + L. *axis,* axis] Situated above or behind an axis.

epencephalon (ĕp″ĕn-sĕf′ă-lŏn) [″ + *enkephalos,* brain] The anterior portion of the embryonic hindbrain (rhombencephalon) from which the pons and cerebellum arise. SYN: *metencephalon*.

ependyma (ĕp-ĕn′dĭ-mă) [Gr. *ependyma,* an upper garment, wrap] The membrane lining the cerebral ventricles and central canal of the spinal cord. **ependymal,** *adj.*

ependymitis (ĕp″ĕn-dĭ-mī′tĭs) [″ + *itis,* inflammation] Inflammation of the ependyma.

ependymoblast (ĕp-ĕn′dĭ-mō-blăst) [″ + *blastos,* germ] An embryonic ependymal cell, or ependymocyte.

ependymocyte (ĕp-ĕn′dĭ-mō-sīt) [″ + *kytos,* cell] Ependymal cell.

ependymoma (ĕp-ĕn″dĭ-mō′mă) [″ + *oma,* tumor] A tumor arising from fetal inclusion of ependymal elements.

ephebiatrics (ĕ-fē-bē-ăt′rĭks) [Gr. *epi,* at, + *hebe,* youth, + *iatrikos,* healing] A branch of medicine dealing with adolescents.

ephedra (ĕf-ĕd′ră) Ma huang

ephedrine (ĕ-fĕd′rĭn, ĕf′ĕ-drēn) A synthetic sympathomimetic alkaloid originally obtained from species of *Ephedra;* first isolated in 1887. In ancient Chinese medicine it was used as a diaphoretic and antipyretic. Its action is similar to that of epinephrine. Its effects, although less powerful, are more prolonged, and it exerts action when given orally, whereas epinephrine is effective only by injection. Ephedrine dilates the bronchial muscles, contracts the nasal mucosa, and raises the blood pressure. It is used chiefly for its bronchodilating effect in asthma, and for its constricting effect on the nasal mucosa in hay fever.

INCOMPATIBILITY: Calcium chloride, iodine, and tannic acid are incompatible with ephedrine.

CAUTION: Ephedrine and ephedra may produce hypertensive crises, myocardial ischemia, and cardiac rhythm disturbances.

---

e. hydrochloride A more soluble salt of ephedrine, having the same action and uses.

e. sulfate The salt of ephedrine and sulfuric acid. It occurs as fine white crystals or as a powder. Its action and uses are the same as those of ephedrine.

ephelis (ĕf-ē′lĭs) *pl.* **ephelides** [Gr. *ephelis,* freckle] A freckle.

ephemeral (ĕ-fĕm′ĕr-ăl) [Gr. *epi,* on, + *hemera,* day] Of brief duration.

epi-, ep- [Gr.] Prefix meaning *upon, over, at, in addition to, after*.

epiandrosterone (ĕp″ē-ăn-drŏs′tĕr-ōn) An androgenic hormone normally present in the urine.

epiblast (ĕp′ĭ-blăst) [Gr. *epi,* upon, + *blastos,* germ] The outer layer of cells of the blastoderm. SYN: *ectoderm*. **epiblastic** (-blăst′ik), *adj.*

epiblepharon (ĕp″ĭ-blĕf′ă-rŏn) [″ + Gr. *blepharon,* eyelid] A fold of skin that passes across the margin of either the upper or lower eyelid so that the eyelashes are pressed against the eye.

epibole, epiboly (ĕ-pĭb′ŏ-lē) [Gr. *epibole,* cover] Inclusion of the hypoblast within the epiblast due to swifter growth of the latter. SEE: *embole*.

epibulbar (ĕp″ĭ-bŭl′băr) Lying on the bulb of any structure; more specifically, located on the eyeball.

epicanthus [Gr. *epi,* upon, + *kanthos,* canthus] A vertical fold of skin extending from the root of the nose to the median end of the eyebrow, covering the inner canthus and caruncle. It is a characteristic of certain races and may occur as a congenital anomaly in others.

epicardia (ĕp″ĭ-kărd′ē-ă) [″ + *kardia,* heart] The abdominal portion of the esophagus extending from the diaphragm to the stomach, about 2 cm in length.

epicardium The serous membrane on the surface of the myocardium; the visceral layer of the pair of serous pericardial membranes.

epichordal (ĕp″ĭ-kord′ăl) [″ + *khorde,* cord] Located dorsad to the notochord.

epichorion (ĕp″ĭ-kō′rē-ŏn) [″ + *chorion*] The portion of the endometrium that covers the implanted early embryo.

epicomus (ē-pĭk′ō-mŭs) [″ + *kome,* hair] A congenital malformation in which the head of a parasitic twin is attached to the summit or vertex of the skull of the larger twin.

epicondylalgia (ĕp″ĭ-kŏn-dĭ-lăl′jē-ă) [″ + *kondylos,* condyle, + *algos,* pain] Pain in the elbow joint in the region of the epicondyles.

epicondyle (ĕp-ĭ-kŏn′dīl) [″ + *kondylos,* condyle] The eminence at the articular end of a bone above a condyle.

epicondylitis (ĕp″ĭ-kŏn″dĭ-lī′tĭs) [″ + ″ + *itis,* inflammation] Inflammation of the epicondyle of the humerus and surrounding tissues.

lateral humeral e. Tennis elbow.

medial humeral e. Golfer's elbow.

epicranium [″ + *kranion,* cranium] The soft tissue covering the cranium.

epicranius (ĕp″ĭ-krā′nē-ŭs) The occipitofrontal muscle and scalp.

epicrisis (ĕp′ĭ-krī″sĭs) [″ + *krisis,* crisis] A secondary turning point following the initial critical stage of a disease.

epicritic (ĕp-ĭ-krĭt′ĭk) [Gr. *epikritikos,* judging] **1.** Pert. to acute sensibility, such as that of the skin when it discriminates among degrees of sensation caused by touch or temperature. **2.** Pert. to an epicrisis. **3.** Something such as pain or itching that is well localized.

epicystotomy (ĕp″ĭ-sĭs-tŏt′ō-mē) [″ + ″ + *tome,* incision] A surgically created opening above the symphysis pubis into the bladder.

epicyte (ĕp′ĭ-sīt) [″ + *kytos,* cell] **1.** An epithelial cell. **2.** A cell membrane.

epidemic (ĕp″ĭ-dĕm′ĭk) [″ + *demos,* people] An infectious disease or condition that attacks many people at the same time in the same geographical area. SEE: *endemic; epizootic; pandemic.*

epidemic intelligence service ABBR: EIS. An epidemiology field training program for postdoctoral fellows at the Centers for Disease Control and Prevention. It provides epidemiological assistance in the investigation and prevention of public health problems and a source of trained field epidemiologists for federal, state, and local health departments around the U.S.

epidemic viral gastroenteropathy Viral gastroenteritis.

epidemiologist (ĕp″ĭ-dē-mē-ŏl′ō-jĭst) A specialist in the field of epidemiology.

epidemiology (ĕp″ĭ-dē-mē-ŏl′ō-jē) [″ + *demos,* people, + *logos,* study] The study of the distribution and determinants of health-related states and events in populations, and the application of this study to the control of health problems. Epidemiology is concerned with the traditional study of epidemic diseases caused by infectious agents, and with health-related phenomena including accidents, suicide, climate, toxic agents such as lead, air pollution, and catastrophes due to ionizing radiation. SEE: *pharmacoepidemiology.* **epidemiological** (-ŏl-ŏ′jĭ-kăl), *adj.*

epidermal growth factor ABBR: EGF. A polypeptide that stimulates growth of several different cells, including keratinocytes. It has been used experimentally to promote wound healing.

epidermatoplasty (ĕp″ĭ-dĕr-măt′ō-plăs-tē) [″ + ″ + *plassein,* to mold] A surgical procedure grafting pieces of epidermis with the underlying layer of the corium.

epidermis (ĕp″ĭ-dĕr′mĭs) [″ + *derma,* skin] The outermost layer of the skin. SEE: *skin.* **epidermal, epidermic,** *adj.*

epidermitis (ĕp″ĭ-dĕr-mī′tĭs) [″ + ″ + *itis,* inflammation] Inflammation of the superficial layers of the skin.

epidermization (ĕp″ĭ-dĕr″mĭ-zā′shŭn) **1.** Skin grafting. **2.** Conversion of the deeper germinative layer of cells into the outer layer of the epidermis.

epidermodysplasia verruciformis (ĕp″ĭ-dĕr″mō-dĭs-plā′sē-ă) Generalized warts of the skin.

epidermoid (ĕp″ĭ-dĕr′moyd) [Gr. *epi,* upon, + *derma,* skin, + *eidos,* form, shape] **1.** Resembling or pert. to the epidermis. **2.** A tumor arising from aberrant epidermal cells. SYN: *cholesteatoma.*

epidermolysis (ĕp″ĭ-dĕr-mŏl′ĭ-sĭs) [″ + ″ + *lysis,* dissolution] Loosening of the epidermis.

e. bullosa A genetically transmitted form of epidermolysis marked by the formation of deep-seated bullae appearing after irritation or rubbing.

epidermomycosis (ĕp-ĭ-dĕr″mō-mī-kō′sĭs) [″ + ″ + *mykes,* fungus, + *osis,* condition] A skin disease caused by a fungus.

Epidermophyton (ĕp″ĭ-dĕr-mŏf′ĭ-tŏn) [″ + ″ + *phyton,* plant] A genus of fungi, similar to *Trichophyton* but affecting the skin and nails instead of the hair.

E. floccosum The causative agent of certain types of tinea, esp. tinea pedis (athlete's foot), tinea cruris, tinea unguium, and tinea corporis.

epidermophytosis (ĕp″ĭ-dĕr-mō-fī-tō′sĭs) [″ + ″ + ″ + *osis,* condition] Infection by a species of *Epidermophyton.*

epididymectomy (ĕp″ĭ-dĭd″ĭ-mĕk′tō-mē) [″ + *didymos,* testis, + *ektome,* excision] Removal of the epididymis.

epididymis (ĕp″ĭ-dĭd′ĭ-mĭs) *pl.* **epididymides** A small oblong organ resting on and beside the posterior surface of a testis, consisting of a convoluted tube 13 to 20 ft (3.97 to 6.1 m) long, enveloped in the tunica vaginalis, ending in the ductus deferens. It consists of the head (caput or globus major), which contains 12 to 14 efferent ducts of the testis, the body, and the tail (cauda or globus minor). It is the first part of the secretory duct of each testis. The epididymis is supplied by the internal spermatic, deferential, and external spermatic arteries; it is drained by corresponding veins. SEE: illus.

epididymitis (ĕp″ĭ-dĭd″ĭ-mī′tĭs) [″ + *didymos,* testis, + *itis,* inflammation] Inflammation of the epididymis, usually as a result of infection, and rarely as a result of trauma or urinary reflux from the urethra. SEE: *Nursing Diagnoses Appendix.*

ETIOLOGY: The causes of epididymitis are age- and activity-dependent. Children may have epididymal infection as a result of congenital malformations of the genitourinary tract. In sexually active young men, chlamydia and gonorrhea are the most common causes. Middle-aged and elderly men typically have infections caused by gram-negative urinary pathogens, such as *Escherichia coli* or other enteric bacteria. Syphilis, tuberculosis, mumps, and

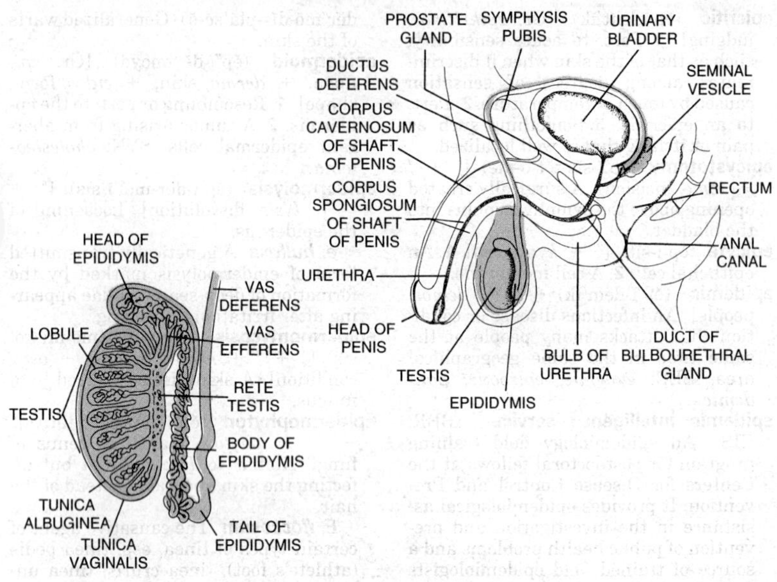

EPIDIDYMIS

other microorganisms are also occasionally responsible for epididymal infection.

SYMPTOMS: The primary symptom in adults is pain and swelling in the scrotum that is usually localized to the superior pole of one of the testicles. Urethral discharge, fever, and chills are also common.

TREATMENT: Antibiotic therapy (such as a tetracycline for sexually active men) and nonsteroidal anti-inflammatory drugs (for pain and fever) are effective. Drug therapy usually begins to relieve symptoms in 2 or 3 days, and eradicates infection in about a week.

PATIENT CARE: The patient is encouraged to rest in bed with his legs slightly apart and with the testes elevated on a towel roll to promote venous return, reduce edema, and relieve pain. Warm compresses or sitz baths, for 15 minutes every 3 hours, may also be used to reduce edema and pain. The patient should wear nonconstrictive, lightweight clothing until the swelling subsides. Straining at stool is minimized through the use of stool softeners. The patient should wear a scrotal support when he sits, stands, or walks. Lifting more than 20 pounds is discouraged. The patient is observed for signs of abscess formation (a localized hot, red tender area) or extension of the infection into the testes. The importance of adhering to the prescribed antibiotic regimen for the full course of therapy is emphasized.

If the patient faces the possibility of sterility, further counseling is suggested and arranged as necessary. If epididymitis is secondary to a sexually transmitted disease, the patient is encouraged to use a condom during sexual intercourse and to notify sexual partners so that they can be treated for the infection.

epididymodeferentectomy (ĕp″ĭ-dĭd″ĭ-mō-dĕf″ĕr-ĕn-tĕk′tō-mē) [″ + ″ + L. *deferens,* carrying away, + Gr. *ektome,* excision] Excision of the epididymis and ductus deferens.

epididymodeferential (ĕp″ĭ-dĭd″ĭ-mō-dĕf″ĕr-ĕn′shăl) Concerning both the epididymis and ductus deferens.

epididymography (ĕp″ĭ-dĭd″ĭ-mŏg′ră-fē) [″ + ″ + *graphein,* to write] Radiography of the epididymis after the introduction of a contrast medium.

epididymo-orchitis (ĕp″ĭ-dĭd″ĭm-ō-or-kī′tis) [″ + *didymos,* testis, + *orchis,* testis, + *itis,* inflammation] Epididymitis with orchitis.

epididymotomy (ĕp″ĭ-dĭd″ĭ-mŏt′ō-mē) [″ + ″ + *tome,* incision] An incision into the epididymis.

epididymovasostomy (ĕp-ĭ-dĭd″ĭ-mō-văs-ŏs′tō-mē) [″ + ″ + L. *vas,* vessel, + Gr. *stoma,* mouth] A surgical anastomosis between the epididymis and the vas.

epididymovesiculography (ĕp″ĭ-dĭd″ĭ-mō-vĕ-sĭk″ū-lŏg′ră-fē) Radiography of the epididymis and seminal vesicle after introduction of a contrast medium.

epidural [Gr. *epi,* upon, + L. *durus,* hard] Located over or on the dura.

epidurogram (ĕp″ĭ-dūr′ō-grăm) A spinal

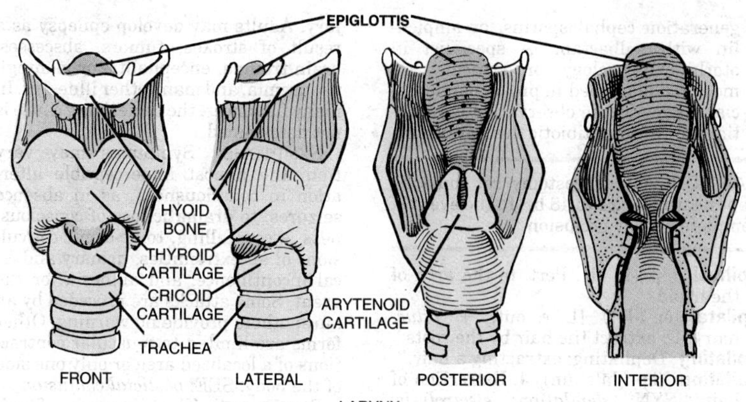

EPIGLOTTIS

x-ray examination that uses injected contrast to provide an outline of compressed nerve roots. This study is sometimes used in the evaluation of back pain.

epiduroscopy (ĕp″ĭ-dūrŏs′kō-pē) The insertion of a fiberoptic scope into the epidural space that surrounds the spinal cord to diagnose and to treat chronic back pain.

epifascial (ĕp″ĭ-făsh′ē-ăl) On or above a fascia.

epifolliculitis (ĕp″ĭ-fŏl-lĭk″ū-lī′tĭs) [″ + L. *folliculus,* follicle, + Gr. *itis,* inflammation] Inflammation of the hair follicles of the scalp.

epigallocatechin gallate (ĕp″ĭ-găl′ō-kăt-ĕ-chĭn găl′lāt) ABBR: EGCg, EGCG. A polyphenol compound present in green tea that inhibits the growth of cancer cells in the laboratory. Its effect on patients with cancer is unknown.

epigaster [″ + *gaster,* belly] An embryonic structure that develops into the large intestine. SYN: *hindgut*.

epigastralgia (ĕp″ĭ-găs-trăl′jē-ă) [″ + ″ + *algos,* pain] Pain in the epigastrium.

epigastric reflex Contraction of the upper portion of the rectus abdominis muscle when the skin of the epigastric region is scratched.

epigastrium (ĕp″ĭ-găs′trē-ŭm) [″ + *gaster,* belly] The region over the pit of the stomach. SEE: *Auenbrugger's sign; precordium*. **epigastric** (-găs′trĭk), *adj.*

epigastrocele (ĕp″ĭ-găs′trō-sēl) [″ + ″ + *kele,* hernia] A hernia in the epigastrium.

epigastrorrhaphy (ĕp″ĭ-găs-tror′ă-fē) [″ + ″ + *rhaphe,* seam, ridge] Suture of an abdominal wound in the epigastric area.

epigenesis (ĕp″ĭ-jĕn′ĕ-sĭs) [″ + *genesis,* generation, birth] In embryology, the development of specific cells and tissues from undifferentiated cells of the early embryo.

epiglottidean (ĕp″ĭ-glŏ-tĭd′ē-ăn) Pert. to the epiglottis.

epiglottidectomy (ĕp″ĭ-glŏt″ĭd-ĕk′tō-mē) [″ + ″ + *ektome,* excision] Excision of the epiglottis.

epiglottiditis Epiglottitis.

epiglottis (ĕp″ĭ-glŏt′ĭs) *pl.* **epiglottides** [Gr.] The uppermost cartilage of the larynx, located immediately posterior to the root of the tongue. It covers the entrance of the larynx when the individual swallows, thus preventing food or liquids from entering the airway. SEE: illus.

epiglottitis (ĕp″ĭ-glŏt-ī′tĭs) [″ + *itis,* inflammation] Inflammation of the epiglottis as the result of infection. The severe swelling above the epiglottis may obstruct air flow and can cause death. Epiglottitis is an emergency and must be treated immediately. SYN: *epiglottiditis; supraglottitis*. SEE: *croup; laryngotracheobronchitis*.

ETIOLOGY: It usually occurs in children, esp. from ages 2 to 5, as a result of infection with bacteria such as *Haemophilus influenzae,* streptococci, and staphylococci. It also can affect adults, usually resulting from group A streptococcal infection.

SYMPTOMS: Children abruptly develop a sore throat, dysphagia, and high fever, usually at night. They are agitated and frightened and want to sit in a tripod position (upright, leaning forward, mouth open). Drooling, dyspnea with substernal and suprasternal retractions, and stridor are common. Severe respiratory distress and cyanosis may develop suddenly. Unlike children with croup, those with epiglottitis have no cough or hoarseness.

TREATMENT: Epiglottitis is treated with intravenous second- or third-generation cephalosporins, or ampicillin with sulbactam. A specialist in otorhinolaryngology or critical care medicine may need to provide an artificial airway. Close observation is essential even after antibiotic therapy begins.

CAUTION: A tracheostomy set must be kept nearby for 24 to 48 hr, in the event of complete airway occlusion.

---

epihyal (ĕp-ĭ-hī′ăl) Pert. to the arch of the hyoid.

epilate (ĕp′ĭ-lāt) [L. *e,* out, + *pilus,* hair] To extract the hair by the roots.

epilating Depilating; extracting a hair.

epilation (ĕp-ĭ-lā′shŭn) **1.** Extraction of hair. SYN: *depilation; electrolysis.* **2.** Loss of hair due to exposure to ionizing radiation.

epilemma (ĕp-ĭ-lĕm′ă) [Gr. *epi,* upon, + *lemma,* husk] A neurilemma of small branches of nerve filaments.

epilepsy (ĕp′ĭ-lĕp″sē) [Gr. *epilepsia,* to seize] A disease marked by recurrent seizures; that is, by repetitive abnormal electrical discharges within the brain. Epilepsy is prevalent; it is found in about 2% or 3% of the population. Its incidence is highest in children (i.e., under age 10) and in elderly people (i.e., over age 70); adolescents and adults are affected less frequently.

The International League Against Epilepsy categorizes epilepsy as either partial, generalized, or unclassified. Generalized seizures result from electrical discharges that affect both hemispheres of the brain. Tonic-clonic seizures (in which there is loss of consciousness with violent movements of the extremities) and absence seizures (in which there are brief interruptions of awareness and activity) are two examples of generalized seizure disorders. Partial seizure disorders typically begin with focal or local discharges in one part of the brain (and body); they may generalize in some instances. When a patient remains awake during a seizure episode, the seizure is said to be simple and partial. If loss of consciousness occurs after a focal seizure, the syndrome is said to be partial and complex.

Patients who suffer recurrent episodes of alcohol withdrawal or from frequent severe hypoglycemia, hypercalcemia, or similar metabolic illnesses may have repetitive seizures but are not considered to have epilepsy if the seizures stop after their underlying illnesses are treated.

ETIOLOGY: Epilepsy may result from congenital or acquired brain disease. Infants born with lipid storage diseases, tuberous sclerosis, or cortical dysplasia, for example, may have recurrent seizures, as may children born with intracranial hemorrhage or anoxic brain injury. Adults may develop epilepsy as a result of strokes, tumors, abscesses, brain trauma, encephalitis or meningitis, uremia, and many other illnesses. In many instances, the underlying cause is not determined.

SYMPTOMS: Symptoms may vary from the almost imperceptible alteration in consciousness, as in absence seizures, to dramatic loss of consciousness, a cry, falling, tonic-clonic convulsions of all extremities, urinary and fecal incontinence, and amnesia for the event. Some attacks are preceded by an aura; others provide no warning. Other forms are limited to muscular contractions of a localized area or only one side of the body. SEE: *postictal confusion.*

DIAGNOSIS: The diagnosis of epilepsy is made by a careful assessment of the patient's history, augmented by diagnostic studies. Typically, these include blood tests to assess for metabolic disarray, brain imaging using magnetic resonance imaging or computed tomography, and electroencephalography. The differential diagnosis of epilepsy includes many other illnesses marked by episodes of loss of consciousness, including pseudoseizures, syncope, transient ischemic attacks, orthostatic hypotension, and narcolepsy, to name a few.

TREATMENT: Medical therapy is available for the prevention and control of recurrent seizures. Antiepileptic agents often include phenytoin or carbamazepine for partial seizures, valproic acid for absence seizures, and any of these agents or phenobarbital, with or without newer drugs, such as gabapentin or lamotrigine, for generalized seizures. All these agents may have significant side effects, and many of them have a range of drug-drug interactions.

Surgical therapy to remove an epileptic focus within the brain is used occasionally to manage seizures that have been difficult to control medically. In specialized neurosurgical centers, this may cure or reduce the impact of epilepsy in about 75% of patients.

Lennox-Gastaut syndrome e. Epilepsy with onset in early childhood. This type of epilepsy is characterized by a variety of seizure patterns and an abnormal electroencephalogram, and is frequently associated with developmental and mental retardation. Seizures are not controlled by the usual antiepileptic drugs; however, adjunctive therapy with felbamate may be beneficial.

photogenic e. Convulsive attacks that occur as a result of intermittent light stimulus.

reflex e. Recurrent epileptic seizures that occur in reaction to a specific stimulus, such as photic stimulation while looking at flashing lights or television, auditory stimulation while listening to specific musical compositions, tactile stimulation, or reading.

sleep e. A term formerly, and improperly, used to signify narcolepsy.

traumatic e. Epilepsy caused by trauma to the brain.

epileptic (ĕp″ĭ-lĕp′tĭk) [Gr. *epileptikos*] **1.** Concerning epilepsy. **2.** An individual suffering from attacks of epilepsy.

epileptiform (ĕp″ĭ-lĕp′tĭ-form) [Gr. *epilepsia,* to seize, + L. *forma,* form] Having the form or appearance of epilepsy.

epileptogenic, epileptogenous (ĕp″ĭ-lĕp-tō-jĕn′ĭk, -tŏj′ĕ-nŭs) [″ + *gennan,* to produce] Giving rise to epileptoid convulsions.

epileptoid [″ + *eidos,* form, shape] Resembling epilepsy. SYN: *epileptiform.*

epileptology [″ + *logos,* word, reason] The study of epilepsy.

epiloia (ĕp″ĭ-lŏy′ă) Tuberous sclerosis.

epimandibular (ĕp″ĭ-măn-dĭb′ū-lăr) [Gr. *epi,* upon, above, + L. *mandibulum,* jaw] Located on the lower jaw.

epimer (ĕp′ĭ-mĕr) One of a pair of isomers that differ only in the position of the hydrogen atom and the hydroxyl group attached to one asymmetrical carbon atom.

epimere (ĕp′ĭ-mēr) [Gr. *epi,* upon, + *meros,* apart] In embryology, the dorsal muscle-forming portion of the somite.

epimerite (ĕp″ĭ-mĕr′īt) [″ + *meros,* part] An organelle of certain protozoa by which they attach themselves to epithelial cells.

epimorphosis (ĕp″ĭ-mor′fō-sĭs) [″ + *morphoun,* to give shape, + *osis,* condition] Regeneration of a part of an organism by growth at the cut surface.

epimysium (ĕp″ĭ-mĭz′ē-ŭm) [″ + *mys,* muscle] The outermost sheath of connective tissue that surrounds a skeletal muscle. It consists of irregularly distributed collagenous, reticular, and elastic fibers, connective tissue cells, and fat cells. SYN: *perimysium externum.*

epinephrine (ĕp″ĭ-nĕf′rĭn) [″ + *nephros,* kidney] $C_9H_{13}NO_3$; a catecholamine produced by the adrenal gland, secreted when the sympathetic nervous system is stimulated. In the physiological response to stress, it is responsible for maintaining blood pressure and cardiac output, keeping airways open wide, and raising blood sugar levels. All these functions are useful to frightened, traumatized, injured, or sick humans and animals. The therapeutic uses of epinephrine are diverse. As one of the key agents used in advanced cardiac life support, it is helpful in treating asystole, ventricular arrhythmias, and other forms of cardiac arrest. It counteracts the effects of systemic allergic reactions and is an effective bronchodilator. It helps control local hemorrhage by constricting blood vessels; because of this action, it prolongs the effects of local anesthesia. SEE: *catecholamine.*

INCOMPATIBILITY: Epinephrine is incompatible with light, heat, air, iron salts, and alkalies. SYN: *adrenaline.*

racemic e. A mixture of dextro and levo-isomers of epinephrine that, when nebulized, can be used in the treatment of croup and bronchiolitis. The drug is usually given with parenteral dexamethasone.

CAUTION: Some infants and children who initially respond to this treatment will relapse. Patients treated with racemic epinephrine should be observed for several hours to determine if they should be admitted to the hospital or are stable enough for discharge to home.

---

epinephritis (ĕp″ĭ-nĕf-rī′tĭs) [″ + *nephros,* kidney, + *itis,* inflammation] Inflammation of an adrenal gland.

epinephroma (ĕp-ĭ-nĕ-frō′mă) [″ + ″ + *oma,* tumor] A lipomatoid tumor of the kidney. SYN: *hypernephroma.*

epineural (ĕp″ĭ-nū′răl) [″ + *neuron,* nerve] Located on a neural arch.

epineurium (ĕp″ĭ-nū′rē-ŭm) The connective tissue sheath of a nerve. SEE: *nerve.*

epiotic (ĕp″ē-ŏt′ĭk) [″ + *ous,* ear] Located above the ear.

epipastic (ĕp″ĭ-păs′tĭk) [″ + *passein,* to sprinkle] Resembling a dusting powder.

epipharynx (ĕp″ĭ-făr′ĭnks) [″ + *pharynx,* throat] Nasopharynx.

epiphenomenon (ĕp″ĭ-fĕ-nŏm′ĕ-nŏn) [″ + *phainomenon,* phenomenon] An exceptional symptom or occurrence in a disease that is not related to the usual course of the disease.

epiphora (ĕ-pĭf′ō-ră) [Gr., downpour] An abnormal overflow of tears down the cheek due to excess secretion of tears or obstruction of the lacrimal duct.

epiphyseolysis (ĕp″ĭ-fĭz″ē-ŏl′ĭ-sĭs) [″ + ″ + *lysis,* dissolution] Separation of an epiphysis. Also spelled *epiphysiolysis.*

epiphyseopathy (ĕp″ĭ-fĭz-ē-ŏp′ă-thē) [″ + ″ + *pathos,* disease, suffering] **1.** Any disease of the pineal gland. **2.** Any disease of the epiphysis of a bone. Also spelled *epiphysiopathy.*

epiphysis (ĕ-pĭf′ĭ-sĭs) *pl.* **epiphyses** [Gr., a growing upon] **1.** In the developing infant and child, a secondary bone-forming (ossification) center separated from a parent bone in early life by cartilage. As growth proceeds (at a different time for each epiphysis), it becomes a part of the larger, or parent, bone. It is possible to judge the biological age of a child from the development of these ossification centers as shown radiographically. **2.** A center for ossification at each extremity of long bones. SEE: *diaphysis.* **3.** The end of a long bone. **epiphyseal, epiphysial** (ĕp″ĭ-fĭz′ē-ăl), *adj.*

epiphysitis (ĕ-pĭf″ĭ-sī′tĭs) [″ + *itis,* inflammation] Inflammation of an epiphysis, esp. that at the hip, knee, or shoulder in an infant.

epipial (ĕp″ĭ-pī′ăl) [″ + L. *pia,* tender] Situated on or above the pia mater.

epiplocele (ĕ-pĭp′lō-sēl) [Gr. *epiploon,* omentum, + *kele,* tumor, swelling] A hernia containing omentum.

epiploenterocele (ĕ-pĭp″lō-ĕn′tĕr-ō-sēl) [″ + *enteron,* intestine, + *kele,* tumor, swelling] A hernia consisting of omentum and intestine.

epiploic (ĕp″ĭ-plō′ĭk) [Gr. *epiploon,* omentum] Pert. to the omentum.

epiploitis (ĕ-pĭp″lō-ī′tĭs) [″ + *itis,* inflammation] Inflammation of the omentum.

epiplomerocele (ĕ-pĭp″lō-mē′rō-sēl) [″ + *meros,* thigh, + *kele,* tumor, swelling] A femoral hernia containing omentum.

epiplomphalocele (ĕ-pĭp″lŏm-făl′ō-sēl) [″ + *omphalos,* navel, + *kele,* hernia] An umbilical hernia with omentum protruding.

epiploon (ĕ-pĭp′lō-ŏn) [Gr., omentum] The omentum, esp. the greater omentum. SYN: *omentum.*

epiplopexy (ĕ-pĭp′lō-pĕks″ē) [″ + *pexis,* fixation] Suturing of omentum to the anterior abdominal wall.

epiplosarcomphalocele (ĕ-pĭp″lō-săr″kŏm-făl′ō-sēl) [″ + *sarx,* flesh, + *omphalos,* navel, + *kele,* tumor, swelling] An umbilical hernia with omentum protruding. SYN: *epiplomphalocele.*

epiploscheocele (ĕ-pĭp″lŏs-kē′ō-sēl) [″ + *oscheon,* scrotum, + *kele,* tumor, swelling] An omental hernia into the scrotum.

epipygus (ĕp″ĭ-pī′gŭs) [Gr. *epi,* upon, + *pyge,* buttocks] A developmental anomaly in which an accessory limb is attached to the buttocks. SEE: *pygomelus.*

episclera (ĕp″ĭ-sklē′ră) [″ + *skleros,* hard] The outermost superficial layer of the sclera of the eye.

episcleral (ĕp″ĭ-sklē′răl) **1.** Pert. to the episclera. **2.** Overlying the sclera of the eye.

episcleritis (ĕp″ĭ-sklē-rī′tĭs) [″ + *skleros,* hard, + *itis,* inflammation] Inflammation of the subconjunctival layers of the sclera.

episioperineoplasty (ĕ-pĭs″ē-ō-pĕr″ĭ-nē′ō-plăs″tē) [″ + *perinaion,* perineum, + Gr. *plassein,* to form] Plastic surgery of the perineum and vulva.

episioperineorrhaphy (ĕ-pĭs″ē-ō-pĕr″ĭ-nē-or′ă-fē) [″ + ″ + *rhaphe,* seam, ridge] Suturing of the vulva and perineum to support a prolapsed uterus.

PATIENT CARE: The perineum is inspected at intervals to assess healing and to observe for indications of hematoma formation or infection. Perineal care is provided as needed, and the patient is taught correct perineal hygiene (i.e., wiping from front to back). To relieve pain, anesthetic sprays or creams are applied as prescribed. Other pain relief measures include local heat using a heat lamp, warm soaks, or sitz baths as prescribed. The patient is taught to apply these therapies.

episioplasty (ĕ-pĭs″ē-ō-plăs′tē) [″ + *plassein,* to form] Plastic surgery of the vulva.

episiostenosis (ĕ-pĭs″ē-ō-stĕ-nō′sĭs) [″ + *stenosis,* narrowing] Narrowing of the vulvar opening.

episiotomy (ĕ-pĭs″ē-ŏt′ō-mē) [″ + *tome,* incision] Incision of the perineum at the end of the second stage of labor to avoid spontaneous laceration of the perineum and to facilitate delivery.

episode An occurrence that is one in a sequence of events.

episome (ĕp′ĭ-sōm) Plasmid.

epispadias (ĕp″ĭ-spā′dē-ăs) [Gr. *epi,* upon, + *spadon,* a rent] A congenital opening of the urethra on the dorsum of the penis.

episplenitis (ĕp″ĭ-splē-nī′tĭs) [″ + *splen,* spleen, + *itis,* inflammation] Inflammation of the splenic capsule.

epistasis (ĕ-pĭs′tă-sĭs) [Gr., stoppage] **1.** A film that forms on urine that has been allowed to stand. **2.** The suppression of any discharge. SEE: *hypostasis.*

epistaxis (ĕp″ĭ-stăk′sĭs) [Gr.] Hemorrhage from the nose; nosebleed. SEE: *Kiesselbach's area.*

ETIOLOGY: Epistaxis may occur spontaneously or secondary to local infections (vestibulitis, rhinitis, sinusitis), systemic infections (scarlet fever, typhoid), drying of nasal mucous membranes, trauma (including picking the nose), tumor of the paranasal sinus or nasopharynx, septal perforation, arteriosclerosis, hypertension, and bleeding tendencies associated with anemia, leukemia, hemophilia, or liver disease.

TREATMENT: Firm, continuous pressure applied by compressing the nostrils against the septum may control epistaxis temporarily. If this is ineffective, the site of the bleeding is determined, and pressure is applied against a clean cloth or tampon impregnated with a vasoconstrictor such as phenylephrine 0.25%. The patient should breathe through the mouth while the pressure is maintained for 5 min. If this fails, the procedure should be repeated for another 5 min. The patient should lie quietly, propped up in bed. SEE: *nosebleed* for illus.

If the bleeding is in the posterior nasal cavity, the area is anesthetized with 2% lidocaine applied topically and then cauterized by using electrocautery or applying 75% silver nitrate.

CAUTION: Cautery should not be used if the nosebleed is due to a bleeding tendency. Pressure is applied against gauze impregnated with petrolatum, to minimize trauma to the adjacent area. Posterior packing of the nasal cavity or balloon tamponade may be needed. The latter is done by inserting a Foley-like catheter into the nose and inflating the balloon after it is placed posteriorly. Traction is then applied to the catheter so that the vessels in the area are compressed.

PATIENT CARE: Airway clearance, level of discomfort and anxiety, and any prior history of nosebleeds are determined. The patient should sit upright and leaning forward to prevent aspiration, and should expectorate blood to limit nausea and vomiting due to swallowed blood. Bleeding is controlled by pinching the nostrils against the nasal septum for 5 to 10 min while the patient breathes through the mouth. Pressure is applied across or under the upper lip, and cold over the nose or the nape of the neck to help stop bleeding. If a posterior packing or balloon tamponade is ordered, the procedure is explained, and the prescribed presedation is administered. Hypoxemia is assessed, and supplemental oxygen by face mask is administered as needed. The nares are inspected for pressure necrosis. The patient should avoid blowing or picking at the nose, and increased humidity may help to prevent repeated bleeding if dryness is a factor. Simple measures, including applying pressure with the fingers, are taught to help the patient stop a nosebleed at home.

episternum Upper portion of the sternum. SYN: *manubrium sterni*. **episternal,** *adj.*

epitendineum (ĕp″ĭ-tĕn-dĭn′ē-ŭm) [″ + L. *tendere,* to stretch] The fibrous sheath enveloping a tendon.

epitenon SEE: *epitendineum.*

epithalamus (ĕp″ĭ-thăl′ă-mŭs) [″ + *thalamos,* chamber] The uppermost portion of the diencephalon of the brain. It includes the pineal body, trigonum habenulae, habenula, and habenular commissure.

epithelia Pl. of *epithelium.*

epithelial cancer Basal cell carcinoma.

epithelial diaphragm The epithelial extension of Hertwig's root sheath that determines the number and size of tooth roots. It induces dentin formation locally as the root elongates. SEE: *Hertwig's root sheath.*

epithelialization (ĕp″ĭ-thē″lē-ăl-ī-zā′shŭn) The growth of skin over a wound.

epitheliitis (ĕp″ĭ-thē″lē-ī′tĭs) Overgrowth and inflammation of the mucosal epithelium following injury such as is caused by ionizing radiation.

epithelioblastoma (ĕp″ĭ-thē″lē-ō-blăs-tō′mă) [″ + *thele,* nipple, + *blastos,* germ, + *oma,* tumor] An epithelial cell tumor.

epitheliogenic, epitheliogenetic (ĕp″ĭ-thē″lē-ō-jĕn′ĭk, -jĕ-nĕt′ĭk) [″ + ″ + *gennan,* to produce] Caused by epithelial proliferation.

epithelioglandular (ĕp″ĭ-thē″lē-ō-glăn′dū-lăr) Concerning the epithelial cells of a gland.

epithelioid (ĕp″ĭ-thē′lē-oyd) [″ + ″ + *eidos,* form, shape] Resembling epithelium.

epitheliolysin (ĕp″ĭ-thē-lē-ŏl′ĭ-sĭn) [″ + ″ + *lysis,* dissolution] A specific lysin formed in blood serum of an animal into which epithelial cells of an animal of a different species were injected. The epitheliolysin destroys the cells of an animal of the same species as that from which the epithelial cells were derived.

epitheliolysis (ĕp″ĭ-thē-lē-ŏl′ĭ-sĭs) Death of epithelial tissue. Destruction or dissolving of epithelial cells by an epitheliolysin.

epithelioma (ĕp″ĭ-thē-lē-ō′mă) [″ + *thele,* nipple, + *oma,* tumor] A malignant tumor consisting principally of epithelial cells; a carcinoma. A tumor originating in the epidermis of the skin or in a mucous membrane. **epitheliomatous** (-mă-tŭs), *adj.*

e. adamantinum An epithelioma of the jaw arising from the enamel organ. It may be solid or partly cystic. SYN: *adamantinoma.*

e. adenoides cysticum A basal cell carcinoma occurring on the surface of the body, esp. the face, and characterized by formation of cysts. SYN: *acanthoma adenoides cysticum; trichoepithelioma.*

basal cell e. basal cell carcinoma.

deep-seated e. An epithelioma that invades and destroys tissue, forming irregular rounded ulcers. SYN: *rodent ulcer.*

epitheliosis (ĕp″ĭ-thē″lē-ō′sĭs) [″ + *thele,* nipple, + *osis,* condition] Trachomatous proliferation of the conjunctival epithelium.

epithelium (ĕp″ĭ-thē′lē-ŭm) *pl.* **epithelia** [″ + *thele,* nipple] The layer of cells forming the epidermis of the skin and the surface layer of mucous and serous membranes. The cells rest on a basement membrane and lie in close approximation with little intercellular material between them. They are devoid of blood vessels. The epithelium may be simple, consisting of a single layer, or stratified, consisting of several layers. Cells making up the epithelium may be flat (squamous), cube-shaped (cuboidal), or cylindrical (columnar). Modified forms of epithelium include ciliated, pseudostratified, glandular, and neuroepithelium. The epithelium may include

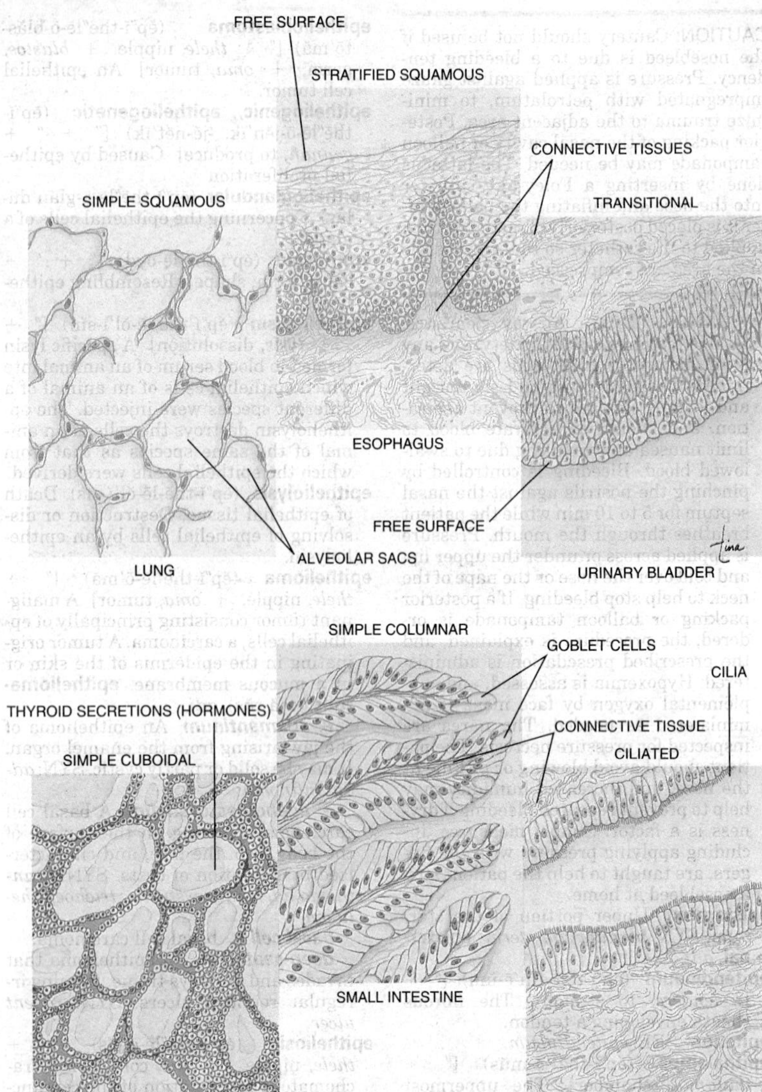

EPITHELIAL TISSUES

(Orig. mag. ×430)

goblet cells, which secrete mucus. Stratified squamous epithelium may be keratinized for a protective function or abnormally keratinized in pathological response. Squamous epithelium is classified as endothelium, which lines the blood vessels and the heart, and mesothelium, which lines the serous cavities. Epithelium serves the general functions of protection, absorption, and secretion, and specialized functions such as movement of substances through ducts, production of germ cells, and reception of stimuli. Its ability to regenerate is excellent; it may replace itself as frequently as every 24 hr. SEE: illus.; *skin*. **epithelial** (-ăl), *adj.*

ciliated e. Epithelium with hairlike processes on the surface that wave actively only in one direction. This type is present in the respiratory tract and fallopian tubes.

columnar e. Epithelium composed of cylindrical cells.

cuboidal e. Epithelium consisting of cube-shaped or prismatic cells with height about equal to their width.

germinal e. **1.** Epithelium that covers the surface of the genital ridge of the urogenital folds of an embryo. It gives rise to the seminiferous tubules of the testes and the surface layer of the ovary. It was once thought to produce the germ cells (spermatozoa and ova). **2.** The epithelium that covers the surface of a mature mammalian ovary.

glandular e. Epithelium consisting of secretory cells.

junctional e. The zone of soft tissue attached to the tooth. SYN: *epithelial attachment; gingival cuff.*

laminated e. Stratified e.

mesenchymal e. Squamous epithelium that lines the subarachnoid and subdural cavities, the chambers of the eye, and the perilymphatic spaces of the ear.

pavement e. Epithelium consisting of flat, platelike cells in a single layer.

pigmented e. Epithelium containing pigment granules.

pseudostratified e. Epithelium in which the bases of cells rest on the basement membrane but the distal ends of some do not reach the surface. Their nuclei lie at different levels, giving the appearance of stratification.

reduced enamel e. Combined epithelial layers of the enamel organ, which form a protective layer over the enamel crown as it erupts and then become the primary epithelial attachment surrounding the tooth.

stratified e. Epithelium with the cells in layers. SYN: *laminated e.*

sulcular e. The nonkeratinized epithelium that lines the gingival sulcus.

transitional e. A form of stratified epithelium in which the cells adjust to mechanical changes such as stretching and recoiling. This type of tissue is found only in the urinary system (renal pelvis, ureter, bladder, and a part of the urethra).

epitope (ĕp′ĭ-tōp) Any component of an antigen molecule that functions as an antigenic determinant by permitting the attachment of certain antibodies. SYN: *antigenic determinant*. SEE: *paratope.*

epitrichial layer Epitrichium.

epitrichium (ĕp″ĭ-trĭk′ē-ŭm) [Gr. *epi,* upon, + *trichion,* hair] The superficial layers of the epidermis of the fetus. SYN: *epitrichial layer; periderm.*

epitrochlea (ĕp″ĭ-trŏk′lē-ă) [″+*trochalia,* pulley] The inner condyle of the humerus. **epitrochlear,** *adj.*

epiturbinate (ĕp″ĭ-tĕr′bĭn-āt) [″+L. *turbo,* top] The tissue on or covering the turbinate bone.

epitympanum (ĕp″ĭ-tĭm′pă-nŭm) [″ + *tympanon,* drum] The attic of the middle ear; the area above the drum membrane.

epizoon (ĕp″ĭ-zō′ŏn) *pl.* **epizoa** [″ + *zoon,* animal] An animal organism living as a parasite on the exterior of the host animal. **epizoic** (-zō′ĭk), *adj.*

epizootic Any disease of animals that attacks many animals in the same area.

epoetin alfa Synthetic human erythropoietin. Trade name is Epogen. SEE: *erythropoietin.*

eponychium (ĕp″ō-nĭk′ē-ŭm) [″ + *onyx,* nail] **1.** The horny embryonic structure from which the nail develops. **2.** The perionychium.

eponym (ĕp′ō-nĭm) [Gr. *eponymos,* named after] A name for anything (disease, organ, function, place) adapted from the name of a particular person or sometimes a geographical location (e.g., Haverhill fever, Lyme disease).

epoophorectomy (ĕp″ō-ō-fō-rĕk′tō-mē) [Gr. *epi,* upon, + *oophoron,* ovary, + *ektome,* excision] Removal of the parovarium.

epoophoron (ĕp″ō-ŏf′ō-rŏn) A rudimentary structure located in the mesosalpinx. Consisting of a longitudinal duct (duct of Gartner) and 10 to 15 transverse ducts, it is the remains of the upper portion of the mesonephros and is the homologue of the head of the epididymis in males. SYN: *parovarium; Rosenmüller's body.*

epoxide (ĕ-pŏk′sīd) Any chemical compound that contains two carbon atoms joined to a single oxygen atom.

epoxy (ĕ-pŏk′sē) A general term for a polymer that contain molecules in which oxygen is attached to two different carbon atoms. These compounds are widely used as adhesives.

epsilon-aminocaproic acid A synthetic substance used to correct an overdose of certain fibrinolytic agents. It is also useful in treating excessive bleeding due to increased fibrinolytic activity in the blood.

EPSP *excitatory postsynaptic potential.*

Epstein-Barr virus [M. A. Epstein, Brit. physician, b.1921; Y. M. Barr, contemporary Canadian physician] ABBR: EBV. A member of the herpes virus family, discovered in 1964. It is one of the causes of infectious mononucleosis. In South African children, it is associated with Burkitt's lymphoma; in Asian populations, with nasopharyngeal carcinoma.

Epstein's pearls [Alois Epstein, Czech. pediatrician, 1849–1918] In infants, benign retention cysts resembling small pearls, which are sometimes present in the palate. They disappear in 1 to 2 months.

epulis (ĕp-ū′lĭs) *pl.* **epulides** [Gr. *epoulis,* a gumboil] **1.** A fibrous sarcomatous tumor having its origin in the periosteum of the lower jaw. **2.** A nonpathological softening and swelling of the gums due to hyperemia that begins during midtrimester pregnancy and subsides after delivery. In susceptible women, this condition tends to recur during subsequent pregnancies. **epuloid,** *adj.*

epulosis (ĕp″ū-lō′sĭs) [Gr. *epoulosis*] Cicatrization. **epulotic,** *adj.*

epulotic (ĕp″ū-lŏt′ĭk) [Gr. *epoulotikos*] Promoting cicatrization.

EQA *External quality assessment.*

Equal Employment Opportunity Commission ABBR: EEOC. A federal agency that enacts and enforces regulations that protect against discrimination in the workplace, esp. on the basis of age, gender, race, religious preference, or functional impairment.

equation [L. *aequare,* to make equal] **1.** The state of being equal. **2.** In chemistry, a symbolic representation of a chemical reaction.

e. of motion A statement of the variables of pressure, volume, compliance, resistance, and flow for respiratory system mechanics.

personal e. SEE: *personal equation.*

equator [L. *aequator*] A line encircling a round body and equidistant from both poles. **equatorial,** *adj.*

e. of cell The boundary of a plane through which the division of a cell occurs.

e. of crystalline lens The line that marks the junction of the anterior and posterior surfaces of the crystalline lens. The fibers of the suspensory ligament are attached to it.

e. oculi An imaginary line encircling the eyeball midway between the anterior and posterior poles.

equi- [L. *aequus,* equal] Prefix meaning *equal.*

equianalgesic A dose of one form of analgesic drug that is equivalent to another analgesic in pain-relieving potential. Knowing this equivalence permits the substitution of analgesics without undesired side effects.

equilibrating (ē-kwĭl′ĭ-brāt-ĭng) [L. *aequilibris,* in perfect balance] Maintaining equilibrium.

equilibration The modification of masticatory forces or occlusal surfaces of teeth to produce simultaneous occlusal contacts between upper and lower teeth, and to equalize the stress of occlusal forces of the supporting tissues of the teeth.

equilibrium [L. *aequus,* equal, + *libra,* balance] A state of balance; a condition in which contending forces are equal.

dynamic e. **1.** The sense of balance while the body or head is in motion. This is maintained by coordinating data from postural (stretch) receptors in the limbs with data from the inner ear and cerebellum. **2.** Homeostasis.

nitrogenous e. A situation where a balance between nitrogen excretion and nitrogen intake are equal.

physiological e. In nutritional theory, a state in which the body's intake and excretion of nutrients are perfectly matched.

static e. The sense of balance while the body or head is not in motion.

thermal e. A condition in which two substances exist at the same temperature and in which heat transfer is therefore in a steady state.

equilin (ĕk′wĭl-ĭn) [L. *equus,* horse] Crystalline estrogenic hormone derived from the urine of pregnant mares.

equimolar In the quantitative comparison of chemical substances, having the same molar concentration.

equine (ē′kwīn) [L. *equus,* horse] Concerning or originating from a horse.

equinovarus (ē-kwī″nō-vā′rŭs) [L. *equinus,* equine, + *varus,* bent inward] A form of clubfoot with a combination of pes equinus and pes varus (i.e., walking without touching the heel to the ground and with the sole turned inward).

equipoise In the design of clinical trials, a state in which the risks and benefits of alternative treatments offered during the trial are balanced, so that no preexisting advantage is known to exist for one treatment arm over the other. This is a required ethical consideration in clinical research.

equipotential (ē″kwĭ-pō-tĕn′shăl) [L. *aequus,* equal, + *potentia,* ability] Having the same electric charge or physical strength.

equivalence (ē-kwĭv′ă-lĕns) [″ + *valere,* to be worth] The quality of being equal in power, force, or value.

equivalent (ē-kwĭv′a-lĕnt) **1.** Equal in power, force, or value. **2.** The amount of weight of any element needed to replace a fixed weight of another body.

anginal e. Any symptom of myocardial ischemia caused by dysfunction of the heart muscle, in which chest pain is absent. The most commonly reported complaints are exertional breathing difficulties and fatigue.

dose e. In radiology, the product of the absorbed dose and the quality factor. Expressed in rems or sieverts, it measures the effects of absorbing different types of radiation. SEE: *factor, quality.*

metabolic e. ABBR: MET. A unit used to estimate the metabolic cost of physical activity. One MET equals the uptake of 3.5 ml of oxygen per kilogram of body weight per minute.

E.R. *external resistance; Emergency Room.*

Er Symbol for the element erbium.

eradication Complete elimination of a disease, esp. one that is epidemic or endemic.

***erb*B-2** (ĕrb-bē too) Member of the *erb*-B family of oncogenes. This oncogene is overexpressed in some human cancers, including breast. Its protein product contains part of the epidermal growth factor (EGF) receptor. Overexpression of this oncogene is associated with progression of human breast cancer. SEE: *oncogene; epidermal growth factor; breast cancer.*

Erben's reflex (ĕrb'ĕnz) [Siegmund Erben, Austrian physician, b. 1863] Retardation of the pulse when the head and trunk are forcibly bent forward.

erbium (ĕr'bē-ŭm) A rare metallic element with atomic number 68, an atomic weight of 167.26, and a specific gravity of 9.051. Its symbol is Er.

Erb's paralysis [Wilhelm Heinrich Erb, Ger. neurologist, 1840–1921] Paralysis of the group of shoulder and upper arm muscles involving the cervical roots of the fifth and sixth spinal nerves. The arm hangs limp, the hand rotates inward, and normal movements are lost. Afflicted newborns fail to exhibit the Moro reflex on the paralyzed side. In general, prognosis is good, and function returns within 3 months. SYN: *Duchenne-Erb paralysis; Erb's palsy.*

Erb's point The point on the side of the neck 2 to 3 cm above the clavicle and in front of the transverse process of the sixth cervical vertebra. Electrical stimulation over this area causes various arm muscles to contract.

ERCP *endoscopic retrograde cholangiopancreatography.*

erectile (ĕ-rĕk'tĭl) [L. *erigere,* to erect] Able to assume an upright position.

erection The state of swelling, hardness, and stiffness observed in the penis and to a lesser extent in the clitoris, generally due to sexual excitement. It is caused by engorgement with blood of the corpora cavernosa and the corpus spongiosum of the penis in men and the corpus cavernosa clitoridis in women.

Erection is necessary in men for the natural intromission of the penis into the vagina but not for the emission of semen. The blood withdraws from the penis after ejaculation and the erection is reduced. Erection of the penis may occur as the result of sexual excitement, during sleep, or due to physical stimulation of the penis. Abnormal persistent erection of the penis due not to sexual excitement but to certain disease states is called priapism. SEE: *nocturnal emission; penile prosthesis; priapism.*

erector [L. *erigere,* to erect] A muscle that raises a body part.

erector spinae reflex Irritation of the skin over the erector spinae muscles causing contraction of the muscles of the back. SYN: *dorsal reflex; lumbar reflex.*

eremophobia (ĕr"ĕm-ō-fō'bē-ă) [Gr. *eremos,* solitary, + *phobos,* fear] Dread of being alone.

erethism, erethism mercurialis (ĕr'ĕ-thĭzm) [Gr. *erethismos,* irritation] A group of psychological signs and symptoms associated with acute mercury poisoning. Included are restlessness, irritability, insomnia, difficulty in concentrating, and impaired memory. In severe cases, delirium and toxic psychosis may develop. SEE: *mercury poisoning.*

erethismic (ĕr"ĕ-thĭz'mĭk) Pert. to or causing erethism.

erethisophrenia (ĕr"ĕ-thĭ-zō-frē'nē-ă) [" + *phren,* mind] Unusual mental excitability.

ereuthrophobia (ĕr"ū-thrō-fō'bē-ă) [Gr. *erythros,* red, + *phobos,* fear] Pathological fear of blushing. SYN: *erythrophobia.*

ERG *electroretinogram.*

erg [Gr. *ergon,* work] In physics, the amount of work done when a force of 1 dyne acts through a distance of 1 cm. One erg is roughly 1/980 gram-centimeter. That is, raising a load of 1 g against gravity the distance of 1 cm requires that a force of 980 dynes operate through a distance of 1 cm, and hence that 980 ergs of work be done.

ergasiomania (ĕr-gā"sē-ō-mā'nē-ă) [Gr. *ergasia,* work, + *mania,* madness] An abnormal desire to be busy at work.

ergasiophobia (ĕr-gā"sē-ō-fō'bē-ă) [" + *phobos,* fear] Abnormal dislike for work of any kind or for assuming responsibility.

ergastic (ĕr-găs'tĭk) [Gr. *ergastikos*] Possessing potential energy.

ergastoplasm SEE: *endoplasmic reticulum.*

ergocalciferol (ĕr-gō-kăl-sĭf'ĕr-ŏl) Vitamin D_2, an activated product of ergosterol. It is used primarily in prophylaxis and treatment of vitamin D deficiency.

ergogenic (ĕr"gō-jĕn'ĭk) [Gr. *ergon,* work, + *gennan,* to produce] Having the ability to increase work, esp. to increase the potential for work output.

ergometer (ĕr-gŏm'ĕ-tĕr) [" + *metron,* measure] An apparatus for measuring the amount of work done by a human or animal subject.

arm e. A hand-driven crank used instead of a bicycle or treadmill to measure cardiopulmonary conditioning or health.

bicycle e. A stationary bicycle used in determining the amount of work performed by the rider.

ergonomic aid In athletic medicine, the questionable and often harmful use of various substances in an attempt to enhance performance. Some of these materials—such as blood transfusions, anabolic steroids, amphetamines, amino acids, and human growth hormone—are standard medicines approved for uses other than those intended by the athlete. Others are not only not indicated for any illness but may be harmful, esp. when the amount of the active ingredient in the product is unknown. Included in this latter group are cyproheptadine, taken to increase appetite, strength, and, allegedly, testosterone production; ginseng; pangamic acid; octacosanol, a 28-carbon straight-chain alcohol obtained from wheat germ oil, the biological effects of which are unknown; guarana, prepared from the seeds of the *Paulliania cupana* tree, used for its alleged ability to increase energy; gamma-oryzanol, an isomer of oryzanol extracted from rice bran oil, allegedly useful in decreasing recovery time after exercise; proteolytic enzymes (e.g., chymotrypsin, trypsin-chymotrypsin, and papain), the safety and efficacy of which have not been established, esp. when used with oral anticoagulants or by pregnant or lactating women; and bee pollen, which has shown no evidence of improving athletic performance. SEE: *anabolic agent; blood doping*.

ergonomics (ĕr″gō-nŏm′ĭks) [″ + *nomikos,* law] The science concerned with fitting a job to a person's anatomical, physiological, and psychological characteristics in a way that enhances human efficiency and well-being.

ergonovine maleate (ĕr″gō-nō′vĭn) An ergot derivative to treat migraine, and in obstetrics, to stimulate postpartum uterine contractions. Trade name is Ergotrate Maleate.

ergophobia (ĕr″gō-fō′bē-ă) [″ + *phobos,* fear] Morbid dread of working.

ergosterol (ĕr-gŏs′tĕr-ŏl) The primary sterol, or fat, found in the cell membranes of fungi. It plays a role similar to that of cholesterol in human cell walls. Most antifungal drugs act on ergosterol to increase permeability of the cell wall of the fungus, promoting its destruction.

ergot (ĕr′gŏt) A drug obtained from *Claviceps purpurea,* a fungus that grows parasitically on rye. Several valuable alkaloids, such as ergotamine, are obtained from ergot.

ergotamine (ĕr-gŏt′ă-mēn) A crystalline alkaloid, $C_{33}H_{35}O_5N_5$, derived from ergot.

e. tartrate A white crystalline substance that stimulates smooth muscle of blood vessels and the uterus, inducing vasoconstriction and uterine contractions. It is used in the treatment of migraine. Trade names are Ergomar, Ergostat, and Gynergen.

ergotherapy (ĕr″gō-thĕr′ă-pē) [″+ *therapeia,* treatment] Using physical exertion as a treatment for disease, (e.g., in the treatment of diabetes mellitus, type 2, or hyperlipidemia).

ergothioneine (ĕr-gō-thī′ō-nēn) $C_9H_{15}N_3O_2S \cdot 2H_2O$; thiolhistidine-betaine. A compound containing crystalline sulfur, it is found in ergot and red blood cells.

ergotism (ĕr′gŏ-tĭzm) ergot poisoning.

ergot poisoning A toxic reaction that may result from eating bread made with grain contaminated with the *Claviceps purpurea* fungus, or from an overdose of ergot. SYN: *ergotism*.

SYMPTOMS: Within several hours of ingestion, the patient may develop anticholinergic symptoms (such as abdominal cramping, bradycardia, pupillary dilation, urinary retention) and vasoconstriction (with ischemia and gangrene of the extremities).

TREATMENT: Sodium nitroprusside may counteract the vascular spasm produced by ergots. SEE: *Poisons and Poisoning Appendix*.

ergotrate (ĕr′gō-trāt) An active principle isolated from ergot.

Erikson, Erik H. [Ger.-born U.S. psychoanalyst, 1902–1993] A psychological theorist who proposed eight developmental stages from birth to late adulthood. In each stage, there is conflict between a specific psychosocial task and an opposing ego threat that must be resolved:

Birth to 1 year: Trust/mistrust

2 to 3 year: Autonomy/shame and doubt

4 to 5 year: Initiative/guilt

6 to 12 year: Industry/inferiority

13 to 18 year: Identity/role confusion

Young adult: Intimacy/isolation

Middle-aged adult: Generativity/self-absorption

Old adult: Ego integrity/despair

Eristalis (ĕrĭs′tă-lĭs) A genus of flies belonging to the family Syrphidae. The larva, called rat-tailed maggot (*E. tenax*), may cause intestinal myiasis in humans.

erode (ē-rōd′) [L. *erodere*] **1.** To wear away. **2.** To eat away by ulceration.

erogenous (ĕr-ŏj′ĕ-nŭs) [Gr. *eros,* love, + *gennan,* to produce] Causing sexual excitement. SYN: *erotogenic*.

eros **1.** In psychoanalysis, the collective instincts for self-preservation. **2.** Eros, the Greek god of love.

E rosette test A laboratory test performed to identify human T lymphocytes. When T lymphocytes combine with sheep red blood cells in a culture, a cluster of cells called a rosette forms. This test is often replaced by the use of monoclonal antibodies that identify the CD4 receptor specific for T cells.

erosion (ē-rō′shŭn) [L. *erodere,* to gnaw away] **1.** An eating away of tissue. **2.** External or internal destruction of a surface layer by physical or inflammatory processes.

e. of cervix uteri The alteration of

the epithelium on a portion of the cervix as a result of irritation or infection.

SYMPTOMS: In the early stages, the epithelium shows necrosis; in healing, there is a downgrowth of epithelium from the endocervical canal. If the growth is a single layer of tissue with a grossly granular appearance, it is called a simple granular erosion. If the growth is excessive and shows papillary tufts, it is called a papillary erosion. Histologically, the papillary erosion shows many branching racemose glands; their epithelium is the mucus-bearing cell with the nucleus at the base. In the healing process, squamous epithelium grows over the eroded area with one of the following results: the squamous cells replace the tissue beneath them completely, giving complete healing; the glands fill with squamous plugs and remain in that state; or the mouths of the glands are occluded by the squamous cells and nabothian cysts form. In the congenital type of erosion, the portio is covered by high columnar epithelium. SEE: *carcinoma in situ; Papanicolaou test.*

TREATMENT: Treatment consists of proper care of the cervix following delivery. Electrocauterization of the early erosion is usually curative. Cryotherapy may be used.

dental e. The wearing away of the surface layer (enamel) of a tooth. SEE: *abrasion; attrition; bruxism.*

erosive (ē-rō′sĭv) **1.** Able to produce erosion. **2.** An agent that erodes tissues or structures.

erotic (ĕ-rŏt′ĭk) [Gr. *erotikos*] **1.** Stimulating sexual desire. **2.** Concerning sexual love. **3.** A person who stimulates sexual desire.

eroticism (ĕ-rŏt′ĭ-sĭzm) [″ + *-ismos,* condition] Sexual desire.

anal e. **1.** Sensations of pleasure experienced through defecation during a stage in the development of children. **2.** In psychiatry, fixation of the libido at the anal-erotic developmental stage. Personality traits associated with anal eroticism include cleanliness, frugality, and neatness, and an unusual interest in regularity of bowel movements.

oral e. **1.** Sexual pleasure derived from use of the mouth. **2.** In psychiatry, fixation of the libido to the oral phase of development.

erotogenic (ĕ-rō″tō-jĕn′ĭk) [Gr. *eros,* love, + *gennan,* to produce] Producing sexual excitement. SEE: *erogenous zone.*

erotology (ĕr″ŏ-tŏl′ō-jē) [″ + *logos,* word, reason] The study of love and its manifestations.

erotomania (ĕ-rō″tŏ-, ĕ-rŏt″ŏ-mā′nē-ă) [″ + *mania,* madness] The delusion in a man or woman that he or she is loved by a particular person. SYN: *erotomonomania.*

erotomonomania Erotomania.

erotophobia (ĕ-rō″tō-, ĕ-rŏt″ō-fō′bē-ă) [″ + *phobos,* fear] An aversion to sexual love or its manifestations.

erratic [L. *errare,* to wander] Wandering, having an unpredictable or fluctuating course or pattern. SYN: *eccentric.*

error A mistake or miscalculation.

inborn e. of metabolism Any inherited metabolic disease caused by the absence or deficiency of specific enzymes necessary to the metabolism of basic substances such as amino acids, carbohydrates, vitamins, or essential trace elements. Examples include phenylketonuria and hereditary fructose intolerance. SEE: *metabolism.*

measurement e. The difference between the true value of something being measured and the value obtained by measurement. Measurement error can be the result of one or more of several different factors, including operational blunders, random error, and systematic error. SEE: *bias; proportional e.; random e.*

proportional e. Systematic error that varies directly with the concentration or activity of the analyte.

random e. The patternless differences observed between successive analytical results or statistical trials. Even though the individual results are patternless and unpredictable, the range of random error can be predicted with a given probability once sufficient experience has been gained. The random error is then quantified by the standard deviation, the coefficient of variation, and other statistics. SEE: *measurement e.; systematic e.*

systematic e. The residual error after random error has been subtracted from total error. SEE: *bias; proportional e.*

type I e. In statistics, experimental medicine, and epidemiology, erroneous rejection of a hypothesis.

type II e. In statistics, experimental medicine and epidemiology, erroneous acceptance of a hypothesis.

ERT *estrogen replacement therapy.*

eructation (ĕ-rŭk-tā′shŭn) [L. *eructare*] Producing gas from the stomach, usually with a characteristic sound; belching.

eruption (ē-rŭp′shŭn) [L. *eruptio,* a breaking out] **1.** A visible breaking out, esp. of a skin lesion or rash accompanying a disease such as measles or scarlet fever. **2.** The appearance of a lesion such as redness or spotting on the skin or mucous membrane. **3.** The breaking of a tooth through the gum; the cutting of a tooth. **eruptive** (-tĭv), *adj.*

active e. Movement of the tooth toward the occlusal plane.

creeping e. A skin lesion marked by a tortuous elevated red line that progresses at one end while fading out at the other. It is caused by the migration into the skin of the larvae of certain nematodes, esp. *Ancylostoma braziliense* and *A. caninum,* which are present in ground exposed to dog or cat feces. SYN: *cutaneous larva migrans*.

delayed e. The most common variation in the tooth eruption pattern. It may be due to crowding or to various genetic, endocrine, or physiological factors.

drug e. Dermatitis produced in some patients by application or ingestion of drugs. Drug rashes are usually not specific for certain drugs.

fixed drug e. A localized red rash with a sharp border, which follows exposure to a drug. The rash usually burns, occurs on the face or the genitals, and, if the offending agent is given again, recurs in the same location (i.e., it is "fixed" in place).

passive e. Increased size of the clinical crown of a tooth by apical migration of the attachment epithelium and periodontium.

seabather's e. Itching red papules that may appear on the skin within a few hours of swimming in saltwater. The rash is caused by the sting of the larval forms of the thimble jellyfish or the sea anemone. The rash is usually more prominent under swimsuits than on exposed skin because the pressure of clothing on the skin releases the stinging barbs of the larvae. The swimsuit should be washed before it is worn again. Treatment is symptomatic, with oral antihistamines or topical corticosteroids.

serum e. An eruption that occurs following the injection of serous fluid. It may be accompanied by chills, fever, and arthritic symptoms.

erysipelas (ĕr″ĭ-sĭp′ĕ-lăs) [Gr. *erythros,* red, + *pella,* skin] An infection of the skin (usually caused by group A streptococci) that is marked by a bright red, sharply defined rash on the face or legs. Systemic symptoms such as fevers, chills, sweats, or vomiting may occur; local tissue swelling and tenderness are common. A toxin released into the skin by *Streptococcus pyogenes* creates many of the signs and symptoms of the infection. SEE: illus.; *cellulitis*.

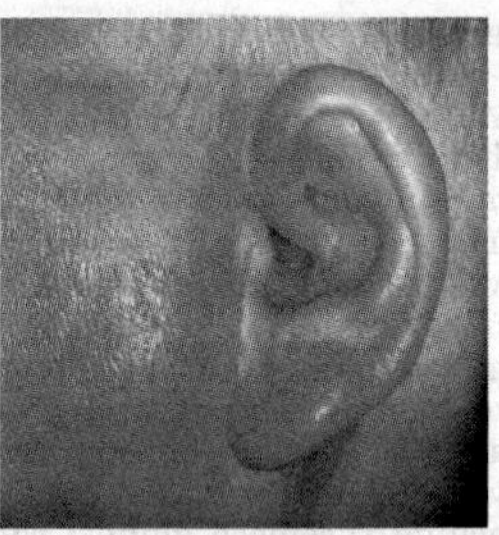

ERYSIPELAS

TREATMENT: Penicillins, erythromycin, first-generation cephalosporins, vancomycin, or clindamycin may effectively eradicate the responsible bacteria. Analgesic and antipyretic drugs, such as acetaminophen or ibuprofen, provide comfort.

PROGNOSIS: The prognosis is excellent with treatment. Without treatment, nephritis, abscesses, and septicemia may develop.

PATIENT CARE: Patients and family members are taught to use thorough handwashing before and after touching the affected area to prevent the spread of infection. The application of cool compresses and elevating the affected parts may reduce discomfort.

erysipelatous (ĕr″ĭ-sĭ-pĕl′ă-tŭs) Of the nature of or pert. to erysipelas.

erysipeloid (ĕr-ĭ-sĭp′ĕ-loyd) [″ + ″ + *eidos,* form, shape] Inflammation of the skin, primarily the hands and fingers, caused by the bacteria *Erysipelothrix rhusiopathiae.* It occurs in butchers, fishermen, and others who handle raw fish and poultry. The infected areas are warm, swollen, and reddish-purple. The infection rarely moves to the bloodstream and is treated with penicillin G or ampicillin, which resolves the infection in approx. 3 weeks. Erysipeloid-like rashes of the hands are sometimes caused by other infectious agents, such as *Leishmania* or fungi.

Erysipelothrix rhusiopathiae (ĕr″ĭ-sĭ-pĕl′ō-thrĭks) [″ + ″ + *thrix,* hair] A species of gram-positive, branching, filamentous, rod-shaped nonmotile bacteria. They cause erysipeloid.

erysipelotoxin (ĕr″ĭ-sĭp″ĕ-lō-tŏk′sĭn) The poisonous substance produced by *Streptococcus pyogenes,* the causative agent of erysipelas.

erysiphake (ĕr-ĭs′ĭ-fāk) A small spoon-shaped device used in cataract surgery to remove the lens by suction.

erythema (ĕr″ĭ-thē′mă) [Gr., redness] Reddening of the skin. Erythema is a common but nonspecific sign of skin irritation, injury, or inflammation. **erythematic, erythematous** (-thĕ-măt′ĭk, -thĕm′ă-tŭs), *adj.*

ETIOLOGY: It is caused by dilation of superficial blood vessels in the skin.

e. ab igne Localized erythema due to exposure to heat.

e. annulare A red, ring-shaped rash.

e. chronicum migrans ABBR: ECM. The hallmark of acute infection with Lyme disease. ECM is an expanding red rash with a sharply defined border and (typically) central clearing. The center of the rash is the site of inoculation (tick bite). The causitive agent is *Borrelia burgdorferi,* a spirochete that may later invade the joints, the central nervous system, or the conducting system of the heart. SEE: *Lyme disease* for illus.

e. induratum Chronic vasculitis of the skin occurring in young women. Hard cutaneous nodules break down to form necrotic ulcers and leave atrophic scars. SYN: *Bazin's disease.*

e. infectiosum A mild, moderately contagious disease seen most commonly in school-age children. SYN: *Fifth disease.*

ETIOLOGY: The causative agent is human parvovirus B-19. Transmission is thought to be via respiratory secretions from infected patients; however, maternal-fetal transmission can occur and hemolytic disease of the newborn may result.

SYMPTOMS: Patients experience a mild, brief illness; complaints include fever, malaise, headache, and pruritus. The characteristic erythema appears about 10 days later. Facial redness is similar to that which occurs when a child is slapped; however, circumoral redness is absent. Several days following initial erythema, a less distinct rash may appear on the extremities and trunk. The rash usually resolves within 1 week but may occur for several weeks when the patient is exposed to heat, cold, exercise, or stress. Adults may also experience arthralgia and arthritis, although these symptoms are less common in children. In addition, mild transient anemia, thrombocytopenia, and leukopenia may develop.

TREATMENT: Most patients require no specific therapy. Patients with coexisting chronic hemolytic anemia may experience transient aplastic crisis (TAC). These patients should be warned of the danger of exposure to parvovirus B-19 infection, informed of the early signs and symptoms, and instructed to seek medical consultation promptly if exposure is suspected. Patients with TAC may develop a life-threatening anemia that requires immediate blood transfusion or partial exchange transfusion.

e. intertrigo Chafing.

e. marginatum A form of erythema multiforme in which the center of the area fades, leaving elevated edges.

e. multiforme ABBR: EM. A rash that is usually caused by an immune response to drugs or to an infection, esp. herpes simplex virus. It may express itself on the skin in "multiform" ways, including macules, papules, blisters, hives, and, characteristically, iris or target lesions. It may involve the palms and soles, the mucous membranes, the face, and the extremities. The disease is usually self-limited. The most severe—and occasionally fatal—variant of the illness, in which the eyes, mouth, and internal organs are involved, is called Stevens-Johnson syndrome, or toxic epidermal necrolysis. SEE: illus.

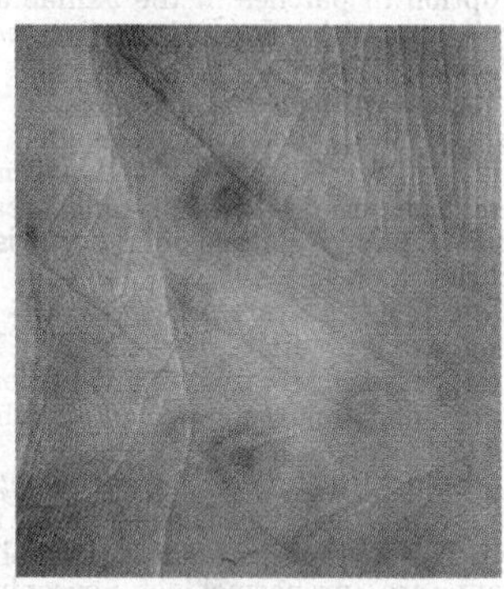

ERYTHEMA MULTIFORME

necrolytic migratory e. The raised red scaly rash characteristic of glucagonoma.

e. nodosum A tender, red, nodular rash on the shins that typically arises in conjunction with another illness, such as a streptococcal, fungal, or tubercular infection; inflammatory bowel disease; occult cancer; or sarcoidosis. Biopsies of the rash reveal inflammation of subcutaneous fat (panniculitis). Because the disease is often associated with other serious illnesses, a diagnostic search for an underlying cause usually is undertaken. In some patients, no cause is identified.

TREATMENT: Therapy is directed at the cause, when it is known. Nonsteroidal anti-inflammatory drugs provide symptomatic relief for many patients.

e. nodosum leprosum ABBR: ENL. A red, nodular vasculitic rash, which may be a complication of the treatment for leprosy. SEE: *lepra.*

TREATMENT: Treatment consists of withdrawing therapy against leprosy (i.e., clofazimine, steroids, or thalidomide).

punctate e. Erythema occurring in minute points, such as scarlet fever rash.

e. toxicum neonatorum A benign, self-limited rash marked by firm, yellow-white papules or pustules from 1 to 2 mm in size present in about 50% of full-term infants. The cause is unknown, and the lesions disappear without need for treatment.

e. venenatum A form of erythema caused by contact with a toxic substance.

erythemogenic (ĕr″ĭ-thē″mō-jĕn′ĭk) [″ +

gennan, to produce] Producing erythema.

erythr- SEE: *erythro-*.

erythralgia (ĕr″ĭ-thrăl′jē-ă) [″ + *algos,* pain] Erythromelalgia.

erythrasma (ĕr″ĭ-thrăz′mă) A red-brown eruption in patches in the axillae and groin caused by *Corynebacterium minutissimum.*

erythremia (ĕr″ĭ-thrē′mē-ă) [″ + *haima,* blood] Polycythemia vera.

erythrism (ĕr′ĭ-thrĭzm) [″ + *-ismos,* condition of] Red hair and beard with a ruddy complexion. **erythristic** (-thrĭs′tĭk), *adj.*

erythrityl tetranitrate (ĕ-rĭth′rĭ-tĭl) A drug used to dilate the coronary arteries, used in treating angina pectoris.

erythro-, erythr- [Gr. *erythros*] Combining form meaning *red.*

erythroblast (ĕ-rĭth′rō-blăst) [″ + *blastos,* germ] Any form of nucleated red cell. The earliest stages in the development are pronormoblast, basophilic normoblast, polychromatic normoblast, and orthochromatic normoblast. Nucleated red cells are not normally seen in the circulating blood. Erythroblasts contain hemoglobin. In the embryo they are found in blood islands of the yolk sac, body mesenchyma, liver, spleen, and lymph nodes; after the third month they are restricted to the bone marrow. **erythroblastic** (-blăs′tĭk), *adj.*

erythroblastemia (ĕ-rĭth″rō-blăs-tē′mē-ă) [″ + ″ + *haima,* blood] An excessive number of erythroblasts in the blood.

erythroblastoma (ĕ-rĭth″rō-blăs-tō′mă) [″ + *blastos,* germ, + *oma,* tumor] A tumor (myeloma) with cells resembling megaloblasts.

erythroblastosis (ĕ-rĭth″rō-blăs-tō′sĭs) [″ + ″ + *osis,* condition] A condition marked by erythroblasts in the blood.

e. fetalis A hemolytic disease of the newborn marked by anemia, jaundice, enlargement of the liver and spleen, and generalized edema (hydrops fetalis). SYN: *hemolytic disease of the newborn.*

erythrochloropia (ĕ-rĭth″rō-klor-ō′pē-ă) [Gr. *erythros,* red, + *chloros,* green, + *ops,* eye] Partial color blindness with ability to see red and green, but not blue and yellow.

erythrochromia (ĕ-rĭth″rō-krō′mē-ă) [″ +*chroma,* color] Hemorrhagic red pigmentation of the spinal fluid.

erythroclasis (ĕr″ĕ-thrŏk′lă-sĭs) The splitting up of red blood cells.

erythroclastic (ĕ-rĭth-rō-klăs′tĭk) [″ + *klasis,* a breaking] Destructive to red blood cells.

erythrocyanosis (ĕ-rĭth-rō-sī″ă-nō′sĭs) [″ + *kyanos,* blue, + *osis,* condition] Red or bluish discoloration on the skin with swelling, itching, and burning.

erythrocyte (ĕ-rĭth′rō-sīt) [″ + *kytos,* cell] A mature red blood cell (RBC). Each is a nonnucleated, biconcave disk averaging 7.7 μm in diameter. An RBC has a typical cell membrane and an internal stroma, or framework, made of lipids and proteins to which more than 200 million molecules of hemoglobin are attached. Hemoglobin is a conjugated protein consisting of a colored iron-containing portion (hematin) and a simple protein (globin). It combines readily with oxygen to form an unstable compound (oxyhemoglobin). The total surface area of the RBCs of an average adult is 3820 sq m, or about 2000 times more than the external total body surface area. SEE: illus. (Normal Erythrocytes); *blood* for illus.

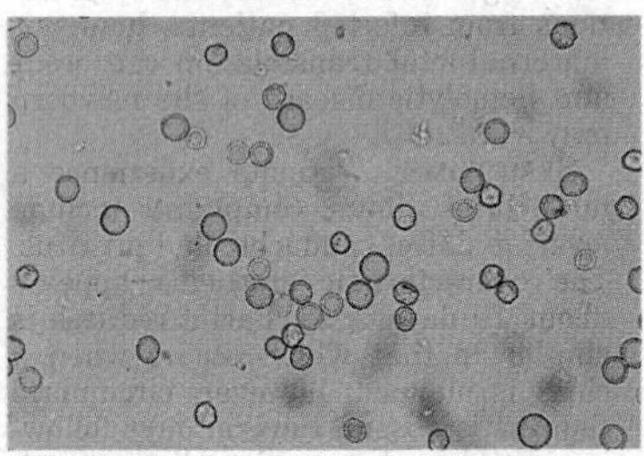

NORMAL ERYTHROCYTES, UNSTAINED

(Orig. mag. ×400)

NUMBER: In a normal person, the number of RBCs averages about 5,000,000 per microliter (5,500,000 for men and 4,500,000 for women). The total number in an average-sized person is about 35 trillion. The number per microliter varies with age (higher in infants), time of day (lower during sleep), activity and environmental temperature (increasing with both), and altitude. Persons living at altitudes of 10,000 ft (3048 m) or more may have an RBC count of 8,000,000 per microliter or more.

If an individual has a normal blood volume of 5 L (70 ml per kilogram of body weight) and 5,000,000 RBCs per mm^3 of blood, and the RBCs have an average life span of about 120 days, the red bone marrow must produce 2,400,000 RBCs per second to maintain this concentration of blood.

PHYSIOLOGY: The primary function of RBCs is to carry oxygen. The hemoglobin also contributes to the acid-base balance of the blood by acting as a buffer for the transport of carbon dioxide in the plasma as bicarbonate ions.

DEVELOPMENT: RBC formation (erythropoiesis) in adults takes place in the bone marrow, principally in the vertebrae, ribs, sternum, diploë of cranial bones, and proximal ends of the humerus and femur. They arise from large nucleated stem cells (promegaloblasts), which give rise to pronormoblasts, in which hemoglobin appears. These produce normoblasts, which extrude their nuclei. RBCs at this stage possess a fine reticular network and are known as reticulocytes. This reticular structure is usually lost before the cells enter circulation as mature RBCs. The proper formation of RBCs depends on several factors, including healthy condition of the bone marrow; dietary substances such as iron, cobalt, and copper, all essential for the formation of hemoglobin; essential amino acids; and certain vitamins, esp. B_{12} and folic acid (pteroylglutamic acid). SEE: illus. (Erythrocyte Development).

The average life span of an RBC is about 120 days. As RBCs age and become fragile, they are removed from circulation by macrophages in the liver, spleen, and red bone marrow. The protein and iron of hemoglobin are reused; iron may be stored in the liver until needed for the production of new RBCs in the bone marrow. The heme portion of the hemoglobin is converted to bilirubin, which is excreted in bile as one of the bile pigments.

VARIETIES: On microscopic examination, RBCs may reveal variations in the following respects: size (anisocytosis), shape (poikilocytosis), staining reaction (achromia, hypochromia, hyperchromia, polychromatophilia), structure (possession of bodies such as Cabot's rings, Howell-Jolly bodies, Heinz bodies; parasites such as malaria; a reticular network; or nuclei), and number (anemia, polycythemia).

achromatic e. An RBC from which the hemoglobin has been dissolved; a colorless cell.

basophilic e. An RBC in which cytoplasm stains blue. The staining may be diffuse (material uniformly distributed) or punctate (material appearing as pinpoint dots).

crenated e. An RBC with a serrated or indented edge, usually the result of withdrawal of water from the cell, as occurs when cells are placed in hypertonic solutions.

immature e. Any incompletely developed RBC.

orthochromatic e. An RBC that stains with acid stains only, the cytoplasm appearing pink.

polychromatic e. An RBC that does not stain uniformly.

erythrocyte reinfusion **1.** Infusion of blood into the person who donated it. This is usually done by obtaining one or two units of blood, separating the red blood cells and infusing them at a later date. **2.** Infusion with his or her own blood by a healthy person in an attempt to enhance athletic performance. SYN: *blood doping*.

erythrocythemia (ĕ-rĭth″rō-sī-thē′mē-ă) [Gr. *erythros,* red, + *kytos,* cell, + *haima,* blood] An obsolete term for polycythemia vera.

erythrocytolysin (ĕ-rĭth″rō-sī-tŏl′ĭ-sĭn) Anything that hemolyzes red blood cells.

erythrocytolysis (ĕ-rĭth″rō-sī-tŏl′ĭ-sĭs) [″ + ″ + *lysis,* dissolution] Dissolution of red blood cells with the escape of hemoglobin.

erythrocytometer (ĕ-rĭth″rō-sī-tŏm′ĕ-tĕr) [″ + ″ + *metron,* measure] An instrument for counting red blood cells.

erythrocyto-opsonin (ĕ-rĭth″rō-sī″tō-ŏp-sō′nĭn) [″ + ″ + *opsonein,* to buy food] A substance opsonic for red blood cells.

erythrocytopenia (ĕ-rĭth″rō-sī″tō-pē′nē-ă) [″ + ″ + *penia,* poverty] A deficiency in the number of red blood cells in the body. SYN: *erythropenia*.

erythrocytopoiesis Erythropoiesis.

erythrocytorrhexis (ĕ-rĭth″rō-sī″tō-

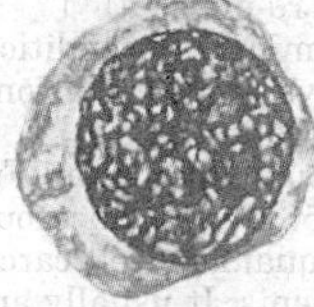
PRONORMOBLAST

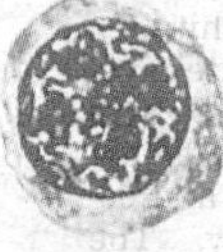
BASOPHILIC NORMOBLAST

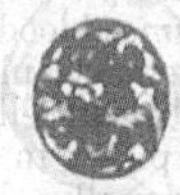
POLYCHROMATIC NORMOBLAST

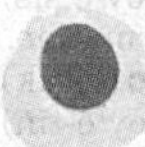
ORTHOCHROMATIC NORMOBLAST

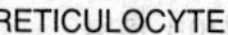
RETICULOCYTE

ERYTHROCYTE

ERYTHROCYTE DEVELOPMENT

rĕk′sĭs) [″ + ″ + *rhexis,* rupture] The breaking up of red blood cells with particles or fragments of the cells escaping into the plasma.

erythrocytosis (ĕ-rĭth″rō-sī-tō′sĭs) [″ + ″ + *osis,* increasing condition] An abnormal increase in the number of red blood cells in circulation, found, for example, in hypoxemic patients or patients with polycythemia vera.

stress e. Gaisböck's syndrome.

erythroderma, erythrodermia (ĕ-rĭth″rō-dĕr′mă) [″ + *derma,* skin] Abnormally widespread redness and scaling of the skin, sometimes involving the entire body. This condition may be seen in patients with extensive psoriasis, cutaneous T-cell lymphoma, drug reactions, seborrheic or atopic dermatitis, or other conditions. SYN: *erythrodermia; exfoliative dermatitis.*

e. desquamativum A disease of breast-fed infants. Resembling seborrhea, it is characterized by redness of the skin and development of scales.

e. ichthyosiforme congenitum A congenital condition characterized by thickening and redness of the skin; it may resemble ichthyosis or lichen.

erythrodermia (ĕ-rĭth″rō-dĕr′mē-ă) Erythroderma.

erythrodontia (ĕ-rĭth″rō-dŏn′shē-ă) [″ + *odous,* tooth] Reddish-brown or yellow discoloration of the dentin of the teeth. This may be present in patients with congenital erythropoietic porphyria.

erythrogenesis (ĕ-rĭth″rō-jĕn′ĕ-sĭs) [″ + *genesis,* generation, birth] The development of red blood cells.

erythroid (ĕr′ĭ-throyd) [″ + *eidos,* form, shape] **1.** Reddish. **2.** Concerning the red blood cells.

erythrokeratodermia (ĕ-rĭth″rō-kĕr″ă-tō-dĕr′mē-ă) [″ + *keras,* horn, + *derma,* skin] Reddening and hardening of the skin.

erythrokinetics (ĕ-rĭth″rō-kĭ-nĕt′ĭks) [″ + *kinesis,* movement] The quantitative description of the production rate of red blood cells and their life span.

erythroleukemia (ĕ-rĭth″rō-loo-kē′mē-ă) [Gr. *erythros,* red, + *leukos,* white, + *haima,* blood] A variant of acute myelogenous leukemia with anemia, bizarre red blood cell morphology, erythroid hyperplasia in the bone marrow, and occasionally hepatosplenomegaly. The leukocyte count may be extremely high or quite low.

erythromelalgia (ĕ-rĭth″rō-mĕl-ăl′jē-ă) [″ + *melos,* limb, + *algos,* pain] Episodic burning, throbbing, and redness of the extremities caused by local dilation of blood vessels. The affected areas (typically the feet or lower legs) become flushed and warm. This condition is a symptom of myeloproliferative diseases, such as polycythemia vera, and of neuritis, multiple sclerosis, and systemic lupus erythematosus. It may also occur as a drug reaction. SYN: *acromelalgia; erythralgia.*

erythromelia (ĕ-rĭth″rō-mē′lē-ă) [″ + *melos,* limb] Painless erythema of the extensor surfaces of the extremities.

erythromycin (ĕ-rĭth″rō-mī′sĭn) [″ + *mykes,* fungus] An antibiotic derived from *Streptomyces erythraeus,* used primarily to treat gram-positive and atypical microorganisms, such as streptococci, mycoplasma, and legionella. Its primary side effects are nausea, vomiting, abdominal pain, bloating, and diarrhea.

erythron (ĕr′ĭ-thrŏn) [Gr. *erythros,* red] The blood as a body system including the circulating red cells and the tissue from which they originate.

erythroneocytosis (ĕ-rĭth″rō-nē″ō-sī-tō′sĭs) [″ + *neos,* new, + kytos, cell, + *osis,* condition] The presence of immature red blood cells in the peripheral blood.

erythroparasite (ĕ-rĭth″rō-păr′ă-sīt) [″ + *parasitos,* parasite] A red blood cell parasite.

erythropenia (ĕ-rĭth″rō-pē′nē-ă) [″ + *penia,* poverty] Erythrocytopenia.

erythrophage (ĕ-rĭth′rō-fāj) [″ + *phagein,* to eat] A phagocyte that destroys red blood cells.

erythrophagia Destruction of red blood cells by phagocytes.

erythrophile (ĕ-rĭth′rō-fīl [″ + *philein,* to love]. An agent that readily stains red. **erythrophilous** (ĕr″ĭ-thrŏf′ĭ-lŭs), *adj.*

erythrophobia (ĕ-rĭth″rō-fō′bē-ă) [″ + *phobos,* fear] **1.** Abnormal dread of blushing or fear of being diffident or embarrassed. **2.** Morbid fear of, or aversion to, anything red.

erythrophose (ĕ-rĭth′rō-fōz) [″ + *phos,* light] Any red subjective perception of a bright spot. SEE: *phose.*

erythropia, erythropsia (ĕr″ĭ-thrō′pē-ă, -thrŏp′sē-ă) [″ + *opsis,* vision] A condition in which objects appear to be red.

erythroplasia (ĕ-rĭth″rō-plā′zē-ă) [″ + *plasis,* molding, forming] A condition characterized by erythematous lesions of the mucous membranes.

e. of Queyrat [Louis A. Queyrat, Fr. physician, 1856–1953] A precancerous lesion or invasive squamous cell carcinoma of the glans penis. It usually appears moist or velvety, and typically arises in uncircumcised middle-aged men.

erythropoiesis (ĕ-rĭth″rō-poy-ē′sĭs) [″ + *poiesis,* making] The formation of red blood cells. **erythropoietic** (-ĕt′ĭk), *adj.*

erythropoietin (ĕ-rĭth″rō-poy′ĕ-tĭn) A cytokine made by the kidneys that stimulates the proliferation of red blood cells. Synthetic erythropoietin (epoetin alfa) is used to treat anemia, esp. in patients with renal or bone marrow failure. Hypertension is a common side effect of the drug. SEE: *blood doping; cytokine; epoetin alfa.*

CAUTION: Athletes have used erythropoietin in an attempt to enhance performance. When the hormone is used without medical supervision and in large doses, it can cause an abnormal increase in red blood cell mass and may lead to death.

erythroprosopalgia (e-rĭth″rō-prō-sō-păl′jē-ă) [″ + *prosopon,* face, + *algos,* pain] Neuropathy marked by redness and pain in the face.

erythropoietin independence A characteristic of red blood cell colonies in polycythemia rubra vera. Normal red blood cell progenitors do not multiply without stimulation by erythropoietin; cells from patients with polycythemia vera can replicate independently of this cytokine because of the intracellular derangement of other growth-promoting proteins.

erythropsia (ĕr-ĭ-thrŏp′sē-ă) [″ + *opsis,* vision] A disorder of color vision in which all objects look red.

erythropsin (ĕ-rĭth-rŏp′sĭn) [″ + *opsis,* vision] A term formerly used to indicate rhodopsin, or visual purple. SYN: *rhodopsin.*

erythrosine sodium A dye used as a dental disclosing agent. It is applied to the teeth in a 2% solution or in soluble tablets, which are chewed. SEE: *disclosing agent.*

erythrosis (ĕr-ĭ-thrō′sĭs) [″ + *osis,* condition] A reddish-purple discoloration of the skin and mucous membranes in polycythemia.

erythrostasis (ē-rĭth″rō-stā′sĭs) [″ + *stasis,* standing still] Accumulation of red blood cells in vessels due to cessation of the blood flow. SEE: *sludged blood.*

erythrotoxin (ĕ-rĭth″rō-tŏk′sĭn) [″ + *toxikon,* poison] An exotoxin that lyses red blood cells.

erythruria (ĕr-ĭ-thrū′rē-ă) [″ + *ouron,* urine] Red color of the urine.

Es Symbol for the element einsteinium.

escape [O. Fr. *escaper*] **1.** To break out of confinement; to leak or seep out. **2.** The act of attaining freedom.

vagal e. An ectopic heartbeat that occurs when the normal rhythm of the heart has been stopped or inhibited by stimulation of the vagus nerve.

ventricular e. Single or repeated ventricular beats that arise from pacemakers in the ventricular muscle when beats from pacemakers in the sinoatrial or atrioventricular nodes fail to appear.

escape phenomenon The development of resistance to the effects of a continuously present stimulus.

eschar (ĕs′kăr) [Gr. *eschara,* scab] Dead matter that is cast off from the surface of the skin, esp. after a burn. The material is often crusty or scabbed. SEE: *escharotic.*

escharotic (ĕs-kăr-ŏt′ĭk) [Gr. *escharotikos*] A caustic agent, such as a strong acid or base, that is used to destroy tissue and cause sloughing. Escharotics may be acids, alkalies, metallic salts, phenol or carbolic acid, carbon dioxide, or electric cautery.

escharotomy (ĕs-kăr-ŏt′ō-mē) [Gr. *eschara,* scab, + *tome,* incision] **1.** Removal of the eschar formed on the skin and underlying tissue of severely burned areas. This procedure can be life-saving when used to allow expansion of the chest and is also used to restore circulation to the extremities of patients in which the eschar forms a tight swollen band around the circumference of the limb. **2.** Excision of dense necrotic skin about a decubitus or ischemic ulcer.

Escherichia (ĕsh-ĕr-īk′ē-ă) A genus of bacteria belonging to the family Enterobacteriaceae, tribe Eschericheae. They are common inhabitants of the alimentary canal of humans and other animals.

Escherichia coli ABBR: E. coli. A gram-negative bacillus in the human colon. These small, plump, aerobic bacilli are normally nonpathogenic in the intestinal tract, but some serotypes may cause diarrheal illnesses, urinary tract infections, sepsis, or the hemolytic uremic syndrome. The bacillus is motile and non-spore forming. Certain enterotoxigenic strains are a principal cause of travelers' diarrhea.

TREATMENT: *E. coli* are sensitive to many antibiotics, including sulfa drugs and quinolones. Diarrhea caused by *E. coli* also should be treated with aggressive fluid and electrolyte replacement to prevent dehydration.

enteroaggregative E.c. ABBR: EAggEC. A type of *E. coli* that causes persistent diarrhea.

enterohemorrhagic E.c. ABBR: EHEC. The strain of *E. coli* that causes colitis with copious bloody diarrhea.

enteroinvasive E.c. ABBR: EIEC. A type of *E. coli* that invades and multiplies in the epithelial cells of the distal ileum and colon causing dysentery.

enteropathogenic E.c. ABBR: EPEC. A type of *E. coli* that produces infantile diarrhea.

enterotoxigenic E.c. ABBR: ETEC. A type of *E. coli* that can cause diarrhea in infants and travelers. Fluid loss may be as severe as in cholera.

E.c. 0157:H7 An enterohemorrhagic *E. coli* serotype that produces verotoxin, also called *Shiga-like* toxin. It was first recognized as a cause of an outbreak of hemorrhagic colitis in 1982. Since that time, a number of outbreaks have occurred in schools, nursing homes, day care centers, families, and communities. The organism may be present in undercooked meat, esp. hamburger; unpreserved apple cider; vegetables grown in cow manure; or contaminated water supplies. The infection may be spread from one person to another through food-to-food cross-contamination.

SYMPTOMS: Asymptomatic infection is common. In other cases, after the 3- to 8-day incubation period, an afebrile and self-limiting diarrhea occurs; however, the infection may progress to hemorrhagic colitis with bloody diarrhea, severe abdominal pain, and low-grade fever. Resolution usually occurs in 1 week. In 2% to 7% of cases, patients will develop hemolytic uremic syndrome (HUS); the mortality among patients who develop HUS ranges from 3% to 5%. The highest incidence of HUS is found among children and the elderly.

DIAGNOSIS: Without a high index of suspicion, diagnosis in either a lone case or an outbreak may be delayed. To prevent unnecessary diagnostic or therapeutic intervention, such as colonoscopy or colectomy, diagnosis should be made as quickly as possible.

PREVENTION: Ground meat should be cooked until it reaches a temperature of 160°F (71.1°C) and the meat should not be pink in the center. Leftovers should be reheated to 165°F (73.3°C). Individuals who change a baby's diapers should thoroughly wash their hands immediately afterward. Food handlers must wash their hands after using the toilet.

Escherich's reflex (ĕsh′ĕr-ĭks) [Theodor Escherich, Ger. physician, 1857–1911] A pursing or muscular contraction of the lips resulting from irritation of the mucosa of the lips.

eschrolalia (ĕs-krō-lā′lē-ă) [Gr. *aischros,* indecent, + *lalia,* babble] Coprolalia.

escorcin (ĕs-kor′sĭn) A stain derived from escalin. It is used to stain and identify defects or injury of the cornea.

esculent (ĕs′kū-lĕnt) Suitable for use as food.

escutcheon (ĕs-kŭch′ăn) [L. *scutum,* a shield] The pattern of pubic hair growth. It is different in males and females.

eserine (ĕs′ĕr-ĭn) [*esere,* African name for the Calabar bean] Physostigmine salicylate.

ESF *erythropoietic stimulating factor.* SEE: *erythropoietin*.

-esis Suffix meaning *condition* or *state.* SEE: *-sis; -asis; -osis*.

Esmarch's bandage (ĕs′mărks) [Johannes F. A. von Esmarch, Ger. surgeon, 1823–1908] **1.** A triangular bandage. **2.** A rubber bandage used to minimize bleeding. Before surgery is begun, the bandage is applied tightly to the limb, commencing at the distal end and reaching above the site of operation, where a pneumatic tourniquet is firmly applied. The bandage is then removed, having rendered the surgical area virtually bloodless. SEE: *bandage*.

esodic (ē-sŏd′ĭk) [Gr. *es,* toward, + *hodos,* way] Pert. to sensory nerves conducting impulses toward the brain and spinal cord. SYN: *afferent; centripetal*.

esoethmoiditis (ĕs″ō-ĕth″moy-dī′tĭs) [Gr. *eso,* inward, + *ethmos,* sieve, + *eidos,* form, shape, + *itis,* inflammation] Inflammation of the membrane of ethmoid cells.

esogastritis (ĕs″ō-găs-trī′tĭs) [″ + *gaster,* belly, + *itis,* inflammation] Inflammation of the gastric mucous membrane.

esoph- SEE: *esophago-*.

esophag- SEE: *esophago-*.

esophagalgia (ē-sŏf-ă-găl′jē-ă) [Gr. *oisophagos,* esophagus, + *algos,* pain] Pain in the esophagus.

esophageal (ē-sŏf″ă-jē′ăl) Pert. to the esophagus.

esophageal apoplexy An intramural hematoma of the esophagus.

esophageal cancer An adenocarcinoma or squamous cell carcinoma of the esophagus. The disease is responsible for more than 10,000 deaths each year in the U.S. It occurs most often in men over the age of 60.

Esophageal tumors usually are fungating and infiltrating, and in most cases, the tumor partially constricts the esophageal lumen. Regional metastasis occurs early by way of submucosal lymphatics, often fatally invading adjacent vital intrathoracic organs. The liver and lungs are the usual sites of distant metastases.

PREDISPOSING FACTORS: The cause of esophageal cancer is unknown; however, several predisposing factors have been identified. These include chronic smoking or excessive use of alcohol; stasis-induced inflammation, as in achalasia or stricture; previous head and neck tumors; and nutritional deficiency, as in untreated sprue and Plummer-Vinson syndrome.

COMPLICATIONS: Direct invasion of adjoining structures may lead to severe complications, such as mediastinitis, tracheoesophageal or bronchoesophageal fistula (causing an overwhelming cough when swallowing liquids), and aortic perforation with sudden exsanguination. Other complications include an inability to control secretions, obstruction of the esophagus, malnutrition, and loss of lower esophageal sphincter control, which can result in aspiration pneumonia.

SIGNS AND SYMPTOMS: Early in the disease, the patient may report a feeling of fullness, pressure, indigestion, or substernal burning and may report using antacids to relieve gastrointestinal upset. Later, the patient may complain of dysphagia and weight loss. The degree of dysphagia varies, depending on the extent of the disease, ranging from mild dysphagia occurring only after eating solid foods (esp. meat) to difficulty in swallowing coarse foods and even liquids. The patient may complain of hoarseness (from laryngeal nerve involvement), a chronic cough (possibly from aspiration), anorexia, vomiting, and regurgitation of food. These latter symptoms result from the tumor size exceeding the limits of the esophagus. The patient may also complain of pain on swallowing or pain that radiates to the back. In the later stages of the disease, the patient will appear very thin, cachectic, and dehydrated.

DIAGNOSTIC TESTS: Radiography of the esophagus, with barium swallow and motility studies; chest radiography or esophagography; esophagoscopy; punch and brush biopsies; and exfoliative cytological tests; bronchoscopy; endoscopic ultrasonography of the esophagus; computed tomography scan; magnetic resonance imaging; liver function studies; a liver scan; and mediastinal tomography may be performed to delineate the tumor, confirm its type, reveal growth into adjacent structures, and reveal distant metastatic lesions.

TREATMENT: Because esophageal cancer usually is advanced when diagnosed, treatment is often palliative rather than curative. Treatment to keep the esophagus patent includes dilation, laser therapy, radiation therapy, and insertion of prosthetic tubes to bridge the tumor. Radical surgery can excise the tumor and resect either the esophagus alone or the stomach and esophagus. Chemotherapy and radiation therapy can slow the growth of the tumor. Gastrostomy or jejunostomy can help provide adequate nutrition. A prosthesis can be used to seal fistulae. Endoscopic laser treatment and bipolar electrocoagulation can help restore swallowing by vaporizing cancerous tissue; however, if the tumor is in the upper esophagus, the laser cannot be positioned properly. Analgesics provide pain control.

PROGNOSIS: Regardless of cell type, the prognosis for esophageal cancer is grim: 5-year survival rates are less than 5%, and most patients die within 6 months of diagnosis.

PATIENT CARE: The patient is assessed for signs and symptoms as above. Food and fluid intake and body weight are monitored. All procedures are explained; the patient is prepared physically and emotionally for surgery and postsurgical care as indicated.

A high-calorie, high-protein diet is provided. Pureed or liquefied foods and commercially available nutritional supplements are offered as necessary. Supplemental parenteral nutrition is administered as prescribed. The patient is placed in Fowler's position for meals and plenty of time is allowed to eat to prevent aspiration. Any regurgitation is documented, and oral hygiene is provided. Prescribed analgesics and noninvasive pain relief measures are provided.

When a gastrostomy tube is used, feedings are administered slowly by gravity in prescribed amounts (usually 200 to 500 ml), and the patient may be given something to chew before and during each feeding to stimulate gastric secretions and promote some semblance of normal eating. The patient and family are taught about nutritional concerns (e.g., care of the feeding tube, including checking patency; administering the feeding; providing skin care at the insertion site; and keeping the patient upright during and immediately after feedings).

After surgery, vital signs and fluid and electrolyte balance (including intake and output) are monitored. The patient is observed for complications, such as infection, fistula formation, pneumonia, empyema, and malnutrition. If surgical resection with an esophageal anastomosis was performed, the patient is observed for signs of an anastomotic leak. If a prosthetic tube was inserted, the patient is monitored for signs of blockage or dislodgement, which can perforate the mediastinum or precipitate tumor erosion.

If chemotherapy is prescribed, the patient is monitored for complications such as bone marrow suppression and gastrointestinal reactions. Adverse reactions are minimized by use of saline mouthwashes. Extra periods of rest are encouraged, and prescribed medications are administered. If radiation therapy is used, the patient is monitored for complications such as esophageal perforation, pneumonitis, pulmonary fibrosis, and spinal cord inflammation (myelitis).

Expected outcomes of the prescribed therapies are explained to the patient and family. Assurance is provided that pain will be managed, and the nurse or other health care providers stay with the patient during periods of anxiety or distress. The patient is encouraged to participate in care decisions.

The patient should resume as normal a routine as possible during recovery to maintain a sense of control and to reduce complications associated with immobility. Both patient and family are referred to appropriate organizations for information and support.

esophagectasia, esophagectasis (ē-sŏf″ă-jĕk-tā′sē-ă, -jĕk′tă-sĭs) [″ + *ektasis,* distention] Dilatation of the esophagus.

esophagectomy (ē-sŏf″ă-jĕk′tō-mē) [″ + *ektome,* excision] Surgical removal of all or a portion of the esophagus.

esophagismus (ē-sŏf-ă-jĭs′mŭs) [″ + *-ismos,* condition] Spasm of the esophagus.

esophagitis (ē-sŏf-ă-jī′tĭs) [″ + *itis,* inflammation] Inflammation of the esophagus. SEE: *acid reflux test.*

reflux e. SEE: *gastroesophageal reflux; reflux disease.*

esophago-, esoph-, esophag- [Gr. *oisophagos,* esophagus] Combining form meaning *esophagus.*

esophagobronchial (ĕ-sŏf″ă-gō-brŏng′kē-ăl) [″ + *bronchos,* windpipe] Concerning the esophagus and bronchus.

esophagocele (ē-sŏf′ă-gō-sēl) [″ + *kele,* tumor, swelling] A hernia of the esophagus.

esophagodynia (ē-sŏf″ă-gō-dĭn′ē-ă) [Gr. *oisophagos,* esophagus, + *odyne,* pain] Pain in the esophagus.

esophagoenterostomy (ē-sŏf″ă-gō-ĕn-tĕr-ŏs′tō-mē) [″ + *enteron,* intestine, + *stoma,* mouth] A surgical opening between the esophagus and intestine following excision of the stomach.

esophagogastrectomy (ĕ-sŏf″ă-gō-găs-trĕk′tō-mē) [″ + *gaster,* belly, + *ektome,* excision] Surgical removal of all or part of the stomach and esophagus.

esophagogastroanastomosis (ĕ-sŏf″ă-gō-găs″trō-ă-năs″tō-mō′sĭs) [″ + ″ + *anastomosis,* opening] A joining of the esophagus to the stomach.

esophagogastroplasty (ĕ-sŏf′ă-gō-găs′trō-plăs″tē) [″ + ″ + *plassein,* to form] Plastic repair of the esophagus and stomach.

esophagogastroscopy (ē-sŏf″ă-gō-găs-trŏs′kō-pē) [″ + ″ + *skopein,* to examine] Inspection of the esophagus and stomach by using an endoscope.

esophagogastrostomy (ē-sŏf″ă-gō-găs-trŏs′tō-mē) [″ + ″ + *stoma,* mouth] Formation of an opening or anastomosis between the esophagus and stomach.

esophagojejunostomy (ē-sŏf″ă-gō-jĕ-jū-nŏs′tō-mē) [″ + L. *jejunum,* empty, + Gr. *stoma,* mouth] The surgical anastomosis of a free end of the divided jejunum to the esophagus. It provides a bypass for food in cases of esophageal stricture.

esophagomalacia (ē-sŏf″ă-gō-mă-lā′sē-ă) [Gr. *oisophagos,* esophagus, + *malakia,* softness] Softening of the esophageal walls.

esophagomycosis (ē-sŏf″ă-gō-mī-kō′sĭs) [″ + *mykes,* fungus, + *osis,* condition] A fungal disease of the esophagus, typically esophageal candidiasis. SEE: *antigenic shift.*

esophagomyotomy (ĕ-sŏf″ă-gō-mī-ŏt′ō-mē) [″ + *mys,* muscle, + *tome,* incision] Cutting of the muscular coat of the esophagus, used in treating stenosis of the lower esophagus. SEE: *achalasia.*

esophagoplasty (ē-sŏf′ă-gō-plăs″tē) [″ + *plassein,* to form] Repair of the esophagus by plastic surgery.

esophagoplication (ē-sŏf″ă-gō-plĭ-kā′shŭn) [″ + L. *abplicare,* to fold] Division of the longitudinal and circular muscles of the distal esophagus.

esophagoptosia, esophagoptosis (ē-sŏf″ă-gŏp-tō′sē-ă, -sĭs) [″ + *ptosis,* a dropping] Relaxation and prolapse of the esophagus.

esophagoscope (ē-sŏf′ă-gō-skōp) [″ + *skopein,* to examine] An endoscope for examination of the esophagus.

esophagospasm (ē-sŏf′ă-gō-spăzm″) [″ + *spasmos,* a convulsion] A spasm of the esophagus.

esophagostenosis (ē-sŏf″ă-gō-stĕn-ō′sĭs) [″ + *stenosis,* act of narrowing] Stricture or narrowing of the esophagus.

esophagostomy (ē-sŏf-ă-gŏs′tō-mē) [″ + *stoma,* mouth] Surgical formation of an opening into the esophagus.

esophagotome (ē-sŏf′ă-gō-tōm) [″ + *tome,* incision] An instrument for forming an esophageal fistula.

esophagotomy (ē-sŏf-ă-gŏt′ō-mē) A surgical incision into the esophagus. SEE: *achalasia; cardiospasm; dysphagia.*

esophagotracheal (ĕ-sŏf″ă-gō-trā′kē-ăl) Concerning the esophagus and the trachea, or a communication between them.

esophagus (ē-sŏf′ă-gŭs) *pl.* **esophagi** [Gr. *oisophagos*] The muscular tube, about 10 to 12 in. (25 to 30 cm) long, that carries swallowed foods and liquids from the pharynx to the stomach. In the upper third of the esophagus, the muscle is striated; in the middle third, striated and smooth; and in the lower third, entirely smooth. Peristalsis is regulated by the autonomic nervous system. At the junction with the stomach is the lower esophageal or cardiac sphincter, which relaxes to permit passage of food, then contracts to prevent backup of stomach contents. SEE: illus.

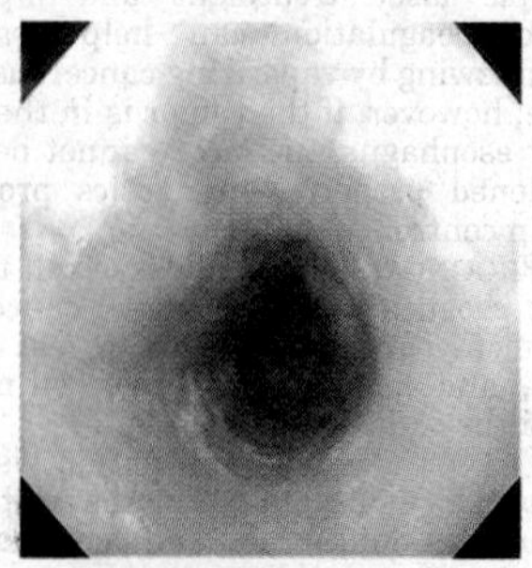

ESOPHAGUS
(as seen through an endoscope)

esophoria (ĕs-ō-fō′rē-ă) [Gr. *eso,* inward, + *phorein,* to bear] **1.** The tendency of visual lines to converge. **2.** An inward turning, or the amount of inward turning, of the eye. Opposite of exophoria. SEE: *heterotropia.*

esosphenoiditis (ĕs″ō-sfē-noyd-ī′tĭs) [″ + *sphen,* wedge, + *eidos,* form, shape, + *itis,* inflammation] Osteomyelitis of the sphenoid bone.

esotropia (ĕs-ō-trō′pē-ă) [″ + *tropos,* turning] Marked turning inward of the eye; crossed eyes.

ESP *extrasensory perception.*

ESR *electron spin resonance; erythrocyte sedimentation rate.*

ESRD *end-stage renal disease.*

essence [L. *essentia,* being or quality] **1.** The spirit or principle of anything. **2.** An alcoholic solution of volatile oil.

essential [L. *essentialis*] **1.** Pert. to an essence. **2.** Indispensable. **3.** Independent of a local abnormal condition; having no obvious external cause. SEE: *idiopathic.*

EST *electroshock therapy.* SEE: *electroconvulsive therapy.*

ester [L. *aether,* ether] In organic chemistry, a fragrant compound formed by the combination of an organic acid with an alcohol. This reaction removes water from the compound.

esterase (ĕs′tĕr-ās) Generic term for an enzyme that catalyzes the hydrolysis of esters.

esterification (ĕs-tĕr″ĭ-fĭ-kā′shŭn) The combination of an organic acid with an alcohol to form an ester.

esthematology (ĕs″thĕm-ă-tŏl′ō-jē) [Gr. *aisthema,* sensation, + *logos,* word, reason] The science of the sense organs and their function.

esthesia (ĕs-thē′zē-ă) [Gr. *aisthesis,* sensation] **1.** Perception; feeling; sensation. **2.** Any disease that affects sensation or perception.

esthesiology (ĕs-thē″zē-ŏl′ō-jē) [″ + *logos,* word, reason] The science of sensory phenomena.

esthesiometer, aesthesiometer (ĕs-thē-zē-ŏm′ĕ-tĕr) [″ + *metron,* measure] A device for measuring tactile sensibility.

esthesioneurosis (ĕs-thē″zē-ō-nū-rō′sĭs) [″ + *neuron,* nerve, + *osis,* condition] Any sensory impairment.

esthesiophysiology (ĕs-thē″sē-ō-fĭs-ē-ŏl′ō-jē) [″ + *physis,* nature, + *logos,* study] The physiology of the sense organs.

esthesioscopy (ĕs-thē″zē-ŏs′kō-pē) [″ + *skopein,* to examine] The testing of tactile and other forms of sensibility.

estheticokinetic (ĕs-thĕt″ĭ-kō-kĭn-ĕt′ĭk) [″ + *kinesis,* movement] Being both sensory and motor.

esthetics (ĕs-thĕt′ĭks) Aesthetics.

esthesioneuroblastoma A malignant glioma of the nasal passages. The tumor is occasionally partially responsive to surgical removal, chemotherapy, or radiotherapy.

estival (ĕs′tĭ-văl) [L. *aestivus*] Pert. to or occurring in summer.

estivoautumnal [″ + *autumnalis,* pert. to autumn] Pert. to summer and autumn, formerly applied to a type of malaria.

estradiol (ĕs-tră-dī′ŏl) $C_{18}H_{24}O_2$, a steroid produced by the ovary and possessing estrogenic properties. Large quantities are found in the urine of pregnant women and of mares and stallions, the latter two serving as sources of the commercial product that is used to treat estrogen deficiencies, e.g. menopause. Estradiol is effective when given subcutaneously or intramuscularly but not when given orally. It is converted to estrone in the body. SEE: *diethylstilbestrol; estrogen.*

e. dipropionate An ester of estradiol.

estrin (ĕs′trĭn) Estrogen.

estrinization (ĕs″trĭn-ĭ-zā′shŭn) The production of vaginal epithelial changes characteristic of estrogen stimulation.

estriol (ĕs′trē-ŏl) $C_{18}H_{24}O_3$, an estrogenic hormone considered to be the metabolic product of estrone and estradiol. It is found in the urine of women.

estrogen (ĕs′trō-jĕn) [Gr. *oistros,* mad desire, + *gennan,* to produce] Any natural or artificial substance that induces estrus and the development of female sex characteristics; more specifically, the estrogenic hormones produced by the ovary; the female sex hormones. Estrogens are responsible for cyclic changes in the vaginal epithelium and endometrium of the uterus. Natural estrogens include estradiol, estrone, and their metabolic product, estriol. When used therapeutically, estrogens are usually given in the form of a conjugate such as ethinyl estradiol, conjugated estrogens, or the synthetic estrogenic substance diethylstilbestrol. These preparations are effective when given by mouth.

Estrogens provide a satisfactory replacement hormone for treating menopausal symptoms and for reducing the risk of osteoporosis and cardiovascular disease in postmenopausal women. It is important to observe patients closely for any malignant changes in the breast or endometrium. Estrogen should be administered intermittently and in the lowest effective dose.

conjugated e. Estrogenic drugs, principally estrone and equilin, used to treat menopausal symptoms, and to prevent osteoporosis. Trade name is Premarin.

estrogenic (ĕs-trō-jĕn′ĭk) Causing estrus; acting to produce the effects of an estrogen.

estrone (ĕs′trōn) $C_{18}H_{22}O_2$, an estrogenic hormone found in the urine of pregnant women and mares. Also prepared synthetically, it is used in the treatment of estrogen deficiencies. It is less active than estradiol but more active than estriol. Trade name is Theelin.

estropipate Estrogen manufactured synthetically from plant sources. The previously used name was *piperazine estrone citrate*. Trade name is Ogen.

estrual (ĕs'troo-ăl) [Gr. *oistros*, mad desire] Pert. to the estrus of animals.

estruation The sexually fertile period in animals; the so-called period of heat.

estrus, oestrus [Gr. *oistros*, mad desire] The cyclic period of sexual activity in nonhuman female mammals, marked by congestion of and secretion by the uterine mucosa, proliferation of vaginal epithelium, swelling of the vulva, ovulation, and acceptance of the male by the female. During estrus, the animal is said to be "in heat."

estrus cycle The sequence from the beginning of one estrus period to the beginning of the next. It includes proestrus, estrus, and metestrus followed by a short period of quiescence called diestrus.

e.s.u. *electrostatic unit*.

état criblé (ā-tă' krēb-lā') [Fr., sievelike state] Multiple irregular perforations of Peyer's patches of the intestines. These patches are characteristic of typhoid fever.

etching (ĕch'ĭng) [Ger. *ätzen*, to feed] Application of a corrosive or abrasive material to a glass or metal surface to create a pattern or design.

acid e. A dental procedure used to roughen the surface of tooth enamel for better mechanical retention in bonding resin to the tooth structure.

ethacrynic acid A diuretic drug. Trade name is Edecrin.

ethambutol hydrochloride (ĕ-thăm'bū-tōl) A drug used to treat tuberculosis and other mycobacterial infections. Trade name is Myambutol.

ethanol (ĕth'ă-nŏl) Ethyl alcohol. SEE: *alcohol*.

ethaverine hydrochloride (ĕth"ă-vĕr'ēn) A drug formerly used to dilate the coronary arteries and treat angina pectoris.

ethchlorvynol (ĕth-klor'vĭ-nŏl) A sedative hypnotic drug that may produce addiction. Trade name is Placidyl.

ethene (ĕth-ēn') Ethylene.

ether (ēth'ĕr) [Gr. *aither*, air] Any organic compound in which an oxygen atom links with carbon chains. The ether used for anesthesia is diethyl ether, $C_4H_{10}O$. As an anesthetic it causes postoperative nausea and profuse salivation.

CAUTION: Ether is highly flammable and should be handled with great care. Also, it should not be stored once its container has been opened because toxic products form when ether is exposed to light.

---

ethereal (ĕ-thē'rē-ăl), *adj*.

ether asphyxia Suffocation during ether anesthetization. SEE: *resuscitation*.

etherization (ē"thĕr-ĭ-zā'shŭn) Administration of ether to induce anesthesia.

etherize (ē'thĕr-īz) To anesthetize by use of ether.

ethics [Gr. *ethos*, moral custom] A system of moral principles or standards governing conduct. SEE: *Declaration of Geneva; Declaration of Hawaii; Hippocratic oath; Nightingale Pledge; Prayer of Maimonides*.

dental e. A system of principles governing dental practice; a moral obligation to render the best possible quality of dental service to the patient and to maintain an honest relationship with other members of the profession and society at large.

medical e. A system of principles governing medical conduct. It deals with the relationship of a physician to the patient, the patient's family, fellow physicians, and society at large. SEE: *advance directive; do not attempt resuscitation; euthanasia; Hippocratic oath; living will*.

nursing e. A system of principles governing the conduct of a nurse. It deals with the relationship of a nurse to the patient, the patient's family, associates and fellow nurses, and society at large. SEE: *Nightingale Pledge*.

ethinamate (ĕ-thĭn'ă-māt) A mild sedative and hypnotic drug.

ethinyl estradiol (ĕth'ĭ-nĭl) SEE: *estradiol*.

ethionamide (ĕ-thī"ŏn-ăm'īd) A "second-line" drug used to treat tuberculosis, typically as part of a drug cocktail made up of several agents.

ethionine (ĕ-thī'ō-nĭn) A progestational agent used in some oral contraceptives.

ethmoid (ĕth'moyd) [Gr. *ēthmos*, sieve, + *eidos*, form, shape] Cribriform.

ethmoidal Pert. to the ethmoid bone or sinuses.

ethmoid bone A sievelike, spongy bone that forms a roof for the nasal fossae and part of the floor of the anterior fossa of the skull. It permits passage of the olfactory nerves to the brain and also contains three groups of air cavities, the ethmoid sinuses, which open into the nasal cavity.

ethmoidectomy (ĕth-moy-dĕk'tō-mē) [" + *eidos*, form, shape, + *ektome*, excision] Excision of the ethmoid sinuses that open into the nasal cavity.

ethmoiditis (ĕth"moy-dī'tĭs) [" + " + *itis*, inflammation] Inflammation of the ethmoidal sinuses. This may be acute or chronic.

SYMPTOMS: Symptoms include headache, acute pain between the eyes, and a nasal discharge.

ethmoid sinus An air cavity or space within the ethmoid bone, opening into the nasal cavity.

ethnic (ĕth′nĭk) [Gr. *ethnikos,* of a nation] Concerning groups of people within a cultural system who desire or are given a distinct classification based on traits such as religion, culture, language, or appearance.

ethnobiology (ĕth″nō-bī-ŏl′ō-jē) [Gr. *ethnos,* race, + *bios,* life, + *logos,* word, reason] The study of the biological characteristics of various races.

ethnocentrism **1.** A belief that one's own way of viewing and experiencing the world is superior to other perspectives; a mindset that judges the actions and beliefs of others according to one's own cultural rules. **2.** In health care, a perspective that supports the worldview of the caretaker, rather than considering the patient's perspective of health and illness. **ethnocentric,** *adj.*

ethnogerontology The study of aging and population groups in reference to race, national origin, and cultural practices. Ethnogerontology addresses the causes, processes, heritage, and consequences specific to these groups.

ethnography (ĕth-nŏg′ră-fē) [″ + *graphein,* to write] The study of the culture of a single society. Data are gathered by direct observation during a period of residence with the group. SEE: *anthropology.*

ethnology (ĕth-nŏl′ō-jē) [″ + *logos,* word, reason] The comparative study of cultures using ethnographic data. SEE: *anthropology.*

ethology (ĕ-, ē-thŏl′ō-jē) [Gr. *ethos,* manners, habits, + *logos,* word, reason] The scientific study of the behavior of animals in their natural habitat and in captivity.

ethosuximide (ĕth″ō-sŭk′sĭ-mīd) An anticonvulsant drug. Trade name is Zarontin.

ethyl (ĕth′ĭl) [Gr. *aither,* air, + *hyle,* matter] In organic chemistry, the radical $C_2H_5^-$, which is contained in many compounds, including ethyl ether, ethyl alcohol, and ethyl acetate.

e. acetate $C_4H_8O_2$; a colorless flammable liquid used as a solvent.

e. aminobenzoate Benzocaine, a topical anesthetic.

e. biscoumacetate An anticoagulant drug.

e. chloride C_2H_5Cl; A volatile anesthetic liquid, used topically. When sprayed on the skin, it evaporates so quickly that the tissue is cooled immediately.

USES: Ethyl chloride is used as a topical local anesthetic in minor surgery. It is used only for very short periods.

ethylamine (ĕth″ĭl-ăm′ĭn) An amine, $CH_3CH_2NH_2$, formed in the decomposition of certain proteins.

ethylcellulose (ĕth″ĭl-sĕl′ū-lōs) An ether of cellulose, used in preparing drugs.

ethylene (ĕth′ĭl-ēn) ABBR: ETO. A flammable, explosive, colorless gas, CH_2CH_2, prepared from alcohol by dehydration. It is present in illuminating gas. It is colorless and has a sweetish taste but a pungent, foul odor. It is lighter than air and diffuses when liberated.

e. glycol The simplest glycol, $C_2H_6O_2$; a colorless alcohol used as an antifreeze. Fomepizole is a specific antidote for intoxications with ethylene glycol. SEE: *Poisons and Poisoning Appendix.*

e. oxide ABBR: EtO. A chemical, C_2H_4O, that in its gaseous state is used to sterilize materials that cannot withstand heat or steam. It is also used as a fumigant.

ethylene anesthesia Ethylene given as a combination of oxygen 20%, cyclopropane 10%, and ethylene 70%. Because it is a rather weak anesthetic, and volatile and inflammable, it is rarely if ever used.

ethylenediamine (ĕth″ĭ-lēn-dī′ă-mēn) Drug used as a solvent for theophylline; it is present in aminophylline injection.

ethylnorepinephrine hydrochloride (ĕth″ĭl-nor-ĕp″ĭ-nĕf″rĭn) An adrenergic drug used in treating asthma. Trade name is Bronkephrine.

ethynodiol diacetate (ĕ-thī″nō-dī′ōl) A progesterone used as an oral contraceptive in combination with an estrogen.

ethynyl (ĕth′ĭ-nĭl) An organic radical, $HC{\equiv}C{-}$.

etic (ē′tĭk) In anthropology and transcultural nursing, related to a kind of analysis that emphasizes the universal or culture-free aspects of disease. The categories of Western medicine may be viewed as etic classifications because objective measures are used to formulate a diagnosis irrespective of the patient's cultural and subjective perspectives. For example, hallucinations are classified as an "illness" from an etic perspective when, in fact, hallucinations may be a component of normal grieving in some cultures. SEE: *emic.*

etio- Combining form meaning *causation.*

etiocholanolone (ē″tē-ō-kō-lăn′ō-lōn) A steroid produced by testosterone catabolism. It is excreted in the urine.

etiology (ē″tē-ŏl′ō-jē) [Gr. *aitia,* cause, + *logos,* word, reason] **1.** The study of the causes of disease. **2.** The cause of a disease. **etiologic, etiological** (-ō-lŏj′ĭk, -ĭ-kăl), *adj.*

etiotropic (ē″tē-ō-trŏp′ĭk) [Gr. *aita,* cause, + *tropos,* turning] Directed against the cause of a disease; used of a drug or treatment that destroys or inactivates the causal agent of a disease. Opposite of nosotropic.

ETO *ethylene oxide.*

etodolac A nonsteroidal anti-inflammatory agent. Trade name is Lodine.

etretinate A tretinoin drug to treat severe recalcitrant psoriasis. Trade name is Tegison.

CAUTION: Etretinate must not be used by women who are pregnant or who intend to become pregnant. It should be prescribed only by physicians knowledgeable in the systemic use of retinoids.

etymology (ĕt″ĭ-mŏl′ō-jē) [L. *etymon,* origin of a word, + *logos,* word, reason] The science of the origin and development of words. Most medical words are derived from Latin and Greek, but many of those from Greek have come through Latin and have been modified by it. Generally, when two Greek words are used to form one word, they are connected by the letter "o." Many medical words have been formed from one or more roots—forms used or adapted from Latin or Greek—and many are modified by a prefix, a suffix, or both. A knowledge of important Latin and Greek roots and prefixes will reveal the meanings of many other words. SEE: *Abbreviations Appendix; Prefixes and Suffixes Appendix.*

Eu Symbol for the element europium.

eu- [Gr. *eus,* good] Combining form meaning *healthy; normal; good; well.*

Eubacteriales (ū″băk-tē-rē-ā′lēz) [Gr. *eus,* good, + *bakterion,* little rod] An order of bacteria that includes many of the microorganisms pathogenic to humans.

Eubacterium (ū″băk-tē′rē-ŭm) A genus of bacteria of the order Eubacteriales.

eubiotics (ū″bī-ŏt′ĭks) [″ + *bios,* life] The science of healthy and hygienic living.

eucalyptol, eucalyptus oil (ū″kă-lĭp′tōl) [″ + *kalyptein,* to cover] Aromatic substances derived from eucalyptus leaves, occasionally used as expectorants.

eucalyptus oil (ū-kă-lĭp′tŭs) Oil distilled from fresh eucalyptus leaves, used as an expectorant.

eucapnia (ū-kăp′nē-ă) [″ + *kapnos,* smoke] The presence of normal amounts of carbon dioxide in the blood.

eucatropine hydrochloride (ū-kăt′rō-pēn) An anticholinergic used as a mydriatic. It is applied topically to the eye.

euchlorhydria (ū″klor-hī′drē-ă) The presence of the normal amount of free hydrochloric acid in gastric juice.

eucholia (ū-kō′lē-ă) [″ + *chole,* bile] The normal condition of bile regarding its constituents and the amount secreted.

euchromatin (ū-krō′mă-tĭn) [″ + *chroma,* color] Unfolded or uncondensed portions of chromosomes during interphase. Transcription of DNA by messenger RNA occurs, and proteins are synthesized. SEE: *heterochromatin.*

eucrasia (ū-krā′sē-ă) [″ + *krasis,* mixture] Normal health; the state of the body in which all activities are in normal balance.

eudiaphoresis (ū″dī-ă-fō-rē′sĭs) [″ + *dia,* through, + *pherein,* to carry] Normal perspiration.

eudiometer (ū″dē-ŏm′ĕ-tĕr) [Gr. *eudia,* good weather, + *metron,* measure] An instrument for testing air purity and analyzing gases.

eugenics (ū-jĕn′ĭks) [″ + *gennan,* to produce] The study of improving a population by selective breeding in the belief that desirable traits will become more common and undesirable traits will be eliminated. Ths practice may have some utility in controlled animal populations, but it is unethical in humans.

eugenol (ū′jĕn-ŏl) A material obtained from clove oil and other sources. It is used as a topical analgesic in dentistry. It is also mixed with zinc oxide to form a material that hardens sufficiently to be used as a temporary dental filling.

euglobulin (ū-glŏb′ū-lĭn) A true globulin, or one that is insoluble in distilled water and soluble in dilute salt solution. SEE: *pseudoglobulin.*

euglycemia A normal concentration of glucose in the blood.

euhydration A normal amount of water in the body.

eukaryon (ū-kăr′ē-ŏn) [″ + *karyon,* nucleus] The nucleus of a eukaryote cell.

eukaryote (ū-kăr′ē-ōt) An organism in which the cell nucleus is surrounded by a membrane. SEE: *prokaryote.*

Eulenburg's disease (oyl′ĕn-bŭrgz) [Albert Eulenburg, Ger. neurologist, 1840–1917] Myotonia congenita.

Eumycetes (ū″mī-sē′tēz) [″ + *mykes,* fungus] A class of Thallophyta that includes all the true fungi.

eunuch (ū′nŭk) [Gr. *eune,* bed, + *echein,* to guard] A castrated man; one who has had his testicles removed, esp. before puberty so that secondary sexual characteristics do not develop. Absence of the male hormones produces a high-pitched voice and loss of hair on the face. In Middle Eastern and some Asian countries, eunuchs were employed to guard the women of a harem.

eunuchism (ū′nŭk-ĭzm) [″ + ″ + *-ismos,* condition] A condition resulting from complete lack of male hormones. It may be due to atrophy or removal of the testicles.

pituitary e. A condition produced by failure of the anterior lobe of the pituitary to secrete gonadotrophic hormones; secondary hypogonadism.

eunuchoid (ū′nŭ-koyd) [″ + ″ + *eidos,* form, shape] Having the characteristics of a eunuch, such as retarded development of sex organs, absence of beard and bodily hair, high-pitched voice, and striking lack of muscular development.

eunuchoidism (ū′nŭk-oyd-ĭzm) [″ + ″ + ″ + *-ismos,* condition] Deficient male hormone production by the testes.

eupancreatism (ū-păn′krē-ă-tĭzm) [Gr. *eus,* good, + *pankreas,* pancreas, + *-ismos,* condition] The normal condition of the pancreas.

eupepsia [″ + *pepsis,* digestion] Normal digestion as distinguished from dyspepsia. **eupeptic,** *adj.*

euphonia (ū-fōn′ē-ă) [″ + *phone,* voice] The condition of having a normal clear voice.

euphoria (ū-for′ē-ă) [″ + *phoros,* bearing] **1.** A condition of good health. **2.** In psychiatry, an exaggerated feeling of well-being; mild elation.

euphoriant Any agent or drug that induces an extraordinary sense of well-being.

euplastic (ū-plăs′tĭk) [″ + *plastikos,* formed] Healing quickly and well.

euploidy (ū-ploy′dē) [″ + *ploos,* fold, + *eidos,* form, shape] In genetics, the state of having complete sets of chromosomes.

europium (ŭ-rō′pē-ŭm) SYMB: EU. A rare element of the lanthanide series with atomic number 63 and an atomic weight of 151.96.

Eurotium (ū-rō′shē-ŭm) [Gr. *euros,* mold] A genus of molds.

eury- (ū′rē) [Gr. *eurys,* wide] Combining form meaning *broad.*

eurycephalic (ū″rē-sĕ-făl′ĭk) [″ + *kephale,* head] Having a broad or wide head.

eustachian (ū-stā′kē-ăn, -shĕn) [Bartolomeo Eustachio (Eustachi), It. anatomist, 1520–1574] Pert. to the auditory tube. SEE: *ear; eustachian tube.*

eustachian catheter An instrument for insertion into the eustachian tube.

eustachianography Radiography of the eustachian tube and middle ear after the introduction of a contrast medium.

eustachian valve The valve at the entrance of the inferior vena cava.

eustachitis (ū″stā-kī′tĭs) Inflammation of the eustachian tube.

eusystole (ū-sĭs′tō-lē) [Gr. *eus,* good, + *systellein,* to draw together] A condition in which the systole of the heart is normal in time and force.

eutectic (ū-tĕk′tĭk) [Gr. *eutektos*] Easily melted.

eutectic mixture A mixture of two or more substances that has a melting point lower than that of any of its constituents.

euthanasia (ū-thă-nā′zē-ă) [Gr. *eus,* good, + *thanatos,* death] **1.** An easy, quiet, and painless death. **2.** The deliberate ending of the life of people (or in veterinary practice, animals) with incurable or terminal illnesses or unbearable suffering. The ethical ramifications are actively debated and unresolved: should patients have the right to choose death? when is death imminent, or suffering intolerable? does participation by a health care provider (e.g., a doctor, nurse, or pharmacist) violate personal, professional, religious, or social mores? SEE: *advance directive; assisted death; assisted suicide; death; death with dignity; do not attempt resuscitation; dying; living will.*

involuntary e. Euthanasia performed without a competent person's consent.

nonvoluntary e. Euthanasia provided to an incompetent person according to a surrogate's decision.

euthenics (ū-thĕn′ĭks) [Gr. *euthenia,* well-being] The science of improvement of a population through modification of the environment.

Eutheria A subclass of mammals with a true placenta.

euthyroid (ū-thī′royd) Having a normally functioning thyroid gland.

Eutrombicula (ū″trŏm-bĭk′ū-lă) A genus of mites.

eutrophication (ū-trŏf″ĭ-kā′shŭn) [Gr. *eutrophein,* to thrive] Alteration of the environment by increasing the nutrients required by one species to the disadvantage of other species in the ecosystem, esp. in an aquatic environment.

euvolemic Having appropriate hydration (neither excessively hydrated nor dehydrated). SYN: normovolemic.

ev, eV, EV *electron volt.*

evacuant (ē-văk′ū-ănt) [L. *evacuans,* making empty] A drug that stimulates the bowels to move. A laxative.

evacuate [L. *evacuatio,* emptying] **1.** To discharge, esp. from the bowels; to empty the uterus. **2.** To move patients from the site of an accident or catastrophe to a hospital or shelter.

evacuation (ē-văk″ū-ā′shŭn) **1.** The act of emptying (e.g., the bowels). In obstetrics, the term refers to emptying the uterus of the products of conception, as in abortion or removal of retained placental fragments. **2.** The material discharged from the bowels; stool. **3.** Removal of air from a closed container; production of a vacuum. **4.** The act of moving people to a safe place, esp. from a disaster or a war-torn area.

evacuator (ē-văk′ū-ā-tor) A device for emptying, as the bowels, or for irrigating the bladder and removing calculi.

evagination (ē-văj-ĭ-nā′shŭn) **1.** Emergence from a sheath. **2.** Protrusion of an organ or part. SEE: *invagination.* **evaginate** (-nāt), *adj.*

evaluation **1.** A rating or assessment, e.g., of the accuracy of a diagnosis, the effectiveness of a plan of care, or the quality of care. **2.** An appraisal of the health or status of an individual, based on specific criteria. **3.** A clinical judgment. SEE: *nursing assessment; nursing intervention; nursing process; planning; problem-oriented medical record.*

evanescent (ĕv″ă-nĕs′ĕnt) [L. *evanescere,* to vanish] Not permanent; of brief duration.

Evans blue [Herbert M. Evans, U.S. anatomist, 1882–1971] A diazo dye occurring as a blue-green powder, very soluble in water. It is used intravenously as a diagnostic agent.

Evans syndrome [Robert S. Evans, U.S. physician, b. 1912] An autoimmune disease characterized by thrombocytopenia and hemolytic anemia.

evaporation [L. *e,* out, + *vaporare,* to steam] **1.** Change from liquid to vapor. **2.** Loss in volume due to conversion of a liquid into a vapor.

evenomation (ē-vĕn″ō-mā′shŭn) [L. *ex,* from, + *venenum,* poison] Removal of venom from a biting insect or reptile; removal of venom from the victim of a bite.

eventration (ē″vĕn-trā′shŭn) [L. *e,* out, + *venter,* belly] **1.** Partial protrusion of the abdominal contents through an opening in the abdominal wall. **2.** Removal of the contents of the abdominal cavity.

eversion (ē-vĕr′zhŭn) [″ + *vertere,* to turn] Turning outward. SEE: *chilectropion.*

evidement (ā-vēd-mŏn′) [Fr., a scooping out] Scraping away of diseased tissue.

evidence In forensic medicine, all the tangible items and record materials pertinent to the legal considerations.

chain of custody of e. In legal and forensic medicine, the procedures for ensuring that specimens, data, or information important to legal proceedings are properly handled, labeled, and stored in a locked and secure place. If a biological specimen is stored, it may be frozen or refrigerated. Only authorized persons are allowed access to the stored material. When a specimen to be tested for drugs (e.g., urine, sputum, blood, or breath) is obtained from an individual, the person must be observed while providing the specimen. In drug testing, samples are stored in duplicate so one is available for retesting at a later date.

material e. In medicolegal considerations, facts or evidence important to proving or disproving matters of dispute.

evil [AS. *yfel*] An infrequently used term for disease or illness.

eviration (ē″vī-rā′shŭn) [L. *e,* out, + *vir,* man] **1.** Castration. **2.** In psychiatry, delusion in a man who thinks he has become a woman.

evisceration (ē-vĭs″ĕr-ā′shŭn) [″ + *viscera,* viscera] **1.** Removal of the viscera or of the contents of a cavity. **2.** Spilling out of abdominal contents resulting from wound dehiscence.

PATIENT CARE: The patient's surgeon should be contacted immediately. The wound is covered with a sterile towel moistened with warm sterile physiological saline solution. Tension on the abdomen is decreased by placing the patient in the low Fowler's position and raising the knees or by instructing the patient to flex the knees and support them with a pillow. Vital signs are monitored, and fluid therapy is initiated via IV line. The patient is reassured and prepared for surgery.

evisceroneurotomy (ē-vĭs″ĕr-ō-nū-rŏt′ō-mē) [″ + ″ + Gr. *neuron,* nerve, + *tome,* incision] Scleral evisceration of the eye with division of the optic nerve.

evocation (ĕv″ō-kā′shŭn) [″ + *vocare,* to call] **1.** Re-creation by recollection or by imagination. **2.** In the embryo, the induction or formation of a tissue in response to an evocator.

evocator A chemical produced by one part of an embryo that stimulates organ and tissue development in another part.

evoked response The electroencephalographic record of electrical activity produced at one of several levels in the central nervous system by stimulation of an area of the sensory nerve system. Analysis of the response can provide important information concerning the function of the peripheral and central nervous systems. SEE: *brainstem auditory evoked potential; somatosensory evoked response; visual evoked response.*

evolution (ĕv″ō-lū′shŭn) [L. *e,* out, + *volvere,* to roll] A process of orderly and gradual change or development. More generally, any orderly and gradual process of modification whereby a system, whether physical, chemical, social, or intellectual, becomes more highly organized.

theory of e. The theory that all species of plants and animals, including humans, have come into existence by gradual continuous change from earlier forms. SEE: *natural selection.*

evulsion avulsion.

Ewing's tumor, Ewing's sarcoma (ū′ĭngz) [James Ewing, U.S. pathologist, 1866–1943] A diffuse endothelioma forming a fusiform swelling on a long bone.

ex- [L., Gr. *ex,* out] Combining form meaning *out; away from; completely.*

exacerbation (ĕks-ăs″ĕr-bā′shŭn) [″ + *acerbus,* harsh] Aggravation of symptoms or increase in the severity of a disease.

exaltation [L. *exaltare,* to lift up] A mental state characterized by feelings of grandeur, excessive joy, elation, and optimism; an abnormal feeling of personal well-being or self-importance.

examination [L. *examinare,* to examine] The act or process of inspecting the body and its systems to determine the presence or absence of disease. Terms employed indicate type of examination: physical, bimanual, digital, oral, rectal, obstetrical, roentgenological, cystoscopic.

Local physical examination includes specific parts and organs. Four procedures used are inspection, palpation, percussion, and auscultation. Laboratory examination includes urinalysis, blood tests, bacteriological cultures, and various special means of visualizing body spaces and organs and their functions. SEE: *abdomen*.

bimanual e. SEE: *pelvic e.*

dental e. Examination of the surfaces of teeth and dental fillings, usually with a sharp-pointed explorer to detect areas of demineralization or caries or failing margins of restorations. The depth of the gingival sulcus is also probed and measured around each tooth to assess the state of health of the periodontium.

double-contrast e. A radiographic examination in which a radiopaque and a radiolucent contrast medium are used simultaneously to visualize internal anatomy.

focused history and physical e. ABBR: FHPE. A combination of the appropriate questions (i.e., SAMPLE, History, and OPQRST) and physical examination vectored to the specific body system (i.e., cardiopulmonary, neurological, musculoskeletal) that the EMS provider suspects may be causing a patient's presenting problem. This assessment is conducted after the initial assessment has been completed and differs for medical or trauma patients.

Folstein Mini Mental Status E. SEE: *Folstein Mini Mental Status Exam*.

oral double-contrast e. A careful and thorough inspection and palpation of the mouth, tongue, cheek, and tissues of the neck to assess their condition. The floor of the mouth may be palpated bimanually to search for nodules or other irregularities. SEE: *oral diagnosis*.

pelvic e. Physical examination of the vagina and adjacent organs. A speculum is used first to permit visualization of anatomical structures. During speculum examination cultures and Pap smear specimens may be obtained. After the speculum is removed, the pelvic organs and rectum are examined manually by the examiner.

rectoabdominal e. Physical examination of the abdomen and rectum; for example, to determine the cause of abdominal pain or to identify occult bleeding.

examinations, National Board Examinations administered to test the qualifications of medical, dental, and other professional students. Successful completion of the basic science and clinical parts of the examinations is required for licensure in most states.

exanthem (ĕks-ăn′thĕm) *pl.* **exanthems** [Gr. *exanthema,* eruption] Any eruption or rash that appears on the skin, as opposed to one that appears on the mucous membranes (enanthem). The term is often used to describe childhood or infectious rashes (e.g., measles or scarlet fever) but also applies to other rashes. **exanthematous** (-ăn-thĕm′ă-tŭs), *adj.*

e. subitum An acute disease of infants, caused by herpesvirus 6. It is marked by high fever for 3 or 4 days and sometimes by convulsions at the onset. A diffuse maculopapular rash usually appears just when the fever suddenly subsides. Treatment is symptomatic. SYN: *roseola infantum*. SEE: *convulsion*.

exanthema (ĕks-ăn-thē′mă) *pl.* **exanthemas** *pl.* **-mata** [Gr.] Exanthem.

exanthrope (ĕks′ăn-thrōp) [Gr. *ex,* out, + *anthropos,* man] A cause or source of a disease originating outside the body.

exarticulation (ĕks″ăr-tĭk-ū-lā′shŭn) [L. *ex,* out, + *articulus,* joint] **1.** Amputation of a limb through a joint. **2.** Excision of a part of a joint.

excavation (ĕks″kă-vā′shŭn) [″ + *cavus,* hollow] **1.** A hollow or depression. **2.** Formation of a cavity.

atrophic e. A hollow or cupped appearance of the optic nerve head as seen by use of an ophthalmoscope.

dental e. The preparation of a cavity in a tooth before filling.

e. of optic nerve A slight depression in the center of the optic papilla, or disk, from which retinal vessels emerge. Depression is total in glaucoma as a result of high intraocular pressure.

rectouterine e. The rectouterine pouch or pouch of Douglas.

excavator (ĕks′kă-vā″tor) An instrument for removing tissue or bone. It may be spoon-shaped if used on soft tissue and spoon-shaped with sharp edges if used in dentistry.

excerebration (ĕk″sĕr-ĕ-brā′shŭn) [″ + *cerebrum,* brain] Removal of the brain, esp. that of the dead fetus to facilitate delivery.

excess, base The difference between the normal and the actual buffer base concentration in a blood sample when titrated by strong acid at pH = 7.4 and P_{CO_2} = 40 mm Hg. The base excess is usually determined indirectly using measured values for pH and P_{CO_2} and then calculated using known relationships.

b. e. of blood The substance concentration of base in whole blood determined at a pH of 7.40 and P_{CO_2} of 40 mm Hg. This measurement helps one assess the relative contribution of respiratory versus metabolic components in acid-base imbalances in the blood.

b. e. of extracellular fluid ABBR: BE (ecf). The substance concentration of base in extracellular fluid determined at a pH of 7.40 and P_{CO_2} of 40 mm Hg. Because this quantity cannot be determined directly, a model of extracellular fluid is used as a basis. The model consists of one volume of blood plus two volumes of plasma. As with the base excess of blood, this quantity helps one assess the respiratory versus metabolic components in acid-base balance. In contrast to the base excess of blood, the base excess of extracellular fluid is said to be more representative of the acid-base status of the accessible fluid compartment and thus more appropriate for deciding on and evaluating therapy.

exchange **1.** To give up or substitute something for something else. **2.** In dietetics, the substitution of an equivalent amount of one food substance for another so that the caloric intake remains the same.

cation e. The transfer of cations between those in a liquid medium and those in a solid polymer. The polymer is termed the cation exchanger. This technique is used in ion-exchange chromatography.

sister chromatid e. The exchange of corresponding parts of homologous maternal and paternal chromosomes during the first meiotic division. This contributes to genetic diversity in the offspring. SYN: *crossing over*.

exchange list A grouping of foods to assist people on special diets. In each group, foods are listed in serving sizes that are interchangeable with respect to carbohydrates, fats, protein, and calories. The groups are starches and bread; meat; vegetables and fruit; milk; and fats. This approach is esp. useful in managing diets for diabetics.

excipient (ĕk-sĭp′ē-ĕnt) [L. *excipiens,* excepting] Any substance added to a medicine so that it can be formed into the proper shape and consistency; the vehicle for the drug.

excise (ĕk-sīz′) [L. *ex,* out, + *caedere,* to cut] To cut out or remove surgically.

excision (ĕk-sĭ′zhŭn) [L. *excisio*] The act of cutting away or taking out.

excitability [L. *excitare,* to arouse] Sensitivity to stimulation.

muscle e. In a muscle fiber, the inducibility to contract. This is a function of the chemical and electrical state of the sarcolemma and the time since a previous stimulus was applied.

nerve e. The property of a neuron to produce an action potential. This is a function of the permeability and the chemical and electrical state of the neuron cell membrane. Also, the intensity of electrical stimuli influences the excitability of the neuron.

reflex e. Sensitivity to reflex irritation.

excitant (ĕk-sīt′ănt) An agent that excites a special function of the body. According to their action, excitants are classified as motor, cerebral, and so forth. Amphetamine, cocaine, and strychnine are examples of medical excitants.

excitation [L. *excitatio*] **1.** The act of exciting. **2.** The condition of being stimulated or excited.

direct e. Stimulation of a muscle physically or by placement of an electrode in it.

indirect e. Stimulation of a muscle via its nerve.

exciting Causing excitement.

excitoglandular (ĕk-sīt″ō-glăn′dū-lăr) [L. *excitare,* to arouse, + *glans,* kernel] Increasing glandular function.

excitometabolic (ĕk-sīt″ō-mĕt″ă-bŏl′ĭk) [″ + Gr. *metabole,* change] Inducing metabolic changes.

excitomotor (ĕk-sīt″ō-mō′tor) [″ + *motor,* moving] Pert. to increasingly rapid muscular activity.

excitomuscular (ĕk-sīt″ō-mŭs′kū-lăr) [″ + Gr. *mys,* muscle] Causing muscular activity.

excitor (ĕk-sī′tor) [L. *excitare,* to arouse] Something that incites to greater activity. SYN: *stimulant*.

excitosecretory (ĕk-sīt″ō-sē′krē-tor-ē) [″ + *secretio,* a hiding] Tending to produce secretion.

excitotoxin A neurotransmitter (e.g., glutamate or aspartate) that can cause brain cell injury or death if its action is unabated. Brain damage is mediated by excitotoxins during prolonged seizure activity and stroke.

excitovascular (ĕk-sī″tō-văs′kū-lăr) [″ + *vascularis,* pert. to a vessel] Increasing circulation activity.

exclusion (ĕks-kloo′zhŭn) [L. *exclusio,* fr. *ex,* out, + *claudere,* to shut] **1.** Shutting off or removing from the main part. **2.** In medical insurance programs, a list of specific hazards, perils, or conditions for which the policy will not provide benefits or coverage payments. Common exclusions include preexisting conditions such as cancer, heart disease, diabetes, hypertension, a pregnancy that began before the effective date of the policy, self-inflicted injuries, combat injuries, plastic surgery for cosmetic reasons, and on-the-job injuries covered by workers' compensation.

excoriation (ĕks-kō-rē-ā′shŭn) [″ + *corium,* skin] An abrasion of the skin or of the surface of other organs by scratching, traumatic injury, chemicals, burns, or other causes. On the skin, the lesion is typically linear and scaly.

excrement (ĕks′krĕ-mĕnt) [L. *excrementum*] Waste material passed out of the body, esp. feces. SEE: *excretion*. **excrementitious** (ĕks″krĕ-mĕn-tĭsh′ŭs), *adj.*

excrescence (ĕks-krĕs'ĕns) [L. *ex,* out, + *crescere,* to grow] Any abnormal growth from the surface of a part.

excreta (ĕks-krē'tă) [L.] Waste matter excreted from the body, including feces, urine, and perspiration. In some diseases, the excreta of the patient contains infectious material. This must be disinfected and handled carefully by hospital personnel. SEE: *Standard and Universal Precautions Appendix.*

Pads made of absorbent materials should be placed under the patient who has involuntary discharges. When disposed of, the pads should be placed in sturdy plastic bags. In handling all infected discharges, the health care worker should wear gloves and a face mask.

CAUTION: Some disinfecting materials such as phenol and chlorinated compounds may be toxic. Direct exposure to skin, mucous membranes, or the eyes should be avoided.

excrete (ĕks-krēt') [L. *excretus,* sifted out] To expel or eliminate waste material from the body, blood, or organs.

excretion (ĕks-krē'shŭn) [L. *excretio*] **1.** Excreta. **2.** The elimination of waste products from the body.

ORGANS: *Intestines:* These produce indigestible residue, water, and bacteria. *Kidneys:* Water, nitrogenous substances (urea, uric acid, creatine, creatinine), mineral salts are excreted. *Respiratory system:* This produces carbon dioxide, water vapor, and other gases. *Skin:* A small amount of material is excreted through perspiration of water, salts, and minute quantities of urea.

excretory (ĕks'krē-tō-rē) [L. *excretus,* sifted out] Pert. to or bringing about excretion.

excursion (ĕks-kŭr'zhŭn) [L. *excursio*] **1.** Wandering from the usual course. **2.** The extent of movement of a part such as the extremities or eyes.

diaphragmatic e. In respiration, the movement of the diaphragm from its level during full exhalation to its level during full inhalation. Normal diaphragmatic excursion is 5 to 7 cm bilaterally in adults. It may be seen during fluorscopic or ultrasonographic examinations of the chest, or percussed during physical examination of the chest wall.

excurvation (ĕks"kŭr-vā'shŭn) [Gr. *ex,* out, + L. *curvus,* bend] A curvature outward.

excystation (ĕk"sĭs-tā'shŭn) [" + *kystis,* cyst] The escape of certain organisms (parasitic worms or protozoa) from an enclosing cyst wall or envelope. This process occurs in the life cycle of an intestinal parasite after the encysted form is ingested.

exencephalia (ĕks"ĕn-sĕf-ā'lē-ă) [" + *enkephalos,* brain] A congenital anomaly in which the brain is located outside the skull; a term for encephalocele, hydrencephalocele, and meningocele.

exenteration (ĕks-ĕn"tĕr-ā'shŭn) [" + *enteron,* intestine] Evisceration.

exercise [L. *exercitus,* having drilled] A physical or mental activity performed to maintain, restore, or increase normal capacity. Physical exercise involves activities that maintain or increase muscle tone and strength, esp. to improve physical fitness or to manage a handicap or disability. SEE: table; *physical fitness; risk factor; sedentary lifestyle.*

Daily physical activity for a minimum of 35 minutes will increase exercise capacity and the ability to use oxygen to

Exercise: Energy Required*

Calories Required per Hour of Exercise	Activity†
80	Sitting quietly, reading
200	Golf with use of powered cart
250	Walking 3 miles/hr (4.83 km/hr); housework; light industry; cycling 6 miles/hr (9.7 km/hr)
330	Heavy housework; walking 3.5 miles/hr (5.6 km/hr); golf, carrying own bag; tennis, doubles; ballet exercises
400	Walking 5 miles/hr (8 km/hr); cycling 10 miles/hr (16.1 km/hr); tennis, singles; water skiing
500	Manual labor; gardening; shoveling
660	Running 5.5 miles/hr (8.9 km/hr); cycling 13 miles/hr (20.9 km/hr); climbing stairs; heavy manual labor
1020	Running 8 miles/hr (12.9 km/hr); climbing stairs with 30-lb (13.61-kg) load

* These estimates are approximate and can serve only as a general guide. They are based on an average person who weighs 160 lb (72.58 kg).

† Energy requirements for swimming are not provided because of variables such as water temperature, whether the water is fresh or salt, buoyancy of the individual, and whether the water is calm or not.

derive energy for work, decrease myocardial oxygen demands for the same level of work, favorably alter lipid and carbohydrate metabolism, prevent cardiovascular disease, and help to control body weight and body composition. An exercise program should include developing joint flexibility and muscle strength, esp. in the arms. This is of particular importance as people age. Exercise can have a beneficial effect in patients with depression or anxiety. It is thought to have a positive effect on mental health.

An exercise program should be neither begun nor continued if the individual or the person prescribing the exercise program has evidence that the activity is painful or harmful. Persons have died while exercising, and heavy physical exertion may precede acute myocardial infarction, particularly in people who are habitually sedentary.

Mental exercise involves activities that maintain or increase cognitive faculties. Daily intellectual stimulation improves concentration, integration, and application of concepts and principles; enhances problem-solving abilities; promotes self-esteem; facilitates self-actualization; counteracts depression associated with social isolation and boredom; and enhances the quality of one's life. This is particularly important during aging. SEE: *reminiscence therapy*.

Most of the negative aspects of aging can be either altered or diminished by a lifelong healthy lifestyle. For example, the loss of physical fitness and strength, an inevitable consequence of aging, can be altered by an individualized fitness and strength program. Progressive loss of bone mass due to osteoporosis either may be prevented or slowed by a program of regular exercise. Loss of cardiac fitness can be forestalled by an ongoing aerobic fitness program. Many cases of type 2 diabetes can be controlled by exercise and an appropriate diet. Arthritic stiffness and loss of flexibility can be influenced favorably by exercise, for example, walking and jogging; for patients who experience joint pain with impact exercise, swimming is an alternative. Obesity and loss of muscle mass can be prevented or minimized.

Exercise stimulates release of endorphins, and people who participate in regular exercise programs express positive feelings toward living. Exercise programs can be adapted for patients who are confined to wheelchairs. An important consideration for any exercise program is that it be enjoyable. No matter how beneficial the program may be, if it is not enjoyable or rewarding, it will not be continued.

e. accumulation Physical exertion that is divided into several short bouts of exercise scattered throughout the day, instead of during a single longer workout.

active e. A type of bodily movement performed by voluntary contraction and relaxation of muscles.

aquatic e. The use of a pool or tank of water for early exercise in the treatment of musculoskeletal injuries and for non- or partial weight-bearing activities in early rehabilitation training. SEE: *hydrotherapy*.

assistive e. A type of bodily movement performed by voluntary contraction and relaxation of muscles with the aid of a therapist.

Bates e. SEE: *Bates exercises*.

blowing e. An exercise in which the patient exhales into a tube with high end-expiratory pressure to open regions of the lung that may have collapsed and to prevent atelectasis. This encourages deep breathing, which tends to aid lung expansion. SEE: *atelectasis; empyema; pneumonia*.

breathing e. Exercise that enhances the respiratory system by improving ventilation, strengthening respiratory muscles, and increasing endurance.

Buerger's postural e. [Leo Buerger, U.S. physician, 1879–1943] An exercise used for circulatory disturbances of the extremities.

Codman's e. A gentle, active exercise of the upper extremity following immobilization to reestablish range of motion and function following fracture. Also called *Codman's movements*. SYN: *pendulum e.*

concentric e. A form of isotonic exercise in which the muscle fibers shorten as tension develops. SEE: *muscle contraction, concentric; muscle contraction, eccentric*.

corrective e. Use of specific exercises to correct deficiencies caused by trauma or inactivity.

dynamic stabilization e. Stabilization e.

eccentric e. An exercise in which there is overall lengthening of the muscle in response to an external resistance. SEE: *muscle contraction, concentric; muscle contraction, eccentric*.

flexibility e. An exercise designed to increase range of motion and extensibility of muscle.

free e. An exercise carried through with no external assistance.

isokinetic e. An exercise, usually using a specially designed machine, that controls the velocity of muscle shortening or lengthening, so that the force generated by the muscle is maximal through the full range of motion.

isometric e. Contraction and relaxation of a skeletal muscle or group of muscles in which the force generated by the muscle is equal to the resistance. There is no change in muscle length, and no movement results. SYN: *muscle-setting e.; static e.*

isotonic e. An active muscle contraction in which the force exerted remains constant and muscle length changes.

Kegel e. SEE: *Kegel exercise.*

kinetic chain e. An exercise that requires the foot to apply pressure against a plate, pedal, or ground. This rehabilitation concept was determined by the anatomical functional relationship in the lower extremities. Kinetic chain exercises are more functional than open-chain exercises, in which the foot is off the ground and the force is generated by the muscles against a shin plate.

muscle-setting e. Isometric e.

neurobic e. Brainteasers, association tasks, calculations, puzzles, and other mental and physical exercises designed to stimulate thinking, problem solving, and other cerebral functions.

passive e. A therapeutic exercise technique used to move a patient's joints through a range of motion without any effort on the part of the patient. It is accomplished by a therapist, an assistant, or the use of a machine. SYN: *passive motion; passive movement.*

pelvic floor e. SEE: *Kegel exercise.*

pendulum e. Codman's e.

range-of-motion e. Movement of a joint through its available range of motion. It can be used to prevent loss of motion. SEE: illus.

resistive e. A form of supervised exercise, with or without apparatus, that offers resistance to muscle action.

stabilization e. The application of fluctuating resistance loads while the patient stabilizes the part being trained in a symptom-free position. Exercises begin easily so that control is maintained, and progress in duration, intensity, speed, and variety. SYN: *dynamic stabilization e.*

static e. Isometric e.

stretching e. A therapeutic exercise maneuver, using physiological principles, designed to increase joint range of motion or extensibility of pathologically shortened connective tissue structures.

therapeutic e. Scientific application of physical activity as an intervention for 1) improving function, general health, and sense of well-being in patients; 2) preventing complications and further functional loss; 3) or improving or maintaining functional performance in healthy clients. Therapeutic exercise interventions may include techniques to improve motion, strength, motor control, muscle and cardiopulmonary endurance, and efficiency, posture, balance, and coordination.

exercise electrocardiogram A record of the electrical activity of the heart taken during graded increases in the rate of exercise. SEE: *stress test.*

exercise prescription An exercise schedule usually intended to increase the physical fitness of a previously sedentary individual who has recently had a serious illness such as myocardial infarction, or who is physically fit and wants to know the amount, frequency, and kind of exercise necessary to maintain fitness. The prescription is individualized, taking into account the person's age, the availability of facilities and adequate supervision, and health, particularly if the person has had chronic diseases of the heart or lungs. SEE: *physical activity and exercise.*

exercise tolerance test A measure of cardiovascular (or cardiopulmonary) fitness, in which people exert themselves while having their heart rate, blood pressure, oxygen saturation, and electrocardiographic response monitored. A treadmill or ergometer is typically used as the testing device. The amount of exercise the patient must perform is increased gradually over several minutes, until the patient experiences excessive symptoms (such as fatigue, shortness of breath, chest pain, or claudication) or until objective findings of cardiopulmonary malfunction are demonstrated (such as arrhythmias, decreases in blood pressure, or ST-segment changes on the electrocardiogram). SYN: *stress test.*

Exercise tests are used most often to help diagnose symptoms or signs suggestive of coronary ischemia. They also are used frequently after patients have suffered a myocardial infarction or an exercise-induced arrhythmia. In these situations, the test may provide patients with important information about their likelihood of suffering further cardiac events or about the efficacy of their medical regimens in controlling their symptoms. When used in the evaluation of patients with cardiovascular disease, exercise testing often is combined with echocardiography or nuclear imaging of the heart to improve the predictive value, sensitivity, and specificity of the assessment.

In sports medicine, exercise testing can be used to help athletes train to achieve peak performance.

exeresis (ěks-ěr′ĕ-sĭs) [Gr. *exairesis,* taking out] Excision of any part.

exergonic (ěk″sěr-gŏn′ĭk) [Gr. *ex,* out, + *ergon,* work] Pert. to a chemical reaction that produces energy.

exflagellation (ěks″flăj-ĕ-lā′shŭn) [″ + L. *flagellum,* whip] The formation of microgametes (flagellated bodies) from the microgametocytes. This process occurs in the malarial organism *(Plasmodium)* in the stomach of a mosquito.

exfoliatin A toxin, produced by certain

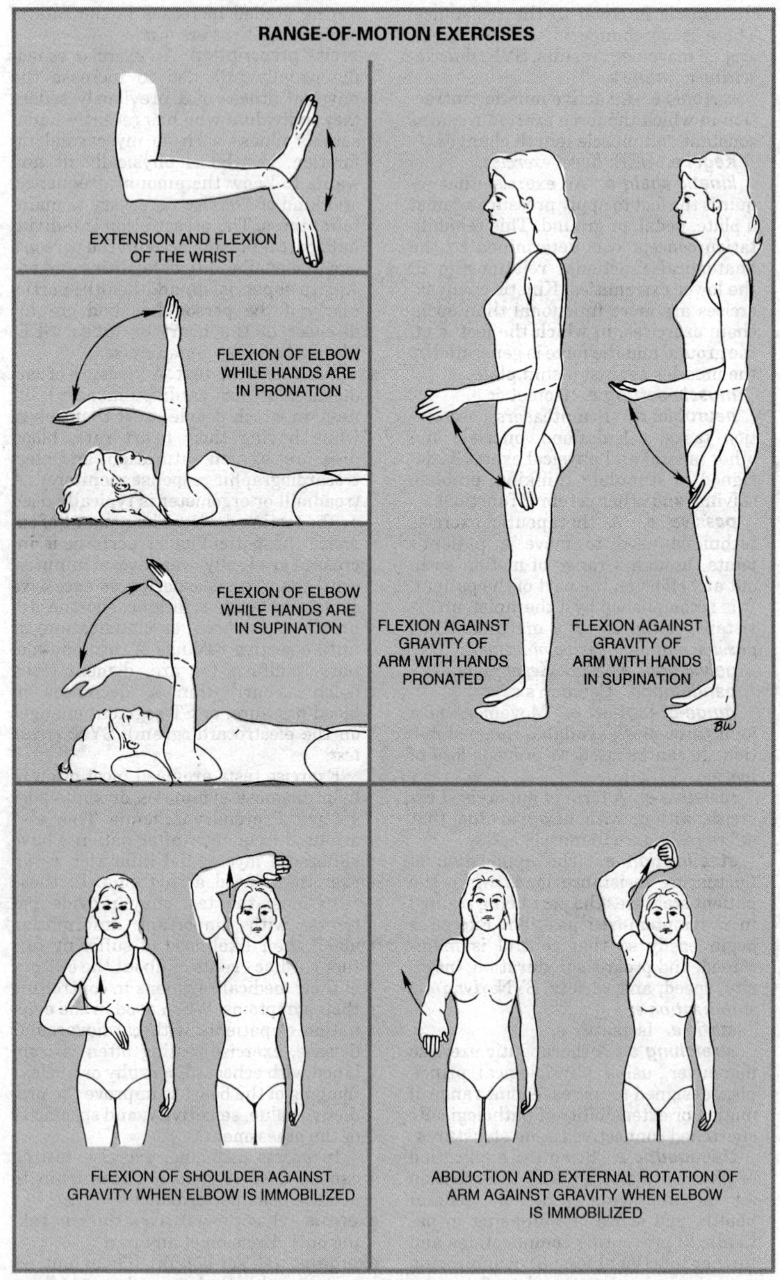

strains of *Staphylococcus aureus,* responsible for the major dermatological changes in staphylococcal "scalded skin" syndrome in neonates and adults.

exfoliation (ěks″fō-lē-ā′shŭn) [″ + L. *folium,* leaf] The shedding or casting off of a body surface (e.g., the outer layer of skin cells, the outer table of bone, the primary set of teeth).

exhalation (ěks″hă-lā′shŭn) [″ + L. *halare,* to breathe] The process of breathing out; emanation of a gas or vapor. Opposite of inhalation.

exhaustion [″ + L. *haurire,* to drain]

1. A state of extreme fatigue or weariness; loss of vital powers; inability to respond to stimuli. **2.** The process of removing the contents or using up a supply of anything. **3.** The act of drawing or letting out.

heat e. An acute reaction to a hot, humid environment marked by profuse sweating, dizziness, nausea, headache, and profound fatigue as the result of excess fluid loss from the body. Heat exhaustion differs from heat stroke in that the body's thermoregulatory system is still functioning; if untreated, heat exhaustion can progress to heat stroke. SEE: table.

SYMPTOMS: The patient's rectal temperature will be elevated to about 102.5°F (39.0°C). The skin feels cool; pulse may be rapid but weak; blood pressure is decreased. The patient may appear disoriented and complain of thirst. Nausea and vomiting may also be noted.

PREVENTION: See heat stroke for preventive measures.

TREATMENT: The patient should be removed from the hot, humid environment to a cooler, well-ventilated location (e.g., indoors, under a shade tree) and placed in a head-low position. Clothing should be loosened and the patient's body cooled by placing cold packs in the axilla, on the neck, groin, and behind the knees. Fluid consumption, in the form of water or electrolyte drinks, should be administered to conscious patients. Intravenous infusion of isotonic saline may be required. Prognosis is favorable if the patient is properly treated

Comparison of Heatstroke and Heat Exhaustion

Heatstroke	Heat Exhaustion
Definition	**Definition**
A derangement of thermoregulation with altered mental status and high body temperature	A state of weakness produced by exposure to heat and excessive loss of fluids and electrolytes
History	**History**
Nonexertional	*Nonexertional*
Exposure to high temperatures and high humidity	Same as for heatstroke
Use of medications that increase heat production or inhibit perspiration	
Absence of fans or air conditioners	
Demographics: urban poor, elderly, obese	
Exertional	*Exertional*
Excessive exercise under tropical conditions	Same as for heatstroke
Demographics: outdoor laborers, athletes, military recruits	
Physical Exam	**Physical Exam**
Temperature: usually >105°F	*Temperature:* 99.5–102.2°F
Pulse: tachycardic	*Pulse:* weak, thready, and rapid
Blood pressure: variable	*Blood pressure:* usually normotensive
Skin: Nonexertional—Absence of sweating is common; Exertional—Signs of profuse sweating may be present	*Skin:* Diaphoretic
Neurological: Altered mental status, possible convulsions or coma	*Neurological:* Normal mental status
Treatment	**Treatment**
Bedrest	Rest
Active cooling by any available means, often by bathing or spraying skin with water, then fanning the patient	Administration of fluids and electrolytes by mouth or by vein
Administration of fluids and electrolytes	
Close monitoring of temperature to avoid excessive cooling and shivering (which generates heat). Avoidance of alcohol bath (risk of intoxication); avoid antipyretics (ineffective)	
Mortality	**Mortality**
Common	Rare

in the acute stages. SYN: *heat prostration*.

exhibitionism [″ + Gr. *-ismos,* condition] **1.** A tendency to attract attention to oneself by any means. **2.** A sexual identity disorder manifesting itself in an abnormal impulse that causes one to expose one's genitals to a stranger.

exhibitionist **1.** A person with an abnormal desire to attract attention. **2.** A person who yields to an impulse to expose the genitals to a stranger.

exhilarant (ĕg-zĭl′ăr-ănt) [L. *exhilarare,* to gladden] Something that is mentally stimulating.

exhumation (ĕks″hū-mā′shŭn) [L. *ex,* out, + *humus,* earth] Removal of a dead body from the grave after it has been buried.

exigency A situation requiring immediate management. SEE: *emergency*.

exitus (ĕk′sĭ-tŭs) [L., going out] Death.

Exner's nerve (ĕks′nĕrz) [Siegmund Exner, Austrian physiologist, 1846–1926] A nerve leading from the pharyngeal plexus to the cricothyroid membranes.

Exner's plexus A plexus of nerve fibers forming a layer near the surface of the cerebral cortex.

exo- [Gr. *exo,* outside] Combining form meaning *without; outside of*.

exobiology (ĕk″sō-bī-ŏl′ō-jē) The biological science of the universe, exclusive of our planet.

exocardia (ĕk″sō-kăr′dē-ă) [″ + *kardia,* heart] A congenitally abnormal position of the heart.

exocardial Occurring outside the heart.

exocataphoria (ĕks″ō-kăt-ă-for′ē-ă) [″ + *kata,* down, + *phoros,* bearing] A condition in which the visual axes are turned downward and outward.

exocolitis (ĕks″ō-kō-lī′tĭs) [″ + *kolon,* colon, + *itis,* inflammation] Inflammation of the peritoneum of the colon.

exocrine (ĕks′ō-krĭn) [″ + *krinein,* to separate] **1.** A term applied to the external secretion of a gland. Opposed to endocrine. **2.** A term applied to glands whose secretion reaches an epithelial surface either directly or through a duct.

exocytosis (ĕks″ō-sī-tō′sĭs) [″ + *kytos,* cell, + *osis,* condition] The discharge of particles from a cell. They are too large to pass through the cell membrane by diffusion. SEE: *pinocytosis*.

exodeviation (ĕk″sō-dē″vē-ā′shŭn) A turning outward. When this condition occurs in the eyes, it is termed exotropia.

exodontia (ĕks-ō-dŏn′shē-ă) [″ + *odous,* tooth] The subdivision of dentistry that specializes in the extraction of teeth. Exodontia is often included with other procedures in a department or division of oral and maxillofacial surgery.

exodontology (ĕks″ō-dŏn-tŏl′ō-jē) [″ + ″ + *logos,* word, reason] The branch of dentistry concerned with extraction of teeth.

exoenzyme (ĕk-sō-ĕn′zīm) [″ + *en,* in, + *zyme,* leaven] An enzyme that does not function within the cells that secrete it.

exoerythrocytic (ĕk″sō-ĕ-rĭth″rō-sī′tĭk) [″ + *erythros,* red, + *kytos,* cell] Occurring outside the red blood cells. Most of the life cycle of the malaria parasite in a human host is inside the red blood cell, where it causes symptoms; the rest is outside the red blood cell, and latent (i.e., exoerythrocytic).

exogamy (ĕks-ŏg′ă-mē) [″ + *gamos,* marriage] **1.** Marriage outside a particular group. **2.** In biology, conjugation between protozoan gametes of different ancestry.

exogastritis (ĕks″ō-găs-trī′tĭs) [″ + *gaster,* belly, + *itis,* inflammation] Inflammation of the peritoneal coat of the stomach.

exogenous (ĕks-ŏj′ĕ-nŭs) [″ + *gennan,* to produce] Originating outside an organ or part.

exohysteropexy (ĕks″ō-hĭs′tĕr-ō-pĕks″ē) [″ + *hystera,* womb, + *pexis,* fixation] Fixation of the uterus by implanting the fundus into the abdominal wall.

exomphalos (ĕks-ŏm′fă-lŭs) [Gr. *ex,* out, + *omphalos,* navel] **1.** An umbilical protrusion. **2.** An umbilical hernia.

exon One of the coding regions of the DNA of genes. SEE: *intron*.

exophasy The expression of thought by spoken or written words and the understanding of spoken or written words of others. It is also called external speech. SEE: *endophasy*.

exophoria (ĕks″ō-fō′rē-ă) [″ + *phoros,* bearing] A tendency of the visual axes to diverge outward. Opposite of esophoria.

exophthalmia (ĕks″ŏf-thăl′mē-ă) [″ + *ophthalmos,* eye] Abnormal protrusion of the eyeball. SYN: *exophthalmos*.

exophthalmometer (ĕk″sŏf-thăl-mŏm′ĕ-tĕr) A device for measuring the degree of protrusion of the eyeballs.

exophthalmos, exophthalmus (ĕks″ŏf-thăl′mŏs, -mŭs) Abnormal protrusion of the eyeball. This may be due to thyrotoxicosis, tumor of the orbit, orbital cellulitis, leukemia, or aneurysm. **exophthalmic** (-mĭk), *adj.*

pulsating e. Exophthalmos accompanied by pulsation and bruit due to an aneurysm behind the eye.

exoplasm (ĕk′sō-plăzm) [″ + LL. *plasma,* form, mold] Ectoplasm.

exoserosis (ĕks″ō-sĕr-ō′sĭs) [″ + *serum,* whey, + Gr. *osis,* condition] An oozing of serum or discharging of an exudate.

exoskeleton (ĕk″sō-skĕl′ĕ-tŏn) [″ + *skeleton,* a dried-up body] The hard outer covering of certain invertebrates such as the mollusks and arthropods. It is composed of chitin, calcareous material, or both.

exosmosis (ĕks″ŏs-mō′sĭs) [″ + *osmos,* a thrusting, + *osis,* condition] Diffusion of a fluid outward, as from a blood vessel.

exosplenopexy (ĕks″ō-splĕn′ō-pĕks-ē) [″ + *splen,* spleen, + *pexis,* fixation] Suturing of the spleen to an opening in the abdominal wall.

exostosis (ĕks″ŏs-tō′sĭs) *pl.* **exostoses** [″ + *osteon,* bone] A bony growth that arises from the surface of a bone, often involving the ossification of muscular attachments. SYN: *hyperostosis; osteoma.*

e. bursata An exostosis arising from the epiphysis of a bone and covered with cartilage and a synovial sac.

e. cartilaginea An exostosis consisting of cartilage underlying the periosteum.

dental e. An exostosis on the root of a tooth.

multiple osteocartilaginous e. A hereditary growth disorder marked by the development of multiple exostoses, usually on the diaphyses of long bones near the epiphyseal lines. It causes irregular growth of the epiphyses and often secondary deformities.

retrocalcaneal e. Abnormal bone growth over the Achilles tendon's attachment on the calcaneus. The colloquial term "pump bumps" is derived from this condition's association with the wearing of tight-fitting, high-heeled shoes.

SYMPTOMS: A hard nodule is present over the Achilles tendon attachment. The area appears inflamed and is sensitive to the touch. Patients often demonstrate hindfoot rigidity and decreased foot pronation. The patient may complain of pain during resisted plantar flexion (e.g., during the toe-off phase of gait). Symptoms may increase when wearing tight-fitting shoes.

TREATMENT: Physical therapy and anti-inflammatory medications are used to minimize the inflammatory response. The patient should be instructed to wear loose-fitting shoes or open-backed shoes such as sandals, whenever practical. Improper foot biomechanics should be corrected, if applicable.

exothermal, exothermic [Gr. *exo,* outside, + *therme,* heat] Pert. to a chemical reaction that produces heat.

exothymopexy (ĕks″ō-thī′mō-pĕks″ē) [″ + *thymos,* thymus, + *pexis,* fixation] Suturing of an enlarged thymus gland to the sternum.

exothyropexy (ĕks″ō-thī′rō-pĕks″ē) Suturing of the thyroid gland and external fixation to induce atrophy.

exotic (ĕg-zŏt′ĭk) [Gr. *exotikos*] Not native; originating in another part of the world.

exotoxin (ĕks″ō-tŏks′ĭn) [Gr. *exo,* outside, + *toxikon,* poison] A poisonous substance produced by bacteria, including staphylococci, streptococci, *Vibrio cholerae, Pseudomonas* species, and *Escherichia coli.* The actions of specific exotoxins vary with the organism. Staphylococcal exotoxins stimulate release of gamma interferon and can cause systemic inflammatory response syndrome. Inactivated exotoxins are used as the basis for diphtheria and tetanus vaccines. SEE: *bacterium; sepsis; systemic inflammatory response syndrome; toxoid.*

exotropia (ĕks″ō-trō′pē-ă) [″ + *tropos,* turning] Divergent strabismus; abnormal turning outward of one or both eyes.

expander (ĕk-spăn′dĕr) [L. *expandere,* to spread out] Something that increases the size, volume, or amount of something.

expected date of confinement ABBR: EDC. The predicted date of childbirth. SEE: *Naegele's rule; pregnancy* for table.

expectorant (ĕk-spĕk′tō-rănt) [Gr. *ex,* out, + L. *pectus,* breast] An agent, such as guaifenesin, that promotes the clearance of mucus from the respiratory tract.

expectoration (ĕk-spĕk″tō-rā′shŭn) **1.** The act or process of spitting out saliva or coughing up materials from the air passageways leading to the lungs. **2.** The expulsion of mucus or phlegm from the throat or lungs. It may be mucoid, mucopurulent, serous, or frothy. In pneumonia, it is viscid and tenacious, sticks to anything, appears rusty, and contains blood. In bronchitis, it is mucoid, often streaked with blood, and greenish-yellow from pus. In advanced tuberculosis, it varies from small amounts of frothy fluid to abundant, offensive greenish-yellow sputum often streaked with blood. SEE: *sputum.*

expel (ĕks-pĕl′) [L. *expellere*] To drive or push out.

experience **1.** To encounter something personally or undergo an event. **2.** The knowledge or wisdom obtained from one's own observations.

experiment [L. *experimentum,* to test] A scientific procedure used to test the validity of a hypothesis, gain further evidence or knowledge, or test the usefulness of a drug or type of therapy that has not been tried previously.

expiration (ĕks″pĭ-rā′shŭn) [Gr. *ex,* out, + L. *spirare,* to breathe] **1.** Expulsion of air from the lungs in breathing. Normally the duration of expiration is shorter than that of inspiration. In general, if expiration lasts longer than inspiration, a pathological condition such as emphysema or asthma is present. SEE: *diaphragm* for illus.; *inspiration; respiration.* **2.** Death.

active e. Expiration accomplished as a result of muscular activity, as in forced respiration. The muscles used in forced expiration are those of the abdominal wall (external and internal oblique, rectus, and transversus abdominis), the internal intercostalis, serratus posterior inferior, platysma, and quadratus lumborum.

passive e. Expiration, performed during quiet respiration, that requires no muscular effort. It is brought about by the elasticity of the lungs, and by the ascent of the diaphragm and the weight of the descending chest wall, which compress the lungs.

expiratory (ěks-pī′ră-tor″ē) Pert. to expiration of air from the lungs.

expiratory center The part of the respiratory center in the medulla that promotes a forced exhalation.

expire **1.** To breathe out or exhale. **2.** To die.

explant (ěks-plănt′) [″ + L. *planta,* sprout] **1.** To remove a piece of living tissue from the body and transfer it to an artificial culture medium for growth, as in tissue culture. Opposite of implant. **2.** To remove a donor organ for transplantation. **3.** An organ removed for transplantation.

explode (ěks-plōd′) [L. *explodere,* fr. *ex,* out, + *plaudere,* to clap the hands] **1.** To burst or to have rapid onset, as an epidemic. **2.** To decompress suddenly, as a cavity. Explosive decompression occurs when the pressure in the cabin of an airplane flying at high altitude is suddenly decreased.

exploration [L. *explorare,* to search out] Examination of an organ or part by various means. **exploratory,** *adj.*

explorer An instrument used in exploration, esp. a device used to locate foreign bodies or to define passageways in body sinuses or cavities.

dental e. A sharp-pointed instrument used to detect unsound enamel, carious lesions, or imperfect margins of restorations in teeth.

exponent (ěks′pō-něnt) In mathematics, the number that indicates the power to which another number is to be raised. It is written as a superscript (e.g., 10^2 or x^2 indicates that 10 and x are to be squared, or multiplied by themselves). The exponent can have any numerical value and may be positive or negative; it does not have to be a whole number. SEE: *Scientific Notation in Units of Measurement Appendix.*

expose **1.** To open, as in surgically opening the abdominal cavity. **2.** To cause someone or something to lack heat or shelter. **3.** To place in contact with an infected person or agent. **4.** To display one's genitals publicly, esp. when members of the opposite sex are present. **5.** To deliver an amount of radiation.

exposure The amount of radiation delivered or received over a given area or to the entire body or object.

acute e. Exposure to radiation that is of short duration and usually of high intensity.

double e. Two exposures on one photographic or radiographic film.

pulp e. An opening in the dentin that exposes the pulp of a tooth to the oral cavity.

express [L. *expressare*] To squeeze out.

expression **1.** Expulsion by pressure. **2.** Facial disclosure of feeling or a physical state. SYN: *facies.* SEE: *face.*

expressivity The extent to which a heritable trait is manifest in the individual carrying the gene.

expulsion rate In gynecology, the rate of spontaneous rejection of intrauterine contraceptive devices in the group of women who use them. It is usually expressed with respect to the time elapsed following implantation.

expulsive [L. *expellere,* to drive out] Having a tendency to expel.

exsanguinate (ěks-săn′gwĭn-āt) [Gr. *ex,* out, + *sanguis,* blood] To lose blood to the point at which life can no longer be sustained.

exsanguination (ěk-săn″gwĭn-ā′shŭn) Massive bleeding.

exsanguine (ěks-săn′gwĭn) Anemic; bloodless.

exsiccant (ěk-sĭk′ănt) [L. *exsiccare,* to dry out] **1.** Absorbing or drying up a discharge. **2.** An agent that absorbs moisture. **3.** A dusting or drying powder.

exsiccation (ěk″sĭ-kā′shŭn) **1.** The process of drying up. **2.** In chemistry, removing the water from compounds or solutions. SYN: *desiccation.*

exsorption (ěk-sorp′shŭn) Movement of material including cells and electrolytes from the blood to the lumen of the intestines. In pathological conditions such as intestinal obstruction, this process may greatly increase pressure inside the affected area of the intestinal tract.

exstrophy (ěks′trō-fē) [″ + *strephein,* to turn] Congenital turning inside out of an organ. SYN: *eversion.*

exsufflation (ěk″sŭ-flā′shŭn) [″ + *sufflatio,* blown up] Forceful expulsion of air from a cavity by artificial means, such as use of a mechanical exsufflator.

ext L. *extractum,* extract.

extemporaneous [LL. *extemporaneus*] Not prepared according to formula but devised for the occasion.

extend (ěk-stěnd′) [Gr. *ex,* out, + L. *tendere,* to stretch] **1.** To straighten a leg or arm. **2.** To move forward. **3.** To increase the angle between the bones forming a joint.

extended care facility A medical care institution for patients who require long-term custodial or medical care, esp. for a chronic disease or one requiring prolonged rehabilitation therapy.

extender (ĕk-stĕn′dĕr) Something that increases duration or effect. The time required for absorption of some medicines given intramuscularly may be increased by injecting them with a substance such as an oil, which slows absorption.

leg e. A device added to lengthen the legs of furniture (e.g., beds, tables, chairs) to accommodate the needs of persons with functional limitations.

extension (ĕks-tĕn′shŭn) [L. *extensio*] **1.** The movement that pulls apart both ends of any part. **2.** A movement that brings the members of a limb into or toward a straight position. Opposite of flexion. **3.** The application of a pull (traction) to a fractured or dislocated limb.

Buck's e. A method of producing traction by applying regular or flannel-backed adhesive tape to the skin and keeping it in smooth close contact by circular bandaging of the part to which it is applied. The adhesive strips are aligned with the long axis of the arm or leg, the superior ends being about 1 in. (2.5 cm) from the fracture site. Weights sufficient to produce the required extension are fastened to the inferior end of the adhesive strips by a rope that is run over a pulley to permit free motion.

extensor [L.] A muscle that extends a part of the body.

exterior [L.] Outside of; external; opposite of interior or internal.

exteriorize **1.** To mobilize without the body, a part temporarily in surgery. SEE: *marsupialization*. **2.** In psychiatry, to turn one's interests outward.

extern (ĕks′tĕrn) [L. *externus,* outside] A medical student, living outside a hospital, who assists in the medical and surgical care of patients. SEE: *intern*.

external Exterior; the opposite of interior or internal.

external fixator A device for holding fractured bones in place by use of external rather than internal fixation.

externalia (ĕks″tĕr-nā′lē-ă) [L. *exter,* outside, + *genitalis,* genital] The external genitals.

externalize (ĕks-tĕr′nă-līz) **1.** In surgery, to provide exposure to the outside. **2.** In psychiatry, to direct one's inner conflicts to the outside rather than keeping them hidden inside.

exteroceptive (ĕks″tĕr-ō-sĕp′tĭv) [L. *externus,* outside, + *receptus,* having received] Pert. to the reception by end organs receiving stimuli from outside.

exteroceptor (ĕks″tĕr-ō-sĕp′tor) A sense organ (e.g., in the eye, ear, or skin) adapted for the reception of stimuli from outside the body.

extima (ĕks′tĭ-mă) [L., outermost] The outer layer of a structure. SEE: *intima*.

extinction [L. *exstinctus,* having extinguished] **1.** The process of extinguishing or putting out. **2.** The complete inhibition of a conditioned reflex through failure to reinforce it.

extinguish (ĕks-tĭng′gwĭsh) [L. *extinguere,* to render extinct] To abolish, esp. to remove a reflex, by surgical, psychological, or pharmacological means, depending on the type of reflex involved.

extirpation (ĕks-tĭr-pā′shŭn) [L. *extirpare,* to root out] Complete removal of a part.

extorsion (ĕks-tor′shŭn) [Gr. *ex,* out, + L. *torsio,* twisting] Rotation of an organ or limb outward.

extra- [L. *extra,* outside] Prefix meaning *outside of; in addition to; beyond*.

extra-articular [″ + *articulus,* joint] Outside a joint.

extra beat Extrasystole.

extracapsular (ĕks″tră-kăp′sū-lăr) Outside a capsule (e.g., a joint capsule or the capsule of the lens of the eye).

extracellular (ĕks″tră-sĕl′ū-lăr) Outside the cell.

extrachromosomal Not connected to the chromosomes; exerting an effect other than through chromosomal action.

extracorporeal (ĕks″tră-kor-por′ē-ăl) [″ + *corpus,* body] Outside the body.

extracorporeal membrane oxygenator ABBR: ECMO. An external device that oxygenates blood delivered to it from the body and then returns it to the patient. It has been used experimentally in patients with acute respiratory failure. It has also been used to treat newborns with meconium aspiration syndrome, pneumonia, and persistent pulmonary hypertension, who have failed to respond to standard treatments.

extracorporeal shock-wave lithotriptor A device that breaks up kidney stones. After the patient is placed in water bath, and given analgesics, electrically generated shock waves are focused on the stones, disintegrating them and permitting their passage in the urine. This technique is also used to treat gallstones. SEE: *calculus, renal; percutaneous ultrasonic lithotriptor*.

extracorticospinal (ĕks″tră-kor″tĭ-kō-spī′năl) Outside the corticospinal tract of the central nervous system.

extracranial (ĕks″tră-krā′nē-ăl) Outside the skull.

extract (ĕks-trăkt′, ĕks′trăkt) [L. *extractum*] **1.** To surgically remove or remove forcibly, as to extract a tooth. **2.** A solid or semisolid preparation made by removing the soluble portion of a compound by using water or alcohol as the solvent and evaporating the solution. **3.** The active principle of a drug obtained by distillation or chemical processes.

alcoholic e. An extract in which alcohol is the solvent.

aqueous e. An extract in which water is the solvent.

aromatic fluid e. An extract made from an aromatic powder.

compound e. An extract prepared from more than one drug or substance.

ethereal e. An extract using ether as the vehicle.

fluid e. An extract of a vegetable drug made into a solution. It contains medicinal components.

liver e. A dry brown powder obtained from mammalian livers that was once used as a crude source of vitamin B_{12} and other vitamins.

powdered e. A dried, crushed extract.

soft e. An extract with the consistency of honey.

solid e. An extract made by evaporating the fluid part of a solution.

extraction [L. *extractum,* drawing out] **1.** Surgical removal, as a tooth. **2.** The removal of the active portion of a drug from its vehicle.

breech e. SEE: *delivery, breech.*

extracapsular e. A surgical technique for cataract removal. The nucleus, cortex, and anterior capsule are removed; the posterior capsule is left intact. This is often done by phacoemulsification under local anesthesia using a microscope.

extractive (ĕks-trăk′tĭv) Something that has been extracted or removed.

extractor An instrument for removing foreign bodies. Varieties include esophageal, throat, bronchial, and tissue extractors.

vacuum e. SEE: *vacuum extractor.*

extractum (ĕks-trăk′tŭm) *pl.* **extracta** [L., a drawing out] An extract. SEE: *fluidextract.*

extracystic (ĕks″tră-sĭs′tĭk) [L. *extra,* outside, + Gr. *kystis,* bladder] Outside or unrelated to a bladder or cystic tumor.

extradural (ĕks-tră-dū′răl) [″ + *durus,* hard] **1.** On the outer side of the dura mater. **2.** Unconnected with the dura mater.

extraembryonic (ĕks″tră-ĕm″brē-ŏn′ĭk) [″ + Gr. *embryon,* something that swells in the body] Apart from and outside the embryo (e.g., concerning the amnion).

extragenital (ĕks″tră-jĕn′ĭ-tăl) [″ + *genitalis,* genital] Outside or unrelated to the genital organs.

extrahepatic (ĕks″tră-hĕ-păt′ĭk) [L. *extra,* outside, + Gr. *hepatos,* liver] Outside or unrelated to the liver.

extraligamentous [″ + *ligare,* to bind] Outside or unrelated to a ligament.

extramalleolus (ĕks″tră-măl-lē′ō-lŭs) [″ + *malleolus,* little hammer] The external or lateral malleolus of the ankle.

extramarginal (ĕks″tră-măr′jĭ-năl) [″ + *margo,* margin] Pert. to subliminal consciousness.

extramastoiditis (ĕks″tră-măs″toyd-ī′tĭs) [″ + Gr. *mastos,* breast, + *eidos,* form, shape, + *itis,* inflammation] Inflammation of outside tissues contiguous to the mastoid process.

extramedullary (ĕks″tră-mĕd′ū-lă-rē) [″ + *medulla,* marrow] Outside the medulla or the bone marrow.

extramural (ĕks″tră-mū′răl) [″ + *murus,* wall] Outside the wall of an organ or vessel.

extraneous (ĕks-trā′nē-ŭs) [L. *extraneus,* external] Outside and unrelated to an organism.

extranuclear [L. *extra,* outside, + *nucleus,* kernel] Outside a nucleus.

extraocular (ĕks″tră-ŏk′ū-lăr) [″ + *oculus,* eye] Outside the eye, as in extraocular eye muscles.

extraocular eye muscle ABBR: EOM. A muscle attached to the eyeball that controls eye movement and coordination. SEE: illus.

extrapolar [″ + *polus,* pole] Outside instead of between poles, as the electrodes of a battery.

extrapolate To infer a point between two given, or known, points on a graph or progression. Thus, if an infant weighed 20 lb at a certain age and 4 months later weighed 23 lb, it could be inferred that at a point halfway between the two time periods, the infant might have weighed 21.5 lb.

extrapyramidal (ĕks″tră-pĭ-răm′ĭ-dăl) Outside the pyramidal tracts of the central nervous system.

extrapyramidal side effects of medications ABBR: EPS. Muscular rigidity, tremor, bradykinesia, and difficulty walking induced by neuroleptic medications; drug-induced parkinsonism.

extrapyramidal syndrome Any of several degenerative nervous system diseases that involve the extrapyramidal system and the basal ganglion of the brain. The symptoms include tremors, chorea, athetosis, and dystonia. Parkinsonism is an extrapyramidal syndrome.

extrasensory Pert. to forms of perception, such as thought transference, that are not dependent on the five primary senses.

extrasystole (ĕks″tră-sĭs′tō-lē) [″ + Gr. *systole,* contraction] Premature contraction of the heart. It may occur in either the presence or absence of organic heart disease. It may be of reflex origin or may be triggered by stimulants (e.g., caffeine, cocaine, or theophylline), hypoxia, psychological stress, electrolyte abnormalities, thyroid disorders, or myocardial infarction.

atrial e. Premature contraction of the atrium.

junctional e. Nodal e.

nodal e. Extrasystole occurring as a result of an impulse originating in the atrioventricular node. SYN: *junctional e.*

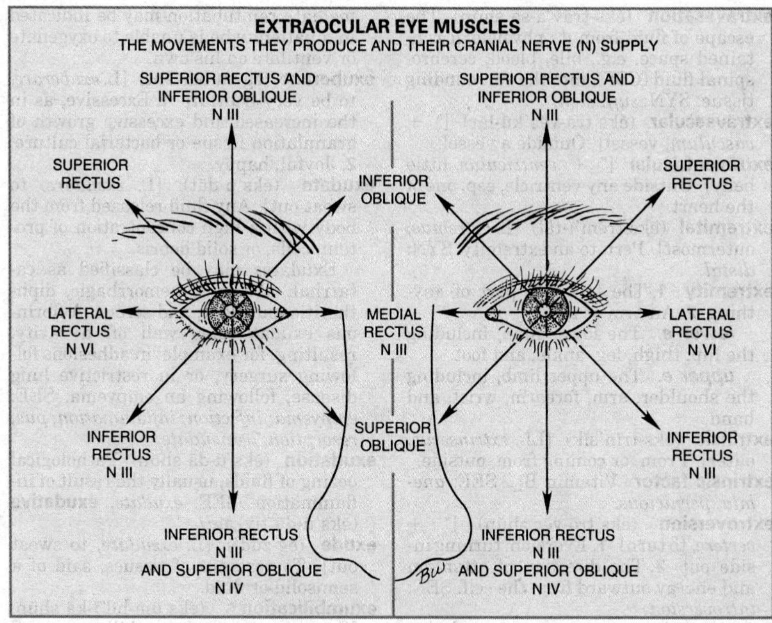

ventricular e. Premature ventricular beat.

extrathoracic Outside the thorax.

extratubal (ĕks″tră-tū′băl) Outside a tube, esp. the uterine tube.

extrauterine (ĕks″tră-ū′tĕr-ĭn) [″ + *uterus,* womb] Outside the uterus.

extravaginal (ĕks″tră-văj′ĭ-năl) [″ + *vagina,* sheath] Outside the vagina.

extravasate (ĕks-trăv′ă-sāt) [″ + *vas,* vessel] **1.** To escape from a vessel into the tissues, said of serum, blood, or lymph. **2.** Fluid escaping from vessels into surrounding tissue.

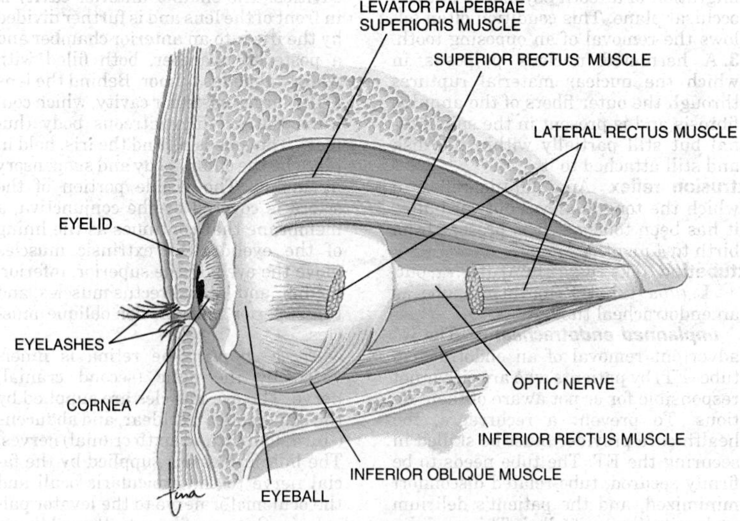

EXTRAOCULAR EYE MUSCLES

Lateral view, left eye (superior oblique and medial rectus not shown)

extravasation (ěks-trăv″ă-sā′shŭn) The escape of fluid from its physiologic contained space, e.g., bile, blood, cerebrospinal fluid (CSF), into the surrounding tissue. SYN: *suffusion.*

extravascular (ěks″tră-văs′kū-lăr) [″ + *vasculum,* vessel] Outside a vessel.

extraventricular [″ + *ventriculus,* little belly] Outside any ventricle, esp. one of the heart.

extremital (ěks-trěm′ĭ-tăl) [L. *extremus,* outermost] Pert. to an extremity. SYN: *distal.*

extremity **1.** The terminal part of anything. **2.** An arm or leg.

lower e. The lower limb, including the hip, thigh, leg, ankle, and foot.

upper e. The upper limb, including the shoulder, arm, forearm, wrist, and hand.

extrinsic (ěks-trĭn′sĭk) [LL. *extrinsecus,* outer] From, or coming from, outside.

extrinsic factor Vitamin B_{12}. SEE: *anemia, pernicious.*

extroversion (ěks″trō-vĕr′zhŭn) [″ + *vertere,* to turn] **1.** Eversion; turning inside out. **2.** The direction of attention and energy outward from the self. SEE: *introversion.*

extrovert An outgoing or extremely sociable person; one who is interested mainly in external objects and actions. The extreme pathological extrovert reaction is seen in bipolar disorders. Opposite of introvert.

extrude (ěks-trūd′) [L. *extrudere,* to squeeze out] To push or force out.

extrusion (ěks-troo′zhŭn) **1.** Something occupying an abnormal external position. **2.** In dentistry, the overeruption or migration of a tooth beyond its natural occlusal plane. This condition often follows the removal of an opposing tooth. **3.** A herniated nucleus pulposus in which the nuclear material ruptures through the outer fibers of the annulus fibrosis and is present in the spinal canal but still partially within the disk and still attached to it.

extrusion reflex An infantile reflex in which the tongue moves outward after it has been touched. It is present from birth to 4 months.

extubation (ěks″tū-bā′shŭn) [Gr. *ex,* out, + L. *tuba,* tube] Removal of a tube, as an endotracheal tube.

unplanned endotracheal e. The inadvertent removal of an endotracheal tube (ET) by patients who are either not responsible for or not aware of their actions. To prevent a recurrence, the health care provider must be skilled in securing the ET. The tube needs to be firmly secured, tube-related discomfort minimized, and the patient's delirium and agitation controlled. This may require careful patient monitoring, or occasionally, sedation, paralysis, or the application of physical restraints. Immediate reintubation may be indicated in a patient who is unable to oxygenate or ventilate on his own.

exuberant (ěg-zū′bĕr-ănt) [L. *exuberare,* to be very fruitful] **1.** Excessive, as in the increased and excessive growth of granulation tissue or bacterial culture. **2.** Joyful, happy.

exudate (ěks′ū-dāt) [L. *exsudare,* to sweat out] Any fluid released from the body with a high concentration of protein, cells, or solid debris.

Exudates may be classified as catarrhal, fibrinous, hemorrhagic, diphtheritic, purulent, and serous. A fibrinous exudate may wall off a cavity, resulting, for example, in adhesions following surgery, or in restrictive lung disease, following an empyema. SEE: *empyema; infection; inflammation; pus; resorption; transudate.*

exudation (ěks″ū-dā′shŭn) Pathological oozing of fluids, usually the result of inflammation. SEE: *exudate.* **exudative** (ěks′ū-dā″tĭv), *adj.*

exude (ěg-zūd′) [L. *exsudare,* to sweat out] To ooze out of tissues; said of a semisolid or fluid.

exumbilication (ěks″ŭm-bĭl″ĭ-kā′shŭn) [Gr. *ex,* out, + L. *umbilicus,* navel] Protrusion of the navel. SYN: *exomphalos.* SEE: *umbilical hernia.*

eye [AS. *eage*] The organ of vision. SEE: illus.

ANATOMY: The eyeball has three layers: the inner retina, which contains the photoreceptors; the middle uvea (choroid, ciliary body, and iris); and the outer sclera, which includes the transparent cornea. The eyeball contains two cavities. The smaller anterior cavity is in front of the lens and is further divided by the iris into an anterior chamber and a posterior chamber, both filled with watery aqueous humor. Behind the lens is the larger posterior cavity, which contains the jellylike vitreous body (humor). The lens is behind the iris, held in place by the ciliary body and suspensory ligaments. The visible portion of the sclera is covered by the conjunctiva, a membrane that continues as the lining of the eyelids. Six extrinsic muscles move the eyeball: the superior, inferior, medial, and lateral rectus muscles, and the superior and inferior oblique muscles.

Nerve supply: The retina is innervated by the optic (second cranial) nerve. The eye muscles are supplied by the oculomotor, trochlear, and abducens (third, fourth, and sixth cranial) nerves. The lid muscles are supplied by the facial nerve to the orbicularis oculi and the oculomotor nerve to the levator palpebrae. Sensory fibers to the orbit are furnished by ophthalmic and maxillary fibers of the fifth cranial (trigeminal) nerve. Sympathetic postganglionic fi-

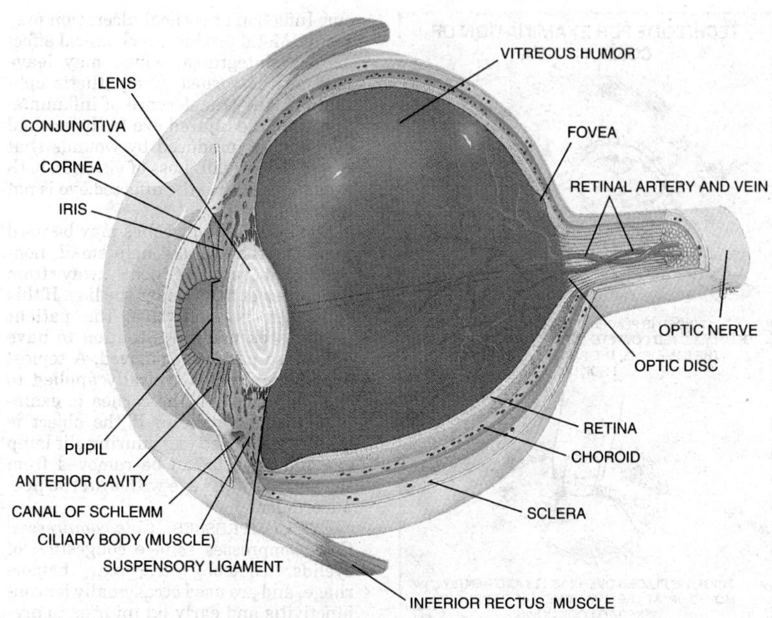

ANATOMY OF THE EYE

bers originate in the carotid plexus, their cell bodies lying in the superior cervical ganglion. They supply the dilator muscle of the iris, lacrimal gland, and smooth muscle fibers in the eyelid. Parasympathetic fibers from the ciliary ganglion pass to the ciliary muscle and constrictor muscles of the iris.

PHYSIOLOGY: Light entering the eye passes through the cornea, then through the pupil, an opening in the iris, and on through the crystalline lens and the vitreous body to the retina. The cornea, aqueous humor, lens, and vitreous body are the refracting media of the eye. Changes in the curvature of the lens are brought about by its elasticity and the contraction of the ciliary muscle. These changes focus light rays on the retina, thereby stimulating the rods and cones, the sensory receptors. The cones are concerned with color vision and the rods with vision in dim light. Sensory impulses pass through the optic nerve to the brain. The visual area of the cerebral cortex, located in the occipital lobe, registers them as visual sensations. The amount of light entering the eye is regulated by the iris; its constrictor and dilator muscles change the size of the pupil in response to varying amounts of light. The eye can distinguish nearly 8 million differences in color. As the eye ages, objects appear greener. The principal aspects of vision are color sense, light sense, movement, and form sense.

DIAGNOSIS: Following trauma to the head and in certain disease states, the size, shape, motion, and reactions of the pupils provide extremely important diagnostic information.

Constricted pupils: This may denote irritative lesions of the third nerve in early stages of some types of anesthesia or during alcoholic excitement, or may result from a therapeutic dose of an opiate such as morphine. Constriction of one pupil indicates an irritative lesion of the opposite side of the brain, situated at the third nerve nuclei, or a paralysis of the sympathetic nerve fibers due to a lesion somewhere in their course.

Dilated pupils: This may be caused by the medicines belladonna or atropine, or by irritation of the sympathetic nerve fibers. It may occur during attacks of dyspnea in the last stages of anesthesia. Dilation of one pupil indicates a paralysis of the third nerve from some brain lesion or an irritation of the cervical sympathetic nerve fibers.

Floating specks: Most people see little specks of material, which are small pieces of tissue, floating in the vitreous humor. These are called *muscae volitantes,* Latin for "flying flies." These specks are the remainder of intraocular embryonic tissue that did not disappear completely. This is not an abnormal condition.

Squint: This is caused by a lack of alignment of the visual axes. It is an un-

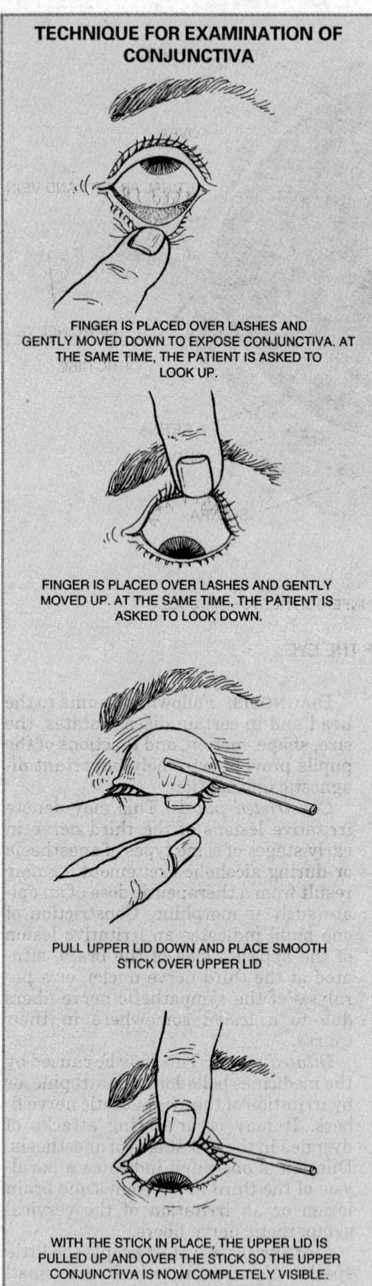

favorable symptom in the course of a brain disease.

TECHNIQUE FOR EXAMINATION OF CONJUNCTIVA
FINGER IS PLACED OVER LASHES AND GENTLY MOVED DOWN TO EXPOSE CONJUNCTIVA. AT THE SAME TIME, THE PATIENT IS ASKED TO LOOK UP.
FINGER IS PLACED OVER LASHES AND GENTLY MOVED UP. AT THE SAME TIME, THE PATIENT IS ASKED TO LOOK DOWN.
PULL UPPER LID DOWN AND PLACE SMOOTH STICK OVER UPPER LID
WITH THE STICK IN PLACE, THE UPPER LID IS PULLED UP AND OVER THE STICK SO THE UPPER CONJUNCTIVA IS NOW COMPLETELY VISIBLE.

FOREIGN BODY IN EYE: This condition is manifested by pain, lacrimation, and spasm of the eye; later, redness, swelling, and occasionally headache occur. Infection or corneal ulceration may result. Metal produces a chemical effect as it disintegrates, which may leave rust on the cornea. Sympathetic ophthalmia, the transference of inflammation from the injured eye to the normal eye, may be produced by wounds that pierce the eyeball. Loss of vision in both eyes may result if the affected eye is not removed.

Eye baths or eyewashes may be used to soothe the eye and help small, nonembedded particles float away from the cornea or from under the lids. If this treatment is ineffective, the patient should seek medical attention to have embedded particles removed. A topical anesthetic drop is typically applied to the eye, and then the cornea is examined with fluoroscein. If the object is readily visualized (e.g., during slit lamp examination), it can be removed from the surface of the eye with a sterile needle or burr.

EYE COMPRESSES: *Cold compresses:* Cold compresses relieve congestion of eyelids, control intraocular hemorrhage, and are used occasionally for conjunctivitis and early lid injuries to prevent hemorrhage into tissues. The hands are scrubbed, and the compresses moistened with isotonic saline solution, wrung out with forceps, and placed on ice to chill. The compresses are placed over the lids and extended over the cheek and are changed every 2 or 3 min. Each compress may be used repeatedly if there is no pus. When pus is present, each compress may be used only once.

Hot compresses: Comfortably warm compresses are used to increase the blood supply to the eyelids and eyeballs and to relieve pain. The hands are scrubbed, and petroleum jelly is applied with a clean swab to the area where the compresses will be applied. The compresses are wrung dry with forceps, tested on the wrist, and applied with as much heat as the patient can tolerate. To increase blood supply to the eyelids, compresses are placed over the lids and extended over the cheeks; to increase blood supply to the eyeballs, they are placed over the lids and extended over the brow. New compresses are used for each application if pus is present. The eyelid is dried when the last compress is removed. SEE: *lacrimal apparatus; Standard and Universal Precautions Appendix.*

PATIENT CARE: When injury to the eye occurs, visual acuity is assessed immediately. If the globe has been penetrated, a suitable eye shield, not an eye patch, is applied. A penetrating foreign body should not be removed. All medications, esp. corticosteroids, are withheld until the patient has seen an ophthalmologist.

The patient is assessed for pain and tenderness, redness and discharge, itching, photophobia, increased tearing, blinking, and visual blurring. When any prescribed topical eye medications (drops, ointments, or solutions) are administered, the health care provider should wash his or her hands thoroughly. The patient's head is turned slightly toward the affected eye, and his or her cooperation is sought in keeping the eye wide open. Drops are instilled in the conjunctival sac (not on the orb), and pressure is applied to the lacrimal apparatus in the inner canthus as necessary to prevent systemic absorption. Ointments are applied along the palpebral border from the inner to the outer canthus, and solutions are instilled from the inner to the outer canthus. Touching the dropper or tip of the medication container to the eye should be avoided, and hands should be washed immediately after the procedure.

Both patient and family are taught correct methods for instilling prescribed medications. Patients with visual defects are protected from injury, and family members taught safety measures. Patients with insufficient tearing or the inability to blink or close their eyes are protected from corneal injury by applying artificial tears and by gently patching the eyes closed. The importance of periodic eye examinations is emphasized. Persons at risk should protect their eyes from trauma by wearing safety goggles when working with or near dangerous tools or substances. Tinted lenses should be worn to protect the eyes from excessive exposure to bright light. Patients should avoid rubbing their eyes to prevent irritation or possibly infection. SEE: *eyedrops; tears, artificial*.

CAUTION: Corticosteroids should not be administered topically or systemically until the patient has been seen by a physician, preferably an ophthalmologist. *A red eye due to herpes simplex plus use of corticosteroids indicates risk for blindness in that eye.*

---

aphakic e. An eye from which the crystalline lens has been removed.

artificial e. A prosthesis for placement in the orbit of an individual whose eye has been removed. SEE: *ocularist*.

black e. Bruising, discoloration, and swelling of the eyelid and tissue around the eye due to trauma.

TREATMENT: Application of ice packs during the first 24 hr will inhibit swelling. Hot compresses after the first day may aid absorption of the fluids that produce discoloration.

crossed e. Strabismus with deviation of the visual axis of one eye toward that of the other eye.

dark-adapted e. An eye that has become adjusted for viewing objects in dim light; one adapted for scotopic, or rod, vision. Dark adaptation depends on the regeneration of rhodopsin, the light-sensitive glycoprotein in the rods of the eye.

e. deviation In eye muscle imbalance and "crossed eyes," the abnormal visual axis of the eye that is not aligned.

dominant e. The eye to which a person unconsciously gives preference as a source of stimuli for visual sensations. The dominant eye is usually used in sighting down a gun or looking through a monocular microscope.

dry e. Insufficient lubrication in the eye and abnormal lack of moisture in the conjunctiva. This condition produces pain and discomfort in the eyes. Dry eye may occur in any disorder that scars the cornea (e.g., erythema multiforme, trachoma, or corneal burns), Sjögren's syndrome, lagophthalmos, Riley-Day syndrome, absence of one or both of the lacrimal glands, paralysis of the facial or trigeminal nerves, medication with atropine, deep anesthesia, and debilitating diseases. Suitably prepared water-soluble polymers are effective in treating this condition.

exciting e. In sympathetic ophthalmia, the damaged eye, which is the source of sympathogenic influences.

fixating e. In strabismus, the eye that is directed toward the object of vision.

lazy e. Amblyopia.

light-adapted e. An eye that has become adjusted to viewing objects in bright light; one adapted for photopic, or cone, vision. In this type of eye, most rhodopsin has been broken down.

squinting e. An eye that deviates from the object of fixation in strabismus.

sympathizing e. In sympathetic ophthalmia, the uninjured eye, which reacts to the pathological process in the injured eye.

trophic ulceration of e. A noninfectious ulceration of the corneal epithelium of the eye due to repeated trauma.

eyeball The globe of the eye. Tension and position of the globe in relation to the orbit should be noted.

PATHOLOGY: Pathological conditions include enophthalmos (recession of the eyeball) and exophthalmos (protrusion of the eyeball).

eyeball, voluntary propulsion of The ability to voluntarily cause the globe of the eye to protrude by as much as 10 mm (0.4 in.). This is not harmful to the eye or visual acuity.

eye bank An organization that collects and stores corneas for transplantation.

eyebrow The arch over the eye; also its covering, esp. the hairs.

eye contact The meeting of the gaze of two persons; a direct look into the eyes of another.

eyecup **1.** The optic vesicle, an evagination of the embryonic brain from which the retina develops. **2.** A small cup that fits over the eye, used for bathing its surface.

eyedrops Any medicinal substance dropped in liquid form onto the conjunctiva.

In applying eyedrops, the head should be held back; the drops will not pass from under the upper lid to under the lower lid or vice versa. The smaller the eyedrops, the better. Too much liquid in the eye causes the patient to blink, and the medication is then washed away by the increased lacrimal secretion.

CAUTION: Many medicines are not absorbed from the conjunctiva; they may be readily absorbed from the nasolacrimal duct. For this reason, esp. in children, it is advisable to close off the duct by applying pressure to the inner canthus of the eye for a few minutes after each instillation.

---

eye-gaze communicator An electronic device that allows a person to control a computer by looking at words or commands on a video screen. A very low intensity light shines into one of the user's eyes. A television camera picks up reflections from the cornea and retina. As the direction of the person's gaze moves, the relative position of the two reflections changes, and the computer uses this information to determine the area at which the person is looking. The computer then executes the selected command.

eyeglass A glass lens used to correct a defect in visual acuity or to prevent exposure to bright light if the lens is tinted. SEE: *glasses*.

eyeground The fundus of the eye, seen with an ophthalmoscope.

eyelash A stiff hair on the margin of the eyelid. SYN: *cilium*.

eyelid One of two movable protective folds that cover the anterior surface of the eyeball when closed. They are separated by the palpebral fissure. The upper (palpebra superior) is the larger and more movable. It is raised by contraction of the levator palpebrae superioris muscle. Angles formed at the inner and outer ends of the lids are known as the canthi. The cilia, or eyelashes, arise from the edges of the eyelids. The posterior surface is lined by the conjunctiva, a mucous membrane.

drooping e. Ptosis of the eyelid.

fused e. A congenital anomaly resulting from failure of the fetal eyelids to separate.

eyelid closure reflex Contraction of the orbicularis palpebrarum muscle with closure of lids resulting from percussion above the supraorbital nerve. SYN: *McCarthy's reflex; supraorbital reflex*.

eye muscle imbalance A pathological condition of the extraocular muscles of one or both eyes. It causes the eyes to be misaligned in one or more axes. SEE: *eye, crossed; esophoria; exophoria; squint; strabismus*.

eyepiece (ī′pēs) The portion of an optical device closest to the viewer's eye.

eye protection Goggles, plastic or glass face masks, or shatterproof glasses to prevent injury to the eye during work or play.

CAUTION: Protective eye wear should be worn in surgery (and other health care settings where splashes or splatters are common), in many sports, and in most vocations or occupations where splinters, cinders, hooks, or other small objects may injure the cornea, lens, or ocular bulb.

---

eye stones Very small stones placed in the conjunctival sac to remove a mobile foreign body from the eye.

eyestrain Tiredness of the eye due to overuse or use of an improper corrective lens.

eyewash Any suitable liquid used to rinse the eyes (e.g., sterile physiological saline or sterile water).

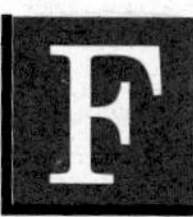

F 1. *Fahrenheit; femto-; field of vision; folic acid; formula; function.* **2.** Symbol for the element fluorine.

F_1 In genetics, the first filial generation, the offspring of a cross between two unrelated individuals.

F_2 In genetics, the second filial generation, the offspring of a cross between two individuals of the F_1 generation.

FA, F.A. *fatty acid; filterable agent; first aid; fluorescent antibody.*

F.A.A.N. *Fellow of the American Academy of Nursing.*

Fab *fragment antigen binding.*

fabella (fă-bĕl′lă) *pl.* **fabellae** [L., little bean] Fibrocartilage or bone that sometimes develops in the head of the gastrocnemius muscle.

fabism (fā′bĭzm) [L. *faba,* bean, + Gr. *-ismos,* condition] Favism.

fabrication (făb″rĭ-kā′shŭn) [L. *fabricatus,* having built] A deliberately false statement told as if it were true.

Fabry's disease (fă′brēz) [J. Fabry, Ger. physician, 1860–1930] An x-linked, recessive metabolic disease in which there is a galactosidase deficiency, which leads to accumulation of glycosphingolipids throughout the body. Clinically, by age 10, there is discomfort of the hands and feet with paresthesia or burning pain. There may be painful abdominal crises resembling other causes of acute abdominal pain. As these patients age, glycolipid deposition in the kidneys, heart, and brain may produce serious organ dysfunction.

F.A.C.C.P. *Fellow of the American College of Chest Physicians.*

F.A.C.D. *Fellow of the American College of Dentists.*

face [L. *facies*] **1.** The anterior part of the head from the forehead to the chin, extending laterally to but not including the ears. SEE: illus.; *facial expression.*

ANATOMY: There are 14 bones in the face. The blood supply is bilateral from the facial, maxillary, and superficial temporal branches of the external carotid artery and the ophthalmic branch of the internal carotid artery. The veins include the external and internal jugular veins.

2. The visage or countenance.

moon f. A full, round face seen in Cushing's syndrome or more often as a side effect of corticosteroid therapy.

face-lift A nonscientific term for plastic surgery of the face. SEE: *rhitidectomy.*

FACEP *Fellow of the American College of Emergency Physicians.*

facet (făs′ĕt) [Fr. *facette,* small face] A small, smooth area on a bone or other hard surface.

wear f. A line or plane worn on a tooth surface by attrition.

facetectomy (făs″ĕ-tĕk′tō-mē) [″ + Gr. *ektome,* excision] Surgical removal of the articular facet of a vertebra.

facet joint One of the zygapophyseal joints of the vertebral column between the articulating facets of each pair of vertebrae.

facial [L. *facialis*] Pert. to the face.

facial bones The 14 bones that make up the face: maxillae (2); nasal (2); palatine (2); inferior nasal conchae (2); mandible (1); zygoma (2); lacrimal (2); vomer (1).

facial expression An appearance of the face conveying emotion or reaction. The human face has a great store and variety of expressions. Expressions may convey different meanings in different cultures. Also, certain disease states (e.g., schizophrenia) may limit the ability to interpret facial expression, and parkinsonism is associated with facial rigidity. In certain cultures a smile is to be expected, but in others it may be an infrequent facial expression.

facial reflex In coma, contraction of facial muscles following pressure on the eyeball. SYN: *bulbomimic reflex; Mondonesi's reflex.*

facial spasm An involuntary contraction of muscles supplied by the facial nerve, involving one side of the face or the region around the eye. SEE: *cranial nerve; tic.*

-facient Suffix meaning *to make happen; to cause.*

facies (fā′shē-ēz) *pl.* **facies** [L] **1.** The face or the surface of any structure. **2.** The expression or appearance of the face.

f. abdominalis A pinched, anxious, shrunken, and drawn expression once thought to be indicative of abdominal diseases.

adenoid f. A dull, lethargic appearance with open mouth, which may be due to hypertrophy of adenoids or to chronic mouth breathing.

f. aortica A facial appearance once thought to be indicative of aortic insufficiency, with bluish sclerae, sunken cheeks, and sallow skin.

f. hepatica The appearance of the face in end-stage liver disease. The skin is sallow, the conjunctivae yellow, and the eyeballs sunken.

f. hippocratica The facial appearance classically described in those dying from long-continued illness or from

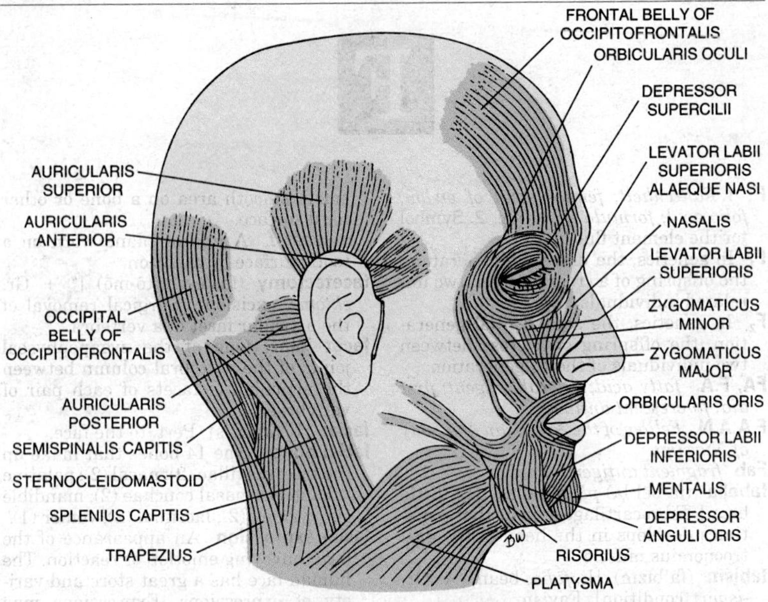

MUSCLES OF FACE AND SCALP

cholera. The cheeks and temples are hollow, the eyes sunken, the complexion leaden, and the lips relaxed.

f. leontina The lion-like facial appearance seen in certain forms of leprosy.

masklike f. An expressionless face with little or no animation, seen in parkinsonism.

f. mitralis The facies seen in advanced mitral insufficiency. Capillaries are more or less visible, and the cheeks are pink, although the patient may be cyanotic.

myopathic f. The facies due to muscular relaxation. The lids drop and the lips protrude.

parkinsonian f. A masklike facies with infrequent eye blinking and decreased facial expressiveness, characteristic of parkinsonism.

facilitation (fă-sĭl″ĭ-tā′shŭn) [L. *facilis,* easy] **1.** The hastening of an action or process; esp., addition of the energy of a nerve impulse to that of other impulses activated at the same time. **2.** In neuromuscular rehabilitation, a generic term referring to various techniques that elicit muscular contraction through reflex activation.

autogenic f. The process of inhibiting the muscle that generated a stimulus while providing an excitatory impulse to the antagonist muscle.

proprioceptive neuromuscular f. ABBR: PNF. An approach to therapeutic exercise directed at relaxing muscles, increasing joint range of motion, and regaining function by using spiral-diagonal patterns of movement. The principles and techniques were created and refined in the 1940s by Dr. Herman Kabat and two physical therapists, Maggie Knott and Dorothy Voss. PNF uses a developmental sequence of mobility, stability, controlled mobility, and skill; it emphasizes precision in patient position, manual contacts, verbal cueing, and timing.

facility, long-term care An institution such as a nursing home that is capable of providing continuous care for elderly or chronically ill patients.

facing [L. *facies,* face] A veneer of restorative material used on a tooth or on a prosthesis to simulate a natural tooth.

faciobrachial (fā″shē-ō-brā′kē-ăl) [″ + Gr. *brachion,* arm] Pert. to the face and arm, esp. to juvenile muscular dystrophy.

faciocervical (fā″shē-ō-sĕr′vĭ-kăl) [″ + *cervix,* neck] Pert. to the face and neck, esp. to progressive dystrophy of facial muscles.

faciolingual (fā″shē-ō-lĭn′gwăl) [″ + *lingua,* tongue] Pert. to the face and tongue, esp. to paralysis of these.

facioplasty (fā″shē-ō-plăs′tē) [″ + Gr. *plassein,* to form] Plastic surgery of the face.

facioscapulohumeral (fā″shē-ō-skăp″ū-lō-hū′mĕr-ăl) [″ + *scapula,* shoulder blade, + *humerus,* shoulder] Pert. to the face, scapula, and upper arm.

F.A.C.O.G. *Fellow of the American College of Obstetricians and Gynecologists.*

F.A.C.P. *Fellow of the American College of Physicians.*

F.A.C.S. *Fellow of the American College of Surgeons.*

F.A.C.S.M. *Fellow of the American College of Sports Medicine.*

factitious (făk-tĭsh′ŭs) [L. *facticius,* made by art] Produced artificially; not natural.

factor [L., maker] **1.** A contributing cause in any action. **2.** In genetics, a gene. **3.** An essential element such as a vitamin or immunoglobulin.

antihemophilic f. ABBR: AHF. Blood coagulation factor VIII. SYN: *antihemophilic globulin*. SEE: *coagulation factor*.

autocrine motility f. A chemical released by cancer cells that induces motility, enabling the cells to metastasize.

coagulation f. One of the various factors involved in blood clotting. The generally accepted terms for the factors and their Roman numeral designations are as follows:

Factor I, fibrinogen; *Factor II,* prothrombin; *Factor III,* tissue; *Factor IV,* calcium ions; *Factor V,* proaccelerin (an unstable protein substance also called labile factor); *Factor VII,* proconvertin; *Factor VIII,* antihemophilic factor; *Factor IX,* Christmas factor (also called plasma thromboplastin component [PTC]); *Factor X,* Stuart factor; *Factor XI,* plasma thromboplastin antecedent (PTA); *Factor XII,* Hageman factor; *Factor XIII,* fibrin-stabilizing factor (FSF); prekallikrein; and HMWK, also called *Fitzgerald, Falujenc,* or *Williams factor,* or *contact activation cofactor*. Factor VI, once called accelerin, is no longer used.

correction f. A number by which a measured value is multiplied, to correct for systematic measurement error.

eosinophil chemotactic f. A mediator released when mast cells are injured. This is in response to inflammation.

heparin-binding epidermal growth f. ABBR: HB-EGF. A cytokine, classed as a monokine, that is involved in immune and inflammatory responses. It is produced by macrophages and stimulates production of smooth muscle cells and fibroblasts.

hepatocyte growth f. ABBR: HGF. A cytokine, classed as a monokine, that is involved in immune and inflammatory responses. It is formed from platelets, fibroblasts, macrophages, endothelial cells, and smooth muscle cells. It stimulates growth of hepatocytes and increases migration and motility of various epithelial and endothelial cells.

intrinsic f. A glycoprotein secreted by the parietal cells of the gastric mucosa. It is necessary for the absorption of ingested vitamin B_{12}. The absence of this factor leads to vitamin B_{12} deficiency and pernicious anemia.

lethal f. A gene or an abnormality in genetic composition that causes death of a zygote or of an individual before the reproductive age.

leukocyte inhibitory f. Leukocyte migration inhibition f.

leukocyte migration inhibition f. ABBR: LMIF. A lymphokine that inhibits movement of neutrophils.

lymphocyte mitogenic f. ABBR: LMF. A lymphokine that stimulates production of lymphocytes and other lymphokines.

magnification f. ABBR: MF. Image size divided by object size; a quantitative expression of the degree of enlargement of an image. In radiography, it is the ratio of the source-to-image-receptor distance to the source-to-object distance.

maturation-promoting f. ABBR: MPF. A complex cellular protein that stimulates cell division in eukaryotic cells. Part of MPF is the protein cyclin, which accumulates during interphase and triggers mitosis or meiosis.

milk f. A substance present in certain strains of mammary cancer-prone mice that is transferred to offspring through milk from the mammary glands. It can induce the development of mammary cancer in suckling mice exposed to the factor.

M-phase promoting f. Maturation-promoting f.

neutrophil chemotactic f. A lymphokine that attracts neutrophils, but not other white blood cells, and causes proteolytic damage in sepsis and trauma.

platelet-activating f. A phospholipid mediator of chemical response to injury. It is an important mediator of bronchoconstriction.

quality f. ABBR: QF. In radiology, a scale used to account for the biological effects of different radiations. Factors include beta, electron, and gamma x-radiation (Q = 1), thermal neutrons (Q = 5), and alpha neutrons and protons (Q = 20).

Rh f. An antigen present on the surface of erythrocytes. SEE: *Rh blood group*.

transforming growth f. ABBR: TGF. Polypeptide growth factor that competitively binds to epidermal growth factor (EGF) receptors. This molecule can promote growth of fibroblasts in cell cultures, thus "transforming" normal cells into those with the abnormal properties of malignant cells. SEE: *cytokine*.

vascular endothelial growth f. ABBR: VEGF. A growth factor produced by endothelial cells that promotes angiogenesis and increases microvascular permeability.

facultative (făk′ŭl-tā″tĭv) [L. *facultas,* capability] **1.** Having the ability to do something that is not compulsory. **2.** In biology and particularly bacteriology, having the ability to live under certain conditions. Thus a microorganism may be facultative with respect to oxygen and be able to live with or without oxygen.

faculty 1. A normal mental attribute or sense; ability to function. 2. Persons employed as teachers at a college or university.

FAD *flavin adenine dinucleotide.*

Faget's sign [Jean C. Faget, Fr. physician, 1818–1884] A pulse slower than would be expected with the elevated temperature present. It may be seen in some viral infections.

Fahrenheit scale (făr'ĕn-hīt") [Daniel Gabriel Fahrenheit, Ger.-Dutch physicist, 1686–1736] A temperature scale with the freezing point of water at 32° and the boiling point at 212°, indicated by F. SEE: table; *Celsius scale; Kelvin scale; thermometer*.

fail safe Problem-free or infallible, said of a device, system, or program manufactured or conceived not to malfunction.

failure (fāl'yĕr) Inability to function, esp. loss of what was once present, as in failing eyesight or hearing.

fulminant hepatic f. Sudden onset of jaundice, coagulopathy, and encephalopathy due to massive liver injury.

heart f. SEE: *heart failure*.

kidney f. Renal f.

liver f. The inability of the liver to function because of a disease process within the liver or because of demands beyond its capability. SEE: *fulminant hepatic f.*

metabolic f. Rapid failure of physical and mental functions ending in death.

multisystem organ f. SEE: *multiple systems organ failure*.

renal f. Inability of the kidneys to function adequately. It may be partial, temporary, chronic, acute, or complete. SYN: *kidney f.* SEE: *end-stage renal disease* .

respiratory f. SEE: *respiratory failure, acute; respiratory failure, chronic.*

adult f. to thrive A progressive functional deterioration of a physical and cognitive nature; the individual's ability to live with multisystem diseases, cope with ensuing problems, and manage his/her care are remarkably diminished. SEE: *Nursing Diagnoses Appendix.*

f. to thrive ABBR: FTT. A condition in which infants and children not only fail to gain weight but also may lose it, or in which elderly persons lose the physiological or psychosocial reserves needed to care for themselves. The causes include almost any chronic and debilitating condition. SEE: *Nursing Diagnoses Appendix.*

faint [O.Fr. *faindre*, to feign] 1. To feel weak as though about to lose consciousness. 2. Weak. 3. Loss of consciousness resulting from vasovagal or vasodepressor mechanisms.

SYMPTOMS: Before the onset, the patient may be pale, weak, and dizzy, with cold perspiration and an uncomfortable abdominal sensation. The patient may fall to the ground. The pulse is usually weak and rapid and is often irregular.

FIRST AID: The individual must be placed in a horizontal position, preferably with the head low to facilitate blood flow to the brain. At the same time, it is essential to ensure that the airway is clear and that clothing is loose, esp. if a tight collar was being worn. It is important to ascertain that respiratory and cardiac functions are within normal limits. Fainting usually is of short duration and is counteracted by the supine posi-

Fahrenheit and Celsius Scales*

F	C	F	C	F	C
500°	260°	203°	95°	98°	36.67°
401	205	194	90	97	36.11
392	200	176	80	96	35.56
383	195	167	75	95	35
374	190	140	60	86	30
356	180	122	50	77	25
347	175	113	45	68	20
338	170	110	43.33	50	10
329	165	109	42.78	41	5
320	160	108	42.22	32	0
311	155	107	41.67	23	−5
302	150	106	41.11	14	−10
284	140	105	40.56	5	−15
275	135	104	40.00	−4	−20
266	130	103	39.44	−13	−25
248	120	102	38.89	−22	−30
239	115	101	38.33	−40	−40
230	110	100	37.78	−76	−60
212	100	99	37.22		

* To convert a Fahrenheit temperature to degrees Celsius, subtract 32 and multiply by 5/9.
To convert a Celsius temperature to degrees Fahrenheit, multiply by 9/5 and add 32.

tion. Nevertheless, the cause of the faint must be established before the episode is dismissed as being of no consequence. If recovery from fainting is not prompt, the patient should be moved to a hospital.

faintness **1.** A sensation of impending loss of consciousness. SYN: *presyncope*. **2.** A sensation of weakness due to lack of food.

faith healing Recovery from illness attributed to the agency of a divine being or power.

falcate (făl′kāt) [L. *falx,* sickle] Sickle-shaped.

falces (făl′sēz) [L.] Plural of falx.

falcial (făl′shăl) Pert. to a falx.

falciform (făl′sĭ-form) [L. *falx,* sickle, + *forma,* form] Sickle-shaped.

falciform ligament The triangular ligament attached to the sides of the sacrum and coccyx by its base.

falciform ligament of the liver A wide, sickle-shaped reflection of the peritoneum that serves as a principal attachment of the liver to the diaphragm and separates the right and left lobes of the liver. Its broad attachment extends from the posterior superior portion of the liver to the anterior convex portion connected to the internal surface of the right rectus abdominis muscle. SYN: *falx ligamentosa*.

falcular **1.** Sickle-shaped. **2.** Pert. to the falx cerebelli.

fall **1.** To drop accidentally to the floor or ground. **2.** An accidental drop, usually caused by slipping or losing one's balance. In the elderly, injuries sustained during falls are a leading cause of death. Approximately 30% of people 65 years of age or older fall each year. It is important for health care providers to search for the cause or causes of the fall. The single biggest predictor of a fall is a history of falls. Other risk factors include reduced visual acuity and hearing, vestibular dysfunction, peripheral neuropathy, musculoskeletal disorders including physical weakness, postural hypotension, and use of medicines such as antidepressants, sedatives, or vasodilators. Other specific risk factors include daily use of four or more prescription drugs, inability to transfer from bed or chair to bathtub or toilet, and being female. By careful clinical investigation, the cause of falls sometimes can be determined and appropriate steps taken to prevent them.

Hazards in the home that increase the chances of falling are scatter rugs that are not secure or slip resistant, out-of-the-way light switches, cluttered access to paths through a room or entrance, poorly lighted steps and stairways, lack of handrails on the entire length of a stairway, and tubs and showers that are not fitted with sturdy grab bars and have slippery floors.

fallectomy (făl-ĕk′tō-mē) The surgical removal of part of a fallopian tube.

falling drop **1.** In physical diagnosis, a metallic tinkle heard over the normal stomach and bowel when they are inflated. **2.** A metallic tinkle heard over large cavities containing fluid and air, as in hydropneumothorax.

fallophobia A colloquial term for the fear of falling and of what it may mean for one's future health and prospects for independent living.

fallopian canal (fă-lō′pē-ăn) [Gabriele Fallopio, It. anatomist, 1523–1562] A canal in the petrous portion of the temporal bone. The facial nerve passes through it.

fallopian ligament The round ligament of the uterus.

falloposcopy (fă-lōp′ŏ-skō-pē) Imaging the interior of the fallopian tube (the endosalpinx) with a flexible fiberoptic endoscope. The procedure is used in the diagnosis and treatment of tubal infertility.

Fallot, tetralogy of (făl-ō′) [Etienne L. A. Fallot, Fr. physician, 1850–1911] A congenital malformation of the heart and great vessels marked by a defect in the interventricular septum, pulmonary artery stenosis, dextroposition of the aorta, and right ventricular hypertrophy. The defect can be repaired surgically.

fallotomy (făl-ŏt′ō-mē) Surgical incision into the fallopian tube. SYN: *salpingotomy*.

fallout Settling of radioactive molecules from the atmosphere after their release into the air following an explosion or radiation accident.

false imprisonment An intentional tort; unlawful intentional confinement of another within fixed boundaries so that the confined person is conscious of the confinement or harmed by it.

false-negative (făwls′nĕg′ă-tĭv) A test result that falsely indicates that a condition is not present when in fact it is. SEE: *Bayes' theorem; false-positive*.

false-positive (făwls′pŏs′ĭ-tĭv) A test or procedure result that falsely indicates that a condition is present when in fact it is not. SEE: *Bayes' theorem; false-negative*.

falsification (făwl″sĭ-fĭ-kā′shŭn) The act of writing or stating what is not true.

retrospective f. Deliberate or unconscious alteration of memory for past events or situations, a mental mechanism for ego preservation.

falx [L.] Any sickle-shaped structure.

f. cerebelli A fold of the dura mater that forms a vertical partition between the hemispheres of the cerebellum.

f. cerebri A fold of the dura mater that lies in the longitudinal fissure and separates the two cerebral hemispheres.

f. inguinalis The conjoined, or conjoint, tendon that forms the origin of the transversus abdominis and internal oblique muscles.

f. ligamentosa Falciform ligament of the liver.

famciclovir (făm-sī′klō-vēr) An antiviral drug used to treat herpes simplex and herpes zoster. Trade name is Famvir.

fames (fā′mēz) [L.] Hunger.

familial [L. *familia,* family] Pert. to or common to the same family (e.g., a disease occurring more frequently in a family than would be expected by chance).

familial Mediterranean fever An inherited autosomal recessive disorder seen most commonly in Middle Eastern ethnic groups. It has also appeared in family clusters in persons of Irish or Italian descent. The attacks, which almost always include fever, first appear between the ages of 5 and 15. The syndrome includes some of the following: abdominal pain resembling peritonitis, chest pain of pleural or pericardial origin, erysipelas-like redness near the ankle, and joint involvement. Duration and frequency of attacks are unpredictable. Some of the patients develop amyloidosis. Otherwise, the prognosis is favorable although there is no specific therapy. SYN: *periodic fever.*

familial periodic paralysis A rare familial disease marked by attacks of flaccid paralysis, often at awakening. This condition is usually associated with hypokalemia, but is sometimes present when the blood potassium level is normal or elevated. In affected individuals the condition may be precipitated by administration of glucose in patients with hypokalemia, and by administation of potassium chloride in those with hyperkalemia.

TREATMENT: Acetazolamide is used to prevent either hypokalemia or hyperkalemia. Oral potassium chloride is given in attacks accompanied by hypokalemia.

family **1.** A group of individuals who have descended from a common ancestor. **2.** In biological classification, the division between an order and a genus. **3.** A group of people living in a household who share common attachments, such as mutual caring, emotional bonds, regular interactions, and common goals, which include the health of the individuals in the family.

blended f. A common contemporary family group including children from previous and current relationships.

extended f. The basic or nuclear family plus close relatives.

single-parent f. A family in which only one of the parents is living with the child or children.

family care leave Permission to be absent from work to care for a family member who is pregnant, ill, disabled, or incapacitated.

family coping, ineffective: compromised A state in which a usually supportive primary person (family member or close friend [significant other]) provides insufficient, ineffective, or compromised support, comfort, assistance, or encouragement that may be needed by the patient to manage or master adaptive tasks related to the patient's health challenge. SEE: *Nursing Diagnoses Appendix.*

family coping, ineffective: disabling A state in which the behavior of a significant person (family member or other primary person) disables his or her own capacities and the patient's capacities to effectively address tasks essential to either person's adaptation to the health challenge. SEE: *Nursing Diagnoses Appendix.*

family coping, potential for growth A state in which the family member has effectively managed adaptive tasks involved with the patient's health challenge and is exhibiting desire and readiness for enhanced health and growth in regard to self and in relation to the patient. SEE: *Nursing Diagnoses Appendix.*

family planning The spacing of conception of children according to the wishes of the parents rather than to chance. It is accomplished by practicing some form of birth control.

symptothermal f.p. A fertility awareness method by which a woman plots her daily basal body temperature, cervical mucus characteristics, and common subjective complaints associated with ovulation (e.g., mittelschmerz) on a graph to identify the days of the menstrual cycle during which there is the highest potential for conception. The validity of this method is controversial.

family practice Comprehensive medical care with particular emphasis on the family unit, in which the physician's continuing responsibility for health care is not limited by the patient's age or sex or by a particular organ system or disease entity.

Family practice is the specialty that builds on a core of knowledge derived from other disciplines, drawing most heavily on Internal Medicine, Pediatrics, Obstetrics and Gynecology, Surgery, and Psychiatry, and establishes a cohesive unit, combining the behavioral sciences with the traditional biological and clinical sciences. The core of knowledge encompassed by the discipline of family practice prepares the family physician for a unique role in patient management, problem solving, counseling, and as a personal physician who coordinates total health care delivery. (Definition supplied by The American Academy of Family Physicians.)

family process, altered: alcoholism The state in which the psychosocial, spiritual, and physiological functions of the family unit are chronically disorganized, leading to conflict, denial of problems, resistance to change, ineffective problem solving, and a series of self-perpetuating crises. SEE: *Nursing Diagnoses Appendix.*

family processes, altered A change in family relationships and/or functioning. SEE: *Nursing Diagnoses Appendix.*

family therapy Treatment of the members of a family together, rather than an individual "patient"; the family unit is viewed as a social system important to all of its members.

famine Pronounced scarcity of food, causing hunger and starvation. The worst famine of the 20th century occurred in China between 1959 and 1961 when between 15 million and 30 million people died. In the 1990s, Angola, Ethiopia, Liberia, Mozambique, Somalia, and Sudan reported famines. Armed conflicts have been the major cause.

famotidine (fă-mō′tĭ-dēn) An H_2 receptor antagonist antihistamine used to treat gastric and duodenal ulcers, gastritis, duodenitis, esophagitis, and gastroesophageal reflux.

Fanconi's syndrome [Guido Fanconi, Swiss pediatrician, 1892–1979] **1.** Congenital hypoplastic anemia. **2.** One of several diseases marked by aminoaciduria associated with failure of the proximal renal tubules. Polyuria, osteomalacia, and growth failure are common findings.

fang [AS., to plunder] **1.** A sharp-pointed tooth. **2.** The root of a tooth.

fango (făn′gō) [Italian, mud] Mud obtained from thermal springs in Battaglia, Italy, used to treat rheumatism and gout.

Fannia (făn′ē-ă) A genus of small houseflies.

fantast (făn′tăst) [Gr. *phantasia,* imagination] A daydreamer.

fantasy (făn′tă-sē) [Gr. *phantasia,* imagination] An imaginary (mental) image; a daydream.

FAOTA *Fellow of the American Occupational Therapy Association.*

FAPTA *Fellow of the American Physical Therapy Association.*

farad (făr′ăd) [Michael Faraday, Brit. physicist, 1791–1867] A unit of electrical capacity. The capacity of a condenser that, charged with 1 coulomb, gives a difference of potential of 1 V. This unit is so large that 1 millionth of it has been adopted as a practical unit called a microfarad.

faraday (făr′ă-dā) The amount of electric charge associated with 1 g equivalent of an electrochemical reaction. It is equal to approx. 96,000 coulombs. SEE: *coulomb; farad.*

faradic Pert. to induced electricity.

faradism Therapeutic use of an interrupted current to stimulate muscles and nerves. Such a current is derived from the secondary, or induction, coil.

faradization **1.** The treatment of nerves or muscles with faradic current. **2.** The condition of nerves or muscles so treated.

faradotherapy Treatment of disease by faradic current.

farcy (făr′sē) [L. *farcire,* to stuff] A chronic form of glanders.

button f. Farcy marked by dermal tubercular nodules.

farina (fă-rē′nă) [L.] Finely ground meal commonly made from wheat or other grain, used as cereal and flour.

farinaceous (făr″ĭ-nā′shŭs) **1.** Starchy. **2.** Pert. to flour.

farmer's lung A form of hypersensitivity alveolitis caused by exposure to moldy hay that has fermented. *Actinomyces micropolyspora faeni* and *Thermoactinomyces vulgaris* are the causative microorganisms. SEE: *alveolitis; bagassosis; hypersensitivity.*

farpoint The greatest distance at which objects can be seen distinctly with the eyes in complete relaxation.

Farre's tubercles (fărz) [John R. Farre, Brit. physician, 1775–1862] Carcinomatous masses on the surface of the liver.

farsightedness An error of refraction in which, with accommodation completely relaxed, parallel rays come to a focus behind the retina. Affected individuals can see distant objects clearly, but cannot see near objects in proper focus. SYN: *hyperopia.* **farsighted,** *adj.*

fascia (făsh′ē-ă) *pl.* **fasciae** [L., a band] A fibrous membrane covering, supporting, and separating muscles (deep fascia); the subcutaneous tissue that connects the skin to the muscles (superficial fascia). **fascial,** *adj.*

Abernethy's f. SEE: *Abernathy's fascia.*

anal f. A fascia of connective tissue covering the levator ani muscle from the perineal aspect.

aponeurotic f. A thick fascia that provides attachment for a muscle.

Buck's f. The fascial covering of the penis, derived from Colles' fascia.

Cloquet's f. The femoral fascia.

Colles' f. The inner layer of the perineal fascia.

cremasteric f. The fascia covering the cremaster muscle of the spermatic cord.

cribriform f. The fascia of the thigh covering the saphenous opening.

crural f. The deep fascia of the leg.

deep f. Fascia that covers an individual muscle.

deep cervical f. The fascia of the neck covering the muscles, vessels, and nerves.

dentate f. The gray matter in the cerebral dentate convolution of the brain. SYN: *gyrus, dentate*.

endothoracic f. The fascia that separates the pleura of the lung from the inside of the thoracic cavity and the diaphragm. SYN: *extrapleural f.*

extrapleural f. Endothoracic f.

intercolumnar f. The fascia derived from the external abdominal ring sheathing the spermatic cord and testis.

f. lata femoris The wide fascia encasing the hips and the thigh muscles.

lumbodorsal f. Thoracolumbar f.

pectineal f. The pubic section of the fascia lata.

pelvic f. The fascia within the pelvic cavity. It is extremely important in maintaining normal strength in the pelvic floor. SEE: *diaphragm, pelvic*.

perineal f. Three layers of tissue between the muscles of the perineum.

pharyngobasilar f. The fascia lying between the mucosal and muscular layers of the pharyngeal wall. SYN: *pharyngeal aponeurosis*.

plantar f. The fascia investing the muscles of the sole of the foot. SYN: *plantar aponeurosis*.

Scarpa's f. The deep layer of the superficial fascia of the abdomen.

superficial f. The areolar connective tissue and adipose tissue below the dermis of the skin. SYN: *subcutaneous tissue*.

superficial cervical f. The fascia of the neck just inside the skin.

thoracolumbar f. The fascia and aponeuroses of the latissimus dorsi, serratus posterior inferior, internal oblique, and transverse abdominis muscles, which provide support and stability for the lumbar spine in postural and lifting activities. The fascia attaches medially to the spinous processes of the vertebral column and inferiorly to the iliac crest and sacrum. SYN: *lumbodorsal f.*

thyrolaryngeal f. The fascia covering the thyroid gland.

f. transversalis The fascia located between the perineum and the transversalis muscle. It lines the abdominal cavity.

fascial reflex Muscular contraction resulting from percussing facial fascia.

fasciaplasty (făsh′ē-ă-plăs″tē) [″ + Gr. *plassein*, to form] Plastic surgery of a fascia.

fascicle (făs′ĭ-kl) [L. *fasciculus*, little bundle] A fasciculus.

fascicular (fă-sĭk′ū-lăr) **1.** Arranged like a bundle of rods. **2.** Pert. to a fasciculus.

fasciculation (fă-sĭk″ū-lā′shŭn) **1.** Formation of fascicles. **2.** Involuntary contraction or twitching of muscle fibers, visible under the skin. **3.** Spontaneous contractions of muscle fibers that do not cause movement at a joint.

fasciculus (fă-sĭk′ū-lŭs) *pl.* **fasciculi** A small bundle, esp. of nerve or muscle fibers; more specifically, a division of a funiculus of the spinal cord comprising fibers of one or more tracts. Sometimes the term is used as a synonym for *tract*. SYN: *fasciola*.

f. cuneatus A triangular bundle of nerve fibers lying in the dorsal funiculus of the spinal cord. Its fibers enter the cord through the dorsal roots of spinal nerves and terminate in the medulla. SYN: *Burdach's tract; column of Burdach; root zone*.

dorsolateral f. SEE: *tract, dorsolateral*.

dorsal longitudinal f. A bundle of association fibers connecting the frontal lobe with the occipital and temporal lobes of the brain.

fundamental f. The portion of the anterior column of the spinal cord continuing into the medulla oblongata.

f. gracilis A bundle of nerve fibers, lying in the dorsal funiculus of the spinal cord medial to the fasciculus cuneatus, that conducts sensory impulses from the periphery to the medulla. SYN: *column of Goll; Goll's tract*.

inferior longitudinal f. A bundle of association fibers connecting the occipital and temporal lobes of the brain.

medial longitudinal f. A nerve fiber bundle running from the spinal cord to the upper portion of the midbrain.

posterior longitudinal f. A nerve fiber bundle running between the corpora quadrigemina and the nuclei of the fourth and sixth spinal nerves.

unciform f. Fibers within the sylvian fissure connecting the frontal and temporosphenoid lobes of the brain. SYN: *uncinate fasciculus*.

fasciectomy (făsh″ē-ĕk′tō-mē) [L. *fascia*, band, + Gr. *ektome*, excision] Excision of strips of fascia.

fasciitis (făs″ē-ī′tĭs) Inflammation of any fascia. SYN: *fascitis*.

eosinophilic f. Inflammation of muscle fascia, associated with eosinophilia, pain, and swelling.

necrotizing f. A rapidly spreading bacterial infection that dissects through the body along superficial or deep fascial planes.

SYMPTOMS: The onset of illness is usually acute and progression is rapid. Initially there is severe pain, fever, chills, and malaise. These symptoms worsen as the infection spreads. If extensive surgical débridement, drainage, and antibiotics are not instituted early, the patient may die.

ETIOLOGY: Bacterial penetration of the skin and subcutaneous tissues (e.g., at a wound or ulcer) may cause necrotizing infection. The germs most commonly responsible are invasive streptococci, *Clostridium perfringens,* oral flora (e.g., after a bite), enteric flora (esp. in the groin or perineum), and *Vibrio vulnificus* (esp. in alcoholics or fishermen).

TREATMENT: Surgical débridement is required.

fasciodesis (făsh″ē-ŏd′ĕ-sĭs) [″ + Gr. *desis,* binding] Surgical attachment of a fascia to a tendon or another fascia.

Fasciola (fă-sī′ō-lă) [L. *fasciola,* a band] A genus of flukes belonging to the class Trematoda.

F. hepatica A species of flukes infesting the liver and bile ducts of cattle, sheep, and other herbivores; the common liver fluke. Infestation of watercress is a rare source of infection in humans. Intermediate hosts are snails belonging to the genus *Lymnaea.* SEE: illus.

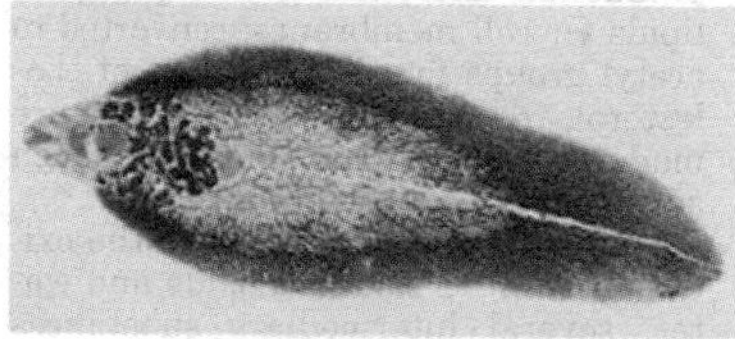

FASCIOLA HEPATICA
(Orig. mag. ×2)

fasciola (fă-sī′ō-lă, fă-sē′ō-lă) *pl.* **fasciolae** [L., a band] A bundle of nerve or muscle fibers.

f. cinerea The upper portion of the dentate gyrus.

fasciolar (fă-sē′ō-lăr) Pert. to the fasciola cinerea.

fasciolopsiasis (făs″ē-ō-lŏp-sī′ă-sĭs) Infection with a genus of trematode worms, *Fasciolopsis buski.* It is contracted by ingestion of plants grown in water infested by the intermediate host, snails.

SYMPTOMS: The symptoms are diarrhea, abdominal pain, anasarca, and eosinophilia.

TREATMENT: Treatment is with praziquantel.

Fasciolopsis buski (făs″ē-ō-lŏp′sĭs) A trematode (fluke) that infests the intestinal tract of certain mammals including humans. Symptoms include vomiting, anorexia, and diarrhea alternating with constipation. The number of flukes present may be sufficient to cause intestinal obstruction. The disease occurs in Asia, including central and southern China. SEE: illus.; *fasciolopsiasis.*

fascioplasty (făsh′ē-ō-plăs″tē) [L. *fasciola,* a band, + Gr. *plassein,* to form] Plastic operation on a fascia.

fasciorrhaphy (făsh-ē-or′ă-fē) [″ + Gr. *rhaphe,* seam, ridge] Suturing of a fascia.

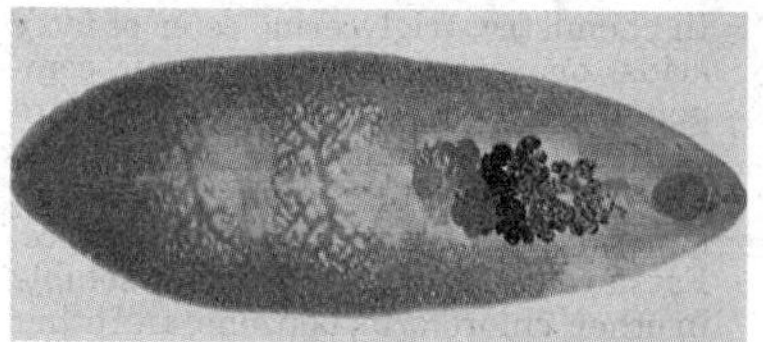

FASCIOLOPSIS BUSKI
(Orig. mag. ×2)

fasciotomy (făsh-ē-ŏt′ō-mē) [″ + Gr. *tome,* incision] Surgical incision and division of a fascia.

fascitis (fă-sī′tĭs) [″ + Gr. *itis,* inflammation] Fasciitis.

FASRT *Fellow of the American Society of Radiologic Technologists.*

fast [AS. *faest,* fixed] Resistant to the effects or action of a chemical substance.

fast [AS. *faestan,* to hold fast] Abstention from food, usually voluntary.

fastidious In microbiology, concerning an organism that has precise nutritional and environmental requirements for growth and survival.

fastidium (făs-tĭd′ē-ŭm) [L., aversion] Aversion to food or eating. SEE: *anorexia nervosa.*

fastigium (făs-tĭj′ē-ŭm) [L., ridge] **1.** The highest point. **2.** The fullest point of development of acute, infectious diseases when the temperature reaches the maximum. **3.** The most posterior portion of the fourth ventricle, formed by the junction of the anterior and posterior medullary vela projecting into the medullary substance of the cerebellum of the brain.

fasting [AS. *faestan,* to hold fast] Going without food or other nutritional support. This forces the body to catabolize its own glycogen, fat and protein reserves in order to produce glucose. Since glycogen reserves are depleted quickly in children, fasting can be esp. hazardous to their health. The products of incomplete fat metabolism (fatty acids, diacetic acid and acetic acid) produce ketosis and mild acidosis. This occurs after utilization of the body's glycogen and as children have little glycogen reserve, it occurs quickly in children.

CAUTION: Unsupervised fasting to lose weight can cause severe health hazards, including cholecystitis, electrolyte disturbances, cardiac dysrhythmias, and occasionally death.

---

fastness [AS. *faest,* fixed] The ability of cells to resist stains or destructive agents.

fat [AS. *faett*] **1.** Adipose tissue of the body, which serves as an energy reserve. SEE: ***heart; obesity.*** **fatty (făt′ē),** ***adj.*** **2.** -

In chemistry, triglyceride ester of fatty acids; one of a group of organic compounds closely associated in nature with the phosphatides, cerebrosides, and sterols. The term *lipid* is applied in general to a fat or fatlike substance. Fats are insoluble in water but soluble in ether, chloroform, benzene, and other fat solvents. During hydrolysis, fats break down into fatty acids and glycerol (an alcohol). Fats are hydrolyzed by the action of acids, alkalies, lipases (fat-splitting enzymes), and superheated steam.

CHEMICAL STRUCTURE: In the fat molecule, one molecule of glycerol is combined with three of fatty acids. Three fatty acids, oleic acid ($C_{18}H_{34}O_2$), stearic acid ($C_{18}H_{36}O_2$), and palmitic acid ($C_{16}H_{32}O_2$), constitute the bulk of fatty acids in neutral fats found in body tissues. According to the fatty acid with which the glycerol is combined, corresponding fats are triolein, tristearin, and tripalmitin. These three fats are the principal fats present in foods.

PHYSIOLOGY: The most important function of fats is as a form of stored or potential energy. In conjunction with carbohydrates, fats are protein sparers—dietary or body protein need not be used for energy production. Glycogen storage is sufficient to supply energy needs for about 12 hr, but in a 70-kg man of average build, 12 kg of stored fat (in the form of triglycerides) can supply energy needs for as long as 8 weeks. Subcutaneous fat provides a small amount of insulation against heat loss, and some organs such as the eyes and kidneys are cushioned by fat. The diglyceride phospholipids are part of all cell membranes. Dietary fat provides the essential fatty acids needed for normal growth.

Because certain fatty acids (linoleic, D-linolenic, and arachidonic) are necessary for formation of other products in the body and because the body does not synthesize them, they are classed as *essential fatty acids.* Linolenic acid can, however, be converted into other fatty acids including arachidonic acid. Arachidonic acid is of particular importance because it is essential to the formation of prostaglandins, thromboxanes, prostacyclins, and leukotrienes. These three essential fatty acids are obtainable in the diet from plant sources.

Animals fed a fat-free diet develop dermatitis and fail to grow; the liver becomes fatty, and there are neurological disturbances. These changes can be prevented or reversed by the addition of linoleic and linolenic acids to the diet. The human diet should consist of about 4% of the calories from linoleic and 1% from linolenic acids.

DIGESTION AND ABSORPTION: In the stomach, emulsified fats such as cream or egg yolk are acted on by gastric lipase; however, most fats undergo digestion in the intestine, where a pancreatic lipase hydrolyzes them to fatty acids and glycerol. The bile salts in bile are not enzymes; they emulsify fats and permit pancreatic lipase to digest them. Bile salts then make fatty acids soluble in water so that they may be readily absorbed. In the intestinal mucosa, fatty acids and glycerol combine to form neutral fats, then join to proteins to form chylomicrons, which enter the lacteals. In this form, they are carried in the lymph through the lymph vessels to the thoracic duct, which empties lymph into the blood.

METABOLISM: Absorbed fats are used in the following ways: oxidized to carbon dioxide and water to produce energy; stored in adipose tissue for energy production later; changed to phospholipids for cell membranes; converted to acetyl groups for the synthesis of cholesterol, from which other steroids are made; and used to make secretions such as sebum.

Intermediary metabolism: In the oxidation of fat to carbon dioxide and water, several intermediary substances (ketones) are formed. The principal ones are acetoacetic acid, betahydroxybutyric acid, and acetone. Excessive production of ketone bodies, which occurs when fats are incompletely oxidized, is called ketosis. This occurs esp. when there is an interference in carbohydrate metabolism, as in diabetes. Ketosis also occurs in starvation, certain fevers, pregnancy toxemias, and hyperthyroidism. Ketosis results in acidosis.

SOURCES: In addition to fat being absorbed from the intestine, body fat may arise from the conversion of carbohydrates (glucose) or excess amino acids into fat. Fatty acids cannot be converted directly to glucose, but they are split into two-carbon acetyl groups that enter the Krebs cycle and thereby have the same energy-producing function as carbohydrates.

NUTRITION: Fats have a high caloric value, yielding about 9 kcal per gram as compared with about 4 kcal per gram for carbohydrates and proteins. The average diet of 3000 kcal may derive 40% of the caloric value from fats. Nutritionists and epidemiologists believe that decreasing dietary fat to 30% would decrease the risk of developing cancer, esp. of the colon, breast, and prostate.

In addition to their nutritive values, fats improve the taste and odor of foods, provide a feeling of satiety, and because of their high caloric content are of special importance in high-calorie diets. Fat-free fat substitutes that have been termed " designer fats" have been inves-

Food Sources of Saturated Fats

Meat products	Visible fat and marbling in beef, pork, and lamb, especially in prime-grade and ground meats, lard
Processed meats	Frankfurters, luncheon meats such as bologna, corned beef, liverwurst, pastrami, and salami
	Bacon, sausage, lard, suet, salt pork
Poultry and fowl	Chicken and turkey (mostly beneath the skin), cornish hens, duck, and goose
Whole milk and whole-milk products	Cheeses made with whole milk or cream, condensed milk, ice cream, whole-milk yogurt, all creams (sour, half-and-half, whipped)
Plant products	Coconut oil, palm-kernel oil, cocoa butter
Miscellaneous	Fully hydrogenated shortening and margarine, many cakes, pies, cookies, and mixes

SOURCE: Lutz, CA and Przytulski, KR: Nutrition and Diet Therapy. FA Davis, Philadelphia, 1994.

tigated for several decades. Whether they will play a major role in providing foods with fewer calories from fat has not been determined. SEE: table.

CONTRAINDICATIONS: Fat intake should be reduced in certain diseases such as hepatitis and in low-calorie diets.

body f. The portion of the human body that consists of fat. This is estimated in several ways: by determining body density by underwater weighing (hydrodensitometry), by calculating the ratio of weight in kilograms to height in meters squared (Quatelet index), and more recently, by estimating bioelectrical impedance of the body. None of these methods provides a precise indicator of body composition; however, bioelectrical impedance is the simplest, least expensive, and most nearly accurate.

brown f. Adipose tissue occurring primarily in the full-term newborn. It is located near major vessels. The fat produces heat metabolically and is therefore an important factor in temperature regulation. As the infant matures, shivering is established as a means of controlling body temperature. The brown fat either involutes or becomes white fat. SEE: *tissue, brown adipose*.

neutral f. Compounds of the higher fatty acids (palmitic, stearic, and oleic) with glycerol. They are the common fats of animal and plant tissues.

fatal (fāt'l) [L. *fatalis*] **1.** Inevitable. **2.** Causing death.

fatality A death, esp. from an accident or a disaster.

father, biological The male who contributes the ovum-fertilizing sperm that subsequently becomes a fetus.

fatigability (făt"ĭ-gă-bĭl'ĭ-tē) The condition of becoming easily tired or exhausted.

fatigue (fă-tēg') [L. *fatigare,* to tire] **1.** An overwhelming sustained sense of exhaustion and decreased capacity for physical and mental work at the usual level. SEE: *Nursing Diagnoses Appendix.* **2.** The condition of an organ or tissue in which its response to stimulation is reduced or lost as a result of overactivity. **3.** To bring about fatigue. Fatigue may be the result of excessive activity, which causes the accumulation of metabolic waste products such as lactic acid; malnutrition (deficiency of carbohydrates, proteins, minerals, or vitamins); circulatory disturbances such as heart disease or anemia, which interfere with the supply of oxygen and energy materials to tissues; respiratory disturbances, which interfere with the supply of oxygen to tissues; infectious diseases, which produce toxic products or alter body metabolism; endocrine disturbances such as occur in diabetes, hyperinsulinism, and menopause; psychogenic factors such as emotional conflicts, frustration, anxiety, neurosis, and boredom; or physical factors such as disability. Environmental noise and vibration contribute to the development of fatigue. SEE: *chronic fatigue syndrome*.

acute f. Fatigue with sudden onset such as occurs following excessive exertion. It is relieved by rest.

chronic f. Long-continued fatigue not relieved by rest, indicative of disease such as tuberculosis, diabetes, or other conditions of altered body metabolism. SEE: *chronic fatigue syndrome*.

muscle f. The reduced capacity of a muscle to perform work as a result of repeated contractions and accumulation of lactic acid in anaerobic cell respiration. Fatigue may be partial or complete.

fat overload syndrome A rare complication of intravenous administration of fat emulsion. Findings include sudden elevation of the serum triglyceride level, fever, hepatosplenomegaly, coagulopathy, and dysfunction of other organs. Specific therapy is not available, but plasma exchange has been used experimentally.

fat replacement, fat substitute Any substance developed to provide the physical characteristics of fats with relatively few or no calories. Fat replacements may be carbohydrate polymers, protein or fat-based materials that are either not absorbed or not digested in human metabolism.

Simplesse is the trade name for a fat replacement made of milk and egg white and provides only 1 to 2 kcal/gram as opposed to the 9 kcal/gram supplied by fat. Olestra is a calorie-free fat replacement made from sucrose and vegetable oil and is suitable for cooking. Overconsumption of Olestra may result in fat-soluble vitamin deficiency.

fatty streak SEE: *atherosclerosis*.

fauces (fŏ′sēz) [L.] The constricted opening leading from the oral cavity to the oropharynx. It is bounded by the soft palate, the base of the tongue, and the palatine arches. The anterior pillars of the fauces are known as the glossopalatine arch, and the posterior pillars as the pharyngopalatine arch. SEE: *fossa*. **faucial** (-shăl), *adj.*

fault In legal medicine, failing to meet an obligation; a legal responsibility for a failed outcome.

fauna (faw′nă) [L. *Faunus*, mythical deity of herdsmen] **1.** Animal life as distinguished from plant life. **2.** All the animals, including microscopic forms, in a specified area. SEE: *flora*.

faveolate (fā-vē′ō-lāt) [L. *faveolus*, little honeycomb] Honeycombed. SYN: *alveolate*.

faveolus (fā-vē′ō-lŭs) [L., little honeycomb] A depression or small pit, esp. on the skin. SYN: *foveola*.

favism (fā′vĭzm) [It. *fava*, bean, + Gr. *-ismos*, condition] A hereditary condition common in Sicily and Sardinia resulting from sensitivity to a species of bean, *Vicia faba*. It is marked by fever, acute hemolytic anemia, vomiting, and diarrhea, and may lead to prostration and coma. It is caused by ingestion of the beans or inhalation of the pollen of the plant by persons who have an inherited deficiency of the enzyme glucose-6-phosphate dehydrogenase.

favus (fā′vŭs) [L., honeycomb] A skin disease caused by the fungus *Trichophyton schoenleinii*. It is marked by pinhead- to pea-sized, cup-shaped, yellowish crusts (scutulum) over the hair follicles of the scalp and is accompanied by musty odor and itching. It may spread all over the body. SEE: *scutulum*.

F.C.A.P. *Fellow of the College of American Pathologists.*

Fc fragment A small piece of an immunoglobulin (an antibody) used by macrophages in processing and presenting foreign antigens to T lymphocytes. SEE: *immune response; macrophage processing*.

Fc receptor A receptor on phagocytes (neutrophils, monocytes, and macrophages) that binds Fc fragments of immunoglobulins G and E. SEE: *immunoglobulin; macrophage processing; phagocytosis*.

F.D. *fatal dose; focal distance.*

F.D.A. *Food and Drug Administration.*

FDP *fibrin degradation products.*

Fe [L. *ferrum*] Symbol for the element iron.

fear [AS. *faer*] Anxiety caused by a perceived threat, real or imagined. Focussed apprehension and fright. SEE: *emotion; Nursing Diagnoses Appendix; Phobias Appendix.*

features Any part of the face.

febrifacient (fĕb-rĭ-fā′sē-ĕnt) [L. *febris*, fever, + *facere*, to make] Producing fever.

febrifuge (fĕb′rĭ-fūj) Something that reduces fever. SYN: *antipyretic*. **febrifugal,** *adj.*

febrile (fē′brĭl, fē′brīl, fĕb′rĭl) [L. *febris*, fever] Feverish; pert. to a fever. SEE: *fever*.

febrile state A term used to describe constitutional symptoms that accompany a rise in temperature. The pulse and respiration rate usually increase, with headache, pains, malaise, loss of appetite, concentrated and diminished urine, chills or sweating, restlessness, insomnia, and irritability.

febriphobia (fĕb″rĭ-fō′bē-ă) [″ + Gr. *phobos*, fear] Anxiety or fear induced by a rise in body temperature.

fecal impaction Constipation caused by a firm mass of feces in the distal colon or rectum. The size or firmness of the mass prevents its passage.

ETIOLOGY: Fecal impaction is relatively common in the elderly, esp. in immobilized residents of nursing homes, and in children with encopresis. It may also result from painful anal conditions that inhibit the patient's desire to defecate; drugs such as narcotics, calcium-channel blockers, retained barium, or anticholinergics that retard bowel movements; neurological diseases such as spinal cord injury; complications of intestinal or obstetrical surgery; dehydration; rectoceles, colon cancers, or other pathological lesions; and functional (psychogenic) disorders.

SYMPTOMS: Abdominal colic and a sensation of fullness, anorexia, and rectal pain are common.

PREVENTION: Impaction of stool may be prevented by following a high-fiber, fluid-rich diet; getting regular exercise; limiting intake of constipating drugs; routinely using stool softeners or laxatives; and learning biofeedback and habit-training.

TREATMENT: A trial of laxatives or enemas may relieve the obstructing feces. If this is unsuccessful, manual extraction is indicated. This may require local anesthesia. The impaction is fragmented by using a scissoring action of the fingers. After the impaction is fragmented, use of mild laxatives, such as mineral oil instilled into the rectum, provides lubrication and assists in passage of the fragments. Surgery is rarely required.

fecalith (fē′kă-lĭth) [″ + Gr. *lithos,* stone] A fecal concretion. SYN: *coprolith.*

fecaloid (fē′kă-loyd) [″ + Gr. *eidos,* form, shape] Resembling feces.

fecaloma (fē″kăl-ō′mă) [″ + Gr. *oma,* tumor] A large mass of accumulated feces in the rectum resembling a tumor. SYN: *scatoma.*

fecaluria (fē″kăl-ū′rē-ă) [″ + Gr. *ouron,* urine] Fecal matter in the urine.

fecal vomit Feces in vomitus. This occurs in strangulated hernia or intestinal obstruction preventing normal bowel movements.

feces (fē′sēz) [L. *faeces*] Body waste such as food residue, bacteria, epithelium, and mucus, discharged from the bowels by way of the anus. Also called *dejecta; excrement; excreta; stool.* **fecal** (fē′kăl), *adj.*

COMPOSITION: The total weight of the feces in a healthy man on a normal diet is 100 to 200 g daily. Of this, 65% is water and the remainder dry matter. Excreted nitrogen is less than 1.7 g daily. The feces are composed of food residue including undigested cellulose; water; secretions from the intestinal glands, stomach, and liver; indole; skatole; cholesterol; mucus and epithelial cells; purine bases; pigment; microorganisms; inorganic salts; and sometimes foreign substances. The normal reaction is neutral or slightly alkaline. The feces of infants usually are acid.

PHYSICAL CHARACTERISTICS OF FECES: Inspection should include color, form, consistency, odor, and the presence of any observable foreign substances.

Color: Color may indicate various disorders. *Black* or *tarry* feces can indicate bleeding or hemorrhage into the gastrointestinal tract. *Tarry* describes feces containing digested blood or affected by drugs such as bismuth, iron, tannin, manganese, or charcoal. *Bloody:* Blood may indicate hemorrhoids, cancer of the rectum or colon, ulcers, fissures, abraded rectal membrane from dry feces, eroded rectal polypus, acute proctitis, foreign bodies, colitis, intussusception or strangulated hernia in children, typhoid fever, or phosphorus poisoning. *Clay-colored:* Clay color may denote impaired bile formation or obstruction, other causes of jaundice, or phosphorus poisoning. *Green:* In general, green feces in children and infants indicate that the bowel contents have passed quickly **through the intestinal tract.**

Form and consistency: Feces are normally soft and formed. They are hard, nodular, or scybalous in constipation and fluid or mushy in diarrhea. Consistently flattened or ribbonlike feces indicate rectal obstruction or spastic colitis.

Frothy, poorly formed stools: They may indicate a spastic colon, the presence of gas, or intestinal inflammation.

Lienteric stools: These contain much undigested food and are noted in inflammatory conditions of the stomach and upper bowel.

Membranous shreds: They may exist in cancer of the colon, dysentery, relapsing fever, acute proctitis, and in sloughing of intestinal mucosa.

Oily or greasy: This may be found in pancreatic insufficiency or intestinal malabsorption.

Mucus: Mucus is present in both abnormal and normal circumstances. It may occur as superficial gelatinous streaks or blobs; mixed with the feces and only apparent after a thin paste is made with water; or mixed with blood as in dysentery. Mucus may be the principal component.

Offensive odor: This occurs in jaundice, acute indigestion, enteritis, typhoid fever, and occasionally constipation. *Putrid odor:* This may be the result of syphilitic or carcinomatous ulceration of the rectum or gangrenous dysentery. *Sour odor:* The feces of infants normally smell sour.

Parasites: The presence of various intestinal parasites can be determined by examination of the feces. Gross examination may reveal nematodes (roundworms) or tapeworms; however, microscopic examination is necessary to determine the presence of protozoa, helminth ova, or larvae. Feces to be examined are collected in clean, dry containers. For microscopic examination, representative bits of feces or mucus are emulsified in saline solution on a clean slide, then spread evenly and covered with a coverglass. Diagnosis of pinworms is by examination of scrapings or contact slides from the anal and perianal regions.

Fechner's law (fĕk′nĕrz) [Gustav Theodor Fechner, Ger. psychologist, 1801–1887] A theory stating that the magnitudes of sensation produced by given stimuli form an arithmetical progression, the stimuli forming a geometrical progression.

$Fe(C_3H_5O_3)_2$ Ferrous lactate; lactate of iron.

$FeCl_2$ Ferrous chloride.

$FeCl_3$ Ferric chloride.

$FeCO_3$ Ferrous carbonate.

fecula (fĕk′ū-lă) [L. *faecula,* dregs] **1.** Sediment. **2.** Starch.

feculent (fĕk′ū-lĕnt) [L. *faeculentus*] **Having sediment.**

fecund Fertile.

fecundate (fē′kŭn-dāt) [L. *fecundare,* to bear fruit] To fertilize, impregnate, or render fertile.

fecundation (fē″kŭn-dā′shŭn) Impregnation; fertilization.

artificial f. Impregnation by mechanical injection of the seminal fluid into the uterus. SYN: *artificial insemination.*

fecundity (fē-kŭn′dĭ-tē) Ability to produce offspring; fertility.

Federal Emergency Management Agency ABBR: FEMA. The agency of the federal government that supervises civil defense, disaster planning, and emergency medical services in communities that have suffered floods, tornados, hurricanes, and other catastrophes.

Federal Register A publication that makes available to the public proposed and final government rules, legal notices, orders, and documents having general applicability and legal effect. It contains published material from all federal agencies.

feedback **1.** The influence of the output or result of a system on the input or stimulus. Feedback may be positive or negative. In positive feedback, the result of the process intensifies the stimulus (e.g., uterine contraction stimulates oxytocin secretion, which brings about increased contractions and increased oxytocin). In negative feedback, the result of the process reverses or shuts off the stimulus (e.g., a high blood glucose level stimulates insulin secretion, which lowers blood glucose, which in turn decreases insulin secretion). **2.** In psychiatry, the expressed verbal reaction or physical reaction (i.e., body language) of one person to another person's actions or behaviors.

feeder cerebral palsy feeder.

feeding [AS. *fedan,* to give food to] Taking or giving nourishment.

artificial f. **1.** Providing a liquid food preparation through a tube passed into the stomach, duodenum, jejunum, or rarely, the rectum or intravenously. This is also done through gastrostomy or duodenostomy. SEE: *hyperalimentation.* **2.** Feeding of an infant with food other than mother's milk.

enteral tube f. Feeding through a tube that extends through the mouth or more commonly, the nostril into the stomach or duodenum. It is indicated for patients who cannot swallow or chew food but who have functioning gastrointestinal tracts. The nasogastric tube is preferred to the orogastric tube, because a much smaller tube can be used, which is less likely to be resisted. A tube lubricated with glycerin is gently passed into the pharynx and avoiding the larynx is passed into the stomach. Entry into the larynx by mistake may compromise oxygenation. SEE: *enteral tube feeding.*

CAUTION: Before feedings it is important to ascertain that the tube is in the gastrointestinal tract and not in the bronchus. This can be determined by aspirating the tube and observing for gastric contents or by listening to the end of the tube. If air comes out of the tube with each expiration, the tube is not in the stomach. If the position of the tube is in doubt, a small amount of air should be injected into it while the stomach area is being auscultated. If the tube is in the stomach, a gurgling should be heard as the air is injected. Foods or nutritional substances are initially infused slowly to maximize their tolerability.

---

forced f. Tube feeding to an individual who does not want to eat or to be fed by this means.

intravenous f. The provision of total or partial nutritional requirements intravenously; essential in treating some diseases. It is accomplished by carefully controlling the composition of fluid given with respect to total calories derived from protein hydrolysates, dextrose, and fat emulsions, and the electrolytes, minerals, and vitamins. Patients unable to safely eat have been completely maintained for extended periods via intravenous nutritional support, usually through a major vein, such as the subclavian or the jugular. SEE: *total parenteral nutrition.*

nasal f. SEE: *enteral tube f.; nasogastric tube f.*

rectal f. The introduction of fluid nutrients into the colon through the rectum, a mode of feeding rarely used because little nourishment other than water is absorbed through the colon. SYN: *nutritive enema.*

fee-for-service Payment for specific health care services provided to a patient (as opposed to payments received for the number of patients seen, the number of hours worked, or the number of patients enrolled in a health care panel). The individual or an insurance carrier may make the payment.

feeling [AS. *felan,* to feel] **1.** The conscious experience of emotion. **2.** A sensory perception.

Feer's disease (fārz) [Emil Feer, Swiss pediatrician, 1864–1955] Acrodynia.

fee splitting The unethical practice of returning to the referring health care provider a portion of the fee received from a patient who is seen in consultation.

feet [AS. *fet*] The pedal extremities of the legs. SEE: *foot.*

Fehling's solution (fā′lĭngz) [Hermann von Fehling, Ger. chemist, 1812–1885] A solution formerly used to detect the presence of glucose in urine.

Feingold diet (fīn′gōld) [Benjamin Feingold, U.S. pediatrician, 1900–1982] A nutritional plan in which all foods containing artificial coloring, flavoring, and preserving materials are excluded. It had been used in treating hyperactive children.

Feiss' line A line that extends from the first metatarsophalangeal joint, over the navicular tubercle, to the apex of the medial malleolus. Changes in the angle formed by this line before and during weightbearing can be used to determine excessive pronation of the foot. If the angle formed by Feiss' line is in the range of 30 to 90 degrees while the foot is weight bearing, it may be considered hyperpronated.

fel (fĕl) [L.] The Latin term for bile.

Feldenkrais method [Dr. Moshe Feldenkrais, Ukrainian physicist, 1904–1984] A form of physiotherapy devoted to improving limitations of range of motion, improving poor posture, and relieving stress.

feline (fē′līn) [L. *feles,* cat] Concerning cats.

fellatio (fĕl-ā′shē-ō) [L. *fellare,* to suck] Oral stimulation of the penis. SEE: *cunnilingus*.

fellatrix, fellatrice A woman who performs fellatio.

felon (fĕl′ŏn) [ME. *feloun,* malignant] An infection or abscess of the soft tissue of the terminal joint of a finger. SYN: *whitlow*.

felony A more serious crime than a misdemeanor with punishment greater than that for misdemeanors; can be grounds for license denial, revocation, or suspension of a healthcare provider. It is punishable by imprisonment or death, depending on state law and the type of crime.

feltwork **1.** A fibrous network. **2.** A plexus of nerve fibrils.

Felty's syndrome (fĕl′tēz) [Augustus Roi Felty, U.S. physician, 1895–1963] Rheumatoid arthritis associated with splenomegaly and neutropenia.

FEMA *Federal Emergency Management Agency*.

female [L. *femella,* little woman] **1.** An individual of the sex that produces ova or bears young. **2.** Characteristic of this sex or gender. SEE: *genitalia, female*.

female genital mutilation A traditional practice in some African, Middle Eastern, and Southeast Asian cultures. The mutilation usually is performed between the ages of 1 week and 14 years. The procedure is performed by nonmedical personnel without benefit of anesthesia or sterile conditions. The most common procedures are removal of the clitoral prepuce, excision of the clitoris, removal of the labia minora and sometimes most of the labia majora; the two sides may be sutured together to occlude the vagina. Possible immediate complications include infection, tetanus, shock, hemorrhage, and death. The possible long-term physical and mental disabilities include chronic pelvic infection, keloids, vulvar abscesses, sterility, incontinence, depression, anxiety, sexual dysfunction, and obstetric complications. SEE: *circumcision, female*.

female sexual arousal disorder According to the DSM-IV, the essential feature of this condition is a persistent or recurrent inability to attain, or to maintain until completion of the sexual activity, an adequate vaginal lubrication-swelling response of sexual excitement. In order to establish this diagnosis, the disturbance must cause marked distress or interpersonal difficulty, and the difficulty cannot be attributed to a medical condition, substance abuse, or medications. SEE: *male erectile disorder*.

feminine (fĕm′ĭ-nĭn) Concerning or being of the female sex.

feminism [L. *femininus*] The development of female secondary sexual characteristics in a man. SEE: *gynecomastia*.

feminization The normal development of female secondary sexual characteristics, or the pathological development of these in a man.

testicular f. The phenotypic appearance of female sexual characteristics in a person who is genetically male (i.e., whose sex chromosomes are XY). This rare condition is caused by cell receptor defects that prevent testosterone and dihydrotestosterone from acting on somatic tissues. The external genitalia are rudimentary, and the testicles may be in the abdomen.

femoral (fĕm′or-ăl) [L. *femoralis*] Pert. to the femur.

femoral artery The artery that begins at the external iliac artery and terminates behind the knee as the popliteal artery on the inner side of the femur.

femoral reflex Extension of the knee and flexion of the foot resulting from irritation of the skin over the upper anterior third of the thigh.

femoral vein A continuation of the popliteal vein upward toward the external iliac vein.

femorotibial (fĕm″ō-rō-tĭb′ē-ăl) [″ + *tibia,* pipe] Pert. to the femur and tibia.

femto- [Danish *femten,* fifteen] In the metric system, a prefix indicating that the number following is to be multiplied by 10^{-15}. Thus a femtogram is 10^{-15} g.

femur (fē′mŭr) *pl.* **femora** [L.] The thigh bone. It extends from the hip to the knee and is the longest and strongest bone in the skeleton. SEE: illus.

fenestra (fĕ-nĕs′tră) *pl.* **fenestrae** [L., window] **1.** An aperture frequently closed by a membrane. **2.** An open area, as in the blade of a forceps. **fenestral** (-trăl), *adj.*

f. cochleae Round window.

f. rotunda Round window.

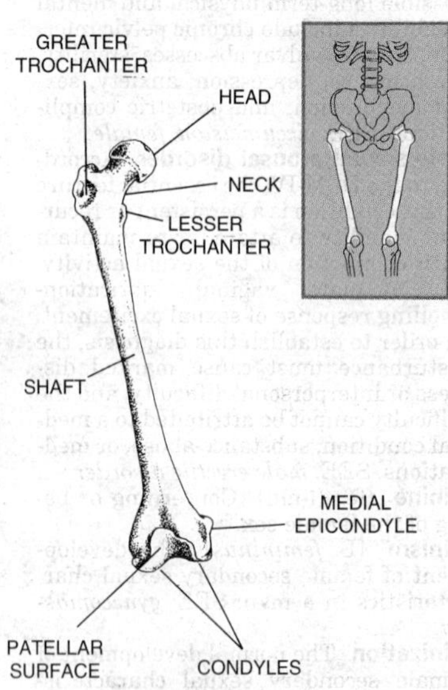

RIGHT FEMUR
Front view

f. vestibuli Oval window.

fenestrated (fĕn′ĕ-strāt-ĕd) Having openings.

fenestration (fĕn″ĕ-strā′shŭn) **1.** The condition of having a fenestra. **2.** An operation in which an artificial opening is made into the labyrinth of the ear. This procedure is performed to treat deafness associated with otosclerosis. **3.** An operation to open the mucoperiosteum and alveolar plate of bone over the root of an infected tooth to remove the inflammatory exudate and relieve pain.

fenfluramine hydrochloride (fĕn-floor′ă-mēn) An amphetamine-like substance that enhances weight loss. When used with phentermine, a similar drug, it has been implicated in the destruction of the pulmonary valve of a small percentage of patients.

feng shui (fŭng shwăy) An ancient Chinese art of interior and architectural design, the object of which is to create a soothing and healthful living environment.

fennel (fĕn′ĭl) A perennial herb (*Foeniculum vulgare*) grown for its foliage, seeds, and aniselike flavor and promoted by alternative and complementary medicine practitioners as a potential source of estrogen-like compounds. (It is said by some to improve sexual drive.) Known side effects of exposure to fennel in some agricultural workers include asthma, rhinitis, and conjunctivitis. Scientific evidence for its clinical effectiveness is sparse.

fentanyl citrate (fĕn′tă-nĭl) A synthetic opioid analgesic. It is used in anesthesia and to manage acute and chronic pain.

feral (fĕr′ŭl) [L. *fera,* wild animal] Existing in a wild, untamed, and undomesticated state.

ferment (fĕr-mĕnt′, fĕr′mĕnt) [L. *fermentum*] **1.** To decompose. **2.** A substance capable of inducing oxidative decomposition in other substances. **3.** An obsolete term for an enzyme.

fermentation The oxidative decomposition, under anaerobic conditions, of complex substances through the action of enzymes or ferments, produced by microorganisms. Bacteria, molds, and yeasts are the principal groups of organisms involved. Fermentations of economic importance are those involved in the production of alcohol, alcoholic beverages, lactic and butyric acids, and bread.

acetic f. Production of acetic acid by the bacterial oxidation of ethyl alcohol under aerobic conditions.

alcoholic f. Production of ethyl alcohol from carbohydrates, usually through the action of yeasts.

amylolytic f. Hydrolysis of starch with the formation of sugar mixtures.

autolytic f. Disintegration of tissues after death due to enzymes present in the tissues.

butyric f. Formation of butyric acid from bacterial action on carbohydrates under anaerobic conditions.

citric acid f. Formation of citric acid from the action of molds on carbohydrates.

invertin f. Conversion of cane sugar into glucose and fructose.

lactic f. Formation of lactic acid from carbohydrates by bacterial action. The genera *Streptococcus* and *Lactobacillus* are the forms usually involved. Bacterial action is responsible for the souring of milk.

oxalic acid f. Formation of oxalic acid from carbohydrates by the action of certain molds, esp. *Aspergillus.*

propionic acid f. Formation of propionic acid from carbohydrates by the action of certain bacteria.

viscous f. Production of gelatinous material by different forms of bacilli.

fermium (fĕr′mē-ŭm) [Enrico Fermi, It. U.S. physicist and Nobel Prize winner, 1901–1954] SYMB: Fm. A radioactive element with atomic number 100 and an atomic weight of 257.

ferning, fern pattern **1.** The palm leaf (arborization) pattern that mid-cycle cervical mucus assumes when it is placed in a thin layer on a glass slide and allowed to dry. The pattern, caused by crystallization of the mucus as it dries, depends on the concentration of electrolytes, esp. sodium chloride, which in turn depends on the amount of estrogen in the mucus. Smears of cervical mucus may be helpful in determining when a woman has ovulated. The mucus has a beaded pattern at other times in the menstrual cycle. SYN: *cervical mucus*. **2.** Arborization found on microscopic examination of a sample of dried vaginal fluid at term; it confirms the rupture of membranes.

-ferous [L. *ferre,* to bear] Suffix meaning *producing*.

ferri-, ferro- [L. *ferrum,* iron] Prefix meaning *iron*.

ferric **1.** Pert. to iron. SYN: *ferruginous*. **2.** Denoting a compound containing iron in its trivalent form.

f. chloride $FeCl_3$, used principally in tincture form as an astringent.

ferritin (fĕr′ĭ-tĭn) An iron-phosphorus-protein complex containing about 23% iron. It is formed in the intestinal mucosa by the union of ferric iron with a protein, apoferritin. Tissues store iron in this form, principally in the reticuloendothelial cells of the liver, spleen, and bone marrow.

ferrokinetics (fĕr″rō-kĭ-nĕt′ĭks) [″ + Gr. *kinesis,* movement] The study of the absorption, use, storage, and excretion of iron.

ferropexia (fĕr-ō-pĕks′ē-ă) Iron fixation.

ferroprotein (fĕr″ō-prō′tē-ĭn) A protein combined with an iron-containing radical. Ferroproteins are important oxygen-transferring enzymes (e.g., nicotinamide adenine dinucleotide dehydrogenase, cytochrome oxidase).

ferrotherapy (fĕr″ō-thĕr′ă-pē) [″ + Gr. *therapeia,* treatment] The use of iron in treating anemia.

ferrous (fĕr′ŭs) [L. *ferrum,* iron] **1.** Pert. to iron. SYN: *ferruginous*. **2.** Denoting a compound containing bivalent iron.

f. fumarate $C_4H_2FeO_4$, an iron preparation used to treat anemias.

f. gluconate $C_{12}H_{22}FeO_{14}$, an iron preparation occurring as a yellowish powder or granules. It is used to treat iron deficiency anemia.

ferruginous (fĕr-ū′jĭ-nŭs) [L. *ferrugo,* iron rust] **1.** Pert. to or containing iron. **2.** Having the color of iron rust.

ferrule (fĕr′ūl) [L. *viriola,* little bracelet] A band or ring of metal applied to the end of the root or crown of a tooth to strengthen it.

ferrum (fĕr′ŭm) [L., iron] Iron.

fertile (fĕr′tĭl) [L. *fertilis*] Capable of reproduction.

fertility (fĕr-tĭl′ĭ-tē) The quality of being productive or fertile.

fertilization [L. *fertilis,* reproductive] **1.** The process that begins with the penetration of the secondary oocyte by the spermatozoon and is completed with the fusion of the male and female pronuclei. This usually takes place in the fallopian tube. Viable spermatozoa have been found in the tube 48 hr after the last coitus. After the ovum is fertilized and the diploid chromosome number is restored in the zygote, cell division begins. The blastocyst then enters the uterus, where it may implant for continued nurture and development. **2.** In botany, the union of the male and female gametes. In higher plants, when the pollen tube enters the ovule, two gametes emerge. One unites with the ovum to form the zygote, from which the embryo develops; the other unites with two endosperm nuclei to form a primary endosperm cell, from which the endosperm (reserve food) develops. SEE: illus.

heterologous f. Assisted fertilization of a woman's ova with donor sperm. SEE: *in vitro f.; artificial insemination*.

homologous f. Artificial fertilization of a woman's ovum by her husband's sperm. The ovum and sperm are united while both are outside the body and then are placed intravaginally during the optimum time for fertilization.

in vitro f. ABBR: IVF. Laboratory-produced conception, used to enable pregnancy in infertile women when sperm access to ova is prevented by structural defects in the fallopian tubes or other factors, or in combination with her partner's sterility. After drug-induced follicle maturation, a sample of ova and follicular fluid is removed surgically and mixed with a specimen of the partner's sperm for incubation. The resulting zygote is introduced into the woman's uterus for implantation. SEE: *embryo transfer; GIFT; ZIFT*.

fester (fĕs′tĕr) [L. *fistula,* ulcer] To become inflamed and suppurate.

festinant (fĕs′tĭ-nănt) Increasing in speed; accelerating.

festination (fĕs″tĭ-nā′shŭn) [L. *festinatio*] festinating gait

festoon (fĕs-toon′) [L. *festus,* festal] A carving in the base material of a denture that simulates the natural indentations of the gums.

FET *forced expiratory time*.

fetal (fē′tăl) Pert. to a fetus.

fetal activity diary A periodic record used to count and compare fetal movements at different times. The woman may record the number of fetal movements in a given time (e.g., 1 hr), the average number of movements occurring during the same length of time at different times during the day, or the amount of time needed for a specified number of movements to occur (e.g., 10). SEE: *Cardiff Count-to-Ten*.

fetal alcohol syndrome ABBR: FAS. Birth defects in an infant born to a mother who consumed alcoholic beverages during gestation. Characteristic findings include a small head with multiple facial abnormalities: small eyes with short slits, a wide, flat nasal bridge, a midface that lacks a groove between the lip and the nose, and a small

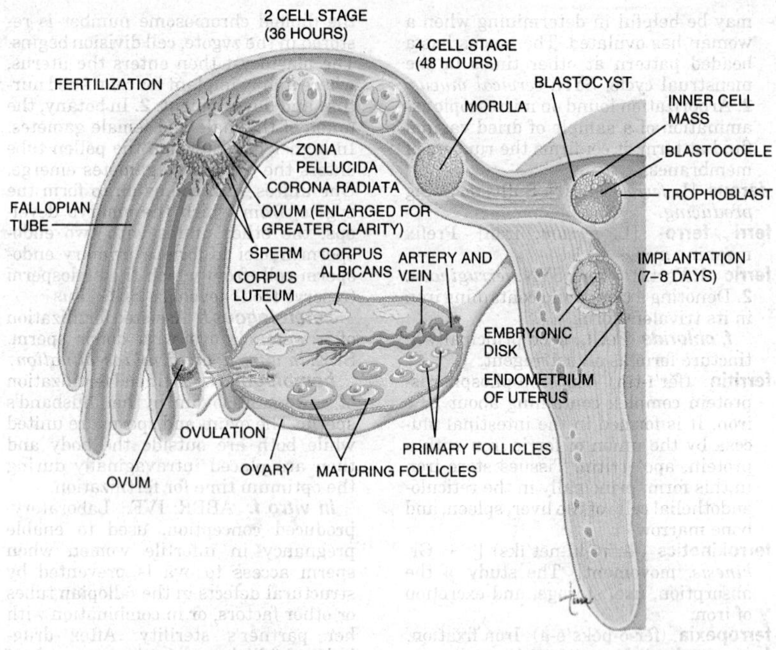

OVULATION, FERTILIZATION, AND EARLY EMBRYONIC DEVELOPMENT

jaw related to maxillary hypoplasia. Affected children often exhibit persistent growth retardation, hyperactivity, and learning deficits and may have signs and symptoms of alcohol withdrawal a few days after birth. SEE: *Nursing Diagnoses Appendix.*

SYMPTOMS: Birth defects that result from FAS are marked by abnormalities in growth, central nervous system function, and facial characteristics. Facial abnormalities detected at birth may become less obvious as the child continues to grow. Even more serious, however, are the developmental delays that affect the child's behaviors, social skills, and learning. Included are hyperactivity, poor social skills and judgment, impulsiveness, poor ego or self-image, sensory processing problems, and high levels of anxiety. Mental retardation (IQ below 79 at age seven) seriously impairs the child's potential, and poor fine motor function (weak grasp and poor hand-to-mouth coordination) adds to the child's handicaps.

PREVENTION: The patient should be taught that when she drinks, her baby also drinks, as alcohol crosses into the baby's bloodstream and affects its developing organs and tissues. No amount of alcohol is known to be safe for the developing fetus; thus, all health care providers should make ongoing efforts to educate women who are planning pregnancy or are pregnant to abstain completely from alcohol. They should suggest effective contraception and referral to abstinence treatment programs to individuals with known alcohol problems. The father's drinking does not directly affect his unborn child; however, his drinking may influence his partner to drink.

PATIENT CARE: Initial infant care is related to clinical problems that include increased respiratory effort, poor sucking ability, irritability, and hypotonia. A patent airway is maintained, and the infant's respiratory effort is monitored, with ventilatory assistance provided if required. Seizure activity must be assessed for, treated, and prevented with medical management. The infant's weight and fluid balance are assessed and recorded. The mother is taught feeding techniques that promote taking and retaining nutrients sufficient for growth. As necessary, the infant's nares and mouth are suctioned, and gavage feedings are provided.

Family members are taught about the child's special needs. They are helped to recognize and eventually accept the child's handicaps and to be aware of their effects on the child's future. Parents and other family members are encouraged to voice their concerns. A social worker evaluates the parent's needs and refers them to appropriate community resources and national support organizations.

fetal assessment Estimating the current status of the fetus. SEE: *amniocentesis; biophysical profile*.

fetal demise Fetal death. SEE: *Nursing Diagnoses Appendix*.

fetal development The growth and maturation of the fetus in utero. This is divided into three periods: the preembryonic period begins with conception and ends on gestational day 14; the embryonic period encompasses gestational weeks 3 through 8; and the remainder of the pregnancy is known as the fetal period. Body organs and systems arise from three primary germ layers (ectoderm, mesoderm, and endoderm) and rudimentary formation of all organ systems is completed by gestational week 16. Systems maturation essential to extrauterine survival begins during week 24 with the formation of pulmonary surfactant. Two critical events occur between weeks 26 and 29: the pulmonary vasculature becomes capable of gas exchange and the central nervous system becomes capable of controlling respiration. SYN: *fetal maturation*. SEE: *preterm birth*.

fetal heart rate monitoring The techniques used to determine the heart rate of the fetus. They include auscultation, use of an electronic device, or Doppler ultrasound. SEE: *deceleration; Doppler echocardiography; fetal monitoring in utero*.

fetal maturation fetal development.

fetal monitoring in utero The techniques used to obtain information on the physical condition of the fetus. They include recording the fetal electrocardiogram, respiratory rate, and, by invasive techniques, blood gas and pH data. SEE: *amniocentesis; chorionic villus sampling; deceleration; Doppler echocardiography; fetal heart rate monitoring; fetal (vibratory) acoustic stimulation*.

fetal scalp blood sampling The process of obtaining a small amount of blood from the fetal scalp for pH testing. When the monitor recording suggests fetal compromise during labor, the physician or nurse-midwife may elect to perform this procedure. The normal finding for fetal pH is at or above 7.25. Findings between 7.20 and 7.24 indicate a preacidotic state; if the pH is below 7.20, acidosis is present.

fetal tissue transplant A controversial experimental technique in which tissue from a dead fetus, severed umbilical cord, or placenta is grafted into a patient in an attempt to treat or cure disease.

fetal viability The ability of a fetus to survive outside of the womb. Historically, a fetus was considered to be capable of living at the end of gestational week 20 when the mother had felt fetal movement (quickening) and the fetal heart tones could be auscultated with a fetoscope. In actuality, even with prompt and intensive neonatal support, a preterm fetus of less than 25 weeks' gestation has little chance of surviving outside of the womb. SEE: *viable*.

feticide (fē′tĭ-sīd) [″ + *cidus*, kill] Killing of a fetus. SEE: *infanticide*.

fetid (fē′tĭd) [L. *fetidus*, stink] Rank or foul in odor.

fetish (fĕ′tĭsh) [Portug. *feitico*, charm, sorcery] **1.** An object, such as an idol or charm, that is thought to have mysterious, magical, and supernatural power. **2.** In psychiatry, the love object of a person who suffers from fetishism.

fetishism (fē′tĭsh-, fĕt′ĭsh-ĭzm) [″ + Gr. *-ismos*, condition] **1.** Belief in some object as possessing power or capable of being a stimulus. **2.** Erotic stimulation or sexually arousing fantasies involving contact with nonliving objects, such as an article of dress or a braid of hair.

fetochorionic (fē″tō-kor-ē-ŏn′ĭk) [L. *fetus* + Gr. *chorion*, membrane] Pert. to the fetus and the chorion, or chorionic membrane, of the placenta.

fetoglobulin (fē″tō-glŏb′ū-lĭn) Fetoprotein.

fetography (fē-tŏg′ră-fē) Radiography of the fetus in utero. This procedure has been virtually replaced by ultrasound.

fetology (fē-tŏl′ō-jē) [″ + Gr. *logos*, word, reason] Study of the fetus.

fetometry (fē-tŏm′ĕ-trē) [L. *fetus* + Gr. *metron*, measure] Estimation of fetal size (e.g., biparietal diameter and crown-rump length), age, and growth, typically using ultrasonography.

fetoplacental (fē″tō-plă-sĕn′tăl) [″ + *placenta*, a flat cake] Pert. to the fetus and its placenta.

fetoprotein (fē″tō-prō′tēn) An antigen present in the human fetus and in certain pathological conditions in adults. The amniotic fluid level can be used to evaluate fetal development. Elevated serum levels are found in adults with certain kinds of liver diseases. SEE: *alpha-fetoprotein*.

fetor (fē′tor) [L.] Stench; an offensive odor.

f. hepaticus A mousy odor in the breath of persons with severe liver impairment. SEE: *hepatic coma*.

f. oris Halitosis.

fetoscope **1.** An optical device, usually flexible and made of fiberoptic materials, used for direct visualization of the fetus in the uterus. SEE: *embryoscopy; fetoscopy*. **2.** Historical name for stethoscope used to auscultate fetal heart sounds.

fetoscopy Direct visualization of the fetus in the uterus through a fetoscope. SEE: *embryoscopy*.

fetotoxic (fē″tō-tŏk′sĭk) [L. *fetus*, fetus, + Gr. *toxikon*, poison] Poisonous to the fetus. Materials considered potentially

Development of Fetal Tissue

Ectoderm	Mesoderm	Endoderm
Nervous tissue	Bone, cartilage, and other connective tissues	Epithelium of respiratory tract except nose; digestive tract except mouth and anal canal; bladder except trigone
Sense organs	Male and female reproductive tracts	Proximal portion of male urethra
Epidermis, nails, and hair follicles	Heart, blood vessels, and lymphatics	Female urethra
Epithelium of external and internal ear, nasal cavity and sinuses, mouth, anal canal	Kidneys, ureters, trigone of bladder	Liver
Distal portion of male urethra	Pleura, peritoneum, and pericardium	Pancreas
	Skeletal muscle	

fetotoxic include alcohol, morphine, cocaine, salicylates, coumarin anticoagulants, sedatives, tetracyclines, thiazides, tobacco smoke, and large doses of vitamin K. SEE: *teratogenic; thalidomide*.

fetus (fē′tŭs) [L.] **1.** The latter stages of the developing young of an animal within the uterus or within an egg. **2.** The developing human, in utero, after completion of the eighth gestational week. Before that time it is called an embryo. SEE: table.

f. amorphus A shapeless fetal anomaly, scarcely recognizable as a fetus.

calcified f. A fetus that has died in utero and become hardened by calcium salts. SYN: *lithopedion*.

harlequin f. A newborn with abnormal skin that resembles a thick horny armor, divided into areas by deep red fissures. These infants die within a few days. The condition is also known as ichthyosis fetalis and ichthyosiform erythroderma, which were once regarded as separate diseases but are now known to represent different degrees of severity of the same entity. SYN: *ichthyosis congenita; ichthyosis fetalis*.

f. in fetu Parasitic f.

mummified f. A dead fetus that has become dried and shriveled after resorption has failed to occur.

f. papyraceus In a twin pregnancy, a dead fetus pressed flat by the development of the living twin.

parasitic f. A small imperfect fetus, called a parasite, contained within the body of another fetus, the autosite. SYN: *f. in fetu*. SEE: *dermoid cyst*.

FEV *forced expiratory volume.*

FEV$_1$ *forced expiratory volume in 1 sec.*

fever [L. *febris*] **1.** Abnormal elevation of temperature. The normal temperature taken orally ranges from about 97.6° to 99.6°F, although there is some individual variation. Rectal temperature is 0.5° **to 1.0°F higher than oral temperature.** Normal temperature fluctuates during the day and is lowest in the morning and highest in the late afternoon; these variations are maintained during a fever. The basal energy expenditure is estimated to be increased about 12% for each degree centigrade of fever. SYN: *pyrexia*. SEE: *basal energy expenditure; temperature*.

ETIOLOGY: Fever involves resetting the temperature set point that the body seeks to maintain at a higher level. It is caused by the release of interleukin-1 (IL-1), interleukin-2 (IL-2), and tumor necrosis factor (TNF) from white blood cells, esp. macrophages, secretion of acute phase proteins, and redistribution of the blood away from the skin by the autonomic nervous system. Elevated temperatures that are caused by inadequate thermoregulatory responses during exercise in very hot weather is called hyperthermia; the set point is not increased. Infections, drugs, tumors, breakdown of necrotic tissue, CNS damage, and collagen diseases are the underlying causes of fevers. Despite common beliefs, fever is not harmful except in patients who cannot tolerate its hypermetabolic effects, some elderly patients in whom it can cause delirium, and children with a history of febrile seizures.

TREATMENT: Fever can be relieved by antipyretics, drugs such as acetaminophen and aspirin, or other nonsteroidal anti-inflammatory agents that inhibit prostaglandins involved in the acute phase response. Recently, emphasis has been placed on not treating fever because of its potentially beneficial effects: enhanced immune function, increasing the effect of antibiotics, and possible changes in the availability of certain nutrients (e.g., iron) that organisms need for growth. SEE: *Reye's syndrome*.

CAUTION: Aspirin and other salicylates are contraindicated for use as antipyretics or analgesics in children because of their association with an increased risk of Reye's syndrome.

2. A disease characterized by an elevation of body temperature, such as typhoid fever, yellow fever.

childbed f. puerperal sepsis.

continuous f. A sustained fever, as in scarlet fever, typhus, or pneumonia, with a slight diurnal variation.

dengue f. SEE: *dengue*.

drug f. Elevated body temperatures caused by the administration of a drug. Because fevers are more often caused by infections, rheumatological illnesses, or malignancies, the diagnosis of drug fever may be overlooked initially.

factitious f. Fever produced artificially by a patient. This is done by artificially heating the thermometer or by self-administered pyrogenic substances. An artificial fever may be suspected if the pulse rate is much less than expected for the degree of fever noted. This diagnosis should be considered in all patients in whom there is no other plausible explanation for the fever. Patients who pretend to have fevers may have serious psychiatric problems. SEE: *factitious disorder; malinger; Munchausen syndrome*.

induced f. Fever produced artificially to treat certain diseases such as central nervous system syphilis. Sustained fever of 105°F (40.5°C), or even higher, maintained for 6 to 8 or 10 hr may be induced by medical diathermy or injection of malarial parasites.

intermittent f. Fever in which symptoms disappear completely between paroxysms. SEE: *malaria; undulant fever*.

neutropenic f. Fever associated with an abnormally low neutrophil level, usually caused by infection. This condition is treated with empirical antibiotic therapy while awaiting the results of cultures. Neutropenia may be caused by many diseases and conditions, including chemotherapy, radiation exposure, aplastic anemia, bone marrow infiltration from malignancy, and complications of bone marrow transplantation. The risk of potentially life-threatening infection is substantial when the absolute neutrophil count is below 500/mm^3.

periodic f. Familial Mediterranean fever.

phlebotomus f. Sandfly fever.

relapsing f. borreliosis.

remittent f. A pattern of fever that varies over a 24-hr period but does not return to normal. SEE: *malaria*.

f. of unknown origin ABBR: FUO. An illness of at least 3 weeks' duration with fever exceeding 38.3°C on several occasions and diagnosis not established after 1 week of hospital investigation. The main causes are systemic and localized infections, neoplasms, or collagen-vascular diseases such as rheumatoid arthritis, disseminated lupus erythematosus, and polyarteritis nodosa. Less common causes are granulomatous disease, inflammatory disease of the bowel, pulmonary embolization, drug fever, cirrhosis of the liver, and rare conditions such as Whipple's disease. Diseases such as AIDS, chronic fatigue syndrome, or Lyme disease may be added to the list of possible causes of FUO; however, better diagnostic methods may eliminate other diseases from the list. Some cases remain undiagnosed. SEE: *factitious fever*.

fever blister A vesicular rash usually appearing on the lips or mucous membrane of the mouth during another infectious illness. The rash is caused by herpes simplex virus. SYN: *cold sore*.

feverfew (fee′vĕr-fū) A perennial herb (*Tanacetum parthenium*) grown as an ornamental plant and used medicinally by alternative medicine practitioners to treat rheumatologic illnesses and to prevent migraines.

FFB *flexible fiberoptic bronchoscope.*

F.F.D. *focal-film distance.*

fFN *Fetal fibronectin.*

FH_4 *5,6,7,8-tetrahydrofolic acid* (folacin).

FHPE *Focused history and physical examination.*

fiat (fī′ăt) [L.] Let there be made, a term used in writing prescriptions.

fiber [L. *fibra*] **1.** A threadlike or filmlike structure, as a nerve fiber. **2.** A neuron or its axonal portion. **3.** An elongated threadlike structure. It may be cellular as nerve fiber or muscle fiber, or may be a cellular product, as collagen, elastic, oxytalan, or reticular fiber. **4.** A slender cellulosic structure derived from plants such as cotton. SEE: *rayon, purified*.

accelerator f. A nerve fiber that carries impulses to increase heart rate.

afferent f. A nerve fiber that carries sensory impulses to the central nervous system from receptors in the periphery.

cholinergic f. Any preganglionic fiber, postganglionic parasympathetic fiber, postganglionic sympathetic fiber to a sweat gland, or efferent fiber to skeletal muscle.

circular f. Collagen bundles in the gingiva that surround a tooth.

dietary f. The components of food that resist chemical digestion, including cellulose, hemicellulose, lignin, gums, mucilages, and pectin. These substances can soften and increase the bulk of the bowel movement.

Dietary fibers are classified according to their solubility in water. Water-insoluble fibers include cellulose, lignin, and some hemicelluloses. Natural gel-forming fibers such as gums, mucilages, and some hemicelluloses are water soluble. Most foods of plant origin contain both soluble and insoluble dietary fiber. Many disease processes including constipation, colonic polyps and colonic cancer gallstones, irritable bowel syndrome, obesity and atherosclerosis have either been shown to be ameliorated by a high fiber diet or there is epidemiological data supporting the existence of an inverse relationship between the disease and dietary fiber consumption.

Foods rich in fiber include whole-grain foods, bran flakes, beans, fruits, leafy vegetables, nuts, root vegetables and their skins.

efferent f. A nerve fiber that carries motor impulses from the central nervous system to effector organs.

gingival f. Collagen fibers that support the marginal or interdental gingiva and are adapted to the tooth surface.

inhibitory f. A nerve fiber that carries impulses to decrease heart rate.

intercolumnar f. An intercrural fiber, part of the superficial inguinal ring.

interradicular f. The collagen fibers of the periodontal ligament in the interradicular area, attaching the tooth to alveolar bone.

intrafusal muscle f. The structural component of the muscle spindle, made up of small skeletal muscle fibers at either end and a central noncontracile region where the sensory receptors are located.

man-made f. A synthetic fiber made from chemicals (e.g., rayon or polyester). SYN: *synthetic f.*

medullated f. Old term for a myelinated neuron.

mossy f. Any of the afferent fibers to the cerebellar cortex. The fibers give off many collaterals, each ending in a tuft of branches.

motor f. Any of the axons of motor neurons that innervate skeletal muscles.

muscle f. A muscle cell in striated, smooth, or cardiac muscle.

myelinated f. A nerve fiber whose axon (dendrite) is wrapped in a myelin sheath.

nerve f. A neuron, although often used to mean *axon*. SEE: *nerve*.

nonmedullated f. Unmyelinated f.

oxytalan f. Bundles of thin, acid-resistant fibrils found in the periodontium.

postganglionic f. The axon of a postganglionic neuron that passes from an autonomic ganglion to a visceral effector.

principal f. The major fiber groups of the functioning periodontium. They attach the tooth to the bone and adjacent teeth.

Purkinje f. Any of the atypical muscle fibers lying beneath the endocardium that form the impulse-conducting system of the heart.

synthetic f. Man-made f.

transseptal f. Any of the collagenous fibers that extend between the teeth and are embedded in the cementum of adjacent teeth.

unmyelinated f. A nerve fiber that lacks a myelin sheath, although a neurilemma may be present in the peripheral nervous system.

fibercolonoscope (fī″bĕr-kō-lŏn′ō-skōp) A fiberoptic endoscope for examining the colon.

fibergastroscope (fī″bĕr-găs′trō-skōp) A fiberoptic endoscope for examining the stomach.

fiberglass Glass spun into fine fibers. It is used in the building industry for insulation. The fibers are irritating to the skin.

fiber-illumination (fī′bĕr-ĭl-loo″mĭn-ā″shŭn) The transmission of light to an object through fiberoptic cables.

fiberoptics The transmission of light through flexible glass or plastic fibers by reflections from the side walls of the fibers. This permits transmission of visual images around sharp curves and corners. Devices that use fiberoptic materials are useful in endoscopic examinations.

fiberscope (fī′bĕr-skōp) A flexible endoscope that uses fiberoptics for visualization.

fibra (fī′bră) *pl.* **fibrae** [L.] A fiber.

fibremia (fī-brē′mē-ă) [″ + Gr. *haima*, blood] Fibrin formed in the blood, causing embolism or thrombosis. SYN: *inosemia*.

fibril (fī′brĭl) [L. *fibrilla*] **1.** A small fiber. **2.** A very small filamentous structure, often the component of a cell or a fiber.

muscle f. Myofibril.

nerve f. A delicate fibril found in the cell body and processes of a neuron. SYN: *neurofibril*.

fibrilla (fī-brĭl′ă) *pl.* **fibrillae** [L.] A fibril or small fiber.

fibrillar, fibrillary Pert. to or consisting of fibrils.

fibrillated (fī′brĭ-lāt′d) [L. *fibrilla*, little fiber] Composed of minute fibers.

fibrillation (fī″brĭl-ā′shŭn) **1.** Formation of fibrils. **2.** Quivering or spontaneous contraction of individual muscle fibers. **3.** An abnormal bioelectric potential occurring in neuropathies and myopathies.

atrial f. ABBR: AF. The most common cardiac arrhythmia, affecting as many as 10% of people age 70 and over. It is marked by rapid, irregular electrical activity in the atria, resulting in ineffective ejection of blood into the ventricles. Blood that eddies in the atria

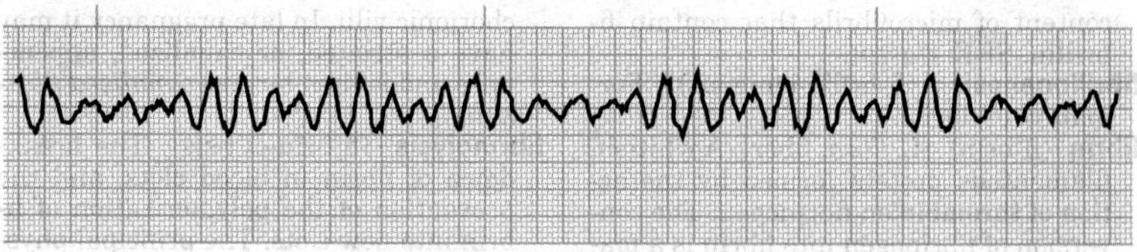

VENTRICULAR FIBRILLATION

may occasionally form clots that may embolize (esp. to the brain, but also to other organs). As a result AF is an important risk factor for stroke. It may also contribute to other diseases and conditions, including congestive heart failure, dyspnea on exertion, and syncope.

ETIOLOGY: AF may occur in otherwise healthy persons with no structural heart disease ("lone" AF) (e.g., during stress or exercise). It may also develop acutely during alcohol withdrawal; in patients with underlying arrhythmias (such as tachybrady syndrome or Wolff-Parkinson-White syndrome); after cardiac surgery; during cocaine intoxication; in hypertensive urgencies, hypoxia, or hypercarbia (carbon dioxide retention); during myocardial infarction; in pericarditis and pulmonary embolism; or as a consequence of thyrotoxicosis or other metabolic disorders. Chronic AF usually occurs in patients with structural abnormalities of the heart, such as cardiomyopathies; enlargement of the left atrium; mitral valve disease; or rheumatic heart disease.

SYMPTOMS: Some patients may not notice rapid or irregular beating of their heart, even though the ventricular rate rises to 200 bpm. Most patients, however, report some of the following symptoms at slower heart rates (100 bpm or greater): dizziness, dyspnea, palpitations, presyncope, or syncope.

DIAGNOSIS: Patients who present with their first episode of atrial fibrillation are typically evaluated with thyroid function tests, cardiac enzymes, a complete blood count, and blood chemistries. In patients with a cardiac murmur or evidence of congestive heart failure, echocardiography is typically performed.

TREATMENT: The acutely ill patient with a rapid ventricular response and signs or symptoms of angina pectoris, congestive heart failure, hypotension, or hypoxia should be prepared for immediate cardioversion. Patients who tolerate the rhythm disturbance without these signs or symptoms are typically treated first with drugs to slow the heart rhythm (e.g., calcium-channel blockers, beta blockers, or digoxin). Anticoagulation (e.g., with warfarin) markedly reduces the risk of stroke and should be given for several weeks before, and about a week after, elective cardioversion, and to patients in chronic AF who do not return to sinus rhythm with treatment. Patients who elect not to use anticoagulants for chronic AF, or in whom anticoagulants pose too great a risk of bleeding, usually are given 325 mg of aspirin daily. AF can also be treated with radiofrequency catheter ablation, or with surgical techniques to isolate the source of the rhythm disturbance in the atria. SEE: *ablation*.

PATIENT CARE: The acutely ill patient is placed on bedrest and monitored closely, with frequent assessments of vital signs, oxygen saturation, heart rate and rhythm, and 12-lead electrocardiography. Supplemental oxygen is supplied and intravenous access established. Preparations for cardioversion (if necessary) and the medications prescribed for the patient are explained. Patients should be carefully introduced to the risks, benefits, and alternatives to stroke prevention with anticoagulation.

lone atrial f. Atrial fibrillation that is not caused by or associated with underlying disease of the heart muscle, heart valves, coronary arteries, pulmonary circulation, or thyroid gland. Prognosis seems better for this type of atrial fibrillation than for that which results from anatomical or metabolic abnormalities.

paroxysmal atrial f. Intermittent episodes of atrial fibrillation.

ventricular f. ABBR: VFIB. A treatable, but lethal dysrhythmia present in nearly half of all cases of cardiac arrest. It is marked on the electrocardiogram by rapid, chaotic nonrepetitive waveforms; and clinically by the absence of effective circulation of blood (pulselessness). Rapid defibrillation (applying unsynchronized electrical shocks to the heart) is the key to treatment. Basic measures, such as opening the airway and providing rescue breaths and chest compressions, should be undertaken until the defibrillator is available. SEE: illus; *defibrillation; advanced cardiac life support*.

fibrillin A protein constituent of connective tissue. It is present in skin, ligaments, tendons, and in the aorta. In Marfan's syndrome, there is reduced content of microfibrils that contain fibrillin. SEE: *elastin*.

fibrillogenesis (fī-brĭl″ō-jĕn′ĕ-sĭs) Formation of fibrils.

fibrin (fī′brĭn) [L. *fibra,* fiber] A whitish, filamentous protein formed by the action of thrombin on fibrinogen. The conversion of fibrinogen into fibrin is a major aspect of blood clotting. The fibrin is deposited as fine interlacing filaments which entangle red and white blood cells and platelets, the whole forming a coagulum, or clot. SEE: *coagulation, blood*. **fibrinous,** *adj.*

fibrin-fibrinogen degradation products A group of soluble protein fragments produced by the proteolytic action of plasmin on fibrin or fibrinogen. These products impair the hemostatic process and are a major cause of hemorrhage in intravascular coagulation and fibrinogenolysis.

fibrin glue Fibrinogen concentrate combined with bovine thrombin. It may be applied topically to stop bleeding, esp. during surgery. It also may be injected into a variety of fistulae with some degree of success. Autologous fibrinogen (as cryoprecipitate) mixed with calcium chloride and bovine thrombin will result in fibrin glue. Commercially available is fibrin sealant composed of human plasma and bovine-derived components.

fibrinocellular (fī″brĭ-nō-sĕl′ū-lăr) Composed of fibrin and cells, as in certain exudates.

fibrinogen (fī-brĭn′ō-jĕn) [″ + Gr. *gennan,* to produce] A protein, also called factor I, synthesized by the liver and present in blood plasma that is converted into fibrin through the action of thrombin in the presence of calcium ions. Fibrin forms the clot. SEE: *blood coagulation; coagulation factor*.

fibrinogenic, fibrinogenous Producing fibrin.

fibrinogenolysis (fī″brĭ-nō-jĕ-nŏl′ĭ-sĭs) [″ + ″ + *lysis,* dissolution] Decomposition or dissolution of fibrin.

fibrinogenopenia (fī-brĭn″ō-jĕn″ō-pē′nē-ă) [″ + Gr. *gennan,* to produce, + *penia,* poverty] Reduction in the amount of fibrinogen in the blood, usually the result of a liver or a coagulation disorder.

fibrinoid (fī′brĭ-noyd) [″ + Gr. *eidos,* form, shape] Resembling fibrin.

fibrinoid change Alteration in connective tissues in response to immune reactions. The tissue becomes swollen, homogeneous, and bandlike.

fibrinoid material A fibrinous substance that develops in the placenta, increasing in quantity as the placenta develops. Its origin is attributed to the degenerating decidua and trophoblast. It forms an incomplete layer in the chorion and decidua basalis and also occurs as small irregular patches on the surface of the chorionic villi. In late pregnancy it may have a striated, or canalized, appearance and is then termed *canalized fibrinoid*.

fibrinolysis (fī″brĭn-ŏl′ĭ-sĭs) The breakdown of fibrin in blood clots, and the prevention of the polymerization of fibrin into new clots. The principal physiological activator of the fibrinolytic system is tissue plasminogen activator. It converts plasminogen in a fibrin-containing clot to plasmin. The fibrin polymer is degraded by plasmin into fragments that are then scavenged by monocytes and macrophages. This process begins immediately after a clot forms. It can be stimulated by administering fibrinolytic drugs, such as recombinant tissue plasminogen activator. **fibrinolytic** (-ō-lĭt′ĭk), *adj.*

fibrinopenia (fī″brĭn-ō-pē′nē-ă) [″ + Gr. *penia,* poverty] Fibrin and fibrinogen deficiency in the blood.

fibrinopeptide (fī″brĭ-nō-pĕp′tīd) The substance removed by thrombin from fibrinogen during blood clotting.

fibrinosis (fī-brĭ-nō′sĭs) [″ + Gr. *osis,* condition] Excess of fibrin in the blood.

fibrin split products The materials released into the bloodstream when the crosslinked fibrin in a blood clot is digested by plasmin.

fibrinuria (fī-brĭn-ū′rē-ă) [″ + Gr. *ouron,* urine] Passage of fibrin in the urine.

fibro- [L. *fibra*] Combining form meaning *fiber; fibrous tissues*.

fibroadenia (fī″brō-ă-dē′nē-ă) [L. *fibra,* fiber, + Gr. *aden,* gland] Fibrous degeneration of glandular tissue.

fibroadenoma (fī″brō-ăd″ĕ-nō′mă) [″ + ″ + *oma,* tumor] An adenoma with fibrous tissue forming a dense stroma.

fibroadipose [″ + *adeps,* fat] Containing fibrous and fatty tissue.

fibroangioma [″ + Gr. *angeion,* vessel, + *oma,* tumor] A fibrous tissue angioma.

fibroareolar Fibrocellular.

fibroblast (fī′brō-blăst) [″ + Gr. *blastos,* germ] Any cell from which connective tissue is developed; it produces collagen, elastin, and reticular protein fibers. SYN: *desmocyte; fibrocyte*.

fibroblast growth factor Polypeptides that stimulate wound healing, new blood vessel growth, and skeletal muscle development. Overactivity of these factors has been associated with neoplasia.

fibroblastoma (fī″brō-blăs-tō′mă) [″ + ″ + *oma,* tumor] A tumor of connective tissue, or fibroblastic, cells.

fibrocalcific (fī″brō-kăl-sĭf′ĭk) Fibrous and partially calcified.

fibrocarcinoma (fī″brō-kăr″sĭ-nō′mă) [″ + Gr. *karkinos,* cancer, + *oma,* tumor] A carcinoma in which the trabeculae are resistant and thickened with granular degeneration of the cells.

fibrocartilage (fī″brō-kăr′tĭ-lĭj) [″ + *cartilago,* gristle] A type of cartilage in which the matrix contains thick bundles of white or collagenous fibers. It is found in the intervertebral disks.

fibrocellular (fī″brō-sĕl′ū-lăr) [″ + *cellula,* little cell] Containing fibrous and cellular tissue. SYN: *fibroareolar.*

fibrochondritis (fī″brō-kŏn-drī′tĭs) [″ + Gr. *chondros,* cartilage, + *itis,* inflammation] Inflammation of fibrocartilage.

fibrochondroma (fī″brō-kŏn-drō′mă) [″ + ″ + *oma,* tumor] A tumor of fibrous tissue and cartilage.

fibrocyst (fī′brō-sĭst) [″ + Gr. *kystis,* cyst] A fibrous tumor that has undergone cystic degeneration or has accumulated fluid in the interspaces.

fibrocystic (fī″brō-sĭs′tĭk) **1.** Consisting of fibrocysts. **2.** Fibrous with cystic degeneration.

fibrocystoma (fī″brō-sĭs-tō′mă) [″ + Gr. *kystis,* cyst, + *oma,* tumor] A fibroma combined with a cystoma.

fibrocyte (fī′brō-sīt) [″ + Gr. *kytos,* cell] A mature, older fibroblast.

fibrodysplasia (fī″brō-dĭs-plā′sē-ă) [″ + Gr. *dys,* bad, + *plassein,* to form] Abnormal development of fibrous tissue.

fibroelastic (fī″brō-ē-lăs′tĭk) [″ + Gr. *elastikos,* elastic] Pert. to connective tissue containing both white nonelastic collagenous fibers and yellow elastic fibers.

fibroelastosis (fī″brō-ē″lăs-tō′sĭs) Overgrowth of fibroelastic tissue.

endocardial f. Fibroelastosis of the endocardium, leading to cardiac failure.

fibroenchondroma (fī″brō-ĕn″kŏn-drō′mă) [″ + Gr. *en,* in, + *chondros,* cartilage, + *oma,* tumor] A benign cartilaginous tumor containing fibrous elements.

fibroepithelioma (fī″brō-ĕp″ĭ-thē″lē-ō′mă) [″ + Gr. *epi,* upon, + *thele,* nipple, + *oma,* tumor] A new growth containing fibrous and epithelial elements.

fibroid (fī′broyd) [″ + Gr. *eidos,* form, shape] **1.** Containing or resembling fibers. SEE: *degeneration.* **2.** A benign tumor of the uterine myometrium. SEE: *uterine leiomyoma.*

fibroidectomy (fī-broyd-ĕk′tō-mē) [″ + ″ + *ektome,* excision] Surgical removal of a fibroid tumor.

fibrolipoma (fī″brō-lĭ-pō′mă) [″ + Gr. *lipos,* fat, + *oma,* tumor] Lipofibroma.

fibroma (fī-brō′mă) *pl.* **fibromata** [″ + Gr. *oma,* tumor] A fibrous, encapsulated connective tissue tumor. It is irregular in shape, slow in growth, and has a firm consistency. Pressure or cystic degeneration may cause pain. It may affect the periosteum, jaws, occiput, pelvis, vertebrae, ribs, long bones, or sternum. SYN: *fibroid.* **fibromatous** (-mă-tŭs), *adj.*

f. of breast A benign, nonulcerative, painless breast tumor.

interstitial f. A tumor in the muscular wall of the uterus that may grow inward and form a polypoid fibroid, or outward and become a subperitoneal fibroid. SEE: *uterine f.*

intramural f. A tumor located in muscle tissue of the uterus between the peritoneal coat and endometrium.

submucous f. A fibroma encroaching on the endometrial cavity. It may be either sessile or pedunculated.

subserous f. A fibroma, often pedunculated, lying beneath the peritoneal coat of the uterus.

uterine f. A fibroid tumor of the uterus. It is the most common tumor found in women.

SYMPTOMS: Fibromata rarely cause symptoms before the age of 30. Although their cardinal symptoms are supposed to be dysmenorrhea, menorrhagia, and leukorrhea, these are found infrequently, and the symptomatology is directly related to the location of the tumor in the uterus. Thus, tumors that encroach on the bladder region cause frequency and dysuria, those pressing on the rectum cause rectal tenesmus, those that encroach on the endometrium may cause menorrhagia and dysmenorrhea, and very large subserous growths may be symptomless.

Use of oral contraceptives reduces the risk for uterine fibroma, as does cigarette smoking; obesity increases the risk. Fibromata may cause infertility because of their size or location. Whether or not fibromata enlarge during pregnancy is unclear. SEE: *dysmenorrhea; dysuria; menorrhagia; tenesmus.*

PATHOLOGY: The tumor may vary in diameter from a few millimeters to a size large enough to fill the entire abdominal cavity. Fibromata may be single or multiple. They usually increase in size during the reproductive years and may regress after menopause. They are completely enclosed by a fibrous connective tissue capsule containing the blood vessels that supply the tumor. They are subjected to numerous benign degenerations such as necrobiotic changes (red and gray degeneration), hyaline changes, telangiectatic and lymphangiectatic changes, calcareous degeneration, fatty degeneration, and infection. Occasionally a fibroma shows sarcomatous degeneration.

TREATMENT: Fibromata producing no symptoms should be left in place and the patient kept under observation. Medical treatment using luteinizing hormone–releasing hormone (LHRH) analogues will cause fibromata to shrink, but the growth returns when LHRH is discontinued. If there is evidence of unusually rapid growth, they **should be removed. Small submucous** tumors may be removed by electrocautery during hysteroscopy. Laser technique has been used to remove these tumors. If pregnancy is a possibility, tumors large enough to interfere with childbearing should be removed.

fibromatosis (fī″brō-mă-tō′sĭs) [L. *fibra,* fiber, + Gr. *oma,* tumor, + *osis,* condition] The simultaneous development of many fibromata.

f. colli Congenital muscular torticollis.

gingival f. An inherited condition marked by hypertrophy of the gums before the eruption of the teeth. Hypertrichosis is usually present.

palmar f. Dupuytren's contracture.

fibromectomy (fī″brō-mĕk′tō-mē) [″ + Gr. *oma,* tumor, + *ektome,* excision] Removal of a fibroma.

fibromembranous (fī″brō-mĕm′bră-nŭs) [″ + *membrana,* web] Having both fibrous and membranous tissue.

fibromuscular (fī″brō-mŭs′kū-lăr) [″ + *musculus,* muscle] Consisting of muscle and connective tissue.

fibromyalgia [″ + Gr. *mys,* muscle, + *algos,* pain] Chronic and frequently difficult to manage pain in muscles and soft tissues surrounding joints. Efforts to classify this condition have resulted in the American College of Rheumatology criteria for classification of fibromyalgia, published in 1990. SYN: *fibromyitis; fibromyositis; fibrositis; tension myalgia.* SEE: table.

TREATMENT: Various approaches have been tried. Essential to the management of this condition are reassurance, elimination of contributing factors, physical therapy with the objective of restoring normal neuromuscular function, institution of a cardiovascular fitness program, and appropriate medications for sleep disturbances. Drug therapies include topical capsaicin, oral anti-inflammatories, antidepressants, trigger point injections, and/or narcotic analgesics. SEE: *trigger point.*

fibromyitis Fibromyalgia.

fibromyoma (fī″brō-mī-ō′mă) [″ + ″ + *oma,* tumor] **1.** A fibrous tissue myoma. **2.** A fibroid tumor of the uterus that contains more fibrous than muscle tissue.

fibromyomectomy (fī″brō-mī″ō-mĕk′tō-mē) [″ + ″ + *ektome,* excision] Removal of a fibromyoma from the uterus, leaving that organ in place.

fibromyositis Fibromyalgia.

fibromyotomy (fī″brō-mī-ŏt′ō-mē) [″ + ″ + *tome,* incision] Surgical incision of a fibroid tumor.

fibromyxoma (fī″brō-mĭk-sō′mă) [″ + Gr. *myxa,* mucus, + *oma,* tumor] An encapsulated fibrous tumor composed of

The American College of Rheumatology 1990 Criteria for Classification of Fibromyalgia*

1. History of widespread pain

Definition: Pain is considered widespread when all the following are present: pain in the left side of the body, pain in the right side of the body, pain above the waist, and pain below the waist. In addition, axial skeletal pain (cervical spine, anterior chest, thoracic spine, or low back) must be present. In this definition, shoulder and buttock pain is considered as pain for each involved side. "Low back" pain is considered lower segment pain.

2. Pain in 11 of 18 tender point sites on digital palpation

Definition: On digital palpation, pain must be present in at least 11 of the following 18 tender point sites:

Occiput—bilateral, at the suboccipital muscle insertions

Low cervical—bilateral, at the anterior aspects of the intertransverse spaces at C5–7

Trapezius—bilateral, at the midpoint of the upper border

Supraspinatus—bilateral, at origins, above the scapular spine near the medial border

Second rib—bilateral, at the second costochondral junctions, just lateral to the junctions on upper surfaces

Lateral epicondyle—bilateral, 2 cm distal to the epicondyles

Gluteal—bilateral, in upper outer quandrants of buttocks in anterior fold of muscle

Greater trochanter—bilateral, posterior to the trochanteric prominence

Knee—bilateral, at the medial fat pad proximal to the joint line

Digital palpation should be performed with an approximate force of 4 kg. For a tender point to be considered "positive," the subject must state that the palpation was painful. "Tender" is not to be considered "painful."

* For classification purposes, patients will be said to have fibromyalgia if both criteria are satisfied. Widespread pain must have been present for at least 3 months. The presence of a second clinical disorder does not exclude the diagnosis of fibromyalgia.

SOURCE: American College of Rheumatology, Multicenter Criteria Committee, Arthritis Rheum 1990; 33(2):160–172, with permission.

large fibroblasts in loose connective tissue.

fibromyxosarcoma (fī″brō-mĭk″sō-săr-kō′mă) [″ + ″ + *sarkos,* flesh, + *oma,* tumor] **1.** A sarcoma containing fibrous and myxoid tissue. **2.** A sarcoma that has undergone mucoid degeneration.

fibronectin Any of a group of opsonic proteins present in blood plasma and extracellular matrix that are involved in wound healing and cell adhesion. The presence of fetal fibronectin in the cervical and vaginal secretions may be a marker for subsequent development of preterm labor. SEE: *fetal fibronectin assay.*

fibroneuroma (fī″brō-nū-rō′mă) [″ + Gr. *neuron,* nerve, + *oma,* tumor] Neurofibroma.

fibro-osteoma (fī″brō-ŏs-tē-ō′mă) [″ + Gr. *osteon,* bone, + *oma,* tumor] A tumor containing bony and fibrous elements. SYN: *osteofibroma.*

fibropapilloma (fī″brō-păp-ĭ-lō′mă) [″ + *papilla,* nipple, + Gr. *oma,* tumor] A mixed fibroma and papilloma sometimes occurring in the bladder.

fibroplasia (fī″brō-plā′sē-ă) [″ + Gr. *plasis,* a molding] The development of fibrous tissue, as in wound healing or by other stimulating factors, e.g., as retrolental fibroplasia in the neonate due to the administration of excessive oxygen.

retrolental f. ABBR: RLF. Retinopathy of prematurity.

fibroplastic (fī″brō-plăs′tĭk) [″ + Gr. *plassein,* to form] Giving formation to fibrous tissue.

fibropurulent (fī″brō-pūr′ū-lĕnt) [″ + *purulentus,* festering] Pert. to pus that contains flakes of fibrous tissue.

fibrosarcoma (fī″brō-săr-kō′mă) [L. *fibra,* fiber, + Gr. *sarkos,* flesh, + *oma,* tumor] A spindle-celled sarcoma containing a large amount of connective tissue.

fibrose (fī′brōs) To form or produce fibrous tissue (e.g., a scar).

fibroserous (fī″brō-sē′rŭs) [″ + *serosus,* serous] Containing fibrous and serous parts, such as the pericardium. The pericardium is such a tissue.

fibrosis (fī-brō′sĭs) [″+ Gr. *osis,* condition] The repair and replacement of inflamed tissues or organs by connective tissues. The process results in the replacement of normal cells by fibroblasts (and eventually, the replacement of normal organ tissue by scar tissue).

arteriocapillary f. Arteriolar and capillary fibroid degeneration.

diffuse interstitial pulmonary f. Idiopathic pulmonary f.

idiopathic pulmonary f. The formation of scar tissue in the parenchyma of the lungs, following inflammation of the alveoli. The disease results in difficulty breathing caused by impaired gas exchange. SYN: *Hamman's syndrome.* SEE: *interstitial lung disorders.*

SYMPTOMS: Dyspnea, cough, exertional fatigue, and generalized weakness are common. Signs of the illness include pulmonary crackles, finger clubbing, cyanosis, and evidence of right ventricular failure (such as lower-extremity swelling). The disease typically progresses to end-stage lung disease and death within 7 years of diagnosis.

DIAGNOSIS: A biopsy of the lung is needed to make the diagnosis.

TREATMENT: Corticosteroids (such as prednisone) may be helpful in 10% to 20% of patients. Lung transplantation can be curative if a donor organ is available.

postfibrinosis f. Development of fibrosis in a tissue in which fibrin has been deposited.

proliferative f. Formation of new fibrous tissue from connective tissue cells.

pulmonary f. idiopathic pulmonary f.

f. uteri Diffuse growth of fibrous tissue throughout the uterus.

fibrositis (fī-brō-sī′tĭs) [″ + Gr. *itis,* inflammation] Fibromyalgia.

fibrotic (fī-brŏt′ĭk) Marked by or pert. to fibrosis.

fibrous plaques SEE: *arteriosclerosis.*

fibula (fĭb′ū-lă) [L., pin] The outer and smaller bone of the leg from the ankle to the knee, articulating above with the tibia and below with the tibia and talus. It is one of the longest and thinnest bones of the body. **fibular,** ***adj.***

fibulocalcaneal (fĭb″ū-lō-kăl-kā′nē-ăl) [L. *fibula,* pin, + *calcaneus,* pert. to the heel] Pert. to the fibula and calcaneus.

ficin (fī′sĭn) [L. *ficus,* fig] Sap from the fig tree. It contains an enzyme capable of hydrolyzing proteins.

Fick, Adolf Eugen German physician, 1829–1901.

F. equation F. principle.

F's. law The rule stating that diffusion through a tissue membrane is directly proportional to the cross-sectional area, driving pressure, and gas coefficient and inversely proportional to tissue thickness.

F. method A method of determining cardiac output by calculating the difference in oxygen content of mixed venous and arterial blood. This figure is then divided into the total oxygen consumption.

F. principle In respiratory physiology, the rule stating that blood flow equals the amount of a substance absorbed in an organ divided by the difference in the amount of the substance entering and leaving the organ. Usually the substance is oxygen or a dye.

F.I.C.S. *Fellow of the International College of Surgeons.*

FID *flame ionization detector.*

field [AS. *feld*] A specific area in relation to an object.

auditory f. The space or distance from the individual within which he or she hears sounds.

high-power f. The portion of an object seen when the high-magnification lenses of a microscope are used.

low-power f. The portion of an object seen when the low-magnification lenses of a microscope are used.

useful f. of view ABBR: UFOV. A test of visual attention that measures the space in which an individual can receive information rapidly from two separate sources. It is a strong predictor of accidents in older drivers. Training can expand the useful field of view and increase the visual processing speed of an elderly person.

fifth cranial nerve SEE: *trigeminal nerve.*

fight-or-flight reaction of Cannon [Walter B. Cannon, U.S. physiologist, 1871–1954] The generalized response to an emergency situation. This includes intense stimulation of the sympathetic nervous system and the adrenal gland. The heart and respiratory rates, blood pressure, and blood flow to muscles are increased. This response prepares the body to either flee or fight.

FIGLU, FIGlu *formiminoglutamic acid.*

FIGLU excretion test An obsolete test for folic acid deficiency. When histidine is administered to a patient with folic acid deficiency, formiminoglutamic (FIGLU) acid in the urine increases.

FIGO staging system The staging system for cancer of the cervix uteri developed by the International Federation of Gynecology and Obstetrics.

figurate (fĭg′ū-rāt) [L. *figuratum,* figured] Having a rounded, curved, circular, or ringed shape. The term is used to describe rashes that leave elaborately embroidered markings on the skin.

figure [L. *figura*] **1.** A body, form, shape, or outline. **2.** A number.

filaceous (fĭ-lā′shŭs) Composed of filaments.

filament [L. *filamentum*] **1.** A fine thread. **2.** A threadlike coil of tungsten found in the x-ray tube that is the source of electrons.

axial f. A fine filament forming the central axis of the tail of a spermatozoon.

filamentous Made up of long, interwoven or irregularly placed threadlike structures.

filar (fī′lăr) [L. *filum,* thread] Filamentous.

Filaria (fĭl-ā′rē-ă) [L. *filum,* thread] Term formerly applied to a genus of nematodes belonging to the superfamily Filarioidea.

F. bancrofti Wuchereria bancrofti.

F. loa Loa loa.

F. medinensis Dracunculus medinensis.

F. sanguinis hominis Wuchereria bancrofti.

filaria (fĭl-ā′rē-ă) *pl.* **filariae** [L. *filum,* thread] A long thread-shaped nematode belonging to the superfamily Filarioidea. The adults live in vertebrates. In humans, they may infect the lymphatic vessels and lymphatic organs, circulatory system, connective tissues, subcutaneous tissues, and serous cavities. Typically, the female produces larvae called microfilariae, which may be sheathed or sheathless. They reach the peripheral blood or lymphatic vessels, where they may be ingested by a blood-sucking arthropod (a mosquito, gnat, or fly). In the intermediate host, they transform into rhabditoid larvae that metamorphose into infective filariform larvae. These migrate to the proboscis and are deposited in or on the skin of the vertebrate host. SEE: *elephantiasis.* **filarial,** *adj.*

filariasis (fĭl-ă-rī′ă-sĭs) [″ + Gr. *-iasis,* condition] A chronic disease due to one of the filaria species. SEE: *elephantiasis.*

filaricide (fĭ-lăr′ĭ-sīd) [″+*caedere,* to kill] Something that destroys *Filaria.* **filaricidal** (-sīd′ăl), *adj.*

Filarioidea (fĭ-lăr″ē-oy′dē-ă) A superfamily of filarial nematodes that parasitize many animal species, including humans. SEE: *filariasis.*

file (fīl) **1.** A metal device with a roughened surface. It is used for shaping bones and teeth. **2.** In computing, data stored in a specifically designated area of the computer's memory.

filgrastim (phĭl-grăs′stĭm) Granulocyte colony-stimulating factor.

filiform (fĭl′ĭ-form) [″ + *forma,* form] **1.** In biology, pert. to a growth that is uniform along the inoculation line in stab or streak cultures. **2.** Hairlike; filamentous.

fillet (fĭl′ĕt) [Fr. *filet,* a band] **1.** A loop of thread, cord, or tape used to provide traction or suspension of tissue during surgery or obstetrical delivery. **2.** Lemniscus.

filling (fĭl′ĭng) [AS. *fyllan,* to fill] **1.** A material inserted into a cavity preparation. Common materials include amalgam, acrylics, resins, and glass ionomers. **2.** The operation of filling tooth cavities. SYN: *restoration.*

film **1.** A thin skin, membrane, or covering. **2.** A thin sheet of material, usually cellulose and coated with a light-sensitive emulsion, used in taking photographs. **3.** In microscopy, a thin layer of blood or other material spread on a slide or coverslip.

bite-wing f. A radiograph taken with a part of the film holder held between the teeth and the film parallel to the teeth. This technique permits films to be taken of several upper and lower teeth at the same time.

spot f. A radiograph of a small anatomical area.

x-ray f. A special photographic film with a sensitive emulsion layer that blackens in response to the light from intensifying screens. The emulsion has silver halide crystals immersed in gelatin. *Single-emulsion film* has the emulsion on one side of the cellulose base. It is used for digital, mammographic, and extremity imaging, in which high detail is necessary. *Duplitized film* has the emulsion on both sides of the cellulose base. It is used for general-purpose radiological studies.

film badge A badge containing film that is sensitive to x-rays. It is used to determine the cumulative exposure to x-rays of persons who work in radiology.

filovaricosis (fī″lō-văr-ī-kō′sĭs) [″ + *varix,* a dilated vein, + Gr. *osis,* condition] Dilatation or thickening of the axis cylinder of a nerve fiber.

filter [L. *filtrare,* to strain through] **1.** To pass a liquid through any porous substance that prevents particles larger than a certain size to pass through. **2.** A device for filtering liquids, light rays, or radiations. SEE: *absorption; osmosis.* **3.** Material, such as aluminum or molybdenum, inserted between the radiation source and the patient to absorb low-level radiation that would increase the dose.

Berkefeld f. A diatomaceous earth filter that removes bacteria from solutions passed through it, but allows virus-sized particles to pass through into the filtrate.

compensating f. In dentistry, a filter that shields less dense areas to produce a more nearly uniform radiographic image.

high efficiency particulate air f. ABBR: HEPA filter. An air filter capable of removing 99.7% of particles greater than O.3 μm in diameter.

infrared f. A filter that permits passage of only infrared waves of a certain wavelength.

membrane f. A filter made from biologically inert cellulose esters, polyethylene, or other porous materials.

Millipore f. Trademark name of a filter usually composed of cellulose acetate with controlled pore size that separates particles above specific sizes from the solutions that flow through.

optical f. A device that passes only a portion of the visible light spectrum. Absorption filters absorb the unwanted wavelengths. Interference filters employ the wave effects of constructive and destructive superposition to pass or inhibit appropriate wavelengths.

Pasteur-Chamberland f. An unglazed porcelain filter capable of retaining bacteria and some viruses. Either pressure or suction is required to force or draw the liquid through the filter.

umbrella f. A filter placed in a blood vessel to prevent emboli from passing that point. Once inserted, the device opens up like an umbrella. This technique has been used most commonly in the vena cava to prevent emboli in the veins from reaching the lungs, but has not been proven to be effective.

vena cava f. A wire apparatus inserted through a catheter into the inferior vena cava to prevent pulmonary emboli. SYN: *umbrella f.*

wedge f. A filter used in radiography and radiation therapy to vary the intensity of the x-ray beam. This compensates for differences in the thicknesses of the parts being exposed to radiation.

Wood's f. An ultraviolet light source used to diagnose some fungal and bacterial skin diseases.

filterable [L. *filtrare,* to strain through] Capable of passing through the pores of a porcelain filter, through which bacteria cannot pass.

filtrate (fĭl′trāt) The fluid that has been passed through a filter. The residue is the precipitate.

glomerular f. The fluid that passes from the blood through the capillary walls of the glomeruli of the kidney. It is similar to plasma but with far less protein; urine is formed from it.

filtration (fĭl-trā′shŭn) The process of removing particles from a solution by allowing the liquid portion to pass through a membrane or other partial barrier. This contains holes or spaces that allow the liquid to pass but are too small to permit passage of the solid particles. SEE: *filter.*

f. of x-ray photons The absorption of some longer-wavelength, low-energy x-ray photons by an absorbing medium placed in the path of the beam. Materials include aluminum, copper, molybdenum, and zinc.

filum (fī′lŭm) *pl.* **fila** [L.] A threadlike structure.

f. coronaria A fibrous band extending from the base of the medial cusp of the tricuspid valve to the aortic annulus.

f. terminale A long, slender filament of connective tissue at the end of the spinal cord.

fimbria (fĭm′brē-ă) *pl.* **fimbriae** [L., fringe] Any structure resembling a fringe or border.

f. ovarica The longest fringelike extremity of a fallopian tube, extending from the infundibulum close to the ovary.

f. tubae The fringelike portion at the abdominal end of a fallopian tube.

fimbriate, fimbriated (fĭm′brē-āt″, fĭm′brē-āt″ĕd) **1.** Having finger-like projections. **2.** Fringed.

fimbriocele (fĭm′brē-ō-sēl″) [″ + Gr. *kele,* tumor, swelling] A hernia including the fimbriated portion of the oviduct.

finasteride (fĭ-năs′tĕr-īd) A 5-alpha-reductase inhibitor used to treat benign prostatic hypertrophy and male hair loss. Trade name is Proscar.

fine motor skill Motor skills that require greater control of the small muscles than large ones, esp. those needed for hand-eye coordination, and those that require a high degree of precision in hand and finger movement. Examples of these motor skills include handwriting, sewing, and fastening buttons. It is important to note that most movements require both large and small muscle groups, and that although there is considerable overlap between fine and gross motor skills, a distinction between the two is useful in rehabilitation settings, special education, adapted physical education tests, motor development tests, and industrial and military aptitude tests.

fineness The proportion of pure gold in a gold alloy.

finger [AS.] One of the five digits of the hand.

baseball f. Permanent flexion resulting from violent posterior dislocation of the terminal phalanx onto the dorsum of the middle phalanx, as when an extended finger is struck on its tip. It is due to damage of the extensor tendon. SYN: *hammer f.; mallet f.*

clubbed f. clubbing.

dislocation of f. Displacement of a finger bone. This occurs only at a joint. If there has been a crushing injury, it should be treated as a fracture until radiography has been performed. Dislocations of a finger usually are easily diagnosed and quite easily reduced. They may be caused by blows, falls, and similar accidents.

First, it is important to ascertain that there is no fracture. Then the patient should be asked to steady and support the wrist (or have somebody else do so) for countertraction. The finger is grasped beyond the dislocated muscles and tendons and, with the free hand, the dislocated bone is slipped into place. A splint is applied from the tip of the finger well into the palm of the hand. The splint may be made of plastic, of tongue depressors, or temporarily of heavy cardboard.

CAUTION: No attempt should be made to reduce a dislocation of any finger joint until radiography has ruled out the possibility of fracture.

---

hammer f. A flexion deformity of the distal joint of a finger, caused by avulsion of the extensor tendon. SYN: *baseball f.*

hippocratic f. clubbing.

jersey f. A traumatic avulsion of the insertion of the flexor digitorum profundus, caused by a forceful extension motion during an active muscular contraction. It is commonly seen in football players. As a tackler grabs a defender's jersey, the defender pulls the jersey out of the tackler's hand.

mallet f. Baseball f.

seal f. An infection of the finger caused by the bite of a seal. The infectious agent, which has not been identified, is carried in the blood of the seal. It is sensitive to tetracycline.

webbed f. A congenital condition in which some or all of the fingers are fused; syndactylism.

finger cot A protective covering for a finger. It is usually made of plastic, rubber, metal, or leather. The injured finger is protected from trauma during the healing process. SYN: *finger-stall.*

finger ladder A device attached to a wall and in which notches are cut along an inclined line. The patient "walks" up this notched ladder by placing the fingertips in the notches. This self-stretching technique assists with shoulder flexion or abduction to maintain range of motion, and may be used to increase shoulder flexibility by stretching the extensors or adductors of the shoulder.

fingernail SEE: *nail.*

fingerprint An imprint made by the cutaneous ridges of the fleshy portion of the distal end of a finger. Fingerprints are used for identification because they are individually unique. SEE: illus.

finger separator Finger spreader.

finger spelling A method of communication used by persons with hearing or visual impairment in which words are spelled out letter by letter rather than depicted with single signs as in American Sign Language. Finger spelling can be done visually as well as tactually.

finger splint A padded strip of malleable metal used to immobilize a fractured finger. As an alternative, the injured finger is often "buddy taped" to an adjoining finger for support.

finger spreader An orthotic device, usually made of foam rubber, used to hold the thumb and fingers in extension while maintaining the normal arches of the hand. SYN: *finger separator*.

finger spring A device for assisting extension or flexion of finger joints.

finger-stall Finger cot.

finger-to-nose test A clinical test of cerebellar function. The patient stands with eyes closed and arms at the side and is asked to touch the nose with the tip of the finger.

finger trapping Using an adjacent digit to provide passive range of motion to an affected (injured, paralyzed) digit.

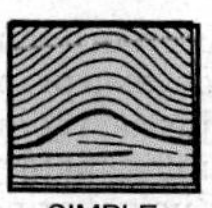

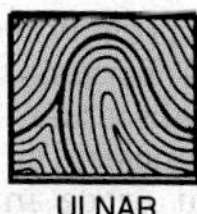

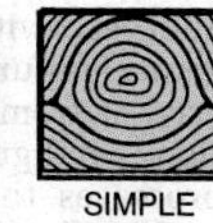

DERMATOGLYPHIC AREAS OF THE HAND

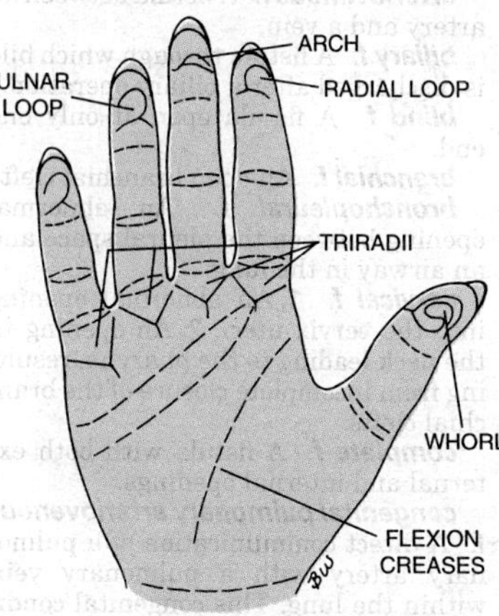

FINGERPRINTS

finite Having limits or boundaries.

Finklestein's test A test used to assist in the diagnosis of de Quervain's disease. The patient tucks the thumb in a closed fist, and the examiner deviates the fist ulnarly. Pain indicates a positive result.

FIO$_2$ *fractional concentration of inspired oxygen.*

fire [AS. *fyr*] **1.** Flame that produces heat. **2.** Fever.

St. Anthony's f. Former term for erysipelas.

fire-damp Methane, CH_4, found in coal mines.

first aid The administration of immediate care to an injured or acutely ill patient before the arrival of a physician or ALS unit and transport to either a physician's office or hospital emergency department. First aid is not a substitute for definitive care. SEE: *basic life support; burn; cardiopulmonary resuscitation; Standard and Universal Precautions Appendix.*

first cranial nerves The nerves supplying the nasal olfactory mucosa. They consist of delicate bundles of unmyelinated fibers, the fila olfactoria, which pass through the cribriform plate and terminate in the olfactory bulb. The fila are the central processes of bipolar receptor neurons of the olfactory mucous membrane. SYN: *olfactory nerves.*

first-degree atrioventricular block Delayed conduction through or from the atrioventricular node, marked on the electrocardiogram by a prolonged PR interval. Usually no treatment is necessary.

first intention healing Healing that takes place when wound edges are held or sutured together without the formation of obvious granulation tissue. SEE: *healing.*

first responder **1.** The first individual to arrive at the scene of an emergency. Many communities have made an effort to train public safety personnel (e.g., police and fire department) or other volunteers to respond to trauma and medical emergencies and provide CPR and first aid. **2.** The U.S. Department of Transportation training curriculum designed for the first arriving personnel on the scene of a medical emergency or traumatic event. The focus of this training is to assess and manage life-threatening emergencies.

Fishberg concentration test (fĭsh′bĕrg) [A. M. Fishberg, U.S. physician, 1898–1992] An obsolete test of the ability of the kidneys to produce urine of high specific gravity.

fishskin disease A skin disease characterized by increase of the horny layer with scaling and dryness. SYN: *ichthyosis.*

fission (fĭsh′ŭn) [L. *fissio*] **1.** Splitting into two or more parts. **2.** Bombardment or splitting of the nucleus of a heavy atom to release energy and neutrons.

binary f. Asexual reproduction, or cell division, in prokaryotic cells. The cell enlarges, duplicates its chromosome, and produces a transverse septum to form two identical daughter cells.

fissiparous (fĭ-sĭp′ă-rŭs) [L. *fissus,* cleft, + *parere,* to bring forth] Reproducing by fission.

fissura (fĭs-ū′ră) *pl.* **fissurae** [L.] A fissure.

fissure (fĭsh′ūr) [L. *fissura*] **1.** A groove, natural division, cleft, slit, or deep furrow in the brain, liver, spinal cord, and other organs. SYN: *fissura; sulcus.* **2.** An ulcer or cracklike sore. **3.** A break in the enamel of a tooth. **fissural,** *adj.*

anal f. A painful linear ulcer on the margin of the anus.

auricular f. A fissure of the petrous portion of the temporal bone.

f. of Bichat The fissure in the brain beneath the corpus callosum and above the diencephalon.

branchial f. SEE: *cleft, branchial.*

Broca's f. The fissure encircling the third left frontal convolution of the brain.

Burdach's f. The fissure connecting the lateral surface of the insula and the inner surface of the operculum of the brain.

calcarine f. The fissure extending from the occipital end of the cerebrum to the the occipitoparietal fissure.

callosomarginal f. A conspicuous fissure in the medial surface of the cerebral hemisphere running above and concentric with the curved upper surface of the corpus callosum.

central f. Rolando's f.

Clevenger's f. The inferior temporal fissure of the brain.

collateral f. The fissure on the inferior surface of the cerebral hemisphere separating the subcalcarine and subcollateral gyri.

Henle's f. Any of the connective tissue areas between the muscular fibers of the heart.

hippocampal f. The fissure extending from the posterior part of the corpus callosum to the tip of the temporal lobe of the brain.

horizontal f. Transverse f. (3).

inferior orbital f. The fissure at the apex of the orbit through which the infraorbital blood vessels and maxillary branch of the trigeminal nerve pass.

interparietal f. The intraparietal sulcus.

longitudinal f. **1.** The fissure on the lower surface of the liver. **2.** A fissure that separates the cerebral hemispheres; at its base is the corpus callosum, which connects the hemispheres.

occipitoparietal f. The fissure between the occipital and parietal lobes of the brain.

palpebral f. The opening separating the upper and lower eyelids.

portal f. The opening into the undersurface of the liver. It continues into the liver as the portal canal.

Rolando's f. The fissure separating the frontal and parietal lobes of the brain.

sphenoidal f. The fissure separating the wings and body of the sphenoid bone.

f. of Sylvius The fissure separating the frontal and parietal lobes from the temporal lobe of the brain.

transverse f. **1.** The fissure between the cerebellum and cerebrum. **2.** The fissure on the lower surface of the liver that serves as the hilum transmitting vessels and ducts to the liver. **3.** The fissure that divides the upper right lobe of the lung from the middle right lobe. SYN: *horizontal f.*

umbilical f. The anterior portion of the longitudinal fissure of the liver. It contains the round ligament, the obliterated umbilical vein.

Wernicke's f. The fissure dividing the temporal and parietal lobes from the occipital lobe of the brain.

zygal f. A transverse cerebral sulcus that connects two parallel sulci. The three sulci are in the form of an H.

fistula (fĭs′tū-lă) [L., *fistula,* pipe] An abnormal tubelike passage from a normal cavity or tube to a free surface or to another cavity. It may result from a congenital failure of organs to develop properly, or from abscesses, injuries, radiation, malignancies, or inflammatory processes that erode into neighboring organs. **fistulous** (-lŭs), *adj.*

anal f. A fistula near the anus.

arteriovenous f. A fistula between an artery and a vein.

biliary f. A fistula through which bile is discharged after a biliary operation.

blind f. A fistula open at only one end.

branchial f. An open branchial cleft.

bronchopleural f. An abnormal opening between the pleural space and an airway in the lung.

cervical f. **1.** An abnormal opening into the cervix uteri. **2.** An opening in the neck leading to the pharynx, resulting from incomplete closure of the branchial clefts.

complete f. A fistula with both external and internal openings.

congenital pulmonary arteriovenous f. A direct communication of a pulmonary artery with a pulmonary vein within the lung. This congenital condition allows blood to bypass the oxygenation process in the lungs.

craniosinus f. A fistula between the intracranial space and a paranasal sinus.

enterovaginal f. An abnormal canal between the bowel and vagina.

fecal f. A fistula in which there is a discharge of feces through the opening.

gastric f. A tract from the stomach to the abdominal wall or another internal organ, such as the small or large bowel.

horseshoe f. A perianal fistula in which the tract goes around the rectum and communicates with the skin at one or more points.

incomplete f. A fistula with only one opening, which leads to the skin (i.e., it does not communicate with an internal cavity or organ).

metroperitoneal f. An abnormal connection between the uterine and peritoneal cavities.

oroantral f. A communicating tract between the oral cavity and the maxillary sinus, occasionally resulting from the extraction of the first or second molar. It may become infected. Treatment varies with the size of the defect. Small lesions heal spontaneously; larger ones may be repaired with flap surgery or with prostheses.

parotid f. A fistula from the parotid gland to the skin surface.

perilymphatic f. A canal through which inner ear fluid may leak into the middle ear that may produce sudden hearing loss, tinnitus, or vertigo. The lesion, which can arise congenitally, after trauma, or by erosion, is one of the few examples of sensorineural hearing loss that can be repaired with surgery to the cochlear aqueduct.

perineovaginal f. An opening from the vagina through the perineum.

pilonidal f. A fistula beneath the skin at the lower end of the spinal column resulting from a pilonidal cyst.

rectovaginal f. An opening between the rectum and the vagina.

thyroglossal f. A midline fistula just above the thyroid that connects the openings in the skin to a persistent embryonic thyroglossal duct.

tracheoesophageal f. A congenital defect linking the trachea and the esophagus, resulting from failure of the lungs to separate from the gastrointestinal tract during embryological development. Surgery is needed to prevent recurring episodes of aspiration pneumonia in the newborn.

umbilical f. An abnormal congenital passageway between the umbilicus and the gut. It is usually due to nonclosure of the urachal duct.

ureterovaginal f. A fistula between the ureter and the vagina.

vesicouterine f. An abnormal connection between the urinary bladder and the uterus.

vesicovaginal f. An abnormal connection between the urinary bladder and the vagina, usually resulting from surgical trauma, irradiation, or malignancy.

fistulatome (fĭs′tū-lă-tōm″) [″ + Gr. *tome,* incision] An instrument for incising a fistula.

fistulectomy (fĭs″tū-lĕk′tō-mē) [″ + Gr. *ektome,* excision] Excision of a fistula.

fistulization (fĭs″tŭ-lī-zā′shŭn) [L. *fistula,* pipe] The process of becoming fistulous by extension of an inflammatory process from one tissue organ to another.

fistuloenterostomy (fĭs″tū-lō-ĕn-tĕr-ŏs′tō-mē) [″ + Gr. *enteron,* intestine, + *stoma,* mouth] Surgical closure of a biliary fistula and formation of a new biliary passage into the intestine.

fit (fĭt) [AS. *fitt*] **1.** A sudden attack, convulsion, or paroxysm. SEE: *convulsion.* **2.** Modification of one structure to that of another, as in dental restoration.

fitness, biological The ability of an individual with a disease to produce children who survive to adult life and are themselves able to reproduce.

fitness, physical SEE: *physical fitness.*

fix **1.** To treat tissues chemically so that the components and products of the cells are preserved for staining and microscopic examination. **2.** Slang for a dose of a drug of abuse. **3.** In film processing, the step that stops the development action, removes the undeveloped silver halide crystals, and makes the image permanent.

fixation [L. *fixatio*] **1.** The act of holding or fastening in a rigid position. The act of immobilizing or making rigid. **2.** Rigidity or immobility. **3.** A phase of Freudian psychosexual development in which the libido is arrested at an early or presexual level. **4.** Staining of microscopic specimens for examination. **5.** The process of making a film-recorded image permanent.

binocular f. Focusing of both eyes on an object.

complement f. The action of complement (a series of plasma proteins) on an antigen-antibody complex. In the body, it brings about lysis of cellular foreign antigens. Complement is the basis for complement fixation tests, which determine the presence of particular antibodies (or antigens) in a patient's serum. SEE: *complement.*

external f. The use of external devices, such as pins, in fractured bone segments to keep them in place.

f. of eyes Movement of the eyes so that the visual axes meet and the image of an object falls on corresponding points of each retina. This provides the most acute visualization of the object.

field of f. The widest limits of vision in all directions within which the eyes can fixate.

internal f. The use of internal wires, screws, or pins applied directly to fractured bone segments to keep them in place.

fixative (fĭk′să-tĭv) [L. *fixus,* fastened] **1.** A substance that firms or makes rigid. **2.** A substance used to preserve normal and pathological specimens for gross examination or for the sectioning and preparation of microscope slides.

fixed-dose combination Combining two or more drugs in one capsule or tablet, in order to simplify drug regimens and improve compliance.

Fl *fluid.*

flaccid (flăk′sĭd) [L. *flaccidus,* flabby] Relaxed; flabby; having defective or absent muscular tone.

flagella (flă-jĕl′ă) [L.] Pl. of flagellum.

flagellant (flăj′ĕ-lănt) [L. *flagellum,* whip] **1.** Pert. to a flagellum. **2.** Pert. to stroking in massage. **3.** One who practices flagellation.

flagellate (flăj′ĕ-lāt) **1.** Having one or more flagella. **2.** A protozoon with one or more flagella.

flagellation (flăj″ĕ-lā′shŭn) **1.** Whipping. **2.** Massage by strokes. **3.** A form of sexual behavior in which the libido is stimulated by whipping oneself, being whipped, or whipping someone else. **4.** The arrangement of flagella on the surface of a microorganism.

flagelliform (flă-jĕl′ĭ-form) [″ + *forma,* shape] Shaped like a flagellum.

flagellum (flă-jĕl′ŭm) *pl.* **flagella** [L., whip] A threadlike structure that provides motility for certain bacteria and protozoa (one, few, or many per cell) and for spermatozoa (one per cell).

flag sign A peculiar change in hair color in which the hair becomes discolored in a band perpendicular to its long axis. This is seen in kwashiorkor and indicates a period of severe malnutrition.

flammable Burning easily.

flange (flănj) **1.** A border that projects above the main structure. **2.** In dentistry, the part of an artificial denture that extends from the embedded teeth to the border of the denture.

flank [O. Fr. *flanc*] The part of the body between the ribs and the upper border of the ilium. The term also refers loosely to the outer side of the thigh, hip, and buttock. SEE: *latus*.

flannelmouth A colloquial and disparaging term for a patient with dysarthria.

flap [Dutch *flappen,* to strike] **1.** A mass of partially detached tissue. **2.** A mass of partially detached tissued incurred by accidental trauma used in plastic surgery of an adjacent area or in covering the end of a bone after resection. **3.** An uncontrolled movement seen in some diseases. SEE: *asterixis*.

amputation f. A flap of skin used to cover the end of a part left after an amputation.

island f. A skin flap or myocutaneous tissue in which the edges are free but the center is attached and contains the vascular supply.

jump f. A skin flap moved from place to place by successively cutting one end and attaching it to a new site once vascularity is established on the stationary portion.

mucoperiosteal f. A flap of mucosal tissue, including the underlying periosteum, reflected from the bone during oral surgery.

pedicle f. In plastic surgery, a type of flap that is attached by a pedicle to its source of blood supply. The other end may be attached to a site from which a new blood supply will develop. This permits the eventual severance of the original pedicle, so the flap may be moved step by step to where it is needed in the plastic surgical procedure. SYN: *pedicle graft*. SEE: *jump f.*

periodontal f. A section of soft tissue surgically separated from underlying bone and removed or repositioned to eliminate periodontal pockets or to correct mucogingival defects.

skin f. A flap containing only skin.

sliding f. Horizontal movement of a flap to cover a nearby denuded area.

tube f. A variety of pedicle flap which is fashioned into a tubular configuration. SEE: *pedicle f.*

flare 1. A flush or spreading area of redness that surrounds a line made by drawing a pointed instrument across the skin. It is the second reaction in the triple response of skin to injury and is due to dilatation of the arterioles. SEE: *triple response*. **2.** Exacerbation of a disease, such as rheumatoid arthritis.

flaring, nasal Dilation of the nostrils during inspiration; a sign of respiratory distress.

flash 1. A hot flash. A flush accompanied by a sensation of heat. It is common during menopause. SYN: *hot flush*. SEE: *menopause*. **2.** Excess material from a mold.

flashback The return of imagery and hallucinations after the immediate effects of a traumatic or hallucinogenic experience. SEE: *hallucinogen*.

flash method 1. A means of pasteurizing milk by rapidly raising its temperature to 178°F (80.1°C), maintaining it there for a few minutes, and rapidly chilling it until the temperature is 40°F (4.4°C). SEE: *pasteurization*. **2.** A fast low-angle shot method of obtaining magnetic resonance images.

flask [LL. *flasco*] A small bottle with a narrow neck.

flatfoot Abnormal flatness of the sole and the arch of the foot. This condition may exist without causing symptoms or interfering with normal function of the foot. The inner longitudinal and anterior transverse metatarsal arches may be depressed. This condition may be acute, subacute, or chronic. SYN: *pes planus; splayfoot*. SEE: illus.

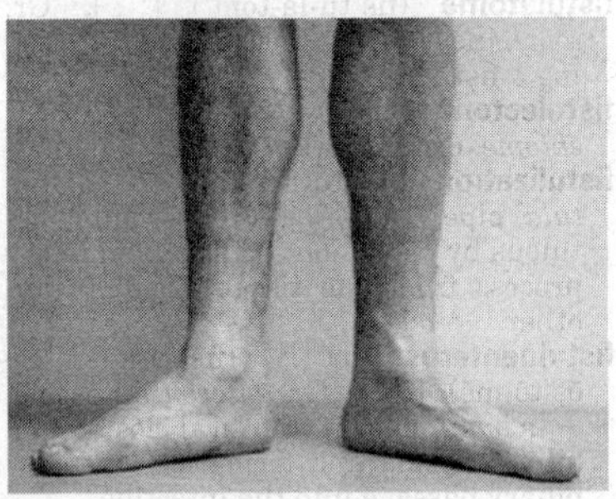

FLATFOOT (PES PLANUS)

spasmodic f. Flatfoot in which the foot is held everted by spasmodic contraction of the peroneal muscle.

flatness Resonance heard on percussion over solid organs or when there is fluid in the thoracic cavity.

flatplate A radiograph requiring a frontal projection of the abdomen or other body part with the patient supine.

flatulence (flăt′ū-lĕns) [L. *flatulentus*] Excessive gas in the stomach and intestines. SEE: *distention; gastrointestinal decompression; paralytic ileus; Wangensteen tube*. **flatulent,** *adj.*

PATIENT CARE: Initial assessment should include auscultation of bowel sounds, percussion, and observation and measurement of abdominal girth. The patient is questioned about the presence and location of any pain or cramping and the passage of flatus. If the situation is acute in onset or associated with severe pain or altered vital signs, x-rays or other investigative studies may be ordered. If the condition is deemed functional, ambulation is encouraged to increase peristalsis. If the patient cannot ambulate or if ambulation is ineffective, the patient is turned from side to side (or as permitted by activity restrictions). If the gaseous accumulation is thought to be intracolonic, laxative suppositories or enemas may be given to help the patient expel flatus and to relieve gaseous distention. If the patient is able to eat, medications containing simethicone may provide some degree of relief. If bowel sounds decrease or abdominal distention increases (as demonstrated by percussion, abdominal girth measurement, and increasing patient discomfort) and flatus is not passed, a diagnosis of ileus is suggested.

flatus (flā′tŭs) [L., a blowing] **1.** Gas in the digestive tract. **2.** Expelling of gas from a body orifice, esp. the anus. The average person excretes 400 to 1200 cc of gas each day. The gas passages may average a dozen a day in some persons and up to a hundred in others. Flatus from the lower intestinal tract contains hydrogen, methane, skatoles, indoles, carbon dioxide, and small amounts of oxygen and nitrogen. SEE: *borborygmus; eructation.*

Foods known for their ability to cause excess intestinal gas include beans, peas, lentils, cabbage, onions, Brussels sprouts, bananas, apples, raisins, apricots, high-fiber cereals, whole wheat products, milk and milk products, and sorbitol present in some dietetic foods.

TREATMENT: Some persons can control excess intestinal gas by avoiding foods they have found to be flatulogenic. Others in whom there is no distinct relationship to foods should be reassured that flatulence, although sometimes socially awkward or embarrassing, is not detrimental to health.

Administration of the enzyme alpha-D-galactosidase derived from *Aspergillus niger* may be effective in treating intestinal gas or bloating due to eating a variety of grains, cereals, nuts, and seeds of vegetables containing sugars such as raffinose or verbacose. This includes oats, wheat, beans, peas, lentils, foods containing soy, pistachios, broccoli, Brussels sprouts, cabbage, carrots, corn, onions, squash, and cauliflower.

vaginal f. Expulsion of air from the vagina. Air can enter the vagina during sexual intercourse.

flatus tube A rectal tube to facilitate expulsion of flatus. It formerly was used in cases of severe distention or before a saline enema.

flatworm A worm belonging to the phylum Platyhelminthes.

flavescent (flă-vĕs′ĕnt) Yellowish.

flavin (flā′vĭn) One of a group of natural water-soluble pigments occurring in milk, yeasts, bacteria, and some plants. All contain the flavin or isoalloxazine nucleus and are yellow. Flavin is present in riboflavin and nicotinamide adenine dinucleotide dehydrogenase.

flavin adenine dinucleotide ABBR: FAD. A hydrogen carrier in the citric acid cycle of cell respiration; it is a derivative of riboflavin.

flavism (flā′vĭzm) [L. *flavus,* yellow, + Gr. *-ismos,* condition] Having a yellow tinge.

flavivirus (flā″vē-vī′rŭs) A genus of Togaviridae. They were previously called group B arboviruses. Viruses that cause yellow fever, certain types of encephalitis, and dengue are species in this genus.

Flavobacterium A genus of rod-shaped bacteria belonging to the Achromobacteraceae. They are found in soil and water and produce an orange-yellow pigment in cultures. *Flavobacterium meningosepticum* is esp. virulent for premature infants, in whom it causes meningitis. The fatality rate is high.

flavone (flā′vōn) $C_{15}H_{10}O_2$; the chemical from which the natural colors of many vegetables are derived.

flavoprotein One of a group of conjugated proteins that contain nicotinamide adenine dinucleotide (NAD) phosphate and NAD dehydrogenase, enzymes that are essential in cellular respiration.

flavor (flā′vor) **1.** The quality of a substance that affects the sense of taste. It may also stimulate the sense of smell. **2.** A material added to a food or medicine to improve its taste.

flaxseed The seed of *Linum usitatissimum.* SYN: *linseed.*

fl. dr. *fluidram.*

flea (flē) [AS. *flea*] Any insect of the order Siphonaptera. Fleas are wingless, suck blood, and have legs adapted for jumping. Usually they are parasitic on warm-blooded animals including humans. Fleas of the genus *Xenopsylla* transmit the plague bacillus *(Yersinia pestis)* from rats to humans. Fleas may transmit other diseases such as tularemia, endemic typhus, and brucellosis. They are intermediate hosts for cat and dog tapeworms. SEE: illus.

f. bite A hemorrhagic punctum surrounded by erythematous and urticarial patches and caused by the injection of flea saliva.

TREATMENT: Ice applied to the site decreases the pain. Application of a cor-

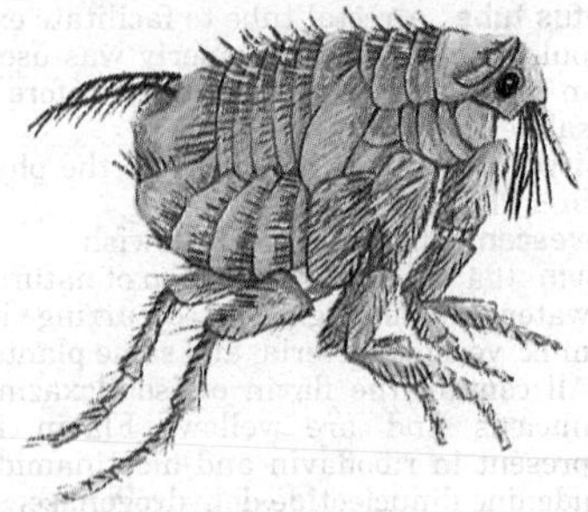

FLEA

Xenopsylla (orig. mag. ×15)

ticosteroid cream may decrease the inflammatory response.

PREVENTION: The skin should be treated with an insect repellent available as a powder, spray, or oil for topical use.

cat f. *Ctenocephalides felis.*

chigger f. *Tunga penetrans.* SYN: *chiggers; jigger.*

dog f. *Ctenocephalides canis.*

human f. *Pulex irritans.*

rat f. *Xenopsylla cheopis.*

flea infestation The harboring of fleas, esp. in a home with dogs or cats. It is possible to kill the flea population by treating the house for 24 hr by using naphthalene, permethrins, and other substances.

CAUTION: Any plants, pets, or humans could suffer adverse effects if they remain in the house during the treatment period. The house should be thoroughly ventilated afterwards to remove the fumes.

flecainide acetate An antiarrhythmic drug. Trade name is Tambocor.

Flechsig's areas (flĕk'zĭgz) [Paul E. Flechsig, Ger. neurologist, 1847–1929] The anterior, lateral, and posterior areas of each lateral half of the medulla of the brain.

fleece of Stilling A meshwork of white fibers that surrounds the dentate nucleus of the cerebellum.

Fleming, Sir Alexander (flĕm'ĭng) A Scottish physician, 1881–1955, who in 1945, along with Ernst B. Chain and Sir Howard W. Florey, was awarded the Nobel Prize in medicine and physiology for the discovery of penicillin.

flesh [AS. *flaesc*] The soft tissues of the animal body, esp. the muscles. SEE: *carnivorous; meat.*

examination of animal f. An obsolete method of examining food to ensure its safety, long promulgated by the U.S. Department of Agriculture. The technique, which cannot identify serious bacterial contamination, relied on gross inspection of food color, consistency, odor, and after cooking, its flavor.

goose f. Cutis anserina.

proud f. Pyogenic granuloma.

Fletcher factor A blood clotting factor, prekallikrein.

fletcherism [Horace Fletcher, U.S. dietitian, 1849–1919] Taking small amounts of food at a time. These small bites are chewed for a prolonged period prior to swallowing. SEE: *psomophagia.*

Fletcher-Suit system The most commonly used applicator for brachytherapy of gynecological malignancies.

flex [L. *flexus,* bent] To bend on itself, as a muscle.

flexibilitas cerea (flĕks″ĭ-bĭl'ĭ-tăs sē'rē-ă) [L.] Waxy flexibility.

flexibility [L. *flexus,* bent] The quality of bending without breaking; adaptability. SYN: *pliability.*

relative f. Increased mobility or frequency of movement in a joint adjacent to a body part with restricted mobility, such as an injured muscle, bone, capsule, tendon, or ligament. This can be a normal relationship between segments, but can cause pathology and impairments. Relative flexibility can account for overuse, sprain, or strain of a joint due to stiffness in an adjacent joint. For example, lumbar spine strain due to short hamstrings limits hip motion.

waxy f. A cataleptic state in which limbs retain any position in which they are placed. It is characteristic of catatonic patients. SYN: *flexibilitas cerea.* **flexible,** *adj.*

flexile (flĕks'ĭl) [L. *flexus,* bent] Pliant, flexible.

flexion (flĕk'shŭn) [L. *flexio*] **1.** The act of bending or condition of being bent in contrast to extension. SEE: *antecurvature.* **2.** Decrease in the angle between the bones forming a joint.

flexor (flĕks'or) [L.] A muscle that brings two bones closer together, causing flexion of the part or a decreased angle of the joint. Opposed to extensor.

flexura (flĕk-shoo'ră) [L.] A flexure.

flexure (flĕk'shĕr) [L. *flexura*] A bend.

dorsal f. A convex curve in the thoracic area of the spine.

duodenojejunal f. A curve at the meeting point of the jejunum and duodenum.

hepatic f. The bend of the colon under the liver; the junction of the ascending and transverse colon. SYN: *right colic f.*

left colic f. A bend at the transition point where the transverse colon becomes the descending colon. SYN: *splenic f.*

right colic f. Hepatic f.

sigmoid f. An S-like curve (in the left iliac fossa) of the descending colon as it joins the rectum. Former name for sigmoid colon. SEE: *colon* for illus.

splenic f. Left colic f.

flicker The visual sensation of alternating intervals of brightness caused by rhythmic interruption of light stimuli.

flicker phenomenon A sensation of continuous light caused by an intermittent light stimulus produced at a certain rate.

flight into disease Ready adoption of a sick status to escape reality.

flight into health Voluntary and temporary suppression of mental or physical symptoms to prevent further psychoanalytic probing into the patient's psyche.

flip-flop A condition in which the reduction in fraction of inspired oxygen to reduce hypoxemia in infants causes a persistent and greater-than-expected decrease in oxygen tension (PaO_2).

floater (flō'tĕr) [AS. *flotian,* float] A translucent speck that passes across the visual field. Floaters vary in size and shape. They are due to small bits of protein or cells floating in the vitreous. Most people have these benign materials in their eyes. SEE: *muscae volitantes.*

floating [AS *flota,* a raft] **1.** Moving about; out of normal location. **2.** A staffing arrangement in which one may be asked to work on any of several hospital wards or units, depending on the immediate needs of the health care institution.

floating ribs The 11th and 12th ribs, which do not articulate with the sternum.

floccillation, floccitation (flŏk"sĭ-lā'shŭn, -tā'shŭn) [L. *floccilatio*] Semiconscious picking at bedclothes in association with fever, stupor, and delirium. SYN: *carphology.*

floccose (flŏk'ōs) [L. *floccosus,* full of wool tufts] In biology, pert. to a growth consisting of short and densely but irregularly interwoven filaments.

flocculence (flŏk'ū-lĕns") Resemblance to shreds or tufts of cotton.

flocculent (flŏk'ū-lĕnt) **1.** Resembling tufts or shreds of cotton. **2.** Pert. to a fluid or culture containing whitish shreds of mucus.

flocculus (flŏk'ū-lŭs) *pl.* **flocculi** [L., little tuft] **1.** A small tuft of woollike fibers. **2.** A lobe below and behind the middle peduncle of the cerebrum on each side of the median fissure. **floccular,** *adj.*

flood **1.** A pathological uterine hemorrhage. **2.** Excessive menstrual bleeding.

flooding (flŭd'ĭng) **1.** A colloquial term for excessive menstrual flow. **2.** In treating phobias, repeated exposure to the disturbing ideas, situations, or conditions until these no longer produce anxiety.

Flood's ligament [Valentine Flood, Ir. surgeon, 1800–1847] A band of ligaments attached to the lower part of the lesser tuberosity of the humerus.

floor [AS. *flor*] The surface that forms the lower limit of a cavity or space, as the floor of the cranial cavity, fourth ventricle, mouth, nasal fossa, pelvis, or a cavity preparation in a tooth.

floppy-valve syndrome Mitral valve prolapse.

flora [L. *flos,* flower] **1.** Plant life as distinguished from animal life. **2.** Microbial life occurring or adapted for living in a specific environment, such as the intestinal, vaginal, oral, urinary tract, or skin flora. SEE: *fauna.*

intestinal f. Bacteria present in the intestines. Bacteria do not exist in the intestines at birth but appear very shortly thereafter. These bacteria produce vitamins, esp. vitamin K, and inhibit the growth of pathogens. Certain antibiotics may cause drastic alterations in the number and kinds of bacteria present. SEE: *Clostridium difficile.*

normal f. Potentially pathogenic organisms that are harmless in certain areas of the body, including bacteria, fungi, and protozoa found on the skin and mucosa of the gastrointestinal and genitourinary tracts, that protect the body from pathogens. When one type of normal flora is destroyed, an overgrowth of others can occur. For example, when the bacteria are killed by antibiotics, fungal growth, usually from *Candida,* appears in the mouth, vagina, and moist skin folds, requiring treatment with an antifungal agent. Destruction of normal flora can also permit infection by more serious agents. SEE: *colitis, pseudomembranous; infection; microorganism.*

The ability of the body to provide an environment that prevents overgrowth of certain species of bacteria is remarkable. The largest concentration of bacteria in humans is in the colon, where more than 400 genera may coexist. In the colon, anaerobic bacteria outnumber aerobic bacteria 1000:1, and there may be 10^{11} per g of fecal material. The anaerobic gram-positive lactobacilli may be concentrated in the vagina at the 10^5 to 10^8/ml level, but 20% of women have no detectable anaerobes in the vagina. In dental plaque and gingival sulci, the bacteria may reach a concentration of 10^{12}/ml.

florid [L. *floridus,* blossoming] **1.** Bright deep-red. The term describes skin coloration. **2.** Complete or full-bodied, as in an illness that is in full flower.

floss **1.** A waxed or unwaxed tape or thread used to clean and remove plaque between teeth and below the gumline. SYN: *dental f.* **2.** To use dental floss or tape to remove plaque and calculus from the otherwise inaccessible dental surfaces between teeth.

dental f. Floss (1).

flour [L. *flos,* flower] Finely ground meal obtained from wheat or other grain; any soft fine powder.

flow [AS. *flowan,* to flow] **1.** Movement with respect to time. **2.** The act of moving or running freely.

laminar f. laminar air flow.

peak f. The maximum volume of air that can be expelled from the lungs during a vigorous exhalation. Its measurement is used to determine the degree of respiratory impairment in patients with obstructive lung diseases.

turbulent f. A movement of gas in disorderly currents, associated with high velocity and high density with increased tubing diameter.

flow cell A type of optical cell employed in photometers and cell counters through which the sample and any standards are passed for detection. SEE: *cytometry*.

flowmeter A device for measuring the movement of a gas or liquid. It is used esp. in monitoring the use of anesthetic gases.

flow state An altered state of consciousness in which the mind functions at its peak, time may seem distorted, and a sense of happiness seems to pervade that period. In such a state the individual feels alive and fully attentive to what is being done. This state is distinguished from strained attention, in which the person forces himself or herself to perform a task in which he or she has little interest.

floxuridine (flŏks-ŭr′ĭ-dēn) An antimetabolite used to treat solid cancers (e.g., adenocarcinomas).

fl. oz. *fluidounce*.

flu (floo) 1. Influenza. **2.**. An imprecise term for any respiratory or gastrointestinal illness.

fluctuant (flŭk′chū-ănt) Varying or unstable. SEE: *fluctuation*.

fluctuation [L. *fluctuatio*] **1.** A variation from one course to another. **2.** A wavy impulse felt in palpation and produced by vibration of body fluid.

DIAGNOSIS: If fluctuation is felt over the lower abdomen, ascites usually is present. Fluctuation may be caused by peritoneal hemorrhage. If it is confined to a limited portion of the abdomen, tuberculous peritonitis may be implicated; over the central portion, bladder distention; in the lower abdomen in women, an ovarian cyst or pregnancy; in the right hypochondrium, a hydatid cyst, liver abscess, or distended gallbladder; over the left hypochondrium, cysts or abscess; above the umbilicus, a dilated colon or stomach partly filled with fluid and gas.

flucytosine (flū-sī′tō-sēn″) An antifungal drug used to treat candida, cryptococci, and other fungi. It is used with amphotericin B to improve the efficacy of therapy against cryptococcal meningitis.

fludrocortisone (floo″drō-kor′tĭ-sōn) A synthetic corticosteroid.

f. acetate A corticosteroid drug. Trade name is Florinef Acetate.

fluency (floo′ĕn-sē) The ease and efficiency of speech; the production of speech without pauses, lapses, or hesitation. **fluent,** *adj.*

fluid [L. *fluidus*] A nonsolid, liquid, or gaseous substance. SEE: *secretion*.

allantoic f. Fluid found in the fetal membrane that develops from the yolk sac.

amniotic f. A clear liquid that fills the amniotic cavity during pregnancy. Its primary functions are to suspend and to protect the growing fetus. Although its origin is uncertain, amniotic fluid may be derived from amnionic secretions and/or maternal vascular transudate. By gestational week 12, fetal urine contributes to it. Volume increases from about 50 ml at 12 gestational weeks to around 1000 ml at 38 weeks. Approximately one-half the total volume (e.g., 500 ml) is replaced hourly through bidirectional maternal-fetal exchange of water. The fluid is 98% water and contains electrolytes, lipids, proteins, urea and creatinine, bilirubin, epidermal cells, lanugo, and vernix caseosa. Samples of amniotic fluid may be collected to identify fetal chromosomal abnormalities or to estimate fetal maturity. SEE: *amniocentesis; oligohydramnios; polyhydramnios*.

cerebrospinal f. ABBR: CSF. A watery cushion that protects the brain and spinal cord from physical impact and bathes the brain in electrolytes and proteins. SEE: *blood-brain barrier; lumbar puncture*.

FORMATION: The fluid is formed by the choroid plexuses of the lateral and third ventricles. That of the lateral ventricles passes through the foramen of Monro to the third ventricle, and through the aqueduct of Sylvius to the fourth ventricle. There it may escape through the central foramen of Magendie or the lateral foramina of Luschke into the cisterna magna and to the cranial and spinal subarachnoid spaces. It is reabsorbed through the arachnoid villi into the blood in the cranial venous sinuses, and through the perineural lymph spaces of both the brain and the cord. SEE: illus. (Formation, Circulation, and Reabsorption of Cerebrospinal Fluid).

CHARACTERISTICS: The fluid is normally watery, clear, colorless, and almost entirely free of cells. The initial pressure of spinal fluid in a side-lying adult is about 100 to 180 mm of water. On average, the total protein is about 15 to 50 mg/dl, and the concentration of

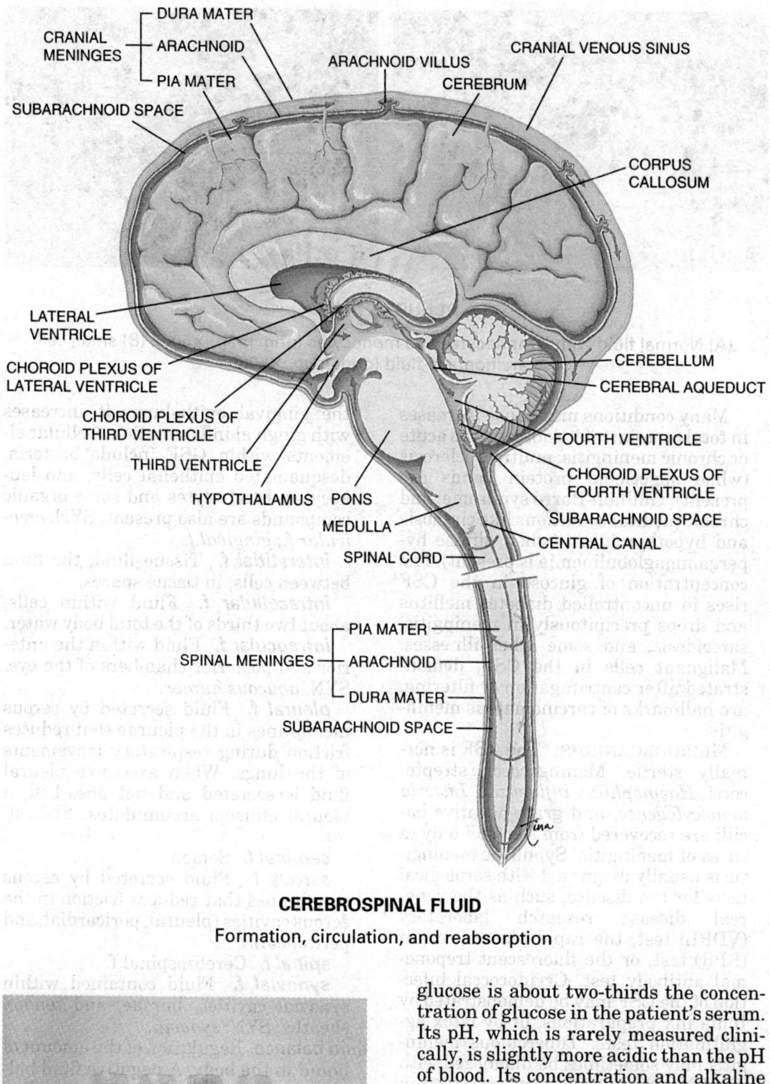

DURA MATER
CRANIAL MENINGES
ARACHNOID
PIA MATER
SUBARACHNOID SPACE
ARACHNOID VILLUS
CEREBRUM
CRANIAL VENOUS SINUS
CORPUS CALLOSUM
LATERAL VENTRICLE
CHOROID PLEXUS OF LATERAL VENTRICLE
CHOROID PLEXUS OF THIRD VENTRICLE
THIRD VENTRICLE
HYPOTHALAMUS
PONS
MEDULLA
SPINAL CORD
CEREBELLUM
CEREBRAL AQUEDUCT
FOURTH VENTRICLE
CHOROID PLEXUS OF FOURTH VENTRICLE
SUBARACHNOID SPACE
CENTRAL CANAL
SPINAL MENINGES
PIA MATER
ARACHNOID
DURA MATER
SUBARACHNOID SPACE

CEREBROSPINAL FLUID

Formation, circulation, and reabsorption

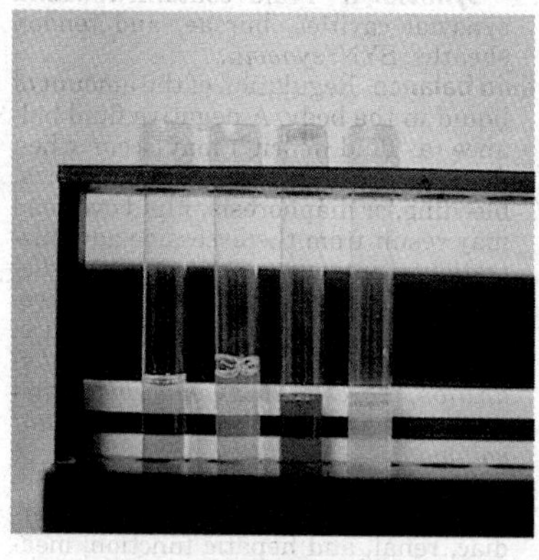

CEREBROSPINAL FLUID

(Left to right) normal, xanthochromic, hemolyzed, cloudy

glucose is about two-thirds the concentration of glucose in the patient's serum. Its pH, which is rarely measured clinically, is slightly more acidic than the pH of blood. Its concentration and alkaline reserve are similar to those of blood. It does not clot on standing. Turbidity suggests an excessively high number of cells in the fluid, typically white blood cells in infection or red blood cells in hemorrhage. SEE: illus. (Cerebrospinal Fluid Specimens).

CSF may appear red following a recent subarachnoid hemorrhage or when the lumbar puncture that obtained the CSF caused traumatic injury to the dura that surround the fluid. Centrifugation of the fluid can distinguish between these two sources of blood in the spinal fluid: the supernatant is usually stained yellow (xanthochromic) only when there has been a recent subarachnoid hemorrhage.

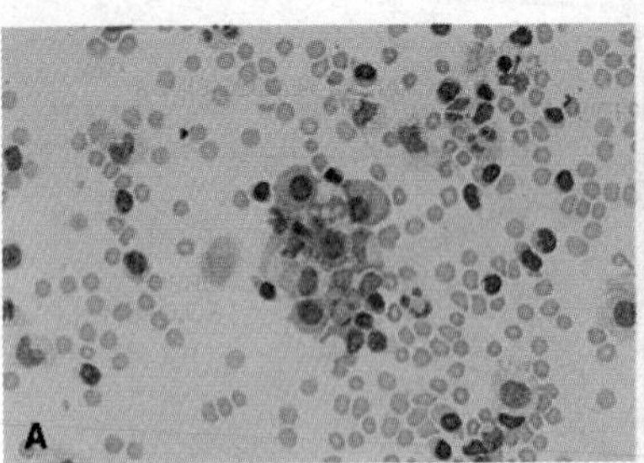

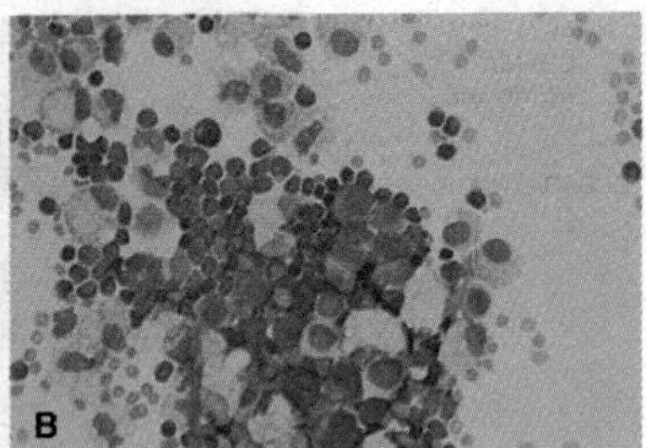

PLEURAL FLUID

(A) Normal fluid with lymphocytes and monocytes (orig. mag. ×500), (B) small cell carcinoma in fluid (orig. mag. ×500)

Many conditions may cause increases in total protein: infections, such as acute or chronic meningitis; multiple sclerosis (when oligoclonal protein bands are present); Guillain-Barré syndrome; and chronic medical conditions like cirrhosis and hypothyroidism (when diffuse hypergammaglobulinemia is present). The concentration of glucose in the CSF rises in uncontrolled diabetes mellitus and drops precipitously in meningitis, sarcoidosis, and some other illnesses. Malignant cells in the CSF, demonstrated after centrifugation or filtering, are hallmarks of carcinomatous meningitis.

MICROORGANISMS: The CSF is normally sterile. Meningococci, streptococci, *Haemophilus influenzae, Listeria monocytogenes,* and gram-negative bacilli are recovered from the CSF only in cases of meningitis. Syphilitic meningitis is usually diagnosed with serological tests for the disease, such as the venereal disease research laboratory (VDRL) test, the rapid plasma reagin (RPR) test, or the fluorescent treponemal antibody test. Cryptococcal infection of the CSF may be demonstrated by India ink preparations, or by latex agglutination tests. Tuberculous meningitis may sometimes be diagnosed with Ziehl-Neelsen stains, but more often this is done with cultures. These last three infections (syphilis, cryptococcosis, and tuberculosis) are much more common in patients who have acquired immunodeficiency syndrome (AIDS) than in the general population.

crevicular f. Gingival sulcular f.

extracellular f. All body fluid outside cells, including tissue fluid, plasma, and lymph.

extravascular f. All the body fluids outside the blood vessels. They include tissue fluid, fluids within the serous and synovial cavities, cerebrospinal fluid, and lymph.

gingival f. Gingival sulcular f.

gingival sulcular f. ABBR: GSF. In dentistry, the fluid that seeps through the gingival epithelium. It increases with gingival inflammation. Cellular elements within GSF include bacteria, desquamated epithelial cells, and leukocytes. Electrolytes and some organic compounds are also present. SYN: *crevicular f.; gingival f.*

interstitial f. Tissue fluid; the fluid between cells, in tissue spaces.

intracellular f. Fluid within cells, about two thirds of the total body water.

intraocular f. Fluid within the anterior and posterior chambers of the eye. SYN: *aqueous humor*.

pleural f. Fluid secreted by serous membranes in the pleurae that reduces friction during respiratory movements of the lungs. When excessive pleural fluid is secreted and not absorbed, a pleural effusion accumulates. SEE: illus.

seminal f. Semen.

serous f. Fluid secreted by serous membranes that reduces friction in the serous cavities (pleural, pericardial, and peritoneal).

spinal f. Cerebrospinal f.

synovial f. Fluid contained within synovial cavities, bursae, and tendon sheaths. SYN: *synovia*.

fluid balance Regulation of the amount of liquid in the body. A negative fluid balance (a "fluid deficit") may occur when fluids are lost by vomiting, diarrhea, bleeding, or diaphoresis. Fluid overload may result from the excessive administration of intravenous fluids, or in diseases marked by impaired fluid excretion, such as congestive heart failure, cirrhosis, or renal failure. SEE: *dehydration; diuresis; fluid replacement;* and entries beginning with the words *fluid volume*.

Treatment of fluid imbalances depends on the cause; the patient's cardiac, renal, and hepatic function; measured serum electrolytes; and acid-base balance.

Useful means of gauging changes in fluid balance are 1) to measure fluid inputs and outputs; or 2) to measure day-to-day variations in body weight.

fluid diet A nutritional plan for persons unable to chew and swallow solid food or for patients whose gastrointestinal tract must be free of solid matter.

fluidextract, fluidextractum [L. *fluidus,* fluid, + *extractum,* extract] A solution of the soluble constituents of vegetable drugs in which each cubic centimeter or milliliter represents 1 g of the drug. Fluidextracts contain alcohol as a solvent or preservative. Many of them form precipitates when water is added.

aromatic cascara f. A liquid preparation of cascara sagrada, magnesium oxide, glycyrrhiza extract, saccharin, anise oil, coriander oil, methyl salicylate, alcohol, and water. It can be used as a laxative.

glycyrrhiza f. A liquid preparation of glycyrrhiza.

fluidounce SYMB: f℥. An apothecaries' measure of fluid volume, equal to 8 fluidrams or 29.57 ml.

fluidram SYMB: fʒ. An apothecaries' measure of fluid volume, equal to 3.697 ml.

fluid replacement Administration of fluids by any route to correct fluid and electrolyte deficits. The deficit may be physiological, as in dehydration due to perspiring in a hot, dry climate during hard physical labor or sports, or due to inadequate intake of fluids. It may be pathological, as in traumatic or septic shock, acute respiratory distress syndrome, severe vomiting or diarrhea or both, or metabolic and endocrine conditions such as diabetic ketosis, chronic renal failure, and adrenal insufficiency. SEE: *intravenous infusion* for illus; *central venous catheter; central line; intravenous infusion; oral rehydration therapy; solution.*

The goal of fluid replacement is to correct fluid, electrolyte, and acid-base imbalances. The oral route of replacement is used if possible. The intravenous, intraperitoneal, or subcutaneous routes are also used, with the intravenous route being used most frequently. Fluids may be isotonic, hypotonic, or hypertonic; may contain certain crystalloids (e.g., sodium, potassium, chloride, or calcium); or may contain osmotically active substances (e.g., glucose, protein, starch, or a synthetic plasma volume expander such as dextran or hetastarch). The composition, rate of administration, and route depend on the clinical condition being treated.

CAUTION: A critically ill patient receiving fluid replacement should be monitored frequently to be certain that fluid overload is prevented and that the solution is flowing and not extravasating. This is esp. important in treating infants, small children, and the elderly.

---

fluid retention Failure to eliminate fluid from the body because of renal, cardiac, or metabolic disease, or combinations of these disorders. Excess salt is another cause of fluid retention, which maintains the proper chemical and physical properties of body fluids. A low-sodium diet is indicated in fluid retention. The advisability of using diuretics, angiotensin-converting enzyme inhibitors, and/or other drug therapies depends on the functional state of the kidneys, heart, and liver.

fluid volume deficit [active loss] The state in which an individual experiences vascular, cellular, or intracellular dehydration (in excess of needs or replacement capabilities owing to active loss); a nursing diagnosis. SEE: *Nursing Diagnoses Appendix.*

fluid volume deficit [regulatory failure] The state in which an individual experiences vascular, cellular, or intracellular dehydration [in excess of needs or replacement capabilities owing to failure of regulatory mechanisms]; a nursing diagnosis. SEE: *Nursing Diagnoses Appendix.*

fluid volume deficit, risk for The state in which an individual is at risk of experiencing vascular, cellular, or intracellular dehydration [due to active or regulatory losses of body water in excess of needs or replacement capability]; a nursing diagnosis. SEE: *Nursing Diagnoses Appendix.*

fluid volume excess The state in which an individual experiences increased isotonic fluid retention; a nursing diagnosis. SEE: *Nursing Diagnoses Appendix.*

fluid volume imbalance, risk for A risk of a decrease, increase, or rapid shift from one to the other of intravascular, interstitial, and/or intracellular fluid; a nursing diagnosis. This refers to the loss or excess or both of body fluids or replacement fluids. SEE: *Nursing Diagnoses Appendix.*

fluke (flook) [AS. *floc,* flatfish] A parasitic worm belonging to the class Trematoda, phylum Platyhelminthes. Those parasitic in humans belong to the order Digenea. Most flukes have complex life cycles including asexual reproductive forms that live in a mollusc (snail or bivalve). Stages of a typical fluke include adult, egg, miracidium, sporocyst, redia, cercaria, and metacercaria.

blood f. A fluke of the genus *Schistosoma,* including *S. haematobium, S. mansoni,* and *S. japonicum.* Adults live principally in the mesenteric and pelvic veins. They cause schistosomiasis.

intestinal f. One of several species of flukes infesting the intestine in humans. They include *Gastrodiscoides* *hominis, Fasciolopsis buski, Heterophyes heterophyes,* and *Metagonimus yokogawai.*

liver f. One of several species of fluke infesting the liver and bile ducts. Those infesting humans include *Clonorchis sinensis, Fasciola hepatica, Dicrocoelium dendriticum,* and *Opisthorchis felineus.* Adult liver flukes infest biliary and pancreatic ducts. The eggs pass from the body with the feces and continue their development in snails of the subfamily Buliminae (family Hydrobiidae). Cercariae emerge and infest numerous species of freshwater fishes in which they encyst. Infestation results from eating raw fish containing encysted metacercariae.

lung f. A fluke that infests lung tissue. Only one species, *Paragonimus westermani,* is common in humans.

flumazenil (floo-măz′ĕn-ĭl) A drug that reverses the sedation caused by benzodiazepines. Occasionally it may trigger acute drug withdrawal symptoms, such as seizures.

flumina pilorum (floo′mĭ-nă pī-lō′rŭm) [L., rivers of hair] **1.** The curved lines along which the hairs of the body are arranged, esp. in the fetus. **2.** Hairs lying in the same direction.

fluo- Combining form meaning *flow.*

fluocinolone acetonide (floo-ō-sĭn′ō-lŏn) A synthetic corticosteroid. Trade names are Fluonid and Synalar.

fluor albus (floo′or ăl′bŭs) [L., white flow] A white discharge from the uterus or vagina. SYN: *leukorrhea.*

fluorescein sodium (floo″ō-rĕs′ē-ĭn) A red crystalline powder used chiefly for diagnostic purposes and for detecting foreign bodies or lesions in the cornea of the eye.

fluorescence (floo″ō-rĕs′ĕnts) The emission of a longer wavelength light by a material exposed to a shorter wavelength light. Fluorescent materials, such as fluorspar, the first material found to have this property, emit light only while a light is shining on them.

fluorescent (floo-ō-rĕs′ĕnt) **1.** In biology, having one color by transmitted light and another by reflected light. **2.** Luminous when exposed to other light rays.

fluorescent polarization immunoassay ABBR: FPIA. An antigen-antibody analysis using fluorescent-tagged antigens. The technique is based on the principle that antigens, which are small molecules, rotate rapidly and therefore emit randomly polarized fluorescence, whereas antigens bound to antibodies, which are large molecules, rotate slowly and produce highly polarized fluorescence. When many unbound antigens are present, there will be less polarized light.

fluorescent screen **1.** A sheet of cardboard, paper, or glass coated with a material that fluoresces visibly, such as calcium tungstate. It is used in fluoroscopy, in which x-rays, radium rays, or electrons cause the object being examined to cast a shadow. **2.** A sheet of cardboard, paper, or glass, coated with anthracene or other fluorescing materials to reveal ultraviolet radiations.

fluorescent treponemal antibody-absorption test ABBR: FTA, FTA-ABS. A test for syphilis using the fluorescent antibody technique that is used to confirm a positive rapid plasma reagin, or Venereal Disease Research Laboratory test.

fluoridation (floo″or-ĭ-dā′shŭn) The addition of fluorides to a water supply to prevent dental caries. The development of dental caries in the deciduous and permanent teeth can be decreased by providing fluoride as a supplement in the drinking water, as a topical application to the teeth, or as a daily medication. There are several important considerations. Fluoride that exceeds the daily dose discolors the teeth if a child ingests fluoride while the teeth are developing (i.e., from birth to 8 or 10 years). If a woman consumes fluoridated water during pregnancy, the deciduous teeth of the fetus, which begin to mineralize during the fourth or fifth month in utero, incorporate that compound and become more resistant to caries. In the adult tooth, when enamel has lost mineral (white spot lesion), fluoride greatly enhances the remineralization, because it leads to the precipitation of calcium phosphate.

The most commonly used method of administering fluoride is by providing drinking water that contains between 0.7 and 1.2 parts per million, depending on the climate. In rural areas without a central water supply, fluoridation of the school's water supply is an alternative to community water fluoridation. Because children spend only 5 to 7 hours a day in school, the advisable concentration of fluoride in the school water supply should be 4.5 times the optimal level recommended for the community water fluoridation for that locale. Persons exposed to chronically high levels of fluoride may develop fluorosis. Acute intoxication with extremely high doses of fluoride may be fatal.

CAUTION: Children drinking fluoridated water should not receive supplemental fluoride medication.

fluoride (floo′ō-rīd) A compound of fluorine, usually with a radical; a salt of hydrofluoric acid. Three preparations of fluoride-containing compounds are available for topical application to teeth for the prevention of decay. They are stannous fluoride, sodium fluoride, and acidulated phosphate fluoride. Considerable evidence shows that fluoride compounds prevent dental caries.

acidulated phosphate f. ABBR: APF. A fluoride compound used to prevent dental caries, available in solution and gel. It has often been used by dentists as a cariostatic agent.

sodium f. A stable, tasteless fluoride compound, NaF, used to prevent dental caries. It is commonly used as a fluoride supplement in commercially available toothpastes, gels, ionomers, and some bone cements.

stannous f. An unstable acidic fluoride solution, SnF_2, used to prevent dental caries. It has traditionally been used in some dentifrices and has a bitter, metallic taste.

fluoride dental treatment The application of a fluoride solution or gel to the teeth as a means of controlling or preventing caries. SEE: *dental sealant.*

fluoride poisoning SEE: *Poisons and Poisoning Appendix.*

fluorine (floo′ō-rēn, floor′ēn) SYMB: F. A gaseous chemical element, atomic weight 18.9984, atomic number 9. It is found in the soil in combination with calcium. SEE: *fluoridation.*

fluoroacetate (floo″or-ō-ăs′ĕ-tāt) A salt of fluoroacetic acid. SEE: *Poisons and Poisoning Appendix.*

fluoroapatite A compound formed when tooth enamel is treated with appropriate concentrations of the fluoride ion. The modified hydroxyapatite is less acid soluble and therefore resistant to caries. Fluoroapatite is formed in bone, as well as in enamel and dentin of teeth, when fluoride is taken systemically.

fluorocarbon A general term for a hydrocarbon in which some of the hydrogen atoms have been replaced with fluorine. The use of such compounds in aerosol sprays was discontinued because of an adverse effect on the atmosphere.

fluorometer (floo-or-ŏm′ĕ-tĕr) **1.** A device for determining the amount of radiation produced by x-rays. **2.** A device for adjusting a fluoroscope to establish the location of the target more accurately and to produce an undistorted image or shadow. **3.** A clinical laboratory instrument used in many types of immunochemistry assays (e.g., fluorescent polarization immunoassay).

fluorometholone (floor″ō-mĕth′ō-lōn) A synthetic corticosteroid used ophthalmically.

fluorophor A substance that tends to fluoresce, such as fluorescein.

fluoroquinolone (flŏr-ō-kwĭn′ō-lōn) A class of antimicrobial agents that kill bacteria by inhibiting their DNA gyrase and topoisomerase enzymes. Antibiotics of this class include norfloxacin, ciprofloxacin, ofloxacin, grepafloxacin, levofloxacin, and sparfloxacin.

CAUTION: Pregnant women should not take these antibiotics because of their adverse effects on the developing fetus.

---

fluoroscope (floo′or-ō-skōp) A device consisting of a fluorescent screen, mounted either separately or in conjunction with an x-ray tube, that shows the images of objects interposed between the tube and the screen. It has been replaced by the image intensifier for performing fluoroscopic studies.

fluoroscopy Examination of the body using a fluoroscope.

fluorosis Chronic fluorine poisoning, sometimes marked by mottling of tooth enamel. It may result from excessive exposure to fluorides from dietary, waterborne, and supplemental sources.

fluorouracil (floor″ō-ŭr′ă-sĭl) An antimetabolite used in treating certain forms of cancer.

fluoxetine hydrochloride A drug used in the treatment of depression, bulimia, and obsessive-compulsive disorder. It is an inhibitor of serotonin reuptake in the central nervous system. Trade name is Prozac.

fluoxymesterone (floo-ŏk″sē-mĕs′tĕr-ōn) An anabolic and androgenic hormone.

fluphenazine enanthate (floo-fĕn′ă-zēn) A phenothiazine-type tranquilizer. Trade name is Prolixin Enanthate.

fluprednisolone (floo″prĕd-nĭs′ō-lōn) A corticosteroid drug.

flurandrenolide (floor″ăn-drĕn′ō-līd) A corticosteroid drug.

flurazepam hydrochloride (floor-ăz′ĕ-păm) A sedative-hypnotic drug.

flush [ME. *flusshen,* to fly up] **1.** Sudden redness of the skin. **2.** Irrigation of a cavity, or a device such as a feeding tube, with water.

hot f. Flash.

malar f. A bright-colored flush over the malar area and cheekbones. It may be associated with any febrile disease.

flutter [AS. *floterian,* to fly about] A tremulous movement, esp. of the heart, as in atrial and ventricular flutter.

atrial f. A cardiac arrhythmia marked by rapid (about 300 beats per minute) regular atrial beating, and usually a regular ventricular response (whose rate may vary depending on the conduction of electrical impulses from the atria through the atrioventricular node). On the electrocardiogram, the fluttering of the atria is best seen in leads II, III, and F as "sawtooth" deflections between the QRS complexes. Atrial flutter usually converts to sinus rhythm with low-voltage direct current (DC) cardioversion or atrial pacing.

SYMPTOMS: Patients may be asymptomatic, esp. when ventricular rates are less than 100 bpm. During tachycardic episodes, patients often report palpitations, dizziness, presyncope, or syncope.

TREATMENT: Radiofrequency catheter ablation of the responsible circuit eliminates the arrhythmia about 90% of the time.

diaphragmatic f. Rapid contractions of the diaphragm. They may occur intermittently or be present for an extended period. The cause is unknown.

mediastinal f. Abnormal side-to-side motion of the mediastinum during respiration.

ventricular f. Ventricular contractions of the heart at 250 per minute, creating a high-amplitude, sawtooth pattern on the surface electrocardiogram. The rhythm is lethal unless immediate life support and resuscitation are provided.

Flutter device A handheld device designed to facilitate clearance of mucus in hypersecretory lung disorders. Exhalation through the Flutter results in oscillations of expiratory pressure and airflow, which vibrate the airway walls, loosening mucus, decrease the collapsibility of the airways, and accelerate airflow. This facilitates movement of mucus up the airways. SEE: *cystic fibrosis.*

flutter-fibrillation Cardiac dysrhythmia alternating between atrial fibrillation and atrial flutter, or showing a pattern that is difficult to distinguish during routine cardiac monitoring.

flux [L. *fluxus,* a flow] **1.** An excessive flow or discharge from an organ or cavity of the body. **2.** In physics, the flow rate of a liquid, particles, or energy. **3.** In dentistry, an agent that lowers the fusion temperature of porcelain. **4.** In metallurgy, a substance used to increase the fluidity of a molten metal and to prevent or reduce its oxidation. **5.** A substance that deoxidizes, cleans, and promotes the union of surfaces to be brazed, soldered, or welded together.

fly [AS. *fleoge*] An insect belonging to the order Diptera, characterized by sucking mouth parts, one pair of wings, and complete metamorphosis, such as the housefly, horsefly, or deerfly. The term is sometimes applied to insects belonging to other orders. SEE: *Diptera.*

black f. A fly of the genus *Simulium* whose bites often cause local bleeding and pain.

flesh f. The Sarcophagidae.

screwworm f. A fly belonging to the families Calliphoridae and Sarcophagidae.

Spanish f. Cantharides.

tsetse f. *Glossina palpalis;* the fly that transmits African sleeping sickness or trypanosomiasis.

warble f. Dermatobia.

Fm Symbol for the element fermium.

f.m. L. *fiat mistura,* let a mixture be made. This abbreviation is used in prescription writing.

FNR *False-negative ratio.*

foam (fōm) [AS. *fam*] A mixture of finely divided gas bubbles interspersed in a liquid.

FOBT *Fecal occult blood test.*

focal (fō′kăl) Pert. to a focus.

focal infection Infection occurring near a focus, such as the cavity of a tooth.

focal spot The area on the x-ray tube target that is bombarded with electrons to produce x-radiation.

foci (fō′sī) [L.] Pl. of focus.

focus *pl.* **foci** [L. *focus,* hearth] **1.** The point of convergence of light rays or sound waves. **2.** The starting point of a disease process.

real f. The point at which convergent rays intersect.

virtual f. The point at which divergent rays would intersect if extended backward.

FOD *focus-object distance.* The distance from the target of an x-ray tube to the surface being radiographed.

fog Droplets suspended in a gas, as minute water droplets in air.

fogging **1.** A method of testing vision, used particularly in testing astigmatism and in postcycloplegic examination, in which accommodation is relaxed by overcorrection. **2.** A method of intense application of an insecticide. The solution is nebulized and appears in the air as a mist. **3.** Unwanted density on radiographic film resulting from exposure to secondary radiation, light, chemicals, or heat.

foil A thin, pliable sheet of metal. In dentistry, various types of gold foil are used for restoring or preparing appliances.

folacin Folic acid.

fold [AS. *fealdan,* to fold] A ridge; a doubling back. SYN: *plica.*

amniotic f. The folded edge of the inner fetal membrane where it rises over and finally encloses the embryo of birds, reptiles, and some mammals.

aryepiglottic f. The ridgelike lateral walls of the entrance to the larynx.

circular f. A macroscopic fold of the mucosa and submucosa of the small intestine that is arranged like accordion pleats.

costocolic f. A ligament, arising from the peritoneum, that attaches the splenic flexure of the colon to the diaphragm.

Douglas' f. A fold of peritoneum extending on each side to the base of the broad ligament. This forms the rectouterine space, called Douglas' pouch.

epicanthal f. Epicanthus.

gastric f. Any of the folds of mucosa, mostly longitudinal, in the empty stomach.

genital f. A fold of skin in the embryo

on each side of the genital tubercle that develops into the labia minora in females.

glossoepiglottidean f. One of three mucous membrane folds between the base of the tongue and the epiglottis. SYN: *epiglottic plica.*

gluteal f. The linear crease in the skin that separates the buttocks from the thighs.

lacrimal f. A valvelike fold in the lower part of the nasolacrimal duct.

mesouterine f. A fold of peritoneum supporting the uterus.

mucobuccal f. The line of flexure where the oral mucosa passes from the maxilla or mandible to the cheek; the vestibule.

mucolabial f. The line of flexure where the oral mucosa passes from the maxilla or mandible to the lip.

mucosal f. A fold of mucosal tissue.

nail f. A groove in the cutaneous tissue surrounding the margins and proximal edges of the nail.

palmate f. Any of the ridges on the cervical canal of the uterus.

semilunar f. of conjunctiva The fold of conjunctiva at the inner angle of the eye.

transverse f. of rectum Any of the transverse mucosal folds of the rectum. SYN: *Houston's valve.*

urogenital f. SEE: *ridge, urogenital.*

ventricular f. The false vocal cord. SYN: *vestibular f.*

vestibular f. Ventricular f.

vestigial f. The ligament of the left side of the superior vena cava. Also known as *Marshall's fold.*

vocal f. The true vocal cord.

Foley catheter [Frederic W. B. Foley, U.S. urologist, 1891–1966] A urinary tract catheter with a balloon attachment at one end. After the catheter is inserted, the balloon is inflated. Thus the catheter is prevented from leaving the bladder until the balloon is emptied.

folia (fō′lē-ă) [L.] Pl. of folium.

foliaceous (fō-lē-ā′shē-ŭs) [L. *folia,* leaves] Resembling or pert. to a leaf.

folie (fō-lē′) [Fr.] Psychosis.

f. à deux The sharing and reinforcement of a delusion, usually of the paranoid type, at the same time by two closely associated persons.

f. du doute Abnormal doubts about ordinary acts and beliefs; inability to decide on a definite course of action or conduct.

f. du pourquoi Unreasonable and unrelenting questioning.

f. gémellaire Psychosis occurring in twins.

folinic acid The active form of folic acid. It is used in counteracting the effects of folic acid antagonists, and in treating anemia due to folic acid deficiency.

folium (fō′lē-ŭm) *pl.* **folia** [L., leaf] A thin, broad, leaflike structure.

f. vermis A fold on the posterior part of the upper surface of the vermis of the cerebellum.

follicle [L. *folliculus,* little bag] A small secretory sac or cavity. **follicular,** *adj.*

aggregated f. Peyer's patch.

atretic f. An ovarian follicle that has undergone degeneration or involution.

dental f. **1.** The connective tissue structure that encloses the developing tooth within the substance of the jaw prior to tooth eruption. **2.** The dental sac and its contents.

gastric f. The glands in the gastric mucosa of the stomach.

graafian f. SEE: *graafian follicle.*

hair f. An invagination of the epidermis that forms a cylindrical depression, penetrating the corium into the connective tissue that holds the hair root. Sebaceous glands, which secrete sebum, and tiny muscles (arrectores pili) that cause the hair to stand are attached to these follicles.

lymph f. The densely packed collection of lymphocytes and lymphoblasts that make up the cortex of lymph glands.

maturing f. SEE: *graafian follicle.*

nabothian f. A dilated cyst of the glands of the cervix uteri.

ovarian f. A spherical structure in the cortex of the ovary consisting of an oogonium or an oocyte and its surrounding epithelial (follicular) cells. The follicles are of three types. The first type, or primary follicle, consists of an oogonium and a single layer of follicular cells. In the second type, or growing follicle, cells proliferate, forming several layers, and the first maturation division occurs. The third type, the vesicular (graafian) follicle, possesses a cavity (antrum) containing the follicular fluid (liquor folliculi). The oocyte lies in the cumulus oophorus, a mass of cells on the inner surface. The cells lining the follicle constitute the stratum granulosum. The follicle is a secretory structure producing estrogen and progesterone. SEE: *corpus luteum.*

primordial f. An ovarian follicle consisting of the ovum enclosed in a single layer of cells.

sebaceous f. Sebaceous gland.

solitary f. A single lymph nodule of the intestine.

thyroid f. A spherical or ovoid structure, found in the thyroid gland, lined with a single layer of cuboidal epithelial cells, which secrete the thyroid hormone. The follicles are filled with colloid, a viscid substance rich in iodine.

vesicular f. A follicle containing a cavity; a mature ovarian (graafian) follicle.

follicular Pert. to a follicle or follicles.

follicular tumor A sebaceous cyst.

folliculitis (fō-lĭk″ū-lī′tĭs) [L. *folliculus,*

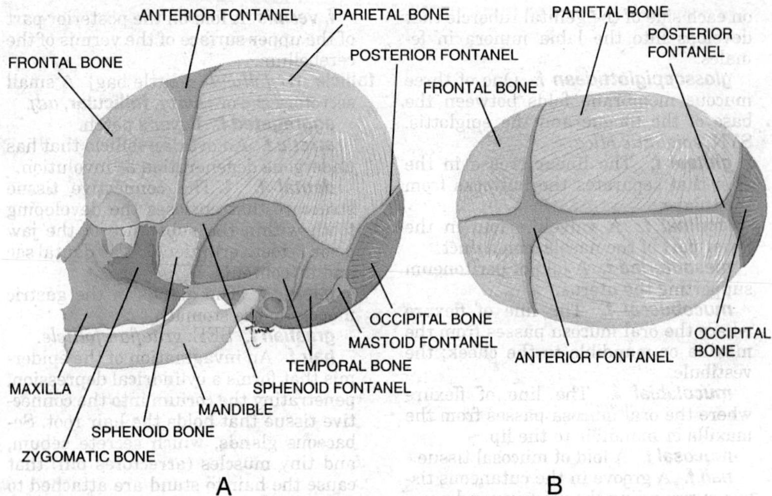

FONTANELS OF INFANT SKULL
(A) lateral view, (B) superior view

little bag, + Gr. *itis,* inflammation] Inflammation of a follicle or follicles.

f. barbae A deep-seated infection of the hair follicles of the beard—usually caused by staphylococcal or fungal infection. SYN: *sycosis barbae*.

f. decalvans Purulent follicular inflammation of the scalp resulting in permanent irregular alopecia and scarring. This rare disease occurs mostly in men. The cause is unknown.

keloidal f. Chronic dermatitis with production of hard papules that join together to form hypertrophied scars.

folliculogenesis, induction of Stimulation of follicle development with drugs (e.g., clomiphene) or hormones (e.g., gonadotropins). SEE: *assisted reproductive technologies; clomiphene citrate; in vitro fertilization; gamete intrafallopian transfer*.

folliculoma (fō-lĭk″ū-lō′mă) [″ + Gr. *oma,* tumor] A tumor of the ovary originating in a graafian follicle in which the cells resemble those of the stratum granulosum.

folliculose (fō-lĭk′ū-lōs) Composed of follicles.

folliculosis (fō-lĭk″ū-lō′sĭs) [″ + Gr. *osis,* condition] The presence of an abnormal number of lymph follicles.

folliculus (fō-lĭk′ū-lŭs) *pl.* **folliculi** [L.] A follicle.

follow-up The continued care or monitoring of a patient after the initial visit or examination.

Folstein Mini Mental Status Exam A screening test of 30 items to assess cognitive function in individuals suspected of having dementia or delirium.

fomentation (fō″mĕn-tā′shŭn) [L. *fomentatio*] A hot, wet application for the relief of pain or inflammation. SEE: *dressing, hot moist; stupe*.

fomepizole 4-methylpyrazole A drug used as an antidote for ethylene glycol (antifreeze) poisoning.

fomes (fō′mēz) *pl.* **fomites** [L., tinder] Any substance that adheres to and transmits infectious material.

fomites (fō′mĭ-tēz) Pl. of fomes.

Fontana's spaces (fŏn-tă′năz) [Felice Fontana, It. scientist, 1730–1805] The spaces between the processes of the ligamentum pectinatum of the iris. These convey the aqueous humor.

fontanel, fontanelle (fŏn″tă-nĕl′) [Fr. *fontanelle,* little fountain] An unossified membrane or soft spot lying between the cranial bones of the skull of a fetus or infant. SEE: illus.

anterior f. The diamond-shaped junction of the coronal, frontal, and sagittal sutures; it becomes ossified within 18 to 24 months.

posterior f. The triangular fontanel at the junction of the sagittal and lambdoid sutures; ossified by the end of the first year.

Fontan procedure [Francois Maurice Fontan, Fr. surgeon, b. 1929] A procedure used to repair complex congenital heart defects such as a single ventricle, that prevent oxygen from reaching the systemic circulation. The superior vena cava (SVC) is divided adjacent to its entry to the right atrium; the pulmonary trunk is divided close to the pulmonic valve and both ends are closed. The distal and cardiac ends of the divided SVC are anastomosed to the right pulmonary artery. The inferior vena cava is connected to the atrial orifice of the SVC, usually by means of a vascular prosthesis. This procedure may be modified.

fonticulus (fŏn-tĭk′ū-lŭs) [L., little fountain] The Latin word for fontanel.

food [AS. *foda*] Any material, including water, that provides the nutritive requirements of an organism to maintain growth and physical well-being. For people, food includes carbohydrates, fats, proteins, vitamins, and minerals. SEE: *carbohydrate; digestion; fat* (2); *nutrition; protein; stomach.*

contamination of f. The presence, introduction, or development of infectious or toxic material in food. Food may cause illness by carrying pathogenic organisms such as those that cause enteritis *(Salmonella)* or tuberculosis, parasites such as those that cause trichinosis, certain types of worms (e.g., roundworms, tapeworms), or poisons (such as botulinum toxin).

convenience f. Food in which one or more steps in preparation have been completed before the product is offered for retail sale. Examples include frozen vegetables, bake mixes, heat-and-serve foods as well as ready-to-eat foods.

dietetic f. Food in which the nutrient content has been modified for use in special diets, esp. for diabetics.

enriched f. Food in which the vitamin and mineral content has been increased by either addition or irradiation.

fast f. Commercially available, ready-to-eat meals (such as hamburgers, hot dogs, pizza, fried chicken, or french fries) with a high fat content, little fiber, and minimal quantities of vitamins or calcium.

functional f. Food products with additives for which, following FDA approval, health claims can be made.

medical f. A food formulated by the selective use of nutrients and manufactured for the dietary treatment of a specific condition.

organic f. A crop or animal product cultivated with specific guidelines that limit the use of petrochemicals, radiation, or genetically engineered technologies in its agriculture.

f. rendering The conversion of the waste products of animal butchery into feeds, bone meal, tallows, oils, and fertilizer. Rendered feed products are sometimes the source of animal and human infections.

textured f. Food products manufactured from various nutritional components made to resemble conventional protein-source foods, such as meat, seafood, or poultry, in texture.

food adulterant A substance that makes food impure or inferior, such as toxins, organisms, pesticide residues, radioactive fallout, any poisonous or deleterious substance, or any substance added to increase bulk or weight.

Food and Drug Administration ABBR: FDA. In the U.S., an official regulatory body for foods, drugs, cosmetics, and medical devices. It is a part of the U.S. Department of Health and Human Services.

food and drug interactions Drugs may interfere with absorption or use of food, or vice versa. Excess intake of food high in vitamin K may interfere with the action of anticoagulants. Prolonged use of antacids may cause phosphate depletion. SEE: *monoamine oxidase inhibitor.*

food ball Phytobezoar.

food-borne disease ABBR: FBD. A disease acquired by the ingestion of food contaminated with pathogenic germs or their toxins. These include *Staphylococcus, Clostridium botulinum, Salmonella, Shigella, Cholera, Campylobacter, Cryptosporidia, Listeria, Yersinia, Entamoeba histolytica, Giardia, Vibrio,* hepatitis A, and *Escherichia.* Symptoms, treatment, and outcome depend on the causative agent and the patient's general health. In the U.S., more than 75 million instances of food-borne illness occur each year. SEE: pathogens mentioned above; *travelers' diarrhea.*

food exchange A grouping of commonly used foods according to similarities in composition so that such foods may be used interchangeably in diet planning.

Food Guide Pyramid Recommendations developed by the U.S. Department of Agriculture for planning a balanced diet. Foods are divided into six groups: bread, cereal, rice, and pasta; fruits; vegetables; milk, yogurt, and cheese; meat, poultry, fish, dry beans, eggs, and nuts; and fats, oils, and sweets. The guide recommends the number of servings for each food group. SEE: illus.

Food Guide Pyramid for the Elderly A modification of the original Food Guide Pyramid, for those over age 70. At its base is eight servings of water, and at its peak is the recommendation for supplements of calcium, vitamin D, and vitamin B_{12}. SEE: *Nutrition Appendix.*

food hypersensitivity reaction SEE: *food allergy.*

food intolerance An abnormal, nonimmunological response to ingested food. The basis for the intolerance may be pharmacological, enzymatic, metabolic, or toxic. Pharmacological intolerance is the body's reaction to a component of the food that produces druglike effects; enzymatic intolerance results in an inability to digest a food because of an inadequate production or the absence of an enzyme necessary for its digestion; metabolic intolerance is due to the effect of the food on the person's metabolism; and food toxicity is due to toxins in the

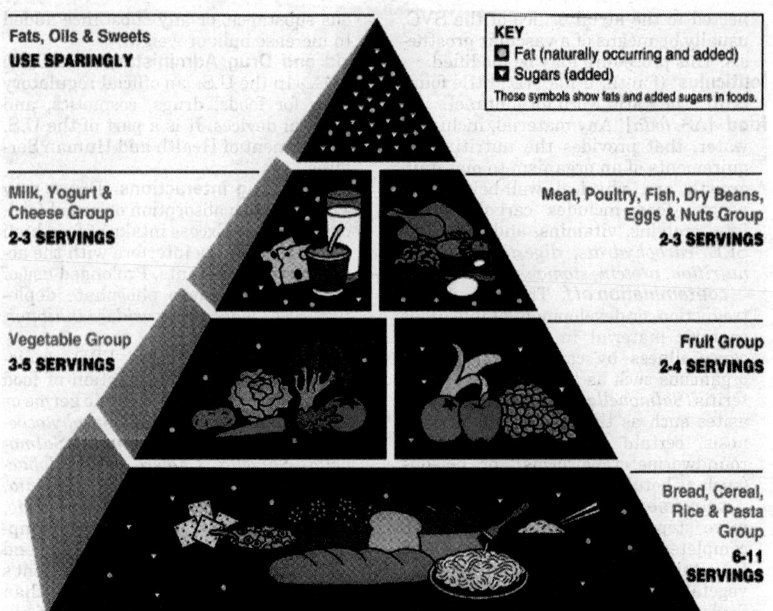

Source: U. S. Department of Agriculture, Human Nutrition Information Services

FOOD GUIDE PYRAMID

food or released by microorganisms contaminating the food.

food label The information provided on a food package indicating the various nutrients, calories, and additives present in the food. U.S. Food and Drug Administration regulations mandate the listing of total fats, calories from fat, cholesterol, saturated fats, total carbohydrates, sugars, sodium, potassium, protein, vitamin and minerals, among other nutritional components.

food requirements The need for various amounts and types of food according to a person's use of energy. It is calculated that an average healthy man (154 lb or 70 kg) performing light to moderate muscular work requires 2700 kcal/day, while an average healthy woman (128 lb or 58 kg) requires 2000 kcal/day. These needs are met through the intake of carbohydrate, protein, and fat. An estimation of the protein requirement for the average adult is 1 g of protein per day for each kilogram of their ideal weight. Generally, a woman requires fewer calories per day than a comparably active man because of her smaller build. Sedentary individuals generally require fewer calories. On a body weight basis, children and pregnant women require more calories than predicted to support growth and development. Febrile patients have an increased basal energy expenditure of about 12% for each degree centigrade of fever. It is generally agreed that a diet that is rich in fruits, vegetables, legumes, and whole grains and has adequate minerals (including calcium) and vitamins is superior to diets that are rich in fats and sugars. SEE: *calorie; diet; energy expenditure, basal; nutrition; Recommended Daily Dietary Allowances Appendix.*

food trap SEE: *trap, food.*

foot [AS. *fot*] ABBR: ft. The terminal portion of the lower extremity. The bones of the foot include the tarsals, metatarsals, and phalanges. SEE: illus.; *leg* for illus.; *skeleton.*

arches of f. The four vaulted structures in the foot: the internal (medial)

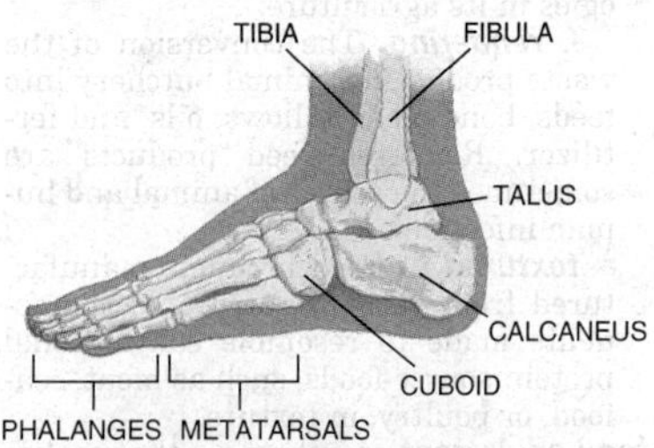

BONES OF FOOT AND ANKLE

Left foot, lateral view

longitudinal, the outer (lateral) longitudinal, and two transverse.

athlete's f. A scaling, cracked, or macerated rash, typically found between the toes and usually caused by a fungal skin infection (e.g., tinea), although bacteria may also be involved. The rash is usually mildly itchy. SYN: *dermatophytosis; tinea pedis.* SEE: illus.; *Nursing Diagnoses Appendix.*

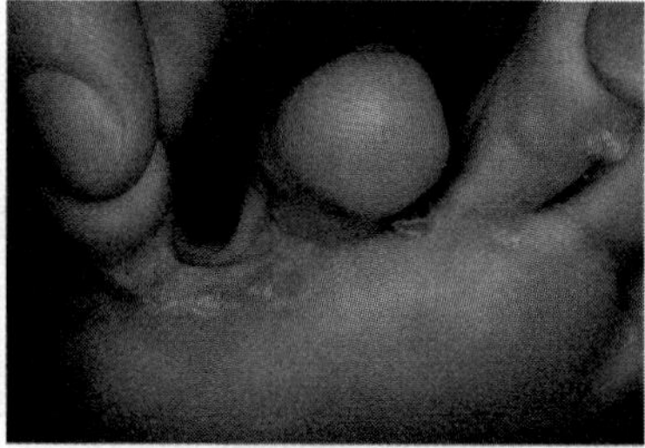

ATHLETE'S FOOT

TREATMENT: The feet, esp. the webbing between the toes, should be carefully dried after bathing. Well-ventilated shoes and absorbent socks should be worn. Topically applied antifungal drugs, such as terbinafine, effectively treat the condition except when maceration is prominent and bacterial infection is also present. In these instances, oral antibiotics are needed.

cleft f. A condition in which a cleft extends between the digits to the metatarsal region, usually due to a missing digit and metatarsal.

immersion f. A condition of the feet, resulting from prolonged immersion in cold water, in which pain and inflammation are followed by swelling, discoloration, and numbness.

Madura f. SEE: *Madura foot.*

march f. A spontaneous fracture of one of the metatarsal bones of the foot.

trench f. Degeneration of the skin of the feet due to prolonged exposure to moisture. The condition, which resembles frostbite, may be prevented by ensuring that clean, dry socks are worn at all times. The feet do not have to be exposed to cold to develop this condition.

foot board A board or similar material placed at the foot end of a patient's bed. It is angled slightly away from the patient and extends up above the mattress. When used properly it helps to prevent footdrop. The patient should be positioned in bed so that when the legs are fully extended the soles of the feet just touch the board.

foot-candle An amount of light equivalent to 1 lumen per square foot.

footdrop Plantar flexion of the foot due to weakness or paralysis of the anterior muscles of the lower leg. It may occur in any patient who is in bed continuously, esp. if comatose. For bedridden patients, a foot board should be used to prevent footdrop.

footplate The flat part of the stapes, a bone in the middle ear.

foot-pound The amount of energy required to lift 1 lb of mass a vertical distance of 1 ft.

footprint An impression of the foot, esp. an ink impression used for identification of infants.

forage (fō-rŏzh′) [Fr., boring] Creation of a channel through an enlarged prostate by use of an electric cautery. This technique may be used in other tissues.

foramen (for-ā′mĕn) *pl.* **foramina** [L.] A passage or opening; an orifice, a communication between two cavities of an organ, or a hole in a bone for passage of vessels or nerves.

anterior condyloid f. The opening above the condyle of the occipital bone. The 12th cranial nerve passes through it.

anterior sacral f. One of the openings on the anterior aspect of the sacrum through which the anterior primary branches of the sacral nerve pass.

apical f. The opening in the end of the root of a tooth through which the blood, lymphatic, and nerve supplies pass to the dental pulp.

f. of Bochdalek A fetal diaphragmatic opening that may not close completely; a site for a congenital diaphragmatic hernia.

epiploic f. The opening connecting the peritoneal cavity to its lesser sac. SYN: *f. of Winslow.*

ethmoidal f. One of the openings in the medial wall of the orbit. The ethmoidal nerve and artery pass through these openings.

external auditory f. The outer auditory meatus, through which sound waves travel to reach the tympanic membrane.

greater sciatic f. The opening bounded by the hip bone, sacrum, and sacrotuberous ligament.

incisive f. One of the small openings sometimes present in the incisive fossa of the hard palate. SYN: *palatine f.*

infraorbital f. The opening in the maxilla through which the infraorbital branch of the maxillary nerve passes.

internal auditory f. The opening in the petrous portion of the temporal bone through which the seventh and eighth cranial nerves pass.

interventricular f. SEE: *Monro's foramen.*

intervertebral f. The opening between adjacent articulated vertebrae for passage of nerves to and from the spinal cord.

jugular f. The opening in the base of the skull through which pass the sigmoid and inferior petrosal sinus and the 9th, 10th, and 11th cranial nerves.

lesser sciatic f. The opening bounded by the hip bone, sacrum, and sacrospinous ligament.

lingual f. A small opening on the lingual surface of the mandible at the midline. It is surrounded by small bony protuberances called genial tubercles. The terminal branches of the mandibular nerve exit the bone through the lingual foramen and innervate the gingiva in the anterior portion of the mandible.

Magendie's f. SEE: *Magendie's foramen.*

f. magnum The opening in the occipital bone through which the spinal cord passes from the brain.

mandibular f. The opening on the medial surface of the mandibular ramus through which the inferior alveolar vessels and nerve enter the mandibular canal.

mastoid f. The opening in the mastoid part of the temporal bone. A small vein passes through it.

mental f. The opening on the ventral surface of the body of the mandible. The mental nerve and artery exit through it for superficial distribution.

Monro's f. SEE: *Monro's foramen.*

obturator f. A large oval foramen below the acetabulum bounded by the pubis and ischium.

olfactory f. An opening in the ethmoid bone for passage of the olfactory nerves.

optic f. An opening in the lesser wing of the sphenoid bone. The optic nerve and ophthalmic artery pass through it.

f. ovale **1.** The opening between the two atria of the fetal heart. It usually closes shortly after birth as a result of hemodynamic changes related to respiration. If it remains open, the defect can be repaired surgically. Patency of the foramen ovale occasionally is a source of paradoxical stroke in patients with lower extremity deep venous thrombosis. SEE: *fetal circulation.* **2.** The oval opening in the posterior margin of the great sphenoidal wing for the mandibular branch of the trigeminal nerve and the small meningeal artery.

palatine f. Incisive f.

palatine (greater and lesser) f. The openings of the palatine canals through which nerves pass to the mucosa of the hard and soft palate.

posterior condyloid f. The opening behind the condyle of the occipital bone. A small vein passes through it.

posterior sacral f. One of the openings on the posterior aspect of the sacrum through which the posterior primary branches of the sacral nerve pass.

f. rotundum The opening in the great sphenoidal wing through which the maxillary branch of the trigeminal nerve passes.

Scarpa's f. The opening behind the upper medial incisor tooth through which the nasopalatine nerve passes. This opening is not always present.

sphenopalatine f. The opening between the palatine and sphenoid bones. It provides a passage from the pterygopalatine fossa to the nasal cavity for the sphenopalatine artery and nasal nerves.

spinous f. The opening in the spine of the sphenoid bone through which the middle meningeal artery passes.

supraorbital f. An opening sometimes present above the superior border of the orbit of the eye. The supraorbital nerve and vessels pass through it.

thebesian f. One of the openings leading directly into the atria and ventricles of the heart. Very small thebesian veins empty into these openings.

transverse f. An opening in the transverse process of a cervical vertebra.

vena caval f. The opening in the diaphragm through which the inferior vena cava and branches of the right vagus nerve pass.

vertebral f. The large opening between the neural arch and the body of the vertebra that contains the spinal cord.

f. of Vesalius An opening sometimes present in the sphenoid bone medial to the foramen ovale. A vein from the cavernous sinus passes through it.

Weitbrecht's f. The opening in the articular capsule of the shoulder joint.

f. of Winslow Epiploic f.

zygomatico-orbital f. A small opening on the outer surface of the zygomatic bone through which the zygomatic nerve passes. There may be one or several openings.

Forbes' disease [Gilbert B. Forbes, U.S. pediatrician, b. 1915] Glycogen storage disease type III.

force An external influence; a push or pull exerted on an object. The metric unit for force is the newton. One newton equals 0.225 lb of force.

catabolic f. Energy produced by metabolism of food.

centrifugal f. The force that impels a thing, or parts of it, outward from the center of rotation. SEE: *centrifuge.*

electromotive f. ABBR: EMF. Energy that causes flow of electricity in a conductor. The energy is measured in volts.

G f. The gravitational constant. In aerospace medicine, the term indicates the forces acting on the human body during acceleration in certain flight maneuvers. Thus a force of 2 positive G means that the aviator is being subjected to a force twice that of gravity with a doubling of weight in that condition (i.e., the force against the seat is

2 G). G force may be in any axis and may be negative or positive.

maximum inspiratory f. ABBR: MIF. The output of the inspiratory muscles measured in centimeters of negative water pressure. It is measured by having the subject inhale from a tube connected to a manometer under conditions of no flow. Also called *maximum inspiratory pressure; negative inspiratory force.*

reserve f. The energy available above that required for normal functioning of the heart.

unit of f. An arbitrary measure of a certain amount of force. For example, a dyne is the amount of force acting continuously on a mass of 1 g that will accelerate the mass 1 cm per second.

forced expiratory time ABBR: FET. The time required to forcibly exhale a specified volume of air from the lung.

forced expiratory volume ABBR: FEV. The volume of air that can be expired after a full inspiration. The expiration is done as quickly as possible and the volume measured at precise times; at ½, 1, 2, and 3 sec. This provides valuable information concerning the ability to expel air from the lungs.

forceps (for′sĕps) [L.] Pincers for holding, seizing, or extracting according to the purpose for which they are intended. It is important to note that forceps may be called by different names, according to geographic location or institution. In obstetrics, forceps application is classified according to the position of the fetal head when the forceps are applied (i.e., outlet forceps, low forceps, and midforceps). SEE: *station.*

alligator f. A straight or angled clamp with jawlike movement at its end.

Allis f. Forceps with curved, serrated edges. They are used to grasp tissue firmly.

artery f. A delicate clamp that will not injure the vessel; used for temporary occlusion of a vessel.

axis-traction f. Obstetrical forceps fitted with a handle that makes it possible to provide traction in line with the direction in which the head must be moved.

bone f. A heavy-duty scissors-like instrument for cutting bone and removing bone fragments.

capsule f. Forceps for removing the capsule of the lens of the eye during cataract surgery.

Chamberlen f. The original obstetrical forceps, named after the inventor Peter Chamberlen (1560–1631) or his son Peter (1601–1683). They kept their development secret until Hugh Chamberlen (1664–1726) disclosed it.

clamp f. Any forceps with an automatic lock.

dental f. Forceps of varying shapes for grasping teeth during extraction procedures.

dressing f. Forceps for general use in dressing wounds and removing dead tissue and drainage tubes.

Halsted's f. A small curved or straight hemostatic forceps.

Magill f. SEE: *Magill forceps.*

mosquito f. A smaller variety of Halsted's forceps with a finely pointed tip.

needle f. Forceps for grasping and holding a needle.

obstetrical f. Forceps used to extract the fetal head from the pelvis during delivery. They serve the dual purpose of allowing withdrawal force to be applied to the fetal head and protecting the head during the passage.

rongeur f. Forceps used for cutting bone.

tissue f. A pincer-like toothed instrument for grasping delicate tissues.

towel f. Sharply pointed clip for holding towels and/or skin.

forcipate (for′sĭ-pāt) [L. *forceps,* tongs] Shaped like forceps.

Fordyce-Fox disease (for′dīs-fŏks′) [John Fordyce, U.S. dermatologist, 1858–1925; George Henry Fox, U.S. dermatologist, 1846–1937] A chronic pruritic papular eruption of areas of the skin that contain apocrine sweat glands. The intraepidermal ducts of the apocrine glands become obstructed and eventually rupture. The disease occurs mostly in persons 13 to 35 years of age and about 10 times more frequently in women than men. It does not occur before puberty. SYN: *Fox-Fordyce disease; miliaria, apocrine.*

TREATMENT: Several agents, including estrogens, corticosteroids, and topical tretinoin cream, have been used, but with little benefit.

Fordyce's disease (for′dī-sĕs) [John Fordyce] Enlarged ectopic sebaceous glands in the mucosa of the mouth and genitals. They appear as small yellow spots, called Fordyce's spots. They are asymptomatic and are present in most people.

Fordyce's spots SEE: *Fordyce's disease.*

forearm [AS. *fore,* in front, + *arm,* arm] The portion of the arm between the elbow and wrist.

forebrain [″ + *bregen,* brain] The anterior portion of the brain of the embryo. SYN: *prosencephalon.*

forefinger The first (index) finger.

forefoot The part of the foot in front of the tarsometatarsal joint.

foregut [″ + *gut,* a pouring] The first part of the embryonic digestive tube from which the pharynx, esophagus, stomach, and duodenum are formed. SYN: *protogaster.*

forehead [AS. *forheafod*] The anterior part of the head below the hairline and above the eyes. SYN: *frons.*

foreign body Anything present at a site where it would not normally be found. Slivers, cinders, dirt, or small objects may lodge in the skin, ears, eyes, or nose or may be taken internally. If not removed, they may cause unsightly marks or tattooing of the skin and inflammation and infection of the tissue involved.

FIRST AID: *In skin:* The areas involved are cleaned carefully. Foreign material can be removed carefully piece by piece or by vigorous swabbing with gauze or a brush and a soapy solution. A sterile dressing should be used.

For removal of a small foreign body, the area is cleaned first with mild soap and warm water. A clean needle can be sterilized by heating it to a dull or bright red in a flame; this can be done with a single match. Because both ends of the needle get hot, it is wise to hold the far end in a nonconductor such as a fold of paper or a cork. The needle is allowed to cool. A black deposit on its surface should be disregarded; it is sterile carbon and does not interfere with the procedure. The needle is introduced at right angles to the direction of the sliver, and the sliver is lifted out. Most people attempt to stick the needle in the direction of the foreign body and consequently thrust many times before they manage to lift the sliver out. When the sliver is removed, an antiseptic is applied and the wound covered with a sterile dressing. Tetanus antitoxin or a tetanus booster may be required, depending on the history of immunization.

In the ear: Water is not introduced if any vegetable matter is in the ear because it may push the foreign body further into the ear or cause it to swell and become firmly embedded. A globule of ordinary glue can be placed on the end of a match stick or an applicator, gently introduced until it touches the foreign body, and removed gently.

If an insect is in the ear, loud buzzing, pain, and dizziness may result. The ear should be flooded with lidocaine to let the insect float out.

In the esophagus: Occasionally, patients present with items trapped in the esophagus (typically fishbones, coins, or unchewed pieces of meat). Parenteral glucagon may help the material pass through the esophageal sphincter to the stomach, but endoscopic retrieval of the material is usually necessary. SEE: illus.

In the vagina: A great variety of foreign bodies may be present in the vagina, esp. in children and in the insane. Also, it is possible to forget to remove a vaginal tampon, pessary, or contraceptive diaphragm. The treatment is to remove the foreign body. Antibiotic therapy is not usually necessary.

forelock A lock of hair that grows on the forehead.

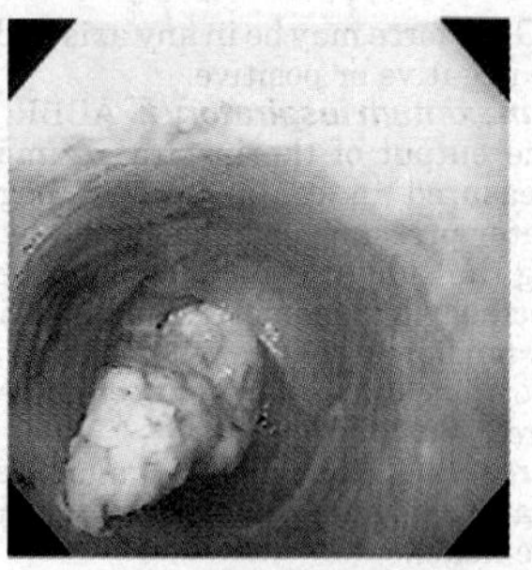

FOREIGN BODY

Meat impaction in the lower esophageal sphincter

white f. A white tuft of hair that grows on the forehead. It is associated with Waardenburg syndrome, and is seen in vitiligo.

forensic (for-ĕn′sĭk) [L. *forensis,* public] Pert. to the law; legal.

foreplay Fondling of the sex partner to produce mutual sexual arousal and pleasure prior to intercourse.

foreskin [AS. *fore,* in front, + O. Norse *skinn,* skin] The prepuce, the loose skin at and covering the end of the penis or clitoris like a hood. Excision of the prepuce constitutes circumcision. Smegma praeputii is secreted by Tyson's glands and collects under the foreskin.

forewaters (for′wăt-ĕrz) A pocket of amniotic fluid that precedes the presenting part of the fetus into the cervical canal. Expulsion or dissolution of the mucus plug (cervical operculum) allows the pocket to descend into the canal during the first stage of labor. SEE: *operculum*.

forgetting Inability to remember something previously known or learned. SEE: *memory*.

fork An elongated instrument that splits at the end to form two or more prongs.

tuning f. A device that vibrates at specific frequencies, e.g., 128, 256, or 512 cycles per second. It is used in simple tests of hearing, including bone conduction and air conduction.

form The distinctive size, shape, and external appearance of anything.

arch f. The shape of the dental arch when viewed in the horizontal plane.

formaldehyde (for-măl′dĕ-hīd) A colorless, pungent, irritant gas (HCOH) commonly made by oxidation of methyl alcohol, the simplest member of the aldehyde group. An aqueous solution of 37% formaldehyde (formalin) is used as a preservative. This chemical has been shown to be carcinogenic in certain animals and may be carcinogenic in humans.

formaldehyde poisoning Poisoning caused by ingestion of formaldehyde.

SYMPTOMS: Symptoms include local

irritation of the eyes, nose, mouth, throat, respiratory and gastrointestinal tracts, and central nervous system disorders, including vertigo, stupor, convulsions, unconsciousness, and renal damage. SEE: *Poisons and Poisoning Appendix.*

formalin (for′mă-lĭn) An aqueous solution of 37% formaldehyde. SEE: *aldehyde.*

formate (for′māt) A salt of formic acid.

formatio (for-mā′shē-ō) *pl.* **formationes** [L.] A structure with definite arrangement and shape.

f. reticularis The dorsal part of the medulla oblongata.

formation **1.** A structure, shape, or figure. **2.** The giving of form or shape to, or the development of, a structure.

reticular f. A meshed structure formed of gray matter and interlacing fibers of white matter found in the medulla oblongata between the pyramids and the floor of the fourth ventricle of the brain. It is also present in the spinal cord, midbrain, and pons. Fibers from this structure are important in controlling or influencing alertness, waking, sleeping, and various reflexes. They are thought to activate the cerebral cortex independently of specific sensory or other neural systems. The reticular formation is part of the reticular activating (alerting) system.

forme fruste (form froost) *pl.* **formes frustes** [Fr., defaced] An aborted or incomplete form of disease arrested before running its course; an atypical and indefinite manifestation of an illness.

formic [L. *formica,* ant] Pert. to ants or to formic acid.

formic aldehyde Formaldehyde.

formication The profoundly disturbing sensation that insects are crawling on one's skin. This is one of the more troublesome side effects of alcohol and cocaine withdrawal.

formiciasis (for″mĭs-ī′ă-sĭs) [L. *formica,* ant, + Gr. *-iasis,* condition] Irritation caused by ant bites.

formilase (for′mĭ-lās) An enzyme that catalyzes conversion of acetic acid to formic acid.

formol (for′mŏl) Formaldehyde solution. SEE: *formalin.*

formula [L., a little form] **1.** A rule prescribing ingredients and proportions for the preparation of a compound. **2.** In chemistry, a symbolic expression of the constitution of a molecule. It consists of letters, each denoting one atom of one element, with subscripted numbers denoting the number of atoms present. Water, or H_2O, consists of two molecules of the element hydrogen and one of oxygen. It may also be written HOH.

Collections of atoms that constitute a group by themselves (radical) are often separated by periods or parentheses. In this case, figures prefixed or appended to the parentheses, or prefixed to an expression contained within periods, apply to all the symbols embraced by the parentheses or periods. In all other cases, a figure prefixed to a symbolic expression for a molecule, such as a coefficient in an algebraic formula, is a multiplier of all the symbols following.

Arneth's f. A method of estimating the number of immature leukocytes by means of an elaborate differential blood count, on the basis of their shape and the number of lobes in the nucleus. It is seldom used.

chemical f. SEE: *formula* (2).

dental f. A brief method of expressing the dentition of mammals in which the numbers of the teeth are given in the form of a fraction, each portion representing one quadrant; the numbers of the upper teeth form the numerator, and those of the lower teeth the denominator.

The first number listed represents the incisors; the second, the canines; the third, the premolars; and the fourth, the molars. The dental formula of the upper and lower right half of the mouth in humans is:

$$\frac{2-1-2-3 \text{ (right upper jaw)}}{2-1-2-3 \text{ (right lower jaw)}}$$

empirical f. The formula of a compound that shows the atoms and their relative numbers in a molecule, as H_2O.

molecular f. The chemical formula indicating the elements and the number of each present, but providing no information concerning their two- or three-dimensional arrangements in the formula. SEE: *stereochemical f.*

official f. A formula in a pharmacopeia.

spatial f. Stereochemical f.

stereochemical f. A method of depicting chemical formulas so that the elements and their number are depicted as well as their position in space in relation to each other. SYN: *spatial f.*

structural f. A formula of a compound that shows the relationship of the atoms in a molecule. The atoms are shown joined by valence bonds (e.g., H—O—H).

formulary [L. *formula,* a little form] **1.** A book of formulas. **2.** A list of drugs available for routine use at a health care facility.

National F. ABBR: NF. A book that provides standards and specifications for drugs. Previously issued by the American Pharmaceutical Association, it is now published by the U.S. Pharmacopeial Convention, Inc.

formyl The radical of formic acid, HCO.

fornicate [L. *fornicatus*] Arched or vault-like; shaped like a fornix.

fornicate [L. *fornicari*] To have sexual intercourse.

fornication Sexual intercourse.

fornices (for′nĭ-sēz) [L.] Pl. of fornix.

fornicolumn [L. *fornix,* arch, + *columna,* column] The anterior pillar of the fornix uteri.

fornicommissure (for-nĭ-kŏm′ĭ-sūr) [″ + *commissura,* a joining together] The commissure or body of the fornix uteri.

fornix [L., arch] **1.** A fibrous vaulted band connecting the cerebral lobes. **2.** Any vaultlike or arched body.

f. conjunctivae The loose folds connecting the palpebral and bulbar conjunctivae.

f. uteri F. vaginae.

f. vaginae Each of the four recesses that surround the cervix. The posterior fornix is deeper than the anterior or lateral (right and left) fornices. SYN: *f. uteri.*

Fort Bragg fever [Fort Bragg, North Carolina, a U.S. military base] Pretibial fever; a form of leptospirosis.

fortification spectrum The appearance of a dark patch with a zigzag outline in the visual field, causing a temporary blindness in that portion of the eye. SYN: *teichopsia.*

fortify In food science technology, to add one or more substances to a food to increase its nutrient density.

fos (făs) A family of cancer-causing genes, first identified in viruses, that function within cells as transcription factors. Members of this family can transform normal cells (e.g., fibroblasts) into cancer cells (e.g., osteosarcomas, chondrosarcomas). SEE: *oncogene; transformation.*

ETIOLOGY: The name is derived from "FBJ osteosarcoma virus," in which these oncogenes were first identified.

Foshay's test [Lee Foshay, U.S. physician, 1896–1961] Intradermal injection of a suspension of killed *Francisella tularensis,* the causative agent of tularemia. The appearance of an area of erythema at the injection site is considered a positive reaction.

fossa (fŏs′ă) *pl.* **fossae** [L.] A furrow or shallow depression.

amygdaloid f. Tonsillar f.

articular f. of mandible Mandibular f.

articular f. of temporal bone Mandibular f.

axillary f. Axilla; armpit.

canine f. The wide, shallow depression on the external surface of the maxilla superolateral to the canine tooth. It serves as the origin of the levator anguli oris muscle.

cerebral f. Any of several depressions on the inside floor of the cranium. SYN: *cranial f.*

Claudius' f. Ovarian f.

condylar f. The depression behind the occipital epicondyle.

coronoid f. The depression on the anterior surface of the lower end of the humerus. During full flexion of the forearm, the coronoid process of the ulna fits into the depression.

cranial f. Cerebral f.

digastric f. The depression behind the lower margin of the mandible at the side of the symphysis menti. The anterior belly of the digastric muscle attaches here.

epigastric f. The pit of the inside of the stomach.

ethmoid f. SYN: *olfactory groove.*

glenoid f. **1.** The depression on the scapula that articulates with the head of the humerus. **2.** Mandibular f.

hyaloid f. The depression on the anterior surface of the vitreous body of the eye. The lens is located there.

hypophyseal f. The deep depression in the sphenoid bone in which the pituitary gland rests. SYN: *pituitary f.; sella turcica.*

iliac f. One of the concavities of the iliac bones of the pelvis.

incisive f. The depression on the anterior surface of the body of the maxilla medial to the root of the canine incisor tooth.

infratemporal f. The shallow depression under and medial to the zygomatic arch. It contains the muscles of mastication, the first two parts of the maxillary artery, the pterygoid venous plexus, and branches of the mandibular nerve, the third division of the trigeminal nerve.

intercondyloid f. The depression on the inferior surface of the femur between the femoral condyles. The cruciate ligaments pass through it.

interpeduncular f. The deep groove in the anterior surface of the midbrain, between the cerebral peduncles. The third cranial nerve emerges here.

ischiorectal f. The space on either side of the lower end of the rectum and anal canal. It is bounded laterally by the obturator internus muscle and the tuberosity of the ischium, medially by the levator ani and coccygeus muscles, and posteriorly by the gluteus maximus muscle.

jugular f. The depression in the petrosal portion of the temporal bone for the jugular vein.

lacrimal f. The hollow of the frontal bone that holds the lacrimal gland.

lenticular f. The depression in the anterior surface of the vitreous for reception of the crystalline lens.

mandibular f. The depression in the temporal bone into which the condyle of the mandible fits. SYN: *articular f. of mandible; articular f. of temporal bone; glenoid f.* (2).

mastoid f. The small triangular area between the posterior wall of the acoustic meatus and the posterior root of the zygomatic process of the temporal bone.

nasal f. The cavity between the anterior opening to the nose and the nasopharynx.

navicular f. The depression between the vulva and fourchette.

olecranon f. The depression on the posterior surface of the lower end of the humerus. During full extension of the forearm, the olecranon process of the ulna fits into this depression.

f. ovalis The opening in the fascia of the thigh through which the large saphenous vein passes.

f. ovalis cordis The remnant of the embryonic foramen ovale in the right cardiac atrium.

ovarian f. The depression in the parietal peritoneum of the pelvis that contains the ovary. SYN: *Claudius' f.*

piriform f. Depressions in the lateral walls of the laryngopharynx.

pituitary f. Hypophyseal f.

popliteal f. The soft tissue depression posterior to the knee.

pterygopalatine f. A space bounded posteriorly by the root of the pterygoid process, medially by the orbital and sphenoidal processes of the palatine bone, and anteriorly by the superomedial aspect of the posterior surface of the maxilla. Also called *sphenomaxillary fossa.*

Rosenmüller's f. The depression in the pharynx posterior to the opening of the eustachian tube.

sublingual f. A shallow depression on the inner surface of the body of the mandible above the anterior part of the mylohyoid ridge. It is occupied by the major salivary gland in the area, the sublingual gland.

submandibular f. An oblong depression between the mylohyoid ridge and the inferior border of the medial surface of the body of the mandible. It is occupied by the submandibular gland. These were previously referred to as the submaxillary fossa and submaxillary gland.

subpyramidal f. A depression in the inferior wall of the middle ear. It is inferior to the round window and posterior to the pyramid.

supraspinous f. The concave triangular area above the spinous process of the posterior surface of the clavicle.

f. supratonsillaris The space between the anterior and posterior pillars of the fauces above the tonsil.

temporal f. The depression on the side of the skull below the temporal lines. It is deep to the zygomatic arch and continuous with the infratemporal fossa.

tonsillar f. The depression in the back of the oral cavity containing the tonsil. SYN: *amygdaloid f.*

fossae (fŏs′ē) [L.] Pl. of fossa.

fossette (fŏ-sĕt′) [Fr.] **1.** A small depression or fossa. **2.** A small but deep corneal ulcer.

fossula (fŏs′ū-lă) A small furrow, depression, or fossa.

foster care The care of individuals who cannot live independently (such as children, homeless families, or frail elderly persons) in a group or private home.

adult f.c. Long-term care for elderly individuals in an adult foster care facility. Typically, such a facility resembles a residence rather than a nursing home and may have fewer regulations than a nursing home.

Fothergill's disease (fŏth′ĕr-gĭlz) [John Fothergill, Brit. physician, 1712–1780] **1.** Scarlatina anginosa, an ulcerative sore throat present in severe scarlet fever. **2.** Trigeminal neuralgia.

foulage (foo-lŏzh′) [Fr.] Massage by kneading with pressure on the muscles.

foundation, denture The area on which a denture rests.

fourchet, fourchette (foor-shĕt′) [Fr. *fourchette,* a fork] A tense band or transverse fold of mucous membrane at the posterior commissure of the vagina, connecting the posterior ends of the labia minora. The fossa navicularis, a cul-de-sac anterior to the fourchette, separates it from the hymen. It disappears after defloration or parturition, leaving a more open vulva below and behind. SYN: *frenulum labiorum pudendi.* SEE: *vestibule of vagina.*

Fournier's gangrene, Fournier's disease (fŏr-nē′āz) Necrotizing fasciitis of the male genitalia that may spread to the thighs or abdomen. This aggressive and life-threatening form of cellulitis typically occurs in patients who have had local trauma to the genitals and patients with diabetes mellitus.

ETIOLOGY: Multiple aerobic and anaerobic bacteria cause the infection.

TREATMENT: Treatment consists of broad-spectrum antibiotics and wide surgical débridement.

fourth cranial nerve A small mixed nerve exiting from the dorsal surface of the midbrain. It contains efferent motor fibers to the superior oblique muscle of the eye and afferent sensory fibers conveying proprioceptive impulses from the same muscle. SYN: *trochlear nerve.*

fovea (fō′vē-ă) *pl.* **foveae** [L.] A pit or cuplike depression. SEE: *fossa.*

f. capitis The depression on the head of the femur for attachment of the ligamentum teres.

f. centralis retinae In the eye, the pit in the middle of the macula lutea that contains only cones.

foveate (fō′vē-āt) [L. *foveatus*] Pitted.

foveation (fō″vē-ā′shŭn) Pitting, as in smallpox.

foveola (fō-vē′ō-lă) *pl.* **foveolae** [L., little pit] A minute pit or depression.

Fowler's position [George R. Fowler, U.S. surgeon, 1848–1906] A semi-sitting position. The head of an adjustable bed can be elevated to the desired height to produce angulation of the body, usually 45° to 60°. The knees may or may not be bent. A wedge support can be used to elevate the patient's head and back if an adjustable bed is not available. The position is used to facilitate breathing and drainage and for the comfort of the bedridden patient while eating or talking.

NOTE: The hips (knees) may or may not be flexed in this position, which has three variations: high (sitting upright in bed), regular (head or torso elevated 45° or more), and low or semi-low (head and torso elevated to 30°).

Fox-Fordyce disease SEE: *Fordyce-Fox disease.*

foxglove (fŏks′glŏv) The common name for the flowering plant *Digitalis purpurea,* from which the drug digitalis is obtained. It was first described by William Withering in a book published in 1785.

FPR *False-positive ratio.*

Fr Symbol for the element francium.

fraction [L. *fractio,* act of breaking] **1.** In biological chemistry, the separable part of a substance such as blood or plasma. **2.** The ratio of a component to the total (e.g., the substance fraction of carboxyhemoglobin [relative to the total hemoglobin]).

f. of inspired oxygen ABBR: FIO_2. The concentration of oxygen in the inspired air, esp. that supplied as supplemental oxygen by mask or catheter. Concentrations of oxygen greater than 50% are toxic if administered for more than a few days.

mass f. The ratio of the mass of a constituent to the total mass of the system in which the constituent is contained. SEE: *substance f.*

substance f. The ratio of the amount (number of moles or entities) of a constituent of a mixture to the total of constituents of the system. SEE: *mass f.*

volume f. The ratio of the volume of a constituent to the volume of the whole. In practice, it may be difficult to determine the volume fraction because differences in the molecular sizes of the constituents may produce a total volume that differs from the sum of the individual volumes of the mixture. When materials of similar physicochemical characteristics (e.g., multiple aqueous solutions) are combined, this is not a problem.

fractional shortening The reduction of the length of the end-diastolic diameter that occurs by the end of systole. Like the ejection fraction, this is a measure of the heart's muscular contractility. If the diameter fails to shorten by at least 28%, the efficiency of the heart in ejecting blood is impaired.

fractional test meal Extended examination of the stomach contents. First the residual contents are removed and then the test meal is given. After the meal, assessments of gastric emptying, gastric acidity, pancreatic secretion, or nutrient absorption may be undertaken.

fractionation **1.** In radiation therapy, the process of spreading the total required treatment dose over an extended period. **2.** In chemistry, the separation of a mixture into its components, usually to isolate a particular substance for use or study.

fracture [L. *fractura,* break] **1.** Sudden breaking of a bone. **2.** A break of a bone. SEE: illus.

CAUSES: *Pathological:* In certain diseases and conditions such as osteomalacia, syphilis, and osteomyelitis, bones break spontaneously without trauma. *Direct violence:* The bone is broken directly at the spot where the force was applied, as in fracture of the tibia by being run over. *Indirect violence:* The bone is fractured by a force applied at a distance from the site of fracture and transmitted to the fractured bone, as fracture of the clavicle by falling on the outstretched hand. *Muscular contraction:* The bone is broken by a sudden violent contraction of the muscles.

SIGNS: Signs include loss of the power of movement, pain with acute tenderness over the site of fracture, swelling and bruising, deformity and possible shortening, unnatural mobility, and crepitus or grating that is heard when the ends of the bone rub together. It is important not to try to obtain these last two signs. Radiography should be used to find the type of fracture and the exact position of the bone fragments.

TREATMENT: In simple fractures, the limb or part must be kept immovable by means of splints. If an upper extremity is fractured, it should be supported in a sling, and the patient may then walk. If a lower limb is injured, the patient should remain supine and make no attempt to walk.

The physician reduces the fracture (places the fragments in proper position). The bone is kept in position by means of a cast until union has taken place. Then the limb is restored to complete function by physical therapy and exercise.

In compound fractures, any bleeding must be arrested before the fracture is treated. Open reduction may be required. The wound is then washed and cleaned with sterile saline. If the area is grossly contaminated, mild soap solution may be used provided it is thoroughly washed away with generous amounts of sterile saline. When the wound is clean, a sterile dressing is se-

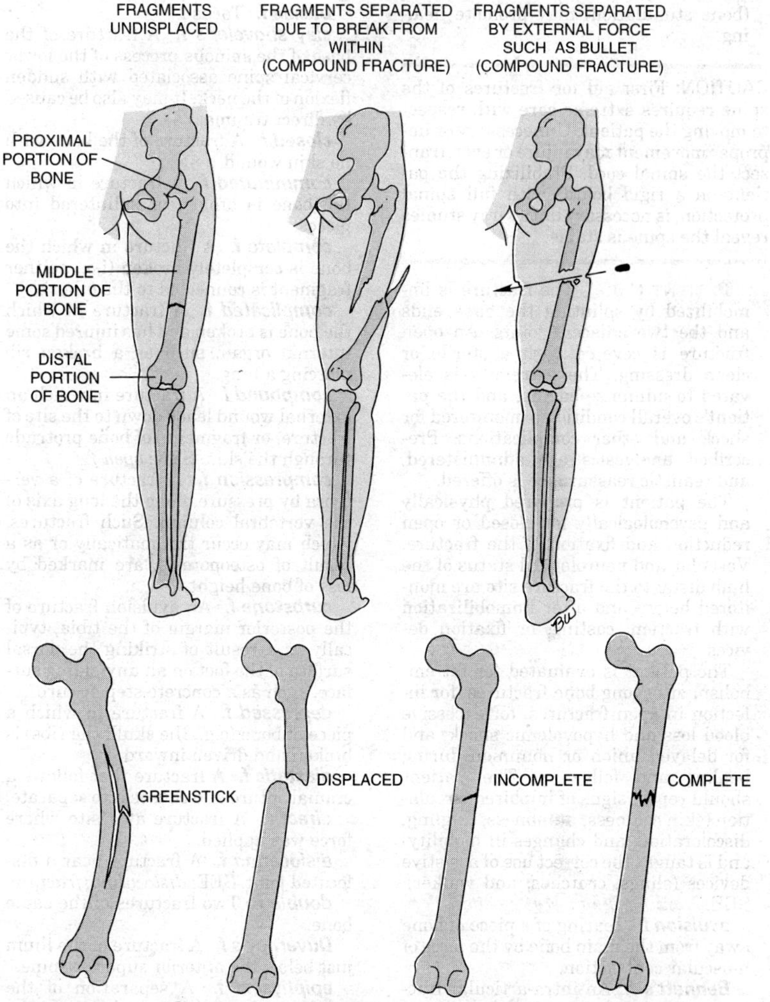

FRAGMENTS UNDISPLACED

FRAGMENTS SEPARATED DUE TO BREAK FROM WITHIN (COMPOUND FRACTURE)

FRAGMENTS SEPARATED BY EXTERNAL FORCE SUCH AS BULLET (COMPOUND FRACTURE)

PROXIMAL PORTION OF BONE

MIDDLE PORTION OF BONE

DISTAL PORTION OF BONE

GREENSTICK

DISPLACED

INCOMPLETE

COMPLETE

COMMINUTED

SEGMENTAL

BUTTERFLY

SPIRAL

HAIR-LINE

TYPES OF FRACTURES AND TERMINOLOGY

cured by a bandage. The bone may then be immobilized by external fixation until the wound heals.

Skeletal traction may be used instead of a cast or external fixator for certain fractures, such as femoral shaft fractures. Pins are placed in the bone and the bone ends are held in place by a system of pulleys and weights until bony union occurs.

If the bone does not heal, a weak electric current applied to the bone ends (bone stimulation) may promote healing.

CAUTION: First aid for fractures of the spine requires extreme care with respect to moving the patient. Unnecessary or improper movement may injure or even transect the spinal cord. Stabilizing the patient on a rigid board, with full spinal protection, is necessary until x-ray studies reveal the spine is stable.

PATIENT CARE: The fracture is immobilized by splinting the bone ends and the two adjacent joints. An open fracture is covered with a sterile or clean dressing. The extremity is elevated to minimize edema, and the patient's overall condition is monitored for shock and other complications. Prescribed analgesics are administered, and realistic reassurance is offered.

The patient is prepared physically and psychologically for closed or open reduction and fixation of the fracture. Vascular and neurological status of the limb distal to the fracture site are monitored before and after immobilization with traction, casting, or fixation devices.

The patient is evaluated for fat embolism after long bone fractures, for infection in open fractures, for excessive blood loss and hypovolemic shock, and for delayed union or nonunion during healing and follow-up. The patient should report signs of impaired circulation (skin coldness, numbness, tingling, discoloration, and changes in mobility) and is taught the correct use of assistive devices (slings, crutches, and walker). SEE: *Nursing Diagnoses Appendix.*

avulsion f. Tearing of a piece of bone away from the main bone by the force of muscular contraction.

Bennett's f. An intra-articular fracture at the base of the first metacarpal with subluxation of the carpometacarpal joint due to traction of the abductor pollicis longus muscle on the first metacarpal. This fracture usually requires percutaneous pinning to maintain reduction.

bimalleolar f. A fracture of the medial and lateral malleoli of the ankle joint.

blow-out f. A fracture of the floor of the orbit in which fragments are displaced downward by a blow to the eye or periorbital area.

bowing f. A bending or curving fracture of a bone (usually a forearm bone) as the result of a traumatic load that compresses the bone along its long axis.

boxer's f. A fracture of the distal end of the fourth or fifth metacarpal with posterior displacement of the proximal structures.

buckle f. Torus f.

clay shoveler's f. A fracture of the base of the spinous process of the lower cervical spine associated with sudden flexion of the neck. It may also be caused by direct trauma.

closed f. A fracture of the bone with no skin wound.

comminuted f. A fracture in which the bone is broken or splintered into pieces.

complete f. A fracture in which the bone is completely broken (i.e., neither fragment is connected to the other).

complicated f. A fracture in which the bone is broken and has injured some internal organ, such as a broken rib piercing a lung.

compound f. A fracture in which an external wound leads down to the site of fracture, or fragments of bone protrude through the skin. SYN: *open f.*

compression f. A fracture of a vertebra by pressure along the long axis of the vertebral column. Such fractures, which may occur traumatically or as a result of osteoporosis, are marked by loss of bone height.

curbstone f. An avulsion fracture of the posterior margin of the tibia, typically as a result of striking the dorsal surface of the foot on an unyielding surface, such as a concrete step or curb.

depressed f. A fracture in which a piece of bone (e.g., the skull, the ribs) is broken and driven inward.

diastatic f. A fracture that follows a cranial suture and causes it to separate.

direct f. A fracture at a site where force was applied.

dislocation f. A fracture near a dislocated joint. SEE: *dislocation; fracture.*

double f. Two fractures of the same bone.

Duverney's f. A fracture of the ilium just below the anterior superior spine.

epiphyseal f. A separation of the epiphysis from the bone between the shaft of the bone and its growing end. It occurs only in young patients.

fatigue f. SEE: *stress f.*

fissured f. A narrow split in the bone that does not go through to the other side of the bone.

hip f. Fracture of the hip.

greenstick f. A fracture in which the bone is partially bent and partially broken, as when a green stick breaks. It occurs in children, esp. those with rickets.

hairline f. A minor fracture in which all the portions of the bone are in perfect alignment. The fracture is seen on a radiograph as a very thin line between the two segments that does not extend entirely through the bone. SEE: *stress f.*

hangman's f. The fracture produced when judicial hanging is done correctly. At the moment when the dropped victim fully extends the rope, the hangman knot causes fracture dislocation of the upper cervical spine and transection of the spinal cord or medulla. If the knot is not made or applied properly, death is usually due to asphyxia.

impacted f. A fracture in which the bone is broken and one end is wedged into the interior of the other.

incomplete f. A fracture in which the line of fracture does not include the whole bone. SEE: *stress f.*

indirect f. A fracture distant from the place where the force was applied.

intracapsular f. A fracture occurring within the capsule of a joint.

intrauterine f. A broken fetal bone.

Jefferson f. Jefferson fracture.

Jones f. A transverse fracture of the proximal diaphysis, approx. three quarters of an inch from the base of the fifth metatarsal. This fracture is commonly confused with an avulsion fracture of the styloid process of the fifth metatarsal. The distinction is important because the true Jones fracture often results in a nonunion.

lead pipe f. A fracture in which the bone is compressed and bent so that one side of the fracture bulges and the other side shows a slight crack.

LeFort f. A fracture usually involving more than one of the facial bones: maxillary, nasal, orbital, and/or zygomatic.

lover's f. A fracture of the calcaneus, due to jumping from a height (e.g., a balcony or second-story window).

march f. A fracture of the lower extremities or bones of the feet as a result of overuse. SEE: *stress f.*

mid-face f. LeFort f.

nightstick f. A nondisplaced transverse fracture of the ulna resulting from a direct blow.

nonunion of f. SEE: *nonunion.*

open f. Compound f.

overriding f. A fracture in which the ends of the fractured bone slide past each other.

pathological f. A fracture of a diseased or weakened bone produced by a force that would not have fractured a healthy bone. The underlying disease may be metastasis from a cancer that originated elsewhere, primary cancer of the bone, or osteoporosis.

PATIENT CARE: The limbs and joints of at-risk patients are gently and carefully supported when repositioning, exercising, or mobilizing. If such patients fall or are otherwise injured, and report limb pain or inability to bear weight, the affected limb should be stabilized and x-rayed.

ping-pong f. A depressed fracture of the skull that resembles the indentation made by pressing firmly on a Ping-Pong ball.

Pott's f. A fracture of the lower end of the fibula with outward displacement of the ankle and foot. The medial malleolus of the fibula may be fractured.

pretrochanteric f. A fracture that passes through the greater trochanter of the femur.

Rolando f. A comminuted intra-articular fracture of the base of the first metacarpal with distal fragment subluxation. This fracture is similar to a Bennett's fracture but with more comminution.

simple f. A fracture without rupture of ligaments and skin.

Smith's f. SEE: *Colles' fracture.*

snowboarder's f. A fracture of the lateral border of the talus caused by inversion and rotation of the talus within the mortise. Signs and symptoms often mimic those of an inversion (lateral) ankle sprain.

spiral f. A fracture that follows a helical line along and around the course of a long bone.

spontaneous f. Pathological f.

stellate f. A fracture with numerous fissures radiating from the central point of injury.

stress f. A fine hairline fracture that appears without evidence of soft tissue injury. This type of fracture is difficult to diagnose by roentgenographical examination and may not become visible until 3 to 4 weeks after the onset of symptoms. It occurs from repetitive microtraumas, as with running, aerobic dancing, or marching; with use of improper shoes on hard surfaces; or with inadequate healing time after stress.

torus f. A fracture in which the bony cortex is not broken but is buckled.

transcervical f. A fracture through the neck of the femur.

transverse f. A fracture in which the fracture line is at right angles to the long axis of the bone.

trimalleolar f. A fracture of the lateral and medial malleoli of the ankle joint with an additional fracture of the posterior edge of the distal tibia.

tripod f. A fracture in which the zygoma is separated from its attachment to the maxilla and the temporal and frontal bones.

fracture dislocation A fracture near a dislocated joint.

fragile X syndrome A chromosomal disease, often associated with mental retardation, in which the tip of the long arm of the X chromosome can separate from the rest of the genetic material. Most males and 30% of females with this syndrome are mentally retarded. Males also develop greatly enlarged testicles (macro-orchidism), enlarged ears, and a prominent jaw.

fragilitas (frā-jĭl′ĭ-tās) [L.] Fragility.

fragility Readily broken, injured, or damaged brittleness.

capillary f. A breakdown of capillaries with hemorrhage into almost any site but most noticeably in the skin.

erythrocyte f. F. of red blood cells.

f. of red blood cells The tendency of red blood cells to rupture. This is determined by subjecting the cells to different concentrations of saline in laboratory tests.

If red blood cells are placed in distilled water, they swell rapidly and burst because they normally are suspended in a solution of much greater osmotic pressure. This phenomenon is called hemolysis. If they are suspended in a solution of normal saline, the cells retain their normal shape and do not burst. If they are placed in successively weaker solutions of saline, a point is reached at which some of the cells burst and liberate their hemoglobin within a given length of time. Finally, at a given dilution, all the cells have burst within the allotted time, which is usually 2 hr. Normal blood cells begin to hemolyze in about 0.44% saline solution, and complete hemolysis occurs in about 0.35% solution.

fragment (frăg′mĕnt) A part broken off a larger entity.

Fab f. Area on an immunoglobulin (antibody) to which antigens bind. The enzyme papain splits antibodies into three fragments, two Fab fragments, each of which is antigen-specific, and an Fc or crystallizable fragment, which is involved in secondary antibody activities such as activating complement.

immunoglobulin f. The portion of the IgG molecule that contains an antibody-combining site. Specific fragments are obtained by treating the molecule with the enzyme papain under specified conditions. The resultant fragments are designated "F(zz) Fragment," where zz represents the specific fragment. SYN: *immunologlobulin isotype*.

fragment antigen binding ABBR: Fab. Area on an immunoglobulin (antibody) to which antigens bind.

fragmentation [L. *fragmentum*, detached part] Breaking up into pieces.

sleep f. Arousals and awakenings that disrupt the normal stages and architecture of sleep. These events, which occur commonly in patients who have sleep apnea or chronic pain, contribute to daytime sleepiness and other health problems.

frail elderly Older persons with medical, nutritional, cognitive, emotional, or activity impairments. These deficits may limit their ability to live independently and predispose them to illnesses and the side effects of treatment.

frailty Weakness; fragility.

frambesia (frăm-bē′zē-ă) [Fr. *framboise*, raspberry] Yaws.

frambesioma (frăm-bē-zē-ō′mă) [″ + Gr. *oma*, tumor] The primary lesion of yaws in the form of a protruding nodule. This mother yaw appears at the site of inoculation of the causative agent, *Treponema pertenue*.

frame A supporting structure.

Balkan f. A framework that fits over a bed. Weights suspended from the frame and connected through ropes and pulleys are used to produce continuous traction while permitting freedom of motion, thus maintaining desired immobilization of the part being treated.

Bradford f. An oblong frame, about 7 × 3 ft (2.13 × 0.91 m), made of 1-in. (2.5-cm) pipe covered with movable canvas strips that run from one side of the frame to the other. It is used for patients with fractures or disease of the hip or spine, permitting them to urinate and defecate without moving the spine or changing position.

quadriplegic standing f. A device for supporting a patient with all four extremities paralyzed.

Stryker f. SEE: *Stryker frame*.

trial f. An eyeglass frame for holding trial lenses while a person is being fitted for glasses.

Franceschetti's syndrome (frăn″chĕs-kĕt′ēz) [Adolphe Franceschetti, Swiss ophthalmologist, 1896–1968] Mandibulofacial dysostosis with hypoplasia of the facial bones, downward angulation of the palpebral fissures, macrostomia, ear defects, and defectively formed extremities. SYN: *Treacher Collins syndrome*.

Franciscella tularensis (frăn″sĭ-sĕl′ă too″lă-rĕn′sĭs) [Edward Francis, Tulare County, California] A short, nonmotile, encapsulated, non–spore-forming, gram-negative bacillus that causes tularemia in humans. Formerly classed as *Pasteurella tularensis*.

francium (frăn′sē-ŭm) [Named for France, the country in which it was discovered] SYMB: Fr. A radioactive metallic element occurring as a natural isotope. Its atomic number is 87; the atomic weight of the most stable isotope is 233.

frank Obvious, esp. in reference to a clinical sign or condition such as blood in the urine, sputum, or feces.

Frankenhäuser's ganglion (frăng′kĕn-hoy″zĕrs) [Ferdinand Frankenhäuser, Ger. gynecologist, 1832–1894] A nerve ganglion sometimes found in the lateral walls of the cervix uteri.

Frankfort horizontal plane A cephalometric plane joining the anthropometric landmarks of porion and orbitale; the reproducible position of the head when the upper margin of the ear openings and lower margin of the orbit of the eye are horizontal.

Franklin glasses [Benjamin Franklin, U.S. statesman and inventor, 1706–1790] Bifocal spectacles.

Frank-Starling law In cardiac physiology, the rule stating that cardiac output increases in proportion to the diastolic stretch of heart muscle fibers.

fratricide (frăt′rĭ-sīd″) [L. *fratricidium*] Murder of one's brother or sister.

Fraunhofer's lines (frown′hōf-ĕrz) [Joseph von Fraunhofer, Ger. optician, 1787–1826] Absorption bands or lines seen in a spectrum, caused by the absorption of groups of light rays in their passage through solids, liquids, or gases.

FRC *functional residual capacity.*

F.R.C.P. *Fellow of the Royal College of Physicians.*

F.R.C.P.(C.) *Fellow of the Royal College of Physicians of Canada.*

F.R.C.S. *Fellow of the Royal College of Surgeons.*

F.R.C.S.(C.) *Fellow of the Royal College of Surgeons of Canada.*

freckle (frĕk′l) [O. Norse *freknur*] A small stained or pigmented spot on sun-exposed skin. SYN: *ephelis; lentigo.*

Hutchinson's f. A noninvasive malignant melanoma.

free base A highly addictive form of cocaine consumed by smoking. It is prepared by alkalinizing the hydrochloride salt, extracting it with an organic solvent such as ether, and then heating the extract to 90°C. The inhaled material is rapidly absorbed from the lung. SEE: *cocaine hydrochloride; crack; freebasing.*

freebasing The inhalation of a form of cocaine called free base. SEE: *cocaine hydrochloride; crack.*

free medical clinic A clinic that is established by the community rather than by a hospital and that provides medical care without expecting payment for services. Typically free clinics combine medical services with patient education, patient empowerment, and social work.

freeze-drying Preservation of tissue by rapidly freezing the specimen and then dehydrating it in a high vacuum. SYN: *lyophilization.*

freezing [AS. *freosan*] **1.** Passing from a liquid to a solid state due to heat loss. **2.** Damaged by exposure to cold temperatures. SEE: *frostbite; hypothermia.*

freezing mixture A combination of 5 oz (150 ml) each of ammonium chloride and potassium nitrate and one part water, used for ice bags.

Freiberg's infraction (frī′bĕrgz) [Albert Henry Freiberg, U.S. surgeon, 1868–1940] Osteochondritis of the head of the second metatarsal bone of the foot.

fremitus (frĕm′ĭ-tŭs) [L.] Vibratory tremors, esp. those felt through the chest wall by palpation. Varieties include vocal or tactile, friction, hydatid, rhonchal or bronchial, cavernous on succussion, pleural, pericardial, tussive, and thrills. SEE: *palpation; thrill.*

hydatid f. A tremulous sensation felt on palpating a hydatid tumor.

tactile f. The vibration or thrill felt while the patient is speaking and the hand is held against the chest.

tussive f. Vibrations felt when the hand is held against the chest when the patient coughs.

vocal f. Vibrations of the voice transmitted to the ear during auscultation of the chest of a person speaking. In determining vocal fremitus, the following precautions should be observed: Symmetric parts of the chest are compared. The same pressure is applied to the stethoscope on each side. Fremitus is decreased in pleural effusions (air, pus, blood, serum, or lymph), emphysema, pulmonary collapse from an obstructed bronchus, pulmonary edema, and cancers of the lung.

French scale A system used to indicate the outer diameter of catheters and sounds. Each unit on the scale is approximately equivalent to one-third mm; thus a 21 French sound is 7 mm in diameter.

frenectomy (frē-nĕk′tō-mē) [L. *fraenum*, bridle, + Gr. *ektome*, excision] Surgical cutting of any frenum, usually of the tongue.

frenotomy (frē-nŏt′ō-mē) [″ + Gr. *tome*, incision] Division of any frenum, esp. for tongue-tie.

frenuloplasty (frĕn′ū-lō-plăs″tē) [″ + Gr. *plassein*, to form] Surgical correction of an abnormally attached frenulum.

frenulum (frĕn′ū-lŭm) *pl.* **frenula** [L., a little bridle] **1.** A small frenum. SYN: *vinculum.* **2.** A small fold of white matter on the upper surface of the anterior medullary velum extending to the corpora quadrigemina of the brain.

f. clitoridis The union of the inner parts of the labia minora on the undersurface of the clitoris.

f. of ileocecal valve The prolongation of the two lips of the ileocecal valve around the inner wall of the colon.

f. labiorum pudendi The fold of membrane connecting the posterior ends of the labia minora.

f. linguae F. of the tongue.

f. of the lips The fold of mucous membrane extending from the middle of the inner surface of the lip to the alveolar mucosa. It is seen in both the upper and lower jaws.

f. preputii The frenulum that unites the foreskin (prepuce) to the glans penis.

f. of the tongue The frenulum that attaches the lower side of the tongue to the floor of the buccal cavity. At birth this may be tight, a condition called tongue-tie. SYN: *f. linguae.*

frenum (frē′nŭm) *pl.* **frena** [L. *fraenum*, bridle] A fold of mucous membrane that connects two parts, one more or less movable, and checks the movement of this part. SEE: *frenulum*. **frenal,** *adj.*

frenzy (frĕn′zē) [ME. *frenesie*] A state of violent mental agitation; maniacal excitement. SEE: *panic*.

Freon Trade name of a group of hydrocarbon gases previously used as a refrigerant and propellant in metered dose inhalers.

frequency [L. *frequens,* often] **1.** The number of repetitions of a phenomenon in a certain period or within a distinct population, such as the frequency of heartbeat, sound vibrations, or a disease. SEE: *incidence*. **2.** The rate of oscillation or alternation in an alternating current circuit, in contradistinction to periodicity in the interruptions or regular variations of current in a direct current circuit. Frequency is computed on the basis of a complete cycle, in which the current rises from zero to a positive maximum, returns to zero, descends to an opposite negative minimum, and returns to zero. **3.** The rate at which uterine contractions occur, measured by the time elapsed between the beginning of one contraction and the beginning of the next.

Fresnel lenses [A. J. Fresnel, Fr. physicist 1788–1827] A magnifying glass that distorts vision, preventing the eye from fixating. Under its influence spontaneous and gaze-specific nystagmus can be precisely evaluated.

F response In electrodiagnostic study of spinal reflexes, the time required for a stimulus applied to a motor nerve to travel in the opposite direction up the nerve to the spinal cord and return.

fretum (frē′tŭm) [L.] A constriction.

Freud, Sigmund (froyd) A famous Austrian neurologist and psychoanalyst (1856–1939) whose teachings involved analysis of resistance and transference, and a procedure for investigating mental function by use of free association and dream interpretation. Freud did not consider psychoanalysis to be scientific. He believed that its purpose was to elucidate the darkest recesses of the mind and to enable individuals to integrate the emotional and intellectual sides of their nature (i.e., the forces of love and death) and to develop better knowledge of self and a level of maturity and peace of mind that would help the individual and others have better lives.

freudian (froy′dē-ăn) Pert. to Sigmund Freud's theories of unconscious or repressed libido, or past sex experiences or desires, as the cause of various neuroses, the cure for which he believed to be the restoration of such conditions to consciousness through psychoanalysis. SEE: *Freud, Sigmund*.

freudian slip [From Freudian psychology] A mistake in speaking or writing that is thought to provide insight into the individual's unconscious thoughts, motives, or wishes.

Freund's adjuvant (froynds) [Jules Thomas Freund, Hungarian-born U.S. immunologist, 1890–1960] A mixture of killed microorganisms, usually mycobacteria, in an oil and water emulsion. The material is administered to induce antibody formation. Because the oil retards absorption of the mixture, the antibody response is much greater than if the killed microorganisms were administered alone.

friable (frī′ă-b′l) [L. *friabilis*] Easily broken or pulverized.

friction [L. *frictio*] **1.** Rubbing. **2.** In massage, strong circular manipulations of deep tissue, always followed by centripetal stroking.

cross-fiber f. Deep transverse f.

deep transverse f. A massage technique in which stroking is applied across the longitudinal direction of the tissues of muscles, tendons, ligaments, or fascia to prevent adhesions, increase mobility of the tissue, and align new fibers along the lines of stress. SYN: *cross-fiber f.*

dry f. Friction using no liquid, or other form of lubricant.

moist f. Friction using a lubricant, such as a liquid or oil.

friction rub The distinct sound heard when two dry surfaces are rubbed together. If the sound is loud enough, the condition producing the sound can also be felt.

pericardial f.r. A friction rub that may be present in pericarditis, particularly when the disease process first starts.

pleural f.r. The creaking, grating sounds made when inflamed pleural surfaces move during respiration. It is often heard only during the first day or two of a pleurisy. SEE: *pericardial friction rub*.

Friedländer's bacillus (frēd′lĕn-dĕrz) [Carl F. Friedländer, Ger. physician, 1847–1887] *Klebsiella pneumoniae,* a species of bacteria that causes pneumonia and is a secondary invader in bronchitis or sinusitis.

Friedländer's disease Endarteritis obliterans.

Friedman's test (frēd′mănz) [Maurice H. Friedman, U.S. physiologist, b. 1903] A pregnancy test in which the urine of the woman is injected into an unmated female rabbit. If the woman is pregnant, corpora lutea and corpora hemorrhagica form in the rabbit after 2 days. Tests that are less difficult to perform are now routinely used.

Friedreich's ataxia (frēd′rĭks) [Nikolaus Friedreich, Ger. neurologist, 1825–1882] An inherited degenerative disease with sclerosis of the dorsal and lateral columns of the spinal cord. It is accompanied by muscular uncoordination, speech impairment, lateral curvature of the spinal column, with muscle paralysis, esp. of the lower extremities. The onset is in childhood or early adolescence.

Friedreich's sign **1.** Sudden collapse of the cervical veins that were previously distended at each diastole. The cause is an adherent pericardium. **2.** Lowering of the pitch of the percussion note that occurs over an area of cavitation during inspiration.

fright [AS. *fryhto*] Extreme sudden fear.

frigid (frĭj'ĭd) [L. *frigidus*] **1.** Cold. **2.** Unresponsive to emotion, applied esp. to the inability of a person to feel sexual desire. SEE: *impotence.*

frigidity (frĭ-jĭd'ĭ-tē) A state of sexual dysfunction marked by the inability to respond to erotic stimuli. SEE: *female sexual arousal disorder; male erectile disorder.*

frigolabile (frĭg"ō-lā'bĭl) [L. *frigor,* cold, + *labilis,* unstable] Capable of being destroyed by low temperature.

frigorific (frĭg"ō-rĭf'ĭk) [L. *frigorificus*] Generating cold.

frigorism [L. *frigor,* cold, + Gr. *-ismos,* condition] Very poor blood circulation caused by long exposure to cold.

frigostabile (frĭg"ō-stā'b'l) [" + *stabilis,* firm] Incapable of being destroyed by low temperature.

frigotherapy (frĭg"ō-thĕr'ă-pē) [" + Gr. *therapeia,* treatment] The use of cold in treatment of disease. SYN: *cryotherapy.*

frit (frĭt) [It. *fritta,* fry] **1.** The material from which glass or the glazed portion of pottery is made. **2.** A similar material for making the glaze of artificial teeth.

frog face Flatness of the face resulting from intranasal disease.

Fröhlich's syndrome (frā'lĭks) [Alfred Fröhlich, Austrian neurologist, 1871–1953] A condition characterized by obesity and sexual infantilism, atrophy or hypoplasia of the gonads, and altered secondary sex characteristics. It is caused by disturbance of the hypothalamus and hypophysis, usually secondary to a neoplasm. SYN: *adiposogenital dystrophy.*

Froin's syndrome (frō-ănz') [Georges Froin, Fr. physician, 1874–1932] The presence of yellow cerebrospinal fluid that coagulates rapidly. This is associated with any condition in which the fluid in the spinal canal is prevented from mixing with the cerebrospinal fluid in the ventricles.

frolement (frōl-mŏn') [Fr.] **1.** Very light friction with the hand in massage. SEE: *massage.* **2.** A sound resembling rustling heard in auscultation.

Froment's sign (frō-măz') [Jules Froment, Fr. physician, 1878–1946] Flexion of the distal phalanx of the thumb when a sheet of paper is held between the thumb and index finger. It indicates ulnar nerve palsy.

Frommann's lines (frŏm'ănz) [Carl Frommann, Ger. anatomist, 1831–1892] Transverse lines in the axon cylinder of myelinated nerve fibers. They are demonstrated by staining with silver nitrate.

frons (frŏnz) [L.] The forehead.

frontad [L. *frons, front-,* brow, + *ad,* toward] Toward the frontal aspect.

frontal [L. *frontalis*] **1.** Anterior. **2.** Pert. to the forehead bone.

frontal bone The forehead bone.

frontal sinuses Two hollow spaces in the frontal bone lying above the orbits. They are lined with mucous membrane, contain air, and communicate with the middle nasal meatus by means of the nasofrontal duct.

fronto- [L. *frons,* brow] Combining form meaning *anterior; forehead.*

frontomalar (frŏn"tō-mā'lăr) [" + *mala,* cheek] Pert. to the frontal and malar bones.

frontomaxillary (frŏn"tō-măx'ĭ-lăr"ē) [" + *maxilla,* jawbone] Pert. to the frontal and maxillary bones.

frontoparietal (frŏn"tō-pă-rī'ĕ-tăl) [" + *parietalis,* pert. to a wall] Pert. to the frontal and parietal bones.

frontotemporal [" + *tempora,* the temples] Pert. to the frontal and temporal bones.

front-tap reflex Contraction of the gastrocnemius muscle when stretched muscles of the extended leg are percussed.

FROPVD *Flow-restricted oxygen-powered ventilation device.*

frost [AS.] A frozen vapor deposit.

uremic f. A deposit of urea crystals on the skin from evaporation of sweat in a patient whose kidneys are severely impaired, as in uremia.

frostbite Severe tissue and cell damage caused by freezing a body part. The injury occurs both because intracellular water turns to ice and because extremely cold temperatures damage and block the blood supply to exposed parts. Exposed areas (e.g., ears, cheeks, nose, fingers, and toes) are most often affected. SEE: illus.; *freezing; frostnip; Nursing Diagnoses Appendix.*

SYMPTOMS: The frozen tissue is usually numb until it is rewarmed, when it may become extremely painful. Signs of frostbite depend on the depth of tissue damage: there may be swelling and hyperemia of the skin (superficial frostbite); blistering or hemorrhagic blistering ("second-" and "third-degree" frostbite); or gangrene of muscles and other subcutaneous tissues ("deep" or "fourth-degree" frostbite).

TREATMENT: After the patient's airway, breathing, and circulation are sta-

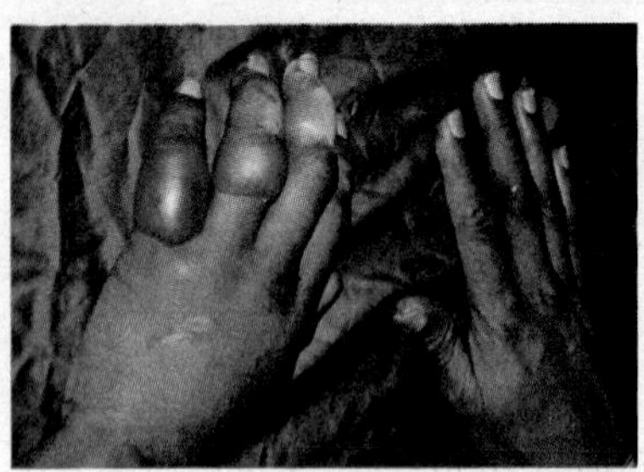

FROSTBITE

bilized, he or she is warmed and rehydrated. Next, the frozen body part is immersed in a warm water bath (40° to 42°C [104° to 108°F]). Tetanus prophylaxis, analgesics, and nonsteroidal anti-inflammatory drugs are given. If tissue sloughing occurs, minimal débridement is performed,unless the patient is septic or otherwise systemically compromised by the injury. Because tissue that appears severely damaged often heals spontaneously, surgery is sometimes delayed for weeks or months. SEE: *freezing* for treatment of frozen parts.

CAUTION: Rubbing or using frozen limbs should be avoided, to minimize injury to the skin and soft tissues.

PATIENT CARE: Emergency department personnel assess for frostbite in any patient who has been exposed to cold and complains of a cold, numb extremity or body part. While the extent of tissue damage depends on the degree of cold and the duration of exposure, the degree of injury may be difficult to determine on initial assessment, and requires ongoing monitoring. A complete history is taken and a thorough physical assessment is conducted to provide baseline information. Any hypothermia that accompanies the frostbite is treated first. Neurovascular status is monitored closely. Preventing infection is an important consideration, and the patient may be placed in protective (reverse) isolation to minimize contact with infectious agents. During rewarming, the patient is assessed frequently for complications (e.g., compartment syndrome).

Depending on the extent of débridement and the necessity for amputation, the physical therapist and occupational therapist work with the patient to manage activities of daily living. Outpatient rehabilitation may be required for an extended period. The patient may require assistance to deal with the emotional stress of the injury. Needs are determined, supportive care is provided, and the patient is referred for further psychological care as necessary.

frost-itch Winter itch.

frostnip A mild form of cold injury, consisting of reversible blanching of the skin, usually on the earlobes, cheeks, nose, fingers, and toes. SEE: *frostbite.*

frottage (frō-tŏzh′) [Fr., rubbing] **1.** A massage technique using rubbing, esp. for sexual gratification. **2.** A surgical treatment sometimes used to treat pneumothorax.

frotteurism Recurrent intense sexual urges and fantasies involving touching and rubbing against a nonconsenting person. These acts are usually performed in crowded places where arrest is unlikely. The perpetrators are usually young men. Persons who have acted on these urges are usually distressed about them.

frozen watchfulness The hopeless reproachful stare of battered children.

F.R.S. *Fellow of the Royal Society.*

F.R.S.C. *Fellow of the Royal Society (Canada).*

fructofuranose (frŭk″tō-fū′ră-nōs) The furanose form of fructose.

fructokinase (frŭk″tō-kī′nās) An enzyme that catalyzes transfer of high-energy phosphate from a donor to fructose.

fructose (frŭk′tōs) [L. *fructus,* fruit] Levulose; fruit sugar. A monosaccharide and a hexose, it has the same empirical formula as glucose, $C_6H_{12}O_6$, and is found in corn syrup, honey, fruit juices, and as part of the disaccharide sucrose. In the liver, fructose is changed to glucose to be used for energy production or to be stored as glycogen. SEE: *disaccharide.*

fructose intolerance Inability to metabolize the carbohydrate fructose due to a hereditary absence or deficiency of the enzyme 1,6-biphosphate aldolase B. Clinical signs develop early in life. They include hypoglycemia, jaundice, hepatomegaly, vomiting, lethargy, irritability, and convulsions. Fructose can be identified in the urine. The fructose tolerance test should not be used because it can induce irreversible coma.

TREATMENT: Acute attacks are treated by glucose administration. For long-term therapy, all foods containing fructose (present in sweet fruits and sugar cane) and sucrose and sorbitol (the latter used as a sweetening agent in foods and drugs) must be eliminated from the diet.

fructosemia (frŭk″tō-sē′mē-ă) [″ + Gr. *haima,* blood] Fructose in the blood.

fructoside (frŭk′tō-sīd) A carbohydrate that yields fructose on hydrolysis.

fructosuria (frŭk″tō-sū′rē-ă) [″ + Gr. *ouron,* urine] Fructose in the urine.

fruit [L. *fructus,* fruit] **1.** The ripened ovary of a seed-bearing plant and the surrounding tissue, such as the pod of a bean, nut, grain, or berry. **2.** The edible product of a plant consisting of ripened seeds and the enveloping tissue. Fruits add vitamins, minerals, and fiber to the diet. They help prevent constipation and vitamin deficiency syndromes. Most people should eat 2 to 3 servings of fruit every day, although people with impaired glucose tolerance or diabetes mellitus should consume just 1 to 2 servings.

COMPOSITION: Carbohydrates in the form of fruit sugars are the chief calorie component of fruits. Seventy-five percent of the calories in most fruit is a mixture of dextrose and fructose. Fruits are a good source of vitamins and minerals.

Pectose bodies: Pectose, the principle in fruits that causes them to jell, is found in unripe fruit; pectin is found in ripe fruit or fruit that has been cooked in a weak acid solution.

Fruit acids: Acetic acid is found in wine and vinegar. Citric acid is found in lemons, oranges, limes, and citrons. Malic acid is found in apples, pears, apricots, peaches, and currants. Oxalic acid is found in rhubarb, sorrel, and cranberries. Tartaric acid is found in grapes, pineapples, and tamarinds. Salicylic acid is found in currants, cranberries, cherries, plums, grapes, and crabapples.

Combined acids: Citric and malic acid are found in raspberries, strawberries, gooseberries, and cherries. Citric, malic, and oxalic acid are found in cranberries.

fruitarian Someone who eliminates all foods from the diet except fruits, vegetable oils, nuts, and honey. SEE: *vegan.*

frumentaceous (froo-mĕn-tā′shŭs) [L. *frumentum,* grain] Resembling or pert. to grain.

frustration [L. *frustratus,* disappointed] **1.** Lack of an adequate outlet for the libido. **2.** The condition that results from the thwarting or prevention of acts that would satisfy or gratify physical or personal needs.

FSH *follicle-stimulating hormone.*

FSH/LHRH *follicle-stimulating hormone and luteinizing hormone–releasing hormone.*

FSH-RF *follicle-stimulating hormone–releasing factor.*

FSH-RH *follicle-stimulating hormone–releasing hormone.*

ft L. *fiat* or *fiant,* let there be made; *florentium,* former name for promethium; *foot.*

FTA-ABS *fluorescent treponemal antibody-absorption test for syphilis.*

FTT *failure to thrive.*

fuchsin (fook′sĭn) A red dye that can be prepared in an acid or basic form.

fucose (fū′kōs) A mucopolysaccharide present in blood group substances and in human milk.

fucosidosis (fū″kō-sī-dō′sĭs) An autosomal recessive disease resulting from absence of the enzyme required to metabolize fucosidase. Clinically, neurological deterioration begins shortly after a period of normal early development. Heart disease, thick skin, and hyperhidrosis develop and are followed by death at an early age.

-fuge [L. *fugare,* to put to flight] Suffix meaning *something that expels or drives away.*

fugitive (fū′jĭ-tĭv) [L. *fugitivus*] **1.** Temporary, transient. **2.** Wandering; pert. to inconstant symptoms.

fugue (fūg) [L. *fuga,* flight] A dissociative disorder in which the person acts normally but has almost complete amnesia for what happened when recovery occurs.

psychogenic f. Sudden, unexpected travel away from one's home or place of work with inability to recall one's past. The individual may assume a partial or complete new identity. The condition is not due to organic brain disease. It may follow severe mental stress such as marital quarrels or a natural disaster. It is usually of short duration but can last for months. Recovery is the usual outcome without recurrences.

fulcrum The object or point on which a lever moves.

fulgurant (fŭl′gū-rănt) [L. *fulgurare,* to lighten] Coming and going intensely like a flash of light, or a shooting pain. SYN: *fulminant.*

fulgurate (fŭl′gū-rāt) To destroy or remove tissue by means of fulguration.

fulguration Destruction of tissue by means of long high-frequency electric sparks. SEE: *electrodesiccation.*

fulling [O. Fr. *fauler,* to fill] A movement in massage: kneading with the limb held between the hands, rolling it backward and forward.

full term In obstetrics, an infant born between the beginning of the 38th and the end of the 41st week of gestation. SYN: *term infant.*

full width half maximum ABBR: FWHM. The width of a peak or the bandpass of an emission or absorption spectrum in a laboratory photometer or spectrophotometer. When combined with other characteristics of the device, this can be used to predict suitability of the photometer or spectrophotometer for specific applications and measurements.

fulminant, fulminating (fool′, fŭl′mĭ-nănt) [L. *fulminans*] **1.** Having a rapid and severe onset. **2.** Coming in lightning-like flashes of pain, as in tabes dorsalis. SYN: *fulgurant.*

fumagillin (fū″mă-jĭl′ĭn) A molecule produced by fungi that prevents new blood vessel formation ("angiogenesis"), and may be useful in treating cancers.

fumarase (fū′mă-rās) An enzyme

present in many plants and animals. It catalyzes the production of L-malic acid from fumaric acid.

fumaric acid $C_4H_4O_4$; one of the organic acids in the citric acid cycle. It is used as a substitute for tartaric acid in beverages and baking powders.

fumes [L. *fumus,* smoke] Vapors, esp. those with irritating qualities.

nitric acid f. The vapors of nitric acid (HNO_3). They are used in various chemical processes. Poisoning is produced by the action of the corrosive fumes on the respiratory tract.

SYMPTOMS: Findings include choking, gasping, swelling of mucous membranes, tightness in the chest, pulmonary edema, cough, and shock. Symptoms may last for 1 week or more.

TREATMENT: The patient must be removed immediately from the fumes and good ventilation of the lungs maintained. Therapy is given for shock and pulmonary edema. Administration of oxygen under pressure using a mask may be required along with analgesics and anxiolytics as needed. Clothes must be removed if they are contaminated. Steroids may help diminish the inflammatory response of the lungs.

fumigant (fū′mĭ-gănt) [L. *fumigare,* to make smoke] An agent used in disinfecting a room. The substance produces fumes that are lethal to insects and rodents. Chemicals used include hydrogen cyanide gas, acrylonitrile, carbon tetrachloride, ethylene oxide, and methyl bromide.

CAUTION: All of these chemicals are highly toxic, potentially lethal, and in some cases explosive. They should be used only by persons skilled in their application.

fumigation (fū″mĭ-gā′shŭn) **1.** The use of poisonous fumes or gases to destroy living organisms, esp. rats, mice, insects, and other vermin. Fumigants are relatively ineffective against bacteria and viruses; consequently, terminal disinfection of the sickroom, formerly a common practice, has been discontinued. **2.** The disinfection of rooms by gases.

fuming [L. *fumus,* smoke] Having a visible vapor.

function (fŭng′shŭn) [L. *functio,* performance] **1.** The action performed by any structure. In a living organism this may pertain to a cell or a part of a cell, tissue, organ, or system of organs. **2.** The act of carrying on or performing a special activity. Normal function is the normal action of an organ. Abnormal activity or the failure of an organ to perform its activity is the basis of disease or disease processes. Structural changes in an organ are pathological and are common causes of malfunction, although an organ may function abnormally without observable structural changes. In humans, function can pertain to the manner in which the individual can perform successfully the tasks and roles required for everyday living.

executive f. Cognitive skills that enable a person to regulate behavior by modifying future behaviors based on consideration of previous actions. Deficits in executive function may lead to difficulties in impulse control, attention to tasks, adaptation, organization, prospective memory, and rehabilitation.

hazard f. A formula used to estimate the prognosis of a person who has already survived an illness for a specific time.

functional **1.** Pert. to function. **2.** A term describing various disturbances of function, such as a disturbance with no organic disease to account for the altered function.

functional bleeding **1.** Loss of blood from the uterus caused by an organic lesion, such as a cyst, fibroid, or malignant tumor. **2.** Metrorrhea.

Functional Independence Measure ABBR: FIM. A clinical tool used to assess the ability of persons needing rehabilitative services to cope independently and perform activities of daily living. These activities include self-care, sphincter control, mobility, locomotion, communication, and social cognition. Data derived from FIM correlate with some outcome measures in rehabilitation, such as the length of time a patient may need to stay in care or the resources the patient will use. The version of FIM for children is called WeeFIM. SEE: *WeeFIM*.

functional overlay The emotional response to physical illness. It may take the form of a conversion reaction, affective overreaction, prolonged symptoms of physical illness after signs of the illness have subsided, or combinations of these. Functional overlay may appear to be the primary disease; skill may be required to determine the actual cause of illness.

functional residual capacity ABBR: FRC. The amount of air remaining in the lungs after a normal resting expiration.

functioning tumor A tumor that is able to synthesize the same product as the normal tissues from which it arises, esp. an endocrine or nonendocrine tumor that produces hormones.

funda (fŭn′dă) [L., sling] A four-tailed bandage. **fundal,** *adj.*

fundament (fŭn′dă-mĕnt) [L. *fundamentum*] **1.** A foundation. **2.** The anus.

fundectomy (fŭn-dĕk′tō-mē) [L. *fundus,* base, + Gr. *ektome,* excision] Removal of the fundus of any organ.

fundic (fŭn′dĭk) Pert. to a fundus.

fundiform (fŭn′dĭ-form) [L. *funda,* sling,+ *forma,* shape] Sling-shaped or looped.

fundoplication (fŭn″dō-plī-kā′shŭn) Procedure used to treat gastroesophageal reflux and/or hiatal hernia by reestablishing a gastroesophageal angle and creating a barrier to intrathoracic gastric displacement. Most of this is accomplished by the Nissen technique by wrapping the fundus about the gastric cardia. This procedure may be performed laparoscopically as well as by open surgery in adults, children, or infants.

Belsey f. A surgical procedure for gastroesophageal reflux that relies on a repair of three quarters of the circumference of the gastroesophageal sphincter.

Nissen f. The surgical correction of an esophageal hiatal hernia or gastroesophageal reflux, by wrapping the gastric cardia with adjacent portions of the gastric fundus. This procedure, which is frequently performed laparoscopically, re-establishes the gastroesophageal angle and prevents intrathoracic displacement of the stomach.

PATIENT CARE: Vital signs, nasogastric tube, and suction (if used) should be checked and recorded. Intake and output is tracked and recorded.

fundoscopy (fŭn-dŏs′kō-pē) [L. *fundus,* base, + Gr. *skopein,* to examine] Examination, esp. visual, of the fundus of any organ. In ophthalmology, visual examination of the fundus of the eye. SYN: *ophthalmoscopy.*

fundus [L., base] **1.** The larger part, base, or body of a hollow organ. **2.** The portion of an organ most remote from its opening. **fundic** (fŭn′dĭk), *adj.*

f. of bladder The base of the urinary bladder, the portion closest to the rectum.

f. of gallbladder The lower dilated portion of the gallbladder.

f. oculi The posterior inner part of the eye as seen with an ophthalmoscope.

f. of stomach The uppermost portion of the stomach, posterior and lateral to the entrance of the esophagus.

f. tympani The floor of the tympanic cavity close to the jugular fossa. It contains the bulb of the internal jugular vein.

f. uteri The area of the uterus above the openings of the fallopian tubes.

funduscope (fŭn′dŭs-skōp) [L. *fundus,* base, + Gr. *skopein,* to examine] A device for examining the fundus of the eye.

fundusectomy (fŭn″dŭs-ĕk′tō-mē) [″ + Gr. *ektome,* excision] Excision of the fundus of the stomach. SYN: *cardiectomy.*

fungal septicemia SEE: *fungemia.*

fungate (fŭn′gāt) [L. *fungus,* mushroom] To grow like a fungus.

fungating (fŭn′gāt-ĭng) Growing rapidly like a fungus; said of certain tumors.

fungemia (fŭn-jē′mē-ă) [″ + Gr. *haima,* blood] The presence of fungi in the blood, most commonly *Candida* or *Aspergillus.* It can be life-threatening, esp. in immunocompromised patients. SYN: *fungal septicemia.* SEE: *amphotericin B; sepsis.*

Fungi (fŭn′jī) [L. *fungus,* mushroom] The kingdom of organisms that includes yeasts, molds, and mushrooms. Fungi grow as single cells, as in yeast, or as multicellular filamentous colonies, as in molds and mushrooms. They do not contain chlorophyll, so they are saprophytic (obtain food from dead organic matter) or parasitic (obtain nourishment from living organisms). Most fungi are not pathogenic, and the body's normal flora contains many fungi. SEE: illus.

Fungi that cause disease come from a group called fungi imperfecti. In immunocompetent humans they cause minor infections of the hair, nails, mucous membranes, or skin. In a person with a compromised immune system due to AIDS or immunosuppressive drug therapy, fungi are a source of opportunistic infections that can cause death.

fungicide (fŭn′jĭ-sīd) [L. *fungi,* mushrooms, + *cidus,* killing] An agent that kills fungi and their spores.

fungiform (fŭn′jĭ-form) [″ + *forma,* shape] Mushroom-shaped.

fungistasis (fŭn-jĭ-stā′sĭs) [″ + Gr. *stasis,* a halting] A condition in which the growth of fungi is inhibited.

fungistat (fŭn′jĭ-stăt) [″ + Gr. *statikos,* standing] An agent that inhibits the growth of fungi. **fungistatic** (-stăt′ĭk), *adj.*

fungitoxic (fŭn″jĭ-tŏk′sĭk) Poisonous to fungi.

fungoid (fŭn′goyd) [″ + Gr. *eidos,* form, shape] Having the appearance of a fungus.

fungosity (fŭn-gŏs′ĭ-tē) A soft, spongy fungus-like growth.

fungus (fŭn′gŭs) *pl.* **fungi** [L., mushroom] **1.** An organism belonging to the kingdom Fungi; a yeast, mold, or mushroom. SEE: *Fungi.* **2.** A spongelike morbid growth on the body that resembles fungi. SEE: *actinomycosis.* **fungal, fungous,** *adj.*

funic (fū′nĭk) [L. *funis,* cord] Pert. to the umbilical cord.

funicle (fū′nĭ-k′l) [L. *funiculus,* little cord] Funiculus (1).

funicular (fū-nĭk′ū-lăr) Pert. to the spermatic or umbilical cord.

funicular process The part of the tunica vaginalis that covers the spermatic cord.

funiculitis (fū-nĭk″ū-lī′tĭs) [″ + Gr. *itis,* inflammation] Inflammation of the spermatic cord.

funiculopexy (fū-nĭk′ū-lō-pĕks″ē) [″ +

Gr. *pexis,* fixation] Suturing of the spermatic cord to the tissues in cases of undescended testicle.

funiculus (fū-nĭk′ū-lŭs) *pl.* **funiculi** [L., little cord] **1.** Any small structure resembling a cord. SYN: *funicle.* **2.** A division of the white matter of the spinal cord consisting of fasciculi, or fiber tracts, lying peripheral to the gray matter. The types of funiculi are dorsal, lateral, and ventral.

funiform (fū′nĭ-form) [L. *funis,* cord, + *forma,* shape] Cordlike.

funipuncture [L. *funis,* a cord, + *punctura,* to prick] Puncture of the umbilical vein in utero, to obtain a sample of fetal blood. The needle is inserted under ultrasonic guidance.

funis (fū′nĭs) [L., cord] A cordlike structure, such as the spermatic cord or the umbilical cord.

funisitis Infection of the umbilical cord.

funnel [L. *fundere,* to pour] A conical device open at both ends for pouring liquid from one vessel into another.

funnel breast, funnel chest A congenital anomaly consisting of sternal depression of the chest walls so that the xiphoid is depressed posteriorly. SYN: *pectus excavatum.*

funny bone The medial epicondyle of the humerus, so termed because pressure applied over this area stimulates the ulnar nerve and produces a buzzing or tingling sensation.

F.U.O. *fever of unknown origin.*

furca SEE: *furcula.*

furcal Forked.

furcation (fŭr-kā′shŭn) The anatomical area of a multirooted tooth where the roots divide. SYN: *furca.*

furcula (fŭr′kū-lă) [L., little fork] The hypobranchial eminence, an elevation in the floor of the embryonic pharynx at the level of the third and fourth branchial arches. It gives rise to the epiglottis and the aryepiglottic folds. SYN: *furca.*

furfur [L., bran] Dandruff scales.

furfuraceous (fŭr-fū-rā′shŭs) Scaly or resembling scales.

furor [L., rage] Extremely violent outbursts of anger, often without provocation.

f. femininus An obsolete term for nymphomania.

furosemide (fū-rō′sĕ-mīd) A loop diuretic. Trade name is Lasix.

furred [O. Fr. *forre,* lining] Covered with a dustlike deposit; used of the tongue.

furrow [AS. *furh*] A groove.

atrioventricular f. The groove demarcating the atria of the heart from the ventricles.

digital f. Any of several transverse lines on the palmar surface of the fingers across the joints.

gluteal f. The vertical groove on the skin between the buttocks.

furuncle (fū′rŭng-k′l) [L. *furunculus*] Boil.

furunculoid (fū-rŭng′kū-loyd) [L. *furunculus,* a boil, + Gr. *eidos,* form, shape] Resembling a furuncle or boil. SYN: *furunculous.*

furunculosis (fū-rŭng″kū-lō′sĭs) [″ +

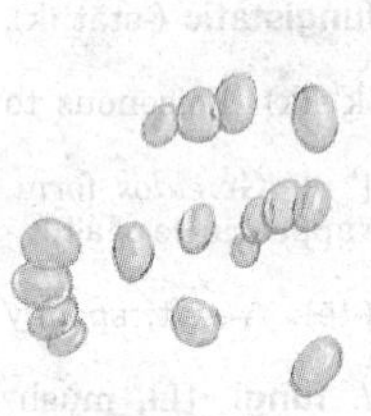
YEAST (×750)

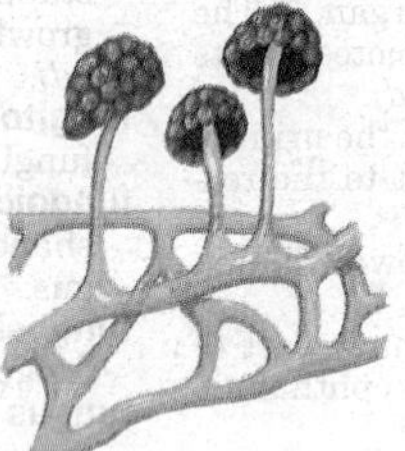
RHIZOPUS (×40)

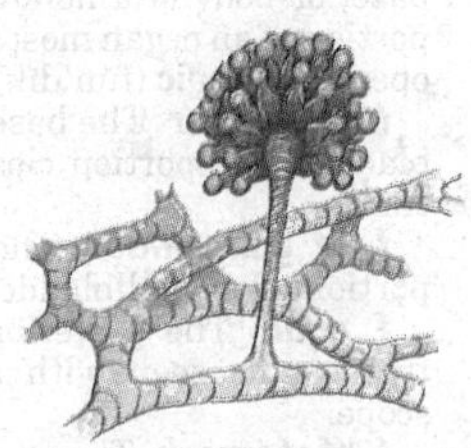
ASPERGILLUS (×40)

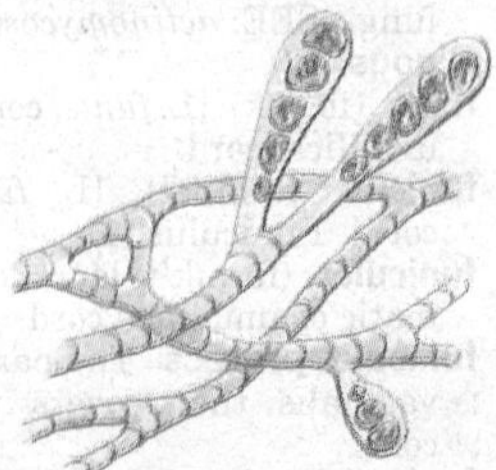
RINGWORM (×750)

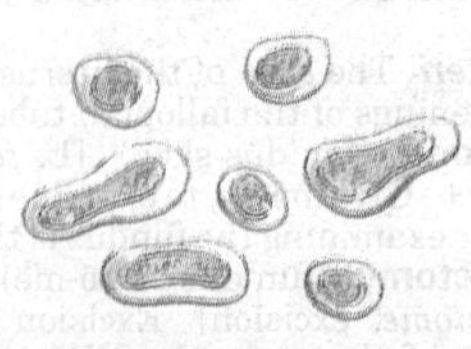
CRYPTOCOCCUS (×500)

FUNGI

Gr. *osis,* condition] A condition resulting from furuncles or boils.

furunculous Pert. to or of the nature of a furuncle or boil.

furunculus (fū-rŭng′kū-lŭs) *pl.* **furunculi** [L., a boil] Furuncle.

Fusarium (fū-zā′rē-ŭm) [L. *fusus,* spindle] A genus of fungi.

fuscin (fŭs′ĭn) [L. *fuscus,* dark brown] A brown pigment, a melanin, present in the outermost layer (pigmented epithelium) of the retina.

fuse (fūz) [L. *fusus,* poured] **1.** A safety device consisting of a strip of wire made from easily meltable metal of predetermined conductance. The metal melts, breaking the circuit when excess current passes through. **2.** To unite or blend together, as the coherence of adjacent body structures.

fusible (fū′zĭ-b'l) Capable of being melted or joined.

fusiform (fū′zĭ-form) [L. *fusus,* spindle, + *forma,* shape] Tapering at both ends; spindle-shaped.

fusimotor (fū″sĭ-mō′tor) Pert. to the motor innervation of the intrafusal muscle fibers originating in the gamma efferent neurons of the anterior gray matter of the spinal cord.

fusion (fū′shŭn) [L. *fusio*] **1.** Meeting and joining together through liquefaction by heat. **2.** The process of fusing or uniting. **3.** The union of adjacent tooth germs to form an oversize tooth of abnormal configuration or two teeth partially fused at the crown or root. **4.** The blending of genetic material of two distinct cells or species.

diaphyseal-epiphyseal f. Surgical obliteration of the epiphyseal line of a bone so that the epiphysis and diaphysis are joined.

nuclear f. Joining of the nucleus of two atoms to form a larger nucleus. It occurs when temperatures reach millions of degrees.

spinal f. Surgical fusion of two or more vertebrae. SYN: *spondylosyndesis*.

Fusobacterium A genus of non–spore-forming, nonencapsulated, nonmotile, gram-negative bacteria usually found in necrotic lesions of the mouth and bowel. *F. nucleatum* has been cultured from lesions of gangrenous stomatitis.

fusocellular [L. *fusus,* spindle, + *cellulus,* little cell] Spindle-celled.

fusospirochetal (fū″sō-spī-rō-kē′tăl) [″ + Gr. *speira,* coil, + *chaite,* hair] Pert. to fusiform bacilli and spirochetes.

fusospirochetosis (fū″sō-spī″rō-kē-tō′sĭs) [″ + ″ + ″ + *osis,* condition] Infection with fusiform bacilli and spirochetes.

fustigation (fŭs″tĭ-gā′shŭn) [L. *fustigatio*] In massage, beating with light rods.

futile care In clinical practice, any intervention that will not improve a patient's health, well-being, comfort, or prognosis. The term is used esp. in the care of patients at the end of life. SEE: *advance directive; hospice*.

FVC *forced vital capacity.*

F wave Flutter waves in atrial fibrillation, detectable on the electrocardiogram at 250 to 350 per minute.

FWB *full weight bearing.*

G

γ **1.** The third letter of the Greek alphabet; gamma is the anglicized equivalent. **2.** Symbol for *microgram; immunoglobulin.*

G **1.** The newtonian constant of gravitation. **2.** Symbol for giga, 10^9, in SI units.

g **1.** Symbol for the standard force of attraction of gravity, 980.665 m/sec^2, or about 32.17 ft/sec^2. **2.** *gingival; gram; gender.*

Ga Symbol for the element gallium.

GABA *gamma-aminobutyric acid.*

gabapentin (gă-bă-pĕn′tĭn) An anticonvulsant drug also used to treat chronic neuropathic pain. Trade name is Neurontin.

gadfly A fly belonging to the family Tabanidae that lays eggs under the skin of its victim, causing swelling simulating a boil. Multiple furuncles appear with hatching of larvae. SEE: *botfly.*

gadolinium (găd″ō-lĭn′ē-ŭm) SYMB: Gd. A chemical element of the lanthanide group, atomic weight 157.25, atomic number 64. Gadolinium is used as a contrast agent in magnetic resonance imaging.

Gaenslen's test, Gaenslen's sign [Frederick J. Gaenslen, U.S. orthopedist] A procedure used to identify the presence of sacroiliac dysfunction. The patient lies supine close to the edge of the examination table, with both legs pulled to the chest. The examiner extends over the side of the table the patient's leg that is closest to the edge and forces it into hyperextension while the patient's other leg remains held against the chest. A positive test result produces pain in the sacroiliac region.

GAF *Global Assessment of Functioning.*

gag **1.** A device for keeping the jaws open during surgery. **2.** To retch or cause to retch.

gag clause An item in a health care provider's contract that prohibits the provider from discussing financial incentives he or she may receive while practicing or withholding treatments.

gage (gāj) Gauge.

gain **1.** To increase in weight, strength, or health. **2.** In electronics, the term used to describe the amplification factor for a given circuit or device. **3.** The real or imagined positive effect of some action or situation. For example, an illness might allow a person to put off going to school or meeting some other obligation such as a court appearance.

flux g. In radiographic image intensification, the ratio of the number of light photons at the output phosphor to the number of photons at the input phosphor.

minification g. In radiographic image intensification, the ratio of the square of the input phosphor diameter to the square of the output phosphor diameter.

primary g. In psychiatry, the relief of symptoms when the patient converts emotional anxiety to what he or she perceives as an organic illness (e.g., hysterical paralysis or blindness).

secondary g. The advantage gained by the patient indirectly from illness, such as attention, care, and release from responsibility.

Gaisböck's syndrome (gīs′bĕks) [Felix Gaisböck, Ger. physician, 1869–1955] Benign erythrocytosis with no clinical findings associated with polycythemia. There is little evidence to support the view that this condition is a true clinical illness. Also called *stress erythrocytosis, spurious erythrocytosis, benign erythrocytosis,* and *pseudopolycythemia vera.*

gait (gāt) [ME. *gait,* passage] A manner of walking.

antalgic g. A gait in which the patient experiences pain during the stance phase and thus remains on the painful leg for as short a time as possible.

ataxic g. An unsteady, staggering gait pattern. If related to cerebellar pathology, the gait is unsteady, irregular, and generally characterized by use of a wide base of support. The deviation is equally severe if the individual walks with eyes open or closed. If the cerebellar lesion is localized to one hemisphere, the individual will sway toward the affected side. Ataxic gait patterns related to spinal ataxia are characterized by a wide base of support, with the feet thrown out. There is a characteristic double tapping sound, as the individual steps on heels first, then on toes. This gait pattern occurs in such conditions as tabes dorsalis and multiple sclerosis and is believed to result from the disruption of the sensory pathways in the central nervous system. SEE: *ataxia* and its subentries.

cerebellar g. An ataxic gait, marked by unsteadiness and staggering movements, that is the result of cerebellar lesions.

double step g. A gait in which alternate steps are of a different length or at a different rate.

drag-to g. A gait in which the crutches are advanced and the feet are dragged, rather than lifted, to the crutches.

equine g. A gait marked by high steps, characteristic of tibialis anterior paralysis. In a rigid equinus posture of the ankle, the person walks on the toes. This is also seen in spastic gait patterns.

festinating g. Festination.

four-point g. A gait in which first the right crutch and the left foot are advanced consecutively, and then the left crutch and the right foot are moved forward.

glue-footed g. A gait in which the individual has difficulty initiating the first step as if the feet were glued to the floor; once the gait is initiated, small, shuffling steps are taken. SYN: *magnetic g.*

gluteus maximus g. A lurching gait, characterized by posterior leaning of the trunk at heel strike in order to keep the hip extended during the stance phase. It is caused by weakness of the gluteus maximus. It also is called hip extensor gait.

gluteus medius g. A gait deviation that occurs with weakness or paralysis of the gluteus medius muscle. In an uncompensated gluteus medius gait, the pelvis drops when the unaffected limb is in swing phase, and there is a lateral protrusion of the stationary affected hip. This is a result of weakness of the gluteus medius muscle, or congenital hip dislocations or coxa vara. A compensated gluteus medius gait appears with paralysis of the muscle, and is characterized by a shifting of the trunk to the affected side during the stance phase. It also is known as Trendelenburg gait.

helicopod g. A gait in which one or both feet describe a half circle with each step, sometimes seen in hysteria.

hemiplegic g. A gait in which the patient abducts the paralyzed limb, swings it around, and brings it forward so that the foot comes to the ground in front. During the stance phase the patient bears very little weight on the involved leg.

magnetic g. Glue-footed g.

Parkinson's g. In patients with Parkinson's disease, a gait marked by short steps with the feet barely clearing the floor in a shuffling and scraping manner. As the steps continue, they may become successively more rapid. The posture is marked by flexion of the upper body with the spine bent forward, head down, and arms, elbows, hips, and knees bent. SEE: *festination.*

quadriceps g. A gait in which the trunk leans forward at the beginning of the stance phase to lock the knee when the quadriceps femoris muscle is weak or paralyzed.

scissor g. A gait marked by excessive hip adduction in swing phase. As a result, the swing leg crosses in front of the stance leg. This gait pattern is seen in patients with an upper motor neuron lesion, and is accompanied by spasticity.

senile g. A gait marked by associated stooped posture, knee and hip flexion, diminished arm swinging, stiffness in turning, and broad-based, small steps. It is usually seen in the elderly.

spastic g. A stiff movement in which the toes seem to catch and drag, the legs are held together, and the hips and knee joints are slightly flexed. It is seen in spastic paraplegia, sclerosis of the lateral pyramidal columns of the cord, tumor of the spinal cord, and arachnoiditis.

spondylitic cervical myelopathic g. A spastic, shuffling gait due to increased muscle tone resulting from deep tendon reflexes below the level of compression.

steppage g. A gait in which the foot is lifted high to clear the toes, there is no heel strike, and the toes hit the ground first. It is seen in anterior tibialis paralysis, peripheral neuritis, late stages of diabetic neuropathy, alcoholism, and chronic arsenic poisoning.

swing-through g. A gait in which the crutches are advanced and the legs are swung between and ahead of the crutches.

swing-to g. A gait in which the crutches are advanced and the legs are advanced to the crutches.

tabetic g. A high-stepping ataxic walk in which the feet slap the ground. It is caused by tabes dorsalis.

three-point g. A gait in which the crutches and the affected leg are advanced first, then the other leg.

toppling g. The tendency of an individual who has suffered a stroke to fall toward the affected side of the brain.

two-point g. A gait in which the right foot and left crutch are advanced simultaneously, then the left foot and right crutch are moved forward.

waddling g. A gait in which the feet are wide apart and the walk resembles that of a duck. It occurs in coxa vara and double congenital hip displacement when lordosis is present. In late pregnancy, hormone-induced softening allows some pelvic movement at the sacroiliac and pubic symphysis articulations on ambulation. Compensatory widening of the stance results in the characteristic waddle.

galact- [Gr. *gala,* milk] SEE: *galacto-.*

galactacrasia [" + *akrasia,* bad mixture] An abnormality of breast milk.

galactagogue (gă-lăk′tă-gŏg) [" + *agogos,* leading] An agent that promotes the flow of milk.

galactase An enzyme of milk.

galactic (gă-lăk′tĭk) Pert. to the flow of milk.

galacto-, galact- Combining form meaning *milk.*

galactoblast (gă-lăk′tō-blăst) [" +

blastos, germ] A body found in mammary acini that contains fat globules.

galactocele (gă-lăk′tō-sēl) [″ + *kele,* tumor, swelling] **1.** A cystic tumor of the female breast caused by occlusion of a milk duct. Fully emptying the breasts during feedings and cleaning the nipples to avoid nipple caking help the cyst resolve. SYN: *galactoma; lactocele.* **2.** A hydrocele containing a milk-like liquid.

galactokinase (gă-lăk″tō-kī′nās) An enzyme that catalyzes the transfer of high-energy phosphate groups from a donor to D-galactose. D-galactose-1-phosphate is produced by this reaction.

galactolipin [″ + *lipos,* fat] A phosphorus-free lipid combined with galactose; a cerebroside.

galactoma (găl-ăk-tō′mă) [″ + *oma,* tumor] SEE: *galactocele* (1).

galactopexy (gă-lăk′tō-pĕk″sē) The fixation of galactose by the liver.

galactophagous (găl″ăk-tŏf′ă-gŭs) [″ + *phagein,* to eat] Feeding on milk.

galactophore (găl-ăk′tō-for) [″ + *pherein,* to bear] A lactiferous duct.

galactophoritis (găl-ăk″tō-for-ī′tĭs) [″ + ″ + *itis,* inflammation] Inflammation of a milk duct.

galactopoiesis (gă-lăk″tō-poy-ē′sĭs) [″ + *poiesis,* forming] Milk production.

galactopoietic (gă-lăk″tō-poy-ĕt′ĭk) [″ + *poiein,* to make] **1.** Pert. to milk production. **2.** A substance that promotes galactopoiesis.

galactorrhea (gă-lăk″tō-rē′ă) [″ + *rhoia,* flow] **1.** The continuation of milk secretion at intervals after nursing has ceased. **2.** Excessive secretion of milk.

galactosamine (gă-lăk″tō-săm′ĭn) A derivative of galactose containing an amine group on the second carbon of the compound.

galactose (gă-lăk′tōs) A dextrorotatory monosaccharide or simple hexose sugar, $C_6H_{12}O_6$. Galactose is an isomer of glucose and is formed, along with glucose, in the hydrolysis of lactose. It is a component of cerebrosides. Galactose is readily absorbed in the digestive tract; in the liver it is converted to glucose and may be stored as glycogen.

galactosemia (gă-lăk″tō-sē′mē-ă) An autosomal recessive disorder marked by an inability to metabolize galactose because of a congenital absence of one of two enzymes needed to convert galactose to glucose. The diagnosis is confirmed by testing the newborn's urine for noncarbohydrate reducing substances or more accurately by tests for the missing enzymes in blood cells. The infant with galactosemia will fail to thrive within a week after birth due to anorexia, vomiting, and diarrhea unless galactose and lactose are removed from the diet. If untreated, the disease may progress to starvation and death. Untreated children who do survive usually fail to grow, are mentally retarded, and have cataracts. If galactose is excluded from the diet early in life, the child may live to adulthood but suffer reproductive and brain disorders. Galactosemia can be diagnosed in utero by amniocentesis. If a pregnant woman is a known carrier, it is advisable that she exclude lactose and galactose from her diet.

galactosidase (gă-lăk″tō-sī′dās) An enzyme that catalyzes the metabolism of galactosides.

galactoside (gă-lăk′tō-sīd) A carbohydrate that contains galactose.

galactostasis (găl″ăk-tŏs′tă-sĭs) [″ + *stasis,* a stopping] The cessation or checking of milk secretion.

galactosuria (găl-ăk″tō-sū′rē-ă) [″ + *ouron,* urine] Galactose in the urine.

galactotherapy (gă-lăk″tō-thĕr′ă-pē) [″ + *therapeia,* treatment] **1.** Treatment of a nursing infant by drugs administered to the mother and excreted in her milk. **2.** Therapeutic use of milk, as a milk diet. SYN: *lactotherapy.*

galactozymase (gă-lăk″tō-zī′mās) [″ + *zyme,* leaven] A starch-hydrolyzing enzyme in milk.

galacturia (găl-ăk-tū′rē-ă) [″ + *ouron,* urine] Chyluria.

galea (gā′lē-ă) [L. *galea,* helmet] **1.** A helmet-like structure. **2.** A type of head bandage.

g. aponeurotica Epicranial aponeurosis.

galeanthropy (gā″lē-ăn′thrō-pē) [Gr. *gale,* cat, + *anthropos,* man] A delusion that one has become transformed into a cat.

Galeazzi's sign [Riccardo Galeazzi, It. orthopedic surgeon, 1866–1952] A clinical indication of congenital hip dislocation in infants and toddlers. With the child lying supine with the knees flexed and hips flexed at 90°, dislocation is present if one knee is higher than the other.

Galen, Claudius A noted Greek physician and medical writer, circa A.D. 130–200, residing in Rome, where he was physician to Emperor Marcus Aurelius. He is called the father of experimental physiology.

G.'s veins The veins running through the tela choroidea formed by the joining of the terminal and choroid veins and forming the great cerebral vein, which empties into the straight sinus of the brain.

galenic (gă-lĕn′ĭk) Pert. to Galen or his teachings.

galenicals, galenics (gă-lĕn′ĭ-kăls, -ĭks) **1.** Herb and vegetable medicines. **2.** Crude drugs and medicinals as distinguished from the pure active principles contained in them. **3.** Medicines prepared according to an official formula.

galeophilia (găl″ē-ō-fĭl′ē-ă) [Gr. *gale,* cat, + *philein,* to love] A fondness for cats.

galeophobia (găl″ē-ō-fō′bē-ă) [″ + *phobos,* fear] An abnormal aversion to cats.

gall [AS. *gealla,* sore place] **1.** An excoriation. **2.** The bitter liver secretion stored in the gallbladder; bile. It has no enzymes, but emulsifies fats to permit digestion by pancreatic lipase, and stimulates peristalsis. Gall is discharged through the cystic duct into the duodenum.

gallamine triethiodide (găl′ă-mīn trī″ē-thī′ō-dīd) A drug that inhibits transmission of nerve impulses across the myoneural junction of voluntary muscles. Trade name is Flaxedil.

Gallant reflex An infantile reflex in which the trunk curves toward the side of stimulation in a prone infant. It is present from birth to age 2 months.

gallate (găl′lāt) A salt of gallic acid.

gallbladder [AS. *gealla,* sore place, + *blaedre,* bladder] A pear-shaped sac on the underside of the right lobe of the liver that stores bile received from the liver. While in the gallbladder, bile is concentrated by removing water. About 500 to 600 ml of bile, approx. 82% water, is secreted each day. The bile is then discharged through the cystic duct, which is 3 to 4 in. (7.6 to 10.2 cm) long. The cystic duct, which is about 0.25 in. (6 mm) in diameter, joins the hepatic duct to form the common bile duct, which empties into the duodenum at the ampulla of Vater.

gallium (găl′ē-ŭm) [L. *Gallia,* Gaul] SYMB: Ga. A rare metal, small amounts of which are found in bauxite and zinc blends; atomic weight 69.72, atomic number 31. Gallium-68 (^{68}Ga) is used in studies involving use of radioactive materials. It has a half-life of 68 min.

gallon [Med. L. *galleta,* jug] Four liquid measure quarts; 231 cu in. or 3.79 L. In England the Imperial liquid gallon is 277.4 cu in. or 4.55 L.

gallop An extra heart sound (i.e., a third or fourth heart sound), typically heard during diastole.

gallstone [AS. *gealla,* sore place, + *stan,* stone] A concretion formed in the gallbladder or bile ducts. Gallstones are found in about 15% of men and 30% of women in the U.S. They may cause pain in the right upper quadrant of the abdomen (biliary colic) or they may be clinically silent. Gallstones typically are made either of crystallized cholesterol deposits or calcium crystals ionized with bilirubin. Cholesterol stones are about 4 times as common as calcium-containing stones (also known as pigment stones). Either type of stone may cause biliary symptoms such as pain or inflammation of the gallbladder; the two types of stones differ in that cholesterol stones are non-radiopaque and may on occasion be dissolved by medication, whereas calcium-containing radiopaque stones are not amenable to chemical dissolution and are therefore visible on plain x-rays of the abdomen. SEE: *Nursing Diagnoses Appendix.* SYN: *biliary calculus.*

SYMPTOMS: Intense pain in the right upper quadrant of the abdomen that may radiate to the right flank, back, or shoulder is typical of biliary colic due to gallstones. The symptoms may occur after a fatty meal and may be associated with nausea or vomiting or fever. Jaundice may be present on physical examination.

TREATMENT: Asymptomatic gallstones are neither removed nor treated. Symptomatic gallstone disease is treated primarily in the U.S. by laparoscopic cholecystectomy which, when successful, avoids prolonged hospitalization. Drug therapy for gallstones may include the use of ursodiol. Stones found in the extrahepatic bile ducts are treated surgically according to the presentation. Cholecystotomy is reserved for patients who are judged to be too ill to tolerate cholecystectomy, usually as a temporizing procedure. Gallstone lithotripsy is infrequently used because it is technically more complex than laparoscopic cholecystectomy (and relatively equipment and labor is intensive, and less universally effective).

CAUTION: Ursodiol (ursodeoxycholic acid), taken orally, is sometimes effective in treating cholesterol gallstones for 1 year. Treatment may need to be continued for 1 year. A similar agent, chenodiol, is no longer available as it caused unacceptable incidence of hepatotoxicity.

GALT *gut-associated lymphoid tissue.*

Galton's whistle [Sir Francis Galton, Brit. scientist, 1822–1911] A whistle used to test hearing.

galvanic [Luigi Galvani, It. physiologist, 1737–1798] Pert. to galvanism.

g. battery A series of cells giving a combined effect of all the units and generating electricity by chemical reaction.

g. current Direct electric current, usually from a battery.

galvanism (găl′vă-nĭzm) In dentistry, an electrochemical reaction occurring in the mouth when dissimilar metals used to restore teeth come into contact, producing a direct electric current that may cause pain.

galvanization (găl″văn-ī-zā′shŭn) Therapeutic use of a galvanic current.

galvanometer (găl″vă-nŏm′ĕ-tĕr) [″ + Gr. *metron,* measure] An instrument that measures electric current by electromagnetic action.

galvanopuncture (găl″vă-nō-pŭng′chūr) [″ + L. *punctura,* puncture] Introduction of needles to complete a galvanic current.

gam- SEE: *gamo-*.

gamete (găm′ēt) [Gr. *gamein,* to marry] A mature male or female reproductive cell; the spermatozoon or ovum. **gametic** (-ĕt′ĭk), *adj.*

gamete intrafallopian transfer ABBR: GIFT. A procedure developed by Ricardo Asch, a contemporary American physician, to help infertile couples conceive. After ovulation is induced, ova are retrieved from a mature follicle via laparoscopy and are transferred along with sperm to the woman's fallopian tube to facilitate fertilization. SEE: *embryo transfer; fertilization, in vitro; zygote intrafallopian transfer.*

gametocide (găm′ĕ-tō-sīd″) [″ + L. *caedere,* to kill] An agent destructive to gametes or gametocytes, particularly those of malaria.

gametocyte (gă-mē′tō-sīt) [″ + *kytos,* cell] A stage in the life cycle of the malarial protozoon (*Plasmodium*) that reproduces in the blood of the Anopheles mosquito.

gametogenesis (găm″ĕt-ō-jĕn′ĕ-sĭs) [″ + *genesis,* generation, birth] Development of gametes; oogenesis or spermatogenesis.

gametogony (găm″ĕ-tŏg′ō-nē) The phase in the life cycle of the malarial parasite (*Plasmodium*) in which male and female gametocytes, which infect the mosquito, are formed.

gametophyte (găm′ĕ-tō-fīt)) [″ + *phyton,* plant] In plants, the sexual (gamete-producing) generation that alternates with the asexual (spore-producing) generation.

gamic (găm′ĭk) [Gr. *gamein,* to marry] Sexual, esp. as applied to eggs that develop only after fertilization in contrast to those that develop without fertilization. SEE: *parthenogenesis.*

gamma **1.** The third letter of the Greek alphabet, γ. **2.** In chemistry, the third of a series (e.g., the third carbon atom in an aliphatic chain).

gamma-aminobutyric acid ABBR: GABA. The brain's principal inhibitory neurotransmitter.

gamma benzene hexachloride (găm′ă bĕn′zēn hĕk″să-klor′īd) A miticide used to treat scabies. Trade names are Kwell and Scabene. SYN: *lindane.*

gammacism An inability to pronounce "g" and "k" sounds correctly.

gamma hydroxy butyrate (găm-ă hī-drŏk-sē bū′tĭ-rāt) ABBR: GHB. A central nervous system depressant used in some countries as an anesthetic agent. It has no approved use in the U.S., where it is sometimes abused as an illicit drug. Its street names include *grievous bodily harm, liquid ecstasy,* and *organic quaalude.*

gamma knife surgery Radiosurgery that can destroy an intracranial target by directing gamma radiation at the lesion, while attempting to spare adjacent healthy tissue. The gamma knife consists of 201 cylindrical gamma ray (cobalt 60) beams designed to intersect at the target lesion, resulting in about 200 times the dose of any single beam aimed at the periphery. The area to be treated is carefully identified with neuroimaging before the gamma knife is used and the proper dose of gamma energy calculated. The procedure takes about 2 to 3 hr, with the patient under mild sedation, given intravenously, and local anesthesia. The gamma knife can be used to treat primary and metastatic brain tumors, trigeminal neuralgia, arteriovenous malformations, and other lesions. Complications include seizures, confusion, paralysis, nausea and vomiting, other radiation reactions, and radiation necrosis of normal brain tissue, but the incidence of side effects is no greater than with other brain irradiation or neurosurgical techniques.

PATIENT CARE: The patient's vital signs and neurological signs must be checked frequently during and after the procedure.

gamma motor neuron A small nerve originating in the anterior horns of the spinal cord that transmits impulses through type A gamma fibers to intrafusal fibers of the muscle spindle for muscle control.

gammopathy (găm-ŏp′ă-thē) Any disease in which serum immunoglobulins are increased, such as multiple myeloma, benign monoclonal gammopathy, and cirrhosis.

monoclonal g. of unclear significance ABBR: MGUS. A condition marked by excessive levels of paraproteins in the blood. It is a precursor of multiple myeloma in roughly 20% of cases.

gamo-, gam- [Gr. *gamos,* marriage] Combining form meaning *marriage* or *sexual union.*

gamogenesis (găm″ō-jĕn′ĕ-sĭs) [″ + *genesis,* generation, birth] Sexual reproduction.

gamont (găm′ŏnt) [″ + *on,* being] A sexual form of certain protozoa. SEE: *gametocyte.*

gamophobia (găm″ō-fō′bē-ă) [″ + *phobos,* fear] A neurotic fear of marriage.

gampsodactylia (gămp″sō-dăk-tĭl′ē-ă) [Gr. *gampsos,* curved, + *daktylos,* digit] Deformity of the toes causing them to resemble claws. SYN: *clawfoot.*

ganciclovir A synthetic antiviral drug used to treat cytomegalovirus infections orally or intravenously. SEE: *cytomegalic inclusion disease.*

CAUTION: Ganciclovir is a potential carcinogen. Because of its mutagenic potential, women of childbearing age must use effective contraception during treatment. Male patients must practice barrier contraception during treatment and for at least 90 days afterward. Persons who care for patients receiving this drug must take appropriate precautions to prevent coming into contact with the drug, the patient's excreta, or the patient's used bed linens.

---

ganglia (găng'glē-ă) Pl. of ganglion.

ganglial (găng'lē-ăl) [Gr. *ganglion,* knot] Ganglionic.

gangliated (găng'lē-ā-tĕd) **1.** Having ganglia. **2.** Intermixed.

gangliectomy (găng"glē-ĕk'tō-mē) [" + *ektome,* excision] Excision of a ganglion.

gangliform (găng'lĭ-form) [" + L. *forma,* shape] Formed like a ganglion.

gangliitis (găng"glē-ī'tĭs) [" + *itis,* inflammation] Inflammation of a ganglion.

ganglioblast (găng'glē-ō-blăst") [" + *blastos,* germ] An embryonic ganglion cell.

gangliocyte (găng'glē-ō-sīt") [" + *kytos,* cell] A ganglion cell.

gangliocytoma (găng"glē-ō-sī-tō'mă) [" + " + *oma,* tumor] SYN: *ganglioneuroma.*

ganglioglioma (găng"glē-ō-glī-ō'mă) [" + *glia,* glue, + *oma,* tumor] A ganglion-cell glioma.

ganglioglioneuroma (găng"glē-ō-glī"ō-nū-rō'mă) [" + " + *neuron,* nerve, + *oma,* tumor] Ganglion cells, glia cells, and nerve fibers in a nerve tumor.

ganglioma (găng-lē-ō'mă) [" + *oma,* tumor] **1.** A tumor of neural or neuroectodermal origin. **2.** A swelling of lymphoid tissue.

ganglion (găng'lē-ŏn) *pl.* **ganglia, ganglions** [Gr.] **1.** A mass of nervous tissue composed principally of neuron cell bodies and lying outside the brain or spinal cord (e.g., the chains of ganglia that form the main sympathetic trunks; the dorsal root ganglion of a spinal nerve). **2.** A cystic tumor developing on a tendon or aponeurosis. It sometimes occurs on the back of the wrist.

abdominal g. Any ganglion located in the abdomen.

aorticorenal g. A ganglion lying near the lower border of the celiac ganglion. It is located near the origin of the renal artery.

Arnold's auricular g. Otic g.

auricular g. Otic g.

autonomic g. A ganglion of the autonomic nervous system.

basal g. A mass of gray matter beneath the third ventricle consisting of the caudate, lentiform, and amygdaloid nuclei and the claustrum.

cardiac g. Superficial and deep cardiac plexuses that contain autonomic nerves and branches of the left vagus nerve. They are located on the right side of the ligamentum arteriosus. SYN: *Wrisberg's ganglia.*

carotid g. A ganglion formed by filamentous threads from the carotid plexus beneath the carotid artery.

celiac g. One of a pair of prevertebral or collateral ganglia located near the origin of the celiac artery. Together they form a part of the celiac plexus.

cephalic g. One of the parasympathetic ganglia (otic, pterygopalatine, and submandibular) in the head.

cervical g. One of the three pairs of ganglia (superior, middle, inferior) in the cervical portion of the sympathetic trunk.

cervicothoracic g. Stellate g.

cervicouterine g. A ganglion near the uterine cervix. SYN: *Frankenhäuser's g.*

ciliary g. A tiny ganglion in the rear portion of the orbit. It receives preganglionic fibers through the oculomotor nerve from the Edinger-Westphal nucleus of the midbrain. Six short ciliary nerves pass from it to the eyeball. Postganglionic fibers innervate the ciliary muscle, the sphincter of the iris, the smooth muscles of blood vessels of these structures, and the cornea. SYN: *lenticular g.; ophthalmic g.*

coccygeal g. A ganglion located in the coccygeal plexus and forming the lower termination of the two sympathetic trunks; sometimes absent.

collateral g. One of several ganglia of the sympathetic nervous system. They are in the mesenteric nervous plexuses near the abdominal aorta and include the celiac and mesenteric ganglia.

Corti's g. A ganglion on the cochlear nerve.

dorsal root g. A ganglion located on the dorsal root of a spinal nerve. It contains the cell bodies of sensory neurons. SYN: *intervertebral g.; spinal g.*

false g. An enlargement on a nerve that does not contain a ganglion.

Frankenhäuser's g. Cervicouterine g.

gasserian g. Trigeminal g.

geniculate g. A ganglion on the pars intermedia, the sensory root of the facial nerve. It lies in the anterior border of the anterior geniculum of the facial nerve.

inferior mesenteric g. A prevertebral sympathetic ganglion located in the inferior mesenteric plexus near the origin of the inferior mesenteric artery.

intervertebral g. Spinal g.

jugular g. A ganglion located on the root of the vagus nerve and lying in the upper portion of the jugular foramen.

lateral g. One of a chain of ganglia forming the main sympathetic trunk.

lenticular g. Ciliary g.

lumbar g. One of the ganglia usually occurring in fours in the lumbar portion of the sympathetic trunk.

nodose g. A ganglion of the trunk of the vagus nerve located immediately below the jugular ganglion. It connects with the spinal accessory nerve, the hypoglossal nerve, and the superior cervical ganglion of the sympathetic trunk.

ophthalmic g. Ciliary g.

otic g. A small ganglion located deep in the zygomatic fossa immediately below the foramen ovale. It lies medial to the mandibular nerve and supplies postganglionic parasympathetic fibers to the parotid gland. SYN: *Arnold's auricular g.; auricular g.*

parasympathetic g. One of the ganglia on the cholinergic nerves of the parasympathetic nervous system, near or in the visceral effector.

petrous g. A ganglion located on the lower margin of the temporal bone's petrous portion.

pharyngeal g. A ganglion in contact with the glossopharyngeal nerve.

phrenic g. One of a group of ganglia joining the phrenic plexus.

renal g. One of a group of ganglia joining the renal plexus.

sacral g. One of the four small ganglia located in the sacral portion of the sympathetic trunk that lie on the anterior surface of the sacrum and are connected to the spinal nerves by gray rami.

Scarpa's g. Vestibular g.

semilunar g. Trigeminal g.

sensory g. One of the ganglia of the peripheral nervous system that transmit sensory impulses.

simple g. A cystic tumor in a tendon sheath. SYN: *wrist g.*

spinal g. Dorsal root g.

spiral g. A long, coiled ganglion in the cochlea of the ear. It contains bipolar cells, the peripheral processes of which terminate in the organ of Corti. The central processes form the cochlear portion of the acoustic nerve and terminate in the cochlear nuclei of the medulla.

stellate g. A ganglion formed by joining of the inferior cervical ganglion with the first thoracic sympathetic ganglion. SYN: *cervicothoracic g.*

submandibular g. A ganglion lying between the mylohyoideus and hyoglossus muscles and suspended from the lingual nerve by two small branches. Peripheral fibers pass to the submandibular, sublingual, lingual, and adjacent salivary glands.

superior mesenteric g. A prevertebral ganglion of the sympathetic nervous system located near the base of the superior mesenteric artery. It lies close to the celiac ganglion and with it forms a part of the celiac plexus.

suprarenal g. A ganglion situated in the suprarenal plexus.

sympathetic g. One of the ganglia of the thoracolumbar (sympathetic) division of the autonomic nervous system. It includes vertebral or lateral ganglia (those forming the sympathetic trunk) and prevertebral or collateral ganglia, more peripherally located.

temporal g. A tiny ganglion joining the anterior branches of the superior cervical ganglion.

terminal g. A ganglion of the autonomic division of the nervous system that lies close to or within the organ innervated.

thoracic g. One of 11 or 12 ganglia of the thoracic area of the sympathetic trunk.

trigeminal g. A ganglion on the sensory portion of the fifth cranial nerve. SYN: *gasserian g.; semilunar g.*

tympanic g. An enlargement on the tympanic portion of the glossopharyngeal nerve.

vestibular g. A bilobed ganglion on the vestibular branch of the acoustic nerve at the base of the internal acoustic meatus. Its peripheral fibers begin in the maculae of the utricle and saccule and in the cristae of the ampullae of the semicircular ducts. SYN: *Scarpa's g.*

Wrisberg's g. Cardiac ganglia.

wrist g. Simple g.

ganglionated Having or consisting of ganglia.

ganglionectomy (găng″lē-ō-nĕk′tō-mē) [Gr. *ganglion,* knot, + *ektome,* excision] Excision of a ganglion.

ganglioneuroma (găng″lē-ō-nū-rō′mă) [″ + *neuron,* nerve, + *oma,* tumor] A neuroma containing ganglion cells. SYN: *gangliocytoma.*

ganglionic (găng-lē-ŏn′ĭk) Pert. to or of the nature of a ganglion. SYN: *ganglial.*

ganglionic blockade Blocking of the transmission of stimuli in autonomic ganglia. Pharmacologically, this is done by using drugs that occupy receptor sites for acetylcholine and by stabilizing the postsynaptic membranes against the actions of acetylcholine liberated from presynaptic nerve endings. The usual effects of drugs that cause ganglionic blockade are vasodilatation of arterioles with increased peripheral blood flow; hypotension; dilation of veins with pooling of blood in tissues, decreased venous return, and decreased cardiac output; tachycardia; mydriasis; cycloplegia; reduced tone and motility of the gastrointestinal tract with consequent constipation; urinary retention; dry mouth; and decreased sweating. Ganglionic blocking drugs are not often used to treat hypertension but are used to treat autonomic hyperreflexia and to produce controlled hypotension during certain types of surgery. Several drugs are available for ganglionic blocking.

ganglionitis (găng″lē-ŏn-ī′tĭs) [″ + *itis,* inflammation] Inflammation of a ganglion.

ganglionostomy (găng″glē-ō-nŏs′tō-mē) [″ + *stoma,* mouth] Surgical incision of a simple ganglion. Ganglionectomy is generally more efficacious when feasible.

ganglioplegia (găng″glē-ō-plē′jē-ă) [″ + *plege,* stroke] The failure of nervous stimuli to be transmitted by a ganglion. SEE: *blockade, ganglionic.*

ganglioplegic Any drug that prevents transmission of nervous impulses through sympathetic or parasympathetic ganglia. Such drugs have limited therapeutic applicability because of undesired side effects. They are useful in treating hypertensive crises. Because they decrease blood pressure, they are used to limit bleeding during certain surgical procedures.

ganglioside (găng′glē-ō-sīd) A particular class of glycosphingolipid present in nerve tissue and in the spleen.

gangliosidosis (găng″glē-ō-sī-dō′sĭs) *pl.* **gangliosidoses** An accumulation of abnormal amounts of specific gangliosides in the nervous system. SEE: *sphingolipidosis.*

gangosa (găng-gō′să) [Sp. *gangosa,* muffled voice] Ulceration of the nose and hard palate, seen in the late stage of yaws, leishmaniasis, or leprosy.

gangrene (găng′grēn) [Gr. *gangraina,* an eating sore] Necrosis or death of tissue, usually resulting from deficient or absent blood supply. SEE: *necrosis.*

ETIOLOGY: Gangrene usually is caused by obstruction of the blood supply to an organ or tissue, possibly resulting from inflammatory processes, injury, or degenerative changes such as arteriosclerosis. It is commonly a sequela of infections, frostbite, crushing injuries, or diseases such as diabetes mellitus and Raynaud's disease. Emboli in large arteries in almost any part of the body can cause gangrene of the area distal to that point. The part that dies is known as a slough (for soft tissues) or a sequestrum (for bone). The dead matter must be removed before healing can take place.

PATIENT CARE: The elderly or diabetic patient is assessed for arterial insufficiency related to decreases in the strength and elasticity of blood vessels. Capillary refill also is assessed. The presence and strength of distal pulses and the patient's normal sensation response to light and deep palpation are checked. Symmetry, color, temperature, and quantitative and qualitative changes in fingernails or toenails, skin texture, and hair patterns also are assessed. Any unusual areas of pigmentation indicating new skin lesions or scarring from past injury or ulceration are observed for and documented, with description given of the extent and nature of gangrene that is present.

If appropriate, prescribed vasodilating and thrombolytic agents are administered, and the patient's response is evaluated. If surgical intervention is required, the patient's understanding of the procedure, its desired effects, and possible complications is evaluated. Health care professionals collaborate with the surgeon to fill in knowledge gaps and to prepare the patient for surgery and the postoperative period. Care required will depend on the particular procedure. If amputation is required, the patient needs to understand that the level of amputation depends on determining the presence of viable tissues to ensure healing, and the requirements for fitting a prosthesis. The entire health care team must understand the patient's perception of the amputation in order to assist with grief resolution and adjustment to a permanent change in body image. Physical and occupational therapists assist the patient to deal with changes in mobility and ability to perform ADL. The multidisciplinary rehabilitation team involves patient, nurse, physician, social worker, psychologist, and prosthetist, as well as physical and occupational therapists. The patient's age and presence of other body system dysfunctions impact his or her immediate and long-term response to treatment.

diabetic g. Gangrene, esp. of the lower extremities, occurring in some diabetics as a result of vascular insufficiency, neuropathy, and infection.

dry g. Gangrene that results when the necrotic part has little blood and remains aseptic. This occurs when the arteries but not the veins are obstructed. The tissues dry and drop off, the process continuing for weeks or months. SEE: *Nursing Diagnoses Appendix.*

SYMPTOMS: Dry gangrene causes pain in the early stages. The affected part is cold and black and begins to atrophy. The most distal parts are generally affected first, the necrosis then spreading proximally. Dry gangrene is usually seen in arteriosclerosis associated with diabetes.

PATIENT CARE: Patient care concerns for dry gangrene are similar to those in which there is liquefied underlying necrotic tissue (wet gangrene). Necrotic matter must be removed and circulation to the remaining tissues ensured before healing can occur. The elderly diabetic patient with micro- and macrovascular disease may experience very little pain because peripheral neuropathy reduces feeling. The condition may come to light only upon inspection. For this reason, all patients with diabetes mellitus or peripheral vascular disease should show their feet to their caregivers at every office visit.

The recommended plan of care often includes removal of gangrenous tissue (amputation). All involved health care professionals need to recognize the patient's right to refuse such treatment. As long as the patient has been informed about the benefits of the planned treatment and the dire risks of refusal (loss of the affected part) and is of sound mind, he or she should be supported in the decision, and the family assisted to achieve acceptance. The gangrenous limb should be kept clean and dry, and protected as much as possible from trauma or infection. Psychological needs may require a psychiatric nurse practitioner, a psychologist, and a spiritual counselor of the patient's choice.

embolic g. Gangrene arising subsequent to an embolic obstruction.

Fournier's g. SEE: *Fournier's gangrene.*

gas g. Gangrene in a wound infected by a gas-forming microorganism, the most common causative agent being *Clostridium perfringens.*

TREATMENT: Gas gangrene is treated with débridement of the wound site, antibiotics, and clostridial antitoxin.

idiopathic g. Gangrene of unknown etiology.

inflammatory g. Gangrene associated with acute infections and inflammation.

moist g. Gangrene that is wet as a result of tissue necrosis and bacterial infection. The condition is marked by serous exudation and rapid decomposition.

SYMPTOMS: At first the affected part is hot and red; later it is cold and bluish, starting to slough. Moist gangrene spreads rapidly and carries a significant risk of local or systemic infection and occasionally death.

primary g. Gangrene developing in a part without previous inflammation.

secondary g. Gangrene developing subsequent to local inflammation.

symmetrical g. Gangrene on opposite sides of the body in corresponding parts, usually the result of vasomotor disturbances. It is characteristic of Raynaud's and Buerger's diseases.

traumatic g. Tissue death caused by serious injuries (e.g., compartment syndrome or crush injury).

gangrenous Pert. to gangrene.

Ganser's syndrome (găn′zĕrz) [Sigbert J. M. Ganser, Ger. psychiatrist, 1853–1931] A factitious disorder in which the individual mimics behavior he or she thinks is typical of a psychosis (e.g., giving nonsense answers and doing things incorrectly). Although there may be amnesia, disturbance of consciousness, and hallucinations, the individual is not psychotic.

gantry (găn′trē) [Gr. *kanthēlios,* pack ass] **1.** The housing for the imaging source and detectors into which the patient is placed for computed tomography and magnetic resonance imaging. **2.** The portion of the radiation therapy machine (linear accelerator, cobalt unit) that houses the source of therapeutic particles.

gap [Old Norse *gap,* chasm] An opening or a break; an interruption in continuity.

auscultatory g. A period of silence that sometimes occurs in the determination of blood pressure by auscultation. It may occur in patients with hypertension or aortic stenosis. SEE: *blood pressure; pulsus paradoxus.*

health care g. A disparity between health care needs and health care services, esp. as it applies to the medically indigent.

gap junction Minute pores between cells that provide pathways for intercellular communication. Originally described in muscle tissue, they are known to be present in most animal cells.

Garcinia cambogia An herbal agent promoted by alternative medicine practitioners for the treatment of obesity.

Gardnerella vaginalis [Herman Gardner, U.S. physician, d. 1947] One of several bacteria implicated in bacterial vaginosis in women. The bacilli are usually gram-negative, but in older cultures the bacilli may stain variably (some gram-negative and some falsely gram-positive). SEE: *bacterial vaginosis.*

Gardnerella vaginalis vaginitis Bacterial vaginosis.

Gardner's syndrome [Eldon J. Gardner, U.S. geneticist, b. 1909] Familial polyposis of the colon associated with a high risk of developing carcinoma of the colon. Also present are multiple osteomas and soft-tissue tumors of the skin. The condition is inherited as an autosomal dominant trait.

gargle [Fr. *gargouille,* throat; but may be onomatopoeia for gargle] **1.** A throat wash. **2.** To wash out the mouth and throat by tipping the head back and allowing the fluid to accumulate in the back of the throat, while agitating it by the forceful expiration of air.

gargoylism (găr′goyl-ĭsm) Hurler's syndrome.

garlic [AS. *gar,* spear, + *leac,* the leek] An edible, strongly flavored bulb of *Allium sativum* used mainly for seasoning. The chemical allicin, responsible for the smell of garlic, is not evident until the clove is cut or crushed. The evidence that garlic has therapeutic properties in cardiovascular disease and cancer prevention is inconclusive. Extracts of garlic contain very little allicin.

garment, front-opening Any female garment that opens from the front rather than the rear to increase dressing convenience for persons with limited function.

Garré's disease (găr-āz′) [Carl Garré, Swiss surgeon, 1858–1928] Chronic sclerosing osteitis or osteomyelitis due to pyogenic cocci.

Garren gastric bubble [Lloyd and Mary Garren, contemporary U.S. gastroenterologists] A deflated bladder that is placed in the stomach and then inflated; used to treat morbid obesity by reducing the effective volume of the stomach and thereby decreasing hunger.

Gartner's duct [Hermann T. Gartner, Danish surgeon and anatomist, 1785–1827] A small duct lying parallel to the uterine tube. It is a vestigial structure representing the persistent mesonephric duct. SYN: *duct of the epoophoron; ductus epoophori longitudinalis*.

GAS **1.** *general adaptation syndrome*. **2.** *Group A streptococci*.

gas One of the basic forms of matter. Gas molecules are free and move swiftly in all directions. Therefore, a gas not only takes the shape of the containing vessel but expands and fills the vessel no matter what its volume. Among the common important gases are oxygen; nitrogen; hydrogen; helium; sewer gas, which contains carbon monoxide; carbon dioxide; the anesthetic gases; ammonia; and the poisonous war gases. Liquids and solids may release toxic fumes when heated. SEE: *war g.; anesthesia*.

binary g. A toxic nerve gas formed by mixing two relatively harmless components. It was devised for use in chemical warfare. SEE: *war g.*

blood g. The principal gases found in the blood: oxygen, nitrogen, and carbon dioxide. They may be dissolved in the plasma or may exist in loose chemical combination with other compounds (e.g., oxygen combined with hemoglobin).

Clayton g. SEE: *Clayton gas*.

coal g. A flammable, explosive, toxic gas produced from the distillation of coal; used for heating and lighting. The principal constituents are methane, carbon monoxide, and hydrogen.

digestive tract g. Intestinal gas.

illuminating g. A mixture of various combustible gases including hydrogen and carbon monoxide. Its poisonous effects are largely due to carbon monoxide.

inert g. A gas that reacts little or not at all with other substances. Examples include helium, argon, neon, and krypton.

intestinal g. One of several gaseous compounds, such as carbon dioxide, oxygen, nitrogen, hydrogen, methane, methylmercaptan, and hydrogen sulfide, present in the intestinal tract. They are produced by digestive processes and intestinal bacteria. SEE: *digestion; flatus*.

laughing g. SEE: *nitrous oxide*.

lewisite g. A poisonous gas that contains arsenic and smells like geraniums. Symptoms of poisoning are similar to those caused by vesicant gas, but begin abruptly and are usually less severe. Arsenic can be recovered from the serum of the blisters, and symptoms of arsenic poisoning may occur. The treatment is similar to that used for vesicant gas poisoning. SEE: *vesicant g.; war g.*

lung irritant g. Any toxic or noxious gas that causes irritation or inflammation of the airways or alveoli. SEE: *Nursing Diagnoses Appendix; war gases*.

SYMPTOMS: Symptoms of exposure include a burning sensation of the eyes, nose, and throat; bronchitis; and pneumonitis. Pulmonary edema sometimes occurs and may cause severe respiratory failure and death.

TREATMENT: Supplemental oxygen and/or mechanical ventilation may be required for hours or days, depending on the extent of lung injury.

marsh g. Methane.

mustard g. Dichlorethyl sulfide, a poisonous gas used in warfare. SEE: *vesicant g.; war g.*

nerve g. A gas that interferes with or prevents transmission of nerve impulses. SEE: *war g.*

nitric oxide g. A toxic gas administered in very small concentrations during mechanical ventilation to treat persistent pulmonary hypertension.

nose irritant g. Diphenylchloroarsine, an irritant smoke. It causes intense pain in the nose, throat, and air passages, sneezing followed by headache and aching in the teeth and jaws, acute mental depression, and sometimes vomiting. The patient must be reassured that no permanent harm is done and should be warned against removing the respirator even though its use may worsen the symptoms. Nasal douching with warm sodium bicarbonate solution is helpful. SEE: *war g.*

sewer g. A gas that is produced by decaying matter in sewage and contains methane and hydrogen sulfide. It is toxic, usually flammable, and explosive. Sewer gas may be used for fuel. SEE: *carbon monoxide*.

suffocating g. Any of several war gases, such as phosgene or diphosgene, made from chlorine compounds. It irritates the bronchi and lungs, resulting in pulmonary edema. SEE: *lung irritant g.; war g.*

tear g. A gas such as bromoacetone that irritates the conjunctiva and produces a flow of tears. Treatment is rarely necessary. When the victim is removed from the contaminated area, the symptoms tend to subside gradually. Irrigating the eyes with large amounts of clear water or physiological saline hastens recovery.

toxic g. Any harmful gas.

vesicant g. A type of gas that blisters the skin. Clothing and boots become contaminated and a source of danger. Mustard and lewisite gases are examples.

SYMPTOMS: Symptoms do not appear at once; their onset may be delayed 6 hr or longer. Eye pain, lacrimation, and discharge may be the first evidence. The eyelids swell and the patient becomes unable to see. A diffuse redness of the skin is followed by blistering and ulceration.

TREATMENT: Decontamination is essential and must be thorough. The eyes should be bathed freely with normal saline or plain water. No bandage should be worn. The patient should be scrubbed, if possible, under a hot or warm shower for 10 min. If blisters arise despite these precautionary measures, they should be treated with a mild antiseptic and a protective dressing.

PROGNOSIS: Healing is very slow, but generally complete if the correct treatment is begun promptly.

vomiting g. A gas, particularly chloropicrin, that induces emesis.

war g's. Any chemical substances, whether solid, liquid, or vapor, used to produce poisonous gases with irritant effects. They can be classified as lacrimators, sternutators (sneeze causing), lung irritants, vesicants, and systemic poisons, such as nerve gas. Some gases have multiple effects.

War gases are known as nonpersistent (diffusing and dispersing fairly rapidly) or persistent (lingering and evaporating slowly).

FIRST AID: When giving first aid, the rescuer avoids becoming a casualty by taking appropriate precautions. All gas masks are checked to ensure that they are in working order. The rescuer first puts on his or her own mask, then fits masks to patients. The rescuer's skin is covered and exposed skin of persons at risk is flooded with water to flush off chemical contaminants if suspected.

PATIENT CARE: Decontamination centers are essential to the rescue effort. Thorough decontamination of patients, clothing, foot coverings, equipment, and even ambulances precedes admitting patients to emergency care areas to prevent unaffected persons in the area from becoming casualties.

gas bacillus SEE: *Clostridium perfringens.*

gas chromotography An analytical technique in which a sample is separated into its component parts between a gaseous mobile phase and a chemically active stationary phase.

gas distention Accumulation of excessive gas within the lumen of the gastrointestinal tract, the peritoneum, or the bowel wall. Treatment may be surgical or nonsurgical, depending on the etiology.

gaseous Having the nature or form of gas.

gas exchange, impaired The state in which the individual experiences a deficit in oxygenation and/or carbon dioxide elimination at the alveolar-capillary membrane, often producing subjective fatigue or anxiety. SEE: *Nursing Diagnoses Appendix.*

gasoline A product of the destructive distillation of petroleum. Commercial gasoline may contain toxic additives.

CAUTION: Using the mouth to produce suction on a tube for siphoning gasoline from a tank is dangerous because the gasoline may be inhaled or swallowed.

---

gasoline poisoning The reaction of the body to ingested or inhaled gasoline.

SYMPTOMS: The most hazardous symptom of gasoline exposure is a potentially fatal inflammation of the lungs, caused by aspiration of even small quantities of distilled petroleum. Symptoms of oral ingestion may also include dizziness, disorientation, seizures, and other neurological difficulties; gastric irritation and vomiting; rashes; and cardiac rhythm disturbances.

PATIENT CARE: The exposed patient should be observed for at least 6 hours. If no evidence of respiratory distress or dysfunction is found, and if a chest x-ray exam shows no signs of chemical pneumonitis, the patient may be safely discharged home.

Patients with strong evidence of chemical pneumonitis should be treated with oxygen and monitored in a hospital. Patients in full respiratory failure will require mechanical ventilation. Those who have deliberately ingested gasoline may benefit from supportive psychotherapy or psychiatric referral.

gasometric (găs″ō-mĕt′rĭk) Pert. to the measurement of gases.

gasometry (găs-ŏm′ĕ-trē) Estimation of the amount of gas in a mixture.

gasp [Old Norse *geispa*] To catch the breath; to inhale and exhale with quick, difficult breaths; the act of gasping.

gasserectomy (găs″ĕr-ĕk′tō-mē) The excision of a gasserian (trigeminal) ganglion. SEE: *ganglion, trigeminal.*

gaster- [Gr. *gaster,* belly] SEE: *gastro-.*

gastero- SEE: *gastro-.*

Gasterophilus (găs″tĕr-ŏf′ĭ-lŭs) A genus

of botflies belonging to the family Oestridae, order Diptera. The larvae infest horses.

G. hemorrhoidalis A species of botflies that infests the noses of horses.

G. intestinalis A species of botflies that infests the stomachs of horses.

G. nasalis The chin fly, which lays eggs on hair shafts on the lower lip and jaw of horses.

gastorrhagia (găs-tor-ā′jē-ă) [″ + *rhegnynai,* to burst forth] Gastrorrhagia.

gastr- SEE: *gastro-*.

gastralgia (găs-trăl′jē-ă) [″ + *algos,* pain] Pain in the stomach from any cause.

gastratrophia (găs″tră-trō′fē-ă) [″ + *atrophia,* atrophy] Atrophy of the stomach.

gastrectasia, gastrectasis [″ + *ektasis,* dilatation] Acute or chronic dilation of the stomach.

gastrectomy (găs-trĕk′tō-mē) [″ + *ektome,* excision] The surgical removal of part or all of the stomach.

gastric (găs′trĭk) [Gr. *gaster,* stomach] Pert. to the stomach. SEE: *digestion; stomach*.

gastric cancer Adenocarcinoma of the stomach. About 50% to 60% of all carcinomas of the stomach occur in the pyloric region. About 20% occur along the lesser curvature; the rest are located in the fundus, particularly along the greater curvature. Although this form of cancer is common throughout the world in people of all races, the incidence of gastric cancer exhibits unexplained geographic, cultural, and gender differences, with the highest incidence in men over age 40 and high mortality in Japan, Iceland, Chile, and Austria.

From 1930 to the 1990s, the incidence of gastric cancer declined from about 38 cases per 100,000 to about 6 cases per 100,000. In 1999, the American Cancer Society estimated there would be 21,900 new cases of gastric cancer and 13,500 deaths from this disease. The prognosis for a particular patient depends on the stage of the disease at the time of diagnosis, but overall the 5-year survival rate is about 15%.

PREDISPOSING CAUSES: Although the cause of gastric cancer is unknown, predisposing factors, such as gastritis with gastric atrophy, increase the risk. Genetic factors have been implicated. People with the type A blood group have a 10% increased risk, and the disease occurs more commonly in people with a family history of such cancer. *Helicobacter pylori* has also been implicated in the pathogenesis of this disease.

COMPLICATIONS: Malnutrition occurs as a result of impaired eating, the metabolic demands of the growing tumor, or obstruction of the GI tract. Iron deficiency anemia results as the tumor causes ulceration and bleeding. The tumor can interfere with the production of the intrinsic factor needed for vitamin B_{12} absorption, resulting in pernicious anemia. As the cancer metastasizes to other structures, related complications occur.

SIGNS AND SYMPTOMS: In the early stages, the patient may experience pain in the back or in the epigastric or retrosternal areas that is relieved with nonprescription analgesics; however, this symptom may not be reported because of failure to recognize its significance. The patient typically reports a vague feeling of fullness, heaviness, and moderate abdominal distention after meals. Depending on the cancer's progression, the patient may report weight loss, resulting from appetite disturbance; nausea; and vomiting. Coffee-ground vomitus may be reported if the tumor is located in the cardia. Weakness and fatigue are common complaints.

If the tumor is located in the proximal area of the stomach, the patient may experience dysphagia. Palpation of the abdomen may disclose a mass. Also, the examiner may be able to palpate enlarged lymph nodes, esp. in the supraclavicular and axillary regions. Other assessment findings depend on the extent of the disease and the location of metastases.

DIAGNOSTIC STUDIES: Gastric cancer is diagnosed by gastroscopy with biopsy. Fluoroscopy of the upper GI tract may be strongly suggestive of tumor. Studies to rule out specific organ metastases include computed tomography scans, chest radiographs, liver and bone scans, and liver biopsy.

TREATMENT: Surgery to remove the tumor often is the treatment of choice. Excision of the lesion with appropriate margins is possible in more than one third of patients. Even in the patient whose disease is not considered surgically curable, resection eases symptoms and improves the potential benefits of the chemotherapy and radiation therapy that usually follow surgery. The nature and extent of the lesion determine the type of surgery. Surgical procedures include gastroduodenostomy, gastrojejunostomy, partial gastric resection, and total gastrectomy. If metastasis has occurred, the omentum and spleen may have to be removed.

Chemotherapy for GI tumors may help to control signs and symptoms and to prolong survival. Gastric adenocarcinomas respond to several agents, including fluorouracil, carmustine, doxorubicin, and mitomycin. Antispasmodics and antacids may help relieve GI distress. Antiemetics can control nausea, which intensifies as the tumor grows. In the more advanced stages, the patient may need sedatives and tranquilizers to control overwhelming anxiety. Opioid analgesics can relieve severe and unremitting pain.

If the patient has a nonresectable or partially resectable tumor, radiation therapy can be effective if combined with chemotherapy. The patient should receive this therapy on an empty stomach. It should not be given preoperatively, because it may damage viscera and impede healing.

PATIENT CARE: Nutritional intake is monitored, and the patient is weighed periodically. If not already done, the health care provider initiates comprehensive clinical and laboratory investigations including serial studies as indicated. The patient is prepared physically and emotionally for surgery or other treatment (radiotherapy) as necessary.

Throughout the course of the illness, a high-protein, high-calorie diet is provided to help the patient avoid or recover from weight loss, malnutrition, and anemia. This diet also helps the patient tolerate surgery, chemotherapy, and radiotherapy; promotes wound healing; and provides enough protein, fluid, and potassium to aid glycogen and body protein synthesis. Frequent small meals are offered, and iron-rich foods are included if the patient has an iron deficiency. Dietary supplements are provided as prescribed.

To stimulate a poor appetite, antidepressant drugs may be administered. Parenteral nutrition is given as prescribed. A prescribed antacid is administered to relieve heartburn and gastric acidity, and a prescribed histamine$_2$-receptor antagonist, such as cimetidine or famotidine, is given to decrease gastric secretions. Prescribed opioid analgesics are also administered. The patient is instructed in use of all drugs.

Complications of radiation therapy may include nausea, vomiting, alopecia, malaise, and diarrhea. Complications of chemotherapy may include infection, nausea, vomiting, mouth ulcers, and alopecia. During radiation or chemotherapy, oral intake is encouraged to help relieve some of the adverse effects; bland fruit juices, ginger ale, or other fluids and prescribed antiemetics are provided to minimize nausea and vomiting; and comfort measures and reassurance are offered as needed. The patient is advised to report persistent adverse reactions.

The patient is encouraged to follow a normal routine as much as possible after recovery from surgery and during radiation therapy and chemotherapy. He or she should stop activities that cause excessive fatigue (at least temporarily) and incorporate rest periods. The patient should avoid crowds and people with known infections.

gastric-inhibitory polypeptide ABBR: GIP. A polypeptide hormone secreted by the duodenum and jejunum that inhibits motility and the secretion of gastric hydrochloric acid and pepsin and that stimulates insulin secretion. SEE: *enterogastrone*.

gastric intramucosal pH An experimental procedure to measure the pH of gastric mucosa to determine the adequacy of its oxygenation. The goal is to obtain an index of tissue oxygenation in general.

gastric lavage SEE: *gastric lavage*.

gastrin A hormone secreted by the mucosa of the pyloric area of the stomach and duodenum in various species of animals, including humans. The hormone is released into gastric venous blood, from which it flows into the liver and into the general circulation. When the hormone reaches the stomach, it stimulates gastric acid secretion. Gastrin causes the lower esophageal sphincter to contract and the ileocecal valve to relax. Also, it has a mild effect on small-intestine and gallbladder motility. Gastrin is released in response to partially digested protein, ethyl alcohol in about 10% concentration, and distention of the antrum of the stomach. SEE: *Zollinger-Ellison syndrome*.

gastrinoma (găs″trĭn-ō′mă) The gastrin-secreting tumor associated with Zollinger-Ellison syndrome. SEE: *Zollinger-Ellison syndrome*.

gastritis (găs-trī′tĭs) [Gr. *gaster*, stomach, + *itis*, inflammation] Acute or chronic inflammation of the lining of the stomach. Worldwide, the most common cause is infection with *Helicobacter pylori*. Other less common causes of gastric inflammation include use of alcohol and tobacco products; injury to the lining of the stomach by nonsteroidal anti-inflammatory drugs (NSAIDs); portal hypertension, with congestion of the stomach lining; autoimmune diseases (such as pernicious anemia); duodenal reflux; and gastric ischemia. SYN: *endogastritis*. SEE: *Helicobacter pylori*.

SYMPTOMS: The inflammation may be asymptomatic, especially in mild chronic gastritis, or it may be acute, with symptoms such as epigastric pain, nausea, vomiting, and hematemesis.

TREATMENT: When *H. pylori* is responsible, antibiotic therapy combined with a potent acid-suppressing agent cures most patients. Abstaining from the use of alcohol, tobacco products, and NSAIDs improves gastritis caused by these agents; typically an H2 blocking drug (such as ranitidine) or proton pump inhibitors (such as omeprazole) also are given to promote healing.

PATIENT CARE: The patient is educated about the disorder. Compliance with multidrug antibiotic regimens is encouraged when the patient is found to have gastritis caused by *H. pylori*. If gastritis is caused by smoking, drinking alcohol, or overusing NSAIDs, abstinence from these substances is encouraged. Patients who are unable to take foods or liquids by mouth or who begin to vomit blood should seek medical attention promptly.

acute g. Acute and sudden irritation of the gastric mucosa. This may be due to ingestion of toxic substances such as alcohol or poisons. The symptoms include moderate fever, anorexia, nausea, intense epigastic pain, persistent vomiting, thirst, and prostration. Therapy includes antisecretory drugs. For severe prolonged bleeding, surgery may rarely be required. SEE: *Nursing Diagnoses Appendix*.

PATIENT CARE: A thorough patient history is conducted to assist in determining and eliminating the cause. If the cause is a toxic substance, the patient is helped to understand that vomiting and diarrhea are the body's ways of ridding itself of the substance. Vital signs, fluid intake and output, appearance, and gastric symptoms are monitored. Symptomatic and supportive therapy is given as prescribed (antiemetics, IV fluids). Prescribed histamine antagonists and barrier agents, such as sucralfate and antacids, are administered; the patient is instructed in their use and the importance of correctly spacing dosages. Antibiotic therapy for *H. pylori* also is discussed if appropriate. The patient is advised to avoid aspirin-containing OTC compounds. The patient is assisted to identify foods that contribute to symptoms, and to eliminate them from the diet. The nurse can provide an initial diet that is bland and contains frequent small servings; referral to a dietician enables further instruction. Emotional support is given to help the patient manage symptoms and to deal with life-style changes (stress reduction, smoking cessation, alcohol elimination) that may be required. If surgery is necessary, the patient receives appropriate preoperative and postoperative care.

atrophic g. Chronic gastritis with atrophied mucosa and glands. Patients with this type often are asymptomatic.

chronic g. Prolonged continual or intermittent inflammation of the gastric mucosa. *Helicobacter pylori* is the most common cause. It typically produces superficial changes in the lining of the antrum of the stomach. Prolonged *H. pylori*-induced gastritis predisposes patients to gastric adenocarcinoma and gastric lymphoma. SEE: *H. pylori; Nursing Diagnoses Appendix*.

PATIENT CARE: A careful history is compiled to help determine the cause. Symptoms may be vague or, in the case of atrophic gastritis, absent. The patient is prepared for diagnostic testing. He or she is instructed to avoid spicy foods and any others noted to exacerbate symptoms, and also is warned to avoid aspirin. If symptoms persist, the patient may take antacids. When pernicious anemia is the underlying cause, the patient (or significant other care provider) is taught to administer vitamin B_{12} parenterally or orally.

giant hypertrophic g. Gastritis probably caused by *Helicobacter pylori*, marked by excessive proliferation of the stomach mucosal folds. SYN: *Ménétrier's disease*.

toxic g. Gastritis due to any toxic agent, including poisons or corrosive chemicals.

gastro-, gaster-, gastero-, gastr- [Gr. *gaster*, stomach] Combining form meaning *stomach*.

gastroanastomosis (găs″trō-ăn-ăs″tō-mō′sĭs) [″ + *anastomosis*, outlet] The formation of a passage between the pyloric and cardiac ends of the stomach for relief of persistent hourglass contraction. SYN: *gastrogastrostomy*.

gastrocamera (găs″trō-kăm′ĕ-ră) A camera, small enough to be swallowed, used to photograph the inside of the stomach.

gastrocardiac (găs″trō-kăr′dē-ăk) [″ + *kardia*, heart] Concerning the stomach and heart.

gastrocele (găs′trō-sēl) [″ + *kele*, hernia] A hernia of the stomach.

gastrocnemius (găs″trŏk-nē′mē-ŭs) [″ + *kneme*, leg] The large muscle of the posterior portion of the lower leg. It is the most superficial of the calf muscles. It plantar flexes the foot and flexes the knee.

gastrocoele (găs′trō-sēl) Archenteron.

gastrocolic (găs″trō-kŏl′ĭk) [″ + *kolon*, colon] Pert. to the stomach and colon.

gastrocolitis (găs″trō-kō-lī′tĭs) [″ + ″ + *itis*, inflammation] Inflammation of the stomach and colon.

gastrocoloptosis (găs″trō-kŏl″ŏp-tō′sĭs) [″ + ″ + *ptosis*, dropping] Downward prolapse of the stomach and colon.

gastrocolostomy (găs″trō-kŏl-ŏs′tō-mē) [″ + ″ + *stoma*, mouth] Establishment of a permanent passage between the stomach and colon.

gastrocolotomy (găs″trō-kō-lŏt′ō-mē) [″ + ″ + *tome*, incision] Incision into the stomach and colon.

gastrocolpotomy (găs″trō-kŏl-pŏt′ō-mē) [″ + *kolpos*, vagina, + *tome*, incision] An incision through the abdominal wall into the upper part of the vagina.

gastrocutaneous (găs″trō-kū-tā′nē-ŭs) [″ + L. *cutis*, skin] A communication between the stomach and the skin.

gastrodialysis (găs″trō-dī-ăl′ĭ-sĭs) [″ + *dia,* through, + *lysis,* dissolution] Dialysis (i.e., washing out) of the stomach to clear both the stomach and the blood of toxic materials secreted into the stomach.

gastrodidymus (găs″trō-dĭd′ĭ-mŭs) [″ + *didymos,* twin] Congenitally deformed twins united by a common abdominal cavity.

gastrodisciasis (găs″trō-dĭs-kī′ă-sĭs) Infestation by a fluke, *Gastrodiscoides hominis.*

Gastrodiscoides (găs″trō-dĭs-koy′dēz) A genus of flukes belonging to the family Gastrodiscidae, suborder Amphistomata.

G. hominis A species of flukes commonly infesting hogs but occasionally found in humans.

gastroduodenal (găs″trō-dū″ō-dēn′ăl) [Gr. *gaster,* stomach, + L. *duodeni,* twelve] Rel. to the stomach and duodenum.

gastroduodenitis (găs″trō-dū-ŏd″ĕn-ī′tĭs) [″ + ″ + Gr. *itis,* inflammation] Inflammation of the stomach and duodenum.

gastroduodenoscopy (găs″trō-dū″ō-dĕ-nŏs′kō-pē) [″ + ″ + *skopein,* to examine] The use of an endoscope to visually examine the stomach and duodenum.

gastroduodenostomy (găs″trō-dū″ō-dĕn-ŏs′tō-mē) [″ + ″ + Gr. *stoma,* mouth] Excision of the pylorus of the stomach with anastomosis of the upper portion of the stomach to the duodenum. SYN: *Billroth I operation.*

Other procedures of gastroduodenostomy do not involve resection of portions of either organ.

gastroenteralgia (găs″trō-ĕn″tĕr-ăl′jē-ă) [″ + *enteron,* intestine, + *algos,* pain] Pain in the stomach and intestines.

gastroenteric (găs″trō-ĕn-tĕr′ĭk) Pert. to the stomach and intestines or to a condition involving both.

gastroenteritis (găs″trō-ĕn-tĕr-ī′tĭs) [″ + *enteron,* intestine, + *itis,* inflammation] Inflammation of the stomach and intestinal tract that causes vomiting, diarrhea, or both. The most common causes are viruses (e.g., rotavirus) and bacteria (e.g., *Salmonella*) in food and water. SEE: *diarrhea; enterocolitis; Nursing Diagnoses Appendix.*

SYMPTOMS: The patient typically suffers episodes of vomiting and diarrhea and may develop symptoms of dehydration (such as thirst and dizziness when standing up), as well as malaise, abdominal cramps, or fever.

TREATMENT: Rehydration, usually with liquids taken by mouth, is the key to avoiding dehydration or electrolyte imbalance. Symptomatic remedies that reduce the frequency or volume of diarrhea (such as kaolin/pectin or loperamide) often are helpful.

PREVENTION: Prevention is emphasized by teaching children and adults correct handwashing techniques and proper care of food. The basic principles of food handling should be taught to all those in the home, including the following topics: the need to wash hands frequently, particularly after using the toilet; use of a meat thermometer to check that meat and dishes containing eggs are adequately cooked; refrigeration of foods (below 40°F) until just before cooking and again within 1 hr after cooking (esp. in warm weather); separation of raw and cooked foods; and use of different utensils and dishes for raw and cooked meats. Travelers, esp. to developing countries, should not eat raw seafood, raw vegetables, or salads and should peel all fruit themselves. Campers should determine if they are in a location where streams are known to be contaminated with protozoa (e.g., New Hampshire, upstate New York, Oregon).

viral g. Gastroenteritis caused by ingested viruses. It may be clinically difficult to confirm these viral infections, and public health interventions needed to control outbreaks caused by these agents usually must be made before results of viral testing are available. The median incubation period is 24 to 48 hr and the median duration of the symptoms is 12 to 60 hr. Most patients will experience diarrhea, nausea, abdominal cramps, and vomiting. There is no specific treatment other than supportive therapy and fluid replacement. SYN: *epidemic viral gastroenteropathy.* SEE: *diarrhea; enterocolitis.*

ETIOLOGY: The rotavirus, which causes more than 100 million cases and approx. 1 million deaths each year worldwide, most frequently strikes children 6 to 24 months of age, causing 3 to 8 days of diarrhea and vomiting. The Norwalk virus causes most food-borne infections in older children and adults and may cause epidemics in schools and institutions. Diarrhea, accompanied by vomiting and abdominal pain, lasts 1 to 3 days.

TREATMENT: Adequate fluid replacement through oral solutions or, when severe, intravenous fluids is the basis for treatment. Prevention is emphasized by teaching children and adults correct handwashing techniques and proper care of food.

PATIENT CARE: Because rotavirus is more prevalent in children under age 2, parents, day-care personnel, and other caregivers require teaching about methods to prevent the spread of infection (which is primarily fecal-oral transmission). Caregivers also must learn proper handling and disposal of diapers. They must understand that, while the illness usually is mild and self-limited (seldom lasting more than 3 days), infected children are at risk for dehydration. Caregivers are taught early indicators of dehydration that necessitate bringing the child to a physician or pediatric nurse practitioner; hospitalization may be required in severe cases.

If the child is hospitalized, he or she is isolated from children without diarrhea, and parents are taught necessary isolation procedures. Intravenous (IV) fluids are administered as prescribed for rehydration; fluid and electrolyte balance, body weight, and other indicators are monitored throughout. If the child is able to ingest oral fluids, an oral rehydration formula is used, with fluids given at room temperature for better tolerance. Age-appropriate foods are reintroduced gradually, once liquids are well tolerated. Protective mouth and skin care to relieve dryness and prevent breakdown is provided and taught to caregivers. Comfort measures are an important part of the child's care, including age-appropriate sensory stimulation and diversion. Additionally, the family requires support and reassurance, with explanations of therapeutic measures and diet. Good hygiene and sanitary measures are emphasized.

In older children or adults, antidiarrheal agents may be used, although antiemetics should be avoided. The patient is encouraged to rest, which relieves symptoms and conserves strength, and to avoid sudden movements, which can increase the severity of nausea. Warm sitz baths, witch hazel compresses, and petroleum jelly as a barrier may help to ease anal irritation. The patient is taught about prescribed treatments, preventive measures, and careful handwashing.

gastroenteroanastomosis (găs″trō-ĕn″tĕr-ō-ă-năs″tō-mō′sĭs) The formation of a passage between the stomach and small intestine.

gastroenterocolitis (găs″trō-ĕn″tĕr-ō-kŏl-ī′tĭs) [″ + ″ + *kolon,* colon, + *itis,* inflammation] Inflammation of the stomach, small intestine, and colon.

gastroenterocolostomy (găs″trō-ĕn″tĕr-ō-kō-lŏs′tō-mē) [″ + ″ + ″ + *stoma,* mouth] The creation of a passage joining the stomach, small intestine, and colon.

gastroenterology (găs″trō-ĕn″tĕr-ŏl′ō-jē) [″ + ″ + *logos,* word, reason] The branch of medical science concerned with the study of the physiology and pathology of the stomach, intestines, and related structures, such as the esophagus, liver, gallbladder, and pancreas.

gastroenteroptosis (găs″trō-ĕn″tĕr-ŏp-tō′sĭs) [″ + ″ + *ptosis,* a dropping] Prolapse of the stomach and intestines.

gastroenterostomy (găs″trō-ĕn-tĕr-ŏs′tō-mē) [″ + *enteron,* intestine, + *stoma,* mouth] Surgical anastomosis between the stomach and small bowel. This operation may be employed for a variety of malignant and benign gastroduodenal diseases.

gastroepiploic (găs″trō-ĕp″ĭ-plō′ĭk) [″ + *epiploon,* omentum] Pert. to the stomach and greater omentum.

gastroesophageal (găs″trō-ĕ-sŏf″ă-jē′ăl) [″ + *oisophagos,* esophagus] Concerning the stomach and esophagus.

gastroesophageal reflux Gastroesophageal reflux disease.

gastroesophageal reflux disease ABBR: GERD. The regurgitation of stomach acid gastric and other contents into the esophagus. This is a common cause of heartburn, chest pain, and esophagitis, and rarely, of cancer of the esophagus. SYN: *acid-reflux disorder*.

gastroesophagitis (găs″trō-ē-sŏf″ă-jī′tĭs) [″ + ″ + *itis,* inflammation] Inflammation of the stomach and esophagus.

gastroesophagostomy (găs″trō-ē-sŏf″ă-gŏs′tō-mē) [″ + ″ + *stoma,* mouth] The formation of a passage from the esophagus to the stomach.

gastrofiberscope (găs″trō-fī′bĕr-skōp) A flexible endoscope using fiberoptics for visual examination of the stomach.

gastrogastrostomy (găs″trō-găs-trŏs′tō-mē) [″ + *gaster,* stomach, + *stoma,* mouth] Gastroanastomosis. Surgical anastomosis between one portion of the stomach and another.

gastrogavage (găs″trō-gă-văzh′) [″ + Fr. *gavage,* cramming] Artificial feeding through an opening into the stomach or a tube passed into the stomach.

gastrogenic (găs″trō-jĕn′ĭk) [″ + *gennan,* to produce] Originating in the stomach.

gastrohepatic [″ + *hepar,* liver] Pert. to the stomach and liver.

gastrohepatitis (găs″trō-hĕp-ă-tī′tĭs) [″ + ″ + *itis,* inflammation] The combination of gastritis and hepatitis.

gastroileac (găs-trō-ĭl′ē-ăk) [″ + L. *ileum,* groin] Pert. to the stomach and ileum.

gastroileitis (găs″trō-ĭl-ē-ī′tĭs) Inflammation of the stomach and ileum.

gastroileostomy (găs″trō-ĭl-ē-ŏs′tō-mē) A surgical anastomosis between the stomach and ileum.

gastrointestinal [″ + L. *intestinalis,* intestine] Pertaining to the entire digestive tract, from the mouth to the anus.

gastrointestinal bleeding Bleeding from the digestive tract; for example, vomiting blood, bleeding from the rectum, or passing melenic (black, tarry) stools. This may be caused by a broad range of problems, including esophagitis, gastritis, ulcers, cancers, vascular malformations, hemorrhoids, and other lesions. The severity of the bleeding is often evident on physical examination. The heavily bleeding patient may be tachycardic, hypotensive, and pale and will often complain of dizziness on rising from a bed or chair. These important findings require prompt medical evaluation.

gastrointestinal decompression The removal of contents of the intestinal tract by use of suction through a tube inserted through the nostrils and into the digestive tract. The tube may be inserted by pharyngostomy or gastrostomy. SEE: *Wangensteen tube*.

gastrojejunostomy (găs-trō-jĕ-jū-nŏs′tō-mē) [″ + L. *jejunum,* empty, + Gr. *stoma,* mouth] A connection, usually constructed surgically, between the stomach and the jejunum. SYN: *Billroth II operation*.

gastrolienal (găs″trō-lī′ĕn-ăl) [″ + L. *lien,* spleen] Concerning the stomach and spleen.

gastrolith (găs′trō-lĭth) [″ + *lithos,* stone] A calculus in the stomach.

gastrolithiasis (găs″trō-lĭth-ī′ă-sĭs) The formation of calculi in the stomach.

gastrology (găs-trŏl′ō-jē) [″ + *logos,* word, reason] The study of function and diseases of the stomach.

gastrolysis (găs-trŏl′ĭ-sĭs) [″ + *lysis,* dissolution] Surgical breaking of adhesions between the stomach and adjoining structures.

gastromalacia (găs-trō-mă-lā′shē-ă) [″ + *malakia,* softening] A softening of the stomach walls.

gastromegaly (găs″trō-mĕg′ă-lē) [″ + *megas,* large] An enlargement of the stomach.

gastromycosis (găs″trō-mī-kō′sĭs) [″ + *mykes,* fungus, + *osis,* condition] A disease of the stomach caused by fungi.

gastromyotomy (găs″trō-mī-ŏt′ō-mē) [″ + *mys,* muscle, + *tome,* incision] An incision of the circular muscle fibers of the stomach.

gastropancreatitis (găs″trō-păn″krē-ă-tī′tĭs) [″ + *pan,* all, + *kreas,* flesh, + *itis,* inflammation] A simultaneous inflammation of the stomach and pancreas.

gastroparalysis (găs″trō-păr-ăl′ĭ-sĭs) [″ + *para,* beyond, + *lyein,* to loosen] Paralysis of the stomach. SYN: *gastroplegia*.

gastroparesis (găs″trō-pă-rē′sĭs) Delayed emptying of food from the stomach into the small bowel. Gastroparesis occurs acutely in patients receiving parenteral nutrition. It may also be a chronic complication of diseases marked by autonomic failure, such as diabetes mellitus, chronic renal failure, and amyloidosis. It may occur during pregnancy, as a result of elevated levels of progesterone.

gastropathy (găs-trŏp′ă-thē) [″ + *pathos,* disease, suffering] Any disorder of the stomach.

hypertrophic g. An uncommon disorder marked by protein loss from the upper gastrointestinal tract and enlarged gastric rugal folds.

gastropexy, gastropexis (găs′trō-pĕk″sē, -sĭs) [″ + *pexis,* fixation] Suturing of the stomach to the abdominal walls for correction of displacement.

gastrophrenic (găs″trō-frĕn′ĭk) [″ + *phren,* diaphragm] Rel. to the stomach and diaphragm.

gastroplasty (găs′trō-plăs″tē) [″ + *plassein,* to form] Plastic surgery of the stomach. This procedure has been used in several ways to decrease the size of the stomach to treat morbid obesity; its success is variable.

gastroplegia (găs″trō-plē′jē-ă) [″ + *plege,* stroke] Gastroparalysis.

gastroplication (găs″trō-plī-kā′shŭn) [″ + L. *plicare,* to fold] Stitching of the walls of the stomach to reduce dilatation.

gastroptosis (găs″trō-tō′sĭs) [″ + *ptosis,* falling] Downward displacement of the stomach, which rarely causes symptoms or illness.

gastropulmonary (găs″trō-pŭl′mō-năr-ē) [″ + L. *pulmo,* lung] Concerning the stomach and lungs.

gastropylorectomy (găs″trō-pī″lor-ĕk′tō-mē) [″ + *pyloros,* pylorus, + *ektome,* excision] Excision of the pyloric part of the stomach.

gastropyloric Rel. to the stomach and pylorus.

gastroradiculitis (găs″trō-ră-dĭk″ū-lī′tĭs) [″ + L. *radix,* root, + Gr. *itis,* inflammation] Inflammation of the posterior spinal nerve roots, the sensory fibers of which supply the stomach.

gastrorrhagia (găs″trō-rā′jē-ă) [″ + *rhegnynai,* to burst forth] Hemorrhage from the stomach.

gastrorrhaphy (găs-tror′ă-fē) [″ + *rhaphe,* seam, ridge] **1.** Suture of an injured stomach wall. **2.** Gastroplication.

gastrorrhexis A rupture or tearing of the stomach.

gastroschisis (găs-trŏs′kĭ-sĭs) [″ + *schisis,* a splitting] A congenital fissure that remains open in the wall of the abdomen.

gastroscope (găs′trō-skōp) [″ + *skopein,* to examine] An endoscope for inspecting the stomach's interior. This rigid instrument has been replaced by a flexible, fiberoptic gastroduodenoscope.

gastroscopy (găs-trŏs′kō-pē) Examination of the stomach using a gastroscope.

gastrospasm (găs′trō-spăzm) [″ + *spasmos,* spasm] A spasm of the stomach.

gastrosplenic (găs″trō-splĕn′ĭk) [″ + *splen,* spleen] Of or pert. to the stomach and spleen.

gastrostenosis (găs″trō-stĕn-ō′sĭs) [″ + *stenosis,* narrowing] Contraction (stenosis) of the stomach.

g. cardiaca Stenosis of the cardiac orifice of the stomach.

g. pylorica Stenosis of the pylorus of the stomach.

gastrostogavage (găs-trŏs″tō-gă-văzh′) [″ + *stoma,* mouth, + Fr. *gaver,* to stuff] Feeding by means of a tube leading from outside the body into the stomach through a gastric fistula. SEE: *gavage.*

gastrostolavage (găs-trŏs″tō-lă-văzh′) [″ + Fr. *lavage,* fr. L. *lavare,* to wash] Irrigation of the stomach through a nasogastric or orogastric tube, or surgically constructed gastrostomy.

gastrostoma (găs-trŏs′tō-mă) [″ + *stoma,* mouth] A fistula, or a passageway created from the stomach through the abdominal wall.

gastrostomy (găs-trŏs′tō-mē) Surgical creation of a gastric fistula through the abdominal wall, necessary in some cases of stricture of the esophagus for the purpose of introducing food into the stomach.

PATIENT CARE: The skin around the tube is inspected for signs of irritation or excoriation and kept clean, dry, and protected from excoriating gastric secretions. Tension on the tube that may cause the incision to widen and allow spillage of gastric secretions on the skin or into surrounding tissues is prevented.

Before the patient is fed, tube patency and position are assessed, and the volume of the remaining stomach contents is measured by aspirating the stomach. If the volume is greater than the amount permitted by protocol or the physician's direction, feeding is withheld. After feedings, the tube is flushed with water.

Assistance is provided with oral hygiene at intervals throughout the day to prevent dryness and parotitis. Both patient and family are taught correct techniques for tube and skin care and for feeding through the gastrostomy tube. SEE: *gastrostomy tube.*

percutaneous endoscopic g. ABBR: PEG. A feeding ostomy. PEG tubes are inserted transorally into the stomach with the aid of an endoscope and then pulled through a stab wound made in the abdominal wall. Commercially prepared kits are available to facilitate this procedure.

gastrotherapy (găs″trō-thĕr′ă-pē) [″ + *therapeia,* treatment] The treatment of gastric diseases.

gastrothoracopagus (găs″trō-thō″ră-kŏp′ă-gŭs) [″ + *thorax,* chest, + *pagos,* thing fixed] Congenitally deformed twins joined at the stomach and thorax.

gastrotome (găs′trō-tōm) [″ + *tome,* incision] An instrument for incising the stomach or abdomen.

gastrotomy (găs-trŏt′ō-mē) [″ + *tome,* incision] A gastric or abdominal incision.

gastrotonometer (găs″trō-tō-nŏm′ĕ-tĕr) [″ + *tonos,* tension, + *metron,* measure] An instrument for measuring intragastric pressure.

gastrotympanites (găs″trō-tĭm″pă-nī′tēz) [″ + *tympanites,* distention] Distention of the stomach by gas or air.

gastrula (găs′troo-lă) [L., little belly] The stage in embryonic development following the blastula in which the embryo assumes a two-layered condition. The outer layer is the ectoderm or epiblast; the inner layer, the endoderm or hypoblast. The latter lines a cavity, the gastrocoele or archenteron, that opens to the outside through an opening, the blastopore.

gastrulation (găs″troo-lā′shŭn) The development of the gastrula in the embryo.

Gatch bed [Willis Dew Gatch, U.S. surgeon, 1878–1962] A bed in which the patient can be raised and held in a half-sitting position by raising the knee section of the bed.

gatekeeper A person who decides whether further medical assistance or care should be sought or allowed. Conflicts and problems may arise owing to the gatekeeper's financial interest in controlling costs (and thus not referring the patient for further care). Ideally, the gatekeeper would be financially neutral and make decisions concerning medical resource allocation based on the best available evidence.

gatekeeping In medical care, deciding the allocation, limitation, or rationing of services. Decisions are based on a variety of factors including need; cost; the potential for success of the proposed therapy; and the availability of facilities, staff, and equipment. SEE: *triage.*

gate theory The hypothesis that painful stimuli may be prevented from reaching higher levels of the central nervous system by stimulation of larger sensory nerves. This is one of the proposed explanations of the action of acupuncture.

gating In radiology, a procedure used to reduce image artifacts caused by involuntary motion.

cardiac g. Medical image information consistently collected during a specific phase of the cardiac cycle.

respiratory g. Medical image information consistently collected during a specific phase of respiration.

gatism (gā′tĭzm) [Fr. *gâter,* to spoil] Urinary or rectal incontinence.

Gaucher, Philippe C. E. (gō-shā′) French physician, 1854–1918.

G.'s cell A large reticuloendothelial cell seen in Gaucher's disease, which contains a small, eccentrically placed nucleus and kerasin. SEE: illus.

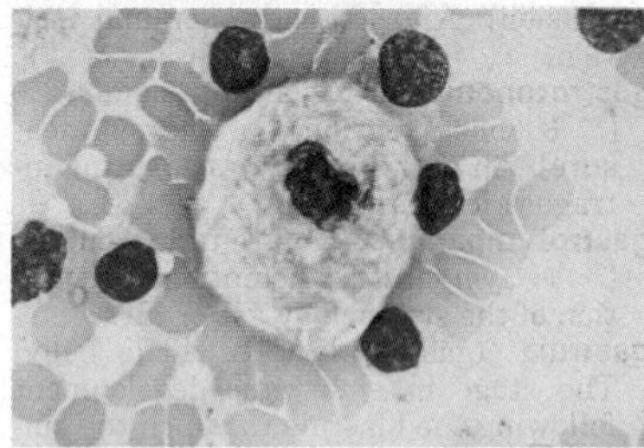

GAUCHER'S CELL IN BONE MARROW
(Orig. mag. ×640)

G.'s disease One of several autosomal recessive disorders of lipid metabolism caused by a deficiency of the enzyme beta-glucocerebrosidase. The severe form is rare, but milder forms frequently occur, esp. in people of Jewish extraction. Fatty substances called *glycosphingolipids* accumulate in the reticuloendothelial cells. SYN: *cerebroside lipoidosis*.

Three clinical subtypes of the disease exist. Type 1, comprising 99% of cases, is associated with an enlarged liver and spleen, increased skin pigmentation, and painful bone marrow lesions. Enzyme replacement therapy is effective in this type but may be prohibitively expensive. Type 2 is characterized by neurological symptoms including oculomotor apraxia, strabismus, and hypertonicity. These symptoms usually occur in the first year of life, with death following by age 18 months. Therapy is symptomatic. Type 3 is similar to type 2, but the onset of symptoms is much later and the course is longer. Therapy is symptomatic.

gauge (gāj) **1.** A device for measuring the size, capacity, amount, or power of an object or substance. **2.** A standard of measurement.

Gault's reflex (gawlts) Contraction of the orbicularis palpebrarum muscle to produce a blinking of the eye following a loud noise close to the ear. This reflex is tested in patients suspected of malingering to feign deafness. SEE: *malingerer*.

gauntlet (gawnt'lĕt) [Fr. *gant,* glove] A glovelike bandage that fits the hand and fingers.

gauss (gows) [Johann Carl F. Gauss, Ger. physicist, 1777–1855] The unit of intensity of a magnetic flux.

Gauss' sign (gows) [Carl J. Gauss, Ger. gynecologist, 1875–1957] An unusual mobility of the uterus in the early weeks of pregnancy.

gauze (gawz) [O.Fr. *gaze,* gauze] Thin, loosely woven muslin or similar material used for bandages and surgical sponges.

absorbent g. Gauze made of absorbent material.

antiseptic g. Gauze containing an antiseptic substance.

aseptic g. Sterilized gauze, often packaged in an aseptic container, usually paper, and ready for use.

petrolatum g. Sterilized absorbent gauze saturated with petrolatum.

petroleum g. Sterilized absorbent gauze saturated with petroleum jelly, used, for example, to cover burns.

gavage (gă-văzh') [Fr. *gaver,* to stuff] Feeding with a stomach tube or with a tube passed through the nares, pharynx, and esophagus into the stomach. The food is in liquid or semiliquid form at room temperature. SEE: *gastrostogavage*.

Gavard's muscle (gă-vărz') [Hyacinthe Gavard, Fr. anatomist, 1753–1802] The oblique muscular fibers of the stomach wall.

gay Homosexual.

gay bowel syndrome Infectious diarrhea in men who have sex with men whose sexual activity includes penile penetration of the anus and rectum. *Shigella* as well as other pathogens have been associated with this syndrome.

Gay's gland [Alexander H. Gay, Russian anatomist, 1842–1907] A large sebaceous circumanal gland.

Gay-Lussac's law (gā"lū-săks') Charles' law.

gaze (gāz) **1.** To look or stare intently in one direction. **2.** The act of looking or staring intently in one direction.

conjugate g. The paired movements of the eyes as they track moving objects.

disconjugate g. Unpaired movements of the eyes. SEE: *ophthalmoplegia*.

ETIOLOGY: Uncoupling of eye movements may occur in many diseases and conditions, including injuries to the oculomotor nerves; fractures of the orbit; strokes affecting the brainstem, frontal lobes, or cerebrum; multiple sclerosis; some nutritional deficiencies (e.g., Wernicke-Korsakoff's syndrome); Bell's palsy; and others.

GB *gallbladder*.

GBS *group B streptococci*.

GCS *Glasgow Coma Scale*.

Gd Symbol for the element gadolinium.

Ge Symbol for the element germanium.

Gee, Samuel J. (gē) British physician, 1839–1911.

G. disease Infantile nontropical sprue. Also called *Gee-Herter disease; Gee-Herter-Heubner disease*. SEE: *celiac sprue*.

Gee-Thaysen disease [Gee; Thorwald E. H. Thaysen, Danish physician, 1883–1936] Adult form of nontropical sprue.

gegenhalten (gā"gĕn-hălt'ĕn) [Ger.] In cerebrocortical disease, involuntary resistance to passive movement.

Geigel's reflex (gī′gĕlz) [Richard Geigel, Ger. physician, 1859–1930] A reflex produced in the female when the inner anterior aspect of the upper thigh is stroked. It involves contraction of muscular fibers adjacent to the superior portion of Poupart's ligaments. This reflex corresponds to the male cremasteric reflex.

Geiger counter (gī′gĕr) [Hans Geiger, Ger. physicist in England, 1882–1945] An instrument for detecting ionizing radiation.

gel (jĕl) [L. *gelare,* to congeal] A semisolid condition of a precipitated or coagulated colloid; jelly; a jelly-like colloid. It contains a large amount of water.

aluminum hydroxide g. A white viscous suspension containing aluminum hydroxide and hydrated aluminum oxide; an antacid esp. useful in treatment of peptic ulcer.

gelasmus (jĕ-lăs′mŭs) [Gr. *gelasma,* a laugh] **1.** Spasmodic laughter of the insane. **2.** Hysterical laughter.

gelate (jĕl′āt) To cause formation of a gel.

gelatin (jĕl′ă-tĭn) [L. *gelatina,* gelatin] **1.** A derived protein obtained by the hydrolysis of collagen present in the connective tissues of the skin, bones, and joints of animals. It is used as a food, in the preparation of pharmaceuticals, and as a medium for culture of bacteria. It is unusual as an animal protein in that it is not a good source of essential amino acids. **2.** The substance on an x-ray film in which the silver halide crystals are suspended in the radiographic emulsion.

nutrient g. A bacterial culture medium composed of broth and gelatin.

gelatinase (jĕl′ă-tĭn-ās) ABBR: MMP-2; MMP-9. Metalloproteinases that cleave gelatin, or nondenatured collagen. Two forms of gelatinase, A and B, have been identified. Gelatinase A (MMP-2) has a molecular weight of about 72,000, and gelatinase B (MMP-9) has a molecular weight of about 92,000. Both are involved in cancer angiogenesis and metastasis and are blocked by a variety of naturally occurring and synthetic inhibitors.

gelatiniferous (jĕl″ăt-ĭn-ĭf′ĕr-ŭs) [″ + *ferre,* to bear] Producing gelatin.

gelatinize (jĕl-ăt′ĭn-īz) [L. *gelatina,* gelatin] To convert into gelatin.

gelatinoid (jĕl-ăt′ĭn-oyd) [″ + Gr. *eidos,* form, shape] Resembling gelatin.

gelatinolytic (jĕl-ăt″ĭn-ō-lĭt′ĭk) [″ + Gr. *lysis,* dissolution] Dissolving or splitting gelatin.

gelatinous (jĕl-ăt′ĭn-ŭs) Containing or of the consistency of gelatin.

gelation (jĕl-ā′shŭn) The transformation of a colloid from a sol into a gel.

Gellé's test (zhĕl-āz′) [Marie Ernst Gellé, Fr. physician, 1834–1923] A test in which a tuning fork is connected with a rubber tube inserted in the ear. Pressure or suction in the tube is produced by an attached bulb. If the ear is normal, vibrations are felt.

gelling In arthritis, becoming stiff and fixed in any position in which movement does not occur for a prolonged period.

gelose (jĕ′lōs) [L. *gelare,* to congeal] **1.** The gelatinous component of agar $(C_6H_{10}O_5)_n$. **2.** A bacterial culture medium.

gelosis (jĕl-ō′sĭs) A hard lump that is so firm as to appear frozen. It occurs esp. in muscle tissue.

gelotherapy (jĕl″ō-thĕr′ă-pē) [Gr. *gelos,* laughter, + *therapeia,* treatment] A method used to treat certain forms of mental illness by inducing laughter.

gelotripsy (jĕl′ō-trĭp″sē) [L. *gelare,* to congeal, + Gr. *tripsis,* a rubbing] The massaging away of indurated swellings.

Gemella morbillorum A gram-positive coccus of the viridans group, formerly called *Streptococcus morbillorum;* it is a cause of septic arthritis, endocarditis, oral abscesses, and peritonitis.

gemellipara (jĕm″ĕl-lĭp′ă-ră) [L. *gemelli,* twins, + *parere,* to produce] One who has borne twins.

gemellology (gĕm″ĕl-ŏl′ō-jē) [L. *gemellus,* twin, + Gr. *logos,* study] The study of twins.

gemellus (jĕm-ĕl′ŭs) *pl.* **gemelli** [L., twin] Either of two muscles inserted in the obturator internus tendon.

gemfibrozil (jĕm-fī′brō-zĭl) A drug used to treat patients with hyperlipidemia; it is esp. effective when used for hypertriglyceridemia. Trade name is Lopid.

geminate (jĕm′ĭ-nāt) [L. *geminatus,* paired] In pairs.

gemination (jĕm-ĭ-nā′shŭn) **1.** The development of two teeth or two crowns within a single root. **2.** A doubling.

gemistocyte (jĕm-ĭs′tō-sīt) [Gr. *gemistos,* laden, full, + *kytos,* cell] In the central nervous system, a swollen astrocyte with an eccentric nucleus, seen adjacent to areas of edema or infarct.

gemma (jĕm′mă) [L., bud] **1.** A small budlike reproductive structure produced by lower forms of life. **2.** Any small budlike structure such as a taste bud or endbulb. SYN: *gemmule.*

gemmation (jĕm-mā′shŭn) [L. *gemmare,* to bud] Cell reproduction by budding. Budlike processes or daughter cells, each containing chromatin, separate from the mother cell from which the bud is projected.

gemmule (jĕm′ūl) [L. *gemmula,* little bud] **1.** A gemma. **2.** One of numerous minute processes present on the dendrites of a neuron.

gen-, -gen [Gr. *genes,* born or producing] Combining form used as a prefix or suffix meaning *that which produces or forms.*

gena (jē′nă) [L.] The side of the face; the cheek.

genal (jē′năl) Buccal.

gender [L. *genus,* kind] The sex of an individual (i.e., male or female).

gender identification Assignment of gender to a newborn. Genetic or chromosomal anomalies may create ambiguous genitalia, as may exposure of a female fetus to an androgenic hormone, or inhibition of androgen production or metabolism in a male fetus. In such cases, it is important to delay the final disposition until the chromosomal studies and endocrinological evaluation have been completed. These studies should be done as soon as possible. SEE: *gender identity.*

mistaken g.i. Assignment of incorrect gender to a newborn. This may lead to the individual's having a gender role opposite of the chromosomal sex.

gender identity The sense of maleness or femaleness experienced by a person, as opposed to sexual identity, which is biological.

gene (jēn) *pl.* **genes** [Gr. *gennan,* to produce] The basic unit of heredity, made of DNA, the code for a specific protein. Each gene occupies a certain location on a chromosome. Genes are self-replicating sequences of DNA nucleotides, subject to random structural changes called mutations. Hereditary traits are controlled by pairs of genes in the same position on a pair of chromosomes. These gene pairs, or alleles, may both be dominant or both be recessive in their expression of that trait. In either of those cases, the individual is homozygous for the trait controlled by that gene pair. If the gene pair consists of one dominant and one recessive gene, the individual is heterozygous for the trait controlled by that gene pair. SEE: illus. (Inheritance of Eye Color); *chromosome; DNA; RNA.*

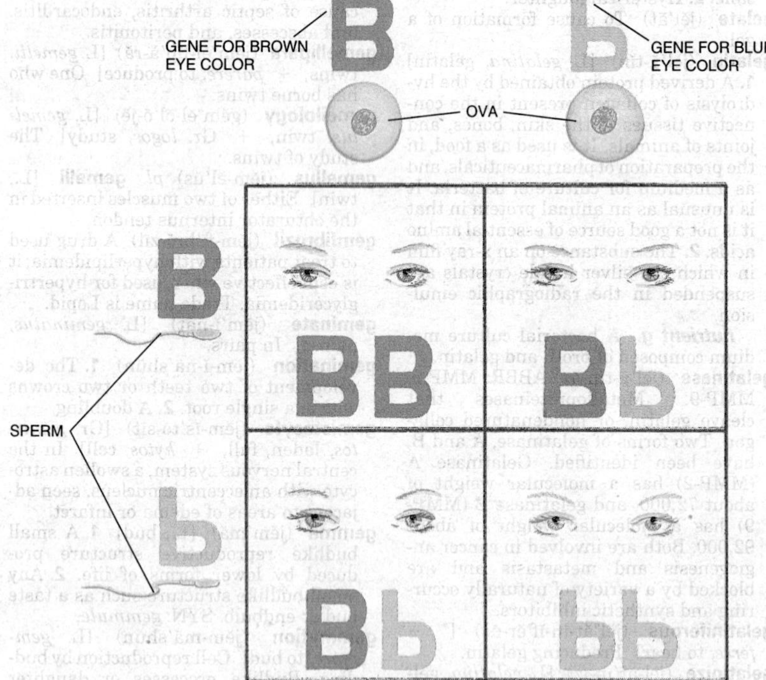

Key

BB	Genotype: homozygous brown (2 dominant genes) Phenotype: brown
Bb	Genotype: heterozygous (1 dominant and 1 recessive gene) Phenotype: brown (since brown is dominant)
bb	Genotype: homozygous blue (2 recessive genes) Phenotype: blue

INHERITANCE OF EYE COLOR

allelic g. Pairs of genes located at the same site on chromosome pairs.

complementary g. Nonallelic, independent genes, neither of which will express its effect without the presence of the other.

dominant g. A gene that expresses a trait without assistance from its allele.

histocompatibility g. One of the genes composing the HLA complex that determine the histocompatibility antigenic markers on all nucleated cells. These genes create the antigens by which the immune system recognizes "self" and determines the "nonself" nature of pathogens and other foreign antigens. These genetic antigens are also important in determining the success of surgical transplantation of organs and tissues. SEE: *histocompatibility locus antigen*.

holandric g. A gene located in the nonhomologous portion of the Y chromosome of males.

immune response g. One of the many genes that control the ability of lymphocytes to respond to specific antigens. SEE: *antigen; B cell; HLA complex; T cell*.

inhibiting g. A gene that prevents the expression of another gene.

lethal g. A gene that, when homozygous, brings about an effect that results in death, usually in utero.

modifying g. A gene that influences or alters the effect of another gene.

mutant g. An altered gene that permanently functions differently than it did before its alteration.

operator g. One of certain genes believed to have a role in controlling the actions of other genes. SEE: *operon*.

g. p53 A gene thought to be important in controlling the cell cycle, DNA repair and synthesis, and programmed cell death (apoptosis). Mutations of p53 have occurred in almost half of all types of cancer, arising from a variety of tissues. Mutant types may promote cancer. The normal, wild-type gene produces a protein that is important in tumor suppression.

pleiotropic g. A gene that has multiple effects.

presenilin g. Rare traits responsible for early-onset Alzheimer's disease.

RB g. Tumor suppressor gene encoding for the retinoblastoma (RB) protein, mutations of which are associated with various human tumors, including retinoblastoma, osteosarcoma, some leukemias, and some adenocarcinomas. SEE: *tumor suppressor g.; retinoblastoma*.

recessive g. A gene that, in the presence of its dominant allele, does not express itself. A recessive trait may be apparent in the phenotype only if both alleles are recessive.

regulator g. A gene that can control some specific activity of another gene.

sex-linked g. A gene contained within the X or Y chromosome. The X and Y chromosomes determine sex but also produce traits unrelated to sex.

structural g. A gene that determines the structure of polypeptide chains by controlling the sequence of amino acids.

tumor suppressor g. A gene that suppresses the growth of malignant cells. When this regulatory system is inadequate or fails, cancer may develop. SEE: *cancer*.

X-linked g. A gene on the X chromosome for which there is no corresponding gene on the Y chromosome. Such a gene is usually recessive, but in males without a corresponding gene to mask it, expression of the trait (e.g., red-green color blindness) occurs with the presence of only one recessive gene.

genealogy The study of the ancestry of an individual or group. Such investigations are particularly important in tracing the inheritance of genetically transmitted conditions or traits. One of the most important collections of genealogical information is in the archives of the Church of Latter Day Saints (i.e., the Mormon Church) in Salt Lake City, Utah.

gene amplification The duplication of regions of DNA to form multiple copies of a specific portion of the original region. This method of gene enhancement is important in increasing a tumor cell's resistance to cytotoxic drugs, and in allowing multiple drug resistance to a wide range of unrelated drugs after resistance to a single agent has developed.

gene expression The process by which genetic information from the DNA is carried to the RNA and translated into proteins.

gene knockout A mutation or deletion leading to loss of function of a gene. In the laboratory, specific genes can be inactivated or removed from mice or other animals to help study, for example, the effects of mutations on tumor growth and suppression. SEE: *gene; mutation; transgenic*.

gene mapping Determining the location of hereditary information carried on chromosomes. In humans, this requires determining the base pairs, or chemical code, of each of the estimated 60,000 to 100,000 human genes. The magnitude of this task can be appreciated by the fact that there are 3.5 billion base pairs in the human genome. Once a human gene is mapped, that information may be used to compare abnormal genes with normal ones; molecular biological techniques then may be used to search for methods of treating and preventing conditions resulting from genetic abnormality. SYN: *genome mapping*. SEE: *gene splicing*.

gene probe In molecular biology, the

technique of matching a short segment of DNA or RNA with the matching sequence of bases on a chromosome. Use of this method permits identification of the precise area on a chromosome responsible for the genetic abnormality being investigated. SEE: *gene splicing*.

genera Pl. of genus.

general adaptation syndrome ABBR: G.A.S. The syndrome described by Hans Selye (Austrian-Canadian endocrinologist, 1907–1982) as the total organism's nonspecific response to stress. The response occurs in the following three stages: (1) The alarm reaction stage, in which the body recognizes the stressor and the pituitary-adrenocortical system responds by producing the hormones essential to "flight or fight." In this stage, heart rate increases, blood glucose is elevated, pupils dilate, and digestion slows. (2) The resistance or adaptive stage, in which the body begins to repair the effect of the arousal. The acute stress symptoms diminish or disappear. If, however, the stress continues, adaptation fails in its attempts to maintain the defense. (3) The exhaustion stage, in which the body can no longer respond to the stress. As a consequence, one or several of a great variety of diseases such as emotional disturbances, cardiovascular and renal diseases, and certain types of asthma may develop. SEE: *stress*.

generalize [L. *generalis*] **1.** To become or render nonspecific. **2.** To become systemic, as a local disease.

general systems framework A conceptual model of nursing developed by Imogene King in which individuals and groups are categorized into three interacting systems—personal, interpersonal, and social—and in which the goal of nursing is to help people remain healthy so that they can function in their social roles. SEE: *Nursing Theory Appendix*.

generation (jĕn″ĕr-ā′shŭn) [L. *generare*, to beget] **1.** The act of reproducing offspring. **2.** A group of animals or plants the same distance removed from an ancestor, as the first filial (F_1) generation. SEE: *filial g.* **3.** The average period of time between the birth of parents and the birth of their children, which could be 16 to 20 years in some cultures and 20 to 25 years in others. Also the time would be different if only mothers were considered in computing this average, unless all marriages occurred between persons of the same age. **4.** The production of an electric current.

alternate g. A mode of reproduction in which sexual generation alternates with an asexual generation, characteristic of all plants above the division Thallophyta. It also occurs in some of the lower animals.

asexual g. Reproduction that occurs without the union of sexual elements or gametes, such as reproduction by fission or spore production.

filial g. In genetics, the first offspring of a specific mating or crossmating. This is abbreviated F_1. Descendants resulting from F_1 matings are known as the F_2, or second, filial generation.

parental g. In genetics, the generation in which a specific study is begun.

sexual g. Reproduction by the union of male and female cells.

generative (jĕn′ĕr-ă-tĭv) Concerned in reproduction of, or affecting, the species.

generator (gĕn′ĕr-ā″tor) That which produces something, esp. a device that produces heat, electricity, or impulses.

aerosol g. A device that produces minute particles from liquid materials such as medicines in solution. These particles may be used in inhalation therapy.

electric g. A device that changes mechanical energy into electrical energy.

flow g. A pneumatic engine that powers life-support equipment and uses a gauge of 5 to 50 lb/sq in. to supply gas to a ventilator circuit, allowing for a constant flow pattern.

pressure g. A pneumatic engine that powers a life-support ventilator and incorporates a proportional meter, a motor-driven piston, or a blower. Pressure generators can adjust flow according to the patient's condition.

pulse g. A device that produces intermittent electrical discharges (e.g., in a cardiac pacemaker).

generic (jĕn-ĕr′ĭk) [L. *genus*, kind] **1.** General. **2.** Pert. to a genus. **3.** Distinctive.

generic drugs Nonproprietary drugs (i.e., not protected by a trademark). In the U.S., generic drugs are required to meet the same bioequivalency test as the original brand name drugs. Manufacturers of brand name drugs produce the majority of generic drugs and allow them to be sold without the original brand name. Generic and brand name drugs may experience manufacturing defects. Nearly half of all proprietary drugs available in the U.S. are also sold less expensively as generic drugs. SYN: *nonproprietary name*.

genesis (jĕn′ĕ-sĭs) **1.** The act of reproducing; generation. **2.** The origin of anything.

gene splicing The insertion of a portion of a gene from one chromosome or one species into a gene from another. This allows the altered gene to function in a new context. Gene splicing can be used to alter the expression of gene products or to produce new proteins in cells. SEE: *recombinant DNA*.

gene testing The study of genetic material, as by amniocentesis, to attempt to diagnose and predict conditions caused by abnormalities of genes or chromosomes. This can be done on both plants and animals. These studies have allowed inherited diseases to be predicted prior to their clinical manifestations and, in some cases, prenatally.

gene therapy The treatment of genetic illnesses, metabolic diseases, cancers, and some infections by introducing nucleic acid sequences into the chromosomes of diseased cells. The goal of gene therapy is to modify the genetic instructions of the diseased cells, so that the cells will express a protein or enzyme that modifies or treats the disease.

somatic g.t. An experimental method of cloning genes and reintroducing them into cells for the purpose of correcting inherited disease. As this form of therapy develops so do ethical questions concerning its use: what diseases should be treated, and whether an individual could be treated to enhance his or her normal condition (e.g., to become a stronger or faster athlete).

genetic (jĕn-ĕt′ĭk) Pert. to reproduction.

genetic burden The number of diseases and deaths that occur as a result of inherited traits.

genetic counseling The application of knowledge about human genetics to prospective parents concerned about the possibility of hereditary diseases.

genetic engineering The synthesis, alteration, replacement, or repair of genetic material by artificial means.

geneticist (jĕn-ĕt′ĭ-sĭst) [Gr. *gennan,* to produce] One who specializes in genetics.

genetics The study of heredity and its variation.

biochemical g. The science of the biochemistry of genes and chemical influences on genes.

clinical g. The study and use of genetics in health and disease.

molecular g. The study of genetics at the molecular level, in contrast to the study of entire genes or chromosomes. SEE: *gene splicing*.

genetotrophic (jĕ-nĕt″ō-trōf′ĭk) Concerning genetics and nutrition.

gene transfer The transfer of a gene from one animal to another to repair an inherited defect in the recipient.

Geneva Convention Regulations concerning the status of those wounded in military action on land, established in 1864 by military powers meeting in Geneva, Switzerland. The sick and wounded and all those involved in their care, including physicians, nurses, corpsmen, ambulance drivers, and chaplains, were declared to be neutral and, therefore, would not be the target of military action. These provisions were expanded in 1868 to include naval military action. Much evidence indicates that warring nations have not always abided by the provisions of the Convention.

genial (jē′nē-ăl) [Gr. *geneion,* chin] Pert. to the chin.

genic (jĕn′ĭk) [Gr. *gennan,* to produce] Relating to or caused by genes.

-genic Suffix meaning *generation* or *production*.

genicular (jĕ-nĭk′ū-lăr) Concerning the knee.

geniculate (jĕ-nĭk′ū-lāt) [L. *geniculare,* to bend the knee] **1.** Bent, like a knee. **2.** Pert. to the ganglion or geniculum of the facial nerve.

geniculate otalgia Pain transmitted from the facial nerve to the ear.

geniculocalcarine tract Optic radiation.

geniculum (jĕn-ĭk′ū-lŭm) [L. *geniculum,* little knee] A structure resembling a knot or a knee, indicating an abrupt bend or angle in a small structure.

genion (jē′nē-ŏn) [Gr. *geneion,* chin] The apex of the mental spine of the mandible.

genioplasty (jē′nē-ō-plăs″tē) [″ + *plassein,* to form] Plastic surgery of the chin or cheek.

genistein A soy isoflavone that has been found to inhibit the activity of enzymes involved in the control of cell proliferation.

genital (jĕn′ĭ-tăl) [L. *genitalis,* belonging to birth] Pert. to the genitals.

genital cutting Female circumcision.

genitalia, genitals (jĕn-ĭ-tāl′ē-ă, jĕn′ĭ-tăls) Organs of generation; reproductive organs.

ambiguous g. External reproductive organs that are not easily identified as male or female.

female g. Reproductive organs of the female sex. The external genitalia collectively are termed the vulva or pudendum and include the mons veneris, labia majora, labia minora, clitoris, fourchet, fossa navicularis, vestibule, vestibular bulb, Skene's glands, glands of Bartholin, hymen and vaginal introitus, and perineum. The internal genitalia are the two ovaries, two fallopian tubes, uterus, and vagina. SEE: illus.

male g. Reproductive organs of the male sex, including two bulbourethral (Cowper's) glands, two ejaculatory ducts, two glands producing spermatozoa (the testes or gonads), the penis with urethra, two seminal ducts (vasa deferentes or ducti deferentes), two seminal vesicles, two spermatic cords, the scrotum, and the prostate gland. SEE: illus.; *penis; prostate*.

genito- [L. *genitivus,* of birth, of generation] Combining form meaning *reproduction*.

genitocrural (jĕn″ĭ-tō-kroo′răl) Concerning the genitalia and leg. SYN: *genitofemoral*.

genitofemoral (jĕn″ĭ-tō-fĕm′or-ăl) Genitocrural.

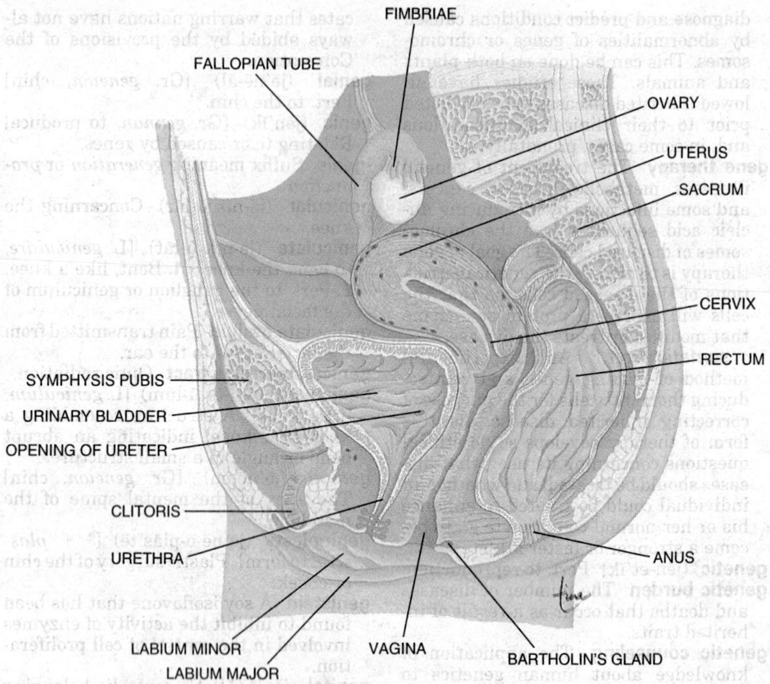

FIMBRIAE
FALLOPIAN TUBE
OVARY
UTERUS
SACRUM
CERVIX
RECTUM
SYMPHYSIS PUBIS
URINARY BLADDER
OPENING OF URETER
CLITORIS
URETHRA
ANUS
LABIUM MINOR
VAGINA
BARTHOLIN'S GLAND
LABIUM MAJOR

FEMALE GENITAL ORGANS
Midsagittal section

SACRUM
OPENING OF URETER
SYMPHYSIS PUBIS
RECTUM
DUCTUS DEFERENS
SEMINAL VESICLE
URINARY BLADDER
EJACULATORY DUCT
CORPUS CAVERNOSUM
PROSTATE GLAND
CORPUS SPONGIOSUM
CAVERNOUS URETHRA
BULBOURETHRAL GLAND
ANUS
GLANS PENIS
PREPUCE
EPIDIDYMIS
MEMBRANOUS URETHRA
SCROTUM
TESTIS

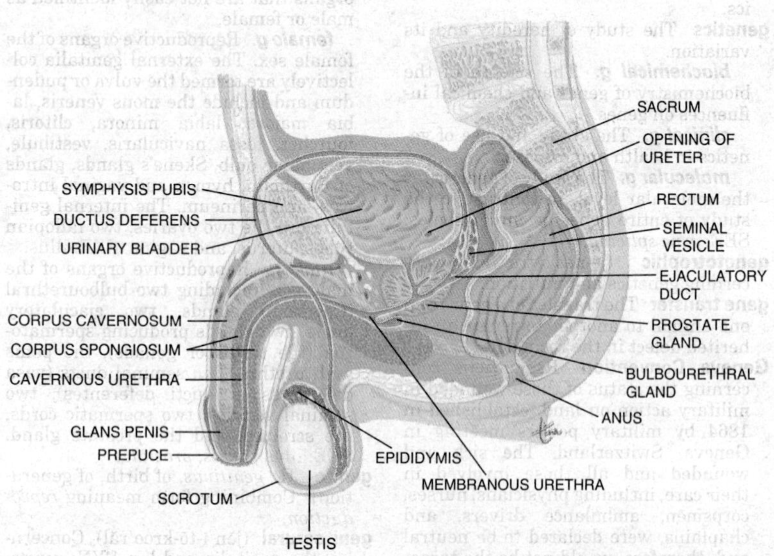

MALE GENITAL ORGANS
Midsagittal section

genitoplasty (jĕn′ĭ-tō-plăs″tē) [L. *genitalis*, genital, + Gr. *plassein*, to form] Reparative surgery on the genital organs.

feminizing g. Surgical reduction in the size of the clitoris, along with construction of a vagina and labia, used to treat female children born with ambiguous genitalia.

genitourinary (jĕn″ĭ-tō-ūr′ĭ-nār-ē) [″ + Gr. *ouron*, urine] Pert. to the genitals and urinary organs.

genius (jēn′yŭs) **1.** The distinctive or inherent character of a disease. **2.** An individual with exceptional physical, mental, or creative power. SEE: *idiot-savant*.

genocide (jĕn′ō-sīd″) [Gr. *genos*, race, + L. *caedere*, to kill] The willful and planned murder of a particular social or ethnic group.

genodermatosis (jĕn″ō-dĕr-mă-tō′sĭs) [Gr. *gennan*, to produce, + *derma*, skin, + *osis*, condition] Any of a group of serious hereditary skin diseases such as hereditary angioedema, hereditary coproporphyria, hereditary telangectasia, tuberous sclerosis, Recklinghausen's disease, and Peutz-Jeghers syndrome.

genogram A family map of three or more generations that records relationships, deaths, occupations, and health and illness history.

genome (jē′nōm) The complete set of chromosomes, and thus the entire genetic information present in a cell.

genome mapping Gene mapping.

genomic Concerning the genome.

genotoxic (jĕn″ō-tŏks′ĭk) [″ + *toxikon*, poison] Toxic to the genetic material in cells.

genotoxic damage Injury to the chromosomes of the cells. This may be determined by noting the number of micronuclei in the target tissues. When a cell with damaged genetic material divides, fragments of chromosomes and micronuclei remain in the cytoplasm.

genotype (jĕn′ō-tīp) [″ + *typos*, type] **1.** The total of the hereditary information present in an organism. **2.** The pair of genes present for a particular characteristic or protein. **3.** A type species of a genus. SEE: *phenotype*.

APOE g. A genetic variant with some use in the diagnosis of Alzheimer's disease and other dementias.

CCR5 delta 32 g. A mutation that confers a survival advantage and substantial resistance to the human immunodeficiency virus (HIV). Homozygosity for this allele protects adults from HIV-1 after blood and body fluid exposure. Heterozygosity may confer some protection against disease progression.

gentamicin (jĕn″tă-mī′sĭn) An antibiotic derived from the fungi of the genus *Micromonospora*.

g. sulfate An aminoglycoside antibiotic obtained from the actinomycete *Micromonospora purpurea*. This agent is active against many gram-negative bacilli and may be used with a primary antibiotic to help treat some gram-positive infections.

gentian (jĕn′shŭn) Dried rhizome and roots of the plant *Gentiana lutea*.

gentianophil(e) (jĕn′shăn-ō-fĭl, -fīl) A cell or cell part that stains readily with gentian violet. **gentianophilic** (-fĭl′ĭk), *adj*.

gentianophobic (jĕn″shăn-ō-fō′bĭk) Not staining well with gentian violet.

genu (jē′nū) *pl.* **genua** [L.] **1.** The knee. **2.** Any structure of angular form resembling a bent knee.

g. recurvatum Hyperextension at the knee joint.

g. valgum Knock-knee.

g. varum Bowleg.

genucubital (jĕn″ū-kū′bĭ-tăl) [″ + *cubitus*, elbow] Pert. to the elbows and knees.

genupectoral (jĕn″ū-pĕk′tor-ăl) [″ + *pectus*, breast] Pert. to the chest and knees.

genus (jē′nŭs) *pl.* **genera** [L. *genus*, kind] In taxonomy, the classification between the family and the species.

genyplasty (jĕn′ĭ-plăs″tē) [Gr. *genys*, jaw, + *plassein*, to form] Genioplasty.

geobiology (jē″ō-bī-ŏl′ō-jē) [Gr. *geo*, earth, + *bios*, life, + *logos*, word, reason] The study of terrestrial life.

geode (jē′ōd) [Gr. *geodes*, earthlike] A subchondral (bony) cyst occasionally found in patients with rheumatological illnesses.

geographic distribution of disease The relationship between the prevalence of a disease and specific geographical-environmental conditions. For example, goiter occurs in inland iodine-deficient areas of the U.S., and pulmonary hypertension occurs in those who reside at high altitude. Certain infectious diseases, such as leprosy, leishmaniasis, and Chagas' disease, are endemic in specific tropical or subtropical areas.

geographic ulceration of the cornea An ulcer of the cornea with an irregular and lobulated border.

geomedicine (jē″ō-mĕd′ĭ-sĭn) [Gr. *geo*, earth, + L. *medicina*, medicine] The study of the influence of geography and climate on health. SYN: *nosochthonography*.

geophagia, geophagism, geophagy (jē-ō-fā′jē-ă, -ŏf′ă-jĭzm, -ŏf′ă-jē) [″ + *phagein*, to eat] A condition in which the patient eats inedible substances such as chalk, clay, or earth. SYN: *geotragia*. SEE: *pica*.

geotaxis (jē″ō-tăk′sĭs) [″ + *taxis*, arrangement] Geotropism.

geotragia (jē″ō-trā′jē-ă) [″ + *trogein*, to chew] Geophagia.

geotrichosis (jē″ō-trī-kō′sĭs) Infection by the fungus *Geotrichum,* which usually attacks the lungs, causing symptoms resembling those of chronic bronchitis or tuberculosis. This infection may also affect the mouth or intestine.

Geotrichum (jē-ŏt′rĭ-kŭm) A genus of fungi belonging to the family Eremascaceae; the causative agent of geotrichosis.

geotropism (jē″ŏt′rō-pĭzm) [″ + *tropos,* a turning] The influence of gravity on living organisms. SYN: *geotaxis.*

gephyrophobia (jē-fī″rō-fō′bē-ă) [Gr. *gephyra,* bridge, + *phobos,* fear] An aversion to bodies of water, to crossing on bridges over water, or to traveling on boats.

GERD *gastroesophageal reflux disease.*

Gerdy's fibers (zhĕr′dēz) [Pierre N. Gerdy, Fr. physician, 1797–1856] The superficial transverse ligament of the palm.

Gerdy's tubercle The attachment site for the iliotibial band, located on the anterolateral portion of the proximal tibia, just lateral to the superior tibial tuberosity.

geriatric day hospital A form of adult day care providing rehabilitative, medical, and personal care services as well as social and recreational services for the elderly. SEE: *care, respite.*

geriatrician A physician who specializes in the care of elderly people.

geriatrics (jĕr″ē-ăt′rĭks) [Gr. *geras,* old age, + *iatrike,* medical treatment] The branch of health care concerned with the care of the aged, including physiological, pathological, psychological, economic, and sociological problems. As life expectancy in society as a whole increases, geriatrics takes on ever greater importance in health care. Also called *geriatric medicine.* SEE: *gerontology.*

dental g. The special area of dentistry dealing with the problems of aging as it relates to dental illness and treatment. SYN: *geriatric dentistry.*

Gerlach's valve (gĕr′lăks) [Joseph von Gerlach, Ger. anatomist, 1820–1896] An inconstant valve present at the opening of the vermiform appendix into the cecum.

germ [L. *germen,* sprout, fetus] **1.** A microorganism, esp. one that causes disease. **2.** The first rudiment of a developing organ or part.

dental g. The embryonic structure that gives rise to the tooth. It consists of the enamel organ, dental papilla, and dental sac. SYN: *tooth bud.* SEE: *enamel organ.*

hair g. The rudimentary structure from which a hair develops. It consists of an ingrowth of epidermal cells called *hair peg,* which pushes into the corium.

wheat g. The vitamin-rich embryo of the wheat seed or kernel. It contains vitamin E, thiamine, riboflavin, and other micronutrients.

germanium (jĕr-mā′nē-ŭm) [L. *Germania,* Germany] SYMB: Ge. A grayish-white metallic element of the silicon group. Atomic weight is 72.59, atomic number is 32, and specific gravity is 5.323 (25°C).

germ epithelium The ridge of epithelium in the embryo which covers the reproductive organs.

germicidal (jĕrm″ĭ-sī′dăl) [L. *germen,* sprout, + *caedere,* to kill] **1.** Destructive to germs. **2.** Pert. to an agent destructive to germs.

germicide (jĕr′mĭ-sīd) A substance that destroys microorganisms. Bacteria may be killed by boiling for 30 min, by dry heat at 160° to 170°C for 1 hr, and by steam at 121°C for 20 min. SEE: *antiseptic; disinfectant.*

germinal [L. *germen,* sprout] Pert. to a germ or reproductive cells (egg or sperm) or to germination.

germinal vesicle Purkinje vesicle.

germination [L. *germinare,* to sprout] **1.** The development of an impregnated ovum into an embryo. **2.** The sprouting of the spore or seed of a plant.

germinoma (jĕr″mĭ-nō′mă) A neoplasm usually arising from germ cells in the testis, ovary, or mediastinum.

germ layers Three primary cell layers in the embryo from which the organs and tissues develop. They are the ectoderm, mesoderm, and endoderm.

germ plasm The reproductive tissues.

gero- [Gr. *geras,* old age] Combining form meaning *old age.*

Gerontological Society of America ABBR: GSA. An organization established in 1945 for the main purpose of promoting scientific study of aging. Researchers, practitioners, and educators are members. The society publishes *The Journal of Gerontology* and *The Gerontologist.* The organization's website is www.geron.org/.

gerontology (jĕ-rŏn-tŏl′ō-jē) [″ + *logos,* word, reason] The scientific study of the effects of aging and of age-related diseases on humans. SEE: *geriatrics.*

gerontophilia (jĕr″ŏn-tō-fĭl′ē-ă) [″ + *philein,* to love] **1.** A fondness or love for old people. **2.** Sexual inclination toward or sexual mistreatment of the elderly.

gerontophobia A fear of aging.

gerontotherapeutics (jĕr-ŏn″tō-thĕr″ă-pū′tĭks) [″ + *therapeia,* treatment] **1.** Treatments (such as antioxidants) designed to slow the aging process. **2.** In traditional Chinese and alternative medicine, walking and bathing in the forest ("shinrin-yoku") for health and the prevention of the effects of aging.

gerontoxon (jĕ-rŏn-tŏks′ŏn) [″ + *toxon,* bow] Arcus senilis.

geropsychiatry A subspecialty of psychiatry dealing with mental illness in the elderly.

Gerota's capsule, Gerota's fascia (gā-rō'tăz) [Dimitru Gerota, Rumanian anatomist, 1867–1939] The perirenal fascia.

Gerstmann syndrome [Josef Gerstmann, Austrian neurologist, 1887–1969] A neurological disorder resulting from a lesion in the left (or dominant) parietal area. Patients are unable to point or name different fingers, have confusion of the right and left sides of the body, and are unable to calculate or write. In addition, they may have word blindness and homonymous hemianopia.

gestagen (jĕs'tă-jĕn) Something that produces progestational effects. This general term is usually applied to natural or synthetic steroid hormones used to alter reproductive physiology.

gestalt (gĕs-tawlt') [Ger. *Gestalt,* form] The concept that the configuration of objects and experience is present as a whole formation that cannot be analyzed by breaking it into its component parts.

g. therapy A form of therapy that emphasizes the treatment of the person as a whole, with a focus on the reality of the present time and place and with an emphasis on personal growth and enhanced self-awareness.

gestation (jĕs-tā'shŭn) [L. *gestare,* to bear] In mammals, the length of time from conception to birth. The average gestation time is a species-specific trait. In humans, the average length, as calculated from the first day of the last normal menstrual period, is 280 days, with a normal range of 259 days (37 weeks) to 287 days (41 weeks). Infants born prior to the 37th week are considered premature and those born after the 41st week, postmature. SEE: *gestational assessment; pregnancy.*

abdominal g. Ectopic pregnancy in which the embryo develops in the peritoneal cavity.

cornual g. Pregnancy in an ill-developed cornu of a bicornuate uterus.

ectopic g. Pregnancy in which the fetus develops outside the uterus.

interstitial g. Tubal pregnancy in which the embryo is developed in a portion of the fallopian tube that traverses the wall of the uterus.

multiple g. The presence of two or more embryos in the uterus. The incidence of this in the U.S. is about 1.5% of all births. Up to 40% of twin gestations are undiagnosed before labor and delivery. When twins are diagnosed by ultrasound early in the first trimester, in about half of these cases one twin will silently abort, and this may or may not be accompanied by bleeding. This phenomenon has been termed the vanishing twin. The incidence of birth defects in each fetus of a twin pregnancy is twice that in singular pregnancies. Triplet, quadruplet, and higher gestation pregnancies are a side effect of commonly used fertility drugs.

prolonged g. Pregnancy that continues past 41 weeks.

secondary g. Pregnancy in which the embryo becomes dislodged from the original seat of implantation and continues to develop in a new situation.

secondary abdominal g. Extrauterine pregnancy in which the embryo, originally situated in the oviduct or elsewhere, has developed in the abdominal cavity.

tubal g. Ectopic pregnancy in which the embryo grows in the fallopian tube.

tuboabdominal g. Extrauterine pregnancy in which the embryonic sac is formed partly in the abdominal extremity of the oviduct and partly in the abdominal cavity.

tubo-ovarian g. Extrauterine pregnancy in which the embryonic sac is partly in the ovary and partly in the abdominal end of the fallopian tube.

uterotubal g. Pregnancy in which the ovum develops partially in the uterine end of the fallopian tube and partially within the cavity of the uterus.

gestational assessment Determination of the prenatal age of the fetus. This information is essential for obstetrical care because it influences the decision to intervene and at what time. The age has been estimated by evaluating the menstrual history, time of initial detection of fetal heart tones, and date the level of the fundus reaches the umbilicus. These methods are not precise, esp. if the date of the last menstrual period is either vaguely remembered or unknown.

Use of ultrasound to measure the crown-rump length in the first trimester, the biparietal diameter in the second trimester, and other measurements permits a more nearly precise estimate of gestational age. Even so, these techniques, because of biological variation of fetal size and early intrauterine growth failure, may not be consistently accurate. SEE: *Dubowitz tool.*

gestation sac The amnion and its contents.

gestation time The duration of a normal pregnancy for a particular species. SEE: *pregnancy* for table.

gestosis (jĕs-tō'sĭs) [L. *gestare,* to bear, + Gr. *osis,* condition] Any disorder of pregnancy.

gesture **1.** A body movement that helps to express or conceal thoughts or emphasize speech. SEE: *body language.* **2.** An act, written or spoken, to indicate a feeling.

geumaphobia (gū″mă-fō′bē-ă) [Gr. *geuma,* taste, + *phobos,* fear] An abnormal dislike or fear of tastes.

GFR *glomerular filtration rate.*

GH *growth hormone.*

Ghon's complex (gănz) [Anton Ghon, Czech. pathologist, 1866–1936] A small, sharply defined shadow in radiographs of the lung seen in certain cases of pulmonary tuberculosis. It represents the necrotic, calcified remains of the primary lesion of tuberculosis. The mycobacteria within the lesion may remain viable and be the source of endogenous and generalized reinfection with tuberculosis. Also called *Ghon's primary lesion.*

Ghon's tubercle Ghon's complex.

GH-RH *growth hormone–releasing hormone.*

GI *gastrointestinal.*

Giannuzzi's cells (jăn-noot′sēz) [Guiseppe Giannuzzi, It. anatomist, 1839–1876] Crescent-shaped groups of serous cells found in the mixed salivary glands. They appear as darkly staining cells forming a caplike structure on the alveoli.

giant [Gr. *gigas,* giant] An individual or structure much larger than normal.

giant cell tumor 1. A malignant or benign bone tumor that probably arises from connective tissue of the bone marrow. Histologically, it contains a vascular reticulum of stromal cells and multinucleated giant cells. **2.** A yellow giant cell tumor of a tendon sheath. **3.** Epulis. **4.** Chondroblastoma.

giantism (jī′ăn-tĭzm) Gigantism.

Giardia (jē-ăr′dē-ă) [Alfred Giard, Fr. biologist, 1846–1908] A genus of protozoa possessing flagella. They inhabit the small intestine of humans and other animals, are pear shaped, and have two nuclei and four pairs of flagella. They attach themselves to the cells of the intestinal mucosa, from which they absorb nourishment. Cysts can survive in water for up to 3 months. The concentration of chlorine routinely used in treating domestic water supplies does not kill *Giardia* cysts, but boiling water inactivates them.

G. lamblia A species of *Giardia* found in humans, transmitted by ingestion of cysts in fecally contaminated water or food. *G. lamblia* organisms are found worldwide. The most common symptoms of *G. lamblia* infection are diarrhea, fever, cramps, anorexia, nausea, weakness, weight loss, abdominal distention, flatulence, greasy stools, belching, and vomiting. Onset of symptoms begins about 2 weeks after exposure; the disease may persist for up to 2 to 3 months.

There is no effective chemoprophylaxis for this disease. Metronidazole or albendazole are preferred treatments. SEE: *water, emergency preparation of safe drinking.*

DIAGNOSIS: Cysts or trophozoites can be identified in feces. Three consecutive negative tests are required before the feces are considered to be negative. Duodenal contents also can be examined by aspiration or string test, in which an ordinary string is swallowed and allowed to remain in the duodenum long enough for the protozoa to attach. On removal, it is examined for the presence of cysts or trophozoites. A stool antigen assay test detects *Giardia.* This involves either immunofluorescence or enzyme-linked immunosorbent assay. SEE: illus.

giardiasis (jī″ăr-dī′ă-sĭs) Infection with the flagellate protozoan *Giardia lamblia.*

giardins (gē-ăr′dĭnz) Specialized proteins found in the sucker disks of *Giardia lamblia* and used by that organism to support its binding to the lining of the small intestine.

Gibbon's hydrocele (gĭb′ŏns) [Quinton V. Gibbon, U.S. surgeon, 1813–1894] A hydrocele and large hernia combined.

gibbosity (gĭ-bŏs′ĭ-tē) [LL. *gebbosus,* humped] **1.** The condition of having a humpback. **2.** A hump or gibbus, as the deformity of Pott's disease.

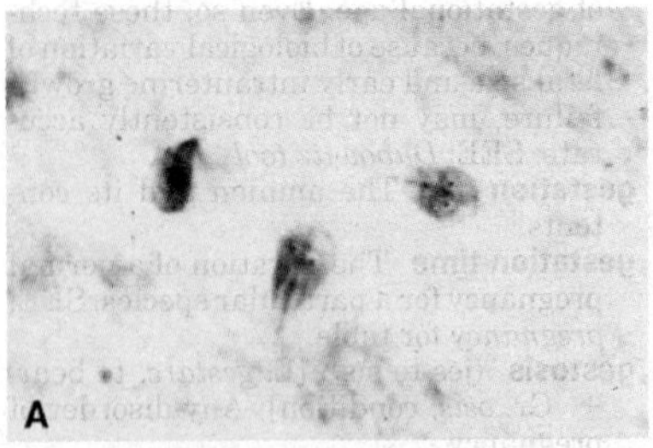

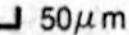

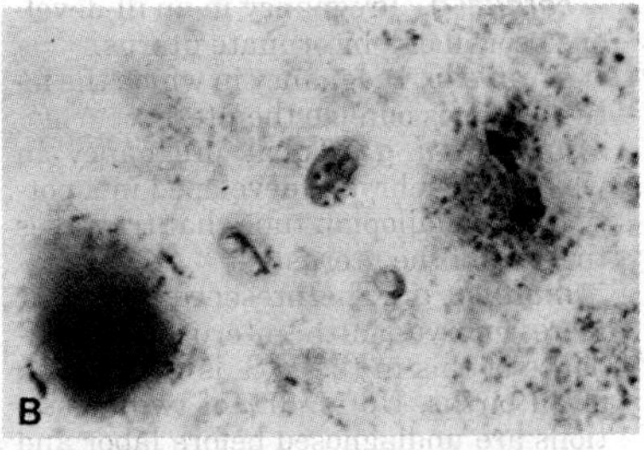

GIARDIA LAMBLIA

(A) trophozoites (orig. mag. ×1000), (B) cysts (orig. mag. ×1000)

gibbous (gĭb′bŭs) Humped; protuberant or hunchbacked.

gibbus (gĭb′ŭs) [L. *gibbosus*] Hump; protuberance. SEE: *protuberance*.

Gibney's boot, Gibney's bandage (gĭb′nēz) [Virgil P. Gibney, U.S. surgeon, 1847–1927] A basket-weave bandage made of adhesive tape, used to treat ankle sprain or to support the ankle.

Gibraltar fever Brucellosis.

Gibson's murmur (gĭb′sŭnz) [George A. Gibson, Scot. physician, 1854–1913] A continuous cardiac murmur that increases in systole, occurring in patients with patent ductus arteriosus. It is heard best at the left of the sternum in the first and second intercostal spaces.

giddiness [AS. *gydig*, insane] Dizziness.

Giemsa's stain (gēm′zăs) [Gustav Giemsa, Ger. chemist, 1867–1948] A stain for blood smears, used for differential leukocyte counts and to detect parasitic microorganisms.

Gifford's reflex (gĭf′fords) [Harold Gifford, U.S. ophthalmologist, 1858–1929] Pupillary contraction resulting from endeavoring forcibly to close eyelids that are held apart.

GIFT *gamete intrafallopian transfer*.

giga- (jĭg′ă, jī′gă) In SI units, a prefix indicating that the entity following is to be multiplied by 10^9.

gigantism (jī′găn-tĭzm) [Gr. *gigas*, giant, + *-ismos*, state of] The excessive development of the body or a body part. SYN: *giantism*.

acromegalic g. Gigantism characterized by overgrowth of the bones of the hands, feet, and face, owing to excessive production of pituitary growth hormone after full skeletal growth has been attained.

eunuchoid g. Gigantism accompanied by eunuchoid features and sexual insufficiency.

normal g. Gigantism in which the bodily proportions and sexual development are normal, usually the result of hypersecretion of growth hormone.

gigantoblast (jī-găn′tō-blăst) [″ + *blastos*, germ] A very large nucleated red blood cell.

gigantocyte (jī-găn′tō-sīt) [″ + *kytos*, cell] **1.** A giant cell. **2.** A very large erythrocyte.

Gigli's saw (jēl′yēz) [Leonardo Gigli, It. gynecologist, 1863–1908] A flexible wire saw with specialized teeth used for cutting bony structures. It is operated manually by pulling its handles back and forth. It was first used to section the symphysis pubis as a way of making difficult deliveries easier.

Gilbert's syndrome (zhēl-bārz′) [Nicolas A. Gilbert, Fr. physician, 1858–1927] A benign, hereditary form of jaundice secondary to glucuronyl-transferase deficiency, resulting in elevated unconjugated bilirubin. There are no hemolytic changes. No treatment is necessary. The presence of jaundice may not be noticed by the patient until it is detected by a laboratory test for bilirubin. Food deprivation increases serum bilirubin in these patients.

Gilchrist's disease (gĭl′krĭsts) [Thomas Caspar Gilchrist, U.S. dermatologist, 1862–1927] Blastomycosis.

Gilles de la Tourette's syndrome SEE: *Tourette's syndrome*.

Gimbernat's ligament (hĭm-bĕr-năts′) [Antonio de Gimbernat, Sp. surgeon, 1734–1790] The pectineal portion of the inguinal ligament. Its lateral free edge forms the medial portion of the femoral ring. SYN: *lacunar ligament*.

ginger A pungent, spicy material obtained from the root (rhizome) of the plant *Zingiber officinale* and used to flavor medicines and foods. It may prevent nausea, vomiting, and motion sickness in patients affected by these conditions.

gingiv- SEE: *gingivo-*.

gingiva (jĭn-jī′vă, jĭn′jĭ-vă) [L.] The gums; the tissue that surrounds the necks of the teeth and covers the alveolar processes of the maxilla and mandible. The gingiva can be divided into three regions: the gingival margin, free gingiva, and attached gingiva. Normal gingival tissue is coral pink, firm, and resilient. The attached gingiva is stippled, the gingival margin and free gingiva are not.

alveolar g. The part of the gums that covers the alveolar processes of the jawbones.

attached g. Gingiva lying between the free gingival groove and the mucogingival line. It is firmly attached by lamina propria to underlying periosteum, bone, and tooth.

free g. The unattached portion of the gingiva. It forms part of the wall of the fissure surrounding the anatomical crown of a tooth.

labial g. Gingiva covering the labial surfaces of the teeth.

lingual g. Gingiva covering the lingual surfaces of the teeth.

marginal g. The crest of the free gingiva surrounding the tooth like a collar. It is about 1 mm wide and forms the soft tissue portion of the gingival sulcus.

gingival (jĭn′jĭ-văl) [L. *gingiva*, gum] Rel. to the gums.

gingivalgia (jĭn″jĭ-văl′jē-ă) [″ + Gr. *algos*, pain] Pain in the gums.

gingivally (jĭn′jĭ-văl″lē) Toward the gums.

gingivectomy (jĭn″jĭ-vĕk′tō-mē) [″ + Gr. *ektome*, excision] Excision of diseased gingival tissue in surgical treatment of periodontal disease.

gingivitis (jĭn-jĭ-vī′tĭs) [″ + Gr. *itis*, inflammation] Inflammation of the gums characterized by redness, swelling, and tendency to bleed. SYN: *ulitis*.

ETIOLOGY: Gingivitis may be local due to improper dental hygiene, poorly fitting dentures or appliances, or poor occlusion. It may accompany generalized stomatitis associated with mouth and upper respiratory infections. It may also occur in deficiency diseases such as scurvy, blood dyscrasias, or metallic poisoning.

g. gravidum Gingivitis of pregnancy. The generalized hypertrophy of the gums characteristic of this disease may progress to tumor formation.

ETIOLOGY: This type of gingivitis is caused by local irritants.

SYMPTOMS: The clinical picture varies considerably. The gingival tissue tends to be bright red or magenta, soft, and friable, with a smooth, shiny surface. Bleeding occurs spontaneously or with little provocation. Lesions are typically generalized and more prominent at interproximal areas.

PATIENT CARE: A dental professional must remove the local irritants. Patients should be referred for a dental prophylaxis.

hyperplastic g. Gum overgrowth associated with an increase in the number of the gingival component cells. This may be idiopathic, or it may be caused by local irritants or by long-term use of phenytoin, nifedipine, or cyclosporine.

SYMPTOMS: The primary lesion starts as a painless enlargement of the gingiva. If left to progress, the lesion may develop into a massive tissue mass that covers the crowns of the teeth.

TREATMENT: Treatment includes avoiding causative factors and surgical removal of enlarged tissue.

PATIENT CARE: The presence of the enlarged gingiva makes plaque removal difficult. Remaining plaque will result in a secondary inflammatory process. Patients should schedule regular dental appointments for dental prophylaxis and oral hygiene instruction.

interstitial g. Inflammation of the gums and alveolar processes that precedes pyorrhea.

necrotizing ulcerative g. ABBR: NUG. A relatively rare and severe form of periodontal disease, marked by destruction of the gingiva and ulcerations of the epithelium of the mouth. It is associated with infection with multiple oral microbes. SYN: *trench mouth; Vincent's angina.*

TREATMENT: This condition is treated by débriding the teeth, and rinsing the mouth with saline or a dilute hydrogen peroxide solution. Chlorhexidine (2%) rinses are also effective. Chemical or physical trauma to the mucosa must be avoided. Fluids should be forced and proper nutrition and dental hygiene provided. Antibiotic therapy with penicillin or metronidazole is effective.

phagedenic g. A rapidly spreading ulceration of the gums accompanied by extensive ulceration and sloughing of tissue.

gingivo-, gingiv- [L. *gingiva,* gum (of the mouth)] Combining form meaning *gums* (of the mouth).

gingivoglossitis (jĭn″jĭ-vō-glŏs-sī′tĭs) [″ + Gr. *glossa,* tongue, + *itis,* inflammation] Inflammation of the gums and tongue. SYN: *stomatitis.*

gingivolabial (jĭn″jĭ-vō-lā′bē-ăl) Concerning the gums and lips.

gingivoplasty (jĭn′jĭ-vō-plăs″tē) [″ + Gr. *plassein,* to form] Surgical correction of the gingival margin.

gingivostomatitis (jĭn″jĭ-vō-stō″mă-tī′tĭs) [″ + Gr. *stoma,* mouth, + *itis,* inflammation] Inflammation of the gingival tissue and the mucosa of the mouth due to herpesvirus types I or II.

ginglymoarthrodial (jĭng″lĭ-mō-ăr-thrō′dē-ăl) [″ + *arthrodia,* gliding joint] Pert. to a joint that is both hinged and arthrodial. SEE: *arthrodia.*

ginglymoid (jĭng′lĭ-moyd) [″ + *eidos,* form, shape] Pert. to or shaped like a hinged joint.

ginglymus (jĭng′lĭ-mŭs) [Gr. *ginglymos,* hinge] Hinge joint. SEE: *joint.*

Ginkgo biloba (geen-kō bĭ-lō′bă) A deciduous gymnosperm tree with fan-shaped leaves and spherical cones. Its extracts have been used medicinally in China for centuries and promoted as a memory aid. Its extracts and metabolites are antioxidants.

ginseng (jĭn′sĕng) [Chinese *jen-shen,* man, man image] An herbal remedy promoted by alternative medicine practitioners for its purported effect on sexual potency. In a recent study of 55 ginseng preparations available in the U. S., only seven were found to be alcohol-free.

giotrogen (gĕ′trō-jĕn) A substance that produces massive enlargement of the thyroid by inhibiting iodide metabolism and thyroid hormone synthesis. It occurs naturally in certain foods including raw turnips, rutabagas, cabbages, and cassava.

Giraldés' organ (hĭr-ăl-dās′) [Joachim A. C. C. Giraldés, Portuguese surgeon in Paris, 1808–1875] Paradidymis.

girdle [AS. *gyrdel,* girdle] **1.** A zone or belt; the waist. **2.** A structure that resembles a circular belt or band.

pelvic g. The portion of the lower extremities to which the lower limbs are attached. It is composed of the two innominate or hip bones.

shoulder g. The portion of the upper extremities to which the upper limbs are attached. It is composed of the two clavicles and two scapulae.

girdle symptom A symptom in tabes as of a tight girdle, such as a feeling of constriction about the chest; also found in compression of the cord owing to collapse of the vertebrae, as in Pott's disease.

gitter cell A macrophage present at sites of brain injury. The cells are packed with lipoid granules from phagocytosis of damaged brain cells. SEE: *microglia*.

gizzard (gĭz′ărd) The very strong muscular stomach of certain birds. Food is mixed with gastric juice and macerated with the aid of small stones, called *grit,* that are ingested and remain in the gizzard.

glabella [L. *glaber,* smooth] The smooth surface of the frontal bone lying between the superciliary arches; the portion directly above the root of the nose. SYN: *intercilium; mesophryon*.

glabrate, glabrous [L. *glaber,* smooth] **1.** Bald. **2.** Smooth.

glacial (glā′shĭl) [L. *glacialis,* icy] **1.** Glassy; resembling ice. **2.** Highly purified.

gladiate (glā′dē-āt) [L. *gladius,* sword] Xiphoid.

glairy Viscous; albuminous; mucoid.

gland [L. *glans,* acorn] An organized cluster of cells or tissues that manufactures a substance to be excreted from or used in the body. Glands may be classified by their anatomical structure (e.g., tubular, saccular, villous, papillary, ductless), their complexity (simple, compound), their function (endocrine, exocrine), the quality of their secretions (mucous, serous, sebaceous, or mixed), or the way in which their secretions are released (e.g., merocrine, apocrine, holocrine, eccrine).

accessory g. A small gland similar in function to another gland of similar structure some distance removed.

acinotubular g. A gland structurally midway between an acinous and a tubular gland.

acinous g. A gland whose secreting units are composed of saclike structures, each possessing a narrow lumen. SYN: *racemose g.*

adrenal g. A triangular gland covering the superior surface of each kidney. SYN: *suprarenal g.* SEE: illus.

EMBRYOLOGY: The adrenal gland is essentially a double organ composed of an outer cortex and an inner medulla. The cortex arises in the embryo from a region of the mesoderm that also gives rise to the gonads, or sex organs. The medulla arises from ectoderm, which also gives rise to the sympathetic nervous system.

ANATOMY: The gland is enclosed in a tough connective tissue capsule from which trabeculae extend into the cortex. The cortex consists of cells arranged into three zones: the outer zona glomerulosa, the middle zona fasciculata, and the inner zona reticularis. The cells are arranged in a cordlike fashion. The medulla consists of chromaffin cells arranged in groups or anastomosing cords. The two adrenal glands are situated retroperitoneally, each embedded in perirenal fat above its respective kidney. In an adult, the average weight of an adrenal gland is 5 g, and the range is 4 to 14 g. It is usually heavier in men than in women.

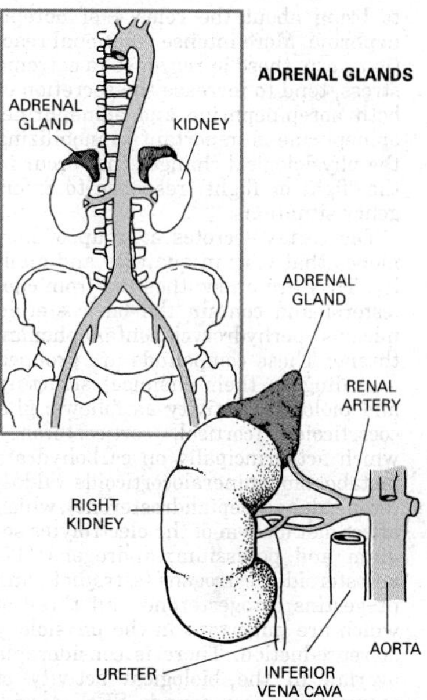

ADRENAL GLANDS

PHYSIOLOGY: The adrenal medulla synthesizes and stores three catecholamines: dopamine, norepinephrine, and epinephrine. Dopamine's chief effects are dilation of systemic arteries, increased cardiac output, and increased flow of blood to the kidneys. The primary action of norepinephrine is to constrict the arterioles and venules, resulting in increased resistance to blood flow, elevated blood pressure, and slowing of the heart. Epinephrine constricts vessels in the skin and viscera, dilates vessels in skeletal muscle, increases heart rate, dilates the bronchi by relaxing bronchial musculature, increases the glucose level in the blood by stimulating the production of glucose from glycogen in the liver, increases the amount of fatty acid in the blood, and diminishes activity of the gastrointestinal system. The three catecholamines are also produced in other parts of the body.

The adrenal medulla is controlled by the sympathetic nervous system and functions in conjunction with it. It is intimately related to adjustments of the body in response to stress and emotional changes. Anticipatory states tend to bring about the release of norepinephrine. More intense emotional reactions, esp. those in response to extreme stress, tend to increase the secretion of both norepinephrine and epinephrine; epinephrine is important in mobilizing the physiological changes that occur in the "fight or flight" response to emergency situations.

The cortex secretes a group of hormones that vary in quantity and quality. They are all synthesized from cholesterol and contain the basic steroid nucleus perhydrocyclopentanophenanthrene. These compounds are grouped according to their chemical structure and biological activity as follows: glucocorticoids (cortisol, corticosterone), which act principally on carbohydrate metabolism; mineralocorticoids (aldosterone, dehydroepiandrosterone), which affect metabolism of the electrolytes sodium and potassium; androgens (17-ketosteroids), estrogens (estradiol), and progestins (progesterone), all three of which are important in the physiology of reproduction. There is considerable overlap in the biological activity of many of these compounds. SEE: *steroid*.

Almost all body systems are influenced by the action of adrenocortical hormones. Cortisol and cortisone are important in carbohydrate, water, muscle, bone, central nervous system, gastrointestinal, cardiovascular, and hematological metabolism. They are also important anti-inflammatory agents. The principal long-term effect of cortisone and cortisol is catabolic.

The 17-ketosteroids act principally as androgenic and anabolic agents. Aldosterone's principal action is to control sodium and potassium levels in the blood.

PATHOLOGY: In the medulla, increased secretion of catecholamines occurs when a pheochromocytoma develops. In this condition, some patients develop classical symptoms such as hypertension, excessive sweating, paroxysmal attacks of blanching or flushing of the skin, episodic tachycardia, headache, anorexia, weight loss, personality changes, and postural hypotension. Diagnosis may be confirmed by determining the level of catecholamines or their metabolic end products in the urine. SEE: *pheochromocytoma*.

Excess secretion of cortical hormones in the cortex may result in a variety of syndromes, depending on which hormone or group of hormones is increased. If cortisol is increased, the signs of Cushing's syndrome result: obesity with striae and redistribution of fat to produce a "buffalo hump" and "moon face," muscle wasting, osteoporosis, decreased glucose tolerance, atherosclerosis, and systolic hypertension. If androgen levels are increased, male sex characteristics are accentuated; in women, this results in deepening of the voice, hirsutism, clitoral enlargement, and increased muscular development. Male pattern hair loss and acne will develop in persons of either sex who have this condition. Puberty that has an early onset due to androgen excess is called the adrenogenital syndrome.

When the adrenal glands overproduce aldosterone, hypertension, hypokalemia, and rarely edema will be present. This condition is called primary aldosteronism. SEE: *primary aldosteronism*.

Adrenocortical deficiency may be acute or chronic. The chronic form is called Addison's disease and is marked by anemia, sluggishness, weakness, weight loss, hypotension, sometimes hypoglycemia, nausea, vomiting, diarrhea, abnormal skin pigmentation, and mental changes. The acute form is called adrenal crisis because it results in circulatory shock. Adrenal crisis due to hemorrhage into the adrenal gland caused by meningococcal infection is called the Waterhouse-Friderichsen syndrome.

aggregate g. A rarely used term for the lymphoid nodules of the small intestine. SEE: *Peyer's patches*.

albuminous g. Glands secreting a fluid containing albumin. SYN: *serous g.*

anal g. Glands in the region of the anus. SYN: *circumanal g.*

apocrine g. A gland whose cells lose some of their cytoplasmic contents in the formation of secretion. Examples include the mammary glands.

areolar g. Sebaceous glands in the areola surrounding the nipple of the female breast. SEE: *Montgomery's glands*.

axillary g. Axillary lymph nodes.

Bartholin's g. SEE: *Bartholin's gland*.

Blandin's g. SEE: *Blandin's glands*.

Bowman's g. SEE: *Bowman's glands*.

brachial g. Lymph nodes in the arm and forearm.

bronchial g. Mixed glands lying in the submucosa of the bronchi and bronchial tubes.

Bruch's g. Conjunctival lymph nodes in the lower lids.

Brunner's g. SEE: *Brunner's glands*.

buccal g. Acinous glands in the mucosa of the cheek.

bulbourethral g. Either of two small, round, yellow glands, one on each side of the prostate gland, each with a duct about 1 in. (2.5 cm) long, terminating in the wall of the urethra. Their alkaline secretion is part of seminal fluid. They correspond to the Bartholin glands in the female. SYN: *Cowper's g.* SEE: *prostate; urethra*.

cardiac g. Glands of the stomach

near the cardiac orifice of the esophagus.

carotid g. Obsolete term for the carotid body.

celiac g. Several lymph nodes anterior to the abdominal aorta.

ceruminous g. Glands in the external auditory canal that secrete cerumen.

cervical g. Lymph nodes in the neck.

ciliary g. SEE: *Moll's glands.*

circumanal g. Anal g.

Cobelli's g. Glands in the esophageal mucosa.

coccygeal g. Luschka's g.

compound g. A gland consisting of a number of branching duct systems that open into the main secretory duct.

compound tubular g. A gland composed of numerous tubules leading to a lone duct.

conglobate g. Obsolete term for a lymph node.

Cowper's g. Bulbourethral g.

cutaneous g. Glands of the skin, esp. the sebaceous and sudoriferous glands. These include modified forms such as the ciliary, ceruminous, anal, preputial, areolar, and meibomian glands.

ductless g. A gland without ducts, secreting directly into capillaries one or more hormones that have specific effects on target organs or tissues. SEE: *endocrine gland; exocrine.*

duodenal g. SEE: *Brunner's glands.*

Ebner's g. Serous glands of the tongue located in the region of the vallate papillae, their ducts opening into the furrows surrounding the papillae.

eccrine g. A simple tubular sweat gland of the skin. SEE: *apocrine g.; eccrine sweat gland.*

endocrine g. A ductless gland that produces an internal secretion discharged into the blood or lymph and circulated to all parts of the body. The endocrine glands include the pituitary gland (which produces thyroid-stimulating hormone, adrenocorticotropic hormone, luteinizing hormone, follicle-stimulating hormone, growth hormone, endorphins, and prolactin); the hypothalamus (which produces thyrotropin-releasing hormone, growth hormone-releasing hormone, somatostatin, dopamine, gonadotropic hormone-releasing hormone, antidiuretic hormone, and oxytocin); the thyroid gland; the parathyroid glands; the adrenal glands; the islets of the pancreas; and the gonads (testes and ovaries). During pregnancy, the placenta has endocrine functions: it releases numerous substances, including human chorionic gonadotropin, that maintain pregnancy. SEE: illus.; table.

The hormones secreted by endocrine glands may exert their specific effects on one or a few target organs or tissues, or on virtually all body tissues, as does thyroxine, which increases metabolic rate. Other processes affected by hormones include cell division, protein syntheses, the use of food molecules for en-

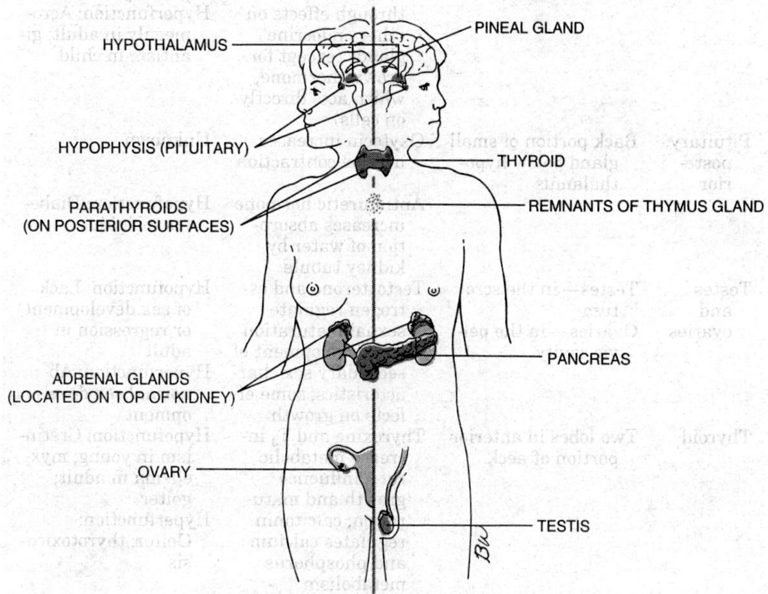

ENDOCRINE SYSTEM

Principal Endocrine Glands

Name	Position	Function	Endocrine Disorders
Adrenal cortex	Outer portion of gland on top of each kidney	Cortisol regulates carbohydrate and fat metabolism; aldosterone regulates salt and water balance	Hypofunction: Addison's disease Hyperfunction: Adrenogenital syndrome; Cushing's syndrome
Adrenal medulla	Inner portion of adrenal gland; surrounded by adrenal cortex	Effects of epinephrine and norepinephrine mimic those of sympathetic nervous system; increases carbohydrate use for energy	Hypofunction: Almost unknown Hyperfunction: Pheochromocytoma
Pancreas (endocrine portion)	Abdominal cavity; head adjacent to duodenum; tail close to spleen and kidney	Secretes insulin and glucagon, which regulate carbohydrate metabolism	Hypofunction: Diabetes mellitus Hyperfunction: If a tumor produces excess insulin, hypoglycemia
Parathyroid	Four or more small glands on back of thyroid	Parathyroid hormone regulates calcium and phosphorus metabolism; indirectly affects muscular irritability	Hypofunction: Hypocalcemia; tetany Hyperfunction: Hypercalcemia; resorption of bone; kidney stones; nausea; vomiting; altered mental status
Pituitary, anterior	Front portion of small gland below hypothalamus	Influences growth, sexual development, skin pigmentation, thyroid function, adrenocortical function through effects on other endocrine glands (except for growth hormone, which acts directly on cells)	Hypofunction: Dwarfism in child; decrease in all other endocrine gland functions except parathyroids Hyperfunction: Acromegaly in adult; gigantism in child
Pituitary, posterior	Back portion of small gland below hypothalamus	Oxytocin increases uterine contraction	Unknown
		Antidiuretic hormone increases absorption of water by kidney tubule	Hypofunction: Diabetes insipidus
Testes and ovaries	Testes—in the scrotum Ovaries—in the pelvic cavity	Testosterone and estrogen regulate sexual maturation and development of secondary sex characteristics; some effects on growth	Hypofunction: Lack of sex development or regression in adult Hyperfunction: Abnormal sex development
Thyroid	Two lobes in anterior portion of neck	Thyroxine and T_3 increase metabolic rate; influence growth and maturation; calcitonin regulates calcium and phosphorus metabolism	Hypofunction: Cretinism in young; myxedema in adult; goiter Hyperfunction: Goiter; thyrotoxicosis

ergy production, secretory activity of other endocrine glands, development and functioning of the reproductive organs, sexual characteristics and libido, development of personality and higher nervous functions, the ability of the body to meet conditions of stress, and resistance to disease.

Endocrine dysfunction may result from hyposecretion, in which an inadequate amount of hormone is secreted, or from hypersecretion, in which an excessive amount of hormone is produced. Secretion of endocrine glands may be controlled by the nervous system, by blood levels of nutrients and minerals, or, in some cases, by other hormones. Many pathological conditions are caused by or associated with malfunction of the endocrine glands.

Fraenkel's g. Tiny glands located below the margin of the vocal cords.

fundic g. Glands of the body and fundus of the stomach; gastric glands, which secrete gastric juice.

gastric g. One of the tubular glands, or gastric pits, of the stomach. SYN: *peptic g.* SEE: *stomach.*

Gay's g. Circumanal sebaceous glands.

genal g. A gland in the buccal submucosa.

genital g. The female ovaries and male testes.

haversian g. Synovial g.

hemal g. Hemal node.

hepatic g. Lymph nodes located in front of the portal vein.

holocrine g. SEE: *holocrine.*

inguinal g. Lymph nodes in the inguinal region.

interscapular g. Brown fat.

interstitial g. Leydig cell.

intestinal g. Simple or branched tubular glands of the intestine that secrete the intestinal juice. These include Brunner's glands and crypts of Lieberkühn.

jugular g. A firm or enlarged lymph node lying beneath the sternocleidomastoid muscle, often associated with malignancy. SEE: *sentinel node* (1).

Krause's g. Small tear-producing glands in the conjunctiva.

labial g. Multiple acinous glands of the mucosa of the lips.

lacrimal g. The gland that secretes tears. It is a tubuloalveolar gland located in the orbit, superior and lateral to the eyeball, and consists of a large superior portion (pars orbitalis) and a smaller inferior portion (pars palpebralis).

lactiferous g. Mammary g.

lenticular g. One of the small masses of lymphatic tissue in the lamina propria of the pyloric region of the stomach.

Lieberkühn's g. Lieberkühn crypt.

lingual g. Glands of the tongue, including the anterior lingual glands (glands of Nuhn), posterior lingual glands (glands of von Ebner), and mucous glands at the root of the tongue.

Littré's g. SEE: *Littré's gland.*

Luschka's g. A gland located near the coccygeal tip. SYN: *coccygeal g.*

lymph g. An obsolete term for lymph node.

mammary g. A compound alveolar gland that secretes milk. In women, these glands are made up of lobes and lobules bound together by areolar tissue. Each of the 15 to 20 main ducts, known as lactiferous ducts, discharges through a separate orifice on the surface of the nipple. The dilatations of the ducts form reservoirs for the milk during lactation. SYN: *lactiferous g.*

meibomian g. Tarsal g.

merocrine g. A gland in which the cells remain intact during the elaboration and discharge of their secretion. SEE: *eccrine sweat gland.*

mixed g. **1.** A gland that has both endocrine and exocrine function (e.g., the pancreas). **2.** A salivary gland that has both mucous and serous secretions, often with both cell types in the same acinus. SEE: *submandibular gland.*

Moll's g. SEE: *Moll's glands.*

Montgomery's g. SEE: *Montgomery's glands.*

Morgagni's g. SEE: *Littré's gland.*

muciparous g. Glands that secrete mucus.

nabothian g. Dilated mucous glands in the uterine cervix.

odoriferous g. Glands exuding odoriferous materials, as those around the prepuce or anus.

olfactory g. Glands in the olfactory mucous membranes.

oxyntic g. Gastric glands found in the fundus and body of the gastric mucosa.

palatine g. Mucous glands in the tissue of the palate.

palpebral g. Tarsal g.

parathyroid g. Several small endocrine glands about 6 mm long by 3 to 4 mm wide, on the back and lower edge of the thyroid gland or embedded within its substance. These glands secrete parathyroid hormone, which regulates calcium and phosphorus metabolism.

paraurethral g. SEE: *Skene's glands.*

parotid g. The largest of the salivary glands, located below and in front of the ear. It is a compound tubuloacinous serous gland. Its secreting tubules and acini are long and branched, and it is enclosed in a sheath, the parotid fascia. Saliva lubricates food and makes it easier to taste, chew, and swallow. SEE: *mumps.*

peptic g. Gastric g.

Peyer's g. Peyer's patch.

pineal g. An endocrine gland in the brain, shaped like a pine cone and located in a pocket near the splenium of the corpus callosum. It is the site of melatonin synthesis, which is inhibited by light striking the retina. SEE: *melatonin.*

pituitary g. SEE: *pituitary gland.*

preputial g. A modified sebaceous gland located on the neck of the penis and the inner surface of the prepuce; its secretion is a component of smegma. SYN: *Tyson's gland.*

prostate g. The male gland that surrounds the neck of the bladder and the urethra. It is partly glandular, with ducts opening into the prostatic portion of the urethra, and partly muscular. It secretes a thin, opalescent, slightly alkaline fluid that forms part of the semen. The prostate consists of a median lobe and two lateral lobes measuring about 2 × 4 × 3 cm and weighing about 20 g; it is enclosed in a fibrous capsule containing smooth muscle fiber in its inner layer. The nerve supply is from the inferior hypogastric plexus.

pyloric g. Gastric glands near the pylorus that secrete gastric juice.

racemose g. Acinous g.

Rivinus' g. Sublingual g.

salivary g. The parotid, sublingual, or submandibular salivary gland of the mouth.

sebaceous g. A simple or branched alveolar gland that secretes sebum. It is found in the skin and its duct usually opens into a hair follicle.

sentinel g. A term formerly used to indicate a sentinel lymph node, i.e., a lymph node that first alerts a clinician to serious pathology (such as a spreading cancer).

seromucous g. A mixed serous and muciparous gland.

serous g. Albuminous g.

sex g. The ovary or testis.

Skene's g. SEE: *Skene's glands.*

sublingual g. The smallest of the major salivary glands, located in the tissue in the floor of the mouth between the tongue and mandible on each side. It is a mixed seromucous gland. Its main duct opens into or near the submandibular duct, but several smaller ducts may open to the oral cavity independently along the sublingual fold. Numerous minor sublingual glands are scattered throughout the mucosa under the tongue, each with its own duct to the oral surface.

submandibular g. One of the salivary glands, a mixed tubuloalveolar gland about the size of a walnut that lies in the digastric triangle beneath the mandible. Its main duct (Wharton's duct) opens at the side of the frenulum linguae.

sudoriferous g. Glands in the skin that secrete perspiration. SYN: *sweat g.* SEE: *sweat gland* for illus.

suprarenal g. Adrenal g.

sweat g. Sudoriferous g.

synovial g. Glands that secrete synovial fluid.

target g. Any gland affected by the action or secretion of another gland (e.g., the thyroid is a target gland of the pituitary).

tarsal g. Glands in the eyelid that secrete a sebaceous substance that keeps the lids from adhering to each other. SYN: *meibomian g.; palpebral g.*

thymus g. The thymus. SEE: *thymus.*

thyroid g. SEE: *thyroid gland.*

tracheal g. Acinous glands of the tracheal mucosa.

tubular g. A gland whose terminal secreting portions are narrow tubes.

Tyson's g. SEE: *Tyson's gland.*

unicellular g. Mucus-secreting cells present in columnar or pseudostratified columnar epithelial tissue layers. They are called *goblet cells.*

urethral g. SEE: *Littré's gland.*

vaginal g. Acinous glands found in the uppermost portion of the vaginal mucosa near the cervix, most of the vaginal mucosa being devoid of glands.

vestibular g. Glands of the vaginal vestibule. They include the minor vestibular glands and the major vestibular glands (Bartholin's glands).

vulvovaginal g. SEE: *Bartholin's gland.*

Waldeyer's g. SEE: *Waldeyer's gland.*

Weber's g. SEE: *Weber's gland.*

g. of Zeis SEE: *Zeis gland.*

Zuckerkandl's g. A tiny yellowish lobe occasionally seen between the geniohyoid muscles. It is an accessory thyroid gland.

glanders (glăn′dĕrz) A contagious infection caused by *Pseudomonas mallei* in horses, donkeys, and mules. It is communicable to humans, but no cases have occurred in the Western Hemisphere since 1938. Experience with the disease is limited, but sulfadiazine is the recommended therapy.

SYMPTOMS: Patients develop fever, inflammation of the skin and mucous membranes (esp. those of the nasal cavity), with formation of ulcers and abscesses. Small subcutaneous nodules develop, break down, and give rise to ulcers. Beginning as small areas, these tend to spread and coalesce and finally involve large areas that exude a viscid, mucopurulent discharge with a foul odor. The infection may occur in an acute or chronic form. In the acute septicemic form, prognosis is grave and the disease is almost invariably fatal.

glandilemma (glăn″dĭ-lĕm′ă) [L. *glans,* acorn, + Gr. *lemma,* sheath] The outer covering or capsule of a gland.

glandula (glăn′dū-lă) *pl.* **glandulae** Glandule.

glandular [L. *glandula,* little acorn] Pert. to or of the nature of a gland.

glandular therapy Treatment of disease with natural or synthetic hormones. SYN: *organotherapy*.

glandule (glăn′dūl) A small gland. SYN: *glandula*.

glans [L. *glans,* acorn] A gland.

g. clitoridis The head of the clitoris. SEE: *clitoris*.

g. penis The bulbous end of the penis. SEE: *penis*.

Glanzmann's thrombasthenia (glănz′mănz) [Edward Glanzmann, Swiss pediatrician, 1887–1959] A rare autosomal recessive abnormality of platelet glycoprotein IIb-IIIa, characterized by easy bruising and epistaxis that sometimes requires blood transfusions. Bleeding is prolonged, clot retraction is diminished, and platelets do not aggregate during blood coagulation or after addition of adenosine diphosphate. Treatments include platelet transfusions, progestational agents, and iron replacement, among others.

glare [ME. *glaren,* to gleam] A condition causing temporary blurring of vision with possible permanent injury to the retina. The condition is caused by intense light (visible radiation) emanating from highly reflective objects (such as sunlight reflected on water or snow), or projected by an automobile headlight or by a therapeutic lamp. SEE: *dazzle*.

glaserian artery (glā-sē′rē-ăn) [Johann Heinrich Glaser, Swiss anatomist, 1629–1679] A branch of the internal maxillary artery that supplies the tympanum.

glaserian fissure A narrow slit posterior to the mandibular fossa of the temporal bone. The chorda tympani nerve passes through it.

Glasgow Coma Scale ABBR: GCS. A scale used to determine a patient's level of consciousness. It is a rating from 3 to 15 of the patient's ability to open his or her eyes, respond verbally, and move normally. The GCS is used primarily during the examination of patients with trauma or stroke. Repeated examinations can help determine if the patient's brain function is improving or deteriorating. Many EMS systems use the GCS for triage purposes and for determining which patients should be intubated in the field. SEE: *coma; Trauma Score*.

Glasgow Outcome Scale A scale that assesses current neurological awareness of the environment, and recovery and disability in all types of brain injury. The scale is to be used during the evaluation of trauma, stupor, or coma, and at prescribed time intervals, such as 3 months, 6 months, and 1 year after injury. The Glasgow group reports the greatest recovery in the 6-month period after injury. The nurse (or other health-care practitioner) notes the patient's abilities at a particular time using this practical scale:

1. *Good outcome:* may have minimal disabling sequelae but returns to independent functioning comparable to preinjury level and a full-time job
2. *Moderate disability:* is capable of independent functioning but not of returning to full-time employment
3. *Severe disability:* depends on others for some aspect of daily living
4. *Persistive vegetative state:* has no obvious cortical functioning
5. *Dead*

glass [AS. *glaes*] A hard, brittle, amorphous, transparent material composed of silica and various bases.

ground g. Abnormal shadowing seen radiographically. In chest x-ray films, it may indicate interstitial fibrosis of the lung; in abdominal films, it suggests ascites.

leaded g. Safety glass that contains lead, used in radiology to help protect technicians from x-rays.

photochromic g. Glass that is manufactured to appear clear until light strikes it. When used in sunglasses, the lens becomes dark and reduces the amount of light transmitted, becoming clear again when no longer exposed to bright light.

polarized g. Glass treated with a medium that permits the exiting light waves to vibrate in only one direction.

safety g. A type of laminated glass that meets specific requirements concerning the force necessary to break it and is designed to break without shattering. Its use in automobiles reduces the risk of injury from broken glass.

tempered g. Glass that has been heat-treated to increase the force required to break it.

ultraviolet transmitting g. Glass designed to admit ultraviolet radiation through it. It transmits about half of the solar radiation, between the wavelengths of 290 and 320 nm.

watch g. A shallow, saucer-like glass dish, resembling the glass cover widely used to cover the face of a large pocket watch.

glasses [AS. *glaes,* glass] **1.** A transparent refractive device worn to correct refraction errors in the patient's eyes. **2.** A device worn to protect eyes from glare or particles in the air. SYN: *eyeglass; spectacles*.

bifocal g. Glasses in which the refracting power of the lower portion differs from that in the upper portion, the lower portion being used for viewing near objects or reading, the upper portion for distant objects. SYN: *Franklin glasses*.

prism g. An optical device, used by persons who must lie supine for extended periods, to allow them to view objects in their environment without eye or neck strain. Prisms mounted on spectacle frames bend the image to make the feet visible while the person is looking straight ahead.

safety g. Glasses using heat-treated glass or impact-resistant plastic lenses. Their use serves to protect the eyes from dangerous slivers of glass that are produced when ordinary lenses are broken in an accident. Use of safety glass in manufacturing eyeglass lenses is mandatory in the U.S.

trifocal g. Glasses with three different corrections in each lens: one each for near, intermediate, and far vision.

glassy Hyaline; vitreous; glasslike, smooth, and shiny.

Glauber's salt (glō'bĕrz) [Johann Rudolf Glauber, Dutch physician, 1604–1668] Sodium sulfate.

glaucoma (glaw-kō'mă) [L., cataract] A group of eye diseases characterized by increased intraocular pressure, resulting in atrophy of the optic nerve and possibly leading to blindness. Glaucoma is the third most prevalent cause of visual impairment and blindness in the U.S. Cataract and macular degeneration of aging are the two principal causes. An estimated 15 million residents of the U.S. have glaucoma; of these, 150,000 have bilateral blindness. The three major categories of glaucoma are closed-angle (acute) glaucoma, which occurs in persons whose eyes are anatomically predisposed to develop the condition; open-angle (chronic) glaucoma, in which the angle that permits the drainage of aqueous humor from the eye seems normal but functions inadequately; and congenital glaucoma, in which the intraocular pressure is increased for an unknown reason. The increased pressure causes the globe of the eye to be enlarged; a condition known as *buphthalmia*. The acute type of glaucoma often is attended by acute pain. The chronic type has an insidious onset. A normal tonometer reading ranges from 13 to 22. An initial visual dysfunction is loss of the mid-peripheral field of vision. The loss of central visual acuity occurs later in the disease. SEE: *visual field* for illus.

ETIOLOGY: Glaucoma occurs when the aqueous humor drains from the eye too slowly to keep up with its production in the anterior chamber. Thus, narrowing or closure of the filtration angle that interferes with drainage through the canal of Schlemm causes intraocular fluid to accumulate, after which intraocular pressure increases. Glaucoma may develop, however, even if the filtration angle is normal and the canal of Schlemm appears to be functioning; the cause of this form of glaucoma is not known.

DIAGNOSIS: Glaucoma may not cause symptoms. It is detected usually by an abnormal intraocular pressure (IOP) measurement. The frequent need to change eyeglass prescriptions, vague visual disturbances, mild headache, and impaired dark adaptation may also be present. The standard for determining visual loss in glaucoma is the visual-field test.

Open-angle glaucoma causes mild aching in the eyes, loss of peripheral vision, haloes around lights, and reduced visual acuity (esp. at night) that is uncorrected by prescription lenses. Acute angle-closure glaucoma (an ophthalmic emergency) causes excruciating unilateral pain and pressure, blurred vision, decreased visual acuity, haloes around lights, diplopia, lacrimation, and nausea and vomiting due to increased IOP. The eyes may show unilateral circumcorneal injection, conjunctival edema, a cloudy cornea, and a moderately dilated pupil that is nonreactive to light.

TREATMENT: Nonoperative treatment includes the use of miotics (eserine, pilocarpine), timolol maleate, intravenous mannitol, and parenteral acetazolamide. Experimental studies indicate that marijuana alleviates the symptoms of severe glaucoma. Control of associated disorders such as diabetes should be maintained. Operative treatment includes paracentesis of the cornea, iridectomy (broad peripheral), cyclodialysis, anterior sclerotomy, sclerotomy with inclusion of the iris, as iridotasis or iridencleisis; sclerectomy. SEE: illus.; *ciliarotomy; trabeculoplasty*.

CAUTION: Acute glaucoma may be precipitated in patients with closed-angle glaucoma by dilating the pupils. In glaucoma patients, cycloplegic drops are given only after trabeculectomy and only in the eye that had the procedure. Administering drops in an eye affected with glaucoma can precipitate an acute attack in an eye already compromised by elevated IOP.

PATIENT CARE: Health care providers should wash their hands thoroughly before touching the patient's eye. Prescribed topical and systemic medications are administered and evaluated.

The patient is prepared physically and psychologically for diagnostic studies and surgery as indicated. If the patient has a trabeculectomy, prescribed cycloplegic drugs are administered to relax the ciliary muscle and decrease iris action.

After any surgery, an eye patch and shield are applied to protect the eye, the patient is positioned with the head slightly elevated, and general safety

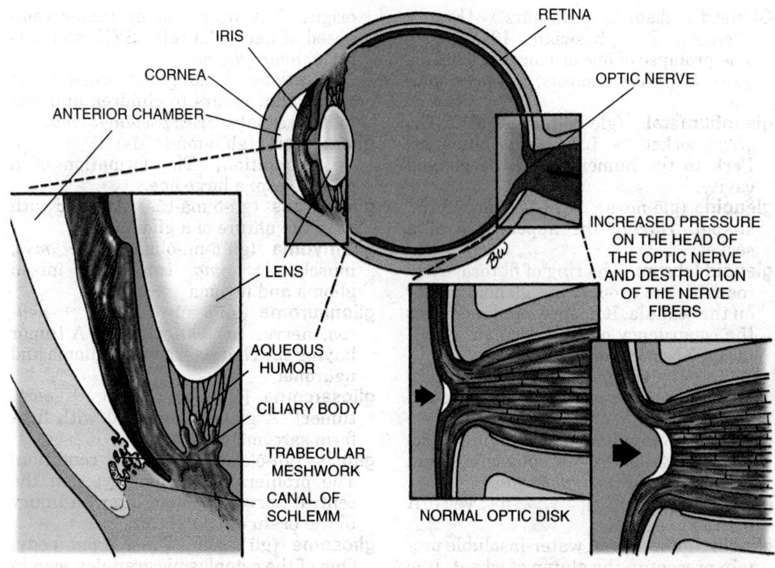

GLAUCOMA

measures geared to the patient's level of sensory alteration are instituted.

Patients with glaucoma need to know that the disease can be controlled, but not cured. Fatigue, emotional upsets, excessive fluid intake, and use of antihistamines may increase IOP. Signs and symptoms such as vision changes or eye pain should be reported immediately. Both patient and family are instructed in correct techniques for eyedrop administration, the importance of strict adherence to the prescribed regimen, and adverse reactions to report. Information is provided to the patient and family as needed. Referral is made to local organizations and support groups.

Public education is carried out to encourage glaucoma screening for early detection of the disease. Written information should be made available about detection and control of glaucoma. SEE: *Nursing Diagnoses Appendix.*

absolute g. An extremely painful form of glaucoma in which the eye is completely blind and hard as stone (as a result of elevated intraocular pressures) with an insensitive cornea, a shallow anterior chamber, and an excavated optic disk.

chronic g. Glaucoma in which the tonometer indicates an intraocular pressure reading of up to 45 or 50, the anterior ciliary veins are enlarged, the cornea is clear, the pupil is dilated, and pain is present. During attacks vision is poor. The visual field may be normal. Cupping of the optic disk is not present in the early stages.

closed-angle g. Glaucoma caused by a shallow anterior chamber and thus a narrow filtration angle through which the aqueous humor normally passes. Because the rate of movement of the aqueous is impaired, intraocular pressure increases. In general, headache, haloes around single sources of light, blurred vision, and eye pain are symptomatic. SYN: *narrow-angle glaucoma.*

narrow-angle g. Closed-angle g.

pigmentary g. Glaucoma produced by the dispersion of organic pigment from the zonula ciliaris to the trabecular meshwork of the eye.

primary open-angle g. The most common type of glaucoma. It usually affects both eyes, and there is a characteristic change in the appearance of the optic disk. The cup (the depression in the center of the disk) is enlarged. Visual loss is determined by the visual-field test. Many patients with glaucoma have increased intraocular pressure but this is not considered essential to the diagnosis because some patients have normal intraocular pressure.

glaucomatous (glaw-kō′mă-tŭs) Pert. to glaucoma.

GLC *gas-liquid chromatography.*

Gleason's score (glē′sŭnz) [Donald F. Gleason, U.S. pathologist, b. 1920] A measure of the cellular differentiation of prostate cancers that uses the microscopic appearance of biopsied tissue to determine the tumor grade and stage. SYN: *Gleason's grade.*

gleet (glēt) A mucous discharge from the urethra in chronic gonorrhea.

Glénard's disease (glā-nărz′) [Frantz Glénard, Fr. physician, 1848–1920] The prolapse of one or more internal organs. SYN: *enteroptosis; splanchnoptosia.*

glenohumeral (glē″nō-hū′mĕr-ăl) [Gr. *glene,* socket, + L. *humerus,* humerus] Pert. to the humerus and the glenoid cavity.

glenoid (glē′noyd) [″ + *eidos,* form, shape] Having the appearance of a socket.

glenoid labrum The ring of fibrocartilaginous tissue around the glenoid cavity on the scapula. It deepens and increases the congruency of the articulating surface. SYN: *glenoid lip.*

glia (glī′ă) [Gr. *glia,* glue] The neuroglia; the nonnervous or supporting tissue of the brain and spinal cord.

glia cells Neuroglia cells, including astrocytes, oligodendroglia (oligoglia), and microglia. SEE: *cell; neuroglia.*

gliacyte (glī′ă-sīt) [″ + *kytos,* cell] A neuroglia cell.

gliadin (glī′ă-dĭn) A water-insoluble protein present in the gluten of wheat. It is deficient in the essential amino acid lysine. The sticky mass that results when wheat flour and water are mixed is due to gliadin. In some individuals the intestinal mucosa lacks the ability to digest this substance, which therefore damages the intestinal lining and causes gluten-induced enteropathy.

glial (glī′ăl) Concerning glia or neuroglia.

gliarase (glī′ă-rās) [Gr. *glia,* glue] An astrocytic mass with incomplete fission of cytoplasm.

glide 1. To move in a smooth, virtually frictionless manner. **2.** Movement in a smooth, virtually frictionless manner. **3.** A joint mobilization technique in which the therapist applies a force to move bones in a direction parallel to the treatment plane. This technique is used to maintain or increase joint play.

mandibular g. The movement of the mandible in any direction as the teeth come into contact.

glioblastoma (glī″ō-blăs-tō′mă) [″ + *blastos,* germ, + *oma,* tumor] A neuroglia cell tumor. SYN: *glioma.*

g. multiforme A type of astrocytoma marked pathologically by the presence of extremely abnormal malignant brain cells. Clinically, this tumor is among the most aggressive of the primary brain tumors. Survival 1 to 2 yr after diagnosis is rare.

gliocyte (glī′ō-sīt) [″ + *kytos,* cell] A neuroglia cell.

gliocytoma (glī-ō-sī-tō′mă) [″ + ″ + *oma,* tumor] A neuroglia cell tumor.

gliogenous (glī-ŏj′ĕ-nŭs) [″ + *gennan,* to produce] Of the nature of neuroglia.

glioma (glī-ō′mă) *pl.* **gliomata** [″ + *oma,* tumor] **1.** A sarcoma of neuroglial origin. **2.** A neoplasm or tumor composed of neuroglia cells. SYN: *glioblastoma; neuroglioma.*

g. retinae A malignant tumor of the retina that occurs in children and metastasizes late. SEE: *pseudoglioma.*

gliomatosis (glī″ō-mă-tō′sĭs) [″ + ″ + *osis,* condition] The formation of a glioma, esp. a large one.

gliomatous (glī-ō′mă-tŭs) Affected with or of the nature of a glioma.

gliomyoma (glī″ō-mī-ō′mă) [″ + *mys,* muscle, + *oma,* tumor] A mixed glioma and myoma.

glioneuroma (glī″ō-nū-rō′mă) [″ + *neuron,* nerve, + *oma,* tumor] A tumor having the characteristics of glioma and neuroma.

gliosarcoma [″ + *sarx,* flesh, + *oma,* tumor] A glioma combined with fusiform sarcoma cells.

gliosis (glī-ō′sĭs) [″ + *osis,* condition] The proliferation of astrocytes in the central nervous system after an injury to the brain or spinal cord.

gliosome (glī′ō-sōm) [″ + *soma,* body] One of the cytoplasmic granules seen in the endoplasmic reticulum of neuroglia cells.

glipizide (glĭp′ĭ-zīd) An oral drug from the class of medications called sulfonylureas used to lower blood sugar levels in type 2 diabetes mellitus. It is used as part of a regimen that includes regular exercise and a calorically restricted diet. Its side effects may include weight gain and hypoglycemia.

Glisson, Francis (glĭs′ŭn) A British physician and anatomist, 1597–1677.

G.'s capsule The outer capsule of fibrous tissue investing the liver.

G.'s disease Vitamin D deficiency. SEE: *osteomalacia; rickets.*

glissonian cirrhosis An inflammation of the peritoneal coat of the liver. SYN: *perihepatitis.*

glissonitis An inflammation of Glisson's capsule.

Global Assessment of Functioning Scale ABBR: GAF scale. A tool for rating an individual's social, occupational, and psychological functioning from high functioning (i.e., highly adapted and integrated to one's environment) to poorly functioning (i.e., self-destructive, homicidal, isolated, or lacking the rudiments of self-care).

Global Assessment of Relational Functioning Scale ABBR: GARF scale. A measure of the degree to which a family meets the emotional and functional needs of its members.

global warming The effect of increasing levels of greenhouse gases, including carbon dioxide, to cause the temperature of the earth to increase. Global warming can adversely affect many biological systems, including that of human health (e.g., by allowing tropical disease vectors to spread to temperate climates). SEE: *greenhouse effect; ozone*.

globi (glō′bī) [L.] Pl. of globus.

globin (glō′bĭn) [L. *globus,* globe] **1.** A protein constituent of hemoglobin. **2.** One of a particular group of proteins.

globoid (glō′boyd) [″ + Gr. *eidos,* form, shape] Resembling a globe. SYN: *spheroid*.

globular (glŏb′ū-lăr) [L. *globus,* a globe] Resembling a globe or globule; spherical.

globule (glŏb′ūl) [L. *globulus,* globule] Any small, rounded body.

globulin (glŏb′ū-lĭn) [L. *globulus,* globule] One of the group of plasma proteins that controls colloidal osmotic pressure (oncotic pressure) within capillaries, participates in the immune response, and binds with substances to transport them in blood. Globulins make up approximately 38% of all plasma proteins. Alpha globulins transport bilirubin and steroids; beta globulins carry copper and iron. Gamma globulins, the most common, are immunoglobulins (antibodies). SEE: *antibody; immunoglobulin; oncotic pressure*.

Ac g. Accelerator globulin; a globulin present in blood serum that speeds up the conversion of prothrombin to thrombin in the presence of thromboplastin and calcium ions.

antihemophilic g. Antihemophilic factor.

antilymphocyte g. ABBR: ALG. A solution containing polyclonal antibodies, created by injecting animals with human lymphocytes, which is used as a nonspecific immunosuppressant in the treatment of transplant rejection. Because it is polyclonal, ALG is active against many antigens; in contrast, monoclonal antibodies act against one specific antigen only. SEE: *polyclonal antibody*.

antithymocyte g. An agent used for immunosuppression in organ transplantation.

gamma g. The name commonly used for immune globulin, a solution containing antibodies (immunoglobulins) to specific organisms that are obtained from human blood plasma of donors; most of these antibodies are gamma class (IgG). It is used to provide immediate, short-term protection against specific infectious diseases, such as measles, diphtheria, hepatitis A and B, varicella, and respiratory syncytial virus (RSV) if antibody-specific immune globulins are unavailable. It also is used to treat autoimmune illnesses, such as idiopathic thrombocytopenic purpura and Guillain-Barré syndrome. Intravenous immune globulin (IVIG) is also called immunoglobulin. SYN: *immune g.* SEE: *antibody; globulin; immunoglobulin*.

immune g. Gamma g.

Rh immune g. A solution of gamma globulin containing anti-Rh; it is given to Rh-negative women at 28 weeks' gestation to minimize the potential for sensitization secondary to transplacental bleeding. The injection is repeated within 72 hours after delivery of an Rh-positive newborn if the mother's indirect and the newborn's direct Coombs tests are negative. The globulin also should be given to Rh-negative women after spontaneous or induced abortion. Previously called *Rho(D) immune globulin*.

Rh_o(D) immune g. Rh immune g.

serum g. Any of the globulins present in blood plasma or serum. By electrophoresis, they can be separated into alpha, beta, and gamma globulins, which differ in their isoelectric points. SEE: *oncotic pressure*.

varicella-zoster immune g. ABBR: VZIG. An immune globulin obtained from the blood of healthy persons found to have high antibody titers to varicella zoster. Administration of this gamma globulin provides passive immunity against chickenpox and shingles. SEE: Prevention under *varicella*.

globulinuria (glŏb″ū-lĭn-ū′rē-ă) [L. *globulus,* globule, + Gr. *ouron,* urine] Globulin in the urine.

globulose (glŏb′ū-lōs) [L. *globulus,* globule] Protein produced by the digestion of globulins.

globus [L.] A globe or sphere.

g. hystericus A lump in the throat felt as a choking sensation in anxiety, hypertension, or panic attacks.

g. major The head of the epididymis.

g. minor The lower end of the epididymis.

g. pallidus A pale section within the lenticular nucleus of the brain. SEE: *paleostriatum*.

glomangioma (glō-măn″jē-ō′mă) [L. *glomus,* a ball, + Gr. *angeion,* vessel, + *oma,* tumor] A benign tumor that develops from an arteriovenous glomus (cluster of blood cells) of the skin.

glomectomy (glō-mĕk′tō-mē) The surgical removal of a glomus.

glomerate (glŏm′ĕr-āt) [L. *glomerare,* to wind into a ball] Conglomerate, clustered, grouped.

glomerular (glō-mĕr′ū-lăr) [L. *glomerulus,* little ball] Pert. to a glomerulus; clustered.

glomerular disease Any of a large group of diseases that affect the glomerulus of the kidneys. They may be classified by clinical severity, by histological changes in the kidney, or by etiology. Etiological factors include *primary glomerular disease;* disease secondary to *systemic disease,* such as lupus erythematosus or polyarteritis; *infectious disease* such as streptococcal infection, malaria, syphilis, or schistosomiasis; *metabolic disease* such as diabetes or amyloidosis; *toxins* such as mercury, gold, or snake venom; *serum sickness;* and drug *hypersensitivity.*

Glomerular disease may also be associated with hereditary disorders (e.g., Alport's syndrome, Fabry's disease). SEE: *glomerulonephritis; kidney; nephritis; nephrotic syndrome.*

Clinical findings are those associated with the primary dysfunction and pathological changes in the glomerulus, which include proteinuria and hypertension. If protein loss exceeds 5 g/day, the nephrotic syndrome will develop.

glomerulitis (glō-mĕr″ū-lī′tĭs) [″ + Gr. *itis,* inflammation] An inflammation of glomeruli, esp. of the renal glomeruli.

glomerulonephritis (glō-mĕr″ū-lō-nĕ-frī′tĭs) [″ + Gr. *nephros,* kidney, + *itis,* inflammation] A form of nephritis in which the lesions involve primarily the glomeruli. This condition may be acute, subacute, or chronic. Acute glomerulonephritis, also known as acute nephritic syndrome, frequently follows infections, esp. those of the upper respiratory tract caused by particular strains of streptococci. It may also be caused by systemic lupus erythematosus, subacute bacterial endocarditis, cryoglobulinemia, various forms of vasculitis including polyarteritis nodosa, Henoch-Schönlein purpura, and visceral abscess. The condition is characterized by hematuria, proteinuria, red cell casts, oliguria, edema, pruritus, nausea, constipation, and hypertension. Investigation of serum complement and renal biopsy facilitates diagnosis and helps to establish the prognosis. SEE: *glomerular disease; glomerulonephritis, rapidly progressive; Nursing Diagnoses Appendix.*

PATIENT CARE: Serum creatinine, blood urea nitrogen, and urine creatinine clearance levels are monitored, and the patient is assessed for electrolyte and acid-base imbalance. Fluid balance is monitored, and changes in the amount of edema, daily weight, and fluid intake and output are documented. Vital signs are monitored every 4 hr or as necessary, and skin is inspected for signs of breakdown. Skin care and frequent repositioning are provided.

The patient is instructed to limit activities during acute periods of hematuria, azotemia, gross edema, and hypertension; but self-care is encouraged as acute symptoms subside, depending on fatigue levels and changes in blood pressure. Appropriate activities are encouraged. Instruction is provided in dietary and fluid restrictions; the importance of low-sodium, high-calorie meals with adequate (though at times restricted) protein content is stressed. Prescribed medications should be taken as scheduled.

The patient should avoid individuals with communicable illnesses and should report signs of infection, particularly urinary tract infections, immediately. The importance of keeping follow-up appointments is stressed. The patient's response is monitored, and the patient with severe renal dysfunction is prepared for dialysis.

rapidly progressive g. ABBR: RPGN. Any glomerular disease in which there is rapid loss of renal function, usually with crescent-shaped lesions in more than 50% of the glomeruli.

glomerulopathy (glō-mĕr″ū-lŏp′ă-thē) Any disease of the renal glomeruli. SEE: *glomerular disease.*

glomerulosclerosis (glō-mĕr″ū-lō-sklē-rō′sĭs) Fibrosis of renal glomeruli associated with protein loss in the urine; the loss of protein may be massive.

diabetic g. A type of glomerulosclerosis seen in some cases of diabetes mellitus. Eosinophilic material is present in various parts of the glomerulus. SYN: *intercapillary g.*

focal segmental g. An irreversible form of glomerular injury often seen in patients with a history of injection drug use or acquired immunodeficiency syndrome.

intercapillary g. Diabetic g.

glomerulus (glō-mĕr′ū-lŭs) *pl.* **glomeruli** [L.] **1.** One of the capillary networks that are part of the renal corpuscles in the nephrons of the kidney. Each is surrounded by a Bowman's capsule, the site of renal (glomerular) filtration, which is the first step in the formation of urine. SEE: *kidney* for illus. **2.** A group of twisted capillaries or nerve fibers.

olfactory g. A neural network found in the olfactory bulb, formed by the dendrites of mitral cells intertwined with the axons of olfactory receptor cells.

glomoid (glō′moyd) Appearing similar to a glomus.

glomus (glō′mŭs) [L., a ball] A small, round swelling made of tiny blood vessels and found in stromata containing many nerve fibers.

g. caroticum Carotid body.

g. choroideum An enlargement of the choroid plexus at its entrance into the lateral ventricle.

g. coccygeum The coccygeal body.

periodontal g. The sensory endings of the periodontal ligament that provide acute sensitivity.

gloss- SEE: *glosso-.*

glossa [Gr. *glossa,* tongue] The tongue.

glossal Rel. to the tongue.

glossalgia (glŏs-săl′jē-ă) [″+ *algos,* pain] Glossodynia.

glossectomy (glŏs-ĕk′tō-mē) [″ + *ektome,* excision] Surgical excision of the tongue.

Glossina (glŏs-sī′nă) A genus of flies called tsetse flies, which includes about 20 species of bloodsucking flies that are confined principally to central and southern Africa. They transmit the trypanosomes *(Trypanosoma gambiense, T. rhodesiense),* the causative agents of sleeping sickness in humans, and other trypanosomes that infect wild and domestic animals. Important species are *Glossina palpalis, G. morsitans, G. tachinoides,* and *G. swynnertoni.* SEE: *sleeping sickness; Trypanosoma.*

glossitis (glŏs-sī′tĭs) [″ + *itis,* inflammation] An inflammation of the tongue.

acute g. Glossitis that develops in hours or days, often associated with stomatitis. The tongue is painful, red, inflamed, and swollen. It may appear smooth or be covered with papular lesions. Fever may be present.

ETIOLOGY: It may be associated with diabetes mellitus, bacterial infections, candidal infections, adverse drug reactions, smoking, and trauma to the tongue. Surrounding structures may be swollen sufficiently to produce asphyxia. Tracheostomy may be necessary to maintain the airway.

TREATMENT: The underlying disorder must be treated. In order to maintain oral cleanliness, patients should rinse the mouth with an anesthetic oral solution, such as 2% xylocaine.

PROGNOSIS: Prognosis is excellent if treatment of the underlying condition is successful.

g. areata exfoliativa A condition of the tongue marked by numerous denuded patches on the dorsal surface coalescing into freeform shapes similar to the geographic areas on a map. SYN: *geographic tongue.*

g. desiccans A painful, raw, and fissured tongue.

herpetic geometric g. Herpes simplex virus type 1 infection of the tongue. This may be seen in immunocompromised patients. High-dose acyclovir is an effective treatment.

median rhomboid g. An inflammatory area, somewhat diamond-shaped, found on the dorsum of the tongue anterior to the vallate papillae.

Moeller's g. [Julius O. L. Moeller, Ger. surgeon, 1819–1887] A chronic superficial glossitis characterized by burning or pain and an increased sensitivity to hot and spicy foods. SYN: *glossodynia exfoliativa.*

g. parasitica SEE: *tongue, hairy.*

glosso-, gloss- [Gr. *glossa,* tongue] Combining form meaning *tongue.*

glossocele (glŏs′sō-sēl) [″ + *kele,* swelling] A swelling and protrusion of the tongue resulting from disease or malformation.

glossodynamometer (glŏs″sō-dī″nă-mŏm′ĕ-tĕr) [″ + *dynamis,* power, + *metron,* measure] A device for measuring the strength of the tongue muscles.

glossodynia (glŏs″ō-dĭn′ē-ă) [″ + *odyne,* pain] Pain in the tongue. SYN: *glossalgia.* SEE: *burning mouth syndrome.*

g. exfoliativa Moeller's glossitis.

glossoepiglottic (glŏs″ō-ĕp-ĭ-glŏt′ĭk) [″ + *epi,* upon, + *glottis,* back of tongue] Pert. to the ligament between the base of the tongue and the epiglottis.

glossoepiglottidean (glŏs″ō-ĕp-ĭ-glŏ-tĭd′ē-ăn) Rel. to the tongue and epiglottis.

glossograph (glŏs′ō-grăf) [″ + *graphein,* to write] An instrument for recording the tongue's movements during speech.

glossohyal (glŏs″ō-hī′ăl) [″ + *hyoeides,* U-shaped] Rel. to the tongue and hyoid bone. SYN: *hyoglossal.*

glossokinesthetic (glŏs″ō-kĭn″ĕs-thĕt′ĭk) [″ + *kinesis,* movement, + *aisthetikos,* perceptive] Pert. to movements of the tongue, esp. those in speech.

glossolabial (glŏs″ō-lā′bē-ăl) [″ + L. *labium,* lip] Pert. to the tongue and lips.

glossolalia (glŏs″ō-lā′lē-ă) [″ + *lalia,* babble] The repetition of senseless remarks not related to the subject or situation involved.

glossology (glŏ-sŏl′ō-jē) [″ + *logos,* word, reason] The study of the tongue and its diseases. SYN: *glottology.*

glossopalatine (glŏs″ō-păl′ă-tīn) Pert. to the tongue and palate.

glossopathy (glŏs-sŏp′ă-thē) [″ + *pathos,* disease, suffering] Any disease of the tongue.

glossopharyngeal (glŏs″ō-fă-rĭn′jē-ăl) [″ + *pharynx,* throat] Rel. to the tongue and pharynx.

glossopharyngeal breathing A technique of breathing in which the patient with inspiratory muscle weakness increases the volume of air breathed in by taking several "gulps" of air, closing the mouth, and forcing air into the lungs.

glossoplasty (glŏs′ō-plăs″tē) [″ + *plassein,* to form] Reparative surgery of the tongue.

glossoplegia (glŏs″ō-plē′jē-ă) [″ + *plege,* stroke] Paralysis of the tongue, usually unilateral, which may result from cerebral hemorrhage, disease, or injury that involves the hypoglossal nerve.

glossoptosis (glŏs″ŏp-tō′sĭs) [″ + *ptosis,* a dropping] A dropping of the tongue downward out of normal position.

glossopyrosis (glŏs″ō-pī-rō′sĭs) [″ + *pyrosis,* a burning] A burning sensation of the tongue. SEE: *burning mouth syndrome.*

glossorrhaphy (glŏ-sor′ă-fē) [″ + *rhaphe,* seam, ridge] Suture of a wound of the tongue.

glossospasm (glŏs′ō-spăzm) [″ + *spasmos,* spasm] The spasmodic contraction of the muscles of the tongue.

glossotomy (glŏ-sŏt′ō-mē) [″ + *tome,* incision] An incision of the tongue.

glossotrichia (glŏs″ō-trĭk′ē-ă) [″ + *thrix,* hair] SEE: *tongue, hairy.*

glossy Smooth and shining.

glottic [Gr. *glottis,* back of tongue] Of or pert. to the tongue or glottis.

glottis (glŏt′ĭs) *pl.* **glottises or glottides** [Gr. *glottis,* back of tongue] The sound-producing apparatus of the larynx consisting of the two vocal cords and the intervening space, the rima glottidis. A leaf-shaped lid of cartilage (the epiglottis) protects this opening. SEE: illus.

edema of the g. Pathological accumulation of fluid in the tissues lining the vocal structures of the larynx. It may result from improper use of the voice, excessive use of tobacco or alcohol, chemical fumes, or viral, bacterial, or fungal infections. Clinically, the patient often presents with hoarseness or, in severe cases, with respiratory distress and stridor. SEE: *epiglottitis.*

SYMPTOMS: Initially hoarseness, and later complete aphonia, characterize this condition. Other symptoms are extreme dyspnea, at first on inspiration only, but later on expiration also; stridor; and a barking cough when the epiglottis is involved.

glottology (glŏ-tŏl′ō-jē) [″ + *logos,* word, reason] Glossology.

glove A protective covering for the hand. In medical care the glove is made of a flexible impervious material that permits full movement of the hand and fingers. Gloves are used to protect both the operative site from contamination with organisms from the health care worker and the health care worker from contamination with pathogens from the patient. These factors are particularly important when the patient has a disease such as hepatitis B or AIDS. SEE: *Standard and Universal Precautions Appendix.*

CAUTION: It is not advisable to wash gloves and wear them again while treating another patient.

---

edema control g. An elastic pressure-gradient glove designed to facilitate tissue healing following hand injury.

gloving Placing of gloves on the hands. During physical examination and invasive procedures, such as phlebotomy or surgery, this is done to protect both caregiver and patient from transmissible diseases.

gluc- SEE: *gluco-.*

glucagon (gloo′kă-gŏn) A polypeptide hormone secreted by the alpha cells of the pancreas that increases the blood glucose level by stimulating the liver to change stored glycogen to glucose. Glucagon opposes the action of insulin, and it is used as an injection in diabetes to reverse hypoglycemic reactions and insulin shock. It also increases the use of fats and excess amino acids for energy production. It is obtained from pork and beef pancreas glands. Parenteral administration of glucagon relaxes the smooth muscle of the stomach, duodenum, small bowel, and colon.

glucagonoma (glū″kă-gŏn-ō′mă) A malignant tumor of the alpha cells of the pancreatic islets of Langerhans. The principal signs and symptoms include weight loss, diabetes mellitus, skin rash, glossitis, elevated serum glucagon levels, and anemia. The treatment is surgical excision or octreotide.

gluco-, gluc- Combining form denoting relationship to sweetness. SEE: *glyco-.*

glucocerebroside (gloo″kō-sĕr′ĕ-brō-sīd″) A cerebroside with the carbohydrate glucose contained in the molecule; ac-

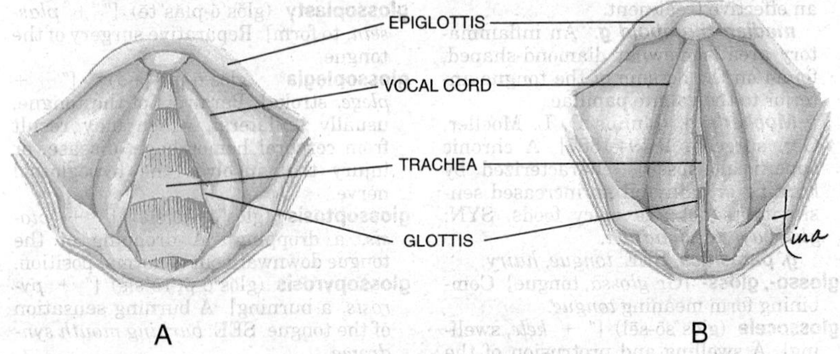

GLOTTIS AND VOCAL CORDS

(A) during breathing, (B) during speaking

cumulates in tissues in individuals with Gaucher's disease.

glucocorticoid (gloo″kō-kort′ĭ-koyd) [Gr. *gleukos,* sweet (new wine), + L. *cortex,* + Gr. *eidos,* form, shape] A general classification of adrenal cortical hormones that are primarily active in protecting against stress and in affecting protein and carbohydrate metabolism. The most important glucocorticoid is cortisol (hydrocortisone). SEE: *mineralocorticoid.*

glucofuranose (gloo″kō-fū′ră-nōs) The form of glucose containing the furanose ring.

glucogenesis (gloo″kō-jĕn′ĕ-sĭs) The formation of glucose.

glucokinase (gloo″kō-kī′nās) An enzyme in liver cells that, in the presence of ATP, catalyzes the conversion of glucose to glucose-6-phosphate. This is the first step in glycolysis, the breakdown of glucose to two molecules of pyruvic acid.

glucokinetic (gloo″kō-kī-nĕt′ĭk) Acting to maintain the blood glucose level.

Glucometer A battery-operated device used to measure blood glucose from a few drops of blood obtained from the finger.

gluconeogenesis (gloo″kō-nē″ō-jĕn′ĕ-sĭs) [″ + *neos,* new, + *genesis,* generation, birth] The formation of glucose from excess amino acids, fats, or other noncarbohydrate sources.

glucopenia, glycopenia (gloo″kō-pē′nē-ă) [″ + Gr. *penia,* lack] Hypoglycemia.

glucopenic brain injury Neuroglycopenia.

glucoprotein (gloo″kō-prō′tē-ĭn) Glycoprotein.

glucopyranose (gloo″kō-pī′ră-nōs) The form of glucose containing the six-carbon pyran ring.

glucosamine (gloo″kō-săm′ēn) A health food supplement used in the treatment of pain caused by osteoarthritis. It has about the same strength as low-dose ibuprofen, but does not cause the same gastrointestinal and renal side effects. This agent has not undergone extensive evaluation by health regulatory agencies in the U.S.

glucose (gloo′kōs) [Gr. *gleukos,* sweet (new wine)] A simple sugar or monosaccharide, $C_6H_{12}O_6$, that is the end product of carbohydrate digestion. Its right-handed (dextrorotatory) isomer (D-glucose) serves as a primary energy source for living organisms. Glucose is found naturally in fruits and other plants. It is also formed during digestion from the hydrolysis of disaccharides and polysaccharides. After absorption by the small intestine, the portal vein carries glucose to the liver, where it may be stored as the starch called glycogen. Within cells, glucose is used to synthesize the pentose sugars, ribose and deoxyribose, for RNA and DNA, respectively. SYN: *dextrose.* SEE: *carbohydrate.*

In healthy people, normal blood glucose levels are maintained at about 70 to 110 mg/dl. Lower blood glucose levels (hypoglycemia) may cause confusion, anxiety, or other neurological complications. Higher blood glucose levels (hyperglycemia) may result in the "sugar-coating" (glycosylation) of body tissues. Hyperglycemia is characteristic of diabetes mellitus (which is diagnosed when a fasting patient has a blood glucose level exceeding 126 mg/dl); hypoglycemia may result from starvation, the treatment of diabetes mellitus, or rarely, insulin-secreting tumors of the pancreas.

GLUCOSE METABOLISM: Within most cells, glucose is the primary energy source and is oxidized in cell respiration to carbon dioxide and water to produce energy in the form of adenosine triphosphate (ATP). The stages of cell respiration are glycolysis, which uses enzymes in the cell cytoplasm, and the Krebs cycle and the cytochrome transport system, which take place in the mitochondria. Insulin enables cells to take in glucose for use in energy production. Excess glucose may be converted to glycogen and stored in the liver and muscles; insulin and cortisol facilitate this process. The hormone glycogen (and epinephrine in stress situations) stimulates the liver to change glycogen back to glucose when the blood glucose level decreases. Any further excess glucose is converted to fat and stored in adipose tissue.

When the glucose level is below normal, fat stores are metabolized. Incomplete metabolism of fats leads to the formation of ketone bodies, also a symptom of diabetes. Blood glucose acts as a protein sparer. Nervous tissue is esp. dependent on glucose as its source of energy, the brain being able to oxidize glucose directly.

blood level of g. The glucose found in the bloodstream. SEE: *glucose.*

capillary blood g. ABBR: CBG. The level of circulating blood glucose as measured by glucometer analysis of a fingerstick sample. Regular measurements of CBG allow diabetic patients to participate actively in their own health management. SYN: *finger stick blood g.*

finger stick blood g. ABBR: FSBG. Capillary blood g.

liquid g. A thick, syrupy, sweet-tasting liquid obtained from the incomplete hydrolysis of starch, containing D-glucose (dextrose), dextrins, and other carbohydrates. It is used for nutritive purposes and in various pharmaceutical and food preparations.

glucose-6-phosphate dehydrogenase ABBR: G6PD. An enzyme that dehydrogenates glucose-6-phosphate to form 6-phospho-D-glucono-δ-lactone. This is the initial step in the pentose phosphate pathway of glucose catabolism.

glucose-6-phosphate dehydrogenase deficiency An inherited disorder that is transmitted as an autosomal recessive trait. It is present in the U.S. in about 13% of black males and 2% of black females. The enzyme deficiency also occurs in Arabic, Mediterranean, and Asian ethnic groups. The enzyme is essential to maintaining the integrity of red blood cells, thus a deficiency of it causes nonimmune hemolytic anemia. There are many variants of the enzyme and great variation in severity of the disease. Some individuals do not have clinical symptoms until they are exposed to certain drugs such as antimalarials, antipyretics, sulfonamides, or to fava beans, or when they contract an infectious disease. In others the condition is present at birth. When present at birth, anemia, hepatomegaly, hypoglycemia, and interference with growth are present. In those who have the deficiency but are not affected until exposed to certain drugs or infections, hemolytic anemia and jaundice occur.

DIAGNOSIS: The clinical condition may not be diagnostic, but laboratory tests for evidence of the enzyme deficiency are available.

TREATMENT: The only treatment is avoidance of drugs known to cause hemolysis and avoidance of fava beans if the individual is known to be sensitive to them.

glucose polymer A glucose saccharide mixture of 3% glucose, 7% maltose, 5% maltotriose, and 85% polysaccharides of 4 to 15 glucose units, used in oral glucose tolerance tests.

glucosidase (gloo-kō′sĭ-dās) An enzyme that catalyzes the hydrolysis of a glucoside.

glucoside (gloo′kō-sīd) A glycoside that on hydrolysis yields a sugar, glucose, and one or two additional products. Glucosides are numerous and widely distributed in plants. Many glucosides have medicinal properties (e.g., digitalin and strophanthin, present in digitalis and strophanthus, respectively, which have a specific effect on the heart). SEE: *glycoside*.

glucosuria (gloo″kō-sū′rē-ă) [″ + *ouron,* urine] Glycosuria.

β-glucuronidase (gloo″kū-rŏn′ĭ-dās) An enzyme that splits glycosidic linkages in glucuronides. It is involved in cell division.

glucuronide (gloo-kū′rŏn-īd) The combination of glucuronic acid with phenol, alcohol, or any acid containing the carboxyl, ⁻COOH, group.

glucuronyl transferase An enzyme that converts unconjugated or indirect bilirubin to conjugated or direct bilirubin.

glue-sniffing The inhalation of vapor from types of glue or solvents that contain toxic chemicals such as benzene, toluene, or xylene. This may produce an altered state of consciousness and occasionally death.

Gluge's corpuscles (gloo′gēz) [Gottlieb Gluge, Ger. pathologist, 1812–1898] Granular cells containing fat droplets, usually found in degenerating nervous tissue.

glutamate (gloo′tă-māt) A salt of glutamic acid that functions as the brain's main excitatory neurotransmitter.

glutaminase (gloo-tăm′ĭ-nās) An enzyme that catalyzes the breakdown of glutamine into glutamic acid and ammonia.

glutamine (gloo′tă-mĭn, -mēn″) A nonessential amino acid thought to play a major role in maintaining the integrity of the gastrointestinal mucosa, esp. during the hypermetabolic phase of the stress response. By enhancing cellular proliferation, it may reduce the incidence of bacterial translocation from the gut and improve absorption from the mucosa.

γ-glutamyl transpeptidase A tissue enzyme that is elevated in patients with many conditions involving hepatic damage, including that induced by alcohol; in patients with renal disease, pancreatitis, diabetes mellitus, coronary artery disease, or carcinoma of the prostate; and in individuals taking phenytoin and barbiturates.

glutaral (gloo′tă-răl) A solution of glutaraldehyde in sterile water.

glutaraldehyde (gloo″tă-răl′dĕ-hīd) **1.** A sterilizing agent effective against all microorganisms including viruses and spores. **2.** An excellent primary fixative agent for electron microscopy, usually followed by osmium in the preparation of material for transmission electron microscopy.

glutathione (gloo-tă-thī′ōn) [″ + Gr. *theion,* sulfur] $C_{10}H_{17}N_3O_6S$; a tripeptide of glutamic acid, cysteine, and glycine. Found in small quantities in active animal tissues, it takes up and gives off hydrogen and is fundamentally important in cellular respiration.

PATIENT CARE: Overdose with acetaminophen depletes glutathione resources in the liver, resulting in hepatic failure. This toxic effect can be reversed by giving acetylcysteine to the intoxicated patient.

reduced g. The form of glutaraldehyde present in red blood cells. It detoxifies hydrogen peroxide that forms either spontaneously or after drug administration, thus protecting red cells from injury due to this substance.

gluteal (gloo′tē-ăl) [Gr. *gloutos,* buttock] Pert. to the buttocks.

gluten [L., glue] Vegetable albumin, a

protein that can be prepared from wheat and other grain.

gluten-sensitive enteropathy Celiac sprue.

glutethimide (gloo-tĕth′ĭ-mīd) A hypnotic drug. Trade name is Doriden.

glutinous (gloo′tĭn-ŭs) [L. *glutinosus*, glue] Adhesive; sticky.

glutitis [Gr. *gloutos*, buttock, + *itis*, inflammation] An inflammation of the muscles of the buttocks.

glyburide (glī′bū-rīd) An oral drug, from the class of medications called sulfonylureas, used to lower blood sugars in type 2 diabetes mellitus. It should be used as part of a coordinated care plan that includes regular exercise and a diabetic diet. The side effects of glyburide include weight gain and excessively low blood sugars.

glyc- SEE: *glyco-*.

glycan Polysaccharide.

glycase (glī′kās) [Gr. *glykys*, sweet] The enzyme that converts maltose into dextrose. SEE: *enzyme*.

glycation (glī′kā-shŭn) The binding of a sugar molecule to an amino acid. In hyperglycemia and poorly controlled diabetes mellitus, sugar molecules become attached to cell surface proteins throughout the body; this sugar coating leads to microvascular damage in nerves, nephrons, and the retina.

advanced g. end products ABBR: AGE. Proteins that have been nonenzymatically modified by the addition of sugar residues to lysine. These altered proteins increase with aging, and in patients with hyperglycemia and diabetes mellitus. **glycated,** *adj.*

glycemia (glī-sē′mē-ă) [″ + *haima*, blood] Sugar or glucose in the blood.

DL-glyceraldehyde (glĭs″ĕr-ăl′dĕ-hīd) An aldose, $CHOCH(OH)CH_2OH$, produced by the metabolism of fructose in the liver.

glyceride (glĭs′ĕr-īd) [Gr. *glykys*, sweet] An ester of glycerin compounded with an acid.

glycerin (glĭs′ĕr-ĭn) $C_3H_8O_3$; a trihydric alcohol, trihydroxy-propane, present in chemical combination in all fats. It is a syrupy colorless liquid, soluble in all proportions in water and alcohol. It is made commercially by the hydrolysis of fats, esp. during the manufacture of soap, and is used extensively as a solvent, a preservative, and an emollient in various skin diseases. Given orally, it reduces intracranial pressure and, preoperatively, reduces intraocular pressure in glaucoma. SYN: *glycerol*.

glycerol (glĭs′ĕr-ŏl) [Gr. *glykys*, sweet] Glycerin.

glyceryl (glĭs′ĕr-ĭl) The trivalent radical C_3H_5 of glycerol.

g. monostearate An emulsifying agent used in preparing creams and ointments.

g. triacetate The previously used name for triacetin.

g. trinitrate Nitroglycerin; a valuable medicine used to treat an angina pectoris attack or to prevent one if given before exercise.

NOTE: Tablets should be stored in tightly sealed, dark containers to prevent loss of potency.

glycine (glī′sēn, -sĭn) [Gr. *glykys*, sweet] NH_2CH_2COOH; a nonessential amino acid. SYN: *aminoacetic acid*.

glyco-, glyc- (glī-kō) [Gr. *glykys*, sweet] Combining form indicating a relationship to sugars or the presence of glycerol or a similar substance. SEE: also *gluco-*.

glycocalyx (glī″kō-kăl′ĭks) **1.** A thin layer of glycoprotein and oligosaccharides on the outer surface of cell membranes that contributes to cell adhesion and forms antigens involved in the recognition of "self." **2.** An adhesive substance secreted by microorganisms such as *Staphylococcus epidermidis* that helps them to adhere to prosthetic material in the body and prevents their phagocytosis by white blood cells.

glycocholate (glī″kō-kŏl′āt) A salt of glycocholic acid.

glycoclastic (glī″kō-klăs′tĭk) [″ + *klan*, to break] Pert. to the hydrolysis and digestion of sugars.

glycogen (glī′kŏ-jĕn) [″ + *gennan*, to produce] A polysaccharide, $(C_6H_{10}O_5)x$, commonly called animal starch, a whitish powder that can be prepared from mammalian liver and muscle and other animal tissues. Formation of glycogen from carbohydrate sources is called glycogenesis; from noncarbohydrate sources, glyconeogenesis. The conversion of glycogen to glucose is called glycogenolysis. SEE: *glycogen storage disease; glyconeogenesis*.

Glycogen is the form in which excess carbohydrate is stored in the liver and muscles; the hormones insulin and cortisol facilitate this process. When the blood glucose level decreases, the liver converts glycogen to glucose; this process is facilitated by the hormone glucagon or, in stressful situations, by epinephrine. In cells, glucose is oxidized to carbon dioxide and water with the release of energy in the forms of ATP and heat. In muscle cells under anaerobic conditions, glucose is metabolized only to lactic acid, and oxygen is needed to convert lactic acid back to glucose, primarily in the liver.

glycogenase (glī-kō′jĕn-ās) A liver enzyme that converts glycogen to glucose.

glycogenesis (glī″kō-jĕn′ĕ-sĭs) [″ + *genesis*, generation, birth] The formation of glycogen from glucose. SEE: *glyconeogenesis*.

glycogenetic Pert. to the formation of glycogen.

glycogenic Rel. to glycogen.
glycogenolysis (glī″kō-jĕn-ŏl′ĭ-sĭs) [″ + *gennan,* to produce, + *lysis,* dissolution] Conversion of glycogen into glucose in the liver and muscles.
glycogenolytic (glī″kō-jĕn″ŏ-lĭt′ĭk) [″ + ″ + *lysis,* dissolution] Pert. to the hydrolysis of glycogen.
glycogenosis (glī″kō-jĕn-ō′sĭs) [″ + ″ + *osis,* condition] A disorder associated with an abnormal accumulation of normal or abnormal forms of glycogen in tissue.
glycogen storage disease Any one of several heritable diseases characterized by the abnormal storage and accumulation of glycogen in the tissues, esp. in the liver. These diseases are grouped into various types according to the enzyme deficiency responsible.

phosphorylase b kinase deficiency g.s.d. A form of glycogen storage disease caused by an x-linked deficiency of the kinase that activates phosphorylase. Previously called type VIa, VIII, or IX.

g.s.d. type Ia A form of glycogen storage disease with onset usually in the first year of life. This autosomal recessive genetic disorder is due to a glucose-6-phosphatase deficiency. SYN: *von Gierke disease.*

g.s.d. type Ib A form of glycogen storage disease similar to type Ia but occurring at only one tenth its frequency. The disorder is due to a deficiency of glucose-6-phosphatase microsomal translocase.

g.s.d. type II A form of glycogen storage disease caused by a deficiency of lysosomal α-glucosidase.

g.s.d. type III A form of glycogen storage disease caused by a deficiency of two debranching enzymes in liver and muscle tissues.

g.s.d. type IV A congenital glycogen storage disease marked by liver failure, muscular weakness, muscular contractures, and death in the first few years of life SYN: *Andersen's disease; branching enzyme deficiency.*

g.s.d. type V A form of glycogen storage disease caused by a muscle phosphorylase deficiency. SYN: *McArdle's disease.*

g.s.d. type VI A form of glycogen storage disease caused by a deficiency of liver phosphorylase and characterized by growth retardation, hepatomegaly, hypoglycemia, and acidosis.

g.s.d. type VII A form of glycogen storage disease caused by a deficiency of muscle phosphofructokinase and characterized by muscular weakness and cramping following exercise.

glycogeusia (glī″kō-jū′sē-ă) [Gr. *glykys,* sweet, + *geusis,* taste] A sweet taste.
glycohemoglobin Glycosylated hemoglobin.
glycol (glī′kōl, -kŏl) [″ + *alcohol*] Any one of the dihydric alcohols related to ethylene glycol, $C_2H_6O_2$.

PATIENT CARE: The glycols, including ethylene and propylene glycol, are found in many antifreezes, solvents, detergents, and lacquers, and their ingestion is a common cause of accidental poisoning in the U.S. The intoxicated patient should be treated by decontaminating the stomach in order to decrease uptake of the chemical. Sodium bicarbonate is also given if metabolic acidosis develops. Seizures, brain damage, ophthalmic injury, and renal failure are common complications of exposure. Support of the patient often includes parenteral administration of thiamine and other vitamins, as well as of alcohol dehydrogenase inhibitors.

glycolipid(e) (glī″kō-lĭp′ĭd) [″ + *lipos,* fat] A compound of fatty acids with a carbohydrate, containing nitrogen but not phosphoric acid. It is found in the myelin sheath of nerves.
glycolysis (glī-kŏl′ĭ-sĭs) [″ + *lysis,* dissolution] **1.** The series of reactions that convert a molecule of glucose into two molecules of pyruvic acid. **2.** The first stage of the cell respiration of a molecule of glucose, releasing a small amount of energy in the form of ATP.
glycolytic Pert. to glucose hydrolysis.
glycometabolism (glī″kō-mĕ-tăb′ŏ-lĭzm) Use of glucose by the body. SEE: *metabolism.*
glyconeogenesis (glī″kō-nē″ŏ-jĕn′ĕ-sĭs) [″ + *neos,* new, + *genesis,* generation, birth] The formation of glycogen from noncarbohydrates such as fat or amino acids from protein. It occurs in the liver under such conditions as low carbohydrate intake or starvation.
glyconucleoprotein (glī″kō-nū″klē-ō-prō′tē-ĭn) [″ + L. *nucleus,* kernel, + Gr. *protos,* first] A nucleoprotein so named to emphasize the presence of glucose units in the substance.
glycopexic (glī″kō-pĕks′ĭk) [″ + *pexis,* fixation] Pert. to the fixing or storing of glucose.
glycopexis (glī″kō-pĕk′sĭs) The storage of glycogen in the liver.
glycophorin (glī″kō-fō′rĭn) A glycoprotein that spans the bilipid layer of the red blood cell membrane. The outside end of this complex substance contains blood group antigens and sites to which some viruses attach. This protein provides the conduit through which anions pass in and out of the red blood cell.
glycopolyuria (glī″kō-pŏl″ē-ū′rē-ă) [″ + *polys,* much, + *ouron,* urine] Diabetes mellitus with moderately increased glucose but greatly increased uric acid in the urine.
glycoprival, glycoprivous (glī″kō-prī′văl, -vŭs) [″ + L. *privus,* deprived of] Lacking in or without carbohydrates.
glycoprotein (glī″kō-prō′tē-ĭn) [″ +

protos, first] A compound consisting of a carbohydrate and protein. SYN: *glucoprotein.*

glycoptyalism (glī″kō-tī′ăl-ĭzm) [″ + *ptyalon,* saliva, + *-ismos,* condition] The excretion of glucose in the saliva. SYN: *melitoptyalism.*

glycopyrrolate (glī″kō-pĭr′rō-lāt) An anticholinergic drug. Trade name is Robinul.

glycorrhachia (glī-kō-rā′kē-ă) [″ + *rhachis,* spine] Glucose in the cerebrospinal fluid.

glycosaminoglycan (glī″kōs-ăme-nō-glī′kăn) A complex polysaccharide found in cartilage, intercellular material, and the basement membranes of epithelial tissues; also called mucopolysaccharide.

glycosecretory (glī″kō-sē-krē′tō-rē) [″ + L. *secretus,* separate] Pert. to or determining the formation of glycogen.

glycosialia (glī″kō-sī-ăl′ē-ă) [″ + *sialon,* saliva] Glucose in the saliva.

glycosialorrhea (glī″kō-sī″ăl-ō-rē′ă) [″ + ″ + *rhoia,* flow] Excessive secretion of saliva containing glucose.

glycoside A substance derived from plants that, on hydrolysis, yields a sugar and one or more additional products. Depending on the sugar formed, glycosides are designated glucosides or galactosides. Digitalis is a commonly used cardiac glycoside. SEE: *glucoside.*

glycosphingolipids (glī″kō-sfĭng″ō-lĭp′ĭds) A group of carbohydrate-containing fatty acid derivatives of ceramide. Three classes of these lipids are cerebrosides, gangliosides, and ceramide oligosaccharides. When the enzymes essential to the metabolism of these compounds are absent, the glycosphingolipids accumulate, particularly in the nervous system. Death is the usual outcome.

glycostatic (glī″kō-stăt′ĭk) [Gr. *glykys,* sweet, + *statikos,* standing] Acting to maintain the level of glucose in the body.

glycosuria (glī″kō-sū′rē-ă) [″ + *ouron,* urine] An abnormal amount of glucose in the urine. Traces of sugar, particularly glucose, may occur in normal urine but are not detected by ordinary qualitative methods. The presence of a reducing sugar found during routine urinalysis is suggestive but not diagnostic of diabetes mellitus. It is found when the blood glucose level exceeds the renal threshold (about 170 mg/dl of blood). The fasting level of blood glucose is normally between 80 and 120 mg/dl of blood. SYN: *glucosuria.* SEE: *diabetes mellitus.*

alimentary g. Glycosuria following ingestion of large amounts of starches or sugars.

diabetic g. Glycosuria resulting from type 1 or type 2 diabetes mellitus.

emotional g. Glycosuria resulting from stress.

phloridzin g. Glycosuria resulting from the injection of phloridzin, which reduces the renal threshold for glucose.

pituitary g. Glycosuria caused by dysfunction of the anterior pituitary.

renal g. Glycosuria occurring when glucose is persistent and not accompanied by hyperglycemia and when the renal threshold for glucose is decreased.

glycosylation (glī″kōs-ī-lā′shŭn) The chemical linkage of sugar molecules to proteins. In diabetes mellitus and some other diseases, excessive levels of glucose in the blood may over time sugar-coat tissues and cells, causing them to function improperly. Glycosylation may injure cytokines, cell receptors, the extracellular matrix, retinas, kidneys, nerves, and arteries, among other tissues.

glycuronuria (glĭ-kū″rō-nū′rē-ă) Glucuronic acid in the urine.

glycyltryptophan (glĭs″ĭl-trĭp′tō-făn) A dipeptide of glycine and tryptophan.

glycyrrhiza (glĭs-ĭ-rī′ză) [″ + *rhiza,* root] The dried root of *Glycyrrhiza glabra,* known commercially as Spanish licorice, used as an ingredient of glycyrrhiza fluidextract and glycyrrhiza syrup, both of which are used as flavoring agents in compounding medicine. This substance has a weak aldosterone-like effect and may therefore increase blood pressure. SEE: *licorice.*

glyoxalase (glē-ōk′să-lās) An enzyme that catalyzes the conversion of methylglyoxal to lactic acid by the addition of water.

glyoxylic acid $C_2H_2O_3$; an acid produced by the action of glycine oxidase on glycine or sarcosine.

GML *glabellomeatal line.*

GNA *geriatric nursing assistant.*

gnashing (năsh′ing) Grinding, as of the teeth. SEE: *bruxism.*

gnat (năt) Any of a number of small insects belonging to the order Diptera, suborder Orthorrhapha, including black flies, midges, and sandflies. It applies generally to insects smaller than mosquitoes.

buffalo g. A small dipterous insect belonging to the genus *Simulium.*

gnath- SEE: *gnatho-.*

gnathalgia (năth-ăl′jē-ă) [Gr. *gnathos,* jaw, + *algos,* pain] Pain in the jaw. SYN: *gnathodynia.*

gnathic (năth′ĭk) [Gr. *gnathos,* jaw] Pert. to an alveolar process or to the jaw.

gnathion (năth′ē-ŏn) The lowest point of the middle line of the lower jaw; a craniometric point.

gnathitis (năth-ī′tĭs) [″ + *itis,* inflammation] Inflammation of the jaw or adjacent soft parts.

gnatho-, gnath- (năth′ō) [Gr. *gnathos,*

jaw] Combining form meaning *jaw* or *cheek*.

gnathocephalus (năth″ō-sĕf′ă-lŭs) [″ + *kephale,* head] A malformed fetus in which the head consists principally of the jaws.

gnathodynamometer (năth″ō-dī″nă-mŏm′ĕ-tĕr) [″ + *dynamis,* power, + *metron,* measure] A device for measuring biting force. SYN: *occlusometer.*

gnathodynia (năth″ō-dĭn′ē-ă) [″ + *odyne,* pain] Gnathalgia.

gnathoplasty (năth′ō-plăs″tē) [″ + *plassein,* to form] Reparative surgery of the jaws or cheek.

gnathoschisis (năth-ŏs′kĭ-sĭs) [″ + *schizein,* to split] A congenital jaw cleft.

Gnathostoma (năth-ŏs′tō-mă) [″ + *stoma,* mouth] A genus of nematode worms that infest the stomach walls of domestic and wild animals. They occasionally infest humans.

gnathostomiasis (năth″ō-stō-mī′ă-sĭs) A form of visceral larva migrans infection of human tissues caused by the nematode parasite of dogs and cats, *Gnathostoma spinigerum.* Acquisition is by ingestion of undercooked fish and poultry containing the larvae. The parasite migrates through various body tissues and causes a transient inflammatory response and possibly abscess formation. If the brain is invaded, eosinophilic meningoencephalitis may develop and can be fatal. Travelers to areas such as the Orient where the condition is endemic are advised to avoid eating raw fish or undercooked fish or poultry.

TREATMENT: Therapy consists of surgical removal of lesions and administration of albendazole.

gnosia (nō′sē-ă) [Gr. *gnosis,* knowledge] The perceptive faculty of recognizing persons, things, and forms.

gnotobiotics (nō″tō-bī-ŏt′ĭks) [Gr. *gnotos,* known, + *bios,* life] The study of animals that have been raised in germ-controlled or germ-free surroundings.

Gn-RH *gonadotropin-releasing hormone.*

goal The desired outcome of actions to alter status or behavior. SEE: *nursing goal.*

Godfrey's test A test to identify a tear of the posterior cruciate ligament. With the patient lying supine and the hips flexed to 90 degrees, the examiner lifts both of the patient's lower legs and holds them parallel to the table. The relative position of the lower legs is then observed. Inferior displacement (a downward sagging) of the involved knee can indicate a tear of the posterior cruciate ligament.

goggle-eyed Exophthalmic. SEE: *exophthalmos.*

goiter (goy′tĕr) [L. *guttur,* throat] Thyroid gland enlargement. An enlarged thyroid gland may be caused by thyroiditis, benign thyroid nodules, malignancy, iodine deficiency, or any condition that causes hyperfunction or hypofunction of the gland. SEE: illus.

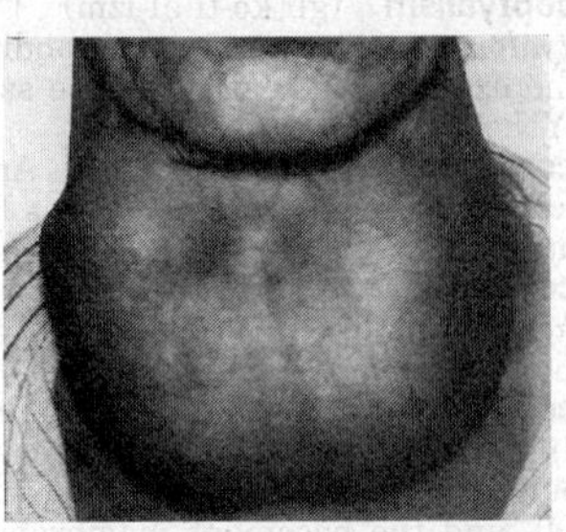

MASSIVE GOITER

aberrant g. A supernumerary goiter.

acute g. A goiter that grows rapidly.

adenomatous g. A goiter caused by the growth of an encapsulated adenoma.

colloid g. A goiter in which there is a great increase of the follicular contents.

congenital g. A goiter present at birth.

cystic g. A goiter in which a cyst or cysts are formed, possibly resulting from the degeneration of tissue or liquefaction within an adenoma.

diffuse g. A goiter in which the thyroid tissue is diffuse, in contrast to its nodular form as in adenomatous goiter.

diving g. A movable goiter, located either below or above the sternal notch.

endemic g. Goiter development in certain geographic localities, esp. where the iodine content in food and water is deficient. Goiters are more prevalent in fresh water and lake areas and less so on the seacoast, owing to the lack of iodine in fresh water. The treatment consists of iodine taken orally or in iodized salt.

fibrous g. A goiter with a hyperplastic capsule.

intrathoracic g. A goiter in which a portion of the thyroid tissue lies within the thoracic cavity.

lingual g. A hypertrophied mass forming a tumor at the posterior portion of the dorsum of the tongue.

nodular g. A goiter that contains nodules.

parenchymatous g. A usually diffuse goiter characterized by multiplication of cells lining the follicles or alveoli. Colloid is usually reduced and the follicular cavities assume various sizes and are often obliterated by the infoldings of their walls. Fibrous tissue may increase markedly. The iodine content of the gland is low.

perivascular g. A goiter surrounding a large blood vessel.

retrovascular g. A goiter that develops behind a large blood vessel.

simple g. A goiter unaccompanied by constitutional symptoms.

substernal g. An enlargement of the lower part of the thyroid isthmus.

suffocative g. A goiter that causes shortness of breath owing to pressure.

toxic g. An exophthalmic goiter or a goiter in which there is an excessive production of the thyroid hormone.

vascular g. A goiter due to distention of the blood vessels of the thyroid gland.

goitrogen (goy'trō-jĕn) [L. *guttur,* throat, + *gennan,* to produce] A substance that produces massive enlargement of the thyroid gland. Goitrogen occurs naturally in certain foods, including turnips, rutabagas, and cabbages.

gold SYMB: Au (from L. *aurum,* gold). A yellow metallic element; atomic weight 196.967; atomic number 79; specific gravity 19.32. Its salts have been used to treat early rheumatoid arthritis not adequately controlled by other anti-inflammatory agents or conservative therapy. Injection of radioactive gold, ^{198}Au, is used to treat certain types of cancer and to help outline certain organs, as in liver scanning. SEE: *scanning.*

g. alloy An alloy of gold with copper, silver, platinum, or other metals added for strength or hardness. Pure gold is rated 24 carats. A gold alloy that contains other metals is less than 24 carats. Thus, 18 parts of gold mixed with 6 parts of another metal would be rated as 18-carat gold.

g. Au 198 injection A sterile colloidal solution of radioactive gold (^{198}Au) used as an antineoplastic.

dental casting g. alloy A hard or extra-hard alloy used principally for dental crowns, inlays, clasps, splints, and orthodontic and prosthetic appliances.

g. sodium thiomalate A water-soluble gold preparation used intramuscularly to treat rheumatoid arthritis with active joint inflammation. Trade name is Myochrysine.

goldbeater's skin A strong, thin membrane prepared from the cecum of the ox and previously used as a surgical dressing.

Goldblatt kidney [Harry Goldblatt, U.S. physician, 1891–1977] Kidney injury and secondary hypertension due to inadequate kidney perfusion. This condition may occur as a result of renal artery stenosis.

golden hour The 60-minute period in which a critically injured person must receive definitive care in an appropriate medical facility to enhance the patient's chance of survival.

goldenseal (gōld'ĕn-sēl) An herbal remedy used by alternative medicine practitioners as an eyewash and as a treatment for irritated mucous membranes. Some illicit-drug users believe the herb will mask the results of drug-screening tests; this use has not been validated.

gold standard In medical care and experimental medicine, a therapeutic action, drug, or procedure that is the best available and with which other therapeutic actions, drugs, or procedures are compared to determine their efficacy.

Golgi apparatus (gŏl'jē) [Camillo Golgi, It. pathologist, 1843–1926] A lamellar membranous structure in almost all cells, best viewed by electron microscopy. It contains curved parallel series of flattened sacs that are often expanded at their ends. In secretory cells, the apparatus concentrates and packages the secretory product. Its function in other cells, although apparently important, is poorly understood.

Golgi cell, Golgi neuron A multipolar nerve cell in the cerebral cortex and posterior horns of the spinal cord. Type I possesses long axons; type II, short axons.

Golgi tendon organ ABBR: GTO. A spindle-shaped structure at the junction of a muscle and a tendon. This structure is thought to function as a feedback system that senses muscle tension through tendon stretch, inhibits muscle contraction of the agonist, and facilitates contraction of the antagonistic muscle. The purpose of this mechanism, known as autogenic facilitation, is to prevent overuse and damage to the muscle and corresponding joint.

Goll's tract (gŏlz) [Friedrich Goll, Swiss anatomist, 1829–1903] The tract in the posterior white column of the spinal cord. SYN: *fasciculus gracilis.*

Golytely Trade name for polyethylene glycol electrolyte for gastrointestinal lavage solution.

gomphosis (gŏm-fō'sĭs) [Gr., bolting together] A conical process fitting into a socket in an immovable joint (e.g., a tooth in its bony socket in the alveolus).

gon- SEE: *gono-.*

gonad (gō'năd, gŏn'ăd) [Gr. *gone,* seed] **1.** The embryonic sex before differentiation into definitive testis or ovary. **2.** A generic term referring to the female ovaries and the male testes. Each forms the cells necessary for human reproduction: spermatozoa from the testes, ova from the ovaries. SEE: *estrogen; ovary; testicle; testosterone.*

HORMONES: *Female:* The follicles of the ovaries secrete estrogen, which helps regulate the menstrual cycle and the development of the secondary sex characteristics. The corpus luteum also produces progesterone, which stimulates growth of blood vessels in the endometrium for the implantation of a fertilized egg. *Male:* The interstitial cells of the testes secrete testosterone, which is essential for maturation of sperm and for development of the secondary sex characteristics.

Hormones from both sexes have been isolated and standardized and are used to treat conditions arising from an insufficiency of these hormones. **gonadal,** *adj.*

gonadectomy (gŏn-ă-dĕk'tō-mē) [Gr. *gonos,* genitals, + *ektome,* excision] The excision of a testis or ovary.

gonadopathy (gŏn"ă-dŏp'ă-thē) [" + *pathos,* disease, suffering] Any disease of the sexual organs.

gonadotrophic, gonadotropic (gŏn"ă-dō-trŏf'ĭk) [" + *trophe,* nourishment] Rel. to stimulation of the gonads.

gonadotrophic hormone Gonadotropin.

gonadotrophin (gŏn"ă-dō-trō'phĭn) Gonadotropin.

gonadotropin (gŏn"ă-dō-trō'pĭn) A gonad-stimulating hormone. SYN: *gonadotrophin.*

anterior pituitary g. One of the two anterior pituitary hormones that affects the ovaries or testes: follicle-stimulating hormone and luteinizing hormone.

human chorionic g. ABBR: hCG. A hormone, secreted in early pregnancy by the trophoblasts of the fertilized ovum, that maintains the corpus luteum during early pregnancy, stimulating it to secrete both estrogen and progesterone. Laboratory tests for hCG in maternal blood or urine are used as pregnancy tests and in follow-up assessments after treatment for hydatid mole and choriocarcinoma.

human menopausal g. ABBR: hMG. A purified form of the pituitary gonadotropins FSH and LH; it may be used therapeutically to treat infertility, hypogonadotropic hypogonadism, polycystic ovary disease, and other conditions. In the management of infertility, it is particularly used for women with ovulatory difficulties, in whom it stimulates follicular growth and maturation, ovulation, and development of the corpus luteum.

gonaduct (gŏn'ă-dŭkt) [" + L. *ductus,* canal] The seminal duct or the oviduct.

gonangiectomy (gŏn"ăn-jē-ĕk'tō-mē) [Gr. *gone,* seed, + *angeion,* vessel, + *ektome,* excision] Vasectomy.

gonarthritis (gŏn"ăr-thrī'tĭs) [Gr. *gony,* knee, + *arthron,* joint, + *itis,* inflammation] Inflammation of the knee joint.

gonarthromeningitis (gŏn-ăr"thrō-mĕn-ĭn-jī'tĭs) [" + " + *meninx,* membrane, + *itis,* inflammation] Synovitis of the knee joint.

gonarthrotomy (gŏn"ăr-thrŏt'ō-mē) [" + " + *tome,* incision] Incision of the knee joint.

gonatocele (gŏn-ăt'ō-sēl) [" + *kele,* tumor, swelling] A tumor of the knee.

gonecyst, gonecystis (gŏn'ĕ-sĭst, gŏn-ĕ-sĭs'tĭs) [Gr. *gone,* seed, + *kystis,* a bladder] A seminal vesicle.

gonecystitis (gŏn"ĕ-sĭs-tī'tĭs) [" + " + *itis,* inflammation] Inflammation of the seminal vesicles.

gonecystolith (gŏn"ĕ-sĭs'tō-lĭth) [" + " + *lithos,* stone] A stone in a seminal vesicle.

Gongylonema (gŏn"jĭ-lō-nē'mă) [Gr. *gongylos,* round, + *nema,* thread] A genus of nematode worms belonging to the suborder Spirurata, usually parasitic in the wall of the esophagus and stomach of domestic animals. Occasionally, they are parasitic in humans. *G. pulchrum* is the species most frequently involved.

goniometer (gō"nē-ŏm'ĕ-ter) [Gr. *gonia,* angle, + *metron,* measure] An apparatus to measure joint movements and angles. Various sizes and types of goniometers are available, including finger goniometers, bubble goniometers, gravity goniometers, and recording electrogoniometers. SEE: illus.

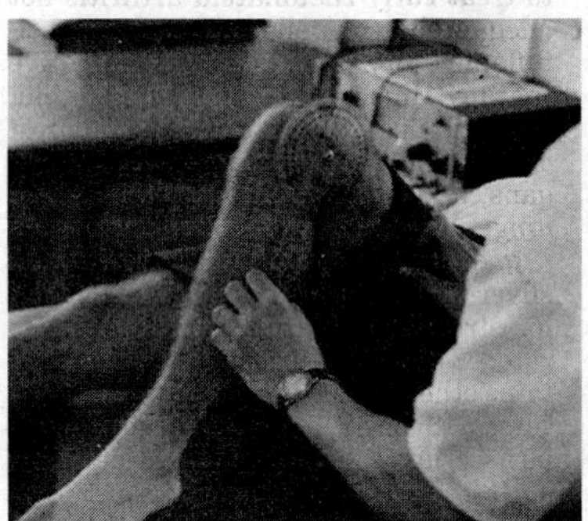

GONIOMETER

gonion (gō'nē-ŏn) [Gr. *gonia,* angle] The point of the angle of the mandible or lower jaw.

goniopuncture (gō"nē-ō-pŭnk'tūr) A surgical procedure for allowing aqueous humor to drain from the eye, used in treating glaucoma.

gonioscope (gō'nē-ō-skōp) [" + *skopein,* to examine] An instrument for inspecting the angle of the anterior chamber of the eye and for determining ocular motility and rotation.

goniosynechia (gō'nē-ō-sĭ-nĕk'ē-ă) Adhesion of the iris to the cornea of the eye.

goniotomy (gō"nē-ŏt'ō-mē) [" + *tome,* incision] A surgical procedure for removing obstructions to the free flow of aqueous humor into the canal of Schlemm of the eye.

gono-, gon- (gŏn'ō) [Gr. *gonos,* genitals] Combining form meaning *generation, genitals, offspring, semen.*

gonococcal (gŏn"ō-kŏk'ăl) [" + *kokkos,* berry] Rel. to or caused by gonococci.

gonococcal conjunctivitis SEE: *gonorrheal conjunctivitis.*

gonococcemia (gŏn″ō-kŏk-sē′mē-ă) [″ + ″ + *haima,* blood] Gonococci in the blood; gonococcal septicemia.

gonococci (gŏn″ō-kŏk′ sī) Pl. of gonococcus.

gonococcic (gŏn″ō-kŏk′sĭk) [″ + *kokkos,* berry] Pert. to the gonococcus.

gonococcic smear A smear using Gram's method and methylene blue. Gonococci, which appear in pairs and tetrads, are gram-negative and intracellular.

gonococcus (gŏn″ō-kŏk′ŭs) *pl.* **gonococci** [Gr. *gonos,* genitals, + *kokkos,* berry] The organism causing gonorrhea, a member of the species *Neisseria gonorrhoeae.* It is a gram-negative intracellular diplococcus that tends to occur in pairs. This bacterium may be found in or on the genitals and in blood, joints, heart, eyes, urine, feces, and pustules. SEE: *gonorrhea.*

gonocyte (gŏn′ō-sīt) [″ + *kytos,* cell] The primitive reproductive cell.

gonorrhea (gŏn″ō-rē′ă) [″ + *rhoia,* flow] A sexually transmitted infection caused by the gram-negative diplococcus *Neisseria gonorrhoeae.* The disease often causes inflammation of the urethra, prostate, cervix, fallopian tubes, rectum, and/or pharynx. Blood-borne infection may spread to the joints and skin, and congenitally transmitted infection to the eyes of a newborn may cause neonatal conjunctivitis. Infection around the liver may result from peritoneal spread of the disease. Although members of either sex with urogenital gonorrhea may be asymptomatic, women are much less likely to notice burning with urination, urethral discharge, or perineal pain than men, in whom these symptoms are present 98% of the time. Coinfection with *Chlamydia trachomatis* is common in both sexes: some studies have shown simultaneous infection with both organisms to be as high as 30%. Even though syphilis rarely accompanies gonorrheal infection, patients with gonorrhea are routinely tested for this disease. Young, sexually active inner-city teens are at highest risk for contracting gonorrhea. Each year in the U.S. roughly 500,000 cases of the disease are reported. SEE: *safe sex; Nursing Diagnoses Appendix; Standard and Universal Precautions Appendix.*

SYMPTOMS: Urethral symptoms in men typically include discomfort with urination (dysuria) accompanied by a yellow, mucopurulent penile discharge. Painful induration of the penis may occur in some cases. Women may have urethral or vaginal discharge, dysuria, urinary frequency, lower abdominal pain, and tender vulvovaginal glands, or fever, dyspareunia, and other symptoms of pelvic inflammatory disease.

DIAGNOSIS: In men, Gram stain of the urethral discharge is very accurate in diagnosing gonorrhea; in men and women, urethral, cervical, or anal swabs for the disease can be used to inoculate Thayer-Martin media, on which the gonococcus specifically grows. Single swabs can be used to identify infections with gonorrhea and/or *Chlamydia.*

PROPHYLAXIS: Safe sexual practices limit the spread of gonorrhea and have decreased the disease's incidence. To prevent gonorrhea in newborns, all babies are treated with a drop of 1% silver nitrate or a thin ribbon of antibiotic ointment in the conjunctival sac of each eye. SEE: *ophthalmia neonatorum.*

TREATMENT: A single dose of a third-generation cephalosporin, such as ceftriaxone or cefixime, is curative in virtually all cases of urogenital gonorrhea. Follow-up cultures are not required unless re-exposure occurs. A week-long course of oral tetracycline, doxycycline, or azithromycin is usually given to patients with gonorrhea, to eradicate any coexisting chlamydial infection. Quinolones are effective therapy for patients who are allergic to cephalosporins. During pregnancy, women must avoid tetracyclines and quinolones because of the risk of fetal malformation; the usual substitute is erythromycin. Gonococcal ophthalmia in newborns is treated with aqueous penicillin or ceftriaxone.

PATIENT CARE: A history of allergies, esp. antibiotic sensitivity, is obtained. Universal precautions are observed.

Antibiotics should be taken as prescribed, and the full course of therapy completed. Moist heat or sitz baths should be taken as directed. The patient should avoid contact with his or her bodily discharges so that the eyes do not become contaminated. The patient should also refrain from sexual intercourse until the disease has been treated, because the infection will continue and can be transmitted until cultures become negative.

The patient's response to therapy is evaluated, and the patient is taught to recognize and report adverse drug reactions. The need for testing for other sexually transmitted diseases is discussed, as well as prevention of future infections and the importance of follow-up testing. All persons with whom the patient has had sexual contact should be tested and receive treatment, even if a culture is negative; and the case and known sexual contacts are reported to the local public health department for appropriate follow-up.

gonorrheal Of the nature of or pert. to gonorrhea.

Gonyaulax (gŏn″ē-aw′lăks) A genus of dinoflagellate that causes certain shellfish that eat them to become toxic. It is also one of the causes of "red tide" when present in massive numbers in the ocean. This condition has occurred on certain beaches of North America. Shellfish present in such water contain the toxin present in the dinoflagellate.

gonycampsis (gŏn″ĭ-kămp′sĭs) [Gr. *gony,* knee, + *kampsis,* bending] An abnormal curvature of the knee.

gonycrotesis (gŏn″ĭ-krō-tē′sĭs) [″ + *krotesis,* knocking] Knock-knee.

gonyectyposis (gŏn″ē-ĕk-tĭ-pō′sĭs) [″ + *ektyposis,* modeling in relief] Bowleg.

gonyocele (gŏn′ē-ō-sēl) [″ + *kele,* swelling] Tuberculous synovitis of the knee.

gonyoncus (gŏn″ē-ŏn′kŭs) [″ + *onkos,* tumor] A tumor of the knee.

Goodell's sign [William Goodell, U.S. gynecologist, 1829–1894] Softening of the cervix; a probable sign of pregnancy that may be present during the second and third months of gestation. Palpation reveals the cervix has altered from a nonpregnant firmness similar to the tip of the nose to a softness similar to the lips. This change is due to increasing uterine vascularity and edema.

Goodpasture's syndrome [Ernest William Goodpasture, U.S. pathologist, 1886–1960] The rare autoimmune illness marked by progressive glomerulonephritis, hemoptysis, and hemosiderosis. Death is usually due to renal failure.

Good Samaritan Law The legal protection given to those who stop and render care in an emergency situation without expectation for remuneration. The necessity for this legislation arose when physicians who assisted in giving emergency care were later accused of malpractice by the patient.

gooseflesh Piloerection.

Gordon's reflex [Alfred Gordon, U.S. neurologist, 1874–1953] The extension of the great toe on sudden pressure on the deep flexor muscles of the calf of the leg. It is present in pyramidal tract disease. SEE: *Babinski's reflex.*

gorget (gor′jĕt) [Fr. *gorge,* throat, because of shape of instrument] An instrument grooved to protect soft tissues from injury as a pointed instrument is inserted in a body cavity.

goserelin acetate A synthetic form of luteinizing hormone–releasing hormone. It is used to treat hormone-sensitive illnesses, including diseases of puberty, and cancers of the breast, ovary, or prostate.

Gossypium (gŏ-sĭp′ē-ŭm) [L.] A genus of perennial shrub of the Malvaceae family, widely grown because of the cotton fiber derived from its seed covering. The bark of some species is diuretic, emmenagogic, and oxytocic. SEE: *cotton; gossypol.*

gossypol A toxic chemical present in cottonseed, which has been used experimentally as an infertility agent in men.

gouge (gowj) An instrument used for cutting away the hard tissue of bone.

goundou (goon′doo) [African] Periostitis of the nasal processes of the maxillae caused by prior infection with yaws or syphilis. The nasal bones become quite enlarged, and the orbit may be involved. The appearance of the nose has been characterized colloquially as "big nose" or "dog nose." SEE: *anakré.*

gout (gowt) [L. *gutta,* drop] A common group of arthritic disorders marked by the deposition of monosodium urate crystals in joints and other tissues. Any joint may be affected, but gout usually begins in the knee or the metacarpaphalangeal joint of the foot. SEE: *tophus; Nursing Diagnoses Appendix.*

SYMPTOMS: Most hyperuricemic persons are asymptomatic between acute attacks. When an attack of acute gouty arthritis does develop, it usually begins at night with moderate pain that increases in intensity to the point where no body position provides relief. Low-grade fever and joint inflammation may be present. SEE: illus. (Uric Acid Crystals and White Blood Cells in Synovial Fluid).

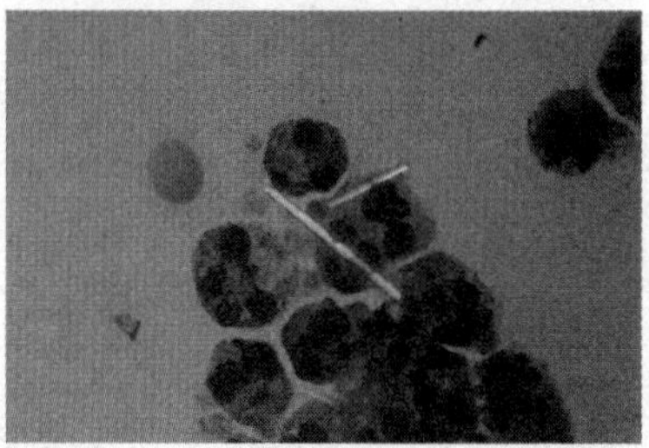

GOUT

Uric acid crystals and white blood cells in synovial fluid (orig. mag. ×500)

TREATMENT: Colchicine, nonsteroidal anti-inflammatory agents, or corticosteroids are used to treat acute gouty attacks. Long-term therapy aims at preventing hyperuricemia by giving uricosuric drugs such as probenecid, or xanthine oxidase inhibitors such as allopurinol. Patients with gout have a tendency to form uric acid kidney stones. To help prevent this, fluids should be encouraged. Low doses of salicylates inhibit uric acid excretion in urine. The diet should be well balanced and devoid of purine-rich foods.

PATIENT CARE: During the acute phase, bedrest is prescribed for at least the first 24 hr, and affected joints are elevated, immobilized, and protected by a bed cradle. Analgesics are administered. The patient is taught about these measures. Colchicine, indomethacin, prednisone, or other prescribed drugs are administered. A low-purine diet is recommended, and the importance of gradual weight reduction is explained if obesity is a factor. If soft-tissue tophi are present, the patient should wear soft clothing to cover these areas and should use meticulous skin care and sterile dressings to prevent infection of open lesions.

Surgery may be required to excise or drain infected or ulcerated tophi, to correct joint deformities, or to improve joint function. Even minor surgery may precipitate gouty attacks (usually within 24 to 96 hr after surgery); therefore, the patient should be instructed about this risk.

abarticular g. Gout that involves structures other than the joints.

chronic g. A persistent form of gout.

lead g. Goutlike symptoms associated with lead poisoning. SYN: *saturnine g.*

saturnine g. Lead g.

tophaceous g. Gout marked by the development of tophi (deposits of sodium urate) in the joints and in the external ear.

gouty Of the nature of or rel. to gout.

Gowers' sign, Gowers' maneuver [Sir William R. Gowers, Brit. neurologist, 1845–1915] A clinical sign of muscular dystrophy in childhood, indicative of weakness of the hip and knee extensors. Children with muscular dystrophy cannot stand up from a kneeling position without using their arms to push themselves erect by moving their hands up their legs and then their thighs.

Gowers' tract (gow'ĕrz) A bundle of fibers from the posterior roots of the lateral tract of the spinal cord, reaching the cerebellum by way of the superior peduncle.

G.P. *general practitioner.*

G6PD *glucose-6-phosphate dehydrogenase.*

gr *grain.*

graafian follicle (grăf'ē-ăn) [Regnier de Graaf, Dutch physician and anatomist, 1641–1673] A mature vesicular follicle of the ovary. Beginning with puberty and continuing until the menopause, except during pregnancy, a graafian follicle develops at approx. monthly intervals. Each follicle contains a nearly mature ovum (an oocyte) that, on rupture of the follicle, is discharged from the ovary, a process called ovulation. Ovulation usually occurs 12 to 16 days before the first day of the next menstrual period. Within the ruptured graafian follicle, the corpus luteum develops. Both the follicle and the corpus luteum are endocrine glands, the former secreting estrogens, and the latter, estrogen and progesterone. SEE: *ovum* for illus.

grab bar A bar attached to the wall to assist in climbing stairs or using the bath, shower, or toilet safely.

gracile (grăs'ĭl) [L. *gracilis,* slender] Slender; slight.

gracile nucleus A mass of medullary gray matter terminating the funiculus gracilis.

gracilis (grăs'ĭ-lĭs) [L., slender] A long slender muscle on the medial aspect of the thigh.

grade (grād) A standard measurement or assessment.

Gleason's g. Gleason's score.

Gradenigo's syndrome (gră-dĕn-ē'gōz) [Giuseppe Gradenigo, It. physician, 1859–1926] A syndrome involving the fifth and sixth cranial nerves. Ear pain, draining middle ear, and paralysis of the sixth cranial nerve are present. The lesion may be caused by inflammation or tumor of the petrous portion of the temporal bone. Appropriate antibiotics should be administered if the condition is due to an infection.

gradient (grā'dē-ĕnt) **1.** A slope or grade. **2.** An increase or decrease of varying degrees or the curve that represents such.

alveolar/arterial g. ABBR: A/a gradient. The difference between the calculated oxygen pressure available in the alveolus and the arterial oxygen tension. It measures the efficiency of gas exchange.

average g. In sensitometry, a measure of the contrast of the film or film-screen system by determination of the slope of the sensitometric curve.

axial g. A gradient of physiological or metabolic activity exhibited by embryos and many adult animals, the principal one of which follows the main axis of the body, being highest at the anterior end and lowest at the posterior end.

concentration g. The difference in the amounts of a substance on either side of a membrane or in two areas of a biological system. Substances diffuse down a concentration gradient, from the area of higher concentration to lower concentration.

pressure g. The difference in hydrostatic pressure on either side of a membrane. As the difference in pressures rises, filtration increases from the area of high pressure to the area of low pressure.

graduate (grăd'ū-āt, -ăt) [L. *gradus,* a step] **1.** A vessel, usually a cylinder with one end closed, and marked by scribed lines for measuring liquids. **2.** One who has been awarded an academic or professional degree from a college or university.

graduated Marked by a series of lines indicating degrees of measurement, weight, or volume.

graduated tenotomy Partial surgical division of a tendon of an eye muscle.

Graefe's sign (grā′fēz) [Albrecht von Graefe, Ger. ophthalmologist, 1828–1870] Failure of the upper lid to follow a downward movement of the eyeball when the patient changes his or her vision from looking up to looking down. This finding, referred to colloquially as "lid lag," is seen in Graves' disease (hyperthyroidism) with exophthalmos.

graft (grăft) [L. *graphium,* grafting knife] **1.** Tissue transplanted or implanted in a part of the body to repair a defect. A homograft (or allograft) is a graft of material from another individual of the same species. A heterograft (or xenigraft) is a graft of material from an individual of another species. **2.** The process of placing tissue from one site to another to repair a defect.

allogeneic g. A graft from a genetically nonidentical donor of the same species as the recipient. SYN: *allograft; homograft.*

autologous g. A graft taken from another part of the patient's body.

avascular g. A graft in which vascular infiltration does not occur.

bone g. A piece of bone usually taken from the tibia and inserted elsewhere in the body to replace another osseous structure. Bone storage banks have been established.

bypass g. A surgical conduit inserted into the vascular system that routes blood around an obstructed vessel. SEE: *coronary artery bypass surgery.*

cable g. A nerve graft made up of bundles of segments from an unimportant nerve. SYN: *rope g.*

cadaver g. Grafting tissue, including skin, cornea, or bone, obtained from a body immediately after death.

delayed g. A skin graft that is partially elevated and then replaced so that it may be moved later to another site.

dermal g. A split-skin or full-thickness skin graft. The graft will grow hair and have active sweat and sebum glands.

endovascular g. A graft implanted within an existing blood vessel.

fascia g. A graft using fascia, usually removed from the fascia lata, for repairing defects in other tissues.

fascicular g. A nerve graft in which each bundle of nerves is separately sutured.

free g. A graft that is completely separated from its original site and then transferred.

full-thickness g. A graft of the entire layer of skin without the subcutaneous fat.

gingival g. A sliding graft employing the gingival papilla as the graft material.

heterodermic g. A skin graft taken from a donor of another species.

heteroplastic g. A graft taken from another person.

heterotopic g. SEE: *transplantation, heterotopic.*

homologous g. A graft taken from a donor of the same species as the recipient.

isologous g. A graft in which the donor and recipient are genetically identical (i.e., identical twins). SYN: *isograft.*

lamellar g. A very thin corneal graft used to replace the surface layer of opaque corneal tissue.

mesh g. A split-skin graft that contains multiple perforations or slits, which allow the graft to be expanded so that a much larger area is covered. The holes in the graft are covered by new tissue as the graft spreads.

nerve g. The transplantation of a healthy nerve to replace a segment of a damaged nerve.

Ollier-Thiersch g. SEE: *Ollier-Thiersch graft.*

omental g. The use of a portion of the omentum to cover or repair a defect in a hollow viscus or to cover a suture line in an abdominal organ.

ovarian g. The implantation of a section of an ovary into the muscles of the abdominal wall.

pedicle g. Pedicle flap.

periosteum g. The application of a piece of bone and its periosteum to another site.

pinch g. A graft consisting of small bits of skin.

postmortem g. Tissue taken from a body after death and stored under proper conditions to be used later on a patient requiring a graft of such tissue.

punch g. A full-thickness graft, usually circular, for transplanting skin containing hair follicles to a bald area.

rope g. Cable g.

sieve g. A graft similar to a mesh graft in which a section of skin is removed except for small, regularly spaced areas that remain. The removed portion is used at the new site. The small remaining areas will grow to cover the entire area at the donor site.

skin g. The use of small sections of skin harvested from a donor site to repair a defect or trauma of the skin, such as a large superficial burn. The skin surface at the receiving site should be clean and raw.

PATIENT CARE: Before surgery, assessments are made of the patient's general status. Confirmation is needed that appropriate laboratory parameters, including hemoglobin and coagulation studies, are acceptable as they may affect the surgical result. The donor and recipient sites are prepared according to protocol. The postsurgical appearance of the wound and dressing and, if applicable, the need to immobilize the part after surgery are explained. Both patient and family receive support and encouragement. The graft is observed at regular intervals postoperatively for swelling or for development of hematoma and signs of purulent drainage. Appropriate aseptic technique is followed in applying dressings and compresses to prevent infection. Prophylactic antibiotics are administered as prescribed, and the graft site is immobilized to allow healing. Analgesics are administered as necessary to relieve pain. Before discharge, the patient learns about wound care and the need to keep the graft site clean, well lubricated, and away from sunlight according to the health care provider's instructions.

split-skin g. A graft of a part of the skin thickness.

sponge g. A small piece of sponge placed over an ulcerating part to stimulate epidermal growth.

thick-split g. A graft of about half or more of the skin's thickness.

Thiersch's g. SEE: *Thiersch's graft.*

Wolfe's g. A graft using the whole skin thickness.

grafting The act of applying a graft of skin or tissue from a healthy site to an injured site.

graft-versus-host disease ABBR: GVH. Immunological injury suffered by an immunosuppressed recipient of a bone marrow transplant. The donated lymphoid cells (the "graft") attack the recipient (the "host"), causing damage, esp. to the skin, liver, and gastrointestinal tract. GVH occurs in about 50% of allogeneic bone marrow transplants. It may develop in the first 60 days after transplantation ("acute" GVH) or many months later ("chronic" GVH).

Graham's law (grā'ămz) [Thomas Graham, Brit. chemist, 1805–1869] A law stating that the rate of diffusion of a gas is inversely proportional to the square root of its molecular mass (molecular weight).

grain [L. *granum*] ABBR: gr. **1.** A weight; 0.065 of a gram. **2.** The seed or seedlike fruit of many members of the grass family, esp. corn, wheat, oats, and other cereals. **3.** Direction of fibers or layers. SYN: *granum.*

gram ABBR: g. A unit of weight (mass) of the metric system. It equals approx. the weight of a cubic centimeter or a milliliter of water. One gram is equal to 15.432 gr or 0.03527 oz (avoirdupois), 1000 g are equal to 1 kg. SEE: table.

fat g. A standard measure of fat and the calories (9 kcal/g) contained. Counting and limiting fat grams is a method used in weight-reduction diets.

gram-equivalent In chemistry, the mass

Gram Conversion into Ounces (Avoirdupois)*

G	Oz	G	Oz	G	Oz	G	Oz
1	0.03	30	1.06	59	2.08	88	3.10
2	0.07	31	1.09	60	2.12	89	3.14
3	0.11	32	1.13	61	2.15	90	3.17
4	0.14	33	1.16	62	2.18	91	3.21
5	0.18	34	1.20	63	2.22	92	3.24
6	0.21	35	1.23	64	2.26	93	3.28
7	0.25	36	1.27	65	2.29	94	3.31
8	0.28	37	1.30	66	2.33	95	3.35
9	0.32	38	1.34	67	2.36	96	3.38
10	0.35	39	1.37	68	2.40	97	3.42
11	0.39	40	1.41	69	2.43	98	3.46
12	0.42	41	1.44	70	2.47	99	3.49
13	0.45	42	1.48	71	2.50	100	3.53
14	0.49	43	1.51	72	2.54	125	4.41
15	0.53	44	1.55	73	2.57	150	5.30
16	0.56	45	1.59	74	2.61	175	6.18
17	0.60	46	1.62	75	2.64	200	7.05
18	0.63	47	1.65	76	2.68	250	8.82
19	0.67	48	1.69	77	2.71	300	10.58
20	0.70	49	1.73	78	2.75	350	12.34
21	0.74	50	1.76	79	2.79	400	14.11
22	0.77	51	1.80	80	2.82	450	15.87
23	0.81	52	1.83	81	2.85	454	16.00
24	0.84	53	1.87	82	2.89	500	17.64
25	0.88	54	1.90	83	2.93	600	21.16
26	0.91	55	1.94	84	2.96	700	24.69
27	0.95	56	1.97	85	3.00	800	28.22
28	0.99	57	2.01	86	3.03	900	30.75
29	1.02	58	2.04	87	3.07	1000	35.27

* g is equal to 0.03527 oz (avoirdupois).

in grams of a substance that will react with 1 g of hydrogen.

gramicidin (grăm″ĭ-sī′dĭn) One of the antibiotics produced by *Bacillus brevis.*

Gram's method Gram stain.

gram molecule The weight in grams of a substance equal to its molecular weight.

gram-negative Losing the crystal violet stain and taking the color of the red counterstain in Gram's method of staining, a primary characteristic of certain microorganisms. SEE: *Gram stain.*

gram-positive Retaining the color of the crystal violet stain in Gram's method of staining. SEE: *Gram stain.*

Gram stain [Hans C. J. Gram, Danish physician, 1853–1938] A method of staining bacteria, important in their identification. SYN: *Gram's method.*

PROCEDURE: A film on a slide is prepared, dried, and fixed with heat. The film is stained with crystal violet for 1 min; rinsed in water, then immersed in Gram's iodine solution for 1 min. The iodine solution is rinsed off and the slide decolorized in 95% ethyl alcohol. The slide is then counterstained with dilute carbolfuchsin or safranine for 30 sec, after which it is rinsed with water, blotted dry, and examined. Gram-positive bacteria retain the violet stain and gram-negative bacteria adopt the red counterstain. SEE: illus.

NOTE: As a simple means of checking on the accuracy of the staining materials, a small amount of material from between one's teeth can be placed on the slide at the opposite end from that of the specimen being examined. As gram-negative and gram-positive organisms are always present in the mouth, that end of the slide should be examined first. If both types of organisms are seen, the specimen may then be examined.

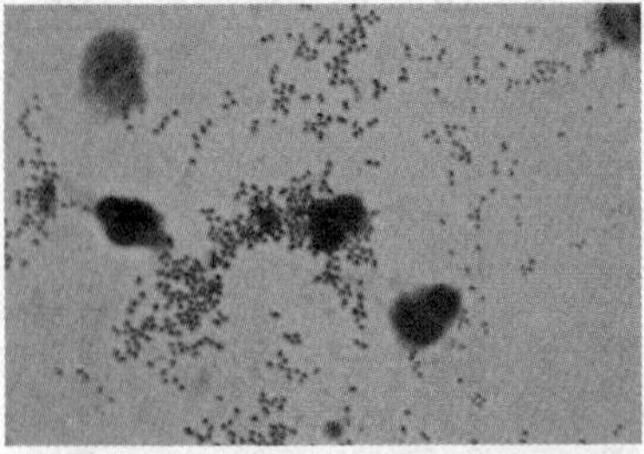

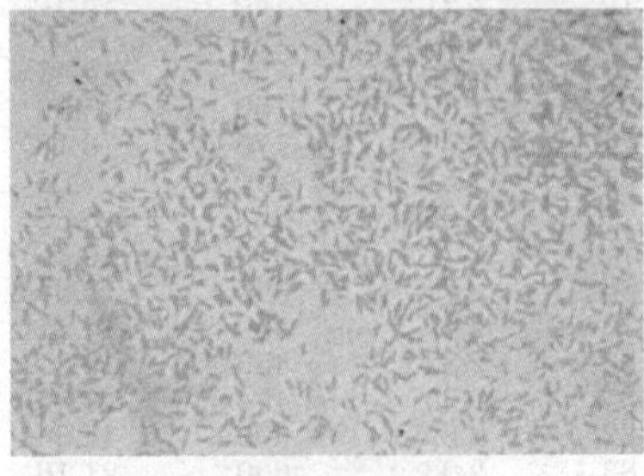

GRAM STAIN

(*Top*) Gram-positive *Staphylococcus aureus* in a pus smear (orig. mag. ×500) (*Bottom*) Gram-negative *Campylobacter jejuni* bacilli (orig. mag. ×500)

Grancher's sign (grăn-shăz′) [Jacques J. Grancher, Fr. physician, 1843–1907] The raised pitch of expiratory murmur in pulmonary consolidation.

grandiose (grăn′dē-ōs) In psychiatry, concerning one's unrealistic and exaggerated concept of self-worth, importance, wealth, and ability.

grandiosity An exaggerated sense of self-importance, power, or status.

grand mal SEE: *epilepsy.*

granular [L. *granulum,* little grain] **1.** Of the nature of granules. **2.** Roughened by prominences like those of seeds.

granulatio (grăn″ū-lā′shē-ō) [L.] Granule.

granulation 1. The formation of granules or the condition of being granular. **2.** Fleshy projections formed on the surface of a gaping wound that is not healing by first intention or indirect union. Each granulation represents the outgrowth of new capillaries by budding from the existing capillaries and then joining up into capillary loops supported by cells that will later become fibrous scar tissue. Granulations bring a rich blood supply to the healing surface.

arachnoid g. Folds of the arachnoid layer of the cranial meninges that project through the inner layer of dura mater into the superior sagittal sinus and other venous sinuses of the brain. Through them, cerebrospinal fluid reenters the bloodstream. SYN: *arachnoid villus; pacchionian body.*

exuberant g. An excessive mass of granulation tissue formed in the healing of a wound or ulcer; proud flesh.

granule (grăn′ūl) [L. *granulum,* little grain] **1.** A small, grainlike mass. **2.** In histology, a minute mass in a cell that has an outline but no apparent structure. SYN: *granulatio.*

acidophil g. A granule that stains readily with acid dyes.

albuminous g. A cytoplasmic granule in many normal cells. It is not affected by ether or chloroform but disappears from view when acetic acid is added.

amphophil g. Beta g.

azurophil g. A small red or reddish-purple granule that easily takes a stain with azure dyes. Found in lymphocytes and monocytes, it is inconstant in number, being present in about 30% of the cells.

basal g. Basal body.

basophil g. A cellular granule that stains with a basic dye.

beta g. An azurophil granule found in beta cells of the hypophysis or islets of Langerhans of the pancreas that stains with both acid and basic dyes. SYN: *amphophil g.*

chromophil g. Nissl bodies.

cone g. The nuclei of the cones, sensory cells of the retina. They form the outer zone of the outer nuclear layer of the retina.

delta g. A small granule in the delta cells of the pancreas.

eosinophil g. One of various granules that react with acid dyes. It is present in eosinophils.

glycogen g. One of the minute particles of glycogen seen in liver cells following fixation.

juxtaglomerular g. One of the granules in the juxtaglomerular cells of the glomerulus of the kidney that excrete renin.

Kölliker's interstitial g. A granule in the sarcoplasm of a striated muscle fiber.

metachromatic g. An irregularly sized granule found in the protoplasm of numerous bacteria. It stains a different color from that of the dye used.

Much's g. [Hans Christian Much, Ger. physician, 1880–1932] The granules sometimes seen in sputum from patients with tuberculosis. They do not stain with acid-fast stain but do take Gram stain. These particles are probably degenerated tubercle bacilli.

neutrophil g. A granule such as those found in neutrophils that stains with both basic and acid dyes, assuming a neutral tint.

Nissl g. Nissl bodies.

pigment g. A granule seen in pigment cells.

Plehn's g. A basophilic granule seen in the conjugating form of *Plasmodium vivax.*

protein g. A minute protein particle found in cells.

rod g. A nucleus of a rod photoreceptor found in the retina.

Schüffner's g. [Wilhelm A.P. Schüffner, Ger. pathologist, 1867–1949] A coarse, red, polychrome methylene blue–staining granule found in erythrocytes infected with *Plasmodium ovale* or *P. vivax* malaria. SYN: *Schüffner's dots.*

secretory g. Zymogen g.

seminal g. One of the minute particles in semen, supposed to derive from disintegrated nuclei in nutritive cells from seminiferous tubules.

zymogen g. A granule present in gland cells, esp. the secretory cells of the pancreas, the chief cells of the gastric glands, and the serous cells of the salivary glands. It is the precursor of the enzyme secreted. SYN: *secretory g.*

granuloblast (grăn′ū-lō-blăst) [″ + Gr. *blastos,* germ] The mother cell of a granulocyte; a myeloblast found in bone marrow.

granulocyte (grăn′ū-lō-sīt″) [″ + Gr. *kytos,* cell] A granular leukocyte; a polymorphonuclear leukocyte (neutrophil, eosinophil, or basophil).

granulocyte colony-stimulating factor ABBR: G-CSF. A naturally occurring cytokine glycoprotein that stimulates the proliferation and functional activity of neutrophils. It is effective in treating bone marrow deficiency following cancer chemotherapy or bone marrow transplantation. The generic name is filgrastim; trade name is Neupogen. SEE: *colony-stimulating factor–1.*

granulocyte-macrophage colony-stimulating factor ABBR: GM-CSF. A naturally occurring cytokine glycoprotein that stimulates the production of neutrophils, monocytes, and macrophages. It is effective in treating bone marrow deficiency following cancer chemotherapy or bone marrow transplantation. The generic name is sargramostim; trade names are Leukine and Prokine. SEE: *colony-stimulating factor–1.*

granulocytopenia (grăn″ū-lō-sī″tō-pē′nē-ă) [″ + ″ + *penia,* poverty] An abnormal reduction of granulocytes in the blood. SYN: *granulopenia.*

granulocytopoiesis (grăn″ū-lō-sī″tō-poy-ē′sĭs) [″ + ″ + *poiein,* to form] The formation of granulocytes. SEE: illus.

granulocytosis (grăn″ū-lō-sī-tō′sĭs) [″ + ″ + *osis,* condition] An abnormal increase in the number of granulocytes in the blood.

granuloma [″ + Gr. *oma,* tumor] An inflammatory response that results when macrophages are unable to destroy foreign substances that have entered or invaded body tissues. Large numbers of macrophages are drawn to the affected area over 7 to 10 days, surround the target, and enclose it. They in turn are surrounded by polymorphonuclear leukocytes, other immune cells, and fibroblasts. Granulomas are common in many conditions, including leprosy, tuberculosis, cat scratch disease, some fungal infections, and foreign body reactions (e.g., reactions to sutures). SEE: *giant cell; tuberculosis; Wegener's granulomatosis.*

g. annulare A circular rash with a raised red border, usually found on the hands, knuckles, or arms of young patients. The cause is unknown. The rash often lasts 1 or 2 years, and then may disappear spontaneously.

apical g. Dental g.

benign g. of the thyroid A lymphadenoma of the thyroid.

coccidioidal g. A chronic, generalized granulomatous disease caused by the fungus *Coccidioides immitis.* SEE: *coccidioidomycosis.*

MYELOID STEM CELL

PROMYELOCYTE (PROGRANULOCYTE)

BASOPHILIC MYELOCYTE NEUTROPHILIC MYELOCYTE EOSINOPHILIC MYELOCYTE

BASOPHILIC METAMYELOCYTE NEUTROPHILIC METAMYELOCYTE EOSINOPHILIC METAMYELOCYTE

BASOPHILIC BAND NEUTROPHILIC BAND EOSINOPHILIC BAND

BASOPHILIC SEGMENTED NEUTROPHILIC SEGMENTED EOSINOPHILIC SEGMENTED

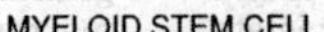

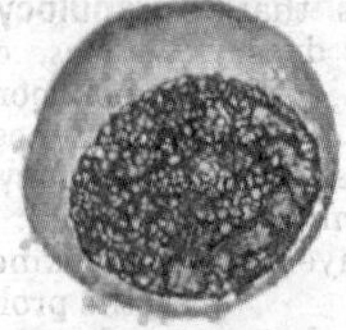

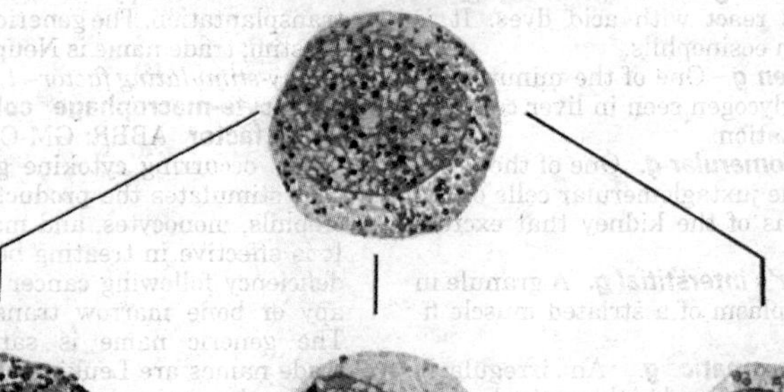

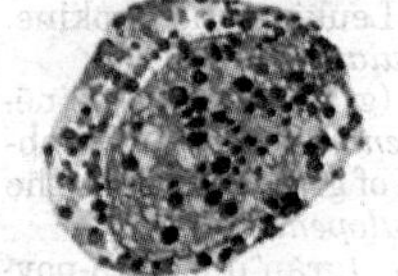

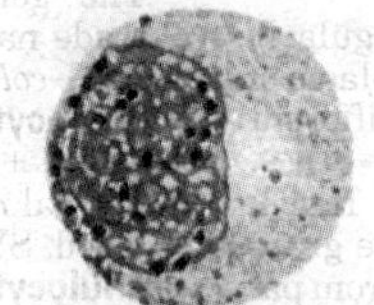

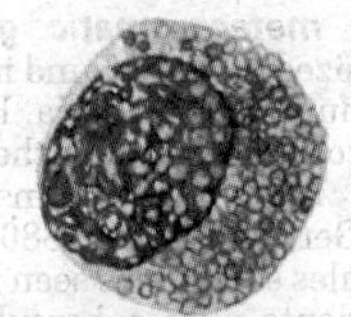

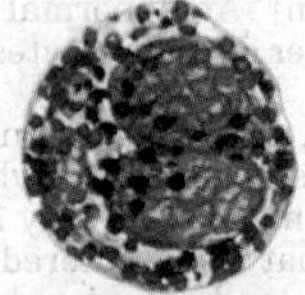

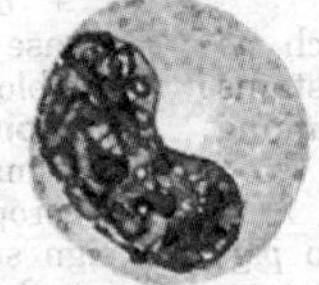

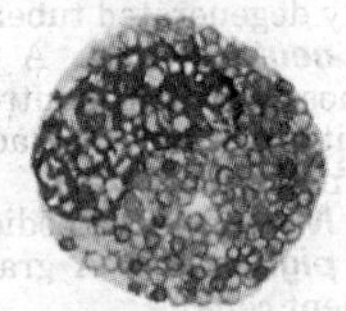

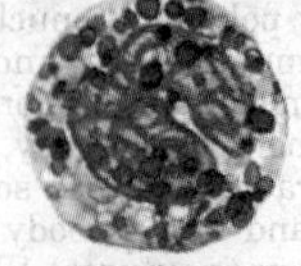

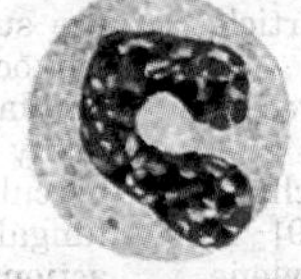

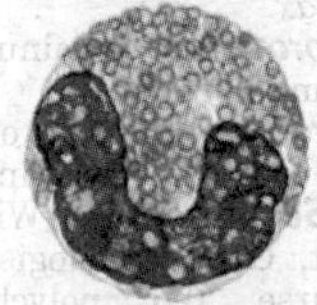

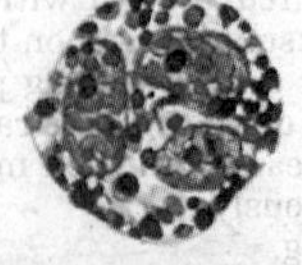

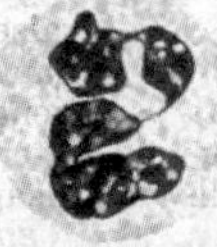

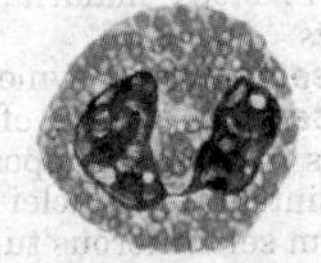

GRANULOCYTOPOIESIS

dental g. A granuloma developing at the tip of a tooth root, usually the result of pulpitis. It consists of a proliferating mass of chronic inflammatory tissue and possibly epithelial nests or colonies of bacteria. It may be encapsulated by fibrous tissue of the periodontal ligament. SYN: *apical g.; apical periodontitis.*

eosinophilic g. A form of xanthomatosis accompanied by eosinophilia and the formation of cysts on bone.

g. fissuratum A circumscribed, firm, fissured, fibrotic tumor caused by chronic irritation. It may occur where hard objects such as dentures or the earpieces of glasses rub against the labioalveolar fold or the retroauricular fold, respectively. The tumor is not malignant and disappears when the irritating object is removed.

foreign body g. Chronic inflammation around foreign bodies such as sutures, talc, splinters, or gravel. SYN: *foreign body reaction.*

g. fungoides Mycosis fungoides.

infectious g. Any infectious disease in which granulomas are formed, such as tuberculosis or syphilis. Granulomas are also formed in mycoses and protozoan infections.

g. inguinale A granulomatous ulcerative disease in which the initial lesion commonly appears in the genital area as a painless nodule.

ETIOLOGY: This type of granuloma is caused by a short, gram-negative bacillus, *Calymmatobacterium granulomatis,* commonly called a Donovan body.

TREATMENT: Erythromycin, trimethoprim-sulfamethoxazole, or tetracyclines are used in treating this disease. Single-dose therapy with intramuscular ceftriaxone or oral ciprofloxacin may be effective.

g. iridis A granuloma that develops on the iris.

lipoid g. A granuloma that contains fatty tissue or cholesterol.

lipophagic g. A granuloma in which the macrophages have phagocytosed the surrounding fat cells.

Majocchi's g. Trichophytic g.

malignant g. Hodgkin's disease.

pyogenic g. A fleshy, polyp-shaped hemangioma that may develop at the site of a wound. It bleeds easily and is usually tender. SYN: *g. pyogenicum.*

g. pyogenicum Pyogenic g.

swimming pool g. Chronic skin infection with *Mycobacterium balnei,* an organism that may be present in unchlorinated swimming pools.

g. telangiectaticum A very vascular granuloma at any site, but esp. in the nasal mucosa or pharynx.

trichophytic g. A granuloma of the skin follicles and follicular areas of the legs. It is caused by fungi, usually *Trichophyton rubrum.* SYN: *Majocchi's g.*

granulomatosis (grăn″ū-lō″mă-tō′sĭs) [L. *granulum,* little grain, + Gr. *oma,* tumor, + *osis,* condition] The development of multiple granulomas.

Wegener's g. A rare vasculitis of unknown etiology characterized by widespread granulomatous lesions of the bronchi, necrotizing arteriolitis, and glomerulonephritis.

granulomatous (grăn″ū-lŏm′ă-tŭs) Containing granulomas.

granulopenia (grăn″ū-lō-pē′nē-ă) [″ + Gr. *penia,* poverty] Granulocytopenia.

granuloplasm (grăn′ū-lō-plăzm) A granular cytoplasm.

granuloplastic (grăn″ū-lō-plăs′tĭk) [″ + Gr. *plassein,* to form] Developing granules.

granulopoiesis (grăn″ū-lō-poy-ē′sĭs) [″ + Gr. *poiein,* to make] The formation of granulocytes.

granulopotent (grăn″ū-lō-pō′tĕnt) [″ + *potentia,* power] Potentially capable of forming granules.

granulosa (grăn″ū-lō′să) A layer of cells in the theca of the graafian follicle.

granulosis (grăn″ū-lō′sĭs) [″ + Gr. *osis,* condition] A mass of minute granules.

g. rubra nasi A disease of the skin of the nose, characterized by a moist erythematous patch on numerous macules. The disease is caused by an inflammatory infiltration about the nose, with slightly elevated papules and dilated sweat glands.

granum (grā′nŭm) [L.] Grain.

granzyme Any of a family of proteases stored in the granules of cytotoxic T lymphocytes. They are involved in cytolytic functions.

grape seed extract (gŏr′p) A mixture of antioxidant oils isolated from the seeds of grapes (*Vitis*) and promoted by alternative and complementary medical practitioners as a potential treatment for coronary artery disease, cancer, and other illnesses produced or worsened by oxidative stresses on body tissues. Scientific evidence for its clinical effectiveness is sparse.

grape sugar Glucose.

graph (grăf) **1.** A visual presentation of statistical, clinical, or experimental data represented by a relationship between two sets of numbers or variables on the ordinate (y) (vertical) axis and the abscissa (x) (horizontal) axis. **2.** Any visual representation of a numerical relationship.

-graph [Gr. *graphos,* drawn or written; one who draws] Combining form used as a suffix meaning an instrument used to make a drawing or written record.

graphesthesia (grăf″ĕs-thē′zē-ă) [″ + *aisthesis,* sensation] The ability to recognize outlines, numbers, words, or symbols traced or written on the skin.

graphite (grăf′īt) [Gr. *graphein,* to write] A soft form of carbon.

grapho- [Gr. *graphein,* to write] Combining form meaning *writing.*

graphology (grăf-ŏl'ō-jē) [" + *logos,* word, reason] The examination of handwriting of patients, as a means of diagnosis or of analyzing a patient's personality.

graphomotor (grăf"ō-mō'tor) [" + L. *motor,* mover] Pert. to movements involved in writing.

graphophobia (grăf"ō-fō'bē-ă) [" + *phobos,* fear] An abnormal fear of writing.

graphorrhea (grăf"ō-rē'ă) [" + *rhoia,* flow] The writing of many meaningless words and phrases.

graphospasm (grăf'ō-spăzm) [" + *spasmos,* spasm] Writer's cramp.

GRAS List A list of food additives *generally recognized as safe* by the U.S. Food and Drug Administration. SEE: *food additive.*

grasp A specific type of prehension involving the fingers, the palmar surface, or both. Types of grasp include cylindrical, as in holding a tubular structure, where the fingers and palmar surface are in opposition; and ball grasp, as in holding a spherical object, where the fingers, thumb, and palmar surface surround an object.

pincher g. The apposition of the thumb and index finger to pick up small objects. This fine motor skill is a developmental milestone usually attained by 10 months of age.

plantar g. A type of prehension involving the toes, which curl forward in response to pressure from the examiner's finger across their base. This normal newborn reflex usually disappears by age 8 to 9 months. The reflex reappears in adults with frontal lobe diseases or dementia.

grating In spectrophotometry, the element used in a monochromator that disperses white light into the visible spectrum.

grattage (gră-tăzh') [Fr., a scraping] The removal of morbid growths by rubbing with a brush or harsh sponge.

grave [L. *gravis,* heavy] Serious; dangerous; severe.

gravel [Fr. *gravelle,* coarse sand] Crystalline dust or concretions of crystals from the kidneys; generally made up of phosphates, calcium, oxalate, and uric acid.

Graves' disease [Robert James Graves, Irish physician, 1796–1853] A distinct type of hyperthyroidism caused by an autoimmune attack on the thyroid gland. It typically produces enlargement of the thyroid gland and also may cause ocular findings (proptosis, lid lag, stare, and pretibial myxedema).

SYMPTOMS: Other findings include nervousness, heat intolerance, hyperdefecation, insomnia, menstrual irregularities, tremor, weight loss, velvety skin, and thinning of the hair.

DIAGNOSIS: The clinical signs and symptoms (goiter, proptosis) in the setting of elevated thyroxine levels and a suppressed thyroid stimulating hormone are diagnostic.

TREATMENT: Drugs that limit the thyroid gland's output of thyroid hormone are effective as therapy. The thyroid gland may be removed surgically or it may be inactivated by use of radioactive iodine therapy.

PATIENT CARE: A history documenting classic symptoms is obtained. Assistance is provided to help the patient to cope with related anxiety, and the patient is encouraged to minimize emotional and physical stress and to balance rest and activity periods. A high-calorie, high-protein diet is recommended to treat increased protein catabolism. The patient is taught comfort measures to deal with elevated body temperature and G.I. complaints (abdominal cramping, frequent bowel movements); safety measures to protect the eyes from injury, including moistening the conjunctiva frequently with isotonic eye drops and wearing sunglasses to protect the eyes from light; and appropriate administration and safety procedures for iodide therapy, beta-blocker therapy, and propylthiouracil and methimazole therapy, as prescribed. Special instructions are provided for therapeutic use of radioactive iodide.

The patient is prepared physically and psychologically for surgery if planned, and postoperative care specific to thyroidectomy is provided. Regular medical follow-up is needed to detect and treat hypothyroidism, which may develop 2 to 4 weeks after surgery and after radioactive iodine therapy. The patient is advised of the possible need for lifelong thyroid hormone replacement therapy, and should wear or carry a medical identification tag and keep a supply of medication with him or her at all times.

Graves' ophthalmopathy Ophthalmopathy associated with hyperthyroidism with the clinical characteristics of exophthalmos, periorbital edema, periorbital and conjunctival inflammation, decreased extraocular muscle mobility, and corneal injury. Accompanying these may be lacrimation, eye pain, blurring of vision, photophobia, diplopia, and loss of vision.

TREATMENT: The underlying hyperthyroidism must be treated. The patient should sleep with the head of the bed elevated. Methylcellulose eyedrops and diuretics will help to relieve eye discomfort. If the condition is severe and progressive, surgical decompression of the orbit will be required to treat impaired retinal function and exposure keratopathy.

gravid (grăv′ĭd) [L. *gravida,* pregnant] Pregnant; heavy with child.

gravida (grăv′ĭ-dă) [L.] A pregnant woman.

gravida macromastia Rapid enlargement of the breasts during pregnancy. This may progress to cause severe distention with sloughing of breast tissue, bleeding, and infection. Surgical therapy may be required.

gravidism [L. *gravida,* pregnant, + Gr. *-ismos,* state of] SYN: *pregnancy.*

gravidity (gră-vĭd′ĭ-tē) [L. *gravida,* pregnant] The total number of a woman's pregnancies.

gravidocardiac (grăv″ĭd-ō-kăr′dē-ăk) [″ + Gr. *kardia,* heart] Pert. to cardiac disorders that result from the physiological changes associated with pregnancy.

gravimetric (grăv″ĭ-mĕt′rĭk) [L. *gravis,* heavy, + Gr. *metron,* measure] Determined by weight.

gravistatic (grăv″ĭ-stăt′ĭk) [″ + Gr. *statikos,* causing to stand] Resulting from gravitation, as in a form of gravistatic pulmonary congestion.

gravitation [L. *gravitas,* weight] The force and movement tending to draw every particle of matter together, esp. the attraction of the earth for bodies at a distance from its center.

gravity **1.** The property of possessing weight. **2.** The force of the earth's gravitational attraction.

specific g. ABBR: sp. gr. The weight of a substance compared with an equal volume of water. Water is used as a standard and is considered to have a specific gravity of 1 (1.000).

gravity-induced loss of consciousness ABBR: GLOC. The loss of consciousness due to positive gravity (G) forces. Certain aviation maneuvers produce increased downward force (i.e., positive G) that is measured as a multiple of the gravitational constant. When these forces are of sufficient intensity, blood flow to the brain is diminished, which, if continued, leads to unconsciousness.

Gravlee jet washer [Leland Clark Gravlee, Jr., U.S. obstetrician and gynecologist, 1928–1984] A proprietary device for irrigating the endometrial cavity with sterile isotonic saline and then removing the solution and dislodged cells. The cells are then stained and examined for evidence of malignancy.

gray ABBR: Gy. A measure of the quantity of ionizing radiation absorbed by any material per unit mass of matter. 1 Gy equals 100 rad. SEE: *radiation absorbed dose.*

gray syndrome of the newborn The appearance of vomiting, lack of sucking response, irregular and rapid respiration, abdominal distention, and cyanosis in newborn infants treated at birth with chloramphenicol. Flaccidity and an ashen-gray color are present within 24 hr. About 40% of the patients die, most frequently on the fifth day of life. Because of the risk of this rare syndrome, chloramphenicol is rarely if ever used in pediatric care in the U.S.

green A color intermediate between blue and yellow, afforded by rays of wavelength between 492 and 575 nm. SEE: words beginning with *chloro-.*

g. blindness Aglaucopsia.

brilliant g. A derivative of malachite green, used in staining bacteria.

indocyanine g. A dye used intravenously to determine blood volume.

malachite g. A dye used as a stain and antiseptic.

g. soap tincture Green soap to which lavender oil and alcohol have been added.

Greenfield's disease [J. Godwin Greenfield, Brit. neuropathologist, 1884–1958] Metachromatic leukodystrophy.

Grey Turner's sign (grā-tŭr′nĕrz) [George Grey Turner, English surgeon, 1877–1951] A blue discoloration of the skin around the flanks or umbilicus in a patient with hemorrhagic pancreatitis.

grid **1.** A chart with an abscissa (x) (horizontal) axis and an ordinate (y) (vertical) axis on which to plot graphs. **2.** A device made of parallel lead strips, used to absorb scattered radiation during radiography of larger body parts.

Fixott-Everett g. A plastic-embedded screen placed over dental radiographic film before x-ray exposure. It facilitates measurement of bone loss and other tissue changes.

grief, chronic Unresolved denial of the reality of a personal loss. Also called *dysfunctional grieving.* SEE: *grief reaction.*

grief reaction The emotional reaction that follows the loss of a love object. Somatic symptoms include easy fatigability, hollow or empty feelings in the chest and abdomen, sighing, hyperventilation, anorexia, insomnia, and the feeling of having a lump in the throat. Psychological symptoms begin with an initial stage of shock and disbelief accompanied by an inner awareness of mental discomfort, sorrow, and regret. These may be followed by tears, sobbing, and cries of pain. The duration of the reaction is variable.

grieving, anticipatory Intellectual and emotional responses and behaviors by which individuals (families, communities) work through the process of modifying self-concept based on the perception of potential loss. SEE: *Nursing Diagnoses Appendix.*

grieving, dysfunctional Extended, unsuccessful use of intellectual and emotional responses by which individuals (families, communities) attempt to work through the process of modifying self-concept based upon the perception of potential loss. SEE: *Nursing Diagnoses Appendix.*

grinder (grīn′dĕr) [AS. *grindan*, to gnash] A molar tooth. SYN: *dens molaris.*

grinders' disease Pneumoconiosis.

grinding A forceful rubbing together, as in chewing. SEE: *bruxism.*

selective g. Altering and correcting the dental occlusion by grinding in accordance with what is required.

grip, grippe (grĭp) [Fr. *gripper*, to seize] Influenza.

gripes (grīps) [AS. *gripan*, to grasp] Intermittent severe pains in the bowels. SYN: *intestinal colic.*

griping An acute intermittent cramplike pain, esp. in the abdomen.

griseofulvin An oral antifungal antibiotic, esp. effective against ringworm.

groin [AS. *grynde*, abyss] The depression between the thigh and trunk; the inguinal region.

grommet (grŏm′ĭt) A device, also known as a ventilation tube, placed in an artificial opening in the tympanic membrane to permit air to flow freely between the inner ear and the external auditory canal. The prosthesis is used as a treatment adjunct in managing chronic otitis media with effusion. The routine use of grommets as part of the initial therapy for otitis media is not advised. Their use should be reserved for persistent or recurrent infections that have failed to respond to appropriate antibiotic therapy.

groove [MD. *groeve*, ditch] A long narrow channel, depression, or furrow. SYN: *sulcus.*

bicipital g. The groove for the long tendon of the biceps brachii located on the anterior surface of the humerus.

branchial g. A groove in the embryo that is lined with ectoderm and lies between two branchial arches.

carotid g. A broad groove on the inner surface of the sphenoid bone lateral to its body. It lodges the carotid artery and the cavernous sinus.

costal g. The groove on the lower internal border of a rib. It lodges the intercostal vessels and nerve. SYN: *subcostal g.*

costovertebral g. A broad groove that extends along each side of a vertebra. It lodges the sacrospinalis muscle and its subdivisions.

Harrison's g. The groove or line extending laterally from the xiphoid process of the sternum. It marks the attachment of the diaphragm to the costal margins and is seen in children with severe rickets.

infraorbital g. The groove on the orbital surface of the maxilla that transmits the infraorbital vessels and nerve.

labial g. The groove that develops in each of the primitive jaws. It gives rise to the vestibule separating the lips from the gums.

lacrimal g. Two grooves, one on the posterior surface of the frontal process of the maxilla, and the other on the anterior surface of the posterior lacrimal crest of the lacrimal bone. These grooves lodge the lacrimal sac.

laryngotracheal g. The groove along the ventral surface of the anterior portion of the embryonic gut that gives rise to the respiratory organs.

malleolar g. The groove on the anterior surface of the distal end of the tibia that lodges tendons of the tibialis posterior and flexor digitorum longus musculi.

meningeal g. One of several depressions on the internal surface of the cranial bones where blood vessels follow the meningeal and osseous structures of the skull.

musculospiral g. Radial g.

mylohyoid g. The groove on the inner surface of the mandible that runs obliquely forward and downward and contains the mylohyoid nerve and artery. In the embryo it lodges Meckel's cartilage.

nasolacrimal g. The groove extending from the inner angle of the eye to the primitive olfactory sac in the embryo. It separates the maxillary and lateral nasal processes; its epithelial lining gives rise to the nasolacrimal duct.

nasopalatine g. The groove on the vomer that lodges the nasopalatine nerve and vessels.

neural g. A longitudinal indentation that forms on the dorsal surface of the embryonic ectoderm. It is bordered by the neural folds, which merge dorsally to form the neural tube, a cylinder around the groove. Superiorly, the groove forms the ventricles of the brain; inferiorly, it becomes the central canal of the spinal cord.

obturator g. The groove at the superior and posterior angle of the obturator foramen through which pass the obturator vessels and nerve.

olfactory g. A shallow groove on the superior surface of the cribriform plate of the ethmoid on each side of the crista galli. It contains the olfactory bulb.

palatine g. One of several grooves on the inferior surface on the palatine process of the maxilla. They contain the palatine vessels and nerves.

peroneal g. A shallow groove on the lateral aspect of the calcaneus and a deep groove on the inferior surface of the cuboid bone. Each transmits the tendon of the peroneus longus muscle.

primitive g. In the embryo, a shallow groove in the primitive streak of the blastoderm, bordered by the primitive folds.

pterygopalatine g. The groove on the maxillary surface of the perpendicular portion of the palatine bone that, with corresponding grooves on the maxilla and pterygoid process of the sphenoid, transmits the palatine nerve and descending palatine artery.

radial g. A broad, shallow, spiraling groove on the posterior surface of the humerus. It transmits the radial nerve and the profunda branchi artery. SYN: *musculospiral g.*

rhombic g. One of seven transverse grooves in the floor of the developing rhombencephalon of the brain. They separate the neuromeres.

sagittal g. A shallow groove on the inner surface of the parietal bones that lodges the superior sagittal sinus. SYN: *sagittal sulcus.*

sigmoid g. The groove on the inner surface of the mastoid portion of the temporal bone. It transmits the transverse sinus.

subcostal g. Costal g.

tympanic g. The groove at the bottom of the exterior auditory meatus that receives the inferior portion of the tympanic membrane.

urethral g. The groove on the caudal surface of the genital tubercle or phallus bordered by the urethral folds. The latter close, transforming the groove into the cavernous urethra.

gross (grōs) [L. *grossus,* thick] **1.** Visible to the naked eye. **2.** Consisting of large particles or components; coarse or large.

gross motor skills The group of motor skills (including walking, running, and throwing) that require large muscle groups to produce the major action, and require less precision than that exerted by small muscles. Most motor activities combine some elements of both fine and gross motor function.

ground **1.** Basic substance or foundation. **2.** Reduced to a powder; pulverized. **3.** In electronics, the negative or earth pole that has zero electrical potential.

ground bundle A bundle of nerve fibers that immediately surrounds the gray matter of the spinal cord. It is divided into three regions, the anterior, lateral, and posterior bundles, which lie in the corresponding funiculi. These consist principally of short descending fibers.

group [It. *gruppo,* knot] A number of similar objects or structures considered together (e.g., bacteria with similar metabolic characteristics). Atomic molecules and compounds with similar structures or properties are classified with certain groups.

alcohol g. The hydroxyl, —OH, which imparts alcoholic characteristics to organic compounds. These may be in three forms: primary, $—CH_2OH$; secondary, =CHOH; and tertiary, ≡COH.

azo g. In chemistry, the group —N=N—.

coli-aerogenes g. Coliform bacteria.

colon-typhoid-dysentery g. The collective term for *Escherichia, Salmonella,* and *Shigella* bacteria.

focus g. An assembly of individuals affected by a specific subject (e.g., a disease, health care delivery system, marketed service, professional or management issue) to solicit and study their opinions, identify interests, and make strategic plans to meet expressed needs.

peptide g. The ⁻CONH radical.

prosthetic g. **1.** In a conjugated protein, the nonprotein portion of the molecule. **2.** The nonprotein component of a coenzyme.

resource utilization g. A grouping of nursing home patients according to diagnosis, treatment, and age for the purpose of providing adequate staff and ascertaining cost data. The primary use is for insurance reimbursement calculations.

saccharide g. The monosaccharide unit, $C_6H_{10}O_5$, which is a component of higher polysaccharides.

support g. Patients or families of patients with similar problems such as breast cancer, multiple sclerosis, alcoholism, or other life experiences, who meet to assist each other in coping with the problems and seeking solutions and ways of coping. The composition and focus of support groups varies. Some groups may be comprised of patients who are experiencing or have experienced the same disorder. Discussions often center on current treatments, resources available for assistance, and what individuals can do to improve or maintain their health. Other groups involve those who have experienced the same psychological and emotional trauma such as rape victims or persons who have lost a loved one. Benefits expressed by members include the knowledge that they are not alone but that others have experienced the same or similar problems and that they have learned to cope effectively.

grouping The classification of individual traits according to a shared characteristic.

blood g. Classification of blood of different individuals according to agglutinating and hemolyzing qualities before making a blood transfusion. SEE: *blood group; blood transfusion.*

group therapy A form of psychiatric treatment in which six to eight patients meet a specific number of times with a therapist. The value of this type of therapy is the opportunity for gaining insight from others into one's life experience.

group transfer An oxidation-reduction chemical reaction involving the exchange of chemical groups. A transferase enzyme is required.

Grover's disease [R. W. Grover, contemporary U.S. dermatologist] A common itchy (pruritic) condition of sudden onset, characterized by a few or numerous smooth or warty papules, vesicles, eczematous plaques, or shiny translucent nodules. The pruritus may be mild or severe and is aggravated by heat. Even though the condition is self-limiting, it may last months or years.

TREATMENT: The patient should be treated symptomatically. Heat and sweat-inducing activities should be avoided. Retinoic acid may be helpful.

growth [AS. *growan,* to grow] Development, maturation, or expansion of physical structures or cognitive and psychosocial abilities. The process may be normal, as in the development of a fetus or a child, or pathological, as in a cyst or malignant tumor.

TYPES:

1. General body growth is seen in the increase in the physical size of the body and increase in the total weight of the muscles and various internal organs. Growth is usually slow and steady but has a marked acceleration just after birth and at the time of puberty (the "growth spurt").

2. Lymphoid organs, such as the thymus and the lymph nodes, grow fastest early in life, reach their peak of development at about the age of 12 years, and then stop growing or regress.

3. The brain, cord, eye, and meninges grow in childhood but reach adult size by the age of 8 years. This size is maintained without regression.

4. The testes, ovaries, and other genitourinary structures grow slowly in infancy, but at puberty they develop rapidly and cause the striking changes in appearance that make up the secondary sex characteristics.

5. Cognitive growth is evidenced by the progressive maturation of thought, reasoning, and intellect, esp. in school-aged children.

6. Psychosocial growth involves the development of personality, judgment, and temperament; it evolves throughout life, as experience in work, play, and emotional interactions with others broaden.

risk for altered g. At risk for growth above the 97th percentile or below the 3rd percentile for age, crossing two percentile channels; disproportionate growth. SEE: *Nursing Diagnoses Appendix.*

growth and development, altered The state in which an individual demonstrates deviations in norms from his/her age group. SEE: *Nursing Diagnoses Appendix.*

growth curve A graph of heights and weights of infants and children of various ages. Using a line to join the data points produces the curve. Usually the changes in height and weight are shown on the same chart.

growth hormone, human synthetic SEE: under *hormone.*

gruel [L. *grutum,* meal] Any cereal boiled in water.

grumose, grumous (groo'mōs, -mŭs) [L. *grumus,* heap] **1.** Made up of coarse granular bodies in the center. **2.** Lumpy, clotted.

Grünfelder's reflex (groon'fĕld-ĕrs) A fanlike spreading of the toes with upward flexion of the great toe, resulting from pressure over the posterior fontanel.

gryposis (grĭ-pō'sĭs) [G. *gryposis,* a crooking] Abnormal curvature of any part of the body, esp. the nails.

GSA *Gerontological Society of America.*

GSR *galvanic skin response.*

G-suit A coverall-type garment designed for use by aviators. It contains compartments that inflate and bring pressure on the legs and abdomen to prevent blood from pooling there. In aviators this helps to prevent unconsciousness caused by positive acceleration with resulting pooling of blood in the lower extremities. The suit has been used in medicine to treat postural hypotension. SEE: *MAST.*

GSW *gunshot wound.*

gt L. *gutta,* a drop.

gtt L. *guttae,* drops.

GU *genitourinary.*

guaiac (gwī'ăk) [NL. *Guaiacum*] A resin obtained from trees of the genus *Guaiacum,* either *G. officinale* or *G. sanctum.* An alcoholic solution of guaiac is used to test for occult blood in feces.

guaiacol (gwī'ă-kōl) O-Methoxyphenol; a substance similar to phenol obtained by fractional distillation of creosote or by synthetic means. It is used as an antiseptic and germicide, intestinal antiseptic, and expectorant.

guaifenesin (gwī-fĕn'ĕ-sĭn) An expectorant. Trade name is Robitussin.

guanidine (gwăn'ĭ-dēn) A crystalline organic compound, $(NH_2)_2C{=}NH$, found among the decomposition products of proteins.

guanidinemia (gwăn"ĭd-ĕn-ē'mē-ă) [*guanidine* + Gr. *haima,* blood] Guanidine in the blood.

guanidoacetic acid A chemical formed in the liver, kidney, and other tissues. It is then metabolized to form creatine.

guanine (gwă'nēn) $C_5H_5N_5O$; one of the purine bases in DNA and RNA. Purine bases are degraded to urate and excreted in the urine.

guanosine (gwăn'ō-sĭn) The nucleoside formed from guanine and ribose. It is a major constituent of RNA and DNA.

guard A device for protecting something (e.g., a mouth guard or a face guard).

guarded prognosis A prognosis given by a physician when the outcome of a patient's illness is in doubt.

guardian ad litem [L.] In cases of child abuse, a guardian for the child appointed by the court to protect the best interests of the child.

guardianship A legal arrangement by which a person or institution assumes responsibility for an individual. When guardians are appointed, the individuals receiving the care are presumed to be incompetent and unable to care for themselves.

guarding A body defense method to prevent movement of an injured part, esp. spasm of abdominal muscles when an examiner attempts to palpate inflamed areas or organs in the abdominal cavity.

gubernaculum (gū″bĕr-năk′ū-lŭm) [L., helm] **1.** A structure that guides. **2.** A cordlike structure uniting two structures.

g. dentis A connective tissue band that connects the tooth sac of an unerupted tooth with the overlying gum.

g. testis A fibrous cord in the fetus that extends from the caudal end of the testis through the inguinal canal to the scrotal swelling. It plays a role in the descent of the testis into the scrotum.

Gubler's line (goob′lĕrz) [Adolphe Gubler, Fr. physician, 1821–1879] The level of superficial origin of the trigeminus or fifth nerve.

Gubler's paralysis A form of alternate hemiplegia in which a brainstem lesion causes paralysis of the cranial nerves on one side and of the body on the opposite side.

Gubler's tumor A fusiform swelling on the wrist in lead palsy.

Gudden's inferior commissure (gūd′ĕnz) [Bernard A. von Gudden, Ger. neurologist, 1824–1886] Nerve fibers that make up part of the supraoptic tract.

Gudden's law A law stating that, in the division of a nerve, degeneration in the proximal portion is toward the nerve cell.

guidance The act of guiding or counseling (e.g., of a patient).

manual g. Physical cueing or prompting by a therapist, to facilitate the mastery of movements needed to perform a specific task or to extinguish or suppress undesired movements.

guide A mechanical aid or device that assists in setting a course or directing the motion either of one's hand or of an instrument one holds.

guide dog A dog specifically trained to assist blind or partially sighted persons with mobility.

guideline An instructional guide or reference to indicate a course of action in a specified situation (e.g., critical care guideline).

guidewire A device used to assist in inserting, positioning, and moving a catheter. These wires vary in size, length, stiffness, composition, and shape of the tip.

guile The use of deception or cunning in order to accomplish something.

Guillain-Barré syndrome (gē-yă′băr-rā′) [Georges Guillain, Fr. neurologist, 1876–1961; J. A. Barré, Fr. neurologist, b. 1880] ABBR: GBS. A rare neurological illness, affecting 1 to 2 persons per 100,000, marked by an ascending paralysis. The loss of motor function begins in the extremities and may quickly rise to include the respiratory muscles, causing respiratory failure. The loss of motor function can occur in a few days to 2 to 3 weeks. Pain in the hips, thighs, and back are commonly experienced. Recovery may take more than a year. The syndrome may produce only limited muscle weakness or complete paralysis, followed by general recovery or partial recovery with residual weakness in the extremities. SYN: *acute inflammatory polyneuropathy; acute inflammatory polyradiculopathy*.

ETIOLOGY: The syndrome often follows an acute infection, esp. with *Campylobacter jejuni,* cytomegalovirus, or Ebstein-Barr virus.

TREATMENT: Some patients need intubation and mechanical ventilation until they can breathe on their own again. Plasma exchange or intravenously infused immunoglobins are also helpful. The goal of other treatments, such as physical therapy and skin care, is to reduce complications of the illness.

PATIENT CARE: The patient is carefully assessed for evidence of impending respiratory failure, through the use of bedside spirometry. If the inspiratory force or vital capacity decline, endotracheal intubation and mechanical ventilation are required.

Pain should be monitored closely to ensure that adequate analgesia is prescribed and administered since the paralysis is not accompanied by sensory loss. Stool softeners or laxatives are necessary to minimize the constipation associated with long-term narcotic use.

Gentle passive range-of-motion exercises (in water if possible) are provided three to four times daily within the patient's pain limits. As the patient's condition stabilizes, gentle stretching and active-assisted exercises are provided.

Skin is inspected for signs of breakdown. To prevent decubiti, a strict 2-hr turning schedule is established, and alternating pressure pads are applied at points of contact. Care should be taken at each repositioning to ensure that the patient is covered sufficiently for warmth, since his or her temperature control center may be defective.

Fluid and electrolyte balance is maintained. To prevent aspiration, the head of the bed is elevated and the gag reflex tested before oral intake. If the gag reflex is impaired, nasogastric enteral feedings are provided until the reflex returns. The nurse encourages adequate fluid intake (2000 ml/day) orally, enterally, or if necessary, parenterally unless contraindicated. The bladder should be palpated and percussed to assess for urine retention. Either urinal or bedpan is offered every 3 to 4 hr, and manual pressure applied over the bladder. Intermittent urinary catheterization is instituted if necessary. To prevent or relieve constipation, prune juice and a high-bulk diet, stool softeners and laxatives, glycerin or bisacodyl suppositories, or enemas (as prescribed) are provided daily or on alternate days.

If the patient has facial paralysis, the nurse provides oral hygiene and eye care every 4 hr, protecting the corneas with shields and isotonic eye drops. If the patient cannot vocalize, establishing alternative methods of communication, such as eye blink or letter boards, is essential to ensure that patient needs are met. Complete explanations of care and frequent contact help reduce the patient's fear and sense of isolation.The patient's legs are inspected regularly for signs of thrombophlebitis, and antiembolism devices are applied and anticoagulants given if prescribed.

Routine care of the paralyzed patient is implemented including range of motion exercises, turning and positioning every 2 hours, and scrupulous skin care. The patient's temperature control center may be defective, requiring adjustments in the amount of bedclothes based on the patient's sensations of warmth or coolness. As patients recover, progressive physical therapy, monitoring closely for postural hypotension, is implemented.

Before discharge, the nurse assists the patient and family to develop an appropriate home care plan and makes appropriate referrals for home care as necessary. The patient and family are also taught the skills required for home care or are referred for instruction. SEE: *Nursing Diagnoses Appendix.*

guillotine (gĭl'ŏ-tēn) [Fr., instrument for beheading] An instrument for excising tonsils and laryngeal growths.

guilt (gĭlt) An emotion resulting from doing what is thought to be wrong, associated with self-reproach and the need for punishment. An excess or absence of guilt characterizes various psychiatric disorders.

guinea pig (gĭn'ē pĭg) **1.** A small rodent used in laboratory research. **2.** A colloquial term for persons used in medical experiments.

guinea worm *Dracunculus medinensis.*

Gull's disease [Sir William W. Gull, Brit. physician, 1816–1890] Atrophy of the thyroid gland, which causes myxedema.

gullet [L. *gula,* throat] The esophagus.

Gullstrand's slit lamp (gŭl'străndz) [Allvar Gullstrand, Swedish ophthalmologist, 1862–1930] A device for illuminating the eye so that its anterior portion can be examined by microscope.

gum 1. A resinous substance given off by or extracted from certain plants. It is sticky when moist but hardens on drying. Roughly, gum is any resin-like substance produced by plants. **2.** The fleshy substance or tissue covering the alveolar processes of the jaws. SYN: *gingiva.*

DIAGNOSIS: *Bleeding:* If the gums bleed easily, conditions such as gingivitis, scurvy, trench mouth, or anticoagulation may be present. Silver poisoning causes the gums to turn *blue;* mercurial stomatitis or lead poisoning turns the gums *bluish red,* with a bluish line at the edge of the teeth. A *greenish line* at the edge of the teeth may indicate copper poisoning. A *purplish line or color* indicates scurvy. In youth, gingivitis, pyorrhea, or scurvy may cause a *red line. Spongy gums and ulceration* may indicate gingivitis, scurvy, stomatitis, leukemia, tuberculosis, or diabetes.

gumboil A gum abscess. SYN: *parulis.*

SYMPTOMS: The gum is red, swollen, tender, and very painful. A fluctuating swelling containing pus may appear, which may point and break or require incision.

ETIOLOGY: The abscess may be caused by a subperiosteal infection associated with a carious tooth. It may also be caused by irritation or injury by a denture.

TREATMENT: The patient should receive hot mouthwashes and applications over the gum or externally. The patient should be warned not to swallow pus. Frequent mouthwashes should continue after the lesion is evacuated.

gumma (gŭm'mă) [L. *gummi,* gum] A soft granulomatous tumor of the tissues characteristic of the tertiary stage of syphilis. Varying from a millimeter to a centimeter or more in diameter, it may be single or multiple and tends to be encapsulated. It consists of a central necrotic mass surrounded by an inflammatory zone and fibrosis. The necrotic portion may be firm or elastic, gelatinous or hyalinized. Infectious organisms may be present. The tumor occurs most frequently in the liver but may occur in other areas, such as the brain, testis, heart, skin, and bone. SEE: *syphilis.*

SYMPTOMS: Symptoms vary depending on the gumma location. Bursting of a gumma leads to a gummatous ulcer that is painless but slow to heal. The base is formed by a "wash-leather" slough, but surrounding tissues are healthy.

gummatous (gŭm'ă-tŭs) Having the character of a gumma.

gummose (gŭm'ōs) $C_6H_{12}O_6$; a sugar from animal gum.

gummy [L. *gummi,* gum] Sticky, swollen, puffy.

Gunn's dots (gŭnz) [Robert Marcus Gunn, Brit. ophthalmologist, 1850–1909] White spots on the retina of the eye, close to the macula.

Gunn's syndrome SEE: *Marcus Gunn syndrome.*

Günther's disease [Hans Günther, Ger. physician, 1884–1956] Congenital erythropoietic porphyria.

gurney (gĕr'nē) A litter, equipped with wheels, used for transporting patients. SYN: *ambulance cot; stretcher.*

gustation (gŭs-tā'shŭn) [L. *gustare,* to taste] The sense of taste.

gustatory (gŭs'tă-tō-rē) Pert. to the sense of taste.

gustometry (gŭs-tŏm'ĕ-trē) [" + Gr. *metron,* measure] The measurement of the acuteness of the sense of taste.

gut [AS.] **1.** The bowel or intestine. **2.** The primitive gut or embryonic digestive tube, which includes the foregut, midgut, and hindgut. **3.** Short term for catgut.

gut-associated lymphoid tissue ABBR: GALT. A term used for all lymphoid tissue associated with the gastrointestinal tract, including the tonsils, appendix, and Peyer's patches. GALT contains lymphocytes, primarily B cells, and is responsible for controlling microorganisms entering the body via the digestive system. SEE: *mucosal immune system.*

Guthrie test [Robert Guthrie, U.S. microbiologist, 1916–1995] A blood test used to detect hyperphenylalaninemia and to diagnose phenylketonuria (PKU) in the newborn. SEE: *phenylketonuria.*

gutta [L., a drop] ABBR: gt. (pl. *gtt.*) A drop. The amount in a drop varies with the nature of the liquid and its temperature. It is therefore not advisable to use the number of drops per minute of a solution as anything more than a general guide to the amount of material being administered intravenously.

gutta-percha (gŭt"ă-pĕr'chă) The purified dried latex of certain trees, used in dentistry as a temporary filling.

guttate [L. *gutta,* drop] Resembling a drop, said of certain cutaneous lesions.

guttatim (gŭt-tā'tĭm) [L.] Drop by drop.

guttering (gŭt'ĕr-ĭng) Cutting a channel or groove in a bone.

guttur (gŭt'ŭr) [L. *gutter,* throat] The throat.

guttural (gŭt'ū-răl) Pert. to the throat.

gutturotetany (gŭt"ŭr-ō-tĕt'ă-nē) [" + Gr. *tetanos,* tension] A laryngeal spasm of the throat with temporary stutter.

Guyon's canal A tunnel on the ulnar side of the wrist formed by the hook of the hamate and pisiform bones. The ulnar nerve may be compressed at this site in long-distance bicyclists, by falling on the wrist, or by repetitive wrist actions.

Guyon's sign (gē-yŏnz') [Felix J. C. Guyon, Fr. surgeon, 1831–1920] Ballottement of the kidney.

GVHD *graft-versus-host disease.*

Gwathmey's method (gwăth'mēz) [James T. Gwathmey, U.S. surgeon, 1863–1944] The use of an anesthetic, consisting of ether and olive oil solution, placed in the rectum and colon, where it is absorbed.

Gy *gray* (unit of measure).

gymnastics [Gr. *gymnastikos,* pert. to nakedness] Systematic body exercise with or without special apparatus.

ocular g. Systematic exercise of the eye muscles to improve muscular coordination and efficiency.

Swedish g. A system of movements made by the patient against a resistance provided by the attendant, once used worldwide in physical training. It influenced the development of modern gymnastics.

gymnophobia (jĭm-nō-fō'bē-ă) [Gr. *gymnos,* naked, + *phobos,* fear] An abnormal aversion to viewing a naked body.

gyn- SEE: *gyneco-.*

gynander (jĭ-năn'dĕr, jī-, gī-) [Gr. *gyne,* woman, + *aner, andros,* man] Pseudohermaphrodite.

gynandrism (jĭ-năn'drĭzm) **1.** Male hermaphroditism. **2.** Partial female pseudohermaphroditism.

gynandroid (jĭ-năn'droyd, jī-, gī-) [" + " + *eidos,* form, shape] An individual having sufficient hermaphroditic sexual characteristics to be mistaken for a person of the opposite sex.

gynatresia (jĭ-nă-trē'zē-ă, jī-, gī-) [" + *a-,* not, + *tresis,* perforation] Congenital absence or closure of the vagina.

gyne- SEE: *gyneco-.*

gynecic (jĭ-nē'sĭk, jī, gī-) [Gr. *gyne,* woman] Pert. to women.

gyneco-, gyno-, gyn-, gyne- [Gr.] Combining form meaning *woman, female.*

gynecogenic (jĭn"ĕ-kō-jĕn'ĭk) [Gr. *gyne,* woman, + *gennan,* to produce] Producing female characteristics.

gynecoid (jĭn'ĕ-koyd) [" + *eidos,* form, shape] Resembling the female of the species.

gynecologic, gynecological (gī"nĕ-kō-lŏj'ĭk, jī", jĭn"ĕ-; -ĭ-kăl) [" + *logos,* word, reason] Pert. to gynecology, the study of diseases specific to women.

gynecological operative procedures Examination and surgery involving the female reproductive tract. Included are pelvic examination, dilation and curettage, hysterectomy, tubal ligation, cautery of the cervix, and cesarean section.

PATIENT CARE: *Preoperative:* The patient is prepared physically and emotionally for the procedure.

Postoperative: Vital signs are monitored frequently in the immediate postoperative period. If they deteriorate, the patient is assessed for shock or internal hemorrhage. Abdominal dressings are inspected for drainage, the presence of surgical drains is noted, the incision is assessed and redressed, and any vaginal drainage or perineal sutures are managed. A calm, quiet environment and light blankets are provided.

Ventilatory function is monitored; the patient is encouraged to breathe deeply and cough, and to use an incentive spirometer if prescribed. Fluid and electrolyte balance is monitored, and intravenous fluid intake is maintained as prescribed until oral intake (clear liquids) is permitted and tolerated.

The urinary bladder is gently palpated and percussed for evidence of urinary retention. The patient is offered the bedpan frequently to encourage urination, and the time and amount of each voiding are documented. Intermittent catheterization is instituted for urinary retention (allowing no more than 12 hr to pass without urine output immediately postoperatively, then no more than 8 hr until the patient is able to void). Closed, continuous drainage is maintained via an indwelling catheter if the surgeon prefers or if the patient continues to be unable to void. Bowel activity is assessed, and stool softeners are provided as prescribed.

Regular assessments are made for signs of thrombophlebitis. Active leg exercises are encouraged, and antiembolism stockings, pneumatic boots, heparins, or warfarin are used as prescribed. Early ambulation is encouraged.

gynecologist (gī″nĕ-kŏl′ō-jĭst, jī″, jĭn″ĕ-) A physician who specializes in gynecology.

gynecology (gī″nĕ-kŏl′ō-jē, jī″, jĭn″ĕ-) [″ + *logos,* word, reason] The study of the diseases of the female reproductive organs and the breasts.

gynecomastia (jī″nĕ-kō-măs′tē-ă, gī″, jĭn″ĕ-) [″ + *mastos,* breast] Enlargement of breast tissue in the male. This may occur during three distinct age periods: transiently at birth, again beginning with puberty and declining during the late teenage years, and finally in adults over age 50 years. In the newborn, it is caused by stimulation from maternal hormones. A milky secretion ("witch's milk") may be produced; the condition disappears within a few weeks. During middle adolescence, as many as 60% of boys may develop some degree of gynecomastia, either unilateral or bilateral and, if bilateral, often with varying degrees of growth between the two sides. It is considered a normal, nonpathological condition and usually disappears within 18 months. Hormonal assays should be performed only if the condition appears before puberty, persists longer than 2 years, or is associated with other signs of endocrine disorders. In older men, the condition can be caused by pituitary or testicular tumors, medications containing estrogens, or cirrhosis of the liver causing enhanced activity (due to delayed liver catabolism) of naturally produced estrogens.

TREATMENT: Therapy depends on the cause. Because gynecomastia has a high rate of spontaneous regression, medical therapies are most effective during the active proliferative phase. To help alleviate the acute embarrassment from the condition adolescent boys may suffer, they should be reassured that the problem will go away. Tender breasts should be treated with analgesics.

gynecopathy (jī-nĕ-kŏp′ă-thē, gī″, jĭn″ĕ-) [″ *pathos,* disease, suffering] Diseases specific to women.

gynecophonus (jī″nĕ-kŏf′ŏn-ŭs, gī″, jĭn″ĕ-) [″ + *phone,* voice] Having a soft, high-pitched voice.

gynephobia (jī″nĕ-fō′bē-ă, gī″, jĭn″ĕ-) [″ + *phobos,* fear] An abnormal aversion to the company of women, or fear of them. **gynephobic,** *adj.*

gynesic (gī-nē′sĭk, jī-, jĭn-ē′) [Gr. *gyne,* woman] Pert. to diseases of the female reproductive organs and breasts.

gyno- SEE: *gyneco-*.

gynopathic [″ + *pathos,* disease, suffering] Pert. to diseases of the female reproductive organs and breasts.

gynoplasty [″ + *plassein,* to form] Reparative surgery of the female genitalia.

gypsum (jĭp′sŭm) [L.; G. *gypsos,* chalk] **1.** A natural form of hydrated calcium sulfate. When heated to 130°C, it loses its water and becomes plaster of Paris. **2.** A hemihydrate of gypsum resulting from heating gypsum and allowing it to dehydrate in the presence of sodium succinate or calcium hydrochloride. This form is used as a dental stone in preparing investments for dental casting.

gyrate (jī′rāt) [Gr. *gyros,* circle] **1.** Ring-shaped, convoluted. **2.** To revolve.

gyration (jī-rā′shŭn) A rotary movement.

gyre (jīr) [Gr. *gyros,* circle] Gyrus.

gyrectomy (jī-rĕk′tō-mē) [″ + *ektome,* excision] Surgical removal of a cerebral gyrus.

gyrencephalic (jī-rĕn-sĕ-făl′ĭk) [″ + *enkephale,* head] Having a brain marked by numerous convolutions.

gyri (jī′rī) Pl. of gyrus.

gyro- [Gr.] Combining form meaning *circle, spiral, ring.*

gyroma (jī-rō′mă) [Gr. *gyros,* circle, + *oma,* tumor] An ovarian tumor consisting of a convoluted mass.

gyrometer (jī-rŏm′ĕ-ter) [″ + *metron,* measure] A device for measuring the cerebral gyri of the brain.

gyrose (jī′rōs) In bacteriology, marked by circular or wavy lines. This term is applied to bacterial colonies.

gyrospasm (jī′rō-spăzm) [″ + *spasmos,* a convulsion] A spasmodic rotary head movement.

gyrus (jī′rŭs) *pl.* **gyri** One of the convolutions of the cerebral hemispheres of the brain. The gyri are separated by shallow grooves (sulci) or deeper grooves (fissures). SYN: *gyre.* SEE: *convolution.*

angular g. A gyrus of the parietal lobe that embraces the posterior end of the superior temporal sulcus.

annectent g. Any of many short folds of gray matter formed as a result of short branches or twigs of sulci extending into adjacent gyri. They are not always present.

anterior central g. A gyrus of the frontal lobe extending vertically between the precentral and central sulci.

g. breves insulae Preinsular gyri of the brain.

Broca's g. Inferior frontal g.

callosal g. A large gyrus on the medial surface of the cerebral hemisphere that lies directly above the corpus callosum and arches over its anterior end.

g. cerebelli A layer of the cerebellum.

cingulate g. An arch-shaped convolution of the cingulum, curved over the surface of the corpus callosum, from which it is separated by the callosal sulcus.

dentate g. A gyrus marked by indentations that lie on the upper surface of the hippocampal gyrus.

g. fornicatus A gyrus on the medial surface of the cerebrum, which includes the gyrus cinguli, isthmus, hippocampus, hippocampal gyrus, and uncus.

fusiform g. A gyrus beneath the collateral fissure joining the occipital and temporal lobes. SYN: *occipitotemporal g.*

Heschl's g. A transverse temporal gyrus.

hippocampal g. A gyrus between the hippocampal and collateral fissures.

inferior frontal g. A convolution on the external surface of the frontal lobe of the cerebrum located between the sylvian fissure and the inferior frontal sulcus. SYN: *Broca's g.*

lingual g. A gyrus between the calcarine and collateral fissures.

g. longus insulae A lengthy gyrus composing the postinsula.

middle frontal g. A gyrus between the superior and inferior frontal sulci.

middle temporal g. A gyrus between the middle temporal sulcus and superior temporal sulcus.

occipital g. Any of the gyri on the lateral surface of the occipital lobe. They are classified roughly into two groups, the inferior or lateral occipital gyri and the superior occipital gyri. They are not always present.

occipitotemporal g. Fusiform g.

orbital g. One of four gyri (anterior, posterior, lateral, and medial) forming the inferior surface of the frontal lobe.

paracentral g. The area on the medial aspect of the cerebrum; the paracentral lobule. It lies above the cingulate sulcus.

parahippocampal g. A gyrus on the lower surface of each cerebral hemisphere between the hippocampal and collateral sulci.

paraterminal g. A small area of the cerebral cortex anterior to the lamina terminalis and below the rostrum of the corpus callosum.

parietal g. A gyrus on the lateral aspect of the parietal lobe. It includes the posterior central gyrus and the superior and inferior parietal gyri.

postcentral g. A gyrus immediately posterior to the central sulcus of the cerebrum. It contains most of the general sensory area of the brain. SYN: *posterior central g.*

posterior central g. Postcentral g.

precentral g. A gyrus immediately anterior to the central sulcus of the cerebrum. It contains the motor area for initiation of voluntary movement.

g. profundus cerebri One of the very deep gyri of the cerebrum.

g. rectus A gyrus on the orbital aspect of the frontal lobe, located between the medial margin and the olfactory sulcus.

Retzius g. The supracallosal and subcallosal gyri.

subcallosal g. A narrow band of gray matter on the medial surface of the hemisphere below the rostrum of the corpus callosum.

superior frontal g. A convolution of the cerebral frontal lobe situated above the superfrontal fissure.

supracallosal g. A rudimentary gyrus on the upper surface of the corpus callosum.

supracallosus g. The gray matter layer covering the corpus callosum.

supramarginal g. A gyrus in the inferior parietal lobule twisting about the upper terminus of the sylvian fissure.

temporal g. One of the three gyri (superior, middle, inferior) on the lateral surface of the temporal lobe.

uncinate g. The anterior hooked portion of the hippocampal gyrus.

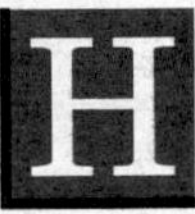

H Symbol for the element hydrogen.

H, h *haustus,* a draft of medicine; *height; henry; hora* or *hour; horizontal; hypermetropia.*

h Symbol for hecto, a term used in SI units.

ħ Symbol for Planck's constant.

H^+, *c*H^+ Symbol for hydrogen ion.

[H^+] Symbol for hydrogen ion concentration.

^1H Symbol for protium.

^2H Symbol for deuterium, an isotope of hydrogen.

^3H Symbol for tritium, an isotope of hydrogen.

Ha Symbol for hahnium.

Haab's reflex (hŏbz) [Otto Haab, Swiss ophthalmologist, 1850–1931] Contraction of pupils without alteration of accommodation or convergence when gazing at a bright object. It may indicate a cortical lesion.

HAAg *hepatitis A antigen.*

HAART *Highly active antiretroviral therapy.*

habena (hă-bē′nă) *pl.* **habenae** [L., rein] **1.** A frenum. **2.** Habenula. **habenal, habenar,** *adj.*

habenula (hă-bĕn′ū-lă) *pl.* **habenulae** [L., little rein, strap] **1.** A frenum or any reinlike or whiplike structure. **2.** A peduncle or stalk attached to the pineal body of the brain. Fibers that travel posteriorly along the dorsomedial border of the thalamus to the habenular ganglia (epithalamus) resemble reins. **3.** A narrow bandlike stricture. **habenular,** *adj.*

h. urethralis One of two whitish bands between the clitoris and meatus urethra in young females.

habenular Pert. to the habenula, esp. the stalk of the pineal body.

h. commissure A band of transverse fibers connecting the two habenular areas.

h. trigone A depressed triangular area located on the lateral aspect of the posterior portion of the third ventricle. It contains a medial and lateral habenular nucleus.

habilitation (hă-bĭl″ĭ-tā′shŭn) The process of educating or training persons with functional limitation to improve their ability to function in society. SEE: *rehabilitation.*

habit [L. *habere, habitus,* to have, hold] **1.** A motor pattern executed with facility following constant or frequent repetition; an act performed at first in a voluntary manner but after sufficient repetition as a reflex action. Habits result from the passing of impulses through a particular set of neurons and synapses many times. **2.** A particular type of dress or garb. **3.** Mental or moral constitution or disposition. **4.** Bodily appearance or constitution, esp. as related to a disease or predisposition to a disease. SYN: *habitus* (1). **5.** Addiction to the use of drugs or alcohol.

chorea h. An obsolete term for tic.

masticatory h. An individual's sequence and pattern of jaw movement in chewing. It is influenced by the type of food, occlusal problems or missing teeth, personal habits, or state of mind and may be unilateral or bilateral. Under some conditions it would be recognized as clenching or bruxing habit. SEE: *bruxism.*

h. spasm An infrequently used term for a tic.

habituation **1.** The act of becoming accustomed to anything from frequent use or exposure. In drug addiction, the mental equivalent of physical tolerance and dependence on drugs. **2.** The newborn's unconscious suppression or extinction of automatic physiological responses to selective levels of commonly experienced stimuli, such as environmental noise.

newborn h. The rapid development of decreased sensitivity to specific common postbirth stimuli, such as environmental noise, light, and heelsticks. This adaptive response protects the newborn against overstimulation.

habitus [L., habit] A physical appearance, body build, or constitution.

hachement (hăsh-mŏn′) [Fr., chopping] In massage, a chopping stroke with the edge of the hand.

haem- SEE: *hem-.*

Haemadipsa (hē″mă-dĭp′să) [Gr. *haima,* blood + *dipsa,* thirst] A genus of terrestrial leeches found in Asia that attach to humans and animals.

H. ceylonica A species of leech found in certain humid, tropical areas.

Haemagogus (hē″mă-gŏg′ŭs) [″ + *agogos,* leading] A genus of mosquitoes that includes species that serve as vectors of yellow fever endemic in the Amazon region of South America. It is similar to *Aedes* species.

Haemaphysalis (hĕm″ă-fis′ă-lĭs) [″ + *physallis,* bubble] A genus of ticks including species that serve as vectors for tick-borne viral diseases including hemorrhagic fever.

Haemophilus (hē-mŏf′ĭl-ŭs) [″ + *philein,* to love] A genus of small, nonmotile, gram-negative bacteria. They may cause a variety of human illnesses, including pneumonia, meningitis, sepsis, and sexually transmitted diseases.

H. aegyptius Koch-Weeks bacillus; the cause of one form of contagious conjunctivitis.

H. ducreyi The causative organism of chancroid or soft chancre. SEE: *chancroid.*

H. influenzae Gram-negative bacteria that cause acute respiratory infections and meningitis, esp. in children. Encapsulated type b is the form most commonly seen, but nonencapsulated forms also cause infections. Infections may be mild (e.g., pharyngitis, tonsillitis, otitis media) or severe and life-threatening (e.g., epiglottitis, septicemia, meningitis, postviral pneumonia, endocarditis). Antibiotic treatment depends on the site infected. The *H. influenzae* type B vaccine, given in three or four doses during infancy, has reduced the incidence of infection in young children significantly. SEE: *epiglottitis; meningitis.*

H. influenzae type b infection ABBR: HIB. An important preventable cause of meningitis. In children, this organism also causes acute epiglottitis, pneumonia, septic arthritis, and cellulitis.

TREATMENT: A cephalosporin that penetrates into the cerebrospinal fluid, such as cefotaxime or ceftriaxone, should be used.

PREVENTION: Administer the HIB vaccine three or four doses beginning at 2 months of age. Because the various forms of HIB vaccine are administered on different schedules, it is important to check the package insert for the appropriate scheduling information. Booster doses may be required. SEE: *vaccine* for table.

H. vaginalis The name formerly used for *Gardnerella vaginalis.*

Haemosporidia (hē″mō-spō-rĭd′ē-ă) An order of sporozoa that live in the blood cells of vertebrates and reproduce sexually in invertebrates; includes the genus *Plasmodium,* which causes malaria in humans.

Haff disease [First described in persons living along the Konigsberg Haff, a German inlet of the Baltic Sea] A rare syndrome of rhabdomyolysis (muscle breakdown) from eating certain kinds of fish. It is believed to result from ingestion of a marine toxin.

hafnium (hăf′nē-ŭm) [L. *Hafnia,* Copenhagen] SYMB: Hf. A rare chemical element; atomic weight 178.49, atomic number 72, specific gravity 13.31.

Hagedorn needle (hă′gĕ-dorn) [Werner Hagedorn, Ger. surgeon, 1831–1894] A curved surgical needle with flattened sides.

Hahnemann, Samuel (hă′nĕ-măn) [German physician, 1755–1843] The founder of homeopathy. He proposed that minuscule doses of medications could cure disease.

hahnium (hăhn′ē-ŭm) [Named after Otto Hahn, Ger. scientist, 1879–1968] SYMB: Ha. Name proposed for the artificially made element 105.

Hailey-Hailey disease [W. H. Hailey, 1898–1967; H. E. Hailey, b. 1909, U.S. dermatologists] Benign familial pemphigus. SEE: *pemphigus.*

hair [AS. *haer*] **1.** A keratinized, threadlike outgrowth from the skin of mammals. **2.** Collectively, the threadlike outgrowths that form the fur of animals or that grow on the human body.

A hair is a thin, flexible shaft of cornified cells that develops from a cylindrical invagination of the epidermis, the hair follicle. Each consists of a free portion or shaft (scapus pili) and a root (radix pili) embedded within the follicle. The shaft consists of three layers of cells: the cuticle or outermost layer; the cortex, forming the main horny portion of the hair; and the medulla, the central axis. Hair color is due to pigment in the cortex. SEE: illus.

Hair in each part of the body has a definite period of growth, after which it is shed. In the adult human there is a constant gradual loss and replacement of hair. Hair of the eyebrows lasts only 3 to 5 months; that of the scalp 2 to 5 years. Baldness or alopecia results when replacement fails to keep up with hair loss. It may be hereditary or due to pathologic conditions such as infections or injury from irradiation. Also cytotoxic agents used in cancer chemotherapy may cause temporary loss of hair. SEE: *alopecia.*

auditory h. The stereocilia of a specialized epithelial cell. These are present in the ear in the spiral organ of Corti, concerned with hearing; and in the crista ampullaris, macula utriculi, and macula sacculi, concerned with equilibrium.

bamboo h. Sparse, brittle hair with bamboolike nodes. These apparent nodes are actually partial fractures of the hair shaft, caused by an atrophic condition of the hair. Also called *trichorrhexis nodosa.*

beaded h. Swellings and constrictions in the hair shaft caused by a developmental defect known as monilethrix.

burrowing h. A hair that grows horizontally under the skin, causing a foreign body reaction.

gustatory h. One of several fine hairlike processes extending from the ends of gustatory cells in a taste bud. They project through the inner pore of a taste bud. SYN: *taste h.*

ingrown h. A hair that reenters the skin, causing a foreign body reaction.

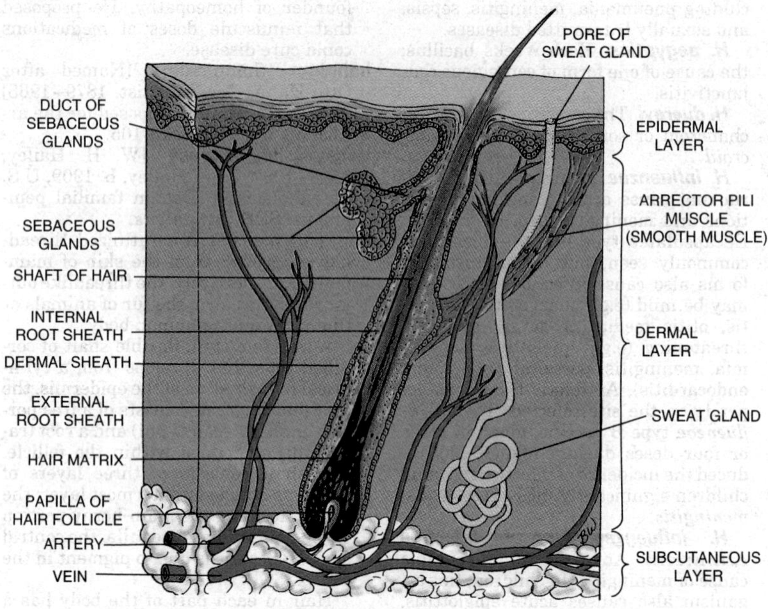

HAIR AND ADJACENT STRUCTURES OF CROSS-SECTION OF SKIN

kinky h. Short, sparse, kinky hair that may be poorly pigmented. The condition is associated with kinky hair disease.

lanugo h. SEE: *lanugo*.

moniliform h. Monilethrix.

moth-eaten h. Patchy areas of baldness, with poorly defined borders. This type of alopecia is one of the cutaneous hallmarks of syphilis.

h. papilla A projection of the corium that extends into the hair bulb at the bottom of a hair follicle. It contains capillaries through which a hair receives nourishment.

pubic h. Hair that appears over the pubes at the onset of sexual maturity.

sensory h. Specialized epithelial cells with hairlike processes.

tactile h. Hair that is capable of receiving tactile or touching stimuli.

taste h. Gustatory h.

terminal h. The long, coarse, pigmented hair of the adult.

twisted h. Congenitally deformed hair that is short, brittle, and twisted.

hairball Trichobezoar.

halal (hă-lăl′) Pert. to food prepared and served according to Muslim dietary laws.

halation (hăl-ā′shŭn) [Gr. *alos,* a halo] A blurring of vision caused by light being scattered to the side of the source.

halazone (hăl′ă-zōn) A chloramine disinfectant. SEE: *water, emergency preparation of safe drinking*.

Haldane effect The oxygenation of hemoglobin, which lowers its affinity for carbon dioxide. SEE: *Bohr effect*.

half-life **1.** Time required for half the nuclei of a radioactive substance to lose their activity by undergoing radioactive decay. **2.** Time it takes for a radioactive substance to reduce to one-half its energy due to metabolism and excretion. **3.** In biology and pharmacology, the time required by the body, tissue, or organ to metabolize or inactivate half the amount of a substance taken in. This is an important consideration in determining the proper amount and frequency of dose of drug to be administered. **4.** Time required for radioactivity of material taken in by a living organism to be reduced to half its initial value by a combination of radioactive decay and biological elimination.

half-value thickness The thickness of a substance that, when placed in the path of a given beam of radiation, will lower its intensity to one half of the initial value.

halfway house A facility to house psychiatric patients who no longer need hospitalization but are not yet ready for independent living.

halide (hăl′īd) A compound containing a halogen (i.e., bromine, chlorine, fluorine, or iodine) combined with a metal or some other radical.

halitosis (hăl-ĭ-tō′sĭs) [L. *halitus,* breath, + Gr. *osis,* condition] Bad breath.

halitus (hăl′ĭ-tŭs) **1.** The breath. **2.** Warm vapor.

Haller's anastomotic circle (hăl′ĕrz) [Albrecht von Haller, Swiss physiologist, 1708–1777] The circle of arteries around the intraocular portion of the optic nerve. It is composed of branches of the posterior ciliary arteries.

Hallervorden-Spatz disease, H.-S. syndrome [Julius Hallervorden, 1882–1965; H. Spatz, 1888–1969, Ger. neurologists] An inherited, progressive, degenerative disease, beginning in childhood, of the globus pallidus, red nucleus, and reticular part of the substantia nigra of the brain. Clinically, characteristics include progressive rigidity, retinal degeneration, athetotic movements, and mental and, late in the disease, emotional retardation. There is no effective therapy.

hallex (hăl'ĕks) *pl.* **hallices** [L.] Hallux.

Hallpike maneuver, Hallpike-Dix maneuver [C. Hallpike, 20th century neurologist] A test performed to diagnose benign positional vertigo. The patient is moved from a sitting position to recumbency with the head tilted down over the end of the bed and turned toward either shoulder. If vertigo develops after a delay of several seconds, the test is subjectively positive. If vertigo is associated with visible nystagmus, it is objectively positive. Vertigo and nystagmus that occur immediately, rather than after a delay, are suggestive of intracranial, rather than labyrinthine, disease. SEE: *benign positional vertigo*.

hallucination (hă-loo-sĭ-nā'shŭn) [L. *hallucinari,* to wander in mind] A false perception having no relation to reality and not accounted for by any exterior stimulus; a dreamlike (or nightmarish) perception occurring while awake. It may be visual (esp. in medical illnesses or drug withdrawal syndromes), auditory (esp. in psychoses), tactile, gustatory, or olfactory. Affected patients typically appear confused and agitated. They are unable to distinguish between the real and the imaginary.

auditory h. An imaginary perception of sounds, usually voices. Auditory hallucinations are a hallmark of psychotic illnesses but are also heard by patients with acquired hearing impairments and by some persons with temporal lobe seizures.

extracampine h. A hallucination that arises from outside the normal sensory field or range, as people having the sensation of seeing something behind them.

gustatory h. The sense of tasting something that is not present.

haptic h. A hallucination pert. to touching the skin or to sensations of temperature or pain.

hypnagogic h. A presleep phenomenon having the same practical significance as a dream but experienced during consciousness. It may include a sense of falling, of sinking, or of the ceiling moving.

kinetic h. A sensation of flying or of moving the body or a part of it.

microptic h. A hallucination in which things seem smaller than they are.

motor h. An imagined perception of movement.

olfactory h. A hallucination involving the sense of smell.

somatic h. A sensation of pain attributed to visceral injury.

stump h. SEE: *phantom limb*.

tactile h. A false sense of touching something or of objects moving on the skin. This abnormal perception is a hallmark of some withdrawal states, such as delirium tremens in alcohol withdrawal. SEE: *formication*.

visual h. The sensation of seeing objects that are not really there. This is a hallmark of alcohol and drug withdrawal and of other medical illnesses that adversely affect the brain.

hallucinogen (hă-loo'sĭ-nō-jĕn) [" + Gr. *gennan,* to produce] A drug that produces hallucinations (e.g., LSD, peyote, mescaline, PCP, and sometimes ethyl alcohol).

hallucinosis (hă-loo"sĭn-ō'sĭs) [" + Gr. *osis,* condition] The state of having hallucinations more or less persistently. SEE: *hallucination*.

acute alcoholic h. Alcohol withdrawal, marked by visual hallucinations, extreme agitation, tachycardia, hypertension, and other signs and symptoms of cerebral and autonomic hyperactivity.

hallus Hallux.

hallux (hăl'ŭks) *pl.* **halluces** [L.] The great toe.

h. dolorosus Pain in the metatarsophalangeal joint of the great toe resulting from flatfoot.

h. flexus H. malleus.

h. malleus Hammertoe of the great toe.

h. rigidus A restriction or loss of motion of the joint connecting the great toe to the metatarsal. Pain occurs upon walking.

h. valgus Displacement of the great toe toward the other toes.

h. varus Displacement of the great toe away from the other toes.

halo [Gr. *halos,* a halo] **1.** The areola, esp. of the nipple. **2.** A ring surrounding the macula lutea in ophthalmoscopic images. **3.** A circle of light surrounding a shining body.

Fick's h. A colored halo around light observed by some persons as a result of wearing contact lenses.

glaucomatous h. The visual perception of rainbow-like colors around lights, caused by glaucoma-induced corneal edema.

senile peripapillary h. A ring of choroidoretinal atrophy around the head of the optic nerve, a condition that may occur in the aged.

h. symptom The perception of one or more colored circles around lights, seen by patients with glaucoma or cataract.

halodermia (hăl″ō-dĕr′mē-ă) A skin eruption caused by exposure to a halogen.

halogen (hăl′ō-jĕn) [Gr. *hals,* salt, + *gennan,* to produce] Any one of the elements (chlorine, bromine, iodine, fluorine, and astatine) forming Group VII of the periodic table. These elements have very similar chemical properties, combining with hydrogen to form acids and with metals to form salts.

haloid (hăl′oyd) [″ + *eidos,* form, shape] Resembling salt or a halogen.

haloperidol (hă″lō-pĕr′ĭ-dŏl) A neuroleptic drug used to treat patients with psychotic illnesses, extreme agitation, or Tourette's syndrome. Trade name is Haldol.

halophilic (hăl″ō-fĭl′ĭk) [″ + *philein,* to love] Concerning or having an affinity for salt or any halogen.

halothane (hăl′ō-thān) A fluorinated hydrocarbon used as a general anesthetic.

halo vest, halo vest orthosis A device used to immobilize the head and cervical spine following vertebral injury or surgery, designed to provide inline traction of the cervical spine while allowing for a moderate amount of functional independence. The halo vest consists of three parts: 1) the halo, which is secured into the skull through the use of four pins or screws; 2) the vest, which is worn over the shoulders and trunk to support the weight of the halo, skull, and cervical spine; and 3) four metal bars that connect the halo to the vest.

PATIENT CARE: The screws attaching the halo to the skull must be kept clean to reduce the risk of infection. Hygiene consists of cleaning each pin two to three times per day with peroxide or other disinfectant prescribed by a physician. The patient should be instructed on how to use a mirror to inspect the sites for signs of infection. The shoulders and thorax should be inspected for signs of irritation from the vest. Additional padding may be required around pressure-sensitive areas.

CAUTION: Although patients can function without assistance, physical or occupational therapy is required to integrate the individual back into the activities of daily living, including bathing techniques. Peripheral vision and the ability to look upward or downward are limited because the head and spine are immobilized. Care should be taken to prevent the patient from bumping the halo, as this may loosen its attachment to the skull.

Halsted's operation (hăl′stĕdz) [William Stewart Halsted, U.S. surgeon, 1852–1922] **1.** An operation for inguinal hernia. **2.** A radical mastectomy for cancer of the breast.

Halsted's suture An interrupted suture for intestinal wounds.

ham [AS. *haum,* haunch] **1.** The popliteal space or region behind the knee. **2.** A common name for the thigh, hip, and buttock.

hamartoma (hăm-ăr-tō′mă) [Gr. *hamartia,* defect, + *oma,* tumor] A tumor resulting from new growth of normal tissues. The cells grow spontaneously, reach maturity, and then do not reproduce. Thus, the growth is self-limiting and benign.

multiple h. A congenital malformation that presents a slowly growing mass of abnormal tissue in multiple sites. The tissues are appropriate to the organ in which the hamartomas are located but are not normally organized. They may appear in blood vessels as hemangiomata, and in the lung and kidney. They are not malignant but cause symptoms because of the space they occupy.

hamartomatosis (hăm″ăr-tō-mă-tō′sĭs) [″ + ″ + *osis,* condition] Existence of multiple hamartomas.

hamate (hăm′ăt) Hooked; unciform. SYN: *hamular.*

h. bone The medial bone in the distal row of carpal bones of the wrist. SYN: *hamatum; os hamatum; unciform bone.*

hamatum (hă-mā′tŭm) [L. *hamatus,* hooked] Hamate bone.

hamaxophobia [Gr. *amaxa,* a carriage, + *phobos,* fear] A fear of riding in a vehicle.

Hamman, Louis (hăm′ăn) U.S. physician, 1877–1946.

H.'s disease Spontaneous mediastinal emphysema with a crunching sound heard during auscultation of the heart.

H.'s syndrome Previously used term for idiopathic pulmonary fibrosis.

hammer **1.** An instrument with a head attached crosswise to the handle for striking blows. **2.** The common name for the malleus, the hammer-shaped bone of the middle ear.

dental h. A mallet or motor-driven hammer used for condensing direct-filling gold or silver amalgam during the placement of fillings in teeth.

percussion h. A hammer with a rubber head used for tapping surfaces of the body in order to produce sounds for diagnostic purposes. SEE: *plexor.*

reflex h. A hammer used for tapping body parts such as a muscle, tendon, or nerve in order to test nerve function.

hammertoe A toe with dorsal flexion of the first phalanx and plantar flexion of the second and third phalanges. SYN: *hallux malleus.*

hamster A rodent, *Cricetus cricetus,* belonging to the family Cricetidae, common in Europe and western Asia. It is extensively used in medical research.

hamstring [AS. *haum,* haunch] **1.** One of the tendons that form the medial and lateral boundaries of the popliteal space. **2.** Any one of three muscles on the posterior aspect of the thigh, the semitendinosus, semimembranosus, and biceps femoris. They flex the leg and adduct and extend the thigh.

inner h. One of the tendons of the semimembranosus, semitendinosus, and gracilis muscles.

outer h. A tendon of the biceps femoris.

Ham test A test for diagnosing paroxysmal nocturnal hemoglobinuria, in which the red cells are assessed for resistance to lysis during incubation with acidified serum.

hamular (hăm'ū-lăr) [L. *hamulus,* a small hook] Hamate.

hamulus (hăm'ū-lŭs) *pl.* **hamuli** [L., a small hook] **1.** Any hook-shaped structure. **2.** The hooklike process on the hamate bone.

h. cochleae The hooklike process at the tip of the osseous spiral lamina of the cochlea.

h. lacrimalis The hooklike process on the lacrimal bone.

h. pterygoideus The hooklike process at the tip of the medial pterygoid process of the sphenoid bone.

hand [AS.] The body part attached to the forearm at the wrist. It includes the wrist (carpus) with its eight bones, the metacarpus or body of the hand (ossa metacarpalia) having five bones, and the fingers (phalanges) with their 14 bones. In some occupations and recreational endeavors, workers use their hands as hammers, which may damage the ulnar nerve and artery, with consequent signs of ischemia and neuropathy. SYN: *manus*. SEE: illus.

ape h. A deformity of the hand in which the thumb is permanently extended, usually caused by a median nerve injury. Paralysis and atrophy of the thenar muscles result.

claw h. Clawhand.

cleft h. A bipartite hand resulting from failure of a digit and its corresponding metacarpal to develop.

diabetic h. Stiffness and fibrotic contractures of the metacarpophalangeal (MCP) and proximal interphalangeal (PIP) joints in patients with advanced diabetes mellitus.

drop h. Wrist drop.

functional position of h. The principle used in splint fabrication whereby the wrist is dorsiflexed 20 to 35 degrees, a normal transverse arch is maintained, and the thumb is in abduction and opposition and aligned with the pads of the four fingers. Proximal interphalangeal joints are flexed 45 to 60 degrees.

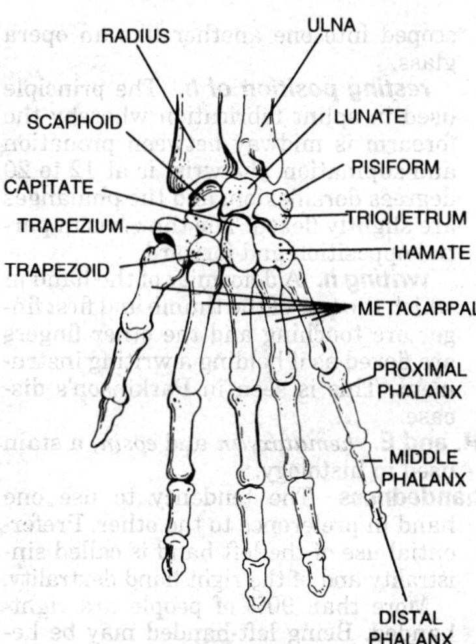

VIEW FROM PALMAR SIDE

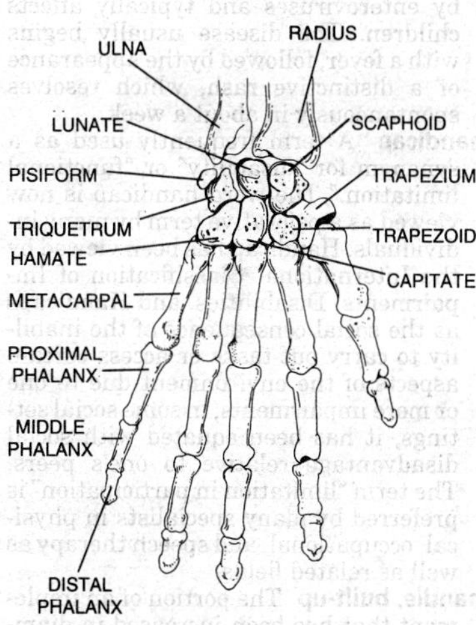

VIEW FROM BACK OF THE HAND

BONES OF THE RIGHT HAND AND WRIST

lobster-claw h. Cleft h.

obstetrician's h. The position of the hand in tetany with extension at the metacarpophalangeal and the interphalangeal joints, and adduction of the thumb. It is named for the position of the obstetrician's hand during vaginal examination.

opera-glass h. A deformity of the hand caused by chronic arthritis in which the phalanges appear to be telescoped into one another like an opera glass.

resting position of h. The principle used in splint fabrication whereby the forearm is midway between pronation and supination, the wrist is at 12 to 20 degrees dorsiflexion, and the phalanges are slightly flexed. The thumb is in partial opposition and forward.

writing h. A deformity of the hand in which the tips of the thumb and first finger are touching and the other fingers are flexed as if holding a writing instrument. This is seen in Parkinson's disease.

H. and E. *hematoxylin* and *eosin,* a stain used in histology.

handedness The tendency to use one hand in preference to the other. Preferential use of the left hand is called sinistrality and of the right hand dextrality.

More than 90% of people are right-handed. Being left-handed may be hereditary or due to disease of the left cerebral hemisphere in early life.

hand-foot-and-mouth disease An infectious disease characterized by painful oral ulcers and vesicles, papules, or pustules on the hands and feet. It is caused by enteroviruses and typically affects children. The disease usually begins with a fever, followed by the appearance of a distinctive rash, which resolves spontaneously in about a week.

handicap A term frequently used as a synonym for "disability" or "functional limitation." The word handicap is now viewed as a pejorative term by many individuals. Handicap has been viewed by the International Classification of Impairments, Disabilities, and Handicaps as the social consequence of the inability to carry out tasks or access certain aspects of the environment due to one or more impairments; in some social settings, it has been equated with social disadvantage relative to one's peers. The term "limitation in participation" is preferred by many specialists in physical, occupational, and speech therapy as well as related fields.

handle, built-up The portion of an implement that has been increased in diameter to accommodate its use by persons with limited or weak grasp.

handpiece, dental (hănd′pēs) A motor-driven device used in dentistry. The three basic designs are based on the shape of the handpiece and include the straight, contra-angle, and right angle handpiece. Handpieces are classified according to the speed of their rotation. They contain a chuck for holding tools used in preparing teeth for restoration, polishing, and condensing. SYN: *drill.*

CAUTION: The Centers for Disease Control recommends that all dental handpieces be heat sterilized after each use.

---

contra-angle d.h. A handpiece with one or more bends so that the shaft of the rotary instrument is at an angle to the handpiece to reach less accessible areas of the mouth for dental work.

high-speed d.h. A dental handpiece that operates at speeds about 100,000 to 800,000 rpm. The high-speed or ultra-speed handpiece operates with a water spray and may have a fiberoptic light to facilitate better visibility. A water spray is necessary to reduce the temperature within the handpiece and surgical site. SYN: *turbine d.h.*

low-speed d.h. A dental handpiece that operates at speeds about 6,000 to 10,000 rpm. Low-speed handpieces are used to polish and finish dental procedures.

turbine d.h. High-speed d.h.

Hand-Schüller-Christian disease (hănd-shĭl′ĕr-krĭs′chăn) [Alfred Hand, Jr., U.S. pediatrician, 1868–1949; Artur Schüller, Austrian neurologist, b. 1874; Henry A. Christian, U.S. physician, 1876–1951] SEE: *histiocytosis, Langerhans cell; islets of Langerhans.*

handsock A type of glove that covers the hand but, because it has no individual spaces for the fingers, makes grasping objects difficult. Use of handsocks during infancy may inhibit the rate of development of hand skills.

handwashing Using soap and water, or alcohol-based solutions, to decrease the number of germs on the hands, a fundamental (and occasionally overlooked) aspect of infection control. SEE: *universal precautions.*

hangnail [AS. *ang-,* tight, painful, + *naegel,* nail] Partly detached piece of skin at root or lateral edge of finger or toenail.

hangover A nontechnical term for describing the malaise that may be present after ingestion of a considerable amount of an alcoholic beverage or other central nervous system depressant. Symptoms usually present upon awakening from a sleep include some if not all of the following: mental depression, headache, thirst, nausea, irritability, fatigue. Symptoms and their severity will vary with the individual. The presence of congeners in alcoholic beverages is thought to be related to the development of a hangover. There is no specific therapy. SEE: *alcoholism, acute; delirium tremens.*

Hansen's bacillus [Gerhard H. A. Hansen, Norwegian physician, 1841–1912] *Mycobacterium leprae,* the cause of leprosy, which Hansen discovered in 1871.

Hansen's disease Leprosy.

Hantavirus A genus of viruses of the family Bunyaviridae; the cause of epidemic hemorrhagic fever and hantavirus pulmonary syndrome. The natural reservoir is rodents.

hantavirus pulmonary syndrome ABBR: HPS. An acute respiratory illness that first appeared in the southwestern U.S. in 1993, characterized by acute noncardiogenic pulmonary edema. It is caused by several newly identified strains of hantaviruses. The Sin Nombre virus is the most common in the U.S., but other pathogenic strains also have been identified throughout the world.

ETIOLOGY: Hantaviruses are single-stranded RNA viruses. They are carried by rodents, of which the deer mouse is the most common in the U.S. Infection usually is the result of inhalation of aerosolized excreta from rodents infected with the virus, but person-to-person transmission was documented in Argentina with infection from the Andes Hantavirus. There have been 185 cases throughout the U.S. as of June 1998, but HPS has been seen worldwide; the incidence rises after warm, wet winters during which few rodents die. All cases originated in rural areas in people who were involved in rodent control activities or hiked in rodent-infested areas.

SYMPTOMS: Patients usually report several days of myalgia, fever, headache, nausea, vomiting, and diarrhea. The abrupt onset of dyspnea and nonproductive cough follows, which rapidly progresses to noncardiogenic pulmonary edema and shock. Disseminated intravascular coagulation and renal failure are common.

DIAGNOSIS: HPS is diagnosed by clinical presentation, the presence of IgM antibodies to the virus in the blood, and Western blot enzyme-linked immunosorbent assays, among other tests.

TREATMENT: No effective antiviral drug therapy has been identified. Patients are given supportive care in the intensive care unit, with oxygen, mechanical ventilation, intravenous fluids, and vasopressors. The mortality rate, however, is approx. 50%. Vaccines against the virus provide a possible source of protection for persons at risk of exposure.

PATIENT CARE: People living in or visiting areas where the disease has been reported need to be educated about being careful under porches, in basements, and in attics or storage areas, where mouse droppings may be present. Mouse droppings should not be vacuumed or swept with a broom; these practices increase the risk of inhalation. Instead, individuals should cover infestations with a 10% solution of household bleach, wipe them up while wearing protective clothing and a HEPA filter mask, and place them in a bag for disposal. Vacation cottages should be aired before anyone enters. Campers should avoid burrows and sleep on cots or mattresses rather than the bare ground. Children must be taught not to try to catch or play with deer mice. A safety pamphlet is available from the Centers for Disease Control.

hapalonychia (hăp″ăl-ō-nĭk′ē-ă) [Gr. *hapalos,* soft, + *onyx,* nail] Onychomalacia.

haphalgesia (hăf″ăl-jē′zē-ă) [Gr. *haphe,* touch, + *algesis,* sense of pain] A sensation of pain upon touching the skin lightly or with a nonirritating object.

haphephobia (hăf″ē-fō′bē-ă) [″ + *phobos,* fear] An aversion to being touched by another person.

haplodont (hăp′lō-dŏnt) [″ + *odous,* tooth] Having teeth without ridges or tubercles on the crown.

haploid [Gr. *haploos,* simple, + *eidos,* form, shape] Possessing half the diploid or normal number of chromosomes found in somatic or body cells. Such is the case of the germ cells—ova or sperm—following the reduction divisions in gametogenesis, the haploid number being 23 in humans. SEE: *chromosome; diploid.*

haploidy (hăp′loy-dē) The state of being haploid.

haplopia (hăp-lō′pē-ă) [″ + *ops,* vision] Single vision; a condition in which an object viewed by two eyes appears as a single object, in contrast to diplopia, in which it appears as two objects.

haplotype The combination of several alleles in a gene cluster.

hapten(e) (hăp′tĕn, -tēn) [Gr. *haptein,* to seize] A substance that normally does not act as an antigen or stimulate an immune response but that can be combined with an antigen and, at a later time, initiate a specific antibody response on its own. SYN: *haptin.*

haptic (hăp′tĭk) [Gr. *haptein,* to touch] Tactile.

haptics The science of the sense of touch.

haptin (hăp′tĭn) Hapten.

haptoglobin (hăp″tō-glō′bĭn) A mucoprotein to which hemoglobin released from lysed red cells into plasma is bound. It is increased in certain inflammatory conditions and decreased in hemolytic disorders.

hardening [AS. *heardian,* to harden] **1.** Rendering a pathological or histological specimen firm or compact, for making thin sections for microscopic study. **2.** The development of increased resistance to extremes of environmental temperature. SEE: *acclimation.*

h. of the arteries Colloquial expression used for arteriosclerosis.

hardness **1.** A quality of water containing certain substances, esp. soluble salts of calcium and magnesium. These react with soaps, forming insoluble compounds that are precipitated out of solution, thus interfering with their cleansing action. **2.** The quality or penetrating power of x-rays. Hardness increases as wavelengths become shorter. **3.** The quality of firmness or density of a material imparted by the cohesion of the particles that compose it.

harelip [AS. *hara,* hare, + *lippa,* lip] Cleft lip.

h. suture A twisted figure-of-eight suture used in the surgical correction of harelip.

harlequin sign A benign transient color change seen in neonates in which one half of the body blanches while the other half becomes redder, with a clear line of demarcation.

harmonic In physics, concerning wave forms, an oscillation or frequency that is a whole number multiple of the basic frequency.

harmony (hăr′mō-nē) The condition of working or living together smoothly.

functional occlusal h. The ideal occlusion of the teeth so that in all mandibular positions during chewing, the teeth will be functioning efficiently and without trauma to supporting tissues.

harness In postamputation rehabilitation, the part of an upper extremity prosthesis that fits around the shoulder and back to permit mechanical control of the terminal device and hold the socket firmly around the stump.

harpoon (hăr-poon′) [Gr. *harpazein,* to seize] A device with a hook on one end for obtaining small pieces of tissue such as muscle for examination.

Harrison Narcotic Act A law enacted in 1914 that classified certain drugs as habit forming and restricted their sale and distribution.

Harrison's groove [Edwin Harrison, Brit. physician, 1779–1847] A depression on the lower edge of the thorax caused by the tug of the diaphragm, seen in rickets and any infant disease that tends to obstruct inspiration.

Hartmann's procedure [Henri Hartmann, Fr. surgeon, 1860–1952] The surgical removal of a diseased portion of the distal colon or proximal rectum with formation of an end colostomy, accompanied by oversewing of the distal colonic or rectal remnant. This procedure may be the first stage of a two-part operation, in which at a later date, the colostomy and the oversewn remnant are reconnected. The Hartmann procedure is most often employed in debilitated patients or in emergent circumstances in which primary anastomosis or complete distal segment excision would not be appropriate.

Hartmann's solution [Alexis F. Hartmann, U.S. pediatrician, 1849–1931] Lactated Ringer's injection used for fluid and electrolyte replacement. A sterile solution of 0.6 g of sodium chloride, 0.03 g of potassium chloride, 0.02 g of calcium chloride, and 0.31 g of sodium lactate diluted with water for injection to make 100 ml.

Hartnup disease [*Hartnup,* the family name of the first reported case] A rare autosomal recessive metabolic disease in which absorption, excretion, and kidney resorption of amino acids, esp. tryptophan, is abnormal. Clinical signs resemble pellagra, with a rash that is worsened by exposure to sunlight.

harvest **1.** To obtain samples or remove bacteria or other microorganisms from a culture. **2.** Removal of donor organs for transplantation.

Harvey, William (hăr′vē) British physician, 1578–1657, who described the circulation of the blood.

Hashimoto's thyroiditis [Hakaru Hashimoto, Japanese surgeon, 1881–1934] A common autoimmune illness in which there is inflammation, and then destruction and fibrosis of the thyroid gland, ultimately resulting in hypothyroidism. Thyroid hormone replacement is required. Women are much more commonly affected than men.

hashish (hăsh′ĭsh) [Arabic, hemp, dried grass] A more or less purified extract prepared from the flowers, stalks, and leaves of the hemp plant *Cannabis sativa.* The gummy substance is smoked or chewed for its euphoric effects. SEE: *cannabis; marijuana.*

Hasner's valve, H.'s fold [Joseph R. Hasner, Prague ophthalmologist, 1819–1892] A fold of the mucous membrane at the opening of the nasolacrimal duct in the inferior meatus of the nasal cavity. SYN: *lacrimal plica.*

Hassall's corpuscle [Arthur H. Hassall, Brit. chemist and physician, 1817–1894] A spherical or oval body present in the medulla of the thymus. It consists of a central area of degenerated cells surrounded by concentrically arranged flattened or polygonal cells.

Hatchcock's sign Tenderness just beyond the angle of the jaws when the finger follows on the undersurface of the mandible toward the angle. This may be found in mumps before any swelling can be detected.

hatchet, enamel A hand-held cutting instrument with a blade set continuous with the handle.

haunch (hawnsh) [Fr. *hanche*] The hips and buttocks.

haustration (haws-trā′shŭn) The formation of segment or recess, esp. in the bowel.

haustrum (haw′strŭm) *pl.* **haustra** [L. *haurire,* to draw, drink] One of the sacculations of the colon caused by longitudinal bands of smooth muscle (taeniae coli) that are shorter than the gut. **haustral** (haw′străl), *adj.*

HAV *hepatitis A virus.*

Haverhill fever (hā′vĕr-ĭl) [Haverhill, MA, U.S., where the initial epidemic occurred] A febrile disease transmitted to humans by rats, usually by rat bite. *Streptobacillus moniliformis* is the etiological agent. SYN: *rat-bite fever*.

Havers, Clopton British physician and anatomist (1650–1702) whose work is particularly remembered for its detailed description of the microscopic structure of bone. SEE: *haversian system*.

haversian canal SEE: under *canal*.

haversian canaliculus One of several delicate canals extending from the lacunae into the matrix of bone. It anastomoses with canaliculi of adjacent lacunae, forming a network of fine channels that communicate with haversian and Volkmann's canals, and transmits nutrient materials.

haversian gland A minute gland projecting from the surface of the synovial tissue into the joint space, that secretes synovial fluid.

haversian system An architectural unit of compact bone consisting of a central tube (haversian canal) with alternate layers of intercellular material (matrix) surrounding it in concentric cylinders. Alternating layers of matrix and cells are called haversian lamellae. SYN: *osteon*. SEE: *bone*.

hay fever A seasonal illness, marked by sneezing, sniffling, runny nose, and itchy or watery eyes. This condition, which affects 10% to 20% of the U.S. population, results from a type I hypersensitivity reaction involving the mucous membranes of the nose and upper air passages. It is the most common manifestation of atopic (inherited) allergy. SYN: *allergic rhinitis; pollinosis*. SEE: *allergen; desensitization; hypersensitivity reaction; Nursing Diagnoses Appendix*.

ETIOLOGY: Airborne pollens, fungal spores, dust, and animal dander cause hay fever. It is most commonly triggered in the spring by pollen from trees, in the summer by grass pollen, and in the fall by pollen from wildflowers, such as ragweed. Nonseasonal rhinitis may result from inhalation of animal dander, dust from hay or straw, or house dust mites.

TREATMENT: Seasonal usage of antihistamines, cromolyn, and corticosteroid nasal sprays provides the mainstay of therapy in the U.S. Prophylaxis through desensitization also is useful, but it is less convenient and usually less cost-effective. Avoiding allergens also is effective but not always possible. Patients may use high-efficiency particulate air (HEPA) face masks outdoors when pollen counts are high, although few will choose to do so.

CAUTION: Overuse of corticosteroids may damage the nasal mucosa, and absorption of the drug can cause adverse side effects.

Hayflick's limit [Leonard Hayflick, U.S. microbiologist, b. 1928] The maximum number of cell divisions that will take place in human cells prior to their death. In 1961 Hayflick and P.S. Moorehead showed that human cells can reproduce themselves a finite number of times. This limited replication ability is postulated to correlate with the aging, failure, and eventual death of organs and individuals. Hayflick's limit is exceeded by some cell lines that exist solely to reproduce themselves, such as blood-forming cells and cancer cells. It can also be extended artificially by manipulation of a cellular enzyme known as telomerase. Experiments on the functions of telomerase may lead to new understanding of the aging process, the replication ability of cancer cells, and mortality.

Haygarth's deformities [John Haygarth, Brit. physician, 1740–1827] Exostoses or bony tumors on joints in rheumatoid arthritis.

hazardous material ABBR: hazmat. A toxic material that may cause personal injury or property damage. The hazard of any material is determined by its chemical, physical, and biological properties and by the possibility of exposure to that material. SEE: *health hazard; permissible exposure limits; right-to-know law; toxic substance*.

hazmat Contraction for hazardous material.

Hb *hemoglobin*.

HB Ag An obsolete term for any one of the hepatitis B antigens. SEE: *hepatitis B*.

HbCo Carboxyhemoglobin.

Hbg *hemoglobin*.

H2 blockers SEE: *H2-receptor antagonists*.

HBV *hepatitis B virus*.

HCFA *Health Care Financing Administration*.

HCG, hCG *human chorionic gonadotropin*.

HCl *hydrochloric acid*.

HCO_3^- Chemical formula for bicarbonate ion.

H_2CO_3 Chemical formula for carbonic acid.

H.D. *hearing distance*.

HCV *hepatitis C virus*.

h.d. L. *hora decubitus,* the hour of going to bed.

HDCV *human diploid cell vaccine* (for rabies).

H. disease. *Hartnup disease*.

HDL *high-density lipoprotein*.

He Symbol for helium.

head [AS. *heafod*] **1.** Caput; the part of the body containing the brain and organs of sight, hearing, smell, and taste and including the facial bones. SEE: illus. **2.** The larger extremity of any organ.

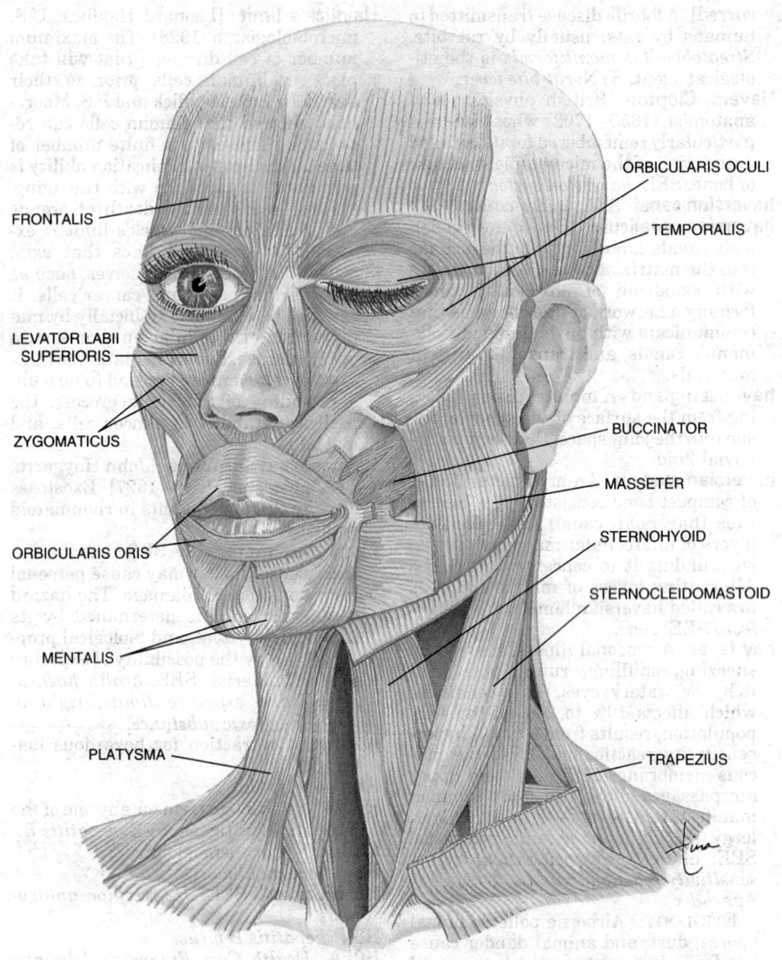

MUSCLES OF THE HEAD AND NECK

(Anterior view)

ABNORMALITIES: *An abnormal fixation* of the head may be caused by postpharyngeal abscess, arthritis deformans, swollen cervical glands, rheumatism, traumatism of the neck, sprains of cervical muscles, congenital spasmodic torticollis, caries of a molar tooth, burn scars, or eye muscle imbalance (hyperphoria). An inability to move the head may be due to caries of the cervical vertebrae and diseases of articulation between the occiput and atlas or paralysis of neck muscles.

Abnormal movements of the head include habit spasms such as nodding. Rhythmical nodding is seen in aortic regurgitation, chorea, and torticollis. A retracted head is seen in acute meningitis, cerebral abscess, tumor, thrombosis of the superior longitudinal sinus, acute encephalitis, laryngeal obstruction, tetanus, hydrophobia, epilepsy, spasmodic torticollis, strychnine poisoning, hysteria, rachitic conditions, and painful neck lesions at the back.

after-coming h. Childbirth with the head delivered last.

articular h. A projection on bone that articulates with another bone.

headache [AS. *heafod,* head, + *acan,* to ache] ABBR: HA. Pain felt in the forehead, eyes, jaws, temples, scalp, skull, occiput, or neck. Headache is exceptionally common; it affects almost every person at some time. From a clinical perspective, benign HA must be distinguished from HA that may be life-threatening. Types of benign HA in-

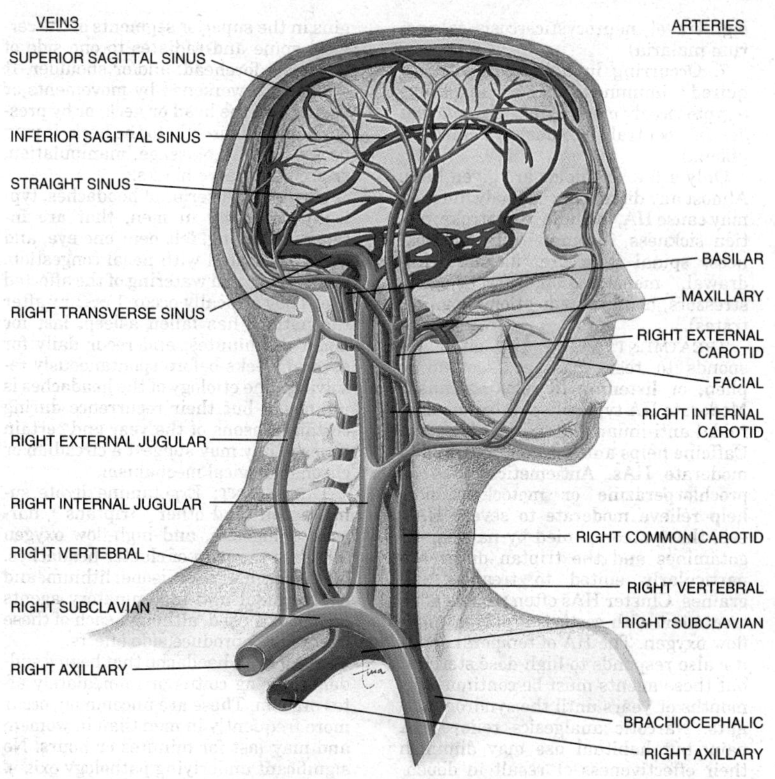

ARTERIES AND VEINS OF THE HEAD

(Right lateral view)

clude tension, migraine, cluster, sinus, and environmentally induced (e.g., "ice cream" HA or "caffeine-withdrawal" HA). Life-threatening HA may be caused by rupture of an intracranial aneurysm, subarachnoid hemorrhage, hemorrhagic stroke, cranial trauma, encephalitis, meningitis, brain tumors, or brain abscesses. SYN: *cephalalgia*. SEE: *migraine*.

Typically, benign HAs have a recurrent or chronic history with which the patient is familiar. The tension HA sufferer, for example, develops bandlike pressure around the head at the end of a difficult or stressful day. The onset of the HA is gradual and progressively worsens but is usually not severe or intense.

The migraine HA sufferer also typically has a history of recurrent HA, often dating back to childhood. Migraine HA is often of rapid onset, unilateral, throbbing, or beating in character. It may be preceded by a visual disturbance (flickering lights or wavy visual disturbances), technically called *scotoma*, and can be associated with nausea, vomiting, or even transient neurological deficits, such as hemibody weakness. The HA may be triggered by eating chocolate or some cheeses, drinking alcohol, or taking certain medications, such as the hormone estrogen. By contrast, an HA that is life-threatening may have some of the following hallmarks:

1. The first, or the worst, HA a patient has ever suffered (e.g., subarachnoid hemorrhage should be suspected)
2. Occurring for the first time in a patient with a history of cancer (metastatic tumor)
3. Accompanied by fever, stiff neck, or photophobia (meningitis, intracranial hemorrhage)
4. Associated with loss of consciousness or severely altered mental status (intracerebral hemorrhage, brain embolism, encephalitis, meningitis)
5. Associated with neurological deficits that do not quickly resolve (intracerebral hemorrhage, brain embolism, brain abscesses)
6. Occurring in a patient with recent head trauma (hemorrhage, carotid artery dissection) or a history of recent for-

eign travel (neurocysticercosis; falciparum malaria)

7. Occurring in a patient with acquired immunodeficiency syndrome (cryptococcal meningitis, *Toxoplasma gondii*, central nervous system lymphoma)

Only a few examples are given here. Almost any disturbance of body function may cause HA, including sunstroke, motion sickness, insomnia, altitude sickness, spinal puncture, alcohol withdrawal, menstruation, psychological stressors, or new medications (e.g., nitrates).

TREATMENT: Mild HA often responds to rest, massage, acetaminophen, or listening to relaxing music. Moderate HA typically requires nonsteroidal anti-inflammatory drug therapy. Caffeine helps ameliorate many mild to moderate HAs. Antiemetics, such as prochlorperazine or metoclopramide, help relieve moderate to severe HAs, esp. those accompanied by nausea; ergotamines and the triptan drugs are particularly suited to treating migraines. Cluster HAs often resolve after treatment with corticosteroids or high-flow oxygen. The HA of temporal arteritis also responds to high-dose steroids, but these agents must be continued for months or years until the syndrome remits. Narcotic analgesics relieve HA pain, but habitual use may diminish their effectiveness or result in dependence.

PATIENT CARE: A description of the headache is obtained and documented, including the character, severity, location, radiation, prodromata, or associated symptoms, as well as any palliative measures that have brought relief. Temporal factors and any relationship of recurring headaches to other activities are also documented. Noninvasive comfort measures and prescribed drug therapy are instituted, and the patient is taught about these and evaluated for desired responses and any adverse reactions.

analgesic-rebound h. A headache that occurs when a patient with chronic or recurring headaches stops using pain relievers. Analgesic rebound is a common cause of daily headache pain; it may respond to treatment with antidepressant medications and withdrawal of the offending analgesics.

caffeine withdrawal h. Headache, usually mild to moderate in intensity, that begins as someone stops drinking coffee, tea, or other caffeinated drinks. This type of headache usually occurs only in persons who habitually consume more than 4 cups of caffeine daily and is often accompanied by fatigue and malaise.

cervicogenic h. A headache that begins in the superior segments of the cervical spine and radiates to one side of the neck, forehead, and/or shoulder. It typically is worsened by movements or postures of the head or neck, or by pressure applied directly to the neck. It may be relieved by massage, manipulation, or occipital nerve blocks.

cluster h. A series of headaches, typically occurring in men, that are intense, recurring, felt near one eye, and often associated with nasal congestion, rhinorrhea, and watering of the affected eye. They typically occur 1 or 2 hr after the patient has fallen asleep, last for about 45 minutes, and recur daily for several weeks before spontaneously resolving. The etiology of the headaches is unknown, but their recurrence during certain seasons of the year and certain times of day may suggest a circadian or chronobiological mechanism.

TREATMENT: Ergotamine titrate, sumatriptan (and other "-triptans"), narcotic analgesics, and high-flow oxygen alleviate the pain of cluster headaches. Methysergide, prednisone, lithium, and nonsteroidal anti-inflammatory agents can also be used, although each of these agents may produce side effects.

coital h. A headache that begins suddenly during coitus or immediately after orgasm. These are uncommon, occur more frequently in men than in women, and may last for minutes or hours. No significant underlying pathology exists.

exertional h. An acute headache of short duration that appears after strenuous physical activity. Usually benign, it is relieved by aspirin and prevented by changing to a less strenuous exercise.

histamine h. A headache resulting from ingestion of histamine (found in some wines), injection of histamine, or excessive histamine in circulating blood. This type of headache is due to dilatation of branches of the carotid artery. SEE: *cluster h.*

hypnic h. A headache that awakens a patient from sleep. Hypnic headaches are typically bilateral, and are experienced more often by the elderly than by other patients. Unlike cluster headaches, which also occur during rest or sleep, the hypnic headache is not felt on one side of the face, and not associated with tearing of the eye or painful congestion of the sinuses.

migraine h. Migraine.

mixed h. Headache that may have features of some combination of migraine headache, tension headache, and analgesic withdrawal.

post–lumbar puncture h. A severe headache that may occur in patients who have had a lumbar puncture, marked by its resolution when the patient is lying flat and its exacerbation when the patient is upright. It is caused by the leakage of spinal fluid through a hole that fails to close when the spinal needle is removed from the dura mater. The headache occurs rarely when a small (e.g., 22-gauge or 24-gauge) spinal needle is used and when the needle's obturator is replaced before the needle is removed from the spinal canal.

TREATMENT: Bedrest in a completely flat and prone position (without a pillow), forced oral and intravenous fluids, and administration of cortical steroids are useful in treating the headache. If the headache persists in spite of therapy, it may be possible to stop the leakage of spinal fluid by injection of 10 ml of the patient's blood in the epidural space at the site of the lumbar puncture. The blood may "patch" the hole in the dura.

tension h. **1.** A headache associated with chronic contraction of the muscles of the neck and scalp. **2.** A headache associated with emotional or physical strain.

thundering h. A sudden acute headache that may accompany intracranial hemorrhage. Its absence, however, does not rule out intracranial hemorrhage.

weight-lifter's h. A form of exertional headache that occurs after straining during workouts with free weights or weight-training machines.

head banging In children, a tension-discharging action in which the head is repeatedly banged against the crib; may be part of a temper tantrum.

headgear **1.** A covering for the head, esp. a protective one, such as a helmet used by soldiers and those who participate in contact sports, auto racing, bicycle riding, or aviation. **2.** Extraoral traction and anchorage used to apply force to the teeth and jaws.

head-tilt chin-lift maneuver A maneuver for opening the airway in cardiopulmonary resuscitation. The head is tilted by gentle pressure to the forehead while the neck is lifted into an arched position by the hand placed behind it. The mandible is then lifted forward with a second hand. This procedure prevents the tongue from blocking the airway.

head trauma Injury to the head, esp. to the scalp and cranium, that may be limited to soft tissue damage or may include the cranial bones and the brain.

heal (hēl) [AS. *hael,* whole] To cure; to make whole or healthy.

healer An individual who cures diseases, eases discomfort, or relieves the suffering of others.

healing The restoration to a normal mental or physical condition, esp. of an inflammation or a wound. Tissue healing usually occurs in predictable stages:

1. Blood clot formation at the wound
2. Inflammatory phase (during which plasma proteins enter the injured part)
3. Cellular repair (with an influx of fibroblasts and mesenchymal cells)
4. Regrowth of blood vessels (angiogenesis)
5. Synthesis and revision of collagen fibers (scar formation)

In skin lesions, regrowth of epithelial tissues also occurs. The many processes involved in the healing of a wound take 3 weeks or more to complete. Many factors may delay tissue healing, including malnutrition, wound infection, and coexisting conditions (e.g., diabetes mellitus, advanced age, tobacco abuse, cancer), as well as the use of several drugs, including corticosteroids. SEE: illus.

COMPLICATIONS: These may result from the formation of a scar that interferes with the functioning of a part and possible deformity; the formation of a keloid, the result of overgrowth of connective tissue forming a tumor in the surface of a scar; necrosis of the skin and mucous membrane that produces a raw surface, which results in an ulcer; a sinus or fistula, which may be due to bacteria or some foreign substance remaining in the wound; proud flesh, which represents excessive growth of granulation tissue.

h. by first intention A process that closes the edge of a wound with little or no inflammatory reaction and in such a manner that little or no scar is left to reveal the site of the injury. New cells are formed to take the place of dead ones, and the capillary walls stretch across the wound to join themselves to each other in a smooth surface. New connective tissue may form an almost imperceptible but temporary scar. In repairing lacerations and surgical wounds, the goal is to produce a repaired area that will heal by first intention.

h. by second intention Healing by granulation or indirect union. Granulation tissue is formed to fill the gap between the edges of the wound with a thin layer of fibrinous exudate. Granulation tissue also excludes bacteria from the wound and brings new blood vessels to the injured part. Healing by second intention takes several days more than healing by primary intention and typically results in the formation of a prominent scar; wounds that heal by second intention show signs of failure if the wound loses the normal red-grey appearance of granulation tissue and becomes pale, dry, or insubstantial. When granulations first form at the top instead of the bottom of the wound, the base of the wound may have to be kept open with wicks or drains to promote healthy tissue repair.

h. by third intention Delayed wound healing that occurs in the base of ulcerated or cavitary wounds, esp. those that

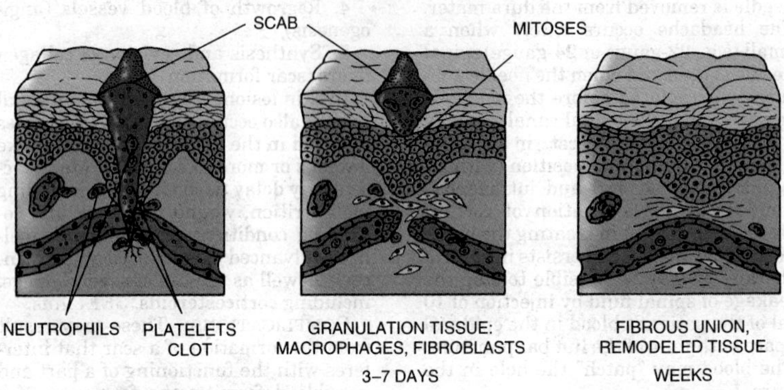

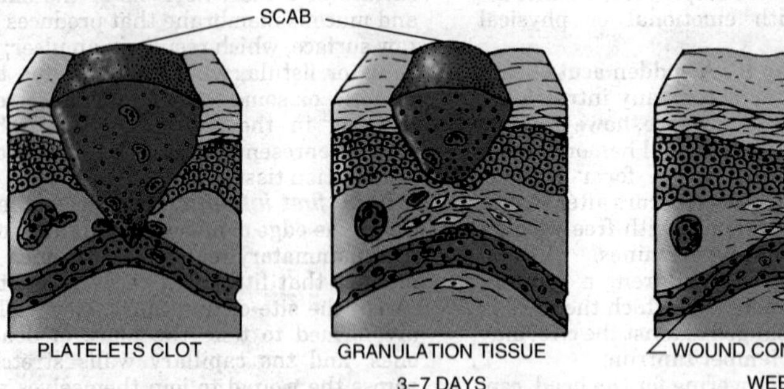

WOUND HEALING

have become infected. The wound fills very slowly with granulation tissue and often forms a large scar.

holistic h. Holism.

health (hĕlth) [AS. *haelth,* wholeness] A condition in which all functions of the body and mind are normally active. The World Health Organization defines health as a state of complete physical, mental, or social well-being and not merely the absence of disease or infirmity.

bill of h. A public health certificate stating that passengers on a public conveyance or ship are free of infectious disease.

board of h. A public body, appointed or elected, concerned with administering the laws pert. to the health of the public.

h. care proxy A legal document that allows individuals to name someone they know and trust to make health care decisions for them if, for any reason and at any time, the individual becomes unable to make or communicate those decisions. Some states limit the age at which such a proxy may be established and prohibit certain persons, such as an estate administrator or an employee of a health care facility in which the person making the proxy is a resident, from being appointed to make health care decisions unless he or she is related to the person by blood, marriage, or adoption. SEE: *advance directive; do not attempt resuscitation; living will; power of attorney, durable, for health care; donor card* for illus.

h. certificate An official statement signed by a physician attesting to the state of health of a particular individual.

department of h. The branch of a government (city, county, or nation) that regulates, coordinates, and oversees food and drug safety, immunization services, control of epidemic diseases, maternal and child care, substance abuse services, elder care, health statistics, and awareness of health improvement strategies.

h. education An educational process or program designed for the improvement and maintenance of health. It is directed to the general public, in contrast to a health education program organized for instructing persons who will become health educators.

h. hazard Any organism, chemical, condition, or circumstance that may cause injury or illness. With respect to chemicals, a substance is considered a health hazard if at least one study, conducted in accordance with established scientific principles, documents that acute or chronic effects may occur in connection with use of or exposure to that chemical. SEE: *hazardous material; permissible exposure limits; right-to-know law; toxic substance.*

industrial h. The health of employees of industrial firms.

h. insurance Indemnification to cover some or all of the costs of treating injury or disease.

mental h. Psychological adjustment to one's circumstance or environment; the ability to cope with or make the best of changing stresses and stimuli. Individuals are considered mentally healthy if they have adjusted to life in such a way that they are comfortable with themselves and, at the same time, are able to live so that their behavior does not conflict with their associates or the rest of society. Inherent in this, for most individuals, are feelings of self-worth and accomplishment and the ability to be gainfully employed with sufficient reward for that employment to satisfy economic needs.

h. promotion Public health efforts to reduce the incidence of disease and its impact on people, communities, and populations. Currently, in the U.S., major health promotion goals include eliminating vaccine-preventable illnesses; improving the early treatment of strokes; decreasing cardiovascular risk factors related to inappropriate diet, high blood pressure, obesity, and tobacco use; and reducing the high-risk behaviors that may contribute to the spread of acquired immunodeficiency syndrome, hepatitis, and other illnesses.

public h. The state of health of an entire community or population, as opposed to that of an individual.

h. risk appraisal An analysis of all that is known about a person's entire life situation including personal and family medical history, occupation, and social environment in order to estimate his or her risk of disability or death as compared with the national averages. The data used for comparison will vary with the patient's age, sex, ethnic background, and income, and the skill of the evaluator and the sensitivity and specificity of the tests used in the evaluation. Assessments should include special diagnostic procedures such as mammography, prostate examination, Pap smear, electrocardiogram, tests for total serum lipids including cholesterol, tests for occult blood in feces, hearing tests, and stress tests as indicated and appropriate for the individual patient (i.e., health screening). SEE: *risk factor.*

h. screening SEE: *h. risk appraisal.*

health care All of the services made available by medical professionals to promote, maintain, or preserve life and well-being. Its major objectives are to relieve pain; treat injury, illness, and disability; and provide comfort and hope.

Health Care Financing Administration ABBR: HCFA. The division of the U.S. Department of Health and Human Services responsible for Medicare funding.

healthful Conducive to good health.

health maintenance, altered Inability to identify, manage, and/or seek out help to maintain health. SEE: *Nursing Diagnoses Appendix.*

Health Maintenance Organization ABBR: HMO. A prepaid health care program of group practice that provides comprehensive medical care, esp. preventive care, while aiming to control health care expenditures.

Health Plan Employer Data and Information Set ABBR: HEDIS. A set of benchmarks used to assess the quality of care provided to patients by managed-care organizations. Included in these benchmarks are the numbers of immunizations administered by the plans and the extent of health screening tests provided by them.

health-seeking behaviors Alterations in personal health habits or the environment in order to move toward a higher level of health. Stable health status is defined as age-appropriate illness prevention measures achieved, client reports good or excellent health, and signs and symptoms of disease, if present, are controlled. SEE: *Nursing Diagnoses Appendix.*

healthy Being in a state of good health.

healthy persons, medical evaluation of The examination of asymptomatic individuals to screen for and prevent future illnesses.

hearing [AS. *hieran*] The sense or perception of sound. The normal human ear can detect sounds with frequencies ranging from about 20 Hz to 20,000 Hz but is most sensitive to sounds in the 1500-Hz to 3000-Hz frequency range, which is the range most often used in speech. Hearing deficits occur when sound waves are not conducted properly to the cochlea, when lesions interrupt the workings of the cochlear nerve, or when central nervous system pathways involved in the processing of auditory stimuli are injured.

FUNCTION TESTS: Hearing acuity can be determined by measuring the distance at which a person can hear a certain sound such as a water tick, by using audiometers, and by bone conduction. In audiometers, electrically produced sounds are conveyed by wires to a receiver applied to the subject's ear. Intensity and pitch of sound can be altered and are indicated on the dials. Results are plotted on a graph known as an audiogram. In bone conduction tests, a device such as a tuning fork or an apparatus that converts an electric current into mechanical vibrations is applied to the skull. This is of value in distinguishing between perceptive and conduction deafness. Conductive hearing loss may be diagnosed with the Weber test. Having the patient hum produces no difference in the sound heard if hearing is normal. The sound is perceived as louder in the ear with conductive hearing loss.

h. distance The distance at which a given sound can be heard.

h. hallucinations A colloquial term for "auditory hallucinations."

h. impaired Having any degree of hearing loss that interferes with communication, development, learning, or interpersonal interactions.

h. loss A decreased ability to perceive sounds as compared with what the individual or examiner would regard as normal. In the U.S., about 1 million school-age children and 25 million adults have some degree of hearing loss. SEE: *audiogram; audiometry*.

sensorineural h. loss Hearing loss caused by permanent or temporary damage to the sensory cells or nerve fibers of the inner ear.

sudden h. loss Hearing loss that occurs in 72 hr or less. It may be temporary or permanent. Some of the most common causes include cerumen impaction, medication toxicities, acute infections, ear trauma, Ménière's disease, and ischemia.

hearsay Statements overheard and repeated, rather than personally witnessed.

cular organ, the pump of the circulatory system. Its wall has three layers: the outer epicardium, a serous membrane; the middle myocardium, made of cardiac muscle; and the inner endocardium, endothelium that lines the chambers and covers the valves. The heart is enclosed in a fibroserous sac, the pericardium; the potential space between the parietal pericardium and the epicardium is the pericardial cavity, which contains serous fluid to prevent friction as the heart beats. SEE: illus. (The Heart); *circulation, coronary* for illus.; *cardiomyopathy, hypertrophic*.

CHAMBERS: The upper right and left atria (singular: atrium) are thin-walled receiving chambers separated by the interatrial septum. The lower right and left ventricles are thick-walled pumping chambers separated by the interventricular septum; normally the right side has no communication with the left. The right side receives deoxygenated blood via the venae cavae from the body and pumps it to the lungs; the left side receives oxygenated blood from the lungs and pumps it via the aorta and arteries to the body. Contraction of the heart chambers is called systole; relaxation with accompanying filling with blood is called diastole. The sequence of events that occurs in a single heartbeat is called the cardiac cycle, with atrial systole followed by ventricular systole. For a heart rate of 70 beats per minute, each cycle lasts about 0.85 sec.

VALVES: In the healthy state, all four cardiac valves prevent backflow of blood. The atrioventricular valves are at the openings between each atrium and ventricle; the tricuspid valve, between the right atrium and ventricle; and the bicuspid or mitral valve, between the left atrium and ventricle. The pulmonary semilunar valve is at the opening of the right ventricle into the pulmonary artery; the aortic semilunar valve is at the opening of the left ventricle into the aorta.

FUNCTION: In adults, the cardiac output varies from 5 L/min at rest to as much as 20 L/min during vigorous exercise. At the rate of 72 times each minute, the adult human heart beats 104,000 times a day, 38,000,000 times a year. Every stroke forces approx. 5 cu in. (82 ml) of blood out into the body, amounting to 500,000 cu in. (8193 L) a day. In terms of work, this is the equivalent of raising 1 ton (907 kg) to a height of 41 ft (12.5 m) every 24 hr.

BLOOD SUPPLY: The myocardium receives its blood supply from the coronary arteries that arise from the ascending aorta. Blood from the myocardium drains into several cardiac veins.

NERVE SUPPLY: The heart initiates its own beat, usually from 60 to 80 beats per minute, but the rate may change due to the cardiac centers in the medulla oblongata. Accelerator impulses are carried by sympathetic nerves. Preganglionic neurons in the thoracic spinal cord synapse with postganglionic neurons in the cervical ganglia of the sympathetic trunk; their axons continue to the heart. Sympathetic impulses are transmitted to the sinoatrial (SA) node, atrioventricular (AV) node, bundle of His, and myocardium of the ventricles, and increase heart rate and force of contraction. Inhibitory impulses are carried by the vagus nerves (parasympa-

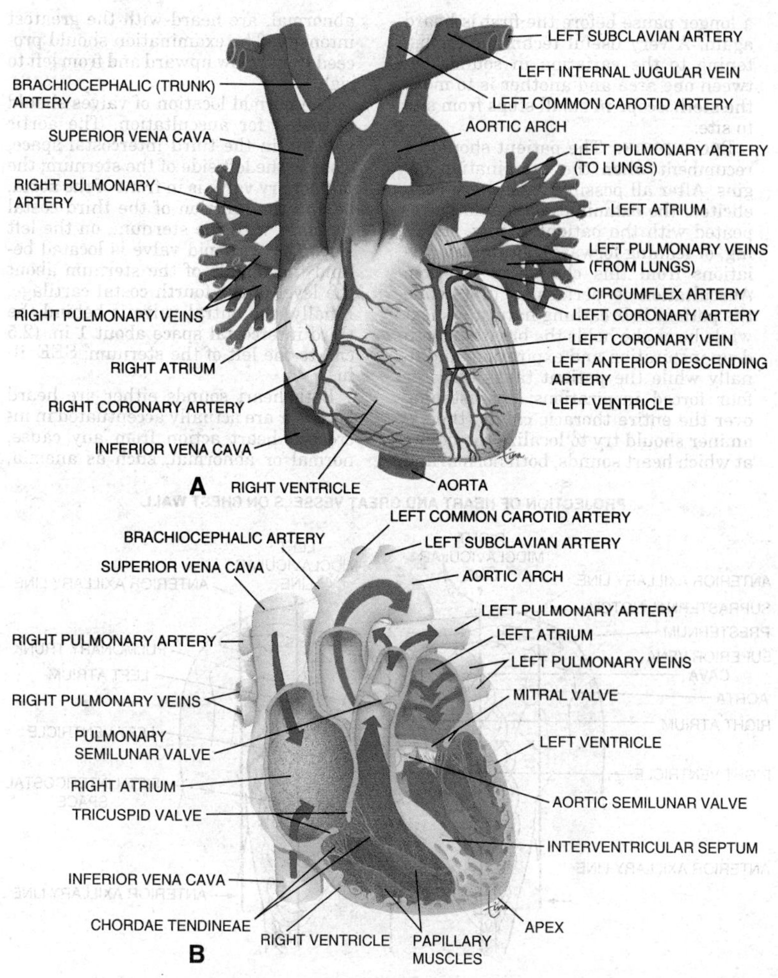

THE HEART

(A) anterior view, (B) frontal section

thetic). Preganglionic neurons (vagus) originating in the medulla synapse with postganglionic neurons in terminal ganglia in the wall of the heart. Parasympathetic impulses are transmitted to the SA and AV nodes and decrease the heart rate. Sensory nerves from the heart are for the sensation of pain, caused by an insufficient supply of oxygen to the myocardium. The sensory nerves for reflex changes in heart rate are the vagus and glossopharyngeal, which arise from pressoreceptors or chemoreceptors in the aortic arch and carotid sinus, respectively.

AUSCULTATION: Listening to the heart with a stethoscope reveals the intensity, quality, and rhythm of the heart sounds and detects any adventitious sounds, such as murmurs or pericardial friction. The two separate sounds heard by the use of a stethoscope over the heart have been represented by the syllables “lubb,” “dupp.” The first sound (systolic), which is prolonged and dull, results from the contraction of the ventricle, tension of the atrioventricular valves, and the impact of the heart against the chest wall, and is synchronous with the apex beat and carotid pulse. The first sound is followed by a short pause, and then the second sound (diastolic) is heard, resulting from the closure of the aortic and pulmonary valves. This sound is short and high pitched. After the second sound there is a longer pause before the first is heard again. A very useful technique for listening to the variation in sounds between one area and another is to move the stethoscope in small steps from site to site.

PROCEDURE: The patient should be recumbent when the examination begins. After all possible signs have been elicited, the examination should be repeated with the patient sitting, standing, or leaning forward, noting any variations from this change of position. Auscultation is performed first while the patient is breathing naturally, next while he or she holds the breath in both deep inspiration and expiration, and finally while the patient takes three or four forced inspirations. By listening over the entire thoracic cavity, the examiner should try to localize the points at which heart sounds, both normal and abnormal, are heard with the greatest intensity. The examination should proceed from below upward and from left to right.

The normal location of valves should be noted for auscultation. The aortic valve is in the third intercostal space, close to the left side of the sternum; the pulmonary valve is in front of the aorta, behind the junction of the third costal cartilage with the sternum, on the left side. The tricuspid valve is located behind the middle of the sternum about the level of the fourth costal cartilage. Finally, the mitral valve is behind the third intercostal space about 1 in. (2.5 cm) to the left of the sternum. SEE: illus.

Both heart sounds either are heard better or are actually accentuated in increased heart action from any cause, normal or abnormal, such as anemia,

PROJECTION OF HEART AND GREAT VESSELS ON CHEST WALL

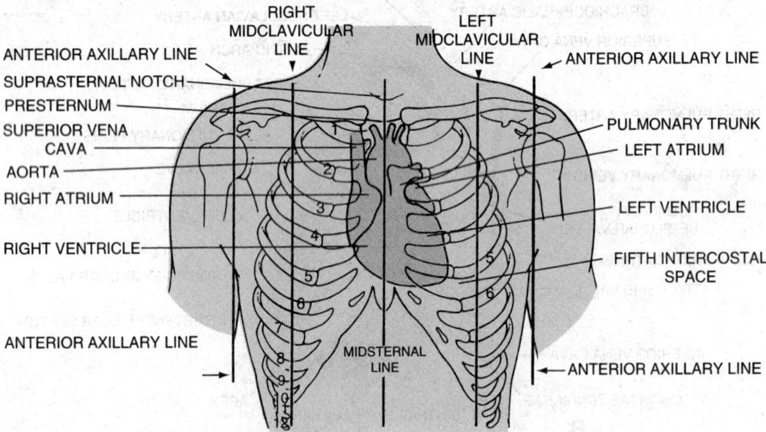

PROJECTION OF HEART AND VALVES ON CHEST WALL

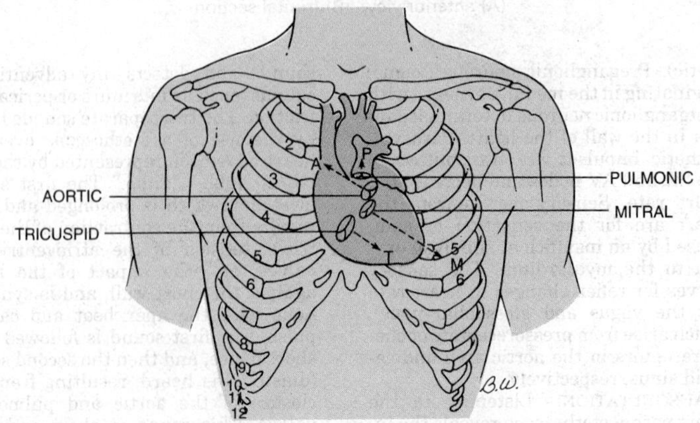

Heart sounds from each valve are heard best over areas shown

vigorous exercise, cardiac hypertrophy, thin chest walls, and lung consolidation as found in pneumonia. Accentuation of the aortic second sound results from hypertrophy of the left ventricle, increased arterial resistance as in arteriosclerosis with hypertension, or aortic aneurysm. Accentuation of the pulmonary second sound results from pulmonary obstruction as in emphysema, pneumonia, or hypertrophy of the right ventricle. Both heart sounds are poorly heard or are actually decreased in intensity in general obesity, general debility, degeneration or dilatation of the heart, pericardial or pleural effusion, and emphysema.

The reduplication of heart sounds is probably due to a lack of synchronous action in the valves of both sides of the heart. It results from many conditions but notably from increased resistance in the systemic or the pulmonary circulation, as in arteriosclerosis and emphysema. It is also frequently noted in mitral stenosis and pericarditis.

A murmur, an abnormal sound heard over the heart or blood vessels, may result from obstruction or regurgitation at the valves following endocarditis; dilatation of the ventricle or relaxation of its walls rendering the valves relatively insufficient; aneurysm; a change in the blood constituents, as in anemia; roughening of the pericardial surfaces, as in pericarditis; and irregular action of the heart. Murmurs produced within the heart are termed endocardial; those outside, exocardial; those produced in aneurysms, bruits; those produced by anemia, hemic murmurs.

Hemic murmurs, which are soft and blowing and usually systolic, are heard best over the pulmonary valves. They are associated with symptoms of anemia.

An aneurysmal murmur, or bruit, is usually loud and booming, systolic, and heard best over the aorta or base of heart. It is often associated with an abnormal area of dullness and pulsation and with symptoms resulting from pressure on neighboring structures.

Pericardial friction sounds are superficial, rough, and creaking, to and fro in time, and not transmitted beyond the precordium. These sounds may be modified by the pressure of the stethoscope.

Murmur intensity and configuration: The intensity (loudness) of murmurs may be graded from I to VI as follows:

1. Grade I–faint, can be heard only with intense listening in a quiet environment.
2. Grade II–quiet but can be heard immediately.
3. Grade III–moderately loud.
4. Grade IV–quite loud; a thrill (like the purring of a cat) is usually felt over the heart.
5. Grade V–loud enough to be heard with the stethoscope not completely in contact with the chest wall.
6. Grade VI–loud enough to be heard with the stethoscope close to but not actually touching the chest.

The configuration of sound intensity of a murmur may begin low and rise in intensity (crescendo) or be relatively loud and then decrease in intensity (decrescendo) or some combination of those features; or may exhibit the same intensity from beginning to end.

PALPATION: This process not only determines position, force, extent, and rhythm of the apex beat, but also detects any fremitus or thrill. A thrill is a vibratory sensation likened to that received when the hand is placed on the back of a purring cat. Thrills at the base of the heart may result from valvular lesions, atheroma of the aorta, aneurysm, and roughened pericardial surfaces as in pericarditis. A presystolic thrill at the apex is almost pathognomonic of mitral stenosis. In children esp., a precordial bulge, substernal thrust, or apical heave suggests cardiac enlargement.

PERCUSSION: This procedure determines the shape and extent of cardiac dullness. The normal area of superficial or absolute percussion dullness (the part uncovered by the lung) is detected by light percussion and extends from the fourth left costosternal junction to the apex beat; from the apex beat to the juncture of the xiphoid cartilage with the sternum; and thence up the left border of the sternum. The normal area of deep percussion dullness (the heart projected on the chest wall) is detected by firm percussion and extends from the third left costosternal articulation to the apex beat; from the apex beat to the junction of the xiphoid cartilage with the sternum; and thence up the right border of sternum to the third rib. The lower level of cardiac dullness fuses with the liver dullness and can rarely be determined. The area of cardiac dullness is increased in hypertrophy and dilation of the heart and in pericardial effusion; it is diminished in emphysema, pneumothorax, and pneumocardium.

abdominal h. A heart that is displaced into the abdominal cavity.

armored h. A dated term for calcific pericarditis.

artificial h. A device that pumps the blood the heart would normally pump. It may be located inside or outside the body. SEE: *heart-lung machine*.

athlete's h. Enlargement of the heart as a result of prolonged physical training (e.g., the aerobic exercise of running). This is not known to be a predisposing factor for any form of heart disease.

beriberi h. Heart failure due to deficiency of the vitamin thiamine.

boatshaped h. A heart in which one ventricle is dilated and hypertrophied as a result of aortic regurgitation.

bony h. A heart with calcified patches in its walls and pericardium.

cervical h. A heart that is displaced into the neck region.

conduction system of the h. Specialized myocytes in the heart that conduct the electrical impulses throughout the heart. It consists of (in order of normal conduction) the sinoatrial node, the intra-atrial tracts, the atrioventricular node, the bundle of His, the right and left bundle branches, and the Purkinje fibers. SEE: illus.

dilation of the h. Enlargement of the chambers of the heart, typically because of diseases of the heart valves or cardiomyopathy. It may result in ineffective ejection of blood into the aorta and secondary congestive heart failure.

fatty degeneration of the h. Fatty infiltration of the heart.

fatty infiltration of the h. An abnormal accumulation of triglycerides in the myocardium seen on pathological examination of biopsy specimens as clear vacuoles or droplets. SYN: *fatty degeneration of the heart.*

fibroid h. Scarring of the myocardium, for example, after myocardial infarction.

hypertrophy of the h. An enlarge-

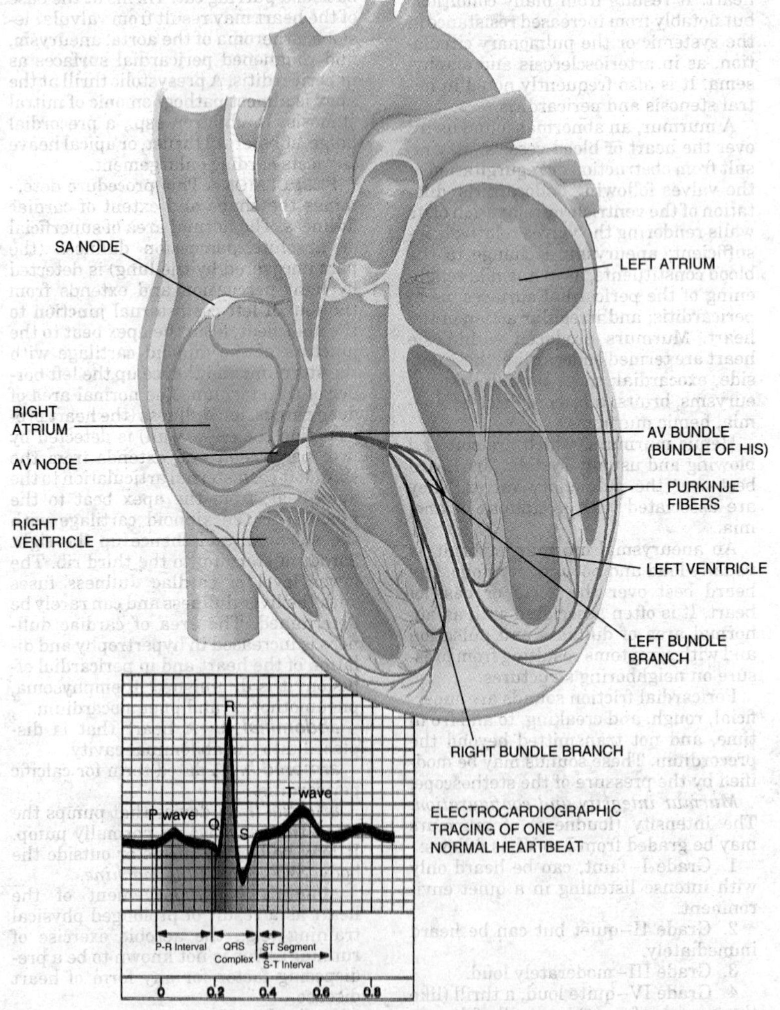

CONDUCTION SYSTEM OF THE HEART

ment of the heart caused by an increased size of the myocardium. It may be caused by exercise, valvular stenosis, and many other conditions. The myocardium increases in size by enlargement of each cell, not by an increase in number of cells. SYN: *cardiac hypertrophy*.

irritable h. An old term for neurocirculatory asthenia or effort syndrome, characterized by breathlessness, palpitation, weakness, and exhaustion.

left h. The left atrium and ventricle. The left atrium receives oxygenated blood from the lungs; the left ventricle pumps this blood into systemic circulation.

right h. The right atrium and ventricle. The right atrium receives deoxygenated blood from the body; the right ventricle pumps this blood to the lungs.

soldier's h. An old term for panic attack.

heart attack Myocardial infarction.

heartbeat The rhythmic contraction of the heart.

heart block Interference with the normal transmission of electrical impulses through the conducting system of the heart. The condition is seen on electrocardiogram as a prolongation of the PR interval, a widening of the QRS complex, a delay in the appearance of an expected beat, the loss of synchrony of atrial and ventricular beats, or dropped (missing) beats.

ETIOLOGY: Heart block may be produced by temporary changes in vagal tone, drugs or toxins (e.g., some antiarrhythmics or antihypertensives), infections (e.g., infective endocarditis or Lyme disease), fibrosis or other degenerative diseases of the conducting system, ischemia or infarction, or other mechanisms.

atrioventricular h.b. SEE: *block, atrioventricular*.

bilateral bundle branch h.b. SEE: *block, atrioventricular*.

bundle branch h.b. A condition in which impulses are blocked in one of the branches of the bundle of His, resulting in ventricles beating out of rhythm with each other, which stimulates one ventricle to beat slightly before the other. SYN: *interventricular h.b.*

complete h.b. A condition in which there is a complete dissociation between atrial and ventricular systoles. Ventricles may beat from their own pacemakers at a rate of 30 to 40 beats per minute while atria beat independently. SYN: *third-degree h.b.* SEE: illus.

congenital h.b. A type of heart block present at birth owing to improper development of the conducting system of the heart.

fascicular h.b. A conduction defect in either or both of the subdivisions of the left bundle branch.

first-degree h.b. A heart block in which the conduction of impulses through the atrioventricular node is delayed but all atrial beats are followed by ventricular beats. It is recognized on the electrocardiogram by a prolonged P-R interval.

interventricular h.b. Bundle branch h.b.

second-degree h.b. A form of atrioventricular block in which only some atrial impulses are conducted to the ventricles. Two variants exist: Mobitz I (Wenckebach) and Mobitz II. In Mobitz I, the PR intervals become progressively longer until a QRS complex is dropped. Because of the dropped beats, the QRS complexes appear to be clustered (a phenomenon called "grouped beating") on the electrocardiogram. In Mobitz II, PR intervals have a constant length, but QRS complexes are dropped periodically, usually every second, third, or fourth beat.

sinoatrial h.b. A partial or complete heart block characterized by interference in the passage of impulses from the sinoatrial node. SEE: *sick sinus syndrome*.

third-degree h.b. Complete heart block.

heartburn A burning sensation felt in the mid-epigastrium, behind the sternum, or in the throat caused by reflux of the acid contents of the stomach into the esophagus. SYN: *brash; pyrosis*. SEE: *gastroesophageal reflux disease*.

TREATMENT: Antacids, H_2-receptor antagonists (e.g., cimetidine), and proton pump inhibitors (e.g., lansoprazole) are all effective remedies.

PATIENT CARE: Patients are helped

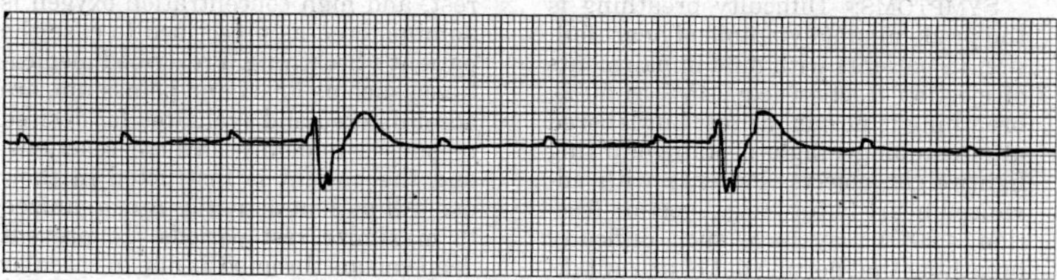

COMPLETE HEART BLOCK

to identify the time of occurrence in relation to food intake, if position changes exaggerate discomfort, precipitating factors (such as type and amount of food), and factors that aggravate the discomfort. For many people mints, chocolates, alcohol, late meals, and anti-inflammatory drugs all worsen the symptom. If antacids are used to treat heartburn, their ability to limit the effect of other oral medications is explained and a schedule established to prevent interactions.

heart disease Any pathological condition of the coronary arteries, heart valves, myocardium, or electrical conduction system of the heart.

ischemic h.d. A lack of oxygen supply to the heart altering cardiac function. The most common cause of myocardial ischemia is atherosclerosis of the coronary arteries. Depending upon several factors, including oxygen demand of the myocardium, degree of narrowing of the lumen of the arteries, and duration of the ischemia, the end result is temporary or permanent damage to the heart. SEE: *risk factors for h.d.; coronary artery; coronary artery disease.*

risk factors for ischemic h.d. Conditions that predispose people to ischemic heart disease (coronary artery disease). These may be divided into those that are not reversible (aging, male gender, menopause, genetic factors) and those that are potentially reversible (tobacco use, hypertension, hyperlipidemia, diabetes mellitus, left ventricular hypertrophy, obesity, and sedentary lifestyle).

heart failure Inability of the heart to circulate blood effectively enough to meet the body's metabolic needs. Heart failure may affect the left ventricle, right ventricle, or both. It may result from impaired ejection of blood from the heart during systole or from impaired relaxation of the heart during diastole. The prognosis for patients with heart failure depends on the ejection fraction, that is, the proportion of blood in the ventricle that is propelled from the heart during each contraction. In healthy patients, the ejection fraction equals about 55% to 78%. SYN: *congestive heart failure*. SEE: *ejection fraction; pulmonary edema*.

SYMPTOMS: Difficulty breathing is the predominant symptom of heart failure. In patients with mild impairments of ejection fraction (e.g., 45% to 50%), breathing is normal at rest but labored after climbing a flight of stairs or lifting lightweight objects. Patients with advanced heart failure (e.g., ejection fraction <20%) may have such difficulty breathing that getting out of bed or taking a few steps is very tiring.

Difficulty breathing while lying flat (orthopnea) or awakening at night with shortness of breath (paroxysmal nocturnal dyspnea) are also hallmarks of heart failure, as are exertional fatigue and lower extremity swelling (edema).

ETIOLOGY: Heart failure may result from myocardial infarction, myocardial ischemia, arrhythmias, heart valve lesions, congenital malformation of the heart or great vessels, constrictive pericarditis, cardiomyopathies, or conditions that affect the heart indirectly, including renal failure, fluid overload, thyrotoxicosis, severe anemia, and sepsis. Of the many causes of heart failure, ischemia and infarction are the most common.

TREATMENT: Diuretics, afterload reducers (e.g., angiotensin-converting enzyme inhibitors), and agents that improve the contractility of the heart (e.g., digoxin, dobutamine) are often combined in the acute and chronic treatment of heart failure. Other drugs that have been shown to be effective are the combination of nitrates and hydralazine, and some beta blockers. In patients with heart failure caused by valvular heart disease, valve replacement surgery may be effective. Cardiac transplantation can be used in advanced heart failure when donor organs are available.

PATIENT CARE: The patient is assessed for signs and symptoms. Vital signs are monitored for increased heart and respiratory rates and for narrowing pulse pressure, and the mental status is evaluated using AVPU. The chest is auscultated for abnormal heart sounds and for lung crackles (rales) or gurgles (rhonchi). Daily weights are obtained to detect fluid retention, and the extremities are inspected for evidence of peripheral edema. If the patient is confined to a bed, the sacral area of the spine is assessed for edema. Fluid intake and output are monitored (esp. if the patient is receiving diuretics). Blood urea nitrogen and serum creatinine, potassium, sodium, chloride, and bicarbonate levels are monitored frequently. Continuous ECG monitoring is provided during acute and advanced disease stages to identify and manage dysrhythmias promptly. The patient is placed in high Fowler's position and on prescribed bedrest, and high concentration oxygen is administered as prescribed to ease the patient's breathing. Prescribed medications, such as Lasix and potassium, are administered and evaluated for desired responses and any adverse reactions, and the patient is instructed in their use. All patient activities are organized to maximize rest periods. To prevent deep venous thrombosis due to vascular congestion, the caregiver assists with range-of-motion exercises and applies antiembolism stockings or uses heparins or warfarin. Any deterioration in the patient's condition is documented and reported immediately. A diet high in potassium (to replace that lost through diuresis) may sometimes be provided, including such potassium-rich foods as bananas, apricots, and orange juice, and the patient is instructed in this type of diet. To help curb fluid overload, the patient should avoid foods high in sodium content, such as canned and commercially prepared foods and dairy products. The importance of regular medical checkups is emphasized, and the patient is advised to notify the health care practitioner if the pulse rate is unusually irregular, falls below 60, or increases above 120, or if the patient experiences palpitations, dizziness, blurred vision, shortness of breath, persistent dry cough, increased fatigue, paroxysmal nocturnal dyspnea, swollen ankles, decreased urine output, or a weight gain of 3 to 5 lb (1.4 to 2.3 kg) in 1 week.

backward h.f. Heart failure in which blood congests the lungs, and often the right ventricle, liver, and lower extremities.

congestive h.f. ABBR: CHF. Heart failure. SEE: *Nursing Diagnoses Appendix.*

forward h.f. Heart failure in which forward flow of blood to the tissues is inadequate because the left ventricle is unable to pump blood with enough force to the systemic circulation (e.g., as a result of cardiomyopathy, muscular stunning, or infarction) or because outflow from the left ventricle is obstructed (e.g., in aortic stenosis).

high output h.f. Heart failure that occurs in spite of high cardiac output, for example, in severe anemia, thyrotoxicosis, arteriovenous fistulae, or other diseases.

left ventricular h.f. Failure of the heart to maintain left ventricular output.

low output h.f. Heart failure.

right ventricular h.f. Failure of the heart to maintain right ventricular output.

heart-lung machine A device that maintains the functions of the heart and lungs while either or both are unable to continue to function adequately. The device pumps, oxygenates, and removes carbon dioxide from the blood. In animal studies and in open heart surgery, these machines take over the function of the heart and lungs while these organs are being treated or possibly replaced. The function of the heart-lung machine is also called heart-lung bypass. SEE: illus.

heart pump, nuclear-powered An artificial heart powered by nuclear energy.

heart rate, target zone A heart rate that is 50% to 75% of an individual's maximum heart rate. Persons who exercise to attain or maintain physical fitness should attempt to exercise vigorously enough to produce a heart rate that is both safe and effective. When an exercise program is begun, the heart rate should be at the lower end of the 50% to 75% range for the first few months. Then it should be gradually built up to 75%.

heart size The dimensions of the cardiac image as seen on radiographs, echocardiographs, computed tomography, angiography, or magnetic resonance imaging of the thorax.

heart valve, prosthetic SEE: under *valve*.

heat [AS. *haetu*] **1.** The condition or sensation of being hot; opposite of cold. **2.** -

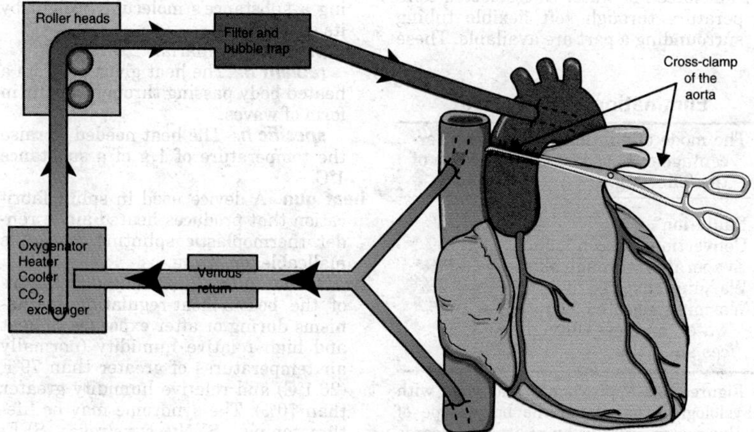

HEART-LUNG MACHINE

Higher than normal body temperature; generalized fever or localized warmth caused by an infection. Calor (fever), dolor (pain), rubor (redness), and tumor (swelling) are the four classic signs of inflammation. SEE: *febrile convulsion; fever*. **3.** Estrus. **4.** Energy that increases the temperature of surrounding tissues or objects by conduction, convection, or radiation. SEE: table.

acclimatization to h. The adjustment of an organism to heat in the environment. Exposure to high environmental temperature requires a period of adjustment in order for the body to function efficiently. The amount of time required depends on the temperature, humidity, and duration of daily exposure. Significant physiological adjustments occur in 5 days and are completed within 2 weeks to a month.

application of h. Placing an object, warmed above body temperature, on a body part to increase blood flow or provide relief of pain.

CAUTION: Heat should not be applied to extremities with reduced blood supply, as could be the case in most forms of arteriosclerosis or advanced diabetes.

Dry or moist heat sources may be used. Dry applications include hot water bottles, radiant heat, electric pads, and diathermy. Moist heat is considered more penetrating than dry heat, but this is due more to the fact that water-soaked materials lose heat slower than dry ones. The application should be approx. 120°F (48.9°C). Compresses may be kept warm by keeping hot water bottles at the proper temperature next to them. Do not use electric heating devices next to moist dressings. Devices that force hot water at a selected temperature through soft flexible tubing surrounding a part are available. These may be used to heat wet or dry compresses.

conductive h. Heat transferred by conduction from a heat source to an object that is cold when the two materials are in contact with each other.

convective h. The flow of heat to an object or part of the body by passage of heated particles, gas, or liquid from the heat source to the colder body.

diathermy h. Diathermy

dry h. Heat that has no moisture. It may take the form of a hot dry pack, hot water bottle, electric light bath, heliotherapy, hot bricks, resistance coil, electric pad or blanket, hot air bath, or therapeutic lamp.

h. of evaporation The heat absorbed per unit of mass when a substance is converted from a liquid to a gas, such as the change of water to steam when it is heated sufficiently. For water, the amount of heat required to transform water into steam is 540 cal/g of water.

initial h. Muscular heat produced during contraction when tension is increasing, during maintenance of tension, and during relaxation when tension is diminishing.

latent h. SEE: *latent heat*.

luminous h. Heat derived from light. This form may be tolerated better than other forms of radiation. Light may be converted into heat. Short infrared rays penetrate subcutaneous tissues to a greater extent than long invisible rays.

mechanical equivalent of h. The value of heat units in terms of work units. One Calorie (kilocalorie) is equal to 4.1855 × 10^4 joules.

moist h. Heat that has moisture content. It may be applied as hot bath pack, hot wet pack, hot foot bath, or vapor bath. The patient should be observed for dizziness, headache, or weakness.

molecular h. The result of multiplying a substance's molecular weight by its specific heat.

prickly h. Miliaria.

radiant h. The heat given off from a heated body passing through the air in form of waves.

specific h. The heat needed to raise the temperature of 1 g of a substance 1°C.

heat gun A device used in splint fabrication that produces heated air to render thermoplastic splinting materials malleable for fitting.

heatstroke A condition caused by failure of the body's heat-regulating mechanisms during or after exposure to heat and high relative humidity (normally air temperatures of greater than 79°F (26.1°C) and relative humidity greater than 70%). The syndrome may be life-threatening. SYN: *sunstroke*. SEE: *Nursing Diagnoses Appendix*.

SYMPTOMS: Heatstroke is marked

Elimination of Body Heat

The mode of elimination and the percentage of heat lost through each of the following is:

Radiation	55%*
Convection and conduction	15%*
Evaporation through skin	24%*
Warming inspired air	2%*
Warming ingested food and water, and loss through feces and urine	1%*

* Figures are approximate and vary with physiological activity of the body, type of clothing worn, relative humidity, and degree of acclimatization to a particular environment.

by high body temperature, usually above 105°F (40.6°C); headache; numbness and tingling; confusion preceding sudden onset of delirium or coma; tachycardia; rapid respiratory rate; and increased blood pressure. Patients with an insidious (non–activity-related) onset of heat stroke may have hot dry skin; the skin of active people may still be damp from perspiration, but sweating will cease as the condition worsens.

TREATMENT: Effective, immediate treatment to lower the body's core temperature can save the patient's life. The patient's clothes should be removed immediately and the patient actively cooled. For several days the patient should be observed for signs of fluid and electrolyte imbalance and renal failure.

PATIENT CARE: The patient suspected of heatstroke is assessed for airway patency, breathing adequacy, circulation, mental status using AVPU, and other associated signs and symptoms such as: shock, weakness, dizziness, nausea, vomiting, blurred vision, infection, and skin findings. Vital signs are obtained and, using a rectal or core probe, the caregiver monitors the patient's temperature; initially it may be extremely elevated. In the hospital setting, laboratory studies, including blood chemistry, arterial blood gases, urinalysis, complete blood count, and appropriate cultures are obtained to aid in treatment management. Cooling procedures are promptly instituted in the field and continued in the hospital. Intravenous therapy is begun to replace fluids in the dehydrated patient and high concentration oxygen is administered. Fluid intakes and urinary outputs are monitored. Invasive hemodynamic monitoring, endotracheal intubation and ventilation, or emergency dialysis may be needed in severe instances.

PREVENTION: Heat-related illness is preventable through education of the public. Athletic personnel are taught to recognize the signs and symptoms of heat problems and the importance of prevention and prompt treatment of symptoms. High-risk patients (those who are elderly, obese, diabetic, or alcoholic, those with cardiac disease and other chronic debilitating illnesses, and those taking phenothiazines or anticholinergics) are advised to take the following precautions: wear loose-fitting, lightweight clothing; take frequent rest breaks, esp. during strenuous activities; ingest adequate amounts of fluids, including electrolyte drinks; avoid hot, humid environments if possible; use proper room cooling or air conditioner and seek air-conditioned areas for relief. As necessary, the patient is referred to a social service agency for assistance with home cooling.

heat unit ABBR: HU. The amount of heat created at the anode during the production of x-ray photons. It is the product of the milliamperage times the seconds of exposure times the kilovoltage peak.

heaves (hēvs) Vomiting.

heavy chain disease ABBR: HCD. Any one of several abnormalities of immunoglobulins in which excessive quantities of alpha, gamma, delta, epsilon, or mu chains are produced. The immunoglobulins formed are incomplete, causing, in some cases, distinct clinical signs and symptoms including weakness, recurrent fever, susceptibility to bacterial infections, lymphadenopathy, hepatosplenomegaly, nephrotic syndrome and renal failure, anemia, leukopenia, thrombocytopenia, and eosinophilia. The disease may be diagnosed with immunoelectrophoresis or biopsy of affected organs.

alpha h.c.d. A form of heavy chain disease that is related to Mediterranean lymphoma and celiac sprue. The principal organ involved is the small intestine, although respiratory tissues are occasionally affected. The symptoms and signs may include malabsorption, diarrhea, abdominal pains, and weight loss. In some patients there is peripheral adenopathy and splenomegaly with no signs of intestinal or respiratory tract changes. Diagnosis is made through tests for the abnormal immunoglobulins. Chemotherapy may produce long-term remissions. SYN: *Seligmann's disease*.

gamma h.c.d. A rare disease whose hallmark is the production of abnormal immunoglobins (made of gamma heavy chains) by malignant B-lymphocytes. Clinical findings may include lymphadenopathy, hepatosplenomegaly, arthritis, edema of the uvula, and infiltration of the skin and thyroid gland. Treatment includes therapy for the underlying disorders, including the particular type of lymphoma present. SEE: *heavy chain disease*.

mu h.c.d. A heavy chain disease with presenting symptoms of a lymphoproliferative malignancy, especially chronic lymphocytic leukemia. Treatment focuses on the underlying disorders.

heavy metals Metals such as mercury, lead, chromium, cadmium, and arsenic that have known toxic effects on internal organs, such as the kidneys, brain, bone, or retina. SEE: *Poisons and Poisoning Appendix*.

Heberden's disease (hē'bĕr-dĕnz) [William Heberden, Brit. physician, 1710–1801] Arthritis with deformity that begins in the fingers and progresses. The concomitant deformity is caused by ankylosis, exostosis, and atrophy of soft parts.

Heberden's nodes Hard nodules or enlargements of the distal interphalangeal joints of the fingers; seen in osteoarthritis.

hebetude [L. *hebet,* dull] Dullness or lethargy.

hebotomy (hē-bŏt'ō-mē) Pubiotomy.

hecateromeric, hecatomeric (hĕk"ă-tĕr"ō-mĕr'ĭk, hĕk"ă-tō-mĕr'ĭk) [Gr. *hekateros,* each of two, + *meros,* part] Having two processes on a spinal neuron, one supplying each side of the spinal cord.

hecto- [Gr. *hekaton,* hundred] In the metric system, a prefix indicating 100 times (10^2) the unit named. Thus, hectoliter (10^2 liters) is 100 L.

hectogram [" + *gramma,* small weight] One hundred grams, or 3.527 avoirdupois ounces.

hectoliter (hĕk'tō-lē"tĕr) [" + *litra,* a pound] One hundred liters.

hectometer (hĕk-tŏm'ĕ-tĕr) [" + *metron,* measure] One hundred meters.

HEDIS *Health Plan Employer Data and Information Set.*

hedonism (hēd'ŏn-ĭzm) [Gr. *hedone,* pleasure, + *-ismos,* condition] A theory or standard of conduct in which the principal object of life is pleasure. SEE: *pleasure principle.*

heel [AS. *huela,* heel] Rounded posterior portion of the foot under and behind the ankle. SYN: *calx.*

h. bone Calcaneus.

h. puncture A method for obtaining a blood sample from a newborn or premature infant.

CAUTION: The puncture should be made in the lateral or medial area of the plantar surface of the heel, while avoiding the posterior curvature of the heel. The puncture should go no deeper than 2.4 mm. Previous puncture sites should not be used.

Thomas h. A corrective shoe in which the heel is approx. 12 mm longer and 4 to 6 mm higher on the medial edge. This produces varus of the foot and prevents depression of the head of the talus.

HEENT *head, eyes, ears, nose, throat.*

Heerfordt's disease (hār'forts) [C. F. Heerfordt, Danish ophthalmologist, 1871–1953] Uveoparotid fever, a form of sarcoidosis, marked by enlargement of the parotid gland, inflammation of the uveal tract, and prolonged low-grade fever.

Hegar's sign (hā'gărz) [Alfred Hegar, Ger. gynecologist, 1830–1914] Softening of the lower uterine segment; a probable sign of pregnancy that may be present during the second and third months of gestation. On bimanual examination, the lower part of the uterus is easily compressed between the fingers placed in the vagina and those of the other hand over the pelvic area. This is due to the overall softening of the uterus related to increasing vascularity and edema and because the fetus does not fill the uterine cavity at this point, so the space is empty and compressible.

Heidenhain's demilunes (hī'dĕn-hīnz) [Rudolph Peter Heinrich Heidenhain, Ger. physiologist, 1834–1897] Crescent-shaped groups of serous cells at the base, or along the sides, of the mucous alveoli of the salivary glands, esp. sublingual and submandibular. SYN: *Giannuzzi's cells.*

height (hīt) [AS. *hiehthu*] The vertical distance from the bottom to the top of an organ or structure.

h. of contour A line encircling a structure, designating its greatest diameter in a specified plane. In dentistry, the term refers to the largest circumferential measurement around a tooth. The height of contour must be maintained during restoration of a tooth to maintain the normal flow of food over the tooth.

fundal h. The distance (in centimeters) from the portion of the uterus above the insertion of the fallopian tubes to the symphysis pubis. *Antepartum:* When compared against gestational norms, this measurement is helpful in confirming the estimated number of weeks elapsed since conception and in monitoring intrauterine fetal growth. The fundus is first palpable at the level of the symphysis pubis during gestational week 12. *Postpartum:* Maintain as presented.

Heimlich maneuver (hīm'lĭk) [H. J. Heimlich, U.S. physician, b. 1920] A technique for removing a foreign body, such as a food bolus, from the trachea or pharynx, where it is preventing air flow to and from the lungs. Also called *abdominal thrust maneuver.*

The maneuver consists of the rescuer applying subdiaphragmatic pressure by: (1) wrapping his or her arms around the victim's waist from behind; (2) making a fist with one hand and placing it against the patient's abdomen between the navel and the rib cage; and (3) clasping the fist with the free hand and pressing in with a quick forceful upward thrust. This procedure should be repeated several times if necessary. If one is alone and experiences airway obstruction caused by a foreign body, this technique may be self-applied.

If the person is supine, the rescuer places the heel of one hand on the abdomen in the same position as described above and then, with the other hand on top of that hand, exerts a sudden upward pressure in the midline.

When the patient is a child and he or she can speak, breathe, or cough, the maneuver is unnecessary. If the maneuver is done it should be applied as gently as possible but still forcibly enough to dislodge the obstruction. The abdominal viscera of children are more easily damaged than those of adults.

This treatment is quite effective in dislodging the obstruction by forcing air against the mass much as pressure from a carbonated beverage forcibly removes a cork or cap from a bottle. The average air flow produced is 225 L/min. SEE: illus; *choking*.

Heineke-Mikulicz pyloroplasty (hī′nĕ-kĕ-mĭk′ū-lĭch) [Walter Hermann Heineke, Ger. surgeon, 1834–1901; Johann von Mikulicz-Radecki, Polish surgeon, 1850–1905] Pyloroplasty performed to enlarge the gastric outlet (pyloric canal) by incising the pylorus longitudinally and suturing the incision transversely. It is most often employed for treatment of peptic ulcer disease that does not respond to medical therapy in conjunction with vagotomy.

Heinz, Robert German pathologist, 1865–1924.

H. bodies Granules in red blood cells usually attached to the red blood cell membrane, seen in blood smears of persons with hemoglobinopathies, thalassemias, and after splenectomy. The bodies are best seen when the blood is stained with a special stain.

H. body anemia Hemolytic anemia associated with the finding of Heinz bodies in the red blood cells.

Heister, spiral valve of (hī′stĕr) [Lorenz Heister, Ger. anatomist, 1683–1758] A spiral fold of the mucous membrane lining the cystic duct of the gallbladder. It keeps the lumen open.

HeLa cells SEE: under *cell*.

helcoid (hĕl′koyd) [Gr. *helkos,* ulcer, + *eidos,* form, shape] Resembling an ulcer.

helcology (hĕl-kŏl′ō-jē) [″ + *logos,* word, reason] The study of ulcers.

helcoma (hĕl-kō′mă) [″ + *oma,* tumor] Ulcer of the cornea.

helcosis (hĕl-kō′sĭs) [″ + *osis,* condition] Ulceration.

helianthine (hē-lē-ăn′thĭn) Methyl orange used as an indicator in determining pH.

helical (hĕl′ĭ-kăl) In the shape of a helix.

helicine (hĕl′ĭ-sĭn) [Gr. *helix,* coil] **1.** Spiral. **2.** Pert. to a helix or coil.

h. arteries Tortuous arteries in the cavernous tissue of the penis, clitoris, and uterus.

Helicobacter pylori A motile, gram-negative bacterium that causes peptic ulcers. It is treated with combined antibiotics and agents to block gastric acid secretion (e.g., omeprazole).

DIAGNOSIS: Noninvasive diagnostic procedures include immunological tests of antibodies to *H. pylori* and urea breath tests. Invasive tests include endoscopy, gastric biopsy, and biopsy with bacterial culture for *H. pylori.*

helicoid (hĕl′ĭ-koyd) [″ + *eidos,* form, shape] Resembling a helix or spiral.

helicopodia (hĕl″ĭ-kō-pō′dē-ă) [″ + *pous,* foot] A peculiar movement in which the foot, when brought forward, drags and describes a partial arc, resulting in a gait such as that seen in spastic hemiplegia.

helicotrema (hĕl″ĭ-kō-trē′mă) [″ + *trema,* a hole] The opening at the tip of the cochlear canal where the scala tympani and scala vestibuli unite.

heliophobia (hē″lē-ō-fō′bē-ă) [Gr. *helios,* sun, + *phobos,* fear] An abnormal fear of the sun's rays, esp. by one who has suffered sunstroke.

heliotaxis (hē-lē-ō-tăk′sĭs) [″ + *taxis,* arrangement] A reaction in plants that causes them to respond negatively or positively to sunlight.

negative h. A turning away from the sun.

positive h. A turning toward the sun.

heliotherapy (hē″lē-ō-thĕr′ă-pē) [″ + *therapeia,* treatment] Exposure to sunlight for therapeutic purposes.

heliotropism (hē″lē-ŏt′rō-pĭzm) [″ + *trepein,* to turn, + *-ismos,* condition] The tendency of living organisms to turn or grow toward the sun.

heliox A therapeutic gas mixture of helium and oxygen.

helium (hē′lē-ŭm) [Gr. *helios,* sun] SYMB: He. A gaseous element; atomic weight 4.0026; atomic number 2. A liter of the gas at sea level pressure and 0°C weighs 0.1785 g. The second lightest element known, it is given off by radium and other radioactive elements in the form of charged helium ions known as alpha rays. Because of its low density, it is mixed with air or oxygen and used in the treatment of various respiratory disorders. Because of its low solubility, it is mixed with air supplied to workers laboring under high atmospheric pressure, as in caissons. When so used, it reduces the time required to adjust to increasing or decreasing air pressure and reduces the danger of bends.

helix (hē′lĭks) [Gr., coil] **1.** A coil or spiral. **2.** The margin of the external ear.

Watson-Crick h. SEE: *Watson-Crick helix.*

Heller's test [Johann F. Heller, Austrian pathologist, 1813–1871] A test formerly used for the presence of albumin in urine. It has been replaced by immunochemical, immunoelectrophoretic, and nephelometric tests. SEE: *urine.*

Hellerwork (hĕl-ĕr-wŏrk) [Joseph Heller, U.S. engineer, b. 1940] A type of body work combining massage therapy with relaxation techniques.

Hellin's law [Dyonizy Hellin, Polish pathologist, 1867–1935] A law stating that twins occur once in 80 pregnancies,

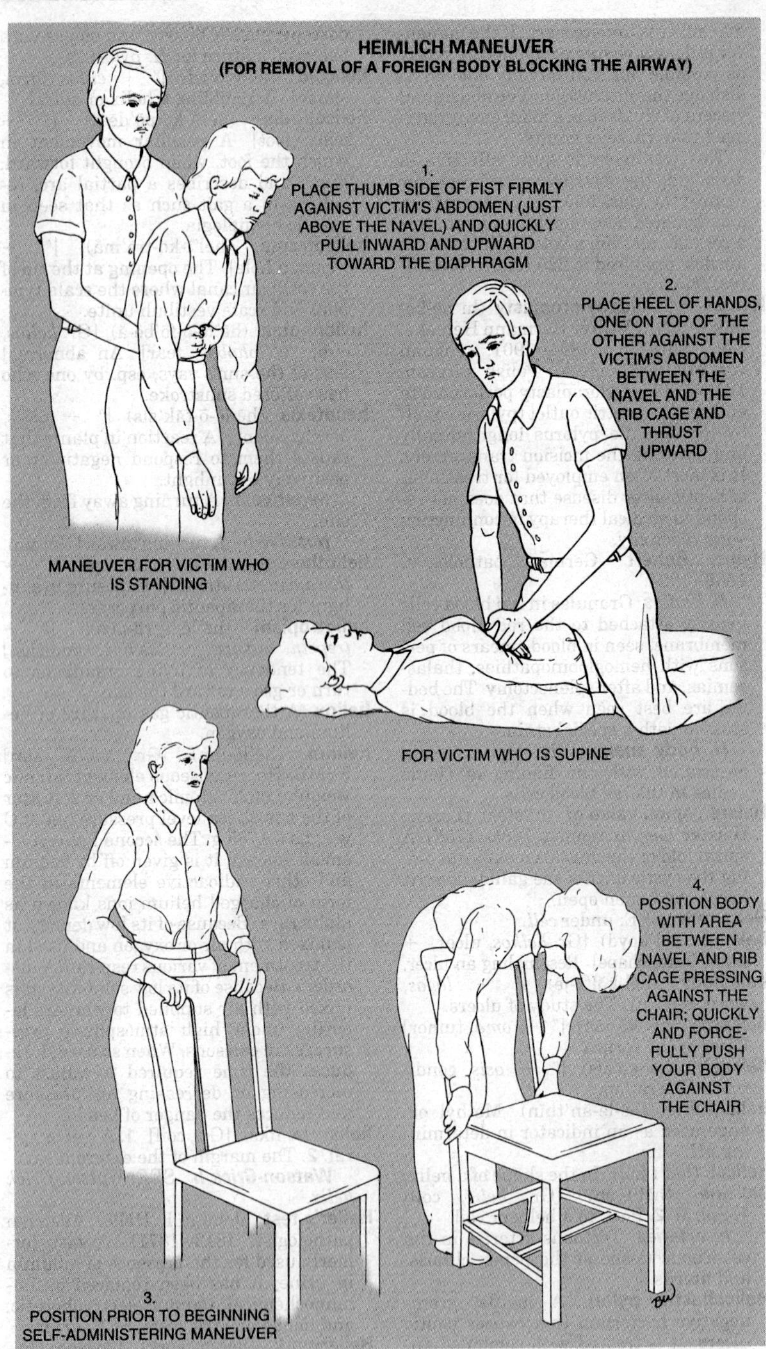

triplets once in 6400 (80^2) pregnancies, quadruplets once in 512,000 (80^3) pregnancies.

HEIMLICH MANEUVER
(FOR REMOVAL OF A FOREIGN BODY BLOCKING THE AIRWAY)
1.
PLACE THUMB SIDE OF FIST FIRMLY AGAINST VICTIM'S ABDOMEN (JUST ABOVE THE NAVEL) AND QUICKLY PULL INWARD AND UPWARD TOWARD THE DIAPHRAGM
MANEUVER FOR VICTIM WHO IS STANDING
2.
PLACE HEEL OF HANDS, ONE ON TOP OF THE OTHER AGAINST THE VICTIM'S ABDOMEN BETWEEN THE NAVEL AND THE RIB CAGE AND THRUST UPWARD
FOR VICTIM WHO IS SUPINE
3.
POSITION PRIOR TO BEGINNING SELF-ADMINISTERING MANEUVER
4.
POSITION BODY WITH AREA BETWEEN NAVEL AND RIB CAGE PRESSING AGAINST THE CHAIR; QUICKLY AND FORCEFULLY PUSH YOUR BODY AGAINST THE CHAIR

HELLP An acronym derived from the first letters of the terms that describe the following laboratory findings: Hemolysis, Elevated Liver enzymes, and Low Platelet count.

HELLP syndrome Severe pre-eclampsia marked by laboratory findings that include *h*emolytic anemia, *e*levated *l*iver function, and *l*ow *p*latelet levels. This potentially life-threatening condition usually arises in the last trimester of pregnancy. Initially, affected patients may complain of nausea, vomiting, and epigastric pain. Between 1% and 25% of affected women die of the syndrome. Complications may include acute renal failure, disseminated intravascular coagulation, liver failure, respiratory failure, or multiple organ system failure. SEE: *pre-eclampsia.*

helmet cell A schistocyte or fragmented blood cell, seen in hemolytic anemias. SEE: illus.

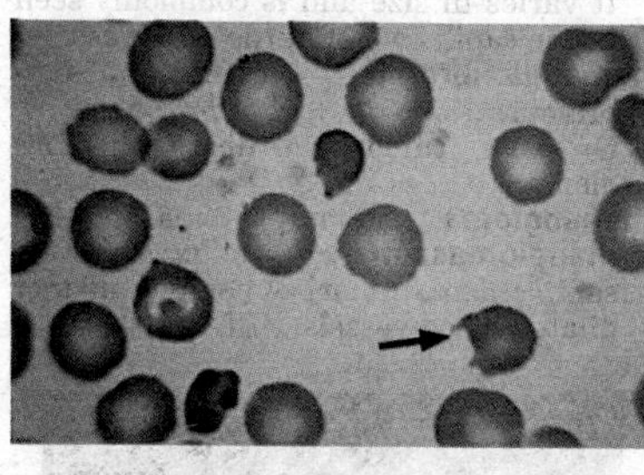

HELMET CELL (ARROW)

(Orig. Mag.×640)

helminth [Gr. *helmins,* worm] **1.** A wormlike animal. **2.** Any animal, either free-living or parasitic, belonging to the phyla Platyhelminthes (flatworms), Acanthocephala (spinyheaded worms), Nemathelminthes (threadworms or roundworms), or Annelida (segmented worms). SEE: illus.

helminthagogue (hĕl-mĭnth′ă-gŏg) [″ + *agogos,* leading] Anthelmintic.

helminthemesis (hĕl-mĭn-thĕm′ĕ-sĭs) [″ + *emesis,* vomiting] The vomiting of intestinal worms.

helminthiasis (hĕl-mĭn-thī′ă-sĭs) [″ + *iasis,* condition] Infestation with worms.

helminthic (hĕl-mĭn′thĭk) **1.** Pert. to worms. **2.** Pert. to that which expels worms. SYN: *anthelmintic; vermifugal.*

helminthicide (hĕl-mĭn′thĭ-sīd) [″ + L. *cidus,* kill] Anthelmintic.

helminthoid (hĕl-mĭn′thoyd) [″ + *eidos,* form, shape] Wormlike or resembling a worm.

helminthology (hĕl″mĭn-thŏl′ō-jē) [″ + *logos,* word, reason] The study of worms.

helminthoma (hĕl″mĭn-thō′mă) [″ + *oma,* tumor] A tumor caused by parasitic worms.

helminthophobia (hĕl-mĭn″thō-fō′bē-ă) [″ + *phobos,* fear] A morbid dread of worms or the delusion of being infested by them.

heloderma (hē″lō-dĕr′mă) Fibromas that form on the extensor surfaces of the proximal interphalangeal joints of the hands.

heloma (hē-lō′mă) [Gr. *helos,* nail, + *oma,* tumor] Clavus.

helotomy (hē-lŏt′ō-mē) [″ + *tome,* incision] The surgical treatment of corns.

helper T cells SEE: *cell, helper T.*

helplessness A feeling of dependence, powerlessness, defenselessness or de-

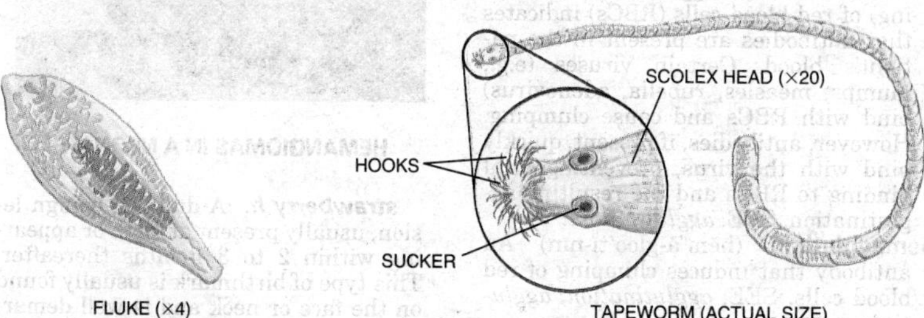

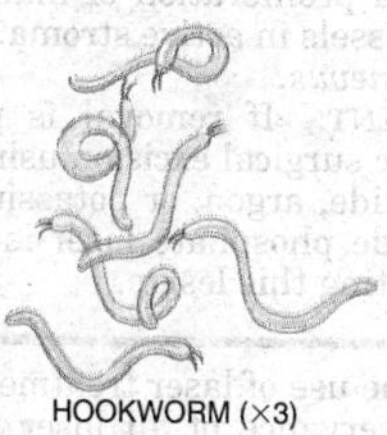

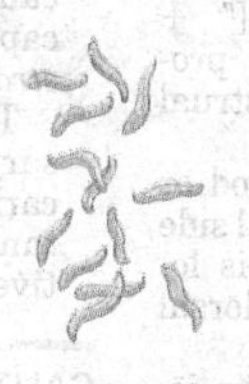

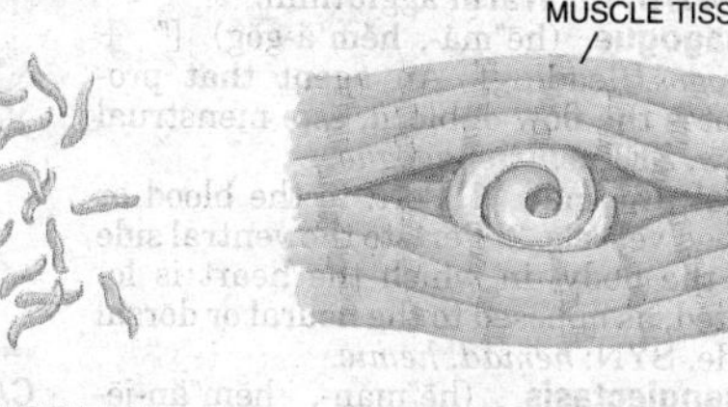

REPRESENTATIVE HELMINTHS

pression, e.g., in the face of crisis or overwhelming circumstances. SEE: *hopelessness; powerlessness*.

learned h. A passive fatalistic behavior that one cannot influence one's environment, or alter one's existence. This condition may sometimes arise in persons who have chronic illnesses, depression, phobias, or loss of functional independence.

Helweg's bundle (hĕl'vĕgz) [Hans K. S. Helweg, Danish physician, 1847–1901] A small tract passing from the olivary body to the anterior horn cells in the cervical region. Part of the extrapyramidal motor system.

hem-, hema-, hemo- [Gr. *haima,* blood] Combining form meaning *blood*. SEE: *hemat-*.

hemachrosis (hē″mă-, hĕm″ă-krō'sĭs) [″ + *chrosis,* coloring] Abnormal redness of blood. It is present in a very small number of cases of carbon monoxide poisoning.

hemacytometer (hē″mă-, hĕm″ă-sī-tŏm'ĭ-tĕr) [″ + *kytos,* cell, + *metron,* measure] Apparatus used in counting blood cells.

hemacytozoon (hē″mă-, hĕm″ă-sī-tō-zō'ŏn) [″ + ″ + *zoon,* animal] A protozoan parasite infesting red blood cells.

hemad (hē'măd) [Gr. *haima,* blood, + L. *ad,* toward] Hemal (2).

hemadsorption (hĕm″ăd-sorp'shŭn) The adherence of red blood cells to other cells or surfaces.

hemagglutination, hemoagglutination (hĕm″ă-gloo-tĭ-nā'shŭn) [″ + L. *agglutinare,* to paste to] The clumping of red blood cells. SEE: *agglutination*.

h. inhibition A laboratory test in which the lack of agglutination (clumping) of red blood cells (RBCs) indicates that antibodies are present in the patient's blood. Certain viruses (e.g., mumps, measles, rubella, adenovirus) bind with RBCs and cause clumping. However, antibodies, if present, quickly bind with the virus, preventing viral binding to RBCs and the resulting agglutination. SEE: *agglutination*.

hemagglutinin (hĕm″ă-gloo'tĭ-nĭn) An antibody that induces clumping of red blood cells. SEE: *agglutination; agglutinin*.

cold h. Cold agglutinin.

warm h. Warm agglutinin.

hemagogue (hē″mă-, hĕm'ă-gŏg) [″ + *agogos,* leading] An agent that promotes the flow of blood, esp. menstrual flow. SEE: *emmenagogue*.

hemal (hē'măl) **1.** Pert. to the blood or blood vessels. **2.** Pert. to the ventral side of the body, in which the heart is located, as opposed to the neural or dorsal side. SYN: *hemad; hemic*.

hemangiectasis (hē″măn-, hĕm″ăn-jē-ĕk'tă-sĭs) [″ + *angeion,* vessel, + *ektasis,* dilatation] Dilatation of the blood vessels.

hemangioblast (hĕ-măn'jē-ō-blăst) [″ + ″ + *blastos,* germ] A mesodermal cell that can form either vascular endothelial cells or hemocytoblasts.

hemangioblastoma (hĕ-măn″jē-ō-blăs-tō'mă) [″ + ″ + *oma,* tumor] A hemangioma of the brain, usually in the cerebellum.

hemangioendothelioblastoma (hĕ-măn″jē-ō-ĕn″dō-thē″lē-ō-blăs-tō'mă) [″ + ″ + *endon,* within, + *thele,* nipple, + *blastos,* germ, + *oma,* tumor] A neoplasm of the epithelial cells that line the blood vessels.

hemangioendothelioma (hē″măn-jē-ō-ĕn″dō-thē-lē-ō'mă) [″ + ″ + ″ + ″ + *oma,* tumor] A tumor of the endothelium of the minute capillary vessels. It varies in size and is commonly seen in the capillary net of the meninges.

hemangiofibroma (hĕ-măn″jē-ō-fī-brō'mă) [″ + ″ + L. *fibra,* fiber, + Gr. *oma,* tumor] A fibrous hemangioma.

hemangioma (hē-măn″jē-ō'mă) *pl.* **hemangiomas, -mata** [″ + *angeion,* vessel, + *oma,* tumor] A benign tumor of dilated blood vessels. SEE: illus.

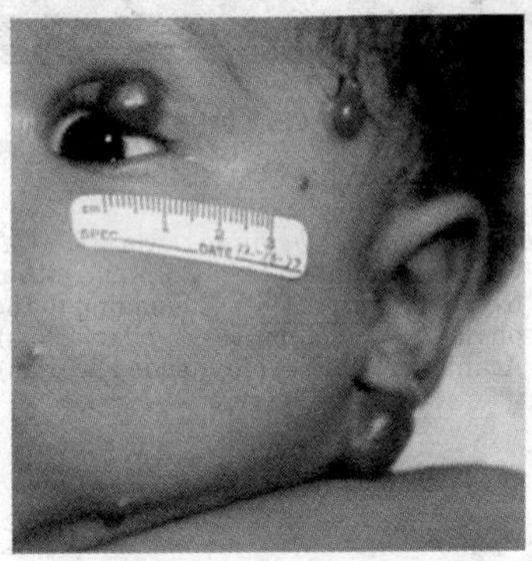

HEMANGIOMAS IN A NEONATE

strawberry h. A dull red benign lesion, usually present at birth or appearing within 2 to 3 months thereafter. This type of birthmark is usually found on the face or neck and is well demarcated from the surrounding skin. It grows rapidly and then regresses. It is caused by a proliferation of immature capillary vessels in active stroma. SYN: *strawberry nevus*.

TREATMENT: If removal is necessary, plastic surgical excision using the carbon dioxide, argon, or potassium titanium oxide phosphate laser is effective in ablating this lesion.

CAUTION: The use of laser treatment necessitates observance of all laser safety precautions.

hemangiomatosis (hē-măn″jē-ō-mă-tō′sĭs) [″ + ″ + ″ + *osis,* condition] Multiple angiomata of the blood vessels.

hemangiopericytoma (hĕ-măn″jē-ō-pĕr″ĕ-sī-tō′mă) A tumor arising in the capillaries, composed of pericytes.

hemangiosarcoma (hē-măn″jē-ō-săr-kō′mă) [″ + ″ + *sarkos,* flesh, + *oma,* tumor] A malignant neoplasm originating from the blood vessels. SYN: *angiosarcoma.*

hemapheresis SEE: *plasmapheresis.*

hemapophysis (hĕm-ă-pŏf′ĭ-sĭs) [″ + *apo,* from, + *physis,* growth] The portion of a developing vertebra that forms a rib and costal cartilage.

hemarthros, hemarthrosis (hĕm-ăr′thrōs, hĕm-ăr-thrō′sĭs) [″ + *arthron,* joint] A bloody effusion within a joint.

hemat-, hemato- [Gr. *haimatos,* blood] Combining form meaning *blood.* SEE: *hem-.*

hematapostema (hĕm″ăt-ă-pŏs-tē′mă) [Gr. *haimatos,* blood, + *apostema,* abscess] An abscess that contains blood.

hematemesis (hĕm-ăt-ĕm′ĕ-sĭs) [″ + *emesis,* vomiting] The vomiting of blood. SEE: *hemoptysis* for table; *hemorrhage.*

ETIOLOGY: The lesions most likely to cause vomiting of blood are duodenal or gastric ulcers; esophageal varices; esophagitis, gastritis, or duodenitis; Mallory-Weiss tears in the esophagus; arteriovenous malformations; or, rarely, fistulae between the aorta and the upper gastrointestinal tract. Typically, the vomiting of blood implies that the responsible lesion is located in the upper gastrointestinal tract (above the ligament of Treitz).

SYMPTOMS: The blood may be clotted, fluid, or mixed with food. Subsequent stools may be black and tarry (melenic). If blood loss is severe enough, shock and collapse may occur.

TREATMENT: The patient should be resuscitated with intravenous fluids. Transfusions are given when blood loss is massive, prolonged, or life-threatening. Endoscopy of the upper gastrointestinal tract may reveal a lesion susceptible to coagulation, sclerosis, ligation, or surgical excision. H_2-receptor antagonists (e.g., famotidine) or proton pump inhibitors (e.g., omeprazole) may be given when bleeding results from peptic disease.

PATIENT CARE: Vital signs and mental status, using AVPU, are monitored. Vomitus is inspected and its character and quantity documented, along with associated signs and symptoms. Management is focused at determining the underlying cause of bleeding. The patient is supported in an upright position (or turned to one side) to prevent aspiration. Oral hygiene is provided after episodes of vomiting and as needed while the patient is not taking anything by mouth.

hematencephalon (hĕm″ăt-ĕn-sĕf′ă-lŏn) [″ + *enkephalos,* brain] A cerebral hemorrhage.

hemathermal (hĕm″ă-, hē″mă-thĕr′măl) [″ + *therme,* heat] Warm blooded; applied to animals whose blood remains at a fairly constant temperature.

hemathidrosis, hematidrosis (hē-măt″hĭ-drō′sĭs) [Gr. *haimatos,* blood, + *hidros,* sweat, + *osis,* condition] A condition in which sweat contains blood. SYN: *hematohidrosis; hemidrosis* (2).

hematic (hē-măt′ĭk) Hematinic.

hematin (hĕm′ă-tĭn) The nonprotein portion of the hemoglobin molecule wherein the iron is in the ferric (Fe^{3+}) rather than the ferrous (Fe^{2+}) state. SEE: *ferritin; heme.*

hematinemia (hē-mă-, hĕm-ă-tĭn-ē′mē-ă) Hematin in the circulating blood.

hematinic (hē-mă-, hĕm-ă-tĭn′ĭk) [Gr. *haima,* blood] **1.** Pert. to blood. **2.** An agent that facilitates blood formation, used in treating anemia. SYN: *hematic.*

hemato- SEE: *hemat-.*

hematobilia (hĕm″ă-tō-bĭl′ē-ă) [″ + L. *bilis,* bile] Blood in the bile or bile ducts.

hematobium (hē″mă-, hĕm″ă-tō′bē-ŭm) [″ + *bios,* life] Hemocytozoon.

hematoblast (hē′mă-, hĕm′ă-tō-blăst) [″ + *blastos,* germ] Hemocytoblast.

hematocele (hē′mă-, hĕm′ă-tō-sēl) [″ + *kele,* tumor, swelling] **1.** A blood cyst. **2.** The effusion of blood into a cavity. **3.** A swelling due to effusion of blood into the tunica vaginalis testis.

parametric h. A tumor formed by blood effusion in the cul-de-sac of Douglas walled off by adhesions.

pudendal h. A blood-filled swollen area of the labium.

hematocelia (hĕm″ă-tō-sē′lē-ă) [″ + *koilia,* cavity] Bleeding into the peritoneal cavity.

hematochezia (hĕm″ă-tō-kē′zē-ă) [″ + *chezein,* to go to stool] The passage of bright red blood in the stool. SEE: *melena.*

hematochromatosis (hĕm″ă-tō-krō″mă-tō′sĭs) [″ + *chroma,* color, + *osis,* condition] Hemochromatosis.

hematochyluria (hē″mă-, hĕm″ă-tō-kī-lū′rē-ă) [″ + *chylos,* juice, + *ouron,* urine] Blood and chyle in the urine.

hematocolpos (hē″mă-, hĕm″ă-tō-kŏl′pŏs) Retention of menstrual blood in the vagina, caused by an imperforate hymen.

hematocrit (hē-măt′ō-krĭt) [″ + *krinein,* to separate] **1.** An obsolete term for a centrifuge for separating solids from plasma in the blood. **2.** The volume of erythrocytes packed by centrifugation in a given volume of blood. The hematocrit is expressed as the percentage of total blood volume that consists of erythrocytes or as the volume in cubic centimeters of erythrocytes packed by centrifugation of blood. Approximate normal values at sea level: men, average 47%, range 40% to 54%; women, average 42%, range 37% to 47%; children, varies with age from 35% to 49%; newborn, 49% to 54%. SEE: *blood*.

hematocyst (hē′mă-, hĕm′ă-tō-sĭst) [Gr. *haimatos,* blood, + *kystis,* a bladder] **1.** Hemorrhage into a cyst or into the urinary bladder. **2.** A blood-filled cyst.

hematocytoblast (hĕm″ă-tō-sī′tō-blăst) [″ + ″ + *blastos,* germ] Hemocytoblast.

hematocytometer (hē″mă-, hĕm″ă-tō-sī-tŏm′ĕ-ter) [″ + ″ + *metron,* measure] A device for counting the number of blood cells in a given quantity of blood. SYN: *hemocytometer*.

hematocytozoon (hē″mă-, hĕm″ă-tō-sī-tō-zō′ŏn) [″ + ″ + *zoon,* animal] A parasite that lives in red blood cells.

hematocyturia (hē″mă-, hĕm″ă-tō-sī-tū′rē-ă) [″ + ″ + *ouron,* urine] Red blood cells in the urine; hematuria, as differentiated from hemoglobinuria.

hematogenesis (hē″mă-, hĕm″ă-tō-jĕn′ĕ-sĭs) [″ + *genesis,* generation, birth] Hematopoiesis.

hematogenic, hematogenous (hē″mă-, hĕm″ă-tō-jĕn′ĭk, -tŏj′ĕ-nŭs) [″ + *gennan,* to produce] **1.** Hematopoietic. **2.** Pert. to or originating in the blood.

hematohidrosis (hē″mă-, hĕm″ă-tō-hī-drō′sĭs) [″ + *hidros,* sweat, + *osis,* condition] Hemathidrosis.

hematoidin (hē″mă-, hĕm-ă-toy′din) The yellow crystalline substance, biliverdin, that remains when red blood cells are destroyed in bruised tissue.

hematologist (hē″mă-, hĕm″ă-tŏl′ō-jĭst) [″ + *logos,* word, reason] A physician who specializes in the diagnosis and treatment of disorders of blood and blood-forming tissues.

hematology (hē″mă-, hĕm″ă-tŏl′ō-jē) The science concerned with blood and the blood-forming tissues.

hematolymphangioma (hē″mă-, hĕm″ă-tō-lĭmf-ăn″jē-ō′mă) [″ + L. *lympha,* lymph, + Gr. *angeion,* vessel, + *oma,* tumor] A tumor consisting of dilated blood vessels and lymphatics. SYN: *hemolymphangioma*.

hematolytic (hĕm-ă-tō-lĭt′ĭk) Hemolytic.

hematoma (hē″mă-, hĕm-ă-tō′mă) [Gr. *haimatos,* blood, + *oma,* tumor] A swelling comprised of a mass of extravasated blood (usually clotted) confined to an organ, tissue, or space and caused by a break in a blood vessel.

h. auris An effusion of blood, causing a hard swelling between perichondrium and the cartilage of the pinna of the ear. Common in fighters and wrestlers. SYN: *othematoma*. SEE: *cauliflower ear*.

epidural h. A hematoma above the dura mater, usually arterial, except in posterior fossa.

intracerebral h. A hemorrhage localized in one area of the brain.

pelvic h. A hematoma present in the cellular tissue of the pelvis.

subarachnoid h. A hemorrhage between the arachnoid membrane and the pia mater; usually caused by the rupture of a congenital intracranial aneurysm or berry aneurysm, hypertension, or trauma.

subdural h. A hematoma located beneath the dura, usually the result of a head injury.

vulvar h. Extravasation of blood into the soft tissues of the external female genitalia. The bleeding may occur after delivery or as a result of trauma. Postpartum bleeding usually is due to the shearing of submucosal tissues during a difficult or forceps-assisted delivery.

PATIENT CARE: The woman usually complains of severe vulvar pain. Inspection may reveal a unilateral firm area of the labia majora that is extremely painful to the touch. Prompt application of an ice pack may limit further bleeding; however, large or enlarging hematomas may require surgical intervention (i.e., ligation and evacuation).

hematomediastinum (hē″mă-, hĕm″ă-tō-mē″dē-ă-stī′nŭm) [″ + L. *mediastinus,* in the middle] Hemomediastinum.

hematometra (hē″mă-, hĕm″ă-tō-mē′tră) [″ + *metra,* uterus] **1.** Hemorrhage in the uterus. **2.** An accumulation of menstrual blood in the uterus. SEE: *hematocolpos; hydrometra; pyometra*.

hematomphalocele (hē″mă-, hĕm″ăt-ŏm-făl′ō-sēl) [″ + *omphalos,* navel, + *kele,* tumor, swelling] The effusion of blood into an umbilical hernia.

hematomyelia (hē″mă-, hĕm″ă-tō-mī-ē′lē-ă) [″ + *myelos,* marrow] Hemorrhage into the spinal cord.

hematomyelitis (hē″mă-, hĕm″ă-tō-mī″ĕl-ī′tĭs) [″ + ″ + *itis,* inflammation] An inflammation of the spinal cord accompanied by bloody effusion.

hematonephrosis (hē″mă-, hĕm″ă-tō-nĕ-frō′sĭs) [″ + *nephros,* kidney, + *osis,* condition] Hemonephrosis.

hematopathology [″ + *pathos,* disease, suffering, + *logos,* word, reason] The study of pathologic conditions of the blood.

hematopericardium (hē″mă-, hĕm″ă-tō-pĕr″ĭ-kăr′dē-ŭm) [″ + *peri,* around, + *kardia,* heart] A bloody effusion into the pericardium.

hematoperitoneum (hē″mă-, hĕm″ă-tō-pĕr″ĭ-tō-nē′ŭm) [″ + *peritonaion,* peritoneum] Hemoperitoneum.

hematophagia (hĕm″ă-tō-fā′jē-ă) The ingestion of blood.

hematophagous (hĕm-ă-tŏf′ă-gŭs) Living on blood.

hematophilia (hĕm″ă-tō-fĭl′ē-ă) [″ + *philein,* to love] Hemophilia.

hematophobia (hē″mă-, hĕm″ă-tō-fō′bē-ă) [″ + *phobos,* fear] Hemophobia.

hematophyte (hē′mă-, hĕm′ă-tō-fīt) [″ + *phyton,* plant] A plant organism or bacterium in the blood.

hematoplastic [″ + *plassein,* to form] Hematopoietic.

hematopoiesis (hē″mă-, hĕm″ă-tō-poy-ē′sĭs) [Gr. *haimatos,* blood, + *poiesis,* formation] The production and development of blood cells, normally in the bone marrow.

extramedullary h. The production of blood cells in tissues other than bone marrow, which occurs in severe anemia and other diseases affecting the blood.

hematopoietic (hē″mă-, hĕm″ă-tō-poy-ĕt′ĭk) **1.** Pert. to the production and development of blood cells. **2.** A substance that assists in or stimulates the production of blood cells. SYN: *hematogenic; hematoplastic.*

h. growth factors A group of at least seven substances involved in the production of blood cells, including several interleukins and erythropoietin.

h. malignancies Cancers that arise from unregulated clonal proliferation of hematopoietic stem cells, such as leukemia and lymphoma. In these disorders, genetically abnormal blood-forming cells (derived from precursors of granulocytes, lymphocytes, platelets, or red blood cells) reproduce in an unchecked fashion, consume nutrients, infiltrate various tissues, and replace the body's normally functioning cells. SEE: *leukemia; lymphoma.*

hematoporphyrin (hē″mă-, hĕm″ă-tō-por′fĭ-rĭn) [″ + *porphyra,* purple] Iron-free heme, a decomposition product of hemoglobin present in the urine in certain conditions.

hematoporphyrinuria (hē″mă-, hĕm″ă-tō-por″fĭ-rĭn-ū′rē-ă) [″ + ″ + *ouron,* urine] Hematoporphyrin in the urine.

hematorrhachis (hĕm-ă-tor′ă-kĭs) [″ + *rhachis,* spine] Hemorrhage into the spinal cord.

hematosalpinx (hē″mă-, hĕm″ă-tō-săl′pinks) [″ + *salpinx,* tube] Retained menstrual fluid in a fallopian tube. SYN: *hemosalpinx.*

hematoscheocele (hĕm-ă-tŏs′kē-ō-sēl) [″ + *oscheon,* scrotum, + *kele,* tumor, swelling] Blood accumulated in the scrotum.

hematospermatocele (hĕm″ă-tō-spĕr-măt′ō-sēl) [″ + *sperma,* seed, + *kele,* tumor, swelling] A blood-filled spermatocele.

hematospermia (hĕm″ă-tō-spĕr′mē-ă) Semen that contains blood. SYN: *hemospermia.*

h. spuria Hematospermia coming from the prostatic urethra.

h. vera Hematospermia coming from the seminal vesicles.

hematostatic (hĕm″ă-tō-stăt′ĭk) [Gr. *haimatos,* blood, + *stasis,* standing] Hemostatic.

hematosteon (hĕm-ă-tŏs′tē-ŏn) [″ + *osteon,* bone] Bleeding into bone marrow.

hematothorax (hĕm″ă-tō-thō′răks) [″ + *thorax,* chest] Hemothorax.

hematotoxic (hĕm″ă-tō-tŏk′sĭk) [″ + *toxikon,* poison] **1.** Pert. to septicemia. **2.** Toxic to blood cells.

hematotropic (hĕm″ă-tō-trŏp′ĭk) [″ + *tropos,* a turning] Having a special affinity for red blood cells.

hematotympanum (hĕm″ă-tō-tĭm′păn-ŭm) [″ + *tympanon,* drum] Hemotympanum.

hematoxylin (hĕm″ă-tŏk′sĭ-lĭn) $C_{16}H_{14}O_6$; a colorless crystalline compound obtained by ether extraction of the wood portion of the tree *Haematoxylon campechianum.* Upon oxidation it is converted into hematein, an oxidation product of hematoxylin, which stains certain structures a deep blue. It is widely used in histology to stain cell nuclei.

hematozoon (hē″mă-, hĕm″ă-tō-zō′ŏn) [″ + *zoon,* animal] Any living organism in the blood. SYN: *hemozoon.*

hematozymosis (hē″mă-, hĕm″ă-tō-zī-mō′sĭs) [″ + *zymosis,* fermentation] Blood fermentation.

hematuria (hē″mă-, hĕm″ă-tū′rē-ă) [″ + *ouron,* urine] Blood in the urine.

ETIOLOGY: Blood may appear in the urine as a result of a wide variety of conditions, including contamination during menstruation or the puerperium; internal trauma or kidney stones; vigorous exercise; urinary tract infections or systemic infections with renal involvement; some cases of glomerulonephritis; vascular anomalies of the urinary tract; or cancers of the urethra, bladder, prostate, ureters, or kidneys.

FINDINGS: The urine may appear tea-colored, slightly smoky, reddish, or frankly bloody.

DIAGNOSIS: The clinical history may help determine the cause of bleeding in the urine. Kidney stones often cause hematuria associated with intense flank pain that radiates into the groin. Hematuria in a child with recent sore throat, new edema, and hypertension may reflect a poststreptococcal glomerulonephritis. Urinary bleeding in a patient with abdominal pain and an enlarged or prosthetic aorta may have a fistulous connection to a ureter—a true surgical emergency. In the laboratory, microscopic examination of the urine also provides clues to the cause of bleeding. Red blood cells from the upper urinary tract often are deformed or misshapen, whereas those from the urethra or bladder have a normal microscopic appearance.

microscopic h. Blood in the urine that is detected only by microscopic examination. It may be a sign of cancer of the genitourinary tract; kidney stones; urinary tract infections, schistosomiasis, or urinary tuberculosis; glomerular diseases; or other conditions. SYN: *microhematuria*.

renal h. Hematuria in which the blood comes from the upper tract. On gross examination, the urine is often smoky, red, or cola-colored. Some causes include: glomerular diseases, kidney tumors, kidney stones, among others.

urethral h. Urinary bleeding that may result from urethral trauma, surgery, adenomas, or other lesions of the lower urinary tract. The voided urine usually is bright red at the onset of urination and more dilute in appearance as the stream continues.

vesical h. Urinary bleeding typically produced by bladder malignancies, stones, or cystitis.

heme (hēm) An iron-containing nonprotein portion of the hemoglobin molecule wherein the iron is in the ferrous (Fe^{2+}) state. SEE: *ferritin; hematin*.

hemeralopia (hĕm″ĕr-ăl-ō′pē-ă) [Gr. *hemera,* day, + *alaos,* blind, + *ops,* eye] Diminished vision in bright light. Term formerly erroneously applied to night blindness or nyctalopia. Nyctalopia indicates inability to see in dim light, though otherwise vision is normal.

In hemeralopia, the sight is poor in sunlight and in good illumination; it is good at dusk, at twilight, and in poor illumination. This is noted in albinism, retinitis with central scotoma, toxic amblyopia, coloboma of the iris and choroid, opacity of the crystalline lens or cornea, and in conjunctivitis with photophobia.

hemi- (hĕm′ē) [Gr.] Prefix meaning *half.*

hemiacephalus (hĕm″ē-ă-sĕf′ă-lŭs) [″ + *a-,* not, + *kephale,* head] A malformed fetus with a markedly defective head. SEE: *anencephalus*.

hemiachromatopsia (hĕm″ē-ă-krō-mă-tŏp′sē-ă) [″ + ″ + *chroma,* color, + *opsis,* vision] Color blindness in one-half, or in corresponding halves, of the vision field. SYN: *hemichromatopsia*.

hemiageusia (hĕm″ē-ă-gū′zē-ă) [″ + ″ + *geusis,* taste] Loss of sense of taste on one side of the tongue.

hemialbumin (hĕm″ē-ăl-bū′mĭn) [″ + L. *albumen,* white of egg] A product resulting from the digestion of albumin.

hemialbumose (hĕm″ē-ăl′bū-mōs) An albumoid product from the digestion of certain proteins. It is found in bone marrow.

hemialbumosuria (hĕm″ē-ăl-bū″mō-sū′rē-ă) [″ + ″ + Gr. *ouron,* urine] Hemialbumose in the urine.

hemialgia (hĕm-ē-ăl′jē-ă) [″ + *algos,* pain] Pain in half of the body.

hemiamaurosis (hĕm″ē-ăm″ō-rō′sĭs) [″ + *amaurosis,* darkness] Hemianopia.

hemiamblyopia (hĕm″ē-ăm″blē-ō′pē-ă) [″ + *amblys,* dim, + *ops,* sight] Hemianopia.

hemiamyosthenia (hĕm″ē-ă″mī-ŏs-thē′nē-ă) [Gr. *hemi-,* half, + *a-,* not, + *mys,* muscle, + *sthenos,* strength] Absence of normal muscular power on one side of the body. SYN: *hemiparesis*.

hemianacusia (hĕm″ē-ăn″ă-kū′zē-ă) [″ + *an-,* not, + *akousis,* hearing] Deafness in one ear.

hemianalgesia (hĕm″ē-ăn-ăl-jē′zē-ă) [″ + ″ + *algos,* pain] Lack of sensibility to pain (analgesia) on one side of the body.

hemianencephaly (hĕm″ē-ăn″ĕn-sĕf′ă-lē) [″ + *an-,* not, + *enkephalos,* brain] Congenital absence of half of the brain.

hemianesthesia (hĕm″ē-ăn-ĕs-thē′zē-ă) [″ + ″ + *aisthesis,* sensation] Anesthesia of half of the body.

hemianopia, hemianopsia (hĕm″ē-ă-nŏ′pē-ă, -nŏp′sē-ă) [″ + *an-,* not, + *ops,* eye] Blindness in one-half of the visual field. SYN: *hemiamaurosis; hemiamblyopia*. **hemianopic,** *adj.*

altitudinal h. Blindness in upper or lower half of the visual field of one or both eyes.

binasal h. Blindness in the nasal half of the visual field in each eye.

bitemporal h. Blindness in the temporal half of visual field in each eye.

complete h. Blindness in half the visual field.

crossed h. Either bitemporal or binasal hemianopsia. SYN: *heteronymous h.*

heteronymous h. Crossed h.

homonymous h. Blindness of nasal half of the visual field of one eye and temporal half of the other, or right-sided or left-sided hemianopsia of corresponding sides in both eyes.

incomplete h. Blindness in less than half of the visual field of each eye.

quadrant h. Blindness of symmetrical quadrant of the field of vision in each eye.

unilateral h. Hemianopsia affecting only one eye.

hemianosmia (hĕm″ē-ăn-ŏs′mē-ă) [Gr. *hemi-,* half, + *an-,* not, + *osme,* smell] Loss of sense of smell in one nostril.

hemiapraxia (hĕm″ē-ă-prăks′ē-ă) [″ + *a-,* not, + *prassein,* to do] Incapacity to exercise purposeful movements on one side of the body.

hemiarthrosis (hĕm″ē-ăr-thrō′sĭs) [″ + *arthron,* joint, + *osis,* condition] A false articulation between two bones. SYN: *synchondrosis*.

hemiasynergia (hĕm″ē-ă″sĭn-ĕr′jē-ă) [″ + *a-,* not, + *syn,* with, + *ergon,* work] A lack of coordination of parts affecting one side of the body.

hemiataxia (hĕm″ē-ă-tăks′ē-ă) [″ + *ataxia,* lack of order] Impaired muscular coordination causing awkward movements of the affected side of the body.

hemiathetosis (hĕm″ē-ăth″ĕ-tō′sĭs) [″ + *athetos,* without fixed position, + *osis,* condition] Athetosis of one side of the body.

hemiatrophy (hĕm-ē-ăt′rō-fē) [″ + *atrophia,* atrophy] Impaired nutrition resulting in atrophy of one side of the body or of an organ or part.

hemiballism (hĕm-ē-băl′ĭzm) [″ + *ballismos,* jumping] Jerking and twitching movements of one side of the body.

hemiblock (hĕm′ĭ-blŏk) In heart block, a failure of conduction in one of the two main divisions of the left bundle branch.

hemic (hē′mĭk, hĕm′ĭk) [Gr. *haima,* blood] Pert. to blood. SYN: *hemal* (1).

hemicanities (hĕm″ē-kăn-ĭsh′ĭ-ēz) [Gr. *hemi-,* half, + L. *canities,* gray hair] Grayness of hair on one side only.

hemicardia (hĕm-ē-kăr′dē-ă) [″ + *kardia,* heart] Half of a four-chambered heart.

hemicastration (hĕm″ē-kăs-trā′shŭn) [″ + L. *castrare,* to prune] The removal of one ovary or testicle. At one time, removal of the left testicle was done on the erroneous assumption that sperm from the right testicle produced only sons.

hemicellulose (hĕm-ē-sĕl′ū-lōs) One of a group of polysaccharides that differ from cellulose in that they may be hydrolyzed by dilute mineral acids, and from other polysaccharides in that they are not readily digested by amylases. The group includes pentosans, galactosans (agar-agar), and pectins.

hemicentrum (hĕm-ē-sĕn′trŭm) [″ + *kentron,* center] Either lateral half of the centrum of a vertebra.

hemicephalia (hĕm″ē-sĕ-fā′lē-ă) [″ + *kephale,* head] The congenital absence of one half of the skull and brain.

hemicephalus (hĕm″ē-sĕf′ă-lus) A congenital deformity in which the child has only one cerebral hemisphere.

hemicerebrum (hĕm″ē-sĕr′ĕ-brŭm) [″ + L. *cerebrum,* brain] Half of the cerebral hemisphere.

hemichorea (hĕm-ē-kō-rē′ă) [″ + *choreia,* dance] Chorea affecting only one side of the body.

hemichromatopsia (hĕm″ē-krō-mă-tŏp′sē-ă) [″ + *chroma,* color, + *opsis,* vision] Hemiachromatopsia.

hemicolectomy (hĕm″ē-kō-lĕk′tō-mē) [″ + *kolon,* colon, + *ektome,* excision] Surgical removal of half (either left or right) or less of the colon.

hemicorporectomy (hĕm″ē-kor″pō-rĕk′tō-mē) [″ + L. *corpus,* body, + Gr. *ektome,* excision] Surgical removal of the lower portion of the body, including the pelvis, pelvic contents, and the lower extremities.

hemicrania (hĕm-ē-krā′nē-ă) [″ + *kranion,* skull] **1.** Unilateral head pain, usually migraine. **2.** A malformation in which only one half of the skull is developed.

hemicraniectomy (hĕm″ē-krā-nē-ĕk′tō-mē) [″ + ″ + *ektome,* excision] The surgical division of the cranial vault from front backward, exposing half of the brain.

hemicraniosis (hĕm″ē-krā-nē-ō′sĭs) [″ + ″ + *osis,* condition] An enlargement of half of the cranium or face.

hemidesmosome The half of a desmosome produced by epithelial cells for attachment of the basal surface of the cell to the underlying basement membrane or the enamel or cementum tooth surface in the case of junctional epithelium.

hemidiaphoresis (hĕm″ē-dī″ă-for-ē′sĭs) [″ + *dia,* through, + *pherein,* to carry] Sweating on one side of the body. SYN: *hemidrosis; hemihidrosis.*

hemidiaphragm (hēm″ĕ-dī′ă-frăm) [″ + ″ + *phragma,* wall] Half of the diaphragm.

hemidrosis (hĕm″ĭ-drō′sĭs) [″ + *hidrosis,* sweating] Hemidiaphoresis.

hemidrosis (hĕm″ĭ-drō′sĭs) [Gr. *haima,* blood, + *hidrosis,* sweating] Secretion of sweat containing blood. SYN: *hemathidrosis.*

hemidysergia (hĕm″ē-dĭs-ĕr′jē-ă) [Gr. *hemi-,* half, + *dys,* bad, + *ergon,* work] A lack of muscular coordination on one side of the body.

hemidysesthesia (hĕm″ē-dĭs-ĕs-thē′zē-ă) [″ + ″ + *aisthesis,* sensation] Impaired sensation of half of the body.

hemidystrophy (hĕm″ē-dis′trō-fē) [″ + ″ + *trophe,* nourishment] An inequality in development of the two sides of the body.

hemiectromelia (hĕm″ē-ĕk-trō-mē′lē-ă) [″ + *ektro,* abortion, + *melos,* limb] Deformed extremities on one side of the body.

hemiepilepsy (hĕm″ē-ĕp′ĭ-lĕp-sē) [″ + *epilepsia,* seizure] Epilepsy with convulsions confined to one side of the body.

hemifacial (hĕm″ē-fā′shăl) [″ + L. *facies,* face] Pert. to one side of the face.

hemigastrectomy (hĕm″ē-găs-trĕk′tō-mē) [″ + *gaster,* belly, + *ektome,* excision] Excision of half of the stomach.

hemigeusia (hĕm-ē-gū′sē-ă) [″ + *geusis,* taste] A loss of the sense of taste on one side of the tongue.

hemiglossal (hĕm″ē-glŏs′săl) [″ + *glossa,* tongue] Concerning one side of the tongue.

hemiglossectomy (hĕm″ē-glŏs-sĕk′tō-mē) [″ + ″ + *ektome,* excision] The surgical removal of one side of the tongue.

hemiglossitis [″ + ″ + *itis,* inflammation] Herpetic vesicular eruption on half of the tongue and the inner surface of the cheek.

hemignathia (hĕm″ē-năth′ē-ă) [″ + *gnathos,* jaw] Congenital absence of one half of the lower jaw.

hemihepatectomy (hĕm″ē-hĕp″ă-tĕk′tō-mē) [″ + *hepatos,* liver, + *ektome,* excision] The surgical removal of half of the liver.

hemihidrosis (hĕm″ē-hī-drō′sĭs) [″+ *hidros,* sweat, + *osis,* condition] Hemidiaphoresis.

hemihydrate A chemical compound with one molecule of water for every two molecules of the other substance. In dentistry, calcium sulfate hemihydrate is mixed with water to produce a hardened plaster or stone (calcium sulfate dihydrate), which, in turn, is commonly used to produce dental models.

hemihypalgesia (hĕm″ē-hī″păl-jē′zē-ă) [″ + *hypo,* under, + *algesis,* sense of pain] Partial anesthesia on one side of the body.

hemihyperesthesia (hĕm″ē-hī-pĕr-ĕs-thē′zē-ă) [″ + *hyper,* over, + *aisthesis,* sensation] Abnormal sensitivity to touch or pain on one side of the body.

hemihyperidrosis, hemihyperhidrosis (hĕm″ē-hī-pĕr-ĭ-drō′sĭs, -hĭ-drō′sĭs) [″ + ″ + *hydrosis,* sweating] Excessive perspiration confined to one side of the body.

hemihyperplasia (hĕm″ē-hī″pĕr-plā′zē-ă) [″ + ″ + *plassein,* to form] The excessive development of one side or one half of the body or of an organ.

hemihypesthesia, hemihypoesthesia (hĕm″ē-hī″pĕs-thē′zē-ă, -pō-ĕs-thē′zē-a) [Gr. *hemi-,* half, + *hypo,* under, + *aisthesis,* sensation] Diminished sensibility on one side of the body.

hemi-inattention Unilateral visual inattention.

hemikaryon (hĕm″ē-kăr′ē-ŏn) [″ + *karyon,* nucleus] A cell nucleus with half the diploid number of chromosomes.

hemilaminectomy (hĕm″ē-lăm″ĭ-nĕk′tō-mē) [″ + L. *lamina,* thin plate, + Gr. *ektome,* excision] The surgical removal of the lamina of the vertebral arch on one side.

hemilaryngectomy (hĕm″ē-lăr″in-jĕk′tō-mē) [″ + *larynx,* larynx, + *ektome,* excision] The surgical removal of the lateral half of the larynx.

hemilateral [″ + L. *latus,* side] Relating to one side only.

hemilesion (hĕm″ē-lē′zhŭn) [″ + L. *laesio,* a wound] A lesion on one side of the body.

hemilingual (hĕm″ē-lĭng′gwăl) [″ + L. *lingua,* tongue] Affecting or concerning one lateral half of the tongue.

hemimacroglossia (hĕm″ē-măk″rō-glŏs′ē-ă) [″+ *makros,* large, + *glossa,* tongue] Enlargement of one lateral half of the tongue.

hemimandibulectomy (hĕm″ē-măn-dĭb-ū-lĕk′tō-mē) [″ + L. *mandibula,* lower jawbone, + Gr. *ektome,* excision] The surgical removal of half of the mandible.

hemimelus (hĕm″ĭ-mē′lŭs) [″+ *melos,* limb] A fetal malformation with defective development of the extremities, esp. the distal portion.

hemin (hē′mĭn) [Gr. *haima,* blood] A brownish-red crystalline salt of heme formed when hemoglobin is heated with glacial acetic acid and sodium chloride. The iron is present in the ferric (Fe^{3+}) state. Hemin is used in testing for presence of blood. SYN: *crystal of hemin.* SEE: *heme.*

heminephrectomy (hĕm″ē-nĕ-frĕk′tō-mē) [Gr. *hemi-,* half, + *nephros,* kidney, + *ektome,* excision] The excision or removal of a portion of a kidney.

hemineurasthenia (hĕm″ē-nū-răs-thē′nē-ă) [″ + *neuron,* nerve, + *astheneia,* weakness] Neurasthenia affecting one side of the body only.

hemiopalgia (hĕm″ē-ŏp-ăl′jē-ă) [″+ *ops,* eye, + *algos,* pain] Pain in one side of the head and the eye on that side.

hemiopia (hĕm-ē-ō′pē-ă) [″ + *ops,* eye] Hemianopia.

hemiopic (hĕm-ē-ŏp′ĭk) [″ + *ops,* eye] Pert. to hemiopia.

hemipagus (hĕm-ĭp′ă-gŭs) [″ + *pagos,* a thing fixed] Twins fused at the navel and thorax.

hemiparalysis (hĕm″ē-pă-răl′ĭ-sĭs) [″ + *paralyein,* to disable] Hemiplegia.

hemiparaplegia (hĕm″ē-păr-ă-plē′jē-ă) [″ +″ + *plege,* stroke] Paralysis of the lower half of one side or of one leg. This term is confusing because paraplegia indicates paralysis of both lower extremities.

hemiparesis (hĕm″ē-păr′ĕ-sĭs, hĕm-ē-păr-ē′sĭs) [″ + *paresis,* paralysis] Hemiplegia.

hemiparesthesia (hĕm″ē-păr-ĕs-thē′zē-ă) [″ + *para,* beyond, + *aisthesis,* sensation] Numbness of one side of the body.

hemipelvectomy (hĕm″ē-pĕl″vĕk′tō-mē) [″ + L. *pelvis,* basin, + Gr. *ektome,* excision] The surgical removal of half of the pelvis, and the corresponding lower extremity.

hemiplegia (hĕm-ē-plē′jē-ă) [″ + *plege,* a stroke] Paralysis of one side of the body, usually resulting from damage to the corticospinal tracts of the central nervous system. SYN: *hemiparalysis; hemiparesis.* SEE: *Benedikt's syndrome; paralysis; thalamic syndrome.*

ETIOLOGY: The most common cause of hemiplegia is stroke caused by thrombosis, brain hemorrhage, or cerebral embolism. Tumors are responsible for hemiplegia in a smaller number of patients.

SYMPTOMS: The patient will be unable to move the arm and/or leg or facial muscles on one side of the body. Usually the paralysis is more complete at the proximal muscles (e.g., at the shoulder or hip muscles) than it is in the more distal muscles of the hands or feet. If the nondominant parietal lobe of the brain is injured (e.g., after an occlusion of the middle cerebral artery on that side), the patient may neglect the paralyzed side of the body. He or she may deny neurological deficits on that side and may be unable to see or feel stimuli presented to the affected hemibody or visual field. SEE: *visual anosognosia*.

PATIENT CARE: Assistance is provided with active range-of-motion exercises to unaffected limbs and passive exercises to affected limbs. Active participation in rehabilitation through physical therapy and occupational therapy is encouraged. The patient is taught to use the unaffected limbs to move and exercise the affected limbs to maintain joint mobility and prevent contractures and to maintain muscle tone and strength. The patient is protected from injury through the use of supportive devices to prevent subluxation or dislocation of affected joints. The patient and the family are taught how to use assistive devices (e.g., slings, splints, walkers), and the goals and processes involved in rehabilitation are explained. Both the patient and family are encouraged to talk about their fears and concerns, and positive strategies for dealing with the change in body function are supported. Accurate information, realistic reassurance, and emotional support are provided to assist with coping.

capsular h. Hemiplegia resulting from a lesion of the internal capsule of the brain.

cerebral h. Hemiplegia caused by a brain lesion.

facial h. Paralysis of the muscles on one side of the face.

pontile h. Hemiplegia due to a lesion of the pons. The arm and leg on one side and the face on the opposite side are affected.

spastic h. Increased muscular tone occurring in half of the body. It results from an upper motor neuron lesion, such as a stroke, central nervous system trauma, or tumor.

spinal h. Hemiplegia resulting from a lesion of the spinal cord. SEE: *Brown-Séquard's syndrome*.

hemiplegic (hĕm-ē-plē′jĭk) **1.** Pert. to hemiplegia. **2.** A colloquial reference to a patient having hemiplegia.

Hemiptera (hĕm-ĭp′tĕr-ă) [Gr. *hemi-*, half, + *pteron,* wing] The true bugs; an order of insects characterized by piercing and sucking mouth parts. The first pair of wings is leathery at the base and membranous at the tip; the second pair is membranous. Metamorphosis is incomplete. The order includes bedbugs, kissing bugs, and several other species that are pests or vectors of pathogenic organisms.

hemipyocyanin (hĕm″ē-pī″ō-sī′ă-nĭn) Antibacterial pigment produced by *Pseudomonas pyocyanea*.

hemirachischisis (hĕm″ē-ră-kĭs′kĭ-sĭs) [″ + *rhachis,* spine, + *schisis,* a splitting] Spina bifida occulta.

hemisacralization (hĕm″ē-sā″krăl-ī-zā′shŭn) The abnormal development of one half of the fifth lumbar vertebra so that it is fused with the sacrum.

hemisection (hĕm″ē-sĕk′shŭn) [″ + L. *sectio,* a cutting] Bisection.

hemisomus (hĕm″ē-sō′mŭs) [″ + *soma,* body] A fetus with the lateral half of the body either missing or malformed.

hemispasm (hĕm′ē-spăzm) [″ + *spasmos,* a convulsion] A spasm of only one side of the body or face.

hemisphere (hĕm′ĭ-sfēr) [″ + *sphaira,* sphere] Either half of the cerebrum or cerebellum.

dominant h. The cerebral hemisphere with which the higher cortical functions, esp. those relating to speech and certain motor activities, are associated (i.e., the left hemisphere in right-handed individuals).

nondominant h. In neurology, the hemisphere of the brain that does not control speech or the predominantly used hand.

hemispheric specialization The control of distinct neurological functions by the right and left hemispheres of the brain. In most people, the left hemisphere controls language use, analytical thought, and abstract thinking, while the right manages visual and spatial relations, musical abilities, and other functions.

hemisyndrome (hĕm″ē-sĭn′drōm) [″ + *syndrome,* a running with] A syndrome indicating a unilateral lesion of the spinal cord.

hemithermoanesthesia (hĕm″ē-thĕr″mō-ăn″ĕs-thē′zē-ă) [Gr. *hemi-,* half, + *therme,* heat, + *an-,* not, + *aisthesis,* sensation] The unilateral loss of sensitivity to heat and cold.

hemithorax (hĕm″ē-thō′răks) [″ + *thorax,* chest] One half of the chest.

hemithyroidectomy (hĕm″ē-thī″roydĕk′tō-mē) [″ + *thyreos,* shield, + *eidos,* form, shape, + *ektome,* excision] The surgical removal of one half of the thyroid gland tissue.

hemitremor (hĕm″ē-trĕm′or) A tremor present in one lateral half of the body.

hemivertebra (hĕm″ē-vĕr′tĕ-bră) The congenital absence of or the failure to develop half of a vertebra.

hemizygosity (hĕm″ē-zī-gŏs′ĭ-tē) [″ + *zygotos,* yoked] Possessing only one of the gene pair that determines a particular genetic trait.

hemlock [AS. *hemleac*] **1.** A species of evergreen plant. **2.** The volatile oil from either *Conium maculatum* or *Cicuta maculata* containing cicutoxin. Ingestion of these hemlock plants, esp. their roots, may cause fatal poisoning.

h. poisoning Poisoning by hemlock ingestion, causing weakness, drowsiness, nausea, vomiting, difficult breathing, paralysis, and death.

TREATMENT: Oral activated charcoal may be given to decrease the absorption of the toxin from the gastrointestinal tract. Respiratory failure should be treated with intubation and mechanical ventilation. The local Poison Control Center should be contacted for additional instructions.

Hemlock Society An organization that publishes information about physician-assisted suicide, and decisions by patients regarding end-of-life choices. Address: P.O. Box 101810, Denver, CO 80250. Telephone: 800-247-7421. Website: www.hemlock.org.

hemo- SEE: *hem-*.

hemoagglutination (hē″mō-ă-gloo″tĭ-nā′shŭn) [Gr. *haima,* blood, + L. *agglutinans,* gluing] The clumping of red blood corpuscles.

hemoagglutinin (hē″mō-ă-gloo′tĭ-nĭn) An agglutinin that clumps the red blood corpuscles.

hemobilia (hē″mō-bĭl′ē-ă) Blood in the bile or bile ducts.

hemobilinuria (hē″mō-bĭl-ĭn-ū′rē-ă) [″ + L. *bilis,* bile, + Gr. *ouron,* urine] Urobilin in the blood and urine.

hemochromatosis (hē″mō-krō″mă-tō′sĭs) [″ + *chroma,* color, + *osis,* condition] A genetic disease marked by excessive absorption and accumulation of iron in the body. The disease is caused by one of several recessive mutations that result in excessive absorption of iron from the gastrointestinal tract. It is not caused by secondary iron overload, as may occur in patients who have received multiple transfusions or who have hemolytic anemia. The disease is often diagnosed before it causes symptoms. SYN: *bronze diabetes*.

SYMPTOMS: At the time of diagnosis, the patient may be asymptomatic. Symptomatic patients may experience weakness, fatigue, arthralgias, abdominal pain, liver failure (cirrhosis), symptoms of heart failure, thyroid disorders, or impotence. These symptoms are caused by the deposition of excess iron into multiple organ systems.

DIAGNOSIS: Physical findings include gray or bronzed skin, enlarged liver, arthritis, signs of congestive heart failure, and in males, testicular atrophy. Laboratory studies used to screen for the disease include the transferrin saturation or ferritin tests. Liver biopsies from affected persons show excessive stainable iron. Genetic testing is available to identify patients with the most common forms of hemochromatosis. SEE: illus.

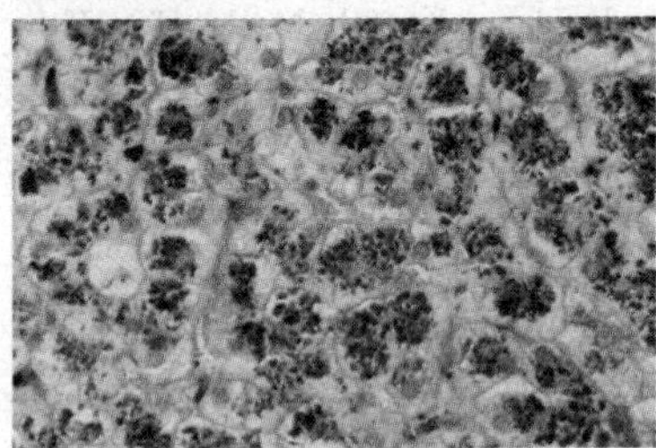

HEMOCHROMATOSIS

Liver biopsy (excess iron stained green)

TREATMENT: Treatment includes phlebotomy (blood drawing) done at regular intervals until the patient's iron stores drop to below normal. Typically, the ferritin level is monitored to ensure that this has occurred. Initially, approximately 1 unit of blood is removed each week until the desired ferritin level is reached. Maintenance therapy consists of removal of blood at 1- to 4-month intervals. Iron chelators are used if phlebotomy is not possible, but they are much less effective at decreasing iron stores than is blood drawing.

CAUTION: Blood removed from patients with iron overload cannot be used for transfusion.

PATIENT CARE: The need for phlebotomy and its role in the removal of excess iron are explained to the patient. To prevent dizziness or hypotension, the patient is encouraged to drink plenty of fluids and to abstain from vigorous exercise for the first 24 hr after the procedure.

hemochromogen (hē″mō-krō′mō-jĕn) [″ + *chroma,* color, + *gennan,* to produce] A compound of heme with nitrogen-containing substances such as a protein.

hemochromoprotein (hē″mō-krō″mō-prō′tē-ĭn) Any protein combined with the blood pigment hemoglobin.

hemoclip A metal clip used to ligate blood vessels. Absorbable polyglycolic acid clips may also be used.

hemoconcentration A relative increase in the number of red blood cells resulting from a decrease in the volume of plasma (e.g., in dehydration).

hemoconia (hē″mō-kō′nē-ă) [Gr. *haima,* blood, + *konis,* dust] Minute colorless bodies in the blood thought to be the products of disintegration of red blood cells. SYN: *blood dust*.

hemoconiosis (hē″mō-kō″nē-ō′sĭs) [″ + ″ + *osis,* condition] Having an abnormal amount of hemoconia in the blood.

hemocuprein (hē″mō-kū′prē-ĭn) A blue copper-containing compound present in red blood cells.

hemocyte (hē′mō-sīt) [″ + *kytos,* cell] **1.** Any blood cell. **2.** A red blood cell.

hemocytoblast (hē″mō-sī′tō-blăst) [″ + ″ + *blastos,* germ] An undifferentiated stem cell found in mesenchymal tissues that may give rise to any type of blood cell. SEE: illus.

hemocytology (hē″mō-sī-tŏl′ō-jē) [″ + ″ + *logos,* word, reason] The study of the structure and function of blood cells.

hemocytometer (hē″mō-sī-tŏm′ĕ-tĕr) [″ + ″ + *metron,* measure] A device for determining the number of cells in a stated volume of blood.

hemocytophagia The phagocytic ingestion of red blood cells.

hemocytotripsis (hē″mō-sī″tō-trĭp′sĭs) [″ + ″ + *tribein,* to rub] The destruction of red blood cells caused by extreme pressure.

hemocytozoon (hē″mō-sī″tō-zō′ŏn) [″ + ″ + *zoon,* animal] A protozoan parasite of the blood cells. SYN: *hematobium.*

hemodiagnosis (hē″mō-dī″ăg-nō′sĭs) [″ + *dia,* through, + *gnosis,* knowledge] Examination of the blood for diagnostic purposes.

hemodialysis (hē″mō-, hĕm″ō-dī-ăl′ĭ-sĭs) [″ + ″ + *lysis,* dissolution] The use of an artificial kidney to clear urea, metabolic waste products, toxins, and excess fluid from the blood. This procedure is used to treat end-stage renal failure, transient renal failure, and some cases of poisoning or drug overdose. In the U.S., more than 200,000 patients undergo hemodialysis regularly for end-stage renal disease. The pri-

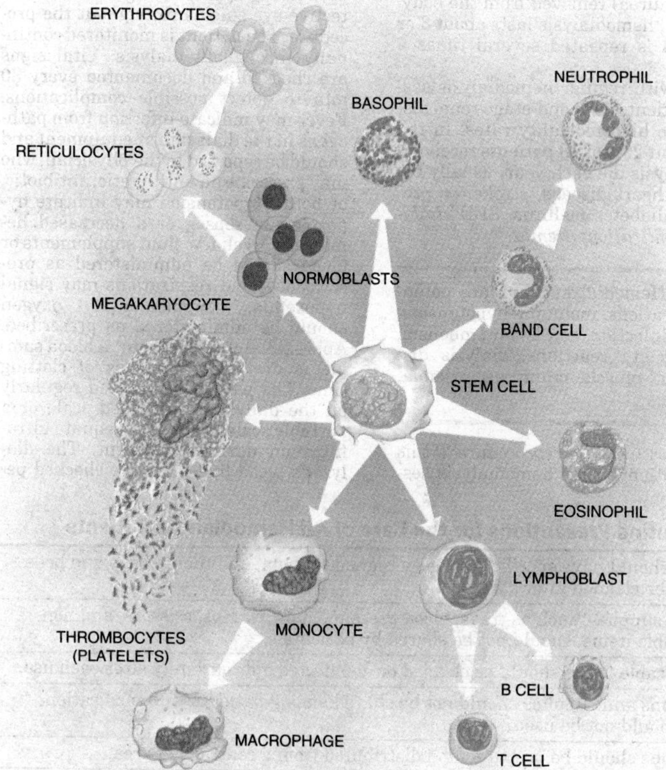

HEMOCYTOBLAST (STEM CELL) AND BLOOD CELLS

mary use of hemodialysis is to manage renal failure, a disorder in which fluids, acids, electrolytes, and many drugs are ineffectively eliminated in the urine. Hyperkalemia, uremia, fluid overload, acidosis, and uremic pericarditis are other indications for hemodialysis. SEE: table; *hemoperfusion; Nursing Diagnoses Appendix.*

The technique of hemodialysis involves the following:

1. Establishing access to the circulation (e.g., via an arteriovenous fistula, graft, or temporary catheter)
2. Anticoagulating the patient's blood to prevent extracorporeal clotting
3. Pumping the blood to a dialysis membrane
4. Adjusting the diffusion of solutes from the blood into a buffered dialysis solution
5. Returning the cleansed and buffered blood to the patient

The adequacy of hemodialysis is determined by the amount of fluid and solute (esp. urea) removed from the body. Typically, hemodialysis lasts about 3 or 4 hr and is repeated several times a week.

Even with regular hemodialysis sessions, patients with end-stage renal disease have high mortality rates. In the U.S., about 25% of all patients receiving hemodialysis die each year, usually because of heart disease, stroke, or preexisting diabetes mellitus. SEE: *dialysis; hemofiltration; uremia.*

CAUTION: Hemodialysis has many potential complications, including hypotension, access site infection, sepsis, air embolism, hypersensitivity reactions, dialysis disequilibrium, muscle cramping, anemia, and bleeding.

PATIENT CARE: *Preprocedure:* If this is the patient's first hemodialysis session, the purpose of the treatment and expected results are explained. First, the patient undergoes a surgical procedure to create a vascular access. After the access site has been created and the patient is ready for dialysis, the patient's weight is obtained and vital signs are checked; blood pressure should be measured in the nonaccessed arm while the patient is in both supine and standing positions. As prescribed, the hemodialysis equipment is prepared according to the manufacturer's guidelines and the institution's protocol. Strict aseptic technique is maintained to avoid introducing pathogens into the patient's bloodstream during treatment. The patient is placed in a supine or low Fowler position and made as comfortable as possible, with the venous access site well supported and resting on a sterile drape or sterile barrier shield.

During the procedure: Health care providers follow Occupational Safety and Health Administration guidelines by wearing appropriate gloves and protective eye shields throughout the procedure. The patient is monitored continually throughout dialysis. Vital signs are checked and documented every 30 min to detect possible complications. Fever may indicate infection from pathogens in the dialysate or equipment and should be reported to the physician, who may prescribe an antipyretic, antibiotic, or both. Hypotension may indicate hypovolemia, sepsis, or a decreased hematocrit level; I.V. fluid supplements or blood should be administered as prescribed. Rapid respirations may signal hypoxemia; supplemental oxygen should be administered as prescribed. Approximately every hour, a blood sample is drawn for analysis of clotting time. The patient is weighed regularly on the dialyzing unit's bed scale or a portable scale to ensure adequate ultrafiltration during treatment. The dialyzer's blood lines also are checked pe-

Routine Precautions for the Care of All Hemodialysis Patients

Patients should have specific stations assigned to them, and their chairs and beds should be cleaned after each use.
Ancillary supplies, such as trays, blood pressure cuffs, clamps, scissors, and nondisposable items, should not be shared by patients.
Nondisposable items should be cleaned or disinfected appropriately after each use.
Medications and supplies should not be shared among patients, and medication carts should not be used.
Medications should be prepared and distributed from a centralized area.
Clean and contaminated areas should be separated (e.g., handwashing, handling of blood samples, and equipment cleaning should be kept distinct from areas for preparation of foods, drink, and medications).

Adapted from Recommendations for prevention and control of hepatitis C virus (HCV) infection and HCV-related chronic disease. Morbidity and Mortality Weekly Report 47(N0. RR-19), Centers for Disease Control and Prevention.

riodically to ensure that all connections are secure, and the lines are monitored for clotting. The patient is assessed for headache, muscle twitching, backache, nausea or vomiting, and seizures, which may indicate disequilibrium syndrome caused by rapid fluid removal and electrolyte changes. If this syndrome occurs, the physician should be notified immediately; he or she may reduce the blood flow rate or stop the dialysis. Muscle cramps also may result from rapid fluid and electrolyte shifts. Cramps may be relieved by injecting prescribed 0.9% sodium chloride solution into the venous line. The patient is observed carefully for signs of internal bleeding; apprehension; restlessness; pale, cold, clammy skin; excessive thirst; hypotension; rapid, weak, thready pulse; increased respirations; and decreased body temperature. Such findings are documented and reported to the physician immediately, and preparations are made to decrease heparinization and possibly to administer blood. Health care providers are esp. alert for signs of air embolism, a potentially fatal complication characterized by sudden hypotension; dyspnea; chest pain; cyanosis; and a weak, rapid pulse. If these signs occur, the patient is turned onto the left side, the head of the bed lowered (to help keep air bubbles on the right side of the body, where they can be absorbed from the pulmonary vasculature), and the physician notified immediately.

Postprocedure: The venous access site is monitored for bleeding. If bleeding is excessive, pressure is maintained on the site and the physician notified. To prevent clotting and other blood flow problems, the arm used for venous access is not used for any other procedures, including I.V. line insertion, blood pressure monitoring, and venipuncture. At least four times daily, circulation at the access site is assessed by auscultating for a bruit and by palpating for a thrill; the patient also is instructed in these assessment techniques. An accurate record of the patient's food and fluid intake is maintained, and the patient is encouraged to cooperate with prescribed restrictions, such as limited protein, potassium, and sodium intake; increased caloric intake; and decreased fluid intake. The patient is instructed in care of the venous access site: cleaning the incision with hydrogen peroxide solution daily and keeping it dry until healing is complete (usually 10 to 14 days). Any pain, swelling, redness, or drainage in the accessed arm should be reported immediately. The patient may use his or her arm fully once the site has healed; however, no treatments or procedures should be performed on the accessed arm, including blood pressure measurements and needle punctures. The patient also should avoid putting excessive pressure on the arm, such as sleeping on it, wearing constricting clothing, or lifting heavy objects. He or she should avoid showering, bathing, or swimming for several hours after dialysis. The patient is instructed in the following exercises to promote venous dilation and to enhance blood flow in the affected arm: One week after access site surgery, squeeze a small rubber ball or other soft object for 15 min, four times each day. Two weeks after surgery, apply a tourniquet on the upper arm above the fistula site, making sure it is snug but not tight. With the tourniquet in place, squeeze the rubber ball for 5 min, repeating four times daily. After the incision has healed completely, perform the exercise with the arm submerged in warm water. If the patient will perform hemodialysis at home, both the patient and a family member must thoroughly understand all aspects of the procedure. They are provided with the phone number of the dialysis center and encouraged to call if any questions or concerns arise. The patient also is advised to arrange for another (trained) person to be present during dialysis in case any problems occur and to contact the National Association of Patients on Hemodialysis and Transplantation or the National Kidney Foundation for information and support.

hemodialyzer (hē″mō-dī′ă-līz″ĕr) A device used in performing hemodialysis.

hemodilution (hē″mō-dī-lū′shŭn) An increase in blood plasma volume resulting in reduced relative concentration of red blood cells.

hemodynamic monitoring A general term for determining the functional status of the cardiovascular system as it responds to acute stress such as myocardial infarction and cardiogenic or septic shock. This may include frequent assessments of blood pressure, pulse, mental status, urinary output, intracardiac pressure changes, and cardiac output. The data obtained permit the critical care team to follow the patient's course carefully and without delay.

hemodynamics (hē″mō-dī-năm′iks) [Gr. *haima,* blood, + *dynamis,* power] A study of the forces involved in circulating blood through the body.

hemoendothelial (hē″mō-ĕn-dō-thē′lē-ăl) Pert. to the relationship between blood of the mother and the endothelium of the chorionic vessels. SEE: *placenta.*

hemofiltration (hē″mō-fĭl-trā′shŭn) An ultrafiltration technique to remove excess metabolic products from the blood. The technical aspects are similar to those of renal dialysis in that the blood flows from the body to the hemofilter and is then returned to the body.

CAUTION: Depending on the type of filter membrane used, essential materials may be removed from the blood. It is important to replace the excess crystalloids removed.

continuous arteriovenous h. ABBR: CAVH. A technique using a hemofilter to facilitate removal of water, electrolytes, and small to medium molecular weight molecules from the vascular space. It is used in patients with renal failure or fluid overload.

hemoflagellate (hē″mō-flăj′ĕ-lāt″) [″ + L. *flagellum*, whip] Any flagellate protozoan of the blood. The most important genera are *Trypanosoma* and *Leishmania.*

hemofuscin (hē″mō-fū′sĭn) [″ + L. *fuscus*, brown] A brown pigment, derived from hemoglobin, which produces a reddish color in urine.

hemoglobin (hē″mō-, hĕm″ō-glō′bĭn) [″ + L. *globus*, globe] ABBR: Hb, Hbg, Hgb. The iron-containing pigment of red blood cells that carries oxygen from the lungs to the tissues. The amount of hemoglobin in the blood averages 12 to 16 g/100 ml in women, 14 to 18 g/100 ml in men, and somewhat less in children. Hemoglobin is a crystallizable, conjugated protein consisting of heme, an iron-containing pigment, and globin, a simple protein. In the lungs, 1 g of hemoglobin combines readily with 1.36 cc of oxygen, by a process called *oxygenation*, to form oxyhemoglobin, an unstable compound. In the tissues where oxygen concentration is low and carbon dioxide concentration is high (low pH), hemoglobin releases its oxygen. Hemoglobin also acts as a buffer for the hydrogen ions produced in red blood cells (RBCs) when carbon dioxide is converted to bicarbonate ions for transport in the plasma.

When old RBCs are phagocytized by macrophages in the liver, spleen, and red bone marrow, the iron of hemoglobin is reused immediately to produce new RBCs or is stored in the liver until needed. The globin is converted to amino acids for the synthesis of other proteins. The heme portion is of no further use and is converted to bilirubin, a bile pigment excreted by the liver in bile.

Hemoglobin combines with carbon monoxide (in carbon monoxide poisoning) to form the stable compound carboxyhemoglobin, which renders hemoglobin unable to bond with oxygen and results in hypoxia of tissues. Oxidation of the ferrous iron of hemoglobin to the ferric state produces methemoglobin.

Hundreds of different types of hemoglobin have been discovered. Some of these, such as hemoglobin S, are described in subentries that follow. SEE: *blood.*

h. A_{1c} ABBR: Hb A_{1c}. Hemoglobin A that contains a glucose group linked to the terminal amino acid of the beta chains of the molecule. The amount of glucose bound to the hemoglobin depends on the average concentration of glucose in the blood over time. In patients with diabetes mellitus, when the blood glucose level is optimally and carefully regulated over 5 to 6 weeks, the Hb A_{1c} level is normal or slightly elevated. If the blood glucose level has not been controlled (and has been abnormally elevated) in the preceding 5 to 6 weeks, the Hb A_{1c} blood level is increased. Hb A_{1c} is a good indicator of long-term glycemic control. The blood test for it may be performed when the patient is not fasting. SYN: *glycohemoglobin; glycated h.; glycosylated h.*

h. C disease A genetic variant of the hemoglobin molecule that causes a chronic hemolytic anemia with splenomegaly, arthralgias, and abdominal pain. SEE: illus.

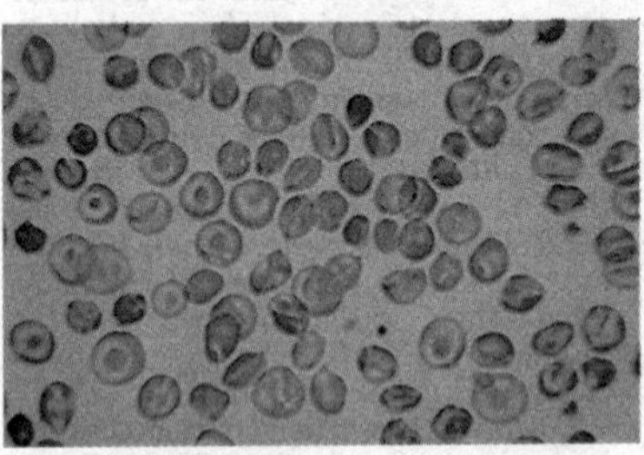

HEMOGLOBIN C DISEASE

h. E disease A genetic variant of hemoglobin that produces a mild form of hemolytic anemia. It is primarily in persons of Southeast Asian origin, in whom it may provide protection against falciparum malaria.

fetal h. The type of hemoglobin found in the erythrocytes of the normal fetus. The induction of fetal hemoglobin in patients with sickle cell anemia often improves their clinical status, because fetal hemoglobin does not deform or "sickle" in the circulation. It is capable of taking up and giving off oxygen at lower oxygen tensions than can the hemoglobin in adult erythrocytes.

glycated h. h. A_{1c}.

glycosylated h. h. A_{1c}.

h. H disease A genetic variant of hemoglobin that causes a chronic hemolytic anemia marked by hypochromic erythrocytes with inclusion bodies. Sometimes called *thalassemia intermedia.*

h. M disorder A genetic variant of hemoglobin that causes cyanosis and methemoglobinemia. The iron in this type of hemoglobin is in the ferric (Fe^{3+}) state and cannot combine with oxygen.

mean corpuscular h. ABBR: MCH. The hemoglobin content of the average red blood cell, usually expressed in picograms per red cell and calculated by multiplying the number of grams of hemoglobin/100 ml by 10 and dividing by the red cell count.

h. S disease A genetic variant of hemoglobin that causes sickle cell trait in heterozygotes, and sickle cell disease in hemozygotes. It is common, esp. in persons of African ancestry in whom sickle cell trait is found in 8–10% of the population. SEE: *sickle cell anemia.*

h. SC disease A disease of persons who have inherited two abnormal forms of hemoglobin, S and C. Affected persons may have vaso-occlusive crises similar to those seen in sickle cell anemia, with bony and visceral infarcts.

hemoglobinemia (hē″mō-glō-bĭn-ē′mē-ă) [Gr. *haima,* blood, + L. *globus,* globe, + Gr. *haima,* blood] The presence of hemoglobin in the blood plasma.

hemoglobinocholia (hē″mō-glō″bĭn-ō-kō′lē-ă) [″ + ″ + Gr. *chole,* bile] Hemoglobin in the bile.

hemoglobinolysis (hē″mō-glō-bĭn-ŏl′ĭ-sĭs) [″ + ″ + Gr. *lysis,* dissolution] The dissolution of hemoglobin.

hemoglobinometer (hē″mō-glō-bĭn-ŏm′ĕ-ter) [″ + ″ + Gr. *metron,* measure] A device for determining the amount of hemoglobin in the blood.

hemoglobinopathy (hē″mō-glō″bĭ-nŏp′ă-thē) Any one of a group of genetic diseases caused by or associated with the presence of one of several forms of abnormal hemoglobin in the blood. SEE: *hemoglobin.*

hemoglobinophilic (hē″mō-glō-bĭn-ō-fĭl′ĭk) [″ + ″ + Gr. *philein,* to love] Pert. to organisms that grow better in the presence of hemoglobin.

hemoglobinous (hē″mō-glō′bĭ-nŭs) Pert. to or containing hemoglobin.

hemoglobinuria (hē″mō-glō-bĭn-ū′rē-ă) [″ + L. *globus,* globe, + Gr. *ouron,* urine] The presence in urine of hemoglobin free from red blood cells. This condition occurs when the amount of hemoglobin from disintegrating red blood cells or from rapid hemolysis of red cells exceeds the ability of the blood proteins to combine with the hemoglobin. **hemoglobinuric,** *adj.*

ETIOLOGY: Causes of this condition include hemolytic anemia, scurvy, purpura, exposure to or ingestion of certain chemicals such as arsenic and phosphorus, typhus fever, and septicemia.

cold h. Hemoglobinuria following local or general exposure to cold. SYN: *paroxysmal h.*

epidemic h. Hemoglobinuria of the newborn characterized by jaundice, cyanosis, and fatty degeneration of heart and liver. SYN: *Winckel's disease.*

intermittent h. Paroxysmal nocturnal hemoglobinuria.

malarial h. Blackwater fever.

march h. Urinary bleeding that occurs following strenuous exercise (e.g., running a marathon).

paroxysmal h. Intermittent, recurring attacks of bloody urine following exposure to cold (cold hemoglobinuria) or strenuous exercise (march hemoglobinuria). Results from increased fragility of red blood cells or presence of a thermolabile autohemolysin.

paroxysmal nocturnal h. ABBR: PNH. A clonal disorder of the red blood cell membrane that predisposes patients to episodic hemolysis.

toxic h. Hemoglobinuria resulting from toxic substances such as muscarine or snake venom; toxic products of infectious diseases such as yellow fever, typhoid fever, syphilis, and certain forms of hemolytic jaundice; organisms such as *Plasmodium malariae,* which destroy red blood cells; foreign protein in blood as may follow blood transfusion.

hemolith (hē′mō-lĭth) [″ + *lithos,* stone] A stone in the wall of a blood vessel.

hemolymph (hē′mō-lĭmf″) [″ + L. *lympha,* lymph] Blood and lymph.

hemolymphangioma (hē″mō-lĭm-făn″jē-ō′mă) Hematolymphangioma.

hemolysate (hē-mŏl′ĭ-sāt) The product of hemolysis.

hemolysin (hē-mŏl′ĭ-sĭn) [″ + *lysis,* dissolution] A toxic agent or condition that destroys red blood cells. SYN: *hemotoxin.*

hemolysis (hē-mŏl′ĭ-sĭs) [″ + *lysis,* dissolution] The destruction of red blood cells (RBCs) because of RBC diseases (e.g., spherocytosis or sickle cell disease) or because of their exposure to drugs, toxins, artificial heart valves, antibodies, some infections, or snake venoms. The cell membranes are destroyed directly or through antibody-mediated lysis. Donor antibodies in blood products cause hemolysis associated with transfusion reactions. Autoantibodies develop as the result of disease (esp. hematological cancers), in response to certain drugs (alpha-methyldopa), or in Rh-negative mothers carrying an Rh-positive fetus. Viral and bacterial infections are frequent causes of hemolysis in children, whose RBC membranes are very fragile.

When the RBCs are destroyed, hemoglobin is released into the surrounding plasma and lost through the kidneys, turning the urine red, a condition called hemoglobinuria. Hemolysis may result from infection by certain disease organisms (e.g., certain streptococci, staphylococci, and the tetanus bacillus). It also occurs in smallpox and diphtheria and following severe burns.

When hemolysis is gradual, patients compensate for the resulting anemia, reporting only fatigue and a slight tachycardia with physical exertion. Laboratory tests show decreased RBC count, hemoglobin, haptoglobin, and hematocrit, as well as elevated levels of lactate dehydrogenase and unconjugated bilirubin. Fragments of RBCs may sometimes be seen under the microscope. SEE: *autoantibody; fragility of red blood cells; hemolytic anemia*.

colloid osmotic h. The swelling and rupture of red blood cells when they become excessively permeable to sodium and fill with water.

hemolytic (hē″mō-lĭt′ĭk) Pert. to the breaking down of red blood cells.

h. disease of the newborn Neonatal disease characterized by anemia, jaundice, liver and spleen enlargement, and generalized edema (hydrops fetalis). SYN: *erythroblastosis fetalis*. SEE: *Rh blood group*.

ETIOLOGY: This disease is due to transplacental transmission of maternal antibody, usually evoked by maternal and fetal blood group incompatibility. Incompatibilities of the ABO system are common but are not severe because maternal antibodies are too large to cross the placenta readily. Rh incompatibility, however, can result in profound fetal anemia, causing death in utero.

Rh incompatibility may develop when an Rh-negative woman carries an Rh-positive fetus. At the time of delivery, fetal red blood cells may enter maternal circulation, stimulating antibody production against the Rh factor. In a subsequent pregnancy, these antibodies cross the placenta to the fetal circulation and destroy fetal red blood cells.

TREATMENT: In cases of Rh incompatibility, the condition can be controlled during pregnancy by following the anti-Rh titer of the mother's blood and the bilirubin level of the fetus by amniocentesis. These indices show whether the pregnancy should be allowed to go to full term and if intrauterine transfusion is indicated; or if labor should be induced earlier. Delivery should be as free of trauma as possible and the placenta should not be manually removed. The infant with hemolytic disease should be immediately seen by a physician who is capable of and has the facilities and blood supplies available for exchange transfusion. The use of Rh (D) immune globulin after abortion, at 28 weeks' gestation, and within 72 hr of delivery has been beneficial.

h. uremic syndrome An acute condition consisting of microangiopathic hemolytic anemia, thrombocytopenia, and acute nephropathy. *Escherichia coli* 0157:H7 is a causative agent that may be acquired from eating contaminated raw or rare hamburger or other meats. Children are most often affected. Onset may initially involve gastroenteritis and diarrhea or an upper respiratory tract infection. An acute phase whose hallmarks are a purpuric rash, irritability, lethargy, and oliguria follows, continuing with splenomegaly, mild jaundice, seizures (in some patients), hepatomegaly, pulmonary edema, and renal failure. The acute phase may last from 1 to 2 weeks in mild cases and much longer in severe cases.

TREATMENT: The treatment of this syndrome is for the renal failure and anemia. Antibiotics are ineffective.

PROGNOSIS: The usual outcome is complete recovery, but about 5% of affected persons die, and 10% of patients develop end-stage renal disease and require life-long hemodialysis.

PATIENT CARE: If the child has been anuric for 24 hours or demonstrates oliguria with seizures and hypertension, the physician places a peritoneal catheter and the nurse institutes peritoneal dialysis as prescribed, with fluid replacement based on estimated sensible and insensible losses. Fluid and electrolyte balance, complete blood count, body weight, sensorium, and vital signs are carefully monitored, and BUN and azotemia levels are followed to evaluate therapy. Hypertension is reported and controlled with antihypertensive drugs. Severe anemia is treated with fresh, washed packed red blood cells; careful assessment is required throughout the transfusion to prevent circulatory overload, hypertension, and hyperkalemia. Seizures are managed by treating specific causes when known (hypertension, hyponatremia, hypocalcemia), and with anticonvulsant drugs as required. The patient is protected from injury during seizure activity, with the airway guarded. Heart and breath sounds are auscultated periodically, as cardiac failure with pulmonary edema can occur in association with hypervolemia. Prevention and treatment include water and sodium restriction and diuretic therapy, if prescribed. Meeting the child's nutritional needs can be difficult, as concentrated foods must be ingested without fluids and the child may be nauseated. The dietician should be consulted for nutrition management. The child who is quite ill also may be irritable, restless, anxious, and frightened by frequent painful and stress-producing tests and treatments. Comfort and stability are provided in this threatening environment. Support and reassurance are given to the parents and significant others, who are stressed by the severity of the illness, and who may experience a degree of guilt if the illness resulted from ingestion of contaminated or raw foods. The family benefits not only from explanations about tests and treatments and information about their child's progress but also from sympathetic listening.

hemolyze (hē′mō-līz) To destroy red blood cells.

hemomediastinum (hē″mō-mē″dē-ă-stī′nŭm) [Gr. *haima,* blood, + L. *mediastinus,* in the middle] Effusion of blood into mediastinal spaces. SYN: *hematomediastinum.*

hemometra (hē″mō-mē′tră) [″ + *metra,* uterus] Hematometra.

hemonephrosis (hē″mō-nĕ-frō′sĭs) [″ + *nephros,* kidney, + *osis,* condition] Accumulation of blood in the renal pelvis. SYN: *hematonephrosis.*

hemopathic (hē″mō-păth′ĭk) [″ + *pathos,* disease, suffering] Relating or due to disease of the blood.

hemopathology (hē″mō-pă-thŏl′ō-jē) [″ + ″ + *logos,* word, reason] The science of blood disorders.

hemoperfusion The perfusion of blood through substances, such as activated charcoal or ion-exchange resins, to remove toxic materials. The blood is then returned to the patient. This technique differs from hemodialysis in that the blood is not separated from the chemicals or solutions by a semipermeable dialysis membrane. SEE: *hemodialysis.*

hemopericardium (hē″mō-pĕr″ĭ-kăr′dē-ŭm) [″ + *peri,* around, + *kardia,* heart] Accumulation of blood in the pericardium.

hemoperitoneum (hē″mō-pĕr″ĭ-tō-nē′ŭm) [″ + *peritonaion,* peritoneum] Bleeding into the peritoneal cavity.

hemophage (hē′mō-fāj) [″ + *phagein,* to eat] A cell that destroys red blood cells by phagocytosis.

hemophagocyte (hē″mō-făg′ō-sīt) [″+ ″ + *kytos,* cell] A phagocyte that ingests red blood cells.

hemophagocytosis (hē″mō-făg″ō-sī-tō′sĭs) [″ + ″ + ″ + *osis,* condition] The ingestion of red blood cells by phagocytes.

hemophil (hē′mŏ-fĭl) [″ + *philein,* to love] A type of bacteria that grows very well on agar that contains blood.

hemophilia (hē″mō-, hĕm″ō-fĭl′ē-ă) [″ + *philein,* to love] A group of hereditary bleeding disorders marked by deficiencies of blood-clotting proteins. Hemophilias are rare. Hemophilia A affects 1 in 5,000 to 10,000 boys; hemophilia B is present in about 1 in 30,000 boys. SEE: *blood; Nursing Diagnoses Appendix.*

ETIOLOGY: There are two principal types: hemophilia A (in which blood clotting factor VIII: C is either missing from the bloodstream or defective) and hemophilia B (in which blood clotting factor IX is deficient or defective). Both of these disorders are sex-linked (i.e., caused by X chromosome mutations) and occur in boys only.

SYMPTOMS: Bleeding after minor trauma is the hallmark of the hemophilias. Typically, bleeding occurs in the joints (hemarthrosis), in soft tissues, and in the urinary tract. Bleeding may also occur during dental procedures and surgery. Intracranial bleeding and bleeding into deep body sites may be life-threatening.

TREATMENT: Deficient clotting factors can be replaced intravenously, but doing so has carried significant risks. In the 1980s, for example, the injection of contaminated clotting factors spread hepatitis C and human immunodeficiency virus to many patients with hemophilia. Before these epidemics, these patients had life expectancies of about 65 years. Acquired immunodeficiency syndrome and other blood-borne infections decreased the average lifespan of patients with hemophilia to about 50 years. Today, the purification of clotting factors has resulted in safer treatment for patients with hemophilia.

Other agents that aid blood clotting, such as desmopressin and epsilon-aminocaproic acid, are also helpful in managing or preventing bleeding episodes.

CAUTION: Patients with hemophilia should avoid drugs that interfere with anticoagulation and trauma. They should also wear bracelets identifying their illness to medical personnel.

PATIENT CARE: In the bleeding patient, vital signs are monitored, and the patient is observed for signs and symptoms of decreased tissue perfusion (i.e., restlessness, anxiety, confusion, pallor, cool and clammy skin, chest pain, decreased urine output, hypotension, tachycardia). The skin, mucous membranes, and wounds are inspected for bleeding. Emergency care is provided for external bleeding; wounds are cleaned; and gentle, consistent pressure is applied to stop the bleeding. Safety measures are instituted to prevent injury, and the patient and family are instructed in these measures. The patient is assessed for development of hemarthrosis, and appropriate care is provided, which includes elevating the affected part, immobilizing the joint in a slightly flexed position, and applying ice intermittently. As necessary, deficient clotting factors or plasma is administered as prescribed until bleeding is controlled. The patient is monitored for adverse reactions to blood products, such as flushing, headache, tingling, fever, chills, urticaria, and anaphylaxis. Movement of the injured part is restricted, and exercise and weight bearing are prohibited for 48 hours until bleeding has stopped and swelling has subsided. Gentle passive range-of-motion exercises are then provided, with gradual progression to active-assisted and then active exercise. Prescribed analgesics are administered to control pain; however, IM injections are avoided as they may result in hematoma formation. Intracranial, muscle, subcutaneous, renal, and cardiac bleeding are monitored and managed according to protocols or as prescribed by the hematologist. Fluid balance is monitored throughout emergencies, and adequate fluid replacement is instituted as needed.

Both the patient and family are encouraged to verbalize their fears and concerns, and accurate information, realistic reassurance, and emotional support are provided. Health care providers remain with the anxious or fearful patient or family. Gentle, careful, but thorough oral care is provided with a soft toothbrush or sponge-stick (toothette) to prevent inflamed and bleeding gums, and the patient is instructed in this method. Regular dental examinations are recommended. Regular isometric exercise is encouraged to strengthen muscles, which in turn protects joints by reducing the incidence of hemarthrosis. Use of safety measures to protect the patient from injury is encouraged, while unnecessary restrictions that impair normal development are discouraged. The patient should remain independent and self-sufficient; assistance is provided to both the patient and family to identify safe activities. Techniques are taught for managing bleeding episodes at home. The use of transfusion therapy is explained, and information is provided on all available methods of obtaining such therapy (including how to administer cryoprecipitate at home if appropriate). The seriousness of head injuries and the need for their immediate treatment are explained. Diversional activities and private time with family and friends are provided to help the patient overcome feelings of isolation. The patient's and family's knowledge of the disease and its treatment, as well as the impact on the patient, siblings, and parents' marital relationship, are continually assessed. The patient and family are encouraged to talk with others in similar circumstances through local support groups and services, and they are referred to the National Hemophilia Foundation for further information.

h. A Hemophilia due to a deficiency of blood coagulation factor VIII. SEE: *hemophilia*.

h. B Hemophilia due to a deficiency of blood coagulation factor IX (plasma thromboplastin component). This condition can be treated with a lyophilized product that contains concentrated factor IX. SYN: *Christmas disease*. SEE: *hemophilia*.

h. C Hemophilia due to a deficiency of blood coagulation factor XI.

hemophiliac (hē″mō-fĭl′ē-ăk) One afflicted with hemophilia.

hemophilic (hē″mō-fĭl′ĭk) **1.** Fond of blood, said of bacteria that grow well in culture media containing hemoglobin. **2.** Pert. to hemophilia or hemophiliacs.

Hemophilus *Haemophilus*.

hemophobia (hē″mō-fō′bē-ă) [Gr. *haima*, blood, + *phobos*, fear] An aversion to seeing blood or to bleeding.

hemophthalmia, hemophthalmus (hē″mŏf-thăl′mē-ă, -mŭs) [″ + *ophthalmos*, eye] An effusion of blood into the eye.

hemopleura (hē″mō-ploo′ră) An outdated term for hemothorax. SEE: *hemothorax*.

hemopneumopericardium (hē″mō-nū″mō-pĕr″ĭ-kăr′dē-ŭm) [″ + *pneuma*, air, + *peri*, around, + *kardia*, heart] Blood and air in the pericardium.

hemopneumothorax (hē″mō-nū-mō-thō′răks) [″ + ″ + *thorax*, chest] Hemorrhage and the release of air into the chest, often as a result of trauma, but occasionally occurring spontaneously.

hemopoiesis (hē″mō-poy-ē′sĭs) [″ + *poiesis*, formation] Hematopoiesis.

hemoprecipitin (hē″mō-prē-sĭp′ĭ-tĭn) A precipitin in the blood.

hemoprotein (hē″mō-prō′tē-ĭn) Any protein combined with the heme blood pigment.

hemopsonin (hē″mŏp-sō′nĭn) [″ + *opsonein*, to buy food] An antibody that makes red blood cells more susceptible to phagocytosis.

hemoptysis (hē-mŏp′tĭ-sĭs) [″ + *ptyein*, to spit] The expectoration of blood that arises from the nasopharynx, larynx, trachea, bronchi, or lungs. Massive hemoptysis, which occurs rarely, should be managed by a pulmonary specialist experienced in bronchoscopy. Small amounts of hemoptysis may occur in many illnesses, including nosebleeds, acute bronchitis, pneumonia, pulmonary tuberculosis, and cancers of the lung. Management depends on the underlying disorder. A careful history and physical examination, along with chest x-ray examination and laboratory studies, often help identify the underlying cause. SEE: table; *bleeding; hematemesis; hemorrhage; Nursing Diagnoses Appendix*.

PATIENT CARE: Vital signs are monitored to determine the patient's stability; special emphasis is placed on evaluations of respiration and hemodynamics. Universal precautions are used when blood and secretions are

Comparison of Hemoptysis and Hematemesis

Hemoptysis	Hematemesis
Blood is coughed up.	Blood is vomited.
Blood is frothy, bright red, and alkaline.	Blood is either dark or bright red, usually not frothy, and acid. It may have a coffee-ground appearance.
Blood may be mixed with sputum.	Blood may be mixed with food or bile.
Dyspnea, pleuritic pain, or other chest discomfort is common.	Nausea or abdominal pain are common.
Underlying diagnoses commonly include bronchitis, pneumonia, tuberculosis, nosebleed, lung cancer, pulmonary embolism or infarct, foreign bodies, and rarely autoimmune illnesses.	Underlying diagnoses commonly include peptic ulcers, gastritis, esophagitis, duodenitis, esophageal varices, upper GI tumors, vascular malformations, nosebleed, tears in the esophagus.

handled, and when the patient is cleansed. Expectorated blood is inspected to assist in determining the site of bleeding. Blood and secretions are saved for the physician's inspection and possible laboratory analysis. A quiet, calm, and reassuring environment is maintained. The patient is placed at bedrest with the head slightly elevated and turned to keep the bleeding side, if known, down. Oral care is provided and fluids are administered as ordered. Excessive coughing is discouraged. Anticoagulants are withheld.

parasitic h. Coughing up blood resulting from infection of the lungs by *Paragonimus westermani,* a parasitic fluke.

hemorrhage (hĕm′ĕ-rĭj) [″ + *rhegnynai,* to burst forth] Blood loss. "Hemorrhage" usually is used to describe episodes of bleeding that last more than a few minutes, compromise organ or tissue perfusion, or threaten life. The most hazardous forms of blood loss result from arterial bleeding, internal bleeding, or bleeding into the cranium. The risk of uncontrolled bleeding is greatest in patients who have coagulation disorders or take anticoagulant drugs. SEE: table.

Common Sites of Bleeding

Location	Descriptive Term
Biliary tract	Hemobilia
Fallopian tubes	Hemosalpinx
Gastrointestinal tract	
• Lower	• Hematochezia; melena
• Upper (vomited)	• Hematemesis
Joints	Hemarthosis
Lungs/Bronchi (coughed up)	Hemoptysis
Nasal passages	Epistaxis
Skin	Ecchymosis
Urinary tract	Hematuria

SYMPTOMS: Orthostatic dizziness, weakness, fatigue, shortness of breath, and palpitations are common symptoms of hemorrhage. Signs of hemorrhage include tachycardia, hypotension, pallor, and cold moist skin.

TREATMENT: Pressure should be applied directly to any obviously bleeding body part, and the part should be elevated. Cautery may be used to stop bleeding from visible vessels. Ligation of blood vessels, surgical removal of hemorrhaging organs, or the instillation of sclerosants is often effective in managing internal hemorrhage. Procoagulants (e.g., vitamin K, fresh frozen plasma, cryoprecipitate, desmopressin) may be administered to patients with primary or drug-induced bleeding disorders. Transfusions of red blood cells may be given if bleeding compromises heart or lung function or threatens to do so because of its pace or volume.

For trauma patients with massive bleeding, the experienced nurse or emergency care provider may apply pneumatic splints or antishock garments during patient transportation to the hospital. These devices may prevent hemorrhagic shock.

CAUTION: Standard precautions should be used for all procedures involving contact with blood or wounds.

antepartum h. Excessive blood loss during the prenatal period, most commonly associated with spontaneous or induced abortion, ruptured ectopic pregnancy, placenta previa, or abruptio placentae.

arterial h. A hemorrhage from an artery. In arterial bleeding, which is bright red, the blood ordinarily flows in waves or spurts; however, the flow may be steady if the torn artery is deep or buried.

FIRST AID: Almost all arterial bleeding can be controlled with direct pressure to the wound. If it cannot be controlled with applied pressure, the responsible artery may need to be surgically ligated. SEE: *arterial b.* for table; *pressure point*.

capillary h. Bleeding from minute blood vessels, present in all bleeding. When large vessels are not injured, capillary bleeding may be controlled by simple elevation and pressure with a sterile dry compress.

carotid artery h. Bleeding from the carotid artery. This type of hemorrhage can be rapidly fatal, because it may be profuse and may deprive the brain of oxygen.

FIRST AID: The wound should be compressed with the thumbs placed transversely across the neck, both above and below the wound, and the fingers directed around the back of the neck to aid in compression. Urgent surgical consultation is required.

cerebral h. Bleeding into the brain, a common cause of stroke. SEE: *stroke*.

ETIOLOGY: It usually results from rupture of aneurysm, extremely high blood pressure, brain trauma, or brain tumors.

SYMPTOMS: This type of hemorrhage may cause symptoms of stroke, such as unconsciousness, apnea, vomiting, hemiplegia, and death. There may be speech disturbance, incontinence of the bladder and rectum, or other findings, depending on the area of brain damage.

TREATMENT: Supportive therapy is needed to maintain airway and oxygenation. Neurosurgical consultation should be promptly obtained. Hydration and fluid and electrolyte balance should be maintained. Rehabilitation may include physical therapy, speech therapy, and counseling.

fibrinolytic h. A hemorrhage due to a defect in the fibrin component in blood coagulation.

gastrointestinal h. Bleeding into or from the stomach, small intestine, or large intestine.

internal h. Hemorrhage into an area where it is not visible. SYN: *occult bleeding*.

intracranial h. Bleeding into the cranium.

h. of the knee Bleeding from the knee.

TREATMENT: If the bleeding is at the knee or below, a pad should be applied with pressure. If the bleeding is behind the knee, a pad should be applied at the site and the leg bandaged firmly. The bandage should be loosened at 12-min to 15-min intervals to prevent arterial obstruction.

lung h. Hemorrhage from the lung, with bright red and frothy blood, frequently coughed up.

petechial h. Hemorrhage in the form of small rounded spots or petechiae occurring in the skin or mucous membranes.

postmenopausal h. Bleeding from the uterus after menopause. It may be a sign of malignancy of the reproductive tract and should be carefully and thoroughly investigated.

postpartum h. Hemorrhage that occurs after childbirth. *Early postpartum hemorrhage* is defined as a blood loss of more than 500 ml of blood during the first 24 hr after delivery. The most common cause is loss of uterine tone caused by overdistention; prolonged or precipitate labor; uterine overstimulation; trauma, rupture, or inversion; lacerations of the lower genital tract; or blood coagulation disorder. *Late postpartum hemorrhage* occurs after the first 24 hr have passed. It usually is caused by retained placental fragments.

CAUTION: Universal precautions are essential. SEE: *Standard and Universal Precautions Appendix*.

PATIENT CARE: The risk is highest within 1 hr after delivery. The woman's prenatal, labor, and delivery records are reviewed. The presence of risk factors is noted, and the woman's pulse, blood pressure, fundal and bladder status, and vaginal discharge are assessed every 15 min. If the fundus is boggy, it is massaged to stimulate uterine contractions, and then the status of the woman's bladder is assessed. If the bladder is distended, the patient is encouraged to void and then postvoiding fundal status is assessed; if the fundus remains firm after massage, the fundus and vaginal flow are reassessed in 5 min. SEE: *fundal massage*.

If bleeding does not respond to the above measures or the fundus remains firm and the patient exhibits bright red vaginal discharge, retained placental fragments or cervical or vaginal laceration should be suspected; the primary caregiver should be notified. Continued massage at this point is contraindicated; the physician or nurse midwife may order oxytocin to stimulate uterine contractions. Pharmacological agents such as methylergonovine or prostaglandin F2 analogs may be administered intramuscularly or intravenously. If blood loss has been extensive, intravenous infusions or blood transfusion may be needed to combat hypovolemic shock. If the patient exhibits signs of a clotting defect, prompt life-saving treatment is vital. SEE: *disseminated intravascular coagulation*.

The patient is prepared for and the primary caregiver is assisted with examination of the uterine cavity, removal of any placental fragments, or repair of any lacerations. To reduce the patient's understandable anxiety and to allay apprehension, all procedures are explained, support and comfort are provided, and the mother is assured that her newborn is receiving good care.

primary h. A hemorrhage immediately following any trauma.

retroperitoneal h. Bleeding into the retroperitoneal space.

secondary h. **1.** A hemorrhage occurring some time after primary hemorrhage, usually caused by sepsis and septic ulceration into a blood vessel. It may occur after 24 hours or when a ligature separates, usually between the 7th and 10th days. **2.** Bleeding from the mother's uterus or the infant's umbilicus, resulting from a septic infection.

subarachnoid h. ABBR: SAH. Bleeding into the subarachnoid space of the brain, usually because of the rupture of an intracranial aneurysm or arteriovenous malformation and occasionally because of hypertensive vascular disease. The bleeding causes intense headache pain, often with nausea and vomiting, loss of consciousness, paralysis, and, in some cases, coma, decerebrate posturing, and brain death. About 30,000 Americans are affected annually. Prompt diagnosis is facilitated by neuroimaging or lumbar puncture. A neurosurgical consultation should be obtained.

subconjunctival h. Rupture of the superficial arteries in the sclera. SEE: illus.

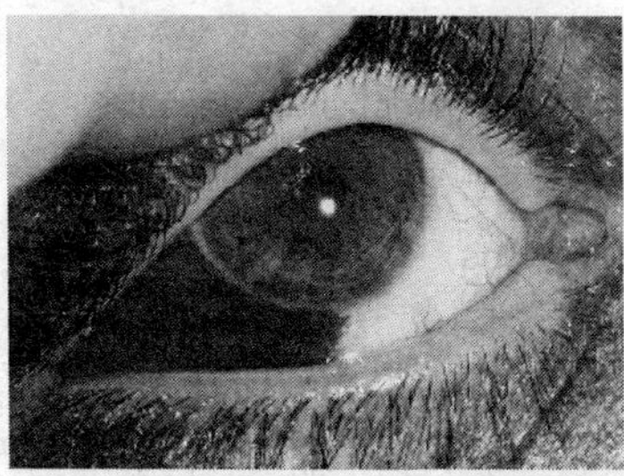

SUBCONJUNCTIVAL HEMORRHAGE

ETIOLOGY: Subconjunctival hemorrhage can result from blunt trauma to the eye or from increased intracranial or intraocular pressure.

SYMPTOMS: Patients have visible bleeding between the sclera and the conjunctiva.

TREATMENT: A subconjunctival hemorrhage normally resolves within 1 to 7 days.

CAUTION: Subconjunctival hemorrhage must be differentiated from hyphema, the collection of blood within the anterior chamber of the eye.

thigh h. Bleeding at the upper part of the thigh, near the groin.

TREATMENT: A pad or gauze should be inserted into the wound and pressure applied. Failure of the bleeding to stop requires surgical consultation.

typhoid h. A gross hemorrhage that occurs in approx. 10% of cases of typhoid that progress to the stage of gastrointestinal ulceration. Blood loss may reach 1000 ml. Single large hemorrhages or smaller successive ones may occur; the latter type are the most serious. Hemorrhages take place at the end of the second week and during the third week of the disease.

uterine h. Hemorrhage into the cavity of the uterus. The three types of pathologic uterine hemorrhage are essential uterine hemorrhage (metropathia haemorrhagica), which occurs with pelvic, uterine, or cervical diseases; intrapartum hemorrhage, which occurs during labor; and postpartum hemorrhage, which occurs after the third stage of labor. The latter may be caused by rupture, lacerations, relaxation of the uterus, hematoma, or retained products of conception including the placenta or membrane fragments.

ETIOLOGY: Common causes are trauma; congenital abnormalities; pathologic processes such as tumors; infections, esp. of the alimentary, respiratory, and genitourinary tracts; and generalized vascular disorders such as purpuras and coagulation defects. Hemorrhage also may result from premature separation of the placenta, particularly with extravasation into the uterine musculature, and from retained products of conception after abortion or delivery. SEE: *abruptio placentae; Couvelaire uterus*.

TREATMENT: Application of an umbrella pack will apply pressure to the uterine arterial supply. When ultrasonography reveals that retained placental fragments are the source of hemorrhage, they are usually removed by suction or surgical curettage. If the uterus is flaccid, it can usually be stimulated to contract by administering intravenous oxytocin. The patient may need transfusion and, in some cases, surgery to prevent fatal hemorrhage.

venous h. Hemorrhage of a vein, characterized by steady, profuse bleeding of rather dark blood.

PATIENT CARE: The patient should be reassured, while direct pressure to the wound is applied, and the affected body part is elevated. If bleeding does not stop after 15 minutes of direct pressure, evaluation by a health care provider is advisable. SEE: *tourniquet*.

vicarious h. Hemorrhage from one part as a result of suppression of bleeding in another part. SEE: *vicarious menstruation*.

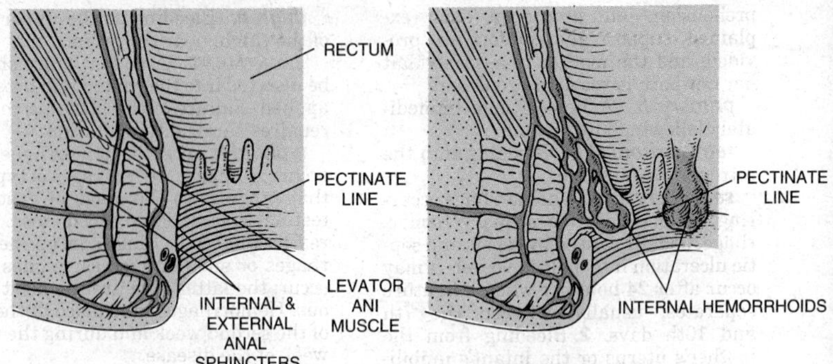

ANATOMY OF RECTUM

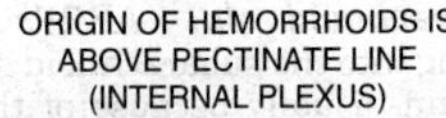

ORIGIN OF HEMORRHOIDS IS ABOVE PECTINATE LINE (INTERNAL PLEXUS)

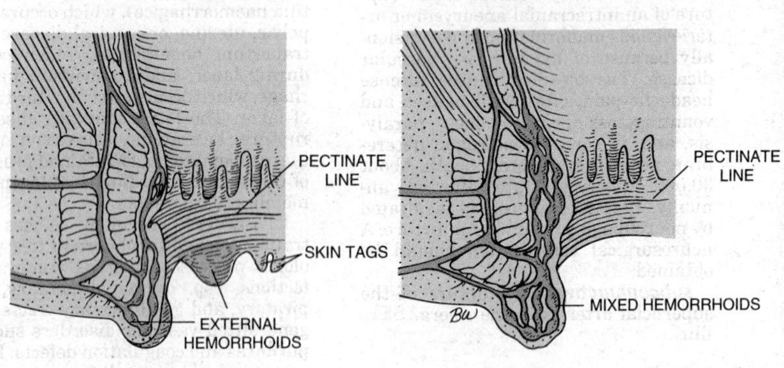

ORIGIN OF HEMORRHOIDS IS BELOW PECTINATE LINE (EXTERNAL PLEXUS)

ORIGIN OF HEMORRHOIDS IS ABOVE AND BELOW PECTINATE LINE (INTERNAL AND EXTERNAL PLEXUS)

HEMORRHOIDS

hemorrhagenic (hĕm″ō-ră-jĕn′ĭk) [″ + *rhegnynai,* to burst forth, + *gennan,* to form] Producing hemorrhage.

hemorrhagic (hĕm-ō-răj′ĭk) Pert. to or marked by hemorrhage.

h. disease of the newborn Hemorrhaging due to an inadequate supply of prothrombin received from the mother or a delay in the establishment of the bacterial intestinal flora that produces vitamin K. Parenteral vitamin K given to the infant within 6 hr of birth prevents this condition.

h. fever with renal syndrome An arthropod-borne viral disease caused by Hanta virus or related viruses. SEE: *hantavirus pulmonary syndrome.*

h. nephrosonephritis An acute infectious disease caused by the Hanta virus, with abrupt onset of fever that lasts 3 to 8 days, conjunctival injection, prostration, anorexia, and vomiting. Renal involvement may be mild or progress to acute renal failure, which may last several weeks. The mode of transmission is unknown but is apparently not from person to person. The incubation period varies from 9 to 35 days. Shock and renal failure should be treated symptomatically. There is no specific therapy. Also known as *epidemic hemorrhagic fever* and *Korean hemorrhagic fever.*

viral h. fever ABBR: VHF. One of a group of diseases caused by arthropod-borne viruses, esp. the Bunyaviridae group, including Lassa, Marburg, Ebola, Rift Valley, and Congo-Crimean hemorrhagic fever viruses.

hemorrhoid (hĕm′ō-royd) [Gr. *haimorrhois*] Veins of the internal or external hemorrhoidal plexuses and the immediately surrounding tissues. Hemorrhoids are most often referred to only when diseased (i.e., enlarged, painful, bleeding). Other anorectal conditions (e.g., anal fissure, condylomata, anal cancers) may produce similar symptoms and must be distinguished from hemorrhoids by appropriate examination. SYN: *piles*. SEE: illus.; *Nursing Diagnoses Appendix*.

TREATMENT: Therapy depends on the severity of the symptoms, not the extent of the hemorrhoids. In many instances, the only therapy required is improvement in anal care, adherence to appropriate fluid intake and diet if necessary, administration of stool softeners to prevent straining to have a bowel movement. Measures to reduce local pain and congestion include the temporary use of local anesthetic agents, lubrication, cold compresses, warm sitz baths, and thermal packs. The necessity of surgery or other modalities of direct intervention (e.g., latex band ligation, sclerotherapy, cryosurgery, infrared photocoagulation, laser surgery) need not be applied until the acute process resolves except in cases of significant bleeding, intractable pain, recurrent episodes, and various individualized considerations. SEE: *hemorrhoidectomy*.

external h. Hemorrhoid located at or distal to the pectinate line (dentate margin), covered by anodermal epithelium or skin and extremely sensitive to most stimuli. SEE: *hemorrhoid* for illus.

internal h. Hemorrhoid located proximal to the pectinate line, covered by mucous membrane and relatively insensitive to direct noxious stimuli. SEE: *hemorrhoid* for illus.

mixed (or combined) h. Hemorrhoid that incorporates both internal and external components.

prolapsed h. The protrusion of an internal hemorrhoid through the anus. SEE: illus.

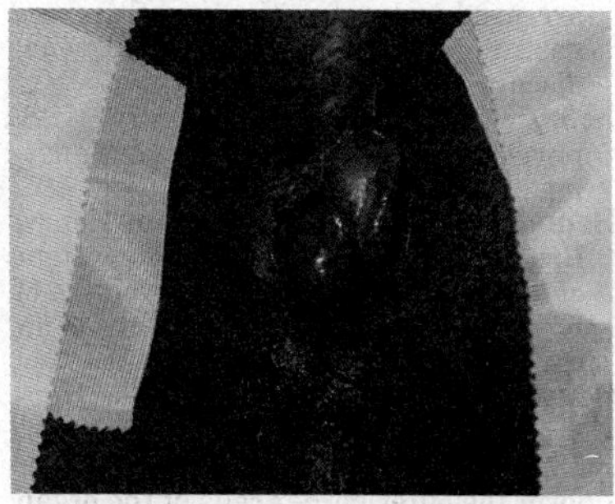

PROLAPSED HEMORRHOIDS

strangulated h. A prolapsed hemorrhoid that is trapped by the anal sphincter, thus compromising blood flow to the vein in the hemorrhoid.

hemorrhoidal (hĕm-ō-roy′dăl) **1.** Relating to hemorrhoids. **2.** Pert. to anal structures, e.g., inferior hemorrhoidal nerve, hemorrhoidal venous plexuses, and inferior hemorrhoidal arteries, etc.

hemorrhoidectomy (hĕm″ō-royd-ĕk′tō-mē) [Gr. *haimorrhois,* vein liable to bleed, + *ektome,* excision] The excision or destruction of hemorrhoids by one of several techniques, including traditional surgery, cryosurgery, laser surgery, infrared photocoagulation, latex band ligation, and sclerotherapy. The latter three modalities are used exclusively for internal hemorrhoids. SEE: *Nursing Diagnoses Appendix*.

PATIENT CARE: Preparation for diagnostic testing is explained. The patient is taught about the use of stool softeners, and is encouraged to increase fluid and fiber intake (unless otherwise restricted) and to exercise to prevent constipation. The patient should not sit on the toilet for longer than necessary in order to avoid venous congestion. The need for good anal hygiene is emphasized, and the patient is cautioned against vigorous wiping and the use of harsh soaps and toilet tissues containing dyes or perfumes.

If hemorrhoidectomy is indicated, physical preparation is conducted; details of postoperative care are explained to the patient. Postoperatively, vital signs and fluid balance are monitored, dressings are checked, and excessive drainage or bleeding is reported. The patient's ability to void within the designated period is ensured. Perianal care is provided and taught to the patient; analgesics and local measures to reduce pain and swelling are provided. The patient is encouraged to assume a prone position for 15 minutes every few hours to reduce edema at the surgical site. When oral intake is tolerated, a bulk-forming or stool-softening laxative is administered as prescribed to ease defecation. Before discharge, anal hygiene and comfort measures are reinforced; the patient is instructed to report increased rectal bleeding, purulent drainage, fever, constipation, or rectal spasm. The patient also is cautioned against overuse of laxatives.

hemosalpinx (hē″mō-săl′pĭnks) [Gr. *haima,* blood, + *salpinx,* tube] Hematosalpinx.

hemosiderin (hē″mō-sĭd′ĕr-ĭn) [″ + *sideros,* iron] An iron-containing pigment derived from hemoglobin from disintegration of red blood cells. It is one form in which iron is stored until it is needed for making hemoglobin.

hemosiderosis (hē″mō-sĭd-ĕr-ō′sĭs) [″ + ″ + *osis,* condition] A condition characterized by the deposition, esp. in the liver and spleen, of hemosiderin. It occurs in diseases associated with excess iron accumulation in the body (e.g., the iron storage diseases) and hemolytic anemias and after multiple transfusions. SEE: *hemochromatosis*.

hemospermia (hē″mō-spĕr′mē-ă) [″ + *sperma,* seed] Hematospermia.

Hemosporida, Hemosporidia (hē-mō-spor-ĭ′dē-ă) [″ + *sporos,* seed] An order of protozoan parasites found in the blood of various animals, including humans.

hemostasis, hemostasia (hē-mŏs′tă-sĭs, hē″mō-stā′zē-ă) [″ + *stasis,* standing still] **1.** An arrest of bleeding or of circulation. **2.** Stagnation of blood.

hemostat (hē′mō-stăt) [″ + *statikos,* standing] **1.** A device or medicine that arrests the flow of blood. **2.** A compressor for controlling hemorrhage of a bleeding vessel.

hemostatic (hē″mō-stăt′ĭk) **1.** Arresting hemorrhage. **2.** Any drug, medicine, surgical device, or blood component that serves to stop bleeding, such as vasopressin, gamma-aminobutyric acid, vitamin K, whole blood, or epinephrine applied locally.

hemostyptic (hē-mō-stĭp′tĭk) [″ + *styptikos,* astringent] An astringent that stops bleeding; a chemical hemostatic.

hemothorax (hē″mō-thō′răks) [″ + *thorax,* chest] Blood or bloody fluid in the pleural cavity caused by rupture of blood vessels resulting from inflammation of the lungs in pneumonia or pulmonary tuberculosis, lung cancer, or trauma. SEE: *Nursing Diagnoses Appendix.*

hemotoxin (hē″mō-tŏks′ĭn) [″ + *toxikon,* poison] Hemolysin.

hemotrophe (hē′mō-trŏf) [″ + *trophe,* nourishment] Nutrition carried to the developing embryo by the maternal blood.

hemotrophic (hē-mō-trŏf′ĭk) [″ + *trophe,* nourishment] Pert. to nutrients carried in the blood.

h. nutrition Transplacental passage of nutrients from the maternal bloodstream to the fetal circulation.

hemotropic (hē-mō-trŏp′ĭk) [″ + *tropos,* turning] Attracted to or having an affinity for blood or blood cells.

hemotympanum (hē″mō-tĭm′pă-nŭm) [″ + *tympanon,* drum] Blood in the middle ear, a finding sometimes identified in serious traumatic brain injury. SYN: *hematotympanum.*

hemozoon (hē″mō-zō′ŏn) Hematozoon.

Henderson, Virginia A nursing educator, 1897–1996, who developed a definition of nursing that was adopted by the International Council of Nurses. SEE: *Nursing Theory Appendix.*

Henderson's Definition of Nursing [Virginia Henderson, U.S. nursing educator, 1897–1996.] A definition, adopted by the International Council of Nurses, stating that the unique function of the nurse is to help sick or well individuals to perform activities that contribute to health, recovery, or a peaceful death. SEE: *Nursing Theory Appendix.*

Henderson-Hasselbalch equation [Lawrence Joseph Henderson, U.S. biochemist, 1878–1942; K. A. Hasselbalch, Danish physician, 1874–1962] An equation that describes the dissociation constant of an acid. In fluid and electrolyte balance, this important equation may be expressed in terms of the bicarbonate (HCO_3^-) system as: pH = 6.095 + log HCO3⁻/α ($PaCO_2$), where α = 0.0307 mM/L/mm Hg at 37°C. At the normal pH of the blood, 7.4, the ratio of HCO_3^- to α ($PaCO_2$) is 20 to 1.

Henle, Friedrich G. J. (hĕn′lē) German anatomist, 1809–1885.

H.'s ampulla Ductus deferens dilatation just above the ejaculatory duct.

H.'s fissure The fibrous tissue between the cardiac muscle fibers.

H.'s layer The outer layer of cells of the inner root sheath of the hair follicle.

H.'s ligament The conjoint tendon of the transversus abdominis muscle.

H.'s loop The U-shaped portion of a renal tubule lying between the proximal and distal convoluted portions. It consists of a thin descending limb and a thicker ascending limb.

H.'s membrane Bruch's layer forming the inner boundary of the choroid of the eye.

H.'s sheath Endoneurium.

H.'s tubules The portion of the nephron following the proximal tubule. SEE: *nephron.*

Henoch-Schönlein purpura (hĕn′ŏk-shān′līn) [Eduard H. Henoch, Ger. pediatrician, 1820–1910; Johann Lukas Schönlein, Ger. physician, 1793–1864] SEE: *Henoch-Schönlein purpura.*

TREATMENT: Joint symptoms respond to rest and administration of nonsteroidal anti-inflammatory drugs. Corticosteroid drugs, such as prednisone, are used to treat patients with severe gastrointestinal involvement or renal disease.

henry (hĕn′rē) [Joseph Henry, U.S. physicist, 1797–1878] A unit designating electrical inductance.

Henry's law (hĕn′rēz) [William Henry, Brit. chemist, 1774–1836] The weight of a gas dissolved by a given volume of liquid at a constant temperature is directly proportional to the pressure.

Hensen's cells (hĕn′sĕns) [Victor Hensen, Ger. anatomist and physiologist, 1835–1924] Tall columnar cells that form the outer border cells of the organ of Corti of the cochlea.

Hensen's disk The band in the center of the A disk of a sarcomere of striated muscle. During contraction it appears lighter than the remaining portion and in its center, a dark stripe, the M line, is seen. SYN: *H band.*

Hensen's stripe A dark band on the undersurface of the tectorial membrane of the inner ear.

HEPA filter *high efficiency particulate air filter.*

hepar (hē′păr) [Gr. *hepatos,* liver] The liver.

heparin (hĕp′ă-rĭn) A parenteral anticoagulant drug with a faster effect than warfarin or its derivatives. It is composed of polysaccharides that inhibit coagulation by forming an antithrombin that prevents conversion of prothrombin to thrombin and by preventing liberation of thromboplastin from platelets. Because heparin is poorly absorbed from the gastrointestinal tract, it is usually administered intravenously or subcutaneously as a sodium or calcium salt.

USES: Heparin is used as an anticoagulant in the prevention and treatment of thrombosis and embolism. It is an important agent in the management of acute coronary syndromes (such as unstable angina pectoris or acute myocardial infarction). Because heparin compounds are too large to cross the placental barrier, they are the preferred anticoagulants in pregnant women. The antagonist for an overdose is protamine sulfate. The most common side effect of heparin is abnormal bleeding.

h. lock An intermittent infusion device that is used episodically for fluid or medication infusion. Heparin solution flushes are used to maintain its patency. Saline locks have replaced heparin locks because of the unacceptable risk of heparin allergy. SEE: *heparin lock flush solution.*

h. lock flush solution A solution of unfractionated heparins that was used in the past to keep intravenous infusion devices from clotting. Heparin flushes now are used infrequently because they pose an unacceptably high risk of heparin-related thrombocytopenia, a potentially life-threatening allergy.

low molecular weight h. The most bioavailable fraction of heparin; it has a more precise anticoagulant effect than unfractionated heparins. It is used to prevent and treat deep venous thrombosis, pulmonary embolism, and unstable coronary syndromes.

h. sulfate A sulfurated mucopolysaccharide that accumulates in the connective tissue in abnormal amounts in some mucopolysaccharidoses. SEE: *mucopolysaccharidosis.*

heparinize (hĕp′ĕr-ĭ-nīz) To inhibit blood coagulation with heparin.

heparinoid A substance that prevents or treats blood clots. Heparinoids have a lower risk for bleeding and thrombocytopenia than heparin.

hepat- SEE: *hepato-*.

hepatalgia (hĕp″ă-tăl′jē-ă) [Gr. *hepatos,* liver, + *algos,* pain] Pain in the liver.
hepatalgic (hĕp″ă-tăl′jĭk), *adj.*

hepatatrophia (hĕp″ăt-ă-trō′fē-ă) [″ + *atrophia,* atrophy] Atrophy of the liver.

hepatectomy (hĕp″ă-tĕk′tō-mē) [″ + *ektome,* excision] Excision of part or all of the liver.

hepatic (hĕ-păt′ĭk) [Gr. *hepatikos*] Pert. to the liver.

h. vein One of three vessels that take blood from the liver to the inferior vena cava.

hepaticoduodenostomy (hĕ-păt″ĭ-kō-dū″ō-dĕ-nŏs′tō-mē) [″ + L. *duodeni,* duodenum, + Gr. *stoma,* mouth] Hepatoduodenostomy.

hepaticoenterostomy (hĕ-păt″ĭ-kō-ĕn-tĕr-ŏs′tō-mē) [″ + *enteron,* intestine, + *stoma,* mouth] An operation to create an artificial opening between the hepatic duct and intestine.

hepaticogastrostomy (hĕ-păt″ĭ-kō-găs-trŏs′tō-mē) [″ + *gaster,* stomach, + *stoma,* mouth] An operation to create a passage between the hepatic duct and the stomach.

hepaticojejunostomy (hĕ-păt′ĭ-kō-jē″jū-nŏs′tō-mē) [″ + L. *jejunum,* empty, + Gr. *stoma,* mouth] The surgical joining of the hepatic duct and the jejunum. SEE: *hepaticoenterostomy*.

hepaticolithotomy (hĕ-păt″ĭ-kō-lĭ-thŏt′ō-mē) The surgical removal of gallstones from the hepatic duct.

hepaticolithotripsy (hĕ-păt″ĭ-kō-lĭth′ō-trĭp-sē) [″ + *lithos,* stone, + *tripsis,* a crushing] Crushing of a biliary calculus in the hepatic duct.

hepaticostomy (hĕ-păt″ĭ-kŏs′tō-mē) [″ + *stoma,* mouth] The establishment of a permanent fistula into the hepatic duct.

hepaticotomy (hĕ-păt″ĭ-kŏt′ō-mē) [″ + *tome,* incision] An incision into the hepatic duct.

hepatitis (hĕp″ă-tī′tĭs) [″ + *itis,* inflammation] Inflammation of the liver, usually caused by exposure to an infectious agent (e.g., a hepatitis virus), a toxin (e.g., alcohol), or a drug (such as acetaminophen). The illness may be mild or life-threatening, chronic or acute. Chronic cases may be detected only by the discovery of elevated liver enzymes in the blood. Acute cases are marked by jaundice, hepatic enlargement, and sometimes bleeding, altered mental status, and multiple organ system failure.

PATHOLOGY: Damage to liver cells (hepatocytes) is caused by direct injury from the causative agent, or indirectly as a result of inflammatory or autoimmune responses. During acute inflammation, the swollen hepatocytes are less able to detoxify drugs; produce clotting factors, cholesterol, plasma proteins, bile and glycogen; store fat-soluble vitamins; and perform other functions. All of the hepatitis viruses may cause severe (“fulminant”) hepatitis, but hepatitis B and D are the most common causes. Drug overdoses, ingestion of toxins, and shock are also responsible for rapid liver deterioration.

PATIENT CARE: Patients generally are not hospitalized unless they experience significant liver damage; the more severely affected need supportive medical and psychological care. Patients at home should be instructed about the nature and course of the illness, its care and treatment, and signs and symptoms of complications. The patient should eat a well-balanced diet and drink adequate fluids, but should avoid alcohol and other liver toxins. When hepatitis is foodborne, scrupulous handwashing, food handling, and cleaning of dishes and silverware are necessary to prevent transmission to household members. The patient should avoid intimate contact until antigen and antibody levels are reduced. Emotional support and reassurance should be offered to the patient, as interference with the patient's habits and lifestyle may be considerable. SEE: *Nursing Diagnoses Appendix; Standard and Universal Precautions Appendix; hepatitis A; autoimmune hepatitis; hepatitis E; fulminant hepatitis.*

h. A Hepatitis caused by hepatitis A virus (HAV), an RNA virus without an envelope. Because it can be contracted through contaminated water or food, young adults and children in institutional settings and travelers in countries with minimal sanitation are at greatest risk for infection; small epidemics have been seen among persons eating at restaurants that served contaminated shellfish. The course of the illness is usually mild, although it can be severe; incubation period is 2 to 6 weeks, the acute stage lasts 2 to 12 weeks, and complete recovery takes weeks to months. The infection affects about 30,000 Americans every year. Hepatitis A does not produce a carrier state and does not cause chronic hepatitis. The two antibodies produced in response to hepatitis A antigen serve as markers for infection; one of these, IgG anti-HAV, provides immunity against reinfection. Hepatitis A previously was called *infectious hepatitis*.

TREATMENT: No drugs specifically treat hepatitis A. Immune globulin containing IgG anti-HAV antibodies may be prescribed for family members; it provides passive immunity for 6 to 8 weeks. Preventive education focuses on good personal hygiene, especially handwashing; use of good judgment in choice of food and eating places; and, in some areas of the world, basic sanitation. Hepatitis A vaccine prevents the infection either before or immediately after exposure to the virus and is recommended for health care workers, travelers to developing countries, day care workers, persons with pre-existing liver disease, and others at high risk.

acute anicteric h. Hepatitis marked by slight fever, gastrointestinal upset, and anorexia, but no jaundice.

amebic h. The syndrome of a tender, enlarged liver; pain over the liver; fever; and leukocytosis in a patient with amebic colitis. This name is a misnomer in that the liver changes are not due to an infestation of that organ with amebae but are a part of the nonspecific reaction to the infection in the intestinal tract. Nevertheless, occasionally a liver abscess will develop and the walls of the abscess will contain amebae.

TREATMENT: Metronidazole plus iodoquinol, or chloroquine phosphate plus either emetine or dehydroemetine, are used to treat amebic hepatitis. These latter two drugs are toxic and should be given only if their course can be carefully observed by a cardiac monitor. The drugs should not be given to a patient who has cardiac disease or is pregnant. Needle aspiration of the abscess may be needed.

h. antigen The original term for the Australian antigen, which is now called hepatitis B surface antigen (HBsAg). Its discovery made possible the differentiation of hepatitis B from other forms of viral hepatitis.

autoimmune h. Persistent hepatic inflammation and necrosis, in the setting of hypergammaglobulinemia and autoantibodies, and in the absence of other common causes of liver injury.

h. B Injury to liver cells caused by hepatitis B virus (HBV), a double-stranded DNA virus. It may appear as an asymptomatic, acute, chronic, or fulminant infection. Acute infection often is marked by jaundice, nausea and vomiting, joint pains, or rashes, associated with marked elevations in serum liver function tests. Chronic infection typically is asymptomatic and may be detected only by blood tests, until it causes late complications such as cirrhosis, portal hypertension, or hepatocellular carcinoma. Fulminant hepatitis B infection is defined as the deterioration of the patient into hepatic encephalopathy within 8 weeks of the onset of the disease.

The virus is transmitted by exposure to the blood or body fluids of an infected individual. The incubation period is approximately 2 to 6 months. Acute infection usually resolves in less than 6 months; when hepatitis B virus surface antigen does not clear from the blood within 6 months, chronic hepatitis is said to have developed. Each year in the U.S. alone, about 300,000 people are infected with hepatitis B virus. Worldwide, chronic hepatitis affects about 300 million people.

Individuals at greatest risk for infection include intravenous drug abusers, individuals with multiple sex partners, men who have sex with men, infants born of HBV-infected mothers, and health care workers. Blood banks now routinely screen for HBV antigens, which has greatly reduced the transmission of infection by transfusion.

CAUTION: Individuals who have not been vaccinated against HBV and receive a needlestick or mucous membrane contact with blood or other body secretions should contact their occupational health department. Hepatitis B virus immune globulin (HBIg) can be given to provide temporary protection.

ANTIGENS AND ANTIBODIES: The primary antigenic markers used to diagnose hepatitis B infection include the following:

1. Hepatitis B surface antigen (HBsAg)—the first marker to appear in the blood. It is sometimes detected before serum levels of hepatic enzymes rise.
2. Hepatitis Be antigen (HBeAg) and hepatitis B DNA—markers of active viral replication and high infectivity.

Protective IgG antibodies to the HB surface antigen (HBsAB), which develop late in the disease, persist for life and protect against reinfection. As hepatitis B surface antibody levels rise, HBsAg levels fall, indicating resolution of acute infection. Antibodies against hepatitis B core antigen, and hepatitis Be antigen are not protective. Approx. 5% to 10% of patients develop chronic infection.

PREVENTION: Hepatitis B vaccine, which contains the HB surface antigen, provides active immunity and is recommended for persons at increased risk (e.g., children, health care workers, hemodialysis patients, intravenous drug abusers). Also, all pregnant women should be screened for infection. Hepatitis B immune globulin, which contains antibodies against HBV, provides passive immunity to those who have not been vaccinated and are exposed to the virus.

TREATMENT: No drug therapy is available that controls acute HBV infection, so treatment for this phase of the illness is supportive. Alpha interferon has been effective in some patients with chronic infection; some antiviral drugs, including lamivudine and ganciclovir, have also been shown to have some beneficial effect, esp. when given until HBsAB levels rise or HBeAg levels fall.

h. B core antigen ABBR: HBcAg. A protein marker found on the core of the hepatitis B virus (HBV). It does not circulate in the blood but is found only in liver cells that have been infected by HBV. HBcAg stimulates the production of a protective antibody, immunoglobulin M (IgM-anti-HBc), which appears in the blood shortly before the onset of symptoms. Tests for this antibody are used with other blood tests in the diagnosis of acute and chronic hepatitis B infection. During the convalescent stage of hepatitis B infection, IgM anti-HBc is replaced by another antibody, IgG anti-HBc, which remains in the blood for years. SEE: *hepatitis B e antigen; hepatitis B surface antigen.*

h. B e antigen ABBR: HBeAg. A polypeptide from the hepatitis B viral core that circulates by itself in the blood of infected persons and indicates that the patient is highly infectious. It is released when viral DNA is actively replicating.

h. B immune globulin ABBR: HBIG. A sterilized solution of antibodies against hepatitis B surface antigen obtained from plasma of human donors who have high titers of antibodies. It provides passive immunity against infection for persons who have not been vaccinated and are exposed to HBV. HBIG is derived from the plasma of HBV carriers who have high titers of antibodies solution. SEE: *h. B; hepatitis B virus vaccine.*

h. B surface antigen ABBR: HBsAg. The glycoprotein found on the surface of the hepatitis B viral envelope. It is the first marker of infection with the hepatitis B virus. If HBsAg is present in the blood after 6 months, the person is chronically infected and can transmit the infection to others. SEE: *h. B core antigen; h. Be antigen.*

h. B virus vaccine A recombinant vaccine used to vaccinate children and persons at high risk for coming in contact with either hepatitis B carriers or blood or fluids from such individuals. It contains noninfectious hepatitis B surface antigen (HBsAg), which stimulates the production of antibodies and provides active immunity. Included in the high-risk group are health care workers, hemodialysis patients, police officers and other public safety workers, persons with other forms of chronic hepatitis, injection drug users, family members and sexual partners of those infected with HBV, and persons who travel extensively abroad. SEE: *hepatitis B immune globulin.*

h. C A chronic blood-borne infection that affects about 4,000,000 people in the U.S. Hepatitis C (formerly known as non-A, non-B hepatitis) is caused by a single-stranded RNA virus that is transmitted from person to person by exposure to blood or body fluids. In the past it was the most common form of hepatitis transmitted by transfusions of blood or blood products and by organ transplantation.

About 28,000 new cases occur each year in the U.S., most of which result from needle sharing during injection drug abuse. A smaller number of infections are acquired as a result of exposure to tainted blood at work (e.g., in health care). About 6% of cases are the result of the transmission of the virus from mother to child during childbirth. Tattooing, body piercing, and intranasal cocaine abuse are associated with some cases. Sexual transmission of the virus (for example, between married couples) seems to occur rarely. The incubation period is usually 6-12 weeks, although it can be longer, and the acute phase lasts approx. 4 weeks. Signs and symptoms of acute infection are often milder than with hepatitis A and B. Approx. 75% to 85% of patients develop chronic hepatitis. Twenty to thirty years after initial infection, there is an increased risk of cirrhosis of liver (occurring in about 20% of the infected) and liver cancer (in about 1-5%).

Infection with hepatitis C virus (HCV) usually is identified when an asymptomatic person is found to have repeatedly elevated liver enzymes on routine blood tests. Antibodies to HCV, or HCV RNA in the blood, confirm the infection. Antibody production is stimulated by HCV RNA, but antibodies against HCV do not destroy the virus or provide immunity.

Antiviral agents, such as interferon alfa (given by injection several times a week) in combination with ribavirin can cure hepatitis C, if given for prolonged courses (e.g., more than a year) to patients who have susceptible viral genotypes. Genotype 1, the type most often found in the U.S., is not very responsive to treatment. Genotypes 2 and 3 respond to combination therapy more than 40% of the time. The treatment can cause significant side effects, including high fevers, chills, malaise, muscle aches, and other flu-like symptoms.

chronic h. Hepatic inflammatory and necrotic changes that continue for more than 6 months. The most common causes are hepatitis B, C, and D viruses. Chronic liver inflammation may also result from abuse of alcohol or other drugs, exposure to toxic chemicals, or autoimmune processes. Patients may be asymptomatic or present with only elevated serum transaminase, fatigue, anorexia, malaise, or mild jaundice. In other patients, the disease actively progresses, eventually leading to liver failure (cirrhosis) and death. Depending on the underlying cause, corticosteroids, alpha interferon, lamivudine (3TC), or other agents may be used to manage chronic hepatitis. In alcoholic patients, abstinence from alcohol may allow the liver to heal.

h. D A form of hepatitis caused by the hepatitis delta virus (HDV). It is considered a "defective" virus because it can produce infection only when hepatitis B virus (HBV) is present and therefore can be prevented through hepatitis B vaccination. It is rare in the U.S. In healthy people, coinfection with HDV and HBV usually causes acute disease and recovery with immunity. In patients with chronic hepatitis B, it may produce severe acute disease or, more commonly, chronic progressive disease that may lead to cirrhosis. Mortality is approx. 10%. Hepatitis D antigens (HDV RNA) are found in the blood and liver and stimulate production of an antibody that is present only briefly during early acute infection. Hepatitis D virus is also sometimes referred to as delta hepatitis. SEE: *hepatitis B*.

h. E A form of hepatitis similar to hepatitis A that occurs primarily in nations with contaminated water supplies, or in travelers returning from abroad. It is caused by an RNA virus which causes acute infection only.

fulminant h. The development of severe liver damage with encephalopathy within eight weeks of the onset of symptoms and jaundice. Coagulopathy, electrolyte imbalance, and cerebral edema are common. Death is likely without liver transplantation.

infectious h. Term previously used for hepatitis A virus infection.

serum h. Term previously used for hepatitis B virus infection.

toxic h. An inflammation of the liver caused by the entry of toxins or drugs into the body. Included in the great number of agents known to be able to cause this type of hepatitis are common drugs and chemicals (e.g., halothane, isoniazid, anabolic steroids, carbon tetrachloride, trichlorethylene) used in either the treatment of disease or in the workplace.

hepatization (hĕp″ă-tĭ-zā′shŭn) The second and third stages in consolidation in lobar pneumonia, in which the lung's surface looks solid, like the liver.

hepato-, hepat- [Gr. *hepatikos*] Combining form meaning *liver.*

hepatoblastoma (hĕp″ă-tō-blăs-tō′mă) [″ + *blastos,* germ, + *oma,* tumor] An aggressive malignant tumor of the liver, typically found in children age 3 or younger, consisting of epithelial cells or a mixture of epithelial and mesenchymal tissues.

hepatocarcinogen Anything that causes cancer of the liver.

hepatocarcinoma (hĕp″ă-tō-kăr″sĭn-ō′mă) [″ + *karkinos,* crab, + *oma,* tumor] Carcinoma of the liver.

hepatocele (hĕp′ă-tō-sēl) [+ *kele,* tumor, swelling] Hernia of the liver.

hepatocellular (hĕp″ă-tō-sĕl′ū-lăr) Concerning the cells of the liver.

hepatocholangiocystoduodenostomy (hĕp″ă-ō-kō-lăn″jē-ō-sĭs″tō-dū″ō-dĕ-nŏs′tō-mē) [″ + *chole,* bile, + *angeion,* vessel, + *kystis,* bladder, + L. *duodenum,* duodenum, + Gr. *stoma,* mouth] The establishment of drainage of bile ducts into the duodenum through the gallbladder.

hepatocholangioduodenostomy (hĕp″ă-tō-kō-lăn″jē-ō-dū-ō-dĕ-nŏs′tō-mē) [″ + ″ + ″ + L. *duodenum,* duodenum, + Gr. *stoma,* mouth] The establishment of drainage of (hepatic) bile ducts into the duodenum.

hepatocholangioenterostomy (hĕp″ă-tō-kō-lăn″jē-ō-ĕn″tĕr-ŏs′tō-mē) [″ + ″ + ″ + *enteron,* intestine, + *stoma,* mouth] The establishment of a passage between the hepatic bile ducts and intestine.

hepatocholangiogastrostomy (hĕp″ă-tō-kō-lăn″jē-ō-găs-trŏs′tō-mē) [″ + ″ + ″ + *gaster,* belly, + *stoma,* mouth] The establishment of drainage of bile ducts into the stomach.

hepatocholangiostomy (hĕp″ă-tō-kō-lăn-jē-ŏs′tō-mē) [″ + ″ + ″ + *stoma,* mouth] The establishment of free drainage by opening into the hepatic bile.

hepatocholangitis (hĕp″ă-tō-kō-lăn-jī′tis) [″ + ″ + ″ + *itis,* inflammation] An inflammation of the cells of the liver and bile ducts.

hepatocolic (hĕp″ă-tō-kŏl′ĭk) [″ + *kolon,* colon] Relating to the liver and colon.

hepatocystic (hĕp″ă-tō-sĭs′tĭk) [″ + *kystis,* bladder] Relating to the gallbladder or to both liver and gallbladder.

hepatocyte (hĕp′ă-tō-sīt) A parenchymal liver cell.

hepatoduodenostomy (hĕp″ă-tō-dū″ō-dĕ-nŏs′tō-mē) [″ + L. *duodenum,* duodenum, + Gr. *stoma,* mouth] The establishment of an opening from the hepatic bile duct into the duodenum. SYN: *hepaticoduodenostomy.*

hepatoenteric (hĕp″ă-tō-ĕn-tĕr′ĭk) [″ + *enteron,* intestine] Relating to the liver and intestines.

hepatogastric (hĕp″ă-tō-găs′trĭk) [Gr. *hepatikos,* liver, + *gaster,* belly] Relating to the liver and stomach.

hepatogenous (hĕp″ă-tŏj′ĕ-nŭs) Originating in the liver.

hepatography (hĕp″ă-tŏg′ră-fē) [″ + *graphein,* to write] Radiography of the liver, usually after injection of a radiographic contrast medium.

hepatojugular (hĕp″ă-tō-jŭg′ū-lăr) Concerning the liver and jugular vein.

hepatolenticular (hĕp″ă-tō-lĕn-tĭk′ū-lăr) [″ + L. *lenticula,* lentil, lens] Relating to the liver and lenticular nucleus of the eye.

hepatolienography (hĕp″ă-tō-lī″ĕ-nŏg′ră-fē) [″ + L. *lien,* spleen, + Gr. *graphein,* to write] Radiography of the liver and spleen, usually after intravenous injection of a contrast medium.

hepatolienomegaly (hĕp″ă-tō-lī″ĕ-nō-mĕg′ă-lē) [″ + ″ + *megas,* large] Hepatosplenography.

hepatolithectomy (hĕp″ă-tō-lĭ-thĕk′tō-mē) [″ + *lithos,* stone, + *ektome,* excision] The surgical removal of a stone from the hepatic duct.

hepatolithiasis (hĕp″ă-tō-lĭ-thī′ă-sĭs) [″ + ″ + *-iasis,* disease condition] A condition characterized by stones in the intrahepatic ducts.

hepatologist (hĕp″ă-tŏl′ō-jĭst) [″ + *logos,* word, reason] A specialist in diseases of the liver.

hepatology (hĕp″ă-tŏl′ō-jē) [″ + *logos,* word, reason] The study of the liver.

hepatolytic (hĕp″ă-tō-lĭt′ĭk) Destructive to tissues of the liver.

hepatoma (hĕp″ă-tō′mă) [″ + *oma,* tumor] Any liver tumor, benign or malignant. The term is usually used to describe a hepatocellular carcinoma.

hepatomalacia (hĕp″ă-tō-mă-lā′sē-ă) [″ + *malakia,* softening] A softening of the liver.

hepatomegaly (hĕp″ă-tō-mĕg′ă-lē) [″ + *megas,* large] An enlargement of the liver.

hepatomelanosis (hĕp″ă-tō-mĕl″ă-nō′sĭs) [″ + *melas,* black, + *osis,* condition] Pigmented deposits or melanosis in the liver.

hepatomphalocele (hĕp″ă-tŏm′fă-lō-sēl″) [Gr. *hepatikos,* liver, + *omphalos,* navel, + *kele,* tumor, swelling] The protrusion of a part of the liver, which is covered by a membrane, through the umbilicus.

hepatonecrosis (hĕp″ă-tō-nĕ-krō′sĭs) [″ + *nekrosis,* state of death] Gangrene of the liver.

hepatonephric (hĕp″ă-tō-nĕf′rĭk) [″ + *nephros,* kidney] Concerning the liver and kidney.

hepatonephritis (hĕp″ă-tō-nĕ-frī′tĭs) [″ + ″ + *itis,* inflammation] An inflammation of the liver and kidneys.

hepatonephromegaly (hĕp″ă-tō-nĕf″rō-mĕg′ă-lē) [″ + ″ + *megas,* large] Hypertrophy of the liver and kidneys.

hepatoperitonitis (hĕp″ă-tō-pĕr″ĭ-tō-nī′tĭs) [″ + *peritonaion,* peritoneum, + *itis,* inflammation] Perihepatitis.

hepatopexy (hĕp′ă-tō-pĕks″ē) [″ + *pexis,* fixation] Fixation of a movable liver to the abdominal wall.

hepatopleural (hĕp″ă-tō-ploo′răl) [″ + *pleura,* side] Concerning the liver and pleura.

hepatopneumonic (hĕp″ă-tō-nū-mŏn′ĭk) [″ + *pneumonikos,* of the lungs] Hepatopulmonary.

hepatoportogram (hĕp″ă-tō-por′tō-grăm) A radiograph of the portal vein and its hepatic branches after injection of a contrast medium.

hepatoptosia, hepatoptosis (hĕp″ă-tŏp-tō′sē-ă, -tō′sĭs) [″ + *ptosis,* a dropping] A downward displacement of the liver.

hepatopulmonary (hĕp″ă-tō-pŭl′mō-năr″ē) [″ + L. *pulmo,* lung] Relating to the liver and lungs. SYN: *hepatopneumonic.*

hepatorenal (hĕp″ă-tō-rē′năl) [″ + L. *renalis,* kidney] Pert. to the liver and kidneys.

hepatorrhaphy (hĕp-ă-tor′ă-fē) [″+ *rhaphe,* seam, ridge] The suturing of a wound of the liver.

hepatorrhexis (hĕp″ă-tō-rĕks′ĭs) [″ + *rhexis,* rupture] A rupture of the liver.

hepatoscan (hĕp′ă-tō-skăn) A radioautograph of the liver.

hepatoscopy [″ + *skopein,* to examine] Inspection of the liver.

hepatosplenitis (hĕp″ă-tō-splĕ-nī′tĭs) [″ + *splen,* spleen, + *itis,* inflammation] An inflammation of the liver and spleen.

hepatosplenography (hĕp″ă-tō-splĕ-nŏg′ră-fē) [″ + ″ + *graphein,* to write] An obsolete radiographic examination of the liver and spleen usually after intravenous injection of a contrast medium. It has been replaced by computed tomography and magnetic resonance imaging.

hepatosplenomegaly (hĕp″ă-tō-splē″nō-mĕg′ă-lē) [″ + ″ + *megas,* large] An enlargement of the liver and spleen.

hepatosplenopathy (hĕp″ă-tō-splĕ-nŏp′ă-thē) [″ + ″ + *pathos,* disease, suffering] A disease that affects the liver and spleen.

hepatotherapy (hĕp″ă-tō-thĕr′ă-pē) [″ + *therapeia,* treatment] **1.** The treatment of liver disease. **2.** The use of liver or liver extract.

hepatotomy (hĕp″ă-tŏt′ō-mē) [″ + *tome,* incision] An incision into the liver.

hepatotoxemia (hĕp″ă-tō-tŏks-ē′mē-ă) [″ + *toxikon,* poison, + *haima,* blood] Autointoxication due to malfunctioning of the liver.

hepatotoxic Toxic to the liver.

hepatotoxin (hĕp″ă-tō-tŏk′sĭn) A cytotoxin specific for liver cells.

heptachromic (hĕp″tă-krō′mĭk) [Gr. *hepta,* seven, + *chroma,* color] Possessing normal color vision.

heptapeptide (hĕp″tă-pĕp′tīd) [″+ *peptein,* to digest] A polypeptide containing seven amino acids.

heptaploidy (hĕp′tă-ploy″dē) [″+ *ploos,* fold] Having seven sets of chromosomes.

heptose (hĕp′tōs) Any sugar containing seven carbon atoms in its molecule.

heptosuria (hĕp″tō-sū′rē-ă) [″+ *ouron,* urine] Heptose in the urine.

herb (ĕrb) [L. *herba,* grass] An annual, biennial, or perennial plant with a soft stem containing little wood, esp. an aromatic plant used in medicine or seasoning. The plant usually produces seeds and then dies back at the end of the growing season.

herbalist One who attempts to promote healing or health through the use of herbs.

herbicide A substance (such as a chemical) that kills plants or inhibits plant growth.

h. poisoning Poisoning due to the use of a toxic herbicide such as 2,4-D.

herbivorous (hĕr-bĭv′ō-rŭs) [″ + *vorare,* to eat] Vegetarian.

herd [AS. *heord*] Any large aggregation of people or animals.

hereditary (hĕ-rĕd′ĭ-tĕr-ē) [L. *hereditarius,* an heir] Pert. to a genetic characteristic transmitted from parent to offspring. SEE: *chromosome; gene.*

heredity (hĕ-rĕd′ĭ-tē) [L. *hereditas,* heir] The transmission of genetic characteristics from parent to offspring.

heredo- [L. *hereditas,* heir] Prefix meaning *heredity.*

heredoataxia (hĕr″ĕ-dō-ă-tăks′ē-ă) [″ + Gr. *ataxia,* lack of order] Friedreich's ataxia.

heredodegeneration (hĕr″ĕ-dō-dē-jĕn″ĕr-ā′shŭn) An inherited degeneration caused by defective or diseased hyaloplasm. It is seen in Marie's ataxia.

heredofamilial (hĕr″ĕ-dō-fă-mĭl′ē-ăl) Referring to any disease that occurs in families owing to an inherited defect.

Hering, Heinrich Ewald German physiologist, 1866–1948.

H.'s nerves Afferent nerve fibers leading from the carotid sinus by way of the glossopharyngeal nerve to the brain. They are pressoreceptor nerves responding to changes in blood pressure that reflexly control heart rate. An increase in pressure diminishes heart rate.

H.'s reflex A reflex inhibition of inspiration resulting from stimulation of pressoreceptors by inflation of the lungs.

heritable Able to be inherited.

heritage The genetic and other characteristics transmitted to offspring.

hermaphrodism (hĕr-măf′rō-dĭzm) Hermaphroditism.

hermaphrodite (hĕr-măf′rō-dīt) [Gr. *Hermaphroditos,* mythical son of Hermes and Aphrodite, who was man and woman combined] An individual possessing genital and sexual characteristics of both sexes. The clitoris is usually enlarged, resembling the male penis. SYN: *androgyne.*

hermaphroditism (hĕr-măf′rō-dīt-ĭzm) A condition in which both ovarian and testicular tissue exist in the same individual, occurring rarely in humans. SYN: *hermaphrodism.* SEE: *intersex.*

bilateral h. A condition in which an ovary and testicle are present on both sides.

complex h. A form of hermaphroditism in which the person has internal and external organs of both sexes.

dimidiate h. Lateral h.

false h. Pseudohermaphroditism.

lateral h. A condition in which a testis is present on one side and an ovary on the other. SYN: *dimidiate h.*

transverse h. Hermaphroditism characterized by having the outward organs of one sex and the internal organs of the other.

true h. Hermaphroditism in which the individual possesses both ovarian and testicular glands.

unilateral h. Hermaphroditism in which an ovary and a testis or an ovotestis is present on one side and either an ovary or a testis is present on the other side.

hermetic (hĕr-mĕt′ĭk) [L. *hermeticus*] Airtight.

hernia (hĕr′nē-ă) [L.] The protrusion of an anatomical structure through the wall that normally contains it. SYN: *rupture* (2). SEE: *herniotomy*.

ETIOLOGY: Hernias may be caused by congenital defects in the formation of body structures, defects in collagen synthesis and repair, trauma, or surgery. Conditions that increase intra-abdominal pressures (e.g., pregnancy, obesity, weight lifting, straining [the Valsalva maneuver], and abdominal tumors) may also contribute to hernia formation.

TREATMENT: Surgical or mechanical reduction is the treatment of choice.

abdominal h. A hernia through the abdominal wall.

acquired h. A hernia that develops any time after birth in contrast to one that is present at birth (congenital hernia). This type of hernia is usually the result of excessive strain on the muscular wall, frequently occurring following injuries or operations.

bladder h. The protrusion of the bladder or part of the bladder through a normal or abnormal orifice. SYN: *cystic h.*

Cloquet's h. A type of femoral hernia. SEE: *femoral h.*

complete h. A hernia in which the sac and its contents have passed through the aperture.

concealed h. A hernia that is imperceptible by palpation.

congenital h. A hernia existing from birth.

crural h. A hernia that protrudes behind the femoral sheath.

cystic h. Bladder h.

diaphragmatic h. Herniation of abdominal contents into the thoracic cavity through an opening in the diaphragm. This may cause respiratory distress or strangulation and gangrene of the fundus of the stomach. The condition may be congenital, acquired (traumatic), or esophageal. In the latter, a portion of the stomach is pushed through the esophageal hiatus into the pleural cavity.

direct inguinal h. Inguinal h.

diverticular h. The protrusion of an intestinal congenital diverticulum.

encysted h. A scrotal protrusion that, enveloped in its own sac, passes into the tunica vaginalis.

epigastric h. A hernia usually composed of fatty tissue through a defect in the linea alba above the umbilicus.

fascial h. Protrusion of muscular tissue through its fascial covering.

fatty h. The protrusion of fatty tissue through the abdominal wall.

femoral h. Any hernia into the femoral canal.

hiatal h. The protrusion of the stomach upward into the chest through the esophageal hiatus of the diaphragm. SEE: illus.; *Nursing Diagnoses Appendix*.

incarcerated h. A hernia in which the presenting content cannot be returned to its site of origin, e.g., a hernia in which a segment of intestine cannot be returned to the abdominal cavity causing pain or obstruction, or if untreated leads to strangulation.

incisional h. A hernia through a surgical scar.

incomplete h. A hernia that has not gone completely through the aperture.

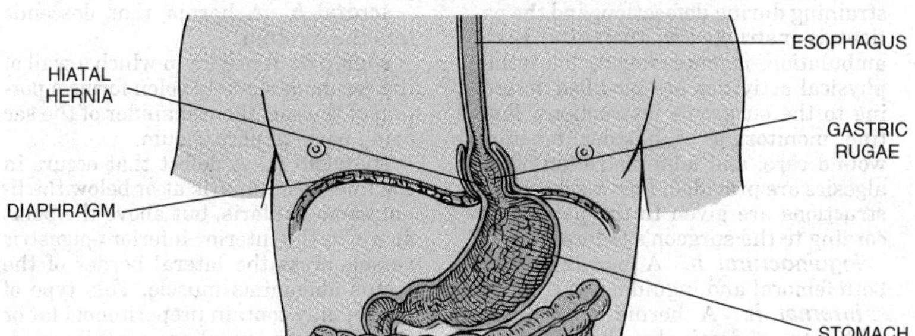

HIATAL HERNIA

indirect inguinal h. Inguinal h.

inguinal h. The protrusion of a hernial sac containing intraperitoneal contents (e.g., intestine, omentum, ovary, etc.) at the superficial inguinal ring. In an indirect inguinal hernia, the sac protrudes through the internal inguinal ring into the inguinal canal, often descending into the scrotum. In a direct inguinal hernia, the sac protrudes through the abdominal wall within Hesselbach's triangle, a region bounded by the rectus abdominus muscle, inguinal ligament, and inferior epigastric vessels. A variety of indirect inguinal hernia is the sliding hernia, in which a portion of the wall of the protruding cecum or sigmoid colon is part of the sac, the remainder, comprised of parietal peritoneum. Indirect and direct inguinal hernias and femoral hernias are collectively referred to as groin hernias. Inguinal hernias account for about 80% of all hernias. SYN: *direct inguinal h.; indirect inguinal h.; lateral h.; medial h.; oblique h.*

PATIENT CARE: *Preoperative:* The surgical procedure and expected postoperative course are explained to the patient; this discussion should be geared to the patient's age, level of comprehension, type of hernia, and planned repair. A signed consent form is obtained. The patient should understand that the surgery will repair the defect caused by the hernia, but that surgical failures can occur. If the patient is undergoing elective surgery, recovery usually is rapid; if no complications occur, the patient probably will return home the same day as surgery and usually can resume normal activity within 4 to 6 weeks. Patients who undergo emergency surgery for a strangulated or incarcerated hernia may remain hospitalized longer commensurate with the degree of intestinal involvement. The patient is prepared for surgery.

Postoperative: Vital signs are monitored. The patient is instructed on the changing of position to avoid undue stress on the wound area. Stool softeners may be administered to prevent straining during defecation, and the patient is instructed in their use. Early ambulation is encouraged, but other physical activities are modified according to the surgeon's instructions. Routine monitoring of bladder function, wound care, and administration of analgesics are provided. Post discharge instructions are given to the patient according to the surgeon's orders.

inguinocrural h. A hernia that is both femoral and inguinal.

internal h. A hernia that occurs within the abdominal cavity. It may be intraperitoneal or retroperitoneal.

interstitial h. A form of inguinal hernia in which the hernial sac lies between the layers of the abdominal muscles.

irreducible h. A hernia that cannot be returned to its original position out of its sac by manual methods. SEE: *incarcerated h.*

labial h. The protrusion of a loop of bowel or other intraperitoneal organ into the labium majus.

lateral h. Inguinal h.

lumbar h. A hernia through the inferior lumbar triangle (Petit) or the superior lumbar triangle (Grynfelt).

medial h. Inguinal h.

mesocolic h. A hernia between the layers of the mesocolon.

Nuckian h. A hernia into the canal of Nuck.

oblique h. Inguinal h.

obturator h. A hernia through the obturator foramen.

omental h. A hernia containing a portion of the omentum.

ovarian h. The presence of an ovary in a hernial sac.

perineal h. Perineocele.

phrenic h. A hernia projecting through the diaphragm into one of the pleural cavities.

posterior vaginal h. A hernia of Douglas' sac downward between the rectum and posterior vaginal wall. SYN: *enterocele* (2).

properitoneal h. A hernia located between the parietal peritoneum and the transversalis fascia.

reducible h. A hernia that can be replaced by manipulation.

retroperitoneal h. A hernia protruding into the retroperitoneal space, e.g., duodenojejunal hernia, Treitz's hernia.

Richter's h. A hernia in which only a portion of intestinal wall protrudes, the main portion of the intestine being excluded from the hernial sac and the lumen remaining open. The patient may present with groin swelling and vague abdominal complaints; when incarcerated or strangulated, the hernia may produce considerable bowel injury or occasionally death, if it is not properly and promptly diagnosed.

scrotal h. A hernia that descends into the scrotum.

sliding h. A hernia in which a wall of the cecum or sigmoid colon forms a portion of the sac, the remainder of the sac being parietal peritoneum.

spigelian h. A defect that occurs in the linea semilunaris at or below the linea semicircularis, but above the point at which the interior inferior epigastric vessels cross the lateral border of the rectus abdominis muscle. This type of hernia may contain preperitoneal fat or may be a peritoneal sac containing intraperitoneal contents. It is rare and difficult to diagnose unless large, because it is typically not palpable when small. Large spigelian hernias may be mistaken for sarcomas of the abdominal wall. Ultrasonography or computed tomography scans are often used in diagnosis.

TREATMENT: Small spigelian hernias are easily repaired; larger ones may require a prosthesis.

PATIENT CARE: After reparative surgery, the patient must void before being discharged.

CAUTION: Patients should be advised not to lift heavy items or to strain in any way.

---

strangulated h. A hernia in which the protruding viscus is so tightly trapped that gangrene results, requiring prompt surgery. Once strangulation of the contents occurs, a non-surgical attempt to reduce it may severely compromise treatment and outcome.

umbilical h. A hernia occurring at the navel, seen mostly in children. Usually it requires no therapy.

uterine h. The presence of the uterus in the hernial sac.

vaginal h. The hernial protrusion of the vaginal wall into the surrounding area, usually the pouch of Douglas.

vaginolabial h. A hernia of a viscus into the posterior end of the labium majus.

ventral h. A hernia through the abdominal wall. SEE: *incisional h.*

hernial (hĕr′nē-ăl) [L. *hernia,* rupture] Pert. to a hernia.

herniated Enclosed in or protruding like a hernia.

herniation (hĕr-nē-ā′shŭn) The displacement of body tissue through an opening or defect.

cerebral h. Downward displacement of the brain (usually as a result of cerebral edema, hematoma, or tumor) into the brainstem. The resulting injury to brainstem functions rapidly leads to coma, nerve palsies, and death if treatment is ineffective.

h. of nucleus pulposus Prolapse of the nucleus pulposus of a ruptured intervertebral disk into the spinal canal. This often results in pressure on a spinal nerve, which causes lower back pain that may radiate down the leg, a condition known as sciatica. SEE: illus.; *Nursing Diagnoses Appendix.*

PATIENT CARE: A history is obtained of any unilateral low back pain that radiates to the buttocks, legs, and feet. When herniation follows trauma, the patient may report sudden pain, subsiding in a few days; then a dull, aching sciatic pain in the buttocks that increases with Valsalva's maneuver, coughing, sneezing, or bending. The patient may also complain of muscle spasms accompanied by pain that subsides with rest. The health care professional inspects for a limited ability to bend forward, a posture favoring the affected side, and decreased deep tendon reflexes in the lower extremity. In later stages, muscle atrophy may be observed. Palpation may disclose tenderness over the region. Tissue tension assessment may reveal radicular pain from straight leg raising (with lumbar herniation) and increased pain from neck movement (with cervical herniation). Thorough assessment of the patient's peripheral vascular status, including posterior tibial and dorsalis pedis pulses and skin temperature of the arms and legs, may help to rule out ischemic disease as the cause of leg numbness or pain.

The patient is prepared for diagnostic testing by explaining all procedures and expected sensations. Tests may include radiographic studies of the spine (to show degenerative changes and rule out other abnormalities), myelography (to pinpoint the level of herniation), computed tomography scanning (to detect bone and soft tissue abnormalities and possibly show spinal compression resulting from the herniation), magnetic resonance imaging (to define tissues in areas otherwise obscured by bone), electromyography (to confirm nerve involvement by measuring the electrical activity of muscles innervated by the affected nerves), and neuromuscular testing (to detect sensory and motor loss as well as leg muscle weakness). If the patient will undergo myelography, a history of allergies to iodides, iodine-containing substances, or seafood is obtained, because such allergies may indicate sensitivity to the radiopaque contrast agent used in the test. Prescribed sedation is administered before the test, fluid intake is encouraged before and after the test, intake and output are monitored, the patient is positioned with the head elevated, and the patient is observed for allergic reactions and seizure activity.

Pain status is monitored, prescribed analgesics are administered, the patient is taught about noninvasive pain relief measures (such as relaxation, transcutaneous nerve stimulation, distraction, heat or ice application, traction, bracing, or positioning), and the patient's response to the treatment regimen is evaluated. During conservative treatment, neurological status is monitored (esp. in the first 24 hr after beginning treatment) for signs of deterioration, which may indicate a need for emergency surgery. Neurovascular assessments of the patient's affected and unaffected extremities (both legs or both arms) are performed to check color, motion, temperature, sensation, and pulses. Vital signs are monitored, bowel

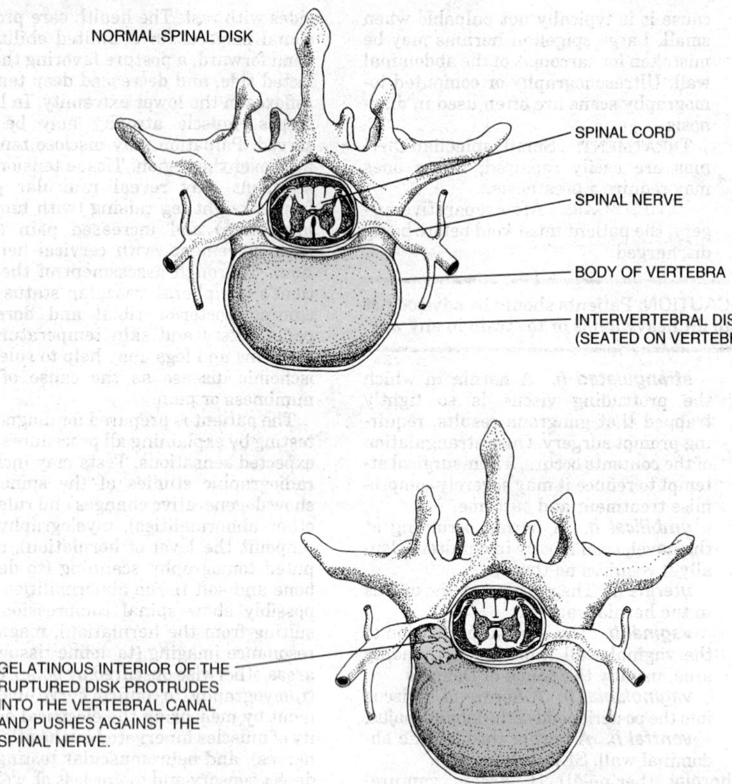

NORMAL AND HERNIATED SPINAL DISKS

sounds are auscultated, and the abdomen is inspected for distention. The disorder and the various treatment options are explained to the patient, including bedrest and pelvic (or cervical) traction, local heat application, an exercise program, antispasmodic and anti-inflammatory drug therapy, and surgery.

Both the patient and family are encouraged to express their concerns about the disorder; questions are answered honestly, and support and encouragement are offered to assist the patient and family to cope with the frustration of impaired mobility and the discomfort of chronic back pain. The patient is encouraged to perform self-care to the extent that immobility and pain allow, to take analgesics before activities, and to allow adequate time to perform activities at a comfortable pace. Assistance is provided to help the patient to identify and perform care activities that promote rest and relaxation.

Antiembolism stockings or medications are applied as prescribed, leg movement and exercises are encouraged as permitted, and a foot board or right-angle foam and Velcro foot support are provided as necessary to prevent footdrop. The health care team works together to ensure a consistent regimen of leg- and back-strengthening exercises. If the patient is restricted to bedrest (or in traction), the patient should increase fluid intake and use incentive spirometry to avoid pulmonary complications. Skin care and a fracture bedpan are provided if the patient is not permitted bathroom or commode privileges.

As necessary, the patient is prepared physically and emotionally for surgery (e.g., laminectomy, spinal fusion, or microdiskectomy) according to institutional or surgeon's protocol, and a signed informed consent form is obtained. After microdiskectomy, bedrest is enforced for the prescribed period, the blood drainage system in use is managed, and the amount and color of drainage is documented. Any colorless moisture or excessive drainage should be reported; the former may indicate cerebrospinal fluid leakage. A log-rolling technique is used to turn the patient from side to side. Analgesics are administered as prescribed, esp. 30 min before early attempts at sitting or walking. The health care professional assists the patient with prescribed mobilization, provides a straight-backed chair, and explains any restrictions.

Before discharge, proper body mechanics are reviewed with the patient: bending at the knees and hips (never the waist), standing straight, and carrying objects close to the body. The patient is advised to lie down when tired and to sleep on the side (never on the abdomen) on an extra-firm mattress or a bed board. All prescribed medications are reviewed, including dosage schedules, desired actions, and adverse reactions to be reported. Referral for home health care or occupational therapy may be necessary to help the patient manage activities of daily living.

tonsillar h. The protrusion of the cerebellar tonsils through the foramen magnum. It causes pressure on the medulla oblongata and may be fatal.

transtentorial h. A herniation of the uncus and adjacent structures into the incisure of the tentorium of the brain. It is caused by increased pressure in the cranium. SYN: *uncal h.*

uncal h. Transtentorial h.

hernioenterotomy (hĕr″nē-ō-ĕn″tĕr-ŏt′ō-mē) [″ + Gr. *enteron,* intestine, + *tome,* incision] Herniotomy and enterotomy done during the same surgical procedure.

herniography (hĕr″nē-ŏg′ră-fē) [″ + Gr. *graphein,* to write] The radiographical examination of a hernia after the introduction of a contrast medium.

hernioid (hĕr′nē-oyd) [″ + Gr. *eidos,* form, shape] Resembling a hernia.

herniolaparotomy (hĕr″nē-ō-lăp″ă-rŏt′ō-mē) [″ + Gr. *lapara,* loin, + *tome,* incision] Abdominal surgery for the treatment of hernia.

hernioplasty (hĕr′nē-ō-plăs″tē) [″ + Gr. *plassein,* to form] Surgical repair of a hernia.

herniopuncture (hĕr″nē-ō-pŭnk′chŭr) [″ + *punctura,* prick] The puncture of a hernia with a hollow needle to withdraw fluid or gas.

herniorrhaphy (hĕr-nē-or′ă-fē) [″ + Gr. *rhaphe,* seam, ridge] A surgical procedure for repair of a hernia.

herniotomy (hĕr-nē-ŏt′ō-mē) [″ + Gr. *tome,* incision] Surgery for the relief of hernia; an operation for the correction of irreducible hernia, esp. strangulated hernia.

heroic measures In medical practice, the undertaking of a procedure or therapy in an attempt to save or sustain a patient's life.

heroin (hĕr′ō-ĭn) An opioid derived from morphine, whose importation, sale, and use are illegal in the U.S. SYN: *diacetylmorphine.* SEE: *drug addiction; endorphin.*

black tar h. A form of illicitly manufactured diacetylmorphine known for its tarry appearance and increased potency relative to "white" heroin.

h. toxicity Poisoning by heroin. SEE: *opiate poisoning* .

heroinism (hĕr′ō-ĭn-ĭzm) [*heroin* + Gr. *-ismos,* condition] An addiction to heroin use. SEE: *drug addiction.*

herpangina (hĕrp-ăn-jī′nă, -ăn′jĭ-nă) [Gr. *herpes,* creeping skin disease, + L. *angina,* a choking] A benign infectious disease of children and, less commonly, of young adults, caused by one of several strains of group A coxsackievirus and rarely other enteroviruses. Epidemics occur worldwide, most often in summer and early fall.

SYMPTOMS: This disease is marked by sudden onset of fever, severe sore throat, nausea, vomiting, excess salivation, and malaise. The throat and posterior area of the mouth are covered with vesicles 1 to 2 mm in diameter that rupture and form ulcers.

TREATMENT: The treatment is symptomatic and supportive. There is no specific therapy, but recovery is prompt, usually within 3 to 6 days.

herpes (hĕr′pēz) [Gr. *herpes,* creeping skin disease] Vesicular eruption caused by a virus, esp. herpes simplex or herpes zoster. SEE: *Nursing Diagnoses Appendix.*

h. corneae An inflammation of the cornea caused by herpesvirus.

h. facialis A form of herpes simplex that occurs on the face.

h. febrilis Herpes simplex of the lips and nasal mucosa.

genital h. A persistent, recurring eruption of the genital or anorectal skin or mucous membranes, caused by herpes simplex virus (usually herpes simplex virus 2). It usually is spread by intimate contact and is classified as a sexually transmitted disease. Worldwide about 85 to 90 million people are infected. SEE: illus.

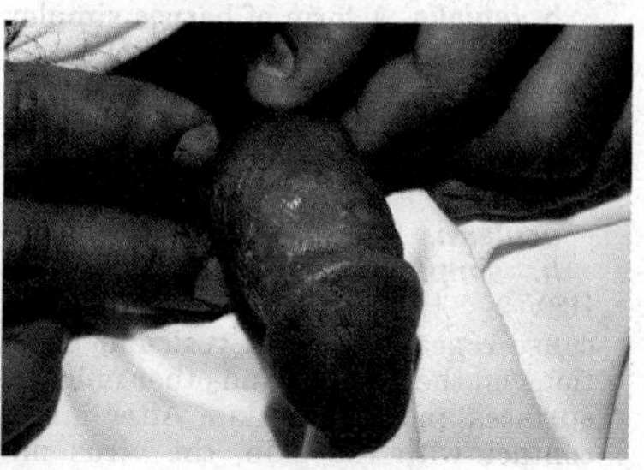

GENITAL HERPES

SYMPTOMS: Patients often experience local pain, itching, burning, dysuria, or other uncomfortable sensations that sometimes begin before a rash appears on the skin. The rash consists of a reddened patch, dotted by small blisters (vesicles) or pustules. It typically takes about 10 days to heal. Systemic symptoms (such as fever and malaise) sometimes accompany the initial outbreak or recurrences. However, asymptomatic shedding of the virus is common, and may represent the most common way in which the virus is transmitted from person to person.

POTENTIAL COMPLICATIONS: Genital herpes may be transmitted to the newborn during childbirth and may cause serious complications, including respiratory illnesses, retinal infection, or encephalitis. Cesarean delivery or maternal suppression of the virus with acyclovir are two methods used to prevent newborn infection.

TREATMENT: Oral acyclovir or its derivatives can treat both the initial outbreak and subsequent recurrences, as well as diminish asymptomatic viral shedding.

CAUTION: The lesions are highly contagious, and persons caring for the patient must avoid contact with the exudates. SEE: *Standard and Universal Precautions Appendix.*

PATIENT CARE: Patients with genital herpes often experience anger, self-doubt, fear, or guilt, esp. at the time of initial diagnosis or during recurrences. Counseling and support may help the patient address these issues. Patient education improves understanding of the prevalence of the disease in the general population, the recurring nature of the eruption, safe sexual practices, and medication use, as well as psychosocial and relationship issues.

human h. virus 8 A herpesvirus thought to cause Kaposi's sarcoma. It has also been implicated in the pathogenesis of some lymphomas and lymphomatoid illnesses.

h. labialis A form of herpes simplex that occurs on the lips. SYN: *cold sore; fever blister*. SEE: illus.

h. menstrualis Herpetic lesions appearing at the time of the menstrual period.

ocular h. Herpes of the eye.

h. simplex virus ABBR: HSV-1, HSV-2. Human DNA viruses that cause repeated painful vesicular eruptions on the genitals and other mucosal surfaces and on the skin. After initial contact with the skin, the virus migrates along nerve fibers to sensory ganglia, where it establishes a latent infection. Under a variety of stimuli, such as sexual contact, exposure to ultraviolet light, febrile illnesses, or emotional stress, it may reappear, traveling back to the site of initial contact. The rash caused by the infection has a red base, on which small blisters cluster. SEE: illus; *Nursing Diagnoses Appendix.*

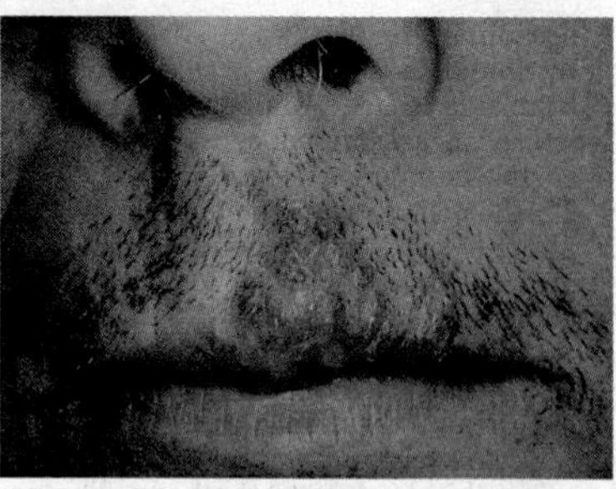

HERPES LABIALIS

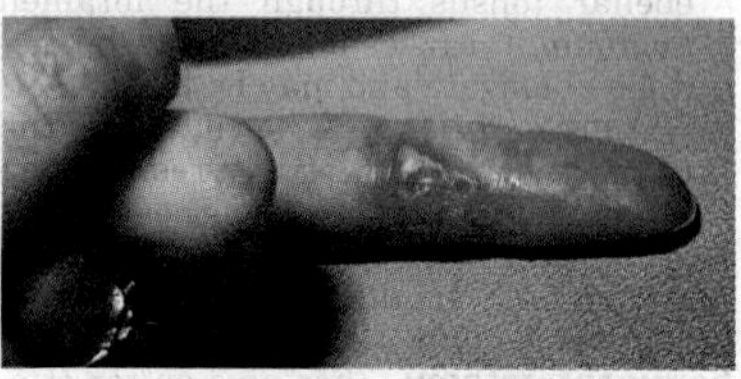

HERPES SIMPLEX

Herpetic whitlow

In immunosuppressed patients, the virus can cause a widely disseminated rash. Some infections with HSV may involve the brain and meninges; these typically cause fevers, headaches, altered mental status, seizures, or coma, requiring parenteral therapy with antiviral drugs. In newborns, infection involving the internal organs also may occur occasionally. Experienced ophthalmologists should manage ocular infection with herpes simplex viruses.

TREATMENT: Acyclovir and related drugs (e.g., famciclovir, valacyclovir) may be used to treat outbreaks of HSV 1 and 2, and are also effective in preventing disease recurrences.

PATIENT CARE: Prescribed antiviral agents and analgesics are administered; their use is explained to the patient, with instruction given about adverse effects to report. The patient's response to therapy is evaluated, and signs of complications are monitored. Adequate rest and nutrition are encouraged.

The patient with HSV-1 is instructed to avoid skin-to-skin contact with uninfected individuals when lesions are present or prodromal symptoms are felt. To decrease the discomfort from oral lesions, the patient is advised to use a soft toothbrush, a saline- or bicarbonate-based mouthwash, and oral anesthetics if necessary. He or she should eat soft foods. Use of lip balm with sunscreen reduces reactivation of oral lesions.

The patient with genital herpes should wash the hands carefully after bathroom use. He or she also should avoid sexual intercourse during the active stage of the disease, and should inform sexual partners of the condition. The female patient with HSV-2 should have a Pap smear yearly if results are normal, and more frequently as advised if results have been abnormal. The pregnant patient must be advised of the potential risk to the infant during vaginal delivery, and the use of cesarean delivery if she has an HSV outbreak when labor begins if her membranes have not ruptured. The patient may experience normal feelings of powerlessness; he or she requires assistance to identify coping mechanisms, strengths, and support resources. The patient with genital herpes is encouraged to voice feelings about perceived changes in sexuality and behavior, and is provided with current information about the disease and treatment options. A referral is made for additional counseling as appropriate.

CAUTION: Caregivers with active oral or cutaneous lesions should not care for patients in high risk groups until their lesions are crusted and dry. They should wear protective coverings including mask and gloves.

---

traumatic h. Herpes at a wound site.

h. zoster Reactivation of varicella virus years after the initial infection with chickenpox. It is marked by inflammation of the posterior root ganglia of only a few segments of the spinal or cranial peripheral nerves. A painful vesicular eruption occurs along the course of the nerve and almost always is unilateral. The trunk is the region most often affected, but the face also may be involved. The virus may cause meningitis or affect the optic nerve or hearing. Chickenpox (varicella zoster) virus incorporates itself into nerve cells and lies dormant there after patients recover from the initial infection. Normally, immunity is boosted by exposure to infected children; as more children are vaccinated against chickenpox, adult immunity against HZV is decreased.

The incubation period is from 7 to 21 days. The total duration of the disease from onset to complete recovery varies from 10 days to 5 weeks. If all the vesicles appear within 24 hr, the total duration is usually short. In general, the disease lasts longer in adults than in children. It is estimated that about 50% of people who live to age 80 will have an attack of herpes zoster. This infection is more common in persons with a compromised immune system: the elderly, those with AIDS or illnesses such as Hodgkin's disease and diabetes, those taking corticosteroids, or those undergoing cancer chemotherapy.

Pain often develops along affected skin and persists for months after resolution of the rash. This discomfort, which may be severe in patients older than 50, is known as postherpetic neuralgia. It may intensify at night or worsen when clothes rub against the skin. SYN: *shingles*. SEE: illus; *h. zoster ophthalmicus; Nursing Diagnoses Appendix.*

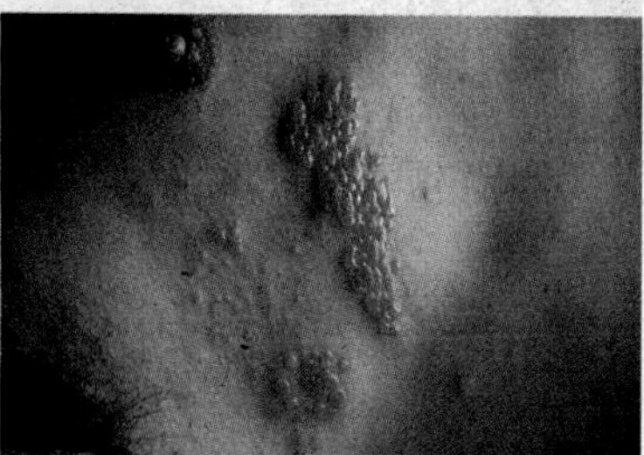

HERPES ZOSTER

TREATMENT: In healthy adults, acyclovir, famciclovir, and valacyclovir are effective in reducing viral shedding and nerve pain damage if administered within 3 days of onset of the rash. Corticosteroids, gabapentin, nonsteroidal anti-inflammatory drugs, tricyclic antidepressants, and narcotics may decrease the pain of postherpetic neuralgia. Itching may be reduced with colloidal oatmeal or other topical treatments. Capsaicin cream (an extract of hot chili peppers) may be applied topically for pain relief, but this should be done only after active lesions have subsided.

PATIENT CARE: The prescribed antiviral agent is administered and explained to the patient, along with information about desired and adverse effects. Skin lesions are inspected daily for signs of healing or secondary infection; the patient's response to treatment is evaluated regularly, and he or she is monitored for associated complications. Prescribed analgesics are given on a schedule to minimize neuralgic pain. Patients experiencing neuralgia following the acute stage of the disease should be referred for ongoing therapy. He or she is reassured that HSV pain will subside eventually, that the prognosis for complete recovery is good, and that the infection seldom recurs.

h. zoster ophthalmicus Herpes zoster affecting the first division of the fifth cranial nerve. The area of the face, eye, and nose supplied by this nerve is affected. Ocular complications may threaten sight. It is important that the eye be treated early with idoxuridine and that therapy be supervised by an ophthalmologist. SEE: illus.

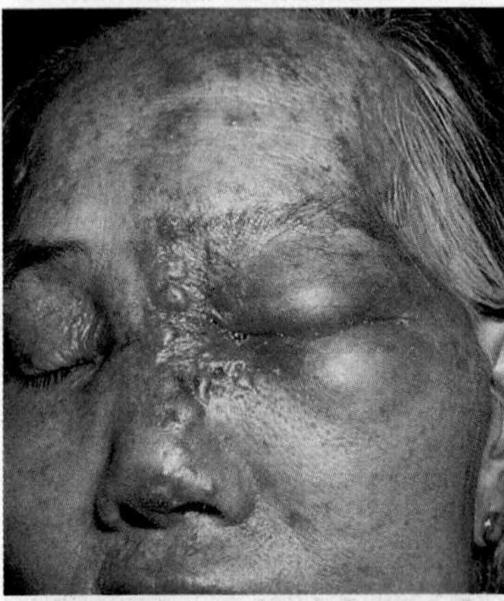

HERPES ZOSTER OPHTHALMICUS

herpesviruses A family, Herpesviridae, of structurally similar DNA viruses, many of which produce chronic infections, and some of which can transform normal cells to malignant ones. Included in this family are a number of viruses important to humans.

herpesvirus simian encephalomyelitis A severe, almost always fatal, encephalomyelitis caused by the herpesvirus simiae (also called B virus). It occurs among veterinarians, laboratory workers, and others who come in contact with infected monkeys.

herpetic (hĕr-pĕt′ĭk) [Gr. *herpes,* creeping skin disease] Pert. to herpes.

h. sore throat Herpetic tonsillitis.

herpetiform (hĕr-pĕt′ĭ-form) [″ + L. *forma,* form] Resembling herpes.

Herring bodies [Percy T. Herring, Brit. physiologist, 1872–1967] Neurosecretory granules in the pars nervosa of the pituitary in the terminal nerve endings of the hypothalamus and hypophyseal tract. The granules are thought to be a protein related to the hormones oxytocin and vasopressin.

hersage (ār-săzh′) [Fr., a harrowing] The splitting of a nerve trunk into separate fibers.

Herter's infantilism [Christian Archibald Herter, U.S. physician, 1865–1910] A form of infantilism resulting from defective fat and calcium absorption. It resembles sprue in adults. SEE: *celiac sprue.*

Hertwig's root sheath [Wilhelm August Oscar Hertwig, Ger. physiologist, 1849–1922] A downgrowth of epithelium from the cervical loop of the enamel organ that induces dentin formation of the forming tooth root and determines its shape. The epithelial diaphragm, a horizontal extension of the Hertwig's root sheath, will determine the number and size of the tooth roots.

hertz [Heinrich R. Hertz, Ger. physicist, 1857–1894] ABBR: Hz. A unit of frequency equal to 1 cycle/sec. (CPS)

hesitancy Involuntary delay in initiating urination. This symptom may be caused by drugs, such as tricyclic antidepressants, by abnormal relaxation of the detrusor muscle of the bladder, by prostatic hyperplasia, and other urinary tract disorders.

hesperidin (hĕs-pĕr′ĭ-dĭn) A bioflavonoid present in orange and lemon peel.

Hesselbach's hernia (hĕs′ĕl-bŏks) [Franz K. Hesselbach, Ger. surgeon, 1759–1816] A lobated hernia that passes through the cribriform fascia.

Hesselbach's triangle SEE: under *triangle.*

hetastarch A synthetic polymer plasma volume expander composed of more than 90% amylopectin molecules. It has an average molecular weight of 450,000. Trade name is Hespan. SEE: *fluid replacement.*

heter- SEE: *hetero-.*

heteradelphia (hĕt″ĕr-ă-dĕl′fē-ă) [Gr. *heteros,* other, + *adelphos,* brother] Congenitally joined fetuses in which one twin is more nearly developed than the other.

heteradenoma (hĕt″ĕr-ăd-ĕ-nō′mă) *pl.* **heteradenomata** [″ + *aden,* gland, + *oma,* tumor] A glandular tumor arising from an area that does not usually contain glands.

heterecious (hĕt″ĕr-ē′shŭs) [″ + *oikos,* house] Denoting a parasite living on different hosts at different stages of development. SYN: *metoxenous.*

heterecism (hĕt″ĕr-ē′sĭzm) The state of being heterecious; the development of different cycles of existence on different hosts, said of certain parasites.

heteresthesia (hĕt″ĕr-ĕs-thē′zē-ă) [″ + *aisthesis,* sensation] The variation in degree (plus or minus) of sensory response to cutaneous stimuli.

hetero-, heter- [Gr. *heteros,* other] Prefix indicating *different; relationship to another.*

heteroagglutination (hĕt″ĕr-ō-ă-gloo″tĭ-nā′shŭn) The agglutination by one animal's serum of the red blood cells of an animal of another species.

heteroagglutinin (hĕt″ĕr-ō-ă-glū′tĭ-nĭn) **1.** Agglutinin formed as the result of an injection of an antigen from an animal of a different species. **2.** Agglutinin capable of agglutinating blood cells of other species of animals.

heteroalbumose (hĕt″ĕr-ō-ăl′bū-mōs) [″ + L. *albumen,* white of egg] Albumose insoluble in water but soluble in saline solutions or in acid or alkaline solutions. SYN: *hemialbumose.*

heteroantibody (hĕt″ĕr-ō-ăn″tĭ-bŏd′ē) An antibody corresponding to an antigen from another species.

heteroantigen (hĕt″ĕr-ō-ăn′tĭ-jĕn) An antigen in one species that produces a corresponding antibody in another species.

heteroblastic (hĕt″ĕr-ō-blăs′tĭk) [″ + *blastos,* germ] Originating in tissue of another kind; the opposite of homoblastic.

heterocellular (hĕt″ĕr-ō-sĕl′ū-lăr) Composed of different kinds of cells.

heterocephalus (hĕt″ĕr-ō-sĕf′ă-lŭs) [″ + *kephale,* head] Congenitally deformed fetus with two heads of unequal size.

heterochiral (hĕt″ĕr-ō-kī′răl) [″ + *cheir,* hand] Reversed as to right and left, but otherwise of the same form and size; said of images in a plane mirror and of the hands.

heterochromatin (hĕt″ĕr-ō-krō′mă-tĭn) [″ + *chroma,* color] Highly condensed or folded portions of chromosomes during interphase. They stain less distinctly than euchromatin. There is apparently no transcription of the DNA by messenger RNA (mRNA); these portions may be inactive genes. SEE: *euchromatin.*

heterochromatosis (hĕt″ĕr-ō-krō-mă-tō′sĭs) [″ + ″ + *osis,* condition] **1.** A pigmentation of the skin from foreign substances. **2.** Heterochromia.

heterochromia (hĕt″ĕr-ō-krō′mē-ă) A difference in color. SYN: *heterochromatosis* (2).

h. iridis Different colors of the iris or sector of the iris in the two eyes. It may occur naturally or as a result of previous disease in the lighter-colored eye. Rarely it is associated with Waardenberg syndrome.

heterochromosome (hĕt″ĕr-ō-krō′mō-sōm) **1.** The X and Y or sex chromosomes. **2.** A chromosome containing material, heterochromatin, that stains differently from the remainder of the chromatin material.

heterochromous (hĕt″ĕr-ō-krō′mŭs) [″ + *chroma,* color] Having an abnormal difference in coloration.

heterochronia (hĕt″ĕr-ō-krō′nē-ă) [″ + *chronos,* time] Denoting an abnormal time for the occurrence of a phenomenon or production of a structure.

heterochronic (hĕt″ĕr-ō-krŏn′ĭk) Occurring at different or at abnormal times.

heterochthonous (hĕt″ĕr-ŏk′thō-nŭs) [Gr. *heteros,* other, + *chthon,* a particular land or country] Originating in a different place from where it was found.

heterocinesia (hĕt″ĕr-ō-sĭ-nē′zē-ă) [″ + *kinesis,* movement] Movements different from those the patient is instructed to make.

heterocyclic (hĕt″ĕr-ō-sĭk′lĭk) [″ + *kyklos,* circle] Pert. to ring compounds that contain one or more elements other than carbon in the ring.

heterodermic (hĕt″ĕr-ō-dĕr′mĭk) [″ + *derma,* skin] Pert. to a method of skin grafting in which grafts are taken from another person.

heterodont (hĕt″ĕr-ō-dŏnt) [″ + *odous,* tooth] Having teeth of various shapes.

heterodromus (hĕt″ĕr-ŏd′rō-mŭs) [″ + *dromos,* running] Acting, arranged, or moving in the opposite direction.

heterogametic (hĕt″ĕr-ō-gă-mĕt′ĭk) [″ + *gamos,* marriage] Pert. to the production of unlike gametes, applied esp. to a male that produces two types of sperm, one containing the X chromosome, the other the Y chromosome. SEE: *homogametic.*

heterogamy (hĕt″ĕr-ŏg′ă-mē) The union of gametes that are dissimilar in size and structure. This union occurs in higher plants and animals. SEE: *isogamy.*

heterogeneity (hĕt″ĕr-ō-jĕ-nē′ĭ-tē) The quality of being heterogeneous.

heterogeneous (hĕt″ĕr-ō-jē′nē-ŭs) [″ + *genos,* type] Of unlike natures; composed of unlike substances; the opposite of homogeneous.

heterogeneous vaccine A vaccine made from some source other than the patient's own tissues or cells; the opposite of autogenous vaccine.

heterogenesis (hĕt″ĕ-rō-jĕn′ĕ-sĭs) [″ + *genesis,* generation, birth] The production of offspring that have different characteristics in alternate generations, as in the regular alternation of asexual with sexual reproduction. This characteristic is found in some fungi. SYN: *metagenesis.* SEE: *homogenesis.*

heterogenetic (hĕt″ĕ-rō-jĕ-nĕt′ĭk) Relative to heterogenesis.

heterogeusia (hĕt″ĕr-ō-gū′sē-ă) [″ + *geusis,* taste] The perception of an inappropriate quality of taste when food is present in the mouth or being chewed. The taste sensation is unexpected and unusual but not necessarily unpleasant.

heterograft (hĕt′ĕ-rō-grăft) [″ + L. *grapheim,* stylus] A graft taken from another individual or an animal of a different species from the one for whom it is intended. SEE: *autograft; graft; isograft.*

heterography (hĕt″ĕr-ŏg′ră-fē) [″ + *graphein,* to write] Writing different words from those the writer intended.

heterohemagglutination (hĕt″ĕr-ō-hĕm″ă-gloo″tĭ-nā′shŭn) The agglutination of red blood cells by hemagglutinins from another species.

heterohemagglutinin (hĕt″ĕr-ō-hĕm″ă-gloo′tĭ-nĭn) Hemagglutinin from one species that will agglutinate red blood cells from another species.

heteroimmunity (hĕt″ĕr-ō-ĭm-mū′nĭ-tē) Having immunity to an antigen from another species.

heterokeratoplasty (hĕt″ĕr-ō-kĕr′ă-tō-plăs″tē) [″ + *keras,* horn, + *plassein,* to form] Plastic surgery of the cornea using tissue from the cornea from another species.

heterolalia (hĕt″ĕr-ō-lā′lē-ă) [″ + *lalia,* babbling] Heterophasia.

heteroliteral (hĕt″ĕr-ō-lĭt′ĕr-ăl) In speaking, pert. to an incorrect letter being substituted for the correct one.

heterologous (hĕt″ĕr-ŏl′ō-gŭs) [″ + *logos,* word, reason] **1.** Made up of cell tissue not normal to the part. **2.** Obtained from a different individual or species, with respect to tissue, cells, or blood. SEE: *autologous; homologous.*

heterolysin (hĕt″ĕr-ŏl′ĭ-sĭn) [″ + *lysis,* solution] A lysin formed from an antigen from an animal of a different species. SEE: *autolysis; hemolysis.*

heteromeric (hĕt″ĕr-ō-mĕr′ĭk) [″ + *meros,* a part] **1.** Pert. to spinal neurons with processes extending to the opposite side of the spinal cord. **2.** Possessing a different chemical composition.

heterometaplasia (hĕt″ĕr-ō-mĕt″ă-plā′zē-ă) [″ + *meta,* beyond, + *plassein,* to form] The transformation of tissue into a type foreign to the part where it was produced.

heterometropia (hĕt″ĕr-ō-mĕ-trō′pē-ă) The ability of one eye to refract differently than the other, which produces perceived images of different sizes. The condition is probably prevalent in many individuals who are completely unaware of it.

heteromorphosis (hĕt″ĕr-ō-mor-fō′sĭs) [″ + *morphe,* form, + *osis,* condition] The regeneration of an organ different from the one that it replaced.

heteromorphous (hĕt″ĕr-ō-mor′fŭs) [″ + *morphe,* form] Deviating from the normal type.

heteronomous (hĕt″ĕr-ŏn′ō-mŭs) [″ + *nomos,* law] Abnormal; differing from type.

heterophasia (hĕt″ĕr-ō-fā′zē-ă) [″ + *phasis,* speech] Expression of meaningless words instead of those intended. SYN: *heterolalia; heterophemia.*

heterophemia, heterophemy (hĕt″ĕr-ō-fē′mē-ă, hĕt-ĕr-ŏf′ĕ-mē) [″ + *pheme,* speech] Heterophasia.

heterophil(e) (hĕt′ĕr-ō-fĭl, -fīl) [″ + *philein,* to love] **1.** In humans, a term formerly used to designate the neutrophil leukocyte. **2.** Pert. to an antibody reacting with other than the specific antigen. **3.** Pert. to a tissue or microorganism that takes a stain other than the ordinary one. **4.** Pert to antigens that occur in more than one species of animal and that may be immunologically related to plant or microbe antigens.

heterophilic (hĕt″ĕr-ō-fĭl′ĭk) [Gr. *heteros,* other, + *philein,* to love] **1.** Having an affinity for something abnormal. **2.** Having an antibody response to an antigen other than the specific one.

heterophonia (hĕt″ĕr-ō-fō′nē-ă) [″ + *phone,* voice] A change of voice, esp. that which occurs at puberty.

heterophoria (hĕt″ĕ-rō-for′ē-ă) [″ + *phoros,* bearing] A tendency of the eyes to deviate from their normal position for visual alignment, esp. when one eye is covered; latent deviation or squint. This tendency is caused by an imbalance or weakness of the ocular muscles. SEE: *phoria.*

Heterophyes (hĕt″ĕr-ŏf′ĭ-ēz) [″ + *phye,* stature] A genus of flukes belonging to the family Heterophyidae.

H. heterophyes A species of intestinal fluke commonly infesting humans. In heavy infestations, it may cause diarrhea, nausea, and abdominal discomfort.

heterophyiasis (hĕt″ĕr-ō-fī-ī′ă-sĭs) [″ + ″ + *-iasis,* diseased condition] Infestation by any fluke belonging to the family Heterophyidae.

Heterophyidae A family of Trematoda (flukes) that infests the intestines of dogs, cats, and other mammals including humans. It includes the genera *Heterophyes, Haplorchis, Diorchitrema,* and *Metagonimus.* Infestations are common in Egypt and in Asia. Intermediate hosts are snails; the cercaria encyst in fish, esp. mullets, or frogs.

heteroplasia (hĕt″ĕr-ō-plā′zē-ă) [″ + *plassein,* to mold] The development of tissue at a location where that type of tissue would not normally occur. SYN: *alloplasia.*

heteroplastic (hĕt″ĕr-ō-plăs′tĭk) Relating to heteroplasia.

heteroploid (hĕt′ĕr-ō-ployd) [″ + *ploos,* fold] Possessing a chromosome number that is not a multiple of the haploid number common for the species.

heteroprosopus (hĕt″ĕr-ō-prō′sō-pŭs) [″ + *prosopon,* face] A congenitally deformed fetus having one head and two faces.

heteropsia (hĕt″ĕr-ŏp′sē-ă) [″ + *opsis,* vision] An inequality of vision in the two eyes.

heteroptics (hĕt″ĕr-ŏp′tĭks) A perversion of vision, such as seeing objects that do not exist or misinterpreting what is seen.

heteropyknosis (hĕt″ĕr-ō-pĭk-nō′sĭs) [″ + *pyknos,* dense, + *osis,* condition] The property whereby various parts of a chromosome stain with varying degrees of intensity. This is thought to be due to variations in the concentration of nucleic acid.

heterosexual (hĕt″ĕr-ō-sĕk′shū-ăl) [″ + L. *sexus,* sex] **1.** Pert. to the opposite sex. **2.** A person who has sexual interest in, or sexual intercourse exclusively with partners of the opposite sex.

heterosexuality (hĕt″ĕr-ō-sĕk″shū-ăl′ĭ-tē) Sexual attraction for one of the opposite sex.

heterosis (hĕt-ĕr-ō′sĭs) [Gr., alteration] Greater strength, size, vigor, and growth rate seen in the first hybrid generation.

heterosmia (hĕt″ĕr-ŏs′mē-ă) [Gr. *heteros,* other, + *osme,* odor] The consistent perception of an inappropriate smell when an odorant is inhaled. The smell perceived is unusual and unexpected but not unpleasant. SYN: *allotriosmia.*

heterotaxia (hĕt″ĕr-ō-tăk′sē-ă) [″ + *taxis,* arrangement] An abnormal position of organs or parts. SEE: *dextrocardia; situs inversus viscerum.*

heterotherm (hĕt″ĕr-ō-thĕrm″) An animal whose temperature varies considerably in different situations. SEE: *heterothermy.*

heterothermy (hĕt′ĕr-ō-thĕr″mē) [″ + *therme,* heat] Condition in which an animal's temperature varies considerably in different situations, but is not poikilothermic.

heterotopia (hĕt″ĕr-ō-tō′pē-ă) [″ + *topos,* place] **1.** The appearance of a cluster of normal cells in an abnormal location (e.g., of a cluster of cells from the adrenal glands found in a tissue specimen taken from the ovaries). **2.** The displacement of an organ or body part from its normal location. **heterotopic,** *adj.*

heterotopy (hĕt″ĕr-ŏt′ō-pē) [″ + *topos,* place] Heterotopia (2).

heterotoxin (hĕt″ĕr-ō-tŏk′sĭn) [″ + *toxikon,* poison] A toxin introduced from outside the patient's body.

heterotransplant (hēt″ĕr-ō-trăns′plănt) [″ + L. *trans,* across, + *plantare,* to plant] An organ, tissue, or structure taken from an animal and grafted into, or on, another animal of a different species. Such transplants usually atrophy.

heterotrichosis (hĕt″ĕr-ō-trĭ-kō′sĭs) [″ + *trichosis,* growth of hair] The growth of different kinds or color of hairs on the scalp or body.

heterotroph (hĕt′ĕr-ō-trōf) [″ + *trophe,* food] An organism such as a human, requiring complex organic food in order to grow and develop; in contrast to plants, which can synthesize food from inorganic materials.

heterotropia (hĕt″ĕr-ō-trō′pē-ă) [″ + *tropos,* a turning] A manifest deviation of the eyes resulting from the absence of binocular equilibrium. SEE: *strabismus.*

heterotypic (hĕt″ĕr-ō-tĭp′ĭk) Concerning something of a different type than that which is being discussed or examined, esp. a tissue.

heterovaccine (hĕt″ĕr-ō-văk′sēn) [″ + L. *vaccinus,* pert. to a cow] A vaccine from a microbial source other than that causing the disease for which it is intended.

heteroxenous (hĕt″ĕr-ŏk′sē-nŭs) [″ + *xenos,* stranger] The property of a parasite that requires two different hosts in order to complete its life cycle.

heterozygosis (hĕt″ĕr-ō-zī-gō′sĭs) [″ + *zygone,* yoke, pair, + *osis,* condition] The state of having different alleles at a specific locus. SEE: *homozygosis.*

heterozygote (hĕt″ĕr-ō-zī′gōt) An individual with different alleles for a given characteristic. SEE: *allele.*

heterozygous (hĕt″ĕr-ō-zī′gŭs) Possessing different alleles at a given locus. SEE: *homozygous.*

Heubner, Johann Otto L (hoyb′nĕr) German pediatrician, 1843–1926.

H. disease Syphilitic endarteritis of the brain.

H.-Herter disease Nontropical sprue in infants.

heuristic (hū-rĭs′tĭk) [Gr. *heuriskein,* to find out, discover] Helping to discover or experiment, esp. the encouragement of students to learn through their own investigation.

H.E.W. U.S. Department of *H*ealth, *E*ducation and *W*elfare. This agency is now the U.S. Department of Health and Human Services.

hex-, hexa- [Gr. *hex,* six] Prefix indicating *six.*

hexabasic [Gr. *hex,* six, + *basis,* base] An acid that contains six hydrogen (H) atoms that can be replaced by six hydroxyl (OH) radicals.

hexachlorophene (hĕks″ă-klō′rō-fēn) An antibacterial compound typically used in soaps and scrubs and experimentally used as a cholinesterase inhibitor.

hexachromic [″ + *chroma,* color] Able to distinguish only six of the seven colors of the spectrum, or unable to distinguish violet from indigo.

hexad (hĕk′săd) **1.** Six similar things. **2.** An element with a valence of six.

hexadactylism (hĕks″ă-dăk′tĭl-ĭzm) [″ + *daktylos,* finger, + *-ismos,* condition] The presence of six fingers or six toes on one hand or foot.

hexadecimal (hĕks″ă-dĕs′ĭ-mŭl) [″ + L. *decimus,* tenth] In computers, a number system using base 16 rather than base 2 (binary) or 10 (decimal).

hexamethonium (hĕks″ă-mĕ-thō′nē-ŭm) A compound that acts as a ganglionic blocking agent, used to treat hypertension.

hexaploidy (hĕk′să-ploy″dē) [″ + *ploos,* fold] A condition of having six sets of chromosomes.

Hexapoda (hĕks-ăp′ō-dă) [″ + *pous,* foot] Insecta.

hexatomic (hĕks″ă-tŏm′ĭk) [″ + *atomos,* indivisible] Pert. to a compound consisting of six atoms or one with six replaceable hydrogen or univalent atoms.

hexavalent (hĕks″ă-vā′lĕnt) [″ + L. *valere,* to have power] Having a chemical valence of six.

hexavitamin A standardized vitamin preparation containing vitamins A, D, C, and B, riboflavin, and niacinamide.

hexokinase (hĕks″ō-kī′nās) [″ + *kinein,* to move, + *-ase,* enzyme] An enzyme in cells that in the presence of ATP catalyzes the conversion of glucose to glucose-6-phosphate, the first step in glycolysis.

hexosamine (hĕk′sōs-ăm″ĭn) A sugar containing an amino group in place of a hydroxyl group (e.g., glucosamine).

hexose (hĕk′sōs) Any monosaccharide of the general formula $C_6H_{12}O_6$; the group includes glucose, fructose, and galactose.

hexosephosphate (hĕks″ōs-fōs′fāt) [Gr. *hex,* six, + *phosphoros,* phosphorus] A phosphoric acid ester of glucose; one of several esters formed in the muscles and other tissues in the metabolism of carbohydrates.

hexylresorcinol (hĕks″ĭl-rĕ-sor′sĭ-nŏl) $C_{12}H_{18}O_2$; white needle-shaped crystals used as an anthelmintic.

Hey's ligament (hāz) [William Hey, Brit. surgeon, 1736–1819] The semilunar lateral margin (falciform margin) of the fossa ovalis, which lies between the iliac and pubic portions of the fascia lata.

HF **1.** *Hageman factor;* blood coagulation factor XII. **2.** *high frequency.*

Hf Symbol for the element hafnium.

HFJV *high-frequency jet ventilation.*

Hg [L. *hydrargyrum*] Symbol for the element mercury.

Hgb *hemoglobin.*

$HgCl_2$ Symbol for mercuric chloride; corrosive sublimate.

Hg_2Cl_2 Symbol for mercurous chloride; calomel.

HGE *human granulocytic ehrlichiosis.*

HGF **1.** *human growth factor.* **2.** *hyperglycemic-glycogenolytic factor* (glucagon).

HgI_2 Symbol for mercuric iodide.

HgO Symbol for mercuric oxide.

HgS Symbol for mercuric sulfide.

HGSIL *high-grade squamous intraepithelial lesion.*

$HgSO_4$ Symbol for mercuric sulfate.

HHb *reduced hemoglobin (deoxyhemoglobin).*

HHS U.S. Department of Health and Human Services.

5-HIAA *5-hydroxyindoleacetic acid.*

hiatus (hī-ā′tŭs) [L., an opening] **1.** An opening, a foramen. **2.** An aperture.

h. aorticus An opening in the diaphragm through which pass the aorta and the thoracic duct.

h. canalis facialis A hiatus of the canal for the greater petrosal nerve. SYN: *h. fallopii.*

h. esophageus The opening in the diaphragm through which the esophagus passes.

h. fallopii H. canalis facialis.

h. maxillaris The opening of the maxillary sinus into the nasal cavity, located on the nasal surface of the maxillary bone.

sacral h. The opening on the inferior-posterior surface of the sacrum into the sacral canal.

h. semilunaris The groove in the external wall of the middle meatus of the nasal fossa into which the frontal sinus, maxillary sinus, and anterior ethmoid sinuses drain.

Hib *Haemophilus influenzae type b.*

hibernation (hī″bĕr-nā′shŭn) [L. *hiberna,* winter] The condition of spending the winter asleep and in an almost comatose state. Some animals adapt to winter by this method.

artificial h. A state of hibernation produced therapeutically by use of drugs alone or drugs and hypothermia. This greatly reduces the metabolic rate during procedures such as open heart surgery.

hibernoma (hī″bĕr-nō′mă) A rare multilobular encapsulated tumor that contains fetal fat tissue closely resembling the fat stored in the foot pads of hibernating animals.

hiccup, hiccough (hĭk′ŭp) [probably of imitative origin] A spasmodic periodic closure of the glottis following spasmodic lowering of the diaphragm, causing a short, sharp, inspiratory cough. Hiccups may occur transiently or may occasionally be intractable, lasting days, weeks, or longer. SYN: *singultus.*

ETIOLOGY: Phrenic nerve or diaphragmatic irritation, distention of the stomach, chest or abdominal surgery, metabolic disorders (e.g., hyponatremia), and intracerebral lesions (e.g., tumors, infections) commonly cause prolonged hiccuping.

TREATMENT: Hiccups may be treated by antiemetic drugs, rebreathing in a paper bag, briefly applying ice cubes to both sides of the neck at the level of the larynx, or inhalation of carbon dioxide. Stimulation of the nasopharynx with a soft rubber tube or placement of a thin coating of dry granulated sugar in the hypopharynx may also be tried. If these are not effective, anesthetization of the phrenic nerve may be helpful.

Hickman catheter A tunneled central venous catheter commonly used to administer solutions by central intravenous therapy for a prolonged period. Applications include total parenteral nutrition, antibiotic therapy, or blood transfusion.

Hicks sign Braxton Hicks contractions.

hidebound disease [AS. *hyd,* a skin, + *bindan,* to tie up] Scleroderma.

hidradenitis (hī-drăd-ĕ-nī′tĭs) [Gr. *hidros,* sweat, + *aden,* gland, + *itis,* inflammation] An inflammation of the sweat glands.

hidradenoma (hī″drăd-ĕ-nō′mă) [″ + ″ + *oma,* tumor] Adenoma of the sweat glands.

hidrocystoma (hī″drō-sĭs-tō′mă) [″ + *kystis,* cyst, + *oma,* tumor] Hydrocystoma.

hidropoiesis (hī″drō-poy-ē′sĭs) [″ + *poiesis,* formation] The formation of sweat. **hidropoietic** (-poy-ĕt′ĭk), *adj.*

hidrosadenitis (hī″drŏs-ăd″ĕ-nī′tĭs) [″ + *aden,* gland, + *itis,* inflammation] Hidradenitis.

hidrosis (hī-drō′sĭs) [″ + *osis,* condition] **1.** The formation and secretion of sweat. **2.** Excessive sweating.

hidrotic (hī-drŏt′ĭk) **1.** Causing the secretion of sweat. SYN: *diaphoretic; sudorific.* **2.** Any drug or medicine that induces sweating.

hierarchy (hī′răr-kē) The ordering or classification of anything in ascending or descending order of importance, or value in the case of numerical data. For example, the needs of a human being might be listed in order of theoretical importance, as air, water, food, health, protection from the elements and predators, security, esteem, and love.

hierolisthesis (hī″ĕr-ō-lĭs-thē′sĭs) [″ + *olisthanein,* to slip] Displacement of the sacrum.

hierophobia (hī″ĕr-ō-fō′bē-ă) [Gr. *hieros,* sacred, + *phobos,* fear] An abnormal fear of sacred things or persons connected with religion.

high colonic (hī kō-lŏn′ĭk) Irrigation of the bowel with large volumes of fluid. It is promoted by alternative medicine practitioners as a form of internal cleansing.

Highmore, antrum of (hī′mor) [Nathaniel Highmore, Brit. surgeon, 1613–1685] The maxillary sinus. SEE: *antrocele.*

Highmore's body Mediastinum testis.

high-takeoff coronary artery A coronary artery that originates more than a centimeter above the sino-tubular junction of the aorta.

hila (hī′lă) [L.] Pl. of hilum.

hilar (hī′lăr) Concerning or belonging to the hilus.

hilitis (hī′lī′tĭs) [L. *hilus,* a trifle, + Gr. *itis,* inflammation] An inflammation of any hilum, esp. the hilum of the lung.

hillock (hĭl′ŏk) [ME. *hilloc*] A small eminence or projection.

anal h. One of two small eminences that lie lateral and posterior to the cloacal membrane and, later, the anal fissure in the embryo.

axon h. A small conical elevation on the cell body of a neuron from which the axon arises.

seminal h. Colliculus seminalis.

Hill-Sachs lesion An indentation fracture of the posterolateral humeral head that occurs following an anterior dislocation of the glenohumeral joint. The lesion involves the cartilage of the humeral head, causing instability that may predispose the individual to subsequent anterior glenohumeral dislocations.

ETIOLOGY: A Hill-Sachs lesion occurs in about 40% of all first-time anterior dislocations and up to 80% of recurrent dislocations. The relative size of the lesion, as determined through an arthroscope or diagnostic imaging, can be used to ascertain the relative magnitude of the original dislocation.

SYMPTOMS: Although many Hill-Sachs lesions are asymptomatic, pain may arise from the posterolateral humeral head when the glenohumeral joint is abducted to 90 degrees and passive external rotation is applied.

TREATMENT: Surgical repair may be needed to increase anterior stability of the glenohumeral joint.

Hill sign [Sir Leonard Erskine Hill, Brit. physiologist, 1866–1952] A physical finding formerly used to determine aortic regurgitation. When the blood pressure in the leg is 20 to 40 mm Hg higher than in the arm, this sign is considered positive and indicative of aortic regurgitation.

Hilton's law [John Hilton, Brit. surgeon, 1804–1878] A law stating that the trunk of a nerve sends branches not only to a particular muscle but also to the joint moved by that muscle and to the skin overlying the insertion of the muscle.

Hilton's line A line at the junction of the anal skin and mucosa, beneath which the intersphincteric groove may be palpable. Because many persons have no visible line in this location, anatomists disagree about the significance of Hilton's line.

Hilton's muscle The aryepiglottic muscle.

Hilton's sac Laryngeal saccule.

hilum (hī′lŭm) *pl.* **hila** [L., a trifle] **1.** A depression or recess at the exit or entrance of a duct into a gland or of nerves and vessels into an organ. **2.** The root of the lungs at the level of the fourth and fifth dorsal vertebrae.

hilus (hī′lŭs) *pl.* **hili** [L.] Hilum.

himantosis (hī″măn-tō′sĭs) [Gr. *himantosis,* a long strap] An abnormal lengthening of the uvula.

hindbrain (hīnd′brān) [AS. *hindan,* behind, + *bragen,* brain] The most caudal of the three divisions of the embryonic brain. It differentiates into the metencephalon, which gives rise to the cerebellum and pons; and the myelencephalon, which develops into the medulla oblongata. SYN: *rhombencephalon.*

hindfoot (hīnd′foot) The posterior part of the foot consisting of the talus and calcaneus.

hindgut (hĭnd′gŭt) The caudal portion of the endodermal tube, which develops into the alimentary canal. It gives rise to the ileum, colon, and rectum.
hind-kidney (hīnd-kĭd′nē) Metanephros.
hip [AS. *hype*] The region lateral to the ilium of the pelvic bone.

anterior h. dislocation A dislocation of the hip through the obturator foramen, on the pubis, in the perineum, or through a fractured acetabulum.

SYMPTOMS: Pain, tenderness, and immobility accompany this condition. Shortening is present in the pubic and suprapubic forms; lengthening in the obturator and perineal forms.

TREATMENT: Hyperextension and direct traction are used to treat this condition, followed by flexion, abduction with inward rotations, and adduction.

congenital dislocation of the h. A congenital defect of the hip joint, probably caused by multifactorial effects of several abnormal genes.

dislocation of the h. Physical displacement of the head of the femur from its normal location in the acetabulum. It is very often accompanied by a fracture.

SYMPTOMS: Pain, rigidity, and loss of function characterize this condition. The dislocation may be obvious by the abnormal position in which the leg is held or by seeing or feeling the head of the femur in an abnormal position.

DIAGNOSIS: The person has great difficulty in straightening the hip and leg. The knee on the injured side resistantly points inward toward the other knee.

FIRST AID: The patient should be placed on a large frame, gurney, or support, such as that used for a fractured back. A large pad such as a pillow should be placed under the knee of the affected side. The patient should be treated for shock if required.

fracture of the h. A very common occurrence in older persons who fall, it is actually a fracture occurring in the proximal third of the femur, including the head, neck, intertrochanteric, and subtrochanteric areas. It is estimated to occur in one of every three white women older than 85. At least 50% of elderly patients who experience a hip fracture die within 1 yr after the injury.

ETIOLOGY: Osteoporosis predisposes an elderly person to hip fracture.

SYMPTOMS: Pain in the knee or groin is the classic presenting sign of a hip fracture. If the femur is displaced, shortening and rotation of the leg may be present.

TREATMENT: Preoperatively, Buck's traction may be used short-term to alleviate muscle spasms. An open reduction, internal fixation of the hip to realign the bone ends for healing is the preferred surgical treatment. The bone takes 6 to 12 weeks to heal in an elderly patient. The patient uses a walker until the bone is completely healed.

PATIENT CARE: Pain relief and prevention and monitoring of postoperative complications, including infection, hip dislocation, and blood clots in the legs, are primary concerns. Prophylactic antibiotics and anticoagulants are administered as ordered, and hip precautions are implemented to prevent dislocation. These precautions include having the patient avoid hip adduction, rotation, and flexion greater than 90 degrees during transfer and ambulation activities.

inferior h. dislocation A rare type of hip dislocation that is treated with traction in the flexed position, followed by outward rotation and extension.

posterior h. dislocation A dislocation of the hip onto the dorsum ilii or sciatic notch. Most posterior hip dislocations occur when the hip is flexed and adducted and a violent longitudinal force is applied to the femur that forces the femoral head posterior relative to the acetabulum. This mechanism is often seen in automobile accidents.

SYMPTOMS: The condition is characterized by an inward rotation of the thigh, with flexion, inversion, adduction, and shortening; pain and tenderness; and a loss of function and immobility.

TREATMENT: The patient should first be anesthetized and then laid in the dorsal position with the leg flexed on the thigh, and the latter upon the abdomen. The thigh is adducted and rotated outward. Circumduction is performed outwardly across the abdomen, and back to the straight position. Traction may be required.

snapping h. A slipping of ligaments around the hip joint, sometimes producing an audible snapping sound. Snapping hip syndrome may be caused by trochanteric or iliopsoas bursitis, but its etiology is often unknown.

total h. replacement Surgical procedure used in treating severe arthritis of the hip. Both the head of the femur and the acetabulum are replaced with synthetic components. SEE: *arthroplasty;* illus.

PATIENT CARE: *Preoperative:* The patient is educated about the procedure, postoperative care, and the expected surgical outcomes. Postoperative limitations, hip abduction methods, use of a trapeze, mobility regimen, gluteal and quadriceps setting, and triceps exercises are also instructed. The importance of respiratory toilet is explained, and the proper technique taught. Prescribed antibiotics and other drugs are administered. Reports of laboratory and radiological studies are reviewed, and the physician is notified of any abnor-

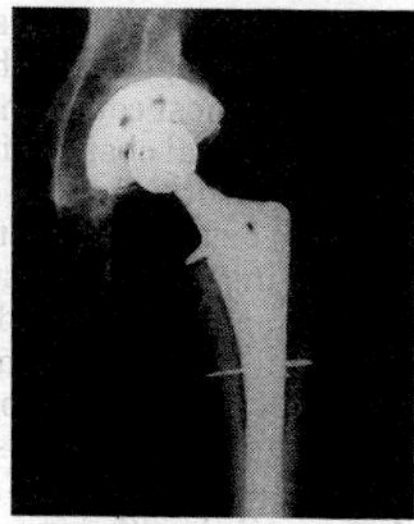

TOTAL HIP REPLACEMENT (Prosthesis)

mal findings. The patient is informed about pain evaluation techniques and the availability of analgesics is explained. Preoperative preparations are carried out (skin, gastrointestinal tract, urinary bladder, and premedication), and their significance is explained to the patient. The patient should be encouraged to verbalize feelings and concerns.

Postoperative: Dressings and drainage devices are monitored for excessive bleeding, and the area beneath the buttocks is inspected for gravity pooling of drainage. Dressings are replaced or reinforced according to the surgeon's protocol and aseptic technique. Vital signs are monitored, and neurovascular status of the affected extremity is checked frequently. Analgesics are administered as prescribed and required, and the patient is evaluated for response. The patient is repositioned frequently in prescribed positions, and the integrity of all supportive equipment (splints, pillows, traction devices) is maintained during repositioning. The patient should avoid leg crossing and internal rotation, which enhance the potential for prosthesis dislocation and interfere with venous return. Respiratory status is assessed, and deep breathing and coughing are encouraged to prevent pulmonary complications. An exercise program and ambulation should begin as prescribed by the surgeon (type and extent of weight bearing on affected limb) and in collaboration with the physical therapist. Raised toilet seats and semireclining chairs are used to prevent hip flexion. A diet high in protein and vitamin C is provided, wound healing assessed, and skin breakdown prevented. Antiembolic devices and anticoagulant drugs are given if prescribed, and the patient is assessed for such complications as thrombophlebitis, embolism, and dislocation. Discharge teaching focuses on the exercise regimen and activity limitations, stressing the importance of swimming and walking programs. Outpatient orthopedic follow-up and therapy are arranged as required. The patient should participate in a weight reduction program if necessary.

hip-joint disease Any disease of the hip joint, esp. tuberculosis.

Hippel's disease, von Hippel-Lindau disease (hĭp′ĕlz, vŏn hĭp′ĕl-lĭn′dow) [Eugen von Hippel, Ger. ophthalmologist, 1867–1939; Arvid Lindau, Swedish pathologist, 1892–1958] Angiomatosis of the retina and various areas of the body including the central nervous system, spinal cord, and visceral organs.

hippocampal (hĭp″ō-kăm′păl) [Gr. *hippokampos,* seahorse] Pert. to the hippocampus.

h. formation Olfactory structures lying along the medial margin of the pallium. It includes the hippocampus, dentate gyrus, supracallosal gyrus, longitudinal striae, subcallosal gyrus, diagonal band of Broca, and hippocampal commissure.

hippocampus An elevation of the floor of the inferior horn of the lateral ventricle of the brain, occupying nearly all of it. The hippocampus seems to be important in establishing new memories.

digitations of h. Three or four shallow grooves on the anterior portion of the hippocampus.

h. minor Calcar avis.

Hippocrates (hĭ-pŏk′ră-tēz) [ca. 460–375 B.C.] A Greek physician referred to as the Father of Medicine because he was the first healer to attempt to record medical experiences for future reference. By so doing he established the foundation for the scientific basis of medical practice. SEE: *Hippocratic oath.*

hippocratic facies The appearance of the face, felt in ancient times to indicate death was imminent, characterized by dark brown, livid, or lead-colored skin; hollow appearance of the eyes; collapse of the temples and sharpness of the nose.

Hippocratic oath The oath exacted of his students by Hippocrates: "I swear by Apollo the physician, and Aesculapius, and Hygeia, and Panacea, and all the gods and goddesses, that according to my ability and judgment, I will keep this oath and its stipulation—to reckon him who taught me this art equally dear to me as my parents, to share my substance with him, and to relieve his necessities if required; to look upon his offspring in the same footing as my own brothers, and to teach them this art if they shall wish to learn it, without fee or stipulation, and that by precept, lecture, and every other mode of instruction, I will impart a knowledge of the art to my own sons, and those of my teachers, and to disciples bound by a stipulation and oath according to the law of medicine, but to none other.

"I will follow that system of regimen which, according to my ability and judgment, I consider for the benefit of my patients, and abstain from whatever is deleterious and mischievous. I will give no deadly medicine to anyone if asked, nor suggest any such counsel; and in like manner I will not give to a woman a pessary to produce abortion. With purity and with holiness I will pass my life and practice my art. I will not cut persons laboring under the stone, but will leave this to be done by men who are practitioners of this work. Into whatever houses I enter, I will go into them for the benefit of the sick, and I will abstain from every voluntary act of mischief and corruption; and, further, from the seduction of females or males, of freemen and slaves. Whatever, in connection with my professional practice, or not in connection with it, I see or hear, in the life of men, which ought not to be spoken of abroad, I will not divulge, as reckoning that all such should be kept secret.

"While I continue to keep this Oath unviolated, may it be granted to me to enjoy life and the practice of this art, respected by all men, in all times. But should I trespass and violate this Oath, may the reverse be my lot." SEE: *Declaration of Geneva; Declaration of Hawaii; Nightingale Pledge; Prayer of Maimonides.*

hippurase (hĭp′ū-rās) Hippuricase.

hippuria (hĭ-pū′rē-ă) [Gr. *hippos,* horse, + *ouron,* urine] Large quantities of hippuric acid in the urine.

hippuric acid $C_6H_5CONHCH_2COOH$; an acid formed and excreted by the kidneys. It is formed in the human body from the combination of benzoic acid and glycine, the synthesis taking place in the liver and, to a limited extent, in the kidneys.

hippuricase (hĭ-pūr′ĭ-kās) An enzyme found in the liver, kidney, and other tissues that catalyzes the synthesis of hippuric acid from benzoic acid and glycine. SYN: *hippurase.*

hippus (hĭp′ŭs) [Gr. *hippos,* horse] The rhythmical and rapid dilatation and contraction of the pupils and spasmodic tremor of the iris seen in an aphakic eye or one with a subluxated lens. SYN: *iridodonesis.*

respiratory h. A dilatation of the pupil during inspiration, and contraction on expiration.

hircismus (hĭr-sĭs′mŭs) A malodorous condition of the axillae caused by bacterial action on the sweat.

hircus (hĭr′kŭs) *pl.* **hirci** [L., goat] An axillary hair.

Hirschberg's reflex (hĭrsh′bĕrgz) [Leonard Keene Hirschberg, U.S. neurologist, b. 1877] Adduction of the foot when the sole at the base of the great toe is irritated.

Hirschsprung's disease (hĭrsh′sprŭngz) [Harald Hirschsprung, Dan. physician, 1830–1916] The most common cause of lower gastrointestinal obstruction in neonates. Patients with this disease exhibit signs of an extremely dilated colon and accompanying chronic constipation, fecal impaction, and overflow diarrhea. It occurs in 1 in 5000 children, with a male-to-female ratio of 4:1. About 15% of cases are diagnosed in the first month of life, 64% by the third month, and 80% by age 1 year. Only 8% remain undiagnosed by 3 years of age. SYN: *aganglionic megacolon.* SEE: *megacolon.*

ETIOLOGY: The condition is caused by congenital absence of some or all the normal bowel ganglion cells, beginning at the anus and extending variable lengths proximally, though 75% of cases are limited to the immediate rectosigmoid area.

DIAGNOSIS: Barium contrast enema (BE) is usually used for diagnosis, but for mild cases when the BE result is negative, rectal biopsy is the diagnostic standard.

TREATMENT: Treatment is surgical excision of the affected segment and reanastomosis of healthy bowel, by any of four procedures.

PATIENT CARE: In the neonatal period, health care providers assist the parents to adjust to their child's congenital defect and foster infant-parent bonding. They prepare the parents intellectually and emotionally for medical-surgical intervention, and teach about care of the child's colostomy after discharge.

Preoperative patient care focuses on ensuring adequate nutrition to withstand surgery and aid healing. Surgical preparation in any baby other than a newborn (whose bowel is sterile) requires bowel cleansing and sterilization, using saline enemas and antibiotic therapy. A nasogastric tube may be inserted to prevent abdominal distention. Progressive distention is a serious problem, so the abdominal circumference is measured at the umbilicus each time that vital signs are checked. Psychological preparation for surgery is dictated by the child's age; spacing explanations appropriately can prevent anxiety and confusion. Parents and older children should be reminded that the colostomy is temporary.

Postoperative care is similar to that for an infant or child experiencing abdominal surgery. Parents are instructed to pin diapers below the area of incision to prevent urine contamination of the wound. Before discharge, the ability of parents to carry out colostomy care and skin protection is evaluated; children from preschool age up can be involved in self-care as appropriate. For continuity of care, the child and family are referred to a home health care agency. The community nurse also assists in preparing the family for subsequent surgery. The family may be referred to a social worker, psychologist, or other service agency as appropriate if financial assistance or further psychological support is required.

hirsute (hŭr′sūt) [L. *hirsutus,* shaggy] Hairy.

hirsuties (hŭr-sū′shē-ēz) Hirsutism.

hirsutism (hŭr′sūt-ĭzm) Condition characterized by the excessive growth of hair or the presence of hair in unusual places, esp. in women. Hirsutism in women is usually caused by abnormalities of androgen production or metabolism. In patients who do not have an adrenal tumor, this condition may be treated symptomatically by shaving, depilatories, or electrolysis. The goal of medical therapy is to decrease androgen production. This may involve the use of various agents including hormones or an antiandrogen (cyproterone acetate).

hirudicide (hĭ-rū′dĭ-sīd) [L. *hirudo,* a leech, + *caedere,* to kill] Any substance that destroys leeches.

hirudin (hĭ-rū′dĭn) A substance present in the secretion of the buccal glands of the leech that prevents coagulation of the blood by inactivating thrombin. Hirudin can be used to treat acute myocardial infarction and unstable angina pectoris.

Hirudinea (hĭr″ū-dĭn′ē-ă) A class of Annelida. This group is hermaphroditic, lacks setae or appendages, usually has two suckers, and includes the blood-sucking leeches. A number of species, including *H. medicinalis,* were formerly used extensively for bloodletting because they produce natural anticoagulants. SEE: *hirudin; leech.*

hirudiniasis (hĭr″ū-dĭn-ī′ă-sĭs) Infestation by leeches. SEE: *leech.*

external h. The attachment of leeches to the skin. After the leeches drop off, bleeding may continue as a result of the action of hirudin. Bites may become infected or ulcerate.

internal h. A condition resulting from accidental ingestion of leeches in drinking water. They may attach themselves to the wall of the pharynx, nasal cavity, or larynx.

Hirudo (hĭ-roo′dō) [L., leech] A genus of leeches belonging to the family Gnathobdellidae.

His, Wilhelm Jr. (hĭs) German physician, 1863–1934.

bundle of H. The atrioventricular (AV) bundle, a group of modified muscle fibers, the Purkinje fibers, forming a part of the impulse-conducting system of the heart. It arises in the AV node and continues in the interventricular septum as a single bundle, the crus commune, which divides into two trunks that pass respectively to the right and left ventricles, fine branches passing to all parts of the ventricles. It conducts impulses from the atria to the ventricles, which initiates ventricular contraction.

H. disease Trench fever.

histaffine (hĭs′tă-fēn) [Gr. *histos,* tissue, + L. *affinis,* having affinity for] Having an affinity for the tissues.

histaminase (hĭs-tăm′ĭ-nās) An enzyme widely distributed in the body that inactivates histamine.

histamine (hĭs′tă-mĭn, -mēn) $C_5H_9N_3$; a substance produced from the amino acid histidine, which causes dilation of blood vessels, increased secretion of acid by the stomach, smooth muscle constriction (e.g., in the bronchi), and mucus production, tissue swelling, and itching (during allergic reactions). The release of histamine from mast cells is a major component of type I hypersensitivity reactions, including asthma.

h. blocking agent Antihistamine.

h. phosphate Water-soluble colorless crystals, sometimes called histamine acid phosphate or histamine diphosphate. It was used in the past to determine the acid-secreting power of the stomach.

histaminemia (hĭs-tăm″ĭ-nē′mē-ă) [*histamine* + Gr. *haima,* blood] Histamine in the blood.

histenzyme (hĭst-ĕn′zīm) [Gr. *histos,* tissue, + *en,* in, + *zyme,* leaven] A renal enzyme that splits up hippuric acid into benzoic acid and glycine. SYN: *histozyme.*

histidase Histidine ammonia-lyase.

histidine (hĭs′tĭ-dĭn, -dēn) An essential amino acid, $C_6H_9N_3O_2$, that is, one that must be consumed in the diet.

h. ammonia-lyase A liver enzyme that catalyzes L-histidine with the resultant formation of urocanic acid and ammonia. Deficiency of this enzyme causes histidinemia.

histidinemia (hĭs″tĭ-dĭ-nē′mē-ă) A hereditary metabolic disease caused by lack of the enzyme histidine ammonia-lyase, which is normally present in the urine.

histidinuria (hĭs″tĭ-dĭ-nū′rē-ă) The presence of histidine in the urine.

histioblast (hĭs′tē-ō-blăst″) A tissue histiocyte.

histiocyte (hĭs′tē-ō-sīt″) [Gr. *histion,* little web, + *kytos,* cell] A monocyte that has become a resident in tissue. SYN: *histocyte; macrophage.*

histiocytoma (hĭs″tē-ō-sī-tō′mă) [″ + ″ + *oma,* tumor] A tumor containing histiocytes.

histiocytosis (hĭs″tē-ō-sī-tō′sĭs) [″ + ″ + *osis,* condition] An abnormal amount of histiocytes in the blood.

Langerhans cell h. A number of clinical conditions, most commonly seen in infants and children, caused by disease of Langerhans cell histiocytes. These cells, which are characteristic of all of the variants of the disease, cause granulomas. The great variation in the signs and symptoms produced depends upon their location and how widely spread they are. Almost any organ system including the skeleton may be involved. These diseases were previously given names such as histiocytosis X, Hand-Schüller-Christian disease, Letterer-Siwe disease, and eosinophilic granuloma. Treatment may consist of surgical removal of bone lesions and radiation therapy for lesions threatening vital functions such as sight and hearing. Corticosteroids or cytotoxic agents are useful in controlling soft tissue disease and multiple skeletal lesions. Bone marrow transplantation has been used in recurrent and progressive Langerhans cell histiocytosis.

lipid h. Niemann-Pick disease.

histiogenic (hĭs-tē-ō-jĕn′ĭk) [″ + *gennan,* to form] Histogenous.

histo- [Gr. *histos,* web, tissue] Combining form meaning *tissue.*

histoblast (hĭs′tō-blăst) [″ + *blastos,* germ] A tissue cell.

histochemistry (hĭs″tō-kĕm′ĭs-trē) The study of chemistry of the cells and tissues. It involves use of both light and electron microscopy and special chemical tests and stains.

histoclastic (hĭs″tō-klăs′tĭk) [″ + *klastos,* breaking] The ability to break down tissues, said of certain cells.

histocompatibility (hĭs″tō-kŏm-păt″ĭ-bĭl′ĭ-tē) Cell-mediated immunological similarity or compatibility.

histocyte (hĭs′tō-sīt) [″ + *kytos,* cell] Histiocyte.

histodiagnosis (hĭs″tō-dī″ăg-nō′sĭs) [″ + *dia,* through, + *gnosis,* knowledge] A diagnosis made from examination of the tissues, esp. by use of microscopy.

histodifferentiation (hĭs″tō-dĭf″ĕr-ĕn″shē-ā′shŭn) The process of cellular maturation in which a primitive cell develops into specific cellular types.

histogenesis (hĭs-tō-jĕn′ĕ-sĭs) [″ + *genesis,* generation, birth] The development into differentiated tissues of a germ layer; the origin and development of tissue. **histogenetic** (hĭs″tō-jĕ-nĕt′ĭk), *adj.*

histogenous (hĭs-tŏj′ĕ-nŭs) Made by the tissues. SYN: *histiogenic.*

histogram (hĭs′tō-gram) [L. *historia,* observation, + Gr. *gramma,* something written] A graph showing frequency distributions.

histohematin (hĭs″tō-hĕm′ă-tĭn) [″ + *haima,* blood] A hemoglobin pigment in various tissues.

histohematogenous (hĭs″tō-hĕm″ă-tŏj′ĕ-nŭs) [″ + ″ + *gennan,* to form] Arising from the tissues and the blood.

histoincompatible Referring to tissues that are immunologically different enough to prevent their use for transplantation.

histokinesis (hĭs-tō-kĭ-nē′sĭs) [″ + *kinesis,* movement] Movement in the tissues of the body.

histologist (hĭs-tŏl′ō-jĭst) [″ + *logos,* word, reason] A specialist in the study of cells and microscopic tissues.

histology (hĭs-tŏl′ō-jē) The study of the microscopic structure of tissue. **histological** (hĭs″tō-lŏj′ĭ-kăl), *adj.*

normal h. The microscopic study of healthy tissue.

pathologic h. Histopathology.

histolysis (hĭs-tŏl′ĭ-sĭs) [″ + *lysis,* dissolution] Disintegration of the tissues. **histolytic** (hĭs″tō-lĭt′ĭk), *adj.*

histoma (hĭs-tō′mă) [″ + *oma,* tumor] A tumor composed of tissue.

histone (hĭs′tŏn, -tōn) [Gr. *histos,* web, tissue] One of the five kinds of proteins that are part of chromatin in eukaryotic cells. Their positive charge attracts the negatively charged DNA that is folded around them into units called nucleosomes. Histones also regulate some of the further folding of DNA in chromosomes about to undergo mitosis.

histonuria (hĭs-tōn-ū′rē-ă) [″ + *ouros,* urine] Excretion of histones in the urine.

histopathology (hĭs″tō-pă-thŏl′ō-jē) [″ + *pathos,* disease, suffering, + *logos,* word, reason] The microscopic study of diseased tissues. SYN: *pathologic histology.*

histophysiology (hĭs″tō-fĭz″ē-ŏl′ō-jē) [″ + *physis,* nature, + *logos,* word, reason] The study of the functions of cells and tissues.

Histoplasma (hĭs″tō-plăz′mă) [″ + LL. *plasma,* form, mold] A genus of parasitic fungi.

H. capsulatum The causative agent of histoplasmosis. SEE: illus.

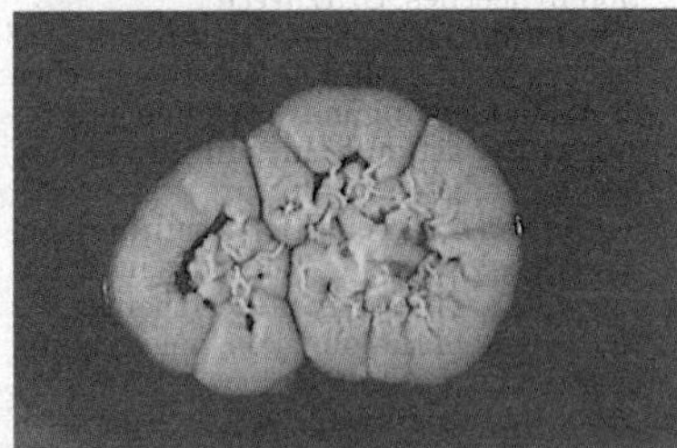

HISTOPLASMA CAPSULATUM IN CULTURE

histoplasmin (hĭs″tō-plăz′mĭn) An antigen prepared from cultures of *Histoplasma capsulatum* and used as a skin test for the diagnosis of histoplasmosis.

histoplasmosis (hĭs″tō-plăz-mō′sĭs) [″ + ″ + Gr. *osis,* condition] A systemic, fungal, respiratory disease caused by

Histoplasma capsulatum. The reservoir for this fungus is in soil with a high organic content and undisturbed bird droppings, esp. that around old chicken houses; caves harboring bats; and starling, blackbird, and pigeon roosts. In the U.S., the infection is endemic in the Ohio River valley. Disseminated histoplasmosis is a common opportunistic infection in patients with acquired immunodeficiency syndrome (AIDS) and other immunosuppressing illnesses.

SYMPTOMS: The signs and symptoms vary from those of a mild self-limited infection to a severe or fatal disease. Immunocompromised persons are esp. susceptible. In the severe form there are fever, anemia, enlarged spleen and liver, leukopenia, pulmonary involvement, adrenal necrosis, and gastrointestinal tract ulcers. The treatment is intravenous amphotericin B.

PATIENT CARE: In patients with severe pneumonia, respiratory status is monitored every 8 hr (or more frequently as necessary) to assess for diminished breath sounds, pleural friction rub, or effusion; cardiovascular status every 8 hr (or more frequently as necessary) to document and immediately report any muffling of heart sounds, jugular vein distention, pulsus paradoxus, or other signs of cardiac tamponade; and neurological status every 8 hr (or more frequently as necessary) to document and report any changes in level of consciousness or any nuchal rigidity. The patient is assessed for signs and symptoms of hypoglycemia and hyperglycemia, indicating adrenal dysfunction. All stools are tested for occult blood, and its presence is documented and reported. Prescribed antifungal therapy (amphotericin B or ketaconazole) is administered and evaluated for desired effects and any adverse reactions. Because amphotericin B may cause pain, chills, fever, nausea, and vomiting, appropriate analgesics, antihistamines, antipyretics, and antiemetics are administered as prescribed. Small doses of meperidine or morphine sulfate may help reduce shaking chills. Such drug therapy should be administered in the early morning or late evening to avoid sedating the patient for the entire day. If needed, oxygen therapy is administered as prescribed, and rest periods are planned to assist the patient to conserve energy. The dietitian is consulted to construct an appetizing and nutritious diet incorporating the patient's food preferences; this diet is best offered in small, frequent meals rather than in three large ones. If the patient has oropharyngeal ulceration, soothing oral hygiene and soft, bland foods are provided. (Parenteral nutrition may be required if ulcerations are severe.) Emotional support is offered to the patient with chronic or disseminated histoplasmosis, and referral to a social worker, psychologist, or occupational therapist for further counseling and support may be necessary to help the patient cope with long-term therapy. The nurse assists parents of a child with this disease to arrange for homebound instruction. The patient is advised that follow-up care on a regular basis will be required for at least a year. Cardiac and pulmonary signs and symptoms that may indicate effusions should be reported to the health care provider immediately. To help prevent histoplasmosis, persons in endemic areas are taught to watch for early signs of this infection and to seek treatment promptly. Persons who risk occupational exposure to contaminated soil are instructed to wear face masks.

history, medical history (hĭs′tō-rē) [Gr. *historia,* inquiry] A systematic record of past events as they relate to a person and his or her medical background. A carefully taken medical, surgical, and occupational history will enable diagnosis in about 80% of patients.

TECHNIQUE: The patient should be given the opportunity to describe his or her symptoms in his/her own words, fully and completely, without interruption. The examiner encourages the patient to speak by maintaining a sympathetic and nonjudgmental attitude. After the patient's explanations are completed, the examiner usually asks carefully chosen questions to elicit details about an illness and gain deeper insights. SEE: *nursing assessment* for illus.

dental h. A record of all aspects of a person's oral health, previous evaluations and treatments, and the state of general physical and mental health. SEE: *oral diagnosis*.

family h. A record of the state of health and medical history of members of the patient's immediate family, which may be of interest to the physician because of genetic or familial tendencies noted.

occupational h. A semistructured interview process used by occupational therapists to determine a person's roles, approach to tasks, and sense of identity.

histothrombin (hĭs″tō-thrŏm′bĭn) [″ + *thrombos,* a clot] A thrombin derived from the connective tissue.

histotoxic (hĭs″tō-tŏk′sĭk) [″ + *toxikon,* poison] Toxic to tissue.

histotropic (hĭs″tō-trŏp′ĭk) [″ + *trope,* a turning] Having attraction for tissue cells, as certain parasites, stains, or chemicals.

histozoic (hĭs″tō-zō′ĭk) [″ + *zoe,* life] Living within or on tissues, said of certain protozoan parasites.

histozyme (hĭs′tŏ-zīm) [″ + *zyme,* leaven] A renal enzyme that converts hippuric acid into benzoic acid and glycine, causing fermentation.

HIV *human immunodeficiency virus.* SEE: *AIDS.*

hives (hīvz) [origin uncertain] Urticaria.

HIV positive SEE: *Nursing Diagnoses Appendix.*

HL, Hl *latent hyperopia.*

hl *hectoliter.*

HLA *histocompatibility locus antigen; human lymphocyte antigen.*

HLA complex SEE: *major histocompatibility complex.*

Hm *manifest hyperopia.*

HMD *hyaline membrane disease.*

HMG *human menopausal gonadotropin.*

HMO *Health Maintenance Organization.*

HNO_2 Symbol for nitrous acid.

HNO_3 Symbol for nitric acid.

Ho Symbol for the element holmium.

H_2O Symbol for water.

H_2O_2 Symbol for hydrogen peroxide.

hoarseness [AS. *has,* harsh] A rough quality of the voice.

ETIOLOGY: Hoarseness may be caused by simple chronic inflammations secondary to chronic nasopharyngitis, chemical irritants, tobacco, or alcohol. Specific causes of chronic laryngitis include syphilis, tuberculosis, leprosy, neoplasms, papilloma, angioma, fibroma, singer's nodes, carcinoma, paralyses, overuse of the vocal cords, and prolapse of ventricle of larynx. Female virilization also usually causes hoarseness.

Hochsinger's sign (hōk′zĭng-ĕrz) [Karl Hochsinger, Austrian pediatrician, b. 1860] Closure of the fist in tetany when the inner side of the biceps muscle is pressed.

Hodgkin's disease (hŏj′kĭns) [Thomas Hodgkin, Brit. physician, 1798–1866] ABBR: HD. A malignant lymphoma whose pathological hallmark is the Reed-Sternberg cell, a giant, multinucleated cell, usually a transformed B lymphocyte. The disease may affect persons of any age but occurs most often in adults in their early 30s. About 7500 new cases of the disease are diagnosed annually in the U.S. The lymphoma typically begins in a single lymph node (esp. in the neck, axilla, groin, or near the aorta) and spreads to adjacent nodes if it is not recognized. It may metastasize gradually to lymphatic tissue on both sides of the diaphragm or disseminate widely to tissues outside the lymph nodes. The degree of metastasis defines the stage of the disease; early disease (stage I or II) is present in one or a few lymph nodes, whereas widespread disease has disseminated to both sides of the diaphragm (stage III) or throughout the body (stage IV). The lower the stage of the disease, the better the prognosis. Patients with stage I Hodgkin's lymphoma have a 90% survival 5 years after diagnosis. SEE: *non-Hodgkin's lymphoma; Reed-Sternberg cell; Nursing Diagnoses Appendix.*

ETIOLOGY: Epstein-Barr virus has been found in the cells of nearly half of all patients with Hodgkin's disease, a fact that suggests a link between the virus and the lymphoma.

SYMPTOMS: Early stage patients may have no symptoms other than a painless lump or enlarged gland in the armpit or neck. Others may develop fevers, night sweats, loss of appetite, and weight loss.

DIAGNOSIS: The presence of the giant polypoid Reed-Sternberg (RS) cell in tissue obtained for biopsy is diagnostic.

TREATMENT: The goal of therapy is cure, not just palliation of symptoms. Combinations of radiation and chemotherapy typically are used. One commonly used drug regimen is identified by the acronym ABVD-MOPP; it consists of eight chemotherapeutic agents, including mechlorethamine, vincristine, procarbazine, prednisone, etoposide, doxorubicin, bleomycin, and lomustine.

PATIENT CARE: All procedures and treatments associated with the plan of care are explained. The patient is assessed for nutritional deficiencies and malnutrition by obtaining regular weights, checking anthropomorphic measurements, and monitoring appropriate laboratory studies (serum protein levels, transferrin levels) and, as necessary, anergy panels. The importance of maintaining good nutrition (aided by eating small, frequent meals of the patient's favorite food) and of drinking plenty of liquids is stressed. A well-balanced, high-calorie, high-protein diet is provided. The patient is observed for complications during chemotherapy, including anorexia, nausea, vomiting, mouth ulcers, alopecia, fatigue, and bone marrow depression; as well as for adverse reactions to radiation therapy, such as hair loss, anorexia, nausea, vomiting, and fatigue. Supportive care is provided as indicated for adverse reactions to chemotherapy or radiation therapy. Comfort measures are provided to promote relaxation, and periods of rest are planned because the patient will tire easily. Antiemetic drugs are administered as prescribed. The importance of gentle but thorough oral hygiene to prevent stomatitis is stressed. To control pain and bleeding, a soft toothbrush or sponge-stick, cotton swabs, and a soothing or anesthetic mouthwash, such as a sodium bicarbonate mixture or viscous lidocaine, are used as prescribed. The patient can apply petroleum jelly to the lips and should avoid astringent mouthwashes.

The patient is advised to pace activities to counteract therapy-induced fatigue and is taught relaxation techniques to promote comfort and rest and reduce anxiety. The patient should avoid crowds and any person with a known infection and should notify the health care provider if any signs or symptoms of infection develop. Health care providers should stay with the patient during periods of stress and anxiety and provide emotional support to the patient and family. Referral to local support groups may be necessary. Women of childbearing age should delay pregnancy until long-term remission occurs, because chemotherapy and radiation therapy can cause genetic mutations and spontaneous abortions. Because sudden withdrawal of prednisone may be life-threatening, the health care provider should not change the dosage or discontinue the drug without consulting with the oncologist. As necessary, both patient and family are referred for respite or hospice care.

Hodgson's disease (hŏj'sŏnz) [Joseph Hodgson, Brit. physician, 1788–1869] Aneurysmal dilatation of the aorta.

Hofbauer cell (hŏf'bow-ĕr) [J. Isfred Isidore Hofbauer, U.S. gynecologist, 1878–1961] A histiocyte, believed to be phagocytic, found in the connective tissue of the chorionic villi.

Hoffmann's reflex, Hoffmann's sign [Johann Hoffmann, Ger. neurologist, 1857–1919] An abnormal reflex found in patients with damaged pyramidal tracts of the brain. Flexion of the distal interphalangeal joint of the middle finger makes the thumb of the same hand flex and adduct.

hol-, holo- [Gr. *holos,* entire] Combining form meaning *complete, entire,* or *homogeneous.*

holandric (hŏl-ăn'drĭk) [" + *aner,* man] Transmitted only by a gene in the nonhomologous portion of the Y chromosome. SEE: *hologynic.*

Holden's line (hōl'dĕnz) [Luther Holden, Brit. anatomist, 1815–1905] A wrinkle or indistinct furrow in the groin at the junction of the thigh and the abdomen.

holding area An Emergency Department area in which patients are kept temporarily before being transferred to an intensive care unit.

holism (hōl'ĭzm) The philosophy based on the belief that, in nature, entities such as individuals and other complete organisms function as complete units that cannot be reduced to the sum of their parts. The philosophy was originally discussed by Jan C. Smuts. SEE: *holistic medicine.* **holistic** (hō-lĭs'tĭk), *adj.*

Hollenhorst plaques, Hollenhorst bodies [R. W. Hollenhorst, U.S. ophthalmologist, b. 1913] Atheromatous plaques that have lodged in the retinal vessels after having been broken off from the lining of other vessels. They appear as shiny irregular patches in the vessels of the retina.

hollow (hŏl'ō) **1.** Having a cavity or space inside. **2.** A depressed area, lower than the surrounding tissue.

Sebileau's h. A depression in the floor of the mouth between the tongue and the sublingual glands.

hollow-back Lordosis.

Holmgren's test (hōlm'grĕnz) [Alarik F. Holmgren, Swedish physiologist, 1831–1897] An obsolete test in which the patient matches colored skeins of yarn to test for color blindness.

holmium (hŏl'mē-ŭm) SYMB: Ho. A rare earth metal, whose atomic weight is 164.930 and atomic number is 67.

holoacardius (hŏl"ō-ă-kăr'dē-ŭs) [Gr. *holos,* entire, + *a-,* not, + *kardia,* heart] A congenitally deformed monozygotic twin fetus with no heart. The in utero circulation is obtained from the heart of the twin to which the deformed fetus is attached.

holocrine (hŏl'ō-krĭn) [" + *krinein,* to secrete] Pert. to a secretory gland or its secretions consisting of altered cells of the same gland, the opposite of merocrine. SEE: *apocrine.*

holodiastolic (hŏl"ō-dī"ă-stŏl'ĭk) [" + *diastellein,* to expand] Relating to the entire diastole, esp. a murmur that occurs during all of diastole.

holoenzyme (hŏl"ō-ĕn'zīm) [" + *en,* in, + *zyme,* leaven] A type of enzyme consisting of a protein portion (apoenzyme) and a non-amino acid portion or prosthetic group. SEE: *apoenzyme; prosthetic group.*

holography (hŏl-ŏg'ră-fē) [" + *graphein,* to write] A method of producing pictures in which the image appears as a three-dimensional representation of the original object. The picture obtained is called a hologram (i.e., whole message).

hologynic (hŏl"ō-jĭn'ĭk) [" + *gyne,* woman] Transmitted only by a gene in the nonhomologous portion of the X chromosome. SEE: *holandric.*

holophrase A single word, usually a verb, used to convey a variety of meanings. It is common in the development of speech in toddlers.

holophytic (hŏl"ō-fĭt'ĭk) [" + *phyton,* plant] Having plantlike characteristics, esp. in reference to protozoa that resemble plants in their metabolic processes.

holoprosencephaly (hŏl"ō-prŏs"ĕn-sĕf'ă-lē) [" + *proso,* before, + *enkephalos,* brain] A congenital defect caused by an extra chromosome, either trisomy 13–15 or trisomy 18, which causes deficiency in the forebrain.

holorachischisis (hŏl"ō-ră-kĭs'kĭ-sĭs) [" + *rhachis,* spine, + *schisis,* a splitting] Complete spina bifida.

holosystolic (hŏl″ō-sĭs-tŏl′ĭk) [″ + *systellein,* to draw together] Relating to the entire duration of systole.

holotetanus, holotonia (hŏl-ō-tĕt′ă-nŭs, hŏl″ō-tō′nē-ah) [″ + *tetanos,* tetanus, ″ + *tonos,* tension] A muscular spasm of the entire body.

holotrichous (hōl-ŏt′rĭ-kŭs) [″ + *thrix,* hair] Covered entirely with flagella, said of certain protozoa and bacteria.

holozoic (hŏl″ō-zō′ĭk) [″ +*zoion,* animal] Resembling an animal as to its method of nutrition in which organic materials serve as a source of energy.

Holter monitor [Norman Jefferis Holter, U.S. biophysicist, 1914–1983] A portable device small enough to be worn by a patient during normal activity. It consists of an electrocardiograph and a recording system capable of storing up to 24 hr of the individual's ECG record. It is particularly useful in obtaining a record of cardiac arrhythmia that would not be discovered by means of an ECG of only a few minutes' duration. Ambulatory electrocardiographic monitoring also can be used to diagnose losses of consciousness or palpitations of unclear etiology, to assess episodes of unrecognized myocardial ischemia, and to evaluate how well therapeutic interventions against such illnesses are working.

Holthouse's hernia (hŏlt′howz-ĕs) [Carsten Holthouse, Brit. surgeon, 1810–1901] An inguinal hernia protruding along the folds of the groin.

Holt-Oram syndrome [Mary Clayton Holt, contemporary Brit. physician; Samuel Oram, contemporary Brit. physician] An inherited disorder, transmitted as an autosomal trait, that is marked by anomalies of the upper limbs and heart. Clinical manifestations vary from minimal radiographic changes to overt structural changes in the hands and arms and single or multiple atrial and ventricular defects that may be life-threatening.

homalocephalus (hŏm″ă-lō-sĕf′ă-lŭs) [Gr. *homalos,* level, + *kephale,* head] A person with a flat skull.

Homans' sign (hō′mănz) [John Homans, U.S. surgeon, 1877–1954] Pain in the calf when the foot is passively dorsiflexed. This is a physical finding suggestive of venous thrombosis of the deep veins of the calf; however, diagnostic reliability is limited, that is, elicited calf pain may be associated with conditions other than thrombosis, and an absence of calf pain does not rule out thrombosis.

homatropine hydrobromide, homatropine methylbromide (hō-măt′rō-pēn) An antimuscarinic drug that acts like belladonna.

homaxial (hō-măk′sē-ăl) [Gr. *homos,* same, + L. *axis,* axis] Having all axes alike, as a sphere.

home assessment An evaluation of the home environment of persons with functional impairment, usually by an occupational therapist or home care specialist, for purposes of identifying architectural barriers and safety hazards and recommending modifications or devices for improving mobility, safety, and independent function. SYN: *home evaluation*.

home evaluation Home assessment.

homeless (hōm′lĕss) Having no permanent or usual domicile. Persons with no fixed home are often economically disadvantaged, socially isolated, unemployed, and/or uninsured. They may have limited access to preventive and acute health care, and may suffer from untreated acute, chronic, or infectious illnesses.

home maintenance management, impaired Inability to independently maintain a safe, growth-promoting immediate environment. SEE: *Nursing Diagnoses Appendix.*

homeo- [Gr. *homoios,* like, similar] Prefix indicating *likeness; resemblance; constant unchanging state.*

homeodynamics A principle within the nursing conceptual system of Martha Rogers, which suggests that human nature is dynamic, everchanging, and holistic. In contrast to homeostasis, in which we adapt to our environment, homeodynamics suggests that we interact with our environment. Nursing assessment then focuses on the patient's pattern, rhythm, and source of energy, rather than on his or her coping mechanisms and modes of adaptation.

homeomorphous (hō″mē-ō-mor′fŭs) [″ + *morphe,* form] Of like shape but different compositions.

homeo-osteoplasty (hō″mē-ō-ŏs′tē-ō-plăs″tē) [″ + *osteon,* bone, + *plassein,* to form] Grafting of a piece of bone that is like the one onto which it is grafted.

homeopathist (hō-mē-ŏp′ă-thĭst) One who practices homeopathy.

homeopathy (hō-mē-ŏp′ă-thē) [Gr. *homoios,* like, + *pathos,* disease] A school of American healing, founded by Dr. Samuel Christian Friedrich Hahnemann (1755–1843) in the late 18th century, based on the idea that very dilute doses of medicines that produce symptoms of a disease in healthy people will cure that disease in affected patients. This is loosely based on the theory that "like cures like." SEE: *allopathy*. **homeopathic** (hō″mē-ō-păth′ĭk), *adj.*

homeoplasia (hō″mē-ō-plā′zē-ă) [″ + *plassein,* to form] The formation of new tissue similar to that already existing in a part.

homeoplastic (hō″mē-ō-plăs′tĭk) Relating to or resembling the structure of adjacent parts.

homeostasis (hō″mē-ō-stā′sĭs) [″ + *stasis,* a standing] The state of dynamic equilibrium of the internal environment of the body that is maintained by the ever-changing processes of feedback and regulation in response to external or internal changes. **homeostatic** (-stăt′ĭk), *adj.*

homeotherapy (hō″mē-ō-thĕr′ă-pē) [″ + *therapeia,* treatment] The treatment or prevention of disease using a substance similar but not identical to the active causative agent, such as jennerian vaccination.

homeothermal (hō″mē-ō-thĕr′măl) [″ + *therme,* heat] Pert. to a homoiotherm.

homeotypical (hō″mē-ō-tĭp′ĭ-kăl) [″ + *typos,* type] Resembling the typical or normal.

home safety checklist A device to evaluate, anticipate, and prevent injuries (usually caused by accidental falls) to an impaired individual in his or her own home.

homesickness [AS. *ham,* home, + *seoc,* ill] Sadness, depression, and anxiety related to being away from home or loved ones.

homicide (hŏm′ĭ-sīd) [L. *homo,* man, + *caedere,* to kill] **1.** Murder. **2.** A murderer. **homicidal,** *adj.*

hominid (hŏm′ĭ-nĭd) [″+ *eidos,* form, shape] A primate of the Hominidae family. Humans are the only surviving species.

Homo (hō′mō) [L., man] A genus of primates of the family Hominidae. The sole existing species is humankind, *Homo sapiens.* Evidence from fossils indicates extinct species (e.g., *H. habilis, H. erectus, H. australopithecus*).

homo- [Gr. *homos,* same] Prefix meaning *the same* or *a likeness.*

homoblastic (hō″mō-blăs′tĭk) [″ + *blastos,* germ] Developing from a single type of tissue; the opposite of heteroblastic.

homocentric (hō″mō-sĕn′trĭk) [″ + *kentron,* center] Having the same center.

homochronous (hō-mŏk-rō′nŭs) [″ + *chronos,* time] Occurring at the same time or at the same age in each generation.

homocysteine (hō″mō-sĭs-tē′ĭn) $HSCH_2CH_2CH(NH_2)COOH$; an amino acid produced by the catabolism of methionine. With serine, it forms a complex that eventually produces cysteine and homoserine. There is evidence that a high level of homocysteine in the blood may be associated with an increased risk of developing atherosclerosis. Blood homocysteine levels may be lowered by eating foods rich in folic acid, such as green leafy vegetables and fruits, and by vitamin B_6 or B_{12} supplementation.

homocystine (hō″mō-sĭs′tĭn) $H_{16}N_2O_4S_2$; a homologue of cystine formed by condensation of two molecules of homocysteine.

homocystinuria (hō″mō-sĭs-tĭn-ū′rē-ă) An inherited disease caused by the absence of the enzyme essential to the metabolism of homocystine. Patients are mentally retarded and have subluxated lenses, a tendency toward seizures, liver disease, an increased risk of atherosclerosis and blood clotting disorders, and growth retardation (short stature).

homocytotropic (hō″mō-sī″tō-trŏp′ĭk) [″ + *kytos,* cell, + *tropos,* a turning] Having an affinity for cells of the same species.

homodromous (hō-mŏd′rō-mŭs) [″ + *dromos,* running] Moving in the same direction or toward the same goal.

homoerotic (hō″mō-ĕ-rŏt′ĭk) Homosexual (2).

homogametic (hō″mō-gă-mĕt′ĭk) [″ + *gamos,* marriage] Pert. to the production of one kind of gamete with regard to the sex chromosome. In humans, the XX female is the homogametic sex, as all ova produced contain the X chromosome. SEE: *heterogametic.*

homogenate (hō-mŏj′ĕ-nāt) The material obtained when something is homogenized.

homogeneous (hō″mŏ-jē′nē-ŭs) [″ + *genos,* kind] Uniform in structure, composition, or nature; the opposite of heterogeneous.

homogenesis (hō-mō-jĕn′ĕ-sĭs) [″ + *genesis,* generation, birth] Reproduction by the same process in succeeding generations; the opposite of heterogenesis.

homogenize (hō-mŏj′ĕ-nīz) To make homogeneous; to produce a uniform emulsion or suspension of two substances normally immiscible.

homogentisuria (hō″mō-jĕn″tĭ-sū′rē-ă) Alkaptonuria.

homograft (hō′mō-grăft) Allograft.

homoiopodal (hō″moy-ŏp′ō-dăl) [Gr. *homoios,* like, + *pous, pod-,* foot] Having only one kind of protruding process, as a dendrite in a nerve cell.

homoiotherm (hō-moy′ō-thĕrm) [″ + *therme,* heat] A warm-blooded organism that maintains a constant body temperature despite fluctuating environmental temperatures; the opposite of poikilotherm.

homokeratoplasty (hō″mō-ker′ă-tō-plăs″tē) A homograft of corneal tissue.

homolateral [Gr. *homos,* same, + L. *latus,* side] Ipsilateral.

homologous (hō-mŏl′ō-gŭs) [″ + *logos,* word, reason] Similar in fundamental structure and in origin but not necessarily in function (e.g., the arm of a man, forelimb of a dog, and wing of a bird). SEE: *heterologous.*

homologous organs Structures that are morphological equivalents, as the arm of a human and the forelimb of a quadruped; the penis of a man and the clitoris of a woman.

homologue (hŏm′ŏ-lŏg) **1.** An organ or part common to a number of species. **2.** One that corresponds to a part or organ in another structure. **3.** In chemistry, any member of a series that resembles the other members in action and general structure but has a constant compositional difference such as a methyl, CH_3, group.

homology (hō-mŏl′ō-jē) [″ + *logos,* word, reason] Similarity in structure but not necessarily in function; the opposite of analogy.

homolysin (hō-mŏl′ĭ-sĭn) [″ + *lysis,* dissolution] An agent in serum destructive to erythrocytes.

Homonidae [L. *homo,* man, + Gr. *ideos,* pert. to] A family of primates that includes ancient and modern humans.

homonomous (hō-mŏn′ō-mŭs) [″ + *nomos,* law] Pert. to parts arranged in a series that are similar in form and structure, as metameres of a segmented animal or the fingers and toes of a mammal.

homonymous (hō-mŏn′ĭ-mŭs) [″ + *onyma,* name] Having the same name.

homophil (hō-mō-fĭl) [″ + *philein,* to love] Pert. to an antibody reacting only with a specific antigen.

homophile (hō-mō-fĭl′) Homosexual (1).

homophobe One who fears or dislikes homosexuals.

homophobia An abnormal fear of homosexuals.

homoplastic (hō″mō-plăs′tĭk) [″ + *plassein,* to form] Having a similar form and structure.

Homo sapiens (hō′mō sā′pē-ĕnz) [L. *homo,* man, + *sapiens,* wise, sapient] The species to which modern humans belong. SEE: *Homo.*

homosexual (hō″mō-sĕks′ū-ăl) [Gr. *homos,* same, + L. *sexus,* sex] A person who has sexual interest in, or sexual intercourse exclusively with members of his or her own sex.

homosexuality (hō″mō-sĕks″ū-ăl′ĭ-tē) A condition in which the libido is directed toward one of the same sex.

homostimulant (hōm″ō-stĭm′ū-lănt) [″ + L. *stimulare,* to arouse] Stimulating the organ from which an extract is derived.

homotherm (hō′mō-thĕrm) [″ + *therme,* heat] An animal whose body temperature remains constant regardless of the temperature of the environment. SYN: *warm-blooded animal.* SEE: *poikilotherm.* **homothermal** (hōm″ō-thĕr′măl), *adj.*

homotopic (hōm″ō-tŏp′ĭk) [″ + *topos,* place] Occurring at the same site on the body.

homotransplantation (hō″mē-ō-trăns″plăn-tā′shŭn) [″ + L. *trans,* across, + *plantare,* to plant] Allotransplantation.

homotype (hō′mō-tīp) [″ + *typos,* type] One organ or part similar in form and function to another, as one of two paired parts or organs.

homotypic (hō′mō-tīp′ĭk) Of the same form and type.

homovanillic acid ABBR: HVA. A catecholamine that is a metabolite of dopamine. It is found in excessive quantities in patients with neuroendocrine tumors, such as pheochromocytoma, or neuroblastoma.

homozygosis (hōm″ō-zī-gō′sĭs) [″ + *zygon,* yoke, pair, + *osis,* condition] The formation of a zygote by the union of gametes that have one or more identical alleles. SEE: *heterozygosis.*

homozygote (hōm″ō-zī′gōt) A homozygous individual; an individual developing from gametes with similar alleles and thus possessing like pairs of genes for a given hereditary characteristic.

homozygous (hōm″ō-zī′gŭs) **1.** Produced by similar alleles. **2.** Said of an organism when germ cells transmit nearly identical alleles as a result of inbreeding.

homunculus (hō-mŭn′kū-lŭs) [L. diminutive of *homo,* man] **1.** A dwarf in whom the body parts develop in their normal proportions. **2.** An anatomic device for representing the innervation of body parts in the central nervous system.

honey [AS. *hunig*] A sweet thick liquid substance produced by bees via the enzymatic digestion of the sucrose in nectar into fructose and glucose. The honey's color and flavor are determined by the flowers from which the nectar was obtained. Honey has been used by humans as a food since ancient times. Honey is composed of mostly fructose and glucose with a typical moisture content of about 17%. It is unsafe for human infants or babies to consume honey because it can contain *Clostridium botulinum* spores. This is usually not an issue for older individuals as their stomach acid is sufficient to inhibit the growth of this organism.

honorific [L. *honorificus,* honor-making] To convey honor upon a person, esp. while writing or speaking about an individual. SEE: *pejorative.*

hook [AS. *hok,* an angle] **1.** A curved instrument. **2.** The terminal device in an upper extremity orthosis.

hookworm A parasitic nematode belonging to the superfamily Strongyloidea, esp. *Ancylostoma duodenale* and *Necator americanus.* SEE: illus.

HOOKWORM DISEASE: Hookworm eggs deposited on the soil in feces mature into larvae capable of penetrating the skin, esp. the bare skin of the foot. An allergic or inflamed rash may develop at the entry site. The larvae pass from the skin into the venous circulation and travel to the alveolar capillaries of the lungs, up the bronchi and trachea, and into the gastrointestinal tract. There they mature, attach to the mucous membrane of the intestine, and begin feeding on host blood. The adults secrete an anticoagulant, which promotes additional bleeding. Eventually,

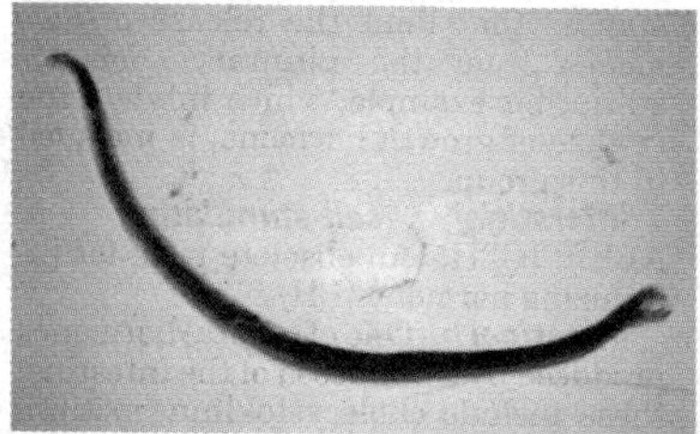

ADULT HOOKWORM

(Orig. Mag. ×10)

the host develops iron-deficiency anemia. Patients sometimes report nausea, colicky abdominal pain, bloating, and pica. Affected children may suffer growth retardation. The adult worms produce eggs that are excreted in the feces, perpetuating the cycle of infection. The detection of these eggs in the stool provides the basis for diagnosis of the disease.

TREATMENT: Mebendazole and pyrantel pamoate are used to eradicate the infection. Iron supplements are needed to treat the anemia.

Hoover sign [Charles F. Hoover, U.S. physician, 1865–1927] A test used in suspected unilateral hysterical paralysis. The examiner places a hand under the heel of the paralyzed leg and asks the patient to raise the normal leg against resistance. In hysterical paralysis, the examiner will feel pressure against the hand under the allegedly paralyzed leg. In true paralysis, no pressure will be felt.

hope The expectation that something desired will occur. One of the bases of professional health care is the presence of hope, while providing accurate information, and realistic reassurance.

hopelessness Despair; loss of faith in the possibility of a positive outcome. Loss of trust in one's prospects may give rise to depression, desperation, or antisocial behaviors. SEE: *grief reaction; helplessness; Nursing Diagnoses Appendix.*

hordeolum (hor-dē′ō-lŭm) [L., barleycorn] Sty(e).

horizontal [L. *horizontalis*] **1.** Parallel to or in the plane of the horizon. **2.** A transverse plane of the body that is at right angles to the vertical axis of the body.

hormesis (hor-mē′sĭs) [Gr. *hormesis,* rapid motion] **1.** The stimulating effect of a small dose of a substance that is toxic in larger doses. **2.** The controversial hypothesis that very low doses of ionizing radiation may not be harmful and may even have beneficial effects.

hormion (hor′mē-ŏn) [Gr., little chain] The junction of the posterior border of the vomer with the sphenoid bone.

hormonagogue (hor-mōn′ă-gŏg) [Gr. *hormon,* urging on, + *agogos,* leading] Stimulating or increasing the production of a hormone.

hormone (hor′mōn) [Gr. *hormon,* urging on] **1.** A substance originating in an organ, gland, or body part that is conveyed through the blood to another body part, chemically stimulating that part to increase or decrease functional activity or to increase or decrease secretion of another hormone. **2.** The secretion of the ductless glands (e.g., insulin from the pancreas). SEE: *endocrine gland.* **hormonal** (hor-mō′năl), *adj.*

adaptive h. A hormone produced in response to adapting to stress or some other powerful stimulus.

adrenocortical h. A hormone secreted by the cortex of the adrenal gland. SEE: *adrenal gland.*

adrenomedullary h. One of several hormones, including epinephrine and norepinephrine, that are produced by the adrenal medulla.

androgenic h. A hormone that regulates the development and maintenance of the male secondary sexual characteristics; an androgen. Androgens are secreted by the interstitial tissue of the testis and by the adrenal cortex of both sexes. Androgens include testosterone, androsterone, and dehydroandrosterone.

anterior pituitary h. One of several hormones secreted by the anterior lobe of the pituitary, including growth hormone; thyrotropic (TSH), gonadotropic, follicle-stimulating (FSH), luteinizing hormone (LH), prolactin; melanocyte-stimulating hormones; and corticotropin.

antidiuretic h. ABBR: ADH. A peptide hormone that plays a crucial role in limiting the amount of water excreted by the kidneys. Deficiencies of this hormone result in central diabetes insipidus. Excesses cause water retention and hyponatremia. SYN: *vasopressin.*

The hormone is produced by the hypothalamus and stored in the posterior pituitary gland; it is secreted when the osmolarity of plasma rises. Secretion of ADH increases the concentration of the urine by preventing water losses from the renal tubules. The hormone also causes constriction of arterioles (raising blood pressure) and increases levels of clotting factor VIII.

calcitonin h. calcitonin.

corpus luteum h. Progesterone. It stimulates development of secretory uterine endometrium and facilitates implantation of the fertilized ovum by reducing uterine motility.

cortical h. Adrenocortical h.

corticotropin-releasing h. ABBR: CRH. A hormone released from the hypothalamus that acts on the anterior pituitary to increase secretion of adrenal corticotropin hormone (ACTH). In response to stress, CRH causes hyperglycemia, increased oxygen consumption, increased cardiac output, and decreased sexual activity; suppresses release of growth hormone; diminishes gastrointestinal function; stimulates respiration; and causes behavioral changes.

counterregulatory h. Any hormone that opposes the effects of insulin. Examples include glucagon, epinephrine, norepinephrine, cortisol, and growth hormone.

digestive h. Any of a group of hormones produced by the stomach or small intestinal mucosa that stimulates various tissues to release enzymes, produce fluids, or affect gastrointestinal motility. The digestive hormones include gastrin, motilin, secretin, cholecystokinin, and vasoactive intestinal peptide, among others.

estrogenic h. A hormone that stimulates the development and maintenance of female sexual characteristics. Estrogens are secreted by the ovaries and the placenta in women and by the adrenal cortex in both sexes. Estrogenic hormones include estradiol, estrone, and estriol.

follicle-stimulating h. ABBR: FSH. A hormone secreted by the anterior lobe of the pituitary that stimulates maturation of the ovarian follicles in women. In men, the hormone is important in maintaining spermatogenesis.

follicle-stimulating h. releasing hormone ABBR: FSHRH. A hormone from the hypothalamus that regulates release of follicle-stimulating hormone.

gastric h. Gastrin.

gonadotropic h. An anterior pituitary hormone (follicle-stimulating hormone or luteinizing hormone) affecting the gonads.

gonadotropin-releasing h. ABBR: GnRH. The hormone produced in the hypothalamus that causes the pituitary to release the gonadotrophic substances luteinizing hormone and follicle-stimulating hormone. This hormone is used in treating endometriosis. SYN: *Luteinizing hormone-releasing h.*

growth h. ABBR: GH. A hormone secreted by the anterior pituitary that regulates the cell division and protein synthesis necessary for normal growth. SYN: *somatotropin.*

growth hormone-releasing h. ABBR: GH-RH. A hormone from the hypothalamus that stimulates the release of growth hormone from the anterior pituitary.

human placental lactogen h. SEE: *lactogen, human placental.*

immunoregulatory h. A hormone that influences components of the immune system, including the number and activity of the white blood cells. Hormones secreted by almost all of the glands in the body, particularly the hypothalamus and adrenal glands, are immunoregulatory.

inhibitory h. One of a group of substances that limit the release of hormones from the pituitary. Somatostatin, for example, which inhibits the release of growth hormone, is included in this group.

interstitial cell-stimulating h. ABBR: ICSH. An obsolete term for luteinizing hormone (LH).

intestinal h. One of several hormones produced by the mucosa of the intestine; these include cholecystokinin, motilin, secretin, vasoactive inhibitory peptide, and others.

lipolytic h. Any hormonal substance that promotes release of free fatty acids from fat tissue (e.g., epinephrine, glucagon, and cortisol).

luteal h. Progesterone.

luteinizing h. ABBR: LH. A hormone produced by the anterior lobe of the pituitary, which stimulates the development of interstitial cells of the testes and the secretion of testosterone by those cells. In women, it stimulates ovulation (i.e., rupture of the mature ovarian follicle, transformation of the follicle into the corpus luteum, and secretion of progesterone and estrogen by the corpus luteum).

luteinizing hormone-releasing h. ABBR: LH-RH. A hormone from the hypothalamus that stimulates the release of luteinizing hormone from the anterior pituitary. SYN: *gonadotropin-releasing h.*

luteotropic h. Luteinizing h.

melanocyte-stimulating h. ABBR: MSH. A hormone of the anterior pituitary gland that causes pigmentation of the skin in humans.

ovarian h. A hormone produced by the ovary. SEE: *estradiol; estriol; estrogen; estrone; progesterone.*

pancreatic h. A hormone produced by the islets of Langerhans of the pancreas. SEE: *glucagon; insulin.*

parathyroid h. A hormone secreted by the parathyroid glands that regulates blood levels of calcium and phosphorus. Its deficiency results in low serum calcium levels (hypoparathyroidism); in excess, it causes hypercalcemia (hyperparathyroidism). SYN: *parathormone.*

placental h. One of the hormones secreted by the placenta; they include estrogen and progesterone, chorionic gonadotropin, a hormone similar to thyroid-stimulating hormone (TSH), melanocyte-stimulating hormone (MSH).

posterior pituitary h. One of the hormones secreted by the posterior lobe of the pituitary, including vasopressin, which produces vasopressor and antidiuretic effects, and oxytocin, which stimulates contraction of smooth muscle of the uterus. SEE: *antidiuretic h.*

progestational h. Progesterone.

releasing h. One of a group of substances secreted by the hypothalamus that control or inhibit the release of various hormones. Thyrotropin-releasing hormone, gonadotropin-releasing hormone, dopamine, growth hormone–releasing hormone, corticotropin-releasing hormone, and somatostatin are included in this group. Dopamine and somatostatin act to inhibit release of the hormones they act upon.

sex h. An androgenic or estrogenic hormone.

somatotropic h. Somatotropin.

somatotropin-releasing h. Growth hormone-releasing h.

synthetic human growth h. A growth hormone made with recombinant DNA techniques.

testicular h. A hormone produced by the interstitial tissue of the testis (e.g., testosterone and inhibin, which is produced by the sustentacular cells).

thyroid h. A hormone secreted by the follicles of the thyroid gland. The two active thyroid hormones are thyroxine (T_4) and triiodothyronine (T_3). They act on receptors in tissues throughout the body to increase the production of cellular proteins, the metabolic rate, and the activities of the sympathetic nervous system. Deficiencies of thyroid hormone produce clinical hypothyroidism; excesses cause hyperthyroidism.

thyrotropic h. Thyrotropin.

thyrotropin-releasing h. ABBR: TRH. A hormone secreted by the hypothalamus that stimulates the anterior pituitary to release thyrotropin.

hormonogenesis (hor″mō-nō-jĕn′ĕ-sĭs) [″ + *genesis,* generation, birth] Hormonopoiesis. **hormonogenic** (-jĕn′ĭk), *adj.*

hormonology (hor″mō-nŏl′ō-jē) [″ + *logos,* word, reason] Clinical endocrinology.

hormonopoiesis (hor″mō-nō-poy-ē′sĭs) [″ + *poiesis,* formation] The production of hormones. SYN: *hormonogenesis.* **hormonopoietic** (-ĕt′ĭk), *adj.*

hormonotherapy (hor″mō-nō-thĕr′ă-pē) The therapeutic use of hormones.

horn A cutaneous outgrowth composed chiefly of keratin; a hornlike projection. SYN: *cornu.*

h. of Ammon Hippocampus.

anterior h. of the spinal cord The horn-shaped portion of the gray matter of the anterior part of the spinal cord. SEE: *spinal cord.*

cicatricial h. A cutaneous horn originating in scar tissue.

cutaneous h. A hard, horny outgrowth from the skin. It is slow-growing, benign, and may be small or large, 10 to 12 cm, in diameter.

dorsal h. The posterior horn of the gray matter of the spinal cord.

posterior h. of the spinal cord The horn-shaped portion of the gray matter of the posterior part of the spinal cord. SEE: *spinal cord.*

sebaceous h. A hard protrusion from a sebaceous gland.

ventral h. The anterior horn of the gray matter of the spinal cord.

warty h. A hard outgrowth from a wart.

Horner's syndrome (hor′nĕrz) [Johann F. Horner, Swiss ophthalmologist, 1831–1886] A syndrome characterized by contraction of the pupil, partial ptosis of the eyelid, enophthalmos, and sometimes loss of sweating over one side of the face. The syndrome is caused by paralysis of the cervical sympathetic nerve trunk, often as a result of an anesthetic mishap, or a tumor in the superior sulcus of the lung.

horopter (hō-rŏp′tĕr) [Gr. *horos,* limit, + *opter,* observer] The sum of all points in space that have a corresponding point on the retina of the eye.

horripilation (hor″ĭ-pĭ-lā′shŭn) [L. *horrere,* to bristle, + *pilus,* hair] Piloerection.

horror Intense fear, revulsion, or dread caused by seeing or hearing something that is terrifying, shocking, or perceived to be life-threatening to the individual or to others.

horsepower A unit of power equal to 745.7 watts, or 550 foot pounds per second.

hospice (hŏs′pĭs) An interdisciplinary program of palliative care and supportive services that addresses the physical, spiritual, social, and economic needs of terminally ill patients and their families. This care may be provided in the home or a hospice center. To obtain information about locating a hospice program, contact the National Hospice Organization (http://www.nho.org/), telephone 800-658-8898; or Hospice Foundation of America (http://www.hospicefoundation.org), telephone 202-638-5419.

hospital [L. *hospitalis,* pert. to a guest] An institution for treatment of the sick and injured.

base h. **1.** A hospital unit within the lines of an army that receives wounded and sick patients from the front and the line. **2.** A hospital that a paramedic unit is assigned to and most frequently calls into for medical control orders.

camp h. An immobile military unit for the care of the sick and wounded in camp.

evacuation h. A mobile advance hospital unit to replace field hospitals and supplement base hospitals.

field h. A portable military hospital beyond the zone of conflict and the dressing stations.

nonprofit h. A hospital that has legal exemption from paying income and property taxes. In these facilities, excess funds are reinvested in the hospital instead of being turned over to shareholders.

teaching h. A hospital concerned with instructing medical students, house officers (residents), and allied health personnel in conjunction with provision of medical care. The teaching programs may or may not be part of degree-granting programs, but most provide practical and didactic training that is needed to gain licensure in the health professions.

hospitalism [L. *hospitalis,* pert. to a guest, + Gr. *-ismos,* condition] **1.** The air of depression and apathy that often surrounds a group of seriously ill patients, esp. if they are in an overcrowded ward. **2.** A neurotic tendency to seek hospitalization and, once hospitalized, to resist being discharged.

hospitalist A physician in charge of caring for hospitalized patients. These practitioners are rarely involved in outpatient care; they concentrate their efforts on caring for emergency patients, critical care patients, and patients confined to wards.

hospitalization The removal of a patient to, and confinement in, a hospital.

host [L. *hospes,* a stranger] **1.** The organism from which a parasite obtains its nourishment. **2.** In embryology, the larger and more relatively normal of conjoined twins. **3.** In transplantation of tissue, the individual who receives the graft.

accidental h. A host other than the usual or normal one.

alternate h. Intermediate h. (1).

h. defense mechanisms A complex interacting system that protects the host from endogenous and exogenous microorganisms. It includes physical and chemical barriers, inflammatory response, reticuloendothelial system, and immune responses. SEE: *cytokine; interleukin-1; interferon.*

definitive h. **1.** The final host or the host in which the parasite reaches sexual maturity. SYN: *final h.* **2.** The vertebrate, when the intermediate host is an invertebrate.

final h. Definitive h. (1).

immunocompromised h. SEE: *immunocompromised.*

intermediate h. **1.** The host in which a parasite passes through its larval or asexual stages of development. SYN: *alternate h.* **2.** The invertebrate host, when the final host is a vertebrate.

h. of predilection The host preferred by a parasite.

reservoir h. A host other than the usual or normal one, in which a parasite is capable of living; it is a source of infestation.

transfer h. An interim host that is not essential for the completion of the life cycle of the parasite.

hostility (hŏ-stĭl′ĭ-tē) In psychiatry, the manifestation of anger, animosity, or antagonism in a situation in which such a reaction is unwarranted. Hostility may be directed toward oneself, others, or inanimate objects. It is almost always a symptom of depression.

hot [AS. *hat,* hot] **1.** Possessing a high temperature. **2.** Actively conducting an electric current. **3.** Contaminated with dangerous radioactive material.

hot flash In women, a common, but not universal symptom of declining ovarian function, falling estradiol levels, and impending menopause, marked by the sensation of sudden, brief flares of heat, followed by sweating. During the event, the face and anterior chest wall flush and radiate warmth. These symptoms may occur during the day, or they may interrupt sleep. In men, these same symptoms often occur during androgen ablation therapy for prostate cancer. SYN: *hot flush.*

TREATMENT: For women, hormone replacement therapy usually is effective in eliminating symptoms within 1 month; however, in the absence of supplemental estrogen, spontaneous resolution occurs in about 2 to 3 years. Men with hot flashes during treatment for prostate cancer may respond to antidepressant medications, such as venlafaxine. SEE: *menopause; estrogen replacement therapy; hormone replacement therapy.*

hotline A continuously managed telephone line for communicating with professionals who can help people experiencing crises, such as abuse or neglect, illicit drug distribution, impending suicide, intoxications and poisoning, domestic violence, or rape.

Hottentot apron [Hottentot, southern African population] An excessive elongation of the labia minora seen in Hottentot women. SYN: *velamen vulvae.*

hottentotism (hŏt′ĕn-tŏt-ĭsm) [*Hottentot* + Gr. *-ismos,* condition] A form of stuttering, initially and incorrectly attributed to the Hottentot tribe of South Africa.

hot water bag Rubber or plastic bag of various shapes and sizes for applying dry heat to circumscribed areas and for keeping moist applications warm.

Hounsfield unit In computed tomography (CT), a number or value that represents the attenuation of x-rays through a voxel (volume element) in the body and is assigned to the corresponding pixel (picture element) on the image. This number is relative to the standard, which is the absorption of x-rays in water on a scale of +1,000 to −1,000. It is also known as a CT unit.

housefly *Musca domestica,* a fly belonging to the order Diptera. It may be a mechanical carrier of pathogenic microorganisms.

house surgeon ABBR: H.S. The senior surgical member of the hospital staff who acts in the absence of the attending surgeon.

Houston's muscle (hūs′tŏns) [John

Houston, Irish surgeon, 1802–1845] The anterior part of the musculus bulbocavernosus of the penis.

Houston's valve One of the normal crescent-shaped folds of mucous membrane, or valves formed by them in the rectum.

Howell-Jolly bodies [William H. Howell, U.S. physiologist, 1860–1945; Justin Jolly, Fr. histologist, 1870–1953] Spherical granules (the remnants of nuclear chrmoatin) seen in erythrocytes in red blood cells of persons who are asplenic, and in hemolytic and pernicious anemias.

Howship's lacuna [John Howship, Brit. surgeon, 1781–1841] One of several small pits, grooves, or depressions found where bone is resorbed by osteoclasts. SEE: *osteoclast*.

Howship's symptom Paresthesia or pain in the obturator hernia on the inner side of the thigh.

Hp *haptoglobin.*

HPG *human pituitary gonadotropin.*

HPL *human placental lactogen.*

HPLC *high-pressure* or *high-performance liquid chromatography.*

HPO_3 Metaphosphoric acid.

H_3PO_2 Hypophosphorous acid.

H_3PO_3 Phosphorous acid.

H_3PO_4 Orthophosphoric acid.

$H_4P_2O_6$ Hypophosphoric acid.

hr *hour.*

H_2-receptor antagonists Drugs that inhibit gastric acid secretion by blocking the effects of histamine or acetylcholine on receptors found on parietal cells. They are used to treat peptic ulcers and gastroesophageal reflux disease. They are also known as H_2 blockers.

H reflex [after Hoffmann, who described it in 1918] In electrodiagnostic studies of spinal reflexes, the time required for a stimulus applied to a sensory nerve to travel to the spinal cord and return down the motor nerve. SEE: *F response*.

H.S. *house surgeon.*

h.s. *hora somni,* at bedtime.

H_2S Hydrogen sulfide.

HSA *human serum albumin.*

H_2SO_3 Sulfurous acid.

H_2SO_4 Sulfuric acid.

HSV *herpes simplex virus.*

5-HT *5-hydroxytryptamine,* serotonin.

Ht *total hypermetropia.*

ht *height.*

HTLV-I *human T-cell lymphotropic virus type I.*

HTLV-II *human T-cell lymphotropic virus type II.*

HTLV-III *human T-cell lymphotropic virus type III.*

Hubbard tank A tank of suitable size and shape for use in active or passive underwater exercises.

Huguier's canal (ū-gē-āz′) [Pierre C. Huguier, Fr. surgeon, 1804–1873] The canal through which the chorda tympani nerve exits from the cranium.

Huhner test (hoon′ĕr) [Max Huhner, U.S. urologist, 1873–1947] Postcoital examination of cervical mucus. Assessments include characteristics of the mucus as correlated with the phase of the woman's menstrual cycle, and the number, morphology, motility, and ability of the sperm to cross the cervical mucus. To maximize potential for coincidental conception, the test may be scheduled 1 to 2 days before the expected date of ovulation and within 2 to 3 hr after intercourse. SEE: *infertility*.

hum A soft continuous sound.

venous h. The sound from large veins in certain anemias.

human [L. *humanus,* human] Pert. to or characterizing men or women.

Human Genome Project An international research effort to map each human gene and to sequence the 3.1 billion chemical bases that make up human DNA. The U.S. National Human Genome Research Institute and Celera Genomics announced the initial deciphering of the genetic code in June 2000. This scientific milestone is expected to improve the way diseases are diagnosed, treated, and prevented, but it presents ethical, legal, and social issues regarding the use of genetic information.

human herpesvirus 6 A DNA virus that causes exanthem subitum (also known as roseola infantum) and childhood febrile seizures. It causes infections in immunocompromised patients (e.g., patients who have received organ transplants, patients with human immunodeficiency virus infection). Among children, infants between 6 months and 2 years of age are at highest risk for this infection, and asymptomatic or unrecognized infection is probably common. The incubation period is about 5 to 15 days.

human immunodeficiency virus ABBR: HIV. A retrovirus of the subfamily lentivirus that causes acquired immunodeficiency syndrome (AIDS). The most common type of HIV is HIV-1, identified in 1984. HIV-2, first discovered in West Africa in 1986, causes a loss of immune function and the subsequent development of opportunistic infections identical to those associated with HIV-1 infections. The two types developed from separate strains of simian immunodeficiency virus. In the U.S., the number of individuals infected with HIV-2 is very small, but blood donations are screened for both types of HIV. SEE: *acquired immunodeficiency syndrome*.

humanism The concept that human interests, values, and dignity are of utmost importance. This is integral to the actions and thoughts of those who care for the sick.

human T-cell lymphotropic virus type I ABBR: HTLV-I. A virus associated with adult T-cell leukemia.

human T-cell lymphotropic virus type II ABBR: HTLV-II. A virus associated with hairy cell leukemia.

human T-cell lymphotropic virus type III ABBR: HTLV-III. The former name for *human immunodeficiency virus.*

humectant (hū-mĕk′tănt) [L. *humectus,* moist] A moistening agent.

humeral (hū′mĕr-ăl) [L. *humerus,* upper arm] Pert. to the humerus.

humeroradial (hū″mĕr-ō-rā′dē-ăl) [″ + *radius,* wheel spoke, ray] Pert. to the humerus and radius, esp. in comparison of their lengths.

humeroscapular (hū″mĕr-ō-skăp′ū-lăr) [″ + *scapula,* shoulder blade] Concerning the humerus and scapula.

humeroulnar (hū″mĕr-ō-ŭl′năr) [″ + *ulna,* elbow] Pert. to the humerus and ulna, esp. in comparison of their lengths.

humerus (hū′mĕr-ŭs) [L., upper arm] The upper bone of the arm from the elbow (articulating with the ulna and radius) to the shoulder joint, where it articulates with the scapula. SEE: illus.

fracture of h. Physical injury of the humerus sufficient to fracture it. If the fracture is of the upper end of the humerus, the arm is abducted and splinted for about 4 weeks. Movements of the elbow and wrist are started early, and active movements of the shoulder are begun in about 3 weeks. SEE: *acromiohumeral; capitellum; cubitus; glenoid cavity.*

In a fracture of the shaft and lower end of the humerus, the limb is put in a plaster cast in a position midway between pronation and supination with the humerus at right angles to the forearm. Movement of the shoulder, wrist, and finger is allowed.

humid [L. *humidus,* moist] Moist, damp, esp. when pert. to air.

humidifier (hū-mĭd′ĭ-fī″ĕr) An apparatus to increase the moisture content of the air in a room.

wick h. A humidification system in which gas flow is exposed to a material saturated with water.

humidity [L. *humiditas*] Moisture in the atmosphere.

The moisture content of air usually is expressed as relative humidity. This indicates the amount of water vapor in the air compared with the maximum amount of moisture the air could contain at that temperature and atmospheric pressure. Air that is fully saturated with moisture has 100% relative humidity. When air that is fully saturated is cooled, the excess moisture condenses as in the case of dew or moisture on a cold glass in the summer.

absolute h. The actual mass of water vapor in a volume of gas, expressed as grams per cubic meter or milligrams per liter. It usually refers to ambient air.

relative h. The ratio of the amount of water vapor present in an air sample to the amount that could be present if the sample were saturated with water vapor. This value depends on the temperature of the air sample.

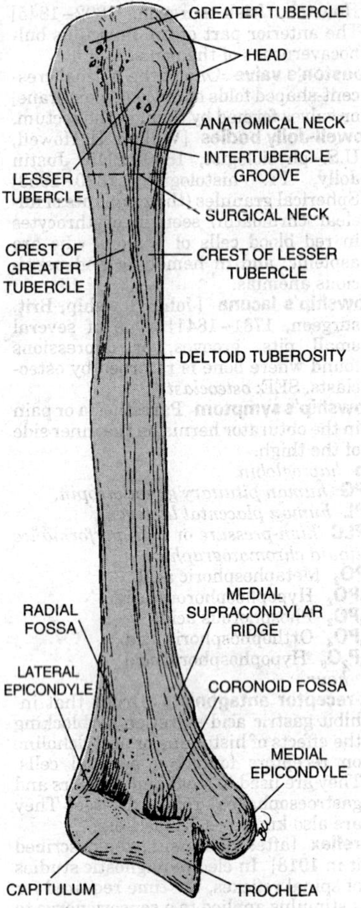

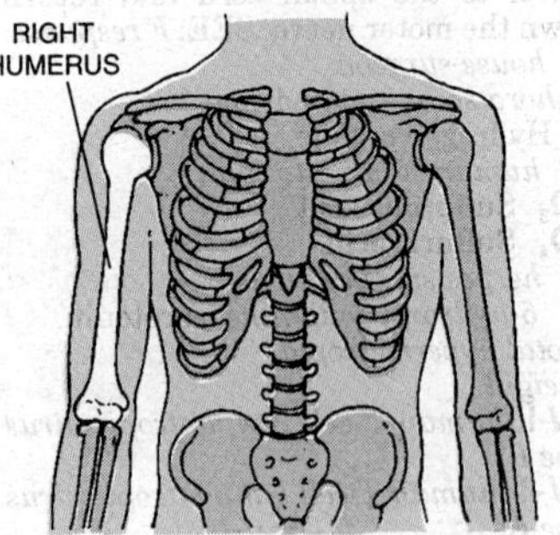

ANTERIOR VIEW OF RIGHT HUMERUS

humor (hū′mor) [L. *humor,* fluid] Any fluid or semifluid in the body. **humoral** (-ăl), *adj.*

aqueous h. The clear, watery fluid in the anterior and posterior chambers of the eye. It is produced by the ciliary processes and passes from the posterior to the anterior chamber, and then to the venous system by way of the canal of Schlemm.

crystalline h. The fluidlike substance of the crystalline lens of the eye.

ocular h. Either of the humors of the eye (aqueous and vitreous).

vitreous h. The vitreous body; a transparent semisolid in the posterior cavity between the lens and retina; one of the four refractive media of the eye.

humpback SEE: *kyphosis.*

hunchback SEE: *kyphosis.*

hunger [AS. *hungur*] **1.** A sensation resulting from lack of food, characterized by a dull or acute pain referred to the epigastrium or lower part of chest. It is usually accompanied by weakness and an overwhelming desire to eat. Hunger pains coincide with powerful contractions of the stomach. Hunger is distinguished from appetite in that hunger is the physical drive to eat while appetite is the psychological drive to eat. Hunger is affected by the physiological interaction of hormones and hormone-like factors while appetite is affected by habits, culture, taste, and many other factors. **2.** To have a strong desire.

air h. Dyspnea; breathlessness.

Hunner's ulcer (hŭn′ĕrz) [Guy LeRoy Hunner, U.S. surgeon, 1868–1957] Interstitial cystitis.

Hunter's canal [John Hunter, Scot. anatomist and surgeon, 1728–1793] Adductor canal.

Hunter's disease [Charles H. Hunter, Canadian physician, 1873–1955] Mucopolysaccharidosis II.

hunterian chancre Indurated, syphilitic chancre. SEE: *chancre.*

Huntington's chorea, Huntington's disease [George Huntington, U.S. physician, 1850–1916] A dominantly inherited disease of the central nervous system, marked by choreoathetosis (involuntary writhing, ballistic, or dance-like movements), gradually worsening emotional and behavioral disturbances, and eventual dementia. This neurodegenerative disease is rare, affecting about 5 persons in 100,000. Symptoms usually become obvious in adulthood, often after individuals who carry the causative gene have already transmitted it to their offspring. The movement disorder, behavioral decline, and loss of cognitive function that are hallmarks of the illness may take decades to come into being fully. Death usually occurs more than 15 yr after diagnosis. Postmortem examination of affected patients reveals atrophy of the putamen and caudate nucleus of the brain.

DIAGNOSIS: The diagnosis is straightforward when typical symptoms develop in a son or daughter of a parent known to have the disease. Genetic testing for the illness is available, although its use presents difficult ethical questions for couples who want to start a family.

TREATMENT: Dopamine agonist drugs, such as haloperidol or risperidone, can help control the movement disorder but must be used carefully because of the potential risk of movement-related side effects. There is no known treatment to stop the degeneration of the affected portions of the brain.

Hunt's neuralgia, Hunt's syndrome [Ramsey Hunt, U.S. neurologist, 1872–1937] Ramsay Hunt syndrome.

Hurler's syndrome (hoor′lĕrz) [Gertrud Hurler, Ger. pediatrician, 1889–1965] Mucopolysaccharidosis I-H.

Hürthle cells (hĕr′tĕl) [Karl Hürthle, Ger. histologist, 1860–1945] Large eosinophil-staining cells occasionally present in the thyroid gland. SEE: *tumor, Hürthle cell.*

Huschke, Emil (hoosh′kē) German anatomist, 1797–1858.

H.'s auditory teeth Tiny, toothlike protuberances at the edge of the cochlear labium vestibulare.

H.'s canal A canal formed by the juncture of the annulus tympanicus tubercules; usually present only during early childhood.

H.'s foramen A perforation found in arrested development near the inner extremity of the tympanic plate.

H.'s valve Lacrimal plica.

Hutchinson, Sir Jonathan British surgeon, 1828–1913.

H.-Gilford disease Progeria.

H.'s patch Salmon patch.

H.'s pupil A condition in which one pupil is dilated and the other is not. The pupil on the side of the lesion is dilated and the other is contracted. This condition is usually due to compression of the third cranial nerve in meningitis.

H.'s teeth A congenital condition marked by pegged, lateral incisors and notched central incisors along the cutting edge. It is a sign of congenital syphilis.

H.'s triad In congenital syphilis, the presence of interstitial keratosis, deafness, and Hutchinson's teeth.

Huxley's layer (hŭks′lēz) [Thomas H. Huxley, Brit. physiologist and naturalist, 1825–1895] The inner layer of nucleated cells forming the inner root sheath of a hair follicle.

HVA *homovanillic acid.*

hyalin (hī′ă-lĭn) [Gr. *hyalos,* glass] **1.** A clear substance present in tissues that have undergone amyloid degeneration. **2.** Material deposited in the glomerulus in certain forms of glomerulonephritis.

hyaline (hī′ă-līn) A histological term

rather than a specific indicator of cell injury, referring to any alteration within cells or in the extracellular space that gives a homogeneous, glassy, pink appearance in reactive histological sections stained with hematoxylin and eosin. SYN: *hyaloid*.

hyaline membrane disease Respiratory distress syndrome of the newborn.

hyalinization (hī″ă-lĭn″ĭ-zā′shŭn) The development of an albuminoid mass in a cell or tissue.

hyalinosis (hī″ă-lĭn-ō′sĭs) [Gr. *hyalos,* glass, + *osis,* condition] Waxy or hyaline degeneration.

hyalinuria (hī″ă-lĭn-ū′rē-ă) [″ + *ouron,* urine] Hyalin present in the urine.

hyalitis (hī-ă-lī′tĭs) [″ + *itis,* inflammation] An inflammation of the hyaloid membrane of the vitreous humor. SYN: *hyaloiditis*.

asteroid h. One of the spherical or star-shaped bodies in the vitreous of the eye, caused by inflammation.

h. punctata A form of hyalitis marked by minute opacities in the vitreous humor.

h. suppurativa A purulent inflammation of the vitreous humor.

hyalo- [Gr. *hyalos,* glass] Combining form indicating resemblance to glass.

hyaloenchondroma (hī″ă-lō-ĕn″kŏn-drō′mă) [″ + *en,* in, + *chondros,* cartilage, + *oma,* tumor] A chondroma composed of hyaline cartilage.

hyalogen (hī-ăl′ō-jĕn) [″ + *gennan,* to produce] A protein in cartilage and the vitreous humor.

hyaloid (hī′ă-loyd) [″ + *eidos,* form, shape] Hyaline.

hyaloiditis (hī″ă-loyd-ī′tĭs) [″ + *eidos,* form, shape, + *itis,* inflammation] Hyalitis.

hyalomucoid (hī″ă-lō-mū′koyd) [″ + L. *mucus,* mucus, + Gr. *eidos,* form, shape] Glycoprotein in the vitreous body.

hyalonyxis (hī″ă-lō-nĭk′sĭs) [″ + *nyxis,* puncture] The surgical procedure of puncturing the vitreous body.

hyalophagia, hyalophagy (hī″ă-lō-fā′jē-ă, -lŏf′ă-jē) [″ + *phagein,* to eat] The eating of glass.

hyalophobia (hī″ă-lō-fō′bē-ă) [″ + *phobos,* fear] A fear of touching glass.

hyaloplasm (hī′ă-lō-plăzm) [″ + LL. *plasma,* form, mold] An old term for cytoplasm.

hyalosis (hī″ă-lō′sĭs) [″ + *osis,* condition] Pathologic changes in the vitreous humor of the eye.

asteroid h. Suspended spherical white bodies, made of calcium salts, in the vitreous humor of the eye.

hyalosome (hī-ăl′ō-sōm) [″ + *soma,* body] An oval or round structure that resembles the nucleolus of a cell but stains only faintly.

hyaluronidase (hī″ă-lūr-ŏn′ĭ-dās) An enzyme that disrupts or destroys the extracellular framework of body tissues. It is found in many animal tissues and can be synthesized for therapeutic use. In the testes and the acrosomes of spermatozoa, along with other acrosomal enzymes, it degrades the hyaluronic acid in the corona radiata, facilitating the entry of sperm. In malignant tumors, it participates in the invasion of cancer cells through the basement membranes of blood vessels. It is also a component of the venoms of several animals (including vipers, stonefish, and bees and wasps) and contributes to the tissue destruction that may follow bites or stings from these animals. Some infectious bacteria that invade fascial planes (e.g., *Clostridia*) release it as an exotoxin.

USES: Synthetic hyaluronidase can be used to facilitate diffusion of injected local anesthetics (e.g., in cataract surgery).

hybrid (hī′brĭd) [L. *hybrida,* mongrel] The offspring of parents that are different, such as different species.

hybridization (hī′brĭd-ī-zā′shŭn) The production of hybrids by crossbreeding.

hybridoma (hī″brĭ-dō′mă) A cell produced by the fusion of a spleen cell from a mouse immunized with a specific antigen and a human multiple myeloma cell (a cancerous plasma B cell that makes antibodies). After the fusion, cells are screened to identify those capable of producing a continuous supply of monoclonal antibodies to the specific antigen. SEE: *monoclonal antibody*.

hydantoin (hī-dăn′tō-ĭn) A colorless base, glycolyl urea, $C_3H_4N_2O_2$, derived from urea or allantoin.

hydatid (hī′dă-tĭd) [Gr. *hydatis,* watery vesicle] **1.** A cyst formed in the tissues, esp. the liver, resulting from the development of the larval stage of the dog tapeworm, *Echinococcus granulosus.* The cyst develops slowly, forming a hollow bladder from the inner surface of which hollow brood capsules are formed. These may be attached to the mother cyst by slender stalks or may fall free into the fluid-filled cavity of the mother cyst. Scolices form on the inner surface of the older brood capsules. Older cysts have a granular deposit of brood capsules and scolices called hydatid sand. Hydatids may grow for years, sometimes to an enormous size. Albendazole, a drug available only from its manufacturer, SmithKline Beecham, has been used to treat this disease. It is poorly absorbed, must be used for a prolonged period, and can be toxic to the liver. The cysts should be removed surgically. SEE: illus.; *echinococcosis*. **2.** A small cystic remnant of an embryonic structure. SEE: *choriocarcinoma; hydatid mole*.

h. of Morgagni A cystlike remnant of the mullerian duct that is attached to the fallopian tube.

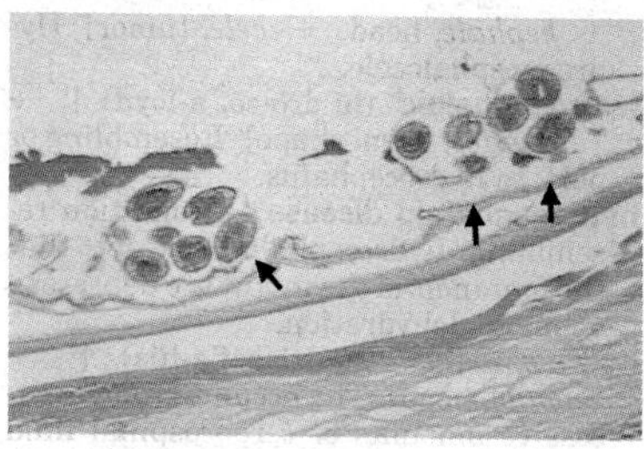

100 μm

HYDATID CYST

Three brood capsules shown (arrows) (orig. mag. ×100)

sessile h. Morgagnian hydatid connected with a testicle.

stalked h. Morgagnian hydatid connected with a fallopian tube.

hydatidocele (hī″dă-tĭd′ō-sēl) [″ + *kele,* tumor, swelling] A hydatid cyst of the scrotum or testicle.

hydatidoma (hī″dă-tĭd-ō′mă) [″ + *oma,* tumor] A tumor consisting of hydatids.

hydatidosis (hī″dă-tĭd-ō′sĭs) [Gr. *hydatis,* watery vesicle, + *osis,* condition] A condition caused by hydatid infestation.

hydatidostomy (hī″dă-tĭ-dŏs′tō-mē) [″ + *stoma,* mouth] The evacuation of a hydatid cyst by means of surgery.

hydatiform (hī-dăt′ĭ-form) [″ + L. *forma,* form] Hydatidiform.

hydatism (hī′dă-tĭzm) [″ + *-ismos,* condition] The sound produced by fluid in a cavity.

hydr- SEE: *hydro-.*

hydradenitis (hī″drăd-ĕn-ī′tĭs) [Gr. *hydros,* sweat, + *aden,* gland, + *itis,* inflammation] Inflammation of a sweat gland.

hydradenoma (hī″drăd-ĕ-nō′mă) [″ + ″ + *oma,* tumor] A tumor of a sweat gland.

hydraeroperitoneum (hī-dră″ĕr-ō-pĕr″ĭ-tō-nē′ŭm) [Gr. *hydor,* water, + *aer,* air, + *peritonaion,* peritoneum] A collection of fluid and gas in the peritoneal cavity.

hydralazine hydrochloride (hī-drăl′ă-zēn) An antihypertensive drug that works by vasodilating arteries and decreasing afterload.

hydramnion, hydramnios (hī-drăm′nē-ŏn, -ŏs) [″ + *amnion,* a caul on a lamb] An excess of amniotic fluid in the uterus.

hydranencephaly (hī″drăn-ĕn-sĕf′ă-lē) [″ + *an-,* not, + *enkephalos,* brain] Internal hydrocephalus caused by congenital absence of the cerebral hemispheres.

hydrarthrosis (hī″drăr-thrō′sĭs) [″ + *arthron,* joint, + *osis,* condition] Serous effusion in a joint; white swelling.

intermittent h. Recurring attacks of swelling of the large joints (esp. the knees), lasting 2 to 5 days and then remitting spontaneously. The condition affects men and women equally. The period between attacks is commonly 2 to 4 weeks, during which time the joint is normal. The knee is the usual joint involved but the elbow, hip, and ankle also may be affected.

hydrase (hī′drās) An enzyme that catalyzes the addition or withdrawal of water from a compound without hydrolysis occurring.

hydrate (hī′drāt) A crystalline substance formed by water combining with various compounds.

hydrated (hī′drā-tĕd) [L. *hydratus*] **1.** Combined chemically with water, forming a hydrate. **2.** Replete with fluids.

hydration (hī-drā′shŭn) **1.** The chemical combination of a substance with water. **2.** The addition of water to a substance, tissue, or patient.

hydraulics (hī-draw′lĭks) [Gr. *hydor,* water, + *aulos,* pipe] The science of fluids.

hydrazine (hī′dră-zēn) **1.** A colorless gas, H_4N_2, with a peculiar odor; soluble in water. **2.** One of a class derived from hydrazine.

h. sulfate A form of rocket fuel promoted by alternative medicine practitioners for the treatment of cancer. It is not effective.

hydremia (hī-drē′mē-ă) [Gr. *hydor,* water, + *haima,* blood] An excess of watery fluid in the blood.

hydrencephalocele (hī″drĕn-sĕf′ă-lō-sēl) [″ + *enkephalos,* brain, + *kele,* tumor] Hydroencephalocele.

hydrencephalomeningocele (hī″drĕn-sĕf″ă-lō-mĕ-nĭng′gō-sēl) [″ + ″ + *meninx,* membrane, + *kele,* tumor, swelling] A herniation through a defect in the skull. It contains brain and cerebrospinal fluid covered by meningeal tissues.

hydrencephalus (hī″drĕn-sĕf′ă-lŭs) Hydrocephalus.

hydrepigastrium (hī″drĕp-ĭ-găs′trē-ŭm) [″ + *epi,* upon, + *gaster,* belly] An accumulation of fluid between the peritoneum and the abdominal muscles.

hydride (hī′drīd) A chemical compound containing hydrogen and an element or radical.

hydrion (hī-drī′ŏn) The hydrogen ion (H^+).

hydro-, hydr- [Gr. *hydor,* water] Combining form pert. to water or to hydrogen.

hydroa (hĭd-rō′ă) Any bullous skin eruption.

hydroappendix (hī″drō-ă-pĕn′dĭks) [″ + L. *appendere,* to hang upon] Watery fluid distending the vermiform appendix.

hydrobilirubin (hī″drō-bĭl″ĭ-roo′bĭn) [″ + L. *bilis,* bile, + *ruber,* red] A brownish-red bile pigment, derived from bilirubin, and thought to be identical with stercobilin and urobilin.

hydrobromate (hī″drō-brō′māt) [″ + *bromos,* stench] A salt of hydrobromic acid.

hydrocalycosis (hī″drō-kăl″ĭ-kō′sĭs) [″ + *kalyx,* cup, + *osis,* condition] Cystic dilation of the renal calyx owing to obstruction.

hydrocarbon (hī″drō-kăr′bŏn) [″ + L. *carbo,* coal] A compound made up primarily of hydrogen and carbon.

alicyclic h. A hydrocarbon that contains cyclic and straight-chain components.

aliphatic h. A straight-chain hydrocarbon that contains no cyclic component.

aromatic h. A hydrocarbon in which the carbon atoms are in a ring, or cyclic, configuration.

cyclic h. A ring-shaped hydrocarbon.

saturated h. A hydrocarbon in which the carbon atoms are linked by a single electron pair and in which all valences are satisfied.

unsaturated h. A hydrocarbon in which carbon atoms share two or three pairs of electrons.

hydrocele (hī′drō-sēl) [″ + *kele,* tumor, swelling] The accumulation of serous fluid in a saclike cavity, esp. in the tunica vaginalis testis.

acute h. The most common hydrocele. The majority of cases occur suddenly between the second and fifth years, usually the result of inflammation of the epididymis or testis.

cervical h. A hydrocele in the neck resulting from the accumulation of serous fluid in the persistent cervical duct or cleft.

chronic h. A hydrocele usually seen in middle-aged men. It may result from filariasis.

congenital h. A hydrocele present at birth, resulting from failure of closure of the vaginal process.

encysted h. A hydrocele in the vaginal process in which openings to the scrotal and peritoneal cavities are closed.

h. feminae A cystlike sac of serous fluid in the labia majora or canal of Nuck. SYN: *h. muliebris.*

h. hernialis A condition in which a hernia accompanies infantile or congenital hydrocele and peritoneal fluid accumulates in a hernial sac.

infantile h. Peritoneal fluid in the tunica vaginalis and vaginal process with the latter closed at the abdominal ring.

h. muliebris H. feminae.

spermatic h. Spermatic fluid in the tunica vaginalis of the testes.

h. spinalis Spina bifida cystica.

hydrocelectomy (hī″drō-sē-lĕk′tō-mē) [″ + ″ + *ektome,* excision] Surgical removal of a hydrocele.

hydrocephalocele (hī″drō-sĕf′ă-lō-sēl) [″ + *kephalc,* head, + *kele,* tumor] Hydroencephalocele.

hydrocephaloid (hī″drō-sĕf′ă-loyd) [″ + ″ + *eidos,* form, shape] Resembling or pert. to hydrocephalus.

hydrocephaloid disease A condition resembling hydrocephalus, except that the fontanels of the infant are depressed owing to dehydration.

hydrocephalus (hī-drō-sĕf′ă-lŭs) [″ + *kephale,* head] The accumulation of excessive amounts of cerebrospinal fluid (CSF) within the ventricles of the brain, resulting from blockage or destruction of the normal channels for CSF drainage. Common causes include congenital lesions (e.g., spina bifida or aqueductal stenosis), traumatic lesions, neoplastic lesions, and infections such as meningoencephalitis. Sometimes the accumulated fluid leads to increased intracranial pressures. In congenital hydrocephalus, the faulty drainage of CSF from the ventricles of the brain often results in malformation of the skull and abnormal development of psychomotor and cognitive or language skills. SYN: *hydrencephalus.* SEE: *Nursing Diagnoses Appendix.* **hydrocephalic,** *adj.*

TREATMENT: Several neurosurgical procedures are available. The most commonly used procedure has been to establish a conduit for CSF (called a "shunt") from the ventricles of the brain to the peritoneal cavity.

PROGNOSIS: In untreated cases of congenital hydrocephalus, the outcome is fatal in about half of the patients. The prognosis for an uncomplicated course is excellent when hydrocephalus is promptly treated by use of a surgically instituted shunt.

PATIENT CARE: Vital signs and neurological status are monitored hourly or as necessary according to institutional protocol or the surgeon's directions. In infants, the anterior fontanel is inspected for bulging or depression. The patient is positioned as directed by the surgeon, usually on the nonoperative side with the head level with the body. Fluid intake and output are monitored, and I.V. fluids are administered as prescribed. The patient is assessed for vomiting (an early sign of increased ICP and shunt malfunction). The patient is monitored for signs of infection (especially meningitis) such as fever, stiff neck, irritability, or tense fontanels. The area over the shunt tract also is inspected for redness, swelling, and other signs of local infection. Dressings are checked for drainage and the wound redressed as necessary using aseptic technique. The patient also is observed for other signs and symptoms of postoperative complications, such as adhesions, paralytic ileus, peritonitis, migration, intestinal perforation (with peritoneal shunt), and dehydration and septicemia. Prescribed analgesics are administered; the dose is carefully titrated to provide pain relief while still permitting adequate neurological assessment. The family is taught postoperative care measures, including watching for signs of shunt malfunction, infection, and paralytic ileus. The parents are informed that shunt insertion requires periodic surgery to lengthen the shunt as the child grows and that surgery also may be necessary to correct malfunctions or treat infection. The parents are assisted to set goals consistent with the patient's ability and potential; the family should focus on the child's strengths rather than weaknesses. Special education programs also are discussed with the parents; the infant's need for sensory stimulation appropriate to age is emphasized.

communicating h. Hydrocephalus that maintains normal communication between the fourth ventricle and subarachnoid space.

congenital h. A chronic type of hydrocephalus occurring in infancy.

external h. An accumulation of fluid in subdural spaces.

h. ex vacuo The appearance on brain imaging of enlarged lateral ventricles, caused by atrophy of the brain.

internal h. An accumulation of fluid within ventricles of the brain.

noncommunicating h. Hydrocephalus in which a blockage at any location in the ventricular system prevents flow of cerebrospinal fluid to the subarachnoid space.

normal pressure h. A type of hydrocephalus with enlarged ventricles of the brain with no increase in the spinal fluid pressure or no demonstrable block to the outflow of spinal fluid. Shunting fluids from the dilated ventricles to the peritoneal cavity may be helpful. The classic triad of symptoms of NPH are disturbances of gait, progressive dementia, and urinary incontinence. SEE: *hydrocephalus*.

secondary h. Hydrocephalus following injury or infections such as meningitis or syphilis.

hydrochlorate (hī″drō-klō′rāt) [Gr. *hydor,* water, + *chloros,* green] Any salt of hydrochloric acid.

hydrochloride (hī″drō-klō′rīd) An alkaloid or other base combined with hydrochloric acid.

hydrochloroquine sulfate An antimalarial, antirheumatic drug, often used as a disease-modifying agent in rheumatoid arthritis, systemic lupus erythematosus, and some dermatological diseases. Trade name is Plaquenil Sulfate.

hydrochlorothiazide (hī″drō-klō″rō-thī′ă-zīd) ABBR: HCTZ. A thiazide diuretic used to treat high blood pressure. A common side effect is hypokalemia.

hydrocholeretic (hī″drō-kō″lĕr-rĕt′ĭk) Any agent that increases the output of bile without increasing the solids secreted in it.

hydrocirsocele (hī″drō-sĭr′sō-sēl) [″ + *kirsos,* varix, + *kele,* tumor, swelling] A hydrocele combined with varicose veins of the spermatic cord.

hydrocodone bitartrate (hī″drō-kō′dōn) A very commonly prescribed opioid pain reliever. Trade name is Vicodin.

hydrocolloid (hī″drō-kŏl′loyd) [″ + *kollodes,* glutinous] A colloidal suspension in which water is the liquid.

irreversible h. A hydrosol of alginic acid whose physical state is changed by an irreversible chemical reaction, forming insoluble calcium alginate. This substance is called alginate or dental alginate. Alginate is used in dentistry as a primary impression material. SYN: *alginate*.

CAUTION: Care should be taken not to inhale the dust created by alginate.

---

hydrocolpos (hī″drō-kŏl′pŏs) [″ + *kolpos,* vagina] Retention cyst of the vagina containing watery, nonsanguineous fluid or mucus.

hydrocortisone (hī″drō-kor′tĭ-sōn) A steroid hormone produced by the adrenal cortex and synthesized for medical use. It has anti-inflammatory, glucocorticoid, and sodium-retaining (mineralocorticoid) properties. It is used clinically to reduce the pain and inflammation of various conditions, including rashes, hemorrhoids, arthritis, and inflammatory bowel disease. It also is used as steroid replacement therapy in patients with adrenal insufficiency. SYN: *cortisol*.

h. acetate A form of corticosteroid that acts slowly over a long period.

hydrocyst (hī′drō-sĭst) [Gr. *hydor,* water, + *kystis,* bladder] A cyst containing watery fluid.

hydrocystoma [″ + ″ + *oma,* tumor] A disease marked by small cysts that originate in the sweat glands. These cysts may appear on the face, esp. in women after middle age. SYN: *hidrocystoma*.

hydrodensitometry The weighing of an object immersed in water and subsequent measurement of the water displaced. The specific gravity of the body can be estimated from that information, and the percentage of the body fat can be estimated. SEE: *lean body mass*.

hydrodiascope (hī″drō-dī′ă-skōp) [″ + *dia,* through, + *skopein,* to examine] A device used to treat astigmatism.

hydrodictiotomy (hī″drō-dĭk″tē-ŏt′ō-mē) [″ + *diktyon,* retina, + *tome,* incision] A surgical procedure to correct retinal displacement.

hydrodissection (hī″drō-dī-sĕk′shŭn)

Technique employing a pressurized fine stream of water (jet) to develop tissue planes or to divide certain soft tissues less traumatically than ordinary sharp dissection. Examples of its use include division of brain, hepatic tissue, etc. without destroying smaller blood vessels and other tubular structures. In abdominal surgery, open or laparoscopic hydrodissection is used to develop tissue planes and separate adhesions. It facilitates dissection of diseased parietal pleura in order to treat malignant pleural effusion. A modification is used in ophthalmologic surgery (e.g., phacoemulsification).

hydrodynamics The study of fluids in motion.

hydroencephalocele (hī″drō-ĕn-sĕf′ă-lō-sēl) [″ + *enkephalos,* brain, + *kele,* tumor, swelling] Brain substance expanded into a watery sac protruding through a cleft in the cranium. SYN: *hydrencephalocele*.

hydroflumethiazide (hī″drō-floo″mĕ-thī′ă-zīd) A diuretic and antihypertensive drug.

hydrogel (hī′drō-jĕl) [″ + L. *gelare,* to congeal] A colloid containing hydrophilic polymers. Hydrogels are used in soft contact lenses and the treatment of burns.

hydrogen [″ + *gennan,* to produce] SYMB: H. An element existing as a colorless, odorless, and tasteless gas, possessing one valence electron; atomic weight 1.0079, atomic number 1, specific gravity 0.069. A liter of the gas at sea level and at 0°C weighs 0.08988 g. Three isotopes of hydrogen (protium, deuterium, and tritium) exist, having atomic weights of approx. 1, 2, and 3, respectively.

OCCURRENCE: Hydrogen is present in the sun and stars. Even though it is the most abundant element in the known universe, its concentration in the earth's atmosphere is only 0.00005%. Hydrogen occurs in its free state (in natural gases and volcanic eruptions) only in minute quantities. It occurs principally on the earth as hydrogen oxide (water, H_2O) and is a constituent of all hydrocarbons. It is present in all acids and in ionic form is responsible for the properties characteristic of acids. It is present in nearly all organic compounds and is a component of all carbohydrates, proteins, and fats.

USES: It is highly flammable and used in the oxyhydrogen flame in welding; in hydrogenation of oils for solidifying purposes; as a reducing agent; and in many syntheses.

h. cyanide Hydrocyanic acid.

h. dioxide Hydrogen peroxide.

h. donor In oxidation-reduction reactions, a substance that gives up hydrogen atoms to another substance, the acceptor. SEE: *h. acceptor*.

h. iodide Hydriodic acid.

h. sulfide H_2S; a poisonous, flammable, colorless compound with a characteristic odor of rotten eggs. SYN: *hydrosulfuric acid*. SEE: *Poisons and Poisoning Appendix*.

hydrogenase (hī′drō-jĕn-ās) An enzyme that catalyzes reduction by molecular hydrogen.

hydrogenate (hī′drō-jĕn-āt″) To combine with hydrogen.

hydrogenation (hī″drō-jĕn-ā′shŭn) A process of changing an unsaturated fat to a solid saturated fat by the addition of hydrogen in the presence of a catalyst.

hydrogen peroxide H_2O_2; a colorless syrupy liquid with an irritating odor and acrid taste. It decomposes readily, liberating oxygen. Because light is particularly effective in decomposing H_2O_2, it should be stored in tightly sealed glass jars in a dark place. SYN: *hydrogen dioxide*.

USES: It is used as a commercial bleaching agent; as an oxidizing and reducing agent; and, in a 3% aqueous solution, as a mild antiseptic, germicide, and cleansing agent.

hydroglossa (hī″drō-glŏs′ă) [Gr. *hydor,* water, + *glossa,* tongue] Ranula.

hydrogymnastics (hī″drō-jĭm-năs′tĭks) A dated term for aquatic therapy.

hydrohematonephrosis (hī″drō-hĕm″ă-tō-nĕf-rō′sĭs) [″ + *haima,* blood, + *nephros,* kidney, + *osis,* condition] Bloody urine distending the pelvis of the kidney.

hydrokinetics (hī″drō-kī-nĕt′ĭks) [″ + *kinesis,* movement] The science of fluids in motion.

hydrolabile (hī″drō-lā′bĭl) Having the tendency to lose weight because of fluid loss possibly owing to gastrointestinal disease, or because of decreased salt or carbohydrate intake.

hydrolase (hī′drō-lās) An enzyme that causes hydrolysis.

hydrology (hī-drŏl′ō-jē) [″ + *logos,* word, reason] The science of water in all its aspects.

hydrolysate (hī-drŏl′ĭ-sāt) That which is produced as a result of hydrolysis.

protein h. The amino acids obtained from splitting proteins by hydrolysis; used as a source of amino acids in certain diets.

hydrolysis (hī-drŏl′ĭ-sĭs) [″ + *lysis,* dissolution] Any reaction in which water is one of the reactants, more specifically the combination of water with a salt to produce an acid and a base, one of which is more dissociated than the other. It involves a chemical decomposition in which a substance is split into simpler compounds by the addition or the taking up of the elements of water. This kind of reaction occurs extremely frequently in life processes. The conversion of starch to maltose, of fat to glycerol and fatty acid, and of protein to amino acids are examples of hydrolysis, as are other reactions involved in digestion. A simple example is the reaction in which the hydrolysis of ethyl acetate yields acetic acid and ethyl alcohol: $C_2H_5C_2H_3O_2 + H_2O = CH_3COOH + C_2H_5OH$. Usually such reactions are reversible; the reversed reaction is called esterification, condensation, or dehydration synthesis. SEE: *assimilation; enzyme.* **hydrolytic** (-drō-lĭt′ĭk), *adj.*

hydrolyze (hī′drō-līz) To cause to undergo hydrolysis.

hydroma (hī-drō′mă) [Gr. *hydor,* water, + *oma,* tumor] Hygroma.

hydromassage A massage produced by a stream of water.

hydromeiosis (hī″drō-mī-ō′sĭs) [″ + *meiosis,* dimunition] The swelling of the epidermis after it is exposed to water, with consequent blockage of the sweat ducts. This phenomenon limits fluid loss from sweating when the body is immersed in water.

hydromeningitis (hī″drō-mĕn″ĭn-jī′tĭs) [″ + *meninx,* membrane, + *itis,* inflammation] **1.** An inflammation of membranes of the brain with serous effusion. **2.** An inflammation of Descemet's membrane.

hydromeningocele (hī″drō-mĕn-ĭn′gō-sēl) [″ + ″ + *kele,* tumor, swelling] Protrusion of the meninges or spinal cord in a sac of fluid.

hydrometer (hī-drŏm′ĕ-tĕr) [″ + *metron,* measure] An instrument that measures the density of a liquid by the depth to which a graduated scale sinks into the liquid. SEE: *urinometer.*

hydrometra (hī″drō-mē′tră) [″ + *metra,* uterus] The collection of watery fluid or mucus in the uterus.

hydrometrocolpos (hī″drō-mē″trō-kŏl′pŏs) [″ + *metra,* uterus, + *kolpos,* vagina] The distention of the uterus by a collection of watery fluid.

hydromicrocephaly (hī″drō-mī″krō-sĕf′ă-lē) [″ + *mikros,* small, + *kephale,* head] A condition in which the head is abnormally small and contains an increased amount of cerebrospinal fluid.

hydromorphone hydrochloride (hī″drō-mor′fōn) An opioid pain reliever.

hydromphalus (hī-drŏm′fă-lŭs) [″ + *omphalos,* navel] Edematous enlargement of the umbilicus.

hydromyelia (hī″drō-mī-ē′lē-ă) [″ + *myelos,* marrow] Increased fluid in the central canal of the spinal cord. SYN: *hydrorrhachis.*

hydromyelocele (hī″drō-mī-ĕl′ō-sēl) [″ + ″ + *kele,* tumor, swelling] The protrusion of a sac with cerebrospinal fluid through a defect in a wall of the spinal canal.

hydromyelomeningocele (hī″drō-mī″ĕ-lō-mĕ-nĭng′gō-sēl) [″ + *myelos,* marrow, + *meninx,* membrane, + *kele,* tumor, swelling] Spinal deformity in which a fluid-filled sac containing spinal cord and surrounding membranes protrudes through the spine.

hydromyoma (hī″drō-mī-ō′mă) [″ + *mys,* muscle, + *oma,* tumor] An encapsulated, benign, cystic tumor of the uterine myometrium. SEE: *intramural fibroma.*

hydronephrosis (hī″drō-nĕf-rō′sĭs) [″ + *nephros,* kidney, + *osis,* condition] Stretching of the renal pelvis as a result of obstruction to urinary outflow. SYN: *nephrydrosis.* SEE: illus.

ETIOLOGY: Anything that obstructs the ureter or bladder may cause hydronephrosis. Lodged kidney stones are a common cause of unilateral hydronephrosis; bilateral hydronephrosis often results from bladder outlet obstruction (e.g., in men who have hyperplasia of the prostate). Neurogenic bladder dysfunction, pregnancy, urogenital cancer, urinary tract inflammation, congenital malformations, ureteral strictures, and even parasites (schistosomiasis) may cause hydronephrosis. If urinary flow is not restored, the kidney tissue dilates and atrophies, and chronic renal failure may occur.

SYMPTOMS: Hydronephrosis often causes no localizing symptoms, except when it is associated with kidney stones (when the primary symptom is severe flank pain).

DIAGNOSIS: Ultrasonography of the urinary tract is used to confirm the diagnosis.

TREATMENT: Unilateral hydronephrosis caused by a kidney stone resolves spontaneously if the stone passes. If the stone does not pass, procedures such as shock wave lithotripsy, surgical removal of the stone, nephrotomy, or nephrostomy tube drainage of the kidney may be needed. Bilateral hydronephrosis caused by prostatic hyperplasia may be relieved if a catheter can be inserted through the obstructed urethra into the bladder. Hydronephrosis caused by other diseases (e.g., tumors) is often treated surgically.

PATIENT CARE: Renal function studies (e.g., blood urea nitrogen, serum creatinine, and serum potassium levels) are monitored daily. As appropriate, urine specific gravity is tested at the bedside. The condition, planned diagnostic procedures, and expected sensations are explained to the patient and family; if the patient is scheduled for a surgical procedure, the surgeon's explanations of the planned procedure are reinforced. Questions are answered, and misconceptions are corrected. The patient is prepared physically for the procedure according to institutional protocol or the surgeon's wishes. Emotional support is provided, postoperative care and activities are explained, a signed informed consent form is obtained, and prescribed preoperative sedation is administered.

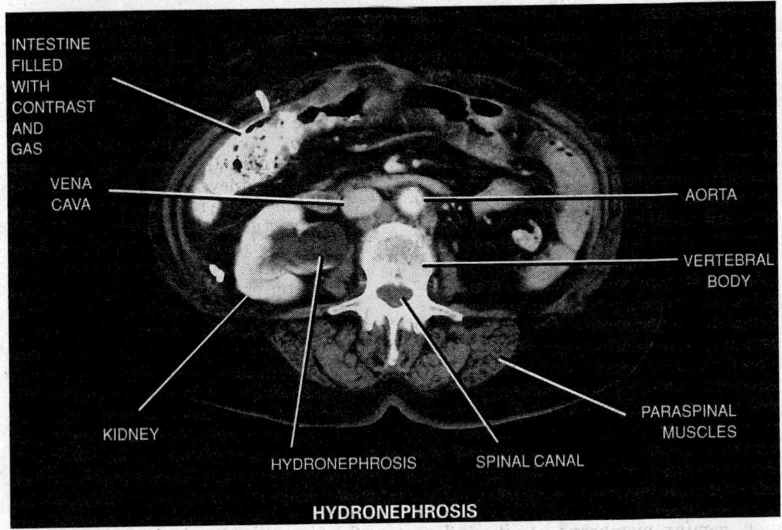

CT scan of abdomen shows kidney with distended pelvis (Courtesy of Harvey Hatch, MD, Curry General Hospital)

Postoperatively, intake and output, vital signs, and fluid and electrolyte balance are monitored (a rising pulse rate and cool, clammy skin may signal impending hypovolemia or hemorrhage and shock). Prescribed analgesics and noninvasive measures are used to relieve pain as necessary. Postobstructive diuresis may cause the patient to lose great volumes of dilute urine over hours or days along with excessive electrolyte loss. If this occurs, I.V. fluids are administered at a prescribed constant rate plus an amount equal to a given percentage of the patient's hourly urine output to safely replace intravascular volume. A dietitian can provide assistance to plan a diet consistent with the treatment plan while including foods that the patient enjoys and will eat. If a nephrostomy tube has been inserted, the tube is irrigated as specifically prescribed, checked for patency, and never clamped or kinked. Meticulous skin care is provided to the tube entry site; if urine leaks around the tube, a protective skin barrier is provided to prevent excoriation, and the wound area is bagged to preserve the patient's dignity and to help prevent infection.

If the patient will be discharged with the nephrostomy tube in place, proper care of the tube and skin at the insertion site is reviewed. Prescribed drug therapies, such as antibiotics, are administered, and the patient is taught about expected outcomes, adverse effects to report, and the necessity to complete the prescribed course of therapy even if feeling better. To prevent the progression of hydronephrosis to irreversible renal disease, older male patients (esp. ones with a family history of benign prostatic hyperplasia or prostatitis) should have routine medical checkups.

hydroparasalpinx (hī″drō-păr″ă-săl′pĭnks) [Gr. *hydor,* water, + *para,* beside, + *salpinx,* tube] An accumulation of serous fluid in the accessory tubes of the fallopian tube.

hydroparotitis (hī″drō-păr″ō-tī′tĭs) [″ + ″ + *ous,* ear, + *itis,* inflammation] An accumulation of fluid in the parotid gland.

hydropenia (hī″drō-pē′nē-ă) [″ + *penia,* poverty] A deficiency of water in the body.

hydropericarditis [″ + *peri,* around, + *kardia,* heart, + *itis,* inflammation] A serous effusion accompanying pericarditis.

hydropericardium (hī″drō-pĕr″ĭ-kăr′dē-ŭm) Pericardial edema; a noninflammatory accumulation of water in the pericardium.

SYMPTOMS: Symptoms may include chest pain or discomfort, diminished cardiac function with signs of heart failure, and dysphagia and dyspnea.

TREATMENT: Pericardiocentesis (drawing fluid from the pericardium with a needle) is used for diagnosis and management. Definitive therapy depends on the cause of the disease.

hydroperinephrosis (hī″drō-pĕr″ĭ-nĕ-frō′sĭs) [″ + *peri,* around, + *nephros,* kidney, + *osis,* condition] An accumulation of the serum of the connective tissue surrounding the kidney.

hydroperion (hī″drō-pĕr′ē-ŏn) [″ + ″ + *oon,* egg] Fluid present between the decidua capsularis and the decidua parietalis, occurring early in pregnancy.

hydroperitoneum (hī″drō-pĕr″ĭ-tō-nē′ŭm) [″ + *peritonaion*, peritoneum] Ascites.

hydrophilia, hydrophilism (hī-drō-fĭl′ē-ă, -drŏf′ĭ-lĭzm) [″ + *philein*, to love] Attracting water molecules, as do molecules with many polar covalent bonds. **hydrophilic**, *adj.*

hydrophilous (hī-drŏf′ĭ-lŭs) Taking up moisture. SYN: *bibulous; hygroscopic.*

hydrophobia (hī-drō-fō′bē-ă) [Gr. *hydor*, water, + *phobos*, fear] **1.** Repelling water molecules, as do molecules with few or no polar covalent bonds. **2.** Fearful or intolerant of water, as in rabies. SEE: *rabies*. **hydrophobic**, *adj.*

hydrophobophobia (hī″drō-fō″bō-fō′bē-ă) [″ + ″ + *phobos*, fear] A morbid fear of contracting hydrophobia (rabies), sometimes resulting in a condition resembling hydrophobia.

hydrophthalmos (hī″drŏf-thăl′mŏs) [″ + *ophthalmos*, eye] Distention of the eyeball owing to an accumulation of fluid within it. SEE: *glaucoma.*

hydrophysometra (hī″drō-fī″sō-mē′tră) [″ + *physa*, air, + *metra*, uterus] The presence of water and gas in the uterus.

hydropic (hī-drŏp′ĭk) [Gr. *hydropikos*] Edematous, or pert. to edema.

hydropneumatosis (hī″drō-nū″mă-tō′sĭs) [″ + *pneumatosis*, inflation] Liquid and gas in the tissues producing combined edema and emphysema.

hydropneumopericardium (hī″drō-nū″mō-pĕr-ĭ-kăr′dē-ŭm) [″ + ″ + *peri*, around, + *kardia*, heart] Serous effusion with gas in the pericardium.

hydropneumoperitoneum (hī″drō-nū″mō-pĕr″ĭ-tō-nē′ŭm) [″ + ″ + *peritonaion*, peritoneum] Gas and serous fluid in the peritoneal cavity.

hydropneumothorax (hī″drō-nū″mō-thō′răks) [″ + ″ + *thorax*, chest] Gas and serous effusion in the pleural cavity. SYN: *pneumohydrothorax.*

hydrops, hydropsy (hī′drŏps, -drŏp′sē) [Gr.] Edema.

h. abdominis Ascites.

endolymphatic h. Labyrinthine h.

h. fetalis The clinical condition in infants of cardiac decompensation with hepatosplenomegaly, respiratory distress, and circulatory distress. This may be caused by erythroblastosis fetalis; infections; tumors; pulmonary, hepatic, or renal disease; diabetes mellitus; Gaucher's disease; or multiple congenital anomalies. SEE: *erythema infectiosum; erythroblastosis fetalis.*

h. folliculi An accumulation of fluid in the graafian follicle of the ovary.

h. gravidarum Edema accompanying pregnancy.

labyrinthine h. Excessive fluid in the organ of balance in the inner ear. It may cause pressure or a sense of fullness in the ears, hearing loss, and vertigo. It often is found in Ménière's disease. SYN: *endolymphatic h.*

h. tubae Hydrosalpinx.

h. tubae profluens Intermittent hydrosalpinx.

hydropyonephrosis (hī″drō-pī″ō-nĕf-rō′sĭs) [Gr. *hydor*, water, + *pyon*, pus, + *nephros*, kidney, + *osis*, condition] Dilatation of the kidney pelvis with pus and urine.

hydroquinone (hī″drō-kwĭn′ōn) A photographic reducing agent known for producing heavy image density.

hydrorheostat (hī″drō-rē′ō-stăt) [″ + *rheos*, current, + *histanai*, to place] A device used to control the flow of electric current by changes in water resistance.

hydrorrhachis (hī-dror′ă-kĭs) [″ + *rhachis*, spine] Hydromyelia.

hydrorrhachitis (hī-dror-ă-kī′tĭs) [″ + ″ + *itis*, inflammation] A serous effusion from the spinal cord or its membranes, with inflammation of the cord.

hydrorrhea (hī″drō-rē′ă) [″ + *rhoia*, flow] Copious watery discharge from any part, as from the nose.

h. gravidarum The discharge of a watery fluid from the vagina during pregnancy.

hydrosalpinx (hī″drō-săl′pĭnks) [″ + *salpinx*, tube] Distention of the fallopian tube by clear fluid. SYN: *hydrops tubae.*

intermittent h. Edema of the fallopian tube in which the distention is so great that the tube is forced by the pressure to empty itself via the uterus. SYN: *hydrops tubae profluens.*

hydrosarcocele (hī″drō-săr′kō-sēl) [″ + *sarx*, flesh, + *kele*, tumor, swelling] A hydrocele with chronic swelling of the testis.

hydroscheocele (hī-drŏs′kē-ō-sēl″) [″ + *oscheon*, scrotum, + *kele*, tumor, swelling] A scrotal hernia that contains serous fluid.

hydrosol (hī′drō-sŏl) The fluid state of a colloidal solution (sol) in which the colloid particles, separated by water in a continuous phase, are free to move about. SEE: *hydrogel.*

hydrostat (hī′drō-stăt) [″ + *statikos*, standing] A device that maintains the water level in a container at a predetermined level.

hydrostatic (hī″drō-stăt′ĭk) [″ + *statikos*, standing] Pert. to the pressure of liquids in equilibrium and to the pressure exerted on liquids.

h. densitometry An underwater weighing technique for the determination of an individual's specific gravity. The amount of water displaced by the body is corrected for the air contained in the lungs. This technique can be used to estimate the percentage of body fat. SYN: *h. weighing.*

h. test A test to determine if a dead infant has breathed prior to death. The infant's lungs are put in water; if they float, prior breathing is proven.

h. weighing H. densitometry.

hydrostatics (hī″drō-stăt′ĭks) The science of the properties of fluids in equilibrium.

hydrosulfuric acid Hydrogen sulfide.

hydrosyringomyelia (hī″drō-sĭr-ĭng″ō-mī-ē′lē-ă) [″ + *syrinx,* tube, + *myelos,* marrow] Distention of the central canal of the spinal cord with effusion of fluid and formation of cavities.

hydrotaxis (hī″drō-tăk′sĭs) [″ + *taxis,* arrangement] The response of an organism or cell toward or away from moisture. SEE: *hydrotropism.*

hydrotherapist (hī″drō-thĕr′ă-pĭst) One who specializes in hydrotherapy.

hydrotherapy (hī-drō-thĕr′ă-pē) [″ + *therapeia,* treatment] The use of water (in baths, jetted, as a douche, packed as ice, heated, etc.) for irrigation, massage, relaxation, or as an anti-inflammatory.

hydrothermic (hī″drō-thĕr′mĭk) Concerning the effect of heated water.

hydrothionammonemia (hī″drō-thī″ō-năm″ō-nē′mē-ă) [″ + *theion,* sulfur, + *ammoniakos,* of Amen, from near whose temple it came, + *haima,* blood] The presence of ammonium sulfide in the blood.

hydrothionemia (hī″drō-thī″ō-nē′mē-ă) [″ + ″ + *haima,* blood] A condition caused by hydrogen sulfide in the blood.

hydrothionuria (hī″drō-thī″ō-nū′rē-ă) [″ + ″ + *ouron,* urine] The presence of hydrogen sulfide in the urine.

hydrothorax (hī″drō-thō′răks) [″ + *thorax,* chest] A noninflammatory collection of fluid in the pleural cavity, causing dyspnea, an absence of vesicular breath sounds, murmur, and decreased resonance to percussion over the location of the fluid.

hydrotis (hī-drō′tĭs) [″ + *ous,* ear] A serous effusion in the internal ear or tympanum.

hydrotropism (hī″drō-trō′pĭzm) [″ + *trope,* a turning] The response of plants toward moisture (positive hydrotropism) or away from it (negative hydrotropism).

hydrotubation Injection of saline solution or liquid medication into the uterus and fallopian tubes to dilate or treat them.

hydrotympanum (hī″drō-tĭm′pă-nŭm) [″ + *tympanon,* drum] Fluid in the middle ear.

hydroureter (hī″drō-ū-rē′tĕr) [″ + *oureter,* ureter] The distention of the ureter with fluid owing to obstruction.

hydrous (hī′drŭs) Containing water. SEE: *anhydrous.*

hydrovarium (hī″drō-vā′rē-ŭm) [″ + LL. *ovarium,* ovary] Edema or cyst of the ovary.

hydroxide (hī-drŏk′sīd) [″ + *oxys,* sour] A compound that contains the OH^- group, such as NaOH (sodium hydroxide, or caustic soda).

hydroxocobalamin (hī-drŏk″sō-kō-băl′ă-mĭn) A naturally occurring form of vitamin B_{12} used to treat B_{12} deficiency.

hydroxyamphetamine hydrobromide (hī-drŏk″sē-ăm-fĕt′ă-mēn hī″drō-brō′mīd) An amphetamine with little ability to stimulate the central nervous system. It is used as a solution placed in the eye, where it has an ephedrine-like action. Trade name is Paredrine.

hydroxyapatite (hī-drŏk″sē-ăp′ă-tīt) $Ca_{10}(PO_4)_6(OH)_2$; the apatite form of calcium phosphate present with calcium carbonate in the bones and skeleton. In teeth it is soluble in the acids of soft drinks or carbohydrate fermentation, but it becomes decay-resistant fluoroapatite after combining with fluoride ions present in fluoridated water or fluoride toothpastes.

hydroxybenzene (hī-drŏk″sē-bĕn′zēn) Phenol.

hydroxybutyric dehydrogenase A serum enzyme whose level is elevated in myocardial infarction. Because other tests (e.g., CK-MB, troponin T, troponin I) are more specific and more sensitive, this test is not commonly performed.

hydroxychloroquine sulfate (hī-drŏk″sē-klō′rō-kwĭn) A drug used to treat both rheumatic illnesses and malaria.

25-hydroxycholecalciferol (hī-drŏk″sē-kō″lē-kăl-sĭf′ĕ-rŏl) A vitamin D derivative.

17-hydroxycorticosterone (hī-drŏk″sē-kor″tĭ-kō-stĕr′ōn) Hydrocortisone.

hydroxyl Hydroxide.

hydroxylase (hī-drŏk′sĭ-lās) Any enzyme that catalyzes the introduction of hydrogen into a substrate.

hydroxylysine (hī″drŏk-sĭl′ĭ-sĭn) An amino acid found in collagen.

hydroxyprogesterone caproate (hī-drŏk″sē-prō-jĕs′tĕr-ōn) A progestational drug.

hydroxyproline (hī-drŏk″sē-prō′lĭn) An amino acid found in collagen.

hydroxypropyl methycellulose Cellulose hydroxypropyl methyl ester; a substance used to increase the viscosity of solutions.

hydroxystilbamidine isethionate (hī-drŏk″sē-stĭl-băm′ĭ-dēn) An antiprotozoal drug used in treating North American blastomycosis.

5-hydroxytryptamine (hī-drŏk″sē-trĭp′tă-mēn) ABBR: 5-HT. Serotonin.

hydroxyurea (hī-drŏk″sē-ū-rē′ă) A cytotoxic drug used to treat solid tumors, leukemias, myeloproliferative diseases, and sickle cell anemia.

hydroxyzine hydrochloride (hī-drŏk′sĭ-zēn) An antihistamine that is used to treat allergies, itch, and anxiety.

hygiene (hī′jēn) [Gr. *hygieinos,* healthful] **1.** Sanitation. **2.** Healthfulness. **3.** The study of health and observance of health rules and the methods and means of preserving health.

community h. That branch of hygiene that deals with the health of a large group of individuals such as in a city, state, or nation, and esp. with the control of communicable diseases.

dental h. Oral h.

industrial h. That branch of hygiene that deals primarily with health of industrial workers, esp. study, treatment, and prevention of occupational diseases.

mental h. The science of developing and maintaining mental health and preventing mental illness.

oral h. Preventive measures to avoid pathological conditions of the teeth and oral cavity. These include discontinuing the use of tobacco products, including "smokeless tobacco" (i.e., snuff); brushing the teeth and using dental floss daily; and removal of impacted food debris. Edentulous persons with partial restorations or false teeth should be sure that their appliances fit properly and are kept clean. An additional oral care measure that is important in the prevention of periodontal disease is the removal of plaque by a dental hygienist at least twice each year. SYN: *dental h.* SEE: *care, mouth; hygienist, dental; toothbrushing.*

hygienic (hī″jē-ĕn′ĭk) **1.** Pert. to health or its preservation. **2.** In a healthy condition.

hygienist (hī-jē′nĭst, hī′jē-ĕn-ĭst) A specialist in hygiene.

dental h. A licensed primary oral health care professional. The dental hygienist is educated to provide dental services that include education, prevention, and therapeutic services. The most common services provided are patient education, oral prophylaxis, dental radiographs, and fluoride applications. The goals of the dental hygienist include the control of oral diseases and the promotion of health. The practice of dental hygiene is regulated by laws called dental practice acts. The laws vary with each licensing jurisdiction.

hygro- Prefix meaning *moisture.*

hygroblepharic (hī″grō-blĕ-făr′ĭk) [″ + *blepharon,* eyelid] Any structure (such as the lacrimal gland) or agent that moistens the eye.

hygroma (hī-grō′mă) *pl.* **hygromas or hygromata** [″ + *oma,* tumor] A sac or bursa containing fluid.

cystic h. A rapidly growing hygroma of lymphatic origin. It is usually located in the neck but may be in the thorax.

hygrometer (hī-grŏm′ĕ-tĕr) [″ + *metron,* measure] An instrument for measuring the amount of moisture in the air.

hygroscopic (hī-grō-skŏp′ĭk) [″ + *skopein,* to examine] **1.** Pert. to hygroscopy. **2.** Absorbing moisture readily. SYN: *bibulous; hydrophilous.*

hygroscopy (hī-grŏs′kō-pē) The estimation of the quantity of moisture in the atmosphere.

hygrostomia (hī-grō-stō′mē-ă) [″ + *stoma,* mouth] Ptyalism.

hyla (hī′lă) A lateral extension of the aqueductus cerebri.

hyloma (hī-lō′mă) [Gr. *hyle,* matter, + *oma,* tumor] A tumor composed of or in the hylic tissues, such as hypohyloma and mesohyloma.

hymen (hī′mĕn) [Gr.] A fold of mucous membrane that partially covers the entrance to the vagina. Contrary to folklore, the presence or absence (or rupture) of the hymen cannot be used to prove or disprove virginity or history of sexual intercourse. Pregnancy has been known to occur even when the hymen is intact. **hymenal** (-ăl), *adj.*

annular h. A hymen with a ring-shaped opening in the center.

h. biforis A vaginal membrane with two openings separated by a thick septum; the structure partially covers the os.

cribriform h. A hymen with many small perforations. SYN: *fenestrated h.*

h. denticulatus A hymen with an opening with serrated edges.

fenestrated h. Cribriform h.

imperforate h. A hymen without an opening. Menstruation occurs, but the blood cannot escape from the vagina because of the obstruction of the hymen. The treatment is surgical incision of the hymen. SYN: *unruptured h.*

lunar h. A hymen shaped like a crescent moon.

ruptured h. A hymen that has been torn by coitus, injury, or surgery.

septate h. A hymen in which the opening is separated by a thin septum.

unruptured h. Imperforate h.

hymenectomy (hī″mĕn-ĕk′tō-mē) [″ + *ektome,* excision] **1.** In surgery and gynecology, the incision or removal of the hymen. **2.** The excision of a membrane.

hymenitis (hī-mĕn-ī′tĭs) [″ + *itis,* inflammation] The inflammation of the hymen or of a membrane.

Hymenolepis (hī″mĕ-nŏl′ĕ-pĭs) [″ + *lepis,* rind] A genus of tapeworm that is parasitic in birds and mammals.

H. nana The dwarf tapeworm, a parasite in the intestine of rats and mice; also commonly found in humans. It averages about 1 in. (2.51 cm) in length and differs from other tapeworms in that it is capable of completing its life cycle within a single host. The parasite, which in humans lives in the proximal ileum, can cause severe toxic symptoms, esp. in children. Included are diarrhea, abdominal pain, irritability, and convulsions that resemble epilepsy. The detection of eggs and gravid segments in the feces confirms the diagnosis of infestation with this parasite. Treatment is with praziquantel. SEE: illus.

hymenology (hī′mĕn-ŏl′ō-jē) [″ + *logos,* word, reason] The science of the membranes and their diseases.

Hymenoptera (hī″mĕn-ŏp′tur-ă) [Gr. *hy-*

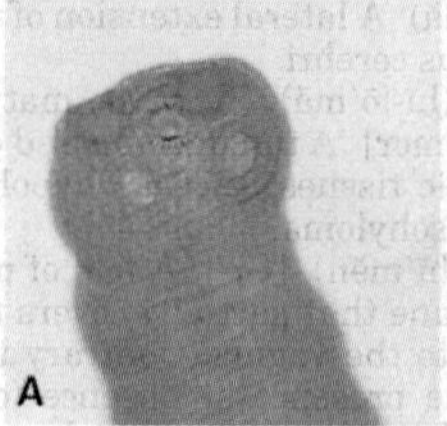

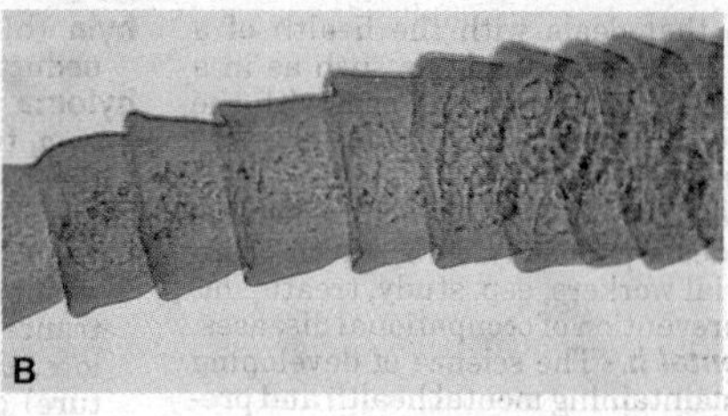

HYMENOLEPIS NANA

(A) Scolex, (B) mature proglottids (orig. mag. ×100)

menopteros, membrane-winged] An order of insects that includes ants, bees, hornets, and wasps. SEE: *bite, insect; sting.*

hymenorrhaphy (hī″mĕn-or′ă-fē) [″ + *rhaphe,* seam, ridge] A plastic operation on the hymen to restore it to the preruptured state.

hymenotome (hī-mĕn′ō-tōm) [″ + *tome,* incision] A knife used to divide membranes.

hymenotomy (hī″mĕn-ŏt′ō-mē) **1.** An incision of the hymen. **2.** A dissection of a membrane.

hyo- [Gr. *hyoeides,* U-shaped] Prefix indicating connection with the hyoid bone.

hyobasioglossus (hī″ō-bā″sē-ō-glŏs′ŭs) [″ + *basis,* base, + *glossa,* tongue] The part of the hyoglossal muscle attached to the hyoid bone.

hyoepiglottic, hyoepiglottidean (hī″ō-ĕp″ĭ-glŏt′ĭk, hī″ō-ĕp″ĭ-glŏt-ĭd′ē-ăn) [″ + *epiglottis,* epiglottis] Relating to the hyoid bone and epiglottis.

hyoglossal (hī″ō-glŏs′ăl) [″ + *glossa,* tongue] **1.** Pert. to the hyoglossus. **2.** Extending to the tongue from the hyoid bone.

hyoglossus (hī″ō-glŏs′ŭs) A muscle arising from the body and greater cornu of the hyoid bone and inserted into the dorsum of the tongue. It draws the sides of the tongue down and retracts it.

hyoid (hī′oyd) [Gr. *hyoeides,* U-shaped] **1.** Shaped like the Gr. letter upsilon (*υ*). **2.** Pert. to the hyoid bone.

hyoid bone The horseshoe-shaped bone at the base of the tongue. SEE: illus.

hyopharyngeus (hī″ō-făr-ĭn′jē-ŭs) [″ + *pharynx,* throat] The middle pharyngeal constrictor.

hyoscine hydrobromide Previous name for scopolamine hydrobromide.

hyoscyamus (hī″ō-sī′ă-mŭs) [Gr. *hys,* a pig, + *kyamos,* bean] The dried leaves of the plant *Hyoscyamus niger;* a narcotic that also acts as an antispasmodic. A relative of atropine, hyoscyamus is also known as henbane.

hyoscyamus poisoning SEE: *atropine in Poisons and Poisoning Appendix.*

hyp- SEE: *hypo-.*

hypacousia, hypacusia, hypacusis (hī″pă-koo′sē-ă, -kū′sē-ă, -sĭs) [Gr. *hypo,* under, + *akousis,* hearing] Impaired hearing. SEE: *hearing; presbyacusia.*

hypalgesia (hī-păl-jē′zē-ă) [″ + *algesis,* sense of pain] A lessened sensitivity to pain; the opposite of hyperalgesia.

hypamnios (hī-păm′nē-ŏs) [″ + *amnion,* caul of a lamb] A deficiency in the amount of amniotic fluid. SEE: *oligohydramnios.*

hypaxial (hī-păks′ē-ăl) [″ + *axon,* axle] Situated beneath the body axis.

hyper- [Gr. *hyper,* over, above, excessive] Prefix meaning *above, excessive,* or *beyond.*

hyperacid (hī″pĕr-ăs′ĭd) [″ + L. *acidus,* sour] Containing too much acid.

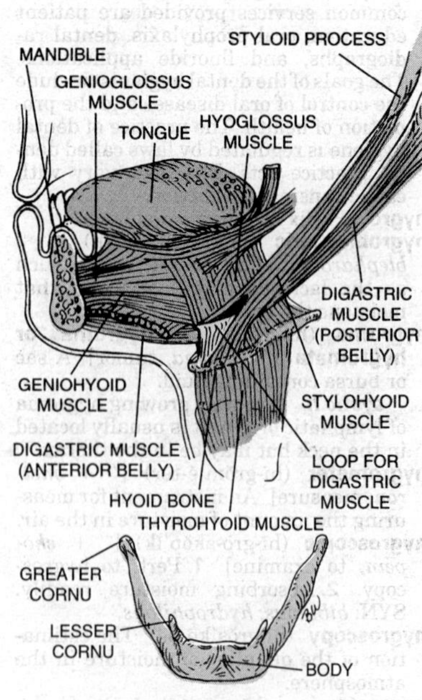

HYOID BONE

hyperacidity (hī″pĕr-ă-sĭd′ĭ-tē) [″ + L. *acidus,* sour] **1.** An excess of acid. **2.** An excess of acid in the stomach. SEE: *hyperchlorhydria.*

hyperactive child syndrome SEE: *attention-deficit hyperactivity disorder; hyperactivity.*

hyperactivity **1.** Increased or excessive activity that may refer to the entire organism or to a particular entity (e.g., hyperactivity of the heart or thyroid). **2.** Excessive muscular activity. **3.** Manifestations of disturbed behavior in children or adolescents characterized by constant overactivity, distractibility, impulsiveness, inability to concentrate, and aggressiveness. Hyperkinetic behavior usually lessens as a child grows older and usually disappears during adolescence. SEE: *attention-deficit hyperactivity disorder.*

Hyperactivity may be caused by emotional disorders, central nervous system dysfunction, mental retardation, or an exaggeration of a normal personality trait.

hyperacuity (hī″pĕr-ă-kū′ĭ-tē) [Gr. *hyper,* over, above, excessive, + L. *acuitas,* sharpness] Abnormal sensitivity to sensory stimulation.

hyperacusis (hī″pĕr-ă-kū′sĭs) [″ + *akousis,* hearing] An abnormal sensitivity to sound. SYN: *oxyacusis.*

hyperacute (hī″pĕr-ă-kūt′) Extremely or excessively acute.

hyperadiposis, hyperadiposity (hī″pĕr-ăd″ĭ-pō′sĭs, -pŏs′ĭ-tē) [″ + L. *adeps,* fat, + Gr. *osis,* condition] Excessive fatness.

hyperadrenalism (hī″pĕr-ă-drē′năl-ĭzm) Increased hormonal secretion from the adrenal gland.

hyperadrenocorticalism (hī″pĕr-ă-drē″nō-kor′tĭ-kăl-ĭzm) Increased hormonal secretion from the cortex of the adrenal gland.

hyperalbuminemia (hī″pĕr-ăl-bū″mĭ-nē′mē-ă) [″ + L. *albumen,* white of egg, + Gr. *haima,* blood] Increased albumin in the blood.

hyperaldosteronism (hī″pĕr-ăl″dō-stĕr′ōn-ĭzm) The excessive production of aldosterone by the adrenal gland. SEE: *aldosteronism.*

hyperalgesia (hī″pĕr-ăl-jē′zē-ă) [″ + *algesis,* sense of pain] An excessive sensitivity to pain; the opposite of hypalgesia. SYN: *hyperalgia.*

hyperalgia (hī-pĕr-ăl′jē-ă) [″ + *algos,* pain] Hyperalgesia.

hyperalimentation (hī″pĕr-ăl″ĭ-mĕn-tā′shŭn) The enteral and parenteral infusion of a solution that contains sufficient amino acids, glucose, fatty acids, electrolytes, vitamins, and minerals to sustain life, maintain normal growth and development, and provide for needed tissue repair. The gastrointestinal tract is the route of choice if it is functional. Intravenous hyperalimentation must utilize less concentrated formulations because of the potential for chemical phlebitis that may result from osmotic stress. Infusion through a central line catheter into the superior vena cava provides a sufficient blood volume to dilute more hypertonic solutions. One crucial draw-back of a central line is the potential for the line to become infected with either bacteria or fungi.

PATIENT CARE: Vital signs, electrolyte values, and fluid balance (intake, output, and daily weight) are monitored for indications of fluid overload or dehydration. Urine specific gravity is measured, and the patient's urine is checked for the presence of glucose and acetone every 6 hours. If the hyperalimentation is enteral, the nurse is aware of the placement of the distal end of the tube (above or below the pyloric sphincter); auscultates for bowel sounds; inspects, percusses, and measures for abdominal distention; and assesses for, documents, reports, and treats nausea, vomiting, or diarrhea. As appropriate, stomach contents are monitored for residual volume. Tube patency as well as volume, rate, and type of feeding are maintained; comfort measures are provided (oral misting, oral hygiene, and analgesic throat sprays); and any indications of infections due to long-term nasal tube placement, such as sinusitis, aspiration reflux chemical pneumonia, and other infections, are assessed. For example, sinusitis can occur because the tube impedes sinus drainage, allowing organisms to colonize the sinuses and resulting in fever and nasopurulent drainage. Chemical aspiration pneumonias often occur because of silent reflux regurgitation, resulting in acidic stomach contents and gram-negative organisms entering the respiratory tract. If hyperalimentation is via peripheral blood vessels, the insertion site is checked frequently for evidence of phlebitis; if via a central line, the site is monitored for signs of inflammation or infection, and the patient is assessed for signs and symptoms of sepsis. The insertion site is redressed and administration sets and connectors are changed according to institutional protocol; strict asepsis is maintained throughout these procedures. For all parenteral hyperalimentation, the flow-rate should never be sped up if an infusion is behind unless this action is specifically prescribed by the physician. The physician is notified if the line becomes occluded or if fluids are stopped or slowed for any reason. The patient is assessed for hypoglycemia or fluid deficit. For all hyperalimentation: The patient is mobilized as possible. Nutritional status is monitored weekly; weight gain or loss, serum protein levels, transferrin levels, and anthropomorphic measurements are documented and reported as directed. Strict asepsis is maintained in handling fluids and equipment, with special vigilance maintained for immobile or paralyzed patients.

hyperalkalinity (hī″pĕr-ăl-kă-lĭn′ĭ-tē) A condition of excessive alkalinity.

hyperaminoacidemia (hī″pĕr-ăm″ĭ-nō-ăs″ĭ-dē′mē-ă) An abnormal amount of amino acids in the blood.

hyperaminociduria (hī′pĕr-am′i-nō-as-i-doo′rē-ă) [″ + ″ + *amine* + Gr. *ouron,* urine] The presence of an excess of amino acids in the urine. SYN: *acidaminuria.*

hyperammonemia (hī″pĕr-ăm″mō-nē′mē-ă) An excess amount of ammonia in the blood. SEE: *ammonia toxicity.*

congenital h. An accumulation of an excess of ammonia in the body due to a congenital deficiency of enzymes, either carbamyl phosphate synthetase or ornithine transcarbamylase, essential to the metabolism of ammonia. Clinical signs of ammonia toxicity are present, including vomiting, lethargy, coma, and eventually death.

hyperamylasemia (hī″pĕr-ăm″ĭl-ās-ē′mē-ă) Increased blood amylase. It is often found in pancreatitis and/or diseases of the salivary glands, but may be present in normal (asymptomatic) persons.

hyperaphia (hī″pĕr-ā′fē-ă) [″ + *haphe,* touch] An excessive sensitivity to touch. SYN: *hyperpselaphesia.* **hyperaphic** (hī-pĕr-ăf′ĭk), *adj.*

hyperazotemia (hī″pĕr-ăz″ō-tē′mē-ă) [″ + L. *azotum,* nitrogen, + Gr. *haima,* blood] An increased amount of nitrogenous substances such as urea in the blood.

hyperazoturia (hī″pĕr-ăz″ō-tū′rē-ă) [″ + ″ + Gr. *ouron,* urine] An excessive amount of nitrogenous matter in the urine.

hyperbarism (hī″pĕr-băr′ĭzm) The consequences of being exposed to gaseous pressure greater than atmospheric pressure. Miners and deep sea divers are subject to this condition. SEE: *bends.*

hyperbetalipoproteinemia (hī″pĕr-bā″tă-lĭp″ō-prō″tē-ĭn-ē′mē-ă) An excessive amount of β-lipoproteins in the blood. SEE: *hyperlipoproteinemia.*

hyperbilirubinemia (hī″pĕr-bĭl″ĭ-roo-bĭn-ē′mē-ă) [Gr. *hyper,* over, above, excessive, + L. *bilis,* bile, + *ruber,* red, + Gr. *haima,* blood] An excessive amount of bilirubin in the blood; the condition is seen in any illness causing jaundice, including diseases in which the biliary tree is obstructed, and those in which blood formation is ineffective. *Pediatrics:* In newborns, high bilirubin levels due to rapid destruction of red blood cells may be caused by maternal factors such as Rh or ABO incompatibility, prenatal use of certain therapeutic drugs, or intrauterine viral infection. Precipitating factors include neonatal sepsis, anoxia, polycythemia, postbirth cold stress and hypoglycemia, and congenital liver or gastrointestinal defects. SEE: *hemolytic disease of the newborn; incompatibility, ABO; isoimmunization; Nursing Diagnoses Appendix.*

PATIENT CARE: Patient care centers on diagnosing the cause of jaundice and addressing it specifically. In newborn infants, desired outcomes include a return of bilirubin to within normal limits and disappearance of signs of hyperbilirubinemia. The infant's skin color is inspected through use of the blanch test. Transcutaneous bilirubinometric or laboratory findings are reviewed, and the infant is assessed for neurologic impairment.

Phototherapy is explained to the parents when bilirubin levels are high enough to merit it. For this measure to be effective, the infant's skin must be exposed to ultraviolet light. Thus, the infant is placed nude under the fluorescent light and is turned frequently to expose all body surfaces. The newborn's head is covered, as evidence suggests it prevents phototherapy-induced hypocalcemia. The eyes are shielded with an opaque mask, which is positioned carefully to exclude the nares. Periodically, the eyes are checked for evidence of discharge, excessive pressure on the lids, or corneal irritation, since the corneas may become excoriated if they contact the dressing. Minor side effects, including loose greenish stools, hyperthermia, increased metabolic rate, increased evaporative water loss, and priapism, are assessed for and documented. The infant's temperature, heart and respiratory rates, and skin (for evidence of dehydration and drying) are monitored. Oily lubricants or lotions are avoided to limit skin tanning. The infant receives up to 25% more fluid volume than usual to compensate for insensible and intestinal fluid losses. Constant reassurance is provided to the parents regarding their infant's progress. They may worry that the baby will be cold or unable to see. They are encouraged to touch the baby and feel that he or she is warm and comfortable under the light. The eye shield may be removed during parental visits, and parents are encouraged to talk to and touch the baby, who benefits from such stimulation. If phototherapy is to continue at home, a home health nurse becomes actively involved in preparing the parents for their role and in supervising the therapy.

Nursing infants may display jaundice that peaks during the third week of life. Treatment involves providing more frequent breast-feeding; however, if bilirubin levels reach 15 to 16 mg/100 ml, the mother may discontinue breastfeeding for 48 hours, substituting water and formula. SEE: *jaundice*.

hyperbrachycephaly (hī″pĕr-brăk″ē-sĕf′ă-lē) [″ + *brachys,* short, + *kephale,* head] An excessive degree of brachycephaly; having a cephalic index above 85.

hypercalcemia (hī″pĕr-kăl-sē′mē-ă) [″ + L. *calx,* lime, + Gr. *haima,* blood] An excessive amount of calcium in the blood. The causes of this condition include primary hyperparathyroidism, lithium therapy, malignancies including solid tumors and hematological malignancies, vitamin D intoxication, hyperthyroidism, vitamin A intoxication, aluminum intoxication; and milk-alkali syndrome.

SYMPTOMS: Clinically, fatigue, depression, mental confusion, nausea, vomiting, constipation, increased urination, and possibly cardiac arrhythmia are present. A short Q-T interval is present on electrocardiographic study.

TREATMENT: Patients initially should be given hydration with saline, followed by diuretics, after dehydration has been resolved. Bisphosphonates, glucocorticoids, and other drugs may be administered to lower serum calcium levels. Therapy is also directed at the underlying cause of the high serum calcium levels, for example, by treating underlying malignancies or by excising overactive parathyroid glands.

idiopathic h. A type of hypercalcemia seen in infants, caused by vitamin D intoxication. SEE: *bends*.

hypercalciuria (hī″pĕr-kăl″sē-ū′rē-ă) [″ + ″ + Gr. *ouron,* urine] An excessive quantity of calcium in the urine.

hypercapnia (hī″pĕr-kăp′nē-ă) [″ + *kapnos,* smoke] An increased amount of carbon dioxide in the blood. Elevated levels of carbon dioxide in the blood result from inadequate ventilation or from massive mismatches between ventilation and perfusion of the blood. When the CO_2 levels are greater than 45 mm Hg, cerebral vasodilation can occur. Some of the common symptoms of hypercapnia include dizziness, drowsiness, confusion, tremors, and twitching.

permissive h. Intentional hypoventilation of a mechanically ventilated patient to minimize intrathoracic pressure.

hypercarbia Hypercapnia.

hypercellularity (hī″pĕr-sĕl″ū-lăr′ĭ-tē) An increased number of cells in any location, but esp. in the bone marrow.

hypercementosis (hī″pĕr-sē″mĕn-tō′sĭs) [″ + L. *cementum,* cement, + Gr. *osis,* condition] An overgrowth of tooth cement (cementum).

hyperchloremia (hī″pĕr-klō-rē′mē-ă) [″ + *chloros,* green, + *haima,* blood] An increase in the chloride content of the blood.

hyperchlorhydria (hī″pĕr-klor-hī′drē-ă) [″ + ″ + *hydor,* water] An excess of hydrochloric acid in the stomach. SEE: *achlorhydria; gastrin; gastritis; H_2-receptor antagonists; hydrochloric acid; hypochlorhydria; peptic ulcer; Zollinger-Ellison syndrome*.

hyperchloridation (hī″pĕr-klō″rĭ-dā′shŭn) A dosing with large amounts of sodium chloride.

hypercholesterolemia (hī″pĕr-kō-lĕs″tĕr-ŏl-ē′mē-ă) [″ + *chole,* bile, + *stereos,* solid, + *haima,* blood] An excessive amount of cholesterol in the blood.

familial h. A type of hyperlipoproteinemia in which low-density lipoproteins are not removed from the bloodstream in normal amounts by lipoprotein receptors in the liver. Affected persons have massively elevated serum lipid levels. SEE: *hyperlipoproteinemia*.

hypercholesterolia (hī″pĕr-kō-lĕs″tĕr-ō′lē-ă) [″ + ″ + *stereos,* solid] Excessive cholesterol in the bile.

hyperchromatic (hī″pĕr-krō-măt′ĭk) [″ + *chroma,* color] Overpigmented.

hyperchromatism (hī″pĕr-krō′mă-tĭzm) [″ + ″ + *-ismos,* condition] **1.** Excessive pigmentation. **2.** The increased staining capacity of any structure.

hyperchromia (hī″pĕr-krō′mē-ă) Hyperchromatism.

hyperchromic (hī-pĕr-krō′mĭk) **1.** Pert. to excessive pigmentation. **2.** Intensely colored.

hyperchylia (hī″pĕr-kī′lē-ă) [Gr. *hyper,* over, above, excessive, + *chylos,* juice] An abnormal secretion of gastric juice.

hyperchylomicronemia (hī″pĕr-kī″lō-mī″krō-nē′mē-ă) The excessive accumulation of fat particles, chylomicrons, in the blood.

hypercoagulability (hīp″ĕr-kō-ăg″ū-lă-bĭl′ĭ-tē) An increased ability of anything to coagulate, but esp. the blood.

hypercorticism (hī″pĕr-kor′tĭ-sĭzm) An excessive production of adrenal cortical hormones in the body.

hypercrinism (hī″pĕr-krī′nĭsm) [″ + *krinein,* to separate, + *-ismos,* condition] A condition due to excessive activity of any endocrine gland.

hypercryalgesia (hī″pĕr-krī″ăl-jē′zē-ă) [″ + *kryos,* cold, + *algesis,* sense of pain] Hypercryesthesia.

hypercryesthesia (hī″pĕr-krī″ĕs-thē′zē-ă) [″ + ″ + *aisthesis,* sensation] An excessive sensitivity to cold. SYN: *hypercryalgesia*.

hypercupremia (hī″pĕr-kū-prē′mē-ă) An increased level of copper in the blood. SEE: *Wilson's disease*.

hypercyanotic (hī″pĕr-sī″ă-nŏt′ĭk) Denoting extreme cyanosis.

hyperdactylia (hī″pĕr-dăk-tĭl′ē-ă) [Gr. *hyper,* over, above, excessive, + *daktylos,* finger] The state of having an excessive number of fingers or toes.

hyperdefecation Increased stool frequency without an increase in stool weight above normal. It may be present in patients with irritable bowel syndrome, hyperthyroidism, or proctitis.

hyperdicrotic (hī″pĕr-dī-krŏt′ĭk) [″ + *dikrotos,* beating double] Abnormally dicrotic. SEE: *dicrotic.*

hyperdynamia (hī″pĕr-dī-nā′mē-ă) [″ + *dynamis,* force] Muscular restlessness or extreme violence.

h. uteri Abnormal uterine contractions in labor.

hypereccrisia, hypereccrisis (hī″pĕr-ĕk-krĭs′ē-ă, -ĕk′krĭ-sĭs) [″ + *ekkrisis,* excretion] An abnormal amount of excretion. **hypereccritic** (-ĕk-krĭt′ĭk), *adj.*

hyperechoic (hī′pĕr-ĕ-kō′ik) In ultrasonography, pertaining to a region of the body that produces more sound echoes than normal.

hyperemesis (hī″pĕr-ĕm′ĕ-sĭs) [″ + *emesis,* vomiting] Excessive vomiting.

h. gravidarum Persistent, continuous, severe, pregnancy-related nausea and vomiting, often accompanied by dry retching. The condition can cause systemic effects such as dehydration, weight loss, fluid-electrolyte and acid-base imbalance leading to metabolic acidosis, and rarely, death. About 2 out of 1000 pregnant women require hospitalization for medical management of the disorder. SEE: *morning sickness; Nursing Diagnoses Appendix.*

SYMPTOMS: This condition of unknown etiology may start as a simple vomiting of early pregnancy, but if it persists, dehydration, chloride depletion, and acidosis occur. With severe and continued vomiting, pathological changes in the liver may be found.

TREATMENT: Early management includes bedrest; small, frequent, high-carbohydrate feedings; moderate fluid restriction; and mild sedation. In severe cases, the patient is hospitalized for complete bedrest and rehydration. Vitamin and electrolyte-enhanced parenteral fluids are administered. Phenothiazine antiemetics, such as prochlorperazine (pregnancy category B), may be administered to control vomiting. Feeding via nasogastric tube or use of total parenteral nutrition is rarely necessary.

When the patient improves, food taken by mouth should consist of a light solid diet given in frequent small feedings, with fruit juice or milk between feedings. Termination of the pregnancy is indicated only when the woman fails to respond to medical measures and is approaching serious physiologic jeopardy.

CAUTION: During therapy the patient's retinas should be monitored for evidence of hemorrhagic retinitis. If it occurs, the pregnancy should be terminated without delay. The death rate in patients with this complication is 50%.

PATIENT CARE: The patient's emotional state is assessed. Environmental stimuli are minimized, with rest, relaxation, and verbalization of concerns encouraged. Prescribed treatments are explained and implemented, and psychological support is provided. Ongoing assessments include vital signs and fetal heart rate; the time, amount, and character of any emesis; fluid intake and output; and the woman's response to treatment. Aspects of complementary medicine may be incorporated by using and teaching techniques that induce the relaxation response, although objective proof of the effectiveness of these interventions is unproven.

hyperemia (hī″pĕr-ē′mē-ă) [″ + *haima,* blood] **1.** Congestion; an unusual amount of blood in a part. **2.** A form of macula; red areas on the skin that disappear on pressure. **3.** In physical therapy, an increase in the quantity of blood flowing through any part of the body, shown by redness of the skin caused by the application of heat.

active h. Hyperemia caused by increased blood inflow. SYN: *arterial h.*

arterial h. Active h.

Bier's h. Passive hyperemia produced by application of an elastic bandage and by suction. SYN: *constriction h.*

constriction h. Bier's h.

leptomeningeal h. Pia-arachnoid congestion.

passive h. Hyperemia caused by decreased drainage of blood. SYN: *venous h.*

reactive h. The increased presence of blood in an area after restoration of blood flow following a decreased supply.

venous h. Passive h.

hyperemotivity (hī″pĕr-ē″mō-tĭv′ĭ-tē) [Gr. *hyper,* over, above, excessive, + L. *emovere,* to disturb] Excessive emotivity or response to stimuli.

hypereosinophilic syndrome, idiopathic Multisystem injury and organ damage caused by excessive numbers of eosinophils in the body. The disease is one of the myelodysplastic disorders. Almost any organ can be affected, but most patients have bone marrow, cardiac, and central nervous system involvement.

TREATMENT: Anticoagulants for patients with thromboembolic complication; corticosteroids. Patients unresponsive to corticosteroids have shown marked improvement when given cytotoxic agents such as hydroxyurea.

hyperequilibrium (hī″pĕr-ē″kwĭ-lĭb′rē-ŭm) [″ + L. *aequus,* equal, + *libra,* balance] A tendency to experience vertigo when making even slight turning movements.

hypererethism (hī″pĕr-ĕr′ĭ-thĭzm) [″ + *erethisma,* stimulation] Excessive irritability.

hyperergasia (hī″pĕr-ĕr-gā′sē-ă) [″ + *ergasia,* work] Unusual functional activity.

hyperergy, hyperergia (hī′pĕr-ĕr″jē) [″ + *ergon,* energy] Hypersensitivity, or a condition in which there is an exaggerated response. SEE: *allergy; anaphylaxis.*

hyperesophoria (hī″pĕr-ĕs″ō-fō′rē-ă) [″ + *eso,* inward, + *phorein,* to bear] A tendency of the visual axis to deviate upward and inward owing to muscular imbalance; a form of heterophoria.

hyperesthesia (hī″pĕr-ĕs-thē′zē-ă) [″ + *aisthesis,* sensation] An increased sensitivity to sensory stimuli, such as pain or touch. SYN: *algesia; oxyesthesia.* **hyperesthetic** (-ĕs-thĕt′ĭk), *adj.*

acoustic h. An abnormal sensitivity to sound.

cerebral h. Hyperesthesia caused by a cerebral lesion.

gustatory h. An oversensitivity of taste.

muscular h. Muscular sensitivity to pain and fatigue.

optic h. An abnormal sensitivity to light.

h. sexualis An abnormal increase in libido.

tactile h. An abnormal sensitivity of touch.

hyperexophoria (hī″pĕr-ĕks″ō-fō′rē-ă) [″ + *exo,* outward, + *phorein,* to bear] A tendency of the visual axis to deviate upward and outward owing to muscular imbalance; a form of heterophoria.

hyperexplexia An excessive reaction to being startled. SEE: *Tourette's syndrome; startle syndrome.*

hyperextension (hī″pĕr-ĕks-tĕn′shŭn) [″ + L. *extendere,* to stretch out] Extreme or abnormal extension.

hyperfibrinogenemia (hī″pĕr-fī-brĭn″ō-jĕ-nē′mē-ă) An increased amount of fibrinogen in the blood; a possible, but unproven, risk factor for cardiovascular disease.

hyperflexion (hī″pĕr-flĕk′shŭn) Increased flexion of a joint, usually resulting from trauma.

hyperfunction [Gr. *hyper,* over, above, excessive, + L. *functio,* performance] Excessive activity.

hypergalactia (hī-pĕr-găl-ăk′shē-ă) [″ + *gala,* milk] Excessive milk secretion after childbirth.

hypergammaglobulinemia (hī″pĕr-găm″ă-glŏb″ū-lĭ-nē′mē-ă) An excessive amount of immunoglobulin G (IgG) in the blood. Excess levels of IgG in the blood may be seen in patients with monoclonal gammopathy, multiple myeloma, and some chronic infections. In women, the excess antibody can produce a bruise-like rash following exercise or alcohol ingestion called benign hypergammaglobulinemia purpura.

hypergamy (hī-pĕr′gă-mē) [″ + *gamos,* marriage] The tendency of women to reproduce with men of equal or higher social standing.

hypergenesis (hī″pĕr-jĕn′ĕ-sĭs) [″ + *genesis,* generation, birth] Hyperplasia.

hypergenitalism (hī″pĕr-jĕn′ĭt-ăl-ĭzm) [″ + L. *genitalis,* genital] An excessive development of the genital organs, caused by disturbances in endocrine secretions of the adrenal gland or gonads or by hypothalamic disorders.

hypergeusesthesia, hypergeusia (hī″pĕr-gūs-ĕs-thē′sē-ă, -gū′sē-ă) [″ + *geusis,* taste + *aisthesis,* perception] An excessive acuteness of the sense of taste.

hyperglandular (hī″pĕr-glăn′dū-lăr) [″ + L. *glandula,* a little acorn] Having excessive glandular secretions.

hyperglobulinemia (hī″pĕr-glŏb″ū-lĭn-ē′mē-ă) [″ + L. *globulus,* a globule, + Gr. *haima,* blood] Excessive globulin in the blood.

hyperglycemia (hī″pĕr-glī-sē′mē-ă) [″ + *glykys,* sweet, + *haima,* blood] Increased blood sugar, as occurs in diabetes. A fasting blood sugar greater than 126 mg/dl on more than one occasion is diagnostic of diabetes mellitus. Sustained high blood sugars result in damage to the retina, the peripheral nerves, and the kidneys, and are reflected in laboratory assays such as the glycosylated hemoglobin test. Patients who are able to reduce their blood sugars below diabetic levels with diet, exercise, or drugs can decrease their risk of complications of diabetes and improve their immune function. SEE: *diabetes.*

hyperglyceridemia (hī″pĕr-glĭs″ĕr-ĭ-dē′mē-ă) Hypertriglyceridemia.

hyperglycinemia (hī″pĕr-glī″sĭ-nē′mē-ă) An accumulation of glycine in the blood. It is caused by a congenital defect in the ability to metabolize the amino acid glycine. There are at least six forms of this disease, all of which are associated with mental and growth retardation.

hyperglycogenolysis (hī″pĕr-glī″kō-jĕn-ŏl′ĭ-sĭs) [″ + ″ + *gennan,* to form, + *lysis,* dissolution] Excessive conversion of glycogen into glucose by hydrolysis.

hyperglycorrhachia (hī″pĕr-glī″kō-rā′kē-ă) [″ + *glykys,* sweet, + *rhachis,* spine] An excess of sugar in the cerebrospinal fluid.

hypergnosia (hī″pĕr-nō′sē-ă) [″ + *gnosis,* knowledge] A distorted or exaggerated perception, influenced by the unconscious projection of emotional subjective experiences.

hypergonadism (hī″pĕr-gō′năd-ĭzm) [″ + *gone,* seed, + *-ismos,* state of] Excessive hormonal secretion of the sex glands.

hyperguanidinemia (hī″pĕr-gwăn″ĭ-dĭn-ē′mē-ă) [″ + Sp. *guano,* dung, + *haima,* blood] An abnormal amount of guanidine in the blood.

hyperhedonia, hyperhedonism (hī″pĕr-hē-dŏ′nē-ă, -hē′dŏn-ĭzm) [Gr. *hyper,* over, above, excessive, + *hedone,* pleasure, + *-ismos,* state of] **1.** Abnormal pleasure in anything. **2.** Abnormal sexual excitement.

hyperhidrosis (hī″pĕr-hī-drō′sĭs) [″ + *hidros,* sweat, + *osis,* condition] Sweating greater than would be expected considering the temperature of the environment. SEE: *bromidrosis; sweat.*

ETIOLOGY: This symptom may be caused by stimulants, sepsis, hyperthyroidism, menopausal hot flashes, obesity, intense activation of the sympathetic nervous system, and other conditions.

TREATMENT: If the sweating is due to a systemic disease, appropriate therapy for that condition is indicated. If localized, application of a 20% solution of aluminum chloride hexahydrate in absolute alcohol at night using occlusive dressings is beneficial. The dressed sites must be dried before application and the salt washed away in the morning.

hyperimmune (hī″pĕr-ĭm-mūn′) A state of greater than normal immunity.

hyperinflation (hī″pĕr-ĭn-flā′shŭn) An excess of air in anything, esp. the lungs.

hyperinosemia (hī″pĕr-ī″nō-sē′mē-ă) [″ + *inos,* fiber, + *haima,* blood] An abnormal coagulability of the blood; an excess of fibrinogen in the blood.

hyperinsulinemia (hī″pĕr-ĭn-sū-lĭn-ē′mē-ă) In patients with type 2 diabetes mellitus (DM), a condition in which hyperglycemia is present despite high levels of insulin in the bloodstream. Insulin resistance and hyperinsulinemia have been linked to hypertension, obesity, hyperlipidemia, and increased cardiovascular mortality in patients with type 2 DM.

TREATMENT: Diet, exercise, and some oral antidiabetic drugs (e.g., metformin) increase the sensitivity of body tissues to the effects of insulin and decrease hyperinsulinemia.

hyperinsulinism (hī″pĕr-ĭn′sū-lĭn-ĭzm) [″ + L. *insula,* island, + Gr. *-ismos,* condition] A relative or absolute excess of insulin in the blood. The condition is commonly found in insulin-resistant patients with type 2 diabetes mellitus and rarely found in patients with insulin secreting tumors of the pancreas. In type 2 diabetes, the condition is marked by hyperglycemia, weight gain, hypertension, and atherosclerosis. The resistance of such patients to the effect of insulin prevents hypoglycemia. By contrast, in patients with insulin-secreting tumors, severe hypoglycemia may be present.

hyperinvolution (hī″pĕr-ĭn″vō-lū′shŭn) [″ + L. *involvere,* to enwrap] **1.** Reduction in the size of the uterus to below normal after childbirth. **2.** Reduction in size to below normal of any organ following hypertrophy. SYN: *superinvolution.*

h. uteri Extreme atrophy of the uterus, seen following prolonged lactation or severe puerperal sepsis.

hyperirritability (hī″pĕr-ĭr″ĭ-tă-bĭl′ĭ-tē) An increased response to a stimulus.

hyperisotonic [″ + *isos,* equal, + *tonos,* tension] Said of one of two solutions that has the greater osmotic pressure. SYN: *hypertonic.*

hyperkalemia (hī″pĕr-kă-lē′mē-ă) [″ + L. *kalium,* potassium, + Gr. *haima,* blood] An excessive amount of potassium in the blood. SEE: *hypokalemia.*

ETIOLOGY: This condition usually is caused by inadequate excretion of potassium or the shift of potassium from tissues. Causes of inadequate secretion include acute renal failure, severe chronic renal failure, renal tubular disorders, hypoaldosteronism, and decreased renin secretion due to kidney disease or drugs (e.g., nonsteroidal anti-inflammatory agents, diuretics) that inhibit potassium excretion. The shift of potassium from tissues occurs in tissue damage due to trauma, hemolysis, digitalis poisoning, acidosis, and insulin deficiency.

SYMPTOMS: Hyperkalemia is often a symptomless condition until very high levels of potassium are present in the blood. The precise level at which cardiac or skeletal muscle toxicities arise varies greatly from patient to patient. Eventually, muscular weakness, electrocardiographic abnormalities (such as peaked T waves), and intractable cardiac rhythm disturbances may result.

PREVENTION: To help prevent hyperkalemia, patients who use salt substitutes containing potassium should be advised to discontinue them if urine output decreases. Predisposed patients, especially those with poor urinary output or taking oral or intravenous potassium supplements, require regular laboratory testing to assess their serum potassium levels.

TREATMENT: Mild hyperkalemia can be treated by eliminating its cause, often a medication or a potassium source in the diet or dietary supplement (e.g., potassium chloride taken as a salt substitute). Severe or progressive hyperkalemia can be treated with infusions of calcium gluconate, sodium bicarbonate, or insulin and glucose, or by the administration of potassium-binding resins orally or rectally. Hemodialysis also is effective.

PATIENT CARE: Cardiac rhythm and serum potassium and other electrolyte levels are monitored. Intake and output are recorded. Prescribed drugs are given and their effects on potassium levels are promptly evaluated. A dietician is consulted to recommend optimal quantities of potassium in foods and fluids. Safety measures are implemented for the patient with muscle weakness. If the patient requires transfused blood, only fresh blood may be used, since older blood contains potassium released by hemolysis.

hyperkeratinization (hī″pĕr-kĕr″ă-tĭn″ĭ-zā′shŭn) [″ + *keras,* horn] A thickening of the horny layers of the skin, esp. of the palms and soles. It may be caused by vitamin A deficiency or chronic arsenic toxicity.

hyperkeratomycosis (hī″pĕr-kĕr″ă-tō-mī-kō′sĭs) [″ + ″ + *mykes,* fungus, + *osis,* condition] Hypertrophy of the horny layer of the epidermis resulting from a parasitic fungus.

hyperkeratosis [″ + ″ + *osis,* condition] **1.** An overgrowth of the cornea. **2.** An overgrowth of the horny layer of the epidermis.

h. congenitalis Hyperkeratosis in the harlequin fetus.

epidermolytic h. A congenital disorder characterized by hyperkeratosis, erythema, and blisters.

hyperketonemia (hī″pĕr-kē″tō-nē′mē-ă) Accumulation of an excess of ketone bodies in the blood.

hyperketonuria (hī″pĕr-kē-tō-nūr′ē-ă) An excessive quantity of ketones in the urine.

hyperkinesia, hyperkinesis (hī″pĕr-kĭ-nē′zē-ă, -nē′sĭs) [Gr. *hyper,* over, above, excessive, + *kinesis,* movement] Increased muscular movement and physical activity. In children it may be due to attention deficit hyperactivity disorder (ADHD). SEE: *hyperactivity.*

hyperlactation (hī″pĕr-lăk-tā′shŭn) [″ + L. *lactare,* to suckle] Excessive milk secretion.

hyperlipemia (hī″pĕr-lĭp-ē′mē-ă) [″ + *lipos,* fat, + *haima,* blood] An excessive quantity of fat in the blood.

hyperlipidemia (hī″pĕr-lĭp-ĕ-dē′mē-ă) An increase of lipids in the blood.

hyperlipoproteinemia (hī″pĕr-lĭp″ō-prō″tē-ĭn-ē′mē-ă) Increased lipids in the blood resulting either from an increased rate of synthesis or from a decreased lipoprotein breakdown rate. The lipoproteins transport triglycerides and cholesterol in the plasma. Clinically, an increased lipoprotein level may cause atherosclerosis and pancreatitis. Hyperlipoproteinemias can develop as a result of a primary and heritable biochemical defect of either lipoprotein lipase activity or one of the cofactors essential to the function of that enzyme. They may also develop secondary to certain endocrine and metabolic disorders such as diabetes mellitus; glycogen storage disease, type I; Cushing's syndrome; acromegaly; hypothyroidism; anorexia; use of drugs such as alcohol, oral contraceptives, and glucocorticoids; renal disease; liver disease; immunological disorders; and stress. The hyperlipoproteinemias have been divided into five different lipoprotein patterns describing the changes found in the plasma. These patterns are not descriptive of specific diseases. SEE: *cholesterol; lipoprotein.*

PATIENT CARE: The patient should receive instruction about, and support for, a high-fiber calorically restricted diet that is low in fat and total cholesterol. A formal consultation with a nutritionist facilitates this process. Regular exercise lasting at least 35 minutes a day also helps the patient to metabolize lipids and raise protective levels of high-density lipoproteins (HDLs) while decreasing levels of low-density lipoproteins (LDLs). Patient education also should include information about serum lipid-lowering drugs, such as niacin or statins, and about their side effects and potential drug interactions and the need for follow-up blood work (esp. liver function tests). Other lifestyle and medical interventions may be indicated for patients with hyperlipoproteinemia and other risk factors for coronary artery disease, such as tobacco abuse or diabetes mellitus.

hyperliposis (hī″pĕr-lĭ-pō′sĭs) [″ + *lipos,* fat, + *osis,* condition] An abnormal amount of fat in the body.

hyperlucency In radiology, increased radiolucency.

hypermastia (hī″pĕr-măs′tē-ă) [″ + *mastos,* breast] **1.** Excessive enlargement of the breast in women or men. This condition may be unilateral. **2.** The presence of an abnormal number of mammary glands.

hypermature (hī″pĕr-mă-tūr′) [″ + L. *maturus,* ripe] **1.** Pert. to anything that has passed the stage of maturity. **2.** Overripe, as a cataract or abscess that has gone past the optimum time for incision.

hypermelanosis One of several disorders of melanin pigmentation resulting in increased melanin in either the epidermis (melanoderma), in which case the coloration is brown, or in the dermis, in which case it is blue or slate gray (ceruloderma). This disorder may be caused by a number of diseases and conditions, including pregnancy, ACTH-producing tumors, Wilson's disease, porphyria, biliary cirrhosis, chronic renal failure, certain drugs, suntanning, and chronic pruritus. SEE: *hypomelanosis.*

hypermenorrhea (hī″pĕr-mĕn″ō-rē′ă) [″ + *men,* month, + *rhoia,* flow] An abnormal increase in the duration or amount of menstrual flow.

hypermetabolic state (hī″pĕr-mĕt″ă-bŏl′ĭk) A condition of an abnormally increased rate of metabolism, seen in fever and in salicylate poisoning.

hypermetabolism (hī″pĕr-mĕ-tăb′ō-lĭzm) An increased rate of metabolism. SEE: *response, stress.*

extrathyroidal h. An increased rate of metabolism not related to thyroid disease.

hypermetaplasia (hī″pĕr-mĕt″ă-plā′sē-ă) [″ + *meta-,* after, + *plassein,* to form] Overactivity in tissue replacement or transformation from one type of tissue to another, as cartilage to bone.

hypermetria (hī″pĕr-mē′trē-ă) [Gr. *hyper,* over, above, excessive, + *metron,* measure] An unusual range of movement; motor incoordination in which muscular movement causes a person to overreach the objective.

hypermetrope (hī″pĕr-mĕt′rōp) [″ + ″ + *ops,* eye] Hyperope.

hypermetropia (hī″pĕr-mē-trō′pē-ă) Hyperopia. **hypermetropic** (-trŏp′ĭk), *adj.*

hypermimia (hī″pĕr-mĭm′ē-ă) [″ + *mimesis,* imitation] The use of a great number of gestures while speaking.

hypermnesia (hī″pĕrm-nē′zē-ă) [″ + *mneme,* memory] **1.** A great ability to remember names, dates, and details. **2.** An exaggeration of memory involving minute details of a past experience. It occurs in the manic phase of manic-depressive psychosis; in delirium and hypnoses; at the moment of shock and fright in life-threatening situations; with fever; during neurosurgical procedures involving temporal lobe stimulation; and following some brain injuries.

hypermobility (hī″pĕr-mō-bĭl′ĭ-tē) Excessive joint play (movement) that permits increased mobility. It is present in certain diseases of connective tissue such as Marfan's or Ehlers-Danlos syndromes.

hypermorph (hī′pĕr-morf) [″ + *morphe,* form] One whose length of limb and consequent standing height is high in proportion to the sitting height. SEE: *hypomorph; somatotype.*

hypermotility (hī″pĕr-mō-tĭl′ĭ-tē) [″ + L. *motio,* motion] Unusual or excessive movement. SYN: *hyperkinesia.*

hypermyatrophy (hī″pĕr-mī-ăt′rō-fē) [″ + *mys,* muscle, + *atrophia,* atrophy] An unusual wasting of muscle.

hypermyesthesia (hī″pĕr-mī″ĕs-thē′sē-ă) [″ + ″ + *aisthesis,* sensation] Muscular hyperesthesia.

hypermyotonia (hī″pĕr-mī″ō-tō′nē-ă) [″ + ″ + *tonos,* tone] Excessive muscular tone.

hypermyotrophy (hī″pĕr-mī-ŏt′rō-fē) [″ + ″ + *trophe,* nourishment] Abnormal muscular development.

hypernatremia (hī″pĕr-nă-trē′mē-ă) [″ + L. *natron,* sodium, + Gr. *haima,* blood] An elevated concentration of sodium in the bloodstream. Hypernatremia is said to be present when the sodium concentration exceeds about 145 mmol/L. In the vast majority of cases, water deficits (and not salt excesses) cause relative sodium levels to rise. Infrequently, hypernatremia results from infusions of concentrated saline.

hypernephroma (hī″pĕr-nĕ-frō′mă) [″ + *nephros,* kidney, + *oma,* tumor] Renal cell carcinoma.

hyperneurotization (hī″pĕr-nū-rŏt″ĭ-zā′shŭn) [″ + *neuron,* nerve] Grafting of a motor nerve into a muscle that has an intact nerve supply.

hypernutrition (hī″pĕr-nū-trĭsh′ŭn) [″ + L. *nutrire,* to nourish] Overfeeding.

hyperonychia (hī″pĕr-ō-nĭk′ē-ă) [″ + *onyx,* nail] An overgrowth (hypertrophy) of the nails.

hyperope (hī′pĕr-ōp) [″ + *ops,* eye] One who is farsighted. SYN: *hypermetrope.*

hyperopia (hī″pĕr-ō′pē-ă) [″ + *ops,* eye] Farsightedness; a defect in vision in which parallel rays come to a focus behind the retina as a result of flattening of the globe of the eye or of an error in refraction. Symptoms include ocular fatigue and poor vision. SYN: *hypermetropia.* SEE: *emmetropia* for illus.

absolute h. Hyperopia in which the eye cannot accommodate.

axial h. Hyperopia caused by shortness of the eye's anteroposterior axis.

facultative h. Hyperopia that can be corrected by accommodation.

latent h. Hyperopia in which the error of refraction is overcome and disguised by ciliary muscle action.

manifest h. Total amount of hyperopia that can be neutralized by a convex lens without interfering with clarity of vision.

relative h. Hyperopia in which vision is clear only when excessive convergence is made.

total h. Complete hyperopia combining both latent and manifest types; the amount of hyperopia present when accommodation is completely suspended by paralyzing the ciliary muscle, which is done by use of a cycloplegic drug.

hyperorchidism (hī″pĕr-or′kĭd-ĭzm) [Gr. *hyper,* over, above, excessive, + *orchis,* testicle, + *-ismos,* state of] An abnormal activity of testicular secretion.

hyperorexia (hī″pĕr-ō-rĕks′ē-ă) [″ + *orexis,* appetite] Abnormal hunger or markedly increased appetite. This occurs in some patients with diabetes mellitus, hyperthyroidism, parasitic infections of the gastrointestinal tract, or bulimia. It also may occur as a side effect of some medications, such as steroids.

hyperorthocytosis (hī″pĕr-or″thō-sī-tō′sĭs) [″ + *orthos,* straight, + *kytos,* cell, + *osis,* condition] Increased white blood cells with normal proportion of various forms and without immature forms.

hyperosmia (hī″pĕr-ŏz′mē-ă) [″ + *osme,* smell] An abnormal sensitivity to odors.

general h. Total h.

partial h. Increased sensitivity to some odors.

total h. Increased sensitivity to all odors. SYN: *general h.*

hyperosmolarity (hī″pĕr-ŏz″mō-lăr′ĭ-tē) Increased osmolarity of the blood.

hyperostosis (hī″pĕr-ŏs-tō′sĭs) [″ + *osteon,* bone, + *osis,* condition] An abnormal growth of osseous tissue. SYN: *exostosis; torus.*

frontal internal h. An osteoma, usually multiple or arising from the internal area of the frontal bone.

infantile cortical h. An increased growth of subperiosteal bone occurring most frequently in the mandible and clavicles, with fever and other systemic manifestations.

hyperovaria [Gr. *hyper,* over, above, excessive, + L. *ovarium,* ovary] Precocious sexual development in young girls owing to excessive ovarian secretion resulting from unusual and premature ovarian development.

hyperovulation The production of a large number of ova, usually in response to hormonal intervention. This is done in an attempt to improve the chance of pregnancy in a patient who has had difficulty conceiving. SEE: *clomiphene citrate; human menopausal gonadotropin.*

hyperoxaluria (hī″pĕr-ŏk″să-lū′rē-ă) Increased oxalic acid in the urine.

enteric h. Hyperoxaluria caused by disease of or surgical removal of the ileum.

primary h. An inherited metabolic disease caused by a defect in glyoxalate metabolism. This causes an increased secretion of oxalate in the urine, renal calculi, renal failure, and generalized deficit of oxalate crystals in tissues.

hyperoxemia (hī″pĕr-ŏk-sē′mē-ă) [″ + *oxys,* sharp, + *haima,* blood] Increased oxygen content of the blood.

hyperoxia (hī″pĕr-ŏk′sē-ă) Increased oxygen in the blood.

hyperoxygenation (hī″pĕr-ŏk″sĭ-jĕn-ā′shŭn) The temporary administration of excess oxygen to a patient to prevent hypoxemia during subsequent therapeutic procedures.

hyperpancreatism (hī″pĕr-păn′krē-ă-tĭzm) [″ + *pankreas,* pancreas, + *-ismos,* condition] An abnormal amount of secretion from the pancreas.

hyperparasitism (hī″pĕr-păr′ă-sī″tĭzm) A condition in which a parasite lives in or upon another parasite.

hyperparathyroidism (hī″pĕr-păr″ă-thī′roy-dĭzm) [″ + *para,* beyond, + *thyreos,* shield, + *eidos,* form, shape, + *-ismos,* condition] A condition caused by excessive levels of parathyroid hormone in the body. Usually this is caused by benign tumors of the parathyroid glands (primary hyperparathyroidism), although occasionally the disease occurs secondary to renal failure or other systemic illnesses. The consequences of excess parathyroid hormone may include symptomatic or unnoticed hypercalcemia, hypophosphatemia, hyperchlorhydria, kidney stone formation, and bone resorption. Mild hyperparathyroidism is managed with medication, but severe primary hyperparathyroidism may require surgical removal of the parathyroid glands. In some cancer patients, malignant tumors release a parathyroid-like hormone with hypercalcemia, which mimics hyperparathyroidism. SEE: *hypercalcemia; parathyroid glands; osteitis fibrosa cystica.*

hyperpathia [″ + *pathos,* disease, suffering] Hypersensitivity to sensory stimuli. Includes hyperesthesia, allodynia, and hyperalgesia.

hyperphagia [″ + Gr. *phagein,* to eat] Eating more food than is required; gluttony or binge eating.

hyperphalangism (hī″pĕr-făl-ăn′jĭzm) [″ + *phalanx,* closely knit row, + *-ismos,* state of] Having an extra phalanx on a finger or toe. SYN: *polyphalangism.*

hyperphasia (hī″pĕr-fā′zē-ă) [″ + *phasis,* speech] An abnormal desire to talk.

hyperphenylalaninemia (hī″pĕr-fĕn″ĭl-ăl″ă-nĭ-nē′mē-ă) An increased amount of phenylalanine in the blood. SEE: *phenylketonuria.*

hyperphonia (hī″pĕr-fō′nē-ă) [″ + *phone,* voice] **1.** Stuttering or stammering due to irritability of the vocal cords. **2.** Explosive speech exhibited by those who stammer.

hyperphoria (hī″pĕr-fō′rē-ă) [″ + *phorein,* to bear] A tendency of one eye to turn upward.

hyperphosphatasemia (hī″pĕr-fŏs″fă-tă-sē′mē-ă) Increased alkaline phosphatase in the blood.

hyperphosphatemia (hī″pĕr-fŏs″fă-tē′mē-ă) [″ + L. *phosphas,* phosphate, + Gr. *haima,* blood] An abnormal amount of phosphorus in the blood. SYN: *hyperphospheremia.*

hyperphosphaturia (hī″pĕr-fŏs-fă-tū′rē-ă) [″ + ″ + Gr. *ouron,* urine] An increased amount of phosphates in the urine.

hyperphospheremia (hī″pĕr-fŏs-fĕr-ē′mē-ă) [″ + ″ + Gr. *haima,* blood] Hyperphosphatemia.

hyperphrenia (hī″pĕr-frē′nē-ă) [Gr. *hyper,* over, above, excessive, + *phren,* mind] **1.** Excessive mental activity, seen in the manic phase of manic-depressive psychosis. **2.** Mental ability and capacity much greater than normal.

hyperpigmentation (hī″pĕr-pĭg″mĕn-tā′shŭn) Increased pigmentation, esp. of the skin.

hyperpituitarism (hī″pĕr-pĭ-tū′ĭ-tăr-ĭsm) [″ + L. *pituita,* mucus, + Gr. *-ismos,* condition] A condition resulting from overactivity of the anterior lobe of the pituitary. SEE: *acromegaly; gigantism.*

hyperplasia (hī″pĕr-plā′zē-ă) [″ + *plassein,* to form] Excessive proliferation of normal cells in the normal tissue arrangement of an organ. SYN: *hypergenesis.* SEE: illus. **hyperplastic** (-plăs′tĭk), *adj.*

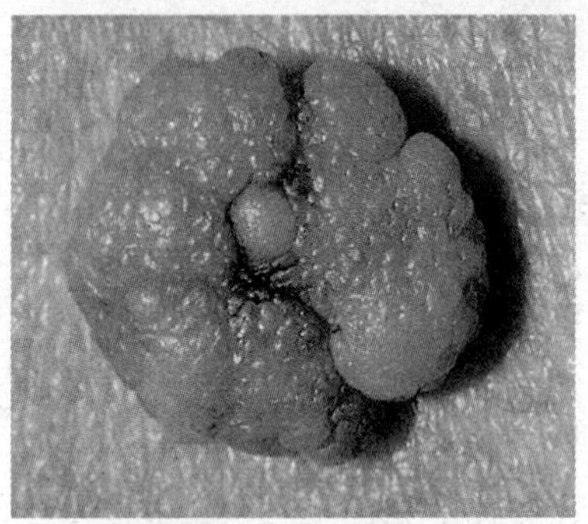

HYPERPLASIA OF A DERMAL MOLE

angiofollicular lymph node h. Castleman's disease.

benign prostatic h. ABBR: BPH. A nonmalignant enlargement of the prostate gland caused by excessive growth of prostatic nodules. It is the most common benign neoplasm of aging men, found on microscopic examination of the prostate in about 70% of men by age 60, and 90% of men by age 70. More than 440,000 men in the U.S. alone have surgery to correct the problem each year. SYN: *benign prostatic hypertrophy*. SEE: *Nursing Diagnoses Appendix; prostate; prostate cancer; transurethral resection of the prostate.*

ETIOLOGY: The prostate gland grows as a result of stimulation of the gland by sex hormones. Dihydrotestosterone (a derivative of the male sex hormone, testosterone) directly stimulates the growth of the gland's epithelial and stromal cells; estrogens, which are found in increasing concentrations in aging men, increase the number of hormone receptors in the prostate, making the gland more susceptible to stimulation by male hormones. Under these influences prostate nodules enlarge around the urethra, and may compress the urinary outlet limiting the flow of urine from the bladder.

SYMPTOMS: Patients often complain of difficulty starting or stopping their urinary stream, frequent urination, urinary urgency, and frequent awakenings at night to urinate. They may also develop urinary tract infections and sudden obstruction of all urinary flow (acute urinary retention). Bladder hypertrophy, hydronephrosis, kidney damage, or sepsis may also develop.

TREATMENT: Men with mild to moderate symptoms often get symptomatic relief from medicines such as alpha-1 adrenergic antagonists (e.g., terazosin); 5-alpha reductase inhibitors (such as finasteride), which block the effect of testosterone on prostatic growth, may reduce the need for prostate surgeries. When patients have recurrent urinary infections, unmanageable urinary symptoms, urinary retention, or damage to the bladder or kidneys, surgery is performed. Transurethral resection of the prostate (TURP) is the most common procedure—it removes hypertrophied prostatic tissue with a loop-shaped resection device. Alternatives to TURP include transurethral incision of the prostate (TUIP), laser or electrothermal reduction in the size of the gland, urethral stent placement, or open prostatectomy.

PATIENT CARE: The patient is evaluated for positive outcomes to the treatment plan, including his ability to effectively empty his bladder, the caliber and force of his urinary stream, reduction in urinary hesitancy and difficulty initiating his stream, dribbling, incontinence, and nocturia.

The importance of annual screening for prostatic cancer is explained to the patient. The patient is prepared for BPH diagnostic testing and for surgical interventions as appropriate. If a urinary tract infection is suspected, the patient is taught how to obtain a midstream urine specimen for culture and sensitivity. Prescribed antibiotic therapy is administered. Antibiotics are also administered as prescribed if the patient is to undergo urethral procedures involving instrumentation.

If urinary retention develops, a urinary catheter is inserted by the nurse or urologist. Sometimes the catheter is inserted with guides. Suprapubic cystotomy is used if a catheter cannot be passed transurethrally. The patient is monitored for rapid bladder decompression and for signs of postobstruction diuresis (increased urine output, hypotension), which may lead to serious dehydration, lowered blood volume, shock, electrolyte losses, and anuria.

The patient with BPH is taught to avoid prescription and over-the-counter drugs that can worsen obstruction (e.g., decongestants, alcohol, anticholinergics, tranquilizers, or antidepressants). The patient also is taught to recognize and report signs of infection, which can worsen obstruction, and to seek medical care immediately if he is unable to void. The patient is advised that regular sexual intercourse will help to relieve prostatic congestion.

fibrous h. An increase in connective tissue cells after inflammation.

hyperploidy (hī″pĕr-ploy′dē) A condition of having one extra chromosome and thus not balanced sets of chromosomes. SEE: *Down syndrome; trisomy 21.*

hyperpnea (hī″pĕrp-nē′ă) [″ + *pnoia,* breath] An increased respiratory rate or breathing that is deeper than that usually experienced during normal activity. A certain degree of hyperpnea is normal after exercise; it may also be caused by pain, respiratory disease, fevers, heart failure, certain drugs, panic attacks, or atmospheric conditions experienced at high altitude.

hyperpolarization (hī-pĕr-pōl″ăr-ĭ-zā′shŭn) An increase in the resting potential of a cell membrane (e.g., a cell membrane of a neuron), causing the inside of the cell to become more negative. This change raises the threshold level for depolarization.

hyperpraxia (hī″pĕr-prăk′sē-ă) Excessive activity and restlessness seen in some mental disorders.

hyperprolactinemia (hī″pĕr-prō-lăk″tĭn-ē′mē-ă) An excess secretion of prolactin thought to be due to hypothalamic-pituitary dysfunction. This is usually associated with amenorrhea with or without galactorrhea.

hyperprolinemia (hī″pĕr-prō″lĭ-nē′mē-ă) An inherited metabolic disease of amino acid metabolism that results in an excess of proline in the body.

hyperproteinemia (hī″pĕr-prō″tē-ĭn-ē′mē-ă) [″ + *protos,* first, + *haima,* blood] An excess of protein in the blood.

hyperproteinuria (hī″pĕr-prō″tē-ĭn-ū′rē-ă) [″ + ″ + *ouron,* urine] An excess of protein in the urine.

hyperpselaphesia (hī″pĕrp-sĕl″ă-fē′zē-ă) [Gr. *hyper,* over, above, excessive, + *pselaphesis,* touch] Hyperaphia.

hyperptyalism (hī″pĕr-tī′ăl-ĭzm) [″ + *ptyalon,* spittle] Ptyalism.

hyperpyrexia (hī″pĕr-pī-rĕks′ē-ă) [″ + *pyressein,* to be feverish] An elevation of body temperature that is markedly abnormal. It may be produced by physical agents such as hot baths, diathermy, or hot air or by reaction to infection caused by microorganisms. SYN: *hyperthermia*. **hyperpyretic, hyperpyrexial** (-rĕt′ĭk, -rĕk′sē-ăl), *adj.*

malignant h. Malignant hyperthermia.

hyperreactive (hī″pĕr-rē-ăk′tĭv) Pert. to an increased response to stimuli.

hyperreflexia (hī″pĕr-rē-flĕk′sē-ă) [″ + L. *reflexus,* bent back] An increased action of the reflexes.

hyperresonance (hī″pĕr-rĕz′ō-năns) [″ + L. *resonare,* to resound] An increased resonance produced when an area is percussed.

hypersalivation (hī″pĕr-săl″ĭ-vā′shŭn) [″ + L. *salivatio,* salivation] Ptyalism.

hypersecretion (hī″pĕr-sē-krē′shŭn) [″ + L. *secretio,* separation] An abnormal amount of secretion.

hypersensibility (hī″pĕr-sĕn″sĭ-bĭl′ĭ-tē) [″ + L. *sensibilitas,* sensibility] Hypersensitivity.

hypersensitive (hī″pĕr-sĕn′sĭ-tĭv) [″ + L. *sensitivus,* sensitive] Excessively and abnormally susceptible to the action of a given agent, as pollen or foreign protein. SYN: *supersensitive*. SEE: *allergy; anaphylaxis; hay fever*.

hypersensitivity (hī″pĕr-sĕn″sĭ-tĭv′ĭ-tē) An abnormal sensitivity to a stimulus of any kind.

hypersensitization (hī″pĕr-sĕn″sĭ-tĭ-zā′shŭn) **1.** Producing or inducing increased sensitivity to an organism or drug. **2.** The condition of being highly sensitive to something.

hypersomnia (hī″pĕr-sŏm′nē-ă) [″ + L. *somnus,* sleep] Sleeping for excessive lengths of time. It may be associated with psychiatric illness, drug or alcohol use, or narcolepsy.

hypersplenism (hī″pĕr-splĕn′ĭzm) An increased activity of the spleen in which increased amounts of all types of blood cells are removed from the circulation.

hypersthenia (hī″pĕr-sthē′nē-ă) [Gr. *hyper,* over, above, excessive, + *sthenos,* strength] Abnormal strength or excessive tension of part or all of the body.

hypersthenic (hī″pĕr-sthĕn′ĭk) **1.** Denoting excessive strength or tension. **2.** Denoting a body habitus characterized by a broad, deep thorax, short thoracic cavity, and a large abdominal cavity; a massive build.

hypersthenuria (hī″pĕr-sthĕn-ū′rē-ă) [″ + *sthenos,* strength, + *ouron,* urine] The passage of abnormally concentrated urine, usually due to dehydration or excess loss of fluids in sweat.

hypersusceptibility (hī″pĕr-sŭ-sĕp″tĭ-bĭl′ĭ-tē) [″ + L. *suscipere,* to take up, + *-bilis,* able] An unusual susceptibility to a disease, pathologic conditions, chemicals, or parasites. SEE: *allergy; anaphylaxis*.

hypersystole (hī″pĕr-sĭs′tō-lē) [″ + *systole,* contraction] Unusual force or duration of systole. **hypersystolic** (-sĭs-tŏl′ĭk), *adj.*

hypertelorism (hī″pĕr-tĕl′or-ĭzm) [″ + *telouros,* distant] Abnormal distance between two paired organs, esp. the eyes.

hypertensinogen (hī″pĕr-tĕn-sĭn′ō-jĕn) An obsolete term for angiotensinogen, the precursor of angiotensin.

hypertension (hī″pĕr-tĕn′shŭn) [″ + L. *tensio,* tension] **1.** Greater than normal tension or tone. **2.** In adults, a condition in which the blood pressure (BP) is higher than 140 mm Hg systolic or 90 mm Hg diastolic on three separate readings recorded several weeks apart. Hypertension also is present in patients under treatment for the disease, in whom the disease has normalized with drug therapy. Hypertension is one of the major risks factors for coronary artery disease, congestive heart failure, stroke, peripheral vascular disease, kidney failure, and retinopathy. It affects about 50 million people in the U.S. alone. Considerable research has shown that controlling hypertension increases longevity and helps prevent cardiovascular illnesses. SYN: *high blood pressure*. SEE: *blood pressure*. **hypertensive,** *adj.*

Although all systems for categorizing

high BP are somewhat arbitrary, the current consensus is that normal BPs are <130 mm Hg systolic and <85 mm Hg diastolic. Borderline (also known as "high normal") BPs are from 130 to 139 mm Hg systolic, and 85 to 89 mm Hg diastolic. Patients with BP readings between 140/90 mm Hg and 160/100 mm Hg are said to have stage 1 hypertension.

Stage 2 hypertension denotes a pressure from 160/100 to 179/109 mm Hg. Stage 3 hypertension begins at 180/110 mm Hg and has no upper limit. At each BP level, cardiovascular risks increase in a predictable fashion. SEE: table.

ETIOLOGY: Hypertension results from many different conditions, some curable and others treatable. Curable forms of hypertension, which are relatively rare, may be caused by coarctation of the aorta, pheochromocytoma, renal artery stenosis, primary aldosteronism, and Cushing's syndrome. Excess alcohol consumption (more than two drinks daily) is a common cause of high BP; abstinence or drinking in moderation effectively lowers BP in these cases. Aortic valve stenosis, pregnancy, obesity, and the use of certain drugs (e.g., cocaine, amphetamines, steroids, or erythropoietin) also may lead to hypertension. Usually, however, the cause is unknown; then high BP is categorized as "essential" or "idiopathic." Essential hypertension may result from the body's resistance to the action of insulin.

SYMPTOMS: Hypertension is usually a "silent" (i.e., asymptomatic) disease in the first few decades of its course. Because most patients are symptom-free until complications arise, they may have difficulty taking seriously a condition from which they perceive no immediate danger. Occasionally, patients with hypertension report headache. When complications result from high BPs, patients mention symptoms referable to the affected organs.

TREATMENT: All patients with high BP should learn about the lifestyle changes they can make to lower their BP without medication. These include increasing the level of exercise, decreasing the amount of calories and fat in the diet, and achieving sensible weight loss. In patients whose BP remains uncontrolled after a trial of lifestyle modification and in patients with other risk factors for cardiovascular disease, antihypertensive medications are added to supplement lifestyle changes. Expert panels have recommended specific recipes for the treatment of hypertension.

PATIENT CARE: BP should be checked at every health care visit, and patients should be informed of their BP reading and its meaning. Positive lifestyle changes should be encouraged. Adherence to medical regimens is also emphasized, and patients are advised to inform their health care providers of any side effects of therapy that they experience. The technique of ambulatory BP monitoring is taught to receptive patients and to those in whom "white coat" hypertension is suspected. SEE: *Nursing Diagnoses Appendix.*

Classification of BP for Adults Age 18 and Older*

Category	Systolic (mm Hg)		Diastolic (mm Hg)
Optimal†	<120	and	<80
Normal	<130	and	<85
High-normal	130–139	or	85–89
Hypertension‡			
Stage 1	140–159	or	90–99
Stage 2	160–179	or	100–109
Stage 3	≥ 180	or	≥ 110

* Not taking antihypertensive drugs and not acutely ill. When systolic and diastolic blood pressures fall into different categories, the higher category should be selected to classify the individual's blood pressure status. For example, 160/92 mm Hg should be classified as stage 2 hypertension, and 174/120 mm Hg should be classified as stage 3 hypertension. Isolated systolic hypertension is defined as SBP of 140 mm Hg or greater and DBP below 90 mm Hg and staged appropriately (e.g., 170/82 mm Hg is defined as stage 2 isolated systolic hypertension). In addition to classifying stages of hypertension on the basis of average blood pressure levels, clinicians should specify presence or absence of target organ disease and additional risk factors. This specificity is important for risk classification and treatment.

† Optimal blood pressure with respect to cardiovascular risk is below 120/80 mm Hg. However, unusually low readings should be evaluated for clinical significance.

‡ Based on the average of two or more readings taken at each of two or more visits after an initial screening.

SOURCE: The Sixth Report of the Joint National Committee on Prevention, Detection, Evaluation, and Treatment of High BP, NIH publication No. 98-4080, November 1997.

accelerated h. Significant increase in blood pressure, with some evidence of vascular damage on funduscopic examination of the retina. Prompt treatment is indicated to prevent organ damage. SEE: *malignant h.*

benign intracranial h. Pseudotumor cerebri.

cuff-inflation h. A marked increase in blood pressure in association with inflation of the sphygmomanometer cuff. This does not represent true hypertension.

drug-resistant h. High blood pressure that does not normalize after treatment with appropriate doses of two or more standard antihypertensive medications.

essential h. Hypertension that develops without apparent cause. SYN: *primary h.*

Goldblatt h. Hypertension that resembles renal hypertension produced in experimental animals by decreasing the blood flow to the kidney.

intracranial h. ABBR: ICH. An increase in the pressure inside the skull from any cause such as a tumor, hydrocephalus, intracranial hemorrhage, trauma, infection, or interference with the venous flow from the brain. SEE: *hydrocephalus*.

CAUTION: Patients with intracranial hypertension should not undergo a lumbar puncture or any other procedure that decreases the cerebrospinal fluid pressure in the vertebral canal.

---

malignant h. A form of hypertension that progresses rapidly, accompanied by severe vascular damage. It may be life-threatening or cause stroke, encephalopathy, cardiac ischemia, or renal failure.

ocular h. Increased intraocular pressure, typically exceeding 21 mm Hg. This condition, present in glaucoma, may predispose affected persons to optic nerve damage and visual field loss.

portal h. Increased pressure in the portal vein caused by an obstruction of the flow of blood through the liver. Portal hypertension is found in diseases such as cirrhosis, in which it is responsible for ascites, splenomegaly, and the formation of varices.

pregnancy-induced h. ABBR: PIH. A complication of pregnancy marked by increasing blood pressure, proteinuria, and edema. Diagnostic criteria include an increase of 30 mm Hg systolic or 15 mm Hg diastolic over the baseline pressure for the individual woman on two assessments with at least a 6-hr interval between measures; edema; and proteinuria. This condition occurs most commonly in the last trimester; however, it may manifest earlier in women with molar pregnancies. It may worsen rapidly and, if untreated, develop into eclampsia. SYN: *pre-eclampsia*. SEE: *eclampsia; HELLP syndrome*.

The cause is unknown; however, the incidence is higher among adolescent and older primigravidas, diabetics, and women with multiple pregnancy. Pathophysiology includes generalized vasospasm, damage to glomerular membranes, and hemoconcentration due to a fluid shift from intravascular to interstitial compartments. Characteristic complaints include sudden weight gain, severe headaches, and visual disturbances. Indications of increasing severity include complaints of epigastric or abdominal pain; generalized, presacral, and facial edema; oliguria; and hyperreflexia.

The treatment consists of bedrest, a high-protein diet, and medications including mild sedatives, antihypertensives, and intravenous anticoagulants if indicated. Complications are HELLP syndrome and eclampsia.

PATIENT CARE: To enable the woman to actively participate in her health maintenance, reduce the potential for development of PIH, and facilitate early diagnosis and treatment, the health care provider should emphasize the importance of regular prenatal visits and good prenatal nutrition. He or she should encourage the patient to eat a well-balanced, high-protein diet and to drink fluids freely. Signs to report promptly are identified with the patient: sudden weight gain, edema of the hands and face, headache, pitting edema of the ankles and legs, and oliguria.

At each prenatal visit, the pregnant woman's blood pressure is monitored for levels greater than 140/90 mm Hg or for increases of 30 mm Hg systolic or 15 mm Hg diastolic (measured on two occasions more than 6 hours apart). The patient also is assessed for albuminuria; weekly weight gain of more than 3 lb (1.36 kg) in the second trimester or more than 1 lb (0.45 kg) in the third trimester; and generalized edema, esp. of the face and hands, and pitting edema of the ankles and legs. Protein intake is monitored to ensure adequate maternal serum protein levels, normal oncotic pressure, limitation of edema formation, and normal fetal development.

As pre-eclampsia progresses, the woman may complain of headaches, blurred vision or other visual disturbances, epigastric pain or heartburn, chest pressure, irritability, emotional tension, and decreased fetal activity. The patient is assessed for hyperreflexia of the deep tendon reflexes and clonus, and, if pre-eclampsia worsens, for oliguria.

Hospitalization may be necessary if

the patient exhibits signs of moderate to severe pre-eclampsia and has failed to respond to home management. Pre-eclampsia can suddenly progress to eclampsia, demonstrated by the onset of seizures, changes in breathing patterns, and onset of coma. Maternal vital signs, level of consciousness, fluid balance (assessing body weight daily in addition to intake and output), deep tendon reflex activity, headache unrelieved by analgesia, and fetal heart tones are monitored. Bedrest in a left side-lying position is prescribed to prevent venal caval and aortic compression and thereby to increase cardiac output and renal and uterine perfusion, and extremities are elevated to promote venous return. A quiet, calm, nonstimulating and nonstressful environment is created, a call bell is provided, full seizure precautions are in effect, and emergency medications and delivery equipment are available on standby.

The clinical status of mother and fetus is continually evaluated; maternal vital signs and fetal heart rate are monitored. The patient is assessed for impending labor, and fetal and maternal responses to labor contractions are evaluated. The obstetrician is notified of any change in the patient's or the fetus's condition. Emergency care is provided during convulsions; prescribed medications are administered as directed, and patient and fetal response are evaluated. Careful monitoring of the administration of magnesium sulfate, intake and output, and the woman's response to the medication is necessary. Health care providers should be esp. alert for signs of toxicity, such as an absence of patellar reflexes (hyporeflexia), flushing, and muscle flaccidity. Calcium gluconate should be available at the bedside to counteract such effects.

Psychological support and assistance to develop effective coping strategies are provided to both patient and family, and they are prepared for possible premature delivery. Although infants of mothers with PIH are usually small for gestational age, they sometimes fare better than other premature infants of similar weight because they have developed adaptive ventilatory and other responses to intrauterine stress. SEE: *Nursing Diagnoses Appendix.*

primary h. Essential h.

pulmonary h. Hypertension in the pulmonary arteries.

rebound h. An increase in blood pressure that follows withdrawal from an antihypertensive drug.

renal h. **1.** Hypertension produced by kidney disease. The mechanism causing an increase in blood pressure is either alteration in the renal regulation of sodium and fluids or alteration in renal secretion of vasoconstrictors, which alter the tone of systemic or local arterioles. **2.** Hypertension produced experimentally by constriction of renal arteries. It is due to a humoral substance (renin) produced in an ischemic kidney.

renovascular h. Hypertension that is caused by decreased blood flow through one or both renal arteries and that normalizes after angioplasty or surgery to open the affected artery. The condition is an uncommon but surgically treatable form of high blood pressure.

white coat h. A colloquial term used to describe an episode of elevated blood pressure when the reading is taken by a health care professional. It is attributed to anxiety regarding medical examination procedures or fear of possible findings.

hypertensive (hī″pĕr-tĕn′sĭv) Marked by a rise in blood pressure.

h. crisis Any severe elevation in blood pressure (usually a diastolic pressure greater than 130 mm Hg) with or without damage to internal organs or other structures (e.g., brain, heart, aorta, kidneys). In hypertensive *emergencies,* end organs are damaged, and antihypertensive drugs usually are given intravenously to try to lower the blood pressure within an hour. Agents used in hypertensive emergencies include sodium nitroprusside, nitroglycerin, labetalol, and enalaprilat.

In hypertensive *urgencies,* the blood pressure is extremely elevated, but there is no sign or immediate threat of organ damage. Typically, oral beta blockers, ACE inhibitors, or clonidine, alone or in combination, are given to lower pressures over 1 or 2 days.

hyperthecosis (hī″pĕr-thē-kō′sĭs) Hyperplasia of the theca interna of the ovary. Hirsutism, amenorrhea, and enlarged clitoris may be present.

hyperthelia (hī″pĕr-thē′lē-ă) [Gr. *hyper,* over, above, excessive, + *thele,* nipple] The presence of more than two nipples.

hyperthermalgesia (hī″pĕr-thĕrm″ăl-jē′zē-ă) [″ + *therme,* heat, + *algesis,* sense of pain] An unusual sensitivity to heat. SYN: *hyperthermoesthesia.*

hyperthermia (hī″pĕr-thĕr′mē-ă) [″ + *therme,* heat] Body temperature elevated above the normal range; an unusually high fever. SYN: *hyperpyrexia.*

ETIOLOGY: Hyperthermia may be caused by heat stroke; central nervous system diseases; thyroid storm; infections including encephalitis, malaria, meningitis, or sepsis, esp. due to gram-negative organisms. To treat some diseases, hyperthermia can be artificially induced by the introduction of the malaria organism, injection of foreign proteins, or physical means.

PATIENT CARE: The patient is placed in a cool environment, and tepid water baths may be used to promote reduction in surface temperature by convection and evaporation. Hypothermia blankets may be used if hyperthermia is the result of neurologic dysfunction. Fluid intake is increased to at least 3 liters per day (unless otherwise restricted by cardiac or renal disorders) to replace fluids lost through diaphoresis, rapid respirations, and increased metabolic activity. Frequent oral hygiene is provided because dehydration dries the oral mucosa. Shivering is prevented through administration of narcotics.

CAUTION: Rubbing alcohol should not be used to reduce fever.

malignant h. A severe and rapid increase in body temperature accompanied by vigorous muscle contractions. It may follow any major stress, but usually occurs as a result of exposure to general anesthetics. Body temperature often exceeds 105°F. SYN: *malignant hyperpyrexia.*

hyperthermia treatment The use of microwave or radiofrequency energy to increase body temperature. This type of therapy, which is usually combined with chemotherapy or radiation, has been used in treating certain malignancies and some autoimmune diseases. SEE: *fever therapy.*

hyperthermoesthesia (hī″pĕr-thĕrm″ō-ĕs-thē′zē-ă) [″ + ″ + *aisthesis,* sensation] Hyperthermalgesia.

hyperthrombinemia (hī″pĕr-thrŏm″bĭn-ē′mē-ă) [″+ *thrombos,* clot, + *haima,* blood] An excess of thrombin in the blood. This tends to promote intravascular clotting.

hyperthymia (hī″pĕr-thī′mē-ă) [″ + *thymos,* mind] Pathological sensitivity or excitability.

hyperthyroidism (hī″pĕr-thī′royd-ĭzm) [″ + *thyreos,* shield, + *eidos,* form, shape, + *-ismos,* state of] A disease caused by excessive levels of thyroid hormone in the body. SEE: *Nursing Diagnoses Appendix.*

ETIOLOGY: The condition may result from various disorders such as nodular goiter and toxic adenomas, hyperemesis gravidarum, excessive thyroid hormone replacement, excessive iodine ingestion, or pituitary adenoma; however, the most common cause is Graves' disease. SEE: *Graves' disease.*

SYMPTOMS: In general, the signs and symptoms of Graves' disease are divided into two categories—those secondary to excessive stimulation of the sympathetic nervous system and those due to excessive levels of circulating thyroxine. The symptoms caused by sympathetic (adrenergic) stimulation include tachycardia, tremor, increased systolic blood pressure, hyperreflexia, eyelid lag (lagophthalmos), staring, palpitations, depression, nervousness, and anxiety. Symptoms caused by increased circulating thyroxine include increased metabolism, hyperphagia, weight loss, and some psychological disturbances. In elderly persons, symptoms of hyperthyroidism are often blunted. SEE: *apathetic h.*

TREATMENT: Definitive therapies include surgical removal of the thyroid gland, radioactive iodine ablation of the gland, or antithyroid drugs. The choice of treatment is individualized for each patient.

PATIENT CARE: Vital signs, fluid balance, and weight are monitored, and activity patterns are documented. Serum electrolyte levels are monitored, blood glucose levels are checked for evidence of hyperglycemia and urine for glycosuria, and the ECG is evaluated for arrhythmias and ST-segment changes. The patient is assessed for classic signs and symptoms (as above) and for indications of thyrotoxic crisis or heart failure. The patient's knowledge of the disorder is determined, misconceptions are corrected, and information on the condition, related problems, and symptom management is provided. Medical treatments, including radioactive iodine, are administered and evaluated for desired response and adverse reactions, and the patient is instructed about these treatments. If the patient has exophthalmos, isotonic eyedrops are instilled to moisten the conjunctivae, and sunglasses or eye patches are recommended to protect the eyes from light. A high-caloric, high-vitamin, high-mineral diet, including between-meal snacks and avoidance of caffeinated beverages, is encouraged. Frequency and characteristics of the patient's stools are checked, and related skin care is provided as needed. The patient should minimize physical and emotional stress, balance rest and activity periods, and wear loose-fitting cotton clothing. A cool, dim, quiet environment also is recommended. The patient is prepared physically and emotionally for surgery if needed. Both patient and family are reassured that mood swings and nervousness will subside with treatment. The patient is encouraged to verbalize feelings about changes in body image. Assistance is provided to help the patient to identify and develop positive coping strategies. Emotional support is offered, and referral for further counseling is arranged as necessary. Life-long thyroid hormone replacement therapy will be necessary after surgical removal or radioactive iodine ablation treatment. The patient should wear or carry a medical identification device describing the condition and treatment and carry medication with him or her at all times.

apathetic h. Overactivity of the thyroid gland, presenting as heart failure, arrhythmias (such as atrial fibrillation), weight loss, or psychological withdrawal. This is more often a presentation of hyperthyroidism in the elderly than in younger patients. Diagnosis is usually easier in the latter group because they present with the classic symptoms of hyperthyroidism. SYN: *subclinical h.*

subclinical h. Apathetic hyperthyroidism.

hyperthyrosis (hī″pĕr-thī-rō′sĭs) Hyperthyroidism.

hyperthyroxinemia (hī″pĕr-thī-rŏk″sĭ-nē′mē-ă) An excess of thyroxine in the blood.

hypertonia (hī″pĕr-tō′nē-ă) [″ + *tonos,* tension] Hypertonicity.

hypertonic (hī″pĕr-tŏn′ĭk) **1.** Pert. to a solution of higher osmotic pressure than another. **2.** In a state of greater than normal tension or of incomplete relaxation, said of muscles; the opposite of hypotonic.

hypertonicity (hī″pĕr-tŏn-ĭ′sĭ-tē) An excess of muscular or arterial tone or intraocular pressure. SYN: *hypertonia.*

hypertonus (hī″pĕr-tō′nŭs) Increased tension, as muscular tension in spasm.

hypertrichophobia (hī″pĕr-trĭk″ō-fō′bē-ă) [″ + ″ + *phobos,* fear] A fear of hair on the body.

hypertrichophrydia (hī″pĕr-trĭk″ō-frĭd′ē-ă) [″ + ″ + *ophrys,* eyebrow] Excessive thickness of the eyebrows.

hypertrichosis (hī″pĕr-trĭ-kō′sĭs) [″ + ″ + *osis,* condition] An excessive growth of hair, possibly caused by endocrine disease, esp. of the adrenal gland, and in women, disease of the ovary. SYN: *polytrichia; polytrichosis.*

hypertriglyceridemia (hī″pĕr-trī-glĭs″ĕr-ī-dē′mē-ă) An increased blood triglyceride level; a possible risk factor for cardiovascular disease.

hypertrophia (hī″pĕr-trō′fē-ă) [Gr. *hyper,* over, above, excessive, + *trophe,* nourishment] Hypertrophy.

hypertrophy (hī-pĕr′trŏ-fē) [″ + *trophe,* nourishment] An increase in the size of an organ or structure, or of the body, owing to growth rather than tumor formation. This term generally is restricted to an increase in size or bulk that results not from an increase in number of cells, but rather from an increase in cellular components, such as proteins. It sometimes is used to apply to any increase in size as a result of functional activity. SYN: *hypertrophia.* SEE: *hyperplasia.* **hypertrophic** (hī″pĕr-trŏf′ik), *adj.*

adaptive h. Hypertrophy in which an organ increases in size to meet increased functional demands, as the hypertrophy of the heart that accompanies valvular disorders.

benign prostatic h. Benign prostatic hyperplasia.

compensatory h. Hypertrophy resulting from increased function of an organ because of a defect or impaired function of the opposite of a paired organ.

concentric h. Hypertrophy in which the walls of an organ become thickened without enlargement but with diminished capacity.

eccentric h. Hypertrophy of an organ with dilatation.

false h. Hypertrophy with degeneration of one constituent of an organ and its replacement by another.

gingival h. Excess growth of the gingival tissue, sometimes associated with prolonged phenytoin therapy.

left ventricular h. ABBR: LVH. An increase in the mass of the left ventricle of the heart to greater than 100 g/m^2 in women or 131 g/m^2 in men. An excessively massive left ventricle is associated with an increased risk of death due to cardiovascular disease, stroke, and other causes. The size of the left ventricle can be reduced through regular exercise, weight loss, and by drugs that control high blood pressure. SYN: *ventricular h.*

Marie's h. Chronic periostitis that causes the soft tissues surrounding the joints to enlarge.

numerical h. Hypertrophy caused by an increase in structural elements.

physiological h. Hypertrophy due to natural rather than pathological factors.

pseudomuscular h. A disease, usually of childhood, characterized by paralysis, depending on degeneration of the muscles, which paradoxically become enlarged from a deposition of fat and connective tissue.

SYMPTOMS: This disease causes muscle weakness. The patient is awkward and often seeks support while walking to prevent falls. As the disease progresses, the muscles, particularly those of the calf, thigh, buttocks, and back, enlarge. The upper extremities are less frequently affected. When the patient stands erect, the feet are wide apart, the abdomen protrudes, and the spinal column shows a marked curvature with convexity forward. Rising from the recumbent position is accomplished by grasping the knees or by resting the hands on the floor in front, extending the legs and pushing the body backward. The gait is characterized by waddling. In a few years the paralysis becomes so marked that the patient is unable to leave the bed, which leads to further generalized muscular atrophy.

TREATMENT: Physical therapy helps

to prevent contractures, but there is no effective therapy. The prognosis for this disease is unfavorable.

simple h. Hypertrophy due to an increase in the size of structural parts.

true h. Hypertrophy caused by an increase in the size of all the different tissues composing a part.

ventricular h. Left or right ventricular hypertrophy.

vicarious h. Hypertrophy of an organ when another organ of allied function is disabled or destroyed.

hypertropia [Gr. *hyper,* over, above, excessive, + *tropos,* turning] Vertical strabismus upward.

hyperuricemia (hī″pĕr-ū″rĭs-ē′mē-ă) [″ + *ouron,* urine, + *haima,* blood] An excessive amount of uric acid in the blood.

hyperuricuria (hī″pĕr-ū″rĭk-ū′rē-ă) [″ + *ouron,* urine] An excessive amount of uric acid in the urine.

hypervalinemia (hī″pĕr-văl″ĭn-ē′mē-ă) An inherited condition caused by a deficiency of the enzymes essential to the metabolism of valine. The condition is marked by mental retardation, nystagmus, vomiting, and failure to thrive.

hypervascular (hī″pĕr-văs′kū-lăr) [″ + L. *vasculus,* vessel] Excessively vascular.

hyperventilation (hī″pĕr-vĕn″tĭ-lā′shŭn) [″ + L. *ventilatio,* ventilation] Increased minute volume ventilation, which results in a lowered carbon dioxide (CO_2) level (hypocapnia). It is a frequent finding in many disease processes such as asthma, metabolic acidosis, pulmonary embolism, and pulmonary edema, and also in anxiety-induced states.

TREATMENT: Treatment is directed at the underlying cause. Immediate therapy in panic attacks consists of coaching the patient to slow down the breathing process to decrease the rate of blowing off CO_2. One way to do this is to have the patient breathe through only one nostril, with the mouth closed. Having the patient breathe in and out of a paper bag is discouraged, as it leads to hypoxemia. After the acute phase of the hyperventilation has been managed, the underlying cause of the problem must be determined.

therapeutic h. The use of carefully controlled but exaggerated ventilation to lower carbon dioxide levels in the blood and reduce cerebral blood flow; used to treat cerebral edema (e.g., after head injury). Its use remains controversial despite decades of research. Typically, the partial pressure of carbon dioxide (CO_2) is lowered to about 28–32 mm Hg. Lower levels of CO_2 produce reductions in cerebral blood flow that may damage the brain.

hyperviscosity (hī″pĕr-vĭs-kŏs′ĭ-tē) [″ + L. *viscosus,* gummy] Excessive resistance to the flow of liquids. Impaired hydraulic behavior, esp. of the plasma. Hyperviscous plasma is found in several hematological illnesses, including multiple myeloma and Waldenström's macroglobulinemia. In the latter illness, it can be treated with plasma exchange therapy.

hypervitaminosis (hī″pĕr-vī″tă-mĭn-ō′sĭs) [″ + L. *vita,* life, + *amine* + Gr. *osis,* condition] A condition caused by an excessive intake of vitamins in the diet or through the consumption of supplements; most commonly due to excessive consumption of fat soluble vitamins.

hypervolemia (hī″per-vŏl-ē′mē-ă) [″ + L. *volumen,* volume, + Gr. *haima,* blood] An abnormal increase in the volume of circulating blood.

hypesthesia (hī″pĕs-thē′zē-ă) [Gr. *hypo,* under, beneath, below, + *aisthesis,* sensation] A lessened sensibility to touch; variant of hypoesthesia.

hypha (hī′fă) *pl.* **hyphae** [Gr. *hyphe,* web] A filament of mold, or part of a mold mycelium.

hyphedonia (hīp″hĕ-dō′nē-ă) [Gr. *hypo,* under, beneath, below, + *hedone,* pleasure] An abnormal diminution of pleasure in acts that should normally give pleasure.

hyphema (hī-fē′mă) [Gr. *hyphaimos,* suffused with blood] Blood in the anterior chamber of the eye, in front of the iris.

Hyphomycetes (hī″fō-mī-sē′tēz) [Gr. *hyphe,* web, + *mykes,* fungus] The fungi imperfecti; filamentous fungi with branched or unbranched threads. They do not have sexual spores.

hypnagogic (hĭp-nă-gŏj′ĭk) [Gr. *hypnos,* sleep, + *agogos,* leading] **1.** Inducing sleep or induced by sleep. SYN: *hypnotic.* SEE: *zone, hypnogenic.* **2.** In psychology, pert. to hallucinations or dreams occurring just before loss of consciousness.

h. state A transitional state between sleeping and waking, and the delusions that may result therefrom.

hypnagogue (hĭp′nă-gŏg) Concerning or causing sleep or drowsiness.

hypno- Prefix meaning *sleep.*

hypnoanalysis (hĭp″nō-ă-năl′ĭ-sĭs) [″ + *analysis,* a dissolving] Combined psychoanalytic therapy and hypnosis.

hypnoanesthesia (hĭp″nō-ăn″ĕs-thē′zē-ă) The use of hypnosis to produce anesthesia.

hypnodontics (hĭp″nō-dŏn′tĭks) The application of controlled suggestion and hypnosis to the practice of dentistry.

hypnogenic (hĭp″nō-jĕn′ĭk) [″ + *gennan,* to produce] Producing sleep.

hypnoidal (hĭp-noy′dăl) [″ + *eidos,* form, shape] Pert. to a condition between sleep and waking, resembling sleep.

hypnoidization (hĭp″noy-dī-zā′shŭn) [″ + *eidos,* form, shape] The induction of hypnosis.

hypnolepsy (hĭp′nŏ-lĕp″sē) [″ + *lepsis,* seizure] Narcolepsy.

hypnonarcoanalysis (hĭp″nō-năr″kō-ă-năl′ĭ-sĭs) A psychiatric interview combining hypnosis with drug-induced sedation or narcosis.

hypnonarcosis (hĭp″nō-năr-kō′sĭs) A combination of hypnosis and narcosis.

hypnophobia (hĭp″nō-fō′bē-ă) [″ + *phobos,* fear] A morbid fear of falling asleep.

hypnopompic (hĭp″nŏ-pŏm′pĭk) [″ + *pompe,* procession] Pert. to dreams or visual images persisting after sleep and before complete awakening.

hypnosis (hĭp-nō′sĭs) [″ + *osis,* condition] A condition resembling sleep in which the objective manifestations of the mind are more or less inactive, accompanied by an increased susceptibility to suggestions. SEE: *autohypnosis; hypnotism; sleepwalking; somnambulism.*

hypnotherapy (hĭp″nō-thĕr′ă-pē) [″ + *therapeia,* treatment] Therapeutic use of hypnotism. It has been used to treat phobias and anxiety, to manage pain, and to extinguish habits and addictions.

hypnotic (hĭp-nŏt′ĭk) [Gr. *hypnos,* sleep] **1.** Pert. to sleep or hypnosis. **2.** An agent that causes an insensitivity to pain by inhibiting afferent impulses or by inhibiting the reception of sensory impressions in the cortical centers of the brain, thus causing partial or complete unconsciousness. Hypnotics include sedatives, analgesics, anesthetics, and intoxicants, and are sometimes called somnifacients and soporifics when used to induce sleep.

hypnotism (hĭp′nō-tĭzm) [″ + *-ismos,* condition] The act of inducing hypnosis.

self-induced h. The use of hypnotism by people who seek to achieve specific goals for themselves (e.g., controlling pain, promoting health, improving relaxation, or quitting tobacco use).

hypnotist (hĭp′nō-tĭst) [Gr. *hypnos,* sleep] One who practices hypnotism.

hypnotize (hĭp′nō-tīz) To put under hypnosis.

hypo (hī′pō) [Gr. *hypo,* under, beneath, below] Popular name for hypodermic syringe or injection.

hypo-, hyp- [Gr. *hypo,* under, beneath, below] Prefix meaning *below, or under, beneath, or deficient.* SEE: *sub-.*

hypoacidity (hī″pō-ă-sĭd′ĭ-tē) [″ + L. *acidus,* sour] A condition of decreased acid in the stomach caused by lowered hydrochloric acid secretion. This condition may occur secondary to other disorders, such as stomach cancer, pernicious anemia, infection with *Helicobacter pylori,* or treatment with acid-suppressing medications or surgeries.

CAUTION: Gastric hypoacidity may alter the uptake and metabolism of many commonly used drugs.

hypoacusis (hī″pō-ă-kū′sĭs) [″ + *akousis,* hearing] Decreased sensitivity to sound stimuli.

hypoadrenalism (hī″pō-ăd-rē′năl-ĭzm) [″ + L. *ad,* to, + *renalis,* pert. to kidney, + Gr. *-ismos,* state of] Adrenal insufficiency.

hypoadrenocorticism (hī″pō-ă-drē″nō-kor′tĭ-sĭzm) Decreased secretion, or the effect of adrenal cortical hormones.

hypoaffectivity (hī″pō-ăf′fĕk-tĭv′ĭ-tē) Decreased responsiveness to emotional stimuli. SEE: *obtund.*

hypoalbuminemia (hī″pō-ăl-bū″mĭn-ē′mē-ă) Decreased albumin in the blood.

hypoaldosteronism (hī″pō-ăl″dō-stĕr′ōn-ĭzm) A condition characterized by decreased aldosterone in the blood associated with hypotension and increased salt excretion.

hypoallergenic [″ + *allos,* other, + *ergon,* work] Diminished potential for causing an allergic reaction.

hypoazoturia (hī″pō-ăz-ō-tū′rē-ă) [″ + L. *azotum,* nitrogen, + Gr. *ouron,* urine] Diminished urea in the urine.

hypobaric (hī″pō-băr′ĭk) [″ + *baros,* weight] Decreased atmospheric pressure. SEE: *bends; edema, high-altitude pulmonary.*

hypoblast (hī′pō-blăst) [″ + *blastos,* germ] The inner cell layer or endoderm, which develops during gastrulation. The external layer is called ectoderm. **hypoblastic** (hī-pō-blăs′tĭk), *adj.*

hypocalcemia (hī″pō-kăl-sē′mē-ă) [″ + L. *calx,* lime, + Gr. *haima,* blood] Abnormally low blood calcium. This condition occurs transiently in patients with severe sepsis, severe pancreatitis, burns, and acute renal failure. It also may result from multiple transfusions with citrated blood, parathyroidectomy, malabsorption, and medications such as protamine, heparin, and glucagon. Chronic hypocalcemia may be caused by chronic renal failure, hypoalbuminemia, and malnutrition. Clinical manifestations in chronic hypocalcemia include muscle spasm, carpopedal spasm, facial grimacing, possible convulsions, and mental changes such as irritability, depression, and psychosis. Treatment consists of calcium infusions and appropriate therapy for the causative disease.

newborn h. Low serum calcium levels present in the first days of life, caused by maternal disease (e.g., gestational diabetes or parathyroid disorders), diseases and conditions of the child (e.g., congenital hypoparathyroidism), or treatments given the newborn (transfusion therapy or phototherapy).

Common symptoms of low calcium in the newborn are tremors or seizures.

hypocalciuria (hī″pō-kăl″sē-ū′rē-ă) Decreased calcium in the urine.

hypocaloric (hī″pō-kăl′ūr-ĭk) **1.** Having few calories (e.g., a hypocaloric meal). **2.** Calorically restricted (e.g., a hypocaloric diet).

hypocapnia (hī″pō-kăp′nē-ă) [Gr. *hypo,* under, beneath, below, + *kapnos,* smoke] A decreased amount of carbon dioxide in the blood. An excessively rapid rate of respiration ("hyperventilation") is usually responsible.

hypocarbia (hī″pō-kăr′bē-ă) Hypocapnia.

hypocellularity (hī″pō-sĕl″ū-lăr′ĭ-tē) Decreased cell content of any tissue.

hypochloremia (hī″pō-klō-rē′mē-ă) [″ + *chloros,* green, + *haima,* blood] Deficiency of the chloride content of the blood. SYN: *chloropenia.*

hypochlorhydria (hī″pō-klor-hī′drē-ă) [″ + ″ + *hydor,* water] Hypoacidity. SEE: *achlorhydria; hyperchlorhydria.*

hypochlorite A salt of hypochlorous acid used in household bleach and as an oxidizer, deodorant, and disinfectant.

hypochlorite salt poisoning SEE: *Poisons and Poisoning Appendix.*

hypochlorization (hī″pō-klō″rī-zā′shŭn) Diminished sodium chloride in the diet; used in treating hypertension and certain kidney diseases.

hypochloruria (hī″pō-klor-ū′rē-ă) [″ + *chloros,* green, + *ouron,* urine] Diminution of chlorides in the urine.

hypocholesteremia (hī″pō-kō-lĕs-tĕr-ē′mē-ă) [″ + *chole,* bile, + *stereos,* solid, + *haima,* blood] Decreased blood cholesterol. As cholesterol has some important functions in the body, excessively low cholesterol levels are not desirable.

hypochondria (hī″pō-kŏn′drē-ă) [″ + *chondros,* cartilage] An abnormal concern about one's health, with the false belief of suffering from some disease, despite medical reassurance to the contrary. This is a common symptom among depressed patients. SYN: *hypochondriasis.* SEE: *somatization.*

hypochondriac (hī″pō-kŏn′drē-ăk) **1.** Pert. to the region of the hypochondrium or the the upper lateral region on each side of the body and below the thorax; beneath the ribs. **2.** An individual with a heightened response to physical stimuli, who believes his or her physical sensations are indicative of disease. **hypochondriacal** (-kŏn-drī′ă-kăl), *adj.*

h. region Hypochondrium.

hypochondriasis (hī″pō-kŏn-drī′ă-sĭs) [″ + *chondros,* cartilage, + *-iasis,* diseased condition] Hypochondria.

hypochondrium (hī″pō-kŏn′drē-ŭm) The part of the abdomen beneath the lower ribs on each side of the epigastrium.

hypochromasia (hī″pō-krō-mā′sē-ă) [″ + *chroma,* color] Decreased hemoglobin in the red blood cells.

hypochromatism (hī″pō-krō′mă-tĭzm) [″ + *chroma,* color] **1.** Decreased or lack of color. **2.** Decreased pigment in a cell, esp. its nucleus. **3.** Decreased hemoglobin in the red cells.

hypochromatosis (hī″pō-krō-mă-tō′sĭs) [″ + ″ + *osis,* condition] The disappearance of the chromatin or nucleus in a cell. SYN: *chromatolysis.*

hypochromia (hī″pō-krō′mē-ă) A condition of the blood in which the red blood cells have a reduced hemoglobin content. **hypochromic** (-krōm′ĭk), *adj.*

hypochylia (hī″pō-kī′lē-ă) [Gr. *hypo,* under, beneath, below, + *chylos,* juice] Lack of normal secretion of gastric juice.

hypocomplementemia (hī″pō-kŏm″plĕ-mĕn-tē′mē-ă) Decreased complement in the blood.

hypocondylar (hī″pō-kŏn′dĭ-lăr) [″ + *kondylos,* condyle] Below a condyle.

hypocone (hī″pō-kōn) [″ + *konos,* cone] The distolingual cusp of an upper molar tooth.

hypoconid (hī″pō-kō′nĭd) The distobuccal cusp of a lower molar tooth.

hypoconulid The distal, or fifth, cusp of the mandibular first molar tooth. SEE: *hypoconid.*

hypocorticism (hī″pō-kor′tĭ-sĭzm) Decreased adrenal cortical hormone.

hypocrinism (hī″pō-krĭ′nĭzm) [″ + *krinein,* to separate, + *-ismos,* condition] Deficient secretion of any gland, esp. an endocrine gland.

hypocupremia (hī″pō-kū-prē′mē-ă) Decreased copper in the blood.

hypocyclosis (hī″pō-sī-klō′sĭs) [″ + *kyklos,* circle] Deficient accommodation of the eye.

ciliary h. A weakness of the ciliary muscle.

lenticular h. A lack of elasticity in the crystalline lens.

hypocythemia (hī″pō-sī-thē′mē-ă) [″ + *kytos,* cell, + *haima,* blood] A decrease in the number of blood cells, esp. red blood cells.

hypodactylia (hī″pō-dăk-tĭl′ē-ă) [″ + *daktylos,* finger] Having less than the normal number of fingers or toes.

Hypoderma (hī″pō-dĕr′mă) [″ + *derma,* skin] A genus of warble flies of the family Oestridae. The larvae of some species attack cattle and, rarely, humans. They cause a subcutaneous channel of inflammation as they burrow under the skin. SEE: *larva migrans, cutaneous.*

hypodermatomy (hī″pō-dĕr-măt′ō-mē) [″ + *derma,* skin, + *tome,* incision] Incision into the subcutaneous tissue, which may be used as an approach for the section of a muscle or tendon.

hypodermiasis (hī″pō-dĕr-mī′ă-sĭs) [″ + ″ + *-iasis,* condition] Infection with *Hypoderma.*

hypodermic (hī″pō-dĕr′mĭk) [″ + *derma,* skin] Under or inserted under the skin, as a hypodermic injection. It may be given subcutaneously (under the skin), intracutaneously (into the skin), intramuscularly (into a muscle), intraspinally (into the spinal canal), or intravascularly (into a vein or artery). It is given to secure prompt action of a drug when the drug cannot be taken by mouth, when it may not be readily absorbed in the stomach or intestines, when it might be changed by the action of the gastric secretions, or to act as an anesthetic about the site of injection. SEE: *anesthesia, local.*

CAUTION: When the injected substance is not intended for intravascular injection, the syringe plunger should be pulled back after the needle is inserted to determine if the needle is in a vein or artery. If blood is obtained, the needle must be repositioned and the procedure repeated. It may be necessary to use a fresh needle and syringe. Because medicines not intended for intravenous injection produce serious undesired effects when given by this route, do not inject the medicine if the needle is in a vessel. If the medicine is to be injected into an artery or vein, it must not be administered unless pulling back on the plunger permits blood freely to enter the syringe.

intracutaneous h. Injection into the skin.

intramuscular h. Injection given in the gluteal or lumbar muscular region. This route is used when a drug is not easily absorbed, when it is irritating, or when a large quantity of liquid is to be used.

intraspinal h. Injection into the spinal canal.

intravenous h. Injection into a vein, the usual site being the median basilic or median cephalic vein of the arm.

subcutaneous h. Injection given just under the skin, usually in the outer surface of the arm and forearm.

hypodermoclysis (hī″pō-dĕr-mŏk′lĭ-sĭs) [Gr. *hypo,* under, beneath, below, + *derma,* skin, + *klysis,* a washing out] The treatment of dehydration by injecting fluids into the subcutaneous tissues (e.g., of the thighs, buttocks, or below the breasts). This practice is sometimes used as a palliative measure to treat elderly patients or cachectic persons with advanced malignancies when other methods of rehydration (oral or intravenous) are not available. Common complications include fluid overload, electrolyte disturbances, and wound infections, among others.

hypodontia (hī″pō-dŏn′shē-ă) Diminished development, or absence, of teeth.

hypodynamia (hī″pō-dī-nā′mē-ă) [″ + *dynamis,* power] Diminished muscular power or energy. SEE: *adynamia.*

hypoeccrisia (hī″pō-ĕk-krĭs′ē-ă) [″ + *ek,* out, + *krisis,* separation] Diminished excretion of waste material.

hypoeccritic (hī″pō-ĕk-krĭt′ĭk) **1.** Retarding normal excretion. **2.** Pert. to insufficient or defective excretion.

hypoechoic (hī′pō-ĕ-kō″ik) In ultrasonography, pertaining to a region of the body that produces fewer sound echoes than normal.

hypoeosinophilia (hī″pō-ē″ō-sĭn″ō-fĭl′ē-ă) [Gr. *hypo,* under, beneath, below, + *eos,* dawn, + *philein,* to love] A diminished number of eosinophils in the blood.

hypoergasia (hī″pō-ĕr-gā′sē-ă) [″ + *ergon,* work] Decreased functional activity.

hypoergia (hī″pō-ĕr′jē-ă) A diminished response to any stimulus. **hypoergic** (-ĕr′jĭk), *adj.*

hypoesophoria (hī″pō-ĕs″ō-fō′rē-ă) [″ + *eso,* inward, + *phorein,* to bear] A downward and inward deviation of the eye.

hypoesthesia (hī″pō-ĕs-thē′zē-ă) [″ + *aisthesis,* sensation] A dulled sensitivity to touch.

hypoexophoria (hī″pō-ĕks-ō-fō′rē-ă) [″ + *exo,* outward, + *phorein,* to bear] A downward and outward deviation of the eye.

hypoferremia (hī″pō-fĕ-rē′mē-ă) Iron deficiency as indicated by diminished iron in the blood.

hypofibrinogenemia (hī″pō-fī-brĭn″ō-jĕ-nē′mē-ă) Decreased fibrinogen in the blood.

hypofunction (hī″pō-fŭnk′shŭn) Decreased function.

hypogalactia (hī″pō-gă-lăk′shē-ă) [″ + *gala,* milk] Deficient milk production.

hypogammaglobulinemia (hī″pō-găm″ă-glŏb″ū-lĭ-nē′mē-ă) The lack of one or more of the five classes of antibodies or immunoglobulins caused by defective B lymphocyte function. Patients are highly susceptible to infections from pyogenic organisms (staphylococci, streptococci, and *Pseudomonas aeruginosa*).

acquired h. A form of hypogammaglobulinemia that usually appears between 15 and 35 years of age. Patients have total immunoglobulin levels of less than 300 mg/dl, IgG levels of less than 250 mg/dl, a propensity to infection, lymphadenopathy, and splenomegaly. The cause is unknown. Patients should not be vaccinated with live attenuated (weakened) vaccines, because of the risk of infection from the injection. Treatment includes intravenous immune globulin (200 to 400 mg/kg) each month and administration of specific antibiotics when needed for specific infections. Although patients often live normal lifespans, chronic lung disease is a common complication and may cause an earlier than expected death.

congenital h. Total immunoglobulin levels that are below 250 mg/dl. Chronic bacterial infections are common. Intravenous immune globulin (beginning at 200 mg/kg per month) usually is effective.

hypogastric (hī″pō-găs′trĭk) [″ + *gaster,* belly] Pert. to the lower middle of the abdomen or to the hypogastrium.

h. artery Internal iliac artery.

h. plexus Sympathetic nerve plexus in the pelvis.

h. region The hypogastrium. SEE: *abdominal regions.*

hypogastrium (hī″pō-găs′trē-ŭm) The region below the umbilicus or navel, between the right and left inguinal regions.

hypogenesis (hī″pō-jĕn′ĕ-sĭs) [Gr. *hypo,* under, beneath, below, + *genesis,* generation, birth] Cessation of growth or development at an early stage, causing defective structure. SEE: *ateliosis.*

hypogenitalism (hī″pō-jĕn′ĭ-tăl-ĭzm) [″ + L. *genitalis,* a genital, + Gr. *-ismos,* condition] A condition in which the genital organs are underdeveloped. It is characterized by reduced size of genital organs, failure of testes to descend in some cases, and incomplete development of secondary sex characteristics. SEE: *hypogonadism.*

hypogeusia (hī″pō-gū′sē-ă) [″ + *geusis,* taste] A blunting of the sense of taste.

idiopathic h. A syndrome of unknown cause, consisting of decreased taste and olfactory acuity, with or without perverted taste (dysgeusia) and smell. Certain trace elements (such as zinc added to the diet) appear to correct some of the symptoms.

hypoglobulinemia, transient Low levels of the immunoglobulin G (IgG) class antibody that occur when an infant is between 5 and 6 months of age. The maternal IgG that has crossed the placenta begins to drop after birth and reaches its lowest level (about 350 mg/dl) at this point. If IgG production is decreased, transient hypogammaglobulinemia develops. Normal blood levels of B cells, IgA, and IgM usually are present, which differentiates this transient disorder from hereditary, X-linked hypogammaglobulinemia. Some infants develop recurrent infections and must be treated with intravenous gamma globulin (IVIG) until IgG production increases.

hypoglossal (hī″pō-glŏs′ăl) [″ + *glossa,* tongue] Situated under the tongue.

h. alternating hemiplegia Medulla lesion paralyzing the tongue by involving the 12th nerve fibers as they course through the uncrossed pyramid. The pathology may extend across the midline or dorsally, involving the medial fillet, causing contralateral anesthesia.

h. nerve A mixed cranial nerve, carrying proprioceptive impulses as well as motor impulses. It originates in the medulla oblongata and is distributed to the extrinsic and intrinsic muscles of the tongue. SYN: *twelfth cranial nerve.*

hypoglottis (hī″pō-glŏt′ĭs) The undersurface of the tongue.

hypoglycemia (hī″pō-glī-sē′mē-ă) [″ + *glykys,* sweet, + *haima,* blood] An abnormally low level of glucose in the blood, often associated with neurological side effects and arousal of the sympathetic nervous system. Medication-induced hypoglycemia is a common occurrence during the treatment of diabetes mellitus. SYN: *glucopenia.* SEE: *brittle diabetes; hypoglycemic coma; diabetes mellitus* for table; *hyperglycemia; neuroglycopenia* Nursing Diagnoses Appendix. **hypoglycemic** (-sē′mĭk), *adj.*

ETIOLOGY: Hypoglycemia may be caused by insulin or oral antidiabetic drug overdoses; failure to eat an adequate number of calories despite diabetic treatments; unusual levels of exercise (again, usually among treated diabetics); extreme starvation; alcoholic depletion of carbohydrate reserves from the liver; salicylate overdoses; and rarely, by an insulin-secreting tumor of the pancreas.

SYMPTOMS: A patient with moderately low blood sugar may feel fatigued, dizzy, restless, hungry, or unusually irritable; have difficulty concentrating; or have spontaneous episodes of sweating, palpitations, tremor, or nausea. Severely low blood sugar produces delirium, violent behaviors, obtundation, seizures, coma, and occasionally death.

DIAGNOSIS: The condition is demonstrated when a symptomatic patient has a capillary blood glucose or plasma glucose level that is less than 3.0 mmol/L (40 mg/dl).

TREATMENT: The acute treatment for hypoglycemia is glucose by mouth or per rectum, dextrose (D50) intravenously, or glucagon intramuscularly or subcutaneously. Treated patients who remain relatively hypoglycemic may require continuous infusions of dextrose during in-hospital observation.

CAUTION: Oral glucose supplements (e.g., juice, or candy) should never be given patients with a severely impaired level of consciousness, because of the risk of aspiration. In the emergency setting, all comatose patients are routinely assumed to be hypoglycemic, and are treated immediately with dextrose infusions.

After a hypoglycemic episode resolves, diabetic management regimens often need adjustment. Patients should be educated to recognize the symptoms that low blood sugar causes and to intervene quickly to reverse low blood sugar in the future. Patients who follow strenuously restricted diets often are encouraged to increase their calorie intake. They may need to reduce doses of insulin or antidiabetic drugs. A patient who suffers repeated hypoglycemic episodes should perform self-monitoring of blood glucose before meals, at bedtime, in the middle of the night, and whenever dietary, exercise, or work routines change.

PATIENT CARE: Signs of hypoglycemia are monitored and reported in high-risk patients. If possible, blood glucose level (with a glucometer at the bedside) is measured to verify the severity of hypoglycemia before providing corrective treatment. The caregiver corrects such episodes quickly and implements measures to protect the unconscious patient, such as maintaining a patent airway. Prescribed medications are administered. The purpose, preparation, procedure, and expected sensations for any diagnostic tests are explained. Hypoglycemic episodes need to be prevented or treated promptly if they do occur to avoid severe complications. The caregiver ensures that the patient understands the signs and symptoms and key dangers of hypoglycemia and urges the patient to note signs and symptoms typically experienced. Once it occurs, the patient may quickly lose his ability to think clearly. If this should happen while the patient drives a car or operates machinery, a serious accident could result. The patient taking beta-blockers may experience only CNS-related symptoms. Family, friends, and coworkers also should be taught to recognize this patient's warning signs so that immediate treatment can be instituted. The caregiver reviews with the patient and family treatment measures they should follow if the patient experiences a hypoglycemic episode. If conscious with a gag reflex, the patient should consume a readily available source of glucose, such as five to six pieces of hard candy; 4 to 6 oz of apple juice, orange juice, cola, or other soft drink; or 1 tbsp of honey or grape jelly. If the patient is unconscious, EMS should be alerted immediately and then the patient should receive a subcutaneous injection of glucagon; the patient's family should also be taught how to administer glucagon injections. If hypoglycemic episodes do not respond to treatment or if they occur frequently, either the patient or family should notify their health care professional. The patient should follow the prescribed diet to prevent a rapid drop in blood glucose levels. A dietitian can help the patient to understand the necessary diet and to develop a dietary plan that includes foods that the patient enjoys while avoiding simple carbohydrates. The patient should eat small meals throughout the day, and bedtime snacks also may be necessary to keep blood glucose at an even level. The patient should avoid delays in mealtimes, as well as alcohol and caffeine, because they may trigger severe hypoglycemic episodes. If the patient is obese and has impaired glucose tolerance, the caregivers suggest ways that the patient can restrict caloric intake and lose weight and assist in finding a weight loss support group as necessary. The patient with fasting hypoglycemia should not postpone or skip scheduled meals or snacks and should call the health care professional for instructions if he or she does not feel well enough to eat. The caregiver helps the patient to identify factors that can precipitate a hypoglycemic episode, such as poor diet, stress, or not cooperating with a diabetes mellitus treatment regimen and suggests ways of changing or avoiding each of these factors. As necessary, the caregiver teaches the patient stress reduction techniques and encourages him or her to join a support group. Precautions need to be taken when the patient exercises; for example, he or she should consume extra calories and not exercise alone or at a time when the blood glucose level is likely to drop. The patient should carry a source of fast-acting carbohydrate, such as hard candy, at all times. The patient should wear or carry a medical identification device describing the condition and emergency treatment measures. For the patient with pharmacological hypoglycemia from insulin or antidiabetic agents, the caregiver reviews the essentials of managing diabetes mellitus. As warranted, the patient is taught about prescribed drug therapy or surgery; when surgery becomes necessary, the patient is prepared physically and emotionally for the procedure and postoperative care provided (as for a patient undergoing other intra-abdominal surgery, with added blood glucose level concerns). Because hypoglycemia may be a recurring problem, the patient should have periodic medical checkups. Both the patient and family are encouraged to discuss their concerns about the patient's condition and treatment, emotional support is offered, and questions are answered honestly.

POSTPRANDIAL "HYPOGLYCEMIA": Many people mistakenly believe that they are hypoglycemic if they become drowsy or fatigued after meals. There is no evidence to support this belief.

newborn h. Blood glucose levels less than 40 mg/dl in infants during the first hours of life.

ETIOLOGY: A high metabolic rate, small glycogen and fat reserves, and limited capacity for gluconeogenesis contribute to the normal newborn's postbirth risk of hypoglycemia. Approximately 8% of normal term infants who were born vaginally, and nearly 16% of those born by cesarean delivery, experience one or more episodes of hypoglycemia. Infants of diabetic mothers and those who are small for gestational age exhibit a higher incidence of low blood sugar. Other factors contributing to the rapid expenditure of glucose by the newborn include postmaturity, macrosomia, cold stress, perinatal asphyxia, sepsis, and respiratory distress syndrome.

PATIENT CARE: Newborns are monitored closely for jitteriness, jerkiness, tremors, seizures, lethargy, poor feeding, vomiting, apnea, and cyanosis. For high-risk infants, glucose levels are assessed every 2 hr for 6 hr, then at 12, 24, and 48 hr after delivery. Prompt treatment with oral or intravenous glucose is necessary.

hypoglycemic agents, oral ABBR: OHA. Any drug taken by mouth that lowers or maintains blood sugar (as opposed to insulin, a drug taken parenterally to control blood sugar). OHAs are typically used, in addition to diet and exercise, to control blood glucose levels in type 2 diabetes mellitus. SEE: table.

hypoglycogenolysis (hī″pō-glī″kō-jĕn-ŏl′ĭ-sĭs) [Gr. *hypo,* under, beneath, below, + *glykys,* sweet, + *gennan,* to produce, + *lysis,* dissolution] Defective hydrolysis of glycogen (glycogenolysis).

hypoglycorrhachia (hī″pō-glī″kō-rā′kē-ă) [″ + ″ + *rhachis,* spine] A decreased amount of glucose in the cerebrospinal fluid. It usually occurs in meningitis.

hypognathous (hī-pŏg′nă-thŭs) [″ + *gnathos,* jaw] Having a lower jaw smaller than the upper jaw.

hypogonadism (hī″pō-gō′năd-ĭzm) [″ + *gone,* semen, + *-ismos,* condition] Inadequate production of sex hormones.

hypogonadotropism (hī″pō-gŏn″ă-dō-trŏp′ĭsm) Low serum levels of gonadotropins. **hypogonadotropic,** *adj.*

hypohepatia (hī″pō-hĕ-pă′tē-ă) [″ + *hepar,* liver] Deficient liver function.

hypohidrosis (hī″pō-hī-drō′sĭs) [″ + *hidros,* sweat, + *osis,* condition] Diminished perspiration.

hypohyloma (hī″pō-hī-lō′mă) [″ + *hyle,* matter, + *oma,* tumor] A tumor formed by embryonic tissue. It is derived from hypoblastic tissue.

hypoinsulinism [″ + L. *insula,* island, + Gr. *-ismos,* condition] **1.** Type 1 diabetes mellitus. **2.** Relative deficiency in insulin secretion or insulin dosing.

hypoisotonic (hī″pō-ī″sō-tŏn′ĭk) [″ + *isos,* equal, + *tonos,* tension] Hypotonic.

hypokalemia (hī″pō-kă-lē′mē-ă) [″ + Mod. L. *kalium,* potash, + Gr. *haima,* blood] An abnormally low concentration of potassium in the blood. SYN: *hypopotassemia*. SEE: *hyperkalemia*. **hypokalemic** (-lē′mĭk), *adj.*

ETIOLOGY: Causes include deficient potassium intake or excess loss of potassium due to vomiting, diarrhea, or fistulas; metabolic acidosis; diuretic therapy; aldosteronism; excess adreno-

Oral Agents That Lower Blood Glucose*

Class of Drug	Activity	Adverse Features	Approximate Cost
Alpha-glucosidase inhibitors (e.g., acarbose)	Delays absorption of glucose from intestinal tract	Flatulence and other abdominal side effects	Expensive
Biguanides (e.g., metformin)	Improves sensitivity to insulin; decreases glucose production by the liver	Less weight gain than with other agents; avoid in patients with renal failure	Very expensive
Sulfonylureas, 1st generation (e.g., tolazamide)	Causes beta cells to release insulin	Resistance to drug may develop over time	Inexpensive
Sulfonylureas, 2nd generation (e.g., glipizide, glyburide, others)	Same as 1st generation; also increase sensitivity to insulin	Same as 1st generation	Moderately expensive
Thiazolidinediones (e.g., rosiglitazone)	Improves sensitivity to insulin; improves lipid profile	Monthly monitoring of liver functions needed for some drugs in this class due to risk of toxicity	Very expensive

* Combinations of these drugs, either with each other or with insulin, may be used in patients with poorly controlled diabetes mellitus.

cortical secretion; renal tubule disease; and alkalosis.

SYMPTOMS: Common manifestations of mild to moderate potassium depletion include muscle aches, fatigue, or mild weakness. As potassium concentrations drop significantly below 3.0 mmol/L, ileus, paralysis, or cardiac conduction and rhythm disturbances may arise. Arrhythmias are particularly likely to affect those patients taking digoxin who become hypokalemic.

PREVENTION: To prevent hypokalemia, patients taking cardiac glycosides or potassium-wasting diuretics are instructed to include potassium supplements in their medical regimens. Potassium-rich foods (such as oranges, bananas, and tomatoes) are not an adequate source of the potassium that is lost by diuresis.

TREATMENT: Therapy consists of oral, intravenous, or combined potassium replacement.

CAUTION: Severely hypokalemic patients may require close electrocardiographic monitoring and frequent assessment of plasma potassium levels.

PATIENT CARE: Potassium and other electrolyte levels are monitored frequently during replacement therapy to avoid overcorrection leading to hyperkalemia. Fluid balance is monitored. A physician must be notified if the patient's urine output is less than 600 ml/day, because 80-90% of potassium is excreted through the kidneys. Cardiac rhythm is monitored, and arrhythmias are reported immediately. Additional care is taken if the patient takes a cardiac glycoside because hypokalemia enhances its action. The patient is assessed for indications of digitalis toxicity. Other signs to watch for include decreased bowel sounds, abdominal distention, and constipation.

Prescribed IV potassium replacement is administered slowly with a volumetric device if the concentration exceeds 40 mEg/liter. The rate should not exceed 200-250 mEg/24 hours, and the drug should never be given as a bolus because it may precipitate cardiac arrest. If the patient is prescribed a liquid oral potassium supplement, he or she is advised to dilute it in a full glass of water or fruit juice and to sip it slowly to prevent gastric irritation. Safety measures are implemented for the patient experiencing muscle weakness due to postural hypotension. The importance of taking potassium supplements as prescribed is emphasized, particularly if the patient also is prescribed a diuretic or digitalis preparation. The patient is taught signs of potassium imbalance to report, including weakness and pulse irregularities.

hypokinesia (hī″pō-kĭ-nē′zē-ă) [″ + *kinesis,* movement] Decreased motor reaction to stimulus. **hypokinetic** (-nĕt′ĭk), *adj.*

hypolactasia (hī″pō-lăk-tāz′ē-ă) Lactase deficiency. The absence of enzymes that break down dietary lactose is common in adults, esp. those of Northern European heritage, in whom it is a common cause of abdominal gas or indigestion.

hypolemmal (hī″pō-lĕm′ăl) [″ + *lemma,* sheath] Situated below a sheath or membrane.

hypoleydigism (hī″pō-lī′dĭg-ĭzm) Decreased secretion of androgen by the interstitial (Leydig) cells of the testicles.

hypolipidemic (hī″pō-lĭp″ĭ-dē′mĭk) Decreasing the lipid concentration of the blood.

hypoliposis (hī″pō-lĭ-pō′sĭs) [″ + *lipos,* fat, + *osis,* condition] A deficiency of fat in the tissues.

hypologia (hī-pō-lō′jē-ă) [″ + *logos,* word, reason] Sparse verbal output; diminished speech.

hypolymphemia (hī″pō-lĭm-fē′mē-ă) [″ + L. *lympha,* lymph, + Gr. *haima,* blood] Decreased amount of lymphocytes in the blood, with a normal number of leukocytes.

hypomagnesemia (hī″pō-măg″nĕ-sē′mē-ă) Decreased magnesium in the blood. Clinically, it is accompanied by increased neuromuscular irritability.

hypomania (hī″pō-mā′nē-ă) [″ + *mania,* madness] Mild mania and excitement, with a moderate change in behavior.

hypomastia (hī-pō-măs′tē-ă) [″ + *mastos,* breast] A condition of having abnormally small breasts. SYN: *hypomazia.*

hypomazia (hī″pō-mā′zē-ă) [″ + *mazos,* breast] Hypomastia.

hypomelanosis One of several disorders of melanin pigmentation in which melanin in the epidermis is decreased or absent. It may be caused by albinism, chronic protein deficiency, burns, trauma, or vitiligo. SEE: *hypermelanosis.*

hypomenorrhea (hī″pō-mĕn-ō-rē′ă) [″ + *men,* month, + *rhoia,* flow] A deficient amount of menstrual flow, but with regular periods. SEE: *oligomenorrhea.*

hypomere (hī′pō-mēr) [″ + *meros,* part] The portion of the mesoderm that later forms the pleuroperitoneal walls. SEE: *epimere; mesomere.*

hypometabolism (hī″pō-mĕ-tăb′ō-lĭzm) [″ + *metabole,* change, + *-ismos,* condition] A lowered metabolism.

hypometria (hī″pō-mē′trē-ă) [″ + *metron,* measure] A shortened range of movement.

hypometropia (hī″pō-mĕ-trōp′ē-ă) [″ +

″ + *ops,* eye] Myopia or nearsightedness.

hypomimia (hī″pō-mĭm′ē-ă) A reduction in the expressiveness of the face, as occurs in patients with Parkinson's disease. It is marked by diminished animation and movement of the facial muscles.

hypomnesia, hypomnesis (hī″pŏm-nē′zē-ă, -nē′sĭs) [″ + *mnesis,* memory] Impaired memory.

hypomobility Restricted joint movement (play) that limits normal range of motion; the opposite of hypermobility.

hypomorph (hī′pō-morf) [″ + *morphe,* form] An individual with disproportionately short legs with respect to the length of the trunk; the opposite of hypermorph. SEE: *somatotype*.

hypomotility (hī″pō-mō-tĭl′ĭ-tē) [″ + L. *motus,* moved] Hypokinesia.

hypomyotonia (hī″pō-mī″ō-tō′nē-ă) [″ + *mys,* muscle, + *tonos,* tension] Lacking in muscular tone.

hypomyxia (hī″pō-mĭks′ē-ă) [″ + *myxa,* mucus] A diminished secretion of mucus.

hyponanosoma (hī″pō-năn-ō-sō′mă) [″ + *nanos,* dwarf, + *soma,* body] Extreme dwarfism.

hyponatremia (hī″pō-nă-trē′mē-ă) [″ + L. *natron,* sodium, + Gr. *haima,* blood] A decreased concentration of sodium in the blood.

hyponeocytosis (hī″pō-nē″ō-sī-tō′sĭs) [″ + *neos,* new, + *kytos,* cell, + *osis,* condition] A decreased number of leukocytes (leukopenia) with immature cells in the blood.

hyponoia (hī″pō-noy′ă) [″ + *nous,* mind] Diminished or sluggish mental activity.

hyponychium (hī-pō-nĭk′ē-ŭm) [Gr. *hypo,* under, beneath, below, + *onyx,* nail] Nailbed. SYN: *matrix unguis*.

hyponychon (hī-pŏn′ĭ-kŏn) [″ + *onyx,* nail] An extravasation of blood beneath the nail.

hypo-orthocytosis (hī″pō-or″thō-sī-tō′sĭs) [″ + *orthos,* regular, + *kytos,* cell, + *osis,* condition] Leukopenia with normal proportions of white blood cells.

hypopallesthesia (hī″pō-păl″ĕs-thē′zē-ă) [″ + *pallein,* to shake, + *aisthesis,* sensation] Decreased ability to perceive vibratory sense.

hypopancreatism (hī″pō-păn′krē-ă-tĭzm) [″ + *pankreas,* pancreas, + *-ismos,* condition] Diminished activity of the pancreas.

hypoparathyreosis (hī″pō-păr-ă-thī-rē-ō′sĭs) [″ + *para,* beside, + *thyreos,* shield, + *osis,* condition] Hypoparathyroidism.

hypoparathyroidism (hī″pō-păr-ă-thī′royd-ĭzm) [″ + ″ + ″ + *eidos,* form, shape, + *-ismos,* condition] A condition caused by an insufficient or absent secretion of the parathyroid glands. SYN: *hypoparathyreosis*. SEE: *Nursing Diagnoses Appendix*.

hypopepsia (hī″pō-pĕp′sē-ă) [″ + *pepsis,* digestion] Impaired digestion owing to lack of pepsin.

hypopepsinia (hī″pō-pĕp-sĭn′ē-ă) Deficient pepsin in the gastric juice.

hypoperfusion (hī″pō-pĕr-fū′shŭn) Inadequate blood flow, for example, to a single organ or through the entire circulatory system.

hypoperistalsis (hī″pō-pĕr″ĭ-stăl′sĭs) Diminished peristalsis. SEE: *paralytic ileus*.

hypophalangism (hī″pō-fă-lăn′jĭzm) The state of having fewer than the normal number of fingers or toes.

hypopharynx (hī″pō-făr′ĭnks) [″ + *pharynx,* throat] The lower portion of the pharynx that opens into the larynx anteriorly and the esophagus posteriorly. SYN: *laryngopharynx*.

hypophonesis (hī″pō-fō-nē′sĭs) [″ + *phone,* voice] A diminished or fainter sound in auscultation or percussion.

hypophonia (hī″pō-fō′nē-ă) An abnormally weak voice resulting from incoordination of speech muscles, including weakness of muscles of respiration.

hypophoria (hī″pō-fō′rē-ă) [″ + *phorein,* to bear] The tendency of one visual axis to fall below the other one.

hypophosphatasia (hī″pō-fŏs″fă-tā′zē-ă) Signs and symptoms of rickets due to a deficiency of alkaline phosphatase. There are four forms of this condition: lethal perinatal, infantile, childhood, and adult. The perinatal and infantile forms are inherited as autosomal recessive traits. The inheritance pattern of the childhood and adult forms is unknown. In the adult form, signs and symptoms may not become apparent until middle age, but there may be a history of early loss of either deciduous or permanent teeth and short stature. No treatment is available.

hypophosphatemia (hī″pō-fŏs″fă-tē′mē-ă) [″ + L. *phosphas,* phosphate, + Gr. *haima,* blood] Abnormally decreased amount of phosphates circulating in the blood.

hypophosphaturia (hī″pō-fŏs″fă-tū′rē-ă) [″ + ″ + Gr. *ouron,* urine] Decreased excretion of phosphate in the urine.

hypophrenia (hī″pō-frē′nē-ă) [″ + *phren,* mind] Mental retardation. **hypophrenic,** *adj.*

hypophrenic (hī″pō-frĕn′ĭk) [″ + *phren,* diaphragm, mind] **1.** Mental retardation. **2.** Below the diaphragm.

hypophyseal (hī″pō-fĭz′ē-ăl) [″ + *physis,* growth] Pert. to the hypophysis or pituitary.

hypophysectomy (hī-pŏf″ĭ-sĕk′tō-mē) [″ + ″ + *ektome,* excision] Excision of the hypophysis cerebri.

hypophyseoportal (hī″pō-fĭz″ē-ō-por′tăl) Concerning the portal system of the pituitary gland. SEE: *system, hypophyseoportal.*

hypophyseoprivic (hī″pō-fĭz″ē-ō-prĭv′ĭk) Deficiency of hormone secretion from the pituitary.

hypophysis (hī-pŏf′ĭ-sĭs) *pl.* **hypophyses** [Gr., an undergrowth] **1.** An undergrowth. **2.** The pituitary gland. An endocrine gland lying in the sella turcica of the sphenoid bone. It consists of two portions, the adenohypophysis (anterior lobe) and the neurohypophysis (posterior lobe), which are attached to the hypothalamus of the brain by the infundibulum. SEE: *pituitary gland.*

h. cerebri Pituitary gland.

pharyngeal h. A small structure anterior to the pharyngeal bursa. It is derived from the lower portion of Rathke's pouch and occasionally gives rise to a cyst or tumor.

hypophysitis (hī-pŏf″ĭ-sī′tĭs) [Gr. *hypo,* under, beneath, below, + *physis,* growth, + *itis,* inflammation] An inflammation of the pituitary body.

hypopigmentation (hī″pō-pĭg″mĕn-tā′shŭn) Diminished pigment in a tissue.

hypopinealism (hī″pō-pĭn′ē-ăl-ĭzm) [″ + L. *pineus,* pert. to pine cone, + Gr. *-ismos,* condition] Diminished secretion of the pineal gland.

hypopituitarism (hī″pō-pĭ-tū′ĭ-tă-rĭzm) [″ + L. *pituita,* mucus, + Gr. *-ismos,* condition] A condition resulting from diminished secretion of pituitary hormones, esp. those of the anterior lobe. SEE: *Sheehan's syndrome.*

hypoplasia (hī″pō-plā′zē-ă) [″ + *plasis,* formation] Underdevelopment of a tissue organ or body. SEE: *tissue.*

hypopnea (hī″pō-nē′ă) [″ + *pnoia,* breath] Decreased rate and depth of breathing. SEE: *apnea.*

hypoporosis (hī″pō-pō-rō′sĭs) [″ + *poros,* callus, + *osis,* condition] Deficient development of a callus at the site of a bone fracture.

hypoposia (hī″pō-pō′zē-ă) [″ + *posis,* drinking] A decreased intake of fluids.

hypopotassemia (hī″pō-pō″tăs-sē′mē-ă) [″ + *potassium* + Gr. *haima,* blood] Hypokalemia.

hypoproteinemia (hī″pō-prō″tē-ĭn-ē′mē-ă) [″ + *protos,* first, + *haima,* blood] A decrease in the amount of protein in the blood.

hypoprothrombinemia (hī″pō-prō-thrŏm″bĭn-ē′mē-ă) [″ + L. *pro,* for, + Gr. *thrombos,* clot, + *haima,* blood] A deficiency of blood clotting factor II (prothrombin) in the blood.

hypopselaphesia (hī″pŏp-sĕl-ă-fē′zē-ă) [″ + *pselaphesis,* touch] Blunted tactile sense.

hypoptyalism (hī″pō-tī′ăl-ĭzm) [″ + *ptyalon,* saliva, + *-ismos,* condition] Decreased salivary secretion.

hypopyon (hī-pō′pē-ŏn) [″ + *pyon,* pus] Pus in the anterior chamber of the eye in front of the iris but behind the cornea, seen in corneal ulcer.

hyporeactive (hī″pō-rē-ăk′tĭv) A decreased response to stimuli.

hyporeflexia (hī″pō-rē-flĕk′sē-ă) [″ + L. *reflexus,* bent back] A diminished function of the reflexes.

hyposalivation (hī″pō-săl″ĭ-vā′shŭn) An abnormal decrease in flow of saliva.

hyposcleral (hī″pō-sklē′răl) Beneath the sclera of the eye.

hyposecretion (hī″pō-sē-krē′shŭn) Lowered amount of secretion.

hyposensitive (hī″pō-sĕn′sĭ-tĭv) [″ + L. *sentire,* to feel] Having a reduced ability to respond to stimuli.

hyposensitization (hī″pō-sĕn″sĭ-tĭ-zā′shŭn) Desensitization.

hyposialadenitis (hī″pō-sī″ăl-ăd-ĕ-nī′tĭs) [Gr. *hypo,* under, beneath, below, + *sialon,* saliva, + *aden,* gland, + *itis,* inflammation] Inflammation of the submandibular salivary gland.

hyposmia (hī-pŏz′mē-ă) [″ + *osme,* smell] Decreased sensitivity to odors.

hyposmolarity (hī-pŏz″mō-lăr′ĭ-tē) Decreased osmolar concentration, esp. of the blood or urine.

hyposomnia (hī″pō-sŏm′nē-ă) A decreased ability to sleep.

hypospadia, hypospadias (hī″pō-spā′dē-ă, -ăs) [″ + *span,* to draw] **1.** An abnormal congenital opening of the male urethra upon the undersurface of the penis. **2.** A urethral opening into the vagina.

hypostasis (hī″pŏs′tă-sĭs) [″ + *stasis,* a standing] **1.** A diminished blood flow or circulation. **2.** A deposit of sediment owing to decreased flow of a body fluid such as blood or urine. **hypostatic,** *adj.*

hypostatic (hī″pō-stăt′ĭk) [″ + *statikos,* standing] **1.** Of or pert. to hypostasis. **2.** In genetics, hidden or suppressed, said of a gene whose effect is suppressed by the presence of another gene.

hyposteatolysis (hī″pō-stē-ă-tŏl′ĭ-sĭs) [″ + *stear,* fat, + *lysis,* dissolution] Diminished emulsification of fats during digestion.

hyposthenic (hī-pŏs-thĕn′ik) **1.** Debilitant. **2.** A body habitus characterized by a long, shallow thorax, a long thoracic cavity, a long, narrow abdominal cavity, and a slender build.

hyposthenuria (hī″pŏs-thĕn-ū′rē-ă) [″ + *sthenos,* strength, + *ouron,* urine] The secretion of urine of low specific gravity, chiefly in chronic nephritis.

tubular h. Hyposthenuria resulting from disease of the renal tubule epithelial cells.

hypostomia (hī″pō-stō′mē-ă) [″ + *stoma,* mouth] A congenital defect in which the mouth is abnormally small.

hypostosis (hĭp″ŏs-tō′sĭs) [″ + *osteon,* bone, + *osis,* condition] Deficient bone development.

hypostypsis (hī″pō-stĭp′sĭs) [″ + *stypsis,* a contracting] The state of being slightly astringent. **hypostyptic** (-stĭp′tĭk), *adj.*

hyposynergia (hī″pō-sĭn-ĕr′jē-ă) [″ + *syn,* together, + *ergon,* work] Poor coordination.

hypotelorism (hī″pō-tĕl′ō-rĭzm) [″ + *telouros,* distant] Abnormally decreased distance between paired organs, esp. the eyes.

hypotension (hī″pō-tĕn′shŭn) [″ + L. *tensio,* tension] **1.** A deficiency in tone or tension. **2.** A decrease of the systolic and diastolic blood pressure to below normal. This occurs, for example, in shock, hemorrhage, dehydration, sepsis, Addison's disease, and in many other diseases and conditions. SEE: *blood pressure, chronic low.*

orthostatic h. Hypotension occurring when a person assumes an upright position after getting up from a bed or chair.

postprandial h. A decrease in systolic blood pressure of 20 mm Hg or more within 2 hr of the start of a meal. This may cause syncope, falls, dizziness, weakness, angina pectoris, or stroke. This condition occurs most often in the elderly and in persons with autonomic failure. Although postural changes may increase the severity of the condition, postprandial hypotension is a different entity from postural hypotension.

hypotensive Characterized by or causing low blood pressure.

hypothalamus (hī″pō-thăl′ă-mŭs) [″ + *thalamos,* chamber] The portion of the diencephalon comprising the ventral wall of the third ventricle below the hypothalamic sulcus and including structures forming the ventricular floor, including the tuber cinereum, infundibulum, and mamillary bodies. It lies beneath the thalamus and laterally is continuous with the subthalamic regions. It produces antidiuretic hormone and oxytocin, both of which are stored in the posterior pituitary gland until needed. It produces releasing hormones, which stimulate hormone production by the anterior pituitary gland: growth hormone, thyroid-stimulating hormone, adrenocorticotropic hormone, follicle-stimulating hormone, luteinizing hormone, and prolactin. For several of these, inhibiting hormones also are produced. The hypothalamus also regulates water balance, body temperature, and appetite. It is the chief region for integration of sympathetic and parasympathetic activities. SEE: *hormone, releasing.*

hypothenar (hī-pŏth′ĕ-năr) [″ + *thenar,* palm] The fleshy prominence on the inner side of the palm next to the little finger. SYN: *hypothenar eminence.*

hypothermal (hī″pō-thĕr′măl) [″ + *therme,* heat] **1.** Tepid. **2.** Subnormal temperature.

hypothermia (hī″pō-thĕr′mē-ă) A body temperature below 35°C (95°F). It may be further classified as mild (32.2°–35°C, 90°–95°F); moderate (27°–32.2°, 80°–90°F); or severe (<27°C, <80°F). Low body temperatures are most likely to affect newborns, the elderly, individuals exposed to wet and cold conditions outdoors, alcoholics, septic patients, trauma patients, and patients with severe hypothyroidism. In these individuals, hypothermia can be life-threatening. SYN: *cold stress.* SEE: *nonshivering thermogenesis.*

PREVENTION: To help prevent hypothermia, patients with multiple traumas receiving treatment in emergency facilities should be maintained under radiant warmers. Individuals who anticipate prolonged exposure to cold should be advised not to smoke or drink alcohol. They should wear layered clothing, two pairs of socks (cotton under wool), mittens (not gloves), and a scarf or hat that covers ears and head (to avoid loss of heat through the head). They also need adequate food and rest. If caught in severe cold weather, the individual should find warmth and shelter as soon as possible and increase physical activity to maintain body warmth.

PATIENT CARE: Emergency department personnel first assess airway, breathing, and circulation. If breathing or pulse is not detected, cardiopulmonary resuscitation (CPR) begins immediately and continues until the patient's core body temperature reaches at least 89.6°F (32°C). Hypothermia helps protect brain tissue from anoxia, which normally accompanies prolonged cardiopulmonary arrest. Significant others should be informed that CPR may resuscitate even the patient who has been unresponsive for a long time, esp. following near drowning. The nurse assists with rewarming techniques as required and prescribed. In moderate to severe hypothermia, only experienced personnel should carry out aggressive rewarming. During rewarming, core body temperature is closely monitored (esophageal or rectal probe). Supportive measures are provided as necessary, including mechanical ventilation, heated humidified ventilatory therapy to maintain tissue oxygenation, and IV fluids warmed to correct hypotension and maintain renal function. Care is taken to avoid rubbing tissues. Cardiac status is carefully and continuously monitored. SEE: *Nursing Diagnoses Appendix.*

CAUTION: Oral thermometers are likely to be inaccurate outdoors. No one should be assumed dead until warming techniques have been used.

Newborn hypothermia is prevented by maintaining the dry but unclothed infant under a radiant warmer with thermistor probe until temperature is stabilized. The initial bath is postponed until skin temperature stabilizes between 97.6° and 99°F (36.5°–37.2°C). Once stabilized, the infant's temperature is maintained by keeping him dry and wrapped in warm blankets, with his head covered, in a nursery unit with an ambient temperature of 75°F (24°C). If the infant has become hypothermic (cold delivery room, birth in a car on the way to the birth center, inadequate drying and wrapping after birth), rewarming is accomplished with great care over a period of 2 to 4 hours, as rapid warming or cooling may result in apneic spells or acidosis.

accidental h. Hypothermia due to exposure to wet and cold conditions (e.g., in skiers, hunters, sailors, swimmers, climbers, the indigent, homeless persons in winter, and alcoholics) rather than diseases (e.g., sepsis or hypothyroidism).

h. blanket A specially designed blanket for cooling patients with hyperthermia. It has flexible tubing between the layers of cloth through which cold water is circulated.

therapeutic h. A technique for lowering body temperature to reduce metabolic rates, oxygen demand, and organ damage in certain diseases (e.g., stroke); to alleviate fever; or to improve surgical outcomes. SEE: *hyperthermia.*

hypothesis (hī-pŏth′ĕ-sĭs) *pl.* **hypotheses** [″ + *thesis,* a placing] **1.** An empirically testable assertion about one or more concepts. It is assumed for the sake of testing its soundness or to facilitate investigation of a class of phenomena. **2.** A conclusion drawn before all the facts are established and tentatively accepted as a basis for further investigation.

null h. The assumption or hypothesis that the observed difference between two groups of patients studied is accidental or due to chance and is not due to one of the groups having received a benefit from treatment.

hypothrombinemia (hī″pō-thrŏm-bĭn-ē′mē-ă) [″ + *thrombos,* clot, + *haima,* blood] A deficiency of thrombin in the blood.

hypothymia (hī″pō-thī′mē-ă) [″ + *thymos,* mind] A decreased emotional response to stimuli.

hypothymism (hī″pō-thī′mĭzm) [″ + ″ + *-ismos,* condition] Decreased activity of the thymus.

hypothyroid (hī″pō-thī′royd) [″ + *thyreos,* shield, + *eidos,* form, shape] Marked by insufficient thyroid secretion.

hypothyroidism (hī″pō-thī′royd-ĭzm) The clinical consequences of inadequate levels of thyroid hormone in the body. When thyroid deficiency is long-standing or severe, it results in diminished basal metabolism, intolerance of the cold temperatures, fatigue, mental apathy, physical sluggishness, constipation, muscle aches, dry skin and hair, and coarsening of features. Collectively, these symptoms are called *myxedema.* In infancy, inadequate levels of thyroid hormone cause *cretinism.* SEE: *thyroid function test; Nursing Diagnoses Appendix.*

ETIOLOGY: Most patients with hypothyroidism have either Hashimoto's thyroiditis or have undergone treatment for hyperthyroidism with thyroidectomy or radioactive iodine. Occasionally, hypothyroidism is drug-induced, e.g., in patients treated with antithyroid drugs or the antiarrhythmic agent amiodarone. Rarely, hypothyroidism results from inadequate stimulation of the thyroid gland by the anterior pituitary or inadequate release of thyrotropin releasing hormone by the hypothalamus.

DIAGNOSIS: Long before the symptoms of hypothyroidism become obvious, the condition can be diagnosed with thyroid function tests. The plasma TSH test is used to screen for the disease; if it is high, hypothyroidism is likely to be present. Other tests, including a low free T4 index, confirm the diagnosis.

TREATMENT: For most patients, the lifelong administration of thyroid hormone restores normal metabolism and well-being. Failure to treat hypothyroidism inevitably results in myxedema, eventual coma, or death. Drug-induced hypothyroidism sometimes requires no treatment other than discontinuation of the offending agent or adjustment of its dose.

PATIENT CARE: The patient is assessed for indications of decreased metabolic rate; easy fatigability; cool, dry, and scaly skin; hypercarotenemia; hair and eyebrow loss; brittle nails, facial puffiness, and periorbital edema; paresthesias; ataxias; cold intolerance; bradycardia; reduced cardiac output; aching muscles and joint stiffness; changes in bowel habits; irregular menses; and decreased libido. Vital signs, fluid intake, urine output, weight, and neurological status are monitored. Diagnostic tests are performed, and the expected sensations of each are explained. Prescribed long-term hormone replacement and other medical therapies aimed at restoring a normal metabolic state are administered and explained.

The patient and family are assisted to deal with the psychosocial and psychomotor effects of decreased metabolism. The patient's activity level is increased gradually as treatment proceeds, while adequate rest is a continual priority to limit fatigue and to decrease myocardial oxygen demand. The patient should wear or carry a medical identification device describing the condition and its treatment and carry medications at all times. Desired outcomes include understanding of and cooperation with treatment regimen, restoration of normal activity level, absence of complications, and restoration of psychological well-being.

hypotonia (hī″pō-tō′nē-ă) [″ + *tonos,* tone] **1.** In physiology, having abnormally low tension (e.g., of the muscles or the arteries). **2.** In chemistry, having a lower osmotic pressure than a reference or isotonic solution. **hypotonic,** *adj.*

hypotrichosis (hī″pō-trĭ-kō′sĭs) [″ + *thrix,* hair, + *osis,* condition] An abnormal deficiency of hair.

hypotrophy (hī-pŏt′rŏ-fē) [″ + *trophe,* nourishment] Atrophy.

hypotropia (hī″pō-trō′pē-ă) [″ + *trope,* a turning] Vertical strabismus downward.

hypotympanotomy (hī″pō-tĭm″pă-nŏt′ō-mē) Surgical incision of the hypotympanum.

hypotympanum (hī″pō-tĭm′pă-nŭm) The part of the middle ear beneath the level of the tympanic membrane.

hypouricuria (hī″pō-ū-rĭ-kū′rē-ă) [″ + *ouron,* urine, + *ouron,* urine] Less than normal amount of uric acid in the urine.

hypovenosity (hī″pō-vĕn-ŏs′ĭ-tē) [″ + L. *venosus,* pert. to a vein] Incomplete development of the venous system in an area, resulting in atrophy or degeneration.

hypoventilation (hī″pō-vĕn″tĭ-lā′shŭn) [″ + L. *ventilatio,* ventilation] Reduced rate and depth of breathing that causes an increase in carbon dioxide.

hypovitaminosis (hī″pō-vī″tă-mĭn-ō′sĭs) [″ + L. *vita,* life, + *amine* + Gr. *osis,* condition] A condition caused by a lack of vitamins in or inadequate uptake of vitamins from the diet.

hypovolemia (hī″pō-vō-lē′mē-ă) [″ + L. *volumen,* volume] A decreased blood volume that may be caused by internal or external bleeding, fluid losses, or inadequate fluid intake.

hypovolia (hī″pō-vō′lē-ă) Decreased water content.

hypoxanthine (hī″pō-zăn′thĭn, -thēn) [″ + *xanthos,* yellow] A purine derivative, $C_5H_4N_4O$, in muscles and tissues in a stage of uric acid formation. It is formed during protein decomposition. Hypoxanthine is normal in urine in small amounts.

hypoxemia (hī-pŏks-ē′mē-ă) [″ + *oxygen* + *haima,* blood] Decreased oxygen tension (concentration) in the blood, measured by arterial oxygen partial pressure (PaO_2) values. It is sometimes associated with decreased oxygen content. SEE: *hypoxia; respiration.*

hypoxia (hī″pŏks′ē-ă) **1.** An oxygen deficiency. **2.** A decreased concentration of oxygen in the inspired air. SEE: *anoxia; hypoxemia; posthypoxia syndrome.*

altitude h. Hypoxia due to insufficient oxygen content of inspired air at high altitudes.

anemic h. Hypoxia due to a decrease in hemoglobin concentration or in the number of erythrocytes in the blood.

anoxic h. Hypoxia due to disordered pulmonary mechanisms of oxygenation; may be due to reduced oxygen supply, respiratory obstruction, reduced pulmonary function, or inadequate ventilation.

cerebral h. Lack of oxygen supply to the brain, usually as a result of either diminished blood flow (e.g., in traumatic childbirth or cardiopulmonary arrest) or diminished oxygenation of the blood (e.g., in high-altitude exposures or patients with advanced cardiopulmonary disease). If nothing is done to treat this condition, irreversible anoxic damage to the brain begins after 4 to 6 minutes and sooner in some cases. If basic resuscitation measures are begun before the end of this period, the onset of cerebral death may be postponed. SEE: *cardiopulmonary resuscitation.*

fetal h. Low oxygen levels in the fetus, commonly as a result of diminished placental perfusion, uteroplacental insufficiency, or umbilical cord compression. The condition often is accompanied by acidosis and is life threatening unless prompt interventions are undertaken to restore well-oxygenated blood to the fetus. Signs of early fetal hypoxia include tachycardia and increased fetal heart rate variability; profound fetal hypoxia is characterized by bradycardia and a sinusoidal fetal heart rate pattern.

histotoxic h. Hypoxia due to inability of the tissues to use oxygen. SEE: *cyanide.*

hypokinetic h. Stagnant h.

stagnant h. Hypoxia due to insufficient peripheral circulation, as occurs in cardiac failure, shock, arterial spasm, and thrombosis. SYN: *hypokinetic h.*

hypoxic lap swimming A practice by competitive swimmers of holding their breath for a number of laps in order to increase the tolerance to oxygen debt during races. The practice is potentially dangerous and may lead to drowning.

hypsarrhythmia (hĭp″săr-ĭth′mē-ă) [Gr. *hypsi,* high, + *a-,* not, + *rhythmos,* rhythm] An abnormal electroencephalographic pattern of persistent generalized slow waves and very high voltage. Clinically it is often associated with infantile spasm and progressive mental deterioration.

hypsibrachycephalic (hĭp″sē-brăk″ē-sĕ-făl′ĭk) [Gr. *hypsi,* high, + *brachys,* broad, + *kephale,* head] Having a broad and high skull.

hypsicephalic (hĭp″sē-sĕ-făl′ĭk) [″ + *kephale,* head] Having a skull with a cranial index greater than 75.1 degrees. SYN: *hypsistenocephalic; hypsocephalous.*

hypsicephaly (hĭp-sē-sĕf′ă-lē) The condition of having a skull with a cranial index greater than 75.1 degrees.

hypsiconchous (hĭp″sē-kŏng′kŭs) [″ + *konche,* shell] Having an orbital index of about 85 degrees.

hypsiloid (hĭp′sĭ-loyd) [Gr. *upsilon,* U or Y, + *eidos,* form] Hyoid.

h. ligament Iliofemoral ligament.

hypsistenocephalic (hĭp″sē-stĕn″ō-sĕ-făl′ĭk) [″ + *stenos,* narrow, + *kephale,* head] Hypsicephalic.

hypsocephalous (hĭp″sō-sĕf′ă-lŭs) [Gr. *hypsos,* height, + *kephale,* head] Hypsicephalic.

hypsokinesis (hĭp″sō-kĭ-nē′sĭs) [″ + *kinesis,* movement] A tendency to fall backward when standing or walking; seen in neurogenerative disorders such as Parkinson's disease.

hypsophobia (hĭp″sō-fō′bē-ă) [″ + *phobos,* fear] Acrophobia.

hyster- SEE: *hystero-.*

hysteralgia (hĭs-tĕr-ăl′jē-ă) [Gr. *hystera,* womb, + *algos,* pain] Uterine pain. SYN: *hysterodynia.*

hysterectomy (hĭs-tĕr-ĕk′tō-mē) [″ + *ektome,* excision] Surgical removal of the uterus. Each year, about 500,000 women undergo hysterectomies. Indications for the surgery include benign or malignant changes in the uterine wall or cavity and cervical abnormalities (including endometrial cancer, cervical cancer, severe dysfunctional bleeding, large or bleeding fibroid tumors, prolapse of the uterus, or severe endometriosis). The approach to excision may be either abdominal or vaginal. The abdominal approach is used most commonly to remove large tumors; when the ovaries and fallopian tubes also will be removed; and when there is need to examine adjacent pelvic structures, such as the regional lymph nodes. Vaginal hysterectomy is appropriate when uterine size is less than that in 12 week gestation, no other abdominal pathology is suspected, and when surgical plans include cystocele, enterocele, or rectocele repair. SEE: illus.; *Nursing Diagnoses Appendix.*

In preparation for abdominal hysterectomy, the patient is placed in the dorsal position. The table is ready to be tipped into the Trendelenburg position. As soon as the incision is made through the peritoneum, the table should be put into Trendelenburg position. This procedure is the same for all abdominopelvic surgery, as the Trendelenburg position allows the abdominal organs to fall away from the pelvis, so that they may be easily packed off and isolated from the surgical field with large pads or a large roll of packing.

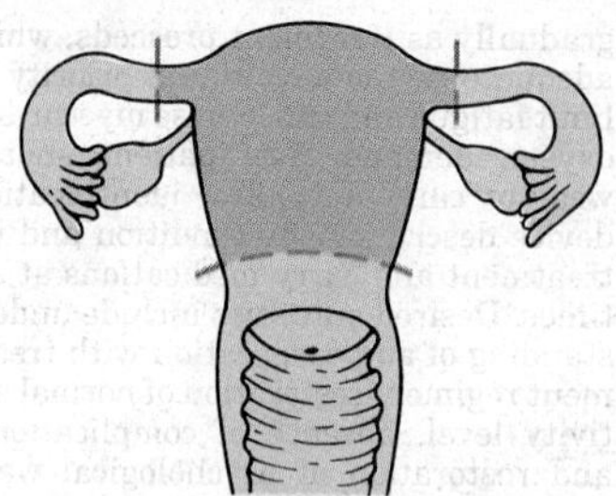

SUBTOTAL HYSTERECTOMY, CERVIX NOT REMOVED

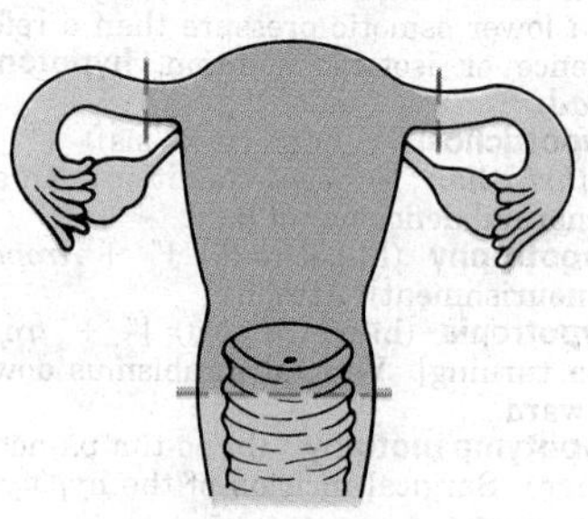

TOTAL HYSTERECTOMY, CERVIX IS REMOVED

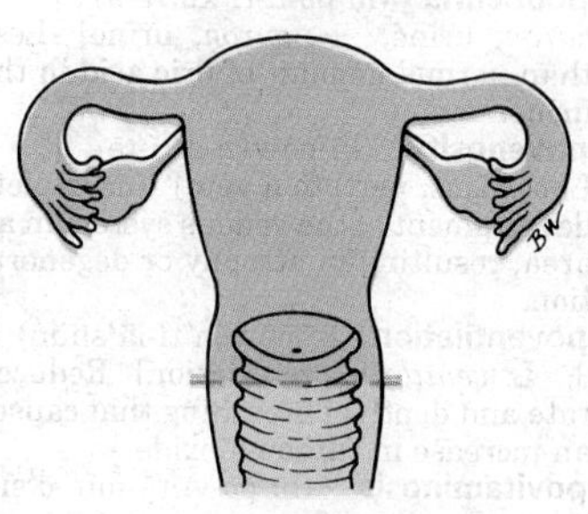

TOTAL HYSTERECTOMY, PLUS BILATERAL SALPINGO-OOPHERECTOMY

HYSTERECTOMY

PATIENT CARE: *Preoperative:* In general, preparations for an abdominal hysterectomy are similar to protocols for any abdominopelvic surgery (e.g., abdominal shave, scrub, insertion of an intravenous line and indwelling catheter).

Vaginal irrigation with antibacterial solution also may be ordered. All procedures are explained to the patient, who is provided with anticipatory guidance for the postoperative period. Misconceptions are clarified, informed consent is validated, and the signing of the operative permit is witnessed. The patient may be encouraged to discuss the personal meaning and implications of the procedure, such as permanent inability to bear children; emotional support is given. Controlled trials that have studied large numbers of women have not shown, in aggregate, any adverse effect of hysterectomy on sexuality or women's perceptions of their femininity.

Postoperative: Initial status assessments include color; vital signs; airway patency and breath sounds; level of consciousness and discomfort; intravenous intake; and nasogastric and indwelling catheter drainage. During the first few hours, assessments usually are made over lengthening intervals, from every 10 to 15 minutes during the first hour to every 30 minutes to hourly. Intervals and assessment priorities may be altered on the basis of current findings, such as bleeding. Color; vital signs; airway patency and lung sounds; level of consciousness and discomfort; intake and output (including intravenous fluids, nasogastric and indwelling catheter drainage); and abdominal dressings (intact, amount and character of any drainage) are monitored. Additional later assessments include bowel sounds; lower extremity circulation (pedal pulses, leg pain); and wound status (redness, edema, ecchymosis, discharge, and approximation). The patient is encouraged to splint the incision, turn from side-to-side, deep breathe and cough every 2 hours, and to use incentive spirometry. Prescribed intravenous fluids and analgesics are administered. The woman is assisted in self-administering patient-controlled analgesia. Antithromboembolitic devices (pneumatic dressings or elastic stockings) are applied as needed. The patient is encouraged and assisted with early ambulation.

Discharge teaching emphasizes self-assessments; self-care procedures; signs to report immediately to the primary caregiver; nutrition; activities; and the potential emotional impact of the implications of the procedure. As appropriate, the rationale for hormone replacement therapy is explained. Effective coping strategies related to anticipated radiation and/or chemotherapy are targeted. Desired outcomes include evidence of incisional healing; absence of complications; return of normal G.I. and bladder function; and understanding of and compliance with the prescribed treatment regimen.

abdominal h. The removal of the uterus through an abdominal incision.

cesarean h. The surgical removal of the uterus at the time of cesarean section.

pan h. Removal of the uterus, fallopian tubes, and ovaries.

Porro h. SEE: *Porro's operation*.

radical h. The surgical removal of the uterus, tubes, ovaries, adjacent lymph nodes, and part of the vagina.

subtotal h. The surgical removal of the uterus, leaving the cervix in place. SYN: *supracervical h.; supravaginal h.*

supracervical h. Subtotal h.

supravaginal h. Subtotal h.

total abdominal h. Removal of the uterus, including the cervix, through an abdominal incision.

vaginal h. The surgical removal of the uterus through the vagina.

hysteresis (hĭs″tĕr-ē′sĭs) [Gr., a coming too late] **1.** The failure of related phenomena to keep pace with each other. **2.** The failure of the manifestation of an effect to keep up with its cause. **3.** The difference between inflation and deflation of the lung, shown as a pressure volume difference.

hystereurynter (hĭs″tĕr-ū-rĭn′tĕr) [Gr. *hystera,* uterus, + *eurynein,* to stretch] Metreurynter.

hysteria (hĭs-tĕ′rē-ă) [Gr. *hystera,* uterus] A pejorative term used in popular speech to mean a conversion reaction, or a widely fluctuating expression of emotions.

NOTE: Currently accepted nomenclature for mental disorders does not include the term *hysteria;* it is included here for historical reasons. SEE: *mass psychogenic illness; somatization disorder.*

SYMPTOMS: Symptoms include emotional instability, sensory disturbances, loss of motor function, or other disorders.

ETIOLOGY: It may be related to emotional or physical stress.

TREATMENT: Rest and reassurance are cornerstones of management.

anxiety h. Hysteria combined with an anxiety neurosis.

conversion h. Conversion disorder.

epidemic h. Mass sociogenic illness.

major h. Agitated behavior, sometimes accompanied by pseudoseizures.

mass h. Mass sociogenic illness.

hysteriac (hĭs-tĕr′ē-ăk) [Gr. *hystera,* womb] A hysterical person.

hysteric, hysterical Pert. to hysteria.

hystericoneuralgic (hĭs-tĕr″ĭk-o-nū-răl′jĭk) [″ + *neuron,* nerve, + *algos,* pain] Pert. to pain of hysterical origin, but resembling neuralgia.

hystero-, hyster- [Gr. *hystera,* womb] Combining form meaning *uterus* or *hysteria.* SEE: *metro-; utero-.*

hysterobubonocele (hĭs″tĕr-ō-bū-bŏn′ō-sēl) [" + *boubon,* groin, + *kele,* tumor, swelling] An inguinal hernia surrounding the uterus.

hysterocele (hĭs′tĕr-ō-sēl) [" + *kele,* tumor, swelling] A hernia of the uterus, esp. when gravid.

hysterocystocleisis (hĭs″tĕr-ō-sĭs″tō-klī′sĭs) [" + *kystis,* a bladder, + *kleisis,* closure] An operation fastening the cervix uteri to the wall of the bladder.

hysterodynia (hĭs″tĕr-ō-dĭn′ē-ă) [" + *odyne,* pain] Hysteralgia.

hysterogastrorrhaphy (hĭs″tĕr-ō-găs-tror′ă-fē) [" + *gaster,* belly, + *rhaphe,* seam, ridge] Fixation of the uterus to the gastric wall.

hysterogenic (hĭs″tĕr-ō-jĕn′ĭk) [" + *gennan,* to produce] Causing hysteria.

hysterogram (hĭs′tĕr-ō-grăm) A radiograph of the uterus after injection of a contrast medium. It has been replaced by ultrasound.

hysterography (hĭs″tĕ-rŏg′ră-fē) [" + *graphein,* to write] A recording of the frequency and intensity of contractions of the uterus.

hysteroid (hĭs′tĕr-oyd) [" + *eidos,* form, shape] Resembling or pert. to hysteria.

hysterolaparotomy (hĭs″tĕr-ō-lăp″ă-rŏt′ō-mē) [" + *lapara,* flank, + *tome,* incision] A uterine incision through the abdominal wall; abdominal hysterectomy.

hysterolith (hĭs′tĕr-ō-lĭth) [" + *lithos,* stone] A calculus in the uterus.

hysterolysis (hĭs″tĕr-ŏl′ĭ-sĭs) [" + *lysis,* dissolution] An operation to loosen the uterus from its adhesions.

hysterometer (hĭs″tĕ-rŏm′ĕ-tĕr) [" + *metron,* measure] A device for measuring the size of the uterus.

hysterometry (hĭs″tĕ-rŏm′ĕ-trē) Measurement of the size of the uterus.

hysteromyoma (hĭs″tĕr-ō-mī-ō′mă) [Gr. *hystera,* womb, + *mys,* muscle, + *oma,* tumor] A myoma or fibromyoma of the uterus.

hysteromyomectomy (hĭs″tĕr-ō-mī″ō-mĕk′tō-mē) [" + " + *ektome,* excision] Excision of a uterine fibroid.

hysteromyotomy (hĭs″tĕr-ō-mī-ŏt′ō-mē) [" + " + *tome,* incision] Uterine incision for removal of a solid tumor.

hystero-oophorectomy (hĭs″tĕr-ō-ō″ŏ-for-ĕk′tō-mē) [" + *oon,* egg, + *phoros,* bearing, + *ektome,* excision] Removal of the uterus and of one or both ovaries.

hysteropathy (hĭs″tĕr-ŏp′ă-thē) [" + *pathos,* disease, suffering] Any uterine disorder.

hysteroptosia, hysteroptosis (hĭs″tĕr-ŏp-tō′sē-ă, -sĭs) [" + *ptosis,* a dropping] Prolapse of the uterus. SYN: *procidentia.*

hysterorrhaphy (hĭs-tĕr-or′ă-fē) [" + *rhaphe,* seam, ridge] Suture of the uterus.

hysterorrhexis (hĭs″tĕr-ō-rĕk′sĭs) [" + *rhexis,* rupture] Rupture of the uterus, esp. when pregnant.

hysterosalpingectomy (hĭs″tĕr-ō-săl″pĭn-jĕk′tō-mē) [" + *salpinx,* tube, + *ektome,* excision] Surgical removal of the uterus and fallopian tubes.

hysterosalpingography (hĭs″tĕr-ō-săl″pĭn-gŏg′ră-fē) [" + " + *graphein,* to write] Radiography of the uterus and oviducts after injection of a contrast medium. This procedure, although sometimes therapeutic in clearing the fallopian tubes, is seldom performed due to the superior imaging possible via ultrasound. SYN: *metrosalpingography.*

hysterosalpingo-oophorectomy (hĭs″tĕr-ō-săl-pĭng″gō-ō″ŏ-for-ĕk′tō-mē) [" + " + *oon,* egg, + *phoros,* bearing, + *ektome,* excision] The surgical removal of the uterus, oviducts, and ovaries.

hysterosalpingostomy (hĭs″tĕr-ō-săl″pĭng-ŏs′tō-mē) [" + " + *stoma,* mouth] Anastomosis of the uterus with the distal end of the fallopian tube after excision of a strictured portion of the tube.

hysteroscope (hĭs′tĕr-ō-skōp) [" + *skopein,* to examine] An instrument for examining the uterine cavity.

hysteroscopy (hĭs″tĕr-ŏs′kō-pē) Inspection of the uterus by use of a special endoscope. SEE: *hysteroscope.*

hysterospasm (hĭs′tĕr-ō-spăzm″) [Gr. *hystera,* womb, + *spasmos,* a convulsion] A uterine spasm.

hysterostomatocleisis (hĭs″tĕr-ō-stō″mă-tō-klī′sĭs) [" + *stoma,* mouth, + *kleisis,* closure] An operation for vesicovaginal fistula, consisting of closure of the cervix uteri and making the vesical and uterine cavities into a common cavity by means of the opening between them.

hysterostomatomy (hĭs″tĕr-ō-stō-măt′ō-mē) [" + " + *tome,* incision] The surgical enlargement of the os uteri; incision of the os or cervix uteri.

hysterotomy (hĭs-tĕr-ŏt′ō-mē) **1.** Incision of the uterus. **2.** Cesarean section.

hysterotracheloplasty (hĭs″tĕr-ō-trā′kĕl-lō-plăs″tē) [" + " + *plassein,* to form] Plastic surgery or repair of the cervix.

hysterotrachelorrhaphy (hĭs″tĕr-ō-trā″kĕl-or′ă-fē) [" + " + *rhaphe,* seam, ridge] Plastic surgery of a lacerated cervix by paring the edges and suturing them together.

hysterotrachelotomy (hĭs″tĕr-ō-trā″kĕl-ŏt′ō-mē) [" + " + *tome,* incision] A surgical incision of the neck of the uterus.

hysterovagino-enterocele (hĭs″tĕr-ō-văj″ĭn-ō-ĕn′tĕr-ō-sēl) [" + L. *vagina,* sheath, + Gr. *enteron,* intestine, + *kele,* tumor, swelling] A hernia surrounding the uterus, vagina, and intestines.

Hz *hertz.*

HZV *herpes zoster virus.*

I

I **1.** Symbol for the element iodine. **2.** Symbol for the quantity of electricity expressed in amperes.

^{131}I Radioactive iodine; atomic weight 131.

^{132}I Radioactive iodine; atomic weight 132.

i *optically inactive.*

-ia Suffix indicating a condition, esp. an abnormal state.

IABC *intra-aortic balloon counterpulsation.*

IABP *intra-aortic balloon pump.*

I.A.D.R. *International Association for Dental Research.*

IAET *International Association for Enterostomal Therapy.*

I and O *intake and output.*

ianthinopsia (ī-ăn″thĭ-nŏp′sē-ă) [Gr. *ianthinos,* violet colored, + *opsis,* vision] An abnormality of vision in which all objects appear to be violet.

-iasis [Gr.] Suffix, the same as or interchangeable with *-osis,* meaning the state or condition of, particularly with respect to a pathological condition. SEE: *-asis; -sis.*

-iatric (ī-ăt′rĭk) [Gr. *iatrikos,* medical] Combining form used as a suffix referring to *medicine, the medical profession,* or *physicians.*

iatro- [Gr. *iatros,* physician] Combining form indicating relationship to medicine or a physician.

iatrogenesis (ī″ăt-rō-jĕn′ĕs-ĭs) [″ + *gennan,* to produce] Any adverse mental or physical condition induced in a patient through the effects of treatment. Some examples: chemotherapy used to treat cancer may cause nausea, vomiting, hair loss, or depressed white blood cell counts. The use of a Foley catheter for incontinence can create a urinary tract infection and urinary sepsis. A guiding principle of health care is to do little harm to patients while effecting cures—but this ideal is not always achieved. In the U.S. in 2000, deaths that result from health care errors and complications of treatment are among the most common causes of mortality. **iatrogenic** (ī″ăt-rō-jĕn′ĭk), *adj.*

iatrology (ī″ă-trŏl′ō-jē) [″ + *logos,* word, reason] Medical science.

IBC *iron-binding capacity.*

IBD *inflammatory bowel disease.*

IBS *irritable bowel syndrome.*

ibuprofen A nonsteroidal anti-inflammatory agent with antipyretic and analgesic properties. It inhibits the synthesis of prostaglandins; this may be responsible for its effects. It is used in treating chronic symptomatic rheumatoid arthritis and osteoarthritis, dysmenorrhea, athletic injuries, and many other diseases and conditions. Trade names are Advil, Motrin, and Nuprin.

CAUTION: All nonsteroidal anti-inflammatory agents may cause bleeding from the gastrointestinal tract and kidney failure.

IBW *ideal body weight.*

IC *inspiratory capacity.*

-ic A suffix indicating *characteristic of* or *relating to.*

ICD *intrauterine contraceptive device; International Classification of Diseases.*

ice (īs) [AS. *is*] A solid form of water. Water becomes ice at a temperature of 32°F (0°C) and may be chilled lower than the freezing point. An ice bag, cap, collar, and cravat are devices for holding ice to be applied to a patient to obtain the effect of continuous cold in a circumscribed area. For patients who have circulatory insufficiency, peripheral vascular disease, or other cold sensitivity, one or two layers of terry cloth toweling should be placed between the skin and the ice pack. Reusable cold packs (e.g., cold packs that are filled with something other than cubed, flaked, or crushed ice) should always be insulated before application.

i. bag A flexible, watertight bag with a sealable opening large enough to permit ice cubes or chipped ice to be added. It is used in any condition requiring local application of cold. In an emergency any sturdy, flexible plastic bag can be used, sealing the open end with a knot. A simple ice pack can be made at home by mixing 3 cups of water and 1 cup of rubbing alcohol in a resealable plastic bag and placing the sealed mixture in the freezer for 8 to 12 hours. The solution will not freeze but will attain a gel-like consistency that molds to the body part on which it is used.

CAUTION: Dry ice should not be placed in an ice bag.

---

dry i. Carbon dioxide cooled to the point at which it becomes solid, which occurs at −110°F (−78.9°C). It is used as a commercial refrigerant and for therapeutic refrigeration in the treatment of certain skin conditions, including warts. SEE: *carbon dioxide.*

i. immersion Technique for administering therapeutic cold treatments to the distal extremities (e.g., the ankle or hand), using a mixture of water and crushed, flaked, or cubed ice with a temperature range of 50° to 60°F (10.0° to 15°C). The liquid medium allows for equal cooling of irregularly shaped body parts. To reduce the amount of discomfort that is initially experienced during this treatment, the fingers or toes can be covered with an insulating material.

Because ice immersion treatments place the body part in a position that does not promote venous return, the treated limb may swell. It should be elevated and a compression wrap applied following the treatment to encourage venous and lymphatic drainage. SYN: *i. slush*. SEE: *cryotherapy*.

CAUTION: This treatment should not be used in patients with cold intolerance or in those for whom cold application is contraindicated.

i. massage Application of ice to obtain a therapeutic numbing effect. Paper cups containing water previously frozen are preferable. The cups are rubbed over a localized area in small circles for 5 to 10 minutes in order to numb the part and prepare it for deep pressure or deep transverse friction massage. Ice massage is also used to treat traumatized tissues and joints.

i. slush i. immersion.

i. treatment The use of ice applied either directly or in a suitable container to cool an injured area. Ice therapy, at least in the first 24 to 48 hours after injury, is believed to be much more beneficial than heat in treating superficial bruises, contusions, and sprains. The application of cold or of ice water in immediate treatment of a burn helps to reduce the extent of inflammation and pain.

iceberg phenomenon The recognition of gross conditions and diseases and failure to recognize the great majority of conditions that are mild and not clinically obvious.

Iceland disease Benign myalgic encephalomyelitis.

Iceland moss An edible lichen of the genus *Cetraria,* which contains a form of starch; a slightly tonic demulcent.

ICF *intracellular fluid.*

ichor (ī'kor) [Gr. *ichor,* serum] Thin, fetid discharge from an ulcer or from a wound.

ichorous (ī'kor-ŭs) [Gr. *ichor,* serum] Resembling ichor or watery pus.

ichthyism, ichthyismus (ĭk'thē-ĭzm, ĭk"thē-ĭz'mŭs) [Gr. *ichthys,* fish, + *-ismos,* condition] Poisoning from eating decomposed or toxic fish. SEE: *tetrodotoxin.*

ichthyo- [Gr. *ichthys,* fish] Combining form meaning *fish.*

ichthyoacanthotoxism (ĭk"thē-ō-ă-kăn"thō-tŏk'sĭzm) [" + *akantha,* thorn, + *toxikon,* poison, + *-ismos,* condition] A toxin or venom present in the sting, spines, or "teeth" of certain venomous fish.

ichthyohemotoxin (ĭk"thē-ō-hē"mō-tŏk'sĭn) [" + *haima,* blood, + *toxikon,* poison] A toxin present in the blood of certain poisonous fish.

ichthyoid (ĭk'thē-oyd) [" + *eidos,* form, shape] Fishlike.

ichthyology (ĭk"thē-ŏl'ō-jē) [" + *logos,* word, reason] The study of fish.

ichthyootoxin (ĭk"thē-ō"ō-tŏk'sĭn) [" + *oon,* egg, + *toxikon,* poison] A toxin present in the roe of certain fish.

ichthyophagous (ĭk"thē-ŏf'ă-gŭs) [" + *phagein,* to eat] Subsisting on fish.

ichthyophobia (ĭk-thē-ō-fō'bē-ă) [" + *phobos,* fear] An abnormal aversion to fish.

ichthyosarcotoxin (ĭk"thē-ō-săr"kō-tŏk'sĭn) [" + *sarx,* flesh, + *toxikon,* poison] A toxin present in the flesh of certain fish.

ichthyosis (ĭk"thē-ō'sĭs) [" + *osis,* condition] A condition in which the skin is dry and scaly, resembling fish skin. Because ichthyosis is so easily recognized, a variety of diseases have been called by this name.

A mild nonhereditary form is called winter itch. This is often seen on the legs of older patients, esp. during dry weather during the winter months. It may be more prevalent in those who bathe frequently, thus causing excessive dryness of the skin.

TREATMENT: The application of lotions or ointments that soften and soothe the skin provide symptomatic relief for all forms of ichthyosis. Dry scales can be removed by applying a combination of 6% salicylic acid in a gel containing propylene glycol, ethyl alcohol, hydroxy propylene cellulose, and water. This is most effective when applied to moistened skin at night, and covered with an occlusive dressing. Soaps should be used sparingly.

i. congenita Harlequin fetus. SEE: under *fetus.*

i. fetalis I. congenita.

i. hystrix Linear nevus. The skin contains bands or lines of rough, thick, warty, hypertrophic papillary growths.

lamellar i. of newborn A rare form of inherited ichthyosis with lamellar desquamation.

i. vulgaris A hereditary form of ichthyosis that includes two genetically distinct types. Dominant ichthyosis vulgaris is produced by an autosomal dominant gene. Characterized by dry, rough, scaly skin, it is not present at birth and is usually noticed between the ages of one and four. Many cases improve in later life.

The second type is sex-linked ichthyosis vulgaris. It is present only in males and is transmitted by the female as a recessive gene. Onset of scattered large brown scales is seen in early infancy. The scalp may be involved, but the face is spared except for the sides and in front of the ear. There is little tendency for this condition to improve with age.

ichthyotic (ĭk″thē-ŏt′ĭk) [Gr. *ichthys,* fish] Relating to ichthyosis.

ichthyotoxicology (ĭk″thē-ō-tŏk″sĭ-kŏl′ō-jē) [″ + *toxikon,* poison, + *logos,* word, reason] The study of poisons and toxins produced by certain fish.

ichthyotoxin (ĭk″thē-ō-tŏk′sĭn) [″ + *toxikon,* poison] Any toxin present in fish.

ICIDH *International Classification of Impairment, Disability and Handicap.*

icing **1.** A technique of cutaneous stimulation using ice (12° to 17°C) to evoke or facilitate reflex muscular responses in patients with central nervous system dysfunction. **2.** Application of ice to a recently traumatized area in order to reduce pain and swelling.

ICN *International Council of Nurses.*

ICP *intracranial pressure.*

ICS **1.** *intercostal space.* **2.** *incident command system.*

I.C.S. *International College of Surgeons.*

ICSH *interstitial cell-stimulating hormone.* Luteinizing hormone.

ictal (ĭk′tăl) [L. *ictus,* a blow or stroke] Pert. to or caused by a sudden attack or stroke such as epilepsy. SEE: *postictal.*

icteric (ĭk-tĕr′ĭk) [Gr. *ikteros,* jaundice] Pert. to jaundice.

icteroanemia (ĭk″tĕr-ō-ă-nē′mē-ă) [″ + *an-,* not, + *haima,* blood] Icterus associated with anemia, hemolysis, and splenic enlargement.

icterogenic, icterogenous (ĭk″tĕr-ō-jĕn′ĭk, -ŏj′ĕn-ŭs) [″ + *gennan,* to produce] Causing jaundice.

icterohemoglobinuria (ĭk″tĕr-ō-hē″mō-glō″bĭ-nū′rē-ă) [″ + *haima,* blood, + L. *globus,* globe, + Gr. *ouron,* urine] Concerning icterus and hemoglobinuria.

icterohepatitis (ĭk″tĕr-ō-hĕp-ă-tī′tĭs) [″ + *hepar,* liver, + *itis,* inflammation] Liver inflammation with jaundice.

icteroid (ĭk′tĕr-oyd) [″ + *eidos,* form, shape] Resembling jaundice; yellow-hued.

icterus (ĭk′tĕr-ŭs) [Gr. *ikteros,* jaundice] Jaundice.

i. gravis neonatorum Hemolytic disease of the newborn. SEE: *erythroblastosis fetalis; exchange transfusion; kernicterus; phototherapy.*

hemolytic i. Hemolytic jaundice.

i. neonatorum Physiologic jaundice of the newborn.

nonobstructive i. Hemolytic jaundice.

obstructive i. Obstructive jaundice.

ictus [L., stroke] A blow or sudden attack.

i. cordis Heartbeat.

i. epilepticus Epileptic seizure.

i. sanguinis A hemorrhagic stroke.

ICU *intensive care unit.*

ID *identification; infective dose; inside diameter; intradermal.*

ID_{50} The infective dose of microorganisms that will produce illness in 50% of the individuals who receive that dose.

id [L. *id,* it; later translators of Freud's writings believed that the word *es* should have been translated to *it* and not to id] In Freudian psychiatry, one of the three divisions of the psyche, the others being the ego and superego. The id, the obscure, inaccessible part of personality, serves as a repository of instinctual drives continually striving for satisfaction. Its existence is unproven.

id L. *idem,* the same.

-id [Gr. *eidos,* form, shape] Suffix indicating certain secondary skin eruptions that appear some distance from the site of primary infection. If the etiological agent of primary infection is known, the secondary lesion is designated by adding the suffix -id, as in tuberculid and trichophytid.

IDDM *insulin-dependent diabetes mellitus.*

idea [Gr., form] A mental image; a concept.

autochthonous i. A thought that comes into the mind independent of a train of thoughts, in an unaccountable way.

compulsive i. A persistent impulse or thought that drives a person to perform or repeat irrational behavior.

dominant i. An idea that controls all one's actions and thoughts.

fixed i. An idea that completely dominates the mind despite evidence to the contrary; a delusion. SYN: *idée fixe.*

flight of i.'s Continuous but fragmented language use; a hallmark of psychosis or mania. The general train of thought can be followed but direction is frequently changed, often by chance stimuli from the environment.

i. of reference An impression that the conversation or actions of others have reference to oneself.

ideal [L. *idea,* model] A goal or endeavor regarded as a standard of perfection.

ideation (ī-dē-ā′shŭn) The process of thinking; formation of ideas. It slows down in dementias, depression, and other organic brain diseases, and in narcotic intoxications; but speeds up in the early stage of some types of intoxication. It is unduly active in manic-depressive states.

idée fixe (ē-dā′ fēks′) [Fr.] Fixed idea. SEE: under *idea.*

identical [L. *identicus,* the same] Exactly alike.

identification [″ + *facere,* to make] **1.** A kind of daydream, as in identification of oneself with the hero of a book or play. **2.** The process of determining the sameness of a thing or person with that described or known to exist. **3.** A defense mechanism, operating unconsciously, by which a person patterns himself or herself after some other person. This plays a major role in personality development.

dental i. The use of the unique characteristics of a person's teeth or dental work as recorded in dental charts, radiographs, and records to establish the person's identity.

palm and sole system of i. A system based on prints of the palmar surface of the hand and the plantar surface of the foot. SEE: *dermatoglyphics.*

identity (ī-dĕn′tĭ-tē) **1.** The concept that each individual has of his or her body in space and his or her thought processes in relation to the social and intellectual environment. **2.** The physical and mental characteristics by which an individual is known and recognized.

ego i. The sense of self that provides a unity of personality.

gender i. One's self-concept with respect to being male or female; a person's sense of his or her true sexual identity.

i. testing SEE: *paternity test.*

ideo- [Gr. *idea,* form] Prefix pert. to mental images.

ideogenous, ideogenetic (ĭd-ē-ŏj′ĕn-ŭs, -ō-jĕ-nĕt′ĭk) [″ + *gennan,* to produce] Stimulated by an idea.

ideology (ī″dē-ŏl′ō-jē) [″ + *logos,* word, reason] **1.** The study of ideas or thought. **2.** A system or schema of ideas; a philosophy.

ideomuscular (ī″dē-ō-mŭs′kū-lăr) [″ + L. *musculus,* muscle] **1.** Indicating muscular activity produced in connection with a thought. **2.** Concerning both ideation and muscular activity.

idio- [Gr. *idios,* own] Prefix indicating *individual, distinct,* or *unknown.*

idiocy [Gr. *idiotes,* ignorant person] A severe mental deficiency, usually due to an arrest in development, or defective development, as opposed to the loss of mental competence. The cause, which occurs either in utero or in the first years after birth, may be genetic or traumatic, or due to severe disease. SEE: *mental retardation.*

cretinoid i. Mental retardation caused by congenital hypothyroidism. SEE: *cretinism.*

hydrocephalic i. Mental redardation accompanied by chronic hydrocephalus.

microcephalic i. Mental retardation accompanied by microcephalia.

traumatic i. An obsolete term for an organic brain syndrome that results from head trauma.

idioglossia (ĭd″ē-ō-glŏs′ē-ă) [″ + *glossa,* tongue] **1.** An inability to articulate properly, so that the sounds emitted are like those of an unknown language. **2.** A unique form of speech that a child with congenital word deafness may utter. It simulates fluent language but does not share its vocabulary, diction, or syntax.

idiogram (ĭd′ē-ō-grăm″) [″ + *gramma,* something written] The graphic representation of the karyotype, or chromosome complement of a cell.

idioisolysin (ĭd″ē-ō-ī-sŏl′ĭ-sĭn) [″ + *isos,* equal, + *lysis,* dissolution] A hemolysin active against the cells of an individual of the same species.

idiolysin (ĭd″ē-ŏl′ĭ-sĭn) [″ + *lysis,* dissolution] A lysin normally present in the blood.

idiopathic (ĭd″ē-ō-păth′ĭk) [″ + *pathos,* disease, suffering] Pert. to conditions without clear pathogenesis, or disease without recognizable cause, as of spontaneous origin.

idiopsychological (ĭd″ē-ō-sī″kō-lŏj′ĭk-ăl) [″ + *psyche,* mind, + *logos,* word, reason] Concerning ideas produced in one's own mind.

idiosyncrasy (ĭd″ē-ō-sĭn′kră-sē) [″ + *syn,* together, + *krasis,* mixture] **1.** Special characteristics by which persons differ from each other. **2.** That which makes one react differently from others; a peculiar or individual reaction to an idea, action, drug, food, or some other substance through unusual susceptibility. **idiosyncratic** (-sĭn-krăt′ĭk), *adj.*

drug i. An unusual response to a drug. It can manifest as an accelerated, toxic, or inappropriate response to the usual therapeutic dose of a drug. SYN: *i. of effect.*

i. of effect Drug i.

idiot [Gr. *idiotes,* ignorant person] Former term for a person with severe mental deficiency. SEE: *idiocy; mental retardation.*

idiotic Like an idiot; said of an idea or action.

idiotope A single antigenic determinant on a variable region of an antibody or T-cell receptor. A set of idiotopes make up the idiotype.

idiotrophic (ĭd″ē-ō-trŏf′ĭk) [Gr. *idios,* own, + *trophe,* nourishment] Capable of securing its own nourishment.

idiotropic (ĭd″ē-ō-trŏp′ĭk) [″ + *trope,* a turning] Egocentric.

idiot-savant (ēd-jō′să-vănt) [Fr., learned idiot] An individual who is generally mentally retarded but has the ability to do complicated tasks such as play instruments, recall dates, or accurately and rapidly perform mathematical calculations. SEE: *autism.*

idiotype (ĭd″ē-ō-tīp′) [Gr. *idios,* own, + *typos,* type] In immunology, the set of antigenic determinants (idiotopes) on an antibody that make that antibody unique. It is associated with the amino acids of immunoglobulin light and heavy chains. **idiotypic** (-tĭp′ĭk), *adj.*

idiovariation (ĭd″ē-ō-văr″ē-ā′shŭn) [″ + L. *variare,* to vary] A mutation that occurs without known cause.

idioventricular (ĭd″ē-ō-vĕn-trĭk′ū-lăr) [″ + L. *ventriculus,* little belly] Pert. to the cardiac ventricle alone when dissociated from the atrium. A heart rhythm that arises in the ventricle is an idioventricular rhythm.

IDM *infant of diabetic mother.*

idoxuridine (ī-dŏks-ūr′ĭ-dēn) ABBR: IDU. 5-iodo-2′deoxyuridine; used to treat herpesvirus infections of the eye.

IDU **1.** *5-iodo-2′deoxyuridine; idoxuridine.* **2.** *Injection drug use.*

IDV Indinavir.

IE *infective endocarditis.*

Ifosfamide A chemotherapeutic drug used to treat many solid tumors, including cancers of the breast, testes, and lung, among others.

IgA *immunoglobulin A.*

IgD *immunoglobulin D.*

IgE *immunoglobulin E.*

IgG *immunoglobulin G.*

IgM *immunoglobulin M.*

ignatia (ĭg-nā′shē-ă) [L.] The seeds of a climbing plant native to the Philippine Islands, which contain about 3% strychnine and brucine.

igniextirpation (ĭg″nē-ĕks″tĭr-pā′shŭn) [L. *ignis,* fire, + *exstirpare,* to root out] Excision by cauterization.

ignis (ĭg′nĭs) [L., fire] Moxa.

i. infernalis Ergotism.

I.H. *infectious hepatitis.*

IHS *Indian Health Service.*

ILD *interstitial lung disorder.*

ilea Plural of ileum.

ileac (ĭl′ē-ăk) **1.** Pert. to the ileum. **2.** Pert. to ileus.

ileal (ĭl′ē-ăl) Pert. to the ileum.

ileal conduit SEE: under *conduit.*

ileectomy (ĭl″ē-ĕk′tō-mē) [L. *ileum,* ileum, + Gr. *ektome,* excision] Excision of the ileum.

ileitis (ĭl″ē-ī′tĭs) [″ + Gr. *itis,* inflammation] Inflammation of the ileum. The most common cause is Crohn's disease (regional ileitis), an inflammatory bowel disease of unknown etiology. SEE: *Crohn's disease; inflammatory bowel disease.*

SYMPTOMS: Patients may have pain in the right lower quadrant of the abdomen, often with diarrhea, nausea, vomiting, weight loss, and fevers. The stool may contain pus, blood, or mucus.

regional i. Crohn's disease.

ileo- (ĭl″ē-ō) [L. *ileum*] Combining form meaning *ileum.*

ileocecal (ĭl′ē-ō-sē′kăl) [″ + *caecus,* blind] Relating to the ileum and cecum.

ileocecostomy (ĭl″ē-ō-sē-kŏs′tō-mē) [″ + ″ + Gr. *stoma,* opening] The surgical formation of an opening between the ileum and cecum.

ileocecum (ĭl″ē-ō-sē′kŭm) The ileum and cecum combined.

ileocolic (ĭl″ē-ō-kŏl′ĭk) [″ + Gr. *kolon,* colon] Pert. to the ileum and colon.

ileocolitis (ĭl″ē-ō-kō-lī′tĭs) [″ + ″ + *itis,* inflammation] Inflammatory bowel disease.

ileocolostomy (ĭl″ē-ō-kō-lŏs′tō-mē) [″ + ″ + *stoma,* mouth] An anastomosis between the ileum and the colon.

ileocolotomy (ĭl″ē-ō-kō-lŏt′ō-mē) [″ + ″ + *tome,* incision] An incision of the ileum and colon.

ileocystoplasty (ĭl″ē-ō-sĭst′ō-plăs″tē) [″ + Gr. *kystis,* bladder, + *plassein,* to form] The use of an isolated ileal segment to increase the size of the bladder.

ileocystostomy (ĭl″ē-ō-sĭs-tŏs′tō-mē) [″ + ″ + *stoma,* mouth] The surgical formation of an opening between the ileum and bladder, used to replace a diseased, absent, or obstructed ureter.

ileoileostomy (ĭl″ē-ō-ĭl″ē-ŏs′tō-mē) [″ + *ileum,* small intestine, + Gr. *stoma,* mouth] The surgical formation of an opening between two parts of the ileum.

ileoproctostomy (ĭl″ē-ō-prŏk-tŏs′tō-mē) [″ + Gr. *proktos,* rectum, + *stoma,* mouth] The establishment of an opening between the ileum and rectum. SYN: *ileorectostomy.*

ileorectal (ĭl″ē-ō-rĕk′tăl) [″ + *rectum,* rectum] Concerning the ileum and rectum.

ileorectostomy (ĭl″ē-ō-rĕk-tŏs′tō-mē) [″ + ″ + Gr. *stoma,* mouth] Ileoproctostomy.

ileorrhaphy (ĭl″ē-or′ă-fē) [″ + Gr. *rhaphe,* seam, ridge] Surgical repair of the ileum.

ileosigmoidostomy (ĭl″ē-ō-sĭg″moyd-ŏs′tō-mē) [″ + Gr. *sigma,* letter S, + *eidos,* form, shape, + *stoma,* mouth] A surgical opening between the ileum and sigmoid flexure.

ileostomy (ĭl′ē-ŏs′tō-mē) [″ + Gr. *stoma,* mouth] A surgical passage through the abdominal wall, through which a segment of ileum is exteriorized. An end stoma or loop stoma may be created. The fecal material drains into a pouch worn on the abdomen. SEE: *Nursing Diagnoses Appendix.*

urinary i. The surgical formation of an opening from the urinary tract to an isolated segment of the ileum, most often by implanting the ureters into an ileal segment fashioned into a continent ileal conduit (e.g., Koch pouch).

ileotomy (ĭl″ē-ŏt′ō-mē) [″ + Gr. *tome,* incision] An incision into the ileum.

ileotransversostomy (ĭl″ē-ō-trăns″vĕr-sŏs′tō-mē) [″ + *transversus,* crosswise, + Gr. *stoma,* mouth] Connection of the ileum with the transverse colon.

ileum (ĭl′ē-ŭm) *pl.* **ilea** [L., ileum] The lower three fifths of the small intestine from the jejunum to the ileocecal valve.

Its length varies from 6 ft (2 m) to 11 ft (3.4 m). SEE: *abdominal regions* and *digestive system* for illus.

duplex i. A congenital doubling of the ileum.

ileus (ĭl′ē-ŭs) [Gr. *eileos,* a twisting] An intestinal obstruction. The term originally meant colic due to intestinal obstruction. It is characterized by loss of the forward flow of intestinal contents, often accompanied by abdominal cramps; constipation; fecal vomiting; abdominal distention; and collapse. SEE: *Nursing Diagnoses Appendix.*

PREVENTION: Prevention of adynamic (paralytic) ileus in postoperative patients occurs by encouraging early ambulation and gradually increasing activity. The patient should receive analgesics so that pain does not interfere with mobilization; however, because opioids slow gastrointestinal (GI) motility, a nonopioid should be used as soon as possible. Enteral feeding also should begin early (especially when surgery did not involve the GI tract). The patient is assessed for abdominal distention. In the absence of evidence of mechanical obstruction, oral intake may begin even before bowel sounds return. (Bowel sounds are an indication of bowel motility, not absorption; even when bowel sounds are absent the small bowel is capable of absorbing nutrients.) The sooner the patient is able to take food, the sooner motility will return. The patient who experiences gas pains should understand that such pains are a sign of recovery, and that walking will stimulate their passage. Since analgesics rarely help to decrease gas pains, heat is applied to the abdomen for relief instead.

PATIENT CARE: If ileus is diagnosed, the patient is told that it usually resolves in 2 to 3 days with mobilization and oral intake. Abdominal girth is measured frequently to detect progressive distention. If resolution does not occur after 48 hours, prescribed medications are administered, and the patient is monitored for the desired response (bowel motility) as well as for adverse effects. A nasogastric (NG) or nasointestinal tube is inserted as prescribed. Characteristics and quantity of drainage from the NG tube are documented, the tube is attached to continuous low suction for decompression, and the pH of drainage from an intestinal tube is measured to help determine its placement level. Since oral intake is withheld because of intubation, oral hygiene and misting are provided to manage dryness and prevent cracking, sordes, and salivary gland obstruction. Lemon and glycerine preparations, which may etch enamel and add to drying, are not used. Intravenous fluids are instituted, renal function is assessed, and fluid and electrolyte balance is monitored to maintain normal hydration. Vital signs also are monitored; any drop in blood pressure must be reported, since it may signify fluid sequestered in the small bowel, reducing plasma volume. The patient also is checked for signs of metabolic alkalosis or acidosis. If colonoscopy or rectal tube is used to aid decompression, the treatment is explained. When ileus develops secondary to another illness, such as severe infection or electrolyte imbalance, the primary problem is treated.

All newborns are observed for passage of meconium. Meconium ileus occurs in about 10% of infants with cystic fibrosis. In this situation, the newborn may pass an initial stool from the rectum with none thereafter. Usually, however, the newborn passes no meconium during the first 24 to 48 hours of life, and his or her abdomen becomes increasingly distended. The newborn with meconium ileus requires a laparotomy for diagnosis and treatment of the condition. In such a case, the infant is prepared for surgery, and the parents are given psychological and emotional support.

adynamic i. Intestinal obstruction resulting from lack of intestinal motility. This causes abdominal distention and interferes with postsurgical recovery, esp. from abdominal surgery. SYN: *i. paralyticus.*

PATIENT CARE: The entire abdomen is auscultated for bowel sounds and is assessed for distention by inspection, measurement of abdominal girth, and percussion for tympanic note every 4 to 8 hr as necessary. Nausea and vomiting, lack of passage of flatus, increases in girth, and changes in bowel sounds are documented and reported. If the ileus is still present after 24 to 48 hr, the patient is prepared for diagnostic tests, such as abdominal radiographs, and for treatment procedures, such as insertion of a nasogastric (NG) or intestinal (Cantor) tube for decompression. Prescribed medications, such as gastrointestinal stimulants or cholinergics, are given, and the patient is warned that intestinal cramping and diarrhea may result. The NG tube is kept open, the amount and character of drainage are recorded, and ambulation is encouraged to stimulate bowel activity. The health care provider evaluates desired therapeutic effects, checking frequently for return of bowel sounds and, if neostigmine (a cholinergic) is prescribed, for adverse cardiovascular effects such as bradycardia and hypotension.

dynamic i. Ileus caused by intestinal muscle contraction.

gallstone i. An obstruction of the

small bowel, occurring typically but not exclusively in elderly female patients and caused by the trapping of a large gallstone at or near the ileocecal valve. Most gallstones responsible for ileus are greater than 2.5 cm in diameter.

mechanical i. Ileus produced by a physical obstruction, such as a hernia, adhesion, or a tumor.

meconium i. Ileus of the newborn owing to obstruction of the bowel with meconium.

i. paralyticus Adynamic i.

postoperative i. Ileus resulting from handling the bowel during surgery, anesthesia, electrolyte imbalance, or intraperitoneal infection.

spastic i. Ileus due to spasm of a segment of the intestine.

ilia Pl. of ilium.

iliac [L. *iliacus,* pert. to ilium] Relating to the ilium.

i. crest The hip; the upper free margin of the ilium.

i. fascia Transversalis fascia over the anterior surface of the iliopsoas muscle.

i. fossa One of the concavities of the iliac bones of the pelvis.

i. region The inguinal region on either side of the hypogastrium.

i. spine One of four spines of the ilium, namely the anterior and posterior inferior spines and the anterior and posterior superior spines.

ilio- [L. *ilium,* flank] Combining form meaning *ilium* or *flank*.

iliococcygeal (ĭl″ē-ō-kŏk-sĭj′ē-ăl) [″ + Gr. *kokkyx,* coccyx] Concerning the ilium and coccyx.

iliocolotomy (ĭl″ē-ō-kō-lŏt′ō-mē) [″ + Gr. *kolon,* colon, + *tome,* incision] An opening into the colon in the iliac or inguinal region.

iliocostal (ĭl″ē-ō-kŏs′tăl) [″ + *costa,* rib] Joining or concerning the ilium and ribs.

iliofemoral (ĭl″ē-ō-fĕm′or-ăl) [″ + *femoralis,* pert. to femur] Pert. to the ilium and femur.

iliohypogastric (ĭl″ē-ō-hī″pō-găs′trĭk) [″ + Gr. *hypo,* under, + *gaster,* stomach] Concerning the ilium and hypogastrium.

ilioinguinal (ĭl″ē-ō-ĭn′gwĭ-năl) [″ + *inguinalis,* pert. to groin] Pert. to the groin and iliac regions.

iliolumbar (ĭl″ē-ō-lŭm′bar) [″ + *lumbus,* loin] Pert. to the iliac and lumbar regions.

iliopagus (ĭl″ē-ŏp′ă-gŭs) [″ + Gr. *pagos,* thing fixed] Twins joined in the iliac region.

iliopectineal (ĭl″ē-ō-pĕk-tĭn′ē-ăl) [L. *ilium,* flank, + *pecten,* a comb] Concerning the ilium and pubes.

iliopelvic (ĭl″ē-ō-pĕl′vĭk) [″ + *pelvis,* basin] Concerning the iliac area and pelvis.

iliopsoas (ĭl″ē-ō-sō′ăs) [″ + Gr. *psoa,* loin] The compound iliacus and psoas magnus muscles.

iliosacral (ĭl″ē-ō-sā′krăl) [″ + *sacralis,* pert. to the sacrum] Concerning the sacrum and ilium.

iliosciatic (ĭl″ē-ō-sī-ăt′ĭk) [″ + *sciaticus,* pert. to the ischium] Concerning the ilium and ischium.

iliospinal (ĭl″ē-ō-spī′năl) [″ + *spinalis,* pert. to the spine] Concerning the ilium and spinal column.

iliothoracopagus (ĭl″ē-ō-thō″ră-kŏp′ă-gŭs) [″ + Gr. *thorax,* chest, + *pagos,* thing fixed] Twins joined from pelvis to thorax.

ilioxiphopagus (ĭl″ē-ō-zī-fŏp′ă-gŭs) [″ + Gr. *xiphos,* sword, + *eidos,* form, shape, + *pagos,* thing fixed] Twins joined from the pelvis to the xiphoid process.

ilium (ĭl′ē-ŭm) *pl.* **ilia** [L., groin, flank] **1.** One of the bones of each half of the pelvis. It is the superior and widest part and serves to support the flank. In the child, before fusion with adjacent pelvic bones, it is a separate bone. SYN: *os ilium*. **2.** The flank. SEE: *sacroiliac*.

Ilizarow method [G. A. Ilizarow, Siberian surgeon, 1921–1992] Lengthening a bone by cutting through the outer layer but not into the marrow cavity. The two ends are held in place for a week and then slowly pulled apart with an external fixator device. This is known as distraction. The bone may be lengthened by about 1 mm/day. After lengthening is complete, the device is left in place for at least a month to allow complete healing of the bone. The bone is radiographically evaluated for completeness of healing before the device is removed.

ill (ĭl) [Old Norse *illr,* bad] Sick; not healthy; diseased.

illaqueation (ĭl″ăk-wē-ā′shŭn) [L. *illaqueare,* to ensnare] Turning an inverted eyelash by drawing a loop of thread behind it.

illiterate Being unable to read and write or to use written language as in understanding graphs, charts, tables, maps, symbols, and formulas.

illness (ĭl′nĭs) [Old Norse *illr,* bad, + AS. *-ness,* state of] **1.** Sickness; disease. **2.** An ailment.

catabolic i. Rapid weight loss with loss of body fat and muscle mass that frequently accompanies short-term, self-limiting conditions such as infection or injury. This condition may be associated with diabetic ketoacidosis, multiple organ system failure, and chemotherapy or radiation therapy for cancer.

TREATMENT: Inflammation should be reduced and appropriate nutrients provided.

catastrophic i. An unusually prolonged or complex illness, esp. one that causes severe organ dysfunction or threatens life. Catastrophic illnesses often make exceptional demands on patients, caregivers, families, and health care resources.

folk i. A disease or condition found only in specific societies, ethnic groups, or cultures. Often the culture has causal explanations for these illnesses, as well as preventive and treatment measures. Several such disorders exist in the Hispanic American culture; these are diagnosed and treated by folk healers called *curandieros.* Other examples of folk illnesses include *amok* and *piblokto,* although there are many others. SEE: *amok; piblokto.*

functional i. An illness for which no organic explanation is present. SYN: *functional disease.* SEE: *somatoform disorder; organic disease.*

heat i. A general term used to describe the harmful effects on the human body of being exposed to high temperature and/or humidity. SEE: *heat cramp; heat exhaustion; heat stroke; syncope.*

mental i. Any disorder that affects mood or behavior.

psychosomatic i. SEE: *somatoform disorder.*

terminal i. An illness that, because of its nature or because of the specific circumstances of the patient, will result in the death of the patient.

illumination (ĭl-lū-mĭn-ā′shŭn) [L. *illuminare,* to light up] The lighting up of a part for examination or of an object under a microscope.

axial i. Light transmitted along the axis of a microscope. SYN: *central i.*

central i. Axial i.

dark-field i. The illumination of an object under a microscope in which the central or axial light rays are stopped and the object is illuminated by light rays coming from the sides, which causes the object to appear light against a dark background. This technique is used to observe extremely small objects such as spirochetes or colloid particles.

direct i. The illumination of an object under a microscope by directing light rays upon its upper surface.

focal i. Concentration of light on an object by means of a mirror or a system of lenses.

oblique i. Illumination of an object from one side.

transmitted light i. Illumination in which the light is directed through the object. Light may come directly from a light source or be reflected by a mirror.

illusion [L. *illusio*] An inaccurate perception; a misinterpretation of sensory impressions, as opposed to a hallucination, which is a perception formed without an external stimulus. Vague stimuli are conducive to the production of illusions. If an illusion becomes fixed, it is said to be a delusion.

optical i. A visual impression that is inaccurately perceived.

illusional Pert. to, or of the nature of, an illusion.

I.M. *intramuscular(ly).*

im- Prefix that is used in place of *in-* before words beginning with *b, m,* or *p.*

ima (ī′mă) [L.] Lowest.

image (ĭm′ĭj) [L. *imago,* likeness] **1.** A mental picture representing a real object. **2.** A more or less accurate likeness of a thing or person. **3.** A picture of an object such as that produced by a lens or mirror. **4.** In radiology, a representation of structures within the body as a result of examination by various physical phenomena (e.g., x-rays, gamma rays, sound, or radio.

body i. **1.** The subjective image or picture people have of their physical appearance based on their own observations and the reaction of others. **2.** The conscious and unconscious perception of one's body at any particular time.

direct i. A picture produced from rays that are not yet focused. SYN: *virtual i.*

double i. A perceived image that occurs in strabismus when the visual axes of the eyes are not directed toward the same object. SYN: *false i.* SEE: *diplopia.*

false i. Double i.

i. intensifier A special vacuum tube used during fluoroscopic imaging that increases the brightness of an image. This increased brightness is controlled by image minification and electron acceleration. The minified image can be viewed directly, coupled with a television camera, or imaged by serial or digital radiography. The quality of the image is better than that of an unintensified fluoroscopic image.

inverted i. An image that is turned upside down.

latent i. **1.** In radiology, the image within the emulsion of an exposed radiograph that is invisible because it has not been developed. **2.** An unprocessed image physically present within an image receptor but not yet visible.

mirror i. An image of an object in which right and left are reversed. The term is also used to indicate the similarity of chemical substances or persons with quite similar personalities and looks (e.g., identical twins).

radiographic i. An x-ray image created on an image receptor (e.g., photographic film) by x-rays passed through a structure.

real i. The image formed by convergence of rays of light from an object.

virtual i. Direct i.

imagery (ĭm′ĭj-rē) [L. *imago,* likeness] **1.** Imagination; the calling up of events or mental pictures. Mental imagery may be of various types. **2.** A form of distraction in which the patient is stimulated to visualize or think about pleasant or desirable feelings, sensations, or events. This is done to divert the patient's attention away from pain or disease.

active i. The conscious formation of a mental picture. This may be used by a patient to counter tense feelings or to imagine that an unwanted symptom is disappearing.

auditory i. A mental image of sounds that can be recalled, as thunder or wind.

smell i. A mental concept of odor previously experienced.

tactile i. A mental image of the way an object feels.

taste i. A mental concept of taste sensations previously experienced.

visual i. A mental concept of an object seen previously. SEE: *afterimage.*

imagination [L. *imago,* likeness] The formation of mental images of things, persons, or situations that are wholly or partially different from those previously known or experienced.

imaging The production of a picture, image, or shadow that represents the object being investigated. In diagnostic medicine the classic technique for imaging is radiographic or x-ray examination. Techniques using computer-generated images produced by x-ray, ultrasound, or magnetic resonance are also available.

digital subtraction i. In radiology, use of electronic means to subtract portions of the radiograph image in order to better visualize the object.

myocardial perfusion i. ABBR: MPI. Using radioactive isotopes, such as ^{201}Tl or ^{99}mTc sestamibi, to gauge the blood supply and viability of the regions or walls of the heart. MPI frequently is used to assess patients with coronary artery disease, often in conjunction with exercise tolerance tests. A patient with a coronary artery that is almost totally blocked, for example, may take up only a small quantity of radioisotope during exercise but much more of the tracer after several hours of rest. By contrast, heart muscle that is fed by a completely blocked artery will take up no radioisotope either during or after exercise.

imago (ĭ-mā'gō) [L., likeness] **1.** An image or shadow. **2.** A memory, esp. of a loved one, developed during childhood that has become clouded by idealism and imagination. **3.** The adult, sexually mature form of an insect.

imbalance [L. *in-,* not, + *bilanx,* two scales] Lack of balance; the state of inequality in power between opposing forces.

autonomic i. An imbalance between sympathetic and parasympathetic divisions of the autonomic nervous system, esp. as pertains to vasomotor reactions.

sympathetic i. Vagotonia.

vasomotor i. Excessive vasoconstriction or vasodilation resulting from impulses to blood vessels.

imbecile (ĭm'bĕ-sĭl) [L. *imbecillus,* feeble] Former term for an individual with severe mental deficiency. SEE: *mental retardation.*

imbecility Former term for a state of severe mental deficiency.

imbed [L. *in,* in, (put) into, + AS. *bedd,* bed] In histology, to surround with a firm substance, such as paraffin, preparatory to cutting sections. SEE: *embedding.*

imbibition (ĭm"bĭ-bĭsh'ŭn) [" + *bibere,* to drink] The absorption of fluid by a solid body or gel.

imbricated, imbrication (ĭm'brĭ-kāt-ĕd, ĭm"brĭ-kā'shŭn) [L. *imbricare,* to tile] **1.** Overlapping, as tiles. **2.** The overlapping of aponeurotic layers in abdominal surgery.

imidazole (ĭm-ĭd-ăz'ōl) An organic compound, $C_3H_4N_2$, characterized structurally by the presence of the heterocyclic ring that occurs in histidine and histamine.

imide (ĭm'ĭd) A compound with the bivalent atom group (—NH).

IMIG *intramuscular immune globulin.*

imipramine hydrochloride (ĭ-mĭp'ră-mēn) A tricyclic antidepressant that can be used to treat depression, panic disorder, agoraphobia, and, because of its anticholinergic side effects, bedwetting. Common side effects include dry mouth, constipation, urinary retention, and drowsiness.

immature (ĭm"mă-tūr') [L. *in-,* not, + *maturus,* ripe] Not fully developed or ripened.

immediate [" + *mediare,* to be in middle] Direct; without intervening steps.

immedicable (ĭ-mĕd'ĭ-kă-b'l) [L. *immedicabilis*] Incurable; pert. to that which cannot be healed.

immersion (ĭm-ĕr'shŭn) [L. *in,* into, + *mergere,* to dip] **1.** Placing a body under water or other fluid. **2.** In microscopy, the act of immersing the objective (then called an immersion lens) in water or oil, preventing total reflection of rays falling obliquely upon peripheral portions of the objective.

i. foot Damage to the foot owing to continued exposure to water or to moisture, e.g., hiking through streams, mud, or puddles. Symptoms of numbness, tingling, and leg cramping are present. The condition can be prevented with waterproof insulated shoes and socks. SEE: *trench foot.*

homogeneous i. Immersion in which the stratum of air between objective and cover glass is replaced by a medium that deflects as little as possible the rays of light passing through the cover glass.

immiscible (ĭ-mĭs'ĭ-bl) [L. *in-,* not, + *miscere,* to mix] Pert. to that which cannot be mixed, as oil and water.

immobilization [″ + *mobilis,* movable] The making of a part or limb immovable. SEE: illus.

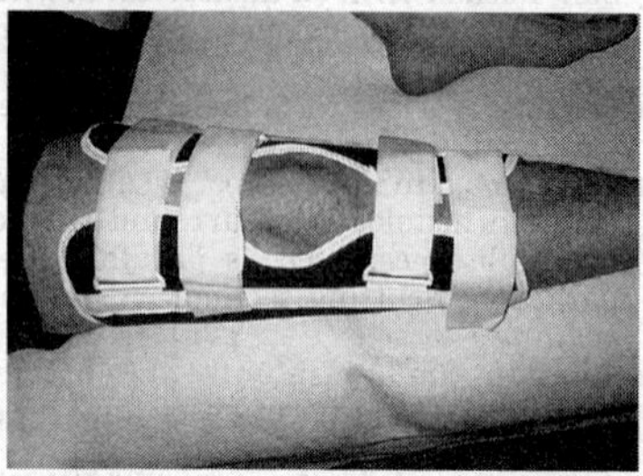

KNEE IMMOBILIZATION

PATIENT CARE: The patient is assessed for development of any of the complications of immobilization, such as pneumonia, thrombophlebitis, urinary tract infections, constipation, decubitus ulcers, and contracture formation. Lung and heart sounds are auscultated, fluid balance and nutritional and dietary fiber intake monitored, bowel sounds auscultated, and bowel and bladder function are assessed. Long-term immobilization will result in the atrophy of skeletal muscle and decreased cardiorespiratory capacity.

Techniques to prevent such complications include having the patient deep breathe and cough every 2 hours, using incentive spirometry if prescribed; completely change position every 2 hours, with lesser position changes in between; wear antithromboembolic devices; do quadriceps setting, gluteal muscle setting, and range-of-motion exercises at least daily; ensure good body hygiene; maintain nutrition, including adequate dietary fiber, protein, and vitamin C intake; and increase fluid intake to 3 liters daily, unless otherwise restricted by renal or cardiac disorders. Skin care is provided, the skin is inspected daily for redness and signs of breakdown, intact areas are gently massaged to increase circulation, and low-pressure foam or flotation pads or mattresses are applied as needed. The health care professional should ensure that blood supply to the extremities is not restricted by any appliance or by tight bedcovers, evaluate distal neurovascular and circulatory status, and note changes in size of extremities, pallor or other changes in color, temperature changes, and pain.

immortality The ability of some cells, particularly cancer cells, to reproduce indefinitely. Normal human cells have a finite life expectancy. They may divide for a few dozen generations, but eventually stop reproducing and die.

immotile cilia syndrome An inherited condition marked by reduced fertility in women and sterility in men. This condition is due to the absence or deficiency of the dynein arms of the cilia, causing them to beat ineffectively. The normal motion of the cilia is 1000 cycles/min. SEE: *dynein; Kartagener's syndrome.*

immune (ĭm-ūn′) [L. *immunis,* safe] Protected from or resistant to a disease or infection by a pathogenic organism as a result of the development of antibodies or cell-mediated immunity.

i. complex A substance formed when antibodies attach to antigens to destroy them. These complexes circulate in the blood and may eventually attach to the walls of blood vessels, producing a local inflammatory response. Immune complexes form in type III hypersensitivity reactions and are involved in the development of glomerulonephritis, serum sickness, arthritis, and vasculitis, which may be called immune-complex diseases.

mucosal i. system Clusters of lymphoid cells beneath the mucosal endothelium of the gastrointestinal, respiratory, and genitourinary tracts that help protect the body from inhaled, consumed, or sexually transmitted infections. The system has two parts: organized and diffuse. The organized part (the mucosal-associated lymphoid tissue of the gastrointestinal and respiratory tracts) is composed of nodules containing lymphocytes and macrophages that are activated by ingested or inhaled microorganisms. The diffuse part is composed of loose clusters of macrophages and mature B and T lymphocytes found within the folds of the intestinal walls. The B cells secrete antibodies, primarily immunoglobulin A; the T cells directly lyse microorganisms.

The mucosal immune system is augmented by the presence of normal microflora; peristalsis and cilia, which move mucus outward; and various chemicals, such as gastric acid and pancreatic enzymes, that destroy pathogens. Normally all of these components must be functioning to prevent infection. SEE: *gut-associated lymphoid tissue; immunoglobulin A.*

primary i. response The initial reaction to an immunogen, during which T and B lymphocytes are activated and antibodies specific to the antigen are produced. This reaction is considered relatively weak but produces large numbers of antigen-specific memory cells.

i. reaction **1.** A demonstrated antigenic response to a specific antibody. **2.** The specific reaction of host cells to antigenic stimulation. SEE: *i. response.*

i. response The body's reaction to foreign antigens so that they are neutralized or eliminated, thus preventing the diseases or injuries these antigens might cause. It requires that the body recognize the antigen as "nonself," or foreign. There are several major components to the immune response. The *nonspecific immune response,* or inflammation, is the response of the body's tissues and cells to injury from any source (e.g., trauma, organisms, chemicals, ischemia). As the initial response of the immune system to any threat, it involves vascular, chemical, and white blood cell activities. The *specific immune response,* involving T cells and B cells, is a reaction to injury or invasion by particular organisms or foreign proteins. The *cell-mediated immune response* refers to the activity of T lymphocytes (T cells) produced by the thymus, in response to antigen exposure. Without T cells, the body cannot protect itself against many disease-causing microbes. The loss of T cells in patients with acquired immunodeficiency syndrome (AIDS), for example, leads to infections with many opportunistic microbes that would otherwise be relatively well tolerated by persons with intact cellular immunity. T-cell activity also is the basis for delayed hypersensitivity, rejection of tissue transplants, and responses to cancers. The *humoral immune response* refers to the production of antigen-specific antibodies by plasma B lymphocytes (B cells); antibodies attach to foreign antigens in the bloodstream, helping to inactivate or remove them. SEE: *cell-mediated i.; humoral i.; inflammation.*

secondary i. response The rapid, strong response by T and B cells to a second or subsequent appearance of an immunogen. This occurs because of the availability of T and B lymphocyte memory cells.

i. system The lymphatic tissues, organs, and physiological processes that identify an antigen as abnormal or foreign and prevent it from harming the body. The skin, mucosa, normal flora of the gastrointestinal tract and skin, and chemicals contained in tears, sebaceous glands, gastric acid, and pancreatic enzymes protect the body from pathogen invasion. The bone marrow produces white blood cells (WBCs), the primary internal defense. Lymphoid tissues, including the thymus gland, spleen, and lymph nodes, influence the growth, maturation, and activation of WBCs; lymphoid tissue in the gastrointestinal and respiratory tracts and mucous membranes contain WBCs for site-specific protection. Finally, physiologically active protein mediators, called cytokines, help regulate the growth and function of immunologically active cells.

Effects of stress: Investigations of the influence of stress on susceptibility to disease have shown that in some, but not all, individuals who experienced undesirable events, the possibility of onset of illness was increased. A decrease in the usual number of pleasant events was a stronger predictor of susceptibility to illness than was an increase in unpleasant ones. Negative experiences included criticism, frustration, irritating encounters with fellow workers, deadlines, heavy workload, and burdensome and unpleasant chores or errands. Even though the concept that stress lowers resistance to disease appears to apply only to some individuals, the explanation of this mechanism has not been established.

immune globulin Drug created from serum containing antibodies (immunoglobulins). It is used to supply necessary antibodies to patients with immunoglobulin deficiencies and to provide passive immunization against common viral infections (e.g., hepatitis A, measles). It also has been used successfully to treat patients with idiopathic thrombocytopenic purpura because it seems to inhibit phagocytosis of platelets coated with autoantibodies, although the exact mechanism of its action is unknown.

cytomegalovirus i.g. intravenous An immune globulin preparation containing cytomegalovirus (CMV)–specific antibodies used to treat or prevent CMV infection after organ or tissue transplantation. Antiviral drugs like ganciclovir may be used for the same purpose.

intramuscular i.g. A preparation of immune globulin that is injected directly into a muscle. It can be used to provide passive immunity to a wide variety of infections including, for example, hepatitis A.

intravenous i.g. ABBR: IVIG. An immune globulin preparation used intravenously in patients with immunodeficiency syndromes and in immunosuppressed recipients of bone marrow transplants. In conjunction with aspirin, it is the standard of care for children during the first 10 days of Kawasaki disease to prevent the development of coronary aneurysms.

IVIG is also used to treat idiopathic thrombocytopenic purpura and Guillain-Barré syndrome, as well as to prevent bacterial infections in patients with hypogammaglobulinemia or recurrent infections associated with B-cell chronic lymphocytic leukemia.

CAUTION: The administration of sucrose-containing IVIGs has been associated with acute renal failure, which in about 10% of patients has proved fatal. Patients should be hydrated before being treated with IVIG.

Rh_0(D) i.g. A solution of immune globulin containing anti-Rh antibodies. It is given to Rh-negative women at 28 weeks' gestation and within 72 hours after delivery of an Rh-positive infant. It prevents hemolytic disease of the newborn (erythroblastosis fetalis) in subsequent pregnancies in which the mother has an Rh-positive fetus by blocking the formation of maternal antibodies against Rh-positive red blood cells. These maternal antibodies would otherwise cross the placenta in subsequent pregnancies, injuring the fetus. SEE: *Rh blood group.*

CAUTION: Rh_0(D) immune globulin should not be injected intravenously.

tetanus i.g. An immune globulin containing tetanus-specific antibodies used for patients with unknown history of tetanus immunization who present with symptoms of tetanus or with wounds that might be contaminated with tetanus spores. SEE: *tetanus.*

varicella-zoster i.g. ABBR: VZIG. An immune globulin, primarily immunoglobulin, used for passive immunization of susceptible immunodeficient individuals after significant exposure to varicella. VZIG does not modify established varicella-zoster infections.

CAUTION: VZIG should not be injected intravenously.

immunifacient (ĭ-mū″nĭ-fā′shĕnt) [″ + *facere,* to make] Making immune.

immunity [L. *immunitas*] Protection from diseases, esp. infectious diseases. SEE: *immune response; immune system; immunization; vaccine.*

acquired i. Immunity that results either from exposure to an antigen or from the passive injection of immunoglobulins.

active i. Immunity resulting from the development within the body of antibodies or sensitized T lymphocytes that neutralize or destroy the infective agent. This may result from the immune response to an invading organism or from inoculation with a vaccine containing a foreign antigen. SEE: *immune response; vaccination.*

B-cell–mediated i. SEE: *humoral i.*

cell-mediated i. The regulatory and cytotoxic activities of T cells during the specific immune response. This process requires about 36 hr to reach its full effect. SYN: *T-cell–mediated i.* SEE: illus.; *humoral i.*

Unlike B cells, T cells cannot recognize foreign antigens on their own. Foreign antigens are recognized by antigen-presenting cells (APCs), such as macrophages, which engulf them and display part of the antigens on the APC's surface next to a histocompatibility or "self" antigen (macrophage processing). The presence of these two markers, plus the cytokine interleukin-1 (IL-1), secreted by the APCs, activates CD4 helper T cells (T_H cells), which regulate the activities of other cells involved in the immune response.

CMI includes direct lysis of target cells by cytotoxic T cells, creation of memory cells that trigger a rapid response when a foreign antigen is encountered for the second time, and delayed hypersensitivity to tissue and organ transplants. T cells also stimulate the activity of macrophages, B cells, and natural killer cells. These functions are controlled largely by the secretion of lymphokines such as the interleukins, interferons, and colony-stimulating factors; lymphokines facilitate communication and proliferation of the cells in the immune system.

congenital i. Immunity present at birth. It may be natural or acquired, the latter depending on antibodies received from the mother's blood.

herd i. The ability of a community to resist epidemic disease. Herd immunity may develop naturally in a society as a result of widespread exposure to disease or it may be stimulated artificially by mass vaccination programs.

humoral i. The protective activities of antibodies against infection or reinfection by common organisms (e.g., streptococci and staphylococci). B lymphocytes with receptors to a specific antigen react when they encounter that antigen by producing plasma cells (which produce antigen-specific antibodies) and memory cells (which enable the body to produce these antibodies quickly should the same antigen appear later). B-cell differentiation also is stimulated by interleukin-2 (IL-2) and secreted by T4 cells and foreign antigens processed by macrophages.

Antibodies produced by plasma B cells, found mainly in the blood, spleen, and lymph nodes, neutralize or destroy antigens in several ways. They kill organisms by activating the complement system, neutralize viruses and toxins released by bacteria, coat the antigen (opsonization), or form an antigen-antibody complex to stimulate phagocytosis, promote antigen clumping (agglutination), and prevent the antigen from adhering to host cells. SYN: *B-cell–mediated i.* SEE: illus.; *cell-mediated i.; immunoglobulin.*

local i. Immunity limited to a given area or tissue of the body.

natural i. Immunity that is genetically determined in specific species, populations, or families. Some pathogens

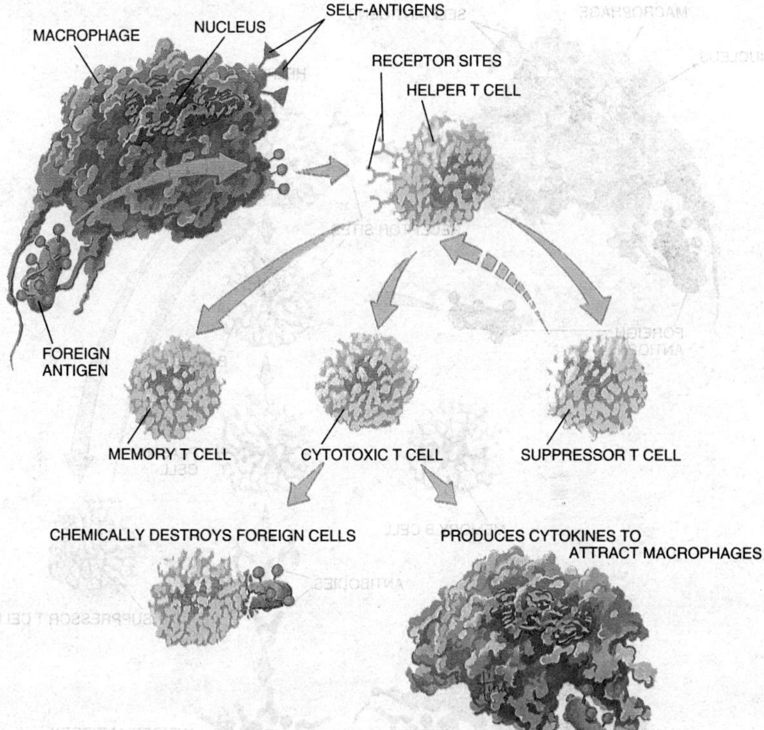

CELL-MEDIATED IMMUNITY

cannot infect certain species because the cells are not suitable environments (e.g., the measles virus cannot reproduce in canine cells; therefore, dogs have natural immunity to measles).

passive i. Immunity acquired by the introduction of preformed antibodies into an unprotected individual. This can occur through intravenous infusion of immune globulin or, in utero, from antibodies that pass from the mother to the fetus through the placenta. Newborns also may acquire immunity through breastfeeding.

T-cell–mediated i. SYN: *cell-mediated i.*

immunization [L. *immunitas,* immunity] The protection of individuals or groups from specific diseases by vaccination or the injection of immune globulins. SEE: *vaccination; vaccine* for table.

immunoablation (ĭm-ū″-nō-ă-blā′shŭn) The systematic destruction of a patient's immune competence. Immunoablation is used to prepare patients for organ transplantation and to treat refractory autoimmune diseases.

PATIENT CARE: Patients who have undergone immunoablation may be easily infected by caregivers. Careful handwashing and reverse isolation techniques should be used to limit exposing these patients to harmful pathogens.

immunoassay (ĭm″ū-nō-ăs′sā) [L. *immunis,* safe, + O.Fr. *assai,* trial] Measuring the protein and protein-bound molecules that are concerned with the reaction of an antigen with its specific antibody. SEE: *immunoelectrophoresis; immunofluorescence; radioimmunoassay.*

cloned enzyme donor i. ABBR: CEDIA. A homogeneous enzyme immunoassay (EIA), based on the modulation of enzyme activity by bound fragments of beta-galactosidase.

end point i. An immunoassay in which the signal is measured as the antigen-antibody complex reaches equilibrium.

enzyme i. ABBR: EIA. A method used to measure immunochemical reactions based on the catalytic properties of enzymes. One heterogeneous EIA technique, enzyme-linked immunosorbent assay (ELISA), and two homoge-

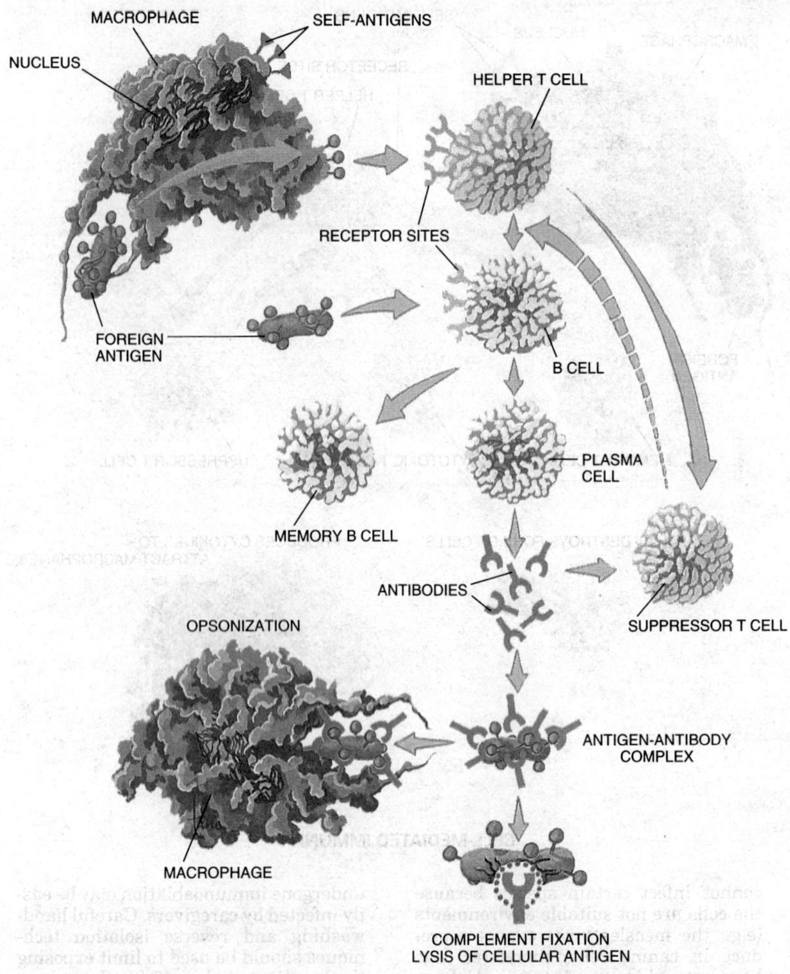

HUMORAL IMMUNITY

neous techniques, enzyme-multiplied immunoassay technique (EMIT) and cloned enzyme donor immunoassay (CEDIA), are widely used.

sandwich i. An immunoassay in which the analyte is bound to a solid phase and a labeled reagent subsequently bound immunochemically to the analyte.

immunobiology (ĭm″ū-nō-bī-ŏl′ō-jē) [″ + Gr. *bios,* life, + *logos,* word, reason] The study of immune phenomena in biological systems, including the immune response to infectious diseases, transplantation of organs, allergy, autoimmunity, and cancer.

immunochemistry (ĭm″ū-nō-kĕm′ĭs-trē) [″ + Gr. *chemeia,* chemistry] The chemistry of immunization; the chemistry of antigens, antibodies, and their relation to each other.

immunocompetence (ĭm″ū-nō-kŏm′pĕ-tĕns) The ability of the body's immune system to respond to pathogenic organisms and tissue damage. This ability may be diminished by drugs specifically developed to inhibit immune cell function (e.g., chemotherapeutic agents used to treat leukemia and drugs used to prevent organ transplant rejections), by diseases that attack elements of the immune system, or overwhelming infections. SEE: *immunocompromised.*

immunocompromised Having an immune system that is incapable of a normal, full reaction to pathogens or tissue damage, as the result of a disease (e.g., diabetes mellitus, overwhelming sepsis, or the acquired immunodeficiency syndrome) or drug therapy with agents that inhibit components of the immune system. SYN: *immunodeficient*. SEE: *immune system*.

immunoconglutinin (ĭm″ū-nō-kŏn-gloo′tĭ-nĭn) [″ + *conglutinare*, to glue together] A protein used in the laboratory to assess the number of immune complexes in blood, which may be related to immunological activity. It acts by binding with complement factor 3, a significant part of an antigen-antibody immune complex.

immunocytoadherence A laboratory test used to identify antibody-bearing cells by the formation of rosettes composed of red blood cells and those cells bearing antibodies.

immunodeficiency (ĭm″ū-nō-dĕ-fĭsh′ĕn-sē) Decreased or compromised ability to respond to antigenic stimuli with an appropriate immune response, as the result of one or more disorders in B-cell–mediated immunity, T-cell–mediated immunity, phagocytic cells, or complement. This state may be genetic or acquired following infections, drug abuse, multiple transfusions, immunosuppressive therapy, or malnutrition. The diagnosis is made through measurement of white blood cell counts or serum immunoglobulin and complement levels. Affected patients develop chronic infections that are difficult to treat and recur frequently; these infections frequently are caused by opportunistic organisms. Other findings related to the type and degree of deficiency in the immune system include failure to thrive, thrombocytopenia, and hepatosplenomegaly. Treatments vary depending on the underlying cause. They may include combinations of antiviral agents in the acquired immunodeficiency syndrome; infusions of immune globulin (IVIG) in disorders of humoral immunity; bone marrow transplantation in patients with malignancies; and antibiotics that specifically treat active infections. Cytokine therapy and gene therapy may play a role in the treatment of patients with defined genetic defects. SEE: *acquired immunodeficiency syndrome; agammaglobulinemia*. **immunodeficient,** *adj.*

immunodeficiency disease, severe combined ABBR: SCID. Any of a group of inherited autosomal or X-linked recessive disorders in which there is partial or complete dysfunction of the immune system. Defects are present in both B- and T-cell–mediated immunity responses and frequently include defective cytokine function. Within 6 months after birth, babies develop infections from bacterial, viral, fungal, or protozoan organisms. Intravenous immune globulin (IVIG) is given to provide antibodies, but a successful bone marrow transplant is required to prevent death. The efficacy of gene therapy is under investigation. SEE: *cytokine; cell-mediated immunity; humoral immunity*.

immunodeficient Immunocompromised.

immunodiagnosis (ĭm″ū-nō-dī″ăg-nō′sĭs) The use of antibody assays, immunocytochemistry, the detection of lymphocyte markers, and other strategies to diagnose infectious and malignant diseases.

immunodiffusion (ĭm″ū-nō-dĭ-fū′zhŭn) A test method in which an antigen and antibody are placed in a gel, where they diffuse toward each other. When they meet, a precipitate is formed.

immunoelectrophoresis (ĭ-mū″nō-ē-lĕk″trō-fō-rē′sĭs) A method of investigating the amount and character of proteins and antibodies in body fluids by using electrophoresis.

immunofluorescence (ĭm″ū-nō-floo″ō-rĕs′ĕns) The detection of antibodies by using special proteins labeled with fluorescein. If the specific organism or antibody that is being searched for is present, it is observed as a fluorescent material when examined microscopically while illuminated with a fluorescent light source.

immunogen (ĭ-mū′nō-jĕn) [″ + Gr. *gennan*, to produce] A substance capable of producing an immune response. Proteins and polysaccharides may be strong immunogens, but lipids and nucleic acids may also be immunogenic. SEE: *antigen*.

immunogenetics (ĭm″ū-nō-jĕ-nĕt′ĭks) [″ + Gr. *gennan*, to produce] The study of the influence of genetic factors on one's susceptibility to infectious diseases (e.g., malaria) and autoimmune illnesses (e.g., rheumatoid arthritis) or on one's suitability for organ transplantation. SEE: *histocompatibility* and its subentries.

immunogenic (ĭm″ū-nō-jĕn′ĭk) Capable of inducing an immune response. This response depends on the properties of both the immunogen and the host. It is essential that the host recognize that the immunogen is foreign (i.e., nonself).

immunogenicity (ĭm″ū-nō-jĕ-nĭs′ĭ-tē) The capacity to induce a detectable immune response.

immunoglobulin (ĭm″ū-nō-glŏb′ū-lĭn) ABBR: Ig. **1.** A diverse group of plasma proteins, made up of polypeptide chains, that are one of the primary mechanisms for protection against organisms. Two different forms exist. The first group of immunoglobulins lie on the surface of mature B cells, enabling them to bind to thousands of antigens. When the antigens are bound, the B plasma cells secrete the second type of immunoglobulins, antigen-specific antibodies, which circulate in the blood and accumulate in lymphoid tissue, esp. the spleen and lymph nodes, binding and destroying specific foreign antigens and stimulating other immune activity. Antibodies also activate the complement cascade, neutralize bacterial toxins and viruses, and function as opsonins, stimulating phagocytosis.

Immunoglobulins are formed by light and heavy (depending on molecular weight) chains of polypeptides made up of about 100 amino acids. These chains determine the structure of antigen-binding sites and, therefore, the specificity of the antibody to one antigen. The five types of immunoglobulins (IgA, IgD, IgE, IgE, IgM) account for approximately 30% of all plasma proteins. Antibodies are one of the three classes of globulins, or plasma proteins, in the blood that contribute to maintaining colloidal oncotic pressure. SYN: *antibody*. SEE: *antigen; B cell*.

2. A name commonly used for immune globulin, a solution containing antibodies to specific organisms that are obtained from donated human plasma.

i. A ABBR: IgA. The principal immunoglobulin in exocrine secretions such as milk, respiratory and intestinal mucin, saliva, and tears. It prevents pathogenic bacteria and viruses from invading the body through the mucosa of the gastrointestinal, pulmonary, and genitourinary tracts. Its presence in colostrum and breast milk helps prevent infection in breastfeeding infants.

i. D ABBR: IgD. An immunoglobulin that is present on the surface of B lymphocytes and acts as an antigen receptor.

i. E ABBR: IgE. An immunoglobulin that attaches to mast cells in the respiratory and intestinal tracts and plays a major role in allergic reactions. About 50% of patients with allergies have increased IgE levels. IgE is also important in the formation of reagin, a type of immunoglobulin gamma E (IgGE), found in the blood of individuals with an atopic hypersensitivity.

i. G ABBR: IgG. The principal immunoglobulin in human serum. Because it moves across the placental barrier, IgG is important in producing immunity in the infant before birth. It is the major antibody for antitoxins, viruses, and bacteria. It also activates complement and serves as an opsonin. As gamma globulin, IgG may be given to provide temporary resistance to hepatitis or other diseases.

intravenous i. ABBR: IVIG. A solution containing concentrated human immunoglobulins (antibodies), primarily IgG. IVIG has numerous uses in health care, including as replacement therapy for patients with primary immune deficiencies; as a treatment for those with Kawasaki disease, bullous pemphigoid, Guillain-Barré syndrome, idiopathic thrombocytopenic purpura, chronic inflammatory demyelinating polyneuropathy, and other immune-mediated illnesses; and as a means of providing patients with passive immunity against infectious diseases.

i. M ABBR: IgM. An immunoglobulin formed in almost every immune response during the early period of the reaction. IgM controls the A, B, O blood group antibody responses and is the most efficient antibody in stimulating complement activity. Its size prevents its moving across the placenta to the fetus.

immunohematology (ĭ-mū-nō-hēm″ă-tŏl′ō-jē) [L. *immunis,* safe, + Gr. *haima,* blood, + *logos,* word, reason] The study of the immunology and genetics of blood groups, blood cell antigens and antibodies, and specific blood proteins (such as complement); esp. important in blood banking and transfusion medicine.

immunoincompetency An inability to produce an immune response. SEE: *immunodeficiency*.

immunological therapy Immunotherapy.

immunologist (ĭm″ū-nŏl′ō-jĭst) An individual whose special training and experience is in immunology.

immunology (ĭm″ū-nŏl′ō-jē) [″ + Gr. *logos,* word, reason] The study of the components of the immune system and their function. SEE: *immune system*. **immunologic** (ĭm″ū-nō-lŏj′ĭk), *adj*.

immunomagnetic technique The use of magnetic microspheres to sort, isolate, or identify cells with specific antigenic markers.

immunomodulation **1.** The alteration of immune responses with monoclonal antibodies, cytokines, glucocorticoids, immunoglobulins, ultraviolet light, plasmapheresis, or related agents known to alter cellular or humoral immunity. SEE: *immunotherapy; biological response modifier*. **2.** In alternative medicine, the use of vitamins, minerals, natural foods, or other nutrients to promote health or prevent degenerative or malignant diseases. SEE: *biotherapy*.

immunonutrition (ĭm″ū-nō-nū-trĭ′shŭn) The study of the effects of nutrients including macronutrients, vitamins, minerals, and trace elements on inflammation, the actions of white blood cells, the formation of antibodies, and the resistance to disease.

immunopathology (ĭm″ū-nō-pă-thŏl′ō-jē) The study of tissue alterations that result from immune or allergic reactions.

immunophenotyping Differentiation among subsets of lymphocytes, using antibodies that select for identifying molecules on their cell membranes.

immunoprecipitation (ĭm″ū-nō-prē-sĭp″ĭ-tā′shŭn) The formation of a precipitate when an antigen and antibody interact.

immunoproliferative (ĭm″ū-nō-prō-lĭf′ĕr-ă-tĭv) The proliferation of cells and tissues involved in producing antibodies.

immunoprotein (ĭm″ū-nō-prō′tē-ĭn) [″ + Gr. *protos,* first] An immunologically active protein, esp. one that is used as a target for immunological probes or therapies.

immunoreactant (ĭ-mū″nō-rē-ăk′tănt) Any of the substances involved in immunologic reactions, including immunoglobulins, complement components, and specific antigens.

immunoreaction (ĭ-mū″nō-rē-ăk′shŭn) The reaction of an antibody to an antigen, exploited in some laboratory tests that stain, isolate, or purify cells that express specific markers on their cell membranes.

immunoselection (ĭm″ū-nō-sĕ-lĕk′shŭn) The selective survival of cell lives owing to their having the least amount of cell surface antigenicity. This aspect allows those cells to escape the destructive activity of either antibodies or immune lymphoid cells.

immunosenescence The age-associated decline of the immune system and host defense mechanisms. Elderly individuals frequently have a decline in cell-mediated immunity and secondary declines in humoral immunity. The clinician caring for an elderly patient can assume that the individual has defective host defenses, is at greater risk for developing an infectious disease, and has an increased risk of morbidity and mortality from infectious diseases.

immunostimulator (ĭm″ū-nō-stĭm′ū-lā-tŏr) SEE: *immunotherapy*.

immunosuppression (ĭm″ū-nō-sū-prĕsh′ŭn) Prevention of the activation of immune responses. **immunosuppressive,** *adj.*

immunosurveillance (ĭm″ū-nō-sĕr-vā′lĕns) The immune system's recognition and destruction of newly developed abnormal cells that arise from mutations of cell lines. This would occur in cancer cells that contained new antigens.

immunotherapy (ĭm″ū-nō-thĕr′ă-pē) [″ + Gr. *therapeia,* treatment] The use of natural and synthetic substances to stimulate or suppress the immune response, to treat deficits, or to interfere with the growth of malignant neoplasms. Therapeutic agents are either antigen specific or non–antigen specific. Immunological therapies include cytokines (e.g., alpha interferon and interleukin-2), monoclonal antibodies, intravenous immune globulin, heat shock proteins, and cancer vaccines, among others. SYN: *immunological therapy*.

adoptive i. The treatment of malignancies with T cells that are taken from patients with cancer, grown and activated in a culture where they are stimulated to react to specific tumor antigens, and then returned to patients by infusion. The adopted T cells invade the cancer and immunologically reject it. Side effects of the treatment include fever and nausea, among others.

passive i. The prevention of disease by administering antibodies in the form of a gamma globulin infusion or injection. Preparations enriched with specific antibodies can be used, for example, to prevent hepatitis B (HBIG), tetanus (Hyper-Tet), and chickenpox (VZIG).

stimulation i. The therapeutic use of agents that stimulate immune function (immunostimulants). These agents include cytokines and cytokine antagonists, monoclonal antibodies, compounds obtained from bacteria, and hormones from the thymus. The most successful immunostimulants have been laboratory-prepared cytokines, the protein mediators of immune responses. Granulocyte colony-stimulating factor (G-CSF) and granulocyte-macrophage colony-stimulating factor (GM-CSF) are used widely to increase white blood cell production in the bone marrow following cancer chemotherapy, bone marrow transplantation, and AIDS. Erythropoietin is effective in treating anemia in patients with chronic renal failure, AIDS, and bone marrow depression following cancer therapy. Transforming growth factor beta seems to enhance wound healing and reduce fibrotic changes following inflammation. Interleukins and interferons are being studied for their beneficial effects in patients with certain leukemias and other malignant tumors. Lymphocyte-activated killer (LAK) cells and tumor-infiltrating lymphocytes (TILs), which are lymphocytes that have been removed from the patient and stimulated with interleukin-2, also show promise in treating malignant tumors. Monoclonal antibodies against mediators of inflammation have been created in the laboratory from hybridomas and are being studied for clinical use.

Bacteria-based compounds, which produce nonspecific stimulation, have been used the longest. Attenuated (weak) solutions of *Mycobacterium bovis* (bacille Calmette-Guérin) and endotoxins from *Staphylococcus aureus* and OK432, prepared from *Streptococcus pyogenes,* are being used as adjunct cancer therapy because of their ability to activate natural killer cells, T cells, and macrophages. New techniques have enabled researchers to isolate hormones from the thymus gland, where T lymphocytes mature, to treat viral infections and cancers. Their clinical effectiveness has not been established. SEE: *cytokine; monoclonal antibody.*

suppressive i. Any treatment used to block abnormal or excessive immune responses.

Corticosteroids, the most widely known anti-inflammatory agents, increase the number of neutrophils in the blood but decrease their aggregation at inflammatory sites, decrease the number and function of other white blood cells, and inhibit cytokine production. They are most effective during an acute flareup of a chronic autoimmune disease and in conjunction with other agents because they do not adequately block autoantibodies when used alone.

Cytotoxic drugs kill all white blood cells and their precursors and were originally developed as anticancer agents. However, low-dose methotrexate is now known to be effective in reducing the symptoms and the need for corticosteroids in chronic inflammatory diseases such as rheumatoid arthritis, Crohn's disease, psoriasis, and asthma.

Cyclosporin and *tacrolimus* are related to the cytotoxic drugs, but these drugs selectively inhibit helper T-cell production of interleukin-2, effectively preventing replication rather than killing them. They are used extensively to prevent rejection of transplanted tissue and graft-versus-host disease.

Intravenous gamma globulin (IVIG) is used routinely to replace antibodies in patients with immunodeficiency disorders. However, it also can be used as an immunosuppressive. IVIG inhibits phagocytosis of platelets in idiopathic thrombocytopenic purpura; it has been most successful in the treatment of children but also can produce a short-term remission in adults. Because it seems to inhibit natural killer cells and augment suppressor T cells, it also has been used to treat other autoimmune diseases, but its clinical effectiveness has not been determined.

Antilymphocyte antibodies inhibit the T-cell–mediated immune response. The two types are monoclonal antibodies, which react with one specific antigen, and polyclonal antibodies, which target several different antigens. Polyclonal antibodies are created by injecting animals (usually mice) with human lymphocytes. The animals' B cells are harvested from lymphoid tissue or peripheral blood and used to create antilymphocyte serum (ALS); isolated antibodies from these B cells are the active agents in antilymphocyte globulin (ALG). Both ALS and ALG are used routinely to treat transplant rejection and graft-versus-host reactions. Because they come from animals, however, they can cause serum sickness. In addition, they are not specific to T cells and also can destroy platelets.

Monoclonal antibodies are laboratory-created antibodies developed from a single cell line that block the receptor molecules that bind and transfer cytokine signals on T cells. OKT3, a monoclonal antibody obtained from mice, is a strong immunosuppressant used in the primary treatment of acute transplant rejection; it also may be effective in preventing rejection. It frequently causes a massive release of cytokines whose effects must be controlled, usually by corticosteroids, after the first or second dose. In addition, over time it stimulates the production of antimouse antibodies that block its effectiveness. SEE: *hybridoma.*

Plasmapheresis, the separation and removal of plasma containing autoantibodies (AAb), is most effective against disorders in which the AAbs are tissue specific, such as myasthenia gravis, and those in which more AAbs are found in the blood than in extravascular spaces.

PATIENT CARE: Many immunosuppressant drugs increase patients' susceptibility to infections, esp. opportunistic infections, and also increase their risk of developing malignant tumors, because of the loss of immunosurveillance. Patients need to learn to minimize their exposure to infectious organisms and consistently to use good handwashing and oral hygiene measures. The medication regimen may be rigorous and should be accompanied by intensive teaching about purpose and side effects of the drugs and the need for frequent bloodwork; written as well as verbal instructions should be provided.

immunotoxin (ĭm″ū-nō-tŏk′sĭn) [″ + Gr. *toxikon,* poison] Toxic agents that can be attached to antibody molecules and, because of this enhanced toxicity, used to combat tumor cells. This technique has been used to eliminate malignant tumors in the bone marrow.

impacted [L. *impactus,* pressed on] Pressed firmly together so as to be immovable. This term may be applied to a fracture in which the ends of the bones are wedged together, a tooth so placed in the jaw bone that eruption is impossible, a fetus wedged in the birth canal, cerumen, calculi, or accumulation of feces in the rectum.

impaction (ĭm-păk′shŭn) [L. *impactio,* a pressing together] A condition of being tightly wedged into a part, as when the eruption of a tooth is blocked by other teeth; the overloading of an organ, as the feces in the bowels.

food i. The forcing of food into the interproximal spaces of teeth by chewing (vertical impaction) or by tongue and cheek pressure (horizontal impaction).

impairment Any loss or abnormality of

psychological, physiological, or anatomical structure or function.

nonsyndromic hereditary hearing i. Hearing loss, or deafness, that is inherited and is not associated with other inherited characteristics.

syndromic hereditary hearing i. Hearing loss or deafness that is genetically transmitted and associated with other inherited diseases or deficits.

impaled object A foreign body that penetrates the skin and remains embedded in tissue. Such objects should be stabilized to prevent movement, and allowed to remain in place while the patient is transported to receive professional care.

impalpable (ĭm-păl′pă-b'l) [L. *in-,* not, + *palpare,* to touch] Felt with difficulty, if at all; hardly perceptible to the touch.

impar (ĭm′păr) [L., unequal] Single; not paired.

imparidigitate (ĭm-păr″ĭ-dĭj′ĭ-tāt) [″ + *digitus,* finger] Having an uneven number of fingers or toes.

impatent (ĭm-pă′tĕnt) [″ + *patere,* to be open] Closed; not patent.

impedance (ĭm-pē′dăns) [L. *impedire,* to hinder] Resistance met by alternating currents in passing through a conductor; consists of resistance, reactance, inductance, or capacitance. The resistance due to the inductive and condenser characteristics of a circuit is called reactance.

acoustic i. Resistance to the transmission of sound waves.

imperative [L. *imperativus,* commanding] Obligatory; not controlled by the will; involuntary.

deontological i. Moral obligation or duty of caregivers, established by tradition and culture.

imperception [L. *in-,* not, + *percipere,* to perceive] The inability to form a mental picture; lack of perception.

imperforate (ĭm-pĕr′fō-rāt) [″ + *per,* through, + *forare,* to bore] Without an opening.

imperforation Atresia.

impermeable [L. *in-,* not, + *permeare,* to pass through] Not allowing passage, as of fluids; impenetrable.

impervious [L. *impervius*] Unable to be penetrated.

impetiginous (ĭm″pĕ-tĭj′ĭ-nŭs) [L. *impetiginosus*] Relating to or resembling impetigo.

impetigo, impetigo contagiosa (ĭm-pĕ-tī′gō, -tē′gō) [L.] A bacterial infection of the skin, caused by streptococci or staphylococci, and marked by yellow to red, weeping and crusted or pustular lesions, esp. around the nose, mouth, and cheeks or on the extremities. The disease is common in children and adults and may develop after trauma or irritation to the skin. SEE: illus. *Nursing Diagnoses Appendix.* **impetiginous,** *adj.*

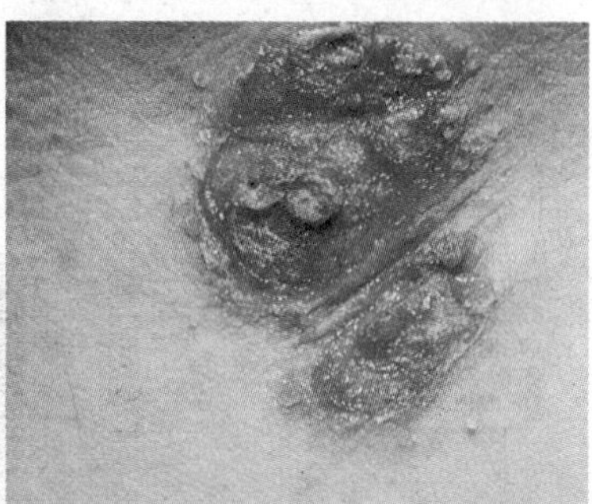

IMPETIGO CONTAGIOSA IN AXILLA

TREATMENT: Topically applied mupirocin ointment or oral agents such as dicloxacillin or cephalexin provide effective therapy.

PATIENT CARE: The appearance, location, and distribution of lesions are documented, along with any associated symptoms (pruritus, pain). Family members are taught to keep the skin clean and dry, removing exudate 2 to 3 times daily by washing the lesions with soap and water; warm saline soaks or compresses may be applied to remove stubborn crusts. Patients and families are taught the importance of not sharing washcloths, towels, or bed linens; the need for thorough hand washing; and the urgency for early treatment of any purulent eruption to limit spread to others.

Non-prescription antihistamines may be used to reduce itching. The fingernails should be cut and, if necessary, mittens applied to prevent further injury if the patient is unable to avoid scratching. Diversional activities appropriate to the patient's developmental stage are encouraged to distract from local discomforts. The school nurse or employer is notified of the infection, and family members are checked for evidence of impetigo. The patient can return to school or work when all lesions have healed.

bullous i. A rare infection, usually occurring in infants, caused by a strain of *Staphylococcus aureus* that produces a toxin that splits the epidermis. SEE: illus.

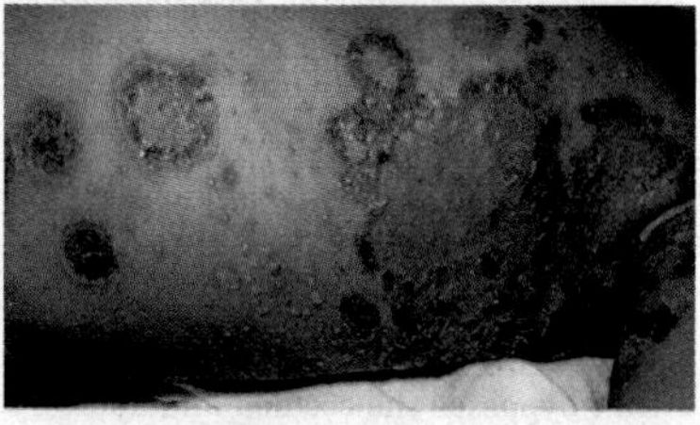

BULLOUS IMPETIGO

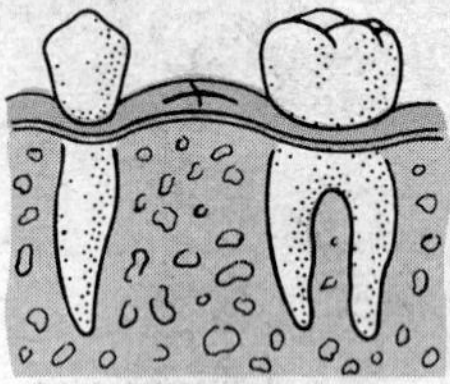
1. INCISION INTO GUM FOR PLACEMENT OF IMPLANT

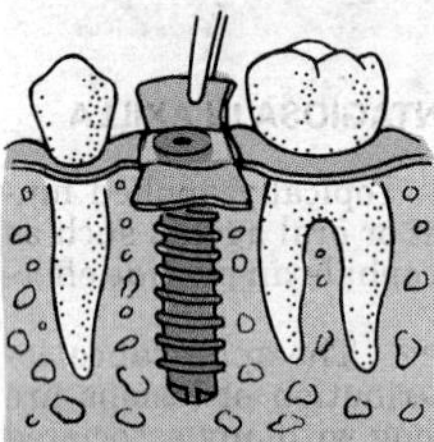
2. SCREW OR PIN FOR PLACEMENT INTO THE ALVEOLAR BONE DIRECTLY

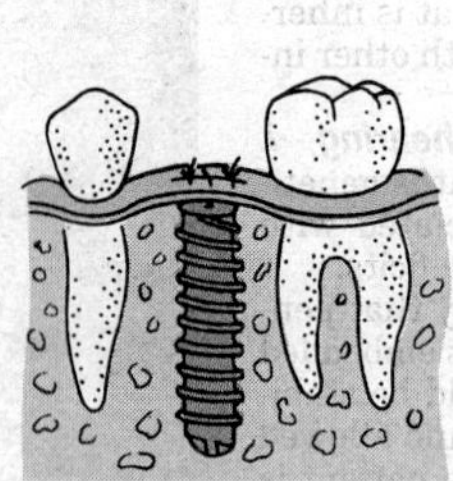
3. THE SOFT TISSUE IS SUTURED TO PERMIT BONE GROWTH AROUND THE IMPLANT

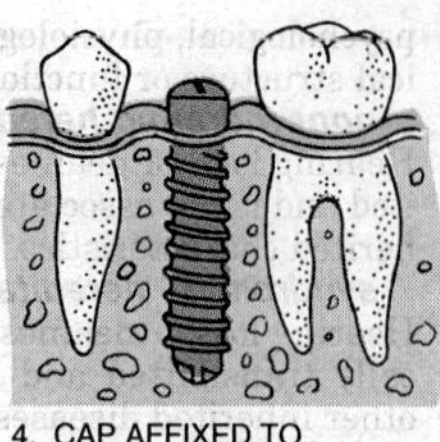
4. CAP AFFIXED TO TOP OF IMPLANT

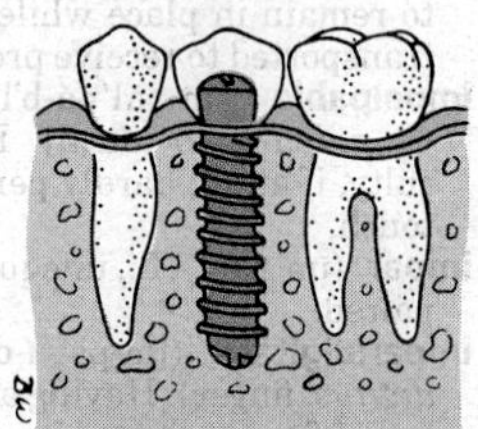
5. RESTORATION APPLIED TO CAP AS SHOWN

ENDOSSEOUS DENTAL IMPLANT

i. herpetiformis A rare and occasionally life-threatening eruption that typically occurs in the third trimester of pregnancy. It is pathologically indistinguishable from pustular psoriasis.

impingement (ĭm-pĭnj'mĕnt) **1.** An area of periodontal tissue traumatized by the occlusal force of a tooth. **2.** An area of tissue overcompaction or displacement by a partial denture.

implant (ĭm-plănt') [L. *in-*, into, + *plantare,* to plant] To transfer a part, to graft, to insert; the opposite of explant.

implant (ĭm'plănt) An object inserted into the body, such as a piece of tissue, a tooth, a pellet of medicine, a tube or needle containing a radioactive substance, liquid and solid plastic materials used to augment tissues or to fill in areas traumatically or surgically removed, and artificial joints. SEE: *mammaplasty, augmentation.*

bone i. The use of implanted materials to repair bone or to cover implanted objects such as artificial hips or tooth implants.

brain i. Transplantation of tissue into the brain to treat a disease. Implantation of tissue from the adrenal gland into the caudate nucleus (of the nondominant side of the brain) has been done experimentally to treat Parkinson's disease.

brainstem i. Auditory prosthesis that bypasses the cochlea and auditory nerve and partially restores hearing by directly stimulating the cochlear nucleus complex. This type of implant helps individuals who have retrocochlear deafness.

dental i. In dentistry, a prosthetic device in any of several shapes. It is implanted into oral tissues beneath the mucosa or the periosteal layer, or within the bone to support or hold a fixed or removable prosthesis. SEE: illus.

Ultrasonic devices should not be used on dental implants.

endosteal i. A dental prosthesis that is partially submerged and anchored within the bone. The blade form and the cylinder form are the two types of endosteal implants used. The cylinder form, which is most common, consists of a screw, a small titanium cylinder, and an abutment surgically inserted into the bone. The blade form consists of one or more abutments. In both forms, the prosthetic device is placed on the abutment(s).

interstitial i. The insertion of an applicator containing a radioactive source directly into a tumor to deliver a high radiation dose while sparing the surrounding tissues.

intracavitary i. The insertion of an applicator containing a radioactive source directly into a hollow organ to deliver a high radiation dose to the organ while sparing the surrounding tissues.

radioactive i. SEE: *brachytherapy; interstitial i.; intracavitary i.*

staple i. Transosteal i.

subperiosteal i. A prosthesis for use in edentulous patients who cannot wear dentures (e.g., because of mandibular atrophy). The implant consists of a metal framework that rests on the residual ridge beneath the periosteum but does not penetrate the mandible.

tooth i. The placement of artificial teeth directly into the maxilla or mandible or into a frame attached to the bone. In some cases, an implant is used to stabilize a loose tooth. This is accomplished by placing an implant through the natural bone into the bone. SEE: *implantation; reimplantation.*

transosteal i. A rarely used type of dental prosthesis that completely penetrates the mandible. Its use is complicated by infection and a high rate of implant failure. SYN: *staple i.*

implantation (ĭm″plăn-tā′shŭn) [″ + *plantare,* to plant] **1.** The grafting of tissue or the insertion of an organ such as tooth, skin, or tendon into a new location in the body. **2.** Embedding of the developing blastocyst in the uterine mucosa 6 or 7 days after fertilization. SYN: *nidation.*

hypodermic i. The introduction of an implant under the skin; usually a solid substance placed by forcing a small amount out of a hypodermic needle.

teratic i. The union of an abnormal fetus with a nearly normal fetus.

implosion A violent collapse inward.

i. flooding A method of treating fear due to a phobia by exposing the person to the worst possible phobic situation. The fear is experienced at maximum intensity for up to an hour until the patient is no longer capable of experiencing further fear. The phobic situation is imagined in the first sessions and later produced in reality. SEE: *phobic desensitization.*

imponderable [L. *in-,* not, + *pondus,* weight] Incapable of being weighed or measured.

impostors, medical Persons who practice medicine without a license and who have not graduated from an accredited medical school.

impotence, impotency [″ + *potentia,* power] A weakness, esp. pert. to the inability of a man to achieve or maintain an erection. SYN: *erectile dysfunction.* SEE: *penile prosthesis; sex therapy; sexual dysfunction; sexual stimulant.*

TREATMENT: Sildenafil (trade name: Viagra), alprostadil, and several other drugs are used to treat erectile dysfunction. Penile vacuum pumps and penile prosthesis are among the nonpharmacological alternatives.

anatomical i. Impotence caused by a genital defect.

atonic i. Impotence resulting from paralysis of nerves supplying the penis.

functional i. Impotence not due to an organic or anatomical defect; usually of psychogenic origin. The individual may experience impotence with one or more sexual partners, but not with others.

neurogenic i. Impotence due to central nervous system lesions, paraplegia, or diabetic neuropathy.

pharmacological i. Impotence due to the side effects of certain drugs and medications (e.g., alcohol, cytotoxic agents, barbiturates, beta blockers, marijuana, cimetidine, clonidine, guanethidine, immunosuppressives, lithium, opiates, phenothiazine, some antihypertensive agents, some diuretics, antidepressants, and anticholinergics).

psychic i. Psychogenic i.

psychogenic i. Impotence caused by emotional factors rather than organic disease. SYN: *psychic i.*

vasculogenic i. Impotence due to an inadequate supply of arterial blood to the corpora cavernosa of the penis.

impotent (ĭm′pō-tĕnt) **1.** Unable to copulate. **2.** Sterile; barren. **3.** Lacking effectiveness.

imprecision (ĭm-prē-sĭ′shŭn) The amount or degree of random error in an assay, research study, or calculation, usually represented by the standard deviation, coefficient of variation, or range.

impregnate (ĭm-prĕg′nāt) [L. *impregnare,* to make pregnant] **1.** To render pregnant; to fertilize an ovum. **2.** To saturate.

impregnation (ĭm″prĕg-nā′shŭn) [L. *impregnare,* to make pregnant] **1.** Fertilization of an ovum. SYN: *fecundation.* **2.** Saturation.

artificial i. Pregnancy resulting from successful assisted reproduction procedures. SEE: *artifical insemination.*

impression [L. *impressio*] **1.** A hollow or depression in a surface. **2.** An effect produced upon the mind by external stimuli. **3.** The imprint of all or part of the dental arch, individual teeth, or cavity preparations, using appropriate dental materials, for the purpose of records or restorative procedures.

addition silicone i. material An elastic final impression material used to construct cast restorations, dental prostheses, and other appliances. It is made from a vinyl polysiloxane paste mixed with a platinum salt catalyst.

CAUTION: Wearing latex gloves inhibits the setting of addition silicone impression material. The contamination is so pervasive that touching the tooth with the latex will inhibit setting.

---

complete dental i. A negative impression of the entire edentulous area (e.g., the area that originally provided the base for the normal teeth).

condensation silicone i. material An elastic final impression material used to construct dental cast restorations, prostheses, and appliances. It is made of two pastes containing siloxane and stannous octoate and has a limited shelf-life.

digitate i. An impression on the inner surface of the frontal bone, allowing for convolutions of the cerebrum. SYN: *impressione digitata.*

final i. An impression that is used for making the master cast for a dental prosthesis.

i. materials A variety of deformable materials used to make a negative reproduction of oral structures. Examples of common impression materials include waxes, polymers, elastomers, reversible hydrocolloids, and irreversible hydrocolloids.

partial dental i. A negative impression of a portion of the maxilla or mandible where teeth were previously present.

polyether i. material The stiffest of the dental final impression materials, used to construct restorations, prosthetics, and other appliances. It is made from a base containing a polyether polymer, silica, filler, and plasticizer, and an accelerator, made of an alkylaromatic sulfonate, filler, and plasticizer.

polysulfide i. material An elastic final dental impression used to construct restorations, prosthetics, and appliances, which is made from a paste composed of polysulfide polymer, filler, sulfur, plasticizer, and an accelerator paste containing lead dioxide (which causes it to turn dark-brown).

i. tray A receptacle or device used to carry the impression material to the mouth and to hold it in apposition to the tissues being recorded.

impressione digitata Digitate impression.

imprinting A special type of learned response that occurs in some animals at a critical period in their development. For example, goslings mothered by a hen may adopt the hen as if she were their mother.

genomic i. The inactivation of a gene by its allele.

impulse (ĭm′pŭls) [L. *impulsus*] **1.** The act of driving onward with sudden force. SEE: *conation.* **2.** An incitement of the mind, prompting an unpremeditated act (e.g., impulse buying). **3.** In physiology, a change transmitted through certain tissues, esp. nerve fibers and muscles, resulting in physiological activity or inhibition.

cardiac i. **1.** The heartbeat felt at the left side of the chest over the apex of the heart; this is a physical impulse. **2.** The electrical impulse transmitted over the conducting pathway of the heart that is responsible for the contraction of the muscular tissue of the heart. SEE: *heart.*

ectopic i. A cardiac impulse arising in some part of the heart other than the sinoatrial node.

enteroceptive i. An afferent nerve impulse arising from stimuli originating in receptors located in internal organs.

excitatory i. An impulse that stimulates activity.

exteroceptive i. An afferent nerve impulse arising from stimuli originating in sense organs located on the body surface.

inhibitory i. An impulse that lessens activity.

nerve i. A self-propagated electrical change transmitted along the membrane of a nerve fiber. At the end of the axon of the nerve fiber, the electrical impulse stimulates the release of a neurotransmitter, which may stimulate or inhibit another electrical impulse in another nerve fiber, cause muscle contraction or glandular secretion, or produce a sensation in the brain. The velocity varies according to the diameter of the fiber and the presence or absence of a myelin sheath. The most rapid conducting mammalian neurons (50 to 80 m/sec) are large, myelinated neurons.

proprioceptive i. An afferent nerve impulse arising from stimuli originating in joints, muscles, or tendons, or other sensory endings that respond to pressure or stretch.

impulsion The idea to do something or commit an act or crime, suddenly imposed on the subject, that tortures him or her until the act is accomplished. Clear consciousness of the proposed act followed by an agonizing struggle, defeat, and sense of relief following the act are characteristics of impulsions, obsessions, and inhibitions. Impulsions may include folie du doute or doubting mania (e.g., repeatedly checking to determine whether something has been done); obsessive fears of contact or delirium of touch; agoraphobia; dipsomania; pyromania; kleptomania; homicidal or suicidal impulsion; onomatomania; arithmomania; exhibitionism.

IMS *incident management system.*

IMV *intermittent mandatory ventilation; intermittent mechanical ventilation.*

In Symbol for the element indium.

in- [L. *in,* into] Prefix indicating *in, inside, within;* and also *intensive action.*

in- [L. *in-,* not] Prefix indicating *negative.*

inaccurate (ĭn-ăk′ūr-ăt) **1.** Mistaken or incorrect; in error. **2.** In quantitative analysis, not in agreement with an accepted value.

inaccuracy (ĭn-ăk′ūr-ăsē) Inexactness as a result of measurement error.

inaction (ĭn-ăk′shŭn) [L. *in-,* not, + *ac-*

tio, act] Failure of or decreased response to a stimulus.

inactivate [″ + *activus,* acting] To render inactive, esp. the alteration or destruction of an enzyme system or a biologically active agent such as a microorganism or antigen.

inactivation Rendering anything inert by using heat or other means.

i. of complement The destruction of complement proteins by pathogens (e.g., herpesviruses or measles virus); allergens (e.g., pollens); or in the laboratory, by heating serum to about 131°F (55°C) for a half hour. The destruction of complement by disease-causing organisms allows them to evade this aspect of the immune system.

inanimate [″ + *animatus,* alive] **1.** Not alive; not animate. **2.** Dull, lifeless.

inanition (ĭn″ă-nĭsh′ŭn) [L. *inanis,* empty] A debilitated condition caused by a lack of sufficient food material essential to the body, such as in starvation or malabsorption syndrome. This condition may also be due to causes other than the food supply, such as malabsorption, or to other diseases of the gastrointestinal system that prevent absorption of food.

inappetence (ĭn-ăp′ĕ-tĕns) [″ + *appetere,* to long for] A lack of craving or desire, esp. for food.

inarticulate [″ + *articulus,* joined] **1.** Not jointed; without joints. **2.** Unable to pronounce distinct syllables or express oneself intelligibly. **3.** Not given to expressing oneself verbally.

in articulo mortis (ĭn ăr-tĭk′ū-lō mor′tĭs) [L.] At the very moment of death.

inassimilable (ĭn″ă-sĭm′ĭ-lă-b′l) [″ + *assimilis,* to make similar] Not capable of being used by the body for nutrition.

inattention **1.** Neglect, e.g., of sensory stimuli. **2.** Distractibility.

unilateral i. An inability to recognize stimulation provided to the side of the body or the visual field damaged by a stroke in the nondominant hemisphere of the brain. Sometimes called visual inattention or visual unilateral inattention. SEE: *altitudinal neglect; hemi-inattention; hemispatial neglect; unilateral spatial agnosia.*

inborn Innate or inherent, said of characteristics both structural and functional that are inherited or acquired during uterine development.

inbreeding [″ + AS. *bredan,* to cherish] Mating of closely related individuals.

incandescent [L. *incandescere,* to glow] Glowing with light; white hot.

incapacitate Being made incapable of some function, act or strength. This may be purely physical or intellectual or both.

incaparina A mixture of cereal grains and oilseed meals of a given range of protein and quality fortified with vitamins and minerals. It was developed at the Institute of Nutrition of Central America and Panama (INCAP) and distributed in Latin American countries for feeding young children to prevent kwashiorkor and other forms of malnutrition.

incarcerated [L. *incarcerare*] Imprisoned, confined, constricted, and confined of blood flow, as an irreducible hernia.

incarceration **1.** Legal confinement. **2.** The imprisonment of a part; constriction, as in a hernia.

incasement Becoming surrounded by a structure or wall.

inception [L. *inceptio,* taking in, beginning] **1.** The beginning of anything. **2.** Ingestion. **3.** Intussusception.

incest (ĭn′sĕst) [L. *incestus,* unchaste, incest] Coitus between close blood relatives.

incidence [L. *incidens,* falling upon] **1.** The frequency of new cases of a disease or condition in a specific population or group. SEE: *prevalence.* **2.** The falling or impinging upon, touching, or affecting in some way.

incident **1.** A happening, event, or occurrence. **2.** Falling or striking, as a ray of light.

multiple casualty i. ABBR: MCI. Medical emergencies that involve more than one patient (e.g., in automobile or plane crashes, bombings, fires, hazardous materials incidents).

incident command system ABBR: ICS. A disaster planning tool designed to standardize management of health-related catastrophes (e.g., multiple car collisions, fires, or plane crashes). The ICS has five key components: command, finance, logistics, operations, and planning. SYN: *incident management system.*

incident management system ABBR: IMS. Incident command system.

incineration (ĭn-sĭn″ĕr-ā′shŭn) [L. *in,* into, + *cineres,* ashes] Destruction by fire; cremation.

incipient (ĭn-sĭp′ē-ĕnt) [L. *incipere,* to begin] Beginning; coming into existence.

incisal (ĭn-sī′zăl) Relating to or involving cutting.

incise (ĭn-sīz′) [L. *incisus*] To cut, as with a sharp instrument.

incised (ĭn-sīzd′) Cut cleanly, as with a knife.

incision (ĭn-sĭzh′ŭn) [L. *incisio*] A cut made with a knife, electrosurgical unit, or laser esp. for surgical purposes.

Pfannenstiel i. SEE: *Pfannenstiel incision.*

incisive (ĭn-sī′sĭv) [L. *incisivus*] **1.** Cutting; having the power of cutting. **2.** Relating to the incisor teeth.

incisive bone An obsolete term for the part of the maxilla that supports the incisor teeth.

incisor (ĭn-sī′zor) [L., a cutter] **1.** That

which cuts. **2.** That which applies to the incisor teeth. **3.** One of the cutting teeth; the four front teeth in each jaw of the adult. SEE: *dentition.*

central i. One of two upper and lower incisors adjacent to the midsagittal plane.

incisura (ĭn-sī-sū′ră) *pl.* **incisurae** [L.] **1.** An incision. **2.** Incisure; notch; emargination; indentation at the edge of any structure.

i. angularis gastrica A fold or notch on the distal end of the lesser curvature of the stomach.

incisure (ĭn-sĭz′ūr) [L. *incisura,* a cutting into] A notch or slit.

i. of Rivinus SEE: *Rivinus' incisure.*

i. of Schmidt-Lanterman Channels of cytoplasm found in myelinated nerve fibers that were once thought to represent breaks in the myelin sheath.

incitant (ĭn-sīt′ănt) [L. *incitarē,* to set in motion] The stimulus that sets off a reaction, disease, or incident.

inclination [L. *inclinere,* to slope] Leaning from the normal or from the vertical, as a tooth or the pelvis.

inclinometer (ĭn″klĭ-nŏm′ĕ-ter) [″ + Gr. *metron,* measure] A device for measuring ocular diameter from vertical and horizontal lines.

inclusion [L. *inclusus,* enclosed] Being enclosed or included.

i. blennorrhea Inclusion conjunctivitis of the newborn.

i. body One of several bodies present in the nucleus or cytoplasm of epithelial or nerve cells in cases of infection by certain viruses such as rabies or herpesviruses. SYN: *cell i.;* SEE: *Negri bodies.*

cell i. Inclusion body.

i. conjunctivitis Inflammation of the conjunctiva of the eye due to the organism *Chlamydia trachomatis.* SEE: *ophthalmia neonatorum.*

dental i. A tooth unable to erupt because of excessive surrounding tissue. SEE: *impacted tooth.*

fetal i. Malformed twins in which one, the parasite, is completely enclosed within the other, its host or autosite. SEE: *teratoma.*

incoagulability (ĭn″kō-ăg″ū-lă-bĭl′ĭ-tē) [L. *in-,* not, + *coagulare,* to congeal] Not coagulable.

incoherence (ĭn″kō-hēr′ĕns) [″ + *cohairens,* adhering] An inability to express oneself coherently or to present ideas in a related order.

incoherent (ĭn″kō-hē′rĕnt) Not coherent or understandable.

incombustible [″ + *combustus,* burned] Incapable of being burned.

incompatibility [L. *incompatibilis*] **1.** The quality of not being suitable for mixture. It can be applied to a state that renders admixture of medicines unsuitable through chemical action or interaction, insolubility, formation of poisonous or explosive compounds, difference in solubility, or antagonistic action. **2.** The quality of not being mixed without chemical changes, or without countering the action of other ingredients in a compound. **3.** The condition of not being in harmony with one's surroundings or associates, esp. a spouse or friend.

ABO i. An antigen-antibody immune response to infusion of another's red blood cells. Transfusion reactions occur most commonly in people with type O blood, which carries no antigens on the red blood cells and contains both anti-A and anti-B antibodies. People with type A blood carry A antigens on their red cells and anti-B antibodies; those with type B blood carry B antigens and anti-A antibodies; those with type AB blood carry both A and B antigens but no antibodies to A or B. The antibodies are called natural antibodies because their formation does not require sensitization by A and B antigens. The antibodies recognize the antigens on the donor cells as foreign and destroy them by agglutination and lysis. ABO incompatibilities are different from Rh incompatibilities, which are most commonly related to the D antigen in the Rh blood group. SEE: table; *blood group.*

Obstetrics: Transplacental fetal-maternal transfusion occurs when fetal blood cells escape into the maternal circulation, eliciting antibody formation. Maternal antibodies then cross the placenta into the fetal circulation, attack, and destroy red blood cells, as evidenced by neonatal hyperbilirubinemia and jaundice.

physiological i. A condition in which one or more substances in a mixture oppose or counteract one of the other compounds being administered.

incompatible **1.** Not capable of uniting.

Blood Type Compatibility

Donor Blood Type	Compatibility with Recipient Blood Type: Type A Blood	Type B Blood	Type AB Blood	Type O Blood
A	yes	no	yes	no
B	no	yes	yes	no
AB	no	no	yes	no
O	yes	yes	yes	yes

2. Antagonistic in action, said of some drugs. **3.** Not being in harmony with one's environment, situation, or associates, esp. a spouse or friend.

incompetence, incompetency [L. *in-*, not, + *competere*, to be suitable] An inadequate ability to perform the function or action normal to an organ or part.

aortic i. Aortic insufficiency.

cervical i. Structural inability of the cervical os to remain closed and support a growing fetus. This problem commonly has been associated with recurrent spontaneous second-trimester abortions. A higher incidence of this structural abnormality is noted after cervical trauma (e.g., previous vaginal or cesarean births, cervical laceration, conization of the cervix). It also has been reported among daughters whose mothers were treated with diethylstilbestrol (DES) during their pregnancies. Traditionally, cerclage has been used for treatment, even though controlled trials of its effectiveness have not been uniformly successful. SEE: *cerclage; Shirodkar operation*.

ileocecal i. An inability of the ileocecal valve to stop the return of the material from the colon to the ileum.

mental i. Legally unable to execute a contract, or to perform necessary activities and tasks expected of one's life roles.

muscular i. An imperfect closure of one of the atrioventricular valves due to weak action of papillary muscles.

pyloric i. A weakness of the pyloric sphincter, which permits undigested food to leave the stomach and enter the duodenum.

relative i. Excessive dilatation of a cardiac cavity, rendering it impossible for the cardiac valves leading in and out of the chamber to close perfectly.

valvular i. The backward flow of blood through a valve, for example, a cardiac valve during the stage of the cardiac cycle when the valve leaflets should be closed.

incompressible [" + *compressus*, pressed together] Compact; not compressible.

incontinence (ĭn-kŏnt'ĭn-ĕns) [" + *continere*, to stop] **1.** Loss of self-control, esp. of urine, feces, or semen. SEE: *bladder drill; continence*. **2.** Loss of neurological or psychological control (e.g., of appetites, habits, or speech).

active i. A discharge of feces and urine in the normal way at regulated intervals but involuntarily.

fecal i. Failure of the anal sphincter to prevent involuntary expulsion of gas, liquid, or solids from the lower bowel. SEE: *encopresis*.

functional urinary i. Inability of a usually continent person to reach the toilet in time to avoid unintentional loss of urine. SEE: *Nursing Diagnoses Appendix*.

giggle i. Involuntary passage of urine induced by laughter. The condition occurs commonly in young girls and women, but tends to improve in the second or third decade of life. It is distinct from stress urinary incontinence, a condition that usually begins after menopause. SEE: *stress urinary i.*

intermittent i. Loss of control of the bladder upon sudden pressure or movement.

i. of milk Galactorrhea.

overflow i. Incontinence characterized by small frequent voidings due to overfilling of the bladder or to a bladder with pathologically decreased volume.

paralytic i. The constant voiding of small amounts of urine and feces owing to defective nervous control of sphincters.

passive i. A form of urinary incontinence; instead of emptying normally, the full bladder allows urine to drip away upon pressure.

reflex urinary i. An involuntary loss of urine at somewhat predictable intervals when a specific bladder volume is reached. SEE: *Nursing Diagnoses Appendix*.

risk for urinary urge i. Risk for involuntary loss of urine associated with a sudden, strong sensation or urinary urgency. SEE: *Nursing Diagnoses Appendix*.

stress urinary i. ABBR: SUI. An inability to prevent escape of small amounts of urine during stress such as laughing, coughing, sneezing, lifting, or sudden movement. SEE: *Nursing Diagnoses Appendix*.

DIAGNOSIS: Direct observation of urine loss while coughing is a reliable method of establishing this diagnosis. The urine should be cultured to rule out urinary tract infection. This phenomenon should be investigated to be certain that it is not caused by a structural abnormality.

TREATMENT: In addition to using devices to absorb urine that escapes, therapy consists of behavioral modification, pharmacological treatment, and surgical management. Behavioral therapy includes bladder training, timed voiding, prompted voiding, and pelvic muscle exercises. Pharmacotherapy includes oxybutynin hydrochloride, propartheline bromide, and imipramine hydrochloride. Surgery may restore anatomic support of the urethra or compensate for a poorly functioning urethral sphincter. SEE: *bladder drill; Kegel exercise*.

PATIENT CARE: The patient is taught Kegel exercises to strengthen pubococcygeal muscles and encouraged to practice the exercises at frequent intervals throughout the day, as well as during urination (by stopping and starting the urinary stream intermittently). The vulva and introitus should be kept clean and dry and odor-free, and commercial barrier products should be used to protect clothing. To avoid isolation, the patient should continue or resume usual activities while using protective barriers. The patient's response to the exercise regimen is periodically evaluated.

total i. The state in which an individual experiences a continuous and unpredictable loss of urine. SEE: *Nursing Diagnoses Appendix.*

urge i. Involuntary passage of urine occurring soon after a strong sense of urgency to void. Drugs that inhibit the detrusor muscle of the bladder, such as oxybutynin, can be used as treatment. SEE: *Nursing Diagnoses Appendix.*

i. of urine Intermittent or complete absence of ability to control loss of urine from the bladder, a problem that affects about 25% of women over the age of 60. It may have significant impact on social, occupational and psychological functioning.

TREATMENT: Therapy will depend upon the cause. Information on this subject may be obtained from Health for Incontinent People at (800) 251-3337. SEE: *Kegel exercise; stress urinary i.*

in control Within an acceptable predetermined range. The limits that define the acceptable range may be set using one or more criteria, depending on the intent. A typical analytical "in-control" limit is based on the calculation of the dispersion of the data measured as standard deviation (SD). Subsequent multiplication of the SD by 2 and then by 3 results in what frequently are used as "warning" and "action" limits, respectively. Other statistical or clinical criteria also can be used to set the limits. SEE: *standard deviation.*

incoordinate [L. *in-*, not, + *coordinare,* to arrange] **1.** Not able to make coordinated muscular movements. **2.** Unable to adjust one's work harmoniously with others.

incoordination (ĭn″kō-or″dĭ-nā′shŭn) An inability to produce harmonious, rhythmic, muscular action that is not due to weakness. The condition is typically caused by a lesion on the cerebellum. SYN: *asynergia.* SEE: *disdiadochokinesia.*

incorporation [L. *in,* into, + *corporare,* to form into a body] Combining two ingredients to form a homogeneous mass.

increment (ĭn′krĕ-mĕnt) [L. *incrementum*] **1.** An increase or addition in number, size, or extent; an enlargement. **2.** Something added or gained. **3.** The beginning portion of a uterine contraction between baseline and acme. Increasing strength of contraction is shown by the upslope record recorded by the fetal monitor.

incrustation [L. *in,* on, + *crusta,* crust] The formation of crusts or scabs.

incubation (ĭn″kū-bā′shŭn) [L. *incubare,* to lie on] **1.** The interval between exposure to infection and the appearance of the first symptom. SYN: *latent period* (2). SEE: table. **2.** In bacteriology, the period of culture development. **3.** The development of an impregnated ovum. **4.** The care of a premature infant in an incubator.

incubator **1.** An enclosed crib, in which the temperature and humidity may be regulated, for care of premature babies. **2.** An apparatus for providing suitable atmospheric conditions for culturing bacteria or for maintaining eggs until they hatch.

incubus (ĭn′kū-bŭs) [L. *incubare,* to lie upon] A nightmare.

incudal (ĭng′kū-dăl) [L. *incus,* anvil] Relating to the incus.

incudectomy (ĭng″kū-dĕk′tō-mē) [″ + Gr. *ektome,* excision] The surgical removal of all or part of the incus of the middle ear.

incudiform (ĭn-kū′dĭ-form) [″ + *forma,* shape] Anvil-shaped.

incudomalleal (ĭng″kū-dō-măl′ē-ăl) [″ + *malleus,* a hammer] Pert. to the incus and malleus and their articulation in the tympanum; in the middle ear.

incudostapedial (ĭn″kū-dō-stă-pē′dē-ăl) [″ + *stapes,* a stirrup] Pert. to the incus and stapes and their articulation in the tympanum; in the middle ear.

incurable [L. *in-*, not, + *curare,* to care for] Not capable of being cured.

incurvation (ĭn″kŭr-vā′shŭn) [L. *incurvare,* to bend in] State of being bent or curved in.

incus (ĭng′kŭs) *pl.* **incudes** [L., anvil] In the middle ear, the middle of the three ossicles in the tympanum; the anvil. SEE: *ear* for illus.

lenticular process of i. The long process of the incus, a middle ear ossicle. It articulates with the head of the stapes.

incyclophoria (ĭn-sī″klō-for′ē-ă) [L. *in-*, not, + Gr. *kyklos,* circle, + *phoros,* bearing] Median or negative cyclophoria in which the affected eye, when covered, turns inward about its anteroposterior axis.

incyclotropia (ĭn-sī″klō-trō′pē-ă) [″ + ″ + *tropos,* turning] Cyclotropia in which the eye turns inward toward the nose even when both eyes are open.

in d [L. *in dies*] daily.

indentation [L. *in,* in, + *dens,* tooth] A depression or hollow.

independent living In rehabilitation, thriving on one's own; living autonomously and actively in one's own home and community.

Incubation and Isolation Periods in Common Infections*

Infection	Incubation Period	Isolation of Patient†
AIDS	Unclear; antibodies appear within 1–3 months of infection	Protective isolation if T cell count is very low; private room only necessary with severe diarrhea, bleeding, copious blood tinged sputum if patient has poor personal hygiene habits
Bloodstream (bacteremia, fungemia)	Variable; usually 2–5 days	
Brucellosis	Highly variable, usually 5–21 days; may be months	None
Chickenpox	2–3 weeks	1 week after vesicles appear or until vesicles become dry
Cholera	A few hours to 5 days	Enteric precautions
Common cold	12 hr–5 days	None
Dysentery, amebic	From a few days to several months, commonly 2–4 weeks	None
Dysentery, bacillary (e.g., shigellosis)	12–96 hr	As long as stools remain positive
Encephalitis, mosquito-borne	5–15 days	None
Giardiasis	3–25 days or longer; median 7–10 days	Enteric precautions
Gonorrhea	2–7 days; may be longer	No sexual contact until cured
Hepatitis A	15–50 days	Enteric (gloves with infected material; gowns as needed to protect clothing)
Hepatitis B	45–180 days	Blood and body fluid precautions (gloves and plastic gowns for contact with infective materials)
Hepatitis C	14–180 days	As for hepatitis B
Hepatitis D	2–8 weeks	As for hepatitis B
Hepatitis E	15–64 days	Enteric precautions
Influenza	1–3 days	As practical
Legionella	2–10 days	None
Lyme disease	3–32 days after tick bite	None
Malaria	7–10 days for *Plasmodium falciparum;* 8–14 days for *P. vivax, P. ovale;* 7–30 days for *P. malariae*	Protection from mosquitoes
Measles (rubeola)	8–13 days from exposure to onset of fever; 14 days until rash appears	From diagnosis to 7 days after appearance of rash; strict isolation from children under 3 years
Meningitis	2–10 days	Until 24 hr after start of chemotherapy
Mononucleosis, infectious	4–6 weeks	None; disinfection of articles soiled with nose and throat discharges
Mumps	12–25 days	Until the glands recede
Paratyphoid fevers	3 days–3 months; usually 1–3 weeks; 1–10 days for gastroenteritis	Until 3 stools are negative
Pneumonia, pneumococcal	Believed to be 1–3 days	Enteric precautions in hospital. Respiratory isolation may be required.

Table continued on following page

Incubation and Isolation Periods in Common Infections* (Continued)

Infection	Incubation Period	Isolation of Patient†
Puerperal fever, streptococcal	1–3 days	Transfer from maternity ward
Rabies	Usually 2–8 weeks; rarely as short as 9 days or as long as 7 years.	Strict for duration of illness; danger to attendants
Rubella (German measles)	16–18 days with range of 14–23 days	None; no contact with nonimmune pregnant women
Salmonellosis	6–72 hr, usually 12–36 hr	Until stool cultures are *Salmonella* free on two consecutive specimens collected in 24 hr period
Scabies	2–6 weeks before onset of itching in patients without previous infections; 1–4 days after reexposed	Patient is excused from school or work until day after treatment
Trachoma	5–12 days	Until lesions disappear, but usually not practical
Tuberculosis	4–12 weeks to demonstrable primary lesion or significant tuberculin reactions	Variable, depending on conversion of sputum to negative after specific therapy and on ability of patient to understand and carry out personal hygiene methods

* SEE: *Standard and Universal Precautions Appendix.*
† Standard precautions and handwashing are assumed.

independent living skills Skills such as shopping, cooking, cleaning, and child care that are necessary for maintaining the home environment.

independent practice association ABBR: IPA. An integrated group of health care professionals who share patients, premiums, and practices to jointly manage costs, risks, and health care delivery.

index (ĭn′dĕks) *pl.* **indexes, indices** [L., an indicator] **1.** The forefinger. **2.** The ratio of the measurement of a given substance with that of a fixed standard.

addiction severity i. A structured assessment tool that evaluates the impact of addictive behaviors on seven areas of living: alcohol use, drug use, employment, family relationships, illegal activities, physical health, and psychological health.

alveolar i. Gnathic i.

ankle-brachial i. ABBR: ABI. A measure of the arterial flow to the lower extremities, derived by dividing the systolic blood pressure at the posterior tibial artery by the systolic pressure at the ipsilateral brachial artery. Diminished flow is demonstrated when the ratio is less than 1.0.

body mass i. ABBR: BMI. An index for estimating obesity, obtained by dividing weight in kilograms by height in meters squared. In adults, a BMI greater than 30 kg/m^2 indicates obesity; a BMI greater than 40 kg/m^2 indicates morbid obesity, and a BMI less than 18.5 kg/m^2 indicates a person is underweight. SEE: illus.

cardiac i. The cardiac output expressed (as liters per minute) divided by the body surface area (expressed in square meters).

i. case The initial individual whose condition leads to the investigation of a hereditary or infectious disease. SEE: *cohort*.

cephalic i. Skull breadth multiplied by 100 and divided by the length of the skull.

cerebral i. The ratio of greatest transverse to the greatest anteroposterior diameter of the cranium.

chemotherapeutic i. The ratio of the toxicity of a drug, expressed as maximum tolerated dose per kilogram of body weight to the minimal curative dose per kilogram of body weight. This index is used in judging the safety and effectiveness of drugs.

DMF i. The index of dental health and caries experience based on the number of DMF teeth or tooth surfaces. D indicates the number of decayed teeth, M the missing teeth, and F the filled or restored teeth.

gas exchange i. One of several measurements of the efficiency of respiration, esp. of the extent of intrapulmonary shunting in respiratory failure. Among the commonly used gas exchange indexes is the alveolar-arterial oxygen tension difference (a measurement derived from an analysis of the

Federal health guidelines in the U.S. call for use of the Body Mass Index (BMI) to help assess overweight and obesity. A BMI of 25 or more is considered overweight. On the chart below your BMI is located at the intersection of your height and weight.

WEIGHT / HEIGHT	100	105	110	115	120	125	130	135	140	145	150	155	160	165	170	175	180	185	190	195	200	205	210	215	220
5'0"	20	21	21	22	23	24	25	26	27	28	29	30	31	32	33	34	35	36	37	38	39	40	41	42	43
5'1"	19	20	21	22	23	24	25	26	26	27	28	29	30	31	32	33	34	35	36	37	38	39	40	41	42
5'2"	18	19	20	21	22	23	24	25	26	27	27	28	29	30	31	32	33	34	35	36	37	37	38	39	40
5'3"	18	19	19	20	21	22	23	24	25	26	27	27	28	29	30	31	32	33	34	35	35	36	37	38	39
5'4"	17	18	19	20	21	21	22	23	24	25	26	27	27	28	29	30	31	32	33	33	34	35	36	37	38
5'5"	17	17	18	19	20	21	22	22	23	24	25	26	27	27	28	29	30	31	32	32	33	34	35	36	37
5'6"	16	17	18	19	19	20	21	22	23	23	24	25	26	27	27	28	29	30	31	31	32	33	34	35	36
5'7"	16	16	17	18	19	20	20	21	22	23	23	24	25	26	27	27	28	29	30	31	31	32	33	34	34
5'8"	15	16	17	17	18	19	20	21	21	22	23	24	24	25	26	27	27	28	29	30	30	31	32	33	33
5'9"	15	16	16	17	18	18	19	20	21	21	22	23	24	24	25	26	27	27	28	29	30	30	31	32	32
5'10"	14	15	16	17	17	18	19	19	20	21	22	22	23	24	24	25	26	27	27	28	29	29	30	31	32
5'11"	14	15	15	16	17	17	18	19	20	20	21	22	22	23	24	24	25	26	26	27	28	29	29	30	31
6'0"	14	14	15	16	16	17	18	18	19	20	20	21	22	22	23	24	24	25	26	26	27	28	28	29	30
6'1"	13	14	15	15	16	16	17	18	18	19	20	20	21	22	22	23	24	24	25	26	26	27	28	28	29
6'2"	13	13	14	15	15	16	17	17	18	19	19	20	21	21	22	22	23	24	24	25	26	26	27	28	28
6'3"	12	13	14	14	15	16	16	17	17	18	19	19	20	21	21	22	22	23	24	24	25	26	26	27	27
6'4"	12	13	13	14	15	15	16	16	17	18	18	19	19	20	21	21	22	23	23	24	24	25	26	26	27

SOURCES: Shape Up America; National Institutes of Health

BODY MASS INDEX

oxygen tension of an arterial blood gas, compared with the atmospheric oxygen content).

glycemic i. A ratio used to describe the ability of a food to increase blood sugar as compared with consumption of either glucose or white bread as the standard. Foods with a low glycemic index result in a slower rise and lower maximum elevation of blood glucose levels than foods with a higher glycemic index. Consumption of low glycemic index foods can contribute to blood glucose regulation in patients with diabetes mellitus. Another use for the index is for choice of food to raise blood sugar levels after, for example, endurance exercise.

gnathic i. A measure of the degree of projection of the upper jaw by finding the ratio of the distance from the nasion to the basion to that of the basion to the alveolar point multiplying by 100. SYN: *alveolar i.*

leukopenic i. A test formerly used to determine hypersensitivity to foods, in which the white blood cell count was checked 90 min after the consumption of a suspected allergen. A precipitous decrease in the white blood cell count within 90 min after ingestion of the test food was thought to indicate that the food was incompatible with that individual.

opsonic i. A ratio of the number of bacteria that are ingested by leukocytes contained in the serum of a normal individual, compared with the number ingested by leukocytes in the patient's own blood serum.

oral hygiene i. ABBR: OHI. A popular indicator developed in 1960 to determine oral hygiene status in epidemiological studies. The index consists of an oral debris score and a calculus score. Six indicator teeth are examined for soft deposits and calculus. Numerical values are assigned to the six indicator teeth according to the extraneous deposits present. The scores are added and divided by the number of surfaces examined to calculate the average oral hygiene score.

Oswestry Disability I. SEE: *Oswestry Disability Index.*

pelvic i. The ratio of pelvic conjugate and transverse diameters.

periodontal (Ramfjord) i. An extensive consideration of the periodontal status of six teeth by evaluating gingival condition, depth of gingival sulcus or pocket, plaque or calculus, attrition, tooth mobility, and extent of tooth contact.

phagocytic i. The average number of bacteria ingested by each leukocyte after incubation of the bacteria in a mixture of serum and bacterial culture.

refractive i. SEE: under *refraction.*

respiratory i. The ratio of the alveolar-arterial oxygen tension gradient to the arterial partial pressure of oxygen.

respiratory disturbance i. A measurement of the number of disordered breathing cycles during sleep. Sleep disordered breathing, which includes both apneas and hypopneas, results in daytime fatigue. It is also associated with an increased prevalence of cardiovascular disease.

sulcus bleeding i. ABBR: SBI. A sensitive measure of gingival condition that involves probing of all sulci. The score is based on six defined criteria. It is calculated by counting the number of sulci with bleeding, dividing by the total number of sulci, and multiplying by 100.

therapeutic i. The maximum tolerated dose of a drug divided by the minimum curative dose.

thoracic i. The ratio of the thoracic anteroposterior diameter to the transverse diameter.

vital i. The ratio of the number of births to the number of deaths in a population over a stated period of time.

Index Medicus A publication of the National Library of Medicine that lists biomedical and health sciences journal articles by title, subject, field, and country of publication. The major medical and biological journals are indexed.

Indian Health Service ABBR: IHS. A bureau of the U.S. Department of Health and Human Services, responsible for providing public health and medical services to American Indians.

indican (ĭn′dĭ-kăn) **1.** Potassium salt of indoxylsulfate, found in sweat and urine, and formed when intestinal bacteria convert tryptophan to indole. **2.** In plants, a yellow glycoside, the precursor of the dye indigo.

indicanemia (ĭn″dĭ-kăn-ē′mē-ă) [*indican* + Gr. *haima,* blood] Indican in the blood.

indicant (ĭn′dĭ-kănt) **1.** Something such as a sign or symptom that points to the presence of a disease. **2.** Something such as loss of a symptom or sign that indicates that the treatment of the disease is proper and effective.

indicanuria (ĭn″dĭ-kăn-ū′rē-ă) [″ + Gr. *ouron,* urine] An excess of indoxylsulfate of potassium, a derivative of indole, in urine. It is found in small quantities in normal urine. SEE: *urocyanosis*.

indication [L. *indicare,* to show] A sign or circumstance that indicates the proper treatment of a disease.

causal i. An indication provided by the knowledge of the cause of a disease.

symptomatic i. An indication provided by the symptoms of a disease rather than because of precise knowledge of the actual disease process (e.g., a patient may be given acetaminophen without knowing the cause of the symptoms of headache or fever).

indicator [L. *indicare,* to show] In chemical analysis, a substance that can be used to determine pH. In a more general sense, any substance that can be used to determine the completeness of a chemical reaction, as in volumetric analysis. Its uses include (1) in the titration of ammonia and other weak bases; (2) in Topfer's reagent, for determining free acid in gastric juice; and (3) in the titration of weak acids and determination of combined acid in gastric juice. SEE: table.

empirical i. An instrument, experimental condition, or clinical procedure that is used for observation, measurement, or protocol writing, esp. in clinical research.

indictment (ĭn-dīt′mĕnt) First step in criminal procedure; a written accusation or charge that identifies the alleged offense that must be proved at trial, beyond a reasonable doubt, in order to convict the defendant.

indifferent [L. *in-,* not, + *differre,* to differ] **1.** Neutral; tending in no specific direction. **2.** Not responsive to normal stimuli; apathetic. **3.** Pert. to cells that have not differentiated.

indigestible (ĭn″dĭ-jĕs′tĭ-bl) [L. *in-,* not, + *digerere,* to separate] Not digestible.

indigestion [″ + *digerere,* to separate] Incomplete or imperfect digestion, usually accompanied by one or more of the following symptoms: pain, nausea and vomiting, heartburn, acid regurgitation, accumulation of gas, and belching. SYN: *dyspepsia.*

indigitation (ĭn-dĭj″ĭ-tā′shŭn) [L. *in,* in, + *digitus,* finger] Intussusception.

indigo A blue dye obtained from plants or made synthetically.

indigotindisulfonate sodium (ĭn″dĭ-gō″tĭn-dī-sŭl′fō-nāt) A dye used in testing renal function. Trade name is Indigo Carmine.

indinavir ABBR: IDV. A protease inhibitor used in the treatment of HIV-1.

indisposition [L. *in-,* not, + *dispositus,* arranged] A mild disorder; any slight or temporary illness.

indium (ĭn′dē-ŭm) [L. *indicum,* indigo] SYMB: In. A rare metallic element; atomic weight 114.82; atomic number 49; specific gravity 7.31.

indium-111 (^{111}In) An isotope of indium with a half-life of 2.8 days; used in radioactive tracer studies.

Colors of Indicators of pH

	Color		
	Toward Acid	**Toward Alkali**	**Range of pH**
Methyl yellow	Red	Yellow	2.9–4.0
Congo red	Blue	Red	3.0–5.2
Methyl orange	Red	Yellow	3.1–4.4
Methyl red	Red	Yellow	4.2–6.2
Litmus	Red	Blue	4.5–8.3
Bromcresol purple	Yellow	Purple	5.2–6.8
Bromothymol blue	Yellow	Blue	6.0–7.6
Phenol red	Yellow	Red	6.8–8.4
Phenolphthalein	Colorless	Pink	8.2–10.0

individuation (ĭn″dĭ-vĭd″ū-ā′shŭn) **1.** During development, the emergence of specific and individual structures and functions. **2.** The process by which a healthy, integrated personality is developed.

indocyanine green A fluorescent contrast agent used for many purposes, including tests of liver function, blood volume, and retinal perfusion (e.g., during angiography).

indolaceturia (ĭn″dō-lăs″ē-tū′rē-ă) [*indole* + L. *acetum,* vinegar, + Gr. *ouron,* urine] The excretion of an increased amount of indoleacetic acid in the urine. This occurs in patients with phenylketonuria (PKU) and may also be increased by eating serotonin-containing foods (e.g., bananas).

indole (ĭn′dōl) C_8H_7N; a substance found in feces. It is the product of bacterial decomposition of tryptophan and is partially responsible for the odor of feces. In intestinal obstruction it is absorbed and eliminated in the urine in the form of indican.

indolent (ĭn′dō-lĕnt) [LL. *indolens,* painless] **1.** Indisposed to action. **2.** Inactive; not developing; sluggish.

indologenous (ĭn″dō-lŏj′ĕn-ŭs) [*indole* + Gr. *gennan,* to produce] Causing the production of indole.

indoluria (ĭn″dōl-ū′rē-ă) [″ + Gr. *ouron,* urine] The presence of indole in the urine.

indomethacin (ĭn″dō-mĕth′ă-sĭn) A potent nonsteroidal anti-inflammatory drug, used to treat gout and other joint diseases. Its side effects may include inflammation and ulceration of the gastrointestinal tract and renal failure.

indoxyl (ĭn-dŏk′sĭl) [Gr. *indikon,* indigo, + *oxys,* sharp] C_8H_7NO; an oily substance sometimes found in the urine of apparently healthy individuals. It is formed from the decomposition of tryptophan by intestinal bacteria.

indoxylemia (ĭn-dŏk″sĭl-ē′mē-ă) [″ + ″ + *haima,* blood] Indoxyl in the blood.

indoxyluria (ĭn″dŏk-sĭl-ū′rē-ă) [″ + ″ + *ouron,* urine] The excretion of indoxyl in the urine.

induced (ĭn-dūsd′) [L. *inducere,* to lead in] Produced; caused.

inducer (ĭn-dūs′ĕr) In chemistry, a compound that increases the concentration of another molecule; in molecular biology, something that facilitates the development of a gene. SEE: *catalyst*.

inductance That property of an electric circuit by virtue of which a varying current induces an electromotive force in that circuit or a neighboring circuit. The unit of inductance, or self-induction, is the henry.

induction (ĭn-dŭk′shŭn) [L. *inductio,* leading in] **1.** The process of causing or producing, as induction of labor with oxytocic drugs in cases of uterine dysfunction. **2.** The generation of an electric current in a conductor by electricity in another conductor near it. **3.** In embryology, the production of a specific morphogenic effect by a chemical substance from one part of the embryo to another. SYN: *evocation*. **4.** In anesthesia, the period from the initial inhalation or injection of an anesthetic gas or drug until optimum level of anesthesia is reached. **5.** Reasoning from the particular to the general. SEE: *deduction*.

rapid-sequence i. Rapid sequence intubation.

inductor (ĭn-dŭk′tĕr) **1.** Any substance that causes cells exposed to it to differentiate into an organized tissue. **2.** In electronics, a component that employs the principles of electromagnetic induction. It is used in filter circuits and transformers.

inductothermy Treatment of disease by artificial production of fever by electromagnetic induction.

indulin (ĭn′dū-lĭn) Any one of a group of dyes used in histology.

indulinophil(e) (ĭn″dū-lĭn′ō-fĭl, -fīl) The state of being readily stained with indulin.

indurate (ĭn′dū-rāt) [L. *in,* in, + *durus,* hard] **1.** To harden. **2.** Hardened.

indurated Hardened.

induration (ĭn′dū-rā″shun) **1.** The act of hardening. **2.** An area of hardened tissue. SEE: *sclerosis; skin*. **indurative** (-dūr-ā″tĭv), *adj.*

black i. Anthracosis of the lung.

brown i. Pigmentation and fibrosis of the lung as a result of chronic venous congestion of the lung.

cyanotic i. Induration from long continued venous hyperemia, pressure on vessels causing transudation of blood and serum, and formation of a dark, hard mass. In the liver or spleen it leads to absorption of the parenchyma with formation of scar tissue.

granular i. Fibrosis of an organ such as the liver or kidney in which small fibrotic granules are present.

gray i. Unresolved pneumonia with fibrosis of the lung, and no pigmentation.

red i. Chronic interstitial pneumonia with severe congestion.

indusium (ĭn-dū′zē-ŭm) [L., tunic] A membranous covering.

i. griseum A rudimentary gyrus located on the upper surface of the corpus callosum. SYN: *supracallosal gyrus*.

indwelling Inside the body; said of invasive diagnostic or therapeutic devices; pert. to a catheter, drainage tube, or other device that remains inside the body for a prolonged time.

inebriant (ĭn-ē′brē-ănt) [L. *inebrius,* drunken] **1.** Any intoxicant. **2.** Making drunk.

inebriate To make drunk or to become intoxicated.

inebriation (ĭn-ē″brē-ā′shŭn) Intoxication.

inelastic [L. *in-,* not, + Gr. *elastikos,* elastic] Not elastic.

inert (ĭn-ĕrt′) [L. *iners,* unskilled, idle] **1.** Not active; sluggish. **2.** In chemistry, having little or no tendency or ability to react with other chemicals.

inertia (ĭn-ĕr′shē-ă) [L., inactivity] **1.** In physics, the tendency of a body to remain in its state (at rest or in motion) until acted upon by an outside force. **2.** Sluggishness; a lack of activity.

uterine i. An absence or weakness of uterine contractions in labor.

in extremis (ĭn ĕks-trē′mĭs) [L.] At the point of death.

infancy The very early period of life in which the child is still unable to walk or to feed itself. SEE: *infant.*

infant [L. *infans*] A child in the first year of life. SEE: *neonate.*

Development: For three days after birth a baby loses weight; in the next four days, however, a baby should regain the loss and weigh as much as at birth.

The average weekly weight gain in the first three months is 210 g for boys and 195 g for girls; from three to six months it is 150 g for both girls and boys; from six to nine months, 90 g for boys and 105 g for girls; from 9 to 18 months 60 g for both sexes; and from 18 to 24 months 45 g, both sexes.

The newborn is aware of shadow, movement, and voice. By the fourth week the infant lifts the head momentarily; by the 16th week, holds the head erect, coos, or laughs; walks with hands held by the 52nd week; and by the 15th month, toddles alone and may have a vocabulary of a few words. SEE: *psychomotor and physical development of infant.*

Respiration: At birth, respirations are 40 to 50/min; during the first year, 20 to 40/min; during the fifth year, 20 to 25/min; during the 15th year, 15 to 20/min. SEE: *pulse; respiration; temperature.*

Temperature: Normal (rectal) temperature may have a daily variation of 1° to 1.5°C (1.8° to 2.7°F). It is usually highest between 5 and 8 P.M. and lowest between 3 and 6 A.M. Therefore, there is no specific normal temperature, but the values given should be regarded as ranging around the value of 37.6°C (99.7°F) when the temperature is taken rectally. Axillary temperatures in the normal newborn range from 36.4° to 37.2°C (97.5° to 99°F). Infants have poorly developed temperature-regulating mechanisms, and need to be protected from chilling and overheating.

i. of substance-abusing mother ABBR: ISAM. All-inclusive term describing a newborn whose birth mother used alcohol, cocaine, opiates, or other potentially hazardous chemicals during pregnancy. These babies are considered to be at high risk for complications during the neonatal period; many also exhibit related long-term disabilities that influence their potential for normal growth and development. *Perinatal complications* include intrauterine growth retardation, infection, asphyxia, congenital abnormalities, low birth weight, low Apgar score, withdrawal-related symptoms, jaundice, and behavioral problems. *Long-term complications* include behavioral problems such as short attention span, delayed development of language-related skills, and sudden infant death syndrome. SEE: *cocaine baby; fetal alcohol syndrome; heroin.*

post-term i. An infant born after the beginning of the 42nd week of gestation (longer than 288 days).

premature i. Preterm i. SEE: *Nursing Diagnoses Appendix.*

preterm i. An infant born before the completion of 37 weeks (259 days) of gestation. SEE: *prematurity.*

i. stimulation The use of various techniques to provide neonates and infants identified with or at risk for developmental delay with an environment that has a rich and diverse range of sensations and experiences.

term i. An infant born between the beginning of the 38th week through the 41st week of gestation (260 to 287 days).

infant feeding pattern, ineffective A state in which an infant demonstrates an impaired ability to suck or to coordinate the suck-swallow response. SEE: *Nursing Diagnoses Appendix.*

infanticide (ĭn-făn′tĭ-sīd) [LL. *infanticidium*] The killing of an infant.

infantile (ĭn′făn-tīl) [Fr. *infantilis*] Pert. to infancy or an infant.

infantilism (in-făn′tĭl-ĭzm, ĭn′făn-tĭl-ĭzm″) [″ + Gr. *-ismos,* condition] **1.** A condition in which the mind and body make slow development and the individual fails to attain adult characteristics. It is characterized by mental retardation, stunted growth, and sexual immaturity. **2.** Childishness.

angioplastic i. Infantilism due to defective development of the vascular system.

Brissaud's i. Cretinism.

cachectic i. Infantilism caused by chronic infection or poisoning.

celiac i. Infantilism caused by intestinal malabsorption due to intolerance to gluten in the diet.

dysthyroidal i. Infantilism caused by a defective thyroid.

hepatic i. Infantilism combined with cirrhosis of the liver.

hypophyseal i. Infantilism resulting from hypofunction of the anterior lobe of the pituitary gland. SYN: *pituitary i.*

intestinal i. Infantilism associated with a chronic intestinal disorder, causing poor growth.

myxedematous i. Cretinism.

pituitary i. Hypophyseal i.

renal i. Infantilism caused by a defect in renal function.

sexual i. The continuation of childish traits, esp. sex characteristics, beyond the age of puberty.

symptomatic i. Infantilism caused by poor tissue development.

universal i. Infantilism marked by dwarfed stature and an absence of secondary sexual characteristics.

infarct [L. *infarctus*] An area of tissue in an organ or part that undergoes necrosis following cessation of the blood supply. This may result from occlusion or stenosis of the supplying artery or, more rarely, from occlusion of the vein that drains the tissue.

anemic i. An infarct in which blood pigment is lacking or decoloration has occurred. SYN: *pale i.; white i.*

bland i. An infarct in which infection is absent.

calcareous i. An infarct in connective tissue in which calcium salts have been deposited.

cicatrized i. An infarct that has been replaced or encapsulated by fibrous tissue.

hemorrhagic i. Red i.

infected i. Infarcted tissue that has been invaded by pathogenic organisms. SYN: *septic i.*

pale i. Anemic i.

red i. An infarct that is swollen and red as a result of hemorrhage. SYN: *hemorrhagic i.*

septic i. Infected i.

uric acid i. An infarct in the kidney caused by obstruction of the renal tubules by uric acid crystals.

white i. Anemic i.

infarction Death of tissue that results from deprivation of its blood supply.

cardiac i. An infrequently used synonym for myocardial infarction.

cerebral i. An infarction in the brain due to loss of blood flow through one of the arteries of the brain; an ischemic stroke.

evolution of i. The normal healing process after myocardial infarction; seen on ECG as progressive changes in the QRS complex and S-T segment.

extension of i. An increase in the size of a myocardial infarction, occurring after the initial infarction and usually accompanied by a return of acute symptoms, such as angina unrelieved by appropriate medicines.

lacunar i. A small stroke deep within the brain (e.g., in the internal capsule, basal ganglia, thalamus, or pons) caused by damage to or a blockage of a tiny penetrating artery. Lacunar infarctions are associated with a kind of vascular damage caused by chronic high blood pressure called lipohyalinosis. They may be asymptomatic, showing up only on brain imaging, or may produce pure motor, pure sensory, ataxic, or mixed motor and sensory symptoms. SYN: *lacunar stroke.*

placental i. A localized necrotic area caused by abruption. SEE: *abruptio placentae.*

pulmonary i. An infarction in the lung usually resulting from pulmonary embolism that may appear on x-rays as a wedge-shaped infiltrate near the pleura. Immediate therapy includes control of pain, oxygen administered continuously by mask, intravenous heparin (unless patient has a known blood clotting defect), and treatment of shock or dysrhythmias, if present.

silent myocardial i. Unrecognized myocardial infarction. The patient may experience difficulty breathing, heartburn, nausea, arm pain, or other atypical symptoms.

infect [ME. *infecten*] To cause pathogenic organisms to be present in or upon, as to infect a wound.

infection (ĭn-fĕk′shŭn) A disease caused by microorganisms, esp. those that release toxins or invade body tissues. Worldwide, infectious diseases (e.g., malaria, tuberculosis, hepatitis viruses, diarrheal illnesses) produce more disability and death than any other cause. Infection differs from colonization of the body by microorganisms in that during colonization, microbes reside harmlessly in the body or perform useful functions for it (e.g., bacteria in the gut that produce vitamin K). By contrast, infectious illnesses typically cause harm. SEE: table.

ETIOLOGY: The most common pathogenic organisms are bacteria (including mycobacteria, mycoplasmas, spirochetes, chlamydiae, and rickettsiae), viruses, fungi, protozoa, and helminths. Life-threatening infectious disease usually occurs when immunity is weak or suppressed (e.g., in the first few months of life, old age, malnourished persons, trauma or burn victims, leukopenic patients, and those with chronic illnesses such as diabetes mellitus, renal failure, cancer, asplenia, alcoholism, heart, lung, or liver disease). Many disease-causing agents, however, may afflict vigorous persons, whether they are young or old, fit or weak. Some examples include sexually transmitted illnesses (e.g., herpes simplex or chlamydia), respiratory illnesses (influenza or varicella), food or waterborne pathogens (cholera, schistosomiasis), and numerous others.

SYMPTOMS: Systemic infections cause fevers, chills, sweats, malaise,

Fungal Infections

Disease	Causative Organisms	Structures Infected	Microscopic Appearances
Superficial Fungal Infections			
Epidermophytosis (dhobie itch, etc.)	*Epidermophyton* (*floccosum,* etc.)	Inguinal, axillary, and interdigital folds; hairs not affected	Long, wavy, branched and segmented hyphae and spindle-shaped cells in stratum corneum
Favus (tinea favosa)	*Trichophyton schödonleini*	Epidermis around a hair; all parts of body; nails	Vertical hyphae and spores in epidermis; sinuous branching mycelium and chains in hairs
Ringworm (tinea, otomycosis)	*Microsporum* (*audouinii,* etc.)	Horny layer of epidermis and hairs, chiefly of scalp	Fine septate mycelium inside hairs and scales; spores in rows and mosaic plaques on hair surface
	Tricophyton (*tonsurans,* etc.)	Hairs of scalp, beard, and other parts; nails	Mycelium of chained cubical elements and threads in and on hairs; often pigmented
Thrush and other forms of candidiasis	*Candida albicans*	Tongue, mouth, throat, vagina, and skin	Yeastlike budding cells and oval thick-walled bodies in lesion
Systemic Fungal Infections			
Aspergillosis	*Aspergillus fumigatus*	Lungs	Y-shaped branching of septate hyphae
Blastomycosis	*Blastomyces brasiliensis, B. dermatitidis*	Skin and lungs	Yeastlike cells demonstrated in lesion
Candidiasis	*Candida albicans*	Esophagus, lungs, peritoneum, mucous membranes	Small thin-walled ovoid cells
Coccidioidomycosis	*Coccidioides immitis*	Respiratory tract	Nonbudding spores containing many endospores, in sputum
Cryptococcosis	*Cryptococcus neoformans*	Meninges, lungs, bone, skin	Yeastlike fungus having gelatinous capsule; demonstrated in spinal fluid
Histoplasmosis	*Histoplasma capsulatum*	Lungs	Oval, budding, uninucleated cells
Nocardiosis	*Nocardia asteroides*	Lungs, brain, subcutaneous tissues	Closely resemble bacteria; found in pus

and occasionally, headache, muscle and joint pains, or changes in mental status. Localized infections produce tissue redness, swelling, tenderness, heat, and loss of function.

TRANSMISSION: Pathogens can be transmitted to their hosts by many mechanisms, namely, inhalation, ingestion, injection or the bite of a vector, direct (e.g., skin-to-skin) contact, contact with blood or body fluids, fetomaternal contact, contact with contaminated articles ("fomites"), or self-inoculation.

In health care settings, infections are often transmitted to patients by the hands of professional staff or other employees. Handwashing before and after patient contact prevents many of these infections.

DEFENSES: The body's defenses against infection begin with mechanisms that block entry of the organism into the skin or the respiratory, gastrointestinal, or genitourinary tract. These defenses include (1) chemicals (e.g., lysozymes in tears, fatty acids in skin, gastric acid, and pancreatic enzymes in the bowel), (2) mucus that traps the organism, (3) clusters of antibody-producing B lymphocytes (e.g., tonsils, Peyer's patches), and (4) bacteria and fungi (normal flora) on skin and mucosal surfaces that destroy more dangerous organisms. In patients receiving immunosuppressive drug therapy, the normal flora can become the source of opportunistic infections. Also, one organism can impair external defenses and permit another to enter; for example, viruses can enhance bacterial invasion by damaging respiratory tract mucosa.

The body's second line of defense is the nonspecific immune response, inflammation. The third major defensive system, the specific immune response, depends on lymphocyte activation, during which B and T cells recognize specific antigenic markers on the organism. B cells produce immunoglobulins (antibodies) and T cells orchestrate a multifaceted attack by cytotoxic cells. SEE: *cell, B; cell, T; inflammation.*

SPREAD: Once pathogens have crossed cutaneous or mucosal barriers and gained entry into internal tissues, they may spread quickly along membranes such as the meninges, pleura, or peritoneum. Some pathogens produce enzymes that damage cell membranes, enabling them to move rapidly from cell to cell. Others enter the lymphatic channels; if they can overcome WBC defenses in the lymph nodes, they move into the bloodstream to multiply at other sites. This is frequently seen with pyogenic organisms, which create abscesses far from the initial entry site. Viruses or rickettsiae, which reproduce only inside cells, travel in the blood to cause systemic infections; viruses that damage a fetus during pregnancy (e.g., rubella and cytomegalovirus) travel via the blood.

DIAGNOSIS: Although many infections (e.g., those that cause characteristic rashes) are diagnosed clinically, definitive identification of infection usually occurs in the laboratory. Carefully collected and cultured specimens of blood, urine, stool, sputum, or other body fluids are used to identify pathogens and their susceptibilities to treatment.

TREATMENT: Many infections, like the common cold, are self-limited and require no specific treatment. Understanding this concept is crucial, because the misuse of antibiotics does not help the affected patient and may damage society by fostering antimicrobial resistance. Many common infections, such as urinary tract infections or impetigo, respond well to antimicrobial products. Others, like abscesses, may require incision and drainage.

acute i. An infection that appears suddenly and may be of brief or prolonged duration.

air-borne i. An infection caused by inhalation of pathogenic organisms in droplet nuclei.

apical i. An infection located at the tip of the root of a tooth.

bacterial i. Any disease caused by bacteria. Bacteria exist in a variety of relationships with the human body. Bacteria colonize body surfaces and provide benefits (e.g., by limiting the growth of pathogens and producing vitamins for absorption (symbiotic relationship). Bacteria can coexist with the human body without producing harmful or beneficial effects (commensal relationship). Bacteria may also invade tissues, damage cells, trigger systemic inflammatory responses, and release toxins (pathogenic, infectious relationship).

blood-borne i. An infection transmitted through contact with the blood (cells, serum, or plasma) of an infected individual. The contact may occur sexually, through injection, or via a medical or dental procedure in which a blood-contaminated instrument is inadvertently used after inadequate sterilization. Examples of blood-borne infections include hepatitis B and C, and AIDS. SEE: *needle-stick injury; Standard and Universal Precautions Appendix.*

chronic i. An infection having a protracted course.

concurrent i. The existence of two or more infections at the same time. SEE: *superinfection.*

cross i. The transfer of an infectious organism or disease from one patient in a hospital to another.

cryptogenic i. An infection whose source is unknown. SEE: *infection.*

deep neck i. An infection that enters the fascial planes of the neck after originating in the oral cavity, pharynx, or a regional lymph node. It may be life-threatening if the infection enters the carotid sheath, the paravertebral spaces, or the mediastinum. Death may also result from sepsis, asphyxiation, or hemorrhage. Aggressive surgical therapy is usually required because antibiotics alone infrequently control the disease.

diabetic foot i. A polymicrobial infection of the bones and soft tissues of the lower extremities of patients with diabetes mellitus, typically those patients who have vascular insufficiency or neuropathic foot disease. Eradication of the infection may require prolonged courses of antibiotics, surgical débridement or amputation, or reconstruction or bypass of occluded arteries.

droplet i. An infection acquired by the inhalation of a microorganism in the air, esp. one added to the air by sneezing or cough.

fungal i. Pathological invasion of the body by yeast or fungi. Fungi are most likely to produce disease in patients whose immune defenses are compromised.

local i. An infection that has not spread but remains contained near the entry site.

low-grade i. A loosely used term for a subacute or chronic infection with only mild inflammation and without pus formation.

nosocomial i. An infection contracted in a hospital, typically with virulent, or drug-resistant germs. Patients in burn units and surgical intensive care units have the highest rates of nosocomial infections, while patients in coronary care units have the lowest. SEE: *infection control.*

PATIENT CARE: Hospital-acquired infections result from the exposure of debilitated patients to the drug-altered environment of the hospital, where indwelling urinary catheters, intravenous lines, and endotracheal tubes enter normally sterile body sites, and allow microbes to penetrate and multiply. *Enterobacter* species, *Pseudomonas* sp., staphylococci, enterococci, *Clostridium difficile,* and fungi often are responsible for the individual and epidemic infectious outbreaks that result.

opportunistic i. **1.** Any infection that results from a defective immune system that cannot defend against pathogens normally found in the environment. Common types include bacterial (*Pseudomonas aeruginosa*), fungal (*Candida albicans*), protozoan (*Pneumocystis carinii*), and viral (cytomegalovirus). Opportunistic infections are seen in patients with impaired defenses against disease, such as those with cystic fibrosis, poorly controlled diabetes mellitus, acquired or congenital immune deficiencies, or organ transplants. **2.** An infection that results when resident flora proliferate and infect a body site in which they are normally present or at some other location. In healthy humans, the millions of bacteria in and on the body do not cause infection or disease. Host defenses and interaction with other microorganisms prevent excess growth of potential pathogens. A great number of factors, many poorly understood, may allow a normal bacterial resident to proliferate and cause disease. SEE: *acquired immunodeficiency syndrome; immunocompromised.*

protozoal i. An infection with a protozoon (e.g., malaria).

pyogenic i. An infection resulting from pus-forming organisms.

risk for i. An immunocompromised state. SEE: *Nursing Diagnoses Appendix.*

secondary i. An infection made possible by a primary infection that lowers the host's resistance (e.g., bacterial pneumonia following influenza).

subacute i. An infection intermediate between acute and chronic.

subclinical i. An infection that is immunologically confirmed but does not produce obvious symptoms or signs.

systemic i. An infection in which the infecting agent or organisms circulate throughout the body.

infectious (ĭn-fĕk′shŭs) [ME. *infecten,* infect] **1.** Capable of being transmitted with or without contact. **2.** Pert. to a disease caused by a microorganism. **3.** Producing infection.

infecundity (ĭn-fē-kŭn′dĭ-tē) [L. *infecunditas,* sterility] Barrenness; an inability to conceive.

inferior (ĭn-fē′rē-or) [L. *inferus,* below] **1.** Beneath; lower. **2.** Used medically in reference to the undersurface of an organ or indicating a structure below another structure.

inferiority complex SEE: under *complex.*

infertility Inability to achieve pregnancy during a year or more of unprotected intercourse. The condition may be present in either or both partners and may be reversible. In the U.S., about 20% of all couples are infertile. In women, infertility may be primary (i.e., present in women who have never conceived) or secondary (i.e., occurring after previous conceptions or pregnancies). Causes of primary infertility in women include ovulatory failure, anatomical anomalies of the uterus, Turner's syndrome, and eating disorders, among many others. Common causes of secondary infertility in women include but are not limited to tubal scarring (e.g., after sexually transmitted infections), endometriosis, cancers, and chemotherapy. In men, infertility usually is caused by failure to manufacture adequate amounts of sperm (e.g., as a result of exposures to environmental toxins, viruses or bacteria, developmental or genetic diseases, varicoceles, or endocrine abnormalities).

DIAGNOSIS: Investigation begins with a comprehensive individual history from both partners, assessment of their usual timing of intercourse, and thorough physical examinations. The initial test for men is semen analysis to assess sperm morphology, motility, and number. This should be done after 2 to 3 days of sexual abstinence. At least two to three ejaculates, obtained at no less than 1-week intervals, should be examined, because of the variability in sperm counts. Female assessment usually begins with evaluation of ovulation by use of a basal body temperature graph. Additional special assessments of the woman may be ordered to evaluate ovarian, tubal, uterine, and cervical factors.

TREATMENT: The specific problems that testing identifies may be managed by either pharmacological or surgically assisted reproduction techniques. SEE: *embryo transfer; in vitro fertilization; gamete intrafallopian transfer; transcervical balloon tuboplasty*.

secondary i. Infertility in which one or more pregnancies have occurred before the present condition of infertility.

infest [L. *infestare,* to attack] To overrun to a harmful extent; said esp. of parasites.

infestation The harboring of animal parasites, esp. macroscopic forms such as worm endoparasites and arthropod ectoparasites.

infibulation (ĭn-fĭb-ū-lā′shŭn) [L. *in,* in, + *fibula,* clasp] The process of fastening, as in joining the lips of wounds by clasps. Also, suturing together of the labia of women to prevent sexual intercourse.

infiltrate (ĭn-fĭl′trāt, ĭn′fĭl-trāt) [″ + *filtrare,* to strain through] **1.** To pass into or through a substance or a space. **2.** The material that has infiltrated. **3.** A shadow seen on a chest x-ray, and assumed to represent blood, pus, or other body fluids in the lung.

alveolar i. Opacification of air spaces, caused by the filling of alveoli with blood, pus, or fluid. Alveolar infiltrates are seen on the chest radiograph as patchy areas of increased density, often surrounding air bronchograms.

lobar i. A well-defined site of lung consolidation, seen on the chest radiograph as an area of increased density confined within a specific lobe or segment. SYN: *lobar pneumonia*.

ETIOLOGY: Lobar infiltrates are usually due to bacterial infection (pneumonia).

TREATMENT: The patient will need antibiotics, oxygen, and bronchial hygiene.

patchy i. A poorly defined area of lung consolidation seen on the chest radiograph as scattered opacification within normal lung tissue. It is usually caused by a mixture of normally aerated and infected lung lobules.

infiltration (ĭn″fĭl-trā′shŭn) The process of a substance passing into and being deposited within the substance of a cell, tissue, or organ. Examples of infiltration include that of a tissue or organ by blood corpuscles and that of a cell by fatty particles. Infiltration must not be confused with degeneration; in the latter condition the foreign substances are from changes within the cell.

amyloid i. The infiltration of tissue or viscera with amyloid, a starchlike glycoprotein. SEE: *amyloid*.

anesthesia i. The injection of an anesthetic solution directly into tissue. SEE: *anesthesia*.

calcareous i. Deposits of calcium or magnesium salts within a tissue.

cellular i. An infiltration of cells, esp. blood cells, into tissues; invasion by cells of malignant tumors into adjacent tissue.

fatty i. A deposit of fat in the tissues, or oil or fat globules in the cells.

glycogenic i. Glycogen deposit in cells.

lymphocytic i. An infiltration of tissue by lymphocytes.

pigmentary i. An infiltration of pigments.

purulent i. Pus in tissue.

serous i. An infiltration with lymph.

urinous i. An infiltration with urine.

waxy i. Amyloid degeneration.

infinite distance **1.** A distance without limits. **2.** In ophthalmology, the assumption that the light rays coming from a point of a distance beyond 20 ft (6.1 m) are practically parallel and accommodation is unnecessary.

infirm [L. *infirmis*] Weak or feeble, esp. from old age or disease.

infirmary [L. *infirmarium*] A small hospital; a place for the care of sick or infirm persons.

infirmity **1.** Weakness. **2.** A sickness or illness.

inflammation [L. *inflammare,* to flame within] An immunological defense against injury, infection, or allergy, marked by increases in regional blood flow, immigration of white blood cells, and release of chemical toxins. Inflammation is one mechanism the body uses to protect itself from invasion by foreign organisms and to repair tissue trauma. Its clinical hallmarks are redness, heat,

Mediating Factors in Inflammation

Factors	Source	Effect
Arachidonic acid metabolites (prostaglandins and leukotrienes)	Phospholipids of cell membranes, especially mast cells	Primary mediators of late-stage (>6 hrs) inflammation; increase dilation and permeability of blood vessels; stimulate neutrophil adhesion to endothelial tissue; bronchoconstriction; anaphylaxis
Bradykinin	Kinin system of plasma proteins	Primary mediator of prolonged (>1 hr) inflammation; vasodilation and increased permeability of blood vessels; pain; release of leukotrienes and prostaglandins
Complement proteins	Macrophages; liver endothelium	Increase vasodilation and vascular permeability; coat antigens to enhance phagocytosis; attract neutrophils; destroy pathogens
Histamine and serotonin	Mast cells Basophils	Primary mediators of early (≤30 min) inflammation; rapid dilation and increase in permeability of venules; bronchoconstriction; stimulation of prostaglandin production
Interleukin 1 (IL-1)	Macrophages; B cells, dendritic cells, neutrophils, other nucleated cells	Increased production and activity of other chemical mediators, phagocytes and lymphocytes; promotes release of acute phase proteins; causes fever
Interleukin 8 (IL-8)	T lymphocytes; monocytes	Attract neutrophils and more T cells
Platelet-activating factor (PAF)	Platelets	Releases chemical mediators; activates neutrophils; dilates and increases permeability of vessels
Transforming growth factor β (TFGβ)	Activated macrophages and T lymphocytes	Attracts neutrophils and monocytes; stimulates growth of connective tissue; inhibits other mediators
Tumor necrosis factors (TFNα)	Activated macrophages and some lymphocytes	Increases synthesis of other cytokines; induces formation of new blood vessels; increases adhesion of neutrophils to endothelium; causes fever and cachexia

swelling, pain, and loss of function of a body part. Systemically, inflammation may produce fevers, joint and muscle pains, organ dysfunction, and malaise. SEE: table; *autoimmune disease; infection*. **inflammatory,** *adj.*

THE INFLAMMATORY PROCESS: Local inflammatory responses begin when traumatized or infected tissues activate the humoral and cellular immune systems. Complement proteins and cytokines are manufactured; these signaling proteins start a cascade of chemical events that result in increases in local blood flow and the attraction of white blood cells to the damaged tissue. White blood cells in turn consume foreign or injured cells and release arachidonic acid metabolites, kinins, histamines, and more complement, thereby amplifying and perpetuating the immune response. The white blood cells also release toxic oxygen radicals, nitric oxide, and tissue-destroying enzymes in an attempt to kill any invading microorganisms. In healthy individuals, the process continues until all damaged tissues or invading pathogens are removed (usually about 5 days); an inpouring of fibroblasts, which repair the injury and form a healed scar, follows.

Systemic inflammatory responses occur when foreign proteins are recognized (e.g., in the bloodstream) and immune complexes are formed or cytotoxic T cells are activated. If sepsis triggers the immune response, these agents may help clear microorganisms from the blood.

Autoimmune illnesses occur when the chemical and cellular tools of inflammation are directed relentlessly against the body's own tissues.

DIAGNOSIS: Nonspecific test results that suggest inflammation include an elevated white blood cell count, erythrocyte sedimentation rate, or C-reactive protein level.

TREATMENT: Mild inflammation (such as the inflammatory change that follows minor injuries) often resolves with the topical application of ice packs or cold water. Nonsteroidal anti-inflammatory drugs (e.g., ibuprofen) and steroids (e.g., prednisone) are useful in managing more severe inflammation, as are many disease-modifying antirheumatic drugs, such as methotrexate or azathioprine.

acute i. The early response to tissue injury, marked by the influx of white blood cells and inflammatory mediators into damaged tissues. The majority of the response takes place in 12–24 hours.

chronic i. Inflammation that persists weeks to months after tissue damage. Its pathological hallmarks include simultaneous tissue repair and destruction.

exudative i. An inflammatory process in which the fluid leaving the capillaries is rich in plasma proteins.

fibrinous i. Inflammation in which the exudate is rich in fibrin.

granulomatous i. An inflammation characterized by granulomas, growths that result when macrophages are unable to destroy foreign bodies after engulfing them; seen esp. in tuberculosis, syphilis, and some fungal infections.

hyperplastic i. Inflammation characterized by excess production of young fibrous tissue. SYN: *proliferative i.*

interstitial i. Inflammation involving principally the noncellular or supporting elements of an organ.

proliferative i. Hyperplastic i.

pseudomembranous i. Inflammation in which a shelf of fibrin and white blood cell debris forms on an epithelial lining, usually as a result of a toxin that necroses tissue. Most often this type of inflammation is seen in colitis caused by *Clostridium difficile;* in the era before vaccinations against diphtheria, it frequently was found in the oral cavity of individuals infected with that germ.

purulent i. Inflammation in which pus is formed. SYN: *suppurative i.*

serous i. Inflammation of a part with serous exudate, or inflammation of a serous membrane.

subacute i. Mild inflammatory process with minimal signs and symptoms. It may become chronic and gradually damage tissues.

suppurative i. Purulent i.

ulcerative i. The formation of an ulcer over an area of inflammation.

inflammatory [L. *inflammare,* to flame within] Pert. to or marked by inflammation.

inflation (ĭn-flā′shŭn) [L. *in,* into, + *flare,* to blow] The distention of a part by air, gas, or liquid.

inflator (ĭn-flā′tor) An apparatus for forcing air or other gas into an organ. This may be done for diagnostic or therapeutic purposes.

inflection (ĭn″flĕk′shŭn) [″ + *flectere,* to bend] **1.** An inward bending. **2.** A change of tone or pitch of the voice; a nuance.

infliximab (ĭn-flĕx′ē-măb) A monoclonal antibody against tumor necrosis factor, used to treat patients with Crohn's disease and rheumatoid arthritis.

influenza (ĭn″floo-ĕn′ză) [It., influence] An acute contagious respiratory infection marked by fevers, muscle aches, headache, prostration, cough, and sore throat. The disease usually strikes during the winter. In patients with serious pre-existing illnesses and people over 65, influenza frequently is fatal. The disease spreads primarily by inhalation of infectious aerosols, although spread by direct personal contact also is possible. Sporadic cases occur each year in the U.S., taking about 20,000 lives. Epidemics or pandemics arise intermittently around the world during periods of viral evolution; in the winter of 1918 to 1919, an influenza pandemic claimed 20,000,000 victims. SYN: *flu.* SEE: *cold; Nursing Diagnoses Appendix.* **influenzal** (-zăl), *adj.*

ETIOLOGY: The responsible virus is either influenza A (about 65% of cases) or influenza B (about 35% of cases).

COURSE: The incubation period of influenza is about 1 to 3 days, and the acute course of the illness typically lasts less than a week. Bacterial superinfection may occur, causing secondary pneumonias, sinusitis, or otitis media. Many patients have a several-week period of malaise during their recuperation from acute infection.

PREVENTION: Worldwide surveillance for new influenza antigens is an ongoing public health project; each year, updated vaccines are developed to counteract new strains of the disease. In the U.S., about 70,000,000 people are vaccinated each year. Vaccination should be offered to people over 65 and individuals with underlying cardiac, pulmonary, renal, or hepatic disease. Vaccination of the general population prevents epidemic disease and prevents significant economic losses caused by employee absenteeism. Influenza vaccines are more than 70% effective in the elderly and about 90% effective in younger recipients.

VACCINATION IN PREGNANCY: Women in the second and third trimesters of pregnancy are among the "target groups" for immunization—that is, they more than other members of the general population should be recruited to receive influenza vaccination. Pregnant women with underlying heart, lung, or other chronic illnesses (e.g., diabetes mellitus) should receive influenza vaccination at *any* stage of pregnancy.

CAUTION: Children with influenza-like illnesses should avoid aspirin products because of the risk of Reye's syndrome. All patients receiving influenza vaccines should review federally mandated Vaccine Information Sheets carefully before getting their injections.

TREATMENT: Influenza A virus is treatable with the antiviral drugs amantadine and rimantadine. Zanamivir and several other antiviral agents have a small impact on the duration of infection with either influenza A or B virus. Symptom-based treatment with acetaminophen, guaifenesin, and other over-the-counter remedies alleviate some of the misery the illness causes.

PATIENT CARE: For the hospitalized patient, respiratory and blood and body fluid precautions are followed. Vital signs and fluid balance are monitored. Respiratory function is assessed for signs and symptoms of developing pneumonia, such as inspiratory crackles, increased fever, pleuritic chest pain, dyspnea, and coughing accompanied by sputum. Prescribed analgesics, antipyretics, and decongestants are administered. Bedrest and increased oral fluid intake are encouraged, and I.V. fluids administered if prescribed. Cool, humidified air is provided, and the humidifier water is changed daily to prevent secondary infection; oxygen therapy is administered if necessary. The patient is assisted to return to normal activities gradually. Mouthwash or warm saline gargles are provided to ease throat soreness. The patient is taught proper disposal of tissues and correct and thorough hand-washing techniques to prevent spread of the virus. The patient treated at home is taught about all of the above supportive care measures as well as about signs and symptoms of serious complications to be reported. Influenza immunizations are discussed with patients; high-risk patients and health-care workers should get an annual inoculation in late fall.

Asian i. Influenza caused by a variant strain of influenza virus type A.

infolding Process of enclosing within a fold; an operation formerly employed in the treatment of stomach ulcer in which the walls on either side of the lesion are sutured together.

infra- [L. *infra,* below, underneath] Prefix meaning *below; under; beneath; inferior to; after.*

infra-axillary (ĭn″fră-ăks′ĭl-ă-rē) [″ + *axilla,* little axis] Below the axilla.

infrabulge (ĭn′fră-bŭlj) The surfaces of the tooth gingival to the height of contour.

infraclavicular (ĭn″fră-klă-vĭk′ū-lăr) [″ + *clavicula,* little key] Below the clavicle.

infracortical (ĭn″fră-kor′tĭ-kăl) [″ + *cortex,* rind] Beneath the cortex of any organ.

infracostal (ĭn″fră-kŏs′tăl) [″ + *costa,* rib] Below the rib.

infracotyloid (ĭn″fră-kŏt′ĭ-loyd) [″ + Gr. *kotyloeides,* cup shaped] Beneath the cotyloid cavity of the acetabulum of the hip.

infraction (ĭn-frăk′shŭn) [L. *infractus,* to destroy] An incomplete fracture of a bone in which parts do not become displaced.

infradentale A craniometric landmark; it is the bony point between the mandibular central incisors. SEE: *cephalometry.*

infradiaphragmatic (ĭn″fră-dī″ă-frăg-măt′ĭk) Subdiaphragmatic.

infraglenoid (ĭn″fră-glē′noyd) [L. *infra,* below, underneath, + Gr. *glene,* cavity, + *eidos,* form, shape] Subglenoid.

infraglottic (ĭn″fră-glŏt′ĭk) [″ + Gr. *glottis,* back of tongue] Below the glottis.

infrahyoid (ĭn″fră-hī′oyd) [″ + Gr. *hyoeides,* U-shaped] Below the hyoid bone.

inframammary [″ + *mamma,* breast] Below the mammary gland.

inframandibular (ĭn″fră-măn-dĭb′ū-lăr) [″ + *mandibula,* lower jawbone] Below the lower jaw (mandible).

inframarginal [″ + *margo,* a margin] Below any edge or margin.

inframaxillary [″ + *maxilla,* jawbone] Below the upper jaw (maxilla).

infranuclear (ĭn″fră-nū′klē-ăr) [″ + *nu-*

cleus, kernel] In the nervous system, peripheral to a nucleus.

infraocclusion [″ + *occlusio,* a shutting up] Location of a tooth below the line of occlusion.

infraorbital (ĭn-fră-or′bĭ-tăl) [″ + *orbita,* track] Beneath the orbit.

infrapatellar (ĭn″fră-pă-tĕl′ăr) [″ + *patella,* a small plate] Below the patella.

infrapsychic (ĭn″fră-sī′kĭk) [″ + Gr. *psyche,* mind] Below the level of consciousness; automatic.

infrapubic [″ + *pubes,* hair covering pubic area] Below the pubis.

infrared Lying outside the red end of the visible spectrum.

infrascapular [″ + *scapula,* shoulder blade] Beneath the shoulder blade.

infrasonic (ĭn″fră-sŏn′ĭk) [L. *infra,* below, underneath, + *sonus,* sound] Sound wave frequency lower than those normally heard.

i. recorder A device that can be used to determine blood pressure by detecting and recording the subaudible oscillations of the arterial wall under an occluding cuff. The resulting values are comparable to those determined by use of an intra-arterial catheter. SEE: *blood pressure, indirect measurement of; pseudohypertension.*

infrasound Sounds of low frequency used for example, in diagnostic and therapeutic technologies.

infraspinous [″ + *spina,* thorn] Beneath the scapular spine.

infrasternal [″ + Gr. *sternon,* chest] Beneath the sternum.

infratemporal (ĭn″fră-tĕm′pō-răl) [″ + *temporalis,* pert. to the temple] Below the temporal fossa of the skull.

infratonsillar (ĭn″fră-tŏn′sĭ-lăr) [″ + *tonsilla,* almond] In the pharynx below the tonsils.

infratrochlear (ĭn″fră-trŏk′lē-ăr) [″ + *trochlea,* pulley] Beneath the trochlea.

infraumbilical (ĭn″fră-ŭm-bĭl′ĭ-kăl) [″ + *umbilicus,* a pit] Below the umbilicus.

infraversion (ĭn″fră-vĕr′zhŭn) [″ + *versio,* a turning] A downward deviation of the eye.

infundibulectomy (ĭn″fŭn-dĭb″ū-lĕk′tō-mē) [L. *infundibulum,* funnel, + Gr. *ektome,* excision] Surgical excision of the infundibulum of any structure or organ, esp. the heart.

infundibuliform (ĭn″fŭn-dĭb′ū-lĭ-form) [″ + *forma,* form] Funnel-shaped.

i. fascia The membranous layer investing the spermatic cord.

infundibulopelvic (ĭn″fŭn-dĭb″ū-lō-pĕl′vĭk) [″ + *pelvis,* basin] Concerning the infundibulum and pelvis of an organ, esp. the kidney.

infundibulum (ĭn″fŭn-dĭb′ū-lŭm) [L.] **1.** A funnel-shaped passage or structure. **2.** The tube connecting the frontal sinus with the middle nasal meatus. **3.** The stalk of the pituitary gland. **4.** Any renal pelvis division. **5.** The cavity formed by the fallopian fimbriae. **6.** The terminus of a bronchiole. **7.** The terminus at the upper end of the cochlear canal. **8.** The conelike upper anterior angle of the right cardiac ventricle from which the pulmonary artery arises. SYN: *conus arteriosus.*

ethmoidal i. The area in the middle meatus of the nose. The anterior ethmoid sinuses and the frontal sinus open into this area.

i. of hypothalamus Infundibulum of the hypothalamus. The stalk that extends from the hypothalamus to the posterior lobe of the pituitary gland.

i. of the uterine tube The funnel-shaped opening at the lateral end of the uterine tube.

infusible [L. *in-,* not, + *fusio,* fusion] Not capable of being fused or melted.

infusible [L. *in,* into, + *fundere,* to pour] Capable of being made into an infusion.

infusion (ĭn-fū′zhŭn) [L. *infusio*] **1.** Steeping a substance in hot or cold water in order to obtain its active principle. **2.** The product obtained from the process of steeping. **3.** Any liquid substance (other than blood) introduced into the body via a vein for therapeutic purposes.

bone marrow i. An old term for intraosseous infusion.

continuous hepatic artery i. ABBR: CHAI. The use of an infusion pump to provide a continuous supply of chemotherapeutic agents to the hepatic artery to control metastases from cancers of the gastrointestinal tract.

continuous i. A controlled method of drug administration in which the rate and quality of drug administration can be precisely adjusted over time. Cancer chemotherapies, insulin, antibiotics, heparins, and many other drugs, fluids, and nutrients can be given by this method.

intravenous i. The injection into a vein of a solution, drugs, or blood components. SEE: illus.

SOLUTIONS: Many liquid preparations are given by intravenous infusion. Those commonly used include isotonic saline, Ringer's lactated, dextrose 5% in water, and potassium chloride 0.2% in 5% dextrose. The quantity depends on the needs of the patient. The solution is usually given continuously at the rate of 1 to 2 or more liters per day. In severe shock, however, rapid infusion of larger volumes may be necessary.

SITE: Intravenous infusion is usually given in the arm, to the median basilic or median cephalic vein, but veins at various other sites may be used. Preparation is the same as for intravenous injection, except that a needle or cannula is used. The vein must be exposed if a cannula is used. Introduction of so-

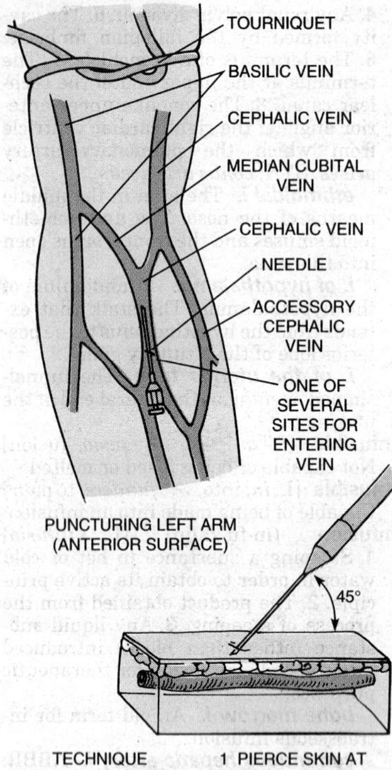

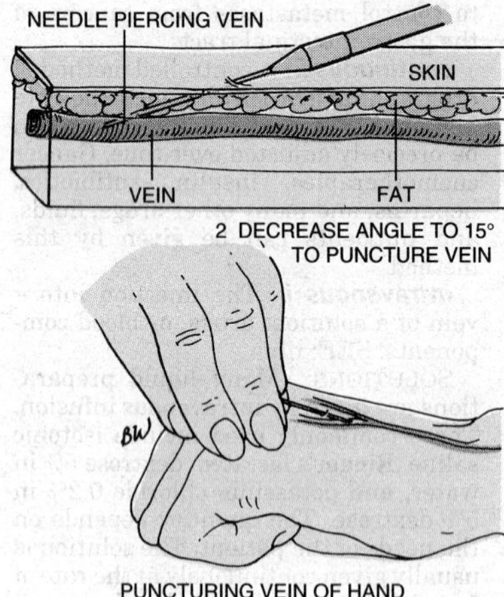

INTRAVENOUS INFUSION TECHNIQUE

lution should be at the rate required to deliver the needed amount of fluid and contained electrolytes, medicines, or nutrients in a prescribed time.

CAUTION: Intravenous infusions should be discontinued or infusion fluid replenished when the solution being administered is depleted. Clotting of blood in the needle occurs when the infusion is not continuous.

PATIENT CARE: Using scrupulous aseptic technique and universal precautions, the nurse prepares the I.V. infusion, selects and prepares a venous site, inserts an I.V. cannula to initiate the infusion (if an I.V. access is not in place), and secures it in place (all according to protocol), restraining joint motion near the insertion site as necessary. The amount of fluid is calculated and the flow of the prescribed fluid (and additive as appropriate) initiated at the desired flow rate. Prior to beginning the infusion, the nurse ensures that the correct fluid is being administered at the designated flow-rate, and observes the infusion site at least every hour for signs of infiltration or other complications, such as thrombophlebitis, fluid or electrolyte overload, and air embolism. The site dressing and administration set are changed according to protocol.

lipid i. Hyperalimentation with a fat-containing solution administered intravenously.

subcutaneous i. The infusion of solutions into the subcutaneous space.

infusion pump A pump used to give fluids into an artery, vein, or enteral tube, beneficial in overcoming arterial resistance or administering thick solutions. The pump can be programmed to set the rate of administration depending on the patient's needs. SEE: *electronic infusion device*. SYN: *intravenous infusion pump*.

electronic implantable i.p. ABBR: EIIP. A type of infusion pump inserted in the body. The pump is placed in a subcutaneous pocket and is connected to a dedicated catheter leading to the appropriate compartment or site. The pump may be programmable or nonprogrammable.

Infusoria (ĭn-fū-sō′rē-ă) The former name of a class of Protozoa, now called Ciliata.

ingesta (ĭn-jĕs′tă) [L. *in*, into, + *gerere*, to carry] Food and drink received into the body through the mouth.

ingestant (ĭn-jĕs′tănt) [″ + *gerere*, to carry] Any substance such as food and drink taken orally.

ingestion **1.** The process of taking material (particularly food) into the gastrointestinal tract. **2.** Phagocytosis.

caustic i. Exposure of the oral cavity, pharynx, larynx, or trachea to acids or alkalis, with resulting tissue damage. SEE: *burn of aerodigestive tract*.

Ingrassia's apophysis (ĭn-gră′sē-ăs) [Giovanni Filippo Ingrassia, It. anatomist, 1510–1580] One of the lesser wings of the sphenoid.

ingredient (ĭn-grē′dē-ĕnt) [L. *ingredi,* to enter] Any part of a compound or a mixture; a unit of a more complex substance.

inert i. In pharmaceutical manufacturing, nonreactive substances (also known as fillers) used to facilitate the manufacturing of pills and other forms of medication.

ingrowing [L. *in,* into, + AS. *growan,* to grow] Growing inward so that a portion that is normally free becomes covered.

inguen (ĭn′gwĕn) *pl.* **inguina** [L.] The groin.

inguinal (ĭng′gwĭ-năl) [L. *inguinalis,* pert. to the groin] Pert. to the region of the groin.

i. canal Canalis inguinalis; a narrow, somewhat elongated opening in the lower lateral portion of the abdominal wall, extending from the abdominal (internal) inguinal ring to the subcutaneous (external) inguinal ring. It is an oblique passageway about 1½ in. (3.8 cm) long. In men it transmits the spermatic cord and the ilioinguinal nerve, and in women, the round ligament of the uterus and the ilioinguinal nerve. It forms a channel through which an indirect inguinal hernia descends. SEE: illus.

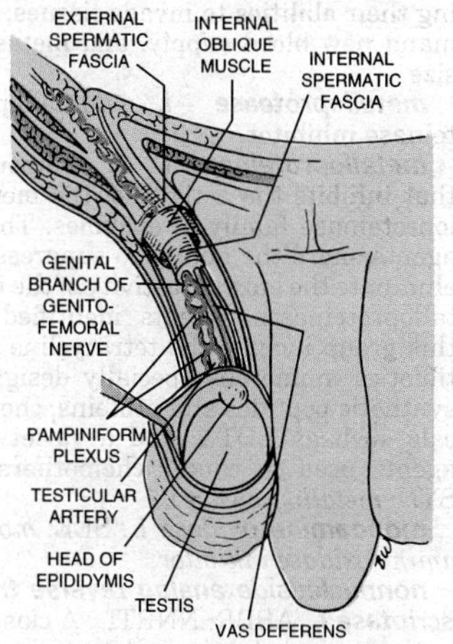

INGUINAL CANAL/SPERMATIC CORD CONTENTS

i. reflex Contractions of the musculature in the female groin when the upper thigh is scratched. SEE: *Geigel's reflex.*

i. region The iliac region on either side of the pubes. SYN: *groin.*

inguinal ring The interior opening of the inguinal canal (abdominal inguinal ring) and the end of the inguinal canal (subcutaneous inguinal ring).

inguinocrural (ĭng″gwĭ-nō-kroo′răl) [L. *inguen,* groin, + *cruralis,* pert. to the leg] Concerning the inguinal and thigh areas.

inguinolabial (ĭng″gwĭ-nō-lā′bē-ăl) [″ + *labialis,* pert. to the lips] Concerning the inguinal and labial areas.

inguinoscrotal (ĭng″gwĭ-nō-skrō′tăl) [″ + *scrotum,* a bag] Concerning the inguinal and scrotal areas.

INH *isoniazid.*

inhalant [L. *inhalare,* to inhale] A medication or compound suitable for inhaling.

inhalation (ĭn″hă-lā′shŭn) [L. *inhalatio*] **1.** The act of drawing breath, vapor, or gas into the lungs; inspiration. **2.** The introduction of dry or moist air or vapor into the lungs for therapeutic purposes, such as metered-dose bronchodilators in the treatment of asthma.

inhale (ĭn-hāl′) [L. *inhalare*] To draw in the breath; to inspire.

inhaler **1.** A device for administering medicines by inhalation. **2.** One who inhales.

metered-dose i. ABBR: MDI. A device used for self-administration of aerosolized drugs.

inherent (ĭn-hĕr′ĕnt) [L. *inhaerens,* to inhere] Belonging to anything naturally, not as a result of circumstance. SYN: *innate* (1); *intrinsic* (1).

inheritance (ĭn-hĕr′ĭ-tăns) [L. *inhereditare,* to inherit] The sum total of all that is inherited; that which is the result of genetic material (DNA) contained within the ovum and sperm.

alternative i. The inheritance of a trait from one parent.

extrachromosomal i. Inherited traits governed by mechanisms other than by chromosomes.

holandric i. Inherited traits carried only by men; thus, the operative gene is on the Y chromosome.

hologynic i. Transmission of traits from mothers only to daughters.

multifactorial i. The inheritance of traits influenced by a number of genetic and nongenetic factors, none of which has a major effect.

sex-influenced i. Inherited traits for which the genes are on autosomes, but their expression is influenced by the sex chromosomes (e.g., the reproductive organs).

sex-limited i. A trait that can be expressed in only one sex.

sex-linked i. The inheritance of traits regulated by either of the sex chromosomes, X or Y.

inherited Body traits and genetic make-up received as a result of genetic transmission rather than acquired.

inhibin (ĭn-hĭb′ĭn) A hormone secreted by the corpus luteum in females and by the testicle in males. It inhibits the secretion of gonadotropin-releasing hormone (GnRH) and human chorionic gonadotropin (hCG). In women, inhibin is secreted throughout the menstrual cycle and during pregnancy, but it normally is not present in postmenopausal women. It is, however, elevated in most postmenopausal women with granulosa or mucinous carcinomas of the ovary. In men, inhibin levels are elevated in prostatic hyperplasia and decreased in cancers of the prostate. SEE: *cancer, ovarian.*

inhibited sexual excitement SEE: *frigidity.*

inhibition (ĭn″hĭ-bĭsh′ŭn) [L. *inhibere*, to restrain] **1.** The repression or restraint of a function. **2.** In physiology, a stopping of an action or function of an organ, as in the slowing or stopping of the heart produced by electrical stimulation of the vagus. **3.** In psychiatry, restraint of one mental process almost simultaneously by another opposed mental process; an inner impediment to free thought and activity.

competitive i. Inhibiting the function of an active material by competing for the cell receptor site. SYN: *selective i.*

contact i. The inhibition of cell division caused by the close contact of similar cells.

noncompetitive i. The inhibition of enzyme activity resulting only from the concentration of the inhibitor.

psychic i. The arrest of an impulse, thought, action, or speech. SYN: *suppression.*

selective i. Competitive i.

inhibitor That which inhibits (e.g., a chemical substance that stops enzyme activity or a nerve that suppresses activity of an organ innervated by it).

ACE i. A drug that blocks the effects of angiotensin-converting enzyme, preventing the formation of angiotensin II and therefore preventing a rise in blood pressure. Drugs from this class are used to treat hypertension, heart failure, myocardial infarction, and in diabetics, kidney failure.

acetylcholinesterase i. ABBR: ACE inhibitor. An agent that prevents the degradation of the neurotransmitter acetylcholine, a chemical involved in memory and learning. Drugs from this class are used in the treatment of Alzheimer's dementia.

alpha-glucosidase i. An oral drug that lowers blood sugars by preventing carbohydrate absorption from the gastrointestinal tract.

aromatase i. Drugs that block the synthesis of estrogen in the body. A number of these agents have been developed to treat breast cancer, which is often a hormone-responsive malignancy.

competitive i. **1.** A chemical that binds to or blocks another reagent from participating in a reaction. **2.** A medication, hormone, or other intercellular messenger that binds and blocks the cellular receptor or target enzyme of another agent. Drugs that act by competitive inhibition may treat or prevent disease by inactivating pathogenic enzymes or by blocking the effects of hormones or precursor molecules. For example, protease inhibitors interfere with production of human immunodeficiency virus (HIV) by binding and inactivating the protease enzyme; selective estrogen-receptor modulators limit the impact of estrogen by replacing this hormone on cells that are sensitive to its effects.

glycoprotein IIB/IIIa receptor i. Drugs that block a receptor on the surface of platelets, which are crucial to blood clotting. Drugs from this class are used to treat acute myocardial infarction, unstable angina pectoris, and other acute coronary syndromes. The most common side effect of treatment with these drugs is bleeding.

HMG CoA enzyme i. One of several medications (e.g., atorvastatin) useful in treating hypercholesterolemia and other lipid disturbances; also called "statins."

matrix metalloproteinase i. An agent that inhibits cancer cells by blocking their abilities to invade tissues, demand new blood supply, and metastasize.

metalloprotease i. Metalloproteinase inhibitor.

metalloproteinase i. A compound that inhibits the activity of the metalloproteinase family of enzymes. These agents share the ability to suppress or eliminate the enzyme activity of the metalloproteinases. Agents identified in this group include the tetracycline antibiotics, numerous specially designed synthetic peptides and proteins, chemicals such as EDTA, and a variety of agents used in cancer chemotherapy. SYN: *metalloprotease i.*

monoamine oxidase i. SEE: *monoamine oxidase inhibitor.*

nonnucleoside analog reverse transcriptase i. ABBR: NNRTI. A class of antiretroviral drugs used to treat patients infected with the human immunodeficiency virus. NNRTIs bind with and inhibit the activity of reverse transcriptase, an enzyme needed to transcribe viral RNA into the host cell DNA. Examples include nevirapine, delavirdine, and efavirenz.

nucleoside reverse transcriptase i. ABBR: NRTI. One of a class of antiretroviral drugs used to treat patients with human immunodeficiency virus infection. NRTIs prevent transcription of viral RNA to host DNA by interfering with the action of the enzyme reverse transcriptase. Azidothymidine, dideoxyinosine, zalcitabine, d4T, and abacavir are NRTIs. SYN: *reverse transcriptase inhibitor*.

proton pump i. A class of medications that eliminate acid production in the stomach. Drugs from this class are used to treat peptic ulcers, gastroesophageal reflux disease, and related disorders. Omeprazole (trade name Prilosec) and lansoprazole (trade name Prevacid) are members of this drug class.

reverse transcriptase i. ABBR: RTI. A class of antiretroviral agents that competitively inhibit the reverse transcriptase enzyme of HIV. SEE: *antiretroviral*.

inhibitory (ĭn-hĭb′ĭ-tō-rē) Restraining, preventing.

iniencephalus (ĭn′ē-ĕn-sĕf′ă-lŭs) [Gr. *inion,* back of the head, + *enkephalos,* brain] A congenitally deformed fetus in which the brain substance protrudes through a fissure in the occiput, so that the brain and spinal cord occupy a single cavity.

inion (ĭn′ē-ŏn) [Gr.] External occipital protuberance. **iniac, inial** (ĭn″ē-ăk, -ăl), *adj.*

iniopagus (ĭn″ē-ŏp′ă-gŭs) [″ + *pagos,* thing fixed] Twins fused at the occiput.

iniops (ĭn′ē-ŏps) [″ + *ops,* eye] A double deformity in which two fetuses are joined from the posterior thorax up, so that one complete face is anterior, with the suggestion of a face posteriorly.

initial (ĭn-ĭsh′ăl) [L. *initium,* beginning] Relating to the beginning or commencement of a thing or process.

initis (ĭn-ī′tĭs) [Gr. *inos,* fiber, + *itis,* inflammation] **1.** An inflammation of fibrous tissue. SYN: *fibrositis*. **2.** An inflammation of a tendon. SYN: *tendinitis*. **3.** An inflammation of a muscle. SYN: *myositis*.

inject [L. *injicere,* to throw in] To introduce fluid into the body or its parts artificially.

injectable Capable of being injected.

injected [L. *injectus,* thrown in] **1.** Filled by injection of fluid. **2.** Congested.

injection (ĭn-jĕk′shŭn) **1.** The forcing of a fluid into a vessel, tissue, or cavity. **2.** A solution introduced in this manner. **3.** The state of being injected; congestion. SEE: *Standard and Universal Precautions Appendix*.

PATIENT CARE: All supplies used in preparing and administering an injection should be sterile. The caregiver chooses the appropriate syringe size for the volume of fluid to be injected, the appropriate needle gauge for the type of fluid, and the appropriate needle length for the administration route and site, considering the amount of muscle and adipose tissue, mobility limitations, and other site-related factors. Hands should be thoroughly washed before and after the procedure, and gloves worn if preparing a chemotherapeutic agent. The prescribed dose is accurately measured. An appropriate site is identified by using anatomical landmarks, and the area is cleansed with an alcohol swab (from the center outward) and time allowed for alcohol evaporation. The needle is inserted at the appropriate angle, given the prescribed route. After insertion into muscle, the syringe plunger is aspirated to ensure that no blood returns to prevent accidental injection into a blood vessel. The prescribed medication is injected slowly, then the needle is removed, and pressure is applied to the site with a dry sponge. When removing a needle after administering an intravenous injection, the caregiver lessens the chance of bleeding into soft tissue by applying firm pressure while elevating the site above heart level for several minutes. The needle should not be recapped; both the needle and syringe should be disposed in a "sharps" container according to protocol. The injection time and site, any untoward responses to the injection, desired effects, and adverse reactions to the particular drug injected are recorded.

depot i. Parenteral administration of a long-acting medication or hormone.

i. drug user An individual who gives himself or herself drugs parenterally, usually to attain a euphoric or altered state of consciousness. The practice is rarely performed aseptically, and may result in the spreading of communicable disease, or self-injury.

epidural i. The injection of anesthetic solution or other medicine into the epidural space of the spinal cord.

fractional i. The process of injecting small amounts at a time until the total injection is complete.

hypodermic i. The term originally indicating injection of a substance beneath the skin. It is preferable, however, to specify the route of administration (e.g., intramuscular). SEE: *anesthesia, local*.

intra-alveolar i. Infiltration method of anesthesia where the anesthetic is introduced into the soft tissues adjacent to the tooth.

intracardial i. Injection into the heart.

intracutaneous i. Injection into the skin, used in giving serums and vaccines when a local reaction is desired.

intracytoplasmic sperm i. ABBR: ICSI. A commonly used assisted reproduction technique, in which spermatozoa, usually from a man with obstructive azoospermia or a low sperm count, are introduced directly into the ova of his partner. Some oocytes become fertilized, and can then be transferred to the woman's uterus, where they mature.

intralingual i. The injection of medicines into the tongue, usually done as an emergency measure when a vein suitable for use is not available because of circulatory collapse.

intramuscular i. Injection into intramuscular tissue, usually the anterior thigh, deltoid, or buttocks. Intramuscular injections are used primarily in the administration of vaccines, immune globulins, corticosteroids, some antibiotics, some hormones, and sedatives. In shock, medications given intramuscularly may not be rapidly absorbed. No more than 4 ml should be injected at one time into an adult with normal musculature; in children and adults with underdeveloped musculature, no more than 2 ml should be injected at one time.

CAUTION: To avoid injury, newborn intramuscular injections should be administered in the middle third of the vastus lateralis muscle using a 5/8-in., 25-gauge needle.

---

intraosseous i. The injection of anesthetic solution directly into the cancellous bone of the alveolar process adjacent to the tooth, to produce a localized effect.

intraperitoneal i. Injection into the peritoneal cavity.

intravenous i. The injection into a vein or more commonly, into an intravenous catheter, of drugs, electrolytes, or fluids. The insertion of a needle directly into a vein (rarely necessary) requires a degree of skill that is easily obtained if proper instruction is obtained. The vein may be distended by applying a tourniquet with sufficient pressure to stop venous return but not arterial flow. The tourniquet is applied several inches above the injection site. If the patient does not have vascular collapse, the arterial pulse can be palpated; if not, the tourniquet is too tight. Heat applied to the area for 15 minutes before starting the injection will also help distend the vessels. The use of a needle attached to a 5- or 10-ml syringe will greatly facilitate controlling the course of the needle. It is best to insert the needle into the vein with the bevel side facing out and then, after the needle is in the vein, to rotate it so that the bevel is face in. There will be resistance as the needle goes through one side of the vein wall. The vein should be entered with the needle making only a narrow angle with the long axis of the vein. This will help to prevent pushing the needle completely through the vein. SEE: *cutdown; intraosseous infusion; Standard and Universal Precautions Appendix.*

SOLUTIONS: Many liquid preparations are given by intravenous infusion. Those commonly used include isotonic saline, Ringer's lactate, dextrose 5% in sterile water, hyperalimentation fluids, lipids, vitamins, and numerous medications. The solution may be given continuously or by intermittent or bolus injection. The rate of infusion varies with the patient's needs.

SITE: Intravenous infusion usually is given in the arm, but central veins or other peripheral veins may be used as indicated.

NOTE: In patients with collapsed veins it may be possible to make the veins apparent by placing a tourniquet around the arm or leg and then inserting a 23- or 25-gauge catheter into a tiny superficial vein. Instillation of sterile intravenous fluid into the vein while the catheter is in place will distend the entire larger vein proximal to the small vein. A larger needle or catheter can then be inserted into the larger vein.

jet i. The technique of injecting medicines and vaccines through the skin or intramuscularly without a needle. A nozzle ejects a fine spray of liquid at such speed as to penetrate but not harm the skin. The procedure is harmless and is esp. useful in immunizing a great number of persons quickly and economically.

rectal i. An instillation (i.e., not an injection) into the rectum; an enema.

sclerosing i. The injection into a vessel or into a tissue of a substance that will bring about obliteration of the vessel or hardening of the tissues used, for example, to manage esophageal varices or malignant pleural effusions.

spinal i. Injection into the spinal canal.

subcutaneous i. Injection beneath the skin. Typical sites include: in the abdomen, upper or outer arm, or the thigh.

vaginal i. A historical term describing the instillation of fluid into the introitus; douche.

Z-track i. An injection technique in which the surface (skin and subcutaneous) tissues are pulled and held to one side before the needle is inserted deep into the tissue in the identified site. The medication is injected slowly, followed by a 10-second delay, at which time the needle is removed and the tissues are quickly permitted to resume their normal position. This provides a Z-shaped track, which makes it difficult for the injected drug to seep back into subcutaneous tissues.

injector A device for making injections.

jet i. SEE: *injection, jet.*

pressure i. A device that delivers a substance to be injected, often controlled by a timing mechanism, at a specified pressure.

injunction A court order prohibiting an individual from performing some act or demanding that a person begin to perform some act.

injury [L. *injurius,* unjust] Trauma or damage to some part of the body. SEE: *transportation of the injured.*

SYMPTOMS: Various symptoms may occur, depending on the nature, extent, and severity of the damage. Mild injury produces pain, tissue swelling, redness, and temporary disruption of tissue function. Severe injury may result in irretrievable loss of the function of an organ, massive hemorrhage, or shock.

blast i. An injury sustained as a result of an explosion. These insults often cause burns and sometimes produce soft tissue injuries, fractures, or injuries to internal organs if the victim is hit by flying debris propelled by the blast.

immersion i. Drowning or near drowning.

internal i. Any injury to the organs occupying the thoracic, abdominal, or cranial cavities.

SYMPTOMS: Symptoms vary depending on the structures involved. Often, shock is present. The patient may be pale, cold, and perspiring freely; and have an altered state of consciousness. Pain is usually intense at first, and may continue or gradually diminish as the patient grows worse. In some injuries, pain may not be manifested.

PATIENT CARE: The patient's vital signs should be monitored carefully and frequently for evidence of shock and altered cerebral function. If the patient is in shock, the shoulders should be lowered and the lower extremities elevated at least 45 degrees. Intravenous infusions, oxygen, airway management, cardiac monitoring, control of hemorrhage, and bony stabilization are quickly begun pending definitive surgical management.

repetitive strain i. Overuse syndrome.

risk for i. A state in which the individual has the potential for physical harm as a result of environmental hazards and/or impairments in an individual's adaptive and defensive resources. SEE: *Nursing Diagnoses Appendix.*

steering wheel i. Blunt trauma to the chest sustained when an unrestrained driver contacts the steering wheel or column. Typical injuries include rib fractures, inflamed cartilage, pneumothorax, hemothorax, or contusion of the heart. Occasionally, the trauma produces dissection of the thoracic aorta.

straddle i. Blunt trauma to the perineum, often with fractures of the pelvis and genital and internal injuries (e.g., to the vagina, penis, testes, bladder, uterus, or other organs).

traumatic brain i. ABBR: TBI. Any injury involving direct trauma to the head, accompanied by alterations in mental status or consciousness. TBI is one of the most common causes of neurological dysfunction in the U.S. Each year about 50,000 Americans die from brain trauma, and an additional 70,000 to 90,000 sustain persistent neurological impairment because of it. The most common causes of TBI are motor vehicle or bicycle collisions; falls; assaults and abuse; and sports-related injuries.

PATIENT CARE: Many traumatic injuries to the head and brain are preventable if simple precautions are followed: motorists should never drive while intoxicated; bicyclists should always wear helmets; frail elderly persons should use sturdy devices to assist them while walking.

CAUTION: If an injury to the brain has occurred or is suspected, the victim should not be moved until spinal precautions are carefully implemented.

---

inlay (ĭn′lā) [L. *in,* in, + AS. *lecgan,* to lay] A solid filling made to the precise shape of a cavity of a tooth and cemented into it; usually the inlay is made of casting alloy, but it may be porcelain.

inlet A passage leading to a cavity.

i. of pelvis The upper pelvic entrance between the sacral promontory and the superior aspect of the symphysis pubis.

INN *International Nonproprietary Names,* a list of pharmaceuticals published periodically by the World Health Organization.

innate (ĭn-nāt′) [″ + *natus,* born] **1.** Belonging to the essential nature of something. SYN: *inherent; intrinsic.* **2.** Existing at birth.

innervate (ĭn-nĕr′vāt, ĭn′ĕr-vāt) [″ + *nervus,* nerve] To stimulate a part, as the nerve supply of an organ.

innervation (ĭn″ĕr-vā′shŭn) **1.** The stimulation of a part through the action of nerves. **2.** The distribution and function of the nervous system. **3.** The nerve supply of a part.

collateral i. Development of the nerve supply in a nerve tract adjacent to the original nerve supply that has been injured or destroyed.

double i. Innervation of an organ with both sympathetic and parasympathetic fibers.

reciprocal i. Innervation of muscles, as around a joint, in which contraction of one set of muscles leads to the relaxation of opposing muscles.

innidiation (ĭn-nĭd-ē-ā′shŭn) The growth of metastasized cells in a new site. SYN: *colonization* (2).

innocent (ĭn′ō-sĕnt) [L. *innocens*] Harmless or benign; clinically unimportant; not pathological (as referring to a heart murmur). SYN: *innocuous.*

innocuous (ĭ-nŏk′ū-ŭs) [L. *innocuus*] Innocent.

innominate (ĭ-nŏm′ĭ-nāt) [L. *innominatus,* unnamed] Nameless.

inochondritis (ĭn″ō-kŏn-drī′tĭs) [Gr. *inos,* fiber, + *chondros,* cartilage, + *itis,* inflammation] The inflammation of a fibrocartilage.

inochondroma (ĭn″ō-kŏn-drō′mă) [″ + ″ + *oma,* tumor] Fibrochondroma.

inoculable **1.** Transmissible by inoculation. **2.** Susceptible to a transmissible disease. **3.** Capable of being inoculated.

inoculate To inject an antigen, antiserum, or antitoxin into an individual to produce immunity to a specific disease. SEE: *vaccine.*

inoculation (ĭn-ŏk″ū-lā′shŭn) **1.** The injection or introduction of an antigen or microbe into a person, animal, or organ or into a solution, growth medium, or other laboratory apparatus. **2.** Vaccination. This can be accomplished parenterally (through the skin), orally, or intranasally; by using an aerosol mist; or by scarification of the skin.

animal i. The injection of serums, microorganisms, or viral organisms into laboratory animals for the purpose of immunizing them or of investigating the effects of the inoculated material on them.

inoculum (ĭn-ŏk′ū-lŭm) [L.] A substance introduced by inoculation.

inocyst (ĭn′ō-sĭst) [Gr. *inos,* fiber, + *kystis,* a bladder] A fibrous capsule.

inocyte (ĭn′ō-sīt) [″ + *kytos,* cell] Fibroblast.

inogenesis (ĭn″ō-jĕn′ĕ-sĭs) [″ + *genesis,* generation, birth] The formation of fibrous tissue.

inogenous (ĭn-ŏj′ĭ-nŭs) [″ + *gennan,* to produce] Forming or produced from fibrous tissue.

inohymenitis (ĭn″ō-hī″mĕn-ī′tĭs) [″ + *hymen,* membrane, + *itis,* inflammation] The inflammation of any fibrous membrane or of an aponeurosis.

inomyositis (ĭn″ō-mī″ō-sī′tĭs) [″ + *mys,* muscle, + *itis,* inflammation] Fibromyositis.

inomyxoma (ĭn″ō-mĭk-sō′mă) [″ + *myxa,* mucus, + *oma,* tumor] Fibromyxoma.

inoneuroma (ĭn″ō-nū-rō′mă) [″ + *neuron,* nerve, + *oma,* tumor] Fibroneuroma.

inoperable [L. *in-,* not, + *operari,* to work] Unsuitable for surgery. In the case of a tumor, the disease may have spread so extensively as to make surgery ineffective, or the patient's general condition may be so poor that surgery could result in the patient's death.

inorganic [L. *in-,* not, + Gr. *organon,* an organ] **1.** In chemistry, occurring in nature independently of living things; sometimes considered to indicate chemical compounds that do not contain carbon. **2.** Not pert. to living organisms.

inosculate [L. *in,* in, + *osculum,* little mouth] Anastomose.

inosculation (ĭn-ŏs″kū-lā′shŭn) Anastomosis.

inose (ĭn′ōs) Inositol.

inosemia (ĭn-ō-sē′mē-ă) [Gr. *inos,* fiber, + *haima,* blood] **1.** An excessive amount of fibrin in the blood. **2.** The presence of inositol in the blood.

inosite (ĭn′ō-sīt) Inositol.

inositis (ĭn″ō-sī′tĭs) [″ + *itis,* inflammation] Inflammation of fibrous tissue.

inositol (ĭn-ŏs′ĭ-tŏl) Hexahydroxycyclohexane, $C_6H_6(OH)_6$; a sugar-like crystalline substance found in the liver, kidney, skeletal muscle, and heart muscle, as well as in the leaves and seeds of most plants. It is part of the vitamin B complex. Deficiency of inositol in experimental animals results in hair loss, eye defects, and growth retardation. Its significance in human nutrition has not been established. SYN: *inose; inosite.*

inosituria (ĭn″ō-sī-tū′rē-ă) [*inositol* + Gr. *ouron,* urine] Inosuria.

inosuria (ĭn-ō-sū′rē-ă) [Gr. *inos,* fiber, + *ouron,* urine] Fibrinous excess in urine.

inosuria (ĭn-ō-sū′rē-ă) [*inositol* + Gr. *ouron,* urine] Inositol in the urine. SYN: *inosituria.*

inotropic (ĭn″ō-trŏp′ĭk) [Gr. *inos,* fiber, + *trepein,* to influence] Influencing the force of muscular contractility.

inpatient A patient who is hospitalized. SEE: *outpatient.*

inquest [L. *in,* into, + *quaerere,* to seek] **1.** In legal medicine, an official examination and investigation into the cause, circumstance, and manner of sudden, unexpected, violent, or unexplained death. **2.** The act of inquiring.

INR *International normalized ratio.*

insalivation [″ + *saliva,* spittle] The process of mixing saliva with food, as in chewing.

insane (ĭn-sān′) [″ + *sanus,* sound] Mentally deranged and therefore, legally incompetent.

insanitary Not conducive to health; unhealthful, unhygienic.

insanity [L. *insanitas,* insanity] **1.** An imprecise term indicating a severe mental disorder such as a psychosis; now obsolete except as a legal term. **2.** In legal medicine, the inability to manage one's own affairs or take responsibility for one's actions as a result of cognitive deficits, absence of impulse control, or psychosis.

i. defense In legal and forensic medicine, the premise that an insane individual who commits a crime is not legally responsible for that act.

insatiable (ĭn-sā′shē-ă-b′l) [L. *insatiabilis*] Incapable of being satisfied or appeased.

inscriptio (ĭn-skrĭp′shē-ō) [L.] **1.** Inscription. **2.** A band or line. SYN: *intersection.*

i. tendinea A tendinous band traversing a muscle.

inscription (ĭn-skrĭp′shŭn) [L. *in,* upon, + *scribere,* to write] The body of a prescription, which gives the names of the drug(s) prescribed and the dosage. SYN: *inscriptio* (1).

insect [L. *insectum*] The common name for any of the class Insecta of the phylum Arthropoda. Insects of medical importance are flies, mosquitoes, lice, fleas, bees, hornets, and wasps. For more information see entries for individual insects.

Insecta A class of the phylum Arthropoda characterized by three distinct body divisions (head, thorax, abdomen), three pairs of jointed legs, trachea, and usually two pairs of wings. Insects are of medical significance in that some are parasitic; some are vectors of pathogenic organisms; and some are annoying pests causing injury by their bites or stings. SYN: *Hexapoda.*

insecticide (ĭn-sĕk′tĭ-sīd) [L. *insectum,* insect, + *caedere,* to kill] **1.** An agent used to exterminate insects. **2.** Destructive to insects.

insectifuge (ĭn-sĕk′tĭ-fūj) [″ + *fugare,* to put to flight] An insect repellent.

Insectivora (ĭn″sĕk-tĭv′ō-ră) [″ + *vorare,* to devour] An order of small mammals, including moles and shrews.

insectivore (ĭn-sĕk′tĭ-vor) A member of the order Insectivora.

insecurity Feelings of helplessness, apprehension, and vulnerability, and an inability to cope with situations or people.

insemination (ĭn-sĕm″ĭn-ā′shŭn) [L. *in,* into, + *semen,* seed] **1.** The discharge of semen from the penis into the vagina during coitus. **2.** The fertilization of an ovum.

artificial i. ABBR: AI. Mechanical placement of semen containing viable spermatozoa into the vagina. SYN: *artificial impregnation.*

donor artificial i. ABBR: AID. Artificial insemination of a woman with sperm from an anonymous donor. This procedure is generally done in cases in which the husband is sterile. SEE: *Standard and Universal Precautions Appendix.*

heterologous artificial i. ABBR: AID. Artificial insemination in which the semen is obtained from a donor other than the husband or partner.

homologous artificial i. ABBR: AIH. Artificial insemination in which the semen is obtained from the husband or partner.

husband artificial i. ABBR: AIH. Use of a husband's sperm to artificially inseminate his wife.

insenescence (ĭn″sĕ-nĕs′ĕns) [″ + *senescens,* growing old] The process of growing old or the approaching of old age.

insensible [L. *in-,* not, + *sensibilis,* appreciable] **1.** Unconscious; without feeling or consciousness. **2.** Not perceptible.

insertion [L. *in,* into, + *serere,* to join] **1.** The movable attachment of the distal end of a muscle, which produces shape changes or skeletal movement when the muscle contracts. **2.** The placement or implanting of something into something else (e.g., in dentistry, the process of placing a filling or inlay in a cavity preparation or placing dentures or other prostheses in the mouth).

velamentous i. The attachment of the umbilical cord to the edge of the placenta.

insheathed (ĭn-shēthd′) [″ + AS. *sceath,* sheath] Enclosed, as by a sheath or capsule. SYN: *encysted.*

insidious (ĭn-sĭd′ē-ŭs) [L. *insidiosus,* cunning] Of gradual, subtle, or indistinct onset; said of some slowly developing diseases.

insight **1.** Self-understanding; comprehension of one's circumstances; the opposite of denial. **2.** In psychiatry, the patient's comprehension that he or she is mentally ill; and awareness of the character of the illness or of the unconscious factors responsible for the emotional conflict involved.

in situ (ĭn sī′tū, sĭt′ū) [L.] **1.** In position, localized. **2.** In the normal place without disturbing or invading the surrounding tissue.

insolation (ĭn″sō-lā′shŭn) [L. *insolare,* to expose to the sun] **1.** Any exposure to the rays of the sun. **2.** Heatstroke or sunstroke. SEE: *heat; heat exhaustion; hyperpyrexia.*

In the past it was felt that exposure to the sunlight was therapeutic. It is now known that exposure to excess sunlight on either an acute or a chronic basis may be unwise. Acute overexposure leads to sunburn. Chronic exposure to the sun increases the likelihood of skin cancers.

insoluble (ĭn-sŏl′ū-b′l) [L. *insolubilis*] Incapable of solution or of being dissolved.

insomnia Prolonged or abnormal inability to sleep. SEE: *sleep disorder.*

fatal familial i. ABBR: FFI. An inherited, rapidly progressive prion disease of middle or later life. Signs and symptoms include intractable insomnia, autonomic dysfunction, endocrine disturbances, dysarthria, myoclonus, coma, and death. There is no specific therapy. SEE: *prion disease.*

insomniac (ĭn-sŏm′nē-ăk) One who has insomnia.

insorption (ĭn-sorp′shŭn) [L. *in,* into, + *sorbere,* to suck in] The passage of material into the blood, as when substances move from the gastrointestinal tract into the bloodstream.

inspect [L. *inspectare,* to examine] To examine visually.

inspection Visual examination of the external surface of the body as well as of its movements and posture. SEE: *abdomen; chest; circulatory system.*

inspiration (ĭn″spĭr-ā′shŭn) [L. *in,* in, + *spirare,* to breathe] Inhalation; drawing air into the lungs; the opposite of expiration. The average rate is 12 to 18 respirations per minute in a normal adult at rest. SEE: *diaphragm* for illus.; *respiration.*

Inspiration may be costal or abdominal, the latter being deeper. The muscles involved in inspiration are the external intercostals, diaphragm, levatores costarum, pectoralis minor, scaleni, serratus posterior, superior sternocleidomastoid, and sometimes the platysma.

crowing i. The peculiar noise heard in stridor or croup. SEE: *croup, spasmodic.*

forcible i. Inspiration in which the muscles of inspiration are assisted by accessory muscles of respiration, such as the sternocleidomastoids, intercostals, and serratus posterior. Forced inspiration is normal during vigorous exercise, but indicative of hypoxia, hypercarbia, or acidosis when it occurs at rest.

full i. Inspiration in which the lungs are filled as completely as possible (voluntarily, as in determining the vital capacity, or involuntarily, as in cardiac dyspnea).

sustained maximal i. A deep-breathing maneuver that mimics the normal physiological sigh mechanism. The patient inspires from a resting expiratory level up to maximum inspiratory capacity, with a pause at end inspiration.

inspirator (ĭn′spĭ-rā″tor) A type of respirator or inhaler.

inspiratory (ĭn-spīr′ă-tor″e) Pert. to inspiration.

i. capacity The maximum amount of air a person can breathe in after a resting expiration.

i. hold A ventilating maneuver in which the delivered volume of gas is held in the lung for a while before expiration; called a plateau or ledge at end inspiration. Also called *grunt breathing.*

inspirometer (ĭn″spĭ-rŏm′ĕ-tĕr) [″ + ″ + Gr. *metron,* measure] A device for determining the amount of air inspired.

inspissate (ĭn-spĭs′āt) [L. *inspissatus,* thickened] To thicken by evaporation or absorption of fluid.

inspissated (ĭn-spĭs′ā-tĕd) Thickened by absorption, evaporation, or dehydration.

inspissation (ĭn-spĭ-sā′shŭn) **1.** Thickening by evaporation or absorption of fluid. **2.** Diminished fluidity or increased thickness.

instability The lack of ability to maintain alignment of bony segments, usually due to torn or lax ligaments and weak muscles.

instar Any one of the various stages of insect development during successive molts.

instep The arched medial portion of the foot.

instillation (ĭn″stĭl-ā′shŭn) [L. *in,* into, + *stillare,* to drop] Slowly pouring or dropping a liquid into a cavity or onto a surface.

instillator An apparatus for introducing, drop by drop, liquids into a cavity.

instinct (ĭn′stĭngkt) [L. *instinctus,* instigation] The inherited tendency for the members of specific species to react to certain environmental conditions and stimuli in a particular way. The nature of the reaction has enabled the individuals and species involved to adapt and survive through many generations. Instincts are best understood when considered against the evolutionary background of the individuals and species being observed. Freud spoke of instinct, but current psychoanalytic terminology would refer to the forces Freud described as drive instead of instinct.

death i. In psychoanalytic theory, the unconscious will to destroy oneself; the counterinstinct for the instinct to live.

herd i. The basic drive to be associated with a group.

instinctive Determined by instinct.

Institute of Electrical and Electronic Engineers ABBR: IEEE. An organization partially responsible for standards regulating electrical devices and equipment.

institutionalization **1.** Residence in or confinement to a nursing home or other long-term care setting for an extended period. **2.** The process of arranging for an individual to be placed in a health care facility. **3.** The process in which individuals who live together gradually develop certain common patterns of behavior and thought (e.g., assumption of illness and depression apathy, behaviors frequently associated with nursing home residency). The current movement in medicine and nursing is away from institutionalism in an attempt to create a more normalized home environment.

institutional review board ABBR: IRB. A medical oversight committee that governs or regulates medical investigations involving human subjects. The purpose of the board is to protect the rights and health of participants in clinical trials. SEE: *informed consent.*

instruction **1.** A direction or command. **2.** The act of teaching or furnishing information.

dental hygiene i. A program in which patients are taught the methods of oral hygiene and the importance of plaque control through proper toothbrushing, flossing, and appropriate nutrition.

instrument (ĭn′stroo-mĕnt) [L. *instrumentum,* tool] **1.** A mechanical device. **2.** A special tool for accomplishing specific tasks. Thus a reflex hammer, microscope, stethoscope, cystoscope, and surgeon's scalpel are all examples of instruments.

dental i. Any instrument used in the practice of dentistry including a variety of hand or machine-driven cutting instruments for soft and calcified tissues, forceps, elevators, clamps, reamers, wire pliers, pluggers, carvers, explorers, and other instruments unique to the dental specialties: oral surgery, endodontics, orthodontics, periodontics, prosthodontics, and restorative dentistry.

instrumental **1.** Pert. to instruments. **2.** Important in achieving a result or goal.

i. activities of daily living ABBR: IADL. Those daily living skills, such as shopping, cooking, cleaning, and child care, that are necessary for maintaining the home environment.

instrumentarium (ĭn′stroo-mĕn-tā′rē-ŭm) Instruments required for a surgical or other procedure.

instrumentation **1.** The use of instruments and their care. **2.** The accomplishment of a task by use of instruments (e.g., removal of a foreign body from the bronchus by means of a bronchoscope).

biomedical i. The use of mechanical and electronic devices in medical diagnosis, therapy, or measurement.

insufficiency (ĭn″sŭ-fĭsh′ĕn-sē) [L. *in-,* not, + *sufficiens,* sufficient] The condition of being inadequate for a given purpose.

active i. The loss of the ability to generate muscle tension because of muscle shortening.

adrenal i. Decreased or abnormally low production of adrenal cortical hormone by the adrenal gland, a condition resulting in Addison's disease.

aortic i. ABBR: AI. An imperfect closure of the aortic semilunar valve at the junction of the left ventricle and the aorta. This causes blood that has been ejected into the aorta to fall back into the left ventricle. It may produce volume overload of the ventricle and congestive heart failure. SYN: *aortic incompetence; aortic regurgitation.*

Chronic aortic insufficiency produces a gradual volume overload of the heart and eventual congestive heart failure. It may occur in patients with poorly controlled hypertension, tertiary syphilis, Marfan's disease, or other disorders that affect aortic valve competence. Management often includes antihypertensive vasodilators, such as nifedipine. If congestive heart failure becomes severe enough, valve replacement may be recommended for patients who are good operative candidates.

SYMPTOMS: Chronic AI may be asymptomatic until congestive heart failure (CHF) occurs. With CHF, patients often report difficulty breathing (e.g., during exercise or sleep) and lower extremity swelling. Patients may occasionally report palpitations or a subjective awareness of their heart beating.

PHYSICAL FINDINGS: The murmur of AI occurs in diastole and is usually described as "blowing" and "decrescendo" (i.e., it begins loudly and gradually softens). It is best heard after the patient exhales and sits forward, holding his or her breath. Patients with AI often have a widened pulse pressure with a waterhammer pulse, and may have head bobbing, bobbing of the uvula, or visible movement of blood under the nails when the tips of the nails are gently compressed (Quincke's pulse).

PATIENT CARE: A history of related cardiac illnesses and symptoms is obtained. Fever and other signs of infection are noted. Vital signs, weight, and fluid intake and output are monitored for indications of fluid overload. Activity tolerance and degree of fatigue are assessed regularly, and the patient is taught to intersperse periods of activity with rest. If bedrest is required, its importance is explained, assistance is offered as necessary, and a bedside commode is provided because it requires less cardiac effort than the use of a bedpan. The patient is encouraged to express concerns about activity restrictions and is reassured of their temporary nature. The patient is placed in an upright position to relieve dyspnea if necessary, and prescribed oxygen is administered to prevent tissue hypoxia. When sitting in a chair, the patient should keep the legs elevated to improve venous return. The diet should consist of foods that the patient enjoys, but prescribed dietary restrictions must be maintained. The patient receives appropriate instruction regarding prescribed medications.

Desired outcomes include adequate cardiopulmonary tissue perfusion and cardiac output, reduced fatigue with exertion, and ability to manage the treatment regimen.

cardiac i. Heart failure.

coronary i. Obstruction to the flow of blood through the coronary arteries, resulting in an inadequate supply of blood relative to the metabolic demands of the heart muscle. SEE: *angina pectoris; coronary artery disease.*

gastric i. An inability of the stomach to empty itself.

hepatic i. An inability of the liver to function properly.

ileocecal i. Ileocecal incompetence.

mitral i. Mitral regurgitation.

muscular i. A condition in which a muscle is unable to exert its normal force and bring about normal movement of the part to which it is attached.

i. of ocular muscles An absence of dynamic equilibrium of ocular muscles.

passive i. Restriction in motion caused by inadequate length of an antagonist muscle or muscles.

pulmonary valvular i. An imperfect closure of the pulmonary semilunar valve at the junction of the right ventricle and the pulmonary artery. The clinical consequences may include right ventricular failure.

renal i. A reduced capacity of the kidney to remove waste products from the blood.

respiratory i. Inadequate oxygen intake or carbon dioxide retention associated with abnormal breathing and signs and symptoms of distress.

thyroid i. Hypothyroidism.

uteroplacental i. Inadequate blood flow through the placental intervillous spaces to enable sufficient transmission of nutrients, oxygen, and fetal wastes. It may be caused by diminished maternal cardiac output due to anemia, heart disease, regional anesthesia, or supine hypotension; vasoconstriction due to chronic or pregnancy-related hypertension or uterine overstimulation; vasospasm due to pregnancy-induced hypertension; vascular sclerosis due to maternal diabetes or collagen disease; or intrauterine infection.

valvular i. Valvular incompetence.

velopharyngeal i. Failure of the palatal sphincter to close, with inadequate separation of the nasopharynx from the oropharynx. This may result in snoring, nasal speech, or inhalation of food into the nasal passages SEE: *cleft palate*.

venous i. A failure of the valves of the veins to function, which interferes with venous return to the heart, and may produce edema.

insufflate [L. *insufflare,* to blow into] **1.** To introduce a gas or air into the lungs. **2.** To blow a medicated powder or medicinal vapor into a cavity.

insufflation The act of blowing a gas, vapor, or powder into a cavity, as the lungs.

perirenal i. The obsolete technique of instilling air into the perirenal space in order to visualize the adrenal gland better on radiographic studies.

tubal i. Test for patency of the fallopian tubes. SEE: *Rubin's test*.

insufflator (ĭn′sŭ-flā″tor) A device for blowing powders or a gas into a cavity.

insula (ĭn′sū-lă) [L.] **1.** The central lobe of the cerebral hemisphere. It is a triangular area of the cerebral cortex lying in the floor of the lateral fissure. SYN: *island of Reil*. **2.** Any structure resembling an island.

insular (ĭn′sū-lăr) [L. *insula,* island] Relating to any insula, as in pancreatic islets.

insulation [L. *insulare,* to make into an island] **1.** The protection of a body or substance with a nonconducting medium to prevent the transfer of electricity, heat, or sound. **2.** The material or substance that insulates.

insulator That which insulates. Specifically, a substance or body that prevents the transmission of electricity to surrounding objects by conduction; anything that exerts great resistance to the passage of an electric current by conduction. The electrical resistance of an insulator is expressed in ohms. SEE: *nonconductor*.

insulin (ĭn′sŭ-lĭn) [L. *insula,* island] A hormone secreted by the beta cells of the pancreas that controls the metabolism and cellular uptake of sugars, proteins, and fats. As a drug, it is used principally to control diabetes mellitus. Insulin therapy is required in the management of type 1 diabetes mellitus because patients with this illness do not make enough insulin on their own to survive. The drug also is used in the care of patients with gestational diabetes to prevent fetal complications caused by maternal hyperglycemia (insulin itself does not cross the placenta or enter breast milk). In type 2 diabetes mellitus, its use typically is reserved for those patients who have failed to control their blood sugars with diet, exercise, and oral drugs. SEE: illus.; *diabetes mellitus*.

Insulin preparations differ with respect to the speed with which they act and their duration and potency following subcutaneous injection. SEE: table.

In the past, insulin for injection was obtained from beef or porcine pancreas. These peptides differed from human insulin by a few amino acids, causing some immune reactions and drug resistance. Most insulin now in use is made by recombinant DNA technology and is equivalent to human insulin from an immunological perspective.

PHYSIOLOGY: In health, the pancreas secretes insulin in response to elevations of blood glucose, such as occur after meals. It stimulates cells, esp. in muscular tissue, to take up sugar from the bloodstream. It also facilitates the storage of excess glucose as glycogen in the liver and prevents the breakdown of stored fats. In type 1 diabetes mellitus, failure of the beta cells to produce insulin results in hyperglycemia and ketoacidosis.

DOSAGE: The insulin dosage should always be expressed in units. There is no average dose of insulin for diabetics;

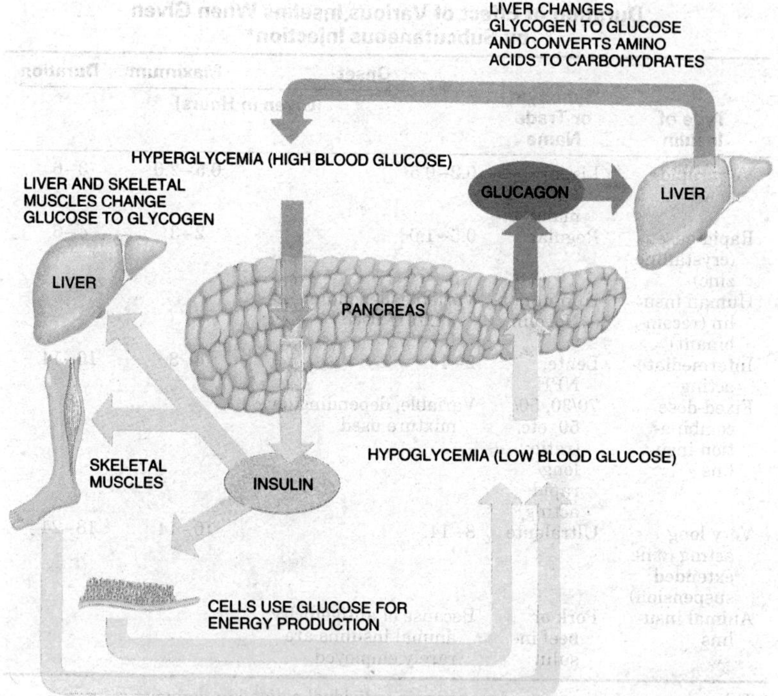

COMPLEMENTARY FUNCTIONS OF INSULIN AND GLUCAGON

each patient must be assessed and treated individually.

STORAGE: The FDA requires that all preparations of insulin contain instructions *to keep in a cold place and to avoid freezing.*

CAUTION: Persons who use insulin should wear an easily seen bracelet or necklace stating that they have diabetes and use the drug. This helps to ensure that patients with hypoglycemic reactions will be diagnosed and treated promptly.

---

i. human Insulin prepared by recombinant DNA technology utilizing strains of *Escherichia coli*. In its effect it is similar to insulins secreted by the human pancreas. Trade names are Humulin and Novolin. SEE: *insulin* for table.

inhaled i. Insulin given by inspiration, with the use of an inhaler.

i. injection site The places on the body that are suitable for injecting insulin. Because insulin is administered at least once daily, it is important to have a plan for selecting the site. The best sites for insulin injection are in the subcutaneous tissue of the abdomen. The arms and legs can also be used, but insulin uptake from these sites is less uniform. It is advisable to map out a number of injection sites in one area, use those and then use other sites.

i. isophane suspension Intermediate-acting insulin with onset in ½ to 1 hr and a duration of 18 to 28 hr. SEE: *insulin* for table.

i. lipodystrophy SEE: under *lipodystrophy*.

i. lispro A synthetic insulin with a very rapid onset and short duration of action. Diabetic patients typically use it immediately before meals to prevent postprandial hyperglycemia. Its absorption is more rapid than regular insulin. It is made by reversing the amino acids lysine and proline in the beta chain of the insulin polypeptide (hence its name *lispro*).

monocomponent i. Single component i.

i. protamine zinc suspension Long-acting insulin with onset in 6 to 8 hr and a duration of 30 to 36 hr. SEE: *insulin* for table.

i. pump A small battery-driven pump that delivers insulin subcutaneously into the abdominal wall. The pump can be programmed to deliver varying doses of insulin as a patient's need for insulin changes during the day (e.g., before exercise or meals, when

Duration of Effect of Various Insulins When Given by Subcutaneous Injection*

Type of Insulin	Synonym or Trade Name	Onset	Maximum	Duration
		(Given in Hours)		
Very rapid onset	Lispro Humalog	0.2–0.5	0.5–2.0	3–6
Rapid onset (crystalline zinc)	Regular	0.5–1.0	2–3	4–6
Human insulin (recombinant)	Humulin, Novolin	Variable, depending on mixture used		
Intermediate-acting	Lente, NPH	2–4	4–8	10–14
Fixed-dose combination insulins	70/30, 50/50, etc. (ratio: long/rapid acting)	Variable, depending on mixture used		
Very long acting (zinc extended suspension)	Ultralente	8–14	10–14	18–24
Animal insulins	Pork or beef insulin	Because of antigenicity, animal insulins are rarely employed		

* These times are estimates and may vary in individual patients.

physical or psychological levels of stress change).

i. shock SEE: under *shock*.

single component i. Highly purified insulin that contains less than 10 parts per million of proinsulin, a substance that is capable of inducing formation of anti-insulin antibodies. SYN: *monocomponent i.*

synthetic i. Insulin made by the use of recombinant DNA methodology.

i. zinc extended suspension Long-acting insulin with onset in 5 to 8 hr and duration of more than 36 hr. SEE: *insulin* for table.

i. zinc prompt suspension Fast-acting insulin with onset less than 1 hr and a duration of 12 to 16 hr. SEE: *insulin* for table.

insulinase (ĭn′sū-lĭn-ās) An enzyme that inactivates insulin.

insulinemia (ĭn-sū-lĭn-ē′mē-ă) [L. *insula,* island, + Gr. *haima,* blood] Hyperinsulinemia.

insulinogenesis (ĭn″sū-lĭn-ō-jĕn′ĕ-sĭs) [″ + Gr. *genesis,* generation] The production of insulin by the pancreas.

insulinogenic (ĭn″sū-lĭn″ō-jĕn′ĭk) [″ + Gr. *gennan,* to produce] **1.** Caused by insulin whether administered therapeutically or produced naturally by the pancreas. **2.** Pert. to the production of insulin.

insulinoid (ĭn′sū-lĭn-oyd) [″ + Gr. *eidos,* form, shape] Resembling or having the properties of insulin.

insulinoma (ĭn″sū-lĭn-ō′mă) [″ + Gr. *oma,* tumor] A tumor of the islets of Langerhans of the pancreas. These rare tumors secrete insulin and cause hypoglycemia. SEE: *hypoglycemia; neuroglycopenia.*

insulitis (ĭn″sū-lī′tĭs) [″ + Gr. *itis,* inflammation] Inflammation of the islets of Langerhans of the pancreas. In insulin dependent diabetes mellitus, the islets in the pancreas contain cells with enlarged nuclei, some degranulated beta cells, and a chronic inflammatory infiltrate.

insulopathic (ĭn″sū-lō-păth′ĭk) [″ + Gr. *pathos,* disease, suffering] Relating to or caused by abnormal insulin secretion.

insult In medicine, an injury or trauma.

insusceptibility (ĭn″sŭ-sĕp″tĭ-bĭl′ĭ-tē) [L. *in,* not, + *suscipere,* to take up] **1.** Immunity or lack of susceptibility to infection or disease. **2.** The resistance of a microorganism to treatment with one or more antibiotic drugs.

intake (ĭn-tāk′) That which is taken in, esp. food and liquids.

i. and output ABBR: I and O. A record of the oral and parenteral intake of foods and fluids; and of all output including urine, feces, vomitus, and, if required, an estimate of fluid loss as a result of perspiration.

integrase (ĭn′tĕ-grās) A retroviral enzyme that incorporates DNA derived from the virus into host cell chromosomes. The enzyme is a target for experimental antiretroviral therapies.

integration (ĭn″tĕ-grā′shŭn) [L. *integrare,* to make whole] The bringing together of various parts or functions so that they function as a harmonious whole.

primary i. The early recognition of the body and its psyche as apart from one's environment.

secondary i. The process involved in developing the adult personality so that the individual coordinates the components into unified and socialized action.

structural i. Rolfing.

integrin The receptor on cell surfaces that links with proteins and chemical mediators to enhance cell-to-cell communication. SEE: *cytokine; interleukin.*

integrity **1.** Having an undiminished or unimpaired state. **2.** Ethical purity.

integument (ĭn-tĕg″ū-mĕnt) [L. *integumentum,* a covering] A covering; the skin, consisting of the corium or dermis, and epidermis.

integumentary (ĭn-tĕg-ū-mĕn′tă-rē) Relating to the integument.

intellect [L. *intelligere,* to understand] The mind, or understanding; conscious brain function.

intellectual **1.** Pert. to the mind. **2.** Possessing intellect.

intellectualization (ĭn″tĕ-lĕk″chū-ăl-ĭ-zā′shŭn) The analysis of personal or social problems on an intellectual basis despite the individual's personal and emotional reactions to those problems.

intelligence [L. *intelligere,* to understand] The capacity to comprehend relationships; the ability to think, to solve problems, and adjust to new situations. The use of a single test to estimate the intelligence of persons from different social, racial, cultural, or economic backgrounds, however, is unreliable.

artificial i. SEE: *Computer Glossary.*

intelligence quotient SEE: under *quotient.*

intensifying [L. *intensus,* intense, + *facere,* to make] Making intense; magnifying or amplifying.

i. screen SEE: under *screen.*

intensity **1.** A state of increased force or energy. **2.** The strength of uterine labor contractions at acme. Palpation identifies contractions as mild, moderate, or strong by indentability. Contraction strength can be measured in millimeters of mercury by insertion of a saline-filled intrauterine pressure catheter attached to a transducer.

signal i. The relative brilliance of a radiographic image, radioactive tracer, or biological marker.

spatial average i. ABBR: SAI. The measure of power per unit area of ultrasound application, expressed in watts per square centimeter (w/cm^2). The spatial average intensity is calculated by dividing the ultrasonic output, expressed in watts, by the effective radiating area of the sound head (e.g., 20 watts/10 cm^2 sound head = 2.0 w/cm^2 SAI).

temporal average i. ABBR: TAI. The amount of therapeutic ultrasonic energy delivered to the tissues over a given time. The temporal average intensity is calculated by multiplying the spatial average intensity by the percent duty cycle (e.g., 20 w/cm^2 × 50% duty cycle = 1 w/cm^2 TAI). The temporal average intensity is meaningful only during the application of pulsed ultrasound.

intensive (ĭn-tĕn′sĭv) Relating to or marked by intensity.

intensive care unit ABBR: ICU. A special hospital unit for patients who, because of the nature of their illness, injury, or surgical procedure, require almost continuous monitoring by specially trained staff. In large hospitals, units may be devoted to a single group of patients such as surgical cases, compromised newborns, or patients with burns, trauma, emergency cardiac care needs, or infectious diseases.

intent (ĭn-tĕnt′) A state of mind of a person who knows that acting in a certain manner will cause or otherwise accomplish a specific result. Intent is the key element and basis for the intentional torts that healthcare providers may come in contact with, e.g., assault and battery.

intention (ĭn-tĕn′shŭn) [″ + *tendere,* to stretch] **1.** A natural process of healing. **2.** Goal or purpose.

first i. Healing by first intention.

second i. Healing by second intention.

third i. Healing by third intention.

intentional infliction of emotional distress Deliberate destruction of a person's peace of mind. The conduct must be outrageous and beyond all bounds of decency; ordinary rude or insulting behavior is not enough. This can be compensable to a plaintiff if it can be proven that the healthcare provider inflicted this upon the patient.

inter- [L.] Prefix meaning *in the midst, between.*

interacinar (ĭn″tĕr-ăs′ĭ-năr) [L. *inter,* between, + *acinus,* grape] Located between acini of a gland.

interaction, dielectric A term used to quantitate the electrical polarity or dipole moment of a molecule. SEE: *dipole.*

interaction, photoelectric The interaction between x-rays and matter that completely absorbs the incoming photon. In radiology, photoelectric absorption is the cause of image contrast as well as increasing patient exposure.

interalveolar (ĭn″tĕr-ăl-vē′ō-lăr) [″ + *alveolus,* little tub] Between the alveoli, esp. the alveoli of the lungs.

interarticular [″ + *articulus,* joint] **1.** Between two joints. **2.** Situated between two articulating surfaces.

interarytenoid (ĭn″tĕr-ăr″ē-tē′noyd) [″ + Gr. *arytaina,* ladle, + *eidos,* form, shape] Between the arytenoid cartilages of the larynx.

interatrial (ĭn″tĕr-ā′trē-ăl) [″+ *atrium,* hall] Between the atria of the heart. SYN: *interauricular.*

interauricular (ĭn″tĕr-aw-rĭk′ū-lăr) [″ + *auricula,* little ear] Interatrial.

interbrain [″ + AS. *braegen,* brain] Diencephalon.

intercadence (ĭn″tĕr-kā′dĕns) [″ + *cadere,* to fall, die] A supernumerary pulse wave between two regular heartbeats.

intercalary, intercalated (ĭn-tĕr′kă-lĕr″ē, -kăl-āt″ĕd) [″ + *calare,* to call] **1.** Inserted or interposed between. SYN: *extraneous; interposed.* **2.** Pert. to an upstroke or cardiac extrasystole that comes between two heartbeats.

intercanalicular (ĭn″tĕr-kăn″ă-lĭk′ū-lăr) [″ + *canalicularis,* pert. to a canaliculus] Between the canaliculi of a tissue.

intercapillary (ĭn″tĕr-kăp′ĭ-lăr-ē) [″ + *capillaris,* hairlike] Between the capillaries.

intercarpal (ĭn″tĕr-kăr′păl) [″ + Gr. *karpalis,* pert. to the carpus] Between the carpal bones.

intercartilaginous (ĭn″tĕr-kăr″tĭ-lăj′ĭ-nŭs) [″ + *cartilago,* cartilage] Connecting or between cartilages. SYN: *interchondral.*

intercavernous (ĭn″tĕr-kăv′ĕr-nŭs) [″ + L. *caverna,* a hollow] Between the cavernous sinuses.

intercellular (ĭn″tĕr-sĕl′ū-lăr) [″ + *cella,* compartment] Between the cells of a structure.

i. junctions The microscopic space between cells. These spaces are important in assisting the transfer of small molecules across capillary walls. These junctions may be widened by chemical or physical factors and are acted on by chemical mediators of inflammation to increase vascular permeability.

intercept (ĭn-tĕr-sĕpt′) The point at which the line representing a function intersects an axis.

intercerebral (ĭn″tĕr-sĕr′ĕ-brăl) [″ + *cerebrum,* brain] Between the two cerebral hemispheres. SYN: *interhemicerebral.*

interchange In dispensing drugs, the use of a generic form of the drug in place of the proprietary form.

interchondral (ĭn″tĕr-kŏn′drăl) [″ + Gr. *chondros,* cartilage] Intercartilaginous.

intercilium (ĭn″tĕr-sĭl′ē-ŭm) [″ + *cilium,* eyelash] Glabella.

interclavicular (ĭn″tĕr-klă-vĭk′ū-lăr) [″ + *clavicula,* clavicle] Between the clavicles.

intercoccygeal (ĭn″tĕr-kŏk-sĭj′ē-ăl) [″ + Gr. *kokkyx,* coccyx] Between the segments of the coccyx.

intercolumnar (ĭn″tĕr-kō-lŭm′năr) [″ + *columna,* column] Between columns.

intercondylar, intercondyloid, intercondylous [″ + Gr. *kondylos,* knuckle] Between two condyles.

intercostal (ĭn″tĕr-kŏs′tăl) [″ + *costa,* rib] Between the ribs.

intercostobrachial (ĭn″tĕr-kŏs″tō-brā′kē-ăl) [″ + ″ + *brachium,* arm] Pert. to the intercostal space and the arm, as the posterior lateral branch of the second intercostal nerve supplying the skin of the arm, or a similar branch of the third intercostal nerve; formerly called intercostohumeralis.

intercostohumeral (ĭn″tĕr-kŏs-tō-hū′mĕr-ăl) [″ + ″ + *humerus,* upper arm] Concerning or connecting an intercostal space and the humerus.

intercourse [L. *intercursus,* running between] The social interaction between individuals or groups; communication.

sexual i. Coitus.

intercricothyrotomy (ĭn″tĕr-krī″kō-thī-rŏt′ō-mē) [L. *inter,* between, + Gr. *krikos,* ring, + *thyreos,* shield, + *tome,* incision] The surgical separation of the cricothyroid membrane in order to incise the larynx.

intercristal (ĭn″tĕr-krĭs′tăl) [″ + *crista,* crest] Between two crests of a bone, organ, or process.

intercrural (ĭn″tĕr-krū′răl) [″ + *crus,* limb] Between two crura.

intercurrent [″ + *currere,* to run] **1.** Intervening. **2.** Pert. to a disease attacking a patient with another disease.

intercuspation [″ + *cuspis,* point] The cusp-to-fossa relation of the upper and lower posterior teeth in occlusion. SYN: *intercusping.* SEE: *occlusion.*

interdent A specially designed knife used for removing interdental tissue.

interdental [″ + *dens,* tooth] Between adjacent teeth in the same arch. SYN: *interproximal.* SEE: *interocclusal.*

interdentium (ĭn″tĕr-dĕn′shē-ŭm) The space between any two contiguous teeth.

interdigit (ĭn″tĕr-dĭ′jĭt) The area between any two contiguous toes or fingers or their associated metatarsals or metacarpals. SEE: *intermetacarpal; intermetatarsal.*

interdigitation [″ + *digitus,* digit] **1.** Interlocking of toothed or finger-like processes. **2.** Processes so interlocked.

interdisciplinary Involving or overlapping of two or more health care professions in a collaborative manner or effort.

interest checklist An assessment approach used by occupational therapists to determine an individual's unique play and leisure interests.

interfascicular (ĭn″tĕr-făs-ĭk′ū-lăr) [″ + *fasciculus,* bundle] Between fasciculi.

interfemoral [″ + *femoralis,* pert. to the thigh] Between the thighs.

interference [″ + *ferire,* to strike] **1.** Clashing or colliding. **2.** A dental occlusion that interferes with harmonious movement of the mandible.

i. of impulses A condition in which two excitation waves, upon approaching each other and meeting in any part of the heart, are mutually extinguished.

interferometer (ĭn″tĕr-fēr-ŏm′ĕ-tĕr) An optical device that acts on the interference of two beams of light, permitting examination of the structure of spectral lines. It is also used in examining prisms of lenses for faults.

interferon (ĭn-tĕr-fēr′ŏn) ABBR: IFN. Any of a group of glycoproteins with antiviral activity. The antiviral type I interferons (alpha and beta interferons) are produced by leukocytes and fibroblasts in response to invasion by a pathogen, particularly a virus. These interferons enable invaded cells to produce class I major histocompatibility complex (MHC) surface antigens, increasing their ability to be recognized and killed by T lymphocytes. They also inhibit virus production within infected cells. Type I alpha interferon is used to treat condyloma acuminata, chronic hepatitis B and C, and Kaposi's sarcoma. Type I beta interferon is used to treat multiple sclerosis.

Type II gamma interferon is distinctly different from and less antiviral than the other interferons. It is a lymphokine, excreted primarily by CD8+ T cells and the helper T subset of CD4+ cells that stimulates several types of antigen-presenting cells, particularly macrophages, to release class II MHC antigens that enhance CD4+ activity. It is used to treat chronic granulomatous disease. SEE: *cell, antigen-presenting; macrophage*.

interfibrillar, interfibrillary (ĭn″tĕr-fĭb′rĭ-lăr, -rĭ-lār″ē) [″ + *fibrilla,* a small fiber] Between fibrils.

interfilamentous (ĭn″tĕr-fĭl″ă-mĕn′tŭs) [″ + *filamentum,* filament] Between filaments.

interfilar (ĭn-tĕr-fī′lăr) [″ + *filum,* thread] Between the fibrils of a reticulum.

interganglionic [″ + *ganglion,* a swelling] Between ganglia.

intergemmal (ĭn″tĕr-jĕm′ăl) [″ + *gemma,* bud] Between taste buds.

interglobular [″+ *globulus,* globule] Between globules.

intergluteal (ĭn″tĕr-gloo′tē-ăl) [″ + Gr. *gloutos,* buttock] Between the buttocks.

intergonial An anthropometric line between the tips of the two angles of the mandible.

intergyral (ĭn″tĕr-jī′răl) [″+ Gr. *gyros,* circle] Between the cerebral gyri.

interhemicerebral (ĭn″tĕr-hĕm″ĭ-sĕr′ĕ-brăl) [″+ Gr. *hemi,* half, + L. *cerebrum,* brain] Intercerebral.

interictal (ĭn″tĕr-ĭk′tăl) [″ + *ictus,* a blow] Between seizures.

interior [L. *internus,* within] The internal portion or area of something; situated within.

interischiadic (ĭn″tĕr-ĭs″kē-ăd′ĭk) [L. *inter,* between, + Gr. *ischion,* hip] Between the ischia of the pelvis.

interkinesis (ĭn″tĕr-kĭ-nē′sĭs) [″ + Gr. *kinesis,* movement] The interval between the first and second meiotic divisions of cells.

interlabial Between the lips or any two labia.

interlamellar (ĭn″tĕr-lă-mĕl′ăr) [″ + *lamella,* layer] Between lamellae.

interleukin ABBR: IL. A type of cytokine that enables communication among leukocytes and other cells active in inflammation or the specific immune response. The result is a maximized response to a microorganism or other foreign antigen. SEE: *cell-mediated immunity; cytokine; inflammation*.

i.-1 ABBR: IL-1. A cytokine released by almost all nucleated cells that activates the growth and function of neutrophils, lymphocytes, and macrophages; promotes the release of additional mediators that influence immune responses; enhances production of cerebrospinal fluid; and modulates certain adrenal, hepatic, bone, and vascular smooth muscle cell activity. Interleukin-1 and tumor necrosis factors, whose actions are almost identical to those of IL-1, are involved in fever production and other systemic effects of inflammation. SEE: *tumor necrosis factor*.

i.-2 ABBR: IL-2. A cytokine released primarily by activated CD4+ helper T lymphocytes. It is a major mediator of T cell proliferation, promotes production of other cytokines, enhances natural killer cell function, and is a cofactor for immunoglobulin secretion. SYN: *T-cell growth factor*.

i.-3 ABBR: IL-3. A cytokine produced by activated T cells that promotes proliferation of bone marrow stem cells.

i.-4 ABBR: IL-4. A cytokine released by activated T cells and mast cells that stimulates B and T lymphocyte production and activity, prevents macrophages from releasing monokines, and promotes mast cell, immunoglobulin E, and eosinophil activity.

i.-5 ABBR: IL-5. A cytokine produced by T cells, eosinophils and mast cells that acts as the primary stimulant for eosinophil production. SEE: *basophil(e); eosinophil*.

i.-6 ABBR: IL-6. A lymphokine produced by many cell types, including mononuclear phagocytes, T cells, and endothelial cells. It mediates the acute phase response, enhances B cell production and differentiation to immunoglobulin secreting plasma cells, and stimulates megakaryocyte production. SEE: *acute phase reaction; lymphokine*.

i.-7 ABBR: IL-7. A cytokine produced by the thymus, spleen, and bone marrow stromal cells. It stimulates growth of B-cell precursors, development of thymocytes, and activity of cytotoxic T-cells.

i.-8 ABBR: IL-8. A cytokine produced by many cell types. It acts as a neutrophil chemoattractant.

i.-9 ABBR: IL-9. A cytokine produced by T cells. Among other functions, it promotes the proliferation and multiplication of mast cells.

i.-10 ABBR: IL-10. A cytokine derived from mononuclear phagocytes, T cells, and keratinocytes. It inhibits cytokine synthesis by macrophages, T cells, and natural killer cells, and enhances B cell growth and secretion of immunoglobulin.

i.-11 ABBR: IL-11. A cytokine produced by bone marrow stromal cells. It mediates acute phase protein synthesis, enhances B cell growth and differentiation to plasma cells, and promotes megakaryocyte production.

i.-12 ABBR: IL-12. A cytokine produced by mononuclear phagocytes and B cells. It induces interferon gamma production from T cells and natural killer cells, and enhances T cell and natural killer cell cytotoxicity.

i.-13 ABBR: IL-13. A cytokine produced by T cells. It induces major histocompatibility class II expression on mononuclear phagocytes and B cells, B cell proliferation, and immunoglobulin production.

i.-14 ABBR: IL-14. A cytokine produced by T lymphocytes and follicular dendritic cells. It stimulates proliferation of activated B lymphocytes and inhibits immunoglobulin secretion from activated B lymphocytes.

i.-15 ABBR: IL-15. A cytokine released by epithelial cells in the kidney, skeletal muscle, liver, lungs, heart, and bone marrow, which stimulates production of T cells, esp. cytotoxic T cells and natural killer cells. It can bind with interleukin-2 receptors and mimic IL-2's effects. SEE: *interleukin-2*.

i.-16 ABBR: IL-16. A cytokine produced by T lymphocytes that stimulates movement of monocytes, CD4+ T cells, and eosinophils to the area. It was previously known as lymphocyte chemoattractant factor (LCF).

interlobar (ĭn″tĕr-lō′băr) [″ + *lobus,* lobe] Between lobes.

interlobitis (ĭn″tĕr-lō-bī′tĭs) [″ + ″ + Gr. *itis,* inflammation] Inflammation of the pleura separating the pulmonary lobes.

interlobular (ĭn″tĕr-lŏb′ū-lăr) [″ + *lobulus,* lobule] Between the lobules of an organ.

intermalleolar (ĭn″tĕr-mă-lē′ō-lăr) [″ + *malleolus,* little hammer] Between the malleoli.

intermammary (ĭn″tĕr-măm′ă-rē) [″ + *mamma,* breast] Between the breasts.

intermamillary (ĭn″tĕr-măm′ĭ-lār″ē) [″ + *mammilla,* nipple] Between the nipples of the breasts.

intermarriage [″ + *maritare,* to marry] **1.** Marriage between persons from two distinct populations. **2.** Marriage between related individuals.

intermaxillary [″ + *maxilla,* jawbone] **1.** Between the two maxillae, as in an intermaxillary suture. **2.** Formerly meaning between the two jaws.

intermediary (ĭn″tĕr-mē′dē-ār-ē) [″ + *medius,* middle] **1.** Situated between two bodies. **2.** Occurring between two periods of time.

intermediate (ĭn″tĕr-mē′dē-ĭt) [″ + *medius,* middle] Between two extremes; sequentially, after the beginning and before the end.

intermedin (ĭn″tĕr-mē′dĭn) A substance secreted by the pars intermedia of the pituitary. It is important in controlling pigment cells of the skin of some reptiles, fish, and amphibians.

intermediolateral [″ + ″ + *latus,* side] Intermediate but not central.

intermedius (ĭn″tĕr-mē′dē-ŭs) [″ + *medius,* middle] The middle of three structures.

intermembranous (ĭn″tĕr-mĕm′bră-nŭs) [″ + *membrana,* membrane] Between membranes.

intermeningeal (ĭn″tĕr-mĕn-ĭn′jē-ăl) [″ + *meninx,* membrane] Between the meninges.

intermenstrual (ĭn″tĕr-mĕn′stroo-ăl) [″ + Gr. *men,* month] Between the menses or menstrual periods.

intermetacarpal (ĭn″tĕr-mĕt″ă-kăr′păl) [″ + Gr. *meta,* beyond, + *karpos,* wrist] Between the metacarpal bones.

intermetatarsal (ĭn″tĕr-mĕt″ă-tăr′săl) The area between any two contiguous metatarsals.

intermission [″ + *mittere,* to send] **1.** The interval between two paroxysms of a disease. **2.** A temporary cessation of symptoms.

intermittence [″ + *mittere,* to send] **1.** A condition marked by intermissions in the course of a disease or of a process. **2.** A loss of one or more pulse beats.

intermittent (ĭn″tĕr-mĭt′ĕnt) Suspending activity at intervals; coming and going.

intermittent positive-pressure breathing SEE: under *breathing*.

intermural (ĭn″tĕr-mū′răl) [L. *inter,* between, + *murus,* wall] Between the walls or sides of an organ.

intermuscular [″ + *musculus,* muscle] Between muscles.

intern (ĭn′tĕrn) [L. *internus,* within] A physician or surgeon on a hospital staff, usually a recent graduate receiving a year of postgraduate training before being eligible to be licensed to practice medicine. SEE: *extern.*

internal [L. *internus,* within] Within the body; within or on the inside; enclosed; inward; the opposite of external.

internal injury SEE: under *injury.*

internalization (ĭn-tĕr″năl-ĭ-zā′shŭn) The unconscious mental mechanism in which the values and standards of society and one's parents are taken as one's own.

internal medicine SEE: under *medicine.*

internarial (ĭn″tĕr-nā′rē-ăl) [L. *inter,* between, + *nares,* nostrils] Between the nares.

internasal (ĭn″tĕr-nā′zăl) [″ + *nasus,* nose] Between the nasal bones.

internatal (ĭn″tĕr-nā′tăl) [″ + *nates,* buttocks] Between the buttocks.

International Association for Dental Research ABBR: I.A.D.R. An association founded in 1920 to provide research in dental science and application of research to develop dental treatment and oral health.

International Classification of Diseases ABBR: ICD. A codification of diseases, injuries, causes of death, and procedures including operations and diagnostic and nonsurgical procedures. The ICD's principal use is to standardize reporting of illness, death, and procedures. The publication is essential to the compilation of statistical information about diseases in a format that allows international comparison of those data.

International Classification of Impairment, Disability and Handicap ABBR: ICIDH. A standard originated by the World Health Organization in 1980 for classifying and coding conditions requiring rehabilitation, superseded by the adoption of ICIDH-2. As its title implies, the major categories of ICIDH were impairment, disability, and handicap, designed to describe a hierarchy of the consequences of pathology on human function. The revised ICIDH, known as ICIDH-2, consists of major changes in terminology and underlying concepts.

ICIDH-2 was developed to provide a scheme that was more reliable, applicable, and useful. It modifies the original classification scheme to better address chronic conditions and to integrate medical and social models of disability. This new version provides operational definitions for classifications that use culturally universal language that is acceptable to people with disabilities. It uses the categories of impairment, activity, and participation, acknowledging that consequences of pathology result from individual, environmental, and situational influences.

International Psychogeriatric Association ABBR: IPA. An organization of health care professionals and scientists with an interest in the behavioral and biological aspects of mental health in the elderly.

International Sensitivity Index ABBR: ISI. A laboratory standard for thromboplastins, the reagents used to determine the prothrombin time (PT). Because thromboplastin contents vary, PT results performed on the same sample of blood in different laboratories can be markedly different, even though the patient's actual level of anticoagulation is a constant. The ISI is used to calculate the international normalized ratio (INR), a standardized measure of anticoagulation, thus enabling health care professionals working with different laboratories to compare results and adjust anticoagulant doses according to a single set of guidelines.

International Symbol of Access A symbol used to identify buildings and facilities that are barrier-free and therefore accessible to disabled persons with restricted mobility, including wheelchair users. SEE: illus.

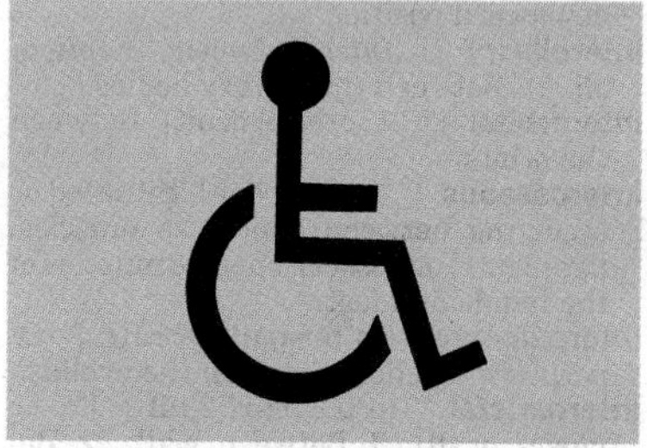

INTERNATIONAL SYMBOL OF ACCESS

International System of Units ABBR: SI. An internationally standardized system of units. The basic quantity measured and the names of the units are meter (length), kilogram (mass), second (time), ampere (electric current), kelvin (temperature), candela (luminous intensity), and mole (amount of a substance). All other units of measurement are derived from these seven basic units. SEE: *SI Units Appendix.*

International Union of Pure and Applied Chemistry ABBR: IUPAC. An organization composed of experts from many countries whose charter is to standardize aspects of the basic science of chemistry, including nomenclature, structural formulae, and so forth.

interneuron (ĭn″tĕr-nū′rŏn) [L. *inter,* between, + Gr. *neuron,* nerve] A neuron of the central nervous system that transmits impulses from sensory to motor neurons or to other interneurons. SYN: *association neuron*.

internist A physician who specializes in internal medicine.

internode [″ + *nodus*, knot] The space between adjacent nodes.

internship (ĭn′tĕrn-shĭp) The period an intern spends in training, usually in a hospital.

internuclear (ĭn″tĕr-nū′klē-ăr) [″ + *nucleus*, a kernel] **1.** Between nuclei. **2.** Between outer and inner nuclear layers of the retina.

internuncial (ĭn″tĕr-nŭn′shē-ăl) [″ + *nuncius*, messenger] Acting as a connecting medium.

interocclusal (ĭn″tĕr-ŏ-kloo′zăl) [L. *inter*, between, + *occlusio*, a shutting up] Between the occlusal surfaces or cusps of opposing teeth of the maxillary and mandibular arches. SEE: *interdental; interproximal*.

interoceptive [L. *internus*, within, + *capere*, to take] In nerve physiology, concerned with sensations arising within the body itself, as distinguished from those arising outside the body.

interofective (ĭn″tĕr-ō-fĕk′tĭv) [″ + *afficere*, to influence] Pert. to that which concerns the interior of an organism.

interoinferior (ĭn″tĕr-ō-ĭn-fē′rē-or) [″ + *inferus*, below] Pert. to an inward and downward position.

interolivary [L. *inter*, between, + *oliva*, olive] Between the olivary bodies.

interorbital [″ + *orbita*, orbit] Between the orbits.

interosseous [″ + *os*, bone] Situated or occurring between bones, as muscles, ligaments, or vessels; specific muscles of the hands and feet.

interpalpebral (ĭn″tĕr-păl′pĕ-brăl) [″ + *palpebra*, eyelid] Between the eyelids.

interparietal (ĭn″tĕr-pă-rī′ĕ-tăl) [″ + *paries*, wall] **1.** Between walls. **2.** Between the parietal bones. **3.** Between the parietal lobes of the cerebrum.

interparoxysmal (ĭn″tĕr-păr″ŏk-sĭz′măl) [″ + Gr. *paroxysmos*, spasm] Between paroxysms.

interpeduncular (ĭn″tĕr-pĕ-dŭnk′ū-lăr) [L. *inter*, between, + *pedunculus*, peduncle] Between peduncles.

interpersonal Concerning the relations and interactions between persons.

interphalangeal (ĭn″tĕr-fă-lăn′jē-ăl) [″ + Gr. *phalanx*, closely knit row] In a joint between two phalanges.

interphase **1.** The stage of a cell between mitotic divisions during which DNA replication takes place. **2.** The area or zone where two phases of a substance, such as a gas and a liquid, contact each other.

interpolation (ĭn-tĕr″pō-lā′shŭn) **1.** In surgery, the transfer of tissues from one site to another. **2.** In statistics, the calculation of an intermediate value from the observed values larger and smaller than the unknown intermediate.

interposed (ĭn′tĕr-pōzd) Inserted between parts.

interpretation **1.** In psychotherapy, the analysis of the meaning and significance of what the patient says or does. It is explained to the patient to help provide insight. **2.** In dentistry or radiology, the study and analysis of a diagnostic radiograph and the integration of the findings with the case history and the laboratory and clinical evidence.

interproximal [″ + *proximus*, next] Between two adjoining surfaces. SYN: *interdental*.

interpubic (ĭn-tĕr-pū′bĭk) [″ + *pubes*, pubes] Between the pubic bones.

interpupillary [″ + *pupilla*, pupil] Between the pupils.

interradicular Between the roots of teeth; the furcation area.

interrenal (ĭn″tĕr-rē′năl) [L. *inter*, between, + *ren*, kidney] Between the kidneys.

interrogatory In law, a written question sent by one party to another requesting information about issues and witnesses surrounding the allegations in a lawsuit.

interscapilium (ĭn″tĕr-skă-pĭl′ē-ŭm) [″ + *scapula*, shoulder blade] The area between the shoulders or scapulae.

interscapular Between the shoulders or scapulae.

intersection The site where one structure crosses another or joins a similar structure.

intersegmental (ĭn″tĕr-sĕg-mĕn′tăl) [″ + *segmentum*, a portion] Between segments.

interseptal (ĭn″tĕr-sĕp′tăl) [″ + *saeptum*, a partition] Between two septa.

intersex (ĭn′tĕr-sĕks) An individual having both male and female secondary sexual characteristics. The term is descriptive but has little or no diagnostic value. Determination of sex in individuals who appear to have both male and female characteristics is complex. The diagnosis should be made after careful study of the chromosomes and of the gross and microscopic anatomical findings. SEE: *hermaphrodite; hermaphroditism*.

female i. A genetic female with external sexual characteristics of both sexes.

male i. A genetic male with external sexual characteristics of both sexes.

true i. An individual whose genetic sex may be either male or female and whose sexual characteristics are of both sexes.

intersexuality (ĭn″tĕr-sĕks″ū-ăl′ĭ-tē) The varying expression of male and female physical and sexual characteristics in the same individual. SEE: *intersex*.

interspace **1.** The space between two similar parts, as between two ribs. **2.** In radiology, the distance between the lead strips in a grid. It may contain organic material or aluminum.

interspinal (ĭn-tĕr-spī′năl) [″ + *spinalis,* pert. to the spine] Between two spinous processes of the spine.

interstice (ĭn-tĕr′stĭs) [L. *interstitium*] The space or gap in a tissue or structure of an organ. SYN: *interstitium.*

interstitial (ĭn″tĕr-stĭsh′ăl) **1.** Placed or lying between. **2.** Pert. to interstices or spaces within an organ or tissue.

i. lung disorders ABBR: ILD. A large group of diseases with different causes but with the same or similar clinical and pathological changes. These are due to chronic, nonmalignant, noninfectious diseases of the lower respiratory tract characterized by inflammation and disruption of the walls of the alveoli. This manifests clinically as a limitation in the ability of the lungs to transfer oxygen from the alveoli to the pulmonary capillary bed. Patients with these disorders are dyspneic first in connection with exercise and, later, as the disease progresses, even at rest.

Approx. 180 different types of ILD exist, many of which are poorly understood. Known causes include inhalation of irritating or toxic environmental agents such as organic dusts, fumes, vapors, aerosols, and inorganic dusts; drugs; radiation; aspiration pneumonia; and the consequences of acute respiratory distress syndrome. SEE: *idiopathic pulmonary fibrosis.*

interstitium (ĭn″tĕr-stĭsh′ē-ŭm) [L.] Interstice.

intersystole (ĭn″tĕr-sĭs′tō-lē) [L. *inter,* between, + Gr. *systole,* contraction] The period between the end of the atrial systole and the commencement of the ventricular systole.

intertarsal (ĭn″tĕr-tăr′săl) [″ + Gr. *tarsos,* a broad, flat surface] Between the tarsal bones of the foot.

intertransverse (ĭn″tĕr-trăns-vĕrs′) [″ + *transversus,* turned across] Between vertebrae; joining the transverse processes of a vertebra.

intertrigo (ĭn″tĕr-trī′gō) [″ + *terere,* to rub] Skin chafing that occurs in or under folds of skin. The irritation and trapped moisture often results in secondary bacterial or fungal infection. SEE: *erythema intertrigo.* **intertriginous,** *adj.*

intertrochanteric (ĭn″tĕr-trō″kăn-tĕr′ĭk) [″ + Gr. *trochanter,* trochanter] Situated between the greater and lesser trochanters of the femur.

intertubular (ĭn″tĕr-tū′bū-lăr) [″ + *tubulus,* tubule] Between or among tubules.

interureteral, interureteric (ĭn″tĕr-ū-rē′tĕr-ăl, ĭn″tĕr-ū″rē-tĕr′ĭk) [″ + Gr. *oureter,* ureter] Between the two ureters.

intervaginal (ĭn″tĕr-văj′ĭ-năl) [″ + *vagina,* sheath] Between sheaths.

interval [″ + *vallum,* a breastwork] **1.** A space or time between two objects or periods. **2.** A break in the course of disease or between paroxysms.

atriocarotid i. In a venous pulse tracing, the interval between the onset of the presystolic wave (a) and that of the systolic wave (c). It indicates the time required for impulses to travel from the SA node to the ventricle, normally about 0.2 sec.

atrioventricular (AV) i. An interval between the beginning of atrial systole and ventricular systole, measured by an electrocardiogram, as the P-R interval.

birth i. The time elapsed between a full-term pregnancy and the termination or completion of the next pregnancy. SYN: *interpregnancy i.*

cardioarterial i. The time between the apex beat and radial pulsation.

confidence i. ABBR: CI. The range of values within which it is expected (with a given probability) that the true value of a parameter will lie. SEE: *confidence level.*

contraction i. The period between uterine contractions. Relaxation of the uterine muscle replenishes the blood flow to the muscle and to the intervillous spaces of the placenta.

focal i. The distance between the anterior and posterior focal points of the eyes.

interpregnancy i. Birth i.

isometric i. Presphygmic i.

lucid i. A brief remission of symptoms in a psychosis, or after a traumatic brain injury.

postsphygmic i. The interval between closure of the semilunar valves and opening of atrioventricular valves.

P-R i. In the electrocardiogram, the period between the onset of the P wave and the beginning of the QRS complex.

presphygmic i. The brief period between the beginning of ventricular systole and opening of the semilunar valves. SYN: *isometric i.*

Q-R i. In the electrocardiogram, the period between the onset of the QRS complex and the peak of the R wave.

QRS i. In the electrocardiogram, the interval that denotes depolarization of the ventricles, between the beginning of the Q wave and the end of the S wave. The normal interval is less than 0.12 sec.

QRST i. The ventricular complex of the electrocardiogram. SEE: *electrocardiogram* for illus.

Q-T i. In the electrocardiogram, the interval between the beginning of the Q wave and the end of the T wave.

intervalvular (ĭn″tĕr-văl′vū-lăr) [L. *inter,* between, + *valva,* leaf of a folding door] Between valves, esp. the heart valves.

intervascular [″ + *vasculum,* a vessel] Between blood vessels.

intervention (ĭn″tĕr-vĕn′shŭn) One or

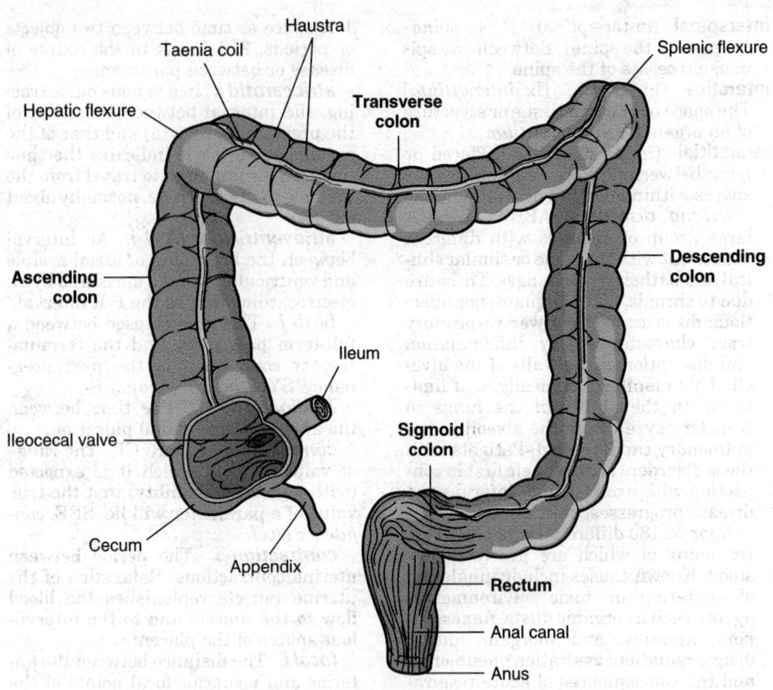

LARGE INTESTINE

more actions taken in order to modify an effect.

crisis i. Problem-solving activity intended to correct or prevent the continuation of a crisis, as in poison control centers or suicide prevention services. Usually these activities are mediated through telephone services operated by professional or paraprofessional workers in the medical and social fields.

life-sustaining i. Any method, medicine, or device used to prolong life. Whether, when, and how to use life-sustaining treatments are difficult topics that require careful consideration by patients, their surrogates, and health care professionals. SEE: *advance directive; living will.*

nursing i. SEE: *nursing intervention.*

interventricular [″ + *ventriculum,* a small cavity] Between the ventricles.

intervertebral (ĭn″tĕr-vĕrt′ĕ-brĕl, -vĕr-tē′brĕl) [″ + *vertebra,* joint] Between two adjacent vertebrae.

intervillous (ĭn″tĕr-vĭl′ŭs) [″ + *villus,* tuft] Between villi.

intestinal [L. *intestinum,* intestine] Pert. to the intestines. SEE: *digestion; intestine.*

i. obstruction SEE: under *obstruction.*

i. perforation SEE: *perforation of stomach or intestine.*

intestine (ĭn-tĕs′tĭn) [L. *intestinum*] The portion of the alimentary canal that extends from the pylorus of the stomach to the anus. It includes the duodenum, jejunum, ileum (small intestine), and colon (large intestine) and is responsible for the absorption of ingested nutrients and fluids. SYN: *bowel; gut* (1). SEE: *abdomen.*

large i. The large intestine extends from the ileum to the anus and is about 1.5 m (5 ft) in length. It absorbs water, minerals, and vitamins from the intestinal contents and eliminates undigested material during defecation. The mucosa has no villi but contains glands that secrete mucus. Hyperactivity of the colon may cause diarrhea. SEE: illus.

The first part of the large intestine is the cecum, a pouch on the right side into which the ileum empties. Attached to the cecum is the vermiform appendix, about 7.5 to 10.4 cm (3 to 4 in.) long. The ascending colon extends from the cecum upward to the undersurface of the liver, where it turns left (hepatic flexure) and becomes the transverse colon, which continues toward the spleen and turns downward (splenic flexure) to become the descending colon. At the level of the pelvic brim, the descending colon turns inward in the shape of the letter S and is then called the sigmoid colon. The rectum, about 10.2 to 12.7 cm (4 to 5 in.) long, is the straight part that continues downward; the last 2.5 cm (1 in.) is called the anal canal, which surrounds the anus.

small i. The first part of the small intestine is the duodenum, approx. 8 to 11 in. (20 to 28 cm) long, which receives chyme from the stomach through the pyloric orifice, and by way of the common bile duct, bile from the liver and gallbladder, and pancreatic juice from the pancreas. The second part is the jejunum, about 9 ft (2.8 m) long. The third part is the ileum, about 13 ft (4 m) long. The ileum opens into the cecum of the large intestine, and the ileocecal valve prevents backup of intestinal contents.

The wall of the small intestine has circular folds (plicae circulares), which are folds of the mucosa and submucosa that look like accordion pleats. The mucosa is further folded into villi, which look like small (0.5 to 1.5 mm long) projections. The free surfaces of the epithelial cells have microscopic folds called microvilli that are collectively called the brush border. All of the folds increase the surface area for absorption of the end products of digestion. Intestinal glands (of Lieberkühn) between the bases of the villi secrete enzymes. The duodenum has submucosal Brunner's glands that secrete mucus. Enzymes secreted by the small intestine are peptidases, which complete protein digestion, and sucrase, maltase, and lactase, which digest disaccharides to monosaccharides. Some of these enzymes function in the brush border rather than in the lumen of the intestine. Hormones secreted by the duodenum are gastric inhibitory peptide, secretin, and cholecystokinin; these influence secretions or motility of other parts of the digestive tract.

The end products of digestion (amino acids, monosaccharides, fatty acids, glycerol, vitamins, minerals, and water) are absorbed into the capillaries or lacteals within the villi. Blood from the small intestine passes through the liver by way of the portal vein before returning to the heart. SEE: *digestive system* for illus.; *duodenum; liver; pancreas.*

intestinum (ĭn″tĕs-tī′nŭm) *pl.* **intestina** [L.] Intestine.

intima (ĭn′tĭ-mă) [L.] The innermost layer of the wall of an artery or vein. It consists of a continuous layer of endothelial cells. Normally these cells are a semipermeable barrier that regulates the entry of substances from the lumen into the wall of the vessel. Materials may cross this barrier by means of transport systems. The endothelial cells are very smooth, which prevents abnormal clotting; they secrete chemicals that are important for normal blood coagulation and for controlling relaxation and contraction of the smooth muscle tissue in the middle layer of the vessel. As the normal artery ages, the intima thickens due to an increase in lipid material.

intimal (ĭn′tĭ-măl) Pert. to the inner layer of a blood vessel, the intima.

intimitis (ĭn″tĭ-mī′tĭs) [L. *intima,* innermost, + Gr. *itis,* inflammation] Inflammation of an intima.

intolerance [L. *in-,* not, + *tolerare,* to bear] An inability to endure, or an incapacity for bearing, pain or the effects of a drug or other substance.

intorsion (ĭn-tor′shŭn) [L. *in,* toward, + *torsio,* twisting] Rotation of the eye inward toward the nose on the anterio-posterior axis of the eye. In this condition, twelve o'clock on the corneal margin would be closer to the nose than normal.

intoxicant (ĭn-tŏks′ĭ-kănt) An agent that produces intoxication.

intoxication [L. *in,* in, + Gr. *toxikon,* poison] **1.** Poisoning by a drug or toxic substance. **2.** Impaired cognitively by alcoholic beverages. Colloquially: drunk.

The determination of alcohol content of the blood (i.e., ethyl alcohol or the alcohol present in commercial beverages such as beer, wine, and whiskey) is sometimes of value in the diagnosis of alcohol intoxication, esp. in differentiating it from other disorders. Normally the alcohol content of body tissues and fluids is negligible. Upon ingestion, alcohols are absorbed slowly or quickly, depending upon the amount swallowed, presence of food in the stomach, the drinker's gender (women become inebriated more easily with the same amount of alcohol consumption than men), and rate of gastric emptying. The amount of alcohol found in each milliliter of blood also depends on body size.

The amount of alcohol present in the blood does not provide valid information about the degree of intoxication because of the ability of the central nervous system, liver, and other organs to adapt to alcohol. SEE: *alcoholism.*

water i. Excess intake or undue retention of water, with symptomatic hyponatremia or hypo-osmolality or both. SEE: *brain edema; hyponatremia.*

SYMPTOMS: Abdominal cramps, nausea, vomiting, dizziness, lethargy, or edema may be present. Severe water intoxication may produce convulsions or coma.

ETIOLOGY: Causes include compulsive water drinking (e.g., in psychogenic polydipsia), massive administration of hypotonic solutions, excesses of antidiuretic hormone, or replacement of fluids and solutes lost by perspiration or vomiting with pure water.

intra- [L.] Prefix meaning *within.*

intra-abdominal [L. *intra,* within, + *abdomen,* belly] Within the abdomen.

intra-acinous (ĭn-tră-ăs′ĭ-nŭs) [″ + *acinus,* grape] Within an acinus.

intra-alveolar Inside the alveoli.

intra-aortic balloon counterpulsation ABBR: IABC. The use of a balloon attached to a catheter inserted through the femoral artery into the descending thoracic aorta to produce alternating inflation and deflation during diastole and systole, respectively. This permits lowering resistance to aortic blood flow during systole and increasing resistance during diastole. The result is to decrease the work of the heart and increase blood flow to the coronary arteries. The balloon is inflated with helium. This method is used to treat cardiogenic shock.

PATIENT CARE: *Patient preparation:* If time permits, the nurse explains to the patient that the cardiologist will place a special catheter into the aorta to help the heart pump more easily, and provide specific procedural and sensation information. The nurse explains that the catheter will be connected to a large console beside the bed that has an alarm system, and that a nurse will promptly answer any alarms. The nurse explains that the console normally makes a pumping sound, and ensures that the patient understands that this does not mean that his heart is not beating. The nurse also explains that because of the catheter, the patient will not be able to sit up, bend the knee, or flex the hip more than 30 degrees. The nurse explains that the patient will continue on the cardiac monitor, and will have a central line (pulmonary artery catheter), arterial line, and peripheral I.V. line in place. If the procedure is to be performed at the bedside, the nurse gathers the appropriate equipment, including a surgical tray for percutaneous catheter insertion, heparin solution, normal saline solution, the IABC catheter, and the pump console. The nurse prepares the femoral insertion site according to institutional protocol, ascertains that a signed informed consent for the procedure has been obtained, and provides the patient with emotional support throughout the procedure.

Monitoring and aftercare: Following institutional protocol or physician orders, the nurse sets the console to regulate the rate of inflation and deflation of the balloon based on the ECG or the arterial waveform. (If the patient has no intrinsic heart rate, the pump may be set to its own intrinsic rate.) The nurse uses strict aseptic technique in caring for the catheter insertion site and connections, and frequently inspects the site for bleeding or inflammation. If bleeding occurs at the insertion site, the nurse applies direct pressure over it and notifies the cardiologist. The nurse maintains the catheterized leg in correct body alignment and prevents hip flexion. The nurse maintains head elevation at no more than 30 degrees, to prevent upward migration of the catheter and occlusion of the left subclavian artery. If the balloon does occlude the artery, the nurse might expect to note a diminished left radial pulse and a patient report of dizziness. (Incorrect balloon placement also may occlude the renal artery, causing flank pain or a sudden drop in urine output.) The nurse also periodically assesses distal pulses, and documents the color, temperature, and capillary refill of the patient's extremities. The nurse assesses the affected leg's warmth, color, pulses, and the patient's ability to move the toes at 30-minute intervals for the first 4 hours after insertion, then hourly for the duration of IABC. (Often, arterial flow to the involved extremity diminishes during insertion, but the pulse should strengthen once pumping begins.)

If the patient is receiving heparin or low-molecular-weight dextran to inhibit thrombosis, the nurse keeps in mind that he or she is still at risk for thrombus formation, and observes for such indications as a sudden weakening of pedal pulses, pain, and motor or sensory loss. The nurse also maintains adequate hydration to help prevent thrombus formation. As prescribed, the nurse applies antiembolism stockings for 8 hours, then removes them, inspects and palpates the legs, and reapplies the stockings (or more recently, pneumatic pulsatiled stockings are used). The nurse encourages active range-of-motion exercises every 2 hours for the arms, the unaffected leg, and the affected ankle.

An alarm on the console may detect gas leaks from a damaged or ruptured balloon. If the alarm sounds, or if the nurse observes blood in the catheter, the nurse should shut down the pump console and immediately place the patient in Trendelenburg's position to prevent an air (gas) embolus from reaching the brain, then notify the cardiologist.

Once the signs and symptoms of left ventricular failure have diminished, and the patient requires only minimal pharmacological support, the patient will be gradually weaned from IABC. Then to discontinue IABC, the cardiologist or a designate will deflate the balloon, clip the sutures, and remove the catheter, allowing the site to bleed for 5 seconds to expel clots. The nurse then applies direct pressure to the site accordingly, followed by a pressure dressing. The nurse evaluates the site for bleeding and hematoma formation hourly for the next 4 hours.

intra-arterial [″ + Gr. *arteria,* artery] Within the artery(ies).

intra-articular (ĭn″tră-ăr-tĭk′ū-lăr) [″ + *articulus,* little joint] Within a joint.

intra-atrial (ĭn″tră-ā′trē-ăl) [″ + Gr. *atrion,* hall] Within one or both atria of the heart.

intrabronchial (ĭn″tră-brŏng′kē-ăl) [″ + Gr. *bronchos,* windpipe] Within a bronchus.

intrabuccal (ĭn″tră-bŭk′ăl) [″ + *bucca,* cheek] Within the tissue of the cheek or within the mouth.

intracanalicular (ĭn″tră-kăn″ă-lĭk′ū-lăr) [″ + *canalicularis,* pert. to a canaliculus] Within a canaliculus.

intracapsular [″ + *capsula,* little box] Within a capsule.

i. extraction The basic surgical technique for cataract removal, in which the nucleus, cortex, and capsule are removed as one unit. SEE: *cataract.*

intracardiac Within the heart.

intracarpal (ĭn″tră-kăr′păl) [″ + Gr. *karpalis,* pert. to the carpus] Within the wrist.

intracartilaginous (ĭn″tră-kăr″tĭ-lăj′ĭn-ŭs) [″ + *cartilago,* gristle] Within a cartilage or cartilaginous tissue.

intracath A device for facilitating the introduction of an intravenous catheter. An inflexible needle is surrounded by a catheter. They are inserted into the vein as a unit; then the needle is removed. This allows the catheter to be inserted further in the vein. The traditional intracath has been replaced by the angiocath or central venous line.

intracellular (ĭn″tră-sĕl′ū-lăr) [″ + *cellula,* cell] Within the cell.

intracerebellar (ĭn″tră-sĕr″ĕ-bĕl′ăr) [″ + *cerebellum,* little brain] Within the cerebellum of the brain.

intracerebral (ĭn″tră-sĕr′ĕ-brăl) [″ + *cerebrum,* brain] Within the main portion of the brain, the cerebrum.

intracervical (ĭn″tră-sĕr′vĭ-kăl) [″ + *cervicalis,* pert. to the neck] Within the neck of the uterus.

intracisternal (ĭn″tră-sĭs-tĕr′năl) [″ + *cisterna,* cavity] Within a cistern of the brain.

intracostal (ĭn″tră-kŏs′tăl) [″ + *costa,* rib] On the inner surface of a rib.

intracoronary (ĭn-tră-kŏr′ō-nă-rē) Within the coronary arteries.

intracranial [″ + Gr. *kranion,* skull] Within the cranium or skull.

intractable (ĭn-trăk′tă-b′l) Incurable or resistant to therapy.

intracutaneous [″ + *cutis,* skin] Within the skin. SYN: *intradermal.*

intracystic [″ + Gr. *kystis,* bladder] Within a bladder or cyst.

intrad (ĭn′trăd) Inwardly; toward the inner part.

intradermal (ĭn″tră-dĕr″măl) [″ + Gr. *derma,* skin] ABBR: ID. Intracutaneous, or more specifically, within the dermis.

intraduct (ĭn′tră-dŭkt) [″ + *ductus,* a canal] Within a duct.

intraduodenal (ĭn″tră-dū″ō-dē′năl) [″ + *duodeni,* twelve] Within the duodenum.

intradural (ĭn-tră-dū′răl) [″ + *durus,* hard] Within or enclosed by the dura mater.

intraepidermal (ĭn″tră-ĕp″ĭ-dĕr′măl) [L. *intra,* within, + Gr. *epi,* upon, + *derma,* skin] Within the epidermis.

intraepithelial (ĭn″tră-ĕp″ĭ-thē′lē-ăl) [″ + ″ + *thele,* nipple] Within the epithelium or located between its cells.

intrafebrile [″ + *febris,* fever] During the febrile stage. SYN: *intrapyretic.*

intrafilar (ĭn-tră-fī′lăr) [″ + *filum,* thread] Within a network or reticulum.

intragastric [″ + Gr. *gaster,* belly] Within the stomach.

i. balloon An inflatable device placed in the stomach in an uninflated state. Once in place, it is inflated. This method of treating obesity has not been effective on a long-term basis.

intragemmal (ĭn″tră-jĕm′ăl) [″ + *gemma,* bud] Within a bud or the expanded ending of a nerve, as a taste bud.

intraglandular [″ + *glans,* acorn] Within a gland.

intragyral (ĭn″tră-jī′răl) [″ + Gr. *gyros,* circle] Within a gyrus of the brain.

intrahepatic (ĭn″tră-hĕ-păt′ĭk) [″ + Gr. *hepatikos,* pert. to the liver] Within the liver.

intraintestinal [″ + *intestinum,* intestine] Within the intestine.

intralaryngeal (ĭn″tră-lă-rĭn′jē-ăl) [″ + Gr. *larynx,* larynx] Within the larynx.

intralesional (ĭn″tră-lē′zhŭn-ăl) [″ + *laesio,* a wound] Within a lesion.

intraligamentary [″ + *ligamentum,* a binding] Within the folds of a ligament; usually used in referring to fibroid tumors or cysts of the ovary that have grown within the broad ligament.

intraligamentous Within a ligament.

intralingual Within the tongue.

intralobar (ĭn″tră-lō′băr) [″ + *lobus,* a lobe] Within a lobe.

intralobular (ĭn″tră-lŏb′ū-lăr) [″ + *lobulus,* a lobule] Within a lobule.

intralocular (ĭn″tră-lŏk′ū-lăr) [″ + *loculus,* a cavity] Within the cavity of any structure.

intralumbar [″ + *lumbus,* loin] Within the lumbar region or portion of the spinal cord.

intraluminal (ĭn″tră-lū′mĭ-năl) [″ + *lumen,* light] Intratubal.

intramastoiditis (ĭn″tră-măs″tŏyd-ī′tĭs) [″ + Gr. *mastos,* breast, + *eidos,* form, shape, + *itis,* inflammation] An inflammation of the antrum and mastoid process. SYN: *endomastoiditis.*

intramedullary (ĭn″tră-mĕd′ū-lăr″ē) [″ + *medullaris,* marrow] **1.** Within the medulla oblongata of the brain. **2.** Within the spinal cord. **3.** Within the marrow cavity of a bone.

intramural [″ + *murus,* a wall] Within the walls of a hollow organ or cavity.

intramuscular [″ + *musculus,* a muscle] ABBR: IM. Within a muscle.

intranasal [″ + *nasus,* nose] Within the nasal cavity.

intranatal [″ + *natalis,* birth] Occurring during birth.

intraocular (ĭn″tră-ŏk′ū-lĕr) [″ + *oculus,* eye] Within the eyeball.

intraoperative (ĭn″tră-ŏp′ĕr-ă″tĭv) [L. *intra,* within, + *operativus,* working] Occurring during surgery.

intraoral [″ + *oralis,* pert. to the mouth] Within the mouth.

intraorbital [″ + *orbita,* mark of a wheel] Within the orbit.

intraosseous (ĭn″tră-ŏs′ē-ŭs) [″ + *os,* bone] Within the bone matrix.

intraosseous infusion A method of obtaining immediate vascular access, esp. in children by percutaneous insertion of a bone marrow aspiration needle into the marrow cavity of a long bone, usually into the proximal tibia. Once access is gained, substances may be injected into the bone marrow where they are absorbed almost immediately into the general circulation. This avenue of access does not collapse in the presence of shock.

intraovarian (ĭn″tră-ō-vā′rē-ăn) [″ + *ovarium,* ovary] Within the ovary.

intraparietal (ĭn″tră-pă-rī′ĕ-tăl) [″ + *paries,* wall] **1.** Within the parietal lobe of the cerebrum. **2.** Intramural.

intrapartal The period from the onset of labor to its termination, marked by delivery of the placenta.

intrapartum (ĭn″tră-păr′tŭm) [″ + *partus,* birth] Happening during childbirth.

intrapelvic (ĭn″tră-pĕl′vĭk) [″ + *pelvis,* basin] Within the pelvis.

intraperitoneal [″ + Gr. *peritonaion,* peritoneum] Within the peritoneal cavity.

intraplacental (ĭn″tră-plă-sĕn′tăl) [″ + *placenta,* a flat cake] Within the placenta.

intrapleural [″ + Gr. *pleura,* rib] Within the pleural cavity.

intrapontine (ĭn″tră-pŏn′tīn) [″ + *pons,* bridge] Within the pons varolii.

intrapsychic, intrapsychical (ĭn″tră-sī′kĭk, -kĭ-kăl) [″ + Gr. *psyche,* mind] Having a mental origin or basis, such as conflicts and complexes.

intrapulmonary [″ + *pulmo,* lung] Within the lungs.

intrapyretic (ĭn″tră-pī-rĕt′ĭk) [″ + Gr. *pyretos,* fever] Intrafebrile.

intrarectal (ĭn″tră-rĕk′tăl) [″ + *rectum,* straight] Within the rectum.

intrarenal (ĭn″tră-rē′năl) [″ + *renalis,* pert. to the kidney] Within the kidney.

intraretinal (ĭn″tră-rĕt′ĭ-năl) [″ + *retina,* retina] Within the retina of the eye.

intrascrotal (ĭn″tră-skrō′tăl) [″ + *scrotum,* a bag] Within the scrotum.

intraspinal [L. *intra,* within, + *spina,* thorn] **1.** Ensheathed; within a sheath. **2.** Within the spinal canal.

intrathecal (ĭn″tră-thē′kăl) [″ + Gr. *theke,* sheath] **1.** Within the spinal canal. **2.** Within a sheath.

intrathoracic (ĭn″tră-thō-răs′ĭk) [″ + Gr. *thorax,* chest] Within the thorax.

intratracheal (ĭn″tră-trāk′ē-ăl) [″ + Gr. *tracheia,* trachea] Introduced into, or inside, the trachea.

intratubal [″ + *tubus,* hollow tube] Within a tube, esp. the fallopian tube. SYN: *intraluminal.*

intratympanic (ĭn″tră-tĭm-păn′ĭk) [″ + Gr. *tympanon,* drum] Within the tympanic cavity.

intrauterine (ĭn″tră-ū′tĕr-ĭn) [″ + *uterus,* womb] Within the uterus.

i. contraceptive device ABBR: IUCD or IUD. A copper or polypropylene artifact that is inserted into the uterine cavity to interfere with conception or implantation. The actual mechanism by which IUDs function is unclear, but they may prevent conception either by inhibiting the intrauterine transit of sperm or by expediting ovum passage through the fallopian tube. The local inflammatory response to the IUD may inhibit nidation. The estimated pregnancy rate is between 2% and 4%.

Although once manufactured in several different shapes and materials, the incidence of uterine perforation, severe pelvic inflammatory disease, or both, led to product liability lawsuits and the discontinuance of many models in the U.S. The two contemporary IUDs are T-shaped. The most commonly used device is the Copper T380A (ParaGard), which may remain in place for as long as 10 years. The Progesterone T (Progestasert) provides protection for women who are allergic to copper, but this slow-release progesterone device must be replaced each year. Common clinical criteria for insertion include primiparity or multiparity; a monogamous relationship; and the absence of vaginal, cervical, or pelvic disease. The device is inserted during menstruation or on the first postpartum visit.

CAUTION: Because of the increased risk of sexually transmitted infections, the IUD is contraindicated for women who have multiple sexual partners.

Patient Care: To help prospective users make informed decisions, patient teaching should include discussing the comparative advantages and disadvantages of the method of contraception under consideration. *Advantages:* Little maintenance is required, other than checking for the presence of the string each week during the first month after insertion and thereafter each month after menses, and having an annual routine pelvic examination. Only 10% of users experience spontaneous expulsion of the device during the first year after insertion. *Disadvantages:* Transient cramping or bleeding for a few weeks after insertion is not uncommon; dysmenorrhea, menorrhagia, and/or metrorrhagia also may occur. An increased risk of ectopic pregnancy (10 times more common) may be related to the increased risk of pelvic inflammatory disease. Uterine perforation is rare. Health care professionals should instruct users to promptly inform their health care providers if they experience delayed menses, abnormal vaginal discharge, dyspareunia, abdominal pain, or signs of infection.

i. growth retardation ABBR: IUGR. A decreased rate of fetal growth; most commonly related to inadequate placental perfusion resulting from pre-existing or coexisting maternal or placental factors. The infant's birth weight is below the 10th percentile on the intrauterine growth curve for the calculated gestation period. Although about 50% of cases of IUGR cannot be linked to any particular cause, certain characteristics are associated with increased fetal jeopardy:

1. *Demographic factors:* Maternal age under 16 or over 40; primiparity or grand multiparity; low socioeconomic status; low weight gain; poor nutrition; and inadequate prenatal care
2. *Maternal medical disorders:* Common pre-existing and coexisting health problems, including cyanotic heart disease, chronic or pregnancy-related hypertensive disease, advanced diabetes mellitus, hemoglobinopathies, substance abuse, and asymptomatic pyelonephritis
3. *Placental factors:* Placenta previa; small placenta; abnormal site of cord insertion; large or multiple infarcts; or thrombosis
4. *Fetal factors:* Congenital infections such as rubella, cytomegalovirus, or toxoplasmosis, particularly when occurring during an early stage of fetal development; chromosomal abnormalities and fetal anomalies; and multiple gestation (i.e., two or more fetuses).

SYMPTOMS: The first prenatal sign of abnormal fetal growth usually is noted during the second trimester, when the increase in fundal height is found to be less than expected for the number of weeks' gestation. Ultrasonography enables comparisons of measurements of the fetal head circumference, biparietal diameter, abdominal circumference, and femur length and the expected norms for the estimated gestational week. IUGR newborns evidence birth weights at or below the 10th percentile on the intrauterine growth curve for an equal number of weeks' gestation. SEE: *gestational age assessment*.

TYPES: *Asymmetric.* There may be a disproportional reduction in size of structures. For example, the biparietal diameter may be within normal limits for gestational age, while the abdominal circumference is less than expected. Asymmetry usually reflects episodic interference with uteroplacental circulation accompanying such events as placental infarction and pre-eclampsia. During the neonatal period, these infants are at high risk for asphyxia, aspiration syndrome, hypocalcemia, polycythemia, and pulmonary hemorrhage. *Symmetric.* A generalized proportional reduction in the size of all structures and organs, other than the brain and heart, reflects diminished cell numbers related to persistent, chronic nutritional deprivation, resulting from substance abuse, congenital anomalies, and early intrauterine infection. SEE: *cocaine baby; parabiosis*.

PROGNOSIS: Asymmetric IUGR infants usually exhibit normal weights within 3 to 6 months of birth. Symmetric IUGR infants exhibit an individual potential for growth; however, their growth usually does not equal that of their peers. Later, these children may exhibit learning disabilities associated with a lessened ability to concentrate and focus on tasks because of their hyperactivity and short attention spans, and they may become frustrated because of their poor fine motor coordination. SEE: *dysmaturity*.

intravasation (ĭn-trăv″ă-zā′shŭn) [″ + *vas,* vessel] Passage into the blood vessels of matter formed outside of them through traumatic or pathological lesions.

intravascular Within blood vessels.

intravenous (ĭn-tră-vē′nŭs) [″ + *vena,* vein] ABBR: IV. Within or into a vein.

i. feeding SEE: under *feeding*.

i. infusion SEE: under *infusion*.

i. infusion pump Infusion pump.

i. injection SEE: under *injection*.

i. treatment Intravenous injection or infusion.

intraventricular [L. *intra,* within, + *ventriculus,* ventricle] Within a ventricle.

intravesical (ĭn″tră-vĕs′ĭ-kăl) [″ + *vesica,* bladder] Within the urinary bladder.

intravital [″ + *vita,* life] During life. SYN: *intra vitam*.

intra vitam (ĭn′tră vī′tăm) [L.] Intravital.

intravitelline (ĭn″tră-vī-tĕl′ĭn) [″ + *vitellus,* yoke] Within the vitelline or yolk.

intravitreous (ĭn″tră-vĭt′rē-ŭs) [″ + *vitreus,* glassy] Within the vitreous of the eye.

intrinsic [L. *intrinsicus,* on the inside] **1.** Belonging to the essential nature of a thing. It is both essential and natural, not merely apparent or accidental. SYN: *inherent; innate*. **2.** In anatomy, structures belonging solely to a certain body part, as intrinsic nerves or muscles. **3.** Due to causes or elements within the body, an organ, or a part.

intro- [L.] Prefix meaning *in* or *into.*

introducer [L. *intro,* into, + *ducere,* to lead] Intubator.

introflexion (ĭn″trō-flĕk′shŭn) [″ + *flexus,* bent] A bending inward.

introitus (ĭn-trō′ĭ-tŭs) [L.] An opening or entrance into a canal or cavity, as the vagina.

i. canalis sacralis The terminal opening of the spinal canal at the end of the sacrum.

i. laryngis The upper opening of the larynx.

i. vaginae The exterior orifice of the vagina.

introjection [″ + *jacere,* to throw] In psychoanalysis, identification of the self with another or with some object, the victim assuming the supposed feelings of the other personality.

intromission (ĭn″trō-mĭsh′ŭn) [″ + *mittere,* to send] An insertion or placing of one part into another, esp. insertion of the penis into the vagina.

intromittent (ĭn-trō-mĭt′ĕnt) Conveying or injecting into a cavity or body.

intron The noncoding space between the discrete coding regions (exons) of the DNA of the gene.

introspection [″ + *spicere,* to look] Looking within, esp. examination of one's own mind.

introsusception (ĭn″trō-sŭ-sĕp′shŭn) [″ + *suscipere,* to receive] Intussusception.

introversion (ĭn″trō-vĕr′shŭn) [″ + *versio,* a turning] **1.** Turning inside out of a part or organ. **2.** The condition of an introvert; preoccupation with one's self.

introvert **1.** A personality-reaction type characterized by withdrawal from reality, fantasy formation, and stress on the subjective side of life adjustments, seen pathologically in extreme form in schizophrenia. **2.** To turn one's psychic energy inward upon oneself.

intubate (ĭn′tū-bāt) [L. *in,* into, + *tuba,* a tube] To insert a tube in a part, such as the larynx.

intubation (ĭn″tū-bā′shŭn) The insertion of a tube into any hollow organ. Intubation of the trachea provides an open airway and thus is an essential step in advanced life support. It also permits the instillation of certain critical care drugs, such as lidocaine, epinephrine, and atropine, which the lungs can absorb directly when other forms of internal access are unavailable. In the patient with no evidence of head or cervical spine trauma, using a head-tilt, chin-lift maneuver to place the patient in a "sniffing" position facilitates intubation of the trachea.

Intubation of other structures, such as the organs of the upper gastrointestinal tract, may permit enteral nutrition, the dilation of strictures, or the visualization of internal anatomy.

endotracheal i. The insertion of an endotracheal tube through the nose or mouth into the trachea to maintain the airway, to administer an anesthetic gas or oxygen, or to aspirate secretions.

nasogastric i. SEE: *gastric lavage.*

nasotracheal i. The insertion of an endotracheal tube through the nose and into the trachea. Unlike orotracheal intubation, the tube is passed "blindly" without using a laryngoscope to visualize the glottic opening. Because this technique may be used without hyperextension of the neck, it is used in patients suspected of having cervical spinal trauma or known to have oral lesions. SEE: *endotracheal i.*

rapid sequence i. An airway control technique that uses powerful sedatives and paralytic drugs to quickly gain control of the airway, e.g., in life-threatening emergencies.

intubator A device for controlling, directing, and placing an intubation tube within the trachea, blood vessel, or heart (as in Swan-Ganz catheter placement). SYN: *introducer*.

intuition **1.** Assumed knowledge; guesswork; a hunch. **2.** Nonrational cognition.

intumesce (ĭn-tū-mĕs′) [L. *intumescere*] To enlarge or swell.

intumescence **1.** A swelling. **2.** The process of enlarging. SYN: *tumefaction.*

intumescent (ĭn-tū-mĕs′ĕnt) Swelling or becoming enlarged.

intussusception (ĭn″tŭ-sŭ-sĕp′shŭn) [L. *intus,* within, + *suscipere,* to receive] The slipping of one part of an intestine into another part just below it; becoming ensheathed. It is noted chiefly in children and usually occurs in the ileocecal region; in adults, an intraintestinal tumor or polyp may become the leading portion of the intussusception. In some instances, the process may be reduced by low pressure contrast enema; ultimately, surgery may be necessary if the process recurs. Prognosis is good if surgery is performed immediately; but mortality is high if this condition is left untreated more than 24 hours. SYN: *introsusception; invagination*. SEE: *ileus*.

intussusceptum (ĭn″tŭ-sŭ-sĕp′tŭm) [L.] The inner segment of intestine that has been pushed into another segment.

intussuscipiens (ĭn″tŭ-sŭ-sĭp′ē-ĕns) [L.] The portion of intestine that receives the intussusceptum.

Inuit [Eskimo people] People native to Arctic America.

inulase (ĭn′ū-lās) An enzyme that converts inulin to levulose.

inulin A polysaccharide found in plants that yields fructose when hydrolyzed. It is used to study renal function.

inunction (ĭn-ŭngk′shŭn) [L. *in,* into, + *unguere,* to anoint] An ointment or medicated substance rubbed into the skin to secure a local or a more general systemic effect.

in utero (ĭn ū′tĕr-ō) [L.] Within the uterus.

in vacuo (ĭn văk′ū-ō) [L.] Within a cavity or a space from which air has been exhausted.

invaginate (ĭn-văj′ĭn-āt) [L. *invaginatio*] **1.** To ensheath. **2.** To insert one part of a structure within a part of the same structure. **3.** In embryology, to grow in or from an ingrowth or inpocketing, esp. the ingrowth of the wall of the blastula, which results in the formation of the gastrula.

invaginated Enclosed in a sheath; ensheathed.

invagination Intussusception.

invalid [L. *in-,* not, + *validus,* strong] **1.** Not well; weak. **2.** A sickly person, particularly one confined to a bed or wheelchair.

invasion [L. *in,* into, + *vadere,* to go] **1.** The penetration of body tissues by infectious organisms or malignant cells.

invasive Tending to spread, esp. the tendency of a malignant process or growth to spread into healthy tissue.

i. procedure A procedure in which the body is penetrated or entered (e.g., by use of a tube, needle, device, or ionizing radiation).

inventory Any list of items, esp. items to describe an individual's personality.

invermination [″ + *vermis,* worm] Infestation by intestinal worms.

inversion (ĭn-vĕr′zhŭn) [L. *inversio,* to turn inward] **1.** The reversal of a normal relationship. **2.** A turning inside out of an organ (e.g., the uterus). **3.** In chemistry, the process of converting sucrose (which rotates the plane of polarized light to the right) into a mixture of dextrose and levulose (which rotates the plane to the left). The resulting mixture is called invert sugar, and the enzyme that catalyzes this conversion is called invertase. SEE: *enzyme*.

uterine i. A condition that may occur during the third stage of labor in which a relaxed uterus is turned inside out, causing the internal surface to protrude into the vagina. Uterine inversion most commonly is caused by traction on an umbilical cord attached to a yet-adherent placenta or to application of forceful fundal pressure to empty the uterus. It is accompanied by profound maternal blood loss if normal anatomical position is not restored immediately. Inversion also can occur during the fourth stage of labor if forceful fundal massage is applied to an uncontracted uterus without support of the lower uterine segment.

invert (ĭn-vĕrt′) To turn inside out or upside down.

invertase (ĭn-vĕr′tās) Sucrase.

invertebrate [L. *in-,* not, + *vertebratus,* vertebrate] **1.** Without a backbone. **2.** Species of animals that do not have a backbone.

invertin (ĭn-vĕr′tĭn) Invertase.

invertor (ĭn-vĕr′tor) A muscle that rotates a part inward.

investing [L. *in,* into, + *vestire,* to clothe] **1.** Ensheathing, encircling with a sheath or coating, as tissue; surrounding. **2.** In dentistry, the complete or partial covering of an object (e.g., a tooth, denture, wax form, or crown) with a suitable material before processing, soldering, or casting.

investment A covering or sheath.

dental casting i. A material combining principally a form of silica and a bonding agent. The bonding substance may be gypsum or silica phosphate according to the casting temperature.

inveterate [″ + *vetus,* old] Chronic; firmly seated, as a disease or a habit.

inviscation (ĭn″vĭs-kā′shŭn) [L. *in,* among, + *viscum,* slime] The mixing of saliva with food during chewing.

in vitro (ĭn vē′trō) [L., in glass] In glass, as in a test tube. An in vitro test is one done in the laboratory, usually involving isolated tissue, organ, or cell preparations. SEE: *in vivo*.

in vivo (ĭn vē′vō) [L., in the living body] In the living body or organism. An in vivo test is one performed on a living organism. SEE: *in vitro*.

involucre, involucrum (ĭn′vō-lū″kĕr, ĭn″vō-lū′krŭm) [″ + *volvere,* to wrap] **1.** A sheath or covering. **2.** The covering of newly formed bone enveloping the sequestrum in infection of the bone.

involuntary [L. *in-,* not, + *voluntas,* will] **1.** Independent of or contrary to volition. **2.** Occurring as a result of a reflex.

involution (ĭn″vō-lū′shŭn) [″ + *volvere,* to roll] **1.** A turning or rolling inward. **2.** The reduction in size of the uterus after childbirth. **3.** The retrogressive change in vital processes after their functions have been fulfilled, such as the change that follows the menopause. **4.** A backward change. **5.** The diminishing of an organ in vital power or in size. **6.** In bacteriology, digression from the usual morphological type such as occurs in certain bacteria, esp. when grown under unfavorable conditions; degeneration.

i. of uterus The return of the uterus to normal size after childbirth.

senile i. The atrophy of an organ as a result of the aging process.

involutional (ĭn-vō-lū′shŭn-ăl) Concerning involution or a turning inward.

Io Symbol for the element ionium.

iocetamic acid A radiopaque agent formerly used in cholecystography.

Iodamoeba (ī″ō-dă-mē′bă) A genus of amebas found in the intestinal tract. Their cysts are peculiar in that they are shaped irregularly, the nucleus usually is single, and they possess a vacuole filled with glycogen that stains brown in iodine.

I. bütschlii A small, sluggish ameba found in the large intestine of humans, as well as in monkeys and pigs. It is usually nonpathogenic.

iodide (ī′ō-dīd) A compound of iodine containing another radical or element, as potassium iodide.

cesium i. A phosphor used in radiographical image intensifiers that emits light when struck by radiation.

sodium i. I 125 solution A standardized solution of radioactive iodide, ^{125}I.

iodinate (ī-ō′dĭ-nāt) To combine with iodine.

iodinated I 131 albumin injection A standardized preparation of albumin iodinated with the use of radioactive iodine, ^{131}I.

iodine (ī′ō-dīn, ī′ō-dēn) [Gr. *ioeides,* violet colored] SYMB: I. A nonmetallic element belonging to the halogen group; atomic weight 126.904; atomic number 53; specific gravity (solid, 20°C) 4.93. It is a black crystalline substance with a melting point of 113.5°C; it boils at 184.4°C, giving off a characteristic violet vapor. Sources of iodine include vegetables, esp. those growing near the seacoast; iodized salt; and seafoods, esp. liver of halibut and cod, or fish liver oils.

FUNCTION: Iodine is part of the hormones triiodothyronine (T_3) and thyroxine (T_4), and prevents goiter by enabling the thyroid gland to function normally. The amount of iodine in the entire body averages 50 mg, of which 10 to 15 mg is found in the thyroid. The adult daily requirement for iodine is from 100 to 150 μg. Growing children, adolescents, pregnant women, and those under emotional strain need more than this amount of iodine.

DEFICIENCY SYMPTOMS: Iodine deficiency in the diet may lead to simple goiter characterized by thyroid enlargement and hypothyroidism. In young children, this deficiency may result in retardation of physical, sexual, and mental development, a condition called cretinism.

i. poisoning SEE: *Poisons and Poisoning Appendix.*

protein-bound i. Iodine that is attached to serum protein.

radioactive i. SYMB: ^{131}I. An isotope of iodine with an atomic weight of 131; used in diagnosis and treatment of thyroid disorders and in the treatment of toxic goiter and thyroid carcinoma.

tincture of i. A solution of 2% iodine and 2.4% sodium iodide diluted in 50% ethyl alcohol. It is used as a disinfectant for the skin and as a germicide. It may be used to make contaminated water safe for drinking. Adding three drops of tincture of iodine to a quart of water will kill amebas and bacteria within 30 minutes, and the water will still be palatable. If water to be treated by this method is cloudy or turbid, it should be allowed to settle; then the clear portion should be decanted and treated with iodine.

iodinophilous (ī″ō-dĭn-ŏf′ĭ-lŭs) [Gr. *ioeides,* violet colored, + *philos,* love] Easily stained with iodine.

iodipamide meglumine injection A radiographic contrast medium combination of iodipamide and meglumine used to aid in x-ray examination of the gallbladder. Trade name is Cholografin Meglumine.

iodipamide sodium I 131 Radioactive chemical used in examining body organs and cavities. Trade name is RadioCholografin.

iodism (ī′ō-dĭzm) A condition induced by prolonged and excessive use of iodine or its compounds.

iodize To administer or impregnate with iodine, most commonly as a fortification of salt.

5-iodo-2′-deoxyuridine ABBR: IDU. Idoxuridine.

iododerma (ī-ō″dō-dĕr′mă) [″ + *derma,* skin] Dermatitis due to iodine.

iodoform (ī-ō′dō-form) [Gr. *ioeides,* violet colored, + L. *forma,* form] CHI_3; a yellow crystalline substance with a disagreeable odor, produced by the action of iodine on acetone in the presence of an alkali. Used topically, it has mild antibacterial action.

iodoformism (ī′ō-dō-form″ĭzm) [″ + ″ + Gr. *-ismos,* state of] Poisoning caused by iodoform.

iodoglobulin (ī″ō-dō-glŏb′ū-lĭn) [″ + L. *globus,* globe] A globulin protein that contains iodine.

iodohippurate sodium I 131 injection (ī-ō″dō-hĭp′ū-rāt) A radioactive contrast medium used in testing renal function. Trade name is Hippuran I 131.

iodophilia (ī″ō-dō-fĭl′ē-ă) [″ + *philein,* to love] A condition in which certain cells, esp. polymorphonuclear leukocytes, when stained, show a pronounced affinity for iodine. These cells turn a brownish-red color. It is seen in pathologic conditions such as acute infections and anemia.

extracellular i. Iodophilia in which substances in the plasma outside the cells are colored.

intracellular i. Iodophilia in which color changes occur within the cells.

iodophor (ī-ō′dō-for) A combination of iodine and a solubilizing agent or carrier that liberates free iodine in solution. Some forms are used as general antiseptics; they are less irritating than elemental forms of iodine. SEE: *povidone-iodine*.

iodopsin In cones of the retina, the photopsin molecule and retinal, the functional photopigment.

iodopyracet (ī-ō″dō-pī′ră-sĕt) A radiopaque contrast medium used in intravenous pyelography and urography. Trade name is Diodrast.

iodoquinol (ī-ō″dō-kwĭn′ŏl) $C_9H_5I_2NO$; an antiamebic agent used in the treatment of amebiasis and *Trichomonas hominis* infection of the intestines. Its previously used name was diiodohydroxyquin.

CAUTION: The use of this drug has been associated with production of a severe disease of the central nervous system called subacute myelo-optic neuropathy.

iodotherapy [Gr. *ioeides,* violet colored, + *therapeia,* treatment] The use of iodine medication, as in treating goiter due to iodine deficiency.

IOML *infraorbitomeatal line.*

ion [Gr. *ion,* going] An atom or group of atoms that has lost one or more electrons and has a positive charge, or has gained one or more electrons and has a negative charge. In aqueous solutions, ions are called electrolytes because they permit the solution to conduct electricity. Positive ions such as sodium, potassium, magnesium, and calcium are called cations; negative ions such as chloride, bicarbonate, and sulfate are called anions. In body fluids, ions are available for reactions (e.g., calcium ions from food may be combined with carbonate ions to form calcium carbonate, part of bone matrix). SEE: *electrolyte* for table.

Ions occur in gases, esp. at low pressures, under the influence of strong electrical discharges, x-rays, and radium; in solutions of acids, bases, and salts.

dipolar i. An ion that contains both positive and negative charges.

hydrogen i. A hydrogen atom that has lost an electron. It has a positive charge, and its symbol is H^+.

ion-exchange resins Synthetic organic substances of high molecular weight. They replace certain negative or positive ions that they encounter in solutions.

ionic [Gr. *ion,* going] Pert. to ions.

ionium (ī-ō′nē-ŭm) A natural radioactive isotope of thorium. It has a mass number of 230.

ionization (ī-ō-nĭ-zā′shŭn) The process of adding or subtracting an electron from an atom. In radiology, ionization is the most common cause of radiobiological damage.

ionize To separate into ions.

ionogen (ī-ŏn′ō-jĕn) [Gr. *ion,* going, + *gennan,* to produce] Anything that can be ionized.

ionophore A chemical material that has a high affinity for ions. Ionophores are used in ion-selective electrode (ISE) membranes.

ionotherapy (ī″ŏn-ō-thĕr′ă-pē) [″ + *therapeia,* treatment] Iontophoresis.

iontophoresis (ī-ŏn″tō-fō-rē′sĭs) [″ + *phorein,* to carry] **1.** The process of electric current traveling through a salt solution, causing migration of the metal (positive) ion to the negative pole and the radical (negative) ion to the positive pole. **2.** The introduction of various ions into tissues through the skin by means of electricity. SYN: *ionic medication; ionotherapy; iontotherapy.* SEE: *electrical patch.*

iontotherapy (ī-ŏn″tō-thĕr′ă-pē) [″ + *therapeia,* treatment] Iontophoresis.

IOP *intraocular pressure.*

iopanoic acid A radiopaque contrast medium used in radiographic studies of the gallbladder.

iophendylate (ī″ō-fĕn′dĭ-lāt) A radiopaque contrast medium used in myelography.

iophobia (ī″ō-fō′bē-ă) [Gr. *ios,* poison, + *phobos,* fear] **1.** Toxicophobia. **2.** Fear of touching any rusty object.

iotacism (ī-ō′tă-sĭzm) [Gr. *iota,* letter i] Defective utterance marked by the constant substitution of an ē sound (Greek iota) for other vowels.

iothalamate meglumine injection (ī-ō-thăl′ă-māt) A radiopaque contrast medium used in investigating arteries of the brain as well as in the rest of the body, and in studying kidney function.

I.P. *intraperitoneal; isoelectric point.*

IPA *independent practice association.*

ipecac (ĭp′ĕ-kăk) A drug that induces vomiting. For many years, it was used to help empty the upper gastrointestinal tract after toxic ingestions and accidental overdoses. It no longer is used for this purpose in hospitals, where activated charcoal and whole bowel irrigation have proved to be more effective and better tolerated. The drug is derived from the dried root of ipecacuanha, a plant that is native to Brazil. It typically is given as a syrup. SEE: *Poisons and Poisoning Appendix.*

I.P.L. *interpupillary line;* the line between the center of both pupils.

ipodate calcium (ī′pō-dāt) A radiopaque contrast medium used in radiographical studies of the gallbladder.

ipodate sodium A radiopaque contrast medium used in radiographical studies of the gallbladder.

IPPB *intermittent positive-pressure breathing.*

IPPV *intermittent positive-pressure ventilation.*

ipratropium bromide An anticholinergic bronchodilator used for bronchoconstriction associated with chronic bronchitis, chronic obstructive pulmonary disease, asthma, and emphysema. It is dispensed via a metered-dose inhaler (MDI) or as a solution for nebulized use, and usually is combined with another bronchodilator such as albuterol. SEE: *asthma.*

iproniazid (ī″prō-nī′ă-zĭd) An antitubercular drug.

ipsi- [L. *ipse,* same] Prefix meaning *same* or *self.*

IPSID *immunoproliferative small intestinal disease.*

ipsilateral (ĭp″sĭ-lăt′ĕr-ăl) [″ + *latus,* side] On the same side; affecting the same side of the body; the opposite of contralateral. For example, when the right patellar tendon is tapped, an ipsilateral knee-jerk is observed on the same side. In paralysis, this term is used to describe findings appearing on same side of the body as the brain or spinal cord lesion producing them. SYN: *homolateral.*

IPSP *inhibitory postsynaptic potential.*

IQ *intelligence quotient.*

IR *infrared.*

I.R. *internal resistance.*

Ir Symbol for the element iridium.

iralgia (ĭr-ăl′jē-ă) [Gr. *iris,* colored circle, + *algos,* pain] Iridalgia.

irascible (ĭ-răs′ĭ-b′l) [LL. *irascibilis*] Marked by outbursts of temper or irritability; easily angered.

IRB *institutional review board.*

irid- [Gr. *iridos,* colored circle] Combining form indicating relationship to the iris of the eye.

iridadenosis (ĭr″ĭd-ăd-ĭn-ō′sĭs) [L. *iris,* colored circle, + Gr. *aden,* gland, + *osis,* condition] A glandular infection of the iris.

iridal (ī′rĭd-ăl) Iridic.

iridalgia (ī″rĭd-ăl′jē-ă) [″ + *algos,* pain] Pain felt in the iris. SYN: *iralgia.*

iridectome (ĭr″ĭ-dĕk′tōm) [″ + *tome,* incision] An instrument for cutting the iris in iridectomy.

iridectomesodialysis (ĭr″ĭ-dĕk″tō-mēs″ō-dī-ăl′ĭ-sĭs) [″ + *ektome,* excision, + *mesos,* middle, + *dialysis,* loosening] The formation of an artificial pupil, by separating adhesions on the inner margin of the iris.

iridectomize (ĭr″ĭd-ĕk′tō-mīz) [″ + *ektome,* excision] To excise a portion of the iris.

iridectomy The surgical removal of a portion of the iris.

optical i. Iridectomy performed to make an artificial pupil.

iridectropium (ĭr-ĭ-dĕk-trō′pē-ŭm) [″ + *ektrope,* a turning aside] Partial eversion of the iris.

iridemia (ĭr-ĭ-dē′mē-ă) [″ + *haima,* blood] Bleeding from the iris.

iridencleisis (ĭr″ĭ-dĕn-klī′sĭs) [″ + *enklein,* to lock in] An operation for relieving increased intraocular pressure, as in glaucoma, in which the iris and a portion of the limbus are excised to allow increased volume of the aqueous humor under the conjunctiva.

iridentropium (ĭr″ĭ-dĕn-trō′pē-ŭm) [″ + *en,* in, + *tropein,* to turn] Partial inversion of the iris.

irideremia (ĭr″ĭd-ĕr-ē′mē-ă) [″ + *eremia,* lack] Aniridia.

irides (ĭr′ĭ-dēz) [Gr.] Plural of iris.

iridescence (ĭr″ĭ-dĕs′ĕns) [L. *iridescere,* to gleam like a rainbow] Having the capability to disperse light into the colors of the spectrum.

iridesis (ĭ-rĭd′ĕ-sĭs) [″ + *desis,* a binding] Repositioning the pupil by bringing a portion of the iris through an incision in the cornea. SYN: *iridodesis.*

iridic (ī-rĭd′ĭk) [Gr. *iris,* colored circle] Relating to the iris. SYN: *iridal; iritic.*

iridium (ī-rĭd′ē-ŭm) [Gr. *iris,* colored circle] SYMB: Ir. A white, hard metallic element; atomic weight, 192.2; atomic weight 77.

irido- [Gr. *iridos,* colored circle] Combining form pert. to the iris.

iridoavulsion (ĭr″ĭ-dō-ăv-ŭl′shŭn) [″ + L. *avulsio,* a pulling away from] A tearing away of the iris.

iridocapsulitis (ĭr″ĭd-ō-kăp-sū-lī′tĭs) [″ + L. *capsula,* little box, + Gr. *itis,* inflammation] Iritis with inflammation of the capsule of the lens.

iridocele (ĭ-rĭd′ō-sēl) [″ + *kele,* tumor, swelling] Protrusion of a portion of the iris through a defect in the cornea.

iridochorioiditis, iridochoroiditis (ĭr″ĭ-dō-kō″rē-oy-dī′tĭs, ĭr″ĭ-dō-kō-roy-dī′tĭs) [″ + *chorioeides,* skinlike, + *itis,* inflammation] An inflammation of both iris and choroid.

iridocoloboma (ĭr″ĭd-ō-kŏl″ō-bō′mă) [″ + *koloboma,* mutilation] Congenital defect or fissure of the iris.

iridoconstrictor (ĭr″ĭ-dō-kŏn-strĭk′tor) A muscle or drug that acts to constrict the pupil of the eye.

iridocyclectomy (ĭr″ĭ-dō-sī-klĕk′tō-mē) [″ + *kyklos,* circle, + *ektome,* excision] Surgical removal of the iris and ciliary body.

iridocyclitis (ĭr″ĭd-ō-sī-klī′tĭs) [″ + ″ + *itis,* inflammation] An inflammation of the iris and ciliary body.

heterochromic i. An inflammation of the iris that leads to depigmentation.

iridocyclochoroiditis (ĭr″ĭ-dō-sī″klō-kō″roy-dī′tĭs) [″ + ″ + *chorioeides,* skinlike, + *itis,* inflammation] An inflammation of the iris, ciliary body, and choroid of the eye.

iridocystectomy (ĭr″ĭ-dō-sĭs-tĕk′tō-mē) [″ + *kystis,* bladder, + *ektome,* excision] Surgical removal of a cyst from the iris.

iridodesis (ĭr-ĭ-dŏd′ĕ-sĭs) [″ + *desis,* a binding] Iridesis.

iridodiagnosis [″ + *dia,* through, + *gnosis,* knowledge] Diagnosis of disease by examination of the iris.

iridodialysis (ĭr″ĭd-ō-dī-ăl′ĭ-sĭs) [″ + *dialysis,* loosening] Separation of the outer margin of the iris from its ciliary attachment.

iridodilator [″ + L. *dilatare,* to dilate] A substance causing dilatation of the pupil.

iridodonesis (ĭr″ĭd-ō-dō-nē′sĭs) [″ + *donesis,* tremor] Hippus.

iridokeratitis (ĭr″ĭ-dō-kĕr″ă-tī′tĭs) [″ + *keras,* horn, + *itis,* inflammation] An inflammation of the iris and cornea.

iridokinesis (ĭr″ĭd-ō-kĭn-ē′sĭs) [Gr. *iridos,* colored circle, + *kinesis,* movement] The contracting and expanding movements of the iris.

iridoleptynsis (ĭr″ĭ-dō-lĕp-tĭn′sĭs) [″ + *leptynsis,* attenuation] Thinning or atrophy of the iris.

iridology (ĭr″ĭ-dŏl′ō-jē) [″ + *logos,* word, reason] A diagnostic method developed by Dr. Ignatz von Peczely, a 19th century physician, and used today by some alternative medicine practitioners, in which disease is indicated by the color of the iris. It has no proven validity.

iridomalacia (ĭr″ĭd-ō-mă-lā′shē-ă) [″ + *malakia,* softness] A softening of the iris.

iridomedialysis (ĭr″ĭd-ō-mē-dē-ăl′ĭ-sĭs) [″ + L. *medius,* in middle, + Gr. *dialysis,* loosening] A separation of the inner marginal adhesions of the iris. SYN: *iridomesodialysis.*

iridomesodialysis (ĭr″ĭd-ō-mĕs″ō-dī-ăl′ĭ-sĭs) [″ + *mesos,* middle, + *dialysis,* loosening] Iridomedialysis.

iridomotor [″ + L. *motor,* that which moves] Relating to movements of the iris.

iridoncus (ĭr-ĭ-dong′kŭs) [″ + *onkos,* bulk] Swelling of the iris.

iridoparalysis [″ + *paralyein,* to disable] Iridoplegia.

iridoparelkysis (ĭr″ĭ-dō-păr-ĕl′kĭ-sĭs) [″ + *parelkysis,* protraction] Surgically induced prolapse of the iris in order to displace the pupil artificially.

iridopathy (ĭr″ĭ-dŏp′ă-thē) [″ + *pathos,* disease, suffering] Disease of the iris.

iridoperiphacitis, iridoperiphakitis (ĭr″ĭ-dō-pĕr″ĭ-fă-sī′tĭs, -pĕr″ĭ-fă-kī′tĭs) [″ + *peri,* around, + *phakos,* lens, + *itis,* inflammation] An inflammation of the iris and anterior portion of the capsule of the lens.

iridoplegia (ĭr″ĭd-ō-plē′jē-ă) [″ + *plege,* stroke] Paralysis of the sphincter of the iris. SYN: *iridoparalysis.*

accommodative i. Noncontraction of the pupils during accommodation.

complete i. Iridoplegia in which the iris fails to respond to any stimulation; seen in Adie's pupil.

reflex i. The absence of light reflex, with retention of the accommodation reflex (Argyll Robertson pupil).

iridoptosis (ĭr″ĭ-dŏp-tō′sĭs) [″ + *ptosis,* a falling] Prolapse of the iris.

iridopupillary (ĭr″ĭ-dō-pū′pĭ-lĕr″ē) [″ + L. *pupilla,* pupil] Concerning the iris and the pupil of the eye.

iridorrhexis (ĭr″ĭd-ō-rĕk′sĭs) [″ + *rhexis,* rupture] Rupture of the iris, or a tearing of the iris away from its attachment.

iridoschisis (ĭr″ĭ-dŏs′kĭ-sĭs) [″ + *schisis,* a splitting] Separation of the stroma of the iris into two layers with disintegration of the anterior layer.

iridosclerotomy (ĭr″ĭd-ō-sklē-rŏt′ō-mē) [″ + *skleros,* hard, + *tome,* incision] Piercing of the sclera and the border of the iris.

iridosteresis (ĭr″ĭ-dō-stē-rē′sĭs) [″ + *steresis,* loss] Removal of the iris or a portion of it.

iridotasis (ĭr-ĭ-dŏt′ă-sĭs) [″ + *tasis,* a stretching] A stretching of the iris in the treatment of glaucoma.

iridotomy (ĭr-ĭ-dŏt′ō-mē) [″ + *tome,* incision] An incision of the iris without excising a portion, done for the purpose of making a new aperture in the iris when the pupil is closed. This is indicated in eyes that had been operated on for cataract but that have lost their sight through subsequent iridocyclitis. SYN: *iritomy; irotomy.*

iris [Gr.] The colored contractile membrane suspended between the lens and the cornea in the aqueous humor of the eye, separating the anterior and posterior chambers of the eyeball and perforated in the center by the pupil. By contraction and dilatation it regulates the amount of light that enters the eye. SEE: *aniridia; choroidoiritis; heterochromia iridis; irid-; iris, chromatic asymmetry of; rubeosis iridis.*

ANATOMY: The free inner edge rests on the lens when the pupil is constricted or partially dilated. The iris contains two sets of smooth muscle fibers, the sphincter pupillae (circular fibers), about 1 mm wide; and the dilator pupillae (meridionally arranged fibers), extending from the sphincter pupillae to the outer edge of the iris. The former, supplied through the oculomotor nerve with parasympathetic fibers derived from the ciliary ganglion, constricts the pupil; the latter, supplied by sympathetic fibers from the superior cervical ganglion, dilates the pupil. The color of the iris depends on the pigment in the stroma cells and in the cells of the retinal layers. However, the color may change due to some medications.

i. bombé A condition seen in annular posterior synechia. The iris is bulged forward by the pressure of the aqueous humor, which cannot reach the anterior chamber.

chromatic asymmetry of i. A difference in color between the two irides (heterochromia). For example, one may be blue or gray and the other brown. The asymmetry may occur in early iritis or cyclitis, or may be present without an associated pathological process.

piebald i. A dark discoloration in an irregularly shaped area. It may be in one or both eyes.

Irish moss Carrageen.

irisopsia (ī″rĭs-ŏp′sē-ă) [Gr. *iris,* colored circle, + *opsis,* vision] A visual defect in which colored circles are seen around lights.

iritic (ĭ-rĭt′ĭk) [Gr. *iris,* colored circle] Iridic.

iritis [″ + *itis,* inflammation] An inflammation of the iris.

SYMPTOMS: In iritis, there are pain, photophobia, lacrimation, and diminution of vision. The iris appears swollen, dull, and muddy; the pupil contracted, irregular, and sluggish in reaction.

TREATMENT: Mydriatic or cyclopegic drugs are used for symptomatic relief. Cortisone or hydrocortisone is used systemically as well as topically. If the primary disease causing the iritis is known, it should be treated; however, the etiological factor is usually not known.

CAUTION: Ophthalmic corticosteroids should be prescribed only by an ophthalmologist, or other physician skilled in their use and side effects.

plastic i. Iritis in which the fibrinous exudate forms new tissue.

purulent i. Iritis with a purulent exudate.

secondary i. Iritis in which the inflammation has spread from neighboring parts, as in diseases of the cornea and sclera.

serous i. Iritis in which serum forms the exudate.

iritoectomy (ī″rĭ-tō-ĕk′tō-mē) [″ + *ektome,* excision] In cataract treatment, excision of the part of the iris that is inflamed and occluding the pupil.

iritomy (ĭ-rĭt′ō-mē) [″ + *tome,* incision] Iridotomy.

iron (ī′ĕrn) [AS. *iren;* L. *ferrum*] SYMB: Fe. A metallic element widely distributed in nature; atomic weight 55.847, atomic number 26. Compounds (oxides, hydroxides, salts) exist in two forms: ferrous, in which iron has a valence of two (Fe^{++}), and ferric, in which it has a valence of three (Fe^{+++}). It is widely used in the treatment of certain forms of anemia. Iron is essential for the formation of chlorophyll in plants, although it is not a constituent of chlorophyll. It is part of the hemoglobin and myoglobin molecules. SEE: *ferritin.*

FUNCTION: Iron, as part of hemoglobin, is essential for the transport of oxygen in the blood; it is also part of some of the enzymes needed for cell respiration. Men's bodies have approx. 3.45 g of iron and women approx. 2.45 g, distributed as follows: 60% to 70% in hemoglobin; 10% to 12% in myoglobin and enzymes; and, as ferritin, 29% in men and 10% in women, stored in the liver, spleen, and bone marrow. Iron is stored in the tissues principally as ferritin. It is absorbed from the food in the small intestine and passes, in the blood, to the bone marrow. There, it is used in making hemoglobin, which is incorporated into red blood cells. A red cell, after circulating in the blood for approx. 120 days, is destroyed, and its iron is used over again.

Men require from 0.5 to 1.0 mg of iron a day. A woman of menstrual age requires about twice this amount. During pregnancy and lactation from 2 to 4 mg of iron per day is required. Before puberty and after menopause, women require no more iron than men. Because only a fraction of the iron present in food is absorbed, it is necessary to provide from 15 to 30 mg of iron in the diet to be certain that 1 to 4 mg will be absorbed.

In the first few months of life, infants will use up most of their iron stores, and the typical diet or formula may not have sufficient iron to replenish those stores. It is therefore important to add iron-containing foods to an infant's diet by age 6 months.

Manganese, copper, and cobalt are necessary for the proper use of iron. Copper is stored in the body and reused repeatedly.

There are two broad types of dietary iron. About 90% of iron from food is in the form of iron salts and is called nonheme iron, which is poorly absorbed. The other 10% of dietary iron is in the form of heme iron, which is derived primarily from the hemoglobin and myoglobin of meat and is well absorbed. Iron absorption is influenced by other dietary factors. About 50% of iron from breast milk is absorbed but only about 10% of iron in whole cow's milk is absorbed. The reasons for the higher bioavailability of iron in breast milk are unknown. Ascorbic acid, meat, fish, and poultry enhance absorption of nonheme iron. Bran, oxalates, vegetable fiber, tannins in tea, and phosphates inhibit absorption of iron. Orange juice doubles the absorption of iron from the meal and tea decreases it by 75%.

DEFICIENCY SYMPTOMS: Iron deficiency is characterized by anemia, lowered vitality, exertional breathlessness, pale complexion, conjunctival pallor, retarded development, and a decreased amount of hemoglobin in each red cell.

NOTE: Sometimes a disturbance in iron metabolism occurs, in which an iron-containing pigment, hemosiderin, and hemofuscin are deposited in the tissues, leading to hemochromatosis. Excessive deposition of hemosiderin in the tissues, such as may occur as a result of excessive breakdown of red cells, is called hemosiderosis. SEE: *hemochromatosis*.

SOURCES: The following foods provide iron in the diet: almonds, asparagus, bran, beans, Boston brown bread, cauliflower, celery, chard, dandelions, egg yolk, graham bread, kidney, lettuce, liver, oatmeal, oysters, soybeans, and whole wheat. Other good sources are apricots, beets, beef, cabbage, cornmeal, cucumbers, currants, dates, duck, goose, greens, lamb, molasses, mushrooms, oranges, parsnips, peanuts, peas, peppers, potatoes, prunes, radishes, raisins, rhubarb, pineapple, tomatoes, and turnips.

iron dextran injection A preparation of iron suitable for parenteral use.

CAUTION: Because of the risk of anaphylaxis, a test dose should be given before starting an infusion of iron.

iron lung Drinker respirator.

iron overload Organ failure that results from excessive accumulation of iron in the body, usually as a result of frequent transfusions or hemochromatosis.

iron poisoning SEE: under *poisoning*.

iron storage disease Hemochromatosis.

irotomy (ī-rŏt′ō-mē) [Gr. *iris*, colored circle, + *tome*, incision] Iridotomy.

irradiate (ĭ-rā′dē-āt) [L. *in*, into, + *radiare*, to emit rays] **1.** To expose to radiation. **2.** To treat with high-energy x-rays or other forms of radiation. SEE: *irradiation*.

irradiating Diverging or spreading out from a common center.

irradiation **1.** The diagnostic or therapeutic application of x-ray photons, nuclear particles, high-speed electrons, ultraviolet rays, or other forms of radiation to a patient. **2.** The application of a form of radiation to an object or substance to give it therapeutic value or increase that which it already has. **3.** A phenomenon in which a bright object on a dark background appears larger than a dark object of the same size on a bright background. **4.** The spreading in all directions from a common center (e.g., nerve impulses, the sensation of pain).

food i. The preservation of foods with ionizing radiation. Radiation extends the shelf life of foods by decreasing the number of germs and insects present in them. The process is expensive, and it has met with considerable resistance from consumers.

interstitial i. Therapeutic irradiation by insertion into the tissues of capillary tubes or beads containing radon (a radioactive isotope). It may be temporary or permanent.

lymphoid i. Exposure of an organ recipient's lymphocytes to ionizing radiation before organ transplantation, in an effort to decrease the likelihood of rejection of the donor graft.

i. of reflexes The spread of a reflex to an increasing number of motor units upon increasing the strength of the stimulus.

irrational Contrary to what is reasonable or logical; used to describe ideas that are unsound, unwise, or extremely intemperate.

irreducible (ĭr″rē-dū′sĭ-bl) [L. *in-*, not, + *re*, back, + *ducere*, to lead] Not capable of being reduced or made smaller, as a fracture or dislocation.

irreversible Not being possible to reverse.

irrigate [L. *in*, into, + *rigare*, to carry water] To wash out with a fluid.

irrigation The cleansing of a canal by flushing with water or other fluids; the washing of a wound. The solutions used for cleansing should be sterile and, for comfort, have an approximate temperature slightly warmer than body temperature (100° to 115°F or 37.8° to 46.1°C). SYN: *lavage*. SEE: illus; *gastric lavage*.

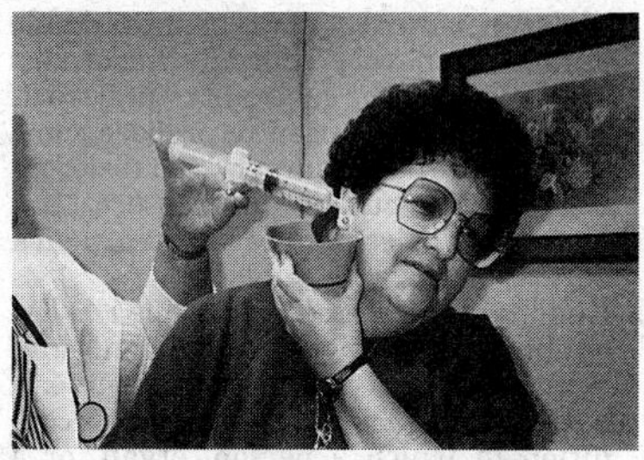

IRRIGATION OF THE EAR CANAL

bladder i. Washing out of the bladder to treat inflammation or infection or to maintain patency of a urinary catheter. The irrigation may be intermittent or continuous. Normal saline is commonly used.

PATIENT CARE: The necessary sterile equipment and the prescribed irrigant are assembled. The patient is prepared physically and emotionally for the procedure: the procedure and expected sensations are explained, and emotional and physical warmth and security are provided by draping the patient to preserve privacy. A catheter is inserted into the urinary bladder according to protocol; placement is determined by onset of urinary drainage. The prescribed volume of irrigant is instilled by bulb syringe; the catheter clamped to allow the solution to remain in the bladder for the prescribed period of time; then the catheter is unclamped to allow the irrigant to flow out of the bladder by gravity drainage into a collecting basin. The irrigation is repeated the prescribed number of times, and the character of the irrigation solution returned and the presence of any mucus, blood, or other material visible in the drainage is noted and then the catheter removed. The time of the procedure, the type and volume of irrigant instilled, the type and volume of return, and the patient's response to the procedure are documented. If intermittent or continuous bladder irrigation is required, the nurse inserts a three-lumen indwelling catheter, in which the first lumen leads to the inflation balloon, the second lumen is for instillation of irrigating fluid, and the third lumen provides a channel to a closed drainage system.

colonic i. Flushing of the colon with water. This procedure is done to cleanse the bowel.

continuous bladder i. ABBR: CBI. A constant flow of normal saline or another bladder irrigant through a three-way urinary catheter to keep the catheter patent. It is typically used postoperatively following a transurethral resection of the prostate gland.

whole bowel i. The administration of large volumes of a nonabsorbable fluid to remove potentially hazardous contents from the gastrointestinal tract. The technique is used to prepare some patients for bowel surgery and to decontaminate the gut after overdose.

irrigator A device used to flush or wash a part or cavity with fluids.

irritability [L. *irritabilis,* irritable] **1.** Excitability. **2.** An ability to respond in a specific way to a change in environment, a property of all living tissue. **3.** A condition in which a person, organ, or a part responds excessively to a stimulus. **4.** A quick response to annoyance; impatience.

muscular i. The normal response of muscle to a stimulus.

nervous i. The response of a nerve to a stimulus.

irritable **1.** Capable of reacting to a stimulus. **2.** Sensitive to stimuli.

irritable bowel syndrome SEE: under *syndrome.*

irritant An agent that, when used locally, produces a more or less local inflammatory reaction. Anything that induces or gives rise to irritation, such as iodine.

irritation [L. *irritatio*] **1.** A reaction to a noxious or unpleasant stimulus. It is important to distinguish between irritation and sensitization. For example, a substance contacting the skin may cause no irritation when initially applied but can cause a sensitization reaction that will not become obvious until the material is applied the second time. SEE: *allergen; sensitization.* **2.** An extreme reaction to pain or pathological conditions. **3.** A normal response to stimulus of a nerve or muscle.

spinal i. A condition characterized by tenderness along the spinal column, numbness and tingling in the limbs, and susceptibility to fatigue.

sympathetic i. The response of an organ to irritation in another organ.

irritative Pert. to that which causes irritation.

ischemia (ĭs-kē′mē-ă) [Gr. *ischein,* to hold back, + *haima,* blood] A temporary deficiency of blood flow to an organ or tissue. The deficiency may be caused by diminished blood flow either through a regional artery or throughout the circulation.

intestinal i. SEE: *angina, intestinal.*

lower limb i. An inadequate blood flow to one or both legs due either to chronic arterial obstruction caused by atherosclerosis or to acute obstruction caused by embolism.

myocardial i. An inadequate supply of blood and oxygen to meet the metabolic demands of the heart muscle. SEE: *angina pectoris; atherosclerosis; coronary artery disease.*

vertebrobasilar i. Insufficient blood flow to the base of the brain. This can cause malfunction of the cerebellum or brain stem, producing difficulties with balance, vertigo, double vision, altered vision, swallowing disorders, dysarthria, and other symptoms.

warm i. The absence of blood flow to a body part or organ intended for transplantation before its removal from a cadaveric donor.

ischesis (ĭs-kē′sĭs) Suppression of a discharge, esp. a normal one.

ischia (ĭs′kē-ă) [L.] Pl. of ischium.

ischiac, ischiadic (ĭs′kē-ăk, ĭs-kē-ăd′ĭk) Sciatic.

ischial (ĭs′kē-ăl) [Gr. *ischion,* hip] Pert. to the ischium.

ischialgia (ĭs″kē-ăl′jē-ă) [″ + *algos,* pain] Sciatica.

ischiatic (ĭs″kē-ăt′ĭk) [Gr. *ischion,* hip] Sciatic.

ischiatitis (ĭs″kē-ă-tī′tĭs) [″ + *itis,* inflammation] Sciatic nerve inflammation.

ischidrosis (ĭs″kĭ-drō′sĭs) [Gr. *ischein,* to hold back, + *hidrosis,* sweat] The suppression of perspiration.

ischio- [Gr. *ischion,* hip] Combining form meaning *ischium.*

ischioanal (ĭs″kē-ō-ā′năl) [″ + L. *anus,* anus] Concerning the ischium and anus.

ischiobulbar (ĭs″kē-ō-bŭl′băr) [″ + L. *bulbus,* bulb] Relating to the ischium and urethral bulb.

ischiocapsular (ĭs″kē-ō-kăp′sū-lăr) [″ + L. *capsula,* capsule] Concerning the ischium and capsule of the hip.

ischiocavernosus (ĭs″kē-ō-kă″vĕr-nō′sŭs) [″ + L. *cavernosus,* cavernous] A muscle extending from the ischium to the penis or clitoris and assisting in their erection.

ischiocele (ĭs'kē-ō-sēl) [" + *kele,* tumor, swelling] A hernia through the sciatic notch.

ischiococcygeus (ĭs"kē-ō-kŏk-sĭj'ē-ŭs) [" + *kokkyx,* coccyx] **1.** The coccygeus muscle. **2.** The posterior portion of the levator ani.

ischiodynia (ĭs"kē-ō-dĭn'ē-ă) [" + *odyne,* pain] Pain in the ischium.

ischiofemoral (ĭs"kē-ō-fĕm'or-ăl) [" + L. *femur,* thigh] Relating to the ischium and femur.

ischiofibular (ĭs"kē-ō-fĭb'ū-lăr) [" + L. *fibula,* pin] Relating to the ischium and fibula.

ischiohebotomy (ĭs"kē-ō-hē-bŏt'ō-mē) [" + *hebe,* pubes, + *tome,* incision] Surgical division of the ascending ramus of the pubes and the ischiopubic ramus. SYN: *ischiopubiotomy.*

ischioneuralgia (ĭs"kē-ō-nū-răl'jē-ă) [" + *neuron,* nerve, + *algos,* pain] Sciatica.

ischionitis (ĭs"kē-ō-nī'tĭs) [" + *itis,* inflammation] Inflammation of the tuberosity of the ischium.

ischiopubic (ĭs"kē-ō-pū'bĭk) [" + L. *pubes,* the pubes] Relating to the ischium and pubes.

ischiopubiotomy (ĭs"kē-ō-pū"bē-ŏt'ō-mē) Ischiohebotomy.

ischiorectal (ĭs"kē-ō-rĕk'tăl) [" + L. *rectus,* straight] Pert. to the ischium and rectum.

ischiosacral (ĭs"kē-ō-sā'krăl) [" + L. *sacralis,* pert. to the sacrum] Concerning the ischium and sacrum.

ischiovaginal (ĭs"kē-ō-văj'ĭ-năl) [" + L. *vagina,* sheath] Concerning the ischium and vagina.

ischium (ĭs'kē-ŭm) *pl.* **ischia** [Gr. *ischion,* hip] The lower portion of the innominate or hip bone.

I.S.C.L.T. *International Society of Clinical Laboratory Technologists.*

iseikonia (īs"ī-kō'nē-ă) [Gr. *isos,* equal, + *eikon,* image] Isoiconia.

island [AS. *igland,* island] A structure detached from surrounding tissues or characterized by difference in structure; an islet.

blood i. A small area of blood accumulation present in the yolk sac of the early embryo.

i.'s of Calleja Groups of densely packed, small cells in the cortex of the gyrus hippocampi. SYN: *islets of Calleja.*

i.'s of Langerhans Islets of Langerhans.

pancreatic i.'s Islets of Langerhans.

i. of Reil The insula, a lobe of the cerebral cortex comprising a triangular area lying in the floor of the lateral or sylvian fissure. It is overlapped and hidden by the gyri of the fissure, which constitute the operculum of the insula.

islet (ī'lĕt) A tiny isolated mass of one kind of tissue within another type.

i. of Calleja Islands of Calleja.

i. of Langerhans Clusters of cells in the pancreas. They are of three types: alpha, beta, and delta cells. The alpha cells secrete glucagon, which raises the blood glucose level; the beta cells secrete insulin, which lowers it; and the delta cells secrete somatostatin, an inhibitor of growth hormone secretion. Destruction or impairment of function of the islets of Langerhans may result in diabetes or hypoglycemia. SYN: *islands of Langerhans; pancreatic islands.*

Walthard's i. Embryological nests of epithelial-like cells in the superficial part of the ovaries, tubes, and uterine ligaments. They may also appear as minute cysts. Brenner's tumor is thought to arise from these islets.

-ism [Gr. *-ismos*] Suffix meaning *condition* or *theory of; principle* or *method.*

I.S.O. *International Organization for Standardization.*

iso- [Gr. *isos,* equal] Prefix meaning *equal.*

isoagglutination (ī"sō-ă-gloo"tĭ-nā'shŭn) [" + L. *agglutinare,* to glue to] Agglutination of red blood cells by agglutinins from the blood of another member of the same species. SYN: *isohemagglutination.*

isoagglutinin (ī"sō-ă-glū'tĭn-ĭn) [" + L. *agglutinare,* to glue to] An antibody in a serum that agglutinates the blood cells of those of the same species from which it is derived. SEE: *agglutinin; blood group; isohemagglutinin.*

isoagglutinogen (ī"sō-ă-glū-tĭn'ō-jĕn) Agglutinin.

isoantibody (ī"sō-ăn'tĭ-bŏd"ē) An antibody produced in response to an isoantigen.

isoantigen (ī"sō-ăn'tĭ-jĕn) [" + L. *anti,* against, + *gennan,* to produce] A substance present in certain individuals that stimulates antibody production in other members of the same species but not in the donor (e.g., blood group isoantigens that are harmless to the donor but may produce severe antibody response in a recipient of a different blood group or type). SYN: *alloantigen.*

isobar (ī'sō-băr) [" + *baros,* weight] **1.** A locus of equal pressure. When pressures are unequal, fluids and gases will flow from a high- to a low-pressure region. **2.** In chemistry, one of two or more chemical bodies having the same atomic weight but different atomic numbers.

isobaric (ī"sō-băr'ĭk) **1.** 1. Specific gravity equal to that with which it is being compared. For example, an anesthetic solution used in spinal anesthesia, if isobaric, would have the same specific gravity as the spinal fluid. **2.** Pressure equal to that with which it is being compared.

isocaloric (ī″sō-kă-lō′rĭk) [″ + L. *calor,* heat] Containing the same number of calories as the food or diet with which it is being compared.

isocellular [″ + L. *cellula,* cell] Composed of equal and similar cells.

isochromatic (ī″sō-krō-măt′ĭk) [″ + *chroma,* color] **1.** Having the same color. **2.** Of uniform color.

isochromatophil(e) (ī″sō-krō-măt′ō-fĭl, -fīl) [″ + ″+ *philein,* to love] Having the same affinity for a dye.

isochromosome (ī″sō-krō′mō-sōm) [″ + ″ + *soma,* body] A chromosome with arms that are morphologically identical and contain the same genetic loci. This is the result of the transverse rather than the longitudinal splitting of a chromosome.

isochronal (ī-sŏk′rō-năl) [″ + *chronos,* time] Acting in uniform time, or taking place at regular intervals.

isochronia (ī″sō-krō′nē-ă) [Gr. *isos,* equal, + *chronos,* time] The correspondence of events with respect to time, rate, or frequency.

isochroous (ī-sŏk′rō-ŭs) [″ + *chroa,* color] Isochromatic (2).

isocitrate dehydrogenase (ī″sō-cĭt′rāt dē″hī-drŏj′ĕn-ās) An enzyme that catalyzes the conversion of isocitric acid to α-ketoglutaric acid.

isocolloid (ī-sō-kŏl′oyd) [″ + *kollodes,* glutinous] A colloid having the same composition in every transformation.

isocoria (ī″sō-kō′rē-ă) [″ + *kore,* pupil] Equality of size of both pupils. SEE: *anisocoria*.

isocortex (ī″sō-kor′tĕks) [″ + L. *cortex,* bark] The nonolfactory portion of the cerebral cortex. It is composed of six layers of neurons and nerve fibers having a similar distribution pattern. Phylogenetically, it is the new part of the cerebral cortex. SYN: *neocortex; neopallium.*

isocytosis (ī″sō-sī-tō′sĭs) [″ + *kytos,* cell, + *osis,* condition] Cells of equal size.

isocytotoxin (ī″sō-sī″tō-tŏk′sĭn) [″ + ″ + *toxikon,* poison] Cytotoxin destructive to homologous cells of the same species.

isodactylism (ī-sō-dăk′tĭl-ĭzm) [″ + *daktylos,* finger] A condition of having fingers or toes of equal length.

isodiametric (ī″sō-dī-ă-mĕt′rĭk) [″ + *dia,* across, + *metron,* measure] Having equal diameters.

isodontic (ī″sō-dŏn′tĭk) [″ + *odous,* tooth] Having teeth of equal size.

isodose (ī′sō-dōs) In radiology, equal doses of radiation received by different areas of the body.

i. curve In radiation therapy, a graph on which the points plot areas or levels of equal radiation dose.

isodynamic (ī″sō-dī-năm′ĭk) [″ + *dynamis,* power] Having equal power.

isoelectric (ī″sō-ē-lĕk′trĭk) [″ + *elektron,* amber] Having equal electric potentials.

isoenergetic [Gr. *isos,* equal, + *energeia,* energy] Showing equal force or activity.

isoenzyme (ī″sō-ĕn′zīm) [″ + *en,* in, + *zyme,* leaven] One of several forms in which an enzyme may exist in various tissues. Although the isoenzymes are similar in catalytic qualities, they may be separated from each other by special chemical tests. SYN: *isozyme*. SEE: *lactic dehydrogenase*.

isoetharine hydrochloride (ī-sō-ĕth′ă-rēn) A sympathomimetic drug used as a bronchodilator.

isoflavone A relatively weak estrogen-like compound. SEE: *phytoestrogen*.

isoflurophate (ī-sō-floo′rō-fāt) An anticholinesterase drug used in treating glaucoma as well as atony of the smooth muscle of the intestinal tract and urinary bladder.

isoform One of several proteins that have the same antigenic structure but may differ in either steric structure or minor amino acid content.

isogamete (ī″sō-găm′ēt) [″ + *gamete,* wife, *gametes,* husband] **1.** A cell that reproduces through conjugation or fusion with a similar cell. **2.** A gamete of the same size as the one with which it fuses or unites.

isogamy (ī-sŏg′ă-mē) [″ + *gamos,* marriage] Reproduction resulting from the conjugation of isogametes or identical cells.

isogeneic (ī″sō-jĕn-ē′ĭk) Syngeneic.

isogeneric (ī″sō-jĕ-nĕr′ĭk) [″ + L. *genus,* kind] Of the same kind; concerning or obtained from members of the same genus.

isogenesis (ī″sō-jĕn′ĕ-sĭs) [″ + *genesis,* generation, birth] A similarity in morphological development.

isogenic (ī″sō-jĕn′ĭk) Isologous.

isograft [″ + L. *graphium,* grafting shoot] A graft taken from another individual or animal of the same genotype as the recipient. SEE: *autograft*.

isohemagglutination (ī″sō-hĕm″ă-gloo″tĭ-nā′shŭn) [″ + *haima,* blood, + L. *agglutinare,* to glue to] Isoagglutination.

isohemagglutinin (ī″sō-hĕm″ă-glū′tĭn-ĭn) [″ + *haima,* blood, + L. *agglutinare,* to glue to] The naturally occurring anti-A and anti-B antibodies against the antigens present on red blood cells. If incompatible blood is given, these antibodies destroy the recipient's red blood cells through agglutination and hemolysis. Patients with type A blood cannot receive blood from a donor with type B or AB blood, because they have anti-B antibodies. Patients with type B blood cannot receive type A or AB blood, because they have anti-A antibodies. Patients with type O blood cannot receive type A, B, or AB blood, because they have anti-A and anti-B antibodies. Type

O patients have no A or B antigens and are called universal donors because they can donate blood to any of the other groups. Type AB patients are universal recipients because they lack both anti-A and anti-B antibodies, and thus can receive blood from donors with any blood type. SEE: *agglutinin; agglutinogen.*

isohemolysis (ī″sō-hē-mŏl′ĭ-sĭs) The destruction of red blood corpuscles produced by an isolysin; the action of an isohemolysin. SEE: *hemolysis.*

isohypercytosis (ī″sō-hī″pĕr-sī-tō′sĭs) [″ + *hyper,* over, above, excessive + *kytos,* cell, + *osis,* condition] A condition in which the total number of white blood cells is increased but the proportions of the polymorphonuclear leukocytes remain stable.

isoiconia (ī″sō-ī-kō′nē-ă) [Gr. *isos,* equal, + *eikon,* image] Equality of both retinal images. SYN: *iseikonia.*

isoiconic (ī″sō-ī-kŏn′ĭk) Having equal retinal images.

isoimmunization [″ + L. *immunis,* safe] Active immunization of an individual against blood from an individual of the same species, esp. the production of anti-Rh antibodies by Rh-negative mothers against red fetal blood cell antigens. During maternal trauma, loss of pregnancy (abortion), or delivery, some of the infant's blood is transferred to the mother, stimulating antibody production. If a second child is Rh-positive, the mother's anti-Rh antibodies will cross the placenta and cause hemolytic disease of the newborn. SEE: *erythroblastosis fetalis.*

isolate [It. *isolato,* isolated] **1.** To separate or detach from other persons, as during an infectious disease. **2.** In chemistry, to obtain a substance in pure form from the mixture or solution that contains it.

isolation 1. Solitude, or the psychological discomfort that accompanies it. SEE: *loneliness.* **2.** The physical separation of infected or contaminated organisms from others to prevent or limit the transmission of disease. In contrast, quarantine applies to restriction on healthy contacts of an infectious agent. SEE: *incubation* for table; *infectious i.; protective i.; quarantine; Standard and Universal Precautions Appendix.*

PATIENT CARE: The rules to be followed for achieving isolation are based on the mode of transmission of the particular organism; for example, if the organism is spread by droplet, then all items that come in contact with the patient's upper respiratory tract are isolated and destroyed or disinfected. Those in contact with the patient also are protected from droplet transmission by wearing protective barriers such as special masks (and if necessary gowns, caps, boots, and gloves), by careful and thorough hand washing, and by keeping the hands away from the nose and mouth, to prevent transmission of infections. On leaving the patient area, the health care provider or family member unties the lower gown tie (if worn); removes gloves (if worn); washes hands; unties the upper gown tie; removes the gown, stripping and folding it inside out as it is removed; removes mask, goggles, boots, and cap, and immediately places them in an appropriate container. The individual then rewashes the hands. Most agencies use disposable equipment as much as possible in the care of an isolated patient. Contaminated disposables are double-bagged for safe disposal, usually by incineration. Contaminated linens and other non-disposable equipment are also double-bagged and marked "isolation," so that they will be properly decontaminated or disinfected on receipt by the laundry or supply service. Laboratory specimens also are double-bagged and marked with the particular type of isolation, so that personnel handle them appropriately. Centers for Disease Control and Prevention recommendations and institutional procedure are followed for the specific type of isolation that is in effect. The purpose of the isolation precautions is explained to the patient and family to decrease their fears and to increase their cooperation, and the family and other visitors are taught how to use and discard the required barriers and especially how to thoroughly wash their hands. When the at-risk patient requires protection from others, equipment going to the patient is disposable or sterilized, and human contacts wear barriers that may be clean or sterile depending on the circumstances and protocol. After use, these items are handled in the agency's usual manner, with no special care necessary beyond that defined in universal precautions.

body substance i. A method of infection control that assumes all body fluids are potentially infectious and that an effective task-specific barrier must always be placed between the medical provider and the patient.

body substance i. precautions The standard precautions that are taken by all health care personnel, such as wearing gloves, goggles, and masks, to avoid contact with potentially infectious body substances such as urine, feces, saliva, vomit, and blood.

infectious i. An isolation technique that protects health care personnel from a patient who has or is suspected of having an infectious disease.

protective i. Isolation in which the patient is being protected from potentially harmful bacteria in the environment. This is particularly important in caring for immunodeficient patients such as those undergoing organ transplantation surgery. SYN: *reverse i.*

reverse i. Protective i.

i. ward A hospital ward in which patients suffering from communicable diseases may be separated from other patients.

isoleucine (ī″sō-lū′sēn) $C_6H_{13}NO_2$; an amino acid formed during hydrolysis of fibrin and other proteins. It is essential in the diet.

isologous (ī-sŏl′ō-gŭs) Genetically identical. In transplantations, being isologous (or isogenic) indicates the absence of any tissue incompatibility between the recipient of tissue and the tissue or organ itself. SYN: *isogenic; syngeneic.*

isolophobia (ī″sō-lō-fō′bē-ă) [It. *isolato,* isolated, + Gr. *phobos,* fear] The fear of being alone. SEE: *agoraphobia.*

isomer (ī′sō-mĕr) [Gr. *isos,* equal, + *meros,* part] One of two or more chemical substances that have the same molecular formula but different chemical and physical properties owing to a different arrangement of the atoms in the molecule. Dextrose is an isomer of levulose. SEE: *polymer.*

isomerase (ī-sŏm′ĕr-ās) Any enzyme that catalyzes the isomerization of its substrate. For example, phosphoglucose isomerase interconverts glucose and fructose-6-phosphate. SEE: *isomerism.*

isomeric (ī″sō-mĕr′ĭk) Pert. to isomerism.

isomerism (ī-sŏm′ĕr-ĭzm) The state of being composed of compounds of the same number of atoms but having different atomic arrangement in the molecule. SEE: *metamerism; polymerism.*

isomerization (ī-sŏm″ĕr-ī-zā′shŭn) The conversion of one chemical substance to an isomer. SEE: *isomer; isomerism.*

isometric [″ + *metron,* measure] Having equal dimensions. SEE: *isotonic* (2).

i. contraction phase The first phase in contraction of the ventricle of the heart in which ventricular pressure increases but there is no decrease in volume of contents because semilunar valves are closed.

isometropia (ī″sō-mĕ-trō′pē-ă) [″ + ″ + *ops,* eye] Same refraction of the two eyes.

isomorphism (ī-sō-mor′fĭzm) [″ + *morphe,* form, + *-ismos,* state of] A condition marked by possession of the same form.

isomorphous (ī″sō-mor′fŭs) Possessing the same shape.

isoniazid (ī″sō-nī′ă-zĭd) ABBR: INH. $C_6H_7N_3O$. An odorless compound occurring as colorless or white crystals or as a white crystalline powder. It is an antibacterial, used principally in treating tuberculosis. Side effects of its use include hepatitis and peripheral neuropathy. The antidote for isoniazid overdose is pyridoxine. SYN: *isonicotinoylhydrazine.*

isonicotinoylhydrazine (ī″sō-nĭk″ō-tĭn″ō-ĭl-hī′dră-zēn) Isoniazid.

isonormocytosis (ī″sō-nor″mō-sī-tō′sĭs) [″ + L. *norma,* rule, + Gr. *kytos,* cell, + *osis,* condition] The state of having the normal amount and proportion of varieties of leukocytes.

isopathy (ī-sŏp′ă-thē) [Gr. *isos,* equal, + *pathos,* disease, suffering] Isotherapy.

isophoria (ī″sō-fō′rē-ă) [″ + *phorein,* to carry] Equal tension of vertical muscles of each eye with visual lines in the same horizontal plane; absence of hyperphoria and hypophoria.

isopia (ī-sō′pē-ă) [″ + *ops,* vision] Equal vision in the eyes.

isoplastic (ī″sō-plăs′tĭk) [″ + *plastos,* formed] Removed from one individual and transplanted to another of the same species, as a graft. SEE: *isograft.*

isopropanol (ī″sō-prō′pă-nŏl) Isopropyl alcohol.

isoproterenol hydrochloride (ī″sō-prō″tĕ-rē′nŏl) A sympathomimetic amine used to relieve bronchoconstriction in asthma and also as a cardiac stimulant in heart block.

CAUTION: Overdosage administered by inhalation can be fatal.

isopters (ī-sŏp′tĕrz) [″ + *opter,* observer] Lines on a chart of the field of vision that connect points of equal visual acuity.

isopyknosis (ī″sō-pĭk-nō′sĭs) [″ + *pyknosis,* condensation] Having uniform density, esp. being in a state of equal condensation as in comparing different chromosomes.

isosexual (ī″sō-sĕks′ū-ăl) Concerning or characteristic of the same sex.

isosmotic (ī″sŏs-mŏt′ĭk) [″ + *osmos,* impulsion] Having the same total concentration of osmotically active molecules or ions in solution as the solution or body fluid to which it is being compared. SEE: *isotonic* (1).

isosorbide dinitrate tablets (ī″sō-sor′bīd) An antianginal drug used orally.

Isospora (ī-sŏs′pō-ră) [″ + *sporos,* spore] A genus of Sporozoa belonging to the order Coccidia.

I. hominis A parasitic, nonpathogenic protozoon inhabiting the small intestine in humans.

isospore (ī′sō-spor) [Gr. *isos,* equal, + *sporos,* spore] A nonsexual spore from plants with only one kind of spore. It grows to maturity without conjugating.

isosthenuria (ī″sŏs-thĕn-ū′rē-ă) [″ + *sthenos,* strength, + *ouron,* urine] Having a uniform urinary specific gravity and osmolarity despite marked variations in plasma osmolarity; a sign of impaired renal tubular function.

isostimulation [″ + L. *stimulare,* to goad] Stimulation of an animal by the use of antigenic material derived from another animal of the same species.

isotherapy (ī″sō-thĕr′ă-pē) [″ + *therapeia,* treatment] The treatment of a disease by administering the active causative agent of the same disease. SYN: *isopathy.*

isothermal [″ + *therme,* heat] Having equal temperature.

isothermognosis (ī″sō-thĕrm″ŏg-nō′sĭs) [″ + ″ + *gnosis,* knowledge] Abnormal perception in which pain, heat, and cold are all felt as heat.

isotone (ī′sō-tōnz) One of several nuclides with the same number of neutrons but a different number of protons.

isotonia (ī″sō-tō′nē-ă) [″ + *tonos,* tone] The state of equal osmotic pressure of two or more solutions or substances.

isotonic (ī″sō-tŏn′ĭk) **1.** Relating to the maintenance of a constant amount of resistive force during muscular contraction. **2.** Having equal pressure. SEE: *isometric.* **3.** Pert. to a solution with the same osmotic pressure as a reference solution.

isotonicity (ī″sō-tō-nĭs′ĭ-tē) The state or condition of being isotonic.

isotope (ī′sō-tōp) [″ + *topos,* place] One of a series of chemical elements that have nearly identical chemical properties but different atomic weights and electric charge. Many isotopes are radioactive.

i. cisternography The use of a radioactive tracer to investigate the circulation of cerebrospinal fluid. A tracer such as ^{131}I serum albumin is injected in the lumbar subarachnoid space. Flow of the tracer toward the head and into areas of the brain can be recorded by means of serial scintillation scanning. This technique is useful in studying hydrocephalus.

radioactive i. An isotope in which the nucleus is unstable.

stable i. An isotope that does not undergo radioactive decay into another element.

isotretinoin A keratolytic agent used in treating acne.

CAUTION: This medicine should not be used by pregnant women or those who are sexually active and at risk of becoming pregnant.

isotropic (ī″sō-trŏp′ĭk) [″ + *tropos,* a turning] **1.** Possessing similar qualities in every direction. **2.** Having equal refraction.

isotropy (ī-sŏt′rō-pē) The state of being isotropic.

isotype In immunology, one of the determinants on the immunoglobulin molecule that distinguish among the main classes of antibodies of a given species. They are the same for all normal individuals of that species. SEE: *idiotype.*

immunoglobulin i. Immunoglobulin fragment.

isotypical (ī-sō-tĭp′ĭ-kăl) [″ + *typos,* mark] Belonging to the same variety or classification.

isovaleric acidemia (ī″sō-vă-lĕr′ĭk-ăs″ĭ-dē′mē-ă) An inherited metabolic disease affecting leucine metabolism. Isovaleric acid accumulates in the blood during periods of increased amino acid metabolism (i.e., during infections or following ingestion of proteins). Coma and death may occur.

isoxsuprine hydrochloride (ī-sŏk′sū-prēn) A vasodilator drug used primarily in veterinary medicine.

isozyme (ī′sō-zīm) Isoenzyme.

issue (ĭsh′ū) [ME.] **1.** Offspring. **2.** A suppurating sore maintained by a foreign body in the tissue to act as a counterirritant. **3.** A discharge of pus or blood. **4.** A matter of conflict or dispute.

isthmectomy (ĭs-mĕk′tō-mē) [Gr. *isthmos,* isthmus, + *ektome,* excision] Excision of an enlarged isthmus, esp. of the thyroid gland.

isthmian (ĭs′mē-ăn) Relating to an isthmus.

isthmitis (ĭs-mī′tĭs) [″ + *itis,* inflammation] An inflammation of the throat or fauces.

isthmoparalysis (ĭs″mō-pă-răl′ĭ-sĭs) [″ + *para,* beyond, + *lyein,* to loosen] Paralysis of the muscles of the fauces. SYN: *isthmoplegia.*

isthmoplegia (ĭs″mō-plē′jē-ă) [″ + *plege,* a stroke] Isthmoparalysis.

isthmospasm (ĭs′mō-spăzm″) [″ + *spasmos,* a convulsion] Sudden muscular contraction of the narrow segment of the fallopian tube at its point of insertion into the uterus.

isthmus (ĭs′mŭs) *pl.* **isthmuses, isthmi** [Gr. *isthmos,* isthmus] **1.** A narrow passage connecting two cavities. **2.** A narrow structure connecting two larger parts. **3.** A constriction between two larger parts of an organ or structure.

aortic i. A constriction in the fetal aorta between the ductus arteriosus and left subclavian artery. The condition sometimes persists to adulthood.

i. of eustachian tube The narrowest portion of the eustachian tube.

i. faucium A constriction connecting the posterior mouth cavity proper with the pharynx.

pharyngeal i. The passageway between the nasopharynx and oropharynx.

i. of thyroid gland A narrow band of thyroid tissue connecting the right and left lobes of the thyroid gland.

i. uteri I. of uterus.

i. of uterine tube The constricted portion (of the medial third) of the fallopian tube.

i. of uterus A slight constriction on the surface of the uterus midway between the uterine body and cervix.

itch, itching [ME. *icchen*] Pruritus; a generally unpleasant sensation in the skin that creates the urge to rub or scratch it. Itch is a frequent manifestation of many inflammatory, infectious, and allergic skin disorders (e.g., most forms of dermatitis); of dry or cracked skin (xerosis); and of systemic illnesses (such as jaundice, hyperbilirubinemia, and some leukemias and lymphomas).

baker's i. A rash that occurs on the hands and forearms of bakers. It may be due to mechanical or chemical factors.

barber's i. Folliculitis of the hair follicles of the beard; usually caused by staphylococcal or fungal infection. SYN: *folliculitis barbae; sycosis barbae.*

dhobie i. Tinea cruris.

grain i. Dermatitis caused by mites in stored grain.

grocer's i. Dermatitis caused either by mites in grain or cheese, or by sugar.

ground i. A local irritation produced by penetration of the skin of the foot by hookworm larvae, esp. *Necator americanus.* SYN: *ancylostomiasis.*

jock i. Tinea cruris.

seven-year i. Scabies.

swimmer's i. The appearance of papules resembling insect bites on the skin of persons who swim in water containing the cercariae of certain schistosomes. It is usually present only on exposed surfaces of the skin. The papules appear from 4 to 13 days after exposure. The disease is self-limited; thus treatment is symptomatic. SYN: *cercarial dermatitis; schistosome dermatitis; seabather's eruption; water i.*

water i. Swimmer's i.

winter i. SEE: *winter itch.*

-ite [Gr.] **1.** Suffix meaning *of the nature of.* **2.** In chemistry, a salt of an acid having the termination *-ous.*

iter (ī'tĕr) [L.] A passageway between two parts. **iteral** (-ăl), *adj.*

iteroparity (ĭt"ĕr-ō-păr'ĭ-tē) [L. *iterare,* to repeat, + *parere,* to bear] The state of reproducing more than once in a lifetime. SEE: *multiparity.*

ithycyphosis, ithyokyphosis (ĭth"ĭ-sī-fō'sĭs, ĭth"ē-ō-kī-fō'sĭs) [Gr. *ithys,* straight, + *kyphos,* humped] Kyphosis with backward projection of the spine.

ithylordosis (ĭth"ĭ-lor-dō'sĭs) [" + *lordosis,* a bending forward] Lordosis without lateral curvature of the spine.

-itis (ī'tĭs) [Gr.] Suffix meaning *inflammation of.*

ITP **1.** *idiopathic thrombocytopenic purpura.* **2.** *immune thrombocytopenic purpura.*

I.U. *immunizing unit; international unit.*

IUCD *intrauterine contraceptive device.*

IUD *intrauterine device.*

IUGR *intrauterine growth retardation.*

IUFD *intrauterine fetal death.*

IUPAC *International Union of Pure and Applied Chemistry.*

IV *intravenous(ly).*

IVC *intravenous cholangiography.*

IVCD *intraventricular conduction defect.*

ivermectin An antiparasitic drug used primarily to treat infestations with worms, such as onchocerciasis (river blindness). It also treats other helminth infections and has been used to treat scabies.

IVF *in vitro fertilization.*

IVIG *intravenous immunoglobulin.*

IVP *intravenous pyelogram.*

IV push The administration of medicine intravenously by quick and forcible injection.

IVT *intravenous transfusion.*

IVU *intravenous urography.*

Ivy method SEE: *bleeding time.*

ivy poisoning SEE: *poison ivy dermatitis.*

Ixodes (ĭks-ō'dēz) [Gr. *ixodes,* like birdlime] A genus of ticks of the family Ixodidae, many of which are parasitic on humans and animals. SEE: illus.

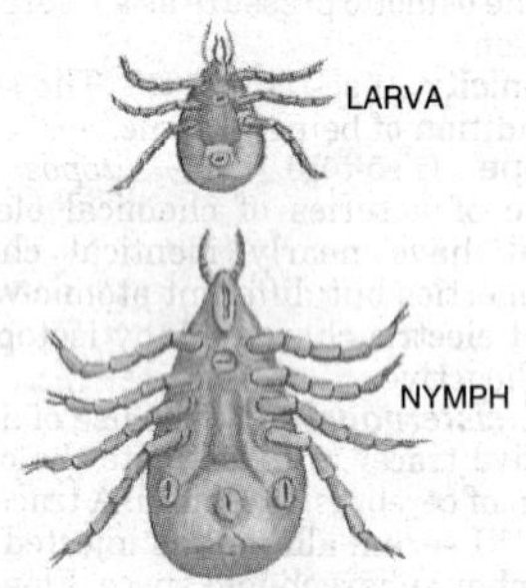

IXODES TICK

(Orig. mag. ×12)

ixodiasis (ĭks"ō-dī'ă-sĭs) **1.** Lesions of the skin caused by tick bites. **2.** Any disease caused by ticks, such as Rocky Mountain spotted fever.

ixodic (ĭks-ŏd'ĭk) Pert. to or caused by ticks.

Ixodidae (ĭks-ŏd'ĭ-dē) A family of ticks belonging to the order Acarina, class Arachnida, comprising the hard-bodied ticks including the genera *Amblyomma, Boophilus, Dermacentor, Haemaphysalis, Hyalomma, Ixodes,* and *Rhipicephalus.* All are parasitic and of significance as pests or as transmitters of disease in domestic animals and humans. Among the diseases transmitted by ticks are Rocky Mountain spotted fever, relapsing fever, tularemia, and Lyme disease.

Ixodides (ĭks-ŏd'ĭ-dēz) Ticks.

Ixodoidea (ĭks"ō-doy'dē-ă) A superfamily of Acarina, the ticks, in which the adults have a thick cuticle.

ixomyelitis (ĭks"ō-mī-ĕ-lī'tĭs) [Gr. *ixodes,* like birdlime, + *myelos,* marrow, + *itis,* inflammation] An inflammation of the spinal cord in the lumbar region.

J

J Symbol for joule.

Jaboulay's amputation (zhă″boo-lāz′) [Mathieu Jaboulay, Fr. surgeon, 1860–1913] Amputation of the thigh and removal of the hip bone.

Jaboulay's button Two cylinders that may be screwed together for lateral intestinal anastomosis without the use of sutures.

jacket [O.Fr. *jacquet,* jacket] A bandage usually applied to the trunk to immobilize the spine or correct deformities.

porcelain j. A jacket crown tooth restoration made of porcelain.

Sayre's j. A plaster-of-Paris jacket used as a support for a deformity of the spinal column.

jackscrew A threaded screw used for expanding the dental arch or for positioning bone fragments after a fracture.

jacksonian epilepsy [John Hughlings Jackson, Brit. neurologist, 1835–1911] A localized form of epilepsy with spasms confined to one part or one group of muscles. SEE: *epilepsy.*

Jackson's syndrome A dysfunction of cranial nerves X through XII caused by medullary lesions, resulting in unilateral muscle paralysis in the head, the mouth including the soft palate, and the vocal cords.

Jacob, Arthur Irish ophthalmologist, 1790–1874.

J. membrane The retinal layer of rods and cones.

J. ulcer A deep ulceration of the facial skin caused by locally invasive basal cell carcinoma.

Jacobson, Ludwig Danish anatomist, 1783–1843.

J. cartilage One of two narrow longitudinal cartilages lying along the anterior inferior border of the nasal septum. They are rudimentary in humans.

J. nerve Tympanic nerve.

J. organ Organ of Jacobson.

J.'s sulcus A portion of the middle ear containing branches of the tympanic plexus.

Jacquemier's sign (zhăk-mē-āz′) [Jean Jacquemier, Fr. obstetrician, 1806–1879] Blue or purple color of the vaginal mucosa; a presumptive sign of pregnancy.

jactatio (jăk-tā′shē-ō) [L., tossing] Restless tossing of the head and body; seen in acute illness. SYN: *jactitation.*

j. capitis nocturna A form of sleep disturbance characterized by nocturnal head-banging.

jactitation (jăk″tĭ-tā′shŭn) [L. *jactitatio,* tossing] Jactatio.

Jaeger's test types (yā′gĕrz) [Eduard Jaeger, Ritter von Jaxtthal, Austrian ophthalmologist, 1818–1884] Lines of type of various sizes, printed on a card for testing near vision. The smallest type read at the closest distance is recorded.

jamais vu (zhăm′ā voo) [Fr., never seen] The subjective mental sensation of being in a completely strange environment when in familiar surroundings; may be associated with temporal lobe lesions. SEE: *déjà vu.*

James fibers [T. N. James, U.S. cardiologist and physiologist, b. 1925] A pathway for conduction of cardiac impulses so that they bypass the atrioventricular node. This alternate fiber pathway permits pre-excitation of the ventricle with resultant tachycardia.

Janeway lesion [Edward Gamaliel Janeway, U.S. physician, 1841–1911] A small, painless, red-blue macular lesion a few millimeters in diameter; found on the palms and soles in patients with subacute bacterial endocarditis. SEE: *Osler's nodes; Roth's spots.*

janiceps (jăn′ĭ-sĕps) [L. *Janus,* a two-faced god, + *caput,* head] A deformed embryo having a face on both the anterior and the posterior aspects of the single head.

Jansky-Bielschowsky syndrome (jăn′skē-bē-ăl-show′skē) [Jan Jansky, Czech physician, 1873–1921; Max Bielschowsky, Ger. neuropathologist, 1869–1940] Early juvenile cerebral sphingolipidosis. SEE: *sphingolipidosis.*

jar **1.** A container made of glass, plastic, or other sturdy material. It is usually taller than it is wide and may be cylindrical, square, or another shape. **2.** To move suddenly, as in a jolt or shock.

bell j. A glass vessel with an opening at only one end.

heel j. The production of pain by having the patient stand on tiptoes and suddenly bring the heels to the floor. This physical finding may be suggestive of spinal disease, pelvic inflammatory disease in women, or kidney stones, among other ailments.

jargon (jăr′gŭn) [O.Fr., a chattering] **1.** Paraphasia. **2.** The technical language or specialized terminology used by those in a specific profession or group.

jaundice (jawn′dĭs) [Fr. *jaune,* yellow] A condition marked by yellow staining of body tissues and fluids, as a result of excessive levels of bilirubin in the bloodstream. Jaundice is not usually visible until the total bilirubin level rises above 3 mg/dl. Jaundice is a symptom of an array of illnesses, including those marked by any of the following: Obstruction of the biliary tract by gallstones, inflammatory masses, or tumors (e.g., cholecystitis, pancreatic carcinoma); Slowing of the release of bile from hepatic portals (e.g., cholestasis); Alteration of bile metabolism at the cellular level (e.g., in genetic diseases such as Gilbert's disease); Release of bilirubin because of liver cell injury by toxins or viruses (e.g., acetaminophen overdose; hepatitis B virus infection); Release of bile pigments as a result of the destruction or ineffective manufacturing of red blood cells (e.g., hemolysis; hereditary spherocytosis); Resorption of bile from hematomas within the body, esp. after trauma. SYN: *icterus*.

SYMPTOMS: Deposits of bilirubin in the skin often cause pruritus. Other symptoms of jaundice depend on whether the bilirubin is direct (conjugated [i.e., soluble in body fluids]) or indirect (unconjugated). Obstructive jaundice, for example, causes conjugated hyperbilirubinemia; in this disease, bile pigments dissolve in the urine, which turns bright green, and the stool appears gray or white owing to the deprivation of bile.

TREATMENT: The precise cause of jaundice must be determined in each patient to provide suitable therapies. For example, patients with gallstones obstructing the cystic duct need surgical treatment, and newborns with severe jaundice may require treatment with ultraviolet light to prevent kernicterus, but jaundiced patients with acute hepatitis A usually heal with symptomatic rather than specific remedies.

DIAGNOSIS: Tests to determine the cause of jaundice include a carefully performed history and physical exam, urinalysis (positive for bilirubin only in conjugated hyperbilirubinemia), liver function tests, blood tests for hepatitis, and abdominal ultrasonography. Invasive diagnostic testing with cholangiography, endoscopic retrograde cholangiopancreatography, or percutaneous transhepatic cholangiography is performed when occult biliary obstruction is suspected.

acholuric j. Jaundice without bile pigment in the urine. That is, jaundice in which the majority of the excess bilirubin is unconjugated.

breastfeeding j. An exaggerated physiological jaundice of the newborn. It may result initially from hemoconcentration due to inadequate fluid intake.

breast milk j. Hyperbilirubinemia resulting from pregnanediol or free fatty acids that inhibit bilirubin conjugation. Serum bilirubin level usually peaks above 20 ml/dl by 14 to 21 days of age. Some pediatricians recommend stopping breastfeeding for 24 to 36 hr if the level exceeds 20 ml/dl. If the infant's bilirubin level drops rapidly, the mother may resume nursing.

cholestatic j. Jaundice produced by failure of bile to flow to the duodenum. It may be caused by intrahepatic bile duct obstruction (e.g., in certain drug reactions), liver cell damage (e.g., in viral hepatitis), or extrahepatic obstruction to the flow of bile (e.g., in cholecystitis).

congenital j. Jaundice occurring at or shortly after birth. SEE: *hyperbilirubinemia*.

hematogenous j. Hemolytic j.

hemolytic j. Jaundice caused by the fragmentation of red blood cells and the release of unconjugated bilirubin in the bloodstream. This finding is associated with hemolytic anemia (HA). Because the bilirubin is not conjugated by the liver, it is not soluble in water and does not discolor the urine. Many conditions may be responsible, including congenital HA; sickle cell anemia; autoimmune HA (e.g., in infectious mononucleosis or *Mycoplasma pneumoniae* infections); microangiopathic HA (e.g., in hemolytic uremic syndrome); or transfusion-associated HA. SYN: *hematogenous j.; hemolytic icterus; nonobstructive icterus*.

hemorrhagic j. Leptospiral j.

hepatocellular j. Jaundice resulting from disease of liver cells, e.g., in acute hepatitis. SYN: *parenchymatous j.*

infectious j. Infectious hepatitis.

leptospiral j. Jaundice caused by leptospirosis. SYN: *hemorrhagic j.*

j. of newborn Nonpathological jaundice affecting newborns. It manifests 48 to 72 hr after birth, lasts only a few days, and does not require therapy. SYN: *icterus neonatorum*.

nonhemolytic j. Jaundice due to abnormal metabolism of bilirubin or to biliary tract obstruction, and not to excessive destruction of red blood cells.

obstructive j. Jaundice caused by a mechanical impediment to the flow of bile from the liver to the duodenum. Gallstones are the most common cause. Cholangitis, obstructing cancers, cysts, parasites in the biliary ducts, or hepatic abscesses are responsible less frequently. SYN: *obstructive icterus; postobstructive j.; regurgitation j.*

SYMPTOMS: The condition is marked by yellow staining of the skin, mucous membranes, sclera, and secretions. The patient may complain of pruritus caused by bile pigments in the skin. The urine is yellow or green, but the stools turn light or clay-colored because of absence of bile pigment in the intestinal tract. Acute obstruction to the flow of bile causes right upper quadrant pain and may be associated with biliary colic due to entrapment of gallstones.

TREATMENT: Cholecystectomy with common bile duct exploration (choledochostomy) is used to resolve obstructive jaundice caused by gallstones. Radical surgeries (e.g., the Whipple procedure) or stenting of the biliary tract with or without external damage may temporarily relieve obstructive jaundice caused by cancer.

pathological j. of newborn Hemolytic disease of the newborn.

parenchymatous j. Hepatocellular j.

postobstructive j. Obstructive j.

regurgitation j. Obstructive j.

retention j. Jaundice resulting from the inability of liver cells to remove bile pigment from circulation.

spirochetal j. Leptospirosis.

toxic j. Jaundice resulting from chemical injury to the liver or sepsis.

Javelle water (zhŭ-vĕl′) [Javel, a city now part of Paris] An aqueous solution of potassium or sodium hypochlorite used as a bleach and disinfectant.

jaw [ME. *iawe*] Either or both of the maxillary and mandibular bones, bearing the teeth and forming the mouth framework. SEE: illus.

cleft j. An early embryonic malformation resulting in lack of fusion of the right and left mandible into a single bone.

crackling j. Noise in the normal or diseased temporomandibular joint during movement of the jaw. SYN: *crepitation.*

dislocation of j. Traumatic or spontaneous displacement of the mandible. Jaw dislocations are uncomfortable and may be psychologically distressing. They may occur on either side, in which instance the tip of the jaw is pointed away from the dislocation. On the unaffected side, just in front of the ear, may be felt a little hollow or depression that is often tender. If both sides of the jaw are dislocated, the jaw is pushed downward and backward. In either event, there is pain and difficulty in speech and the condition is often accompanied by shock. Backward dislocation of the jaw is rare.

CAUSES: Jaw dislocation is usually caused by a blow to the face or by keeping the mouth open for long periods as in dental treatment, but occasionally may be caused by chewing large chunks of food, yawning, or hearty laughing. A fall or blow on the chin could cause dislocation, but backward dislocation seldom occurs without fracture or extreme trauma.

REDUCTION: These dislocations are reduced by placing well-padded thumbs inside of the mouth on the lower molar (back) teeth with the fingers running along the outside of the jaw as a lever. The thumbs should press the jaw downward and backward. The jaw will glide posteriorly over the ridge of bone (articular eminence), which can be felt, and

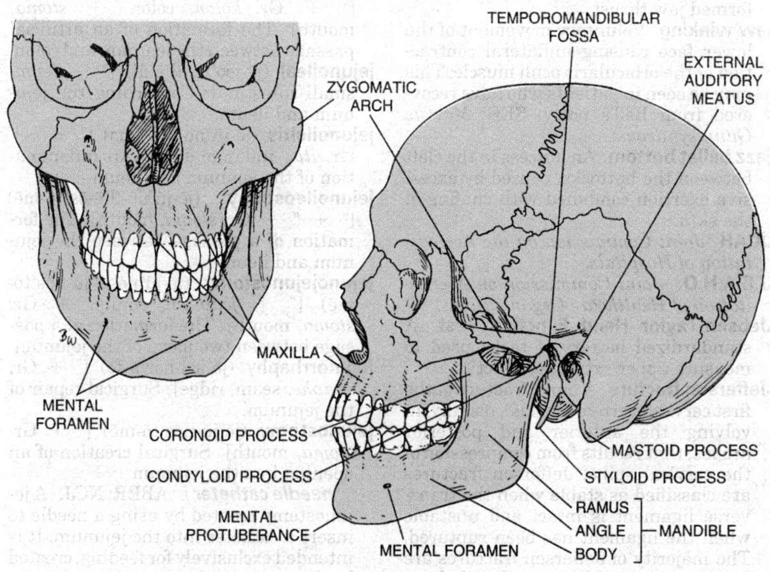

JAW

just as this occurs the jaw usually snaps into place. When this motion is noted, the thumbs should be moved laterally toward the cheeks to keep them from being crushed between the molars.

This snapping into place is due to an involuntary spasm of the muscles, which pulls the jaw as though an overstretched rubber band were attached to it. Following the reduction, an immobilizing bandage or double cravat should be applied.

CAUTION: It is important that the hands be protected by heavy gloves to prevent trauma by the teeth. SEE: *Standard and Universal Precautions Appendix.*

---

lumpy j. Actinomycosis.

swelling of j. In the lower jaw, a condition that may be due to alveolar abscess, a cyst, gumma, sarcoma, or actinomycosis. In the upper jaw, this sign may occur in alveolar abscess, parotid tumor, parotitis, carcinoma, sarcoma, necrosis of bone, or disease of antrum.

jawbone Unscientific term used to indicate the maxilla or mandible.

jaw thrust A maneuver used to open the airway of unconscious patients or of patients who cannot control their own airway, by jutting the patient's jaw forward, which in turn moves the tongue away from the back of the throat. This procedure is used especially in opening the airway of patients with suspected spinal injury, because the cervical spine is not moved during a properly performed jaw thrust.

jaw winking Voluntary movement of the lower face causing unilateral contraction of the orbicularis oculi muscle. This may be seen in patients who have recovered from Bell's palsy. SEE: *Marcus Gunn syndrome.*

jazz ballet bottom An abscess in the cleft between the buttocks, caused by excessive exertion combined with chafing of the skin.

JCAH *Joint Commission on the Accreditation of Hospitals.*

J.C.A.H.O. *Joint Commission on Accreditation of Healthcare Organizations.*

Jebsen-Taylor Hand Function Test A standardized battery of tasks used to measure upper extremity function.

Jefferson fracture A burst fracture of the first cervical vertebra (atlas), usually involving the anterior and posterior arches, that results from compression of the cervical spine. Jefferson fractures are classified as stable when the transverse ligament is intact and unstable when the ligament has been ruptured. The majority of Jefferson fractures are associated with other spinal pathology, esp. fractures of the second cervical vertebra (axis). SEE: *halo vest.*

SYMPTOMS: The patient may complain of pain arising from the upper cervical spine but may not demonstrate signs or symptoms of neurological impairment. On x-ray examination, odontoid views may demonstrate displacement of the C1-C2 facets. Lateral and flexion-extension views are needed to ascertain the status of the transverse ligament.

TREATMENT: For unstable fracture, cranial traction, skeletal traction, and/or halo vest are applied for a total of 3 months. A nondisplaced stable fracture may be treated with the use of a soft cervical collar. Stable fractures with less than 7 mm displacement require the use of a rigid cervical collar. Follow-up evaluations should be performed regularly, to rule out insidious subluxation of the first cervical vertebra.

jejunal (jē-jū'năl) [L. *jejunum,* empty] Relating to the jejunum.

jejunectomy (jē"jū-něk'tō-mē) [" + Gr. *ektome,* excision] Excision of part or all of the jejunum.

jejunitis (jē"jŭ-nī'tĭs) [" + Gr. *itis,* inflammation] An inflammation of the jejunum, caused by one of many possible diseases, including bacterial infections, celiac sprue, Crohn's disease, ischemia, radiation, injury, or vasculitis.

jejuno- [L.] Combining form meaning *jejunum.*

jejunocecostomy (jě-joo"nō-sē-kŏs'tō-mē) [" + *caecum,* blindness, + Gr. *stoma,* mouth] The formation of a passage between the cecum and jejunum.

jejunocolostomy (jē-jū"nō-kōl-ŏs'tō-mē) [" + Gr. *kolon,* colon, + *stoma,* mouth] The formation of an artificial passage between the jejunum and colon.

jejunoileal (jě-joo"nō-ĭl'ē-ăl) [" + *ileum,* small intestine] Concerning the jejunum and ileum.

jejunoileitis (jē-jū"nō-ĭl"ē-ī'tĭs) [" + " + Gr. *itis,* inflammation] An inflammation of the jejunum and ileum.

jejunoileostomy (jē-jū"nō-ĭl"ē-ŏs'tō-mē) [" + " + Gr. *stoma,* mouth] The formation of a passage between the jejunum and ileum.

jejunojejunostomy (jē-jū"nō-jē"jū-nŏs'tō-mē) [" + *jejunum,* empty, + Gr. *stoma,* mouth] The formation of a passage between two parts of the jejunum.

jejunorrhaphy (jě"joo-nor'ă-fē) [" + Gr. *rhaphe,* seam, ridge] Surgical repair of the jejunum.

jejunostomy (jē"jū-nŏs'tō-mē) [" + Gr. *stoma,* mouth] Surgical creation of an opening into the jejunum.

needle catheter j. ABBR: NCJ. A jejunostomy created by using a needle to insert a catheter into the jejunum. It is intended exclusively for feeding, created by direct surgical approach or percutaneously. SEE: *percutaneous endoscopic j.*

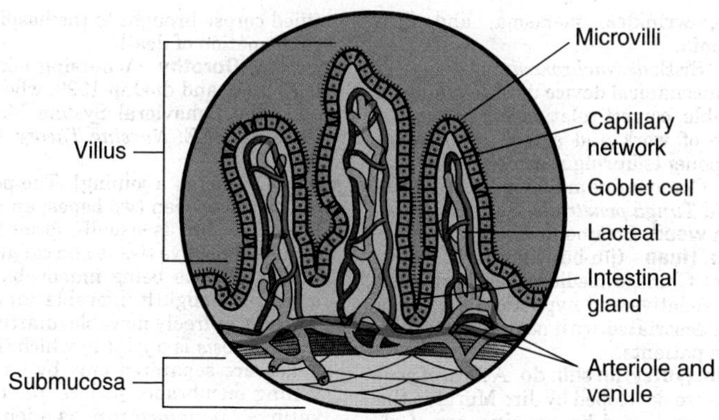

JEJUNUM

percutaneous endoscopic j. ABBR: PEJ. A jejunostomy created for feeding purposes with the use of an endoscope and guide wire.

jejunotomy (jē″jū-nŏt′ō-mē) [″ + Gr. *tome,* incision] Surgical incision into the jejunum.

jejunum (jē-jū′nŭm) [L., empty] The second portion of the small intestine extending from the duodenum to the ileum. It is about 8 ft (2.4 m) long, two fifths of the small intestine. SEE: illus.

inflammation of j. Jejunitis.

jelly [L. *gelare,* to freeze] A thick, semisolid, gelatinous mass.

contraceptive j. Gel introduced into the vagina for the prevention of conception. It serves as a vehicle for spermicidal substances. SEE: *contraceptive.*

mineral j. Petrolatum.

petroleum j. Petrolatum.

vaginal j. Gel introduced into the vagina for therapeutic or contraceptive purposes.

Wharton's j. Soft, gelatinous, connective tissue that constitutes the matrix of the umbilical cord.

Jendrassik's maneuver (yĕn-dră′sĭks) [Ernö Jendrassik, Hungarian physician, 1858–1921] A method used to facilitate elicitation of the deep tendon reflexes of the lower extremities. The patient hooks together the fingers of the hands and attempts to pull them apart. While this pressure is maintained, the patellar or Achilles tendon reflex is tested.

Jenner, Edward British physician (1749–1823) who invented the vaccination for smallpox. Jenner observed that individuals exposed to cowpox, such as those who milked cows, would develop a minor skin lesion and then be immune to smallpox. From this observation, he developed a vaccine from cowpox lesions, which provides immunity to smallpox.

Jenner's stain [Louis Jenner, Brit. physician, 1866–1904] Eosin methylene blue stain.

jerk (jĕrk) **1.** A sudden muscular movement. **2.** Certain reflex actions resulting from striking or tapping a muscle or tendon. SEE: *reflex.*

Achilles j. Ankle j.

ankle j. Contraction of the calf muscles produced by tapping the stretched Achilles tendon. SYN: *Achilles j.*

biceps j. A reflex contraction of the biceps brachii produced by tapping over the insertion of the tendon at the head of the radius. Usually, the evaluator places a thumb against the tendon and taps the nail of the thumb to elicit the reflex.

elbow j. Elbow reflex.

jaw j. A movement resulting from tapping the mandible when the jaw is half open. It may be increased when there are bilateral supranuclear cerebral lesions.

knee j. The extension of the lower leg upon striking the patellar tendon when the knee is flexed at a right angle. Knee jerk is absent in locomotor ataxia, infantile paralysis, meningitis, destructive lesions of the lower part of the spinal cord, and certain forms of paralysis. It is increased in lesions of pyramidal areas, brain tumors, spinal irritability, and cerebrospinal sclerosis. SYN: *patellar reflex.* SEE: *reflex, knee-jerk.*

tendon j. The contraction of a muscle after tapping its tendon.

triceps surae j. Ankle j.

Jerusalem syndrome A temporary or permanent delusional disorder following a pilgrimage to the capital of Israel, characterized by extreme religious preoccupations or the belief that the pilgrim has become the embodiment or incarnation of an important Biblical character.

Jessner's solution (jĕs′nĕrz) A topical liquid used as a chemical peel to treat acne, wrinkles, melasma, and dyschromia.

jet lag SEE: *desynchronosis*.

jig A mechanical device used to maintain a stable, correct relationship between a piece of work and a tool, or between components during assembly.

jigger Common name for parasitic fleas called *Tunga penetrans*. SEE: *chiggers*.

jimson weed Stramonium.

Jin Bu Huan (jĭn-bū-whăn′) In traditional Chinese medicine, an herb used as a sedative and hypnotic. Its use has been associated with acute hepatitis in some patients.

Jin shin, jyutsy, jin shin do A form of acupressure developed by Jiro Murai in the 1900s and used by practitioners of alternative medicine to treat selected health problems.

jitters (jĭt′ĕrz) Shakes.

Jobst pressure garment An elastic garment fabricated to apply varying pressure gradients to an area. It may be worn over severely burned areas for the purpose of reducing hypertrophic scarring as wounds heal or may be used to prevent or control lymphedema in the arms or legs.

Job's syndrome [Job, Biblical character] Recurrent staphylococcal infections of the skin related to impaired immune defenses.

Jocasta complex (jō-kăs′tă) [Jocasta, mythical character who was the wife and mother of Oedipus] The psychological or emotional fixation of a mother toward her son. SEE: *Oedipus complex*.

Joffroy's reflex (zhŏf-rwhăz′) [Alexis Joffroy, Fr. physician, 1844–1908] A twitching of the gluteal muscles when pressure is made against the buttocks.

Joffroy's sign **1.** The absence of facial muscle contraction when the eyes turn upward in exophthalmic goiter. **2.** An inability to do simple sums in arithmetic; an early sign of general paralysis in organic brain syndrome.

jogger's heel An irritation of the fibrous and fatty tissue covering the heel. The condition is due to the type of running characteristic of jogging, in which the heel strikes the surface first, rather than that of sprinting, in which the toes strike first. Persons prone to develop this may diminish the risk by wearing pads on their heels and by running on surfaces softer than wood, concrete, or asphalt.

jogging Running for enjoyment or to maintain physical fitness. In contrast to running, jogging is not a competitive exercise.

John Doe **1.** In law, a fictitious name used when that of the actual defendant is unknown. **2.** Name assigned to an unidentified patient (e.g., one admitted to a hospital in a coma), or to an unidentified corpse brought to the hospital for confirmation of death.

Johnson, Dorothy A nursing educator, born 1919 and died in 1999, who developed the Behavioral System Model of Nursing. SEE: *Nursing Theory Appendix*.

joint [L. *junctio*, a joining] The point of juncture between two bones; an articulation. A joint is usually formed of fibrous connective tissue and cartilage. It is classified as being immovable (synarthrosis), slightly movable (amphiarthrosis), or freely movable (diarthrosis). *Synarthrosis* is a joint in which the two bones are separated only by an intervening membrane, such as the cranial sutures. *Amphiarthrosis* is a joint having a fibrocartilaginous disk between the bony surfaces (symphysis), such as the symphysis pubis; or one with a ligament uniting the two bones (syndesmosis), such as the tibiofibular articulation. *Diarthrosis* is a joint in which the adjoining bone ends are covered with a thin cartilaginous sheet and joined by a joint capsule lined by a synovial membrane, which secretes synovial fluid, a lubricant. SYN: *arthrosis* (1). SEE: illus.

MOVEMENT: Joints are also grouped according to motion: ball and socket (enarthrosis); hinge (ginglymus); condyloid; pivot (trochoid); gliding (arthrodia); and saddle joint.

Joints can move in four ways: *gliding*, in which one bony surface glides on another without angular or rotatory movement; *angular*, occurring only between long bones, increasing or decreasing the angle between the bones; *circumduction*, occurring in joints composed of the head of a bone and an articular cavity, the long bone describing a series of circles, the whole forming a cone; and *rotation*, in which a bone moves about a central axis without moving from this axis. Angular movement, if it occurs forward or backward, is called flexion or extension, respectively; away from the body, abduction; and toward the median plane of the body, adduction.

Because of their location and constant use, joints are prone to stress, injury, and inflammation. The main diseases affecting the joints are rheumatic fever, rheumatoid arthritis, osteoarthritis, and gout. Injuries are contusions, sprains, dislocations, and penetrating wounds.

amphidiarthrodial j. A joint that is both ginglymoid and arthrodial.

j. approximation A rehabilitation technique whereby joint surfaces are compressed together while the patient is in a weight-bearing posture for the purpose of facilitating cocontraction of muscles around a joint.

arthrodial j. Diarthrosis permitting a gliding motion. SYN: *gliding j.*

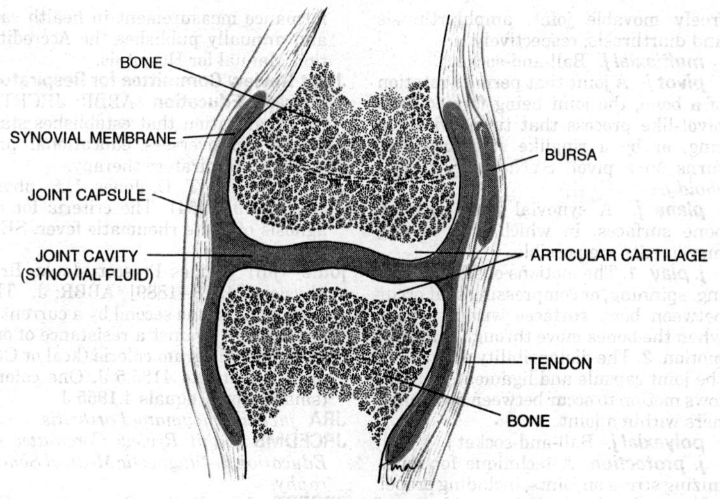

SYNOVIAL JOINT

ball-and-socket j. A joint in which the round end of one bone fits into the cavity of another bone. SYN: *enarthrodial j.; multiaxial j.; polyaxial j.*

biaxial j. A joint possessing two chief movement axes at right angles to each other.

bilocular j. A joint separated into two sections by interarticular cartilage.

bleeders' j. Hemorrhage into joint space in hemophiliacs. SYN: *hemophilic j.*

Budin's j. A congenital cartilaginous band between the squamous and condylar parts of the occipital bone.

cartilaginous j. A joint in which there is cartilage connecting the bones.

Charcot's j. SEE: *Charcot's joint.*

Chopart's j. The union of the remainder of the tarsal bones with the calcaneus and talus.

cochlear j. A hinge joint permitting lateral motion. SYN: *spiral j.*

compound j. A joint made up of several bones.

condyloid j. A joint permitting all forms of angular movement except axial rotation.

craniomandibular j. The encapsulated, double synovial joints between the condylar processes of the mandible and the temporal bones of the cranium. The double synovial joints are separated by an articular disk and function as an upper gliding joint and a lower modified hinge or ginglymoid joint. SYN: *temporomandibular j.*

diarthrodial j. A joint characterized by the presence of a cavity within the capsule separating the bones, thus permitting considerable freedom of movement.

dry j. Arthritis of the chronic villous type.

elbow j. The hinge joint between the humerus and the ulna.

ellipsoid j. A joint having two axes of motion through the same bone.

enarthrodial j. Ball-and-socket j.

false j. False joint formation subsequent to a fracture.

fibrous j. Joints connected by fibrous tissue.

flail j. A joint that is extremely relaxed, the distal portion of the limb being almost beyond the control of the will.

ginglymoid j. A synovial joint having only forward and backward motion, as a hinge. SYN: *hinge j.; ginglymus.*

gliding j. Arthrodial j.

hemophilic j. Bleeders' j.

hinge j. Ginglymoid j.

hip j. A stable ball-and-socket joint in which the head of the femur fits into the acetabulum of the hip bone.

immovable j. Synarthrosis.

intercarpal j. Articulations formed by the carpal bones in relation to one another.

irritable j. A recurrent joint inflammation of unknown cause.

knee j. The joint formed by the femur, patella, and tibia.

j. mice Free bits of cartilage or bone present in the joint space, esp. the knee joint. These are usually the result of previous trauma, and may or may not be symptomatic.

midcarpal j. A joint separating the navicular, lunate, and triangular bones from the distal row of carpal bones.

mortise j. The ankle joint.

movable j. A slightly movable or

freely movable joint, amphiarthrosis and diarthrosis, respectively.

multiaxial j. Ball-and-socket j.

pivot j. A joint that permits rotation of a bone, the joint being formed by a pivot-like process that turns within a ring, or by a ringlike structure that turns on a pivot. SYN: *rotary j.; trochoid j.*

plane j. A synovial joint between bone surfaces, in which only gliding movements are possible.

j. play **1.** The motions of sliding, rolling, spinning, or compressing that occur between bony surfaces within a joint when the bones move through ranges of motion. **2.** The distensibility or "give" of the joint capsule and ligaments that allows motion to occur between bony partners within a joint.

polyaxial j. Ball-and-socket j.

j. protection A technique for minimizing stress on joints, including proper body mechanics and the avoidance of continuous weight-bearing or deforming postures.

receptive j. Saddle j.

rotary j. Pivot j.

saddle j. A joint in which the opposing surfaces are reciprocally concavo-convex. SYN: *receptive j.*

shoulder j. The ball-and-socket joint between the head of the humerus and the glenoid cavity of the scapula.

simple j. A joint composed of two bones.

spheroid j. A multiaxial joint with spheroid surfaces.

spiral j. Cochlear j.

sternoclavicular j. The joint space between the sternum and the medial extremity of the clavicle.

subtalar j. The three articular surfaces on the inferior surface of the talus.

synarthrodial j. Synarthrosis.

synovial j. A joint in which the articulating surfaces are separated by synovial fluid. SEE: *joint* for illus.

tarsometatarsal j. A joint composed of three arthrodial joints, the bones of which articulate with the bases of the metatarsal bones.

temporomandibular j. Craniomandibular j.

trochoid j. Pivot j.

ulnomeniscal-triquetral j. The functional articulation of the distal ulna, articular disc, and triquetrum. The disc may subluxate following injury or with arthritis and block supination of the forearm.

uniaxial j. A joint moving on a single axis.

unilocular j. A joint with a single cavity.

Joint Commission on Accreditation for Healthcare Organizations ABBR: JCAHO. Group that oversees and establishes standards of quality and performance measurement in health care and annually publishes the Accreditation Manual for Hospitals.

Joint Review Committee for Respiratory Therapy Education ABBR: JRCRTE. An organization that establishes standards and oversees educational programs in respiratory therapy.

Jones criteria [T. D. Jones, U.S. physician, 1899–1954] The criteria for diagnosis of acute rheumatic fever. SEE: *rheumatic fever*.

joule (jūl) [James Prescott Joule, Brit. physicist, 1818–1889] ABBR: J. The work done in one second by a current of one ampere against a resistance of one ohm. One kilogram calorie (kcal or Calorie) is equal to 4185.5 J. One calorie (small calorie) equals 4.1855 J.

JRA *juvenile rheumatoid arthritis.*

JRCEDMS *Joint Review Committee on Education in Diagnostic Medical Sonography.*

JRCERT *Joint Review Committee on Education in Radiologic Technology.*

JRCRTE *Joint Review Committee for Respiratory Therapy Education.*

judgment The use of available evidence or facts to formulate a rational opinion or to make socially acceptable choices or decisions. Judgment may be impaired by conditions such as mental illness, medications, delirium, fatigue, or bias.

substituted j. Instructions regarding patients' wishes from significant others, usually with respect to their preferences for life support, drug therapy, fluid infusions, or supplemental nutrition. Substituted judgments are relied upon when patients are unable to advocate for themselves, and are generally respected by health care workers, but their validity in representing the actual desires of patients has been questioned.

jugal [L. *jugalis,* of a yoke] **1.** Connected or united as by a yoke. **2.** Pert. to the malar or zygomatic bone.

jugale (jū-gā′lē) The point at the margin of the zygomatic process.

jugomaxillary (joo″gō-măk′sĭ-lār″ē) Concerning the maxilla and the zygomatic bone.

jugular (jŭg′ū-lăr) [L. *jugularis*] Pert. to the throat.

j. vein Any of the two pairs of bilateral veins that return blood to the heart from the head and neck. The external jugular vein receives the blood from the exterior of the cranium and the deep parts of the face. It lies superficial to the sternocleidomastoid muscle as it passes down the neck to join the subclavian vein. The internal jugular vein receives blood from the brain and superficial parts of the face and neck. It is directly continuous with the transverse sinus, accompanying the internal carotid artery as it passes down the neck, and joins with the subclavian vein to form the innominate vein. The jugular veins are more prominent during expiration than during inspiration and are also prominent during cardiac decompensation.

When the patient is sitting or in a semirecumbent position, the height of the jugular veins and their pulsations can provide an accurate estimation of central venous pressure and give important information about cardiac compensation.

jugulate (jŭg′ū-lāt) [L. *jugulare*, to cut the throat] To quickly arrest a process or disease by therapeutic measures.

jugulation (jŭg″ū-lā′shŭn) The sudden arrest of a disease by therapeutic means.

jugulum (jŭg′ū-lŭm) [L.] Neck or throat.

jugum (jū′gŭm) *pl.* **juga** [L., a yoke] **1.** A ridge or furrow connecting two points. **2.** A type of forceps.

j. penis A forceps for temporarily compressing the penis.

j. petrosum An eminence on the petrous section of the temporal bone showing the position of the superior semicircular canal. SYN: *arcuate eminence.*

juice [L. *jus*, broth] Liquid excreted, secreted, or expressed from any part of an organism.

alimentary j. Digestive secretion.

gastric j. The digestive secretion of the gastric glands of the stomach. It is a thin, colorless fluid; is mostly water; and contains mucus, intrinsic factor, hydrochloric acid, the enzyme pepsin, and the enzyme lipase. The pH is 1–2, strongly acidic, which destroys pathogens and changes pepsinogen to the active pepsin. Pepsin begins the digestion of proteins. Gastric lipase has little effect on unemulsified fats; most fat digestion takes place in the small intestine. The amount of gastric juice secreted in 24 hr varies with food intake. SEE: *stomach.*

grapefruit j. A drink derived from a fruit rich in chemicals called flavonoids, which impair the metabolism of drugs processed by the liver's cytochrome P 450 system. Patients should be advised that the juice alters the performance of several important drugs, including warfarin, steroids, calcium channel blockers, statins, second-generation antihistamines, protease inhibitors, and others.

intestinal j. Alkaline secretion that contains peptidases and enzymes to complete the digestion of disaccharides. SEE: *digestion.*

pancreatic j. A clear, viscid, alkaline digestive juice of the pancreas poured into the duodenum. It contains the enzymes trypsin, amylase, and lipase.

juicing (joo′sĭng) The conversion of vegetables and fruits into consumable liquids.

Julian date [Julius Caesar, Roman general, ca 44 B.C., who devised the Julian calendar] In medical records, identifying a calendar date by using a code for the day of the year. Each day is numbered sequentially from 1 through 365, or 366 on leap years.

Jumping Frenchmen of Maine A condition characterized by a sudden, single, sometimes violent movement or cry that occurs in response to a sharp unexpected sound or touch. The individual may also blurt out whatever was being thought of at the time of the stimulus. The condition may begin in childhood and be lifelong. It has been most frequently described in persons of French descent living in Maine, but may occur in a person of almost any nationality or geographic location. The cause is unknown and there is no effective therapy. SEE: *Tourette's syndrome; miryachit; startle syndrome.*

jun (joon) A family of oncogenes that can transform some normal cells (e.g., rat embryo cells) into cancer cells. All members of this family can bind to activating protein-1 (AP-1) sites and to specific DNA sequences. SEE: *oncogene; transformation.*

junction (jŭnk′shŭn) [L. *junctio*, a joining] The place of union or coming together of two parts or tissue layers.

amelodentinal j. Dentinoenamel j.

atrioventricular j. The area of cardiac conduction pathway composed of the AV node and bundle of His.

cementodentinal j. The interface of dentin and cementum of the tooth. SYN: *dentinocemental j.*

cementoenamel j. The line around the tooth that marks the boundary between the crown and root of the tooth; the interface between enamel and cementum.

dentinocemental j. Cementodentinal j.

dentinoenamel j. The plane or interface between the dentin of the tooth and the enamel crown; histological sections show it to be a scalloped boundary at the site of the basement membrane which separated the cell layers that formed the calcified enamel and dentin. SYN: *amelodentinal j.*

dentogingival j. The interface and zone of attachment between the gingiva and enamel or cementum of the tooth. It holds in place the junctional or attachment epithelium.

interneuronal j. Synapse.

liquid j. The point in a potentiometric reference electrode measurement system at which the reference solution makes contact with the test solution. An example is pH reference electrode.

mucocutaneous j. The junction between the skin and a mucous membrane.

mucogingival j. A scalloped, indistinct boundary between the gingiva and the oral mucosa on the alveolar process. The coral color of gingiva may be contrasted with the more vascular oral mucosa. Also called the mucogingival line.

myoneural j. The axon terminal of a motor neuron, synaptic cleft, and sarcolemma of a muscle cell. SYN: *neuromuscular j.* SEE: illus.; *motor endplate.*

neuromuscular j. Myoneural j.

sclerocorneal j. The meeting point between the sclera and the cornea marked on the external surface of the eyeball by the outer scleral sulcus.

squamocolumnar j. The point in the cervical canal at which the squamous and columnar epithelia meet. As most cervical cancers begin in this area, it is important to obtain cells from this location for the Pap test.

tight j. A part of the junctional complex at the lateral interface between epithelial cells; also called zonula occludens.

junctura (jŭnk-tū′ră) *pl.* **juncturae** [L., a joining] Suture of bones. SYN: *articulation* (1).

Jung, Carl Gustav [Swiss psychiatrist, 1875–1961] The founder of the Jungian school of analytic psychology. In his early career, Jung was associated with Sigmund Freud. Later he proposed his own theory of the unconscious mind, based on his belief that all human beings share common myths and symbols. This concept has not been objectively validated.

juniper tar (joo′nĭ-pĕr) A volatile oil obtained from the wood of *Juniperus oxycedrus.* It is used in shampoos and bath emulsions.

jurisdiction The authority and power of courts to hear and render judgments on the parties and subject matter of a case.

jurisprudence (joor″ĭs-proo′dĕns) [L. *juris prudentia,* knowledge of law] The scientific study or application of the principles of law and justice.

dental j. The application of the principles of law as they relate to the practice of dentistry, to the obligations of the practitioners to their patients, and to the relations of dentists to each other and to society in general. This term and forensic dentistry are sometimes used

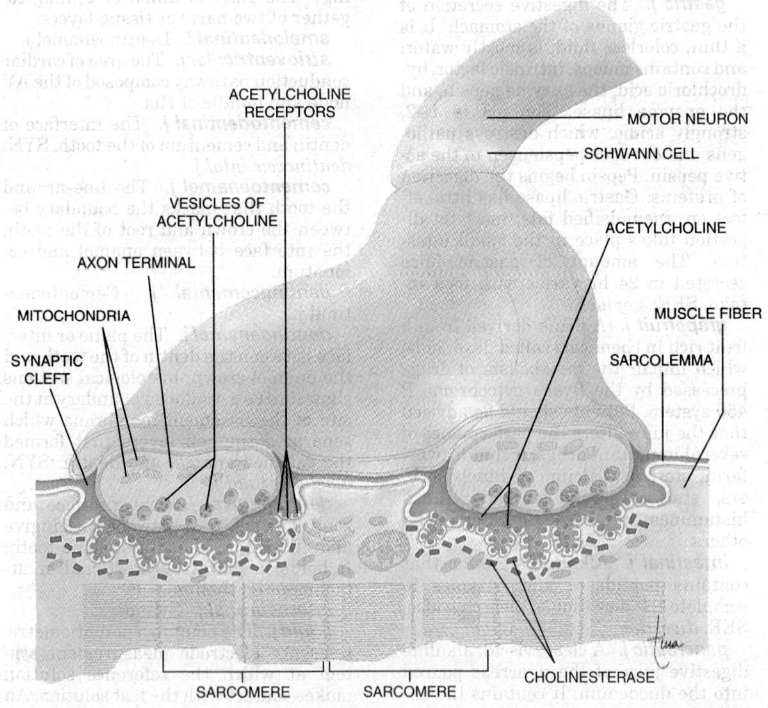

MYONEURAL JUNCTION

as synonyms, but some authorities consider the first as a branch of law and the second as a branch of dentistry.

medical j. The application of the principles of law as they relate to the practice of medicine, to the obligations of the practitioners to their patients, and to the relations of physicians to each other and to society in general.

nursing j. The application of the principles of law as they relate to the practice of nursing, to the obligations of nurses to their patients, and to the relations of nurses with each other and with other health care professionals.

jury-mast (jūr′ē-măst) [L. *jurare,* to be right, + AS. *masc,* a stick] An apparatus for support of the head in diseases of the spine.

Juster's reflex [Emile Juster, 20th century Fr. neurologist] Finger extension instead of flexion when the palm of the hand is irritated.

justo major (jŭs′tō mā′jor) [L.] Bigger than normal, as a pelvis.

justo minor (jŭs′tō mī′nor) [L.] Smaller than normal, as a pelvis.

juvenile (jū′vě-nīl″) [L. *juvenis,* young] **1.** Pert. to youth or childhood. **2.** Young; immature.

juxta- [L., near] Prefix indicating *proximity.*

juxta-articular (jŭks″tă-ăr-tĭk′ū-lăr) [″ + *articulus,* joint] Situated close to a joint.

juxtaglomerular (jŭks″tă-glō-mĕr′ū-lăr) [″ + *glomus,* ball] Near or adjacent to a glomerulus.

juxtaposition (jŭks″tă-pō-zĭ′shŭn) [″ + *positio,* place] Apposition.

juxtapyloric (jŭks″tă-pī-lor′ĭk) [″ + Gr. *pyloros,* pylorus] Near the pylorus or pyloric orifice.

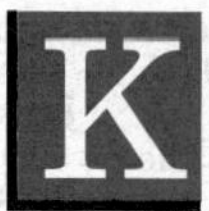

K [L. *kalium*] Symbol for the element potassium.

K, k **1.** Symbol for the Greek letter *kappa.* **2.** Used in some formulas in chemistry and physics to indicate a constant or value that does not change. **3.** Kelvin temperature scale. **4.** Symbol for kilo.

Kader's operation (kă'děrs) [Bronislaw Kader, Polish surgeon, 1863–1937] The surgical formation of a gastric fistula with the feeding tube inserted through a valvelike flap.

kaif (kĭf) [Arabic, quiescence] A dreamy, tranquil state induced by drugs.

kainophobia (kī-nō-fō'bē-ă) [Gr. *kainos,* new, + *phobos,* fear] Neophobia.

kaiserling (kī'zěr-lĭng) [Karl Kaiserling, Ger. pathologist, 1869–1942] A solution used in preserving pathological specimens.

kakidrosis (kăk-ī-drō'sĭs) [Gr. *kakos,* bad, + *hidrosis,* sweat] Bromidrosis.

kakke (kŏk'kā) [Japanese] Beriberi.

kakosmia (kăk-ŏz'mē-ă) [Gr. *kakos,* bad, + *osme,* smell] Cacosmia.

kala azar (kă'lă ă-zăr') [Hindi, black fever] An infectious disease caused by *Leishmania donovani,* an intracellular protozoan. It is marked by fevers, splenic enlargement, and decreased blood cell counts. The disease is common in the rural parts of tropical and subtropical areas of the world, where it is often fatal. SYN: *visceral leishmaniasis.*

kaligenous (kā-lĭj'ĕ-nŭs) [" + Gr. *gennan,* to produce] Forming potash.

kalimeter (kă-lĭm'ĕ-ter) [" + Gr. *metron,* measure] An obsolete term for a device for measuring the degree of alkalinity of a mixture.

kaliopenia (kă"lē-ō-pē'nē-ă) [L. *kalium,* potassium, + Gr. *penia,* poverty] Hypokalemia; decreased potassium in the blood.

kaliuresis (kă"lē-ū-rē'sĭs) [L. *kalium,* potassium, + Gr. *ouresis,* urination] The excretion of potassium in the urine.

kallidin (kăl'ĭ-dĭn) A plasma kinin. SEE: *kinin.*

kallikrein (kăl-ĭ-krē'ĭn) [Gr. *kallikreas,* pancreas] An enzyme normally present in blood plasma, urine, and body tissue in an inactive state. When activated, kallikrein has many actions: it dilates blood vessels, influences blood pressure, modulates salt and water excretion by the kidneys, and influences cardiac remodeling after myocardial infarction.

kallikreinogen (kăl"ĭ-krī'nō-jěn) [" + *gennan,* to produce] The precursor of kallikrein in blood plasma.

Kallmann's syndrome [Franz Josef Kallman, U.S. psychiatrist, 1897–1965] A disorder whose hallmarks are congenital absence of the sense of smell and decreased functional activity of the sex organs, resulting from insufficient production of gonadotropin-releasing hormone. Affected individuals also may have hearing loss and other deficits caused by intracranial, sinus, or facial abnormalities.

Kanner syndrome [Leo Kanner, Austrian psychiatrist in the U.S., b. 1894] Infantile autism.

kaolin (kā'ō-lĭn) [Fr., from Mandarin Chinese *kao,* high, + *ling,* mountain] A yellow-white or gray clay powder occurring in a natural state as a form of hydrated aluminum silicate. It is used internally as an absorbent, e.g., in treating diarrhea, externally as a protective by absorbing moisture. SYN: *China clay.*

kaolinosis (kā"ō-lĭn-ō'sĭs) Pneumonoconiosis caused by inhaling kaolin particles.

Kaposi, Moritz K. (kăp'ō-sē") Austrian physician, 1837–1902. Originally his name was Moritz Kohn.

K.'s disease Xeroderma pigmentosum.

K.'s sarcoma ABBR: KS. A vascular malignancy, composed of multiple red or purple macules, papules, or nodules, that is first apparent on the skin or mucous membranes, but may involve the internal organs. Once a rare disease seen primarily in elderly men of Mediterranean, African, or Ashkenazi Jewish descent (so-called classic KS), it has become a common marker of the acquired immunodeficiency syndrome (AIDS). In patients with AIDS, KS is believed to be sexually acquired as a result of the acquisition of human herpes virus 8. When KS is associated with AIDS, it progresses and disseminates rapidly to multiple skin sites, as well as the lymph nodes and visceral organs. SEE: illus.; *AIDS.*

SYMPTOMS: The lesions are typically painless but may be cosmetically disfiguring. They are found most often on the dorsa of the feet and lower extremities in patients with classic KS, and on the face, trunk, oral cavity, and internal organs in immunosuppressed patients (the "epidemic" variant). In advanced

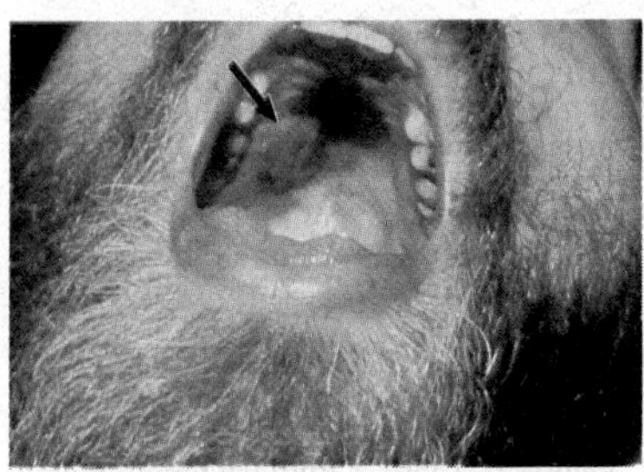

KAPOSI'S SARCOMA

As seen on the hard palate of a patient with AIDS

disease, the lesions may merge into large plaques, sometimes blocking lymphatics and causing localized swelling. Involvement of internal organs, such as the gastrointestinal tract or the lungs, may result in dyspepsia or dyspnea, among other symptoms.

DIAGNOSIS: Characteristic tumors on the skin suggest the diagnosis, which should be confirmed by tissue biopsy.

TREATMENT: Options include radiation therapy, cancer chemotherapies, hormone therapies, and interferon alfa.

PATIENT CARE: Epidemic KS may profoundly alter the patient's appearance. Emotional support to the patient and family may help them cope with the diagnosis and its effects on body image.

K.'s varicelliform eruption Eczema herpeticum.

karaya gum (kăr′ā-ă) The dried gum from *Sterculia* plants, which becomes gelatinous when moist. It is used as an adhesive and as a bulk laxative.

karelian fever An infectious disease marked by influenza-like symptoms (headache, body aches, fever, nausea, vomiting) and rashes (esp. blistering rashes on the hands and feet). A postinfectious arthritis sometimes follows.

ETIOLOGY: It is caused by the Sindbis virus, an alphavirus that mosquitoes transmit to people.

Karman catheter [Harvey Karman, U.S. psychologist, b. 1924] A catheter used for suction curettage of the uterus.

Karnofsky Index, Karnofsky Scale [D. A. Karnofsky, 1914–1969, American oncologist] A tool to estimate clinically a patient's physical state, performance, and prognosis. The scale is from 100%, perfectly well and active, to 0%, completely inactive, or dead. It has been used in studying cancer and chronic illness. Lower Karnofsky scores are generally associated with poorer treatment response and prognosis. SEE: table.

Kartagener's syndrome (kăr′tă-gā″nĕrz) [Manes Kartagener, Swiss physician, 1897–1975] A hereditary syndrome consisting of abnormal ciliary movement, bronchiectasis, maldevelopment of the sinuses, and transposition of the viscera. SEE: *immotile cilia syndrome*.

Karvonen formula A calculation of the optimal range of heart rate for achieving physical fitness during cardiovascular endurance exercise. The calculation is based on a percentage of predicted maximum heart rate of 220 minus the person's age (HR_{max}) and the resting heart rate (HR_{rest}). The formula that determines the best physical training range is: $HR = HR_{rest} + (HR_{max} - HR_{rest})$ (.60 to .80).

karyo-, kary- [Gr. *karyon,* kernel] Prefix referring to a cell's nucleus.

karyochromatophil (kăr″ē-ō-krō-măt′ō-fĭl) [″ + *chroma,* color, + *philein,* to love] Having a nucleus that stains.

karyochrome (kăr′ē-ō-krōm″) A neuron with an easily staining nucleus.

karyocyte (kăr′ē-ō-sīt) [″ + *kytos,* cell] An immature normoblast.

karyogamy (kăr-ē-ŏg′ă-mē) [″ + *gamos,* marriage] The union of nuclei in cell conjugation.

karyogenesis (kăr″ē-ō-jĕn′ĕ-sĭs) [″ + *genesis,* generation, birth] The formation and development of a cell nucleus.

karyokinesis (kăr″ē-ō-kĭn-ē′sĭs) [″ + *ki-*

Karnofsky Index

100%	Normal, no complaints; no evidence of disease
90%	Able to carry on normal activity; minor signs or symptoms of disease
80%	Normal activity with effort, some signs or symptoms of disease
70%	Cares for self; unable to carry on normal activity or do active work
60%	Requires occasional assistance, but is able to care for most personal needs
50%	Requires considerable assistance and frequent medical care
40%	Disabled; requires special care and assistance
30%	Severely disabled; hospitalization is indicated, although death not imminent
20%	Very sick; hospitalization is necessary; active supportive treatment is required
10%	Terminally ill; fatal processes progressing rapidly
0%	Dead

nesis, movement] The equal division of nuclear material that occurs in cell division. SEE: *cytokinesis; mitosis.*

karyokinetic (kăr″ē-ō-kĭ-nĕt′ĭk) **1.** Pert. to karyokinesis. **2.** Ameboid.

karyoklasis (kăr″ē-ŏk′lă-sĭs) [″ + *klasis,* a breaking] Disintegration of the cell nucleus.

karyolobism (kăr″ē-ō-lō′bĭzm) [″ + L. *lobus,* lobe, + Gr. *-ismos,* state of] A condition in which the nucleus of a cell is lobed, as in polymorphonuclear leukocytes.

karyolymph [″ + L. *lympha,* lymph] Fluid in meshes of the nucleus; now known to contain active submicroscopic components of the nucleoplasm. Thus the terms karyolymph and nuclear sap do not describe clearly definable entities and should not be used. SEE: *cell; organelle.*

karyolysis (kăr-ē-ŏl′ĭ-sĭs) [″ + *lysis,* dissolution] Chromatolysis. **karyolytic** (-ō-lĭt′ĭk), *adj.*

karyomegaly (kăr″ē-ō-mĕg′ă-lē) [″ + *megas,* large] An abnormal enlargement of the cell nucleus.

karyomere (kăr′ē-ō-mēr″) [″ + *meros,* part] **1.** Chromomere. **2.** A vesicle containing only a small portion of the nucleus.

karyomicrosome (kăr″ē-ō-mī′krō-sōm) [″ + *mikros,* small, + *soma,* body] Any one of the small particles or segments of chromatin in the nucleoplasm. **2.** Any one of the small tangible bodies or segments of chromatin fiber.

karyomitosis (kăr″ē-ō-mī-tō′sĭs) [″ + *mitos,* thread, + *osis,* condition] Karyokinesis.

karyomorphism (kăr-ē-ō-mor′fĭzm) [″ + *morphe,* form, + *-ismos,* state of] The form of a cell nucleus.

karyon (kăr′ē-ŏn) [Gr.] The nucleus of a cell.

karyophage (kăr′ē-ō-fāj) [Gr. *karyon,* kernel, + *phagein,* to eat] An intracellular protozoan parasite that destroys the nucleus of a cell.

karyopyknosis (kăr″ē-ō-pĭk-nō′sĭs) [″ + *pyknos,* thick, + *osis,* condition] Shrinkage of the nucleus of the cell with condensation of the chromatin.

karyorrhexis (kăr″ē-ō-rĕk′sĭs) [″ + *rhexis,* rupture] Fragmentation of the chromatin in nuclear disintegration.

karyosome (kăr′ē-ō-sōm) [″ + *soma,* body] Irregular clumps of nondividing chromatin material seen in the nuclei of cells. SYN: *chromocenter.*

karyostasis (kăr″ē-ŏs′tă-sĭs) [″ + *stasis,* standing] The resting stage of a cell nucleus.

karyotheca (kăr″ē-ō-thē′kă) [″ + *theke,* sheath] The enveloping membrane of a cell nucleus.

karyotype (kăr′ē-ō-tīp) [″ + *typos,* mark] A photomicrograph of the chromosomes of a single cell, taken during metaphase, when each chromosome is still a pair of chromatids. The chromosomes are then arranged in numerical order, in descending order of size. SEE: *chromosome* for illus.

karyozoic (kăr″ē-ō-zō′ĭk) [″ + *zoon,* animal] Living in the cell nucleus, as would occur with an intracellular protozoal parasite.

Kasabach-Merritt syndrome [Haig H. Kasabach, U.S. pediatrician, 1898–1943; Katherine K. Merritt, U.S. physician, b. 1886] Capillary hemangioma associated with thrombocytopenic purpura.

Kasai procedure [Morio Kasai, Japanese surgeon] A procedure performed to treat biliary atresia in the newborn. SYN: *hepatic portoenterostomy.*

Kashin-Beck disease [N. I. Kashin, Russian physician, 1825–1872; E. V. Beck (Bek)] Endemic polyarthritis limited to certain areas of Asia. It is believed to be a form of mycotoxicosis caused by eating grain contaminated with the fungus *Fusarium sporotrichiella.*

kata- [Gr. *kata,* down] Prefix meaning *down, reversing process, wrongly, back, destruction, against.* SEE: *cata-.*

katathermometer (kăt″ă-thĕr-mŏm′ĕ-ter) [″ + *therme,* heat, + *metron,* measure] A device consisting of two thermometers, one a dry bulb and the other a wet bulb. Both are heated to 110°F (43.3°C) and the time required for each thermometer to fall from 100° to 90°F (37.8° to 32.2°C) is noted. The dry bulb gives the cooling power by radiation and convection, the wet bulb by radiation, convection, and evaporation.

katayama fever A systemic allergic reaction to invasion of the body by *Schistosoma* larvae. It is marked by fevers, an urticarial rash, cough, enlargement of the lymph nodes and viscera, and eosinophilia. It is named for the Katayama River Valley in Japan, where the disease was first identified.

kathisophobia (kăth″ĭ-sō-fō′bē-ă) [Gr. *kathizein,* to sit down, + *phobos,* fear] A fear of sitting down, and subsequent inability to sit still.

katophoria (kăt″ō-fō′rē-ă) Katotropia.

katotropia (kăt″ō-trō′pē-ă) [Gr. *kata,* down, + *tropos,* a turning] A tendency of the eyeball to deviate downward. SYN: *katophoria.*

katzenjammer (kăts′ĕn-yăm′ĕr) [Ger. *katzen,* cats, + *jammer,* distress, misery] German word meaning hangover.

kava (kă′vă) [Tongan, bitter] *Piper methysticum,* a plant native to the Pacific islands, whose dried roots are used medicinally to treat anxiety and stress. It can produce stomach upset and side effects similar to those produced by alcohol. It is also known as kava kava.

kavalactone (kă′vă-lăk-tōn) A central nervous system depressant derived from the kava plant.

Kawasaki disease [Tomsaku Kawasaki, contemporary Japanese pediatrician] An acute febrile disease of children, marked acutely by fever, rashes, lymphadenopathy, and irritability, and chronically by late cardiac complications, including coronary artery aneurysms and myocardial infarction. The fever is present on the first day of the illness and may last from 1 to 3 wk. The child is irritable, lethargic, and has bilateral congestion of the conjunctivae. The oral mucosa is deep red, and strawberry tongue is prominent. Lips are dry, cracked, and red. On the third to fifth day, the palms and soles are distinctly red, the hands and feet are edematous. The skin on the tips of the fingers and toes peels in layers. A macular erythematous rash free of crusts and vesicles spreads from the extremities to the trunk. Cervical lymphadenopathy is present in the first 3 days and lasts more than 3 weeks. The disease is rarely fatal in the acute phase, but children may die suddenly from coronary artery disease some years later. This disease was previously called *mucocutaneous lymph node syndrome.* SEE: *toxic shock syndrome; Nursing Diagnoses Appendix.*

EPIDEMIOLOGY: In 80% of the children, diagnosis takes place before age 5, and usually the younger the age at onset, the more severe the disease. In Japan, the incidence is 67 out of every 100,000 children under age 5, which is the equivalent of 5000 to 6000 cases annually. By comparison, about 3000 cases occur annually in the U.S.

DIAGNOSIS: Because of the similarities of this disease to others (i.e., scarlet fever and toxic shock syndrome), diagnostic criteria are strict. There must be fever and at least four of the following five findings: conjunctivitis; oral lesions like those described above; redness, swelling, and peeling of the fingers and toes; rash similar to that described above; cervical lymphadenopathy.

ETIOLOGY: Although the clinical presentation suggests an infectious etiology, none has been found as yet.

COMPLICATIONS: Formation of giant aneurysms of the coronary artery (esp. in infants and very young children) is the major complication and can lead to sudden death or myocardial infarction later in life. Other findings may include arthritis, otitis media, diarrhea, uveitis, pyelonephritis (sterile), and hepatic dysfunction.

TREATMENT: If given within 10 days of onset of fever, high-dose intravenous immunoglobulin (IVIG) therapy over 12 to 24 hours can dramatically relieve the symptoms and prevent coronary artery dilation. Daily aspirin therapy will also decrease the risk of coronary artery dilation but must be continued for about a year. Antibiotics are not useful, and corticosteroids have not been used since the introduction of IVIG therapy. Frequent follow-up care, including repeat echocardiograms to detect or monitor heart disease, is essential.

PATIENT CARE: Medications are administered as prescribed, and the child is observed for salicylate toxicity. Both child and family benefit from psychological support during the acute period of illness and require continued support through the chronic phase. Parents learn about aspirin administration, the importance of following the prescribed regimen, and early signs of toxicity. The child requires careful monitoring during the acute phase and conscientious follow-up thereafter. The child's progress is monitored; parents must understand the importance of normal activity, sound nutrition, and good hygiene. The family may have difficulty facing the possibility of the child's death from coronary thrombosis or severe scar formation and stenosis of the main coronary artery. Referral to a mental health practitioner or spiritual counselor may assist them in dealing with this possibility.

Kayser-Fleischer ring A pigmented ring seen within the limbus of patients with Wilson's disease and some other liver disorders. SEE: *Wilson's disease.*

KBr Potassium bromide.

kc *kilocycle.*

K cells A type of T lymphocyte activated by an antigen-antibody reaction that directly lyses (kills) infected cells.

$KC_2H_3O_2$ Potassium acetate.

KCl Potassium chloride.

KClO Potassium hypochlorite.

$KClO_3$ Potassium chlorate.

K_2CO_3 Potassium carbonate.

kc.p.s., kc/s *kilocycles per second.*

KED *Kendrich extrication device.*

K-edge In radiography, the sharp increase in characteristic x-ray production resulting when the incoming x-ray beam matches the K-shell-binding energy of an atom. K-edge production can cause problems in predicting radiation exposure, i.e., when kilovolts peak is decreased and the K-edge is matched by the incoming x-ray photons, image density may increase.

keep vein open ABBR: kvo. An order indicating that the patency of an intubated vessel be maintained so that subsequent intravenous (IV) solutions or medicines can be administered. This is done using the lowest possible infusion rate.

kefir, kefyr (kĕf'ĕr) [Caucasus region of Russia] A preparation of curdled milk made originally in the Caucasus by adding kefir grains to milk.

Kegel exercise [A. H. Kegel, contemporary U.S. physician] An exercise for strengthening the pubococcygeal and levator ani muscles. The patient should repeatedly and rapidly alternate contracting and relaxing the muscles for 10 seconds; relax for 20 seconds, then sustain the contraction for 10 to 20 seconds; the patient should then rest for 10 seconds and repeat the routine until fatigued. The number of repetitions should be increased gradually to 150 per day. SEE: *incontinence, stress urinary.*

Kehr's sign (kĕrz) [Hans Kehr, German surgeon, 1862–1916] Pain that radiates into the shoulder during respiration. The sign points to a diaphragmatic or peridiaphragmatic lesion.

Keith's bundle, Keith's node (kēths) [Sir Arthur Keith, Brit. anatomist, 1866–1955] Sinoatrial node of the heart.

Keith-Wagener-Barker classification Classification of the funduscopic findings in hypertensive patients. Grades 1 to 4 indicate progressive pathological changes. Grade 1 is moderate narrowing of the retinal arterioles; grade 2 indicates retinal hemorrhages in addition to arteriolar narrowing; in grade 3 there are cotton-wool exudates; grade 4 shows papilledema, that is, edema of the optic disk.

kelis (kē'lĭs) [Gr., blemish] Keloid.

Kell blood group One of the human blood groups. It is composed of three forms of antigens present on the surface of the red blood cells. SEE: *blood group.*

keloid (kē'lŏyd) [Gr. *kele,* tumor, + *eidos,* form, shape] An exuberant scar that forms at the site of an injury (or an incision) and spreads beyond the borders of the original lesion. The scar is made up of a swirling mass of collagen fibers and fibroblasts. Grossly it appears to have a shiny surface and a rubbery consistency. The most common locations for keloid formation are on the shoulders, chest, and back. SEE: illus.

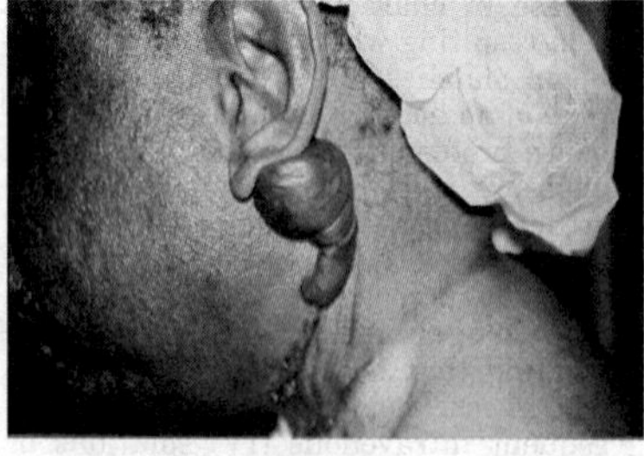

KELOIDS

TREATMENT: The injection of a corticosteroid sometimes helps the lesion regress. Freezing the tissue with liquid nitrogen, applying pressure dressings, treating it with lasers, excising it surgically, or a combination of these treatments, may be used, but recurrences are frequent.

acne k. A keloid that develops at the site of an acne pustule.

keloidosis (kē"loy-dō'sĭs) [" + " + *osis,* condition] The formation of keloids.

kelotomy (kē-lŏt'ō-mē) [" + *tome,* incision] An operation for strangulated hernia through tissues of the constricting neck.

kelp **1.** Any member of the brown seaweeds of the order Laminariales. **2.** The ash of seaweed from which potassium and iodine salts are prepared.

Kelvin scale [Lord (William Thompson) Kelvin, Brit. physicist, 1824–1907] ABBR: K. The temperature scale in which absolute zero is equal to minus 273° on the Celsius scale. On the Kelvin scale the freezing point of water is 273°K, and the boiling point 373°K.

Kempner rice-fruit diet (kĕmp'nĕr) [Walter Kempner, U.S. physician, b. 1903] A rigid salt-restriction diet used in treating hypertension. It consists of rice, fruit, and sugar for no more than 2000 kcal/day and 7 mEq of sodium per day.

Kendrick Extrication Device ABBR: KED. A vest-type immobilizer designed to limit movement of the cervical and thoracic spine in seated patients with suspected spinal cord injuries.

Kenny treatment [Sister Elizabeth Kenny, Australian nurse, 1886–1952] Type of physical therapy that was used to treat poliomyelitis. The regimen consisted of application of hot, moist packs to affected muscles and early re-education of muscles, first through passive exercise and then by active movements as soon as possible. Rigid fixation of paralyzed limbs was discouraged.

kenophobia (kĕn"ō-fō'bē-ă) [Gr. *kenos,* empty, + *phobos,* fear] A fear of empty spaces.

Kent's bundles [Albert Frank Stanley Kent, Brit. physiologist, 1863–1958] Accessory conduction fiber bundles in the heart which rapidly convey atrial impulses across the atrioventricular tissue. They are usually present in the Wolff-Parkinson-White syndrome.

kerasin (kĕr'ă-sĭn) A cerebroside isolated from brain tissue.

keratalgia (kĕr"ă-tăl'jē-ă) [Gr. *keras,* horn, + *algos,* pain] Neuralgia of the cornea.

keratectasia (kĕr"ă-tĕk-tā'sē-ă) [" + *ektasis,* extension] Conical protrusion of the cornea.

keratectomy (kĕr-ă-tĕk'tō-mē) [" + *ektome,* excision] Excision of a portion of the cornea.

photorefractive k. ABBR: PRK. The

removal of microscopic layers of corneal cells and the resculpting of the cornea with an excimer laser. The procedure is used to correct myopia. Its complications may include corneal haze, keratitis, retinal tears, and a delay in refractive stabilization.

Only one eye is treated at a time. This allows the patient to function during the 24 to 48 hours that the corrected eye may be covered. Frequently, the treated patient does not need glasses after the procedure.

CAUTION: Potential complications include corneal swelling, double vision, shadow images, light sensitivity, tearing, and pupil enlargement. Possible long-term adverse effects are as follows: anterior stromal reticular haze, glare, halo, loss of previously corrected vision, improper correction, induced astigmatism, increased intraocular pressure, and night vision difficulties.

keratiasis (kĕr-ă-tī′ă-sĭs) [″ + *-iasis,* condition] Horny wart formations on the skin.

keratic (kĕr-ăt′ĭk) **1.** Horny. **2.** Relating to the cornea.

k. precipitates ABBR: KP. Inflammatory cells of the anterior chamber of the eye that adhere to the endothelial surface of the cornea. These precipitates are present in uveitis.

keratin (kĕr′ă-tĭn) A family of durable protein polymers that are found only in epithelial cells. They provide structural strength to skin, hair, and nails. The fibrous protein is produced by keratinocytes and may be hard or soft.

hard k. Keratin found in the hair and nails.

soft k. Keratin found in the epidermis of the skin as the flexible, tough stratum corneum in the form of flattened non-nucleated scales which slough continually.

keratinase (kĕr′ă-tĭ-nās) An enzyme that hydrolyzes the protein keratin.

keratinization The process of keratin formation that takes place within the keratinocytes as they progress upward through the layers of the epidermis of skin to the surface stratum corneum. This process may occur normally on moist oral mucosa during chewing. Pathological changes (keratoses) may occur due to an autosomal dominant gene, or environmental trauma (e.g., the heat or toxins of tobacco or other carcinogens).

keratinize (kĕr′ă-tĭn-īz) [Gr. *keras,* horn] To become hard or horny; usually said of tissue.

keratinocyte (kĕ-răt′ĭ-nō-sīt) [″ + *kytos,* cell] Any one of the cells in the skin that synthesize keratin.

cultured k. Keratinocytes that are grown in the laboratory so that a small biopsy sample from uninjured skin may grow as a sheet and expand to have a surface area 1,000 to 10,000 times the area of the sample. The sheet can be used to cover wounds such as burns. The culture technique requires 2 to 3 wk and the regeneration of tissue below the sheet may not be complete for 5 to 6 months.

keratinous (kĕr-ăt′ĭ-nŭs) Pert. to or composed of keratin.

keratitis (kĕr-ă-tī′tĭs) [″ + *itis,* inflammation] Inflammation and ulceration of the cornea, which is usually associated with decreased visual acuity. Eye pain, tearing, and light sensitivity are the most common symptoms.

ETIOLOGY: The inflammation may be caused by microorganisms, trauma, drugs, vitamin A deficiency, exposure, or immune-mediated reactions.

TREATMENT: Therapy depends upon the underlying cause. Infections respond to antibacterial medications, while exposure keratitis, as in Bell's palsy, is preventable with topical lubricants.

PATIENT CARE: Because of the seriousness of this condition, patients experiencing eye inflammation or pain should seek immediate medical attention. The patient is assessed for a history of recent upper respiratory infection accompanied by cold sores; pain; central vision loss; sensitivity; the sensation of a foreign body in the eye; photophobia, and blurred vision. The eye is inspected for loss of normal corneal luster and inflammation. A slit lamp examination is often used for optimal viewing of the eye. The patient should refrain from rubbing the eye, which can cause complications. Prescribed therapies are administered, and the patient is instructed in their use. Warm compresses are applied as prescribed to relieve pain. If the patient complains of photophobia, the use of dim lighting or sunglasses is recommended. The patient should follow the prescribed treatment regimen carefully for the entire course and return for follow-up examination. In patient-teaching, the correct instillation of prescribed eye medications and the importance of thorough handwashing are emphasized. A well-balanced diet is recommended because nutritional deficiencies can increase susceptibility to this condition. Stress, traumatic injury, fever, colds, and overexposure to the sun may trigger flare-ups. Both patient and family are taught about safety precautions pertaining to visual sensory or perceptual alterations.

They are encouraged to verbalize their fears and concerns. Appropriate information and emotional support and reassurance are provided.

CAUTION: Because many common forms of keratitis are infectious, examiners should use standard precautions during the evaluation of the eye.

band-shaped k. A white or gray band extending across the cornea.

k. bullosa The formation of large, quite resistant blebs with increased tension in the cornea of blind trachomatous eyes.

chlamydial k. Corneal ulcerations that accompany chlamydial infection of the conjuctiva.

dendritic k. Superficial branching corneal ulcers.

k. disciformis A gray, disk-shaped opacity in the middle of the cornea.

exposure k. Ulceration of the cornea that results from inadequate protection of the eye by the eyelids, as in Bell's palsy.

fascicular k. A corneal ulcer resulting from phlyctenules that spread from limbus to the center of cornea accompanied by fascicle of blood vessels.

herpetic k. Vesicular keratitis in herpes zoster or herpes simplex infections.

hypopyon k. A serpent-like ulcer with pus in the anterior chamber of the eye.

interstitial k. A deep form of nonsuppurative keratitis with vascularization, occurring usually in syphilis and rarely in tuberculosis. It commonly occurs between ages 5 and 15. Symptoms include pain, photophobia, lacrimation, and loss of vision. SYN: *parenchymatous k.*

lagophthalmic k. Drying due to air exposure of the cornea resulting from a defective closure of the eyelids.

mycotic k. Keratitis produced by fungi.

neuroparalytic k. The dull and slightly cloudy insensitive cornea seen in lesions of the fifth nerve. SYN: *neurotrophic k.*

neurotrophic k. Neuroparalytic k.

parenchymatous k. Interstitial k.

phlyctenular k. Circumscribed inflammation of the conjunctiva and cornea accompanied by the formation of small projections called phlyctenules, which consist of accumulations of lymphoid cells. The phlyctenules soften at the apices, forming ulcers. SEE: *phlyctenular k.*

punctate k. Cellular deposits on the posterior surface of the cornea seen in diseases of the uveal tract.

purulent k. Keratitis with the formation of pus.

sclerosing k. A triangular opacity in the deeper layers of the cornea, associated with scleritis.

superficial punctate k. Small gray spots in the superficial layers of the cornea beneath Bowman's membrane. This occurs in young persons.

trachomatous k. A form of chlamydial keratitis. SEE: *pannus.*

traumatic k. Keratitis caused by a wound of the cornea.

xerotic k. Softening, desiccation, and ulceration of cornea resulting from dryness of the conjunctiva.

kerato-, kerat- [Gr. *keras*, horn] Combining form indicating *horny substance* or *cornea.*

keratoacanthoma (kĕr″ă-tō-ăk″ăn-thō′mă) [″ + *akantha*, thorn, + *oma*, tumor] A common benign tumor that has a mound-shaped body with a central keratin-filled crater. The lesion clinically and histologically resembles squamous cell carcinoma of the skin, and may be related to this cancer. SEE: illus.

TREATMENT: Spontaneous healing of the tumor is common. Lesions that do not heal on their own can be surgically excised.

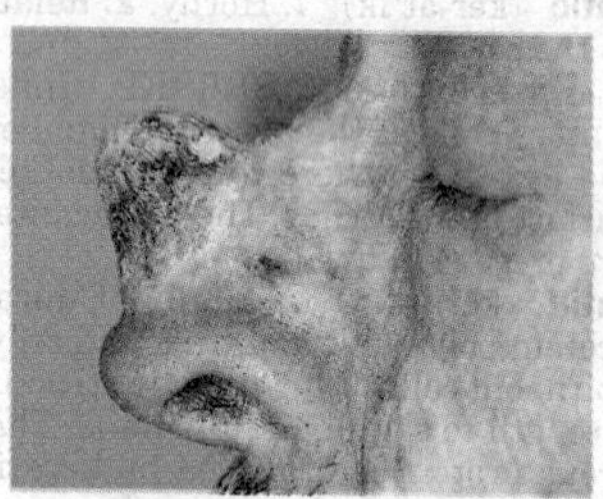

KERATOACANTHOMA

keratocele (kĕr-ăt′ō-sēl) [″ + *kele*, tumor, swelling] The protrusion or herniation of Descemet's membrane through a weakened or absent corneal stroma as a result of injury or ulcer.

keratoconjunctivitis (kĕr″ă-tō-kŏn-jŭnk″tĭ-vī′tĭs) Inflammation of the cornea and the conjunctiva.

epidemic k. An acute, self-limited keratoconjunctivitis caused by a highly infectious adenovirus.

flash k. Painful keratoconjunctivitis resulting from exposure of the eyes to intense ultraviolet irradiation. Arc welders whose eyes are not properly protected will develop this acute condition.

phlyctenular k. A delayed hypersensitivity response (type IV) to antigens in the conjunctiva. The disease may be caused by *Chlamydia*, *Mycobacterium tuberculosis*, and *Staphylococcus aureus*. Symptoms include pain and photophobia; in severe cases, perforation of the cornea can occur. Treatment depends on the underlying cause.

k. sicca Dryness with hyperemia of the conjunctiva in Sjögren's syndrome owing to autoimmune-mediated decreased lacrimal function. The corneal epithelium may be thickened and visual acuity impaired. The condition is treated by use of artificial tears and other ocular lubricants. SYN: *dry eye; xerophthalmia*. SEE: *Schirmer's test; Sjögren's syndrome*.

keratoconus (kĕr-ă-tō-kō'nŭs) [" + *konos,* cone] Conical protrusion of the center of the cornea with blurring of vision, but without inflammation. This occurs most often in persons aged 20–60, and is often an inherited disease.

keratocyte (kĕr'ă-tō-sīt) **1.** A corneal connective tissue cell. **2.** A spiculated or spindle-shaped red blood cell, sometimes seen in peripheral blood smears in patients with hemolytic anemias.

keratoderma (kĕr"ă-tō-dĕr'mă) [" + *derma,* skin] A localized or disseminated disease of the horny layer of the skin.

k. blennorrhagicum Prominent hyperkeratotic scaling lesions of the palms, soles, and penis; around the nails; and occasionally in other areas. This condition is associated with Reiter's syndrome.

k. climactericum Hyperkeratosis of the palms and soles of women, which may occur during menopause.

keratodermatitis (kĕr"ă-tō-dĕr"mă-tī'tĭs) [" + " + *itis,* inflammation] Inflammation of the horny layer of the skin with proliferation.

keratodermia Hypertrophy of the stratum corneum or horny layer of the epidermis, esp. on the palms of hands and soles of feet, producing a horny condition of the skin. SYN: *hyperkeratosis*.

keratogenous (kĕr-ă-tŏj'ĕ-nŭs) [" + *gennan,* to produce] Causing horny tissue development.

keratoglobus (kĕr"ă-tō-glō'bŭs) [" + L. *globus,* circle] A globular protrusion and enlargement of the cornea, seen in congenital glaucoma.

keratohelcosis (kĕr"ă-tō-hĕl-kō'sĭs) [" + *helkosis,* ulceration] Corneal ulceration.

keratohemia (kĕr"ă-tō-hē'mē-ă) [" + *haima,* blood] Deposits of blood in the cornea.

keratohyalin The precursor of keratin, present in the form of granules in the cytoplasm of cells in the stratum granulosum of keratinized mucosa or epidermis of the skin.

keratoid (kĕr'ă-toyd) [" + *eidos,* form, shape] Horny; resembling corneal tissue.

keratoiditis (kĕr"ă-toyd-ī'tĭs) [" + " + *itis,* inflammation] Inflammation of the cornea.

keratoiritis (kĕr"ă-tō-ī-rī'tĭs) [" + *iris,* iris, + *itis,* inflammation] Inflammation of the cornea and iris.

keratoleptynsis (kĕr"ă-tō-lĕp-tĭn'sĭs) [" + *leptynein,* to make thin] A cosmetic operation performed on a sightless eye. The procedure involves removing the corneal surface and covering the area with bulbar conjunctiva.

keratoleukoma (kĕr"ă-tō-lū-kō'mă) [" + *leukos,* white, + *oma,* tumor] White corneal opacity.

keratolysis (kĕr-ă-tŏl'ĭ-sĭs) [" + *lysis,* dissolution] **1.** A loosening of the horny layer of the skin. **2.** Shedding of the skin at regular intervals.

pitted k. Hyperkeratotic areas of the soles and palms with erosion and pitting. The etiology is unknown but may involve infection with *Corynebacterium* or *Actinomyces*. It occurs mostly in barefooted adults in the tropics.

keratolytic (kĕr"ă-tō-lĭt'ĭk) **1.** Relating to or causing keratolysis. SYN: *desquamative*. **2.** An agent that causes or promotes keratolysis.

keratoma (kĕr"ă-tō'mă) [" + *oma,* tumor] Keratosis (2).

keratomalacia (kĕr"ă-tō-mă-lā'shē-ă) [" + *malakia,* softness] Softening of the cornea seen in early childhood owing to deficiencies of vitamin A. SYN: *xerotic keratitis*.

keratome (kĕr'ă-tōm) [" + *tome,* incision] A knife for incising the cornea. SYN: *keratotome*.

keratometer (kĕr-ă-tŏm'ĕ-ter) [" + *metron,* measure] An instrument for measuring the curves of the cornea that is used to prepare conact lenses.

keratometry (kĕr"ă-tŏm'ĕ-trē) [" + *metron,* measure] Measurement of the cornea.

keratomileusis (kĕr"ă-tō-mĭ-loo'sĭs) [" + *smileusis,* carving] Plastic surgery of the cornea in which a portion is removed and frozen and its curvature reshaped; then it is reattached to the cornea.

laser-assisted in-situ k. A surgical treatment for nearsightedness, farsightedness, and other refractive errors of vision. In this procedure, a microtome is used to cut a thin flap on the surface of the cornea and a laser is used to resculpt the deeper tissue and correct refractive errors. Many patients have a marked improvement in their visual acuity as a result of the procedure. Complications can include infections, hazy vision, double vision, visual halos, the need for reoperation, corneal burns requiring corneal transplant, and blindness.

keratomycosis (kĕr"ă-tō-mī-kō'sĭs) [" + *mykes,* fungus, + *osis,* condition] Fungal infection of the cornea.

keratonosis (kĕr″ŭ-tō-nō′sĭs) [″ + *nosos,* disease] Any noninflammatory disease or deformity of the horny layer of the skin.

keratonyxis (kĕr″ă-tō-nĭks′ĭs) [″ + *nyssein,* to puncture] A corneal puncture, esp. surgical puncture.

keratopathy (kĕr″ă-tŏp′ă-thē) [″ + *pathos,* disease] Any disease of the cornea.

band k. Band-shaped calcium deposits in the superficial layer of the cornea and Bowman's membrane. This occurs with chronic intraocular inflammation such as in juvenile rheumatoid arthritis, and with systemic diseases in which there is hypercalcemia.

bullous k. Blistering of the cornea, accompanied by corneal swelling.

keratoplasty (kĕr′ă-tō-plăs″tē) [″ + *plassein,* to form] Corneal grafting. The replacement of a cloudy cornea with a transparent one, typically derived from an organ donor. SEE: *lens, corneal contact.*

optic k. The removal of a corneal scar and replacement with corneal tissue.

refractive k. Treatment of myopia or hyperopia by removing a portion of the cornea, freezing it in order to reshape it surgically to correct refractive error, and then replacing it after it has thawed. SEE: *keratomileusis.*

tectonic k. Use of corneal tissue to replace that lost because of trauma or disease.

keratoprosthesis A corneal implant, used to replace a clouded portion of the cornea.

keratoprotein (kĕr″ă-tō-prō′tē-ĭn) [″ + *protos,* first] The protein of the hair, nails, and epidermis. SYN: *keratin.*

keratorrhexis (kĕr″ă-tō-rĕks′ĭs) [″ + *rhexis,* rupture] Corneal rupture.

keratoscleritis (kĕr″ă-tō-sklĕr-ī′tĭs) [″ + *skleros,* hard, + *itis,* inflammation] Inflammation of both cornea and sclera.

keratoscope (kĕr′ăt-ō-skōp) [″ + *skopein,* to examine] An instrument for examination of the cornea.

keratoscopy Examination of the cornea and its reflection of light.

keratose (kĕr′ă-tōs) [Gr. *keras,* horn] Horny.

keratosis (kĕr-ă-tō′sĭs) *pl.* **keratoses** [″ + *osis,* condition] **1.** Horny growth. **2.** Any condition of the skin characterized by the formation of horny growths or excessive development of the horny growth. SYN: *keratoma.*

actinic k. A rough, sandpaper-textured, premalignant macule or papule caused by excess exposure to ultraviolet light. AKs often appear on facial skin (e.g., near the eyes, on the nose, on the ears, or the lips), the parts of the body that receive the most sunlight exposure. Prevention of AKs depends on limiting one's exposure to sunlight, beginning in childhood and continuing throughout life.

TREATMENT: Liquid nitrogen destroys these lesions and prevents them from progressing to squamous cell cancers of the skin. SYN: *solar k.* SEE: *sunscreen.*

k. follicularis Darier's disease.

k. nigricans Acanthosis nigricans.

oral k. Keratinization of the mucosa of the mouth to an unusual extent, or in locations normally not keratinized, as a result of an inherited autosomal dominant gene or the more common effect of tobacco and other carcinogens.

k. palmaris et plantaris A congenital abnormality of the palms and soles, characterized by a dense thickening of the keratin layer in these regions.

k. pharyngis Horny projections from the pharyngeal tonsils and adjacent lymphoid tissue.

k. pilaris Chronic inflammatory disorder of area surrounding the hair follicles. The etiology is unknown.

SYMPTOMS: The disorder is characterized by an accumulation of horny material at follicular orifices of persons with rough, dry skin. It is most pronounced in winter on lateral aspects of thighs and upper arms with possible extension to legs, forearms, and scalp.

TREATMENT: There is no specific therapy, but keratolytic lotions may be of some value.

k. punctata Discrete horny projections from the sweat pores of the palms and soles.

seborrheic k. A benign skin tumor that may be pigmented. It is composed of immature epithelial cells and is quite common in the elderly. Its etiology is unknown.

SYMPTOMS: Keratoid, nevoid, acanthoid, or verrucose types occur in the elderly and in those with longstanding dry seborrhea, on the face, scalp, interscapular or sternal regions, and backs of the hands. The yellow, gray, or brown sharply circumscribed lesions are covered with a firmly adherent scale, greasy or velvety on the trunk or scalp but harsh, rough, and dry on the face or hands.

TREATMENT: Thorough curettage is effective. This leaves a flat surface that becomes covered with normal skin within about one week. Pedunculated lesions can be removed surgically. Cautery may produce scarring and should not be used. SYN: *wart, seborrheic.*

k. senilis An inaccurate synonym for actinic keratosis, which is caused by accumulated ultraviolet light exposure, not by aging.

solar k. Actinic k.

keratotome (kĕr-ăt′ō-tōm) [″ + *tome,* incision] Keratome.

keratotomy (kĕr-ă-tŏt′ō-mē) Incision of the cornea.

radial k. Surgical therapy for nearsightedness. Very shallow, bloodless, hairline, radial incisions are made (e.g., using a laser) in the outer portion of the cornea where they will not interfere with vision. This allows the cornea to flatten and helps to correct the nearsightedness. About two thirds of patients undergoing this procedure will be able to eliminate the use of glasses or contact lenses.

keraunoneurosis (kĕ-raw″nō-nū-rō′sĭs) [Gr. *keraunos,* lightning, + *neuron,* nerve, + *osis,* condition] A neurosis caused by fear of a thunderstorm or stroke of lightning.

keraunophobia (kĕ-raw″nō-fō′bē-ă) [″ + *phobos,* fear] Fear of thunder and lightning.

Kerckring's folds (kĕrk′rĭngz) [Theodorus Kerckring, Dutch anatomist, 1640–1693] Circular plica.

kerectomy (kē-rĕk′tō-mē) [Gr. *keras,* horn, + *ektome,* excision] Excision of a portion of the cornea.

kerion (kē′rē-ŏn) [Gr., honeycomb] An inflamed, boggy mass that appears on the scalp of some patients with tinea capitis. It is believed to represent a hypersensitivity reaction to fungal antigens. It may result in a localized area of permanent hair loss. SEE: illus.

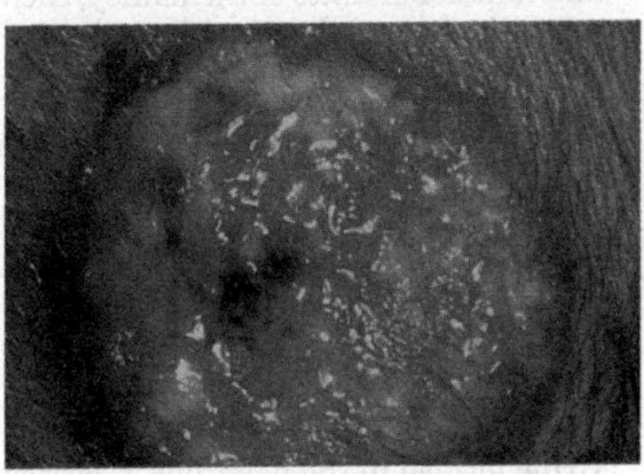

KERION

Kerley lines [P. J. Kerley, Brit. radiologist, b. 1900] Lines present on chest radiographs of patients with any disease that causes thickening or infiltration of the interlobular septa. Those in the costophrenic angle area are called Kerley B lines, and those extending peripherally from the hilum are termed Kerley A lines. Kerley C lines are fine lines in the middle of pulmonary tissue.

kerma (kĕr′mŭh) A measure of the energy imparted directly to the electrons of an atom per unit of mass.

kernicterus (kĕr-nĭk′tĕr-ŭs) [Ger.] A form of jaundice occurring in newborns during the second to eighth day after birth. The basal ganglia and other areas of the brain and spinal cord are infiltrated with bilirubin, a yellow substance produced by the breakdown of hemoglobin. The disorder is treated aggressively by phototherapy and exchange transfusion to limit neurological damage. The prognosis is quite poor if the condition is left untreated. For prevention and treatment, SEE: *erythroblastosis fetalis; hemolytic disease of the newborn; hyperbilirubinemia; icterus gravis neonatorum; phototherapy.*

Kernig's sign (kĕr′nĭgz) [Vladimir Kernig, Russ. physician, 1840–1917] A sign of meningeal irritation evidenced by reflex contraction and pain in the hamstring muscles, when attempting to extend the leg after flexing the hip.

kerosene (kĕr′ō-sēn) A flammable liquid fuel distilled from petroleum. It is used as a solvent as well as a fuel source. SEE: *Poisons and Poisoning Appendix.*

ketamine hydrochloride A nonbarbiturate medication, $C_{13}H_{16}ClNO \cdot HCl$, that is used intravenously or intramuscularly to produce anesthesia. The patient becomes cataleptic and may seem awake but is unaware of the environment and unresponsive to pain. Because the laryngeal reflexes are depressed, an endotracheal tube is used to prevent aspiration. It is used most often for diagnostic procedures and minor operations in which muscle relaxation is not required. SEE: *anesthesia, dissociative.*

PATIENT CARE: Ketamine should be administered on an empty stomach to prevent vomiting and possible aspiration and after administration of a prescribed anticholinergic to reduce salivation. The patient should reawaken in a quiet area with minimal stimulation to reduce the risk of postoperative hallucinations and delirium. Premedication with prescribed diazepam or a narcotic also may reduce the severity of symptoms during the recovery period. The patient is cautioned about the possibility of flashback-type hallucinations within 24 hr of having received ketamine anesthesia. The patient is monitored for hypertension, and respiratory status for airway patency, depressed laryngeal and pharyngeal reflexes, and respiratory depression (rare with this drug). Resuscitative equipment is made (or kept) readily available. The patient should not be discharged after recovery from anesthesia unless accompanied by a responsible adult. The patient should not drive or operate other motorized equipment for 24 hr after anesthesia.

ketoacidosis (kē″tō-ă″sĭ-dō′sĭs) [Ger. *keton,* alter. of *azeton,* acetone, + L. *acidus,* sour, + Gr. *osis,* condition] Acidosis due to an excess of ketone bodies.

ketoaciduria (kē″tō-ăs″ĭ-dū′rē-ă) [″ + ″ + Gr. *ouron,* urine] The presence of keto acids in the urine.

ketogenesis (kē-tō-jĕn′ĕ-sĭs) [″ + Gr.

genesis, generation, birth] The production of acetone or other ketones.

ketolysis (kē-tŏl′ĭ-sĭs) [″ + Gr. *lysis,* dissolution] The dissolution of acetone or ketone bodies. **ketolytic,** *adj.*

ketone (kē′tōn) A substance containing the carbonyl group (C=O) attached to two carbon atoms. Acetone, C_3H_6O, is an example of a simple ketone.

k. body SEE: under *body.*

k. threshold The level of ketone in the blood above which ketone bodies appear in the urine.

ketonemia (kē″tō-nē′mē-ă) [″ + Gr. *haima,* blood] The presence of acetone bodies in the blood, which causes the characteristic fruity breath odor in ketoacidosis.

ketonuria (kē-tō-nū′rē-ă) [″ + Gr. *ouron,* urine] Acetone bodies in the urine.

ketoplasia (kē-tō-plā′sē-ă) [″ + Gr. *plassein,* to form] The formation or excretion of ketones.

ketoplastic [″ + Gr. *plastikos,* formed] Pert. to ketoplasia or to the formation of ketones.

ketose A carbohydrate containing the ketones.

ketosis (kē-tō′sĭs) [″ + Gr. *osis,* condition] The accumulation in the body of the ketone bodies: acetone, beta-hydroxybutyric acid, and acetoacetic acid. It is frequently associated with acidosis. Ketosis results from the incomplete metabolism of fatty acids, usually from carbohydrate deficiency or inadequate use, and is commonly observed in starvation, high-fat diet, and pregnancy; following ether anesthesia; and most significantly in inadequately controlled diabetes mellitus. Large quantities of these ketone bodies may be eliminated in the urine (ketonuria). Ketosis is easily determined by testing for the presence of ketones in blood specimens. **ketotic,** *adj.*

17-ketosteroid One of a group of neutral steroids having a ketone group in carbon position 17. They are produced by the adrenal cortex and gonads and appear normally in the urine. Among them are androsterone, dehydroisoandrosterone, corticosterone, and 11-hydroxyisoandrosterone. A greater than normal or less than normal excretion in the urine is indicative of certain endocrine disorders such as adrenal adenomas or Cushing's syndrome. SEE: *perhydrocyclopentanophenanthrene.*

ketosuria (kē″tō-sū′rē-ă) Presence of ketone bodies in the urine. SEE: *ketosis.*

keV *kiloelectron volts.*

Key-Retzius foramina (kē′rĕt′zē-ŭs) [Ernst A. H. Key, Swedish physician, 1832–1901; Gustav Magnus Retzius, Swedish anatomist, 1842–1919] Passages in the pia mater carrying the choroid plexus to the fourth ventricle.

kg *kilogram.*

kg-m *kilogram-meter.*

$KHCO_3$ Potassium bicarbonate.

$KHSO_4$ Potassium bisulfate.

kHz *kilohertz.*

KI Potassium iodide.

kidney [ME. *kidenei*] One of a pair of purple-brown organs situated at the back (retroperitoneal area) of the abdominal cavity; each is lateral to the spinal column. The kidneys form urine from blood plasma. They are the major regulators of the water, electrolyte, and acid-base content of the blood and, indirectly, all body fluids.

ANATOMY: The top of each kidney is opposite the 12th thoracic vertebra; the bottom is opposite the third lumbar vertebra. The right kidney is slightly lower than the left one. Each kidney weighs 113 to 170 g (4 to 6 oz), and each is about 11.4 cm (4½ in.) long, 5 to 7.5 cm (2 to 3 in.) broad, and 2.5 cm (1 in.) thick. The kidneys in the newborn are about three times as large in proportion to body weight as they are in the adult.

Each kidney is surrounded by adipose tissue and by the renal fascia, a fibrous membrane that helps hold the kidney in place. On the medial side of a kidney is an indentation called the hilus or hilum, at which the renal artery enters and the renal vein and ureter emerge. The microscopic nephrons are the structural and functional units of the kidney; each consists of a renal corpuscle and renal tubule with associated blood vessels. In frontal section, the kidney is composed of two areas of tissue and a medial cavity. The outer renal cortex is made of renal corpuscles and convoluted tubules. The renal medulla consists of 8 to 18 wedge-shaped areas called renal pyramids; they are made of loops of Henle and collecting tubules. Adjacent to the hilus is the renal pelvis, the expanded end of the ureter within the kidney. Urine formed in the nephrons is carried by a papillary duct to the tip (papilla) of a pyramid, which projects into a cuplike calyx, an extension of the renal pelvis. SEE: illus. (Kidney).

NEPHRON: The nephron consists of a renal corpuscle and renal tubule. The renal corpuscle is made of a capillary network called a glomerulus surrounded by Bowman's capsule. The renal tubule extends from Bowman's capsule. The parts, in order, are as follows: proximal convoluted tubule, loop of Henle, distal convoluted tubule, and collecting tubule, all of which are surrounded by peritubular capillaries. SEE: illus. (Nephron and Blood Vessels).

FORMATION OF URINE: Urine is formed by filtration, reabsorption, and secretion. As blood passes through the glomerulus, water and dissolved sub-

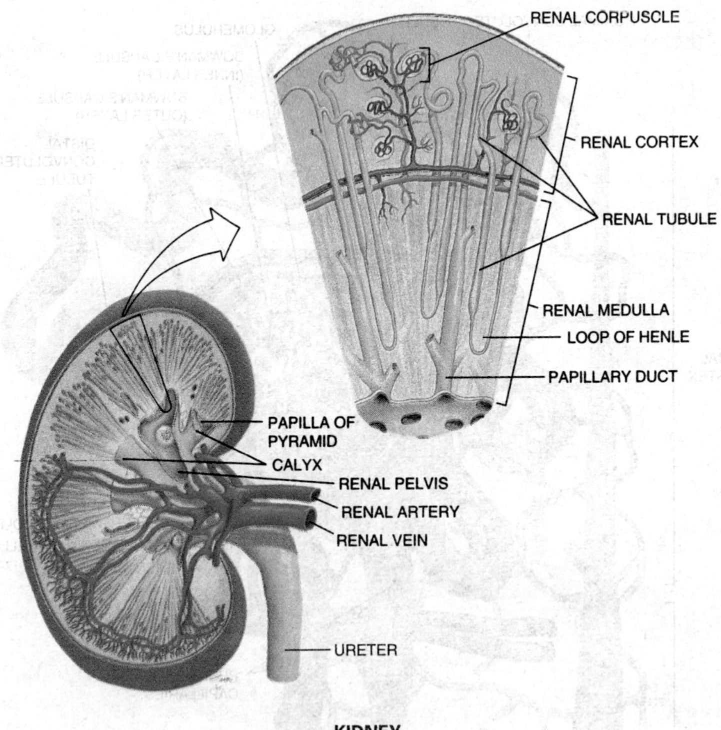

KIDNEY

Frontal section

stances are filtered through the capillary membranes and the inner or visceral layer of Bowman's capsule; this fluid is now called glomerular filtrate. Blood cells and large proteins are retained within the capillaries. Filtration is a continuous process; the rate varies with blood flow through the kidneys and daily fluid intake and loss. As the glomerular filtrate passes through the renal tubules, useful materials such as water, glucose, amino acids, vitamins, and minerals are reabsorbed into the peritubular capillaries. Most of these have a renal threshold level, that is, a limit to how much can be reabsorbed, but this level is usually not exceeded unless the blood level of these materials is above normal. Reabsorption of water is regulated directly by antidiuretic hormone and indirectly by aldosterone. Most waste products remain in the filtrate and become part of the urine. Hydrogen ions, creatinine, and the metabolic products of medications may be actively secreted into the filtrate to become part of the urine. The collecting tubules unite to form papillary ducts that empty urine into the calyces of the renal pelvis, from which it enters the ureter and is transported to the urinary bladder. Periodically the bladder is emptied (a reflex subject to voluntary control) by way of the urethra; this is called micturition, urination, or voiding. If a normally hydrated individual ingests a large volume of aqueous fluids, in about 45 minutes a sufficient quantity will have been excreted into the bladder to cause the urge to urinate. SEE: illus. (Formation of Urine).

URINE: Urine is about 95% water and about 5% dissolved substances. The dissolved materials include minerals, esp. sodium, the nitrogenous waste products urea, uric acid, and creatinine, and other metabolic end products. The volume of urine excreted daily varies from 1000 to 2000 ml (averaging 1500 ml). The amount varies with water intake, nature of diet, degree of body activity, environmental and body temperature, age, blood pressure, and many other factors. Pathological conditions may affect the volume and nature of the urine excreted. However, patients with only one kidney have been found to have normal renal function even after half of that kidney was removed because of cancer. There is no evidence that forcing fluids is detrimental to the kidneys.

NERVE SUPPLY: The nerve supply

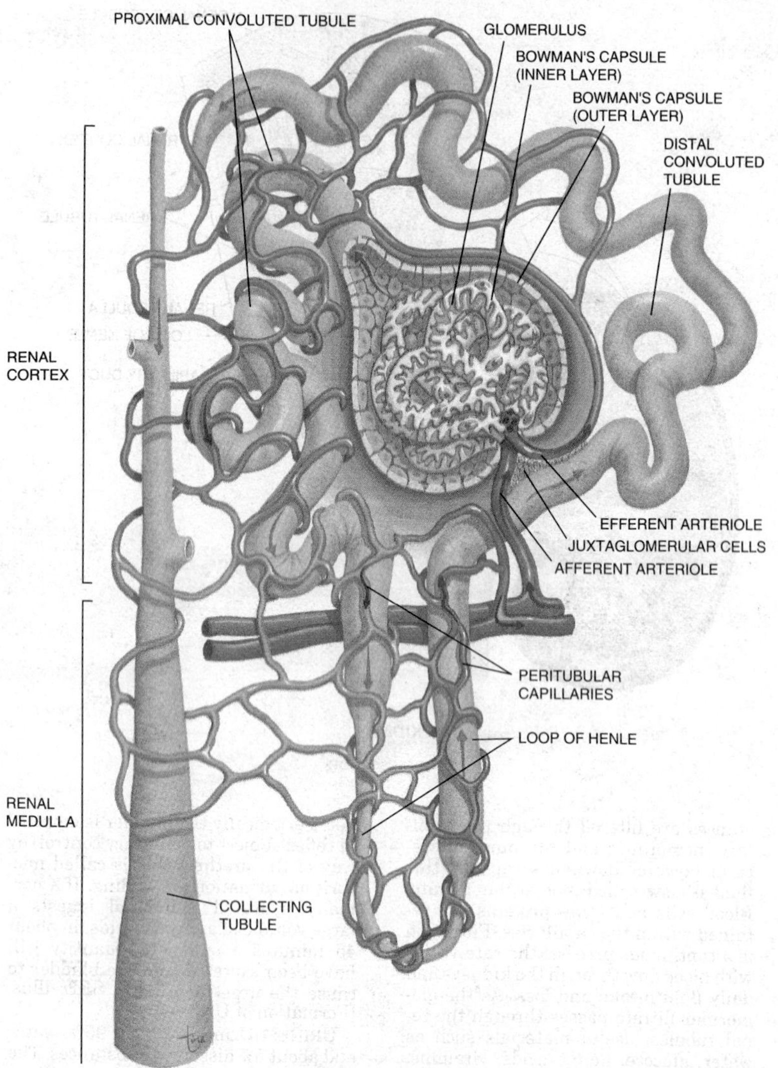

NEPHRON AND BLOOD VESSELS

consists of sympathetic fibers to the renal blood vessels. These promote constriction or dilation, esp. of arteries and arterioles.

DISORDERS: Frequently encountered diseases of the kidney include infection (pyelonephritis), stone formation (nephrolithiasis), dilation (hydronephrosis), protein loss (nephrosis), cancer (hypernephroma), and acute or chronic renal failure. SEE: *dialysis; glomerulonephritis; nephropathy; nephritis; renal failure.*

EXAMINATION: The kidneys are examined by palpation, intravenous pyelography, ultrasonography, CT scan, cystoscopy, retrograde cystoscopy, or magnetic resonance imaging. Kidney function is also frequently examined with blood tests (e.g., for electrolytes, blood urea nitrogen, and creatinine) and by urinalysis or timed collections of urine.

amyloid k. An enlarged, firm, smooth kidney usually associated with systemic amyloidosis. SYN: *waxy k.*

SYMPTOMS: Infected persons typically lose large quantities of protein in

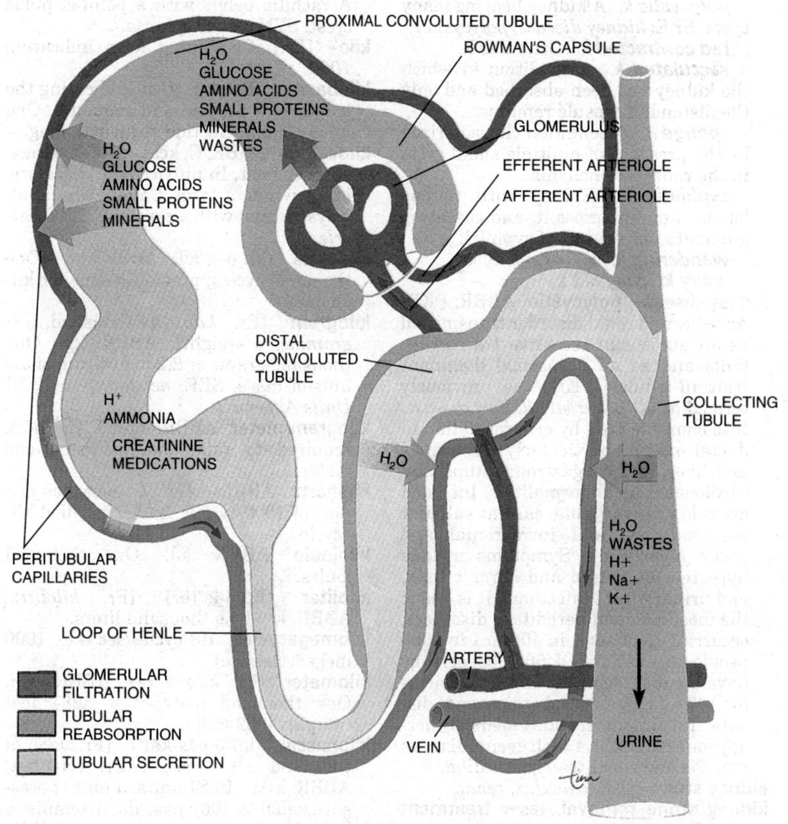

FORMATION OF URINE

the urine, and may present with edema or symptoms of fluid overload, nephrosis, or renal failure.

artificial k. Hemodialyzer.

cake k. Congenitally fused kidneys.

contracted k. The abnormally small kidney found in end-stage renal disease.

cystic k. A kidney that has undergone cystic degeneration. SEE: *polycystic kidney disease.*

embolic contracted k. A kidney in which embolic infarction of the renal arterioles produces degeneration of renal tissue and hyperplasia of fibrous tissues produces irregular contraction.

fatty k. A kidney with fatty infiltration or degeneration of tubular, glomerular, or capsular epithelium, or of vascular connective tissue.

flea-bitten k. A kidney with small petechiae covering the surface, a pathological finding in bacterial endocarditis, and some other systemic illnesses.

floating k. A kidney that is displaced and movable.

fused k. A condition in which the kidneys are joined into one anomalous organ.

Goldblatt k. A kidney with impaired blood supply and resultant hypertension; named after the U.S. physician Harry Goldblatt, who produced the same type of kidney experimentally in animals.

granular k. A slow form of chronic nephritis characterized by diminishing size; by redness; and by a hard, fibrous, and granular texture. SYN: *red contracted k.*

horseshoe k. A congenital malformation in which the superior or inferior extremities are united by an isthmus of renal or fibrous tissue, forming a horseshoe shape.

hypermobile k. A freely movable kidney. SYN: *wandering k.*

movable k. A kidney that is not firmly attached owing to lack of support of fatty tissue and perinephric fascia. SYN: *nephroptosis.*

polycystic k. A kidney bearing many cysts. SEE: *kidney disease, polycystic.*

red contracted k. Granular k.

sacculated k. A condition in which the kidney has been absorbed and only the distended capsule remains.

sponge k. A condition characterized by the presence of multiple small cysts in the renal parenchyma.

syphilitic k. Kidney with fibrous bands running across it, and caseating gummata, as a result of syphilis.

wandering k. Hypermobile k.

waxy k. Amyloid k.

kidney disease, polycystic ABBR: PKD. An inherited renal disorder transmitted as an autosomal recessive trait in infants and as an autosomal dominant trait in adults. PKD was previously termed *adult polycystic kidney disease.* It is characterized by cyst formation in ductal organs, particularly the kidney and liver, and by gastrointestinal and cardiovascular abnormalities. Included are colonic diverticula, cardiac valvular abnormalities, and intracranial and aortic aneurysms. Symptoms include hypertension, acute and chronic pain, and urinary tract infections. It is one of the most common hereditary disorders, occurring in about 1 in 400 to 1 in 1000 people. An estimated 500,000 persons have the disease in the U.S. It accounts for 10% of cases of end-stage renal disease. Treatment includes medical therapy for renal failure with eventual renal dialysis and renal transplantation.

kidney stone SEE: *calculus, renal.*

kidney stone removal, laser treatment for The use of a laser to disintegrate renal calculi. A fiberoptic device is inserted via the urethra, bladder, and ureter to the calculus. The laser is activated and the stone is destroyed without injuring adjacent tissues. SEE: *extracorporeal shock-wave lithotriptor.*

Kienböck's disease (kēn′běks) [Robert Kienböck, Austrian physician, 1871–1953] Osteochondrosis or slow degeneration of the lunate bone of the wrist; usually resulting from trauma. Radiographic evidence includes sclerosis and collapse of the lunate. Treatment goals are to reduce pain, maintain motion, and prevent carpal collapse and ultimately arthritis.

Kiernan's space (kēr′nănz) [Francis Kiernan, Brit. physician, 1800–1874] Any of the spaces between the lobes of the liver.

Kiesselbach's area (kē′sěl-bŏks) [Wilhelm Kiesselbach, Ger. laryngologist, 1839–1902] A rich network of veins on the anteroinferior portion of the nasal septum. Because of its abundant supply of capillaries, it is a common site of nosebleed.

Kilian's pelvis (kĭl′ē-ănz) [Hermann F. Kilian, Ger. gynecologist, 1800–1863] A rachitic pelvis with a pointed pubic crest. SYN: *pelvis spinosa.*

kilo- [Fr.] Combining form indicating *1000.*

kilobase ABBR: kb. Unit indicating the length of a nucleic acid sequence. One kb is 1000 nucleotide sequences long.

kilocalorie ABBR: C, kcal. A unit of measure for heat. In nutrition, a kilocalorie is known as a large Calorie and is always written with a capital C. SEE: *calorie.*

kilocycle (kĭl′ō-sī″k′l) ABBR: kc. One thousand cycles; previous name for kilohertz.

kilogram [Fr. *kilo,* a thousand, + *gramme,* a weight] ABBR: kg. One thousand grams or 2.2 lb avoirdupois. A unit of mass. SEE: *newton; pascal; SI Units Appendix.*

kilogram-meter ABBR: kg-m. The work required to raise one kilogram one meter.

kilohertz ABBR: kHz. In electricity, a unit of 1000 cycles; formerly called kilocycle.

kilojoule ABBR: kJ. One thousand joules.

kiloliter (kĭl′ō-lē″tĕr) [Fr. *kilolitre*] ABBR: kl. One thousand liters.

kilomegacycles 10^9 cycles/sec (i.e., 1000 megacycles/sec).

kilometer [Fr. *kilometre*] ABBR: km. One thousand meters, or 3281 feet (roughly 0.62 mile).

kilopascal (kĭl″ō-păs-kăl′) [Fr. *kilo,* a thousand, + *Pascal,* Fr. scientist] ABBR: kPa. In SI units, a unit of pressure equal to 1000 pascals. Attempts to have blood pressure expressed in kPa have not been accepted. SEE: *pascal.*

kilounit (kĭl″ō-ū′nĭt) One thousand units.

kilovolt [Fr. *kilo,* a thousand, + *volt*] ABBR: kV. One thousand volts.

kilovoltage peak ABBR: kVp. The highest voltage occurring during an electrical cycle.

kilowatt ABBR: kW. A unit of electrical energy equal to 1000 watts.

Kimmelstiel-Wilson syndrome [Paul Kimmelstiel, Ger. physician, 1900–1970; Clifford Wilson, Brit. physician, b. 1906] A syndrome that may develop in patients in whom diabetes mellitus has been present for several years. Hypertension, glomerulonephrosis, edema, and retinal lesions are present and arteriosclerosis of the renal artery is a common complication. SEE: *diabetes.*

kinanesthesia (kĭn-ăn-ĕs-thē′zē-ă) [Gr. *kinesis,* movement, + *an-,* not, + *aisthesis,* sensation] The inability to perceive the extent of a movement or direction, resulting in ataxia.

kinase (kĭn′ās) An enzyme that catalyzes the transfer of phosphate from ATP to an acceptor.

cyclin-dependent k. ABBR: CDK. A

family of enzymes involved in regulation of the cell cycle. They serve as targets for pharmacological manipulation of this cycle, particularly during the unregulated proliferation of tumor cells.

myosin light chain k. An enzyme in smooth muscle cells that catalyzes the transfer of a phosphate group from adenosine triphosphate (ATP) to myosin, which initiates contraction.

protein k. SEE: *protein kinase.*

kindling The triggering of seizures as a result of repetitive low-amplitude electrical stimulation of the brain. This phenomenon is typical of seizures in persons suffering alcohol (and other forms of drug) withdrawal.

kinematics [Gr. *kinematos,* movement] The branch of biomechanics concerned with description of the movements of segments of the body without regard to the forces that caused the movement to occur. SEE: *arthrokinematics; osteokinematics.*

kinematograph (kĭn″ĕ-măt′o-grăf) A device for viewing photographs of objects in motion; used in studying the motion of organs such as the heart and lungs, and the gastrointestinal tract.

kineplastic (kĭn″ĭ-plăs′tĭk) [Gr. *kinein,* to move, + *plastikos,* formed] Pert. to kineplasty.

kineplasty A form of amputation enabling the muscles of the stump to impart motion to an artificial limb. SEE: *Boston arm; cineplastics.*

kinesalgia (kĭn″ĕ-săl′jē-ă) [Gr. *kinesis,* movement, + *algos,* pain] Pain associated with muscular movement.

kinescope (kĭn′ĕ-skōp) [″ + *skopein,* to examine] A device for testing the refraction of the eye. A slit of variable width moves as the patient observes a fixed object.

kinesia (kī-nē′sē-ă) **1.** Sickness caused by motion (e.g., seasickness, carsickness). **2.** Movement.

kinesiatrics (kĭ-nē″sē-ăt′rĭks) [″ + *iatrikos,* curative] Kinesiotherapy.

kinesics (kī-nē′sĭks) Systematic study of the body and the use of its static and dynamic position as a means of communication. SEE: *body language.*

kinesimeter (kĭn″ĕ-sĭm′ĕ-tĕr) [″ + *metron,* measure] An apparatus for determining the extent of movement of a part.

kinesiodic (kĭ-nē″sē-ŏd′ĭk) [″ + *hodos,* path] Pert. to paths through which motor impulses pass.

kinesiology (kĭ-nē″sē-ŏl′ō-jē) [″ + *logos,* word, reason] The study of muscles and body movement. SEE: *biomechanics.*

kinesioneurosis (kĭ-nē″sē-ō-nū-rō′sĭs) [″ + *neuron,* nerve, + *osis,* condition] A functional disorder marked by tics and spasms. SEE: *Tourette's syndrome.*

external k. Kinesioneurosis affecting external muscles.

vascular k. Kinesioneurosis of the vasomotor system.

visceral k. Kinesioneurosis affecting muscles of internal organs.

kinesiotherapy (kĭ-nē″sē-ō-thĕr′ă-pē) [″ + *therapeia,* treatment] A rehabilitative treatment that uses exercise or movement, formerly known as corrective therapy. This form of treatment was conceived by the Armed Forces to assist physical therapists with the large number of injured soldiers following World War II. SYN: *kinesiatrics.*

kinesis (kĭn-ē′sĭs) [Gr.] Motion.

kinesitherapy [″ + *therapeia,* treatment] Kinesiotherapy.

kinesthesia (kĭn″ĕs-thē′zē-ă) [″ + *aisthesis,* sensation] The ability to perceive extent, direction, or weight of movement. **kinesthetic,** *adj.*

kinesthesiometer (kĭn″ĕs-thē-zē-ŏm′ĕ-tĕr) [″ + ″ + *metron,* measure] An instrument for testing the ability to determine the position of the muscles.

kinetic (kĭ-nĕt′ĭk) [Gr. *kinesis,* motion] Pert. to or consisting of motion.

kinetics **1.** The branch of mechanics that examines the forces acting on the body during movement and the motion with respect to time and forces. **2.** The turnover rate or rate of change of a factor, esp. a chemical process.

kinetochore A protein disk attached to the DNA of the centromere that connects a pair of chromatids during cell division. A spindle fiber is in turn attached to the kinetochore.

kinetotherapy (kĭ-nĕt″ō-thĕr′ă-pē) [″ + *therapeia,* treatment] Kinesitherapy.

King, Imogene A nursing educator who developed the General Systems Framework and Theory of Goal Attainment. SEE: *Nursing Theory Appendix.*

Kingella (kĭng-ĕl′lăh) A genus of gram-negative, rod-shaped bacilli from the family Neisseriaceae.

kingdom [AS. *cyningdom*] The largest category in the classification of living organisms. There are five kingdoms: Procaryotae (Monera), Protista, Fungi, Plantae, and Animalia. SEE: *taxonomy.*

kinin (kī′nĭn) [Gr. *kinesis,* movement] A general term for a group of polypeptides that have considerable biological activity. They are capable of influencing smooth muscle contraction; inducing hypotension; increasing the blood flow and permeability of small blood capillaries; and inciting pain.

kininases, plasma Plasma carboxypeptidases that inactivate plasma kinins.

kininogen A substance that produces a kinin when acted on by certain enzymes.

kink [Low Ger. *kinke,* a twist in rope] An unnatural angle or bend in a duct or tube such as the intestine, umbilical cord, or ureter.

kino- (kī′nō) [Gr. *kinein,* to move] Combining form meaning *movement.*

kinocilium (kī″nō-sĭl′ē-ŭm) [″ + L. *cilium,* eyelash] Protoplasmic filament on the cell surface.

kinship (kĭn′shĭp) The descendants of a common ancestor.

Kirschner wire (kērsh′nĕr) [Martin Kirschner, Ger. surgeon, 1879–1942] Steel wire placed through a long bone in order to apply traction to the bone.

Kisch's reflex (kĭsh′ĕs) [Bruno Kisch, Ger. physiologist, 1890–1966] Closure of an eye resulting from stimulation by heat or some tactile irritant on the auditory meatus.

KJ *knee jerk.*

KK *knee kick* (knee jerk).

kl *kiloliter.*

Klatskin tumor [Gerald Klatskin, American physician, 1910–1986] A cholangiocarcinoma that arises in the large intrahepatic biliary ducts.

Klebsiella (klĕb″sē-ĕl′ă) [T. A. Edwin Klebs, Ger. bacteriologist, 1834–1913] A genus of bacteria of the family Enterobacteriaceae. These short, plump, gram-negative bacilli form capsules but not spores. They are frequently associated with respiratory infections and may cause urinary tract infections.

K. ozaenae A species found in ozena.

K. pneumoniae Friedländer's bacillus.

K. rhinoscleromatis A species that can cause rhinoscleroma, a destructive granuloma of the nose and pharynx.

Kleiger test (klĭg′ĕr) A test used to determine stability of the distal tibiofibular syndesmosis and rotatory instability of the ankle mortise. With the patient sitting with the knee flexed over the table's edge, the examiner stabilizes the patient's lower leg, slightly dorsiflexes the ankle, and externally rotates the foot. Pain along the lateral ankle indicates a sprain of the distal tibiofibular syndesmosis. Medial ankle pain or a palpable subluxation of the talus within the ankle mortise is indicative of ankle rotatory instability.

Klein-Bell ADL Scale In rehabilitation, an objectively scored measure of functional independence, which includes items related to self-care, mobility, and communication.

klepto- (klĕp′tō) [Gr. *kleptein,* to steal] Combining form meaning *stealing, theft.*

kleptolagnia (klĕp″tō-lăg′nē-ă) [″ + *lagneia,* lust] Sexual gratification derived from stealing.

kleptomania (klĕp-tō-mā′nē-ă) [″ + *mania,* madness] Impulsive stealing, the motive not being in the intrinsic value of the article to the individual. In almost all cases, the individual has enough money to pay for the stolen goods. The stealing is done without prior planning and without the assistance of others. There is increased tension before the theft and a sense of gratification while committing the act.

kleptomaniac **1.** Pert. to kleptomania. **2.** An individual who repeatedly steals objects that he or she does not need.

kleptophobia (klĕp-tō-fō′bē-ă) [″ + *phobos,* fear] Morbid fear of stealing.

Klieg eye (klēg) [after John H. Kliegl, Ger. manufacturer, 1869–1959] Conjunctivitis, lacrimation, and photophobia from exposure to the intense lights used in making motion pictures or television films.

Klinefelter's syndrome (klīn′fĕl-tĕrs) [Harry F. Klinefelter, Jr., U.S. physician, b. 1912] The most common sex chromosome syndrome, marked by primary testicular failure. The classic form is associated with the presence of an extra X chromosome. Affected persons have small, firm testes, gynecomastia, abnormally long legs, minimal body and facial hair, and infertility. In variant forms the chromosomal abnormalities vary and the severity and number of abnormal findings are diversified. The syndrome is estimated to occur in one of 500 live male births. Diagnosis may be confirmed by chromosomal analysis of tissue culture which usually demonstrates a 47, XXY genotype.

Klippel's disease (klĭ-pĕlz′) [Maurice Klippel, Fr. neurologist, 1858–1942] Weakness or pseudoparalysis due to generalized arthritis.

Klippel-Feil syndrome [Maurice Klippel; André Feil, Fr. physician, b. 1884] A congenital anomaly characterized by a short wide neck; low hairline, esp. on the back of the neck; reduction in the number of cervical vertebrae; and fusion of the cervical spine. The central nervous system also may be affected.

klismaphilia The derivation of sexual pleasure by receiving enemas.

Klumpke's paralysis (kloomp′kĕz) [Madame Augusta Déjérine-Klumpke, Fr. neurologist, 1859–1927] Atrophic paralysis of the forearm.

Klüver-Bucy syndrome [Heinrich Klüver, Ger.-born U.S. neurologist, 1897–1979; Paul C. Bucy, U. S. neurologist, b. 1904] Behavioral syndrome usually following bilateral temporal lobe removal. It is characterized by loss of recognition of people, loss of fear, rage reactions, hypersexuality, uncontrolled appetite, memory deficit, and overreaction to certain stimuli.

km *kilometer.*

kMc *kilomegacycle.*

$KMnO_4$ Potassium permanganate.

Knapp's forceps (năps) [Herman J. Knapp, U.S. ophthalmologist, 1832–1911] A forceps with roller-like blades for expressing trachomatous granulations on the palpebral conjunctiva.

kneading (nēd'ĭng) [AS. *cnedan*] Pétrissage.

knee [AS. *cneo*] **1.** The anterior aspect of the leg at the articulation of the femur and tibia and the articulation itself, covered anteriorly with the patella or kneecap. It is formed by the femur, tibia, and patella. SEE: illus. **2.** Any structure shaped like a semiflexed knee. SYN: *geniculum.*

Brodie's k. Osteomyelitis of the knee. SYN: *Brodie's abscess.*

dislocation of k. Displacement of the knee, an uncommon injury, universally complicated by tearing of the cruciate ligament, and often associated with peroneal nerve or popliteal artery damage. Dislocations should be reduced by an orthopedic surgeon as soon as is feasible to preserve circulation to the lower extremity.

game k. A lay term for internal derangement of the knee joint, characterized by pain or instability, locking, and weakness. It is usually the result of a torn internal cartilage, a fracture of the tibial spine, or an injury to the collateral or cruciate ligaments.

FIRST AID: The knee should be immobilized with a posterior splint.

DIAGNOSIS: Arthroscopy and/or magnetic resonance imaging may be necessary for a definitive diagnosis.

housemaid's k. An inflammation of the bursa anterior to the patella, with accumulation of fluid. It may be seen in those who have to kneel frequently or continually while working.

k. of internal capsule The curve at the meeting place of the anterior and posterior limbs of the internal capsule of the brain.

jumper's k. An overuse syndrome, marked by chronic inflammation and infrapatellar tendinitis, resulting from repetitive jumping or leg extension exercises. The usual treatment is nonsteroidal anti-inflammatory drugs, rest, and phonophoresis.

locked k. A condition in which the leg cannot be extended. It is usually due to displacement of meniscal cartilage.

replacement of k. Orthopedic implantation of a prosthetic knee joint, particularly useful in treating patients with severe disabling arthritis of the knee. SYN: *arthroscopy.*

runner's k. A general term describing several overuse conditions resulting from excessive running. These may involve the extensor mechanism and other musculotendinous insertions. Patellar tendinitis (jumper's knee), patellofemoral dysfunction, iliotibial band syndrome, and pes anserinus tendinitis or bursitis have all been called by this term.

kneecap Patella.

kneeling bus A specially designed bus to transport elderly persons and disabled individuals. The front of the bus can be lowered to facilitate getting on and off the bus. A ramp usually is provided to facilitate wheelchair access.

Kneipp cure, kneippism (nīp) [Rev. Father Sebastian Kneipp, Ger. priest, 1821–1897] The application of water in various forms and degrees of temperature in the cure of disease, esp. wading in cold, dewy grass. SEE: *hydrotherapy.*

knemometry (nē-mŏm'ĕt-rē) [Gr. *kneme,* shinbone, + *metron,* measure] A precise method of determining the length of a limb, esp. the lower leg. It has been used to assess infant and childhood growth and development (e.g., in premature infants or children treated with corticosteroids).

knife (nīf) [AS. *cnif*] A cutting device.

electric k. A knife that functions by use of a high-frequency cutting current.

gamma k. A radiosurgical device first used in 1968 that relies on gamma rays from radioactive cobalt to cut or excise diseased tissue, esp. in the brain. The radioactive energy emitted by the knife is focused stereotactically to limit injury to healthy tissue.

gold k. A special contra-angle knife used to trim a gold filling in a tooth.

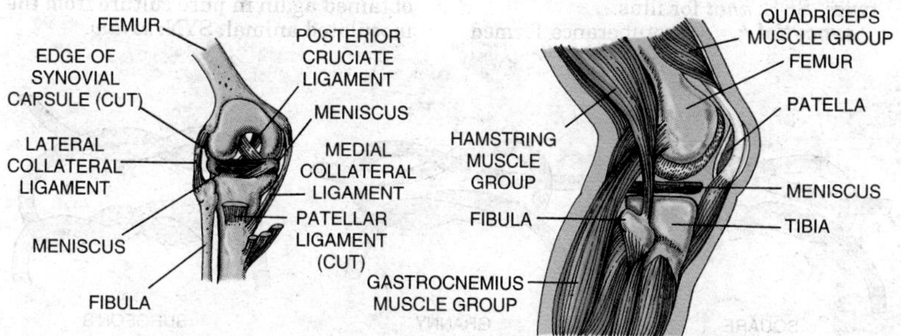

ANATOMY OF THE SUPPORTING STRUCTURES OF THE KNEE

interdental k. A double-ended knife used in periodontal surgery for removing tissue between teeth.

periodontal k. A surgical knife with a scaler-shaped blade whose entire perimeter is a cutting edge. It is used in gingivectomy and other periodontal surgery.

plaster k. A stout knife used for cutting and trimming plaster study models in dental practice.

knitting [AS. *cnyttan,* to make knots] The process of healing by uniting pieces of a fractured bone.

KNO_3 Potassium nitrate; niter; saltpeter.

knob (nŏb) [ME. *knobbe*] A protuberance on a surface or extremity; a mass or nodule.

knock-knee A condition in which knees are very close to each other and the ankles are apart. SYN: *genu valgum.*

Knoop hardness test ABBR: KHN. A test of surface hardness, using a stylus with a pyramidal diamond indenter. The long diagonal of the resulting indentation determines the hardness of the substance.

knot [AS. *cnotta*] **1.** An intertwining of a cord or cordlike structure to form a lump or knob. **2.** In surgery, the intertwining of the ends of a suture, ligature, bandage, or sling so that the ends will not slip or become separated. SEE: illus.; *square knot.* **3.** In anatomy, an enlargement forming a knoblike structure.

false k. An external bulging of the umbilical cord, resulting from the coiling of the umbilical blood vessels.

granny k. A double knot in which the ends of the cord do not lie parallel, but alternate being over and under each other. This knot is not as secure as a square knot. SEE: *knot* for illus.

Hensen's k. A knoblike structure at the anterior end of the primitive streak.

primitive k. Hensen's k.

square k. A double knot in which the ends of the second knot are in the same place as the ends of the first knot. SEE: *knot* for illus.; *square knot.*

surgeon's k. A double knot in which the cord is passed through the first loop twice. SEE: *knot* for illus.

syncytial k. A protuberance formed by many nuclei of the syntrophoblast and found on the surface of a chorionic villus.

true k. A knot formed by the fetus slipping through a loop of the umbilical cord.

knowledge deficit Lack of specific information necessary for the patient and significant other(s) to make informed choices regarding condition/therapies/treatment plan. SEE: *Nursing Diagnoses Appendix.*

knowledge, fund of Information that a person has stored in memory about people, places, and things. The fund of stored memories increases with education and decreases in dementia.

knuckle (nŭk′ĕl) [Middle Low Ger. *knokel*] Prominence of the dorsal aspect of any of the phalangeal joints, esp. of the distal heads of the metacarpals when the fist is clenched.

k. pad A discrete fibromatous pad appearing over a finger joint. It usually appears between the ages of 15 and 30. The etiology is unknown but trauma is not a significant factor.

K.O.C. *cathodal opening contraction.*

Koch, Heinrich Herman Robert (kōk) German bacteriologist, 1843–1910.

K.'s bacillus *Mycobacterium tuberculosis.*

K.'s law Koch's postulate.

K.'s phenomenon A local inflammatory reaction resulting from injection of tuberculin into the skin of a person who has been previously exposed to the tubercle bacillus. The test represents the clinical application of a type IV (delayed-type) hypersensitivity reaction. In contemporary skin tests for tuberculosis, Koch's, or "old," tuberculin has been replaced by tuberculin purified protein derivative. SEE: *tuberculosis.*

K.'s postulate The criterion used in proving an organism is the cause of a disease or lesion: the microorganism in question is regularly found in the lesions of the disease; pure cultures can be obtained from it. When inoculated into susceptible animals, pure cultures can reproduce the disease or pathological condition; and the organism can be obtained again in pure culture from the inoculated animal. SYN: *k. law.*

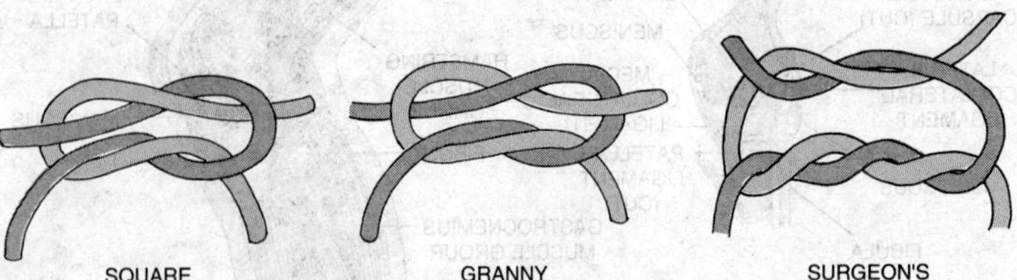

KNOTS

Koch, Walter (kōk) German surgeon, b. 1880.

K.'s node Atrioventricular node.

kocherization (kōk″ĕr-ī-zā′shŭn) An operative technique used in opening the duodenum to expose the ampulla of the common bile duct.

Kocher's reflex (kō′kĕrz) [Theodor Kocher, Swiss surgeon, 1841–1917] A contraction of abdominal muscles following moderate compression of the testicle.

Koebner phenomenon [Heinrich Koebner, Ger. dermatologist, 1838–1904] The appearance of a skin lesion as a result of nonspecific trauma (e.g., sunlight, burn, operative wound). It will appear at the trauma site and may be of a type found elsewhere on the skin. It may be seen in lichen planus or eczema but is particularly characteristic of psoriasis. The lesion must be sufficient to act on the papillary and epidermal layers of the skin and will appear in 3 to 18 days following the trauma.

KOH Symbol for potassium hydroxide.

Köhler's disease (kă′lĕrz) [Alban Köhler, Ger. physician, 1874–1947] **1.** Aseptic necrosis of the navicular bone of the wrist. **2.** Osteochondrosis of the head of the second metatarsal bone of the foot.

Kohler's syndrome Pain in the midfoot with accompanying point tenderness over the navicular bone, with increased density and narrowing of the tarsal navicular on radiographs. Most patients respond to 6 weeks' cast immobilization without long-term sequelae.

Kohlman Evaluation of Living Skills ABBR: KELS. A standard assessment for determining the ability of an individual to perform self-care and community living tasks. The assessment includes an interview and tasks that measure self-care, safety and health, money management, transportation and telephone use, and work and leisure behaviors.

Kohlrausch's fold (kōl′rowsh-ĕs) [Otto L. B. Kohlrausch, Ger. physician, 1811–1854] The rectal valve; one of the horizontal folds of the mucosa of the rectum. SYN: *Houston's valve; transverse plica of the rectum.*

Kohnstamm's phenomenon (kōn′stămz) [Oscar Kohnstamm, Ger. physician, 1871–1917] Aftermovement.

koilocyte (koy′lō-sīt) [Gr. *koilos,* hollow, + *kytos,* cell] An abnormal cell of the squamous epithelium of the cervix. It is associated with infection with human papillomavirus and the eventual development of cervical intraepithelial neoplasia.

koilocytotic atypia (koy″lō-sī-tŏt′ĭk ā-tĭp′ē-ă) [″ + ″ + *osis,* condition, + *a-,* not, + *typicalis,* typical] Abnormality of the top layers of the epithelium of the uterine cervix wherein the cells undergo vacuolization and enlargement. SEE: *koilocyte.*

koilonychia (koy-lō-nĭk′ē-ă) [″ + *onyx,* nail] Dystrophy of the fingernails in which they are thin and concave with raised edges. This condition is sometimes associated with iron-deficiency anemia. It is often called *spooning of nails.* SEE: illus.

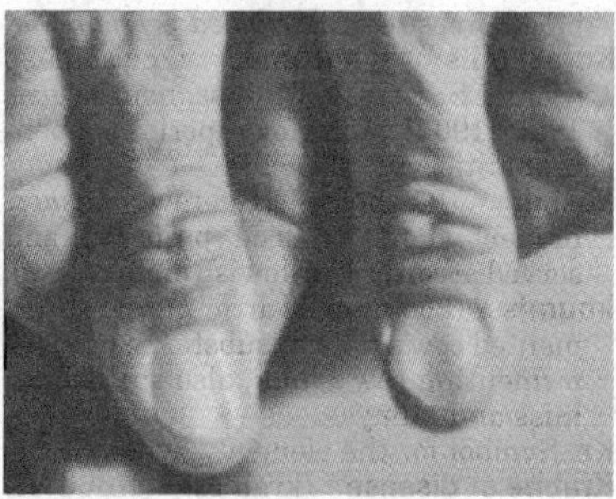

KOILONYCHIA

koilosternia (koy″lō-stĕr′nē-ă) [″ + Gr. *sternon,* sternum] Condition in which the chest has a funnel-like depression in the middle of the thoracic wall.

kolp- SEE: *colpo-.*

kolpo- SEE: *colpo-.*

Kondoleon's operation (kŏn-dō′lē-ŏnz) [Emmanuel Kondoleon, Gr. surgeon, 1879–1939] The surgical removal of layers of subcutaneous tissue to relieve elephantiasis.

koniocortex (kō″nē-ō-kor′tĕks) [Gr. *konis,* dust, + L. *cortex,* rind] The cortex of the sensory areas, so named because of its granular appearance.

koniology [″ + *logos,* word, reason] Coniology.

koniometer (kō-nē-ŏm′ĕ-ter) [″ + *metron,* measure] A device for estimating amount of dust in the air.

koniosis (kō-nē-ō′sĭs) [″ + *osis,* condition] Coniosis.

Koplik's spots [Henry Koplik, U.S. pediatrician, 1858–1927] Small red spots with blue-white centers on the oral mucosa, particularly in the region opposite the molars; a diagnostic sign in measles before the rash appears. Not infrequently, the spots disappear as the rash develops.

kopophobia (kŏp″ō-fō′bē-ă) [Gr. *kopos,* fatigue, + *phobos,* fear] Abnormal fear of fatigue or exhaustion.

Korányi's sign (kō-răn′yēz) [Friedrich von Korányi, Hung. physician, 1828–1913] Increased resonance on percussion of the dorsal spine, a sign of pleural effusion.

koro (kō′rō) In China and Southeast Asia, a phobia that the penis will retract into the abdomen (or in females, that the nipples or vulva will retract into the chest or pelvis). The individual believes that once the sexual organ disappears completely, he or she will die.

koronion (kō-rō′nē-ŏn) [Gr. *korone,* crest] Apex of coronoid process of the mandible.

Korotkoff's sounds (kō-rŏt′kŏfs) [Nikolai S. Korotkoff, Russ. physician, 1874–1920] Sounds heard in auscultation of blood pressure. SEE: *blood pressure.*

Korsakoff's syndrome (kor′să-kŏfs) [Sergei S. Korsakoff, Russ. neurologist, 1854–1900] Anterior superior polioencephalitis.

kosher (kō′shĕr) [Hebrew *kasher,* proper] Pert. to food prepared and served according to Jewish dietary laws.

koumiss (koo′mĭs) [Tartar *kumyz*] Fermented cow's milk or substance used for fermenting cow's milk; also spelled kumiss and kumyss.

Kr Symbol for the element krypton.

Krabbe's disease (krăb′ēz) [Knud H. Krabbe, Danish neurologist, 1885–1961] Globoid cell leukodystrophy due to the accumulation of galactocerebroside in the tissues, resulting from a deficiency of galactocerebrosidase. Clinically, affected infants develop seizures, deafness, blindness, cachexia, paralysis, and marked mental deficiency. Survival beyond 2 years is rare.

Kraepelin's classification (krā′pā-lĭnz) [Emil Kraepelin, Ger. psychiatrist, 1856–1926] An obsolete classification of mental illness into two groups: the manic-depressive and the schizophrenic.

krait (krāt) A small venomous snake of the genus *Bungarus,* indigenous to India.

kraurosis (krŏ-rō′sĭs) [Gr. *krauros,* dry] Atrophy and dryness of the skin and any mucous membrane, esp. of the vulva. The subcutaneous fat of the mons pubis and labia disappears, clitoris and prepuce atrophy, and stenosis of the vaginal orifice is common. Fissures may develop.

k. penis Kraurosis in which the glans penis atrophies and becomes shriveled.

k. vulvae Lichen sclerosis et atrophicus.

Krause, Karl (krowz) German anatomist, 1797–1868.

K.'s gland A small mucous acinous gland located beneath the fornix conjunctivae. This accessory lacrimal gland opens into the fornix.

K.'s valve A fold of mucous membrane of the lacrimal sac at the junction of the lacrimal duct.

Krause, Wilhelm (krowz) German anatomist, 1833–1910.

K.'s end bulb One of the widely distributed encapsulated nerve endings present superficially in the skin, cornea, and organs such as the testicles.

K.'s membrane A thin, dark disk that transversely crosses through and bisects the clear zone of a striated muscle and bisects the clear zone (isotropic disk) of a striated muscle fiber. The portion between two disks constitutes a sarcomere. SYN: *Z disk.*

Krebs cycle [Sir Hans Krebs, Ger. biochemist, 1900–1981, co-winner of a Nobel prize in 1953.] A complicated series of reactions in the body involving the oxidative metabolism of pyruvic acid and liberation of energy. It is the main pathway of terminal oxidation in the process of which not only carbohydrates but proteins and fats are utilized. SYN: *citric acid cycle; tricarboxylic acid cycle.* SEE: illus.

kringle A subunit of plasminogen consisting of 80 amino acids in a loop structure.

Krönig's area (krā′nĭgz) [Georg Krönig, Ger. physician, 1856–1911] Resonant region in the thorax over the apices of the lungs.

Krukenberg's chopsticks [Hermann Krukenberg, Ger. surgeon, 1863–1935] A condition occurring after surgical separation of the remaining ulna and radius of a forearm stump after traumatic removal of a lower arm. This allows the ulna and radius to act as crude pincers (i.e., chopsticks).

Krukenberg's tumor (kroo′kĕn-bĕrgz) [Frederick Krukenberg, Ger. pathologist, 1871–1946] A malignant tumor of the ovary, usually bilateral and frequently secondary to malignancy of the gastrointestinal tract. Histologically, these tumors consist of myxomatous connective tissue and cells having a signet ring arrangement of their nuclei. The epithelial tissue resembles malignancy of the original site.

krypton (krĭp′tŏn) [Gr. *kryptos,* hidden] SYMB: Kr. A gaseous element found in small amounts in the atmosphere; atomic weight 83.80; atomic number 36.

K_2SO_4 Potassium sulfate.

K-space In magnetic resonance imaging, the computer memory where multiecho data can be stored prior to full reconstruction of the image.

KT-2000 A testing device that measures the laxity of the anterior cruciate ligament and determines clinical instability by comparison with the normal opposite knee.

KUB *kidneys, ureters, bladder;* pert. to anteroposterior projection films of the abdomen.

kubisagari (koo-bĭs″ă-gă′rē) [Japanese, hang-head] Ptosis and bulbar weakness in nutritionally deficient children; endemic in Japan. A similar disorder was observed in prisoners of war in Japan. Parenteral administration of thiamine has been beneficial.

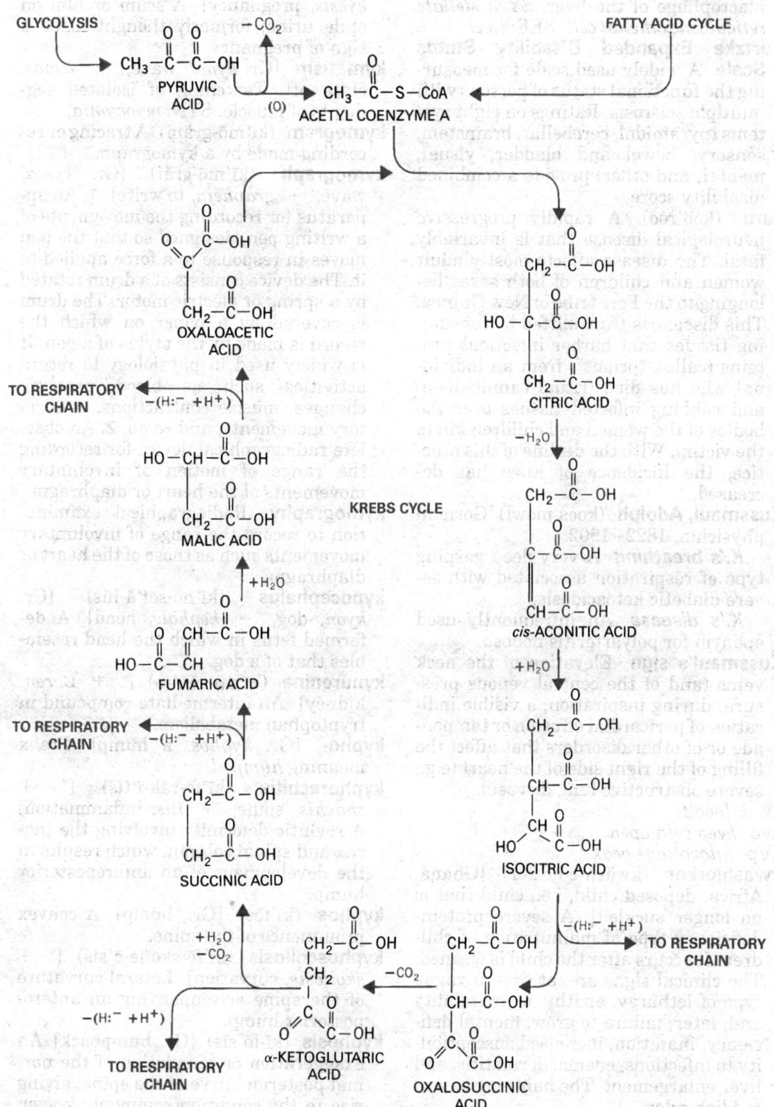

KREBS CYCLE
(TRICARBOXYLIC ACID CYCLE)

Kufs' disease [H. Kufs, Ger. psychiatrist, 1871–1955] The adult form of cerebral sphingolipidosis. The onset of symptoms is between 21 and 26 years of age. The disease is diagnosed by the development of dementia, myoclonic jerks, blindness, and retinitis pigmentosa.

Kugelberg-Welander disease [Eric Klaus Henrik Kugelberg, 1913–1983; L. Welander, b. 1909; Swedish neurologists] Juvenile spinal muscular atrophy.

kumiss, kumyss (koo'mĭs) [Tartar *kumyz*] Koumiss.

Kümmell's disease, Kümmell's spondylitis (kĭm'ĕlz) [Hermann Kümmell, Ger. surgeon, 1852–1937] Spondylitis following compression fracture of the vertebrae.

Kupffer cell (koop'fĕr) [Karl W. von

Kupffer, Ger. anatomist, 1829–1902] A macrophage of the liver. SYN: *stellate reticuloendothelial cell*. SEE: *liver*.

Kurtzke Expanded Disability Status Scale A widely used scale for measuring the functional status of persons with multiple sclerosis. Ratings on eight systems (pyramidal, cerebellar, brainstem, sensory, bowel and bladder, visual, mental, and other) provide a combined disability score.

kuru (koo′roo) A rapidly progressive neurological disease that is invariably fatal. The disease affects mostly adult women and children of both sexes belonging to the Fore tribe of New Guinea. This disease is transmitted by consuming tissues that harbor infectious proteins (called "prions") from an individual who has died (ritual cannibalism) and rubbing infected tissues over the bodies of the women and children kin to the victim. With the decline of this practice, the incidence of kuru has decreased.

Kussmaul, Adolph (koos′mowl) German physician, 1822–1902.

K.'s breathing A very deep gasping type of respiration associated with severe diabetic ketoacidosis.

K.'s disease An infrequently used eponym for polyarteritis nodosa.

Kussmaul's sign Elevation of the neck veins (and of the central venous pressure) during inspiration, a visible indication of pericardial effusion or tamponade or of other disorders that affect the filling of the right side of the heart (e.g., severe obstructive lung disease).

kv *kilovolt.*

kvo *keep vein open.*

kVp *kilovoltage peak.*

kwashiorkor (kwăsh-ē-or′kor) [Ghana, Africa, deposed child, i.e., child that is no longer suckled] A severe protein-deficiency type of malnutrition of children. It occurs after the child is weaned. The clinical signs are, at first, a vague type of lethargy, apathy, or irritability and, later, failure to grow, mental deficiency, inanition, increased susceptibility to infections, edema, dermatitis, and liver enlargement. The hair may have a reddish color.

TREATMENT: In addition to dietary therapy, the acute problems of infections, diarrhea, poor renal function, and shock need immediate attention. At first the diet must be carefully supervised to prevent overloading the system with calories or protein. In the first weeks of therapy, the child may lose weight owing to the loss of edema. If the disease has been severe and longstanding, the child may never attain full growth and mental development.

Kyasanur Forest disease One of the Russian tick-borne encephalitides.

kyestein, kiestein (kī-ĕs′tē-ĭn) [Gr. *kyesis,* pregnancy] A scum or film on stale urine; formerly thought to be a sign of pregnancy.

kymatism [Gr. *kyma,* wave, + *-ismos,* state of] Twitching of isolated segments of muscle. SYN: *myokymia*.

kymogram (kī′mō-grăm) A tracing or recording made by a kymograph.

kymograph (kī′mō-grăf) [Gr. *kyma,* wave, + *graphein,* to write] **1.** An apparatus for recording the movements of a writing pen, designed so that the pen moves in response to a force applied to it. The device consists of a drum rotated by a spring or electric motor. The drum is covered by a paper on which the record is made by the stylus of a pen. It is widely used in physiology to record activities such as blood pressure changes, muscle contractions, respiratory movements, and so on. **2.** An obsolete radiographical device for recording the range of motion of involuntary movements of the heart or diaphragm.

kymography Radiographical examination to record the range of involuntary movements such as those of the heart or diaphragm.

kynocephalus (kī″nō-sĕf′ă-lŭs) [Gr. *kyon,* dog, + *kephale,* head] A deformed fetus in which the head resembles that of a dog.

kynurenine (kī″nū-rĕn′ĭn) [″ + L. *ren,* kidney] An intermediate compound in tryptophan metabolism.

kypho- [Gr. *kyphos,* a hump] Prefix meaning *humped.*

kyphorachitis (kī″fō-răk-ī′tĭs) [″ + *rhachis,* spine, + *itis,* inflammation] A rachitic deformity involving the thorax and spinal column, which results in the development of an anteroposterior hump.

kyphos (kī′fŏs) [Gr., hump] A convex prominence of the spine.

kyphoscoliosis (kī″fō-skō″lē-ō′sĭs) [″ + *skoliosis,* curvation] Lateral curvature of the spine accompanying an anteroposterior hump.

kyphosis (kī-fō′sĭs) [Gr., humpback] An exaggeration or angulation of the normal posterior curve of the spine, giving rise to the condition commonly known as humpback, hunchback, or Pott's curvature. It may be due to congenital anomaly, disease (tuberculosis, syphilis), malignancy, or compression fracture. This term also refers to an excessive curvature of the spine with convexity backward, which may result from osteoarthritis or rheumatoid arthritis, rickets, or other conditions. SYN: *humpback; spinal curvature*. **kyphotic** (-fŏt′ĭk), *adj.*

kysth- SEE: *kystho-*.

kystho-, kysth- Combining form meaning *vagina*.

L

Λ, λ The Greek letter for lambda.

L, l *Lactobacillus; Latin; left; left eye; length; lethal; light sense; liter.*

L_+ Symbol for limes tod.

L1, L2, etc. *first lumbar nerve, second lumbar nerve,* and so forth.

L_0 Symbol for limes nul.

L- In biochemistry, a symbol used as a prefix to indicate that the carbon atom is symmetrical (or achiral) and that only three dissimilar groups attach to it. The names of such compounds would be preceded by L-. SEE: *D-*.

LA *left atrium.*

La Symbol for the element lanthanum.

lab Colloquial for laboratory.

Labbé's vein (lăb-āz′) [Léon Labbé, Fr. surgeon, 1832–1916] The vein that connects the superficial middle cerebral vein and the transverse sinus of the brain.

label The attachment of a radioactive marker or other chemical to a biologically active substance such as a drug or body chemical (such as glucose, protein, or fat). The metabolic fate of the labeled material may be investigated by detecting the presence of the label in various body sites or in excretions. The labeling material is chosen so that it does not alter the metabolism or action of the substance being investigated. SEE: *tracer.*

labeling SEE: *tag, radioactive; tagging.*

la belle indifference [Fr., beautiful indifference] A disproportionate degree of indifference to, or complacency about, symptoms such as paralysis or loss of sensation in a part of the body. It is seen in the conversion reaction.

labetalol hydrochloride An alpha- and beta-adrenergic blocking agent used in treating hypertension. SEE: *hypertensive crisis.*

labia (lā′bē-ă) [L.] Plural of labium.

l. majora The two folds of skin and adipose tissue on either side of the labia minora and vaginal opening; they form the lateral borders of the vulva. Their medial surfaces unite anteriorly above the clitoris to form the anterior commissure; posteriorly they are connected by a poorly defined posterior commissure. They are separated by a cleft, the rima pudendi, into which the urethra and vagina open. In young girls, their medial surfaces are in contact with each other, concealing the labia minora and vestibule. In older women, the labia minora may protrude between them.

l. minora The two thin folds of integument that lie between the labia majora. They enclose the vestibule. Anteriorly each divides into two smaller folds that unite with similar folds from the other side and enclose the clitoris, the more anterior one forming the prepuce (preputium clitoridis) of the clitoris and the posterior one the frenulum clitoridis. In young girls, they are hidden entirely by the labia majora.

labial (lā′bē-ăl) [L. *labialis*] Pert. to the lips.

labialism (lā′bē-ăl-ĭzm) [L. *labium,* lip, + Gr. *-ismos,* state of] Defective speech in which sounds influenced by the position of the lips are stressed.

labile (lā′bīl) [L. *labi,* to slip] Not fixed; unsteady; easily disarranged.

heat l. Destroyed or changed easily by heat; unstable. Also called *thermolabile.*

lability (lă-bĭl′ĭ-tē) The state of being unstable or changeable.

emotional l. Excessive emotional reactivity associated with frequent changes or swings in emotions and mood.

labioalveolar (lā″bē-ō-ăl-vē′ō-lăr) [L. *labium,* lip, + *alveolus,* little hollow] Pert. to the lips and tooth sockets.

labiocervical (lā″bē-ō-sĕr′vĭ-kl) [″ + *cervix,* neck] Pert. to the buccal surface of the lips and the neck of a tooth.

labiochorea (lā″bē-ō-kō-rē′ă) [″ + Gr. *choreia,* dance] A spasm of the lips in chorea, causing stammering.

labioclination (lā″bē-ō-klī-nā′shŭn) [″ + Gr. *klinein,* to slope] In dentistry, deviation of a tooth from the normal vertical toward the labial side.

labiodental (lā″bē-ō-dĕn′tăl) [″ + *dens,* tooth] **1.** Concerning the lips and teeth, esp. the labial surface of a tooth. **2.** Referring to the pronunciation of certain letters that require interaction of the teeth and lips.

labiogingival (lā″bē-ō-jĭn′jĭ-văl) [″ + *gingiva,* gum] Concerning the lips and gums or referring to the labial and gingival surfaces of a tooth.

labioglossolaryngeal (lā″bē-ō-glŏs″ō-lăr-ĭn′jē-ăl) [″ + Gr. *glossa,* tongue, + *larynx,* larynx] Pert. to the lips, tongue, and larynx.

labioglossopharyngeal (lā″bē-ō-glŏs″ō-făr-ĭn′jē-ăl) [″ + ″ + *pharynx,* throat] Pert. to the lips, tongue, and pharynx.

labiomental (lā″bē-ō-mĕn′tăl) [″ + *mentum,* chin] Pert. to the lower lip and chin.

labiomycosis (lā″bē-ō-mī-kō′sĭs) [″ + Gr. *mykes,* fungus, + *osis,* condition] Any disease of the lips caused by the presence of a fungus.

labionasal (lā″bē-ō-nā′zăl) [″ + *nasus,* nose] Concerning the nose and lips.

labiopalatine (lā″bē-ō-păl′ă-tīn) [″ + *palatum,* palate] Relating to the lips and palate.

labioplasty (lā′bē-ō-plăs″tē) [″ + Gr. *plassein,* to form] Cheiloplasty.

labiotenaculum (lā″bē-ō-tĕn-ăk′ū-lŭm) [″ + *tenaculum,* a hook] An instrument for holding the lips during an operation.

labioversion (lā″bē-ō-vĕr′zhŭn) [″ + *versio,* a turning] The state of being twisted in a labial direction, esp. a tooth.

labium (lā′bē-ŭm) *pl.* **labia** [L.] A lip or a structure like one; an edge or fleshy border.

l. cerebri The margin of the cerebral hemispheres overlapping the corpus callosum.

l. inferius oris The lower lip.

l. majus SEE: *labia majora.*

l. minus SEE: *labia minora.*

l. minus pudendi SEE: *labia minora.*

l. oris The skin and muscular tissue surrounding the mouth; the lips of the mouth.

l. superius oris The upper lip.

l. tympanicum The outer edge of the organ of Corti.

l. urethrae The lateral margin of the meatus urinarius externus.

l. uteri The thickened margin of the cervix uteri.

l. vestibulare The vestibular or inner edge of the organ of Corti.

labor [L., work] In pregnancy, the process that begins with the onset of repetitive and forceful uterine contractions sufficient to cause dilation of the cervix and ends with delivery of the products of conception. SYN: *childbirth; parturition.* SEE: illus.

Traditionally, labor is divided into three stages. The *first stage of labor,* progressive cervical dilation, is completed when the cervix is fully dilated, usually 10 cm. This stage is subdivided into the latent phase and the active phase.

First Stage (stage of dilatation): This is the period from the onset of regular uterine contractions to full dilation and effacement of the cervix. This stage averages 12 hours in primigravidas and 8 hours in multiparas.

The identification of this stage is particularly important to women having their first baby. Its diagnosis is complicated by the fact that many women experience false labor pains, which may begin as early as 3 to 4 weeks before the onset of true labor. False labor pains are quite irregular, are usually confined to the lower part of the abdomen and groin, and do not extend from the back around the abdomen as in true labor. False labor pains do not increase in frequency with time and are not made more intense by walking. The conclusive distinction is made by determining the effect of the pains on the cervix. False labor pains do not cause effacement and dilatation of the cervix as do true labor pains. SEE: *Braxton Hicks contractions.*

A reliable sign of impending labor is *show.* The appearance of a slight amount of vaginal blood-tinged mucus is a good indication that labor will begin within the next 24 hours. The loss of more than a few milliliters of blood at this time, however, must be regarded as being due to a pathological process. SEE: *placenta previa.*

Second Stage (stage of expulsion): This period lasts from complete dilatation of the cervix through the birth of the fetus, averaging 50 minutes in primigravidas and 20 minutes in multigravidas. Labor pains are severe, occur at 2- or 3-minute intervals, and last from a little less than 1 minute to a little more than 1½ minutes.

Rupture of the membranes (bag of water) usually occurs during the early part of this stage, accompanied by a gush of amniotic fluid from the vagina. The muscles of the abdomen contract involuntarily during this portion of labor. The patient directs all her strength to bearing down during the contractions. She may be quite flushed and perspire. As labor continues the perineum bulges and, in a head presentation, the scalp of the fetus appears through the vulvar opening. With cessation of each contraction, the fetus recedes from its position and then advances a little more when another contraction occurs. This continues until more of the head is visible and the vulvar ring encircles the head. This is called *crowning.*

At this time the decision is made concerning an incision in the perineum (i.e., episiotomy) to facilitate delivery. If done, it is most commonly a midline posterior episiotomy. When the head is completely removed from the vagina it falls posteriorly; later the head rotates as the shoulders turn to come through the pelvis. There is usually a gush of amniotic fluid as the shoulders are delivered.

Third Stage (placental stage): This is the period following the birth of the fetus through expulsion of the placenta and membranes. As soon as the fetus is delivered, the remainder of the amniotic fluid escapes. It will contain a small amount of blood. Uterine contractions return, and usually within 8 to 10 minutes the placenta and membranes are delivered. After this, there is a certain amount of bleeding from the uterus. The amount may vary from 100 to 500 ml or more, but the average is 200 ml.

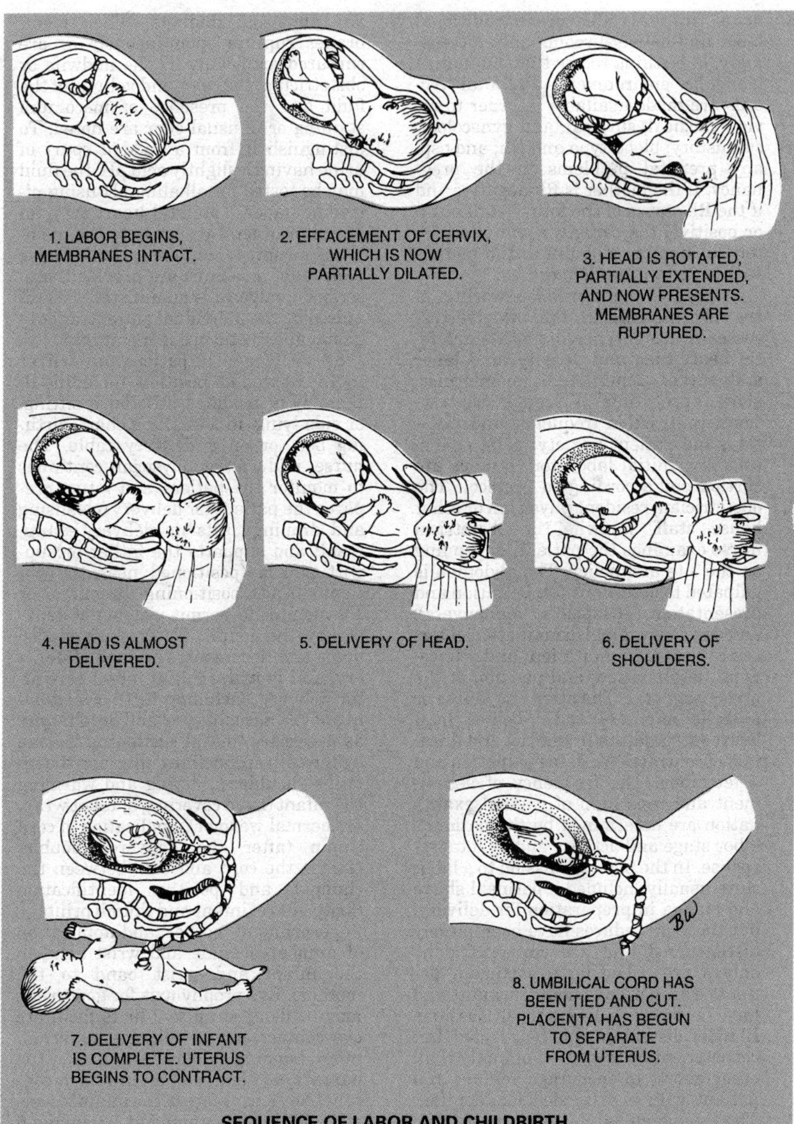

1. LABOR BEGINS, MEMBRANES INTACT.
2. EFFACEMENT OF CERVIX, WHICH IS NOW PARTIALLY DILATED.
3. HEAD IS ROTATED, PARTIALLY EXTENDED, AND NOW PRESENTS. MEMBRANES ARE RUPTURED.
4. HEAD IS ALMOST DELIVERED.
5. DELIVERY OF HEAD.
6. DELIVERY OF SHOULDERS.
7. DELIVERY OF INFANT IS COMPLETE. UTERUS BEGINS TO CONTRACT.
8. UMBILICAL CORD HAS BEEN TIED AND CUT. PLACENTA HAS BEGUN TO SEPARATE FROM UTERUS.

SEQUENCE OF LABOR AND CHILDBIRTH

The amount of blood loss will vary directly with the size of the fetus. The probability that blood loss will exceed 500 ml is less than 5% if the fetus weighs 5 lb (2268 gm) or less. The chances that blood loss will exceed 500 ml is 25% if the fetus weighs more than 9 lb (4082 gm). Other factors such as episiotomy or perineal laceration will also affect the amount of blood loss. SEE: *birthing chair; Credé's method* for assisting the expulsion of the placenta.

PATIENT CARE: Most frequently, prenatal classes taught by obstetrical nurses prepare the patient and family for labor, delivery, and care of the newborn. Such classes teach exercises; breathing techniques; supportive care measures for labor, delivery, and the postpartum period; and neonatal care and feeding techniques. Expectant couples (or the pregnant woman and a support person) should attend classes together. The goals of expectant parent education are the birth of a healthy infant and a positive experience for the couple. Labor and delivery may take place in a hospital, birthing center, or at home. Hospitals offer care in traditional labor and delivery rooms and, increasingly, in birthing rooms that simulate a homelike environment. Prenatal records are made available in order to review medical, surgical, and gynecological history; blood type and Rh; and esp. any prenatal problems in the pregnancy. If the mother is Rh negative and if the Rh status of the fetus is unknown or positive, the caregiver will administer Rh immune globulin to the mother within 72 hr after delivery.

As part of the admission workup of the laboring woman, the caregiver assesses vital signs, height and weight, fetal heart tone and activity, and labor status (i.e., condition of membranes, show, onset time of regular contractions, contraction frequency and duration, and patient anxiety, pain, or discomfort). Initial laboratory studies are carried out according to protocol. The obstetrician, resident physician or other house staff, midwife, or obstetrical nurse examines the patient, depending on the site and policy. The abdomen is palpated to determine fetal position and presentation (Leopold's maneuvers), and a sterile vaginal examination determines cervical dilatation and effacement, fetal station, and position of the presenting part. The attending nurse or midwife monitors and assesses fetal heart rate and the frequency and duration of contractions, using palpation and a fetoscope. The frequency of assessment and repetition of vaginal examination are determined by the patient's labor stage and activity and by fetal response. In the past, admission to a labor suite usually included a perineal shave and enema in preparation for delivery, but these procedures have been largely discontinued and are currently done only if prescribed for a particular patient. The patient should urinate and have a bowel movement, if possible. Bladder distention is to be avoided, but catheterization is carried out only if all other efforts to encourage voiding in a patient with a distended bladder fail. The perineum is cleansed (protecting the vaginal introitus from entry of cleansing solutions) and kept as clean as possible during labor. Special cleansing is performed before vaginal examination and delivery, as well as after expulsion of urine or feces.

First stage: The patient may be alert and ambulating, depending on membrane status, fetal position, and labor activity. Electrolyte-rich oral liquids may be prescribed, or I.V. therapy initiated. The caregiver supports the patient and her husband or other support person and monitors the progress of the labor and the response of the fetus, notifying the obstetrician or midwife of any abnormal findings. When membranes rupture spontaneously or are ruptured artificially by the midwife or obstetrician, the color and volume of the fluid and the presence of meconium staining or unusual odor are noted. To distinguish it from a sudden spurt of urine having a slightly acid pH, the fluid may be tested for alkaline pH using nitrazine paper. The fetal heart rate, an indicator of fetal response to the membrane's rupture, is noted. Noninvasive pain relief measures are provided, prescribed analgesia is administered as required by the individual patient, and regional anesthetic use is monitored.

Second stage: The patient may deliver in any agreed-on position, including lithotomy or modified lithotomy, sitting, or side lying, in a birthing chair, birthing bed, or on a delivery table. The nurse, midwife, or physician continues to monitor the patient and fetus; prepares the patient for delivery (cleansing and draping); sets up delivery equipment; and supports the father or support person (positioned near the patient's head), positioning the mirror or TV monitor to permit viewing of delivery by the couple. The caregiver also notes and documents the time of delivery, and provides initial infant care after delivery, including further suctioning of the nasopharynx and oropharynx as necessary (initial suctioning is done by the deliverer before delivering the infant's shoulders), drying and warming the infant (head covering, blanket wrap, or thermal warmer), application of cord clamp (after the deliverer double-clamps the cord and cuts between the clamps), and positive identification (footprints of infant and thumb prints or fingerprints of mother, and application of numbered ankle and wrist band to the infant and wrist band to the mother). Eye prophylaxis for gonorrhea may be delayed up to 2 hr to facilitate eye contact and to enhance maternal-infant bonding, or may be refused by the parents, on signing of an informed consent. An Apgar score of the infant's overall condition is obtained at 1 min and 5 min after the birth. The infant in good condition is placed on the mother's chest or abdomen or put to the breast, and the couple is encouraged to inspect and interact with the infant. An infant in distress is hurried to the nursery, usually with the father attending, so that specialized care can be provided by nursery and neonatal-nurse specialists, and a pediatrician. In extreme cases (and at parental request), the infant may be baptized by the nurse or by a chaplain or other Christian minister, and photographs may be taken to assist the parents in dealing with the life, critical time, and possible death of the infant.

Third stage: The caregiver continues to monitor the status of the patient and the fundus through delivery of the placenta and membranes (documenting the time), examination of the vagina and uterus for trauma or retained products, and repair of any laceration or surgical episiotomy. The placenta is examined to ascertain that no fragments remain in the uterus. The perineal area is cleansed and the mother is assisted to a comfortable position and covered with a warm blanket.

Fourth stage: The caregiver continues to observe the patient closely and is alert for hemorrhage or other complications through frequent assessment, including monitoring vital signs, palpating the fundus for firmness and position in relation to the umbilicus at intervals (determined by agency policy or patient condition), and massaging the fundus gently or administering prescribed oxytocic drugs to maintain uterine contraction and to limit bleeding. The character (including presence, size, and number of clots) and volume of vaginal discharge or lochia are assessed periodically; the perineum is inspected and ice applied as prescribed, and the bladder is inspected, palpated, and percussed for distention. The patient is encouraged to void, and catheterization is performed only if absolutely necessary. The nurse notifies the obstetrician or midwife if any problems occur or persist. This period also is used for parent-infant bonding, because the infant is usually awake for the first hour or so after delivery. The mother can breast-feed if desired, and the couple can inspect the infant. The nurse supports the couple's responses to the newborn, as well as to the labor and delivery experience. The infant is then taken to the nursery for initial infant care.

Early postpartum period: Once the infant's temperature has stabilized, measurements have been taken (length, head and chest circumference, weight), and other prescribed care carried out, the infant may be returned to the mother's side (in its crib carrier). The caregiver continues to assess the mother's physical and psychological status after delivery, checking the fundus, vulva, and perineum according to policy; inspects the mother's breasts and assists the mother with feeding or measures to prevent lactation as desired; helps the mother to deal with other responsibilities of motherhood; and carries out the mandated maternal teaching program, including providing written information for later review by the patient. In hospitals or birthing centers, the caregiver prepares the mother for early discharge to the home setting and arranges for follow-up care as needed and available. In many settings, the nurse makes follow-up calls or visits to the mother during the early postpartum period or encourages the patient to call in with concerns, or the patient may receive follow-up visits by a caregiver from her health maintenance organization. The mother may also be referred to support groups, such as the La Leche League, Nursing Mothers' Club, and others as available in the particular community.

active l. Regular uterine contractions that result in increasing cervical dilation and descent of the presenting part. This encompasses the active phase of stage 1, as well as stages 2 and 3 of labor.

arrested l. Failure of labor to proceed through the normal stages. This may be due to uterine inertia, obstruction of the pelvis, or systemic disease.

artificial l. Induction of labor.

augmented l. Induction of labor.

back l. Labor involving malposition of the fetal head with the occiput opposing the mother's sacrum. The laboring woman experiences severe back pain. SEE: *occiput posterior, persistent.*

complicated l. Labor occurring with an accompanying abnormal condition such as hemorrhage or inertia.

dry l. Labor associated with extensive loss of amniotic fluid related to premature rupture of membranes.

dysfunctional l. Abnormal progress of dilation and/or descent of the presenting part.

false l. Uterine contractions that occur before the onset of labor (i.e., that do not result in dilation of the cervix). They may resolve spontaneously or continue until effective contractions occur and labor begins. SEE: under *labor; Braxton Hicks contractions.*

hypertonic l. Condition in which frequent, painful, but poor-quality contractions fail to accomplish effective cervical effacement and dilation. Hypertonicity usually occurs in the latent phase of labor and most often is related to fetal malpresentation and cephalopelvic disproportion.

hypotonic l. Condition in which fewer than one to three contractions occur within 10 minutes. Hypotonicity usually occurs after the woman has entered the active phase of labor and most often is related to uterine overdistention, fetal macrosomia, multiple pregnancy, or grand multiparity.

induction of l. The use of pharmacological, mechanical, or operative interventions to assist the progression of a previously dysfunctional labor. Induction may be considered when the risks of expectant management outweigh the benefits, placing the fetus and/or the mother in jeopardy. Among the more common indications are preeclampsia or eclampsia, premature rupture of membranes, fetal compromise, maternal medical diseases, chorioamnionitis, intrauterine fetal demise, postdate pregnancy, as well as some psychosocial factors. Contraindications include placenta previa, vasa previa, umbilical cord prolapse, history of classic uterine incision, and transverse fetal lie, as well as many relative contraindications. SYN: *artificial l.; augmented l.* SEE: *Nursing Diagnoses Appendix.*

CAUTION: Oxytocin should be used only intravenously, using a device that permits precise control of flow rate. While oxytocin is being administered, the fetal heart rate and uterine contractions should be monitored electronically.

instrumental l. Labor completed by mechanical means, such as the use of forceps.

missed l. **1.** False l. **2.** Labor in which true labor pains begin but subside. This may be a sign of a dead fetus or extrauterine pregnancy.

normal l. Progressive dilatation and effacement of the cervix with descent of the presenting part.

obstructed l. Interference with fetal descent related to malposition, malpresentation, and cephalopelvic disproportion.

precipitate l. Labor marked by sudden onset, rapid cervical effacement and dilation, and delivery within 3 hours of onset.

premature l. SYN: *preterm l.*

preterm l. Labor that begins before completion of 37 weeks from the last menstrual period. The condition affects 7% to 10% of all live births and is one of the most important risk factors for preterm birth, the primary cause of perinatal and neonatal mortality. Although associated risk factors do exist, in most cases the cause is unknown. SYN: *premature l.* SEE: *premature rupture of membranes; prematurity; Nursing Diagnoses Appendix.*

PATIENT CARE: *In-hospital management:* The patient is prepared for the use of cardiac, uterine, and fetal monitors during IV therapy. Maternal vital signs and fetal heart rate (FHR) are monitored. The prescribed tocolytic agent dose is administered intravenously; the infusion rate is increased every 10 to 30 min, depending on uterine response, but never exceeds a rate of 125 ml/hr. Uterine activity is monitored continuously; vital signs and FHR are checked every 15 min. Maternal pulse should not exceed 140/min; FHR should not exceed 180 bpm. Breath sounds when counting respiratory rate are noted, and the lungs are auscultated at least every 8 hours. The patient is assessed for desired response and adverse effects and is taught about symptoms she may expect and should report. If signs of drug toxicity occur, the medication is stopped. The IV line is kept open with a maintenance solution, and the prescribed beta-blocker as an antidote is prepared and administered. The patient is placed in high Fowler's position, and oxygen is administered. Cardiac rate and rhythm, blood pressure, respiratory rate, auscultatory sounds, and FHS are closely monitored to evaluate the patient's response to the antidote. If no complications are present, absolute bed rest is maintained throughout the infusion, with the patient in a left-lateral position or supine with a wedge under the right hip to prevent hypotension. Antiembolism stockings are applied, and passive leg exercises are performed. A daily fluid intake of 2 to 3 liters is encouraged to maintain adequate hydration, and fluid intake and output are measured. The patient is weighed daily to assess for overhydration. The patient is instructed in methods to deal with stress. Health care providers should respond to parental concern for the fetus with empathy, but never with false reassurance. Fetal fibronectin enzyme immunoassay may be carried out on a sample of vaginal secretions taken from the posterior vaginal fornix; the patient should understand that this test can help assess the risk of preterm delivery within 7 days from the sampling date. As prescribed, a glucocorticoid is administered to stimulate fetal pulmonary surfactant production.

Home management: Patients who undergo in-house therapy often receive magnesium sulfate, which helps restore the patient's beta-2 receptor sensitivity (thus improving the effectiveness of terbutaline) and decrease uterine contractions. The patient may be discharged on oral or subcutaneous tocolytic therapy. IV therapy may be employed using a portable micropump that can deliver a basal rate or programmed intermittent bolus doses at predetermined times when the patient's circadian rhythms are known to increase uterine activity. The plan for at-home care must target individuals whom the woman can call upon to help with home management. A social service referral can help the family access available community and financial assistance. Home health care nurses assist the patient to carry out the plan, provide ongoing emotional support, and evaluate the patient's response to therapy.

The treatment regimen is reviewed with the family, and written instructions are provided to help those involved to cooperate. The patient is maintained on bed rest (left-side, supine, with head on small pillow, feet flat or elevated) to increase uterine perfusion and to keep fetal pressure off the cervix. The patient usually is allowed out of bed only to go to the bathroom. The women's physical and psychological rest have the highest priority, as anxiety is known to compromise uterine blood flow. Paid or voluntary helpers must care for other children and all household chores. The patient's tocolytic therapy (most frequently using terbutaline) is scheduled around the clock (with food if desired), and the patient is taught about its action and adverse effects. The patient must be able to count her pulse, and is instructed to report a rate above 120/min. The patient also is taught about symptoms to report (palpations, tremors, agitation, nervousness) and how to palpate for contractions twice each day. Home uterine activity monitoring may be employed, with the patient or home health care provider recording uterine activity for an hour twice daily. The perinatal nurse analyzes the results. If contractions exceed a predetermined threshold, the patient is advised to drink 8 to 12 ounces of water, rest, then empty her bladder and monitor uterine activity for another hour. The process can reduce unnecessary visits to the medical setting, and increase the patient's peace of mind. The patient is encouraged to drink water throughout the day to prevent dehydration and reduce related uterine irritability. She also is warned not to take OTC drugs without her obstetrician's approval. The patient is taught how to use sedation, if prescribed. Avoidance of activities that could stimulate labor is emphasized; these include sexual and nipple stimulation. Personal hygiene is reviewed, and the patient is made aware of signs of infection to report. A nonstress test may be performed weekly at home or in a medical setting, depending on the acuity of the situation and on maternal health factors (diabetes, PIH). The patient usually is provided with a 24-hour phone link to perinatal nurses in the health care system, who may contact her twice daily to discuss her situation. She is taught what to do in an emergency (bright red bleeding, membrane rupture, persisting contractions, decreased or absent fetal activity). If labor is inevitable, it is carried out as for a low-birth-weight, readily compromised fetus. During the post-partum period, care focuses on helping the family to understand their infant's special needs, and to participate as fully as possible in care, or, in a worst-case scenario, to come to terms with the baby's death. In such a case, the family is assisted in their grieving, with encouragement to hold the swaddled infant, and look at pictures of the child if they are able. Psychological counseling may be required.

primary dysfunctional l. Abnormally slow dilation of the cervix in the active phase of labor; defined as less than 1.2 cm/hr in a nullipara and 1.5 cm/hr in a multipara. SYN: *protraction disorder.* SEE: *arrested l; precipitate l.*

prodromal l. The initial changes that precede actual labor, usually occurring 24 to 48 hr before the onset of labor. Some women report a surge of energy. Findings include lightening, excessive mucoid vaginal discharge, softening and beginning effacement of the ripe cervix, scant bloody show associated with expulsion of the mucus plug, and diarrhea.

prolonged l. Abnormally slow progress of labor, lasting more than 20 hr. SEE: *dystocia.*

prolonged latent phase l. Abnormally slow progress of the latent phase, lasting more than 20 hr in a nullipara or 14 hr in a multipara. SEE: *dystocia.*

spontaneous l. Labor that begins and progresses without pharmacological, mechanical, or operative intervention.

stage I l. SEE: *labor; Nursing Diagnoses Appendix.*

stage II l. SEE: *labor; Nursing Diagnoses Appendix.*

trial of l. Permitting labor to continue long enough to determine if normal vaginal birth appears to be possible (e.g., in vaginal birth after cesarean delivery).

laboratory (lăb′ră-tor″ē) [L. *laboratorium*] A room or building equipped for scientific experimentation, research, testing, or clinical studies of materials, fluids, or tissues obtained from patients.

Laborde's method (lă-bordz′) [Jean B. V. Laborde, Fr. physician, 1830–1903] Stimulation of the respiratory center in asphyxiation by a series of rhythmical traction movements upon the tongue.

labret (lā′brĕt) [L. *labrum,* lip] Among some primitive peoples, a distinctive plug of ivory, bone, stone, or bottle top worn in a hole artificially produced in the lips of adolescent boys.

labrocyte (lăb′rō-sīt) [Gr. *labros,* greedy, + *kytos,* cell] A mast cell.

labrum (lā′brŭm) *pl.* **labra** [L., lip] **1.** Lip or liplike structure. **2.** The upper lip of an insect.

labyrinth (lăb′ĭ-rĭnth) [Gr. *labyrinthos,* maze] **1.** A series of intricate communicating passages. **2.** The inner ear, the bony and membranous labyrinths, which contain the receptors for hearing and equilibrium. SEE: illus.

bony l. Osseous l.

ethmoidal l. The lateral mass of the

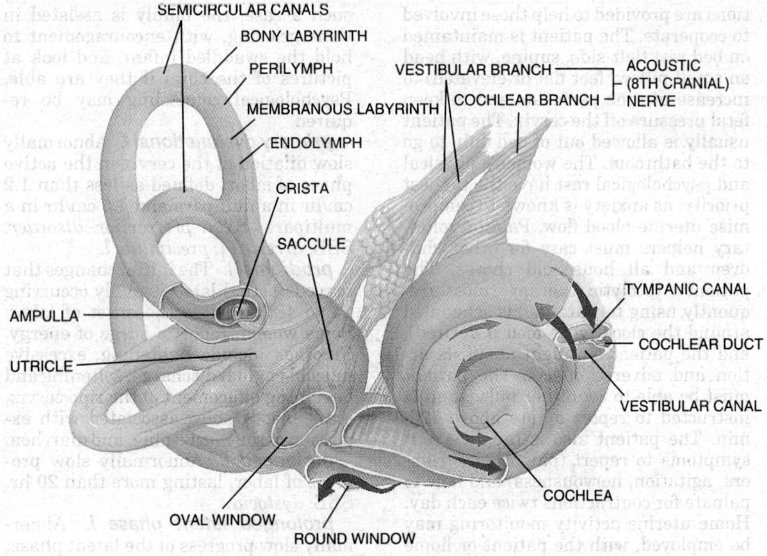

LABYRINTHS OF INNER EAR

Arrows in cochlea indicate path of vibrations

ethmoid bone, which includes the superior and middle conchae and encloses the ethmoid sinuses. SYN: *olfactory l.*

membranous l. The structure in the osseous labyrinth consisting of the utricle and saccule of the vestibule, three semicircular ducts, and the cochlear duct, all filled with endolymph.

olfactory l. Ethmoidal l.

osseous l. The labyrinth in the temporal bone that consists of the vestibule, three semicircular canals, and cochlea, all filled with perilymph. SYN: *bony l.*

labyrinthectomy (lăb-ĭ-rĭn-thĕk′tō-mē) [″ + *ektome,* excision] Excision of the labyrinth.

labyrinthine (lăb-ĭ-rĭn′thīn) **1.** Pert. to a labyrinth. **2.** Intricate or involved, as a labyrinth. **3.** Pert. to speech that wanders aimlessly and unconnectedly from subject to subject, as seen in schizophrenia.

labyrinthitis (lăb″ĭ-rĭn-thī′tĭs) [″ + *itis,* inflammation] An inflammation (acute or chronic) of the labyrinth. Symptoms include vertigo, vomiting, and nystagmus. It may result from such conditions as viral infections, bacterial infections, or head trauma. SEE: *Ménière's disease; otitis interna.*

labyrinthotomy (lăb″ĭ-rĭn-thŏt′ō-mē) [″ + *tome,* incision] Surgical incision into the labyrinth.

labyrinthus (lăb″ĭ-rĭn′thŭs) [L., Gr. *labyrinthos,* maze] A labyrinth.

lac (lăk) [L.] **1.** Milk. **2.** Milky medicinal substance.

lacerate (lăs′ĕr-āt) [L. *lacerare,* to tear] To tear, as into irregular segments. **lacerated,** *adj.*

laceration (lăs″ĕ-rā′shŭn) A wound or irregular tear of the flesh. **lacerable** (lăs′ĕr-ă-b'l), *adj.*

l. of cervix Bilateral, stellate, or unilateral tear of the cervix uteri caused by childbirth.

l. of perineum An injury of the perineum caused by childbirth. If it extends through the sphincter ani muscle, it is considered complete or fourth degree. SEE: *episiotomy.*

stellate l. A tear in the skin or in an internal organ caused by blunt trauma. Several lines emanate outward from the tear's center.

lacertus (lă-sĕr′tŭs) [L., lizard] **1.** The muscular part of the arm. **2.** A muscular or fibrous band.

l. cordis A muscular tissue band on the inner cardiac surface. SYN: *trabecula carnea cordis.*

l. fibrosus An aponeurotic band from the biceps tendon to the bicipital or semilunar fascia of forearm.

Lachman test A sensitive test to evaluate the integrity of the anterior cruciate ligament of the knee. The examiner stands on the side being examined and grasps the tibia at the level of the tibial tubercle while stabilizing the femur with the other hand. The patient relaxes the leg while the examiner holds the knee flexed at 30° and pulls forward on the tibia. Excessive motion and no discernible end point determine a positive result.

laciniate (lă-sĭn′ē-āt) [L. *lacinia,* fringe] Being jagged or fringed.

lacrima (lăk′rĭ-mă) [L.] Tear fluid from eye.

lacrimal (lăk′rĭm-ăl) [L. *lacrima,* tear] Pert. to the tears.

l. apparatus Structures concerned with the secretion and conduction of tears. It includes the lacrimal gland and its secretory ducts, lacrimal canaliculi, lacrimal sac, and nasolacrimal duct, which empties into the nasal cavity. SEE: illus.

Patency of the lacrimal duct may be tested by placing a dilute solution of sugar in the conjunctival sac; if the duct is patent, the individual will report the sensation of sweetness in the mouth; if not, the sugar will not be perceived.

lacrimation [L. *lacrima,* tear] The secretion and discharge of tears.

test for l. Schirmer's test.

lacrimator A substance that increases the flow of tears.

lacrimatory (lăk′rĭ-mă-tō″rē) Causing the production of tears.

lacrimonasal (lăk″rĭ-mō-nā′zăl) [″ + *nasus,* nose] Concerning the nose and lacrimal apparatus.

lacrimotome (lăk′rĭ-mō-tōm) [″ + Gr. *tome,* incision] A cutting instrument used for incising the lacrimal sac or duct.

lacrimotomy (lăk″rĭ-mŏt′ō-mē) [″ + Gr. *tome,* incision] Incision of lacrimal duct.

lactacid Lactic acid.

lactacidemia (lăk-tăs″ĭ-dē′mē-ă) [″ + ″ + Gr. *haima,* blood] An accumulation of an excess of lactic acid in the blood. It occurs normally following strenuous and prolonged exercise. SYN: *lacticemia.*

lactaciduria (lăkt-ă-sĭd-ū′rē-ă) [″ + ″ + Gr. *ouron,* urine] Lactic acid excreted in the urine.

lactagogue (lăk′tă-gŏg) [″ + Gr. *agogos,* leading] Galactagogue.

lactalbumin [″ + *albumen,* coagulated white of egg] The albumin of milk and cheese; a soluble simple protein. Lactalbumin is present in higher concentration in human milk than in cow's milk. When milk is heated, the lactalbumin coagulates and appears as a film on the surface of the milk.

lactam (lăk′tăm) An organic chemical that contains the —NH—CO group in a ring form. It is formed by the removal of a molecule of water from certain amino acids.

***β*-lactamase-resistant antibiotics** Antibiotics that are resistant to the action of *β*-lactamase. This property makes them effective against microbial organisms that produce *β*-lactamase.

***β*-lactamases** (bā″tă-lăk′tă-mās) A group of enzymes that act on certain antibiotics to inactivate them.

lactase [″ + *-ase,* enzyme] An intestinal sugar-splitting enzyme converting lactose into dextrose and galactose; found in intestinal juice. SEE: *enzyme; maltase; sucrase; sugar.*

lactate (lăk′tāt) **1.** Any salt derived from lactic acid. **2.** To secrete milk.

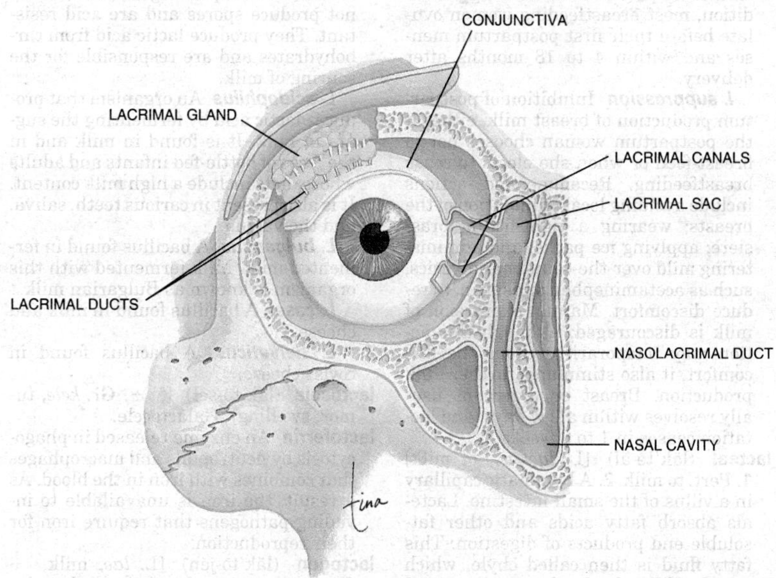

LACRIMAL APPARATUS

Anterior view of right eye

lactate dehydrogenase Lactic dehydrogenase.

lactation (lăk-tā′shŭn) [L. *lactatio,* a sucking] **1.** The production and release of milk by mammary glands. **2.** The period of breastfeeding after childbirth, beginning with the release of colostrum (the nutrient-rich substance that precedes milk production) and continuing until the infant is weaned. Many hormonal factors are involved in lactation. The process depends on secretion of the hormone prolactin by the pituitary gland, but it begins only after the marked decreases in estrogen and progesterone that follow childbirth. Nursing by the infant stimulates pulsatile increases in prolactin secretion. Oxytocin, secreted by the hypothalamus, also contributes to the release of milk by stimulating the contraction of muscular cells in the milk ducts and mammary glands.

DIET: The dietary needs of the mother are increased during lactation, usually by about 500 kcal daily. In addition, maternal needs for calcium, folate, and other vitamins increase while breastfeeding. SEE: *breastfeeding; colostrum.*

l. amenorrhea method ABBR: LAM. The method of causing decreased fertility in a woman by nursing a child for a lengthy period (several years or more). In general, the longer a woman breastfeeds, the longer ovulation is delayed. The questionable reliability of this method of contraception is compromised further by partial breastfeeding. In addition, most breastfeeding women ovulate before their first postpartum menses and within 4 to 18 months after delivery.

l. suppression Inhibition of postpartum production of breast milk, either if the postpartum woman chooses not to breast-feed or when she elects to cease breastfeeding. Recommended actions include avoiding local stimulation of the breasts; wearing a tight-fitting brassiere; applying ice packs; and administering mild over-the-counter analgesics, such as acetaminophen or aspirin, to reduce discomfort. Manual expression of milk is discouraged; although this action may temporarily reduce the discomfort, it also stimulates further milk production. Breast engorgement usually resolves within a few days, and lactation ceases in 1 to 2 weeks.

lacteal (lăk′tē-ăl) [L. *lacteus,* of milk] **1.** Pert. to milk. **2.** A lymphatic capillary in a villus of the small intestine. Lacteals absorb fatty acids and other fat-soluble end products of digestion. This fatty fluid is then called chyle, which travels through the larger intestinal lymphatic vessels and, by way of the thoracic duct, to the left subclavian vein. SEE: *lymph.*

lactic (lăk′tĭk) [L. *lac,* milk] Pert. to milk.

lactic dehydrogenase ABBR: LD. An enzyme present in various tissues and serum that is important in catalyzing the oxidation of lactate. In humans, LD is present in several molecular forms called isoenzymes. Some LD isoenzymes are present in certain tissues to a greater extent than in others. When one of these particular tissues is damaged, an isoenzyme of LD is released into the blood. In that case, determination of the pattern of LD isoenzymes in serum may help to identify which tissue has been damaged. SYN: *lactate dehydrogenase.*

lacticemia (lăk-tĭ-sē′mē-ă) [″ + Gr. *haima,* blood] Lactacidemia.

lactiferous (lăk-tĭf′ĕr-ŭs) [″ + *ferre,* to bear] Secreting and conveying milk.

lactification (lăk″tĭ-fĭ-kā′shŭn) [″ + *facere,* to make] Lactic acid production.

lactifuge (lăk′tĭ-fūj) [″ + *fugare,* to expel] **1.** Stopping milk secretion. **2.** An agent stopping milk secretion.

lactigenous (lăk-tĭj′ĕn-ŭs) [″ + Gr. *gennan,* to produce] Producing milk.

lactigerous (lăk-tĭj′ĕr-ŭs) [″ + *gerere,* to carry] Secreting or conveying milk.

lactinated (lăk′tĭ-nāt″ĕd) Containing or prepared with lactose, or milk sugar.

lactivorous (lăk-tĭv′or-ŭs) [″ + *vorare,* to devour] Living on milk.

Lactobacillus (lăk-tō-bă-sĭl′ŭs) [″ + *bacillus,* little rod] A genus of bacteria belonging to the family Lactobacillaceae. These bacteria are gram-positive, nonmotile, rod-shaped organisms that do not produce spores and are acid resistant. They produce lactic acid from carbohydrates and are responsible for the souring of milk.

L. acidophilus An organism that produces lactic acid by fermenting the sugars in milk. It is found in milk and in the feces of bottle-fed infants and adults whose diets include a high milk content. It is also present in carious teeth, saliva, and the vagina.

L. bulgaricus A bacillus found in fermented milk. Milk fermented with this organism is known as Bulgarian milk.

L. casei A bacillus found in milk and cheese.

L. helveticus A bacillus found in Swiss cheese.

lactocele (lăk′tō-sēl) [″ + Gr. *kele,* tumor, swelling] Galactocele.

lactoferrin An enzyme released in phagocytosis by neutrophils and macrophages that combines with iron in the blood. As a result, the iron is unavailable to invading pathogens that require iron for their reproduction.

lactogen (lăk′tō-jĕn) [L. *lac,* milk, + Gr. *gennan,* to produce] Any substance that stimulates milk production. SEE: *prolactin.*

human placental l. ABBR: HPL. A

hormone produced by the placenta and released to maternal blood. It acts in the last stage of gestation to prepare the breasts for milk production. It is no longer present in the maternal circulation 2 days after delivery.

lactogenic [″ + Gr. *gennan,* to produce] Inducing the secretion of milk.

lactoglobulin (lăk″tō-glŏb′ū-lĭn) [″ + *globulus,* globule] A protein found in milk. Casein and lactoglobulin are the most common proteins in cow's milk.

immune l. Antibodies present in the colostrum.

lactometer (lăk-tŏm′ĕ-tĕr) [″ + Gr. *metron,* measure] A device for determining the specific gravity of milk.

lacto-ovo-vegetarian (lăk″tō-ō″vō-vĕj″ĕ-tā′rē-ăn) A person consuming a vegetarian diet that includes eggs and dairy products.

lactophosphate (lăk″tō-fŏs′fāt) [″ + *phosphas,* phosphate] A salt derived jointly from lactic and phosphoric acids.

lactoprotein (lăk″tō-prō′tē-ĭn) [″ + Gr. *protos,* first] Any protein present in milk.

lactorrhea (lăk-tō-rē′ă) [″ + Gr. *rhoia,* flow] The discharge of milk between nursings and after weaning of offspring. SYN: *galactorrhea.*

lactose **1.** A disaccharide that on hydrolysis yields glucose and galactose. Bacteria can convert it into lactic and butyric acids, as in the souring of milk. The milk of mammals contains 4% to 7% lactose. Its presence in the urine may be indicative of obstruction to flow of milk after cessation of nursing. Commercial lactose is a fine white powder that will not dissolve in cold water. **2.** A sugar, $C_{11}H_{22}O_{11}$, obtained from evaporation of cow's milk. It is used in manufacturing tablets and as a diluent.

l. intolerance An inability to digest milk and some dairy products, leading to abdominal bloating, cramping, and diarrhea. The intolerance may be congenital or may begin in childhood, adolescence, or young adulthood. SYN: *lactase deficiency syndrome.*

ETIOLOGY: A deficiency of the enzyme lactase, which digests lactose in the small intestine, causes this intolerance.

TREATMENT: The patient should limit consumption of milk and other lactose containing foods as determined by the patient's reaction. Yogurt may be consumed instead of milk and may lessen the limitation on consumption of lactose. Enzyme tablets containing lactase prior to consuming lactose containing foods may be helpful.

lactose tolerance test A test for deficiency of lactase in the small intestine that consists of the administration of a weighed amount of lactose, followed by successive measurements of blood glucose at timed intervals. Low levels of glucose indicate a lactase deficiency.

lactosuria (lăk-tō-sū′rē-ă) [″ + Gr. *ouron,* urine] The presence of milk sugar (lactose) in the urine, a condition that occurs frequently during pregnancy and lactation.

lactotherapy (lăk-tō-thĕr′ă-pē) [″ + Gr. *therapeia,* treatment] SYN: *galactotherapy.*

lactovegetarian **1.** Pert. to milk and vegetables. **2.** One who lives on a diet of milk, other dairy products, and vegetables.

lactulose A synthetic disaccharide, 4-*O*-β-D-galactopyranosyl-D-fructofuranose, that is not hydrolyzed or absorbed in humans. It is metabolized by bacteria in the colon with the production of organic acids and is used to treat constipation and the encephalopathy that develops in patients with advanced cirrhosis of the liver. The unabsorbed sugar produces diarrhea, and the acid pH helps to contain ammonia in the feces.

lacunae (lă-koo′nē) [L.] Pl. of lacune.

lacune, lacuna (lă-koo′n) *pl.* **lacunae** [L., a pit] **1.** A small pit, space, or cavity. **2.** The space occupied by cells of calcified tissues (e.g., cementocytes, chondrocytes, and osteocytes). **3.** A focal loss of brain tissue due to a stroke involving a small penetrating artery in the brain. **lacunar** (-năr), *adj.*

absorption l. Howship's l.

Howship's l. A pit or groove in bone where resorption or dissolution of bone is occurring; usually contains osteoclasts. SYN: *absorption l.*

intervillous l. A space in the placenta occupied by maternal blood and into which fetal placenta villi project.

l. laterales Irregular diverticula on either side of the superior sagittal sinus of the brain into which the arachnoid villi project.

l. magna The largest pitlike recess in the fossa navicularis of the distal end of the male urethra.

l. pharyngis Pit at pharyngeal end of the eustachian tube.

trophoblastic l. An irregular cavity in the syntrophoblast that develops into intervillous spaces or lacunae. SEE: *intervillous l.*

l. of the urethra One of several recesses in the mucous membrane of the urethra, esp. along the floor and in the bulb. They are the openings of the urethral glands.

l. vasorum Space for passage of femoral vessels to the thigh.

lacunula, lacunule (lă-kū′nū-lă, -nūl) [L., little pit] A small or minute lacuna.

lacus (lā′kŭs) [L., lake] A collection of fluid in a small hollow or cavity.

l. lacrimalis The space at the medial canthus of the eye where tears collect.

LAD *left anterior descending* (branch of the left coronary artery).

L.A.D.A. *Left acromion-dorsal-anterior fetal position.*

L.A.D.P. *Left acromion-dorsal-posterior fetal position.*

Laënnec's cirrhosis (lā″ĕ-nĕks′) [René T. H. Laënnec, Fr. physician and the inventor of the stethoscope, 1781–1826] Cirrhosis of the liver associated with chronic excessive alcohol ingestion. SYN: *hobnail liver*. SEE: *liver, cirrhosis of*.

Laënnec's pearls Round gelatinous masses seen in asthmatic sputum.

Laënnec's thrombus Globular thrombus in the heart.

Laetrile Amygdalin; a glycoside derived from pits or other seed parts of plants, including apricots and almonds. Amygdalin contains sufficient cyanide to be fatal when taken in large doses. It has no known therapeutic or nutritional value. There is no evidence that it is effective in treating cancer. It is also known as *vitamin* B_{17}.

CAUTION: Complications of Laetrile treatment may include acute or chronic cyanide poisoning.

Lafora, Gonzalo R (lă-fō′ră) Spanish physician, 1887–1971.

L.'s bodies Cytoplasmic inclusion bodies that are made of acid mucopolysaccharides and are present in neuronal tissue of the brain in familial myoclonus epilepsy.

L.'s disease Familial progressive epilepsy.

lag **1.** The period of time between the application of a stimulus and the resulting reaction. **2.** The early period following bacterial inoculation into a culture medium, characterized by slow growth. SYN: *lag phase; latent period*.

lageniform (lă-jĕn′ĭ-form) [L. *lagena*, flask, + *forma*, shape] Flask-shaped.

lagophthalmos, lagophthalmus (lăg″ŏf-thăl′mōs, -mŭs) [Gr. *lagos*, hare, + *ophthalmos*, eye] An incomplete closure of the palpebral fissure when an attempt is made to shut the eyelids. This results in exposure and injury to the bulbar conjunctiva and cornea. This condition is caused by contraction of a scar of the eyelid, facial nerve injury, atony of the orbicularis palpebrarum, or exophthalmos.

TREATMENT: Artificial tears or other ocular lubricants are needed to prevent corneal ulceration.

nocturnal l. Failure of the eyelids to remain closed during sleep, which may be due to chronic keratitis.

la grippe (lă grĭp′) [Fr.] Influenza.

laity (lā′ĭ-tē) [Gr. *laos*, the people] Individuals who are not members of a particular profession such as law, dentistry, medicine, or the ministry.

LAK cell *lymphokine-activated killer cell*. SEE: under *cell*.

lake [L. *lacus*] A small cavity of fluid. SYN: *lacus*.

lacrimal l. The small pouch formed by the junction of the conjunctiva at the medial canthus of the eye.

venous l. A small subcutaneous bleb filled with blood. It may be present on the lips, mouth or ears.

laked A term used to describe the blood in hemolysis or disintegration of the red blood cells, freeing the hemoglobin into the blood plasma.

laking The freeing of hemoglobin from red blood cells.

LAL *limulus amebocyte lysate*.

La Leche League An organization whose purpose is to promote breastfeeding. Street address: 1400 N. Meacham Road, Schaumberg, IL 60173-4048. Website: www.lalecheleague.org

laliatry (lăl-ī′ă-trē) [Gr. *lalia*, talk, + *iatria*, therapy] The study and treatment of speech disorders and defects.

lallation (lă-lā′shŭn) [L. *lallatio*] A babbling form of stammering; an infantile form of speech.

lalopathology (lăl″ō-pă-thŏl′ō-jē) [″ + *pathos*, disease, + *logos*, word, reason] The medical area concerned with speech pathology.

lalopathy (lă-lŏp′ă-thē) [″ + *pathos*, disease] Any disorder of the speech.

lalophobia (lăl″ō-fō′bē-ă) [″ + *phobos*, fear] A morbid reluctance to speak owing to fear of stammering or committing errors.

laloplegia (lăl-ō-plē′jē-ă) [″ + *plege*, a stroke] A paralysis of the speech muscles without affecting the action of the tongue.

lalorrhea (lăl″ō-rē′ă) [″ + *rhoia*, flow] An abnormal flow of speech.

Lamarck's theory (lă-mărks′) [Jean Baptiste P. A. Lamarck, Fr. naturalist, 1744–1829] The theory, popular in the 19th century but now rejected, that evolutionary changes are the result of environmental changes, and that acquired characteristics are inherited and passed on to descendants. SEE: *natural selection*.

Lamaze technique, Lamaze method (lă-măz′) [Fernand Lamaze, Fr. obstetrician, 1890–1957] A method of psychoprophylaxis for childbirth in which the mother is instructed in breathing techniques that permit her to facilitate delivery by relaxing at the proper time with respect to the involuntary contractions of abdominal and uterine musculature. Those who are able to use the method require little if any anesthesia during delivery. SEE: *labor*.

lambda (lăm′dă) [Gr.] **1.** A letter in the Greek alphabet (Λ, λ); also signified by the letter L or l. **2.** The point or angle of junction of the lambdoid and sagittal sutures.

lambdacism (lăm′dă-sĭzm) [Gr. *lambdakismos*] **1.** Stammering of the "l" sound. **2.** An inability to pronounce the "l" sound properly. **3.** Substitution of "l" for "r" in speaking.

lambdoid, lambdoidal (lăm′doyd, lăm-doyd′ăl) [Gr. *lambda,* + *eidos,* form, shape] Shaped like the Greek letter Λ.

lambert [Johann H. Lambert, Ger. physicist, 1728–1777] A unit of brightness equal to that seen when a perfectly diffusing surface radiates or reflects one lumen of light per square centimeter. SEE: *lumen* (2).

Lambert-Eaton myasthenia syndrome [Edward Howard Lambert, U.S. physiologist, b. 1915; Lee McKendree Eaton, U.S. physician, 1905–1958] A syndrome of muscle weakness, hyporeflexia, and autonomic dysfunction. About half of the cases are associated with small cell carcinoma of the lung.

lame [AS. *lama*] Disabled in one or more limbs, esp. in a leg or foot, impairing normal locomotion. It may also be applied to a weak or painful condition, such as a lame back.

lamella (lă-mĕl′ă) *pl.* **lamellae** [L., a little plate] **1.** A thin plate or scale. **2.** A medicated disk of gelatin inserted under the lower eyelid and against the eyeball; used as a local application to the eye.

bone l. A thin layer of ground substance of osseous tissue.

circumferential l. A layer of bone that underlies the periosteum.

concentric l. The plate of bone surrounding a haversian canal. SYN: *haversian l.*

enamel l. Microscopic cracks or calcification imperfections in the enamel surface of a tooth. They may be shallow or extend into the underlying dentin and occur as a developmental defect or a microfracture caused by temperature change or shearing forces.

ground l. Interstitial l.

haversian l. Concentric l.

interstitial l. The bone lamella filling the irregular spaces within the haversian system. SYN: *ground l.*

medullary l. An osseous lamella surrounding and forming the wall of the marrow cavity of long bones.

periosteal l. The bone lamella next to and parallel with the periosteum, forming the external portion of bone.

triangular l. The small fibrous lamina between the choroid plexuses of the third ventricle of the brain.

vitreous l. Bruch's membrane.

lamellar (lă-mĕl′ăr) **1.** Arranged in thin plates or scales. **2.** Pert. to the lamella.

lameness Limping, abnormal gait, or hobbling resulting from partial loss of function in a leg. The symptom may be due to maldevelopment, injury, or disease.

lamina (lăm′ĭ-nă) *pl.* **laminae** [L.] **1.** A thin flat layer or membrane. **2.** The flattened part of either side of the arch of a vertebra.

alar l. The alar plate of the spinal cord in the human embryo, which later becomes the sensory portion.

anterior elastic l. Bowman's membrane.

basal l. **1.** The basal plate of the spinal cord in the human embryo, which later becomes the motor portion. **2.** A mucopolysaccharide layer on the basal surface of epithelial cells which separates them functionally from the underlying connective tissue of the body.

l. basalis choroideae Bruch's membrane.

l. basilaris ductus cochlearis The membranous portion of the spiral lamina of the cochlea of the inner ear.

Bowman's l. Bowman's membrane.

l. cartilaginis cricoideae The posterior portion of the cricoid cartilage.

l. choriocapillaris The middle layer of the choroid, containing a dense mesh of capillaries.

l. cribrosa The cribriform plate of the ethmoid bone.

l. cribrosa sclerae The portion of the sclera forming a sievelike plate through which pass fibers of the optic nerve to the retina.

dental l. A U-shaped internal growth of the oral epithelium in the embryonic maxillary and mandibular regions that forms into enamel organs which produce the teeth. SEE: *enamel organ.*

l. dura A radiographical term describing the compact bone (alveolar bone proper) that surrounds the roots of teeth. In a state of health, it appears on a radiograph as a dense radiopaque line.

epithelial l. The epithelial layer covering the choroid layer of the eye.

l. fusca sclerae The layer of thin pigmented connective tissue on the inner surface of the sclera of the eye.

internal medullary l. The layer of white matter that divides the gray matter of the thalamus into three parts: anterior, medial, and lateral.

interpubic fibrocartilaginous l. Part of the articulation of the pubic bones, connecting the opposing surfaces of these bones.

labial l. A thickened band of epithelium that grows from the ectodermal covering of the embryonic jaw. The ectodermal plate splits and separates the lip from the gum. SYN: *vestibular l.*

l. multiformis The polymorphic layer of the isocortex of the cerebral cortex.

l. papyracea A thin, smooth plate of bone on the lateral surface of the ethmoid bone; it forms part of the orbital plate.

perpendicular l. A thin sheet of bone forming the perpendicular plate of the ethmoid bone. It supports the upper portion of the nasal septum.

l. propria mucosae The thin layer of areolar connective tissue, blood vessels, and nerves that lies immediately beneath the surface epithelium of mucous membranes.

pterygoid l. One of the internal and external laminae that make up the pterygoid process of the sphenoid bone. They are areas of attachment for the muscles of mastication.

rostral l. A continuation of the rostrum of the corpus callosum and the terminal lamina of the third ventricle of the brain.

l. suprachoroidea The outermost layer of the choroid.

terminal l. The thin sheet of tissue forming the anterior border of the third ventricle.

l. of vertebral arch One of the laminae extending from the pedicles of the vertebral arches and fusing together to form the dorsal portion of the arch. The spinous process extends from the center of these laminae.

vestibular l. Labial l.

l. vitrea Bruch's membrane.

l. zonalis The outer or plexiform layer of the isocortex of the brain.

laminae (lăm′ĭ-nē) Pl. of lamina.

laminagram (lăm′ĭ-nă-grăm) [L. *lamina,* thin plate, + Gr. *gramma,* something written] A radiograph taken of a section of the body, so that the area being investigated appears as if only a slice through the tissue is depicted. SEE: *tomogram.*

laminagraph (lăm′ĭ-nă-grăf) [″ + Gr. *graphein,* to write] An x-ray technique for producing a laminagram.

laminagraphy (lăm″ĭ-năg′ră-fē) [″ + Gr. *graphein,* to write] An outdated technique for the study of body tissues by use of laminagrams. SEE: *tomography.*

laminar Made up of or pert. to laminae.

l. air flow Filtered air moving along separate parallel flow planes to surgical theaters, patient rooms, nurseries, bacteriology work areas, or food preparation areas. This method of air flow helps to prevent bacterial contamination and collection of hazardous chemical fumes in areas where they would pollute the work environment.

Laminaria digitata (lăm-ĭ-nār′ē-ă dĭj-ĭ-tā′tă) A genus of kelp or seaweed that, when dried, has the ability to absorb water and expand with considerable force. It has been used to dilate the uterine cervical canal in induced abortion and to induce cervical ripening. Hazards associated with the use of seaweed include cervical lacerations, accidental rupture of membranes, and infection.

laminarin (lăm″ĭ-nă′rĭn) A polysaccharide obtained from *Laminaria* species of seaweed. It consists principally of glucose residues.

laminated (lăm′ĭn-āt″ĕd) [L. *lamina,* thin plate] Arranged in layers or laminae.

lamination (lăm″ĭn-ā′shŭn) Layer-like arrangement.

laminectomy (lăm″ĭ-nĕk′tō-mē) [″ + Gr. *ektome,* excision] The excision of a vertebral posterior arch, usually to remove a lesion or herniated disk. SEE: *Nursing Diagnoses Appendix.*

PATIENT CARE: *Preoperative:* The patient's knowledge of the procedure is determined, misconceptions are corrected, additional information is provided as necessary, and a signed informed consent form is obtained. A baseline assessment of the patient's neurological function and of lower extremity circulation is documented. Health care providers discuss postoperative care concerns, demonstrate maneuvers such as log-rolling, assure the patient of the availability of pain medications on request, and prepare the patient for surgery according to the surgeon's or institutional protocol.

Postoperative: Vital signs and neurovascular status (motor, sensory, and circulatory) are monitored, antiembolism stockings or pneumatic dressings are applied, and anticoagulants are given if prescribed. The dressing is inspected for bleeding or cerebrospinal fluid leakage; either problem is documented and reported immediately, and the incision is redressed as necessary and directed with the use of scrupulous aseptic technique. The patient is maintained in a supine position, with the head flat or no higher than 45 degrees according to the surgeon's preference, for the prescribed time (usually 1 to 2 hr), then repositioned side to side every 2 hr by log-rolling the patient with a pillow between the legs to prevent twisting and hip adduction and to maintain spinal alignment. Deep breathing (with use of an inspirometer if prescribed) is encouraged, and assistance is provided with range-of-motion, gluteal muscle setting, and quadriceps setting exercises. Adequate assistance should be available when the patient is permitted to dangle, stand, and ambulate in the early postoperative period. Prescribed anti-inflammatory, muscle-relaxant, and antibiotic agents are administered, and noninvasive measures in addition to prescribed analgesia are provided to prevent and relieve incisional discomfort. Fluid balance is monitored by administering prescribed I.V. fluids and by assessing urine output. The patient is encouraged to void within 8 to 12 hr postsurgery and is assessed for bladder distention, which may indicate urinary retention; however, catherization is instituted only after other measures to promote voiding have been attempted. The abdomen is auscultated for return of bowel sounds, and adequate oral nutrition is provided when G.I. function has returned.

Rehabilitative and home care: Incisional care techniques are taught to the patient and family, and the importance of checking for signs of infection (increased local pain and tenderness, redness, swelling, and changes in the amount or character of any drainage) and of reporting these to the surgeon is stressed. A gradual increase in the patient's activity level is encouraged, which usually includes a walking regimen and rest periods as prescribed by the surgeon and physical therapist. Any prescribed exercises (pelvic tilts, leg raising, toe pointing) are reviewed, and prescribed activity restrictions are reinforced. Such restrictions usually include sitting for prolonged periods, lifting heavy or moderately heavy objects, bending over, and climbing long flights of stairs. Proper body mechanics are taught to lessen strain and pressure on the spine; these include maintaining proper body alignment and good posture and sleeping on a firm mattress. Involvement in an exercise program is encouraged after 6 wk, beginning with gradual strengthening of abdominal muscles. The patient should schedule and keep a follow-up appointment with the surgeon and communicate any concerns to the surgeon (if necessary) before that visit.

laminin (lăm′i-nĭn) A glycoprotein found in all basement membranes that is involved in the binding of cells to the extracellular matrix, particularly to type IV collagen. It contributes to the growth and cellular organization of tissues and is involved in angiogenesis, invasion, and metastasis of tumor cells, and cellular attachment. SEE: *glycoprotein; extracellular matrix.*

laminitis (lăm-ĭn-ī′tĭs) [″ + Gr. *itis,* inflammation] The inflammation of a lamina.

laminotomy (lăm″ĭ-nŏt′ō-mē) [″ + Gr. *tome,* incision] A division of one of the vertebral laminae.

lamivudine (lă-mē′voo-dīn) A nucleoside analogue reverse transcriptase inhibitor used in the treatment of HIV-1 and chronic viral hepatitis. Trade name is Epivir.

lamotrigine (lă-mō′trĭ-jēn) A drug used to treat seizure disorders.

lamp [Gr. *lampein,* to shine] A device for producing and applying light, heat, radiation, and various forms of radiant energy for the treatment of disease, resolution of impairments, or palliation of pain.

infrared l. Heat lamp; a lamp that develops a high temperature, emitting infrared rays. The rays penetrate only a short distance (5 to 10 mm) into the skin. Its principal effect is to cause heating of the skin.

slit l. A lamp constructed so that an intense light is emitted through a slit; used for examination of the eye. SEE: illus.

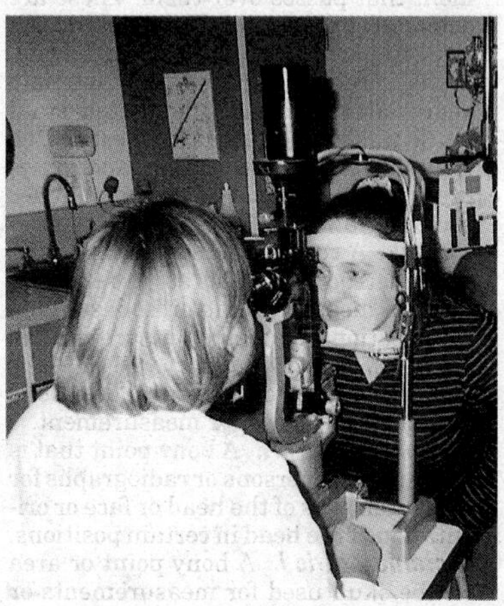

SLIT LAMP EXAMINATION

sun l. A lamp that produces ultraviolet light used in therapeutic doses for treatment of skin diseases, such as psoriasis and cutaneous T-cell lymphoma. SYN: *ultraviolet l.*

ultraviolet l. Sun l.

Wood's l. Wood's filter.

lamprophonia (lăm″prō-fō′nē-ă) [Gr. *lampros,* clear, + *phone,* voice] A marked distinctness or clearness of voice.

lamprophonic (lăm″prō-fŏn′ĭk) Possessing a clear voice.

lanatoside C (lăn-ăt′ō-sīd) A glycoside of *Digitalis lanata;* an agent used for atrial fibrillation and congestive heart failure.

lance (lăns) [L. *lancea*] **1.** A two-edged surgical knife. **2.** To incise with a lancet or other cutting instrument.

Lancefield classification (lăns′fēld) [Rebecca Craighill Lancefield, U.S. bacteriologist, 1895–1981] A classification of hemolytic streptococci into various groups according to antigenic structure.

lancet (lăn′sĕt) [L. *lancea,* lance] **1.** A pointed surgical knife with two edges. **2.** A spring-loaded or manual blade used to make a limited skin incision as for collection of blood specimen.

lancinating (lăn′sĭ-nāt″ĭng) [L. *lancinare,* to tear] Sharp or cutting, as pain.

L and A Abbreviation for the reaction of the pupils of the eye to *light* and *accommodation.*

Landau reflex An infantile reflex in which the body flexes when the head is passively flexed forward in a prone position. It appears normally at 3 months and is absent in children with cerebral palsy and gross motor retardation.

land mines Explosive devices placed in or on the ground for the purpose of destroying humans, animals, or equipment that passes over them. These are activated on contact. They remain active after armed conflict has ceased and, if they are not removed, can detonate years later, causing unexpected traumatic injury and death. It is estimated that about 65 to 110 million land mines are scattered throughout 60 countries around the world.

landmark A recognizable skeletal or soft tissue structure used as a reference point in measurements or in describing the location of other structures. SEE: *cephalometry; craniometry*.

bony l. A structure or spot on a bone used as a reference for measurement.

cephalometric l. A bony point that is used in living persons or radiographs for measurements of the head or face or orientation of the head in certain positions.

craniometric l. A bony point or area on the skull used for measurements or orientation of the skull.

orbital l. A cephalometric point located at the lowest point of the orbital margin.

radiographic l. A cephalometric, craniometric, or soft tissue landmark used for orientation or measurements.

soft tissue l. An area or point on a soft tissue used as a point of reference for measurements of the body or its parts.

Landouzy-Déjérine dystrophy (lăn-dū-zē′ dĕ″zhĕ-rēn′) [Louis T. J. Landouzy, Fr. physician, 1845–1917; Joseph Jules Déjérine, Fr. neurologist, 1849–1917] A slowly progressive dystrophy involving principally the musculature of the face and shoulders. It is marked by atrophic changes in the muscles of the shoulder girdle and face, inability to raise the arms above the head, myopathic facies, eyelids that remain partly open in sleep, and inability to whistle or purse the lips. SYN: *dystrophy, facioscapulohumeral muscular; Landouzy-Déjérine atrophy*.

TREATMENT: Therapy is supportive; for example, orthopedic devices can be used to prevent functional losses at the shoulder girdle. The patient should be encouraged to maintain as full and normal a life as possible and to avoid prolonged bed rest.

Landry-Guillain-Barré syndrome Guillain-Barré syndrome.

Landsteiner's classification (lănd′stī-nĕrz) [Karl L. Landsteiner, Austrian-born U.S. biologist, 1868–1943; Nobel prize winner in medicine in 1930] A classification of blood types designating O, A, B, and AB based on the presence of antigens on the erythrocytes.

Lane's kinks [Sir William Arbuthnot Lane, Brit. surgeon, 1856–1943] Bending or twisting of the last few centimeters of the ileum with external adhesions between the folded loops of intestines. This may cause intestinal obstruction.

Langerhans' islands SEE: *islets of Langerhans*.

Langer's lines (lăng′ĕrz) [Carl (Ritter von Edenberg) Langer, Austrian anatomist, 1819–1887] The structural orientation of the fibrous tissue of the skin, forming the natural cleavage lines that, though present in all body areas, are visible only in certain sites such as the creases of the palm. These lines are of particular importance in surgery. Incisions made parallel to them make a much smaller scar upon healing than those made at right angles to the lines. SEE: illus.

Langer's muscle Muscular fibers from insertion of the pectoralis major muscle, over the bicipital groove to the insertion of the latissimus dorsi.

Lange's test (lăng′ĕz) [Carl Lange, Ger. physician, 1883–1953] An obsolete test for diagnosis of cerebrospinal syphilis by the degree of gold precipitation in varying concentrations of colloidal gold solution and spinal fluid.

Langhans' layer (lăng′hăns) [Theodor Langhans, Ger. pathologist, 1839–1915] A cellular layer present in the chorionic villi of the placenta. SYN: *cytotrophoblast*.

language The spoken or written words or symbols used by a population for communication.

languor (lăng′gĕr) [L. *languere,* to languish] A feeling of weariness or exhaustion as from illness; lack of vigor or animation; lassitude.

laniary (lăn′ē-ā″rē) [L. *laniare,* to tear to pieces] Adapted or designed for tearing, as the canine teeth.

lanolin (lăn′ŏ-lĭn) [L. *lana,* wool] The purified, fatlike substance obtained from the wool of sheep; used as an ointment base.

anhydrous l. Wool fat containing not more than 0.25% water; used as an ointment base that has the ability to absorb water.

lansoprazole (lan-soh′pra-zohl) A proton pump inhibitor that decreases gastric acid production and is used to treat peptic ulcers, gastroesophageal reflux, *Helicobacter pylori* infections, and related diseases. Trade name is Prevacid.

lanthanum (lăn′thă-nŭm) SYMB: La. A metallic element; atomic weight 138.906; atomic number 57. It is one of a group of elements called lanthanides.

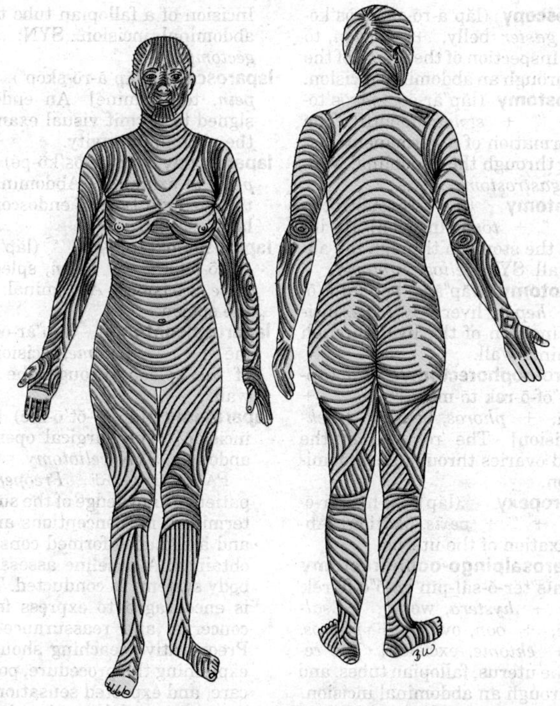

LANGER'S LINES

lantibiotic (lan′tī-bī-ŏt-ĭk) Any peptide antibiotic whose chemical structure includes a bridge maintained by the rare amino acid lanthionine. Subtilin and nisin are examples of lantibiotics.

lanuginous (lă-nū′jĭn-ŭs) Covered with lanugo.

lanugo (lă-nū′gō) [L. *lana,* wool] **1.** Downy hair covering the body. **2.** Fine downy hairs that cover the body of the fetus, esp. when premature. The presence and amount of lanugo aids in estimating the gestational age of preterm infants. The fetus first exhibits lanugo between weeks 13 and 16. By gestational week 20, it covers the face and body. The amount of lanugo is greatest between weeks 28 and 30. As the third trimester progresses, lanugo disappears from the face, trunk, and extremities.

LAO *left anterior oblique* position.

laparectomy (lăp″ă-rĕk′tō-mē) [Gr. *lapara,* flank, + *ektome,* excision] Excision of strips or gores in the abdominal wall to relieve extreme weakness of the abdominal muscles.

laparo- [Gr. *lapara,* flank] Combining form pert. to the flank and to operations through the abdominal wall.

laparocele (lăp′ă-rō-sēl) [″ + *kele,* tumor, swelling] An abdominal hernia.

laparocholecystotomy (lăp″ăr-ō-kōl″ē-sĭs-tŏt′ō-mē) [″ + *chole,* bile, + *kystis,* bladder, + *tome,* incision] An incision into the gallbladder through the abdominal wall.

laparocolectomy (lăp″ă-rō-kō-lĕk′tō-mē) [″ + *kolon,* colon, + *ektome,* excision] Colectomy.

laparocolostomy, laparocolotomy (lăp″ăr-ō-kō-lŏs′tō-mē, lăp″ăr-ō-kō-lŏt′ō-mē) [″ + ″ + *stoma,* mouth] The formation of a permanent opening into the colon through the abdominal wall.

laparocystectomy (lă″pă-rō-sĭs-tĕk′tō-mē) [″ + *kystis,* bladder, + *ektome,* excision] The removal of an extrauterine fetus or a cyst through an abdominal incision.

laparocystidotomy (lăp″ăr-ō-sĭst-ĭ-dŏt′ō-mē) [″ + ″ + *tome,* incision] An incision of the bladder through the abdominal wall.

laparocystotomy (lăp″ăr-ō-sĭs-tŏt′ō-mē) An incision of the abdomen to remove the contents of a cyst or an extrauterine fetus.

laparoenterostomy (lăp″ă-rō-ĕn″tĕr-ŏs′tō-mē) [″ + *enteron,* intestine, + *stoma,* mouth] The formation of an artificial opening into the intestine through the abdominal wall.

laparoenterotomy (lăp″ăr-ō-ĕn″tĕr-ŏt′ō-mē) [″ + ″ + *tome,* incision] An opening into the intestinal cavity by incision through the loins.

laparogastroscopy (lăp″ă-rō-găs-trŏs′kō-pē) [″ + *gaster,* belly, + *skopein,* to examine] Inspection of the inside of the stomach through an abdominal incision.

laparogastrostomy (lăp″ăr-ō-găs-trŏs′tō-mē) [″ + ″ + *stoma,* mouth] The surgical formation of a permanent gastric fistula through the abdominal wall. SYN: *celiogastrostomy.*

laparogastrotomy (lăp″ă-rō-găs-trŏt′ō-mē) [″ + ″ + *tome,* incision] An incision into the stomach through the abdominal wall. SYN: *celiogastrotomy.*

laparohepatotomy (lăp″ăr-ō-hĕp″ă-tŏt′ō-mē) [″ + *hepar,* liver, + *tome,* incision] An incision of the liver through the abdominal wall.

laparohystero-oophorectomy (lăp″ăr-ō-hĭs″tĕr-ō-ō″ŏf-ō-rek′tō-mē) [″ + ″ + *oon,* ovum, + *phoros,* bearer, + *ektome,* excision] The removal of the uterus and ovaries through an abdominal incision.

laparohysteropexy (lăp″ăr-ō-hĭs′tĕr-ō-pĕks-ē) [″ + ″ + *pexis,* fixation] Abdominal fixation of the uterus.

laparohysterosalpingo-oophorectomy (lăp″ăr-ō-hĭs″tĕr-ŏ-săl-pĭn″gō-ō″ŏ-fō-rĕk′tō-mē) [″ + *hystera,* womb, + *salpinx,* tube, + *oon,* ovum, + *phoros,* bearer, + *ektome,* excision] The removal of the uterus, fallopian tubes, and ovaries through an abdominal incision.

laparohysterotomy (lăp″ăr-ō-hĭs″tĕr-ŏt′ō-mē) [″ + ″ + *tome,* incision] Surgery of the uterus through an abdominal incision. SEE: *cesarean section.*

laparoileotomy (lăp″ăr-ō-ĭl-ē-ŏt′ō-mē) [″ + L. *ileum,* ileum, + Gr. *tome,* incision] An abdominal incision into the ileum.

laparomyitis (lăp″ăr-ō-mī-ī′tĭs) [″ + *mys,* muscle, + *itis,* inflammation] Inflammation of the muscular portion of the abdominal wall.

laparomyomectomy (lăp″ăr-ō-mī″ō-mĕk′tō-mē) [″ + ″ + *oma,* tumor, + *ektome,* excision] Abdominal excision of a muscular tumor.

laparonephrectomy (lăp″ăr-ō-nĕ-frĕk′tō-mē) [″ + *nephros,* kidney, + *ektome,* excision] Renal excision through the loin.

laparorrhaphy (lăp-ă-ror′ă-fē) [″ + *rhaphe,* seam, ridge] Suture of a wound in the abdominal wall. SYN: *celiorrhaphy.*

laparosalpingectomy (lăp″ăr-ō-săl-pĭn-jek′tō-mē) [″ + *salpinx,* tube, + *ektome,* excision] Excision of a fallopian tube through an abdominal incision.

laparosalpingo-oophorectomy (lăp″ăr-ō-săl-pĭn″gō-ō″ŏf-ō-rĕk′tō-mē) [″ + ″ + *oon,* ovum, + *phoros,* bearer, + *ektome,* excision] The removal of the fallopian tubes and ovaries through an abdominal incision.

laparosalpingotomy (lăp″ăr-ō-săl-pĭn-gŏt′ō-mē) [″ + ″ + *tome,* incision] Incision of a fallopian tube through an abdominal incision. SYN: *celiosalpingectomy.*

laparoscope (lăp′ă-rō-skōp″) [″ + *skopein,* to examine] An endoscope designed to permit visual examination of the abdominal cavity.

laparoscopy (lăp-ăr-ŏs′kō-pē) [″ + *skopein,* to examine] Abdominal exploration using a type of endoscope called a laparoscope.

laparosplenectomy (lăp″ăr-ō-splēn-ĕk′tō-mē) [″ + *splen,* spleen, + *ektome,* excision] Abdominal excision of the spleen.

laparosplenotomy (lăp″ăr-ō-splēn-ŏt′ō-mē) [″ + ″ + *tome,* incision] Incision of the spleen through the abdominal wall.

laparotomy (lăp-ăr-ŏt′ō-mē) [″ + *tome,* incision] The surgical opening of the abdomen. SYN: *celiotomy.*

PATIENT CARE: *Preoperative:* The patient's knowledge of the surgery is determined, misconceptions are clarified, and a signed informed consent form is obtained. A baseline assessment of all body systems is conducted. The patient is encouraged to express feelings and concerns, and reassurance is offered. Preoperative teaching should focus on explaining the procedure, postoperative care, and expected sensations. Physical preparation of the patient is carried out according to institutional or surgeon's protocol regarding diet; shaving of abdomen and pubic area; enemas, douches, and collecting of urine specimens. Antithrombotic medications and antiembolic measures are applied as prescribed.

Postoperative: Vital signs and dressing status are monitored; the latter includes checking any drains in place and for the presence of vaginal bleeding if applicable. Ventilatory status is assessed by auscultating for adventitious or decreased breath sounds, and respiratory toilet (deep breathing, coughing, incentive spirometry, oral hygiene, and repositioning) is provided as determined by the patient's response. The nurse assists the patient to use noninvasive pain relief measures and prescribed analgesia for pain relief or monitors patient-controlled analgesia for effectiveness. Fluid balance is monitored, and prescribed fluid and electrolyte replacement therapy is administered. The patient is encouraged to void after surgery; the bladder assessed for distention, which may indicate urinary retention; and catheterization is instituted only when nursing measures are unsuccessful. The abdomen is auscultated for the return of bowel sounds, and a high-protein, high vitamin C diet is initiated when G.I. function has returned. Leg mobilization, turning, and early ambulation are encouraged, to promote gastrointestinal activity and prevent venous thrombosis. The hospital staff initiates early discharge planning, which includes carrying out patient teaching focused on incisional care, complications to report, and activity resumption and restrictions; arranging referral for home care as appropriate; and ensuring that the patient has scheduled (and plans to keep) a follow-up appointment with the surgeon.

laparotrachelotomy (lăp″ăr-ō-trā-kĕl-ŏt′ō-mē) [″ + *trachelos,* neck, + *tome,* incision] A cesarean section with the incision through the lower segment of the uterus.

laparotyphlotomy (lăp″ăr-ō-tĭ-flŏt′ō-mē) [″ + *typhlon,* cecum, + *tome,* incision] Incision of the cecum through a lateral abdominal incision.

lap board A wheelchair attachment serving as a tray or platform over the lap to support the hands and arms or to permit manual activities.

lapinization (lăp″ĭn-ī-zā′shŭn) [Fr. *lapin,* rabbit] In virology, the serial passage of a virus through rabbits in order to modify the virus.

Laplace, law of [Pierre-Simon Laplace, Fr. scientist, 1749–1827] A law stating that pressure within a tube is inversely proportional to the radius. The larger the diameter of a tubular structure, the less chance that it will rupture when subjected to an increase in pressure. So, for example, when pressure in the colon is increased due to obstruction, the right colon, which has a larger diameter than the left colon, would be at less risk of perforation than the left.

lard [L. *lardum,* fat] Purified fat from the hog. The sole nutrient is fat; a 100-g portion contains 902 kcal.

benzoinated l. Lard containing 1% benzoin, used as a vehicle for certain types of topically applied medicines.

lardaceous (lăr-dā′shŭs) [L. *lardum,* fat] Resembling lard; waxy, fatty.

large for gestational age ABBR: LGA. Term used of a newborn whose birth weight is above the 90th percentile on the intrauterine growth curve. Such babies should be monitored for signs of hypoglycemia during the first 24 hr after birth.

large loop excision of the transformation zone ABBR: LLETZ. Obtaining a biopsy of the uterine cervix in patients in whom the colposcopic examination or Pap smear indicates the area is abnormal. The tissue is obtained by use of an electrically heated wire loop. This procedure is used in treating noninvasive carcinoma of the cervix. SYN: *loop electrode excision procedure.*

Larmor frequency In magnetic resonance imaging (MRI), the frequency of the radio wave that will resonate with all the protons in the nucleus of a given element. The Larmor radio frequency induces the magnetic resonance used to create MRI images.

larva [L., mask] **1.** General term applied to the developing form of an insect after it has emerged from the egg and before it transforms into a pupa, from which it emerges as an adult. **2.** The immature forms of other invertebrates such as worms. **larval** (lăr′văl), *adj.*

l. currens A type of larva migrans. The organism, *Strongyloides stercoralis,* travels subcutaneously at the rate of about 10 cm an hour rather than at the slow rate of larva migrans.

cutaneous l. migrans A skin lesion characterized by a tortuous elevated red line that progresses at one end while fading out at the other. It is caused by the subcutaneous migration of the larvae of certain nematodes, esp. *Ancylostoma braziliense* and *A. caninum,* that occur as parasitic infections in humans.

visceral l. migrans Toxocariasis.

larvate [L. *larva,* mask] Hidden, concealed, as a hidden symptom.

larvicide [″ + *caedere,* to kill] An agent that destroys insect larvae.

larviphagic (lăr″vĭ-fā′jĭk) [″ + Gr. *phagein,* to eat] Consuming larva, as is done by certain fish.

laryngalgia (lăr-ĭn-găl′jē-ă) [Gr. *larynx,* larynx, + *algos,* pain] Laryngeal pain.

laryngeal (lăr-ĭn′jē-ăl) [Gr. *larynx,* larynx] Pert. to the larynx.

laryngectomee (lăr″ĭn-jĕk′tō-mē) [″ + *ektome,* excision] An individual whose larynx has been removed.

laryngectomy (lăr″ĭn-jĕk′tō-mē) [″ + *ektome,* excision] Removal of all or part of the larynx, to treat cancers of the larynx, most of which are squamous cell carcinomas. Additional treatment may include radiation, chemotherapy, or both. The procedure may cure the cancer if it is confined to the organ. Common complications of the surgery are loss of voice, gastroesophageal reflux, and adjustment disorders or depression as a result of the changes in body image produced by the operation. SEE: *Nursing Diagnoses Appendix.*

PATIENT CARE: *Preoperative:* The patient is prepared for vocal and airway changes and for other functional losses after surgery. Explanations are supplemented with diagrams and samples of required equipment. Postsurgical communication methods most appropriate for and agreeable to the particular patient (e.g., simple sign language, flash cards, magic slate, alphabet board) are explained. The postoperative setting and care are described to the patient, including assessment measures, therapies, equipment, procedures, and expected sensations. Nutritional modalities (parenteral, enteral via tube feeding, then oral feeding) also are explained. Both patient and family are encouraged to verbalize their feelings and concerns, and realistic reassurance and information are provided. The patient is supported during anticipatory grieving and referred as necessary for further psychological or religious support. Once the signed informed consent form is obtained, the patient is prepared for surgery according to the surgeon's or institutional protocol.

Postoperative: Vital signs are monitored, especially ventilatory rate and effort, as well as level of consciousness, arterial blood gas values, peripheral oxygen saturation levels, and the status of dressings and drains. The airway is assessed for patency; the laryngostomy tube is gently (but not deeply) suctioned, as are the oral cavity and nose, as needed. Crust formation is prevented by increasing humidity and fluid intake, and frequent oral hygiene and assistance in managing saliva are provided. The patient usually is positioned on one side, with the head elevated to 30 to 45 degrees. Support is provided to the patient's neck posteriorly during movement. Fluid balance is monitored, prescribed replacement therapy is provided, and urination is encouraged. The patient is assessed for early complications such as respiratory distress due to edema, infection, dehydration, and hemorrhage (remembering to check the posterior aspect of the neck, as well as dressings, drains, and vital signs); and for later ones such as fistula formation, tracheal stenosis, and carotid artery rupture. Protein-rich, high–vitamin C nutrition is provided, via the prescribed route, to aid healing. Noninvasive measures and prescribed analgesics to relieve pain are provided. The patient is allowed time for communication and is reassured that verbal communication ability will be reestablished through surgically implanted prostheses, speech therapy for esophageal speech, or external mechanical or electronic voice boxes. Professional staff supports the patient and family through their grief over losses (including loss of voice, whistling, sucking ability, sense of smell, nose blowing, activities such as swimming) and damage to self-esteem. The patient is prepared for possible follow-up therapies, such as radiation and chemotherapy. Patient education also should include self-care activities and instructions about important complications. A list of the resources in the community should be provided for support, counseling, and further education. Patients are encouraged to join local branches of groups such as the American Speech-Learning-Hearing Association, American Cancer Society, International Association of Laryngectomees, or Lost Chord Club. A rapid return to employment is encouraged. Tobacco smokers and alcohol users are encouraged to seek help in quitting.

laryngismal (lăr″ĭn-jĭs′măl) [″ + *-ismos,* condition] Concerning or resembling laryngeal spasm.

laryngismus (lăr″ĭn-jĭs′mŭs) [″ + *-ismos,* condition] Spasm of the larynx.

laryngitic (lăr-ĭn-jĭt′ĭk) [Gr. *larynx,* larynx] **1.** Resulting from laryngitis. **2.** Relating to laryngitis.

laryngitis (lăr-ĭn-jī′tĭs) [″ + *itis,* inflammation] Inflammation of the larynx. SEE: *croup; Nursing Diagnoses Appendix.*

acute l. Acute congestive laryngitis; inflammation of laryngeal mucosa and the vocal cords. It is characterized by hoarseness and aphonia and occasionally pain on phonation and deglutition. It may be caused by improper use or overuse of the voice, exposure to cold and wet, extension from infections in nose and throat, inhalation of irritating vapors and dust, or systemic diseases such as whooping cough or measles.

TREATMENT: Treatment includes vocal rest, liquid or soft diet, steam inhalations, and codeine or nonnarcotic cough suppressants for pain and cough. If the laryngitis is viral, no specific therapy exists; if bacterial, appropriate antibiotics should be given. If acute or chronic bronchitis is present, treatment of that condition will help control laryngitis.

atrophic l. Laryngitis leading to diminished secretion and atrophy of the mucous membrane. Symptoms are a tickling sensation in the throat, hoarseness, cough, and dyspnea when the crusts are thick and accumulate on the vocal cords, narrowing the breathing aperture. Inhalants and medicated sprays should be used to loosen the crusts, along with strict attention to associated nose and throat pathology.

chronic l. A type of laryngitis caused by a recurrent irritation, or following the acute form. It is often secondary to sinus or nasal pathology, improper use of the voice, excessive smoking or drinking, or neoplasms. The patient experiences a tickling in the throat, huskiness of the voice, and dysphonia. The treatment involves correcting the preexisting nose and throat pathology, discontinuing alcohol and tobacco use, and avoiding excessive use of the voice.

croupous l. Laryngitis occurring mainly in infants and young children and characterized by a barky cough, hoarseness, and stridor.

diphtheritic l. Invasion of the larynx by diphtheria, usually with formation of a membrane.

membranous l. Laryngitis characterized by inflammation of the larynx, with the formation of a false, nondiphtheritic membrane.

syphilitic l. A chronic form of laryngitis caused by syphilis. It is characterized by hoarseness, cough, formation of broad condylomata, follicular hyperplasia, syphiloma, and syphilitic perichondritis. In secondary syphilis, mucous patches may involve large areas of the larynx. In tertiary syphilis, gumma may be present. Scarring and deformity follow healing of gumma. The appropriate antibiotic therapy (e.g., penicillin or ceftriaxone) should be given.

tuberculous l. Laryngitis secondary to pulmonary tuberculosis. Patients have hoarseness, aphonia, pain in swallowing, and cough. Lesions may be located in the interarytenoid area, vocal cords, epiglottis, or false cords. Lesions are relatively pale; ulceration occurs early.

laryngo- [Gr. *larynx,* larynx] Combining form pert. to the larynx.

laryngocele (lăr-ĭn′gō-sēl) [″ + *kele,* tumor, swelling] A congenital air sac connected to the larynx. Its presence is normal in some animals but abnormal in humans.

laryngocentesis (lăr-ĭn″gō-sĕn-tē′sĭs) [″ + *kentesis,* puncture] Incision or puncture of the larynx.

laryngofissure (lăr-ĭng″gō-fĭsh′ūr) [″ + L. *fissura,* a cleft] The operation of opening the larynx by a median line incision through the thyroid cartilage.

laryngogram (lă-rĭng′gō-grăm) [″ + *gramma,* something written] A radiograph of the larynx.

laryngograph (lăr-ĭng′ō-grăf) [″ + *graphein,* to write] A device for making a record of laryngeal movements.

laryngography (lăr″ĭn-gŏg′ră-fē) **1.** A description of the larynx. **2.** Radiography of the larynx using a radiopaque contrast medium.

laryngologist (lăr″ĭn-gŏl′ō-jĭst) [″ + *logos,* word, reason] A specialist in laryngology.

laryngology The specialty of medicine concerned with the pharynx, throat, larynx, nasopharynx, and tracheobronchial tree.

laryngomalacia (lăr-ĭng″gō-mă-lā′shē-ă) [″ + *malakia,* softness] A softening of the tissues of the larynx.

laryngometry (lăr″ĭn-gŏm′ĕ-trē) [″ + *metron,* measure] The systematic measurement of the larynx.

laryngoparalysis (lăr-ĭn″gō-păr-ăl′ĭ-sĭs) [″ + *paralyein,* to disable at one side] Paralysis of the muscles of the larynx.

laryngopathy (lăr″ĭn-gŏp′ă-thē) [″ + *pathos,* disease] Any disease of the larynx.

laryngopharyngeal (lăr-ĭn″gō-făr-ĭn′jē-ăl) [″ + *pharynx,* throat] Relating jointly to the larynx and pharynx.

laryngopharyngectomy (lăr-ĭn″gō-făr-ĭn-jĕk′tō-mē) [″ + ″ + *ektome,* excision] Removal of the larynx and pharynx.

laryngopharyngeus (lă-rĭng″gō-fă-rĭn′jē-ŭs) The muscle that constricts the inferior pharynx.

laryngopharyngitis (lăr-ĭn″gō-făr-ĭn-jī′tĭs) [″ + ″ + *itis,* inflammation] Inflammation of the larynx and pharynx.

laryngopharyngography (lă-rĭng″gō-fă-rĭn-jŏg′ră-fē) [″ + ″ + *graphein,* to write] Radiographical examination of the larynx and pharynx when filled with air.

laryngopharynx (lăr-ĭn″gō-făr′ĭnks) [Gr. *larynx,* larynx, + *pharynx,* throat] Hypopharynx.

laryngophony (lăr″ĭn-gŏf′ō-nē) [″ + *phone,* voice] Voice sounds heard in auscultating the pharynx.

laryngophthisis (lăr″ĭng-gŏf′thĭ-sĭs) [″ + *phthisis,* a wasting] Tuberculosis of the larynx.

laryngoplasty (lăr-ĭn′gō-plăs″tē) [″ + *plassein,* to form] Plastic reparative surgery of the larynx.

laryngoplegia (lă-rĭng″gō-plē′jē-ă) [″ + *plege,* stroke] Paralysis of the laryngeal muscles.

laryngorhinology (lăr-ĭn″gō-rīn-ŏl′ō-jē) [″ + *rhis,* nose, + *logos,* word, reason] The branch of medical science concerned with diseases of the larynx and nose.

laryngorrhagia (lăr″ĭn-gō-rā′jē-ă) [″ + *rhegnynai,* to flow forth] Laryngeal hemorrhage.

laryngorrhea (lăr″ĭn-gō-rē′ă) [″ + *rhoia,* flow] Excessive discharge of laryngeal mucus.

laryngoscleroma (lăr-ĭn″gō-sklĕ-rō′mă) [″ + *skleros,* hard, + *oma,* tumor] Scleroma affecting the larynx.

laryngoscope (lăr-ĭn′gō-skōp) [″ + *skopein,* to examine] An instrument, consisting of a blade and a fiberoptic light source, used to examine the larynx (e.g., during endotracheal intubation).

laryngoscopic (lăr″ĭn-gō-skŏp′ik) [″ + *skopein,* to examine] Pert. to observation of the interior of the larynx with the aid of a small long-handled mirror. SEE: *laryngoscopy.*

laryngoscopist (lăr″ĭng-gŏs′kō-pĭst) [″ + *skopein,* to examine] An individual trained in laryngoscopy.

laryngoscopy (lăr″ĭn-gŏs′kō-pē) Visual examination of the interior of the larynx to determine the cause of hoarseness, obtain cultures, manage the upper airway, or take biopsies.

PATIENT CARE: The patient's knowledge of the procedure is determined, misconceptions are corrected, and additional information about the procedure and expected sensations is provided as necessary. Once the signed informed consent form has been obtained, the patient is prepared for the procedure according to the institutional or surgeon's protocol. After the procedure, the patient is placed in the semi-Fowler position, and vital signs are monitored until stable. Oral intake is withheld until the patient's swallowing reflex has returned, usually within 2 to 8 hr. An emesis basin is provided for spitting saliva, and sputum is inspected for blood and excessive bleeding reported. Application of an ice collar helps to minimize edema; subcutaneous crepitus around the face or neck should be reported immediately, because it may indicate tracheal perforation. The patient should not cough, clear the throat, or smoke for at least 24 hr to prevent irritation.

direct l. Laryngoscopy using a laryngeal speculum or laryngoscope.

indirect l. Laryngoscopy using a mirror.

laryngospasm (lăr-ĭn′gō-spăzm) [″ + *spasmos,* a convulsion] Spasm of the laryngeal muscles.

laryngostenosis (lăr-ĭng″gō-stĕ-nō′sĭs) [″ + *stenosis,* a narrowing] Stricture of the larynx.

compression l. Stricture of the larynx owing to outside causes such as abscess, tumor, or goiter.

occlusion l. Stricture of the larynx owing to congenital bands or membranes, foreign bodies, tumors, scarring following ulceration as in diphtheria and tertiary syphilis, penetrating wounds, or corrosive fluid. Patients experience dyspnea, esp. on inspiration and exertion, often accompanied by stridor. Treatment depends on the cause. Tracheotomy is often necessary.

laryngostomy (lăr-ĭn-gŏs′tō-mē) [″ + *stoma,* mouth] Establishing a permanent opening through the neck into the larynx.

laryngostroboscope (lăr″ĭn-gō-strō′bō-skōp) [″ + *strobos,* whirl, + *skopein,* to view] An instrument for inspecting vibration of the vocal cords.

laryngotomy (lăr-ĭn-gŏt′ō-mē) [″ + *tome,* incision] Incision of the larynx.

inferior l. Surgical incision of the larynx through the cricoid cartilage.

median l. Surgical incision of the larynx through the thyroid cartilage.

subhyoid l. Surgical incision of the larynx through the thyroid membrane. SYN: *superior l.*

superior l. Subhyoid l.

laryngotracheal (lă-rĭng″gō-trā′kē-ăl) [″ + *tracheia,* trachea] Concerning the larynx and trachea.

laryngotracheitis (lăr-ĭn″gō-trā-kē-ī′tĭs) [″ + ″ + *itis,* inflammation] An inflammation of the larynx and trachea.

laryngotracheobronchitis (lă-rĭng″gō-trā″kē-ō-brŏng-kī′tĭs) [″ + ″ + *bronchos,* windpipe, + *itis,* inflammation] Inflammation of the larynx, trachea, and bronchi.

laryngotracheotomy (lăr-ĭn″gō-trā-kē-ŏt′ō-mē) [″ + ″ + *tome,* incision] Incision of the larynx with section of upper tracheal rings.

laryngoxerosis (lăr-ĭn″gō-zĕr-ō′sĭs) [″ + *xeros,* dry, + *osis,* condition] Abnormal dryness of the larynx.

larynx (lăr′ĭnks) *pl.* **larynges** [Gr.] A musculocartilaginous organ at the upper end of the trachea, below the root of the tongue, lined with ciliated mucous membrane, that is part of the airway and the vocal apparatus. SEE: illus.

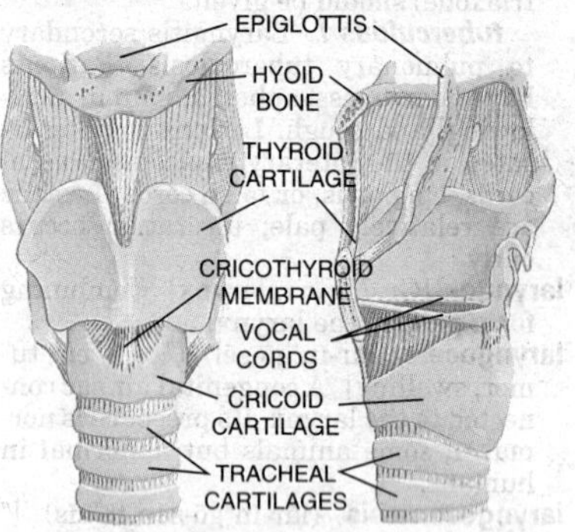

LARYNX

(A) anterior view, (B) midsagittal section

ANATOMY: The larynx consists of nine cartilages bound together by an elastic membrane and moved by muscles. The cartilages include three single (cricoid, thyroid, and epiglottic) and three paired (arytenoid, corniculate, and cuneiform). The thyroid cartilage pushes soft tissue forward, forming the Adam's apple. The extrinsic muscles include the omohyoid, sternohyoid, sternothyroid, and several others; intrinsic muscles include the cricothyroid, external and internal thyroarytenoid, transverse and oblique arytenoid, and external and internal thyroarytenoid. The cavity of the larynx contains two pairs of folds—the ventricular folds (false vocal cords) and the vocal folds (true vocal cords)—and is divided into three regions—the vestibule, ventricle, and inferior entrance to the glottis. An opening between the true vocal folds forms a narrow slit, the rima glottidis or glottis.

The larynx is innervated from the interior and external branches of the superior laryngeal nerve. Blood supply is provided by the inferior thyroid, a branch of the thyroid axis, and the superior thyroid, a branch of the external carotid.

NERVES: The larynx is innervated from the interior and external branches of the superior laryngeal nerve.

BLOOD SUPPLY: Inferior thyroid,

branch of thyroid axis and superior thyroid, branch of external carotid.

foreign bodies in l. An inhaled or aspirated solid object, such as a piece of meat, hard candy, safety pin, or coin, in the larynx—of great concern because of the risk of airway obstruction.

SYMPTOMS: Symptoms may include coughing, choking, dyspnea, fixed pain, or loss of voice.

PATIENT CARE: If the patient is able to speak or cough, the rescuer should not interfere with the patient's attempts to expel the object. If the patient is unable to speak, cough, or breathe, the rescuer should apply the Heimlich maneuver 6 to 10 times rapidly in succession. Using air already in the lungs, the thrusts create an artificial cough to propel the obstructing object out of the airway. If the patient loses consciousness, the rescuer lowers him or her carefully to the floor, while protecting the head and neck, and continues the effort by applying abdominal thrusts 6 to 10 times from a position kneeling astride the victim's thighs. The rescuer also initiates CPR for unconscious pulseless patients, based on assessment of airway, breathing, and circulation. After the abdominal thrusts, the rescuer opens the airway and attempts to remove visible obstructions by sweeping the airway and then attempts to ventilate the patient. For an obese or pregnant patient or a child, the rescuer administers chest thrusts applied to the middle of the sternum rather than abdominal thrusts. For an infant, the rescuer uses back blows before chest thrusts. Direct laryngoscopy and the use of Magill forceps may be required to remove a foreign object. If the object cannot be readily removed with these measures, an emergency cricothyrotomy, or emergency tracheotomy may be required. SEE: *Heimlich maneuver*.

Lasègue's sign (lă-sĕgz′) [Ernest C. Lasègue, Fr. physician, 1816–1883] In lumbar disk disease, pain that radiates into the leg after the hips and knees are flexed and the knee is extended.

laser (lā′zĕr) Acronym for *l*ight *a*mplification by *s*timulated *e*mission of *r*adiation. A device that emits intense heat and power at close range. The instrument converts various frequencies of light into one small and extremely intense unified beam of one wavelength radiation. The laser can be focused on a very small target. Lasers that provide short pulses of light rather than a continuous beam have been found to cause less damage to normal tissue. Lasers have multiple treatment applications. In ophthalmology, they are used, for example, in treating retinal detachment and diabetic retinopathy; in cardiology, experimentally to vaporize arterial blockage; in dermatology, to obliterate blood vessels, for superficial removal of warts and skin cancers, to remove excess tissue in enlarged noses, for superficial removal of pigmented conditions (brown spots) and port-wine nevus, and for removal of tattoos; in gynecology, to remove vulval lesions, including genital warts; in gastroenterology, to control bleeding in the gastrointestinal tract; in surgery and dentistry, to remove tumors. A variety of lasers are used depending upon the wavelength and power required, including argon, carbon dioxide, copper vapor, dye, excimer, helium-neon, ion, krypton, neodymium:yttrium-aluminum garnet, and ruby lasers.

argon l. A gas-produced light (in the blue and green visible light spectrum) with a wavelength spectrum of 488 nm to 633 nm, which coagulates tissues, is used in photodynamic therapy, and can be absorbed by oxyhemoglobin in blood vessels. Argon lasers have been used to treat skin lesions, bleeding ulcers, hemangiomas, periodontal disease, glaucoma, retinal diseases, and other conditions.

carbon dioxide l. ABBR: CO_2 laser. A gas-produced colorless light with a wavelength of 10,600 nm (infrared), used, for example, in dermatological surgeries to remove scars, wrinkles, and solar skin damage. It can also be used as a scalpel in stereotactic neurosurgeries, gynecological surgeries, and many other applications.

PATIENT CARE: Laser precautions must be observed. The patient is given support by answering questions and explaining the need for eye covering during the procedure. The procedure is documented in a laser log.

CAUTION: Laser safety precautions must be observed. For example, warning signs should be posted indicating that a laser is being used; equipment must be checked before the procedure; conventional endotracheal tubes must be wrapped with aluminum foil tape or flexible metallic endotracheal tubes insulated with silicone may be used; skin preparation solution may not contain combustible agents; and towels draped around the site must be kept wet. The laser equipment must be moved carefully, to avoid jarring the mirrors out of alignment. Alcohol-based skin preparations should not be used.

---

cutaneous l. Any of several lasers (e.g. argon, CD_2, etc.) employed for cosmetic and plastic surgery, including the treatment of pigmented lesions, wrinkles, vascular malformations, and other cosmetic skin surface irregularities.

diode l. A compact laser designed

with semiconductors, which has many medical applications, including use in skin, eye, urological, and other surgeries. Wavelengths are from 800 to 1000 nm.

PATIENT CARE: Care involves general support, giving explanations, and answering questions. Equipment must be checked and regulations followed. The surgeon is given assistance, as needed.

CAUTION: Laser safety precautions must be observed. The fiber must not be permitted to kink. The manufacturer's directions explain care, use, and cleaning protocol.

---

dye l. A laser whose energy is applied in pulses, primarily to manage skin lesions. Wavelengths are 510 nm for green, and 577 nm to 600 nm for yellow.

PATIENT CARE: Care involves giving general emotional support, explanations, and answering questions regarding the procedure. The equipment is checked, and all rules are observed. The needs of the surgeon are anticipated and the procedure is recorded in the laser log.

excimer l. An ultraviolet laser used clinically to remove plaque from arteries. This rare gas (halide) energy source laser breaks chemical bonds instead of destroying tissue with heat; it penetrates less than 1 mm into tissue. The rare gas (halide) combines with an active medium (an excited dimer), from which it derives its name. The dimeric media are excited, emitting laser energy. The chemical composition of the medium determines the ultraviolet wavelength. The four most popularly used are: the argon fluoride (ArF) laser at 193 nm, the krypton fluoride (KrF) at 248 nm, the xenon chloride (XeCl) at 308 nm, and the xenon fluoride (XeFl) at 351 nm.

l. safety Rules and regulations designed to minimize health, electrical, fire, and safety hazards posed by the use of lasers. Warning signs are posted, indicating that a laser is being used, on the operating room's doors. Equipment must be checked before the procedure. Only personnel trained to use the equipment may participate. A master key for the laser must be obtained before and returned after the procedure. The laser is set on "standby" or "stop" when use is interrupted. Eye protection is mandatory for patient and personnel when applicable. Only nonflammable anesthetics are to be used. Conventional endotracheal tubes must be wrapped with aluminum foil tape or flexible metallic endotracheal tubes insulated with silicone may be used. Skin preparation solution may not contain combustible agents. Gowns and drapery should be flame retardant. Towels draped around the site must be kept wet for some lasers (e.g., CO_2). Special fire extinguishers (e.g., Halon) can be used in case of flash fire. A smoke plume evacuator and special masks may be necessary.

Yttrium-aluminum-garnet l. ABBR: YAG laser. A laser with a crystal made of yttrium, aluminum, and garnet that can be used for skin resurfacing, or tissue penetration in oral, urological, ophthalmic, cardiac, orthopedic, or other applications. The depth of the penetration of the laser energy, its tissue absorption, and tissue-sparing characteristics vary with the materials used as additives to the crystal, such as erbium, holmium, or neodymium.

PATIENT CARE: Care involves general support, giving explanations, and answering questions. All equipment must be checked and all rules observed. The nurse assists the surgeon as necessary.

CAUTION: Laser precautions, as well as the manufacturer's directions for usage, care, and storage, must be followed. Care must be taken not to bend the fibers of the laser.

Lassa fever [Lassa, city in Africa] A potentially lethal viral illness marked by hemorrhage, extreme muscle pain, and in some cases shock. It is contracted solely in Africa. The responsible agent, an arenavirus, is spread to people after contact with infected rodents or their excretions. Each year, approx. 300,000 people are infected.

SYMPTOMS: Patients have abrupt onset of high fever that is continuous or intermittent and spiking, with generalized myalgia, chest and abdominal pain, headache, sore throat, cough, dizziness with flushing of the face, conjunctival injection, nausea, diarrhea, and vomiting. Hemorrhagic areas of the skin and mucous membranes may appear on the fourth day. Mortality of those in Africa with this disease varies from 16% to 45%.

TREATMENT: Ribavirin given in the first week of illness and continued for 10 days has been very effective in reducing the death rate. This medicine should also be given orally for 10 days prophylactically to those who have been percutaneously exposed to the virus. Patients are isolated in special isolation units that filter the air leaving the room and maintain negative pressure. All sputum, blood, excreta, and objects that the patient has contacted are disinfected. SEE: *Standard and Universal Precautions Appendix.*

lassitude (lăs'ĭ-tūd) [L. *lassitudo,* weariness] Weariness; exhaustion.

LAT *licensed athletic trainer.*

latah (lă'tă) A type of mental disorder that occurs in people of Southeast Asia, esp. in women, marked by imitative behavior, coprolalia, echolalia, and automatic obedience. It may be provoked by startling, tickling, or frightening the patient.

LATC *licensed athletic trainer, certified.*

latchkey children Children who have a key to their home, needed for when they return home when no adult is present to supervise them. These children are at a higher risk of accidents, abusing drugs, and smoking cigarettes.

latency (lā'tĕn-sē) [L. *latens,* lying hidden] State of being concealed, hidden, inactive, or inapparent.

sleep l. The amount of time between reclining in bed and the onset of sleep.

latent **1.** Lying hidden. **2.** Quiet; not active.

l. content In psychoanalysis, that part of a dream or unconscious mental content that cannot be brought into the objective consciousness through any effort of will to remember.

latent heat The caloric or heat energy absorbed by matter changing from solid to liquid or from liquid to vapor with no change in temperature.

l.h. of fusion The heat required to convert 1 g of a solid to a liquid at the same temperature. For example, the process of converting 1 g of ice at 0°C to water at 0°C requires 80 cal, and until it is completed there will be no rise in the temperature.

l.h. of vaporization The heat required to change 1 g of a liquid at its boiling point to vapor at the same temperature. The latent heat of steam is 540 cal; therefore, when steam cools to liquid, each gram gives out 540 cal. This explains why a scald from steam is much more severe than one caused by boiling water.

laterad (lăt'ĕr-ăd) [L. *latus,* side, + *ad,* toward] Toward a side or lateral aspect.

lateral (lăt'ĕr-ăl) [L. *lateralis*] Pert. to the side.

lateralis (lăt″ĕr-ā'lĭs) [L.] Located away from the mid-plane of the body.

laterality (lăt″ĕr-ăl'ĭ-tē) Relating to one side of the body, i.e., the left or right; used, for example, to specify which side of the body or brain is dominant.

crossed l. Mixed dominance of certain body parts so that the left arm and right leg would be dominant.

dominant l. Preferential dominance and use of the parts of one side of the body such as the eye, arm, leg, or hand.

latericeous, lateritious (lăt″ĕr-ĭsh'ŭs) [L. *later,* brick] Resembling brick dust.

lateroabdominal (lăt″ĕr-ō-ăb-dŏm'ĭ-năl) [L. *lateralis,* pert. to side, + *abdomen,* belly] Concerning the side of the body and the abdominal area.

laterodeviation (lăt″ĕr-ō-dē″vē-ā'shŭn) [″ + *deviare,* to turn aside] Deviation or displacement to one side.

lateroduction (lăt″ĕr-ō-dŭk'shŭn) [″ + *ducere,* to lead] Movement to one side, esp. of the eye.

lateroflexion (lăt″ĕr-ō-flĕk'shŭn) [″ + *flexis,* bending] Bending or curvature toward one side.

laterognathism Asymmetry of the mandible owing to retarded growth, fractures, tumors, or soft tissue atrophy or hypertrophy.

lateroposition (lăt″ĕr-ō-pō-zĭsh'ŭn) [″ + *positio,* position] Displacement to one side.

lateropulsion (lăt″ĕr-ō-pŭl'shŭn) [L. *lateralis,* pert. to side, + *pulsus,* driving] In cerebellar and labyrinthine disease, the involuntary tendency to fall to one side.

laterotorsion (lăt″ĕr-ō-tor'shŭn) [″ + *torsio,* a twisting] Twisting to one side.

lateroversion (lăt″ĕr-ō-vĕr'shŭn) [″ + *versio,* a turning] A tendency or a turning toward one side.

lathyrism (lăth'ĭ-rĭzm) [Gr. *lathyros,* vetch] A neurotoxic disorder caused by eating the grass pea, *Lathyrus sativus.* Its hallmarks are irreversible muscular paralysis and spasticity.

lathyrogen (lăth'ĭ-rō-jĕn) [″ + *gennan,* to produce] Something that produces lathyrism.

Latino A Latin American.

latissimus (lă-tĭs'ĭ-mŭs) [L., widest] Denoting a broad structure such as a muscle.

latitude In radiology, a range of exposure that would produce a technically correct radiograph.

latrine (lă-trēn') [L. *latrina*] A toilet, particularly one in a military camp.

pit l. A type of latrine installed outdoors and used where it is impractical to provide a standard, flushing-type toilet. The structure may be manufactured and installed so that odors and flies are not a problem.

latrodectism (lăt″rō-dĕk'tĭzm) [*Latrodectus* + Gr. *-ismos,* condition] The toxic reaction to the bite of spiders of the genus *Latrodectus.* SEE: *spider, black widow.*

Latrodectus (lăt″rō-dĕk'tŭs) [L. *latro,* robber, + Gr. *daknein,* biting] A genus of black spiders belonging to the family Theridiidae.

L. mactans Black widow spider.

LATS *long-acting thyroid stimulator.*

lattice (lăt'ĭs) **1.** A network or framework formed by structures intertwined usually at right angles with each other. **2.** In physics, the arrangement of atoms in a crystal.

latus (lā'tŭs) *pl.* **latera** [L., broad] The side; the flank.

latus, lata, latum (lā'tŭs, lā'tă, lăt'ŭm) [L., broad] Broad, as the uterine broad ligament.

laudable [L. *laudabilis,* praiseworthy] Commendable; healthy; normal; formerly said erroneously of pus.

laudanum (lăw'dăn-ŭm) Tincture of opium. SEE: *morphine*.

laugh (lăf) [ME. *laughen,* to laugh] **1.** The sound produced by laughing. SYN: *risus*. **2.** To express emotion, usually happiness or mirth, by a series of inarticulate sounds. Typically the mouth is open and a wide smile is present.

sardonic l. Risus sardonicus.

laughing gas SEE: *nitrous oxide*.

laughter (lăf'tĕr) A series of inarticulate sounds produced as an expression of emotion, usually happiness or mirth. The role of humor and laughter in promoting a positive attitude and health and in preventing the progress of some diseases has been documented esp. when it is combined with proven medical therapies.

compulsive l. Laughter without cause, occurring in certain psychoses, esp. schizophrenia.

pathological l. Uncontrolled laughter (occasionally accompanied by, or alternating with, uncontrolled crying), caused by pseudobulbar lesions of the brain. These lesions may result from lacunar strokes, multiple sclerosis, anoxic brain injury, and other forms of brain injury.

l. reflex Uncontrollable laughter resulting from tickling or the fear of tickling.

Laurence-Moon-Biedl syndrome (law'rĕns-moon'bē'dĕl) [John Zachariah Laurence, Brit. ophthalmologist, 1829–1870; Robert C. Moon, U.S. ophthalmologist, 1844–1914; Arthur Biedl, Prague endocrinologist, 1869–1933] The combination of girdle-type obesity, sexual underdevelopment, mental retardation, retinal degeneration, polydactyly, and deformity of the skull. The condition is inherited as an autosomal recessive trait.

lavage (lă-văzh') [Fr., from L. *lavare,* to wash] Washing out of a cavity. SYN: *irrigation*.

gastric l. Rinsing or irrigating the stomach to remove or dilute irritants or poisons or to cleanse the organ before or after surgery. Gastric lavage is used most often to manage patients who have ingested potentially toxic pills. Its use in overdose is controversial. It has not been shown to improve clinical outcomes, except perhaps in those instances in which the patient presents for care within an hour of a toxic ingestion, and the patient has consumed a life-threatening amount of poison. The procedure has some risks: the trachea, instead of the stomach, may be intubated; gastric contents may be aspirated; and the mouth, teeth, pharynx, or esophagus may be injured.

PATIENT CARE: The following equipment is assembled: plastic or rubber large-lumen nasogastric tube; ice in a bowl if a rubber tube is to be used; water-soluble lubricant; disposable irrigation set with bulb syringe; adhesive tape or other device; clamp, safety pins, and rubber band; gloves and stethoscope; tissues; glass of water with straw; emesis basin; container for aspirant; at least 500 to 1000 ml of prescribed irrigating solution; and any specified antidote.

Physical restraints are applied only if prescribed and required. The patient's clothing is removed and a hospital gown put on. If conscious and cooperative, the patient is placed in the high Fowler's position (head elevated 80 to 90 degrees), and the chest is covered with a water-impermeable bib or drape. If unconscious, the patient is positioned to prevent aspiration of stomach contents, and suction equipment is readily available.

The distance for tube insertion is measured by placing the tip of the tube at the tip of the patient's nose and extending the tube to the ear lobe and then to the xiphoid process. This location or the length of tubing that will remain outside the patient after insertion is marked on the tube. Nostril patency is checked and the nostril with the least obstruction used for the procedure. While the patient holds the emesis basin, the nurse lubricates the tip of the tube and inserts it. A downward and backward motion aids passage through the back of the nose and down into the nasopharynx, thus avoiding producing a gag reflex. The patient is instructed to dry-swallow during this phase of passage. The tube should not be forced. If obstruction is met, the tube is removed, the patient permitted to rest briefly, the tube relubricated, and the procedure attempted again. If the tube cannot be passed without traumatizing the mucosa, the physician is notified.

When the tube is in the nasopharynx, the patient is instructed to flex the neck slightly to bring the head forward. The glass of water (if permitted) is given to the patient, and the patient is encouraged to swallow the tube with small sips of water (or to dry swallow if water is not permitted). Rotating the tube toward the opposite nostril often helps direct toward the esophagus and away from the trachea. Placing the nondominant hand on the nose to secure the tube, the nurse advances it with the dominant hand as the patient swallows.

The back of the throat is periodically

inspected for any evidence of coiled tubing, esp. if the patient is gagging or uncomfortable, or unconscious. When the tube has been passed, placement is verified by aspirating gastric contents with the bulb syringe or by injecting a small volume of air and auscultating over the epigastrium for a whooshing sound. The tube is then secured to the nostrils with adhesive tape or another securing device according to protocol.

CAUTION: Gastric lavage should never be performed on a patient who has ingested hydrocarbons. It also should never be performed on patients who cannot protect their own airways, unless they are already intubated.

The irrigation fluid is instilled, and care is taken to prevent the entrance of air. A Y connector can be attached to the nasogastric tube, with one tubing exiting to the bulb syringe or irrigant container and the other to a drainage set. The return line is clamped, and the solution, usually 500 ml or more, instilled to distend the stomach and expose all areas to the solution. The large volume also dilutes harmful liquids and thins or dissolves other materials.

The patient is monitored throughout for retching. If retching occurs, the flow is stopped, suction is applied to the bulb syringe, or the drainage line is opened to remove some of the instilled fluid. The stomach is then drained, and the procedure repeated as necessary to cleanse and empty the stomach of harmful materials and irrigant. An antidote or activated charcoal slurry is then instilled as appropriate and prescribed.

A specimen of the aspirant is sent to the laboratory for analysis as directed. The tube may remain in place, attached to intermittent low suction as required, or be removed immediately after the procedure.

For removal, the tube is clamped securely. Any securing devices are removed, and the tube is rotated gently to ensure that it is freely moveable and then gently but steadily pulled outward and folded. The nurse's glove is then pulled off over the tube, and the second glove over the closed fist to effectively "double-bag" the tube. The patient is handed tissues to wipe the eyes and blow the nose and is assisted with oral hygiene. A fresh gown or linens are provided as necessary. The patient continues to be monitored for adverse effects of the toxic material.

The tube and prescribed suction are maintained as necessary, drainage is documented, comfort measures (oral misting, anesthetic throat sprays) are provided, and the patient is assessed for any complications.

peritoneal l. Irrigation of the peritoneal cavity (e.g., to diagnose blunt abdominal trauma; to diagnose, by obtaining cytologic specimens, or treat tumors of the peritoneum with chemotherapeutic agents; and to treat peritonitis, assist in evacuation of blood, fecal soilage, and/or purulent secretions as in hemorrhage or peritonitis).

law [AS. *laga,* law] **1.** A scientific statement that is found to apply to a class of natural occurrences. **2.** A body of rules, regulations, and legal opinions of conduct and action that are made by controlling authority and are legally binding.

administrative l. Body of law in the form of decisions, rules, regulations, and orders created by administrative agencies under the direction of the executive branch of the government used to carry out the duties of such agencies. Regulations of nursing practice, for example, are considered administrative laws.

all-or-none l. The weakest stimulus capable of producing a response produces the maximum contraction of cardiac and skeletal muscle cells, and the maximal impulse transmission rate in neurons.

Avogadro's l. SEE: *Avogadro's law.*

Bell's l. SEE: *Bell's law.*

biogenetic l. Ontogeny recapitulates phylogeny (i.e., an individual in its development recapitulates stages in its evolutionary development). SYN: *Haeckel's l.*

Boyle's l. SEE: *Boyle's law.*

Charles' l. SEE: *Charles' law.*

common l. Law that evolves from the judiciary branch of the government through court decisions. It is the most frequent source of legal precedent for malpractice issues.

Courvoisier's l. SEE: *Courvoisier's law.*

criminal l. Area of the law relating to violations of statutes that pertain to public offenses or acts committed against the public. A healthcare provider for example, can be prosecuted for criminal acts such as assault and battery, fraud, and abuse.

l. of definite proportions Two or more elements when united to form a new substance do so in a constant and fixed proportion by weight.

Fechner's l. SEE: *Fechner's law.*

fraud and abuse l. A statute that regulates the appropriateness of health care provider behavior in billing practices, receipt of payments, and provision of medically necessary services.

Gay-Lussac's l. SEE: *Charles' law.*

Good Samaritan l. SEE: *Good Samaritan law.*

Graham's l. SEE: *Graham's law.*

l. of Grotthus-Draper The inverse relationship between the amount of energy absorption and the depth of penetration of the energy. Energy that is absorbed by superficial layers is no longer available to deeper-lying tissues.

Haeckel's l. Biogenetic l.

l. of the heart Other things being equal, the stroke volume of the heart varies as the extent of diastolic filling, that is, the energy of contraction is a function of the initial length of the muscle fibers.

Hilton's l. SEE: *Hilton's law*.

Hooke's l. The stress used to stretch or compress a body is proportional to the strain as long as the elastic limits of the body have not been exceeded.

l. of the intestine Moderate distention of the intestine at a point causes relaxation below (aborally to the point) and contraction above.

inverse-square l. A law stating that the intensity of radiation or light at any distance is inversely proportional to the square of the distance between the irradiated surface and a point source. Thus, a light with a certain intensity at a 4-ft distance will have only one-fourth that intensity at 8 ft and would be four times as intense at a 2-ft distance.

Koch's l. SEE: *Koch's law*.

l. of Magendie SEE: *Bell's law*.

Marey's l. The heart rate varies inversely with arterial blood pressure (i.e., a rise or fall in arterial blood pressure brings about, respectively, a slowing or speeding up of heart rate).

Mariotte's l. SEE: *Boyle's law*.

l. of mass action In any chemical reaction, the law that states that the ratio of the mathematical products of the concentrations of the products to the mathematical products of the concentrations of the reactants is constant at a given temperature.

Mendel's l.'s SEE: *Mendel's laws*.

l. of multiple proportions When two substances unite to form a series of chemical compounds, the proportions in which they unite are simple multiples of one another or of one common proportion.

Nysten's l. SEE: *Nysten's law*.

periodic l. The physical and chemical properties of chemical elements are periodic functions of atomic weight. A natural classification of elements is made according to their atomic weight. When arranged in order of their atomic weight or atomic number, elements show regular variations in most of their physical and chemical properties.

l. of reciprocal proportions In chemistry, the proportions in which two elementary bodies unite with a third one are simple multiples or simple fractions of the proportions in which these two bodies unite with each other.

reciprocity l. Any milliamperage multiplied by an exposure time setting that gives the same milliamperage-second outcome should give the same density to the film. For example, 100 mA at 1 sec should give a density equivalent to that produced by 200 mA at 0.5 sec. In radiographic film screen technology, the reciprocity law does not hold at long exposure times because of lesser film density.

Rubner's l.'s **1.** Law of constant energy consumption: rapidity of growth is proportional to intensity of the metabolic process. **2.** Law of constant growth quotient: the same proportional part, or growth quotient, of total energy is used for growth.

Sutton's l. SEE: *Sutton's law*.

Waller's l. of degeneration If a spinal nerve is completely divided, the distal portion undergoes fatty degeneration.

Weber's l. The increase in stimulus necessary to produce the smallest perceptible increase in sensation bears a constant ratio to the strength of the stimulus already acting.

Wolff's l. Law that states that bones adapt structurally to resist the specific forces acting on them.

lawrencium (lă-rĕn'sē-ŭm) [Ernest O. Lawrence, U.S. physicist, 1901–1958] SYMB: Lr. A synthetic transuranic chemical element; atomic weight of most stable isotopes is 260; atomic number is 103.

lax (lăks) [L. *laxus,* slack] **1.** Without tension. **2.** Loose and not easily controlled; said of bowel movements.

laxative (lăk'să-tĭv) [L. *laxare,* to loosen] A food or chemical substance that acts to loosen the bowels (i.e., facilitate passage of bowel contents at time of defecation), and, therefore, to prevent or treat constipation. Laxatives may act by increasing peristalsis by irritating the intestinal mucosa, lubricating the intestinal walls, softening the bowel contents by increasing the amount of water in the intestines, and increasing the bulk of the bowel contents. Many individuals feel that it is essential to have one or more bowel movements a day, and if they do not, they may develop the habit of taking some form of laxative daily. They should be instructed that missing a bowel movement is not harmful and bowel movements do not necessarily occur at regular intervals. SYN: *aperient; cathartic; purgative*. SEE: *constipation; enema*.

CAUTION: A sudden change in bowel habits may be the first sign of a malignancy of the intestinal tract. When this happens, the individual should consult a physician without delay.

---

l. regimen A diet modified to avoid chronic constipation by maintaining an adequate volume of food; eating high-bulk foods that contain a high fiber content; eating foods that tend to stimulate bowel activity such as stewed fruits and vegetables; maintaining adequate fluid intake; and participating in regular exercise. In addition, foods that the individual has found to cause constipation should be avoided. Some persons are esp. liable to be constipated by certain cheeses.

laxator (lăk-sā'tor) [L. *laxare,* to loosen] That which has a relaxing effect.

l. tympani One of two muscles or ligaments of the malleus of the inner ear.

layer (lā'ĕr) [ME. *leyer*] A stratum; a thin sheetlike structure of more or less uniform thickness.

ameloblastic l. The enamel layer of the tooth. SYN: *enamel l.*

bacillary l. The rod and cone layer of the retina of the eye.

basal l. The outermost layer of the uterine endometrium lying next to the myometrium.

blastodermic l. Germ l.

choriocapillary l. Lamina choriocapillaris.

claustral l. The layer of gray matter between the external capsule and insula.

clear l. The stratum lucidum of the skin.

columnar l. A layer of tall, narrow epithelial cells forming a covering or lining.

compact l. The compact surface layer of the uterine endometrium.

cuticular l. of epithelium A layer of dense cytoplasm at the luminal end of some epithelial cells, esp. that at the surface of columnar epithelium of the intestine.

enamel l. Ameloblastic l.

ependymal l. The inner layer of cells of the embryonic neural tube.

functional l. The portion of the endometrium adjacent to the uterine cavity; after it is shed in menstruation it is regenerated by the basilar layer.

ganglionic l. **1.** The fifth layer of the cerebral cortex. **2.** The inner layer of ganglion cells in the retina whose axons form the fibers of the optic nerve.

germ l. One of the three primary layers of the developing embryo from which the various organ systems develop. SYN: *blastodermic l.* SEE: *ectoderm; endoderm; mesoderm.*

germinative l. The innermost layer of the epidermis, consisting of a basal layer of cells and a layer of prickle cells (stratum spinosum). SYN: *malpighian l.; stratum germinativum.*

granular exterior l. The second layer of the cerebellar cortex, lying within the molecular layer and separated from it by a single row of Purkinje cells; consists principally of granule cells.

granular interior l. The fourth layer of the cerebral cortex, consisting principally of closely packed stellate cells.

half-value l. ABBR: HVL. The amount of lead, copper, cement, or material that would dissipate the beam of radiation by 50%. The number of half-value layers required for safety in blocking the area on a patient is five, because that represents 50% of 50% and 50% of that, and so forth. For example, 50% + 25% + 12.5% + 6.23%+ 3.12% = 96.9%. Thus the patient would be shielded from all but about 3% of the radiation. (Examples of the thickness of material required to protect from radiation are 2 in. [5 cm] of lead or 2 ft [61 cm] of cement.)

Henle's l. SEE: *Henle's layer.*

horny l. Outermost layer of the skin, consisting of clear, dead, scalelike cells, those of the surface layer being constantly desquamated. SYN: *stratum corneum.*

Huxley's l. SEE: *Huxley's layer.*

Langhans' l. SEE: *Langhans' layer.*

malpighian l. Germinative l.

mantle l. The middle layer of the neural tube of the developing embryo.

molecular l. **1.** The outermost layer of the cerebral or cerebellar cortex. **2.** The inner or outer plexiform layer of the retina.

nervous l. The nerve-containing portion of the retina of the eye.

odontoblastic l. The layer of connective tissue cells at the outer edge of the pulp where they produce the dentin of the tooth.

osteogenic l. The inner layer of the periosteum; it contains osteoblasts that become active during repair of fractures. SYN: *Ollier layer.*

outer nuclear l. The layer of the retina containing the nuclei of the visual cells (rods and cones).

papillary l. The superficial layer of the corium lying immediately under the epidermis into which it extends, forming dermal papillae.

pigment l. The outermost layer of the retina. Cells contain a pigment called fuscin.

prickle cell l. Stratum spinosum epidermidis; the layer between the granular and basal layers of the skin. Prickle cells are present in this layer. SYN: *spinous l.*

Purkinje l. SEE: *Purkinje layer.*

l. of pyramidal cells The exterior pyramidal layer; the third layer of the cerebral cortex.

reticular l. The inner layer of the corium lying beneath the papillary layer.

l. of rods and cones The layer of the retina of the eye next to the pigment layer. It contains the rods and cones.

somatic l. In the embryo, a layer of extraembryonic mesoderm that forms a part of the somatopleure, the outer wall of the coelom.

spinous l. Prickle cell l.

splanchnic l. In the embryo, a layer of extraembryonic mesoderm that with the endoderm forms the splanchnopleure.

spongy l. Middle layer of the uterine endometrium; contains dilated portions of uterine glands. SYN: *stratum spongiosum*.

subendocardial l. The layer of loose connective tissue immediately under the endocardium that binds it to the myocardium; contains fibers of the conducting system of the heart.

subendothelial l. The layer of fine fibers and fibroblasts lying immediately under the endothelium of the tunica intima of larger arteries and veins.

Tomes' granular l. The layer of interglobular dentin beneath the dentinocemental junction in the root of a tooth.

Weil's basal l. A relatively cell-free zone just below the odontoblastic layer in the dental pulp. It is also called subodontoblastic layer; cell-free zone of Weil; cell-poor zone.

zonal l. of thalamus The layer of myelinated fibers covering the thalamus of the brain.

Lazarus sign (lăz′ăr-ŭs sīn) [Biblical figure in the New Testament] Dramatic movements of the arms across the torso, which are occasionally observed in brain-dead patients after they have been disconnected from mechanical life support. These movements may be misinterpreted as signs of life, when in fact they are merely involuntary reflexes.

lb *pound*.

LBBB *left bundle branch block*.

LD *lethal dose*.

LD_{50} The *median lethal dose* of a substance, which will kill 50% of the animals receiving that dose. Dose is usually calculated on amount of material given per gram or kilogram of body weight or amount per unit of body surface area.

LDH *lactic dehydrogenase*.

LDL *low-density lipoprotein*.

L-dopa L-3,4-dihydroxyphenylalanine; a drug used in the treatment of Parkinson's disease. SYN: *levodopa*.

LDRP An acronym for Labor, Delivery, Recovery, Postpartum that describes a maternity unit designed for family-centered care. Women in labor and their families complete normal childbearing experiences in one homelike room. The newborn may remain at the bedside thoughout the stay.

L.E. *lupus erythematosus*.

leachate **1.** A contaminated liquid that leaves soil after water percolates through earth (e.g., in waste disposal sites), farmlots, or landfills. **2.** Any product of percolation.

leaching (lēch′ĭng) [AS. *leccan,* to wet] Extraction of a substance from a mixture by washing the mixture with a solvent in which only the desired substance is soluble. SYN: *lixiviation*.

lead (lēd) [AS. *laedan,* to guide] **1.** Insulated wires connecting a monitoring device to a patient. **2.** A conductor attached to an electrocardiograph. The three limb leads are lead I, right arm to left arm; lead II, right arm to left leg; lead III, left arm to left leg. These are also known as standard leads, bipolar limb leads, or indirect leads. SEE: *electrocardiogram* for illus.

bipolar l. In electrocardiography, any lead that consists of one electrode at one body site and another at a different site. A standard limb lead, I, II, or III, is a bipolar lead.

esophageal l. A lead that is placed in the esophagus.

limb l. Any lead, unipolar or bipolar, in which a limb is the location of one of the electrodes.

precordial l. A lead having one electrode placed over the precordium, the other over an indifferent region.

unipolar l. In electrocardiography, any lead that consists of one electrode placed on the chest wall overlying the heart, where potential changes are of considerable magnitude, and the other (distant or indifferent electrode) placed in a site where potential changes are of small magnitude.

lead (lĕd) [L. *plumbum*] SYMB: Pb. A metallic element whose compounds are poisonous; atomic weight 207.2, atomic number 82, specific gravity 11.35. Accumulation and toxicity occur if more than 0.5 mg/day is absorbed. Any level of lead in the blood is abnormal. Most cases of lead poisoning occur in children who live in homes in which the paint contains lead. Children who eat the paint develop signs of lead toxicity. SEE: *acute l. encephalopathy; lead poisoning, acute; lead poisoning, chronic; pica*.

l. acetate A lead compound that is used in solution as an astringent.

acute l. encephalopathy A syndrome seen mostly in children, following the rapid absorption of a large amount of lead. Initially there is clumsiness, vertigo, ataxia, headache, insomnia, restlessness, and irritability. As the syndrome progresses, vomiting, agitation, confusion, convulsions, and coma will occur. A sudden and marked increase in intracranial pressure accompanies these symptoms. Sequelae include permanent damage to the central nervous system, causing mental retardation, EEG abnormalities, cerebral palsy, and optic atrophy.

TREATMENT: Lead exposure should be discontinued. Corticosteroids and intravenous mannitol, 20% solution, will relieve increased intracranial pressure.

Lead can be removed from the body by giving dimercaprol (BAL) and calcium disodium edetate in a carefully administered dose schedule. Convulsions may be controlled with phenobarbital, hydantoin, or diazepam. Hydration should be maintained with intravenous administration of fluids, while avoiding sodium-containing materials. Oral fluids or food should not be given for at least 3 days.

l. line SEE: under *line*.

l. monoxide A reddish-brown compound used to prepare lead subacetate.

l. pipe contraction Cataleptic condition during which limbs remain in any position in which placed.

lead poisoning, acute The ingestion or inhalation of a large amount of lead, causing abdominal pain, metallic taste in mouth, anorexia, vomiting, diarrhea, headache, stupor, renal failure, convulsions, and coma. SEE: *Nursing Diagnoses Appendix.*

TREATMENT: Adequate urine flow should be established; convulsions may be controlled with diazepam. Calcium disodium edetate and dimercaprol are administered to remove lead from the body. After acute therapy is completed, penicillamine is given orally for 3 to 6 months for children and up to 2 months for adults. The exposure to lead should be reduced or eliminated.

CAUTION: Patients receiving penicillamine therapy must be monitored weekly for adverse reactions, including diffuse erythematous rashes, angioneurotic edema, proteinuria, and neutropenia. Penicillamine is contraindicated in patients with a history of penicillin sensitivity, renal disease, or both.

---

lead poisoning, chronic The chronic ingestion or inhalation of lead, damaging the central and peripheral nervous systems, kidneys, the blood-forming organs, and the gastrointestinal tract. Early symptoms include loss of appetite, weight loss, anemia, vomiting, fatigue, weakness, headache, lead line on gums, apathy or irritability, and a metallic taste in the mouth. Later, symptoms of paralysis, sensory loss, incoordination, and vague pains develop. Laboratory diagnosis is made through evidence of anemia; blood lead level above 5 μg/dl; elevated free erythrocyte protoporphyrin (FEP); increased excretion of lead in urine; characteristic x-ray changes in the ends of growing bones. SEE: *Nursing Diagnoses Appendix.*

TREATMENT: Lead exposure should be eliminated and an adequate diet with added vitamins provided. Chelating agents, such as dimercaprol, dimercaptosuccinic acid (succimer), or EDTA are given to reduce lead levels to normal.

PATIENT CARE: A history is obtained to determine environmental, work-related, or folk remedy related sources of lead ingestion or inhalation, and preparations are made for their removal. (In many states, removal of household lead must be done by licensed specialists, not homeowners, following state regulations. The Centers for Disease Control and Prevention and local poison control centers provide relevant information. A 1-cm square chip of lead-based paint may contain a thousand times the usual safe daily ingestion of lead.) A history is obtained of pica; recent behavioral changes, particularly disinterest in play; and behavioral problems such as aggression and hyperirritability. The patient is assessed for developmental delays or loss of acquired skills, esp. speech. Central nervous system signs indicative of lead toxicity may be irreversible. The younger child is assessed for at-risk characteristics such as the high level of oral activity in late infancy and toddlerhood; small stature, which enhances inhalation of contaminated dust and dirt in areas heavily contaminated with lead; and nutritional deficiencies of calcium, zinc, and iron, the single most important predisposing factor for increased lead absorption. Older children are assessed for gasoline sniffing, which is esp. prevalent among children in some cultures. The parent-child interaction is assessed for indications of inadequate child care, including poor hygienic practices, insufficient feeding to promote adequate nutrition, infrequent use of medical facilities, insufficient rest, less use of resources for child stimulation, less affection, and immature attitudes toward maintaining discipline. Prescribed chelating agent(s) are administered to mobilize lead from the blood and soft tissues by enhancing its deposition in bones and its excretion in urine. A combination of drugs may result in fewer side effects and better removal of lead from the brain. If encephalopathy is present, fluid volume is restricted to prevent additional cerebral edema. Injections are administered intramuscularly, and injection sites are rotated for painful injections (which may include simultaneous procaine injection for local anesthesia). The child is allowed to express pain and anger, and physical and emotional comfort measures are provided to relieve related distress. In the absence of encephalopathy, injections are administered intravenously, and hydration is maintained. The patient is evaluated for desired drug effects measured by blood levels and urinary excretion of lead (Note: special blood collection and urine collection containers are necessary for some of the monitoring tests. The laboratory should be consulted prior to collection) and for signs of toxicity from the chelating agents. As necessary, prescribed anticonvulsants are administered to control seizures, which are often severe and protracted, an antiemetic for nausea and vomiting, an antispasmodic for muscle cramps, and analgesic and muscle relaxant agents for muscle and joint pain. Serum electrolytes are monitored daily, and renal function is evaluated frequently. Whole bowel irrigation is used when lead is visible in the G.I. tract (or for episodes of acute lead ingestion). Adequate nutrition is provided, and coexisting nutritional deficiencies are corrected, by administering prescribed supplemental iron, for example. An active, active-assisted, or passive range-of-motion exercise program is established to maintain joint mobility and prevent muscle atrophy. Parents are taught and supported to prevent recurrence and the public is educated about the dangers of lead ingestion, the importance of screening young (esp. preschool) children at risk, the signs and symptoms indicative of toxicity, and the need for treatment.

leak, air Any injury to the lung in which air escapes the tracheobronchial tree. Pneumothorax, pneumomediastinum, pneumopericardium, pulmonary interstitial edema, and subcutaneous emphysema are examples.

lean (lēn) [AS. *hlaene,* without flesh] Without excess fat; as applied by the USDA it indicates that a meat or poultry product contains less than 10 g of fat, 4.5 g of saturated fat and 95 mg of cholesterol per serving.

l. body mass The weight of the body minus the fat content.

learning A change in behavior or skill level that follows gaining experience and practice.

educative l. The concept of learning as a process in which the learner makes judgments, gains foresights and insights, identifies patterns, and finds meanings. It is characteristic of the paradigm shift in nursing education and health teaching.

latent l. Learning that is inapparent to the individual at the time it occurs but later becomes evident when the learning is facilitated beyond what would be expected in the area of the original learning.

motor l. The processes related to the acquisition and retention of skills associated with movement. They are influenced by practice, experience, and memory.

programmed l. An interactive system of education in which information is presented in small increments. As each new fact or concept is introduced, the student is required to use what he or she has learned by responding to a prescribed series of questions. Mastery of each topic must be demonstrated before the student can proceed to more advanced subject matter. SEE: *Skinner box.*

LEAS *Lower extremity arterial studies.* SEE: *ankle-brachial index.*

Leber's disease (lā'bĕrz) [Theodor Leber, Ger. ophthalmologist, 1840–1917] A hereditary form of atrophy of the optic nerve that affects males.

Leber's plexus A plexus of venules in the eye between Schlemm's canal and Fontana's spaces.

Leboyer method (lĕ-boy-yā') [Frederick Leboyer, Fr. obstetrician, b. 1918] An approach to childbirth that employs a darkened, quiet, and peaceful environment. Central to this method is the physical contact between the mother and the child immediately after delivery. The newborn is supported in a warm bath at this time. Caressing and massaging the infant begins immediately and is continued daily for several months. The method is believed to facilitate the child's mental and physical development.

Lecat's gulf (lā-kăz') [Claude Nicholas Lecat, Fr. surgeon, 1700–1768] The hollow of the bulbous portion of the urethra.

L.E. cell Abbreviation for *lupus erythematosus* cell, a mature neutrophilic polymorphonuclear leukocyte that contains the phagocytosed nucleus of another cell. It is characteristic but not diagnostic of lupus erythematosus.

This distinctive cell may form when the blood of patients with systemic lupus erythematosus is incubated and further processed according to a specified protocol. The plasma of some patients contains an antibody to the nucleoprotein of leukocytes. These altered nuclei, which are swollen, pink, and homogeneous, are ingested by phagocytes. These are the L.E. cells. The ingested material, when stained properly, is lavender and displaces the nucleus of the phagocyte to the edge of the cell wall. The L.E. cell phenomenon can be demonstrated in most patients with systemic lupus erythematosus but is not essential for diagnosis. SEE: illus.; *lupus erythematosus, systemic.*

lecithal (lĕs'ĭ-thăl) [Gr. *lekithos,* egg yolk] Concerning the yolk of an egg.

lecithin (lĕs'ĭth-ĭn) [Gr. *lekithos,* egg yolk] A phospholipid (phosphoglyceride) that is part of cell membranes; also found in blood and egg yolk. On hydrolysis, it yields stearic acid, glycerol, phosphoric acid, and choline on hydrolysis.

lecithinase (lĕs'ĭ-thĭn-ās) An enzyme that catalyzes the decomposition of lecithin.

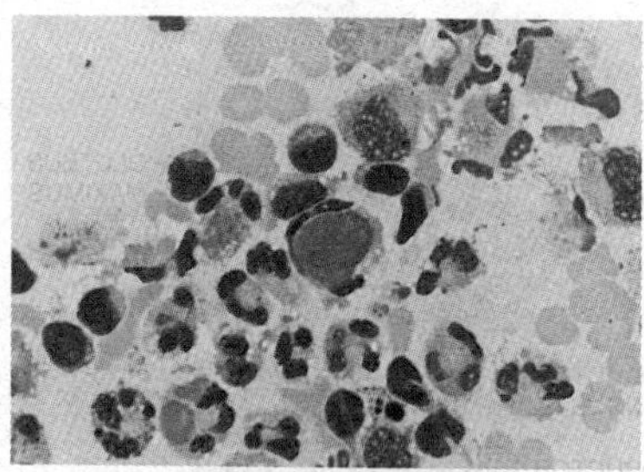

L.E. CELL (center)

(Orig. mag. ×1000)

cobra l. An enzyme present in certain snake venoms.

lecithin : sphingomyelin ratio ABBR: L : S ratio. The ratio of lecithin to sphingomyelin in the amniotic fluid. It is used to assess maturity of the fetal lung. Until about the 34th week of gestation the lungs produce less lecithin than sphingomyelin. As the fetal lungs begin to mature, they produce more lecithin than sphingomyelin. Delivery before the reversal of the ratio is associated with an increased risk of hyaline membrane disease in the infant. The use of this test enables the obstetrician to determine the optimum time for elective termination of pregnancy. SEE: *amniocentesis*.

lecithoblast (lĕs′ĭ-thō-blăst″) [″ + *blastos*, germ] One of the cells that proliferates to form the yolk sac.

lecithoprotein (lĕs″ĭ-thō-prō′tē-ĭn) [″ + *protos*, first] A protein in which lecithin is part of the conjugate.

lectin (lĕk′tĭn) [L. *legere*, to pick and choose] One of several plant proteins that stimulate lymphocytes to proliferate. Phytohemagglutinin and concanavalin A are lectins. SEE: *mitogen*.

lectual (lĕkt′ū-ăl) [L. *lectus*, bed] Pert. to a bed or couch.

LED *light-emitting diode.*

leech (lētch) [AS. *laece*] A bloodsucking water worm, belonging to the phylum Annelida, class Hirudinea. It is parasitic on humans and other animals. Leeches were used as a means of bloodletting, a practice common up to the middle of the 19th century but now almost completely abandoned. The worms are a source of hirudin, an anticoagulant secreted by their buccal glands. In modern times leeches have been used to evacuate periorbital hemorrhage (black eye) and to remove congested venous blood from the suture lines of reimplanted fingers. In addition to hirudin, leech saliva contains several active substances including inhibitors of platelet aggregation, that have been synthesized for use as anticoagulants in clotting disorders. SEE: *Hirudinea; hirudiniasis*.

artificial l. Cup and suction pump or syringe for drawing blood.

LEEP *loop electrocautery excision procedure.*

Lee's ganglion (lēz) [Robert Lee, Brit. gynecologist and obstetrician, 1793–1877] Cervical uterine ganglion formed from the third and fourth sacral nerves and the hypogastric and ovarian plexuses.

Leeuwenhoek's disease (lū′ĕn-hōks) [Antoni van Leeuwenhoek, Dutch microscopist, 1632–1723] Repetitive involuntary contractions of the diaphragm and accessory muscles of respiration. The patient complains of shortness of breath and epigastric pulsations. The disease is caused by an abnormality of the respiratory control system of the brainstem.

TREATMENT: Diphenylhydantoin may be effective. If not, section of the phrenic nerve may be necessary. SYN: *respiratory myoclonus*.

left The opposite of right. SYN: *sinistral*.

left-handedness Using the left hand as the dominant hand, e.g., for writing, work, or sports. SYN: *sinistrality*.

leg (lĕg) [ME.] One of the two lower extremities, including the femur, tibia, fibula, and patella; specifically, the part between the hip and ankle. SEE: illus.

badger l. Inequality in the length of the legs.

baker l. Knock-knee.

bandy l. Bowleg.

Barbados l. Elephantiasis of the legs.

bayonet l. An uncorrected backward displacement of the knee bones, followed by ankylosis at the joint.

milk l. Phlegmasia alba dolens.

restless l. A sense of uneasiness and uncomfortableness of the legs that comes on at bedtime. Moving the legs tends to relieve the condition. This syndrome is often associated with other sleep disturbances, such as sleep apnea.

scissor l. Crossed-leg deformity, a result of double hip disease, in which the patient walks with the legs swinging across the midline with each step.

white l. Phlegmasia alba dolens.

legal Pert. to or according to the law.

Legg-Calvé-Perthes disease (lĕg′kăl-vā′pĕr′tĕz) [Arthur T. Legg, U.S. surgeon, 1874–1939; Jacques Calvé, Fr. orthopedist, 1875–1954; Georg C. Perthes, Ger. surgeon, 1869–1927] Legg's disease.

Legg's disease (lĕgz) [Arthur T. Legg] Osteochondritis of the upper femoral epiphysis. SYN: *coxa plana; Legg-Calvé-Perthes disease*.

leggings (lĕg′gĭngs) [ME. *leg*, leg] Sterile leg coverings used on patients while in the operating room.

Legionella pneumophila The gram-negative, rod-shaped bacterium that

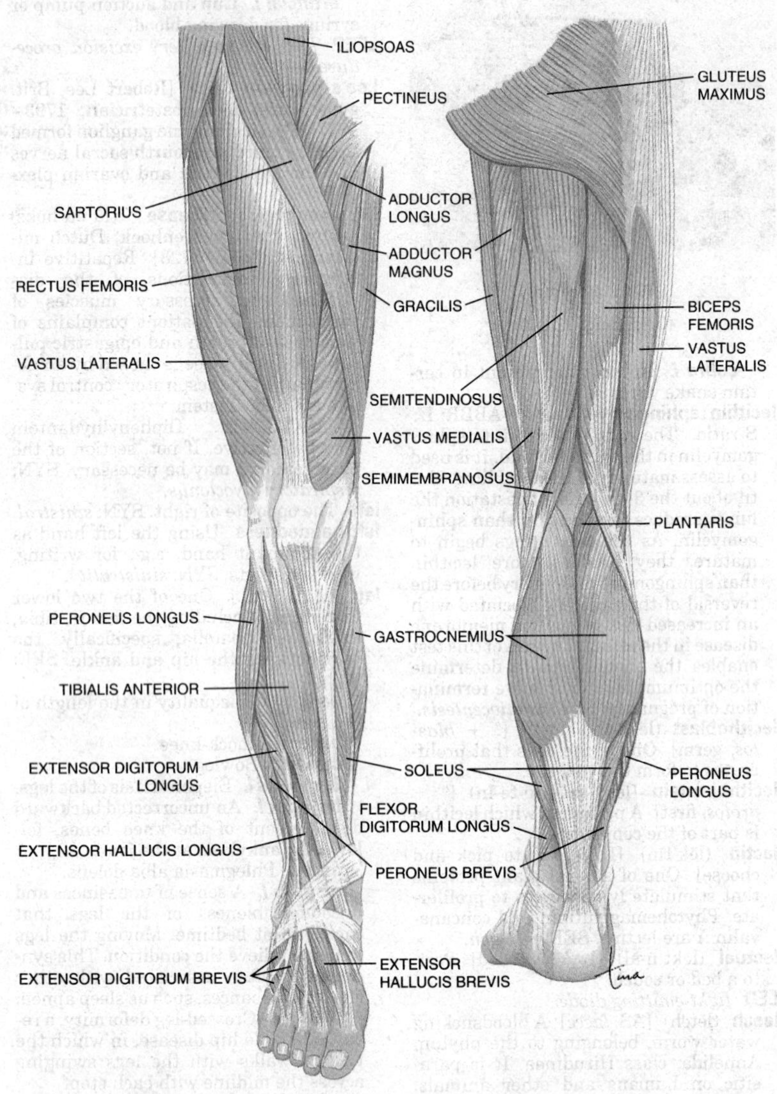

MUSCLES OF THE LEG

causes Legionnaires' disease. SEE: *Legionnaires' disease*.

legionellosis Legionnaires' disease.

Legionnaires' disease [after individuals stricken while attending an American Legion convention in Philadelphia, PA, in 1976] A severe, sometimes fatal disease characterized by pneumonia, dry cough, myalgia, and sometimes gastrointestinal symptoms. It may occur in epidemics or sporadically and has become an important cause of nosocomial pneumonia. Approx. 12,000 people are infected each year in the U.S. Persons at risk include middle-aged or older adults who smoke cigarettes or have chronic lung disease and those whose immune systems are compromised by diabetes, renal failure, cancer, or AIDS. The disease is responsible for about 5% of all pneumonias. SYN: *legionellosis*.

ETIOLOGY: The infection is caused by bacteria of the genus *Legionella*, a group of gram-negative, aerobic bacilli. The bacteria may be inhaled from contaminated water supplies, such as

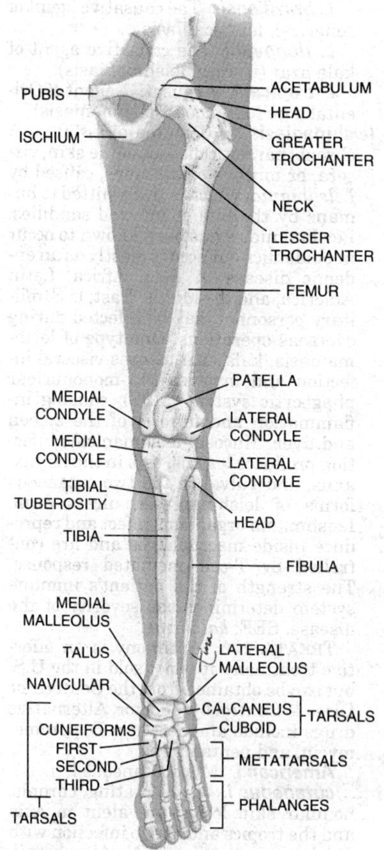

BONES OF THE LEG AND FOOT

Anterior view

water cooling towers, humidifiers, air conditioning vents, or contaminated respiratory therapy equipment.

SYMPTOMS: The signs and symptoms of Legionnaire's disease are similar to those of other pneumonias: fever, chills, and dry or productive cough. Fatigue, anorexia, headache, myalgia, and diarrhea also may be present. The incubation period is 2–10 days. A mild infection with *L. pneumophila* marked by fever and muscle aches and requiring no treatment is called Pontiac fever.

DIAGNOSIS: It is diagnosed by growing the bacteria on a special medium and silver staining; the bacteria also can be identified in sputum and a Legionella antigen is seen in urine.

TREATMENT: Erythromycin given early in the course of the disease and for a prolonged period is the drug of choice. Rifampin also is of benefit. Newer macrolides, such as clarithromycin and azithromycin, as well as fluoroquinolones, are effective therapeutic options.

PATIENT CARE: Respiratory status is monitored, including chest wall expansion, depth and pattern of ventilations, cough and chest pain, and restlessness, which may indicate hypoxemia. Vital signs, arterial blood gas levels, hydration, and color of lips and mucous membranes are also monitored. The health care providers are alert for signs of shock (decreased blood pressure; tachycardia with weak, thready pulse; diaphoresis; and cold, clammy skin). Level of consciousness is monitored for signs of neurological deterioration, and seizure precautions are instituted as needed. Prescribed antibiotic therapy is administered and evaluated for desired effects and adverse reactions. Respiratory care is provided, including prescribed oxygen therapy, repositioning, postural drainage, chest physiotherapy, and suctioning as prescribed and warranted by the patient's condition. As required, the respiratory therapist assists with endotracheal intubation and the provision and management of mechanical ventilation or other prescribed respiratory therapies. The patient is kept comfortable and protected from drafts. Antipyretics are administered and tepid sponge baths given. A cooling blanket may be used as prescribed to control fever. Frequent oral hygiene is provided, and a soothing cream is applied to irritated nostrils if necessary. Fluid and electrolyte balance is monitored, and replacement therapy initiated as needed and prescribed. Prescribed antiemetics are administered as necessary. The respiratory therapist or nurse teaches the patient about pulmonary hygiene, explaining how to perform deep-breathing and coughing exercises and chest physiotherapy and postural drainage. The patient should continue these measures until completely recovered. The patient is also taught how to dispose of soiled tissues to prevent disease transmission. SEE: *pneumonia*.

legume (lĕ′gūm) [L. *legumen,* pulse, bean] Fruit or pod of beans, peas, or lentils.

COMPOSITION: The nitrogen content of legumes is almost equal to that of meat. Legumin, a globulin, is present.

VITAMINS: Sprouted beans are a good source of vitamin B complex. Vitamin A and ascorbic acid are present in small amounts.

CARBOHYDRATES: Generally, carbohydrate is present in the form of starch in about the same proportion as in the cereals but with more cellulose.

legumelin (lĕg-ū′mĕl-ĭn) [L. *legumen,* pulse, bean] An albumin present in many leguminous seeds, as in peas. SEE: *legume*.

Leiner's disease (lī'nĕrz) [Karl Leiner, Austrian pediatrician, 1871–1930] Exfoliative dermatitis.

Leininger, Madeleine The founder and leader of transcultural nursing; developed the Theory of Cultural Care Diversity and Universality. SEE: *Nursing Theory Appendix.*

leio- [L. *leios,* smooth] Combining form meaning *smooth.*

leiodermia (lī″ō-dĕr'mē-ă) [Gr. *leios,* smooth, + *derma,* skin] Dermatitis characterized by abnormal glossiness and smoothness of the skin.

leiomyofibroma (lī″ō-mī″ō-fī-brō'mă) [″ + *mys,* muscle, + L. *fibra,* fiber, + Gr. *oma,* tumor] A benign tumor composed principally of smooth muscle and fibrous connective tissue.

leiomyoma (lī″ō-mī-ō'mă) [″ + ″ + *oma,* tumor] A myoma consisting principally of smooth muscle tissue.

epithelioid l. A smooth muscle tumor, usually of the stomach.

uterine l. A benign fibrous tumor of the uterus. Single or multiple tumors may range in size from one mm to 20 cm in diameter. Leiomyomas may be within the uterine wall or protrude into the endometrial cavity. They are the most common neoplasms of the female pelvis. They are present in 40% of women by age 40. SYN: *fibroid tumor; uterine fibroma.*

SYMPTOMS: Leiomyomas usually are asymptomatic. When present, symptoms are related to the size and site of the tumor. The most common symptom seen in women 40 to 45 years of age is abnormal uterine bleeding. SEE: *menorrhagia.*

TREATMENT: It is unusual for a leiomyoma to be large enough to interfere with delivery. If symptoms persist and preservation of fertility is not important then hysterectomy is indicated. In persons who wish to maintain the potential for fertility, myomectomy is indicated. Preoperative treatment of large symptomatic leiomyomas with gonadotropin-releasing hormone agonists can facilitate surgery.

leiomyosarcoma (lī″ō-mī″ō-săr-kō'mă) [″ + ″ + *sarx,* flesh, + *oma,* tumor] A combined leiomyoma and sarcoma.

leiotrichous (lī-ŏt'rĭ-kŭs) [″ + *thrix,* hair] Possessing smooth or straight hair.

Leishman-Donovan bodies SEE: under *body.*

Leishmania (lēsh-mā'nē-ă) [Sir William B. Leishman, Brit. medical officer, 1865–1926] A genus of parasitic flagellate protozoa that occur as typical leishmanian forms in vertebrate hosts but as leptomonad forms in invertebrate hosts or in cultures. These organisms are transmitted by the bite of the female sandflies.

L. braziliensis The causative agent of American leishmaniasis.

L. donovani The causative agent of kala azar (visceral leishmaniasis).

L. tropica The causative agent of Oriental sore (cutaneous leishmaniasis).

leishmaniasis (lēsh″mă-nī'ă-sĭs) A chronic parasitic disease of the skin, viscera, or mucous membranes, caused by *Leishmania,* which is transmitted to humans by the bite of infected sandflies. Leishmaniasis has been known to occur in epidemics but occurs mostly as an endemic disease in Asia, Africa, Latin America, and the Middle East; U.S. military personnel may be infected during overseas operations. One type of leishmaniasis, kala azar, causes visceral infection and involves the mononuclear phagocytic system (MPS), causing inflammation and fibrosis of the spleen and liver. Mucosal leishmaniasis infection produces lesions, esp. in the larynx, anus, and vulva. In the two cutaneous forms of leishmaniasis, ulcers form. Leishmania organisms infect and reproduce inside macrophages and are controlled by T-cell–mediated response. The strength of the patient's immune system determines the severity of the disease. SEE: *kala azar.*

TREATMENT: Antimony is an effective treatment; it is not sold in the U.S. but can be obtained from the Centers for Disease Control by a doctor. Alternative drugs include amphotericin B, paromomycin, and pentamidine.

American l. Mucocutaneous l.

cutaneous l. An ulcerating, chronic, nodular skin lesion prevalent in Asia and the tropics and due to infection with *Leishmania tropica.* SYN: *Aleppo boil; Oriental sore.*

mucocutaneous l. A form of cutaneous leishmaniasis, involving principally the nasopharynx and mucocutaneous membranes, found in parts of Central and South America. The causative organism is *Leishmania braziliensis* transmitted by sandflies, usually of the genus *Lutzomyia.* SYN: *American leishmaniasis.* SEE: illus.

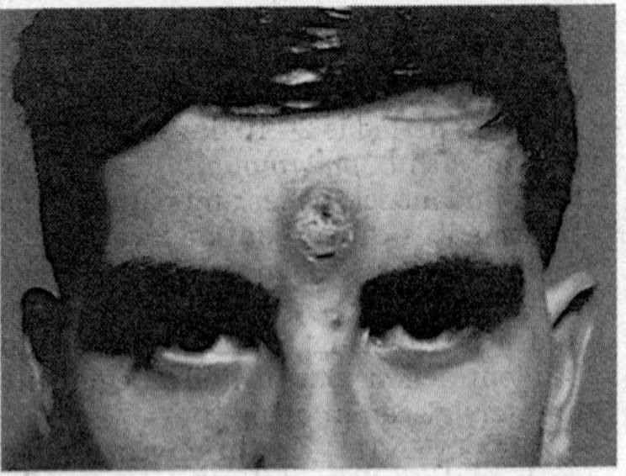

MUCOCUTANEOUS LEISHMANIASIS

Cutaneous lesion caused by *L. Braziliensis*

visceral l. Kala azar.

lema (lē′mă) [Gr. *leme*] The dried secretion of the tarsal glands that collects in the inner canthus of the eye. SYN: *sebum palpebrale*.

lemmocyte (lĕm′ō-sīt) [Gr. *lemma*, husk, + *kytos*, cell] A cell that becomes a neurilemma cell. SEE: *nerve fiber*.

lemniscus (lĕm-nĭs′kŭs) *pl.* **lemnisci** [Gr. *lemniskos*, a ribbon] A bundle of sensory fibers (lateral or exterior and median or interior) in the medulla and pons.

lemon [Persian *limun*, lemon] Fruit of the tree *Citrus limon*, containing citric acid. Lemons contain enough vitamin C to prevent or treat scurvy. Lemon may be used in place of vinegar, spices, and aromatic substances by those who cannot use such items.

CAUTION: Food faddists who drink large quantities of lemon juice by sucking directly from the raw fruit may develop erosion of the enamel of their teeth.

lemostenosis [″ + *stenosis*, act of narrowing] Stricture of the esophagus.

Lenegre's disease (Le-neh′gres) [Jean Lenegre, 20th century Fr. cardiologist] Atrioventricular or intraventricular conduction abnormalities resulting from fibrosis of the His-Purkinje fibers of the heart.

length The measurement of the distance between two points.

basialveolar l. The distance from the basion of the foramen magnum of the skull to the intermaxillary suture of the jaw.

basinasal l. The distance from the basion of the foramen magnum of the skull to the center of the suture between the frontal and nasal bones.

crown-heel l. In the embryo, fetus, or newborn, the distance from the crown of the head to the heel.

crown-rump l. In the embryo, fetus, or newborn, the distance from the crown of the head to the apex of the buttocks. The measurement can be used to estimate gestational age.

focal l. In optics, the distance from the lens to the point of focus of light rays passing through the lens.

l. of stay The number of days between admission and discharge from an inpatient care facility.

wave l. In the line of progression of a wave, the distance from one point on the wave to the same point on the next wave. The length of a wave determines whether or not the wave is a visible light, x-ray, gamma, or radio wave.

Lennox-Gastaut syndrome A form of early childhood epilepsy marked by atypical absence and tonic clonic seizures, slow-spike electroencephalographic waves, and a high incidence of mental retardation.

lens (lĕnz) [L. *lens*, lentil] **1.** A transparent refracting medium; usually made of glass. **2.** The crystalline lens of the eye.

achromatic l. Lens that transmits light without separating it into the colors of the visual spectrum.

aplanatic l. A lens that corrects spherical aberrations.

apochromatic l. A lens that corrects both spherical and chromatic aberrations.

biconcave l. A lens that has a concave surface on each side. SEE: *biconcave* for illus.

biconvex l. A lens that has a convex surface on each side. SEE: *biconcave* for illus.

bifocal l. A corrective lens containing upper and lower segments, each with a different power. The main lens is for distant vision; the secondary lens is for near vision.

bifocal contact l. A contact lens that contains two corrections in the same lens.

concave spherical l. A lens formed of prisms with their apices together, which is, therefore, thin at the center and thick at the edge. This type of lens is used in myopia.

contact l. A device made of various materials, either rigid or flexible, that fits over the cornea or part of the cornea to supplement or alter the refractive ability of the cornea or the lens of the eye. Contact lenses of any type require special care with respect to storage when they are not being worn, directions for insertion and removal, and the length of time they can be worn. The manufacturer's or dispensing health care worker's instructions should be read and followed. Failure to do this could result in serious eye diseases. Wearing contact lenses while swimming is inadvisable.

convexoconcave l. A lens with a convex surface on one side and a concave surface on the opposite side.

convex spherical l. A lens formed of prisms with their bases together, which is, therefore, thick at the center and thin at the edge. This type of lens is used in hyperopia.

corneal contact l. A type of contact lens that adheres to and covers only the cornea.

crystalline l. A transparent colorless biconvex structure in the eye, enclosed in a capsule, and held in place just behind the pupil by the suspensory ligament. It consists principally of lens fibers that at the periphery are soft, forming the cortex lentis, and in the center of harder consistency, forming the nucleus lentis. Beneath the capsule on the anterior surface is a thin layer of cells, the lens epithelium. The shape is changed by the ciliary muscle to focus light rays on the retina.

cylindrical l. A segment of a cylinder parallel to its axis, used in correcting astigmatism.

disposable contact l. A soft contact lens worn for a week or two and then discarded.

extended wear contact l. A contact lens made of materials that permit permeation of gas (i.e., oxygen) so that there is less chance for corneal irritation.

hard contact l. A contact lens made of rigid translucent materials.

implanted l. Intraocular l.

intraocular l. ABBR: IOL. An artificial lens usually placed inside the capsule of the lens to replace the one that has been removed. A lens is removed because of abnormalities such as cataracts. If the original lens capsule is present and an IOL is placed inside it, the surgical procedure is called *posterior chamber IOL implantation.* If the capsule has been removed in a previous surgical procedure, the IOL may be placed in front of the iris, directly adjacent to the cornea. This is called *anterior chamber IOL implantation.* In another procedure, the IOL is implanted behind the iris. Which method of IOL implantation produces the best results is being investigated. SYN: *implanted l.* SEE: *cataract.*

oil immersion l. A special lens with oil placed between the lens and the object being visualized. This eliminates a layer of air between the microscope slide and the lens, producing a clearer image than would be the case if the oil were not used.

omnifocal l. An eyeglass lens whose power to alter light rays varies from the top to the bottom of the lens, permitting a smooth transition from one power lens to the other as one moves the eyes. This is in contrast to an eyeglass lens with the usual two-component bifocal lens.

orthoscopic l. A lens that produces no distortion of the periphery of the image.

soft contact l. A contact lens made of flexible, translucent materials. These lenses are more comfortable, can be worn longer, and are harder to displace than hard lenses, but there are disadvantages. They may not provide the same degree of visual acuity as hard lenses and they require more cleaning and disinfection. Tear production may be decreased, esp. in older patients. The soft lenses may need to be replaced every 6 to 18 months. Corneal infections can prevent further use of soft lenses, as well as causing permanent loss of vision.

spherical l. A lens in which all surfaces are spherical.

trial l. Any lens used in testing the vision.

trifocal l. A corrective eyeglass lens containing three segments—for near, intermediate, and distant vision.

lentectomy (lĕn-tĕk′tō-mē) [L. *lens,* lentil, + Gr. *ektome,* excision] Surgical removal of the lens of the eye.

lenticonus (lĕn″tĭ-kō′nŭs) [″ + *conus,* cone] Conical protrusion of the anterior or posterior surface of the lens.

lenticular [L. *lenticularis,* lentil] **1.** Lens shaped. SYN: *lentiform.* **2.** Pert. to a lens.

lenticulostriate (lĕn-tĭk″ū-lō-strī′āt) [″ + *striatus,* streaked] Relating to the lenticular nucleus and corpus striatum.

lenticulothalamic Pert. to the lenticular nucleus and the thalamus.

lentiform (lĕnt′ĭ-form) [L. *lens,* lentil, + *forma,* shape] Lenticular (1).

lentiginosis (lĕn-tĭj″ĭ-nō′sĭs) [L. *lentigo,* freckle, + Gr. *osis,* condition] The presence of multiple lentigines. SEE: *lentigo.*

lentiginous (lĕn-tĭj′ĭn-ŭs) [L. *lentigo,* freckle] **1.** Affected by lentigo. **2.** Covered with very small dots.

lentiglobus (lĕn″tĭ-glō′bŭs) [L. *lens,* lentil, + *globus,* sphere] A lens of the eye that has extreme anterior spherical bulging.

lentigo (lĕn-tī′gō) *pl.* **lentigines** [L., freckle] Freckle.

l. maligna A noninvasive malignant melanoma. SYN: *Hutchinson's freckle.*

l. senilis SYN: *solar l.*

solar l. A flat brown spot usually appearing on sun-exposed skin, such as the face or the back of the hands. They are commonly found on the skin of elderly individuals. Although they are popularly referred to as "liver spots," they are not caused by diseases of the liver. SYN: *l. senilis.* SEE: illus.

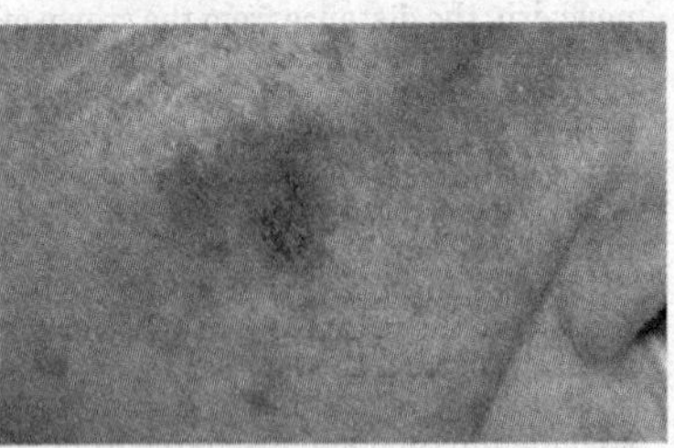

LENTIGO OF SUN-EXPOSED SKIN

lentitis (lĕn-tī′tĭs) [L. *lens,* lentil, + Gr. *itis,* inflammation] Phakitis.

lentivirus [L. *lentus,* slow] A group of retroviruses that cause slowly developing diseases. Human immunodeficiency virus (HIV), the virus that causes acquired immunodeficiency syndrome

(AIDS), is included in this group of viruses.

leontiasis (lē″ŏn-tī′ă-sĭs) [Gr. *leon,* lion, + *-iasis,* condition] Lionlike appearance of the face seen in certain diseases, esp. lepromatous leprosy. SYN: *facies leontina.*

l. ossea Enlargement and distortion of facial bones, giving one the appearance of a lion. It can occur as a complication of hyperparathyroidism, Paget's disease, uremia, and other conditions.

Leopold's maneuver [Christian Gerhard Leopold, Ger. physician, 1846–1911] In obstetrics, the use of four steps in palpating the uterus in order to determine the position and presentation of the fetus.

leper (lĕp′ĕr) [Gr. *lepros,* scaly] A person afflicted with leprosy.

lepidic (lĕ-pĭd′ĭk) [Gr. *lepis,* scale] Concerning scales, or a scaly covering.

lepido- [Gr. *lepis,* scale] Combining form meaning *flakes* or *scales.*

Lepidoptera (lĕp″ĭ-dŏp′tĕr-ă) [″ + *pteron,* feather, wing] An order of the class Insecta that includes the butterflies, moths, and skippers; characterized by scaly wings, sucking mouth parts, and complete metamorphosis.

lepidosis (lĕp″ĭ-dō′sĭs) [″ + *osis,* condition] Any scaly or desquamating eruption such as pityriasis.

lepirudin A recombinant form of hirudin, the leech anticoagulant, which directly inhibits the action of thrombin to prevent clotting. It is used as an alternative to heparin (an indirect thrombin inhibitor) to treat myocardial ischemia and infarction, as well as heparin-induced thrombocytopenia. The primary side effect of this drug is bleeding.

lepothrix (lĕp′ō-thrĭks) [″ + *thrix,* hair] A condition in which the shaft of the hair is encased in hardened, scaly, sebaceous matter.

lepra (lĕp′ră) [Gr. *lepra,* leprosy] A term formerly used for leprosy. It is now used to indicate a reaction that occurs in leprosy patients consisting of aggravation of lesions accompanied by fever and malaise. It can occur in any form of leprosy and may be prolonged.

l. alba A form of lepra in which the skin is anesthetic and white, associated with different forms of paralysis.

l. Arabum True or nodular leprosy.

l. maculosa A form of lepra with pigmented cutaneous areas.

leprechaunism (lĕp′rĕ-kŏn″ĭzm) A hereditary disease in which the elfin features of the face are accompanied by retardation of physical and mental development, a variety of endocrine disorders, emaciation, and susceptibility to infections. SYN: *Donohue's syndrome.*

leprid (lĕp′rĭd) [Gr. *lepra,* leprosy, + *eidos,* form, shape] A leprous cutaneous lesion.

leprology (lĕp-rŏl′ō-jē) [″ + *logos,* word, reason] The study of leprosy and methods of treating it.

leproma (lĕp-rō′mă) [″ + *oma,* tumor] A cutaneous nodule or tubercle characteristic of leprosy.

lepromatous (lĕp-rō′mă-tŭs) Concerning lepromas. SEE: *leprosy.*

leprosarium An outmoded term for a hospital that provides care for persons with Hansen's disease (leprosy).

leprostatic (lĕp″rō-stăt′ĭk) [″ + *statikos,* standing] **1.** Inhibiting the growth of *Mycobacterium leprae.* **2.** An agent that inhibits the growth of *M. leprae.*

leprosy (lĕp′rō-sē) [Gr. *lepros,* scaly] A chronic infectious disease of the skin and peripheral nerves, caused by *Mycobacterium leprae.* In chronically infected persons, it may produce characteristic ring-shaped, nodular, or erosive skin changes, esp. on or near the face, and sensory and motor dysfunction, esp. of the hands and feet. Approx. 12 million people are infected worldwide; leprosy is endemic in India and other tropical countries. It occasionally is reported in the U.S., for example, in Hawaii, where it was once endemic, and in the Gulf Coast states, where it is carried by an animal host, the nine-banded armadillo. SYN: *Hansen's disease.* SEE: *granuloma.*

The *lepromatous* (LL) form is characterized by skin lesions and symmetrical involvement of peripheral nerves with anesthesia, muscle weakness, and paralysis. In this form, the lesions are limited to the cooler portions of the body such as skin, upper respiratory tract, and testes. In *tuberculoid* (TT) leprosy, which is usually benign, the nerve lesions are asymmetrical and skin anesthesia is an early occurrence. Visceral involvement is not seen. Because of the anesthesia, rats have been able to remove digits while the patient sleeps. For some time this loss of digits was thought, erroneously, to be due to spontaneous amputation as a part of the disease process.

Lepromatous leprosy is much more contagious than the tuberculoid form. In the latter, *M. leprae* are found in lesions only rarely except during reactions.

Between the two major forms are *borderline* (BB) and *indeterminate* leprosy. In the borderline group, the clinical and bacteriological features represent a combination of the two principal types. In the indeterminate group, there are fewer skin lesions and bacteria are much less abundant in the lesions. In many respects, this infection resembles tuberculosis and for many years was regarded as incurable; this is no longer considered to be valid.

ETIOLOGY: The disease-producing

bacterium, *M. leprae,* grows only at 32° to 34°C, the temperature of skin. A normal T cell response by the host produces tuberculoid leprosy, which can be transmitted by respiratory droplets. Once inhaled, the organisms produce granulomas in the lungs and move through the bloodstream to the skin.

In contrast, lepromatous (anergic) leprosy occurs in persons who have an abnormal T-lymphocyte response to the organism. Transmission requires contact between material from a skin lesion and the blood of a recipient, which is reached through cuts on the skin. Genetic differences have been identified in those who develop the two forms of leprosy. Other intermediate or borderline forms of the disease are well-known, such as borderline lepromatous, borderline tuberculoid, and tuberculoid leprosy.

SYMPTOMS: In tuberculoid leprosy, skin lesions initially are flat and red, but later become large, hard, irregular, and swollen, with pale depressed centers. Granulomas infiltrate the peripheral nerves, which gradually degenerate, producing loss of feeling in the skin, muscle atrophy, and contractures. Lepromatous leprosy produces large macular (flat), papular (raised), or nodular lesions without sensation on the skin, particularly on the face, hands, knees, and feet. The eyes, mucosa of the upper airway, and testes also are commonly involved. The lesions contain large numbers of infected macrophages. Infection of peripheral nerves causes loss of sensation and muscle atrophy. Nonprotective antibodies are formed, which bind with bacterial antigens; the resulting immune complexes may cause vasculitis and glomerulonephritis. In all patients with leprosy, loss of sensation leads to inadvertent trauma and skin ulcers; autoamputation may occur. The disease has a slow course and rarely causes death.

DIAGNOSIS: Biopsy of a suspected skin lesion is used for diagnosis. The bacilli may not be present in tuberculoid lesions. In vitro tests of the immunological response can be accomplished by the lymphocyte transformation test and the leukocyte migration inhibition test.

COMPLICATIONS: Bacterial skin infections, ulcers, and traumatic amputation of fingers owing to anesthesia may occur. Tuberculosis is a much more common complication in untreated cases of lepromatous leprosy than in the tuberculoid form. Amyloidosis may be the cause of death in advanced cases.

TREATMENT: Tuberculoid leprosy is treated with multiple drug therapies, such as daily oral dapsone plus one dose of rifampin each month for 6 months. Daily dapsone and clofazimine plus monthly doses of rifampin for 24 months are required to treat lepromatous leprosy. Directly observed therapy (DOT) is recommended, esp. for the rifampin doses. There is concern that *M. leprae* is becoming resistant to these drugs. Treatment is complicated in pregnant women and in persons with glucose-6-phosphate dehydrogenase enzyme deficiency, because of drug intolerance. Despite effective treatments for many patients, the incidence of leprosy worldwide has not diminished in recent years.

PROGNOSIS: With proper therapy, esp. if given at the earliest time possible, the outlook is favorable.

leprotic (lĕp-rŏt′ĭk) [Gr. *lepra,* leprosy] Leprous.

leprous (lĕp′rŭs) **1.** Pert. to leprosy. **2.** Affected by leprosy. SYN: *leprotic.*

leptin A peptide hormone that influences the storage of body fat. It also acts on the hypothalamus to affect food consumption, sympathetic responses, insulin secretion by the pancreas, and gonadal activity (e.g., the onset of puberty).

lepto- [Gr. *leptos,* thin, fine, slim] A combining form meaning *thin, fine, slight, delicate.*

leptocephalia (lĕp″tō-sĕ-fā′lē-ă) [Gr. *leptos,* slender, + *kephale,* head] Having an abnormally vertically elongated, narrow skull.

leptocephalus An individual possessing an abnormally vertically elongated, narrow skull.

leptochromatic (lĕp″tō-krō-măt′ĭk) [″ + *chromatin*] Having a fine chromatin network.

leptocyte (lĕp′tō-sīt) [″ + *kytos,* cell] Target cell.

leptocytosis (lĕp″tō-sī-tō′sĭs) [″ + ″ + *osis,* condition] The presence of target cells in the blood.

leptodactyly (lĕp″tō-dăk′tĭ-lē) [″ + *daktylos,* finger] Abnormally slim fingers.

leptomeninges (lĕp″tō-mĕn-ĭn′jēs) *sing.,* **leptomeninx** [″ + *meninx,* membrane] The pia mater and arachnoid as distinct from the dura mater, because of their thinner and more delicate structure.

leptomeningitis (lĕp″tō-mĕn-ĭn-jī′tĭs) [″ + ″ + *itis,* inflammation] Meningitis in which infection, carcinoma, or inflammation involves only the pia mater and arachnoid membranes of the brain, not the dura mater. SEE: *meningitis.*

SYMPTOMS: Patients have an acute headache, pain in the back, spinal rigidity, irritability, and drowsiness ending in coma. Clinically, it cannot be distinguished from pachymeningitis. SYN: *piarachnitis.*

leptomeningopathy (lĕp″tō-mĕn″ĭn-gŏp′ă-thē) [″ + ″ + *pathos,* disease] A disease of the leptomeninges of the brain.

leptomeninx Sing. of leptomeninges.

leptonema (lĕp″tō-nē′mă) [″ + *nema,* thread] The early stage of prophase in meiosis. At this stage the chromatin coils into visible filaments. SEE: *cell division.*

leptophonia (lĕp″tō-fō′nē-ă) [″ + *phone,* voice] Weakness of the voice.

leptoprosopia (lĕp″tō-prō-sō′pē-ă) [″ + *prosopon,* face] Narrowness of the face.

leptorhine, leptorrhine (lĕp′tor-rīn) [″ + *rhis,* nose] Having a very thin or slender nose.

leptoscope (lĕp′tō-skōp) [″ + *skopein,* to examine] An optical device for measuring the thickness of cell membranes.

Leptospira (lĕp-tō-spī′ră) [″ + *speira,* coil] A genus of thin, spiral, and hook-ended spirochetes.

L. interrogans icterohaemorrhagiae Serotype causing infectious, hemorrhagic, spirochetal jaundice (Weil's disease).

leptospire (lĕp′tō-spīr) Any organism belonging to the genus *Leptospira.*

leptospirosis (lĕp″tō-spī-rō′sĭs) [″ + ″ + *osis,* condition] Condition resulting from *Leptospira* infection. SYN: *spirochetal jaundice.*

leptospiruria (lĕp″tō-spĭr-ū′rē-ă) [″ + ″ + *ouron,* urine] The presence of *Leptospira* organisms in the urine.

leptotene (lĕp′tō-tēn) [″ + *tainia,* ribbon] The initial stage of the prophase of cell division. The chromosomes become visible as separate entities but are not yet paired.

leptothricosis (lĕp″tō-thrī-kō′sĭs) [″ + *thrix,* hair] Disease caused by the gram-negative bacillus *Leptothrix.*

Leptus autumnalis Parasitic mite larvae causing itch and sometimes wheals. SEE: *chiggers.*

Leriche's syndrome (lĕ-rēsh′ĕz) [René Leriche, Fr. surgeon, 1879–1955] Occlusion of the abdominal aorta by a thrombus at its bifurcation. This causes intermittent ischemic pain (i.e., claudication) in the lower extremities and buttocks, impotence, and absent or diminished femoral pulses.

Leri's pleonosteosis (lā′rēz) [André Leri, Fr. physician, 1875–1930] A form of hereditary physical malformation characterized by upward slanting palpebral fissures, broad thumbs, short stature, and flexion contractures of the fingers.

lesbian (lĕs′bē-ăn) [Gr. *lesbios,* pert. to island of Lesbos] **1.** Pert. to lesbianism or sexual intercourse between women. SEE: *bisexual; homosexual.* **2.** A women who has sex exclusively with women.

lesbianism Sexual congress preferentially or exclusively between women. It was named for the Island of Lesbos, where the practice of lesbianism was reputed to have been widespread in ancient Greek history. SYN: *sapphism.*

Lesch-Nyhan disease [M. Lesch, b. 1939, William Leo Nyhan, b. 1926, U.S. pediatricians] An inherited metabolic disease that affects only males, in whom mental retardation, aggressive behavior, self-mutilation, and renal failure are exhibited. Biochemically there is excess uric acid production owing to a virtual absence of an enzyme essential for purine metabolism.

lesion (lē′zhŭn) [L. *laesio,* a wound] **1.** A circumscribed area of pathologically altered tissue. **2.** An injury or wound. **3.** A single infected patch in a skin disease.

Primary or initial lesions include macules, vesicles, blebs or bullae, chancres, pustules, papules, tubercles, wheals, and tumors. Secondary lesions are the result of primary lesions. They may be crusts, excoriations, fissures, pigmentations, scales, scars, and ulcers.

coin l. Solitary pulmonary nodule.

degenerative l. A lesion caused by or showing degeneration.

diffuse l. A lesion spreading over a large area.

discharging l. **1.** A brain lesion that discharges nervous impulses. **2.** A lesion that discharges an exudate.

focal l. A lesion of a small definite area.

gross l. A lesion visible to the eye without the aid of a microscope.

indiscriminate l. A lesion affecting separate systems of the body.

initial l. of syphilis A hard chancre. SEE: *chancre; syphilis.*

irritative l. A lesion that stimulates or excites activity in the part of the body where it is situated.

local l. A lesion of nervous system origin giving rise to local symptoms.

lower motor neuron l. An injury occurring in the anterior horn cells, nerve roots, or peripheral nervous system that results in diminished reflexes, flaccid paralysis, and atrophy of muscles.

peripheral l. A lesion of the nerve endings.

primary l. The first lesion of a disease, esp. used in referring to chancre of syphilis.

reverse Hill Sachs l. An indentation fracture of the anteromedial humeral head that occurs following a posterior dislocation of the glenohumeral joint. The cartilage of the humeral head is damaged, causing instability that may predispose the individual to subsequent posterior glenohumeral dislocations.

TREATMENT: Usually no surgical intervention is required when less than approx. 25% of the articular surface is involved in the fracture. When the glenoid fossa is also fractured, shoulder arthroplasty may be required.

structural l. A lesion that causes a change in tissue.

systemic l. A lesion confined to organs of common function.

toxic l. A lesion resulting from poisons or toxins from microorganisms.

vascular l. A lesion of a blood vessel.

LET *linear energy transfer.* A measure of the rate of energy transfer from ionizing radiation to soft tissue.

lethal [Gr. *lethe,* oblivion] Pert. to or that which causes death.

lethargy (lĕth′ăr-jē) [Gr. *lethargos,* drowsiness] Sleepiness, drowsiness, somnolence, or mental sluggishness.

African l. Sleeping sickness. SEE: *encephalitis lethargica.*

induced l. A hypnotic trance. **lethargic,** *adj.*

lethe (lē′thē) [Gr., oblivion] Amnesia.

lethologica (lĕth-ō-lŏj′ĭ-kă) [Gr. *lethe,* forgetfulness, + *logos,* word, reason] The temporary inability to remember a word, name, or intended action.

Letterer-Siwe disease (lĕt′ĕr-ĕr-sī′wē) [Erich Letterer, Ger. physician, b. 1895; S. August Siwe, Ger. physician, 1897–1966] The most common of three distinct histiocytosis syndromes collectively known as Langerhans cell histiocytosis, marked by proliferation of histiocytes in the viscera, bones, and skin. It is believed that this disease and the other two forms—eosinophilic granuloma of bone and Hand-Schüller-Christian syndrome—share a common pattern of granulomatous lesions with histiocyte proliferation.

The cutaneous lesions often develop during infancy or early childhood and in some cases are present at birth. These lesions include papulovesicular eruptions; inflamed, pruritic diaper area rashes; and scaly scalp lesions, all of which can be misdiagnosed as "cradle cap" (seborrheic dermatitis of the scalp) or severe diaper rash. When the disease is confined to the skin, spontaneous resolution in infancy may occur. In systemic presentations, the spleen and liver are enlarged, pulmonary infiltration is widespread, and bone marrow failure is accompanied by fever and infections. The cause of the disease is unknown.

DIAGNOSIS: Diagnosis is based on results of a skin biopsy performed with special staining techniques.

TREATMENT: No specific treatment exists. Corticosteroids and antineoplastic drugs are used in the more severe forms of the disease, but many children die of pulmonary failure or overwhelming infections despite treatment. SEE: *histiocytosis, Langerhans cell.*

Leu Conventional symbol for the amino acid leucine.

leuc- SEE: *leuko-.*

leucine (loo′sĭn) [Gr. *leukos,* white] An essential amino acid, $C_6H_{13}NO_2$; it cannot be synthesized by the liver and must be present in the diet; required for protein synthesis. It is present in body tissues and is essential for normal growth and metabolism.

leucine aminopeptidase ABBR: LAP. A proteolytic enzyme present in the pancreas, liver, and small intestine. Its serum level is elevated in disease of the pancreas, esp. acute pancreatitis, and in obstruction of the common bile duct.

leucinosis (loo″sĭn-ō′sĭs) [″ + *osis,* condition] An excess of leucine in the body, thus producing leucine in the urine.

leucinuria (loo″sĭn-ū′rē-ă) [″ + *ouron,* urine] The presence of leucine in urine.

leucitis (loo-sī′tĭs) [″ + *itis,* inflammation] Scleritis.

leucovorin calcium (loo″kō-vō′rĭn) The calcium salt of folinic acid. It is used in the treatment of megaloblastic anemias, and to antagonize the effect of methotrexate on normal cells when methotrexate is being used to treat malignancies.

leuk- SEE: *leuko-.*

leukapheresis (loo″kă-fĕ-rē′sĭs) [″ + *aphairesis,* removal] The separation of leukocytes from blood, which are then transfused back into the patient.

leukemia (loo-kē′mē-ă) [Gr. *leukos,* white, + *haima,* blood] A class of hematological malignancies in which immortal clones of immature blood cells multiply at the expense of normal blood cells. As normal blood cells are depleted from the body, anemia, infection, hemorrhage or death result. The leukemias are categorized as acute or chronic; by the cell type from which they originate; and by the genetic, chromosomal, or growth factor aberration present in the malignant cells.

Chronic leukemias, which have a relatively slow course, include chronic lymphocytic, chronic myelogenous, and hairy cell leukemia. Median survival in these illnesses is about 4 yr.

Acute leukemias include acute lymphocytic and acute myeloid (myelogenous) leukemia. If untreated, these diseases are fatal within weeks or months. SEE: *Nursing Diagnoses Appendix.*

ETIOLOGY: All the different molecular events leading to the development of unchecked cellular reproduction in the leukemias result from genetic or chromosomal lesions in blood-forming cells. Duplications of genetic material (hyperdiploidy), loss of genetic information (hypodiploidy), inactivation of genes that normally suppress tumor development, chromosomal translocations, and the release of abnormal fusion proteins can all cause leukemia. These genetic lesions in turn can be produced by viruses, ionizing radiation, chemotherapeutic drugs, and toxic chemicals. Rarely, leukemias are caused by familial genetic syndromes, such as ataxia telangiectasia, Bloom's syndrome, or Fanconi's syndrome.

SYMPTOMS: Clinical findings such as anemia, fatigue, lethargy, fever, and bone and joint pain may be present. Physical findings include combinations of pallor, petechiae, or purpura; mucous membrane bleeding; enlarged liver, spleen, and kidneys; and tenderness over the sternum and other bones.

DIAGNOSIS: Examination of peripheral blood and specimens of bone marrow are used to establish the diagnosis.

TREATMENT: Chemotherapy, bone marrow transplantation, or both are used to treat leukemias. New regimens are devised regularly and are tailored to specific illnesses. Treatment often is given in several phases, with a period of induction chemotherapy to induce remission, followed by consolidation and maintenance phases. This multiphase treatment is designed to further deplete malignant cells from the bone marrow and to achieve complete cure.

PATIENT CARE: Patient care measures focus on comfort, attempts to minimize the effects of chemotherapy, preservation of veins, management of complications, education, and psychological support. The specific needs of patients (some of whom are children) and their families must be considered. Instruction is provided about drugs the patient will receive, including any adverse reactions and measures that can be taken to prevent or alleviate these effects. Prescribed chemotherapy is administered with special precautions when indicated for infusion and drug disposal. If the chemotherapy causes weight loss or anorexia, nutritional guidance is provided. Oral, skin, and rectal care must be meticulous. The nurse, for example, thoroughly cleans the skin before all invasive procedures, inspects the patient for perirectal erosions, uses strict aseptic technique when starting an IV line, and changes sets (i.e., intravenous tubing and associated equipment) according to chemotherapeutic protocols. If the patient is receiving intrathecal chemotherapy, the lumbar puncture site is checked frequently for bleeding or oozing. The patient and family are taught to recognize signs of infection (fevers, chills, sore throat, cough, urinary difficulties) and are urged to report these to the oncologist promptly. To prevent infection in neutropenic patients, strict handwashing protocols, special diets, and laminar airflow or other isolation measures are instituted. The patient is monitored for bleeding. If bleeding occurs, compresses are applied and the bleeding site is elevated. Transfusions of platelets and other blood cells often are needed. Prescribed analgesics are administered as needed, and noninvasive pain relief techniques and comfort measures such as position changes, cutaneous stimulation, distraction, relaxation breathing, and imagery may be used. Complications of care such as nausea, vomiting, oral ulcerations, fevers, and altered mental status are promptly brought to the attention of the attending physician. Patient care routines and visiting hours should be flexible. Both the patient and family are encouraged to participate in care as much as possible. Referrals are made to social service agencies, home health care agencies, and support groups. If the patient does not respond to treatment and has reached the terminal phase of the disease, supportive nursing or hospice care may be appropriate.

acute lymphoblastic l. SYN: *acute lymphocytic l.*

acute lymphocytic l. ABBR: ALL. A hematological malignancy marked by the unchecked multiplication of immature lymphoid cells in the bone marrow, blood, and body tissues. ALL affects more than 2000 children and 1000 adults in the U.S. each year. It is rapidly fatal if left untreated. SYN: *acute lymphoblastic l.* SEE: illus; *leukemia*.

ETIOLOGY: A wide range of acquired or congenital chromosomal abnormalities can cause ALL, including lesions that result in the release of excess

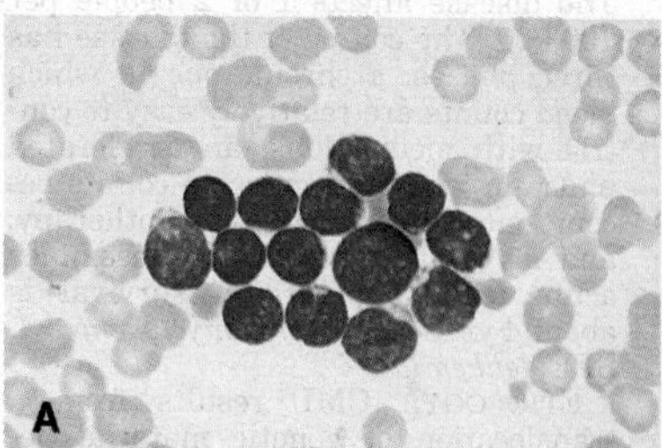

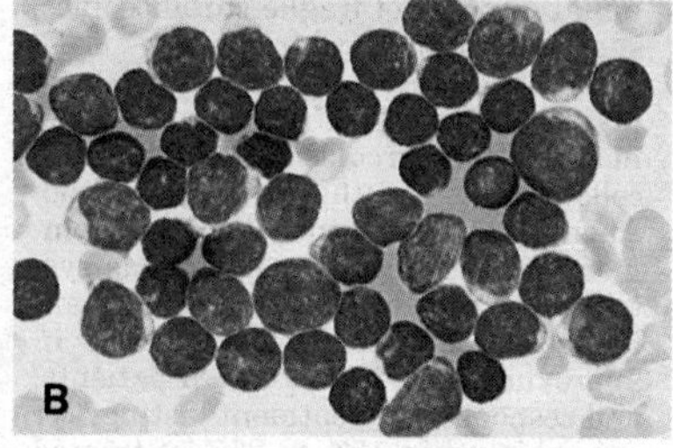

ACUTE LYMPHOCYTIC LEUKEMIA

(A) Peripheral blood (orig. mag. ×640), (B) bone marrow (orig. mag. ×640)

growth factors from cells and those that cause the loss of cancer-suppressing genes.

SYMPTOMS: Fatigue, lethargy, bleeding, bone and joint pain, and a predisposition to fever and infection are characteristic of ALL and other leukemias.

DIAGNOSIS: The disease is suggested by the presence of abnormalities on the complete blood count or peripheral blood smear, and confirmed by immunophenotyping.

TREATMENT: In childhood, ALL induction chemotherapy often begins with steroids, vinca alkaloids, and asparaginase. This is followed, after bone marrow recovery, by consolidation chemotherapy with multidrug regimens, including high-dose methotrexate. Maintenance therapies, which may last 1 to 2 yr, include methotrexate, mercaptopurines, and other cytotoxic agents. Prophylaxis against central nervous system disease is accomplished by intrathecal drug administration. In referral hospitals, allogeneic stem cell transplantation is sometimes used for refractory disease. About 90% of children achieve remission, and nearly 80% of children with ALL are cured. Adult ALL is much less responsive to therapy; only about a third of adult patients are cured. In both childhood and adult ALL, allopurinol and hydration precede induction chemotherapy to prevent hyperuricemia caused by tumor lysis.

PROGNOSIS: Nearly 80% of children and one third of adults will be cured, but late complications of therapy are not uncommon.

acute myelogenous l. ABBR: AML. SYN: *acute myeloid l.*

acute myeloid l. ABBR: AML. A group of hematological malignancies in which neoplastic cells develop from myeloid, monocytic, erythrocytic, or megakaryocytic precursors. AML is four times more common in adults than acute lymphocytic leukemia (ALL). It occasionally follows a myelodysplastic disorder or aplastic anemia, and sometimes occurs as a consequence of a familial disorder of fragile chromosomes, such as Fanconi's syndrome.

All forms of AML are marked by neoplastic replacement of normal bone marrow and circulation of immature cells ("blasts") in the peripheral blood. Anemia and thrombocytopenia commonly occur. The central nervous system and other organs occasionally are invaded. Complete remissions occur in approximately 65% of treated patients, and responses to treatment lasting 5 yr are achieved in 15% to 25% of treated patients. SYN: *acute myelogenous l.; acute nonlymphocytic l.*

ETIOLOGY: Genetic and chromosomal aberrations, such as those found in other leukemias, are characteristic.

SYMPTOMS: Exertional fatigue as a result of anemia, bleeding due to thrombocytopenia, and infections due to a lack of normal white blood cells are common.

TREATMENT: Cytotoxic chemotherapies, with an induction phase followed by consolidation, are used. Typically, cytosine arabinoside and an anthracycline are used during induction for AML. Allogeneic bone marrow transplantation is used when a matching donor is available; stem cell transplantation is an option for some patients with specific cytogenetic abnormalities.

acute nonlymphocytic l. ABBR: ANLL. SYN: *acute myeloid l.*

chronic lymphocytic l. ABBR: CLL. A malignancy in which abnormal lymphocytes, usually B cells, proliferate and infiltrate body tissues, often causing lymph node enlargement and immune dysfunction. Infectious complications are common. Median life expectancy is about 4 yr. Chronic lymphocytic leukemia is the most common leukemia in industrialized nations. It usually occurs in people age 60 or older. Its incidence rises to 20 cases per 100,000 in people over age 80. The timing of treatment and the prognosis in CLL depend on the stage of the disease. Staging includes such factors as the number of abnormal lymphocytes in the bloodstream, how quickly they double, and the presence of lymphadenopathy, organomegaly, or cytopenias. SEE: illus.

TREATMENT: Patients with advanced stages of the illness often are treated with chlorambucil, fludarabine, or other cytotoxic agents. Patients with early-stage disease are not usually given therapy.

chronic myelogenous l. ABBR: CML. SYN: *chronic myeloid l.*

chronic myeloid l. ABBR: CML. A hematological malignancy marked by a sustained increase in the number of granulocytes, splenic enlargement, and a specific cytogenetic anomaly—the Philadelphia chromosome—in the bone marrow of more than 90% of patients. The disease affects 1 or 2 people per 100,000. The course of the disease has three phases: a chronic one in which blood counts are relatively easy to control with medications; an accelerated phase in which granulocyte counts become more resistant to chemotherapy; and a "blast" crisis, which resembles acute leukemia. Median survival is about 4 yr. SYN: *chronic myelogenous l.* SEE: *leukemia.*

ETIOLOGY: CML results from a translocation of genetic material between chromosomes 9 and 22. The translocation results in the production of an abnormal tyrosine kinase that makes affected cells immortal.

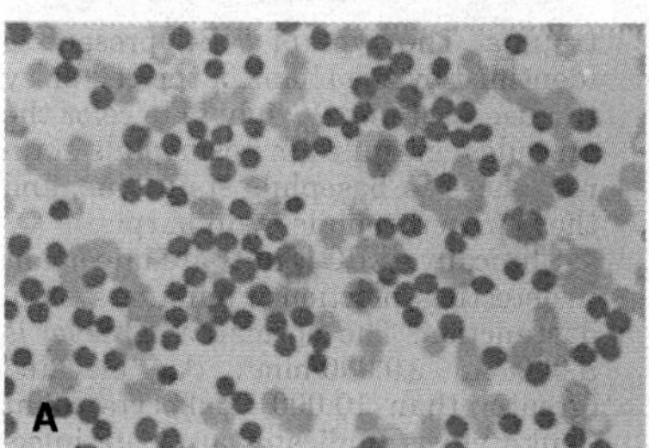

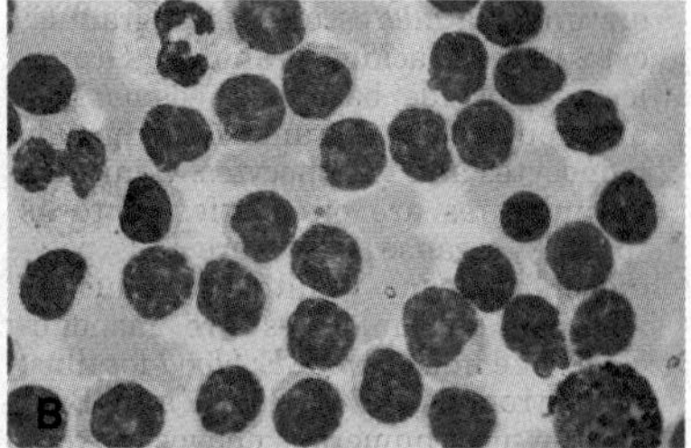

CHRONIC LYMPHOCYTIC LEUKEMIA

(A) Peripheral blood (orig. mag. ×400), (B) bone marrow (orig. mag. ×640)

SYMPTOMS: CML often is diagnosed in asymptomatic patients who are found to have an unexplained leukocytosis when their complete blood counts are checked. Subsequent evaluation, including bone marrow aspiration and biopsy with cytogenetic analysis, reveal the Philadelphia chromosome.

TREATMENT: Busulfan, hydroxyurea, interferon alpha, and bone marrow transplantation all have been used.

hairy cell l. ABBR: HCL. A chronic, low-grade hematological malignancy of abnormally shaped B lymphocytes ("hairy cells"). The disease is marked by pancytopenia and splenomegaly. Median survival in untreated patients is about 5 yr. The disease is rare, comprising only 1% to 2% of all leukemias. The median age of patients is 50 yr; men are affected more commonly than women by a 4-to-1 ratio. SEE: illus.

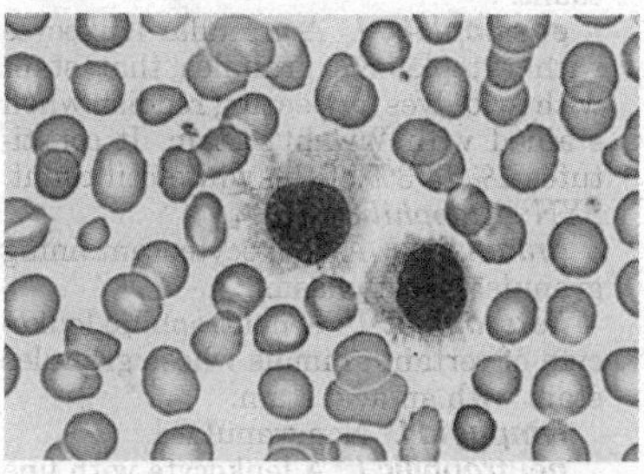

LYMPHOCYTES IN HAIRY CELL LEUKEMIA

(Orig. mag. ×640)

SYMPTOMS: Weight loss, hypermetabolism, infectious complications, and abdominal discomfort due to splenic enlargement are common.

TREATMENT: Cladribine, pentostatin, 2-chlorodeoxyadenosine, and fludarabine have been used.

PROGNOSIS: Prior to the availability of the chemotherapeutic agents, the mean survival time was 4.6 years for nonsplenectomized patients and 6.4 for those who had splenectomy. The use of chemotherapy in HCL patients may permit longer survival times.

leukemic (loo-kēm′ĭk) [″ + *haima,* blood] **1.** Relating to leukemia. **2.** Affected with leukemia.

leukemid (loo-kē′mĭd) Any nonspecific skin lesion associated with leukemia. The lesions may or may not contain leukemic cells.

leukemogenesis (loo-kē″mō-jĕn′ĕ-sĭs) [″ + ″ + *genesis,* generation, birth] The induction of leukemia.

leukemoid (loo-kē′moyd) [″ + ″ + *eidos,* form, shape] Having a markedly elevated white blood cell count (e.g., about 50,000 cells/mm³). The extreme leukocytosis initially may be confused with leukemia, but after more careful study is found to be the result of other stressful illnesses, such as tuberculosis, abscesses, Ebstein-Barr virus infection, osteomyelitis, severe burns, or diabetic ketoacidosis, among others.

leukin (loo′kĭn) A thermostable bactericidal substance present in leukocytes.

leuko-, leuk-, leuc- [Gr. *leukos,* white] Combining form meaning *white* or *white corpuscle.*

leukoagglutinin (loo″kō-ă-gloo′tĭ-nĭn) [″ + L. *agglutinans,* gluing] An antibody that agglutinates white blood cells.

leukoareosis (loo-koh-ar-ee-oh′sis) An abnormal appearance of the periventricular white matter of the brain, seen in patients with chronic and poorly controlled high blood pressure.

leukocidin (loo-kō-sī′dĭn) [″ + L. *caedere,* to kill] A bacterial toxin that destroys leukocytes.

leukocoria, leukokoria White or abnormal pupillary reflex. This reflex may be present in infants and children who have retinoblastoma, cataract, retinal detachment, and intraocular infections. Patients with this reflex should be referred to an ophthalmologist without delay.

leukocyte (loo′kō-sīt) [″ + *kytos,* cell] A white blood cell or corpuscle (WBC). There are two types: granulocytes (those possessing, in their cytoplasm, large granules that stain different colors under a microscope) and agranulocytes (those lacking granules). Granulocytes include basophils, eosinophils, and neutrophils. Agranulocytes include monocytes and lymphocytes. Clinically, granulocytes are often referred to as "polys" because they are all polymorphonuclear (multilobed nuclei); whereas agranulocytes are mononuclear (one nucleus). SEE: *blood* for illus.

Neutrophils, 55% to 70% of all WBCs, are the most numerous phagocytic cells and are a primary effector cell in inflammation. Eosinophils, 1% to 3% of total WBCs, destroy parasites and are involved in allergic reactions. Basophils, less than 1% of all WBCs, contain granules of histamine and heparin and are part of the inflammatory response to injury. Monocytes, 3% to 8% of all WBCs, become macrophages and phagocytize pathogens and damaged cells, esp. in the tissue fluid. Lymphocytes, 20% to 35% of all WBCs, have several functions: recognizing foreign antigens, producing antibodies, suppressing the immune response to prevent excess tissue damage, and becoming memory cells.

Leukocytes are formed from the undifferentiated stem cells, that give rise to all blood cells. Those in the red bone marrow may become any of the five kinds of WBCs. Those in the spleen and lymph nodes may become lymphocytes or monocytes. Those in the thymus become lymphocytes called T lymphocytes.

FUNCTION: Leukocytes are the primary effector cells against infection and tissue damage. They not only neutralize or destroy organisms, but also act as scavengers, cleaning up damaged cells by phagocytosis to initiate the repair process. Leukocytes travel by ameboid movement and are able to penetrate tissue and then return to the bloodstream. Their movement is directed by chemicals released by injured cells, a process called chemotaxis. After coming in contact with and recognizing an antigen, neutrophils or macrophages phagocytize (engulf) it in a small vacuole that merges with a lysosome, to permit the lysosomal enzymes to digest the phagocytized material. When leukocytes are killed along with the pathogenic organisms they have destroyed, the resulting material is called pus, commonly found at the site of localized infections. Pus that collects because of inadequate blood or lymph drainage is called an abscess.

Microscopic examination: Leukocytes can be measured in any bodily secretion. They are normally present in blood and, in small amounts, in spinal fluid and mucus. The presence of WBCs in urine, sputum, or fluid drawn from the abdomen is an indication of infection or trauma. The type of WBC present is identified by the shape of the cell or by the use of stains (Wright's) to color the granules: granules in eosinophils stain red, those in basophils stain blue, and those in neutrophils stain purple.

Clinically, WBC counts are important in detecting infection or immune system dysfunction. The normal WBC level is 5,000 to 10,000/mm^3. An elevated (greater than 10,000) leukocyte count (leukocytosis) indicates an acute infection or disease process (such as certain types of leukemia), whereas a decrease in the number of leukocytes (less than 5,000) indicates either immunodeficiency or an overwhelming infection that has depleted WBC stores. In addition to the total WBC count, the differential count is also frequently important. A differential count measures the percent of each type of WBC (e.g., neutrophils, monocytes, lymphocytes). The differential also measures the number of immature cells of each cell type as an indication of production by the bone marrow. Immature cells are called "blasts" (e.g., lymphoblasts, myeloblasts). During infections or in certain types of leukemia, blasts may be present in peripheral blood. SEE: *inflammation*.

acidophilic l. Eosinophilic l.

agranular l. Nongranular l.

basophilic l. A leukocyte with cytoplasmic granules that stain with basic dyes, turning a deep purple with Wright's stain. This leukocyte constitutes 0% to 0.75% of the white cell count.

eosinophilic l. A granular leukocyte with cytoplasmic granules that stain with acid dyes, appearing reddish when stained with Wright's stain. It constitutes 1% to 3% of the white cell count. SYN: *acidophilic l.*

granular l. A leukocyte containing granules in cytoplasm.

heterophilic l. A neutrophilic leukocyte of certain animals whose granules stain with an acid stain.

lymphoid l. Nongranular l.

neutrophilic l. A leukocyte with fine cytoplasmic granules that do not stain with acid or basic stains but have an affinity for neutral stains.

nongranular l. An agranulocyte; a lymphocyte or monocyte. SYN: *agranular l.*

polymorphonuclear l. ABBR: PMN. A white blood cell that possesses a nucleus composed of two or more lobes or parts; also called a *granulocyte* (neutrophil, eosinophil, basophil). Neutrophils, the most numerous polymorphonuclear leukocytes, are important phagocytic cells. Clinically, polymorphonuclear leukocytes are often referred to as "polys."

leukocytic (loo″kō-sĭt′ĭk) [″ + *kytos,* cell] Pert. to leukocytes.

leukocytoblast (loo″kō-sī′tō-blast) [″ + ″ + *blastos,* germ] A cell from which a leukocyte arises.

leukocytogenesis (loo″kō-sī″tō-jĕn′ĕ-sĭs) [″ + *kytos,* cell, + *genesis,* generation, birth] Leukopoiesis.

leukocytoid (loo′kō-sī″toyd) [″ + ″ + *eidos,* form, shape] Resembling a leukocyte.

leukocytolysin A lysin that destroys leukocytes. SEE: *leukocidin.*

leukocytolysis (loo″kō-sī-tŏl′ĭ-sĭs) [″ + *kytos,* cell, + *lysis,* dissolution] Destruction of leukocytes.

leukocytoma (loo″kō-sī-tō′mă) [″ + ″ + *oma,* tumor] **1.** A tumor composed of cells resembling leukocytes. **2.** A tumorlike mass of leukocytes.

leukocytopenia (loo″kō-sī″tō-pē′nē-ă) [″ + ″ + *penia,* want] Leukopenia.

leukocytopoiesis (loo″kō-sī″tō-poy-ē′sĭs) [″ + ″ + *poiein,* to make] The formation of white blood cells.

leukocytosis (loo″kō-sī-tō′sĭs) [″ + *kytos,* cell, + *osis,* condition] An increase in the number of leukocytes (usually above 10,000/mm^3) in the blood. It occurs most commonly in disease processes involving infection, inflammation, trauma, or stress, but it also can result occasionally from the use of some medications (e.g., corticosteroids). SEE: *leukemoid; leukocyte; leukopenia.*

It usually is caused by an increase in one particular type of white blood cell (WBC). For example, neutrophils increase in acute bacterial infections and inflammation, monocytes increase in chronic infections, lymphocytes increase in viral and chronic bacterial infections, and eosinophils increase in allergic disorders, such as asthma. Leukemias often cause a huge increase in circulating cells, owing to the unchecked reproduction of a single clone of malignant cells.

basophilic l. An increase in the basophils in the blood.

mononuclear l. An increase in the monocytes in the blood.

pathological l. Leukocytosis due to a disease such as an infection.

leukocytotaxis (loo″kō-sī″tō-tăk′sĭs) [Gr. *leukos,* white, + *kytos,* cell, + *taxis,* arrangement] The movement of leukocytes either toward or away from an area such as a traumatized or infected site.

leukocytotoxin (loo″kō-sī″tō-tŏk′sĭn) [″ + ″ + *toxikon,* poison] A toxin that destroys leukocytes.

leukocyturia (loo″kō-sī-tū′rē-ă) [″ + ″ + *ouron,* urine] Leukocytes in the urine.

leukoderma (loo-kō-dĕr′mă) [″ + *derma,* skin] Deficiency of skin pigmentation, esp. in patches. SEE: *vitiligo.*

syphilitic l. Macular depigmentation, esp. of the skin of the neck and shoulders, seen in late syphilis.

leukodystrophy (loo″kō-dĭs′trō-fē) Any disease (such as globoid cell leukodystrophy, adrenoleukodsytrophy, or metachromatic leukodystrophy) whose hallmarks are metabolic defects in the formation of myelin. Bone marrow transplantation can cure some affected children.

metachromatic l. A type of hereditary leukodystrophy caused by a deficiency of the enzyme cerebroside sulfatase, an enzyme that is essential for the degradation of sulfatide. Deficiency of the enzyme allows excess deposition of sulfatide in nerve tissues. Clinical signs of this disease usually appear at about 1 year of age. They include gait disturbance, inability to learn to walk, spasticity of the limbs, hyperreflexia, dementia, and eventually death. The disease, for which there is no specific therapy, is usually fatal by age 10.

leukoedema (loo″kō-ĕ-dē′mă) [″ + *oidema,* swelling] A benign leukophakia-like abnormality of the mucosa of the mouth or tongue. The affected areas are opalescent or white, and wrinkled.

leukoencephalitis (loo″kō-ĕn-sĕf-ă-lī′tĭs) [″ + *enkephalos,* brain + *itis,* inflammation] Inflammation of the white matter of the brain.

acute hemorrhagic l. A neurological syndrome marked by rapidly progressive neurological findings, associated with asymmetric inflammatory pathological changes in the brain, and bleeding. SYN: *Weston Hurst syndrome.*

leukoencephalopathy, progressive multifocal ABBR: PML. Widespread demyelinating lesions of the brain, brainstem, and cerebellum caused by the JC virus (the initials of the first patient from whom the virus was isolated). It is usually associated with chronic neoplastic diseases including Hodgkin's disease, chronic lymphocytic leukemia, and lymphosarcoma. It also occurs as a complication of AIDS and in immunocompromised patients. Clinically there is paralysis, blindness, aphasia, ataxia, dysarthria, dementia, confusional states, and coma. There is no treatment. Death occurs 3 to 6 months after onset of neurological symptoms.

leukoerythroblastosis (loo″kō-ĕ-rĭth″rō-blăs-tō′sĭs) [″ + *erythros,* red, + *blastos,* germ, + *osis,* condition] Anemia due to any condition that causes the bone marrow to be infiltrated and thus inactivated.

leukokeratosis (loo″kō-kĕr-ă-tō′sĭs) [″ + *keras,* horn, + *osis,* condition] Leukoplakia.

leukokoria (loo″kō-kō′rē-ă) [″ + *kore,* pupil] Leukocoria.

leukokraurosis (loo″kō-kraw-rō′sĭs) [″ +

krauros, dry, + *osis,* condition] Lichen sclerosis et atrophicus.

leukolymphosarcoma (loo″kō-lĭm″fō-săr-kō′mă) [″ + L. *lympha,* lymph, + Gr. *sarx,* flesh, + *oma,* tumor] Lymphosarcoma cell leukemia.

leukoma (loo-kō′mă) [″ + *oma,* tumor] A white, opaque corneal opacity.

l. adherens A corneal scar with incarcerated iris tissue.

leukomatous (loo-kō′mă-tŭs) [Gr. *leukos,* white, + *oma,* tumor] **1.** Pert. to leukoma. **2.** Suffering from leukoma.

leukomyelitis (loo″kō-mī-ĕ-lī′tĭs) [″ + *myelos,* marrow, + *itis,* inflammation] Inflammation of the white matter of the spinal cord.

leukomyelopathy (loo″kō-mī-ĕl-ŏp′ă-thē) [″ + ″ + *pathos,* disease] Disease involving the white matter of the spinal cord.

leukonecrosis (loo″kō-nĕ-krō′sĭs) [″ + *nekrosis,* state of death] Dry, light-colored, or white gangrene.

leukonychia (loo″kō-nĭk′ē-ă) [″ + *onyx,* nail] White spots or streaks on the nails. SYN: *canities unguium.*

leukopathia (loo″kō-păth′ē-ă) [″ + *pathos,* disease] **1.** The absence of pigment in the skin. SEE: *leukoderma.* **2.** A disease involving leukocytes.

l. unguium Leukonychia.

leukopedesis (loo″kō-pĕ-dē′sĭs) [″ + *pedan,* to leap] The passage of leukocytes through the walls of the blood vessels.

leukopenia (loo″kō-pē′nē-ă) [″ + *penia,* lack] Abnormal decrease of white blood cells usually below 5000/mm^3. A great number of drugs may cause leukopenia, as can failure of the bone marrow. SYN: *granulocytopenia; leukocytopenia.*

leukoplakia (loo″kō-plā′kē-ă) [″ + *plax,* plate] Formation of white spots or patches on the mucous membrane of the tongue or cheek. The spots are smooth, irregular in size and shape, hard, and occasionally fissured. The lesions may become malignant.

l. buccalis Leukoplakia of the mucosa of the cheek.

oral hairy l. Leukoplakia of the tongue. SEE: illus.

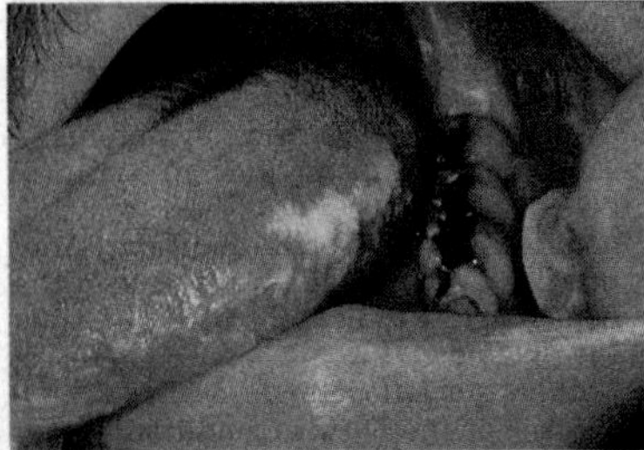

ORAL HAIRY LEUKOPLAKIA

In a patient with AIDS

l. vulvae Lichen sclerosis et atrophicus.

leukoplasia (loo-kō-plā′zē-ă) Leukoplakia.

leukopoiesis (loo″kō-poy-ē′sĭs) [″ + *poiesis,* formation] Leukocyte production. SYN: *leukocytogenesis.*

leukopoietic (loo″kō-poy-ĕt′ĭk) [″ + *poiein,* to make] Forming leukocytes.

leukopsin A substance formed in the rods of the retina from rhodopsin under the influence of light.

leukorrhagia (loo″kō-rā′jē-ă) [″ + *rhegnynai,* to burst forth] Leukorrhea.

leukorrhea (loo″kō-rē′ă) [″ + *rhoia,* flow] A white, estrogen-related, scant-to-moderate, odorless, physiological vaginal discharge, normally preceding menarche and occurring during ovulation, during pregnancy, and in response to sexual excitement. Some women note an increased discharge related to oral contraceptive or hormone replacement therapy. Chronic cervicitis and vaginal infections are the most common causes of abnormal genital discharge. Signs of infection include increased discharge, change in color and consistency, odor, vulvar irritation, dysuria, and itching. SEE: *vaginitis.*

leukosarcoma (loo″kō-săr-kō′mă) [Gr. *leukos,* white, + *sarx,* flesh, + *oma,* tumor] A variant of malignant lymphoma in which the blood cells become leukemic.

leukotactic (loo″kō-tăk′tĭk) [″ + *taxis,* arrangement] Possessing the power of attracting leukocytes.

leukotaxis (loo″kō-tăks′ĭs) Possessing the power of attracting (positive leukotaxis) or repelling (negative leukotaxis) leukocytes.

leukotomy (loo-kŏt′ō-mē) [″ + *tome,* incision] Lobotomy.

leukotoxic (loo″kō-tŏks′ĭk) [″ + *toxikon,* poison] Destructive to leukocytes.

leukotoxin (loo″kō-tŏk′sĭn) [″ + *toxikon,* poison] Leukocytotoxin.

leukotrichia (loo″kō-trĭk′ē-ă) [″ + *thrix,* hair] Whiteness of the hair. SYN: *canities.*

leukotriene Any of a group of arachidonic acid metabolites that functions as a chemical mediator of inflammation. Leukotrienes C4, D4, and E4 are derived from the precursor molecule leukotriene A4. All are synthesized by cells in response to inflammation or tissue injury. Leukotrienes have been implicated in the development of the inflammation responses in asthma, psoriasis, rheumatoid arthritis, and inflammatory bowel disease. They are extremely powerful bronchoconstrictors and vasodilators and mediate the adverse vascular and bronchial effects of systemic anaphylaxis.

leukous (loo′kŭs) [Gr. *leukos,* white] White, esp. relating to the skin.

levallorphan tartrate (lĕv″ăl-lor′făn) A narcotic antagonist used to counteract morphine or opioid-induced respiratory depression.

levamisole hydrochloride An antihelminthic drug originally used in veterinary medicine and now as adjuvant therapy in treating metastatic colorectal cancer.

levarterenol bitartrate (lĕv″ăr-tĕ-rē′nŏl bī-tăr′trāt) Previously used name for norepinephrine bitartrate. A sympathomimetic agent that, due to its vasopressor effect, may be useful in treating hypotension that accompanies shock. It is usually administered intravenously because it is rapidly inactivated. Trade name is Levophed.

levator (lē-vā′tor) *pl.* **levatores** [L., lifter] **1.** A muscle that raises or elevates a part; opposite of depressor. **2.** An instrument that lifts depressed portions.

l. ani A broad muscle that helps to form the floor of the pelvis.

l. palpebrae superioris A muscle that elevates the upper eyelid.

LeVeen shunt [Harry LeVeen, U.S. surgeon, b. 1917] A shunt from the peritoneal cavity to the venous circulation used to help control ascites by allowing ascitic fluid to enter the venous circulation.

level of activities In the nervous system, the levels corresponding to different stages of development into which connector neurons are grouped: spinal cord level, medullary level, midbrain level, basal ganglial level, and cortical level. Each level is responsible for certain activities but is controlled by the one above it.

level of health care SEE: *system, health care.*

lever (lĕv′ĕr, lē′vĕr) [L. *levare,* to raise] A rigid bar used to modify direction, force, and motion. A type of simple machine that provides the user with a mechanical advantage. Levers are used to facilitate the moving and lifting of objects too heavy or awkward for one to move unassisted.

Levey-Jennings chart A graphical representation of control data, arranged in chronological order, that shows a mean or target value and one or more sets of acceptable limits.

Levine, Myra A nursing educator who developed the Conservation Model of Nursing. SEE: *Nursing Theory Appendix.*

Levin's tube (lĕ-vĭnz′) [Abraham L. Levin, U.S. physician, 1880–1940] A catheter that is usually introduced through the nose and extends into or through the stomach. It is used to help prevent accumulation of intestinal liquids and gas during and after intestinal surgery. This tube is often referred to as a nasogastric tube.

levitation [L. *levitas,* lightness] The subjective sensation of rising in the air or moving through the air unsupported. It occurs in dreams, altered states of consciousness, and certain mental disorders.

levocardia (lē″vō-kăr′dē-ă) [L. *laevus,* left, + Gr. *kardia,* heart] A term describing the normal position of the heart when other viscera are inverted. SEE: *dextrocardia.*

levocarnitine An amino acid-derived drug used in treating primary carnitine deficiency. SEE: *carnitine.*

levoclination (lē″vō-klī-nā′shŭn) [″ + *clinatus,* leaning] Torsion or twisting of the upper meridians of the eyes to the left. SYN: *levotorsion* (2).

levocycloduction (lē″vō-sī″klō-dŭk′shŭn) [″ + Gr. *kyklos,* circle, + L. *ducere,* to lead] Levoduction.

levodopa L-3,4-dihydroxyphenylalanine; a drug used in the treatment of Parkinson's disease. Also called L-dopa.

levoduction (lē″vō-dŭk′shŭn) [L. *laevus,* left, + *ducere,* to lead] Movement or drawing toward the left, esp. of an eye. SYN: *levocycloduction.*

levophobia (lĕv″ō-fō′bē-ă) [″ + Gr. *phobos,* fear] A morbid dread of objects on the left side of the body.

levorotation (lē″vō-rō-tā′shŭn) [″ + *rotare,* to turn] Levotorsion (1).

levorotatory (lē″vō-rō′tă-tor-ē) Causing to turn toward the left, applied esp. to substances that turn polarized light rays to the left.

levorphanol tartrate (lēv-or′fă-nōl) A synthetic analgesic that acts similarly to morphine.

levothyroxine sodium (lē″vō-thī-rŏk′sēn) ABBR: T_4. The sodium salt of the natural isomer of thyroxine used in treating thyroid deficiency.

levotorsion, levoversion (lē″vō-tor′shŭn, lē″vō-vĕr′shŭn) [″ + *torsio,* a twisting] **1.** A twisting to the left. SYN: *levorotation.* **2.** Levoclination.

levulinic acid $CH_3COCH_2CH_2COOH$; An acid formed when certain simple sugars are acted on by dilute hydrochloric acid.

levulose SEE: *fructose.*

levulosemia (lĕv″ū-lō-sē′mē-ă) [″ + Gr. *haima,* blood] The presence of fructose in the blood.

levulosuria (lĕv″ū-lō-sū′rē-ă) [″ + Gr. *ouron,* urine] The presence of fructose in the urine.

lewisite (lū′ĭ-sīt) [Warren Lee Lewis, U.S. chemist, 1878–1943] A toxic gas similar in action to mustard gas, used in warfare to disable and kill. It acts as a vesicant in the lungs. Dimercaprol is the treatment drug of choice.

Lewy bodies [Frederic H. Lewy, Ger. neurologist, 1885–1950] Neuronal cells with pigmented inclusion bodies. They are found in the brain in the substantia nigra and locus ceruleus, esp. in Parkinson's disease.

Leydig cell (lī′dĭg) [Franz von Leydig, Ger. anatomist, 1821–1908] One of the interstitial cells in the testicles that produce testosterone.

L.F.A. *left frontoanterior* fetal position.

L-forms [named for *Lister* Institute] Spontaneous variants of bacteria that replicate as filterable spheres with defective or absent cell walls. They are filterable because of their flexibility rather than their size. Stable forms may grow for an indefinite time in a wall-less state. Organisms of the unstable form are capable of regenerating their cell walls and reverting to their antecedent bacterial form. The ability of L-forms to cause disease is unknown. SYN: *L-phase variants.*

L.F.P. *left frontoposterior* fetal position.

L.F.T. *left frontotransverse* fetal position.

LGA *large for gestational age.*

LGSIL Low-grade squamous intraepithelial lesions.

LH *luteinizing hormone.*

Lhermitte's sign (lār′mĭts) [Jacques Jean Lhermitte, Fr. neurologist, 1877–1959] The symptom (rather than a sign) of a pain resembling a sudden electric shock throughout the body produced by flexing the neck. It is caused by trauma to the cervical portion of the spinal cord, multiple sclerosis, cervical cord tumor, or cervical spondylosis.

LHRH *luteinizing hormone–releasing hormone.*

Li Symbol for the element lithium.

liability Legal responsibility. A health care provider is legally responsible for actions that fail to meet the standards of care or are grossly negligent, thereby causing harm to the patient.

school-specific l. The legal standard that holds licensed practitioners liable only for those actions that violate the standards of their own education and training. As a result, chiropractic liability is judged based on standards of care in the school of chiropractic, while surgical liability is based on the standards set forth among surgeons.

strict l. In health law, a health care provider's responsibility, even if not at fault, for any harm or injury done to a patient.

vicarious l. Legal responsibility of a health care professional or health care institution for the negligent actions of its trainees and employees.

Liberty Mutual elbow Boston arm.

libidinous (lĭ-bĭd′ĭ-nŭs) [L. *libidinosus,* pert. to desire] Characterized by sexual desires.

libido (lĭ-bī′dō, -bē′dō) [L., desire] **1.** The sexual drive, conscious or unconscious. **2.** In psychoanalysis, the energy or force that is the driving force of human behavior. It has been variously identified as the sex urge, desire to live, desire for pleasure, or satisfaction.

Some Classes of Drugs That Inhibit Libido

Class	Examples
alcohol	beer, liquor, wine
antidepressants	amitriptyline, fluoxetine
alpha blockers	clonidine
beta blockers	atenolol, propranolol
drugs of abuse	amphetamines, cocaine, heroin
histamine$_2$ blockers	cimetidine
major tranquilizers	clozapine, fluphenazine, thioridazine
oral contraceptives	many types
sedative/hypnotics	benzodiazepines

low l. A sexual dysfunction marked by inhibited sexual desire and inability to sustain arousal during sexual activities. Diminished sexual drive may be related to advanced age, psychogenic causes, general illness, side effects of some medications, or substance abuse.

In men it manifests as partial or complete failure to attain or maintain erection until completion of the sex act. In women there is partial or complete failure to attain or maintain the vaginal lubrication-swelling response of sexual excitement until completion of the sex act. SEE: table.

Libman-Sacks disease (lĭb′măn-săks′) [Emanuel Libman, U.S. physician, 1872–1946; Benjamin Sacks, U.S. physician, 1896–1939] Verrucous, nonbacterial endocarditis. SEE: *endocarditis.*

lice Pl. of louse.

licensure In the health care professions, the granting of permission—official, legal, or both—to perform professional actions in various fields such as medicine or nursing that may not be legally done by persons who do not have such permission. Qualification for a license in health care is usually determined by an official body representing the state or federal government.

individual l. In the health care profession, licensure of an individual to perform certain medical actions.

institutional l. In the health care industry, the authorization of hospitals, clinics, or corporations to provide specific forms of care.

mandatory l. Licensure that regulates the practice of a profession such as nursing or medicine by requiring compliance with the licensing statute if an individual engages in activities defined within the scope of that profession.

multistate nurse l. In the U.S., authority or permission to practice nursing in several states, granted after making a single application.

licentiate (lī-sĕn′shē-ăt) **1.** An individual who practices a profession by the authority granted by a license. **2.** In some countries, a medical practitioner who has no medical degree.

lichen (lī′kĕn) [Gr. *leichen,* lichen] **1.** Any form of papular skin disease; usually denoting lichen planus. **2.** In botany, any one of numerous plants consisting of a fungus growing symbiotically with certain algae. They form characteristic scaly or branching growths on rocks or barks of trees.

myxedematous l. Generalized eruption of asymptomatic nodules caused by mucinous deposits in the upper layers of the skin and in vessels and organs.

l. nitidus A rare skin condition characterized by small, chronic, asymptomatic papules that are usually pink and are usually located only on the penis, abdomen, and flexor surfaces of the elbows and palms.

l. pilaris L. spinulosus.

l. planopilaris A form of lichen planus in which white shiny follicular papules are present along with the usual plane papules.

l. planus An inflammatory rash marked by the presence of itchy, red to violet, polygon-shaped papules, which typically appear on the scalp, in the oral cavity, or on the limbs. The papules may merge into plaques crisscrossed by faint lines called "Wickham's striae." Typically, the rash persists for 1 to 2 years and then spontaneously improves, although about one in five patients will suffer a recurrence. SEE: illus.

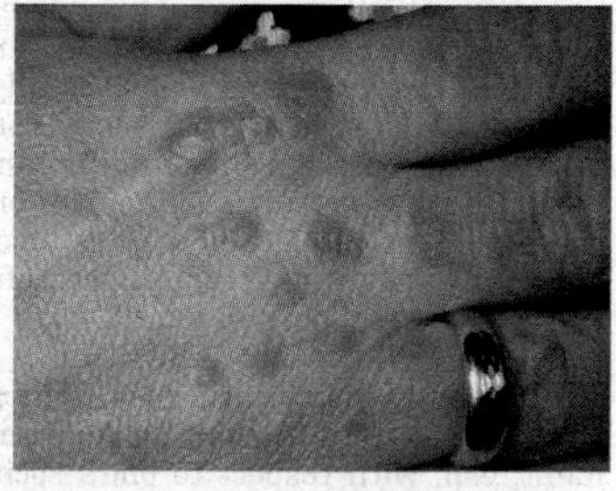

LICHEN PLANUS

ETIOLOGY: The cause of the rash is not known, but it is occasionally associated with the use of certain chemicals (e.g., photoprocessing compounds, gold) or medications (e.g., beta blockers, diuretics, nonsteroidal anti-inflammatory drugs).

TREATMENT: Corticosteroids, applied topically, taken orally, or injected into the lesions, often are effective.

l. ruber moniliformis Large verrucous lesions of lichen planus arranged as the beads in a necklace.

l. ruber planus L. planus.

l. sclerosus et atrophicus A chronic, atrophic skin disorder marked by the appearance of discrete, flat-topped, white papules, which may coalesce and degenerate. The skin affected by the rash, which occurs most often on the vulva, is often thin, shiny, and scarred. Although this condition is not considered precancerous, squamous cell carcinomas arise in 1% to 5% of cases.

SYMPTOMS: Itching of the vulva, which may be intractable, is the most common complaint.

TREATMENT: Potent topical corticosteroids produce remission, but not cure, in the great majority of patients.

l. scrofulosus An eruption of tiny punctate reddish-brown papules arranged in circles or groups in young persons with tuberculosis. The lesions are caused by the spread of the tubercle bacilli through the blood to the skin.

l. simplex chronicus An itching papular eruption that is circumscribed and located on skin that has become thickened and pigmented as a result of scratching. SEE: illus; *neurodermatitis* for illus.

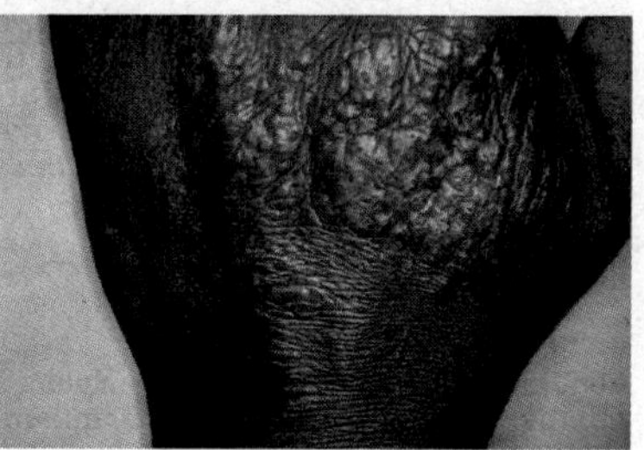

LICHEN SIMPLEX CHRONICUS

l. spinulosus A form of lichen with a spine developing in each follicle. SYN: *l. pilaris; keratosis pilaris.*

l. striatus A papular eruption usually seen on one extremity of a child. It is arranged in linear groups and consists of pink papules. The disease, though self-limiting, may last for a year or longer.

l. tropicus A form of lichen with redness and inflammatory reaction of the skin. SYN: *miliaria.*

lichenification (lī-kĕn″ĭ-fĭ-kā′shŭn) [Gr. *leichen,* lichen, + L. *facere,* to make] **1.** Cutaneous thickening and hardening from continued irritation. **2.** The changing of an eruption into one resembling a lichen.

lichenoid (lī′kĕn-oyd) [″ + *eidos,* form, shape] Resembling lichen.

Lichtheim's syndrome (lĭkt′hīmz) [Ludwig Lichtheim, Ger. physician, 1845–

1928] Subacute combined degeneration of the spinal cord associated with pernicious anemia.

licorice (lĭk′ĕr-ĭs, -ĕr-ĭsh) [ME.] A dried root of *Glycyrrhiza glabra* used as a flavoring agent, demulcent, and mild expectorant. Glycyrrhiza is prepared from licorice. Ingestion of large amounts of licorice can cause salt retention, excess potassium loss in the urine, and elevated blood pressure. SYN: *glycyrrhiza.*

lid [ME.] An eyelid.

lidocaine (lī′dō-kān) A local anesthetic drug. Trade name is Xylocaine.

l. hydrochloride A local anesthetic that is also used intravenously to treat certain cardiac arrhythmias, esp. ventricular dysrhythmias.

lie, transverse A position of the fetus in utero in which the long axis of the fetus is across the long axis of the mother. SEE: *presentation* for illus.

Lieberkühn crypt (lē′bĕr-kēn) [Johann N. Lieberkühn, Ger. anatomist, 1711–1756] One of the simple tubular glands present in the intestinal mucosa. In their epithelium are found goblet cells, cells of Paneth, and argentaffin cells. The glands form minute invaginations opening between the bases of the villi. They lie in the lamina propria, their blind ends extending to the muscularis mucosa. In the large intestine they are longer and contain few if any Paneth cells and more goblet cells. They are arranged vertically with much regularity. SYN: *intestinal glands; Lieberkühn's glands.*

lie detector SEE: *polygraph.*

lien (lī′ĕn) [L.] The spleen.

l. accessorius Accessory spleen.

l. mobilis Floating spleen.

lienal (lī-ē′năl) [L. *lien,* spleen] Splenic.

lienitis (lī″ĕ-nī′tĭs) [″ + Gr. *itis,* inflammation] Splenitis.

lienocele (lī-ē′nō-sēl) [″ + Gr. *kele,* tumor, swelling] Splenocele.

lienography (lī″ē-nŏg′ră-fē) [″ + Gr. *graphein,* to write] An obsolete radiographical examination of the spleen after introduction of a contrast medium.

lienomalacia (lī-ē″nō-mă-lā′shē-ă) [″ + Gr. *malakia,* softening] Splenomalacia.

lienomedullary (lī-ē″nō-mĕd′ū-lăr-ē) [″ + *medulla,* marrow] Relating to both spleen and bone marrow.

lienomyelogenous (lī-ē″nō-mī-ĕl-ŏj′ĕ-nŭs) [″ + Gr. *myelos,* marrow, + *gennan,* to produce] Derived from both spleen and bone marrow.

lienomyelomalacia (lī-ē″nō-mī″ĕl-ō-mă-lā′shē-ă) [″ + ″ + *malakia,* softening] Softening of the spleen and bone marrow.

lienopancreatic (lī-ē″nō-păn″krē-ăt′ĭk) [″ + Gr. *pankreas,* pancreas] Relating to the spleen and pancreas.

lienorenal (lī-ē″nō-rē′năl) [″ + *renalis,* pert. to kidney] Relating to the spleen and kidney.

life (līf) [AS.] **1.** The capability of using metabolic or biochemical processes to grow, reproduce, and adapt to the environment. **2.** The time between the birth or inception and the death of an organism. Biologically, the life of a system begins at the moment of conception and ends at death; however, for legal and other reasons the definition of when life begins and death occurs has been subject to a variety of interpretations. SEE: *death.* **3.** The sum total of those properties that distinguish living things (animals or plants) from nonliving inorganic chemical matter or dead organic matter.

l. expectancy The number of years that an average person of a given age may be expected to live. Numerous factors influence life expectancy, including habits (e.g., smoking); chronic illnesses (e.g., congestive heart failure, end-stage renal disease, or cancers); gender (women live longer than men); and socioeconomic status. In the U.S., the average life expectancy at birth is about 76 years. SEE: tables; *years of life lost.*

l. extension The concept that certain types of intervention may allow a person to live longer than would have been the case if those interventions had not been used (e.g., proper nutrition, exercise, abstinence from cigarettes, and limiting alcohol intake).

l. review therapy A type of insight-oriented therapy that was first described by Robert Butler in 1964. The therapy has a psychoanalytical theoretical base and is focused on conflict resolution. It is usually conducted with persons who are near the end of their life cycle. The therapeutic process allows the patients to review their lives, come to terms with conflict, gain meaning from their lives, and die peacefully.

l. satisfaction One's attitudes concerning one's present life situation and the extent to which one is either content or discontent. It is sometimes used simultaneously with morale, successful aging, and well-being.

l. satisfaction index ABBR: LSI. A self-reporting instrument used to measure personal fulfillment or contentment, esp. with respect to one's social relationships, occupation, maturation, or aging. A total of five rating scales are used.

l. span The maximal obtainable age by a member of a species.

l. table A statistical table that estimates the life expectancy of individuals in a particular population. The data used to establish the table come from records of the age of death of the individuals in that same population.

lifestyle The pattern of living and behavior of an individual, society, or culture, esp. as it distinguishes individuals con-

Expectation of Life in Years, by Race, Sex, and Age: 1996

	White		Black	
Age in 1990 (years)	**Male**	**Female**	**Male**	**Female**
Birth	73.9	79.7	66.1	72.2
5	69.5	75.2	62.4	70.3
10	64.5	70.2	57.5	65.4
15	59.6	65.3	52.6	60.5
20	54.9	60.4	48.0	55.7
25	50.2	55.6	43.7	50.9
30	45.6	50.7	39.4	46.2
35	40.9	45.9	35.1	41.6
40	36.4	41.1	31.5	37.1
45	31.9	36.4	27.1	32.8
50	27.5	31.7	23.4	28.5
55	23.3	27.3	19.9	24.5
60	19.4	23.0	16.7	20.7
65	15.8	19.1	13.9	17.2
70	12.6	15.4	11.2	13.9
75	9.8	12.0	9.0	11.2
80	7.3	8.9	7.0	8.5
85 and over	5.3	6.3	5.3	6.2

SOURCE: Adapted from U.S. Bureau of the Census: Statistical Abstract of the United States: 1999, 119th edition. Washington, DC, 1999.

Expectation of Life at Birth, 1970 to 1997, and Projections, 1995 to 2010*

	Total		White		Black and Other	
Year	**Male**	**Female**	**Male**	**Female**	**Male**	**Female**
1970	67.1	74.7	68.0	75.6	61.3	69.4
1975	68.8	76.6	69.5	77.3	63.7	72.4
1980	70.0	77.4	70.7	78.1	65.3	73.6
1981	70.4	77.8	71.1	78.4	66.2	74.4
1982	70.8	78.1	71.5	78.7	66.8	74.9
1983	71.0	78.1	71.6	78.7	67.0	74.7
1984	71.1	78.2	71.8	78.7	67.2	74.9
1985	71.1	78.2	71.8	78.7	67.0	74.8
1986	71.2	78.2	71.9	78.8	66.8	74.9
1987	71.4	78.3	72.1	78.9	66.9	75.0
1988	71.4	78.3	72.2	78.9	66.7	74.8
1989	71.7	78.5	72.5	79.2	66.7	74.9
1990	71.8	78.8	72.7	79.4	67.0	75.2
1991	72.0	78.9	72.9	79.6	67.3	75.5
1992	72.3	79.1	73.2	79.8	67.7	75.7
1993	72.2	78.8	73.1	79.5	67.4	75.5
1994	72.3	79.0	73.2	79.6	67.5	75.8
1995	72.5	78.9	73.4	79.6	67.9	75.7
1996	73.0	79.0	73.8	79.6	68.9	76.1
1997	73.6	79.2	74.3	73.9	(NA)	(NA)
Projection†:						
1995	72.5	79.3	73.6	80.1	(NA)	(NA)
2000	73.0	79.7	74.2	80.5	(NA)	(NA)
2005	73.5	80.2	74.7	81.0	(NA)	(NA)
2010	74.1	80.6	75.5	81.6	(NA)	(NA)

* In years. Excludes deaths of nonresidents of the United States.
† Based on middle mortality assumptions.
‡ NA = Not available.
SOURCE: Adapted from U.S. Bureau of the Census: Statistical Abstract of the United States: 1999, 119th edition. Washington, DC, 1999.

cerned or included in the groups from other individuals or groups.

life support The use of any technique, therapy, or device to assist in sustaining life. SEE: *basic l.s.*

advanced cardiac l.s. ABBR: ACLS. **1.** The resuscitation of dying patients; a process that involves management of the airway, reestablishment of breathing, and the restoration of spontaneous heart rhythm, blood pressure, and organ perfusion. ACLS begins with the recognition of cardiac or respiratory emergencies, and includes basic life support, defibrillation, endotracheal intubation, oxygenation and ventilation, the use of medications that restore normal cardiac rhythms and cardiac output, cardiac pacing (when needed), and post-resuscitation care. It may begin in the out-of-hospital setting, or take place in the hospital. **2.** A training program offered by the American Heart Association, commonly called ACLS. SEE: *basic life support; cardiopulmonary resuscitation; emergency cardiac care*.

advanced trauma l.s. ABBR: ATLS. **1.** Treatment measures needed to stabilize a critically injured patient. **2.** A continuing education course taught by the American College of Surgeons.

basic cardiac l.s. ABBR: BLS. The phase of cardiopulmonary resuscitation (CPR) and emergency cardiac care that either (1) prevents circulatory or respiratory arrest or insufficiency by prompt recognition and early intervention or by early entry into the emergency care system or both; or (2) externally supports the circulation and respiration of a patient in cardiac arrest through CPR. When cardiac or respiratory arrest occurs, BLS should be initiated by anyone present who is familiar with CPR. SEE: *advanced cardiac life support; bag-valve-mask resuscitator; cardiopulmonary resuscitation; emergency cardiac care; Heimlich maneuver*.

prehospital trauma l.s. ABBR: PHTLS. A continuing education course developed by the National Association of Emergency Medical Technicians, designed to improve the assessment and management of trauma patients in the field.

withholding l.s. Removal of or not giving medical interventions during end-of-life care, with the expectation that the patient will die as a result.

life-sustaining therapy Therapy of a critically ill patient that, if discontinued, would cause the patient to die. SEE: *life support*.

Li-Fraumeni syndrome (lē′frō-mē-nē) [Fredrick Li, Epidemiologist; Joseph Fraumeni, Epidemiologist] Inherited condition in which individuals develop multiple primary tumors, including breast cancer, osteosarcoma, chondrosarcoma, soft tissue sarcoma, brain tumors, adrenal cortex tumors, etc. Mutations of the p53 gene on chromosome 17 are responsible for this disease.

ligament (lĭg′ă-mĕnt) [L. *ligamentum*, a band] **1.** A band or sheet of strong fibrous connective tissue connecting the articular ends of bones, binding them together and facilitating or limiting motion. **2.** A thickened portion or fold of peritoneum or mesentery that supports a visceral organ or connects it to another viscus. **3.** A band of fibrous connective tissue connecting bones, cartilages, and other structures and serving to support or attach fascia or muscles. **4.** A cordlike structure representing the vestigial remains of a fetal blood vessel.

accessory l. A ligament that supplements another, esp. one on the lateral surface of a joint. This type of ligament lies outside of and independent of the capsule of a joint.

acromioclavicular l. The ligament supporting the acromioclavicular joint; it joins the acromial process of the scapula and the distal end of the clavicle and, in combination with the coracoclavicular ligaments, holds the clavicle down.

alar l. One of a pair of ligaments that stabilize the dens of the second vertebra to the occipital bone of the skull, limiting side flexion and rotation of the head.

annular l. A circular ligament, esp. one enclosing a head or radius or one holding the footplate of the stapes in the oval window.

anterior talofibular l. The ligament of the ankle that connects the lateral talus and fibular malleolus, preventing anterior displacement of the talus in the mortise. This ligament is injured with an inversion movement and is the most commonly injured ligament of the ankle.

anterior tibiofibular l. A broad ligament located on the anterior half of the distal fibula, superior to the lateral malleolus, that binds the fibula to the tibia. The anterior tibiofibular ligament is part of the distal ankle syndesmosis. SEE: *crural interosseous l.; posterior tibiofibular l.*

anterior tibiotalar l. Ligament of the ankle that connects the anteromedial portion of the talus to the anterior portion of the medial malleolus, preventing anterior displacement of the talus within the mortise, esp. when the ankle is plantar flexed. The anterior tibiotalar ligament is categorized as part of the ankle's deltoid ligament complex. SEE: *deltoid l.*

apical l. A single median ligament extending from the odontoid process to the occipital bone.

arcuate l. The lateral, medial, and exterior ligaments that extend from the

12th rib to the transverse process of the first lumbar vertebra, to which the diaphragm is attached.

arterial l. A fibrous cord extending from the pulmonary artery to the arch of the aorta, the remains of the ductus arteriosus of the fetus.

auricular l. The anterior, posterior, and superior auricular ligaments uniting the external ear to the temporal bone.

broad l. of liver A wide, sickle-shaped fold of peritoneum, attached to the lower surface of the diaphragm, the internal surface of the right rectus abdominis muscle, and the convex surface of the liver.

broad l. of uterus The folds of peritoneum attached to lateral borders of the uterus from insertion of the fallopian tube above to the pelvic wall. They consist of two layers between which are found the remnants of the wolffian ducts, cellular tissues, and the major blood vessels of the pelvis.

calcaneofibular l. ABBR: CFL. An extracapsular ligament of the lateral ankle joint. The calcaneofibular ligament originates from the inferior apex of the lateral malleolus and courses at approximately a 133-degree angle to attach to the calcaneus. It is the primary restraint against talar inversion when the ankle is in its neutral position.

capsular l. Heavy fibrous structures, lined with synovial membrane and surrounding articulations.

carpal l. The ligaments uniting the carpal bones.

caudal l. The ligament formed by bundles of fibrous tissue uniting dorsal surfaces of the two lower coccygeal vertebrae and superjacent skin.

check l. A ligament that restrains the motion of a joint, esp. the lateral odontoid ligaments.

collateral l. One of the ligaments that provide medial and lateral stability to joints. They include the medial (ulnar) and lateral (radial) collateral ligaments at the elbow, the medial (tibial) and lateral (fibular) collateral ligaments at the knee, the medial (deltoid) and lateral collateral ligaments at the ankle, and the collateral ligaments of the fingers.

conoid l. The posterior and inner portion of the coracoclavicular ligament.

coracoacromial l. The broad triangular ligament attached to the outer edge of the coracoid process of the scapula and the tip of the acromion.

coracoclavicular l. The ligament uniting the clavicle and coracoid process of the scapula.

coracohumeral l. The broad ligament connecting the coracoid process of the scapula to the greater tubercle of the humerus.

coronary l. of liver A fold of peritoneum extending from the posterior edge of the liver to the diaphragm.

costocolic l. The ligament attaching the splenic flexure of the colon to the diaphragm.

costocoracoid l. The ligament joining the first rib and coracoid process of the scapula.

costotransverse l. The ligaments uniting the ribs with the transverse processes of the vertebrae.

costovertebral l. Ligaments uniting the ribs and vertebrae.

cricopharyngeal l. A ligamentous bundle between the upper and posterior border of the cricoid cartilage and the anterior wall of the pharynx.

cricothyroid l. The ligament uniting cricoid and thyroid cartilages and the location for the horizontal incision (called coniotomy) to prevent choking.

cricotracheal l. The ligamentous structure uniting the upper ring of the trachea and the cricoid cartilage.

cruciate l. **1.** The ligament of the ankle passing transversely across the dorsum of the foot that holds tendons of the anterior muscle group in place. **2.** A cross-shaped ligament of the atlas consisting of the transverse ligament and superior and inferior bands, the former passing upward and attaching to the margin of the foramen magnum, the latter passing downward and attaching to the body of the atlas. **3.** The ligament of the knee that originates on the anterior portion of the femur in the intercondylar notch and inserts on the posterior aspect of the tibial plateau. It prevents posterior translation of the tibia on the femur and, in combination with the anterior cruciate ligament, provides rotary stability to the knee.

SYMPTOMS: A torn or ruptured anterior cruciate ligament (ACL) causes instability and pain in the knee.

TREATMENT: Arthroscopic surgery is usually necessary to repair torn ACLs. Sometimes open surgery, or arthrotomy, is necessary for particularly complex repairs.

cruciform l. A structure consisting of one ligament crossing another.

crural l. Inguinal l.

crural interosseous l. A thickening of the interosseous membrane as it extends into the space between the distal tibia and fibula, allowing only a slight amount of spreading between the two bones. SEE: *anterior tibiofibular l.; posterior tibiofibular l.*

deltoid l. The collective term for the medial ankle ligaments, formed by the anterior tibiotalar, tibionavicular, tibiocalcaneal, and posterior tibiotalar ligaments. As a group, the deltoid ligament limits eversion and rotation of the talus within the ankle mortise. SEE: illus.

dentate l. Lateral extensions of the

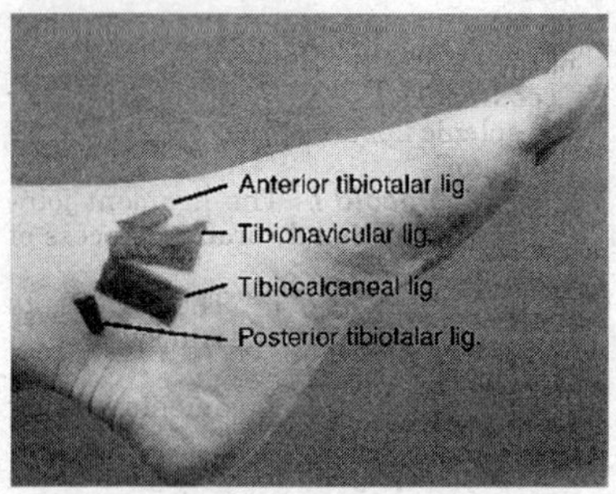

DELTOID LIGAMENTS
Surface anatomy

spinal pia mater between the nerve roots; they fuse with the arachnoid and dura mater, and hold the spinal cord in place in the dural sheath. They have a scalloped appearance as they pierce the arachnoid to attach to the dura mater at regular intervals.

dentoalveolar l. Periodontal l.

falciform l. of liver A wide, sickle-shaped fold of peritoneum attached to the lower surface of the diaphragm, internal surface of the right rectus abdominis muscle, and convex surface of the liver.

fundiform l. of penis The ligament extending from the lower portion of the linea alba and Scarpa's fascia to the dorsum of the penis.

gastrophrenic l. A fold of peritoneum between the esophageal end of the stomach and the diaphragm.

Gimbernat's l. SEE: *Gimbernat's ligament.*

gingivodental l. The part of the periodontal ligament that extends into the gingiva and blends with the connective tissue lamina propria.

glenohumeral l. One of the fibers of the coracohumeral ligament passing into the joint and inserted into the inner and upper part of the bicipital groove.

glenoid l. The ligament that extends between the palmar surfaces of phalanges and the corresponding metacarpal bone.

glossoepiglottidean l. The elastic band from the base of the tongue to the epiglottis in the middle glossoepiglottidean fold.

Henle's l. The lateral extension of the tendinous insertion of the rectus abdominis muscle. It is posterior to the falx inguinalis.

hepaticoduodenal l. A fold of peritoneum from the transverse fissure of the liver to the vicinity of the duodenum and right flexure of colon, forming the anterior boundary of the epiploic foramen.

iliofemoral l. The bundle of fibers forming the upper and anterior portion of the capsular ligament of the hip joint. This ligament extends from the ilium to the intertrochanteric line. SYN: *Y ligament.*

iliolumbar l. The ligament extending from the fourth and fifth lumbar vertebrae to the iliac crest.

iliopectineal l. A portion of the pelvic fascia attached to the iliopectineal line and to the capsular ligament of the hip joint.

infundibulopelvic l. Suspensory l. of ovary.

inguinal l. The ligament extending from the anterior superior iliac spine to the pubic tubercle. It forms the lower margin of aponeurosis of the exterior oblique muscle. SYN: *crural l.; Poupart's l.*

interclavicular l. The bundle of fibers between the sternal ends of the clavicles, attached to the interclavicular notch of the sternum.

interspinal l. The ligament extending from the superior margin of a spinous process of one vertebra to the lower margin of the one above.

ischiocapsular l. In the hip, the ligament extending from the ischium to the ischial border of the acetabulum.

lacunar l. SEE: *Gimbernat's ligament.*

lateral occipitoatlantal l. The ligament on each side between the transverse processes of the atlas and the jugular process of the occipital bone.

lateral odontoid l. One of the ligaments extending between the sides of the odontoid process of the axis of the spinal column and the inner sides of condyles of the occipital bone.

lateral l. of liver Folds of peritoneum extending from the lower surface of the diaphragm to adjacent borders of the right and left lobes of the liver. SYN: *triangular l. of liver.*

lateral umbilical l. The fibrous cord extending from the bladder to the umbilicus. It represents the obliterated interior iliac artery of the fetus.

Lisfranc's l. SEE: *Lisfranc's ligament.*

Lockwood's l. SEE: *Lockwood's ligament.*

Mackenrodt's l. SEE: *Mackenrodt's ligament.*

medial l. A broad ligament that connects the medial malleolus of the tibia to the tarsal bones.

median umbilical l. The fibrous cord extending from the apex of the bladder to the umbilicus. It represents the remains of the urachus of the fetus.

meniscofemoral l. Two small ligaments of the knee, one anterior and one posterior. The anterior one attaches to the posterior area of the lateral meniscus and the anterior cruciate ligament. The posterior one attaches to the posterior area of the lateral meniscus and the medial condyle of the femur.

middle costotransverse l. A ligament consisting of parallel fibers extending between a vertebra and its adjacent rib.

nephrocolic l. Fibrous strands that connect the kidneys with the ascending and descending colon.

nuchal l. The upward continuation of the supraspinous ligament, extending from the seventh cervical vertebra to the occipital bone.

palpebral l. Two ligaments, medial and lateral, extending from tarsal plates of the eyelids to the frontal process of the maxilla and the zygomatic bone respectively.

patellar l. A strong, flat band securing the patella to the tibia. It is a continuation of the tendon of the quadriceps femoris muscle.

pectineal l. A triangular-shaped ligament that extends from the medial end of the inguinal ligament and the pectineal line of the pubis.

periodontal l. ABBR: PDL. The connective tissue attached to the cementum on the outer surface of a dental root and the osseous tissue of the alveolar process. The periodontal ligament holds the teeth in the sockets of the bone. SYN: *dentoalveolar l.; alveolar periosteum.*

Petit's l. SEE: *Petit's ligament.*

phrenicocolic l. A fold of peritoneum joining the left colic flexure of the colon to the adjacent costal portion of the diaphragm.

popliteal arcuate l. The ligament on the posterolateral side of the knee, extending from the head of the fibula to the joint capsule.

posterior talofibular l. ABBR: PTL. A ligament of the lateral ankle that attaches the posterior portion of the talus, and a portion of the posterolateral calcaneus, to the medial malleolus. The posterior talofibular ligament limits the excessive dorsiflexion and inversion of the talus within the ankle mortise.

posterior tibiofibular l. A broad ligament that binds the fibula to the tibia; located on the posterior half of the distal fibula, superior to the lateral malleolus. The posterior tibiofibular ligament is part of the distal ankle syndesmosis. SEE: *anterior tibiofibular l.; crural interosseous l.*

posterior tibiotalar l. Ligament of the ankle that connects the posteromedial portion of the talus to the posterior portion of the medial malleolus, preventing posterior displacement of the talus within the mortise, esp. when the ankle is dorsiflexed. The anterior tibiotalar ligament is categorized as part of the ankle's deltoid ligament complex. SEE: *deltoid l.*

Poupart's l. Inguinal l.

pterygomandibular l. The ligament between the apex of the internal pterygoid plate of the sphenoid bone and the posterior extremity of the internal oblique line of the mandible.

pubic arcuate l. The ligaments connecting the pubic bones at the symphysis pubis, including anterior and superior pubic ligaments and the arcuate (inferior) ligament.

pulmonary l. A fold of pleura that extends from the hilus of the lung to the base of the medial surface of the lung.

rhomboid l. of clavicle A ligament extending from the tuberosity of the clavicle to the outer surface of the cartilage of the first rib.

round l. of femur The ligament of the head of the femur that is attached to the anterior superior part of the fovea of the head of the femur and to the sides of the acetabular notch.

round l. of liver A fibrous cord extending upward from the umbilicus and enclosed in lower margin of the falciform ligament; represents obliterated left umbilical vein of the fetus.

round l. of uterus The pair of ligaments attached to the uterus immediately below and in front of the entrance of the fallopian tubes. Each extends laterally in the broad ligament to the pelvic wall, where it passes through the inguinal ring, terminating in the labium majora.

sacroiliac l. Two ligaments, the anterior and posterior, that connect sacrum and ilium.

sacrospinous l. The ligament extending from the spine of the ischium to the sacrum and coccyx in front of the sacrotuberous ligament.

sacrotuberous l. The ligament extending from the tuberosity of the ischium to the posterior superior and inferior iliac spines and to the lower part of the sacrum and coccyx.

sphenomandibular l. The ligament attached superiorly to the spine of the sphenoid and inferiorly to the lingula of the mandible.

spiral l. of cochlea The thickened periosteum of the peripheral wall of the osseous cochlear canal. The basilar membrane is attached to its inner surface.

stylohyoid l. A thin fibroelastic cord between the lesser cornu of the hyoid bone and the apex of the styloid process of the temporal bone.

stylomandibular l. A thin fibrous band of tissue extending between the styloid process of the temporal bone and the lower part of the posterior border of the ramus of the mandible. SYN: *stylomaxillary l.*

stylomaxillary l. Stylomandibular l.

suprascapular l. A thin fibrous band

of tissue extending from the base of the coracoid process of the scapula to the inner margin of the suprascapular notch.

supraspinal l. A ligament uniting the apices of the spinous processes of the vertebrae.

suspensory l. A ligament suspending an organ.

suspensory l. of axilla The continuation of the clavipectoral fascia down to attach to the axillary fascia.

suspensory l. of lens The zonula ciliaris (ciliary zonule); the fibers holding the crystalline lens in position.

suspensory l. of ovary A ligament extending from the tubal end of the ovary laterally to the pelvic wall. It lies in the layers of the broad ligament in which the ovarian artery is found. SYN: *infundibulopelvic l.*

suspensory l. of penis A triangular bundle of fibrous tissue extending from the anterior surface of the symphysis pubis and adjacent structures to the dorsum of the base of the penis.

suspensory l. of uterus The broad ligaments, the round ligaments, and the rectouterine folds of the uterus.

sutural l. Thin, fibrous layers interposed between articulating surfaces of bones united by suture.

temporomandibular l. The thickened portion of the joint capsule that passes from the articular tubercle at the root of the zygomatic arch to attach to the subcondylar neck of the mandible.

tendinotrochanteric l. A ligament that forms a part of the capsule of the hip joint.

transverse crural l. The ligament lying on the anterior surface of the leg just above the ankle.

transverse humeral l. A fibrous band that bridges the bicipital groove of the humerus in connecting the lesser and greater tuberosities.

transverse l. of atlas A ligament passing over the odontoid process of the axis.

transverse l. of hip joint A ligamentous band extending across the cotyloid notch of the acetabulum.

transverse l. of knee joint A fibrous band extending from the anterior margin of the external semilunar fibrocartilage of the knee to the extremity of the internal semilunar fibrocartilage.

trapezoid l. The anterior exterior portion of the coracoclavicular ligament.

triangular l. of liver Lateral l. of liver.

uterorectosacral l. One of the ligaments that arise from the sides of the cervix and pass upward and backward, passing around the rectum, to the second sacral vertebra. They are enclosed within the rectouterine folds, which demarcate the borders of the rectouterine pouch.

uterosacral l. SEE: *Petit's ligament.*

venous l. of liver A solid fibrous cord representing the obliterated ductus venosus of the fetus. It lies between the caudate and left lobes of the liver and connects the left branch of the portal vein to the inferior vena cava.

ventricular l. of larynx The lateral free margin of the quadrangular membrane. It is enclosed within and supports the ventricular fold.

vesicouterine l. The ligament that attaches the anterior aspect of the uterus to the bladder.

vestibular l. A thin fibrous band attached anteriorly to the lamina of the thyroid cartilage and posteriorly to the anterior portion of the arytenoid cartilage.

vocal l. The thickened free edges of the elastic cone extending from the thyroid angle to the vocal processes of arytenoid cartilages. They support the vocal folds.

Weitbrecht's l. SEE: *Weitbrecht's ligament.*

yellow l. One of the ligaments connecting the laminae of adjacent vertebrae.

ligamenta Pl. of ligamentum.

ligamentopexis (lĭg″ă-mĕn″tō-pĕks′ĭs) [L. *ligamentum,* band, + Gr. *pexis,* fixation] Suspension of the uterus on the round ligament.

ligamentous (lĭg″ă-mĕn′tŭs) [L. *ligamentum,* band] **1.** Relating to a ligament. **2.** Like a ligament.

ligamentum (lĭg″ă-mĕn′tŭm) *pl.* **ligamenta** [L., a band] Ligament.

ligand (lī′gănd, lĭg′ănd) [L. *ligare,* to bind] **1.** In chemistry, an organic molecule attached to a central metal ion by multiple bonds. **2.** In immunology, a small molecule bound to another chemical group or molecule.

ligase (lī′gās, lĭg′ās) The general term for a class of enzymes that catalyze the joining of the ends of two chains of DNA.

ligate (lī′gāt) To apply a ligature.

ligation (lī-gā′shŭn) The application of a ligature.

rubber-band l. The application of a rubber band around a superficial bit of tissue, such as a hemorrhoid or an esophageal varix. Because its blood supply is thereby cut off, the tissue dies and sloughs off.

ligature (lĭg′ă-chūr) [L. *ligatura,* a binding] **1.** Process of binding or tying. **2.** A band or bandage. **3.** A thread or wire for tying a blood vessel or other structure in order to constrict or fasten it. The cord or material used may be catgut, synthetic suture materials such as nylon or Dacron, polyglycolic acid, or natural fibers such as silk or cotton. Sometimes strips of fascia obtained from the patient are used as a ligature. SEE: *suture.*

light (līt) [AS. *lihtan,* to shine] The sensation produced by electromagnetic radiation that falls on the retina. Radiant energy producing a sensation of luminosity on the retina is limited to a wavelength of about 400 nm (extreme violet) to 770 nm (extreme red). SEE: *laser; ray; seasonal affective disorder*.

l. adaptation Changes that occur in a dark-adapted eye in order for vision to occur in moderate or bright light. Principal changes are contraction of the pupil and breakdown of rhodopsin. Bright sunlight is 30,000 times the intensity of bright moonlight, but the eye adapts so that visual function is possible under both conditions. SEE: *night vision; vision*.

axial l. Light with rays parallel to each other and to the optic axis.

cold l. Any form of light that is not perceptibly warm. The heat of ordinary light rays is dissipated when they are passed through some medium such as quartz.

l. difference The difference between the two eyes with respect to sensitivity to light intensity.

diffused l. Rays broken by refraction.

idioretinal l. The sensation of light when there are no retinal stimuli to produce that sensation. SYN: *intrinsic l.*

intrinsic l. Idioretinal l.

oblique l. Light that strikes a surface obliquely.

polarized l. Light in which waves vibrate in one direction only.

reflected l. Light rays that are thrown back by an illuminated object such as a mirror.

refracted l. Rays bent from their original course.

l. sense One of the three parts of visual function, the other parts being color sense and form sense. It is tested by visual field examination. SEE: *color sense; form sense*.

l. therapy Phototherapy.

transmitted l. Light that passes through an object.

white l. Light that contains all of the visible wavelengths of light.

Wood's l. SEE: *Wood's rays*.

lightening [AS. *leohte,* not heavy] The descent of the presenting part of the fetus into the pelvis. This often occurs 2 to 3 weeks before the first stage of labor begins. It may not occur in multiparas until active labor begins. SYN: *engagement*. SEE: *labor*.

light-headedness The feeling of dizziness or of being about to faint; a nonspecific symptom of many conditions, including for example, anemia, anxiety, cardiac rhythm disturbances, fever, low blood pressure, many infections, and some drugs. SEE: *vertigo, benign positional*.

lightning The discharge of atmospheric electricity from cloud to cloud or from cloud to earth. About 100 lightning strokes hit the earth every second. In the U.S. each year, about 500 to 1000 persons are struck by lightning; 100 of these persons die as a result of being struck. SEE: *lightning safety rules*.

lightning safety rules Rules that, if followed, could reduce the estimated 100 deaths that occur annually in the U.S. from electrocution due to lightning. During a lightning storm one should remain indoors, but should not stay near open doors, fireplaces, radiators, or appliances. Plug-in electric equipment such as hair dryers, electric toothbrushes, or electric razors should not be used. One should not take laundry off clotheslines or work on fences, computers or word processors, telephones or telephone lines, power lines, pipelines, or structural steel construction, or use metal objects such as fishing rods or golf clubs. When outdoors if lightning is spotted nearby, one should plan an evacuation to a safe, substantial building or an enclosed metal vehicle. Hilltops should be avoided. In a forest, shelter should be sought in a low area under a thick growth of small trees. Open spaces, wire fences, metal clotheslines, exposed sheds, and all electrically conductive elevated objects should be avoided. Persons should get out of water and off small boats, but stay in an automobile if driving. If an electrical charge is evidenced by hair standing on end or tingling of the skin, one should immediately squat with feet touching each other and hands clasped around the knees. No part of the rest of the body should touch the ground. It is important to be aware that when lightning strikes, the charge may be as much as 100 million volts. Trees conduct electricity better than air, and metal and water conduct better than trees. Lightning will strike the tallest object.

lignan (lĭg′năn) A steroid-like chemical found in flaxseed and related plants that may be beneficial in the management of hormone-sensitive illnesses. SEE: *phytoestrogen*.

lignin (lĭg′nĭn) A polymer present in plants that combines with cellulose to form the cell walls.

lignocaine (lĭg′nō-kān) The British word for "lidocaine."

lignoceric acid A saturated, naturally occurring fatty acid, $C_{24}H_{48}O_2$, present in certain foods, including peanuts.

limb (lĭm) [AS. *lim*] **1.** An arm or leg. **2.** An extremity. **3.** A limblike extension of a structure.

anacrotic l. The ascending portion of the pulse wave.

anterior l. of internal capsule The lenticulocaudate portion that lies between the lenticular and caudate nuclei.

ascending l. of renal tubule The portion of the tubule between the bend in

Henle's loop and the distal convoluted section.

catacrotic l. The descending portion of the pulse wave.

descending l. of renal tubule The portion of the tubule between the proximal convoluted section and the bend in Henle's loop.

pectoral l. The arm.

pelvic l. The lower extremity.

phantom l. SEE: *sensation, phantom.*

l. replantation The surgical reattachment of a traumatically amputated limb or part.

thoracic l. The upper extremity.

limbic (lĭm′bĭk) [L. *limbus,* border] Pert. to a limbus or border. SYN: *marginal.*

l. system A group of brain structures, including the hippocampus, amygdala, dentate gyrus, cingulate gyrus, gyrus fornicatus, the archicortex, and their interconnections and connections with the hypothalamus, septal area, and a medial area of the mesencephalic tegmentum. The system is activated by motivated behavior and arousal, and it influences the endocrine and autonomic motor systems. SEE: illus.

limbus (lĭm′bŭs) *pl.* **limbi** [L., border] The edge or border of a part.

l. alveolaris **1.** The upper free edge of the alveolar process of the mandible. **2.** The lower free edge of the alveolar process of the maxilla. SYN: *arcus alveolaris maxillae.*

l. conjunctivae The edge of the conjunctiva overlapping the cornea.

l. corneae The edge of the cornea where it unites with the sclera.

corneoscleral l. In the eye, a transitional dome 1 or 2 mm wide where the cornea joins the sclera and conjunctiva.

l. fossae ovalis The thickened margin of the fossae ovalis, esp. the rim of the septum secundum bounding the fossa.

l. laminae spiralis osseae A thickening of the periosteum of the osseous spiral lamina of the cochlea to which the tectorial membrane is attached.

l. palpebrales anteriores The anterior margin of the free edge of the eyelids from which the cilia or eyelashes grow.

l. palpebrales posteriores The posterior margin of the free edge of the eyelids; the region of transition of skin to conjunctival mucous membrane.

l. sphenoidalis Ridge on the anterior portion of upper surface of sphenoid bone.

lime (līm) [AS. *lim,* glue] Calcium oxide, CaO. A substance obtained from limestone. Calcium oxide is prepared from limestone, $CaCO_3$, by heating it sufficiently to drive off the carbon dioxide. When lime is mixed with water, heat is produced. Lime is an ingredient of cement and mortar. SYN: *calcium oxide; quicklime.* SEE: *calcium.*

CAUTION: Lime should not come into contact with one's eyes or be inhaled.

chlorinated l. A substance resulting from chlorination of slaked lime, consisting chiefly of calcium chloride and

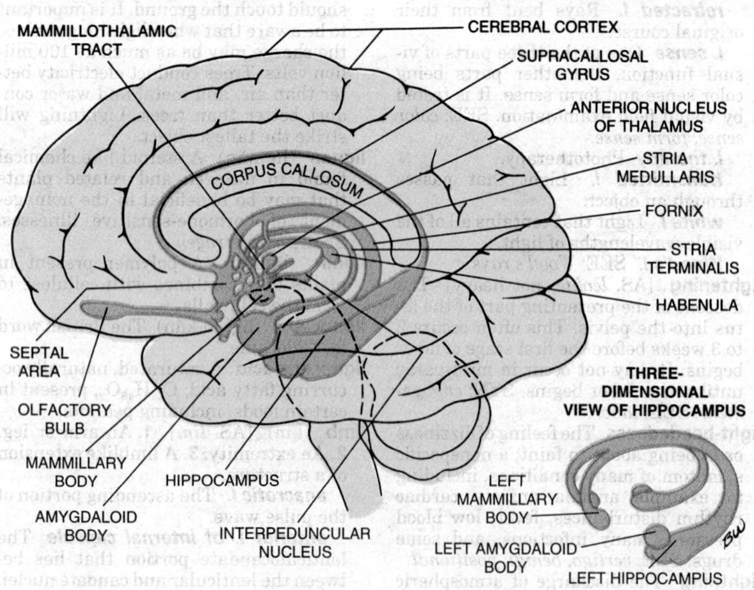

THE LIMBIC SYSTEM OF THE BRAIN

calcium hypochlorite. It is used principally as a disinfectant and in aqueous solution as a bleaching agent.

slaked l. The substance produced when lime is allowed free access to water and carbon dioxide from the atmosphere. It is a mixture of calcium hydroxide, $Ca(OH)_2$, and calcium carbonate, $CaCO_3$.

soda l. A combination of calcium oxide and sodium hydroxide.

sulfurated l. A solution of lime, sublimated sulfur, and water, used as a topical solution in treating skin disease.

l. water Alkaline solution of calcium hydroxide, $Ca(OH)_2$, in water; a weak base formerly used as an antacid.

lime [Fr.] The fruit of *Citrus aurantifolia,* which contains vitamin C.

limen (lī′mĕn) *pl.* **limina** [L.] Entrance; threshold.

l. nasi The boundary line between the bony and cartilaginous portion of the nasal cavity. It is also at this point that the nasal cavity proper and the vestibule of the nose meet.

l. of insula The portion of the cortex of the brain that provides a threshold to the insula. The middle cerebral artery passes over this threshold to extend to the insula.

limes nul SYMB: L_0. The greatest amount of toxin that, when mixed with 1 unit of antitoxin and injected into a guinea pig weighing 250 g, will cause no local reaction.

limes tod SYMB: L_+. The least amount of toxin that, when mixed with 1 unit of antitoxin and injected into a guinea pig weighing 250 g, will kill it within 96 hr.

limestone A rock formed of organic fossil remains of shells, composed mostly of calcium carbonate. SEE: *lime*.

liminal (lĭm′ĭ-năl) [L. *limen,* threshold] Hardly perceptible; relating to a threshold as of consciousness or vision.

limit (lĭm′ĭt) **1.** A boundary. **2.** A point or line beyond which something cannot or may not progress.

acceptance l. In radiology, the range of images within the diagnostic range of quality (i.e., density, contrast, detail).

assimilation l. The amount of carbohydrate that can be absorbed or ingested without causing glycosuria.

audibility l. The limits of sound frequencies at both the low and high ends of the sound scale beyond which sound cannot be heard by humans. The lower limit is approx. 8 to 16 Hz (cycles per second) and the upper limit between 12,000 and 20,000 Hz, depending on various factors, including age. In general, the upper limit of audible sound decreases with age.

l. of detection The smallest amount of an analyte that can be detected by an analytical system.

elastic l. The extent to which something may be stretched or bent and still be able to retain its original shape.

l. of flocculation The amount of a toxin or toxoid that causes the most rapid flocculation when combined with its antitoxin.

Hayflick's l. SEE: *Hayflick's limit.*

l. of perception The smallest object that can be detected by the eye. Such an object usually subtends a visual image of 1 minute. This produces a retinal image slightly larger than the diameter of a retinal cone (i.e., about 0.004 mm). Also called *normal limit of visual acuity.*

l. of quantitation ABBR: LOQ. The smallest amount of analyte that can be measured with stated and acceptable imprecision and inaccuracy. SEE: *l. of detection; sensitivity*.

quantum l. The minimum wavelength present in the spectrum produced by x-rays.

ventilator l. A secondary ventilator alarm or stop mechanism that prevents a specific variable from exceeding a preset parameter.

limitans (lĭm′ĭ-tăns) [L. *limitare,* to limit] **1.** A term used in conjunction with other words to denote limiting. **2.** Membrane limitans.

limitation (lĭm″ĭ-tā′shŭn) The condition of being limited.

activity l. Functional limitation.

functional l. In rehabilitation science, any restriction in the performance of activities resulting from disease, injury, or environmental restrictions. SYN: *activity l.; disability.*

l. of motion The restriction of movement or range of motion of a part or joint, esp. that imposed by disease or trauma to joints and soft tissues.

limnology [Gr. *limne,* pool, + *logos,* study] The scientific study of fresh water in the environment (i.e., potability, pH, degree of pollution, mineral content, and variation with seasonal and climatic changes).

limonene (lĭm′ō-nēn) An essential oil derived from orange or lemon peel. It is used as a flavoring agent in cough syrups.

limp To walk with abnormal, jerky movements.

lincomycin hydrochloride (lĭn″kō-mī′sĭn) An antibiotic obtained from *Streptomyces lincolnensis.*

lincture, linctus (lĭnk′tūr, -tŭs) [L. *linctus,* a licking] A thick, sweet, syrupy medicinal preparation given for its effect on the throat, usually sipped but may be licked or sucked as with a throat lozenge.

lindane (lĭn′dān) SYN: *gamma benzene hexachloride*.

Lindau's disease (lĭn′dowz) [Arvid Lindau, Swedish pathologist, 1892–1958] Lindau–von Hippel disease.

Lindau–von Hippel disease (lĭn′dow-vŏn-hĭp′ĕl) [Arvid Lindau; Eugen von Hippel, Ger. ophthalmologist, 1867–1939] Angiomata of the retina and cysts and angiomata of the brain and certain visceral organs.

line (līn) [L. *linea*] **1.** Any long, relatively narrow mark. **2.** A boundary or outline. **3.** A wrinkle. **4.** In anthropometry or cephalometry, an imaginary line connecting two anatomical points. This is necessary to establish a plane or an axis. **5.** A catheter attached to a patient, as an intravenous line or arterial line.

abdominal l. A line indicating abdominal muscle boundaries.

absorption l. A black line in the continuous spectrum of light passing through an absorbing medium.

alveolobasilar l. The line from basion to alveolar point.

alveolonasal l. The line from alveolar point to nasion.

auriculobregmatic l. The line from auricular point to bregma.

axial l. A line running in the main axis of the body or part of it. The axial line of the hand runs through the middle digit; the axial line of the foot runs through the second digit.

axillary l. Anterior, posterior, and midaxillary lines that extend downward from the axilla.

base l. The line from the infraorbital ridge through the middle of the external auditory meatus to midline of occiput.

basiobregmatic l. The line from basion to bregma.

Baudelocque's l. SEE: *Baudelocque's diameter*.

Beau's l. SEE: *Beau's lines*.

biauricular l. A line over the vertex from one auditory meatus to the other.

blue l. Lead l.

canthomeatal l. An imaginary line extending from the canthus of the eye to the center of the external auditory meatus. SYN: *orbitomeatal line*.

cement l. The refractile boundary of an osteon in compact bone.

cervical l. **1.** A line of junction of cementum and enamel of a tooth. **2.** A line on the neck of the tooth where the gum is attached.

cleavage l. Langer's lines.

costoarticular l. The line from sternoclavicular joint to a point on the 11th rib.

costoclavicular l. The line midway between the nipple and the sternum border.

l. of demarcation A line of division between healthy and diseased tissue.

Douglas' l. A crescent-shaped line at the lower limit of the posterior sheath of the rectus abdominis muscle. It is sometimes indistinct.

epiphyseal l. A line at the junction of the epiphysis and diaphysis of a long bone. It is at this junction that bone growth occurs. SYN: *epiphyseal disk*.

Feiss' l. SEE: *Feiss' line*.

l. of fixation An imaginary line drawn from the subject viewed to the fovea centralis.

gingival l. A line determined by the extent of coverage of the tooth by gingiva. The shape of the gingival line is similar to the curvature of the cervical line but they rarely coincide. It is also called the free gingival margin.

glabelloalveolar l. An imaginary line through the glabella on the frontal bone and the alveolar process of the maxilla.

glabellomeatal l. An imaginary line that extends from the glabella to the center of the external auditory meatus and is used for radiographical positioning of the skull.

gluteal l. Three lines—anterior, posterior, and inferior—on the exterior surface of the ilium.

gum l. Gingival l.

iliopectineal l. The bony ridge marking the brim of the pelvis.

incremental l. One of the lines seen in a microscopic section of tooth enamel. They resemble growth lines in a tree.

incremental l. of Retzius Periodic dark lines seen in the enamel of a tooth that represent occasional metabolic disturbances of mineralization.

incremental l. of von Ebner Very light lines in the dentin of a tooth that represent the boundary between the layers of dentin produced daily.

inferior nuchal l. One of two curved ridges on the occipital bone extending laterally from the exterior occipital crest. SEE: *superior nuchal l.*

infraorbitomeatal l. An imaginary line from the inferior orbital margin to the external auditory meatus, used for radiographical positioning of the skull.

interauricular l. A line joining the two auricular points.

intercondylar l. The transverse ridge joining condyles of the femur above the intercondyloid fossa.

intermediate l. of ilium The ridge on the crest of the ilium between the inner and outer lips.

interpupillary l. An imaginary line between the centers of the eyes, used for radiographical positioning of the skull.

intertrochanteric l. The ridge on the posterior surface of the femur exterior between the greater and lesser trochanters.

intertuberal l. The line joining the inner borders of the ischial tuberosities below the small sciatic notch.

Langer's l. SEE: *Langer's lines*.

lateral supracondylar l. One of two ridges on the posterior surface of the distal end of the femur, formed by diverging lips of the linea aspera. SEE: *medial supracondylar l.*

lead l. An irregular dark line in the gingival margin. The line is present in chronic lead poisoning and is caused by the deposition of lead in that portion of the gum. SYN: *blue l.*

lip l. The highest or lowest point the lips reach on the teeth or gums during a broad smile.

M l. In striated muscle, the thin, dark line in the center of an H band of a sarcomere. It contains the protein that connects the thick (myosin) filaments. SYN: *M disk.*

mamillary l. An imaginary vertical line through the center of the nipple.

mammary l. An imaginary horizontal line from one nipple to the other.

medial supracondylar l. One of two ridges on the posterior surface of the distal end of the femur, formed by diverging lips of the linea aspera. SEE: *lateral supracondylar l.*

median l. An imaginary line joining any two points in the periphery of the median plane of the body or one of its parts.

mentomeatal l. An imaginary line from the mental point of the mandible to the external auditory meatus, used in radiography of the skull.

milk l. SEE: *ridge, mammary.*

mucogingival l. SEE: *junction, mucogingival.*

mylohyoid l. A ridge on the inner surface of the mandible. It extends from a point beneath the mental spine upward and back to the ramus past the last molar. The mylohyoid muscle and the superior constrictor muscle of the pharynx attach to this ridge.

nasobasilar l. A line through the basion and nasion.

oblique l. of fibula The medial crest of posteromedial border; a line extending from the medial side of the head and terminating distally at the interosseous crest.

oblique l. of mandible The ridge on the outer surface of the lower jaw.

oblique l. of radius The faint ridge on the anterior surface passing downward and laterally from the radial tuberosity.

orbitomeatal l. The imaginary line running through the mid-orbit and external auditory meatus.

l. of Owen [Sir Richard Owen, Brit. anatomist, 1804–1892] Occasional prominent growth lines or bands in the dentin of a tooth. They provide a record of the growth of the coronal or radicular dentin.

parasternal l. The line midway between the nipple and the border of the sternum.

pectineal l. The line on the posterior surface of the femur extending downward from the lesser trochanter. It is the portion of the iliopectineal line formed by the os pubis.

popliteal l. of femur An oblique line on the posterior surface of the femur.

popliteal l. of tibia A line on the posterior surface of the tibia, extending obliquely downward from the fibular facet on the lateral condyle to the medial border of the bone.

resting l. A smooth cement line seen in microscopic sections that separates old bone from newly formed bone.

reversal l. A cement line seen in microscopic sections of bone that shows scallops and irregularites representing earlier bone resorption. Resorption to that point occurred before the process reversed and new bone was formed by apposition. SEE: *Howship's lacuna.*

scapular l. The line extending downward from the lower angle of the scapula.

semilunar l. Spigelian line.

Shenton's l. SEE: *Shenton's line.*

sight l. The line from the center of the pupil to a viewed object.

spigelian l. SEE: *spigelian line.*

sternal l. The medial line of the sternum.

sternomastoid l. The line from between the heads of the sternomastoid muscle to the mastoid process.

superior nuchal l. One of two curved ridges on the occipital bone extending laterally from the exterior occipital crest. SEE: *inferior nuchal l.*

supraorbital l. The line across the forehead above the root of the exterior angular process of the frontal bone.

temporal l. of frontal bone Two curved lines on the lateral surface of the skull, passing upward and backward from the zygomatic process of the frontal bone and terminating posteriorly at the supramastoid crest.

umbilicopubic l. The portion of median line extending from the umbilicus to the symphysis pubis.

visual l. The line that extends from object to macula lutea passing through the nodal point. SYN: *visual axis.*

Z l. In striated muscle, the end boundary of a sarcomere to which the thin filaments (actin) are directly attached. SYN: *Z disk.*

Zöllner's l. Parallel lines, usually three long ones, with a series of short lines drawn at regular intervals across one of the lines at approx. 60 degrees. Similar lines are drawn across the second line at the angle of approx. 120 degrees. Short lines are drawn across the third at the same angle as on the first lines. These lines produce the optical illusion that the long lines are converging or diverging.

linea (lĭn′ē-ă) *pl.* **lineae** [L. *linea,* line] An anatomical line.

l. alba The white line of connective tissue in the middle of the abdomen from sternum to pubis.

l. albicantes Lines seen on the abdomen, buttocks, and breasts, frequently caused by pregnancy, obesity, or prolonged adrenal cortical hormone therapy but may occur as the result of abdominal distention from any cause.

l. aspera A longitudinal ridge on the posterior surface of the middle third of the femur.

l. costoarticularis A line between the sternoclavicular articulation and the point of the 11th rib.

l. nigra A dark line or discoloration of the abdomen that may be seen in pregnant women during the latter part of term. It runs from above the umbilicus to the pubes.

l. semilunaris Spigelian line.

l. splendens A thickening of the pia mater extending along the anterior median surface of the spinal cord.

l. sternalis The median line of the sternum.

l. striae atrophicae Stria atrophica.

l. terminalis A bony ridge on the inner surface of the ilium continued on to the pubis that divides the true and false pelvis.

l. transversae ossis sacri Ridges formed by lines of union of the five sacral vertebrae.

linear (lĭn′ē-ăr) [L. *linea,* line] Pert. to or resembling a line.

l. energy transfer A measure of the rate of energy transfer from ionizing radiation to soft tissue.

linearity In radiography, the production of a constant amount of radiation for different combinations of milliamperage and exposure time, commonly used as a quality management benchmark.

line pairs per millimeter ABBR: lp/mm. A measurement of fine radiographic image detail.

liner (līn′ĕr) Anything applied to the inside of a hollow body or structure.

cavity l. A layer of material applied to a cavity preparation to protect the pulp of the tooth. It is usually a suspension of zinc phosphate or calcium hydroxide and is used to neutralize the acidity of the base or cement material.

soft l. The material applied to the underside of a denture to provide a soft surface contact with the oral tissues. Some acrylic or silicone resins have been made resilient and are used as liners.

lingua (lĭng′gwă) *pl.* **linguae** [L.] The tongue or a tonguelike structure.

l. frenata Ankyloglossia.

l. geographica Geographic tongue.

l. nigra Hairy tongue.

l. plicata Fissured tongue.

lingual (lĭng′gwăl) [L. *lingua,* tongue] **1.** Pert. to the tongue. **2.** Tongue-shaped. SYN: *linguiform.* **3.** In dentistry, pert. to the tooth surface that is adjacent to the tongue.

linguiform (lĭng′gwĭ-form) [″ + *forma,* shape] Tongue-shaped. SYN: *lingual* (2).

lingula (lĭng′gū-lă) [L., little tongue] A tongue-shaped process, esp. lingula cerebelli.

l. cerebelli A tonguelike process of the cerebellum projected forward on the upper surface of the superior medullary velum.

l. of lung The projection of lung that separates the cardiac notch from the inferior margin of the left lung.

l. of mandible The projection of bone that forms the medial boundary of the mandibular foramen and gives attachment to the sphenomandibular ligament.

l. of sphenoid The ridge between the body and the greater wings of the sphenoid.

lingulectomy (lĭng″gū-lĕk′tō-mē) [L. *lingula,* little tongue, + Gr. *ektome,* excision] Surgical removal of the lingula of the upper lobe of the left lung.

linguo- [L. *lingua,* tongue] Combining form meaning *tongue.*

linguoclination (lĭng′gwō-klī-nā′shŭn) [″ + *clinatus,* leaning] Angulation of a tooth in its vertical axis toward the tongue.

linguodental Relating to the tongue and teeth, such as the speech sound “th,” which is produced with the aid of the tongue and teeth.

linguodistal (lĭng″gwō-dĭs′tăl) [″ + *distare,* to be distant] Concerning the distal part of a tooth and the tongue.

linguogingival (lĭng″gwō-jĭn′jĭ-văl) [″ + *gingiva,* gum] Concerning the tongue and the gingiva, or pert. to the lingual and gingival walls of a cavity preparation.

linguomesial Pert. to the lingual and mesial surfaces of a tooth or the lingual and mesial walls of a cavity preparation.

linguo-occlusal (lĭng″gwō-ŏ-kloo′zăl) [″ + *occludere,* to shut up] Concerning or bounded by the lingual and occlusal surfaces of a tooth.

linguopapillitis (lĭng″gwō-păp″ĭ-lī′tĭs) [″ + *papilla,* nipple, + Gr. *itis,* inflammation] Small ulcers of the papillae of the edge of the tongue.

linguopulpal Pert. to the lingual and pulpal surfaces of a cavity preparation.

linguoversion (lĭng″gwō-vĕr′zhŭn) [″ + *versio,* a turning] Displacement of a tooth toward the tongue.

liniment [L. *linimentum,* smearing substance] A liquid vehicle (usually water, oil, or alcohol) containing a medication to be rubbed on or applied to the skin. It may be applied by the friction method or on a bandage.

camphor l. A preparation of camphor and a suitable vehicle, such as an oil, that is used topically as an irritant.

medicinal soft soap l. A tincture of green soap.

linimentum (lĭn-ĭ-mĕn′tŭm) [L.] Liniment.

linitis (lĭn-ī′tĭs) [Gr. *linon,* flax, + *itis,* inflammation] Inflammation of the lining of the stomach.

l. plastica An infiltrating cancer of the stomach wall. SYN: *leather-bottle stomach.*

linkage In genetics, the association between distinct genes that occupy closely situated loci on the same chromosome. This results in an association in the inheritance of these genes.

sex l. A genetic characteristic that is located on the X or Y chromosome.

linseed [AS. *linsaed*] Seed of the common flax, *Linum usitatissimum;* the source of linseed oil. Linseed is used as a demulcent and emollient. SYN: *flaxseed.*

lint (lĭnt) [L. *linteum,* made of linen] **1.** Linen scraped until soft and wooly for dressing wounds. **2.** Cotton fiber. **3.** Household dust.

lintin (lĭn′tĭn) Prepared absorbent cotton; fabric used in dressings.

liothyronine sodium (lī″ō-thī′rō-nēn) ABBR: T_3. Sodium salt of triiodothyronine; used in treating hypothyroidism. SEE: *thyroid function test.*

lip- SEE: *lipo-.*

lip [AS. *lippa*] **1.** A soft external structure that forms the boundary of the mouth or opening to the oral cavity. SYN: *labium oris.* **2.** One of the lips of the pudendum (labia majora or minora). SEE: *labia; labium.* **3.** A liplike structure forming the border of an opening or groove.

PATHOLOGY: *Chancre:* It is not unusual to have the initial lesion of syphilis appear on the lip of the mouth as an indurated base with a thin secretion and accompanied by enlargement of the submaxillary glands. *Condyloma latum:* This appears as a mucous patch, flattened, coated with gray exudate, with strictly delimited area, usually at the angle of the mouth. *Eczema:* This is characterized by dry fissures, often covered with a crust, bleeding easily, and occurring on both lips. *Epithelioma:* This may be confused with chancre. It seldom appears before the age of 40, but there are exceptions. It may appear as a common cold sore, a painless fissure, or other break of the lower lip. A crust or scab covers the lesion, leaving a raw surface if removed. Pain does not appear until the lesion is well advanced. It is much more common on the lower lip than on the upper. *Herpes:* These lesions may appear on the lips in pneumonia, typhoid, common cold, and other febrile diseases. *Tuberculous ulcer:* This type of ulcer is located at the inner portion of the lip, close to the angle of the mouth. Pathological examination is necessary for verification.

DIAGNOSIS: Examination is considered to be incomplete unless the lips are everted to expose buccal surfaces. *Bluish or purplish:* This sign may appear in the aged, in those exposed to great cold, and in hypoxemia. *Dry:* Mouth dryness may be seen in fevers or be caused by drugs such as atropine, by thirst, or by mouth breathing. *Fissured:* This may occur after exposure to cold, in avitaminosis, and in children with congenital syphilis. *Pale:* Pallor may be seen in anemia and wasting diseases, in prolonged fever, and after a hemorrhage. *Rashes:* These may be manifestations of typhoid fever, meningitis, or pneumonia. Mucous patches may appear in secondary syphilis, chancre, cancer, and epithelioma.

cleft l. A vertical cleft or clefts in the upper lip. This congenital condition, resulting from the faulty fusion of the median nasal process and the lateral maxillary processes, is usually unilateral and on the left side, but may be bilateral. It may involve either the lip or the upper jaw, or both, and often accompanies cleft palate. Nongenetic factors may also be responsible for causing this condition. The incidence of cleft lip is from one in 600 to one in 1250 births. SYN: *harelip.*

double l. A redundant fold of mucous membrane in the mouth on either side of the midline of the lip.

glenoid l. SYN: *glenoid labrum.*

Hapsburg l. A thick, overdeveloped lower lip.

oral l. Upper and lower lips that surround the mouth opening and form the anterior wall of the buccal cavity.

tympanic l. The lower border of the sulcus spiralis internus of the cochlea.

vestibular l. The upper border of the sulcus spiralis internus of the cochlea.

lipacidemia (lĭp″ăs-ĭ-dē′mē-ă) [Gr. *lipos,* fat, + L. *acidus,* acid, + Gr. *haima,* blood] Excess fatty acids in the blood.

lipaciduria (lĭp″ăs-ĭ-dū′rē-ă) [″ + ″ + Gr. *ouron,* urine] Fatty acids in the urine.

liparocele (lĭp′ă-rō-sēl) [″ + *kele,* tumor, swelling] **1.** A scrotal hernia containing fat. **2.** A fatty tumor.

lipase (lī′pās, lĭ′pās) [″ + *-ase,* enzyme] A lipolytic or fat-splitting enzyme found in the blood, pancreatic secretion, and tissues. Emulsified fats of cream and egg yolk are changed in the stomach to fatty acids and glycerol by gastric lipase. SEE: *digestion; enzyme.*

pancreatic l. The pancreatic enzyme that digests emulsified (by bile salts) fats to fatty acids and glycerol.

lipasuria (lĭp″ăs-ū′rē-ă) [″ + ″ + Gr. *ouron,* urine] Lipase in the urine.

lipectomy (lĭ-pĕk′tō-mē) [″ + *ektome,* excision] Excision of fatty tissues.

suction l. SEE: *liposuction.*

lipedema (lĭp″ĕ-dē′mă) [″ + *oidema*, swelling] Swelling of the skin, esp. of the lower extremity, owing to accumulation of fat and fluid subcutaneously.

lipemia (lĭ-pē′mē-ă) [″+ *haima*, blood] An abnormal amount of fat in the blood.

alimentary l. An accumulation of fat in the blood after eating.

l. retinalis A condition in which retinal vessels appear reddish white or white; found in cases of hyperlipidemia. SEE: *hyperlipoproteinemia*.

lipid(e) (lĭp′ĭd, -īd) [Gr. *lipos*, fat] Any one of a group of fats or fatlike substances, characterized by their insolubility in water and solubility in fat solvents such as alcohol, ether, and chloroform. The term is descriptive rather than a chemical name such as protein or carbohydrate. It includes true fats (esters of fatty acids and glycerol); lipoids (phospholipids, cerebrosides, waxes); and sterols (cholesterol, ergosterol). SEE: *fat; lipoprotein*.

lipidemia Lipemia. SEE: *atherosclerosis; cholesterol*.

lipid histiocytosis Niemann-Pick disease.

lipidosis Any disorder of fat metabolism.

arterial l. Arteriosclerosis.

cerebroside l. Gaucher's disease.

lipiduria (lĭp″ĭ-dū′rē-ă) [″+ Gr. *ouron*, urine] Lipids in the urine.

lipo-, lip- [Gr. *lipos*, fat] Combining form meaning *fat*. SEE: *adipo-; steato-*.

lipoarthritis (lĭp″ō-ărth-rī′tĭs) [″+ *arthron*, joint, + *itis*, inflammation] Presence of lipid particles in joint fluid.

lipoatrophia, lipoatrophy (lī″pō-ă-trō′fē-ă, lī″pō-ăt′rō-fē) [″ + *a-*, not, + *trophe*, nourishment] Atrophy of subcutaneous fatty tissue. This may occur, for example, at the site of insulin injection. SEE: *lipodystrophy*.

lipoblast (lĭp′ō-blăst) [″ + *blastos*, germ] An immature fat cell.

lipoblastoma (lĭp″ō-blăs-tō′mă) [″ + ″ + *oma*, tumor] A benign tumor of the fatty tissue. SYN: *lipoma*.

lipocardiac (lĭp″ō-kăr′dē-ăk) [″ + *kardia*, heart] **1.** Pert. to fatty heart degeneration. **2.** One who suffers from fatty degeneration of the heart.

lipocele (lĭp′ō-sēl) [″ + *kele*, tumor, swelling] The presence of fatty tissue in a hernia sac. SYN: *adipocele; liparocele*.

lipochondrodystrophy (lĭp″ō-kŏn″drō-dĭs′trō-fē) [″ + *chondros*, cartilage, + *dys*, bad, + *trephein*, to nourish] Mucopolysaccharidosis IH.

lipochondroma (lĭp″ō-kŏn-drō′mă) [″ + ″ + *oma*, tumor] A tumor that is both fatty and cartilaginous.

lipochrome (lĭp′ō-krōm) [″ + *chroma*, color] Any one of a group of fat-soluble pigments (e.g., carotene, the fat-soluble yellow pigment found in carrots, sweet potatoes, egg yolk, butter, body fat and corpus luteum).

lipocyte (lĭp′ō-sīt) SEE: *cell, fat*.

lipodystrophy (lĭp″ō-dĭs′trō-fē) [″ + *dys*, bad, + *trophe*, nourishment] Disturbance of fat metabolism.

insulin l. A complication of insulin administration characterized by changes in the subcutaneous fat at the site of injection. The changes may take the form of atrophy or hypertrophy; rarely are both types present in the same patient. Atrophy develops in as many as one third of children and women who use insulin regularly, but rarely in men. The defect in subcutaneous fat leaves a saucer-like depression. Hypertrophy at the injection site occurs in the form of a spongy localized area. This complication of insulin administration is slightly more common in males than in females. It is usually associated with a history of repetitive use of one injection site.

intestinal l. A disease characterized principally by fat deposits in intestinal and mesenteric lymphatic tissue, fatty diarrhea, loss of weight and strength, and arthritis.

progressive l. A pathological condition in which there is progressive, symmetrical loss of subcutaneous fat from the upper part of the trunk, face, neck, and arms.

trochanteric l. Excess accumulation of fatty tissue over the thighs, commonly known as saddlebag thighs.

lipofibroma (lĭp″ō-fī-brō′mă) [″ + L. *fibra*, fiber, + Gr. *oma*, tumor] A lipoma having much fibrous tissue. SYN: *fibrolipoma*.

lipofuscin (lĭp″ō-fŭs′sĭn) [″+ L. *fuscus*, brown] An insoluble fatty pigment found in aging cells. It is the residue of cellular or extracellular material that the cells have ingested but not completely digested. SEE: *atrophy, brown; free radical*.

lipofuscinosis (lĭp″ō-fū″sĭn-ō′sĭs) [″ + ″ + Gr. *osis*, condition] Abnormal deposition of lipofuscin in tissues.

lipogenesis (lĭp″ō-jĕn′ĕ-sĭs) [Gr. *lipos*, fat, + *genesis*, generation, birth] Fat formation.

lipogenetic, lipogenic (lĭp″ō-jĕ-nĕt′ĭk, lĭp″ō-jĕn′ĭk) Producing fat. SYN: *lipogenous*.

lipogenous (lĭp-ŏj′ĕ-nŭs) Lipogenetic.

lipogranuloma (lĭp″ō-grăn-ū-lō′mă) [″ + L. *granulum*, granule, + Gr. *oma*, tumor] Inflammation of fatty tissue with granulation and development of oily cysts.

lipogranulomatosis (lĭp″ō-grăn″ū-lō-mă-tō′sĭs) [″ + ″ + ″ + *osis*, condition] A disorder of fat metabolism in which a nodule of fat undergoes central necrosis and the surrounding tissue becomes granulomatous.

lipohyalinosis (lī-pō-hī′ă-lĭn-ō-sĭs) Degenerative changes in small blood vessels, marked by the accumulation of a glassy- or waxy-appearing lipid within the vessel wall. This type of vascular degeneration occurs in hypertension and atherosclerosis, and predisposes patients to small infarcts, esp. in penetrating arteries of the brain.

lipoid (lĭp′oyd) [″ + *eidos,* form, shape] **1.** Similar to fat. **2.** Lipid(e).

lipoidosis (lĭp-oy-dō′sĭs) [″ + ″ + *osis,* condition] Excessive lipid accumulation. SYN: *lipidosis.* SEE: *xanthomatosis.*

arterial l. Arteriosclerosis.

cerebroside l. A familial disease characterized by deposition of glucocerebroside in cells of the reticuloendothelial system. SYN: *Gaucher's disease.*

lipoiduria (lĭp″oy-dū′rē-ă) [″ + ″ + *ouron,* urine] Lipoids in the urine.

lipolipoidosis (lĭp″ō-lĭp″oy-dō′sĭs) [″ + *lipos,* fat, + *eidos,* form, shape, + *osis,* condition] Infiltration of fats and lipoids into a tissue.

lipolysis (lĭp-ŏl′ĭ-sĭs) [″ + *lysis,* dissolution] The decomposition of fat.

lipolytic (lĭp-ō-lĭt′ĭk) Relating to lipolysis.

l. digestion The conversion of neutral fats by hydrolysis into fatty acids and glycerol; fat splitting.

lipoma (lĭ-pō′mă) [Gr. *lipos,* fat, + *oma,* tumor] A fatty tumor. It is frequently found in multiple but is not metastatic. SEE: *chondrolipoma.*

l. arborescens An abnormal treelike accumulation of fatty tissue in a joint.

cystic l. A lipoma containing cysts.

diffuse l. A lipoma not definitely circumscribed.

l. diffusum renis A condition in which fat displaces parenchyma of the kidney.

l. durum A lipoma in which there is marked hypertrophy of the fibrous stroma and capsule.

nasal l. A fibrous growth of the subcutaneous tissue of the nostrils.

osseous l. A lipoma in which the connective tissue has undergone calcareous degeneration.

l. telangiectodes A rare form of lipoma containing a large number of blood vessels.

lipomatoid (lĭ-pō′mă-toyd) [″ + ″ + *eidos,* form, shape] Similar to a lipoma.

lipomatosis (lĭp″ō-mă-tō′sĭs) [″ + *oma,* tumor + *osis,* condition] A condition marked by the excessive deposit of fat in a localized area. SYN: *liposis; obesity.*

l. renis Lipoma diffusum renis.

lipomatous (lĭp-ō′mă-tŭs) **1.** Of the nature of lipoma. **2.** Affected with lipoma.

lipomeningocele (lĭp″ō-mĕ-nĭng′gō-sēl) [″ + *meninx,* membrane, + *kele,* tumor, swelling] A meningocele associated with lobules of fat tissue.

lipomeria (lī″pō-mē′rē-ă) [Gr. *leipein,* to leave, + *meros,* a part] In a deformed fetus, the congenital absence of a limb.

lipometabolism (lĭp-ō-mĕ-tăb′ŏl-ĭzm) [″ + ″ + *-ismos,* condition] Fat metabolism.

lipomyoma (lĭp″ō-mī-ō′mă) [″ + *mys,* muscle, + *oma,* tumor] A myoma containing fatty tissue.

lipomyxoma (lĭp″ō-mĭks-ō′mă) [″ + *myxa,* mucus, + *oma,* tumor] A mixed lipoma and myxoma. SYN: *myxolipoma.*

lipopenia (lĭp″ō-pē′nē-ă) [″ + *penia,* poverty] A deficiency of lipids. **lipopenic** (-nĭk), *adj.*

lipopeptid, lipopeptide (lĭp″ō-pĕp′tĭd, -tīd) A complex of lipids and amino acids.

lipophagia, granulomatous (lĭp″ō-fā′jē-ă) Intestinal lipodystrophy.

lipophagy (lĭ-pŏf′ă-jē) The ingestion of fat cells by phagocytes.

lipophanerosis (lĭp″ō-făn″ĕ-rō′sĭs) [″ + *phaneros,* visible, + *osis,* condition] The alteration of fat in a cell so that it becomes visible as droplets.

lipophil (lĭp′ō-fĭl) [″ + *philein,* to love] **1.** Having an affinity for fat. **2.** Absorbing fat.

lipophilia (lĭp″ō-fĭl′ē-ă) [″ + *philos,* love] Affinity for fat.

lipopolysaccharide (lĭp″ō-pŏl″ē-săk′ă-rīd) The linkage of molecules of lipids with polysaccharides.

lipoprotein Conjugated chemicals in the bloodstream consisting of simple proteins bound to fat. Cholesterol, phospholipids, and triglycerides are all fatty components of lipoproteins. Analyzing the concentrations and proportions of lipoproteins in the blood can provide important information about patients' risks of atherosclerosis, coronary artery disease, and death.

Lipoproteins are classified as very low-density (VLDL), low-density (LDL), intermediate-density (IDL) and high-density (HDL). Increased levels of LDL and total cholesterol directly raise one's chances of having coronary heart disease (CHD). For this reason LDL has been referred to colloquially as "bad" cholesterol. By contrast, increased levels of HDL ("good" cholesterol) are linked with a lowered risk of CHD. The National Cholesterol Education Program has designated 100 mg/dl or less as a desirable level of LDL in persons already affected by CHD; for people without CHD, a desirable level of LDL is 130 mg/dl or less. SEE: *atherosclerosis; coronary artery disease; hyperlipoproteinemia; statins.*

ETIOLOGY: Elevated levels of lipoproteins usually are the result of a diet that is excessively rich in fats, saturated fats, and cholesterols. In a small number of patients with extremely high lipoprotein levels, genetic diseases play a part.

SYMPTOMS: High lipoprotein levels may cause no symptoms of their own until patients develop arterial blockages. If arteries become blocked by lipoproteins, ischemic symptoms may develop.

TREATMENT: Abnormal lipoprotein levels normalize in many patients who consume less dietary fat and increase their level of exercise. When lipoproteins do not reach expected levels despite diet and exercise, medications to improve lipoprotein profiles are prescribed. These include drugs such as niacin, bile-acid binding resins, and the statins.

l. (a) A lipid-protein complex that is found normally in the plasma in small amounts in all people, but in very high concentrations in some persons with familial forms of atherosclerosis.

alpha l. High-density l.

high-density l. ABBR: HDL. Plasma lipids bound to albumin, consisting of lipoproteins. They contain more protein than either very low-density lipoproteins or low-density lipoproteins. High-density lipoprotein cholesterol is the so-called good cholesterol; therefore a high level is desirable. SYN: *alpha l.*

intermediate-density l. ABBR: IDL. Plasma lipids bound to albumin, consisting of lipoproteins with less protein than high-density, but more than low-density, lipoproteins.

l. lipase ABBR: Lp(a). An enzyme produced by many cells. On the surface of cells lining the vasculature, it hydrolyzes fat (chylomicrons) and very low-density lipoprotein (VLDL) to monoglycerides to free fatty acids and intermediate-density lipoprotein (IDL). This enzyme, similar to plasminogen, is an important regulator of lipid and lipoprotein metabolism. Even though the physiological functions of Lp(a) and apo(a) are not fully understood, there is a positive association of plasma Lp(a) with premature myocardial infarction. Deficiency of this enzyme leads to an increase in chylomicrons and VLDLs, and to low levels of high-density lipoproteins (HDL). Diseases associated with acquired causes of decreased lipoprotein lipase include acute ethanol ingestion, diabetes mellitus, hypothyroidism, chronic renal failure, and nephrotic syndrome.

low-density l. ABBR: LDL. Plasma lipids that carry the majority of the cholesterol in plasma. Bound to albumin, LDLs are a proven cause of atherosclerosis; lowering LDLs with a low-fat diet or with drugs helps to prevent and treat coronary artery disease.

very low-density l. ABBR: VLDL. Plasma lipids bound to albumin and consisting of chylomicrons and prelipoproteins. This class of plasma lipoproteins contains a greater ratio of lipid than the low-density lipoproteins and is the least dense.

liposarcoma (lĭp″ō-săr-kō′mă) [Gr. *lipos,* fat, + *sarx,* flesh, + *oma,* tumor] A malignant tumor derived from embryonal fat cells.

liposhaver (li′pō-shā-ver) A device used in plastic surgery to carve out unwanted fat and create smooth contours beneath the skin.

liposis (lĭ-pō′sĭs) [″ + *osis,* condition] Adiposis.

liposoluble (lĭp″ō-sŏl′ū-b′l) [″ + L. *solubilis,* soluble] Soluble in fats.

liposome (lĭp′ō-sōm) [″ + *soma,* body] The sealed concentric shells formed when certain lipid substances are in an aqueous solution. As it forms, the liposome entraps a portion of the solution in the shell. Liposomes may be manufactured and filled with a variety of medications. These have been used to deliver substances to particular organs. These drug forms may be more effective and less toxic than drugs given by other means.

lipostomy (lī-pŏs′tō-mē) [Gr. *leipein,* to fail, + *stoma,* mouth] Congenital absence or extreme smallness of the mouth.

liposuction The removal of subcutaneous fat tissue with a blunt-tipped cannula introduced into the fatty area through a small incision. Suction is then applied and fat tissue removed. Liposuction is a form of plastic surgery intended to remove adipose tissue from localized areas of fat accumulation as on the hips, knees, buttocks, thighs, face, arms, or neck. To be cosmetically successful, the skin should be elastic enough to contract after the underlying fat has been removed. Liposuction will not benefit dimpled or sagging skin or flabby muscles. There are no health benefits to liposuction, and as with any surgery there may be risks such as infection, severe postoperative pain, cardiac arrhythmias, shock, and even death. There is also the possibility the results will be unsatisfactory to the patient. SYN: *suction lipectomy.*

lipotropic (lĭp-ō-trŏp′ĭk) [″ + *trope,* a turning] Having an affinity for lipids, as with certain dyes (e.g., Sudan III, which stains fat readily).

l. factors Compounds that promote the transportation and use of fats and help to prevent accumulation of fat in the liver.

lipotropism, lipotropy (lĭ-pŏt′rō-pĭzm, -pē) [″ + *trope,* a turn, + *-ismos,* condition] **1.** Having the action of removing fat deposits in the liver. **2.** An agent that acts to remove fat from the liver.

lipovaccine (lĭp″ō-văk′sēn) A vaccine suspended in vegetable oil.

lipoxidase (lĭ-pŏk′sĭ-dās) An enzyme that catalyzes the oxidation of the double bonds of an unsaturated fatty acid.

lipoxin A group of arachidonic acid metabolites (eicosanoids) formed by the action of phospholipases on cell membrane phospholipids, some of which have anti-inflammatory effects and some of which promote inflammation and hypersensitivity reactions. SEE: *leukotriene; prostaglandin.*

lipoxygenase (lĭ-pŏks′ĭ-jĕ-nās) Lipoxidase.

Lippes loop (lĭ′pēz) [Jacob Lippes, U.S. obstetrician, b. 1924] A type of intrauterine contraceptive device.

lipping (lĭp′ĭng) A growth of bony tissue beyond the joint margin in degenerative joint disease.

lippitude (lĭp′ĭ-tūd) [L. *lippitudo,* fr. *lippus,* blear-eyed] Blepharitis.

lip reading Interpreting what is being said by watching the speaker's lip and facial movements and expression. This method is used as a means of speech discrimination by people with hearing impairments.

lipuria (lĭ-pū′rē-ă) [Gr. *lipos,* fat, + *ouron,* urine] Fat in the urine.

liquefacient (lĭk″wĕ-fā′shĕnt) [L. *liquere,* to flow, + *facere,* to make] **1.** An agent that converts a solid substance into a liquid. **2.** Converting a solid into a liquid.

liquefaction (lĭk″wĕ-făk′shŭn) **1.** The conversion of a solid into a liquid. **2.** The conversion of solid tissues to a fluid or semifluid state.

liquescent (lĭk-wĕs′sĕnt) [L. *liquescere,* to become liquid] Becoming liquid.

liquid (lĭk′wĭd) [L. *liquere,* to flow] **1.** Flowing easily. **2.** The state of matter in which a substance flows without being melted. SEE: *emulsion; liquefacient; liquefaction.*

l. measure A measure of liquid capacity.

liquid crystal display ABBR: LCD. A type of electronic display unit used on devices from watches to clinical laboratory instruments. It is very efficient and consumes little energy or power.

liquor (lĭk′ĕr) [L.] **1.** Any liquid or fluid. **2.** An alcoholic beverage. **3.** A solution of medicinal substance in water.

l. amnii The amniotic fluid, a clear watery fluid that surrounds the fetus in the amniotic sac. SEE: *hydramnion.*

l. folliculi The fluid contained in the graafian follicle.

l. sanguinis Blood serum or plasma.

l. solution An aqueous solution of nonvolatile substances formerly used to prepare medicines.

Lisch nodule [K. Lisch, contemporary Ger. scientist] A melanocytic hamartoma projecting from the surface of the iris of the eye. It is a well-defined, dome-shaped elevation that is clear to yellow or brown. These growths, which do not cause ophthalmological complications, may be seen without magnification, but examination with use of a slit lamp is needed to differentiate them from nevi of the iris. Lisch nodules are found only in patients with neurofibromatosis, type 1.

Lisfranc's dislocation (lĭs-frănks′) [Jacques Lisfranc, Fr. surgeon, 1790–1847] A dislocation of the tarsometatarsal joints of the foot by direct or indirect mechanisms. Accompanying fracture is common.

Lisfranc's ligament The ligament joining the first cuneiform bone of the ankle to the second metatarsal.

lisinopril (lī-sĭn′ō-prĭl) An angiotensin-converting enzyme inhibitor, used for example, to treat high blood pressure and congestive heart failure. Trade names are Zestril and Prinivil.

lisping (lĭsp′ĭng) [AS. *wlisp,* lisping] A substitution of sounds owing to a defect in speech, as of the "th" sound for "s" and "z."

lissencephalous (lĭs″sĕn-sĕf′ă-lŭs) [Gr. *lissos,* smooth, + *enkephalos,* brain] Pert. to a condition in which the brain is smooth owing to failure of cerebral gyri to develop.

lissotrichy (lĭs-sŏt′rĭ-kē) [″ + *thrix,* hair] The condition of having straight hair.

Lister, Lord Baron Joseph (lĭs′tĕr) British surgeon, 1827–1912, who developed the technique of antiseptic surgery, subsequently evolving into aseptic surgery, without which modern surgery would not be possible. Lister is also associated with various pharmacological compounds and anatomical structures.

Listeria A genus of gram-positive, non–spore-forming coccobacilli that may be found singly or in filaments. They are normal soil inhabitants.

Listeria monocytogenes The causative agent of listeriosis. This species lives in soil or the intestines of animals and may contaminate food, esp. milk or meat. Its growth is not inhibited by refrigeration.

listeriosis, listerosis (lĭs-tĕr″ē-ō′sĭs, lĭs″tĕr-ō′sĭs) Infection with *Listeria monocytogenes,* an intracellular bacterium found in soil that causes mild food poisoning in healthy persons and severe systemic disease in immunosuppressed patients, the elderly, pregnant women, and neonates. The organism may be found in meat or dairy products from infected animals, vegetables contaminated by soil or water containing the organism, or processed foods, such as lunch meats, contaminated after production. Unlike other food-borne pathogens, *Listeria* grows in food even when it is refrigerated; it also grows on the walls of refrigerators and can infect other foods. The organism is destroyed by heat, thus the danger lies in foods served cold or not heated to 158°F for at least 2 minutes. The Department of Agriculture recommends people at risk for infection should not eat hot dogs, lunch meats, dried sausage, raw milk, and soft cheese (e.g., brie, blue cheese) or cheese made from raw milk. In pregnant women, *Listeria* infects the amniotic fluid and causes spontaneous abortion; in immunosuppressed adults and neonates, it most commonly causes meningitis.

TREATMENT: Ampicillin plus ceftriaxone or cefotaxime or ampicillin plus an aminoglycoside have proven effective against *Listeria* meningitis. If the patient is allergic to penicillin, then trimethoprim or sulfamethoxazole should be used. Dexamethasone may be given before antibiotic therapy to decrease cerebral edema.

PATIENT CARE: Public education is needed to inform pregnant women, the elderly, persons on immunosuppressive drug therapy, or those with HIV infection of the danger of ready to eat foods such as cold cuts and soft cheeses. Safe food handling techniques to minimize the risk of infection include washing hands well (at least 20 seconds) when handling ready to eat cold foods, washing cutting boards and other utensils with hot soapy water before using them for another food, keeping uncooked foods separated from cooked foods, and washing all fruits and vegetables before eating, even those that come from a personal garden.

liter (lē′tĕr) [Fr. *litre,* liter] SI (metric) fluid measure; equivalent to 1000 mL, 270 fl drams, 61 cu in., 33.8 fl oz, or 1.0567 qt. The volume occupied by 1 kg of water at 4°C and 760 mm Hg pressure. SEE: *metric system*.

NOTE: It is common to define a liter as 1000 cc. This is not quite correct because 1 ml equals 1.000028 cc. Thus, liquid volume should be expressed in milliliters rather than in cubic centimeters.

literate Being able to read and write, and to use written language as in understanding graphs, charts, tables, maps, symbols, and formulas.

lith- SEE: *litho-*.

lithectasy (lĭth-ĕk′tă-sē) [Gr. *lithos,* stone, + *ektasis,* dilatation] The removal of a kidney stone from the bladder through the dilated urethra.

lithectomy (lĭ-thĕk′tō-mē) [″ + *ektome,* excision] The surgical removal of a calculus.

lithemia (lĭth-ē′mē-ă) [″ + *haima,* blood] An excess of lithic or uric acid in the blood owing to imperfect metabolism of the nitrogenous substances.

lithiasis (lĭth-ī′ă-sĭs) **1.** The formation of stones. **2.** Uric acid diathesis.

l. biliaris Gallstone.

l. nephritica SYN: *kidney stone*.

l. renalis SYN: *kidney stone*.

lithic acid (lĭth′ĭk) Uric acid.

lithicosis (lĭth″ĭ-kō′sĭs) [Gr. *lithikos,* made of stone] Silicosis.

lithium (lĭth′ē-ŭm) [Gr. *lithos,* stone] SYMB: Li. A metallic element; atomic weight 6.941; atomic number 3.

l. carbonate A drug that is used to treat bipolar disorder. Given orally it is readily absorbed and eliminated at a fast rate for 5 to 6 hr and much more slowly over the next 24 hr. It is essential to monitor the blood level of the drug in patients taking this therapy; samples should be taken 8 to 10 hr after the last dose and at intervals after medication. SEE: *bipolar disorder*.

The dose is adjusted as needed to produce a plasma level of 0.8 mEq/L. When the dose has been found to produce the optimal plasma concentration, blood analysis is done every 3 months unless symptoms suggestive of toxicity are present. Plasma levels of 2 mEq/L or more cause serious toxic effects including stupor or coma, muscular rigidity, marked tremor, and, in some cases, epileptic seizure.

Side effects including fatigue, weakness, fine tremor of the hands, nausea and vomiting, thirst, dry mouth, and polyuria may be noticed in the first week of therapy. Most will disappear, but the thirst, polyuria, and tremor tend to persist. Dry mouth may be severe enough to promote dental decay.

CAUTION: Decreased dietary sodium intake lowers the excretion rate of lithium. It should not be administered to patients following a salt-free diet. The risk of toxicity is very high in patients with significant renal or cardiovascular disease, severe debilitation, dehydration, sodium depletion, or in patients receiving diuretics or nonsteroidal anti-inflammatory drugs.

litho-, lith- [Gr. *lithos,* stone] Combining form meaning *stone* or *calculus*.

lithocenosis (lĭth″ō-sĕn-ō′sĭs) [″ + *kenosis,* evacuation] The removal of crushed fragments of kidney stones from the bladder.

lithoclast (lĭth′ō-klăst) [″ + *klastos,* broken] Forceps for breaking up large calculi.

lithoclasty (lĭth′ō-klăs″tē) The crushing of a stone into fragments that may pass through natural channels.

lithocystotomy (lĭth″ō-sĭs-tŏt′ō-mē) [″ + *kystis,* bladder, + *tome,* incision] Incision of the bladder to remove a kidney stone.

lithogenesis (lĭth″ō-jĕn′ĕ-sĭs) [″ + *gennan,* to produce] Formation of calculi.

lithokelyphopedion (lĭth″ō-kĕl″ĭ-fō-pē′dē-ŏn) [″ + *kelyphos,* sheath, + *paidion,* child] Calcification of both the fetus and the membranes of a lithopedion.

lithokelyphos (lĭth″ō-kĕl′ĭ-fŏs) [″ + *kelyphos,* sheath] A type of lithopedion in which only the membranes are calcified.

lithokonion (lĭth″ō-kō′nē-ŏn) [″ + *konios,* dusty] Lithomyl.

litholabe (lĭth′ō-lāb) [″ + *lambanein,* to hold] A device for holding a stone during its removal.

litholapaxy (lĭth-ŏl′ă-păks″ē) [Gr. *lithos,* stone, + *lapaxis,* evacuation] The operation of crushing a stone in the bladder followed by immediate washing out of the crushed fragments through a catheter. SEE: *percutaneous ultrasonic lithotriptor*.

lithology (lĭth-ŏl′ō-jē) [″ + *logos,* word, reason] The science dealing with calculi.

litholysis (lĭth-ŏl′ĭ-sĭs) [″ + *lysis,* dissolution] Dissolving of stones.

lithometer (lĭth-ŏm′ĕ-tĕr) [″ + *metron,* measure] An instrument for estimating the size of calculi.

lithometra (lĭth-ō-mē′tră) [″ + *metra,* uterus] Uterine tissue ossification.

lithomyl (lĭth′ō-mĭl) [″ + *myle,* mill] An instrument for crushing a bladder stone. SYN: *lithokonion.*

lithonephritis (lĭth″ō-nĕ-frī′tĭs) [″ + *nephros,* kidney, + *itis,* inflammation] An inflammation of the kidney because of a stone.

lithonephrotomy (lĭth″ō-nē-frŏt′ō-mē) [″ + *nephros,* kidney, + *tome,* incision] An incision of the kidney for removal of a kidney stone.

lithopedion (lĭth″ō-pē′dē-ŏn) [″ + *paidion,* child] A uterine or extrauterine fetus that has died and become calcified. SYN: *ostembryon; osteopedion.*

lithotome (lĭth′ō-tōm) [″ + *tome,* incision] An instrument for performing lithotomy.

lithotomy (lĭth-ŏt′ō-mē) [″ + *tome,* incision] The incision of a duct or organ, esp. of the bladder, for removal of a stone. SEE: *lithotomy p.*

PATIENT CARE: A dietary history is obtained to identify factors contributing to stone formation. Noninvasive measures and prescribed analgesic agents are provided to relieve pain. Fluid balance is monitored, and unless otherwise contraindicated by cardiac or renal status, fluid intake of 4 L/day is recommended to maintain a urine output of 3 to 4 L/day, which aids in the passage of small calculi (up to 5 mm in diameter) and prevents ascending infections. Supplemental I.V. fluids are provided if the patient is unable to tolerate the required volume by mouth. Vital signs and laboratory studies are monitored for signs of infection, and prescribed antibiotics are administered. The nurse prepares the patient for lithotripsy or surgery, as indicated, by explaining postoperative equipment, care procedures, and expected sensations. Any incisions are assessed for drainage and healing, the character and amount of drainage are documented, and a ureteral catheter or nephrotomy tube, if prescribed, is irrigated. Using aseptic techniques, the nurse protects surrounding skin from excoriation by redressing frequently. All urine is strained for evidence of stones and any solid material is sent for analysis. Based on laboratory analysis of the stone, treatments are prescribed to prevent recurrence.

bilateral l. A lithotomy performed with the incision across the perineum.

high l. A lithotomy performed through a suprapubic incision.

lateral l. A lithotomy performed with the incision from the front of the rectum to one side of the raphe.

median l. A lithotomy performed with the incision in the median line in front of the anus.

rectal l. A lithotomy performed through the rectum.

vaginal l. A lithotomy performed with the incision through the vaginal wall.

lithotony (lĭth-ŏt′ō-nē) [Gr. *lithos,* stone, + *teinein,* to stretch] The removal of a kidney stone through a small bladder incision that is instrumentally dilated.

lithotresis (lĭth″ō-trē′sĭs) [″ + *tresis,* boring] The drilling or boring of holes in a calculus to facilitate crushing. More recently, an ultrasonic probe is employed.

lithotripsy (lĭth′ō-trĭp″sē) [″ + *tribein,* to rub] **1.** The application of the physical force of sound waves to crush a stone in the bladder or urethra. **2.** The production of shock waves by use of an external energy source in order to crush renal stones.

lithotriptic (lĭth-ō-trĭp′tĭk) **1.** Pert. to lithotripsy. **2.** An agent that dissolves stones.

NOTE: There are no substances that have this capability and are harmless to the patient.

lithotriptor (lĭth′ō-trĭp″tor) [″ + *tripsis,* friction] A device for breaking up kidney stones.

percutaneous ultrasonic l. A device that uses ultrasound to break up kidney stones and gallstones. The sound waves are applied to the outside of the body and penetrate to the calculi.

lithotriptoscopy (lĭth″ō-trĭp-tŏs′kō-pē) [″ + ″ + *skopein,* to examine] The crushing of a kidney stone under direct vision by using a lithotriptoscope.

lithotrity (lĭth-ŏt′rĭ-tē) The crushing of a kidney stone to small fragments in the bladder.

lithous (lĭth′ŭs) [Gr. *lithos,* stone] Relating to a stone. SYN: *calculous.*

lithoxiduria (lĭth″ŏks-ĭ-dū′rē-ă) [″ + L. *oxidum,* oxide, + Gr. *ouron,* urine] The presence of xanthic oxide in the urine.

lithuria (lĭth-ū′rē-ă) [″ + *ouron,* urine]

An excess of uric acid or urates in the urine.

litigation A lawsuit or legal action that determines the legal rights and remedies of the person or party.

litmus (lĭt′mŭs) A blue dyestuff made by treating coarsely powdered lichens, such as those of the genus *Roccella,* with ammonia.

l. paper Chemically prepared blue paper that is turned red by acids and remains blue in alkali solutions; pH range is 4.5 to 8.5. SEE: *indicator*.

litter (lĭt′tĕr) [O.Fr. *litiere,* offspring at birth, bed] **1.** A stretcher for carrying the wounded or the sick. **2.** The young produced at one birth by a multiparous mammal.

Little's disease [William John Little, Brit. physician, 1810–1894] Congenital spastic paralysis on both sides (diplegia), although it may be paraplegic or hemiplegic in form.

SYMPTOMS: The child may be delayed in developing sphincter control and is usually mentally normal. Symptoms include stiff, awkward movements; legs crossed and pressed together; arm(s) adducted; forearm(s) flexed; hand(s) pronated; scissors gait.

ETIOLOGY: The cause is unknown. Efforts to implicate hypoxemia in utero have not been successful.

Littré's gland (lē′trz) [Alexis Littré, Fr. surgeon, 1658–1725] Urethral glands.

littritis (lĭt-trī′tĭs) An inflammation of the urethral glands.

Litzmann's obliquity [Karl K. T. Litzmann, Ger. gynecologist, 1815–1890] Posterior parietal presentation of the fetal head during labor. SYN: *posterior asynclitism*.

lived experience The subjective perception of one's health or illness experience. Associated with Rosemarie Parse's Nursing Theory of Human Becoming, it emphasizes the nurse's need to understand the personal health experience of patients, rather than to collect data from patients as objects. SEE: *Nursing Theory Appendix*.

livedo (lĭv-ē′dō) [L. *livedo,* lividness] A mottled staining of the skin, often blue or purple, as may be seen in a bruise. SYN: *lividity*.

l. reticularis Semipermanent bluish mottling of the skin of the legs and hands. It is aggravated by exposure to cold.

liver (lĭv′ĕr) [AS. *lifer*] The largest solid organ in the body, situated on the right side below the diaphragm. The liver occupies the right hypochondrium (the epigastrium) and part of the left hypochondrium, and is level with the bottom of the sternum. Its undersurface is concave and covers the stomach, duodenum, hepatic flexure of colon, right kidney, and adrenal capsule. The liver secretes bile and is the site of numerous metabolic functions. SEE: illus.

ANATOMY: The liver has four lobes, five ligaments, and five fissures and is covered by a tough fibrous membrane, Glisson's capsule, which is thickest at the transverse fissure. At this point the capsule carries the blood vessels and hepatic duct, which enter the organ at the hilus. Strands of connective tissue originating from the capsule enter the liver parenchyma and form the supporting network of the organ and separate the functional units of the liver, the hepatic lobules.

The many intrahepatic bile ducts converge and anastomose, finally forming the secretory duct of the liver, the hepatic duct, which joins the cystic duct from the gallbladder to form the common bile duct or the ductus choledochus, which enters the duodenum at the papilla of Vater. A ring of smooth muscle at the terminal portion of the choledochus, the sphincter of Oddi, permits the passage of bile into the duodenum by relaxing. The bile leaving the liver enters the gallbladder, where it undergoes concentration principally through loss of water absorbed by the gallbladder mucosa. When bile is needed in the small intestine for digestive purposes, the gallbladder contracts and the sphincter relaxes, thus permitting escape of the viscid gallbladder bile. Ordinarily, the sphincter of Oddi is contracted, shutting off the duodenal entrance and forcing the bile to enter the gallbladder after leaving the liver.

The functional units of the liver are the liver lobules, six-sided aggregations of hepatocytes permeated by capillaries called sinusoids. Lining these sinusoids are Kupffer cells, the macrophages of the liver.

BLOOD SUPPLY: The blood supply consists of oxygenated blood from the hepatic artery, a branch of the celiac artery, and blood from all the digestive organs and spleen by way of the portal vein. The end products of digestion and other materials thus pass through the liver before entering general circulation.

NERVE SUPPLY: The nerve supply consists of parasympathetic fibers from the vagi and sympathetic fibers from the celiac plexus via the hepatic nerve.

FUNCTION: The liver is one of the most metabolically active organs of the body. *Amino acid metabolism:* It synthesizes nonessential amino acids, deaminates excess amino acids for use in energy production, and forms urea, which the kidneys excrete. *Bile production:* It is responsible for the production of bile salts, which emulsify fats in the small intestine; 800 to 1000 ml of bile is secreted in 24 hr, and the secretion rate is

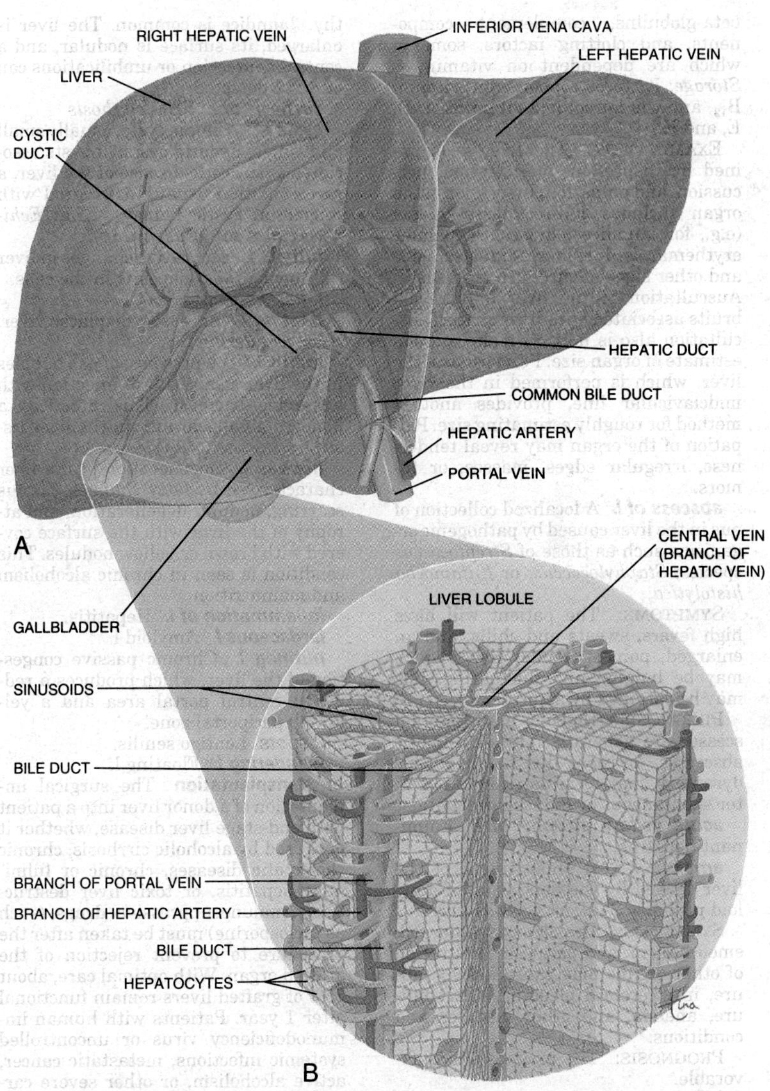

(A) LIVER AND GALLBLADDER, (B) LOBULE

increased greatly during digestion of meals rich in fats. *Carbohydrate metabolism:* It converts monosaccharides other than glucose to glucose, and stores excess glucose as the starch glycogen, until such energy is needed. *Detoxification:* It produces enzymes to metabolize potentially harmful substances found in the portal circulation (e.g., alcohol, ammonia, indole, many medications, and skatole) into less toxic ones. *Endocrine functions:* It facilitates the conversion of levothyroxine to the more metabolically active thyroid hormone, triiodothyronine. *Excretion:* It discharges the breakdown products of hemoglobin (bilirubin and biliverdin) into the bile; these are eliminated in feces. *Fat metabolism:* It synthesizes cholesterol as well as lipoproteins for the transport of fat to other body tissues; it converts fatty acids to acetyl groups or ketones, so they may be used as energy sources. *Phagocytosis:* Its macrophages (Kupffer cells) scavenge bacteria, other pathogens, and senescent red blood cells from the portal circulation. *Protein syntheses:* It manufactures albumin, alpha-globulins and beta-globulins, complement components, and clotting factors, some of which are dependent on vitamin K. *Storage:* It stores copper, iron, vitamin B_{12}, and the fat-soluble vitamins A, D, E, and K.

EXAMINATION: The liver is examined by inspection, auscultation, percussion, and palpation. Inspection of the organ includes indirect assessments (e.g., for jaundice [skin color], palmar erythema, and spider telangiectasias and other signs of chronic liver disease. Auscultation of the liver may reveal bruits associated with liver cancer; auscultation also is used to make a crude estimate of organ size. Percussion of the liver, which is performed in the right midclavicular line, provides another method for roughly estimating size. Palpation of the organ may reveal tenderness, irregular edges, masses, or tumors.

abscess of l. A localized collection of pus in the liver caused by pathogenic organisms such as those of *Streptococcus* species; *Staphylococcus;* or *Entamoeba histolytica*.

SYMPTOMS: The patient will have high fevers; sweats and chills; and an enlarged, painful, tender liver, which may be bulging and fluctuating. Pus may be obtained by aspiration.

PROGNOSIS: Embolic (multiple) abscesses are generally fatal. Traumatic abscesses, or those due to an amebic dysentery, may terminate favorably after spontaneous or induced evacuation.

acute yellow atrophy of l. Fulminant hepatitis.

amyloid l. An enlargement of the liver caused by the deposition of amyloid proteins. SYN: *lardaceous liver*.

SYMPTOMS: The liver is enlarged, smooth, firm, and painless. Infiltration of other organs may cause kidney failure, intercerebral bleeding, heart failure, anemia, and other diseases and conditions.

PROGNOSIS: The prognosis is unfavorable.

biliary cirrhotic l. Cirrhosis of the liver caused by fibrous tissue formed, as a result of infection or obstruction of the bile ducts.

cancer of l. Malignancy of the liver that results either from spread from a primary source or from primary tumor of the liver itself. The former is the more frequent cause. Male sex, hepatitis B or C, cirrhosis, and other liver diseases are predisposing factors. The liver is the most common site of metastatic spread of tumors that disseminate through the bloodstream. The prognosis for survival is from a few months to 1 yr.

SYMPTOMS: The disease may cause severe pain and tenderness; cachexia (i.e., loss of weight); and encephalopathy. Jaundice is common. The liver is enlarged, its surface is nodular, and a central depression or umbilications can often be detected.

cirrhosis of l. SEE: *cirrhosis*.

cysts of l. Simple cysts, usually small and single; hydatid cysts; or cysts associated with cystic disease of the liver, a rare condition usually associated with congenital cystic kidneys. SEE: *Echinococcus granulosus; hydatid*.

fatty l. Degenerative changes in liver cells owing to fat deposits in the cells.

l. flap Asterixis.

floating l. An easily displaced liver. SYN: *wandering l.*

foamy l. The presence of gas bubbles in the liver as a result of infection with anaerobic bacteria. This produces a honeycomb appearance in the liver tissue.

hobnail l. Degeneration of the liver characterized by fatty changes, fibrous scarring, nodular degeneration, and atrophy of the liver with the surface covered with brown or yellow nodules. This condition is seen in chronic alcoholism and malnutrition.

inflammation of l. Hepatitis.

lardaceous l. Amyloid l.

nutmeg l. Chronic passive congestion of the liver, which produces a reddened central portal area and a yellowish periportal zone.

l. spots Lentigo senilis.

wandering l. Floating l.

liver transplantation The surgical implantation of a donor liver into a patient with end-stage liver disease, whether it is caused by alcoholic cirrhosis, chronic cholestatic diseases, chronic or fulminant hepatitis, or toxic liver destruction. Immunosuppressive drugs (such as cyclosporine) must be taken after the procedure to prevent rejection of the grafted organ. With optimal care, about 75% of grafted livers remain functional after 1 year. Patients with human immunodeficiency virus or uncontrolled systemic infections, metastatic cancer, active alcoholism, or other severe cardiac, pulmonary, or neurological illnesses are not candidates for the procedure. In the U.S. about 4000 liver transplants are performed annually.

livid (lĭv′ĭd) [L. *lividus,* lead-colored] **1.** Ashen, cyanotic. **2.** Discolored, black and blue.

lividity (lĭ-vĭd′ĭ-tē) **1.** Skin discoloration, as from a bruise or venous congestion. SYN: *livor*. **2.** The state of being livid.

postmortem l. A dark blue staining of the dependent surface of a cadaver, resulting from the pooling and congestion of blood.

living will An advance directive, prepared when an individual is alive, competent, and able to make decisions, regarding that person's specific instructions about end-of-life care. Living wills allow people to specify whether they would want to be intubated, ventilated, treated with pressor drugs, shocked with electricity (to stop life-threatening heart rhythms), and fed or hydrated intravenously (if unable to take food or drink). Some also specify the person or persons who have power of attorney to make health care decisions on the patient's behalf, if the patient is no longer competent to make choices for himself or herself. SEE: *advance directive*.

livor (lī'vor) [L., a black-and-blue spot] Lividity (1).

l. mortis SYN: *Postmortem l.*

lixiviation (lĭks"ĭv-ē-ā'shŭn) [L. *lixivia*, lye] Leaching.

L.L.E. *left lower extremity*.

LLETZ *large loop excision of the transformation zone*.

LLQ *left lower quadrant* (of abdomen).

L.M.A. *left mentoanterior* fetal position. SEE: *presentation* for illus.

L.M.P. *left mentoposterior* fetal position; *last menstrual period*. SEE: *presentation* for illus.

L.M.T. *left mentotransverse* fetal position. SEE: *presentation* for illus.

L.O.A. *left occipitoanterior* fetal position. SEE: *presentation* for illus.

load **1.** The weight supported or force imposed. **2.** A substance given to test body function, esp. metabolic function. SEE: *loading test*.

viral l. A measure of the total body burden of viral particles present in human blood; the greater the number, usually, the sicker the patient. Testing for viral loads has aided the treatment of several illnesses, including AIDS and hepatitis C. In these illnesses, antiviral therapies are initiated at certain levels of viral load and continued if anticipated reductions in viremic burden are achieved.

loading The rapid or repeated administration of a drug to quickly achieve a therapeutic level.

loading, bicarbonate The ingestion of sodium bicarbonate in an effort to neutralize excessive lactic acid produced in the muscles during exercise or to treat acidosis in chronic renal failure.

loading, carbohydrate SEE: *carbohydrate loading*.

loading, glycogen A dietary regimen used to fill the body's glycogen storage areas (i.e., the liver and muscles). SEE: *carbohydrate loading*.

loaiasis Loiasis.

Loa loa (lō'ă) [W. African] The African eyeworm, a species of filarial worm that infests the subcutaneous tissues and conjunctiva of humans. Its migration causes itching and a creeping sensation. Sometimes it causes itchy edematous areas known as Calabar swellings. It is transmitted by flies of the genus *Chrysops*. SEE: illus.

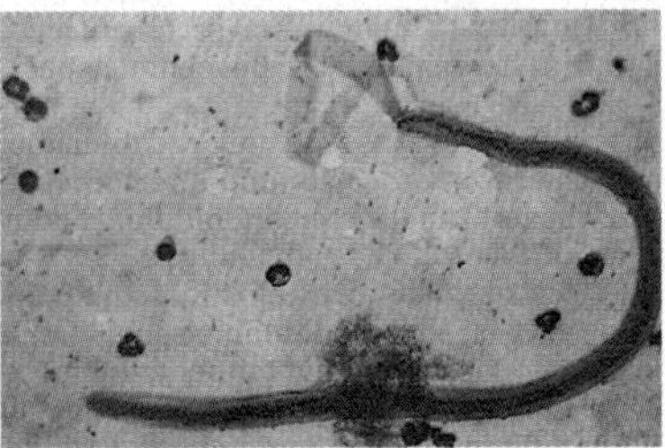

LOA LOA IN BLOOD

(Orig. mag. ×400)

lobar (lō'băr) [Gr. *lobos*, lobe] Pert. to a lobe.

lobate (lō'bāt) [L. *lobatus*, lobed] **1.** Pert. to a lobe. **2.** Having a deeply undulated border. **3.** Producing lobes.

lobbying Attempting to shape legislation, influence legislators, or mold public opinion.

lobe (lōb) [Gr. *lobos*, lobe] **1.** A fairly well-defined part of an organ separated by boundaries, esp. glandular organs and the brain. **2.** A major part of a tooth formed by a separate calcification center.

accessory l. of parotid A small lobe, variable in size, on the anterior surface of the parotid gland superior to the exit of the parotid duct.

anterior l. of hypophysis The anterior portion of the pituitary gland, consisting of the pars distalis and pars tuberalis.

azygos l. An anomalous lobe at the apex of the right lobe of the lung.

caudate l. of liver The irregular quadrangular portion of liver behind the fissure for the portal vein and between the fissures for the vena cava and ductus venosus. SYN: *spigelian l.*

central l. The island of Reil, which forms the floor of the lateral cerebral fossa. SYN: *insular l.*

l. of cerebrum The frontal, parietal, occipital, and temporal lobes and the insula or island of Reil (central lobe).

l. of ear The lower portion of the auricle that has no cartilage.

flocculonodular l. The lobe of the cerebellum consisting of the flocculi, nodulus, and their connecting peduncles.

frontal l. The anterior part of a cerebral hemisphere in front of the central and sylvian fissures.

hepatic l. A lobe of the liver.

insular l. Central l.

lateral l. of prostate The portions of the prostate located on each side of the urethra.

lateral l. of thyroid gland The two main portions of the thyroid, one on each side of the trachea, united below by the thyroid isthmus.

limbic l. The marginal section of a cerebral hemisphere on the medial aspect. SYN: *gyrus fornicatus*.

l. of lungs One of the large divisions of the lungs: superior and inferior lobes of the left lung; superior, middle, and inferior lobes of the right lung.

l. of mamma One of the 15 to 20 divisions of the glandular tissue of the breast separated by connective tissue and each possessing a duct (lobar duct) opening via the nipple.

occipital l. The posterior region of a cerebral hemisphere that is shaped like a three-sided pyramid.

olfactory l. The olfactory bulb and tract. SYN: *rhinencephalon*. SEE: *olfactory nerve* for illus.

orbital l. The convolutions above the orbit.

l. of pancreas A round aggregation of glandular tissue separated by connective tissue.

parietal l. The division of each cerebral hemisphere lying beneath each parietal bone.

posterior l. of hypophysis The posterior portion of the pituitary gland, consisting of the pars intermedia and the processus infundibuli (pars nervosa).

prefrontal l. The frontal portion of the frontal lobe of the brain.

l. of prostate The lateral lobes and the middle lobe of the prostate gland.

pyramidal l. of thyroid A portion of the thyroid gland extending upward from the isthmus. It is extremely variable in size.

quadrate l. of liver An oblong elevation on the lower surface of the liver.

Riedel's l. An anomalous tonguelike extension from the right lobe of the liver to the gallbladder.

spigelian l. Caudate l. of liver.

temporal l. The portion of the cerebral hemisphere lying below the lateral fissure of Sylvius. It is continuous posteriorly with the occipital lobe.

lobectomy (lō-bĕk′tō-mē) [Gr. *lobos*, lobe, + *ektome*, excision] The surgical removal of a lobe of any organ or gland.

lobeline (lŏb′ĕ-lēn) The chief constituent of lobelia.

lobi Pl. of lobus.

lobitis (lō-bī′tĭs) [″ + *itis*, inflammation] Inflammation of a lobe.

Loboa loboi Fungus that causes keloidal blastomycosis (Lobo's disease). It has been identified in tissues but has not been cultured.

Lobo's disease Keloidal blastomycosis. SEE: *blastomycosis*.

lobotomy (lō-bŏt′ō-mē) [Gr. *lobos*, lobe, + *tome*, incision] The incision of a lobe; this procedure was used at one time to treat some forms of mental disturbances that did not respond to other treatments. It is accomplished by a small bilateral trephination in the plane of the coronal suture through which the white matter of the brain is sectioned; the diencephalon, esp. the hypothalamic area, is disconnected from the prefrontal cortex by section of the white fiber connecting pathways subcortically in a plane passing adjacent to the anterior tip of the lateral ventricle and the posterior margin of the sphenoid wing.

Lobstein's disease (lōb′stīnz) [John Georg Friedrich Lobstein, Ger. surgeon, 1777–1835] Osteogenesis imperfecta.

lobular (lŏb′ū-lăr) [L. *lobulus*, small lobe] Lobulate.

lobulate, lobulated (lŏb′ū-lāt, -lāt-ĕd) **1.** Consisting of lobes or lobules. **2.** Pert. to lobes or lobules. **3.** Resembling lobes. SYN: *lobular*.

lobule (lŏb′ūl) [L. *lobulus*, small lobe] A small lobe or primary subdivision of a lobe. It is typical of the pancreas and major salivary glands and may be represented on the surface by bumps or bulges as seen on the thyroid gland.

central l. of cerebellum A small lobe at the anterior part of the superior vermiform process.

l. of breast Subdivisions of the lobes of the mammary glands. They are composed of multiple alveoli surrounding tiny ducts that secrete breast milk components. The lactiferous ducts are formed from the merging of the secretory ducts from several lobules.

l. of epididymis Conelike divisions of the head of the epididymis formed by the much-coiled distal ends of the efferent ducts of the testis.

l. of kidney Subdivision of the renal cortex consisting of a medullary ray and surrounding nephrons.

l. of liver A structural unit consisting of hepatic cells arranged in irregular, branching, and interconnected groups and anastomosing blood channels (sinusoids) surrounding a central vein. It is polyhedral and contains branches of portal vein, hepatic artery, and interlobular bile ducts at its periphery.

l. of lung Physiological units of the lung consisting of a respiratory bronchiole and its branches (alveolar ducts, alveolar sacs, and alveoli).

paracentral l. The superior convolution of the ascending frontal and parietal convolutions of the brain, forming a union of both.

parietal l. One of two subdivisions of the parietal lobe of the brain. The superior parietal lobule is the posterior part of the upper portion, and the inferior parietal lobule is a lateral area continuous with temporal and occipital lobes.

primary pulmonary l. l. of lung.

l. of testis Pyramidal divisions separated from each other by incomplete partitions called septa. Each consists of one to three coiled seminiferous tubules.

l. of thymus Subdivisions of a lobe, each consisting of a cortex and medulla.

lobuli Pl. of lobulus.

lobulus (lŏb′ū-lŭs) *pl.* **lobuli** [L.] A lobule or small division of a lobe.

lobus (lō′bŭs) *pl.* **lobi** [L.] Lobe.

LOC **1.** *levels of consciousness.* **2.** *loss of consciousness.*

local (lō′kăl) [L. *locus,* place] Limited to one place or part.

localization (lō-kăl-ĭ-zā′shŭn) **1.** Limitation to a definite area. **2.** Determination of the site of an infection. **3.** Relation of a sensation to its point of origin.

cerebral l. Determination of centers of various faculties and functions in particular parts of the brain.

localized (lō′kăl-īzd) Restricted to a limited region.

localizer An apparatus, usually opaque or laser, used for finding foreign bodies or exact anatomical locations during radiography.

locator (lō′kā-tĕr) A device for locating or discovering an object such as a foreign body.

lochia (lō′kē-ă) [Gr. *lochia*] The puerperal discharge of blood, mucus, and tissue from the uterus. The character of the discharge progresses through three stages as the normal autolytic healing process proceeds: 1) *lochia rubra or cruenta:* For the first 2 to 4 days, the discharge is distinctly blood-tinged. 2) *lochia serosa:* Between days 7 and 10, the woman usually exhibits a serous pink discharge. 3) *lochia alba or purulenta:* On or about the 10th postpartum day, the discharge becomes white. An offensive odor indicates contamination by saprophytic organisms. **lochial** (-ăl), *adj.*

l. alba The white postpartum vaginal discharge that is no longer blood-tinged. SYN: *l. purulenta.*

l. cruenta The bloody postpartum vaginal discharge. SYN: *l. rubra.*

l. purulenta L. alba.

l. rubra L. cruenta.

l. serosa A thin, watery postpartum vaginal discharge.

lochiocolpos (lō″kē-ō-kŏl′pŏs) [Gr. *lochia,* discharge following childbirth, + *kolpos,* vagina] Distention of the vagina resulting from retention of lochia.

lochiometra (lō″kē-ō-mē′tră) [″ + *metra,* uterus] Retention of lochia in the uterus.

lochiometritis (lō″kē-ō-mē-trī′tĭs) [″ + ″ + *itis,* inflammation] Puerperal inflammation of the uterus.

lochiorrhagia (lō′kē-ō-rā′jē-ă) [″ + *rhegnynai,* to break forth] Excessive flow of lochia.

lochiorrhea (lō″kē-ō-rē′ă) [″ + *rhoia,* flow] Abnormal flow of lochia.

lochioschesis (lō″kē-ŏs′kĕ-sĭs) [″ + *schesis,* retention] Retention or suppression of the lochia.

lochometritis (lō″kō-mē-trī′tĭs) [″ + *metra,* uterus, + *itis,* inflammation] Lochiometritis.

loci [L.] Pl. of locus.

Locke's solution, Locke-Ringer's solution [Frank S. Locke, Brit. physician, 1871–1949; Sydney Ringer, Brit. physiologist, 1835–1910] A solution used in experiments in physiology. It contains sodium, potassium, calcium, and magnesium chlorides; sodium bicarbonate, dextrose, and water.

lockjaw Tonic spasm of muscles of jaw. SEE: *tetanus; trismus.*

lock, saline An intravenous portal, usually placed and left in a vein in one of the patient's arms, that is used episodically for fluid or medication infusions. Salt water flushes are used to maintain its patency. Saline locks replaced heparin locks in the 1990s because the latter posed an unacceptable risk of heparin-related allergies (esp. heparin-related thrombocytopenia).

Lockwood's ligament [Charles B. Lockwood, Brit. surgeon, 1856–1914] The suspensory ligament of the eyeball.

locomotion (lō″kō-mō′shŭn) [L. *locus,* place, + *movere,* to move] Movement or the capacity to move from one place to another.

locomotor (lō″kō-mō′tor) Pert. to locomotion.

locomotorium (lō″kō-mō-tō′rē-ŭm) The locomotor apparatus of the body.

locoweed (lō′kō-wēd) A poisonous plant from the bean family that causes behavioral, visual, and gait disturbances, usually in cattle.

locular (lŏk′ū-lăr) [L. *loculus,* a small space] Loculated.

loculated (lŏk′ū-lāt-ĕd) Containing or divided into loculi. SYN: *locular.*

loculi (lŏk′ū-lī) Pl. of loculus.

loculus (lŏk′ū-lŭs) *pl.* **loculi** [L.] A small space or cavity.

locum tenens (lō′kŭm tĕn′ĕns) [L. *locus,* place, + *tenere,* to hold] A substitute; a physician who temporarily substitutes for another.

locus (lō′kŭs) *pl.* **loci** [L. *locus,* a place] **1.** A spot or place. **2.** In genetics, the site of a gene on a chromosome.

l. ceruleus A dark-colored depression in the floor of the fourth ventricle of the brain at its upper part.

l. of control A term used in reference to an individual's sense of mastery or control over events. Persons with an internal locus of control are more apt to believe that they can influence events, whereas those with an external locus of control tend to believe that events are dictated by fate. These respective orientations can influence a person's practice of health-related behaviors.

l. niger Substantia nigra.

LOD Limit of detection.

Loeffler's bacillus (lĕf′lĕrz) [Friedrich August Johannes Loeffler (Loffler), Ger.

bacteriologist, 1852–1915] *Corynebacterium diphtheriae.*

Löffler's endocarditis (lĕf′lĕrz) [Wilhelm Löffler, Swiss physician, 1887–1972] Endocarditis associated with hypereosinophilia and fibroplastic thickening of the endocardium.

log A continuously kept record of important events, such as medical records or progress notes.

logadectomy (lŏg″ă-dĕk′tō-mē) [Gr. *logades,* the whites of the eyes, + *ektome,* excision] Excision of a portion of the conjunctiva.

logaditis (lŏg″ă-dī′tĭs) [″ + *itis,* inflammation] Scleritis.

logagnosia (lŏg″ăg-nō′sē-ă) [Gr. *logos,* word, reason, + *a-,* not, + *gnosis,* knowledge] A type of aphasia in which words are seen but not identified with respect to their meaning. SEE: *aphasia.*

logagraphia (lŏg-ă-grăf′ē-ă) [″ + ″ + *graphein,* to write] Agraphia.

logamnesia (lŏg-ăm-nē′zē-ă) [″ + *amnesia,* forgetfulness] Aphasia of a sensory character; the inability to recognize spoken or written words.

logaphasia (lŏg″ă-fā′zē-ă) [″ + *a-,* not, + *phasis,* speaking] Motor aphasia, usually the result of a cerebral lesion.

logasthenia (lŏg″ăs-thē′nē-ă) [″ + ″ + *sthenos,* strength] Mental impairment characterized by a defective ability to understand the spoken word.

logoklony (lŏg′ō-klŏn-ē) [″ + *klonein,* to agitate] Intermittent repetition of the last syllable of a word.

logokophosis (lŏg″ō-kō-fō′sĭs) [″ + *kophosis,* deafness] Wernicke's aphasia.

logomania (lŏg-ō-mā′nē-ă) [″ + *mania,* madness] Logorrhea.

logoneurosis (lŏg″ō-nū-rō′sĭs) [″ + *neuron,* nerve, + *osis,* condition] Any neurosis marked by speech disorders.

logopathia (lŏg-ō-păth′ē-ă) [″ + *pathos,* disease, suffering] Any disorder of speech arising from derangement of the central nervous system.

logopedia (lŏg″ō-pē′dē-ă) [″ + *pais,* child] The science dealing with speech defects and their correction.

logoplegia (lŏg-ō-plē′jē-ă) [″ + *plege,* stroke] Paralysis of the speech organs.

logorrhea (lŏg″ō-rē′ă) [″ + *rhoia,* flow] The repetitious, continuous, and excessive flow of speech seen in insanity. SYN: *logomania.*

logospasm (lŏg′ō-spăzm) [″ + *spasmos,* a convulsion] Spasmodic word enunciation.

-logy [Gr. *logos,* word, reason] Combining form used as a suffix meaning *science or study of.* SEE: *-ology.*

loiasis (lō-ī′ă-sĭs) Infection with the African eyeworm, *Loa loa.* SEE: *Loa loa* for illus.

loin (loyn) [O.Fr. *loigne,* long part] The lower part of the back and sides between the ribs and pelvis. SYN: *lumbus.*

lomustine (lō-mŭs′tēn) A chemotherapeutic agent used in treating certain neoplastic conditions; also called *CCNU.*

loneliness The anxious, depressed, or dysphoric mood that occurs as a result of physical or psychic isolation.

risk for l. A subjective state in which an individual is at risk of experiencing subjective isolation. SEE: *Nursing Diagnoses Appendix.*

Long, Crawford Williamson U.S. physician, 1815–1878, who in 1842 first administered an anesthetic during surgery.

long-acting thyroid stimulator ABBR: LATS. An IgG autoantibody that binds to the thyroid-stimulating hormone receptor, stimulating the excessive production of thyroid hormones and causes hyperthyroidism. This immunoglobulin is found in the blood of about 75% of patients with Graves' disease but is used rarely for diagnostic purposes, because the diagnosis usually can be established on clinical grounds, i.e., on finding a patient with hyperthyroidism with a diffuse, nontender goiter, exophthalmos, and/or pretibial myxedema.

longevity (lŏn-jĕv′ĭ-tē) [L. *longaevus,* aged] Long duration of life.

longing A persistent desire or craving for something, usually that which is remote or unattainable.

longissimus (lŏn-jĭs′ĭ-mŭs) [L.] An anatomical term indicating a long structure.

longitudinal (lŏn″jĭ-tū′dĭ-năl) [L. *longitudo,* length] Parallel to the long axis of the body or part.

longsightedness Hyperopia.

longus (lŏng′gŭs) [L.] An anatomical term indicating a long structure.

loop [ME. *loupe*] A curve or bend in a cord or cordlike structure, forming roughly an oval.

l. of capillary Minute blood vessels in the papillae of the skin.

cervical l. The part of an enamel organ in which the inner enamel epithelium is continuous with the outer enamel epithelium. This establishes the limit of enamel formation and therefore represents the site of the cementoenamel junction. The cells of the cervical loop become Hertwig's epithelial root sheath, induce dentinogenesis, and determine the number, size, and shape of the tooth roots.

closed l. A biological system in which a substance produced affects the output of the substance by a feedback mechanism.

flow-volume l. A graphic record of lung function in which the amount of gas inhaled and exhaled is recorded on the horizontal axis and the rate at which the gas moves on the vertical axis. It is used to detect abnormalities in pulmonary function such as those accompanying restrictive or obstructive lung disease.

Henle's l. Portion of a nephron formed by the descending and ascending limbs of the renal tubule.

Lippes l. SEE: *Lippes loop.*

loop electrode excision procedure ABBR: LEEP. A technique for resecting abnormal cervical tissue. Following an abnormal Pap smear, thin wire loop electrodes are used to excise the affected or suspicious area. LEEP provides a specimen suitable for histologic evaluation.

loosening of association A sign of disordered thought processes in which the person speaks with frequent changes of subject, and the content is only obliquely related, if at all, to the subject matter. This may be seen in mania or schizophrenia.

L.O.P. *left occipitoposterior* fetal position. SEE: *presentation* for illus.

loperamide hydrochloride Generic name for Imodium.

lophotrichea (lŏf-ō-trĭk′ē-ă) [Gr. *lophos,* tuft, + *thrix,* hair] Microorganisms possessing flagella in tufts.

lophotrichous (lŏf-ŏt′rĭ-kŭs) Having bunches of flagella at one end.

LOQ *limit of quantitation.*

loratadine (lor-ăh′tă-dēn) An antihistamine (H2-receptor antagonist) used to treat seasonal allergies and urticaria. Like other second-generation antihistamines (e.g., fexofenadine, cetirizine), it is less likely to cause sedation than traditional agents like diphenhydramine or hydroxyzine. Trade name is Claritin.

lorazepam (lō-rā′zĕ-pam) A relatively short-acting benzodiazepine used to treat anxiety, insomnia, seizures, and alcohol withdrawal. Trade name is Ativan.

lordoscoliosis (lor″dō-skō″lē-ō′sĭs) [Gr. *lordosis,* bending, + *skoliosis,* curvation] Forward curvation of the spine complicated by lateral curvature.

lordosis (lor-dō′sĭs) [Gr.] Abnormal anterior convexity of the lumbar spine.

loss 1. The basis of claim on the part of the insurance carrier. **2.** Destruction, degeneration, or the wasting of cells, tissues, organs, or capabilities.

pregnancy l. Spontaneous abortion.

loss, bone Osteoporosis.

loss of consciousness Syncope.

lost to follow-up In clinical medicine and research, a person who has not returned for continued care or evaluation (e.g., because of death, disability, relocation, or drop-out).

L.O.T. *left occipitotransverse* fetal position. SEE: *presentation* for illus.

lotion (lō′shŭn) [L. *lotio*] A liquid medicinal preparation for local application to, or bathing of, a part.

calamine l. SEE: *calamine.*

white l. A combination of 4% zinc sulfate with 4% sulfurated potash.

LOTR *Licensed Occupational Therapist.*

loudness Sound intensity. SEE: *decibel.*

Louis-Bar syndrome (loo-wē′băr) [Denise Louis-Bar, 20th century European physician] Ataxia-telangiectasia.

loupe (loop) [Fr.] A magnifying lens used in the form of a monocular or binocular lens. Surgeons, dentists, jewelers, and watchmakers frequently use this device.

louse [AS. *lus*] Pediculus.

body l. *Pediculus humanus corporis.*

crab l. *Phthirus inguinalis* and *Phthirus pubis;* the louse that infests the pubic region and other hairy areas of the body. SEE: *pediculosis.*

head l. *Pediculus humanus capitis.* SEE: illus.

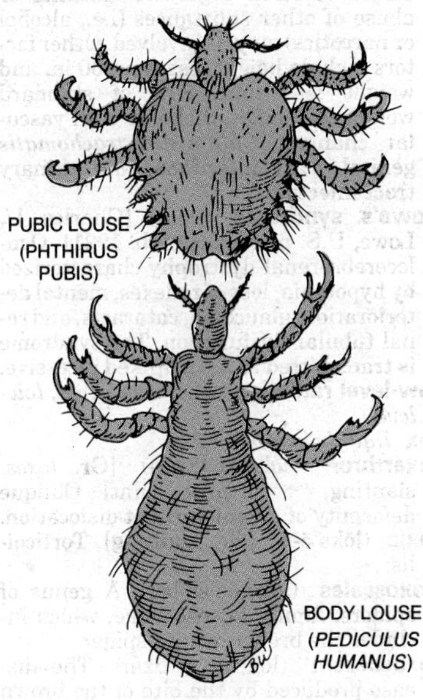

LOUSE

lousiness Pediculosis.

lovastatin A drug used to control the level of cholesterol in the blood by inhibiting the synthesis of cholesterol. This medication is an inhibitor of the enzyme HMG CoA-reductase (3-hydroxy-3-methylglutaryl-coenzyme A reductase) and belongs to a class of medications called the "statins." Trade name is Mevacor.

love [ME.] **1.** Profound concern and affection for another person. **2.** In psychoanalysis, love may be equated with pleasure, particularly as it applies to the gratifying sexual experiences between individuals.

Loven's reflex (lō-vānz′) [Otto Christian

Loven, Swed. physician, 1835–1904] Vasodilation with a corresponding increase in blood pressure in an organ, resulting from stimulation of an afferent nerve.

low birth weight ABBR: LBW. Abnormally low weight of a newborn, usually less than 2500 g. A 280-g infant has survived, but with physical and mental impairment.

Identifying mothers at risk for delivery of LBW infants involves careful assessment. Demographic factors include maternal age (adolescence) and nonwhite race; the highest risk occurs in primiparas under the age of 15. A review of the mother's history often finds low birth weight or prepregnancy weight, previous preterm delivery or spontaneous abortion, delivery of other LBW newborns, or fetal exposure to diethylstilbestrol. Cigarette smoking or abuse of other substances (i.e., alcohol or narcotics) may be involved. Other factors include height less than 60 in. and weight less than 80% of standard weight for height, diabetes with vascular changes, *Chlamydia trachomatis* genital tract infections, and urinary tract infections.

Lowe's syndrome (lōz) [Charles U. Lowe, U.S. pediatrician, b. 1921] Oculocerebrorenal dystrophy characterized by hypotonia, loss of reflexes, mental deterioration, glaucoma, cataracts, and renal tubular dysfunction. The syndrome is transmitted as a sex-linked recessive.

low-level radiation SEE: *radiation, low-level.*

lox *liquid oxygen.*

loxarthron (lŏks-ăr'thrŏn) [Gr. *loxos,* slanting, + *arthron,* joint] Oblique deformity of a joint without dislocation.

loxia (lŏks'ē-ă) [Gr., slanting] Torticollis.

Loxosceles (lŏks-ŏs'sĕ-lēz) A genus of spiders, family Loxoscelidae, which includes the brown recluse spider.

loxoscelism (lŏk-sŏs'sĕ-lĭzm) The disease produced by the bite of the brown recluse spider, *Loxosceles laeta* or *L. reclusa.* Symptoms include a painful red vesicle that eventually becomes necrotic, leaving a skin ulcer. Rarely, the spider bite may produce hemolytic anemia or renal failure.

loxotomy (lŏks-ŏt'ō-mē) [" + *tome,* incision] Amputation by oblique section.

lozenge (lŏz'ĕnj) [Fr.] A small, dry, medicinal solid to be held in the mouth until it dissolves. SYN: *troche.*

Lp(a) *lipoprotein (a).*

L-phase variants L-forms.

L.P.N. *licensed practical nurse.*

LPO *left posterior oblique* position.

Lr Symbol for the element lawrencium.

L.R.C.P. *licentiate of the Royal College of Physicians.*

L.R.C.S. *licentiate of the Royal College of Surgeons.*

LRF *luteinizing hormone releasing factor.*

L.S.A. *left sacroanterior* fetal position. SEE: *presentation* for illus.

L.Sc.A. *left scapuloanterior* fetal position. SEE: *presentation* for illus.

L.Sc.P. *left scapuloposterior* fetal position. SEE: *presentation* for illus.

LSD *lysergic acid diethylamide.*

LSI *life satisfaction index.*

L.S.P. *left sacroposterior* fetal position.

L/S ratio *lecithin/sphingomyelin ratio.*

L.S.T. *left sacrotransverse* fetal position.

l.t.c. *long-term care.*

LTH *luteotropic hormone.*

Lu Symbol for the element lutetium.

lubb-dupp (lŭb-dŭp') The two sounds heard in auscultation of the heart technically referred to as S_1 ("lubb") and S_2 ("dupp"). The pause following the sounds is slightly longer than that between the two sounds. SEE: *auscultation.*

lubricant (loo'brĭ-kănt) [L. *lubricans*] An agent, usually a liquid oil, that reduces friction between parts that brush against each other as they move. Joints are lubricated by synovial fluid.

Lucas-Championnière's disease (lū-kă' shaw"pē-ŏn-ē-ayrz') [J. M. M. Lucas-Championnière, Fr. surgeon, 1843–1913] Pseudomembranous bronchitis.

lucent [L. *lucere,* to shine] Shining, translucent, clear.

lucid (lū'sĭd) [L. *lucidus,* clear] Clear, esp. applied to clarity of the mind.

l. interval **1.** A brief remission of symptoms in a psychosis. **2.** Following a head injury, a brief period when the patient appears alert before the mental status deteriorates further. **3.** A brief period of mental clarity between seizures, or between a seizure and a postictal psychosis.

lucidity (lū-sĭd'ĭ-tē) The quality of clearness or brightness, esp. with regard to mental conditions.

luciferase (loo-sĭf'ĕr-ās) An enzyme that acts on luciferins to oxidize them and cause bioluminescence. It is present in certain organisms (e.g., fireflies, other insects) that emit light either continuously or intermittently.

luciferin (loo-sĭf'ĕr-ĭn) The general term for substances present in some organisms, which become luminescent when acted on by luciferase.

lucifugal (loo-sĭf'ū-găl) [L. *lux,* light, + *fugere,* to flee from] Repelled by bright light.

lucipetal (loo-sĭp'ĭ-tăl) [" + *peter,* to seek] Attracted by bright light.

lucotherapy (lū"kō-thĕr'ă-pē) [" + Gr. *therapeia,* treatment] Phototherapy.

Ludwig's angina (lūd'vĭgz) [Wilhelm F. von Ludwig, Ger. surgeon, 1790–1865] A suppurative inflammation of subcutaneous connective tissue adjacent to a submaxillary gland.

L.U.E. *left upper extremity.*

lues (lū′ēz) [L.] Syphilis.

luetic (lū-ĕt′ĭk) Syphilitic.

Lugol's solution (lū′gŏlz) [Jean G. A. Lugol, Fr. physician, 1786–1851] A strong iodine solution used in iodine therapy, consisting of iodine 5 g, potassium iodide 10 g, and water to make 100 ml.

LUL *left upper lobe* (of the lung).

lumbago (lŭm-bā′gō) [L. *lumbus,* loin] A general nonspecific term for dull, aching pain in the lumbar region of the back. SYN: *lumbodynia.*

lumbar (lŭm′băr) [L. *lumbus,* loin] Pert. to the loins; the part of the back between the thorax and pelvis.

l. puncture Gaining entry into the subarachnoid space of the meningeal sac below the end of the spinal cord, usually at the level of the fourth intervertebral space with a hollow needle. This procedure is done to obtain cerebrospinal fluid (CSF) for analysis (e.g., in the diagnosis of severe headache or in suspected central nervous system infection or bleeding); to administer drugs to the brain or spinal cord (e.g. anesthetics or chemotherapeutic agents); or to relieve the CSF of excess pressure or fluid (e.g., in pseudotumor cerebri). SYN: *spinal puncture.* SEE: illus.; *cisternal puncture; headache; Queckenstedt's sign.*

CAUTION: The procedure is contraindicated in patients with increased intracranial pressure because of the risk of herniation of the brain through the foramen magnum at the base of the skull.

PROCEDURE: Informed consent for the procedure is obtained, except in dire emergencies, when clinical judgment prevails. Next, the patient's skin is prepared with antiseptic solution and a sterile fenestrated barrier placed over the proposed puncture site. Local anesthetic is given, the patient is placed to facilitate access to the spinal canal, and then the spinal needle, with its stylet in place, is slowly advanced between the vertebra to and through the dura and arachnoid membranes. The stylet that fills the needle is removed, and spinal fluid is collected. Initial measurements are made of the opening pressure with a manometer. When the procedure is performed for diagnosis, about 8 to 10 ml of fluid are collected and sent to the laboratory. SEE: illus.

COMPLICATIONS: Pain at the puncture site, infection, bleeding, neurological injury, death, and post–spinal tap headaches are all potential complications. Of these, postural headache, caused by chronic leakage from the puncture site, is the complication most often brought to the attention of health care professionals. It may be treated with the injection of a small amount of the patient's own blood epidurally, to form a "blood patch." SEE: *cerebrospinal fluid.*

PATIENT CARE: The procedure, ex-

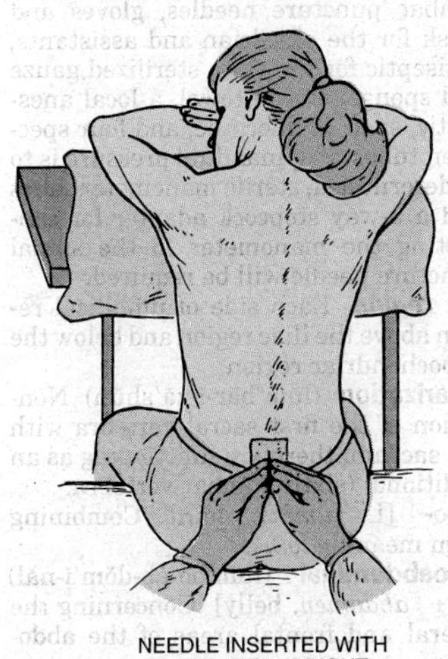
NEEDLE INSERTED WITH PATIENT IN UPRIGHT POSITION WITH HEAD AND SPINE BENT FORWARD

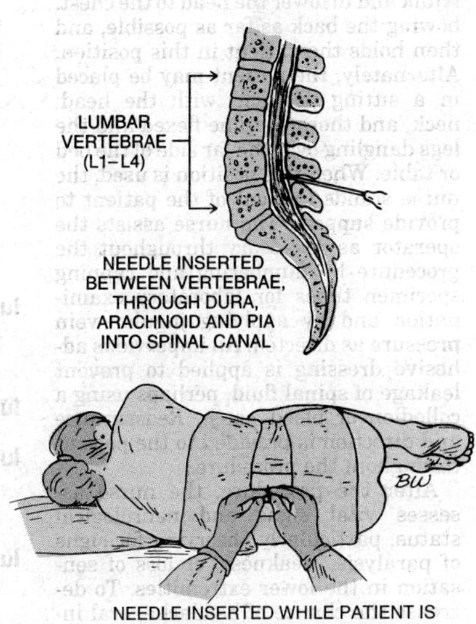

NEEDLE INSERTED WHILE PATIENT IS ON FIRM SURFACE AND WITH HEAD AND SPINE BENT FORWARD

LUMBAR PUNCTURE

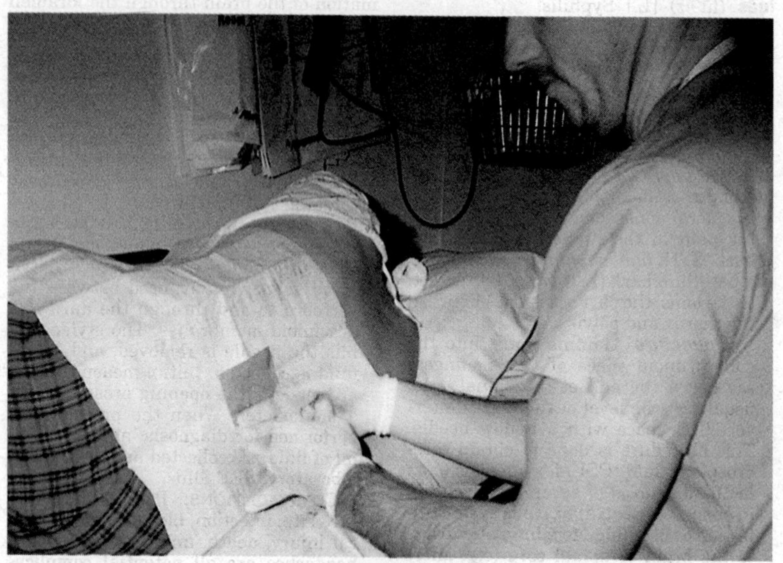

LUMBAR PUNCTURE

pected sensations, and the patient's role are explained to reassure the patient, and a signed informed consent form is obtained. Required equipment is assembled and prepared. The patient is positioned on the left side near the right edge of the bed or examining table, with the back to the operator. The nurse assists the patient to flex the thighs on the trunk and to lower the head to the chest, bowing the back as far as possible, and then holds the patient in this position. Alternately, the patient may be placed in a sitting position, with the head, neck, and thoracic spine flexed and the legs dangling over the far side of the bed or table. When this position is used, the nurse stands in front of the patient to provide support. The nurse assists the operator as necessary throughout the procedure by numbering and capping specimen tubes for laboratory examination and by applying jugular vein pressure as directed. An impervious adhesive dressing is applied to prevent leakage of spinal fluid, perhaps using a collodion or blood patch. Reassurance and direction is provided to the patient throughout the procedure.

After the procedure, the nurse assesses vital signs and neurological status, particularly observing for signs of paralysis, weakness, or loss of sensation in the lower extremities. To decrease the chance of headache, oral intake (for spinal fluid replacement and equalization of pressures) is encouraged, and the patient should remain in bed in a prone position for 4 to 24 hr (per operator or institutional protocol). While the patient should not lift the head, he or she can move it (and himself or herself) from side to side. Noninvasive pain relief measures and prescribed analgesia are provided if headache occurs.

ARTICLES NECESSARY: Sterilized lumbar puncture needles, gloves and mask for the physician and assistants, antiseptic for the skin, sterilized gauze and sponge, sterile towel, a local anesthetic, such as lidocaine, and four specimen tubes. If spinal fluid pressure is to be determined, sterile manometer tubes and a 3-way stopcock adapter for connecting the manometer to the spinal puncture needle will be required.

l. region Each side of umbilical region above the iliac region and below the hypochondriac region.

lumbarization (lŭm″băr-ĭ-zā′shŭn) Nonfusion of the first sacral vertebra with the sacrum, therefore functioning as an additional (sixth) lumbar vertebra.

lumbo- [L. *lumbus,* loin] Combining form meaning *loins*.

lumboabdominal (lŭm″bō-ăb-dŏm′ĭ-năl) [″ + *abdomen,* belly] Concerning the lateral and frontal areas of the abdomen.

lumbocolostomy (lŭm″bō-kō-lŏs′tō-mē) [″ + Gr. *kolon,* colon, + *stoma,* mouth] Colostomy by lumbar incision.

lumbocolotomy (lŭm″bō-kō-lŏt′ō-mē) [″ + ″ + *tome,* incision] Incision into the colon through the lumbar region.

lumbocostal (lŭm″bō-kŏs′tăl) [″ +

costa, rib] Relating to the loins and ribs.

lumbodynia (lŭm″bō-dĭn′ē-ă) [″ + Gr. *odyne,* pain] Lumbago.

lumboiliac (lŭm″bō-ĭl′ē-ăk) [″ + *iliacus,* pert. to ilium] Concerning the lumbar and inguinal areas. SYN: *lumboinguinal.*

lumboinguinal (lŭm″bō-ĭng′gwĭ-năl) [″ + *inguinalis,* pert. to the groin] Lumboiliac.

lumbosacral Pert. to the lumbar vertebrae and the sacrum.

lumbrical (lŭm′brĭ-kăl) [L. *lumbricus,* earthworm] Vermiform.

lumbricalis One of the worm-shaped muscles of the hand or foot.

lumbricide (lŭm′brĭ-sīd) [″ + *caedere,* to kill] An agent that kills lumbricoid worms (i.e., ascarides or intestinal worms).

lumbricoid (lŭm′brĭ-koyd) [″ + Gr. *eidos,* form, shape] Resembling a roundworm.

lumbricosis (lŭm″brĭ-kō′sĭs) [″ + Gr. *osis,* condition] The state of being infested with lumbricoid worms.

Lumbricus (lŭm-brī′kŭs) A genus of worms that includes earthworms.

lumbricus (lŭm-brī′kŭs) *Ascaris lumbricoides.*

lumbus [L.] The loin; the part of the back between the thorax and pelvis.

lumen (lū′mĕn) *pl.* **lumina** [L., light] **1.** The space within an artery, vein, intestine, or tube. **2.** A unit of light, the amount of light emitted in a unit solid angle by a uniform point source of one international candle. SEE: *light unit; candela.*

luminal (lū′mĭ-năl) Relating to the lumen of a tubular structure, such as a blood vessel.

luminescence (loo″mĭ-nĕs′ĕns) **1.** Production of light without production of heat. SEE: *bioluminescence.* **2.** In radiology, the light produced by a fluorescent phosphor when exposed to radiation.

luminiferous (loo″mĭ-nĭf′ĕr-ŭs) [L. *lumen,* light, + *ferre,* to bear] Producing or conveying light.

luminometer A luminescence photometer used to assay chemluminescent and bioluminescent reactions. It is used clinically to assay for bacteria and living cells.

luminophore (loo′mĭ-nō-for″) [″ + Gr. *phoros,* bearing] A chemical present in organic compounds that permits luminescence of those compounds.

luminous (loo′mĭ-nŭs) Emitting light.

lumirhodopsin (loo″mĭ-rō-dŏp′sĭn) A chemical in the retina of the eye, intermediate between rhodopsin and all-*trans*-retinal plus opsin, formed during the bleaching of rhodopsin by exposure to light.

lumpectomy (lŭm-pĕk′tō-mē) [*lump* + Gr. *ektome,* excision] Surgical removal of a tumor from the breast, esp. to remove only the tumor and no other tissue or lymph nodes.

lunacy (lū′nă-sē) [L. *luna,* moon] An obsolete term for insanity. Insanity was formerly thought to be affected by the moon.

lunar Pert. to the moon, a month, or silver.

lunate **1.** Moon-shaped or crescent. **2.** A bone in the proximal row of the carpus. SYN: *semilunar bone.*

lunatic (lū′nă-tĭk) [L. *luna,* moon] An obsolete term for a person with an unsound mind. SEE: *lunacy.*

lung (lŭng) [AS. *lungen*] One of two cone-shaped spongy organs of respiration contained within the pleural cavity of the thorax. SEE: illus.; *alveolus* for illus.

Anatomy: The lungs are connected with the pharynx through the trachea and larynx. The base of each lung rests on the diaphragm and each lung apex rises from 2.5 to 5 cm above the sternal end of the first rib, the collarbone, supported by its attachment to the hilum or root structures. The lungs include the lobes, lobules, bronchi, bronchioles, alveoli or air sacs, and pleural covering.

The right lung has three lobes and the left two. In men, the right lung weighs approx. 625 g, the left 570 g. The lungs contain 300,000,000 alveoli and their respiratory surface is about 70 sq m. Respirations per minute are 12 to 20 in an adult. The total capacity of the lung varies from 3.6 to 9.4 L in men and 2.5 to 6.9 L in women.

The left lung has an indentation, called the cardiac depression, for the normal placement of the heart. Behind this is the hilum, through which the blood vessels, lymphatics, and bronchi enter and leave the lung.

Air travels from the nasal passage to the pharynx and the trachea. Two primary bronchi, one on each side, extend from the trachea. The primary bronchi divide into secondary bronchi, one for each of five lobes. These further divide into a great number of smaller bronchioles. The pattern of distribution of these into the segments of each lobe is important in pulmonary and thoracic surgery. There are about 10 bronchopulmonary segments in the right lung and eight in the left, the actual number varying. There are 50 to 80 terminal bronchioles in each lobe. Each of these divides into two respiratory bronchioles, which in turn divide to form two to 11 alveolar ducts. The alveolar sacs and alveoli arise from these ducts. The spaces between the alveolar sacs and alveoli are called atria.

In the alveolus, blood and inspired air are separated only by the cell of the al-

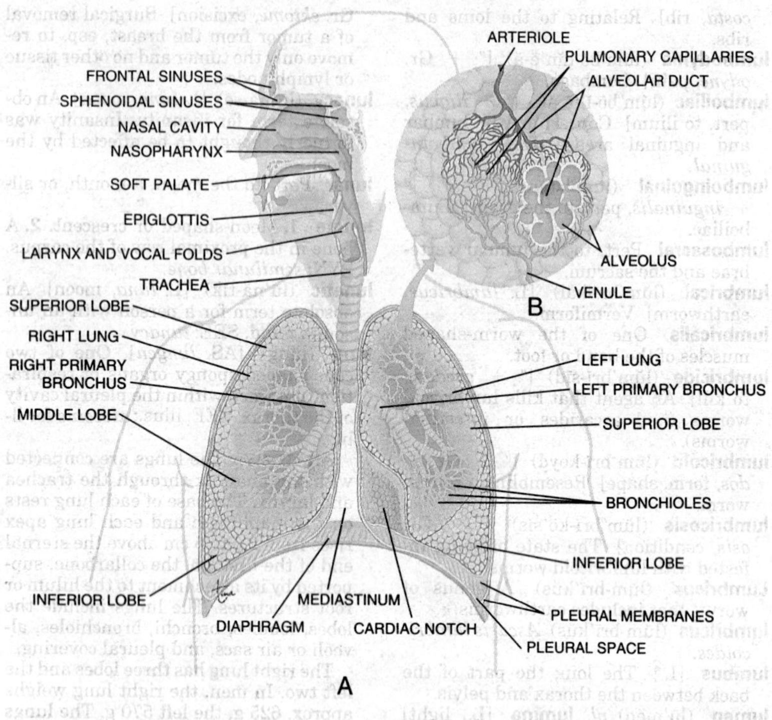

LUNGS

(A) anterior view of upper and lower respiratory tracts, (B) alveoli and pulmonary capillaries

veolus and that of the pulmonary capillary. This respiratory membrane is thin (0.07 to 2.0 μm) and permits oxygen to diffuse into the blood and carbon dioxide to diffuse from the blood to the air.

NERVE SUPPLY: The lungs are innervated by parasympathetic fibers via the vagus nerve and sympathetic fibers from the anterior and posterior pulmonary plexuses to the smooth muscle in the walls of the bronchial tree.

BLOOD VESSELS: The bronchial arteries and veins circulate blood to the bronchial tree. The pulmonary arteries and veins circulate the blood involved in gas exchange.

FUNCTION: The primary purpose of the lung is to bring air and blood into intimate contact so that oxygen can be added to the blood and carbon dioxide removed from it. This is achieved by two pumping systems, one moving a gas and the other a liquid. The blood and air are brought together so closely that only approx. 1 μm (10^{-6} m) of tissue separates them. The volume of the pulmonary capillary circulation is 150 ml, but this is spread out over a surface area of approx. 750 sq ft (69.68 sq m). This capillary surface area surrounds 300 million air sacs called alveoli. The blood that is low in oxygen but high in carbon dioxide is in contact with the air that is high in oxygen and low in carbon dioxide for less than 1 second. SEE: *respiratory defense function*.

PHYSICAL EXAMINATION: *Inspection:* The examiner determines the respiratory rate by unobtrusively watching the patient's chest rise and fall and counting the number of breaths per minute. In adults a normal respiratory rate at rest is about 12 breaths per minute. While counting the respiratory rate, the examiner can observe other breathing characteristics. Dyspneic patients breathe rapidly, often laboring to draw breath even when at rest. Retractions of the intercostal and supraclavicular spaces are visible during inspiration. Sleep apnea is characterized by episodes of stalled breathing followed by periods of respiratory compensation. Regular slow breathing is normal.

Palpation: In health, the chest and lung transmit a vibration, called fremitus, during speech. Fremitus abnormalities may be felt in chronic obstructive lung diseases or obesity, in which the vibration is diminished, and in pneumonia, in which it is increased over the infected lobe.

Percussion: Tapping on the chest wall over healthy lung results in a hollow resonant sound. The hollow character of the resonance sometimes is exaggerated in emphysematous lungs or in pneumothorax, and muffled by pleural effusions or pulmonary consolidation.

AUSCULTATION: *Normal breath sounds:* In the healthy person, breath sounds are low-pitched and have a frequency of 200 to 400 cycles per second (cps); frequency rarely exceeds 500 cps. These sounds are called vesicular breath sounds when heard over the lungs. They are produced by air passing in and out of the airways.

Bronchial and tracheal breath sounds: These are higher-pitched and louder than vesicular sounds, and are produced by air passing over the walls of the bronchi and trachea. These sounds are normally heard only over the bronchi and trachea.

Amphoric and cavernous breathing: These two nearly identical sounds are loud, with a prolonged, hollow expiration. The pitch of amphoric breathing is slightly higher than that of the cavernous type, and may be imitated by blowing over the mouth of an empty jar. It is heard in bronchiectatic cavities or pneumothorax when the opening to the lung is patulous; in the consolidation area near a large bronchus; and sometimes over a lung compressed by a moderate effusion.

Harsh inspiratory sounds are typical of stridor, a medical emergency. Expirations that are prolonged and musical are characteristic of wheezing.

Friction: This sound is produced by the rubbing together of roughened pleural surfaces. It may be heard in both inspiration and expiration. Friction often resembles crackles, but is more superficial and localized than the latter and is not modified by cough or deep inspiration.

Metallic tinkling: A silvery bell-like sound heard at intervals over a hydropneumothorax or large cavity. Speaking, coughing, and deep breathing usually induce this sound. It must not be confused with a similar sound produced by liquids in the stomach.

Crackles: Abnormal bubbling sounds heard in air cells or bronchi.

Succussion-splash or hippocratic succussion: A splashing sound produced by the presence of air and liquid in the chest. It may be elicited by gently shaking the patient during auscultation. This sound nearly always indicates either a hydropneumothorax or a pyopneumothorax, although it has also been detected over very large cavities. The presence of air and liquid in the stomach produces similar sounds.

l. abscess Circumscribed suppuration of the lung, caused by infectious microorganisms. SEE: *empyema*.

SYMPTOMS: This condition is characterized by high and irregular fever, rigors, sweats, and pallor; dyspnea, cough, and purulent expectoration. On exam, there may be bubbling rales, cavernous breathing and pectoriloquy.

TREATMENT: The basic cause of the abscess should be treated. Antimicrobial therapy is given. Surgical drainage of the abscess is rarely necessary.

acute edema of l. Pulmonary edema.

blast l. The shredding-type effect that takes place in the alveolar surfaces of the lung caused by the shock of an explosion or blast, which can cause alveolar contusion.

brewer's l. An allergic respiratory condition caused by the mold *Aspergillus*.

compliance of l. A measure of the distensibility of the lungs. It is expressed as the change in volume of the lungs in liters when the transpulmonary pressure is changed by 1 cm of water pressure. Normally this measure is between 0.08 and 0.33 L/cm of water. It is reduced by abnormalities that stiffen the lungs or chest wall.

flock worker's l. Interstitial lung disease that results from the inhalation of airborne nylon fibers at work. Nylon fibers, which can cause inflammatory damage to the lungs, are used in making products for upholstery, automobiles, carpet, and apparel.

l. inflammation Pneumonia.

honeycomb l. An abnormal appearance of the lungs seen on chest x-ray exam, in which small cystic spaces alternate with coarsely increased interstitial markings. This pattern is typical of pulmonary injury caused by inhalation of dusts, minerals, toxic gases, or fibers; rheumatological diseases; and interstitial pneumonitis.

iron l. Drinker respirator.

shock l. A diffuse lung injury, causing reduced perfusion, pulmonary edema, and alveolar collapse, associated with acute respiratory distress syndrome. SYN: *wet l.*

l. surfactant Pulmonary surfactant.

l. transplantation Grafting of a donor lung into a recipient with end-stage lung disease, usually caused by pulmonary fibrosis, chronic obstructive lung disease, or pulmonary hypertension. Lung transplantation may be performed as a single-organ operation or as part of a combined heart-lung transplantation (e.g., in congenital heart disease). Immunosuppressive therapy with cyclosporine or tacrolimus, azathioprine, and corticosteroids is necessary to minimize the risk of rejection, which is caused by T lymphocyte activity against the donor tissue. Rejection is diagnosed through the use of bronchial biopsies and pulmonary function tests. Acute rejection, characterized by dyspnea, fever, hypoxemia, rales, and tachypnea, must be differentiated from infection. Chronic rejection, a problem in 25% to 50% of cases, presents as bronchiolitis obliterans and occurs 6 to 14 months after the transplant. Flow rates progressively decrease, with few additional symptoms; bronchodilator therapy is not effective, and giving higher doses of immunosuppressives has mixed success. Sixty percent of lung transplant recipients live 2 years.

wet l. Shock l.

lung collapse **1.** Atelectasis. **2.** Compression of lung caused by pneumothorax, hydrothorax, or hemothorax.

TREATMENT: Bronchial hygiene, postural drainage, and percussion are used to assist in mucus removal for those patients with atelectasis due to mucus plugging. Bronchoscopy may also be useful in these patients. Chest tubes are inserted to drain air or fluid from the pleural cavity when present.

lungworm (lŭng′wĕrm) Any of the nematodes that infest the lungs of humans and animals.

lunula (lū′nū-lă) *pl.* **lunulae** [L., little moon] **1.** A crescent-shaped area. **2.** An active area of nailbed growth at the base of the fingernails and toenails. The cells develop and keratinize to form nails.

l. of valves of heart One of two narrow portions on the free edges of the semilunar valves on each side of the nodulus.

lupiform (lū′pĭ-form) [L. *lupus,* wolf, + *forma,* shape] Resembling lupus.

lupoid (loo′poyd) [″ + Gr. *eidos,* form, shape] **1.** Resembling lupus. **2.** Boeck's sarcoid.

lupous (lū′pŭs) **1.** Pert. to lupus. **2.** Affected with lupus.

lupus (lū′pŭs) [L., wolf] Originally any chronic, progressive, usually ulcerating, skin disease. In current usage when the word is used alone, it has no precise meaning.

discoid l. erythematosus ABBR: DLE. A chronic skin disease characterized by periodic acute appearances of a scaling, red, macular rash. DLE is caused by an autoimmune process involving both B-cell– and T-cell–mediated mechanisms that destroy the skin's basal cells. DLE is treated with topical corticosteroids. It is found in about 5% to 30% of patients who have systemic lupus erythematosus (SLE) (esp. those who smoke) but also may occur alone (without other findings of SLE). SEE: *autoimmune d.; systemic l. erythematosus.*

TREATMENT: The patient should avoid exposure to the sun. Skin lesions should be treated with topical corticosteroids, but overuse of these preparations should be avoided.

drug-induced systemic l. erythematosus A group of signs and symptoms similar to those of systemic lupus erythematosus, caused by an adverse reaction to drugs, esp. procainamide, hydralazine, and isoniazid. Joint inflammation and pain, skin rash, pleurisy, and fever are the most common manifestations; kidney and central nervous system involvement are rare. Antinuclear antibodies, specifically against the histones that fold DNA, are common. Some patients develop antinuclear antibodies but do not develop lupus-like symptoms. The lupus-like syndrome usually disappears when the drug causing it is discontinued. SEE: *antinuclear antibodies; systemic lupus erythematosus.*

l. pernio Skin lesions sometimes present in sarcoidosis. They are hard, blue-purple, swollen, shiny lesions of the nose, cheeks, lips, ears, fingers, and knees.

systemic l. erythematosus ABBR: SLE. A chronic autoimmune inflammatory disease involving multiple organ systems and marked by periodic acute episodes. Its name is derived from the characteristic erythematous "butterfly" rash over the nose and cheeks, which resembles a wolf's snout. The disease is most prevalent in women of childbearing age. SEE: *Nursing Diagnoses Appendix.*

ETIOLOGY AND PATHOLOGY: SLE is classified as an autoimmune disease in which the body seems to be unable to maintain normal mechanisms of tolerance to self-antigens. Activation of T helper cells and B cells results in the production of autoantibodies that attack antigens in the cytoplasm and nucleus of cells and on the surface of blood cells. The exact etiology of SLE is unknown; genetic defects, hormonal changes, and environmental triggers are possible predisposing factors. SEE: *autoimmune d.; glomerulonephritis.*

Autoantibodies can react with self-antigens to form immune complexes in such large numbers that they cannot be completely excreted; the immune complexes may precipitate within blood vessels, producing inflammation at the site and disrupting the flow of blood and oxygen to tissues. These deposits are particularly damaging in the glomeruli. Autoantibodies also promote the destruction of cells by stimulating neutrophil and macrophage phagocytic activity, which increases cell destruction from trauma, infection, or drugs.

DIAGNOSIS: In 1997, revised criteria

for diagnosis of SLE were established. The diagnosis can be made if four or more of the following criteria are present, either at one time or sequentially: 1. butterfly rash; 2. raised, scaly discoid skin lesions; 3. antinuclear antibodies seen by immunofluorescence; 4. immunological disorders including lupus erythematosus (LE) cells or other autoantibodies; 5. pleuritis or pericarditis; 6. hemolytic anemia, leukopenia (white blood cell count less than 4,000 mm^3), lymphopenia (lymphocyte count less than $1,500/mm^3$), or thrombocytopenia of less than $100,000/mm^3$; 7. oral or nasopharyngeal ulcers; 8. nonerosive arthritis; 9. psychosis or convulsions without clear cause; 10. photosensitivity skin rash; 11. proteinuria greater than 0.5 g/day or cellular casts in the urine.

Some drugs can cause a lupus-like syndrome; the most common of these are procainamide, isoniazid, and hydralazine. SEE: *drug-induced systemic l. erythematosus*.

SYMPTOMS: Patients have a wide diversity of clinical symptoms, signs, and laboratory findings, but anemia, thrombocytopenia, polyarthritis, skin rashes, glomerulonephritis, fever, malaise, weight loss, and low blood levels of complement are the most common. Other signs include pleuritis, pericarditis, myocarditis, gastrointestinal ulcerations, Raynaud's phenomenon, and other problems caused by inflammatory changes of the blood vessels or connective tissue. Most patients are prone to infection.

TREATMENT: No cure for SLE exists, and complete remission is rare. About 25% of patients have mild disease, demonstrating only minor skin and hematological signs, and can be treated with nonsteroidal anti-inflammatory drugs. Rashes may respond to antimalarials (e.g., Plaquenil), but patients must be observed closely for the possibility of drug-induced retinal damage. Other treatments for skin rash include sunscreens, quinacrine, retinoids, and dapsone. Life-threatening and severely disabling conditions should be treated with high doses of corticosteroids and supplemental calcium to minimize osteoporosis, which may be an undesired side effect of long-term glucocorticoid use. Immunosuppressive drugs are used for severe exacerbations and to reduce steroid dosage.

PROGNOSIS: The prognosis depends on which organ systems are involved, how severely they are damaged, and how rapidly the disease progresses. Ten-year survival rates are high (80%). Renal failure and infections are the most common causes of death.

PATIENT CARE: Patient education related to the disease and treatment is essential in any chronic disease. The purpose, proper dosage, use, and side effects of drugs should be taught. Patients need emotional support to help cope with changes in appearance because of skin lesions or when high-dose corticosteroids are given. Patients should be taught to wear clothing and hats that block direct sunlight and to maintain a diet high in potassium and protein. The nurse should help establish a regimen for adequate relief of both the musculoskeletal pain and chronic fatigue experienced by most patients. Additional support and teaching depend on the organ system most affected by the disease. Over time, patients with severe progressive disease need assistance in coping with the probability of an early death.

l. vulgaris Tuberculosis of the skin; characterized by patches that break down and ulcerate, leaving scars on healing.

LUQ *left upper quadrant* of abdomen.

Luque wires Wires used in the surgical stabilization of scoliosis. Transverse traction on each vertebra is accomplished by wrapping flexible wires around the affected vertebrae and attaching the wires to flexible rods.

Lust's reflex (lŭsts) [Franz Alexander Lust, Ger. pediatrician, b. 1880] Dorsal flexion and abduction of the foot resulting from percussion of the external branch of the sciatic nerve.

lute, luting agent (LOOT) A compound used in dentistry to bond surfaces together and make them impermeable. Compounds identified as luting agents may be cements, resins, or glass ionomers.

luteal [L. *luteus,* yellow] Pert. to the corpus luteum, its cells, or its hormones.

lutein (lū′tē-ĭn) Yellow pigment derived from the corpus luteum, egg yolk, and fat cells or lipochromes.

luteinic (loo″tē-ĭn′ĭk) Concerning the corpus luteum of the ovary.

luteinization (lū″tē-ĭn-ĭ-zā′shŭn) The process of development of the corpus luteum within a ruptured graafian follicle.

Lutembacher's syndrome (loo′tĕm-băk″ĕrz) [René Lutembacher, Fr. physician, 1884–1916] Atrial septal defect of the heart with mitral stenosis.

luteolysin (loo″tē-ō-lī′sĭn) [L. *luteus,* yellow, + Gr. *lysis,* dissolution] Something that promotes death of the corpus luteum.

luteoma (lū″tē-ō′mă) [L. *luteus,* yellow, + Gr. *oma,* tumor] An ovarian tumor containing lutein cells.

luteotropin (loo″tē-ō-trō′pĭn) Luteinizing hormone.

lutetium (lū-tē′shē-ŭm) SYMB: Lu. A rare element; atomic weight 174.97; atomic number 71.

luteum (lū'tē-ŭm) [L.] Yellow.

luting (lut-in) Cementation.

Lutz-Splendore-Almeida disease [A. Lutz, Brazilian physician, 1855–1940; A. Splendore, contemp. Italian physician; Floriano P. de Almeida, Brazilian physician, b. 1898] South American blastomycosis.

lux (lŭks) [L., light] A unit of light intensity equivalent to 1 lumen/sq m.

luxatio erecta (lūks-ă'sē-ō ē-rĕk'tah) Subglenoid displacement of the head of the humerus associated with disruption of the rotator cuff.

luxation (lŭks-ā'shŭn) [L. *luxatio,* dislocation] **1.** Displacement of organs or articular surfaces; complete dislocation of a joint. SEE: *subluxation.* **2.** In dentistry, injury to supporting tissues that results in the loosening of the teeth with rotation or partial displacement.

Luys' body (lū-ēz') [Jules-Bernard Luys, Fr. physician, 1828–1898] A small mass of gray matter lying on the dorsal surface of the peduncle dorsolateral to the substantia nigra of the brain. Luys' nucleus is located in the posterior portion of the thalamus.

LV *left ventricle.*

LVEDP *left ventricular end-diastolic pressure.*

L.V.N. *licensed vocational nurse.*

lyase (lī'ās) The class name for enzymes (such as decarboxylase, aldolase, and synthases) that remove chemical groups other than by hydrolysis.

lycanthropy (lī-kăn'thrō-pē) [Gr. *lykos,* wolf, + *anthropos,* man] A mania in which one believes oneself to be a wild beast, esp. a wolf.

lycopene (lī'kō-pēn) An antioxidant red carotenoid pigment found in tomatoes and other red fruits and berries.

lycopenemia (lī"kō-pĕ-nē'mē-ă) [*lycopene* + Gr. *haima,* blood] A type of carotenemia caused by eating excessive amount of foods that contain lycopene.

lycoperdonosis (lī"kō-pĕr"dŏn-ō'sĭs) [Gr. *lykos,* wolf, + *perdesthai,* to break wind, + *osis,* condition] A respiratory disease caused by inhaling large quantities of spores from the mature mushroom commonly called puffball. *Lycoperdon* is the genus of fungi to which most puffballs belong.

lycopodium (lī-kō-pō'dē-ŭm) A yellow powder formed from spores of *Lycopodium clavatum,* a club moss. It is used as a dusting powder and as a desiccant, and absorbent.

lye (lī) [AS. *leag*] **1.** Liquid from leaching of wood ashes. **2.** Any strong alkaline solution, esp. sodium or potassium hydroxide. SEE: *alkali; potassium hydroxide; sodium hydroxide.*

lye poisoning SEE: *Poisons and Poisoning Appendix.*

lying-in **1.** Historical term for the puerperal state. **2.** Being hospitalized for the purpose of childbearing.

Lyme disease [Lyme, CT, where the disease was originally described] ABBR: LD. A multisystem disorder caused by the spirochete *Borrelia burgdorferi* that is the most common tick-borne disease in the U.S. The disease is endemic in New England, on Long Island, and in the Pacific Northwest. It occurs most often in the spring and summer, when its deer tick vectors (from the genus *Ixodes*) are most active. Prompt removal of ticks from the skin before they become attached or gain access to the bloodstream (i.e., in the first 24 to 48 hr) decreases the risk of transmission. SEE: *Nursing Diagnoses Appendix.*

DIAGNOSIS: The disease is best diagnosed by the presence of a characteristic rash called erythema chronicum migrans, which begins as a red ring at the site of the tick bite and expands, leaving a clear center. Antibody tests for *Borrelia burgdorferi* nonprotective antibodies, using an enzyme-linked immunosorbent assay (ELISA) test, also are used for diagnosis in patients with an appropriate history of exposure and signs and symptoms of Lyme disease, but no evidence of rash. The antibodies are developed against flagellar and outer surface proteins on the spirochete. SEE: illus.

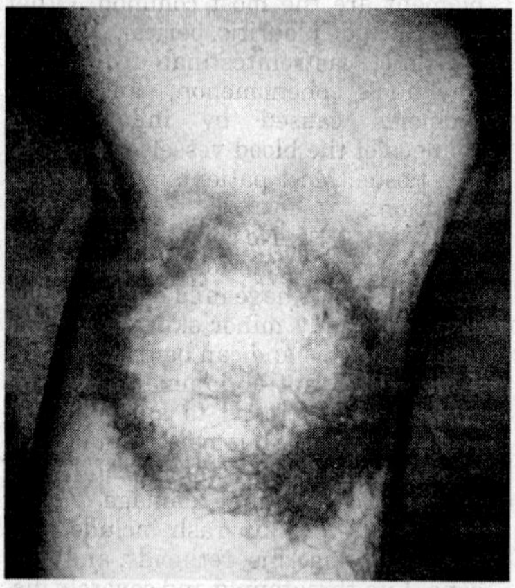

LYME DISEASE

Erythema chronicum migrans rash

SYMPTOMS: The course of Lyme disease is divided into three stages. Stage 1 (localized infection) begins with the tick bite. After an incubation period of 7 to 14 days, patients may develop erythema migrans at the site of the bite, headache, stiff neck, and muscle and joint pains. The nymph or adult tick may be so small and the initial bite so mild that the patient may not recall having been bitten. Stage 2 (disseminated infection) lasts from weeks to months. The spirochetes spread to the rest of the body through the blood, in some cases causing arthritis (esp. of the knee joints), muscle pain, cardiac dysrhythmias, pericarditis, lymphadenopathy, or meningoencephalitis. Nonprotective antibodies develop during this stage. Stage 3 (chronic infection) begins 2 to 3 years after the initial bite. Patients develop mild to severe arthritis, encephalitis, or both, which rarely are fatal.

TREATMENT: Oral doxycycline or ampicillin treatment for 3 to 4 weeks has been effective in eradicating the infection if they are given very early in the disease. Erythromycin or cefuroxime axetil may be administered to patients who are allergic to penicillin. Cardiac and neurological involvement requires treatment with intravenous ceftriaxone or cefotaxime for 4 weeks or more.

PROGNOSIS: When the disease is treated early, results are good. If treated late, convalescence is prolonged, but complete recovery is the usual outcome in most patients.

PREVENTION: A recombinant vaccine against the outer surface protein of *Borrelia* may help prevent Lyme disease. The Centers for Disease Control recommends that people should discuss with their health care providers the possibility of getting a Lyme disease vaccination if they are 15 to 70 years of age; live, work, or vacation in endemic areas; or frequently go into wooded or grassy areas. The vaccine is not recommended for children, pregnant women, and those who do not live in or visit endemic areas.

When planning to spend time in places where ticks may be located, individuals should wear light-colored clothing, hats, long sleeves, pants tucked into socks, heavy shoes, and a tick repellent containing DEET (N,N-diethyltoluamide). They should check clothing carefully for ticks when leaving those areas. Once home, individuals should remove and wash clothing, checking the entire body, especially the hairline and ankles, for ticks or nymphs. If a tick or nymph is found, it should be carefully removed with tweezers, making certain to remove the head and mouth parts from the skin. The bite site should then be cleansed with alcohol, and monitored for indications of Lyme disease. Prophylactic antibiotics generally should not be requested (or given). While pet dogs may receive Lyme vaccine, they still should be checked to prevent them from bringing ticks into the house.

CAUTION: Tick repellent should be applied to clothing, not directly to a child's skin, because of the danger of neurotoxicity.

PATIENT CARE: The patient is checked for any drug allergies. Prescribed pharmacologic therapy is explained to the patient, including dosing schedule, the importance of completing the course of therapy even if he or she feels better, and adverse effects. The few patients who develop a Jarisch-Herxheimer-like reaction within hours of therapy's initiation need reassurance that the condition will resolve within six months and does not require any treatment. Patients being treated for Lyme disease often require antibiotics for a prolonged period, especially in advanced stages, which increases their risk for developing adverse effects (e.g., diarrhea). Methods for dealing with these problems are explained. Patients with chronic Lyme disease often require assistance to deal with changes in lifestyle, family interactions, and ability to perform activities of daily living. Available local and national support groups can assist with such problems. Patients should be made aware that one occurrence of Lyme disease does not prevent recurrences.

lymph (lĭmf) [L. *lympha*] The name given to tissue fluid that has entered lymph capillaries and is found in larger lymph vessels. It is alkaline, clear, and colorless, although lymph vessels from the small intestine appear milky from the absorbed fats (chyle). The protein content of lymph is lower than that of plasma, osmotic pressure is slightly higher, and viscosity slightly less. Specific gravity is 1.016 to 1.023.

Lymph is mostly water, and contains albumin, globulins, salts, urea, neutral fats, and glucose. Its cells are mainly lymphocytes and monocytes, formed in the lymph nodes and nodules.

Lymph capillaries, found in most tissue spaces, collect tissue fluid, which is then called lymph. Lymph from the lower body flows to the cisterna chyli in the abdomen and continues upward through the thoracic duct, which receives intercostal lymph vessels, the left subclavian trunk from the left arm, and the left jugular trunk from the left side of the head. The thoracic duct empties lymph into the blood in the left subclavian vein near its junction with the left jugular vein. The right lymphatic duct drains lymph from the upper right quadrant of the body and empties into the right subclavian vein. SEE: *lymphatic system* for illus.

As lymph flows through the lymph vessels toward the subclavian veins, it passes through lymph nodes, which contain macrophages to phagocytize bacteria or other pathogens that may be present.

l. channel L. sinus.

l. follicle A densely packed collection

of immature and mature lymphocytes and dendritic cells in the cortex of the lymph node. SEE: *germinal center l. node*.

inflammatory l. An exudate due to inflammation.

l. node One of thousands of small kidney-shaped organs of lymphoid tissue that lie at intervals along the lymphatic vessels. SYN: *lymph gland*. SEE: illus; *immune response; inflammation; lymph; lymphocyte*.

ANATOMY AND PHYSIOLOGY: It contains large numbers of lymphocytes and macrophages connected by a network of reticular fibers and grouped into follicles. Lymph enters a node through the afferent vessels along the larger outer rim and passes through the subcapsular sinus lined with macrophages and into the follicles of the cortex. Follicles contain immature and mature B cells and T cells, which produce the humoral and the cellular immune responses, respectively.

As lymph flows through channels between and within the follicles, macrophages destroy microorganisms and abnormal cells by direct lysis or phagocytosis, activated T lymphocytes multiply, and B lymphocytes proliferate and manufacture antigen-specific antibodies. Lymph then passes through the paracortex and the medulla of the node, which contain mature T and B cells, B memory cells, and macrophages, before exiting through the efferent vessel. Antibodies produced in the node travel via

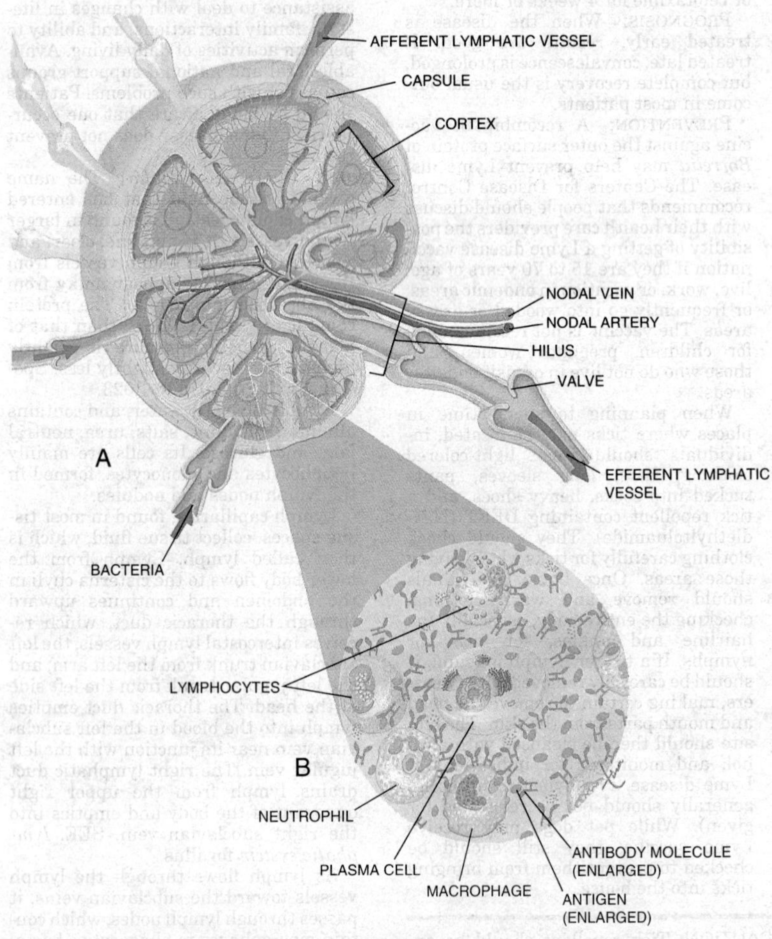

LYMPH NODE

(A) section through a lymph node, (B) microscopic detail of destruction of bacteria the lymph to the blood for distribution throughout the body.

An increase in the size of the node (lymphadenopathy) indicates a high level of activity (e.g., while combating infection or cancer or when participating in local inflammatory reactions).

Lymph nodes occur singly or in closely connected chains, which receive lymph from a single organ or region of the body. Prominent chains in the neck, axilla, groin, and mesentery remove foreign antigens from the lymph coming from the head, arms, legs, and the gastrointestinal tract, respectively.

lymphadenectasis (lĭm-făd″ĕ-nĕk′tă-sĭs) [L. *lympha,* lymph, + Gr. *aden,* gland, + *ektasis,* dilatation] Dilatation or distention of a lymph node.

lymphadenectomy (lĭm-făd″ĕ-nĕk′tō-mē) [″ + ″ + *ektome,* excision] Surgical removal of a lymph node, as in a biopsy.

lymphadenitis (lĭm-făd″ĕn-ī′tĭs) [″ + ″ + *itis,* inflammation] Inflammation of lymph nodes, caused by the activation of phagocytes and lymphocytes, which encounter large numbers of microorganisms, cancer cells, or other antigenic material. Local swelling and pain are common symptoms and often help clinicians diagnose regional diseases (e.g., the anterior cervical lymph nodes become tender and enlarged in people with strep throat; the inguinal lymph nodes enlarge and hurt in some sexually transmitted diseases).

Lymph node inflammation sometimes is associated with inflammation of the lymphatic vessels (lymphangitis) leading into the node. Lymphatic inflammation subsides when the underlying infection is treated. Lymphadenitis of unknown cause may require lymph node biopsy (e.g., excisional or needle biopsies) or aspiration. SEE: *inflammation; lymphangitis.*

SYMPTOMS: The disease is characterized by a marked increase of tissue, with possible suppuration. Swelling, pain, and tenderness are present. The disease usually accompanies lymphangitis.

ETIOLOGY: The condition is caused by drainage of bacteria or toxic substances into the lymph nodes. The etiology may be specific, as when caused by the organisms of typhoid, syphilis, or tuberculosis, or nonspecific, in which the causative organism is not identified.

TREATMENT: Hot, moist dressings should be applied. Incision and drainage are necessary if abscesses occur. Antibiotics should be given as indicated.

tuberculous l. Lymph node inflammation caused by *Mycobacterium tuberculosis* (MTB), with granuloma formation and caseating necrosis within the node. The most common presentation is the finding of a neck mass in a febrile patient (a condition called "scrofula"), although MTB and other mycobacteria also can invade lymph nodes in other parts of the body. SEE: *tuberculosis.*

lymphadenocele (lĭm-făd′ĕ-nō-sēl″) [″ + ″ + *kele,* tumor, swelling] A cyst of a lymph node.

lymphadenogram (lĭm-făd′ĕ-nō-grăm″) [″ + ″ + *gramma,* something written] A radiograph of a lymph gland.

lymphadenography (lĭm-făd″ĕ-nŏg′ră-fē) [″ + ″ + *graphein,* to write] Radiography of the lymph glands after injection of radiopaque material.

lymphadenoid (lĭm-făd′ĕ-noyd) [″ + ″ + *eidos,* form, shape] Resembling a lymph node or lymph tissue.

lymphadenopathy (lĭm-făd″ĕ-nŏp′ă-thē) [″ + ″ + *pathos,* disease] Enlargement of lymph nodes (LN), typically to greater than 1.5 cm. The increased size is caused by activation and proliferation of lymphocytes and phagocytic white blood cells within the node or by invasion of the node by tumor. Most often, lymphadenopathy is found in nodes involved in local, regional, or systemic infections; it results occasionally from cancers. Lymphadenopathy may also be found in an array of other, less common illnesses, including thyroiditis, thyrotoxicosis, autoimmune diseases (e.g., rheumatoid arthritis), sarcoidosis, and drug reactions (e.g., phenytoin).

Enlarged LNs may be tender or not; tenderness often is present when lymph nodes swell rapidly (e.g., in response to infections, hypersensitivity reactions, or some fulminant lymphomas). Rock-hard, enlarged, and immobile LNs are typical of metastatic cancer, whereas rubbery LNs are found in lymphomas. LNs that do not resolve spontaneously within 4 to 6 weeks, or for which no obvious explanation exists, usually are sampled by biopsy or aspiration.

dermatopathic l. Widespread lymphadenopathy secondary to various skin disorders.

lymphadenosis benigna cutis (lĭm-făd″ĕ-nō′sĭs bē-nī′nă cū′tĭs) A benign collection of lymphocytes in the skin.

lymphadenotomy (lĭm-făd″ĕ-nŏt′ō-mē) [″ + ″ + *tome,* incision] Surgical incision of a lymph node.

lymphadenovarix (lĭm-făd″ĕ-nō-vā′rĭks) [″ + ″ + L. *varix,* a twisted vein] Enlargement of lymph nodes due to increased pressure in the lymph vessels.

lymphagogue (lĭmf′ă-gŏg) [″ + Gr. *agogos,* leading] An agent that stimulates the production or flow of lymph.

lymphangial (lĭm-făn′jē-ăl) [″ + Gr. *angeion,* vessel] Concerning lymph vessels.

lymphangiectasis (lĭm-făn″jē-ĕk′tă-sĭs) [″ + ″ + *ektasis,* dilatation] Benign swelling in all or part of an extremity, as the result of dilation of the subcutaneous and deep lymphatic vessels. It occurs mostly in children and may be severe enough to cause deformity. Acquired lymphangiectasis can occur as a complication of surgery or radiation therapy for cancer. SYN: *lymphectasia*.

lymphangiectomy (lĭm-făn″jē-ĕk′tō-mē) [″ + ″ + *ektome,* excision] Surgical removal of lymph vessels.

lymphangiitis (lĭm-făn″jē-ī′tĭs) [″ + ″ + *itis,* inflammation] Inflammation of lymph vessels.

lymphangioendothelioma (lĭm-făn″jē-ō-ĕn″dō-thē-lē-ō′mă) [″ + ″+ *endon,* within, + *thele,* nipple, + *oma,* tumor] Endothelioma originating from lymph vessels. SYN: *lymphendothelioma*.

lymphangiofibroma (lĭm-făn″jē-ō-fī-brō′mă) [″ + Gr. *angeion,* vessel, + L. *fiber,* fiber, + Gr. *oma,* tumor] Fibroma and lymphangioma combined.

lymphangiography (lĭm-făn″jē-ŏg′ră-fē) [″ + ″ + *graphein,* to write] Immediate radiological investigation of the lymphatic vessels after injection of a contrast medium via cutdown, usually on the dorsum of the hand or foot. Delayed films are taken to visualize the nodes. This technique has been replaced by computed tomography and magnetic resonance imaging. SYN: *lymphography*.

lymphangiology (lĭm-făn″jē-ŏl′ō-jē) [″ + ″ + *logos,* word, reason] The branch of medical science concerned with the lymphatic system.

lymphangioma (lĭm-făn″jē-ō′mă) [″ + ″ + *oma,* tumor] A tumor composed of lymphatic vessels.

cavernous l. Dilated lymph vessels filled with lymph.

cystic l. Multilocular cysts filled with lymph. The condition is usually congenital.

lymphangiophlebitis (lĭm-făn″jē-ō-flē-bī′tĭs) [″ + ″ + *phleps,* vein, + *itis,* inflammation] Inflammation of the lymphatic vessels and veins.

lymphangioplasty (lĭm-făn′jē-ō-plăs″tē) [″ + Gr. *angeion,* vessel, + *plassein,* to form] The formation of artificial lymphatics or the use of microsurgical technique to reestablish lymphatic or lymphogenous continuity. SYN: *lymphoplasty*.

lymphangiosarcoma (lĭm-făn″jē-ō-săr-kō′mă) [″ + ″ + *sarx,* flesh, + *oma,* tumor] A malignant neoplasm that develops from the endothelial lining of lymphatics.

lymphangiotomy (lĭm-făn″jē-ŏt′ō-mē) [″ + ″ + *tome,* incision] **1.** Dissection of the lymphatics. **2.** Anatomy of the lymphatics.

lymphangitis (lĭm″făn-jī′tĭs) [″ + Gr. *angeion,* vessel, + *itis,* inflammation] Inflammation of the lymphatic vessels draining a body part that is inflamed or infected. Red streaks are present along the inflamed vessels and are accompanied by heat, pain, and swelling; lymph nodes in the area are enlarged and tender. Treatment consists of antibiotics specific to the organism causing the infection, most commonly group A beta-hemolytic streptococci (occasionally staphylococci). If the infection is not contained, it can spread into the venous system and produce septicemia.

SYMPTOMS: The condition is characterized by the onset of chills and high fever, with moderate swelling and pain. There is a deep general flush with a raised border on the affected area if infection is in the deep layers of skin. The red inflamed area is commonly known as blood poisoning by lay persons.

PATIENT CARE: Elevating the affected part of the body so that local lymphatics can drain reduces pain and helps the underlying infection to resolve rapidly.

lymphatic (lĭm-făt′ĭk) [L. *lymphaticus*] **1.** Of or pert. to lymph. **2.** A vessel that carries lymph.

ANATOMY: A lymph vessel carries lymph toward a subclavian vein. Plasma that leaves blood capillaries and becomes tissue fluid is collected by lymph capillaries. The larger lymph vessels resemble veins in that they have valves to prevent backflow of lymph. These larger vessels unite to form either the thoracic duct or the right lymphatic duct, which empty lymph into the blood in the left and right subclavian veins, respectively. The lymph capillaries within the villi of the small intestine (lacteals) absorb the fat-soluble end products of digestion, which are transported in the form of chylomicrons to the blood by the larger lymphatic vessels.

afferent l. Any of the small vessels carrying lymph to a lymph node.

l. capillary One of the smallest lymphatic vessels. These thin-walled tubes consist of a single layer of endothelium ending blindly in a swollen or rounded end, and form a dense network in most tissues of the body. They are generally slightly larger in diameter than blood capillaries. Because they collect interstitial fluid, the composition of the lymph varies according to the tissue being drained. Intestinal lymphatics contain fatty materials during digestion; those from the liver contain proteins. SEE: illus.

efferent l. Any of the small vessels carrying lymph from a lymph node.

l. system The system that includes all the lymph vessels that collect tissue fluid and return it to the blood (lymph capillaries, lacteals, larger vessels, the thoracic duct, and the right lymphatic duct). SEE: illus.; *lymph*.

lymphaticostomy (lĭm-făt″ĭ-kŏs′tō-mē)

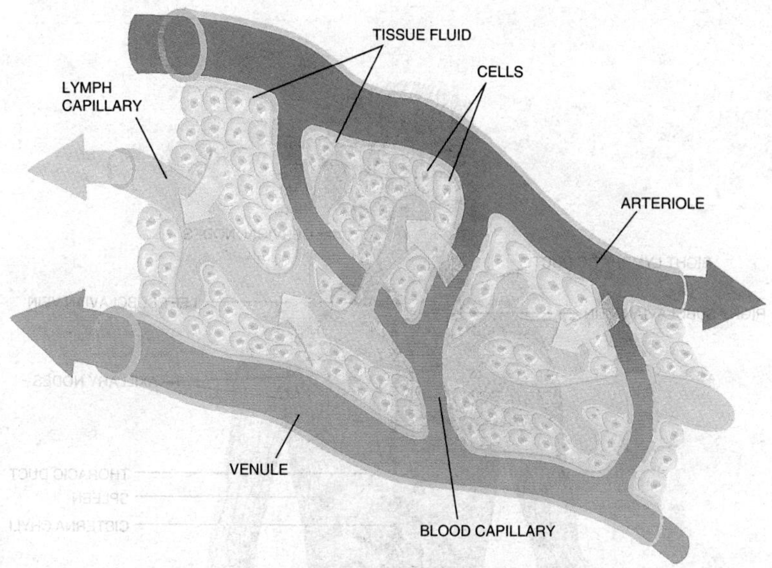

LYMPHATIC CAPILLARIES

Arrows indicate movement of plasma, lymph, and tissue fluid

[L. *lymphaticus,* lymphatic, + Gr. *stoma,* mouth] The making of a permanent aperture into a lymphatic duct, e.g., thoracic duct shunt.

lymphatitis (lĭm″fă-tī′tĭs) [″ + Gr. *itis,* inflammation] An inflammation of the lymphatic system.

lymphatolysis (lĭm″fă-tŏl′ĭ-sĭs) [″ + Gr. *lysis,* dissolution] Destruction of lymphatic vessels or tissue.

lymphatolytic (lĭm″fă-tō-lĭt′ĭk) Destructive to lymphatics.

lymphectasia (lĭmf″ĕk-tā′zē-ă) [L. *lympha,* lymph, + Gr. *ektasis,* dilatation] Lymphangiectasis.

lymphedema (lĭmf-ĕ-dē′mă) [″ + Gr. *oidema,* swelling] An abnormal accumulation of tissue fluid (potential lymph) in the interstitial spaces. The mechanism for this is either impairment of normal uptake of tissue fluid by the lymphatic vessels or the excessive production of tissue fluid caused by venous obstruction that increases capillary blood pressure. Stagnant flow of tissue fluid through body structures may make them prone to infections that are difficult to treat; as a result lymphedematous limbs should be protected from cuts, scratches, burns, and blood drawing.

Common causes of lymphedema include neoplastic obstruction of lymphatic flow (e.g., in the axilla, in metastatic breast cancer); postoperative interference with lymphatic flow (e.g., after axillary dissection); infectious blockade of lymphatics (e.g., in filariasis); radiation damage to lymphatics (e.g., after treatment of pelvic or lung cancers). SEE: *blockade, lymphatic; elephantiasis; pump, lymphedema.*

congenital l. Chronic pitting edema of the lower extremities. SYN: *Milroy's disease.*

lymphedema praecox Obstruction of the lymphatic channels, producing edema, which occurs primarily in women between the ages of 10 and 25; its cause is unknown. The interstitial fluid that accumulates first appears in the feet but can travel proximally to the trunk; it continues to accumulate throughout life. When the edema becomes severe, it predisposes the patient to chronic ulcers and superimposed infections of the legs.

lymphendothelioma (lĭmf″ĕn-dō-thē-lē-ō′mă) [″ + Gr. *endon,* within, + *thele,* nipple, + *oma,* tumor] Tumor from proliferation and dilatation of lymphatics with overgrowth of myxomatous tissue.

lymphization (lĭm″fĭ-zā′shŭn) Production of lymph.

lymphoblast (lĭm′fō-blăst) [″ + Gr. *blastos,* germ] An immature cell that gives rise to a lymphocyte. SYN: *lymphocytoblast.* **lymphoblastic,** *adj.*

lymphoblastoma (lĭm″fō-blăst-ō′mă) [″ + ″ + *oma,* tumor] Lymphosarcoma.

lymphoblastomatosis (lĭm″fō-blăs″tō-mă-tō′sĭs) [″ + ″ + *oma,* tumor, + *osis,* condition] A condition produced by lymphoblastomas.

lymphoblastosis (lĭm″fō-blăs-tō′sĭs) [″

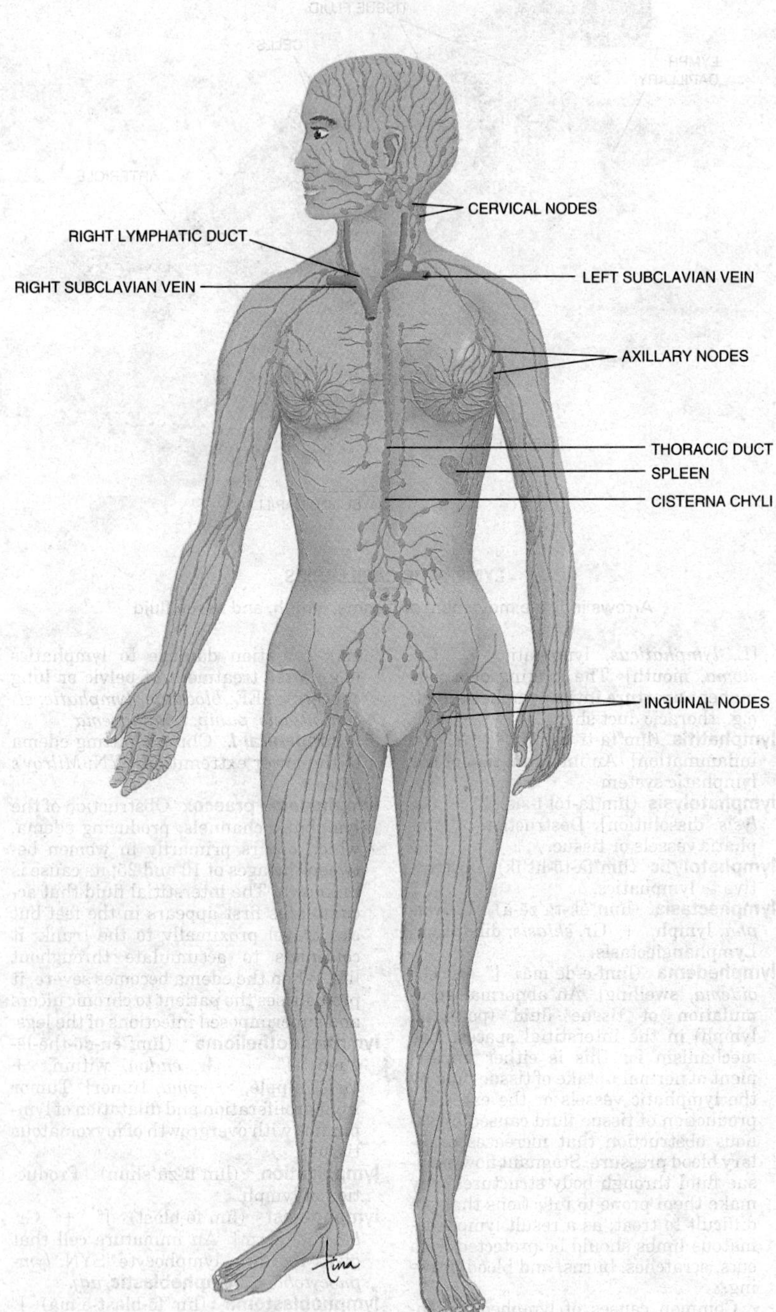

THE LYMPHATIC SYSTEM

+ " + *osis,* condition] An excessive number of lymphoblasts in the blood.

lymphocele (lĭm′fō-sēl) [L. *lympha,* lymph, + Gr. *kele,* tumor, swelling] A cyst that contains lymph.

lymphocytapheresis [" + Gr. *aphairesis,* removal] Removal of lymphocytes from the blood after it has been withdrawn. The blood is then returned to the donor.

lymphocyte (lĭm′fō-sīt) [L. *lympha,* lymph, + Gr. *kytos,* cell] A white blood cell responsible for much of the body's immune protection. Fewer than 1% are present in the circulating blood; the rest lie in the lymph nodes, spleen, and other lymphoid organs, where they can maximize contact with foreign antigens. SEE: illus.; *B cell; T cell; blood* for illus.; *cell, natural killer; cell, plasma; immunity, cell-mediated; immunity, humoral.*

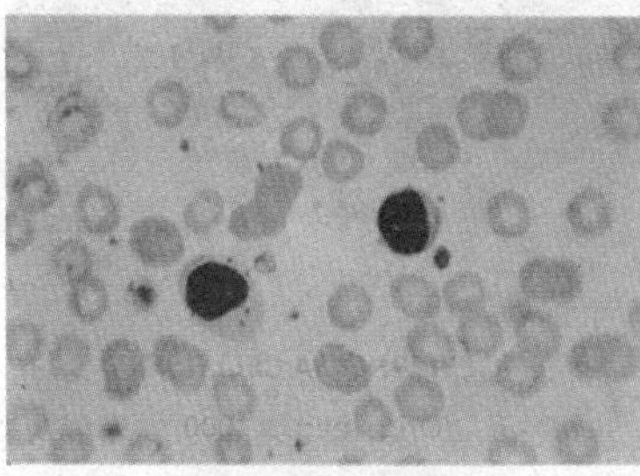

NORMAL LYMPHOCYTES

(Orig. mag. ×1000)

Lymphocytes vary from 5 to 12 μm in diameter; subpopulations can be identified by unique protein groups on the cell surface called clusters of differentiation. T cells, derived from the thymus, make up approx. 75% of all lymphocytes; B cells, derived from the bone marrow, 10%. A third classification is natural killer cells. In the blood, 20% to 40% of the white cells are lymphocytes.

activated l. A lymphocyte that has been stimulated by exposure to a specific antigen or by macrophage processing so that it is capable of responding to a foreign antigen by neutralizing or eliminating it.

l. activation The use of an antigen (or mitogen in vitro) to stimulate lymphocyte metabolic activity.

B l. A lymphocyte formed from pluripotent stem cells in the bone marrow that migrates to the spleen, lymph nodes, and other peripheral lymphoid tissue where it comes in contact with foreign antigens and becomes a mature functioning cell. Mature B cells are able to independently identify foreign antigens and differentiate into antibody-producing plasma cells or memory cells; their activity also may be stimulated by IL-2 (previously called B-cell growth factor). Plasma cells are the only source of immunoglobulins (antibodies). Memory cells enable the body to produce antibodies quickly when it is invaded by the same organism at a later date. SYN: *B cell.* SEE: *humoral immunity; immune response.*

T l. T cell.

lymphocytoblast (lĭm″fō-sī′tō-blăst″) [" + " + *blastos,* germ] Lymphoblast.

lymphocytopenia (lĭm″fō-sīt″ō-pē′nē-ă) [" + " + *penia,* lack] A deficiency of lymphocytes in the blood.

lymphocytopoiesis (lĭm″fō-sīt″ō-poy-ē′sĭs) [" + " + *poiesis,* production] Lymphocyte production.

lymphocytosis (lĭm″fō-sī-tō′sĭs) [" + " + *osis,* condition] An excess of lymph cells in the blood.

lymphocytotoxin (lĭm″fō-sīt″ō-tŏks′ĭn) [" + " + *toxikon,* poison] A toxin destructive to lymphocytes.

lymphoduct (lĭm′fō-dŭkt) [" + *ducere,* to lead] A rarely used term for a lymphatic vessel.

lymphoepithelioma (lĭm″fō-ĕp″ĭ-thē-lē-ō′mă) [" + Gr. *epi,* at, + *thele,* nipple, + *oma,* tumor] A poorly differentiated squamous cell carcinoma that involves the lymphoid tissue of the tonsils and nasopharynx.

lymphogenesis (lĭm″fō-jĕn′ĕ-sĭs) [" + Gr. *genesis,* generation, birth] Production of lymph.

lymphogenous (lĭm-fŏj′ĕn-ŭs) [" + Gr. *gennan,* to produce] **1.** Forming lymph. **2.** Derived from lymph.

lymphoglandula (lĭm″fō-glăn′dū-lă) [" + *glandula,* little gland] A term formerly used to signify a lymph node.

lymphogranuloma inguinale Lymphogranuloma venereum.

lymphogranulomatosis (lĭm″fō-grăn-ū-lō″mă-tō′sĭs) [" + *granulum,* granule, + Gr. *oma,* tumor, + *osis,* condition] **1.** Infectious granuloma of the lymphatics. **2.** Hodgkin's disease.

lymphogranuloma venereum (lĭm″fō-grăn″ū-lō′mă) [" + " + Gr. *oma,* tumor] ABBR: LGV. A sexually transmitted disease, affecting about 300 patients per year in the U.S., caused by *Chlamydia* species. It has an incubation period of about 3 to 30 days. Its hallmarks are a painless, red erosion on the genitals or rectum, followed 1 to 2 weeks later by inguinal lymph node enlargement (historically called "buboes"). These may cause fistulous tracts or obstruct lymphatic channels if the infection is left untreated. Perirectal lymph nodes may scar and produce late rectal obstruction. Tetracyclines cure the disease in its initial stages but do not resolve complications brought on by scarring or lymphatic obstruction. SYN: *lymphogranuloma inguinale; lymphopathia venereum.* SEE: *pelvic inflam-*

matory disease; sexually transmitted disease.

SYMPTOMS: Because up to 75% of women and 50% of men have no symptoms, patients do not know they have the disease, continue to spread it, and develop more severe infection. Symptomatic patients may develop ulcerating vesicles on the genitals, urethral inflammation, abdominal pain, and swollen lymph nodes in the groin and rectum; men often have swollen testicles. Approx 40% of women develop pelvic inflammatory disease (PID), leading to chronic pain, infertility, and an increased risk of having a tubal pregnancy.

The Centers for Disease Control recommend that all sexually active women under 20 years of age should be screened yearly for *Chlamydia;* sexually active women over age 20 with multiple sex partners who do not use condoms also should be screened yearly. The infection is diagnosed using fluorescent anti-*Chlamydia* antibodies. Women, rather than men, are targeted for screening because of their increased use of health care and the risk of developing PID associated with this disease.

TREATMENT: The disease can be treated effectively with a 3-week course of doxycycline; erythromycin is used in pregnant women. Recurrent infection is common if barrier contraception is not used during intercourse.

l.v. antigen An antigen used in a skin test for lymphogranuloma venereum.

lymphography (lĭm-fŏg′ră-fē) [L. *lympha,* lymph, + Gr. *graphein,* to write] Lymphangiography.

lymphoid (lĭm′foyd) [″ + Gr. *eidos,* form, shape] **1.** Consisting of lymphocytes. **2.** Resembling lymphatic tissue.

l. cell A term formerly used to designate a lymphocyte.

lymphoidectomy (lĭm″foyd-ĕk′tō-mē) [″ + ″ + *ektome,* excision] Surgical removal of lymphoid tissue.

lymphokine (lĭm′fō-kīn) A cytokine released by lymphocytes, including many of the interleukins, gamma interferon, tumor necrosis factor beta, and chemokines. SEE: *cytokine.*

lymphokinesis (lĭm″fō-kī-nē′sĭs) [″ + Gr. *kinesis,* motion] **1.** Circulation of lymph in the lymphatic system. **2.** Movement of lymph in the semicircular canals of the inner ear.

lymphology (lĭm-fŏl′ō-jē) [″ + Gr. *logos,* word, reason] The science of the lymphatics.

lymphoma A malignant neoplasm originating from lymphocytes. SEE: *Hodgkin's disease.*

Burkitt's l. A form of malignant, non-Hodgkin's lymphoma that causes bone-destroying lesions of the jaw. The Epstein-Barr virus is the causative agent. It was initially reported from central Africa.

cutaneous T cell l. ABBR: CTCL. A malignant non-Hodgkin's lymphoma, with a predilection for infiltrating the skin. In its earliest stages, it often is mistaken for a mild, chronic dermatitis because it appears as itchy macules and patches, often on the chest or trunk. Later, the lesions may thicken, become nodular, or spread throughout the entire surface of the skin, the internal organs, or the bloodstream.

non-Hodgkin's l. ABBR: NHL. A group of malignant tumors of B or T lymphocytes that are newly diagnosed in about 45,000 Americans annually. SEE: illus.; *Hodgkin's disease.*

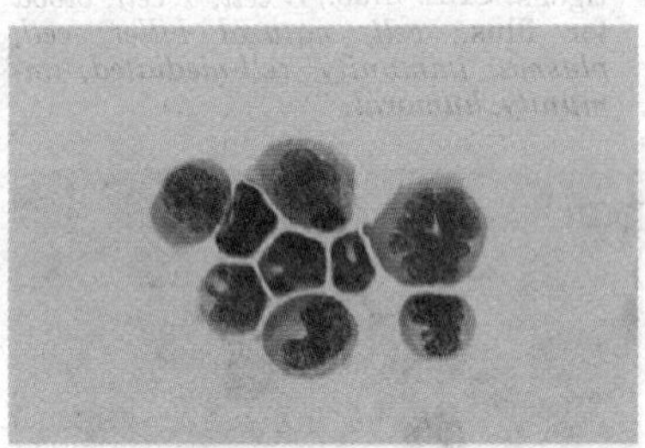

LYMPHOMA CELLS

(Orig. mag. ×1000)

SYMPTOMS: Painless lymphadenopathy in two thirds of patients is the most frequent presenting symptom. Others have fever, night sweats, loss of 10% or more of body weight in the 6 months before presenting with symptoms of infiltration into nonlymphoid tissue. Additional involvement is in peripheral areas such as epitrochlear nodes, the tonsillar area, and bone marrow. NHL is 50% more frequent in men than in women of similar age. In most cases the cause of NHL is unknown, but patients who have received immunosuppressive agents have a more than 100 times greater chance of developing NHL, probably owing to the immunosuppressive agents activating tumor viruses.

TREATMENT: Specific therapy depends on the type, grade, and stage of the lymphoma. Combination chemotherapies, bone marrow transplantation, radiation therapy, and photochemotherapy may be given, depending on the specific diagnosis.

lymphomatoid (lĭm-fō′mă-toyd) [L. *lympha,* lymph, + Gr. *oma,* tumor, + *eidos,* form, shape] Resembling lymphoma.

lymphomatosis (lĭm″fō-mă-tō′sĭs) [″ + ″ + *osis,* condition] Dissemination of lymphoma throughout the body.

lymphomatous (lĭm-fō′mă-tŭs) **1.** Pert.

to a lymphoma. **2.** Affected with lymphomata.

lymphomyxoma (lĭm″fō-mĭk-sō′mă) [″ + Gr. *mys,* muscle, + *oma,* tumor] A soft, nonmalignant tumor that contains lymphoid tissue.

lymphopathia venereum Lymphogranuloma venereum.

lymphopathy (lĭm-fŏp′ă-thē) [″ + Gr. *pathos,* disease] Any disease of the lymphatic system.

lymphopenia (lĭm-fō-pē′nē-ă) [″ + Gr. *penia,* a lack] A deficiency of lymphocytes in the blood.

lymphoplasmapheresis [″ + Gr. *aphairesis,* removal] The removal of lymphocytes and plasma from the blood after it has been withdrawn. The blood is then returned to the donor.

lymphoplasty (lĭm′fō-plăs″tē) [″ + Gr. *plassein,* to form] Lymphangioplasty.

lymphopoiesis (lĭm″fō-poy-ē′sĭs) [″ + Gr. *poiesis,* production] The formation of lymphocytes or of lymphoid tissue.

lymphopoietic (lĭm″fō-poy-ĕt′ĭk) [″ + Gr. *poiein,* to produce] Forming lymphocytes.

lymphoproliferative (lĭm″fō-prō-lĭf′ĕr-ă-tĭv) Concerning the proliferation of lymphoid tissue.

lymphoreticular (lĭm″fō-rĕ-tĭk′ū-lăr) [″ + *reticula,* net] Pert. to the lymphocyte, to the mononuclear phagocyte system, and to the tissues that support their growth.

l. disorder Any benign or malignant disease in which lymphocytes or lymphatic tissues proliferate. Included are self-limited proliferation of lymph glands, lymphocytes, and monocytes; infectious mononucleosis; benign abnormalities of immunoglobulin synthesis; leukemias; lymphomas such as Hodgkin's disease, lymphosarcoma, reticulum cell sarcoma, and mycosis fungoides; malignant proliferative response or abnormal immunoglobulin synthesis such as plasma cell myeloma, macroglobulinemia, and amyloidosis; histiocytosis; and lipid storage disease.

lymphoreticulosis, benign, of inoculation (lĭm″fō-rē-tĭk″ū-lō′sĭs) [″ + ″ + Gr. *osis,* condition] Cat scratch disease.

lymphorrhagia (lĭm″fō-rā′jē-ă) [″ + Gr. *rhegnynai,* to burst forth] Flow of lymph from ruptured lymph vessels. SYN: *lymphorrhea.*

lymphorrhea (lĭm″fō-rē′ă) [″ + Gr. *rhoia,* flow] Lymphorrhagia.

lymphorrhoid (lĭm′fō-royd) Dilated lymph channels that resemble hemorrhoids.

lymphosarcoma (lĭm″fō-săr-kō′mă) [″ + Gr. *sarx,* flesh, + *oma,* tumor] An infrequently used term for lymphoma, used most often in veterinary medicine. SYN: *lymphoblastoma.*

lymphoscintigraphy (lĭm″fō-sĭn-tĭ′gră-fē) The use of radioactive tracers to identify the lymphatic drainage basin of a tumor. The technique is used to guide the surgeon in performing biopsies and in the removal of tumors.

lymphostasis (lĭm″fŏs′tă-sĭs) [″ + Gr. *stasis,* a stoppage] Stoppage of the flow of lymph.

lymphotaxis (lĭm″fō-tăk′sĭs) [″ + Gr. *taxis,* arrangement] The effect of attracting or repelling lymphocytes.

lymphotome (lĭm′fō-tōm) [″ + Gr. *tome,* incision] An instrument for removing glandular growths from tonsils and adenoids.

lymphotoxin (lĭm″fō-tŏk′sĭn) [″ + Gr. *toxikon,* poison] A lymphokine that is produced by activated lymphocytes. The toxin affects a variety of cells.

lymphotrophy (lĭm-fŏt′rō-fē) [″ + Gr. *trophe,* nourishment] Lymph nourishment of cells in regions devoid of blood vessels.

lymphotropic Attracted to lymph cells. For example, human immunodeficiency virus and human T-cell leukemia-lymphoma virus are lymphotropic for CD4+ lymphocytes and Epstein-Barr virus is lymphotropic for B lymphocytes.

lymphuria (lĭm-fū′rē-ă) [″ + Gr. *ouron,* urine] Lymph in the urine.

Lynch syndrome An autosomal dominant predisposition to colon cancer and other solid tumors. People with Lynch I syndrome are susceptible to colon cancer alone, whereas those with Lynch II syndrome have an additional tendency to get cancers of the colon, ovaries, breasts, and/or uterus.

lyo- [Gr. *lyein,* a loosening or dissolution] Combining form meaning to *loosen* or *dissolve.*

lyochrome (lī′ō-krōm) [″ + *chroma,* color] Flavin.

lyoenzyme (lī″ō-ĕn′zīm) [″ + *en,* in, + *zyme,* leaven] An extracellular enzyme.

Lyon hypothesis (lī′ŏn) [Mary Lyon, Brit. geneticist, b. 1925] The idea that one of the X chromosomes of the female is inactivated during embryogenesis and becomes hyperpyknotic. This chromosome forms, in the cell nucleus, the sex chromatin mass, or Barr body. This X chromosome remains in this state throughout the cell's progeny so that in the adult only one X chromosome is active in each cell.

lyophilization (lī-ŏf″ĭ-lĭ-zā′shŭn) The process of rapidly freezing a substance at an extremely low temperature and then dehydrating the substance in a high vacuum. SYN: *freeze-drying.*

lyosorption (lī″ō-sorp′shŭn) [″ + *sorbere,* to suck in] The absorption, in a colloid, of a substance on the surface of the particles in the dispersed phase.

lypressin (lī-prĕs′ĭn) A posterior pituitary hormone obtained from the pituitary glands of healthy pigs. It is used as an antidiuretic. Trade name is Diapid. SEE: *vasopressin.*

lyra (lī′ră) [L., Gr., *lyre*] One of several anatomical structures so called because of their resemblance to the shape of a lyre.

lysate (lī′sāt) **1.** The products of hydrolysis. **2.** Material produced when cells are lysed by the actions of agents such as chemicals, enzymes, or physical agents.

lyse (līz) [Gr. *lysis,* dissolution] To kill.

lysemia (lī-sē′mē-ă) [″ + *haima,* blood] Lysis of red blood cells with release of hemoglobin into the plasma.

lysergic acid diethylamide ABBR: LSD. A hallucinogenic derivative of an alkaloid in ergot. LSD is used legally only for experimental purposes.

lysimeter (lī-sĭm′ĕ-tĕr) [Gr. *lysis,* dissolution, + *metron,* measure] An apparatus for determining solubilities of various substances.

lysin (lī′sĭn) A substance that causes cell destruction and death. SEE: *antibody*.

lysine (lī′sēn) An amino acid that is a hydrolytic cleavage product of digested protein. It is essential for growth and repair of tissues.

l. acetate An amino acid.

l. hydrochloride An amino acid.

lysinogen (lī-sĭn′ō-jĕn) [Gr. *lysis,* dissolution, + *gennan,* to produce] An antibody that forms lysins.

lysis (lī′sĭs) [Gr., dissolution] **1.** The gradual decline of a fever or disease; the opposite of crisis. **2.** The death of cells or microorganisms, caused by antibodies, complement, enzymes, or other substances.

-lysis **1.** Suffix meaning to *loosen* or *dissolve*. **2.** In medicine, combining form indicating *reduction* or *relief of*.

lysocephalin (lī″sō-sĕf′ă-lĭn) Partial hydrolysis of a cephalin. It can be caused by the action of cobra venom.

lysogen (lī′sō-jĕn) [″ + *gennan,* to produce] Something capable of producing a lysin.

lysogenesis (lī″sō-jĕn′ĕ-sĭs) [″ + *genesis,* generation, birth] The production of lysin, a cell-destroying antibody.

lysogenic (lī-sō-jĕn′ĭk) [″ + Gr. *gennan,* to produce] Producing lysins.

lysogeny (lī-sŏj′ĕ-nē) A special type of virus-bacterial cell interaction maintained by a complex cellular regulatory mechanism. Bacterial strains freshly isolated from their natural environment may contain a low concentration of bacteriophage. This phage will lyse other related bacteria. Cultures that contain these substances are said to be lysogenic.

lysolecithin (lī″sō-lĕs′ĭ-thĭn) A substance obtained from lecithin through the action of an enzyme present in cobra venom. It demyelinates nerves and destroys red blood cells.

lysosome (lī′sō-sōm) A cell organelle that is part of the intracellular digestive system. Inside its limiting membrane, it contains a number of hydrolytic enzymes capable of breaking down proteins and certain carbohydrates. Lysosomal enzymes contribute to the digestion of pathogens phagocytized by a cell, and also to the tissue damage that accompanies inflammation.

lysozyme (lī′sō-zīm) [Gr. *lysis,* dissolution, + *zyme,* leaven] An enzyme found in phagocytes, neutrophils, and macrophages, and in tears, saliva, sweat, and other body secretions, that destroys bacteria by breaking down their walls.

lyssa (lĭs′să) [Gr., frenzy] Obsolete term for rabies.

Lyssavirus The genus of the family Rhabdoviridae, which includes the rabies virus.

lyssoid (lĭs′oyd) [Gr. *lyssa,* frenzy, + *eidos,* form, shape] Resembling lyssa or rabies.

lyssophobia (lĭs-ō-fō′bē-ă) [″ + *phobos,* fear] **1.** Hysteria resembling that of rabies. **2.** Fear of rabies.

lytic (lĭt′ĭk) Relating to lysis (cellular destruction) or a lysin.

lyze (līz) [Gr. *lysis,* dissolution] To bring about lysis.

LZ Landing zone for a helicopter, usually a minimum of 100 × 100 feet in size and free of overhead obstructions such as trees and powerlines.

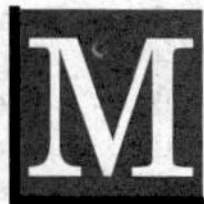

μ [*mu,* the twelfth letter of the Greek alphabet] Symbol for micro-, a prefix indicating one-millionth (10^{-6}) of the quantity (e.g., μg or 0.000001 g).

μμ Symbol for micromicro-; micromicron.

μm Symbol for micrometer.

M *master* or *medicine* in professional titles; *mille,* a thousand; *misce,* mix; *molar.*

m *meter* and *minim;* in chemistry, for *meta-,* and for *mol* or *mole.*

mμ Symbol for millimicron.

MA *mental age.*

M.A. *Master of Arts.*

ma *milliampere.*

MAC *maximum allowable concentration.*

Mace A proprietary substance derived from the spice *myristica fragrans.* Its name is an acronym for *me*thylchloroform chloro-*ace*tophenone, a chemical compound used at one time in riot control because of its ability to irritate the eyes. Now it is considered too toxic for that purpose because it has occasionally caused death when used in poorly ventilated areas. SEE: *IDU.*

TREATMENT: Treatment includes a 0.1% aqueous solution of idoxuridine (IDU) instilled into the affected eye. Water is used to dilute the toxin and flush the eyes or skin. Contact lenses must be removed immediately.

macerate (măs′ĕr-āt) To soften by steeping or soaking in water; usually pertains to the skin.

maceration (măs-ĕr-ā′shŭn) [L. *macerare,* to make soft] **1.** The process of softening a solid by steeping in a fluid. **2.** The dissolution of the skin of a dead fetus retained in utero.

Mache unit (mă′kĕ) [Heinrich Mache, Austrian physicist, 1876–1954] ABBR: M.u., or German, M.E. A unit of measurement of radioactivity.

machine Any mechanical device or apparatus.

Machover test SEE: *Draw-a-Person test.*

macies (mā′shē-ēz) [L., wasting] Atrophy.

Mackenrodt's ligament [A. K. Mackenrodt, Ger. gynecologist, 1859–1925] The uterine suspensory ligaments that are attached to the sides of the pelvic wall, the fornix of the vagina, and the cervix. They support both the uterus and the upper vagina. SEE: *prolapse of uterus.*

macr- SEE: *macro-.*

macrencephalia, macrencephaly (măk-rĕn″sĕ-fā′lē-ă, -sĕf′ă-lē) [Gr. *makros,* large, + *enkephalos,* brain] Abnormally large size of the brain.

macro-, macr- [Gr. *makros,* large] Combining form meaning *large* or *long.*

macroamylase (măk″rō-ăm′ĭ-lās) A form of amylase with a molecular weight much greater than ordinary amylase. The macroamylase molecule is too large to be excreted by the glomerulus of the kidney. It is clinically important because its presence in the bloodstream may falsely suggest the diagnosis of pancreatitis. In patients with macroamylasemia, the urinary amylase would be within normal limits, which would not be true if the elevation of blood amylase were due to an increase in pancreatic amylase.

macroamylasemia (măk″rō-ăm″ĭl-ă-sē′mē-ă) Macroamylase in the serum. The presence of increased amounts of macroamylase in the blood has not been correlated with disease.

macrobiosis (măk″rō-bī-ō′sĭs) [Gr. *makros,* large, + *biosis,* life] Longevity.

macrobiota (măk″rō-bī-ō′tă) The macroscopic living organisms, flora and fauna, of an area.

macroblepharia (măk″rō-blĕ-fā′rē-ă) [Gr. *makros,* large, + *blepharon,* eyelid] Abnormal largeness of the eyelid.

macrobrachia (măk″rō-brā′kē-ă) [″ + *brachion,* arm] Abnormal size or length of the arm.

macrocardius (măk″rō-kăr′dē-ŭs) [″ + *kardia,* heart] An individual with an abnormally large heart; caused by congenital heart disease.

macrocephalia, macrocephaly (măk″rō-sĕ-fā′lē-ă, -sĕf′ă-lē) [″ + *kephale,* head] Abnormally large size of the head. It is found in acromegaly, hydrocephalus, rickets, osteitis deformans, leontiasis ossea, myxedema, leprosy, and pituitary disturbances. **macrocephalic, macrocephalous** (-sĕf′ă-lŭs), *adj.*

macrocheilia (măk″rō-kī′lē-ă) [″ + *cheilos,* lip] Abnormal size of a lip characterized by swelling of the glands of the lip. It is a congenital condition. SYN: *macrolabia.*

macrocheiria (măk-rō-kī′rē-ă) [″ + *cheir,* hand] Excessive size of the hands.

macroconidium (măk″rō-kō-nĭd′ē-ŭm) A large conidium or exospore.

macrocornea (măk-rō-kor′nē-ă) [″ + L. *cornu,* horn] Abnormal size of the cornea. SYN: *megalocornea.*

macrocyst (măk′rō-sĭst) [″ + *kystis,* bladder] A large cyst.

macrocyte [″ + *kytos,* cell] Abnormally large erythrocyte exceeding 10 microns in diameter.

macrocythemia, macrocytosis (măk″rō-sī-thē′mē-ă, măk″rō-sī-tō′sĭs) [″ + ″ + *haima*, blood] Condition in which erythrocytes are larger than normal, (e.g., in folate or vitamin B_{12} deficiencies).

macrodactylia (măk″rō-dăk-tĭl′ē-ă) [″ + *daktylos*, finger] Excessive size of one or more digits.

macrodontia (măk″rō-dŏn′shē-ă) [″ + *odous*, tooth] Abnormal increase in size of the teeth.

macroesthesia (măk″rō-ĕs-thē′zē-ă) [Gr. *makros*, large, + *aisthesis*, sensation] State in which objects seen or felt appear to be greatly magnified.

macrofauna (măk″rō-faw′nă) The animal life visible to the naked eye in a particular location or area.

macroflora (măk″rō-flō′ră) The plant life visible to the naked eye in a particular location or area.

macrogamete (măk″rō-găm′ĕt) [″ + *gamete*, wife] A large immobile reproductive cell formed in certain protozoa and simple plants. It corresponds to the ovum in higher forms.

macrogametocyte (măk″rō-gă-mē′tō-sīt) A large nonmotile reproductive cell developing from the merozoite of certain protozoans and fungi. Macrogametocytes are found in red blood cells infected with malaria. SEE: *Plasmodium*.

macrogenitosomia praecox (măk″rō-jĕn″ĭ-tō-sō′mē-ă prē′kŏks) [″ + L. *genitalis*, genital, + Gr. *soma*, body, + L. *praecox*, early] Abnormal size of genitalia in the developing fetus due to excess androgens (male hormones) from the fetal adrenal. In the female, this causes pseudohermaphroditism, and in the male, enlarged external genitalia.

macrogingivae (măk″rō-jĭn-jī′vē) [″ + L. *gingiva*, gum] Hypertrophy of the gums.

macroglia (măk-rŏg′lē-ă) [″ + *glia*, glue] Astrocyte.

macroglobulin (măk″rō-glŏb′ū-lĭn) A globulin of high molecular weight over about 400,000. Macroglobulin is normally present in the blood but is increased in disease states such as multiple myeloma, connective tissue disease, cirrhosis of the liver, and amyloidosis.

alpha-2 m. Plasma glycoprotein made principally by the liver that inhibits serine proteases, leukocyte elastase, and proteinase 3, but not matrix metalloproteinases.

macroglobulinemia (măk-rō-glŏb″ū-lĭn-ē′mē-ă) Presence of globulins of high molecular weight in serum.

Waldenström's m. Macroglobulinemia marked by excess production of immunoglobulin M (IgM). Peak incidence is in the sixth and seventh decades. The disease is more common in men. Findings include anemia due to infiltration of the bone marrow with lymphocytes and plasma cells, weight loss, neurological disturbances, blurred vision, bleeding disorders, cold sensitivity, generalized lymphadenopathy, and hyperviscosity of the blood.

TREATMENT: Plasma exchange therapy decreases the viscosity of the blood in patients with Waldenström's macroglobulinemia by removing excess IgM from the blood. The procedure may need to be performed every 4 to 6 weeks in some patients. Other specific treatments include the use of chemotherapeutic drugs to decrease the production of IgM by abnormal clones of B lymphocytes.

macroglossia [Gr. *makros*, large, + *glossa*, tongue] Hypertrophy of the tongue.

macrognathia (măk-rō-nā′thē-ă) [″ + *gnathos*, jaw] Abnormal size of the jaw.

macrography (măk-rŏg′ră-fē) [″ + *graphein*, to write] Writing with large letters.

macrogyria [″ + *gyros*, circle] Excessively large size of convolutions (gyri) of the cerebral hemispheres.

macrolabia (măk-rō-lā′bē-ă) [″ + L. *labium*, lip] Abnormal size of a lip. SYN: *macrocheilia*.

macroleukoblast (măk″rō-lū′kō-blăst) [″ + *leukos*, white, + *blastos*, germ] A large leukoblast.

macrolide (măk′rō-līd) A class of antibiotics that inhibits protein synthesis by bacteria at the 50S ribosome. They are usually used for respiratory tract, skin, and genitourinary infections. Examples of macrolides are erythromycin, clarithromycin, and azithromycin.

macrolymphocyte (măk″rō-lĭmf′ō-sīt) [″ + L. *lympha*, lymph, + Gr. *kytos*, cell] A large lymphocyte.

macromastia (măk-rō-măs′tē-ă) [″ + *mastos*, breast] Abnormally large breasts.

macromelia [″ + *melos*, limb] Abnormally large size of the limbs.

macromelus (măk-rŏm′ĕ-lŭs) [″ + *melos*, limb] An individual with abnormally large extremities.

macromere (măk′rō-mēr) [″ + *meros*, a part] A blastomere of large size.

macromethod (măk′rō-mĕth″ŏd) Chemical examinations or analyses wherein ordinary quantities of the material being studied are used.

macromolecule (măk″rō-mŏl′ĕ-kūl) A large molecule such as a protein, polymer, or polysaccharide.

macromonocyte (măk″rō-mŏn′ō-sīt) A large monocyte.

macromyeloblast (măk″rō-mī′ĕ-lō-blăst) [″ + *myelos*, marrow, + *blastos*, germ] A large myeloblast.

macronormoblast (măk″rō-nor′mō-blăst) [″ + L. *norma*, rule, + Gr. *blastos*, germ] A large nucleated red blood cell.

macronucleus (măk″rō-nū′klē-ŭs) The

larger of the two nuclei of ciliated protozoa.

macronutrient Any essential nutrient required in large amounts in a balanced diet, such as carbohydrates, proteins, and fats. SEE: *micronutrient; trace element.*

macronychia (măk″rō-nĭk′ē-ă) [″ + *onyx,* nail] Abnormal length or thickness of the fingernails or toenails.

macropathology (măk″rō-pă-thŏl′ō-jē) Pathological changes in gross anatomical structures.

macrophage, macrophagus (măk′rō-fāj, măk-rŏf′ă-gŭs) [″ + *phagein,* to eat] A monocyte that has left the circulation and settled and matured in a tissue. Macrophages are found in large quantities in the spleen, lymph nodes, alveoli, and tonsils. About 50% of all macrophages are found in the liver as Kupffer cells. They are also present in the brain as microglia, in the skin as Langerhans cells, in bone as osteoclasts, as well as in serous cavities and breast and placental tissue. Along with neutrophils, macrophages are the major phagocytic cells of the immune system. They have the ability to recognize and ingest foreign antigens through receptors on the surface of their cell membranes; these antigens are then destroyed by lysosomes. Their placement in the peripheral lymphoid tissues enables macrophages to serve as the major scavengers of the blood, clearing it of abnormal or old cells and cellular debris as well as pathogenic organisms.

Macrophages also serve a vital role by processing antigens and presenting them to T cells, activating the specific immune response. They also release many substances that participate in inflammation, including chemokines and cytokines, lytic enzymes, oxygen radicals, coagulation factors, and growth factors. SEE: illus.; *chemokine; cytokine; inflammation; oxygen radical.*

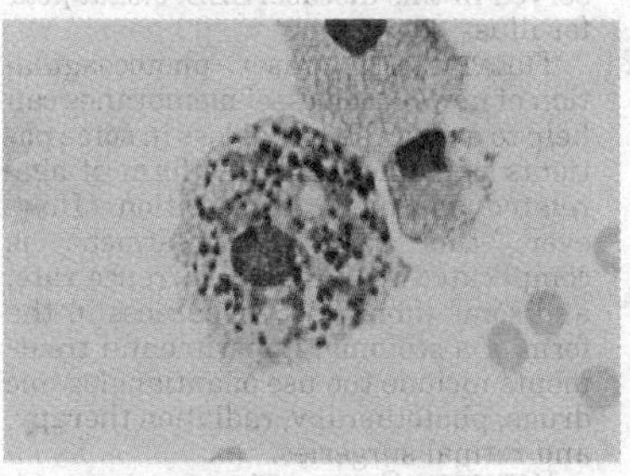

MACROPHAGE
With hemosiderin granules
(orig. mag. ×1000)

m. activating factor ABBR: MAF. A lymphokine that stimulates macrophages to become more effective killers of certain microbial cells. Macrophages stimulated by MAF can kill tumor cells.

m. chemotactic factor ABBR: MCF. A lymphokine released by T and B cell lymphocytes in response to an antigen. It attracts macrophages to the site of the invading antigen.

m. colony stimulating factor ABBR: M-CSF. A hematopoietic growth factor that stimulates monocytes to form colonies.

m. A cytokine that blocks the movement and activity of macrophages during inflammation. SEE: *cytokine.*

m. migration inhibiting factor ABBR: MIF. A lymphokine that blocks the migration of macrophages in culture.

m. processing The mechanism by which foreign antigens are taken into the macrophage by phagocytosis and broken up. Part of the antigen is then displayed on the surface of the macrophage next to a histocompatibility or "self" antigen activating T lymphocytes and the specific immune response. T lymphocytes are unable to recognize or respond to most antigens without macrophage assistance.

macrophagocyte (măk″rō-făg′ō-sīt) A large phagocyte.

macrophallus (măk″rō-făl′ŭs) [Gr. *makros,* large, + *phallos,* penis] Abnormally large penis.

macrophthalmia (măk″rŏf-thăl′mē-ă) [″ + *ophthalmos,* eye] Abnormally large eyeball.

macroplasia (măk″rō-plā′zē-ă) [″ + *plasis,* forming] Abnormally large size of a part or specific tissue.

macropodia (măk-rō-pō′dē-ă) [″ + *pous,* foot] Abnormally large feet.

macropolycyte (măk″rō-pŏl′ē-sīt) [″ + *polys,* many, + *kytos,* cell] A large polymorphonuclear leukocyte with a multisegmented nucleus.

macropromyelocyte (măk″rō-prō-mī′ĕ-lō-sīt) A large promyelocyte.

macroprosopia (măk″rō-prō-sō′pē-ă) [″ + *prosopon,* face] Large facial features.

macropsia (măk-rŏp′sē-ă) [″ + *opsis,* vision] Macroesthesia.

macrorhinia (măk-rō-rīn′ē-ă) [″ + *rhis,* nose] Excessive size of the nose, either congenital or pathological.

macroscelia (măk-rō-sē′lē-ă) [″ + *skelos,* leg] Abnormally large legs.

macroscopic (măk-rō-skŏp′ĭk) [″ + *skopein,* to examine] Large enough to be seen by the naked eye. Opposite of microscopic.

macroscopy (măk-rŏs′kō-pē) Examination of an object with the naked eye.

macrosigmoid (măk″rō-sĭg′moyd) Abnormally large sigmoid colon.

macrosmatic (măk″rŏs-măt′ĭk) [″ + *osmasthai,* to smell] Having an abnormally keen sense of smell.

macrosomatia, macrosomia (măk″rō-sō-mā′shē-ă, măk-rō-sō′mē-ă) [Gr. *makros,* large, + *soma,* body] Abnormally large body.

fetal m. In a newborn, birth weight above the 90th percentile on the intrauterine growth curve. SEE: *large for gestational age*.

macrospore (măk′rō-spor) The larger spore type in certain fungi and protozoa with two spores.

macrostereognosis (măk″rō-stē″rē-ō-nō′sĭs) [″ + *stereos,* solid, + *gnosis,* knowledge] A misperception that objects appear to be larger than they are.

macrostomia (măk-rō-stō′mē-ă) [″ + *stoma,* mouth] Excessively large mouth.

macrostructure (măk′rō-strŭk″tūr) The gross structure of an entity.

macrothrombocyte [″ + *thrombos,* clot, + *kytos,* cell] A large platelet seen in some leukemias and rare disorders of platelets.

macrothrombocytopenia [″ + ″ + ″ + *penia,* lack] Deficiency of macrothrombocytes. SEE: *Alport's syndrome*.

macrotia (măk-rō′shē-ă) [″ + *ous,* ear] Abnormally large ears.

macrotooth An abnormally enlarged tooth.

macula (măk′ū-lă) *pl.* **maculae** [L., spot] **1.** A small spot or colored area. SEE: *roseola*. **2.** Macule. **macular** (-lăr), *adj.*

m. acusticae The site of the hair cells (receptors) in the wall of the saccule and utricle of the inner ear. These receptors respond to changes in the pull of gravity (position of the head) and generate impulses carried by the vestibular branch of the acoustic nerve. They include the macula sacculi and macula utriculi.

m. acustica sacculi M. sacculi.

m. acustica utriculi M. utriculi.

m. albida A white mark found on the visceral layer of the peritoneum or epicardium in some contagious diseases.

m. atrophica A glistening white spot on the skin due to atrophy.

m. caerulea A steel-gray or blue stain of epidermis without elevation. It does not disappear on pressure and occurs esp. with pediculosis pubis or flea bites.

cerebral m. A reddened line that becomes deeper and persists for some time when the fingernail is drawn across the skin, esp. in tuberculous meningitis. SYN: *tache cérébrale*.

m. corneae An opaque spot in the cornea.

m. cribrosa One of several tiny foramina in the wall of the vestibule of the bony labyrinth of the ear through which pass filaments of the acoustic nerve.

m. densa A group of cells in the wall of the distal renal tubule, next to the juxtaglomerular cells, that are sensitive to changes in the salt concentration of the filtrate in the tubule.

m. flava laryngis A small yellow spot at the ventral end of each vocal cord formed by a small mass of elastic tissue or, sometimes, cartilage.

m. folliculi The point on the ovarian follicle where it ruptures.

m. germinativa The germinal area in eggs with large yolks.

m. gonorrhoeica A red spot at the orifice of Bartholin's gland; seen in gonococcal vulvitis.

m. lutea retinae A yellow spot in the center of the retina approx. 2 mm lateral to the exit of the optic nerve. It contains a pit, fovea centralis, where the retina is reduced to a layer of closely packed cones, which functions as the area of most acute vision (central vision).

m. sacculi The site of the hair cells in the saccule; receptors stimulated by the pull of gravity. These cells generate impulses carried by the vestibular branch of the acoustic nerve. SYN: *m. acustica sacculi*.

m. utriculi The site of the hair cells in the utricule; receptors stimulated by the pull of gravity. These cells generate impulses carried by the vestibular branch of the acoustic nerve. SYN: *m. acustica utriculi*.

macular degeneration, age-related macular degeneration Loss of pigmentation in the macular region of the retina, usually affecting persons over age 50; a common disease of unknown etiology that produces central visual field loss and is the leading cause of permanent visual impairment in the U.S. Evidence suggests that key contributing factors to this disease may include sunlight exposure, smoking, alcohol use, and a diet low in carotenoids.

SYMPTOMS: The central visual loss that marks this illness can make reading, working with the hands (e.g., sewing), driving, or recognizing people's faces difficult. Peripheral vision is preserved in this disease. SEE: *visual field* for illus.

TREATMENT: Laser photocoagulation of new blood vessel membranes can help to arrest the visual loss in some patients with the exudative form of age-related macular degeneration. However, this form of treatment is complicated by a high recurrence rate, and some immediate visual loss in the form of a scotoma. Experimental treatments include the use of antiangiogenic drugs, phototherapy, radiation therapy, and retinal surgeries.

PATIENT CARE: The Amsler grid, and other testing devices such as a tangent screen, can be used to test patients for visual distortions due to retinal disease, but the validity and reproducibility of Amsler grid testing is poor.

maculate(d) (măk′ū-lāt, -lāt-ĕd) Spotted, as with macules.

maculation (măk-ū-lā′shŭn) [L. *macula,* spot] Process of becoming maculate; development of macules.

macule (măk′ūl) [L. *macula,* spot] A flat spot on the skin whose color may be lighter or darker than the surrounding skin. Some common examples are freckles, petechiae, and vitiligo. SYN: *macula.*

maculopapular (măk″ū-lō-păp′ū-lăr) A rash that has both flat stained regions (macules) and small elevated bumps or pimples (papules).

maculopathy (măk″ū-lŏp′ă-thē) [″ + Gr. *pathos,* disease] Retinal pathology involving the macula of the eye.

mad **1.** Not rational. SYN: *insane.* **2.** Angry. **3.** Rash, foolish, frantic. **4.** Suffering from infection with rabies. SYN: *rabid.*

madarosis (măd-ă-rō′sĭs) [Gr. *madaros,* bald] Loss of eyelashes or eyebrows.

madder (măd′ĕr) Root of the plant *Rubia tinctorum,* a source of the red dye alizarin.

Madelung's deformity [Otto W. Madelung, Strasbourg surgeon, 1846–1926] Displacement of the hand to the radial side due to relative overgrowth of the ulna.

Madelung's disease Generalized symmetrical deposits of fatty tissue (lipomas) on the upper back, shoulders, and neck. SYN: *Madelung's neck.*

madescent (măd-ĕs′ĕnt) [L. *madescere,* to become moist] Slightly moist or becoming so.

Madura foot [from Madur district in India where disease was first described in 1842] A local painless lesion—called a mycetoma—of an exposed area, such as bare feet. It consists of swollen infected tissues with sinus tracts and a purulent, grainy discharge. Mycetomas may occur in any body part. It is usually found in adult males who work outside and have poor footwear or inadequate wound care. SYN: *maduromycosis.*

ETIOLOGY: Various fungi including eumycetoma and actinomycetes. In the U.S., the most frequent cause is *Pseudallescheria boydii.*

TREATMENT: The antibiotic given depends on the specific organism involved. Clindamycin is used for actinomycetoma. Ketoconazole or itraconazole have been used in eumycetomas. Surgery should not be necessary, but drug treatment often takes several months.

maduromycosis (măd-ū″rō-mī-kō′sĭs) A chronic fungal infection of the foot or hand characterized by marked swelling and development of nodules, vesicles, abscesses, and sinuses. A type of mycetoma.

mafenide acetate (măf′ĕn-īd) An antibacterial of the sulfonamide class, used topically in cream form for treating burns.

magaldrate (măg′ăl-drāt) Aluminum magnesium hydroxide sulfate; used as an antacid.

magenblase syndrome [Ger. *Magen,* stomach, + *Blase,* bubble] Accumulation of swallowed air in the stomach that leads to postprandial fullness and pressure. Radiograph of the stomach will reveal a large gastric bubble.

Magendie's foramen (mă-jĕn′dēz) [François Magendie, Fr. physiologist, 1783–1855] The median of three openings in the roof of the 4th ventricle. It is in front of the cerebellum and behind the pons varolii, connecting the ventricle with the subarachnoid space.

magenstrasse (măg″ĕn-străs′ĕ) [″ + *Strasse,* street] A groove along the lesser curvature of the stomach from cardia to pylorus.

magenta (mă-jĕn′tă) The dye basic fuchsin.

maggot Larva of an insect, esp. the soft-bodied footless larva of flies (order Diptera). Many are parasitic, giving rise to myiasis.

maggot treatment A method of treating septic wounds. In the 1930s, scientific studies indicated that neglected and infected compound fractures were aided in healing when blackbottle fly, bluebottle fly, and blowfly maggots accidentally infested the wounds. The maggots removed necrotic tissue and left healthy granulating tissue. Modern therapy, including antibiotics, has made this method of treating wounds and osteomyelitis obsolete. Nevertheless, it is possible to culture sterile blowfly maggots for this use. In severe skin infections when all other forms of therapy have failed, this method has been used.

magical thinking The feeling that one's thoughts or actions have the ability to cause actions or effects that would defy the normal laws of cause and effect.

Magill forceps Angulated forceps used during direct laryngoscopy to remove a foreign body from an obstructed airway.

magistery (măj′ĭs-tĕr″ē) [L. *magister,* master] **1.** Specially compounded remedy. **2.** A precipitate.

magma (măg′mă) [Gr.] **1.** Mass left after extraction of principal. **2.** Salve or paste. **3.** A suspension of finely divided material in a small amount of water.

magnesia (măg-nē′zē-ă) [magnetic stone found in Magnesia, region of ancient Thessaly] Magnesium oxide; MgO.

milk of m. Aperient composed of magnesium hydroxide and water.

magnesia and alumina (tablets) An antacid preparation composed of aluminum hydroxide and magnesium hydroxide. Trade name is Maalox.

magnesium [L.] SYMB: Mg. A white mineral element found in soft tissue, muscles, bones, and to some extent in the body fluids. It has an atomic mass of 24.312, an atomic number of 12, and a specific gravity of 1.738. It is a naturally occurring element, being extracted from well and sea water. The human body contains approx. 25 g of magnesium, most of which is in the bones. Muscles contain less of it than they do of calcium. Concentration of magnesium in the blood serum is between 1.5 and 2.5 mEq/L.

Magnesium is widely distributed in foods; therefore, deficiency rarely occurs. It is obtained in sufficient quantities in whole grains, fruits, and vegetables. A typical diet contains 200 to 400 mg, but very little of this is absorbed. Deficiency may be present in patients with chronic diarrhea or diseases that interfere with absorption.

FUNCTION: Magnesium is a component of enzymes required for synthesis of adenosine triphosphate (ATP) and for the release of energy from ATP. It is also a component of enzymes involved in muscle contraction and protein synthesis.

DEFICIENCY: Tetany quite similar to that produced by hypocalcemia, weakness, and mental depression.

EXCESS: An excess is usually caused by intravenous magnesium replacement or decreased renal excretion due to renal disease. Bradycardia, hypotension, decreased level of consciousness, and muscle weakness are common symptoms. In severe hypermagnesemia, cardiac arrest may occur. Treatment includes withholding magnesium and administering diuretics.

m. carbonate $MgCO_3 \cdot 3H_2O$; a bulky, white, odorless powder. Taken by mouth to neutralize acid in stomach.

m. chloride $MgCl_2 \cdot 6H_2$; used in treating electrolyte disturbances and in dialysis solutions.

m. gluconate A medicine used to replace magnesium in the body.

m. hydroxide $Mg(OH)_2$; a bulky white powder that, in aqueous suspension, is called milk of magnesia. Used as a laxative and an antacid.

m. oxide MgO; calcined magnesia; light magnesia. A white, very bulky powder. In Great Britain, it is called light magnesium oxide. It is used as an antacid and laxative.

m. salicylate An antipyretic and analgesic. Trade name is Magan.

m. sulfate $MgSO_4 \cdot 7H_2O$; small colorless crystals with a bitter saline taste. It is used as a cathartic, anticonvulsant, and topically as an anti-inflammatory agent. The intravenous form is used to manage pregnancy-induced hypertension, to halt preterm labor, and to treat torsade de pointes. SYN: *epsom salt.*

INCOMPATIBILITY: Ammonium chloride, soapsuds enema, quinine, ferric chloride, sulfanilamide.

magnet [Gr. *magnes,* magnet] Any body that has the property of attracting iron. This may be a natural iron oxide or a mass of iron or steel that has this property given to it artificially. A piece of iron may be magnetized by passage of an electric current through an insulated wire wound around it. **magnetic,** *adj.*

magnetic cortical stimulation The induction of painless electrical current within the brain to detect abnormalities in cortical motor neuron function.

magnetic field The space permeated by the magnetic lines of force surrounding a permanent magnet or coil of wire carrying electric current.

magnetic lines of force The lines indicating the direction of the magnetic force in the space surrounding a magnet or constituting a magnetic field.

magnetic resonance cholangiopancreatography ABBR: MRCP. Visualization of the pancreatic and biliary ducts with magnetic resonance imaging. MRCP provides a noninvasive alternative to endoscopic retrograde cholangiopancreatography (ERCP), esp. if biopsies are not needed and direct visualization of the ampulla of Vater is not required.

magnetic resonance imaging ABBR: MRI. A type of diagnostic radiography that uses the characteristic behavior of protons (and other atomic nuclei) when placed in powerful magnetic fields to make images of tissues and organs. Certain atomic nuclei with an odd number of neutrons, protons, or both are subjected to a radiofrequency pulse, causing them to absorb and release energy. The resulting current passes through a radiofrequency receiver and is then transformed into an image. This technique is valuable in providing soft-tissue images of the central nervous and musculoskeletal systems. Imaging techniques allow visualization of the vascular system without the use of contrast agents. However, agents are available for contrast enhancement. Magnetic resonance imaging is contraindicated in patients with cardiac pacemakers or ferromagnetic aneurysmal clips in place. SEE: illus.; *brain* for illus.; *positron emission tomography.*

PATIENT CARE: Metal may become damaged during testing; therefore, health care providers must establish whether the patient has metal anywhere on or in the body. Patients should not wear metal objects such as jewelry, hair ornaments, or watches, for example. Patients who have had surgical procedures after which metal clips, pins, or other hardware remain in the body should not have the test. During testing, the patient lies on a flat surface that is moved inside a tube encompassing a magnet. The patient must lie as still as possible. No discomfort occurs as a re-

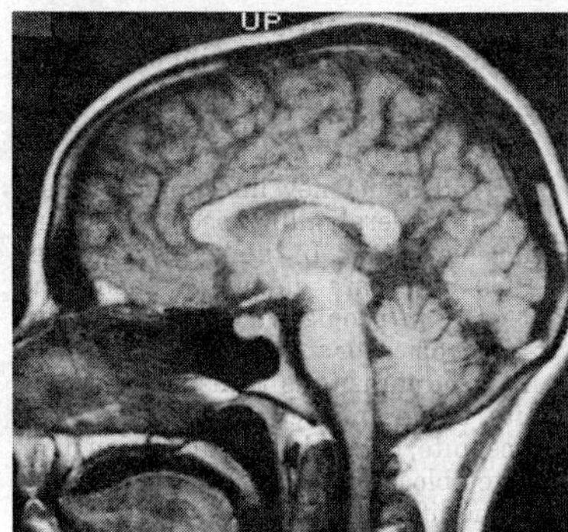

MAGNETIC RESONANCE IMAGIMG

Midsagittal section of brain of normal young subject

sult of the test. Sounds heard during the test come from the pulsing of the magnetic field as it scans the body. Confinement during the 30 to 90 min required for testing may frighten the patient, but the patient can talk to staff by microphone. Relaxation techniques are also taught for use during the test.

magnetism (măg′nĕ-tĭzm) [Gr. *magnes,* magnet, + *-ismos,* condition] The property of repulsion and attraction of certain substances that have magnetic properties. SEE: *magnet.*

magnetoelectricity (măg-nē″tō-ē″lĕk-trĭs′ĭ-tē) [″ + *elektron,* amber] Electricity generated by use of magnets.

magnetometer (măg″nĕ-tŏm′ĕ-tĕr) [″ + *metron,* measure] Device for measuring magnetic fields.

magneton (măg′nĕ-tŏn) The unit of nuclear magnetic force.

magnetotherapy (măg-nē″tō-thĕr′ă-pē) [″ + *therapeia,* treatment] Application of magnets or magnetism in treating diseases. There is no evidence that such therapy is effective.

magnetropism (măg-nĕt′rō-pĭzm) [″ + *trope,* a turn] The change in direction of growth of a plant or organism in response to the action of a magnetic field.

magnification (măg-nĭ-fĭ-kā′shŭn) [L. *magnus,* great, + *facere,* to make] Process of increasing apparent size of an object, esp. under a microscope.

magnitude Size, extent, or dimensions.

magnum [L.] **1.** Large or great. **2.** Old term for capitate bone (os magnum), the largest of the carpals.

Mahaim fibers [I. Mahaim, contemporary Fr. physician] Fibers for conducting cardiac impulses. They connect the proximal main atrioventricular bundle to the septal myocardium and permit ventricular pre-excitation with resultant tachycardia.

ma huang (mă wŏng) An herbal remedy recommended by alternative medicine practitioners for dieting, weight loss, or increased energy. Its main ingredient is the stimulant ephedrine, which may be hazardous to patients with hypertension, vascular disease, or other conditions.

maim (mām) [ME. *maymen,* to cripple] **1.** To injure seriously; to disable. **2.** To deprive of the use of a part, such as an arm or leg.

main (măn) [Fr.] Hand.

m. en griffe Clawhand.

mainstreaming The practice of educating children with disabling conditions in the general classroom instead of within specialized institutions, so as not to deprive them of normal social experiences and conditions.

maintainer Something that supports or keeps another thing in existence or continuity.

space m. Device fashioned to keep teeth separated when placed across an edentulous segment of the dental arch. It may consist of bands, bars, springs, or other materials, and is cemented or soldered to orthodontic bands or crowns on the adjacent teeth.

Majocchi's disease (mă-yŏk′ēz) [Domenico Majocchi, It. physician, 1849–1929] Ring-shaped purple eruption of lower limbs. SYN: *purpura annularis telangiectodes.*

Majocchi's granuloma Allergic skin growth due to fungal infections.

major histocompatibility complex ABBR: MHC. A group of genes on chromosome 6 that code for the antigens that determine tissue and blood compatibility. In humans, histocompatibility antigens are called human leukocyte antigens (HLA) because they were originally discovered in large numbers on lymphocytes. There are thousands of combinations of HLA antigens. Class I MHC antigens (HLA-A, HLA-B, and HLA-C) are found on all nucleated cells and platelets. Class II antigens (HLA-DR, HLA-DQ, and HLA-DP) are found on lymphocytes and antigen processing cells and are important in the specific immune response. In tissue and organ transplantation, the extent to which the HLA or "tissue type" of the donor and recipient match is a major determinant of the success of the transplant.

majority, age of The age–usually 18 or 21 years–at which a person achieves full legal rights to make one's own decisions, enter into contracts, and be held personally accountable for the consequences of one's actions.

mal (măl) [Fr., from L. *malum,* an evil] A sickness or disorder.

m. de mer Seasickness.

mal- Prefix meaning *bad, poor,* or *abnormal.*

mala (mā′lă) [L. *mala,* cheek] **1.** The cheek. **2.** The cheekbone. **malar** (mā′lăr), *adj.*

malabsorption syndrome Disordered or inadequate absorption of nutrients from the intestinal tract, esp. the small intestine. The syndrome may be associated with or due to a number of diseases, including those affecting the intestinal mucosa, such as infections, tropical sprue, celiac disease, pancreatic insufficiency, or lactase deficiency. It may also be due to surgery such as gastric resection and ileal bypass or to antibiotic therapy such as neomycin.

malacia (mă-lā′shē-ă) [Gr. *malakia,* softening] Abnormal softening of tissues of an organ or of tissues themselves.

malacoplakia (măl″ă-kō-plā′kē-ă) [Gr. *malakos,* soft, + *plax,* plaque] Existence of soft patches in mucous membrane of a hollow organ.

m. vesicae Soft, fungus-like patches on mucosa of the bladder and ureters.

malacosarcosis (măl″ă-kō-săr-kō′sĭs) [″ + *sarx,* flesh, + *osis,* condition] Softness of tissue, esp. muscular.

malacosteon (măl-ă-kŏs′tē-ŏn) [″ + *osteon,* bone] Softening of the bones. SYN: *osteomalacia.*

malacotomy (măl-ă-kŏt′ō-mē) [Gr. *malakos,* soft, + *tome,* incision] Incision of soft areas of the body, esp. of the abdominal wall.

maladie de Roger (măl″ă-dē′) [Henry L. Roger, Fr. physician, 1809–1891] Congenital interventricular septal defect.

maladjusted Poorly adjusted; unhappy or unsuccessful because of inability or failure to adjust to life's stresses. Marked by depression, anxiety, and irritability.

malady (măl′ă-dē) [Fr. *maladie,* illness, from L. *malum,* an evil] A disease or disorder. SYN: *disease.*

malaise (mă-lāz′) [Fr.] A subjective sense of discomfort, weakness, fatigue, or feeling rundown that may occur alone or accompany other symptoms and illnesses.

malalignment (măl″ă-līn′mĕnt) Improper alignment of structures such as teeth or the portions of a fractured bone. SEE: *malocclusion.*

malar bone A four-pointed bone on each side of the face, uniting the frontal and superior maxillary bones with the zygomatic process of the temporal bone. SYN: *cheekbone; zygoma; zygomatic bone.*

malaria (mă-lā′rē-ă) [It. *malaria,* bad air] A febrile hemolytic disease caused by protozoa of the genus *Plasmodium.* There are four species of malaria: the "benign" malarias: *P. vivax, P. ovale,* and *P. malariae;* and the potentially "malignant" malaria, *P. falciparum.* Each has its own geographic distribution, incubation period, symptoms, and treatment. **malarial, malarious** (-ăl, -ŭs), *adj.*

Although malaria has been virtually eliminated from temperate climates, it is widespread throughout the tropics. As many as half a billion people may be infected with the disease worldwide; at least 50 million new infections occur annually. Several million people die of malaria each year. In the U.S., fewer than 1000 cases are diagnosed each year, usually in people who have just come from tropical or subtropical regions. The malaria parasite is transmitted by the bite of an infected female *Anopheles* mosquito, or rarely by transfusion of infected blood products.

The life cycle of the parasite is complex. Once the parasitic sporozoite enters the bloodstream, it quickly invades organs such as the liver (this is the "tissue phase" of the infection). There, the organism matures as a schizont. After an incubation period ranging from about 10 to 30 days, multiple malarial merozoites are released into the blood, where they invade red blood cells (the "erythrocytic phase" of the infection). Some dormant forms, called hypnozoites, remain in the liver in *P. vivax* and *P. ovale* malaria, where they may serve as a reservoir for relapse. In the red blood cells, the organisms mature into ring forms and feeding forms (trophozoites). When the parasites break out of red cells to infect other cells in the circulation, they cause hemolysis and periodic symptoms (see below).

After several reproductive cycles, microgametocytes and macrogametocytes develop. Mosquitoes consume these when the parasites take their blood meal from infected humans. Further developmental stages occur within the mosquitoes, resulting in the production of the infectious sporozoites that are injected into human hosts when the mosquitoes feed again. SEE: illus.

SYMPTOMS: Initially, the symptoms are nonspecific and resemble those of a minor febrile illness with malaise, headache, fatigue, abdominal discomfort, and muscle aches, followed by fever and chills. The three stages of the malarial paroxysm are the defining characteristics of the illness. In the first (or chill) stage, patients complain of feeling cold and experience shaking chills that last from a few minutes to several hours. During the second (or hot) stage, minimal sweating occurs, although temperature rises to as high as 106°F; this stage lasts for several hours, and patients are at risk for febrile convulsions and hyperthermic brain damage. The patient also may exhibit tachycardia, hypotension, cough, headache, backache, nausea, abdominal pain, vomiting, diarrhea, and altered consciousness. The third (sweating) stage begins within 2 to 6 hr. In this period, the

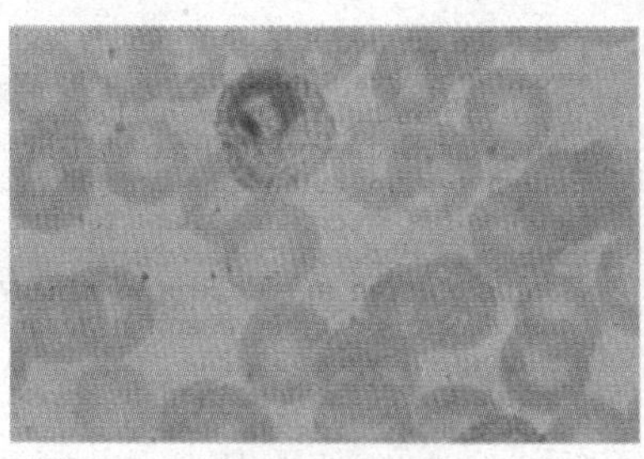

10μm

PLASMODIUM VIVAX SPOROZOITE

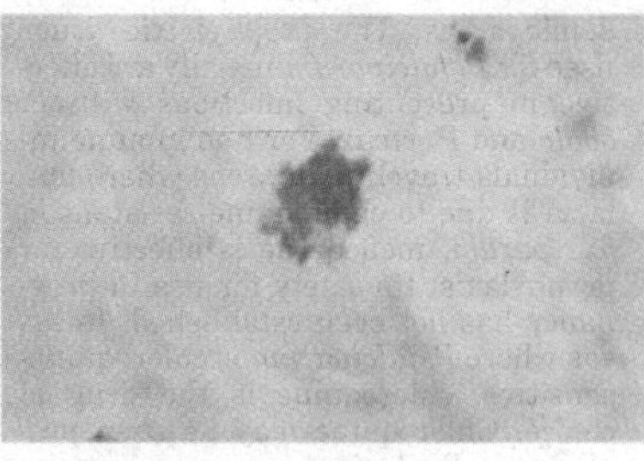

10μm

PLASMODIUM VIVAX SCHIZONT FORMING MEROZOITES

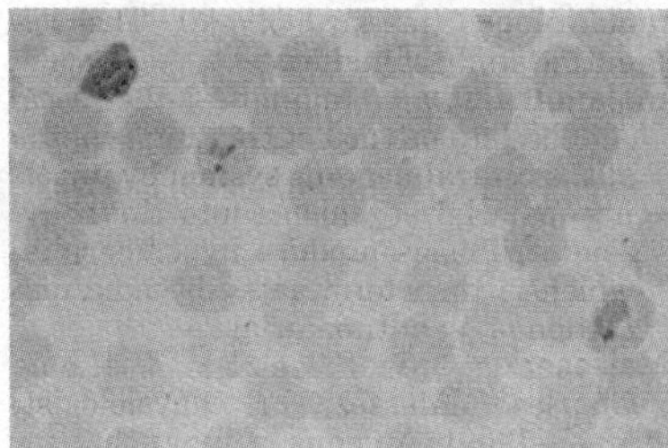

10μm

PLASMODIUM MALARIAE MEROZOITES

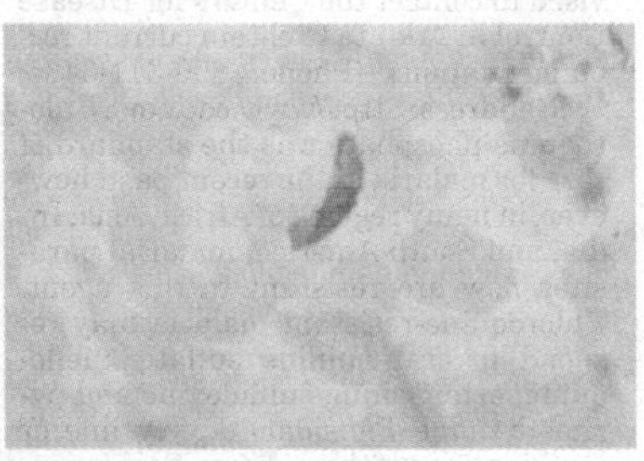

10μm

PLASMODIUM FALCIPARUM GAMETOCYTE

MALARIA - CAUSING ORGANISMS

sweating is marked as the fever subsides, and is followed by profound fatigue and by sleep. If untreated, malarial paroxysms caused by *P. ovale* or *P. vivax* will occur cyclically every 48 hr. If due to *P. malariae,* paroxysms will occur every 72 hr. Infections with *P. falciparum* may have a 48-hr cycle of paroxysms, but continuous fever is more characteristic. A severe form of falciparum malaria (cerebral malaria) is characterized by coma and, in spite of treatment, is associated with a 20% mortality rate in adults and 15% in children. About 10% of children who survive cerebral malaria have persistent neurologic deficits. Residual deficits in adults who survive this form of malaria are unusual. Progressive, possibly severe anemia and enlargement of the spleen are characteristic of all forms of malaria.

A rare but serious hematologic complication of malaria is acute intravascular hemolytic anemia, associated with infection with *P. falciparum*. This condition is called blackwater fever because of the accompanying hemoglobinuria.

DIAGNOSIS: Malaria should be suspected in any febrile person who has returned from an endemic region in the last several months. Giemsa-stained thick and thin blood films are examined to confirm the diagnosis.

PREVENTION: In endemic areas, pools of standing or stagnant water, in which mosquitoes breed, should be eliminated. Individuals traveling to the tropics should wear protective clothing to which insect repellent has been applied. Protective screen netting should cover beds. Individuals should apply DEET or other effective insect repellents to exposed skin, especially between dusk and dawn, when mosquitoes feed most actively.

PROPHYLAXIS: Chemoprophylaxis is begun 1 week before arriving in an endemic area and is continued throughout the stay and for 4 weeks after leaving the area. Chemoprophylaxis is never entirely effective; thus, malaria always should be considered when treating patients who have a febrile illness and who have traveled to an endemic area, even if they have taken prophylactic antimalaria drugs. The drug(s) advised for prophylaxis depend on the sensitivity of local parasites and whether infection is likely. Because of the changing sensitivity of the malaria parasites to drugs, it is not possible to be certain that a particular drug will be effective in all endemic areas. The prophylactic drugs used for *P. falciparum* usually are effective in preventing infections with *P. ovale* and *P. vivax*. For nonimmune individuals traveling in areas where malaria is due to chloroquine-resistant *P. falciparum,* mefloquine is effective for prophylaxis. Its safety for use in pregnancy has not been established. In areas where *P. falciparum* is chloroquine-sensitive, chloroquine is the drug of choice. Chloroquine may be used prophylactically during pregnancy.

TREATMENT: The parasites that cause malaria constantly evolve, making drug treatment difficult. Patients and health care professionals are advised to contact the Centers for Disease Control in Atlanta to obtain current recommendations (Phone: 800-311-3435; Web address: http://www.cdc.gov). Chloroquine phosphate was the standard of care for malaria in the recent past; however, in many regions of Africa, Asia, India, and South America, malarial parasites now are resistant to this agent. Chloroquine-resistant malaria may respond to oral quinine sulfate, mefloquine, artemisinin, sulfadoxine and pyrimethamine (Fansidar), doxycycline, or combinations of these drugs. Severe malaria due to chloroquine-resistant *P. falciparum* has been treated with intravenous quinidine gluconate plus doxycycline. Effective non-antibiotic therapy for malaria sometimes includes exchange transfusion and iron chelation.

PATIENT CARE: Health care providers in endemic areas need to work toward prompt detection and effective treatment of malaria. In such areas, suppressive and prophylactic drugs may be needed to control the disease.

cerebral m. Falciparum malaria in which the brain is affected. This fulminant disease often produces coma, shock, or sudden death.

double quartan m. Malaria in which two concurrent cycles result in fever occurring on two successive days.

falciparum m. Malaria caused by *Plasmodium falciparum*. It is more prevalent in the tropics. Symptoms are more severe than in other types but it runs a shorter course without relapses.

quartan m. Malaria with short and less severe paroxysms. Sporulation occurs each 72 hr, causing seizures every 4 days. It is caused by *Plasmodium malariae.*

quotidian m. Malaria in which paroxysms occur with daily periodicity due to 24-hr sporulation of two groups of *P. vivax*. Temperature rises and falls abruptly.

tertian m. Malaria in which sporulation occurs each 48 hr. Symptoms are more common during the day. Paroxysms are divided into chill, fever, and sweating stages. Cold stage is usually 10 to 15 min but may last an hour or more. Febrile stage varies from 4 to 6 hr. Benign tertian malaria is caused by *Plasmodium vivax,* malignant tertian malaria by *Plasmodium falciparum.*

triple quartan m. Malaria in which three concurrent cycles result in fever occurring every day.

vivax m. Malaria caused by *Plasmodium vivax*. It is the most common form of malaria, marked by frequent recurrence.

malariacidal (mă-lā″rē-ă-sī′dăl) [It. *malaria,* bad air, + L. *caedere,* to kill] Having the property of killing malaria parasites.

malariology (mă-lār-ē-ŏl′ō-jē) The scientific study of malaria.

malariotherapy (mă-lār-ē-ō-thĕr′ă-pē) An obsolete method of treating syphilis of the central nervous system by injecting malarial organisms into the body. The organisms produce hyperthermia, which is then terminated by administration of an antimalarial.

Malassezia (măl″ă-sē′zē-ă) [Louis Charles Malassez, Fr. physiologist, 1842–1909] A genus of fungi that infect animals and humans. The organisms are lipophilic. In hospitals malassezian infections tend to occur in patients receiving lipid infusions. Malassezian infections of the bloodstream result in sepsis.

malassimilation (măl″ă-sĭm-ĭ-lā′shŭn) [L. *malus,* ill, + *assimilatio,* making like] Defective, incomplete, or faulty assimilation, esp. of nutritive material. SEE: *malabsorption syndrome*.

malate (mā′lāt) A salt or ester of malic acid.

malathion (măl″ă-thī′ŏn) An effective pesticide.

maldigestion (măl″dī-jĕs′chŭn) Disordered digestion.

male [O.Fr.] **1.** Masculine. **2.** The sex that has organs for producing sperm for fertilization of ova.

male erectile disorder The persistent or recurrent inability to attain, or to maintain until completion of the sexual activity, an adequate erection. The disturbance causes marked distress or interpersonal difficulty. The difficulty cannot be attributed to a medical condition, substance abuse, or medications. SEE: *erectile dysfunction; female sexual arousal disorder*.

malemission (măl″ē-mĭsh′ŭn) [L. *malus,* evil, + *e,* out, + *mittere,* to send] Failure of semen to be ejaculated from the urinary meatus during coitus.

maleruption (măl-ē-rŭp′shŭn) Incorrect eruption of teeth.

malformation (măl-for-mā′shŭn) [″ + *formatio,* a shaping] Deformity; abnormal shape or structure, esp. congenital.

tooth m. Abnormalities of size and shape that usually occur during the morphodifferentiation stage of tooth formation. Incomplete matrix formation or mineralization will also result in defective teeth that may or may not be abnormal in shape initially.

malfunction (măl-fŭnk′shŭn) Defective function.

malic (mā′lĭk, măl′ĭk) [L. *malum,* apple] Pert. to apples.

malice (măl′ĭs) [L. *malus,* bad] Desire or intent to harm someone or to see others suffer.

malign (mă-līn′) [ME. *maligne*] Tending to injure or harm; malignant.

malignancy (mă-lĭg′năn-sē) [L. *malignus,* of bad kind] **1.** State of being malignant. **2.** A neoplasm or tumor that is cancerous as opposed to benign. SYN: *virulence.*

malignant (mă-lĭg′nănt) Growing worse; resisting treatment, said of cancerous growths. Tending or threatening to produce death; harmful. SYN: *virulent.*

malignant angioendotheliomatosis Intravascular large cell lymphoma that is typically found in the blood vessels of the skin and central nervous system and is often rapidly fatal.

TREATMENT: Current treatment is based on polychemotherapy.

malinger (mă-lĭng′ĕr) [Fr. *malingre,* weak, sickly] To feign illness, usually to arouse sympathy, to escape work, or to continue to receive compensation. SEE: *factitious disorder; Munchausen syndrome.*

malingerer (mă-lĭng′gĕr-ĕr) **1.** One who pretends to be ill or suffering from a nonexistent disorder to arouse sympathy. **2.** One who pretends slow recuperation from a disease once suffered in order to continue to receive benefits of medical insurance and work absence.

malinterdigitation (măl″ĭn-tĕr-dĭj″ĭ-tā′shŭn) Abnormal intercuspal relation of the upper and lower teeth. SEE: *overbite; underbite.*

malleable (măl′ē-ă-bl) [L. *mallere,* to hammer] Having the property of being shaped by pressure.

malleation (măl-lē-ā′shŭn) Spasmodic action of the hands in which they seem drawn to strike any near object, as spasmodic rapping against thighs or furniture. SEE: *tic.*

malleoincudal (măl″ē-ō-ĭng′kū-dăl) [L. *malleus,* hammer, + *incus,* anvil] Concerning or pert. to the malleus and incus.

malleolus (măl-ē′ō-lŭs) *pl.* **malleoli** [L. *malleolus,* little hammer] The protuberance on both sides of the ankle joint; the lower extremity of the fibula is the lateral malleolus and lower end of the tibia is the medial malleolus. **malleolar** (-ō-lăr), *adj.*

external m. Process on outer edge of fibula at lower end.

internal m. Round process on inner edge of tibia at lower end.

malleotomy (măl″ē-ŏt′ō-mē) [″ + Gr. *tome,* incision] **1.** Division of the malleus of the inner ear. **2.** Severing the ligaments attached to the malleoli of the ankle.

mallet A hammer-like tool to condense amalgam or direct filling gold.

mallet finger SEE: *hammer finger.*

mallet toe SEE: *hammertoe.*

malleus (măl′ē-ŭs) *pl.* **mallei** [L., hammer] The largest of the three auditory ossicles in the middle ear. It is attached to the eardrum and articulates with the incus. SEE: *ear.*

Mallophaga (măl-ŏf′ă-gă) [Gr. *mallos,* wool, + *phagein,* to eat] An order of insects that includes biting lice.

Mallory-Weiss syndrome [G. Kenneth Mallory, U.S. pathologist, b. 1900; Soma Weiss, U.S. internist, 1898–1942] Hemorrhage from the upper gastrointestinal tract due to a tear in the mucosa of the esophagus or gastroesophageal junction. Violent retching usually precedes the bleeding. SEE: *Nursing Diagnoses Appendix.*

malnutrition (măl″nū-trĭ′shŭn) Any disease-promoting condition resulting from either an inadequate or excessive exposure to nutrients (i.e., undernutrition or overnutrition, respectively). Common causes of malnutrition are inadequate calorie consumption; inadequate intake of essential vitamins, minerals, or other micronutrients; improper absorption and distribution of foods within the body; overeating; and intoxication by nutrient excesses. SEE: table; and names of specific nutritional disorders (e.g., obesity, pellegra, scurvy).

Worldwide, malnutrition is a disease that results typically from inadequate consumption of foods, esp. proteins, iron, and vitamins (e.g., vitamin A). In industrialized nations, overnutrition is more common than undernutrition. In the U.S., for example, 50% of the population is considered to be overweight, and 22% have a body mass index greater than 30 kg/m^2 and are frankly obese. Undernutrition in Western nations typically results from poverty, alcoholism, chronic illnesses, or extreme dieting.

protein-energy m. ABBR: PEM. Malnutrition due to inadequate intake of calories or protein, or both. It usually is seen in children under age 5 or in patients undergoing the stress of a major illness. In the critically ill patient, hypoalbuminemia results from the depletion of stored protein and/or hepatic dysfunction. It may increase a patient's vulnerability to the toxicities of drugs, skin breakdown, infections, gastrointestinal ulcerations, and other illnesses. SYN: *protein-calorie malnutrition.* SEE: *kwashiorkor.*

Infants and Children	Adolescents and Adults
Lack of subcutaneous fat	Red swollen lingual papillae
Wrinkling of skin on light stroking	Glossitis
Poor muscle tone	Papillary atrophy of tongue
Pallor	Stomatitis
Rough skin (toad skin)	Spongy, bleeding gums
Hemorrhage of newborn, vitamin K deficiency	Muscle tenderness in extremities
Bad posture	Poor muscle tone
Nasal area is red and greasy	Loss of vibratory sensation
Sores at angles of mouth, cheilosis	Increase or decrease of tendon reflexes
Rapid heartbeat	Hyperesthesia of skin
Red tongue	Purpura
Square head, wrists enlarged, rib beading	Dermatitis: facial butterfly, perineal, scrotal, vulval
Vincent's angina, thrush	Thickening and pigmentation of skin over bony prominences
Serious dental abnormalities	Nonspecific vaginitis
Corneal and conjunctival changes	Follicular hyperkeratosis of extensor surfaces of extremities
Adolescents and Adults	Rachitic chest deformity
Nasolabial sebaceous plugs	Anemia not responding to iron
Sores at angles of mouth, cheilosis	Fatigue of visual accommodation
Vincent's angina	Vascularization of cornea
Minimal changes in tongue color or texture	Conjunctival changes

SOURCE: Committee on Medical Nutrition, National Research Council, with permission.

SYMPTOMS: Symptoms of PEM include generalized muscle wasting and weakness. In the elderly, these symptoms are sometimes incorrectly attributed to advanced age. As a result, PEM is underdiagnosed in older individuals.

malocclusion Malposition and imperfect contact of the mandibular and maxillary teeth.

classification of m. The designation by angle of the types of malocclusion based on the relative positions of the first molar in the two arches when in occlusion: *Class I*—normal anteroposterior relationship but with crowding and rotated teeth. *Class II*—the lower arch is distal to the upper arch on one or both sides; the lower first molar is distal to the upper first molar. *Class III*—the lower arch is anterior to the upper arch on one or both sides; the lower first molar is anterior to the upper first molar.

malonylurea (măl″ō-nĭl-ū′rē-ă) Barbituric acid. SEE: *acid, barbituric.*

malpighian body (măl-pĭg′ē-ăn) [Marcello Malpighi, It. anatomist, founder of histology, 1628–1694] Lymph nodule found in the spleen.

malpighian capsule Old term for a renal corpuscle. SEE: *nephron.*

malpighian layer Inner layer of the epidermis that includes both stratum germinativum and stratum spinosum.

malposition (măl-pō-zĭ′shŭn) [L. *malus,* evil, + *positio,* placement] **1.** Faulty or abnormal position or placement, esp. of the body or one of its parts. **2.** Abnormal position of the fetal presenting part in relation to the maternal pelvis. SEE: *occiput posterior, persistent.*

malpractice [″ + Gr. *praxis,* an action] Incorrect or negligent treatment of a patient by persons responsible for health care, such as physicians, dentists, and nurses.

malpresentation [″ + *praesentatio,* a presenting] Abnormal position of the fetal presenting part, making natural delivery difficult or impossible. Labor is longer, and fetal descent may be impaired. SEE: *presentation* for illus.

cephalic m. A head presentation in which the presenting part is the face, brow, or chin.

malreduction (măl-rē-dŭk′shŭn) Imperfect replacement of a dislocated or fractured bone.

malrotation (măl″rō-tā′shŭn) Failure during embryogenesis of normal rotation of all or a portion of an organ or system, esp. the viscera.

MALT *mucosa-associated lymphoid tissue.*

malt [AS. *mealt*] Germinated grain, usually barley, used in manufacture of ale and beer. Contains carbohydrates (dextrin, maltose), a diastase, and proteins. Used as a food, esp. in wasting diseases.

Malta fever Brucellosis.

maltase (mawl′tās) [AS. *mealt,* grain] An enzyme of the small intestine that digests maltose, converting it by hydrolysis to glucose. SEE: *digestion; enzyme.*

malt extract A viscous, light brown fluid obtained from malt steeped in water.

maltose (mawl'tōs) A disaccharide, $C_{12}H_{22}O_{11}$, that is present in malt, malt products, and sprouting seeds. It is formed by the hydrolysis of starch and is converted into glucose by the enzyme maltase. SYN: *malt sugar*. SEE: *carbohydrate*.

maltosuria (mawl"tō-sūr'ē-ă) [" + Gr. *ouron,* urine] Presence of maltose in urine.

malt sugar Maltose.

malturned Abnormally turned, said of a tooth having turned on its long axis.

malunion [L. *malus,* evil, + *unio,* oneness] The joining of the fragments of a fractured bone in a faulty position, forming an imperfect alignment, shortening, deformity, or rotation.

mamanpian (mă-măn"pē-ăn') [Fr. *maman,* mother, + *pian,* yaw] A mother yaw.

mamelon (măm'ĕ-lŏn) [Fr., nipple] One of three rounded protuberances present on the cutting edge of an incisor tooth when it erupts. These are worn away by use.

mamill- SEE: words beginning with *mammill-*

mamm- (măm) SEE: *masto-*.

mamma (măm'ă) *pl.* **mammae** [L., breast] A glandular structure beneath the skin in the female that secretes milk. In the human female, there are normally two, situated over the anterolateral area between the third and sixth ribs. The nipple of each breast extends from the glandular tissue through the surface of the skin. SYN: *breast; mammary gland*.

mammal (măm'ăl) An animal of the class Mammalia, marked by having hair and by having mammary glands that produce milk to nourish the newborn.

mammalgia (măm-ăl'jē-ă) [L. *mamma,* breast, + Gr. *algos,* pain] Pain in the breast. SYN: *mastalgia; mastodynia*.

mammaplasty (măm'ă-plăs"tē) [" + Gr. *plassein,* to form] Plastic reconstructive surgery of the breast. Also spelled *mammoplasty*.

augmentation m. Surgical breast enlargement, either to increase breast size or to make an artificial breast to replace one surgically removed; performed by inserting autogenous tissue with mobilization of myocutaneous flap or a prosthesis filled with gel or saline.

CAUTION: The long-term health risks of some of the implant materials are unknown.

reduction m. Plastic surgery of the breast to decrease and reshape the breast(s).

mammary (măm'ă-rē) [L. *mamma,* breast] Pert. to the breast.

mammary glands Compound glands of the female breast that can secrete milk. They are made up of lobes and lobules bound together by areolar tissue. The main ducts number 15 to 20 and are known as lactiferous ducts, each one discharging through a separate orifice upon the surface of the nipple. The dilatations of the ducts form reservoirs for the milk during lactation. The pink, or dark-colored, skin around the nipple is called the areola. SYN: *mammae*.

mammectomy SEE: *mastectomy*.

mammillated (măm'mĭl-lā-tĕd) Having protuberances like a nipple.

mammilliplasty (măm-mĭl'ĭ-plăs"tē) [" + Gr. *plassein,* to form] Plastic operation on a nipple. SYN: *theleplasty*.

mammillitis (măm"mĭl-ī'tĭs) [" + Gr. *itis,* inflammation] Inflammation of a nipple. SYN: *acromastitis; thelitis*.

mammitis SEE: *mastitis*.

mammo- (măm'ō) SEE: *masto-*.

mammogram (măm'ō-grăm) [" + Gr. *gramma,* something written] X-ray of the breast.

mammography (măm-ŏg'ră-fē) [" + Gr. *graphein,* to write] Radiographic imaging of the breast to screen for (and detect) breast cancer. Mammography detects about 85% to 90% of existing breast cancers and, along with breast self-examination and regular professional check-ups, increases the rate of early breast cancer detection. Mammography detects more cancers when more than one radiologist interprets each image, a technique called "double reading." The American Cancer Society and expert panels convened by the federal government publish guidelines for the frequency of mammographic evaluation in the U.S. Although these guidelines change occasionally, evidence shows that mammographic screening can reduce the risk of dying from breast cancer in women aged 40 to 69 years. SEE: illus.

Palpable abnormalities of the breast that appear mammographically benign should nonetheless be further evaluated (e.g., with ultrasonography, fine-needle or core biopsy, or close follow-up examinations by skilled professionals).

mammoplasty SEE: *mammaplasty*.

mammose (măm'ōs) [L. *mammosus*] **1.** Having unusually large breasts. **2.** Shaped like a breast.

mammotome (măm'ō-tōm) A minimally invasive vacuum core biopsy instrument used to collect breast tissue for pathological analysis. It consists of a probe with an opening in the tip that connects to a vacuum source, a thumbwheel that controls the direction of the opening, a hollow, high-speed rotating cutter, and a tissue collection chamber. SEE: *percutaneous breast biopsy*.

mammotomy SEE: *mastotomy*.

mammotrophic (măm"ō-trŏf'ĭk) [" +

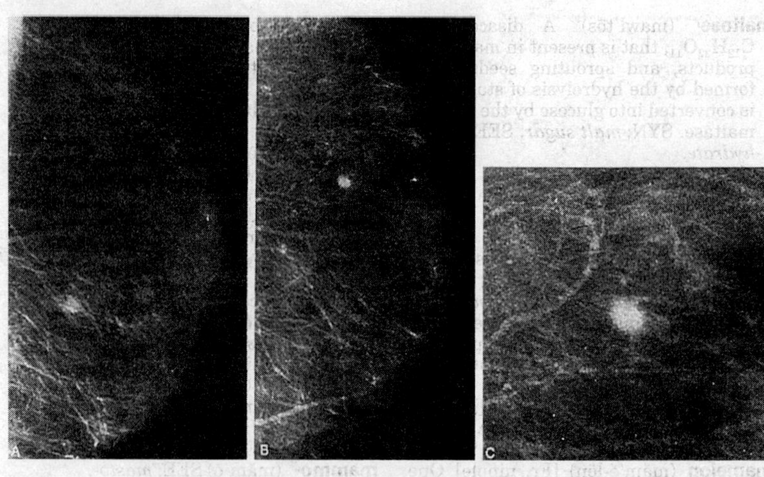

MAMMOGRAPHY SHOWING BREAST CANCER

Gr. *trophe,* nourishment] To have the effect of stimulating size or function of the breast.

man [AS. *mann*] **1.** Member of the human species, *Homo sapiens.* **2.** Male member of the species as distinguished from female. **3.** The human race, collectively; mankind.

managed care A variety of methods of financing and organizing the delivery of health care in which costs are contained by controlling the provision of benefits and services. Physicians, hospitals, and other health care agencies contract with the system to accept a predetermined monthly payment for providing services to patients enrolled in a managed care plan. Enrollee access to care may be limited to the physicians and other health care providers who are affiliated with the plan. In general, managed care attempts to control costs by overseeing and altering the behavior of their providers. Clinical decision making is influenced by a variety of administrative incentives and constraints. Incentives affect the health care provider's financial return for professional services. Constraints include specific rules, regulations, practice guidelines, diagnostic and treatment protocols, or algorithms. Care is overseen by quality assurance procedures and utilization reviews. SEE: *cost awareness; cost-effectiveness; gatekeeper; Health Maintenance Organization; managed competition; resource-based relative value scale.*

managed competition In health care practice, the requirement that health care organizations compete with each other in terms of price and quality of delivered services. SEE: *managed care; resource-based relative value scale.*

manchette (măn-chĕt′) [Fr., a cuff] A circular band consisting of microtubules around the caudal pole of developing sperm.

manchineel (măn″kĭ-nēl′) [Sp. *manzanilla,* small apple] A tree, *Hippomane mancinella,* native to tropical America that contains a milky, poisonous sap. Contact with the sap causes blistering of the skin. The fruit is also poisonous.

mancinism (măn′sĭn-ĭzm) [L. *mancus,* crippled] State of being left-handed.

mandala An ancient Hindu and Buddhist representation of the universe, occasionally used in the practice of complementary medicine as a focal point for meditation.

mandate (măn′dāt) **1.** A legal, ethical, or political requirement to execute actions or orders. **2.** An order from a higher authority to an officer of a lower court.

mandible (măn′dĭ-bl) [L. *mandibula,* lower jawbone] The horseshoe-shaped bone forming the lower jaw. SYN: *mandibula.* SEE: illus. **mandibular** (măn-dĭb′ū-lăr), *adj.*

mandibula SEE: *mandible.*

mandibulopharyngeal (măn-dĭb″ū-lō-fă-rin′jē-ăl) [″ + Gr. *pharynx,* throat] Concerning the mandible and pharynx.

mandrel, mandril (măn′drĕl) Handle that holds a dental tool so that it may be easily positioned by the operator. A spindle or shaft designed to fit a dental handpiece for the purpose of using a variety of tools for grinding, polishing or buffing.

mandrin (măn′drĭn) [Fr.] A guide or stylet for a flexible catheter in order to give it shape and firmness, especially for use in the urinary meatus.

maneuver [Fr. *manoeuvre,* from L. *manu operari,* to work by hand] **1.** Any dexterous or skillful procedure. **2.** In obstetrics, manipulation of the fetus to aid in delivery. SEE: *labor.*

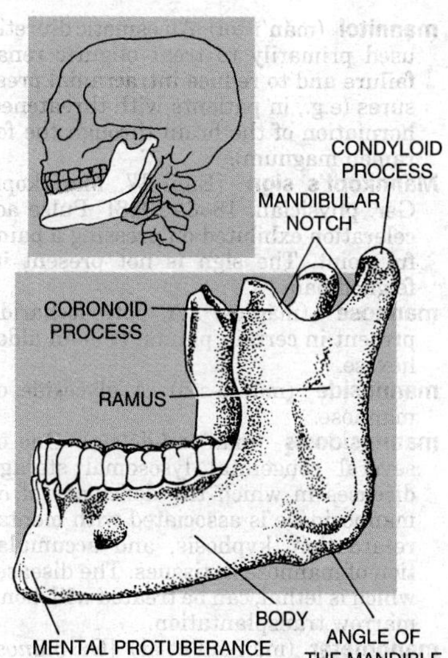

MANDIBLE—LEFT LATERAL VIEW

canalith repositioning m. Use of the Hallpike maneuver to reposition a canalith in the semicircular canal(s) to relieve benign positional vertigo. SEE: *Hallpike maneuver.*

Credé's m. SEE: *Credé's method.*

Heimlich m. SEE: *Heimlich maneuver.*

Leopold's m. SEE: *Leopold's maneuver.*

Mauriceau-Smellie m. [François Mauriceau, Fr. obstetrician, 1637–1709; William Smellie, Brit. obstetrician, 1697–1763] A technique of delivering the aftercoming head in a breech presentation in which traction is applied to the baby's maxilla and shoulders until the occiput appears under the symphysis pubis. The child's body is then raised to the mother's abdomen while the mouth, nose, brow, and occiput are successively brought over the perineum. The maneuver is used rarely, because most breech presentations are delivered by cesarean surgery.

Müller's m. SEE: *Müller's maneuver.*

Munro Kerr m. [John Munro Kerr, Scot. obstetrician, 1868–1955] A method used before the advent of ultrasonography to assess cephalopelvic disproportion, by manually comparing the size of the fetal head with that of the maternal pelvic brim.

Pinard's m. [Adolph Pinard, Fr. obstetrician, 1844–1934] A method of delivering a breech presentation, involving manipulation of the lower extremities of the fetus. Cesarean delivery has largely replaced it.

Prague m. Method for the delivery of the aftercoming head in a breech delivery when the occiput is posterior. It is rarely used in the era of cesarean deliveries.

Scanzoni m. [Friedrich W. Scanzoni, Ger. obstetrician, 1821–1891] Double application of forceps, the first to rotate the fetal occiput from a posterior to an anterior position, and the second to assist fetal descent and birth.

vagal m. Any physical action that increases parasympathetic tone and decreases the conduction of the electrical impulses of the heart. Vagal maneuvers may be used as first-line interventions in the evaluation or management of supraventricular tachycardias. Examples include bearing down or straining; massaging the carotid sinus; coughing; gagging; or immersing the face or neck in ice water. SEE: *Valsalva's m.*

Valsalva's m. SEE: *Valsalva's maneuver.*

manganese (măn′gă-nēz) [L. *manganesium*] SYMB: Mn. A metallic element found in many foods, some plants, and in the tissues of the higher animals. It has an atomic weight of 54.938, an atomic number of 25, and a specific gravity of 7.21. It is an essential element needed for normal bone metabolism and many enzyme reactions. Deficiency in humans has not been demonstrated.

SOURCES: Bananas, bran, beans, beets, blueberries, chard, chocolate, peas, leafy vegetables, and whole grains.

manganese poisoning A rather uncommon cause of toxicity in workers exposed to manganese on a regular basis.

SYMPTOMS: Muscular weakness, difficulty walking, tremors, central nervous system disturbances, salivation.

mange (mānj) A cutaneous communicable disease of domestic animals, including dogs and cats. A number of mites, such as *Chorioptes, Demodex, Psoroptes,* and *Sarcoptes* are causative agents. In humans, this condition is known as scabies.

mania (mā′nē-ă) [Gr., madness] **1.** Mental disorder characterized by excessive excitement. **2.** A form of psychosis characterized by exalted feelings, delusions of grandeur, elevation of mood, psychomotor overactivity, and overproduction of ideas. SEE: *bipolar I mood disorder; bipolar II mood disorder; manic-depressive psychosis.*

histrionic m. Dramatic gestures, expressions, and speech in certain psychiatric states.

religious m. Mania resulting from excessive religious fervor.

transitory m. Attacks of severe frenzy, of short duration.

unproductive m. Behavior characteristic of mania with lack of spontaneity in speech or muteness, sometimes seen in manic-depressive psychosis. SEE: *alcoholism*.

-mania Suffix meaning *frenzy* or *madness*.

maniac (mā'nē-ăk) Person afflicted by mania.

maniacal (mă-nī'ă-kl) **1.** Relating to or characterized by mania. **2.** Afflicted with mania.

manic (măn'ĭk) Mood state characterized by excessive energy, poor impulse control, psychosis, agitation, flight of ideas, frenzied movement, and decreased sleep.

manic-depressive psychosis SEE: under *psychosis*.

manifest To reveal in an obvious manner.

manifestation The demonstration of the presence of a sign, symptom, or alteration, esp. one that is associated with a disease process.

manifest squint Tropia.

manikin [D. *manneken,* little man] A model of the human body or its parts, used esp. in teaching anatomy and emergency medical and nursing procedures.

man-in-a-barrel syndrome A stroke involving watershed regions of the brain, in which movements of the face, legs, and feet are preserved, but those of the arms and hips are lost.

maniphalanx (măn"ĭ-fā'lănks) [L. *manus,* hand, + Gr. *phalanx,* closely knit row] A phalanx, or finger, of the hand. SEE: *pediphalanx*.

manipulation [L. *manipulare,* to handle] **1.** Conscious or unconscious process by which one person attempts to influence another person in order to obtain his or her own needs or desires. **2.** A joint mobilization technique, sometimes involving a rapid thrust or the stretching of a joint, with or without anesthesia. SEE: *joint manipulation*. **3.** A method of realigning a fractured long bone with manual pressure, traction, or angulation.

joint m. Passive therapeutic techniques used to stretch restricted joints or reposition a subluxation. The techniques are sometimes applied with rapid thrust movements and may be applied with the patient under anesthesia to ensure maximum relaxation. SEE: *mobilization, joint*.

spinal m. In chiropractic, a thrusting of the spine to reduce subluxation. It is a standard, effective treatment of uncomplicated acute low back pain.

manna (măn'ă) [L.] **1.** The sweet juice obtained from the flowering ash, *Fraxinus ornus*. **2.** General term applied to sweetish juices obtained from a variety of plants.

mannans (măn'ănz) Any of several polysaccharides of mannose.

mannerism A peculiar modification or exaggeration of style or habit of dress, speech, or action.

mannitol (măn'ĭ-tŏl) An osmotic diuretic used primarily to treat oliguric renal failure and to reduce intracranial pressures (e.g., in patients with threatened herniation of the brain through the foramen magnum).

Mannkopf's sign [Emil W. Mannkopf, Ger. physician, 1836–1918] Pulse acceleration exhibited on pressing a painful point. The sign is not present in feigned pain.

mannose (măn'ōs) A polysaccharide present in certain plants. It is an aldohexose.

mannoside (măn'ō-sīd) A glycoside of mannose.

mannosidosis (măn"ōs-ĭ-dō'sĭs) One of several congenital lysosomal storage diseases in which the deficiency of α-mannosidase is associated with mental retardation, kyphosis, and accumulation of mannose in tissues. The disease, which is lethal, can be treated with bone marrow transplantation.

manometer (măn-ŏm'ĕt-ĕr) [Gr. *manos,* thin, + *metron,* measure] Device for determining liquid or gaseous pressure. The measurement is expressed in millimeters of either mercury or water.

saline m. Manometer that uses a special hollow tube shaped like the letter U and open at both ends. The tube is partially filled with saline. Pressure is determined by connecting one end of the U tube to the system in which pressure is to be measured. The pressure, in millimeters of saline, is the measured distance between the fluid level in one side of the U tube and that in the other side.

strain gauge m. A device attached to an intra-arterial catheter, which is used to measure blood pressures within arteries.

manslaughter (măn"slăw-tĕr) A form of homicide in which the killing of another person is not the result of malice. On occasion, health care professionals who have withheld certain forms of treatment have been charged and convicted of manslaughter. Patients also may be liable to a charge of manslaughter (e.g., if failure to follow medical advice not to drive an automobile results in a fatal crash).

Mansonella (măn"sō-nĕl'ă) A genus of filarial nematodes.

M. ozzardi A species found in humans in Central and South America and the Caribbean. It is transmitted by blackflies and midges. The parasites are unsheathed and most patients are asymptomatic.

mansonelliasis (măn"sō-nĕl-ī'ă-sĭs) [*Mansonella* + Gr. *-iasis,* condition] Infection in humans with *Mansonella ozzardi*.

Mansonia (măn-sō'nē-ă) A genus of mosquitoes found in tropical countries that transmit microfilariae to humans.

mantle [AS. *mentel,* a garment] A covering structure or layer.

dentin m. The narrow zone of dentin that is first formed in the crown and root of a tooth.

Mantoux test (măn-tū′) [Charles Mantoux, Fr. physician, 1877–1947] An intradermal (intracutaneous) injection of 0.1 ml of intermediate strength purified protein derivative (PPD). The needle is removed after a brief delay in order to minimize leakage of the PPD at the puncture site. Within 48 to 72 hours, hardening (induration) of the injected area, whose diameter is greater than 10 mm Hg, provides unequivocal evidence of current or previous infection with tuberculosis. In persons infected with the human immunodeficiency virus (HIV), an indurated area whose diameter is 5 mm or more should be considered evidence of a positive test result. HIV-infected patients who do not react to PPD or to control antigens (i.e., persons who are anergic) should be considered positive as well, esp. if they come from demographic groups known to have high rates of infection with tuberculosis (e.g., homeless people, Asian-born individuals, among many others). SEE: *tuberculosis.*

mantra (măn-tră) A word, phrase, or sound repeated to oneself to focus the mind or reduce stray thoughts during meditation.

manual (măn′ū-ăl) [L. *manus,* hand] **1.** Pert. to the hands. **2.** Performed by or with the hands.

manual lymphatic drainage ABBR: MLD. Gentle massage techniques used to correct localized lymphedema (e.g., in patients who have swelling of the arm after mastectomy). Superficial massage is used; the direction of applied pressure depends on the treatment area.

manual muscle test A technique for estimating the relative strength of specific muscles. Rating categories and values include normal (5), good (4), fair (3), poor (2), trace (1), and absent (0). A grade of fair is based on the ability of the muscle to move the part through its full range of motion against gravity; a grade of poor is based on the ability to move through the range with gravity eliminated.

manubrium (mă-nū′brē-ŭm) *pl.* **manubria** [L., handle] Any handle-shaped structure.

m. sterni The upper segment of the sternum articulating with the clavicle and first pair of costal cartilages.

manudynamometer (măn″ū-dī″nă-mŏm′ĕ-tĕr) [L. *manus,* hand, + Gr. *dynamis,* force, + *metron,* measure] A device for measuring the force of a thrust.

manus (mā′nŭs) *pl.* **manus** [L.] The hand.

MAO *monoamine oxidase.*

map A graphic presentation in two dimensions of the location of all or part of an area.

genetic m. SEE: *gene mapping.*

linkage m. Map of chromosomes indicating the relationship of genes to each other on the chromosome.

maple bark disease A hypersensitivity pneumonitis caused by inhalation of spores from the mold *Cryptostroma corticale,* which is present under the bark of logs cut from maple trees.

maple syrup urine disease An autosomal recessive metabolic disease involving defective metabolism of branched chain amino acids; so named because of the characteristic odor of the urine and sweat. The amino acids involved are leucine, isoleucine, valine, and alloisoleucine. Clinically there is rapid deterioration of the nervous system in the first few months of life and then death at an early age.

TREATMENT: Treatment includes controlling the dietary intake of the involved amino acids, exchange transfusion, peritoneal dialysis, and occasionally, liver transplantation.

mapping Location of the genes on a chromosome.

lymphatic m. In the staging of cancers, injection of a tracer material near a tumor to determine the regional lymph nodes into which metastatic disease might first spread.

MAR *medication administration record.*

marasmus (măr-ăz′mŭs) Emaciation, generalized wasting, and absence of subcutaneous fat caused by malnutrition. The condition results from caloric deficiency secondary to acute diseases, esp. diarrheal diseases of infancy, deficiency in nutritional composition, inadequate food intake, malabsorption, child abuse, failure-to-thrive syndrome, deficiency of vitamin D, or scurvy. SYN: *wasting.* SEE: *kwashiorkor; malnutrition, protein-energy.* **marantic, marasmic** (mă-răn′tĭk, mă-răz′mĭk), *adj.*

SYMPTOMS: Signs include loss of muscle mass and other soft tissues and a wizened, sunken face, resembling that of an elderly person, from loss of temporal and buccal fat pads. Failure to gain weight is followed by a loss of weight. Brain and skeletal growth continues, resulting in a long body and a head that is too large in proportion to weight. Subcutaneous fat is minimal, the eyes are sunken, and tissue turgor is lost. The skin appears loose and sags. The infant is not active, muscles are flabby and relaxed, and the cry is weak and shrill. The absence of pitting edema of the hands and feet and of a protuberant abdomen differentiate this condition from kwashiorkor, but in marasmic kwashiorkor, features of both conditions are combined.

TREATMENT: Initial feedings should be small and low in calories because digestive capacity is poor and a "refeeding" syndrome can occur, marked by hypophosphatemia, congestive heart failure, respiratory distress, convulsions, coma, and death. Diluted formula or breast milk is best. The amount of calories and protein, carbohydrates, and fat should be increased gradually. The goal for protein intake is 5 g/kg of body weight per day. If diarrhea due to disaccharidase deficiency is present, a low-lactose diet is beneficial. Parenteral fluid therapy is indicated if shock or fluid and electrolyte imbalance exists.

PROGNOSIS: Death occurs in 40% of affected children.

marble bone disease Osteopetrosis.

Marburg virus disease [Marburg, Germany] A frequently fatal disease caused by a virus classed as a member of the family Filoviridae. Clinically this disease is identical to that caused by the Ebola virus. SEE: *Ebola virus hemorrhagic fever*.

marc (mărk) [Fr.] The residue remaining after a drug has been percolated. SEE: *percolation*.

Marchiafava-Micheli syndrome (măr″kē-ă-fă′vă-mē-kā′lē) [Ettore Marchiafava, It. pathologist, 1847–1935; F. Micheli, It. clinician, 1872–1937] A rare hemolytic anemia associated with paroxysmal nocturnal hemoglobinuria.

Marcus Gunn pupil [Robert Marcus Gunn, Brit. ophthalmologist, 1850–1909] A pupil of the eye that responds by constricting more to an indirect than a direct light.

Marcus Gunn syndrome [Robert Marcus Gunn] A congenital condition in which a ptotic eyelid retracts briefly when the mouth is opened or the jaw moved to one side. The person appears to wink each time the jaw is opened. SEE: *jaw winking*.

Marfan's syndrome [Bernard-Jean Antonin Marfan, Fr. physician, 1858–1942] A hereditary disorder of connective tissue, bones, muscles, ligaments, and skeletal structures. It affects about one person in 7500.

SYMPTOMS: Distinguishing features include tall lean body type with long extremities including fingers and toes, abnormal joint flexibility, flat feet, stooped shoulders, and dislocation of the optic lens. The aorta usually will be dilated and may become sufficiently weakened to allow an aneurysm to develop. SEE: *arachnodactyly*.

ETIOLOGY: The disease is caused by a defect in the manufacture of fibrillin molecules in the extracellular matrix.

PATIENT CARE: Patients with this condition are encouraged to seek medical attention promptly for complications, which can be serious. The patient's lifestyle requires ongoing monitoring, and reassurance and support should be given continually.

margarine Butter substitute made from refined vegetable oils or a combination of vegetable oils and fats. Coloring material and vitamins A and D are added. It contains 9 kcal/g.

margin [L. *marginalis,* border] **1.** A boundary, such as the edge of a structure. SYN: *margo*. **2.** In dentistry, the apical extent or boundary of enamel adjacent to the cementum of the tooth root; the junction of a restoration with the cavosurface angle of a prepared cavity in enamel.

gingival m. The most coronal part of the gingiva surrounding a tooth.

marginal (măr′jĭn-ăl) Concerning a margin or border. SYN: *limbic*.

margination (măr″jĭ-nā′shŭn) Adhesion of leukocytes to the walls of blood vessels in the first stages of inflammation.

marginoplasty (mar-jĭn′ō-plăs″tē) [L. *marginalis,* border, + Gr. *plassein,* to mold] Plastic surgery of a border, as of an eyelid.

margo (măr′gō) *pl.* **margines** [L.] A border or edge.

m. acutus Sharp margin of the heart extending from the apex to the right.

m. obtusus Portion of a line extending from apex to root of the pulmonary artery that lies along the rounded left side of the left ventricle.

Marie's ataxia (mă-rēz′) [Pierre Marie, Fr. neurologist, 1853–1940] Hereditary cerebellar ataxia caused by bilateral cortical atrophy of the cerebellum.

Marie's disease Acromegaly.

Marie's sign Hand tremor seen in exophthalmic goiter.

marijuana, marihuana (măr″ĭ-wă′nă) The dried flowering tops of *Cannabis sativa,* the hemp plant. SYN: *cannabis*. SEE: *hashish*.

Its psychoactive ingredient, delta-9-tetrahydrocannabinol (THC), may produce euphoria, alterations in mood and judgment, changes in sensory perception, cognition, and psychomotor coordination. Driving and other machine-operating skills may therefore be seriously affected. Users of marijuana have impaired short-term memory; its use also slows learning. Depending on the dose of the drug and the underlying psychological conditions of the user, marijuana may cause transient episodes of confusion, anxiety, or delirium. Its use may exacerbate pre-existing mental illness, esp. schizophrenia. Long-term, relatively heavy use may be associated with behavioral disorders and a kind of ennui called the amotivational syndrome, but it is not known whether use of the drug is a cause or a result of this condition. Transient symptoms occur on withdrawal, indicating that the drug can lead to physical dependence. There has been considerable interest in the effects of marijuana on pregnancy and fetal growth but because substance abusers often abuse more than a single substance, it is difficult to evaluate the effects of individual substances on the outcome of pregnancy or fetal development.

There is no definitive evidence that prolonged heavy smoking of marijuana leads to impaired pulmonary function. The possibility that chronic marijuana use is associated with an increased risk of developing head and neck cancer exists, but it has not been proven.

THC, also known as dronabinol, is approved for use in treating nausea and vomiting associated with cancer chemotherapy in patients who have failed to respond adequately to conventional antiemetic treatment, and treatment of anorexia associated with weight loss in patients with acquired immunodeficiency syndrome. Marijuana has also been approved for other medical uses in some states, although such use violates federal drug enforcement administration standards.

CAUTION: Dronabinol is a controlled substance. Prescriptions are limited to the amount necessary for a single cycle of chemotherapy.

mark [AS. *mearc*] Any nevus, bruise, cut, or spot on the surface of a body.

birth-m. SEE: *birthmark; nevus.*

port-wine m. Nevus flammeus.

strawberry m. Nevus vascularis.

marker **1.** A device or substance used to indicate or mark something. **2.** An identifying characteristic or trait that allows apparently similar materials or disease conditions to be differentiated.

fecal m. A substance, such as carmine, ingested to mark the beginning and end of fecal collection periods.

genetic m. An identifiable physical location on a chromosome (e.g., a gene or segment of DNA with no known coding function) whose inheritance can be monitored.

surrogate m. An indirect indicator of a disease state or of its response to therapy. Such markers often include laboratory tests thought to represent clinical progress accurately. For example, in diabetes mellitus, the glycosylated hemoglobin level is used as a marker of glycemic control; in AIDS the level of HIV RNA is used as a marker of disease progression.

Marlex mesh A monofilament, biologically inert mesh used in surgical procedures to help cover or strengthen areas, as in hernia repair.

Maroteaux-Lamy syndrome Mucopolysaccharidosis VI.

marrow [AS. *mearh*] Bone marrow.

gelatinous m. Yellow marrow of old or emaciated persons, almost devoid of fat and having a gelatinous consistency.

red m. Marrow found in spongy bone that produces all the types of blood cells. SEE: illus.

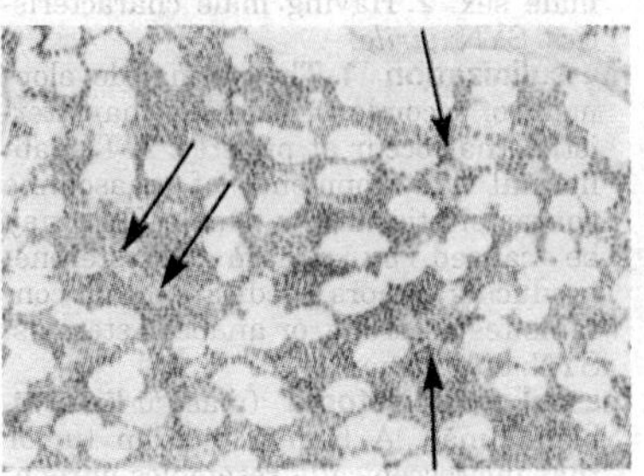

NORMAL RED BONE MARROW

Arrows indicate megakaryocytes (orig. mag. ×200)

spinal m. An obsolete term for the spinal cord.

yellow m. Marrow found in the medullary canal of long bones. Consists principally of fat cells and connective tissue. It does not participate in hematopoiesis.

marrow aspiration Procedure using a special aspirating needle to obtain a specimen of bone marrow for examination. The material is usually obtained from the upper portion of the sternum or the iliac crest. Examination of the stained marrow is helpful in diagnosing a great number of blood disorders, infections, and malignant diseases.

Marshall-Marchetti-Krantz procedure A surgical procedure used to treat urinary stress incontinence in women, in whom the incontinence is caused by a weakness in the support of the bladder neck and proximal urethra. The sutures that are placed periurethrally in the vaginal wall are brought out and anchored to the perichondrium of the pubic symphysis offering a better cystourethral angle and firm support.

PATIENT CARE: Vital signs are checked and the drain examined. Intake and output are monitored, and fluids encouraged.

Marsh's test [James Marsh, Brit. chemist, 1789–1846] A test to detect the presence of arsenic.

marsupialization (măr-sū″pē-ăl-ĭ-zā′shŭn) [L. *marsupium,* pouch] The process of raising the borders of an evacuated tumor or abscess to the edges of the surgical wound and stitching them there to form a pouch. The interior of the sac suppurates and gradually closes by granulation.

marsupium (măr-sū′pē-ŭm) [L., pouch]

1. Scrotum. 2. A sac or pouch that serves to hold the young of a marsupial.

MAS, mAs *milliampere-second.*

masculation (măs-kū-lā′shŭn) [L. *masculus,* a male] Development of male secondary sexual characteristics.

masculine (măs′kū-lĭn) 1. Pert. to the male sex. 2. Having male characteristics. SYN: *virile.*

masculinization 1. The normal development of secondary male sex characteristics that occur at puberty. 2. The abnormal development of masculine characteristics in the female. This may be caused by certain testosterone-producing tumors, medication that contains testosterone, or anabolic steroids. SYN: *virilization.*

masculinovoblastoma (măs″kū-lĭn-ō″vō-blăs-tō′mă) A benign ovarian tumor that microscopically resembles adrenocortical tissue and usually results in masculinization.

maser Acronym for *m*icrowave *a*mplification by *s*timulation *e*mission of *r*adiation. A device that produces a small, nondiverging radiation beam. SEE: *laser.*

mask [Fr. *masque*] 1. A covering for the face that serves as a protective barrier. SEE: *Standard and Universal Precautions Appendix.* 2. The immobile appearance of the face occurring in certain pathological conditions. 3. To conceal or prevent detection.

aerosol m. A mask used for the therapeutic administration of a nebulized solution, humidity, or high airflow with oxygen enrichment. It has a large-bore inlet and an exhalation port.

BLB m. A mask invented by Boothby, Lovelace, and Bulbulian, working at the Mayo Clinic. It is used for administering oxygen to persons at high altitudes (e.g., aviators) or to patients during anesthesia.

death m. A plaster cast of the face molded soon after death.

ecchymotic m. Cyanotic facies accompanying traumatic asphyxia.

face m. A plastic device molded to fit over the face for administration of gases or humidified air.

HAFOE m. *high air flow with oxygen enrichment m.*

high air flow with oxygen enrichment m. ABBR: HAFOE mask. Term applied to Venturi-type devices. SEE: *Venturi mask.*

Hutchinson's m. A feeling of compression over the face as though one is wearing a mask.

laryngeal m. airway ABBR: LMA. A temporary airway management device used to resuscitate patients who require endotracheal intubation but in whom intubation has failed or is unlikely to be successful. Untrained personnel find the device easier to use than standard intubation equipment because direct visualization of laryngeal anatomy is unnecessary. The LMA can be used in the field as well as in critical care settings or in the operating room. Its ease of use must be balanced against its risks: the device provides a less secure airway than endotracheal intubation and its use has occasionally been associated with injuries to the mouth, pharynx, or vocal cords.

luetic m. Blotchy brown pigmentation of cheeks, forehead, and temples, seen in tertiary syphilis.

nonrebreathing m. An oxygen administration device with one-way valves for inspiration and expiration and a reservoir bag; used to attain high concentrations of oxygen.

oxygen m. A device that fits over the mouth and nose and provides oxygen or other therapeutic gas. It includes a simple, partial rebreathing type and a nonrebreathing type.

Parkinson's m. Immobile, expressionless facial appearance resulting from paralysis agitans (Parkinson's disease).

pocket face m. A folding mask that can be carried in a pocket and used for artificial ventilation. Some pocket face masks have an inlet for oxygen and a one-way valve for infection control.

m. of pregnancy Sharply defined and symmetrically distributed areas of increased pigment that arise on the faces of some pregnant women. SYN: *chloasma gravidarum.* SEE: under *chloasma gravidarum* for illus.

ventilation m. A face mask device that applies mechanical ventilation.

masked Concealed, esp. as in masked infection. For example, women exposed to rubella during the first trimester of pregnancy may be given immune globulin. This may prevent clinical symptoms of rubella in the mother, yet the fetus may be adversely affected and born with congenital defects.

Maslach Burnout Inventory ABBR: MBI. A self-reporting questionnaire that measures the frequency and intensity of burnout in the allied health professions. It assesses three aspects of burnout: emotional exhaustion, dehumanization, and lack of a sense of personal accomplishment. It is used to assess professionals who work extensively with cognitively impaired people.

Maslow, Abraham H. [U.S. psychologist, 1908–1970] Articulator of a theory of human motivation based on a synthesis of holistic and dynamic principles. A contemporary of Carl Rogers, Maslow is considered one of the major theorists of humanistic psychology.

M.'s theory of human motivation A theory stating that human existence is based on needs that arise in hierarchal order: physiological needs such as hunger; safety needs; love, affection, and belonging needs; self-respect and self-esteem needs; and self-actualization. Although the term *self-actualization* was coined by Kurt Goldstein in 1939, Maslow believed that the ultimate destiny of mankind was self-actualization or a tendency to become everything that one is capable of becoming. Humans' realization of themselves occurs not only by thinking but also by the realization of all instinctive and emotional capacities as they move toward optimal physical, emotional, and spiritual health, which he called transcendence.

masochism (măs'ō-kĭzm) [Leopold von Sacher-Masoch, Austrian novelist, 1835–1895] A general orientation to life based on the belief that suffering relieves guilt and leads to a reward. Opposite of sadism. SEE: *algolagnia; flagellation.*

sexual m. Sexual excitement produced in an individual by being humiliated or hurt by another.

masochist (măs'ō-kĭst) A person who derives pleasure from masochism.

mass [L. *massa*] **1.** A quantity of material, such as cells, that unite or adhere to each other. **2.** Soft solid preparation for internal use and of such consistency that it may be molded into pills. **3.** A fundamental scalar property of an object that describes the amount of acceleration an object will have when a given force is applied to it. The metric unit of mass is the kilogram. One kilogram equals 2.205 pounds. SEE: *weight.*

cell m. An aggregation of cells that serves as the precursor of a future organ or part.

epithelial m. Inner portion of a developing gonad enclosed within the germinal epithelium.

inner cell m. In embryology, the group of cells within the blastocyst from which the embryo, yolk sac, and amnion develop. SEE: *blastocyst.*

interfilar m. An obsolete term for the cytosol.

intermediate cell m. A plate of nonsegmented mesoderm lying lateral to the segments (somites) and connecting them to the nonsegmented lateral mesoderm. SYN: *nephrotome.*

lateral m. of the atlas The parts of the first cervical vertebra that articulate with the occipital bone superiorly and the axis inferiorly.

molecular m. Molecular weight.

massa [L.] Mass.

m. intermedia The middle commissure of the brain, an inconstant mass of gray matter extending across the third ventricle and connecting adjacent surfaces of the thalamus.

massage [Gr. *massein,* to knead] Manipulation, methodical pressure, friction, and kneading of the body.

auditory m. Massage of the eardrum.

cardiac m. Manual compression of the heart to restore heartbeat after the heart has stopped. This is accomplished by applying pressure over the sternum (closed chest massage) or through an incision in the chest wall (open chest massage), forcing blood out of the heart and, when pressure is removed, allowing the heart to fill as if it were beating. SEE: *cardiopulmonary resuscitation.*

electrovibratory m. Massage by means of an electric vibrator.

fundal m. Manual stimulation of a boggy postpartum uterus to generate effective contractions, express clots, and limit postpartum hemorrhage. To relax the patient's abdominal muscles, the birth attendant places the patient in the lithotomy position. Cupping the dominant hand around the fundus and placing the other hand just above the pubic symphysis to support the lower uterine segment, the attendant gently massages the uterine fundus. When the fundus is firm, gentle downward pressure expresses any clots that have accumulated in the uterine cavity. SEE: *postpartum hemorrhage; uterine inversion.*

CAUTION: Exerting downward pressure on an uncontracted fundus may cause uterine inversion and massive hemorrhage.

general m. Centripetal stroking in connection with some muscular kneading from the toes upward. Used in connection with baths lasting 30 to 40 min. As soon as a part is massaged, it should be given a few passive rotary movements and afterwards covered up.

introductory m. Massage consisting of centripetal strokings around an affected part when it is impossible to apply treatment directly to the part.

local m. Massage confined to particular body parts.

Swedish m. Massage combined with active and passive exercise. These techniques were developed in Sweden by Per Henrik Ling (1776–1839).

vapor m. Treatment of a cavity by a medicated and nebulized vapor under interrupted pressure.

vibratory m. Massage by rapidly repeated tapping of the affected surface by means of a vibrating hammer or sound.

masseter (măs-sē'tĕr) [Gr. *maseter,* chewer] The muscle that closes the mouth and is the principal muscle in mastication.

masseur (mă-soor') [Fr.] **1.** A man who gives massages. **2.** An instrument for massaging.

masseuse (mă-sooz') [Fr.] A woman who gives massages.

mass fraction The ratio of the mass of a

component to the mass of the system of which the component is a part.

massive (măs′sĭv) [Fr. *massif*] Bulky; consisting of a large mass; huge.

massive collapse of the lung Deflation or compression of lung tissues caused either by obstruction of a main bronchus by a mucus plug, tumor, or foreign body; major trauma; or a tension pneumothorax. SEE: *lung; pneumothorax.*

SYMPTOMS: This condition is marked by dyspnea, cyanosis, shock, and chest pain.

TREATMENT: If caused by mucus or foreign body, therapy consists of bronchoscopy, pulmonary toilet, antibiotics, and oxygen.

mass psychogenic illness Mass sociogenic illness.

mass sociogenic illness ABBR: MSI. An unexplained, self-limiting illness characterized by nonspecific symptoms in persons in a social setting such as a school, work place, church, or military group. The onset is usually rapid and may occur after an unusual or peculiar odor is detected. Symptoms may include dizziness, weakness, headache, abdominal pain, rash, itching, blurred vision, nausea and vomiting, and fainting. There are no laboratory studies to confirm an etiologic agent. Resolution of the mass illness may occur when those affected are reassured that it is not due to a toxic substance or disease. SYN: *mass psychogenic illness.*

MAST *medical antishock trousers; military antishock trousers.* SEE: *anti-G suit.*

mast- (măst) SEE: *masto-.*

mastadenitis (măst-ăd-ĕ-nī′tĭs) [Gr. *mastos,* breast, + *aden,* gland, + *itis,* inflammation] A mammary gland inflammation.

mastadenoma (măst″ă-dĕ-nō′mă) [″ + ″ + *oma,* tumor] A tumor of the breast.

mastalgia (măst-ăl′jē-ă) [″ + *algos,* pain] Pain in the breast. SYN: *mammalgia; mastodynia.*

mastatrophia, mastatrophy (măst-ă-trō′fē-ă, măst-ăt′rō-fē) [″ + *atrophia,* want of nourishment] Atrophy of breasts.

mast cell [Gr. *masten,* to feed] A large tissue cell resembling a basophil, which is essential for inflammatory reactions mediated by immunoglobulin E (IgE) but does not circulate in the blood. Mast cells are present throughout the body in connective tissue but also are concentrated beneath the skin, mucosal membranes of the respiratory system, and gastrointestinal mucosa. Mast cells are covered with IgE molecules, which bind with foreign antigens and stimulate degranulation, releasing such mediators as histamine, prostaglandins, leukotrienes, and proteinases from densely packed granules within the cytoplasm. These mediators produce type I (immediate) hypersensitivity reactions (e.g., urticaria, allergic rhinitis, asthma, angioedema, and systemic anaphylaxis). SEE: illus.

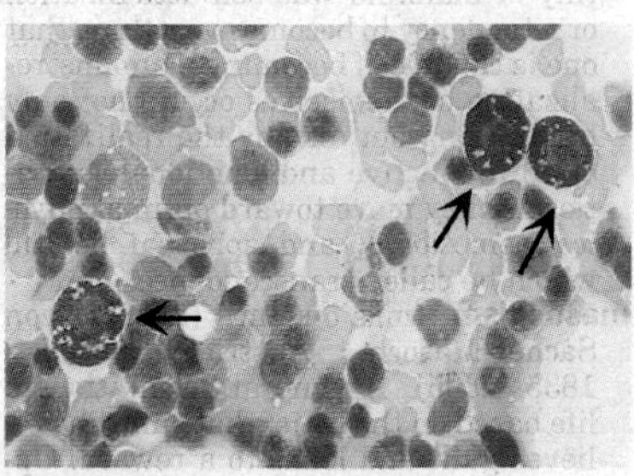

MAST CELLS IN BONE MARROW

(Orig. mag. ×640)

mastectomy (măs-tĕk′tŏ-mē) [Gr. *mastos,* breast, + *ektome,* excision] Surgical removal of the breast. The procedure usually is performed as treatment for or prophylaxis against breast cancer, and can be curative in more than 90% of cases in which the disease is histologically noninvasive and grossly confined to the breast. In patients with more extensive disease, it is one part of a treatment strategy for breast cancer that also may include chemotherapy, radiation therapy, and/or hormone therapy. Radical mastectomy (no longer performed) involved the removal of the breast tissue as well as the pectoralis major muscle, pectoral fascia, axillary contents, nipple, and areola. In modified radical mastectomy, the pectoral fascia is removed but the pectoralis major muscle is left intact. The rest of the operation mimics radical mastectomy. In simple mastectomy, only breast tissue, pectoral fascia, nipple, areola, and axillary fat pad are removed. In the management of breast cancer, because none of these techniques has been proven superior to lumpectomy followed by radiation treatment, patient and practitioner preferences often determine which therapy is used. Mastectomy still is preferred in some breast cancer patients (e.g., pregnant women) who should not receive radiation therapy. SEE: *breast cancer; lumpectomy; Nursing Diagnoses Appendix.*

PATIENT CARE: The patient is encouraged to discuss treatment options. Vital signs and the quantity and character of wound drainage are monitored. Postoperatively, the patient is positioned with the arm on the affected side elevated on a pillow, until drains are removed. Active and passive exercise of the arm is encouraged to prevent joint contracture and muscle shortening. Prescribed pain medication is provided as ordered. Support is provided to help the patient and family to cope with the diagnosis and subsequent grief response and to adjust to changes in body image and self-concept. The patient is taught protective measures for lymphedema and is offered information about breast prostheses and reconstructive surgery.

preventive m. Prophylactic m.

prophylactic m. The removal of one or both breasts in an attempt to prevent the development of breast cancer. This controversial form of treatment sometimes is used for patients who have a very strong family history of breast cancer in first-degree female relatives. SYN: *preventive m.*

radical m. Treatment of breast cancer in which the breast, involved skin, pectoral muscles, axillary lymph nodes, and subcutaneous fat are removed. SEE: *lumpectomy*.

simple m. Treatment of breast cancer in which the breast, nipple, areola, and the involved overlying skin is removed. SEE: *lumpectomy*.

Master two-step test [Arthur Matthew Master, U.S. physician, 1895–1973] A standardized exercise test formerly used to assess cardiopulmonary function. It has been replaced by exercise treadmill testing, pharmacological stress testing, and other tests of fitness and cardiovascular reserve. SEE: *exercise tolerance test*.

masthelcosis (măs″thĕl-kō′sĭs) [Gr. *mastos,* breast, + *helkosis,* ulceration] Ulceration of the breast.

mastic (măs′tĭk) A resin obtained from the tree *Pistacia lentiscus.* It has been used in industry and in coating tablets.

mastication (măs-tĭ-kā′shŭn) [L. *masticare,* to chew] Chewing. Coordination of the large temporal, masseter, pterygoid muscles, and other smaller muscles of the mandible and tongue is required, under the influence of the mandibular division of cranial nerve V. **masticatory** (măs′tĭk-ă-tō″rē), *adj.*

Mastigophora (măs″tĭ-gŏf′ō-ră) Formerly a division of protozoa characterized by one or more flagella. Now called Zoomastigophora, a phylum of the kingdom Protista.

mastigote (măs′tĭ-gōt) A member of the protozoon group formerly called Mastigophora.

mastitis (măs-tī′tĭs) [Gr. *mastos,* breast, + *itis,* inflammation] Inflammation of the breast. This condition is most common in women during breastfeeding in the second or third postpartum week; however, it may occur at any age. SEE: *Nursing Diagnoses Appendix.*

ETIOLOGY: Infection may be due to entry of disease-producing germs through cracks in the nipple. Most commonly, the offending microorganism is *Staphylococcus aureus*. Infection begins in one lobule but may extend to other areas.

SYMPTOMS: The woman complains of breast swelling and tenderness and shooting pains during and between feedings, in addition to headache and malaise. A triangular flush underneath the affected breast is an early sign. Abnormal vital signs include fever and tachycardia.

TREATMENT: Heat should be applied locally; appropriate antibiotics, such as beta-lactamase–stable penicillins, are prescribed; and analgesics are given for discomfort. Frank abscesses require incision and drainage; pumping the breasts may be recommended to avoid engorgement and maintain lactation.

PATIENT CARE: Health care professionals should encourage mothers to get adequate rest and hydration. Patient teaching emphasizes personal hygiene, breast care, wearing a supportive bra, and feeding the infant frequently to empty the breast. The mother is taught to recognize early signs of potential infection such as nipple redness and cracking. SEE: *breastfeeding*.

cystic m. Mastitis resulting in formation of cysts that give the breast a nodular feeling upon palpation.

granulomatous m. A rare inflammatory disease of the breast, often presenting as a tender breast mass. Even with mammography or ultrasonography, it may be difficult to distinguish from breast cancer without biopsy. Once the diagnosis is definitively established, the disease is treated with corticosteroids or by surgically removing the mass.

interstitial m. Inflammation of connective tissue of the breast.

parenchymatous m. Inflammation of the secreting tissue of the breast.

puerperal m. Mastitis, often accompanied by suppuration, occurring in the later portion of puerperium. The breast may become indurated due to retention of milk.

stagnation m. Painful distention of the breast occurring during early lactation. SYN: *caked breast.*

masto-, mast-, mammo-, mamm- (măs′tō) [Gr. *masto,* breast] Combining form meaning *breast.*

mastocarcinoma (măst″ō-kăr-sĭn-ō′mă) [″ + *karkinos,* crab, + *oma,* tumor] Carcinoma of the breast.

mastochondroma (măst″ō-kŏn-drō′mă) [″ + *chondros,* cartilage, + *oma,* tumor] Cartilaginous breast tumor.

mastocyte (măs′tō-sīt) [Gr. *masten,* to feed, + *kytos,* cell] Mast cell.

mastocytoma (măs″tō-sī-tō′mă) [″ + ″ + *oma,* tumor] An accumulation of mast cells that resembles a neoplasm.

mastocytosis (măs″tō-sī-tō′sĭs) [″ + ″ + *osis,* condition] A general term for a variety of rare disorders in which there is proliferation of excessive numbers of normal mast cells systemically or in the skin. Lesions present on the skin are termed urticaria pigmentosa. Firm stroking of the skin lesion will cause the area to become raised and pruritic with surrounding erythema; this is Darier's sign.

Systemic mastocytosis is marked by infiltration of mast cells into the bone marrow, abdominal organs, and lymph nodes. Many of the signs and symptoms of this illness are due to the mast cells releasing granules containing histamine, prostaglandins, and arachidonic metabolites. SEE: *Darier's sign* for illus.

mastodynia (măst-ō-dĭn′ē-ă) [Gr. *mastos,* breast, + *odyne,* pain] Pain in the breast. SYN: *mammalgia; mastalgia.*

mastography [″ + *graphein,* to write] Roentgenography of the breasts. SYN: *mammography.*

mastoid (măs′toyd) [″ + *eidos,* form, shape] **1.** Shaped like a breast. **2.** The mastoid process of temporal bone. **3.** Pert. to mastoid process. **mastoidal** (măs-toy′dăl), *adj.*

mastoidale (măs-toy-dā′lē) The lowest point of the mastoid process.

mastoidalgia (măs-toyd-ăl′jē-ă) [Gr. *mastos,* breast, + *eidos,* form, shape, + *algos,* pain] Pain in the mastoid.

mastoid antrum Old name for mastoid sinuses.

mastoid cells Old name for mastoid sinuses.

mastoidectomy [″ + ″ + *ektome,* excision] Surgical excision of the mastoid sinuses; rarely needed since the advent of antibiotics. It may be simple, involving complete removal of the mastoid sinuses, or radical, involving the middle ear. SEE: *Nursing Diagnoses Appendix.*

PATIENT CARE: Wound dressing is inspected daily and changed as necessary. Aseptic technique is used during dressing changes. The patient is observed postoperatively for bleeding, fever, neck stiffness, vomiting, dizziness, disorientation, headache, or facial paralysis.

mastoideocentesis (măs-toyd″ē-ō-sĕn-tē′sĭs) [″ + ″ + *kentesis,* puncture] Surgical puncture of the mastoid process and subsequent paracentesis of mastoid cells.

mastoiditis (măs-toyd-ī′tĭs) [″ + ″ + *itis,* inflammation] Inflammation of the mastoid sinuses, usually as a result of the spread of infection from acute otitis media (OM). The disease is relatively rare, now that effective antibiotics for otitis media are generally available. The causative organisms usually are the same as those that cause OM: streptococcal species, *Haemophilus influenzae,* and *Staphylococcus aureus,* although on some occasions mycobacteria or fungi may cause the disease.

SYMPTOMS: The patient complains of pain behind the ear, and sometimes of fever and systemic symptoms, such as malaise and chills. Physical examination may reveal redness and tenderness behind the affected ear, with swelling of the external auditory canal.

TREATMENT: Early in the course of the infection, patients may be treated with several days of intravenous antibiotics followed by outpatient medications and close follow-up. Mastoidectomy or other neurosurgical procedures may be needed if the infection has spread to beneath the periosteum, or if intracranial infection or thrombosis of neighboring veins develops. All these complications may be detected with imaging (e.g., computerized tomographic scanning of the head).

Bezold's m. Abscess underneath insertion of the sternocleidomastoid muscle due to pus breaking through the mastoid tip.

m. externa Inflammation of the periosteum of the mastoid process.

sclerosing m. Mastoiditis in which there is thickening and hardening of trabeculae between mastoid cells.

mastoidoscopy (măs-toyd-ŏs′cō-pē) The use of an endoscope to inspect or operate on the middle ear and mastoid sinuses.

mastoidotomy (măs-toyd-ŏt′ō-mē) [″ + ″ + *tome,* incision] Incision into the mastoid process.

mastoid portion of temporal bone Portion of the temporal bone lying behind the external opening of the ear and below the temporal line and containing mastoid cells and antrum. Its inner surface bears a deep, curved, sigmoid groove that contains a part of the transverse sinus in which the opening of the mastoid foramen is visible.

mastoid process Nipple-shaped process of mastoid portion of temporal bone extending downward and forward behind the external auditory meatus. It serves for attachment of the sternocleidomastoid, splenius capitis, and longissimus capitis muscles.

mastology (măs-tŏl′ō-jē) [″ + *logos,* word, reason] The branch of medicine concerned with study of the breast.

mastomenia (măs-tō-mē′nē-ă) [″ + *menes,* menses] Vicarious menstruation from the breast.

mastoncus (măst-ŏng′kŭs) [″ + *onkos,* bulk] Any tumor of the breast.

masto-occipital (măs″tō-ŏk-sĭp′ĭ-tăl) Relating to the mastoid process and occipital bone.

mastoparietal (măs″tō-pă-rī′ĕ-tăl) Concerning the mastoid process and the parietal bone.

mastopathy (măs-tŏp′ă-thē) [Gr. *mastos,* breast, + *pathos,* disease] Any disease of the mammary glands.

mastopexy (măs′tō-pĕks-ē) [″ + *pexis,* fixation] Correction of a pendulous breast by surgical fixation and plastic surgery. SYN: *mazopexy.*

mastoplasia (măst-ō-plā′zē-ă) [″ + *plassein,* to form] Enlargement of mammary gland tissue. SYN: *mazoplasia.*

mastoplasty (măs′tō-plăs″tē) [″ + *plassein,* to form] Plastic surgery of the breast. SYN: *mammoplasty.*

mastoptosis (măs″tō-tō′sĭs) [″ + *ptosis,* a dropping] Pendulous breasts.

mastorrhagia (măs-tor-ā′jē-ă) [″ + *rhegnynai,* to burst forth] Hemorrhage from the breast.

mastoscirrhus (măs-tō-skĭr′ŭs) [″ + *skirros,* hardness] Hardening of the breast.

mastosquamous (măs-tō-skwā′mŭs) Relating to the mastoid process and the squamous portion of the temporal bone.

mastostomy (măs-tŏs′tō-mē) [″ + *stoma,* mouth] Incision into the breast in order to drain a cyst or obtain tissue for microscopic study.

mastotomy (măs-tŏt′ō-mē) Surgical incision of a breast. SYN: *mammotomy.*

masturbate (măs′tĕr-bāt) [L. *masturbari,* fr. *manus,* hand, + *stuprare,* to defile] To practice masturbation.

masturbation (măs″tĕr-bā′shŭn) Stimulation of genitals or other erogenous areas, usually to orgasm, by some means other than sexual intercourse.

At one time practicing masturbation was believed to cause a great variety of mental and physical disorders. There is no scientific basis for such beliefs.

match [ME. *macche,* lamp wick] A narrow strip of wood tipped with a compound that ignites by friction. Lucifer matches usually are made of phosphorus and potassium chlorate. Safety matches contain antimony, sulfide, and potassium chlorate and must be lit by striking a rough surface.

matching **1.** Comparison in order to select objects or persons with similar characteristics. **2.** Being identical, equal, or exactly alike.

cross-m. of blood Technique and procedure for determining the immunologic and genetic characteristics of the patient's blood so that appropriate blood may be used for transfusion.

m. of controls In medical research, ensuring that the group of actively treated subjects has as many relevant similarities as possible to a group of untreated or placebo-treated persons. Matching subjects with controls increases the likelihood that the findings demonstrated by the study are the result of the treatment itself and not another variable.

human leukocyte antigen m. ABBR: HLA matching. In organ transplantation, determining the compatibility of the antigens present on donor organs with those of the patient who will receive the organ. In general, the more closely the donor and recipient match, the greater the likelihood of a successful graft. Mismatching of organ and recipient increases the chances of organ rejection.

residency m. The assignment of medical students to postgraduate medical residency training programs.

treatment m. Using patient profiles and preferences to individualize and optimize therapeutic regimens for patients (e.g., in the management of psychiatric or substance abuse disorders).

match poisoning Gastrointestinal irritation caused by ingesting or sucking on the heads of matches (usually by children).

FIRST AID: The child should be treated supportively (e.g., with oral fluids as tolerated and antiemetics if they are needed). SEE: *phosphorus poisoning.*

maté (mă-tā′) [Sp., vessel for preparing leaves] Tea made from the leaves of *Ilex paraguayensis.* Contains caffeine and tannin.

USES: Diaphoretic and diuretic when taken in large quantities.

mater (mā′tŭr) [L., mother] The tissue coverings of the brain and spinal cord. SYN: *meninges.*

dura m. A fibrous connective tissue membrane, the outermost of the meninges covering the spinal cord (dura mater spinalis) and brain (dura mater cerebri or dura mater encephali). SEE: *pia mater; tentorium cerebelli.*

pia m. SEE: *pia mater.*

materia alba (mă-tē′rē-ă ăl′bă) [L., white matter] Yellow or grayish white, soft, sticky deposit that collects along the junction between the teeth and gingiva. Materia alba consists of microorganisms, desquamated epithelial cells, leukocytes, and a mix of salivary proteins and lipids, with few or no food particles. Materia alba lacks the regular structure of plaque and is clearly visible without the use of disclosing agents.

material The substance from which something may be made, constructed, or created.

base m. The basic ingredient in a denture. It may be a polymer, shellac, or metal.

impression m. Any material used to make an impression of teeth.

spent m. Any material that has been used in medical care (or other industries) which cannot be reused without reprocessing, reclamation, or decontamination.

material safety data sheet ABBR: MSDS. Descriptive sheet required by U.S. federal law, and by laws of other countries and states, that accompanies a chemical or a chemical mixture. The sheet provides identity of the material, physical hazards (e.g., flammability), and acute and chronic health hazards associated with contact with or exposure to the compound. It is estimated that there are almost 600,000 hazardous chemical products in American workplaces. SEE: *right-to-know law*.

materia medica (mă-tē′rē-ă mĕd′ĭ-kă) [L., medical matter] **1.** Pharmacology. **2.** A substance used to treat disease.

maternal [L. *maternus*] **1.** Relating to the mother. **2.** From a mother.

maternal deprivation syndrome Emotional, physical, and nutritional neglect of an infant or young child as a result of the premature loss or absence of the mother. Children suffering from this syndrome are emotionally disturbed, withdrawn, apathetic, and retarded in growth and development.

maternal mortality rate SEE: under *rate*.

maternal serum alpha-fetoprotein Alpha-fetoprotein present in the blood of a pregnant woman. SEE: *alpha-fetoprotein*.

maternity (mă-tĕr′nĭ-tē) **1.** Motherhood. **2.** The obstetrical department of a hospital.

mating [ME. *mate,* companion] Pairing of male and female, esp. for reproduction.

assortative m. Pairing of male and female that is controlled in some manner.

random m. Pairing of male to female when each individual has the same chance of mating with those of other genetic make-up.

matricide [L. *mater,* mother, + *caedere,* to kill] Killing one's mother.

matrilineal (mā″trĭ-lĭn′ē-ăl) [L. *mater,* mother, + *linea,* line] Concerning descent through the female line.

matrilysin A member of the matrix metalloproteinase enzyme family that is expressed by many tumor cells and plays a part in tissue invasion and metastasis.

matrix (mā′trĭks) *pl.* **matrices** [L.] **1.** The basic substance from which a thing is made or develops. **2.** The intercellular material of a tissue. **3.** Mold for casting amalgams in dental restoration.

extracellular m. ABBR: ECM. The network of fibrous and fluid material that is excreted by, surrounds, and supports living cells. The material exterior to cells is critical to their growth and maintenance. Through this milieu, nutrients, hormones, inflammatory mediators, and intercellular signals are delivered to cells and wastes are extruded. This material also provides cushioning to protect cells from physical injury and serves as a barrier to invasion by cancers.

m. unguis Nailbed.

matrixitis (mā-trĭks-ī′tĭs) Inflammation of the nailbed. SYN: *onychia*. SEE: *paronychia*.

matter **1.** Anything that occupies space. May be gaseous, liquid, or solid. **2.** Pus.

gray m. Nerve tissue composed mainly of the cell bodies of neurons rather than their myelinated processes. The term is generally applied to the gray portions of the central nervous system, which include the cerebral cortex, basal ganglia, and nuclei of the brain, and the gray columns of the spinal cord, which form an H-shaped region surrounded by white matter. Sympathetic ganglia and nerves may also be gray. SYN: *substantia grisea*.

white m. Nerve tissue of the spinal cord and brain, composed mainly of myelinated nerve fibers. SYN: *substantia alba*.

maturate (măt′ū-rāt) [L. *maturus,* ripe] **1.** To ripen; to mature. **2.** To suppurate.

maturation (măt″ū-rā′shŭn) **1.** Maturing; ripening, as a graafian follicle. **2.** Suppuration. **3.** The process in the development of germ cells (spermatozoa and ova) occurring in spermatogenesis or oogenesis in which the number of chromosomes is reduced from the diploid number to the haploid number (one half of diploid). Includes two cell divisions. SEE: *oogenesis; spermatogenesis*. **4.** The completion of the mineralization pattern or crystalline structure of calcified tissues.

enamel m. The process of changing from about 30% inorganic mineral in enamel matrix of the teeth to the 96% inorganic content in mature enamel; maturation is accomplished by the ameloblast cells over a long period, with a decrease in water and organic content, and an increase in mineral content and size or density of hydroxyapatite crystals.

in vitro m. ABBR: IVM. An assisted reproduction technique in which an immature oocyte is nurtured in the laboratory until fertilized.

mature (mă-tūr′) **1.** Fully developed or ripened. **2.** To become fully developed.

mature minor rule Regulations in some states that allow the practitioner to treat minors without parental consent if the minor is deemed to be capable of understanding the nature and consequences of the treatment and if the treatment is of benefit to the minor.

maturity **1.** State of completed growth or development. **2.** Stage of growth at which an individual becomes capable of reproducing.

fetal lung m. The ability of the developing lung to oxygenate and ventilate effectively outside the womb. The readiness of the fetal lung can be assessed with several invasive and noninvasive tests. Two predictors of mature lungs are the presence of a well-developed colon on ultrasonography and an adequate number of lamellar bodies in the amniotic fluid. Other tests of fetal lung maturity include the lecithin: sphingomyelin ratio and assays for phosphatidyl glycerol.

PATIENT CARE: Premature infants born with immature lungs have a high likelihood of developing infantile respiratory distress syndrome. Treatment with glucocorticoids improves most amniotic fluid indices of fetal lung maturity.

matutinal (mă-tū′tĭ-năl) [L. *matutinalis,* morning] Pert. to morning or occurring early in the day, such as morning sickness.

Maurer's dots (mow′ĕrz) [Georg Maurer, Ger. physician in Sumatra, b. 1909] Coarse stippling of the red cells seen in malaria, caused by *Plasmodium falciparum.*

maxilla [L., jawbone] A paired bone with several processes that forms most of the upper face, roof of the mouth, sides of the nasal cavity, and floor of the orbit. The alveolar process of the maxilla supports the teeth, which is the basis for calling the maxilla the upper jaw. SEE: *skull* for illus; *skeleton.*

maxillary (măk′sĭ-lĕr″ē) Pert. to the upper jaw.

maxillitis (măks″ĭl-ī′tĭs) [L. *maxilla,* jawbone, + Gr. *itis,* inflammation] Inflammation of the maxilla.

maxillodental (măk-sĭl″ō-dĕn′tăl) [″ + *dens,* tooth] Concerning the maxilla and the teeth it supports.

maxillofacial (măks-ĭl″ō-fā′shăl) Pert. to the maxilla and face.

maxillofacial syndrome Facial defects resulting from improper ossification of the fetal cartilages in the facial area.

maxillojugal (măk-sĭl″ō-jū′găl) Concerning the maxilla and zygomatic bone.

maxillomandibular (măk-sĭl″ō-măn-dĭb′ū-lăr) [″ + *mandibula,* lower jawbone] Concerning the maxilla and mandible.

maxillopalatine (măk-sĭl″ō-păl′ă-tīn) Concerning the maxilla and palatine bone.

maxillotomy (măk″sĭ-lŏt′ō-mē) [″ + Gr. *tome,* incision] Surgical incision of the maxilla.

maximum (măks′ĭ-mŭm) *pl.* **maxima** [L. *maximus,* greatest] **1.** The greatest quantity or effect. **2.** Height of a disease.

repetition m. ABBR: RM. The greatest amount of weight a person can lift "n" number of times. The amount of weight that can be lifted exactly 10 times is 10 RM. The greatest amount of weight that can be lifted once is 1 RM. Repetition maximum can be used as a comparative measure of strength or as a technique in exercise prescription and strength training. During strength training 8 RM or 10 RM is used to develop strength, power, and muscle mass. **maximal** (-măl), *adj.*

maximum allowable concentration ABBR: MAC. The upper limit of concentration of certain atmospheric contaminants allowed in the workplace.

maximum breathing capacity ABBR: MBC. The greatest amount of air that can be breathed in a specified period, usually 30 sec. It is expressed in liters of air per minute.

May Hegglin anomaly An autosomal-dominant inherited blood disorder marked by the presence of Dohle bodies in granulocyte leukocytes. Platelets vary in size and may be decreased in number. Purpura and excessive bleeding may occur, although some affected persons are asymptomatic.

mayhem (mā′hĕm) **1.** Interpersonal violence or disfigurement. **2.** Chaos (e.g., in the organization of the workplace, in the administration of clinical, managerial, or research activities). **3.** Physiological disruption (e.g., by a virulent infection or a severe metabolic illness).

Mayo-Robson's point [Arthur Mayo-Robson, Brit. surgeon, 1853–1933] A point just above and to the right of the umbilicus where pressure causes tenderness in pancreatic disease.

maze A labyrinth of communicating paths.

mazopexy SEE: *mastopexy.*

mazoplasia SEE: *mastoplasia.*

M.B. *Bachelor of Medicine.*

m.b. Prescription sign meaning L. *misce bene,* mix well.

MBC *maximum breathing capacity.*

MBD *minimal brain dysfunction; minimal brain damage.*

M.C. **1.** *Master of Surgery.* **2.** *Medical Corps.*

mc Former abbreviation for *millicurie.*

McArdle's disease [Brian McArdle, Brit. pediatrician, b. 1911] One of the glycogen storage diseases (type V) in which there is an abnormal accumulation of glycogen in muscle tissue due to deficiency of myophosphorylase B. Symptoms include pain, fatigability, and muscle stiffness after prolonged exertion.

McBurney's incision [Charles McBurney, U.S. surgeon, 1845–1913] Abdominal incision employed in appendectomy. The incision is made parallel to the path of the external oblique muscle, 1 to 2 in. (2.5 to 5.1 cm) away from the anterosuperior spine of the right ilium, through the external oblique to the internal oblique and transversalis, separating their fibers.

McBurney's point Point 1 to 2 in. (2.5 to

5.1 cm) above the anterosuperior spine of the ilium, on a line between the ilium and umbilicus, where pressure produces tenderness in acute appendicitis.

McBurney's sign Tenderness and rigidity at McBurney's point, probably indicative of appendicitis.

McCarthy's reflex [Daniel J. McCarthy, U.S. neurologist, 1874–1958] Contraction of orbicularis palpebrarum with closure of lids resulting from percussion above the supraorbital nerve.

McCormac's reflex Adduction of one leg resulting from percussion of the patellar tendon of the opposite leg.

McCune-Albright syndrome Albright's disease.

mcg *microgram.*

McGill Pain Questionnaire [McGill University, Montreal, Canada, where the questionnaire was developed] ABBR: MPQ. An instrument used to quantify the perceived location, type, and magnitude of pain. A typical McGill Pain Questionnaire consists of three parts: location of the source of pain as depicted by marking one or more X's on a diagram; the intensity of pain as indicated by a visual analog scale; and the magnitude of pain by selecting words from a pain rating index.

MCH **1.** *mean corpuscular hemoglobin.* **2.** *maternal-child health.*

mc.h. *millicurie hour.*

MCHC *mean corpuscular hemoglobin concentration.*

μCi *microcurie.*

MCi *megacurie.*

mCi *millicurie.*

McMurray's sign [Thomas P. McMurray, Brit. orthopedic surgeon, 1887–1949] Production of a pronounced click during manipulation of the tibia with the leg flexed when the meniscus has been injured.

MCP *metacarpophalangeal joint.*

MCS *multiple chemical sensitivity.*

MCV *mean corpuscular volume.*

M.D. [L. *Medicinae,* Doctor] *Doctor of Medicine.*

Md Symbol for the element mendelevium.

MDI *metered-dose inhaler.*

MDR *multiple drug resistance.*

meal (mēl) [AS. *mael,* measure, meal] **1.** Portion of food eaten at a particular time to satisfy the appetite. **2.** The edible portion of any cereal grain that has been coarsely ground, as in corn meal.

Meals on Wheels Programs that provide to the elderly and infirmed home-delivered meals that meet federally mandated criteria.

mean In statistics, the average of the values. SEE: *arithmetic mean; median.*

arithmetic m. The result obtained by adding all of the values given and dividing by the number of items that were added. SYN: *average; mean.* SEE: *median.*

means testing The determination of a person's financial eligibility for health care services.

measles (mē′zls) [Dutch *maselen*] A highly communicable disease caused by the rubeola virus and marked by fever, general malaise, sneezing, nasal congestion, brassy cough, conjunctivitis, spots on the buccal mucosa (Koplik's spots), and a maculopapular eruption over the entire body. The occurrence of measles before age 6 months is relatively uncommon, because of passively acquired maternal antibodies from the immune mother. SYN: *rubeola.*

An attack of measles almost invariably confers permanent immunity. Active immunization can be produced by administration of measles vaccine, preferably that containing the live attenuated virus, although measles vaccine containing the inactivated virus is available for individuals in whom the live attenuated type is contraindicated. Passive immunization is afforded by administration of gamma globulin. SEE: *Nursing Diagnoses Appendix.*

SYMPTOMS: The onset of symptoms is gradual and includes coryza, rhinitis, drowsiness, loss of appetite, and gradually increasing temperature for the first 2 days up to 101° to 103°F (38.3° to 39.4°C). Koplik's spots appear on the buccal mucosa opposite the molars on the second or third day. The fever peaks about the fourth day, at times as high as 104° to 106°F (40° to 41.1°C). Photophobia and cough soon develop, and when this happens the temperature may fall somewhat.

At this time, the rash appears, first on the face as small maculopapular lesions that grow rapidly and coalesce in places, often causing a swollen, mottled appearance. The rash extends outward to the body and extremities and in some areas may resemble the rash of scarlet fever.

Ordinarily, the rash lasts 4 to 5 days; as it subsides, the temperature declines. Consequently, 5 days after the appearance of the rash, the temperature should be normal or about normal in uncomplicated cases. Early in the disease, leukopenia may be present.

COMPLICATIONS: Encephalitis is a grave complication; of those who develop this, about one in eight will die, about half will have permanent central nervous system injury, and the remainder will recover completely. Bronchopneumonia is a serious complication. Otitis media, followed by mastoiditis, brain abscess, or even meningitis, is not rare, and unilateral or bilateral nerve deafness may be a permanent consequence. Cervical adenitis, with marked cellulitis, sometimes proves fatal. Tracheitis and laryngeal stenosis, due to edema of the glottis, are sometimes seen in the course of measles. A marked conjunctivitis usually occurs.

DIFFERENTIAL DIAGNOSIS: Signs and symptoms of scarlet fever and German measles may mimic those of measles. Koplik's spots are pathognomonic for measles, however, and if seen, virtually rule out other diagnoses.

INCUBATION: Incubation ranges from 7 to 18 days (10 days on average).

PROGNOSIS: The prognosis is favorable in the healthy child, but the seriousness of the possible complications of measles should not be minimized. An attack of measles confers lifelong immunity.

PREVENTION: Active immunization is available with live attenuated virus vaccine; an inactivated virus vaccine is used in individuals for whom the live type is contraindicated. All children who have not had measles or who have been vaccinated before age 12 months should be immunized with live attenuated measles vaccine at 12 months of age. A second dose is recommended at the start of school (5 to 6 yr) or at junior high school age (11 to 12 yr). Measles vaccine is often given in conjunction with mumps and/or rubella virus vaccines. SEE: under *vaccine*.

Live attenuated vaccine is contraindicated in persons who are pregnant or have leukemia, lymphomas, and other generalized neoplasms; in those taking resistance-lowering agents such as steroids and antimetabolites; in persons with active, untreated tuberculosis or other severe illness; in individuals with neomycin, duck, or egg sensitivity; and after blood transfusion or injection of immune serum globulin. In the latter situation, a 12-week waiting period is necessary before administering the vaccine.

Persons born after 1956 who travel to foreign countries should be vaccinated with live attenuated measles vaccine 1 to 2 weeks before departure unless they've already had measles.

Measles immune serum globulin is used for passive protection in unimmunized, high-risk patients (e.g., those who have cancer or are taking antimetabolic drugs); if given later than the third day of the incubation period, however, it may only extend the incubation period instead of preventing the disease.

PATIENT CARE: The importance of immunization of children to prevent measles should be emphasized to parents and family caregivers. Patients who contract the disease remain isolated from diagnosis until 4 days after the rash appears. Bedrest and a quiet, calm environment are provided. A dimly lit room can help to counteract the effects of photophobia, should it occur. Eye secretions are removed with warm saline or water. The child should avoid rubbing the eyes. Supportive care includes adequate fluid intake, antipyretics as necessary, a cool mist vaporizer to relieve cough and coryza, and antipruritic medication to prevent itching. The parents are taught about the importance of handwashing and care of contaminated articles. Assessments are made for complications of otitis media, pneumonia, brochiolitis, laryngotracheitis with obstructive edema, and encephalitis.

black m. A severe form of measles in which the eruption is dark due to an effusion of blood into the skin.

German m. Rubella.

measly (mē′zlē) Description of pork that is infected with the cysticerci of *Taenia solium* or *saginata*.

measurand Any quantity subject to measurement.

measure (mĕ′zhūr) [L. *mensura,* a measuring] **1.** The dimensions, capacity, or quantity of anything that can be so evaluated. Length, area, volume, and mass are basic properties of matter and materials that can be measured. **2.** To determine the extent of length, area, mass, or volume of a substance or object. SYN: *mensuration*. **3.** A device used in measuring, for example, a marked tape or a graduated beaker. SEE: *Weights and Measures Appendix*.

meat [AS. *mete,* food] The flesh of animals, including that of cows, pigs, poultry, and others. Meat is a concentrated source of proteins, fats, cholesterol, calories, and many vitamins and micronutrients. It contains significant amounts of B complex vitamins (thiamine, riboflavin, niacin), iron, and other minerals. It has limited amounts of calcium and fiber. Its metabolic byproducts include organic acids.

Western diets contain far more meat than is needed for growth and development. Excessive consumption of meats and of other calorically dense, high-fat foods contributes to obesity and atherosclerotic heart disease. SEE: *Food Guide Pyramid*.

meatometer (mē-ă-tŏm′ĕt-ĕr) [L. *meatus,* passage, + Gr. *metron,* measure] Device for measuring the size of a passage or opening.

meatoplasty (mē-ăt′ō-plăs-tē) Surgical construction of an external auditory canal.

meatorrhaphy (mē″ă-tor′ăf-ē) [″ + Gr. *rhaphe,* seam, ridge] Suture of the severed end of the urethra to the glans penis following surgical procedure to enlarge the meatus.

meatoscope (mē-ăt′ō-skōp) [″ + Gr. *skopein,* to examine] A speculum for examining a meatus.

meatoscopy (mē-ă-tŏs′ko-pē) [″ + Gr. *skopein,* to examine] Instrumental examination of a meatus, esp. the meatus of the urethra.

meatotome (mē-ăt′ŏ-tōm) [″ + Gr. *tome,* incision] Knife with probe or guarded point for enlarging a meatus by direct incision.

meatotomy (mē″ă-tŏt′ō-mē) Incision of urinary meatus to enlarge the opening.

meatus (mē-ā′tŭs) *pl.* **meatus** [L.] A passage or opening. **meatal** (mē-ā′tăl), *adj.*

m. acusticus externus External auditory canal from the eardrum to the external ear.

m. acusticus internus Canal in the petrous portion of temporal bone, through which pass the cochlear and vestibular nerves.

external auditory m. The lateral, outer opening of the external auditory canal.

internal auditory m. The most medial opening of the internal auditory canal, located on the posterior surface of the petrous portion of the temporal bone.

m. nasi communis Common nasal cavity on either side of septum, into which three meatus open.

m. nasi inferior Space beneath inferior turbinate or concha of the nose.

m. nasi medius Space beneath middle turbinate or concha of the nose.

m. nasi superior Space beneath superior turbinate or concha of the nose.

m. nasopharyngeus Posterior portion of nasal cavity, which communicates with the nasopharynx.

m. urinarius External opening of the urethra.

mebendazole (mĕ-bĕn′dă-zōl) A broad-spectrum antihelmintic. It is used in treating tapeworm infections and is the drug of choice in treating *Ascaris lumbricoides, Trichuris trichuria,* hookworm, and *Strongyloides stercoralis.*

CAUTION: This drug should not be used during pregnancy.

mecamylamine hydrochloride (mĕk″ă-mĭl′ă-mĭn) An antihypertensive of the ganglionic blocking agent type.

mechanical rectifier A device that, by changing contacts at the proper moment in a cycle, changes alternating current into pulsating direct current.

mechanics [Gr. *mechane,* machine] The science of force and matter.

dynamic m. The continuous automated analysis of simultaneous measurements of lung variables affecting mechanical ventilation.

mechanism **1.** Involuntary and consistent response to a stimulus. **2.** A habit or response pattern formed to achieve a result. **3.** A machine or machine-like structure.

countercurrent m. Mechanism used by the kidneys, making it possible to excrete excess solutes in the urine with little loss of water from the body.

cycling m. The component of a ventilator that ends or begins the inspiratory phase of mechanical ventilation of the lungs.

defense m. SEE: *defense mechanism.*

Duncan's m. Delivery of the placenta when separation begins at the outer margins and progresses inward, presenting the rough maternal side first.

m. of injury ABBR: MOI. The manner in which a traumatic event occurred (e.g., fall from a height, ground-level fall, high- or low-speed motor vehicle accident, ejection from a vehicle, vehicle rollover). The MOI is used to estimate the forces involved in trauma and, thus, the potential severity for wounding, fractures, and internal organ damage that a patient may suffer as a result of his or her injury.

mechanoreceptor (mĕk″ă-nō-rē-sĕp′tor) A receptor that receives mechanical stimuli such as pressure from sound or touch.

mechanotherapy (mĕk″ăn-ō-thĕr′ă-pē) [Gr. *mechane,* machine, + *therapeia,* treatment] Use of various types of mechanical apparatus to perform passive movements and to exercise various parts of the body.

mechlorethamine (mĕk″lor-ĕth′ă-mēn) A cytotoxic of the nitrogen mustard type.

Mecholyl test A test of parasympathetic nervous system function. A 2% solution of methacholine (Mecholyl) is instilled in the conjunctival sac. The pupil constricts if the patient has a parasympathetic disorder, such as familial dysautonomia.

Meckel, Johann Friedrich (the elder) (mĕk′ĕl) German anatomist, 1724–1774.

M.'s ganglion Ganglion located in the sphenomaxillary fossa giving off nerves to eyes, nose, and palate.

M.'s space Area in dura holding the gasserian (trigeminal) ganglion.

Meckel, Johann Friedrich (the younger) (mĕk′ĕl) German anatomist, 1781–1833, grandson of J. F. Meckel, the elder.

M.'s cartilage A cartilaginous bar about which the mandible develops.

M.'s diverticulum A congenital sac or blind pouch sometimes found in the lower portion of the ileum. It represents the persistent proximal end of the yolk stalk. Sometimes it is continued to the umbilicus as a cord or as a tube forming a fistulous opening at the umbilicus. Strangulation may cause intestinal obstruction. SEE: *diverticulitis.*

meckelectomy (mĕk-ĕl-ĕk′tō-mē) Excision of Meckel's ganglion.

meclizine hydrochloride (mĕk′lĭ-zēn) Antiemetic esp. effective for control of nausea and vomiting of motion sickness.

meclocycline sulfosalicylate An antibacterial used topically.

meconium (mĕ-kō′nē-ŭm) [Gr. *mekonion,* poppy juice] **1.** Opium; poppy juice. **2.** First feces of a newborn infant, made up of salts, amniotic fluid, mucus, bile, and epithelial cells. This substance is greenish black, almost odorless, and tarry. The first meconium stool should appear during the first 24 hr. Meconium should persist for about 3 days.

meconium aspiration syndrome ABBR: MAS. Fetal inhalation of meconium in utero during episodes of severe fetal hypoxia or with the first few breaths after birth. Symptoms and signs, which occur to varying degrees, include respiratory distress, tachypnea, rales, and wheezes throughout the lung fields. Chest x-ray examination may show areas of increased density from the aspirated meconium, evidence of chemical pneumonitis, as well as areas of atelectasis caused by bronchiolar obstruction and collapse of alveoli distally. A pneumothorax also may occur from the ball-valve effect of meconium obstruction in the small bronchioles. These complications can produce hypoxia, acidosis, and a persistence of the fetal circulation and persistent pulmonary hypertension of the newborn (PPHN). SEE: *meconium.*

ETIOLOGY: Pre-eclampsia, pregnancy-induced hypertension, postmaturity (with oligohydramnios), intrauterine hypoxia and asphyxia, or other forms of stress on the fetus may be contributory factors. Fetal stress may produce increased intestinal peristalsis, anal sphincter relaxation, and expulsion of meconium into the amniotic fluid. When the fetus gasps in utero, or with the first few breaths of air after delivery, the fluid enters the respiratory tree.

PREVENTION: Preventive measures include gentle suctioning of the baby's nose and mouth by the obstetrician while the baby's head is still on the mother's perineum, followed by immediate tracheal suctioning via endotracheal intubation to remove as much airway meconium as possible before the baby's first breath.

TREATMENT: Oxygen, endotracheal intubation, and assisted ventilation may be required for severe cases. Instillation of pulmonary surfactant via the endotracheal tube may somewhat lessen the respiratory distress.

meconium ileus Ileus due to impacted meconium in the intestines. It is usually associated with newborn children with cystic fibrosis.

meconium staining, meconium show Fetal defecation while in utero at time of labor that occurs with fetal distress. It is composed of thick, mucous-pasty material that must be suctioned before the newborn takes a first breath or the material may be aspirated.

M.E.D. *minimal effective dose; minimal erythema dose.*

Medevac The evacuation of injured persons from the scene of an emergency by air ambulance, usually a helicopter. Air transport of trauma patients is esp. useful in rural locations, to provide definitive care as quickly as possible. SEE: *golden hour.*

medi- SEE: *medio-.*

media (mē′dē-ă) [L.] **1.** Pl. of medium. **2.** The middle or muscular layer of an artery or vein. SYN: *tunica media.*

mediad (mē′dē-ăd) [L. *medium,* middle, + *ad,* toward] Toward the median line or plane of the body.

medial (mē′dē-ăl) [L. *medialis*] **1.** Pert. to middle. **2.** Nearer the medial plane.

medialis (mē″dē-ā′lĭs) [L.] Term indicating something is close to the midline of the body.

medial tibial syndrome Shinsplints.

median (mē′dē-ăn) [L. *medianus*] **1.** Middle; central. **2.** In statistics, a number obtained by arranging the given series in order of magnitude and taking the middle number; one then has an equal number of values above and below that number. Thus, in the series 5, 7, 8, 9, 10, the median is 8. SYN: *mesial.* SEE: *mean.*

mediastinal (mē″dē-ăs-tī′năl) [L. *mediastinalis*] Relating to the mediastinum.

mediastinal crunch A rasping sound, similar to the noise made when leather rubs against leather, that is heard on listening to the heart of a patient with air in the mediastinum. The sound usually is detected during cardiac systole but also may vary in intensity with breathing.

mediastinitis (mē″dē-ăs″tĭ-nī′tĭs) [″ + Gr. *itis,* inflammation] Inflammation or infection of the mediastinum, such as may occur after injury to the neck, perforation of the esophagus, or after surgical procedures on the heart or lungs.

mediastinography (mē″dē-ăs″tĭ-nŏg′ră-fē) [″ + Gr. *graphein,* to write] X-raying of the mediastinum.

mediastinopericarditis (mē-dē-ăs″tĭ-nō-pĕr″ĭ-kăr-dī′tĭs) [″ + Gr. *peri,* around, + *kardia,* heart, + *itis,* inflammation] Inflammatory condition of the mediastinum and pericardium.

mediastinoscopy (mē″dē-ăs″tĭ-nŏs′kō-pē) [″ + *skopein,* to examine] Endoscopic examination of the mediastinum.

mediastinotomy (mē″dē-ăs″tĭ-nŏt′ō-mē) [″ + *tome,* incision] Surgical incision of the mediastinum.

mediastinum (mē″dē-ăs-tī′nŭm) *pl.* **mediastina** [L., in the middle] **1.** A septum or cavity between two principal portions of an organ. **2.** The mass of organs and tissues separating the lungs. It contains the heart and its large vessels, trachea, esophagus, thymus, lymph nodes, and connective tissue.

m. testis The thickened portion of the tunica albuginea on posterior surface of the testis. SYN: *corpus highmorianum.*

mediate (mē′dē-āt) **1.** Accomplished by indirect means. **2.** Between two parts or sides.

mediation (mē″dē-ā′shŭn) The action of a mediating agent.

mediator (mē′dē-ā″tŏr) **1.** Any substance or anatomical structure that transmits information between two reagents, cells, tissues, or organs. **2.** Neutral third party who facilitates agreements by helping disputing parties to identify their needs and work toward mutually agreeable solutions.

medic **1.** Medical corpsman. SEE: *corpsman.* **2.** Slang for paramedic.

medicable (mĕd′ĭ-kă-bl) [L. *medicari,* to heal] Possibly responsive to therapy; curable.

Medicaid A federally aided, but state operated and administered, program for providing medical care for certain low-income individuals.

medical (mĕd′ĭ-kăl) **1.** Pert. to medicine or the study of the art and science of caring for those who are ill. **2.** Requiring therapy with medicines as distinct from surgical treatment.

medical access The right or ability of an individual to obtain medical and health care services.

medical assistance In the U.S., a state-administered program designed to pay for health care provided to medically indigent patients. SEE: *Medicaid.*

medical assistant An individual who assists a qualified physician in an office or other clinical setting, performing administrative tasks (such as those of secretary, receptionist, or bookkeeper) and technical duties (vital signs, height, weight, laboratory tests) as delegated and in accordance with state laws governing medical practice.

medical audit A systematic approach to reviewing, analyzing, and evaluating medical care in order to identify discrepancies in the quality of care and to provide a mechanism for improving that quality. SEE: *medical outcomes study.*

medical corpsman SEE: *corpsman.*

medical device Any health care product intended for use in the diagnosis, treatment, or prevention of disease that is in or on the human body, but neither metabolized nor chemically altered by it.

medical direction Physician input to and overseeing of policies, protocols, medical procedures, training, and quality assurance for an emergency medical service system.

Medic Alert A nonprofit foundation that provides a bracelet or pendant with an emblem on which is contained crucial information about a patient's medical history and a warning in case of emergency. The company also keeps a file of the medical information and provides an emergency phone number that medical personnel can call collect. The goal is to prevent a serious or fatal mistake in rendering aid or medical care to an injured or unconscious person who may have an additional condition or allergy (e.g., diabetes, penicillin allergy). Applications may be obtained from Medic Alert, 2323 Colorado Ave, Turlock, CA 95382. Telephone: 1-800-IDALERT. Website: www.medicalert.org. Persons wishing to donate organs may also acquire an emblem from the Medic Alert company stating that fact. SEE: illus.

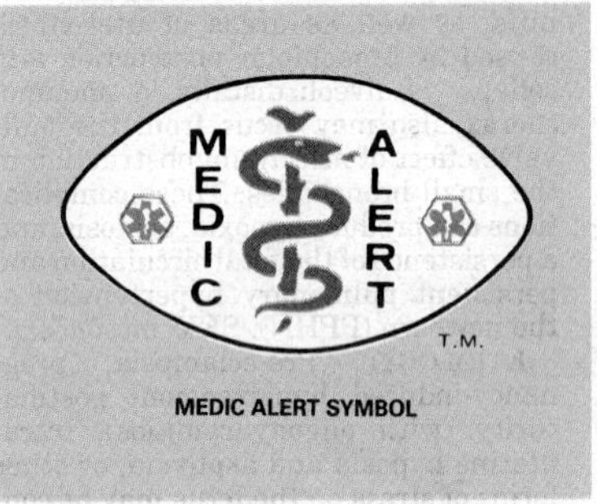

MEDIC ALERT SYMBOL

medical examiner A physician who is trained and qualified for the task of investigating the cause of death and the circumstances surrounding it. Training usually includes study of pathology and forensic medicine. The examiner is empowered by governmental agencies to represent them, and is expected to make a comprehensive report of findings to judicial or police authorities. The skill of a medical examiner is esp. important in investigating deaths wherein malpractice, homicide, suicide, or other criminal actions are suspected of being a contributing factor. SEE: *coroner; death investigation; medicine, forensic.*

medical grand rounds SEE: *grand rounds.*

medical informatics The application of information technology and processing to all aspects of medical knowledge, practice, and management, including medical education and research. This process is facilitated by computer technology.

medical jurisprudence SEE: *jurisprudence, medical.*

medical outcomes study ABBR: MOS. Studies designed to provide valid comparisons between medical care processes and outcomes as they are affected by system of care and clinician's specialty, as well as by patients' diagnoses and the levels of severity of illness. Thus, MOS provides a model for monitoring the results of medical care. SEE: *medical audit.*

medical preparations Preparation (3).

medical problems of musicians SEE: *musicians, medical problems of.*

medical record A written transcript of information obtained from a patient, guardian, or medical professionals concerning a patient's health history, diagnostic tests, diagnoses, treatment, and prognosis.

medical record, problem-oriented SEE: *problem-oriented medical record.*

medical transcriptionist A person who makes a typed record from the data and information available from the physician's dictated material concerning the patient's medical records. An individual who has met the requirements of the American Association of Medical Transcription is certified by that body as a Certified Medical Transcriptionist.

medical waste Infectious or physically dangerous medical or biological waste. Included are discarded blood and blood products; waste from the pathology department, including body parts, tissues, or fluids discarded during surgery or at autopsy; contaminated animal carcasses; animal body parts and bedding; sharps; discarded preparations made from genetically altered living organisms and their products. SEE: *sharps; Standard and Universal Precautions Appendix.*

medicament [L. *medicamentum*] A medicine or remedy.

medicamentosus (mĕd″ĭ-kă-mĕn-tō′sŭs) Concerning drugs.

Medicare In the U.S., a federally sponsored health insurance program for people over age 65, some younger disabled persons, and persons with end-stage renal disease. American Medicare consists of two parts: Medicare Part A provides hospital insurance, and Part B (an option some participants choose to purchase) provides general medical insurance. In the U.S., Medicare also administers its own managed care plan. In Canada, Medicare is administered by the provinces.

medicate (mĕd′ĭ-kāt) [L. *medicatus*] **1.** To treat a disease with drugs. **2.** To permeate with medicinal substances.

medication (mĕd-ĭ-kā′shŭn) **1.** Medicinal substance; a drug. **2.** Treatment with remedies. **3.** Impregnation with medicine.

hypodermic m. Treatment by injection of medicine into the body through the skin, using a syringe and needle.

intravenous m. The injection of a sterile solution of a drug or an infusion into a vein.

ionic m. Introduction of ions of drugs into body tissues through the skin by means of electricity. SEE: *cataphoresis; iontophoresis* (2).

sublingual m. Treatment with an agent, usually in tablet form, placed under the tongue.

substitutive m. Medical therapy to cause a nonspecific inflammation to counteract a specific one.

medication errors Administering the wrong medicine, administering an incorrect dose of a medicine, failing to administer a prescribed medicine, or administering the medicine either at the incorrect time or via the incorrect route. Every effort should be made to prevent errors in medication. It is essential that the nurse, physician, and pharmacist cooperate and communicate concerning medication. In addition, the following will help to avoid errors: Administer no drug without an order; identify drug and amount in each dose unit; be certain that the name of the medicine ordered is spelled precisely as that on the label—if in doubt, do not administer until the question is resolved; do not use outdated medicines; if drug appears unusual due to discoloration or precipitation, do not use; administer medicine at the time specified or as close to that time as possible—if there is a delay, document it; identify patient; do not leave medication at bedside; permit patient to self-administer medicines only if permitted by physician's written order; unless authorized by physician, do not use drugs patient brought to hospital; if an alert patient questions the drug's identity or appropriateness for use, recheck the identity of the patient and the drug; if patient refuses medication, document this on chart and notify the physician responsible for the care of the patient at that time. SEE: *drug handling.*

medication pass The administering of prescribed drugs by nurses or aides to a group of patients or residents, in accordance with state and federal standards.

medication route The way that a drug is introduced into the body. The route of administration is chosen according to the speed of absorption desired and the site of action of the medication. Some medications are formulated for a specific route only and must be given in that manner. It is important that medicines be administered as directed by the manufacturer. Various routes of administration used are as follows:

Oral and *enteral* administration require that the medication not be destroyed by the environment of the stomach and digestive enzymes. It is too slow if rapid absorption is required, and cannot be used if the patient is vomiting. Rectal administration in the form of liquids or suppositories circumvents this problem in enteral administration.

Mucosal routes of administration other than the above include absorption through the nasal mucosa, the buccal mucosa, sublingually, or the bronchioles, the latter usually achieved through inhalation of an aerosol. Vaginal and rectal administration are also mucosal routes of medication.

Percutaneous administration is used for iontophoresis or by direct absorption through the skin.

Parenteral administration is used when a drug cannot be given by mouth. The speed of absorption varies greatly with the specific route used, which may be subcutaneous, intravenous, intramuscular, intra-arterial, intraperitoneal, intrathecal, intracardiac, or intrasternal.

medicinal (mĕ-dĭ′sĭn-ăl) [L. *medicina*, medicine] Pert. to medicine.

medicine 1. A drug or remedy. **2.** The act of maintenance of health, and prevention and treatment of disease and illness. **3.** Treatment of disease by medical, as distinguished from surgical, treatment.

aerospace m. Branch of medicine concerned with the selection of individuals for duty as pilots or crew members for flight and space missions. Includes study of the pathology and physiology of persons and animals who travel in airplanes and spacecraft in the earth's atmosphere and in outer space.

alternative m. Approaches to medical diagnosis and therapy that have not been developed by use of generally accepted scientific methods. Forms of alternative medicine include acupressure, acupuncture, aromatherapy, ayurveda, biofeedback, Christian Science, faith healing, guided imagery, herbal medicine, holistic medicine, homeopathy, hypnosis, macrobiotics, manipulative medicine, massage therapy, naturopathy, ozone therapy, reflexotherapy, relaxation response, Rolfing, shiatsu, and yoga, among others. Some of these techniques and practices are clinically or personally useful, while others are not, and a few are fraudulent or hazardous.

The interest of the American public in alternative approaches to health maintenance, the treatment of illness, and the restoration of health has increased over the last several decades. Individuals seeking medical care from either conventional or unconventional practitioners should be advised to inform the caregiver about all behaviors and therapies in recent or current use. The placebo effect and the natural history of the particular disease must be considered in evaluating the efficacy of alternative therapies. In 1992, the Office of Alternative Medicine was established at the National Institutes of Health to investigate the scientific merits of alternative medicine. It is now known as the National Center for Complementary and Alternative Medicine (NCCAM). SEE: *Integrative Therapies: Complementary and Alternative Medicine Appendix; complementary m.; herbal remedy.*

CAUTION: Individuals who use alternative medicines should be aware that few, if any, of those products are subjected to formulation specifications and manufacturing controls. In their absence the consumer has no assurance of their purity or efficacy. The possible interaction of pharmacological agents with nutritional and/or herbal preparations must be considered by both allopathic and alternative medical providers.

---

clinical m. Observation and treatment at the bedside; the practice of medicine in the clinical setting as distinguished from laboratory science.

community m. Medical care directed toward service of the entire population of the community, with emphasis on preventive medicine.

complementary m. Therapies proven to promote health and well-being but traditionally considered outside the scope of Western allopathic medical practice. The effectiveness of complementary therapies has been validated by the results of experimental trials. Alternative medical practices differ from complementary practices in that their effectiveness is unproven, and they are anecdotal, traditional, ritualistic, or based solely on belief. SEE: *Integrative Therapies: Complementary and Alternative Medicine appendix; alternative m.*

cookbook m. The use of algorithms (in place of individualized care) in medicine. The reliance by practitioners on guidelines and rules rather than on a comprehensive, holistic approach to the medical needs of a patient.

correctional m. Health care provided to inmates of prisons and jails.

dental m. Branch of medicine concerned with the preservation and treatment of the teeth and other orofacial tissues. It includes preventive measures such as oral hygiene, as well as restorative procedures or prostheses and surgery. The results are widespread, including better nutrition and digestion from restored and balanced occlusion, and improved mental health from the control of oral and dental infections that often are overlooked but jeopardize the success of other medical treatments.

disaster m. Large-scale application of emergency medical services in a community, following a natural or man-made catastrophe. The aim is to save lives and restore every survivor to maximum health as promptly as possible. Its success depends on prompt sorting of patients according to their immediate needs and prognosis. SEE: *triage*.

emergency m. Branch of medicine specializing in emergency care of the acutely ill and injured. Board-certified physicians who successfully complete a residency and qualifying examination and who meet other requirements of the American College of Emergency Physicians may use the abbreviation FACEP (Fellow of the American College of Emergency Physicians). SEE: *certified emergency nurse; Emergency Nurses Association; FACEP*.

environmental m. Branch of medicine concerned with the effects of the environment (temperature, rainfall, population size, pollution, radiation) on humans.

evidence-based m. The concept that practice of medicine should be based on firm data rather than anecdote, tradition, intuition, or belief.

experimental m. The scientific study of disease or pathological conditions through experimentation on laboratory animals or through clinical research.

family m. Area of medical specialization concerned with providing or supervising the medical care of all members of the family.

folk m. Use of home remedies for treatment of diseases.

forensic m. Medicine in relation to the law; as in autopsy proceedings, or the determination of time or cause of death, or in the determination of sanity. Also, the legal aspects of medical ethics and standards. SYN: *legal m.*

gender-specific m. Health care that pertains only to men or to women but not to individuals of both genders, for example, diseases and conditions produced by sex hormones.

group m. **1.** Practice of medicine by a group of physicians, usually consisting of specialists in various fields who pool their services and share laboratory and x-ray facilities. Such a group is commonly called a clinic. **2.** Securing of medical services by a group of individuals who, on paying definite sums of money, are entitled to certain medical services or hospitalization in accordance with prearranged rules and regulations.

high-tech m. Engineered advances in medical knowledge and technique that have resulted in improved diagnostic, therapeutic, and rehabilitative procedures.

holistic m. The comprehensive and total care of a patient. In this system, the needs of the patient in all areas, such as physical, emotional, social, spiritual, and economic, are considered and cared for. SEE: *holism*.

industrial m. Occupational and environmental m.

integrative m. Alternative m.

internal m. The medical specialty concerned with the overall health and well-being of adults. The internist uses the tools of history taking, physical examination, and diagnostic testing to diagnose and prevent disease. Patient education, lifestyle modification, psychological counseling, use of medications, inpatient medical care, and referral to other specialists are responsibilities of the internist.

legal m. Forensic m.

mind-body m. Branch of medicine that recognizes the importance of mind-body interrelationship in all illnesses, on which therapy and management are based. SYN: *psychosomatic*.

naturopathic m. The philosophy and practice of healing that relies primarily on the use of nutrition, herbal remedies, homeopathy, massage, and counseling to promote wellness and healthy lifestyles. Other modalities used include such disciplines as astrology, aromatherapy, color therapy, traditional Chinese medicine, and iridology.

nuclear m. Branch of medicine involved with the use of radioactive substances for diagnosis, therapy, and research.

occupational and environmental m. ABBR: OEM. The branch of medicine concerned with work-related diseases, hazards, and injuries; working conditions; employee rehabilitation; and the regulations that pertain to these issues.

patent m. A drug or medical preparation that is protected by patent and sold without a physician's prescription. The law requires that it be labeled with names of active ingredients, the quantity or proportion of the contents, and directions for its use, and that it not have misleading statements as to curative effects on the label. SEE: *nonproprietary name; prescription; proprietary medicine*.

physical m. Treatment of disease by physical agents such as heat, cold, light, electricity, manipulation, or the use of mechanical devices.

preclinical m. **1.** Preventive medicine. **2.** Medical education that takes place in classes, laboratories, and symposia, preceding the training that occurs through the direct care of patients.

preventive m. SEE: *preventive medicine*.

proprietary m. SEE: *proprietary medicine*.

psychosomatic m. Mind-body m.

socialized m. A health care delivery system in which the provision of services is controlled by the government.

sports m. Field of medicine concerned with all aspects of physiology, pathology, and psychology as they apply to persons who participate in sports, whether at the recreational, amateur, or professional level. An important facet of sports medicine is the application of medical knowledge to the prevention of injuries in those who participate in sports.

tropical m. Branch of medical science that deals principally with diseases common in tropical or subtropical regions, esp. diseases of parasitic origin.

veterinary m. Branch of medical science that deals with diagnosis and treatment of diseases of animals.

medicine man Shaman.

medicinerea (mĕd″ĭ-sĭn-ē′rē-a) [L. *medius,* middle, + *cinerea,* ashen] Internal gray matter of the claustrum and lenticula of the brain.

medicochirurgical (mĕd″ĭ-kō-kī-rŭr′jĭ-kăl) [L. *medicus,* medical, + Gr. *cheir,* hand, + *ergon,* work] Concerning both medicine and surgery.

medicolegal (mĕd″ĭ-kō-lē′găl) [″ + *legalis,* legal] Relating to medical jurisprudence or forensic medicine.

medicomechanical (mĕd″ĭ-kō-mĕ-kăn′ĭ-kăl) Concerning both medical and mechanical aspects of treating patients.

medicopsychology (mĕd″ĭ-kō-sī-kŏl′ō-jē) The relationship of medicine to the mind or to mental illness.

medicornu (mĕd″ĭ-kor′nū) [L. *medius,* middle, + *cornu,* horn] The inferior horn of the lateral ventricle of the brain.

Medigap One of several optional, supplemental insurance programs that augment a Medicare beneficiary's health care coverage. The costs and benefit structures of these programs vary. Some provide comprehensive health care services for relatively high prices; others provide more limited benefits for lower costs.

Medina worm *Dracunculus medinensis.*

medio-, medi- [L. *medius,* middle] Prefix meaning *middle.*

mediocarpal (mē″dē-ō-kăr′păl) Concerning the middle part of the carpus.

mediolateral (mē″dē-ō-lăt′ĕr-ăl) Concerning the middle and side of a structure.

medionecrosis (mē″dē-ō-nē-krō′sĭs) [″ + *nekrosis,* state of death] Necrosis of the tunica media of a blood vessel.

mediopontine (mē″dē-ō-pŏn′tīn) [″ + *pons,* bridge] Relating to the center of the pons varolii.

mediotarsal (mē″dē-ō-tăr′săl) Relating to the middle of the tarsus.

medisect (mē′dĭ-sĕkt) [″ + *secare,* to cut] To cut on the median line of the body or structure.

meditation The art of contemplative thinking. In alternative and complementary medicine, it is used to control stress and improve relaxation, focus attention (for example on positive outcomes during an illness), and lower heart rate and blood pressure.

transcendental m. ABBR: TM. A type of meditation based on ancient Hindu practices in which an individual tries to relax by sitting quietly for regular periods while repeating a mantra. The value of TM in treating various conditions is under investigation. SEE: *relaxation response.*

Mediterranean fever, familial A recessively inherited illness characterized by 3- to 5-day attacks of fever, peritonitis, pleuritis, and arthritis. In the past, the most frequent cause of death from familial Mediterranean fever was amyloidosis, which occurred as the disease progressed. The use of prophylactic colchicine has greatly reduced the number of attacks and prevents amyloidosis. SYN: *recurrent polyserositis.*

medium (mēd′ē-ŭm) *pl.* **media** **1.** An agent through which an effect is obtained. **2.** Substance used for the cultivation of microorganisms or cellular tissue. SYN: *culture m.* **3.** Substance through which impulses are transmitted.

clearing m. A substance that renders histological specimens transparent.

culture m. A substance on which microorganisms may grow. Those most commonly used are broths, gelatin, and agar, which contain the same basic ingredients.

defined m. In bacteriology, a medium in which the composition is accurately defined and carefully controlled. One use of this culture medium is to investigate the influence of altering ingredients on bacterial cell growth characteristics.

dispersion m. A liquid in which a colloid is dispersed.

nutrient m. A fortified culture medium with added nutrient materials.

radiolucent m. A substance injected into an anatomical structure to decrease the density, producing a dark area on the radiograph.

radiopaque m. A substance injected into a cavity or region or passed through the gastrointestinal tract to increase the density, producing an image with enhanced contrast between solid and hollow structures.

refracting m. The fluids and transparent tissues of the eye that refract light rays passing through them toward the retina: the cornea, aqueous humor, lens, and vitreous humor.

separating m. In dentistry, a substance applied to the surface of an impression or mold to prevent interaction of the materials and to facilitate their separation after casting.

medium-chain triglycerides SEE: under *triglycerides*.

medius (mē′dē-ŭs) [L.] Middle. Indicating the middle one of three similar structures.

MEDLARS [*Med*ical *L*iterature *A*nalysis and *R*etrieval *S*ystem] A computerized system of databases and data banks available from the National Library of Medicine. A person may search the computer files to produce a list of publications (bibliographic citations) or retrieve factual information on a specific question. MEDLARS databases cover medicine, nursing, dentistry, veterinary medicine, and the preclinical sciences. They are used by universities, medical schools, hospitals, government agencies, commercial and nonprofit organizations, and private individuals. MEDLARS includes two computer subsystems, ELHILL and TOXNET, comprising in the year 2000 more than 40 on-line databases with about 18 million references.

MEDLINE [*MED*LARS on *line*] The computer-accessible bibliographic database of the National Library of Medicine. It is the system that links telephone lines to the MEDLARS databases. It includes references that appear in more than 3,800 research, medical, dental, veterinary, and nursing journals. SEE: *MEDLARS.*

medrogestone SEE: *progestin* (2).

medroxyprogesterone acetate (mĕd-rŏk″sē-prō-jĕs′tĕr-ōn) A progestational agent used to treat secondary amenorrhea, abnormal uterine bleeding related to hormone imbalance, and advanced endometrial and renal malignancies. It also is used with estrogens in hormone replacement therapy and administered intramuscularly as a long-term contraceptive (it is effective for up to 90 days).

medrysone (mĕd′rĭ-sōn) A corticosteroid used in a 1% suspension in ophthalmology.

medulla (mĕ-dŭl′lă) *pl.* **medullae** [L.] **1.** Marrow. **2.** Inner or central portion of an organ in contrast to the outer portion or cortex. **medullary** (mĕd′ū-lār-ē), *adj.*

adrenal m. Inner portion of the adrenal gland. It is composed of chromaffin tissue and secretes epinephrine and norepinephrine. SEE: *adrenal gland.*

m. of hair Central axis of a hair.

m. of kidneys SEE: *pyramid, renal.*

m. nephrica SEE: *pyramid, renal.*

m. oblongata The lowest part of the brainstem, continuous with the spinal cord above the level of the foramen magnum of the occipital bone. It regulates heart rate, breathing, blood pressure, and other reflexes, such as coughing, sneezing, swallowing, and vomiting.

m. ossium Marrow in bone.

m. of ovary Central portion of the ovary composed of loose connective tissue, blood vessels, lymphatics, and nerves.

m. spinalis Latin term for spinal cord.

medullated (mĕd′ū-lāt″ĕd) **1.** Containing marrow. **2.** An old term for myelinated.

medullation A term once used to indicate myelination (the acquisition of myelin by a nerve).

medullectomy (mĕd″ū-lĕk′tō-mē) [L. *medulla,* marrow, + Gr. *ektome,* excision] Surgical excision of a part of the medulla of the brain.

medullitis (mĕd-ū-lī′tĭs) [″ + Gr. *itis,* inflammation] Inflammation of marrow. SYN: *myelitis.*

medullization (mĕd″ū-lī-zā′shŭn) Abnormal conversion of bone to marrow.

medulloadrenal (mē-dŭl″ō-ă-drē′năl) [″ + *ad,* to, + *ren,* kidney] Concerning the medulla of the adrenal gland.

medulloarthritis (mĕ-dŭl″ō-ăr-thrī′tĭs) [L. *medulla,* marrow, + Gr. *arthron,* joint, + *itis,* inflammation] Inflammation of marrow elements of bone ends.

medulloblast (mĕ-dŭl′ō-blăst) [″ + Gr. *blastos,* germ] An immature cell of the neural tube that may develop into either a nerve or neuroglial cell.

medulloblastoma (mĕ-dŭl″ō-blăs-tō′mă) [″ + Gr. *blastos,* germ, + *oma,* tumor] A soft infiltrating malignant tumor of the roof of the fourth ventricle and cerebellum. The tumor often invades the meninges.

medulloepithelioma (mĕ-dŭl″ō-ĕp″ĭ-thēl-ē-ō′mă) [″ + Gr. *epi,* upon, + *thele,* nipple, + *oma,* tumor] Tumor composed of retina epithelium and of neuroepithelium. SYN: *glioma; neuroepithelioma.*

MedWatch A voluntary and confidential program of the Food and Drug Administration (FDA) for monitoring the safety of drugs, biologicals, medical devices, and nutritional products such as dietary supplements, medical foods, and infant formulas. The FDA provides forms for reporting adverse events associated with any of these products. Health professionals may obtain the form by calling 1-800-332-1088. Information may be faxed to the FDA by calling 1-800-332-0178.

Mees lines [R. A. Mees, 20th century Dutch scientist] Transverse white lines that appear above the lunula of the fingernails about 5 weeks after exposure to arsenic.

mefenamic acid An analgesic and antipyretic that also has anti-inflammatory action.

mefipristone An oral agent used to induce abortions. It is typically administered for this purpose with misoprostol or methotrexate. The drug was formerly known as RU-486.

mega- [Gr. *megas,* large] **1.** SEE: *megalo-*. **2.** Indicates 1 million (10^6) when used in combination with terms indicating units of measure; thus a megaton is 1 million tons.

megabladder (mĕg″ă-blăd′ĕr) [″ + AS. *blaedre,* bladder] Permanent abnormal enlargement of the urinary bladder. SYN: *megalocystis.*

megacardia Cardiomegaly.

megacephalic SEE: *megalocephalic.*

megacolon (mĕg-ă-kō′lŏn) [″ + *kolon,* colon] Massive dilation of the colon, which, if left untreated, may result in perforation and peritonitis.

aganglionic m. Hirschsprung's disease.

toxic m. Marked enlargement of the colon, esp. the transverse colon. Clinically, tachycardia, fever, and leukocytosis occur. There may be abdominal tenderness, a palpable abdominal mass, confusion, cramping, and change in number of bowel movements per day. SYN: *toxic dilatation of colon.*

ETIOLOGY: The most common causes of toxic megacolon in adults are ulcerative colitis, pseudomembranous colitis, Crohn's disease, drugs that slow intestinal motility (such as narcotics), and severe electrolyte disturbances. Megacolon in children may result from Hirschsprung's disease.

TREATMENT: Patients with toxic megacolon are treated by withholding oral intake, providing nasogastric suction, giving broad-spectrum antibiotics (and corticosteroids, in inflammatory bowel disease), and carefully resuscitating fluids and electrolytes. Surgery is required if the patient fails to improve or deteriorates.

megacurie (mĕg″ă-kū′rē) [″ + *curie*] ABBR: Mc. A unit of radioactivity equal to 10^6 curies.

megadontia (mĕg″ă-dŏn′shē-ă) [″+ *odous, odont-,* tooth] Macrodontia.

megadose A dose of a nutrient, such as a vitamin supplement, that is 10 times greater than the recommended daily allowance for that nutrient.

megadyne (mĕg′ă-dīn) A unit equal to 1 million dynes. SEE: *dyne.*

megaesophagus (mĕg″ă-ĕ-sŏf′ă-gŭs) [″ + *oisophagos,* esophagus] A grossly dilated esophagus usually associated with achalasia.

megahertz (mĕg′ă-hĕrtz) ABBR: MHz. One million cycles per second, or 10^6 hertz.

megakaryoblast (mĕg″ă-kăr′ē-ō-blăst) An immature megakaryocyte.

megakaryocyte (mĕg″ă-kăr′ē-ō-sīt″) [″ + *karyon,* nucleus, + *kytos,* cell] Large bone marrow cell with large or multiple nuclei from which platelets are derived. SEE: *platelet;* illus.

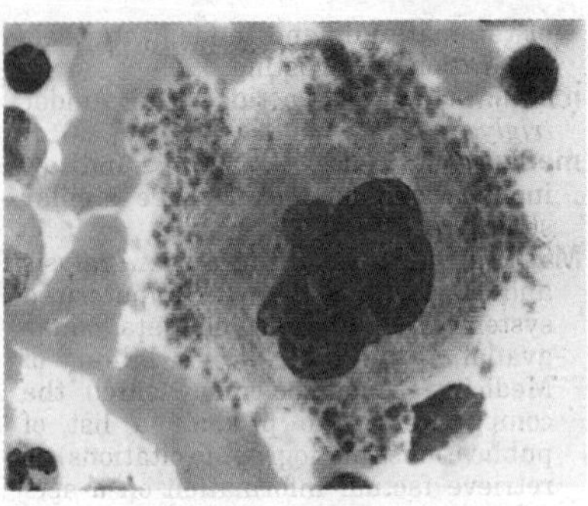

MEGAKARYOCYTE

(Orig. mag. ×640)

megakaryocytosis (mĕg″ă-kăr″ē-ō-sī-tō′sĭs) [″ + ″ + ″ + *osis,* condition] An increased number of megakaryocytes in the bone marrow; presence of megakaryocytes in the blood.

megalencephaly (mĕg″ăl-ĕn-sĕf′ă-lē) [″ + *enkephalos,* brain] Abnormally large size of the brain, usually accompanied by mental deficiency.

megalo-, mega- [Gr. *megas,* large] Combining form meaning *large* or *huge.*

megaloblast (mĕg′ă-lō-blăst) [″ + *blastos,* germ] A large, nucleated, abnormal red blood cell, from 11 to 20 μm in diameter, oval and slightly irregular. It is found in the blood in cases of pernicious anemia. SEE: illus.

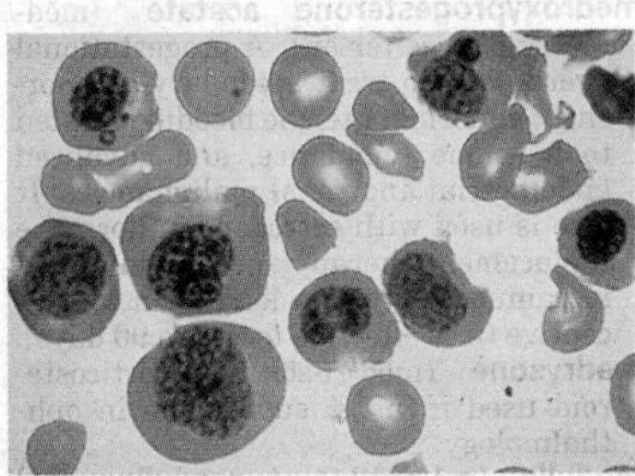

MEGALOBLASTS

megalocephalic (mĕg-ă-lō-sĕf-ăl′ĭk) [″ + *kephale,* head] Having an abnormally large head. SYN: *macrocephalia; megacephalic.*

megalocephaly (mĕg″ă-lō-sĕf′ă-lē) [″ + *kephale,* head] **1.** Abnormal size of the head. SYN: *macrocephalia.* **2.** A rare disease characterized by hyperostosis of bones of the skull. SYN: *leontiasis ossea.*

megalocheiria (mĕg″ă-lō-kī′rē-ă) [″ + *cheir,* hand] Abnormally large hands.

megalocornea (mĕg″ă-lō-kor′nē-ă) [″ + L. *cornu,* horn] Abnormally enlarged cornea due to a developmental anomaly. SYN: *macrocornea.*

megalocystis SEE: *megabladder.*

megalocyte (mĕg'ă-lō-sīt) [" + *kytos,* cell] A larger than average red blood corpuscle.

megalodactyly (mĕg"ă-lō-dăk'tĭ-lĕ) [" + *daktylos,* finger] Having very large fingers or toes.

megalodontia (mĕg"ă-lō-dŏn'shē-ă) [" + *odous,* tooth] Macrodontia.

megaloesophagus Megaesophagus.

megalomania (mĕg"ă-lō-mā'nē-ă) [" + *mania,* madness] A psychosis characterized by ideas of personal exaltation and delusions of grandeur.

megalonychosis (mĕg'ă-lō"nĭ-kō'sĭs) [" + *onyx,* nail] Hypertrophy of the nails.

megalophthalmus (mĕg"ă-lŏf-thăl'mŭs) [" + *ophthalmos,* eye] Abnormally large eyes.

megalopodia (mĕg"ă-lō-pō'dē-ă) [" + *pous,* foot] Abnormally large feet.

megaloscope (mĕg'ă-lō-skōp") [" + *skopein,* to examine] A large magnifying lens; a speculum fitted with a magnifying lens.

megalosyndactyly (mĕg'ă-lō-sĭn-dăk'tĭl-ē) [" + *syn,* with, + *daktylos,* finger] A condition in which the fingers or toes are of large size and webbed.

megaloureter (mĕg"ă-lō-ū-rē'tĕr, -ūr'ĕ-tĕr) [" + *oureter,* ureter] Increase in diameter of the ureter.

-megaly [Gr. *megas,* large] Combining form indicating an enlargement of a specified body part.

megaprosopia (mĕg"ă-prŏs'ō-pŭs) [" + *prosopon,* face] Possessing a large face.

megarectum (mĕg-ă-rĕk'tŭm) [" + L. *rectum,* straight] Excessive dilatation of the rectum.

megaseme (mĕg'ă-sēm) [" + *sema,* sign] Having an orbital aperture with an index exceeding 89, said of a skull.

megavitamin (mĕg"ă-vī'tă-mĭn) A dose of one or more vitamins that is much in excess of the normal daily requirements.

megavolt (mĕg'ă-vōlt) One million, 10^6, volts.

megestrol acetate (mĕ-jĕs'trōl) A synthetic progestin that is used in treating certain neoplasms (such as breast cancer) and wasting syndromes (e.g., in patients with AIDS). Trade name is Megace.

meglumine (mĕg'lū-mēn) A radiopaque compound used in x-ray studies.

m. antimonate A drug used in treating leishmaniasis.

megohm (mĕg'ōm) One million, 10^6, ohms.

megophthalmos Megalophthalmus.

meibomian cyst (mī-bō'mē-ăn) [Heinrich Meibom, Ger. anatomist, 1638–1700] Chalazion.

meibomian gland SEE: *tarsal glands.*

meibomitis (mī-bō"mī'tĭs) Inflammation of the meibomian glands.

Meige syndrome [Henri Meige, French physician, 1866-1940] A dystonic movement disorder that can involve dry eyes and excessive eye blinking, with involuntary movements of the jaw muscles, neck, lips, and tongue.

Meigs' syndrome [Joe V. Meigs, U.S. gynecologist, 1892–1963] Benign tumor of the ovary associated with ascites and pleural effusion.

meio- [Gr. *meioun,* diminution] SEE: *mio-.*

meiogenic (mī"ō-jĕn'ĭk) [Gr. *meiosis,* diminution, + *gennan,* to produce] Causing meiosis.

meiosis (mī-ō'sĭs) [Gr., diminution] A process of two successive cell divisions, producing cells, egg or sperm, that contain half the number of chromosomes in somatic cells. When fertilization occurs, the nuclei of the sperm and ovum fuse and produce a zygote with the full chromosome complement. SEE: illus.; *chromosome; mitosis; oogenesis* for illus.

Meissner's corpuscle (mīs'nĕrz) [Georg Meissner, Ger. histologist, 1829–1905] An encapsulated end-organ of touch found in dermal papillae close to the epidermis. Each is an ovoid body containing endings of myelinated and unmyelinated nerve fibers. They are most numerous in the hairless portions of the skin, esp. the volar surface of hands, fingers, feet, and toes; they are also present in the lips, eyelids, nipples, and the tip of the tongue.

Meissner's plexus An autonomic plexus in the submucosa of the alimentary tube that regulates secretions of the mucosa.

melagra (mĕl-ă'gră) [Gr. *melos,* limb, + *agra,* seizure] Pain of muscular origin in the limbs.

melalgia (mĕl-ăl'jē-ă) [" + *algos,* pain] Pain of neural origin in the limbs.

melancholia (mĕl-ăn-kō'lē-ă) [Gr. *melankholia,* sadness] A severe depression with a dull, uninterested affect and lack of interest in activities that would normally be pleasurable. There may be agitation or retardation. Weight loss, anorexia, insomnia, and worsening of the symptoms may occur in the early morning.

affective m. Melancholia observed in depressed phase of manic-depressive psychoses. SEE: *psychosis, manic-depressive.*

climacteric m. Depression occurring at the time of menopause.

panphobic m. Melancholia accompanied by extraordinary fearfulness.

suicidal m. Impulse to commit suicide combined with melancholia.

melanephidrosis, melanidrosis (mĕl"ăn-ĕf"ĭ-drō'sĭs, mĕl"ăn-ĭd-rō'sĭs) [" + *ephidrosis,* sweating] A form of chromidrosis in which the sweat is black.

melaniferous (mĕl"ăn-ĭf'ĕr-ŭs) [" + L. *ferre,* to carry] Containing melanin or some other black pigment.

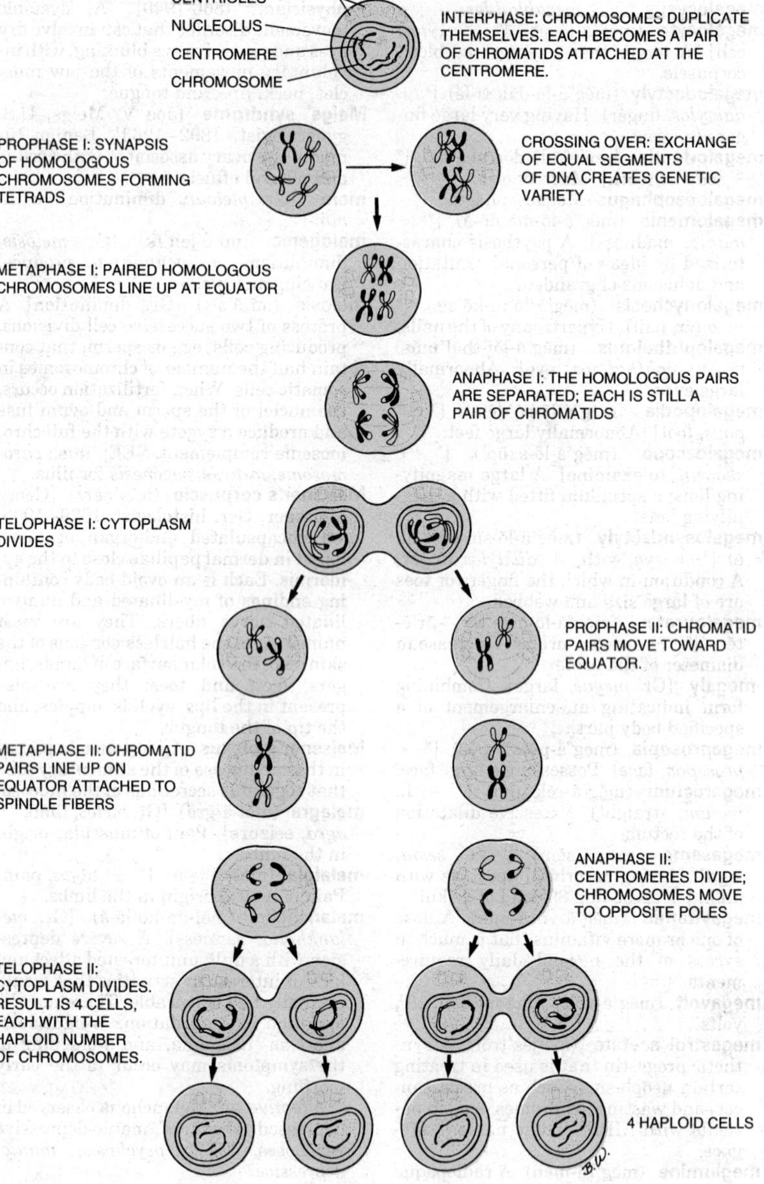
CENTRIOLES
NUCLEOLUS
CENTROMERE
CHROMOSOME
INTERPHASE: CHROMOSOMES DUPLICATE THEMSELVES. EACH BECOMES A PAIR OF CHROMATIDS ATTACHED AT THE CENTROMERE.
PROPHASE I: SYNAPSIS OF HOMOLOGOUS CHROMOSOMES FORMING TETRADS
CROSSING OVER: EXCHANGE OF EQUAL SEGMENTS OF DNA CREATES GENETIC VARIETY
METAPHASE I: PAIRED HOMOLOGOUS CHROMOSOMES LINE UP AT EQUATOR
ANAPHASE I: THE HOMOLOGOUS PAIRS ARE SEPARATED; EACH IS STILL A PAIR OF CHROMATIDS
TELOPHASE I: CYTOPLASM DIVIDES
PROPHASE II: CHROMATID PAIRS MOVE TOWARD EQUATOR.
METAPHASE II: CHROMATID PAIRS LINE UP ON EQUATOR ATTACHED TO SPINDLE FIBERS
ANAPHASE II: CENTROMERES DIVIDE; CHROMOSOMES MOVE TO OPPOSITE POLES
TELOPHASE II: CYTOPLASM DIVIDES. RESULT IS 4 CELLS, EACH WITH THE HAPLOID NUMBER OF CHROMOSOMES.
4 HAPLOID CELLS
B.W.

MEIOSIS

melanin (mĕl′ă-nĭn) [Gr. *melas,* black] The pigment produced by melanocytes that gives color to hair, skin, the substantia nigra of the brain, and the choroid of the eye. Exposure to sunlight stimulates melanin production; melanin protects skin cells from ultraviolet radiation. **melanoid** (mĕl′ă-noyd), *adj.*

melano- [Gr. *melas,* black] Prefix meaning *black, black color,* or *darkness.*

melanoameloblastoma (mĕl″ă-nō-ă-mĕl″ō-blăs-tō′mă) [″ + O.Fr. *amel,* enamel, + Gr. *blastos,* germ, + *oma,* tumor] Melanotic neuroectodermal tumor.

melanoblast (mĕl′ăn-ō-blăst″, mĕl-ăn′ō-blăst) [″ + *blastos,* germ] A cell originating from the neural crest that differentiates into a melanocyte.

melanoblastoma (mĕl″ă-nō-blăs-tō′mă) [″ + ″ + *oma,* tumor] A tumor containing melanin.

melanocyte (mĕl′ăn-ō-sīt, mĕl-ăn′ō-sīt) [″ + *kytos,* cell] A melanin-forming cell. Those of the skin are found in the lower epidermis.

melanocytoma (mĕl″ă-nō-sī-tō′mă) [″ + *kytos,* cell, + *oma,* tumor] A rare pigmented benign tumor of the optic disk.

melanoderma (mĕl″ăn-ō-dĕr′mă) A patchy or generalized skin discoloration caused by either an increase in the production of melanin by the normal number of melanocytes or an increase in the number of melanocytes. SYN: *melanopathy.*

melanodermatitis (mĕl″ă-nō-dĕr″mă-tī′tĭs) [″ + ″ + *itis,* inflammation] Dermatitis in which an excess of melanin is deposited in the involved area.

melanoepithelioma (mĕl″ăn-ō-ĕp″ĭ-thē-lē-ō′mă) [″ + *epi,* upon, + *thele,* nipple, + *oma,* tumor] A malignant epithelioma containing melanin.

melanogen (mĕ-lăn′ō-jĕn) [″ + *gennan,* to produce] A colorless substance that can be converted into melanin.

melanogenesis (mĕl″ăn-ō-jĕn′ĕ-sĭs) [″ + *genesis,* generation, birth] Formation of melanin.

melanoglossia (mĕl″ăn-ō-glŏs′ē-ă) [″ + *glossa,* tongue] Black tongue.

melanoleukoderma (mĕl″ăn-ō-lū″kō-dĕr′mă) [″ + *leukos,* white, + *derma,* skin] Mottled skin.

m. colli Mottled skin of the neck sometimes seen in syphilis. SYN: *collar of Venus; syphilitic leukoderma; venereal collar.*

melanoma (mĕl″ă-nō′mă) [″ + *oma,* tumor] A malignant tumor of melanocytes that often begins in a darkly pigmented mole and can metastasize widely. The incidence of melanoma is rising more rapidly than that of any other cancer. In the U.S. in 1997, approximately 40,000 new cases of melanoma were diagnosed; in the year 2000, the disease affects 1 in 75 Americans. In 1999 the American Cancer Society estimated there would be 44,200 new cases of the disease. More than 90% of melanomas develop on the skin; about 5% occur in the eye, and 2.5% occur on mucous membranes. SEE: illus.

The likelihood of long-term survival depends on the depth of the lesion at diagnosis (thicker lesions are more hazardous), the histological type (nodular and acral lentiginous melanomas are worse than superficial spreading or lentigo malignant melanomas), and the patient's age (older patients do more poorly) and gender (men tend to have a worse prognosis than women). SEE: *ABCD; skin cancer.*

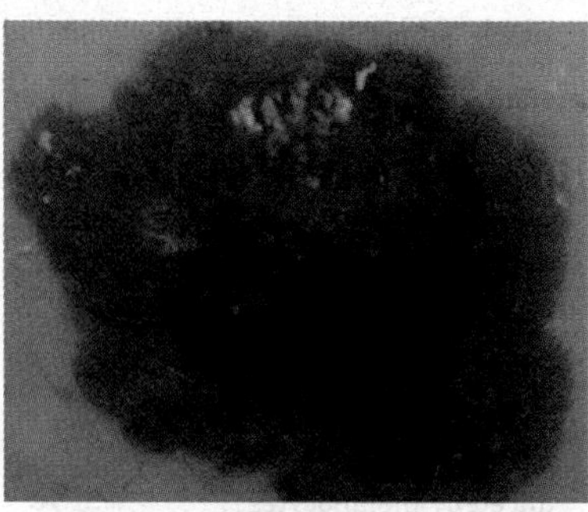

MELANOMA

ETIOLOGY: Excessive exposure to ultraviolet light, especially sunlight, causes melanoma. It is more common in whites than blacks, and it appears as a genetic illness in some families.

SYMPTOMS: Melanomas are marked by their asymmetry, irregular border, and varied color. The diameter usually is greater than 6 mm (about 1/4 in.). A change in the surface appearance or size of a mole often brings the lesion to medical attention.

PREVENTION: Suntanning should be discouraged. Persons spending considerable time outside should wear protective clothing to shield against ultraviolet radiation and use sunscreens on exposed skin.

TREATMENT: Melanomas are treated with surgery, to remove the primary cancer, along with adjuvant therapies to reduce the risk of metastasis. Interferon alpha and levamisole have been used as immunotherapeutics. Vaccines have been developed against melanoma; they appear to improve prognosis in affected patients.

melanomatosis (mĕl″ă-nō″mă-tō′sĭs) [″ + ″ + *osis,* condition] Formation of numerous melanomas on or beneath the skin.

melanonychia (mĕl″ă-nō-nĭk′ē-ă) [″ + *onyx,* nail] Black pigmentation of the nails.

melanopathy Melanoderma.

melanophage (mĕl′ă-nō-fāj″) [″ + *phagein,* to eat] A phagocytic cell that contains ingested melanin.

melanophore (mĕl′ăn-ō-for) [″ + *phoros,* bearing] Cell containing dark pigment.

melanoplakia (mĕl″ăn-ō-plā′kē-ă) [″ + *plax,* a flat plain] Condition marked by pigmented patches on the tongue and buccal mucosa.

melanosarcoma (mĕl″ă-nō-săr-kō′mă) [″ + *sarx,* flesh, + *oma,* tumor] Sarcoma containing melanin.

melanoscirrhus (mĕl″ă-nō-skĭr′ŭs) [Gr. *melas,* black, + *skirros,* hardness]

Black-pigmented cancer; an unusual form of melanoma.

melanosis (mĕl-ăn-ō'sĭs) [" + *osis,* condition] **1.** Unusual deposit of black pigment in different parts of body. **2.** Disorder of pigment metabolism.

m. coli A benign brown or black discoloration of the colon that results from the use of laxatives, such as senna derivatives.

m. lenticularis Xeroderma pigmentosum.

melanosome (mĕl'ă-nō-sōm") [" + *soma,* body] The pigment granule produced by melanocytes.

melanotic **1.** Black. **2.** Pert. to melanosis.

melanotic macule A small, brown to black lesion of the oral mucosa that is usually less than 1 cm in diameter, solitary, and asymptomatic. In most instances, this type of macule is benign and requires no therapy. It can, however, be due to melanoma, which will require vigorous therapy without delay. When it is benign, it may be due to Peutz-Jeghers syndrome, physiologic pigmentation, Addison's disease, or healing of traumatic lesions, or may be secondary to a variety of medications.

melanotrichia linguae (mĕl"ăn-ō-trĭk'ē-ă lĭng'gwē) [" + *thrix,* hair, + L. *linguae,* tongue] Black, hairy tongue.

melanotroph (mĕl'ă-nō-trōf") [" + *trophe,* nutrition] A cell of the pituitary that produces melanocyte-stimulating hormone.

melanuria (mĕl-ăn-ū'rē-ă) [" + *ouron,* urine] Dark pigment in urine.

melasma (mĕl-ăz'mă) [Gr., a black spot] Chloasma.

melatonin (mel"ă-tō'nĭn) A peptide hormone produced by the pineal gland that influences sleep-wake cycles and other circadian rhythms. It has a sedative effect and has been used to treat sleep disorders and jet lag, even though its impact on these conditions remains unclear.

melena (mĕl'ĕ-nă, mĕl-ē'nă) [Gr. *melaina,* black] Black tarry feces caused by the digestion of blood in the gastrointestinal tract. It is common in the newborn and in adult patients with gastrointestinal bleeding from the esophagus, stomach, or proximal small intestine. **melenic, melenotic** (mĕl-ĕ-nŏt'ĭk), *adj.*

m. neonatorum Melena in the newborn.

Meleney's ulcer An infection of an operative site that typically appears 1 to 2 weeks after surgery, and festers as a result of the combined action of multiple different microorganisms. It is characterized by areas of reddened and inflamed skin surrounding necrotic centers, with communicating tracts or tunnels that ulcerate through the outer layer of skin at neighboring locations.

melicera, meliceris (mĕl-ĭ-sēr'ă, -ĭs) [Gr. *meli,* honey, + *keros,* wax] **1.** Cyst containing matter of honey-like consistency. **2.** Viscid, syrupy.

melioidosis (mē"lē-oy-dō'sĭs) [Gr. *melis,* a distemper of asses, + *eidos,* form, shape, + *osis,* condition] An acute or chronic disease due to *Pseudomonas pseudomallei* (formerly called *Malleomyces pseudomallei).* Acute form causes pneumonia, multiple abscesses, septicemia, and occasionally death.

melissophobia (mĕ-lĭs"ō-fō'bē-ă) [Gr. *melissa,* bee, + *phobia,* fear] Abnormal fear of bees.

melitemia (mĕl-ĭ-tē'mē-ă) [+ *haima,* blood] Abnormal amount of sugar in the blood.

melitensis (mĕl-ĭ-tĕn'sĭs) Brucellosis.

melitis (mĕl-ī'tĭs) [Gr. *melon,* cheek, + *itis,* inflammation] Inflammation of the cheek.

melitoptyalism (mĕl"ĭ-tō-tī'ăl-ĭzm) [Gr. *meli,* honey, + *ptyalon,* saliva] Excretion of saliva containing glucose. SYN: *glycoptyalism.*

melituria (mĕl-ĭ-tū'rē-ă) [" + *ouron,* urine] Presence of sugar in the urine.

mellitum (mĕ-lī'tŭm) [L.] A pharmaceutical preparation with honey as the vehicle or excipient.

melo-, mel- [Gr. *melon,* cheek] Combining form meaning *cheek.*

melo-, mel- [Gr. *melos,* limb] Combining form meaning *extremity.*

melo-, mel- [Gr. *meli,* honey] Combining form meaning *honey.*

melomelus (mē-lŏm'ē-lŭs) [Gr. *melos,* limb, + *melos,* limb] A malformed fetus with a rudimentary limb attached to a normal limb.

meloncus (mĕl-ŏn'kŭs) [Gr. *melon,* cheek, + *onkos,* bulk] Tumor of the cheek.

melonoplasty (mĕl'ŏn-ō-plăs"tē) [" + *plassein,* to form] Plastic surgery of the cheek.

meloplasty (mĕl'ō-plăs-tē) [" + *plassein,* to form] Plastic surgery of the face.

melorheostosis (mĕl"ō-rē"ŏs-tō'sĭs) [Gr. *melos,* limb, + *rhein,* to flow, + *osteon,* bone, + *osis,* condition] A rare disease of long bones in which new bone formation resembles a candle with wax dripping down the sides.

meloschisis (mĕ-lŏs'kĭ-sĭs) [Gr. *melon,* cheek, + *schistos,* divided] A congenitally cleft cheek.

melotia (mĕ-lō'shē-ă) [" + *ous,* ear] Congenital displacement of the ear on the cheek.

melphalan (mĕl'fă-lăn) An antineoplastic drug of the nitrogen mustard class.

melting point Temperature at which conversion of a solid to a liquid begins.

member [L. *membrum*] **1.** An organ or part of the body, esp. a limb. **2.** In managed care, a person who contracts with a prepaid health care program to receive medical services.

membrane (mĕm′brān) [L. *membrana*] A thin, pliable layer of tissue that lines a tube or cavity, covers an organ or structure, or separates one part from another.

alveolocapillary m. The structures and substances through which gases must pass as they diffuse from air to blood (oxygen) or blood to air (carbon dioxide), including the alveolar fluid and surfactant, cell of the alveolar wall, interstitial space (tissue fluid), and cell of the capillary wall. SEE: illus.

alveolodental m. SEE: *periodontium.*

arachnoid m. The thin, delicate, intermediate membrane of the meninges that encloses the brain and spinal cord. It is separated from the pia mater, the inner membrane, by the subarachnoid space and from the dura mater, the outer membrane, by the subdural space. SEE: *arachnoid.*

atlanto-occipital m. A single midline ligamentous structure that extends from the arch of the atlas to the borders of the foramen magnum.

basement m. A delicate, noncellular membrane underlying a layer of epithelial cells and providing their support and attachment. SYN: *basement lamina.*

basilar m. The membrane extending from the tympanic lip of the osseous spiral lamina to the crest of the spiral ligament in the cochlea of the ear. It separates the tympanic canal from the cochlear duct and supports the organ of Corti. SEE: illus. under *organ of Corti.*

Bowman's m. SEE: *Bowman's membrane.*

Bruch's m. SEE: *Bruch's membrane.*

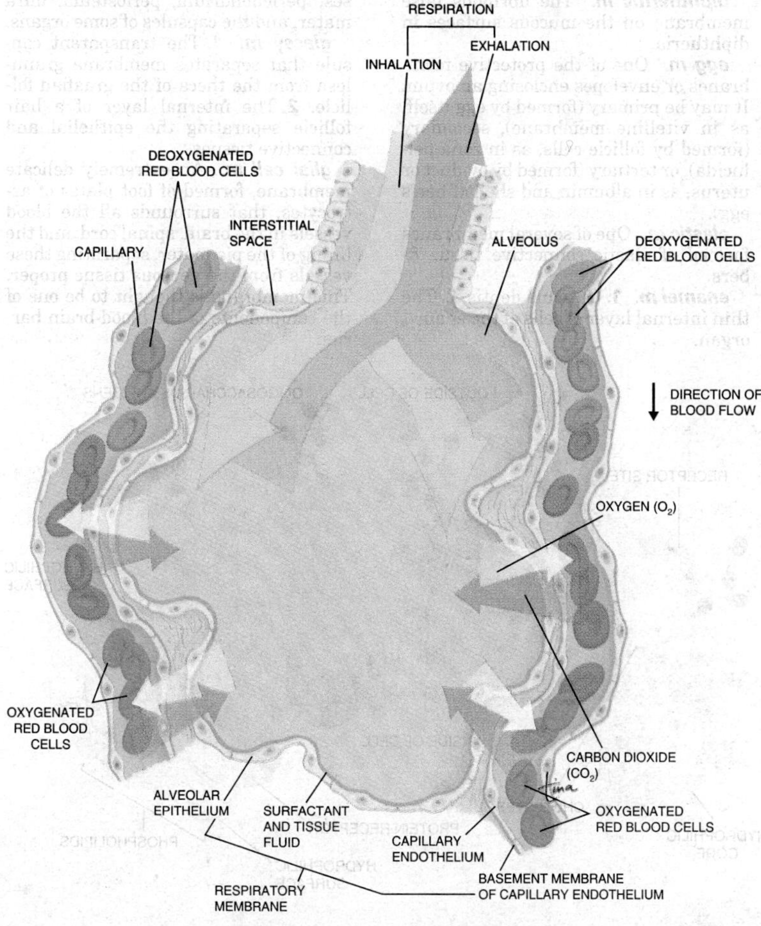

ALVEOLOCAPILLARY MEMBRANE

buccopharyngeal m. In the embryo, the membrane that separates the oral cavity from the foregut until the fourth week of development. SYN: *oral m.; pharyngeal m.*

cell m. The membrane that forms the outer boundary of a cell; it is made of phospholipids, protein, and cholesterol, with carbohydrates on the outer surface. SYN: *plasma m.* SEE: illus.

choroid m. SEE: *choroid.*

costocoracoid m. The dense fascia between the pectoralis minor and subclavius muscles.

cricothyroid m. The membrane connecting the thyroid and cricoid cartilages of the larynx.

croupous m. False m.

decidual m. One of the membranes formed in the endometrium of a pregnant uterus. SEE: *decidua.*

Descemet's m. SEE: *Descemet's membrane.*

diphtheritic m. The fibrinous false membrane on the mucous surfaces in diphtheria.

egg m. One of the protective membranes or envelopes enclosing an ovum. It may be primary (formed by egg itself, as in vitelline membrane), secondary (formed by follicle cells, as in zona pellucida), or tertiary (formed by oviduct or uterus, as in albumin and shell of hen's egg).

elastic m. One of several membranes formed of elastic connective tissue fibers.

enamel m. **1.** Cuticula dentis. **2.** The thin internal layer of cells of the enamel organ.

external limiting m. **1.** The outer layer of cells of the embryonic neural tube. **2.** The membrane in the retina of the eye separating the rods and cones from their cell bodies.

false m. Fibrinous exudate on a mucous surface of a membrane, as in croup or diphtheria.

fenestrated m. A layer of elastic connective tissue possessing minute round or oval openings. Found in the tunica intima and tunica media of medium-sized and large arteries. SYN: *Henle's elastic m.*

fetal m. One of the membranous structures that protect and support the embryo and provide its nutrition, respiration, and excretion. The structures are yolk sac, allantois, amnion, chorion, decidua, and placenta.

fibrous m. A membrane composed entirely of fibrous connective tissue. Examples include the fasciae, aponeuroses, perichondrium, periosteum, dura mater, and the capsules of some organs.

glassy m. **1.** The transparent capsule that separates membrana granulosa from the theca of the graafian follicle. **2.** The internal layer of a hair follicle separating the epithelial and connective tissues.

glial cell m. An extremely delicate membrane, formed of foot plates of astrocytes, that surrounds all the blood vessels in the brain, spinal cord, and the lining of the pia mater, separating these vessels from the nervous tissue proper. This membrane is thought to be one of the components of the blood-brain barrier.

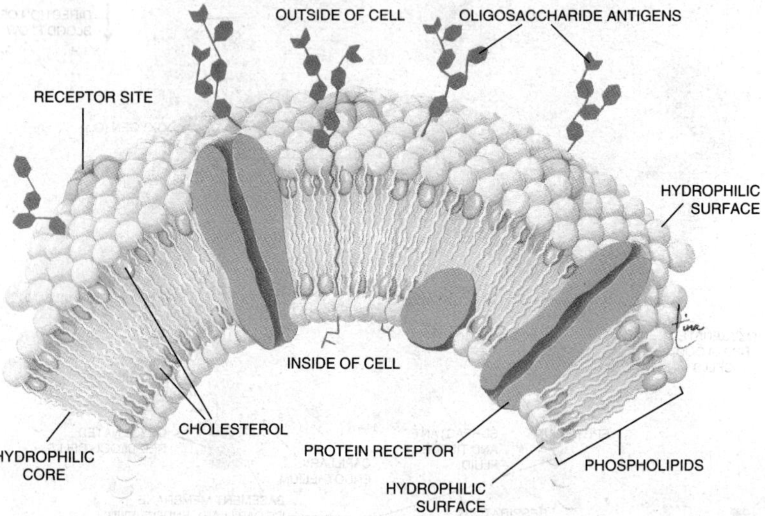

CELL MEMBRANE

Henle's elastic m. Fenestrated m.

homogeneous m. A fine membrane covering villi of the placenta.

Huxley's m. Huxley's layer.

hyaline m. **1.** Basement lamina. **2.** The membrane between the outer root sheath of a hair follicle and the inner fibrous layer.

hyaloid m. The membrane that envelops the vitreous humor.

hyoglossal m. A transverse fibrous membrane uniting tongue to hyoid bone.

interosseous m. **1.** A fibrous membrane in the arm connecting ulna to radius. **2.** A fibrous membrane in the leg connecting tibia to fibula.

internal limiting m. **1.** The inner layer of ependymal cells lining the embryonic neural tube. **2.** The glial membrane forming the innermost layer of the retina and the iris.

ion-selective m. The ion-selective component in an ion-selective electrode. It uses a modified and highly selective ion-exchange mechanism.

Krause's m. SEE: *Krause's membrane.*

laryngeal mucous m. The mucous membrane, glands, and cilia that characterize the lining of the larynx.

lingual mucous m. The mucosa covering the tongue.

masticatory mucous m. The mucosa of the mouth involved in the masticatory process. It is characterized by a keratinized surface epithelium, and includes the hard palate, gingiva, and dorsum of the tongue.

medullary m. Endosteum.

mucous m. SEE: *mucous membrane.*

nasal mucous m. The mucosa lining the nasal cavity and characterized by pseudostratified ciliated columnar epithelium with goblet cells.

Nasmyth's m. SEE: *Nasmyth's membrane.*

nictitating m. A third eyelid present in lower vertebrates and represented in humans by a fold of the conjunctiva, the plica semilunaris.

nuclear m. Either of two layered membranes surrounding the nucleus of a cell. Prior to the advent of electron microscopy, the nucleus was thought to be surrounded by a single thin membrane. SEE: *nuclear envelope.*

obturator m. A fibrous membrane closing the obturator foramen.

olfactory m. The membrane in the upper part of the nasal cavity that contains olfactory receptors.

oral m. Buccopharyngeal m.

oronasal m. A double epithelial layer separating the nasal pits from the embryonic oral cavity.

otolithic m. A layer of gelatinous substance containing otoconia or otoliths, found on the surface of maculae in the inner ear.

palatal mucous m. The lining of the mouth on the hard and soft palates. The hard palate has heavily keratinized epithelium and copious mucous glands or fat in the submucosa. The mobile soft palate contains muscle in addition to mucous glands, and is much less keratinized on the surface.

peridental m. An old term used to describe the periodontal ligament.

periodontal m. Periodontium.

permeable m. A membrane that permits passage of water and certain substances in solution. SEE: *osmosis; selectively permeable m.; semipermeable m.*

pharyngeal m. Buccopharyngeal m.

pharyngeal mucous m. The lining of the pharynx. The mucosa of the nasopharynx is pseudostratified ciliated epithelium; the mucosa of the oropharynx and laryngopharynx is stratified squamous epithelium.

placental m. The membrane of the placenta that separates the maternal blood from fetal blood.

plasma m. Cell m.

pseudoserous m. A membrane resembling a serous membrane but differing in structure as the endothelium.

pupillary m. The transparent membrane closing the fetal pupil. If it persists after birth, it is known as persistent pupillary membrane.

pyogenic m. The granular lining of an abscess or fistula.

pyophylactic m. The lining membrane of an abscess cavity separating it from healthy tissue.

quadrangular m. The upper portion of the elastic membrane of the larynx extending from the aryepiglottic folds to the level of the ventricular folds below.

Reissner's m. SEE: *Reissner's membrane.*

respiratory m. Alveolocapillary m.

Ruysch's m. SEE: *lamina choriocapillaris.*

Scarpa's m. SEE: *Scarpa's membrane.*

schneiderian m. SEE: *schneiderian membrane.*

Schwann's m. SEE: *Schwann cell.*

selectively permeable m. A membrane that allows one substance, such as water, to pass through more readily than another, such as salt or sugar.

semipermeable m. A membrane that allows passage of water but not substances in solution. SEE: *osmosis.*

serous m. A membrane consisting of mesothelium lying on a thin layer of connective tissue that lines the closed cavities (peritoneal, pleural, and pericardial) of the body and is reflected over the organs in the cavity. Serous fluid, similar to lymph, decreases friction between the two layers.

Shrapnell's m. SEE: *Shrapnell's membrane.*

submucous m. Submucosa.

synovial m. The membrane lining the capsule of a joint and secreting synovial fluid. SYN: *synovium.*

tectorial m. The thin, jelly-like membrane projecting from the vestibular lip of the osseous spiral lamina and overlying the spiral organ of Corti of the ear.

thyrohyoid m. The membrane joining the hyoid bone and the thyroid cartilage.

tympanic m. The membrane at the inner end of the external auditory canal, forming the lateral boundary of the middle ear cavity. SYN: *eardrum.* SEE: *ear thermometry; tympanum.*

unit m. The three-layered structure of cell membranes and intracellular membranes.

vestibular m. The membrane in the cochlea of the inner ear that separates the cochlear duct from the vestibular canal.

vestibular mucous m. The mucosa of the oral vestibule with its nonkeratinized stratified squamous epithelium, elastic lamina propria, and seromucous labial glands.

virginal m. An outdated term for the hymen.

vitelline m. The membrane that forms the surface layer of an ovum. SYN: *yolk m.; zona pellucida.*

vitreous m. **1.** The inner membrane of the choroid. **2.** The innermost layer of the connective tissue sheath surrounding a hair follicle. SYN: *Descemet's m.*

yolk m. Vitelline m.

membranectomy (mĕm″brăn-nĕk′tō-mē) [L. *membrana,* membrane, + Gr. *ektome,* excision] Surgical removal of a membrane.

membranelle (mĕm″bră-nĕl′) A thin membrane composed of fused cilia and present in the buccal area of some ciliated protozoa.

membrane potential SEE: under *potential.*

membraniform (mĕm-brā′nĭ-form) Membranoid.

membranocartilaginous (mĕm″brăn-ō-kăr-tĭ-lăj′ĭ-nŭs) **1.** Pert. to both membrane and cartilage. **2.** Derived from both membrane and cartilage.

membranoid (mĕm′bră-noyd) [L. *membrana,* membrane, + Gr. *eidos,* form, shape] Resembling a membrane. SYN: *membraniform; membranous.*

membranous Membranoid.

memory [L. *memoria*] **1.** The mental registration, retention, and recollection of past experiences, sensations, or thoughts. This group of functions relies on the coordinated activities of the association regions of the cerebral cortex, specific sensory areas of the brain, subcortical centers, the hypothalamus, the midbrain, and a wide array of neurochemicals and neurotransmitters. Injury or damage to any of these regions of the brain (e.g., as a result of intoxication, stroke, atrophy, or infection) impairs the ability to incorporate new memories or recall and use prior ones. **2.** The capacity of the immune system to respond to antigens to which it has previously been exposed. Immunological memory depends on the activities of T and B lymphocytes, macrophages, major histocompatibility molecules, adhesion molecules, chemokines, and many other biochemicals.

anterograde m. Ability to remember events occurring in the remote past but not those occurring recently. SYN: *anterograde amnesia.*

declarative m. The conscious recollection of learned information—a memory function that is improved by the association of learning with highly charged emotional experiences.

false m. An inaccurate or incomplete remembrance of a past event. Memory accuracy, validity, and reliability are affected by the following factors: age; serious illness, injury, or psychological trauma; prolonged medication therapy or use of a substance of abuse; mental retardation; mental illness; anxiety; preoccupation; fatigue; guilt and fear of penalty; coercion; or the incentive to testify falsely. These factors must be considered when evaluating the reliability of patient-reported memories.

immediate m. Memory for events or information in the immediate past. Brain damage that limits one's ability to store new information may impair immediate memory but have no effect on memories of the distant past. SYN: *short-term m.* SEE: *digit span test.*

impaired m. The state in which an individual experiences the inability to remember or recall bits of information or behavioral skills. Impaired memory may be attributed to pathophysiological or situational causes that are either temporary or permanent. SEE: *Nursing Diagnoses Appendix.*

implicit m. Recall that is preserved when the patient is given a cue to help retrieve information but deficient without such cues. This type of memory deficit is found in patients whose ability to learn and store new information is intact, but whose ability to retrieve stored memories is impaired.

incidental m. The mental storage of information that occurs passively, that is, without conscious effort.

long-term m. Recall of experiences, or of information gained, in the distant past.

procedural m. The memory capability that permits an individual to perform activities. This type of memory is usually preserved when other memory functions are lost. SEE: *declarative m.*

recovered m. A memory recalled after having been forgotten. Recall may be the result of psychotherapy or suggestion. Not all instances of recovered memory are accurate (some are the result of suggestion). SEE: *false m.*

remote m. Recollection of information that was stored in the distant past.

retrograde m. Ability to recall events of recent occurrence but lacking ability to recall knowledge with which the patient had previously been familiar. SYN: *retrograde amnesia.*

selective m. Limited recall; the recollection only of particular aspects of an event or experience.

short-term m. Immediate m.

MEN *multiple endocrine neoplasia.*

menacme (măn-ăk′mē) [Gr. *men,* month, + *akme,* top] **1.** The time between menarche and menopause. **2.** The height of the menstrual activity of a woman.

menadiol sodium diphosphate A synthetic water-soluble vitamin with the same activity as natural vitamin K. It is used as an antihemorrhagic agent in hypoprothrombinemia or hemorrhagic disorders due to hypoprothrombinemia.

menadione (mĕn″ă-dī′ōn) A synthetic drug that acts like vitamin K. It is used parenterally in oil or orally in tablet form.

CAUTION: Menadione powder is irritating to the respiratory tract and skin. In alcoholic solution, it is a vesicant.

m. sodium bisulfite Synthetic vitamin K.

menarche (mĕn-ăr′kē) [Gr. *men,* month, + *arche,* beginning] The initial menstrual period, normally occurring between the 9th and 17th year. SEE: *adrenarche; puberty.* **menarchal, menarcheal, menarchial,** *adj.*

mendelevium (mĕn-dĕ-lē′vē-ūm) SYMB: Md. A transuranium element; atomic weight 256, atomic number 101.

mendelism (mĕn′dĕl-ĭzm) The principles of heredity expressed in Mendel's laws.

Mendel's laws [Gregor Johann Mendel, Austrian monk, 1822–1884] The laws governing the genetic transmission of dominant and recessive traits. By carefully studying the heredity characteristics of garden peas, Mendel was able to explain the transmission of certain traits from one generation to the next.

Many inherited characteristics are controlled by the interaction of two genes, one from each parent. During meiosis, parent cells divide and contribute half their chromosome complement to the egg or sperm. After fertilization, the zygote contains a pair of each chromosome; each pair has genes for the same traits at corresponding locations. Alternate forms of the gene for a specific trait are called *alleles,* which may be dominant or recessive. SEE: *allele; chromosome; gamete; gene; meiosis.*

Mendel's law of segregation states that as the gametes are formed, the gene pairs separate and do not influence each other.

Mendel's law of dominance resulted from his observation that crossing a tall strain of peas with a short strain resulted in the expression of the dominant trait, in this case tallness. Thus, some alleles will dominate others in physical expression.

Mendel's law of independent assortment states that traits controlled by different gene pairs (such as height and color) pass to the offspring independently of each other.

Mendel's reflex [Kurt Mendel, Ger. neurologist, 1874–1946] Dorsal flexion of second to fifth toes upon percussion of the dorsum of the foot.

Ménétrier's disease (mān″ā-trē-ārz′) [Pierre Ménétrier, Fr. physician, 1859–1935] Giant hypertrophic gastritis.

menhidrosis, menidrosis (mĕn-hī-drō′sĭs, mĕn″ĭ-drō′sĭs) [Gr. *men,* month, + *hidros,* sweat] Vicarious menstruation through the sweat glands.

Ménière's disease (mān″ē-ārz′) [Prosper Ménière, Fr. physician, 1799–1862] A recurrent and usually progressive group of symptoms including progressive deafness, ringing in the ears, dizziness, and a sensation of fullness or pressure in the ears. Attacks occur suddenly and may last for as long as 24 hr. When one ear is affected, the other ear will become involved in approx. 50% of the cases.

ETIOLOGY: The etiology is unknown, but edema of the membranous labyrinth has been found in autopsy studies.

TREATMENT: In acute attacks, bedrest is the most effective treatment. Also effective are antihistamines, sedatives, discontinuation of smoking, and, rarely, surgical treatment. A low-salt diet (less than 2 g/day) and diuretics may be of benefit.

mening- SEE: *meningo-.*

meningeocortical (mĕ-nĭn″jē-ō-kor′tĭ-kăl) [Gr. *meninx,* membrane, + L. *corticalis,* pert. to cortex] Concerning the meninges and cortex of the brain.

meningeorrhaphy (mĕ-nĭn″jē-or′ă-fē) [″ + *rhaphe,* seam, ridge] Suture of membranes, esp. those of the brain and spinal cord.

meninges (mĕn-ĭn′jēz) *sing.,* **meninx** [Gr.] **1.** Membranes. **2.** The three membranes covering the spinal cord and brain: dura mater (external), arachnoid (middle), and pia mater (internal). SEE: illus. **meningeal** (mĕn-ĭn′jē-ăl), *adj.*

meningioma (mĕn-ĭn″jē-ō′mă) [Gr. *me-*

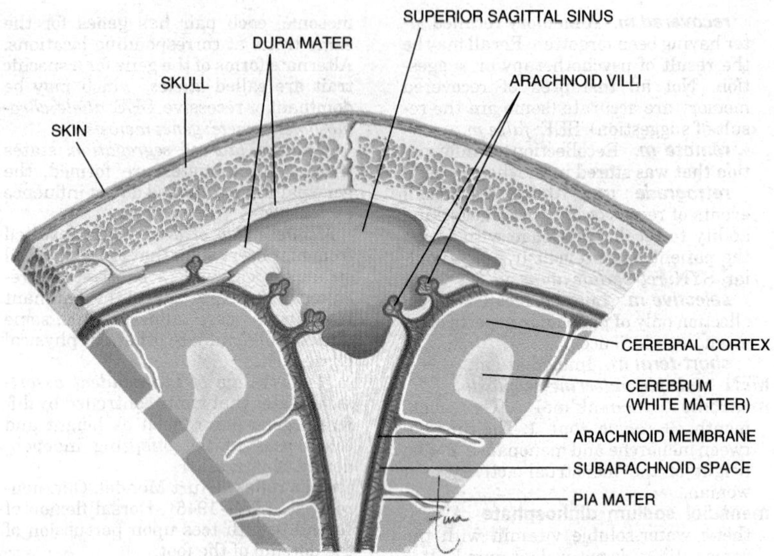

MENINGES

Frontal section of top of skull

ninx, membrane, + *oma,* tumor] A slow-growing tumor that originates in the meninges.

meningiomatosis (mĕ-nĭn″jē-ō-mă-tō′sĭs) [″ + ″ + *osis,* condition] Multiple meningiomas.

meningism (mĕn-ĭn′jĭzm) [″ + *-ismos,* condition] Irritation of the brain and spinal cord with symptoms simulating meningitis, but without actual inflammation.

meningismus Meningism.

meningitis (mĕn-ĭn-jī′tĭs) *pl.* **meningitides** [Gr. *meninx,* membrane, + *itis,* inflammation] Inflammation of the membranes of the spinal cord or brain, usually but not always caused by an infectious illness. Infectious meningitis is a medical emergency that must be treated and diagnosed quickly to obtain the best outcome. It is fatal in 10% to 40% of cases, even with optimal therapy, and may result in persistent neurological injury in about 10% of patients who survive the initial infection. In the U.S., infectious meningitis formerly affected infants and children more than adults; the demographics of the disease changed in the 1990s, after vaccines against *Haemophilus influenzae* were introduced into pediatric care. Infectious meningitis now is largely a disease of adults and usually is caused by *Streptococcus pneumoniae* or *Neisseria meningitidis,* although many other microbes may be responsible. SEE: illus.; *Standard and Universal Precautions Appendix.* **meningitic** (mĕn-ĭn-jĭt′ĭk), *adj.*

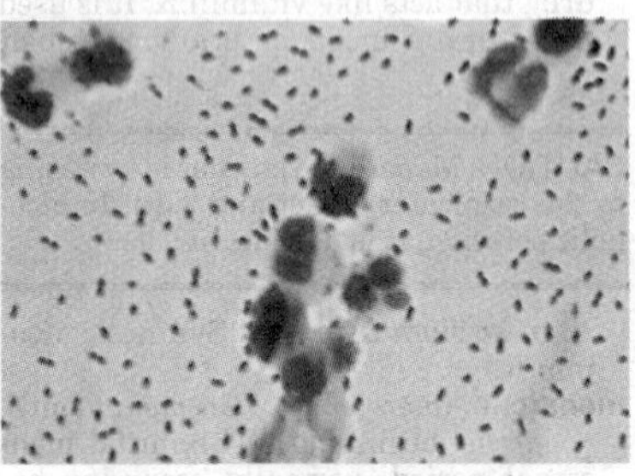

MENINGITIS

Streptococcus pneumoniae in cerebrospinal fluid (orig. mag. ×400)

ETIOLOGY: Meningitis may result from infection with bacteria, viruses, mycobacteria, fungi, and amebas or from noninfectious causes, such as chemical irritation to the meninges. Occasionally, infectious meningitis follows head trauma or sinus or ear infection. It also may result from the spread of blood-borne infection to the meninges.

SYMPTOMS: The hallmarks of meningitis include fever, headache, stiff neck, altered mental status, and photophobia. Many patients with meningitis present with only two or three of these clinical indicators. Acute bacterial meningitis and meningitis caused by some fungi and amebas also may cause rapid deterioration in mental status, seizures, shock, and death.

DIAGNOSIS: Cerebrospinal fluid must be examined. A cell count to assess the level of inflammation, a Gram stain to look for infectious organisms, and levels of bacterial antigens, glucose, and protein typically are obtained.

PREVENTION: All children in the U.S. now are given vaccinations against *H. influenzae* type b (Hib) as primary prevention against the disease. Meningococcal polysaccharide vaccines are highly effective in preventing the disease during epidemic outbreaks with this organism. Close family contacts of patients with meningitis caused by *N. meningitidis* are treated with rifampin or other prophylactic drugs.

TREATMENT: Definitive treatment depends on identification of the underlying causes, but empirical therapies for infectious meningitis must be given immediately, hours before the diagnosis is confirmed. The evolution of penicillin-resistant strains of pneumococci has altered traditional empirical treatments. Third-generation cephalosporins, ampicillin and gentamicin, chloramphenicol, or vancomycin plus rifampin have been given, depending on the patient's age, level of immune function, or clinical presentation. Intravenous corticosteroids are used in children to prevent hearing loss as a result of the disease.

PATIENT CARE: Supportive measures for shock and other complications, such as disseminated intravascular coagulation, metabolic acidosis, or seizures, should be initiated when indicated. The patient with infectious meningitis may need monitoring in an intensive care unit.

acute aseptic m. A nonpurulent form of meningitis often due to viral infection. It usually runs a short, benign course (marked by fever and headache) ending with recovery.

aseptic m. Inflammation of the meninges without obvious evidence of bacterial infection. It typically results from a viral infection (e.g., coxsackievirus or other enteroviruses).

SYMPTOMS: Patients report fever, headache, stiff neck, malaise, and sometimes altered mental status or photophobia.

PATIENT CARE: Antipyretics and tepid sponge baths are administered as ordered. Contaminated articles are disposed of in a double bag. Neurological status is monitored for changes in level of consciousness and for increases in intracranial pressure. Personal hygiene is provided, and measures to prevent complications due to immobility are implemented. Gentle position changes are performed to reduce excessive stimulation. Artificial airway, suction, and oxygen are readily available. A quiet, dark atmosphere is provided, and siderails are padded to reduce the risk of injury. Prescribed analgesics are administered, and cool compresses are applied to the forehead to relieve headache. Intravenous fluids or tube feedings are administered as ordered, and intake and ouput are monitored. Assessments are made for complications such as shock, respiratory distress, and disseminated intravascular coagulation.

basal m. Inflammation of the meninges at the base of the brain, usually due to tuberculosis.

carcinomatous m. Infiltration of the meninges by metastatic tumor cells. It may produce symptoms such as headache, backache, confusion, nerve palsies, or seizures and should be suspected when these symptoms arise in patients with known cancers. The diagnosis is confirmed by lumbar puncture with analysis of the cerebrospinal fluid for tumor cells.

cerebral m. Acute or chronic inflammation of the meninges of the brain.

cerebrospinal m. Inflammation of the meninges of the brain and spinal cord.

chronic m. Inflammation of the meninges, marked by persistent fever, headache, and stiff neck (associated, on lumbar puncture, with cerebrospinal fluid pleocytosis and elevated spinal fluid pressure). The underlying cause of this cluster of findings may be initially difficult to determine. Syphilis, cryptococcosis, human immunodeficiency virus infection, or invasion of the meninges by cancer cells may be responsible. Occasionally, repeated lumbar punctures reveal a vasculitis of the central nervous system or a partially treated bacterial meningitis.

cryptococcal m. Fungal meningitis due to *Cryptococcus neoformans*. A rare cause of disease in healthy hosts, cryptococcal meningitis is an opportunistic infection usually seen in patients with advanced AIDS or patients taking high-dose steroids. It usually presents with gradually progressive headache and fever. The serum cryptococcal antigen test is a useful screening test. The diagnosis is established by the results of analysis and culture of cerebral spinal fluid.

TREATMENT: Treatment options include amphotericin B, often with flucytosine. Fluconazole and/or related antifungals are sometimes used for maintenance therapy.

meningococcal m. Meningitis caused by various serogroups of *Neisseria meningitidis,* a gram-negative diplococcus. SEE: *Nursing Diagnoses Appendix.*

Mollaret's m. SEE: *Mollaret's meningitis.*

pneumococcal m. Meningitis due to

Streptococcus pneumoniae, a deadly disease predominantly found in adults. In the U.S., about 20% of affected patients die. Because of the worldwide emergence of streptococcal resistance to penicillins, chloramphenicol, and cephalosporins, vancomycin, rifampin, and other antibacterial agents are used to treat this infection.

m. serosa circumscripta Meningitis accompanied by the formation of cystic accumulations of fluid that simulate tumors.

serous m. Meningitis with serous exudation into the cerebral ventricles.

spinal m. Inflammation of the spinal cord membranes.

traumatic m. Meningitis resulting from trauma to the meninges.

tuberculous m. Meningitis resulting from the spread of *Mycobacterium tuberculosis* to the central nervous system, usually from a primary focus of infection in the lungs.

viral m. Inflammation of the meninges as a result of infection with adenovirus, coxsackievirus, echovirus, human immunodeficiency virus, mumps virus, lymphocytic choriomeningitis virus, polio viruses, and others. Patients report fever, headache, and stiff neck, and the lumbar puncture reveals an excessive number of lymphocytes, typically without a decrease in cerebrospinal fluid glucose levels. Viral meningitis is a subset of "aseptic" (nonbacterial) meningitis.

meningitophobia (mĕn″ĭn-jĭt″ō-fō′bē-ă) [Gr. *meninx,* membrane, + *phobos,* fear] A condition simulating meningitis, caused by the fear of contracting meningitis.

meningo-, mening- (mĕn-ĭn′gō) [Gr. *meninx,* membrane] Combining form denoting relationship to the meninges (membranes covering the spinal cord or brain).

meningoarteritis (mĕn-ĭn″gō-ăr″tĕr-īt′ĭs) [″ + *arteria,* artery, + *itis,* inflammation] Inflammation of the meningeal arteries.

meningocele (mĕn-ĭn′gō-sēl) [″ + *kele,* tumor, swelling] Congenital hernia in which the meninges protrude through a defect in the skull or spinal column.

meningococcal (mĕn-ĭn-jō-kŏk′ŭl) Pert. to meningococcus.

meningococcemia (mĕn-ĭn″gō-kŏk-sē′mē-ă) [″ + *kokkos,* berry, + *haima,* blood] Meningococci in the blood, a serious illness that may cause a disseminated rash, altered mental status, shock, and death.

meningococcidal (mĕ-nĭng″gō-kŏk-sī′dăl) [″ + ″ + L. *caedere,* to kill] Lethal to meningococci.

meningococcus (mĕn-ĭn″gō-kŏk′ŭs) *pl.* **meningococci** A microorganism of the species *Neisseria meningitidis,* one of the causative agents of meningitis.

meningocortical (mĕn-ĭn″gō-kor′tĭ-kăl) Pert. to the meninges and the cortex of the brain.

meningocyte (mĕ-nĭng′gō-sīt) [″ + *kytos,* cell] A macrophage of the meninges of the brain.

meningoencephalitis (mĕn-ĭn″gō-ĕn-sĕf″ă-lī′tĭs) [″ + *enkephalos,* brain, + *itis,* inflammation] Inflammation of the brain and its meninges. SEE: *encephalitis; meningitis.*

primary amebic m. Inflammation of brain and meninges caused by free-living amebae ordinarily found in water, soil, and decaying vegetation. Organisms that can cause primary amebic meningoencephalitis include *Naegleria fowleri, Acanthamoeba culbertsoni,* and other species of *Acanthamoeba.* The amebae are acquired by swimming in freshwater lakes and sniffing water into the nasal cavities.

SYMPTOMS: Similar to those of acute meningococcal meningitis.

TREATMENT: For *Naegleria* infections, amphotericin B, miconazole, and rifampin are effective if given early in the disease, but diagnosis of this rare disease is often delayed and few patients survive. *Acanthamoeba* species are sensitive to pentamidine, propamidine, ketoconazole, miconazole, neomycin, and flucytosine.

meningoencephalocele (mĕn-ĭn″gō-ĕn-sĕf′ăl-ō-sēl) [″ + ″ + *kele,* tumor, swelling] Hernial protrusion of brain and meninges through a defect in the skull.

meningoencephalomyelitis (mĕn-ĭn″gō-ĕn-sĕf″ăl-ō-mī-ĕl-ī′tĭs) [″ + ″ + *myelos,* marrow, + *itis,* inflammation] Inflammation of the brain and spinal cord, and their meninges.

meningoencephalopathy (mĕ-nĭng″gō-ĕn-sĕf″ă-lŏp′ă-thē) [″ + ″ + *pathos,* disease] Disease of the meninges and brain.

meningomalacia (mĕn-ĭn″gō-mă-lā′shē-ă) [″ + *malakia,* softening] Softening of any membrane.

meningomyelitis (mĕn-ĭn″gō-mī″ĕl-ī′tĭs) [″ + *myelos,* marrow, + *itis,* inflammation] Inflammation of spinal cord and its enveloping membranes.

meningomyelocele (mĕ-nĭng″gō-mī′ĕ-lō-sēl″) [″ + ″ + *kele,* tumor, swelling] Hernia of the spinal cord and membranes through a defect in the vertebral column.

meningomyeloradiculitis (mĕ-nĭng″gō-mī″ĕ-lō-ră-dĭk″ū-lī′tĭs) [″ + ″ + L. *radicula,* radicle, + Gr. *itis,* inflammation] Inflammation of the meninges and the roots of spinal or cranial nerves.

meningo-osteophlebitis (mĕ-nĭng″gō-ŏs″tē-ō-flĕ-bī′tĭs) [″ + *osteon,* bone, + *phleps,* vein, + *itis,* inflammation] Parosteitis and inflammation of the veins of the bone.

meningopathy (mĕn-ĭn-gŏp′ă-thē) [″ + *pathos,* disease, suffering] Any pathological condition of the meninges.

meningoradicular (mĕ-nĭng″gō-ră-dĭk′ū-lăr) [″ + L. *radicula,* radicle] Concerning the meninges and spinal and cerebral nerve roots.

meningoradiculitis (mĕ-nĭng″gō-ră-dĭk″ū-lī′tĭs) [″ + ″ + Gr. *itis,* inflammation] Inflammation of the meninges and roots of the spinal nerves.

meningorhachidian (mĕn-ĭn″gō-ră-kĭd′ē-ăn) [″ + *rhachis,* spine] Concerning the spinal cord and meninges.

meningorrhagia (mĕn-ĭn″gō-rā′jē-ă) [″ + *rhegnynai,* to burst forth] Hemorrhage of the cerebral or spinal membrane.

meningorrhea (mĕn-ĭn″gō-rē′ă) [″ + *rhoia,* flow] Effusion of blood on or between the meninges.

meningotyphoid (mĕn-ĭn″gō-tī′foyd) Typhoid fever with symptoms of meningitis.

meningovascular (mĕn-ĭn″gō-văs′kū-lăr) Pert. to blood vessels of the meninges.

meninx (mē′nĭnks) *pl.* **meninges** [Gr., membrane] **1.** Membrane. **2.** Any of the three membranes investing the spinal cord and brain: dura mater (external), arachnoid (middle), and pia mater (internal).

meniscectomy (mĕn″ĭ-sĕk′tō-mē) [″ + *ektome,* excision] Removal of meniscus cartilage of the knee. SEE: *Nursing Diagnoses Appendix.*

PATIENT CARE: The patient's dressing, peripheral pulses, and sensory and motor status of the affected area are evaluated every 2 hr after surgery. Knee immobility is maintained for a specified period. Use of crutches with partial weight bearing may often begin in 1 to 2 days. The affected leg is kept elevated to prevent or reduce swelling, and ice is applied to control swelling. On discharge, the patient is advised to continue to perform appropriate exercises at home and begin a gradual return to normal activities. Therapy to help restore muscle strength and range of motion is also indicated.

meniscitis (mĕn″ĭ-sī′tĭs) [Gr. *meniskos,* crescent, + *itis,* inflammation] Inflammation of an interarticular cartilage, esp. the medial and lateral menisci of the knee joint.

meniscocyte (mĕn-ĭs′kō-sīt) [″ + *kytos,* cell] A crescent-shaped red blood cell. SYN: *sickle cell.*

meniscus (mĕn-ĭs′kŭs) *pl.* **menisci** [Gr. *meniskos,* crescent] **1.** Convexoconcave lens. **2.** Interarticular fibrocartilage of crescent shape, found in certain joints, esp. the lateral and medial menisci (semilunar cartilages) of the knee joint. **3.** The curved upper surface of a liquid in a container.

m. articularis Crescent-shaped interarticular fibrocartilage found in certain synovial joints.

Menkes disease Metabolic defect resulting from a mutation on the X chromosome that alters the transport of copper within the human body, resulting in neurological degeneration, connective tissue disorders, and premature death. SEE: *kinky hair disease.*

meno- Pert. to menses or menstruation.

menometrorrhagia (mĕn″ō-mĕt-rō-rā′jē-ă) [Gr. *men,* month, + *metra,* womb, + *rhegnynai,* to burst forth] Excessive bleeding during and between menstrual periods. SEE: *menorrhagia.*

menopause (mĕn′ō-pawz) [″ + *pausis,* cessation] The period that marks the permanent cessation of menstrual activity, usually occurring between the ages of 35 and 58. The menses may stop suddenly, there may be a decreased flow each month until a final cessation, or the interval between periods may be lengthened until complete cessation is accomplished. Natural menopause will occur in 25% of women by age 47, 50% by age 50, 75% by age 52, and 95% by age 55. Menopause due to surgical removal of the ovaries has occurred in almost 30% of U.S. women who are 50 years of age or older. Women with short menstrual cycles may reach menopause as much as two years earlier than women with long cycles. Cigarette smoking has an effect on menopause, causing it to occur 1 to 2 years prematurely. SYN: *change of life; climacteric.* SEE: *osteoporosis; perimenopause.*

SYMPTOMS: The symptoms associated with menopause begin soon after the ovaries stop functioning, whether menopause occurs naturally or is due to surgical removal of the ovaries or failure of the pituitary gland to function. Symptoms, which may last from a few months to years, vary from hardly noticeable to severe. Included are vasomotor instability, nervousness, hot flashes (flushes), chills, excitability, fatigue, apathy, mental depression, crying episodes, insomnia, palpitation, vertigo, headache, numbness, tingling, myalgia, urinary disturbances (such as frequency and incontinence), and various disorders of the gastrointestinal system. The long-range effects of lower estrogen levels are osteoporosis and atherosclerosis.

Hot flashes (flushes) may start with an aura preceding abdominal discomfort and perhaps a chill, quickly followed by a feeling of heat moving toward the head. Next the face becomes red, then there is sweating followed by exhaustion. The cause of hot flashes is not understood completely. Although the popular myth is that sexual desire and activity inevitably decrease following menopause, there is little to support this. Sexual desire may remain at the premenopause level or be increased due to the lack of fear of pregnancy.

TREATMENT: Hormone replacement therapy (HRT) is recommended for many postmenopausal women. This therapy consists of estrogen alone (in patients who have had hysterectomy) and estrogen combined with progesterone (in patients with an intact uterus). HRT is contraindicated in women with a history of an estrogen-dependent breast cancer, endometrial cancer, thromboembolic disease, acute liver disease, and vaginal bleeding of unknown etiology. Many women with a strong family history of breast cancer also will avoid HRT. Decisions regarding use of HRT are based on the relative benefits and risks of treatment for the individual woman. Important benefits may include reducing the risk of osteoporosis, lowering the likelihood of Alzheimer's dementia, improving the lipid profile, and decreasing symptomatic hot flashes. Whether HRT impacts heart attack and stroke is uncertain. Significant adverse effects may include increased potential for developing estrogen-related malignancies and resumption of menses. SEE: *estrogen replacement therapy; hormone replacement therapy*.

PATIENT CARE: Because women may experience a variety of symptoms during this period, their nature, severity, and personal impact need to be determined. Menopause is explained as a normal phase in the reproductive cycle. If the woman experiences severe symptoms, a physician may need to assess the patient. The woman is encouraged to maintain a diet high in calcium, vitamins, and minerals. The advantages and disadvantages of HRT are discussed. Health care providers offer emotional support and reassurance, as symptoms can be distressing and frightening, and provide written follow-up information and self-help resources.

artificial m. Menopause occurring subsequent to surgical removal of ovaries, x-ray irradiation, or radium implantation into the uterus.

male m. SEE: *climacteric*.

premature m. Natural or artificial menopause occurring before age 35.

surgical m. Artificial m.

menoplania (mĕn-ō″plā′nē-ă) [″ + *plane,* deviation] Menstruation through other than the normal outlet, as through the nose. SYN: *vicarious menstruation*.

menorrhagia (mĕn″ō-rā′jē-ă) [″ + *rhegnynai,* to burst forth] Menstrual bleeding that is excessive in number of days or amount of blood, or both. SYN: *hypermenorrhea*. SEE: *uterine hemorrhage*.

ETIOLOGY: Menorrhagia may be caused by endocrine disturbances (e.g., diabetes mellitus or disorders of the adrenal glands, ovaries, or pituitary), hypertension, blood dyscrasias, chronic nephritis, retroversion or retroflexion of the uterus, intramural or submucous fibroids of the uterus, uterine adenomyosis, fibrosis of the uterus with hyperplastic changes of the endometrium, erosions or polyps of the cervix uteri, acute salpingitis, acute or chronic metritis, or acute endometritis.

menorrhalgia (mĕn-ō-răl′jē-ă) [″ + *rhoia,* flow, + *algia,* pain] Painful menstruation or pelvic pain accompanying menstruation, sometimes a symptom of endometriosis. SYN: *dysmenorrhea*.

menostasis (mĕn-ŏs′tă-sĭs) [″ + *stasis,* standing still] Suppression of the menses.

menostaxis (mĕn″ō-stăk′sĭs) [″ + *staxis,* dripping] Prolonged menstruation.

menotropins (mĕn″ō-trō′pĭns) A combination of follicle-stimulating hormone (FSH) and luteinizing hormone (LH) used to treat infertility by promoting growth and maturation of the follicle of the ovary. Menotropins is obtained from the urine of postmenopausal women. A standard extract is used with human chorionic gonadotropin (HCG) to induce ovulation. Trade name is Pergonal.

menoxenia (mĕn-ŏk-sē′nē-ă) [″ + *xenos,* strange] Abnormal menstruation.

menses (mĕn′sēz) [L., month] The monthly flow of bloody fluid from the endometrium.

menstrual cramps SEE: *cramps, menstrual; dysmenorrhea*.

menstrual cycle The periodically recurrent series of changes occurring in the uterus and associated sex organs (ovaries, cervix, and vagina) associated with menstruation and the intermenstrual period. The human cycle averages 28 days in length, measured from the beginning of menstruation. The menstrual cycle is, however, quite variable in length, even in the same person from month to month. Variations in the length of the cycle are due principally to variation in the length of the proliferative phase. SEE: illus.

The menstrual cycle is divided into four phases characterized by histological changes that take place in the uterine endometrium. They are:

Proliferative Phase: Following blood loss from the endometrium, the uterine epithelium is restored to normal; the endometrium becomes thicker and more vascular; the glands elongate. During this period, the ovarian follicle is maturing and secreting estrogens; with the estrogen stimulation, the endometrium hypertrophies, thickening and becoming more vascular, and the glands elongate. The phase is terminated by the

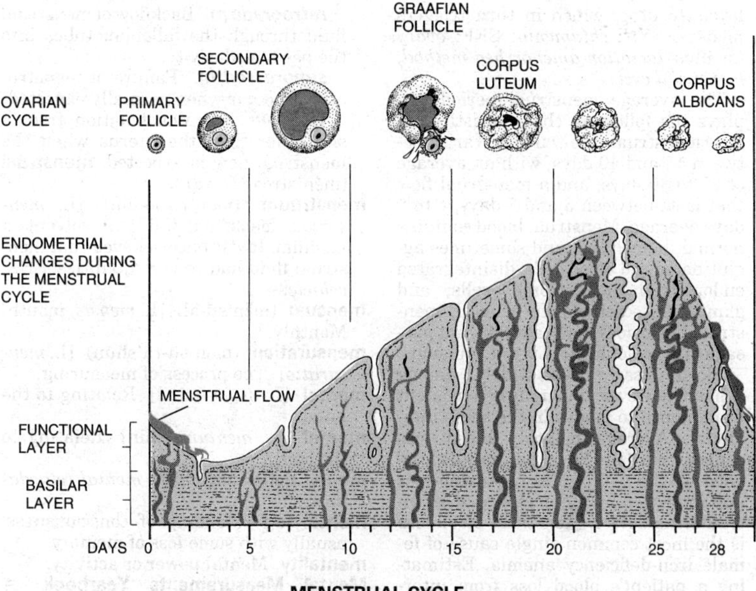

MENSTRUAL CYCLE

rupture of the follicle and the liberation of the ovum at about 14 days before the next menstrual period begins. Fertilization of the ovum is most likely to occur in the days immediately following ovulation.

Luteal or Secretory Phase: After releasing the ovum, the corpus luteum secretes progesterone. With the progesterone stimulation, the endometrium becomes even thicker; the glands become more tortuous and produce an abundant secretion containing glycogen. The coiled arteries make their appearance; the endometrium becomes edematous; the stroma becomes compact. During this period, the corpus luteum in an ovary is developing and secreting progesterone. This phase lasts 10 to 14 days.

Premenstrual or Ischemic Phase: If pregnancy has not occurred, the coiled arteries constrict and the endometrium becomes anemic and shrinks a day or two before menstruation. The corpus luteum of the ovary begins involution. This phase lasts about 2 days and is terminated by the opening up of constricted arteries, the breaking off of small patches of endometrium, and the beginning of menstruation with the flow of menstrual fluid.

Menstruation: The menstrual cycle is altered by pregnancy, the use of contraception, intercurrent illnesses, diet, and exercise.

menstrual epilepsy Epileptic convulsions that tend to occur at certain times during the menstrual period. SEE: *epilepsy*.

menstrual extraction Vacuum or suction curettage of the uterus done just prior to the date of the next menstrual period. The procedure, performed using carefully controlled suction and a soft flexible catheter, is used to be certain the menstrual period is induced, even though the uterus may contain a fertilized ovum.

menstrual regulation Vacuum or suction curettage of the uterus done within the first two weeks following the expected date of the onset of menstruation. If the amenorrhea was due to pregnancy, the procedure is classed as a form of fertility control.

menstrual synchrony The simultaneous occurrence of ovulatory cycles and menstrual bleeding among women who live or work together or socialize closely with one another.

menstruant (mĕn′stroo-ănt) [L. *menstruare*, to discharge the menses] **1.** In the condition of menstruating. **2.** One who menstruates.

menstruate (mĕn′stroo-āt) To discharge menses.

menstruation (mĕn-stroo-ā′shŭn) [L. *menstruare*, to discharge the menses] The cyclic, hormonally generated sloughing of the uterine endometrium, which occurs between puberty and menopause and is accompanied by bloody vaginal discharge. The onset of menstruation (menarche) usually occurs during puberty (9 to 17 years of age). When a woman's ovum is not fertilized, the corpus luteum undergoes involution, which causes progesterone levels to drop, which in turn triggers menses. SYN: *catamenia*. SEE: *ovary* for illus; *lactation amenorrhea method; menstrual cycle*.

The average menstrual period displays the following characteristics: an intermenstrual interval that varies between 18 and 40 days, with an average of 27 to 30 days; and a menstrual flow that lasts between 3 and 7 days, 4 to 5 days average. Menstrual blood contains normal, hemolyzed, and sometimes agglutinated red blood cells; disintegrated endometrial and stromal cells; and glandular secretions. In general, menstrual blood does not coagulate, but passage of occasional clots is not unusual.

Blood loss varies widely among women; however, it usually is consistent from month to month in the same individual. Average monthly blood loss ranges from 44 to 80 ml but may be lessened by the use of oral contraceptives and increased by the presence of an intrauterine device. Menstrual blood loss is the most common single cause of female iron-deficiency anemia. Estimating a patient's blood loss from interviewing is difficult because many women are poor judges of the volume of their flow. A rough estimate of blood loss may be made by querying the number, type, and amount of saturation of tampons or sanitary pads used each day of the period. When noting the number of pads or tampons used daily, the historian should determine the reason for changes; some women may change for reasons other than pad saturation.

Indications of excessive or abnormal menstrual flow include a need to change saturated tampons or pads hourly; passage of clots, esp. when larger than 2 cm in diameter or occurring on other than the first full day of menses; and duration of flow exceeding 7 days in one or more cycles. Menstruation normally ceases during pregnancy, may or may not occur during lactation, and permanently ceases with menopause. SEE: *sanitary napkin; tampon, menstrual*.

Menstrual irregularities: Failure to menstruate may be caused by congenital abnormalities; physical disorders (e.g., obesity, malnutrition, or disease); excessive exercise; emotional and hormonal disturbances affecting the ovaries, pituitary, thyroid, or adrenal glands. An absence of flow when normally expected is called *amenorrhea;* scanty flow is known as *oligomenorrhea;* painful menstruation is *dysmenorrhea.* Excessive loss of blood is termed *menorrhagia;* loss of blood during intermenstrual periods is known as spotting or *metrorrhagia.*

anovulatory m. Menstruation occurring without discharge of ovum from ovary, i.e., without ovulation.

retrograde m. Backflow of menstrual fluid through the fallopian tubes into the peritoneal cavity.

suppressed m. Failure of menstruation to occur when normally expected.

vicarious m. Menstruation from a site other than the uterus when the menstrual flow is expected. **menstrual** (mĕn′stroo-ăl), *adj.*

menstruum (mĕn′stroo-ŭm) [L. *menstruus,* menstrual fluid] A solvent; a medium. It was once believed that menstrual fluid had solvent qualities. SEE: *vehicle*.

mensual (mĕn′sū-ăl) [L. *mensis,* month] Monthly.

mensuration (mĕn-sū-rā′shŭn) [L. *mensuratio*] The process of measuring.

mental [L. *mens,* mind] Relating to the mind.

mental [L. *mentum,* chin] Relating to the chin.

mental deficiency SEE: *mental retardation.*

mental fog Clouding of consciousness, usually with some loss of memory.

mentality Mental power or activity.

Mental Measurements Yearbook A widely used index of commercially published, standardized tests.

mental retardation Below-average intellectual function that is evident before the age of 18 and is associated with impaired learning or communication; poor social, community, or interpersonal adjustment; or inability to function independently (e.g., to support oneself, to live safely and healthfully).

ETIOLOGY: In many persons, the cause is not identified. Injuries that occur during fetal or embryonic development (e.g., exposure to infections or toxins in utero); genetic syndromes (e.g., Tay-Sachs disease or Down syndrome); childhood exposure to toxins (e.g., lead); or social and emotional deprivation during infancy or childhood all may contribute to impairments in intellectual development.

DIAGNOSIS: Tests of intelligence ("intelligence quotient" or IQ tests) are used to diagnose mental retardation, esp. when poor scores on these tests correlate with observed difficulties in adaptation to the environment.

mentally ill Affected by any condition that affects mood or behavior, such as depression, dysphoria, personality disorders, phobias, schizophrenia, or substance abuse, among others.

mentation (mĕn-tā′shŭn) Mental activity.

menthol $C_{10}H_{20}O$; an alcohol obtained from oil of peppermint or other mint oils. Menthol may be prepared synthetically. It occurs in crystalline form. When applied to the skin in a 0.25% to 2% solution, it is an antipruritic.

menton (mĕn′tŏn) [L. *mentum,* chin] A

craniometric landmark, being the lowest point of the mandibular symphysis seen in a lateral radiograph. Similar to, but not necessarily the same as, gnathion, which is the lowest point of the mandible in the midline as palpated in the living.

mentoplasty (mĕn′tō-plăs-tē) Cosmetic surgery designed to enhance the appearance of the chin.

mentulagra (mĕn″tū-lăg′ră) [L. *mentula,* penis, + Gr. *agra,* seizure] Painful involuntary erection of the penis, sometimes curved. SYN: *priapism.* SEE: *chordee; Peyronie's disease.*

mentulate (mĕn′tū-lāt) [L. *mentula,* penis] Possessing a large penis.

mentulomania (mĕn″tū-lō-mā′nē-ă) [″ + Gr. *mania,* madness] Mental state characterized by addiction to masturbation.

mentum [L.] The chin. SYN: *genion.*

MEOS *microsomal ethanol oxidizing system.*

mepacrine hydrochloride (mĕp′ă-krĭn) Quinacrine hydrochloride. An antimalarial drug.

meperidine hydrochloride (mĕ-pĕr′ĭ-dēn) A narcotic analgesic sold under the trade name of Demerol.

mephenytoin (mĕ-fĕn′ĭ-tō-ĭn) An anticonvulsive that is used in the lowest concentration possible in combination with other drugs. This is done because of its toxicity.

mephitic [L. *mephiticus, mephitis,* foul exhalation] Noxious, foul, as a poisonous odor.

mephobarbital (mĕf″ō-băr′bĭ-tăl) An anticonvulsant and sedative of the barbiturate class.

mepivacaine hydrochloride (mĕ-pĭv′ă-kān) A local anesthetic.

meprednisone (mĕ-prĕd′nĭ-sōn) An adrenocorticosteroid.

meprobamate (mĕ-prō′bă-māt) A tranquilizing agent, used for relief of anxiety and mental tension. SEE: *Poisons and Poisoning Appendix.*

mEq Symbol for milliequivalent.

meralgia (mĕr-ăl′jē-ă) [Gr. *meros,* thigh, + *algos,* pain] Pain in the thigh.

m. paresthetica Pain and hyperesthesia on the outer femoral surface from lesion or disease of the lateral cutaneous nerve of the thigh.

mercaptan (mĕr-kăp′tăn) Any organic chemical that contains the —SH radical. It is formed when the oxygen of an alcohol is replaced by sulfur.

mercaptopurine (mĕr-kăp″tō-pū′rēn) An antineoplastic and immunosuppressive agent used, for example, in treating acute leukemia.

Mercier's bar (mĕr-sē-āz′) [Louis A. Mercier, Fr. urologist, 1811–1882] A curved fold at the neck of the bladder forming the posterior margin of the trigonum vesicae.

mercurial (mĕr-kū′rē-ăl) [L. *mercurialis*] **1.** Pert. to mercury. **2.** A substance containing mercury.

mercurial diuretics A class of organic mercurial compounds formerly used to promote urination. They are no longer used because of their toxicity.

mercurialism (mĕr-kū′rē-ăl-ĭzm) [L. *mercurius,* mercury, + Gr. *-ismos,* condition] Chronic poisoning by mercury. Seen as a result of continuous administration of mercury or occurs in persons who work with the metal or inhale its vapors.

SYMPTOMS: Chronic mercury poisoning causes soreness of gums and loosening of teeth; increased salivation; tremor; and behavioral mood disorders.

mercurialized (mĕr-kū′rē-ăl-īzd) **1.** Impregnated with mercury. **2.** Influenced by or treated with mercury.

mercuric (mĕr-kū′rĭk) Relating to bivalent mercury.

m. chloride $HgCl_2$; a highly toxic inorganic salt of mercury. SYN: *mercury bichloride.*

yellow m. oxide HgO; a yellow to orange powder used in the past, in ointments as an antibacterial agent.

mercuric chloride poisoning Acute toxic reaction to ingested or inhaled salt of mercury. This form of mercury may also be absorbed through the skin.

SYMPTOMS: Severe gastrointestinal irritation with pain, cramping, constriction of the throat, vomiting, and a metallic taste in the mouth. Abdominal pain may be severe. Bloody diarrhea, bloody vomitus, scanty or absent urine output, prostration, convulsions, and unconsciousness may follow. Death from uremia is the usual outcome unless treatment is begun immediately.

TREATMENT: Oxygen and intravenous fluids are given. Gastric lavage (not emesis) is used to empty the gastrointestinal tract. Dimercaprol or D-penicillamine is used for chelation. Similar treatment is given for mercurous chloride poisoning. SEE: *Poisons and Poisoning Appendix.*

mercurous (mĕr-kū′rŭs, mĕr′kū-rŭs) Relating to monovalent mercury.

m. chloride HgCl; a heavy white powder previously used in small doses in medicine as a laxative. It is also used as a component of certain reference electrodes used in electrical analysis. SYN: *calomel.*

mercurous chloride poisoning Acute toxic reaction to ingestion or absorption through the skin of the mercury salt, mercurous chloride. Acute poisoning is rare because it is poorly absorbed. Symptoms include increased salivation, abdominal discomfort, and diarrhea. SEE: *mercuric chloride* in *Poisons and Poisoning Appendix.*

mercury (mĕr′kū-rē) [L. *mercurius*]

SYMB: Hg. A metallic element with an atomic weight of 201 and an atomic number of 80. It is insoluble in ordinary solvents but soluble in hydrochloric acid on boiling. (NOTE: This process would result in the release of highly toxic and irritating fumes into the atmosphere.) It is a silvery liquid at room temperature. Mercury forms two series of salts: mercurous, in which it has a valence of one (univalent), and mercuric, in which it has a valence of two (bivalent). SEE: *dental amalgam*.

ammoniated m. A topical antiseptic used in treating certain skin diseases.

CAUTION: Chronic use can cause mercury poisoning. Use should be avoided in infants.

m. bichloride Mercuric chloride.

mercury poisoning Systemic toxicity produced by inhalation, ingestion, or skin contact with organic or inorganic mercury. SEE: *erethism mercuric chloride poisoning; mercuric salts* in *Poisons and Poisoning Appendix*.

mercy (mĕr'sē) [L. *merces,* reward] In medicine, the compassionate provision of relief or mitigation of physical pain, mental suffering, or psychological distress.

meridian (mĕ-rĭd'ē-ăn) **1.** An imaginary line encircling a globular body at right angles to its equator and passing through the poles, or half of such a line. **meridional,** *adj.* **2.** In complementary medicine, traditional Chinese medicine, and acupuncture, one of several pathways that is believed to conduct energy between the surface of the body and the internal organs. Blockage along these pathways is believed to disrupt energy flow (chi or qi) and to cause imbalances that are reflected in symptoms or disease. Using Western scientific methods, meridians and the energy flows they are thought to direct have eluded identification.

m. of eye A circle passing through anterior and posterior poles of the eyeball.

merinthophobia (mĕr-ĭn″thō-fō'bē-ă) [Gr. *merinthos,* a cord, + *phobia,* fear] Morbid fear of being tied.

merispore (mĕr'ĭ-spor) [Gr. *meros,* a part, + *sporos,* seed] A secondary spore resulting from the division of another spore.

meristic (mĕr-ĭs'tĭk) [Gr. *meristikos,* fit for dividing] Bilaterally symmetrical.

meroacrania (mĕr″ō-ă-krā'nē-ă) [Gr. *meros,* a part, + *a-,* not, + *kranion,* skull] Congenital absence of a part of the cranium.

meroblastic (mĕr-ō-blăst'ĭk) [″ + *blastos,* germ] Pert. to a type of ovum containing considerable yolk or a type of cleavage in which cleavage divisions are restricted to the protoplasmic region of the animal pole.

merocele (mĕr'ō-sēl) [″ + *kele,* tumor, swelling] Femoral hernia.

merocoxalgia (mĕr″ō-kŏk-săl'jē-ă) [″ + L. *coxa,* hip, + Gr. *algos,* pain] Painful condition of the thigh and hip.

merocrine (mĕr'ō-krīn) [″ + *krinein,* to separate] Denoting a type of secretion in which the glandular cell remains intact during the process of elaborating and discharging its product. SEE: *apocrine; eccrine; holocrine*.

merodiastolic (mĕr″ō-dī-ă-stŏl'ĭk) Concerning a part of the diastole of the cardiac cycle.

merogenesis (mĕr″ō-jĕn'ĕ-sĭs) [Gr. *meros,* a part, + *genesis,* generation, birth] Multiplication or reproduction by segmentation.

merogony (mĕ-rŏg'ō-nē) [″ + *gonos,* procreation] Incomplete development of fragments of an ovum.

meromelia (mĕr″ō-mē'lē-ă) [″ + *melos,* limb] Partial absence of a limb.

meromicrosomia (mĕr″ō-mī″krō-sō'mē-ă) [″ + *mikros,* small, + *soma,* body] Abnormal smallness of some part or structure of the body.

meromyosin (mĕr″ō-mī'ō-sĭn) Either of the subunits produced by tryptic digestion of myosin.

meropia (mĕr-ō'pē-ă) [″ + *ops,* vision] Partial blindness.

merorhachischisis (mĕ″rō-ră-kĭs'kĭ-sĭs) [″ + *rhachis,* spine, + *schisis,* a splitting] Fissure of a portion of the spinal cord. SYN: *mesorhachischisis*.

merosmia (mĕr-ŏs'mē-ă) [″ + *osme,* odor] Inability to detect certain odors.

merosystolic (mĕr″ō-sĭs-tŏl'ĭk) [″ + *systole,* a contraction] Concerning a portion of the systole of the cardiac cycle.

merotomy (mĕr-ŏt'ō-mē) [″ + *tome,* incision] Division into sections or segments.

merozoite (mĕr″ō-zō'īt) [″ + *zoon,* animal] A body formed by segmentation or breaking up of a schizont in asexual reproduction of certain sporozoans, such as *Plasmodium*. When formed, merozoites are liberated and invade other corpuscles, where they repeat the process of schizogony or develop into gametocytes.

merozygote (mĕr″ō-zī'gōt) [″ + *zygotos,* yoked together] A bacterial mechanism of gene transfer in which part of the genome, or chromosome complement, is transferred into an intact recipient cell.

mesad Mesiad.

mesal Mesial.

mesangium (mĕs-ăn'jē-ŭm) The suspensory structure of the renal glomerulus. **mesangial,** *adj.*

mesaortitis (mĕs″ā-or-tī'tĭs) [″ + *aorte,*

aorta, + *itis,* inflammation] Inflammation of the middle aortic layer.

mesarteritis (mĕs-ăr-tĕr-ī′tĭs) Inflammation of the tunica media or middle layer of an artery.

mesaticephalic (mĕs-ăt″ĭ-sĕf-ăl′ĭk) [Gr. *mesatos,* medium, + *kephale,* brain] Having a skull with a cephalic index of 75 to 79.9.

mesatipellic, mesatipelvic (mĕs-ăt″ĭ-pĕl′lĭk, -pĕl′vĭk) [″ + *pella,* bowl] Having a pelvis of medium size with an index between 90 and 95.

mescaline (mĕs′kă-lēn) A poisonous alkaloid, the active ingredient of the mescal buttons of the cactus plant *Lophophora williamsii,* that causes hallucinations, esp. those involving color and sound.

mescalism (mĕs′kă-lĭzm) Intoxication produced by ingesting mescal.

mesectoderm (mĕs-ĕk′tō-derm) Migratory cells derived from ectoderm, esp. from the neural crest of the cephalic area in young embryos, that become pigment cells.

mesencephalitis (mĕs″ĕn-sĕf″ă-lī′tĭs) [″ + *enkephalos,* brain, + *itis,* inflammation] Inflammation of the mesencephalon.

mesencephalon (mĕs-ĕn-sĕf′ă-lŏn) [″ + *enkephalos,* brain] The midbrain. One of three primitive cerebral vesicles from which develop the corpora quadrigemina, the crura cerebri, and the aqueduct of Sylvius. **mesencephalic,** *adj.*

mesencephalotomy (mĕs″ĕn-sĕf″ă-lŏt′ō-mē) [″ + ″ + *tome,* incision] Surgical incision of the midbrain, usually done to relieve intractable pain.

mesenchyme (mĕs′ĕn-kīm) [″ + *enchyma,* infusion] A diffuse network of cells forming the embryonic mesoderm and giving rise to connective tissues, blood and blood vessels, the lymphatic system, and cells of the mononuclear phagocyte system. **mesenchymal, mesenchymatous,** *adj.*

mesenchymoma (mĕs″ĕn-kī-mō′mă) A neoplasm containing a mixture of mesenchymal and fibrous tissue.

mesenterectomy (mĕs″ĕn-tē-rĕk′tō-mē) [″ + *enteron,* intestine, + *ektome,* excision] Surgical removal of the mesentery.

mesenteriopexy (mĕs″ĕn-tĕr′ē-ō-pĕk″sē) [″ + *enteron,* intestine, + *pexis,* fixation] Surgical attachment of a torn mesentery.

mesenteriorrhaphy (mĕs″ĕn-tĕr-ē-or′ă-fē) [″ + ″ + *rhaphe,* seam, ridge] Suturing of the mesentery. SYN: *mesorrhaphy.*

mesenteriplication (mĕs″ĕn-tĕr″ĭ-plĭ-kā′shŭn) [″ + ″ + L. *plicare,* to fold] Shortening the mesentery by taking tucks in it surgically.

mesenteritis (mĕs″ĕn-tĕr-ī′tĭs) [″ + ″ + *itis,* inflammation] Inflammation of the mesentery.

mesenteron (mĕs-ĕn′tĕr-ŏn) Middle portion of the embryonic digestive tract.

mesentery (mĕs′ĕn-tĕr″ē) [″ + *enteron,* intestine] Commonly, the peritoneal fold that encircles the small intestine and connects it to the posterior abdominal wall. Other abdominal organs, however, also have a mesentery. **mesenteric** (mĕs″ĕn-tĕr′ĭk), *adj.*

MESH *Me*dical *S*ubject *H*eadings. A list of the medical words used in storing and retrieving medical references by the U.S. National Library of Medicine. SEE: *MEDLARS.*

mesh A prosthetic patch or fabric used to repair or reinforce hernias, burns, and other defects. A split-thickness skin graft may be formed into a mesh which may be applied to a burn or other cutaneous defects requiring extensive covering. SEE: *mesh graft.*

mesiad, mesad (mē′zē-ăd, mē′săd) [Gr. *mesos,* middle, + L. *ad,* toward] Toward the median plane of a body or part.

mesial, mesal (mē′zē-ăl, mē′săl) **1.** Toward the middle point or midline plane. **2.** In dentistry, ventral or nearer to the center of the dental arch.

mesial drift The natural tendency for teeth to move in a mesial direction within the dental arch to maintain tight interproximal contacts between adjacent teeth. Also called physiological tooth movement. SEE: *tooth migration, pathological; tooth migration, physiological; tooth movement.*

mesio- [Gr. *mesos,* middle] **1.** A combining form meaning *toward the middle.* **2.** In dentistry, a combining form pert. to the ventral surface of teeth or ventrally toward the center of the dental arch.

mesiobuccal (mē″zē-ō-bŭk′kăl) Concerning the mesial and buccal surfaces of a tooth or the surfaces involved in a cavity in the tooth.

mesiobucco-occlusal (mē″zē-ō-bŭk″kō-ŏ-kloo′zăl) Concerning the mesial, buccal, and occlusal surfaces of a tooth.

mesiobuccopulpal (mē″zē-ō-bŭk″kō-pŭl′păl) Concerning the mesial, buccal, and pulpal sides of a tooth cavity.

mesiocervical (mē″zē-ō-sĕr′vĭ-kăl) Concerning the mesial surface of the neck of a tooth.

mesioclusion (mē″zē-ō-kloo′zhŭn) Malocclusion of the lower teeth. They are located in front of their normal position with respect to the upper teeth.

mesiodens (mē′zē-ō-dĕnz) A supernumerary tooth, often paired, which typically appears between the maxillary central incisors.

TREATMENT: Surgical removal of the mesiodens is usually indicated.

mesiodistal (mē″zē-ō-dĭs′tăl) Concerning the mesial and distal surfaces of a tooth.

mesiogingival (mē′zē-ō-jĭn′jĭ-văl) Concerning the mesial and gingival walls of a tooth cavity.

mesiolabial (mē″zē-ō-lā′bē-ăl) Concerning the mesial and labial surfaces of a tooth or cavity.

mesiolingual (mē″zē-ō-lĭng′gwăl) Concerning the mesial and lingual surfaces of a tooth or cavity.

mesiolinguo-occlusal (mē″zē-ō-lĭng′gwō-ŏ-kloo′zăl) Concerning the mesial, lingual, and occlusal surfaces of a tooth.

mesiolinguopulpal (mē′zē-ō-lĭng″gwō-pŭl′păl) Concerning the mesial, lingual, and pulpal sides of a tooth cavity.

mesion (mē′sē-ŏn) [Gr. *mesos,* middle] The imaginary plane dividing the body into right and left symmetric halves. SYN: *meson* (2).

mesiopulpal (mē″zē-ō-pŭl′păl) Concerning the mesial and pulpal sides of a tooth cavity.

mesioversion (mē″zē-ō-vĕr′zhŭn) Displacement of a tooth posteriorly in the dental arch.

mesiris (mĕs-ī′rĭs) Middle portion of the iris.

mesmerism (mĕs′mĕr-ĭzm) [Franz Anton Mesmer, Austrian physician, 1734–1815] Originally Mesmer's theory of animal magnetism, mesmerism now means therapeutics employing hypnotism or hypnotic suggestion. **mesmeric** (mĕs-mĕr′ĭk), *adj.*

mesna A detoxifying agent used to inhibit the hemorrhagic cystitis induced by ifosfamide. SEE: *ifosfamide.*

meso- [Gr. *mesos,* middle] **1.** Combining form meaning *middle.* **2.** In anatomy, combining form pert. to a mesentery. **3.** In medicine, combining form meaning *secondary* or *partial.*

mesoappendicitis Inflammation of the mesoappendix.

mesoappendix (mĕs″ō-ă-pĕn′dĭks) [Gr. *mesos,* middle, + L. *appendix,* an appendage] Mesentery of the vermiform appendix.

mesoblast (mĕs′ō-blăst) [″ + *blastos,* germ] Mesoderm.

mesobronchitis (mĕs″ō-brŏng-kī′tĭs) Inflammation of the middle layer of the bronchi.

mesocardia (mĕs″ō-kăr′dē-ă) [″ + *kardia,* heart] Location of the heart in the midline of the thorax. This position is normal in the fetal stage, but a malposition after birth.

mesocardium (mĕs-ō-kăr′dē-ŭm) An embryonic mesentery supporting the heart. The dorsal mesocardium connects the heart to the foregut, and the ventral mesocardium connects the heart to the central body wall.

mesocarpal (mĕs″ō-kăr′păl) Mediocarpal.

mesocecum (mĕs″ō-sē′kŭm) [″ + L. *caecum,* blindness] Part of the mesentery that connects the cecum to the right iliac fossa.

mesocele (mĕs′ō-sēl) [″ + *koilia,* hollow] Sylvian aqueduct in the brain.

mesocephalic (mĕs″ō-sĕ-făl′ĭk) [″ + *kephale,* head] **1.** Pert. to the midbrain. **2.** Having a medium-sized head, with a cranial index of 76.0 to 80.9.

mesocephalon (mĕs″ō-sĕf′ă-lŏn) Mesencephalon.

mesocolon (mĕs″ō-kō′lŏn) [″ + *kolon,* colon] Mesentery of the colon. **mesocolic** (mĕs″ō-kŏl′ĭk), *adj.*

mesocolopexy (mĕs″ō-kō′lō-pĕk″sē) [″ + ″ + *pexis,* fixation] The suturing of tucks in the mesocolon to shorten it in order to correct unneeded mobility and ptosis.

mesocoloplication (mĕs″ō-kō″lō-plī-kā′shŭn) [″ + ″ + L. *plicare,* to fold] Plication of the mesocolon for stabilization.

mesocord A portion of umbilical cord attached to the placenta by means of an amniotic fold.

mesocuneiform (mĕs″ō-kū′nē-ĭ-form) The intermediate cuneiform bone of the ankle.

mesoderm (mĕs′ō-dĕrm) [″ + *derma,* skin] A primary germ layer of the embryo lying between ectoderm and endoderm. From it arise all connective tissues; muscular, skeletal, circulatory, lymphatic, and urogenital systems; and the linings of the body cavities. SEE: *ectoderm; endoderm.* **mesodermic, mesodermal,** *adj.*

axial m. Portion of the mesoderm that gives rise to the notochord and prechordal plate.

extraembryonic m. Mesoderm lying outside the embryo proper and involved in the formation of amnion, chorion, yolk sac, and body stalk.

intermediate m. Mesoderm lying between somite and lateral mesoderm, and giving rise to embryonic and definitive kidneys and their ducts. SYN: *mesomere; nephrotome.*

lateral m. Unsegmented mesoderm lying lateral to the intermediate mesoderm. In it develops a cavity (coelom), separating it into layers (somatic and splanchnic mesoderm). SYN: *hypomere.*

paraxial m. Mesoderm lying immediately lateral to the neural tube and notochord.

somatic m. The outer layer of the lateral mesoderm. It becomes intimately associated with the ectoderm, forming the somatopleure, from which the ventral and lateral walls of the embryo develop.

splanchnic m. The inner layer of the lateral mesoderm. It becomes intimately associated with the endoderm, forming the splanchnopleure, from which the gut and the lungs and their coverings arise.

mesodiastolic (mĕs″ō-dī″ă-stŏl′ĭk) Mid-diastole of the heartbeat sequence.

mesodont (mĕs′ō-dŏnt) Having teeth of medium size; a dental index of 42 to 43.9.

mesoduodenum (mĕs″ō-dū″ō-dē′nŭm) Mesentery connecting the duodenum to the abdominal wall.

mesoepididymis (mĕs″ō-ĕp″ĭ-dĭd′ĭ-mĭs) A fold of the tunica vaginalis that is not always present. It binds the epididymis to the testicle.

mesogastrium (mĕs″ō-găs′trē-ŭm) [″ + *gaster,* belly] **1.** The umbilical region. **2.** The part of the mesentery of the embryo attached to the primitive stomach. **mesogastric** (-trĭk), *adj.*

mesoglia (mĕ-sŏg′lē-ă) A term formerly used to signify the microglia (phagocytic cells of the central nervous system).

mesogluteus (mĕs″ō-gloo′tē-ŭs) The gluteus medius muscle. **mesogluteal** (-ăl), *adj.*

mesognathion (mĕs-ŏg-nā′thē-ŏn) A point in the lateral portion of the intermaxillary bone or premaxilla.

mesognathous Having a facial profile that protrudes slightly from the vertical line between nasion and gnathion. SEE: *prognathous.*

mesohyloma (mĕs″ō-hī-lō′mă) [″ + *hyle,* matter, + *oma,* tumor] Tumor derived from the mesothelium.

mesoileum (mĕs″ō-ĭl′ē-ŭm) The mesentery of the ileum.

mesojejunum (mĕs″ō-jē-jū′nŭm) The mesentery of the jejunum.

mesolymphocyte (mĕs″ō-lĭm′fō-sīt) A medium-sized lymphocyte.

mesomere (mĕs′ō-mēr) [″ + *meros,* part] **1.** Portion of the mesoderm between epimere and hypomere. SYN: *mesoderm, intermediate; nephrotome.* **2.** A blastomere that is intermediate in size between a micromere and a macromere.

mesometritis (mĕs-ō-mē-trī′tĭs) [″ + *metra,* uterus, + *itis,* inflammation] Myometritis.

mesometrium (mĕs″ō-mē′trē-ŭm) **1.** The uterine musculature. **2.** The broad ligament below the mesovarium. **mesometric, mesometrial,** *adj.*

mesomorph (mĕs′ō-morf) A body build characterized by predominance of tissues derived from the mesoderm (i.e., muscle, bone, and connective tissues); a well-proportioned individual. SEE: *ectomorph; endomorph; somatotype.*

meson (mĕs′ŏn, mē′sŏn) [Gr. *mesos,* middle] **1.** Particle of mass intermediate between that of the electron and that of the proton. Mesons of more than one variety and of positive, neutral, and negative charges occur. SYN: *mesotron.* **2.** Mesion.

mesonasal (mĕs″ō-nā′zăl) In the middle of the nose.

mesonephric (mĕs-ō-nĕ′rĭk) Pert. to mesonephros.

mesonephroma (mĕs″ō-nē-frō′mă) [″ + *nephros,* kidney, + *oma,* tumor] A relatively rare tumor derived from mesonephric cells developing in reproductive organs, esp. the ovary, or the genital tract.

mesonephros (mĕs″ō-nĕf′rŏs) *pl.* **mesonephroi** A type of kidney that develops in all vertebrate embryos of classes above the Cyclostomes. It is the permanent kidney of fishes and amphibians but is replaced by the metanephros in reptiles and mammals. SYN: *wolffian body.* **mesonephric** (mĕs″ō-nĕf′rĭk), *adj.*

mesoneuritis (mĕs-ō-nū-rī′tĭs) [″ + *neuron,* nerve, + *itis,* inflammation] Inflammation of a nerve or of its lymphatics.

meso-ontomorph (mĕs″ō-ŏn′tō-morf) A broad, husky body type.

mesopexy (mĕs′ō-pĕks″ē) [″ + *pexis,* fixation] Surgery to attach a torn mesentery.

mesophile (mĕs′ō-fīl) [″ + *philein,* to love] Organisms preferring moderate temperatures, as some bacteria, which develop best at temperatures between 15° and 43°C. **mesophilic** (mĕs-ō-fĭl′ĭk), *adj.*

mesophlebitis (mĕs″ō-flĕ-bī′tĭs) Inflammation of the medial layer of the wall of a vein.

mesophragma (mĕs″ō-frăg′mă) [″ + *phragmos,* a fencing in] A band in the center of the A band in the myofibrils of a striated muscle.

mesophryon (mĕs-ŏf′rē-ŏn) [″ + *ophrys,* eyebrow] The smooth surface of the frontal bone lying between the superciliary arches; the portion directly above the root of the nose. SYN: *glabella; metopion.*

mesopia (mĕs-ŏp′ē-ă) Ability to see at low levels of light (e.g., at twilight). **mesopic** (mĕs-ŏp′ĭk), *adj.*

mesopneumon (mĕs″ō-nū′mŏn) [″ + *pneumon,* lung] Meeting point of two pleural layers at the hilus of the lung.

mesoporphyrin $C_{34}H_{38}O_4N_4$; an iron-free derivative of hemin.

mesoprosopic (mĕs″ō-prō-sŏp′ĭk) [″ + *prosopon,* face] Having a face of moderate width with a facial index of 90.

mesopulmonum (mĕs″ō-pŭl-mō′nŭm) The embryonic mesentery of the lung.

mesorchium (mĕs-or′kē-ŭm) [″ + *orchis,* testicle] Peritoneal fold that holds the fetal testes in place.

mesorectum (mĕs″ō-rĕk′tŭm) Mesentery of the rectum.

mesorhachischisis (mĕs″ō-ră-kĭs′kĭ-sĭs) [″ + *rhachis,* spine, + *schisis,* a splitting] Merorhachischisis.

mesoridazine (mĕs″ō-rĭd′ă-zēn) An antipsychotic.

mesoropter (mĕs-ō-rŏp′tĕr) [″ + *horos,* boundary, + *opter,* observer] Normal eye position with muscles at rest.

mesorrhaphy (mĕs-or′ă-fē) [″ + *rhaphe,* seam, ridge] Surgical repair of the mesentery. SEE: *mesenteriorrhaphy.*

mesorrhine (mĕs′ō-rīn) [″ + *rhis,* nose] Having a nasal index variously quoted to range between 48 and 53.
mesosalpinx (mĕs″ō-săl′pĭnks) [″ + *salpinx,* tube] The free margin of the upper division of the broad ligament within which lies the oviduct.
mesoseme (mĕs′ō-sēm) [″ + *sema,* sign] Possessing an orbital index between 83 and 89.
mesosigmoid (mĕs-ō-sĭg′moyd) Mesentery of the sigmoid colon.
mesosigmoiditis (mĕs″ō-sĭg″moy-dī′tĭs) Inflammation of the sigmoid colon.
mesosigmoidopexy (mĕs″ō-sĭg-moy′dō-pĕk″sē) Surgical fixation of the mesosigmoid to treat prolapse of the rectum.
mesoskelic (mĕs-ō-skĕl′ĭk) [″ + *skels,* leg] Having legs of medium length.
mesosome (mĕs′ō-sōm) [″ + *soma,* body] In some bacteria, one or more large irregular convoluted invaginations of the cytoplasmic membrane.
mesosternum (mĕs″ō-stĕr′nŭm) [″ + *sternon,* chest] The middle (second) section of the sternum.
mesosystolic (mĕs″ō-sĭs-tŏl′ĭk) Midsystolic portion of the cardiac cycle.
mesotarsal (mĕs″ō-tăr′săl) Mediotarsal.
mesotendineum (mĕs″ō-tĕn-dĭn′ē-ŭm) The part of the synovial sheath of a tendon that connects the lining of the tendon sheath to the fibrous sheath covering the tendon. SYN: *mesotendon.*
mesotendon Mesotendineum.
mesothelioma (mĕs″ō-thē-lē-ō′mă) A malignant tumor derived from the mesothelial cells of the pleura, peritoneum, or pericardium. It is found most often in smokers or persons with a history of exposure to asbestos.
mesothelium (mĕs″ō-thē′lē-ŭm) [″ + *epi,* at, + *thele,* nipple] The layer of cells derived from the mesoderm lining the primitive body cavity. It becomes the epithelium of the serous membranes. **mesothelial** (mĕs″ō-thē′lē-ăl), *adj.*
mesothenar (mĕs″ō-thē′năr) [″ + *thenar,* palm] The adductor pollicis muscle.
mesothorium (mĕs″ō-thō′rē-ŭm) The first two disintegration products of thorium.
mesotron A subatomic particle of weight intermediate between light particles (electrons) and heavy particles (protons). SYN: *meson* (1).
mesouranic (mĕs″ō-ū-răn′ĭk) Having a palatal index between 110 and 114.9.
mesovarium (mĕs″ō-vā′rē-ŭm) The portion of the peritoneal fold that connects the anterior border of the ovary to the posterior layer of the broad ligament.
mestranol (mĕs′tră-nōl) An estrogen used in combination with progestational drugs in some birth control pill formulations.
MET *metabolic equivalent.*
meta- (mĕt′ă) [Gr. *meta,* after, beyond, over] **1.** Prefix denoting change or transformation, or following something in a series. **2.** In chemistry, a prefix indicating the 1,3 position of benzene derivatives.
meta-analysis The combining of data from several different research studies to gain a better overview of a topic than what was available in any single investigation. Data obtained from combined studies must be compatible in order to be evaluated by this method.
metabiosis (mĕt′ă-bī-ō′sĭs) [″ + *biosis,* way of life] Dependence of an organism for its existence on another. SYN: *commensalism.* SEE: *symbiosis.*
metabolic (mĕt″ă-bŏl′ĭk) Pert. to metabolism.
metabolic body size Body weight in kilograms to the three-fourths power ($kg^{0.75}$), representative of the active tissue mass or metabolic mass of an individual.
metabolic gradient A gradient in metabolic activity that exists in certain structures, such as the small intestine from duodenum to ileum or in embryos from animal to vegetal poles, in which metabolic activity is highest in one region and becomes progressively lower away from this region.
metabolic rate The rate of utilization of energy. This is usually measured at a time when the subject is completely at rest and in a fasting state. Energy used is calculated from the amount of oxygen used during the test. SEE: *basal metabolic rate; metabolism, basal.*
metabolism [Gr. *metaballein,* to change, + *-ismos,* state of] All energy and material transformations that occur within living cells; the sum of all physical and chemical changes that take place within an organism. It includes material changes (i.e., changes undergone by substances during all periods of life, such as growth, maturity, and senescence) and energy changes (i.e., all transformations of chemical energy of foodstuffs to mechanical energy or heat). Metabolism involves two fundamental processes: anabolism (assimilation or building-up processes) and catabolism (disintegration or tearing-down processes). Anabolism is the conversion of food molecules into living cells and tissue; catabolism is the breakdown of complex chemicals into simpler ones, often producing waste products to be excreted. Catabolism also includes cell respiration for the formation of ATP and release of heat energy. **metabolic** (mĕt″ă-bŏl′ĭk), *adj.*

basal m. Lowest level of energy expenditure. It is determined when the body is at complete rest. For an average person, basal metabolism is measured in various ways. In terms of large calories (Cal), measurement is about 1500 to 1800 per day; in terms of body weight, measurement is 1 Cal/kg per hour; in terms of body surface, measurement is 40 Cal/m_2 per hour.

carbohydrate m. The sum of the physical and chemical changes involved in the breakdown and synthesis of carbohydrates in the body. All carbohydrates are digested to monosaccharides and absorbed as such principally in the form of hexoses, of which glucose is the principal one. In the liver and muscles, glucose may be converted to glycogen. In all cells, glucose is oxidized to carbon dioxide and water, with energy released in the forms of ATP and heat. These reactions require the presence of insulin and other hormones such as thyroxine, glucagon, and corticosteroids. In the process, many intermediate compounds are formed, among them lactic acid.

constructive m. The building-up processes by which complex substances are synthesized from simple carbohydrates, amino acids, fats, and other nutrients. SYN: *anabolism; assimilation.*

destructive m. The breakdown or decomposition of substances into their simple constituents. SYN: *catabolism.*

fat m. The digestion of fats to fatty acids and glycerol. Following absorption they may be reconverted to neutral fats and stored as adipose tissue or oxidized to carbon dioxide and water with the release of energy. Fats may be formed from excess carbohydrates or excess dietary amino acids. In the utilization of fats, the liver plays an important role in the desaturation of fatty acids. Fat metabolism also involves the formation and utilization of substances related to fats, such as sterols and phospholipids.

intermediary m. The series of intermediate compounds formed during digestion before the final excretion or oxidation products are formed or eliminated from the body.

muscle m. SEE: *muscle metabolism.*

protein m. The chemical breakdown of proteins to amino acids and absorption. In the body, amino acids are reformed into body proteins; they are essential for normal growth, development, and repair of tissues. Amino acids in excess of protein synthesis requirements are deaminated; the NH_2 group is removed and converted to urea, which is excreted by the kidneys. The remaining carbon chain may be converted to a simple carbohydrate and oxidized to produce energy.

purine m. Metabolism involving nucleic acids, present in nuclei of cells, in which they are combined with proteins to form nucleoproteins. In the breakdown of nucleic acid, uric acid, one of the end products, is formed.

metabolite (mĕ-tăb′ō-līt) Any product of metabolism.

metabolize (mĕ-tăb′ō-līz) [Gr. *metaballein,* to change] **1.** To alter the character of a food substance biochemically. **2.** To break down a compound to its constituents, by biological mechanisms.

metacarp- SEE: *metacarpo-.*

metacarpal [Gr. *meta,* after, beyond, over, + *karpos,* wrist] **1.** Pert. to the bones of the metacarpus. **2.** Any of the bones of the metacarpus. SEE: *hand.*

metacarpectomy (mĕt″ă-kăr-pĕk′tō-mē) [″ + ″ + *ektome,* excision] Surgical excision or resection of one or more metacarpal bones.

metacarpo-, metacarp- (mĕt-ă-căr″pō) [Gr. *meta,* after, beyond, over + Gr. *karpos,* wrist] Combining form meaning *metacarpus* (bones of the hand).

metacarpophalangeal (mĕt″ă-kăr″pō-fă-lăn′jē-ăl) Concerning the metacarpus and the phalanges.

metacarpus (mĕt″ă-kăr′pŭs) [″ + *karpos,* wrist] The five metacarpal bones of the palm of the hand. SEE: *carpometacarpal.*

metacentric (mĕt″ă-sĕn′trĭk) Term indicating a chromosome with the centromere in the median position, making the arms of the chromosome equal in length.

metacercaria (mĕt″ă-sĕr-kā′rē-ă) The encysted stage in the life of a trematode. This stage occurs in an intermediate host prior to transfer to the definitive host.

metachromasia, metachromatism (mĕt″ă-krō-mā′zē-ă, -krōm′ă-tĭzm) [Gr. *meta,* change, + *chroma,* color] Condition in which different components of the same tissue stain different colors or shades of color. The colors are different from that of the dye used. **metachromatic** (mĕt″ă-krō-măt′ĭk), *adj.*

metachromatic granules SEE: *granule, metachromatic.*

metachromatic leukodystrophy SEE: under *leukodystrophy.*

metachromophil (mĕt-ă-krōm′ō-fĭl) [″ + *chroma,* color, + *philein,* to love] Not reacting normally to staining.

metachrosis (mĕt-ă-krō′sĭs) The ability to change color in some animals, as in the chameleon.

metacognition (mĕt-ă-kŏg-nĭsh′ŭn) *pl.* **metacognitions** Awareness of the knowledge one possesses and one's ability to apply that knowledge. SEE: *insight.*

metacone [Gr. *meta,* after, beyond, over, + *konos,* cone] The distobuccal cusp of an upper molar tooth.

metaconid (mĕt-ă-kŏn′ĭd) The mesiolingual cusp of a lower molar tooth.

metaconule (mĕt-ă-kŏn′ūl) The distal intermediate cusp of an upper molar tooth.

metagenesis [″ + *genesis,* generation, birth] Alternation of generations, esp. involving regular alternation of sexual with asexual reproduction, as seen in some fungi.

Metagonimus (mĕt″ă-gŏn′ĭ-mŭs) [″ + *gonimos,* productive] A genus of flukes belonging to the family Heterophyidae.

M. yokogawai A species of intestinal flukes common in the Middle and Far East that normally infests the intestines of dogs, cats, and other animals, but is also commonly found in humans. Intermediate hosts are snails and fish, esp. a species of trout, *Plecoglossus altivelis.*

metainfective (mĕt″ă-ĭn-fĕk′tĭv) Occurring subsequent to an infection.

metakinesis (mĕt″ă-kĭ-nē′sĭs) Moving apart, esp. the moving of the two chromatids of each chromosome away from each other as they move to opposite poles in the anaphase of mitosis.

metalbumin (mĕt-ăl-bū′mĭn) The mucin present in ovarian cysts. SYN: *pseudomucin.*

metal fume fever A syndrome resembling influenza produced by inhalation of excessive concentrations of metallic oxide fumes such as zinc oxide or antimony, arsenic, brass, cadmium, cobalt, copper, iron, lead, magnesium, manganese, mercury, nickel, or tin. It occurs in persons whose occupations lead to exposure to these metals. This disorder is also called brass founder's fever (brass chills) and spelter's fever (zinc chills). SEE: *polymer fume fever.*

SYMPTOMS: The onset of symptoms is usually delayed. There are chills, weakness, lassitude, and profound thirst, followed some hours later by sweating and anorexia. Occasionally, there is mild inflammation of the eyes and respiratory tract. The symptoms are more acute at the beginning of the work week than at the end. This is felt to be due to the individual's adapting to the fumes as exposure continues.

FIRST AID: Therapy includes analgesics, antipyretics, and rest.

metallesthesia (mĕt″ăl-ĕs-thē′sē-ă) [Gr. *metallon,* metal, + *aisthesis,* sensation] Recognition of metals by touching them.

metallic **1.** Pert. to metal. **2.** Composed of or resembling a metal.

metallic tinkling A peculiar ringing or bell-like auscultatory sound in pneumothorax over large pulmonary cavities.

metalloenzyme (mĕ-tăl″ō-ĕn′zīm) An enzyme that contains a metal ion in its structure.

metallophilia (mĕ-tăl″ō-fĭl′ē-ă) [″ + *philein,* to love] The property of some tissues of binding certain metal salts.

metallophobia (mĕ″tăl-ō-fō′bē-ă) [″ + *phobos,* fear] Abnormal fear of metals and metallic objects and of touching them.

metalloporphyrin (mĕ-tăl″ō-por′fĭ-rĭn) Porphyrin combined with a metal, such as iron to form hemoglobin, or with magnesium to form chlorophyll.

metalloprotein (mĕ-tăl″ō-prō′tē-ĭn) A protein bound to metal ions.

metallotherapy (mĕt″ăl-ō-thĕr′ă-pē) [″ + *therapeuein,* to heal] Treatment of disease by applying metals to the affected part.

metallurgy (mĕt″ăl-ŭr′jē) [″ + *ergon,* work] Science of obtaining metals from their ores, refining them, and making them into various shapes and forms.

metamer (mĕt′ă-mĕr) Something similar to but different from something else (e.g., isomers of chemical compounds).

metamere (mĕt′ă-mēr) [Gr. *meta,* after, beyond, over, + *meros,* part] One of a series of similar segments arranged in a linear series and making up the body of an animal such as an earthworm.

metamerism (mĕ-tăm′ĕr-ĭzm) **1.** Isomerism. **2.** Isomerism consisting of segments or metameres. **metameric** (mĕt-ă-mĕr′ĭk), *adj.*

metamorphopsia (mĕt″ă-mor-fŏp′sē-ă) [Gr. *meta,* after, beyond, over, + *morphe,* form, + *opsis,* vision] **1.** Distortion of a visual image. **2.** Distorted vision.

metamyelocyte (mĕt″ă-mī-ĕl′ō-sīt) A transitional cell intermediate in development between a myelocyte and a mature granular leukocyte. SYN: *juvenile cell.*

metanephrine (mĕt″ă-nĕf′rĭn) An inactive metabolite of epinephrine.

metanephrogenic (mĕt″ă-nĕf′rō-jĕn′ĭk) [″ + *nephros,* kidney, + *gennan,* to produce] Concerning the part of the caudal mesoderm of the embryo that forms metanephric tubules of the kidney.

metanephros (mĕt″ă-nĕf′rŏs) *pl.* **metanephroi** [″ + *nephros,* kidney] The permanent kidney of amniotes (reptiles, birds, and mammals). Part of the metanephros develops from the caudal portion of the intermediate cell mass or nephrotome; the remaining portion is derived from a bud of the mesonephric duct.

metaneutrophil (mĕt-ă-nū′trō-fĭl) [″ + L. *neuter,* neither, + Gr. *philein,* to love] Not staining normally with neutral dyes.

metaparadigm (mĕt-ă-păr-ă-dīm′) The concepts that identify the phenomena of central interest to a discipline; the propositions that describe those concepts and their relationships to each other.

metaphase (mĕt′ă-fāz) [″ + *phasis,* an appearance] The second stage of mitosis in which the pairs of chromatids line up on the equator of the cell. Each pair is connected at the centromere, which is attached to a spindle fiber. Metaphase follows prophase and precedes anaphase, in which the chromatids become chromosomes and are pulled to opposite poles of the cell. SEE: *cell division* for illus; *mitosis.*

metaphrenia (mĕt″ă-frē′nē-ă) [″ + *phren,* mind] The mental state of turning away from family interests toward personal goals such as business.

metaphysis (mĕ-tăf′ĭ-sĭs) *pl.* **metaphyses** [Gr. *meta,* after, beyond, over, + *phyein,* to grow] The portion of a developing long bone between the diaphysis, or shaft, and the epiphysis; the growing portion of a bone. **metaphyseal,** *adj.*

metaphysitis (mĕt″ă-fĭs-ī′tĭs) [″ + ″ + *itis,* inflammation] Inflammation of the metaphysis of a bone.

metaplasia (mĕt″ă-plā′zē-ă) [″ + *plassein,* to form] Conversion of one kind of tissue into a form that is not normal for that tissue. **metaplastic** (mĕt-ă-plăs′tĭk), *adj.*

myeloid m. Development of marrow tissue at sites in which it would not normally occur.

metapophysis (mĕt″ă-pŏf′ĭ-sĭs) [″ + *apophysis,* a process] Mammillary process on the superior articular processes of a vertebra.

metaprotein Derived protein resulting from the action of acid or alkali, in which the molecule is changed to form a protein that is insoluble in neutral solvents but is soluble in alkali or weak acid. SEE: *protein.*

metaproterenol sulfate (mĕt″ă-prō-tĕr′ĕ-nōl) An adrenergic stimulant used to treat bronchospasm and bronchial asthma. It is effective when given by inhalation.

metaraminol bitartrate (mĕt″ă-răm′ĭ-nŏl) A drug used for its pressor effect in treating hypotension.

metarteriole (mĕt″ăr-tē′rē-ōl) A small vessel connecting an arteriole to a venule from which true capillaries are given off. SYN: *precapillary.*

metarubricyte A normoblast, the last nucleated stage in the development of an erythrocyte. SEE: *erythrocyte* for illus.

metastasis (mĕ-tăs′tă-sis) *pl.* **metastases** [″ + *stasis,* stand] **1.** Movement of bacteria or body cells (esp. cancer cells) from one part of the body to another. **2.** Change in location of a disease or of its manifestations or transfer from one organ or part to another not directly connected. SEE: illus.

The usual application is to the manifestation of a malignancy as a secondary growth arising from the primary growth in a new location. The malignant cells may spread through the lymphatic circulation, the bloodstream, or avenues such as the cerebrospinal fluid. **metastatic** (mĕt″ă-stăt′ĭk), *adj.*

metastasize (mĕ-tăs′tă-sīz) To invade distant structures of the body. To disseminate widely.

metastatic survey Procedure in which various structures of the body are investigated, esp. by x-ray or imaging, to demonstrate any spread of cancer.

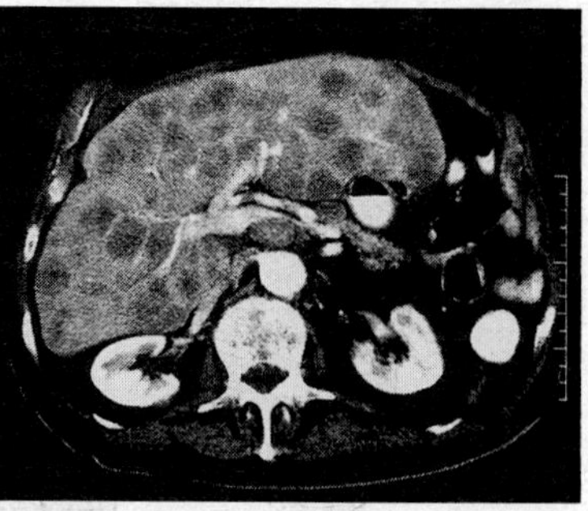

METASTASES

CT scan of liver (upper left) with round metastatic tumors (Courtesy of Harvey Hatch, MD, Curry General Hospital)

metasternum (mĕt″ă-stĕr′nŭm) Xiphoid process of the sternum.

metatarsal (mĕt″ă-tăr′săl) ABBR: MT. **1.** Concerning the metatarsal arch of the foot. **2.** Any of the bones of the metatarsus.

metatarsalgia (mĕt″ă-tăr-săl′jē-ă) [″ + *tarsos,* a broad flat surface, + *algos,* pain] Pain that emanates from the heads of the metatarsal bones and worsens with weight bearing or palpation.

metatarsectomy (mĕt″ă-tăr-sĕk′tō-mē) [″ + ″ + *ektome,* excision] Removal of the metatarsus or a metatarsal bone.

metatarsophalangeal (mĕt″ă-tăr″sō-fă-lăn′jē-ăl) [″ + ″ + *phalanx,* closely knit row] ABBR: MTP. Concerning the metatarsus and phalanges of the toes.

metatarsus (mĕt″ă-tăr′sŭs) [″ + *tarsos,* a broad flat surface] The region of the foot between the tarsus and phalanges that includes the five metatarsal bones. SEE: *foot.*

metatarsus primus varus Inturning of the first metatarsal bone of the foot.

metatarsus varus A congenital deformity of the foot involving adduction of the forefoot. When the child walks, the foot toes in. SEE: illus.

metathalamus (mĕt″ă-thăl′ă-mŭs) [″ + *thalamos,* a chamber] The posterior part of the thalamus including the two geniculate bodies.

metathesis (mĕ-tăth′ĕ-sĭs) [″ + *thesis,* placement] **1.** A changing of places. **2.** Forcible transference of a disease process from one part to another, where it will be more accessible for treatment or where it causes less inconvenience. **3.** Double decomposition of two chemical compounds.

metatrophia (mĕt-ă-trō′fē-ă) [″ + *trophe,* nourishment] **1.** A wasting due to malnutrition. **2.** A change in diet.

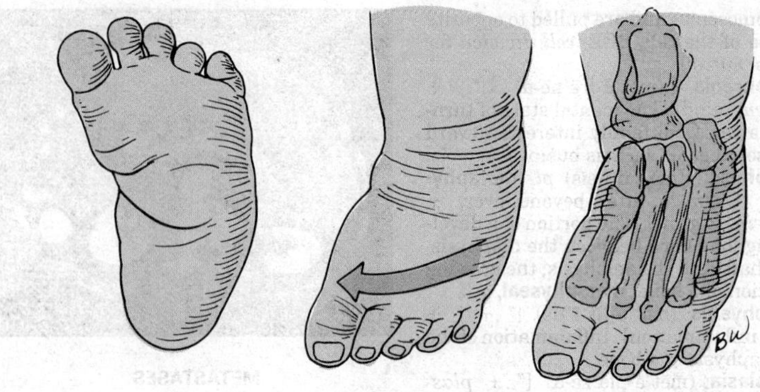

METATARSUS VARUS

metatypical (mĕt″ă-tĭp′ĭ-kăl) Tissue elements similar to those of other tissues at the same site, but having components that are disorganized.

metaxalone (mĕ-tăks′ă-lōn) A centrally acting skeletal muscle relaxant.

metazoa [″ + *zoon,* animal] A term used for the multicellular animals, in contrast to unicellular forms called protozoa.

Metchnikoff's theory (mĕch′nĭ-kŏfs) [Elie Metchnikoff, Russian biologist and zoologist in France, 1845–1916] The theory, developed in 1883, that the body is protected against infection by cells, such as leukocytes and phagocytes, that attack and destroy invading microorganisms. SEE: *phagocytosis.*

metencephalon (mĕt″ĕn-sĕf′ă-lŏn) [Gr. *meta,* after, beyond, over, + *enkephalos,* brain] The anterior portion of the embryonic rhombencephalon, from which the cerebellum and pons arise. SEE: *hindbrain.*

meteorism (mē′tē-or-ĭzm) [Gr. *meteorizein,* to raise up] Distention of the abdomen or intestines due to the presence of gas. SYN: *tympanites.*

meteoropathy (mē″tē-ĕ-rŏp′ă-thē) [″ + *pathos,* disease, suffering] Illness due to climatic conditions.

meteorotropism (mē″tē-ō-rŏt′rō-pĭzm) The influence of meteorological events on biological conditions and events, such as death rate, disease incidence, and birth rate. **meteorotropic** (mē″tē-ō-rō-trŏp′ĭk), *adj.*

meter (mē′tĕr) [Gr. *metron,* measure] ABBR: M. A linear standard of measurement in the Système International d' Unités (SI system) that is equal to about 39.37 inches. Also spelled *metre* in certain European countries.

metergasis (mĕt″ĕr-gā′sĭs) [Gr. *meta,* change, + *ergon,* work] Change or alteration in function.

metestrus (mĕ-tĕs′trŭs) [″ + L. *oistros,* mad desire] Period following estrus and preceding diestrus. SEE: *estrus.*

metformin An oral antidiabetic agent used to treat elevated blood sugar levels in patients with type 2 (adult-onset) diabetes mellitus. It normalizes blood sugar levels by reducing the production of glucose by the liver and by increasing sensitivity of peripheral tissues to the effects of insulin. Trade name is Glucophage.

CAUTION: This agent should not be used in patients with renal failure, because of the risk of metabolic acidosis.

methacholine chloride (mĕth″ă-kō′lēn) A parasympathomimetic bronchoconstrictor similar to acetylcholine, used as an aerosol in different strengths in airway challenge tests.

CAUTION: This substance should be used only for diagnostic purposes under the supervision of a physician trained in and thoroughly familiar with all aspects to the technique. Emergency resuscitation devices and medication should be available to treat respiratory distress.

methadone hydrochloride A synthetic opioid analgesic with a long duration of action, used primarily to treat pain and to detoxify or maintain patients who are addicted to narcotic pain relievers. Methadone is habit-forming and subject to abuse; its use should be carefully supervised. In well-run treatment programs, its use has been associated with reductions in illegal drug use, transmission of human immunodeficiency virus, and criminal behaviors.

methamphetamine hydrochloride (měth″ăm-fĕt′ă-mēn) A sympathomimetic drug used as a stimulant or weight-loss promoter. It is a controlled substance that causes euphoria and has a high potential for abuse.

methane CH_4; a colorless, odorless, inflammable gas. It is produced as a result of putrefaction and fermentation of organic matter. SYN: *marsh gas*.

methanol CH_3OH; a poisonous, volatile, inflammable alcohol, distilled from wood products and found in many solvents, gasolines, and antifreeze. It is toxic if ingested and may cause serious neurological consequences, visual impairment, or death. SYN: *methyl alcohol; wood alcohol*. SEE: *methyl alcohol* in *Poisons and Poisoning Appendix*.

methaqualone hydrochloride (mĕ-thă′kwă-lōn) A hypnotic and sedative that has become a drug of abuse. Because of the potential for abuse of this drug, it is no longer distributed in the U.S.

methazolamide (měth″ă-zō′lă-mīd) A carbonic acid inhibitor used in treating glaucoma.

methemalbumin (mĕt″hĕm-ăl-bū′mĭn) The abnormal combination of heme with albumin instead of globulin. It is present in blackwater fever and paroxysmal nocturnal hemoglobinuria.

methemoglobin (mĕt-hē″mō-glō′bĭn) [Gr. *meta,* across, + *haima,* blood, + L. *globus,* globe] SYMB: metHb. A form of hemoglobin in which the ferrous iron has been oxidized to ferric iron. Methemoglobin cannot transport oxygen. The presence of metHb in the blood may be due to toxic substances such as aniline dyes, potassium chlorate, or nitrate-contaminated water and to atypical responses to benzocaine-like analgesics, among other causes. Methemoglobin also is present in patients with a hereditary deficiency of methemoglobin reductase.

m. reductase An enzyme found in significant amounts in erythrocytes that catalyzes the reduction of methemoglobin in conjunction with the coenzyme nicotine adenine dinucleotide phosphate and other enzymes.

methemoglobinemia (mĕt″hē-mō-glōb″ĭ-nē′mē-ă) [″ + ″ + ″ + *haima,* blood] The clinical condition in which more than 1% of hemoglobin in blood has been oxidized to the ferric (Fe^{3+}) form. The most common sign is cyanosis, because the oxidized hemoglobin does not transport oxygen. Very high concentrations of methemoglobin in the blood (i.e., greater than 30%) may produce dizziness, drowsiness, headache, or more severe neurological symptoms. Coma, seizures, and cardiac arrhythmias may occur with levels greater than 55%. Methylene blue is used as an antidote.

congenital m. Elevated levels of methemoglobin in the blood, resulting from one of several hereditary deficiencies of methemoglobin reductase. Affected persons may appear mildly cyanotic but are rarely symptomatic.

methemoglobinuria (mĕt″hē-mō-glōb″ĭ-nū′rē-ă) [″ + ″ + ″ + *ouron,* urine] Presence of methemoglobin in the urine.

methenamine (měth-ĕn′ă-mēn) A urinary antiseptic. Methenamine was previously called hexamethylenamine.

m. mandelate A urinary antiseptic that derives its activity from the release of formaldehyde. Trade name is Mandelamine.

methene Methylene.

methicillin-resistant Staphylococcus aureus ABBR: MRSA. *Staphylococcus aureus* organisms that are resistant to the antibacterial action of methicillin, a penicillinase-resistant penicillin antibiotic. These pathogens are resistant to all penicillins and cephalosporins. Vancomycin is the drug of choice.

methicillin sodium (měth″ĭ-sĭl′ĭn) A semisynthetic penicillinase-resistant penicillin.

methimazole (měth-ĭm′ă-zōl) A drug that inhibits the synthesis of thyroid hormones. It is used in treating hyperthyroidism.

methiodal sodium (měth-ī′ō-dăl) A radiopaque compound used in x-ray examination of the urinary tract.

methionine (měth-ī′ō-nīn) A sulfur-containing essential amino acid.

methocarbamol (měth″ō-kăr′bă-mŏl) A centrally acting muscle relaxant.

method [Gr. *methodos*] The systematic manner, procedure, or technique in performing details of an operation, tests, treatment, or any act. SEE: *algorithm; maneuver; stain; test; treatment*.

Feldenkrais m. SEE: *Feldenkrais method*.

methodology (měth″ŏ-dŏl′ō-jē) [″ + *logos,* word, reason] The system of principles and procedures used in scientific endeavors.

methohexital sodium (měth″ō-hĕk′sĭ-tăl) An ultrashort-acting barbiturate used as an anesthetic.

methotrexate (měth″ō-trĕk′sāt) An inhibitor of dihydrofolate reductase that is used to treat rheumatoid arthritis, Crohn's disease, psoriasis, and several cancers. It also has been used, with misoprostol, to induce abortion. Side effects to the use of this drug may include suppression of bone marrow production of blood cells, hepatitis, and others.

methotrimeprazine (měth″ō-trī-mĕp′ră-zēn) A tranquilizer and analgesic.

methoxamine hydrochloride (mĕ-thŏk′să-mēn) An adrenergic used to maintain blood pressure in hypotensive states by causing vasoconstriction. It is also used to end attacks of paroxysmal atrial tachycardia.

methoxsalen (mĕ-thŏk′să-lĕn) A psoralen used in treating vitiligo, eczema, mycosis fungoides, and psoriasis. Trade name is Oxsoralen. SEE: *psoralen; psoriasis; PUVA therapy; trioxsalen*.

methoxyflurane (mĕ-thŏk″sē-floo′rān) A general anesthetic administered by inhalation for procedures of short duration. Its renal toxicity prevents its being used for prolonged anesthesia.

methscopolamine bromide (mĕth″skō-pŏl′ă-mēn) An anticholinergic drug rarely used in treating gastric hyperacidity and hypermotility.

methsuximide (mĕth-sŭk′sĭ-mīd) An anticonvulsant used in treating epilepsy.

methyclothiazide (mĕth″ĭ-klō-thī′ă-zīd) An antihypertensive and diuretic.

methyl (mĕth′ĭl) [Gr. *methy,* wine, + *hyle,* wood] In organic chemistry, the radical CH_3^-, seen, for instance, in the formula for methyl alcohol, CH_3OH.

m. alcohol SEE: under *alcohol*.

m. mercury An organic mercury compound produced by marine and soil bacteria. The level of methyl mercury increases in fish as it increases in polluted water. It is toxic to humans, esp. children.

m. orange A dye used as a pH indicator.

m. purine An oxidation product of purine. Includes caffeine, theophylline, and theobromine. SEE: *aminopurine; oxypurine*.

m. salicylate Wintergreen oil. It is produced synthetically or from distillation of leaves of sweet birch, has a characteristic odor, and is commonly used in liniment or ointment form for use as a topical analgesic balm and counterirritant.

m. violet Stain employed in histology and bacteriology.

methyl alcohol poisoning Intoxication with methanol (methyl alcohol). The initial primary consequences are depression of central nervous system function (including coma or convulsions), visual disturbances (including permanent blindness) due to the concentration of the toxin in the vitreous humor and optic nerve, headache, abdominal cramping, nausea, weakness, and an anion-gap metabolic acidosis.

TREATMENT: Fluids and electrolyte and acid-base balance should be carefully monitored and adjusted. Methanol may be removed from the bloodstream by hemodialysis. SEE: *Poisons and Poisoning Appendix*.

methylate (mĕth′ĭ-lāt) **1.** A compound of methyl alcohol and a base. **2.** To introduce the methyl group, CH_3, into a chemical compound. **3.** To mix with methyl alcohol.

methylation (mĕth″ĭ-lā′shŭn) The addition of methyl groups to a compound.

methylcellulose A tasteless powder that becomes swollen and gummy when wet. Methylcellulose is used as a bulk substance in foods and laxatives and as an adhesive or emulsifier.

methylcytosine (mĕth″ĭl-sī′tō-sĭn) A derivative of pyrimidine present in some nucleic acids.

methyldopa (mĕth″ĭl-dō′pă) An antihypertensive used in treating essential hypertension.

methyldopate hydrochloride (mĕth″ĭl-dō′pāt) An antihypertensive used in treating essential hypertension. Trade name is Aldomet.

methylene (mĕth′ĭ-lēn) The chemical radical $=CH_2^-$.

methylene blue (mĕth′ĭ-lēn) A dark green dye available as a crystalline powder. It produces a distinct blue stain. It is used for treatment of severe methemoglobinemia.

methylenophil (mĕth″ĭ-lĕn′ō-fĭl) Something that stains easily with methylene blue.

methylergonovine maleate (mĕth″ĭl-ĕr″gō-nō′vēn) A drug of the ergot alkaloid type. It is used to stimulate uterine contractions and to treat migraine. Trade name is Methergine.

methylmalonic acidemia An inherited metabolic disease caused by inability to convert methylmalonic acid to succinic acid. Clinically, signs are failure to grow, mental retardation, and severe metabolic acidosis. One form of the disease will respond to vitamin B_{12} given either in utero or to the mother prior to delivery.

methylmercury (mĕ-thĭl-mĕr′kū-rē) An esp. toxic form of mercury that is readily taken into the body through the skin or the respiratory tract. SEE: *mercury poisoning*.

methyl methacrylate (mĕth″ĭl-mĕth-ăk′crē-layt) A polymer, made from methacrylic acid, used as a bone cement, bonding agent, drug-delivery vehicle, and tissue adhesive. Its use is sometimes associated with hypotension, fat or air embolism, or other complications.

PATIENT CARE: Care depends on the location of the cemented site. Hospital policy for documenting prosthesis insertion should be followed.

CAUTION: Glue polymeric mixture may harden before the prosthesis has been appropriately placed.

---

methylparaben (mĕth″ĭl-păr′ă-bĕn) An antifungal agent used as a preservative in pharmaceuticals.

methylphenidate hydrochloride (mĕth″ĭl-fĕn′ĭ-dāt) A drug that is chemically related to amphetamine. It is used in treating narcolepsy and attention deficit disorder.

methylprednisolone (mĕth″ĭl-prĕd′nĭ-sō-lōn) An adrenal corticosteroid.

4-methylpyrazole (mĕ-thĭl-pĭr′ă-zōl) An intravenous antidote for ethylene glycol poisoning.

methylrosaniline chloride (mĕth″ĭl-rō-zăn′ĭ-lĭn) Previously used name for gentian violet.

methyltestosterone (mĕth″ĭl-tĕs-tŏs′tĕr-ōn) An androgenic steroid hormone.

methyltransferase (mĕth″ĭl-trăns′fĕr-ās) An enzyme that catalyzes the transfer of a methyl group from one compound to another.

methylxanthine A group of naturally occurring agents present in caffeine, theophylline, and theobromine. They act on the central nervous system, stimulate the myocardium, relax smooth muscle, and promote diuresis. A commonly prescribed methylxanthine is theophylline, which is used primarily to treat asthma and chronic obstructive pulmonary disease.

methysergide maleate (mĕth″ĭ-sĕr′jīd) A vasoconstrictor used to prevent and treat vascular headaches. If it is used regularly, it may cause retroperitoneal fibrosis. SEE: *carcinoid syndrome; serotonin.*

metmyoglobin (mĕt-mī″ō-glō′bĭn) Myoglobin with the ferrous ion in the heme oxidized to the ferric ion.

metocurine iodide (mĕt″ō-kū′rēn) A skeletal muscle relaxant occasionally used in surgery or electroconvulsive therapy.

metol Monomethy-*p*-aminophelol sulfate, one of two developing agents used in dental radiographic developing solutions. Its primary function is to act quickly to bring out the shades of gray in a radiographic image.

metonymy (mĕ-tŏn′ĭ-mē) [Gr. *meta,* after, beyond, over, + *onyma,* name] Mental confusion exhibited by an individual's use of a word that is not the precise term intended but instead has a loosely related meaning (e.g., rifle in place of war; apple in place of ball).

metopagus (mĕ-tŏp′ă-gŭs) [Gr. *metopon,* forehead, + *pagos,* thing fixed] Conjoined twins united at the forehead.

metopic (mē-tŏp′ĭk) [Gr. *metopon,* forehead] Relating to the forehead.

metopion (mē-tō′pē-ŏn) Craniometric point in forehead midway between frontal eminences. SYN: *glabella.*

metopism (mĕt′ō-pĭzm) Persistence of the metopic suture in an adult.

metoprolol tartrate A beta-1 selective beta blocker that lowers blood pressure, slows the heart rate, and reduces the heart's contractility but is less likely than nonselective beta blockers to cause wheezing.

metoxenous (mĕt″ŏk-sē′nŭs) [Gr. *meta,* change, + *xenos,* host] Denoting a parasite living on different hosts at different stages of development. SYN: *heterecious.*

metoxeny (mĕt-ŏk′sĕ-nē) Condition of being metoxenous.

metr- (mē′tr) [Gr.] SEE: *metro-.*

metralgia (mē-trăl′jē-ă) [Gr. *metra,* uterus, + *algos,* pain] Uterine pain. SYN: *hysteralgia; hysterodynia; uteralgia.*

metratonia (mē″tră-tō′nē-ă) Uterine atony occurring after childbirth.

metre (mē′tĕr) [Gr. *metron,* measure] Meter.

metrectasia (mē″trĕk-tā′zē-ă) [Gr. *metra,* uterus, + *ektasis,* extension] Dilatation of a nonpregnant uterus.

metrectopia (mē″trĕk-tō′pē-ă) [″ + *ektopos,* displaced] Displacement of the uterus.

metreurynter (mē-troo-rĭn′tĕr) [″ + *eurynein,* to stretch] An inflatable bag that is inserted in the os uteri and distended to dilate the cervix. SYN: *hystereurynter.*

metreurysis (mē-troo′rĭ-sĭs) Dilatation of the cervix uteri with the metreurynter.

metria (mē′trē-ă) Inflammation of the uterus during pregnancy.

metric system A system of weights and measures based on the meter (about 39.37 in.) as the unit of measurement, the gram (about 15.432 gr) as the unit of weight, and the liter (about 1.057 qt liquid or 0.908 qt dry measure) as the unit of volume.

CONVERSION RULES: (Approximate) To change grams (g) to grains (gr), multiply grams by 15. To change grains to grams, divide by 15. To change grams to avoirdupois ounces (oz), divide by 28.35. To change fluid ounces to milliliters, multiply by 30. SEE: *avoirdupois measure; troy weight; Weights and Measures Appendix.*

metriocephalic (mĕt″rē-ō-sĕ-făl′ĭk) [Gr. *metrios,* moderate, + *kephale,* head] A skull with a vertical index of 72 to 76.9.

metritis (mĕ-trī′tĭs) [Gr. *metra,* uterus, + *itis,* inflammation] Inflammation of the uterus. Metritis is designated endometritis if the endometrium is involved and myometritis if the musculature (myometrium) is involved.

chronic m. Metritis with an increase in fibrous tissue and infiltration of lymphocytes.

metrizamide (mĕ-trĭ′ză-mīd) A water-soluble radiographic contrast medium used to outline structures in the spinal canal during myelography. It occasionally may cause the patient to have seizures after the procedure.

metro-, metr- [Gr. *metra,* uterus] Combining form meaning *uterus.*
metrocarcinoma (mē″trō-kăr-sĭ-nō′mă) [″ + *karkinos,* cancer, + *oma,* tumor] Uterine carcinoma.
metrocele (mē′trō-sēl) [″ + *kele,* tumor, swelling] Uterine hernia.
metrocolpocele (mē″trō-kŏl′pō-sēl) [″+ *kolpos,* vagina, + *kele,* tumor, swelling] Protrusion of the uterus into the vagina, which pushes the vaginal wall downward. SEE: *procidentia.*
metrocystosis (mē″trō-sĭs-tō′sĭs) [″+ *kystis,* cyst, + *osis,* intensive] Formation of uterine cysts.
metrofibroma (mē-trō-fī-brō′mă) [″ + L. *fibra,* fiber, + *oma,* tumor] Uterine fibroma.
metromalacia (mē″trō-măl-ā′shē-ă) [″ + *malakia,* softness] Softening of the uterus.
metromalacosis (mē″trō-măl-ă-kō′sĭs) [″ + ″ + *osis,* condition] Softening of uterine tissues.
metronidazole An antibiotic used to treat infections caused by *Trichomonas vaginalis, Giardia lamblia,* amebic dysentery, anaerobic bacterial infections, and colitis caused by *Clostridium difficile.* Trade name is Flagyl.

CAUTION: This drug may depress the white blood cell count. Drinking alcohol while taking it may cause abdominal pain, nausea, or vomiting, as well as central nervous system symptoms such as vertigo, dizziness, and ataxia.

metronoscope (mĕ-trŏn′ō-skōp) A device for exposing written material to the eye at timed intervals in order to facilitate development of reading skills and speed.
metroparalysis (mē″trō-pă-răl′ĭ-sĭs) [Gr. *metra,* uterus, + *paralyein,* to disable] Uterine paralysis during or immediately following childbirth.
metroperitoneal (mē″trō-pĕr″ĭ-tō-nē′ăl) [″ + *peritonaion,* peritoneum] Concerning the uterus and the peritoneum.
metroperitonitis (mē″trō-pĕr″ĭ-tō-nī′tĭs) [″ + ″ + *itis,* inflammation] Inflammation of the uterus and surrounding peritoneum.
metrophlebitis (mē″trō-flē-bī′tĭs) [″ + *phleps,* vein, + *itis,* inflammation] Inflammation of the uterine veins.
metroplasty (mē″trō-plăs′tē) [″ + *plastikos,* formed] Plastic surgery on the uterus. SYN: *uteroplasty.*
metroptosis (mē-trō-tō′sĭs) [″ + *ptosis,* a dropping] Downward displacement or prolapse of the uterus.
metrorrhagia Intermenstrual bleeding. Bleeding between regular menses may be associated with either benign or malignant conditions and warrants further investigation.
metrorrhea (mē″trō-rē′ă) [″ + *rhoia,* flow] Abnormal uterine discharge.
metrorrhexis (mē″trō-rĕk′sĭs) [″+ *rhexis,* rupture] Rupture of the uterus.
metrosalpingitis (mē″trō-săl″pĭn-jī′tĭs) [″ + *salpinx,* tube, + *itis,* inflammation] Inflammation of the uterus and oviducts.
metrosalpingography (mē″trō-săl″pĭng-gŏg′ră-fē) [″ + ″ + *graphein,* to write] Hysterosalpinography.
metrostenosis (mē″trō-stĕn-ō′sĭs) [″ + *stenosis,* contraction] Contraction or narrowing of the uterine cavity.
metrotomy (mē-trŏt′ō-mē) Incision of the uterus. SYN: *hysterotomy.*
metrourethrotome (mĕt″rō-ū-rē′thrō-tōm) [Gr. *metron,* measure, + *ourethra,* urethra, + *tome,* incision] Device for incising the urethra and measuring depth to be incised.
-metry [Gr. *metrein,* to measure] Suffix meaning *to measure.*
metyrapone (mĕ-tēr′ă-pōn) A drug that inhibits adrenocortical secretion from the adrenal gland. It is used to treat excessive adrenocortical hormone secretion and to test the function of the adrenal gland.
metyrapone test One of several diagnostic tests to assess the integrity of the pituitary-adrenal axis, esp. used in the diagnosis of ACTH deficiencies and Cushing's disease. The drug metyrapone, which inhibits the secretion of cortisol by the adrenal glands, may be given at timed intervals during the day, or as a single nighttime dose. Depending on the method of administration, plasma levels of cortisol, 11-deoxycortisol, or adrenocorticotropic hormone, or urinary levels of 17-hydroxysteroid, are evaluated to assess the patient's response.
Mev, mev *million electron volts.*
Meynert's commissure (mī′nĕrts) [Theodor H. Meynert, Austrian neurologist, 1833–1892] Fibrous tract extending from the subthalamic body to the base of the third ventricle.
Meynet's nodes (mā-nāz′) [Paul C. H. Meynet, Fr. physician, 1831–1892] In rheumatic disease, nodules attached to the tendon sheaths and joints.
M.F.D. *minimum fatal dose.*
μg *microgram.*
Mg Symbol for the element magnesium.
mg *milligram.*
mgh *milligram hour.* Dosage of radiation obtained by application of 1.0 mg radium for 1 hr.
MGUS Monoclonal gammopathy of unclear significance.
MHC *major histocompatibility complex.*
mho (mō) [ohm spelled backward] Siemens.
MHz *megahertz.*
MI *myocardial infarction.*
MIC *minimal inhibitory concentration.*

mica (mī'kă) [L.] **1.** A crumb. **2.** A mineral composed of various silicates of metals. It occurs in thin, laminated scales.

micella, micelle (mī-sĕl'ă, mī-sĕl') A sphere of bile salt molecules, essential for the absorption of fatty acids in the small intestine, composed of a water-soluble exterior and a lipid-rich core.

miconazole nitrate (mĭ-kŏn'ă-zōl) An antifungal agent used for vaginal infections. Trade name is Monistat.

micr- SEE: *micro-*.

micra Pl. of micron.

micrencephalon (mī"krĕn-sĕf'ă-lon) [Gr. *mikros,* small, + *enkephalos,* brain] **1.** Cerebellum. **2.** Smallness of the brain. SEE: *cretinism*.

micrencephaly (mī"krĕn-sĕf'ă-lē) Abnormal smallness of the brain. **micrencephalous** (mī"krĕn-sĕf'ă-lŭs), *adj.*

micro-, micr- [Gr. *mikros,* small] SYMB: μ. Combining form meaning small.

microabscess (mī'krō-ăb'sĕs) [" + L. *abscessus,* a going away] A very small abscess.

microaerophilic (mī"krō-ā'ĕr-ō-fĭl"ĭk) [" + *aer,* air, + *philein,* to love] Growing at low amounts of oxygen; said of certain bacteria.

microaerosol A fine aerosol whose particles are of uniform size, usually less than 1 μm in diameter.

microalbuminuria The excretion of 30 mg or less of albumin in the urine per day. This level of urinary albumin loss is a risk factor for progressive renal failure in patients with diabetes. Angiotensin converting enzyme inhibitors have renally protective effects in patients with this finding.

microanalysis An analytical examination of minute amounts of material.

microanatomy Histology.

microaneurysm (mī"krō-ăn'ū-rĭzm) [" + *aneurysma,* a widening] A microscopic aneurysm.

microangiitis (mī"krō-ăn"jē-ī'tĭs) An inflammation of very small blood vessels.

microangiopathy (mī"krō-ăn"jē-ŏp'ă-thē) [" + *angeion,* vessel, + *pathos,* disease, suffering] Pathology of small blood vessels.

thrombotic m. The formation of blood clots in small blood vessels, such as occurs in thrombotic thrombocytopenic purpura and hemolytic uremic syndrome.

microangioscopy (mī"krō-ăn"jē-ŏs'kō-pē) [" + " + *skopein,* to examine] The use of microscopy to diagnose pathological changes in capillaries.

microarray (mī'krō-ăr-rā) A biological semiconductor or a microscopic integrated circuit that uses DNA instead of silicon to make biochemical calculations, esp. those involving genes.

microatelectasis Microscopic collapse of alveoli that does not involve the airways and may not appear on radiographic examination.

microbalance (mī'krō-băl"ăns) A scale or balance for measuring very small weight changes.

microbe (mī'krōb) [" + *bios,* life] A unicellular or small multicellular organism including bacteria, protozoa, some algae and fungi, viruses, and some worms. SEE: *microorganism*. **microbial, microbic** (mī-krō'bē-ăl, mī-krōb'ĭk), *adj.*

microbicide (mī-krō'bĭ-sīd) [" + *bios,* life, + L. *cidus,* kill] An agent that kills microbes. **microbicidal** (mī-krō"bĭ-sī'dăl), *adj.*

microbiological antagonism SEE: under *antagonism*.

microbiology (mī"krō-bī-ŏl'ō-jē) [" + *bios,* life, + *logos,* word, reason] Scientific study of microorganisms.

microbiophobia (mī"krō-bī"ō-fō'bē-ă) [" + " + *phobos,* fear] Abnormal fear of microbes.

microbiota (mī"krō-bī-ō'tă) Microscopic organisms of an area. SEE: *macrobiota*. **microbiotic** (mī"krō-bī-ŏt'ĭk), *adj.*

microblepharism, microblephary (mī"krō-blĕf'ăr-ĭzm, -ăr-ē) [" + *blepharon,* eyelid] Condition of having abnormally small eyelids.

microbrachia (mī"krō-brā'kē-ă) [" + *brachion,* arm] Abnormally small arms.

microbrachius (mī"krō-brā'kē-ŭs) [" + *brachion,* arm] A fetus with abnormally small arms.

microcardia (mī"krō-kăr'dē-ă) [Gr. *mikros,* small, + *kardia,* heart] Unusual smallness of the heart.

microcentrum (mī"krō-sĕn'trŭm) [" + *kentron,* center] **1.** Centrosome. **2.** Motor or dynamic center of a cell.

microcephalia (mī"krō-sĕf-ā'lē-ă) [" + *kephale,* head] Microcephaly.

microcephalus (mī"krō-sĕf'ă-lŭs) Individual with an exceptionally small head.

microcephaly (mī"krō-sĕf'ă-lē) Abnormal smallness of head (below 1350 cc capacity) often seen in mental retardation. **microcephalic, microcephalous** (mī"krō-sĕf-ăl'ĭk, mī"krō-sĕf'ă-lŭs), *adj.*

microcheilia (mī"krō-kī'lē-ă) [Gr. *mikros,* small, + *cheilos,* lip] Abnormal smallness of the lips.

microchemistry (mī"krō-kĕm'ĭs-trē) [" + *chemeia,* chemistry] Branch of chemistry analyzing specimens of minute quantity.

microcheiria, microchiria (mī"krō-kī'rē-ă) [" + *cheir,* hand] Abnormal smallness of the hands.

microcinematography (mī"krō-sĭn"ē-mă-tŏg'ră-fē) [" + *kinema,* motion, + *graphein,* to write] Motion pictures of microscopic objects.

microcirculation (mī"krō-sĭr"kū-lā'shŭn) Blood flow in the very small vessels (arterioles, capillaries, and venules). **microcirculatory,** *adj.*

Micrococcaceae (mī″krō-kŏk-ā′sē-ē) A family of bacteria belonging to the order Eubacteriales and containing the genera *Micrococcus, Sarcina,* and *Staphylococcus.*

Micrococcus (mī″krō-kŏk′ŭs) [Gr. *mikros,* small, + *kokkos,* berry] A genus of spherical gram-positive bacteria belonging to the family Micrococcaceae. Cells occur singly or in irregular groups.

micrococcus (mī″krō-kŏk′ŭs) *pl.* **micrococci** An organism of the genus *Micrococcus.*

microcolon Abnormally small colon.

microcoria (mī″krō-kō′rē-ă) [″ + *kore,* pupil] Smallness of the pupil of the eye.

microcornea Abnormally small cornea.

microcoulomb (mī″krō-koo′lŏm) A microunit of current electricity; one-millionth part (10^{-6}) of a coulomb.

microcrystalline (mī″krō-krĭs′tăl-īn, -ēn) Composed of microscopic crystals.

microcurie-hour The radiation produced by radioactive decay at the rate of 3.7×10^4 atoms per second.

microcyst (mī′krō-sĭst) A very small cyst.

microcyte A small erythrocyte (red blood cell) less than 5 μm in diameter.

microdactylia, microdactyly (mī″krō-dăk-tĭl′ē-ă, -dăk′tĭ-lē) [″ + *daktylos,* digit] Abnormal smallness of the fingers or toes.

microdissection (mī″krō-dī-sĕk′shŭn) [″ + L. *dissectio,* a cutting apart] Dissection with the aid of a microscope, esp. by utilization of a micromanipulator.

microdont (mī′krō-dŏnt) [″ + *odous,* tooth] Possessing very small teeth.

microdontia (mī″krō-dŏn′shē-ă) [″ + *odous,* tooth] Having abnormally small teeth or a single small tooth.

microdontism (mī″krō-dŏn′tĭzm) [″ + ″ + *-ismos,* condition] Microdontia.

microelectrophoresis Electrophoresis of minute quantities of a solution.

microembolus (mī″krō-ĕm′bō-lŭs) [″ + *embolos,* plug] A very small embolus.

microencapsulation Insertion of a drug or other active substance within a coating to improve the delivery of the active agent to a particular organ or tissue.

microencephaly (mī″krō-ĕn-sĕf′ă-lē) [″ + *enkephalos,* brain] Micrencephaly.

microenvironment The environment at the microscopic or cellular level.

microerythrocyte (mī″krō-ĕ-rĭth′rō-sīt) [″ + *erythros,* red, + *kytos,* cell] Microcyte.

microfarad (mī-krō-făr′ăd) A microunit of electrical capacity; one millionth of a farad.

microfauna (mī″krō-faw′nă) In a specific location, the animal life that is microscopic in size.

microfibril (mī″krō-fī′brĭl) A very small fibril.

microfiche (mī′krō-fēsh″) [Gr. *mikros,* small, + Fr. *fiche,* index card] A sheet of microfilm that enables a large number of library data and medical records to be stored in a small space.

microfilament (mī″krō-fĭl′ă-mĕnt) Submicroscopic fibrils of the protein actin that help give shape to a cell and contribute to movement, either within the cell or of the cell itself.

microfilaremia (mī″krō-fĭl″ă-rē′mē-ă) Presence of microfilariae in the blood.

microfilaria (mī″krō-fĭ-lā′rē-ă) The embryos of filarial worms. Microfilariae are present in the blood and tissues of one infected with filariasis and are of importance in the diagnosis of filarial infections.

microfilm A film containing a greatly reduced photoimage of printed or graphic matter.

microflora (mī″krō-flō′ră) In a specific area, the plant life that is microscopic in size.

microgamete (mī-krō-găm′ēt) [″ + *gametes,* spouse] Male reproductive cell in conjugation of protozoa.

microgamy (mī-krŏg′ă-mē) Union of male and female cells in certain lower forms.

microgastria (mī″krō-găs′trē-ă) [″ + *gaster,* stomach] Unusual smallness of the stomach.

microgenia (mī″krō-jĕn′ē-ă) [″ + *geneion,* chin] Abnormal smallness of the chin.

microgenitalism (mī″krō-jĕn′ĭ-tăl-ĭzm) [″ + L. *genitalia,* genitals, + Gr. *-ismos,* condition] Abnormal smallness of the external genitalia.

microglia (mī-krŏg′lē-ă) [″ + *glia,* glue] Cells of the central nervous system (CNS) present between neurons or next to capillaries. These cells may function as macrophages when they migrate to damaged CNS tissue. SEE: *gitter cell.*

microgliacyte (mī″krŏg′lē-ă-sīt) [″ + ″ + *kytos,* cell] An embryonic cell of the microglia.

microglioma (mī″krō-glī-ō′mă) [″ + ″ + *oma,* tumor] A tumor composed of microglial cells.

microglossia (mī-krō-glŏs′ē-ă) [″ + *glossa,* tongue] Abnormally small tongue.

micrognathia (mī-krō-nā′thē-ă) [″ + *gnathos,* jaw] Abnormal smallness of jaws, esp. the lower jaw.

microgonioscope (mī″krō-gō′nē-ō-skōp) [″ + *gonia,* angle, + *skopein,* to examine] Device for measuring the angles of the anterior chamber of the eye. It is used in studying glaucoma.

microgram ABBR: μg or mcg. One-millionth part of a gram; one-thousandth part of a milligram.

micrograph (mī′krō-grăf) [Gr. *mikros,* small, + *graphein,* to write] **1.** Apparatus for magnifying and recording minute movements. **2.** Photograph of an object seen through a microscope. SYN: *photomicrograph.*

micrography (mī-krŏg′ră-fē) **1.** Study of the physical appearance and characteristics of microscopic objects. **2.** Study of an object by use of a microscope.

microgyria (mī-krō-jĭr′ē-ă) [″ + *gyros,* circle] Abnormal smallness of cerebral convolutions.

microgyrus (mī″krō-jī′rŭs) [″ + *gyros,* circle] A small, malformed gyrus of the brain.

microhematuria Red blood cells that are not grossly obvious but are found instead on microscopic examination of a urine specimen. They may be found in patients with tumors of the urinary tract (kidneys, ureters, or bladder); glomerular diseases; kidney or ureteral stones; urinary tract infections; trauma; or in patients without obvious or demonstrable pathology. SYN: *microscopic hematuria.*

microhepatia (mī″krō-hē-păt′ē-ă) [″ + *hepar,* liver] Abnormally small size of the liver.

microhm (mī′krōm) A microunit of electrical resistance; one-millionth of an ohm.

microincineration Determination of the presence and distribution of inorganic matter in tissues by subjecting a microscopic section of tissue to high temperatures, which destroys organic matter and leaves mineral matter as ash.

microinjection Injection of substances into cells or minute vessels by means of a micropipette.

microinvasion (mī″krō-ĭn-vā′zhŭn) Invasion of the tissue adjacent to a carcinoma in situ. **microinvasive,** *adj.*

microleakage The microscopic seepage of oral fluids between the interface of the tooth and a dental restoration. Microleakage may lead to sensitivity or discoloration of the tooth. Caused by discrepancies between the coefficient of thermal expansion of the tooth structure and the restorative material, microleakage is an inherent weakness of many restorative materials, although it is minimal with glass ionomer and polycarboxylate cements.

microlentia (mī″krō-lĕn′shē-ă) Microphakia.

microlesion (mī″krō-lē′zhŭn) A very small lesion.

microliter (mī′krō-lē″tĕr) ABBR: μl. One-millionth part of a liter.

microlith (mī′krō-lĭth) [″ + *lithos,* stone] A very tiny stone.

microlithiasis (mī″krō-lĭ-thī′ă-sĭs) [″ + ″ + *-iasis,* process] The development of minute stones.

pulmonary alveolar m. Deposition of microscopic concretions throughout the lungs.

micromanipulation The use of minute instruments and magnification aids to perform surgical or other procedures on tissues. SEE: *gene splicing; micromanipulator; microsurgery.*

micromanipulator An apparatus by which extremely minute pipettes or needles can be manipulated under a microscope for microdissection, microinjection, or microsurgery.

micromazia (mī-krō-mā′zē-ă) [Gr. *mikros,* small, + *mastos,* breast] Abnormally small size of the breasts.

micromelia (mī″krō-mē′lē-ă) [″ + *melos,* limb] Abnormally small or short limbs.

micromelus (mī-krŏm′ĕ-lŭs) [″ + *melos,* limb] One who has abnormally small or short limbs.

micromere (mī′krō-mēr) [″ + *meros,* part] A small blastomere.

micrometastases Foci of tumor cells that are invisible to the naked eye or by routine imaging techniques but may be seen using microscopy with special stains or antibodies, or by other laboratory techniques.

micrometer (mī′krō-mē-ter) ABBR: μm. One millionth of a meter (10^{-6}); one thousandth of a millimeter (0.001 mm). SYN: *micron.*

micrometer (mī-krŏm′ĕ-tĕr) ABBR: μm. Device used for measuring small distances.

micromethod (mī″krō-mĕth′ŏd) Any chemical or physical procedure involving small amounts of material or tissue.

micrometry (mī-krŏm′ĕ-trē) [″ + *metron,* measure] Use of device, esp. a micrometer, to measure small objects or thickness.

micromicro- ($\mu\mu$**)** Prefix formerly used to indicate one trillionth (10^{-12}). The term currently used is *pico.*

micromicrogram (mī″krō-mī′krō-grăm) ABBR: $\mu\mu$g. Obsolete term for 1 millionth of a microgram; now called a picogram, or 10^{-12}gram.

micromicron (mī″krō-mī′krŏn) ABBR: $\mu\mu$. Obsolete term for picometer or 10^{-12} meter.

micromillimeter (mī-krō-mĭl′ĭ-mē-tĕr) ABBR: μmm. One millionth of a millimeter. SYN: *millimicron.*

micromole (mī′krō-mōl) One millionth, 10^{-6}, of a mole. SEE: *mole* (1).

micromolecular (mī″krō-mō-lĕk′ū-lăr) Composed of small molecules.

Micromonospora (mī″krō-mō-nŏs′por-ă) A genus of actinomycetes belonging to the family Streptomycetaceae.

micromyelia (mī″krō-mī-ē′lē-ă) [″ + *myelos,* marrow] Abnormally small-sized or short spinal cord.

micromyeloblast (mī-krō-mī′ĕl-ō-blăst) [″ + *myelos,* marrow, + *blastos,* germ] A small, immature myelocyte, often the predominating cell in myeloblastic leukemia.

micromyelolymphocyte (mī″krō-mī″ĕ-lō-lĭm′fō-sīt) [″ + ″ + L. *lympha,* lymph, + Gr. *kytos,* cell] Micromyeloblast.

micron An obsolete term for micrometer.

microneedle Extremely minute needle used in a micromanipulator for microdissection.

micronize To pulverize a substance into particles only a few micra in size.

micronodular (mī″krō-nŏd′ū-lăr) Having small nodules.

micronucleus (mī-krō-nū′klē-ŭs) *pl.* **micronuclei** [″ + L. *nucleus,* kernel] **1.** A small nucleus. **2.** The smaller of the two nuclei of ciliated protozoa; it contains the chromosomes.

micronutrient (mī″krō-nū′trē-ĕnt) A vitamin or mineral required by the body in very small amounts (micrograms or milligrams daily), such as beta carotene, biotin, chromium, copper, folate, manganese, selenium, and others.

micronychia (mī″krō-nĭk′ē-ă) [″ + *onyx,* nail] Possessing abnormally small nails.

microorganism (mī-krō-or′găn-ĭzm) [″ + *organon,* organ, + *-ismos,* condition] A living organism too small to be perceived with the naked eye, esp. a virus, bacterium, fungus, protozoan, or intracellular parasite, and some helminths. SYN: *germ; microbe.*

pathogenic m. Any microorganism capable of injuring its host; for example, by competing with it for metabolic resources, destroying its cells or tissues, or secreting toxins. The injurious microorganisms include viruses, bacteria, mycobacteria, fungi, protozoans, and some helminths. Pathogenic microorganisms may be carried from one host to another as follows: *Animal sources:* Some organisms are pathogenic for animals as well as humans and may be communicated to humans through direct, indirect, or intermediary animal hosts. *Airborne:* Pathogenic microorganisms (such as rhinoviruses, mycobacteria, or varicella) may be discharged into the air and inhaled by exposed persons. *Contact infections:* Direct transmission of microorganisms can occur by skin-to-skin contact, as in many sexually transmitted diseases. *Foodborne:* Food and water may contain pathogenic organisms acquired from the handling of the food by infected persons or through fecal or insect contamination. *Fomites:* Inanimate objects such as linens, books, cooking utensils, or clothing that can harbor microorganisms and could serve to transport them from one location to another. *Human carriers:* Asymptomatic individuals (e.g., "typhoid Mary") may harbor microorganisms without injury but transmit disease to others. *Insects:* Arthropoda or mosquitoes may transmit diseases by biting their hosts and depositing microorganisms into the bloodstream. Flies may deposit germs in food, water, or wounds. *Soilborne:* Spore-forming organisms (such as tetanus) in the soil may enter the body through a cut or wound. Vegetables and fruits, esp. root crops, may transmit microorganisms to the gastrointestinal tract.

PATIENT CARE: In health care settings, handwashing after patient contact can do more than any other intervention to limit the spread of pathogenic microorganisms to patients. A

micropannus Pathological condition in which a vascular sheet of tissue covers the corner of the eye. SEE: *pannus.*

microparasite (mī″krō-păr′ă-sīt) A parasitic microorganism.

micropathology (mī″krō-păth-ŏl′ō-jē) [Gr. *mikros,* small, + *pathos,* disease, + *logos,* word, reason] The use of a microscope to study diseases caused by microorganisms.

micropenis (mī″krō-pē′nĭs) An abnormally small penis. SYN: *microphallus.*

microphage, microphagus (mī′krō-fāj, mī-krŏf′ă-gŭs) [″ + *phagein,* to eat] A small phagocyte.

microphagocyte (mī″krō-făg′ō-sīt) [″ + ″ + *kytos,* cell] Microphage.

microphakia (mī″krō-fā′kē-ă) [″ + *phakos,* lens] Abnormally small crystalline lens. SYN: *microlentia.*

microphallus (mī-krō-făl′ŭs) [″ + *phallos,* penis] Micropenis.

microphobia (mī-krō-fō′bē-ă) [″ + *phobos,* fear] Abnormal fear of small objects.

microphone (mī′krō-fōn) [″ + *phone,* voice] Device for detecting and converting sound energy into an electronic signal, which is then transmitted.

microphonia (mī-krō-fō′nē-ă) Weakness of the voice.

microphonoscope (mī″krō-fō′nō-skōp) [Gr. *mikros,* small, + *phone,* voice, + *skopein,* to examine] Form of binaural stethoscope for magnifying sound.

microphotograph (mī″krō-fō′tō-grăf) [″ + *phos,* light, + *graphein,* to write] **1.** A photograph of extremely small size. **2.** A photograph on microfilm. **3.** Photomicrograph.

microphthalmia, microphthalmus (mī-krŏf-thăl′mē-ă, -mŭs) [″ + *ophthalmos,* eye] Abnormally small size of one or both eyes.

micropipette, micropipet An extremely small pipette used for measuring small amounts of fluid substances.

microplasia (mī″krō-plā′zē-ă) [″ + *plassein,* to form] Failure to attain full size, as in dwarfism.

microplethysmography (mī″krō-plĕth″ĭs-mŏg′ră-fē) [″ + *plethysmos,* increase, + *graphein,* to write] Detection of small changes in the volume of a part due to alteration in blood flow.

micropodia (mī-krō-pō′dē-ă) [″ + *pous,* feet] Unusually small size of the feet.

micropolariscope (mī″krō-pōl-ăr′ĭ-skōp) A microscope with a polarizer.

microprobe (mī′krō-prōb) A very small probe, suitable for use in microsurgery.

microprojection Projection of images of microscopic objects upon a screen.

microprosopia (mī″krō-prō-sō′pē-ă) [″ + *prosopon,* face] Abnormal smallness of the face.

micropsia (mī-krŏp′sē-ă) [″ + *opsis,* vision] Visual disorder in which objects seem smaller than they actually are. Seen in paralysis of accommodation, retinitis, and choroiditis.

micropuncture (mī″krō-pŭnk′chŭr) A very small incision or puncture of a structure such as a single cell.

micropus (mī-krō′pŭs) [″ + *pous,* feet] One with unusually small feet.

micropyle (mī′krō-pīl) [″ + *pyle,* gate] The opening in the ovum for entrance of the spermatozoon. Seen in the ova of some animals.

microradiography (mī″krō-rā″dē-ŏg′ră-fē) Technique of x-raying microscopic objects. The pictures are usually enlarged.

microrefractometer (mī″krō-rē″frăk-tŏm′ĕ-tĕr) Refractometer used to study cells, esp. red blood cells.

microrespirometer (mī″krō-rĕs″pĭ-rŏm′ĕ-tĕr) Device for measuring oxygen consumption of minute amounts of tissue.

microrhinia (mī″krō-rĭn′ē-ă) [″ + *rhis,* nose] Abnormal smallness of the nose.

microscelous (mī-krŏs′kĕ-lŭs) [″ + *skelos,* leg] Having abnormally short legs.

microscope (mī′krō-skōp) [″ + *skopein,* to examine] Optical instrument that greatly magnifies minute objects. **microscopic, microscopical** (mī-krō-skŏp′ĭk, -ĭ-kăl), *adj.*

binocular m. A microscope possessing two eyepieces or oculars.

compound m. A microscope with two or more objective lenses with different magnifications.

dark-field m. A microscope by which objects invisible through an ordinary microscope may be seen by means of powerful side illumination. SYN: *ultramicroscope.* SEE: *illumination, darkfield.*

electron m. A microscope that uses streams of electrons deflected from their course by an electrostatic or electromagnetic field for the magnification of objects. The final image is viewed on a fluorescent screen or recorded on a photographic plate. Because of greater resolution, images may be magnified up to 400,000 diameters. SEE: *scanning electron m.*

light m. A microscope that uses visible light to allow viewing of the object.

operating m. A microscope designed for use during surgery involving small tissue such as nerves, vessels, the inner ear, eye, or fallopian tubes. SEE: *microsurgery.*

phase m. A compound microscope to which a diffraction or phase plate and a specialized condenser diaphragm have been added. These make it possible to view details of objects characterized by differences in refractive index and thus delineate a change of phase, such as brightness or color. This microscope is particularly useful for viewing living cells and observing cytoplasmic organelles.

polarization m. A microscope for examining specimens that polarize light or have double refraction.

scanning electron m. ABBR: SEM. An electron microscope that scans the image point by point and displays the image on a photographic film or television screen. The SEM, unlike other types of microscopes, allows a three-dimensional view of the tissue, and tissues do not need to be extensively handled and prepared in order to be visualized. The magnification ranges from 20 to 100,000 times.

simple m. A microscope with a single magnifying lens.

slit-lamp m. A microscope with slit illumination for examining the eye, esp. the cornea.

stereoscopic m. A binocular microscope with an objective lens for each eyepiece, permitting objects to be viewed stereoscopically.

ultraviolet m. A microscope using ultraviolet radiations as a light source and having an optical system for transmitting them. Used in observing specimens that fluoresce, such as tissues stained with a fluorescent dye.

x-ray m. A microscope using x-rays to reveal the structure of objects through which light cannot pass. The image is usually reproduced on film.

microscopy (mī-krŏs′kōp-ē) Inspection with a microscope.

confocal m. Type of microscopy that permits high-resolution analysis of serial optical sections (microscopic tomograms) into the depths of tissues or cells.

microsecond (mī′krō-sĕk″ŭnd) One-millionth (10^{-6}) of a second.

microseme (mī′krō-sēm) [Gr. *mikros,* small, + *sema,* sign] Possessing an orbital index of less than 83.

microsmatic (mī″krŏs-măt′ĭk) [″ + *osmasthai,* to smell] Having a poorly developed sense of smell.

microsome (mī′krō-sōm) Ribosome.

microspectrophotometry (mī″krō-spĕk″trō-fō-tŏm′ĕ-trē) Method for the histochemical study of substances present in cells, such as nucleic acid, based on absorption in the ultraviolet spectrum. This method permits quantitative and qualitative studies of certain cellular components.

microspectroscope [″ + L. *spectrum,* image, + Gr. *skopein,* to examine] A combined spectroscope and microscope.

microsphere Minute container suitable

for implantation or injection into the body or circulatory system. Microspheres may be used for delivering medicines to certain sites or, if radioactive, to study the blood flow to an area. If microspheres are used as a drug-delivery system, the container is designed to be dissolved in body fluids.

magnetic m. Microscopic magnetic particles that are used experimentally in autologous bone marrow transplant. The particles are coated with or coupled to antibodies and exposed to certain types of malignant cells in order to bind to them. The microspheres so bound can be removed by passing the cells through a magnetic field.

microspherocyte (mī″krō-sfē′rō-sīt) [″ + *sphaira,* globe, + *kytos,* cell] Small, sphere-shaped red blood cells seen in certain kinds of anemia.

microspherocytosis (mī″krō-sfē″rō-sī-tō′sĭs) [″ + ″ + *osis,* condition] Spherocytosis; marked by an excessive number of microspherocytes.

microsplanchnic (mī″krō-splănk′nĭk) Having a relatively small abdominal cavity in comparison with the rest of the body.

microsplenia (mī-krō-splē′nē-ă) [″ + *splen,* spleen] Abnormal smallness of the spleen.

microsporid (mī-krŏs′pō-rĭd) A skin eruption distant from the site of infection with *Microsporum* and due to hypersensitivity to the organism.

microsporidiosis Intracellular spore-forming protozoa that infect many animals and are known to cause human disease, esp. in those with AIDS. The genera of microsporidia implicated are *Encephalitozoon, Pleistophora, Septata, Nosema,* and *Enterocytozoon.* They cause a variety of pathological conditions, including diarrhea, wasting, keratoconjunctivitis, peritonitis, myositis, and hepatitis.

microsporosis (mī″krō-spō-rō′sĭs) Ringworm infection due to fungi of the genus *Microsporum.*

Microsporum (mī″krŏs′por-ŭm) A genus of fungi that causes disease of the skin, hair, and nails.

M. audouini The causative agent of tinea capitis (ringworm of scalp).

M. canis The causative agent of ringworm in cats and dogs. It may be easily transmitted to children.

microstomia (mī-krō-stō′mē-ă) [″ + *stoma,* mouth] Abnormal smallness of the mouth.

microstrabismus (mī″krō-stră-bĭs′mŭs) [″ + *strabismos,* a squinting] Movement of the eyes in divergent directions or at different speeds. These movements are too small and too quick to be seen, but they have been detected through analysis of high-speed motion pictures.

microstreaming The flow of interstitial fluids, or the pulsation of tissue particles associated with the application of therapeutic ultrasound. In physical medicine, microstreaming can promote soft-tissue healing. In dentistry, it is used in the removal of plaque and scale. SEE: *cavitation.*

microsurgery Surgery in which various types of magnification, specialized instrumentation, fine sutures, and meticulous techniques are used to repair, anastomose, or restore delicate tissues.

microthelia (mī″krō-thē′lē-ă) [″ + *thele,* nipple] Abnormal smallness of nipples.

microtia (mī-krō′shē-ă) [″ + *ous,* ear] Unusually small size of the auricle or external ear.

microtome (mī′krō-tōm) [″ + *tome,* incision] Instrument for preparing thin sections of tissue for microscopic study.

freezing m. Microtome equipped to cut frozen tissues.

sliding m. Microtome in which the tissue being sectioned slides along a track.

microtomy (mī-krŏt′ō-mē) The process of incising thin sections of tissues.

microtonometer (mī″krō-tō-nŏm′ĕ-tĕr) Device for determining oxygen and carbon dioxide concentration in blood.

microtrauma (mī″krō-traw′mă) A very small injury.

microtropia (mī″krō-trō′pē-ă) [″ + *trope,* a turning] Strabismus with very small deviation, usually less than 4°.

microtubule (mī″krō-tū′būl) An elongated (200 to 300 Å), hollow or tubular structure present in the cell. Microtubules are important in helping certain cells maintain their rigidity, in converting chemical energy into work, and in providing a means of transporting substances in different directions within a cell. They increase in number during mitosis.

microtus (mī-krō′tŭs) [″ + *ous,* ear] Individual with very small ears.

microvasculature (mī″krō-văs′kū-lă-chur) The very fine blood vessels of the body. **microvascular** (mī″krō-văs′kū-lăr), *adj.*

microvillus (mī″krō-vĭl′ŭs) *pl.* **microvilli** [L., tuft of hair] A microscopic fold from the free surface of a cell membrane. Microvilli greatly increase the exposed surface area of the cell. SEE: *border, brush.*

microvolt One millionth of a volt.

microwave (mī′krō-wāv) That portion of the radio wave spectrum between a wavelength of 1 mm and 30 cm.

m. oven An oven that uses microwave energy for cooking food. This method of food preparation may not kill microorganisms, esp. when used to reheat.

miction (mĭk′shŭn) Urination.

micturate (mĭk′tū-rāt) [L. *micturire*] To

pass urine from the bladder. SYN: *urinate.*

micturition (mĭk-tū-rĭ′shŭn) Urination.

micturition syncope SEE: under *syncope.*

MICU *medical intensive care unit.*

MID *minimum infective dose.*

midazolam hydrochloride A benzodiazepine used to produce sedation for brief diagnostic or endoscopic procedures and as sedation prior to general anesthesia. Use of this drug has been associated with respiratory depression and respiratory arrest.

CAUTION: It should only be used in a setting in which continuous monitoring of respiratory and cardiac function is done. Resuscitative drugs and trained personnel should be immediately available.

midbody (mĭd′bŏd-ē) Microtubules that appear as a granule between daughter cells during telophase of mitosis.

midbrain [AS. *mid,* middle, + *braegen,* brain] The corpora quadrigemina, the crura cerebri, and aqueduct of Sylvius, which connect the pons and cerebellum with the hemispheres of the cerebrum. It contains reflex centers for eye and head movements in response to visual and auditory stimuli. SYN: *mesencephalon.*

midcarpal (mĭd-kăr′păl) **1.** Between the two rows of carpal bones. **2.** Mediocarpal.

middle age An imprecise term that refers to the period of life that begins roughly at age 40 and ends at about age 64. During middle age in Western societies, many medical problems begin to increase in frequency, including degenerative arthritis, cancer, diabetes mellitus, high blood pressure, myocardial ischemia and infarction, obesity, and visual accommodative disorders.

middle lobe syndrome Atelectasis, bronchiectasis, or chronic pneumonitis of the middle lobe of the right lung, possibly due to calcified lymph nodes compressing the right middle lobe bronchus.

midfoot The area of the foot surrounding the cuboid, cuneiform, and navicular bones that lies between the forefoot and hindfoot.

midge (mĭj) [ME. *migge*] Small, gnatlike flies including those from the families Chironomidae and Ceratopogonidae. Some cause painful bites.

midget A nontechnical term for a very small person; an adult who is perfectly formed but has not attained and will not attain normal size.

midgut [AS. *mid,* middle, + *gut,* intestine] The midportion of the embryonic gut that opens ventrally into the yolk stalk.

midline (mĭd′līn) Any line that bisects a structure that is bilaterally symmetrical.

midoccipital (mĭd″ŏk-sĭp′ĭ-tăl) In the middle of the occiput.

midpain (mĭd′pān) Intermenstrual pain. SEE: *mittelschmerz.*

midplane (mĭd′plān) **1.** The plane bisecting a symmetrical structure. **2.** In obstetrics, the plane of least dimensions in the pelvic outlet.

midriff (mĭd′rĭf) [″ + *hrif,* belly] The diaphragm; the middle region of the torso.

midsection (mĭd-sĕk′shŭn) [″ + L. *secare,* to cut] A section through the middle of a structure.

midsternum (mĭd-stĕr′nŭm) The largest and middle portion of the sternum.

midstream specimen A urine specimen collected during the passage of the urine after the flow has begun and prior to the end. It is done to obtain a specimen with little contamination from bacteria in the urethra.

midtarsal (mĭd-tăr′săl) Between the two rows of bones that make up the tarsus of the foot.

midwife [″ + *wif,* wife] SEE: *nurse midwife.*

midwifery (mĭd-wĭf′ĕr-ē) The practice of assisting at childbirth. SEE: *obstetrics.*

MIF *maximum inspiratory force.*

mifepristone An abortifacient used in some countries. It is not used more than 47 days after the last menstrual period. A prostaglandin is administered by injection or as a suppository as an adjunct to mifepristone.

migraine (mī′grān) [Fr. from Gr. *hemikrania,* half skull] A familial disorder marked by periodic, usually unilateral, pulsatile headaches that begin in childhood or early adult life and tend to recur with diminishing frequency in later life. There are two closely related syndromes comprising what is known as migraine. They are classic migraine (migraine with aura) and common migraine (migraine without aura). The classic type may begin with aura, which consists of episodes of well-defined, transient focal neurologic dysfunction that develops over the course of minutes and may last an hour. Visual symptoms include seeing stripes, spots, or lines and scotomata. In most people, the aura precedes the headache; however, occasionally the aura will appear or recur at the height of the headache. Prior to the onset of symptoms, some persons experience mood changes, fatigue, difficulty thinking, depression, sleepiness, hunger, thirst, urinary frequency, or altered libido. Others report a feeling of well-being, increased energy, clarity of thought, and increased appetite, esp. for sweets. The headache follows. Pain usually is confined on one side but occasionally is bilateral. Nausea and vomiting may be present and may last a few hours or a day or two. Common migraine has a similar onset with or without nausea. Light and noise sensitivity are present in both types. In the general population, migraine is present in an estimated 3.5% of males and 7.4% of females. During their reproductive years, women experience a much higher rate of migraine, and their headaches tend to occur during periods of premenstrual tension and fluid retention. Many patients link their attacks to ingesting certain foods, exposure to glare, or to sudden changes in barometric pressure. SYN: *migraine headache*.

ETIOLOGY: A family history of migraine will be found in over half of the patients. Migraine may be precipitated by allergic hypersensitivity or emotional disturbances. In cases of migraine with aura, there is reduced regional cerebral blood flow in the posterior portion of the cerebral hemisphere, usually on the same side as the headache.

DIAGNOSIS: The International Headache Society (IHS) defines migraine without aura as at least five attacks unrelated to organic disease, with a duration of 4 to 72 hr, and pain characterized by at least two of the following: unilateral location, pulsating quality, moderate to severe intensity, or aggravation by routine physical activity; and at least one associated symptom: nausea and vomiting, or photophobia and phonophobia (sensitivity to noise). The IHS defines migraine with aura as at least two attacks unrelated to organic disease with at least one reversible aura symptom indicating focal cerebral cortical or brainstem dysfunction; at least one symptom developing over more than 4 min, or two or more symptoms in succession; and no single aura symptom lasting more than 60 min. The headache may precede, be concurrent with, or follow (within 60 min) the aura.

TREATMENT: Many medications help migraine sufferers. For most mild-to-moderate headaches, nonsteroidal anti-inflammatory drugs (e.g., acetaminophen or high-dose ibuprofen) alleviate pain and restore the patient to normal functioning within a few hours. These agents work best when combined with antiemetic drugs such as metoclopromide or promethazine, as well as rest or relaxation. Triptan drugs (e.g., sumatriptan), ergotamine derivatives, prednisone, and many other agents also are helpful, although each has its own side effect profile. Patients who experience multiple migraine headaches each month may benefit from preventive medications such as beta-blocking drugs (e.g., propranolol), calcium channel blocking drugs (e.g., verapamil), or tricyclic antidepressants taken on a regular basis. Narcotics (e.g., meperidine) are given to abort some severe migraine attacks; however, habitual use of narcotics may result in tolerance to their effects and drug dependence.

PATIENT CARE: The nurse monitors the nature and character of the patient's pain, helps the patient to relax by creating a quiet environment, and teaches the patient techniques for coping with discomfort. Prescribed medications are administered and evaluated for desired effects and any adverse reactions. To enhance the effects of medications and pain relief, noninvasive pain relief measures should be instituted before pain becomes severe.

migration (mī-grā'shŭn) [L. *migrare,* to move from place to place] Movement from one location to another. **migratory,** *adj.*

clot m. The movement of a venous thrombosis from a distal location to one that is closer to the right side of the heart or pulmonary artery. This may increase the chances of pulmonary embolism, and typically requires renewed anticoagulation.

internal m. of ovum Passage of the ovum from the ovary through the fallopian tube to the uterus.

m. of leukocytes Passage of white blood cells through walls of capillaries. SYN: *diapedesis*.

m. of teeth The movement of teeth during eruption or out of their normal position in the dental arch because of periodontal disease or missing adjacent teeth.

m. of testicle Descent of testicle into the scrotum. SYN: *descensus testis*.

milk thistle (mĭlk thĭs'ĭl) *Silybum marianum,* an herbal remedy used by alternative medicine practitioners for liver diseases.

mikro- SEE: words beginning with *micro-*.

Mikulicz's drain (mĭk'ū-lĭch"ĕs) [Johann von Mikulicz-Radecki, Polish surgeon, 1850–1905] A large-scale capillary drain that also serves as a tampon to arrest bleeding. It consists of a tubular piece of iodoform gauze of requisite size, placed in a cavity and filled with narrow strips of plain gauze until the necessary degree of compression is secured. This is used if there is parenchymatous oozing. SYN: *Mikulicz's tampon*.

Mikulicz's mask Gauze-covered frame worn over nose and mouth during performance of an operation.

Mikulicz's pad Folded gauze pad for packing off the viscera in abdominal operations and used as a sponge in general.

Mikulicz's syndrome Chronic infiltration with lymphocytes and painless enlargement of lacrimal and salivary glands.

mildew [AS. *mildeaw*] Lay term for a discoloration or superficial coating on various materials caused by the growth of fungi. Occurs in damp conditions.

milia (mĭl′ē-ă) Pl. of milium.

miliaria (mĭl-ē-ā′rē-ă) [L. *milium,* millet] An inflamed papular or vesicular rash that results from obstruction of the flow of sweat from sweat glands, esp. by occlusive clothing in warm and humid conditions. Miliaria rubra (heat rash or prickly heat) often affects athletes and military troops. SEE: illus.

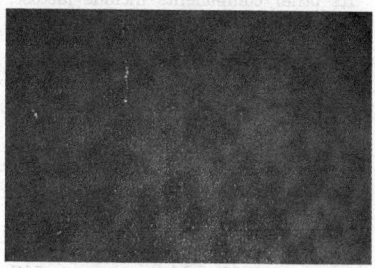

MILIARIA

TREATMENT: The rash often improves after the patient returns to a cooler climate or the affected area is cooled and dried.

apocrine m. Fordyce-Fox disease.

m. crystallina Sudamen.

m. profunda Form of miliaria seen almost exclusively in the tropics, frequently following attacks of miliaria rubra. The affected area is covered with pale, firm, painless papules 1 to 3 mm across. These papules do not cause itching. **miliary** (mĭl′ē-ă-rē), *adj.*

miliary tubercle SEE: under *tubercle.*

miliary tuberculosis SEE: under *tuberculosis.*

milieu (mē-lyŭ′) [Fr.] Environment.

m. interieur Internal environment of the extracellular fluids of the body.

military antishock trousers ABBR: MAST. SEE: *antishock garment.*

milium (mĭl′ē-ŭm) *pl.* **milia** [L., millet seed] White pinhead-size, keratin-filled cyst. Treatment consists of the use of mechanical keratolytics (pumice stone, soap), salicylic acid and sulfur ointment, or incision and expression of contents. In the newborn, milia occur on the face and, less frequently, on the trunk, and usually disappear without treatment within several weeks.

colloid m. Tiny papule formed beneath the epidermis due to colloid degeneration.

milk [AS. *meolc*] A secretion of the mammary glands for the nourishment of the young.

COMPOSITION: Milk from cows consists of water, organic substances, and mineral salts. *Organic substances:* Proteins: The principal proteins are caseinogen, lactoalbumin, and lactoglobulin; in the presence of calcium ions, soluble caseinogen is converted into insoluble casein by the action of acids, rennet, or pepsin. This brings about the curdling of milk. Lactoglobulin is identical with serum globulin of the blood and hence contains maternal antibodies. Carbohydrates: Lactose (milk sugar) is the principal sugar, although small quantities of other sugars are present. Fats: The principal fats are glycerides of oleic, palmitic, and myristic acids. Smaller quantities of stearic acid and short-chain fatty acids with carbon chains of $C_4$to C_{24} are present. Sterols and phosphatides (lecithin and cephalin) are also present. Churning causes the fat globules to unite into a solid mass and separate from the whey to form butter. *Mineral salts:* The principal cations are calcium, potassium, and sodium; the principal anions are phosphate and chloride. Citrates and lactates are present in small quantities. Milk is low in iron and magnesium.

Vitamins: Vitamin A and those of the B complex (thiamine, riboflavin, and pantothenic acid) are present in adequate quantities to meet the needs of a growing child. Milk is low in vitamins C and D.

Milk contains antibodies that are present in the mother's blood and a number of enzymes (catalase, oxidase, reductase, phosphatase).

acidophilus m. Milk inoculated with *Lactobacillus acidophilus,* a bacterium that grows best in an acid medium. Acidophilus milk is used to modify the bacterial flora of the digestive tract in persons with gastrointestinal disorders.

breast m. Milk obtained from the mammary glands of the human breast. It is the ideal source of nutrition for most infants, since it contains maternal antibodies that protect the child from infection, and other substances that promote development of the brain and the gastrointestinal tract, among other organs. Human breast milk that is collected and refrigerated immediately may be used for up to 5 days. If it is collected, frozen, and stored at −17.7°C (0°F), it is safe for 6 months.

CAUTION: Breastfeeding by mothers with human immunodeficiency virus (HIV) is not recommended, because of the risk of transmission of HIV to the child.

butter m. That portion of milk left after removal of butter following churning. It contains 2% fat.

casein m. Milk prepared with a large quantity of casein and fat but little sugar and salts.

condensed m. Partly evaporated and sweetened milk.

cow's m. Milk obtained from cows.

evaporated m. Cow's milk that has been concentrated by evaporating some of the water. It can be canned after pasteurization and stored for long periods of time. SEE: *lactic acid evaporated m.*

fore m. Milk released at the beginning of each breastfeeding that contains a high percentage of water, protein, and vitamins but a lower percentage of fat than the hind milk that is released later.

goat's m. Milk obtained from goats, which, like cow's milk, should be pasteurized before use.

hind m. Milk released late in breastfeeding, distinguished by its high fat content.

homogenized m. Milk that has been processed in such as manner that fats are combined with the body of the milk and the cream does not separate.

instant dry nonfat m. Dried skimmed milk that may be stored at room temperature until needed and then reconstituted by adding water to the granules.

lactic acid evaporated m. Evaporated milk to which sugar and lactic acid have been added. To prepare this milk, add 17 oz (503 ml) of water to 13 oz (384 ml) of evaporated milk, 2 level tbsp (1 oz or 28 g) of granulated sugar, and 3 tbsp (45 ml) of vinegar.

low-fat m. 1% Cow's milk with 1% fat, which represents 22% of the calories.

low-fat m. 2% Cow's milk with 2% fat, which represents 35% of the calories.

mature m. Milk released once lactation has become fully established. SEE: *fore m.; hind m.*

modified m. Milk altered so that its composition more closely approximates that of human milk.

mother's m. Breast m.

nonfat m. Skim m.

pasteurized m. Milk heated to a specified temperature for a precise length of time and then cooled rapidly. This process kills pathogenic bacteria without appreciably altering the taste of the milk. SEE: *pasteurization.*

protein m. Milk modified to be high in protein and low in carbohydrate and fat content.

red m. Milk contaminated by blood, chromogenic bacteria, or plant pigments.

ropy m. Milk that has become viscid due to formation of vegetable gums from carbohydrates or mucin-like substances from proteins as a result of bacterial action.

skim m. Cow's milk from which the fat has been removed.

sour m. Milk with lactic acid caused either by lactic acid–producing bacteria or by the addition of vinegar. It is most commonly used in baked goods.

soy m. Milk product derived from soybeans. It causes fewer allergic reactions than cow-based milk products.

sterilized m. Milk that has been boiled to kill bacteria.

transitional m. The first milk produced as colostrum production fades. It has more triglyceride and medium-chain fatty acid content than colostrum. Its other components include lactose, water-soluble vitamins, and immunoglobulins.

vegetable m. **1.** The latex of plants. **2.** A synthetic milk prepared from juices of various plants, such as soybean.

vitamin D m. Milk in which vitamin D content has been increased by addition of concentrates, ultraviolet irradiation, or feeding of irradiated yeast to milk-producing animals.

whole m. Milk that has not been altered except for pasteurization. The fat content is 3.8%, which represents 51% of the calories present.

witch's m. Milk secreted by the newly born infant's breast, stimulated by the lactating hormone circulating in the mother.

milk-alkali syndrome Elevated blood calcium without an increase in calcium or phosphate in the urine, renal insufficiency, and alkalosis due to prolonged intake of excessive amounts of milk and soluble alkali. This condition is usually found as an undesired side effect of treating a peptic ulcer with calcium-containing antacids. SYN: *Burnett's syndrome.*

milk fever A colloquial term for an elevation in body temperature that occurs after childbirth. It may be caused by genitourinary infection, noninfectious inflammation of the lactating breasts, or infectious mastitis. SEE: *caked breast; mastitis.*

milking Removal of the contents of a tubular structure, such as the urethra, by compressing the tube with the fingers and moving them along the course of the tube and away from the origin of the urethra. This maneuver forces material out of the tube that might not otherwise be seen or available for study. SEE: *strip.*

milk leg Phlegmasia alba dolens.

milk of bismuth A suspension of bismuth hydroxide and bismuth subcarbonate in water, used as an antacid.

milk of magnesia Magnesium hydroxide in suspension, used as an antacid and a cathartic.

Milkman's syndrome (mĭlk′mănz) [Louis A. Milkman, U.S. roentgenologist, 1895–1951] Failure of reabsorption of phosphate by the renal tubules.

This failure causes a special type of demineralization of bones that produces a transverse striped area of multiple pseudofractures in roentgenograms of the bones.

milk tumor A colloquial term for a galactocele. SYN: *galactocele* (1). SEE: *caked breast*.

Miller-Abbott tube [Thomas Grier Miller, U.S. physician,1886–1981; William Osler Abbott, U.S. physician, 1902–1943] A double-channel intestinal tube used to relieve intestinal obstruction. Inserted through a nostril, the tube is passed through the stomach into the small intestine.

Miller Assessment for Preschoolers [Lucy Jane Miller, Ph.D., contemporary occupational therapist] ABBR: M.A.P. A widely used standardized developmental screening test for youngsters from 2 to 5 years of age. It contains sensory, motor, and cognitive performance items.

milli- [L. *milli,* thousand] Prefix used in the metric system to denote one-thousandth (10^{-3}).

milliammeter Ammeter registering in milliamperes. SEE: *ammeter*.

milliampere (mĭl″ē-ăm′pēr) ABBR: ma. One-thousandth of an ampere.

milliampere minute An electrical unit of quantity, equivalent to that delivered by 1 milliampere in 1 min.

milliampere seconds ABBR: MAS. In radiography, the milliamperage of the exposure multiplied by the time of the exposure in seconds. This factor determines the exposure of the radiograph.

millibar (mĭl′ĭ-băr) One thousandth of a bar, which is 100 newtons/sq m. The normal atmospheric pressure of 14.7 lb/sq in. is equal to 1013 millibars.

millicoulomb (mĭl″ĭ-koo′lŏm) ABBR: mC. A unit of electric current, one thousandth (10^{-3}) of a coulomb.

millicurie (mĭl″ĭ-kū′rē) ABBR: mCi. One thousandth of a curie. A practical unit of dosage for a radioactive source: 1 mCi of a radioactive substance applied for 1 hr.

millicurie-hour ABBR: mCi-hr. A practical unit of dosage for radon: 1 mCi of radon applied for 1 hr. The biological effect depends on time, filtration, and distance.

milliequivalent ABBR: mEq. One thousandth of a chemical equivalent. The concentration of electrolytes in a certain volume of solution is usually expressed as milliequivalent per liter (mEq/L). It is calculated by multiplying the milligrams per liter by the valence of the chemical and dividing by the molecular weight of the substance.

milligram (mĭl′ĭ-grăm) ABBR: mg. One thousandth of a gram.

millilambert (mĭl″ĭ-lăm′bĕrt) One thousandth of a lambert, a unit of light intensity. About one foot-candle, but more accurately, it is 0.929 lumens per square foot.

milliliter ABBR: ml. One thousandth of a liter. For practical purposes, a milliliter is equivalent to 1 cu cm. The term milliliter (ml) is used when referring to *liquid* volume; cubic centimeter (cc) is used when referring to the volume of a gas.

millimeter ABBR: mm. One thousandth of a meter.

millimicro- (mμ) Prefix formerly used to indicate one billionth (10^{-9}). The term currently used is *nano.*

millimicrocurie (mĭl″ĭ-mī″krō-kū′rē) A nanocurie, or 10^{-9} curie.

millimicrogram (mĭl″ĭ-mī′krō-grăm) A nanogram, or 10^{-9} g.

millimicron (mĭl-ĭ-mī′krŏn) ABBR: mμ. An obsolete term for distance in the metric system, usually applied to light wavelength. SEE: *nanometer*.

millimole (mĭl′ĭ-mōl) ABBR: mM or mmol. One thousandth of a mole.

milling-in A method of adjusting the occlusion of teeth by moving them against each other while an abrasive substance is between them.

millinormal (mĭl″ĭ-nor′măl) The strength of a solution equal to one-thousandth normal.

milliosmole (mĭl″ē-ŏs′mōl) One thousandth of an osmole. The osmotic pressure equal to one thousandth of the molecular weight of a substance divided by the number of ions that the substance forms in a liter of solution.

millipede (mĭl′ĭ-pēd) A wormlike arthropod with two pairs of legs on each body segment. Some produce an irritating venom.

millirem ABBR: mrem. One thousandth of a rem.

milliroentgen ABBR: mR. One thousandth of a roentgen.

millisecond (mĭl″ĭ-sĕk′ŏnd) One thousandth of a second.

millivolt (mĭl′ĭ-vōlt) One thousandth of a volt.

milphae (mĭl′fē) [Gr. *milphai*] Loss of eyebrow hair.

milphosis (mĭl-fō′sĭs) [Gr.] Loss of eyelashes.

Milroy's disease (mĭl′roys) [William Forsyth Milroy, U.S. physician, 1855–1942] Chronic hereditary lymphedema of the legs.

Milwaukee brace A brace made of strong, lightweight materials. It extends from a chin cup with neck pad to the pelvis, and is used to correct minimal-curve scoliosis.

mimesis [Gr.] Imitation, mimicry. Term applied to a disease that exhibits symptoms of another disease or to conditions in functional illnesses that simulate organic disease. **mimetic, mimic** (mī-mĕt′ĭk, mĭm′ĭk), *adj.*

mimmation (mī-mā′shŭn) A form of stuttering in which the "m" sound is inappropriately used.

min *minim; minimum; minute.*

Minamata disease (mĭn″ă-maw′tă) [Minamata Bay, Japan] A neurological disease due to ingestion of alkyl mercury, an organic mercury compound used in industrial processes. SYN: *yushi.*

SYMPTOMS: Clinical findings are paresthesias, loss of peripheral vision, dysarthria, ataxia, tremors, excessive salivation, sweating, and mental disturbances.

ETIOLOGY: This condition is caused by the ingestion of contaminated seafood.

PROGNOSIS: The prognosis is poor; death may occur.

mind [AS. *gemynd*] Psyche. Integration and organization of functions of the brain resulting in the ability to perceive surroundings, to have emotions, imagination, memory, and will, and to process information in an intelligent manner. The quality and quantity of the functions of the mind vary with experience and development.

mineral [L. *minerale*] **1.** An inorganic element or compound occurring in nature, esp. one that is solid. **2.** Inorganic; not of animal or plant origin. **3.** Impregnated with minerals, as mineral water. **4.** Pert. to minerals.

mineral acid Inorganic acid.

mineral compound One of many compounds of mineral elements. Many such chemicals are present in the body. SEE: *acid-base balance; buffer.*

FUNCTION: Minerals are essential constituents of all cells; they form the greater portion of the hard parts of the body (bone, teeth, nails); they are essential components of respiratory pigments, enzymes, and enzyme systems; they regulate the permeability of cell membranes and capillaries; they regulate the excitability of muscular and nervous tissue; they are essential for regulation of osmotic pressure equilibria; they are necessary for maintenance of proper acid-base balance; they are essential constituents of secretions of glands; they play an important role in water metabolism and regulation of blood volume.

DAILY REQUIREMENTS:: Because mineral salts and water are excreted daily from the body, they must be replaced through food intake. Daily requirements for principal minerals for a healthy adult are as follows: calcium and phosphorus, 800 to 1200 mg; copper, 1.5 to 3 mg; iodine, 150 μg (micrograms); magnesium, 280 to 400 mg; potassium, 2000 mg; sodium, about 500 mg. Daily intake of sodium chloride should be limited to 6 g (2.4 g of sodium) or less each day. Requirements are greater for growing children and pregnant women and in certain pathological conditions. SEE: *Recommended Daily Dietary Allowances Appendix.*

mineralization (mĭn″ĕr-ăl-ī-zā′shŭn) **1.** Normal or abnormal deposition of minerals in tissues. **2.** In the food chain, the degradation by bacteria and fungi of complex organic molecules to simpler organics and inorganics.

mineralocorticoid (mĭn″ĕr-ăl-ō-kor′tĭ-koyd) A steroid hormone (e.g., aldosterone) that regulates the retention and excretion of fluids and electrolytes by the kidneys. SEE: *aldosterone.*

mineral oil SEE: *petrolatum, liquid.*

mineral spring A spring in which water contains mineral salts that are thought to have a therapeutic value in certain diseases, but usually the principal action is as a cathartic. SYN: *spa.*

mineral water Water that contains sufficient inorganic salts to cause it to have therapeutic properties.

minification In radiography, the reduction in the size of a fluoroscopic image to intensify the brightness of that image.

minilaparotomy A limited incision of the abdominal wall into the peritoneum that is less than 5 cm long.

minim (mĭn′ĭm) [L. *minimum,* least] ABBR: m; min. One sixtieth of a fluidram, or 0.06 ml.

minimal (mĭn′ĭ-măl) Least; the smallest possible.

minimal brain damage SEE: *attention-deficit hyperactivity disorder.*

minimal brain dysfunction ABBR: MBD. SEE: *attention-deficit hyperactivity disorder.*

minimal cerebral dysfunction SEE: *attention-deficit hyperactivity disorder.*

minimal change disease The form of nephrotic syndrome most often found in children, in which renal biopsies reveal little if any pathological change under the light microscope. With electron microscopy, effacement of the foot processes of the glomerulus becomes evident. SEE: *nephrotic syndrome.*

Mini–Mental State Examination ABBR: MMSE. A commonly used assessment tool to quantify a person's cognitive ability. It assesses orientation, registration, attention and calculation, and language. Scoring is from 0 to 30, with 30 indicating intact cognition.

minimum (mĭn′ĭ-mŭm) *pl.* **minima** Least quantity or lowest limit. SEE: *threshold.*

minimum daily requirements ABBR: MDR. The daily requirements of vitamins and minerals needed to prevent symptoms of deficiency. SEE: *Recommended Daily Dietary Allowances Appendix.*

Minimum Data Set ABBR: MDS. A comprehensive computer-compatible form for assessment of nursing home residents covering 13 key clinical areas. It was developed as a result of the Omnibus Reconciliation Act of 1987 and mandated for use in nursing homes in the U.S. Resident assessment protocols are used to identify multiple "triggers" for the assessment of various conditions. Under the current prospective payment system, the form must be completed and sent electronically to the federal government within 7 days of admission to a nursing home and at frequent intervals thereafter. SEE: *Nursing Minimum Data Set*.

Minin light (mĭn'ĭn) [A. V. Minin, early 20th century Russian surgeon] A special lamp that produces violet or ultraviolet light.

mini-stroke Transient ischemic attack.

Minnesota Multiphasic Personality Inventory ABBR: MMPI. SEE: *personality testing*.

minocycline hydrochloride (mĭ-nō-sī'klēn) An antibiotic of the tetracycline class.

minor A person not of legal age and thus requiring consent for medical, surgical, or dental care. The legal age in the U.S. varies from state to state.

emancipated m. A person not of legal age who is in the armed services, married, the mother of a child whether married or not, or has left home and is self-sufficient. Some state legislatures do not require such an individual to have parental consent to receive medical or surgical care, or advice on contraception or abortion.

Minot-Murphy diet (mī'nŏt) [George R. Minot, U.S. physician, 1885–1950; William P. Murphy, U.S. physician, b. 1892] Diet for pernicious anemia containing large quantities of liver.

minoxidil A drug used to promote hair growth and to treat hypertension. Trade name is Rogaine.

mio-, meio- (mī'ō) [Gr. *meion,* less] Combining form meaning *less* or *fewer*.

miocardia (mī-ō-kăr'dē-ă) [" + *kardia,* heart] Decreasing heart volume during systolic contraction. SYN: *systole*.

miodidymus (mī"ō-dĭd'ĭ-mŭs) [" + *didymos,* twin] A fetus with two heads joined at the occiput.

miolecithal (mī"ō-lĕs'ĭ-thăl) [" + *lekithos,* egg yolk] Pert. to an egg with a small amount of yolk.

miopus (mī'ō-pŭs) [" + *ops,* face] Conjoined twins with one having a rudimentary face.

miosis (mī-ō'sĭs) [Gr. *meiosis,* a lessening] Abnormal contraction of the pupils, possibly due to irritation of the oculomotor system or paralysis of dilators. Pupillary contraction may occur after a stroke that affects the brainstem or after administration of drugs such as opiates or eyedrops that inactivate acetylcholinesterase.

miotic **1.** An agent that causes the pupil to contract, such as eserine or pilocarpine. **2.** Pert. to or causing contraction of the pupil. **3.** Diminishing.

MIP *maximum inspiratory pressure*.

miracidium (mī"ră-sĭd'ē-ŭm) *pl.* **miracidia** [Gr. *meirakidion,* lad] The ciliated free-swimming larva of a digenetic fluke. On emerging from an ovum, it penetrates a snail of a particular species and metamorphoses into a sporocyst. SEE: *fluke*.

miracle, medical The unexplained spontaneous regression of a medical condition thought to be invariably fatal or incurable or both.

mire (mēr) [L. *mirari,* to look at] A test object on the ophthalmometer, the images of which denote the amount of astigmatism.

mirror [Fr. *miroir*] A polished surface that reflects light and thus reproduces visible images of objects in front of it.

dental m. An instrument commonly used for viewing occlusal and distal surfaces of teeth.

mirror writing Writing in which letters and words are reversed and appear as in a mirror.

miryachit (mĭr-ē'ă-chĭt) [Russian] A type of "jumping disorder" seen in Siberia, the symptoms of which are similar to those of the Jumping Frenchmen of Maine. Also spelled myriachit. SYN: *saltatory spasm*.

misandry [Gr. *miso,* hatred, + *andros,* man] Aversion to or hatred of males. SEE: *misogyny*.

misanthropy (mĭs"ăn'thrō-pē) [" + Gr. *anthropos,* man] Hatred of mankind.

misarticulation Inaccurately produced speech.

miscarriage [" + L. *carrus,* cart] Lay term for termination of pregnancy at any time before the fetus has attained the potential for extrauterine viability. SYN: *abortion, spontaneous*.

misce (mĭs'ē) [L., mix] ABBR: M. A direction on prescriptions that instructs the pharmacist to mix the ingredients.

miscegenation (mĭs"ĕ-jē-nā'shŭn) [L. *miscere,* to mix, + *genus,* race] Sexual relations or marriage between those of different races.

miscible (mĭs'ĭ-bl) Capable of being mixed.

misconduct, sexual (mĭs-kŏn'dŭkt) Inappropriate sexual contact, speech, or behaviors between health care providers and their patients.

misdemeanor A lesser crime than a felony, usually punishable by fines, imprisonment, penalty, or forfeiture.

misery Extreme mental or emotional unhappiness.

misfeasance The performance of a legal act in an improper or unlawful manner.

misinformation Data or information concerning a patient that may be assumed erroneously to be accurate (e.g., laboratory data that are inaccurate, historical data from the patient or the family that are unreliable, and transcription errors in recording data). In some instances, misinformation is knowingly presented to, or the truth withheld from, the physician by the patient in order to conceal something that would be personally embarrassing or incriminating.

misogamy (mĭ-sŏg′ă-mē) [″ + *gamos,* marriage] Aversion to marriage.

misogynist (mĭs-ŏj′ĭ-nĭst) [″ + *gyne,* woman] One who hates women.

misogyny (mĭs-ŏj′ĭn-ē) Aversion to or hatred of females. SEE: *misandry.*

misologia (mĭs-ō-lō′jē-ă) [Gr. *miseio,* to hate, + *logos,* word, reason] Aversion to mental activity.

misoneism (mĭ-sō-nē′ĭzm) [″ + *neos,* new] Aversion to new things or new ideas; conservatism.

misopedia (mĭ-sō-pē′dē-ă) [″ + Gr. *pais,* child] Abnormal dislike of children or the young.

misrepresentation An incorrect, dishonest, or false represenation of facts.

mist A collection of small aerosol particles for inhalation.

Mister In England and other parts of the British Commonwealth, the title of address of a surgeon.

mistura (mĭs-tū′ră) Mixture.

Mitchell's disease (mĭch′ĕlz) [Silas Weir Mitchell, U.S. neurologist, 1829–1914] Erythromelalgia.

mite (mīt) [AS.] A minute arachnid, a member of the order Acarina. Some mites are parasitic and cause conditions such as asthma, mange, and scabies; some serve as vectors of disease organisms and as intermediate hosts for certain Cestodes.

dust m. A type of mite, *Dermatophagoides pteronyssinum* or *D. farinae,* that ingests shed human skin cells. They are a common cause of allergic reactions, including asthma.

follicle m. A mite that lives in hair follicles and sebaceous glands. SYN: *Demodex folliculorum.*

harvest m. A mite, similar in appearance to scabies, that lives in grain stems, grasses, and bushes. It is common in the southern U.S. The larvae attach to the skin and inject a secretion that causes itching. SYN: *chiggers.*

itch m. *Sarcoptes scabiei.* SEE: *scabies.*

mange m. A mite belonging to the families Sarcoptidae and Psoroptidae, and causing mange in many species of animals. SEE: *mange; scabies.*

red m. Redbug or chigger; a member of the family Thrombiculidae. SEE: *chiggers.*

mithridatism (mĭth′rĭ-dāt″ĭzm) [Mithridates, king of Pontus, 132–63 B.C., supposed to have acquired immunity in this fashion] Immunity to a poison acquired by taking it in doses of gradually increasing size.

miticide (mī′tĭ-sīd) [AS. *mite,* mite, + L. *caedere,* to kill] A substance that kills mites.

mitigated (mĭt′ĭ-gāt-ĕd) [L. *mitigare,* to soften.] Diminished in severity. SYN: *allayed; moderated.*

mitis (mī′tĭs) [L.] Mild.

mitochondrion (mīt″ō-kŏn′drē-ŏn) *pl.* **mitochondria** [Gr. *mitos,* thread, + *chondros,* cartilage] Cell organelles of rod or oval shape 0.5 μm in diameter. They can be seen by using phase-contrast or electron microscopy. They contain the enzymes for the aerobic stages of cell respiration and thus are the sites of most ATP synthesis. SEE: *cell; organelle* for illus.

mitogen (mī′tō-jĕn) A plant-derived protein substance that is used in the laboratory to stimulate cell division (mitosis). It is frequently used in vitro to study the proliferation of lymphocytes from blood drawn during a research study. The most commonly used mitogens are phytohemagglutinin and concanavalin A. SEE: *concanavalin A; lectin; phytohemagglutinin.*

pokeweed m. ABBR: PWM. A mitogen isolated from the pokeweed plant, *Phytolacca americana.* In the presence of T lymphocytes, it has the capacity to induce primed B lymphocytes to proliferate and differentiate into plasma cells.

mitogenesis (mī″tō-jĕn′ĕ-sĭs) [″ + *osis,* condition, + *genesis,* generation, birth] The production of cell mitosis.

mitoma, mitome [Gr. *mitos,* thread] A fine network support or framework of protoplasm in a cell.

mitomycin (mī″tō-mī′sĭn) An antibiotic with antineoplastic action.

mitoplasm (mī′tō-plăzm) [″ + *plassein,* to form] The chromatic substance in a cell nucleus.

mitosis (mī-tō′sĭs) *pl.* **mitoses** [″ + *osis,* condition] Type of cell division of somatic cells in which each daughter cell contains the same number of chromosomes as the parent cell. Mitosis is the process by which the body grows and dead somatic cells are replaced. Mitosis is a continuous process divided into four phases: prophase, metaphase, anaphase, and telophase. SEE: illus.; *meiosis.*

Prophase: The chromatin granules of the nucleus stain more densely and become organized into chromosomes. These first appear as long filaments, each consisting of two identical chromatids, the result of DNA replication. Each pair of chromatids is joined at a region called the centromere, which may be central or toward one end. As

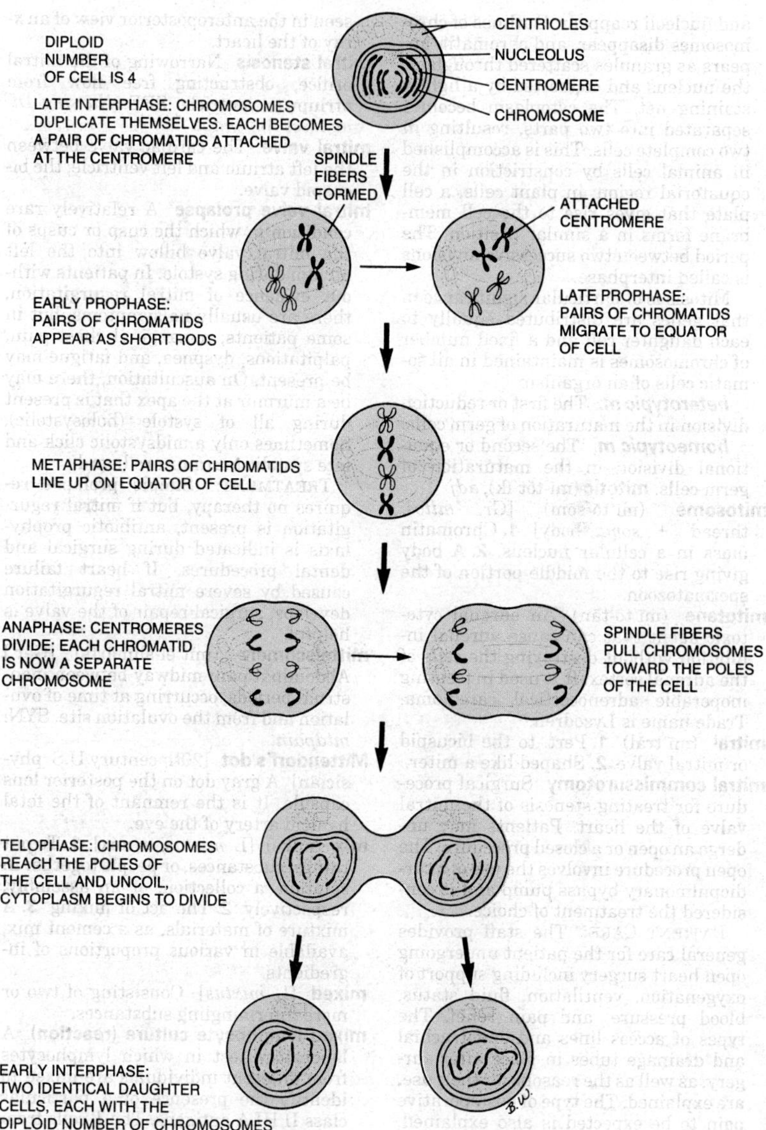
DIPLOID
NUMBER
OF CELL IS 4
CENTRIOLES
NUCLEOLUS
CENTROMERE
CHROMOSOME
LATE INTERPHASE: CHROMOSOMES
DUPLICATE THEMSELVES. EACH BECOMES
A PAIR OF CHROMATIDS ATTACHED
AT THE CENTROMERE
SPINDLE
FIBERS
FORMED
ATTACHED
CENTROMERE
EARLY PROPHASE:
PAIRS OF CHROMATIDS
APPEAR AS SHORT RODS
LATE PROPHASE:
PAIRS OF CHROMATIDS
MIGRATE TO EQUATOR
OF CELL
METAPHASE: PAIRS OF CHROMATIDS
LINE UP ON EQUATOR OF CELL
ANAPHASE: CENTROMERES
DIVIDE; EACH CHROMATID
IS NOW A SEPARATE
CHROMOSOME
SPINDLE FIBERS
PULL CHROMOSOMES
TOWARD THE POLES
OF THE CELL
TELOPHASE: CHROMOSOMES
REACH THE POLES OF
THE CELL AND UNCOIL,
CYTOPLASM BEGINS TO DIVIDE
EARLY INTERPHASE:
TWO IDENTICAL DAUGHTER
CELLS, EACH WITH THE
DIPLOID NUMBER OF CHROMOSOMES
B.W.

MITOSIS

prophase progresses, the chromosomes become shorter and more compact and stain densely. The nuclear membrane and the nucleoli disappear. At the same time, the centriole divides and the two daughter centrioles, each surrounded by a centrosphere, move to opposite poles of the cell. They are connected by fine protoplasmic fibrils, which form an achromatic spindle.

Metaphase: The chromosomes (paired chromatids) arrange themselves in an equatorial plane midway between the two centrioles.

Anaphase: The chromatids (now called daughter chromosomes) diverge and move toward their respective centrosomes. The end of their migration marks the beginning of the next phase.

Telophase: The chromosomes at each pole of the spindle undergo changes that are the reverse of those in the prophase, each becoming a long, loosely spiraled thread. The nuclear membrane re-forms and nucleoli reappear. Outlines of chromosomes disappear, and chromatin appears as granules scattered throughout the nucleus and connected by a lightly staining net. The cytoplasm becomes separated into two parts, resulting in two complete cells. This is accomplished in animal cells by constriction in the equatorial region; in plant cells, a cell plate that gives rise to the cell membrane forms in a similar position. The period between two successive divisions is called interphase.

Mitosis is of particular significance in that genes are distributed equally to each daughter cell and a fixed number of chromosomes is maintained in all somatic cells of an organism.

heterotypic m. The first or reduction division in the maturation of germ cells.

homeotypic m. The second or equational division in the maturation of germ cells. **mitotic** (mī-tŏt′ĭk), *adj.*

mitosome (mī′tō-sōm) [Gr. *mitos,* thread, + *soma,* body] **1.** Chromatin mass in a cellular nucleus. **2.** A body giving rise to the middle portion of the spermatozoon.

mitotane (mī′tō-tān) An adrenal cytotoxic agent that can cause adrenal inhibition without destroying the cells of the adrenal cortex. It is used in treating inoperable adrenocortical carcinoma. Trade name is Lysodren.

mitral (mī′trăl) **1.** Pert. to the bicuspid or mitral valve. **2.** Shaped like a miter.

mitral commissurotomy Surgical procedure for treating stenosis of the mitral valve of the heart. Patients may undergo an open or a closed procedure. The open procedure involves the use of a cardiopulmonary bypass pump and is considered the treatment of choice.

PATIENT CARE: The staff provides general care for the patient undergoing open heart surgery including support of oxygenation, ventilation, fluid status, blood pressure, and pain relief. The types of access lines and endotrachial and drainage tubes in place after surgery, as well as the reasons for their use, are explained. The type of postoperative pain to be expected is also explained, and the patient is encouraged to report pain before it becomes severe to maintain a comfortable state necessary for healing. The caregivers support the patient and family throughout recovery. After discharge, the patient begins a gradual return to activity. Regular medical follow-up and participation in a cardiac rehabilitation program, if recommended by the physician, should be encouraged.

mitral disease Disease of the mitral valve. SEE: *heart.*

mitralization (mī″trăl-ī-zā′shŭn) Straightening of the left border of the heart due to mitral valve disease, as seen in the anteroposterior view of an x-ray of the heart.

mitral stenosis Narrowing of the mitral orifice, obstructing free flow from atrium to ventricle. SEE: *Nursing Diagnoses Appendix.*

mitral valve The cardiac valve between the left atrium and left ventricle; the bicuspid valve.

mitral valve prolapse A relatively rare condition in which the cusp or cusps of the mitral valve billow into the left atrium during systole. In patients without evidence of mitral regurgitation, there are usually no symptoms, but in some patients, nonanginal chest pain, palpitations, dyspnea, and fatigue may be present. On auscultation, there may be a murmur at the apex that is present during all of systole (holosystolic). Sometimes only a midsystolic click and late systolic murmur are heard.

TREATMENT: Simple prolapse requires no therapy, but if mitral regurgitation is present, antibiotic prophylaxis is indicated during surgical and dental procedures. If heart failure caused by severe mitral regurgitation develops, surgical repair of the valve is helpful.

mittelschmerz (mĭt′ĕl-shmārts) [Ger.] Abdominal pain midway between menstrual periods, occurring at time of ovulation and from the ovulation site. SYN: *midpain.*

Mittendorf's dot [20th century U.S. physician] A gray dot on the posterior lens capsule. It is the remnant of the fetal hyaloid artery of the eye.

mix (mĭks) [L. *mixtus,* to mix] **1.** To put things, substances, or people together in solution, a collection, or an assembly, respectively. **2.** The act of mixing. **3.** A mixture of materials, as a cement mix, available in various proportions of ingredients.

mixed [L. *mixtus*] Consisting of two or more intermingling substances.

mixed lymphocyte culture (reaction) A laboratory test in which lymphocytes from different individuals are mixed to identify the presence of a particular class II HLA antigens. The T cells from the "responder" will synthesize DNA and proliferate only if they do not have the same histocompatibility antigens as the "donor cells," homozygous cells with known HLA types. The donor cells are irradiated to prevent their proliferation during the test.

mixture (mĭks′tūr) [L. *mistura*] A combination of two or more substances with or without chemical union. SYN: *mistura.*

eutectic m. of local anesthetics ABBR: EMLA. A cream preparation of lidocaine and prilocaine. A thick layer is applied to the skin to be anesthetized 1 hr before procedures in which needles penetrate the skin. The cream is also used before superficial biopsies and skin grafts and is esp. helpful when such procedures are performed on pediatric patients.

MKS, mks *meter-kilogram-second.* It indicates a measurement system using meter for length, kilogram for weight, and second for time.

ml *milliliter.*

M.L.A. *Medical Library Association.*

M.L.D., MLD *minimum lethal dose.*

mM Symbol for millimole.

mm *millimeter.*

mm Hg *millimeters of mercury.*

MMPI *Minnesota Multiphasic Personality Inventory.*

MMPR *medical malpractice payment report.*

MMR *measles, mumps, rubella* (vaccine).

MMV *mandatory minute ventilation.*

MMWR *Morbidity and Mortality Weekly Report.*

Mn Symbol for the element manganese.

mnemic (nē′mĭk) Relating to memory.

mnemonic (nē-mŏn′ĭk) *pl.* **mnemonics** [Gr. *mnemonikos,* pert. to memory] Anything intended to aid memory.

MNL *mononuclear leukocyte* (e.g., monocytes and macrophages).

M.O. *Medical Officer.*

Mo Symbol for the element molybdenum.

mo *month.*

mobile [L. *mobilis*] Movable.

mobile arm support A device for support of the forearm, usually mounted on a wheelchair, that assists weak shoulder and elbow muscles in positioning the hand, as in feeding. SYN: *balanced forearm orthosis; ball bearing feeder.*

mobile spasm Athetosis.

mobility [L. *mobilitas*] State or quality of being mobile; facility of movement. In rehabilitation, mobility refers to an individual's ability to move within a living environment, including the community.

abnormal tooth m. Excessive tooth movement within the bony socket due to degenerative changes in the supporting alveolar bone and periodontal ligament as a result of poor oral hygiene, hormone balance changes, or trauma. SEE: *tooth movement.*

functional m. The ability to move from one place to another to complete an activity or task.

impaired bed m. Limitation of independent movement from one bed position to another. SEE: *Nursing Diagnoses Appendix.*

This diagnosis was approved at the NANDA 13th Conference, 1998.

impaired wheelchair m. Limitation of independent operation of wheelchair within one's environment. SEE: *Nursing Diagnoses Appendix.*

This diagnosis was approved at the NANDA 13th Conference, 1998.

normal tooth m. Normal movement of teeth horizontally and, to a lesser extent, occlusally in response to various forces. SYN: *physiological tooth migration.*

powered m. Assistive devices—such as adapted vehicles, electrically powered wheelchairs, and scooters—that enhance or improve the movement of functionally impaired persons.

mobility training Techniques and equipment provided to persons with functional deficits to assist them in moving safely from one location to another. For people with blindness or low vision, the term orientation and mobility (O&M) training is used. Orientation involves knowing where in space one is located. Mobility involves enacting a plan to get to a desired location. For blindness and vision deficits, O&M training involves developing sensory awareness and using devices such as long canes, guide dogs, or electronic sensing aids.

mobilization (mō″bĭl-ĭ-zā′shŭn) The process of making a fixed part movable or releasing stored substances, as in restoring motion to a joint, freeing an organ, or making available substances held in reserve in the body as glycogen or fat.

early controlled m. A method of rehabilitating flexor and extensor injuries, using splinting and active exercises, beginning the first week after injury or surgical repair.

joint m. Passive therapeutic techniques that improve joint play or accessory motion or treat joint pain. SYN: *joint manipulation.*

soft-tissue m. The therapeutic manipulation of connective tissue, including muscle, fascia, tendons, and ligaments, for mechanical and physiological effects on blood flow, temperature, metabolism, and autonomic reflex activity. It includes techniques such as myofascial release, muscle energy, Rolfing, and traditional massage.

stapes m. Surgical procedure performed to restore mobility to the stapes. Used in treatment of deafness.

mobilize (mō′bĭl-īz) **1.** To incite to physiological action. **2.** To render movable; to put in movement.

modal (mōd′l) [L. *modus,* mode] Pert. to, or characteristic of, a mode. In statistics, pert. to the most frequent, common, or typical measure of the variables being investigated.

modality **1.** A method of application or the employment of any therapeutic agent; limited usually to physical agents and devices. **2.** Any specific sensory stimulus such as taste, touch, vision, pressure, or hearing.

physical agent m. A form of therapy used in rehabilitation that produces a change in soft tissue through light, water, temperature, sound, or electricity.

It includes transcutaneous electrical nerve stimulation units, ultrasound, whirlpool, hot and cold packs, and other medical devices.

mode (mōd) [L. *modus,* measure, mode] **1.** In statistics, the value or item of the class occurring most frequently in a series of variables. **2.** In respiratory therapy, any of several approaches to continuous mechanical ventilation including volume- and pressure-targeted application with full or partial ventilatory support.

assist-control m. A type of mechanical ventilation with a minimum frequency of respirations determined by ventilator settings. It also permits the patient to initiate ventilation.

control m. Continuous mandatory ventilation using a preset pattern that does not require patient intervention.

model **1.** A pattern or form used to make a replica, as a cast or impression of teeth in dentistry. **2.** A person or thing worthy of emulation or imitation. **3.** A framework or system for organizing concepts into a meaningful schema (e.g., conceptual model of nursing). SEE: *Nursing Theory Appendix.*

animal m. The study of anatomy, physiology, or pathology in laboratory animals in order to apply the results to human function and disease.

conceptual m. A set of abstract and general concepts and statements about those concepts. Also called *conceptual framework, conceptual system,* and *paradigm.*

conceptual m. of nursing Nursing m.

fluid mosaic m. A representation of the structure of the cell membrane, in which protein molecules are dispersed in a lipid bilayer.

m. of human occupation A conceptual framework for viewing occupational therapy practice, aimed at improving the patient's organization of time, overall function, and adaptation as reflected in the performance of occupations. Within this framework, intervention includes strategies for fostering skill development and habit changes through role acquisition, improved self-image, and environmental changes.

Nagi disablement m. SEE: *Nagi disablement model.*

nursing m. A conceptual model that refers to global ideas about people, their environments and health, and nursing.

study m. A diagnostic cast of an impression of the dental arches or a part thereof, trimmed with the arches articulated and the edges perpendicular to the occlusal plane. The study model serves as the basis for construction of dental appliances, dentures, or orthodontic treatment.

modeling A form of behavior therapy involving the patient's acquisition of social behavior and mental response by following the example of associates, esp. parents and siblings.

moderated Mitigated.

modification (mŏd″ĭ-fĭ-kā′shŭn) The act or result of changing something, such as the shape or character of an object or structure.

modifier In medicine, esp. in therapeutics and clinical medicine, use of or addition of something that alters that to which it is added.

biological response m. ABBR: BRM. **1.** An agent that intensifies normal immune responses. Examples include interferon, interleukin-2, and monoclonal antibodies. **2.** A nutrient with hormonal or anti-inflammatory effects. Examples include phytochemicals and phytonutrients, enzymes, botanical medicines, and plant hormones. Usually, these agents are used as adjuncts to other pharmacological agents and therapies in the management of selected malignancies, immunodeficiency and autoimmune disorders, and certain viral infections such as hepatitis C. SEE: *biotherapy.*

modiolus (mō-dī′ō-lŭs) [L., hub] Central pillar or axial part of cochlea extending from the base to the apex.

modulation (mŏd″ū-lā′shŭn) **1.** The alteration in function or status of something in response to a stimulus or altered chemical or physical environment. **2.** In electronics, the manner in which a signal is used to vary either the amplitude, frequency, or phase of a normally constant carrier signal; a method of coding information onto a carrier.

modulus (mŏj′ŭ-lŭs) [L., a small measure] In physics, a constant or coefficient that indicates to what extent a substance possesses some property.

modus operandi Method of performing an act.

Moebius' (Möbius') disease (mē′bē-ŭs) [Paul J. Moebius, Ger. neurologist, 1853–1907] Migraine accompanied by paralysis of the oculomotor nerves.

Moebius' sign A symptom of Graves' disease in which one eye converges and the other diverges when one looks at the tip of one's nose.

Moebius syndrome Congenital paralysis of the facial nerve, occurring in the absence of other neurological deficits. It may be unilateral or bilateral.

mogilalia (mŏj-ĭ-lā′lē-ă) [Gr. *mogis,* with difficulty, + *lalia,* chatter] Any speech defect, such as stuttering.

mogiphonia (mōj-ĭ-fō′nē-ă) [″ + *phone,* voice] Difficulty in emitting vocal sounds.

Mohrenheim's space (mor′ĕn-hīmz) [Baron J. J. Freiherr von Mohrenheim, Austrian surgeon, 1759–1799] Space between the pectoralis major and deltoid muscles just beneath the clavicle.

Mohs' chemosurgery technique [Frederic Edward Mohs, U.S. surgeon, 1910–1979] A method of excising tumors of the skin. The tumor tissue is fixed in place and a layer is removed. That portion is then examined microscopically. This procedure is repeated until the entire tumor is removed. Use of this technique ensures complete removal. It is esp. useful in treating basal cell epitheliomas.

MOI *mechanism of injury.*

moiety (moy'ĕ-tē) [Fr. *moitié,* fr. L. *medietas,* middle] **1.** One of two equal parts. **2.** A portion of something that has been divided.

moist (moyst) Damp, wet.

mol Mole (1).

molal (mō'lăl) One mole of solute per kilogram of solvent. SEE: *mole* (1).

molality (mō-lăl'ĭ-tē) The number of moles of a solute per kilogram of solvent.

molar [L. *moles,* a mass] **1.** Pert. to a mass; not molecular. **2.** Pert. to a mole. **3.** Gram-molecule. SYN: *mole* (1).

molar [L. *molaris,* grinding] A grinding or back tooth, one of three on each side of each jaw. The first permanent molar erupts between 6 and 7 years; the second between the 13th and 16th years. The third molars (wisdom teeth) are extremely variable, usually erupting between the 18th and 25th years; however, they may erupt later or not at all. SEE: *dentition* for table; *teeth.*

impacted m. A tooth that is unable to erupt into its place in normal occlusion, usually due to crowding by other teeth. This condition is commonly related to the third molar, or wisdom tooth.

mulberry m. A malformed first molar with dwarfed cusps and aggregations of enamel globules around the surface so that the crown has the appearance of a berry. This condition is seen in congenital syphilis and other diseases.

molariform (mŏl-ăr'ĭ-form) Resembling a molar tooth.

molarity The number of gram molecular mass (moles) of a substance per liter of solution. Thus 1/M (also expressed as 1 M) means 1 mole of a substance per liter, and 0.1/M indicates 0.1 mole/L.

molar solution SEE: under *solution.*

mold **1.** A fuzzy coating due to growth of a fungus on the surface of decaying vegetable matter or on nonorganic objects. **2.** Any one of a group of parasitic or saprophytic fungi that cause mold, such as black molds (Mucorales) and blue and green molds (Aspergillales), the latter including *Penicillium,* the source of the antibiotic penicillin. **3.** To shape a mass or the container in which the mass is shaped.

molding **1.** Shaping of the fetal head to adapt itself to the dimensions of the birth canal during its descent through the pelvis. **2.** A protective border used in plastic surgery. **3.** The casting of a reproduction.

border m. In dentistry, the shaping of impression material at the edges by the oral tissues.

mole (mōl) [Ger. *Mol,* abbr. for *Molekulargewicht,* molecular weight] In the Système International d' Unités (SI system), 1 mole of a substance contains as many atoms as exist in 0.012 kg of carbon 12.

mole [L. *moles,* a shapeless mass] A uterine mass arising from a poorly developed or degenerating ovum.

blood m. A mass made up of blood clots, membranes, and placenta, retained following abortion.

Breus m. [Karl Breus, Austrian physician, 1852–1914] Malformation of the ovum; a decidual tuberous subchorional hematoma.

carneous m. Blood mole that assumes a fleshlike appearance when retained in the uterus for some time. SYN: *fleshy m.*

false m. Mole formed from a uterine tumor or polypus.

fleshy m. Carneous m.

hydatid m. A polycystic mass in which the chorionic villi have undergone cystic degeneration, resulting in rapid growth of the uterus with hemorrhage. It is thought to be caused by abnormal postfertilization replication of spermatozoal chromosomes. Complete and partial moles differ in karyotype. Complete moles show an absence of maternal chromosomes and a duplication of spermatozoal chromosomes. Partial moles exhibit either karyotype 69 XXY or karyotype 69 XYY due to the presence of the maternal X chromosome. SEE: *gestational trophoblastic disease.*

stone m. A fleshy mole that has undergone calcific degeneration in the uterus.

true m. A mole representing the degenerated embryo or fetus.

vesicular m. Hydatid m.

mole [AS. *mael*] A birthmark or nevus. SEE: illus.

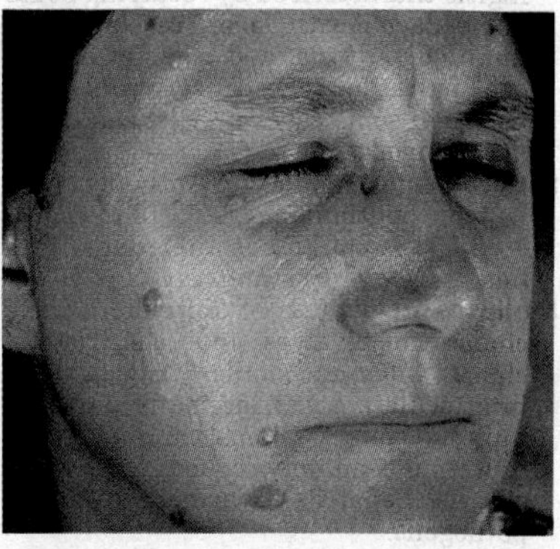

MOLES

CAUTION: Removal of a mole by tying a thread around it should not be attempted. Removal should be done by a physician.

PATIENT CARE: The patient is encouraged to regularly inspect areas of the skin that have moles and consult a physician about any mole that changes color or shows signs of growth or changes in appearance, as such changes may indicate neoplasm.

pigmented m. Nevus pigmentosus.

vascular m. Hemangioma.

molecular (mō-lĕk′ū-lăr) Pert. to molecules.

molecular disease Disease due to a defect in a single molecule. An example is sickle cell anemia, in which a single amino acid substitution in the hemoglobin molecule causes the abnormally shaped red cells characteristic of this disease. SYN: *molecular lesion*.

molecular lesion Molecular disease.

molecule (mŏl′ĕ-kūl) [L. *molecula,* little mass] Any electrically neutral aggregate of atoms held together strongly enough to be considered as a unit. The individual atoms in the molecule may be of the same type or different. Combinations of dissimilar atoms form chemical compounds. The positive and negative electrical charges balance exactly. Excess or deficiency of either positive or negative charge by the loss or acquisition of electrons results in the formation of an ion.

A molecule is designated by the number of atoms it contains, as monatomic (one atom); diatomic (two); triatomic (three); tetratomic (four); pentatomic (five); or hexatomic (six). **molecular** (mō-lĕk′ū-lăr), *adj.*

molimen (mō-lī′mĕn) *pl.* **molimina** [L., effort] Effort to establish any normal function, esp. that necessary to establish the menstrual flow.

Mollaret's meningitis [Pierre Mollaret, Fr. physician, b. 1898.] Form of meningitis characterized by recurring bouts of headache with fever, cerebrospinal fluid leukocytosis, and signs of meningeal irritation. The cause is unknown although some cases may be caused by herpesviruses.

Moll's glands [Jacob Anthoni Moll, Dutch ophthalmologist, 1832–1914] Modified sweat glands at border of eyelids. SYN: *ciliary glands*.

Mollusca A phylum of animals that includes the bivalves (mussels, oysters, clams), slugs, and snails. Snails serve as intermediate hosts for many parasitic flukes. Oysters, clams, and mussels, esp. if inadequately cooked, may transmit the hepatitis A virus or bacterial pathogens.

molluscum (mŏ-lŭs′kŭm) [L., soft] A mildly infective skin disease marked by tumor formations on the skin. **molluscous** (mŏ-lŭs′kŭs), *adj.*

m. contagiosum A rash composed of small dome-shaped papules with a central crater that is said to be "umbilicated" (dimpled or belly button–shaped). Cheesy (caseous) material fills the dimple's core. A pox virus causes the rash, which is commonly spread by person-to-person contact among children and young adults. Widespread lesions are sometimes identified on the skin of immunosuppressed patients (e.g., patients with AIDS). Lesions in the groin, on the genitals, or on the upper thighs usually are sexually transmitted. SEE: illus.

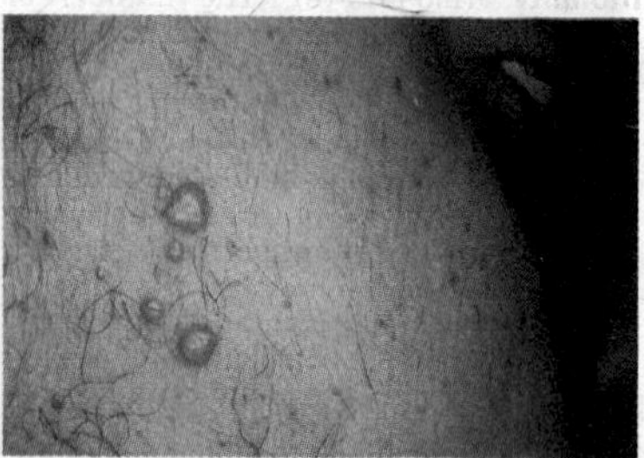

MOLLUSCUM CONTAGIOSUM

TREATMENT: Some lesions may heal spontaneously and require no therapy. Persistent papules can be removed with curettage or frozen with liquid nitrogen.

mollusk, mollusc Any member of the phylum Mollusca.

molt To shed a covering such as feathers or skin that is replaced by new growth.

mol. wt. *molecular weight.*

molybdenum (mō-lĭb′dĕ-nŭm) SYMB: Mo. A hard, heavy, metallic element; atomic weight 95.94, atomic number 42.

molysmophobia (mō-lĭz″mō-fō′bē-ă) [Gr. *molysma,* stain, + *phobia,* fear] Abnormal fear of contamination or infection. SYN: *mysophobia*.

momentum (mō-mĕn′tŭm) [L.] **1.** In physics, the description of a quantity obtained by multiplying the mass of a body by its linear velocity. **2.** Force of motion acquired by a moving object as a result of continuance of its motion; impetus.

momism [Coined by Phillip Wylie in his book *A Generation of Vipers*] In American culture, undue dependence on one's mother, esp. in very early life. This was alleged to cause the individual to be immature.

monad [Gr. *monas,* a unit] **1.** A univalent element. **2.** A unicellular organism. **3.** One of the four components of a tetrad.

monamide (mŏn-ăm′īd) Monoamide.

monamine (mŏn-ăm′ĭn) Monoamine.

monarthric (mŏn-ăr′thrĭk) [Gr. *monos,* single, + *arthron,* joint] Monarticular.

monarticular (mŏn-ăr-tĭk′ŭ-lăr) Concerning or affecting one joint. SYN: *monarthric*.

monaster (mŏn-ăs′tĕr) [″ + *aster*, star] Single starlike figure formed in mitosis.

monathetosis (mŏn″ăth-ē-tō′sĭs) [″ + *athetos*, not fixed, + *osis*, condition] Athetosis affecting a single limb.

monatomic (mŏn″ă-tŏm′ĭk) [″ + *atomos*, indivisible] **1.** Concerning a single atom. **2.** Univalent.

monaural (mŏn-aw′răl) Concerning or affecting one ear.

Mondonesi's reflex (mŏn-dō-nā′zēz) [Filippo Mondonesi, It. physician] In coma, contraction of facial muscles following pressure on the eyeball. SYN: *bulbomimic reflex; facial reflex*.

Mondor's disease (mŏn′dorz) [Henri Mondor, Fr. physician, 1885–1962] Thrombosis and sclerosis of a subcutaneous vein or veins in the breast or chest wall sometimes extending from the axilla to the epigastrium. The condition may occur after trauma or appear without apparent cause. Although a benign, self-limiting disease, its appearance may be confused with breast cancer.

Monera Prokaryotae.

monesthetic (mŏn″ĕs-thĕt′ĭk) [Gr. *monos*, single, + *aisthesis*, sensation] Affecting only one of the senses.

monestrous (mŏn-ĕs′trŭs) Having a single estrous cycle in a single sexual season.

Monge's disease [Carlos Monge, Peruvian physician, 1884–1970] SEE: *mountain sickness, chronic*.

mongolism (mŏn′gōl-ĭzm) An inaccurate and inappropriate term for Down syndrome.

mongoloid (mŏn′gō-loyd) **1.** Concerning Mongols. **2.** Characterized by mongolism (i.e., Down syndrome).

monilethrix (mŏn-ĭl′ĕ-thrĭks) [L. *monile*, necklace, + Gr. *thrix*, hair] A genetic defect of the hair shaft in which the hair becomes beaded and brittle. The defect usually appears by the second month of life. There is no effective treatment.

Monilia [L. *monile*, necklace] Former name for the genus of fungi now called *Candida*. **monilial** (mō-nĭl′ē-ăl), *adj.*

moniliasis (mō″nĭ-lī′ă-sĭs) Candidiasis.

moniliform (mŏn-ĭl′ĭ-form) [″ + *forma*, shape] Resembling a necklace or string of beads.

moniliid (mō-nĭl′ē-ĭd) A skin eruption due to hypersensitivity to a *Candida* infection in another part of the body.

monitor (mŏn′ĭ-tor) [L., one who warns] **1.** One who observes a condition, procedure, or apparatus, esp. one responsible for detecting and preventing malfunction. **2.** A device that provides a warning if that which is being observed fails or malfunctions. **3.** To check by using an electronic device.

apnea m. SEE: *apnea monitoring*.

Beck airway airflow m. A device that produces a whistling sound when an endotracheal tube is correctly placed into the lower airways.

blood pressure m. A device that automatically obtains and usually records the blood pressure at certain intervals, using the direct or indirect method of determining pressure. In some models, an alarm or light signal is activated if the pressure rises or falls to an abnormal level.

cardiac m. Monitor of heart function, providing visual and audible record of heartbeat.

continuous ambulatory electrocardiographic m. SEE: *Holter monitor*.

fetal m. **1.** Monitor that detects and displays fetal heartbeat. **2.** Assessment of fetus in utero with respect to its heart rate by use of electrocardiogram or by chemical analysis of the amniotic fluid or fetal blood. SEE: *fetal heart rate monitoring; fetal monitoring in utero*.

Holter m. SEE: *Holter monitor*.

impedance m. A device used to detect variations in respiratory rate and volume, by measuring changes in the electrical impedance of the chest as the patient breathes. It may be used in intensive care units to monitor critically ill patients or in private residences to detect apnea, esp. in sleeping infants.

peak flow m. A hand-held device used to assess the maximum expiratory flow (in liters/minute) in patients with asthma and chronic obstructive lung disease.

personal radiation m. Small device carried by an individual to measure the accumulated radiation dosage over a period of time. SEE: *dosimeter*.

respiratory m. SEE: *respiratory function monitoring*.

temperature m. Monitor for measuring and recording temperature of the body or some particular portion of the body.

unit m. In radiation therapy, a calibrated unit of dose that determines the length of the treatment.

uterine activity m. An electronic device applied to the abdomen to note and record uterine contractions.

PATIENT CARE: If home monitoring is instituted, patients at high risk for preterm labor are taught to apply the monitor for 1 hour twice daily and transmit the data by telephone to a health care professional for analysis. After analyzing the data, a telephone assessment for symptoms and signs of preterm labor is conducted, with necessary advice given to the patient. Studies that compare the effectiveness of home monitoring with invasive intrauterine pressure catheters show that ambulatory monitoring is imperfect. Improper application of the monitor and incorrect data interpretation may diminish its accuracy.

monitrice (mŏn′ĭ-trĭs) [Fr. *female,* instructor] In the Lamaze technique of childbearing, a labor coach or doula.

monkeypox (mŭn′kē-pŏks) A poxviral illness clinically similar to smallpox.

mono-, mon- [Gr. *monos,* single] Prefix meaning *one, single.*

monoacidic (mŏn″ō-ă-sĭd′ĭk) Having one replaceable hydroxyl (OH) group.

monoamide An amide with only one amide group.

monoamine An amine with only one amine group.

monoamine oxidase inhibitor ABBR: MAOI. One member of a group of drugs that can be used to treat depression and Parkinson's disease. Nonselective versions of these medications produced hypertensive crises and other severe side effects when they were taken with tyramine-containing foods (some cheeses) and several other drugs. Newer members of this class of drugs do not have these effects, but should be used with caution, esp. in persons who take selective serotonin reuptake inhibitors. SEE: *tyramine.*

monoarthritis (mŏn″ăr-thrī′tĭs) [″ + ″ + *itis,* inflammation] Arthritis affecting a single joint.

monobacillary (mŏn″ō-băs′ĭ-lă″rē) Concerning a single species of bacilli.

monobactam (mŏn′ō-băk-tăm) A beta-lactam antibiotic, similar in structure to penicillins and cephalosporins, except with respect to its nucleus: monobactams have a single cyclical nucleus, while penicillins and cephalosporins have two linked cyclical nuclei.

monobacterial (mŏn″ō-băk-tē′rē-ăl) Concerning a single species of bacteria.

monobasic (mŏn-ō-bā′sĭk) [″ + *basis,* a base] Having only one hydrogen atom replaceable by a metal or positive radical.

monoblast (mŏn′ō-blăst) [″ + *blastos,* germ] A cell that gives rise to a monocyte.

monoblastoma (mŏn″ō-blăs-tō′mă) [″ + ″ + *oma,* tumor] A neoplasm that contains both monoblasts and monocytes.

monoblepsia (mŏn-ō-blĕp′sē-ă) [″ + *blepsis,* sight] **1.** Condition in which vision is more distinct when only one eye is used, hence tendency to close one eye to see clearly. **2.** A type of color blindness in which only one color can be seen.

monobrachius (mŏn″ō-brā′kē-ŭs) [″ + *brachion,* arm] **1.** State of having only one arm. **2.** Fetus with only one arm.

monobromated (mŏn″ō-brō′māt-ĕd) Pert. to chemical compound with only one atom of bromine in each molecule.

monocalcic (mŏn-ō-kăl′sĭk) Pert. to a chemical compound containing only one atom of calcium in the molecule.

monocardian (mŏn-ō-kăr′dē-ăn) [″ + *kardia,* heart] An animal possessing a heart with only one atrium and one ventricle.

monocelled (mŏn′ō-sĕld) Composed of a single cell.

monocephalus (mŏn″ō-sĕf′ă-lŭs) [″ + *kephale,* head] A congenitally deformed fetus with duplicated parts except for the head.

monochord (mŏn′ō-kord) [″ + *chordc,* cord] A single-string instrument used for testing upper tone audition.

monochorea (mŏn″ō-kō-rē′ă) [″ + *choreia,* dance] Chorea affecting a single part.

monochorionic (mŏn-ō-kor″ē-ŏn′ĭk) Possessing a single chorion, as in the case of identical twins.

monochromasy (mŏn″ō-krō-mā′sē) Monochromatism.

monochromatic (mŏn″ō-krō-măt′ĭk) [″ + *chroma,* color] **1.** Having one color. **2.** A color-blind person to whom all colors appear to be of one hue.

monochromatism (mŏn″ō-krō′mă-tĭzm) [Gr. *monos,* single, + *chroma,* color, + *-ismos,* condition] Complete color blindness in which all colors are perceived as shades of gray. SYN: *monochromasy.*

monochromatophil (mŏn″ō-krō-măt′ō-fĭl) [″ + ″ + *philein,* to love] A cell or tissue that accepts only one stain.

monochromator (mŏn-ō-krō′mā-tor) A spectroscope modified for selective transmission of a narrow band of the spectrum.

monoclinic (mŏn″ō-klin′ĭk) [″ + *klinein,* to incline] Pert. to crystals in which the vertical axis is inclined to one lateral axis but at right angles to the other.

monoclonal (mŏn″ō-klōn′ăl) Arising from a single cell.

monoclonal antibody A type of antibody, specific to a certain antigen, created in the laboratory from hybridoma cells. Because they are derived from a single cell line and raised against a single antigen, monoclonal antibodies are highly specific. Diagnostically, they are used to identify microorganisms, white blood cells, hormones, and tumor antigens. In patient care, they are used to treat transplant rejection, certain cancers, and autoimmune diseases.

Hybridoma cells, the living factories that are used to produce monoclonal antibodies, are formed by the fusion of a spleen cell from a mouse immunized with an antigen and a multiple myeloma cell (a cancerous plasma B cell). The fused cells are screened to identify those that secrete antibodies against a specific antigen. A continuous supply of these antigen-specific monoclonal antibody secreting cells can then be grown in cultures. SEE: *antibody; B cell; hybridoma.*

monoclonal antibody therapy The use of monoclonal antibodies to suppress immune function, kill target cells, or treat specific inflammatory diseases. Because of their high level of specificity, they

Monoclonal Antibodies and Their Potential Uses

Name of Antibody	Condition Treated or Prevented
Edrecolomab	Solid tumors
Enlimomab	Organ transplant rejection
Infliximab	Crohn's disease; rheumatoid arthritis
OKT3	Organ transplant rejection
Palivizumab	Respiratory syncytial virus
Rituximab	Leukemias and lymphomas
RhuMAbVEGF	Solid tumors
Transtuzumab	Metastatic breast cancer

bind to precise cellular or molecular targets. A potential problem associated with the use of monoclonal antibodies is an allergic reaction to the foreign antigens in the antibody, since they are created from mouse cells. Monoclonal antibodies have numerous uses in health care. SEE: table; *hybridoma; monoclonal antibody*.

monococcus (mŏn-ō-kŏk′ŭs) [″ + *kokkos,* berry] A form of coccus existing singly instead of as part of the usual group or chain.

monocontaminated (mŏn″ō-kŏn-tăm′ĭ-nāt″ĕd) Infected with a single species of organism.

monocrotic (mŏn″ō-krŏt′ĭk) [″ + *krotos,* beat] Indicating a single pulse wave with no notches in it.

monocular (mŏn-ŏk′ū-lar) [″ + L. *oculus,* eye] **1.** Concerning or affecting one eye. **2.** Possessing a single eyepiece, as in a monocular microscope.

monoculus (mŏn-ŏk′ū-lŭs) **1.** A bandage for shielding one eye. **2.** A fetus with only one eye. SYN: *cyclops*.

monocyclic (mŏn″ō-sī′klĭk) Concerning one cycle.

monocyesis (mŏn″ō-sī-ē′sĭs) [″ + *kyesis,* pregnancy] Pregnancy with a single fetus.

monocyte (mŏn′ō-sīt) [″ + *kytos,* cell] A mononuclear phagocytic white blood cell derived from myeloid stem cells. Monocytes circulate in the bloodstream for about 24 hr and then move into tissues, at which point they mature into macrophages, which are long lived. Monocytes and macrophages are one of the first lines of defense in the inflammatory process. This network of fixed and mobile phagocytes that engulf foreign antigens and cell debris previously was called the reticuloendothelial system and is now referred to as the mononuclear phagocyte system (MPS). SEE: illus.; *blood* for illus.; *macrophage*. **monocytic** (mŏn-ō-sĭt′ĭk), *adj.*

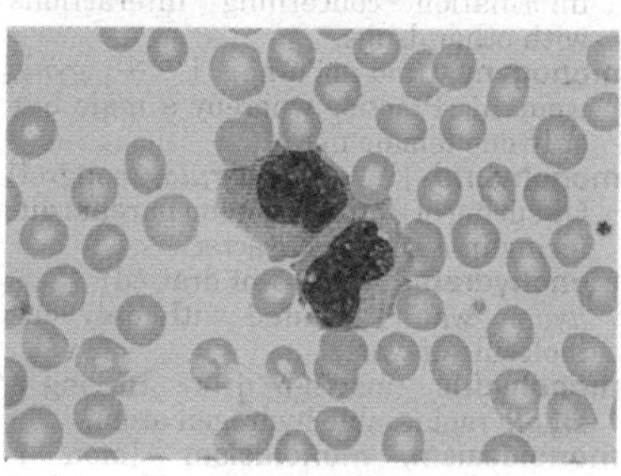

MONOCYTES

(Orig. mag. ×640)

monocytopenia (mŏn″ō-sī″tō-pē′nē-ă) [″ + *kytos,* cell, + *penia,* lack] Diminished number of monocytes in the blood.

monocytosis (mŏn″ō-sī-tō′sĭs) [″ + ″ + *osis,* condition] Excessive number of monocytes in the blood.

monodactylism (mŏn-ō-dăk′tĭl-ĭzm) [″ + *daktylos,* digit] Condition, usually congenital, of having only one digit on a hand or foot. Also called monodactyly or monodactylia.

monodal (mŏn-ō′dăl) [″ + *hodos,* road] Connected with one terminal of a resonator so that the patient acts as a capacitor for entrance and exit of high-frequency currents.

monodermoma (mŏn″ō-dĕr-mō′mă) [″ + *derma,* skin, + *oma,* tumor] A neoplasm originating in one germinal layer.

monodiplopia (mŏn″ō-dĭ-plō′pē-ă) [″ + *diploos,* double, + *ops,* eye] Double vision in one eye only.

monoecious (mŏn-ē′shŭs) [″ + *oikos,* house] Pert. to the presence of functioning male and female sex organs in the same individual.

monogamy (mō-nŏg′ă-mē) [″ + *gamos,* marriage] A long-term exclusive sexual affiliation.

monogenesis (mŏn″ō-jĕn′ĕ-sĭs) [Gr. *monos,* single, + *genesis,* generation, birth] **1.** Production of offspring of only one sex. **2.** The theory that all organisms arise from a single cell. **3.** Asexual reproduction.

monogerminal (mŏn″ō-jĕr′mĭ-năl) Produced from a single ovum.

monogony (mō-nŏg′ō-nē) [″ + *gone,* seed] Asexual reproduction.

monograph (mŏn′ō-grăf) [″+ *graphein,* to write] A treatise dealing with a single subject.

drug m. A publication that specifies for a drug (or class of related drugs) the kinds and amounts of ingredients it may contain, the conditions and limitations for which it may be offered, directions for use, warnings, and other information that its labeling must contain. The monograph may contain important information concerning interactions with other drugs.

monogyny (mō-nŏj′ă-nē) [″ + *gyne,* woman] Practice whereby a male has only one female mate.

monohybrid [″ + L. *hybrida,* mongrel] Offspring of a cross between parents differing in a single character.

monohydrated (mŏn-ō-hī′drāt-ĕd) [″ + *hydor,* water] United with only one molecule of water.

monohydric (mŏn″ō-hī′drĭk) Having a single replaceable hydrogen atom.

monoideaism, monoideism (mŏn″ō-ī-dē′ă-ĭzm, -dē′ĭzm) [″ + *idea,* idea] Preoccupation with only one idea; a slight degree of monomania.

monoinfection (mŏn″ō-ĭn-fĕk′shŭn) Infection with a single species of organism.

monoiodotyrosine (mŏn″ō-ī-ō″dō-tī′rō-sēn) An amino acid intermediate in the synthesis of thyroxine and triiodothyronine.

monokine A chemical mediator released by monocytes and macrophages during the immune response. Monokines affect the growth and activity of other white blood cells. Interleukin-1 is an important monokine. SEE: *cytokine; inflammation; interleukin-1; lymphokine; paracrine.*

monolayer (mŏn″ō-lā′ĕr) A single layer, esp. of cells growing in culture.

monolocular (mŏn″ō-lŏk′ū-lar) [″ + L. *loculus,* a small chamber] Having only one cell or cavity. SYN: *unilocular.*

monomania (mŏn-ō-mā′nē-ă) [″ + *mania,* madness] Mental illness characterized by distortion of thought processes concerning a single subject or idea.

monomaniac One afflicted with monomania.

monomastigote (mŏn-ō-măs′tĭ-gōt) [″ + *mastix,* whip] Mastigote possessing only one flagellum.

monomelic (mŏn-ō-mĕl′ĭk) [″ + *melos,* limb] Affecting a single limb.

monomer (mŏn′ō-mĕr) Any molecule that can be bound to similar molecules to form a polymer.

monomeric (mŏn-ō-mĕr′ĭk) [″ + *meros,* part] Consisting of, or affecting, a single piece or segment of a body.

monometallic (mŏn″ō-mĕ-tăl′ĭk) Containing a single atom of a metal per molecule.

monomicrobic (mŏn″ō-mī-krō′bĭk) Concerning organisms of a single species.

monomolecular (mŏn″ō-mō-lĕk′ū-lăr) Concerning one molecule.

monomorphic (mŏn-ō-mor′fĭk) [″ + *morphe,* form] Unchangeable in form; keeping the same form throughout every stage of development.

monomyoplegia (mŏn″ō-mī″ō-plē′jē-ă) [″ + *mys,* muscle, + *plege,* stroke] Paralysis of only one muscle.

monomyositis (mŏn″ō-mī-ō-sī′tĭs) [″ + ″ + *itis,* inflammation] Inflammation of only one muscle.

mononeural (mŏn-ō-nū′răl) [″ + *neuron,* nerve] Supplied by or concerning a single nerve.

mononeuritis (mŏn″ō-nū-rī′tĭs) [″ + ″ + *itis,* inflammation] Inflammation of a single nerve.

m. multiplex Inflammation of nerves in separate body areas.

mononeuropathy (mŏn″ō-nū-rŏp′ă-thē) [″ + ″ + *pathos,* disease, suffering] Disease of a single nerve.

hypertrophic m. Neuropathy associated with enlargement and tenderness of two or three nerves of the head and neck area. The nerves may appear to be a neurofibroma, but biopsy will provide the correct diagnosis.

mononuclear (mŏn-ō-nū′klē-ăr) [″ + L. *nucleus,* kernel] Having one nucleus, particularly a blood cell such as a monocyte or lymphocyte. SYN: *uninuclear.*

mononuclear phagocyte system ABBR: MPS. The system of fixed macrophages and circulating monocytes that serve as phagocytes, engulfing foreign substances in a wide variety of immune responses. This system formerly was called the reticuloendothelial system. SEE: *macrophage.*

mononucleosis (mŏn-ō-nū″klē-ō′sĭs) [″ + *nucleus,* kernel, + *osis,* condition] Presence of an abnormally high number of mononuclear leukocytes in the blood. SEE: illus.

infectious m. An acute infectious disease caused by the Epstein-Barr virus (EBV), a member of the herpesvirus group. It is most common in the U.S. in persons between 15 and 25 years of age (i.e., in high school- and college-age adolescents and young adults); beyond that age, most persons are immune to EBV. The disease sometimes is referred to colloquially as the "kissing disease." SEE: *Epstein-Barr virus; Nursing Diagnoses Appendix.*

ETIOLOGY: The virus is transmitted in saliva and infects the epithelial cells of the oropharynx, nasopharynx, and salivary glands before spreading to lymphoid tissue (e.g., lymph nodes, spleen, liver) via infected B lymphocytes. The incubation period is 30 to 45 days.

SYMPTOMS: Typically, infectious mononucleosis causes a sudden or gradual onset (7 to 14 days) of flulike symptoms, including a severe sore throat, fatigue, headache, chest pain, and myalgia. Findings include enlarged tender lymph nodes (lymphadenopathy), exudative tonsillitis, and an enlarged spleen. Leukocytosis with atypical lymphocytes are present. The infection usually lasts 2-4 weeks.

Rarely, infectious mononucleosis is complicated by hemolytic anemia, hepatomegaly, jaundice, meningoencepha-

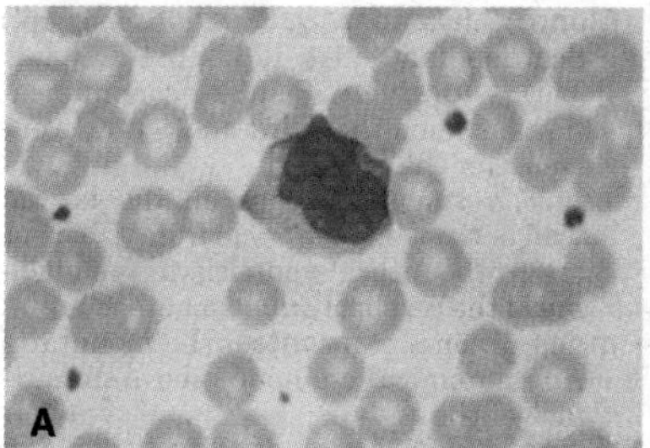

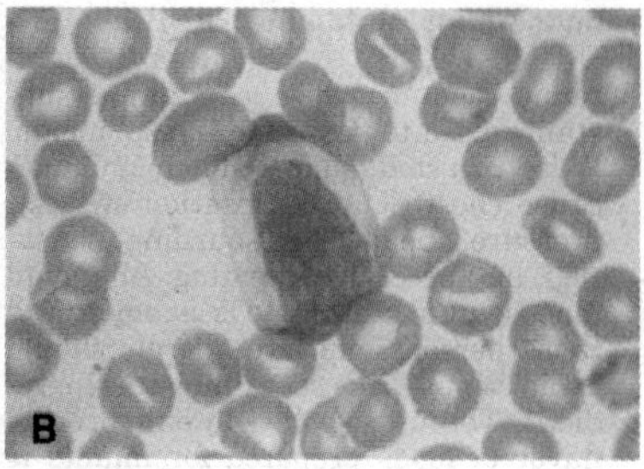

MONONUCLEOSIS

Atypical lymphocytes

litis, or pneumonitis. In Africa, latent EBV infection may be associated with the development of Burkitt's lymphoma.

DIAGNOSIS: The diagnosis of infectious mononucleosis is based on assessment of signs and symptoms, the presence of atypical lymphocytes and IgM antibodies in the blood, and a positive heterophil reaction with sheep red blood cells (Monospot test). Differential diagnoses include cytomegalovirus infection, cat scratch disease, *Toxoplasma gondii* infection, and the acute onset of infection with HIV.

TREATMENT: There is no specific therapy for infectious mononucleosis; NSAIDs are used to treat fever, headache, sore throat, and myalgias. Corticosteroids may be used for complications. Full recovery is usual.

PATIENT CARE: During the acute phase, the patient is encouraged to refrain from activity and to maintain adequate rest to reduce fatigue. Generally, patients may resume activity that does not involve heavy exertion after 1 to 2 weeks and their normal activity level in 4 to 6 weeks. If the spleen is enlarged, patients should avoid contact sports and not lift more than 10 lb until cleared by their health care provider to prevent traumatizing or rupturing the spleen.

mononucleotide (mŏn″ō-nū′klē-ō-tīd″) A product resulting from hydrolysis of nucleic acid, containing phosphoric acid combined with a glucoside or pentoside. SYN: *nucleotide*.

monoparesis (mŏn-ō-păr-ē′sĭs) [Gr. *monos,* single, + *paresis,* weakness] Paralysis of a single part of the body.

monoparesthesia (mŏn″ō-păr-ĕs-thē′sē-ă) [″ + *para,* beside, + *aisthesis,* sensation] Paresthesia of only one region or limb.

monophagia (mŏn-ō-fā′jē-ă) [″ + *phagein,* to eat] **1.** Appetite for only one kind of food. Said esp. of insects. **2.** The habit of eating only one meal a day.

monophasia (mŏn-ō-fā′zē-ă) [″ + *phasis,* speech] Inability to utter anything but one word or phrase repeatedly.

monophobia (mŏn-ō-fō′bē-ă) [″ + *phobos,* fear] Abnormal fear of being alone.

monophyletic (mŏn″ō-fīl-ĕt′ĭk) [″ + *phyle,* tribe] Originating from a single source. Opposite of polyphyletic.

monophyletism (mŏn″ō-fī′lĕ-tĭzm) Concerning the concept that all blood cells are derived from a single stem cell.

monophyodont (mŏn″ō-fī′ō-dŏnt) [″ + *phyein,* to grow, + *odous,* tooth] Having a single, permanent set of teeth.

monoplasmatic (mŏn″ō-plăz-măt′ĭk) [″ + LL. *plasma,* form, mold] Made up of a single substance or tissue.

monoplast (mŏn″ō-plăst) [″ + *plastos,* formed] A single-cell type of organism that does not change during its life cycle.

monoplegia (mŏn-ō-plē′jē-ă) [″ + *plege,* stroke] Paralysis of a single limb or a single group of muscles. **monoplegic,** *adj.*

monopodia (mŏn″ō-pō′dē-ă) [″ + *pous,* foot] Condition of having only one foot; usually the two feet are fused.

monopolar (mŏn-ō-pōl′ăr) [″ + L. *polus,* pole] **1.** Having one pole. SYN: *unipolar.* **2.** In therapeutic electrical stimulation, the application of a current using large dispersive electrodes and smaller active electrodes under which the treatment effects occur.

monopsychosis (mŏn″ō-sī-kō′sĭs) [Gr. *monos,* single, + *psyche,* mind, + *osis,* condition] Monomania.

monorchia (mŏn-or′kē-ă) Monorchidism.

monorchid (mŏn-or′kĭd) [″ + *orchis,* testicle] Person having only one testicle.

monorchidism, monorchism (mŏn-or′kĭd-ĭzm, mŏn′or-kĭzm) Condition in which there is only one descended testicle.

monorhinic (mŏn″ō-rĭn′ĭk) [″ + *rhis,* nose] **1.** Having a single nose, as in conjoined twins. **2.** Having a single fused nasal cavity.

monosaccharide (mŏn-ō-săk′ă-rīd) [″ + Sanskrit *sarkara,* sugar] A simple sugar that cannot be decomposed by hydrolysis, such as fructose, galactose, or glucose.

monosodium glutamate ABBR: MSG. $C_5H_8NNaO_4 \cdot H_2O$; sodium salt of glutamic acid; a white crystalline substance used to flavor foods, esp. meats. When ingested in large amounts, it may cause chest pain, a sensation of facial pressure, headaches, burning sensation, and excessive sweating. Allergy to monosodium glutamate is common, and those persons who are allergic should avoid eating foods containing this ingredient. The use of MSG to enhance the flavor of foods prepared for infants is controversial. MSG is sold under various trade names, such as Ajinomoto, Accent, Vetsin.

monosome (mŏn′ō-sōm) [″ + *soma,* body] An unpaired sex chromosome, X or Y, sometimes called an accessory chromosome.

monosomy (mŏn′ō-sō″mē) Condition of having only one of a pair of chromosomes, as in Turner's syndrome, in which there is one X chromosome rather than the normal pair.

monospasm (mŏn′ō-spăzm) [″ + *spasmos,* convulsion] Spasm of a single limb or part.

monospermy (mŏn′ō-spĕr″mē) [″ + *sperma,* seed] Fertilization by a single spermatozoon entering an ovum.

monostotic (mŏn″ŏs-tŏt′ĭk) [″ + *osteon,* bone] Concerning a single bone.

monosubstituted (mŏn″ō-sŭb′stĭ-tūt″ĕd) Having only a single molecule replaced.

monosymptomatic (mŏn″ō-sĭmp-tō-măt′ĭk) [″ + *symptomatikos,* pert. to symptom] Having only one dominant symptom.

monosynaptic (mŏn″ō-sĭ-năp′tĭk) Transmitted through only a single synapse.

monosyphilide (mŏn-ō-sĭf′ĭl-ĭd) [″ + Fr. *syphilide,* syphilitic lesion] Characterized by a single syphilitic lesion.

monotherapy (mŏn′ō-thĕr-ă-pē) Treatment with a single drug, for example, a single antihypertensive agent.

monotocous (mō-nŏt′ō-kŭs) [Gr. *monos,* single, + *tokos,* birth] Producing a single offspring per birth.

monotricha (mō-nŏt′rĭ-kă) [″ + *thrix,* hair] Bacteria having a single flagellum at one pole.

monotrichous (mŏn-ŏt′rĭ-kŭs) Pert. to or having a single flagellum.

monovalent (mŏn-ō-vā′lĕnt) [″ + L. *valere,* to have power] Having the combining power of a single hydrogen atom. SYN: *univalent* (1).

monoxenous (mō-nŏks′ĕn-ŭs) [″ + *xenos,* stranger] Said of a parasite that requires only one species as a host.

monoxide (mŏn-ŏk′sīd) An oxide having only one atom of oxygen.

monozygotic (mŏn″ō-zī-gŏt′ĭk) [″ + *zygotos,* yoked] Originating from a single fertilized ovum, said of identical twins.

Monro, Alexander (Secundus) (mŏn-rō′) Scottish anatomist, 1733–1817.

M.'s foramen Point of communication between the third and lateral ventricles of the brain.

M.'s sulcus Groove on the lateral wall of the third ventricle from the opening to the lateral ventricle to the opening of the cerebral aqueduct of the brain.

mons (mŏns) *pl.* **montes** [L., mountain] An anatomical eminence above the surface of the body.

m. pubis A pad of fatty tissue and skin overlying the symphysis pubis. After puberty it is covered with coarse hair.

m. veneris M. pubis.

Monteggia's fracture (mŏn-tĕj′ăz) [Giovanni B. Monteggia, It. surgeon, 1762–1815] Fracture of the upper portion of the ulna with dislocation of the radial head.

montelukast (mŏn-tē-lūk′ăst) An oral leukotriene inhibitor used to treat asthma.

Montgomery, William F. Irish obstetrician, 1797–1859.

M.'s glands Areolar glands.

Montgomery straps Paired adhesive straps applied to either side of a wound (usually abdominal), the central sections of which are folded back on themselves with several perforations at the leading edges. This provides a method of securing a bandage and subsequently changing it without having to replace the tape each time. SEE: illus.

month, lunar Four calendar weeks (28 days), a measurement of time used in obstetrics. Pregnancy is calculated in terms of 10 lunar months.

monticulus (mŏn-tĭk′ū-lŭs) *pl.* **monticuli** [L., little mountain] A protuberance.

m. cerebelli In the cerebellum, protuberance of the superior vermis, the anterior portion of which is called the culmen and the posterior portion, the declive.

mood [AS. *mod,* mind, feeling] A pervasive and sustained emotion that may have a major influence on a person's perception of the world. Examples of mood include depression, joy, elation, anger, and anxiety. SEE: *affect.*

mood disorder Any mental disorder that has a disturbance of mood as the predominant feature. In DSM-IV, these have been divided into mood episodes, mood disorders, and specifications describing either the most recent mood episode or the course of recurrent episodes. Mood disorders, including dysthymic disorder, are divided into the depressive disorders (unipolar depression), the bipolar disorders, and two disorders based on etiology (i.e., those due to a general medical condition or substance-induced mood disorder). Depressive disorders are distinguished from the bipolar disorders by the fact that

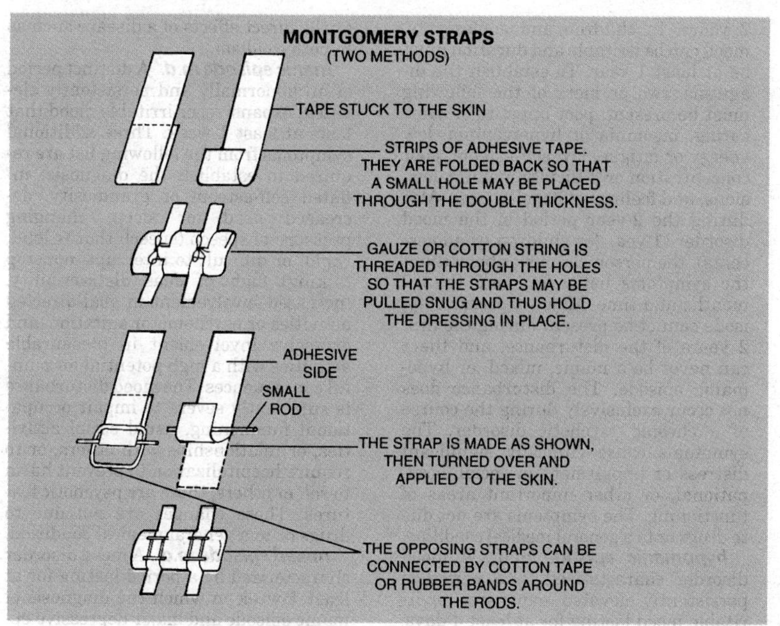
MONTGOMERY STRAPS
(TWO METHODS)
TAPE STUCK TO THE SKIN
STRIPS OF ADHESIVE TAPE. THEY ARE FOLDED BACK SO THAT A SMALL HOLE MAY BE PLACED THROUGH THE DOUBLE THICKNESS.
GAUZE OR COTTON STRING IS THREADED THROUGH THE HOLES SO THAT THE STRAPS MAY BE PULLED SNUG AND THUS HOLD THE DRESSING IN PLACE.
ADHESIVE SIDE
SMALL ROD
THE STRAP IS MADE AS SHOWN, THEN TURNED OVER AND APPLIED TO THE SKIN.
THE OPPOSING STRAPS CAN BE CONNECTED BY COTTON TAPE OR RUBBER BANDS AROUND THE RODS.

there is no history of ever having had a manic, mixed, or hypomanic episode. Bipolar I disorder and bipolar II disorder involve the presence of or history of manic episodes, mixed episodes, or hypomanic episodes usually with presence of or history of major depressive episodes. SEE: *Nursing Diagnoses Appendix.*

bipolar I m.d. A mood disorder characterized by the presence of only one manic episode and no past major depressive episodes that is not better accounted for by a psychotic disorder. The classes or specifiers of bipolar I disorder include mild, moderate, severe without psychotic features, severe with psychotic features, in partial remission, in full remission, with catatonic features, and with postpartum onset.

bipolar II m.d. A mood disorder characterized by the occurrence of one or more major depressive episodes accompanied by at least one hypomanic episode. If manic or mixed episode mood disorders are present, the diagnosis of bipolar I cannot be supported. Episodes of substance-induced mood disorder or a mood disorder due to drugs or toxin exposure preclude the diagnosis of bipolar II mood disorder. In addition, the symptoms must cause clinically significant distress or impairment in social, occupational, or other important areas of functioning. The specifiers "hypomanic" or "depressed" are used to indicate the current or most recent episode.

cyclothymic m.d. A diagnosis of exclusion in which for at least 2 years there has been the presence of numerous periods of hypomanic symptoms and numerous periods with depressive symptoms that do not meet the criteria for major depressive episode. During the 2-year period, the person cannot be without the symptoms mentioned for more than 2 months at a time. In addition, no major depressive episode, manic episode, or mixed episode can be present during the first 2 years of the disturbance. The symptoms cannot be accounted for by a psychosis and are not due to drugs or a general medical condition. The symptoms cause clinically significant distress or impairment in social, occupational, or other important areas of functioning.

m.d. due to a general medical disorder A prominent and persistent disturbance in mood characterized by either or both of the following: markedly diminished interest or pleasure in all, or almost all, activities and elevated, expansive, or irritable mood. The clinical and laboratory findings are consistent with attributing the cause to a direct physiological consequence of the general medical condition. The condition is not better accounted for by another mental disorder. The disturbance does not occur exclusively during the course of a delirium. The symptoms cause clinically significant distress or impairment in social, occupational, or other important areas of functioning.

dysthymic m.d. A chronically depressed mood that occurs for most of the day for more days than not for at least

2 years. In children and adolescents, mood can be irritable and duration must be at least 1 year. To establish the diagnosis, two or more of the following must be present: poor appetite or overeating, insomnia or hypersomnia, low energy or fatigue, low self-esteem, poor concentration or difficulty making decisions, and feelings of hopelessness. Also during the 2-year period of the mood disorder (1 year for children or adolescents), the person can never be without the symptoms listed for more than 2 months at a time. Major depressive episode cannot be present during the first 2 years of the disturbance, and there can never be a manic, mixed, or hypomanic episode. The disturbance does not occur exclusively during the course of a chronic psychotic disorder. The symptoms cause clinically significant distress or impairment in social, occupational, or other important areas of functioning. The symptoms are not due to drugs or to a general medical condition.

hypomanic episode m.d. A mood disorder characterized by a period of persistently elevated, expansive, or irritable mood lasting for at least 4 days. Three or more of the following must be present: inflated self-esteem, decreased need for sleep, talking more than usual, flight of ideas or feeling that thoughts are racing, distractibility, increase in goal-directed activities, and excessive involvement in pleasurable activities with a high potential for painful consequences. The episode is not severe enough to cause marked impairment in social or occupational functioning or to necessitate hospitalization; there are no psychotic features. These changes are not due to drugs or to a general medical condition.

luteal dysphoric m.d. Premenstrual dysphoric disorder.

major depressive episode m.d. A mood disorder characterized by a period of at least 2 weeks of depressed mood or the loss of interest or pleasure in nearly all activities. In children and adolescents, the mood may be irritable rather than sad. Establishing the diagnosis requires the presence of at least four of the following: changes in appetite, weight, sleep, and psychomotor activity; decreased energy; feelings of worthlessness or guilt; difficulty thinking, concentrating, or making decisions; or recurrent thoughts of death, or plans for or attempts to commit suicide. The symptoms must persist for most of the day, nearly every day, for at least 2 consecutive weeks. The episode must be accompanied by clinically significant distress or impairment in social, occupational, or other important areas of functioning. Also, the disorder must not be due to bereavement, drugs, alcohol, or the direct effects of a disease such as hypothyroidism.

manic episode m.d. A distinct period of an abnormally and persistently elevated, expansive, or irritable mood that lasts at least 1 week. Three additional symptoms from the following list are required to establish the diagnosis: inflated self-esteem or grandiosity, decreased need for sleep, changing pressure of speech (speech that is loud, rapid, or difficult to interrupt; nonstop talking), flight of ideas, distractibility, increased involvement in goal-directed activities or psychomotor agitation, and excessive involvement in pleasurable activities with a high potential for painful consequences. The mood disturbance is sufficiently severe to impair occupational functioning, usual social activities, or relationships with others, or to require hospitalization to prevent harm to self or others; there are psychotic features. These changes are not due to drugs or to a general medical condition.

mixed episode m.d. A mood disorder characterized by a period lasting for at least 1 week in which the diagnosis of manic episode and major depressive episode are met nearly each day. SEE: *major depressive episode m.d.; manic episode m.d.*

substance-induced m.d. A prominent and persistent disturbance in mood characterized by either or both of the following: depressed mood or markedly diminished interest or pleasure in all, or almost all, activities and elevated, expansive, or irritable mood. The clinical and laboratory findings must support that either the symptoms developed during, or within a month of, substance intoxication or withdrawal, or that the medication (i.e., substance) is etiologically related to the disturbance. The condition cannot be better accounted for by a mood disorder that is not substance induced. The disturbance does not occur exclusively during the course of a delirium. The symptoms cause clinically significant distress or impairment in social, occupational, or other important areas of functioning.

mood swings Periods of variation in how one feels, changing from a sense of well-being to one of depression. This occurs normally, but may become abnormally intense in persons with manic-depressive states.

moon face SEE: under *face*.

Moore's lightning streaks [Robert F. Moore, Brit. ophthalmologist, 1878–1963] The perception of zigzag flashes of light in the peripheral field of vision that occurs in the dark, esp. in older persons. These flashes are due to vitreous tags on the retina. The condition is benign. SEE: *coruscation*.

Moraxella (mor-ăx-ĕl'ă) A genus of

gram-negative coccobacilli in the family Neisseriaceae; most are nonpathogenic inhabitants of mammalian mucous membranes.

M. catarrhalis A species that is a frequent cause of upper and lower respiratory tract infections, including otitis media in children and bronchitis and pneumonia in the elderly. It is resistant to beta-lactam antibiotics such as most penicillins, but can be treated with many cephalosporins, macrolides, and sulfa drugs.

M. lacunata A species that is a cause of conjunctivitis in humans.

morbid (mor'bĭd) [L. *morbidus,* sick] **1.** Diseased. **2.** Pert. to disease. **3.** Preoccupied with unwholesome ideas and circumstances.

morbidity [L. *morbidus,* sick] **1.** State of being diseased. **2.** The number of sick persons or cases of disease in relationship to a specific population. SEE: *incidence.*

compression of m. Shortening of the period or proportion of long-term disability by elimination of a chronic disease.

expansion of m. Increase in the number of years and proportion of disability by the elimination of a fatal disorder, such as cancer or heart disease.

Morbidity and Mortality Weekly Report ABBR: MMWR. The weekly report of illness and death rates for a variety of diseases and conditions, published by the Centers for Disease Control and Prevention, Atlanta, Georgia. Prominent in the material are statistics on communicable diseases in each state, territory, and 121 major cities in the U.S. Articles concerning outbreaks of disease or accidents appear in the MMWR, sometimes including reports of importance to public health as a result of an international event.

morbidity rate SEE: under *rate.*

morbific (mor-bĭf'ĭk) [" + *facere,* to make] Causing or producing disease.

morbilli (mor-bĭl'ī) [L. *morbillus,* little disease] Measles. **morbillous** (mor-bĭl'ŭs), *adj.*

morbilliform [" + *forma,* shape] Resembling measles or its rash.

morcellation, morcellement (mor-sĕl-ā'shŭn, -ā-mŏn') [Fr. *morceller,* to subdivide] Method of removing a fetus, tumor, or organ by pieces.

mordant (mor'dănt) [L. *mordere,* to bite] A substance that fixes a stain or dye, as alum and phenol.

mores (mō'rāz) [L.] Habits and customs of society; usually those that come to be regarded as being essential to the survival and well-being of the society.

Morgagni, Giovanni B (mor-găn'yē) Italian pathological anatomist, 1682–1771. **morgagnian** (mor-găn'yē-ăn), *adj.*

M.'s caruncle The middle prostatic lobe.

M.'s cataract Cataract that is hypermature with a softened cortex and a hard nucleus.

M.'s hydatid Cystlike remains of müllerian duct attached to testicle or oviduct.

M.'s hyperostosis Hyperostosis of the frontal bones of the head, possibly associated with obesity, headache, amenorrhea, diabetes, multiple endocrine abnormalities, and various neuropsychiatric disturbances. SYN: *frontal internal hyperostosis.*

M.'s rectal columns Vertical ridges in the upper half of the anal canal produced by infolding mucosa over a venous plexus.

M.'s ventricle Ventriculus laryngis. SEE: *ventricle of larynx.*

morgagnian cyst SEE: under *cyst.*

Morganella morganii [Harry de R. Morgan, Brit. physician, 1863–1931] A gram-negative bacillus that may cause urinary tract infections, wound infections, bacteremia, meningitis, keratitis, and acute enteritis.

morgue (morg) [Fr.] A place for holding dead bodies until they are identified or claimed for burial.

moria (mō'rē-ă) [Gr. *moria,* folly] **1.** Simple dementia. **2.** Foolishness. SEE: *witzelsucht.*

moribund (mor'ĭ-bŭnd) [L. *moribundus*] In a dying condition; dying.

morning care Care provided for a patient, which includes taking temperature, pulse, and respiration, assistance with oral hygiene and bathing, changing bed linen, and providing breakfast.

morning sickness The nausea and vomiting that affects many women during the first few months of pregnancy. The condition typically starts about 4 to 6 weeks after conception, peaks in incidence and severity between 8 and 11 weeks, and subsides spontaneously between 12 and 16 weeks of gestation. Occurring in 50% to 88% of pregnancies, nausea is the most common complaint in the first trimester; it probably is caused by the high level of human chorionic gonadotropin, low blood sugars related to fasting while asleep, and altered carbohydrate metabolism. SYN: *nausea gravidarum.*

SYMPTOMS: Patient complaints vary from mild nausea on arising to severe intermittent nausea and vomiting throughout the day. The woman also may experience headache, vertigo, and exhaustion. Severe persistent vomiting with retching between meals should be reported and investigated. SEE: *hyperemesis gravidarum.*

TREATMENT: In most cases of simple morning sickness, dietary management will minimize or eliminate symptoms.

The woman is advised to eat dry crackers or toast before rising; to eat something every 2 hours; to drink fluids between meals; and to avoid spicy, greasy, or fried foods and foods with strong odors. Rarely will the patient need antiemetics.

CAUTION: The use of any drug during pregnancy should be carefully evaluated prior to its administration to avoid possible damage to the fetus.

---

morning stiffness Limitations of joint and muscle movement that are present on awakening or after resting, but which subside with activity. This is one of the principal symptoms of inflammatory, rather than degenerative arthritis.

moron [Gr. *moros,* stupid] An obsolete term for someone who is mildly mentally retarded. SEE: *mental retardation.*

Moro reflex [Ernst Moro, Ger. pediatrist, 1874–1951] A reflex seen in infants in response to stimuli, such as that produced by suddenly striking the surface on which the infant rests. The infant responds by rapid abduction and extension of the arms followed by an embracing motion (adduction) of the arms. SYN: *embrace reflex; startle reflex.*

morphea (mor-fē′ă) [Gr. *morphe,* form] Localized or widespread sclerotic plaques of the skin, often arrayed in lines or bands. The lesions typically have an ivory-colored to yellow slightly firm center, with a violet border. SEE: *progressive systemic sclerosis.*

generalized m. A severe form of localized morphea. There are multiple indurated plaques, hyperpigmentation, and possible muscle atrophy. It is not associated with systemic disease. The disease may become inactive in 3 to 5 years.

localized m. A localized form of scleroderma that does not progress to the systemic form of the disease.

morpheme (mor′fēm) The smallest meaningful unit in phonetics. SEE: *phoneme.*

morphia Morphine.

morphine (mor′fēn) [L. *morphina,* from *Morpheus,* god of dreams or sleep] The principal alkaloid found in opium, occurring as bitter colorless crystals.

m. sulfate An opiate commonly used in oral or injectable form to control severe acute or chronic pain. Its side effects may include sedation, respiratory depression, constipation, itching, hallucinations, tolerance, and dependence.

CAUTION: Like other narcotic analgesics, morphine sulfate is a controlled substance with a high potential for abuse.

---

morphine poisoning Acute intoxication by injected, inhaled, or orally consumed morphine sulfate. SEE: *opiate poisoning; Poisons and Poisoning Appendix.*

morphinism (mor′fĭn-ĭzm) [L. *morphina,* morphine, + *-ismos,* condition] Morbid condition due to habitual or excessive use of morphine. SEE: *morphine poisoning.*

morphodifferentiation The stage of tooth formation that determines the shape and size of the tooth crown. SEE: *enamel organ.*

morphogenesis (mor″fō-jĕn′ĕ-sĭs) [Gr. *morphe,* form, + *genesis,* generation, birth] Various processes occurring during development by which the form of the body and its organs is established. SYN: *morphosis.* **morphogenetic** (mor″fō-jĕn-ĕt′ĭk), *adj.*

morphogenetic process Any of the processes by which morphogenesis is accomplished, including cell migration, cell aggregation, localized growth, splitting (delamination and cavitation), and folding (invagination and evagination).

morphogenetic substance Chemical present in eggs or early embryos that induces cellular differentiation. SEE: *induction.*

morphography (mor-fŏg′ră-fē) [″ + *graphein,* to write] The classification of organisms by form and structure.

morphology (mor-fŏl′ō-jē) [Gr. *morphe,* form, + *logos,* word, reason] The science of structure and form of organisms without regard to function.

morphometry (mor-fŏm′ĕ-trē) [″ + *metron,* measure] The measurement of forms.

morphosis (mor-fō′sĭs) Morphogenesis.

morphovar [*morpho*logical *var*iation] Variants within a species defined by variation in morphological characteristics. SEE: *biovar; serovar.*

morpio, morpion (mor′pē-ō, -pē-ŏn) [L.] The crab louse, *Phthirus pubis,* that infests the pubic area. SEE: *lice.*

Morquio's syndrome (mor-kē′ōz) [Louis Morquio, Uruguayan physician, 1867–1935] Mucopolysaccharidosis IV.

morsal (mor′săl) [L. *morsus,* bite] Involved in biting and chewing, as the occlusal surfaces of teeth.

morsulus (mor′sū-lŭs) [L. dim. of *morsus,* bite] Troche.

mortal [L. *mortalis*] **1.** Causing death. **2.** Subject to death.

mortality **1.** The condition of being mortal. **2.** The number of deaths in a population. In the U.S. about 2,300,000 people die each year. The most common causes of death, according to the National Center for Health Statistics, are (in descending order) heart disease, cancer, stroke, chronic obstructive lung disease, accidents, pneumonia and influenza, diabetes mellitus, suicide, kidney failure, cirrhosis, and other chronic liver diseases. The causes of death vary by age group: accidents are the most common cause of death among infants, children, adolescents, and young adults, whereas cancers are the most common cause of death among people ages 45 to 64. Heart disease predominates after age 65.

fetal m. The number of fetal deaths per 1000 live births, usually per year.

infant m. The number of deaths of children younger than 1 year of age per 1000 live births per year.

maternal m. The number of deaths of women during childbearing per 100,000 births.

neonatal m. The number of deaths of infants younger than 28 days of age per 1000 live births per year.

perinatal m. The number of fetal deaths plus the number of deaths of infants younger than 7 days of age per 1000 live births per year.

mortality table A compilation in tabular form of the death rate at specific ages of the population being studied. Tables also may be constructed to include other demographic data (e.g., race or a causative agent or event such as childbearing or accident). This information allows comparison of the death rates of different populations.

mortar [L. *mortarium*] Vessel with a smooth interior in which crude drugs are crushed or ground with a pestle.

mortician [L. *mors,* death] Undertaker; person trained to prepare the dead for burial.

mortification SEE: *gangrene; necrosis.*

mortinatality (mor″tĭ-nā-tăl′ĭ-tē) [″ + *natus,* birth] Natimortality.

mortise joint Ankle.

Morton's neuralgia [Thomas G. Morton, U.S. surgeon, 1835–1903] Pain in the metatarsal area due to a fallen transverse arch with pressure on the lateral plantar nerve. SYN: *metatarsalgia.*

Morton's neuroma A neuroma-like mass of the neurovascular bundle of the intermetatarsal spaces.

Morton's toe (mor′tŭnz) [Dudley J. Morton, U.S. orthopedist, 1884–1960] Congenital short, hypertrophied second metatarsal bone with tenderness over the head of that bone, callosities under the second and third metatarsals, and pain and tenderness of the metatarsal area. Also called *Morton's disease* or *Morton's syndrome.* SEE: illus.

mortuary (mor′chū-ā-rē) [L. *mortuarium,* a tomb] **1.** Temporary place for keeping dead bodies before burial. SYN: *morgue.* **2.** Relating to the dead or to death.

morula (mor′ū-lă) [L. *morus,* mulberry] **1.** Solid mass of cells, resembling a mulberry, resulting from cleavage of an ovum. **2.** A mulberry-shaped body found in white blood cells in patients afflicted with human granulocyte ehrlichiosis. SEE: *fertilization* for illus.

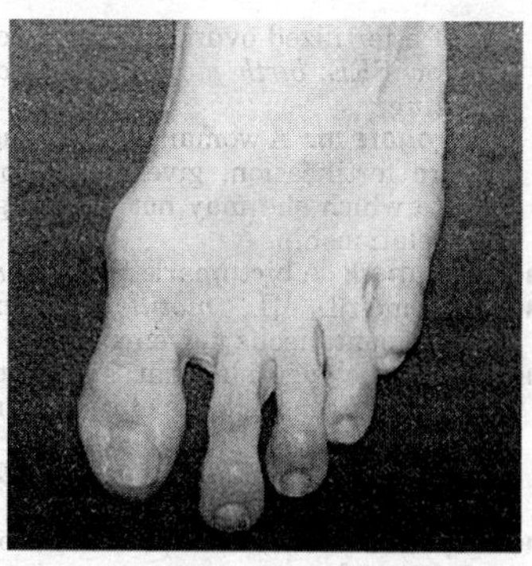

MORTON'S TOE

morulation (mor″ū-lā′shŭn) The formation of morula.

moruloid (mor′ū-loyd) [″ + Gr. *eidos,* form, shape] **1.** A bacterial colony made up of a mass resembling a mulberry. **2.** Resembling a mulberry.

Morvan's disease (mor′vănz) [Augustin M. Morvan, Fr. physician, 1819–1897] A form of syringomyelia, in which there are trophic changes in the extremities with formation of slowly healing lesions.

MOS *medical outcomes study.*

mosaic **1.** A pattern made up of many small segments. **2.** Genetic mutation wherein the tissues of an organism are of different genetic kinds even though they were derived from the same cell. SEE: *chimera.*

mosaicism (mō-zā′ĭ-sĭzm) Presence of cells of two different genetic materials in the same individual.

mOsm Symbol for milliosmol(e).

mosquito [Sp., little fly] A blood-sucking insect belonging to the order Diptera, family Culicidae. Important genera are *Anopheles, Culex, Aedes, Haemagogus, Mansonia,* and *Psorophora.* They are vectors of many diseases, including malaria, filariasis, yellow fever, dengue, viral encephalitis, and dermatobiasis. Illnesses carried by mosquitoes cause millions of deaths annually, especially in underdeveloped countries.

mosquitocide [″ + L. *caedere,* to kill] An agent that is lethal to mosquitoes or their larvae.

moss Any low-growing green plant of the class Musci.

sphagnum m. Peat moss. It has been used as a surgical bandage and by some primitive people as a form of external menstrual protection.

mother [AS. *modor*] **1.** Female parent. **2.** A structure that gives rise to others.

biological m. A woman whose ovum was fertilized and became a fetus. This term does not apply to an individual who provided the uterus for the gestation of a fertilized ovum obtained from a donor. SEE: *birth mother; surrogate parenting.*

surrogate m. A woman who, through in vitro fertilization, gives birth to a child to which she may not have a genetic relationship.

mother's mark A birthmark. SEE: *mark.*

motile (mō′tĭl) [L. *motilis,* moving] Having spontaneous movement.

motilin A polypeptide that stimulates and controls contractions of the gastrointestinal tract. Motilin is secreted by the mucosa of the small intestine. SEE: *secretin.*

motility (mō-tĭl′ĭ-tē) The power to move spontaneously.

motion (mō′shŭn) [L. *motio,* movement] **1.** A change of place or position; movement. **2.** Evacuation of the bowels. **3.** Matter evacuated from bowels. SEE: words beginning with *cine-* and *kine-*.

active m. Movement caused by the patient's own intention.

continuous passive m. ABBR: CPM. The use, usually postsurgical, of an electromechanical device to move a joint or joints repeatedly through a prescribed range of motion. The purpose is to prevent joint stiffness and adhesions and promote circulation and healing.

CAUTION: Patients should be monitored closely during use of these devices.

---

passive m. Movement as the result of an external force; that is, without voluntary muscle contraction.

motion sickness A syndrome, marked primarily by nausea and/or vomiting, as a result of a conflict between the true vertical axis and the subjective or perceived vertical axis. Motion sickness is a common illness experienced by car, boat, plane, or space travelers. It also is felt sometimes during motion picture viewing. Susceptibility to motion sickness is greatest between the ages of 2 and 12; it lessens with age but can be provoked in most individuals if the inciting stimulus is strong enough.

TREATMENT: Antimotion sickness medications include diazepam, diphenhydramine, meclizine, and scopolamine. Some patients with motion sickness benefit by eating small quantities of food when they begin to feel ill.

motivation (mō″tĭ-vā′shŭn) The internal drive or externally arising stimulus to action or thought.

motive (mō′tĭv) The mental condition or state that affects, alters, or stimulates behavior.

motofacient (mō″tō-fā′shĕnt) Producing motion.

motoneuron (mō″tō-nū′rŏn) Motor neuron.

lower m. Lower motor neuron.

peripheral m. Peripheral motor neuron.

upper m. Upper motor neuron.

motor [L. *motus,* moving] **1.** Causing motion. **2.** A part or center that induces movements, as nerves or muscles. **motorial** (mō-tor′ē-ăl), *adj.*

motor neuron disease One of several types of disease of the motoneurons, including progressive muscular atrophy, primary lateral sclerosis, progressive bulbar paralysis, and amyotrophic lateral sclerosis. These diseases are characterized by degeneration of anterior horn cells of the spinal cord, the motor cranial nerve nuclei, and the corticospinal tracts. They occur principally in males. In the U.S., amyotrophic lateral sclerosis is better known as Lou Gehrig's disease.

motorpathy (mō-tor′păth-ē) [L. *motus,* moving, + Gr. *pathos,* disease, suffering] Kinesitherapy.

motor sense SEE: *sense, muscular.*

motor speech area SEE: *Broca's area.*

motor test meal The use of various techniques to monitor the progress of food through the gastrointestinal tract.

mottled enamel SEE: under *enamel.*

mottling (mŏt′lĭng) [ME. *motteley,* many colored] Condition that is marked by discolored areas.

moulage (moo-lăzh′) [Fr.] **1.** A wax model or reproduction of the configuration of some part of the anatomy such as the face or nose, or of a pathological skin lesion. **2.** Molding of a wax model.

mounding [origin uncertain] The rising of a lump, as the mounding of a wasting muscle when struck a quick, firm blow. SYN: *myoedema* (1).

mount (mownt) [ME. *mounten,* to mount] **1.** To place on a support or backing. **2.** To place specimens or sections in special containers or on slides for study.

x-ray m. A stiff cardboard folder with windows in which radiographs of teeth in the dental arches are placed in sequence for examination and diagnosis.

mountain fever Condition occurring in individuals ascending to high altitudes (over 10,000 ft or 3,048 m) or to those subjected to rarefied atmospheres. It is due to anoxia resulting from reduced oxygen tension. SEE: *bends.*

SYMPTOMS: Euphoria, tachycardia, headache, nausea, increased respiratory rate, pulmonary edema, fatigue, and cerebral disorders (loss of memory, errors of judgment).

mountain sickness, chronic The slow onset of symptoms in persons who reside at high altitude for several years. Included are apathy, fatigue, and headache. Laboratory studies often reveal hypoxia and polycythemia. Persons between ages 40 and 60 are most likely to be affected. The symptoms subside when the person returns to sea level. SYN: *Monge's disease.*

mounting (mownt'ĭng) **1.** The arrangement of specimens on slides, frames, chart boards, display boards, or any background for study. **2.** In dentistry, the attachment of a cast of the mandible or maxilla to an articulator.

mourning [AS. *murnan*] Normal grief usually produced by the death of a loved one. Mourning is not synonymous with depression or melancholia. SEE: *grief reaction.*

mouse (mows) **1.** A small rodent of the genus *Mus.* Mice are used extensively in research. **2.** A small piece of tissue that has become free or unattached, esp. in a body cavity or joint.

joint m. Fragment of synovial membrane or cartilage found free in the joint space due to trauma or osteoarthritis.

New Zealand black m. ABBR: NZB m. A mouse bred for the genetic trait of spontaneously developing autoimmune hemolytic anemia.

nude m. A mutant mouse, completely devoid of hair and lacking T lymphocytes, bred for use in immunological investigations.

mouse unit SEE: *Allen-Doisy unit.*

mouth [AS. *muth*] **1.** The opening of any cavity. **2.** The cavity within the cheeks, containing the tongue and teeth, and communicating with the pharynx. SYN: *buccal cavity; oral cavity.* SEE: illus.

ABNORMALITIES: *Tongue:* dry, coated, smooth, strawberry, large, pigmented, geographic, deviated, tremulous, sore. *Gums and teeth:* gingivitis, sordes, lead line, pyorrhea, atrophy, hypertrophy, dental caries, alveolar abscesses. *Mucous membranes and other parts of mouth:* eruptions accompanying exanthematous diseases, stomatitis, canker sores, herpes simplex, thrush, trench mouth, cysts, tumors, carcinoma, lesions of syphilis such as chancre, mucous patches, gumma, lesions of tuberculosis, abscesses.

Disorders of the mouth cavity may be indications of purely local diseases or they may be symptoms of systemic disturbances such as dehydration, pernicious anemia, and nutritional deficiencies, esp. avitaminosis.

Rashes of the mouth may indicate stomatitis, measles, or scarlet fever. Rashes on lips may indicate typhoid fever, meningitis, or pneumonia. In secondary syphilis, chancre, cancer, and epithelioma, mucous patches appear.

EXAMINATION: In addition to visual examination, careful digital examination should be made because it reveals areas of tenderness and alterations of texture characteristic of leukoplakia, cancer, cystic swellings, and lymphadenopathy.

Excessive moisture of the mouth is seen in stomatitis, irritation of the vagus nerve, ingestion of irritating drugs or foods, nervous disorders, teething, seeing appetizing foods, and smelling pleasant odors. SEE: *burning mouth syndrome.*

trench m. Necrotizing ulcerative gingivitis.

mouth guard A removable dental appliance used to protect the teeth and investing tissues during contact sports. SEE: *occlusal guard.*

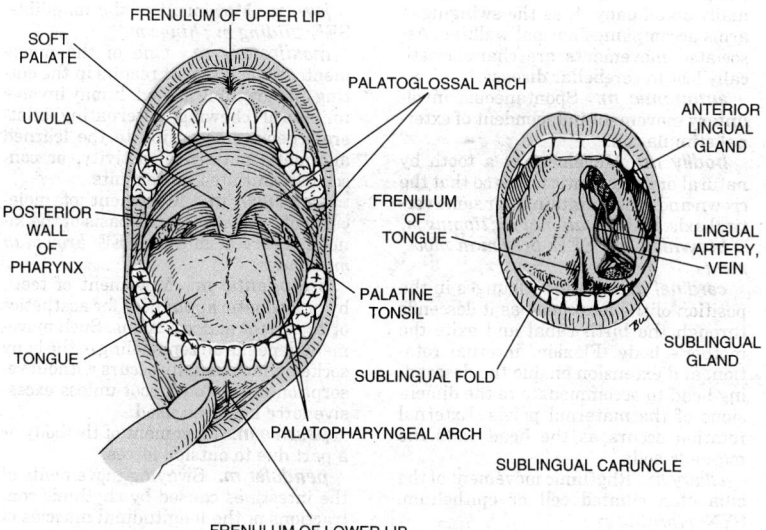

MOUTH, TONGUE, AND PHARYNX

mouthrinse Mouthwash.

mouthstick Adapted device consisting of a stick attached to a molded dental mouthpiece that permits page turning and other tasks through head movement.

mouthwash A medicated solution used to cleanse or treat diseases of the oral mucosa, reduce halitosis, or add fluoride to the teeth for control or prevention of dental caries. It may contain various chemical compounds, such as fluoride or zinc chlorides, alcohol, glycerin, detergents, essential oils for flavoring, and coloring agents. According to the composition and proposed function, mouthwashes may be described as antibacterial, astringent, buffered, concentrated, cosmetic, deodorizing, or therapeutic. SYN: *mouthrinse*.

MOV *minimal occluding volume.*

movement [L. *movere,* to move] **1.** The act of passing from place to place or changing position of the body or its parts. **2.** The act of evacuating feces.

active m. Voluntary movement accomplished without external assistance.

ameboid m. Cellular movement much like that of an ameba. A protoplasmic pseudopod extends, and then the remaining cell contents flow into the pseudopod, which swells gradually. This type of movement allows cells such as leukocytes to move through very small openings. SEE: *diapedesis*.

angular m. Voluntary muscular movement resulting in change in the angle between the involved bones.

associated m. Synchronous correlation of two or more muscles or muscle groups that, although not essential for the performance of some function, normally accompany it, as the swinging of arms accompanies normal walking. Associated movements are characteristically lost in cerebellar disease.

autonomic m. Spontaneous, involuntary movement independent of external stimulation.

bodily m. Movement of a tooth by natural or orthodontic forces so that the crown and root maintain their same vertical axis. SEE: *rotational m.; tipping m.*

brownian m. SEE: *brownian movement*.

cardinal m. of labor Changes in the position of the fetal head as it descends through the birth canal and exits the mother's body. Flexion, internal rotation, and extension enable the descending head to accommodate to the dimensions of the maternal pelvis. External rotation occurs as the head exits the mother's body.

ciliary m. Rhythmic movement of the cilia of a ciliated cell or epithelium. SYN: *vibratile m.*

circus m. **1.** A phenomenon appearing after injury to a corpus striatum, optic thalamus, or crus cerebri, and causing an odd circular gait. **2.** In cardiac rhythm disturbances caused by reentry, the conduction of electrical activity cyclically through tissue, a process that continues indefinitely as long as the tissue ahead of the electrical wave has adequate time to recover before the electrical stimulus reappears.

disorders of m. Hemiplegia, ataxia, monoplegia, tremors, rigors, chorea, athetosis, convulsions, spasm (clonic or tonic), reflex (hysterical, habit spasm, tics), and spastic paralysis. These disorders may be due to injury or disease of muscle, nerve ending, motor nerve, spinal cord, or the brain.

fetal m. Muscular movements performed by the fetus in utero.

gliding m. Movement of one surface over another without angular or rotatory movement, as well. This type of movement occurs in the temporomandibular joint after opening when the condyles and disks move forward, as in protrusion of the jaw.

hinge m. Movement in a joint around a transverse axis, as occurs in the lower compartment of the temporomandibular joints at the beginning of jaw opening when the occluding teeth are separated or in the final stage of wide opening of the mouth.

independent living m. A collective term for societal programs that support a philosophy of full participation, self-reliance, and social integration of persons with functional impairment. Emphasis on self-help, environmental accessibility, freedom of choice, and programs to enable community living characterize this movement.

jaw m. Movement of the mandible. SEE: *gliding m.; hinge m.*

masticatory m. One of the movements of the jaw that results in the cutting and grinding of food. It may involve unilateral chewing, alternating bilateral chewing according to the learned automatic pattern of activity, or consciously initiated movements.

molecular m. Movement of molecules of a substance, the basis of the kinetic theory of matter. SEE: *brownian movement*.

orthodontic m. Movement of teeth by orthodontic appliances for aesthetics or to correct malocclusions. Such movement depends on remodeling of the bony socket, which usually occurs without resorption of the tooth root unless excessive force has been used.

passive m. Movement of the body or a part due to outside forces.

pendular m. Swaying movements of the intestines caused by rhythmic contractions of the longitudinal muscles of the walls of the intestines.

peristaltic m. Peristalsis.

physiological m. A movement that is

normally executed by muscles that are under voluntary control such as flexion, extension, abduction, adduction, and rotation. It is also known as physiological motion.

respiratory m. Any movement resulting from the contraction of respiratory muscles or occurring passively as a result of elasticity of the thoracic wall or lungs. SEE: *compliance* (1); *expiration; inspiration; respiration.*

m. of restitution Alteration in position that aligns the fetal head with the fetal spine.

rotational m. Movement around an axis, as in hinge movement of the temporomandibular joint or rotation of a tooth around its longitudinal axis in tooth movement or extraction. SEE: *bodily m.; tipping m.*

saccadic m. Jerky movements of the eyes as they move from one point of fixation to another.

segmenting m. Movement of the intestine in which annular constrictions occur, dividing the intestine into ovoid segments.

tipping m. Movement of a tooth crown while the root apex remains essentially stationary, resulting in an inclination of the axis of the tooth in one direction. SEE: *bodily m.; rotational m.*

triplanar m. Movement occurring around an oblique axis in all three body planes.

vermicular m. The wormlike movements of peristalsis.

vibratile m. Ciliary m.

moxa (mŏk′sa) [Japanese] A soft, combustible substance to be burned on skin, popular in eastern Asia, Japan, and complementary medicine as a cautery and counterirritant. SEE: *moxibustion.*

moxalactam disodium An antibacterial drug.

moxibustion (mŏks-ĭ-bŭs′chŭn) [″ + L. *combustus,* burned] In traditional Asian and alternative medicine, cauterization and counterirritation used to treat disease by means of a cylinder or cone of cotton wool, called a moxa, placed on the skin and fired at the top.

Mozart ear [Wolfgang Amadeus Mozart, Austrian composer, 1756–1791. Alleged to have had this deformity] Deformity of the ear in which the antihelix is fused with the crura of the helix.

M.P.D. *maximum permissible dose.*

M.P.H. *Master of Public Health.*

M.P.N. *most probable number* (of bacteria present in a quantity of solution, esp. water).

MPS *mucopolysaccharidosis; mononuclear phagocytic system*

MR *magnetic resonance.*

mR *milliroentgen.*

MRCP *Member of the Royal College of Physicians.*

MRCP(C) *Member of the Royal College of Physicians of Canada.*

MRCS *Member of the Royal College of Surgeons.*

MRCS(C) *Member of the Royal College of Surgeons of Canada.*

mrem *millirem.*

MRI *magnetic resonance imaging.*

M.R.L. *Medical Record Librarian.*

mRNA *messenger RNA.*

MRSA *methicillin-resistant* Staphylococcus aureus.

μs Symbol for microsecond.

MS *multiple sclerosis.*

M.S. *Master of Surgery; Master of Science.*

ms *millisecond.*

MSAFP *Maternal serum alpha-fetoprotein.*

MSDS *Material safety data sheets.*

msec *millisecond.*

MSH *melanocyte-stimulating hormone.*

M.S.N. *Master of Science in Nursing.*

MSVC *maximum sustainable ventilatory capacity.* SEE: *ventilation, maximum sustainable.*

M.T. *medical technologist.*

M.u. *Mache unit.*

mu (mū) [Gr. μ, letter m] SYMB: μ; u. Symbol used for the prefix *micro-* which stands for multiplication by 10^{-6}. Thus, μm would stand for 10^{-6} m.

m.u. *mouse unit.*

muc- SEE: *muco-.*

muci- SEE: *muco-.*

muciform (mū′sĭ-form) [″ + *forma,* shape] Appearing similar to mucus.

mucigen (mŭ′sĭ-jĕn) [″ + Gr. *gennan,* to produce] A substance present in mucous cells that, upon being extruded from the cell, is converted into mucin.

mucigenous (mū-sĭj′ĕn-ŭs) Muciparous.

mucilage (mū′sĭ-lĭj) [L. *mucilago,* moldy juice] Thick, viscid, adhesive liquid, containing gum or mucilaginous principles dissolved in water, usually employed to suspend insoluble substances in aqueous liquids or as a demulcent. **mucilaginous** (mū-sĭl-ăj′ĭn-ŭs), *adj.*

mucilloid (mū′sĭl-loyd) A mucilaginous preparation.

psyllium hydrophilic m. Mucilloid prepared from psyllium seeds. It is used as a bulk-type laxative.

mucin (mū′sĭn) [L. *mucus,* mucus] A glycoprotein found in mucus. It is present in saliva, bile, skin, glandular tissues, connective tissues, tendon, and cartilage. Mucin is formed from mucigen and forms a slimy solution in water. **mucinoid** (mū′sĭn-oyd), *adj.*

mucinase (mū′sĭ-nās) Any enzyme that acts on mucin.

mucinemia (mū″sĭn-ē′mē-ă) [″ + Gr. *haima,* blood] Accumulation of mucin in the blood.

mucinogen (mū-sĭn′ō-jĕn) [″ + Gr. *gennan,* to produce] A glycoprotein that forms mucin.

mucinolytic (mū″sĭ-nō-lĭt′ĭk) [″ + Gr. *lysis,* dissolution] Capable of hydrolyzing or dissolving mucin.

mucinuria (mū-sĭn-ū′rē-ă) [″ + Gr. *ouron,* urine] Presence of mucin in the urine.

muciparous (mū-sĭp′ăr-ŭs) [″ + *parere,* to bring forth, to bear] Producing or secreting mucus. SYN: *mucigenous.*

muco-, muc-, muci [L. *mucus,* mucus] Combining form meaning *mucus.*

mucocele (mū′kō-sēl) [″ + Gr. *kele,* tumor, swelling] **1.** Enlargement of the lacrimal sac. **2.** A mucous cyst. **3.** A mucous polypus. **4.** Cystic disease of the air cavities of the cranial bones causing erosion of the bone.

mucociliary Pert. to ciliated mucosa.

mucocutaneous (mū″kō-kū-tā′nē-ŭs) [″ + *cutis,* skin] Concerning mucous membrane and the skin. SYN: *mucodermal.*

mucocutaneous lymph node syndrome Kawasaki disease.

mucodermal (mū-kō-dĕr′măl) Mucocutaneous.

mucoenteritis (mū″kō-ĕn-tĕr-ī′tĭs) [″ + Gr. *enteron,* intestine, + *itis,* inflammation] Inflammation of intestinal mucosa.

mucoglobulin (mū″kō-glŏb′ū-lĭn) [″ + *globulus,* globule] A type of glycoprotein.

mucoid (mū′koyd) [″ + Gr. *eidos,* form, shape] **1.** Glycoprotein similar to mucin. **2.** Muciform, similar to mucus.

mucokinesis Any therapeutic technique that removes excessive or abnormal secretions from the respiratory tract.

mucolytic Pert. to a class of agents that liquefy sputum or reduce its viscosity. SEE: *cystic fibrosis.*

mucomembranous (mū″kō-mĕm′bră-nŭs) [″ + *membrana,* membrane] Concerning mucous membrane.

mucoperiosteum (mū″kō-pĕr″ē-ŏs′tē-ŭm) Periosteum that has a mucous surface, as in the middle ear.

mucopolysaccharidase (mū″kō-pŏl″ē-săk′ă-rī-dās) An enzyme that catalyzes the hydrolysis of polysaccharides.

mucopolysaccharide (mū″kō-pŏl″ī-săk′ă-rīd) A group of polysaccharides, containing hexosamine and sometimes proteins, that forms chemical bonds with water. The thick gelatinous material is found in many places in the body, forming intercellular ground substance and basement membranes of cells and found in mucous secretions and synovial fluid.

mucopolysaccharidosis ABBR: MPS. A group of inherited disorders characterized by a deficiency of enzymes that are essential for the degradation of the mucopolysaccharides heparan sulfate, dermatan sulfate, and keratan sulfate. These chemicals are excreted in excess quantities in the urine, and they usually accumulate in macrophages, the central nervous system, endothelial cells, intimal smooth muscle cells, and fibroblasts throughout the body. Clinical changes are not usually apparent at birth, but the inherited defect can be diagnosed prior to birth by culturing amniotic fluid cells and testing them for specific enzyme activity. After birth, the conditions may be diagnosed by testing cultured skin fibroblasts for specific enzymes. Some MPS may be treated with bone marrow transplantation.

m. IH MPS due to a deficiency of the enzyme α-L-iduronidase with accumulation of dermatan sulfate and heparan sulfate. Clinically, there are lens opacities, coarse facies, skeletal dysplasia, hepatosplenomegaly, and mental retardation. SYN: *Hurler's syndrome.*

m. IHS Hurler-Scheie syndrome. An intermediate form of MPS between MPS IH and MPS IS, due to the same enzyme deficiency. Mental development may be normal.

m. IS MPS due to the same enzyme defect as MPS IH and with similar clinical characteristics, except mental retardation is absent. SYN: *Scheie's syndrome.*

m. II MPS due to a deficiency of the enzyme L-iduronosulfate sulfatase. Clinically, there are retinal degeneration without corneal clouding, mental retardation, joint stiffness, skeletal dysplasia, cardiac lesions, and deafness. SYN: *Hunter's disease.*

m. III MPS that has been further differentiated into Sanfilippo A, B, C, or D, on the basis of the specific enzyme deficiency present in each form. Clinically, it may not be possible to distinguish the types. Present are moderate coarse facies, severe mental retardation, and mild hepatosplenomegaly. Corneal clouding is absent and growth is normal. SYN: *Sanfilippo's disease.*

m. IV MPS due to a deficiency of the enzyme *N*-acetylgalactosamine-6-sulfatase. Clinically, there are dwarfism, thoracolumbar gibbus (hunchback), kyphoscoliosis, coarse facies, cardiac lesions, moderate hepatosplenomegaly, and joint hypermobility. SYN: *chondroosteodystrophy; Morquio's syndrome.*

m. V Former designation for mucopolysaccharidosis IS.

m. VI Maroteaux-Lamy syndrome. MPS due to a deficiency of the enzyme *N*-acetylgalactosamine-4-sulfatase. Clinically, MPS VI is similar to MPS IH, except intelligence is normal.

m. VII MPS due to a deficiency of β-glucuronidase. Clinically, MPS VII is quite similar to MPS IH, except intelligence may be normal. SYN: *glucuronidase deficiency disease.*

mucopolysacchariduria (mū″kō-pŏl″ē-săk′ă-rĭ-dū′rē-ă) Mucopolysaccharides in the urine.

mucoprotein (mū″kō-prō′tē-ĭn) A complex of protein and mucopolysaccharide. Usually, the polysaccharide contains hexosamine.

Tamm-Horsfall m. SEE: *Tamm-Horsfall mucoprotein.*

mucopurulent (mū-kō-pūr′ū-lĕnt) [L. *mucus,* mucus, + *purulentus,* made up of pus] Consisting of mucus and pus.

Mucor (mū′kor) [L.] A genus of mold fungi seen on dead and decaying matter. Some species can cause infections of external ear, skin, and respiratory passageways. SEE: *mucormycosis.*

mucoriferous (mū″kor-ĭf′ĕr-ŭs) [L. *mucor,* mold, + *ferre,* to carry] Covered with mold or a moldlike substance.

mucormycosis (mū″kor-mī-kō′sĭs) [″ + Gr. *mykes,* fungus, + *osis,* condition] Mycosis usually caused by fungi of the family Mucoraceae of the class Zygomycetes. These fungi have an affinity for blood vessels, in which they cause thrombosis and infarction. The form of this disease that affects the head and face usually causes paranasal sinus infections, esp. during periods of ketoacidosis in persons with diabetes mellitus. This form may also disseminate to the brain. The pulmonary form of the disease causes infarcts of the lung; the gastrointestinal form causes mucosal ulcers and gangrene of the stomach. The disease is contracted by inhalation or ingestion of the fungus by susceptible individuals. Most persons have a natural resistance to the fungus, accounting for the rarity of the disease. SYN: *zygomycosis.*

TREATMENT: Control or prevention of diabetic acidosis, administration of amphotericin B, and resection of necrotic tissue.

mucorrhea [″ + *rhoia,* to flow] Increased cervical discharge at ovulation, usually covering a span of 3 to 4 days. The discharge has the character and appearance of raw egg white. SEE: *spinnbarkeit.*

mucosa (mū-kō′să) *pl.* **mucosae** [L., mucous] A mucous membrane or moist tissue layer that lines the hollow organs and cavities of the body that open to the environment. It consists of an epithelial layer on a basement membrane and a connective tissue layer called the lamina propria. The tissue lining the alimentary canal also contains a smooth muscle layer called the muscularis mucosae. The type of epithelium, thickness, and presence or absence of glands vary with the function or location of the mucosa. **mucosal** (mū-kō′săl), *adj.*

alveolar m. A thin, nonkeratinized mucosal layer covering the alveolar process of maxillae and mandible and loosely attached to underlying bone. It is continuous with the mucosa of the cheek, lips, tongue, and palate.

buccal m. The lining of the cheeks of the oral cavity. It is characterized by stratified squamous nonkeratinized epithelium that may become keratinized in local areas due to cheek-biting. It may also contain ectopic sebaceous glands. SEE: *Fordyce's disease.*

lingual m. The keratinized, papillated covering of the dorsum of the tongue that contains nerve endings for the sense of taste.

masticatory m. Those areas of the mucosa of the mouth that have become keratinized due to the friction and abrasion of the masticatory process, esp. the gingivae and hard palate.

nasal m. The mucosa lining the nasal cavity and paranasal sinuses, characterized by pseudostratified ciliated columnar epithelium with goblet cells. Nasal mucosa functions to warm and hydrate the air inspired and by ciliary action sweep mucus-entrapped dust and debris to the pharynx.

oral m. The mucous membrane lining the oral cavity and described by its location on the gingiva, hard palate, soft palate, cheek, vestibule, lip, tongue, and pharyngeal area.

mucosanguineous (mū″kō-săn-gwĭn′ē-ŭs) [″ + *sanguineus,* bloody] Containing mucus and blood.

mucoserous (mū″kō-sēr′ŭs) Composed of mucus and serum.

mucositis (mū″kō-sī′tĭs) [″ + Gr. *itis,* inflammation] Inflammation of a mucous membrane.

chemotherapy-induced m. Oral inflammation caused by medications, especially those used to treat cancers or autoimmune diseases.

radiation-induced m. Inflammation of the lining of the mouth due to radiation injury to the head and/or neck. SEE: *gingivitis, acute necrotizing ulcerative.*

mucosocutaneous (mū-kō″sō-kū-tā′nē-ŭs) Concerning a mucous membrane and the skin.

mucostatic (mū″kō-stăt′ĭk) [″ + *statikos,* standing] Stopping the secretion of mucus.

mucous (mū′kŭs) **1.** Having the nature of or resembling mucus. **2.** Secreting mucus. **3.** Depending on presence of mucus.

mucous colitis An old term for inflammatory bowel disease.

mucous membrane The membrane lining passages and cavities communicating with the air, consisting of a surface layer of epithelium, a basement membrane, and an underlying layer of connective tissue (lamina propria). Mucus-secreting cells or glands are usually present in the epithelium but may be absent. In humans, mucous membranes and the skin provide effective mechanisms for preventing the entry of pathogens. Mucous membranes are normally colonized with nonpathogenic organisms that discourage colonization by pathogens because the resident organisms compete for the nutrients essential to their survival. Some mucosal surfaces in the digestive tract have special characteristics that tend to repel or kill organisms, such as the extremely high acid level on the mucosa of the stomach. SEE: *bacterial adherence*.

Noninvasive examination of membranes should reveal the degree of moisture, cyanosis, pallor, hyperemia, pigmentation, lesions or their absence, and hemorrhage. Pallor is seen in all anemias. If temporary, it may indicate shock or vasomotor spasm, or it may occur in severe hemorrhages. Blanching and flushing alternately accompany aortic regurgitation.

Hyperemia or excessive redness of the mucous membranes is indicative of certain pathological changes in particular tissues. For example: *Buccal mucous membrane:* Due to decayed teeth, traumatism, stomatitis. SEE: *mouth*. *Nasal mucosa:* Ulceration of nose, rhinitis, inflammation. SEE: *nose*. *Eyes (local irritation):* Foreign body, ulcer, inflammation. SEE: *jaundice*. Dryness is seen in fevers, chronic gastritis, some liver disturbances, excitement, shock, prostration, fatigue, thirst, and certain drugs.

mucous polyp Small growth from mucous lining of the cervix or uterus.

mucoviscidosis (mū″kō-vĭs″ĭ-dō′sĭs) Cystic fibrosis.

mucus (mū′kŭs) [L.] A viscid fluid secreted by mucous membranes and glands, consisting of mucin, leukocytes, inorganic salts, water, and epithelial cells. A good example is the almost ropy secretion from the sublingual and submandibular glands.

cervical m. The discharge secreted by the endocervical glands of the uterine cervix. Characteristic assessment findings correlate with normal hormonal changes of the menstrual cycle that influence the type and amount of mucus secreted. Immediately before ovulation, high estrogen levels stimulate secretion of a large amount of thin, watery mucus that is hospitable to sperm transit. After ovulation, high progesterone levels stimulate secretion of a thick, viscous mucus that is less hospitable to sperm. SEE: *ferning; spinnbarkeit*.

mugwort (mŭg′wŏrt) A perennial herb (*Artemisia vulgaris*) that is burned on the skin by acupuncturists during moxibustion. It is toxic if eaten.

mull (mŭl) To grind or pulverize.

Müller, Heinrich (mül′ĕr) German anatomist, 1820–1864.

M. fibers Fine fibers of neuroglia cells that form supporting elements of the retina.

M. muscle **1.** Circular fibers of ciliary muscle. **2.** The superior tarsal muscle of the eyelid. **3.** Smooth muscle covering the sphenomaxillary fissure.

M. trigone Portion of tuber cinereum folding over the optic chiasm.

Müller, Johannes P. (mül′ĕr) German physician, 1801–1858.

M. ducts Embryonic tubes from which the oviducts, uterus, and vagina develop in the female; in the male, they atrophy. SYN: *müllerian duct*.

M. maneuver Inspiratory effort with a closed glottis at the end of expiration. This technique is used during radiographic studies to produce negative intrathoracic pressure and cause engorgement of blood vessels, thus allowing visualization of esophageal varices.

M. ring Muscular ring at the junction of the cervical canal and the gravid uterus.

M. tubercle Projection on the dorsal wall of the cloaca at which Müller's ducts terminate.

mult-, multi- [L. *multus*] Prefix meaning *many, much*.

multangular Having many angles.

multangular bone, greater The first or outermost of the distal row of carpal bones. SYN: *trapezium*.

multangular bone, lesser The second in distal row of carpal bones. SYN: *trapezoid bone*.

multiallelic (mŭl″tē-ă-lĕl′ĭk) Concerning a large number of genes affecting hereditary characteristics.

multiarticular (mŭl″tē-ăr-tĭk′ū-lăr) [L. *multus*, many, + *articulus*, joint] Concerning, having, or affecting many joints. SYN: *polyarticular*.

multicapsular (mŭl″tĭ-kăp′sū-lăr) [″ + *capsula*, a little box] Composed of many capsules.

multicellular (mŭl″tĭ-sĕl′ū-lăr) [″ + *cellula*, small chamber] Consisting of many cells.

Multiceps A genus of tapeworms.

multicuspid, multicuspidate (mŭl″tĭ-kŭs′pĭd, -pĭ-dāt) [″ + *cuspis*, point] Having several cusps.

multidisciplinary Relating to multiple fields of study involved in the care of patients. The term suggests that the various disciplines are working in collaboration, but in a parallel mode of interaction. Each distinctive discipline is accountable and responsible for its tasks and functions regarding patient care.

multifactorial The result of many factors, as in a disease resulting from the combined effects of several components.

multifamilial (mŭl″tĭ-fă-mĭl′ē-ăl) Concerning a familial disease that affects children in several generations.

multifid (mŭl′tĭ-fĭd) [″ + *fidus*, from *findere*, to split] Divided into many sections.

multifocal (mŭl″tĭ-fō′kăl) Concerning or arising from many locations.

multiform (mŭl′tĭ-form) [″ + *forma*, shape] Having many forms or shapes. SYN: *polymorphic; polymorphous*.

multiglandular (mŭl″tĭ-glănd′ū-lar) [″ + *glandula,* a little acorn] Concerning several glands.

multigravida (mŭl″tĭ-grăv′ĭ-dă) [″ + *gravida,* pregnant] A woman who has been pregnant more than once. The number of pregnancies may be recorded as gravida II, gravida III, and so on. SEE: *multipara.*

multi-infarct dementia SEE: under *dementia.*

multi-infection (mŭl″tĭ-ĭn-fĕk′shŭn) [L. *multus,* many, + *infectio,* an infection] A mixed infection with several organisms developing at the same time.

Multilevel Assessment Instrument A questionnaire (used primarily for community-based geriatric patients) that evaluates instrumental activities of daily living. It assesses cognitive and physical limitations in activities such as telephone use, shopping, housework, and money management.

multilobular (mŭl″tĭ-lŏb′ū-lar) [″ + *lobulus,* a small lobe] Formed of or possessing many lobules.

multilocular (mŭl″tĭ-lŏk′ū-lar) [″ + *loculus,* a cell] Having many cells or compartments.

multimammae (mŭl″tĭ-măm′mē) [″ + *mamma,* breast] Polymastia.

multinodal (mŭl-tĭ-nō′dăl) Having many nodes or knots.

multinodular (mŭl-tĭ-nŏd′ū-lar) [″ + *nodulus,* little knot] Possessing many nodules or small knots.

multinuclear, multinucleate (mŭl-tĭ-nū′klē-ăr, -āt) Possessing several nuclei. SYN: *polynuclear.*

multipara (mŭl-tĭp′ă-ră) [″ + *parere,* to bring forth, to bear] A woman who has carried more than one fetus to viability, regardless of whether the offspring were born alive. The number of deliveries may be recorded as para II, para III, and so on. SEE: *multigravida.*

grand m. A woman who has given birth seven or more times.

multiparity (mŭl-tĭ-păr′ĭ-tē) The condition of having carried one or more fetuses to viability, regardless of whether the infants were alive at birth. SEE: *multipara.*

multiparous (mŭl-tĭp′ăr-ŭs) Having borne more than one child.

multiphasic screening SEE: *screening test, multiphasic.*

multiple (mŭl′tĭ-pl) [L. *multiplex,* many folded] **1.** Consisting of or containing more than one; manifold. **2.** Occurring simultaneously in various parts of the body.

multiple drug resistance A lack of expected therapeutic response to several disease-specific pharmaceutical agents, esp. antibiotics. In cancer therapy, resistance to a wide range of unrelated drugs may occur after resistance to a single agent has developed. SEE: *gene amplification.*

multiple-ejaculate resuspension and centrifugation ABBR: MERC. A method of isolating viable sperm from men previously thought to be sterile for in vitro fertilization. The patient ejaculates three or four times in a 24-hour period, and the semen is collected and concentrated. The small number of sperm isolated from the specimens can be used to impregnate the man's partner.

multiple endocrine neoplasia ABBR: MEN. One of several inherited syndromes caused by a defect in tumor suppressor genes that produces benign and malignant tumors of many endocrine glands. Angiofibromas and collagenomas of the skin also are common findings. This group of diseases has been classed according to the glands affected. In MEN type I (MEN I), there are tumors of the parathyroid, pituitary, and islet cells of the pancreas. SYN: *Wermer's syndrome.* MEN type II (MEN II) is characterized by medullary thyroid carcinoma, pheochromocytoma, and parathyroid hyperplasia. SYN: *Sipple syndrome.* MEN type III (MEN III) is quite similar to MEN II, but there are marked facial aberrations with neuromas of the conjunctiva, labial mucosa, tongue, larynx, and gastric intestinal tract.

multiple malformation syndrome Developmental anomalies of two or more systems in the fetus. These may be caused by chromosome and genetic abnormalities, or by teratogens including certain drugs and chemicals. In attempting to determine the etiology, it is important to obtain a complete family history and history of exposure to known teratogens and infectious diseases. SEE: *amniotic band disruption sequence syndrome.*

multiple myeloma SEE: under *myeloma.*

multiple organ dysfunction syndrome ABBR: MODS. Progressive failure of two or more organ systems, resulting from acute, severe illnesses or injuries (i.e., sepsis, systemic inflammatory response, trauma, burns) and mediated by the body's inability to sufficiently activate its defense mechanisms. SYN: *multiple systems organ failure.*

PATIENT CARE: Patients at risk should be closely monitored to help prevent MODS by prompt recognition and correction of perfusion problems, infection, and organ dysfunction. Indicators of hypermetabolic hyperdynamic state should be assessed for as the body tries to compensate for the initial insult. This will be followed by a hypodynamic, decompensated state with imbalances in oxygen supply and demand, maldistribution of circulating volume, and metabolic abnormalities, resulting in organ failure. Common problems are pulmonary, cardiovascular, renal, and hepatic, often followed or accompanied by gram-negative sepsis and disseminated intravascular coagulation. Appropriate medical interventions will be initiated for each failing system's problems. Nursing responsibilities include monitoring vital signs and assessing diagnostic study results, coordinating and carrying out prescribed therapies and evaluating patient responses while simultaneously assessing for adverse effects, protecting the patient from nosocomial infections and environmental stressors, and providing emotional support for the patient and family through this type of devastating illness, which has a 90% mortality rate.

The respiratory therapist assists the physician in determining when to intubate the patient and initiate mechanical ventilation. The patient may develop shock lung and need mechanical ventilation with positive end-expiratory pressure to maintain adequate oxygenation. Mechanical ventilation in these patients also serves to rest the muscles of breathing and reduce oxygen consumption. The health care provider often measures arterial blood gases and pulse oximetry to ensure adequate oxygenation at the lowest possible concentration of inhaled oxygen to prevent oxygen toxicity.

multiple personality A term formerly used for dissociative identity disorder.

multiple sclerosis SEE: under *sclerosis*.

Multiple Sleep Latency Test SEE: *narcolepsy*.

multiple systems organ failure ABBR: MSOF. Multiple organ dysfunction syndrome.

multipolar (mŭl-tĭ-pōl′ăr) [L. *multus,* many, + *polus,* a pole] **1.** Possessing more than two poles. **2.** Possessing more than two processes, said of neurons.

multirooted In dentistry, referring to a tooth having several roots.

multisynaptic (mŭl″tē-sĭ-năp′tĭk) Polysynaptic.

multiterminal [″ + Gr. *terma,* a limit] Providing several sets of terminals, making possible the use of several electrodes.

multivalent (mŭl-tĭ-vā′lĕnt) [″ + *valere,* to have power] **1.** Having ability to combine with more than two atoms of a univalent element or radical. **2.** Active against several strains of an organism.

mummification (mŭm″mĭ-fĭ-kā′shŭn) [Arabian *mumiyaa,* mummy, + L. *facere,* to make] **1.** Mortification producing a hard, dry mass. SYN: *dry gangrene.* **2.** Drying and shriveling of a body, as a dead and retained fetus.

mumps (mŭmps) An acute, contagious disease caused by the mumps paramyxovirus, which results in inflammation of the salivary glands and other organs. The incidence in the U.S. is extremely low because of childhood immunization with the measles, mumps, and rubella vaccine. SEE: *Nursing Diagnoses Appendix.*

SYMPTOMS: Following an incubation period of 12 to 25 days, patients develop a fever, malaise, headache, and swollen salivary glands, esp. the parotid glands. Occasionally, involvement of other organs results in deafness, pancreatitis, meningitis, or in boys, infertility as a result of inflammatory destruction of the testes—a condition known as mumps orchitis.

TREATMENT: Treatment is generally supportive, with bedrest, antipyretics, and analgesics, and intravenous fluids if they are needed. Interferon-alpha 2B may protect against virus-induced testicular atrophy.

PATIENT CARE: Immunization with trivalent measles, mumps, and rubella vaccine (MMR) is encouraged for all children between ages 12 and 15 months and again between ages 4 and 6 years to prevent the disease. If mumps occur, the patient is kept in isolation to prevent transmission of the disease to others. The patient's temperature is monitored closely and fluids are encouraged. Analgesics, local application of heat or cold, and a liquid or soft diet help reduce pain from swollen glands. The patient is observed for signs and symptoms of complications, and is encouraged to gradually resume activity as symptoms subside.

mumps skin test antigen A standardized suspension of sterile formaldehyde-inactivated mumps virus. It is used in diagnosing mumps.

mumps virus vaccine live A sterile preparation of attenuated mumps virus used to immunize against mumps.

Munchausen syndrome (mĕn-chow′zĕn) [Baron Karl F. H. von Munchausen, fictional 18th century baron created by Rudolph Raspe] A type of malingering or factitious disorder in which the patient may practice self-multilation or deception in order to feign illness. When detected, such patients leave one hospital and appear in the emergency room of another. Patients of this type are seldom recognized in time to receive psychiatric diagnoses and therapy, which they need. SEE: *disorder, factitious.*

Munchausen syndrome by proxy The fabrication of symptoms or physical evidence of another's illness, or the deliberate causing of another's illness, to gain medical attention.

mupirocin (mū-pĕr′rō-sĭn) An antibacterial ointment used to treat infections caused by staphylococcal species. It often is used in the treatment of impetigo, in place of oral drugs.

mural (mū′răl) [L. *murus,* a wall] Pert. to a wall of an organ or part.

muramidase An enzyme found in blood

cells of the granulocytic and monocytic series. Its serum and urine level is increased in patients with acute or chronic leukemia. It is also normally present in saliva, sweat, and tears. Also called lysozyme.

Murchison-Pel-Ebstein fever (mŭr′chĭ-sŏn-pĕl-ĕb′stīn) [Charles Murchison, Brit. physician, 1830–1879; Pieter K. Pel; Wilhelm Ebstein] Pel-Ebstein fever.

muriate (mūr′ē-āt) [L. *muria,* brine] Former term for chloride.

muriatic acid (mū″rē-ăt′ĭk) Obsolete term for hydrochloric acid.

murine (mū′rĭn) [L. *mus,* mouse] Concerning rodents, esp. rats and mice.

murmur (mŭr′mŭr) [L.] An abnormal sound heard on auscultation of the heart and adjacent large blood vessels. Murmurs range in sound from soft and blowing to loud and booming and may be heard during systole, diastole, or both. A murmur does not necessarily indicate organic pathology, and heart disease may not be associated with the production of a murmur. Air in the lungs may simulate sounds similar to heart murmurs. SEE: *heart.*

anemic m. Hemic m.

aneurysmal m. A whizzing systolic sound heard over an aneurysm.

aortic obstructive m. A harsh systolic murmur heard with and after the first heart sound. It is loudest at the base.

aortic regurgitant m. A blowing or hissing following the second heart sound.

apex m. An inorganic murmur over the apex of the heart.

arterial m. A soft flowing murmur that is synchronous with the pulse.

Austin Flint m. SEE: *Austin Flint murmur*.

bronchial m. A murmur heard over large bronchi, resembling respiratory laryngeal murmur.

cardiac m. A sound arising due to blood flow through the heart.

cardiopulmonary m. A murmur caused by movement of the heart against the lungs.

continuous m. A murmur that extends throughout systole and diastole.

crescendo m. A murmur that progressively builds up in intensity and then suddenly subsides.

Cruveilhier-Baumgarten m. A murmur heard on the abdominal wall over the collateral veins connecting the caval and portal veins.

diastolic m. A murmur occurring during relaxation of the heart.

Duroziez′ m. SEE: *Duroziez′ murmur.*

ejection m. A systolic murmur that is most intense at the time of maximum flow of blood from the heart. This murmur is associated with pulmonary and aortic stenosis.

endocardial m. An abnormal sound produced by any cause and arising within the heart.

exocardial m. A cardiac murmur produced outside the cavities of the heart.

extracardiac m. Exocardial m.

friction m. A murmur caused by an inflamed mucous surface rubbing against another, as in pericarditis.

functional m. A murmur occurring in the absence of any pathological change in the structure of the heart valves or orifices. It does not indicate organic disease of the heart, and may disappear upon a return to health. It may be mistaken for a pathological murmur by an inexperienced listener.

Gibson's m. SEE: *Gibson's murmur.*

Graham Steell's m. [Graham Steell, Brit. physician, 1867–1942] A high-pitched diastolic murmur heard best along the left sternal border. It is caused by backflow (regurgitation) of blood through the dilated pulmonary valve of the heart. This type of murmur is usually associated with severe pulmonary hypertension.

heart m. Cardiac m.

hemic m. A sound heard on auscultation of anemic persons without valvular lesions and resulting from an abnormal, usually anemic, blood condition.

holosystolic m. Pansystolic m.

machinery m. Gibson's murmur.

mitral m. A murmur produced at the orifice of the mitral (bicuspid) valve.

musical m. A cardiac murmur with sounds that have an intermittent harmonic pattern.

organic m. A murmur due to structural changes.

pansystolic m. A heart murmur heard throughout systole.

pericardial m. A friction sound produced within the pericardium.

physiologic m. Functional m.

prediastolic m. Systolic m.

presystolic m. A murmur occurring just before systole, due to mitral or tricuspid obstruction.

pulmonary m. A murmur produced at the orifice of the pulmonary artery.

regurgitant m. A murmur due to leakage or backward flow of blood through a dilated valvular orifice.

seagull m. A murmur that resembles the cry of a seagull; sometimes associated with aortic insufficiency.

Still's m. A benign, functional midsystolic murmur heard in children. The maximum sound is heard over the left lower sternal border.

systolic m. A murmur heard during contraction of the heart due to obstruction of the flow of blood at one or several of the heart valves or in the aorta.

to-and-fro m. A pericardial murmur heard during both systole and diastole.

tricuspid m. A murmur produced at the orifice of the tricuspid valve and caused by stenosis or incompetency of the valve.

vascular m. A murmur occurring over a blood vessel.

vesicular m. Normal breath sounds.

Murphy's button [John B. Murphy, U.S. surgeon, 1857–1916] Mechanical device used for intestinal anastomosis consisting of two button-like hollow cylinders. Each cylinder is sutured to an open end of the intestine, then they are fitted together. After firm union of the ends of the intestine, the sutures separate and the cylinders are passed in stools.

Murphy's sign Pain on deep inspiration when an inflamed gallbladder is palpated by pressing the fingers under the rib cage.

Mus (mŭs) [L., mouse] A genus of rodents including mice and rats.

M. musculus The common house mouse.

Musca (mŭs′kă) [L., fly] A genus of flies belonging to the order Diptera, family Muscidae.

M. domestica The common house fly. It may transmit typhoid fever, bacillary and amebic dysentery, cholera, trachoma, and many other diseases to humans.

muscae volitantes (mŭs′sē vŏl-ĭ-tăn′tēz) [L., flitting flies] The latin term for a "floater."

muscarine (mŭs′kă-rĭn) [L. *muscarius,* pert. to flies] A highly toxic organic compound present in *Amanita muscaria* (fly agaric mushroom). SEE: *mushroom and toadstool poisoning; amanita* in *Poisons and Poisoning Appendix.*

muscarinic Pert. to the effect of acetylcholine on parasympathetic ganglionic effector sites.

muscegenetic (mŭs″ē-jĕ-nĕt′ĭk) [L. *musca,* fly, + Gr. *genesis,* generation, birth] Causing floating objects to appear in the visual fields.

muscicide (mŭs′ĭ-sīd) [″ + *cidus,* killing] Lethal to flies.

muscle (mŭs′ĕl) [L. *musculus*] A type of tissue composed of contractile cells or fibers that effects movement of an organ or part of the body. The outstanding characteristic of muscular tissue is its ability to shorten or contract. It also possesses the properties of irritability, conductivity, and elasticity. Muscle tissue possesses little intercellular material; hence, its cells or fibers lie close together. SYN: *musculus.* SEE: illus. (Muscles of the Trunk); *leg* for illus; *arm; cell; face.*

TYPES: Three types of muscle occur in the body, differentiated on the basis of histologic structure. These muscle types are smooth, skeletal (striated), and cardiac. SEE: illus. (Muscle Tissues); table.

Smooth (Involuntary): Smooth muscle is found principally in the internal organs, esp. the digestive tract, respiratory passages, urinary and genital ducts, urinary bladder, gallbladder, and walls of blood vessels. It lacks the cross striations characteristic of other types of muscle. This type of muscle tissue is called involuntary because it is not under conscious control. Smooth muscle cells are fusiform or spindle-shaped, each containing a central nucleus. The cells are usually arranged in sheets or layers, but may occur as isolated units in connective tissue.

Striated, Skeletal (Voluntary): Striated muscle is found in all skeletal muscles. It also occurs in the tongue, pharynx, and upper portion of esophagus. Since movement is under conscious control, this type of muscle tissue is called voluntary. The cytoplasm (sarcoplasm) contains numerous myofibrillae. The cell membrane is called the sarcolemma. Muscle fibers are grouped into bundles called fasciculi, each of which is surrounded by a sheath or connective tissue called perimysium. The fibers within a fasciculus are surrounded by and held together by delicate reticular fibrils forming the endomysium.

Cardiac: Cardiac muscle fibers branch and anastomose, forming a continuous network or syncytium. At intervals, prominent bands or intercalated disks cross the fibers. Specialized fibers called Purkinje form the impulse-conducting system of the heart.

ANATOMY: Muscle is a contractile organ consisting of tissue that allows movement of parts of the body, especially a structure composed of striated (voluntary) muscle that is attached to a part of the skeleton. A typical muscle consists of a central fleshy portion or belly and its attachments. One end called the head is attached to a fixed structure termed the origin; the other end is attached to a movable part called the insertion. Some muscles are spindle-shaped; others form flat sheets or bands. Muscles may be attached directly to the periosteum of the bones, or they may be attached by means of tough cords of connective tissue (tendons) or broad flat sheets (aponeuroses). The connective tissue enclosing a muscle is called epimysium; it is continuous with the deep fascia. SEE: illus. (Skeletal Muscle).

BLOOD SUPPLY: Obtained from small blood vessels that enter the muscular tissue and subdivide into capillaries that permeate throughout.

NERVE SUPPLY: *Voluntary:* These muscles are innervated by somatic

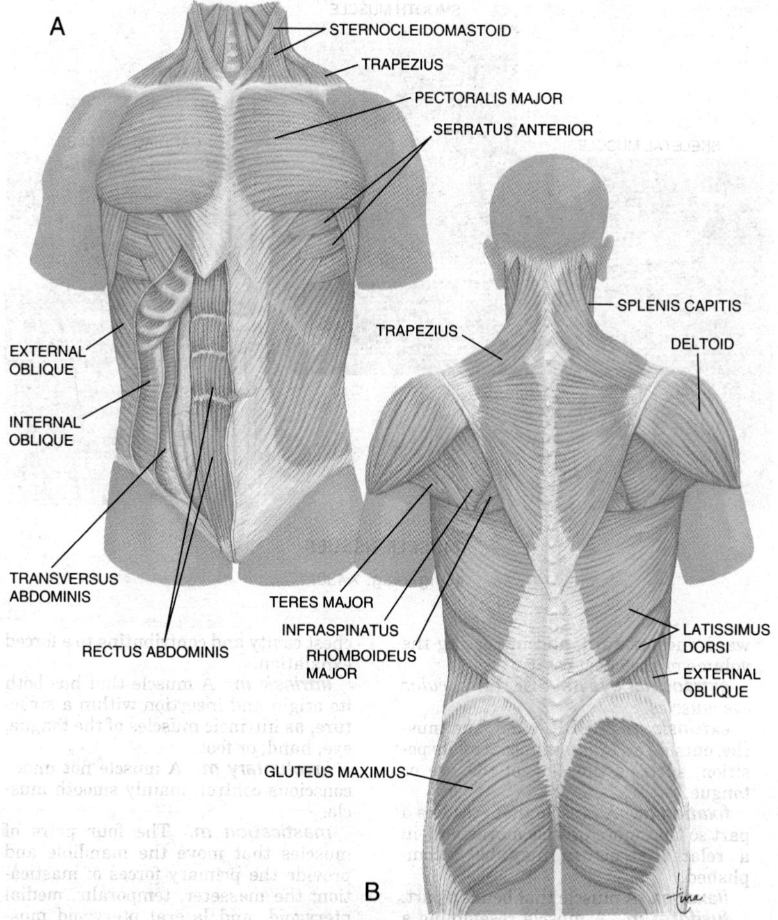

MUSCLES OF THE TRUNK

(A) anterior, (B) posterior

branches of cranial or spinal nerves; it is because of this that the skeletal muscles are under conscious control. *Involuntary:* Smooth and cardiac muscles receive their nerve supply from autonomic nervous system and function involuntarily without conscious control.

abductor m. A muscle that draws away from the midline.

adductor m. A muscle that draws toward the midline.

agonist m. A muscle that is the prime mover.

antagonist(ic) m. A muscle that counteracts the action of another muscle.

antigravity m. Muscles that pull against the constant force of gravity to maintain posture.

appendicular m. One of the skeletal muscles of the limbs.

arrector pili m. Arrector pili.

articular m. A muscle attached to the capsule of a joint.

axial m. A skeletal muscle of the head or trunk.

bipennate m. A muscle in which the fibers converge toward a central tendon on both sides. SEE: illus.

constrictor m. of pharynx A muscle that constricts the pharynx.

digastric m. A muscle that lowers the jaw. SEE: *bipennate m.* for illus.

extensor m. A muscle that extends a part.

external intercostal m. The outer layer of muscles between the ribs, originating on the lower margin of each rib and inserted on the upper margin of the next rib. During inspiration, they draw adjacent ribs together, pulling them up-

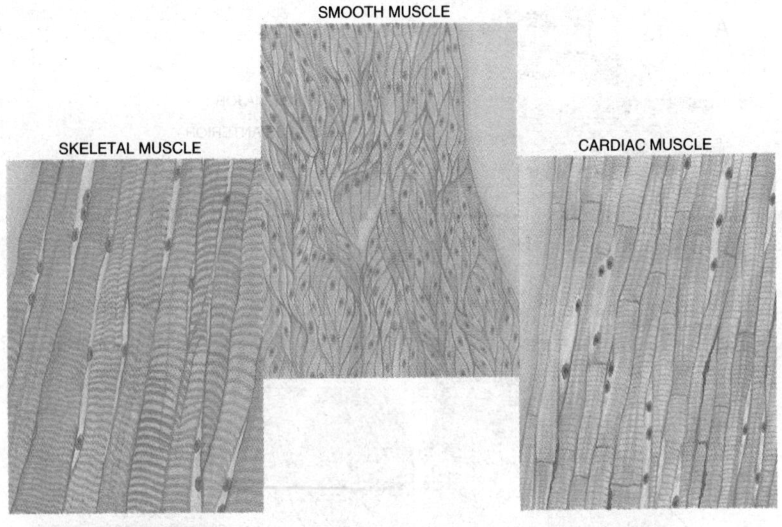

MUSCLE TISSUES

(Orig. mag. ×430)

ward and outward, and increasing the volume of the chest cavity.

extraocular eye m. SEE: *extraocular eye muscles.*

extrinsic m. ABBR: e.m. The muscles outside an organ that control its position, such as the e.m. of the eye or tongue.

fixation m. A muscle that steadies a part so that more precise movements in a related structure may be accomplished.

flexor m. A muscle that bends a part.

fusiform m. A muscle resembling a spindle. SEE: *bipennate m.* for illus.

internal intercostal m. The muscles between the ribs, lying beneath the external intercostals. During expiration, they pull the ribs downward and inward, decreasing the volume of the chest cavity and contributing to a forced exhalation.

intrinsic m. A muscle that has both its origin and insertion within a structure, as intrinsic muscles of the tongue, eye, hand, or foot.

involuntary m. A muscle not under conscious control; mainly smooth muscle.

mastication m. The four pairs of muscles that move the mandible and provide the primary forces of mastication; the masseter, temporalis, medial pterygoid, and lateral pterygoid muscles.

mimetic m. Superficial muscles of the facial region controlling skin movement that produce the facial expressions. Also called *muscles of facial expression.*

Comparison of Properties of Three Types of Muscle

	Smooth	Cardiac	Striated
Synonyms	Involuntary Nonstriated Visceral	Myocardium	Voluntary Skeletal
Fibers			
Length (in μm)	50–200		25,000
Thickness (in μm)	4–8		75
Shape	Spindles		Cylinders
Markings	No striation	Striation	Marked striation
Nuclei	Single	Single	Multiple
Effects of cutting related nerve	Slight	Regulation of heart rate is lost	Complete paralysis

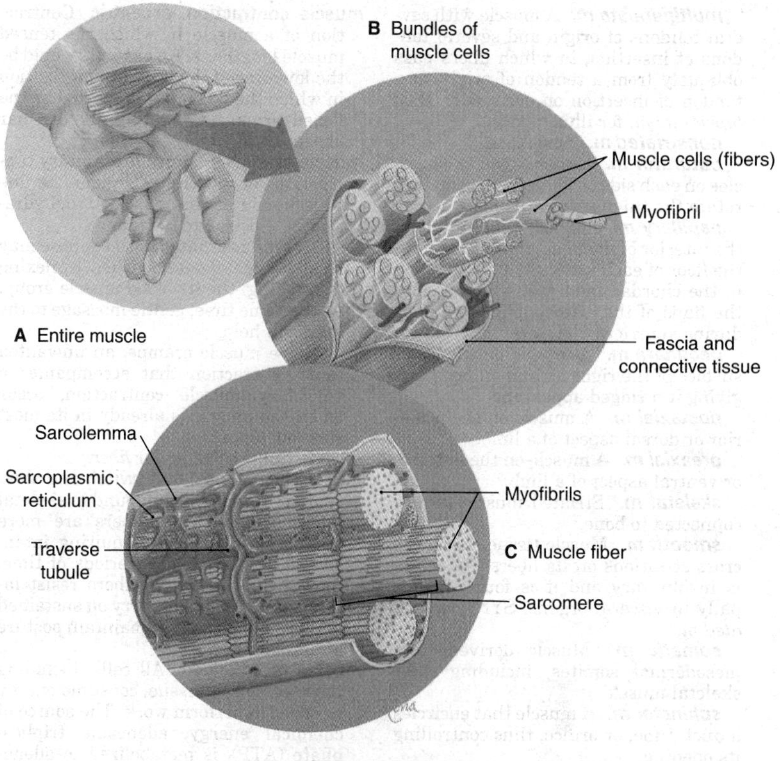

B Bundles of muscle cells
Muscle cells (fibers)
Myofibril
A Entire muscle
Fascia and connective tissue
Sarcolemma
Sarcoplasmic reticulum
Myofibrils
Traverse tubule
C Muscle fiber
Sarcomere

SKELETAL MUSCLE

FUSIFORM
DIGASTRIC
TRICIPITAL
TRIANGULAR
UNIPENNATE
BIPENNATE
MULTIPENNATE

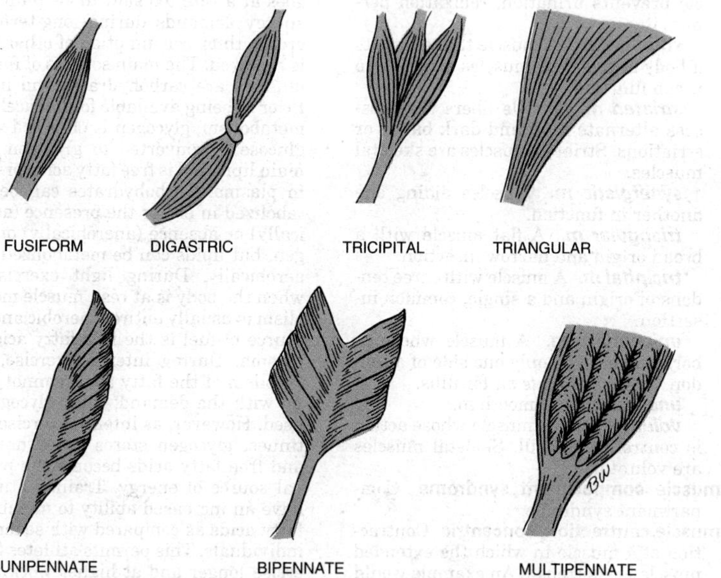

MORPHOLOGICAL FORMS OF MUSCLE

multipennate m. A muscle with several tendons of origin and several tendons of insertion, in which fibers pass obliquely from a tendon of origin to a tendon of insertion on each side. SEE: *bipennate m.* for illus.

nonstriated m. Smooth m.

obturator m. Either of the two muscles on each side of the pelvic region that rotate the thighs outward.

papillary m. A cylindrical muscle of the interior of the heart that arises from the floor of each ventricle. It is attached to the chordae tendinae, which anchor the flaps of the atrioventricular valves during ventricular systole.

pectinate m. A muscle on the inner surface of the right atrium of the heart, giving it a ridged appearance.

postaxial m. A muscle on the posterior or dorsal aspect of a limb.

preaxial m. A muscle on the anterior or ventral aspect of a limb.

skeletal m. Striated muscle that is connected to bone.

smooth m. Muscle tissue that lacks cross striations on its fibers. Its action is involuntary and it is found principally in visceral organs. SYN: *nonstriated m.*

somatic m. Muscle derived from mesodermal somites, including most skeletal muscle.

sphincter m. A muscle that encircles a duct, tube, or orifice, thus controlling its opening.

sphincter m. of urinary bladder The smooth muscle fibers around the origin of the urethra. Contraction of this muscle prevents urination; relaxation permits it.

stabilizer m. A muscle that supports a body segment so muscles attached to it can function.

striated m. Muscle fibers that possess alternate light and dark bands or striations. Striated muscles are skeletal muscles.

synergistic m. Muscles aiding one another in function.

triangular m. A flat muscle with a broad origin and narrow insertion.

tricipital m. A muscle with three tendons of origin and a single, common insertion.

unipennate m. A muscle whose fibers converge on only one side of a tendon. SEE: *bipennate m.* for illus.

unstriated m. Smooth m.

voluntary m. A muscle whose action is controlled by will. Skeletal muscles are voluntary.

muscle compartment syndrome Compartment syndrome.

muscle contraction, concentric Contraction of a muscle in which the extended muscle is shortened. An example would be pulling the body up by grasping a bar over the head.

muscle contraction, eccentric Contraction of a muscle in which the tensed muscle lengthens. An example would be the lowering of the body from a position in which the body was supported by the flexed arms, i.e., holding on to a bar above the head.

muscle cramps Painful involuntary contractions of muscles. They may be due to ischemia of the muscle(s), dehydration, or electrolyte imbalance.

Cramps associated with exercise may be alleviated, if not abolished, by flexing (stretching) the involved muscle group. At the same time, gentle massage to the area will help.

Active muscle cramps, an unwanted tonic contraction that accompanies a voluntary muscle contraction, occur when the muscle is already in its most shortened position.

muscle fiber SEE: under *fiber*.

muscle fiber types, fast twitch and slow twitch Types of fibers found in skeletal muscle. Fast twitch fibers are more abundant in muscles requiring intensive activity for short periods of time. Slow twitch oxidative fibers resist fatigue and are able to carry on sustained activities as needed to maintain posture or aerobic exercise.

muscle metabolism All cells, including those of muscle tissue, consume energy in order to perform work. The source of chemical energy, adenosine triphosphate (ATP), is metabolized to adenosine diphosphate (ADP). If the energy requirement is short term, the ADP is converted back to ATP. This process goes at a rate too slow to keep up with energy demands during long-term exercise; thus, consumption of other fuels is required. The main sources of fuel for muscles are carbohydrates and lipids. Prior to being available for intracellular metabolism, glycogen is obtained when glucose is converted to glycogen. The main lipid fuel is free fatty acids present in plasma. Carbohydrates can be metabolized in either the presence (aerobically) or absence (anerobically) of oxygen, but lipids can be metabolized only aerobically. During light exercise or when the body is at rest, muscle metabolism is usually entirely aerobic and the source of fuel is the free fatty acids in plasma. During intense exercise, metabolism of the fatty acids cannot keep up with the demand; thus, glycogen is used. However, as intense exercise continues, glycogen stores are exhausted and free fatty acids become the principal source of energy. Trained athletes have an increased ability to metabolize fatty acids as compared with sedentary individuals. This permits athletes to exercise longer and at higher work rates than would be the case if they were not trained. Athletic trainers found that muscle glycogen stores could be increased by what is known as carbohydrate loading. This regimen will permit the athlete to exercise for a much longer period than would be possible if carbohydrate loading had not been done prior to exercising. SEE: *carbohydrate loading*.

muscle soreness A nonspecific term used to describe general discomfort in a muscle or muscle group that is the result of disease, trauma, or exertion. SEE: *delayed onset m.s.*

delayed-onset m.s. ABBR: DOMS. Muscle tenderness, decreased strength, and decreased range of motion that develops 12 to 24 hr following strenuous exercise and peaks in intensity between 24 to 48 hr, although symptoms may persist 72 hr or more. DOMS may result from microtearing of muscular fibers, lactic acid accumulation, local inflammatory response, and/or physiochemical changes within the muscle fibers. Muscle soreness is most pronounced following eccentric exercise. SEE: *eccentric exercise; inflammation*.

muscular (mŭs′kū-lăr) [L. *muscularis*] **1.** Pert. to muscles. **2.** Possessing well-developed muscles.

muscular contractions, graduated **1.** The mechanism by which all smooth, coordinated muscle activity occurs. Normally controlled involuntarily by the central nervous system, motor units are recruited and stimulated at an intensity needed to accomplish a desired activity. **2.** Contractions accomplished by use of electric current of varying strength and duration. This method is used in muscles with an intact nerve supply when muscles are atonic, wasted away, or when voluntary exercise is not feasible, and in denervated muscles, as in cases following nerve injury or poliomyelitis.

muscular dystrophy One of nine distinct genetic syndromes that affect muscular strength and action, some of which first become obvious in infancy, and others of which develop in adolescence or young adulthood. The syndromes are marked by either generalized or localized muscle weakness, difficulties with walking or maintaining posture, muscle spasms, and in some instances, neurological, behavioral, cardiac, or other functional limitations. Detailed information about the disease can be obtained from the Muscular Dystrophy Association website at www.mdausa.org.

muscularis (mŭs-kū-lā′rĭs) [L.] The smooth muscle layer of an organ or tubule.

m. mucosae Smooth muscle tissue of a mucous membrane.

musculature [L. *musculus,* muscle] The arrangement of muscles in the body or its parts.

musculo- [L. *musculus,* muscle] Combining form meaning *muscle.*

musculoaponeurotic (mŭs-kū-lō-ăp″ō-nū-rŏt′ĭk) Composed of muscle and an aponeurosis of fibrous connective tissue.

musculocutaneous (mŭs″kū-lō-kū-tān′ē-ŭs) [″ + *cutis,* skin] **1.** Pert. to the muscles and skin. **2.** Supplying or affecting the muscles and skin. **3.** The specific nerve from the brachial plexus that innervates the coracobrachialis, biceps branchii, and brachialis muscles and provides cutaneous sensory distribution to the forearm.

musculofascial (mŭs″kū-lō-făsh′ē-ăl) Composed of muscle and fascia.

musculomembranous (mŭs″kū-lō-mĕm′brān-ŭs) Pert. to or consisting of muscle and membrane.

musculophrenic (mŭs″kū-lō-frĕn′ĭk) Pert. to muscles of the diaphragm.

musculoskeletal (mŭs″kū-lō-skĕl′ĕ-tăl) Pert. to the muscles and skeleton.

musculospiral (mŭs″kū-lō-spī′răl) [″ + *spira,* coil] Concerning the musculospiral (radial) nerve.

musculotendinous Composed of both muscle and tendon.

musculotropic (mŭs″kū-lō-trŏp′ĭk) [″ + Gr. *tropikos,* turning] Affecting, acting on, or having an affinity for muscular tissue.

musculus [L.] Muscle.

mushroom [Fr. *mousseron*] Umbrella-shaped fungus belonging to the class Basidiomycetes. Mushrooms grow on decaying vegetable matter and are generally found in woods and dark, damp places. Some of the poisonous varieties include *Amanita* species and toadstools. SEE: *amanita; toadstool*.

COMPOSITION: Mushrooms are low in carbohydrates and fats, and high in protein. Their relationship and similarity to poisonous fungi are so close that only those who are thoroughly capable of distinguishing the poisonous varieties from the edible ones should attempt to gather and eat them.

mushroom and toadstool poisoning Poisoning resulting from ingestion of mushrooms such as *Amanita muscaria,* which contains muscarine, or other species that contain phalloidine, a component of the amanita toxin. SEE: *amanita* in *Poisons and Poisoning Appendix.*

musicians, medical problems of Profession-related injuries, most commonly overuse injuries involving muscle-tendon units. The pain associated with this type of injury may be mild or severe enough to prevent use of the affected part. Those who play string instruments have more difficulty than those who use percussion instruments; women are more commonly affected than men. Focal dystonias may involve the hands or the muscles of the face and lips, and may be severe. Stress and anxiety may interfere with or prevent performing.

TREATMENT: Treatment consists of rest for physical difficulties and beta-adrenergic blocking agents for stress and anxiety.

musicogenic (mū″zĭ-kō-jĕn′ĭk) [L. *musica,* music, + *gennan,* to produce] Caused by music, esp. epileptic convulsions.

musicogenic epilepsy Epilepsy in which the convulsive attacks are induced by music. SEE: *epilepsy*.

musicomania [″ + Gr. *mania,* madness] Insane love of music.

music therapy [″ + *therapeia,* treatment] Treatment of disease, esp. mental illness, with music.

musk (mŭsk) [Sanskrit *muska,* testicle] An oily secretion obtained from a gland beneath the abdominal skin of male mammals. It has a strong odor and plays a part in animal communication. It is commercially used in manufacturing perfume.

mussel A bivalve mollusc belonging to the class Pelecypoda.

mussel poisoning Poisoning common on the Pacific coast of the United States resulting from eating mussels or clams that have ingested a poisonous dinoflagellate that is not destroyed by cooking. Mussel poisoning typically occurs from June to October.

Musset's sign (mū-sāz′) [Louis C. A. de Musset, Fr. poet, 1810–1857] Repetitive jerking movements of the head and neck, in synchrony with ventricular contractions of the heart, seen in advanced aortic regurgitation or aortic aneurysm.

mustard [Fr. *moustarde*] Yellow powder of mustard seed used as a counterirritant, rubefacient, emetic, stimulant, and condiment. SEE: *plaster*.

nitrogen m. SEE: *nitrogen mustards*.

mustard gas Dichlorodiethyl sulfide, a war gas that causes burns and destruction of tissue either topically or if inhaled.

Mustard procedure A surgical procedure to repair transposition of the great vessels, in which a baffle is placed to shunt blood between the right and left atria, allowing more oxygenated blood to be circulated systemically.

mutacism (mū′tă-sĭzm) A form of speech impediment in which the "m" sound is often substituted for other sounds.

mutagen (mū′tă-jĕn) [L. *mutare,* to change, + Gr. *gennan,* to produce] Any agent that causes genetic mutations. Many medicines, chemicals, and physical agents such as ionizing radiations and ultraviolet light have this ability. SEE: *teratogen*.

mutagenesis (mū″tă-jĕn′ĕ-sĭs) The induction of genetic mutation. SEE: *mutation; teratogenesis*.

mutant (mū′tănt) [L. *mutare,* to change] A variation of genetic structure that breeds true.

mutase (mū′tās) [″ + *ase,* enzyme] **1.** Enzyme that accelerates oxidation-reduction reactions through activation of oxygen and hydrogen. **2.** A food preparation made from leguminous plants high in protein content.

mutation (mū-tā′shŭn) **1.** Change; transformation; instance of such change. **2.** Permanent variation in genetic structure with offspring differing from parents in a characteristic; differentiated from gradual variation through many generations. **3.** A change in a gene potentially capable of being transmitted to offspring.

factor V Leiden m. An autosomal dominant mutation in coagulation factor V that is found in about 5% of all whites. It produces a hypercoagulable state as a result of inherited resistance to activated protein C. Clinically, it is found in many patients with deep venous thrombosis.

founder m. An altered gene that proliferates in a kinship or community from a single identifiable ancestor.

germline m. A mutation in the genetic content of a sperm or egg.

induced m. Mutation resulting from exposure to x-rays, radioactive substances, and certain drugs and chemicals.

natural m. Mutation occurring without artificial external intervention. Natural mutation is thought to be a primary factor in evolutionary change.

somatic m. Mutation occurring in somatic cells.

mute (mūt) [L. *mutus,* dumb] **1.** One who is unable to speak. **2.** Without the ability to speak.

deaf m. One who is unable to hear or speak.

mutilate [L. *mutilatus,* to maim] To deprive of a limb or a part; to maim or disfigure.

mutilation (mū″tĭ-lā′shŭn) Maiming; the act of removing or destroying a conspicuous or essential part or organ.

mutism (mū′tĭzm) [L. *mutus,* dumb] **1.** Condition of being unable to speak. **2.** Persistent inhibition of speech seen in some severe forms of mental illness.

akinetic m. The condition of being immobile and silent while partially or fully awake. This may be caused by lesions of the frontal lobes of the brain or by hydrocephalus.

elective m. Selective m.

hysterical m. Inability to speak due to a conversion disorder.

selective m. A form of social phobia, typically first identified in young children, in which the child fails to speak in certain public settings but has normal speech at other times. SYN: *elective m.*

mutualism (mū′tū-ăl-ĭzm) [L. *mutuus,* exchanged] A form of symbiosis in which organisms of two different species live in close association to the mutual benefit of each.

mutualist (mū′tū-ăl-ĭst) Organism associated with another organism to the mutual benefit of each.

***μ*V** Symbol for microvolt.

M.V. *Medicas Veterinarius.* Latin for veterinary physician.

mv *millivolt.*

M.W.I.A. *Medical Women's International Association.*

my-, myo- [Gr. *mys,* muscle] Prefix denoting *muscle.*

myalgia (mī-ăl′jē-ă) [″ + *algos,* pain] Tenderness or pain in the muscles; muscular rheumatism. SYN: *myodynia.*

tension m. Fibromyalgia.

myasis (mī-ā′sĭs) [Gr. *myia,* a fly] Myiasis.

myasthenia (mī-ăs-thē′nē-ă) [Gr. *mys,* muscle, + *astheneia,* weakness] Muscular weakness and abnormal fatigue. **myasthenic,** *adj.*

angiosclerotic m. An old term for intermittent claudication.

m. gravis ABBR: MG. A motor disorder marked by muscular fatigue that develops with repetitive muscle use and improves with rest. It is caused by antibodies to the acetylcholine receptor in the neuromuscular junction and a decrease in receptor sites for acetylcholine. Because the smallest concentration of acetylcholine receptors in the body is in the cranial nerves, weakness and fatigue of the eye muscles, muscles of mastication, and pharyngeal muscles are the most prominently affected in most patients. The disease is rare, affecting about 60 persons out of a million. SEE: *Nursing Diagnoses Appendix.*

SYMPTOMS: Clinical signs include drooping of the upper eyelid (ptosis) and double vision (diplopia) due to fatigue and weakness in the extraocular muscles, and difficulty chewing and swallowing from impaired facial and pharyngeal muscles.

TREATMENT: The primary treatment is with anticholinesterases (drugs that prevent the breakdown of acetylcholine at the neuromuscular junction) and immunosuppressive agents. In selected patients, removal of the thymus, plasmapheresis, or immunoglobulin therapy is used.

PATIENT CARE: The diagnosis, nature of the disease process, and treatment are explained. Emotional support and reassurance are given. Activity-planning commensurate with capabilities is encouraged to help the patient conserve energy. Positive coping behaviors are reinforced. Regular medical follow-up, early reporting of any untoward symptoms, and family assistance and support are encouraged.

myatonia (mī-ă-tō′nē-ă) Deficiency or loss of muscular tone.

m. congenita Myotonia congenita.

myatrophy (mī-ăt′rō-fē) Muscular wasting.

myc- SEE: *myco-.*

mycelioid (mī-sē′lē-oyd) [″ + *helos,* nail, + *eidos,* form, shape] Moldlike; resembling mold colonies in which filaments radiate from a center, said of bacterial colonies.

mycelium (mī-sē′lē-ŭm) [Gr. *mykes,* fungus, + *helos,* nail] The mass of filaments (hyphae) that constitutes the vegetative body of fungi such as molds.

mycetes (mī-sē′tēz) The fungi.

mycethemia (mī-sĕ-thē′mē-ă) [″ + *haima,* blood] Fungi in the blood.

mycetism, mycetismus (mī′sĕ-tĭzm, mī-sĕ-tĭz′mŭs) [″ + *-ismos,* condition] Poisoning from eating fungi, esp. poisonous mushrooms.

mycetogenetic (mī-sē″tō-jĕn-ĕt′ĭk) [″ + *gennan,* to produce] Induced by fungi.

mycetoma (mī-sĕ-tō′mă) [″ + *oma,* tumor] A syndrome caused by a variety of aerobic actinomycetes and fungi. It is characterized by swelling and suppuration of subcutaneous tissues and formation of sinus tracts, with granules present in the pus draining from the tracts. These tracts usually appear on the lower body.

TREATMENT: Sulfones, trimethoprim and sulfamethoxazole, or sulfonamides may benefit lesions caused by actinomycetes. If lesions are due to fungi, there is no specific therapy.

myco, myc- [Gr. *mykes,* fungus] Combining form meaning *fungus.*

mycobacteriosis (mī″kō-băk-tē″rē-ō′sĭs) An infection caused by any mycobacterium.

Mycobacterium [″ + *bakterion,* little rod] A genus of acid-fast organisms, belonging to the Mycobacteriaceae family, which includes the causative organisms of tuberculosis and leprosy. The organisms are slender, nonmotile, gram-positive rods and do not produce spores or capsules.

Species include *M. africanum, M. avium intracellulare, M. bovis, M. chelonei, M. fortuitum, M. gastri, M. gordonae, M. kansasii, M. marinum, M. scrofulaceum, M. terrae, M. triviale, M. smegmatis,* and *M. xenopi.*

m. avium complex ABBR: MAC, MAI. An atypical mycobacterium that causes systemic bacterial infection in patients with advanced immunosuppression (esp. those with acquired immunodeficiency syndrome [AIDS]). It occasionally causes lung infections in patients with chronic obstructive lung disease. SYN: *m. avium-intracellulare complex.*

SYMPTOMS: MAC infection in persons with AIDS can cause fatigue, fever, weight loss, cachexia, pancytopenia, and death.

TREATMENT: Multiple antimicrobial agents, given at the same time and for long courses, are required to treat MAC. Combination therapy may include a macrolide with drugs such as rifabutin, ethambutol, ciprofloxacin, amikacin, and/or clofazimine.

m. avium-intracellulare complex m. avium complex.

M. bovis The organism that causes tuberculosis in cows and less commonly in humans.

M. kansasii A cause of tuberculosis-like pulmonary disease in humans.

M. leprae The causative agent of leprosy.

M. marinum An atypical mycobacterium that produces skin infection resembling sporotrichosis. The organism has been cultured from tropical fish aquariums. SEE: *swimming pool granuloma.*

M. tuberculosis The causative agent of tuberculosis in humans. SEE: *tuberculosis;* illus.

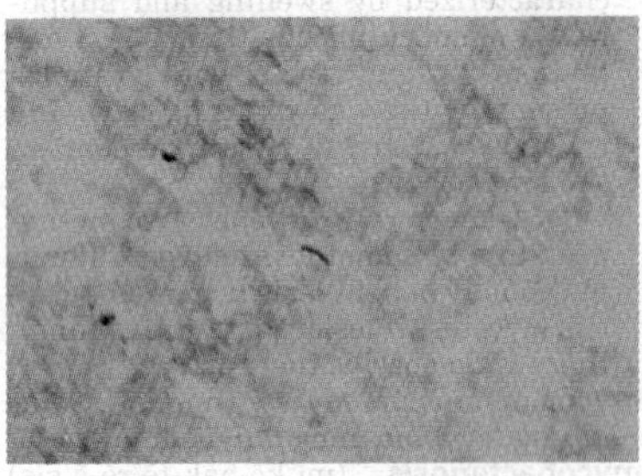

MYCOBACTERIUM TUBERCULOSIS

Acid-fast bacillus in sputum (orig. mag. ×500)

mycocidin (mī″kō-sī′dĭn) An antibiotic derived from molds of the family Aspergillaceae.

mycoderma [Gr. *mykos,* mucus, + *derma,* skin] Mucous membrane.

mycoid (mī′koyd) [″ + *eidos,* form, shape] Fungus-like.

mycology (mī-kŏl′ō-jē) [″ + *logos,* word, reason] The science and study of fungi.

mycophenolate (mī-kō-fē′-nō-lāt) An immunosuppressive drug used to prevent organ rejection after transplantation.

mycophthalmia (mī-kŏf-thăl′mē-ă) Ophthalmia resulting from fungus infection.

Mycoplasma A group of bacteria that lack cell walls and are highly pleomorphic. There are more than 70 organisms in this group, including 12 species that infect humans. *M. hominis* can cause genital tract infections; *M. pneumoniae* can cause infections of the upper respiratory tract and the lungs (i.e., mycoplasma pneumonia).

TREATMENT: Tetracycline or erythromycin are effective for treatment of *M. pneumoniae* and *M. hominis* infections. Other treatment choices include clarithromycin, azithromycin, and the fluoroquinolones.

mycosis (mī-kō′sĭs) [″ + *osis,* condition] Any disease induced by a fungus, or resembling a fungal disease.

m. fungoides ABBR: MF. Cutaneous T-cell lymphoma, esp. when the disease is first clinically apparent on the skin. The skin is marked by irregularly shaped macules, plaques, or nodules, which usually first appear on the trunk and may sometimes cause considerable itching. The rash may be difficult to diagnose or may be misdiagnosed as another form of dermatitis. Biopsy specimens may reveal atypical-appearing lymphocytes in the epidermis or collections of malignant lymphocytes in clusters called Pautrier's microabscesses. Eventually (e.g., 10 or more years after diagnosis), the malignant cells disseminate throughout the skin and into lymph nodes and internal organs.

TREATMENT: Topical nitrogen mustard, phototherapy with psoralens and ultraviolet light, systemic chemotherapy, interferons, extracorporeal phototherapy, and electron beam radiation of the skin have all been used. The disease may be curable when treated in its very earliest stage.

NOTE: The name "mycosis fungoides" is deceptive, as the disease is not fungal in origin.

superficial m. Any of a group of fungus infections of the skin. Included in this group are erythrasma, tinea barbae, tinea capitis, tinea corporis, tinea cruris, tinea favosa, tinea pedis, tinea unguium, and trichomycosis axillaris.

systemic m. Any of a group of deep fungus infections involving various bodily systems or regions. Included in this group are aspergillosis, blastomycosis, chromoblastomycosis, coccidioidomycosis, cryptococcosis, geotrichosis, histoplasmosis, maduromycosis, moniliasis, mucormycosis, nocardiosis, penicilliosis, rhinosporidiosis, and sporotrichosis. SEE: illus.

mycostasis (mī-kŏs′tă-sĭs) [Gr. *mykes,* fungus, + *stasis,* standing] Stopping the growth of fungi.

mycostat (mī′kō-stăt) [″ + *statikos,* standing] Any agent that stops the growth of fungi.

mycotic (mī-kŏt′ĭk) Caused by or infected with fungus; concerning mycosis.

mycotoxicosis (mī″kō-tŏk″sĭ-kō′sĭs) [″ + *toxikon,* poisoning, + *osis,* condition] Disease either caused by toxins on molds or produced by molds.

mycotoxins Substances produced by mold growing in food or animal feed and causing illness or death when ingested by humans or animals. SEE: *ergotism.*

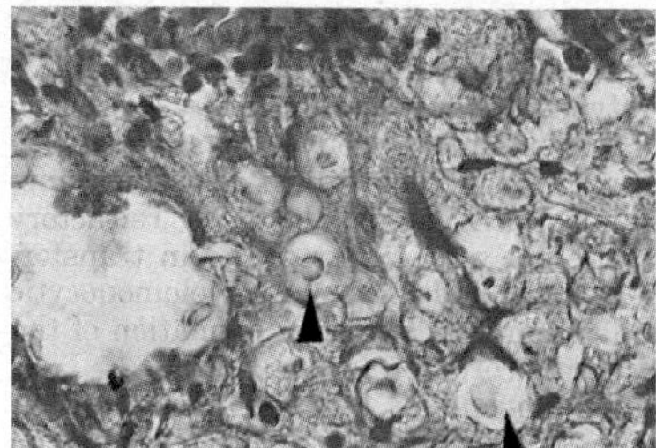

SYSTEMIC MYCOSIS

Cryptococcosis of lung; arrows indicate fungus (orig. mag. ×450)

mycterophonia (mĭk″tĕr-ō-fō′nē-ă) [Gr. *mykter,* nostril, + *phone,* voice] Phonation in which the voice possesses a nasal quality.

mydaleine (mīd-ā′lē-ēn) [Gr. *mydaleos,* moldy] A poisonous ptomaine formed in putrefied visceral organs, acting mainly on the heart.

mydriasis (mĭd-rī′ă-sĭs) [Gr.] Pronounced or abnormal dilation of the pupil.

ETIOLOGY: Causes include fright and other causes of sympathetic nervous system activation, first and third stages of anesthesia, drugs, coma, botulism, and irritation of the cervical sympathetic nerve.

alternating m. Mydriasis that affects one eye, then the other.

paralytic m. Mydriasis resulting from paralysis of the oculomotor nerve.

spastic m. Mydriasis resulting from overactivity of the dilator muscle of the iris or of sympathetic nerves supplying that muscle.

spinal m. Mydriasis resulting from irritation of, or a lesion in, the ciliospinal center of spinal cord.

mydriatic (mĭd-rē-ăt′ĭk) **1.** Causing pupillary dilatation. **2.** A drug that dilates the pupil, such as atropine, cocaine, ephedrine, euphthalmine, and homatropine. In certain eye diseases, it is essential that the pupil be dilated during the course of treatment to prevent adhesions of the pupils.

myectomy (mī-ĕk′tō-mē) [Gr. *mys,* muscle, + *ektome,* excision] Excision of a portion of a muscle.

myel- SEE: *myelo-*.

myelalgia (mī-ĕl-ăl′jē-ă) [Gr. *myelos,* marrow, + *algos,* pain] Pain in the spinal cord or its membranes.

myelapoplexy (mī″ĕl-ăp′ō-plĕks-ē) [″ + *apoplexia,* stroke] Hemorrhagic effusion into the spinal cord.

myelatelia (mī″ĕl-ă-tē′lē-ă) [″ + *ateleia,* imperfection] Myelodysplasia.

myelauxe (mī-ĕl-awks′ē) [″ + *auxe,* increase] Abnormal enlargement of spinal cord.

myelencephalon (mī″ĕl-ĕn-sĕf′ă-lŏn) [Gr. *myelos,* marrow, + *enkephalos,* brain] The most posterior portion of the embryonic hindbrain (rhombencephalon), which gives rise to the medulla oblongata.

myelic Pert. to the spinal cord.

myelin The phospholipid-protein of the cell membranes of Schwann cells (peripheral nervous system) and oligodendrocytes (central nervous system) that forms the myelin sheath of neurons. It acts as an electrical insulator and increases the velocity of impulse transmission. SEE: *neuron* for illus. **myelinic** (mī-ĕl-ĭn′ĭk), *adj.*

myelination (mī″ĕl-ĭn-ā′shŭn) [Gr. *myelos,* marrow] Process of growth of a myelin sheath around nerve fibers. SYN: *myelinization.*

myelinization (mī″ĕl-ĭn-ĭ-zā′shŭn) Myelination.

myelinoclasis (mī″ĕ-lĭn-ŏk′lă-sĭs) [″ + *klasis,* breaking] Process of destruction of myelin.

myelinogenetic (mī″ĕl-ĭn-ō-jĕn-ĕt′ĭk) [″ + *gennan,* to produce] Producing myelin or a myelin sheath.

myelinolysis (mī″ĕ-lĭn-ŏl′ĭ-sĭs) [″ + *lysis,* dissolution] Destruction of the myelin sheaths of nerves.

myelinopathy Degeneration of the myelin sheaths of neurons, esp. in the central nervous system. SEE: *multiple sclerosis.*

myelinosis (mī″ĕl-ĭn-ō′sĭs) [″ + *osis,* condition] Fatty degeneration during which myelin is produced.

myelitis (mī-ĕ-lī′tĭs) [″ + *itis,* inflammation] **1.** Inflammation of the spinal cord, resulting from either an infection (e.g., a viral or bacterial infection) or a noninfectious necrosing or demyelinating lesion of the cord. Patients often exhibit flaccid limb paralysis, incontinence, weakness or numbness of the limbs, and other symptoms. SEE: *poliomyelitis.* **2.** Inflammation of bone marrow. SEE: *osteomyelitis.*

acute m. Myelitis that develops rapidly, that is, in hours or days. Myelitis of rapid onset is more likely to be reversible than chronic or slowly developing inflammation of the spinal cord.

acute ascending m. Myelitis that moves progressively upward in the spinal cord.

acute transverse m. An acute form of myelitis involving the entire thickness of the spinal cord, developing, for example, subsequent to injury to the spinal cord.

bulbar m. Myelitis involving the medulla oblongata.

central m. Inflammation of the gray matter of the spinal cord.

compression m. Myelitis caused by pressure on the spinal cord, as by a hemorrhage or tumor.

descending m. Myelitis affecting successively lower areas of the spinal cord.

disseminated m. Inflammation of several separate areas of the spinal cord.

focal m. Myelopathy of small areas of the spinal cord.

hemorrhagic m. Myelitis with hemorrhage.

sclerosing m. Myelopathy wherein there is hardening of the spinal cord.

transverse m. Myelitis involving the whole thickness of the spinal cord, but limited longitudinally.

traumatic m. Myelitis due to spinal cord injury. **myelitic** (mī-ĕl-ĭt′ĭk), *adj.*

myelo-, myel- [Gr. *myelos,* marrow] Combining form meaning *spinal cord, bone marrow.*

myeloblast (mī′ĕl-ō-blăst) [″ + *blastos,* germ] Immature bone marrow cell that develops into a myelocyte. It matures to develop into a promyelocyte, and eventually into a granular leukocyte.

myeloblastemia (mī″ĕl-ō-blăst-ē′mē-ă) [″ + ″ + *haima,* blood] The occurrence of myeloblasts in the blood.

myeloblastoma (mī″ĕl-ō-blăst-ō′mă) [″ + ″ + *oma,* tumor] Chloroma.

myeloblastosis (mī″ĕ-lō-blăs-tō′sĭs) [″ + ″ + *osis,* condition] Excess production of myeloblasts and their presence in circulating blood.

myelocele (mī′ĕ-lō-sēl) [″ + *kele,* tumor, swelling] A form of spina bifida with spinal cord protrusion.

myelocyst (mī′ĕl-ō-sĭst) [″ + *kystis,* bladder] Cyst arising from the rudimentary vertebral canal enclosing the spinal cord.

myelocystocele (mī″ĕl-ō-sĭst′ō-sēl) [″ + ″ + *kele,* tumor, swelling] Protrusion of the spinal cord through a defect in the vertebral canal.

myelocystomeningocele (mī″ĕl-ō-sĭst″ō-mĕn-ĭn′gō-sēl) [″ + *kystis,* bladder, + *meninx,* membrane, + *kele,* tumor, swelling] Combined myelocystocele and meningocele.

myelocyte (mī′ĕl-ō-sīt) [″ + *kytos,* cell] A large cell in red bone marrow from which leukocytes are derived.

myelocythemia (mī″ĕl-ō-sī-thē′mē-ă) [″ +″ + *haima,* blood] Myelocytosis.

myelocytic (mī″ĕl-ō-sĭt′ĭk) Characterized by presence of, or pert. to, myelocytes.

myelocytosis (mī″ĕl-ō-sī-tō′sĭs) [″ + ″ + *osis,* condition] Presence of an excess number of myelocytes in the blood. SYN: *myelocythemia.*

myelodysplasia (mī″ĕl-ō-dĭs-plā′zē-ă) [″ + *dys,* bad, + *plassein,* to form] **1.** A group of hematological diseases, which primarily affect people over 60, in which there is inadequate bone marrow production of normal blood cells. These conditions begin when an abnormal clone of cells dominates the marrow; they may evolve into acute leukemia. The five types of myelodysplasia are 1) refractory anemia; 2) refractory anemia with ringed sideroblasts; 3) refractory anemia with excess blasts; 4) refractory anemia with excess blasts in transformation; and 5) chronic myelomonocytic leukemia. **2.** Defective formation of the spinal cord.

myeloencephalic (mī″ĕl-ō-ĕn-sĕf-ăl′ĭk) [″ + *enkephalos,* brain] Concerning the spinal cord and the brain.

myeloencephalitis (mī″ĕl-ō-ĕn-sĕf″ă-lī′tĭs) [″ + ″ + *itis,* inflammation] Inflammation of the spinal cord and the brain.

myelofibrosis (mī″ĕ-lō-fī-brō′sĭs) A myeloproliferative disorder marked by the overproduction of a single stem cell clone and reactive bone marrow fibrosis. SEE: illus.

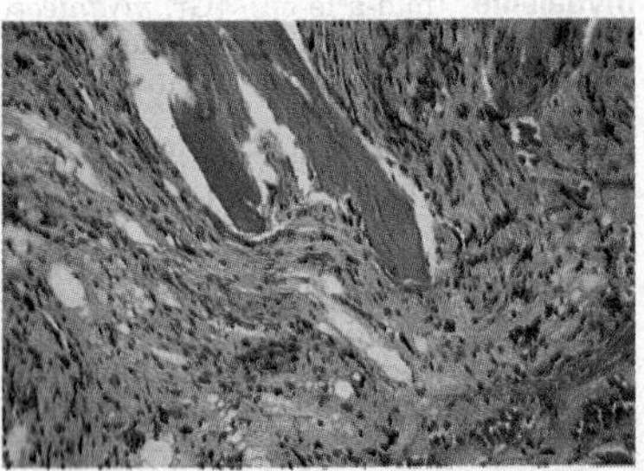

MYELOFIBROSIS

myelogenesis (mī″ĕl-ō-jĕn′ĕ-sĭs) [″ + *genesis,* generation, birth] **1.** Development of the brain and the spinal cord. **2.** Development of the myelin sheath of nerve fiber.

myelogenic, myelogenous (mī-ĕ-lō-jĕn′ĭk, -lŏj′ĕn-ŭs) [″ + *gennan,* to produce] Producing or originating in marrow.

myelogeny (mī″ĕ-lŏj′ĕ-nē) Maturation of the myelin sheaths during the development of the central nervous system.

myelogram (mī′ĕ-lō-grăm) [″ + *gramma,* something written] **1.** A radiograph of the spinal cord and associated nerves. **2.** A differential count of bone marrow cells.

myelography (mī-ĕ-lŏg′ră-fē) [″ + *graphein,* to write] Radiography of the spinal cord and associated nerves after intrathecal injection of a radiopaque, water-soluble contrast medium. This technique has limited use, owing to computed tomography and magnetic resonance imaging.

air m. Myelography using a radiolucent contrast medium, usually air or oxygen.

myeloid (mī′ĕ-loyd) [″ + *eidos,* form, shape] **1.** Medullary; marrow-like.

2. Resembling a myelocyte, but not necessarily originating from bone marrow.

myeloidosis (mī″ĕ-loy-dō′sĭs) [″ + ″ + *osis,* condition] Development of myeloid tissue.

myelolysis (mī″ĕ-lŏl′ĭs-sĭs) [″ + *lysis,* dissolution] Dissolution of myelin.

myeloma (mī-ĕ-lō′mă) [″ + *oma,* tumor] A tumor originating in cells of the hematopoietic portion of bone marrow.

multiple m. A malignant disease characterized by the infiltration of bone and bone marrow by neoplastic plasma cells. The condition is usually progressive and generally fatal within a few years. Findings include anemia, renal failure, pathological fractures, and high globulin levels in blood. Multiple myeloma is common in the sixth decade of life and occurs more frequently in males than in females by a ratio of 3 : 1. SEE: illus.

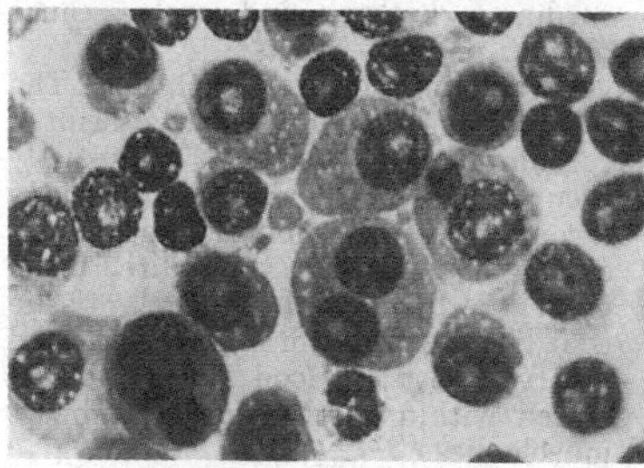

MULTIPLE MYELOMA

Numerous plasma cells replace normal bone marrow (orig. mag. ×600)

TREATMENT: Standard chemotherapy includes the use of melphalan and prednisone. Dialysis can be used to treat renal failure; bisphosphonates prevent bony metastases.

myelomalacia (mī″ĕ-lō-mă-lā′shē-ă) [Gr. *myelos,* marrow, + *malakia,* softening] Abnormal softening of the spinal cord.

myelomatosis (mī″ĕl-ō-mă-tō′sĭs) [″ + *oma,* tumor, + *osis,* intensive] An old term for multiple myeloma.

myelomeningocele (mī″ĕ-lō-mĕn-ĭn′gō-sēl) [″ + ″ + *kele,* tumor, swelling] Spina bifida with a portion of the spinal cord and membranes protruding.

myelomere (mī′ĕ-lō-mēr) [″ + *meros,* part] A segment of the developing spinal cord.

myeloneuritis (mī″ĕ-lō-nū-rī′tĭs) [″ + *neuron,* nerve, + *itis,* inflammation] Neuromyelitis.

myelopathy (mī-ĕ-lŏp′ă-thē) [″ + *pathos,* disease, suffering] Any pathological condition of the spinal cord.

ascending m. Myelopathy that ascends along the spinal cord toward the head.

descending m. Myelopathy that descends along the spinal cord toward the feet.

focal m. Myelopathy of small areas.

sclerosing m. Myelopathy in which there is hardening of the spinal cord.

transverse m. Myelopathy extending across the spinal cord.

traumatic m. Myelopathy due to trauma to the spinal cord.

myelopetal (mī-ĕ-lŏp′ĕt-ăl) [″ + L. *petere,* to seek for] Proceeding toward the spinal cord, said of certain nerve impulses.

myelophthisis (mī-ĕ-lŏf′thĭ-sĭs) [″ + *phthisis,* a wasting] **1.** Atrophy of the spinal cord. **2.** Replacement of the bone marrow by a disease process such as a neoplasm.

myeloplegia (mī″ĕl-ō-plē′jē-ă) [Gr. *myelos,* marrow, + *plege,* stroke] Paralysis of spinal origin.

myelopoiesis (mī″ĕl-ō-poy-ē′sĭs) [″ + *poiein,* to form] Development of bone marrow or formation of cells derived from bone marrow.

ectopic m. Extramedullary m.

extramedullary m. Development of myeloid elements (erythrocytes and granular leukocytes) in regions other than bone marrow. SYN: *ectopic myelopoiesis.*

myelopore An opening in the spinal cord.

myeloproliferative (mī″ĕ-lō-prō-lĭf″ĕr-ā′tĭv) Concerning abnormal proliferation of hematological stem cells.

myeloradiculitis (mī″ĕ-lō-ră-dĭk″ū-lī′tĭs) [″ + L. *radiculus,* rootlet, + Gr. *itis,* inflammation] Inflammation of the spinal cord and the dorsal roots of spinal nerves.

myeloradiculodysplasia (mī″ĕ-lō-ră-dĭk″ū-lō-dĭs-plā′sē-ă) [″ + ″ + Gr. *dys,* bad, + *plassein,* to form] Congenital abnormality of the spinal cord and spinal nerve roots.

myeloradiculopathy (mī″ĕ-lō-ră-dĭk″ū-lŏp′ă-thē) [″ + ″ + Gr. *pathos,* disease, suffering] Disease of the spinal cord and spinal nerves.

myelorrhagia (mī-ĕ-lō-rā′jē-ă) [″ + *rhegnynai,* to burst forth] Hemorrhage into the spinal cord.

myelorrhaphy (mī-ĕl-or′ă-fē) [″ + *rhaphe,* seam, ridge] Suture of a cut or wound of the spinal cord.

myelosarcoma (mī″ĕl-ō-săr-kō′mă) [″ + *sarx,* flesh, + *oma,* tumor] Sarcoma composed of bone marrow cells and tissue. SYN: *osteosarcoma.*

myelosarcomatosis (mī″ĕ-lō-săr-kō″mă-tō′sĭs) [″ + ″ + ″ + *osis,* condition] Disseminated myelosarcomas.

myeloschisis (mī″ĕ-lŏs′kĭ-sĭs) [″ + *schisis,* a splitting] Cleft spinal cord resulting from failure of the neural tube to close. SEE: *rachischisis; spina bifida cystica.*

myelosclerosis (mī″ĕ-lō-sklĕr-ō′sĭs) [″ + *sklerosis,* hardening] Sclerosis of the spinal cord.

myelosis (mī-ĕ-lō′sĭs) [″ + *osis,* condition] Formation of a myeloma or medullary tumor.

erythremic m. A malignancy involving the erythropoietic tissue. Symptoms and signs include anemia, fever, hepatosplenomegaly, bleeding tendency, and abnormal cells in the circulating blood. Also known as Di Guglielmo syndrome.

myelospongium (mī″ĕ-lō-spŏn′jē-ŭm) [Gr. *myelos,* marrow, + *spongos,* sponge] Embryonic network from which the neuroglia arises.

myelosuppression (mī″ĕ-lō-sŭ-prĕsh′ŭn) Inhibition of bone marrow function.

myelotome (mī-ĕl′ō-tōm) [″ + *tome,* incision] Instrument used to dissect the spinal cord.

myelotomy (mī-ĕl-ŏt′ō-mē) Surgical severance of nerve fibers of the spinal cord.

myelotoxic (mī-ĕl-ō-tŏk′sĭk) [″ + *toxikon,* poison] **1.** Destroying bone marrow. **2.** Pert. to or arising from diseased bone marrow.

myelotoxin (mī″ĕl-ō-tŏk′sĭn) Toxin that destroys marrow cells.

myenteric reflex SEE: under *reflex*.

myenteron (mī-ĕn′tĕr-ŏn) The smooth muscle layer of the intestine. **myenteric** (mī″ĕn-tĕr′ĭk), *adj.*

Myerson's sign [Abraham Myerson, U.S. neurologist, 1881–1948] In Parkinson's disease, repeated blinking of the eyes in response to tapping the forehead, nasal bridge, or maxilla.

myesthesia (mī″ĕs-thē′zē-ă) [Gr. *mys,* muscle, + *aisthesis,* sensation] Muscle sense; consciousness of muscle contraction.

myiasis (mī′ă-sĭs) [Gr. *myia,* fly, + *-sis,* condition] Condition resulting from infestation by the larvae (maggots) of flies. Infestation may be cutaneous, intestinal, atrial (within a cavity such as mouth, nose, eye, sinus, vagina, urethra), via a wound, or external.

myiocephalon (mī″yō-sĕf′ă-lŏn) [″ + *kephale,* head] Extrusion of a part of the iris through a tear in the cornea.

myiodesopsia (mī″ē-ō-dĕs-ŏp′sē-ă) [Gr. *myiodes,* flylike, + *opsis,* vision] Condition in which spots are seen before the eyes. SEE: *floater*.

myiosis (mī-yō′sĭs) [″ + *osis,* condition] Myiasis.

mylodus A molar tooth.

mylohyoid (mī″lō-hī′oyd) [Gr. *myle,* mill, + *hyoid,* U-shaped] **1.** Pert. to the hyoid bone and the molar teeth. **2.** The paired muscles attached to the mandible that fuse in the midline and form the floor of the mouth.

myo- [Gr. *mys,* muscle] Combining form meaning *muscle.*

myoalbumin (mī″ō-ăl-bū′mĭn) [″ + L. *albus,* white] Albumin found in muscular tissue.

myoarchitectonic (mī″ō-ăr″kĭ-tĕk-tŏn′ĭk) [Gr. *mys,* muscle, + *architekton,* master workman] Pert. to or resembling structural arrangement of muscle or of fibers.

myoatrophy (mī-ō-ăt′rō-fē) Muscular wasting.

myoblast (mī′ō-blăst) [″ + *blastos,* germ] An embryonic cell that develops into muscle cell.

myoblastoma (mī″ō-blăs-tō′mă) [″ + ″ + *oma,* tumor] A tumor consisting of cells resembling myoblasts.

myobradia (mī″ō-brā′dē-ă) [″ + *bradys,* slow] Slow muscular reaction to stimulation.

myocardial, myocardiac (mī-ō-kăr′dē-ăl, -ăk) [″ + *kardia,* heart] Concerning the myocardium.

m. contusion Cardiac injury resulting from blunt or penetrating trauma to the chest. It is an occasional cause of cardiac arrhythmia and rarely a cause of rupture of the heart.

myocardial infarction ABBR: MI. The loss of living heart muscle as a result of coronary artery occlusion. MI usually occurs when an atheromatous plaque in a coronary artery ruptures, and the resulting clot obstructs the injured blood vessel. Perfusion of the muscular tissue that lies downstream from the blocked artery is lost. If blood flow is not restored within a few hours, the heart muscle dies.

Hundreds of thousands of MIs occur in the U.S. every year, many of them resulting in sudden death. The probability of dying from MI is related to the patient's underlying health, whether arrhythmias such as ventricular fibrillation or ventricular tachycardia occur, and how rapidly the patient receives appropriate therapies, such as thrombolytic drugs, angioplasty, antiplatelet drugs, beta blockers, and intensive electrocardiographic monitoring. SEE: *advanced cardiac life support; atherosclerosis; cardiac arrest; sudden death; unstable angina.*

ETIOLOGY: Plaque rupture causes the vast majority of MIs, occurring in patients with a history of atherosclerosis. The risk factors for MI are: tobacco use, diabetes mellitus, hyperlipidemia, hypertension, male gender, advanced age, obesity, and sedentary lifestyle, among others. Rarely, emboli that lodge in the coronary arteries, spasm of coronary musculature, myocardial bridges, severe anemia, or profoundly low blood pressure result in MI.

SYMPTOMS: Classic symptoms of MI are a gradual onset of pain or pressure, felt most intensely in the center of the chest, radiating into the neck, jaw, shoulders, or arms, and lasting more than a half hour. Pain typically is dull or heavy rather than sharp or stabbing, and often is associated with difficult breathing, nausea, vomiting, and profuse sweating. Clinical presentations, however, vary considerably. Many patients believe they are having indigestion, intestinal gas, or muscular aches; many women and elderly persons experience difficulty breathing more prominently than chest pain or pressure. About a third of all MIs are clinically silent. Often patients suffering MI have had angina pectoris for several weeks before and simply did not recognize it.

DIAGNOSIS: A compatible history in a patient whose ECG reveals ST segment elevation in two or more contiguous leads establishes the diagnosis of acute MI. When the history and ECG are not diagnostic, an analysis of cardiac muscle enzymes (troponins, creatine kinase) can establish the diagnosis, often within a few hours of presentation. The differential diagnosis of chest pain must always be carefully considered because other serious illnesses, such as pulmonary embolism, aortic dissection, esophageal rupture, acute cholecystitis, esophagitis, or splenic rupture, to name a few, may mimic MI.

TREATMENT: MI is a medical emergency; diagnosis and treatment must not be delayed. Typical treatment for the patient includes the following:

1. administering oxygen immediately, and giving aspirin and beta blockers as soon as the disease is recognized;
2. ordering thrombolytic drugs (like streptokinase or tissue plasminogen activator) or emergency angioplasty;
3. administering nitrates and morphine for vasodilation and pain;
4. administering antiplatelet agents such as heparin or abciximab.

Angiotensin converting enzyme inhibitors also are helpful. In some instances (for example, when shock is present), massive infusions of fluids, or pressors, are required. In MI complicated by pulmonary edema, high doses of diuretics are administered. Occasionally, sustained ventricular arrhythmias mandate the use of defibrillation, lidocaine, or other antiarrhythmic drugs.

With contemporary care, about 95% of patients with acute MI who arrive at the hospital in time will survive. These patients are referred to nutrition therapists to learn how to use low-fat, low-cholesterol diets, and to cardiac rehabilitation programs for exercise training, tobacco cessation, and psychosocial support.

PATIENT CARE: All diagnostic and treatment procedures are explained briefly to reduce stress and anxiety. Cardiac rhythm, rate, and conduction are monitored on a lead that provides easily identifiable P and R waves (a 12-lead ECG should be included). Location, radiation, quality and severity, and frequency of chest pain are documented. Prescribed oxygen and analgesic medications (mainly IV) are administered and evaluated for desired effects. Vital signs and hemodynamic status are monitored according to protocol or as the patient requires. An IV access is established and maintained for emergency therapy, such as administration of cardiac and diuretic drugs and implementation of other emergency measures according to protocol or as prescribed for the patient's problems. As the patient recuperates from MI, both the patient and family are taught about the need for long-term drug therapy, a low-fat, low-cholesterol diet, and regular exercise. Stress tests, coronary angiography, cardiac imaging procedures, and other interventions are explained. The patient receives assistance in coping with changes in health status and self-concept.

exercise-related m.i. A myocardial infarction whose symptoms begin within an hour of vigorous physical exercise.

myocardial insufficiency Inability of the heart to perform its usual function, eventually resulting in cardiac failure.

myocardial ischemia SEE: under *ischemia.*

myocardiograph (mī″ō-kăr′dē-ō-grăf) [″ + ″ + *graphein,* to write] Instrument for recording heart movements.

myocardiopathy (mī″ō-kăr″dē-ŏp′ă-thē) [″ + ″ + *pathos,* disease, suffering] Any disease of the myocardium.

myocarditis (mī″ō-kăr-dī′tĭs) [″ + *kardia,* heart, + *itis,* inflammation] Inflammation of the heart muscle, usually as a consequence of *infections* (e.g., viruses, Lyme disease, rheumatic fever, trypanosomes, or toxoplasmosis); *immunological-rheumatological conditions* (e.g., systemic lupus erythematosus, hypersensitivity reactions, or transplant rejection); *toxins* (e.g., cocaine, doxorubicin); *nutritional or metabolic abnormalities* (e.g., thiamine deficiency or hypophosphatemia); or *radiation.* Inflammatory damage to heart muscle fibers may resolve spontaneously or may cause progressive deterioration of the heart. SEE: *cardiomyopathy.*

SYMPTOMS: Patients may be entirely asymptomatic or may seek medical attention because of the sudden onset of palpitations, chest pain, shortness of breath, edema, congestive heart failure, or arrhythmias.

TREATMENT: Any identifiable causes are corrected or treated. Symptomatic management also may include drugs such as angiotensin-converting enzyme inhibitors or diuretics (for heart failure), beta blocking agents, and supplemental oxygen when it is needed.

PATIENT CARE: Hospitalization may be required so that patients can be monitored for dysrhythmias and signs of congestive heart failure (e.g., increasing dyspnea, edema, weight gain, fatigue). Bed rest is maintained to decrease the work of the heart and to minimize myocardial damage. Stool softeners may be used to decrease straining, which can increase the risk of dysrhythmias. Elastic or pneumatic stockings and passive and resistive exercises are used to decrease the risk of venous thrombosis. Activity is increased gradually after the acute phase, and a progressive exercise program is developed for use after recovery. Patients are cautioned to stop exercising if shortness of breath occurs. The patient is taught to recognize and report signs of congestive heart failure.

myocardium (mī-ō-kăr′dē-ŭm) [″ + *kardia,* heart] The middle layer of the walls of the heart, composed of cardiac muscle.

myocele (mī′ō-sēl) [″ + *kele,* tumor, swelling] Muscular protrusion through a muscle sheath.

myocelitis (mī″ō-sē-lī′tĭs) [″ + ″ + *itis,* inflammation] Inflammation of abdominal muscles.

myocellulitis (mī″ō-sĕl-ū-lī′tĭs) [″ + L. *cellula,* little chamber, + Gr. *itis,* inflammation] Myositis combined with cellulitis.

myocerosis (mī″ō-sē-rō′sĭs) [″ + *keros,* wax] Waxy degeneration of a muscle or muscular tissue. SYN: *myokerosis*.

myochorditis (mī″ō-kor-dī′tĭs) [″ + *chorde,* cord, + *itis,* inflammation] Inflammation of the muscles of the vocal cord.

myochosis of the colon Muscular thickening of the bowel wall, with a decrease in the width of the taenia coli. This pathological change in the intestines sometimes is seen in diverticular disease.

myochrome (mī′ō-krōm) [″ + *chroma,* color] **1.** Any muscle pigment. **2.** Cytochrome C.

myochronoscope (mī″ō-krō′nō-skōp) [″ + *chronos,* time, + *skopein,* to examine] Device used for timing a muscular contraction.

myoclonia (mī-ō-klō′nē-ă) Myoclonus.

myoclonus (mī-ŏk′lō-nŭs) [″ + *klonos,* tumult] Twitching or clonic spasm of a muscle or group of muscles.

m. multiplex Condition marked by persistent and continuous muscular spasms in unrelated muscles. SYN: *paramyoclonus multiplex*.

nocturnal m. Involuntary limb movements (e.g., twitching) during the night. SEE: *restless legs syndrome*.

palatal m. Rapid clonus of one or both sides of the palate.

myocoele (mī′ō-sēl) [″ + *koila,* hollow] Cavity within a somite of an embryo.

myocolpitis (mī″ō-kŏl-pī′tĭs) [″ + *kolpos,* vagina, + *itis,* inflammation] Inflammation of vaginal muscular tissue.

myocomma (mī-ō-kŏm′mă) *pl.* **myocommata** [″ + *komma,* cut] Septum dividing the myotomes.

myocyte (mī′ō-sīt) [″ + *kytos,* cell] A muscle tissue cell.

myocytoma (mī″ō-sī-tō′mă) [″ + ″ + *oma,* tumor] Tumor containing muscle cells.

myodemia (mī-ō-dē′mē-ă) [″ + *demos,* fat] Fatty degeneration of muscular tissue. Muscular fiber cells become filled with fat and are ultimately destroyed.

myodiastasis (mī″ō-dī-ăs′tă-sĭs) [Gr. *mys,* muscle, + *diastasis,* separation] Division or rupture of a muscle.

myodiopter (mī″ō-dī-ŏp′tĕr) The force of ciliary muscle contraction needed to increase the refraction of the eye one diopter more than when the eye is at rest.

myodynamia (mī″ō-dī-năm′ē-ă) [″ + *dynamis,* force] Muscular force or strength.

myodynamometer (mī″ō-dī″nă-mŏm′ĕt-ĕr) [″ + ″ + *metron,* measure] Device for measurement of muscular strength.

myodynia (mī″ō-dĭn′ē-ă) [″ + *odyne,* pain] Muscle pain. SYN: *myalgia*.

myodystrophy (mī″ō-dĭs′trō-fē) [″ + ″ + *trophe,* nutrition] SEE: *spinal muscular atrophy*.

myoedema (mī″ō-ĕ-dē′mă) [″ + *oidema,* swelling] **1.** Mounding. **2.** Edema of a muscle.

myoelastic Pert. to muscle and elastic tissue.

myoelectric Pert. to the electrical properties of muscles.

myoelectric prosthesis SEE: under *prosthesis*.

myoendocarditis (mī″ō-ĕn″dō-kăr-dī′tĭs) [″ + *endon,* within, + *kardia,* heart, + *itis,* inflammation] Inflammation of the cardiac muscular wall and membranous lining.

myoepithelial cell SEE: under *cell*.

myoepithelioma (mī″ō-ĕp″ĭ-thē″lē-ō′mă) [″ + *epi,* upon, + *thele,* nipple, + *oma,* tumor] A slow-growing tumor of the sweat gland.

myoepithelium (mī″ō-ĕp″ĭ-thē′lē-ŭm) [″ + ″ + *thele,* nipple] Tissue containing contractile epithelial cells. **myoepithelial** (mī″ō-ĕp″ĭ-thē′lē-ăl), *adj.*

myofasciitis (mī″ō-făs″ē-ī′tĭs) [″ + L. *fascia,* band, + Gr. *itis,* inflammation] Inflammation of a muscle and its fascia.

myofibril, myofibrilla (mī-ō-fī′brĭl, -fī-brĭl′lă) [″ + L. *fibrilla,* a small fiber] A microscopic fibril found in muscle cells, grouped into bundles that run parallel to the long axis of the cell. It is made of myofilaments of myosin and actin, the contractile proteins.

myofibroma (mī″ō-fī-brō′mă) [″ + L. *fibra,* fiber, + Gr. *oma,* tumor] Tumor containing muscular and fibrous tissue.

myofibrosis (mī″ō-fī-brō′sĭs) [″ + ″ + Gr. *osis,* condition] Increase of connective or fibrous tissue with degeneration of muscular tissue.

myofibrositis (mī″ō-fī″brō-sī′tĭs) [Gr. *mys,* muscle, + L. *fibra,* fiber, + Gr. *itis,* inflammation] Inflammation of the perimysium, the fibrous tissue that encloses muscle tissue.

myofilament (mī″ō-fĭl′ă-mĕnt) A filament within the myofibrils of muscle cells. Thick ones are made of myosin; thin ones are made of actin, troponin, and tropomyosin.

myofunctional (mī″ō-fŭnk′shŭn-ăl) Concerning muscle function.

myogelosis (mī″ō-jē-lō′sĭs) [″ + L. *gelare,* to congeal] Abnormal hardening of a portion of muscle.

myogenesis (mī-ō-jĕn′ĕ-sĭs) [″ + *genesis,* generation, birth] Formation of muscular tissue, esp. in embryos.

myogenetic, myogenic (mī-ō-jĕ-nĕt′ĭk, mī-ō-jĕn′ĭk) [″ + *gennan,* to produce] Originating in muscle.

myoglia (mī-ŏg′lē-ă) [″ + *glia,* glue] In embryology, a fibrous network that forms briefly during muscle development.

myoglobin The iron-containing protein found in muscle cells that stores oxygen for use in cell respiration.

myoglobinuria (mī″ō-glō″bĭn-ū′rē-ă) Myoglobin in the urine. It may occur following muscular activity, trauma, or as a result of a deficiency of muscle phosphorylase.

myoglobulin (mī″ō-glŏb′ū-lĭn) [″ + L. *globulus,* globule] A coagulable globulin present in muscular tissue.

myognathus (mī-ŏg′nă-thŭs) [″ + *gnathos,* jaw] Deformed individual with a rudimentary conjoined twin.

myogram [″ + *gramma,* something written] Tracing made by the myograph of muscular contractions.

myograph (mī′ō-grăf) [″ + *graphein,* to write] Instrument for tracing movements caused by muscular contractions. **myographic** (mī-ō-grăf′ĭk), *adj.*

myographic tracing A myogram or muscular tracing.

myography (mī-ŏg′ră-fē) **1.** Recording of muscular contractions by a myograph. **2.** Description of the muscles and their action.

myohematin (mī″ō-hĕm′ă-tĭn) Cytochrome C.

myohemoglobin (mī″ō-hē″mō-glō′bĭn) Myoglobin.

myoid (mī′oyd) [Gr. *mys,* muscle, + *eidos,* form, shape] Resembling muscle.

myoidema (mī-oy-dē′mă) [″ + *oidema,* swelling] Myoedema.

myoischemia (mī″ō-ĭs-kē′mē-ă) [″ + *ischein,* to hold back, + *haima,* blood] Localized deficiency of blood supply in muscle tissue.

myokerosis (mī″ō-kē-rō′sĭs) [″ + *keros,* wax, + *osis,* condition] Myocerosis.

myokinase (mī″ō-kĭn′ās) An enzyme present in muscle that catalyzes the synthesis of adenosine triphosphate.

myokinesimeter (mī″ō-kĭn″ĕ-sĭm′ĕ-tĕr) [″ + *kinesis,* movement, + *metron,* measure] A device for measuring muscle activity.

myokinesis (mī″ō-kĭn-ē′sĭs) [″ + *kinesis,* movement] **1.** Muscular activity. **2.** Surgical displacement of muscular fibers.

myokymia (mī-ō-kĭm′ē-ă) [″ + *kyma,* wave] Twitching of isolated segments of muscle. The condition may be functional; however, it is also seen in organic diseases and general paresis. SYN: *kymatism.*

myolemma (mī″ō-lĕm′ă) [″ + *lemma,* sheath] Sarcolemma.

myolipoma (mī″ō-lī-pō′mă) [″ + *lipos,* fat, + *oma,* tumor] Muscle tissue tumor containing fatty elements.

myology (mī-ŏl′ō-jē) [″ + *logos,* word, reason] The science or study of the muscles and their parts.

myolysis (mī-ŏl′ĭ-sĭs) [″ + *lysis,* dissolution] Fatty degeneration and infiltration with destruction of muscular tissue accompanied by separation and disappearance of muscle cells.

myoma (mī-ō′mă) *pl.* **myomas or myomata** [″ + *oma,* tumor] A tumor containing muscle tissue. SEE: *chondromyoma; leiomyoma.* **myomatous** (-tŭs), *adj.*

m. striocellulare Rhabdomyoma.

m. telangiectoides Angiomyoma.

m. uteri Fibroid tumor of the uterus.

myomalacia (mī″ō-mă-lā′sē-ă) [Gr. *mys,* muscle, + *malakia,* softening] Softening of muscular tissue.

m. cordis Softening of the heart muscle.

myomatosis (mī″ō-mă-tō′sĭs) [″ + *oma,* tumor, + *osis,* condition] The development of multiple myomas.

myomectomy (mī″ō-mĕk′tō-mē) [″ + *oma,* tumor, + *ektome,* excision] **1.** Removal of a portion of muscle or muscular tissue. **2.** Removal of a myomatous tumor, generally uterine, usually by abdominal section, leaving the uterus in place.

myomelanosis (mī″ō-mĕl-ă-nō′sĭs) [″ + *melanosis,* blackening] Abnormal darkening of muscle tissue.

myomere (mī′ō-mēr) [″ + *meros,* part] Myotome (2).

myometer (mī-ŏm′ĕt-ĕr) [″ + *metron,* measure] Device for measurement of muscular contractions.

myometrial Concerning the myometrium.

myometritis (mī″ō-mē-trī′tĭs) [″ + *metra,* uterus, + *itis,* inflammation] Inflammation of the muscular wall of the uterus. SYN: *mesometritis.*

myometrium (mī″ō-mē′trē-ŭm) The smooth muscle layer of the uterine wall, forming the main mass of the uterus.

myomotomy (mī″ō-mŏt′ō-mē) [″ + ″ + *tome,* excision] Myomectomy (2).

myon [Gr. *mys,* muscle] A single muscle unit.

myonecrosis (mī″ō-nĕ-krō′sĭs) [″ + *nekrosis,* state of death] Necrosis of muscle tissue.

myonephropexy (mī″ō-nĕf′rō-pĕk″sē) [″ + *nephros,* kidney, + *pexis,* fixation] Fixation of a movable kidney by attaching it to a portion of muscular tissue with sutures.

myoneural Pert. to muscle and nerve, esp. nerve terminations in muscles.

myoneuralgia (mī″ō-nū-răl′jē-ă) [″ + *neuron,* nerve, + *algos,* pain] Muscle pain.

myoneural junction SEE: under *junction.*

myoneurasthenia (mī″ō-nūr″ăs-thē′nē-ă) [″ + ″ + *astheneia,* weakness] An obsolete term for weakness associated with neurasthenia.

myoneuroma (mī″ō-nū-rō′mă) [″ + ″ + *oma,* tumor] Neuroma partially composed of muscular elements.

myonymy (mī-ŏn′ĭ-mē) [″ + *onoma,* name] Nomenclature of muscles.

myoparalysis (mī″ō-pă-răl′ĭ-sĭs) Paralysis of a muscle.

myoparesis (mī″ō-păr′ĕ-sĭs) Weakness or incomplete paralysis of a muscle.

myopathic facies SEE: under *facies.*

myopathy (mī-ŏp′ă-thē) [″ + *pathos,* disease, suffering] Any congenital or acquired muscle disease, marked clinically by focal or diffuse muscular weakness. **myopathic** (mī-ō-păth′ĭk), *adj.*

centronuclear m. Myopathy in which the muscle fibers resemble those seen in fetal development. The nuclei of the cells are surrounded by a clear zone. SYN: *myotubular myopathy.*

distal m. Myopathy of the hands.

myotubular m. Centronuclear myocerosis. SEE: *myocerosis.*

nemaline m. Congenital nonprogressive weakness, esp. of the proximal muscles. The muscles are thin and resemble rods.

ocular m. Hereditary dystrophy of the extraocular muscles. This may progress to complete paralysis of these muscles.

thyrotoxic m. A progressive muscular weakness and atrophy as a result of hyperthyroidism.

myope (mī′ōp) [Gr. *myein,* to shut, + *ops,* eye] One afflicted with myopia (nearsightedness).

myopericarditis (mī″ō-pĕr-ĭ-kar-dī′tĭs) [Gr. *mys,* muscle, + *peri,* around, + *kardia,* heart, + *itis,* inflammation] Inflammation of the pericardium and cardiac muscular wall.

myopia (mī-ō′pē-ă) [Gr. *myein,* to shut, + *ops,* eye] An error in refraction in which light rays are focused in front of the retina, enabling the person to see distinctly for only a short distance. A negative (concave) lens of proper strength will correct this condition. SYN: *nearsightedness.* SEE: *emmetropia* for illus. **myopic** (mī-ŏp′ĭk), *adj.*

axial m. Myopia due to elongation of the axis of the eye.

chromic m. Color blindness only when viewing distant objects.

curvature m. Myopia due to the curvature of the eye's refracting surfaces.

index m. Myopia resulting from abnormal refractivity of the media of the eye.

malignant m. Progressive myopia leading to retinal detachment and blindness. SYN: *pernicious m.*

pernicious m. Malignant m.

prodromal m. Myopia, seen in incipient cataract, in which reading without glasses becomes possible.

progressive m. Myopia that increases steadily during adult life.

space m. Myopia occurring when the eye is attempting to focus on an object but all that is visible is a complete noncontrasting material, such as may occur when looking into dense fog (e.g., while piloting an airplane). No image is produced on the retina.

stationary m. Myopia that ends after adult growth is attained.

transient m. Myopia seen in spasm of accommodation, as in acute iritis or iridocyclitis.

myoplasm (mī′ō-plăzm) [Gr. *mys,* muscle, + LL. *plasma,* form, mold] The contractile part of the muscle cell, as differentiated from the sarcoplasm.

myoplastic (mī′ō-plăs′tĭk) [″ + *plassein,* to form] Pert. to the plastic use of muscle tissue or plastic surgery on muscles.

myoplasty (mī-ō-plăs″tē) Plastic surgery of muscle tissue.

myoporthosis (mī″ŏp-or-thō′sĭs) Correction of myopia (nearsightedness).

myopsychopathy (mī″ō-sī-kŏp′ă-thē) [″ + *psyche,* mind, + *pathos,* disease, suffering] Any muscle dysfunction associated with mental disorder.

myoreceptor (mī″ō-rē-sĕp′tor) A proprioceptor in the muscle.

myorrhaphy (mī-or′ă-fē) [Gr. *mys,* muscle, + *rhaphe,* a sewing] Suture of a muscle. SYN: *myosuture.*

myorrhexis (mī-or-ĕk′sĭs) [″ + *rhexis,* a rupture] Rupture of a muscle.

myosalpingitis (mī″ō-săl-pĭn-jī′tĭs) [″ + *salpinx,* tube, + *itis,* inflammation] Inflammation of the muscular tissue of a fallopian tube.

myosarcoma (mī″ō-sar-kō′mă) [″ + *sarx,* flesh, + *oma,* tumor] A malignant tumor derived from myogenic cells.

myosclerosis (mī″ō-sklĕr-ō′sĭs) [″ + *skleros,* hardening] Hardening of muscle.

myosin [Gr. *mys,* muscle] A protein

present in muscle fibrils and constituting about 65% of total muscle protein. It consists of long chains of polypeptides joined to each other by side chains. Myosin and actin are the contractile proteins in muscle fibers. Myosin also is an enzyme that catalyzes the removal of the third phosphate from ATP, thereby releasing the energy needed for contraction. SEE: *sarcomere*.

myosinose (mī-ŏs′ĭn-ōs) A protease resulting from the hydrolysis of myosin.

myosinuria (mī″ō-sĭn-ū′rē-ă) The presence of myosin in the urine. SYN: *myosuria*.

myositis (mī-ō-sī′tĭs) [″ + *itis,* inflammation] Inflammation of muscle tissue, esp. voluntary muscles caused, for example, by infection, trauma, autoimmunity, or infestation by parasites. SEE: *fibromyalgia*.

epidemic m. Bornholm disease.

m. fibrosa Myositis accompanied by infiltration of fibrous tissue.

interstitial m. Myositis with hyperplasia of connective tissue.

multiple m. Polymyositis.

m. ossificans Myositis marked by ossification of muscles.

parenchymatous m. Myositis of the substance of a muscle.

m. purulenta Suppurative myositis with abscesses; caused by bacterial infection.

traumatic m. Myositis due to physical injury. The condition may be simple, with accompanying pain and swelling, or may be suppurative.

m. trichinosa Myositis due to infestation with trichinae. SYN: *trichinous myositis*.

myospasm (mī′ō-spăzm) [″ + *spasmos,* a convulsion] Spasmodic contraction of a muscle.

myostatin (mī′ō-stāt′ĭn) A growth-regulating protein that contributes to the size of muscles by inhibiting excessive growth.

myosteoma (mī-ŏs″tē-ō′mă) [″ + *osteon,* bone, + *oma,* tumor] A bony growth found in muscle tissue.

myosthenometer (mī″ō-sthĕn-ŏm′ĕ-tĕr) [″ + *sthenos,* strength, + *metron,* measure] Device for measuring muscle power.

myostroma (mī″ō-strō′mă) [″ + *stroma,* mattress] The framework of muscle tissue.

myosuria (mī-ō-sū′rē-ă) [″ + *ouron,* urine] Myosinuria.

myosuture (mī″ō-sū′chūr) [″ + L. *sutura,* sewing] Myorrhexis.

myotactic (mī″ō-tăk′tĭk) [″ + L. *tactus,* touch] Pert. to muscle or kinesthetic sense.

myotasis (mī-ŏt′ă-sĭs) [″ + *tasis,* stretching] Stretching of a muscle. **myotatic,** *adj.*

myotatic reflex Stretch reflex.

myotenontoplasty (mī″ō-tĕn-ŏn′tō-plăst″ē) [″ + *tenon,* tendon, + *plassein,* to form] Tenomyoplasty.

myotenositis (mī″ō-tĕn-ō-sī′tĭs) [″ + ″ + *itis,* inflammation] Inflammation of a muscle and its tendon.

myotenotomy (mī″ō-tĕn-ŏt′ō-mē) [″ + ″ + *tome,* incision] Division of the tendon of a muscle.

myotherapy A method for relaxing muscle spasm, improving circulation, and alleviating pain. The therapist applies finger pressure to "trigger points," usually in the muscle tissue or area surrounding joints. The success of this method, developed by Bonnie Prudden in 1976, depends on the use of specific corrective exercise of the freed muscles.

myothermic (mī″ō-thĕrm′ĭk) [Gr. *mys,* muscle, + *therme,* heat] Pert. to rise in muscle temperature due to its activity.

myotome (mī′ō-tōm) [″ + *tome,* incision] **1.** Instrument used for cutting muscles. **2.** That portion of an embryonic somite that gives rise to somatic (striated) muscles. SYN: *myomere*.

myotomy (mī-ŏt′ō-mē) Surgical division or anatomical dissection of muscles.

myotonia (mī″ō-tō′nē-ă) [″ + *tonos,* tension] Tonic spasm of a muscle or temporary rigidity after muscular contraction. **myotonic,** *adj.*

m. atrophica M. dystrophica.

m. congenita A benign disease characterized by tonic spasms of the muscles induced by voluntary movements. The condition is usually congenital and is transmitted by either dominant or recessive genes. SYN: *Oppenheim's disease; paramyotonia; Thomsen's disease*.

SYMPTOMS: The disease appears in early childhood and is manifested by a tonic spasm of the muscles every time the muscles are used. In a few minutes, rigidity wears away and the movements become free from repeated contractions, the muscles becoming firm and extremely well developed.

TREATMENT: Quinine or procainamide are indicated for relief of myotonia. Neostigmine is contraindicated. Avoidance of obesity is important.

PROGNOSIS: The disease is incurable, but may improve with age.

m. dystrophica A hereditary disease characterized by muscular wasting, myotonia, and cataract. SYN: *m. atrophica; Steinert's disease*.

myotonic Pert. to tonic muscular spasm, as differentiated from myokinetic spasm.

myotonus (mī-ŏt′ō-nŭs) A tonic muscle spasm with temporary rigidity.

myotrophy (mī-ŏt′rō-fē) [″ + *trophe,* nourishment] Nutrition of muscle tissues.

myotropic (mī″ō-trŏp′ĭk) [″ + *trope,* a turn] Attracted to muscle tissue.

myotube (mī′ō-tūb) The developing stage of skeletal muscle. The central nucleus occupies most of the cell.

myovascular (mī″ō-văs′kū-lăr) Concerning muscles and their blood supply.

myriachit (mĭr-ē′ă-chĭt) [Russian] Miryachit.

Myriapoda (mĭr-ē-ăp′ō-dă) [Gr. *myrios,* numberless, + *pous,* foot] Group of arthropods including millipedes and centipedes.

myriapodiasis (mĭr″ē-ăp-ō-dī′ă-sĭs) Infestation with one of the Myriapoda class of arthropods.

myricin (mĭr′ĭ-sĭn) A chemical obtained from beeswax.

myring- SEE: *tympano-*.

myringa (mĭr-ĭn′gă) [L.] The tympanic membrane.

myringectomy (mĭr-ĭn-jĕk′tō-mē) [″ + Gr. *ektome,* excision] Myringodectomy.

myringitis (mĭr-ĭn-jī′tĭs) [L. *myringa,* drum membrane, + Gr. *itis,* inflammation] Inflammation of the tympanic membrane (eardrum).

m. bullosa Myringitis with serous or hemorrhagic blebs or vesicular inflammation of the eardrum and adjacent wall. A sign of infection with *Mycoplasma pneumoniae*.

myringo- SEE: *tympano-*.

myringodectomy (mĭr-ĭn″gō-dĕk′tō-mē) [″ + Gr. *ektome,* excision] Excision of a part of or the entire tympanic membrane. SYN: *myringectomy*.

myringomycosis (mĭr-ĭn″gō-mī-kō′sĭs) [″ + Gr. *mykes,* fungus, + *osis,* condition] Inflammation of the tympanic membrane resulting from infection by parasitic fungi. SYN: *otomycosis*.

myringoplasty (mĭr-ĭn′gō-plăst″ē) [″ + Gr. *plassein,* to form] Plastic surgery of the tympanic membrane.

myringotome (mĭ-rĭn′gō-tōm) [″ + Gr. *tome,* incision] Surgical knife used for incising the tympanic membrane.

myringotomy (mĭr-ĭn-gŏt′ō-mē) Incision of the tympanic membrane. This procedure is most often performed on children with acute otitis media. Tympanostomy tubes are often placed in the opening made by the incision. SEE: *Nursing Diagnoses Appendix*.

PATIENT CARE: Because this procedure is most often performed on young children in response to a recurring condition, parents are taught to recognize the signs of otitis media and to seek medical assistance when their child complains of pain or when they observe the child experiencing pain to prevent spontaneous rupture of the eardrum. The parents are advised that tubes inserted after myringotomy gradually come out of the eardrum, and that the child should not swim in the early period after surgery.

myrmecia (mŭr-mē′shē-ă) [Gr. *myrmex,* ant] A dome-shaped wart.

myrmecology Study of ants.

myrrh (mŭr) [Gr. *myrra*] A gum resin used in antiquity as a constituent of incense and perfume. Its most important use today is as an aromatic astringent mouthwash. Tincture of myrrh provides symptomatic relief when applied to canker sores.

mysophilia (mī″sō-fĭl′ē-ă) Erotic interest in body excretions.

mysophobia (mī″sō-fō′bē-ă) [Gr. *mysos,* filth, + *phobos,* fear] Abnormal aversion to dirt or contamination. SYN: *molysmophobia*.

mytacism (mī′tă-sĭzm) [Gr. *mytakismos* from Gr. letter μ] Excessive or incorrect use of the letter *m* in writing, or the *m* sound in speaking.

mythomania (mĭth″ō-mā′nē-ă) [Gr. *mythos,* myth, + *mania,* madness] Abnormal tendency to lie and exaggerate.

mythophobia (mĭth″ō-fō′bē-ă) [″ + *phobos,* fear] Abnormal dread of making a false or incorrect statement.

mytilotoxin (mĭt″ĭ-lō-tŏk′sĭn) A neurotoxin present in certain mussels.

myxadenitis (mĭks″ăd-ĕn-ī′tĭs) [Gr. *myxa,* mucus, + *aden,* gland, + *itis,* inflammation] Inflammation of a mucous gland.

m. labialis Painless inflammation of the mucous glands of the lips.

myxadenoma (mĭks″ăd-ē-nō′mă) [″ + ″ + *oma,* tumor] **1.** A tumor with the structure of a mucous gland. SYN: *myxoadenoma*. **2.** A tumor of glandular structure containing mucous elements.

myxangitis (mĭks″ăn-jī′tĭs) [″ + *angeion,* vessel, + *itis,* inflammation] Inflammation of mucous gland ducts.

myxedema (mĭks-ĕ-dē′mă) [Gr. *myxa,* mucus, + *oidema,* swelling] **1.** Infiltration of the skin by mucopolysaccharides, giving it a waxy or coarsened appearance. Myxedematous skin is seen particularly in patients with hypothyroidism. **2.** The clinical and metabolic manifestations of hypothyroidism in adults, adolescents, and children. **myxedematous** (mĭks-ĕ-dĕm′ă-tŭs), *adj.*

SYMPTOMS: The patient with hypothyroidism often complains of sluggishness, cold intolerance, apathy, fatigue, and constipation. Findings may include infiltration of the subcutaneous layers of the skin by mucopolysaccharides, which coarsen the features and create nonpitting edema. The hair may become dry and brittle. If the syndrome is left untreated, hypothermia, coma, and death may result.

TREATMENT: Thyroid hormone replacement reverses the symptoms and re-establishes normal metabolic function.

childhood m. Myxedema occurring before puberty.

operative m. Myxedema following removal of the thyroid gland.

pituitary m. Myxedema occurring secondary to anterior pituitary hypofunction.

pretibial m. Edema of the anterior surface of the legs following hyperthyroidism and exophthalmos.

myxedematoid (mĭks-ĕ-dēm′ă-toyd) [Gr. *myxa,* mucus, + *oidema,* swelling, + *eidos,* form, shape] Resembling myxedema.

myxo-, myx- [Gr. *myxa*] Combining form denoting *mucus.*

myxoadenoma (mĭks″ō-ăd-ē-nō′mă) [″ + *aden,* gland, + *oma,* tumor] Myxadenoma (1).

Myxobacterales (mĭks″ō-băk-tĕ-rā′lēz) An order of bacteria found in soil and dung. It is characterized by a slimy spreading colony.

myxochondrofibrosarcoma (mĭks″ō-kŏn″drō-fī″brō-săr-kō′mă) A malignant tumor composed of myxomatous, chondromatous, fibrous, and sarcomatous elements.

myxochondroma (mĭks″ō-kŏn-drō′mă) A benign tumor composed of myxomatous and chondromatous elements.

myxocystoma (mĭks″ō-sĭs-tō′mă) [Gr. *myxa,* mucus, + *kystis,* cyst, + *oma,* tumor] A benign cystic tumor containing mucus.

myxocyte (mĭk′sō-sīt) [″ + *kytos,* cell] A characteristic cell of mucous tissue.

myxoedema (mĭks″ĕ-dē′mă) [″ + *oidema,* swelling] Myxedema.

myxoenchondroma (mĭks″ō-ĕn-kŏn-drō′mă) [″ + *en,* in, + *chondros,* cartilage, + *oma,* tumor] A cartilaginous tissue tumor that has undergone partial mucous degeneration.

myxofibroma (mĭks″ō-fī-brō′mă) [″ + L. *fibra,* fiber, + Gr. *oma,* tumor] Tumor composed of mucous and fibrous elements.

myxofibrosarcoma (mĭk″sō-fī″brō-săr-kō′mă) [″ + ″ + Gr. *sarx,* flesh, + *oma,* tumor] Fibrosarcoma that contains primitive mesenchymal tissue.

myxoglioma (mĭk″sō-glī-ō′mă) [Gr. *myxa,* mucus, + *glia,* glue, + *oma,* tumor] Tumor composed of myxomatous and gliomatous elements.

myxoid (mĭk′soyd) [″ + *eidos,* form, shape] Similar to or resembling mucus.

myxolipoma (mĭk″sō-lĭ-pō′mă) [″ + *lipos,* fat, + *oma,* tumor] Mucous tumor with fatty tissue elements. SYN: *lipomyxoma.*

myxoma (mĭk-sō′mă) *pl.* **myxomas** or **myxomata** [″ + *oma,* tumor] Tumor composed of mucous connective tissue similar to that present in the embryo or umbilical cord. Cells are stellate or spindle-shaped and separated by mucoid tissue. The tumors are usually soft, gray, lobulated, and translucent and are not completely encapsulated. Myxomas may be pure or of mixed types involving other types of tissue.

cartilaginous m. Chondromyxoma.

cystic m. A tumor with parts fluid enough to resemble cysts.

enchondromatous m. A tumor with nodules of hyaline cartilage.

erectile m. Myxoma containing an excess of vessels, resembling an angioma.

fibrous m. Fibromyxoma.

intracanalicular m. Myxoma that develops in the interstitial connective tissue of the breasts.

odontogenic m. A tumor of the jaw that appears to arise from mesenchymal tissue.

telangiectatic m. Myxoma of highly vascular structure. SYN: *vascular m.*

vascular m. Telangiectatic m.

myxomatosis (mĭk″sō-mă-tō′sĭs) [″ + ″ + *osis,* condition] **1.** Formation of multiple myxomas. **2.** Myxomatous degeneration.

Myxomycetes (mĭk″sō-mī-sē′tēz) [Gr. *myxa,* mucus, + *mykes,* fungus] A class of organisms that includes slime molds. The organisms are of uncertain classification, but are thought to be fungus-like. SEE: *Myxobacterales.*

myxoneuroma (mĭks″ō-nū-rō′mă) [″ + *neuron,* nerve, + *oma,* tumor] Tumor made of mucous membrane and nerve.

myxopapilloma (mĭk″sō-păp″ĭl-ō′mă) [″ + L. *papilla,* nipple, + Gr. *oma,* tumor] A tumor containing myxomatous and papillomatous components.

myxorrhea (mĭk-sō-rē′ă) [″ + *rhoia,* flow] Free discharge from mucous surfaces. SYN: *blennorrhea.*

m. gastrica Excessive mucus secretion in the stomach.

m. intestinalis Excessive secretion of mucus from the bowels.

myxosarcoma (mĭk″sō-săr-kō′mă) [″ + *sarx,* flesh, + *oma,* tumor] Tumor containing myxomatous and sarcomatous components, having undergone partial degeneration. **myxosarcomatous** (mĭk″sō-săr-kō′mă-tŭs), *adj.*

myxospore (mĭks′ō-spor) [″ + *sporos,* seed] A spore embedded in a gelatinous mass; seen in some fungi and protozoa.

Myxosporidia (mĭks-ō-spor-ĭd′ē-ă) Parasitic sporozoans most commonly found in the epithelial cells of lower vertebrates.

myxovirus Any of a family of viruses including those that cause influenza. SEE: *paramyxovirus.*

Myzomyia (mī″zō-mī′ă) [Gr. *myzan,* to suck, + *myia,* fly] Subgenus of anopheline mosquitoes. Some species transmit malarial parasites.

Myzorhynchus (mī″zō-rĭng′kŭs) [″ + *rhynchos,* snout] Subgenus of anopheline mosquitoes. Some species transmit malarial parasites.

N **1.** Symbol for the element nitrogen. **2.** *normal,* esp. with reference to solutions.

n **1.** Symbol for *index of refraction.* **2.** *nasal; number.*

^{15}N Symbol for radioactive isotope of nitrogen.

NA *nicotinic acid; Nomina Anatomica; numerical aperture; nurse's aide.*

Na [L. *natrium*] Symbol for the element sodium.

NAACOG *Nurses Association of the American College of Obstetricians and Gynecologists.*

nabothian cyst (nă-bō'thē-ăn) [Martin Naboth, Ger. anatomist and physician, 1675–1721] A cyst caused by closure of the ducts of the nabothian glands in the uterine cervix as a result of healing of an erosion.

NaBr Sodium bromide.

NaCl Sodium chloride.

NaClO Sodium hypochlorite.

Na_2CO_3 Sodium carbonate.

nacreous (nā'krē-ŭs) [L. *nacer,* mother of pearl] Having an iridescent pearl-like luster, as bacterial colonies.

N.A.D. *no appreciable disease.*

NAD *nicotinamide adenine dinucleotide.*

NAD^+ *nicotinamide adenine dinucleotide,* oxidized form.

NADH *nicotinamide adenine dinucleotide,* reduced form.

NADP *nicotinamide adenine dinucleotide phosphate.*

$NADP^+$ *nicotinamide adenine dinucleotide phosphate,* oxidized form.

NADPH *nicotinamide adenine dinucleotide phosphate,* reduced form.

Naegele, Franz Carl (nā'gĕ-lē) German obstetrician, 1777–1851.

N.'s obliquity Anterior parietal presentation of the fetal head in labor. SYN: *anterior asynclitism.*

N.'s pelvis An obliquely contracted pelvis in which the conjugate diameter assumes an oblique direction. The condition is caused by disease in infancy.

N.'s rule A numerical formula for estimating the date labor will begin; by subtracting 3 months from the first day of the last menstrual period and adding 7 days to that date, a provisional date of delivery is identified.

Naegleria A genus of amebic protozoa present in soil, ground water, and sewage. One species, *N. fowleri,* is the causative agent of a lethal form of meningoencephalitis. SEE: *acanthamebiasis; meningoencephalitis.*

N.A.E.M.S.P. *National Association of EMS Physicians.*

N.A.E.M.T. *National Association of Emergency Medical Technicians.*

NaF Sodium fluoride.

nafcillin sodium (năf-sĭl'ĭn) A semisynthetic penicillin that is penicillinase-resistant. Trade names are Nafcil and Unipen.

Nagi disablement model A descriptive scheme that describes the progression from pathology or disease to disability. The components are pathology, impairment, functional limitation, and disability. Physical therapists use this model to make diagnoses and to help direct intervention.

$NaHCO_3$ Sodium bicarbonate.

$NaHSO_3$ Sodium bisulfite.

nail [AS. *naegel*] **1.** A rod made of metal, bone, or solid material used to attach the ends or pieces of broken bones. **2.** A horny cell structure of the epidermis forming flat plates upon the dorsal surface of the fingers and toes. SYN: *onyx; unguis.* SEE: illus.

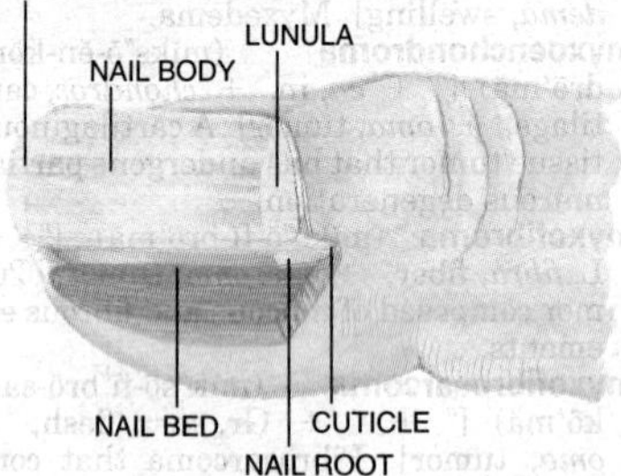

NAIL
Longitudinal section

A fingernail or toenail consists of a body composed of keratin (the exposed portion) and a root (the proximal portion hidden by the nail fold), both of which rest on the nailbed (matrix). The latter consists of epithelium and corium continuous with the epidermis and dermis of the skin of the nail fold. The crescent-shaped white area near the root is called the lunula. The epidermis extending from the margin of the nail fold over the root is called eponychium; that underlying the free border of the distal portion is called hyponychium.

A nail grows in length and thickness through cell division in the stratum germinativum of the root. The average rate of growth in fingernails is about 1 mm per week. Growth is slower in toenails and slower in summer than in winter. Nail growth varies with age and is affected by disease and certain hormone deficiencies. The onset of a disease that briefly interferes with nail growth and development may be estimated by measuring the distance of the line (Beau's line) across the nail from the root of the nail.

DIFFERENTIAL DIAGNOSIS: Changes in the nails, such as ridges, may occur after a serious illness or indicate defective nutrition. In achlorhydria and hypochromic anemia, excessively spoon-shaped nails that are depressed in the center may occur. In chronic pulmonary conditions and congenital heart disease, a spongy excess of soft tissue at the base of the nails may be associated with clubbed fingers. Atrophy may occur as a result of hereditary or congenital tendencies. Permanent atrophy may follow injuries, scars from disease, frostbite, nerve injuries, and hyperthyroidism. Nail shedding is due to the same causes. Fragile or split nails often occur as a congenital condition or may be due to prolonged contact with chemicals or too frequent buffing or filing of the flat surface of the nail during manicuring. In a healthy person brittle nails are usually caused by exposure to solvents, detergents, and soaps. The brittleness disappears when the external causes are avoided. Dry, malformed nails may be due to trophic changes resulting from injury to a nerve or a finger or from neuritis, Raynaud's disease, pulmonary osteoarthropathy, syphilis, onychia, scleroderma, acrodermatitis, or granuloma fungoides of the fingers. Transverse lines (Beau's lines) may result from previous interference of nail matrix growth. These lines may be caused by local or systemic conditions. The approximate date of the lesion may be determined, because it takes 4 to 6 months for the fingernail to be replaced. Chancre may be suspected if a small indolent ulcer appears near the nail, esp. if indurated and associated with enlarged lymph glands above the inner condyle. Quincke's capillary pulsation, indicated by a rhythmic flushing and blanching under the nails, is seen most frequently in aortic regurgitation and often in anemia.

Discoloration of nails is seen in various medical conditions. *Black* discoloration may be seen in diabetic as well as some other forms of gangrene. *Blue-black* discoloration is a common condition due to hemorrhage caused by bleeding diseases, such as hemophilia, or trauma. This condition may be painful and can be relieved by drilling a small hole in the nail at the site of the hemorrhage. A dental drill, the heated tip of a paper clip, or a similar rigid wire of small diameter may be used. *Brown* discoloration may be due to arsenic poisoning. *Brownish-black* discoloration often indicates chronic mercury poisoning, due to the formation of sulfide of mercury in the tissues. *Cyanosis* of the nails usually indicates anemia, poor circulation, or venous stasis. *Green* staining of the nail fold or under the nail is associated with the growth of *Pseudomonas* in a wet area. *Slate* discoloration is an early manifestation of argyria, and intake of silver should be stopped at once. *White* spots or striate lesions may be due to trauma and are more frequently seen in women. Transverse white bands in all nails may be a sign of acute or chronic arsenic poisoning or, rarely, of thallium acetate poisoning. SEE: *Mees lines*.

clubbing of n. SEE: *clubbing*.

eggshell n. A condition in which the nail plate is soft and semitransparent, bends easily, and splits at the end. The condition is associated with arthritis, peripheral neuritis, leprosy, and hemiplegia. It may be the only visible sign of late syphilis.

fungal infection of n. Infection of a nail by one of a number of fungi. Systemic therapy with antifungal drugs may eradicate the infection.

habit deformity n. Disruption of the nail surface by the habit of abrading or stroking that area. This produces a wavy or washboard-like nail surface.

hang n. Broken epidermis at the edge of a nail.

ingrown n. Growth of the nail edge into the soft tissue, causing inflammation and sometimes an abscess. Ingrown nails may be due to improper paring of the nails or pressure on a nail edge from improperly fitted shoes. In many cases, this condition may be prevented by cutting the nails straight across.

intermedullary n. A surgical rod inserted into the intermedullary canal to act as an immobilization device to hold the two ends of a fractured long bone in position.

reedy n. A nail marked by longitudinal fissures.

Smith-Petersen n. A three-flanged nail employed to fix fractures of the neck of the femur.

splitting n. A troublesome condition in which the brittle nails split easily. Polishing, buffing, or abrading the nail surface will weaken the nail; thus, these practices should be discouraged. Brittle nails should be soaked, preferably in bath oil, prior to cutting them.

spoon n. A nail with a depressed center and elevated lateral edges. This condition may follow trauma to the nail fold or iron deficiency anemia or may develop naturally. SYN: *koilonychia*. SEE: *koilonychia* for illus.

nailbed The portion of a finger or toe covered by the nail. SYN: *nail matrix*.

nail biting An anxious behavior in which

the free edges of the nails are bitten down as a means of expressing or relieving stress. SYN: *onychophagy*.

nail fold SEE: under *fold*.

nail groove The space between the nail wall and the nailbed.

nailing Fixing fragments of bone by use of a nail.

nail matrix Nailbed.

nail-patella syndrome Onycho-osteodysplasia.

nail root Proximal portion of nail covered by nail fold.

nail wall Epidermis covering edges of the nail. SYN: *vallum unguis*.

naked (nā′kĕd) [AS *naced,* nude] Uncovered, exposed to view, nude, bare, devoid of clothing.

nalidixic acid An antibiotic used in treating urinary tract infections.

nalorphine hydrochloride (năl-or′fēn) A narcotic antagonist used in the treatment of narcotic overdose.

naloxone hydrochloride (năl-ŏks′ōn) A drug that prevents or reverses the action of morphine and other opioid drugs. Its most important use is treatment of narcotic overdose.

naltrexone An opioid antagonist used to treat addiction to opium-derived drugs. It is also approved to treat alcohol dependence.

CAUTION: Naltrexone may cause liver damage when given in large doses.

NANDA *North American Nursing Diagnosis Association.*

nandrolone decanoate (năn′drō-lōn) An anabolic androgenic steroid.

nandrolone phenpropionate An anabolic androgenic steroid.

nanism (nā′nĭzm) [L. *nanus,* dwarf, + Gr. *-ismos,* condition] Dwarfism.

symptomatic n. Nanism with deficient dentition, sexual development, and ossification.

nano- (nā′nō) [L. *nanus,* dwarf] **1.** Prefix indicating one billionth (10^{-9}) of the unit following; thus, a nanogram is one billionth (10^{-9}) of a gram. **2.** Combining form indicating dwarfism (nanism).

nanobacteria (nă′nō-băk-tēr-ē-ă) The smallest known bacteria with intact gram-negative cell walls. These microbes produce biologically available apatite crystals that mineralize into structures similar to those found in kidney stones. The organisms have been isolated from nearly all kidney stones and are suspected of being a causative agent in stone formation.

nanocephaly (nā-nō-sĕf′ă-lē) [″ + Gr. *kephale,* head, + *-ismos,* condition] Microcephaly. **nanocephalous** (nā-nō-sĕf′ă-lŭs), *adj.*

nanocormia (nā″nō-kor′mē-ă) [L. *nanus,* dwarf, + Gr. *kormos,* trunk] Abnormal smallness of thorax or body.

nanocurie (nā″nō-kū′rē) A unit of radioactivity equal to 10^{-9} curie.

nanogram (năn′o-grăm) One billionth (10^{-9}) of a gram.

nanoid (nā′noyd) [″ + Gr. *eidos,* form, shape] Dwarflike.

nanomelus (nā-nŏm′ĕ-lŭs) [″ + Gr. *melos,* limb] Micromelus.

nanometer (nā″nō-mē′tĕr) A unit of length equal to 10^{-9} meter.

nanomole One billionth (10^{-9}) mole.

nanophthalmia (năn″ŏf-thăl′mē-ă) [″ + Gr. *ophthalmos,* eye] Microphthalmia.

nanosecond (nā″nō-sĕk′ŏnd) A unit of time measurement equal to 10^{-9} second.

nanosoma, nanosomia (nā″nō-sō′mă, nā-nō-sō′mē-ă) [L. *nanus,* dwarf, + Gr. *soma,* body] Dwarfism.

nanosomus (nā-nō-sō′mŭs) A person of stunted size; a dwarf.

nanous (nā′nŭs) [L. *nanus,* dwarf] Dwarfed or stunted.

nanukayami (nă″nū-kă-yă′mē) A form of leptospirosis present in Japan.

NaOH Sodium hydroxide.

nap (năp) [AS. *hnappian,* nap] **1.** To slumber. **2.** A short sleep; a doze. SEE: *sleep.*

napalm (nā′pălm) [from *na*phthene + *palm*itate] Gasoline made thick or jelly-like for use in incendiary bombs and flame throwers.

nape (nāp, năp) The back of the neck. SYN: *nucha.*

napex (nā′pĕks) Scalp beneath the occipital protuberance.

naphazoline hydrochloride (năf-ăz′ō-lēn) A vasoconstrictor drug used topically as a nasal decongestant and as an ophthalmic mydriatic or vasoconstrictor.

naphtha (năf′thă) **1.** A volatile inflammable liquid distilled from carbonaceous substances. **2.** Petroleum, esp. more volatile varieties.

naphthalene (năf′thă-lēn) A hydrocarbon, $C_{10}H_8$; one of principal constituents of coal tar. It is used as a disinfectant, in moth balls, and in the manufacture of dyes and explosives. SEE: *Poisons and Poisoning Appendix.*

naphthol (năf′thōl) $C_{10}H_8O$; a petroleum substance used as an antiseptic and in certain dyes. It is prepared from naphthalene.

N.A.P.N.A.P. *National Association of Pediatric Nurse Associates and Practitioners.*

N.A.P.N.E.S. *National Association for Practical Nurse Education and Services.*

narcissism (năr′sĭs-ĭzm) [Narcissus, a Gr. mythical character who fell in love with his own reflection] **1.** Self-love or self-admiration. **2.** Sexual pleasure derived from observing one's own naked body. **narcissistic** (năr-sĭs-sĭst′ĭk), *adj.*

narcissistic object choice Selection of another like one's own self as the object of love, friendship, or liking.

narco- [Gr. *narke,* numbness] Combining form meaning *numbness, stupor.*

narcoanalysis (năr″kō-ă-năl′ĭ-sĭs) [″ + *analysis,* a dissolving] A form of psychotherapy used in the past, in which light anesthesia was produced by use of I.V. barbiturates. Patients were encouraged to talk about their experiences and discuss events that would ordinarily be suppressed. SYN: *narcosynthesis*.

narcoanesthesia (nar″kō-ăn-ĕs-thē′zē-ă) Anesthesia produced by a narcotic, as scopolamine and morphine.

narcohypnia (năr″kō-hĭp′nē-ă) [Gr. *narke,* numbness, + *hypnos,* sleep] Numbness following sleep.

narcohypnosis (năr″kō-hĭp-nō′sĭs) Stupor or deep sleep produced by hypnosis.

narcolepsy (năr′kō-lĕp″sē) [Gr. *narke,* numbness, + *lepsis,* seizure] A disorder marked by recurrent, uncontrollable attacks of daytime sleepiness, often associated with temporary muscular paralysis (cataplexy), that may occur after powerful emotional experiences. People affected by this condition may have several sleep attacks each day. Typically, narcoleptic patients arouse from sleep relatively easily. SEE: *sleep disorder*. **narcoleptic** (năr-kō-lĕp′tĭk), *adj.*

ETIOLOGY: The cause of the disorder is unknown, but genetic factors are thought to contribute to it because it occurs in families and in some breeds of animals, and because human leukocyte antigen (HLA) testing shows HLA-DR2 and HLA-DQw6 in about 90% of affected people.

TREATMENT: Scheduled naps during the day may prevent sleep attacks, especially if the naps are timed to occur when the patient usually experiences sleep attacks. Drugs used to treat narcolepsy include stimulants such as dextroamphetamine sulfate, pemoline, or methylphenidate hydrochloride.

CAUTION: Narcoleptics should avoid activities that require constant alertness (e.g., driving or flying). At the first sign of drowsiness, affected patients should seek a safe place to sleep. In many states in the U.S., loss of consciousness is grounds for revocation of driving privileges. Patients with narcolepsy should review their motor vehicle usage with their health care professionals.

PATIENT CARE: Patients with this condition are taught to enhance safety through care in driving and other activities in which falling asleep may endanger both the patient's and others' lives.

narcosis [Gr. *narkosis,* a benumbing] Unconsciousness or stupor produced by drugs.

basal n. Initial narcosis produced by sedatives used prior to administration of a general anesthetic.

carbon dioxide n. Personality changes, confusion, and coma due to an increase in carbon dioxide content of the blood. This may occur during oxygen therapy of patients with chronic obstructive pulmonary disease, or in patients receiving inadequate levels of artificial respiration.

medullary n. General anesthesia induced by a local anesthetic injected into the sheath of the spinal cord in lumbar region. SYN: *spinal anesthesia*.

narcosynthesis (năr″kō-sĭn′thĕ-sĭs) [″ + *synthesis,* synthesis] Narcoanalysis.

narcotic [Gr. *narkotikos,* benumbing] **1.** Producing stupor or sleep. **2.** A drug that depresses the central nervous system, thus relieving pain and producing sleep. Most narcotics are habit-forming. Excessive doses produce unconsciousness, stupor, coma, respiratory depression, pulmonary edema, and sometimes death. Opium, morphine, codeine, papaverine, and heroin are examples of narcotics. A more precise term is *opioid analgesic*. SEE: *pain*.

narcotic addict One who has become physiologically or psychologically dependent upon narcotics. SEE: *drug addiction*.

narcotic poisoning Poisoning caused by narcotic or sleep-producing drugs such as opium and its derivatives.

SYMPTOMS: The patient may experience brief exhilaration followed by drowsiness, respiratory depression, or coma, or in massive overdoses, death.

TREATMENT: An airway should be established and ventilation provided. A narcotic antagonist such as naxolene should be given.

narcotism (năr′kō-tĭzm) [Gr. *narke,* stupor, + *-ismos,* condition] An addiction to the use of narcotics. Addiction may be said to exist when discontinuance causes abstinence symptoms that are speedily relieved by a dose of the drug.

TREATMENT: Treatment is ordinarily successful only during hospitalization. Relapses are frequent. Participation in group therapy (e.g., in a program such as Narcotics Anonymous) may be helpful.

narcotize [Gr. *narkotikos,* benumbing] To place under the influence of a narcotic.

naris (nā′rĭs) *pl.* **nares** [L.] The nostril. SEE: *nose*.

anterior n. External nostril.

posterior n. The opening between the nasal cavity and the nasopharynx.

narrowing Decreasing the width or diameter of some space or channel (e.g., narrowing of the size of the coronary arteries), usually due to some pathological process.

NASA *National Aeronautics and Space Administration.*

nasal (nā′zl) [L. *nasus,* nose] **1.** Pert. to the nose. **2.** Uttered through the nose. **3.** A nasal bone.

nasal bleeding Epistaxis.

nasal bone Either of the two small bones forming the bridge of the nose.

nasal cartilage Any of the cartilages forming the principal portion of the subcutaneous framework of the nose.

nasal cavity One of two cavities between the floor of the cranium and the roof of the mouth, opening to the nose anteriorly and the nasopharynx posteriorly. Its lining of ciliated epithelium warms and moistens inhaled air, and traps dust and pathogens on mucus that is then swept toward the pharynx. The nasal septum (ethmoid and vomer) separates the nasal cavities, and the olfactory receptors are in the upper part of each cavity. The paranasal sinuses (frontal, maxillary, sphenoidal, and ethmoidal) open into the meatus below the conchae. The orifices of the frontal, anterior ethmoidal, and maxillary sinuses are in the middle meatus. The orifices of the posterior ethmoidal and sphenoidal sinuses are in the superior meatus. The nasal mucosa is highly vascular; blood is supplied by the maxillary arteries from the external carotid arteries, and by the ethmoidal arteries from the internal carotid arteries. SEE: illus; *nose*.

nasal feeding SEE: *feeding, tube*.

nasal flaring Intermittent outward movement of the nostrils with each inspiratory effort; indicates an increase in the work of breathing.

nasal gavage SEE: *feeding, tube*.

nasal hemorrhage Epistaxis.

nasal height Distance between the lower border of the nasal aperture and the nasion.

nasal index The greatest width of the nasal aperture in relation to a line from the lower edge of the nasal aperture to the nasion.

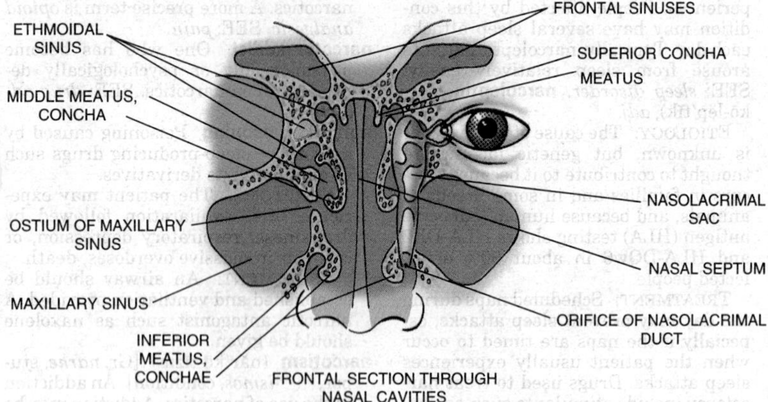

FRONTAL SECTION THROUGH NASAL CAVITIES

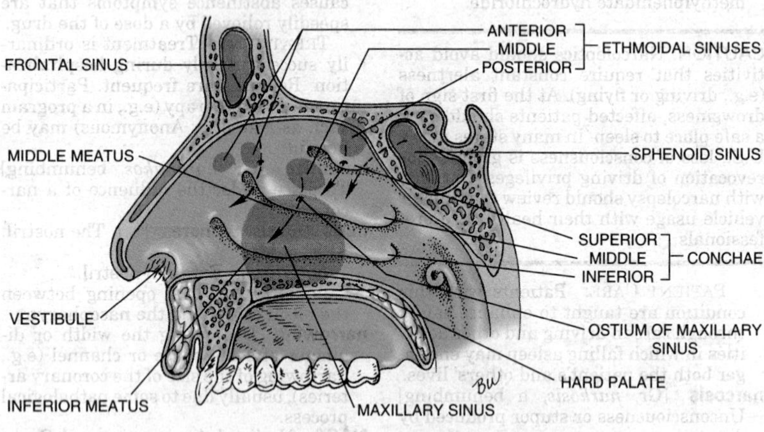

VIEW FROM THE NASAL SEPTUM TOWARD THE LATERAL AREA OF THE NASAL CAVITY

TWO VIEWS OF NASAL CAVITY

nasal line A line from the lower edge of the ala nasi curving to the outer side of the orbicularis oris muscle.

nasal meatus SEE: *meatus*.

nasal obstruction Blockage of the nasal passages. Common causes of nasal obstruction in adults are irregular septum, enlarged turbinates, and nasal polyps. In children, a common cause is a foreign body, such as food, buttons, or pins. Complications such as infections, sinusitis, and otitis may develop.

TREATMENT: Depending upon the cause of the obstruction, nasal douches, inhalations, or operative care, including resection of septum, turbinectomy, removal of polyp, opening and draining sinuses, or removal of foreign body.

nasal polyp A pedunculated polyp of the nasal mucosa. SEE: illus.

Nasal polyps are the most commonly identified nonmalignant tumor of the nasal passages. They are more commonly identified in men than in women.

SYMPTOMS: The most common symptom of nasal polyposis is obstruction to the flow of air into and out of the nasal passages. SEE: illus.

TREATMENT: Steroid nasal sprays may improve airflow through the nasal passages. Surgical removal of polyps may occasionally be necessary when medical treatment is unsuccessful.

nasal reflex Sneezing resulting from irritation of nasal mucosa.

nasal septum SEE: *septum, nasal*.

nasal sinuses, accessory SEE: *sinus, accessory nasal*.

nasal width The maximum width of the nasal aperture.

nascent (năs′ĕnt; nā′sĕnt) [L. *nascens*, born] **1.** Just born; incipient or beginning. **2.** Pert. to a substance being set free from a compound.

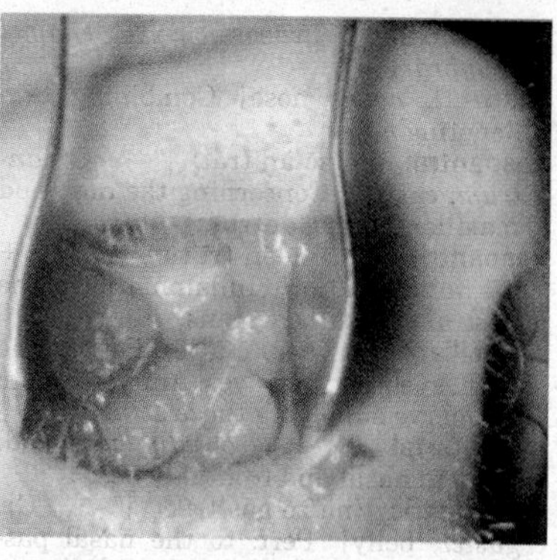

NASAL POLYPS

nasioiniac (nā″zē-ō-ĭn′ē-ăk) [L. *nasus*, nose, + Gr. *inion*, back of the head] Concerning the nasion and inion.

nasion (nā′zē-ōn) [L. *nasus*, nose] The point at which the nasofrontal suture is cut across by the median anteroposterior plane.

Nasmyth's membrane (năz′mĭths) [Alexander Nasmyth, Scottish dental surgeon, d. 1847] A thin cuticle consisting of the cellular remnants of the enamel organ and the mucopolysaccharide basement membrane that attaches them to the enamel surface. This covering is very friable and usually lost after eruption of the tooth into the oral cavity; however, it may persist in protected areas, such as the labial surface

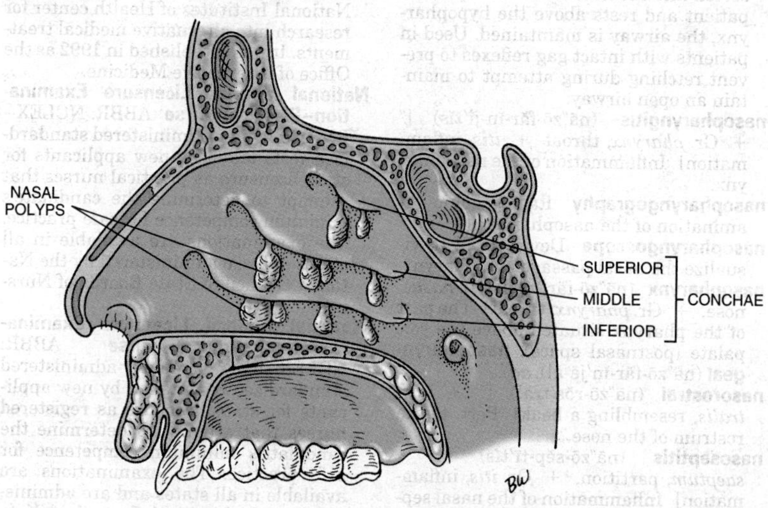

NASAL POLYPS

of maxillary incisors. SYN: *enamel membrane*.

naso- [L. *nasus,* nose] Combining form denoting *nose.*

nasoantral (nā″zō-ăn′trăl) [″ + Gr. *antrum,* cavity] Concerning the nose and maxillary sinus (antrum).

nasoantritis (nā″zō-ăn-trī′tĭs) [″ + ″ + *itis,* inflammation] Inflammation of the nose and maxillary sinus.

nasociliary (nā″zō-sĭl′ē-ār-ē) Pert. to the nose, eyebrow, and eyes. Applied esp. to the nerve supplying these structures.

nasofrontal [″ + *frontalis,* forehead] Pert. to nasal and frontal bones.

nasogastric (nā″zō-găs′trĭk) [″ + Gr. *gaster,* belly] Pert. to the nasal passages and the stomach, esp. relating to intubation.

nasolabial [″ + *labium,* lip] Pert. to the nose and lip.

nasolacrimal (nā″zō-lăk′rĭm-ăl) [″ + *lacrima,* tear] Pert. to the nose and lacrimal apparatus.

nasology (nā-zŏl′ō-jē) [″ + Gr. *logos,* word, reason] Study of the nose and its diseases.

nasomental (nā″zō-mĕn′tăl) [″ + *mentum,* chin] Pert. to the nose and chin.

nasomental reflex Contraction of mentalis muscle with elevation of lower lip and wrinkling of skin of chin. The reflex is elicited by percussion of the side of the nose.

naso-oral (nā″zō-ō′răl) [″ + *oralis,* pert. to the mouth] Pert. to the nose and oral cavity.

nasopalatine (nā″zō-păl′ă-tīn) [L. *nasus,* nose, + *palatum,* palate] Pert. to the nose and palate.

nasopharyngeal airway, maintenance of By means of a flexible tube that is inserted into the nose of an unresponsive patient and rests above the hypopharynx, the airway is maintained. Used in patients with intact gag reflexes to prevent retching during attempt to maintain an open airway.

nasopharyngitis (nā″zō-făr-ĭn-jī′tĭs) [″ + Gr. *pharynx,* throat + *itis,* inflammation] Inflammation of the nasopharynx.

nasopharyngography Radiographic examination of the nasopharynx.

nasopharyngoscope Device used to visualize the nasal passage and pharynx.

nasopharynx (nā″zō-făr′ĭnks) [L. *nasus,* nose, + Gr. *pharynx,* throat] The part of the pharynx situated above the soft palate (postnasal space). **nasopharyngeal** (nā″zō-făr-ĭn′jē-ăl), *adj.*

nasorostral (nā″zō-rŏs′trăl) [″ + *rostralis,* resembling a beak] Pert. to the rostrum of the nose.

nasoseptitis (nā″zō-sĕp-tī′tĭs) [″ + *saeptum,* partition, + Gr. *itis,* inflammation] Inflammation of the nasal septum.

nasosinusitis (nā″zō-sī″nū-sī′tĭs) [″ + *sinus,* cavity] Inflammation of the nasal cavities and paranasal sinuses.

nasospinale (nā″zō-spīn′ăl-ē) The point at which the median sagittal plane intersects the line joining the lowest points on the nasal margins.

nasotracheal intubation SEE: *intubation.*

nasus (nā′sŭs) [L.] The nose.

NATA *National Athletic Trainers Association, Inc.*

NATABOC *National Athletic Trainers Association Board of Certification, Inc.*

natal (nā′tăl) [L. *natus,* birth] Pert. to birth or the day of birth.

natal (nā′tăl) [L. *nates,* buttocks] Pert. to the buttocks.

natality [L. *natalis,* birth] The birth rate; the ratio of births to population of a given community.

natamycin (năt″ă-mī′sĭn) A topical antifungal agent used in treating blepharitis, conjunctivitis, and keratitis caused by fungi.

nates (nā′tēz) *sing.,* **natis** [L.] **1.** The buttocks. **2.** The anterior, superior, or upper two corpora quadrigemina.

natimortality (nā″tī-mor-tăl′ĭ-tē) [L. *natus,* birth, + *mortalitas,* death] Rate of stillbirths in proportion to birth rate.

National Board for Certification in Occupational Therapy An independent agency recognized to certify the eligibility of occupational therapists and occupational therapy assistants to practice in the U.S.

National Board for Respiratory Care ABBR: NBRC. The national accrediting agency for pulmonary function technologists and respiratory care practitioners.

National Center for Complementary and Alternative Medicine ABBR: NCCAM. National Institutes of Health center for research into alternative medical treatments. It was established in 1992 as the Office of Alternative Medicine.

National Council Licensure Examination–Practical Nurse ABBR: NCLEX–PN. Computer-administered standardized tests taken by new applicants for state licensure as practical nurses that attempt to determine the candidate's minimum competence for safe practice. The examinations are available in all states and are administered by the National Council of State Boards of Nursing.

National Council Licensure Examination–Registered Nurse ABBR: NCLEX–RN. Computer-administered standardized tests taken by new applicants for state licensure as registered nurses that attempt to determine the candidate's minimum competence for safe practice. The examinations are available in all states and are administered by the National Council of State Boards of Nursing.

National Formulary ABBR: NF. Collection of officially recognized drug names originally issued by the American Pharmaceutical Association, but now published by the U.S. Pharmacopeial Convention. Included in the NF are drugs of established usefulness that are not listed in the U.S. Pharmacopeia.

National Highway Traffic Safety Administration ABBR: NHTSA. The division of the U.S. Department of Transportation that conducts research on driver behavior and traffic safety, and investigates and enforces safety standards for motor vehicles and their operation. Established in 1970, it is also responsible for developing the national standard emergency medical services training curriculum. Website: http://www.nhtsa.dot.gov/.

National Institute on Aging ABBR: NIA. An institute created by Congress in 1974. Under the National Institutes of Health, the NIA conducts and supports biomedical, social, and behavioral research and training related to aging.

National Institute of Arthritis and Musculoskeletal and Skin Diseases An agency that supports research in diseases associated with aging. These include osteoporosis, Paget's disease, degenerative joint diseases, and skin diseases such as psoriasis.

National Institute of Environmental Health Sciences ABBR: NIEHS. An agency that conducts research on aging, the effects of environmental agents, and the combined effects of aging and exposure to environmental agents.

National Institute of Mental Health ABBR: NIMH. The division of the National Institutes of Health that sponsors and promotes research, education, and training in the study of the brain and behavioral science. The stated goals of the organization are to understand, treat, and prevent mental illness. The website address is www.nimh.nih.gov/.

National Institute of Neurological Disorders and Stroke ABBR: NINDS. An agency that conducts research on nervous system disorders, including Alzheimer's disease, Parkinson's disease, and stroke, that occur with greater frequency in the elderly.

National Institute of Occupational Safety and Health ABBR: NIOSH. A research branch of the Centers for Disease Control and Prevention that investigates workplace hazards and makes recommendations for the prevention of worker injuries, illnesses, and disabilities.

National League for Nursing ABBR: NLN. An organization originally formed by the merging of three other nursing organizations. The principal concern of the League is improvement of nursing education and service.

Nationally Registered Emergency Medical Technician ABBR: N.R.E.M.T. The designation awarded after successful completion of written and practical examinations administered by the National Registry of Emergency Medical Technicians.

National Marrow Donor Program ABBR: NMDP. The coordinating center for bone marrow donors. Phone 1-800-654-1247. Website: www.marrow.org/2nd_page.html

National Organization for Rare Disorders ABBR: NORD. An organization created by a group of voluntary agencies, medical researchers, and individuals concerned about orphan diseases and orphan drugs. Orphan diseases are rare, debilitating illnesses that strike small numbers of people. Orphan drugs are therapies that alleviate symptoms of some rare diseases, but have not been developed by the pharmaceutical industry because they are unprofitable.

NORD's address is P.O. Box 8923, New Fairfield, CT 06812, phone (203) 746-6518. Website: www.rarediseases.org

National Practitioner Data Bank ABBR: NPDB. A national databank, created by the Health Care Quality Improvement Act of 1986, that receives, stores, and disseminates records on the conduct and competence of medical professionals. Health care facilities use the information contributed to the databank during hiring and credentialing. The databank stores:

1. Information relating to medical malpractice payments made on behalf of health care practitioners
2. Information relating to adverse actions taken against clinical privileges of physicians, osteopaths, or dentists
3. Information concerning actions by professional societies that adversely affect membership.

National Safety Council A nonprofit organization whose mission is to promote and influence safety and health at work, on the road, at home, and in the environment.

National Stroke Association A nonprofit organization devoted to stroke prevention, treatment, rehabilitation, and research and to the support of people who have had strokes, as well as their partners and families. Website: http://www.stroke.org/. Phone: 1-800-STROKES.

native (nā′tĭv) [L. *nativus*] **1.** Born with; inherent. **2.** Natural, normal. **3.** Belonging to, as place of one's birth.

natremia (nă-trē′mē-ă) [L. *natrium,* sodium, + Gr. *haima,* blood] Sodium in the blood.

natrium (nā′trē-ŭm) [L.] SYMB: Na. Sodium.

natriuresis (nā″trē-ū-rē′sĭs) [″ + Gr. *ouresis,* make water] The excretion of abnormal amounts of sodium in the urine. SEE: *aldosterone*.

natriuretic (nā″trē-ūr-ĕt′ĭk) A drug that increases rate of excretion of sodium in the urine. SEE: *diuretic*.

natural [L. *natura,* nature] Not abnormal or artificial.

natural childbirth SEE: under *childbirth*.

natural killer cells SEE: under *cell*.

natural selection SEE: *selection, natural*.

nature and nurture The combination of an individual's genetic constitution and the environmental conditions to which he or she is exposed. The interplay of these forces produces physical and mental characteristics that make each human being different from another. In many cases, it is not readily apparent which of these effects is the more important in producing a particular characteristic.

naturopath (nā′tūr-ō-păth) [″ + Gr. *pathos,* disease, suffering] One who practices naturopathic medicine.

naturopathy (nā″tūr-ŏp′ă-thē) Naturopathic medicine.

nausea (naw′sē-ă) [Gr. *nausia,* seasickness] An unpleasant, wave-like sensation in the back of the throat, epigastrium, or throughout the abdomen. This sensation may or may not lead to vomiting. SEE: *Nursing Diagnoses Appendix.*

This diagnosis was accepted at the NANDA 13th Conference, 1998.

PATIENT CARE: Any materials or environmental factors that precipitate the nausea should be removed. Frequency, time, amount, and characteristics of nausea-associated emesis are noted. Vomitus is tested for blood when indicated. Oral hygiene and comfort measures are provided. If nausea persists, professional evaluation may be advisable.

n. gravidarum Morning sickness. SEE: *hyperemesis gravidarum*.

nauseant (naw′shē-ănt, naw′sē-ănt) **1.** Provoking nausea. **2.** An agent that causes nausea.

nauseate (naw′shē-āt, naw′sē-āt) To cause nausea.

nauseous (naw′shŭs, naw′shē-ŭs) **1.** Producing nausea, disgust, or loathing. **2.** Affected with nausea.

navel (nā′vĕl) [AS. *nafela*] Umbilicus.

navicula (nă-vĭk′ū-lă) [L. *navicula,* boat] Navicular fossa.

navicular (nă-vĭk′ū-lăr) **1.** Shaped like a boat. **2.** Scaphoid bones in the carpus (wrist) and in the tarsus (ankle). SEE: *skeleton*.

navicular fossa SEE: under *fossa*.

Nb Symbol for the element niobium.

nCi *nanocurie*.

N.C.I. *National Cancer Institute.*

NCLEX–PN *National Council Licensure Examination–Practical Nurse.*

NCLEX–RN *National Council Licensure Examination–Registered Nurse.*

Nd Symbol for the element neodymium.

N.D.A. *National Dental Association.*

NDDK *National Institute of Diabetes and Digestive and Kidney Diseases.*

Ne Symbol for the element neon.

near-death experience ABBR: NDE. The perception held by certain individuals that they have glimpsed an afterlife when coming close to death. Whether these experiences represent dreams, hallucinations, or other phenomena is unknown. SEE: *out-of-body experience*.

near-drowning Survival after immersion in water. About 330,000 persons, most of whom are children, adolescents, or young adults, survive an immersion injury in the U.S. each year; of these, about 10% receive professional attention. Many who suffer near-drowning do so because of preventable or avoidable conditions, such as the use of alcohol or drugs in aquatic settings or the inadequate supervision of children by adults. Water sports (e.g., diving, swimming, surfing, or skiing) and boating or fishing accidents also are common causes of near-drowning. A small percentage of near-drowning episodes occur when patients with known seizure disorders convulse while swimming or boating. SEE: *drowning*.

ETIOLOGY: The injuries suffered result from breath holding ("dry drowning"), the aspiration of water into the lungs ("wet drowning"), and/or hypothermia.

SYMPTOMS: Common symptoms of near-drowning result from oxygen deprivation, retention of carbon dioxide, or direct damage to the lungs by water. These include cough, dyspnea, coma, and seizures. Additional complications of prolonged immersion may include aspiration pneumonitis, noncardiogenic pulmonary edema, electrolyte disorders, hemolysis, disseminated intravascular coagulation, and arrhythmias.

TREATMENT: In unconscious patients rescued from water, the airway is secured, ventilation is provided, and cardiopulmonary resuscitation is begun. Oxygen, cardiac, and blood pressure monitoring, rewarming techniques, and other forms of support are provided (e.g., anticonvulsants are given for seizures; electrolyte and acid-base disorders are corrected).

PROGNOSIS: Most patients who are rapidly resuscitated from a dry drowning episode recover fully. The recovery of near-drowning victims who have inhaled water into the lungs depends on the underlying health of the victim, the duration of immersion, and the speed and efficiency with which oxygenation, ventilation, and perfusion are restored.

near point ABBR: n.p. Closest point of distinct vision with maximum accommodation. This point becomes more distant with age, varying from about 3 in. (7.62 cm) at age 2 to 40 in. (101.60 cm) at age 60. SYN: *punctum proximum*.

nearsighted Able to see clearly only those objects held close to the eye. SEE: *myopia*.

nearsightedness Myopia.

nearthrosis (nē″ăr-thrō′sĭs) [Gr. *neos,* new, + *arthron,* joint, + *osis,* condition] A false joint or abnormal articulation, as one developing after a fracture that has not united. SYN: *neoarthrosis; pseudarthrosis*.

nebula (nĕb′ū-lă) *pl.* **nebulae** [L., mist, cloud] **1.** Slight haziness on the cornea. **2.** Cloudiness in urine. **3.** Aqueous or oily substance for use in an atomizer.

nebulization Production of particles such as a spray or mist from liquid. The size of particles produced depends upon the method used. SEE: *nebulizer*.

nebulizer (nĕb′ū-lī″zĕr) [L. *nebula,* mist] An apparatus for producing a fine spray or mist. This may be done by rapidly passing air through a liquid or by vibrating a liquid at a high frequency so that the particles produced are extremely small. SEE: *aerosol; atomizer; vaporizer;* illus.

ultrasonic n. An aerosol produced by the action of a vibrating ultrasonic transducer under water.

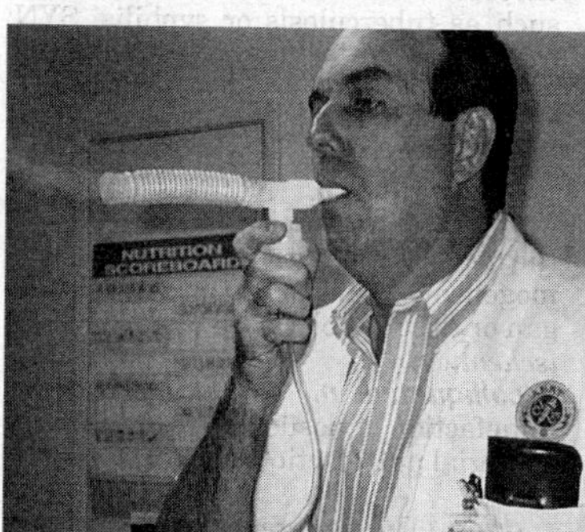

NEBULIZER

NEC *necrotizing enterocolitis.*

Necator (nē-kā′tor) [L., murderer] A genus of parasitic hookworms belonging to the family Ancylostomidae.

N. americanus A parasitic hookworm found worldwide that is responsible for iron-deficiency anemia and impaired growth in children. SEE: *hookworm;* illus.

necatoriasis (nē-kā″tō-rī′ă-sĭs) Hookworm.

neck [AS. *hnecca,* nape] **1.** The part of the body between the head and shoulders. SEE: illus.; *muscle* for illus. **2.** The constricted portion of an organ, or that resembling a neck. **3.** The region between the crown and the root of a tooth.

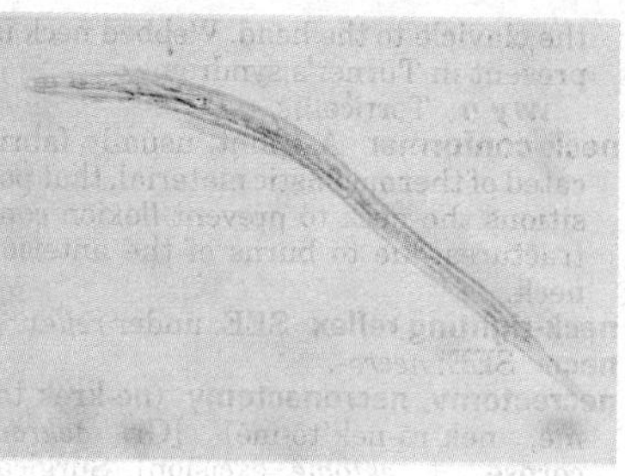

NECATOR

Infective filariform larva (orig. mag. ×100)

anatomical n. of the humerus The constriction just below the head of the humerus.

n. of the femur The heavy column of bone that connects the head of the femur to the shaft.

Madelung's n. Madelung's disease.

n. of the mandible The constricted area below the articular condyle; the area of attachment for the articular capsule and the lateral pterygoid muscle.

surgical n. of the humerus The narrow part of the humerus below the tuberosity. Fracture is common at this location.

n. of the tooth The constricted area that connects the crown of a tooth to the root of a tooth.

n. of the uterus Cervix uteri.

webbed n. A broad neck as seen anteriorly or posteriorly. The breadth is due to a fold of skin that extends from

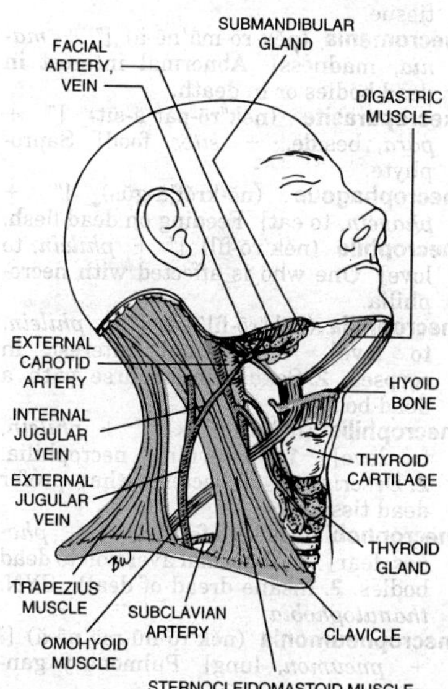

LATERAL ASPECT OF THE NECK

the clavicle to the head. Webbed neck is present in Turner's syndrome.

wry n. Torticollis.

neck conformer A splint, usually fabricated of thermoplastic material, that positions the neck to prevent flexion contractures due to burns of the anterior neck.

neck-righting reflex SEE: under *reflex*.

necr- SEE: *necro-*.

necrectomy, necronectomy (nĕ-krĕk′tō-mē, nĕk-rō-nĕk′tō-mē) [Gr. *nekros,* corpse, + *ektome,* excision] Surgical removal of necrotic tissue.

necro-, necr- [Gr. *nekros,* corpse] Combining form meaning *death, necrosis.*

necrobiosis (nĕk-rō-bī-ō′sĭs) [″ + *biosis,* life] Gradual degeneration and swelling of collagen bundles in the dermis. SEE: *necrosis*. **necrobiotic** (nĕ″krō-bī-ŏt′ĭk), *adj.*

n. lipoidica diabeticorum A skin disease marked by necrotic atrophy of connective and elastic tissue. The lesions have a central yellowish area surrounded by a brownish border and are usually present on the anterior surface of the legs. The disease is commonly found in people who have diabetes mellitus for many years.

necrocytotoxin (nĕk″rō-sī″tō-tŏks′ĭn) A toxin that causes the death of cells.

necrogenic, necrogenous (nĕ-krō-jĕn′ĭk, -krŏj′ĕn-ŭs) [″ + *gennan,* to produce] Caused by, pert. to, or originating in dead matter.

necrology (nĕk-rŏl′ō-jē) The study of mortality statistics.

necrolysis (nĕ-krŏl′ĭ-sĭs) [″ + *lysis,* dissolution] Necrosis and dissolution of tissue.

necromania (nĕk-rō-mā′nē-ă) [″ + *mania,* madness] Abnormal interest in dead bodies or in death.

necroparasite (nĕk″rō-păr′ă-sīt) [″ + *para,* beside, + *sitos,* food] Saprophyte.

necrophagous (nĕ-krŏf′ă-gŭs) [″ + *phagein,* to eat] Feeding on dead flesh.

necrophile (nĕk′rō-fīl) [″ + *philein,* to love] One who is affected with necrophilia.

necrophilia (nĕk″rō-fĭl′ē-ă) [″ + *philein,* to love] **1.** Abnormal interest in corpses. **2.** Sexual intercourse with a dead body.

necrophilic (nĕk″rō-fĭl′ĭk) [″ + *philein,* to love] **1.** Concerning necrophilia. **2.** Descriptive of bacteria that prefer dead tissue.

necrophobia (nĕk-rō-fō′bē-ă) [″ + *phobos,* fear] **1.** Abnormal aversion to dead bodies. **2.** Insane dread of death. SYN: *thanatophobia*.

necropneumonia (nĕk″rō-nū-mō′nē-ă) [″ + *pneumon,* lung] Pulmonary gangrene.

necropsy (nĕk′rŏp-sē) [″ + *opsis,* view] Autopsy.

necrosadism (nĕk″rō-sā′dĭzm) [″ + *sadism*] Sexual gratification derived from the mutilation of dead bodies.

necroscopy (nĕ-krŏs′kō-pē) [″ + *skopein,* to examine] Autopsy.

necrose (nĕk-rōs′) [Gr. *nekroun,* to make dead] To cause or to undergo necrosis.

necrosis (nĕ-krō′sĭs) *pl.* **necroses** [Gr. *nekrosis,* state of death] The death of cells, tissues, or organs. SEE: *gangrene; mortification*. **necrotizing** (nĕk′rō-tīz″ĭng), *adj.*

The causes of necrosis include insufficient blood supply, physical agents such as trauma or radiant energy (electricity, infrared, ultraviolet, roentgen, and radium rays), chemical agents acting locally, acting internally following absorption, or placed into the wrong tissue. Some medicines cause necrosis if injected into the tissues rather than the vein, and some, such as iron dextran, cause necrosis if injected into areas other than deep muscle or vein.

anemic n. Necrosis caused by inadequate blood flow to a body part.

aseptic n. Necrosis occurring without infection, e.g., as a result of trauma or drug use.

Balser's fatty n. SEE: *Balser's fatty necrosis*.

caseous n. Necrosis with soft, dry, cheeselike formation, seen in diseases such as tuberculosis or syphilis. SYN: *cheesy n.*

central n. Necrosis that affects only the center of a body part.

cheesy n. Caseous n.

coagulation n. Necrosis occurring esp. in infarcts. Coagulation occurs in the necrotic area, converting it into a homogeneous mass and depriving the organ or tissue of blood. SYN: *fibrinous n.; ischemic n.*

colliquative n. Necrosis caused by liquefaction of tissue due to autolysis or bacterial putrefaction. SYN: *liquefactive n.*

dry n. Dry gangrene.

embolic n. Necrosis resulting from an embolic occlusion of an artery.

fat n. Destruction or dissolution of fatty tissues, as seen, for example, in patients with severe cases of pancreatitis.

fibrinous n. Coagulation n.

focal n. Necrosis in small scattered areas, often seen in infection.

gummatous n. Necrosis forming a dry rubbery mass, resulting from syphilis.

ischemic n. Coagulation n.

liquefactive n. Colliquative n.

medial n. Necrosis of cells in the tunica media of an artery.

moist n. Necrosis with softening and wetness of the dead tissue.

postpartum pituitary n. Necrosis of the pituitary gland following childbirth. SEE: *Sheehan's syndrome*.

putrefactive n. Necrosis caused by bacterial decomposition.

radiation n. Necrosis caused by radiation exposure.

subcutaneous fat n. of newborn An inflammatory disorder of fat tissue that may occur in the newborn at the site of application of forceps during delivery, and occasionally in premature infants. The cause is unknown.

superficial n. Necrosis affecting only the outer layers of bone or any tissue.

thrombotic n. Necrosis due to thrombus formation.

total n. Necrosis affecting an entire organ or body part.

Zenker's n. SEE: *Zenker's degeneration.*

necrotic [Gr. *nekrosis,* state of death] Relating to, or descriptive of death of a portion of tissue.

necrotomy (nĕ-krŏt'ō-mē) [" + *tome,* incision] **1.** Dissection of a cadaver. **2.** Excision of a sequestrum or other necrotic tissue.

need Something required or essential. Certain things are essential for the physical and mental health of humans. Included in physical needs are oxygen, water, food, shelter, clothing, and warmth. Most human beings seem to need some form of physical exercise over and above that required for ordinary daily living. Mental health needs include some form of human (loving) relationship, a feeling of self-worth and the choice of and pursuit of some personal goal, no matter how trivial or grandiose, and the feeling that the goal is socially acceptable and is being attained.

certificate of n. ABBR: CON. A declaration from a government planning agency indicating that the construction or alteration of an existing health facility is justified. Designed initially in the 1970s to prevent the construction of duplicate health care facilities in local or regional markets, some analysts have suggested that CONs have instead defended existing hospitals from unwanted competition.

needle [AS. *naedl*] A pointed instrument for stitching, ligaturing, puncturing, or cannulating. It may be straight, half-curved, full-curved, semicircular, double-curved (sometimes called "S-" or sigmoid-shaped), double-ended, sharp or blunt-tipped, solid, or hollow. Cutting edge and round point are the two classifications of needles. Cutting edge needles are used in skin and dense tissue, while round point needles are used for more delicate operations, esp. on soft tissues. When a needle is used for stitching, the suture material may be attached via an eye, french eye, or more commonly, a swedged-on which is easily detachable.

aneurysm n. A blunt, curved needle with an eye in the tip used for passing a suture around a vessel.

aspirating n. A long, hollow needle, usually fitted to a syringe, for withdrawing fluids from a cavity.

atraumatic n. A needle of smaller diameter than the suture material. Use of this type of needle causes minimal damage to the tissue being sutured.

cataract n. A needle used in removing a cataract.

discission n. A special cataract needle for making multiple cuts into the lens capsule.

Hagedorn n. A curved, flattened needle with a cutting edge near the end.

hypodermic n. A hollow needle used for administration of hypodermic solutions.

knife n. A narrow needle-pointed knife.

ligature n. Aneurysm n.

obturator n. A device that fits into the lumen of a needle to prevent blockage during the puncture procedure.

Reverdin's n. A needle used to carry a suture. It has an eye at the tip that can be opened and closed by a lever.

scalp vein n. A specially designed needle for the administration of intravenous fluids, with a flat flange on each side to facilitate anchoring it after its placement in a small vein.

stop n. A needle with an eye at its tip, with a flange or shelf extending out from its shank end that prevents the needle from being inserted farther than the shelf.

needle-stick injury Accidental puncturing of the skin with an unsterilized needle. Health care workers are esp. at risk for injury while handling needles. Prevention of needle-stick injury is essential because of the danger of exposure of those involved to infection from diseases transmitted by blood (e.g., AIDS, hepatitis B or C). SEE: *sharps; Standard and Universal Precautions Appendix.*

NEFA *nonesterified fatty acids.*

negation (nē-gā'shŭn) [L. *negare,* to deny] Denial.

negative (nĕg'ă-tĭv) [L. *negare,* to deny] **1.** Possessing a numerical value that is less than zero. **2.** Lacking results or indicating an absence, as in a test result. **3.** Marked by resistance or retreat.

negative sign Minus sign (−) used in subtraction, to denote something that is below zero, or to indicate a lack.

negative study An investigation in which no benefit of a treatment, or no association between a risk factor and an outcome, is demonstrated; also called negative trial. Such studies may be important in disproving misconceptions about a disease, treatment, or presumed associations between risk factors and outcomes.

negativism A behavior peculiarity marked by not performing suggested actions (passive negativism) or in doing the opposite of what one has been asked to do (active negativism), as seen in some forms of mental illness.

neglect (nĕ-glĕkt) **1.** In neurology, absence of perception of—or disregard for—the nondominant part of the body in patients who have had a stroke that has damaged the nondominant hemisphere of the brain. **2.** Inattention to one's responsibilities, esp. to those dependent on one's care.

altitudinal n. Unilateral visual inattention.

hemispatial n. Unilateral visual inattention.

negligence The failure of a health care professional to meet his or her responsibilities to a patient, with resultant injury to the patient. There are four elements of negligence: duty owed, breach of duty or standard of care, proximate cause or causal connection (between the breach and damages), and damages or injuries. Medical professionals are legally liable for their own negligence or can be held liable for negligence of others of which they have knowledge but fail to report or intercede.

corporate n. Failure of a corporation to meet its legal obligations to its clients. With regard to health care facilities, responsibilities included under the doctrine of corporate negligence are 1) monitoring and supervision of the competence of medical and nursing personnel within the facility; 2) investigating physicians' credentials before granting staff privileges; and 3) negligent hiring of health care professionals (including failure to conduct appropriate background investigations).

gross n. Any voluntary, intentional, and conscious act or omission committed by an individual, with reckless disregard for the consequences, esp. how they may affect another person's life or property.

ordinary n. Failure to exercise the care that an ordinary prudent person would exercise under similar circumstances.

Negri bodies (nā'grē) [Adelchi Negri, It. physician, 1876–1912] Inclusion bodies found in the cells of the central nervous system of animals infected with rabies. They are acidophilic masses appearing in large ganglion cells or in cells of the brain, esp. those of the hippocampus and cerebellum. Their presence is considered conclusive proof of rabies.

NEI *National Eye Institute.*

Neisseria (nī-sē'rē-ă) [Albert Neisser, Ger. physician, 1855–1916] A genus of bacteria belonging to the family Neisseriaceae. They are gram-negative cocci and usually occur in pairs with flattened sides but may occur singly or in irregular groups. The two species most often associated with disease in humans are the meningococcus (*Neisseria meningitidis*) and gonococcus (*Neisseria gonorrhoeae.*)

N. catarrhalis A nonpathogenic species found in the upper respiratory tract. It may be mistaken for meningococci.

N. gonorrhoeae The species causing gonorrhea. SYN: *gonococcus*. SEE: illus.; *gonorrhea*.

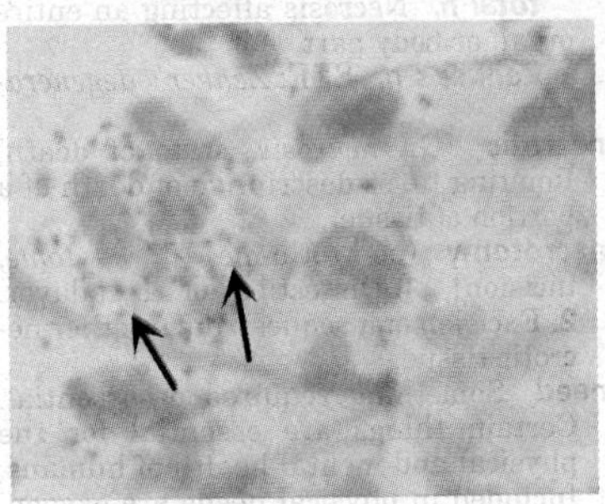

NEISSERIA GONORRHOEAE

(Orig. mag. ×500)

N. meningitidis The species causing epidemic cerebrospinal meningitis. SEE: *meningitis*.

N. sicca Species found in mucous membrane of the respiratory tract. Occasionally, this species may cause bacterial endocarditis.

Neisseriaceae (nīs-sē"rē-ā'sē-ē) A family of bacteria that are spherical, gram-negative, and nonmotile.

Nélaton's line (nā-lă-tŏnz') [Auguste Nélaton, Fr. surgeon, 1807–1873] Line from the anterior superior spine of the ilium to tuberosity of the ischium.

nelfinavir (nĕl-fĭn'ă-vēr) A protease inhibitor used in the treatment of HIV-1. Trade name is Viracept.

nemathelminth (nĕm"ă-thĕl'mĭnth) [Gr. *nema,* thread, + *helmins,* worm] A roundworm belonging to the phylum Nemathelminthes.

Nemathelminthes (nĕm"ă-thĕl-mĭn'thēz) The phylum of the roundworms.

nematocide (nĕm'ă-tō-sīd") [Gr. *nema,* thread, + L. *caedere,* to kill] An agent that kills nematodes.

nematocyst (nĕm'ă-tō-sĭst) [" + *kystis,* bladder] The small stinging barb present in jellyfish and some other coelenterates. It can penetrate the skin upon contact and inflict painful lesions. In some cases, multiple contact can be fatal.

Nematoda (nĕm"ă-tō'dă) [" + *eidos,* form, shape] A class of the phylum Nemathelminthes that includes the true roundworms or threadworms, many species of which are parasitic. They are cylindrical or spindle-shaped worms that possess a resistant cuticle, have a complete alimentary canal, and lack a true coelom. The sexes usually are separate, and development usually is direct and simple.

nematode (nĕm′ă-tōd) [Gr. *nema,* thread, + *eidos,* form, shape] A member of the class Nematoda.

nematodiasis (nĕm″ă-tō-dī′ă-sĭs) [″ + ″ + *-iasis,* condition] Infestation by a parasite belonging to the class Nematoda.

nematoid (nĕm′ă-toyd) Threadlike, like a nematode.

nematology (nĕm″ă-tŏl′ō-jē) The division of parasitology that deals with worms belonging to the class Nematoda.

neo- [Gr. *neos*] Combining form meaning *new, recent.*

neoadjuvant therapy In treating cancer, the use of chemotherapy before radiation or surgery.

neoantigen (nē″ō-ăn′tĭ-jĕn) [″ + *anti,* against, + *gennan,* to produce] A nonspecific term for various tumor antigens.

neoarthrosis (nē″ō-ăr-thrō′sĭs) [″ + *arthron,* joint, + *osis,* condition] Nearthrosis.

neobladder (nē-ō-blăd′dĕr) A surgically constructed urinary reservoir, usually made from a segment of small bowel, that is used to replace a bladder removed during radical cystectomy. It is surgically connected to the patient's native urethra and typically maintains urinary continence, while limiting or eliminating the need for self-catheterization. Neobladders are often used after bladder cancer surgery as an alternative to a urostomy. They cannot be used in patients whose malignancy involves the distal urethra.

neoblastic [″ + *blastos,* germ] Pert. to or constituting a new growth of tissue.

neocerebellum (nē″ō-sĕr-ĕ-bĕl′ŭm) [Gr. *neos,* new, + L. *cerebellum,* little brain] The portion of the corpus cerebelli of the cerebellum that lies between the primary and prepyramidal fissures and consists principally of the ansiform lobules. Phylogenetically, it develops last, in conjunction with cerebral cortex, and is concerned with the integration of voluntary movements. It is the posterior lobe of the cerebellum.

neocortex (nē″ō-kor′tĕks) Isocortex.

neodymium (nē″ō-dĭm′ē-ŭm) SYMB: Nd. A shiny, silvery, rare-earth chemical element, atomic weight 144.24, atomic number 60.

neoenterocystoplasty A neobladder formed surgically from bowel wall and bladder muscle.

neofetus (nē-ō-fē′tŭs) [″ + L. *foetus,* offspring] The embryo during the eighth or ninth week of intrauterine life.

neoformation (nē″ō-for-mā′shŭn) [″ + L. *formatio,* a shaping] **1.** Regeneration. **2.** A neoplasm or new growth.

neogenesis (nē-ō-jĕn′ĕ-sĭs) [″ + *genesis,* generation, birth] Regeneration; reformation, as of tissue. **neogenetic** (nē″ō-jĕn-ĕt′ĭk), *adj.*

neokinetic (nē″ō-kĭ-nĕt′ĭk) [″ + *kinetikos,* pert. to movement] Concerning the portion of the nervous system that regulates voluntary muscular control.

neolalism (nē″ō-lăl′ĭzm) [″ + *laleo,* to chatter] The use of neologisms in speech, esp. that associated with schizophrenia.

neologism (nē-ŏl′ō-jĭzm) [″ + *logos,* word, reason, + *-ismos,* state] **1.** A newly invented word. **2.** A nonsensical word, or verbal tic, the use of which is sometimes associated with neuropsychiatric disorders, such as psychoses or Tourette's syndrome.

neomembrane (nē-ō-mĕm′brān) [″ + L. *membrana,* membrane] Pseudomembrane.

neomorph (nē′ō-morf) [″ + *morphe,* form] A new formation or development that is not inherited from a similar structure in an ancestor.

neomycin sulfate (nē″ō-mī′sĭn) [″ + *mykes,* fungus] An antibiotic from a species of *Streptomyces,* isolated from soil. Active against gram-positive and gram-negative bacteria, as well as streptomycin-resistant strains of *Mycobacterium tuberculosis.* It is toxic to kidneys and to the eighth nerve and may cause renal failure or hearing difficulties.

neon (nē′ŏn) [Gr. *neos,* new] SYMB: Ne. A rare, inert, gaseous element in the air. Only 18 parts per million parts of air are neon. Neon's atomic mass is 20.183, and its atomic number is 10.

n. gas A colorless gas that makes a reddish-orange glow when an electric charge strikes it.

neonatal (nē″ō-nā′tăl) [″ + L. *natus,* born] Concerning the first 28 days after birth.

neonatal mortality rate SEE: under *rate.*

neonate (nē′ō-nāt) A newborn infant up to 1 month of age. SEE: *Nursing Diagnoses Appendix.*

neonate, killing of a SEE: *infanticide.*

neonatologist (nē″ō-nā-tŏl′ō-jĭst) [″ + ″ + Gr. *logos,* word, reason] A physician who specializes in the study, care, and treatment of neonates.

neonatology (nē″ō-nā-tŏl′ō-jē) The study, care, and treatment of neonates.

neopallium (nē″ō-păl′ē-ŭm) [Gr. *neos,* new, + L. *pallium,* cloak] Isocortex.

neopharynx (nē-ō-făr′ĭnks) A surgically reconstructed pharynx. The surgery reestablishes the integrity of the throat tract after laryngectomy.

neophilism (nē-ŏf′ĭl-ĭzm) [″ + *philein,* to love, + *-ismos,* condition] Abnormal love of novelty and new persons and scenes.

neophobia (nē″ō-fō′bē-ă) [″ + *phobos,* fear] Fear of new scenes or novelties; aversion to all that is unknown or not understood. SYN: *kainophobia.*

neoplasia (nē″ō-plā′zē-ă) [″ + *plassein,* to form] The development of neoplasms.

neoplasia, cervical intraepithelial SEE: *cervical intraepithelial neoplasia.*

neoplasm (nē′ō-plăzm) [″ + LL. *plasma,* form, mold] A new and abnormal formation of tissue, as a tumor or growth. It serves no useful function, but grows at the expense of the healthy organism. **neoplastic** (nē″ō-plăs′tĭk), *adj.*

benign n. Growth not spreading by metastases or infiltration of tissue.

histoid n. Neoplasm in which structure resembles the tissues and elements that surround it.

malignant n. Growth that infiltrates tissue, metastasizes, and often recurs after attempts at surgical removal. SYN: *cancer.*

mixed n. Neoplasm composed of tissues from two of the germinal layers.

noninvasive n. A tumor that has not spread or does not spread.

organoid n. Neoplasm in which the structure is similar to some organ of the body.

neoplasty (nē′ō-plăs-tē) [″ + *plassein,* to form] Surgical formation or restoration of parts.

neostigmine (nē-ō-stĭg′mĭn) A cholinergic drug used clinically in the form of a bromide or methylsulfate.

n. bromide A preparation of neostigmine used for oral administration in the treatment of myasthenia gravis. Ophthalmic solution used for glaucoma.

n. methylsulfate A preparation of neostigmine used for parenteral administration in treatment of myasthenia gravis.

neostomy (nē-ŏs′tō-mē) [″ + *stoma,* mouth] Surgical formation of artificial opening into an organ or between two organs.

neostriatum (nē″ō-strī-ā′tŭm) [″ + L. *striatum,* grooved] The caudate nucleus and the putamen considered together.

neoteny (nē-ŏt′ĕ-nē) [″ + *teinein,* to extend] In zoology, maturation during the larval stage.

neothalamus (nē″ō-thăl′ă-mŭs) [″ + L. *thalamus,* thalamus] The lateral and dorsomedial nuclei of the thalamus.

nephelometer (nĕf″ĕl-ŏm′ĕ-ter) [Gr. *nephele,* mist, + *metron,* measure] A device used in nephelometry to measure the number of particles in a solution. For example, it is used to measure the turbidity of a fluid and also may be used to estimate the degree of contamination of air by particulate matter.

nephelometry (nĕf″ĕl-ŏm′ĕ-trē) A technique for detecting proteins in body fluids, based on the tendency of proteins to scatter light in identifiable ways. SEE: *nephelometer.*

nephelopia (nĕf″ĕ-lō′pē-ă) [Gr. *nephele,* mist, + *ops,* eye] Dim or cloudy vision from lessened transparency of the ocular media.

nephr- [Gr. *nephros,* kidney] SEE: *nephro-.*

nephradenoma (nĕf″răd-ĕ-nō′mă) [Gr. *nephros,* kidney, + *aden,* gland, + *oma,* tumor] Renal adenoma.

nephralgia (nĕ-frăl′jē-ă) [″ + *algos,* pain] Renal pain. **nephralgic** (nĕ-frăl′jĭk), *adj.*

nephrapostasis (nĕf″ră-pŏs′tă-sĭs) [″+ *apostasis,* suppuration] Renal abscess or purulent inflammation of the kidney.

nephrectasia, nephrectasis, nephrectasy (nĕf-rĕk-tā′zē-ă, -rĕk′tă-sĭs, -tă-sē) [Gr. *nephros,* kidney, + *ektasis,* distention] Distention of the kidney.

nephrectomize (nĕ-frĕk′tō-mīz) [″ + *ektome,* excision] To remove, surgically, one or both kidneys.

nephrectomy (nĕ-frĕk′tō-mē) [″ + *ektome,* excision] Surgical removal of a kidney, for example, to remove a renal cell carcinoma or injured organ. Complications include spontaneous pneumothorax, infection, azotemia, or secondary hemorrhage. SEE: *Nursing Diagnoses Appendix.*

PATIENT CARE: Adequate preoperative and postoperative instruction is provided. The patient is prepared physically according to protocol, including skin preparation, laboratory studies, and administration of preoperative medications. Activities are provided that are interesting but not tiring. Fluid and electrolyte imbalances are prevented, and daily weight is obtained. The patient is encouraged to verbalize feelings and concerns and is given support and reassurance. Vital signs are checked every 2 to 4 hr. Analgesics and other medications are administered as prescribed. Any excessive bleeding is recorded and reported. The patient is turned frequently. The operative site and dressing are observed, and the dressing is changed as necessary. Frequent position changes also help to prevent complications of immobility. The patient is assisted with deep-breathing and coughing exercises. Range-of-motion exercises are instituted. Drainage tubes are checked frequently for patency. Intake and output are monitored and recorded. Frequent mouth care is provided while the patient takes nothing by mouth. A progressive diet is encouraged on return of normal bowel sounds. Discharge teaching focuses on diet; activities, particularly those that could injure the remaining kidney; incision care; and medications.

abdominal n. Nephrectomy through an incision in the abdominal wall.

paraperitoneal n. Removal of a kidney through an extraperitoneal incision.

nephrelcosis (nĕf-rĕl-kō′sĭs) [Gr. *nephros,* kidney, + *helkosis,* ulceration] Ulceration of the mucosa of the kidney.

nephrelcus (nĕf-rĕl′kŭs) Renal ulcer.

nephremphraxis (nĕf″rĕm-frăks′ĭs) [″ + *emphraxis,* obstruction] Obstruction in the renal vessels.

nephric (nĕf′rĭk) [Gr. *nephros,* kidney] Pert. to the kidney or kidneys. SYN: *renal.*

nephridium (nĕ-frĭd′ē-ŭm) [Gr. *nephridios,* pert. to the kidney] A segmented excretory tubule present in many invertebrates.

nephritic (nĕ-frĭt′ĭk) **1.** Relating to the kidney. **2.** Pert. to nephritis. **3.** An agent used in nephritis.

nephritis (nĕf-rī′tĭs) *pl.* **nephritides** [Gr. *nephros,* kidney, + *itis,* inflammation] Inflammation of the kidneys caused by bacteria or their toxins (e.g., pyelonephritis), autoimmune disorders (e.g., poststreptococcal glomerulonephritis, lupus nephritis), or toxic chemicals (e.g., mercury, arsenic, alcohol, nonsteroidal anti-inflammatory drugs). The glomeruli, tubules, and interstitial tissue may be affected. The condition may be either acute or chronic.

PATIENT CARE: Renal function is assessed, and signs of renal failure (oliguria, azotemia, acidosis) are reported. Hemoglobin, hematocrit, and electrolyte levels are monitored. Aseptic technique is used in handling catheters. The health care provider observes, records, and reports hematuria and monitors blood pressure using the same cuff, arm, and position each time. He or she also observes or questions the patient concerning headache, restlessness, lethargy, convulsions, tachycardia, and arrhythmias. Antihypertensive drugs are administered as prescribed. The patient is encouraged to maintain adequate hydration and follow the prescribed dietary restrictions. Intravenous fluid intake is monitored. Complications of hypertension are anticipated and prevented.

acute n. An inflammatory form of nephritis involving the glomeruli, the tubules, or the entire kidney. It may be called degenerative, diffuse, suppurative, hemorrhagic, interstitial, or parenchymal, depending upon the portion of the kidney involved.

analgesic n. Chronic nephritis caused by excess intake of almost any of the anti-inflammatory analgesics (e.g., salicylates, acetaminophen, nonsteroidal anti-inflammatory agents).

chronic n. A progressive form of nephritis in which the entire structure of the kidney or only the glomerular or tubular processes may be affected.

glomerular n. Glomerulonephritis.

interstitial n. Nephritis associated with pathological changes in the renal interstitial tissue that in turn may be primary or due to a toxic agent such as a drug or chemical. The end result is the destruction of the nephrons and serious impairment of renal function.

scarlatinal n. Acute glomerulonephritis complicating scarlet fever.

suppurative n. Nephritis associated with abscesses in the kidney.

transfusion n. Renal failure and tubular disease caused by transfusion of incompatible blood.

nephritogenic (nĕ-frĭt″ō-jĕn′ĭk) [″ + *gennan,* to produce] Causing nephritis.

nephro-, nephr- [Gr. *nephros,* kidney] Combining form meaning *kidney.*

nephroabdominal (nĕf″rō-ăb-dŏm′ĭ-năl) [″ + L. *abdominalis,* abdomen] Concerning the kidney and abdomen.

nephroblastoma (nĕf″rō-blăs-tō′mă) [″ + *blastos,* germ, + *oma,* tumor] Wilms' tumor.

nephrocalcinosis (nĕf-rō″kăl″sĭn-ō′sĭs) [″ + L. *calx,* lime, + Gr. *osis,* condition] Calcinosis of the kidney characterized by deposits of calcium phosphate in renal tubules.

nephrocapsectomy (nĕf″rō-kăp-sĕk′tō-mē) [″ + L. *capsula,* capsule, + Gr. *ektome,* excision] Excision of the renal capsule.

nephrocardiac (nĕf″rō-kăr′dē-ăk) [″ + *kardia,* heart] Concerning the kidney and the heart.

nephrocele (nĕf′rō-sēl) [″ + *kele,* tumor, swelling] Renal hernia.

nephrocolic (nĕf″rō-kŏl′ĭk) [Gr. *nephros,* kidney, + *kolikos,* colic] **1.** Renal colic. **2.** Concerning the kidney and the colon.

nephrocolopexy (nĕf″rō-kŏl′ō-pĕks″ē) [″ + *kolon,* colon, + *pexis,* fixation] Surgical suspension of the kidney and the colon using the nephrocolic ligament.

nephrocoloptosis (nĕf″rō-kō″lŏp-tō′sĭs) [″ + ″ + *ptosis,* a dropping] Condition in which the kidney and the colon are displaced downward.

nephrocystanastomosis (nĕf″rō-sĭst-ă-năs″tō-mō′sĭs) [″ + *kystis,* bladder, + *anastomosis,* outlet] Surgical formation of an artificial connection between the kidney and the bladder where there is permanent ureteral obstruction.

nephrocystitis (nĕf″rō-sĭs-tī′tĭs) [″ + ″ + *itis,* inflammation] Inflammation of the kidneys and the bladder.

nephrocystosis (nĕf″rō-sĭs-tō′sĭs) [″ + ″ + *osis,* condition] Formation of renal cysts.

nephrogenetic (nĕf″rō-jĕn-ĕt′ĭk) [″ + *gennan,* to produce] Arising in or from the renal organs; capable of giving rise to kidney tissue.

nephrography (nĕ-frŏg′ră-fē) [″ + *graphein,* to write] Radiography of the kidneys, usually after intravenous injection of a contrast medium.

nephrohypertrophy (nĕf″rō-hī-pĕr′trō-fē) [″ + *hyper,* over, + *trophe,* nourishment] Increased size of kidneys.

nephroid (nĕf′royd) [″ + *eidos,* form, shape] Resembling a kidney; kidney-shaped. SYN: *reniform.*

nephrolithiasis (nĕf″rō-lĭth-ī′ă-sĭs) The presence of calculi in the kidney. SEE: *calculus, renal.*

nephrolithotomy (nĕf″rō-lĭth-ŏt′ō-mē) [″ + *lithos,* stone, + *tome,* incision] Renal incision for removal of kidney stones.

nephrology (nĕ-frŏl′ō-jē) [″ + *logos,* word, reason] The branch of medical science concerned with the structure and function of the kidneys.

nephrolysis (nĕ-frŏl′ĭ-sĭs) [″ + *lysis,* dissolution] **1.** Surgical detachment of an inflamed kidney from paranephric adhesions. **2.** Destruction of kidney tissue by the action of a nephrotoxin.

nephroma (nĕ-frō′mă) [″ + *oma,* tumor] Renal tumor.

nephromalacia (nĕf″rō-mă-lā′sē-ă) [″ + *malakia,* softening] Abnormal renal softness or softening.

nephromegaly (nĕf″rō-mĕg′ă-lē) [″ + *megas,* great] Extreme enlargement of a kidney.

nephromere (nĕf′rō-mēr) [″ + *meros,* part] The intermediate mesoderm in an embryo from which the kidney develops. SYN: *nephrotome.*

nephron (nĕf′rŏn) [Gr. *nephros,* kidney] The structural and functional unit of the kidney, consisting of a renal (malpighian) corpuscle (a glomerulus enclosed within Bowman's capsule), the proximal convoluted tubule, the loop of Henle, and the distal convoluted tubule. These connect by arched collecting tubules with straight collecting tubules. Urine is formed by filtration in renal corpuscles and selective reabsorption and secretion by the cells of the renal tubule. There are approx. one million nephrons in each kidney. SEE: *kidney* for illus.; *malpighian capsule; urine.*

nephropathy (nĕ-frŏp′ă-thē) [″ + *pathos,* disease, suffering] Disease of the kidney. This term includes inflammatory (nephritis), degenerative (nephrosis), and sclerotic lesions of the kidney.

analgesic n. Analgesic nephritis.

hypercalcemic n. Renal damage due to hypercalcemia. It is usually caused by hyperparathyroidism, sarcoidosis, excess vitamin D intake, excess ingestion of milk and alkali, multiple myeloma, malignant disease, and, occasionally, by immobilization or Paget's disease. Correction of the primary disease is indicated. If the underlying cause is allowed to persist, the damage to the renal tubules may be permanent.

hypokalemic n. Renal damage due to abnormal depletion of potassium, regardless of the basic cause of the electrolyte abnormality. Characteristically, there are multiple vacuoles in microscopic sections of the renal tubular epithelium. Clinically, the patient is unable to concentrate urine. Therapy for the primary cause of the hypokalemia may allow the kidney lesions to become completely reversed.

membranous n. A glomerular disease of unknown etiology that produces nephrotic syndrome. It may be distinguished from lipoid nephrosis by the use of immunofluorescence and electron microscopy. SEE: *glomerular disease; nephrotic syndrome.*

TREATMENT: Treatment consists of corticosteroids with or without other immunosuppressive drugs.

radiocontrast-induced n. Nephropathy caused by the use of radio contrast media. In normal patients, use of such agents rarely causes nephropathy. However, in some individuals, esp. those with conditions that cause diminished renal blood flow, diabetic renal failure, jaundice, or multiple myeloma, acute renal failure may result.

nephropexy (nĕf′rō-pĕks-ē) [″ + *pexis,* fixation] Surgical fixation of a floating kidney.

nephrophthisis (nĕ-frŏf′thĭ-sĭs) [″ + *phthisis,* a wasting] **1.** Tuberculosis of the kidney with caseous degeneration. **2.** Suppurative nephritis with wasting of the kidney substance.

nephroptosis (nĕf″rŏp-tō′sĭs) [″ + *ptosis,* a dropping] Downward displacement of the kidney.

nephropyelitis (nĕf″rō-pī-ĕl-ī′tĭs) [″ + *pyelos,* pelvis, + *itis,* inflammation] Pyelonephritis.

nephropyelography (nĕf″rō-pī″ĕ-lŏg′ră-fē) [″ + *pyelos,* pelvis, + *graphein,* to write] Radiography of the kidney and renal pelvis after injection of a contrast medium.

nephropyeloplasty (nĕf″rō-pī′ĕ-lō-plăs″tē) [″ + ″ + *plassein,* to form] Plastic surgery on the kidney and renal pelvis.

nephropyosis (nĕf″rō-pī-ō′sĭs) [″ + *pyosis,* suppuration] Purulence of a kidney.

nephrorrhagia (nĕf-ror-ā′jē-ă) [″ + *rhegnynai,* to burst forth] Renal hemorrhage into the pelvis and tubules.

nephrorrhaphy (nĕf-ror′ă-fē) [″ + *rhaphe,* seam, ridge] Surgical procedure of suturing the kidney.

nephros (nĕf′rŏs) [Gr.] The kidney.

nephrosclerosis (nĕf″rō-sklĕ-rō′sĭs) [″ + *sklerosis,* a hardening] Renal sclerosis, that is, hardening of the connective tissues of the kidneys.

arterial n. Arteriosclerosis of the renal arteries resulting in ischemia, atrophy of parenchyma, and fibrosis of the kidney.

arteriolar n. Sclerosis of the smaller renal arterioles, esp. the afferent glomerular arterioles with resulting fibrosis, ischemic necrosis, and glomerular degeneration and failure. This type of nephrosclerosis occurs in most cases of essential hypertension.

malignant n. Nephrosclerosis that develops rapidly in patients with severe hypertension. SEE: *hypertension*.

nephrosis (nĕf-rō′sĭs) *pl.* **nephroses** [Gr. *nephros,* kidney, + *osis,* condition] **1.** Condition in which there are degenerative changes in the kidneys, esp. the renal tubules, without the occurrence of inflammation. **2.** Clinical classification of kidney disease in which protein loss is so extensive that edema and hypoproteinemia are produced. SEE: *nephrotic syndrome*.

lipoid n. Idiopathic nephrotic syndrome.

nephrosonephritis (nĕ-frō″sō-nĕ-frī′tĭs) [″ + *osis,* condition, + *nephros,* kidney, + *itis,* inflammation] Renal disease with characteristics of nephritis and nephrosis.

nephrostoma (nĕ-frŏs′tō-mă) [″ + *stoma,* mouth] The internal orifice of a wolffian tubule, connected with the coelom in the human embryo.

nephrostomy (nĕ-frŏs′tō-mē) The formation of an artificial fistula into the renal pelvis, for example, to drain an obstructed kidney or relieve hydronephrosis.

percutaneous n. The placement of a catheter into the renal pelvis from the posterolateral aspect of the body below the 11th rib by using ultrasound or fluoroscopy.

nephrotic (nĕ-frŏt′ĭk) [Gr. *nephros,* kidney] Relating to, or caused by, nephrosis.

nephrotic syndrome ABBR: NS. A condition marked by increased glomerular permeability to proteins, resulting in massive loss of proteins in the urine, edema, hypoalbuminemia, hyperlipidemia, and hypercoagulability. Several different types of glomerular injury can cause the syndrome, including membranous glomerulopathy, minimal-change disease, focal segmental glomerulosclerosis, glomerulonephritis, and membranoproliferative glomerulonephritis. These pathological findings in the kidney result from a broad array of diseases such as diabetic injury to the glomerulus, amyloidosis, immune-complex deposition disease, vasculitis, systemic lupus erythematosus, and toxic injury to the kidneys by drugs. The disease's prognosis depends on the cause. For example, if the cause is exposure to a drug or toxin, the removal of that substance may be curative. When the disease results from glomerulosclerosis caused by AIDS, death may occur within months. Renal biopsy usually is needed to determine the precise histological cause, treatment, and prognosis. SYN: *nephrosis*. SEE: *proteinuria; Nursing Diagnoses Appendix*.

Idiopathic NS is diagnosed when the known causes of NS have been excluded. It is usually diagnosed in adults by use of renal biopsy. Causes are classified according to the changes found in the capillaries of the glomerulus when examined by use of electron microscopy.

SYMPTOMS: Patients with nephrotic syndrome may initially present with fluid retention in the legs or symptoms caused by blood clotting (e.g., in the renal vein). The hyperlipidemia that often accompanies the syndrome may lead to symptoms caused by atherosclerosis.

TREATMENT: Diuretics are used to treat symptomatic edema. Anticoagulants may be used to treat and prevent clotting. Lipid-lowering medications are used to prevent atherosclerosis. Renally tailored diets, with defined quantities of sodium, potassium, and protein, often are recommended.

Corticosteroids and immunosuppressive drugs (e.g., cyclophosphamide) are used to manage nephrosis caused by some histological subtypes. When renal failure accompanies nephrotic syndrome, dialysis may be required.

PATIENT CARE: Symptoms of proteinuria and fluid and electrolyte balance are monitored (intake and input, weight). Adequate nutritional intake is encouraged. The patient is assisted with skin care. Trauma is prevented, and activities are planned to provide periods of rest and to prevent fatigue and weakness. The patient is protected from infection. Support is offered to patients who have difficulty coping with the consequences of the illness (e.g., edema, the need for intensive medical therapies, or the need for dialysis).

nephrotome (nĕf′rō-tōm) [″ + *tome,* incision] The embryonic bridge of cells connecting primitive segments along the neural tube to the somatic and splanchnic mesoderm from which arises the urogenital system. SYN: *mesomere; nephromere*.

nephrotomogram (nĕf″rō-tō′mō-grăm) A tomogram of the kidney.

nephrotomography (nĕf″rō-tō-mŏg′ră-fē) [″+ ″ + *graphein,* to write] Tomograph of the kidney after the intravenous injection of a radiopaque contrast medium that is excreted by the kidney.

nephrotomy (nĕ-frŏt′ō-mē) [″ + *tome,* incision] Surgical incision of the kidney.

nephrotoxin (nĕf″rō-tŏk′sĭn) [″ + *toxikon,* poison] A toxic substance that damages kidney tissues. Commonly encountered nephrotoxins include aminoglycoside antibiotics (e.g., gentamicin, tobramycin, or amikacin), nonsteroidal anti-inflammatory drugs (e.g., indomethacin), lead (e.g., in "moonshine" whiskey and some paints), and some ionic radiocontrast agents.

nephrotropic (nĕf″rō-trŏp′ĭk) [″ + *tropos,* turning] **1.** Affecting the kidneys. **2.** An agent or drug that exerts its effect principally on the kidney or renal function.

nephrotuberculosis (nĕf″rō-tū-bĕr″kū-lō′sĭs) [″ + *tuberculum,* a little swelling, + *osis,* condition] Infection of the kidney due to *Mycobacterium tuberculosis.*

nephroureterectomy (nĕf″rō-ū-rē″tĕr-ĕk′tō-mē) [″ + *oureter,* ureter, + *ektome,* excision] Surgical excision of the kidney with all or part of the ureter.

nephrydrosis (nĕf″rĭ-drō′sĭs) [″ + *hydor,* water, + *osis,* condition] Hydronephrosis.

neptunium [planet Neptune] SYMB: Np. An element obtained by bombarding uranium with neutrons. Its atomic weight is 237 and its atomic number is 93.

nerve [L. *nervus,* sinew; Gr. *neuron,* sinew] A fiber made of linked neurons that transmit electrical and chemical signals between the central nervous system and body tissues. Afferent nerves conduct sensory impulses from receptors to the CNS; efferent nerves conduct motor impulses from the CNS to effector organs and tissues. The fibers of peripheral nerves are the axons and dendrites of neurons whose cell bodies are located within the brain, the spinal cord, or ganglia. A bundle of nerve fibers is called a fasciculus. The fibers within a fasciculus are surrounded and held together by delicate connective tissue fibers forming the endoneurium. Each fasciculus is surrounded by a sheath of connective tissue (perineurium). The entire nerve is enclosed in a thick sheath of connective tissue (epineurium), which may contain numerous fat cells. Small nerves may lack an epineurium. SYN: *nervus.* SEE: *cell* and *nerve cell* for illus.

SYMPTOMS: A broad array of insults may damage nerves, including direct trauma, repetitive motion injuries, compression by neighboring structures, glycosylation, infections, drugs, toxins, and paraneoplastic syndromes, to name a few. Symptoms of nerve injury include paresthesias, loss of sensation and position sense, impaired motor function, cranial nerve malfunction, changes in reflexes, and impairments in glandular secretion.

TESTS FOR LOSS OF FUNCTION: The assessment of nerve injury includes a careful neurological examination, sometimes accompanied by such tests as electromyography or nerve conduction studies.

accelerator n. A sympathetic nerve to the heart that carries impulses that speed the heart rate.

acoustic n. The eighth cranial nerve. SEE: *vestibulocochlear nerve* for illus.

adrenergic n. A sympathetic nerve that releases norepinephrine at a synapse when it transmits a stimulus.

afferent n. Any nerve that transmits impulses from receptors to the central nervous system. SYN: *sensory nerve.*

autonomic n. SEE: *autonomic nervous system.*

cholinergic n. A parasympathetic nerve that releases acetylcholine, not a synapse, when it transmits a stimulus.

cranial n. One of the 12 pairs of nerves originating in the brainstem, that mainly controls the activities of the face and head. In addition to these cranial nerves, there is a small combined efferent and afferent nerve that goes from the olfactory area of the brain to the nasal septum. This nerve, which is thought by some anatomists to be the first cranial nerve, is called the terminal nerve. SEE: illus.

DIAGNOSIS: Lesions of the cranial nerves give rise to the following alteration(s) (lesions are described as if one of each pair of nerves were diseased): *First* (olfactory): Loss or disturbance of the sense of smell. *Second* (optic): Blindness of various types, depending on the exact location of the lesion. *Third* (oculomotor): Ptosis (drooping) of the eyelid, deviation of the eyeball outward, dilatation of the pupil, double vision. *Fourth* (trochlear): Rotation of the eyeball upward and outward, double vision. *Fifth* (trigeminal): Sensory root: Pain or loss of sensation in the face, forehead, temple, and eye. Motor root: Deviation of the jaw toward the paralyzed side, difficulty in chewing. *Sixth* (abducens): Deviation of the eye outward, double vision. *Seventh* (facial): Paralysis of all the muscles on one side of the face; inability to wrinkle the forehead, to close the eye, to whistle; deviation of the mouth toward the sound side. *Eighth* (vestibulocochlear): Deafness or ringing in the ears; dizziness; nausea and vomiting; reeling. *Ninth* (glossopharyngeal): Disturbance of taste; difficulty in swallowing. *Tenth* (vagus): Disease of the vagus nerve is usually limited to one or more of its divisions. Paralysis of the main trunk on one side causes hoarseness and difficulty in swallowing and talking. The commonest disease of the vagus is of its left recurrent branch, which causes hoarseness as its principal manifestation. *Eleventh* (spinal accessory): Drooping of the shoulder; inability to rotate the head away from the affected

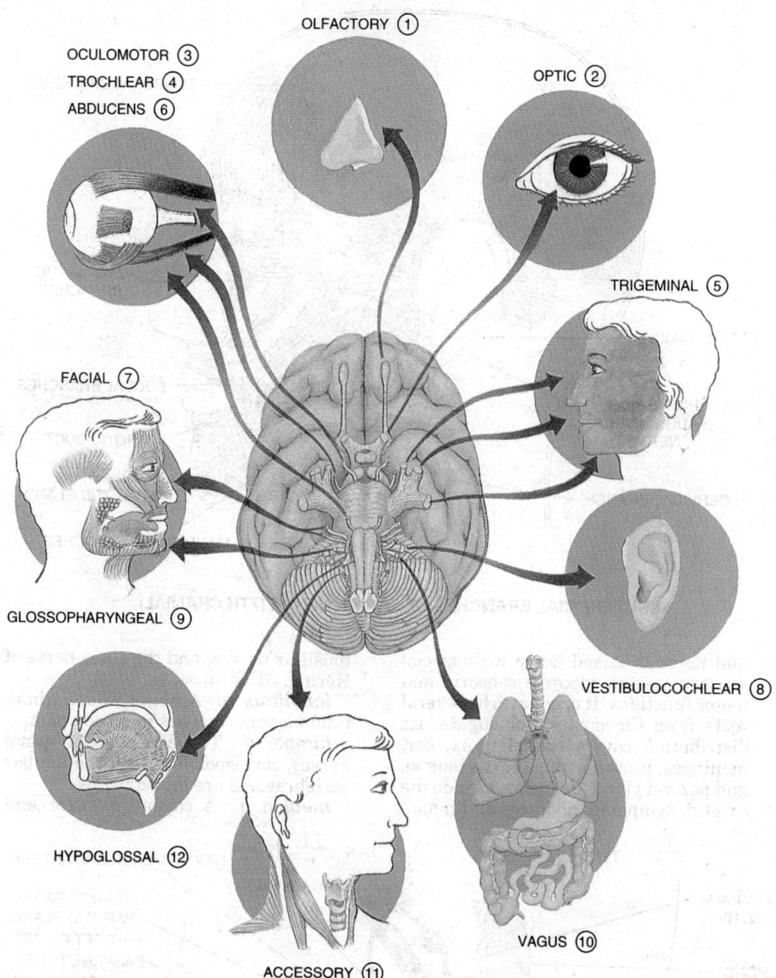

CRANIAL NERVES AND THEIR DISTRIBUTIONS

side. *Twelfth* (hypoglossal): Paralysis of one side of the tongue; deviation of the tongue toward the paralyzed side; thick speech.

depressor n. Any nerve whose stimulation depresses the activity of an organ or nerve center.

efferent n. A nerve that carries impulses having one of the following effects: motor, causing contraction of muscles; secretory, causing glands to secrete; and inhibitory, causing some organs to become quiescent. SYN: *motor nerve.*

excitatory n. A nerve that transmits impulses that stimulate function.

excitoreflex n. A visceral nerve whose stimulation causes reflex action.

facial n. The seventh cranial nerve. A mixed nerve, it consists of efferent fibers supplying the facial muscles, the platysma muscle, the submandibular and sublingual glands; and afferent fibers from taste buds of the anterior two thirds of the tongue and from the muscles. The afferent fibers originate from the geniculate ganglion, and the motor and secretory fibers from nuclei in the pons. They are distributed throughout the ear, face, palate, and tongue. Branches are the tympanic, chorda tympani, posterior auricular, digastric, stylohyoid, temporal, zygomatic, malar, buccal, mandibular, and cervical. SEE: illus.; *cranial nerve.*

gangliated n. Any nerve of the sympathetic nervous system.

glossopharyngeal n. The ninth cra-

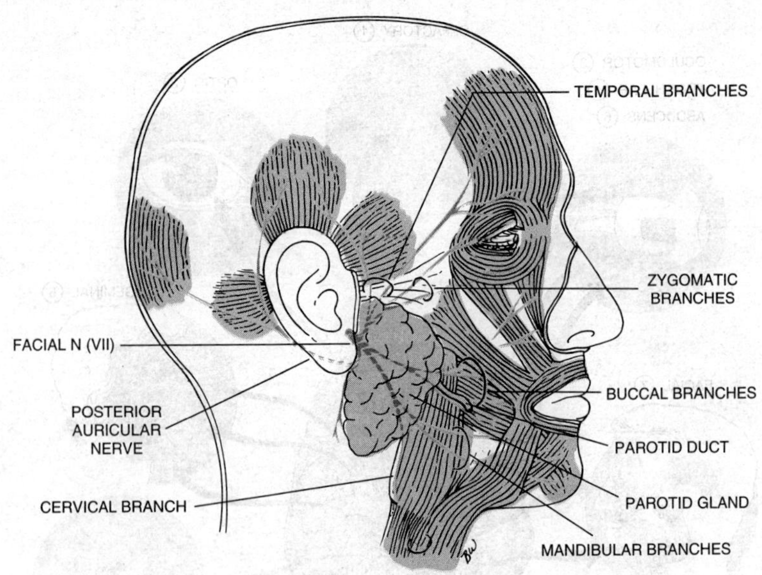

SUPERFICIAL BRANCHES OF FACIAL NERVE (7TH CRANIAL)

nial nerve, a mixed nerve with special sensory (taste), visceral sensory, and motor functions. It originates by several roots from the medulla oblongata. Its distribution covers the pharynx, ear, meninges, posterior third of the tongue, and parotid gland. Branches include the carotid, tympanic, pharyngeal, lingual, tonsillar nerves, and the sinus nerve of Hering. SEE: illus.

inhibitory n. A nerve whose stimulation lessens activity in a body part.

lumbar n. The five pairs of spinal nerves, corresponding with the lumbar vertebrae. All are mixed nerves.

median n. A combined motor and

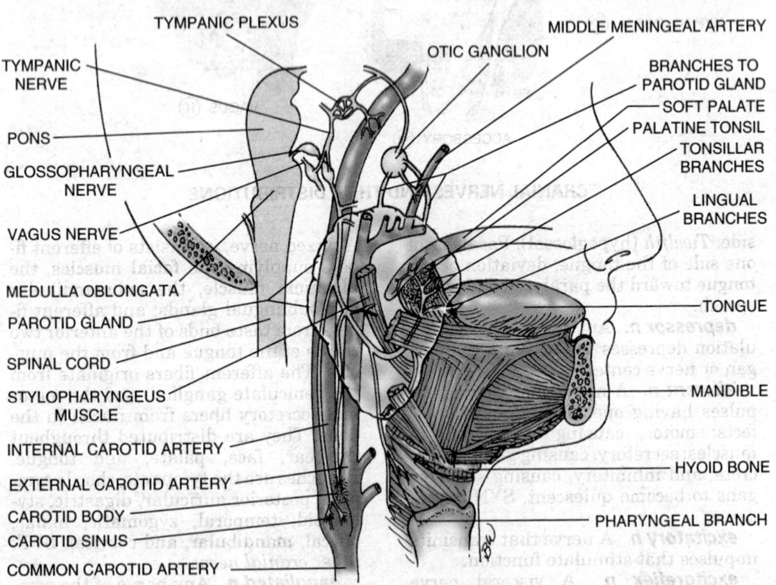

GLOSSOPHARYNGEAL NERVE

sensory nerve of the arm having its origin in the brachial plexus.

mixed n. A nerve containing both afferent (sensory) and efferent (motor) fibers.

motor n. A nerve that transmits impulses from the central nervous system to an effector. SYN: *efferent nerve.*

olfactory n. The first pair of cranial nerves. SEE: *olfactory nerves*.

optic n. The second pair of cranial nerves.

parasympathetic n. SEE: *parasympathetic nervous system.*

peripheral n. Any nerve that connects the brain or spinal cord with peripheral receptors or effectors.

phrenic n. A nerve arising in the cervical plexus, entering the thorax, and passing to the diaphragm; a motor nerve to the diaphragm with sensory fibers to the pericardium.

pilomotor n. A nerve that innervates the arrectores pilorum muscles of hair follicles.

pressor n. An afferent nerve whose stimulation excites the vasoconstrictor center, thus increasing the blood pressure.

secretory n. A nerve whose stimulation excites secretion in a gland or a tissue.

sensory n. A nerve conveying impulses from receptors to the central nervous system, or one composed of sensory neurons. SYN: *afferent nerve.*

somatic n. A nerve that innervates somatic structures. These include skeletal muscle (motor nerves) and receptors in skin, joints, and skeletal muscle (sensory nerves).

spinal n. One of 31 pairs of peripheral nerves that emerge from the spinal cord. Includes 8 cervical, 12 thoracic, 5 lumbar, 5 sacral, 1 coccygeal. SEE: *spinal nerve.*

splanchnic n. Any of the nerves from the thoracic sympathetic ganglia that supply the visceral organs.

sudomotor n. One of the nerves that supply sweat glands.

sympathetic n. Nerve of the sympathetic division of the autonomic nervous system. SEE: *autonomic nervous system*.

thoracic n. The 12 pairs of spinal nerves that emerge from the foramina between the thoracic vertebrae. All are mixed nerves.

trigeminal n. The fifth cranial and the most important sensory and motor nerve of the oral area. SEE: *cranial nerve.*

vagus n. The tenth cranial nerve. SEE: *vagus* for illus.

vasoconstrictor n. A nerve conducting impulses that bring about constriction of a blood vessel.

vasodilator n. A nerve conducting impulses that bring about dilation of a blood vessel.

vasomotor n. A nerve that controls the caliber of a blood vessel; a vasoconstrictor or vasodilator nerve.

vasosensory n. Any nerve providing sensory fibers for a vessel.

nerve block SEE: *block, nerve.*

nerve cell Neuron. The nerve cell consists of a cell body and its processes (an axon and one or more dendrites) extending from the cell body. The axon transmits nerve impulses and the dendrite(s) receives impulses and transmits them to the cell body. SEE: illus.

nerve ending The termination of a nerve fiber (axon or dendrite) in a peripheral structure. It may be sensory (receptor) or motor (effector). Sensory endings can be nonencapsulated (e.g., free nerve endings, peritrichal endings, or tactile corpuscles of Merkel) or they can be encapsulated (e.g., end-bulbs of Krause, Meissner's corpuscles, Vater-Pacini corpuscles, or neuromuscular and neurotendinous spindles).

nerve entrapment syndrome Compression of a nerve or nerves resulting in nerve damage. This may cause anesthesia or pain if a sensory nerve is affected and paralysis if a motor nerve is involved. The compression may be due to physical pressure on the nerve (i.e., sleeping in a position in which a nerve is pressed upon by surrounding tissue), or to swelling of tissue in a compartment through which the nerve passes. SEE: *carpal tunnel syndrome; muscle compartment syndrome.*

nerve fiber **1.** A neuron. **2.** The elongated process of a neuron, often the axon, concerned with the transmission of impulses. Nerve fibers form the major portion of the white matter of the brain and spinal cord and all nerves. Most fibers in peripheral nerves are myelinated; the myelin sheath is the layer of Schwann cell membranes wrapped around the process. Myelin is an electrical insulator. Spaces between adjacent Schwann cells are called nodes of Ranvier. The cytoplasm and nuclei of Schwann cells, outside the myelin sheath, are called the neurilemma, which is important in the regeneration of damaged neurons. Nerve fibers without a myelin sheath are called unmyelinated; such peripheral fibers may still have a neurilemma. Schwann cells are not found in the central nervous system (the myelin sheath is made by oligodendrocytes), so central nervous system fibers do not have a neurilemma.

adrenergic n.f. A nerve fiber that releases norepinephrine at its synapse when an impulse is transmitted. Most postganglionic fibers of the sympathetic division are adrenergic.

arcuate n.f. Any of the arch-shaped

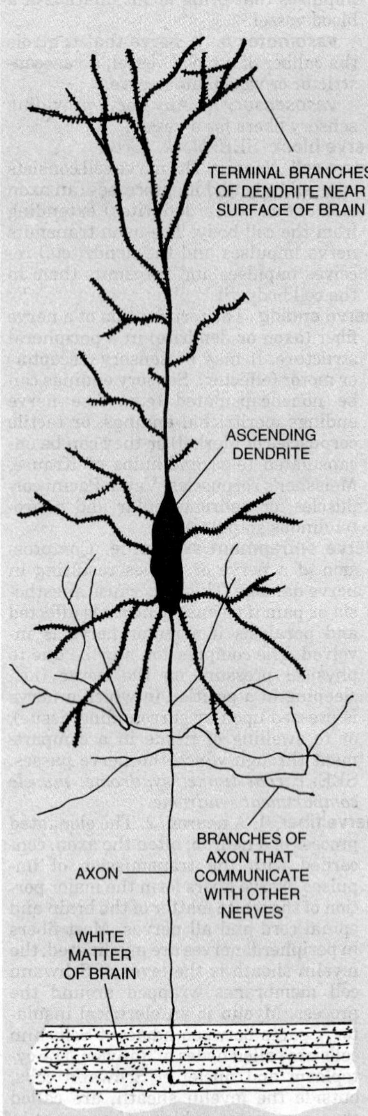

NERVE CELL FROM CEREBRAL CORTEX

nerve fibers in the medulla. They comprise three groups, the external dorsal, external ventral, and internal.

association n.f. A nerve fiber that connects one region of the cerebral cortex with another region in the same hemisphere.

cholinergic n.f. A nerve fiber that releases acetylcholine at its synapse when an impulse is transmitted. Sympathetic and parasympathetic preganglionic fibers, parasympathetic postganglionic fibers, and efferent somatic fibers ending in skeletal muscle are cholinergic.

climbing n.f. of the cerebellum **1.** Afferent nerve fibers entering the cortex and synapsing with dendrites of Purkinje cells. SYN: *mossy fibers*. **2.** Collateral branches of Purkinje cell axons that return to the molecular layer terminating about Purkinje or basket cell dendrites.

collateral n.f. A small branch extending at a right angle from an axon.

commissural n.f. A nerve fiber that passes from one cerebral hemisphere to the other.

medullated n.f. Myelinated nerve fiber.

myelinated n.f. A nerve fiber with a myelin sheath. SYN: Medullated *n.f.*

nonmyelinated n.f. A nerve fiber without a myelin sheath.

postganglionic n.f. A nerve fiber of the autonomic nervous system that terminates in smooth or cardiac muscle or in a gland. Its cell body lies in an autonomic ganglion.

preganglionic n.f. A nerve fiber of the autonomic nervous system that terminates and synapses in one of the autonomic ganglia. Its cell body lies in the brain or spinal cord.

projection n.f. **1.** A nerve fiber arising in the diencephalon and passing to the cerebral cortex. **2.** A nerve fiber arising in the cerebral cortex and terminating in lower portions of the brain or in the spinal cord.

nerve fibril Neurofibril.

nerve gas Gaseous materials used in chemical warfare. The agents may be stored in liquid form but are aerosolized at the time of use. These chemicals are readily absorbed through the skin. Some forms (organophosphates that inhibit acetylcholinesterase) cause copious secretions from the nose, eyes, mouth, lungs, and intestines. Muscle fasiculations, twitching, and miosis will result from exposure. A large dose may cause sudden unconsciousness, convulsions, flaccid paralysis, apnea, and death. With some agents, only a few breaths of the vapor may cause death.

PROTECTION: Charcoal-lined suits offer barrier protection. The agents will penetrate ordinary clothing worn with a gas mask.

TREATMENT: Pretreatment with pyridostigmine and concurrent treatment at the time of exposure with atropine, pralidoxime, and diazepam may be life-saving. Artificial respiration is mandatory. The skin should be decontaminated with household bleach diluted with water at a ratio of 1:10, or with soap and water, and the eyes should be irrigated with plain water. Military personnel carry small towels impregnated with chloramine, hydroxide, and phenol.

CAUTION: Gas masks should cover face and eyes and be proven to be adequately effective. Persons treating patients must protect themselves from contact with toxic chemicals on clothing, hair, and skin.

---

nerve growth factor ABBR: NGF. A protein necessary for the growth and maintenance of sympathetic and certain sensory neurons.

nerve impulse SEE: *impulse, nerve*.

nerve plexus SEE: under *plexus*.

nerve trunk The main stem of a peripheral nerve.

nervimotor (něr″vĭ-mō′tor) [″ + *motus*, moving] Pert. to a motor nerve.

nervone A cerebroside present in brain tissue. It contains nervonic acid.

nervous (něr′věs) [L. *nervosus*] **1.** Anxious. **2.** Characterized by excitability. **3.** Pert. to the nerves.

n. breakdown A lay term for any mental illness, esp. one with acute onset, that interferes with normal function, thought, or action.

n. debility Nervous fatigue with resultant physical exhaustion. SYN: *neurasthenia*.

n. prostration Neurasthenia.

n. tissue Tissue that makes up the nervous system, including neurons and neuroglia (Schwann cells, oligodendrocytes, and astrocytes).

nervousness Anxiety; tension.

nervous system One of the regulatory systems, made of millions of neurons in precise pathways to transmit electrochemical impulses, and of neuroglial cells that have several functions, including formation of myelin sheaths of neurons. It consists of the brain and spinal cord (central nervous system [CNS]) and the cranial nerves and spinal nerves (peripheral nervous system), which include the nerves of the autonomic nervous system and its ganglia. SEE: *autonomic nervous system; central nervous system*.

FUNCTION: Receptors detect external and internal changes and transmit impulses along sensory nerves to the CNS. Receptors are found in the skin, muscles and joints, viscera, and the organs of special sense: the eye, the ear, and the organs of taste and smell. The CNS uses this sensory information to initiate appropriate responses to changes; reflexes involving muscle contraction or glandular secretion, or voluntary movement, all mediated by motor nerves. A function specific to the brain is the integration, analysis, and storage of information for possible later use; this function is learning and memory.

nervus [L.] Nerve.

n. erigens A bundle of parasympathetic autonomic fibers originating from the 2nd to 4th sacral nerves and passing to terminal ganglia from which postganglionic fibers pass to the pelvic organs (bladder, colon, rectum, prostate gland, seminal vesicles, external genitalia).

n. intermedius A branch of the facial nerve consisting principally of sensory fibers.

n. nervorum Nerve fibers that innervate sheaths of nerves.

n. terminales A terminal nerve accompanying the olfactory nerve to the brain and consisting principally of sensory fibers from the mucosa of the nasal septum.

n. vasorum Nerve fibers that innervate the walls of blood vessels.

nesidioblastoma (nē-sĭd″ē-ō-blăs-tō′mă) [″ + *blastos*, germ, + *oma*, tumor] Islet-cell tumor of the pancreas.

nest A small cluster of unusual cells found within normal tissue. SYN: *rest* (4).

cancer n. A mass of cells extending from a common center seen in cancerous growths.

cell n. A mass of epithelial cells set apart from surrounding cells by connective tissue.

nesteostomy (něs″tē-ŏs′tō-mē) [Gr. *nestis*, jejunum, + *stoma*, mouth] Jejunostomy.

n. et m. *nocte et mane*, night and morning.

net reproductive rate ABBR: NRR. A measure of whether a population is reproducing at a greater or lesser rate than needed for its replacement. It is determined by calculating the average number of surviving daughters born to the women in that population during their reproductive years. An NRR of 1 indicates that each woman in the population has one surviving daughter during her lifetime.

ne tr. s. num. *ne tradas sine nummo*, do not deliver unless paid.

nettle [AS. *netel*] Any plant of the genus *Urtica*. A nettle's sawtoothed leaves contain hairs that secrete a fluid that irritates the skin.

n. rash A skin rash with intense itching, resembling the condition produced by stinging with nettles. SYN: *hives; urticaria*.

network [AS. *net*, net, + *wyrcan*, to work] Fiber arrangement in a structure resembling a net. SYN: *rete; reticulum*.

neural n. A form of artificial intelligence that relies on a group of interconnected mathematical equations that accept input data and that calculate an output. The more often the equations are used, the more reliable and valuable they become in drawing conclusions from data. Neural networks have been used in health care to interpret electrocardiograms and to make and suggest diagnoses.

Neuman, Betty Nursing educator, born 1924, who developed Neuman's systems model, a conceptual model of nursing. SEE: *Nursing Theory Appendix.*

N.'s systems model A conceptual model of nursing developed by Betty Neuman in which individuals and groups are considered client systems made up of physiological, psychological, sociocultural, developmental, and spiritual variables. The goal of nursing is to facilitate optimal wellness through retention, attainment, or maintenance of client system stability.

Neumann's disease (noy'mănz) [Isidor Neumann, Austrian dermatologist, 1832–1906] Pemphigus vegetans.

neur-, neuri-, neuro- Combining form denoting *nerve, nervous system.*

neurad (nū'răd) [Gr. *neuron,* nerve, sinew, + L. *-ad,* toward] Toward a nerve or its axis.

neuragmia (nū-răg'mē-ă) [Gr. *neuron,* nerve, sinew, + *agmos,* break] The tearing or rupturing of a nerve trunk.

neural (nū'răl) [L. *neuralis*] Pert. to nerves or connected with the nervous system.

n. crest A band of cells extending longitudinally along the neural tube of an embryo from which cells forming cranial, spinal, and autonomic ganglia arise, as well as to cells (ectomesenchyme) that migrate into the forming facial region and become odontoblasts, which form the dentin of the teeth.

n. fold One of two longitudinal elevations of the neural plate of an embryo that unite to form the neural tube.

n. grafting An experimental procedure for transplanting tissue into the brain and spinal cord. Possible sources of material to be used include human fetal tissue, cultured and genetically engineered cells, and tissues from the patient's own body.

n. plate A thickened band of ectoderm along the dorsal surface of an embryo. The nervous system develops from this tissue.

n. spine Spinous process of vertebrae.

neuralgia (nū-răl'jē-ă) [Gr. *neuron,* nerve, sinew, + *algos,* pain] Severe pain occurring along the course of a nerve. It is caused by pressure on nerve trunks, faulty nerve nutrition, toxins, or inflammation. SYN: *neurodynia.* SEE: *sciatica.* **neuralgic** (nū-răl'jĭk), *adj.*

cardiac n. Angina pectoris.

facial n. Trigeminal n.

geniculate n. Neuralgia characterized by pain over all or any area supplied by sensory fibers of the facial nerve. The pain may be deep in facial muscles, within the ear, or in the pharynx. SYN: *Hunt's n.*

glossopharyngeal n. Neuralgia along the course of the glossopharyngeal nerve, characterized by severe pain in back of the throat, tonsils, and middle ear.

hallucinatory n. An impression of local pain without an actual stimulus to cause the pain.

Hunt's n. Geniculate n.

idiopathic n. Neuralgia without structural lesion or pressure from a lesion.

intercostal n. Pain between the ribs. It is frequently associated with eruption of herpes zoster on the chest, and with costochondritis, an inflammatory condition of the ribs and their cartilage. SYN: *pleuralgia.*

mammary n. Neuralgia of the breast. SYN: *mastodynia.*

Morton's n. Neuralgia of the joint of the third and fourth toes. SYN: *metatarsalgia.*

nasociliary n. Neuralgia of the eyes, brows, and root of the nose.

occipital n. Neuralgia involving the upper cervical nerves. A spot of tenderness is found between the mastoid process and the upper cervical vertebrae. It may be due to spinal caries.

otic n. Geniculate n.

postherpetic n. Neuralgia following an attack of herpes zoster (shingles). It is caused by irritation of the nerve roots of the spinal cord. Treatments include gabapentin. SEE: *herpes zoster.*

reminiscent n. Continued mental perception of pain after neuralgia has ceased.

sphenopalatine n. Neuralgia of the sphenopalatine ganglion, causing pain in the area of the upper jawbone and radiating into the neck and shoulders. There is pain on one side of the face radiating to the eyeball, ear, and occipital and mastoid areas of the skull, and sometimes to the nose, upper teeth, and shoulder on the same side.

stump n. Neuralgia due to irritation of nerves at the site of an amputation.

symptomatic n. Neuralgia not primarily involving the nerve structure but occurring as a symptom of local or systemic disease.

trifacial n. Former term for trigeminal neuralgia.

trigeminal n. A disease of the trigeminal nerve marked by brief attacks of severe lightning-like stabs along the distribution of one or more of its branches, but usually along the maxillary nerve. The attacks last from a few seconds to 2 min, and may be triggered by touch, cold, chewing, brushing teeth, smiling, or talking. It occurs most frequently in persons over 40 and in women more often than men. SYN: *facial n.; tic doulou-*

reux. SEE: *Nursing Diagnoses Appendix.*

SYMPTOMS: Symptoms include episodes of facial pain, often accompanied by painful spasms of facial muscles. In long-standing cases, the hair on the affected side sometimes becomes coarse and bleached.

ETIOLOGY: The cause is thought to be the pressure of blood vessels on the trigeminal nerve root at its point of entrance into the brainstem.

TREATMENT: Carbamazepine in gradually increasing doses is often effective. If this is ineffective or unsuitable because of toxicity, then other anticonvulsant drugs may be used. Nerve block provides temporary relief. Surgical therapy may include techniques such as decompression of the nerve roots.

PATIENT CARE: The characteristics of each attack are observed and recorded. Analgesic drugs are administered as prescribed and observed for side effects. Before surgery is contemplated, an effort should be made to reduce factors that make symptoms worse (e.g., by having the patient use a cotton pad to cleanse the face and a blunt-toothed comb to comb the hair).

After surgery, sensory deficits are assessed to prevent trauma to the face and affected areas. The patient who has had an ophthalmic branch resection should examine the eye for foreign substances with a hand mirror frequently. The patient who has had a mandibular or maxillary branch resection should eat carefully to avoid oral injuries (e.g., by eating food on the unaffected side to prevent inner cheek injury). Frequent dental examinations detect abnormalities that the patient cannot feel.

neuralgiform (nū-răl′jĭ-form) [″ + ″ + L. *forma,* form] Similar to neuralgia.

neural tube Tube formed from fusion of the neural folds from which the brain and spinal cord arise.

n.t. defect ABBR: NTD. A group of congenital structural disorders that result from a failure of the embryonic neural tube to close during development. Cranial fusion disorders, including anencephaly and encephalocele, or spinal fusion disorders, including spina bifida, lumbar meningomyelocele, and meningocele, may occur as a consequence of this failure. The incidence of NTD in the U.S. is 1:1500 births. Although there may be a family history of such disorders, roughly 85% of affected infants are born to women who have not been considered at risk. Prenatal folic acid deficiency has been implicated in NTD, but other predisposing factors may be involved as well. To reduce the risk of NTDs, the U.S. Public Health Service recommends a daily folic acid intake of 0.4 mg for all women of childbearing age who are capable of getting pregnant. The importance of an adequate intake before pregnancy is predicated on the fact that damage to the developing embryo often occurs before the woman knows she is pregnant. The neural tube develops from the neural plate at 3 weeks' gestation. At 4 weeks' gestation, closure has been achieved except at the cranial and caudal ends; cranial closure occurs at 24 days and caudal closure at 26 days' gestation. SEE: *microencephaly; spina bifida cystica; spina bifida occulta.*

Elevated levels of maternal serum alpha-fetoprotein (MSAFP) are found in NTDs such as fetal anencephaly. Screening for MSAFP is done between 15 and 19 weeks' gestation. Alpha-fetoprotein also is found in amniotic fluid. The prognosis for infants born with NTDs depends on the area and the degree of involvement. Despite supportive care, some defects (such as anencephaly) are fatal shortly after birth. Others, such as myelomeningocele, may benefit from surgery done within 24 to 48 hr after birth; in some cases, however, surgery does not improve the deformity, disability, and chronic health problems that compromise the individual's quality of life.

neuraminidase (nūr-ăm′ĭn-ĭ-dās″) An enzyme present on the surface of influenza virus particles. The activity of this enzyme enables the virus to separate itself from cells. Persons with increased levels of antibodies against neuraminidase in their serum have increased resistance to influenza infection.

neurapophysis (nū″ră-pŏf′ĭ-sĭs) [″ + *apo,* from, + *physis,* growth] Either of the two sides of a vertebra that unite to form the neural arch.

neurarchy (nū′răr-kē) [″ + *arche,* rule] The domination of the nervous system over the body.

neurarthropathy (nū″răr-thrŏp′ă-thē) [″ + *arthron,* joint, + *pathos,* disease, suffering] Neuroarthropathy.

neurasthenia (nū″răs-thē′nē-ă) [″ + *astheneia,* weakness] An old term occasionally used to signify functional (psychosomatic) illness, marked by symptoms such as chronic fatigue, weakness, lassitude, noncardiogenic chest pain, panic attacks, irritability, anxiety, depression, headache, insomnia, joint and muscle discomfort, and sexual disorders. Contemporary terms that encompass the idea of neurasthenia include chronic fatigue, anxiety, fibromyalgia, depression, and dysphoria.

neurasthenic (nū-răs-thē′nĭk) **1.** Individual suffering from neurasthenia. **2.** Suffering from or concerning neurasthenia.

neuraxis (nū-răk′sĭs) [″ + L. *axon,* axis] The cerebrospinal axis.

neuraxon, neuraxone (nū-răks′ōn) A term that was formerly used to signify an axon.

neurectasia, neurectasis, neurectasy (nū″rĕk-tā′sē-ă, -rĕk′tă-sĭs, -rĕk′tă-sē) [″ + *ektasis,* a stretching] Surgical stretching of a nerve. SYN: *neurotension.*

neurectomy (nū-rĕk′tō-mē) [″ + *ektome,* excision] Partial or total excision or resection of a nerve.

presacral n. Surgical procedure for removing the hypogastric (presacral) nerve plexus. This is done to treat conditions such as dysmenorrhea and chronic idiopathic pelvic pain.

neurectopia, neurectopy (nū-rĕk-tō′pē-ă, nūr-ĕk′tō-pē) [″ + *ek,* out, + *topos,* place] Displacement or abnormal position of a nerve.

neurenteric (nū-rĕn-tĕr′ĭk) [″ + *enteron,* intestine] Relating to the neural canal and intestinal tube of the embryo.

n. canal A temporary canal in the vertebrate embryo between the neural and intestinal tubes. In human development, the temporary communication between cavities of the yolk sac and the amnion.

neurepithelium (nūr″ĕp-ĭ-thē′lē-ŭm) [″ + *epi,* upon, + *thele,* nipple] Neuroepithelium.

neurexeresis (nūr″ĕks-ĕr′ĕ-sĭs) [″ + *exairein,* to draw out] The tearing out of a nerve to relieve neuralgia.

neurilemma (nū′rĭ-lĕm″mă) [″ + *lemma,* husk] In the peripheral nervous system, the cytoplasm and nuclei of Schwann cells wrapped around the myelin sheath or the unmyelinated processes of nerve fibers. This contributes to regeneration of damaged nerve fibers by producing growth factors and serving as a tunnel or guide for regrowth. SYN: *neurolemma; Schwann's sheath.* SEE: *nerve fiber; neuron* for illus.

neurilemmitis (nū″rĭ-lĕm-mī′tĭs) [″ + ″ + *itis,* inflammation] Inflammation of a neurilemma.

neurilemmoma, neurilemoma (nū″rĭ-lĕm-ō′mă) [″ + *eilema,* tight sheath, + *oma,* tumor] A firm, encapsulated fibrillar tumor of a peripheral nerve. SYN: *neurinoma; neurofibroma; schwannoma.*

neurilemmosarcoma (nū″rĭ-lĕm″ō-săr-kō′mă) A malignant neurilemmoma.

neurimotor [″ + L. *motor,* a mover] Concerning a motor nerve.

neurinoma (nū-rĭ-nō′mă) [″ + *oma,* tumor] Neurilemmoma.

neurinomatosis (nū″rĭ-nō-mă-tō′sĭs) [″ + ″ + *osis,* condition] Neurofibromatosis.

neurite (nū′rīt) [Gr. *neuron,* nerve, sinew] Former word for axon.

neuritis (nū-rī′tĭs) [″ + *itis,* inflammation] Inflammation of a nerve, usually associated with a degenerative process. SEE: *Guillain-Barré syndrome; polyneuritis; Nursing Diagnoses Appendix.*

SYMPTOMS: There are many forms of neuritis, which produce a variety of symptoms, including neuralgia in the part affected, hyperesthesia, paresthesia, dysesthesia, hypesthesia, anesthesia, muscular atrophy of the body part supplied by the affected nerve, paralysis, and lack of reflexes.

ETIOLOGY: Neuritis may be caused by mechanical factors, such as compression or contusion of the nerve, or localized infection involving direct infection of a nerve. It may accompany diseases such as leprosy, tetanus, tuberculosis, malaria, or measles. Toxins, esp. poisoning by heavy metals (arsenic, lead, mercury), alcohol, or carbon tetrachloride, may be the causative factor. Neuritis may accompany thiamine deficiency, gastrointestinal dysfunction, diabetes, toxemias of pregnancy, or peripheral vascular disease.

PATIENT CARE: Changes in motor and sensory function are monitored. Correct positioning and prescribed analgesic drugs are used to relieve pain. Rest is provided, and affected extremities are rested by limiting their use and using supportive appliances. Passive range-of-motion exercises are performed to help prevent contracture formation. Skin care is provided, and proper nutrition and dietary therapy are prescribed for metabolic disorders. Health care providers remove causative factors or counsels the patient about their avoidance. After pain subsides, prescribed activities are performed, such as massage, electrostimulation, and exercise.

adventitial n. Inflammation of a nerve sheath.

ascending n. Neuritis moving upward along a nerve trunk away from the periphery.

axial n. Inflammation of the inner portion of a nerve.

degenerative n. Neuritis with rapid degeneration of a nerve.

descending n. Neuritis that leads away from the central nervous system toward the periphery.

diphtheritic n. Neuritis following diphtheria.

disseminated n. Neuritis involving a large group of nerves.

interstitial n. Neuritis involving the connective tissue of a nerve.

intraocular n. Neuritis of the retinal fibers of the optic nerve causing disturbed vision, contracted field, enlarged blind spot, and fundus findings such as exudates, hemorrhages, and abnormal condition of the blood vessels. Treatment depends on the etiology (e.g., brain tumor, meningitis, syphilis, nephritis, diabetes).

n. migrans Ascending or descending neuritis that passes along a nerve trunk, affecting one area and then another.

multiple n. Simultaneous impairment of a number of peripheral nerves. SYN: *polyneuritis*.

SYMPTOMS: Symptoms are related to the suddenness of onset and severity. Usually, lower limbs are affected first, with weakness that may progress until the entire body is affected. Muscle strength, deep tendon reflexes, sensory nerves, and autonomic nerves become involved.

ETIOLOGY: Causes include infectious diseases (e.g., diphtheria), metabolic disorders (e.g., alcoholism, diabetes, pellagra, beriberi, sprue), and various poisons, including lead. In some instances, the disease arises without apparent cause.

TREATMENT: Causative factors should be removed, if possible. Treatment includes skilled nursing, with particular care taken to prevent bedsores, and dietary therapy (depending upon the etiology).

n. nodosa Neuritis with formation of nodes on nerves.

optic n. Neuritis of the optic nerve with blindness, a finding that often precedes the development of multiple sclerosis.

parenchymatous n. Neuritis of nerve fiber substance.

peripheral n. Neuritis of terminal nerves or end organs.

retrobulbar n. Neuritis of the portion of the optic nerve behind the eyeball.

SYMPTOMS: The main symptom is acute loss of vision in one or both eyes. Pain may be absent or it may be unbearable, lasting for only a brief period or for days.

ETIOLOGY: This type of neuritis may be caused by a variety of illnesses, but in adults it is most frequently associated with multiple sclerosis.

rheumatic n. Neuritis with symptoms of rheumatism.

sciatic n. Inflammation of the sciatic nerve. SEE: *sciatica*.

segmental n. Neuritis affecting segments of a nerve interspersed with healthy segments.

sympathetic n. Neuritis of the opposite nerve without attack of the nerve center.

tabetic n. Neuritis in locomotor ataxia caused by syphilis.

toxic n. Neuritis resulting from metallic poisons (e.g., arsenic, mercury, and thallium) or nonmetallic poisons, such as various hydrocarbons and organic solvents.

traumatic n. Neuritis following an injury.

vestibular n. A condition marked by vertigo, nausea and vomiting, and gait disturbance of relatively acute onset, usually caused by inflammatory processes within the bony labyrinth of the ear.

neuro- [Gr. *neuron,* nerve, sinew] Combining form denoting *nerve, nervous tissue, nervous system.*

neuroablation The destruction or inactivation of nerve tissue, with surgery, cautery, injections of sclerosing agents, lasers, or cryotherapy.

neuroanastomosis (nū″rō-ă-năs″tō-mō′sĭs) [″ + *anastomosis,* opening] Surgical attachment of one end of a severed nerve to the other end.

neuroanatomy (nū″rō-ăn-ăt′ō-mē) The anatomy of the nervous system.

neuroarthropathy (nū″rō-ăr-thrŏp′ă-thē) [″ + ″ + *pathos,* disease, suffering] Disease of a joint associated with disease of the central nervous system.

neuroastrocytoma (nū″rō-ăs″trō-sī-tō′mă) [″ + *kytos,* cell, + *oma,* tumor] A tumor of the central nervous system composed of neurons and glial cells.

neuroaugmentation Any method used to increase the function of a nerve, esp. in managing pain. Transcutaneous electrical nerve stimulation has been used for this purpose.

neurobiology (nū″rō-bī-ŏl′ō-jē) [″ + *bios,* life, + *logos,* word, reason] Biology of the nervous system.

neurobiotaxis (nū″rō-bī-ō-tăk′sĭs) [″ + *bios,* life, + *taxis,* order] The phenomenon involving the growth of dendrites and the migration of nerve-cell bodies during development toward the region from which their dominant impulses are initiated.

neuroblast (nū′rō-blăst) [″ + *blastos,* germ] An embryonic cell derived from the neural tube or neural crest, giving rise to a neuron.

neuroblastoma (nū″rō-blăs-tō′mă) [″ + ″ + *oma,* tumor] A malignant hemorrhagic tumor composed principally of cells resembling neuroblasts that give rise to cells of the sympathetic system, esp. adrenal medulla. This tumor occurs chiefly in infants and children. The primary sites are in the mediastinal and retroperitoneal regions.

neurocanal (nū″rō-kă-năl′) [″ + L. *canalis,* passage] The central canal of the spinal cord.

neurocardiac (nū″rō-kăr′dē-ăk) [″ + *kardia,* heart] **1.** Pert. to the nerves supplying the heart or nervous system and the heart. **2.** Concerning a cardiac neurosis.

neurocardiogenic syncope SEE: *syncope, vasodepressor*.

neurocentral (nū″rō-sĕn′trăl) [″ + *kentron,* center] Pert. to the centrum of a vertebra and the neural arch.

neurocentrum (nū″rō-sĕn′trŭm) The body of a vertebra.

neurochemistry (nū″rō-kĕm′ĭs-trē) The chemistry of the nervous system.
neurochorioretinitis (nū″rō-kō″rē-ō-rĕ″tĭn-ī′tĭs) [Gr. *neuron,* nerve, sinew, + *chorion,* skin, + L. *retina,* retina, + Gr. *itis,* inflammation] Inflammation of choroid and retina combined with optic neuritis.
neurochoroiditis (nū″rō-kō-roy-dī′tĭs) [″ + ″ + *eidos,* form, shape, + *itis,* inflammation] Inflammation of the choroid coat and optic nerve.
neurocirculatory (nū″rō-sŭr′kū-lă-tō″rē) [″ + L. *circulatio,* circulation] Pert. to circulation and the nervous system.
neurocirculatory asthenia SYN: *asthenia.*
neurocladism (nū-rŏk′lă-dĭzm) [″ + *klados,* a young branch, + *-ismos,* condition] Phenomenon occurring after a nerve is severed, where an outgrowth of axons meet to re-establish the nerve's integrity. SYN: *odogenesis.*
neuroclonic (nū″rō-klŏn′ĭk) [″ + *klonos,* spasm] Marked by spasms of neural origin.
neurocranium (nū″rō-krā′nē-ŭm) [″ + *kranion,* skull] The part of the skull enclosing the brain.
neurocrine (nū′rō-krĭn) [″ + *krinein,* to secrete] **1.** Indicating an endocrine influence on nerves or the influence of nerves on endocrine tissue. **2.** A chemical transmitter.
neurocutaneous (nū″rō-kū-tā′nē-ŭs) [″ + L. *cutis,* skin] Pert. to the nervous system and skin.
neurocyte (nū′rō-sīt) [″ + *kytos,* cell] An outdated term for neuron.
neurocytolysis (nū″rō-sī-tŏl′ĭ-sĭs) [″ + *kytos,* cell, + *lysis,* dissolution] Dissolution or destruction of nerve cells.
neurocytoma (nū″rō-sī-tō′mă) [″ + ″ + *oma,* tumor] A tumor formed of cells of nervous origin (usually ganglionic). SEE: *neuroma.*
neurodealgia (nū-rō″dē-ăl′jē-ă) [Gr. *neurodes,* retina, + *algos,* pain] Pain in the retina.
neurodegenerative Concerning wasting, necrosis, or deterioration of nerves, neurons, or the nervous system.
neurodendrite, neurodendron (nū″rō-dĕn′drīt, -drŏn) [Gr. *neuron,* nerve, sinew, + *dendron,* tree] Cytoplasmic branched process of a nerve cell. SYN: *dendrite; dendron.* SEE: *dendrite* for illus.
neurodermatitis (nū″rō-dĕr-mă-tī′tĭs) [″ + *derma,* skin, + *itis,* inflammation] Cutaneous inflammation with itching that is associated with, but not entirely due to, emotional stress. After an initial irritant, scratching becomes a habit and prolongs the condition. Treatment is corticosteroid ointment or cream. Circumscribed neurodermatitis is used as a synonym for lichen simplex chronicus. SEE: illus.

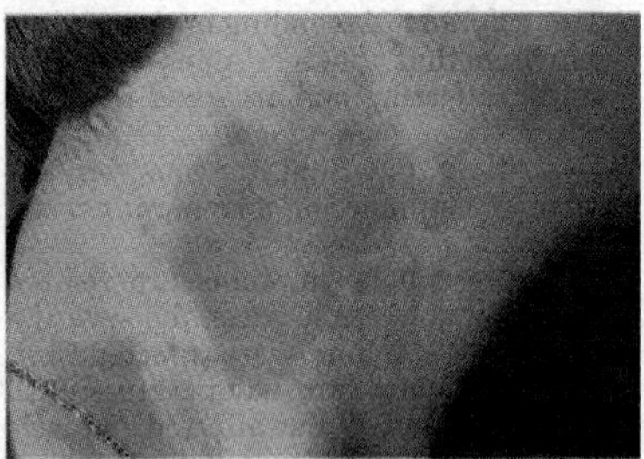

NEURODERMATITIS ON NECK

disseminated n. Chronic superficial inflammation of the skin characterized by thickening, excoriation, and lichenification, usually beginning in infancy. It is common in families with a high incidence of allergic diseases. SYN: *atopic dermatitis.*
neurodermatosis (nū″rō-dĕr-mă-tō′sĭs) [″ + ″ + *osis,* condition] Any skin disease of neural origin, including neurofibromatosis, von Hippel-Lindau disease, Sturge-Weber syndrome, and tuberous sclerosis. SYN: *phacomatosis.*
neurodermatrophia (nū″rō-dĕrm″ă-trōf′ē-ă) Atrophy of the skin from nervous disease.
neurodevelopmental treatment ABBR: NDT. A rehabilitation treatment approach for cerebral palsy, hemiplegia, and other central nervous system deficits that emphasizes the use of carefully considered handling to inhibit abnormal reflexes and movement patterns and facilitate higher level reactions and patterns in order to attain normal movement. This method was developed by Karel and Bertha Bobath, contemporary German physiotherapists working in England.
neurodiagnosis (nū″rō-dī-ăg-nō′sĭs) Diagnosis of neurological disorders.
neurodynamic (nū″rō-dī-năm′ĭk) Pert. to nervous energy.
neurodynia (nū″rō-dĭn′ē-ă) [Gr. *neuron,* nerve, + *odyne,* pain] Pain in a nerve. SYN: *neuralgia.*
neuroectoderm (nū″rō-ĕk′tō-dĕrm) [″ + *ektos,* outside, + *derma,* skin] The embryonic tissue that gives rise to nerve tissue.
neuroencephalomyelopathy (nū″rō-ĕn-sĕf″ă-lō-mī″ĕ-lŏp′ă-thē) [″ + *enkephalos,* brain, + *myelos,* marrow, + *pathos,* disease, suffering] Disease of the brain, spinal cord, and nerves.
neuroendocrine (nū″rō-ĕn′dō-krĭn) Pert. to the nervous and endocrine systems as an integrated functioning mechanism.
n. carcinoma A diverse group of tumors, such as carcinoid, islet cell tumors, neuroblastoma, and small-cell carcinomas of the lung. All have dense core granules and produce polypeptides

that can be identified by immunochemical methods.

neuroendocrinology (nū″rō-ĕn″dō-krĭ-nŏl′ō-jē) [″ + *endon,* within, + *krinein,* to secrete, + *logos,* word, reason] The study of the relationship between the nervous and endocrine systems.

neuroenteric (nū″rō-ĕn-tĕr′ĭk) Concerning the nervous system and the intestines.

neuroepidermal (nū″rō-ĕp-ĭ-dĕr′măl) [″ + *epi,* upon, + *derma,* skin] Pert. to or giving rise to the nervous system and epidermis.

neuroepithelioma (nū″rō-ĕp″ĭ-thē-lē-ō′mă) [″ + ″ + *thele,* nipple, + *oma,* tumor] A relatively rare tumor of the neuroepithelium in a nerve of special sense.

neuroepithelium (nū″rō-ĕp″ĭ-thē′lē-ŭm) **1.** A specialized epithelial structure forming the termination of a nerve of special sense, including gustatory cells, olfactory cells, hair cells of the inner ear, and the rods and cones of the retina. **2.** The embryonic layer of the epiblast from which the cerebrospinal axis is developed. SYN: *neurepithelium.*

neurofibril, neurofibrilla (nū-rō-fī′brĭl, -fī-brĭl′ă) [″ + L. *fibrilla,* a small fiber] Any of the many tiny fibrils that extend in every direction in the cytoplasm of the nerve cell body. They extend into the axon and dendrites of the cell. SEE: *neuron.*

neurofibroma (nū″rō-fī-brō′mă) *pl.* **neurofibromata, -mas** [Gr. *neuron,* nerve, + L. *fibra,* fiber, + Gr. *oma,* tumor] A tumor of the connective tissue (esp. Schwann cells) of a nerve. SYN: *fibroneuroma.*

neurofibromatosis (nū″rō-fī-brō″mă-tō′sĭs) [″ + ″ + ″ + *osis,* condition] A group of genetic disorders that affects the cell growth of neural tissues. For those persons with affected family members, genetic assessment and counseling of parents may be indicated. Genetic assessment and counseling can identify the parents' risk of being a gene carrier and passing the disease on to subsequent offspring. SYN: *Recklinghausen's disease.*

type 1 n. ABBR: NF-1. An autosomal dominant disease that affects about 1 in 3000 persons. Its clinical hallmarks include hyperpigmented macules on the skin (café au lait spots) and multiple cutaneous and subcutaneous tumors that appear in late childhood (there may be only a few or thousands). When the tumors are pressed, they pass through a small opening in the skin, leaving the space previously occupied vacant. This characteristic, called buttonholing, helps to distinguish these tumors from lipomas. In about 2% to 5% of cases, the tumors become malignant. No cure has yet been found. Tumors that give rise to symptoms or those that become malignant should be excised; however, if the tumor is on a vital nerve, excision may be impossible. Radiation therapy and surgery are of benefit.

type 2 n. ABBR: NF-2. An autosomal dominant disease, affecting 1 in 50,000 persons, that causes intracranial and spinal tumors, esp. of the eighth cranial nerve. Although the disease is incurable, its symptoms can be palliated with multidisciplinary care.

neurofibrosarcoma (nū″rō-fī″brō-săr-kō′mă) [″ + ″ + Gr. *sarx,* flesh, + *oma,* tumor] A malignant neurofibroma.

neurofibrositis (nū″rō-fī″brō-sī′tĭs) [″ + ″ + Gr. *itis,* inflammation] Inflammation of nerve fibers and sensory nerve fibers in muscular tissue.

neurogangliitis (nū″rō-găn-glē-ī′tĭs) [″ + *ganglion,* knot, + *itis,* inflammation] Inflammation of a neuroganglion.

neuroganglion (nū″rō-găn′glē-ōn) A group of neuron cell bodies outside the central nervous system.

neurogastric (nū″rō-găs′trĭk) [″ + *gaster,* belly] Concerning the nerves of the stomach.

neurogenesis (nū″rō-jĕn′ĕ-sĭs) [″ + *genesis,* generation, birth] **1.** Growth or development of nerves. **2.** Development from nervous tissue. **neurogenetic** (nū″rō-jĕn-ĕt′ĭk), *adj.*

neurogenic, neurogenous (nū-rō-jĕn′ĭk, -rŏj′ĕn-ŭs) **1.** Originating from nervous tissue. **2.** Due to or resulting from nerve impulses.

neuroglia (nū-rŏg′lē-ă) [″ + *glia,* glue] The interstitial and supporting tissue of the nervous system, also called glia. The cells, of ectodermal origin, are astrocytes, oligodendrocytes, satellite cells, ependymal cells, and Schwann cells. Microglia are phagocytic cells that defend nerve tissue from injury or infection. **neuroglial** (nū-rŏg′lē-ăl), *adj.*

neurogliacyte (nū-rŏg′lē-ă-sīt) [″ + ″ + *kytos,* cell] Any of the cells found in neuroglial tissue. SYN: *glia cell.*

neuroglioma (nū″rō-glī-ō′mă) [Gr. *neuron,* nerve, + *glia,* glue, + *oma,* tumor] A tumor composed of neuroglial tissue. SYN: *glioma.*

n. ganglionare A glioma containing ganglion cells. SYN: *ganglioneuroma.*

neurogliomatosis (nū″rō-glī″ō-mă-tō′sĭs) [″ + ″ + ″ + *osis,* condition] Multiple glioma formation in the nervous system.

neurogliosis (nū-rŏg″lē-ō′sĭs) [″ + ″ + *osis,* condition] Development of numerous neurogliomas.

neuroglycopenia Hypoglycemia of sufficient duration and degree to interfere with normal brain metabolism. Patients with an insulinoma or hypoglycemia due to an insulin overdose may have this condition, which produces confusion, agitation, coma, or brain damage. SYN: *glucopenic brain injury.*

neurohistology (nū″rō-hĭs-tŏl′ō-jē) [″ + *histos,* tissue, + *logos,* study] Branch of histology concerned with the study of the microscopic anatomy of nervous tissue.

neurohypophysis (nū″rō-hī-pŏf′ĭs-ĭs) [″ + *hypo,* under, + *physis,* growth] Posterior pituitary gland (pars nervosa).

neurokeratin (nū″rō-kĕr′ă-tĭn) [″ + *keras,* horn] The type of keratin found in myelinated nerve fibers.

neurolemma Neurilemma.

neurolemmitis (nū″rō-lĕ-mī′tĭs) [″ + *lemma,* husk, + *itis,* inflammation] Neurilemmitis.

neurolemmoma (nū″rō-lĕ-mō′mă) [″ + ″ + *oma,* tumor] Neurilemmoma.

neuroleptanesthesia (nū″rō-lĕp″tăn-ĕs-thē′zē-ă) [″ + *leptos,* slender, + *-an,* not, + *aisthesis,* sensation] General anesthesia involving intravenous administration of a neuroleptic drug and an analgesic.

neuroleptic (nū″rō-lĕp′tĭk) [″ + *lepsis,* a taking hold] **1.** Any drug that modifies or treats psychotic behaviors, usually by blocking dopamine receptors in the brain. Examples include haloperidol (a butyrophenone), thorazine (a phenothiazine), and clozapine (a tricylic dibenzodiazepine). **2.** A condition produced by a neuroleptic agent.

n. anesthesia SEE: *anesthesia, neuroleptic.*

n. malignant syndrome ABBR: NMS. A potentially fatal syndrome marked by hyperthermia, catatonic rigidity, altered mental status, profuse sweating, and occasionally rhabdomyolysis, renal failure, seizures, and death. It typically occurs after exposure to drugs that alter levels of dopamine in the brain (such as antipsychotic agents) or after the withdrawal of agents that increase central nervous system dopamine levels (such as levodopa/carbidopa). The mortality rate may be as high as 30%. Antipyretics, curare-based paralytic drugs, bromocriptine, and dantrolene are used to treat the syndrome. SEE: *hyperpyrexia, malignant.*

neurologist (nū-rŏl′ō-jĭst) A specialist in diseases of the nervous system.

neurology (nū-rŏl′ō-jē) [″ + *logos,* word, reason] The branch of medicine that deals with the nervous system and its diseases. **neurologic, neurological** (nū-rō-lŏj′ĭk, -ĭ-kăl), *adj.*

clinical n. The branch of medicine concerned with the study and treatment of people with diseases of the nervous system.

neurolymphomatosis (nū″rō-lĭm″fō-mă-tō′sĭs) [″ + L. *lympha,* lymph, + Gr. *oma,* tumor, + *osis,* condition] Malignant lymphoma involving the nervous system.

neurolysin (nū-rŏl′ĭs-ĭn) [″ + *lysis,* dissolution] A substance that destroys nerve cells.

neurolysis (nū-rŏl′ĭs-ĭs) **1.** The stretching of a nerve to relieve pain. **2.** The loosening of adhesions surrounding a nerve. **3.** The disintegration or destruction of nerve tissue. **neurolytic** (nū-rō-lĭt′ĭk), *adj.*

neuroma (nū-rō′mă) [″ + *oma,* tumor] Former term for any type of tumor composed of nerve cells. Classification is now made with respect to the specific portion of the nerve involved. SEE: *ganglioneuroma; neurilemmoma.* **neuromatous** (nū-rō′mă-tŭs), *adj.*

acoustic n. A benign tumor of the eighth cranial nerve. The symptoms may include hearing loss, balance disturbances, pain, headache, and tinnitus. SEE: illus.

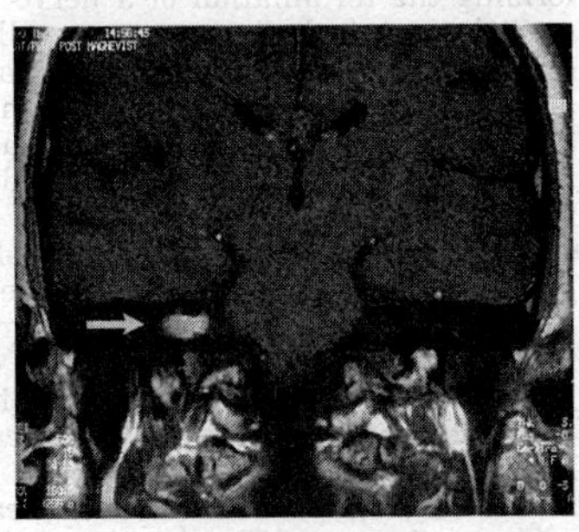

ACOUSTIC NEUROMA

Coronal section

amputation n. Neuroma occurring on the nerves of a stump after amputation.

amyelinic n. Neuroma composed principally of unmyelinated nerve fibers.

appendiceal n. Neuroma found in the mucosa and submucosa of the appendix.

n. cutis Neuroma in the skin.

cystic n. Neuroma with cystic formations.

false n. A tumor arising from the connective tissue of nerves, including the myelin sheath. SYN: *neurofibroma; pseudoneuroma.*

ganglionated n. Neuroma composed of true nerve cells.

multiple n. Neurofibromatosis.

myelinic n. Neuroma composed of medullated nerve fibers.

plexiform n. Neuroma of nerve trunks that appear to be twisted.

n. telangiectodes Neuroma containing an abundance of blood vessels.

traumatic n. An unorganized mass of nerve fibers occurring in wounds or on an amputation stump, resulting after accidental or intentional incision of the nerve.

neuromalacia (nū″rō-măl-ā′sē-ă) [″ + *malakia,* softening] Pathological softening of neural tissue.

neuromatosis (nū-rō″mă-tō′sĭs) [″ + *oma,* tumor, + *osis,* condition] A condition characterized by the occurrence of multiple neuromas in the body.

neuromere (nū′rō-mēr) [″ + *meros,* part] One of a series of segmental elevations on the ventrolateral surface of the rhombencephalon. SYN: *rhombomere.*

neuromodulator Biologically active substances produced by neurons that enhance or diminish the effects of neurotransmitters. Some neuromodulators are substance P, cholecystokinin, and somatostatin. SEE: *neuron; neurotransmitter.*

neuromuscular (nū″rō-mŭs′kū-lăr) [″ + L. *musculus,* a muscle] Concerning both nerves and muscles.

n. blocking agent A drug that causes muscle paralysis by blocking the transmission of nerve stimuli to muscles. It is esp. useful as an adjunct to anesthesia to induce skeletal muscle relaxation, to facilitate the management of patients undergoing mechanical ventilation, and to facilitate tracheal intubation. It is also used to treat status epilepticus and to reduce metabolic demands by preventing shivering or muscle rigidity.

CAUTION: This drug may cause respiratory depression and should be administered only by persons who regularly manage respiratory failure with artificial ventilation.

---

neuromyasthenia (nū″rō-mī″ăs-thē′nē-ă) [″ + *mys,* muscle, + *astheneia,* weakness] An obsolete term for muscular weakness due to an emotional disorder.

neuromyelitis (nū″rō-mī-ĕl-ī′tĭs) [″ + *myelos,* marrow, + *itis,* inflammation] Inflammation of nerves and the spinal cord.

n. optica A rare syndrome in which there is a severe transverse myelitis and optic nerve damage, probably as a result of immunological injury to the optic nerve and spinal cord. It shares some features with multiple sclerosis (predilection for young women, demyelination of nerve cells) but is believed to be a distinct disease.

neuromyopathy (nū″rō-mī-ŏp′ă-thē) [″ + *mys,* muscle, + *pathos,* disease, suffering] Pert. to pathological conditions involving both muscles and nerves.

neuromyositis (nū″rō-mī″ō-sī′tĭs) [″ + ″ + *itis,* inflammation] Neuritis complicated by inflammation of muscles that come in contact with the affected nerves.

neuron (nū′rŏn) [Gr. *neuron,* nerve, sinew] A nerve cell, the structural and functional unit of the nervous system. A neuron consists of a cell body (perikaryon) and its processes, an axon and one or more dendrites. Neurons function in initiation and conduction of impulses. They transmit impulses to other neurons or cells by releasing neurotransmitters at synapses. Alternatively, a neuron may release neurohormones into the bloodstream. SYN: *nerve cell.* SEE: illus. **neuronal** (nū′rō-năl), *adj.*

afferent n. A neuron that conducts sensory impulses toward the brain or spinal cord.

associative n. A neuron that mediates impulses between a sensory and a motor neuron.

bipolar n. **1.** A neuron that bears two processes. **2.** A neuron of the retina that receives impulses from the rods and cones and transmits them to a ganglion neuron. SEE: *retina* for illus.

central n. A neuron confined entirely to the central nervous system.

commissural n. A neuron whose axon crosses to the opposite side of the brain or spinal cord.

efferent n. A neuron that conducts motor impulses away from the brain or spinal cord.

ganglion n. A neuron of the retina that receives impulses from bipolar neurons. Axons of ganglion neurons converge at the optic disk to form the optic nerve. SEE: *retina* for illus.

internuncial n. Interneuron.

lower motor n. A peripheral motor neuron that originates in the ventral horns of the gray matter of the spinal cord and terminate in skeletal muscles. Lesions of these neurons produce flaccid paralysis of the muscles they innervate. SYN: *lower motoneruon.*

motor n. A neuron that carries impulses from the central nervous system either to muscle tissue to stimulate contraction or to glandular tissue to stimulate secretion. SYN: *motoneuron.*

multipolar n. A neuron with one axon and many dendrites.

peripheral n. A neuron whose process constitutes a part of the peripheral nervous system (cranial, spinal, or autonomic nerves).

peripheral motor n. A motor neuron that transmits impulses to skeletal muscle. SYN: *peripheral motoneuron.*

postganglionic n. A neuron whose cell body lies in an autonomic ganglion and whose axon terminates in an effector organ (smooth or cardiac muscle or glands).

preganglionic n. A neuron of the autonomic nervous system whose cell body lies in the central nervous system and whose axon terminates in a peripheral ganglion.

sensory n. An afferent neuron that

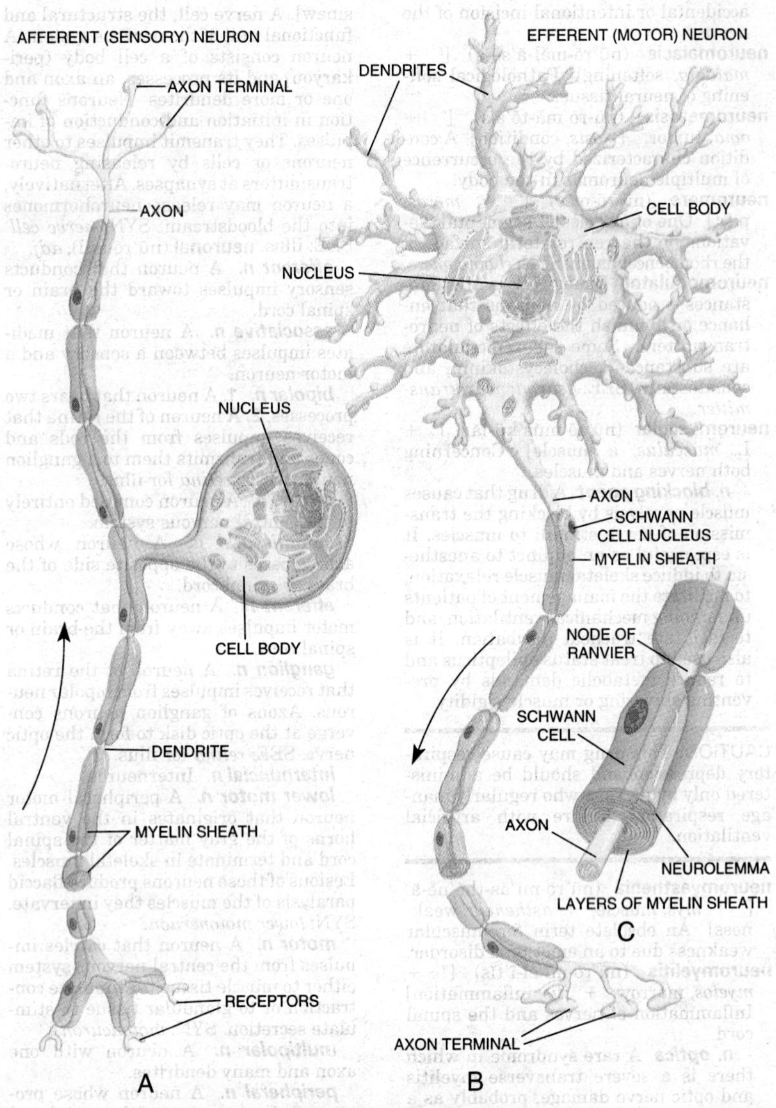

NEURON STRUCTURE

(A) sensory neuron, (B) motor neuron (arrows indicate direction of impulse transmission), (C) myelin sheath and neurolemma formed by Schwann cells

carries impulses from receptors to the central nervous system.

unipolar n. A neuron whose cell body bears one process.

upper motor n. A motor neuron (actually an interneuron) found completely within the central nervous system, that synapses with or regulates the actions of lower motor neurons in the spinal cord and cranial nerves. Lesions of these neurons produce spastic paralysis in the muscles they innervate. SYN: *upper motoneuron.*

neuronephric (nū″rō-něf′rĭk) [″ + *nephros,* kidney] Concerning the nervous and renal systems.

neuronevus (nū″rō-nē′vŭs) An intradermal nevus.

neuronitis (nū-rō-nī′tĭs) [Gr. *neuron,* nerve, + *itis,* inflammation] Inflammation or degenerative inflammation of nerve cells.

neuronophage (nū-rŏn′ō-făj) [″ + *phagein,* to eat] A phagocyte that destroys tissue in the nervous system.

neuronophagia, neuronophagy (nū-rŏn″ō-fā′jē-ă, -ŏf′ă-jē) Destruction of nerve cells by phagocytes.

neuro-ophthalmology (nū″rō-ŏf″thăl-mŏl′ŏ-jē) [″ + *ophthalmos,* eye, + *logos,* word, reason] The branch of ophthalmology concerned with the neurology of the visual system.

neuro-optic (nū″rō-ŏp′tĭk) [″ + *optikos,* pert. to vision] Concerning the central nervous system and the eye.

neuropacemaker An implantable device used to stimulate the brain or spinal cord (e.g., in the management of motor movement disorders or chronic and intractable pain). The electrical energy is provided in pulses at an appropriate rate to inhibit the perception of pain.

neuropapillitis (nū″rō-păp″ĭ-lī′tĭs) [″ + L. *papilla,* nipple, + Gr. *itis,* inflammation] Optic neuritis.

neuropathogenesis (nū″rō-păth″ō-jĕn′ĕ-sĭs) [″ + *pathos,* disease, suffering, + *genesis,* generation, birth] The origin and development of a neural disease.

neuropathogenicity (nū″rō-păth″ō-jĕ-nĭs′ĭ-tē) [″ + *pathos,* disease, suffering, + *gennan,* to produce] The ability to cause pathological changes in nerves.

neuropathology (nū″rō-pă-thŏl′ō-jē) [″ + ″ + *logos,* word, reason] The study of diseases of the nervous system and the structural and functional changes occurring in them. The diseases are divided into (1) congenital defects in development, those in which a degeneration reveals itself only after a period of time, and (2) those in which destructive influences act upon a brain that was initially normal. The latter are mainly vascular, inflammatory, toxic, traumatic, mechanical, or neoplastic.

neuropathy (nū-rŏp′ă-thē) Any disease of the nerves. **neuropathic** (nū-rō-păth′ĭk), *adj.*

ascending n. Pathological condition of the nervous system that ascends from the lower part of the body to the upper.

descending n. Pathological condition of the nervous system that descends from the upper part of the body to the lower.

diabetic n. Damage to autonomic, motor, and/or sensory nerves that results from metabolic or vascular derangements in patients with long-standing diabetes mellitus. Symptoms of this condition may include loss of sensation (or unpleasant sensations) in the feet, loss of the ability to maintain postural blood pressures, or focal sensory or motor deficits. Sensory loss in the feet may result in undetected injuries that become infected or gangrenous.

TREATMENT: Tight control of blood sugar levels may prevent some neuropathic symptoms in patients with diabetes mellitus.

entrapment n. Nerve entrapment syndrome.

glue-sniffer's n. Malfunction of sensory and motor nerves, as a result of inhaling toxic hydrocarbons. The lower extremities and trigeminal nerve are most often damaged.

multifocal motor n. An asymmetrical motor weakness occasionally found in middle-aged men.

optic n. Pathological injury to the optic nerves or the blood supply to them. Usually, only one eye is affected. Several forms have been described, including ischemic optic neuropathy, which if prolonged leads to blindness in the affected eye, optic neuritis due to acute demyelination of optic nerve fibers, infiltrative optic neuropathy, in which the optic nerve is compressed by a tumor or aneurysm, and optic neuropathy due to toxic nutritional factors (e.g., methanol or a combined nutritional and vitamin deficiency).

peripheral n. Any syndrome in which muscle weakness, paresthesias, impaired reflexes, and autonomic symptoms in the hands and feet are common. This syndrome occurs in patients with diabetes mellitus, renal or hepatic failure, alcoholism, or in persons who take certain medications such as phenytoin and isoniazid. Also called *polyneuritis; polyneuropathy.*

neuropharmacology (nū″rō-făr″mă-kŏl′ō-jē) [″ + *pharmakon,* drug, + *logos,* word, reason] The branch of pharmacology concerned with the effects of drugs on the nervous system.

neurophilic (nū″rō-fĭl′ĭk) [″ + *philos,* fond] Having an affinity for nervous tissue.

neurophonia (nū″rō-fō′nē-ă) [Gr. *neuron,* nerve, + *phone,* voice] A tic or spasm of the muscles of speech resulting in an involuntary cry or sound.

neurophthalmology (nū″rŏf-thăl-mŏl′ō-jē) [″ + *ophthalmos,* eye, + *logos,* word, reason] Neuro-ophthalmology.

neurophysin (nū″rō-fī′zĭn) Proteins secreted by the hypothalamus that are involved in the transport of oxytocin and antidiuretic hormone (vasopressin).

neurophysiological treatment approach In occupational and physical therapy, various techniques used in sensorimotor rehabilitation that rely on voluntary and involuntary activation, facilitation, and inhibition of muscle action through the reflex arc.

neurophysiology (nū″rō-fĭz-ē-ŏl′ō-jē) [″ + *physis,* growth, + *logos,* word, reason] Physiology of the nervous system.

neuropil (nū′rō-pĭl) [″ + *pilos,* felt] A network of unmyelinated fibrils into which the nerve processes of the central nervous system divide.

neuroplasm (nū′rō-plăzm) [″ + LL. *plasma,* form, mold] The cytoplasm of a neuron. **neuroplasmic** (nū″rō-plăz′mĭk), *adj.*

neuroplasticity (nū′rō-plăs-tĭs″ĭ-tē) The ability of the nervous system to adapt to trauma or disease; the ability of nerve cells to grow and form new connections to other neurons.

neuroplasty (nū′rō-plăs″tē) [″ + *plassein,* to form] Plastic surgery of the nerves.

neuropodium (nū″rō-pō′dē-ŭm) *pl.* **neuropodia** [″ + *podion,* little feet] The expanded tips of the axon terminals at a synapse.

neuropore (nū′rō-por″) [″ + *poros,* an opening] Embryonic opening from the neural canal to the exterior.

neuroprotection The science of minimizing secondary neurologic damage following stroke or trauma. Certain drugs, enzymes, hormones, and physical agents such as hypothermia may act as neuroprotectors.

neuropsychiatrist (nū″rō-sī-kī′ă-trĭst) [″ + *psyche,* mind, + *iatreia,* healing] A specialist in neuropsychiatry.

neuropsychiatry (nū″rō-sī-kī′ă-trē) The branch of medicine concerned with the study and treatment of both neurological and psychiatric diseases.

neuropsychopharmacology (nū″rō-sī″kō-făr″mă-kŏl′ō-jē) [″ + ″ + *pharmakon,* drug, + *logos,* word, reason] The study of the effects of drugs on mental illness.

neuroradiography (nū″rō-rā″dē-ŏg′ră-fē) [″ + L. *radius,* ray, + Gr. *graphein,* to write] Radiography of the structures of the nervous system.

neuroradiology (nū″rō-rā″dē-ŏl′ō-jē) [″ + ″ + Gr. *logos,* word, reason] The branch of medicine that utilizes radiography for diagnosis of pathology of the nervous system.

neuroretinitis (nū″rō-rĕt″ĭn-ī′tĭs) [″ + L. *retina,* retina, + Gr. *itis,* inflammation] Inflammation of the optic nerve and retina.

neuroretinopathy (nū″rō-rĕt″ĭ-nŏp′ă-thē) [″ + ″ + Gr. *pathos,* disease, suffering] Pathology of the retina and optic nerve.

neurorrhaphy (nū-ror′ă-fē) [″ + *rhaphe,* seam, ridge] The suturing of the ends of a severed nerve.

neurosarcocleisis (nū″rō-săr″kō-klī′sĭs) [″ + *sarx,* flesh, + *kleisis,* closure] Operation for the relief of neuralgia by resection of a wall of the osseous canal carrying a nerve and transplanting the nerve to soft tissues.

neurosarcoma (nū″rō-săr-kō′mă) [″ + ″ + *oma,* tumor] A sarcoma containing neuromatous components.

neuroscience (nū″rō-sī′ĕns) Any one of the various branches of science (e.g., embryology, anatomy, physiology, histopathology, biochemistry, pharmacology) concerned with the growth, development, and function of the nervous system.

neurosclerosis (nū″rō-sklĕ-rō′sĭs) [″ + *sklerosis,* a hardening] Hardening of nerves.

neurosecretion (nū″rō-sē-krē′shŭn) [″ + L. *secretio,* separation] The manufacture and discharge of chemicals by neurons, such as the secretion of hormones by cells of the hypothalamus or anterior pituitary.

neurosensory (nū″rō-sĕn′sō-rē) [″ + L. *sensorius,* pert. to a sensation] Concerning a sensory nerve.

neurosis (nū-rō′sĭs) *pl.* **neuroses** [″ + *osis,* condition] **1.** In traditional (e.g., Freudian) psychiatry, an unconscious conflict that produces anxiety and other symptoms and leads to maladaptive use of defense mechanisms. **2.** An unpleasant or maladaptive psychological disorder that may affect personality, mood, or certain limited aspects of behavior but that does not distract the affected individual from carrying out most activities of daily living. **3.** A term formerly used to describe anxiety disorders, phobias, obsessions and compulsions, or somatoform disorders. SYN: *psychoneurosis.*

TREATMENT: Psychotherapy, cognitive therapy, behavioral therapy, family therapy, minor tranquilizers, and/or sedatives may be used. Many neuroses are chronic and debilitating; others are minor, compensable, or adaptive. Treatment may be difficult in some cases.

anxiety n. Neurosis marked by excessive tension or apprehension that is not restricted to specific situations or objects, unlike the normal anxiety occurring in genuinely threatening situations. Anxiety neurosis is often associated with somatic symptoms, such as palpitation, heart pain, dyspepsia, constriction of the throat, bandlike pressure about the head, or cold, sweaty, tremulous extremities, manifesting in an individual free of organic disease, during clear consciousness. SEE: *effort syndrome.*

cardiac n. Neurasthenia.

compensation n. A form of malingering that develops subsequent to an injury in the belief that financial or other forms of compensation can be obtained or will be continued by being ill. SEE: *factitious disorder.*

compulsion n. A neurosis marked by the overpowering impulse to perform certain acts or rituals repetitively (e.g., hand-washing, counting, touching).

expectation n. Condition in which anticipation of an event produces nervous symptoms.

hysterical n. An outmoded term for a conversion reaction or somatization disorder.

obsessional n. Neurosis in which recurrent and persistent thoughts dominate the victim's behavior, such as reluctance to shake hands for fear of contamination.

war n. Neurosis brought on by conditions of war, seen in soldiers.

neuroskeleton (nū″rō-skĕl′ĕ-tŏn) [Gr. *neuron,* nerve, + *skeleton,* a dried-up body] That portion of the skeleton that surrounds and protects the nervous system (i.e., the cranium, and spinal column). **neuroskeletal** (-tăl), *adj.*

neurosonography (nū″rō-sō-nŏg′ră-fē) The use of ultrasound to obtain diagnostic images of the brain, cranial bones, intracranial and extracranial vascular structures, ventricles, and spinal cord.

neurospasm (nū′rō-spăzm) [″ + *spasmos,* a convulsion] Spasmodic muscular twitching due to a neurological disorder.

neurosplanchnic (nū″rō-splăngk′nĭk) [″ + *splanchnikos,* pert. to the viscera] Concerning the sympathetic and parasympathetic nervous system.

neurospongioma (nū″rō-spŏn″jē-ō′mă) [″ + *spongos,* sponge, + *oma,* tumor] Spongioblastoma.

Neurospora (nū-rŏs′pō-ră) Genus of fungi belonging to the Ascomycetes class. It includes certain bread molds.

neurosurgeon (nū″rō-sŭr′jŭn) A physician specializing in surgery of the nervous system.

neurosurgery [Gr. *neuron,* nerve, sinew, + L. *chirurgia,* hand, + *ergon,* work] Surgery of the brain, spinal cord, cranial nerves, or peripheral nerves.

neurosyphilis (nū″rō-sĭf′ĭ-lĭs) Infection of the central nervous system with *Treponema pallidum,* the spirochete that causes syphilis. It may produce acute or chronic meningitis, dementia, damage to the posterior columns, gummatous lesions, myelopathy, or dementia. The disease is diagnosed most often when cerebrospinal fluid tests positive for syphilis on standard serological testing with VDRL. In patients with AIDS, neurosyphilis is more common and more difficult to eradicate than in persons with intact immunity.

asymptomatic n. Neurosyphilis that is clinically occult. It is diagnosed by changes in spinal fluid.

meningovascular n. A form of neurosyphilis involving the meninges and vascular structures in the brain or spinal cord, or in both.

paretic n. Dementia paralytica.

tabetic n. Tabes dorsalis.

neurotendinous (nū″rō-tĕn′dĭ-nŭs) [″ + L. *tendinosus,* tendinous] Concerning a nerve and tendon.

neurotension (nū″rō-tĕn′shŭn) [″ + L. *tensio,* a stretching] Surgical stretching of a nerve. SYN: *neurectasia.*

neurothecitis (nū″rō-thē-sī′tĭs) [″ + *theke,* sheath, + *itis,* inflammation] Inflammation of a nerve sheath.

neurothele (nū″rō-thē′lē) [″ + *thele,* nipple] A nerve papilla.

neurotic (nū-rŏt′ĭk) [Gr. *neuron,* nerve, sinew] **1.** One suffering from a neurosis. **2.** Pert. to neurosis. **3.** Nervous.

neurotic disorder Neurosis.

neuroticism (nū-rŏt′ĭ-sĭzm) [″ + *-ismos,* condition] A condition or trait of neurosis.

neurotization (nū″rŏt-ĭ-zā′shŭn) [Gr. *neuron,* nerve, sinew] **1.** Regeneration of a nerve after division. **2.** Surgical introduction of a nerve into a paralyzed muscle.

neurotmesis (nū″rŏt-mē′sĭs) [″ + *tmesis,* cutting] Nerve injury with complete loss of function of the nerve even though there is little apparent anatomic damage.

neurotology (nū″rŏ-tŏl′ō-jē) [″ + *ous,* ear, + *logos,* word, reason] Otoneurology.

neurotome (nū′rō-tōm) A fine knife used in the division of a nerve.

neurotomy (nū-rŏt′ō-mē) [″ + *tome,* an incision] Division or dissection of a nerve.

neurotonic (nū″rō-tŏn′ĭk) [″ + *tonos,* tension] **1.** Concerning neural stretching. **2.** Having a stimulating effect upon nerves or the nervous system.

neurotony (nū-rŏt′ō-nē) Nerve stretching, usually to ease pain.

neurotoxicity (nū″rō-tŏk-sĭs′ĭ-tē) [″ + *toxikon,* poison] Having the capability of harming nerve tissue.

neurotoxin (nū″rō-tŏks′ĭn) A substance that attacks or damages nerve cells. SYN: *neurolysin.* **neurotoxic** (-ĭk), *adj.*

neurotransmitter (nū″rō-trăns′mĭt-ĕr) A substance (e.g., norepinephrine, acetylcholine, or dopamine) that is released when the axon terminal of a presynaptic neuron is excited and acts by inhibiting or exciting a target cell. Disorders of neurotransmitters have been implicated in the pathogenesis of a variety of neurological and psychiatric illnesses. SEE: *substance P.*

neurotrauma (nū-rō-traw′mă) [″ + *trauma,* wound] Injury of a nerve.

neurotripsy (nū″rō-trĭp′sē) [″ + *tripsis,* a rubbing] Surgical crushing of a nerve.

neurotubule (nū″rō-too′būl) [″ + L. *tubulus,* a tubule] A microtubule in nerve cells, dendrites, and axons that may be seen by use of electron microscopy.

neurovaccine (nū″rō-văk′sĭn) A standardized vaccine virus of specific strength, usually prepared by cultivation in a rabbit's brain.

neurovascular (nū″rō-văs′kū-lăr) [″ + L. *vasculus,* a small vessel] Concerning both the nervous and vascular systems.

neurovegetative (nū″rō-vĕj′ĕ-tā″tĭv)

Concerning the autonomic nervous system.

neurovirus (nū″rō-vī′rŭs) Virus that has been modified by its growth in nervous tissue and used in preparing vaccines.

neurovisceral (nū″rō-vĭs′ĕr-ăl) [″ + L. *viscera,* body organs] Neurosplanchnic.

neurula (nū′roo-lă) The stage in the development of an embryo (esp. amphibian embryos) during which the neural plate develops and axial embryonic nervous structures are elaborated.

neurulation (nū″roo-lā′shŭn) Formation of the neural plate in the embryo and the development and closure of the neural tube.

neutral (nū′trăl) [L. *neutralis,* neither] **1.** Neither alkaline nor acid. **2.** Indifferent; having no positive qualities or opinions. **3.** Pert. to electrical charges that are neither positive nor negative.

n. fat SEE: *fat.*

n. point A point on the pH scale (pH 7.0) that represents neutrality (i.e., the solution is neither acid or alkaline in reaction).

n. red SEE: *red.*

neutralization (nū″trăl-ĭ-zā′shŭn) **1.** The opposing of one force or condition with an opposite force or condition to such degree as to cause counteraction that permits neither to dominate. **2.** In chemistry, the process of destroying the peculiar properties or effect of a substance (e.g., the neutralization of an acid with a base or vice versa). **3.** In medicine, the process of checking or counteracting the effects of any agent that produces a morbid effect.

neutralize (nū′trăl-īz) **1.** To counteract and make ineffective. **2.** In chemistry, to destroy peculiar properties or effect; to make inert.

neutrino (nū-trē′nō) In physics, a subatomic particle at rest, with no mass and no electric charge. These particles are constantly flowing through the universe and are not known to affect the matter through which they pass.

neutroclusion (nū″trŏ-kloo′zhŭn) [L. *neuter,* neither, + *occludo,* to close] A state in which the anteroposterior occlusal positions of the teeth or the mesiodistal positions are normal but malocclusion of other teeth exists.

neutron (nū′trŏn) [L. *neuter,* neither] A subatomic particle equal in mass to a proton but without an electric charge. It is believed to be a particle of all nuclei of mass number greater than one. As a free particle, it has an average life of about 12 minutes.

neutron capture analysis The use of the ability of a neutron to be absorbed (captured) by an atomic nucleus to detect the presence of various substances.

neutropenia (nū-trō-pē′nē-ă) [″ + Gr. *penia,* lack] The presence of an abnormally small number of neutrophils in the blood, usually less than 1500 to 2000 per microliter. Severely low levels of neutrophils predispose patients to infection.

malignant n. Agranulocytosis.

neutrophil, neutrophile (nū′trō-fĭl, -fīl) [″ + Gr. *philein,* to love] A granular white blood cell (WBC), the most common type (55% to 70%) of WBC. Neutrophils are responsible for much of the body's protection against infection. They play a primary role in inflammation, are readily attracted to foreign antigens (chemotaxis), and destroy them by phagocytosis. Neutrophils killed during inflammation release destructive enzymes and toxic oxygen radicals that eradicate infectious microorganisms. An inadequate number of neutrophils (neutropenia) leaves the body at high risk for infection from many sources and requires protective precautions on the part of health care workers. Cancer patients receiving chemotherapy, which destroys all leukocytes, must be carefully protected from infections during the course of therapy and until the bone marrow produces additional leukocytes.

As part of a severe inflammatory response or autoimmune disorder, neutrophils may begin attacking normal cells and cause tissue damage. This occurs in adult respiratory distress syndrome, inflammatory bowel disease, myocarditis, and rheumatoid arthritis. Corticosteroids are the most commonly used drugs to minimize the damage caused by severe inflammation. SYN: *polymorphonuclear leukocyte.* SEE: illus.; *blood* for illus.

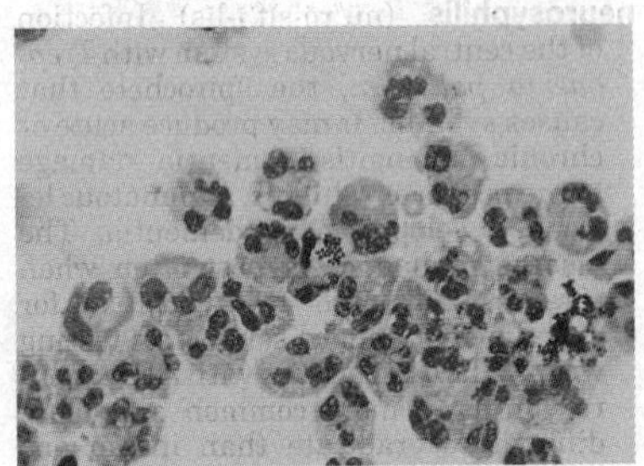

NEUTROPHILS

With ingested bacteria (orig. mag. ×1000)

neutrophilia (nū″trō-fĭl′ē-ă) Increase in the number of neutrophils in the blood (e.g., as a result of inflammation, infection, corticosteroid drugs, or malignancies).

neutrophilic, neutrophilous (nū-trō-fĭl′ĭk, -trŏf′ĭ-lŭs) [″ + Gr. *philein,* to love] Staining readily with neutral dyes.

neutrotaxis (nū″trō-tăk′sĭs) [*neutrophil*

+ Gr. *taxis,* arrangement] The phenomenon in which neutrophils are repelled by or attracted to a substance.

nevocarcinoma (nē″vō-kăr″sĭ-nō′mă) [L. *naevus,* birthmark, + Gr. *karkinos,* crab, + *oma,* tumor] Malignant melanoma.

nevoid (nē′voyd) [″ + Gr. *eidos,* form, shape] Resembling a nevus.

nevolipoma (nē″vō-lĭ-pō′mă) [″ + Gr. *lipos,* fat, + *oma,* tumor] Nevus lipomatodes.

nevose (nē′vōs) [L. *naevus,* birthmark] Spotted or marked with nevi. SEE: *nevus.*

nevoxanthoendothelioma (nē″vō-zăn″thō-ĕn″dō-thē″lē-ō′mă) [″ + Gr. *xanthos,* yellow, + *endon,* within, + *thele,* nipple, + *oma,* tumor] Juvenile xanthogranuloma. SEE: *xanthogranuloma.*

nevus (nē′vŭs) *pl.* **nevi** [L. *naevus,* birthmark] **1.** A congenital discoloration of a circumscribed area of the skin due to pigmentation. SYN: *birthmark; mole.* **2.** A circumscribed vascular tumor of the skin, usually congenital, due to hyperplasia of the blood vessels. SEE: *angioma.*

n. araneus Acquired or congenital dilatation of the capillaries, marked by red lines radiating from a central red dot. SYN: *spider nevus.*

blue n. A dark blue nevus covered by smooth skin. It is composed of melanin-pigmented spindle cells in the middermis.

blue rubber bleb n. An erectile, easily compressible, bluish, cavernous hemangioma that is present in the skin and gastrointestinal tract.

capillary n. A nevus of dilated capillary vessels elevated above the skin. It is usually treated by ligature and excision.

n. comedonicus A horny nevus that contains a hard plug of keratin. It is caused by failure of the pilosebaceous follicles to develop normally.

compound n. Clusters of melanocytes found both in the epidermis and the dermis.

connective tissue n. A nevus composed of collagenous tissue.

cutaneous n. A nevus formation on the skin.

dysplastic n. A nevus composed of cells having some malignant characteristics.

epidermal n. Raised lesions present at birth. They may be hyperkeratotic and widely distributed.

faun tail n. At birth, a tuft of hair over the lower spinal column. It may be associated with spina bifida occulta.

n. flammeus A large reddish-purple discoloration of the face or neck, usually not elevated above the skin. It is considered a serious deformity due to its large size and color. In children, these have been treated with the flashlamp-pulsed tunable dye laser. SYN: *port-wine stain.*

hairy n. A nevus covered by a heavy growth of hair. It is usually darkly pigmented.

halo n. A papular brown nevus with an oval halo occurring in the first three decades of life. This type of nevus is usually benign, but should be evaluated for malignancy.

intradermal n. A nevus in which the melanocytes are found in nests in the dermis and have no connection with the deeper layers from which they were formed.

Ito's n. Mongolian spot–like cutaneous lesion over the shoulders, supraclavicular areas, sides of the neck, scapula areas, and upper arms. It is present at birth and tends to disappear with time, usually by age 4 or 5. Although cosmetically undesirable, the lesion is benign.

junction n. A nevus in the basal cell zone at the junction of the epidermis and dermis. It is slightly raised, pigmented, and does not contain hair. This type of nevus may become malignant. SEE: illus.

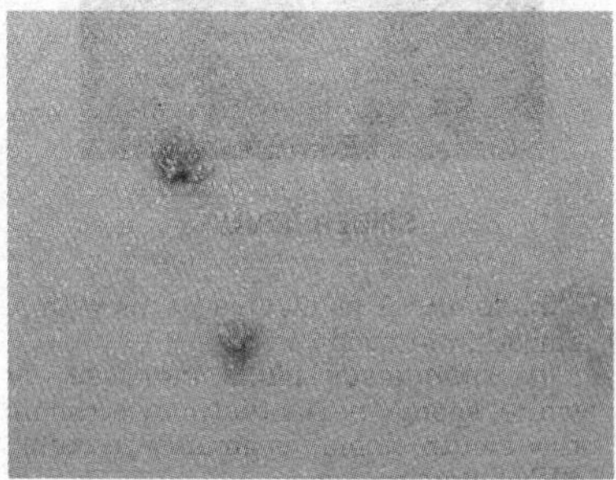

JUNCTION NEVI

n. lipomatodes A tumor composed of fatty connective tissue. It is probably a degenerated nevus containing numerous blood vessels. SYN: *nevolipoma.*

melanocytic n. Any nevus that contains melanocytes.

nevocytic n. A common mole. Moles may appear at any age. They are classified according to their stage of growth and whether or not they are still growing.

Ota's n. Blue, gray, or black macular discoloration of the skin, typically above or just below the eyes. It may be congenital or appear in childhood or adolescence. Close follow-up of this lesion is needed because malignant melanoma may develop in it. SEE: *mongolian spot.*

n. pigmentosus A congenital pigment spot varying in color from light yellow to black. Intradermal or nevocytic nevi are benign. Other types of nevi may become malignant.

TREATMENT: Malignant or suspicious lesions should be treated by wide surgical excision. Benign lesions do not require treatment except when located at sites of friction causing bleeding or ulceration. Some nevi are removed for cosmetic reasons.

sebaceous n. An epidermal nevus containing sebaceous gland tissue.

spider n. A branched growth of dilated capillaries on the skin, resembling a spider. This abnormality may be associated with cirrhosis of the liver. SYN: *nevus araneus*. SEE: illus.

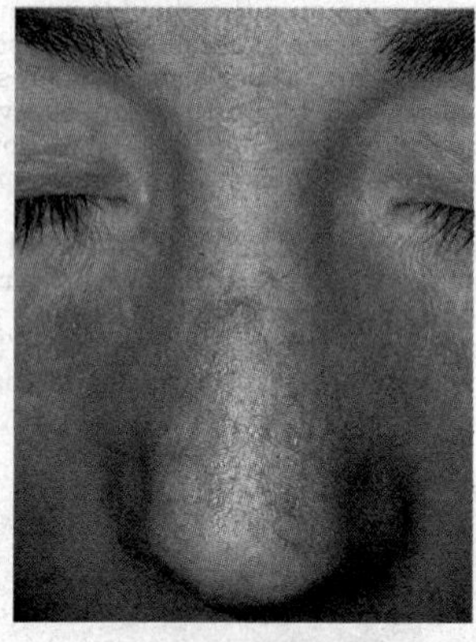

SPIDER NEVUS

n. spilus A pigmented nevus with a smooth, unraised surface.

n. spongiosus albus mucosae A white, spongy nevus that may occur in the mouth, labia, vagina, or rectum. SYN: *white sponge n.*

strawberry n. N. vascularis.

telangiectatic n. A nevus containing dilated capillaries.

n. unius lateris A congenital nevus that occurs in streaks or linear bands on one side of the body. It usually occurs between the neurotomes of the lumbar or sacral area.

n. vascularis A nevus in which superficial blood vessels are enlarged. Nevi of this type are usually congenital. They are of variable size and shape, slightly elevated, and red or purple in color. They generally appear on the face, head, neck, and arms, though no region is exempt. The nevi usually disappear spontaneously, but wrinkling, pigmentation, and scarring are sometimes seen. SYN: *strawberry n.; strawberry mark*.

n. venosus A nevus formed of dilated venules.

n. verrucosus A nevus with a raised, wartlike surface.

white sponge n. N. spongiosus albus mucosae.

newborn **1.** Born recently. **2.** A term applied to human infants less than 28 days old. SYN: *neonate*.

Newcastle disease (nū′kăs-ĕl) [Newcastle, England] An acute viral disease of birds, particularly chickens. It occasionally produces incidental infections in humans, usually in the form of a mild conjunctivitis.

new drug application ABBR: NDA. An application requiring approval by the Food and Drug Administration before any new drug is marketed to the general public. Before approval, the manufacturer must provide the FDA with scientifically acceptable evidence of the new drug's safety and efficacy.

Newman, Margaret Nursing educator, born 1933, who developed the Theory of Health as Expanding Consciousness. SEE: *Nursing Theory Appendix*.

newton SYMB: N. The name of a measure of force derived from the base units used in SI units of measurement. It is equal to the force that will accelerate one kilogram a meter per second squared, 10^5 dynes. SEE: *SI Units Appendix*.

newton meter SYMB: Nm. In SI units, one newton per square meter. This is called one pascal (Pa). Thus 1 Pa = 1N/M^2.

nexus (nĕk′sŭs) *pl.* **nexus** [L., bond] A connection or link; a binding together. It is used to designate a bond between components of a group.

NF *National Formulary*.

N.F.L.P.N. *National Federation of Licensed Practical Nurses.*

NFPA *National Fire Protection Association.*

ng *nanogram*.

NG tube *nasogastric* tube.

NH_3 Ammonia.

NH_4^+ The univalent ammonium radical.

NH_4Br Ammonium bromide.

NH_4Cl Ammonium chloride.

N.H.I. *National Heart Institute.*

NHL *non-Hodgkin's lymphoma.*

N.H.L.I. *National Heart and Lung Institute.*

NH_4NO_3 Ammonium nitrate.

NH_4OH Ammonium hydroxide.

NHTSA *National Highway Traffic Safety Administration.*

Ni Symbol for the element nickel.

NIA *National Institute on Aging.*

NIAAA *National Institute on Alcohol Abuse and Alcoholism.*

niacin (nī′ă-sĭn) A B vitamin existing in two forms, nicotinic acid (niacin) and nicotinamide, both of which are modified within cells to form NAD and NADP, coenzymes that are essential for cellular metabolic processes. It naturally occurs in mushrooms, wheat bran, fish, poultry, meat, asparagus, and peanuts. The many products made with flour fortified with niacin are good sources of this nutrient. As tryptophan is readily converted to niacin, foods such as eggs and milk that lack niacin are good sources of this vitamin. Niacin is the form used orally or parenterally for the treatment of pellagra; oral administration of niacin is used to treat hyperlipidemia. SYN: *nicotinic acid.*

CAUTION: The use of niacin is sometimes associated with nausea, vomiting, flushing, abnormal liver function tests, hyperglycemia, dry skin, itching, muscle injury, and rarely liver failure.

niacinamide (nī″ă-sĭn-ăm′īd) Nicotinamide.

N.I.A.I.D. *National Institute of Allergy and Infectious Diseases.*

N.I.A.M.D. *National Institute of Arthritis and Metabolic Diseases.*

NIAMSD *National Institute of Arthritis and Musculoskeletal and Skin Diseases.*

nib (nĭb) In dentistry, the smooth or serrated blade of a condensing instrument that contacts the restorative material placed in a cavity preparation.

nicardipine A calcium channel blocker.

niche (nĭch) [Fr.] **1.** A depression or recess on a smooth surface, esp. an erosion in the wall of a hollow organ, detected by radiography. **2.** In biology, a habitat to which a particular genetic trait adapts.

enamel n. One of two depressions that develop between the dental lamina and the enamel organ.

N.I.C.H.H.D. *National Institute of Child Health and Human Development.*

nickel SYMB: Ni. A metallic element with an atomic mass of 58.70 and an atomic number of 28.

n. carbonyl $Ni(CO)_4$; an industrial chemical used in plating metals. It is toxic when inhaled, causing pulmonary edema.

nicking, A-V nicking **1.** Compression of the retinal vessels of the eye at the point where a vein and an artery cross, seen in hypertensive cardiovascular disease. **2.** To notch a tissue.

niclosamide (nĭ-klō′să-mīd) An anthelminthic esp. effective against the cestodes that infect humans.

Nicolas-Favre disease (nē″kō-lă-făv′r) [Josef Nicolas, b. 1868, and M. Favre, 1876–1954, Fr. physicians] Lymphogranuloma venereum.

nicotinamide (nĭk″ō-tĭn′ă-mīd) A basic amide that is a member of the vitamin B complex, used in the prophylaxis and treatment of pellagra. The peripheral flush that often accompanies therapy with nicotinic acid is avoided with nicotinamide. SYN: *niacinamide.*

n. adenine dinucleotide ABBR: NAD. An enzyme that is important in accepting electrons in the course of metabolic reactions. In its oxidized form, NAD^+ gives up its electron and is converted to the reduced form, NADH.

n. adenine dinucleotide-dehydrogenase SEE: *nicotinamide adenine dinucleotide phosphate.*

n. adenine dinucleotide phosphate ABBR: NADP. A coenzyme that contains adenosine, nicotinamide, and phosphoric acid. When in its oxidized form ($NADP^+$), it serves as an electron carrier in catabolic and anabolic reactions. In its reduced form (NADPH or NADPH-diaphorase), it is important in reducing the ferric iron (Fe^{+++}) to its ferrous (Fe^{++}) form, thus converting methemoglobin (which is unable to transport oxygen) to hemoglobin (which can transport oxygen). Deficiency of NADPH-diaphorase causes congenital methemoglobinemia. SYN: *methemoglobin reductase.*

nicotine (nĭk′ō-tēn, -tĭn) [L. *nicotiana,* tobacco] A poisonous and highly addictive alkaloid found in all parts of the tobacco plant, but esp. in the leaves. When pure, it is a colorless oily fluid with little odor but a sharp burning taste. On exposure to air or in crude materials, it becomes deep brown with the characteristic tobacco-like smell. Cigarettes, cigars, and chewing tobacco contain varying amounts of nicotine. During cigarette smoking, the blood nicotine level rises 10 to 15 sec after each puff. A person's average daily nicotine intake varies with the number and type of tobacco products used, the depth of inhalation during smoking, and any exposure to second-hand smoke. Many smokers experience withdrawal symptoms when their daily nicotine exposures fall below 5 mg/day. SEE: *cancer, lung; cotinine; nicotine chewing gum; nicotine poisoning, acute; patch, nicotine; smokeless tobacco.*

Smoking during pregnancy is associated with high risk for low-birth-weight infants, prematurity, and perinatal respiratory infections.

SYMPTOMS: In healthy subjects who are not accustomed to using nicotine, nausea, vomiting, dizziness, headache, sleep disturbances, and sweating are commonly reported.

TREATMENT: Nicotine replacement therapy, administered by chewing gum, nasal spray, transdermal patch, or inhaler, can help motivated smokers to abstain from tobacco use. This type of therapy should be offered to patients who have specific plans to quit and who have received some form of structured counseling about smoking cessation.

Nicotine replacement is sometimes helpful in managing active ulcerative colitis, esp. in former smokers with the disease.

nicotine chewing gum The oral form of nicotine, used primarily as an aid to stop smoking. Although the success rate is low unless the product is used in conjunction with a smoking cessation program, some individuals who wish to discontinue the use of tobacco products use it alone. Trade name is Nicorette. SEE: *tobacco*.

nicotine patch SEE: under *patch*.

nicotine poisoning, acute Excessive stimulation of the autonomic nervous system resulting from nicotine exposure. Usually nicotine poisoning occurs when young children accidentally consume nicotine chewing gum or patches found in the home. SEE: *Poisons and Poisoning Appendix*.

SYMPTOMS: Nausea, salivation, abdominal pain, vomiting, diarrhea, sweating, dizziness, and mental confusion. If the dose is sufficient, the patient will collapse, develop shock, convulse, and die of respiratory failure due to paralysis of respiratory muscles.

TREATMENT: Activated charcoal may be given to conscious patients who are not vomiting. Unconscious patients should be intubated and supported in an intensive care unit. Anticonvulsants are used to treat seizures.

nicotinic Pert. to the stimulating effect of acetylcholine on the parasympathetic and sympathetic ganglionic or somatic skeletal muscle receptors.

nicotinic acid Niacin.

nicotinism (nĭk′ō-tĭn-ĭzm) Poisoning from excessive use of tobacco or nicotine.

nictitate (nĭk′tĭ-tāt) To wink.

nictitating (nĭk′tĭ-tāt-ĭng) Winking.

n. membrane SEE: *membrane, nictitating*.

n. spasm Clonic spasm of the eyelid with continuous winking.

NICU *neonatal intensive care unit*.

nidation (nī-dā′shŭn) Implantation (2).

NIDA *National Institute on Drug Abuse*.

NIDDM *non-insulin dependent diabetes mellitus*.

N.I.D.R. *National Institute of Dental Research*.

N.I.D.R.R. *National Institute of Disability and Rehabilitation Research*.

nidus (nī′dŭs) *pl.* **nidi** [L., nest] **1.** A nestlike structure. **2.** Focus of infection. **3.** A nucleus or origin of a nerve. **nidal** (nī′dăl), *adj*.

n. avis cerebelli A deep sulcus on each side of the inferior vermis, separating it from the adjacent lobes of the hemispheres.

n. hirundinis Cerebral depression between the uvula and the posterior velum. SYN: *swallow's nest*.

Niemann-Pick cell A foamy, lipid-filled cell present in the spleen and bone marrow in Niemann-Pick disease.

Niemann-Pick disease (nē′măn-pĭk) [Albert Niemann, Ger. pediatrician, 1880–1921; Ludwig Pick, Ger. physician, 1868–1944] A disturbance of sphingolipid metabolism characterized by enlargement of liver and spleen (hepatosplenomegaly), anemia, lymphadenopathy, and progressive mental and physical deterioration. It is an autosomal recessive lysosomal storage disease, with its onset in early infancy and death usually occurring before the third year. A typical cell, having a foamy appearance and filled with a lipoid believed to be sphingomyelin, can be found in the bone marrow, spleen, or lymph nodes, and aids in establishing the diagnosis.

night blindness Decreased ability to see at night. It is caused by a lack of rhodopsin in the rods of the retina, or by slow resynthesis of rhodopsin after exposure to light. Night blindness may result from vitamin A deficiency or hereditary factors. SYN: *nyctalopia* (1). SEE: *night vision*.

nightguard A dental prosthesis worn at night to prevent traumatic grinding of the teeth during sleep. SEE: *bruxism; occlusal guard*.

Nightingale, Florence (nīt′ĭn-gāl) A British philanthropist, 1820–1910, who is considered the founder of nursing as a profession, a formidable statistician, and a pioneering hospital reformer. She was one of many trained nurses to serve in Crimea and dramatically lowered the death rate in the British army by advocating cleanliness and reform of sanitary conditions in hospitals at the battlefront. The astonishing decrease in morbidity and mortality at the front riveted the public both in Britain and in the rest of the West, and the Nightingale Fund gained large contributions from donors around the world. The fund was used to establish a school of nursing at St. Thomas' Hospital in London, England, in 1860. The school became a model for nursing schools around the world, and the first nursing school based on the Nightingale model to be established in the U.S. was at Bellevue Hospital in New York.

Nightingale Pledge An oath used by nurses on graduation as a pledge of commitment and integrity. The pledge was formulated by a committee of the Farrand School of Nursing, Harper Hospital, Detroit, Michigan, of which Lystra Gretter was the chairperson, and was first administered to the graduating class in 1893.

"I solemnly pledge myself before God and in the presence of this assembly to pass my life in purity and to practice my profession faithfully. I will abstain from whatever is deleterious and mischievous, and will not take or knowingly administer any harmful drug. I will do all in my power to maintain and elevate the standard of my profession, and will hold in confidence all personal matters committed to my keeping and all family affairs coming to my knowledge in the practice of my calling. With loyalty will I endeavor to aid the physician in his work, and devote myself to the welfare of those committed to my care." SEE: *Declaration of Hawaii; Declaration of Geneva; Hippocratic Oath; Prayer of Maimonides.*

nightmare (nīt′mār) [AS. *nyht,* night, + *mara,* a demon] A frightening dream. SYN: *incubus; oneirodynia*. SEE: *sleep disorder*.

nightshade (nīt′shād) [AS. *nihtscada*] Any of several of the poisonous plants of the genus *Solanum,* which contain atropine-like toxins.

deadly n. Belladonna.

night sweat [AS. *nyht,* night, + *swat,* sweat] Profuse sweating during sleep. It is a symptom of many infectious and inflammatory disorders. In perimenopausal women, it is a common vasomotor response to fluctuating hormone levels. The patient should be bathed (if he or she so desires) and changed into dry clothing.

night terrors [″ + L. *terrere,* to frighten] A form of nightmare in children causing them to awaken screaming in terror. The fear continues for a period after the return to consciousness. SYN: *pavor nocturnus*. SEE: *sleep disorder*.

night vision The ability to see at night or in light of low intensity. It results from dark adaptation in which the pupil dilates, rhodopsin increases, and the intensity threshold of the retina is lowered. Any decrease in the oxygen content of the blood is accompanied by some loss of night vision. Thus, smoking cigarettes or being in an atmosphere with decreased oxygen content decreases night vision. SYN: *scotopic vision*.

nightwalking Sleepwalking. SEE: *sleep disorder*.

night work, maladaptation to Difficulty in adapting to sleeping during the day and working at night. In the U.S. about 7.3 million people work at night and are forced to attempt to readjust their day-night schedule for working and sleeping. Adaptation may be facilitated by making the work space as light as possible and scheduling the sleep period (8 hours) in a totally dark environment. SEE: *clock, biological; shift work*.

N.I.G.M.S. *National Institute of General Medical Sciences*. A division of the National Institutes of Health of the U.S. Department of Health and Human Services.

nigra (nī′gră) [L., black] Substantia nigra.

nigricans (nī′grĭ-kăns) Blackened.

nigrities (nī-grĭsh′ĭ-ēz) Blackness; black pigmentation.

n. linguae A black pigmentation of the tongue.

nigrostriatal (nī″grō-strī-ā′tăl) Concerning a bundle of nerve fibers that connect the substantia nigra of the brain to the corpus striatum.

NIH *National Institutes of Health* (of the U.S. Department of Health and Human Services).

nihilism (nī′ĭ-lĭzm) [L. *nihil,* nothing, + Gr. *-ismos,* condition] **1.** Disbelief in efficacy of medical therapy. **2.** In psychiatry, a delusion in which everything is unreal or does not exist. SYN: *therapeutic n.* **nihilistic,** *adj.*

therapeutic n. Nihilism.

nikethamide (nĭ-kĕth′ă-mīd) A drug designed to stimulate selectively central respiratory centers. When used for this purpose in treating respiratory depression due to poisoning from sedative-hypnotic drugs, it is ineffective.

Nikolsky's sign (nĭ-kŏl′skēz) [Pyotr Nikolsky, Russ. dermatologist, 1855–1940] A condition seen in pemphigus, where the external layer of the skin can be detached from the basal layer and rubbed off by slight friction or injury.

N.I.M.H. *National Institute of Mental Health,* a division of the National Institutes of Health of the U.S. Department of Health and Human Services.

NINCDS *National Institute of Neurological and Communicative Disorders and Stroke.*

N.I.N.D.B. *National Institute of Neurological Diseases and Blindness,* a division of the National Institutes of Health of the U.S. Department of Health and Human Services.

ninth cranial nerve Glossopharyngeal nerve.

niobium (nī-ō′bē-um) [Mythological Gr. woman, Niobe, who was turned into stone] SYMB: Nb. A chemical element, formerly called columbium, with an atomic number of 41 and an atomic weight of 92.906.

niphotyphlosis (nĭf″ō-tĭf-lō′sĭs) [Gr. *nipha,* snow, + *typhlosis,* blindness] Snow blindness.

nipple (nĭp′l) [AS. *neble,* a little protuberance] **1.** The erectile protuberance at the tip of each breast from which the lactiferous ducts discharge. The nipple projects from the center of the more heavily pigmented areola; both the nipple and the areola contain small sebaceous glands (Montgomery's glands), which secrete a protective, oily substance. SYN: *mammae papilla; teat*. SEE: *breast* for illus.

PATIENT CARE: *Assessment:* Instructions and demonstrations to help patients examine their own breasts should include inspecting the nipples and areolae for symmetry of shape, size, color, and texture and reporting any sign of retraction or evidence of discharge.

Pregnancy-related: Prenatal instructions about breastfeeding and postpartum breast care emphasize signs to report promptly to the health care provider (e.g., nipple cracking, inversion, redness, or bleeding). SEE: *breast cancer; breastfeeding.*

2. An artificial substitute for a female nipple, used for bottle-feeding infants. Nipple-shaped pacifiers may be used to satisfy infant needs for sucking as a self-consoling activity

crater n. Retracted n.

retracted n. A nipple whose tip lies below the level of the surrounding skin. Retraction is caused by deficiency of muscle tissue or the flattening of erectile tissue.

n. shield A device consisting of an artificial nipple used by some nursing mothers to protect the natural nipple.

nisin (nī′sĭn) A lantibiotic that is active against gram-positive germs; it is used primarily as a food preservative.

Nissl body (nĭs′l) [Franz Nissl, Ger. neurologist, 1860–1919] A large granular body found in nerve cells. They can be demonstrated by selective staining. They are rough endoplasmic reticulum (with ribosomes) and are the site of protein synthesis. Nissl bodies show changes under various physiological conditions, and in pathological conditions they may dissolve and disappear (chromatolysis). SYN: *Nissl granules; tigroid bodies.*

NIST *National Institute of Standards and Technology.*

nit (nĭt) [AS. *hnitu*] The egg of a louse or any other parasitic insect. SEE: *Pediculus.*

nitr- [Gr. *nitron,* salt] Combining form denoting combination with nitrogen or presence of the group NO_2.

nitrate (nī′trāt) [L. *nitratum*] A salt of nitric acid. Agents in this class include isosorbide dinitrate or mononitrate and nitroglycerin. They are arteriovenous dilators and are used to treat angina pectoris, hypertension, and congestive heart failure, among other conditions.

nitrated Combined with nitric acid or a nitrate.

nitration Combination with nitric acid or a nitrate.

nitremia (nī-trē′mē-ă) Azotemia.

nitric acid HNO_3; a colorless, corrosive, poisonous liquid in concentrated form, employed as a caustic. It is widely used in industry and in chemical laboratories.

fuming n.a. Concentrated nitric acid that emits toxic fumes that cause choking if inhaled. SEE: *fumes.*

n.a. poisoning Injury sustained from contact with nitric acid. Symptoms include pain, burning, vomiting, thirst, and shock.

TREATMENT: Emergency measures include oral administration of activated charcoal and large volumes of water. Emetics and stomach tubes should be avoided because they may cause rupture of the esophagus or stomach.

nitric oxide ABBR: NO. A soluble gas that is normally produced in the human body and is present in expired air at a concentration of about 10 parts per billion. Produced by endothelial cells, neurons in the brain, and macrophages during inflammation, it is a potent vasodilator. Nitric oxide (NO) has many other roles: it inhibits the adhesion, activation, and aggregation of platelets and the inflammatory process induced by mast cells; controls chemotaxis of lymphocytes; regulates smooth muscle cell proliferation, penile erection, and other sexual functions; participates in programmed cell death; and interacts with oxygen radicals to form metabolites that destroy pathogens. When NO is given as part of a mixture of inhaled gas, it decreases recruitment of lymphocytes. NO is being studied as a means of reducing inflammation in the treatment of patients with adult respiratory distress syndrome and as a vasodilator in pulmonary hypertension. Previously, NO was called endothelium-derived relaxing factor (EDRF). SEE: *oxygen radical; phagocytosis.*

nitride (nī′trīd) A binary compound formed by direct combination of nitrogen with another element (e.g., lithium nitride [Li_3N]), formed from nitrogen and lithium.

nitrification (nī″trĭ-fĭ-kā′shŭn) The process by which the nitrogen of ammonia or other compounds is oxidized to nitric or nitrous acid or their salts (nitrates, nitrites). This process takes place continually in the soil through the action of nitrifying bacteria.

nitrifying bacteria Bacteria that induce nitrification, including the nitrite bacteria of the genus *Nitrosomonas,* which convert ammonia to nitrites, and nitrate bacteria of the genus *Nitrobacter,* which convert nitrites to nitrates.

nitrile (nī′trĭl) An organic compound in which trivalent nitrogen is attached to a carbon atom. It is used to make latex-free gloves for use in health care.

nitrite (nī′trīt) [Gr. *nitron,* salt] A salt of nitrous acid. Nitrites dilate blood vessels, reduce blood pressure, depress motor centers of the spinal cord, and act as antispasmodics.

nitritoid crisis A syndrome characterized by symptoms resembling those produced by the use of a nitrite, and usually occurring after arsphenamine injection.

nitrituria (nī-trĭ-tū′rē-ă) [″ + *ouron,* urine] Nitrites present in the urine.

nitro- [Gr. *nitron,* salt] Combining form denoting combination with nitrogen or presence of the group NO_2.

nitrobenzene (nī″trō-bĕn′zēn) A toxic derivative of benzene used esp. in making aniline.

nitroblue tetrazolium test A test of the ability of leukocytes to reduce nitroblue tetrazolium from a colorless state to a deep blue. It is used as a marker of nitric oxide synthase. The reduction of NBT may be used in the rapid diagnosis of urinary tract infections and in the study and diagnosis of chronic granulomatous disease and other illnesses in which there are defects in the oxidative metabolism of phagocytic white blood cells.

nitrocellulose (nī″trō-sĕl′ū-lōs) Pyroxylin.

nitrofurantoin (nī″trō-fū-răn′tō-ĭn) An antibacterial drug used in treating urinary tract infections.

nitrofurazone (nī″trō-fū′ră-zōn) An antibacterial agent used topically.

nitrogen (nī′trō-jĕn) [Fr. *nitrogene*] SYMB: N. A colorless, odorless, tasteless, gaseous element occurring free in the atmosphere, forming approx. 80% of its volume. Its atomic number is 7 and its atomic weight is 14.0067.

A component of all proteins, nitrogen is essential to plant and animal life for tissue building. Generally it is found organically only in the form of compounds such as ammonia, nitrites, and nitrates. These are transformed by plants into proteins and, being consumed by animals, are converted into animal proteins of the blood and tissues.

n. balance The difference between the amount of nitrogen ingested and that excreted each day. If intake is greater, a positive balance exists; if less, there is a negative balance.

n. cycle A natural cycle in which nitrogen is discharged from animal life into the soil; it is then taken up from soil into plants for their nourishment; and in turn nitrogen returns to animal life through plants eaten.

n. equilibrium Condition during which nitrogen excreted in the urine, feces, and sweat equals amount taken in by the body in food.

n. fixation The conversion of atmospheric nitrogen into nitrates through the action of bacteria in the soil.

n. lag The extent of time required after a given protein is ingested before an amount of nitrogen equal to that in the protein has been excreted.

n. monoxide Nitrous oxide.

n. mustards **1.** Alkylating drugs (including such drugs as melphalan, cyclophosphamide, and chlorambucil) used to treat a variety of solid and hematological malignancies such as Hodgkin's disease, multiple myeloma, and some leukemias. Nitrogen mustards include mechlorethamine, cyclophosphamide, uracil mustard, melphalan, and chlorambucil. **2.** Gases used in chemical warfare (e.g., mustard gas, vesicant gas).

n. narcosis A condition of euphoria, impaired judgment, and decreased coordination and motor ability seen in persons exposed to high air pressure (e.g., divers and submariners). The effects, caused by the increased concentration of nitrogen gas in body tissues (including the brain), are similar to those produced by alcoholic intoxication.

nonprotein n. A nitrogen-containing constituent of blood or milk that is neither a protein nor an amino acid. Most nonprotein nitrogen in the human body is in the form of urea.

nitrogenase (nī′trō-jĕn-ās) [*nitrogen* + *-ase,* enzyme] An enzyme that catalyzes the reduction of nitrogen to ammonia.

nitrogenous (nī-trŏj′ĕn-ŭs) Pert. to or containing nitrogen. Foods that contain nitrogen are the proteins; those that do not contain nitrogen are the fats and carbohydrates. The retention of nitrogenous waste products such as urea in the blood indicates kidney disease.

nitroglycerin (nī″trō-glĭs′ĕr-ĭn) [Gr. *nitron,* salt, + *glycerin*] Any nitrate of glycerol, but specifically the trinitrate—a heavy, oily, explosive, colorless liquid obtained by treating glycerol with nitric and sulfuric acids. Well known as the explosive constituent of dynamite, in medicine it is used as an arterial and venous dilator, esp. to treat angina pectoris, congestive heart failure, and acute pulmonary edema.

It is available as an intravenous infusion (in critical care), as an ointment that can be rubbed on the chest, as transdermal patches, and as an oral drug (either a tablet that dissolves under the tongue or a spray that can be applied to the mucous membranes of the mouth). Its most common side effects include lowering of blood pressure and headache.

PATIENT CARE: Nitroglycerin used at home should be stored in a tightly sealed dark glass container and replaced every 6 months to ensure that the drug maintains optimal activity. Patients using nitroglycerin during episodes of angina pectoris should take a single dose and sit quietly or lie down for 5 minutes while waiting for relief of chest discomfort. If after 5 minutes the discomfort has not abated, the patient may take a second dose. He or she may take a third dose of the medication if symptoms have not resolved in another 5 minutes, but if this dose is also ineffective, the patient or a family member should call for emergency assistance (dial 911).

CAUTION: Topical nitroglycerin should be removed from the chest wall before attempting cardioversion or defibrillation, to avoid sparking or explosions.

nitromersol (nī″trō-mĕr′sŏl) An organic mercurial antiseptic.

Nitrosomonas A genus of gram-negative, aerobic bacteria that oxidize ammonia to nitrate.

nitrous (nī′trŭs) [Gr. *nitron,* salt] Containing nitrogen in its lowest valency.

nitrous acid HNO_2; a chemical reagent used in biological laboratories.

nitrous oxide An inhaled, flammable anesthetic and analgesic gas, first developed in the 1840s, and used in both general and outpatient dental anesthesia. Some observers have associated its use with miscarriage, organ injuries, and dependence and abuse, although the data linking N_2O to these problems are controversial. SYN: *laughing gas.*

Nitrous oxide has little or no effect on body temperature, metabolism, blood pressure, volume, or composition, or the genitourinary system. Diaphoresis, increased muscle tone, or both may occur with induction of anesthesia with nitrous oxide.

Asphyxiation may occur if it is not administered properly. Prolonged administration of nitrous oxide will cause depression of bone marrow.

SYMPTOMS: Signs of deep nitrous oxide anesthesia include a slight increase in respirations and some dyspnea. The eyeballs become fixed and dilated and there is muscular rigidity and cyanosis that increases to a grayish pallor.

TREATMENT: The patient who suffers from an overdose should be oxygenated and ventilated.

NK cells *natural killer cells.*

N.L.N. *National League for Nursing.*

nm *nanometer.*

N.M.D.P. *National Marrow Donor Program.*

NMRI *Naval Medical Research Institute* (U.S. Navy); *nuclear magnetic resonance imaging.*

NMR spectroscopy *nuclear magnetic resonance spectroscopy.*

N.M.S.S. *National Multiple Sclerosis Society.*

N.N.D. *New and Nonofficial Drugs,* a former publication of the American Medical Association, which described new drugs that had not been admitted to the U.S. Pharmacopeia.

NNRTI Nonnucleoside analog reverse transcriptase inhibitor.

NO Nitric oxide.

N_2O Nitrous oxide.

N_2O_3 Nitrogen trioxide.

N_2O_5 Nitrogen pentoxide.

No Symbol for the element nobelium.

no [L. *numero*] Abbreviation meaning *to the number of.*

nobelium (nō-bē′lē-ŭm) [Named for Nobel Institute, where it was first isolated] SYMB: No. An element obtained from the bombardment of curium. Its atomic number is 102. The atomic mass of the most stable isotope of nobelium is 254; other isotopes vary in weight from 252 through 256.

Nobel Prize [Alfred B. Nobel, Swedish chemist and philanthropist who developed nitroglycerin, 1833–1896, whose will provided funds for awarding the annual prizes] Awards given almost every year since 1901 to honor distinguished contributions to world peace, chemistry, physics, literature, economics, and physiology and medicine.

Nocardia [Edmund I. E. Nocard, Fr. veterinary pathologist, 1850–1903] A genus of gram-positive aerobic bacilli that often appear in filaments. Some species are acid-fast and thus may be confused with the causative organism for tuberculosis when stained. A species pathogenic for humans causes the disease nocardiosis. **nocardial** (nō-kăr′dē-ăl), *adj.*

N. asteroides A species pathogenic for humans in which abscesses called mycetomas arise in the skin. The invasion site may be the lungs or skin. SEE: illus.

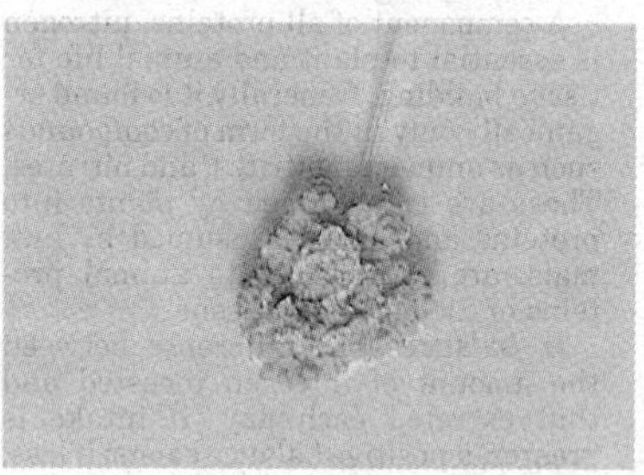

NOCARDIA ASTEROIDES **IN CULTURE**

N. brasiliensis A species pathogenic for humans in which chronic subcutaneous abscesses are formed.

nocardiosis A pulmonary or brain infection caused by the bacteria *Nocardia asteroides* or, less commonly, by other *Nocardia* species that are found in soil. It primarily is considered an opportunistic pathogen, infecting patients with a compromised immune system (e.g., patients with the acquired immunodeficiency syndrome [AIDS] or end-stage renal disease), but approx. 15% of cases occur in healthy persons. Inhalation of contaminated dust causes the infection. SEE: illus; *maduromycosis; opportunistic infection.*

SYMPTOMS: Infection occurs in the lungs in 75% of patients, causing pneumonia characterized by a productive cough, hemoptysis, and, at times, abscesses; pleural invasion may occur, producing pain. The remaining 25% of patients develop brain abscesses marked by headache, nausea, vomiting, and changes in mental status.

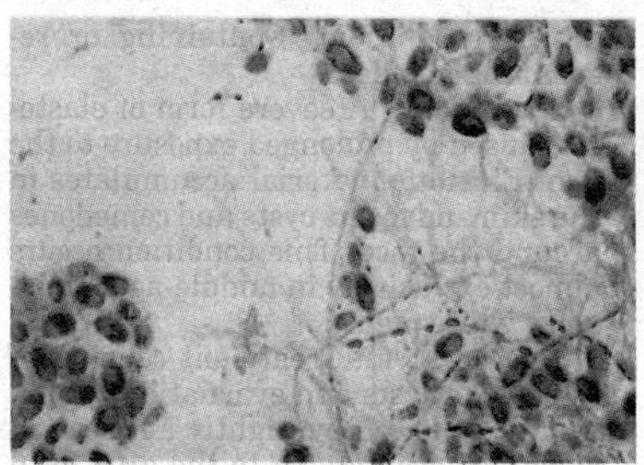

NOCARDIOSIS

Nocardia (chains of bacilli) in tissue (orig. mag. ×500)

DIAGNOSIS: Infection is diagnosed through cultures of sputum or transtracheal aspirates, which may require 4 weeks of growth.

TREATMENT: Nocardiosis usually is treated with 6 months of oral sulfasoxazole or trimethoprim/sulfamethoxazole; persons with AIDS need lifelong suppressive therapy. Pneumonia producing severe respiratory distress is treated with intravenous cefotaxime plus imipenem, followed by oral therapy. In patients with brain abscesses, mortality is approx. 40%; in patients with pneumonia, it ranges from 10% to 30%.

nocebo [L., I will harm] A substance (such as a sugar pill) or an exposure (such as to an odor or fragrance) that makes a person feel ill, even though it has no measurable negative effects. The nocebo effect can be contagious as in cases of mass sociogenic illness. SEE: *placebo*.

noci- (nō′sē) [L. *nocere,* to injure] Combining form indicating *pain, injury*.

nociassociation (nō″sē-ă-sō″sē-ā′shŭn) [″ + *ad,* to, + *socius,* companion] The involuntary release of nervous energy during surgical shock or following trauma.

nociception The stimulus-response process involving the stimulation of peripheral pain-carrying nerve fibers (e.g., C-fibers, A-delta fibers) and the transmission of impulses along peripheral nerves of the central nervous system, where the stimulus is perceived as pain. SEE: *nociceptor; nociceptive impulse*.

nociceptive impulse Impulse giving rise to sensations of pain.

nociceptor (nō″sē-sĕp′tor) [″ + *receptor,* receiver] A free nerve ending that is a receptor for painful stimuli. **nociceptive** (nō″sĭ-sĕp′tĭv), *adj.*

nociperception (nō″sĭ-pĕr-sĕp′shŭn) [″ + *perceptio,* apprehension] The perception by the nerve centers of injurious influences or painful stimuli.

"no code" orders An indication on the chart of a patient that he or she does not want heroic or life-saving measures to be instituted when death is imminent.

noct L. *nocte,* night.

noctiphobia (nŏk″tĭ-fō′bē-ă) [L. *nocte,* at night, + Gr. *phobos,* fear] Abnormal fear of the night and darkness. SYN: *nyctophobia; scotophobia*.

nocturia (nŏk-tū′rē-ă) [″ + Gr. *ouron,* urine] Excessive or frequent urination after going to bed, typically caused by excessive fluid intake, congestive heart failure, uncontrolled diabetes mellitus, urinary tract infections, diseases of the prostate, impaired renal function, or the use of diuretics. Less often, diabetes insipidus is the cause. SYN: *nycturia*. SEE: *enuresis*.

PATIENT CARE: Safety is emphasized for patients who need to get up to go to the bathroom at night because they may not be fully awake or alert. Specific recommendations include strategic placement and use of night lights and removal of objects blocking the route from the bedroom to bathroom, because these may cause the patient to trip or fall.

nocturnal [L. *nocturnus,* at night] Pert. to or occurring in the night. Opposed to diurnal. See words beginning with *nyct-*.

n. emission Harmless involuntary discharge of semen during sleep, usually occurring in conjunction with an erotic dream. SYN: *wet dream*.

n. enuresis SEE: under *enuresis*.

n. myoclonus SEE: under *myoclonus*.

n. penile tumescence ABBR: NPT. Erection occurring during sleep. In the normal male, these erections occur beginning in early childhood and continue to at least the eighth decade. The total time of NPT averages 100 minutes per night. In evaluating erectile dysfunction (ED), the presence of NPT suggests the patient has psychogenic rather than neurogenic or vascular ED.

nocuous (nŏk′ū-ŭs) [L. *nocuus*] Noxious, injurious, harmful, poisonous.

nodal (nō′dăl) [L. *nodus,* knot] Pert. to a protuberance.

n. rhythm Cardiac rhythm with origin at the atrioventricular node.

nodding (nŏd′ĭng) Involuntary motion of the head downward, as when momentarily dozing. SYN: *nutation* (1).

nodding spasm SEE: *spasm, nodding*.

node (nōd) [L. *nodus,* knot] **1.** A knot, knob, protuberance, or swelling. **2.** A constricted region. **3.** A small rounded organ or structure.

Aschoff's n. Atrioventricular n.

atrioventricular n. ABBR: AV node. Specialized cardiac muscle fibers in the lower interatrial septum that receive impulses from the sinoatrial node and transmit them to the bundle of His. SEE: *bundle, atrioventricular; conduction system of the heart* for illus.

AV n. Atrioventricular n.

Bouchard's n. In osteoarthritis, bony enlargement of the proximal interphalangeal joints.

Haygarth's n. Joint swelling seen in rheumatoid arthritis.

Heberden's n. SEE: *Heberden's nodes.*

hemal n. A body resembling a lymph node in structure but composed of blood vessels instead of lymphatic vessels; present in certain ungulates. SYN: *hemal gland.*

Hensen's n. A mass of rapidly proliferating cells at the anterior end of the primitive streak of the embryo.

lymph n. SEE: *lymph node.*

Meynet's n. SEE: *Meynet's nodes.*

neurofibril n. Ranvier's node.

Osler's n. SEE: *Osler's nodes.*

Parrot's n. SEE: *Parrot's nodes.*

piedric n. A node on the hair shaft seen in piedra.

Ranvier's n. SEE: *Ranvier's node.*

Schmorl's n. Node seen in radiographs of the spine. It is caused by prolapse of the nucleus pulposus into the end-plate of the vertebra.

sentinel n. **1.** A lymph node that receives drainage from a tumor, and is likely to harbor metastatic disease before cancer cells have the opportunity to spread elsewhere. **2.** Signal node.

signal n. Enlargement of one of the supraclavicular lymph nodes; usually indicative of primary carcinoma of thoracic or abdominal organs. SYN: *sentinel n.* (2)

singer's n. Noncancerous, callus-like growths on the inner parts of the vocal cords, usually caused by voice abuse or overuse. Hoarseness and an inability of singers to produce the desired sounds mark this condition. It is treated by resting the voice. Surgical removal of the nodules is necessary if they do not respond to conservative therapy. SYN: *chorditis nodosa; laryngeal nodule.*

sinoatrial n. ABBR: SA node. A specialized group of cardiac muscle cells in the wall of the right atrium at the entrance of the superior vena cava. These cells depolarize spontaneously and rhythmically to initiate normal heartbeats. SYN: *pacemaker* (2); *sinus n.*

sinus n. Sinoatrial n.

syphilitic n. Circumscribed swelling at the end of long bones due to congenital syphilis. The nodes are sensitive and painful during inflammation, esp. at night. SEE: *Parrot's nodes.*

Troisier's n. SEE: *signal n.*

Virchow n. SEE: *signal n.*

nodose (nō′dōs) [L. *nodosus,* knotted] Swollen or knotlike at intervals; marked by nodes or projections.

nodosity (nō-dŏs′ĭ-tē) [L. *nodositas,* a knot] **1.** A protuberance or knot. **2.** Condition of having nodes.

nodular (nŏd′ū-lăr) Containing or resembling nodules.

n. elastosis A severe form of elastosis caused by prolonged exposure to the sun. Elastotic material accumulates in the skin and forms cysts and comedones around the face. This condition occurs almost exclusively in middle-aged or elderly white men.

TREATMENT: Treatment consists of removal of cysts and evacuation of comedones, followed by nightly application of retinoic acid cream to the area for 6 to 8 weeks. The patient should avoid sun exposure to prevent recurrence.

nodule (nŏd′ūl) [L. *nodulus,* little knot] **1.** A small node. **2.** A small cluster of cells.

aggregate n. A group of solitary lymph nodules, such as Peyer's patches of the small intestine.

Albini's n. SEE: *Albini's nodules.*

apple jelly n. The jelly-like lesion of lupus vulgaris.

Arantius' n. SEE: *Arantius' body.*

Aschoff's n. SEE: *Aschoff's nodules.*

cortical n. Lymph nodules located in the cortex of a lymph node.

laryngeal n. Singer's node.

lymph n. A mass of compact, densely staining lymphocytes forming the structural unit of lymphatic tissue. These nodules may occur singly, in groups (as in Peyer's patches), or in encapsulated organs such as lymph nodes. Each contains a lighter-staining germinal center where new lymphocytes are formed.

miliary n. Small round density, 1 to 5 mm in diameter as seen on the chest radiograph (e.g., in disseminated tuberculosis).

milker's n. Painless smooth or warty lesions due to a poxvirus that is transmitted from the udders of infected cows to the hands of milkers. SEE: *paravaccinia.*

n. of the semilunar valve SEE: *Arantius' body.*

rheumatic n. Subcutaneous nodes of fibrous tissue that may be present in patients with rheumatic fever.

Schmorl's n. Schmorl's node.

siderotic n. Small brown nodules seen in the spleen and other organs and consisting of necrotic tissue encrusted by iron salts.

solitary n. An isolated nodule of lymphatic tissue such as occurs in mucous membranes.

solitary pulmonary n. Any isolated mass lesion found in the lung, usually during an x-ray study performed for another reason. Most small masses that are identified in this way are benign, although smokers, patients already known to have cancer in another organ system, and older patients have an increased risk that a solitary nodule will be a new malignancy, or a metastasis from another source.

Typical Noise Levels in Decibels and Their Effect

Situation	Level Decibels	Effect
Jet engine (close by)*	140	Harmful to hearing
Jet takeoff*	130	
Propeller aircraft*	120	
Live rock band	110	Risk of hearing loss
Jackhammer	100	
Heavy-duty truck	90	
Private car; business office	70	Probably no risk of permanent damage to hearing
Wooded residential area	50	No harm
Whisper	30	No harm
Rustle of leaf	10	No harm

* Outside aircraft

Patient Care: The first step in evaluating a solitary lung nodule is to search for prior chest x-ray films. If the nodule can be found on films done many months or years earlier, and has not changed in size, shape, or calcification, then it is likely to be benign and can be followed conservatively. Newly identified lesions within the lung that were not previously present usually are evaluated with further studies, such as computed tomography of the lungs, sputum studies, or biopsies.

subcutaneous n. Small, nontender swellings resembling Aschoff's bodies and found over bony prominences in persons with rheumatic fever or rheumatoid arthritis (in rheumatoid arthritis, they are called rheumatoid nodules).

surfer's n. Nodular swelling and possible bone changes of the area of the lower leg and foot exposed to pressure and trauma while on a surfboard. The nodules may be painful. SYN: *surfer's knots.*

thyroid n. A visible or palpable mass in the thyroid gland, benign about 90% to 95% of the time. A history of radiation to the head or neck increases the likelihood that the lesion will be malignant, as does the appearance of the nodule in the first decades of life. Fine-needle aspiration biopsy is the first, and often the definitive, diagnostic test.

typhoid n. Nodules characteristic of typhoid fever and found in the liver.

typhus n. Small nodules of the skin seen in typhus. They are composed of mononuclear cell infiltration around vessels.

nodulus (nŏd'ū-lŭs) *pl.* **noduli** [L.] **1.** Nodule. **2.** The anterior portion of the vermis of the cerebellum.

nodus (nō'dŭs) *pl.* **nodi** [L.] **1.** Node. **2.** Anatomically, a small circumscribed mass of undifferentiated tissue.

noesis (nō-ē'sĭs) [Gr. *noesis,* thought] The act of thinking; cognition.

Noguchia (nō-goo'chē-ă) [Hideyo Noguchi, Japanese bacteriologist in U.S., 1876–1928] A genus of microorganisms of the family Brucellaceae. They are slim, gram-negative, flagellated rods present in the conjunctiva of humans and animals with follicular conjunctivitis.

noise [O.Fr. *noise,* strife, brawl] **1.** Sound of any sort, including that which is loud, harsh, confused, or senseless. SEE: table; *acoustic trauma; pollution, noise.* **2.** In electronics or physics, any electronic disturbance that interferes with the signal being recorded or monitored. In electrocardiography, the 60-cycle alternating current used to power the machine may be inadvertently recorded. This obscures the signal from the electrical activity of the heart. **3.** Unwanted information on a radiograph caused by fogging, or scattered radiation.

n. pollution A level of environmental noise of such nature or intensity as to cause mental or physical discomfort or damage to the hearing system.

noli me tangere (nō"lē mē tăn'jĕ-rē) [L., touch me not] A cancerous ulcer, generally of the face, that eats away bone and soft tissue. SYN: *rodent ulcer.*

noma (nō'mă) [Gr. *nome,* a spreading] Cancrum oris.

n. pudendi An infected ulcer affecting the labia majora, esp. in young children.

nomadism [Gr. *nomas,* roaming about] Having a constantly migratory lifestyle, as is practiced by some animals and humans.

nomenclature (nō'mĕn-klā"chūr) [L. *nomen,* name, + *calare,* to call] A classified system of technical or scientific names. SYN: *terminology.*

binomial n. The system of classifying living organisms by the use of two Latin-derived words to indicate the genus and species.

Nomina Anatomica (nō'mĭ-nă ăn-ă-tŏm'ĭ-kă) [" + Gr. *anatome,* dissection] ABBR: NA. The collected anatomical terminology adopted as official by the International Congress of Anatomists at meetings held periodically since 1955.

nomogram (nŏm′ō-grăm) [Gr. *nomos,* law, + *gramma,* something written] Representation by graphs, diagrams, or charts of the relationship between numerical variables.

Rumack n. A nomogram that predicts both the severity of acetaminophen overdose and the need for specific treatment.

weight-based n. A nomogram used to prescribe medications based on patient size.

nomography (nō-mŏg′ră-fē) [″ + *graphein,* to write] The construction of a nomogram.

nonabandonment The ethical obligation of a health care provider to remain in a continuous caring partnership with his or her patient. This partnership remains in place during periods of health and illness and is particularly important when the patient has a chronic or life-threatening disease. Several aspects of modern medical care, in which the patient's choice of physician may be limited and disrupt the continuity of the physician-patient relationship, make carrying out this obligation difficult. SEE: *abandonment.*

noncompliance The failure or refusal of a patient to cooperate by carrying out that portion of the medical care plan under his or her control (e.g., not taking prescribed medicines or not adhering to the diet or rehabilitation procedures ordered). SEE: *Nursing Diagnoses Appendix.*

non compos mentis (nŏn kŏm′pŏs mĕn′tĭs) [L.] Not of sound mind; mentally incompetent to handle one's affairs.

nonconductor [L. *non,* not, + *con,* with, + *ductor,* a leader] Any substance that does not transmit heat, sound, or electricity or that conducts it with difficulty. Strictly speaking, there is no perfect nonconductor. On the application of a sufficiently high voltage, current may be caused to flow through materials usually spoken of as nonconductors. SEE: *insulator.*

nondisclosure The act of withholding relevant information. Health care providers have a legal and an ethical obligation to ensure that patients have access to information regarding their health and health management. Failure to provide data concerning diagnosis, prognosis, or treatment options and implications, and the projected consequences of choices denies the patient the right to make an informed decision.

nondisjunction The failure of a pair of chromosomes to separate during meiosis, allowing one daughter cell to have two chromosomes and the other to have none.

nondominant In neurology, that hemisphere of the brain that does not control speech or the preferentially used hand. SEE: *cerebral dominance.*

nonelectrolyte [″ + Gr. *elektron,* amber, + *lytos,* dissolved] A solution that will not conduct electricity because its chemical constituents are not sufficiently dissociated into ions.

nongonococcal urethritis SEE: under *urethritis.*

non-Hodgkin's lymphoma SEE: under *lymphoma.*

nonigravida (nō″nĭ-gră′vĭ-dă) [L. *nonus,* ninth, + *gravida,* pregnant] A woman pregnant for the ninth time. Written gravida IX. SEE: *nonipara.*

noninvasive 1. Not tending to spread, as certain tumors. **2.** A device or procedure that does not penetrate the skin or enter any orifice in the body.

nonipara (nō-nĭp′ăr-ă) [″ + *parere,* to bring forth, to bear] A woman who has given birth nine times. Written para IX.

nonlaxative diet A low-residue diet containing boiled milk and toasted crackers. No strained oatmeal, vegetable juice, or fruit juice is given. Fats and concentrated sweets are restricted.

nonmaleficence The principal of not doing something that causes harm. Hippocrates felt this was the underpinning of all medical practice. He advised his students, *primum non nocere* ("first, do no harm").

nonmedullated (nŏn-mĕd′ū-lāt″ĕd) [L. *non,* not, + *medulla,* marrow] Nonmyelinated.

nonmyelinated (nŏn-mī′ĕ-lĭ-nāt″ĕd) [″ + Gr. *myelos,* marrow] Containing no myelin.

nonnucleated (nŏn-nū′klē-āt″ĕd) [″ + *nucleatus,* having a kernel] Containing no nucleus.

nonocclusion (nŏn″ŏ-kloo′zhŭn) [″ + *occlusio,* occlusion] A type of malocclusion in which the teeth fail to make contact.

nonopaque (nŏn″ō-pāk′) Not opaque, esp. to x-rays.

nonose (nŏn′ōs) [L. *nonus,* ninth] A nine-carbon carbohydrate.

nonoxynol (nō-nŏks′ĭ-nŏl) A general class of surface-active agents with the basic formula of $C_{15}H_{24}O(C_2H_4O)_n$, named with respect to the value of *n.* Nonoxynol 9 is a spermicide.

nonpolar [″ + *polus,* a pole] Not having separate poles; sharing electrons.

n. compound A compound formed by the sharing of electrons.

nonprogressor An individual infected with the human immunodeficiency virus who does not develop worsening immune function or symptoms of active disease.

nonproprietary name The name of a drug other than its trademarked (proprietary) name. The nonproprietary name for a new drug is usually the same as that selected by the United States Adopted Name (USAN) Council. The official names for older drugs may differ from the nonproprietary names. In some cases, the generic name is the same as the nonproprietary name. Drugs also have chemical names; in most cases those names are too long and complex to permit their use. The use of a USAN-selected name simplifies and standardizes drug nomenclature. SYN: *generic drugs*. SEE: *proprietary medicine*.

nonprotein [L. *non,* not, + Gr. *protos,* first] Any substance not derived from protein.

nonprotein nitrogen SEE: *nitrogen*.

non rep [L. *non repetatur*] Abbreviation meaning *do not repeat*.

nonresectable Not removable by surgery.

nonresponder **1.** An individual who does not achieve an immunological response to a vaccine. **2.** A person who does not respond in the expected way to therapy, particularly medication.

nonrestraint (nŏn″rē-strānt′) [L. *non,* not, + *re,* back, + *stringere,* to bind back] Treatment of the uncooperative without using mechanical restraints.

nonrotation (nŏn″rō-tā′shŭn) [″ + *rotare,* to turn] Failure of a part or organ to rotate, esp. during embryological development.

n. of the intestine In embryonic development, failure of the gut to turn to its normal position, often reversing the location of the right and left sides of the bowel, changing the relationship of the superior mesenteric vessels, and leading to other anomalies, including polysplenia and/or aplasia of the uncinate process of the pancreas. SYN: *malrotation of the intestine*.

nonsecretor (nŏn″sē-krē′tor) [″ + *secretio,* separation] An individual whose saliva and other body fluids do not contain the ABO blood antigens.

nonseptate (nŏn-sĕp′tāt) [″ + *septum,* a partition] Having no dividing walls.

nonsexual (nŏn-sĕk′shū-ăl) Asexual.

nonspecific **1.** Inexact, imprecise, not well delimited or defined. **2.** Vague. **3.** Poorly identified; described without certainty.

nonsteroidal anti-inflammatory drug ABBR: NSAID. A drug that has analgesic, anti-inflammatory, and antipyretic actions. NSAIDs are used to treat acute and chronic pain, including the pain of injuries, arthritis, and dysmenorrhea; to reduce inflammation; and to prevent complications in serious illness, such as sepsis.

Many patients experience side effects of these medications, including upper gastrointestinal inflammation or bleeding. These side effects occur most often in elderly people, tobacco users, and people who drink alcohol. Other potential complications include acute and chronic renal failure, liver function abnormalities, and aseptic meningitis.

Members of this class of drugs include acetaminophen, aspirin, and ibuprofen, among many others.

Patient Care: Patients who are sensitive to NSAID therapy are told to inform caregivers so they will not be given NSAIDs. Patients are instructed to watch for adverse effects when taking a drug of this category and report any gastrointestinal pain or bleeding. The patient should be cautioned not to take NSAIDs on an empty stomach.

nontoxic (nŏn-tŏk′sĭk) [L. *non,* not, + Gr. *toxikon,* poison] Not poisonous or productive of poison.

nontoxic substances Any substance characteristic of being nonpoisonous as ordinarily encountered. For those involved in patient care, it is important to know that some of the common materials that children and adults can accidentally ingest are not dangerous. A list of substances considered generally nontoxic is provided in the Appendix.

nonunion (nŏn-ūn′yŭn) [″ + *unio,* oneness] Failure to unite, as a fractured bone that fails to heal completely. Diagnosis of nonunion is established when a minimum of 9 months has elapsed since the injury and the fracture site shows no progressive signs of healing for a minimum of 3 months and is not complicated by a synovial pseudoarthrosis.

nonus [L.] **1.** Ninth. **2.** An out-of-date name for the hypoglossal nerve, once thought to be the ninth cranial nerve.

nonviable (nŏn-vī′ă-b′l) [L. *non,* not, + *via,* life] Incapable of life or of living. This term is frequently used to indicate a fetus that has died in utero, born prior to 20th week of gestation.

nonyl A univalent radical, $CH_3(CH_2)_8-$, that contains nine carbon atoms.

nookleptia (nō-ō-klĕp′tē-ă) [Gr. *nous,* mind, + *kleptein,* to steal] An obsession that one's thoughts are being stolen by others.

Noonan's syndrome [Jacqueline A. Noonan, U.S. cardiologist, b. 1921] An autosomal dominant syndrome, occurring in about 1 in 1800 births, marked by cardiac valve and aortic anomalies. Other findings include low-set ears, webbing of the neck, cubitum valgum, and sometimes severe mental retardation.

noopsyche (nō′ō-sī″kē) [Gr. *nous,* mind, + *psyche,* soul] Mental processes.

NORD *National Organization for Rare Disorders.*

norepinephrine (nor-ĕp″ĭ-nĕf′rĭn) **1.** A

hormone produced by the adrenal medulla, similar in chemical and pharmacological properties to epinephrine, but chiefly a vasoconstrictor with little effect on cardiac output. **2.** A neurotransmitter released by most sympathetic postganglionic neurons and by some neurons of the brain. A disturbance in its metabolism at important brain sites has been implicated in affective disorders. It is used to manage severe hypotension, esp. in patients with neurogenic or septic shock.

n. bitartrate A standardized preparation of norepinephrine. The former name was levarterenol bitartrate.

norethindrone (nor-ĕth′ĭn-drōn) A steroid hormone that is similar in action to progesterone and that is used in progestational agents for birth control.

norethynodrel (nor″ĕ-thī′nō-drĕl) A progestational agent used in certain birth control pills.

norflurane (nor-floor′ān) An inhalation anesthetic.

norgestrel (nor-jĕs′trĕl) A progestational agent used in certain birth control pills.

norm [L. *norma,* rule] **1.** A standard or ideal for a specific group. **2.** Normal.

norma [L., rule] A view or aspect, esp. with reference to the skull.

anterior n. N. frontalis.

n. basilaris N. ventralis.

n. facialis N. frontalis.

n. frontalis The outline of the skull viewed from the front. SYN: *anterior n.; n. facialis.*

inferior n. N. ventralis.

n. lateralis A view of the skull as seen from the side; a profile view.

n. occipitalis A view of the skull as seen from behind.

n. sagittalis A view of the skull as seen in sagittal section.

superior n. N. verticalis.

n. ventralis A view of the inferior surface of skull. SYN: *n. basilaris; inferior n.*

n. verticalis A view of the skull as seen from above. SYN: *superior n.*

normal (nor′măl) [L. *normalis,* according to pattern] **1.** Standard; performing proper functions; natural; regular. **2.** In biology, not affected by experimental treatment; occurring naturally and not because of disease or experimentation. **3.** In psychology, free from mental disorder; of average development or intelligence.

n. distribution SEE: under *distribution.*

n. salt SEE: under *salt.*

n. solution A solution in which 1 L contains 1 g equivalent of the solute.

normalization (nor″măl-ī-zā′shŭn) [L. *normalis,* according to pattern] Modification or reduction to the normal standard.

normergic (nor-mĕr′jĭk) Reacting, or pert. to that which reacts, in a normal manner.

normetanephrine (nor-mĕt″ă-nĕf′rĭn) A metabolite of epinephrine.

normoblast (nor′mō-blăst) [″ + Gr. *blastos,* germ] An immature nucleated red blood cell similar in size to a mature erythrocyte, usually found in the bone marrow. **normoblastic** (-blăs-tĭk), *adj.*

normoblastosis (nor″mō-blăs-tō′sĭs) [″ + ″ + *osis,* condition] Increased production and circulation of normoblasts. This indicates a need for greater oxygen-carrying capacity of the blood, as when mature erythrocytes are being rapidly destroyed.

normocalcemia (nor″mō-kăl-sē′mē-ă) Normal level of blood calcium.

normocapnia (nor″mō-kăp′nē-ă) The presence of a normal concentration of carbon dioxide in the blood and serum. **normocapnic** (-kăp′nĭk), *adj.*

normocholesterolemia (nor″mō-kō-lĕs″tĕr-ō-lē′mē-ă) The presence of a normal concentration of cholesterol in the blood.

normochromasia (nor″mō-krō-mā′zē-ă) [″ + Gr. *chroma,* color] Average staining capacity in a cell or tissue.

normocyte (nor′mō-sīt) [″ + Gr. *kytos,* cell] An average-sized red blood cell. SYN: *erythrocyte.*

normoglycemia (nor″mō-glī-sē′mē-ă) [″ + Gr. *glykys,* sweet, + *haima,* blood] Normal sugar content of the blood. **normoglycemic** (-sē′mĭk), *adj.*

normokalemia (nor″mō-kă-lē′mē-ă) Normal level of blood potassium.

normospermic (nor″mō-spĕr′mĭk) [″ + Gr. *sperma,* seed] Producing normal spermatozoa.

normosthenuria (nor″mō-sthĕn-ū′rē-ă) [″ + Gr. *sthenos,* strength, + *ouron,* urine] Urination which is of a normal amount and specific gravity.

normotensive (nor″mō-tĕn′sĭv) **1.** Normal blood pressure. **2.** A person with normal blood pressure.

normothermia (nor″mō-thĕr′mē-ă) [″ + Gr. *therme,* heat] Normal body temperature.

normotopia (nor″mō-tō′pē-ă) [″ + Gr. *topos,* place] Situation in the normal place. **normotopic** (nor″mō-tŏp′ĭk), *adj.*

normovolemia (nor″mō-vō-lē′mē-ă) [″ + *volumen,* volume, + Gr. *haima,* blood] Normal blood volume. **normovolemic,** *adj.*

Norplant Trade name for a contraceptive system that prevents pregnancy for up to 5 yr. Six matchstick-sized silicone plastic capsules containing levonorgestrel are inserted in a fanlike pattern just under the skin of a woman's arm. The procedure takes approx. 15 min and is performed in a physician's office under a local anesthetic. When the implant is removed, fertility is restored. Some problems with removal have been reported.

Norplant, like all drugs, is not free of

side effects. Some users report amenorrhea, menstrual irregularities, weight change, mood swings, and headache. Some of these side effects are the same as would serve to identify early pregnancy. Thus, tests should be performed whenever pregnancy is suspected.

Norrie's disease [Gordon Norrie, Danish ophthalmologist, 1855–1941] A rare form of x-linked hereditary blindness due to retinal malformation. Also present are peripheral vascular pathology, vitreous opacities, microphthalmia, and sometimes mental retardation and loss of hearing.

Norton scale (nor-tan′) A scale used to predict patients at high risk for pressure sores. The patient is rated from 1 to 4 on five risk factors. Individuals with a score of 14 are considered at risk for decubitus ulcers; those who score below 12 are at high risk for skin breakdown. SEE: *pressure sore* for table.

nortriptyline hydrochloride (nor-trĭp′tĭ-lēn) A tricyclic antidepressant.

Norwalk agent [virus first identified in Norwalk, Ohio, U.S.A.] A calicivirus that is the causative organism in over half of the reported cases of epidemic viral gastroenteropathy. The incubation period ranges from 18 to 72 hr. The outbreaks are usually self-limiting and the intestinal signs and symptoms last for 24 to 48 hr. Treatment, if required, is supportive and directed to maintaining hydration and electrolyte balance. SEE: *Calicivirus.*

Norwegian itch SEE: *scabies, Norwegian.*

nose [AS. *nosw*] The projection in the center of the face that is the organ of smell and the entrance to the nasal cavities. The nose is a triangle composed of and bounded by bone and cartilage covered with skin and lined with mucous membrane. Hairs just inside the nostrils block the entrance of dusts and small insects. SYN: *nasus; organum olfactus.*

EXAMINATION: Note the shape, size, color, and state of the alae nasi, and any discharge, interference with respiration, evidence of injury, deflected or perforated septum, enlarged turbinates, and tenderness over frontal and maxillary sinuses.

DIAGNOSIS: *Chronic red nose:* Dilated capillaries as a result of alcoholism, lupus erythematosus, acne rosacea, pustules, and boils. *Superficial ulceration:* Basal cell carcinoma, tuberculosis, syphilis, tuberculous ulcer, epithelioma. *Broad and coarse:* Cretinism, myxedema, acromegaly. *Sunken:* Syphilis or injury. *Pinched with small nares:* Hypertrophied adenoid tissue or chronic obstructions; tumors. *Inoffensive watery discharge:* Allergic rhinitis, the common cold, early stages of measles. *Offensive discharge:* Nasopharyngeal diphtheria, lupus, local infection, impacted foreign bodies, caries, rhinitis, glanders, syphilitic infection.

bridge of the n. The superior portion of the external nose formed by the union of the two nasal bones.

foreign body in the n. Presence of material in the nasal cavity that was either inhaled or accidentally placed there. A child may place a foreign object in his or her own or another child's nose.

SYMPTOMS: Coughing or watery or purulent discharge; occasionally pain and obstruction of nose. The foreign body may cause a nasal obstruction and infection, often with a foul-smelling discharge. If the foreign body is very small, symptoms may be absent.

TREATMENT: Vigorous nose blowing should be discouraged because it may spread infection to the various cavities and sinuses about the nose or to the middle ear. The foreign body should be removed by a health care professional.

hammer n. Rhinophyma.

saddle n. A nose with a depressed bridge due to congenital absence of bony or cartilaginous support, to a disease such as leprosy or congenital syphilis, or to postoperative complications of suppuration and destruction of the supporting framework.

nosebleed Hemorrhage from the nose. SEE: illus.; *epistaxis; Kiesselbach's area.*

Nosema (nō-sē′mă) A genus of parasites of the order Microsporidia. SEE: *microsporidiosis.*

nosepiece (nōz′pēs) The portion of a microscope to which the objective lenses attach.

nose springs A springlike device applied to the bridge of the nose that pulls the nostrils open slightly. The device may reduce nasal airway resistance, thereby improving sleep quality and decreasing snoring.

noso- [Gr. *nosos,* disease] Combining form denoting *disease.*

nosochthonography (nŏs″ŏk-thō-nŏg′ră-fē) [″ + *chthon,* earth, + *graphein,* to write] Study of geographical distribution of diseases. SYN: *geomedicine.*

nosocomial (nŏs″ō-kō′mē-ăl) [Gr. *nosokomos,* one who tends the sick] Pert. to or occurring in a hospital or infirmary.

nosocomial infection Infection acquired in a healthcare facility.

nosology (nō-sŏl′ō-jē) [″ + *logos,* word, reason] The science of description or classification of diseases.

nosomycosis (nŏs″ō-mī-kō′sĭs) [″ + *mykes,* fungus, + *osis,* condition] Any disease caused by a parasitic fungus or schizomycete.

nosophobia (nō″sō-fō′bē-ă) [″ + *phobos,* fear] An abnormal aversion to illness or to a particular disease.

nosophyte (nŏs′ō-fīt) [″ + *phyton,* plant] A disease-causing plant microorganism.

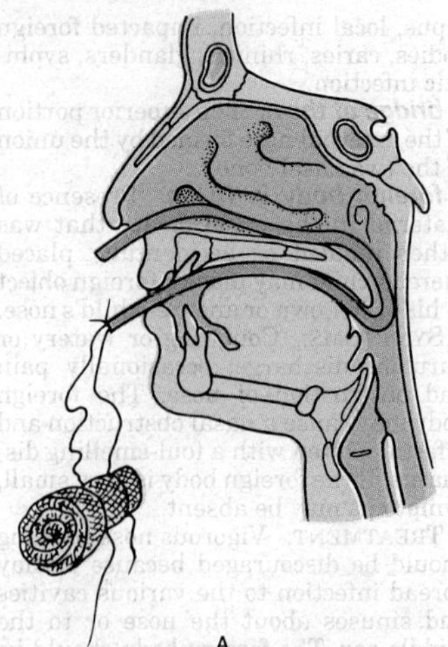

A.
INSERT SOFT FLEXIBLE CATHETER INTO NOSE AND BRING DISTAL TIP OUT THROUGH THE MOUTH. ATTACH MOISTENED PACK TO CATHETER

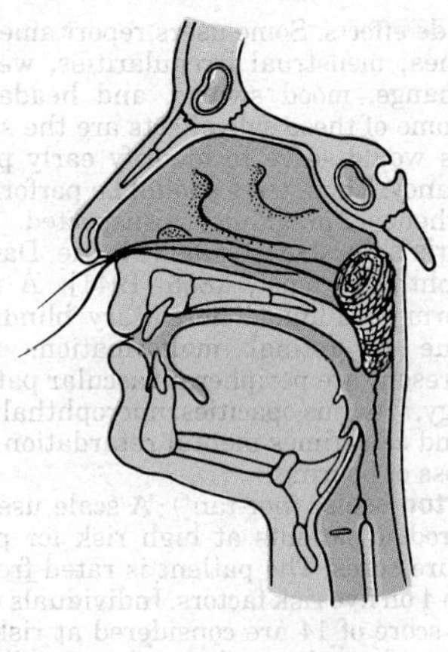

B.
BY PULLING ON CATHETER DRAW PACK IN PLACE SO IT IS PLACED SECURELY IN POSTERIOR NASAL CAVITY

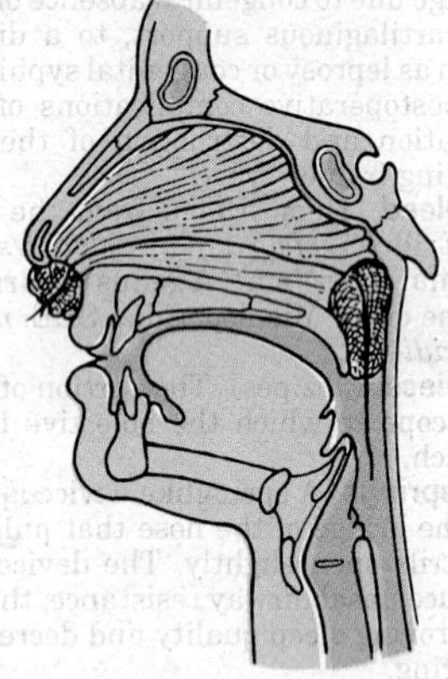

C.
REMOVE CATHETER AND USE STRING TO ATTACH TO A SOFT CUSHION OF SUFFICIENT SIZE TO PREVENT ITS PASSING INTO THE NOSTRIL

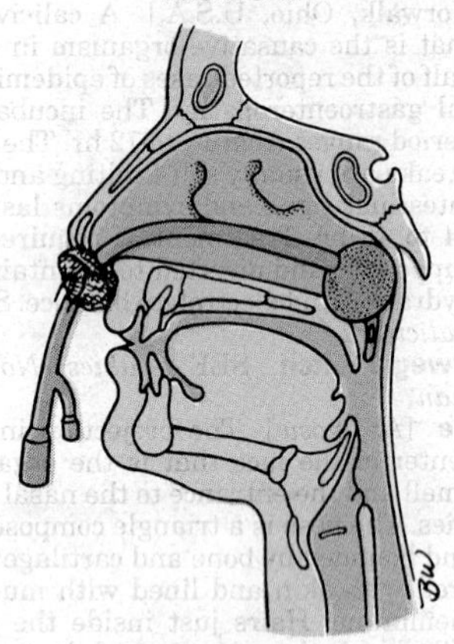

D.
ALTERNATIVELY, A FOLEY CATHETER MAY BE USED. THE INFLATED TIP IS HELD SECURELY IN PLACE AS IN PREVIOUS ILLUSTRATIONS

TECHNIQUE FOR CONTROL OF HEMORRHAGE FROM POSTERIOR NASAL CAVITY

Nosopsyllus (nŏs″ō-sĭl′ŭs) [″ + *psylla,* flea] A genus of fleas belonging to the order Siphonaptera.

N. fasciatus A species of rat fleas responsible for transmission of murine typhus and possibly plague.

nostalgia (nŏs-tăl′jē-ă) [Gr. *nostos,* a return home, + *algos,* pain] Homesickness; longing to return home.

nostril [AS. *nosu,* nose, + *thyrel,* a hole] One of the external apertures of the nose. SYN: *naris*. SEE: *nose*.

n. reflex Reduction of the opening of the naris on the affected side in lung disease in proportion to lessened alveolar air capacity on the affected side.

nostrum (nŏs′trŭm) [L., our] A patent, secret, or quack remedy.

notalgia (nō-tăl′jē-ă) [Gr. *noton,* back, + *algos,* pain] Pain in the back. SYN: *dorsalgia*.

notancephalia (nō″tăn-sĕ-fā′lē-ă) [″ + *-an,* not, + *kephale,* head] Congenital absence of the back of the skull.

notanencephalia (nō″tăn-ĕn-sĕ-fā′lē-ă) [″ + ″ + *enkephalos,* brain] Absence of the cerebellum.

notch (nŏch) A deep indentation or narrow gap in the edge of a structure. SYN: *incisure*.

acetabular n. The notch in the inferior border of the acetabulum.

antigonial n. A depression in the inferior border of the mandible at the anterior edge of the insertion of the masseter muscle.

aortic n. The notch in a sphygmogram caused by rebound at aortic valve closure.

cardiac n. The concavity on the anterior border of the left lung into which the heart projects.

cerebellar n. Either of two deep notches (anterior and posterior) separating the hemispheres of the cerebellum.

clavicular n. A notch at the upper angle of the sternum with which the clavicle articulates.

costal n. Any of seven pairs of indentations on the lateral surfaces of the sternum, for articulation with costal cartilages.

ethmoidal n. The notch separating the two orbital portions of the frontal bone.

frontal n. The notch on the supraorbital arch that transmits the frontal artery and nerve.

greater sciatic n. A large notch on the posterior border of the hip bone between the posterior inferior iliac spine and the spine of the ischium.

interclavicular n. A rounded notch at the top of the manubrium of the sternum between the surfaces articulating with the clavicles.

jugular n. (of occipital bone) A notch that forms the posterior and middle portions of the jugular foramen.

jugular n. (of sternum) A notch on the upper surface of the manubrium of the anterior superior chest between the two clavicular notches.

labial n. A notch in the labial flange of a denture at the point where it crosses the frenum.

lesser sciatic n. A notch immediately below the spine of the ischium on the posterior border of the hip bone, which is converted into a foramen by the sacrotuberous ligament.

mandibular n. A notch on the superior border of the ramus of the mandible separating the coronoid and condyloid processes.

manubrial n. A depression on the superior edge of the sternum.

nasal n. **1.** A deep notch on the anterior surface of the maxilla, forming the lateral border of the piriform aperture. **2.** A notch between the internal angular processes of the frontal bone.

pancreatic n. A notch on the lateral surface of the head of the pancreas for the superior mesenteric artery and vein. It separates the uncinate process of the head from the remaining portion.

parotid n. The space between the ramus of the mandible and the mastoid process of the temporal bone.

radial n. A notch on the lateral surface of the coronoid process of the ulna for receiving the circumference of the head of the radius.

n. of Rivinus SEE: *Rivinus' incisure*.

scapular n. A deep notch on the superior border of the scapula that transmits the suprascapular nerve.

semilunar n. A notch on the anterior aspect of the proximal end of the ulna for articulation with the trochlea of the humerus. SYN: *trochlear n.*

sphenopalatine n. A notch between the orbital and sphenoidal processes of the palatine bone.

tentorial n. An arched cavity in the free border of the tentorium cerebelli through which the brainstem passes.

thyroid n. A deep notch on the superior border of the thyroid cartilage of the larynx that separates the two laminae.

trochlear n. Semilunar notch.

tympanic n. The notch in the upper part of the tympanic portion of the temporal bone.

ulnar n. The notch on the distal end of the radius that receives the head of the ulna.

umbilical n. A notch on the anterior border of the liver where it is crossed by the falciform ligament.

vertebral n. A concavity on the inferior surface of the vertebral arch for transmission of a spinal nerve.

notchplasty A surgical procedure to enlarge the intercondylar notch and space available for an anterior cruciate ligament graft during knee reconstruction. The lateral wall of the notch, which is the medial portion of the lateral femoral condyle, may be removed by various means.

note [L. *nota*, a mark] **1.** A sound of definite pitch. **2.** A brief comment or condensed report.

n. blindness The inability to recognize musical notes, due to a lesion of the central nervous system.

notencephalocele (nō″tĕn-sĕf′ăl-ō-sēl) [Gr. *noton*, back, + *enkephalos*, brain, + *kele*, tumor, swelling] Protrusion of the brain from the back of the head.

notencephalus (nō″tĕn-sĕf′ă-lŭs) [″ + *enkephalos*, brain] A deformed fetus with notencephalocele.

nothing by mouth An instruction used in patient care to indicate that the patient is not to take or receive food, solids, liquid, or medicine orally. This order is usually indicated by the abbreviation *n.p.o.*

noto- [Gr. *noton*, back] Combining form indicating a relationship to the back.

notochord (nō′tō-kord) [″ + *chorde*, cord] A rod of cells lying dorsal to the intestine and extending from the anterior to the posterior end. The notochord forms the axial skeleton in embryos of all chordates. In vertebrates it is replaced partially or completely by the bodies of vertebrae. A remnant persists in humans as a portion of the nucleus pulposus of the intervertebral disk.

notogenesis (nō″tō-jĕn′ĕ-sĭs) [″ + *genesis,* generation, birth] Development of the notochord.

notomelus (nō-tŏm′ĕ-lŭs) [″ + *melos,* limb] A deformed fetus with one or more accessory limbs attached to the back.

nourishment [L. *nutrire,* to nurse] **1.** Sustenance; nutriment; food. **2.** The act of nourishing or of being nourished. SEE: *trophic.*

noxa (nŏk′să) *pl.* **noxae** [L., injury] Anything harmful to health.

noxious (nŏk′shŭs) [L. *noxius,* injurious] Harmful; not wholesome.

NP *nucleoprotein; nurse practitioner; nursing practice; nursing procedure; neuropsychiatrist; neuropsychiatry.*

Np Symbol for the element neptunium.

NPC *nodal premature complex.*

NPDB *National Practitioner Data Bank.*

NPH insulin *neutral protamine Hagedorn* insulin.

NPN *nonprotein nitrogen.*

NPO, n.p.o. [L.] *non per os,* nothing by mouth.

NPT *normal pressure and temperature; nocturnal penile tumescence.*

NREM *nonrapid eye movement.* SEE: under *sleep.*

N.R.E.M.T. *Nationally Registered Emergency Medical Technician.*

N.R.M.S. *National Registry of Medical Secretaries.*

NRTI Nucleoside reverse transcriptase inhibitor.

ns 1. *nanosecond.* **2.** *nonsignificant.*

NSA *Neurosurgical Society of America.*

NSAID *nonsteroidal anti-inflammatory drug.*

NSCC *National Society for Crippled Children.*

NSD in ret *nominal standard dose* in *radiation equivalent therapy.* SEE: *ret.*

nsec *nanosecond.*

N.S.N.A. *National Student Nurses' Association.*

NSR *normal sinus rhythm.*

nth (ĕnth) Used in medical statistics to indicate the continuation of data or subjects to large numbers in a progression or series. Thus, one would indicate patients numbered P1, P2, P3, and so forth through Pnth. Pnth would be the last patient indicated.

nubile (nū′bĭl) [L. *nubere,* to marry] Of marriageable age; pert. to a girl who has attained puberty.

nucha (nū′kă) [L.] The nape (back) of the neck. **nuchal** (nū′kăl), *adj.*

Nuck's canal (nŭks) [Anton Nuck, Dutch anatomist, 1650–1692] A persistent peritoneal pouch that accompanies the round ligament of the uterus through the inguinal canal.

nuclear (nū′klē-ăr) [L. *nucleus,* a kernel] Concerning or pertaining to a cellular, atomic, or anatomical nucleus. SEE: *nucleus; nuclear m.; n. medicine scanning test;* names of specific anatomic nuclei.

n. antigen An antigen present in the cells of patients with certain types of connective tissue disorders. Corticosteroids can be very helpful in treating patients with high concentrations of extractable nuclear antigen.

n. arc Spiral patterns on the surface of the lens due to a concentric pattern of fiber growth.

n. envelope SEE: under *envelope.*

n. family The basic family unit consisting of parents and their children.

n. magnetic resonance imaging ABBR: NMRI. SEE: *magnetic resonance imaging.*

n. medicine SEE: under *medicine.*

n. medicine scanning test Any test that relies on the use of radioactive tracers to diagnose disease. The substances (radioactive isotopes) are either injected into the body or inhaled, the dose of radiation is minimal, and the substances used either lose their radioactivity in a short time or are excreted. This technique, called a "scan," may be used to diagnose tumors, biliary disease, gastrointestinal emptying or bleeding, coronary artery disease, valvular heart disease, red blood cell survival time, renal dysfunction, deep vein thrombosis, thyroid function, osteomyelitis, fractures, and cardiac ejection fraction. Isotopes of thallium, iodine, or other metals are used.

n. transfer The removal of DNA from a cell for placement into an egg (e.g., during cloning).

nuclease (nū′klē-ās) [L. *nucleus,* kernel, + *-ase,* enzyme] Any enzyme in animals or plants that facilitates hydrolysis of nuclein and nucleic acids.

nucleate (nū′klē-āt) [L. *nucleatus,* having a kernel] **1.** Having a nucleus. **2.** To form a nucleus.

nucleic acid Any one of a group of high-molecular-weight chemicals that carry the genetic information crucial to the replication of cells and the manufacturing of cellular proteins. They have a complex structure formed of sugars (pentoses), phosphoric acid, and nitrogen bases (purines and pyrimidines). Most important are ribonucleic acid (RNA) and deoxyribonucleic acid (DNA). SEE: illus.

nuclein (nū′klē-ĭn) [L. *nucleus,* a kernel] A normal chemical constituent of a cell nucleus that is a colorless, shapeless substance obtained by hydrolysis of nucleoproteins to form nucleic acid and proteins.

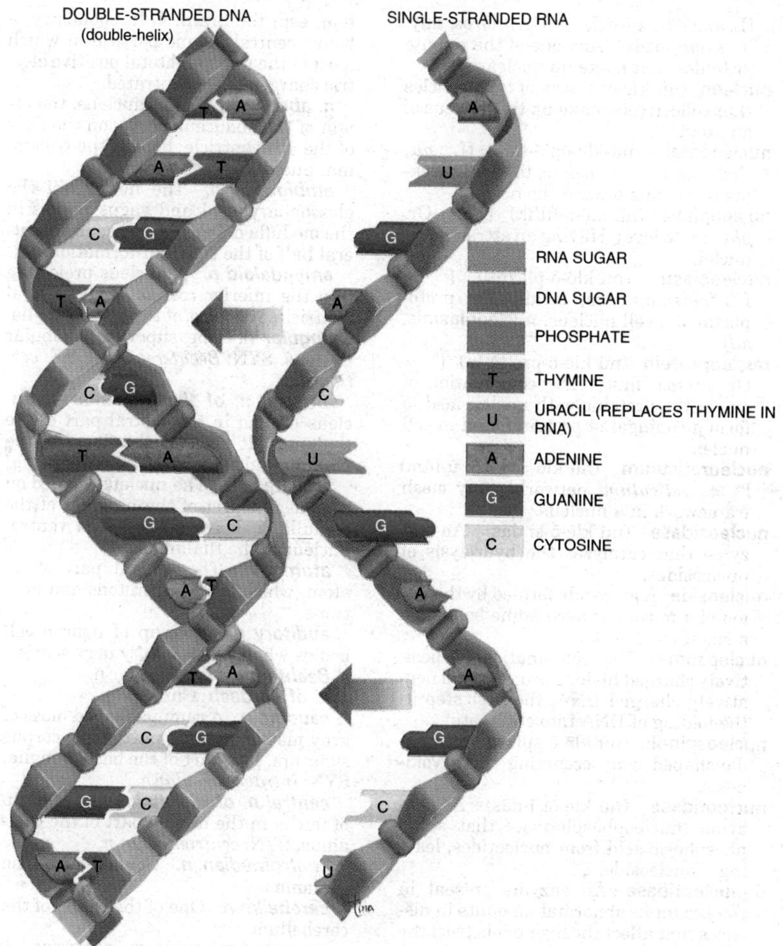

NUCLEIC ACID
DNA and RNA

nuclein base Any of the bases formed from decomposition of nuclein, such as adenine, guanine, xanthine, hypoxanthine.

nucleo- [L. *nucleus,* kernel] Pert. to a nucleus.

nucleocapsid (nū″klē-ō-kăp′sĭd) In a virus, the protein coat and the viral nucleic acid.

nucleofugal (nū-klē-ŏf′ū-găl) [″ + *fugere,* to flee] Directed or moving away from a nucleus.

nucleohistone (nū″klē-ō-hĭs′tŏn, -tōn) [″ + Gr. *histos,* tissue] A substance composed of nuclein and histone, found in sperm of various animals.

nucleoid (nū′klē-oyd) [″ + Gr. *eidos,* form, shape] Resembling a nucleus.

nucleoliform (nū-klē-ō′lĭ-form) [[L. *nucleolus,* a little kernel, + *forma,* shape] Like a nucleolus.

nucleoloid (nū′klē-ō-loyd) Similar to a nucleus.

nucleolonema (nū″klē-ō″lō-nē′mă) [″ + Gr. *nema,* thread] A fine network in the nucleolus of a cell.

nucleolus (nū-klē′ō-lŭs) *pl.* **nucleoli** [L., little kernel] A spherical structure in the nucleus of a cell made of DNA, RNA, and protein. It is the site of synthesis of ribosomal RNA (rRNA); a cell may have more than one. Embryonic cells and those in malignancies actively synthesize rRNA; therefore, their nucleoli are larger than those of cells that do not require increased amounts of rRNA. **nucleolar** (nū-klē′ō-lăr), *adj.*

nucleomicrosome (nū″klē-ō-mī′krō-sōm)

[L. *nucleus,* kernel, + Gr. *mikros,* tiny, + *soma,* body] Any one of the minute granules that make up nuclear fibers.

nucleon (nū′klē-ŏn) Any of the particles that collectively make up the nucleus of an atom.

nucleopetal (nū-klē-ŏp′ĕ-tăl) [L. *nucleus,* kernel, + *petere,* to seek] Seeking or moving toward the nucleus.

nucleophilic (nū″klē-ō-fĭl′ĭk) [″ + Gr. *philein,* to love] Having an attraction to nuclei.

nucleoplasm (nū′klē-ō-plăzm″) [″ + LL. *plasma,* form, mold] The protoplasm of a cell nucleus. **nucleoplasmic,** *adj.*

nucleoprotein (nū″klē-ō-prō′tē-ĭn) [″ + Gr. *protos,* first] The combination of one of the proteins with nucleic acid to form a conjugated protein found in cell nuclei.

nucleoreticulum (nū″klē-ō-rē-tĭk′ū-lŭm) [″ + *reticulum,* network] Any mesh framework in a nucleus.

nucleosidase (nū″klē-ō-sī′dās) An enzyme that catalyzes the hydrolysis of nucleosides.

nucleoside A glycoside formed by the union of a purine or pyrimidine base with a sugar (pentose).

nucleosome The combination of positively charged histone proteins and negatively charged DNA; the first step in the folding of DNA into chromatin.

nucleospindle (nū″klē-ō-spĭn′d'l) A spindle-shaped body occurring in karyokinesis.

nucleotidase (nū″klē-ŏt′ĭ-dās) An enzyme (nucleophosphatase) that splits phosphoric acid from nucleotides, leaving a nucleoside.

5′-nucleotidase An enzyme present in the serum in abnormal amounts in diseases that affect the liver or obstruct the biliary tree.

nucleotide (nū′klē-ō-tīd) [L. *nucleus,* kernel] A compound formed of phosphoric acid, a pentose sugar, and a base (purine or pyrimidine), all of which constitute the structural unit of nucleic acid. SYN: *mononucleotide.*

nucleotidyl (nū″klē-ō-tīd′ĭl) The residue of a nucleotide.

nucleotidyltransferase (nū″klē-ō-tīd″ĭl-trăns′fĕr-ās) An enzyme that transfers nucleotidyls from nucleosides into dimer or polymer forms.

nucleotoxin [″ + Gr. *toxikon,* poison] A toxin acting upon or produced by cell nuclei.

nucleus (nū′klē-ŭs) *pl.* **nuclei** [L., kernel] **1.** A central point about which matter is gathered, as in a calculus. **2.** The structure within a cell that contains the chromosomes. It is responsible for the cell's metabolism, growth, and reproduction. SEE: *cell.* **3.** A group of neuron cell bodies, which form a mass of gray matter in the central nervous system, esp. the brain. **4.** In chemistry, a heavy central atomic particle in which most of the mass and total positive electric charge are concentrated.

n. abducens A gray nucleus, the origin of the abducens nerve, on the floor of the 4th ventricle, behind the trigeminal nucleus.

ambiguous n. The nucleus of the glossopharyngeal and vagus nerves in the medulla oblongata. It lies in the lateral half of the reticular formation.

amygdaloid n. A nucleus projecting into the inferior cornua of the lateral ventricle. It is part of the basal ganglia.

angular n. The superior vestibular nucleus. SYN: *Bechterew's n.* SEE: *vestibular n.*

anterior n. of the thalamus A nucleus located in the rostral part of the thalamus. It receives the fibers of the mamillothalamic tract.

arcuate n. **1.** The nucleus located on the basal aspect of the pyramid of the medulla. **2.** The posteromedial ventral nucleus of the thalamus.

atomic n. The central part of an atom, which contains protons and neutrons.

auditory n. A group of neuron cell bodies where the auditory nerves arise.

Bechterew's n. Angular n.

n. of Burdach Cuneate n.

caudate n. A comma-shaped mass of gray matter forming part of the corpus striatum. It is part of the basal ganglia. SYN: *intraventricular n.*

central n. of the thalamus A group of nuclei in the middle part of the thalamus. SYN: *centromedian n.*

centromedian n. Central n. of the thalamus.

cerebellar n. One of the nuclei of the cerebellum.

cornucommissural n. posterior A column of cells that extends the entire length of the spinal cord and lies along the medial border of the posterior column near the posterior gray commissure.

cuneate n. A nucleus in the inferior portion of the medulla oblongata in which fibers of the fasciculus cuneatus terminate. SYN: *n. of Burdach.*

Deiters' n. The lateral vestibular nucleus. SEE: *vestibular n.*

dentate n. A large convoluted mass of gray matter in the lateral portion of the cerebellum. It is folded so as to enclose some of the central white matter and gives rise to the fibers of the superior cerebellar peduncle.

diploid n. A nucleus containing the normal double complement of chromosomes.

dorsal cochlear n. The nucleus in the medulla oblongata lying dorsal to the restiform body and receiving fibers from the cochlear nerve.

dorsal motor n. of vagus A column of cells in the medulla oblongata lying lateral to the hypoglossal nucleus. Its cells give rise to most of the efferent fibers of the vagus nerve.

dorsal sensory n. of vagus A nucleus lying lateral to the dorsal motor nucleus of the vagus. It receives the fibers of the solitary tract.

dorsal n. of the spinal cord A column of gray matter lying at the base of the dorsal horn of the gray matter and extending from the seventh cervical to the third lumbar segments. These cells give rise to fibers of the dorsal spinocerebellar tract. SYN: *Clarke's column.*

ectoblastic n. A nucleus in the cells of the epiblast.

Edinger-Westphal n. A nucleus of the midbrain located dorsomedially to the oculomotor nucleus. It gives rise to the visceral efferent fibers terminating in the ciliary ganglion, the axons from which innervate the ciliary muscle and the sphincter iridis of the eye.

emboliform n. A nucleus of the cerebellum lying between the dentate and globose nuclei. It receives the axons of Purkinje cells and sends efferent fibers into the brachium conjunctivum.

facial motor n. A nucleus in the medulla oblongata in the floor of the fourth ventricle giving rise to efferent fibers of the facial nerve.

fastigial n. A nucleus in the medullary portion of the cerebellum that receives afferent fibers from the vestibular nerve and superior vestibular nucleus. The afferent fibers form the fasciculus uncinatus and the fastigiobulbar tract.

fertilization n. A nucleus produced by the joining of the male and female nuclei in the fertilization of the ovum.

free n. A nucleus that is no longer surrounded by the other cellular components.

n. funiculi gracilis An elongated mass of gray matter in the dorsal pyramid of the medulla oblongata of the brain. SYN: *postpyramidal n.*

germinal n. A nucleus resulting from the union of male and female pronuclei.

globose n. A nucleus of the cerebellum located medial to the emboliform nucleus.

gonad n. Micronucleus (2).

n. gracilis A nucleus in the medulla oblongata in which fibers of the fasciculus gracilis terminate.

habenular n. A nucleus of the diencephalon located in the habenular trigone. It is an olfactory correlation center.

haploid n. A cell nucleus with half the normal number of chromosomes, as in germ cells (ova and sperm) following the normal reduction divisions in gametogenesis.

hypoglossal n. An elongated mass of gray matter in the medulla oblongata in the floor of the fourth ventricle, giving rise to the motor fibers of the hypoglossal nerve.

hypothalamic n. One of the nuclei occurring in four groups found in the hypothalamus. Hypothalamic nuclei include the dorsomedial, intercalatus, lateral, mamillary (lateral and medial), paraventricular, posterior, supraoptic, tuberal, and ventromedial. The cells of these nuclei secrete oxytocin and antidiuretic hormone. These hormones pass through the efferent fibers of the infundibular stalk to the posterior lobe of the pituitary gland, where they are stored until they are released. SYN: *subthalamic n.*

inferior olivary n. A large convoluted mass of gray matter lying in the ventral part of the medulla oblongata and forming part of the reticular system. It gives rise to fibers of the olivocerebellar tract.

inferior salivatory n. A nucleus located in the pons near the level of the dorsal motor nucleus of the vagus. It gives rise to preganglionic parasympathetic fibers that pass to the otic ganglion via the glossopharyngeal nerve. Impulses regulate secretions of the parotid gland.

interpeduncular n. A nucleus of the midbrain near the superior border of the pons. It receives fibers of the habenulopeduncular tract.

interstitial n. of Cajal A nucleus in the superior portion of the midbrain. It receives fibers from the vestibular nuclei, basal ganglia, and occipital regions of cerebral cortex. The efferent fibers pass to the ipsilateral and contralateral fasciculi and the interstitiospinal tracts.

intraventricular n. Caudate n.

lenticular n. One of the nuclei forming part of the basal ganglia of the cerebrum, consisting of the globus pallidus and putamen. With the caudate nucleus, it forms the corpus striatum.

n. lentis The core or inner dense section of the crystalline lens.

masticatory n. Motor n. of the trigeminal nerve.

mesencephalic tract n. The only site of primary sensory neurons within the central nervous system for proprioceptive impulses from the trigeminal nerve.

mother n. A nucleus that divides into two or more parts to form daughter nuclei.

motor n. A nucleus giving rise to the motor fibers of a nerve.

motor n. of the trigeminal nerve A nucleus in the medulla oblongata near the first margin of the superior part of the 4th ventricle. It gives rise to the motor fibers of the trigeminal nerve, which innervates the muscles of mastication, tensor tympani, tensor palatini, and the anterior digastric muscle. SYN: *masticatory nucleus.*

oculomotor n. A nucleus in the central gray matter of the midbrain lying below the rostral end of the cerebral aqueduct.

n. of origin Any of the collection of nerve cells giving rise to the fibers of a nerve or nerve tract.

paraventricular n. A nucleus of the hypothalamus lying in the supraoptic portion. Its axons with those of the supraoptic nucleus form the supraopticohypophyseal tract. SEE: *hypothalamic n.*

pontine n. One of several groups of nerve cells located in the pons. It transmits afferent fibers to the cerebral cortex; efferent fibers pass through the brachium pontis to the cerebellum.

postpyramidal n. N. funiculi gracilis.

principal trigeminal sensory n. The site of sensory neurons of the trigeminal nerve associated with discriminatory touch. It is located in the pons.

n. pulposus The center cushioning gelatinous mass lying within an intervertebral disk; the remains of the notochord.

pyramidal n. A band of gray matter near the olivary nucleus in the medulla.

red n. A large, oval, pigmented mass in the upper portion of the midbrain extending upward into the subthalamus. It receives fibers from the cerebral cortex and cerebellum; the efferent fibers give rise to the rubrospinal tracts. SYN: *n. ruber.*

reproductive n. Micronucleus (2).

reticular n. A column of neurons in the spinal cord, brainstem, and thalamus affecting local reflex activity, muscle tone, and wakefulness.

n. ruber Red n.

segmentation n. The nucleus of a zygote formed by fusion of the male and female pronuclei.

sensory n. The nucleus of termination of the afferent fibers of a peripheral nerve.

sensory n. of the trigeminal nerve A group of nuclei in the pons and medulla oblongata consisting of the spinal nucleus, which extends inferiorly into the spinal cord, the main nucleus, which lies dorsal and lateral to the motor nucleus, and the mesencephalic nucleus, which lies in the lateral wall of the 4th ventricle.

sperm n. The head of the spermatozoon.

subthalamic n. Hypothalamic n.

superior olivary n. A small nucleus located in the mid-lateral tegmental region of the pons. It receives fibers from the ventral cochlear nucleus.

superior salivatory n. An ill-defined nucleus in the pons lying dorsomedial to the facial nucleus. It gives rise to preganglionic parasympathetic fibers passing through the chorda tympani and lingual nerve to the submaxillary ganglion. Impulses regulate secretions of the submaxillary and sublingual glands.

supraoptic n. The nucleus of the hypothalamus lying above the rostral ends of the optic tracts and lateral to the optic chiasma. SEE: *hypothalamic n.*

n. of termination Any of thc clusters of cells in the brain and medulla in which fibers of a nerve or nerve tract terminate.

thalamic n. Any of the nuclei of the thalamus, including a large number belonging to the anterior, intralaminar, lateral, and medial thalamic nuclei groups.

thoracic n. A column of large neurons in the posterior gray column of the spinal cord. These cells give rise to the dorsal spinocerebellar tract on the same side.

trigeminal spinal n. The site of sensory neurons of the trigeminal nerve associated with pain, temperature, and light touch. It is located in the pons and upper spinal tract.

ventral cochlear n. The nucleus in the medulla oblongata lying anterior and lateral to the restiform body and receiving fibers from the cochlear nerve.

vesicular n. A nucleus having a deeply staining membrane and a pale center.

vestibular n. One of four nuclei in the medulla oblongata in which fibers of the vestibular nerve terminate. These four nuclei are the medial (Schwalbe's), superior (Bechterew's), lateral (Deiters'), and inferior nuclei.

vitelline n. Nucleus formed by union of male and female pronuclei within the vitellus; a part of the cytoplasm of an ovum in which the initial process of accumulation of food supplies is probably located. SYN: *yolk n.*

white n. The central white matter of the corpus dentatum of the olive.

yolk n. Vitelline n.

nuclide (nū′klīd) An atomic nucleus identified by its atomic number, mass, and energy state.

nude [L. *nudus,* naked] **1.** Bare; naked; unclothed. **2.** An unclothed body.

nude mouse SEE: under *mouse.*

nudism **1.** In psychiatry, morbid desire to remove clothing. **2.** The cult or practice of living without clothing.

nudomania (nū″dō-mā′nē-ă) [L. *nudus,* naked + Gr. *mania,* madness] Abnormal desire to be naked.

nudophobia (nū″dō-fō′bē-ă) [″ + Gr. *phobos,* fear] Abnormal fear of being naked. SEE: *gymnophobia.*

Nuel's space (nū′ĕlz) [Jean-Pierre Nuel, Belg. physician, 1847–1920] The space in the organ of Corti between the outer pillar and the outer phalangeal cells (Deiters' cells).

NUG *necrotizing ulcerative gingivitis.*

Nuhn's glands (noonz) [Anton Nuhn, Ger. anatomist, 1814–1889] Blandin's glands.

nuisance Anything that causes inconvenience, annoyance, or disturbance of normal physiology.

null cell SEE: under *cell.*

null hypothesis SEE: under *hypothesis.*

nulligravida A woman who has never conceived a child.

nullipara (nŭl-ĭp′ă-ră) [L. *nullus,* none, + *parere,* to bear] A woman who has never produced a viable offspring.

nulliparity (nŭl″ĭ-păr′ĭ-tē) Condition of not having given birth to a child.

nulliparous (nŭl-lĭp′ăr-ŭs) Never having borne a child.

numb (nŭm) **1.** Insensible; lacking in feeling. **2.** Deadened or lacking in the power to move.

number [L. *numerus,* number] **1.** A total of units. **2.** A symbol graphically representing an arithmetical sum.

atomic n. The number of negatively charged electrons in an uncharged atom, or the number of protons in the nucleus. This number determines the position of elements in the periodic table of elements.

Avogadro's n. SEE: *Avogadro's number.*

hardness n. A number on a calibrated scale indicating the relative hardness as determined by a particular system of testing (e.g., Knoop, Mohs, Rockwell, Vickers hardness tests). A steel ball or diamond point is applied with a known variable load for a determined period of time to produce an indent whose depth or diameter can be measured.

mass n. The mass of the atom of a specific isotope relative to the mass of hydrogen. In general, this number is equal to the total of the protons and neutrons in the atomic nucleus of that specific isotope.

number needed to harm The number of patients who would need to be exposed to a noxious agent or medical intervention in order that one might be harmed. This concept is important in the assessment of the relative hazard of medical interventions, the relative toxicities of poisons, or the relative value of certain experimental interventions. Generally, the smaller the value, the more dangerous the therapy or noxious agent.

number needed to treat The number of patients who must receive a specific therapy (or undergo a specific medical test) so that one of them will benefit. This concept is important in assessing the relative values and costs of interventions for specific illnesses. For example, to prevent one death from breast cancer the number of patients who need annual mammography can be calculated. Similarly, the number of patients with cancer who will survive because of the use of a particular chemotherapy regimen can be assessed. Generally, the smaller the number needed to treat, the greater the value of the intervention. This comparative information can be used to decide how to allocate resources, plan studies, or make recommendations to patients about their care.

numbness Lack of sensation in a part, esp. from cold. SEE: *narcohypnia.*

numeral (nū′mĕr-ăl) [L. *numerus,* number] **1.** Denoting or pert. to a number. **2.** A conventional symbol expressing a number.

nummiform (nŭm′mĭ-form) [L. *nummus,* a coin, + *forma,* shape] **1.** Coin-shaped, said of some mucous sputum. **2.** Arranged like a stack of coins.

nummular (nŭm′ū-lăr) [L. *nummus,* coin] **1.** Coin-shaped. **2.** Stacked like coins, as in a rouleau of red blood cells.

nunnation (nŭn-ā′shŭn) [Heb. *nun,* letter N] The frequent and abnormal use of the "n" sound.

Nuremberg Code A set of principles established after World War II to protect the rights of research participants (subjects).

nurse [L. *nutrix,* nurse] **1.** An individual who provides health care. The extent of participation varies from simple patient care tasks to the most expert professional techniques necessary in acute life-threatening situations. The ability of a nurse to function in making self-directed judgments and to act independently will depend on his or her professional background, motivation, and opportunity for professional development. The health care team includes the technical nurse, who is technique-oriented, deals with commonly recurring nursing problems, and knows standardized procedures and medically delegated techniques. Also included is the professional nurse, who is prepared to assume responsibility for the care of individuals and groups through a colleague relationship with a physician. The roles of nurses constantly change in response to the growth of biomedical knowledge, changes in patterns of demand for health services, and the evolution of professional relationships among nurses, physicians, and other health care professionals. **2.** To feed an infant at the breast. **3.** To perform the duties of caring for an invalid. **4.** To care for a young child.

advanced practice n. A registered nurse with additional education, skill, and specialization in various fields of medicine. SEE: *n. anesthetist; clinical n. specialist; n. midwife; n. practitioner.*

n. anesthetist ABBR: CRNA. A registered nurse who administers anesthesia to patients in the operating room and delivery room. The knowledge and skill required to provide this service are attained through an organized program of study recognized by the American Association of Nurse Anesthetists.

charge n. A nurse who is responsible for supervising the nursing staff on a hospital or nursing home unit. This nurse reports to the nurse manager.

clinical n. specialist A nurse with particular competence in certain areas such as intensive care, cardiology, oncology, obstetrics, or psychiatry. A clinical nurse specialist holds a master's degree in nursing, preferably with emphasis in clinical nursing.

n. clinician A registered nurse with preparation in a specialized educational program. At present this preparation may be in the context of a formal continuing education program, a baccalaureate nursing program, or an advanced-degree nursing program. The nurse clinician is capable of working independently in solving patient-care problems and is able to teach and work successfully with others on the medical care team. The term was first used by Frances Reiter, R.N., M.A., Dean, Graduate School of Nursing, New York Medical College.

community health n. A nurse who combines the principles and practices of nursing and public health to provide care to the people in a community rather than in an institution.

dental n. A dental auxiliary trained to provide oral hygiene instruction and dental health care to school children. Formerly, the term applied to dental hygienists, but now it refers to persons trained according to a program developed in New Zealand.

epidemiologist n. A registered nurse with special training and certification in the prevention of hospital-acquired infections in patients. SEE: *infection control n.*

flight n. A nurse who cares for patients being transported in an aircraft.

general duty n. A nurse not specializing in a particular field but available for any nursing duty.

graduate n. A nurse who is a graduate of a state-approved school of nursing but has not yet passed the National Council Licensure Examination.

head n. Outdated term for nurse manager.

health n. A community or visiting nurse whose duty is to give information on hygiene and prevention of disease. SEE: *community health n.*

home health n. A nurse who visits patients in their homes to provide skilled nursing services, such as assessment and patient and family teaching.

infection control n. A registered nurse employed by an agency to monitor the rate and causes of nosocomial infections and to promote measures to prevent such infections.

licensed practical n. ABBR: L.P.N. A graduate of a school of practical nursing who has passed the practical nursing state board examination and is licensed to administer care, usually working under direction of a licensed physician or a registered nurse.

licensed vocational n. ABBR: L.V.N. Licensed practical n.

n. manager A nurse who has responsibility for a unit within a hospital, nursing home, or ambulatory care setting. The nurse manager supervises staff performance and patient care.

n. midwife A registered nurse who has completed specialized theory and clinical courses in obstetrics and gynecology and is certified by the American College of Nurse Midwives. The nurse midwife's scope of practice includes providing primary obstetric, neonatal, and preventive gynecological care to essentially healthy women and their normal newborns, usually in collaboration with an obstetrician-gynecologist.

n. practitioner ABBR: NP. A licensed registered nurse who has had advanced preparation for practice that includes 9 to 24 months of supervised clinical experience in the diagnosis and treatment of illness. The NP concept was developed in 1965 by Henry Silver, M.D., and Loretta Ford, R.N. Most contemporary NP programs are at the master's degree level; graduates are prepared for primary care practice in family medicine, women's health, neonatology, pediatrics, school health, geriatrics, or mental health. NPs may work in collaborative practice with physicians or independently in private practice or in nursing clinics. Depending upon state laws, NPs may be allowed to write prescriptions for medications. SEE: *n. clinician; n. midwife; nursing, advanced practice.*

prescribing n. A nurse who is allowed to prescribe drugs. Certain states in the U.S. permit nurses to prescribe only certain types and classes of drugs; most states require that prescribing nurses work with a supervising or collaborating physician; and approval for prescribing is granted only to nurse practitioners.

private duty n. A nurse who cares for a patient on a fee-for-service basis, usually in an institution. The nurse is not a staff member of the institution.

psychiatric n. practitioner A registered nurse with advanced preparation who combines medical and nursing skills in the care and treatment of psychiatric or mental health patients.

public health n. Community health n.

registered n. ABBR: RN. A nurse who has graduated from a state-approved school of nursing, has passed the professional nursing state board examination, and has been granted a license to practice within a given state.

school n. A nurse working in a school or college who is responsible for the health of children, adolescents, and young adults in school.

scrub n. An operating room nurse who directly assists the surgeon, primarily by passing instruments and supplies.

special n. Private duty n.

specialist n. Clinical n. specialist.

visiting n. Community health n.

wet n. A woman who breast-feeds a child that is not her own.

nursery A hospital department in which the newborn are cared for.

day n. SEE: *day care center.*

nurse's aide An individual who assists nurses by performing the patient-care procedures that do not require special technical training, such as feeding and bathing patients.

nursing **1.** The care and nurturing of healthy and ill people, individually or in groups and communities. The American Nurses Association identifies four essential features of contemporary nursing practice: attention to the full range of human experiences and responses to health and illness without restriction to a problem-focused orientation; integration of objective data with knowledge gained from an understanding of the patient or group's subjective experience; application of scientific knowledge to the processes of diagnosis and treatment; and provision of a caring relationship that facilitates health and healing. SEE: *nurse*. **2.** Breastfeeding.

advanced practice n. Primary medical care provided by nurses who have been prepared as practitioners and are competent to provide that level of care. These practitioners may act independently or under the supervision of a physician.

barrier n. The use of special gloves, masks, gowns, and so forth, to prevent contact between sources of infection and medical personnel caring for critically ill patients. Situations in which one would use these precautions include care of the patient with tuberculosis, gas gangrene, fulminant sepsis, and other highly contagious conditions. SYN: *isolation*.

director of n. ABBR: DON, DN. The nursing manager or chief executive officer.

PROFESSIONAL ORGANIZATION: The National Association of Directors of Nursing–Long-term Care (NADONA-LTC) addresses the needs of directors of nursing and assistant directors of nursing, and provides educational conferences.

forensic n. A subspecialty of nursing in which the nursing process is applied to public health, occupational health, mental health, or legal proceedings.

gerontological n. The art and science of nursing care of the elderly.

holistic n. The art and science of caring for and nurturing the whole person. SEE: *holism*.

nursing assessment The systematic collection of all data and information relevant to the care of patients, their problems, and needs. The initial step of the assessment consists of obtaining a careful and complete history from the patient. If this cannot be done because the mental or physical condition of the patient makes communication impossible, the nursing history is obtained from those who have information about the patient and the reason(s) for his or her need of medical and nursing care. Obtaining an accurate and comprehensive history requires skill in communicating with individuals who are ill, including those who are reluctant or unable to share important life experiences and medical data. The skilled nurse will be able to obtain the essential information despite resistance. Next in the assessment is the physical examination of the patient in order to determine how the disease has altered physical and mental status. To do this requires that the nurse be capable of performing visual and tactile inspection, palpation, percussion, and auscultation and have knowledge of what represents deviation from the norm and how disease and trauma alter the physical and mental condition of a patient. After these two steps have been completed, the nurse will be able to establish a nursing diagnosis. SEE: illus. *evaluation; nursing process.*

nursing assistant ABBR: N.A. An unlicensed nursing staff member who assists with basic patient care such as giving baths, checking vital signs, bedmaking, and positioning. Nursing assistants usually must complete a training course, including classroom instruction and clinical practice under supervision. Each state regulates nursing assistant practice.

geriatric n. ABBR: GNA. An unlicensed caregiver who provides basic care needs, such as bathing and feeding, to residents in nursing homes or other health care facilities. According to federal regulations, GNAs must successfully complete at least a prescribed training course and register in the state in which they are practicing. SEE: *nursing assistant.*

NURSING ASSESSMENT TOOL (Medical/Surgical)

This adult medical-surgical assessment tool is a suggested guide for creating a database reflecting a nursing focus. It can be adapted to meet the needs of specific patient populations.

General Information

Name: ______

Age: ______ DOB: ______ Gender: ______ Race: ______

Admission Date: ______ Time: ______ From: ______

Source of Information: ______

Reliability (1–4 with 4 = very reliable): ______

Activity/Rest

SUBJECTIVE (REPORTS)

Occupation: ______ Usual activities: ______

Leisure time activities/hobbies: ______

Limitations imposed by condition: ______

Sleep: Hours: ______ Naps: ______ Aids: ______

Insomnia: ______ Related to: ______

Rested on awakening: ______

Excessive grogginess: ______

Feelings of boredom/dissatisfaction: ______

OBJECTIVE (EXHIBITS)

Observed response to activity: Cardiovascular: ______

Respiratory: ______

Mental status (i.e., withdrawn/lethargic): ______

Neuro/muscular assessment:

Muscle mass/tone: ______

Posture: ______ Tremors: ______

ROM: ______ Strength: ______ Deformity: ______

Circulation

SUBJECTIVE (REPORTS)

History of:

Hypertension: ______ Heart trouble: ______

Rheumatic fever: ______ Ankle/leg edema: ______

Phlebitis: ______ Slow healing: ______

Claudication: ______

Dysreflexia: ______

Bleeding tendencies/episodes: ______

Palpitations: ______ Syncope: ______

Extremities: Numbness: ______ Tingling: ______

Cough/hemoptysis: ______

Change in frequency/amount of urine: ______

OBJECTIVE (EXHIBITS)

BP: R and L: Lying/sit/stand: ______

Pulse pressure: ______ Auscultatory gap: ______

Pulses (palpation): Carotid: ______ Temporal: ______

Jugular: ______ Radial: ______ Femoral: ______

Popliteal: ______ Post-tibial: ______ Dorsalis pedis: ______

Cardiac (palpation): Thrill: ______ Heaves: ______

Heart sounds: Rate: ______ Rhythm: ______ Quality: ______

Friction rub: ______ Murmur: ______

Vascular bruit: ______ Jugular vein distention: ______

Breath sounds: ______

SOURCE: Doenges, Marilynn E., et al: Nursing Care Plans: Guidelines for Individualizing Patient Care, ed 5. FA Davis, Philadelphia, 2000.

(continued)

(continued from previous page)

Extremities: Temperature: ____________ Color: ____________
Capillary refill: ____________
Homans' sign: ____________ Varicosities: ____________
Nail abnormalities: ____________ Edema: ____________
Distribution/quality of hair: ____________
Trophic skin changes: ____________
Color: General: ____________
Mucous membranes: ____________ Lips: ____________
Nailbeds: ____________ Conjunctiva: ____________ Sclera: ____________
Diaphoresis: ____________

Ego Integrity

SUBJECTIVE (REPORTS)

Stress factors: ____________
Ways of handling stress: ____________
Financial concerns: ____________
Relationship status: ____________
Cultural factors/ethnic ties: ____________
Religion: ____________ Practicing: ____________
Lifestyle: ____________ Recent changes: ____________
Sense of connectedness/harmony with self: ____________
Feelings of: Helplessness: ____________ Hopelessness: ____________
Powerlessness: ____________

OBJECTIVE (EXHIBITS)

Emotional status (check those that apply):
Calm: ____________ Anxious: ____________ Angry: ____________
Withdrawn: ____________ Fearful: ____________ Irritable: ____________
Restive: ____________ Euphoric: ____________
Observed physiological response(s): ____________
Changes in energy field:
Temperature: ____________ Color: ____________ Distribution: ____________
Movement: ____________
Sounds: ____________

Elimination

SUBJECTIVE (REPORTS)

Usual bowel pattern: ____________
Laxative use: ____________
Character of stool: ____________ Last BM: ____________
Diarrhea: ____________ Constipation: ____________
History of bleeding: ____________ Hemorrhoids: ____________
Usual voiding pattern: ____________
Incontinence/when: ____________ Urgency: ____________
Frequency: ____________ Retention: ____________
Character of urine: ____________
Pain/burning/difficulty voiding: ____________
History of kidney/bladder disease: ____________
Diuretic use: ____________

OBJECTIVE (EXHIBITS)

Abdomen: Tender: ____________ Soft/firm: ____________
Palpable mass: ____________ Size/girth: ____________
Bowel sounds: Location: ____________ Type: ____________
Hemorrhoids: ____________ Stool guaiac: ____________
Bladder palpable: ____________ Overflow voiding: ____________
CVA tenderness: ____________

(continued)

(continued from previous page)

Food/Fluid

SUBJECTIVE (REPORTS)

Usual diet (type): __________

Carbohydrate/Protein/Fat intake: g/d __________

Vitamin/food supplement use: __________

Food preferences: __________ Prohibitions: __________

No. of meals daily: __________

Dietary pattern/content: B: __________ L: __________ D: __________

Last meal/intake: __________

Loss of appetite: __________ Nausea/vomiting: __________

Heartburn/indigestion: __________

Related to: __________ Relieved by: __________

Allergy/food intolerance: __________

Mastication/swallowing problems: __________

Dentures: __________

Usual weight: __________ Changes in weight: __________

Diuretic use: __________

OBJECTIVE (EXHIBITS)

Current weight: __________ Height: __________ Body build: __________

Skin turgor: __________ Mucous membranes moist/dry: __________

Breath sounds: Crackles: __________ Wheezes: __________

Edema: General: __________ Dependent: __________

Periorbital: __________ Ascites: __________

Jugular vein distention: __________

Thyroid enlarged: __________

Condition of teeth/gums: __________

Appearance of tongue: __________

Mucous membranes: __________ Halitosis: __________

Bowel sounds: __________

Hernia/masses: __________

Urine S/A or Chemstix: __________

Serum glucose (glucometer): __________

Hygiene

SUBJECTIVE (REPORTS)

Activities of daily living: Independent/dependent (level):

Mobility: __________ Feeding: __________

Hygiene: __________ Dressing/Grooming: __________

Toileting: __________

Preferred time of personal care/bath: __________

Equipment/prosthetic devices required: __________

Assistance provided by: __________

OBJECTIVE (EXHIBITS)

General appearance: __________

Manner of dress: __________ Personal habits: __________

Body odor: __________ Condition of scalp: __________

Presence of vermin: __________

Neurosensory

SUBJECTIVE (REPORTS)

Fainting spells/dizziness: __________

Headaches: Location: __________ Frequency: __________

Tingling/numbness/weakness (location): __________

Stroke/brain injury (residual effects): __________

Seizures: Type: __________ Aura: __________

Frequency: __________ Postictal state: __________

How controlled: __________

(continued)

(continued from previous page)

Eyes: Vision loss: ______ Last examination: ______
Glaucoma: ______ Cataract: ______
Ears: Hearing loss: ______ Last examination: ______
Sense of smell: ______ Epistaxis: ______

OBJECTIVE (EXHIBITS)

Mental status (note duration of change):
Oriented/disoriented: Time: ______ Place: ______
Person: ______ Situation: ______
Check all that apply:
Alert: ______ Drowsy: ______ Lethargic: ______
Stuporous: ______ Comatose: ______
Cooperative: ______ Combative: ______
Delusions: ______ Hallucinations: ______
Affect (describe): ______
Memory: Recent: ______ Remote: ______
Glasses: ______ Contacts: ______ Hearing aids: ______
Pupil: Shape: ______ Size/reaction: R/L: ______
Facial droop: ______ Swallowing: ______
Handgrasp/release, R/L: ______
Posturing: ______
Deep tendon reflexes: ______ Paralysis: ______

Pain/Discomfort

SUBJECTIVE (REPORTS)

Primary focus: ______ Location: ______
Intensity (0–10 with 10 = most severe): ______
Frequency: ______ Quality: ______
Duration: ______ Radiation: ______
Precipitating/aggravating factors: ______
How relieved: ______
Associated symptoms: ______
Effect on activities: ______
Relationships: ______
Additional focus: ______

OBJECTIVE (EXHIBITS)

Facial grimacing: ______ Guarding affected area: ______
Posturing: ______ Behaviors: ______
Emotional response: ______ Narrowed focus: ______
Change in BP: ______ Pulse: ______

Respiration

SUBJECTIVE (REPORTS)

Dyspnea/related to: ______
Cough/sputum: ______
History of: Bronchitis: ______ Asthma: ______
Tuberculosis: ______ Emphysema: ______
Recurrent pneumonia: ______
Exposure to noxious fumes: ______
Smoker: ______ pk/day: ______ No. of pk-yrs: ______
Use of respiratory aids: ______ Oxygen: ______

OBJECTIVE (EXHIBITS)

Respiratory: Rate: ______ Depth: ______ Symmetry: ______
Use of accessory muscles: ______ Nasal flaring: ______
Fremitus: ______
Breath sounds: ______ Egophony: ______
Cyanosis: ______ Clubbing of fingers: ______

(continued)

(continued from previous page)

Sputum characteristics: ______

Mentation/restlessness: ______

Safety

SUBJECTIVE (REPORTS)

Allergies/sensitivity: ______ Reaction: ______

Exposure to infectious diseases: ______

Previous alteration of immune system: ______

Cause: ______

History of sexually transmitted disease (date/type): ______

Testing: ______ High-risk behaviors: ______

Blood transfusion/number: ______ When: ______

Reaction: ______ Describe: ______

Geographic areas lived in/visited: ______

Seat belt/helmet use: ______

History of accidental injuries: ______

Fractures/dislocations: ______

Arthritis/unstable joints: ______

Back problems: ______

Changes in moles: ______ Enlarged nodes: ______

Delayed healing: ______

Cognitive limitations: ______

Impaired vision/hearing: ______

Prosthesis: ______ Ambulatory devices: ______

OBJECTIVE (EXHIBITS)

Temperature: ______ Diaphoresis: ______

Skin integrity (mark location on diagram): ______

Scars: ______ Rashes: ______ Lacerations: ______

Ulcerations: ______ Ecchymoses: ______ Blisters: ______

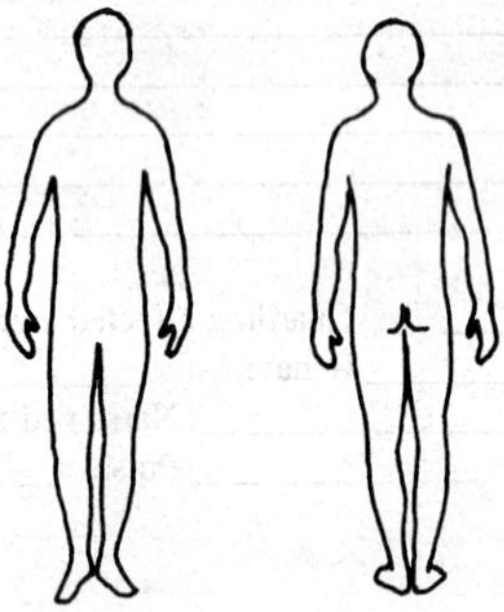

Burns (degree/percent): ______

Drainage: ______

General strength: ______ Muscle tone: ______

Gait: ______ ROM: ______

Paresthesia/paralysis: ______

Results of cultures: ______ Immune system testing: ______

Tuberculosis testing: ______

Sexuality (Component of Ego Integrity and Social Interactions)

SUBJECTIVE (REPORTS)

Sexually active: ______ Use of condoms: ______

Birth control method: ______

Sexual concerns/difficulties: ______

Recent change in frequency/interest: ______

(continued)

(continued from previous page)

OBJECTIVE (EXHIBITS)

Comfort level with subject matter: ____

FEMALE: SUBJECTIVE (REPORTS)

Age at menarche: ____ Length of cycle: ____
Duration: ____ No. of pads used/day: ____
Last menstrual period: ____ Pregnant now: ____
Bleeding between periods: ____
Menopause: ____ Vaginal lubrication: ____
Vaginal discharge: ____
Surgeries: ____
Hormonal therapy/calcium use: ____
Practices breast self-examination: ____
Last mammogram: ____ PAP smear: ____

OBJECTIVE (EXHIBITS)

Breast examination: ____
Genital warts/lesions: ____ Discharge: ____

MALE: SUBJECTIVE (REPORTS)

Penile discharge: ____ Prostate disorder: ____
Circumcised: ____ Vasectomy: ____
Practice self-examination: Breast: ____ Testicles: ____
Last proctoscopic/prostate examination: ____

OBJECTIVE (EXHIBITS)

Breast: ____ Penis: ____ Testicles: ____
Genital warts/lesions: ____ Discharge: ____

Social Interactions

SUBJECTIVE (REPORTS)

Marital status: ____ Years in relationship: ____
Perception of relationship: ____
Living with: ____
Concerns/stresses: ____
Extended family: ____
Other support person(s): ____
Role within family structure: ____
Perception of relationships with family members: ____
Feelings of: Mistrust: ____ Rejection: ____
Unhappiness: ____
Loneliness/isolation: ____
Problems related to illness/condition: ____
Problems with communication: ____
Genogram: ____

OBJECTIVE (EXHIBITS)

Speech: Clear: ____ Slurred: ____
Unintelligible: ____ Aphasic: ____
Unusual speech pattern/impairment: ____
Use of speech/communication aids: ____
Laryngectomy present: ____
Verbal/nonverbal communication with family/SO(s): ____
Family interaction (behavioral) pattern: ____

Teaching/Learning

SUBJECTIVE (REPORTS)

Dominant language (specify): ____ Second language: ____
Literate: ____ Education level: ____
Learning disabilities (specify): ____
Cognitive limitations: ____

(continued)

(continued from previous page)

Where born: ____________ If immigrant, how long in this country? ____________

Health and illness beliefs/practices/customs: ____________

Special healthcare concerns (e.g., impact of religious/cultural practices): ____________

Health goals: ____________

Familial risk factors (indicate relationship):

Diabetes: ____________ Thyroid (specify): ____________

Tuberculosis: ____________ Heart disease: ____________

Strokes: ____________ High BP: ____________

Epilepsy: ____________ Kidney disease: ____________

Cancer: ____________ Mental illness: ____________

Other: ____________

Prescribed medications:

Drug: ____________

Dose: ____________ Times (circle last dose): ____________

Take regularly: ____________ Purpose: ____________

Side effects/problems: ____________

Nonprescription drugs: OTC drugs: ____________

Street drugs: ____________ Tobacco: ____________

Smokeless tobacco: ____________

Alcohol (amount/frequency): ____________

Use of herbal supplements (specify): ____________

Admitting diagnosis per provider: ____________

Reason per patient: ____________

History of current complaint: ____________

Patient expectations of this hospitalization: ____________

Previous illnesses and/or hospitalizations/surgeries: ____________

Evidence of failure to improve: ____________

Last complete physical examination: ____________

Discharge Plan Considerations

DRG projected mean length of stay: ____________

Date information obtained: ____________

Anticipated date of discharge: ____________

Resources available: Persons: ____________

Financial: ____________ Community: ____________

Support groups: ____________

Socialization: ____________

Areas that may require alteration/assistance:

Food preparation: ____________ Shopping: ____________

Transportation: ____________ Ambulation: ____________

Medication/IV therapy: ____________ Treatments: ____________

Wound care: ____________ Supplies: ____________

Self-care (specify): ____________

Homemaker/maintenance (specify): ____________

Physical layout of home (specify): ____________

Anticipated changes in living situation after discharge: ____________

Living facility other than home (specify): ____________

Referrals (date, source, services):

Social services: ____________ Rehab services: ____________

Dietary: ____________ Home care: ____________

Resp/O_2: ____________ Equipment: ____________

Supplies: ____________

Other: ____________

nursing audit A procedure to evaluate the quality of nursing care provided for a patient. Established criteria for care are the yardstick for the evaluation. SEE: *nursing process; problem-oriented medical record*.

nursing care plan SEE: under *plan*.

nursing diagnosis The patient problem identified by the nurse for nursing intervention by analysis of assessment findings in comparison with what is considered to be normal. Nurses, esp. those involved in patient care, are in virtually constant need to make decisions and diagnoses based on their clinical experience and judgment. In many instances, that process dictates a course of action for the nurse that is of vital importance to the patient. As the nursing profession evolves and develops, nursing diagnosis will be defined and specified in accordance with the specialized training and experience of nurses, particularly for nurse practitioners and clinical nurse specialists. SEE: *nursing process; planning*.

nursing goal A specific expected outcome of nursing intervention as related to the established nursing diagnosis. A goal is stated in terms of a desired, measurable change in patient status or behavior. Nursing goals provide direction for selection of appropriate nursing interventions and evaluation of patient progress.

nursing history The first step of the assessment stage of the nursing process that leads to development of a nursing care plan. Valuable information can be obtained from this history, and reactions to previous hospitalization can be recorded and utilized in managing the patient's care during the current stay.

nursing home An extended-care facility for patients who need continued health care, usually after a hospital stay. Nursing homes provide 24-hr nursing supervision, rehabilitation services, activity and social services, a safe environment, careful attention to nutritional needs, and measures to prevent complications of decreased mobility. In addition, some nursing homes have specialty units for patients with dementia, chronic ventilator support, or head injuries. Some nursing homes provide subacute units for patients who are not as medically stable as patients in the typical nursing home setting.

Most nursing homes are licensed and certified to provide an intermediate or skilled level of care or both. Medicare reimbursement is available for patients receiving skilled care in a skilled nursing facility.

Patients who are admitted to nursing homes are called residents. The nursing home must provide a homelike environment for each resident. Residents vary from 18 to over 100 years of age. Many facilities have younger residents who stay for several days or weeks to receive rehabilitation services (e.g., for orthopedic surgeries and strokes). Other residents may remain in the nursing home for the remainder of their lives.

The number of people who reside in a nursing home is expected to increase as the generation of "baby boomers" becomes older and requires more health care services. About 1.5 million Americans live in nursing homes, and that number is expected to triple in 30 yr.

nursing informatics The use of computer science, information technology, and nursing science to help manage, process, and analyze nursing data, information, and knowledge to support the practice of nursing and the delivery of patient care.

nursing intervention In the nursing process, the step after planning. This step involves all aspects of actual caring for the patient and requires full knowledge of the assessment and planning stages of the nursing process. The goals of nursing intervention will have been stated in the planning step of the nursing process. Included in this step are patient care in the areas of hygiene and mental and physical comfort, including assistance in feeding and elimination, controlling the physical aspects of the patient's environment, and instructing the patient about the factors important to his or her care and what actions to take to facilitate recovery. After the patient's acute and immediate needs are met, he or she should be instructed concerning actions that could be taken to help prevent a recurrence of the condition. SEE: *nursing process; planning; problem-oriented medical record*.

Nursing Minimum Data Set ABBR: NMDS. An abstracting system designed to collect minimal, comparable standardized nursing care information. It may be used in different settings and for different types of patients. Among its purposes are to identify trends and emerging needs in nursing care, to guide nursing research, and to use statistics to influence decisions in health care policy. It provides data for multiple users in the health care system. SEE: *Minimum Data Set*.

nursing model SEE: under *model*.

nursing process An orderly, logical approach to administering nursing care so that the patient's needs for such care are met comprehensively and effectively. The objective of health care is to provide total, comprehensive care of patients. Nursing has always been dedicated to this concept and, from the holistic viewpoint, has formalized the scientific processes that contribute to the prevention of illness as well as restoration and maintenance of health. In so doing, the traditional approaches used in problem solving have been used. Therefore the nurse needs skills in the following five areas to provide comprehensive care of patients: (1) *Assessment:* The systemic collection of all data and information relevant to the patients, their problems, and needs. (2) *Problem identification:* The analysis and interpretation of the information obtained during assessment that establishes the nursing diagnosis. (3) *Planning:* The use of skills to determine individualized patient-centered goals and the optimum course of action to solve the problem. (4) *Planning:* The use of skills to determine individualized expected patient-centered outcomes, objective methods of evaluating patient progress toward the contributory goals, and optimum courses of action to resolve the problems identified and achieve the outcomes desired. (5) *Evaluation:* The ongoing process of assessing the effectiveness of the plan in terms of measurable progress toward established nursing goals, and altering the approach and goals as needed. SEE: *evaluation; nursing assessment; nursing intervention; planning; problem-oriented medical record.*

nursing protocol A specific written procedure that prescribes nursing actions in a given situation. Health agencies and physicians establish protocols to ensure consistency and quality of care. A protocol may describe mandatory nursing asessments, behaviors, and documentation for establishing and maintaining invasive appliances; methods of administering specific drugs; special-care modalities for patients with certain disorders; other components of patient care; lines of authority; or channels of communication under particular circumstances.

nursing research A formal, systematic, and rigorous process of inquiry used by nurses to generate and test the concepts and propositions that constitute middle-range nursing theories, which are derived from or linked with a conceptual model of nursing. The theories include: *Grand:* Health belief model; Transactional model of stress and coping; Life process interactive person-environment model; Roy's adaptation model; Interacting systems conceptual framework. *Middle-Range:* Theory of self-care deficit; Theory of health promotion; Theory of self-regulation; Theory of uncertainty in illness; Theory of acute pain management; Theory of families, children, and chronic illness. *Practice:* Theory of interpersonal relations; Theory of representativeness heuristic; Theory of communicative action; Theory of clinical reasoning in nursing practice; Theory of end-of-life decision making.

nursing standards The criteria established by professional nursing organizations that describe peer expectations for safe, competent, ethical performance of professional responsibilities. Documents such as the American Nurses' Association Standards of Clinical Practice and Standards of Professional Performance describe general behaviors expected of all professional nurses. Criteria established by specialty nursing organizations, such as the Standards for the Nursing Care of Women and Newborns developed by the Associaton of Women's Health, Obstetric, and Neonatal Nurses, contain both universal and specialty-specific expectations. Standards are used to develop nursing curricula and job descriptions and to evaluate nursing effectiveness and accountability. SEE: *Code for Nurses; standard of care.*

nursing student An individual enrolled in a school of nursing.

nursing supervisor A substitute for the director or vice president of nursing. This position is seen most commonly, but not exclusively, in nursing home settings. Also called *house supervisor.*

nursing theorist An individual who develops conceptual models and/or theories regarding the purpose, meaning, structure, and functions of the profession and discipline of nursing. SEE: under *theory.*

nursing theory SEE: under *theory.*

NURSYS A centralized nationwide nursing databank that contains information about nursing licensure.

nutation (nū-tā′shŭn) [L. *nutare,* to nod] **1.** Nodding, as of the head. SEE: *nodding.* **2.** A complex movement of the sacrum.

nutgall (nŭt′gawl) A growth on certain oak trees produced by insect eggs and larvae. Gallic and tannic acids are obtained from these growths.

nutraceutical (nū-tră-sū′tĭ-kŭl) Any herb used for medicinal purposes. Rules for the sale and promotion of these agents have been set forth in the Dietary Supplement Health and Education Act of 1994. This legislation permits marketing of these products in the U.S. without proof of their safety or effectiveness, and without preauthorization by the U.S. Food and Drug Administration.

nutrient (nū′trē-ĕnt) [L. *nutriens*] Foods or liquids that supply the body with the chemicals necessary for metabolism. Essential nutrients are those entities that the body either cannot synthesize or cannot synthesize quantities sufficient to meet needs. Nutrients can be subdivided into the macronutrients, consisting of protein, carbohydrate, and fat; the micronutrients, which include vitamins and minerals; and water.

nutrilite (nū′trĭ-līt) Any essential nutrient, esp. ones that are required by bacteria in only trace quantities.

nutriment (nū'trĭ-mĕnt) [L. *nutrimentum,* nourishment] That which nourishes; nutritious substance; food.

nutrition (nū-trĭ'shŭn) [L. *nutritio,* nourish] **1.** All the processes involved in the taking in and utilization of food by which growth, repair, and maintenance of activities in the body as a whole or in any of its parts are accomplished. These processes include ingestion, digestion, absorption, and cellular metabolism. The body is able to store some nutrients (glycogen, calcium, iron) for times when food intake is insufficient. Vitamin C is an example of a nutrient that is not stored. **2.** The professional discipline that includes both the scientific study and the practical use of nutrients in health. **nutritional** (nū-trĭsh'ŭn-ăl), *adj.*

n., altered: less than body requirements The state in which an individual has an intake of nutrients insufficient to meet metabolic needs. SEE: *Nursing Diagnoses Appendix.*

n., altered: more than body requirements The state in which an individual has an intake of nutrients which exceeds metabolic needs. SEE: *Nursing Diagnoses Appendix.*

n., altered: risk for more than body requirements The state in which an individual is at risk of experiencing an intake of nutrients that exceeds metabolic needs. SEE: *Nursing Diagnoses Appendix.*

enteral n. Nutrition provided by introducing nutritional substances into the intestines. This is usually done via a nasogastric tube, but oral insertion is required for intubated patients.

partial enteral n. Supplemental tube feeding or oral feeding of foods that are rich in protein, calories, and other nutrients, to patients receiving partial parenteral nutrition. SEE: *enteral n.*

partial parenteral n. ABBR: PPN. Intravenous administration of nutrients to patients whose nutritional requirements cannot be fully met via the enteral route. An amino acid–dextrose solution (usually 10%) and a lipid emulsion (10% to 20%) are delivered into a peripheral vein through a cannula or catheter.

total enteral n. Enteral tube feeding.

nutritional adequacy The relationship between intake of nutrients and individual requirements.

nutritious (nū-trĭsh'ŭs) [L. *nutritius*] Affording nourishment.

nutritive (nū'trĭ-tĭv) **1.** Pert. to the process of assimilating food. **2.** Having the property of nourishing.

nux vomica (nŭks vŏm'ĭ-kă) The poisonous seed from an East Indian tree that contains several alkaloids, the principal ones being brucine and strychnine.

NWB Non–weight bearing.

nyct- SEE: *nycto-*.

nyctalbuminuria (nĭk"tăl-bū"mĭn-ū'rē-ă) [Gr. *nyx,* night, + L. *albus,* white, + Gr. *ouron,* urine] A cyclic albuminuria occurring at night.

nyctalgia (nĭk-tăl'jē-ă) [" + *algos,* pain] Pain occurring at night.

nyctalopia (nĭk-tă-lō'pē-ă) [" + *alaos,* blind, + *ops,* eye] **1.** Inability to see well in a faint light or at night. This condition occurs in retinitis pigmentosa and choroidoretinitis, or it may be due to vitamin A deficiency. Smoking tobacco may impair the ability to see at night. Hypoxia associated with being above sea level in an aircraft will also decrease night vision. SYN: *night blindness.* **2.** Incorrectly used to indicate the ability to see better at night or in semidarkness than by day.

nyctamblyopia (nĭk"tăm-blē-ō'pē-ă) [Gr. *nyx,* night, + *amblyopia,* poor sight] Reduction or dimness of vision at night without visible eye changes.

nyctaphonia, nyctophonia (nĭk"tă-fō'nē-ă, nĭk"tō-fō'nē-ă) [" + *a,* not, + *phone,* voice] Loss of voice during the night.

nycterine (nĭk'tĕr-īn) [Gr. *nykterinos,* by night] **1.** Nocturnal. **2.** Obscure.

nycto-, nyct- (nĭk'tō) [Gr. *nyx,* night] Combining form indicating *night, darkness.*

nyctohemeral, nycthemerus (nĭk"tō-hĕm'ĕr-ăl, nĭk-thĕm'ĕ-rŭs) Relating to both day and night.

nyctophilia (nĭk"tō-fĭl'ē-ă) [Gr. *nyx,* night, + *philein,* to love] A preference for darkness or night.

nyctophobia (nĭk"tō-fō'bē-ă) [" + *phobos,* fear] Abnormal dread of the night or of darkness. SYN: *scotophobia.*

nyctotyphlosis (nĭk"tō-tĭf-lō'sĭs) [" + *typhlosis,* blindness] Nyctalopia.

nycturia (nĭk-tū'rē-ă) [" + *ouron,* urine] Nocturia.

nymph (nĭmf) [Gr. *nymphe,* a maiden] The immature stage of insect development in which wings and genitalia have not fully developed.

nympha [Gr. *nymphe,* a maiden] One of the labia minora; the small folds of mucous membrane forming the inner lips of the vulva. SYN: *labium minus pudendi.*

nymphectomy (nĭm-fĕk'tō-mē) [" + *ektome,* excision] Excision of hypertrophied nymphae.

nymphitis (nĭm-fī'tĭs) [" + *itis,* inflammation] Inflammation of the nymphae.

nympholepsy (nĭm'fō-lĕp"sē) [Gr. *nymphe,* a maiden, + *lepsis,* a seizure] **1.** Frenzied ecstasy, usually erotic in nature. **2.** Obsession for something that is unattainable.

nymphomania (nĭm"fō-mā'nē-ă) [" + *mania,* madness] Abnormally excessive sexual desire in a female. SYN: *furor femininus.* SEE: *satyriasis.*

nymphomaniac (nĭm"fō-mā'nē-ăk) [" +

mania, madness] **1.** One who is afflicted with excessive sexual desire. **2.** Affected with or characterized by excessive sexual desire.

nymphoncus (nĭm-fŏn′kŭs) [″ + *onkos,* a swelling] Swelling or tumor of the nymphae.

nymphotomy (nĭm-fŏt′ō-mē) [″ + *tome,* incision] **1.** Removal of the nymphae. SYN: *nymphectomy.* **2.** Incision into a nympha or clitoris.

nystagmic (nĭs-tăg′mĭk) [Gr. *nystagmos,* to nod] Relating to or suffering from nystagmus.

nystagmiform (nĭs-tăg′mĭ-form) [″ + L. *forma,* shape] Resembling nystagmus. SYN: *nystagmoid.*

nystagmograph (nĭs-tăg′mō-grăf) [″ + *graphein,* to write] An apparatus for recording the oscillations of the eyeball in nystagmus.

nystagmoid (nĭs-tăg′moyd) [″ + *eidos,* form, shape] Resembling nystagmus.

nystagmus (nĭs-tăg′mŭs) [Gr. *nystagmos,* to nod] Involuntary back-and-forth or cyclical movements of the eyes. The movements may be rotatory, horizontal, or vertical and often are most noticeable when the patient gazes at objects moving by rapidly or at fixed objects in the peripheral field of view.

ETIOLOGY: Lesions of the labyrinth, vestibular nerve, cerebellum, and brainstem commonly produce rhythmic eye movements. Drug intoxications (e.g., with alcohol or phenytoin) also may be responsible.

aural n. Nystagmus due to a disorder in the labyrinth of the ear. Eye movement is spasmodic.

Cheyne's n. Rhythmic nystagmus that resembles the rhythm of Cheyne-Stokes breathing.

convergence n. Slow abduction of eyes followed by rapid adduction. This type of nystagmus usually accompanies other types.

dissociated n. Nystagmus in one eye that is not synchronized with that in the other eye.

end-position n. Nystagmus that occurs when eyes are turned to extreme positions. It may occur normally in debilitation or fatigue, or it may be due to pathology of the subcortical centers for conjugate gaze.

fixation n. Nystagmus that occurs only when the eyes gaze at an object.

gaze-evoked n. Nystagmus upon holding the eyes in an eccentric position. It is due to dysfunction of the brainstem, or it may be caused by drugs such as sedatives or anticonvulsants. The direction of the nystagmus may change when the individual is fatigued or returns fixation to the primary position. This is called *rebound nystagmus.*

jerk n. Rhythmic n.

labyrinthine n. Nystagmus due to disease of the labyrinthine vestibular apparatus.

latent n. Nystagmus that occurs only when one eye is covered.

lateral n. Horizontal movement of the eyes from side to side.

miner's n. Nystagmus occurring in those who work in comparative darkness for long periods.

opticokinetic n. A rhythmic jerk nystagmus occurring when one is looking at constantly moving objects (e.g., viewing telephone poles from a moving car or train).

pendular n. Nystagmus characterized by movement that is approx. equal in both directions. It is usually seen in those who have bilateral congenital absence of central vision or who lost it prior to the age of two.

postrotatory n. A form of vestibular nystagmus that occurs when the body is rotated and then the rotation is stopped. If, while sitting upright in a chair that can be swiveled, the body is rapidly rotated to the right, the nystagmus during rotation has its slow component to the left. When the rotation stops, the slow component is to the right. Stimulation of the semicircular canals causes this type of nystagmus, and it is a normal reaction.

rebound n. SEE: *gaze-evoked n.*

retraction n. Nystagmus associated with the drawing of the eye backward into the orbit.

rhythmic n. Nystagmus in which the eyes move slowly in one direction and then are jerked back rapidly. SYN: *jerk n.*

rotatory n. Nystagmus in which eyes rotate about the visual axis.

seesaw n. Nystagmus in which the inturning eye moves up and the opposite eye moves down, and then both eyes move in the opposite direction.

vertical n. Involuntary up-and-down ocular movements.

vestibular n. Nystagmus caused by disease of the vestibular apparatus of the ear, or due to normal stimuli produced when the semicircular canals are tested by rotating the body. SEE: *postrotatory n.*

voluntary n. A rare type of pendular nystagmus in persons who have learned to oscillate their eyes rapidly, usually by extreme convergence.

nystatin (nĭs′tă-tĭn) An antifungal agent.

nystaxis (nĭs-tăk′sĭs) [Gr.] Nystagmus.

Nysten's law (nē-stănz′) [Pierre Hubert Nysten, Fr. pediatrician, 1774–1817] A law stating that rigor mortis begins with the muscles of mastication and progresses from the head down the body, affecting the legs and feet last.

nyxis (nĭk′sĭs) [Gr.] Puncture or piercing. SYN: *paracentesis.*

NZB mouse SEE: under *mouse.*

O

ω Omega, the twenty-fourth letter in the Greek alphabet.
Ω Capital of the Greek letter omega. Symbol for ohm.
O **1.** Symbol for the element oxygen. **2.** *oculus,* eye. **3.** Symbol for a particular blood type.
o- *ortho-*.
O_2 Symbol for the molecular formula for oxygen.
O_3 Symbol for ozone.
O.A. *anterior.*
OAF *osteoclast activating factor.*
oak bark (ōk bark) The external layer of woody plants of the genus *Quercus,* sometimes used by alternative medicine practitioners as an anti-inflammatory and antidiarrheal. Clinical studies of its effects on humans and their health are sparse.
OAM *Office of Alternative Medicine.*
oarialgia (ō″ăr-ē-ăl′jē-ă) [Gr. *oarion,* little egg, + *algos,* pain] Ovaralgia.
oasis (ō-ā′sĭs) *pl.* **oases** [Gr., a fertile area in an arid region] An area of healthy tissue surrounded by a diseased portion.
oasthouse urine disease Methionine malabsorption syndrome, which is associated with mental retardation, diarrhea, convulsions, phenylketonuria, and a peculiar urinary odor. The odor is due to the absorption from the intestinal tract of fermentation products of methionine. SYN: *Smith-Strang disease.*
oat [AS. *ate,* oat] Grain or seed of a cereal grass used as food.
oath [AS. *ooth*] A solemn attestation or affirmation. SEE: *Hippocratic oath; Nightingale Pledge.*
oatmeal [AS. *ate,* oat, + *mele,* meal] Rolled or ground oats from which a cereal can be made. Oatmeal has several therapeutic uses. In the diet, it provides fiber, lowers cholesterol levels, and can safely be consumed by patients with wheat allergies or celiac sprue because it has no gliaden. Oatmeal is also sometimes used in tepid baths or soaps to sooth inflamed or irritated skin.
OB *obstetrics.*
obelion (ō-bē′lē-ŏn) [Gr. *obelos,* a spit] A craniometric point on the sagittal suture between the two parietal foramina.
Ober test A clinical test for tightness of the iliotibial band. The patient lies on the uninvolved side and abducts the hip maximally in neutral flexion. The examiner stands behind the patient, with the patient's foot resting on the examiner's arms with the thigh supported. The thigh is then released. The result is negative if the abducted knee falls into adduction. It is positive if the knee does not fall into adduction.
obese (ō-bēs′) [L. *obesus*] Overweight, as defined by a body mass index ≥30.
obesity (ō-bē′sĭ-tē) [L. *obesitas,* corpulence] An unhealthy accumulation of body fat. In adults, damaging effects of excess weight are seen when the body mass index exceeds 25 kg/m². Obesity is defined as having a body mass index of >30 kg/m². A person who stands 5′7″ tall, for example, would be obese by this standard if he or she weighed more than 191 lb. SYN: *adiposity; corpulence.* SEE: *body mass index* for table; *Nursing Diagnoses Appendix; Recommended Daily Dietary Allowances Appendix; weight.*

Obesity is the most common metabolic/nutritional disease in the U.S. More than 50% of the adult population is overweight. Obesity is more common in women, minorities, and the poor. Obese individuals have an increased risk of developing diabetes mellitus, hypertension, heart disease, stroke, and other illnesses. In addition, obese individuals may suffer psychologically and socially.

ETIOLOGY: Obesity is the end result of an imbalance between food eaten and energy expended, but the underlying causes are more complex. Genetic, hormonal, and neurological influences all contribute to weight gain and loss. In addition, some medications (e.g., tricyclic antidepressants, insulin, and sulfonylurea agents) may cause patients to gain weight.

TREATMENT: Attempts to lose weight are often unsuccessful. Nonetheless, mild caloric restriction, an increase in physical activity, and supportive therapies each have a role. Medications to enhance weight loss, such as amphetamines or amphetamine-like agents, have had unacceptable side effects (e.g., cardiac valvular injuries with fenfluramine/phentermine, addiction with other anorexiants). Surgical remedies are available for some patients. SEE: *gastroplasty.*

DIET: Caloric intake should be less than maintenance requirements, but all essential nutrients must be included in any weight-loss regimen. Severe caloric restriction is unhealthy and should be avoided unless undertaken under strict supervision. For many patients of average size and activity, consumption of 1200 to 1600 calories per day will result in gradual loss of weight. Most fad diets provide temporary results at best.

EXERCISE: Dietary changes should be accompanied by a complementary program of regular exercise. Exercise improves adherence to weight loss diets and consumes stored fat. For many individuals 35 minutes of low-level exercise performed daily (either in one long workout session or in several shorter intermittent sessions) will aid weight loss and improve other cardiovascular risk factors. Exercise programs may be hazardous for some patients; professional supervision may be recommended for some people who start an exercise program (e.g., people with a history of heart or lung disease, arthritis, or diabetes mellitus, among others).

abdominal o. Android obesity.

adult-onset o. Obesity first appearing in the adult years. Also known as *recent obesity*.

android o. Obesity in which fat is located largely in the waist and abdomen. It is associated with an increased risk of heart disease, hypertension, and diabetes. SYN: *abdominal o.*

endogenous o. Obesity associated with some metabolic or endocrine abnormality.

exogenous o. Obesity due to an excessive intake of food.

gluteal-femoral o. Obesity in which fat deposits are located primarily below the waist in the hips and thighs. The health risks of gluteal-femoral fat appear to be less than those associated with abdominal obesity. SYN: *gynecoid o.*

gynecoid o. Gluteal-femoral o.

hypothalamic o. Obesity resulting from dysfunction of the hypothalamus, esp. the appetite-regulating center.

juvenile o. Obesity that occurs before adulthood. It is associated with an increased risk of obesity in adulthood. Also known as *developmental obesity*.

morbid o. Having a body mass index >40. SEE: *pickwickian syndrome*.

obex (ō′bĕks) [L., a band] A thin, crescent-shaped band of tissue covering the calamus scriptorius at the point of convergence of nervous tissue at the caudal end of the fourth ventricle of the brain.

obfuscation (ŏb-fŭs-kā′shŭn) [L. *obfuscare,* to darken] **1.** The act of making obscure or confusing. **2.** Mental confusion.

OB/GYN, OB-GYN *obstetrics* and *gynecology.*

object [L. *objectus*] That which is visible or tangible to the senses.

object, sex **1.** An individual regarded as being of little interest except for providing sexual pleasure. **2.** A person to whom one is sexually attracted.

objective (ŏb-jĕk′tĭv) **1.** Perceptible to other persons, said of symptoms. Opposite of subjective. **2.** Directed toward external things. **3.** The lens of a microscope that is closest to the object.

achromatic o. A microscope objective in which chromatic aberration is corrected for red and blue light.

apochromatic o. A microscope objective in which chromatic aberration is corrected for red, blue, and green light.

immersion o. A microscope objective designed so that the space between the objective lens and the specimen is filled with oil or water.

object permanence The thought process, first described by Piaget, whereby infants perceive that objects have constancy. This process normally develops by 6 to 12 months.

object relations Emotional attachment for other persons or objects.

object span test A test of the temporal-sequential organization of a child. The child is asked to point to or tap a series of objects in the order demonstrated by the examiner. SEE: *digit span test; temporal-sequential organization.*

obligate (ŏb′lĭ-gāt) [L. *obligatus*] Necessary or required; without alternative. SEE: under *anaerobe*.

oblique (ō-blēk′, ō-blīk′) [L. *obliquus*] Slanting, diagonal.

obliquimeter (ŏb″lĭ-kwĭm′ĕt-ĕr) [″ + Gr. *metron,* measure] An apparatus for determining the angle of the pelvic brim with the upright body.

obliquity (ŏb-lĭk′wĭ-tē) [L. *obliquus,* slanting] The state of being oblique or slanting.

Litzmann's o. SEE: *Litzmann's obliquity*.

Naegele's o. SEE: *Naegele's obliquity*.

o. of the pelvis Inclination of pelvis.

Roederer's o. Presentation of the fetal head with the occiput at the pelvic brim.

obliteration (ŏb-lĭt″ĕr-ā′shŭn) [L. *obliterare,* to remove] Extinction or complete occlusion of a part or a reflex by degeneration, disease, or surgery.

Oblomov syndrome [After Ilya Ilych Oblomov, a character in Ivan Goncharov's 19th century novel who would not get out of bed] Refusal to resume normal activity after an illness or during depression.

oblongata (ŏb″lŏng-gă′tă) [L. *oblongus,* long] Medulla oblongata.

obscure (ŏb-skūr′) [L. *obscurus,* hide] **1.** Hidden, indistinct, as the cause of a condition. **2.** To make less distinct or to hide.

obsession [L. *obsessus,* besiege] A neurotic mental state in which an individual has an uncontrollable desire to dwell on an idea or an emotion. The individual is usually aware of the abnormality and attempts to resist these thoughts. SEE: *obsessive-compulsive disorder*.

obsessive-compulsive disorder ABBR: OCD. A disorder characterized by recurrent obsessions or compulsions that are severe enough to be time consuming or cause marked distress or significant impairment. The person recognizes that the obsessions or compulsions are excessive or unreasonable. The most common obsessions are repeated thoughts about being contaminated as could occur with shaking hands, repeated doubts concerning having failed to lock a door or having hurt someone in a traffic accident, the need to have things in a particular order, aggressive or horrific impulses, and sexual imagery. These obsessions are unlikely to be related to a real-life problem. Compulsions are repetitive behavior (e.g., hand washing, ordering, checking) or mental acts (e.g., praying, counting, repeating words silently) the goal of which is to prevent or reduce anxiety or distress, not to provide pleasure or gratification. This diagnosis is established if distress is present, the acts are time consuming (i.e., take more than an hour a day), or the illness significantly interferes with the individual's normal routine, occupation, or social activities. In the general population, the lifetime prevalence of this disorder is approximately 2.5%. It is estimated to be present in 35% to 50% of patients with Tourette's syndrome. SEE: *Tourette's syndrome; personality disorder, obsessive-compulsive; trichotillomania.*

TREATMENT: Drugs such as clomipramine and fluoxetine have been used to treat OCD. In addition, behavior therapy has been found to be effective. The patient is exposed to a feared object or idea and then discouraged or prevented from carrying out the usual compulsive response. If successful, repeated sessions gradually decrease the anxiety and the patient may be able to refrain from the compulsive actions.

obstetrician (ŏb-stĕ-trĭsh′ăn) A physician who treats women during pregnancy and parturition and delivers infants.

obstetrics (ŏb-stĕt′rĭks) [L. *obstetrix,* midwife] The branch of medicine that concerns management of women during pregnancy, childbirth, and the puerperium. **obstetric** (ŏb-stĕt′rĭk), *adj.*

obstipation (ŏb-stĭ-pā′shŭn) Severe obstruction to the normal flow of feces through the bowels.

obstruction (ŏb-strŭk′shŭn) **1.** Blockage of a structure that prevents it from functioning normally. **2.** A thing that impedes; an obstacle.

aortic o. Blockage of the aorta, thereby preventing the flow of blood.

foreign body airway o. Blockage of the free passage of air from the mouth and nose to the lungs by any object accidentally inhaled into the trachea, bronchus, or pharynx. Common causes of this type of obstruction are red meat, hard candy, hot dogs, coins, and marbles. SEE: *Heimlich maneuver.*

intestinal o. A partial or complete blockage of the lumen of the large or small intestine.

Acute: The small intestine is usually involved. This condition may be due to intussusception, strangulation, volvulus (twists), foreign bodies, adhesions, tumors, stricture, and gallstones in the intestines. Auscultation of the abdomen may reveal a high-pitched tinkle or no sound at all. SEE: *Nursing Diagnoses Appendix.*

SYMPTOMS: Characteristics of intestinal obstruction are pain, localized and intense; temperature, subnormal or normal; vomiting; constipation; and abdominal distention.

TREATMENT: Intestinal and gastric distention is relieved by use of gastric and intestinal suction tubes. Fluid balance must be maintained. Surgical exploration may be necessary to determine the cause. Parenteral antibodies are indicated for peritonitis.

Chronic: This type involves the large intestine and may be due to stricture, inflammation, abscesses, tumors, fecal matter, or chronic peritonitis. Gallstones also may obstruct feces. Constipation gradually develops, with pain becoming more severe in a few days. Acute symptoms follow.

PATIENT CARE: In partial obstruction, nonsurgical interventions include decompression with a nasogastric (NG) or nasointestinal (NI) tube, correction of fluid and electrolyte deficits, and administration of a broad-spectrum antibiotic. Throughout nonsurgical treatment, the patient's condition is monitored closely, and bowel sounds are auscultated periodically. Abdominal girth is measured for signs of distention, and vital signs and fluid and electrolyte balance are monitored. The patient is assessed for signs of dehydration and is given frequent oral hygiene. Prescribed pain medications are administered. The patient must alert health care providers if pain changes from colicky to constant, as this may signal perforation. Throughout, the patient receives support and encouragement.

If conservative treatment fails or the obstruction initially is diagnosed as complete, the patient is prepared physically and psychologically for surgery; the type of surgery depends on the cause of the blockage. Preparation includes correction of fluid and electrolyte imbalances; bowel decompression to relieve vomiting and distention and to prevent aspiration; treatment of shock and peritonitis; and administration of prescribed broad-spectrum antibiotics. If the patient will require a colostomy or ileostomy, an enterostomal therapist makes recommendations regarding stoma location and provides further positive reinforcement and emotional support. Postoperative care is explained; if the patient is well enough to understand, he or she is taught exercises to aid ventilation and prevent immobility complications. Following surgery, all necessary postoperative care is given, including care of the surgical wound, maintenance of ventilatory status and fluid and electrolyte balance, and relief of pain and discomfort. Any necessary postoperative activity limitations are discussed with the patient. Before discharge, any medications, their proper use, desired responses, and adverse effects are reviewed. The importance of following a structured bowel regimen is emphasized (particularly if the cause of obstruction was a fecal impaction). The patient is encouraged to eat a high fiber diet, drink plenty of fluids, and exercise daily.

obstruent (ŏb′stroo-ĕnt) [L. *obstruens*] **1.** Blocking up. **2.** That which closes a normal passage in the body. **3.** Any agent or agency causing obstruction.

obtund (ŏb-tŭnd′) [L. *obtundere,* to beat against] To dull or blunt, as sensitivity or pain. SEE: *consciousness, levels of.*

obtunded Having diminished arousal and awareness, often as the result of intoxication, metabolic illness, infection, or neurological catastrophe.

obtundent (ŏb-tŭn′dĕnt) [L. *obtundens*] **1.** Having the capacity to deaden sensibility of a part or reduce irritability. **2.** A soothing agent.

obturation (ŏb-tūr-ā′shŭn) [L. *obturare,* to stop up] Closure of a passage or opening, as in intestinal obstruction.

obturator (ŏb′tū-rā″tor) **1.** Anything that obstructs or closes a cavity or opening. **2.** A prosthetic bridge used for spanning the gap in a cleft palate. **3.** A device for closing the end of an instrument for purposes of introduction of a taper-tipped device into a cavity (e.g., sigmoidoscope). **4.** Denoting the obturator foramen, the occluding membrane of same and other related structures as obturator muscles, nerve, and plexus.

obturator sign Pain on inward rotation of the hip, a maneuver that stretches the obturator internus muscle. This test result may be positive in acute appendicitis.

obtuse (ŏb-tūs′) [L. *obtusus*] **1.** Not pointed or acute; dull or blunt. **2.** Of dull mentality.

obtusion (ŏb-tū′zhŭn) Blunting or weakening of normal sensation, as in certain diseases.

O.C. *oral contraceptive.*

Occam's razor (ŏck′hăms) [William of Occam, or Ockham, Brit. Franciscan and philosopher, c. 1285–1349] The concept that the simplest explanation for a phenomenon is the best one, that is "what can be done with fewer (assumptions) is done in vain with more."

occipit- SEE: *occipito-.*

occipital (ŏk-sĭp′ĭ-tăl) [L. *occipitalis*] Concerning the back part of the head.

occipital bone A bone in the lower back part of the skull between the parietal and temporal bones.

occipitalis (ŏk-sĭp″ĭ-tā′lĭs) [L.] The posterior portion of the occipitofrontalis muscle at the back of the head.

occipitalization (ŏk-sĭp″ĭ-tăl-ī-zā′shŭn) Fusion of the atlas and occipital bones.

occipito-, occipit- [L. *occiput*] Combining form meaning *occiput.*

occipitoatloid (ŏk-sĭp″ĭ-tō-ăt′loyd) Concerning the occipital and atlas bones.

occipitoaxoid (ŏk-sĭp″ĭ-tō-ăk′soyd) Concerning the occipital and axis bones.

occipitobregmatic (ŏk-sĭp″ĭ-tō-brĕg-măt′ĭk) Concerning the occiput and the bregma.

occipitocervical (ŏk-sĭp″ĭ-tō-sĕr′vĭ-kăl) Concerning the occiput and the neck.

occipitofacial (ŏk-sĭp″ĭ-tō-fā′shăl) Concerning the occiput and the face.

occipitofrontal (ŏk-sĭp″ĭ-tō-frŏn′tăl) Concerning the occiput and the forehead.

occipitomastoid (ŏk-sĭp″ĭ-tō-măs′toyd) Concerning the occiput and the mastoid process.

occipitomental (ŏk-sĭp″ĭ-tō-mĕn′tăl) Concerning the occiput and the chin.

occipitoparietal (ŏk-sĭp″ĭ-tō-pă-rī′ĕ-tăl) Concerning the occipital and parietal bones or lobes of the brain.

occipitotemporal (ŏk-sĭp″ĭ-tō-tĕm′pō-răl) Concerning the occipital and temporal bones.

occipitothalamic (ŏk-sĭp″ĭ-tō-thă-lăm′ĭk) Concerning the occiput and the thalamus.

occiput (ŏk′sĭ-pŭt) [L.] The back part of the skull. On the fetal head, it is used to determine the position of cephalic presentations in relation to the maternal pelvis.

persistent o. posterior A fetal malposition; a cephalic presentation with the occiput directed toward the mother's sacrum. Labor often is longer and the woman complains of back pain.

occlude (ŏ-klūd′) [L. *occludere,* to shut up] To close up, obstruct, or join together, as bringing the biting surfaces of opposing teeth together.

occlusal (ŏ-kloo′zăl) Pert. to the closure of an opening.

o. adjustment Reshaping the occlusal surface of teeth by grinding to create a harmonious contact relationship between upper and lower teeth. This is done to equalize the stress of occlusal forces on the supporting tissues of the teeth, thereby eliminating pain, root resorption, and periodontal problems.

o. equilibration The modification of the occlusal forms of teeth by grinding with the intent of equalizing occlusal forces or producing simultaneous occlusal contacts and harmonious cuspal relations.

o. guard A removable dental appliance that covers one or both arches and is designed to minimize the damaging effects of bruxism, jaw and head trauma during contact sports, or any occlusal habits that are detrimental.

o. surface The masticating surface of the premolar and molar teeth.

o. wear The attritional loss of substance on opposing occlusal surfaces in natural or artificial teeth; the modification of tooth cusps, ridges, and grooves by functional use.

occlusion (ŏ-kloo′zhŭn) [L. *occlusio*] **1.** The acquired or congenital closure, or state of being closed, of a passage. SYN: *imperforation*. **2.** Alignment of the mandibular and maxillary teeth when the jaw is closed or in functional contact (i.e., dental occlusion). SEE: *malocclusion*.

abnormal o. Malocclusion of the teeth.

adjusted o. The alteration of occlusal contacts by dental restorations in order to achieve a balanced or functional occlusion.

anatomical o. A dental occlusion in which the posterior teeth of a denture have masticatory surfaces that resemble natural, healthy dentition and articulate with the surfaces of similar or opposing teeth. The opposing teeth may be artificial or natural.

arterial o. A blockage of blood flow through an artery. It may be acute or chronic and occurs, for example, in coronary or in peripheral arteries. Patients with acute arterial occlusion have severe pain (e.g., angina pectoris), decreased or absent pulses, and mottling of the skin of an affected extremity. The occlusion is removed and blood flow restored if possible.

balanced o. The ideal and equal contact of the teeth of the working side of the jaw by the complementary contact of the teeth on the opposite side of the jaw. SYN: *balanced bite*.

centric o. The position of the mandible, vertically and horizontally, that produces maximal interdigitation of the cusps of the maxillary and mandibular teeth. This is the ideal position or type of occlusion. It is also described as intercuspal position, tooth-to-tooth position, habitual centric, or acquired centric.

coronary o. Complete or partial obstruction of a coronary vessel by thrombosis or as a result of spasm. SYN: *coronary thrombosis*. SEE: *myocardial infarction*.

eccentric o. Any dental occlusion other than centric.

habitual o. The usual relationship between the teeth of the maxilla and mandible that represents the maximum contact; this varies from individual to individual and is seldom ideal or true centric occlusion.

traumatic o. Injury to the tissues that support the teeth due to malocclusion, missing teeth, improper chewing habits, or a pathological condition that causes an individual to chew in an abnormal way.

working o. The usual method of contact of teeth as the mandible is moved to one side during chewing.

occlusive (ŏ-kloo′sĭv) Concerning occlusion.

occlusive dressing SEE: under *dressing*.

occlusometer (ŏk″loo-sŏm′ĕ-tĕr) Gnathodynamometer.

occult (ŭ-kŭlt′) [L. *occultus*] Obscure; not easily understood; mysterious; concealed, as a hemorrhage.

o. blood Blood in such minute quantity that it can be recognized only by microscopic examination or by chemical means.

o. blood test A chemical test or microscopic examination for blood, esp. in feces, that is not apparent on visual inspection. It is used as a screening test for cancer of the colon.

PATIENT CARE: The importance of the test in identifying gastrointestinal bleeding is explained. Because the patient often must collect a specimen at home, instruction is given in specimen collection. The test procedure may be affected by red meat in the diet, so the patient should be instructed to avoid red meat for 3 days prior to sample collection. The patient should place plastic wrap or some other means of collection over the toilet bowl. (The patient should be taught to place the plastic wrap so that it is loose enough to avoid spillage, and allows for urine flow into the commode). The patient should be instructed to use the wooden spatula enclosed with the specimen receptacles to obtain a feces sample from the middle of the specimen. The patient is told that specimens are collected 3 days in succession and should be returned to the laboratory as soon as possible after collection.

occupation An ordinary, everyday goal-directed pursuit. Although the term is often used interchangeably with "vocation," the latter is the preferred term for paid employment.

occupational Relating to source of income or livelihood.

certified o. therapy assistant ABBR: COTA. An occupational therapy assistant who has passed the national certification examination. SEE: *o. therapy assistant*.

o. illness Any acute or chronic disorder associated with or caused by an individual's occupation. SEE: table; *chronic lead poisoning*.

o. performance A term used by occupational therapists to refer to a person's ability to perform the required activities, tasks, and roles of living.

o. science The systematic study of

Representative Occupational Illnesses

Condition	Exposed Workers
Anemia	Lead (battery reclaimers, shipyard workers)
Asbestosis	Shipyard workers and others exposed to asbestos fibers
Asthma	Meat wrappers, wood workers, those exposed to platinum, nickel, solder, ammonia, cotton dust, formaldehyde, pesticides
Byssinosis	Cotton textile workers
Cancer	People who work with radioactive materials (health care, lab workers), x-ray workers (industrial and health care), miners
Carpal tunnel syndrome	Typists, computer programmers, and other people who work with their hands
Contact dermatitis	Healthcare workers using latex gloves and florists
Decompression sickness	Divers, marine salvage workers
Hearing impairment	People who work in noisy environments without adequate ear protection
Leptospirosis	Veterinarians
Pneumoconiosis	Coal miners
Pneumonitis	Wood workers (esp. red cedar), mushroom growers, cheese handlers
Silicosis	Miners, foundry workers
Skin granulomas	Beryllium workers (e.g., in auto or aircraft industries)
Tennis or golfer's elbow	Carpenters, plumbers, and athletes
Vibration syndrome, including Raynaud's phenomenon	Truck drivers, hand-vibrating drill operators, jackhammer workers

the occupational nature of humans. Its goal is to understand how and why people select, organize, perform, and derive meaning from everyday occupations or pursuits.

o. therapist SEE: *under therapist.*

o. therapy assistant ABBR: OTA. One who works under the supervision of an occupational therapist to assist with patient or client assessment and intervention. The degree and scope of supervision required depends on practice statutes and the levels of competency the assistant is able to provide.

occupational therapy aide An individual with on-the-job training or experience in occupational therapy who performs routine tasks under the direction of an occupational therapist.

ochlophobia (ŏk″lō-fō′bē-ă) [Gr. *ochlos,* crowd, + *phobos,* fear] Abnormal fear of crowds or populated places. SYN: *agoraphobia.*

ochronosis (ō-krō-nō′sĭs) [″ + *nosos,* disease] A rare inherited disease caused by the absense of the oxidase of homogentisic acid. It is marked by dark pigmentation of the ligaments, cartilage, fibrous tissues, skin, and urine. This condition is often associated with alkaptonuria, an inborn error of metabolism, or may be the result of chronic phenol poisoning.

OCT *oxytocin challenge test.*

octa-, octo- [Gr. *okto,* L. *octo*] Combining form meaning *eight.*

octahedron (ŏk-tă-hē′drŏn) An eight-sided solid figure.

octan (ŏk′tăn) [L. *octo,* eight] Reappearing every eighth day, as a fever.

octane (ŏk′tān) C_8H_{18}; a hydrocarbon of the paraffin series.

octapeptide (ŏk″tă-pĕp′tīd) A peptide that contains eight amino acids.

octaploid (ŏk′tă-ployd) **1.** Concerning octaploidy. **2.** Having eight pairs of chromosomes.

octaploidy (ŏk′tă-ploy″dē) The condition of having eight sets or pairs of chromosomes.

octavalent (ŏk″tă-vā′lĕnt) [L. *octo,* eight, + *valeo,* to have power] Having a valence of eight.

octigravida (ŏk″tĭ-grăv′ĭ-dă) [″ + *gravida,* pregnant] A woman who has been pregnant eight times.

octipara (ŏk-tĭp′ă-ră) [″ + L. *parere,* to bring forth, to bear] A woman who has given birth to eight children.

octogenarian (ŏk″tō-jĕn-ĕr′ē-ĕn) [L. *octogenarius,* containing eighty] A person who is 80 to 89 years old.

octreotide acetate A synthetic drug that mimics the action of somatostatin and is used in treating acromegaly, carcinoid tumors, vasoactive intestinal peptide tumors, pancreatitis, and gastrointestinal bleeding.

ocular (ŏk′ū-lăr) [L. *oculus,* eye] **1.** Concerning the eye or vision. **2.** The eyepiece of a microscope.

ocularist An allied health specialist who is prepared by training and experience to make and fit artificial eyes.

oculi (ŏk′ū-lī) Pl. of oculus.

oculist (ŏk′ū-lĭst) Obsolete term for ophthalmologist, a physician who is a specialist in diseases of the eye.

oculo- (ŏk′ū-lō) [L. *oculus,* eye] Combining form denoting *eye.*

oculocerebrorenal syndrome A sex-linked hereditary condition characterized by hydrophthalmia, cataracts, mental retardation, aminoaciduria, impaired renal ammonia production, and vitamin D-resistant rickets.

oculocutaneous (ŏk″ū-lō-kū-tā′nē-ŭs) Concerning the eyes and the skin.

oculofacial (ŏk″ū-lō-fā′shē-ăl) Concerning the eyes and the face.

oculogyration (ŏk″ū-lō-jī-rā′shŭn) [″ + Gr. *gyros,* circle] The circular motion of the eyeball around its anterior-posterior axis. SEE: *nystagmus.*

oculogyria (ŏk″ū-lō-jī′rē-ă) The limits of rotation of the eyeballs.

oculogyric (ŏk″ū-lō-jī′rĭk) Producing or concerning movements of the eye. SYN: *oculomotor.*

oculogyric crisis A spasm of involuntary deviation and fixation of the eyeballs, usually upward, often occurring as an adverse reaction to the use of phenothiazine medications. It may last for only several minutes or for hours. This condition is one of the "dystonic" reactions. SEE: *dystonia.*

oculomotor (ŏk″ū-lō-mō′tor) [″ + *motor,* mover] Relating to eye movements. SYN: *oculogyric.*

oculomotor nerve The cranial nerve that originates in the medial surface of the cerebral peduncle of the midbrain and consists of general somatic efferent, general visceral efferent, and general somatic afferent fibers. It is distributed through all extrinsic muscles of the eye except the exterior rectus and superior oblique, through the levator palpebrae superioris of the eyelid, through the ciliary muscle, and through the sphincter muscle of the iris. Its function is primarily motor, but it also contains proprioceptive fibers. SYN: *third cranial nerve.*

oculomycosis (ŏk″ū-lō-mī-kō′sĭs) [″ + Gr. *mykes,* fungus, + *osis,* condition] Any disease of the eye or its parts caused by fungus.

oculonasal (ŏk″ū-lō-nā′săl) [″ + *nasus,* nose] Concerning the eyes and the nose.

oculopupillary (ŏk″ū-lō-pū′pĭ-lăr-ē) Concerning the pupil of the eye.

oculoreaction (ŏk″ū-lō-rē-ăk′shŭn) [L. *oculus,* eye, + *re,* back, + *actus,* acting] Ophthalmic reaction.

oculovestibular test Caloric test.

oculozygomatic (ŏk″ū-lō-zī″gō-măt′ĭk) [″ + Gr. *zygon,* yoke] Pert. to the eye and the zygoma.

o. line A line appearing between the inner canthus of the eye and the cheek, supposedly indicative of neural disorders.

oculus (ŏk′ū-lŭs) *pl.* **oculi** [L.] Eye; the organ of vision made up of the eyeball and optic nerve.

o. dexter ABBR: O.D. The right eye.

o. sinister ABBR: O.S. The left eye.

o. uterque ABBR: O.U. Each eye.

O.D. *Doctor of Optometry; overdose;* [L.] *oculus dexter,* right eye.

OD'd Slang term for a death or illness due to a drug overdose, esp. a drug of abuse.

odaxesmus (ō″dăk-sĕz′mŭs) [Gr. *odaxesmos,* an irritation] The biting of the tongue, lip, or cheek during an epileptic attack.

odaxetic (ō″dăk-sĕt′ĭk) Producing a stinging or itching sensation.

Oddi's sphincter (ŏd′ēz) [Ruggero Oddi, It. physician, 1864–1913] A contracted region at the opening of the common bile duct into the duodenum at the papilla of Vater. It is commonly referred to as the sphincter of Oddi.

odditis (ŏd-dī′tĭs) [*Oddi* + Gr. *itis,* inflammation] Inflammation of the sphincter of Oddi.

odogenesis (ŏ″dō-jĕn′ĕ-sĭs) [Gr. *hodos,* pathway, + *genesis,* generation, birth] Neural regeneration.

odont-, odonto- [Gr. *odous,* tooth] Combining form denoting *tooth, teeth.*

odontagra (ō-dŏn-tă′gră) [Gr. *odous,* tooth, + *agra,* seizure] Toothache, esp. when originating from gout.

odontalgia (ō-dŏn-tăl′jē-ă) [″ + *algos,* pain] Toothache.

phantom o. Pain felt in the area from which a tooth has been pulled. SYN: *odontia; odontodynia.*

odontatrophy (ō″dŏn-tăt′rō-fē) [″ + *atrophia,* atrophy] Imperfect development of the teeth.

odontectomy (ō-dŏn-tĕk′tō-mē) [″ + *ektome,* excision] Surgical removal of a tooth.

odonterism (ō-dŏn′tĕr-ĭzm) [″ + *erismos,* quarrel] Chattering of the teeth.

odontia (ō-dŏn′shē-ă) [Gr. *odous,* tooth] **1.** Pain in a tooth. SYN: *odontalgia; odontodynia.* **2.** Condition or abnormality of the teeth.

odontic (ō-dŏn′tĭk) [Gr. *odous,* tooth] Concerning the teeth.

odontitis (ō″dŏn-tī′tĭs) [″ + *itis,* inflammation] Inflammation of a tooth.

odontoblast (ō-dŏn′tō-blăst) [″ + *blastos,* germ] One of the cells forming the surface layer of the dental papilla that is responsible for the formation of the dentin of a tooth. After a tooth is formed, the odontoblasts line the pulp cavity and continue to produce dentin for years after the tooth has erupted.

odontoblastoma [" + " + *oma,* tumor] A tumor composed principally of odontoblasts.

odontobothritis [" + " + *itis,* inflammation] Inflammation of alveolar process of the tooth.

odontocele (ō-dŏn'tō-sēl) [" + *kele,* tumor, swelling] An alveolodental cyst.

odontochirurgical (ō-dŏn"tō-kī-rŭr'jĭ-kăl) [" + *chirurgia,* surgery] Pert. to dental surgery.

odontoclasis (ō"dŏn-tŏk'lă-sĭs) [" + *klasis,* fracture] The breaking or fracture of a tooth.

odontodynia (ō-dŏn"tō-dĭn'ē-ă) [" + *odyne,* pain] Toothache. SYN: *odontalgia; odontia.*

odontogenesis, odontogeny (ō-dŏn"tō-jĕn'ĕ-sĭs, -tŏj'ĕn-ē) [" + *genesis,* generation, birth] The origin and formation of the teeth.

o. imperfecta A congenital anomaly of the developing teeth in which there is deficient production of enamel and dentin in affected teeth, producing decreased density and enlarged pulp chambers.

odontograph (ō-dŏn'tō-grăf) [" + *graphein,* to write] Device for determining the degree of uneven surface of tooth enamel.

odontography (ō-dŏn-tŏg'ră-fē) Descriptive anatomy of the teeth.

odontoid (ō-dŏn'toyd) [" + *eidos,* form, shape] Toothlike.

odontolith (ō-dŏn'tō-lĭth) [" + *lithos,* stone] Tartar.

odontolysis (ō-dŏn-tŏl'ĭ-sĭs) [" + *lysis,* dissolution] Loss of calcium from a tooth.

odontoma (ō"dŏn-tō'mă) [" + *oma,* tumor] A tumor originating in the dental tissue.

ameloblastic o. A neoplasm that contains enamel, dentin, and odontogenic tissue that does not develop to form enamel.

composite o. A tumor in which the epithelial and mesenchymal cells are completely differentiated. This causes enamel and dentin to be formed in an abnormal manner.

coronary o. A bony tumor at the crown of a tooth.

follicular o. A bony shell in the gums below the tooth margin, usually appearing after the second dentition. It is due to an excessive number of dental follicles. The tumor often involves one or more teeth and is crepitating to pressure. SYN: *dentigerous cyst.*

radicular o. Odontoma close to or on the root of a tooth.

odontonecrosis (ō-dŏn"tō-nĕ-krō'sĭs) [" + *nekros,* corpse, + *osis,* condition] Extensive decay of a tooth.

odontonomy (ō"dŏn-tŏn'ō-mē) [" + *onoma,* name] Dental nomenclature.

odontophobia (ō-dŏn"tō-fō'bē-ă) [" + *phobos,* fear] Abnormal fear of teeth.

odontoprisis (ō-dŏn"tō-prī'sĭs) [" + *prisis,* sawing] Bruxism.

odontorrhagia (ō-dŏn"tō-rā'jē-ă) [" + *rhegnynai,* to burst forth] Hemorrhage from a tooth socket following extraction.

odontoschism (ō-dŏn'tō-skĭzm) [" + *schisma,* cleft] Fissure of a tooth.

odontoscopy (ō"dŏn-tŏs'kō-pē) [" + *skopein,* to examine] **1.** Examination of the teeth and oral cavity by use of an odontoscope. **2.** An impression made of the biting marks made by teeth. These are used as a means of identification.

odontosis (ō-dŏn-tō'sĭs) [" + *osis,* condition] The development or eruption of the teeth.

odontotherapy (ō-dŏn"tō-thĕr'ă-pē) [" + *therapeia,* treatment] The care of diseased teeth.

odor (ō'dĕr) [L.] That quality of a substance that renders it perceptible to the sense of smell.

Odors have been classed as (1) pure, (2) those mixed with sensations from the mucous membrane, and (3) those mixed with the sensation of taste. Although classification attempts are useful, it is important to realize that most complex substances do not produce a single odor.

In the past, body and breath odors were sometimes relied on to suggest diagnoses; this is rarely done in contemporary health care. Examples are a "mousy" odor present in the breath of patients with liver failure (liver breath); an odor of stale urine (uremic breath) in uremia, and the sweet smell of acetone in diabetic ketoacidosis. The characteristic smell of some alcoholic beverages can be detected in the breath. In some hospitals, the employees and staff who work in the presence of patients are asked to refrain from wearing scented substances such as perfumes, hair sprays, underarm deodorants, or aftershave lotions. This is done to prevent olfactory discomfort to patients. Individuals who have just returned from surgery, or who have asthma or other respiratory problems, are particularly sensitive to odors. Electronic devices for detecting and characterizing odors have been developed. SEE: *breath; odorimetry; pheromone.*

odorant (ō'dor-ănt) Something that stimulates the sense of smell.

odoriferous (ō"dor-ĭf'ĕ-rŭs) [L. *odor,* smell, + *ferre,* to bear] Bearing an odor; fragrant; perfumed.

odorimetry The measurement of odors.

odoriphore (ō-dor'ĭ-for) [" + Gr. *phoros,* bearing] The portion of a molecule that imparts odor to the substance.

odorography (ō"dor-ŏg'ră-fē) [" + Gr. *graphein,* to write] A description of odors.

odorous [L. *odor,* smell] Having an odor, scent, or fragrance.

odynacusis (ō"dĭn-ă-kū'sĭs) [Gr. *odyne,*

pain, + *akousis,* hearing] A condition in which noise causes pain in the ear.

-odynia, odyno- (ō-dĭn′ē-ă, ō-dĭn′ō) [Gr. *odyne,* pain] Combining form denoting *pain.*

odynometer (ō″dĭn-om′ĕt-ĕr) [″ + *metron,* measure] A device for measuring pain.

odynophagia (ŏd″ĭn-ō-fā′jē-ă) [″ + *phagein,* to eat] Pain upon swallowing.

odynophobia (ŏd″ĭn-ō-fō′bē-ă) [″ + *phobos,* fear] Abnormal fear of pain.

Oedipus complex (ĕd′ĭ-pŭs) [Oedipus, a character in Gr. tragedy who unwittingly killed his father and married his mother] Abnormally intense love of the child for the parent of the opposite sex. This love continues in adulthood, and usually involves jealous dislike of the other parent. Most often, it is the love of a son for his mother. SEE: *Electra complex; Jocasta complex.*

oersted (ĕr′stĕd) [Hans Christian Oersted, Danish physicist, 1777–1851] A unit of magnetic field intensity. An oersted is the magnetism that exerts a force of one dyne on a unit magnetic pole. This term has largely been replaced by the SI unit amperes per meter.

oesophagostomiasis (ē-sŏf″ă-gō-stō-mī′ă-sĭs) [Gr. *oisophagos,* esophagus, + *stoma,* mouth, + *-iasis,* state] Infection with the nematode of the genus *Oesophagostomum.*

Oesophagostomum (ē-sŏf″ă-gŏs′tō-mŭm) [Gr. *oisophagos,* esophagus, + *stoma,* mouth] A genus of nematodes belonging to the suborder Strongylata that is parasitic in the intestinal walls of animals and humans.

O. apiostomum The nodular nematode worm parasitic to monkeys that occasionally infests humans.

oestrus Estrus.

Oestrus ovis A botfly that may cause ocular myiasis in humans.

OFD *object-film distance.* Distance from the radiographic film to the object being radiographed.

offal (of′fel) Animal parts discarded during the process of butchering or slaughtering, typically including the brain, viscera, skin, hooves, and blood. These by-products have been implicated in the transmission of some infectious illnesses, like mad cow disease.

Office of Alternative Medicine ABBR: OAM. The former name of the National Center for Complementary and Alternative Medicine (NCCAM), a division of the National Institutes of Health.

official Said of medicines authorized as standard in the U.S. Pharmacopeia and in the National Formulary.

off-label drug use The use of a drug to treat a condition for which it has not been approved by the U.S. Food and Drug Administration (FDA), esp. when such use may relieve unpleasant symptoms, or prove compassionate. During the drug approval process in the U.S., drug manufacturers present carefully accumulated data to the FDA about the safety and effectiveness of their products. Drugs are labeled for specific uses when manufacturers make an application to the FDA with data that describe their drug's performance during clinical trials. If this data withstands rigorous scrutiny the drug is labeled for a specific use. Drug effects that have been observed but not specifically proven (and for which no application has been made) may be exploited for unproven, or "off-label" uses by licensed medical practitioners.

Ogilvie's syndrome [Sir William Heneage Ogilvie, Brit. physician, 1887–1971] Acute intestinal pseudo-obstruction due to intestinal dilatation, mostly of the colon. An individual displaying this syndrome has usually undergone recent severe surgical or medical stress (e.g., myocardial infarction, sepsis, or respiratory failure), may be hospitalized or in intensive care, may have metabolic and electrolyte disturbances, and may have received narcotics.

TREATMENT: Treatment consists of therapy for the underlying disease, correction of electrolyte disturbances, avoidance of drugs that inhibit intestinal motility, and intubation of small intestine for decompression. Cecostomy may be required in order to avoid ischemic necrosis and perforation of the bowel.

Oguchi's disease (ō-goot′chēz) [Chuta Oguchi, Japanese ophthalmologist, 1875–1945] Hereditary night blindness with onset in infancy. Commonly found in Japan, the disease is rare in the U.S.

$^{-}$OH Symbol for the hydroxyl ion.

OHA *Oral hypoglycemic agent.*

ohm (ōm) The unit of electrical resistance equal to that of a conductor in which a current of one ampere is produced by a potential of one volt across the terminals. SEE: *electromotive force.*

ohmammeter (ōm′ăm-mē″tĕr) A combined ohmmeter and ammeter.

Ohm's law [Georg S. Ohm, Ger. physicist, 1789–1854] The strength of an electric current, expressed in amperes, is equal to the electromotive force, expressed in volts, divided by the resistance, expressed in ohms. SEE: *electricity.*

ohmmeter (ōm′mē-tĕr) A device for determining the electrical resistance of a conductor.

-oid [Gr. *eidos,* form, shape] Suffix indicating resemblance to the item designated in the first part of the word.

oikofugic (oy″kō-fū′jĭk) [Gr. *oikos,* house, + L. *fugere,* to flee] Having a compulsion to leave home.

oikomania (oy″kō-mā′nē-ă) [″ + *ma-*

nia, madness] A nervous disorder induced by unhappy home surroundings.

oikophobia (oy″kō-fō′bē-ă) Morbid dislike of the home.

oil (oyl) [L. *oleum*] A greasy liquid not miscible with water, usually obtained from and classified as mineral, vegetable, or animal. According to character, oils are subdivided principally as fixed (fatty) and volatile (essential).

Examples of fixed oils are castor oil, olive oil, and cod liver oil. Examples of volatile oils are oils of mustard, peppermint, and rose.

canola o. A light, clear oil derived from the pods of an oilseed plant in the rapeseed family. The oil is composed of 7% saturated fat (the lowest saturated fat content of any vegetable oil), 61% monounsaturated fat, and 22% polyunsaturated fat.

coconut o. A colorless cooking oil, derived from the nut of the *Cocos nucifera* palm tree. Of all cooking oils, it has the highest level of saturated fat (about 91%).

essential o. Volatile oil, esp. one that has an odor and produces taste sensations, obtained from certain plants by various means of extraction. Some of these oils have been used since antiquity as preservatives and antiseptics (e.g., thymol and eugenol); some are used in flavorings, perfumes, and medicines. They are usually complex chemicals that are difficult to purify.

evening primrose o. An herbal remedy used by alternative medicine practitioners for its purported anti-inflammatory effects.

fixed o. Oils in plants and animals that are glyceryl esters of fatty acids. These oils serve as food reserves in animals. They are nonvolatile and contain no acid.

halibut liver o. An oil obtained from the liver of the halibut fish that is rich in vitamins A and D.

medium-chain triglyceride o. A cooking oil of medium-chain triglycerides, used therapeutically as a source of calories and fatty acids. These triglycerides are more readily absorbed from the gut than are most long-chain triglycerides.

peanut o. A refined oil obtained from the seed kernels of one or more of the cultivated varieties of *Arachis hypogaea;* may be used as a solvent for some medicines that are injected intramuscularly.

safflower o. A clear cooking oil derived from the saffron thistle; it has a higher level of polyunsaturated fats than other cooking oils.

silicone o. Injectable silicone.

volatile o. Essential o.

ointment (oynt′měnt) [Fr. *oignement*] A viscous, semisolid vehicle used to apply medicines to the skin. Ointments differ from creams or lotions in their superior ability to occlude the skin and improve the uptake of drugs. The base or vehicle of an ointment typically includes petrolatum, fats, oils, resins, or water-based or water-soluble compounds. SYN: *salve; unguent.*

hydrophilic o. An oil-in-water emulsion in the form of a standardized ointment preparation used topically as an emollient.

white o. Ointment containing white wax and white petrolatum.

yellow o. Ointment containing yellow wax and petrolatum.

OKT3 An immunosuppressive drug used in organ transplantation.

O.L. L. *oculus laevus,* left eye.

ol L. *oleum,* oil.

O.L.A. L. *occipitolaeva anterior* (fetal presentation). SYN: *L.O.A.* SEE: *position.*

olanzapine An atypical antipsychotic agent used to treat psychosis and schizophrenia. It controls both the "positive" symptoms of schizophrenia (delusions, hallucinations) and the "negative" symptoms (passivity, blunted affect, social isolation). Extrapyramidal side effects are less commonly associated with the use of olanzapine than with conventional neuroleptic drugs, such as haloperidol. Common side effects include drowsiness, dizziness, and weight gain. Trade name is Zyprexa.

olea (ō′lē-ă) [L.] **1.** Olive. **2.** Pl. of oleum.

oleaginous (ō-lē-ăj′ĭ-nŭs) [L. *oleaginus*] Greasy; oily; unctuous.

oleander (ō″lē-ăn′dĕr) A poisonous ornamental evergreen shrub, *Nerium oleander.*

oleate (ō′lē-āt) [L. *oleatum*] **1.** Any salt of oleic acid. **2.** A salt of oleic acid dissolved in an excess of the acid and used as an ointment.

oleatum (ō-lē-ā′tŭm) [L.] Preparation made by dissolving metallic salts or alkaloids in oleic acid. SYN: *oleate* (2).

olecranarthritis (ō-lĕk″răn-ăr-thrī′tĭs) [Gr. *olekranon,* elbow, + *arthron,* joint, + *itis,* inflammation] Inflammation of the elbow joint.

olecranarthrocace (ō-lĕk″răn-ăr-thrŏk′ă-sē) [″ + ″ + *kake,* badness] Tuberculous ulceration of the elbow joint.

olecranarthropathy (ō-lĕk″răn-ăr-thrŏp′ă-thē) [″ + ″ + *pathos,* disease, suffering] Any disease of the elbow joint.

olecranoid (ō-lĕk′ră-noyd) [″ + *eidos,* form, shape] Similar to the olecranon.

olecranon (ō-lĕk′răn-ŏn) [Gr., elbow] A large process of the ulna projecting behind the elbow joint and forming the bony prominence of the elbow. In treating a fracture of the olecranon, it is important to prevent spasm of triceps muscle (to avoid separation of the fracture fragments by placing the arm in a sling or bandaging the arm to the side).

The fragments may have to be wired. SEE: *elbow; skeleton; ulna.* **olecranal** (ō-lĕk′răn-ăl), *adj.*

oleic (ō-lē′ĭk) [L. *oleum,* oil] Derived from or pert. to oil.

olein (ō′lē-ĭn) [L. *oleum,* oil] An oleate of glyceryl found in nearly all fixed oils and fats; an important part of oils. SYN: *triolein.*

oleo- [L. *oleum,* oil] Combining form meaning *oil.*

oleogranuloma (ō″lē-ō-grăn″ū-lō′mă) [″ + L. *granulum,* little grain, + Gr. *oma,* tumor] A granuloma caused by continuous contact with oil, or at sites of subcutaneous injection of oily substances.

oleoresin (ō″lē-ō-rĕz′ĭn) [″ + *resina,* resin] An extract of a plant containing a resinous substance and oil, which is prepared by dissolving the crude extract in ether, acetone, or alcohol.

oleosaccharum (ō-lē-ō-săk′ă-rŭm) [″ + *saccharum,* sugar] A compound of sugar and volatile oil used to mitigate the bad taste of some drugs.

oleotherapy (ō″lē-ō-thĕr′ă-pē) [L. *oleum,* oil, + Gr. *therapeia,* treatment] The therapeutic injection of oil.

oleothorax (ō-lē-ō-thō′răks) [″ + Gr. *thorax,* chest] The therapeutic injection of oil into the pleural cavity, used in the distant past to treat pulmonary tuberculosis.

oleovitamin (ō″lē-ō-vī′tă-mĭn) A vitamin preparation in an edible oil.

o. A and D A standardized preparation of vitamins A and D.

Olestra Trade name for a synthetic mixture of sucrose and fatty acids that pass through the digestive tract without absorption. While this fat replacement has been approved for use in savory snacks, it can interfere with uptake of fat-soluble vitamins, such as A, D, E, and K and may result in loose stools.

oleum (ō′lē-ŭm) *pl.* **olea** [L.] Oil.

o. ricini Castor oil.

olfaction (ŏl-făk′shŭn) [L. *olfacere,* to smell] **1.** The sense of smell. **2.** The act of smelling.

olfactometer (ŏl″făk-tŏm′ĕt-ĕr) [″ + Gr. *metron,* measure] Apparatus for testing the power of the sense of smell.

olfactory (ŏl-făk′tō-rē) Pert. to smell.

o. esthesioneuroma Esthesioneuroblastoma.

o. membrane SEE: under *membrane.*

o. nasal sulcus An anterior-posterior groove in the wall of the nasal cavity. It passes from the anterior area to the lamina cribrosa.

o. nerve Any of the nerves supplying the nasal olfactory mucosa. These nerves consist of delicate bundles of unmyelinated fibers (fila olfactoria) that pass through the cribriform plate and terminate in olfactory glomeruli of the olfactory bulb. The fila are central processes of bipolar receptor neurons of the olfactory mucous membrane. SEE: illus.; *cranial nerve.*

o. organ The nose.

olig- SEE: *oligo-.*

oligo-, olig- [Gr. *oligos,* little] Combining form meaning *small, few.*

oligodactylia (ŏl-ĭ-gō-dăk-tĭl′ē-ă) [″ + *daktylos,* digit] Subnormal number of fingers or toes.

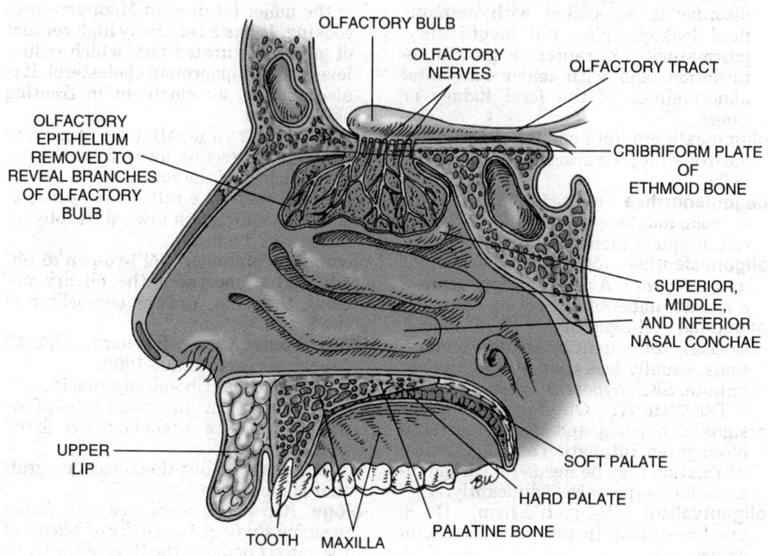

RIGHT OLFACTORY NERVE
(1ST CRANIAL)

oligodendroblast (ŏl″ĭ-gō-dĕn′drō-blăst) [″ + Gr. *dendron,* tree, + *blastos,* germ] A primitive precursor cell of the oligodendrocyte.

oligodendroblastoma (ŏl″ĭ-gō-dĕn″drō-blăs-tō′mă) [″ + ″ + ″ + *oma,* tumor] A neoplasm derived from oligodendroblasts.

oligodendrocyte [″ + ″ + *kytos,* cell] Neuroglial cells having few and delicate processes. SEE: *oligodendroglia.*

oligodendroglia (ŏl″ĭ-gō-dĕn-drŏg′lē-ă) [″ + ″ + *glia,* glue] A neuroglial cell of ectodermal origin that, in the central nervous system, forms or maintains the myelin sheath of neural processes. This type of cell has long, slender processes and is often found associated with nerve cells or satellites.

oligodendroglioma (ŏl″ĭ-gō-dĕn″drō-glī-ō′mă) [″ + ″ + ″ + *oma,* tumor] A malignant tumor of unknown etiology that consists mostly of oligodendrocytes and occurs principally in the cerebrum.

oligodontia (ŏl″ĭ-gō-dŏn′shē-ă) [″ + *odont,* tooth] A hereditary developmental anomaly characterized by fewer teeth than normal.

oligohydramnios (ŏl″ĭg-ō-hī-drăm′nē-ōs) [″ + *hydor,* water, + *amnion,* amnion] An abnormally small amount of amniotic fluid. It is a rare condition in which the volume of amniotic fluid during the third trimester is <300 ml. Insufficient fluid surrounding the fetus increases the potential for cord compression, fetal hypoxia, fetal malformation, perinatal demise, and for dysfunctional and prolonged labor. Although the etiology is unknown, the disorder is associated with amniotic fluid leakage, placental insufficiency, postmaturity, intrauterine growth retardation, and with major congenital abnormalities of the fetal kidney or lungs.

oligomastigate (ŏl″ĭ-gō-măs′tĭ-gāt) [″ + *mastix,* whip] Characterized by two flagella.

oligomenorrhea (ŏl″ĭ-gō-mĕn″ō-rē′ă) [″ + *men,* month, + *rhoia,* flow] Scanty or infrequent menstrual flow.

oligonucleotide (ŏl″ĭ-gō-nū′klē-ō-tīd) [″ + *nucleotide*] A compound made up of a small number of nucleotide units.

oligopnea (ŏl-ĭ-gŏp′nē-ă) [″ + *pnoia,* breath] Infrequent or shallow respirations, usually less than 10 breaths per minute. SEE: *hypoventilation.*

TREATMENT: Observe patient for signs of hypoxia and monitor arterial blood gases. Intubation and mechanical ventilation may be needed if carbon dioxide levels increase significantly.

oligoptyalism (ŏl-ĭ-gō-tī′ă-lĭzm) [″ + *ptyalon,* saliva] Insufficient secretion of saliva.

oligosaccharide (ŏl″ĭ-gō-săk′ă-rīd) A compound made up of a small number of monosaccharide units. Some are found on the outer surface of cell membranes as part of antigens.

oligospermia, oligozoospermatism (ŏl″ĭ-gō-spĕr′mē-ă, -zō″ō-spĕr′mă-tĭzm) [″ + *sperma,* seed] A temporary or permanent deficiency of spermatozoa in seminal fluid.

oligotrichia (ŏl″ĭ-gō-trĭk′ē-ă) [″ + *thrix,* hair] Congenital scantiness of hair.

oliguria (ŏl-ĭg-ū′rē-ă) [″ + *ouron,* urine] Urinary output of less than 400 ml/day. Oliguria results in renal failure if it is not reversed.

ETIOLOGY: Diminished urinary output may result from inadequate perfusion of the kidneys (e.g., in shock or dehydration), from intrarenal diseases (e.g., acute tubular necrosis), or from obstruction to renal outflow (as in bilateral hydronephrosis).

oliva (ō-lī′vă) *pl.* **olivae** [L., olive] An oval body located behind the anterior pyramid of the medulla oblongata and consisting of a convoluted sheet of gray matter enclosing white matter. SYN: *olivary body.* **olivary,** *adj.*

olivary body Oliva.

olive (ŏl′ĭv) [L. *oliva,* olive] **1.** Oliva. **2.** An ovoid device small enough to fit on the tip of a vein stripper. This prevents damaging the vein as the stripper is pushed into it.

accessory o. One of two masses of gray matter lying adjacent to the inferior olive of the brain.

inferior o. Oliva.

superior o. The superior olivary nucleus. SEE: under *nucleus.*

olive oil A monosaturated oil obtained by pressing ripe olives (*Olea europaea*). It is the major fat used in Mediterranean cooking. It has a relatively high content of monounsaturated fats, which reduce levels of low lipoprotein cholesterol. It is also used as an emollient in treating skin disease.

olivifugal (ŏl″ĭ-vĭf′ū-găl) [″ + *fugere,* to flee] In a direction away from the olivary nucleus of the brain.

olivipetal (ŏl″ĭ-vĭp′ĕ-tăl) [″ + *peter,* to seek] In a direction toward the olivary nucleus of the brain.

olivopontocerebellar (ŏl″ĭ-vō-pŏn″tō-sĕr″ĕ-bĕl′ăr) Concerning the olivary nucleus, the pons, and the cerebellum of the brain.

Ollier, Louis Xavier Edouard (ŏl″ē-ā′) French surgeon, 1830–1900.

O.'s disease Chondrodysplasia.

O.'s layer The innermost layer of the periosteum. The osteoblasts are found in this layer.

O.'s graft A split-thickness skin graft that is quite thin.

-ology [Gr. *logos,* word, reason] Suffix meaning *study of, knowledge of, science of* the subject noted in the body of the word.

O.L.P. L. *occipitolaeva posterior* (fetal presentation). SYN: *L.O.P.* SEE: *position.*

olsalazine A drug used to treat ulcerative colitis. It is esp. useful in treating adult patients who cannot tolerate sulfasalazine.

o.m. L. *omni mane,* every morning.

-oma [Gr.] Suffix meaning *tumor.*

omagra (ō-mă′gră) [Gr. *omos,* shoulder, + *agra,* seizure] Gout in the shoulder.

omalgia (ō-măl′jē-ă) [″ + *algos,* pain] Neuralgia of the shoulder.

ombrophobia (ŏm-brō-fō′bē-ă) [Gr. *ombros,* rain, + *phobos,* fear] Fear and anxiety induced by storms or rain.

ombudsman In medicine, an advocate, esp. for patients or clients of health care institutions (e.g. nursing homes, hospitals). The ombudsman verifies complaints and advocates for their resolution. SEE: *Patient's Bill of Rights.*

omega-3 (ω3) fatty acids SEE: under *acid.*

omental (ō-mĕn′tăl) [L. *omentum,* covering] Pert. to the omentum.

omentectomy (ō-mĕn-tĕk′tō-mē) [″ + Gr. *ektome,* excision] Surgical removal all or part of the omentum.

omentitis (ō-mĕn-tī′tĭs) [″ + Gr. *itis,* inflammation] Inflammation of the omentum.

omentopexy (ō-mĕn′tō-pĕks″ē) [″ + Gr. *pexis,* fixation] Fixation of the omentum to the abdominal wall or adjacent organ.

omentoplasty (ō-mĕn′tō-plăs″tē) [L. *omentum,* covering, + Gr. *plassein,* to form] The use of tissue from the greater omentum as a graft in reinforcing tissues.

omentorrhaphy (ō-mĕn-tor′ră-fē) [″ + Gr. *rhaphe,* seam, ridge] Suturing of the omentum.

omentosplenopexy (ō-mĕn″tō-splē′nō-pĕks-ē) [″ + Gr. *splen,* spleen, + *pexis,* fixation] Fixation of the spleen and omentum. Combined omentopexy and splenopexy.

omentotomy (ō-mĕn-tŏt′ō-mē) [″ + Gr. *tome,* incision] Surgical incision of the omentum.

omentovolvulus (ō-mĕn″tō-vŏl′vū-lŭs) [″ + *volvere,* to roll] Twisting of the omentum.

omentum (ō-mĕn′tŭm) *pl.* **omenta** [L., a covering] A double fold of peritoneum attached to the stomach and connecting it with certain of the abdominal viscera. It contains a cavity, the omental bursa (lesser peritoneal cavity). SEE: illus.

PALPATION: Infiltration of the omentum by any kind of new growth, either inflammatory or malignant, can be distinguished by the fact that upon palpation the changes found are limited to the omentum and thus do not extend to the posterior portion of the abdominal cavity, but extend across the abdomen, cannot be traced backward, do not ascend behind the ribs, and are rough, hard, and uneven.

gastrocolic o. Greater o.

gastrohepatic o. Lesser o.

greater o. The portion of the omentum that is suspended from the greater curvature of the stomach and covers the intestines like an apron. It dips in among the folds of the intestines and is attached to the transverse colon and mesocolon. It contains fat, prevents friction, and aids in localizing infections.

lesser o. The portion of the omentum that passes from the lesser curvature of the stomach to the transverse fissure of the liver. **omental** (ō-mĕn′tăl), *adj.*

omeprazole A potent inhibitor of the formation of gastric acid. It is useful in the treatment of erosive esophagitis, gastritis, and peptic ulcer.

OML *orbitomeatal line.*

Ommaya reservoir [A. K. Ommaya, contemporary U.S. neurosurgeon] A mushroom-shaped infusion port, implanted in the ventricles of the brain, to allow access to cerebrospinal fluid (CSF), measurement of CSF pressure, or intrathecal drug administration (e.g., antibiotics, cancer-fighting drugs, or opiates). The reservoir may be used to help treat malignancies or infections of the central nervous system, or control chronic cancer pain. It may occasionally become infected or clogged during use.

omn. bih. L. *omni bihora,* every 2 hours.

omn. hor. L. *omni hora,* every hour.

omnipotence of thought In psychiatry, the infantile concept of reality in which one expects all of one's wishes to be instantly accomplished.

omnivorous (ŏm-nĭv′ō-rŭs) [L. *omnis,* all, + *vorare,* to eat] Consuming foods of both vegetable and animal origin.

omn. noct. L. *omni nocte,* every night.

omn. quad. hor. L. *omni quadrante hora,* every quarter of an hour.

omo- [Gr. *omos,* shoulder] Combining form meaning *shoulder.*

omoclavicular (ō″mō-klă-vĭk′ū-lăr) Concerning the shoulder and clavicle.

omodynia (ō-mō-dĭn′ē-ă) [Gr. *omos,* shoulder, + *odyne,* pain] Pain in the shoulder.

omohyoid (ō-mō-hī′oyd) **1.** Concerning the scapula and the hyoid bone. **2.** The muscle attached to the hyoid bone and the scapula.

omophagia (ō-mō-fā′jē-ă) [Gr. *omos,* raw, + *phagein,* to eat] The custom of eating raw foods, esp. raw flesh.

omphal- SEE: *omphalo-.*

omphalectomy (ŏm-făl-ĕk′tō-mē) [Gr. *omphalos,* navel, + *ektome,* excision] Surgical removal of the umbilicus.

omphalic (ŏm-făl′ĭk) [Gr. *omphalos,* navel] Concerning the umbilicus.

omphalitis (ŏm-făl-ī′tĭs) [″ + *itis,* inflammation] Inflammation of the umbilicus.

omphalo-, omphal- [Gr. *omphalos,* navel] Combining form denoting *navel.*

omphaloangiopagus (ŏm″fă-lō-ăn″jē-ŏp′ă-gŭs) [″ + *angeion,* vessel, + *pagos,* thing fixed] Conjoined twins

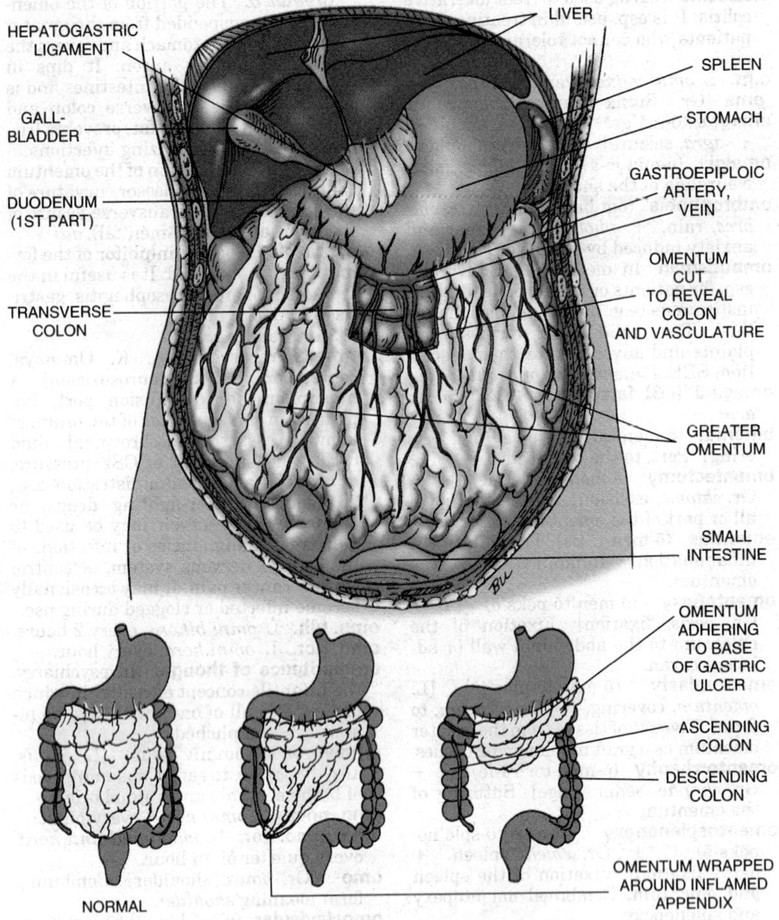

RELATIONSHIP OF GREATER OMENTUM TO ABDOMINAL ORGANS

united by the vessels of the umbilical cord.

omphalocele (ŏm-făl′ō-sēl) [″ + *kele,* tumor, swelling] Congenital hernia of the umbilicus. SEE: *hernia.*

omphalochorion (ŏm″fă-lō-kō′rē-ŏn) A chorion supplied with blood by the omphalomesenteric blood vessels of the yolk sac.

omphalomesenteric (ŏm″făl-ō-mĕs-ĕn-tĕr′ĭk) [″ + *mesenterion,* mesentery] Concerning the umbilicus and mesentery.

omphaloncus (ŏm″făl-ŏn′kŭs) [″ + *onkos,* tumor] An umbilical tumor or swelling.

omphalopagus (ŏm″fă-lŏp′ă-gŭs) [″ + *pagos,* thing fixed] Conjoined twins united at the abdomen.

omphalophlebitis (ŏm″făl-ō-flē-bī′tĭs) [″ + *phleps,* vein, + *itis,* inflammation] Inflammation of the umbilical veins.

omphalorrhagia (ŏm″făl-ō-rā′jē-ă) [″ + *rhegnynai,* to burst forth] Umbilical hemorrhage.

omphalorrhea (ŏm″făl-ō-rē′ă) [″ + *rhoia,* flow] The discharge of lymph from the umbilicus.

omphalorrhexis (ŏm″făl-ō-rĕk′sĭs) [″ + *rhexis,* rupture] Rupture of the umbilicus.

omphalos (ŏm′făl-ŏs) [Gr.] Umbilicus.

omphalosite (ŏm′fă-lō-sīt″) [″ + *sitos,* food] The underdeveloped member of a pair of omphaloangiopagus twins.

omphalospinous (ŏm″făl-ō-spī′nŭs) [″ + L. *spina,* thorn] Concerning the umbilicus and the anterior superior spine of the ilium.

omphalotomy (ŏm-făl-ŏt′ō-mē) [″ + *tome,* incision] Division of the umbilical cord at birth.

omphalotripsy (ŏm″făl-ō-trĭp′sē) [″ + *tripsis,* a rubbing] Severing of the umbilical cord by crushing, rather than cutting.

ON *orthopedic nurse.*

o.n. L. *omni nocte,* every night.

onanism (ō′năn-ĭzm) [So named because it was practiced by the biblical character Onan, son of Judah] Coitus interruptus; withdrawal before ejaculation. The term is erroneously used to designate masturbation.

Onanoff's reflex (ŏn-ă-nŏfs′) [Jacques Onanoff, Fr. physician, b. 1859] Contraction of the bulbocavernous muscle resulting from compression of the glans penis.

Onchocerca (ŏng″kō-sĕr′kă) [Gr. *onkos,* hook, + *kerkos,* tail] A genus of filarial worms that live in the subcutaneous and connective tissues of their hosts, usually enclosed in fibrous cysts or nodules.

O. volvulus A species of *Onchocerca* that infests humans, frequently invading the tissues of the eye. The parasites are transmitted by species of the black fly *Simulium* and *Eusimulium.* SEE: illus.

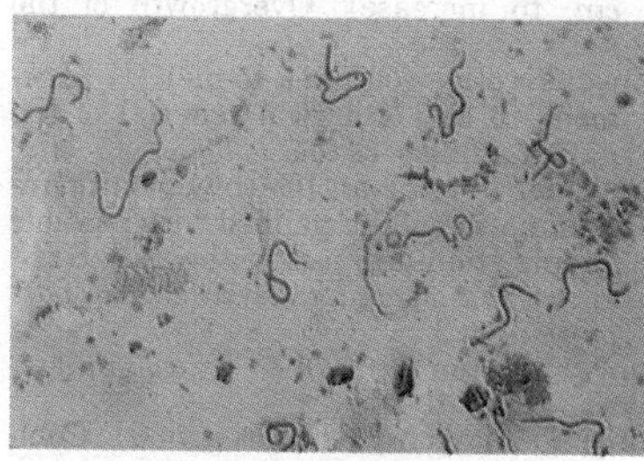

ONCHOCERA VOLVULUS

In skin nodule (orig. mag. ×100)

onchocerciasis (ŏng″kō-sĕr-kī′ă-sĭs) [″ + ″ + *iasis,* infestation] A condition produced by parasitic infestation with one of the filarial worms of the genus *Onchocerca.* It is marked by a nodular swelling of skin and ocular disease ("river blindness"). The microfilariae present in the nodules eventually affect the eyes and cause blindness. The disease is spread by the bites of black flies of the genus *Simulium.* In some areas of Africa, half or more of the middle-aged men are blind from this disease. Treatment includes a single annual dose of ivermectin. SYN: *river blindness.* SEE: illus.

onco- [Gr. *onkos,* bulk, mass] Combining form meaning *tumor, swelling, mass.*

Oncocerca Onchocerca.

oncocercosis Onchocerciasis.

oncocyte (ŏn′kō-sīt) [″ + *kytos,* cell] A large columnar cell with granular, acidophilic cytoplasm and a large number of mitochondria. They may become neoplastic.

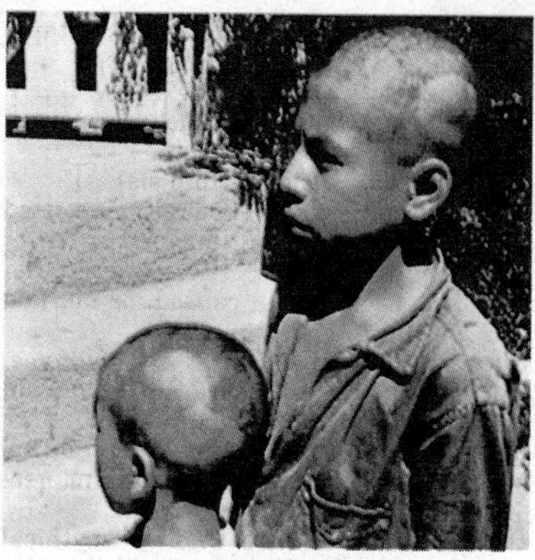

ONCHOCERCIASIS

Cutaneous nodules of onchocerciasis

oncocytoma (ŏng″kō-sī-tō′mă) [″ + ″ + *oma,* tumor] A benign adenoma composed of eosinophilic epithelial cells, esp. one of the salivary or parathyroid glands.

oncofetal (ŏng″kō-fē′tăl) Concerning tumors in the fetus.

oncogene (ŏng′kō-jēn) [″ + *gennan,* to produce] A gene in a virus that has the ability to induce a cell to become malignant. Oncogenes have been identified in human tumors. In addition to genes that can induce tumor formation, there are anti-oncogenes that suppress tumors.

oncogenesis (ŏng″kō-jĕn′ĕ-sĭs) [″ + *genesis,* generation, birth] Tumor formation and development. **oncogenic** (-jĕn′ĭk), *adj.*

oncoides (ŏng-koy′dēz) [″ + *eidos,* form, shape] Turgescence.

oncologist [Gr. *onkos,* bulk, + *logos,* word] A specialist in oncology.

oncology (ŏng-kŏl′ō-jē) [″ + *logos,* word, reason] The branch of medicine dealing with tumors.

radiation o. The branch of medicine in which radioactive rays are used to cure or palliate cancers. The objective is to deliver a therapeutic dose of radiation to malignant tissue, leaving healthy, surrounding tissues unharmed. Radiation therapy is used to treat many cancers, including cancers of the bone, brain, breast, cervix, lymphoid tissues, and uterus.

oncolysis (ŏng-kŏl′ĭ-sĭs) [″ + *lysis,* dissolution] The absorption or dissolution of tumor cells.

oncolytic (ŏng″kō-lĭt′ĭk) Destructive to tumor cells.

oncometry The measurement of variations in size of internal organs.

oncornaviruses A group of RNA viruses that can cause cancer in humans or animals.

oncosphere (ŏng′kō-sfēr) [″ + *sphaira,*

sphere] The embryonic stage of a tapeworm in which it has hooks.

oncotherapy (ŏng″kō-thĕr′ă-pē) [″ + *therapeia,* treatment] The treatment of tumors.

oncothlipsis (ŏng″kō-thlĭp′sĭs) [″ + *thlipsis,* pressure] The pressure caused by the presence of a tumor.

oncotic (ŏng-kŏt′ĭk) [Gr. *onkos,* bulk, mass] Concerning, caused, or marked by swelling.

oncotomy (ŏng-kŏt′ō-mē) [″ + *tome,* incision] The incision of a tumor, abscess, or boil.

oncovirus (ŏn′kō-vī″rŭs) [″ + *virus*] Any virus that causes malignant neoplasms.

Ondine's curse [Fr. Undine, mythical water nymph whose human lover was cursed to continuous sleep] **1.** Primary alveolar hypoventilation caused by reduced responsiveness of the respiratory center to carbon dioxide. **2.** Loss of automatic respiratory function owing to a lesion in the cervical portion of the spinal cord.

oneiric (ō-nī′rĭk) [Gr. *oneiros,* dream] Resembling, relating to, or accompanied by dreams.

oneirism (ō-nī′rĭzm) [″ + *-ismos,* state of] A dreamlike hallucination in a waking state.

oneirodynia (ō-nī″rō-dĭn′ē-ă) [″ + *odyne,* pain] Painful dreaming; nightmare.

oneirology (ō″nī-rŏl′ō-jē) [Gr. *oneiros,* dream, + *logos,* word, reason] The scientific study of dreams.

oniomania (ō″nē-ō-mā′nē-ă) [Gr. *onios,* for sale, + *mania,* madness] A psychoneurotic urge to spend money.

onion (ŭn′yŭn) [AS. *oignon*] The edible bulb of the onion plant, cultivated as a vegetable. Latin name for the common onion is *Allium cepa.* The characteristic odor of onions is due to several volatile chemicals, some of which contain sulfur. The ability of onions to cause persons who peel them to shed tears is probably caused by the chemical propanethial *S*-oxide. When this material comes in contact with tears, sulfuric acid is formed.

onlay **1.** A graft applied to the surface of a tissue, esp. a bone graft applied to bone. **2.** In dentistry, a cast metal restoration that overlays the cusps of the tooth, thereby providing additional strength to the restored tooth.

onomatology (ŏn″ō-mă-tŏl′ō-jē) [Gr. *onoma,* name, + *logos,* word, reason] The science of names. SYN: *nomenclature; terminology.*

onomatomania (ŏn″ō-mă″tō-mā′nē-ă) [″ + *mania,* madness] A mental illness characterized by an abnormal impulse to dwell upon or repeat certain words or by attaching significance to their imagined hidden meanings.

onomatophobia (ŏn″ō-mă″tō-fō′bē-ă) [″ + *phobos,* fear] An abnormal fear of hearing a certain name or word because of an imagined dreadful meaning attached to it.

onomatopoiesis (ŏn″ō-mă″tō-poy-ē′sĭs) [Gr. *onoma,* name, + *poiein,* to make] **1.** The formation of words that imitate the sounds with which they are associated (e.g., hiss, buzz). **2.** In psychiatry, imitative words and sounds created by patients with schizophrenia.

on site Available at an institution. Many medical or surgical services are available in specialized or tertiary care facilities but not in smaller, rural, or less technologically developed hospitals or clinics.

ontogeny (ŏn-tŏj′ĕn-ē) [Gr. *on,* being, + *gennan,* to produce] The history of the development of an individual.

onych- SEE: *onycho-.*

onychalgia (ŏn″ĭ-kăl′jē-ă) [Gr. *onyx,* nail, + *algos,* pain] Pain in the nails.

o. nervosa Extreme sensitivity of the nails.

onychatrophia (ō″nĭk-ă-trō′fē-ă) [″ + *trophe,* nourishment] Atrophy of the nails.

onychauxis (ŏn″ĭ-kawk′sĭs) [″ + *auxein,* to increase] Overgrowth of the nails.

onychectomy (ŏn″ĭ-kĕk′tō-mē) [″ + *ektome,* to cut] Surgical removal of the nail of a finger or toe.

onychia (ō-nĭk′ē-ă) [Gr. *onyx,* nail] Inflammation of the nailbed with possible suppuration and loss of the nail. SYN: *matrixitis; onychitis; onyxitis.* SEE: *paronychia.*

onychitis (ŏn″ĭ-kī′tĭs) [″ + *itis,* inflammation] Onychia.

onycho-, onych- [Gr. *onyx,* nail] Combining form meaning *fingernail, toenail.*

onychodystrophy (ŏn″ĭ-kō-dĭs′trō-fē) [″ + *dys,* bad, + *trophe,* nutrition] Any maldevelopment of a nail.

onychogenic (ŏn″ĭ-kō-jĕn′ĭk) [″ + *gennan,* to produce] Concerning nail formation.

onychograph (ŏn-ĭk′ō-grăf) [″ + *graphein,* to write] A device used for making a record of capillary pulse under the fingernails.

onychogryposis (ŏn″ĭ-kō-grĭ-pō′sĭs) [″ + *gryposis,* a curving] Abnormal overgrowth of the nails with inward curvature.

onychoheterotopia (ŏn″ĭ-kō-hĕt″ĕr-ō-tō′pē-ă) [″ + *heteros,* other, + *topos,* place] Abnormally located nails.

onychoid (ŏn′ĭ-koyd) [″ + *eidos,* form, shape] Similar to a nail, esp. a fingernail.

onycholysis (ŏn″ĭ-kŏl′ĭ-sĭs) [″ + *lysis,* dissolution] Loosening or detachment of the nail from the nailbed. SEE: *photoonycholysis.*

onychoma (ŏn-ĭ-kō′mă) [″ + *oma,* tumor] A tumor of the nail or nailbed.

onychomadesis (ŏn′ĭ-kō-mă-dē′sĭs) [Gr. *onyx,* nail, + *madesis,* loss of hair] The complete loss of the nails.

onychomalacia (ŏn″ĭ-kō-mă-lā′sē-ă) [″ + *malakia,* softening] Abnormal softening of the nails. SYN: *hapalonychia.*

onychomycosis (ŏn″ĭ-kō-mī-kō′sĭs) [″ + *mykes,* fungus, + *osis,* condition] A fungal infection of the nails usually caused by tinea species and occasionally by *Candida.* The hallmarks of the disease are thickening, scaling, and discoloration of the nailbed.

TREATMENT: Antifungal medications like griseofulvin, itraconazole, and terfenabine are relatively effective. However, griseofulvin may cause liver dysfunction and the other two drugs are extremely expensive. SYN: *tinea unguium.* SEE: illus.

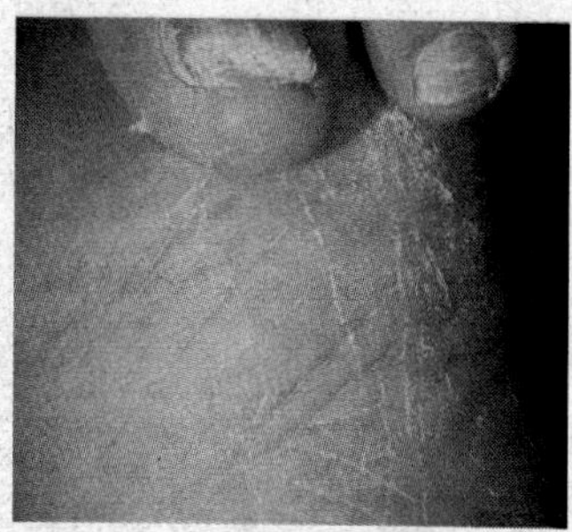

ONYCHOMYCOSIS

onycho-osteodysplasia (ŏn″ĭ-kō-ŏs″tē-ō-dĭs-plā′zē-ă) A genetic disease involving ectodermal and mesodermal tissues. The nails and patellae may be absent; other bones and joints are affected. SYN: *nail-patella syndrome.*

onychopathology (ŏn″ĭ-kō-pă-thŏl′ō-jē) [″ + *pathos,* disease, suffering, + *logos,* word, reason] The study of diseases of the nails.

onychopathy (ŏn-ĭ-kŏp′ăth-ē) [″ + *pathos,* disease, suffering] Any disease of the nails. SYN: *onychosis.*

onychophagy (ŏn-ĭ-kŏf′ă-jē) [″ + *phagein,* to eat] Nail biting.

onychophosis (ŏn″ĭk-ō-fō′sĭs) An accumulation of horny layers of epidermis under the toenail.

onychophyma (ŏn″ĭ-kō-fī′mă) [″ + *phyma,* a growth] Painful degeneration of the nail with hypertrophy.

onychoptosis (ŏn″ĭk-ŏp-tō′sĭs) [″ + *ptosis,* a dropping] Dropping off of the nails.

onychorrhexis (ŏn″ĭ-kō-rĕk′sĭs) [″ + *rhexis,* a rupture] Abnormal brittleness and splitting of the nails.

onychoschizia (ŏn″ĭ-kō-skĭz′ē-ă) [″ + *schizein,* to split] Loosening and eventual separation of the nail from its bed.

onychosis (ŏn-ĭ-kō′sĭs) [″ + *osis,* disease] Onychopathy.

onychotillomania (ŏn″ĭ-kō-tĭl″ō-mā′nē-ă) [″ + *tillein,* to pluck, + *mania,* insanity] A neurotic tendency to pick at the nails.

onychotomy (ŏn″ĭ-kŏt′ō-mē) [″ + *tome,* incision] Surgical incision of a fingernail or toenail.

onychotrophy (ŏn-ĭ-kŏt′rō-fē) [″ + *trophe,* nourishment] Nourishment of the nails.

onyx (ŏn′ĭks) [Gr., nail] **1.** A fingernail or toenail. **2.** Pus collection between the corneal layers of the eye. SYN: *hypopyon.*

onyxitis (ŏn-ĭk-sī′tĭs) [Gr. *onyx,* nail, + *itis,* inflammation] Onychia.

oo- (ō-ō) [Gr. *oon,* egg] Combining form meaning *egg* or *ovary.*

ooblast (ō′ō-blăst) [″ + *blastos,* germ] The primitive cell from which the ovum is developed.

oocyesis (ō″ō-sī-ē′sĭs) [″ + *kyesis,* pregnancy] Ectopic pregnancy in an ovary.

oocyst (ō′ō-sĭst) [Gr. *oon,* egg, + *kystis,* bladder] The encysted form of a zygote occurring in certain sporozoa. SEE: *ookinete.*

oocyte (ō′ō-sīt) [″ + *kytos,* cell] The early or primitive ovum before it has developed completely.

primary o. An oocyte at the end of the growth period of the oogonium and before the first maturation division has occurred.

secondary o. The larger of two oocytes resulting from the first maturation division. SEE: *body, polar.*

oogenesis (ō″ō-jĕn′ĕ-sĭs) [″ + *genesis,* generation, birth] The developmental process by which the mature human ovum (the female reproductive cell) is formed. Formation begins during the first 3 months of female embryonic life with the development of ovarian follicles. Each follicle contains one oogonium which, through the process of mitosis, becomes a primary oocyte containing 46 chromosomes. The oocyte then undergoes the first meiotic reduction division, resulting in formation of a secondary oocyte and a polar body, each containing 22 autosomes (half the number of chromosomes that are found in nongerm cells) and one X heterosome. Further division is arrested in prophase until the female reaches puberty. The second meiotic division begins at ovulation and reaches metaphase where, once again, division is arrested until the ovum is fertilized. The second meiotic division is completed at fertilization, ending with formation of the mature haploid ovum and one polar body. SYN: *ovigenesis.* SEE: illus.; *meiosis.* **oogenetic** (-jĕ-nĕt′ĭk), *adj.*

oogonium (ō″ō-gō′nē-ŭm) *pl.* **oogonia** [″ + *gone,* seed] **1.** The primordial cell from which an oocyte originates. **2.** A descendant of the primordial cell from which the oocyte arises.

ookinesis (ō″ō-kĭn-ē′sĭs) [″ + *kinesis,* movement] The mitosis of oogonia in the embryonic ovary to form primary oocytes.

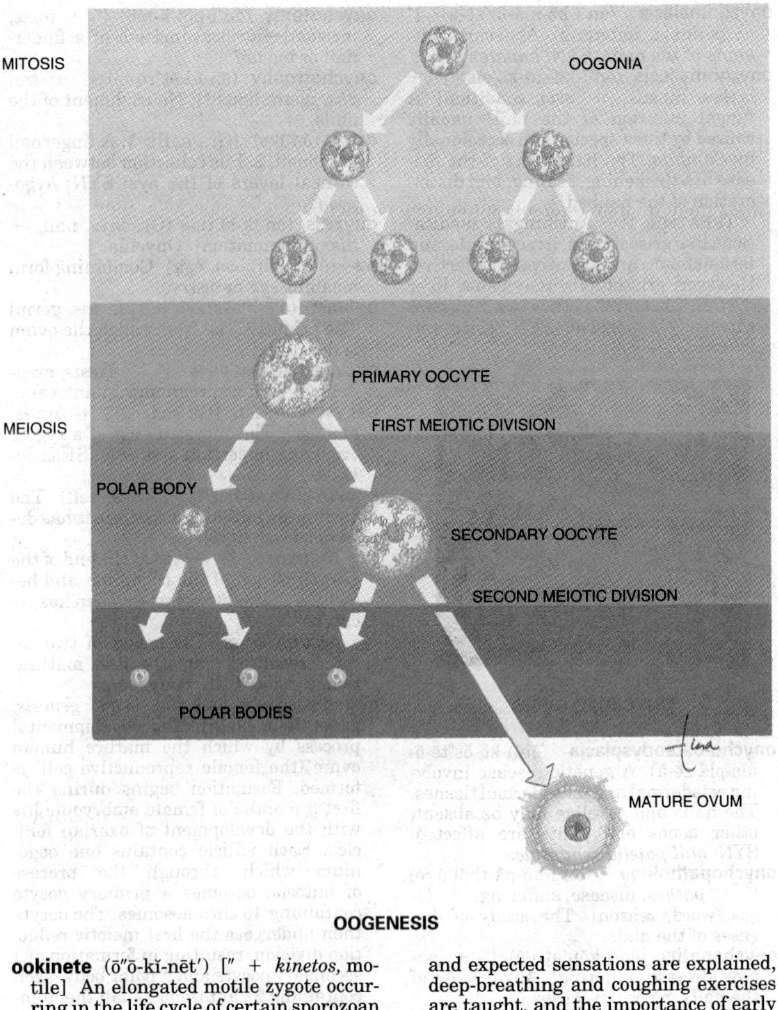

OOGENESIS

ookinete (ō″ō-kĭ-nēt′) [″ + *kinetos*, motile] An elongated motile zygote occurring in the life cycle of certain sporozoan parasites, esp. those of the genus *Plasmodium.* It penetrates the stomach wall of a mosquito and gives rise to an oocyst.

oolemma (ō″ō-lĕm′ă) [″ + *lemma*, sheath] The plasma membrane of the oocyte.

oophagy (ō-ŏf′ă-jē) [″ + *phagein*, to eat] Eating of eggs.

oophor- SEE: *oophoro-*.

oophorectomy (ō″ŏf-ō-rĕk′tō-mē) [Gr. *oophoros*, bearing eggs, + *ektome*, excision] Excision of an ovary. SYN: *ovariectomy*.

PATIENT CARE: Teaching is individualized according to the reason for removal of the ovary. Often the procedure is carried out to remove a benign ovarian cyst, but it may also be performed to remove a tumor of the ovary or an ovary that has twisted. Care before and after surgery is similar to that for other types of abdominal surgery. The procedure and expected sensations are explained, deep-breathing and coughing exercises are taught, and the importance of early ambulation and other activity after surgery is emphasized. After removal of a large cyst, the decrease in intra-abdominal pressure may result in abdominal distention. Use of an abdominal binder may help to prevent this. The effectiveness of care is evaluated. If further treatment is required, the patient is given the opportunity to ask questions and to verbalize her feelings and concerns. Support and reassurance are offered.

oophoritis (ō″ŏf-ō-rī′tĭs) [″ + *itis*, inflammation] Inflammation of an ovary. SYN: *ovaritis*.

follicular o. Inflammation of the graafian follicles.

oophoro-, oophor- [Gr. *oophoros*, bearing eggs] Combining form meaning *ovary.*

oophorocystectomy (ō-ŏf″ō-rō-sĭs-tĕk′tō-mē) [″ + *kystis*, cyst, + *ektome*, excision] Surgical removal of an ovarian cyst.

oophorocystosis (ō-ŏf″ō-rō-sĭs-tō′sĭs) [Gr. *oophoros,* bearing eggs, + *kystis,* cyst, + *osis,* condition] Development of an ovarian cyst.

oophorohysterectomy (ō-ŏf″ō-rō-hĭs″tĕr-ĕk′tō-mē) [″ + *hystera,* womb, + *ektome,* excision] Surgical removal of the uterus and ovaries.

PATIENT CARE: Removal of the uterus and ovaries is a major procedure that may be carried out because of the presence of benign or malignant tumors. Care and teaching are individualized on this basis. Care before and after surgery is similar to that for other types of abdominal surgery. The procedure and expected sensations are explained, deep-breathing and coughing exercises are taught, and the importance of early ambulation and other activity after surgery is emphasized. Pain control measures are discussed, and the patient is advised to seek pain relief in the early postoperative period before pain becomes severe. The effectiveness of care is evaluated. If further treatment is required, the patient is given the opportunity to ask questions and to verbalize feelings and concerns. Support and reassurance are offered to the patient and family.

oophoroma (ō-ŏf″ō-rō′mă) [″ + *oma,* tumor] A malignant ovarian tumor.

oophoropexy (ō-ŏf″ō-rō-pĕk′sē) [″ + *pexis,* fixation] Fixation of a displaced ovary.

oophoroplasty (ō-ŏf′ō-rō-plăs″tē) [″ + *plassein,* to form] Plastic surgery on an ovary.

oophorosalpingectomy (ō-ŏf″ō-rō-săl-pĭn-jĕk′tō-mē) [″ + *salpinx,* tube, + *ektome,* excision] Salpingo-oophorectomy. SYN: *ovariosalpingectomy.*

oophorosalpingitis (ō-ŏf″or-ō-săl″pĭn-jī′tĭs) [″ + ″ + *itis,* inflammation] Inflammation of an ovary and oviduct.

oophorotomy (ō-ŏf″ō-rŏt′ō-mē) [″ + *tome,* incision] Surgical incision of an ovary.

oophorrhagia (ō″ŏf-ō-rā′jē-ă) [″ + *rhegnynai,* to burst forth] Hemorrhage from an ovulatory site severe enough to cause clinical symptoms or signs.

oophorrhaphy (ō-ŏf-or′ă-fē) [″ + *rhaphe,* seam, ridge] Suture of a displaced ovary to the pelvic wall.

ooplasm (ō′ō-plăzm) [Gr. *oon,* egg, + LL. *plasma,* form, mold] The cytoplasm of an ovum.

oosperm (ō′ō-spĕrm) [″ + *sperma,* seed] A cell formed by the union of the spermatozoon with the ovum; a fertilized ovum. SYN: *zygote.*

oosporangium (ō″ō-spō-răn′jē-ŭm) The female portion in the sexual formation of oospores.

oospore (ō′ō-spor) [″ + *sporos,* seed] A spore formed by the union of opposite sexual elements.

ootid (ō′ō-tĭd) The ovum after first maturation has been completed and the second meiotic division has begun.

OP *operative procedure; outpatient.*

O.P. *occiput posterior.*

opacification (ō-păs″ĭ-fĭ-kā′shŭn) [L. *opacitas,* shadiness, + *facere,* to make] **1.** The process of making something opaque. **2.** The formation of opacities.

opacity (ō-păs′ĭ-tē) [L. *opacitas,* shadiness] **1.** The state of being opaque. **2.** An opaque area or spot. **3.** The ratio of incident light to transmitted light in a specific area or on a radiograph.

opalescent (ō″păl-ĕs′ĕnt) Iridescent; similar to an opal with respect to the colors produced.

opaque (ō-pāk′) [L. *opacus,* dark] **1.** Impenetrable by visible light rays or by other forms of radiant energy such as x-rays. **2.** Not transparent or translucent.

OPC *outpatient clinic.*

OPD *outpatient department.*

open [AS.] **1.** Not closed. **2.** Uncovered or exposed, as a wound to air. **3.** To puncture, as to open a boil. **4.** Interrupted, as in an electric circuit when current cannot pass because a switch is open.

opening **1.** The act of making or becoming open. **2.** A hole, aperture, entrance, or open space.

aortic o. The opening in the diaphragm through which the aorta passes.

cardiac o. The opening of the esophagus into the cardiac end of the stomach.

pyloric o. The opening between the stomach and duodenum.

opening snap An abnormal early diastolic extra heart sound usually associated with stenosis of one of the atrioventricular valves. Most commonly, the sound reflects mitral valve stenosis. The brief, high-pitched snapping sound is unaffected by respiration and is heard best between the apex and the lower left sternal border.

open-label study An experimental study involving the use of a medicine, the identity of which is known to the patient.

operable (ŏp′ĕr-ă-bl) [L. *operor,* to work] **1.** Practicable. **2.** Subject to treatment by surgery with reasonable expectation of cure.

operant Producing effects.

operant conditioning SEE: under *conditioning.*

operate (ŏp′ĕr-āt) [L. *operatus,* worked] **1.** To perform an excision or incision, or to make a suture on the body or any of its organs or parts to restore health. **2.** To produce an effect, as a drug.

operation (ŏp-ĕr-ā′shŭn) [L. *operatio,* a working] **1.** The act of operating. **2.** A surgical procedure. **3.** The effect or method of action of any type of therapy. SEE: *surgery.*

Preoperative shaving of the skin over the surgical site may be unnecessary insofar as bacterial considerations are concerned; nevertheless, it is still used to facilitate access to the operative site.

Morrow's o. Surgical excision of a segment of heart muscle (myocardium) of the basil anterior ventricular septum below the aortic valve to treat hypertrophic obstructive cardiomyopathy.

operative (ŏp'ĕr-ă-tĭv) [L. *operativus,* working] **1.** Effective, active. **2.** Pert. to or brought about by an operation.

operative dentistry SEE: under *dentistry.*

operculitis (ō-pĕr"kū-lī'tĭs) [L. *operculum,* a cover, + Gr. *itis,* inflammation] Inflammation of the gingiva over a partially erupted tooth.

operculum (ō-pĕr'kū-lŭm) *pl.* **opercula** [L., a cover] **1.** Any lid or covering. **2.** The narrow opening at the top of the thoracic cage bordered by the sternum and first ribs. **3.** The plug of mucus that fills the opening of the cervix on impregnation. **4.** The convolutions of the cerebrum, the margins of which are separated by the lateral cerebral (sylvian) fissure. The opercula cover the insula. **opercular** (ō-pĕr'kū-lăr), *adj.*

dental o. The soft tissue overlying the crown of a partially erupted tooth.

trophoblastic o. The plug of fibrin that covers the opening in the endometrium made by the implanting zygote.

operon (ŏp'ĕr-ŏn) A group of linked genes and regulatory elements that produces a messenger RNA molecule during transcription in response to a change in the intracellular environment.

ophiasis (ō-fī'ă-sĭs) [Gr. *ophis,* snake] Baldness occurring in winding streaks across the head.

ophidiophobia (ō-fĭd"ē-ō-fō'bē-ă) [Gr. *ophidion,* snake, + *phobos,* fear] Abnormal fear of snakes.

ophidism (ō'fĭd-ĭzm) [" + *-ismos,* condition] Poisoning from snake bite.

ophritis, ophryitis (ŏf-rī'tĭs, -rē-ī'tĭs) [Gr. *ophrys,* eyebrow, + *itis,* inflammation] Inflammation of the eyebrow.

ophryon (ŏf'rē-ŏn) The meeting point of the facial median line with a transverse line across the forehead's narrowest portion.

ophryosis (ŏf"rē-ō'sĭs) [" + *osis,* condition] Eyebrow spasm.

ophthalm- SEE: *ophthalmo-.*

ophthalmagra (ŏf"thăl-măg'ră) [Gr. *ophthalmos,* eye, + *agra,* seizure] Sudden development of eye pain.

ophthalmalgia (ŏf"thăl-măl'jē-ă) [" + *algos,* pain] Pain in the eye. SYN: *ophthalmodynia.*

ophthalmatrophy (ŏf-thăl-măt'rō-fē) [" + *atrophia,* a wasting] Atrophy of the eyeball.

ophthalmectomy (ŏf-thăl-mĕk'tō-mē) [" + *ektome,* excision] Surgical excision of an eye.

ophthalmencephalon (ŏf"thăl-mĕn-sĕf'ă-lŏn) [" + *enkephalos,* brain] The vision apparatus from the retina to the optic nerves, optic chiasm, optic tract, and the visual centers of the brain.

ophthalmia (ŏf-thăl'mē-ă) [Gr. *ophthalmos,* eye] Severe inflammation of the eye, usually including the conjunctiva.

catarrhal o. Conjunctivitis of a severe, frequently purulent, form.

Egyptian o. Trachoma.

electric o. Ophthalmia marked by eye pain, intolerance to light, and tearing (lacrimation). The condition occurs following prolonged exposure to intense light such as that encountered in arc welding.

gonococcal o. Purulent conjunctivitis due to infection with gonococcus.

granular o. Trachoma.

metastatic o. Sympathetic inflammation of the choroid due to pyemia or metastasis.

o. neonatorum Severe purulent conjunctivitis in the newborn.

ETIOLOGY: Infection of the birth canal at the time of delivery. *Neisseria gonorrhoeae* and *Chlamydia trachomatis* are responsible for the great majority of cases. Symptoms are present 12 to 48 hr after birth when due to gonorrhea and 1 week or more after birth for chlamydia infections.

PROPHYLAXIS: Erythromycin ophthalmic ointment is introduced into the conjunctival sac of each eye of the newborn to prevent gonorrheal or chlamydial conjunctivitis. SEE: *Credé's method* (2).

neuroparalytic o. Ophthalmia resulting from injury or disease involving the semilunar ganglion or the branches of the trigeminal nerve supplying the affected eye.

phlyctenular o. Vesicular formations on the epithelium of the conjunctiva or cornea.

purulent o. Purulent inflammation of the eye, usually due to gonococcus.

spring o. Conjunctivitis occurring in the spring, usually due to an allergic reaction to pollen. SYN: *vernal conjunctivitis.*

sympathetic o. A rare bilateral granulomatous inflammation of the entire uveal tract of both eyes. The condition occurs in the untraumatized eye following perforation of the globe of the other eye.

SYMPTOMS: Photophobia, lacrimation, pain, blurring of vision, eyeball tenderness, and deposits on posterior surface of cornea are present. Exudate appears in pupillary area with posterior synechia, seclusio pupillae, and secondary atrophy with blindness.

TREATMENT: Mydriatics, analgesics, and topical and systemic corticosteroids are used to treat this condition. Enucleation of the traumatized eye may reduce the chances of developing this condition. However, if sympathetic ophthalmia does occur, enucleation may be beneficial regardless of the time elapsed since injury.

varicose o. Inflammation that accompanies varicosities of the conjunctival veins.

ophthalmic (ŏf-thăl′mĭk) Pert. to the eye.

o. nerve A branch of the trigeminal (5th cranial) nerve. It is sensory and has lacrimal, frontal, and nasociliary branches.

ophthalmic reaction Reaction of the eye following instillation into the eye of toxins of typhoid or tuberculosis. SYN: *oculoreaction*.

ophthalmitis (ŏf″thăl-mī′tĭs) [″ + *itis,* inflammation] Inflammation of the eye.

ophthalmo-, ophthalm- [Gr. *ophthalmos,* eye] Combining form meaning *eye.*

ophthalmoblennorrhea (ŏf-thăl″mō-blĕn″ō-rē′ă) [″ + *blenna,* mucus, + *rhoia,* flow] Purulent inflammation of the eye or conjunctiva, usually due to gonococcus.

ophthalmocopia (ŏf-thăl″mō-kō′pē-ă) [″ + *kopos,* fatigue] Asthenopia.

ophthalmodesmitis (ŏf-thăl″mō-dĕs-mī′tĭs) [″ + *desmos,* ligament, + *itis,* inflammation] Inflammation of the tendons of the eye.

ophthalmodiaphanoscope (ŏf-thăl″mō-dī-ă-făn′ō-skōp) [″ + ″ + *phainein,* to appear, + *skopein,* to examine] A device for examining the retina by transillumination.

ophthalmodonesis (ŏf-thăl″mō-dō-nē′sĭs) [″ + *donesis,* trembling] Tremor or oscillatory movement of the eye.

ophthalmodynamometer (ŏf-thăl″mō-dī″nă-mŏm′ĕ-tĕr) [″ + *dynamis,* power, + *metron,* measure] An instrument for determining the pressure in the ophthalmic arteries. The device is placed against the conjunctiva of the eye. If the pressure is higher on one side than on the other, appropriate studies to attempt to define the cause are indicated.

ophthalmodynamometry (ŏf-thăl″mō-dī″nă-mŏm′ĕ-trē) Determination of pressure in the ophthalmic artery by use of an instrument that produces pressure on the eyeball until pulsations in the ophthalmic artery are seen through the ophthalmoscope, indicating the diastolic pressure. As the pressure is increased, the vessel collapses and the systolic pressure is obtained.

ophthalmodynia (ŏf-thăl″mō-dĭn′ē-ă) [″ + *odyne,* pain] Pain in the eye. SYN: *ophthalmalgia.*

ophthalmoeikonometer (ŏf-thăl″mō-ī″kō-nŏm′ĕ-tĕr) [″ + *eikon,* image, + *metron,* measure] A device for measuring the relative size of the two ocular images.

ophthalmofundoscope (ŏf-thăl″mō-fŭn′dō-skōp) [″ + L. *fundus,* base, + Gr. *skopein,* to examine] An apparatus used in examining the fundus of the eye.

ophthalmography (ŏf″thăl-mŏg′ră-fē) [″ + *graphein,* to write] Description of the eye.

ophthalmolith (ŏf-thăl′mō-lĭth) [″ + *lithos,* stone] A calculus of the lacrimal duct.

ophthalmologist (ŏf-thăl-mŏl′ō-jĭst) [″ + *logos,* word, reason] A physician who specializes in the treatment of disorders of the eye. SEE: *optician; optometrist.*

ophthalmology (ŏf-thăl-mŏl′ō-jē) [″ + *logos,* word, reason] The health science dealing with the eye and its diseases.

ophthalmomalacia (ŏf-thăl″mō-măl-ā′sē-ă) [″ + *malakia,* softening] Abnormal shrinkage or softening of the eyeball.

ophthalmometer (ŏf-thăl-mŏm′ĕt-ĕr) [″ + *metron,* measure] **1.** An instrument for measuring errors of eye refraction. **2.** An instrument for measuring the volume of various chambers of the eye. **3.** An instrument for measuring the anterior curvatures of the eye. **4.** An instrument for measuring the size of the eye.

ophthalmomycosis (ŏf-thăl″mō-mī-kō′sĭs) [″ + *mykes,* fungus, + *osis,* condition] Any fungal disease of the eye.

ophthalmomyiasis (ŏf-thăl″mō-mī-ī′yă-sĭs) [Gr. *ophthalmos,* eye, + *myia,* a fly, + *-iasis,* condition] Infestation of the eye by larvae of the fly *Oestrus ovis.*

ophthalmomyitis (ŏf-thăl″mō-mī-ī′tĭs) [″ + *mys,* muscle, + *itis,* inflammation] Inflammation of the ocular muscles.

ophthalmomyotomy (ŏf-thăl″mō-mī-ŏt′ō-mē) [″ + *mys,* muscle, + *tome,* incision] Surgical section of the muscles of the eyes.

ophthalmoneuritis (ŏf-thăl″mō-nū-rī′tĭs) [″ + *neuron,* sinew, + *itis,* inflammation] Inflammation of the optic nerve.

ophthalmopathy Any disease of the eye.

ophthalmophlebotomy (ŏf-thăl″mō-flĕ-bŏt′ō-mē) [″ + *phleps,* vein, + *tome,* incision] Incision of the conjunctiva of the eye to overcome congestion of conjunctival veins.

ophthalmoplasty (ŏf-thăl′mō-plăs″tē) [″ + *plassein,* to form] Ocular plastic surgery.

ophthalmoplegia (ŏf-thăl″mō-plē′jē-ă) [″ + *plege,* stroke] Paralysis of ocular muscles.

o. externa Paralysis of extraocular muscles.

o. interna Paralysis of the iris and ciliary muscle.

internuclear o. ABBR: INO. Loss of the normal paired movements of the eyes when tracking an object to the left or right. An INO is marked by the failure of one eye (e.g., the left) to cross the midline during an attempt to see an object on the opposite side of the body (e.g., the right).

ETIOLOGY: This failure of adduction of the affected eye is caused by a lesion of the medial longitudinal fasciculus of the brain.

nuclear o. Paralysis due to a lesion of the nuclei of the ocular motor nerves.

Parinaud's o. SEE: *Parinaud's ophthalmoplegia syndrome.*

o. partialis Incomplete paralysis involving only one or two of the ocular muscles.

o. progressiva Ocular muscle paralysis in which all the muscles become involved slowly, due to deterioration of the motor nerve nuclei.

o. totalis Paralysis that affects both internal and external ocular muscles.

ophthalmorrhagia (ŏf-thăl″mō-rā′jē-ă) [″ + *rhegnynai,* to burst forth] Ocular hemorrhage.

ophthalmorrhea (ŏf-thăl″mō-rē′ă) [″ + *rhoia,* flow] Discharge from the eye.

ophthalmorrhexis (ŏf-thăl″mō-rĕk′sĭs) [″ + *rhexis,* rupture] Rupture of an eyeball.

ophthalmoscope (ŏf-thăl′mō-skōp) [″ + *skopein,* to examine] An instrument used for examining the interior of the eye, esp. the retina.

ophthalmoscopy (ŏf-thăl-mŏs′kō-pē) Examination of the interior of the eye.

medical o. The use of ophthalmoscopy to diagnose systemic disease.

metric o. **1.** The use of ophthalmoscopy to determine the refractive error of the lens of the eye. **2.** The use of ophthalmoscopy to measure the height of the head of the optic nerve in cases of papilledema.

ophthalmospasm (ŏf-thăl′mō-spăsm) Spasm of the ocular muscles.

ophthalmostat (ŏf-thăl′mō-stăt) [″ + *statikos,* standing] An instrument used to hold the eye still during surgery.

ophthalmostatometer (ŏf-thăl″mō-stăt-ŏm′ĕ-tĕr) [″ + ″ + *metron,* measure] An instrument used for determining the presence or absence of exophthalmos.

ophthalmosynchysis (ŏf-thăl″mō-sĭn′kĭ-sĭs) [″ + *synchisis,* a mixing] Effusion into one of the cavities of the eye.

ophthalmotomy (ŏf″thăl-mŏt′ō-mē) [″ + *tome,* incision] Surgical incision of the eyeball.

ophthalmotonometer (ŏf-thăl″mō-tō-nŏm′ĕ-tĕr) [″ + *tonos,* tension, + *metron,* measure] An instrument used for determining tension within the eye.

ophthalmotoxin (ŏf-thăl″mō-tŏk′sĭn) [″ + *toxikon,* poison] Any substance that has a toxic effect on the eyes.

ophthalmotropometer (ŏf-thăl″mō-trō-pŏm′ĕ-tĕr) [″ + ″ + *metron,* measure] An instrument used for measuring the movements of the eye.

ophthalmovascular (ŏf-thăl″mō-văs′kū-lăr) [″ + L. *vasculum,* a small vessel] Pert. to the blood vessels of the eye.

ophthalmoxyster (ŏf-thăl″mŏks-ĭs′tĕr) [″ + *xyster,* scraper] An instrument used to scrape the conjunctiva.

-opia Suffix denoting *vision.*

opiate (ō′pē-ăt) Any drug containing or derived from opium.

opiate poisoning Intoxication by injected, inhaled, dermal, or orally consumed opiate or opioid analgesics.

SYMPTOMS: The patient may experience brief mental exhilaration followed by drowsiness, respiratory depression, pulmonary edema, coma, or in massive overdoses, death.

TREATMENT: An airway should be established and ventilation provided. A narcotic antagonist such as naloxone is given, and may be repeated periodically if symptoms return. Pulmonary edema may be treated with diuretics, nitrates and/or positive pressure ventilation. SEE: *Poisons and Poisoning Appendix.*

opiate receptor A specific site on a cell surface that interacts in a highly selective fashion with opiate drugs. These receptors mediate the major known pharmacological actions and side effects of opiates and the physiologic functions of the endogenous opiate-like substances—endorphins and enkephalins.

opiate withdrawal syndrome Physiological responses to abrupt cessation of the use of addictive substances. The symptoms include chills, runny nose, yawning, irritability, insomnia, and cramping. Physical signs of withdrawal include elevated blood pressure, diaphoresis, diarrhea, and muscle spasms. Discomfort peaks at 48 to 72 hr; however, symptoms persist for 7 to 10 days. Treatment includes methadone and psychological support and counseling.

opioid (ō′pē-oyd) [L. *opium,* opium, + Gr. *eidos,* form, shape] **1.** Any synthetic narcotic not derived from opium. **2.** Indicating substances such as enkephalins or endorphins occurring naturally in the body that act on the brain to decrease the sensation of pain.

opioid peptide, endogenous Any of a group of more than 15 substances present in the brain, certain endocrine glands, and the gastrointestinal tract. They have morphine-like analgesic properties, behavioral effects, and neurotransmitter and neuromodulator functions. Included in this group of chemicals are endorphins, enkephalins, and dynorphin.

opisth- SEE: *opistho-.*

opisthenar (ō-pĭs′thē-năr) [Gr. *opisthen,* behind, in the rear, + *thenar,* palm] The back (dorsum) of the hand.

opisthiobasial (ō-pĭs″thē-ō-bā′sē-ăl) Concerning the opisthion and basion of the skull.

opisthion (ō-pĭs′thē-ŏn) [NL. fr. Gr. *opisthen,* back, in the rear] The craniometric point at the middle of the lower border of the foramen magnum.

opisthionasial (ō-pĭs″thē-ō-nā′zē-ăl) Concerning the opisthion and nasion of the skull.

opistho-, opisth- [Gr. *opisthen,* behind, in the rear] Combining form meaning *backward, behind.*

opisthognathism (ō″pĭs-thō′nă-thĭzm) [″ + *gnathos,* jaw, + *-ismos,* state of] A skull abnormality marked by a receding lower jaw.

opisthoporeia (ō-pĭs″thō-pō-rē′ă) [″ + *poreia,* walk] Involuntary walking backward. SYN: *retropulsion* (2).

opisthorchiasis (ō″pĭs-thor-kī′ă-sĭs) Infestation of the liver by flukes of the genus *Opisthorchis.*

Opisthorchis (ō″pĭs-thor′kĭs) [″ + *orchis,* testicle] A genus of parasitic flukes characterized by having testicles near the posterior end of the tapered body.

O. felineus A species of liver flukes found in cats and other mammals, including humans. Infestation occurs through ingesting raw or partially cooked fish.

O. sinensis A common liver fluke found in humans, esp. in Asia. It develops in those who eat inadequately cooked fish infected with the larval form of the fluke.

opisthotic (ō″pĭs-thŏt′ĭk) [Gr. *opisthen,* behind, in the rear, + *ous,* ear] Located behind the ear.

opisthotonos (ō″pĭs-thŏt′ō-nŏs) [″ + *tonos,* tension] A tetanic spasm in which head and heels are bent backward and the body is bowed forward. This type of spasm is seen in strychnine poisoning, tetanus, epilepsy, the convulsions of rabies, and in severe cases of meningitis. In the latter case, the patient's neck is rigid and the head retracted, seeming to press into the pillow. SEE: illus.; *emprosthotonos; pleurothotonos.* **opisthotonic,** *adj.*

opium (ō′pē-ŭm) [L.] **1.** The substance obtained by air-drying the juice from the unripe capsule of the poppy, *Papaver somniferum.* It contains a number of important alkaloids, such as morphine, codeine, heroin, and papaverine. The growing and transportation of the poppy as well as the manufacture of drugs from the juice are controlled by national and international laws. **2.** A standardized preparation of the air-dried milky exudate from unripe capsules of the poppy, *Papaver somniferum* or *P. album.* It contains not less than 9.5% anhydrous morphine.

opium poisoning SEE: *Opiate poisoning.*

opo- [Gr. *opos,* juice] Prefix meaning *juice;* used in trade names of some organic extracts.

opo- [Gr. *ops,* face] Prefix denoting *face.*

opocephalus (ō″pō-sĕf′ă-lŭs) [Gr. *ops,* face, + *kephale,* head] A congenitally deformed fetus without nose or mouth, fused at the ears. There is either a single orbit or two orbits very close together.

opodidymus (ō″pō-dĭd′ĭ-mŭs) [″ + *didymos,* twin] Congenitally deformed twins in which there is a single body, two fused heads, and partial fusion of the sense organs.

Oppenheim, Hermann (ŏp′ĕn-hīm) German neurologist, 1858–1919.

O.'s disease Myotonia congenita.

O.'s gait Manner of walking in which there is a wide swinging motion of the head, body, and extremities. It is a variation of the gait seen in multiple sclerosis.

opponens (ō-pō′nĕns) [L.] Opposing, a term applied to muscles of hand or foot by which one of the lateral digits may be opposed to one of the other digits.

opportunistic infection SEE: under *infection.*

opposition The ability to move the thumb into contact with the other fingers.

OspA The outer surface protein A of the spirochete *Borrelia burgdorferi.* It is used as an antigen in Lyme disease immunization.

opsialgia (ŏp″sē-ăl′jē-ă) [Gr. *ops,* face, + *algos,* pain] Neuralgic pain of the face.

opsin (ŏp′sĭn) The protein portion of the rhodopsin molecule in the retina of the eye.

opsinogen (ŏp-sĭn′ō-jĕn) An antigen that causes the production of opsonins.

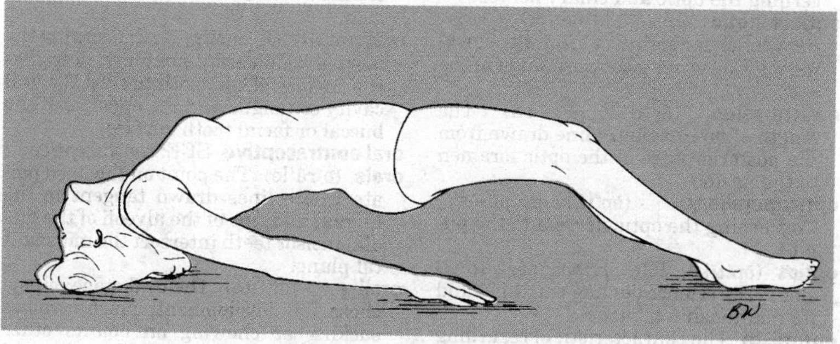

OPISTHOTONOS

opsoclonus Conjugate irregular and nonrhythmical jerking movements of the eyes. The eyes move in any linear or rotating direction at a rate of up to 10 times per second. Any one of several areas of the brain, including the cerebellum and brainstem, may be diseased and cause this condition.

opsomania (ŏp″sō-mā′nē-ă) [Gr. *opson,* food, + *mania,* madness] Craving for some special type of food.

opsonification (ŏp-sŏn″ĭ-fĭ-kā′shŭn) Opsonization.

opsonin (ŏp-sō′nĭn) [Gr. *opsonein,* to purchase food] A substance that coats foreign antigens, making them more susceptible to macrophages and other leukocytes, thus increasing phagocytosis of the organism. Complement and antibodies are the two main opsonins in human blood. **opsonic** (-sŏn′ĭk), *adj.*

immune o. Opsonin formed after stimulation by a specific antigen.

opsonization (ŏp″sō-nī-zā′shŭn) The action of opsonins to facilitate phagocytosis. SYN: *opsonification.*

opsonocytophagic (ŏp″sŏn-ō-sī″tō-fā′jĭk) [″ + *kytos,* cell, + *phagein,* to eat] Pert. to the phagocytic action of the blood when serum opsonins are present.

opsonophilia (ŏp″sō-nō-fĭl′ē-ă) [″ + *philein,* to love] Affinity for opsonins. **opsonophilic,** *adj.*

opsonotherapy (ŏp″sō-nō-thĕr′ă-pē) Treatment by stimulation of a specific opsonin with bacterial vaccines. SEE: *vaccine.*

optic (ŏp′tĭk) [Gr. *optikos*] Pert. to the eye or to sight.

optical (ŏp′tĭ-kăl) [Gr. *optikos;* L. *opticus*] Pert. to vision, the eye, or optics.

o. tweezers A laser device used to alter or manipulate microorganisms, molecules, or living cells.

optician (ŏp-tĭsh′ăn) One who is a specialist in filling prescriptions for corrective lenses for eyeglasses and contact lenses.

optic nerve Second cranial nerve.

optico- [Gr. *optikos*] Combining form denoting *eye, vision.*

opticociliary (ŏp″tĭ-kō-sĭl′ē-ăr-ē) Concerning the optic and ciliary nerves.

opticokinetic (ŏp″tĭ-kō-kĭ-nĕt′ĭk) [Gr. *optikos,* of or for sight, + *kinesis,* movement] Concerning the movement of the eye.

opticonasion (ŏp″tĭ-kō-nā′sē-ŏn) The length of an imaginary line drawn from the posterior edge of the optic foramen to the nasion.

opticopupillary (ŏp″tĭ-kō-pū′pĭl-ĕr″ē) Concerning the optic nerve and the pupil.

optics (ŏp′tĭks) [Gr. *optikos,* pert. to vision] The science dealing with light and its relationship to vision.

optimism The characteristic of regarding only the bright side of a condition or event. SEE: *pessimism.*

optimum (ŏp′tĭ-mŭm) *pl.* **optima** [L. *optimus,* best] Most conducive to a function.

o. temperature The temperature that is most suitable for a procedure or operation, esp. the development of bacterial cultures.

opto- [Gr. *optos,* seen] Combining form meaning *vision, eye.*

optogram (ŏp′tō-grăm) [Gr. *optos,* seen, + *gramma,* something written] The image of an external object that is fixed on the retina by the photochemical bleaching action of light on the visual purple.

optokinetic (ŏp″tō-kĭ-nĕt′ĭk) [″ + *kinesis,* movement] Concerning the appearance of a twitching movement of the eyes, as in nystagmus when the eyes gaze at moving objects.

optometer (ŏp-tŏm′ĕ-tĕr) [″ + *metron,* measure] An instrument used to measure the eye's refractive power.

optometrist (ŏp-tŏm′ĕ-trĭst) A doctor of optometry (O.D.); a primary health care provider who practices optometry, as regulated and permitted by state laws. Most states permit optometrists to prescribe drugs for the treatment of certain eye diseases. SEE: *optometry.*

optometry (ŏp-tŏm′ĕ-trē) The science of diagnosing, managing, and treating conditions and diseases of the human eye and visual system as permitted by state laws.

optomyometer (ŏp″tō-mī-ŏm′ĕ-tĕr) [″ + *mys,* muscle, + *metron,* a measure] An instrument used for determining the strength of the muscles of the eye.

optostriate (ŏp-tō-strī′āt) [″ + L. *striatus,* grooved] Concerning the optic thalamus and the corpus striatum.

optotype (ŏp′tō-tīp) The variable-sized type used in testing visual acuity.

OPV *oral poliovirus vaccine.*

OR *operating room.*

ora (ō′ră) [L.] Plural of os.

ora (ō′ră) *pl.* **orae** [L.] A border or margin.

o. serrata retinae Notched anterior edge of sensory portion of retina.

orad (ō′răd) [L. *oris,* mouth, + *ad,* toward] Toward the mouth or oral region.

oral (or′ăl) [L. *oralis*] **1.** Concerning the mouth. **2.** In dental anatomy, describes the surface of the tooth toward the oral cavity or tongue and the opposite of the buccal or facial tooth surface.

oral contraceptive SEE: *contraceptive.*

orale (ō-rā′lē) The point on the hard palate where lines drawn tangent to the lingual margins of the alveoli of the medial incisor teeth intersect the midsagittal plane.

orality (ō-răl′ĭ-tē) The oral stage of psychosexual development, which involves sucking or chewing on objects other than food.

oral mucous membrane, altered Disruptions of the lips and soft tissue of the oral cavity. SEE: *Nursing Diagnoses Appendix.*

oral rehydration solution ABBR: ORS. A solution used in oral rehydration therapy. The World Health Organization recommends that the solution contain 3.5 g sodium chloride; 2.9 g potassium chloride; 2.9 g trisodium citrate; and 1.5 g glucose dissolved in each liter (approx. 1 qt) of drinking water.

oral rehydration therapy ABBR: ORT. The administration by mouth of a solution of electrolytes in sufficient quantity to correct the deficits produced by dehydration due to diarrhea. The earlier this therapy is begun, the more effective it is (i.e., the fluid should be given before the patient is dehydrated). Because this therapy is simple and economical and can be supervised by nonprofessionals, it has been extremely effective in treating diarrhea in countries lacking health care resources.

In many parts of the world, commercially prepared ORT solutions are not available or are too expensive. In these areas, very inexpensive and effective solutions can be prepared from sources such as cooled water from a pot in which rice is boiled or two pinches of salt and one ounce of molasses added to a quart of boiled water. SEE: *oral rehydration solution; viral gastroenteritis.*

orb [L. *orbis,* circle, disk] A spherical body, esp. the eyeball.

orbicular (or-bĭk′ū-lăr) [L. *orbiculus,* a small circle] Circular.

o. bone The rounded end of the long process of the incus, a middle ear ossicle. It probably represents a secondary ossification center in the long or lenticular process.

o. muscle Muscle encircling an opening.

o. process Lenticular process.

o. sign SEE: *wink.*

orbiculus (or-bĭk′ū-lŭs) *pl.* **orbiculi** [L., little circle] Muscle surrounding an orifice; a sphincter muscle.

o. ciliaris The portion of the ciliary body consisting of a bandlike zone lying directly anterior to the ora serrata. SYN: *ciliary ring.*

o. oris The circular muscle surrounding the mouth.

orbit (or′bĭt) [L. *orbita,* track] The bony pyramid-shaped cavity of the skull that contains and protects the eyeball. It is pierced posteriorly by the optic foramen (which transmits the optic nerve and ophthalmic artery), the superior and inferior orbital fissures, and several foramina. It is formed by the frontal, zygomatic, ethmoid, maxillary, lacrimal, sphenoid, and palatine bones. **orbital** (-bĭ-tăl), *adj.*

orbitale An anthropometric landmark, being the lowest point along the inferior margin of the orbit. It is one of two landmarks (the other is the porion) used to establish the Frankfort horizontal plane, most frequently in positioning the head for radiographs or measurements.

orbitonasal (or″bĭ-tō-nā′zăl) Concerning the orbit and nasal cavity of the skull.

orbitopagus (or″bĭ-tŏp′ă-gŭs) [L. *orbita,* track, + Gr. *pagos,* thing fixed] Conjoined twins in which the smaller fetus is attached to the orbit of the larger fetus.

orbitopathy (ŏr-bĭ-tŏp′ăthē) Disease of the orbit.

dysthyroid o. Ocular dysfunction present in Graves' disease, including protrusion of the eyeball, exposure of the cornea, lid retraction, and occasionally, optic neuropathy. SEE: *Graves' disease.*

orbitotomy (or-bĭ-tŏt′ō-mē) [″ + Gr. *tome,* incision] Surgical incision into the orbit.

orcein (or-sī′ĭn) A chemical used as a histological stain.

orchectomy (or-kĕk′tō-mē) [Gr. *orchis,* testicle, + *ektome,* excision] Orchiectomy.

orcheoplasty (or′kē-ō-plăs″tē) [″ + *plassein,* to form] Orchioplasty.

orchi- SEE: *orchio-.*

orchialgia (or-kē-ăl′jē-ă) [″ + *algos,* pain] Pain in the testes. SYN: *orchiodynia.*

orchichorea (or″kĭ-kō-rē′ă) [″ + *choreia,* a dance] Involuntary jerking movements of the testicles.

orchid- SEE: *orchido-.*

orchidectomy (or″kĭ-dĕk′tō-mē) [″ + *ektome,* excision] Orchiectomy.

orchidic (or-kĭd′ĭk) Concerning or relating to the testes.

orchiditis (or″kĭ-dī′tĭs) [″ + *itis,* inflammation] Orchitis.

orchido-, orchid- [Gr. *orchidion*] Combining form meaning *testicle.*

orchidoncus (or-kĭ-dŏng′kŭs) [″ + *onkos,* bulk, mass] Orchioncus.

orchidopexy (or′kĭd-ō-pĕk″sē) [″ + *pexis,* fixation] Orchiopexy.

orchidoplasty (or′kĭd-ō-plăs″tē) [″ + *plassein,* to form] Orchioplasty.

orchidoptosis (or″kĭd-ŏp-tō′sĭs) [″ + *ptosis,* a dropping] Downward displacement of the testes.

orchidorrhaphy (or″kĭ-dor′ă-fē) [″ + *rhaphe,* seam, ridge] Orchiopexy.

orchidotomy (or-kĭd-ŏt′ō-mē) [″ + *tome,* incision] Orchiotomy.

orchiectomy (or″kē-ĕk′tō-mē) [Gr. *orchis,* testicle, + *ektome,* excision] Surgical excision of a testicle. SYN: *castration, male; orchectomy; orchidectomy.*

PATIENT CARE: The plan of care and expected outcome of the surgery are explained, and information is provided about placing oblate spheroidal prostheses in the scrotum. Patient teaching is modified according to the extent of surgery. Deep-breathing and coughing exercises are taught, and the importance of early ambulation and activity after surgery is emphasized. Pain control measures are discussed, and the patient is advised to seek pain relief in the postoperative period before pain becomes severe. If only one testicle is removed and the other one is healthy, impotence does not occur. Support and reassurance are offered to the patient and family.

orchiepididymitis (or″kē-ĕp″ĭ-dĭd″ĭ-mī′tĭs) [″ + *epi,* upon, + *didymos,* testis, + *itis,* inflammation] Inflammation of a testicle and epididymis.

orchilytic (or″kĭ-lĭt′ĭk) [″ + *lysis,* dissolution] Destructive to testicular tissue. SYN: *orchitolytic.*

orchio-, orchi- Combining form meaning *testicle.*

orchiodynia (or″kē-ō-dĭn′ē-ă) [″ + *odyne,* pain] Orchialgia.

orchioncus (or″kē-ŏng′kŭs) [″+ *onkos,* bulk, mass] A neoplasm of the testicle. SYN: *orchidoncus.*

orchiopathy (or″kē-ŏp′ăth-ē) [″ + *pathos,* disease, suffering] Any disease of the testes.

orchiopexy (or″kē-ō-pĕk′sē) [″ + *pexis,* fixation] The suturing of an undescended testicle to fix it in the scrotum. SYN: *orchidopexy; orchiorrhaphy.*

orchioplasty (or′kē-ō-plăs″tē) [″+ *plassein,* to form] Plastic repair of the testicle.

orchiorrhaphy (or″kē-or′ră-fē) [″+ *rhaphe,* seam, ridge] Orchiopexy.

orchioscheocele (or″kē-ōs′kē-ō-sēl) [″ + *oscheon,* scrotum, + *kele,* tumor, swelling] A scrotal hernia with enlargement or tumor of the testicle.

orchioscirrhus (or″kē-ō-skĭr′rŭs) [″ + *skirros,* hard] Testicular hardening due to tumor formation.

orchiotomy (or″kē-ŏt′ō-mē) [″ + *tome,* incision] Surgical incision of a testicle. SYN: *orchidotomy; orchotomy.*

orchis (or′kĭs) [Gr.] Testis.

orchitis (or-kī′tĭs) [Gr. *orchis,* testicle, + *itis,* inflammation] Inflammation of a testis due to trauma, ischemia, metastasis, mumps, or infection elsewhere in the body.

SYMPTOMS: The symptoms of orchitis include swelling, severe pain, chills, fever, vomiting, hiccough, and in some patients, delirium. Atrophy of the organ may be an end result.

INCIDENCE AND PREVALENCE: With the widespread use of the mumps vaccine in childhood, infectious orchitis is uncommon, as is the atrophy and infertility resulting from it.

TREATMENT: The patient is confined to bed with the organ elevated and supported. An ice bag is applied. Nonsteroidal anti-inflammatory drugs are given.

gonorrheal o. Orchitis due to gonococcus.

metastatic o. Orchitis due to a blood-borne infection that spreads to the testicle.

syphilitic o. Orchitis due to syphilis. This type of orchitis usually begins painlessly in the body of the gland and is apt to be bilateral. It causes dense, irregular, knotty induration but little enlargement in size.

tuberculous o. A rare form of orchitis generally arising in the epididymis. It may be accompanied by formation of chronic sinuses and destruction of tissues. With the widespread use of antituberculosis drugs for primary pulmonary tuberculosis, this condition is rarely seen.

SYMPTOMS: There is little or no pain. It begins with hard, irregular enlargement at the lower and posterior aspects of the gland that gradually increases and sometimes extends along the vas deferens. Later, the whole gland undergoes caseous degeneration.

TREATMENT: INH, pyrazinamide, and rifampin are the drugs of choice; rarely, orchiectomy is needed. **orchitic** (-kĭt′ĭk), *adj.*

orchitolytic (or″kĭt-ō-lĭt′ĭk) [″ + *lysis,* dissolution] Orchilytic.

orchotomy (or-kŏt′ō-mē) [″ + *tome,* incision] Orchiotomy.

orcin, orcinol (or′sĭn, -ŏl) A white, crystalline substance derived from lichens and used as a reagent.

order [L. *ordo,* a row, series] **1.** Instructions from a health care provider specifying patient treatment and care. A directive mandating the delivery of specific patient care services. **2.** An arrangement or sequence of events; rules; regulations; procedures. **3.** In biological classification, the main division under class, superior to family.

stop o. A standing medical order in a patient's chart requiring discontinuation of a specific drug or treatment after a specified time. The order may be reinstated by a health care provider authorized to write orders in the patient's chart.

orderly (or′dĕr-lē) An attendant in a hospital who does general work to assist nurses. Orderlies are responsible for lifting and transporting patients and preparing them for surgery (e.g., shaving, catheterizing, or administering enemas).

ordinate (or′dĭ-năt) The vertical line parallel to the y-axis in a graph in which horizontal and perpendicular lines are crossed in order to provide a frame of reference. The abscissa is the horizontal line parallel to the x-axis. SEE: *abscissa* for illus.

ordure (or′dūr) Feces or other excrement.

Orem, Dorothea Nursing educator, born 1914, who developed the Self-Care Framework, also known as the Self-Care Deficit Theory of Nursing. SEE: *Nursing Theory Appendix.*

oreximania (ō-rĕk″sĭ-mā′nē-ă) [″ + *mania,* madness] Abnormal desire for food because of the fear of losing weight.

orexogen Any substance that stimulates appetite.

orf A contagious pustular dermatitis caused by the orf virus, a DNA virus of the Parapoxvirus genus, which is related to the vaccinia-variola subgroup of poxviruses. Orf mainly affects lambs and occurs in the spring. The disease rarely occurs in humans. When it does, it is usually confined to a single pustular lesion on a finger, which encrusts and finally heals. Antibiotics are not indicated except for secondary bacterial infections.

organ (or′găn) [Gr. *organon;* L. *organum*] A part of the body having a special function. Many organs occur in pairs. In such pairs, one organ may be extirpated and the remaining one can perform all necessary functions peculiar to it. One third to two fifths of some organs may be removed without loss of function necessary to support life. SEE: table.

accessory o. An organ that has a subordinate function.

acoustic o. Organ of Corti.

o. of Corti SEE: under *Corti.*

o. donation Making an anatomical gift of transplantable organs (e.g., heart, lung, kidney, cornea) to persons who will most probably die if transplantation is not performed. The United Network for Organ Sharing (UNOS) maintains a list of patients waiting for organ transplantation and a registry of patients who have received organs. In 1998, more than 21,100 organ transplants were performed in the U.S. In February 2000, more than 67,000 patients were waiting for donor organs.

enamel o. A cup-shaped structure that forms on the dental lamina of an embryo. It produces the enamel and serves as a mold for the remainder of the tooth. SEE: *morphogenesis.*

end o. The expanded end of a nerve fiber in a peripheral structure.

excretory o. An organ that is concerned with the excretion of waste products from the body. SEE: *excretion.*

o. of Giraldés Paradidymis.

Golgi tendon o. SEE: *Golgi tendon organ.*

gustatory o. The organ of taste; a taste bud. SYN: *organum gustus.*

o. of Jacobson A blind tubular sac that develops in the medial wall of the nasal cavity, becoming a functional olfactory organ in lower animals, but degenerating or remaining rudimentary in humans. SYN: *vomeronasal o.*

lymphatic o. A structure composed principally of lymphatic tissue. It includes the lymph nodes, spleen, tonsils, and thymus.

lymphoid o.'s The spleen, lymph nodes, thymus, Peyer's patches, and tonsils, where more than 98% of T lymphocytes are found. SEE: *T cell.*

neuromuscular end o. A spindle-shaped bundle of specialized fibers in which sensory nerve fibers terminate in muscles.

neurotendinous end o. A specialized tendon fasciculus in which sensory nerve fibers terminate in the tendon. SYN: *tendon spindle.*

reproductive o. Any organ concerned with the production of offspring. These include the primary organs (testes and ovaries) and accessory structures (penis and spermatic cord in the male and fallopian tubes, uterus, and vagina in the female). SYN: *sex o.*

o. of Ruffini SEE: *Ruffini's corpuscle.*

sense o. A sensory receptor; a structure consisting of specialized sensory nerve endings that are capable of reacting to a stimulus (an external or internal change) by generating nerve impulses that pass through afferent nerves to the central nervous system. These impulses may give rise to sensations or reflexly bring about responses in the body.

sensory end o. An encapsulated termination of a nerve fiber that serves as a receptor. SEE: *sensory receptor.*

sex o. Reproductive o.

special sense o. The organs of smell, taste, sight, and hearing.

spiral o. Organ of Corti.

target o. An organ upon which a chemical or hormone acts.

vestigial o. An organ that is immature or underdeveloped in humans but is fully functional in some animals.

vomeronasal o. O. of Jacobson.

Weber's o. [Moritz I. Weber, Ger. anatomist, 1795–1875] The residual prostatic pouch in the male, the remains of the müllerian ducts.

o.'s of Zuckerkandl [Emil Zuckerkandl, Hungarian anatomist working in Germany, 1849–1910] A pair of organs containing chromaffin tissue present in the embryo and persisting until shortly after birth. They are located adjacent to the anterior surface of the abdominal aorta. The cells secrete epinephrine. SYN: *corpora para-aortica.*

organelle (or″găn-ĕl′) A specialized part of a cell that performs a distinctive function.

organic (or-găn′ĭk) [Gr. *organikos*] **1.** Pert. to an organ or organs. **2.** Structural. **3.** Pert. to or derived from animal or vegetable forms of life. **4.** Denoting chemical substances containing carbon.

organic brain syndrome Any of a large group of acute and chronic mental disorders associated with brain damage or impaired cerebral function.

SYMPTOMS: The clinical characteristics vary not only with the nature and severity of the underlying organic dis-

Size, Weight, and Capacity of Various Organs and Parts of the Adult Body ♂ Male ♀ Female

Description	Size	Weight	Capacity
Adrenal gland	5 cm high 3 cm across 1 cm thick	5 g	
Bladder	12 cm in diameter		500 ml (when moderately full)
Blood volume			♂ 4–6 L ♀ 3–5 L
Brain		♂ 1240–1680 g ♀ 1130–1570 g	
Ear, external canal	2.5 cm long (from concha)		
Esophagus	23–25 cm		
Eye	23.5 mm vertical diameter 24 mm anteroposterior diameter		
Fallopian tube	10 cm		
Gallbladder	7–10 cm long 3 cm wide		30–50 ml
Heart	12 × 8–9 × 6 cm	♂280–340 g ♀230–280 g	
Intestines—small	Variable 6–7 m long		
Intestines—large	1.5 m long		
Intestines—vermiform appendix	2–20 cm long Average 9 cm		
Intestines—rectum	12 cm long		
Kidney	11 cm long 6 cm broad 3 cm thick	♂ 150 g ♀ 135 g	
Larynx	♂ 44 × 43 × 36 mm ♀ 36 × 41 × 26 mm		
Liver		♂ 1.4–1.8 kg ♀ 1.0–2.5 kg	6500 cc
Lung		Right 625 g Left 565 g	
Ovaries	3 × 1.5 × 1 cm	2–3.5 g	
Pancreas	15 cm long	♂ 74–106 g ♀ 70–100 g	
Parathyroid	6 × 3–4 × 1–2 mm	50 mg	
Pharynx	12.5 cm long		
Prostate	2 × 4 × 3 cm	8 g	
Skeleton		Average adult male, 4957 g	
Skull		Average (without teeth), 642 g	Variable ♂ 406 ml ♀ 207 ml
Spinal cord	42–45 cm long	30 g	
Spleen	12 × 7 × 3–4 cm	150 g 80–300 g Decreases with age	
Stomach	Variable 25 cm long 10 cm wide		Variable 1500 ml
Testes	4–5 × 2.5 × 3 cm	10.5–14 g	
Thoracic duct	38–45 cm long		
Thymus		Newborn, 10.9 g 10–15 yr, 29.5 g 20–25 yr, 18.6 g	

Size, Weight, and Capacity of Various Organs and Parts of the Adult Body ♂ Male ♀ Female (Continued)

Description	Size	Weight	Capacity
Thyroid	Each lobe 5 × 3 × 2 cm	30 g total	
Trachea	11 cm long 2–2.5 cm in diameter		
Ureter	28–34 cm long		
Urethra	♂ 17.5–20 cm long ♀ 4 cm long		
Uterus	7.5 × 5.0 × 2.5 cm	30–40 g (nonpregnant)	
Vagina	Anterior wall length 7.5 cm Posterior wall length 9.0 cm		

SOURCE: Adapted from Gray's Anatomy, ed 27. Lea & Febiger, Philadelphia, 1959; Gray's Anatomy, ed 37. Churchill Livingstone, London, 1987; Growth. Federation of American Societies for Experimental Biology, Washington, DC, 1962; Jandl, JH, Blood. Little, Brown and Co., Boston, 1987.

order but also occasionally between individuals. Consciousness, orientation, memory, intellect, judgment and insight, and thought content may be impaired (e.g., hallucinations, illusions).

ETIOLOGY: Any acute or chronic disease or injury that interferes with cerebral function may trigger symptoms. Possible causes include infection, intoxication, trauma, circulatory disturbance, epilepsy, metabolic and endocrine diseases, or intracranial trauma or neoplasms.

DIAGNOSIS: Difficulty in diagnosis may be encountered because of the possibility of attributing all of the signs and symptoms to a psychiatric disorder, thereby ignoring the possibility of organic disease.

TREATMENT: Treatment of the basic organic disease and provision of psychiatric care are indicated.

organic dust toxic syndrome ABBR: ODTS. A nonallergenic, noninfectious, respiratory disorder caused by inhalation of organic dusts. The most important sources are cotton dust, which causes byssinosis; grain dust; and exposure to moldy hay, called "farmer's lung." SEE: *byssinosis; pneumonitis, hypersensitivity.*

organism (or′găn-ĭzm) [Gr. *organon,* organ, + *-ismos,* condition] Any living thing, plant or animal. An organism may be unicellular (bacteria, yeasts, protozoa) or multicellular (all complex organisms including humans).

decomposer o. Bacteria and fungi that degrade dead organic matter to simple organic and inorganic molecules. SEE: *biodegradation.*

fastidious o. In microbiology, an organism that has precise nutritional and environmental requirements for growth and survival.

organization (or″găn-ĭ-zā′shŭn) **1.** The process of becoming organized. **2.** Systematic arrangement. **3.** That which is organized; an organism.

o. center **1.** An embryonic group of cells that induces the development of another structure. **2.** A region in an ovum that is responsible for the mode of development of the fertilized ovum.

organize (or′găn-īz) To develop from an amorphous state to that having structure and form.

organo- (or′gă-nō) A combining form meaning *organ.*

organoferric (or″gă-nō-fĕr′ĭk) Concerning iron and an organic molecule.

organogel (or-găn′ō-jĕl) A water-in-oil emulsion used, for example, as a drug delivery vehicle.

organogenesis (or″găn-ō-jĕn′ĕ-sĭs) [″ + *genesis,* generation, birth] The formation and development of body organs from embryonic tissues.

It is important that a fetus not be exposed to harmful chemicals, particularly during organogenesis. The first critical period for the effects of teratogenic drugs on the human fetus is between the 13th and 56th days of gestation. The second period of high risk is during the last trimester when metabolic enzyme systems are beginning to be defined.

organoid [″ + *eidos,* form, shape] **1.** Resembling an organ. **2.** An organelle.

organoleptic (or″găn-ō-lĕp′tĭk) [″ + *lepsis,* a seizure] **1.** Affecting an organ, esp. the organs of special sense. **2.** Susceptible to sensory impressions.

organoma (or-gă-nō′mă) [″ + *oma,* tumor] A neoplasm containing cellular elements that can be definitely identified as being specific to certain tissues and organs.

organomegaly (or″gă-nō-mĕg′ă-lē) [″ + *megas,* large] The enlargement of visceral organs.

organometallic (or-gă-nō-mĕ-tăl′ĭk) A compound containing a metal combined with an organic molecule.

organonomy (or″gă-nŏn′ō-mē) [″ + *nomos,* law] The laws regulating the biological processes of living organisms.

organopexy (or′găn-ō-pĕk″sē) [″ + *pexis,* fixation] The surgical fixation of an organ that is detached from its proper position.

organotherapy (or″găn-ō-thĕr′ă-pē) [″ + *therapeia,* treatment] The treatment of disease by preparations of the endocrine glands of animals or by extracts made from them.

organotrope, organotropic (or-găn′ō-trōp, -găn-ō-trŏp′ĭk) [″ + *tropos,* turning] Having affinity for tissues or certain organs.

organotropism (or″gă-nŏt′rō-pĭzm) [″ + *trope,* a turn, + *-ismos,* condition] The attraction or affinity of chemicals or biological agents for body organs or tissues.

organ perfusion system A mechanical device equipped to supply metabolic, oxygen, and electrolyte needs to an organ obtained from a cadaver or donor in order to keep it viable for transplantation. The organ and the perfusion solution pumped through it can be kept at the ideal temperature for organ survival. They can be transported as necessary.

organ-specific (or′găn-spĕ-sĭf′ĭk) Originating in a single organ or affecting only one specific organ.

organum [L.] An organ.

o. auditus O. vestibulocochleare.

o. gustus The organ of taste.

o. olfactus The organ of smell; the olfactory region in the nasal cavity.

o. spirale Organ of Corti.

o. vestibulocochleare The organ of hearing. SYN: *o. auditus*. SEE: *ear*.

o. visus The organ of sight; the eye and its adnexa.

o. vomeronasale The canal opening into the nasal septum. SYN: *organ of Jacobson*.

orgasm (or′găzm) [Gr. *orgasmos,* swelling] A state of physical and emotional excitement that occurs at the climax of sexual intercourse. In the male it is accompanied by the ejaculation of semen. SYN: *climax*.

Oriental sore Cutaneous leishmaniasis. SYN: *Aleppo boil*. SEE: *leishmaniasis*.

orientation (or″ē-ĕn-tā′shŭn) [L. *oriens,* to arise] The ability to comprehend and to adjust oneself with regard to time, location, and identity of persons. This ability is partially or completely lost in some neurological and psychiatric disorders.

Orientia tsutsugamushi An intracellular parasite, formerly known as *Rickettsia tsutsugamushi,* that is the causative agent of scrub typhus. It is transmitted to humans from the bites of infected trombiculid mites, which prey in the wild on rodents.

orifice (or′ĭ-fĭs) [L. *orificium,* outlet] The mouth, entrance, or outlet of any anatomical structure. **orificial** (-fĭ′shăl), *adj.*

anal o. The anus.

atrioventricular o. The opening between the atrium and the ventricle on each side of the heart.

cardiac o. The opening of the esophagus into the stomach.

external urethral o. The exterior opening of the urethra. In the male, it is located at the tip of the glans penis; in the female, it is located anterior and cephalad to the vaginal opening.

ileal o. ileocecal valve.

internal urethral o. The opening from which the urethra makes its exit from the bladder.

mitral o. The opening between the left atrium and the left ventricle.

pyloric o. Pylorus.

ureteric o. The opening of the ureter into the bladder.

origin (or′ĭ-jĭn) [L. *origo,* beginning] **1.** The source of anything; a starting point. **2.** The beginning of a nerve. **3.** The more fixed attachment of a muscle.

deep o. The region within the brain where the fibers that make up a cranial nerve terminate.

superficial o. The point where a cranial nerve exits from the brain.

Orlando, Ida Jean Nursing educator, born 1926, who developed the Theory of the Deliberative Nursing Process. SEE: *Nursing Theory Appendix*.

Ormond's disease [John K. Ormond, U.S. physician, b. 1886] Retroperitoneal fibrosis.

ornithine (or′nĭ-thĭn) An amino acid formed when arginase hydrolyzes arginine. It is not present in proteins.

Ornithodoros (or″nĭ-thŏd′ō-rōs) A genus of ticks (family Argasidae) that infests mammals, including humans. Several species are vectors of the causative agents of disease, including spotted fever, tick fever, Q fever, tularemia, Russian encephalitis, and relapsing fever.

ornithosis (or″nĭ-thō′sĭs) [Gr. *ornithos,* bird, + *osis,* condition] Any acute, generalized, infectious disease of birds and domesticated fowls sometimes communicated to humans. SEE: *Chlamydia psittaci*.

oro- Combining form meaning *mouth*.

orodiagnosis (or″ō-dī-ăg-nō′sĭs) [Gr. *oros,* serum, + *dia,* through, + *gnosis,* knowledge] Serodiagnosis.

orofacial (or″ō-fā′shē-ăl) [L. *oris,* mouth, + *facies,* face] Concerning the mouth and face.

orofaciodigital syndrome An inherited disorder characterized by mental retardation and deformities of the mouth, tongue, fingers, and sometimes the face.

orolingual (or″ō-lĭng′gwăl) [L. *oris,* mouth, + *lingua,* tongue] Concerning the mouth and tongue.

oronasal (or″ō-nā′zăl) [″ + *nasus,* nose] Concerning the mouth and nose.

oropharyngeal airway SEE: under *airway.*

oropharynx (or″ō-făr′ĭnks) [″ + Gr. *pharynx,* throat] The central portion of the pharynx lying between the soft palate and the upper portion of the epiglottis.

orosomucoid (or″ŏ-sō-mū′koyd) An alpha 1-globulin in blood plasma.

orotic aciduria SEE: under *aciduria.*

orotracheal Pert. to the passageway between the mouth and the trachea.

Oroya fever [Oroya, a region of Peru] The first clinical stage of bartonellosis. An acute infectious disease endemic in Peru and other South American countries and characterized by intermittent fever, lymphadenopathy, severe anemia, and pains in the joints and long bones. SEE: *bartonellosis.*

orphan [L. *orphanus,* destitute, without parents] A child whose parents have died or are unknown.

o. disease A type of illness that, because of its rarity, has received minimal attention from medical researchers. SEE: *National Organization for Rare Disorders.*

o. drug Any drug that is effective for certain illnesses but, for a variety of reasons, is not profitable for manufacturers to produce. SEE: *National Organization for Rare Disorders.*

orphenadrine citrate (or-fĕn′ă-drēn) An antiparkinsonism drug.

orrhomeningitis (or″ō-mĕn″ĭn-jī′tĭs) [″ + *meninx,* membrane, + *itis,* inflammation] Inflammation of a serous membrane.

orris root (or′ĭs) The powder made from the root of certain varieties of iris. It is used in making some types of cosmetics. It may be a sensitizer by contact or inhalation.

ORS *oral rehydration solution.*

ORT *oral rehydration therapy.*

orth- SEE: *ortho-.*

ortho-, orth- [Gr. *orthos,* straight] Combining form meaning *straight, correct, normal, in proper order;* commonly used in chemical terminology.

orthoacid (or″thō-ăs′ĭd) An acid with as many hydroxyl groups as the number of valences of the acid-forming portion of the molecule.

orthobiosis (or″thō-bī-ō′sĭs) [″ + *bios,* life] Right living; a term used by Metchnikoff to encompass all the factors that may affect longevity and well-being.

orthocephalic (or″thō-sĕ-făl′ĭk) [″ + *kephale,* head] Having a well-proportioned head with a cephalic index between 70 and 75.

orthochorea (or″thō-kō-rē′ă) [″ + *choreia,* dance] A type of chorea in which attacks appear mainly when the person is in an erect position.

orthochromatic (or″thō-krō-măt′ĭk) [″ + *chroma,* color] Having normal color or staining normally.

orthochromophil (or″thō-krō′mō-fĭl) [″ + ″ + *philein,* to love] Staining normally with neutral dyes.

orthodentin (or″thō-dĕn′tĭn) Tubular dentin, as seen in human teeth.

orthodeoxia Decreased arterial oxygen concentration while in an upright position. The condition improves when the patient assumes the supine position. SEE: *syndrome, hepatopulmonary.*

orthodiagraph (or″thō-dī′ă-grăf) [″ + *dia,* through, + *graphein,* to write] An instrument for accurate recording of the outlines and positions of organs or foreign bodies as seen by radiographic apparatus.

orthodigita (or″thō-dĭj′ĭ-tă) [″ + L. *digitus,* finger] **1.** The division of podiatry that deals with the correction of deviated toes. **2.** The prevention and correction of deformities of the fingers or toes.

orthodontia, orthodontics (or″thō-dŏn′shē-ă, -dŏn′tĭks) [″ + *odous,* tooth] The division of dentistry dealing with the prevention and correction of abnormally positioned or aligned teeth.

orthodontist (or″thō-dŏn′tĭst) A dental specialist who has received graduate training in orthodontia. An orthodontist specializes in the treatment of malocclusions of dental and/or skeletal origins.

orthodromic (or″thō-drŏm′ĭk) [Gr. *orthodromein,* to run straight forward] Moving in the normal direction; said of nerve and cardiac impulses. SEE: *antidromic.*

orthogenesis (or″thō-jĕn′ĕ-sĭs) [Gr. *orthos,* straight, + *genesis,* generation, birth] An erroneous biological principle that the evolution of an animal species is in a given direction, governed by intrinsic factors, and independent of external factors.

orthogenic Pert. to, or related to, the correction, treatment, or rehabilitation of children with mental or emotional difficulties.

orthogenics (or″thō-jĕn′ĭks) Eugenics.

orthograde (or′thō-grād) [″ + L. *gradi,* to walk] Walking with the body vertical or upright; pert. to bipeds, esp. humans. Opposite of pronograde.

orthokeratology Use of special hard contact lenses to treat myopia by altering the curvature of the cornea. The lens presses on the center of the cornea, thus decreasing the protrusion.

orthokinetics Various tactile stimulation techniques used to stimulate the proprioceptors of muscles and tendons and thereby enhance motor performance in rehabilitation.

orthomelic (or″thō-mē′lĭk) [″ + *melos,* limb] Correcting deformed arms and legs.

orthomolecular (or″thō-mō-lĕk′ū-lăr)

Indicating the normal chemical constituents of the body or the restoration of those constituents to normal.

orthomyxovirus (or″thō-mĭk″sō-vī′rŭs) Any of the family of viruses including the viruses of influenza.

orthopantograph A panoramic radiographic device that images the entire dentition, alveolar bone, and other contiguous structures on a single extraoral film.

orthopedic, orthopaedic (or″thō-pē′dĭk) Concerning orthopedics; concerning the prevention or correction of musculoskeletal deformities.

orthopedics, orthopaedics (or″thō-pē′dĭks) [″ + *pais,* child] The branch of medical science that deals with prevention or correction of disorders involving locomotor structures of the body, esp. the skeleton, joints, muscles, fascia, and other supporting structures such as ligaments and cartilage.

orthopedist, orthopaedist (or″thō-pē′dĭst) A specialist in orthopedics.

orthopercussion (or″thō-pĕr-kŭsh′ŭn) [″ + L. *percussio,* a striking] Percussion with the distal phalanx of the percussing finger held perpendicularly to the surface percussed.

orthophoria (or″thō-fō′rē-ă) [″ + *pherein,* to bear] Parallelism of visual axes, the normal eye muscle balance.

orthopnea (or″thŏp′nē-ă) [″ + *pnoia,* breath] Labored breathing that occurs when lying flat and is relieved by sitting up. This is one of the classical symptoms of left ventricular heart failure.

SYMPTOMS: The respiratory rate is usually rapid with the muscles of respiration forcibly used in the struggle to inhale and exhale. A sitting or standing posture is necessary to ease breathing. Patients often feel the necessity to brace themselves in order to breathe. On physical examination, the patient appears anxious and may be cyanotic and actively sweating.

ETIOLOGY: Orthopnea is seen in heart failure, bronchial and cardiac asthma, pulmonary edema, severe emphysema, pneumonia, angina pectoris, and spasmodic cough.

orthopneic position (or″thŏp-nē′ĭk) The upright or nearly upright position of the upper trunk of a patient in a bed or chair. It facilitates breathing in those with congestive heart failure and some forms of pulmonary disease.

Orthopoxvirus A genus of virus that includes the virus causing smallpox (variola) and monkeypox.

orthopraxis (or″thō-prăk′sĭs) [″ + *prassein,* to make] The mechanical correction of deformities.

orthopsychiatry (or″thō-sī-kī′ă-trē) [″ + *psyche,* soul, + *iatreia,* treatment] The branch of psychiatry concerned with mental and emotional development. It encompasses child psychiatry and mental hygiene.

orthoptic (or-thŏp′tĭk) [″ + *optikos,* pert. to vision] Pert. to or producing normal binocular vision.

orthoptics **1.** The science of correcting defects in binocular vision resulting from defects in optic musculature. **2.** The technique of eye exercises for correcting faulty eye coordination affecting binocular vision. The technique is also referred to as orthoptic training.

orthoroentgenography (or″thō-rĕnt-gĕn-ŏg′ră-fē) A technique for obtaining accurate measurement of the size and position of the internal organs using radiographic apparatus. A radiographic procedure used for the accurate measurement of long bones. SEE: *orthodiagraph.*

orthoscopic (or″thō-skŏp′ĭk) **1.** Having correct and undistorted vision. **2.** Made to correct optical distortion.

orthoscopy (or-thŏs′kō-pē) Ocular examination with an orthoscope.

orthosis [Gr., straightening] Any device added to the body to stabilize or immobilize a body part, prevent deformity, protect against injury, or assist with function. Orthotic devices range from arm slings to corsets and finger splints. They may be made from a variety of materials, including rubber, leather, canvas, rubber synthetics, and plastic. **orthotic,** *adj.*

balanced forearm o. Mobile arm support.

orthostatic (or″thō-stăt′ĭk) [Gr. *orthos,* straight, + *statikos,* causing to stand] Concerning or caused by an erect position.

o. vital signs determination The measurement of blood pressure and pulse rate first in supine, then in sitting, and finally in standing positions. A significant change in both of these vital signs signifies hypovolemia or dehydration. A positive test result occurs 1. if the patient becomes dizzy or loses consciousness; or 2. if the pulse increases by 20 or more beats per minute and the systolic blood pressure drops by 20 mm Hg or more 2 min after arising from supine to sitting or from sitting to standing.

orthotast (or′thō-tăst) [″ + *tassein,* to arrange] An instrument used for straightening bone curvatures.

orthotic [Gr. *orthosis,* straightening] Relating to orthosis.

orthotics (or-thŏt′ĭks) **1.** The science pert. to mechanical appliances for orthopedic use. **2.** The use of orthopedic appliances.

orthotist (or′thō-tĭst) [Gr. *orthosis,* straightening] One skilled in orthotics.

orthotonos, orthotonus (or-thŏt′ō-nŏs, -nŭs) [″ + *tonos,* tension] Tetanic spasm marked by rigidity of the body in a straight line. SEE: illus.

orthotopic (or″thō-tŏp′ĭk) **1.** In the correct place. **2.** Pert. to a tissue graft to a site where that tissue would normally be present.

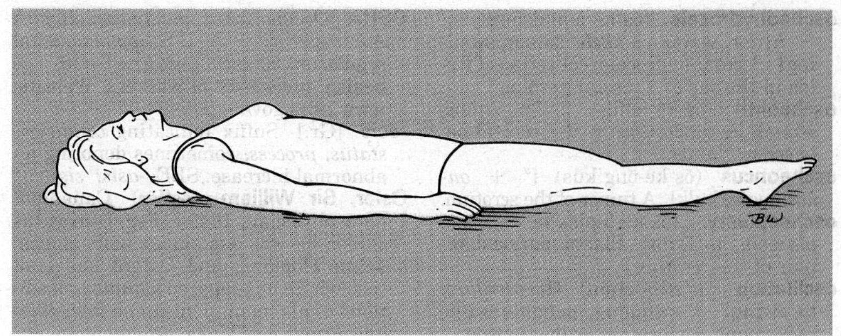

ORTHOTONOS

orthovoltage (or″thō-vŏl′tĭj) The median voltage used in x-ray therapy, approx. 250 kilovolts.

orthropsia (or-thrŏp′sē-ă) [Gr. *orthros,* time near dawn, + *opsis,* sight] A characteristic of human vision by which sight is better at dawn or dusk than in bright sunlight.

Ortner's syndrome (ŏrt′nĕrs) [Norbert Ortner, Austrian physician, 1865–1935] Vocal paralysis caused by pressure from an enlarged heart on the recurrent laryngeal nerve.

Ortolani's maneuver [Marius Ortolani, 20th century Italian orthopedic surgeon] The assessment maneuver designed to detect congenital subluxation or dislocation of the hip. The examiner places the infant on the back with hips and knees flexed while abducting and lifting the femurs. A palpable click is felt as the femur enters the dysplastic joint.

O.S., o.s. L. *oculus sinister,* left eye. SEE: *O.D.*

Os Symbol for the element osmium.

os (ōs) *pl.* **ora** [L.] Mouth, opening.
incompetent cervical o. A uterine cervix that cannot maintain a diameter small enough to support the increasing weight of the fetus. This condition usually results in early second trimester abortion. The cause is a congenital structural defect or previous trauma to the cervix. It is treated with a purse-string ligature that encircles, encloses, and reinforces the cervix.
o. uteri The mouth of the uterus.
o. uteri externum The opening of the cervical canal of the uterus into the vagina.
o. uteri internum The internal opening of the cervical canal into the uterus.
o. ventriculi The cardia of the stomach.

os (ŏs) *pl.* **ossa** [L.] Bone.
o. calcis The heel bone. SYN: *calcaneus.*
o. coxae Innominate bone.
o. hamatum The hooked bone on the ulnar side of the distal row of the carpus (wrist). SYN: *unciform bone.*
o. hyoideum The horseshoe-shaped bone lying at the base of the tongue. SYN: *hyoid bone.*
o. ilium The ilium.
o. innominatum The innominate (hip) bone.
o. magnum The third bone in the second distal row of the carpus. SYN: *capitatum.*
o. orbiculare The tiny bone in the ear that becomes attached to the incus, forming the lenticular process.
o. peroneum A bone occasionally found in the tendon of the peroneus longus muscle.
o. planum **1.** Flat bone; any bone that has only a slight thickness. **2.** The orbital plate of the ethmoid bone.
o. pubis The pubic bone; the anteroinferior part of the hip bone. In the adult, it unites the innominate bone with the ilium and ischium to form the pelvis. It is irregular in shape, divided into a horizontal, ascending, and descending ramus. The outer extremity constitutes approx. one fifth of the acetabulum. The inner ramus forms the symphysis pubis.
o. scaphoideum A proximal boat-shaped bone of the carpus or the tarsus. SYN: *scaphoid.*
o. temporale Temporal bone.
o. trigonum A bone of the foot that develops from an extra center of ossification along the posterior surface of the talus.
o. unguis Lacrimal bone.
o. vesalianum A bone that develops from the ossification of the posterior tubercle of the fifth metatarsal.

osazone (ō′sā-zōn) Any of a series of compounds resulting from heating sugars with acetic acid and phenylhydrazine.

oscheal (ŏs′kē-ăl) [Gr. *oscheon,* scrotum] Scrotal.

oscheitis (ŏs-kē-ī′tĭs) [″ + *itis,* inflammation] Inflammation of the scrotum.

oschelephantiasis (ŏsk″ĕl-ĕ-făn-tī′ă-sĭs) Elephantiasis of the scrotum.

oscheo- [Gr. *oscheon*] Combining form meaning *scrotum.*

oscheocele (ŏs′kē-ō-sēl) [″ + *kele,* tumor, swelling] A scrotal swelling or tumor.

oscheohydrocele (ŏs″kē-ō-hī′drō-sēl) [″ + *hydor,* water, + *kele,* tumor, swelling] Scrotal hydrocele; collection of fluids in the sac of a scrotal hernia.

oscheolith (ŏs′kē-ō-lĭth) [″ + *lithos,* stone] A concretion in the scrotal sebaceous glands.

oscheoncus (ŏs″kē-ŏng′kŭs) [″ + *onkos,* mass, bulk] A tumor of the scrotum.

oscheoplasty (ŏs′kē-ō-plăs″tē) [″ + *plassein,* to form] Plastic surgical repair of the scrotum.

oscillation (ŏs″sĭl-ā′shŭn) [L. *oscillare,* to swing] A swinging, pendulum-like movement; a vibration or fluctuation.

oscillator (ŏs′ĭ-lā″tor) **1.** Device for producing oscillations. **2.** An electronic circuit that will produce an oscillating current of a certain frequency.

oscillogram (ŏs′ĭl-ō-grăm) [″ + Gr. *gramma,* something written] A graphic record made by the oscillograph.

oscillograph (ŏs′ĭl-ō-grăf) [″ + Gr. *graphein,* to write] An electronic device used for detecting, displaying, and recording variations in electrical phenomena. In medicine, it is used for recording electrical activity of the brain, the heart, and other muscular tissues. Electrocardiographs and electroencephalographs are examples of the application of this technique. SEE: *oscilloscope.*

oscillometer (ŏs-ĭl-ŏm′ĕ-tĕr) [″ + Gr. *metron,* measure] A machine used to measure oscillations, esp. those of the bloodstream.

oscillometry (ŏs-ĭl-ŏm′ĕ-trē) The measurement of oscillations with an instrument.

oscillopsia The visual perception that stationary objects are moving. This perception is an illusion, and is usually associated with vestibular dysfunction.

oscilloscope (ŏ-sĭl′ō-skōp) [L. *oscillare,* to swing, + Gr. *skopein,* to examine] An instrument that makes visible the presence, nature, and form of oscillations or irregularities of an electric current. SEE: *oscillograph.*

Oscinidae The eye flies. A family of small hairless flies that includes the genera *Hippelates, Siphunculina,* and *Oscinis.* They are serious pests and transmit a number of infectious diseases.

osculation [L. *osculum,* little mouth, kiss] **1.** The union of two vessels or structures by their mouths. **2.** Kissing.

osculum (ŏs′kū-lŭm) *pl.* **oscula** [L.] A tiny aperture or pore.

-ose **1.** Chemical suffix indicating that a substance is a carbohydrate, such as glucose. **2.** Suffix indicating a primary alteration product of a protein, such as proteose.

Osgood-Schlatter disease (ŏz-good-shlăt′ĕr) [Robert B. Osgood, U.S. orthopedist, 1873–1956; Carl Schlatter, Swiss surgeon, 1864–1934] Osteochondritis of the epiphysis of the tibial tuberosity.

OSHA *Occupational Safety and Health Administration.* A U.S. governmental regulatory agency concerned with the health and safety of workers. Website: www.osha.gov/.

-osis [Gr.] Suffix indicating *condition, status, process,* sometimes denoting an abnormal increase. SEE: *-asis; -sis.*

Osler, Sir William (ŏs′lĕr) Canadian-born physician, 1849–1919. During his career he was associated with McGill, Johns Hopkins, and Oxford Universities, where he prepared a number of editions of his monumental *The Principles and Practice of Medicine.*

O.'s disease **1.** Polycythemia vera. **2.** Hereditary hemorrhagic telangiectasia.

O.'s maneuver An attempt to compress the radial artery sufficiently to prevent palpation of the radial pulse past the point of compression. If this pulse is still palpable, then the artery is sclerosed. This could lead to the diagnosis of hypertension when, in fact, the blood pressure could be normal.

O.'s nodes Small, tender cutaneous nodes, usually present in the fingers and toes, that may be seen in subacute bacterial endocarditis. The nodes are due to infected emboli from the heart.

osmatic (ŏz-măt′ĭk) [Gr. *osmasthai,* to smell] Pert. to, or having, a keen sense of smell.

osmesis (ŏz-mē′sĭs) [Gr. *osmesis,* smelling] **1.** The sense of smell. **2.** The act of smelling. SYN: *olfaction.*

osmesthesia (ŏz″mĕs-thē′zē-ă) [Gr. *osme,* odor, + *aisthesis,* sensation] Olfactory sensibility; the power of perceiving and distinguishing odors.

osmic acid (ŏz′mĭk) OsO_4; a volatile, colorless compound formed by heating osmium in air. It is used as a caustic, a stain for fats, and a tissue fixative for electron microscopy. SYN: *osmium tetroxide.*

CAUTION: Vapors are extremely toxic to the eyes, skin, and respiratory tract.

osmicate (ŏz′mĭ-kāt) To impregnate or stain with osmic acid.

osmidrosis (ŏz-mĭ-drō′sĭs) [″ + *hidros,* sweat] Bromidrosis.

osmiophilic (ŏz″mē-ō-fĭl′ĭk) Having an affinity for the staining material osmium tetroxide.

osmiophobic (ŏz″mē-ō-fō′bĭk) Having resistance to the staining material osmium tetroxide.

osmium (ŏz′mē-ŭm) [Gr. *osme,* smell] SYMB: Os. A metallic element with an atomic mass of 190.2 and the atomic number 76.

o. tetroxide Osmic acid.

osmo- [Gr. *osme,* odor] A combining form indicating *odor, smell.*

osmo- [Gr. *osmos,* impulse] A combining form meaning *a thrusting forth.*

osmo- [Gr. *osmos,* impulse] Pert. to osmosis.

osmol, osmole The standard unit of osmotic pressure based on a one molal concentration of an ion in a solution.

osmodysphoria (ŏz-mō-dĭs-fō′rē-ă) [Gr. *osme,* odor, + *dys,* bad, + *pherein,* to bear] A deep-seated and abnormal dislike of certain odors.

osmolagnia (ŏz″mō-lăg′nē-ă) [″ + *lagneia,* lust] Erotic excitement derived from odors, usually of the body. SYN: *osphresiolagnia*.

osmolality (ŏs″mō-lăl′ĭ-tē) Osmotic concentration; the characteristic of a solution determined by the ionic concentration of the dissolved substances per unit of solvent.

fecal o. The concentration of solutes in stool. In health, this is equivalent to the concentration of solutes in plasma.

plasma o. The osmotic concentration of plasma. Normally the ionic concentration in the plasma is maintained within a narrow range: 275 to 295 mOsm/kg. When plasma osmolality increases above normal, antidiuretic hormone (ADH, also called vasopressin) is released. ADH prevents loss of water by the kidney and thus decreases plasma osmolality. An increase in plasma osmolality also produces the sensation of thirst, which stimulates the person to drink fluids; this, too, serves to decrease plasma osmolality.

serum o. The osmotic concentration of the serum.

urine o. The osmotic concentration of the urine.

osmolar (ŏz-mō′lăr) Concerning the osmotic concentration of a solution.

osmolarity (os″mō-lăr′ĭ-tē) The concentration of osmotically active particles in solution.

osmology (ŏz-mŏl′ō-jē) [Gr. *osme,* odor, + *logos,* word, reason] **1.** The study of odors. SYN: *osphresiology*. **2.** The study of osmosis.

osmometer (ŏz-mŏm′ĕt-ĕr) [Gr. *osme,* odor, + *metron,* measure] A device for measuring the acuity of the sense of smell.

osmometer (ŏz-mŏm′ĕt-ĕr) [Gr. *osmos,* impulse, + *metron,* measure] A device for measuring osmotic pressure either directly or indirectly. It was formerly used to assess the extent of dehydration or blood loss.

osmometry **1.** The study of osmosis. **2.** The measurement of osmotic forces using an osmometer.

osmonosology (ŏz″mō-nō-sŏl′ō-jē) [Gr. *osme,* odor, + *nosos,* disease, + *logos,* word, reason] The branch of medicine dealing with diseases and disorders of the organs of smell.

osmophore (ŏz′mō-for) [Gr. *osme,* odor, + *phoros,* bearing] The portion of a chemical responsible for the odor of the compound.

osmoreceptor (ŏz″mō-rē-sĕp′tor) **1.** A receptor in the hypothalamus that is sensitive to the osmotic pressure of the serum. **2.** A receptor in the brain that is sensitive to olfactory stimuli.

osmoregulation (ŏz″mō-rĕg″ū-lā′shŭn) The regulation of osmotic pressure.

osmose (ŏz′mōs) [Gr. *osmos,* impulse] **1.** To subject to osmosis. **2.** To undergo osmosis.

osmosis (ŏz-mō′sĭs) [Gr. *osmos,* impulse, + *osis,* condition] The passage of solvent through a semipermeable membrane that separates solutions of different concentrations. The solvent, usually water, passes through the membrane from the region of lower concentration of solute to that of a higher concentration of solute, thus tending to equalize the concentrations of the two solutions. The rate of osmosis is dependent primarily upon the difference in osmotic pressures of the solutions on the two sides of a membrane, the permeability of the membrane, and the electric potential across the membrane and the charge upon the walls of the pores in it. SEE: illus.

reverse o. A form of water treatment that removes infectious particles and dissolved ions more effectively than other water purification techniques. Water so purified can be used in hemodialysis. **osmotic** (-mŏt′ĭk), *adj.*

osmostat The area in the anterior region of the hypothalamus that contains cells that control osmolality.

osmotherapy (ŏz″mō-thĕr′ă-pē) [″ + *therapeia,* treatment] Intravenous administration of hypertonic solutions in order to increase the osmolar concentration of the serum. This therapy is used in treating cerebral edema.

osmotic pressure **1.** Pressure that develops when two solutions of different concentrations are separated by a semipermeable membrane. **2.** Pressure that would develop if a solution were enclosed in a membrane impermeable to all solutes present and surrounded by pure solvent. Osmotic pressure varies with concentration of the solution and with temperature increase. Animal cells have an osmotic pressure approx. equal to that of the circulating fluid, the blood. Solutions exerting this osmotic pressure are said to be isotonic or isosmotic; stronger solutions that cause cells to shrink are hypertonic; weaker solutions that cause cells to swell are hypotonic.

osphresiolagnia (ŏs-frē″zē-ō-lăg′nē-ă) [Gr. *osphresis,* smell, + *lagneia,* lust] Erotic excitement produced by odors. SYN: *osmolagnia*.

osphresiology (ŏs″frē-zē-ŏl′ō-jē) [″ + *logos,* word, reason] Science of odors and the sense of smell. SYN: *osmology* (1)

osphresiometer (ŏs″frē-zē-ŏm′ĕ-tĕr) [″ + *metron,* measure] An apparatus for measuring the acuteness of the sense of smell. SYN: *osmometer*.

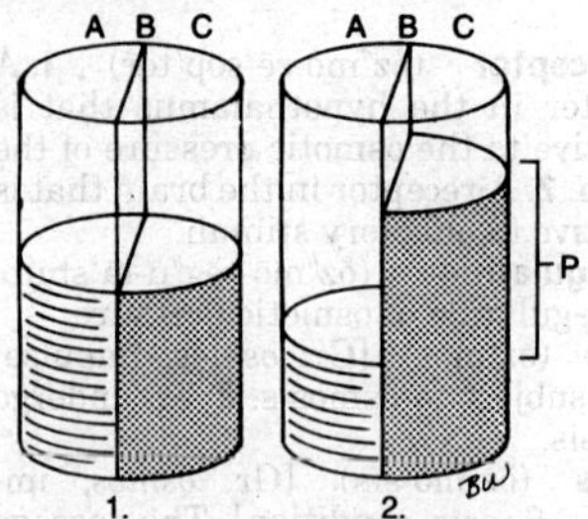

A. CHAMBER CONTAINING WATER.
B. MEMBRANOUS PARTITION SEPARATING TWO CHAMBERS.
C. CHAMBER CONTAINING A SOLUTION OF SALT IN WATER.
1. MEMBRANE B IS PERMEABLE TO WATER AND SALT.
2. MEMBRANE B IS SEMIPERMEABLE IN THAT IT IS IMPERMEABLE TO SALT BUT PERMEABLE TO WATER.
P. OSMOTIC PRESSURE CAUSES THE DIFFERENCE IN LEVELS BETWEEN CHAMBERS A AND C WHEN SEPARATED BY A SEMIPERMEABLE MEMBRANE

OSMOSIS IN WHOLE BLOOD AND IN SALT SOLUTIONS THAT HAVE INCREASED OR DECREASED SALT CONCENTRATION

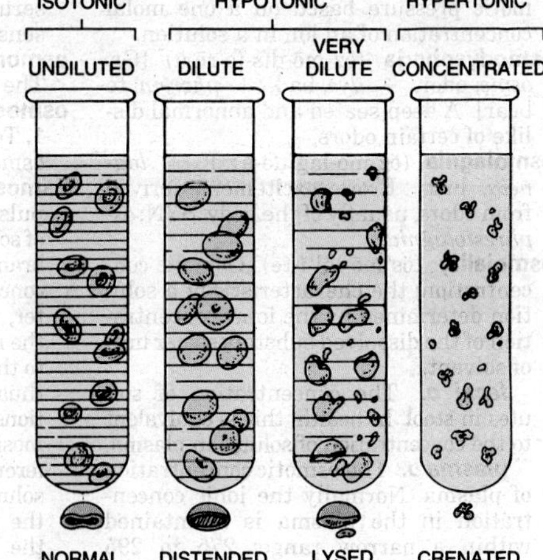

THE ERYTHROCYTES SWELL IN HYPOTONIC AND SHRINK (BECOME CRENATED) IN HYPERTONIC SALT SOLUTION

OSMOSIS

osphresis (ŏs-frē′sĭs) [Gr.] The sense of smell. SYN: *olfaction*. **osphretic** (-frĕt′ĭk), *adj.*

osphyalgia (ŏs-fē-ăl′jē-ă) [Gr. *osphys,* loin, + *algos,* pain] Pain in the hips. SEE: *lumbago; sciatica.*

osphyitis (ŏs-fē-ī′tĭs) [″ + *itis,* inflammation] Inflammation of the lumbar region.

osphyomyelitis (ŏs″fē-ō-mī″ĕl-ī′tĭs) [″ + *myelos,* marrow, + *itis,* inflammation] Inflammation of the lumbar region of the spinal cord.

ossa (ŏs′ă) [L., bones] Pl. of os.

ossein (ŏs′ē-ĭn) [L. *ossa,* bones] The collagen of bone. It forms the framework of bone.

osseocartilaginous (ŏs″ē-ō-kăr″tĭ-lăj′ĭ-nŭs) Concerning bone and cartilage.

osseofibrous (ŏs″ē-ō-fī′brŭs) [″ + *fibra,* fiber] Composed of bone and fibrous tissue.

osseointegration A stable, compatible interface between a dental implant and the bone. It is devoid of fibrous connective tissue. The interface is created by the growth of living bone into direct contact and potential bonding with the implant.

osseous (ŏs′ē-ŭs) [L. *osseus,* bony] Bonelike; concerning bones. SYN: *bony*.

ossicle (ŏs′ĭ-kl) [L. *ossiculum,* little bone] Any small bone, esp. one of the three bones of the ear.

auditory o. One of the three bones of the inner ear: malleus, incus, and stapes. SEE: *ear* for illus.

ossiculectomy (ŏs″ĭk-ū-lĕk′tō-mē) [L. *ossiculum,* little bone, + Gr. *ektome,* excision] Excision of an ossicle, esp. one of the ear.

ossiculotomy (ŏ″sĭk-ū-lŏt′ō-mē) [″ + Gr. *tome,* incision] Surgical incision of one or more of the ossicles of the ear.

ossiculum (ŏ-sĭk′ū-lŭm) *pl.* **ossicula** [L.] Tiny bone, esp. one of the three in the middle ear.

ossific (ŏs-ĭf′ĭk) [″ + *facere,* to make] Producing or becoming bone.

ossification (ŏs″ĭ-fĭ-kā′shŭn) [″ + *facere,* to make] **1.** The formation of bone substance. **2.** The conversion of other tissue into bone. SYN: *osteogenesis*.

endochondral o. The formation of bone in cartilage, as in the formation of long bones, involving the destruction and removal of cartilage and the formation of osseous tissue in the space formerly occupied by the cartilage. SEE: illus.

intramembranous o. The formation of bone in or underneath a fibrous membrane, such as occurs in the formation of the cranial bones.

pathologic o. The formation of bone in abnormal sites or abnormal development of bone.

periosteal o. The formation of successive thin layers of bone by osteoblasts between the underlying bone or cartilage and the cellular and fibrous layer that covers the forming bone. Also called subperiosteal ossification.

ossiform (ŏs′ĭ-form) Resembling bone. SYN: *osteoid* (1).

ossify (ŏs′ĭ-fī) [″ + *facere,* to make] To turn into bone.

ostalgia (ŏs-tăl′jē-ă) [Gr. *osteon,* bone, + *algos,* pain] Pain in a bone.

oste- SEE: *osteo-*.

osteal (ŏs′tē-ăl) Pert. to bone.

osteanagenesis (ŏs″tē-ăn-ă-jĕn′ĕ-sĭs) [″

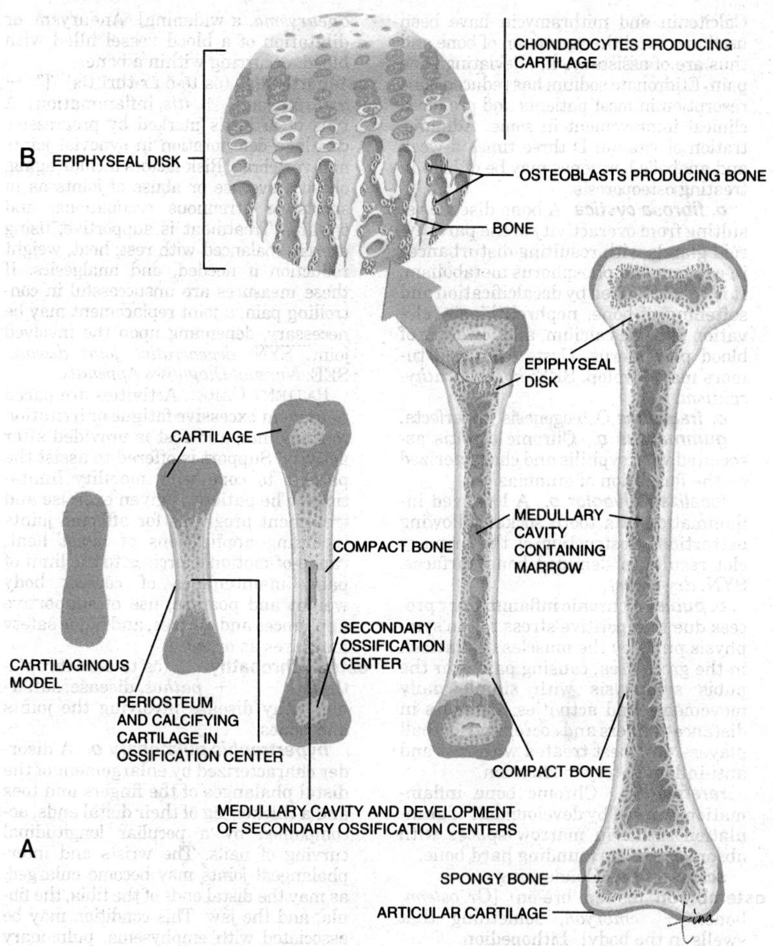

ENDOCHONDRAL OSSIFICATION

Ossification process in a long bone; (A) progression from embryo to young adult, (B) microscopic view of an epiphyseal disk

+ *ana,* on, + L. *genesis,* generation, birth] Osteoanagenesis.

ostearthrotomy (ŏs″tē-ăr-thrŏt′ō-mē) [″ + *arthron,* joint, + *tome,* incision] Osteoarthrotomy.

ostectomy, osteectomy (ŏs-tĕk′tō-mē, -tē-ĕk′tō-mē) [″ + *ektome,* excision] Surgical excision of a bone or a portion of one.

osteectopia (ŏs″tē-ĕk-tō′pē-ă) [″ + *ektopos,* out of place] Displacement of a bone.

osteitis (ŏs-tē-ī′tĭs) [″ + *itis,* inflammation] Inflammation of a bone.

condensing o. Osteitis in which the marrow cavity becomes filled with osseous tissue, causing the bone to become denser and heavier. SYN: *sclerosing o.*

o. deformans A skeletal disease of unknown etiology that affects older people; a chronic form of osteitis with thickening and hypertrophy of the long bones and deformity of the flat bones. SYN: *Paget's disease.*

ETIOLOGY: The disease may be caused by a virus.

SYMPTOMS: Symptoms are insidious in onset and include pain in the lower limbs (esp. the tibia), frequent fractures, waddling gait, and shortened stature. The skull becomes enlarged, so that the face appears small and triangular with the head pushed forward.

TREATMENT: Asymptomatic cases should not be treated. Aspirin or other nonsteroidal anti-inflammatory drugs are given for pain. There is no specific curative therapy, but male and female sex hormones, fluoride, and x-ray therapy have been used to control the pain.

Calcitonin and mithramycin have been used to control the resorption of bone and thus are of assistance in alleviating bone pain. Etidronate sodium has reduced bone resorption in most patients and produced clinical improvement in some. Administration of vitamin D three times a week and anabolic hormones may be of help in treating osteoporosis.

o. fibrosa cystica A bone disease resulting from overactivity of the parathyroid glands with resulting disturbances in calcium and phosphorus metabolism. It is characterized by decalcification and softening of bone, nephrolithiasis, elevation of blood calcium, and lowering of blood phosphorus. Cysts form and tumors may develop. SEE: *hyperparathyroidism.*

o. fragilitans Osteogenesis imperfecta.

gummatous o. Chronic osteitis associated with syphilis and characterized by the formation of gummas.

localized alveolar o. A localized inflammation of a tooth socket following extraction. Destruction of the primary clot results in denuded bone surfaces. SYN: *dry socket.*

o. pubis A chronic inflammatory process due to repetitive stress to the symphysis pubis by the muscles that attach in the groin area, causing pain over the pubis symphysis with simple daily movements and activities. It occurs in distance runners and soccer and football players. It is best treated with rest and anti-inflammatory medication.

rarefying o. Chronic bone inflammation marked by development of granulation tissue in marrow spaces with absorption of surrounding hard bone.

sclerosing o. Condensing o.

ostembryon (ŏs-tĕm′brē-ŏn) [Gr. *osteon,* bone, + *embryon,* something that swells in the body] Lithopedion.

ostempyesis (ŏs″tĕm-pī-ē′sĭs) [″ + *empyesis,* suppuration] Purulent inflammation within a bone.

ostensible agency In malpractice law, the responsibility an employer bears for the negligent actions of professional employees or contractors; among other duties, the employer is assumed to have researched diligently the credentialing, licensure, and suitability to provide care of his or her agents. SYN: *ostensible authority.*

ostensible authority Ostensible agency.

osteo-, oste- [Gr. *osteon,* bone] Combining form meaning *bone.*

osteoanagenesis (ŏs″tē-ō-ăn″ă-jĕn′ĕ-sĭs) [″ + Gr. *ana,* again, + L. *genesis,* generation, birth] Regeneration of bone.

osteoanesthesia (ŏs″tē-ō-ăn″ĕs-thē′zē-ă) [″ + *an-,* not, + *aisthesis,* sensation] The condition of the bone being insensitive, esp. to stimuli that would normally produce pain.

osteoaneurysm (ŏs″tē-ō-ăn′ū-rĭzm) [″ + *aneurysma,* a widening] Aneurysm, or dilatation of a blood vessel filled with blood, occurring within a bone.

osteoarthritis (ŏs″tē-ō-ăr-thrī′tĭs) [″ + *arthron,* joint, + *itis,* inflammation] A type of arthritis marked by progressive cartilage deterioration in synovial joints and vertebrae. Risk factors include aging, obesity, overuse or abuse of joints as in sports or strenuous occupations, and trauma. Treatment is supportive, using exercise balanced with rest, heat, weight reduction if needed, and analgesics. If these measures are unsuccessful in controlling pain, a joint replacement may be necessary, depending upon the involved joint. SYN: *degenerative joint disease.* SEE: *Nursing Diagnoses Appendix.*

PATIENT CARE: Activities are paced to prevent excessive fatigue or irritation to the joints, and rest is provided after activity. Support is offered to assist the patient to cope with mobility limitations. The patient is given exercise and treatment programs for affected joints including applications of moist heat, range-of-motion exercises to the limit of pain, maintenance of correct body weight and posture, use of supportive appliances and devices, and home safety measures as ordered.

osteoarthropathy (ŏs″tē-ō-ăr-thrŏp′ă-thē) [″ + ″ + *pathos,* disease, suffering] Any disease involving the joints and bones.

hypertrophic pulmonary o. A disorder characterized by enlargement of the distal phalanges of the fingers and toes and a thickening of their distal ends, accompanied by a peculiar longitudinal curving of nails. The wrists and interphalangeal joints may become enlarged, as may the distal ends of the tibia, the fibula, and the jaw. This condition may be associated with emphysema, pulmonary tuberculosis, chronic bronchitis, bronchiectasis, and congenital heart disease.

osteoarthrotomy (ŏs″tē-ō-ăr-thrŏt′ō-mē) [″ + ″ + *tome,* incision] Surgical excision of the articular end of a bone. SYN: *ostearthrotomy.*

osteoblast (ŏs′tē-ō-blăst) [Gr. *osteon,* bone, + *blastos,* germ] A cell of mesodermal origin concerned with the formation of bone.

osteoblastoma (ŏs″tē-ō-blăs-tō′mă) [″ + ″ + *oma,* tumor] A large, benign tumor of osteoblasts in a patchy osteoid matrix. It occurs mostly in the vertebral columns of young people.

osteocampsia (ŏs″tē-ō-kămp′sē-ă) [″ + *kamptein,* to bend] Curvature of a bone, as in osteomalacia.

osteocarcinoma (ŏs″tē-ō-kăr-sĭn-ō′mă) [″ + *karkinos,* cancer, + *oma,* tumor] **1.** Combined osteoma and carcinoma. **2.** Carcinoma of a bone.

osteocartilaginous (ŏs″tē-ō-kăr″tĭ-lăj′ĭ-nŭs) Concerning bone and cartilage.

osteocele (ŏs′tē-ō-sēl) [″ + *kele,* tumor,

swelling] **1.** A testicular or scrotal tumor that contains bony tissue. **2.** A bone-containing hernia.

osteochondral (ŏs″tē-ō-kŏn′drăl) Concerning bone and cartilage.

osteochondritis (ŏs″tē-ō-kŏn-drī′tĭs) [″ + *chondros,* cartilage, + *itis,* inflammation] Inflammation of bone and cartilage.

o. deformans juvenilis Chronic inflammation of the head of the femur in children, resulting in atrophy and shortening of the neck of femur with a wide flat head. SYN: *Perthes' disease; Waldenström's disease.*

o. dissecans A condition affecting a joint in which a fragment of cartilage and its underlying bone become detached from the articular surface. It commonly occurs in the knee joint.

osteochondrodystrophy (ŏs″tē-ō-kŏn″drō-dĭs′trō-fē) [″ + ″ + *dys,* bad, + *trephein,* to nourish] A disorder of skeletal growth resulting from bone and cartilage malformation. The condition produces a form of dwarfism. SYN: *Morquio's syndrome.*

familial o. Morquio's syndrome. SEE: *mucopolysaccharidosis IV.*

osteochondrolysis (ŏs″tē-ō-kŏn-drŏl′ĭ-sĭs) [″ + ″ + *lysis,* dissolution] Osteochondritis dissecans.

osteochondroma (ŏs″tē-ō-kŏn-drō′mă) [″ + ″ + *oma,* tumor] A tumor composed of both cartilaginous and bony substance.

osteochondromatosis (ŏs″tē-ō-kŏn″drō-mă-tō′sĭs) [″ + ″ + ″ + *osis,* condition] A disease in which there are multiple osteochondromata.

osteochondrosarcoma (ŏs″tē-ō-kŏn″drō-săr-kō′mă) [″ + ″ + *sarx,* flesh, + *oma,* tumor] Chondrosarcoma occurring in bone.

osteochondrosis (ŏs″tē-ō-kŏn-drō′sĭs) [″ + ″ + *osis,* condition] A disease causing degenerative changes in the ossification centers of the epiphyses of bones, particularly during periods of rapid growth in children. The process may result in aseptic necrosis of bone, or there may be gradual healing and repair.

PATIENT CARE: Bedrest is encouraged, and support is offered through disruption of normal activity. The patient learns the correct use of crutches. Neurocirculatory function distal to supportive device (splint, elastic support, or cast) is evaluated. Joint mobility and limitation of motion are assessed daily.

o. deformans tibiae Degeneration or aseptic necrosis of the medial condyle of the tibia.

osteochondrous (ŏs″tē-ō-kŏn′drŭs) Concerning bone and cartilage.

osteoclasia, osteoclasis (ŏs″tē-ō-klā′zē-ă, -ŏk′lă-sĭs) [″ + *klasis,* a breaking] **1.** Surgical fracture of a bone in order to remedy a deformity. SYN: *diaclasis.* **2.** Bony tissue absorption and destruction.

osteoclast (ŏs′tē-ō-klăst) [″ + *klan,* to break] **1.** A device for fracturing bones for therapeutic purposes. **2.** A giant multinuclear cell formed in the bone marrow of growing bones. Osteoclasts are found in depressions (called Howship's lacunae) on the surface of the bone. By absorbing calcium salts, it removes excess bone tissue as in the remodeling of growing bones, or damaged bone in the repair of fractures. SEE: illus. **osteoclastic** (-klăs′tĭk), *adj.*

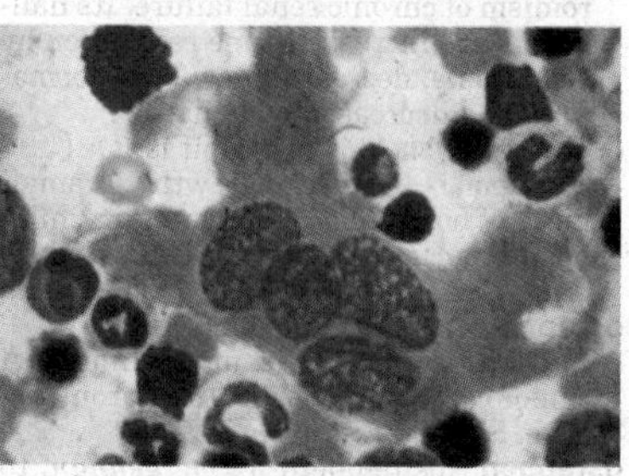

OSTEOCLAST

With multiple nuclei (orig. mag. ×640)

osteoclast activating factor ABBR: OAF. A lymphokine produced in certain conditions associated with resorption of bone, including periodontal disease and lymphoid malignancies such as multiple myeloma and malignant lymphoma. Interleukin-1 is an OAF, as are other substances produced by T lymphocytes and prostaglandins.

osteoclastoma (ŏs″tē-ō-klăs-tō′mă) [″ + ″ + *oma,* tumor] Giant cell tumor of bone.

osteocope (ŏs′tē-ō-kōp) [″ + *kopos,* pain] Extreme pain in the bones, esp. in syphilitic bone disease. **osteocopic** (-kŏp′ĭk), *adj.*

osteocranium (ŏs″tē-ō-krā′nē-ŭm) [″ + *kranion,* skull] The portion of the cranium formed of membrane bones in contrast to that formed of cartilage (chondrocranium).

osteocystoma (ŏs″tē-ō-sĭs-tō′mă) [″ + *kystis,* sac, bladder, + *oma,* tumor] Cystic tumor of a bone.

osteocyte (ŏs′tē-ō-sīt″) [″ + *kytos,* cell] A mesodermal bone-forming cell that has become entrapped within the bone matrix. It lies within a lacuna with processes extending outward through canaliculi and, by its metabolic activity, helps to maintain bone as a living tissue.

osteodensitometer A device used for determining the density of bones.

osteodentin Dentin that forms very rapidly or in response to severe trauma so that cells and blood vessels are incorporated, resembling bone.

osteodermia (ŏs″tē-ō-dĕr′mē-ă) [″ + *derma,* skin] The formation of bony deposits in the skin.

osteodesmosis (ŏs″tē-ō-dĕs-mō′sĭs) [″ +

desmos, tendon, + *osis,* condition] The transformation of tendon into bone.

osteodiastasis (ŏs″tē-ō-dī-ăs′tă-sĭs) [″ + *diastasis,* separation] The separation of two adjacent bones.

osteodynia (ŏs″tē-ō-dĭn′ē-ă) [″ + *odyne,* pain] Ostalgia.

osteodystrophy (ŏs″tē-ō-dĭs′trō-fē) [″ + *dys,* ill, + *trophe,* nourishment] Defective bone development.

renal o. Bony degeneration that results from the secondary hyperparathyroidism of chronic renal failure. Its hallmarks are increased bone resorption by osteoclasts, decreased new bone formation, and decreased bone mass.

osteoepiphysis (ŏs″tē-ō-ē-pĭf′ĭs-ĭs) [″ + *epi,* upon, + *physis,* growth] A small piece of bone that is separated in childhood from a larger bone by cartilage; during later growth, the two bones join.

osteofibroma (ŏs″tē-ō-fī-brō′mă) [″ + L. *fibra,* fiber, + Gr. *oma,* tumor] A tumor composed of bony and fibrous tissues. SYN: *fibro-osteoma.*

osteogen (ŏs′tē-ō-jĕn) [″ + *gennan,* to produce] The substance of the inner periosteal layer from which bone is formed.

osteogenesis, osteogeny (ŏs″tē-ō-jĕn′ĕ-sĭs, -ŏj′ĕ-nē) The formation and development of bone taking place in connective tissue or in cartilage. SYN: *ossification.* **osteogenic,** *adj.*

o. imperfecta An inherited disorder of the connective tissue marked by defective bone matrix, short stature, and abnormal bony fragility. Additional clinical findings are multiple fractures with minimal trauma, blue sclerae, early deafness, opalescent teeth, a tendency to capillary bleeding, translucent skin, and joint instability. Although the disease is heterogeneous, two different classifications of osteogenesis imperfecta are used for clinical distinction. *Osteogenesis imperfecta congenita* manifests in utero or at birth. *Osteogenesis imperfecta tarda* occurs later in childhood with delayed onset of fracturing and much milder manifestations. The healing of bone fractures progresses normally. Later in life, the tendency to fracture decreases and often disappears. The vast majority of cases are inherited as an autosomal dominant trait, although a small percentage of congenital cases are transmitted as an autosomal recessive. There is no known cure for osteogenesis imperfecta; therefore, treatment is supportive and palliative.

osteogenic Pert. to osteogenesis.

osteography (ŏs″tē-ŏg′răf-ē) [Gr. *osteon,* bone, + *graphein,* to write] A descriptive treatise of the bones.

osteohalisteresis (ŏs″tē-ō-hăl-ĭs″tĕr-ē′sĭs) [″ + *hals,* salt, + *sterein,* to deprive] Softening of the bones caused by a deficiency of mineral constituents of the bone.

osteoid (ŏs′tē-oyd) [″ + *eidos,* form, shape] **1.** Resembling bone. SYN: *ossiform.* **2.** The noncalcified matrix of young bone. Also called prebone.

osteokinematics The branch of biomechanics concerned with the description of bone movement when a bone swings through a range of motion around the axis in a joint, such as with flexion, extension, abduction, adduction, or rotation.

osteolipochondroma (ŏs″tē-ō-lĭ-pō″kŏn-drō′mă) [″ + *lipos,* fat, + *chondros,* cartilage, + *oma,* tumor] A cartilaginous tumor containing fatty and bony tissue.

osteologist (ŏs″tē-ŏl′ō-jĭst) [″ + *logos,* word, reason] A specialist in the study of the bones.

osteology (ŏs-tē-ŏl′ō-jē) [″ + *logos,* word, reason] The science concerned with the structure and function of bones.

osteolysis (ŏs″tē-ŏl′ĭ-sĭs) [″ + *lysis,* dissolution] A softening and destruction of bone without osteoclastic activity. Osteolysis occurs within compact bone and results from a breakdown of the organic matrix and subsequent leaching out of the inorganic fraction. The condition is probably caused by localized metabolic disturbances, vascular changes, or the release of hydrolytic enzymes by osteocytes.

osteolytic (ŏs″tē-ō-lĭt′ĭk) Causing osteolysis.

osteoma (ŏs-tē-ō′mă) *pl.* **osteomata, osteomas** [″ + *oma,* tumor] A benign bony tumor; a bonelike structure that develops on a bone or at other sites. SYN: *exostosis.*

cancellous o. A soft and spongy tumor. Its thin and delicate trabeculae enclose large medullary spaces similar to that in cancellous bone.

cavalryman's o. A bony outgrowth of the femur at the insertion of the adductor femoris longus.

o. cutis A benign formation of bone nodules in the skin.

dental o. A bony outgrowth of the root of a tooth.

o. durum A very hard osteoma in which the bone is ivorylike.

o. medullare A bony tumor containing medullary spaces.

osteoid o. A rare benign bone tumor composed of sheets of osteoid tissue that is partially calcified and ossified. The condition occurs esp. in the bones of the extremities of the young.

o. spongiosum A spongy tumor in the bone. SYN: *osteospongioma.*

osteomalacia (ŏs″tē-ō-măl-ā′shē-ă) [Gr. *osteon,* bone, + *malakia,* softening] A vitamin D deficiency in adults that results in a shortage or loss of calcium salts, causing bones to become increasingly soft, flexible, brittle, and deformed. An adult form of rickets, osteomalacia can also be traced to liver disease, cancer, or other ailments that inhibit the normal metabolism of vitamin D. **osteomalacic** (-măl-ā′sĭk), *adj.*

SYMPTOMS: Clinical findings are rheumatic pains in the limbs, spine, thorax, and pelvis, anemia, signs of deficiency disease, and progressive weakness.

ETIOLOGY: The disease is caused by any of the many vitamin D disorders or by deranged phosphorus metabolism.

TREATMENT: In patients with vitamin D–deficient diets, nutritional supplements are helpful.

osteomatosis (ŏs″tē-ō″mă-tō′sĭs) [″ + ″ + *osis,* condition] The formation of multiple osteomas.

osteomere (ŏs′tē-ō-mēr) [″ + *meros,* part] One in a series of similar bony segments, such as the vertebrae.

osteometry (ŏs-tē-ŏm′ĕt-rē) [″ + *metron,* measure] The study of the measurement of parts of the skeletal system.

osteomyelitis (ŏs″tē-ō-mī″ĕl-ī′tĭs) [″ + *myelos,* marrow, + *itis,* inflammation] Inflammation of bone and marrow, usually caused by infection (and less often by radiation or other causes). It most commonly occurs in the long bones or spine. SEE: *bone scan*; *Nursing Diagnoses Appendix.*

ETIOLOGY: Infections may reach the bone by several routes. Usually disease-causing germs are carried to the bone as a result of a bloodborne infection (hematogenous spread). Organisms also may invade bone from an adjacent site such as a decubitus ulcer or an infected tooth socket (contiguous infection), or be introduced during traumatic injury or bone surgery. Pyogenic bacteria, esp. *Staphylococcus aureus*, are the most common cause, but gram-negative bacteria, mycobacteria, fungi, and viruses also cause bone infection; no organism can be identified in approx. 50% of patients. Peripheral vascular disease, sickle cell disease, urinary tract infections, prosthetic joints, inadequate nutrition, diabetes mellitus, aging, and soft tissue infections increase the risk of osteomyelitis.

SYMPTOMS: Clinical presentation of osteomyelitis may be overt or very subtle. Severe throbbing pain over the affected part, fever, and malaise are commonly seen in hematogenous infection. However, only mild pain, swelling, and redness, with or without fever, are seen in more localized infection. Purulent drainage may be present.

DIAGNOSIS: Laboratory studies may reveal an elevated white blood cell count or erythrocyte sedimentation rate; x-ray studies or nuclear medical scans may show bone destruction. Biopsies and bone cultures are necessary to determine the causative organism.

TREATMENT: All forms of osteomyelitis require long courses of treatment with high-dose antibiotics, although many of them, including most cases of osteomyelitis that are found in the limbs of diabetics and many infections associated with prosthetic hardware, will not be cured without surgery. SEE: *diabetic foot infection.*

PATIENT CARE: The patient may be hospitalized initially for intravenous antibiotics and débridement, or cared for at home. Activity and weight-bearing may be restricted to minimize the risk of pathological fractures. The affected part is immobilized and elevated, and adequate analgesics are given to relieve the severe pain and muscle spasms. Gentle passive range of motion is performed on the joints above and below the site of infection. Warm soaks may be applied to enhance blood flow and, thus, delivery of antibiotics to the area. If surgery has been performed and/or drainage is present, the site is monitored for healing and all dressings are disposed of carefully. If the patient is at home, family members are taught the principles of infection control and the need for follow up.

osteon (ŏs′tē-ŏn) [Gr., bone] The microscopic unit of compact bone, consisting of a haversian canal and the surrounding lamellae.

osteonecrosis (ŏs″tē-ō-nē-krō′sĭs) [″ + *nekrosis,* state of death] The death of a segment of bone usually caused by insufficient blood flow to a region of the skeleton. This is a relatively common disorder and an estimated 10% of total joint replacements are for osteonecrosis. From 5% to 25% of patients receiving prolonged therapy with corticosteroids will develop this condition. Treatment is symptomatic, but in some cases of osteonecrosis of the knee or hip joint, prosthetic replacement is required.

osteonectin A glycoprotein present in the noncollagenous portion of the matrix of bone.

osteoneuralgia (ŏs″tē-ō-nū-răl′jē-ă) [″ + *neuron,* nerve, + *algos,* pain] Bone pain.

osteopath (ŏs′tē-ō-păth) [″ + *pathos,* disease] A practitioner of osteopathy.

osteopathic (ŏs″tē-ō-păth′ĭk) Concerning osteopathy.

osteopathology (ŏs″tē-ō-păth-ŏl′ō-jē) [″ + *pathos,* disease, + *logos,* word, reason] **1.** Any bone disease. SYN: *osteopathy* (1). **2.** The study of bone diseases.

osteopathy (ŏs-tē-ŏp′ă-thē) [″ + *pathos,* disease, suffering] **1.** Any bone disease. **2.** A system of medicine founded by Dr. Andrew Taylor Still (1828–1917). It is based upon the theory that the human body is a vital organism in which structural and functional states are of equal importance and that the body is able to rectify toxic conditions when it has favorable environmental circumstances and satisfactory nourishment.

Although manipulation is the primary method used to restore structural and functional balance, osteopaths also rely upon physical, medicinal, and surgical methods. Osteopathy is recognized as a standard method or system of medical and surgical care. Physicians with a degree in osteopathy use the designation D.O.

osteopedion (ŏs″tē-ō-pē′dē-ŏn) [″ + *paidion,* child] Lithopedion.

osteopenia (ŏs″tē-ō-pē′nē-ă) [″ + *penia,* lack] **1.** Any decrease in the amount of bone tissue, regardless of the cause. **2.** Decreased bone density caused by failure of the rate of osteoid tissue synthesis to keep up with the normal rate of bone lysis. SEE: *osteoporosis.*

osteoperiosteal (ŏs″tē-ō-pĕr″ē-ŏs′tē-ăl) [″ + *peri,* around, + *osteon,* bone] Concerning bone and its periosteum.

osteoperiostitis (ŏs″tē-ō-pĕr″ē-ŏs-tī′tĭs) [″ + ″ + ″ + *itis,* inflammation] Inflammation of a bone and its periosteum.

osteopetrosis (ŏs″tē-ō-pĕ-trō′sĭs) [″ + *petra,* stone, + *osis,* condition] A rare hereditary bone disorder of two types: the infantile (malignant) form, which is transmitted as an autosomal recessive trait, and the adult (benign) form, which is transmitted as an autosomal dominant trait. In both types of osteopetrosis, normal bone metabolism is disrupted. Although bone continues to be formed, normal resorption diminishes; the result is that bones become increasingly dense. Radiographs reveal the spotted, marble-like appearance of abnormally calcified bone. In severe cases, this process leads to cranial nerve entrapment, bone marrow failure, and recurrent fractures. SYN: *Albers-Schönberg disease; marble bone disease.*

PROGNOSIS: If untreated, the infantile form is usually fatal during the first decade of life.

TREATMENT: Some infants have responded to bone marrow transplants. Children who are not candidates for bone marrow transplants have improved considerably with long-term administration of interferon gamma-1b. Therapy for the adult type is symptomatic.

osteophage (ŏs′tē-ō-fāj) [″ + *phagein,* to eat] An outdated term for osteoclast.

osteophlebitis (ŏs″tē-ō-flē-bī′tĭs) [″ + *phleps, phleb-,* vein, + *itis,* inflammation] Inflammation of the veins of a bone.

osteophone (ŏs′tē-ō-fōn″) [Gr. *osteon,* bone, + *phone,* voice] A device used by the deaf for conducting sound through facial bones.

osteophony (ŏs″tē-ŏf′ō-nē) Bone conduction of sound.

osteophore (ŏs′tē-ō-for) [″ + *pherein,* to carry] A forceps for crushing bone.

osteophyte (ŏs′tē-ō-fīt) [″ + *phyton,* plant] A bony excrescence or outgrowth, usually branched in shape.

osteoplaque (ŏs′tē-ō-plăk) Any layer of bone.

osteoplast (ŏs′tē-ō-plăst) [″ + *plastos,* formed] An outdated term for osteoblast.

osteoplastic (ŏs″tē-ō-plăs′tĭk) [″ + *plastikos,* formed] **1.** Pert. to bone repair by plastic surgery or grafting. **2.** Concerning bone formation.

osteopoikilosis (ŏs″tē-ō-poy″kĭ-lō′sĭs) [″ + *poikilos,* spotted] A benign, hereditary disease of the bones marked by excessive calcification in spots less than 1 cm in diameter.

osteoporosis (ŏs″tē-ō-por-ō′sĭs) [″ + *poros,* a passage, + *osis,* condition] Loss of bone mass that occurs throughout the skeleton, predisposing patients to fractures. Healthy bone constantly remodels itself by taking up structure elements from one area and patching others. In osteoporosis, more bone is resorbed than laid down, and the skeleton loses some of the strength that it derives from its intact trabeculation. Aging causes bone loss in both men and women, predisposing them to vertebral and hip fractures. This is called type II osteoporosis (formerly "senile" osteoporosis). Type I osteoporosis (also known as "involutional" bone loss) occurs as a result of the loss of the protective effects of estrogen on bone that takes place at menopause. SEE: illus.; *bone scan; fracture of the hip; hormone replacement therapy; osteomalacia; Nursing Diagnoses Appendix.* **osteoporotic** (-por-ŏt′ĭk), *adj.*

ETIOLOGY: Multiple modifiable factors contribute to bone mass and strength: increased body weight, higher levels of sex hormones, higher amounts of calcium and vitamin D in the diet, and frequent weight-bearing exercise all build up bone and prevent fractures. Bone loss and the risk of fractures increase with age, immobilization, thyroid hormone excess, the use of corticosteroids and some anticonvulsant drugs, the consumption of alcohol, tobacco and caffeine, and after menopause. Genetics (a non-modifiable risk factor) also contributes to osteoporosis. SEE: table.

SYMPTOMS: Bone loss progresses for many years without causing symptoms. When it results in fractures, bony pain and loss of mobility may be disabling. Signs of osteoporosis include deformities of the skeleton, such as kyphosis (the so-called "dowager's hump"), and loss of height, especially if vertebral compression fractures occur.

TREATMENT: Supplemental calcium and regular exercise help slow or prevent the rate of bone loss and are recommended for most men and women. Bisphosphonate drugs (such as alendronate), calcitonin, sodium fluoride, and other agents are useful for patients of either gender. In menopausal women, estrogen supplementation or the selective estrogen receptor modulators help prevent bone loss and fractures.

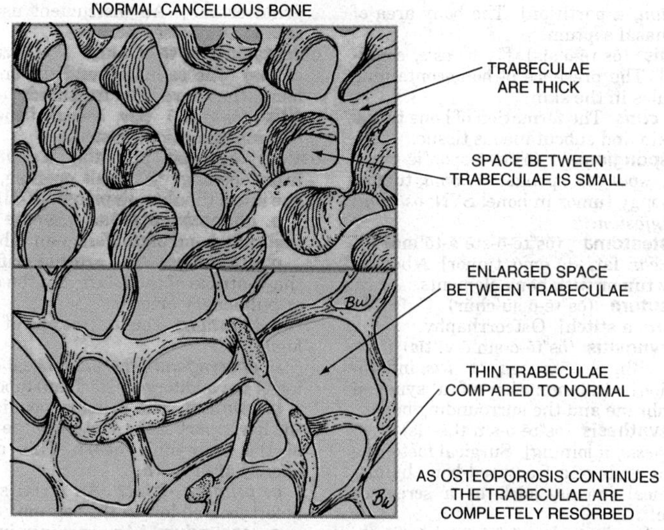

OSTEOPOROSIS

PATIENT CARE: The patient is encouraged to participate in an exercise program, including proper body mechanics and range-of-motion exercises. The patient is taught to use a firm mattress and assistive safety devices at home. A diet high in vitamin D, calcium, and protein to prevent further bone loss is encouraged. The patient is instructed to seek regular gynecological follow-up examinations if maintained on estrogen therapy, to maintain good nutrition and an adequate weight, and to engage in moderate exercise throughout her life.

Risk Factors for Osteoporosis

Female
Advanced age
White or Asian
Thin, small-framed body
Positive family history
Low calcium intake
Early menopause (before age 45)
Sedentary lifestyle
Nulliparity
Smoking
Excessive alcohol or caffeine
High protein intake
High phosphate intake
Certain medications, when taken for a long time (high doses of glucocorticoid, phenytoin, thyroid medication)
Endocrine diseases (hyperthyroidism, Cushing's disease, acromegaly, hypogonadism, hyperparathyroidism

SOURCE: Stanley, M and Beare, PG: Gerontological Nursing, FA Davis, Philadelphia, 1995.

DIAGNOSIS: Dual energy x-ray absorptiometry (DEXA scanning) is recommended by the World Health Organization for the early diagnosis of bone loss. Dual photon absorptiometry, and quantitative computerized tomographic scanning of bone, can also be used.

o. circumscripta cranii Localized osteoporosis of the skull associated with Paget's disease.

o. of disuse Osteoporosis due to the lack of normal functional stress on the bones. It may occur during a prolonged period of bedrest or as the result of being exposed to periods of weightlessness (e.g., astronauts in outer space).

glucocorticoid o. Osteoporosis secondary to long-term therapy with glucocorticoid agents.

posttraumatic o. Loss of bone tissue following trauma, esp. when there is damage to a nerve supplying the injured area. The condition may also be caused by disuse secondary to pain.

osteoradionecrosis (ŏs″tē-ō-rā″dē-ō-nē-krō′sĭs) [Gr. *osteon,* bone, + L. *radiatio,* radiation, + Gr. *nekrosis,* state of death] Death of bone following irradiation.

osteorrhaphy (ŏs-tē-or′ă-fē) [″ + *rhaphe,* seam, ridge] The suturing or wiring of bone fragments. SYN: *osteosuture.*

osteosarcoma (ŏs″tē-ō-săr-kō′mă) [″ + *sarx,* flesh, + *oma,* tumor] A malignant sarcoma of bone. SYN: *myelosarcoma.*

osteosclerosis (ŏs″tē-ō-sklē-rō′sĭs) [″ + *skleros,* hard, + *osis,* condition] An abnormal increase in thickening and density of bone.

o. fragilis Osteopetrosis.

osteoseptum (ŏs″tē-ō-sĕp′tŭm) [″ + L.

septum, a partition] The bony area of the nasal septum.

osteosis (ŏs″tē-ō′sĭs) [″ + *osis,* condition] The presence of bone-containing nodules in the skin.

o. cutis The formation of bone tissue in skin and subcutaneous tissue.

osteospongioma (ŏs″tē-ō-spŏn″jē-ō′mă) [″ + *spongos,* sponge, + *oma,* tumor] A spongy tumor in bone. SYN: *osteoma spongiosum.*

osteosteatoma (ŏs″tē-ō-stē″ă-tō′mă) [″ + *stear,* fat, + *oma,* tumor] A benign fatty tumor with bony elements.

osteosuture (ŏs″tē-ō-sū′chŭr) [″ + L. *sutura,* a stitch] Osteorrhaphy.

osteosynovitis (ŏs″tē-ō-sĭn″ō-vī′tĭs) [″ + *syn,* with, + *oon,* egg, + *itis,* inflammation] Inflammation of a synovial membrane and the surrounding bones.

osteosynthesis (ŏs″tē-ō-sĭn′thĕ-sĭs) [″ + *synthesis,* a joining] Surgical fastening of the ends of a fractured bone by mechanical means, such as a screw or plate.

osteotelangiectasia (ŏs″tē-ō-tĕl-ăn″jē-ĕk-tā′zē-ă) [″ + *telos,* end, + *angeion,* vessel, + *ektasis,* a stretching] A sarcomatous, heavily vascularized tumor of bone.

osteothrombosis (ŏs″tē-ō-thrŏm-bō′sĭs) [″ + *thrombosis,* a clotting] The formation of a blood clot in the veins of a bone.

osteotome (ŏs′tē-ō-tōm) [″ + *tome,* incision] A chisel beveled on both sides for cutting through bones.

osteotomoclasis (ŏs″tē-ō-tō-mŏk′lă-sĭs) [Gr. *osteon,* bone, + *tomos,* section, + *klasis,* breaking] Correction of a pathologically curved bone by bending it after a wedge has been chiseled out of it by use of an osteotome.

osteotomy (ŏs-tē-ŏt′ō-mē) [″ + *tome,* incision] The operation of cutting through a bone.

C-form o. A C-shaped cut through the ramus of the mandible to allow forward placement of the mandible in correcting a retrognathic condition.

condylar neck o. Surgery on the condylar neck of the mandible to correct prognathism.

cuneiform o. The excision of a wedge of bone.

linear o. The lengthwise division of a bone.

Macewen's o. Supracondylar section of the femur for correction of knock-knee.

subtrochanteric o. Division of the shaft of the femur below the lesser trochanter to correct ankylosis of the hip joint.

transtrochanteric o. Section of the femur through the lesser trochanter for correction of a deformity about the hip joint.

osteotribe (ŏs′tē-ō-trīb″) [″ + *tribein,* to rub] A bone rasp.

osteotrite (ŏs′tē-ō-trīt) [″ + *tribein,* to grind or rub] An instrument used to scrape away diseased bone.

osteotylus (ŏs″tē-ŏt′ĭ-lŭs) [″ + *tylos,* callus] The callus around the ends of bones that have been fractured.

ostitis (ŏs-tī′tĭs) [Gr. *osteon,* bone, + *itis,* inflammation] Osteitis.

ostium (ŏs′tē-ŭm) *pl.* **ostia** [L. *ostium,* a little opening] A small opening, esp. one into a tubular organ. **ostial** (-ăl), *adj.*

o. abdominale tubae uterinae The fimbriated end of the fallopian tube.

o. arteriosum The arterial orifice of the ventricle of the heart into the aorta or pulmonary artery.

o. internum The uterine end of a fallopian tube.

o. pharyngeum The pharyngeal opening of the auditory (eustachian) tube.

o. primum The primary opening in the lower part of the septum of the atria of the embryonic heart. This closes shortly after birth.

o. primum defect An atrial septal defect located low in the septum.

o. secundum An opening in the higher part of the septum of the atria of the embryonic heart. This closes shortly after birth.

o. secundum defect An atrial septal defect located high in the septal wall.

o. tympanicum The tympanic opening of the auditory (eustachian) tube.

o. urethrae externum The external opening of the urethra.

o. uteri The opening from the uterus to the vagina. Also called *cervical os.*

o. uterinum tubae The opening of the uterine tube into the uterus.

o. vaginae The external opening of the vagina.

ostomate (ŏs′tō-māt) [L. *ostium,* little opening] One who has a surgically formed fistula connecting the bowel or intestine to the outside, usually through the abdominal wall. SEE: *colostomy; ileostomy.*

ostomy (ŏs′tō-mē) The surgically formed fistula connecting a portion of the intestine to the exterior (usually through the abdominal wall). SEE: *colostomy; ileostomy.*

OSTOMY CARE: Whether the ostomy is temporary or permanent, the patient should be assured that it will be possible to carry on normal activities with a minimum of inconvenience. Prior to being discharged from the hospital, the patient should be provided full explanation and demonstration of ostomy care. It is esp. important to have the patient and family become involved in ostomy care as soon as possible. This will promote confidence that a normal life will be possible. Consultation with another patient who has become competent in ostomy care will be esp. helpful. Those individuals may be contacted through ostomy clubs that have been organized in various cities. The patient should be provided with precise directions concerning places that sell ostomy care equipment. Detailed instructions for care and use of ostomy devices are included in the package.

Specific care involves the stoma (enterostomal care) and irrigation of the bowel, when appropriate, leading to the stoma. In caring for a double-barrel colostomy, it is important to irrigate only the proximal stoma.

STOMA CARE: The character of the material excreted through the stoma will depend on the portion of the bowel to which it is attached. Excretions from the ileum will be fluid and quite irritating to skin, those from the upper right colon will be semifluid, those from the upper left colon are partly solid, and those from the sigmoid colon will tend to be solid. Care of the stoma, whether for ileostomy or colostomy, is directed toward maintaining the peristomal skin and mucosa of the stoma in a healthy condition. This is more difficult to achieve with an ileostomy than with a lower colon colostomy. The skin surrounding the stoma can be protected by use of commercially available disks (washers) made of karaya gum or hypoallergenic skin shields. The collecting bag or pouch can be attached to the karaya gum washer or skin shield so that a watertight seal is made. The karaya gum washers can be used on weeping skin, but the skin shields cannot. New skin will grow beneath the karaya gum. The stoma may require only a gauze pad covering in the case of a sigmoid colostomy that is being irrigated daily or every other day. If a plastic bag is used for collecting drainage, it will need to be emptied periodically and changed as directed. At each change of the bag, meticulous but gentle skin care will be given. The stoma should not be digitally dilated except by those experienced in enterostomal care.

IRRIGATION OF COLOSTOMY: Many individuals will be able to regulate the character of their diet so that the feces may be removed from the digital colonic stoma at planned intervals. The stoma is attached to a plastic bag held in place with a self-adhering collar or a belt. Tap water at 40°C (104°F), is introduced slowly through a soft rubber catheter or cone. The catheter is inserted no further 10 to 15 cm, and the irrigating fluid container is hung at height that will allow fluid to flow slowly. The return from the irrigation may be collected in a closed or open-ended bag. The latter will allow the return to empty into a basin or toilet. The return of fluid and feces should be completed in less than one-half hour after irrigating fluid has entered the bowel.

At the completion of the irrigating process, the skin and stoma should be carefully cleaned and the dressing or pouch replaced. The equipment should be cleaned thoroughly and stored in a dry, well-ventilated space. When irrigation of an ostomy is provided for a hospitalized patient, charting is done on the amount and kind of fluid instilled, the amount and character of return, the care provided for the stoma, the condition of the stoma, and if a pouch or bag is replaced.

MISCELLANEOUS CONSIDERATIONS: Odor may be controlled by avoiding foods that the individual finds to cause undesirable odors. Gas may be controlled by avoiding foods known to produce gas, which will vary from patient to patient. The diet should be planned to provide a stool consistency that will be neither hard and constipating nor loose and watery. The patient may learn this by trial and error and by consulting with nutritionists and ostomy club members. Daily physical activity, sexual relations, and swimming are all possible.

ostosis (ŏs-tō′sĭs) Osteogenesis.

ostraceous (ŏs-trā′shŭs) Shaped like an oyster shell.

Oswestry disability index, Oswestry disability scale, Oswestry disability score (ŏs-wĕs′trē) A questionnaire that requires the patient to rate the effect of back pain on 10 different activities, each having 6 levels of disability. This test was designed to assess patients with failed back surgery but is widely used for patients with other spinal conditions.

ostreotoxism (ŏs″trē-ō-tŏks′ĭzm) [Gr. *ostreon,* oyster, + *toxikon,* poison] Poisoning from eating oysters containing toxic microorganisms.

O.T. *occupational therapy; occupational therapist.* SEE: *therapist, occupational.*

ot- SEE: *oto-.*

otacoustic (ō″tă-koo′stĭk) [Gr. *otakousteo,* to listen] **1.** Aiding or concerning the hearing. **2.** A device to aid hearing; an ear trumpet.

otalgia (ō-tăl′jē-ă) [Gr.] Pain in the ear. SYN: *earache; otodynia.*

TREATMENT: Local treatment consists of application of heat in the form of compresses or a hot water bottle, or instillation of warm glycerin in the affected ear. Generally, nasal astringents help maintain the patency of the eustachian tube, and appropriate systemic antibiotics may be used if there is an infection.

CAUTION: Medicines should not be placed in the external auditory canal unless the eardrum is intact.

otantritis (ō″tăn-trī′tĭs) [Gr. *otos,* ear, + L. *antrum,* sinus, + Gr. *itis,* inflammation] Inflammation of the mastoid antrum.

O.T.(C) *occupational therapist (Canada);* one who is a member of the Canadian Association of Occupational Therapists.

O.T.C. *over the counter;* refers to drugs and devices available without a prescription.

OTD *organ tolerance dose;* the maximum amount of radiation tolerated by specific tissues.

otectomy (ō-tĕk′tō-mē) [Gr. *otos,* ear, + *ektome,* excision] Surgical excision of the contents of the middle ear.

othematoma (ōt″hē-mă-tō′mă) [″ + *haima,* blood, + *oma,* tumor] Hematoma auris.

otic (ō′tĭk) [Gr. *otikos*] Concerning the ear.

otitis (ō-tī′tĭs) [Gr. *otos,* ear, + *itis,* inflammation] Inflammation of the ear. It is differentiated as externa, media, and interna, depending upon which portion of the ear is inflamed. **otitic** (ō-tĭt′ĭk), *adj.*

acute o. media The presence of fluid in the middle ear accompanied by signs and symptoms of intense local or systemic infection. In the U.S. 12,000,000 cases of otitis media are estimated to occur each year.

ETIOLOGY: The most common causes are viruses, such as respiratory syncytial virus (RSV) and influenza virus, and bacteria, including *Streptococcus pneumoniae, Haemophilus influenzae,* and *Moraxella catarrhalis*.

SYMPTOMS: There may be pain in the ear, drainage of fluid from the ear canal, and hearing loss. The systemic signs include fever, irritability, headache, lethargy, anorexia, and vomiting.

TREATMENT: Nasal decongestants may provide some comfort to patients with upper respiratory congestion, but will not alter the course of the illness. Antibiotics are usually prescribed empirically to cover the most common bacterial pathogens, although they may be mis- and over-used in this syndrome. Pain is usually treated with acetaminophen or ibuprofen. Some evidence suggests that vaccinations against common viral illnesses (such as influenza and RSV) will diminish the incidence of acute o.m.

DIAGNOSIS: Definitive diagnosis relies on tympanocentesis, that is, puncturing the eardrum with a needle to aspirate and culture the fluid in the middle ear. This test is rarely performed in routine outpatient care.

PATIENT CARE: Because some children are prone to recurrences, parents are taught to recognize signs of otitis media and to seek medical assistance when their child complains of pain or they observe the child experiencing pain. Failure to treat acute and chronic ear infections may lead to spontaneous rupture of the eardrum, temporary or permanent hearing loss in children, and subsequent communication disorders; therefore, parents must understand the importance of proper medical follow-up.

allergic o. media O. media with effusion.

o. externa Infection or inflammation of the external auditory canal. It may be caused by a contact allergy, an acute bacterial infection, or by fungi. In diabetics and the immunosuppressed, the infection may invade the base of the skull, resulting in deep bone infection.

furuncular o. A furuncle formation in the external meatus of the ear.

o. interna Labyrinthitis.

o. labyrinthica Inflammation of the labyrinth of the ear.

o. mastoidea Inflammation of the middle ear, involving the mastoid spaces.

o. media Acute o. media.

o. media with effusion The presence of fluid in the middle ear without signs or symptoms of acute infection. This causes retraction of the eardrum. Upon examination, a level of air fluid may be seen through the tympanic membrane. The cause of the obstruction may be enlarged adenoid tissue in the pharynx, inflammation in the pharynx, tumors in the pharyngeal area, or allergy. SYN: *allergic otitis media; nonsuppurative otitis media; secretory otitis media; serous otitis media.*

TREATMENT: Nasal decongestants may afford symptomatic relief. The use of antibiotics is controversial. Adenoidectomy and bilateral myringotomy may be necessary if conservative measures, including insertion of a ventilation or tympanostomy tube, are not effective. Adenoidectomy is not advisable in children under 4 years of age. SEE: *tympanocentesis; tympanostomy tube.*

CAUTION: The routine use of grommets, also called ventilation tubes, as part of the initial therapy for otitis media is not advised. Their use should be reserved for persistent or recurrent infections that have failed to respond to appropriate therapy.

---

o. mycotica Inflammation of the ear caused by a fungal infection.

necrotizing o. externa Infection of the base of the skull that originates in the external auditory canal. It is usually caused by infection with the bacterium *Pseudomonas aeruginosa*. The disease occurs most often in diabetic and other immunocompromised patients. It may be life-threatening and requires prolonged antibiotic therapy. Hyperbaric oxygen treatments are used in patients with the most advanced and refractory disease.

nonsuppurative o. media O. media with effusion.

o. parasitica Inflammation of the ear caused by a parasite.

o. sclerotica Inflammation of the inner ear accompanied by hardening of the aural structures.

secretory o. media O. media with effusion.

serous o. media O. media with effusion.

oto-, ot- [Gr. *otos,* ear] Combining form meaning *ear.*

otoantritis (ō″tō-ăn-trī′tĭs) [″ + *antron,* cavity, + *itis,* inflammation] Inflammation of the mastoid antrum and tympanic attic.

otocephalus (ō″tō-sĕf′ă-lŭs) One with otocephaly.

otocephaly (ō″tō-sĕf′ă-lē) [″ + *kephale,* head] A congenital absence of the lower jaw and fusion or near fusion of the ears on the front of the neck.

otocyst (ō′tō-sĭst) [″ + *kystis,* sac, bladder] A primordial chamber from which arises the membranous labyrinth.

otodynia (ō″tō-dĭn′ē-ă) [″ + *odyne,* pain] Otalgia.

otogenic, otogenous (ō″tō-jĕn′ĭk, ō-tŏj′ĕn-ŭs) [″ + *gennan,* to produce] Originating in the ear.

otolaryngologist (ō″tō-lar″ĭn-gŏl′ō-jĭst) [″ + *larynx,* larynx, + *logos,* word, reason] A specialist in otolaryngology.

otolaryngology (ō″tō-lar″ĭn-gŏl′ō-jē) The division of medical science that includes otology, rhinology, and laryngology.

otological (ō″tō-lŏj′ĭ-kăl) [″ + *logos,* word, reason] Relating to study of diseases of the ear.

otologist (ō-tŏl′ō-jĭst) One knowledgeable in the anatomy, physiology, and pathology of the ear; a specialist in diseases of the ear.

otology (ō-tŏl′ō-jē) [Gr. *otos,* ear, + *logos,* word, reason] The science dealing with the ear, its function, and its diseases.

otomucormycosis (ō″tō-mū″kor-mī-kō′sĭs) [″ + L. *mucor,* mold, + Gr. *mykes,* fungus, + *osis,* condition] Mucormycosis of the ear.

otomyces (ō″tō-mī′sēz) [″ + *mykes,* fungus] Any fungal infection of the ear.

otomycosis (ō″tō-mī-kō′sĭs) [″ + ″ + *osis,* condition] An infection of the external auditory meatus of the ear caused by a fungus. SYN: *myringomycosis; otitis mycotica.*

otoncus (ō-tŏng′kŭs) [″ + *onkos,* tumor] A tumor of the ear.

otonecrectomy, otonecronectomy (ō″tō-nē-krĕk′tō-mē, ō″tō-nē″krō-nĕk′tō-mē) [″ + *nekros,* corpse, + *ektome,* excision] Excision of necrosed areas from the ear.

otoneurology (ō″tō-nū-rŏl′ō-jē) [″ + ″ + *logos,* word, reason] The division of otology that deals with the inner ear, esp. its nerve supply, nerve connections with the brain, and auditory and labyrinthine pathways and centers within the brain. SYN: *neurotology.*

otopharyngeal (ō″tō-făr-ĭn′jē-ăl) [″ + *pharynx,* throat] Concerning the ear and pharynx.

otoplasty (ō′tō-plăs″tē) [″ + *plassein,* to form] Plastic surgery of the ear to correct defects and deformities.

otorhinolaryngology (ō″tō-rī″nō-lăr″ĭn-gŏl′ō-jē) [″ + *rhis,* nose, + *larynx,* larynx, + *logos,* word, reason] The science of the ear, nose, and larynx, and their functions and diseases.

otorhinology (ō″tō-rī-nŏl′ō-jē) [″ + ″ + *logos,* word, reason] The branch of medicine dealing with the ear and nose and their diseases.

otorrhea (ō″tō-rē′ă) [″ + *rhein,* flow] Inflammation of ear with purulent discharge. SEE: *otitis.*

cerebrospinal fluid o. Leakage of cerebrospinal fluid from the external auditory canal. It is usually the result of prior surgery to the ear or mastoid bone or of trauma to the skull, and may predispose patients to meningitis.

otoscleronectomy (ō″tō-sklē″rō-nĕk′tō-mē) [″ + *skleros,* hard, + *ektome,* excision] Surgical excision of sclerosed and ankylosed ear ossicles.

otosclerosis (ō″tō-sklē-rō′sĭs) [″ + *sklerosis,* hardening] A condition characterized by chronic progressive deafness, esp. for low tones. It is caused by the formation of spongy bone, esp. around the oval window, with resulting ankylosis of the stapes. In the late stages of this condition, atrophy of the organ of Corti may occur. The cause of this condition is unknown; however, it may be familial. It is more common in women, and may be made worse by pregnancy.

TREATMENT: Various surgical procedures, including stapedectomy, have been used with considerable improvement in hearing. Because the three bones of the middle ear become fused, patients with this condition cannot normally transmit sound to the inner ear from the vibrations of the tympanic membrane. The excellent results achieved from removing the stapes and inserting a stapes implant to allow the bones to function normally again make identification of children and adults who could benefit from this procedure especially important.

otoscope (ō′tō-skōp) [″ + *skopein,* to examine] A device for examination of the ear.

otoscopy (ō-tŏs′kō-pē) The use of the otoscope in examining the ear.

otosteal (ō-tŏs′tē-ăl) [″ + *osteon,* bone] Concerning the bones or ossicles of the ear.

ototomy (ō-tŏt′ō-mē) [″ + *tome,* incision] Incision or dissection of the ear.

ototoxic (ō″tō-tŏk′sĭk) [″ + *toxikon,* poison] Having a detrimental effect on the eighth nerve or the organs of hearing.

O.T.R. *Occupational Therapist, Registered.*

OTR/L *Licensed Occupational Therapist.*

Otto pelvis (ŏt′ō) [Adolph W. Otto, Ger. surgeon, 1786–1845] The protrusion of the acetabulum into the pelvic cavity. This condition may occur in association with severe osteoarthritis of the hip.

O.U., o.u. L. *oculus uterque,* each eye.

ouabain (wă-bā′ĭn) A glycoside prepared

from *Strophanthus gratus.* Its action is similar to that of digitalis.

oulitis (oo-lī′tĭs) [Gr. *oulon,* gum, + *itis,* inflammation] Inflammation of the gums.

oulorrhagia (oo-lō-rā′jē-ă) [″ + *rhegnynai,* to burst forth] Hemorrhage from the gums.

-ous **1.** Suffix meaning *possessing, full of.* **2.** Suffix meaning *pertaining to.*

outbreak The sudden increase in the incidence of a disease or condition in a specific area.

outcome Any result or consequence (e.g., of a disease, an interpersonal interaction, a chemical reaction, drug, or operation).

o. criteria Quality assurance program guidelines in which the adequacy of the program is judged by the achievement of predetermined goals.

functional o. In rehabilitation therapy, a long-term goal toward which a therapeutic program is directed to help a patient return to or achieve a specific activity level.

positive o. In health care, the remediation of functional limitations or disability; the prevention of illness or injury; or an improvement in patient satisfaction.

outflow In neurology, the passage of impulses outwardly from the central nervous system.

craniosacral o. Impulses passing through parasympathetic nerves.

thoracolumbar o. Impulses passing through sympathetic nerves.

outlet A vent or opening through which something can escape.

pelvic o. The lower pelvic opening between the tip of the coccyx, the ischial tuberosities, and the lower margin of the symphysis pubis.

quick-connect o. A device that allows a compressed gas container to be quickly connected to and disconnected from the delivery unit.

out-of-body experience The perception of being away from and overlooking oneself; the feeling that the mind has separated from the body.

outpatient One who receives treatment at a hospital, clinic, or dispensary but is not hospitalized.

outpocketing Evagination.

output (owt′poot) That which is produced, ejected, or expelled.

cardiac o. The amount of blood discharged from the left or right ventricle per minute. For an average adult at rest, cardiac output is approx. 3.0 L per sq m of body surface area each minute. Cardiac output is determined by multiplying the stroke volume by the heart rate. SYN: *minute volume.*

energy o. The work expended by the body per unit of time.

stroke o. The amount of blood pumped in a single heartbeat.

urinary o. The amount of urine produced by the kidneys.

outrigger An attachment for hand splints that permits the fingers to be placed in elastic traction.

outsourcing A method in which services usually provided by the health care agency are now allocated to an outside firm or agency.

ova (ō′vă) [L. *ovum,* egg] Pl. of ovum.

oval (ō′văl) [L. *ovalis,* egg shaped] **1.** Concerning an ovum, the reproductive cell of the female. **2.** Having an elliptical shape like an egg.

ovalbumin (ō″văl-bū′mĭn) [″ + *albumen,* white of egg] Albumin occurring in egg white.

ovalocyte (ō′văl-ō-sīt″) [″ + Gr. *kytos,* cell] An elliptical red blood corpuscle.

ovalocytosis (ō-văl″ō-sī-tō′sĭs) [″ + ″ + *osis,* condition] An abnormally large amount of elliptical red blood cells in the blood.

oval window An oval-shaped aperture in the middle ear into which fits the base of the stapes.

ovaralgia, ovarialgia (ō″văr-ăl′jē-ă, -ē-ăl′jē-ă) [LL. *ovarium,* ovary, + Gr. *algos,* pain] Ovarian pain. SYN: *oarialgia.*

ovari- SEE: *ovario-.*

ovarian (ō-vā′rē-ăn) [LL. *ovarium,* ovary] Concerning or resembling the ovary.

ovarian cyst A fluid-filled sac that develops in the ovary and consists of one or more chambers. Although nonmalignant, the cyst may have to be removed surgically because of twisting of the pedicle, which causes gangrene, or because of pressure. SEE: *polycystic ovary syndrome.*

ovariectomy (ō″vā-rē-ĕk′tō-mē) [″ + Gr. *ektome,* excision] The partial or complete excision of an ovary. SYN: *oophorectomy.*

ovario-, ovari- [LL. *ovarium,* ovary] Combining form meaning *ovary.*

ovariocele (ō-vā′rē-ō-sēl) [″ + Gr. *kele,* tumor, swelling] An ovarian tumor or hernia.

ovariocentesis (ō-vā″rē-ō-sĕn-tē′sĭs) [″ + Gr. *kentesis,* puncture] Surgical puncture and drainage of an ovarian cyst.

ovariocyesis (ō-vā″rē-ō-sī-ē′sĭs) [″ + Gr. *kyesis,* pregnancy] An ectopic pregnancy in an ovary. SEE: *gestation, ectopic.*

ovariogenic (ō-vā″rē-ō-jĕn′ĭk) [″ + *gennan,* to produce] Originating in the ovary.

ovariopexy (ō-vā″rē-ō-pĕk′sē) [″ + *pexis,* fixation] Surgical fixation of the ovary to the abdominal wall.

ovariorrhexis (ō-vā″rē-ō-rĕk′sĭs) [″ + Gr. *rhexis,* a rupture] Rupture of an ovary.

ovariosalpingectomy (ō-vā″rē-ō-săl″pĭn-jĕk′tō-mē) [″ + Gr. *salpinx,* tube, + *ektome,* excision] Salpingo-oophorectomy.

ovariostomy (ō-vā″rē-ŏs′tō-mē) [″+

Gr. *stoma,* mouth] The creation of an opening in an ovarian cyst for the purpose of drainage.

ovariotomy (ō-vā″rē-ŏt′ō-mē) [LL. *ovarium,* ovary, + Gr. *tome,* incision] **1.** The incision or removal of an ovary. **2.** The removal of a tumor of the ovary.

ovariotubal (ō-vā″rē-ō-tū′băl) [″ + *tuba,* a narrow duct] Concerning the ovary and oviducts.

ovariprival (ō-vā″rĭ-prī′văl) [″ + *privare,* to remove] Resulting from loss of the ovaries.

ovaritis (ō″vă-rī′tĭs) [″ + Gr. *itis,* inflammation] The acute or chronic inflammation of an ovary, usually secondary to inflammation of the oviducts or pelvic peritoneum. It may involve the substance of the organ (oophoritis) or its surface (perioophoritis).

ovarium (ō-vā′rē-ŭm) *pl.* **ovaria** [LL.] The ovary.

ovary (ō′vă-rē) [LL. *ovarium,* ovary] One of two almond-shaped glands in the female that produces the reproductive cell, the ovum, and three hormones: estrogen, progesterone, and inhibin. The ovaries lie in the fossa ovarica on either side of the pelvic cavity, attached to the uterus by the utero-ovarian ligament, and close to the fimbria of the fallopian tube. Each ovary is about 4 cm long, 2 cm wide, and 8 mm thick, and is attached to the broad ligament by the mesovarium and to the side of the pelvis by the suspensory ligament. At menarche, the surface of the ovary is smooth; at menopause, the rupture and atrophy of follicles make it markedly pitted.

Each ovary consists of two parts. The outer portion (cortex) encloses a central medulla, which consists of a stroma of connective tissue containing nerves, blood and lymphatic vessels, and some smooth muscle tissue at region of hilus. The cortex consists principally of follicles in various stages of development (primary, growing, and mature or graafian). Its surface is covered by a single layer of cells, the germinal epithelium, beneath which is a layer of dense connective tissue, the tunica albuginea. Each of the 400,000 follicles present in the ovaries at birth has the potential for maturity but fewer than 600 mature during a woman's reproductive years (usually one per cycle). Other structures (corpus luteum, corpus albicans) may be present. The blood supply is mainly derived from the ovarian artery, which reaches the ovary through the infundibulopelvic ligament. SEE: *fertilization* for illus.; *oogenesis* for illus.

PHYSIOLOGY: The functional activity of the ovary is controlled primarily by gonadotropins of the hypophysis, esp. the follicle-stimulating hormone (FSH) and luteinizing hormone (LH). The two functions of the ovaries are the production of ova and hormones. The hormones produced are estrogen, progesterone, and inhibin. Estrogen is produced by the developing follicle; it stimulates development of the secondary sexual characteristics, growth of the mammary glands, and growth of the endometrium for possible implantation of a fertilized egg. Progesterone is secreted by the corpus luteum; it contributes to growth of the endometrium and mammary glands. Inhibin is secreted by cells of the follicle and the corpus luteum; it decreases the secretion of FSH.

overbite The vertical extension of the incisal ridges of the upper teeth over the incisal ridges of the lower anterior teeth when the jaws are in occlusion.

overclosure A form of defective bite in which the mandible closes too far before the teeth make contact.

overcompensation The process by which a person substitutes an opposite trait or exerts effort in excess of that needed to compensate for, or conceal, a psychological feeling of guilt, inadequacy, or inferiority. May lead to maladjustment.

overcorrection The use of too powerful a lens to correct a defect in the refractive power of the eye.

overdenture A denture supported by the soft tissue and whatever natural teeth remain. These have been altered so the denture will fit over them.

overdetermination The idea in psychoanalysis that every symptom and dream may have several meanings, being determined by more than a single association.

overdose ABBR: OD. An excessive, and potentially toxic amount of a medication, given in error, or taken intentionally (for example by patients making suicide gestures or suicide attempts).

overeruption A condition in which the occluding surface of a tooth projects beyond the line of occlusion.

overexertion Physical exertion to a state of abnormal exhaustion.

overextension **1.** Extension beyond that which usually occurs. SYN: *hyperextension.* **2.** In dentistry, the assessment of the vertical extent of a root canal filling, denoting an extrusion beyond the apical foramen.

overflow The continuous escape of fluid from a vessel or viscus, as of urine or tears.

overgrowth **1.** Excessive growth. SYN: *hyperplasia; hypertrophy.* **2.** In bacteriology, the growth of one type of microorganism on a culture plate so that it covers and obscures the growth of other types.

overhang The undesirable extension beyond the margins of a cavity of the excess filling material used.

overhydration An excess of fluids in the body.

overjet Horizontal overlap of the teeth.

overlap Something that covers the tissue or object but also extends past the border.

overlay **1.** An addition superimposed upon an already existing state. **2.** In dentistry, a cast restoration for the occlusal surface of one or more cusps of a tooth but not a three-quarter- or full-cast crown.

psychogenic o. The emotional component of a symptom or illness that has an organic basis.

overmedication Side effects, drug interactions, or other potential problems that result from the excessive use or excessive prescription of medications. Overmedication is a common problem in the elderly, who may have multiple diseases and conditions, and multiple health care providers.

overpressure A force applied passively to a joint and surrounding soft tissue at the end of the range of motion in order to determine the end feel of the tissues.

overproduction Excessive output of an organic element during the reparative process, as excessive callus development after a bone fracture. SEE: *keloid.*

overresponse An abnormally intense reaction to a stimulus; an inappropriate degree of response.

overriding The slipping of one end of a fractured bone past the other part.

overshoot A response to a stimulus that is greater than would normally be expected.

overtoe Hallux varus of the great toe to the extent that it rests over the other toes.

overtone In music and acoustics, a harmonic.

overuse syndrome An injury to musculoskeletal tissues typically affecting the upper extremity or cervical spine, resulting from repeated movement, temperature extremes, overuse, incorrect posture, or sustained force or vibration. Resulting disorders include carpal tunnel syndrome, tenosynovitis, tendinitis, pronator syndrome, peritendinitis, thoracic outlet syndrome, and cervical syndrome, each of which often results from demands of the work environment. Treatment for these conditions often involves surgery or immobilization. There is a growing awareness of the importance of prevention through education, task modification, and workplace design based on ergonomic principles. SYN: *cumulative trauma syndrome; repetitive motion injury; repetitive strain injury.* SEE: *ergonomics.*

overvalued idea An unreasonable and strongly held belief or idea. Such a belief is beyond the norm of beliefs held or accepted by other members of the person's culture or subculture.

overweight (ō-vur-wāt′) Having weight in excess of what is normal for a person's age, height, and build.

ovi- [L. *ovum,* egg] Combining form meaning *egg.*

ovi albumin (ō″vē-ăl-bū′mĭn) [L.] Ovalbumin.

ovicide (ō′vĭ-sīd) [L. *ovum,* egg, + *caedere,* to kill] An agent destructive to ova.

oviduct (ō′vĭ-dŭkt) [″ + *ductus,* a path] Fallopian tube.

oviferous (ō-vĭf′ĕr-ŭs) [″ + *ferre,* to bear] Containing or producing ova.

oviform (ō′vĭ-form) [″ + *forma,* shape] **1.** Having the shape of an egg. SYN: *ovoid.* **2.** Resembling an ovum.

ovigenesis [″ + Gr. *gennan,* to produce] Oogenesis.

ovigerm (ō′vĭ-jĕrm) [″ + *germen,* a bud] The cell that produces or develops into an ovum.

ovination (ō″vĭ-nā′shŭn) [L. *ovinus,* of a sheep] Inoculation with the sheep-pox virus.

ovine (ō′vīn) [L. *ovinus,* of a sheep] Concerning sheep.

oviparity (ō″vĭ-păr′ĭ-tē) The quality of being oviparous.

oviparous (ō-vĭp′ăr-ŭs) [L. *ovum,* egg, + *parere,* to produce] Producing eggs that are hatched outside the body; egg laying; the opposite of ovoviviparous.

oviposition [″ + *ponere,* to place] The laying of eggs as in oviparous reproduction.

ovipositor (ō″vĭ-pŏs′ĭ-tor) A specialized tubular structure found in many female insects, through which they lay their eggs in plants or soil.

ovisac (ō′vĭ-săk) A dated term for a graafian follicle.

ovo- [L. *ovum,* egg] Combining form meaning *egg.*

ovocenter The centrosome of a fertilized ovum.

ovocyte (ō′vō-sīt) [″ + *kytos,* cell] Oocyte.

ovoflavin (ō″vō-flā′vĭn) [″ + *flavus,* yellow] A flavin derived from eggs; identical to riboflavin.

ovogenesis (ō″vō-jĕn′ĕ-sĭs) [″ + Gr. *genesis,* generation, birth] Production of ova. SYN: *oogenesis.*

ovoglobulin (ō″vō-glŏb′ū-lĭn) [″ + *globulus,* globule] The globulin found in egg white. SEE: *albumin; protein, simple.*

ovoid (ō′voyd) [L. *ovum,* egg, + Gr. *eidos,* form, shape] **1.** Shaped like an egg. SYN: *oviform.* **2.** A cylindrical apparatus attached to a handle, used as a pair to hold a radioactive source during brachytherapy of the cervix.

ovomucin (ō″vō-mū′sĭn) A glycoprotein in the white of an egg.

ovomucoid (ō″vō-mū′koyd) [″ + *mucus,* mucus, + Gr. *eidos,* form, shape] A glycoprotein principle derived from egg white.

ovoplasm (ō′vō-plăzm) [″ + LL. *plasma,* form, mold] The protoplasm of an unfertilized egg. SEE: *ooplasm.*

ovotestis (ō″vō-tĕs′tĭs) A gonad that contains both testicular and ovarian tissue.

ovovitellin (ō″vō-vī-tĕl′ĭn) [″ + *vitellus,* yolk] A protein found in an egg yolk.

ovoviviparous (ō″vō-vī-vĭp′ă-rŭs) [″ + *vivus,* alive, + *parere,* to bring forth, to bear] Reproducing by eggs that have a well-developed membrane and that hatch inside the maternal organism; opposite of oviparous.

ovular (ō′vū-lăr) [L. *ovulum,* little egg] Concerning an ovule or ovum.

ovulation (ŏv″ū-lā′shŭn) [L. *ovulum,* little egg] The periodic ripening and rupture of the mature graafian follicle and the discharge of the ovum from the cortex of the ovary. Under the influence of follicle-stimulating hormone secreted by the anterior pituitary, the follicle matures. The enlarging and maturing follicle causes a slight protrusion of the ovarian surface. Final follicular maturation and rupture occur in response to a sudden surge of luteinizing hormone. The ovum is expelled, captured by the fimbriae, and guided into the fallopian tube. Rapid changes occur in the ruptured follicle as it becomes the corpus luteum and secretes large amounts of progesterone. In the absence of fertilization, the corpus luteum degenerates within about a week, forming a fibrous scar known as corpus albicans. SEE: *conception; fertilization* for illus; *menstrual cycle* for illus.

ovulation induction Stimulating ovulation by the use of drugs such as clomiphene citrate, bromocriptine, human menopausal gonadotropin, or gonadotropin-releasing hormone. SEE: *fertilization, in vitro; syndrome, ovarian hyperstimulation.*

ovulatory (ŏv′ū-lă-tō″rē) Concerning ovulation.

ovule (ō′vūl) [L. *ovulum*] **1.** The ovum in the graafian follicle. **2.** A small egg.

ovulogenous (ō-vū-lŏj′ĕn-ŭs) **1.** Giving rise to ovules or ova. **2.** Originating from an ovule or ovum.

ovum (ō′vŭm) *pl.* **ova** [L., egg] **1.** The female reproductive or germ cell. **2.** A cell that is capable of developing into a new organism of the same species. Usually fertilization by a spermatozoon is necessary, although in some lower animals ova develop without fertilization (parthenogenesis). SEE: illus.; *conception; fertilization; menstrual cycle; menstruation.*

alecithal o. An ovum with a small yolk portion that is distributed throughout the protoplasm. SYN: *isolecithal o.*

centrolecithal o. An ovum having a large central food yolk, as in a bird's egg.

holoblastic o. An ovum that undergoes complete cleavage, as opposed to partial or meroblastic cleavage.

human o. The female gamete, that is, germ cell, required for reproduction. The ovum develops from an oogonium within the graafian follicle of the ovary and matures through the meiotic process of oogenesis. A mature ovum is about 0.13 to 0.14 mm (0.0051 to 0.0055 in.) in diameter. At ovulation, the ova is bounded by a translucent cellular membrane, the zona pellucida, which is connected to a layer of

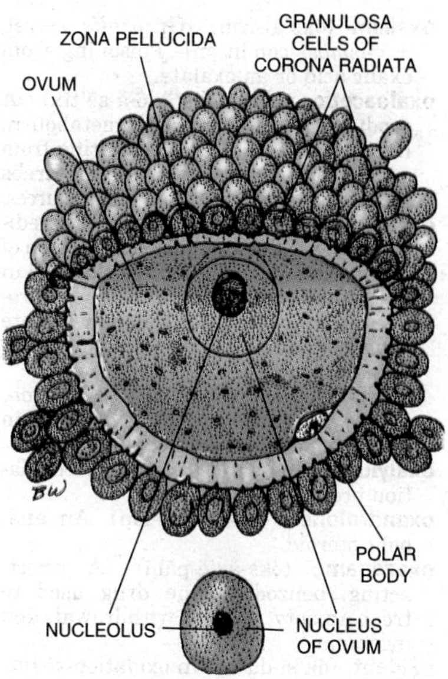

HUMAN OVUM

follicular cells, the corona radiata, which enclose the cytoplasm, nuclei, and chromatin material. The exact time during which a human ovum is capable of fertilization and further development before degenerating is not known; however, it is probably 24 hr. SEE: *oogenesis; ovulation.*

isolecithal o. Alecithal o.

meroblastic o. An ovum in which only the protoplasmic region undergoes cleavage; characteristic in ova containing a large amount of yolk.

permanent o. An ovum that is ready for fertilization.

primordial o. A germ cell that arises very early in the development of the embryo, usually in the yolk sac endoderm, migrates into the urogenital ridge, and possibly serves as the progenitor of the functional sex cell.

telolecithal o. An ovum in which the yolk is fairly abundant and tends to concentrate in one hemisphere.

Owren's disease [Paul A. Owren, Norwegian hematologist, b. 1905] Congenital deficiency of clotting factor V.

ox- Combining form indicating *oxygen.*

oxa- Combining form indicating the presence of oxygen in place of carbon.

oxacillin (ŏks″ă-sĭl′ĭn) A semisynthetic penicillin.

o. sodium An antibiotic drug.

oxal-, oxalo- Combining form indicating derivation from oxalic acid.

oxalate (ŏk′să-lāt) [Gr. *oxalis,* sorrel] A salt of oxalic acid.

potassium o. The potassium salt of oxalic acid.

oxalemia (ŏk″să-lē′mē-ă) [″ + *haima,* blood] Excess oxalates in the blood.

oxalism (ŏks'ăl-ĭzm) [Gr. *oxalis,* sorrel, + *-ismos,* condition] Poisoning from oxalic acid or an oxalate.

oxaloacetic acid (ŏks"ă-lō-ă-sē'tĭk) A product of carbohydrate metabolism $HOOC \cdot CH_2 \cdot CO \cdot COOH$ resulting from oxidation of malic acid during the Krebs cycle. May be derived from other sources.

oxalosis An autosomal recessive hereditary disease due to faulty metabolism of glyoxylic acid. Oxalic acid is elevated in the urine because of the increased production of oxalic acid. Calcium oxalate is deposited in body tissues, esp. in the kidneys.

oxaluria (ŏk-să-lū'rē-ă) [" + *ouron,* urine] Excess excretion of oxalates in the urine, esp. calcium oxalate.

oxalylurea (ŏk"săl-ĭl-ū-rē'ă) An oxidation product of uric acid.

oxandrolone (ŏk-săn'drō-lōn) An anabolic steroid.

oxazepam (ŏks-ăz'ĕ-păm) A short-acting, benzodiazepine drug used to treat anxiety, alcohol withdrawal, and insomnia.

oxidant (ŏk'sĭ-dănt) In oxidation-reduction reactions, the acceptor of an electron.

oxidase (ŏk'sĭ-dās) [Gr. *oxys,* sharp] A class of enzymes present in animal and vegetable life that catalyzes an oxidation reaction; a respiratory enzyme.

cytochrome o. An enzyme present in most cells that oxidizes reduced cytochrome back to cytochrome.

oxidation (ŏk'sĭ-dā'shŭn) [Gr. *oxys,* sharp] **1.** The process of a substance combining with oxygen. **2.** The loss of electrons in an atom with an accompanying increase in positive valence. SEE: *reduction* (2).

oxidation-reduction reaction A chemical interaction in which one substance is oxidized and loses electrons, and thus is increased in positive valence, while another substance gains an equal number of electrons by being reduced and thus is decreased in positive valence. This is called a redox system or reaction.

oxide (ŏk'sīd) Any chemical compound in which oxygen is the negative radical.

oxidize (ŏk'sĭ-dīz) **1.** To combine with oxygen. **2.** To increase the positive valence, or to decrease the negative valence, by bringing about a loss of electrons. SYN: *oxygenize.* SEE: *oxidation-reduction reaction.*

oxidoreductase (ŏk"sĭ-dō-rē-dŭk'tās) An enzyme that catalyzes oxidation-reduction reactions.

oxim, oxime (ŏk'sĭm) Any compound produced by the action of hydroxylamine on an aldehyde or ketone. When an aldehyde is involved, the general formula RCH = NOH is produced. When a ketone is acted upon, R_2CH = NOH is produced.

oximeter (ŏk-sĭm'ĕ-tĕr) [Gr. *oxys,* sharp, + *metron,* measure] An electronic device for determining the oxygen concentration in arterial blood. The oximeter is usually attached to the tip of a finger, preferably the index, middle, or ring finger, but may sometimes be placed on a toe (if there is adequate circulation to the foot) or the bridge of the nose, the forehead, or an ear lobe.

CAUTION: The oximeter should not be so tight that it prevents circulation to the finger, toe, or ear lobe.

ear o. A clip-on device that determines the oxygen saturation of the blood flowing through the ear.

finger o. A pulse oximeter that attaches to the finger.

pulse o. Finger o.

oximetry The use of an oximeter to determine the oxygen saturation of blood.

oxindole (ŏk'sĭn-dōl) Natural derivatives of tryptophan that are present in high concentrations in the brains of patients with hepatic encephalopathy. Chemicals from this class have sedative and antioxidant effects. Some evidence suggests oxindoles may be useful in the treatment of Alzheimer's dementia.

oxisensor An old term for oximeter.

oxy- [Gr. *oxys*] **1.** Combining form indicating *sharp, keen, acute, acid, pungent.* **2.** Combining form indicating the presence of oxygen in a compound. **3.** Combining form indicating the presence of a hydroxyl group.

oxyacusis (ŏk"sē-ă-kū'sĭs) [Gr. *oxys,* sharp, + *akousis,* hearing] Hyperacusis.

oxybenzene (ŏk"sē-bĕn'zēn) Phenol.

oxyblepsia (ŏk"sē-blĕp'sē-ă) [Gr. *oxys,* sharp, + *blepsis,* vision] Extraordinary acuteness of vision.

oxybutyria (ŏk"sē-bū-tĭr'ē-ă) Oxybutyric acid in the urine.

oxycalcium (ŏk"sē-kăl'sē-ŭm) Of or pert. to oxygen and calcium.

oxycellulose Cellulose that has undergone oxidation.

oxycephalous (ŏk-sē-sĕf'ă-lŭs) [Gr. *oxys,* sharp, + *kephale,* head] Denoting a head that is pointed and conelike.

oxycephaly (ŏk"sē-sĕf'ă-lē) Acrocephaly.

oxychloride (ŏk"sē-klō'rīd) [Gr. *oxys,* sharp, + *chloros,* green] A compound consisting of an element or radical combined with oxygen and chlorine or the hydroxyl radical (OH) and chlorine.

oxychromatic (ŏk"sē-krō-măt'ĭk) [" + *chroma,* color] Staining readily with acid dyes.

oxychromatin (ŏk"sē-krō'mă-tĭn) The part of chromatin that stains readily with acid dyes.

oxyecoia (ŏk"sē-ē-koy'ă) [" + *akoe,* hearing] Abnormal sensitivity to noises.

oxyesthesia (ŏk"sē-ĕs-thē'zē-ă) [" + *aisthesis,* sensation] Abnormal acuteness of sensation. SYN: *algesia; hyperesthesia.*

oxygen (ŏk′sĭ-jĕn) [Gr. *oxys,* sharp, + *gennan,* to produce] **1.** A medicinal gas used in the management of anemia, bleeding, ischemia, shock, pulmonary edema, pneumonia, respiratory distress, ventilatory failure, obstructive lung diseases, pulmonary embolism, myocardial infarction, mountain sickness, smoke inhalation, carbon monoxide or cyanide poisoning, gangrene, and other illnesses where its presence in the body is temporarily or chronically insufficient. SEE: *oxygen therapy*. **2.** SYMB: O. A nonmetallic element occurring freely in the atmosphere (approx. 21% at sea level) as a colorless, odorless, tasteless gas; atomic weight 15.9994, atomic number 8. It is a constitutent of animal, vegetable, and mineral substances, and is essential to respiration for most living organisms. At sea level, it represents 10% to 16% of venous blood and 17% to 21% of arterial blood.

Oxygen is absorbed by most living organisms. During photosynthesis it is produced by green plants from carbon dioxide and water. When oxygen is used in cell respiration, the end products are water and carbon dioxide, the latter of which is returned to the atmosphere.

Oxygen combines readily with other elements to form oxides. When it combines with another substance, the process is called oxidation. When combination takes place rapidly enough to produce light and heat, the process is called combustion.

ADMINISTRATION: Oxygen is administered by mask, nasal tube, tent, or in an airtight chamber in which pressure may be increased. No matter how much oxygen is given, it is important to have it adequately humidified. It is desirable to administer oxygen at whatever rate is necessary to increase the oxygen content of inspired air to 50%. SEE: *hypoxia*.

hyperbaric o. The administration of oxygen under greater than normal atmospheric pressure (usually 2 to 3 times absolute atmospheric pressure). It has been used to treat air embolism, decompression sickness, severe carbon monoxide poisoning, and some anaerobic infections. SEE: *hyperbaric oxygenation*.

singlet o. A highly active form of oxygen produced during reactions of hydrogen peroxide with superoxide and hypochlorite ions. It is believed that this free radical is bactericidal.

transtracheal o. The delivery of oxygen to the lungs via a cannula placed directly into the trachea. SEE: *transtracheal oxygenation*.

oxygenase (ŏk′sĭ-jĕn-ās″) [Gr. *oxys,* sharp, + *gennan,* to produce, + *-ase,* enzyme] An enzyme that enables an organism to use atmospheric oxygen in respiration.

oxygenate (ŏk′sĭ-jĕn-āt) To combine or supply with oxygen.

oxygenation (ŏk″sĭ-jĕn-ā′shŭn) Saturation or combination with oxygen, as the aeration of the blood in the lungs.

hyperbaric o. Administration of oxygen under increased pressure while the patient is in an airtight chamber. Pressure chambers in which the oxygen is hyperbaric have been used to treat carbon monoxide poisoning, anaerobic infections such as gas gangrene, necrotizing fasciitis, crush injuries with acute ischemia of tissues, compromised skin grafts and flaps, mixed soft tissue reactions, burns, smoke inhalation, carbon monoxide poisoning, soft tissue radiation necrosis, chronic refractory osteomyelitis, decompression sickness (bends), and gas embolism.

CAUTION: Hyperbaric oxygenation should not be used in untreated pneumothorax or premature infants.

---

tissue o. The oxygen level in tissues. Measurement of the oxygen concentration in body fluids is not as important as knowing the oxygen level in the tissues themselves. Determining the gastrointestinal interstitial pH provides an indication of the adequacy of tissue oxygenation. Decreased oxygen supply leads to anaerobic metabolism in cells, which produces a fall in pH. Thus the tissue pH serves as a marker for the adequacy of oxygen supply in the tissues.

transtracheal o. The application of oxygen via a catheter system inserted into the trachea.

oxygenator (ŏk″sĭ-jĕ-nā′tor) A device for mechanically oxygenating anything, but esp. blood, e.g. during thoracic surgery or open-heart surgery.

bubble o. A device for bubbling oxygen through the blood during extracorporeal circulation.

rotating disk o. A device for oxygenating blood during extracorporeal circulation. A thin film of blood attaches to a disk as it dips into the blood flow. The portion of the disk not in the blood is rotating in an atmosphere of oxygen.

screen o. A device for oxygenating blood during extracorporeal circulation. The blood passes over a series of screens that are in an oxygen atmosphere. Oxygen is exchanged in the thin film of blood on the screens.

oxygen capacity The maximum amount of oxygen expressed in volume percent (cc per 100 ml) that a given amount of blood will absorb. For normal blood it is about 20 cc.

oxygen concentrator A device used for home oxygen therapy that removes most of the nitrogen from room air and delivers the oxygen at a low flow rate. SYN: *oxygen enricher*.

oxygen content The amount of oxygen in volume percent that is present in the blood at any one moment.

oxygen debt After strenuous (i.e., anaerobic) physical activity, the oxygen required in the recovery period, in addition to that required while resting, to oxidize the excess lactic acid produced and to replenish the depleted stores of adenosine triphosphate and phosphocreatinase.

oxygen-derived free radical SEE: *oxygen radical; superoxide.*

oxygen enricher Oxygen concentrator.

oxygenic (ŏk″sĭ-jĕn′ĭk) [″ + *gennan,* to produce] Concerning, resembling, containing, or consisting of oxygen.

oxygenize Oxidize.

oxygen radical Hydrogen peroxide (H_2O_2) or the superoxide radical (O_2^-) produced by the incomplete reduction of oxygen. Oxygen free radicals are released during the "respiratory burst" phase of phagocytosis by neutrophils and macrophages during the inflammatory process. They cause direct cell damage, increase vascular permeability through damage to the capillary endothelium, and promote chemotaxis. Oxygen free radicals are normally contained by antioxidant protective measures; however, with severe inflammation they cause significant damage. They are believed to be responsible for much of the cellular damage involved in adult respiratory distress syndrome (ARDS), in which massive neutrophil aggregation and phagocytosis occur. SEE: *oxygen, singlet.*

oxygen therapy The administration of oxygen at higher levels than are normally found in the atmosphere to patients needing enhanced tissue oxygen uptake. Oxygen can be administered via nasal prongs, Venturi masks, nonrebreathing devices, positive pressure masks, endotracheal tubes, Ambu bags, mist tents, or in airtight or hyperbaric chambers, depending on the needs of the patient. Each of these modes of therapy has its own benefits and limitations. Nasal cannulae facilitate speaking and eating, but can only deliver oxygen concentrations of about 40%. Venturi masks can deliver somewhat more oxygen (approximately 50%) and they can deliver oxygen concentrations more precisely than nasal devices, but they interfere with some communication and oral intake. The highest levels of noninvasive oxygen therapy are delivered by nonrebreather masks (about 90%). One hundred percent oxygen can be given through endotracheal tubes, but patients often are uncomfortable or hemodynamically unstable with these devices, and may need sedation, or paralytic or pressor drugs to support them. Positive pressure masks are useful for oxygen delivery in sleep apnea, or in the prevention of respiratory failure, but they are not tolerated by some patients due to claustrophobia and poor adaptation to the fit of the mask. Supplemental oxygen is also available for home use through an oxygen concentrator which uses a method called a "molecular sieve" to remove nitrogen from room air. SEE: *hyperbaric oxygen; oximeter.*

CAUTION: Inhalation of high concentrations of oxygen, esp. at pressures of more than one atmosphere, may produce deleterious effects such as irritation of respiratory tract, reduced vital capacity, and sometimes neurological symptoms. Serious eye defects may result if premature infants are exposed to a high concentration of oxygen as part of their therapy. Because oxygen provides a perfect environment for combustion, it should not be used in the presence of oil, lighted cigarettes or open flames, or where there is the possibility of electrical or spark hazards.

transtracheal o.t. The delivery of oxygen via a small plastic cannula inserted directly into the trachea through a small surgical opening in the cricothyroid membrane of the neck. SEE: illus.

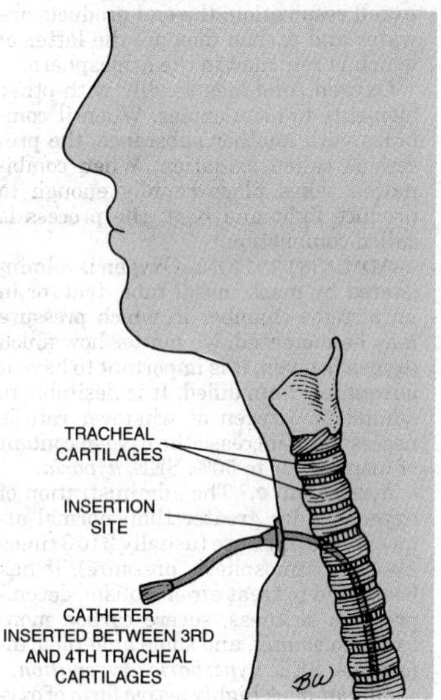

TRANSTRACHEAL OXYGEN THERAPY

oxygen toxicity Progressive respiratory failure that develops when high oxygen concentrations (more than 60%) are breathed for a prolonged period. Respiratory failure leads to decreased oxygen tension in the blood.

Prolonged exposure to a high oxygen concentration can cause blindness or damage to lung tissue in a preterm newborn.

oxygeusia (ŏk″sē-gū′sē-ă) [Gr. *oxys,* sharp, + *geusis,* taste] Abnormally keen sense of taste.

oxyhematin (ŏk″sē-hĕm′ă-tĭn) An iron compound that constitutes the coloring matter in oxyhemoglobin. When oxidized, it yields hematinic acid; when reduced, hematoporphyrin.

oxyhematoporphyrin (ŏk″sē-hĕm″ă-tō-por′fĭ-rĭn) A derivative of hematoporphyrin sometimes present in urine.

oxyhemoglobin (ŏk″sē-hē″mō-glō′bĭn) [″ + *haima,* blood, + L. *globus,* a sphere] The combined form of hemoglobin and oxygen. Hemoglobin with oxygen is found in arterial blood and is the oxygen carrier to the body tissues.

fractional o. SYMB: FO_2Hb. The ratio of the substance fraction of oxyhemoglobin to the substance fraction of all forms of hemoglobin. This quantity takes into account the effects of abnormal hemoglobins such as carboxyhemoglobin, methemoglobin, or sulfhemoglobin. Thus, in the presence of abnormal hemoglobins, the fractional oxyhemoglobin may be decreased while the oxygen saturation is normal.

oxyhemoglobin dissociation curve The mathematical relationship between the partial pressure of oxygen and the percentage of saturation of hemoglobin with oxygen (i.e., the proportion of oxyhemoglobin to reduced hemoglobin). Factors that favor a shift of the curve to the right, accelerating the decomposition of hemoglobin, are a rise in temperature and an increase of H ions that results from liberation of CO_2 and formation of lactic acid. SEE: illus.

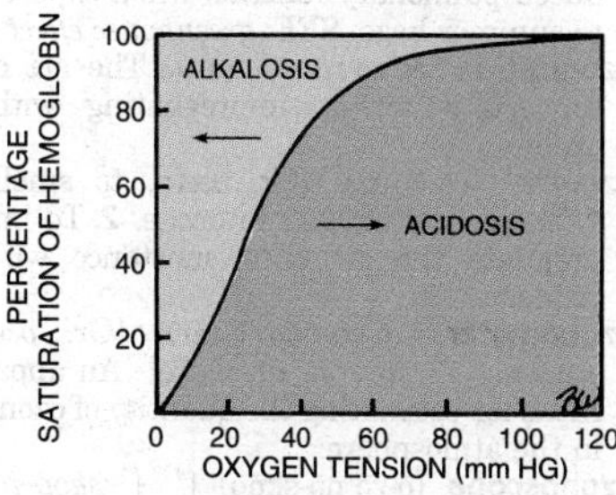

OXYHEMOGLOBIN DISSOCIATION CURVE

oxyhemoglobinometer (ŏk″sē-hē″mō-glō″bĭn-ŏm′ĕ-tĕr) [″ + ″ + ″ + Gr. *metron,* measure] An apparatus for measurement of the amount of oxygen in the blood.

oxyhydrocephalus (ŏk″sē-hī-drō-sĕf′ăl-ŭs) [″ + *hydor,* water, + *kephale,* brain] A type of hydrocephalus in which the head has a pointed shape.

oxyiodide (ŏk″sē-ī′ō-dīd) [″ + *ioeides,* violet colored] A compound of iodine and oxygen with an element or radical.

oxylalia (ŏk″sē-lā′lē-ă) [″ + *lalein,* to speak] Abnormal rapidity of speech.

oxymetazoline hydrochloride (ŏk″sē-mĕt-ăz′ō-lēn) A vasoconstrictor drug used topically for nasal decongestion.

oxymetholone (ŏk″sē-mĕth′ō-lōn) An anabolic steroid.

oxymorphone hydrochloride (ŏk″sē-mor′fōn) A semisynthetic analgesic narcotic similar in action to morphine.

oxymyoglobin (ŏk″sē-mī″ō-glō′bĭn) The compound formed when myoglobin is exposed to oxygen.

oxyntic (ŏk-sĭn′tĭk) [Gr. *oxynein,* to make acid] Producing or secreting acid.

oxyopia (ŏk″sē-ō′pē-ă) [Gr. *oxys,* sharp, + *ops,* sight] Abnormal acuteness of vision.

oxyopter (ŏk″sē-ŏp′tĕr) A unit of measuring visual acuity; the reciprocal of the visual angle expressed in degrees.

oxyosmia (ŏk″sē-ŏz′mē-ă) [″ + *osme,* odor] Unusual acuity of the sense of smell.

oxyosphresia (ŏk″sē-ŏs-frē′zē-ă) [″ + *osphresis,* smell] Abnormal acuity of the sense of smell.

oxypathia, oxypathy (ŏk″sē-păth′ē-ă, -sĭp′ă-thē) [″ + *pathos,* disease, suffering] **1.** Unusual acuity of sensation. **2.** An acute condition. **3.** A condition in which the body is unable to eliminate unoxidizable acids, which combine with fixed alkalies of the tissues and harm the organism.

oxyperitoneum (ŏk″sĭ-pĕr-ĭ-tō-nē′ŭm) [″ + *peritonaion,* peritoneum] The introduction of oxygen into the peritoneal cavity.

oxyphil(e) (ŏk′sē-fĭl, -fīl) [″ + *philein,* to love] **1.** Staining readily with acid dyes. **2.** A cell that stains readily with acid dyes.

oxyphonia (ŏk″sē-fō′nē-ă) An abnormally sharp or shrill pitch to the voice.

oxypurine (ŏk″sē-pū′rēn) [″ + L. *purus,* pure, + *urina,* urine] An oxidation product of purine; includes hypoxanthine, xanthine, and uric acid. SEE: *aminopurine; methyl purine.*

oxyrhine (ŏk′sē-rīn) [″ + *rhis,* nose] **1.** Having a sharp-pointed nose. **2.** Possessing an acute sense of smell.

oxytalan (ŏks-ĭt′ă-lăn) A type of connective tissue fiber present in periodontal tissues.

oxytetracycline (ŏks″ē-tĕt″ră-sī′klēn) One of a group of broad-spectrum antibiotic substances called tetracyclines. It combines with sites of calcification so that teeth forming in children or the unborn fetus may be stained as a result of extensive medication with this group of antibiotics. Originally obtained from a strain of *Streptomyces,* it is now prepared synthetically.

oxytocic (ŏk″sē-tō′sĭk) **1.** Agent that stimulates uterine contractions. **2.** Accelerating childbirth.

oxytocin [injection] (ŏk″sē-tō′sĭn) A pituitary hormone that stimulates the uterus to contract, thus inducing parturition. It also acts on the mammary gland to stimulate the release of milk.

oxytocin challenge test ABBR: OCT. The intravenous infusion of 10 very small doses of oxytocin in order to determine whether contraction of the uterus in response to the oxytocin will cause signs of fetal distress. The results of the test provide a basis of making a decision concerning continuation of high-risk pregnancies. Uterine contractions can also be induced by manual stimulation of the nipple. This process stimulates the hypothalamus, which causes the posterior lobe of the pituitary to release oxytocin. SYN: *contraction stress test*.

Criteria for Interpretation: Negative result: The monitor records a minimum of three uterine contractions and an absence of late decelerations within 10 min. The fetal heart rate exhibits average baseline variablity and acceleration associated with movement. *Positive result:* The monitor records late decelerations with more than 50% of uterine contractions. *Suspicious result:* The monitor records late decelerations associated with fewer than 50% contractions. *Hyperstimulation:* The monitor records uterine hypertonus and uterine contractions occurring more often than every 2 min or lasting longer than 90 sec.

PATIENT CARE: The test is explained, and the patient is supported through the procedure. Oxytocin solution is piggybacked into the tubing of the main intravenous line and delivered via infusion pump or controller to ensure accurate dosing. Uterine contractions and fetal heart rate are monitored until three uterine contractions occur in a 30-min period. The fetal heart rate pattern is then interpreted for the absence or presence of late decelerations. The infusion of oxytocin is then discontinued, the intravenous line is removed, and the patient is assisted with discharge preparations.

oxyuriasis (ŏk″sē-ū-rī′ăs-ĭs) [Gr. *oxys,* sharp, + *oura,* tall, + *iasis,* infection] Infestation with *Enterobius vermicularis* (pinworm). SYN: *enterobiasis*.

oxyuricide (ŏk″sē-ū′rĭ-sīd) [″ + ″ + L. *caedere,* to kill] An agent that is destructive to pinworms.

Oxyuris [″ + *oura,* tail] The former name for the genus of nematode intestinal worms that includes the pinworms or seatworms. SEE: *Enterobius*.

O. vermicularis *Enterobius vermicularis*.

Oxyuroidea (ŏk″sē-ū″roy-dē′ă) A superfamily of nematodes that includes the pinworm *Enterobius vermicularis.*

oyster [AS. *oistre*] A shellfish that, when eaten raw or only partially cooked, may be a source of hepatitis A virus and bacterial pathogens. SEE: *diarrhea, travelers'*.

oz *ounce.*

oz. ap. *ounce apothecary's* (pharmaceutical term).

oz. av. *ounce avoirdupois.*

ozena (ō-zē′nă) [Gr. *oze,* stench] A disease of the nose characterized by atrophy of the turbinates and mucous membrane accompanied by considerable crusting, discharge, and an offensive odor. It is present in various forms of rhinitis.

ozone (ō′zōn) [Gr. *ozein,* to smell] A form of oxygen, present in the stratosphere, in which three atoms of the element combine to form the molecule O_3. Depletion of the ozone in the stratosphere permits increased exposure to ultraviolet light. This favors the development of skin cancers and cataracts, and may impair cellular immunity.

Persons exposed to arc welding, flour bleaching, fumes from copying equipment, or photochemical air pollutants may be in contact with toxic levels of ozone. The signs and symptoms include asthma, mucous membrane irritation, pulmonary hemorrhage and edema, and transient reduced pulmonary function when exposed to summer haze. SEE: *greenhouse effect*.

ozonization (ō″zō-nĭ-zā′shŭn) The act of converting to, or impregnating with, ozone.

ozonize (ō′zō-nīz) [Gr. *ozein,* to smell] **1.** To convert oxygen to ozone. **2.** To impregnate the air of a substance with ozone.

ozonometer (ō″zō-nŏm′ĕ-tĕr) [Gr. *oze,* stench, + *metron,* measure] An apparatus for estimating the quantity of ozone in the atmosphere.

ozonoscope (ō-zō′nō-skōp) [″ + *skopein,* to examine] A device for showing the presence or amount of ozone.

ozostomia (ō″zō-stō′mē-ă) [″ + *stoma,* mouth] Fetid breath; halitosis.

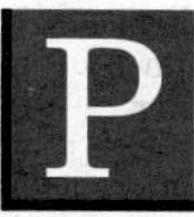

P **1.** *position; posterior; postpartum; pressure; pulse; pupil.* **2.** Symbol for the element phosphorus. **3.** Symbol for partial pressure, preferably italicized.

p *page; probability* (in statistics); *pupil.*

p- *para-* in chemical formulas.

p̄ *after-* or *post-*.

P_1 *first parental generation* (in genetics); *first pulmonic heart sound.*

P_2 *pulmonic second sound.*

^{32}P Symbol for radioactive isotope of phosphorus.

p53 A protein, produced by a tumor-suppressor gene, that is believed to play an important role in the birth and death of cells.

PA *pulmonary artery.*

P.A. *physician assistant.*

Pa **1.** Symbol for the element protactinium. **2.** Pascal.

P-A, p-a *posteroanterior.*

P & A *percussion and auscultation.*

$P(A-a)O_2$ The oxygen pressure gradient between the alveoli and the arterial blood.

pabular (păb′ū-lăr) [L. *pabulum,* food] Pert. to nourishment.

pabulum (păb′ū-lŭm) [L.] Food or nourishment; esp. in an absorbable solution.

PAC *premature atrial contraction.*

pacchionian depressions Small pits produced on the inner surface of the skull by protuberance of the pacchionian bodies.

PACE *Patient Advise and Consent Encounter.*

pacemaker (pās′māk-ĕr) [L. *passus,* a step, + AS. *macian,* to make] **1.** Anything that influences the rate and rhythm of occurrence of some activity or process. **2.** In cardiology, a specialized cell or group of cells that automatically generates impulses that spread to other regions of the heart. The normal cardiac pacemaker is the sinoatrial node, a group of cells in the right atrium near the entrance of the superior vena cava. **3.** A generally accepted term for artificial cardiac pacemaker.

artificial cardiac p. A device that can trigger mechanical contractions of the heart by emitting periodic electrical discharges. If the device delivers electricity through the chest wall, it is called a transcutaneous pacemaker; if it works via electrodes inserted inside the body, it is called an internal or implantable pacemaker. Pacemakers are used most often to treat patients with very slow heart rates or long pauses between heart beats (e.g., patients with third-degree heart block, symptomatic second-degree heart block, bifascicular block with first-degree heart block, carotid sinus hypersensitivity, and tachy-brady syndrome. Occasionally, though, they also are used for other purposes, such as to capture and override some tachyarrhythmias.

All artificial cardiac pacemakers have a pulse generator (a device that gives off an electrical impulse at prescribed intervals), electrical leads (which transmit the impulse to the myocardium), and a battery (usually made of lithium iodide). They typically have the ability to pace the ventricle, the atrium, or both; to sense electrical discharges coming from cardiac chambers; and to respond to sensed beats. Most pacemakers in the U.S. also are programmable, and many are rate responsive.

After pacemaker implantation, follow-up care is provided to ensure that the device is working optimally. Follow-up care typically includes monitoring the pacemaker's performance, either in the cardiologist's office or by telephonic link-up to ensure, for example, that the pulse generator is triggering a heart rate that is appropriate for the patient's needs, that the leads are working, and that the battery's strength is adequate.

PATIENT CARE: *Preoperative:* Health care professionals should monitor the cardiac rate and rhythm for evidence of failure of the heart's pacemaker and treat using the hospital protocol. They should teach the patient and family about cardiac function and pacemaker insertion and function, encourage verbalization of fears and concerns, answer questions, dispel myths, correct misconceptions, and provide routine preoperative preparation.

Postoperative: Health care professionals should ascertain the type of pacemaker employed and expectations for its function; monitor the cardiac rate and rhythm for evidence of pacemaker function; assess the patient for evidence of pacemaker failure or noncapture (vertigo, loss of consciousness, hypotension, chest discomfort, dyspnea) and evaluate the patient for effects on cardiac output; teach the patient technique and rationale for monitoring own pulse rate, and care and protection of insertion site; counsel concerning telephone monitoring check-up, battery replacement, medication regimen, physical activity, and follow-up care. They should encourage the patient to wear or carry medical identification and information indicating the presence and type of pacemaker implanted, along with an electrocardiogram rhythm strip showing pacemaker activity and capture.

breathing p. A device that stimulates breathing by delivering electrical pulses to both phrenic nerves from an external radio transmitter to an implanted receiver. It is used in patients with quadriplegia or sleep apnea.

DDD p. A rate-adaptive implanted pacing device. It senses and paces both atrial and ventricular events, triggering the atrioventricular (AV) interval so that AV synchrony is maintained over a wide range of heart rates. This type of pacing has reduced the incidence of pacemaker syndrome. It is the most versatile pacing device used. SEE: *pacing code; pacemaker syndrome.*

DDI p. An implanted pacing device that senses both atrial and ventricular events but can inhibit only atrial impulses. This type of pacing is used only when atrioventricular conduction is intact. It may be suitable when frequent atrial tachyarrhythmias cause rapid ventricular rates.

demand p. An implanted pacemaker that is designed to permit its electrical output to be inhibited by the heart's electrical impulses. This decreases the chances for the pacemaker to induce discomfort or dysrhythmias.

dual-chamber p. A pacemaker that is also known as an atrioventricular sequential pacemaker because it stimulates both atria and ventricles sequentially.

ectopic p. Any endogenous cardiac pacemaker other than the sinoatrial node.

failure of artificial p. A defect in a pacemaker device caused by either a failure to sense the patient's intrinsic beat or a failure to pace. Failure to pace can be caused by a worn-out battery, fracture or displacement of the electrode, or pulse generator defect.

fixed rate p. A pacemaker that stimulates the heart at a predetermined rate.

internal p. A cardiac pacemaker placed within the body.

permanent p. An electronic device for permanent cardiac pacing. The leads are usually inserted transvenously through the subclavian or cephalic veins with leads positioned in the right atrium for atrial pacing or in the right ventricular apex for ventricular pacing. The leads are connected to the pulse generator, which is implanted in a subcutaneous pocket below the clavicle.

programmable p. An electronic permanent pacemaker in which one or more settings can be changed from outside the patient by use of an electronic device.

rate-responsive p. An electronic pacemaker that senses changes in the body's need for adjustment of the cardiac rate as can occur in sleeping, waking, sitting, walking, or running. The device alters cardiac rate by sensing body motion, changes in breathing, or slight changes in blood temperature, which improves the quality of life for active patients. It is also called a *rate-adaptive pacemaker.*

temporary p. An electronic device for temporary cardiac pacing (e.g., during emergencies). The device consists of an electrode catheter inserted transvenously in the right ventricular apex that receives impulses from an external generator.

transcutaneous p. An artificial cardiac pacemaker that is located outside the body. The electrodes for delivering the stimulus are located on the chest wall.

transthoracic p. A cardiac pacemaker connected to electrodes passed through the chest wall, usually used only in emergency situations, on a temporary basis.

uterine p. One or more areas in the uterus that stimulate contraction of the myometrium.

wandering p. A cardiac arrhythmia in which the site of origin of the pacemaker stimulus shifts from one site to another, usually from the atrioventricular node to some other part of the atrium.

pacemaker syndrome A group of unpleasant symptoms associated with unsynchronized atrioventricular timing in patients who have single-chamber (ventricular) pacemakers. The symptoms may include syncope or presyncope, orthostatic dizziness, cough, dyspnea, palpitations, and others. The symptoms are produced by the contraction of the atria against closed atrioventricular valves and by the loss of cardiac output that the atria would normally contribute to ventricular filling during diastole. DDD pacing has reduced the incidence of this condition by allowing restoration of atrioventricular synchrony.

pacer Pacemaker.

pachometry (păk-ŏm′ĕ-trē) Measurement of the thickness of the cornea, either with a slit lamp or ultrasonographically.

pachy-, pach- [Gr. *pachys,* thick] Combining form meaning *thick.*

pachyblepharosis (păk″ē-blĕf″ă-rō′sĭs) Chronic thickening of the eyelid.

pachycephalic (păk″ē-sĕ-făl′ĭk) [″ + *kephale,* brain] Possessing an abnormally thick skull.

pachycheilia (păk″ē-kī′lē-ă) [″ + *cheilos,* lip] Unusual thickness of the lips.

pachychromatic (păk″ē-krō-măt′ĭk) [″ + *chroma,* color] Possessing a coarse chromatin network.

pachydactylia, pachydactyly (păk″ē-dăk-tĭl′ē-ă, -dăk′tĭ-lē) [″ + *daktylos,* digit] A condition marked by unusually large fingers and toes.

pachyderma (păk-ē-dĕr′mă) [″ + *derma,* skin] Unusual thickness of the skin. SEE: *elephantiasis.*

p. lymphangiectatica A diffuse form of skin thickening caused by blocked or defective lymph drainage.

occipital p. A disease in which the skin of the scalp, esp. in the occipital region, falls into thickened folds.

pachydermatocele (păk″ē-dĕr-măt′ō-sēl) [″ + ″ + *kele,* tumor, swelling] **1.** A pendulous state of the skin with thickening. SYN: *cutis laxa; dermatolysis.* **2.** Huge neurofibroma.

pachydermoperiostosis (păk″ē-dĕr″mō-pĕr″ē-ŏs-tō′sĭs) A hereditary form of osteoarthropathy of unknown origin marked by thickening of the skin over the face and extremities. If associated with an underlying disease, treatment of the disease may cause the symptoms and signs of this condition to disappear.

pachyglossia (păk″ē-glŏs′sē-ă) [″ + *glossa,* tongue] Unusual thickness of the tongue.

pachygnathous (pă-kĭg′năth-ŭs) [″ + *gnathos,* jaw] Having a thick or large jaw.

pachygyria (păk-ē-jī′rē-ă) [″ + *gyros,* a circle] Flat, broad formation of the cerebral convolutions.

pachyleptomeningitis (păk-ē-lĕp″tō-mĕn″ĭn-jī′tĭs) [″ + *leptos,* thin, + *meninx,* membrane, + *itis,* inflammation] Inflammation of the pia and dura of the brain and spinal cord.

pachymenia (păk-ē-mē′nē-ă) [″ + *hymen,* membrane] A thickening of the skin or membranes.

pachymeningitis (păk-ē-mĕn″ĭn-jī′tĭs) [″ + *meninx,* membrane, + *itis,* inflammation] Inflammation of the dura mater. Inflammation of any of three membranes—the pia, dura, or arachnoid—is sure to extend to one or both of the other two membranes, and the consequence in any form is suppuration, abscess, effusion into the ventricles, and softening of cerebral tissue if brain is involved. SYN: *perimeningitis.*

external p. Inflammation of the outer layer of the dura mater.

hemorrhagic p. Circumscribed effusion of blood on the inner surface of the dura with inflammation.

SYMPTOMS: Symptoms include intermittent headache, altered mental status, hemiparesis, and unconsciousness.

ETIOLOGY: This condition is usually the result of traumatic brain injury, resulting in a venous tear. Blood oozes into subdural space, and a blood clot is formed, becomes encysted, and gives rise to a hematoma. SEE: *hematoma, subdural.*

internal p. Inflammation of the inner layer of the dura mater.

spinal p. Inflammation of the dura of the spinal cord.

pachymeningopathy (păk″ē-mĕn″ĭn-gŏp′ă-thē) [″+ ″ + *pathos,* disease] Any noninflammatory disease of the dura mater.

pachymeninx (păk-ē-mē′nĭnks) [″ + *meninx,* membrane] The dura mater.

pachymeter [″ + *metron,* to measure] A device to determine the thickness of a material or object, such as the cornea.

pachyonychia (păk″ē-ō-nĭk′ē-ă) [Gr. *pachys,* thick, + *onyx,* nail] Abnormal thickening of the fingernails or toenails.

p. congenita A congenital condition characterized by thickening of the nails, thickening of the skin on the palms of the hands and the soles of the feet, follicular keratosis at the knees and elbows, and corneal dyskeratosis.

pachyostosis (păk″ē-ŏs-tō′sĭs) [″ + *osteon,* bone, + *osis,* condition] A benign condition of thickening of the bones.

pachyotia (păk-ē-ō′shē-ă) [″+ *ous,* ear] Abnormal thickness of the ears.

pachypelviperitonitis (păk″ē-pĕl″vĭ-pĕr″ĭ-tō-nī′tĭs) [″+ L. *pelvis,* basin, + Gr. *peritonaion,* peritoneum, + *itis,* inflammation] Inflammation of the pelvic and peritoneal membranes with hypertrophy and thickening of their surfaces.

pachyperiostitis (păk″ē-pĕr″ē-ŏs-tī′tĭs) [″ + *periosteon,* periosteum, + *itis,* inflammation] Thickening of the periosteum caused by inflammation.

pachyperitonitis (păk″ē-pĕr″ĭ-tō-nī′tĭs) [″ + ″ + *itis,* inflammation] Inflammation of the peritoneum with thickening of the membrane.

pachypleuritis (păk-ē-plū-rī′tĭs) [″ + *pleura,* side, + *itis,* inflammation] Inflammation of the pleura with thickening.

pachypodous (pă-kĭp′ō-dŭs) [″ + *pous,* foot] Having abnormally thick feet.

pachyrhinic (păk″ē-rī′nĭk) [″ + *rhis,* nose] Having a thick, flat nose.

pachytene (păk′ē-tēn) [″ + *tainia,* band] The stage in meiosis following zygotene, in which the paired homologous chromosomes become shorter, thicker, and form tetrads; crossing over may take place.

pachytrichous Presence of enlarged hair fibers.

pachyvaginalitis (păk″ē-văj″ĭn-ă-lī′tĭs) [″ + L. *vagina,* sheath, + Gr. *itis,* inflammation] Inflammation of the tunica vaginalis of the testes.

pachyvaginitis (păk″ē-văj″ĭn-ī′tĭs) Chronic inflammation of the vagina with thickening of the vaginal walls.

pacifier An artificial nipple, usually made of plastic, provided for infants to satisfy their need to suck.

pacing (pās′ĭng) [L. *passus,* a step] Setting the rate or pace of an event, esp. the heartbeat. SEE: *pacemaker*.

asynchronous p. Cardiac pacing that is set at a rate that is independent of the heart's own pacemakers. This allows pacemaking at heart rates that are faster or slower than the patient's diseased pacemaker.

epicardial p. Electrical pacing of the heart by conductive leads inserted surgically, usually during bypass graft or valvular operations. The leads are used in the postoperative period for the management of heart blocks or dysrhythmias and are removed as the patient stabilizes.

overdrive p. Using a pacemaker to generate a heart rate that is faster than the spontaneous heart rate of the patient. This is used in attempts to capture and terminate tachycardias or, in some cases, to try to trigger and study tachycardias in patients who have suffered them in the past.

synchronous p. Cardiac pacing set at a rate matching the underlying rate of one of the heart chambers.

transcutaneous p. The application of an electrical current between electrodes placed on the skin to stimulate the heart to beat. Typically, the electrodes are placed on the anterior and posterior chest, or to the right of the sternum and below the clavicle and on the midaxillary line at the level of the sixth to seventh ribs. Also called *external pacing, noninvasive pacing, external thoracic pacing,* and *transchest pacing.*

pacing code A code of 3 to 5 letters used for describing pacemaker type and function. The first letter indicates the chamber or chambers paced: V for ventricle, A for atrium, or D (dual) for pacing of both chambers. The second letter, which may also be V, A, or D, indicates the chamber from which electrical activity is sensed. The third letter indicates the response to the sensed electrical activity. O indicates no response to the electrical activity sensed; I, inhibition of the pacing action; T, triggering of the pacemaker function; and D, that a dual response of spontaneous atrial and ventricular activity will inhibit atrial and ventricular pacing. The fourth letter, previously used to describe programmable functions, is now used to designate variability of the pace rate with metabolic need. A fifth letter may indicate antitachycardia-pacing capability, but this is more usually incorporated into automatic implantable defibrillators. SEE: *pacemaker; artificial cardiac pacemaker.*

pacing wire Pacemaker electrode.

pacinian corpuscles (pă-sĭn′ē-ăn) [Filippo Pacini, It. anatomist, 1812–1883] Encapsulated sensory nerve endings found in subcutaneous tissue and many other parts of the body (pancreas, penis, clitoris, nipple). These corpuscles are sensitive to deep or heavy pressure. SYN: *Vater's corpuscles.*

pack (păk) [AS. *pak*] **1.** A dry or moist, hot or cold blanket or sheet wrapped around a patient and used for treatment. **2.** To fill up a cavity with cotton, gauze, or a similar substance.

cold p. **1.** A bulky dressing containing icewater, cubed or crushed ice, or gel, which is refrigerated and used topically to control pain or inflammation. SYN: *ice p.* **2.** A rarely used form of physical restraint, once popular in psychiatric practice. The restless, insomniac, or uncooperative patient was wrapped in two or more sheets that had been placed in cold water and wrung out before application, and then in heavy blankets to prevent loss of cooling and evaporation of moisture.

dry p. A procedure used in combination with a hot bath to induce perspiration. When leaving the hot bath, the patient is placed in a dry warm sheet and wrapped in several warm blankets.

full p. Any pack that enwraps the entire body.

half p. A wet-sheet pack extending from the axillae to below the knees.

hot p. A type of superficial moist heat applied to reduce pain and promote muscle relaxation. The pack is heated to 65° to 90°C in hot water. The pack is then wrapped with terrycloth prior to application.

ice p. Cold pack.

partial p. A wet pack that covers a portion of the body.

periodontal p. A surgical dressing applied over an area involved in periodontal surgery to enhance healing and tissue recovery. Components may include eugenol, resin, zinc oxide, tannic acid, cocoa butter, paraffin, olive oil, and an antibiotic.

posterior nasal p. SEE: *epistaxis.*

wet-dry p. A pack placed in a healing area, esp. an ulcer, to facilitate débridement. The pack, which may contain a topical antiseptic, is moistened, placed in the ulcer, and changed when it becomes dry. Also called *wet-dry dressing.*

wet-sheet p. The envelopment of a patient in one, two, or three linen or soft cotton sheets that have been wrung out of water. They are held against the body by large woolen blankets. The temperature of the water used for the sheets varies, depending on the purpose.

package insert An informational leaflet placed inside the container or package of prescription drugs. The Food and Drug Administration requires that the drug's generic name, indications, contraindications, adverse effects, dosage, and route of administration be described in the leaflet.

packed cells Red blood cells that have been separated from the plasma, used in treating conditions that require red blood cells but not the liquid components of whole blood. This prevents excess hydration of the vascular system.

packer (păk'ĕr) A device for packing a cavity or a wound.

packing (păk'ĭng) **1.** The process of filling a cavity or wound with gauze sponges or gauze strips. **2.** Material used to fill a cavity or wound.

pack-year The consumption of a pack of cigarettes daily for a year (approximately 365 packs of cigarettes annually). The number of pack-years that people smoke correlates closely with the amount of damage that tobacco does to their hearts, lungs, and other organs.

$Paco_2$ Partial pressure of carbon dioxide in the arterial blood; arterial carbon dioxide concentration or tension. It is usually expressed in millimeters of mercury (mm Hg).

pad (păd) **1.** A cushion of soft material, usually cotton or rayon, used to apply pressure, relieve pressure, or support an organ or part. **2.** A fleshlike or fatty mass.

abdominal p. A dressing for absorbing discharges from surgical wounds of the abdomen.

dinner p. A pad placed on the stomach before application of a plaster cast. The pad is then removed, leaving space for abdominal distention after meals.

fat p. **1.** Sucking p. **2.** The pad of fat behind and below the patella.

kidney p. An air or water pad fixed on an abdominal belt for compression over a movable kidney.

knuckle p. A congenital condition in which small nodules appear on the dorsal side of fingers.

Malgaigne's p. [Joseph François Malgaigne, Fr. physician, 1806–1865] A mass of fat in the knee joint on either side of the patella's upper end.

perineal p. A pad covering the perineum; used to cover a wound or to absorb the menstrual flow.

sucking p. A mass of fat in the cheeks, esp. well developed in an infant, aiding sucking. SYN: *fat p.* (1). SEE: *buccal fat pad*.

surgical p. A soft rubber pad with an apron and inflatable rim for drainage of escaping fluids; used in surgery and obstetrics.

paed-, paedo- SEE: *pedo-*.

PAF *platelet aggregating factor.*

Paget, Sir James (păj'ĕt) British surgeon, 1814–1899.

extramammary P.'s disease A plaque with a definite margin found in the anogenital area and in the axilla. It is a rare malignant disease and is treated by surgical excision.

mammary P.'s disease Carcinoma of the mammary ducts.

P.'s disease Osteitis deformans.

pagetoid (paj'ĕ-toyd) [*Paget* + Gr. *eidos,* form, shape] Similar to Paget's disease.

page turner An assistive device for persons with limited or absent upper extremity movement; used to turn the pages of a book.

pagophagia [Gr. *pagos,* frost, + *phagein,* to eat] A form of pica characterized by excessive consumption of ice or ice drinks. Causally associated with iron-deficiency anemia.

-pagus [Gr. *pagos,* thing fixed] A terminal combining form indicating twins joined together at the site indicated in the initial part of the word. SEE: *craniopagus*.

PAH, PAHA *para-aminohippuric acid.*

pain (pān) [L. *poena,* a fine, a penalty, punishment] As defined by the International Association for the Study of Pain, an unpleasant sensory and emotional experience arising from actual or potential tissue damage or described in terms of such damage. Pain includes not only the perception of an uncomfortable stimulus but also the response to that perception. Approx. one half of the persons who seek medical help do so because of the primary complaint of pain. Pain may arise in nearly any organ system and have different characteristics in each. Musculoskeletal pain often is exacerbated by movement and may be accompanied by joint swelling or muscle spasm. Myofascial pain is marked by trigger-point tenderness. Visceral pain often is diffuse or vaguely localized, whereas pain from the lining of body cavities often is localized precisely, very intense, and exquisitely sensitive to palpation or movement. Neuropathic pain usually stings or burns. Colicky pain fluctuates in intensity from severe to mild, and usually occurs in waves. Referred pain results when an injury or disease occurs in one body part but is felt in another.

Several factors influence the experience of pain. Among these are the nature of the injury or illness causing the symptom; the physical and emotional health of the patient; the acuity or chronicity of the symptom; the social milieu and/or cultural upbringing of the patient; neurochemistry; memory; personality; and other features. SEE: table.

SYMPTOMS: Many clinicians use the mnemonic "COLDER" to aid the diagnosis of painful diseases. They will ask the patient to describe the *C*haracter, *O*nset, *L*ocation, and *D*uration of their painful symptoms, as well as the features that *E*xacerbate or *R*elieve it. For example: The pain of pleurisy typically is sharp in character, acute in onset, located along the chest wall, and long-lasting; it is worsened by deep breathing

Usual Adult Doses and Intervals of Drugs for Relief of Pain

Nonopioid Analgesics

Generic Name	Dose, mg*	Interval	Comments
Acetylsalicylic acid	325–650	4–24 hr	Enteric-coated preparations available
Acetaminophen	650	4 hr	Avoid in liver failure
Ibuprofen	400–800	4–8 hr	Available without prescription
Indomethacin	25–75	8 hr	Gastrointestinal and kidney side effects common
Naproxen	250–500	12 hr	Delayed effects may be due to long half-life
Ketorolac	15–60 IM	4–6 hr	Similar to ibuprofen but more potent

Opioid Analgesics

Generic Name	Parenteral Dose (mg)	PO Dose (mg)	Comments
Codeine	30–60 every 4 hr	30–60 every 4 hr	Nausea common
Hydromorphone	1–2 every 4 hr	2–4 every 4 hr	Shorter acting than morphine sulfate
Levorphanol	2 every 6–8 hr	4 every 6 hr	Longer acting than morphine sulfate; absorbed well PO
Methadone	10–100	6–24 hr	Delayed sedation due to long half-life
Meperidine	25–100	300 every 4 hr	Poorly absorbed PO; normeperidine is a toxic metabolite
Morphine	10 every 4 hr	60 every 4 hr	
Morphine, sustained release	30–90	60–180 2 or 3 times daily	
Oxycodone	—	5–10 every 4–6 hr	Usually available with acetaminophen or aspirin

* By mouth unless indicated otherwise.

PO—by mouth only.

SOURCE: Adapted from Isselbacher, K.J., et al.: Harrison's Principles of Internal Medicine, ed 13. McGraw-Hill, New York, 1994.

or coughing, and relieved by analgesics or holding still. By contrast, the pain of myocardial ischemia usually is dull or heavy, gradual in onset, and located substernally. It may be worsened by activity (but not by taking a breath or coughing) and relieved by nitroglycerin.

PATIENT CARE: Because pain is a subjective and intensely personal problem, sympathetic care is an important part of its relief. In addition to administering analgesic drugs, health care professionals should use a wide range of techniques to help alleviate pain, including tactile stimulation, relaxation techniques, diversion, and active listening, among others.

acute p. Pain that typically is produced by sudden injury (e.g., fracture) or illness (e.g., acute infection) and is accompanied by physical signs such as increased heart rate, elevated blood pressure, pupillary dilation, sweating, or hyperventilation. Depending on the severity of the underlying stimulus, acute pain may be managed with acetaminophen or anti-inflammatory drugs, immobilization and elevation of the injured body part, or the topical application of heat or ice. Severe acute pain, such as that of broken ribs or of an ischemic part, may require narcotics, often with adjunctive agents like hydroxyzine for relief, or antiemetics. SEE: *Nursing Diagnoses Appendix.*

adnexal p. Discomfort arising from the fallopian tubes and ovaries; usually due to inflammation, infection, or ectopic pregnancy.

back p. Pain felt in or along the spine or musculature of the posterior thorax. It is usually characterized by dull, continuous pain and tenderness in the muscles or their attachments in the lower lumbar, lumbosacral, or sacroiliac regions. Pain is often referred to the leg, following the distribution of the sciatic nerve.

ETIOLOGY: Common causes of back pain include pain caused by muscular or tendon strain, herniated intervertebral disk, lumbar spinal stenosis, or spondylolisthesis. Patients with a history of cancer may have back pain caused by metastatic tumors to the vertebrae and should be evaluated to be certain that damage to the spinal cord is not imminent. Patients with back pain and fever (esp. those with a history of injection drug use, tuberculosis, or recent back surgery) should be evaluated for epidural abscess or osteomyelitis.

TREATMENT: Depending on the underlying cause of the back pain, treatment may include drugs, brief bedrest, massage, physical therapy, chiropractic, stretching exercises, surgery, and/or radiation. Most nonmalignant causes of back pain improve with a few days of rest, followed by 2 to 4 weeks of anti-inflammatory treatment, appropriate muscle strengthening, and patience. Pain caused by an osteoporotic fracture may prove more debilitating and longer-lasting. Back pain produced by a spinal metastasis can improve with radiation therapy, the use of which also decreases the likelihood of spinal cord compression and subsequent paralysis. Patients with a spinal epidural abscess will need surgical drainage of the infection and antibiotics.

PATIENT CARE: Prolonged bedrest is inadvisable in most patients with back pain. Local heat is applied as directed. The treatment regimen is explained, implemented, and reinforced. Factors that precipitate symptoms are identified and preventive actions are discussed.

bearing-down p. Rectal pressure and discomfort occurring during the second stage of labor, related to fetal descent and the woman's straining efforts to expel the fetus.

boring p. Pain deep in the tissues that gives the sensation of being produced by a boring instrument.

Brodie's p. Pain caused near a joint affected with neuralgia when the skin is folded near it.

burning p. Pain experienced in heat burns, superficial skin lesions, herpes zoster, and circumscribed neuralgias.

causalgic p. Causalgia.

central p. Pain due to a lesion in the central nervous system.

chest p. Discomfort felt in the upper abdomen, thorax, neck, or shoulders. Chest pain is one of the most common potentially serious complaints offered by patients in emergency departments, hospitals, and physicians' offices. A broad array of diseases and conditions may cause it, including (but not limited to) angina pectoris or myocardial infarction; anxiety and hyperventilation; aortic dissection; costochondritis or damaged ribs; cough, pneumonia, pleurisy, pneumothorax, or pulmonary emboli; esophageal diseases, such as reflux or esophagitis; gastritis, duodenitis, or peptic ulcer; and stones in the biliary tree.

chronic p. Long-lasting discomfort, with episodic exacerbations, that may be felt in the back, one or more joints, the pelvis, or other parts of the body. It is often described by sufferers as being intolerable, disabling, or alienating. Studies have shown a high correlation between chronic pain and depression or dysphoria, but it is unclear whether the psychological aspects of chronic pain precede or develop as a result of a person's subjective suffering. SEE: *acute p.; Nursing Diagnoses Appendix.*

PATIENT CARE: The management of chronic, nonmalignant pain is often difficult and may be frustrating for both sufferer and caregiver. The best results are usually obtained through multimodality therapy that combines sympathetic guidance with drugs (e.g., nonsteroidal anti-inflammatories, narcotic analgesics, and/or antidepressants), physical therapy, occupational therapy, physiatry, psychological or social counseling, and alternative medical therapies (e.g., acupuncture, massage, or relaxation techniques).

cramplike p. Cramp.

dental p. Pain in the oral area, which, in general, may be of two origins. Soft tissue pain may be acute or chronic, and a burning pain is due to surface lesions and usually can be discretely localized; pulpal pain or tooth pain varies according to whether it is acute or chronic, but it is often difficult to localize.

dilating p. Discomfort accompanying rhythmic uterine contractions during the first stage of labor.

dull p. A mild discomfort, often difficult to describe, that may be associated with some musculoskeletal injuries or some diseases of the visceral organs.

eccentric p. Pain occurring in peripheral structures owing to a lesion involving the posterior roots of the spinal nerves.

epigastric p. Pain located between the xiphoid process and the umbilicus. It may suggest a problem in one of many different organs, including the stomach, pancreas, gallbladder, small or large bowel, pleura, or heart. SYN: *gastralgic p.* SEE: *cardialgia.*

expulsive p. Discomfort during the second stage of labor, associated with bearing-down efforts to expel the fetus. Women may experience a similar pain during delivery of the placenta.

false p. Abdominal discomfort associated with Braxton Hicks contractions, which occur during the last trimester of pregnancy. Characteristically, the woman complains of irregular, lower abdominal pains, which are relieved by walking. Vaginal examination shows no change in cervical effacement or dilation. SEE: *Braxton Hicks contractions.*

fulgurant p. Lightning p.

gallbladder p. Biliary colic.

gas p. Pain in the intestines caused by an accumulation of gas therein.

gastralgic p. Epigastric p.

girdle p. Zonesthesia.

growing p. An imprecise term indicating ill-defined pain, usually in the shin or other areas of the legs, typically occurring after bedtime in children age 5 to 12. There is no evidence that the pain is related to rapid growth or to emotional problems. If these symptoms occur during the daytime, are accompanied with other symptoms, or become progressively more severe, evaluation for infection, cancer, and other diseases of muscle and bone should be undertaken. In the majority of cases, this evaluation is not necessary.

TREATMENT: The child should be reassured and given acetaminophen or ibuprofen; heat and massage can be applied locally. Children with growing pains benefit from concern and reassurance from their parents and health care providers.

heterotopic p. Referred p.

homotopic p. Pain felt at the point of injury.

hunger p. Pain in the epigastrum that occurs before meals.

inflammatory p. Pain in the presence of inflammation that is increased by pressure.

intermenstrual p. Episodic, localized pelvic discomfort that occurs between menstrual periods, possibly accompanying ovulation. SYN: *midpain*. SEE: *mittelschmerz*.

intractable p. Chronic pain that is difficult or impossible to manage with standard interventions. Common causes include metastatic cancer, chronic pancreatitis, radiculopathy, spinal cord transection, or peripheral neuropathy. Intractable pain may also accompany somatoform disorders, depression, fibromyalgia, irritable bowel syndrome, and opiate dependence. Various combinations of the following management strategies are often used to treat intractable pain: antidepressant medications, counseling, deep brain stimulation, injected anesthetics, narcotic analgesics, neurological surgery, and pain clinic consultations.

labor p. Uncomfortable, intermittent, rhythmic, girdling sensations associated with uterine contractions during childbearing. The frequency, duration, and intensity of the events increase, climaxing with the delivery of the fetus.

lancinating p. Acute p.

lightning p. A sudden brief pain that may be repetitive, usually in the legs but may be at any location. It is associated with tabes dorsalis and other neurological disorders. SYN: *fulgurant p.*

lingual p. Pain in the tongue that may be due to local lesions, glossitis, fissures, or pernicious anemia. SYN: *tongue p.*

lung p. Sharp pain in the region of the lungs.

menstrual p. Dysmenorrhea.

mental p. Psychogenic p.

middle p. Intermenstrual p.

mobile p. Pain that moves from one area to another.

movement p. Kinesalgia.

neuropathic p. Pain that originates in nerves themselves rather than in other damaged organs that are innervated by them. A hallmark of neuropathic pain is its localization to specific dermatomes or nerve distributions. Some examples of neuropathic pain are the pain of shingles (herpes zoster), diabetic neuropathy, radiculopathy, and phantom limb pain.

TREATMENT: Gabapentin provides effective relief of neuropathic pain for many patients. Other treatments include (but are not limited to) regional nerve blocks, tricyclic antidepressants, acupuncture, transcutaneous electrical nerve stimulation, and physical therapy.

night p. Pain that awakens the patient at night or interferes with sleep; may be due to infection, inflammation, neurovascular compromise, or severe structural damage.

noise p. Odynacusis.

objective p. Pain induced by some external or internal irritant, by inflammation, or by injury to nerves, organs, or other tissues that interferes with the function, nutrition, or circulation of the affected part. It is usually traceable to a definite pathologic process.

paresthesic p. A stinging or tingling sensation manifested in central and peripheral nerve lesions. SEE: *paresthesia*.

periodontal p. A discrete, well-localized pain caused by inflammation of tissues surrounding a tooth. This may be contrasted with the throbbing, nonlocalized pain typical of a toothache or pulpal pain.

phantom limb p. The sensation of pain felt in the nerve distribution of a body part that has been amputated. Severe phantom pain can lead to difficulties in prosthetic training. SYN: *phantom sensation*.

postprandial p. Abdominal pain after eating.

precordial p. Pain felt in the center of the chest (e.g., below the sternum) or in the left side of the chest.

premonitory p. Ineffective contractions of the uterus before the beginning of true labor. SEE: *false p.*

pseudomyelic p. The false sensation of movement in a paralyzed limb or of no movement in a moving limb; not a true pain.

psychogenic p. Pain having mental, as opposed to organic, origin.

referred p. Pain that arises in one body part or location but is perceived in another. For example, pain caused by inflammation of the diaphragm often is felt in the shoulder; pain caused by myocardial ischemia may be referred to the neck or jaw; and pain caused by appendicitis may first be felt near the umbilicus rather than in the right lower quadrant, where the appendix lies. SYN: *heterotopic p.; sympathetic p.*

remittent p. Pain with temporary abatements in severity; characteristic of neuralgia and colic.

rest p. Pain due to ischemia that comes on when sitting or lying.

root p. Cutaneous pain caused by disease of the sensory nerve roots.

shooting p. Pain that seems to travel like lightning from one place to another.

standards for p. relief Standards for the Relief of Acute Pain and Cancer Pain developed by the American Pain Society. These are summarized as follows:

1. In order to increase the clinician's responsiveness to complaints of pain, it is now considered by some health care professionals to be the fifth vital sign.

2. Acute pain and cancer pain are recognized and effectively treated. Essential to this process is the development of a clinically useful and easy-to-use scale for rating pain and its relief. Patients will be evaluated according to the scales and the results recorded as frequently as needed.

3. Information about analgesics is readily available. This includes data concerning the effectiveness of various agents in controlling pain and the availability of equianalgesic charts wherever drugs are used for pain.

4. Patients are informed on admission of the availability of methods of relieving pain, and that they must communicate the presence and persistence of pain to the health care staff.

5. Explicit policies for use of advanced analgesic technologies are defined. These advances include patient-controlled analgesia, epidural analgesia, and regional analgesia. Specific instructions concerning use of these techniques must be available for the health care staff.

6. Adherence to standards is monitored by an interdisciplinary committee. The committee is responsible for overseeing the activities related to implementing and evaluating the effectiveness of these pain standards. In 1999 the Joint Commission on the Accreditation of Healthcare Organizations published a revision of these standards. These are available on the Internet at www.jcaho.org.

starting p. A pain accompanied by muscular spasm during the early stages of sleep.

subdiaphragmatic p. A sharp stitch-like pain occurring during breathing caused, for example, by an abscess or tumor beneath the diaphragm. When the breath is held, the pain ceases. Pressure against the lower rib cage eases the pain.

subjective p. Psychogenic p.

sympathetic p. Referred p.

tenesmic p. Tenesmus.

terebrant p. A boring or piercing type of pain.

thalamic p. SEE: *thalamic syndrome.*

thermalgesic p. Pain caused by heat.

thoracic p. Chest pain.

throbbing p. Pain found in dental caries, headache, and localized inflammation.

tongue p. Lingual p.

tracheal p. Trachealgia.

vascular p. Pain that throbs or pulses, such as the pain of a migraine headache.

wandering p. Pain that changes its location repeatedly.

painful arc During active movement of an extremity, a portion of the range of motion in which pain is perceived. Pain is usually due to pinching of soft tissues at only a specific portion of the range of motion. A painful arc may be caused by tendinitis or bursitis.

paint (pānt) **1.** A solution of medication for application to the skin. **2.** To apply a medicated liquid to the skin.

painters' colic Colic accompanying lead poisoning. SEE: *lead* in *Poisons and Poisoning Appendix.*

pair Two of anything similar in shape, size, and conformation.

base p. In the double-stranded helical arrangement of DNA, the purine bases (i.e., base pairs) that are either an adenine-thymine pair or a guanine-cytosine pair. These base pairs connect the helical strands of DNA like the steps of a spiral staircase.

ion p. Two particles of opposite charge, usually an electron and a proton.

PAL *posterior axillary line.*

palatable (păl′ăt-ă-b'l) [L. *palatum,* palate] Pleasing to the palate or taste, as food.

palatal (păl′ă-tăl) Pert. to the roof of the mouth, the palate.

palate (păl′ăt) [L. *palatum,* palate] The horizontal structure separating the mouth and the nasal cavity; the roof of the mouth, supported anteriorly by the maxillae and palatine bones. SEE: *mouth* for illus.

DIFFERENTIAL DIAGNOSIS: *Koplik's*

spots: This rash is frequently seen on the palate in measles. *Secondary syphilis:* This is indicated by mucous patches on the palate. *Herpes of the throat:* This is characterized by vesicles on the pharyngeal walls and soft palate. *Swelling of uvula:* This is noted in inflammations of pharynx and tonsil, in nephritis, severe anemia, and angioneurotic edema. In diphtheria and Vincent's angina, a membranous exudate appears. In some hemorrhagic diatheses, bloody extravasation appears. *Kaposi's sarcoma:* Dark purplish-red lesions may be found on the hard and soft palate. *Paralysis:* This may result from diphtheria, bulbar paralysis, neuritis, basal meningitis, or a tumor at the base of the brain. *Anesthesia:* This is seen in pathological conditions of the second division of the fifth nerve.

artificial p. A prosthetic device molded to fill a cleft in the palate.

bony p. Hard p.

cleft p. A congenital fissure in the roof of the mouth forming a communicating passageway between mouth and nasal cavities. It may be unilateral or bilateral and complete or incomplete.

gothic p. An excessively high palatal arch.

hard p. The anterior part of the palate supported by the maxillary and palatine bones. SYN: *bony p.*

incomplete p. A cleft involving only a part of the hard or soft palate.

pendulous p. Uvula.

primary p. In the embryo, the partition between the nasal cavities and mouth.

secondary p. In the embryo, the palate formed from the maxillary arches and frontonasal processes.

soft p. The posterior musculomembranous fold partly separating the mouth and pharynx. It elevates during swallowing to block the nasopharynx. SYN: *velum palatinum*.

palate bone Palatine bone.

palatiform (pă-lăt′ĭ-form) [L. *palatum,* palate, + *forma,* form] Resembling the palate.

palatine (păl′ă-tīn) [L. *palatinus*] **1.** Concerning the palate. **2.** The palate bones.

palatine arches Two archlike folds of mucous membrane (glossopalatine and pharyngopalatine arches) that form the lateral margins of faucial and pharyngeal isthmuses. They are continuous above with the soft palate.

palatine artery, greater The branch of the maxillary artery that supplies the palate, upper pharynx, and auditory tube.

palatine bone One of the bones forming the posterior part of the hard palate and lateral nasal wall between the interior pterygoid plate of the sphenoid bone and maxilla. SYN: *palate bone.*

palatitis (păl-ăt-ī′tĭs) [L. *palatum,* palate, + Gr. *itis,* inflammation] Inflammation of the palate.

palatoglossal (păl″ă-tō-glŏs′ăl) Concerning the palate and tongue.

palatoglossus (păl″ă-tō-glŏs′ŭs) [″ + Gr. *glossa,* tongue] The muscle arising from the sides and undersurface of the tongue. Fibers pass upward through glossopalatine arch and are inserted in palatine aponeurosis. It constricts the faucial isthmus by raising the root of the tongue and drawing the sides of the soft palate downward.

palatognathous (păl″ă-tŏg′nă-thŭs) [″ + Gr. *gnathos,* jaw] Having a congenital cleft in the palate.

palatography (păl″ă-tŏg′ră-fē) [″ + Gr. *graphein,* to write] **1.** Recording of the movements of the palate in speech. **2.** Radiographical examination of the soft palate after injection of a contrast medium.

palatomaxillary (păl″ă-tō-măk′sĭ-lĕr″ē) Concerning the palate and maxilla.

palatopharyngeal (păl″ă-tō-fă-rĭn′jē-ăl) Concerning the palate and pharynx.

palatopharyngeus (păl″ăt-ō-fă″rĭn′jē-ŭs) [″ + Gr. *pharynx,* throat] The muscle arising from thyroid cartilage and pharyngeal wall, extending upward in posterior pillar, and inserting into aponeurosis of soft palate. It constricts the pharyngeal isthmus, raises the larynx, and depresses the soft palate.

palatopharyngoplasty Plastic surgical procedure for decreasing the size of the opening of the nasopharyngeal passageway. It has been used to treat chronic snoring.

palatoplasty (păl′ăt-ō-plăs″tē) [″ + Gr. *plassein,* to form] Plastic surgery of the palate, usually to correct a cleft. SEE: *staphylorrhaphy*.

palatoplegia (păl″ă-tō-plē′jē-ă) [″ + Gr. *plege,* stroke] Paralysis of muscles of the soft palate. SEE: *palate*.

palatorrhaphy (păl-ă-tor′ă-fē) [″ + Gr. *rhaphe,* seam, ridge] An operation for uniting a cleft palate. SYN: *staphylorrhaphy*.

palatosalpingeus (păl″ă-tō-săl-pĭn′jē-ŭs) [″ + Gr. *salpinx,* tube] The tensor veli palatini muscle.

palatoschisis (păl-ă-tŏs′kĭ-sĭs) [″ + *schisis,* a splitting] Palate with a cleft in it.

palatum (păl-ă′tŭm) *pl.* **palata** [L.] Palate.

paleencephalon, paleoencephalon (pā″lē-ĕn-sĕf′ă-lŏn, -ō-ĕn-sĕf′ă-lŏn) [Gr. *palaios,* old, + *enkephalos,* brain] The phylogenetically older portion of the brain; includes all of it except the cerebral cortex and its allied structures.

paleocerebellum (păl″ē-ō-sĕr″ĕ-bĕl′ŭm) [Gr. *palaios,* old, + L. *cerebellum,* little brain] Phylogenetically, the older portion of the cerebellum including the flocculi, certain parts of the vermis (lingula, nodulus, uvula), and the lobulus centralis (culmen, pyramis, uvula, and simple lobule). These parts are concerned primarily with equilibrium and coordination of locomotion.

paleogenesis (pā″lē-ō-jĕn′ĕ-sĭs) [″ + *genesis,* generation, birth] Atavism.

paleogenetic (pā″lē-ō-jĕn-ĕt′ĭk) [″ + *gennan,* to produce] Originating in a previous generation.

paleokinetic (pā″lē-ō-kĭ-nĕt′ĭk) [″ + *kinetikos,* concerning movement] Regarding a peripheral motor nervous system controlling automatic associated movements. It is older phylogenetically than the system controlling voluntary movement.

paleontology (pā″lē-ŏn-tŏl′ō-jē) [″ + *onta,* existing things, + *logos,* word, reason] The branch of biology dealing with ancient plant and animal life of the earth.

paleopathology (pā″lē-ō-pă-thŏl′ō-jē) [″ + *pathos,* disease, + *logos,* word, reason] The study of diseases in the remains of bodies and fossils of ancient times.

paleostriatal (pā″lē-ō-strī-ā′tăl) [″ + L. *striatus,* ridged] Concerning the primitive portion of the corpus striatum.

paleostriatum (pā″lē-ō-strī-ā′tŭm) The primitive portion of corpus striatum, the globus pallidus. SEE: *neostriatum.*

paleothalamus (pā″lē-ō-thăl′ă-mŭs) [″ + *thalamos,* chamber] The medial portion of the thalamus (the medullary or noncortical part), which is older phylogenetically. SEE: *thalamus.*

pali-, palin- [Gr. *palin,* backward, again] Prefix meaning *recurrence, repetition.*

palilalia (păl-ĭ-lā′lē-ă) [″ + *lalein,* to speak] Involuntary repetition of words or phrases.

palindromia (păl-ĭn-drō′mē-ă) [″ + *dromos,* a running] The recurrence of a disease or a relapse.

palindromic (păl-ĭn-drŏm′ĭk) Relapsing.

palinesthesia (păl″ĭn-ĕs-thē′zē-ă) [Gr. *palin,* again, + *aisthesis,* sensation] The return of the power of sensation, as after recovery from anesthesia or coma.

palingenesis (păl″ĭn-jĕn′ĕ-sĭs) [″ + *genesis,* generation, birth] **1.** Regeneration or restoration of an organism or part of one. **2.** Atavism.

palingraphia (păl″ĭn-grăf′ē-ă) [″ + *graphein,* to write] Pathologic repetition of words or phrases in writing.

palinopsia [″ + *opsis,* vision] Persistence of a visual image after the object has been removed. It may be associated with a lesion in the occipital lobe of the brain. SEE: *afterimage.*

palladium (pă-lā′dē-ŭm) [L.] SYMB: Pd. A metallic element used in dentistry and surgical instruments; atomic weight 106.4; atomic number 46.

pallesthesia (păl-ĕs-thē′zē-ă) [Gr. *pallein,* to shake, + *aisthesis,* sensation] The sensation of vibration felt in the skin or bones, as that produced by a tuning fork held against the body.

palliate (păl′ē-āt) [L. *palliatus,* cloaked] To ease or reduce effect or intensity, esp. of a disease; to allay temporarily, as pain, without curing.

palliative (păl′ē-ā″tĭv) **1.** Relieving or alleviating without curing. **2.** An agent that alleviates or eases a painful or uncomfortable condition.

pallid (păl′ĭd) [L. *pallidus,* pale] Lacking color, pale, wan.

pallidal (păl′ĭ-dăl) Concerning the pallidum of the brain.

pallidectomy (păl″ĭ-dĕk′tō-mē) [L. *pallidum,* pallidum, + Gr. *ektome,* excision] Surgical, chemical, electrical, or cryogenic removal or inactivation of the globus pallidus of the brain.

pallidoansotomy (păl″ĭ-dō-ăn-sŏt′ō-mē) [″ + *ansa,* a handle, + Gr. *tome,* incision] Production of lesions in the globus pallidus and ansa lenticularis of the brain.

pallidotomy (păl″ĭ-dŏt′ō-mē) [″ + Gr. *tome,* incision] Surgical destruction of the globus pallidus done to treat involuntary movements or muscular rigidity. The procedure is used experimentally in treating patients with Parkinson's disease.

pallidum (păl′ĭ-dŭm) [L.] The globus pallidus of the lenticular nucleus in the corpus striatum.

pallium (păl′ē-ŭm) [L., cloak] The cerebral cortex and its adjacent white matter.

pallor (păl′or) [L.] Lack of color; paleness. SEE: *skin.*

palm [L. *palma,* hand] The anterior or flexor surface of the hand from the wrist to the fingers. SYN: *palma; vola manus.* SEE: *antithenar; thenar.*

palma (păl′mă) [L.] Palm.

palmar (păl′măr) Concerning the palm of the hand.

p. cuff SEE: *universal cuff.*

palmaris (păl-mā′rĭs) One of two muscles, palmaris brevis and palmaris longus.

palmature (păl′mă-tūr) [L. *palma,* hand] A pathological condition in which the fingers are joined or united.

palmitin (păl′mĭ-tĭn) An ester of glycerol and palmitic acid, derived from fat of both animal and vegetable origin.

palmoplantar (păl″mō-plăn′tăr) Pert. to the palms of the hands and soles of the feet.

palmus (păl′mŭs) [Gr. *palmos,* pulsation, quivering] **1.** Palpitation; a throb. **2.** Jerking; a disease with convulsive nervous twitching of the leg muscles, similar to jumping. **3.** Heartbeat.

palpable (păl′pă-b′l) [L. *palpabilis,* stroke, touch] Perceptible, esp. by touch.

palpate (păl′pāt) [L. *palpare,* to touch] To examine by touch; to feel.

palpation (păl-pā′shŭn) [L. *palpatio*] **1.** Examination by application of the hands or fingers to the external surface of the body to detect evidence of disease or abnormalities in the internal organs. **2.** In obstetrics, a technique used to evaluate fetal presentation and position; frequency, duration, and strength of uterine contractions; status of membranes; cervical effacement and dilation; and fetal station.

light-touch p. The process of determining the outline of abdominal organs by lightly palpating the abdominal wall with the fingers.

palpatopercussion (păl″pă-tō-pĕr-kŭsh′ŭn) Palpation combined with percussion.

palpebra (păl′pĕ-bră) *pl.* **palpebrae** [L.] An eyelid.

p. inferior The lower eyelid.

p. superior The upper eyelid.

palpebral (păl′pĕ-brăl) Concerning an eyelid.

palpebral cartilage One of the thin plates of connective tissue resembling cartilage that form the framework of the eyelid. SYN: *tarsal cartilage.*

palpebral commissure The union of the eyelids at each end of the palpebral fissure.

palpebral muscles **1.** Palpebral portion of the orbicularis oculi. **2.** Levator palpebrae superioris.

palpitate (păl′pĭ-tāt) [L. *palpitatus,* throbbing] **1.** To cause to throb. **2.** To throb or beat intensely or rapidly, usually said of the heart.

palpitation (păl-pĭ-tā′shŭn) A sensation of rapid or irregular beating of the heart. The beating may be described as a thudding sensation, a fluttering, or a throbbing that is felt beneath the sternum or in the neck. In clinical practice, most palpitations are felt by patients with benign premature ventricular or atrial contractions. In these patients, the sensation, although disturbing, is not associated with serious heart disease. Occasionally palpitations are caused by sustained arrhythmias, such as atrial fibrillation, atrial flutter, paroxysmal supraventricular tachycardia, or ventricular tachycardia. Electrocardiography, outpatient cardiac monitoring, or cardiology consultation may be needed to determine whether a patient's symptoms are benign or hazardous. SEE: *heart.* **palpitant,** *adj.*

arterial p. Palpitation felt in the course of an artery.

PALS *pediatric advanced life support.*

palsy (pawl′zē) [ME. *palesie,* from L. *paralysis*] Paralysis.

birth p. Palsy arising from an injury received at birth.

brachial p. In newborns, unilateral partial or total paralysis of the arm related to trauma to the brachial plexus during delivery. The extent of paralysis is determined by the nerve roots involved.

bulbar p. Palsy caused by degeneration of the nuclear cells of the lower cranial nerves. This causes progressive muscular paralysis.

cerebral p. ABBR: CP. An "umbrella" term for a group of nonprogressive, but often changing, motor impairment syndromes secondary to lesions or anomalies of the brain arising in the early stages of its development. CP is a symptom complex rather than a specific disease. For the vast majority of children born at term in whom CP later develops, the disorder cannot reasonably be ascribed to birth injury or hypoxic-ischemic insults during delivery. CP rarely occurs without associated defects such as mental retardation (60% of cases) or epilepsy (50% of cases).

Risk factors have been divided into three groups: those occurring prior to pregnancy, such as an unusually short interval (less than 3 months) or unusually long interval since the previous pregnancy; those occurring during pregnancy, including physical malformations, twin gestation, abnormal fetal presentation, fetal growth retardation, or maternal hypothyroidism; and perinatal factors such as prematurity, premature separation of the placenta, or newborn encephalopathy. Of infants with one or more of these risk factors, 95% do not have CP.

The disorder is classified by the extremities involved and the type of neurological dysfunction, such as spastic, hypotonic, dystonic, athetotic, or a combination of these. It is not possible to diagnose CP in the neonatal period, and early clinical diagnosis is complicated by the changing pattern of the disease in the first year of life.

All infants and children, especially those with risk conditions for cerebral palsy (CP), are assessed for delays in attaining developmental milestones. This type of assessment can provide valuable clues to recognizing CP. Early recognition and promotion of optimal development assist the child to realize his or her potential within the limits of dysfunction.

TREATMENT: Therapy is directed to maximizing function and preventing secondary handicaps. Essential to the outcome of patients with CP is establishing good hand function, which will help compensate for other motor deficits. Broad therapeutic goals include establishing locomotion, communication, and self help; gaining optimum appearance and integration of motor functions; correcting associated deficits as effectively as possible; and providing educational opportunities adapted to the individual child's needs and capabilities. Antianxiety agents may be employed to relieve excessive motion and tension. Skeletal muscle relaxants may be given on a short-term basis for older children and adolescents. Anticonvulsants may provide relief for children experiencing seizure activity, and dextroamphetamine may improve performance in hyperactive, dyskinetic children. SEE: *Nursing Diagnoses Appendix.*

PATIENT CARE: The individualized therapeutic plan usually involves a variety of settings, facilities, and specially trained personnel, including the parents, who are taught to handle their child's condition properly. A specially trained physical therapist designs an individualized program of exercises and other treatment modalities to meet the child's specific problems and needs and to stimulate the child to achieve functional goals. A speech therapist is an important team member, initiating speech training early, before the child develops poor communication habits. Eye and ear specialists deal with visual and auditory deficits. Dental care is especially important, and should start as soon as teeth erupt. Braces and other mobilizing devices are used to help prevent or reduce deformities, control alignment, and permit self-propulsion. An orthopedic surgeon intervenes when spasticity causes progressive deformities. Nurses in pediatric facilities and community settings are involved in all aspects of therapeutic management, and provide support and encouragement. They teach the child (as appropriate) and the parents about the desired and adverse effects of any medications used in the therapeutic regimen.

A wide variety of technical aids are available to help improve the child's function. They include electromechanical toys, microcomputers, voice synthesizers, and other devices the child can control. Passive range of motion, stretching, and elongation exercises are valuable at any age. Training in ADLs and manual skills is based on the child's developmental level and functional abilities. Hand activities are started early to improve the child's motor function and to provide sensory experiences and environmental information. Play is incorporated into the therapeutic program.

The child's needs and potential determine his or her educational requirements, which range from attendance at regular school to special classes or facilities designed to meet his or her needs. The teaching team develops an individual educational prescription (IEP) which they communicate to parents and any others involved in the child's learning. Special Olympics and other community programs can enable the child to participate in competitive sports, adding an extra dimension to physical activities. The child also should be encouraged to participate in artistic programs, games, and other activities. A most valuable intervention on the part of health care professionals is providing the family with emotional support, helping them to cope with the disorder and to connect with other families. Parent groups share concerns and problems and provide practical information, as well as comfort. United Cerebral Palsy Association Inc. provides a variety of services for children with CP and their families; it can be accessed through a local telephone directory or health department.

Throughout treatment, health care providers and the child's family continually reassess and evaluate the child's status by observing movements and speech, self-care and other activities, school attendance and performance, interactions with others and choice of activities, and behaviors and responses to challenges. The child and family are interviewed regularly about their feelings and concerns and are supported to cope with the condition.

crutch p. Paralysis resulting from pressure on nerves in the axilla from use of a crutch.

diver's p. Bends.

Erb's p. Erb's paralysis.

facial p. Bell's palsy.

lead p. Paralysis of the extremities in lead poisoning.

mercurial p. Paralysis induced by mercury poisoning.

night p. A form of paresthesia characterized by numbness, esp. at night.

peroneal nerve p. Paralysis of the peroneal nerve, often caused by automobile accidents in which a pedestrian's leg is injured, by fractures of the tibia, or by other causes of nerve disruption or compression. It produces footdrop.

pressure p. Temporary paralysis due to pressure on a nerve trunk.

progressive supranuclear p. A chronic progressive degenerative disease of the central nervous system that has its onset in middle age. Conjugate ocular palsies, dystonia of the neck, and widespread rigidity occur.

Saturday night p. Musculospiral paralysis.

scrivener's p. Writer's cramp.

shaking p. An archaic term for Parkinson's disease.

wasting p. Progressive muscular atrophy.

palynology [Gr. *palumein,* to sprinkle, + *logos,* word, reason] The study of pollens, spores, or microscopic segments of organisms present in sediments.

pamidronate disodium A drug used to treat hypercalcemia associated with malignancy, with or without bone metastases, and moderate to severe Paget's disease. In the U.S., it is approved for intravenous use.

CAUTION: This drug should not be mixed with calcium-containing solutions such as Ringer's solution.

pampiniform (păm-pĭn'ĭ-form) [L. *pampinus,* tendril, + *forma,* shape] Convoluted like a tendril.

pan- [Gr.] Combining form indicating *all.*

panacea (păn-ă-sē'ă) [Gr. *panakeia,* universal remedy] A remedy for all ills; a cure-all.

panagglutinable (păn"ă-gloo'tĭ-nă-b'l) [Gr. *pan,* all, + L. *agglutinare,* to glue to] Referring to blood cells that are agglutinable by every blood group serum of the species.

panagglutinin (păn"ă-glū'tĭn-ĭn) [Gr. *pan,* all, + L. *agglutinare,* to glue to] A substance capable of agglutinizing corpuscles of every blood group.

panangiitis (păn"ăn-jē-ī'tĭs) [" + *angeion,* vessel, + *itis,* inflammation] Inflammation of all three layers of a blood vessel (intima, media, and adventitia).

panaris (păn'ă-rĭs) [L. *panaricium,* disease of the fingernail] Paronychia.

panarteritis (păn"ăr-tĕ-rī'tĭs) [Gr. *pan,* all, + *arteria,* artery, + *itis,* inflammation] Inflammation of all three layers of an artery (intima, media, and adventitia).

panarthritis (păn"ăr-thrī'tĭs) [" + *arthron,* joint, + *itis,* inflammation] **1.** Inflammation of all parts of a joint. **2.** Inflammation of all or most of the joints of the body.

panasthenia (păn"ăs-thē'nē-ă) [" + *astheneia,* weakness] Neurasthenia.

panatrophy (păn-ăt'rō-fē) [" + *a-,* not, + *trophe,* nourishment] Localized or generalized wasting away.

panblastic (păn-blăs'tĭk) [" + *blastos,* germ] Concerning all the layers of the blastoderm.

pancarditis (păn-kăr-dī'tĭs) [" + *kardia,* heart, + *itis,* inflammation] Inflammation of all the structures of the heart.

Pancoast's syndrome [Henry Khunrath Pancoast, U.S. physician, 1875–1939] A cluster of signs and symptoms that include: (1) upper extremity or shoulder pain; (2) Horner's syndrome; and (3) atrophy of muscle or bone of the affected arm. It almost always is caused by a malignant neoplasm invading the brachial plexus and cervical sympathetic nerves. Rarely, it results from a tubercular or fungal infection of the same nerves.

Pancoast's tumor [Henry Khunrath Pancoast, U.S. physician, 1875–1939] A tumor (usually from lung cancer) that spreads from the superior pulmonary sulcus into the brachial plexus and cervical sympathetic chain, producing Pancoast's syndrome.

pancolectomy (păn"kō-lĕk'tō-mē) [Gr. *pan,* all, + *kolon,* colon, + *ektome,* excision] Surgical excision of the entire colon.

pancreas (păn'krē-ăs) *pl.* **pancreata** [" + *kreas,* flesh] A compound acinotubular gland located behind the stomach and in front of the first and second lumbar vertebrae. The head lies within the curve of the duodenum, the tail lies near the spleen, and the middle portion constitutes the body. The pancreas is both an exocrine and an endocrine organ. The exocrine glands are acini, each with its own duct; these ducts anastomose to form the main pancreatic duct or duct of Wirsung, which joins the common bile duct and empties into the duodenum at the hepatopancreatic ampulla. An accessory pancreatic duct or duct of Santorini is often present and opens into the duodenum directly. Scattered throughout the exocrine glandular tissue are masses of cells called islets of Langerhans, endocrine glands that secrete hormones. SEE: illus.

FUNCTION: The exocrine secretion of the pancreas consists of powerful enzymes, which contribute to the digestion of all food types in the small intestine. SEE: *pancreatic juice.*

The islets of Langerhans contain alpha, beta, and delta cells. Alpha cells secrete glucagon, which raises blood glucose; beta cells secrete insulin, which lowers blood glucose; delta cells secrete somatostatin, which inhibits the secretion of insulin, glucagon, growth hormone from the anterior pituitary, and gastrin from the stomach.

DISEASES OF THE PANCREAS: Autoimmune damage to the islets of Langerhans results in type 1 diabetes mellitus, a disease in which insulin secretion is insufficient or completely absent. Insulin-secreting tumors of the pancreas, called insulinomas, produce hypoglycemia; they are exceptionally rare. Inflammation of the pancreas, known as pancreatitis, is a common condition that often results from excessive use of alcohol or from obstruction of the exocrine secretions of the pancreas by gallstones. Pancreas divisum is a common congenital anomaly in which the main duct of the exocrine pancreas drains into an accessory pancreatic papilla instead of the duodenal papilla; it has been associated with recurring episodes of pancreatitis. SEE: *diabetes mellitus; insulin; pancreatic function test.*

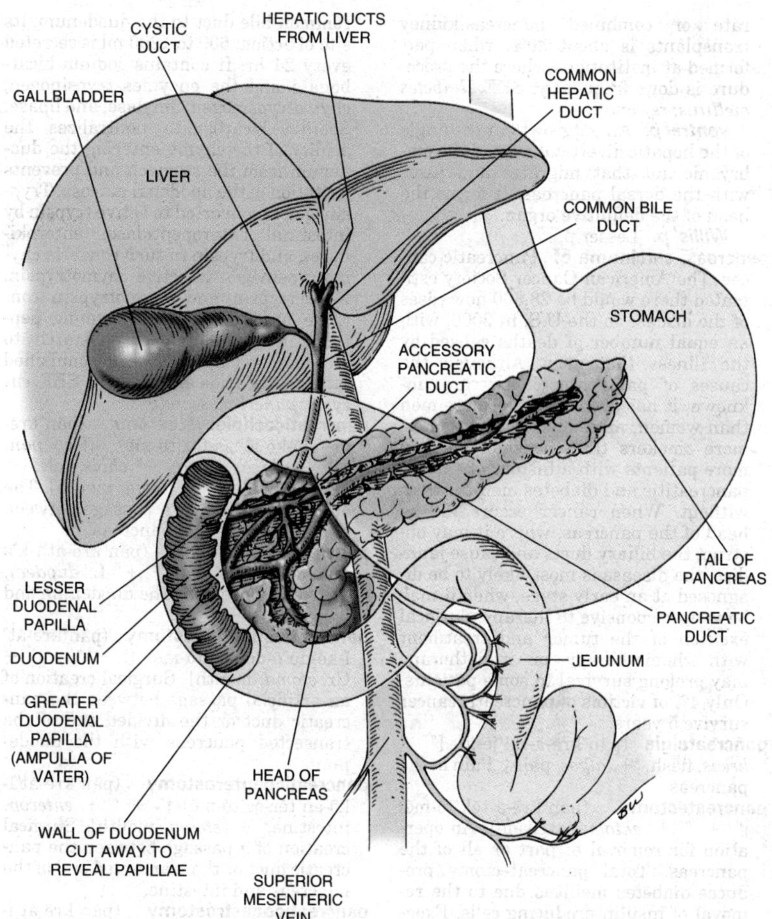

PANCREAS AND ITS RELATIONSHIP TO THE DUODENUM

accessory p. A small mass of pancreatic tissue close to the pancreas but detached from it.

annular p. An anomalous condition in which a portion of the pancreas encircles the duodenum.

p. divisum A congenital anomaly in which the dorsal and ventral pancreatic ducts fail to unite during embryonic development. It has been associated with pancreatitis.

dorsal p. A dorsal outpocketing of the embryonic gut that gives rise to the body and tail of the adult pancreas.

lesser p. The semidetached lobular part of the posterior surface of a head of the pancreas, sometimes having a separate duct opening into the principal one. SYN: *Willis' p.*

transplantation of the p. The implantation of a part of the pancreas (e.g., cells of the islets of Langerhans) or the entire gland from a donor into a patient whose own pancreas is no longer functioning. In the diabetic patient, pancreas transplantation provides an endogenous source of insulin and may be combined with kidney transplantation. The risks of the surgery and the immunosuppression associated with transplantation must be weighed against the kidney, nerve, and retinal damage associated with uncontrolled diabetes mellitus. Some potential complications of the procedure include infections, blood clotting in the vessels that supply the graft, hypoglycemia, bladder injury, and organ rejection. To prevent rejection, immunosuppressive drugs, such as tacrolimus, mycophenolate mofetil, cyclosporine, and corticosteroids, may be used. Episodes of rejection are treated with the monoclonal antibody OKT3. The 1-year survival rate of combined pancreas-kidney transplants is about 80%, when performed at institutions where the procedure is done frequently. SEE: *diabetes mellitus; rejection*.

ventral p. An outgrowth at the angle of the hepatic diverticulum and the embryonic gut that migrates and fuses with the dorsal pancreas. It forms the head of the definitive organ.

Willis' p. Lesser p.

pancreas, carcinoma of Pancreatic cancer. The American Cancer Society estimated there would be 28,300 new cases of the disease in the U.S. in 2000, with an equal number of deaths caused by the illness that year. Although the causes of pancreatic cancer are unknown, it has been found in more men than women, more blacks than whites, more smokers than nonsmokers, and more patients with a history of chronic pancreatitis and diabetes mellitus than without. When cancer occurs in the head of the pancreas, where it may obstruct the biliary ducts and cause jaundice, the disease is most likely to be diagnosed at an early stage, when it may be most responsive to therapy. Surgical excision of the tumor and treatment with chemotherapy or radiotherapy may prolong survival in some patients. Only 4% of victims of pancreatic cancer survive 5 years.

pancreatalgia (păn″krē-ă-tăl′jē-ă) [″ + *kreas,* flesh, + *algos,* pain] Pain in the pancreas.

pancreatectomy (păn″krē-ă-tĕk′tō-mē) [″ + ″ + *ektome,* excision] An operation for removal of part or all of the pancreas. Total pancreatectomy produces diabetes mellitus due to the removal of insulin-producing cells. Exogenous insulin must be administered. After a subtotal (or partial) pancreatectomy, diabetes may develop some time later because the remaining islets may be unable to take care of the increased demands placed on them. SEE: *diabetes.*

pancreatic (păn″krē-ăt′ĭk) [Gr. *pan,* all, + *kreas,* flesh] Concerning the pancreas.

pancreatic function test A test for the exocrine function of the pancreas (i.e., production of pancreatic juice) involving stimulation of the pancreas and measurement of the enzymes present in the duodenal contents obtained from a tube inserted per os into the duodenum. The endocrine function may be tested by the ability of the pancreas to secrete insulin in response to the intake of glucose.

pancreatic juice A clear, viscid, alkaline fluid (pH 8.4 to 8.9); its secretion is stimulated by two hormones, secretin and cholecystokinin, produced by the duodenal mucosa. Pancreatic juice flows through the main pancreatic duct to the common bile duct to the duodenum, its site of action; 500 to 1200 ml is secreted every 24 hr. It contains sodium bicarbonate and the enzymes trypsinogen, chymotrypsinogen, amylase, and lipase. Sodium bicarbonate neutralizes the acidity of the chyme entering the duodenum from the stomach and prevents irritation of the duodenal mucosa. Trypsinogen is converted to active trypsin by intestinal enteropeptidase (enterokinase), and trypsin in turn converts chymotrypsinogen to active chymotrypsin. Both trypsin and chymotrypsin continue protein digestion, forming peptides. Amylase hydrolyzes starch to maltose, and lipase digests emulsified fats to fatty acids and glycerol. SEE: *enzyme; pancreas; secretion.*

pancreaticocholecystostomy (păn″krē-ăt″ĭ-kō-kō″lē-sĭs-tŏs′tō-mē) [Gr. *pan,* all, + *kreas,* flesh, + *chole,* bile, + *kystis,* bladder, + *stoma,* mouth] The surgical creation of a passage between the gallbladder and pancreas.

pancreaticoduodenal (păn″krē-ăt″ĭ-kō-dū-ō-dē′năl) [″ + ″ + L. *duodeni,* twelve] Concerning the duodenum and pancreas.

pancreaticoduodenostomy (păn″krē-ăt″ĭ-kō-dū″ō-dē-nŏs′tō-mē) [″ + ″ + ″ + Gr. *stoma,* mouth] Surgical creation of an artificial passage between the pancreatic duct or the divided end of the transected pancreas with the duodenum.

pancreaticoenterostomy (păn″krē-ăt″ĭ-kō-ĕn″tĕr-ŏs′tō-mē) [″ + ″ + *enteron,* intestine, + *stoma,* mouth] Surgical creation of a passage between the pancreatic duct or the transected end of the pancreas and intestine.

pancreaticogastrostomy (păn″krē-ăt″ĭ-kō-găs-trŏs′tō-mē) [″ + ″ + *gaster,* belly, + *stoma,* mouth] Surgical creation of a passage between the transected end of the pancreas and the stomach. Pancreaticocystogastrostomy is the anastomosis of pancreatic pseudocyst and the stomach.

pancreaticojejunostomy (păn″krē-ăt″ĭ-kō-jĕ″jū-nŏs′tō-mē) [″ + ″ + L. *jejunum,* empty, + Gr. *stoma,* mouth] Surgical creation of a passage between the pancreatic duct or the transected end of the pancreas and jejunum.

pancreatin (păn′krē-ă-tĭn) [Gr. *pan,* all, + *kreas,* flesh] **1.** One of the enzymes of the pancreas. **2.** A mixture of enzymes, chiefly amylase, lipase, and protease.

ACTION/USES: It is used chiefly in patients with chronic pancreatitis, who do not secrete adequate amounts of their own pancreatic enzymes.

pancreatitis (păn″krē-ă-tī′tĭs) [″ + ″ + *itis,* inflammation] Inflammation of the pancreas. SEE: *acute p.; chronic p. Nursing Diagnoses Appendix.*

acute p. Pancreatitis of sudden onset, marked clinically by epigastric pain, nausea, vomiting, and elevated serum pancreatic enzymes. Varying degrees of pancreatic inflammation, necrosis, hemorrhage, gangrene, or pseudocyst formation may develop. The disease may be relatively mild, resolving in 3 or 4 days, or severe enough to cause multiple organ system failure, shock, and death (in about 5% of patients).

ETIOLOGY: Alcohol abuse and obstruction of the pancreatic duct by gallstones are the most common causes of the disease; less often, pancreatitis results from exposure to drugs (e.g., thiazide diuretics, pentamidine, and many others); hypertriglyceridemia; hypercalcemia; abdominal trauma; or viral infections (e.g., mumps or coxsackievirus).

TREATMENT: The patient receives nothing by mouth until pain, nausea, and vomiting have resolved and diagnostic markers (e.g., serum lipase level) show evidence of normalizing. Standard supportive measures include the administration of fluids and electrolytes, sometimes in massive quantities if dehydration or third-spacing of fluids in the abdomen occurs.

CAUTION: Refeeding patients before pancreatic inflammation has resolved frequently results in relapse.

---

calcareous p. Pancreatitis accompanied by calculi formation in the pancreas.

centrilobar p. Pancreatitis located around divisions of the pancreatic duct.

chronic p. A form of pancreatitis that results from repeated or massive pancreatic injury, marked by the formation of scar tissue, which leads to malfunction of the pancreas.

SYMPTOMS: The pain may be mild or severe, tending to radiate to the back. Jaundice, weakness, emaciation, malabsorption of proteins and fats, and diarrhea are present.

gallstone p. Inflammation of the pancreas, caused by the obstruction of the ampulla of Vater by a biliary stone.

interstitial p. Pancreatitis with overgrowth of interacinar and intra-acinar connective tissue.

perilobar p. Fibrosis of the pancreas between acinous groups.

purulent p. Pancreatitis with abscess formation. SYN: *suppurative p.*

suppurative p. Purulent pancreatitis.

pancreatoduodenectomy (păn″krē-ă-tō-dū″ō-dē-nĕk′tō-mē) [Gr. *pan,* all, + *kreas,* flesh, + L. *duodeni,* twelve, + Gr. *ektome,* excision] Excision of the head of the pancreas and the adjacent portion of the duodenum.

pancreatoduodenostomy (păn″krē-ă-tō-dū″ō-dĕ-nŏs′tō-mē) [″ + ″ + ″ + *stoma,* mouth] Surgical anastomosis of the pancreatic duct, or a pancreatic fistula, to the duodenum.

pancreatogenic, pancreatogenous (păn″krē-ă-tō-jĕn′ĭk, -tŏj′ĕ-nŭs) [″ + ″ + *gennan,* to produce] Produced in or by the pancreas; originating in the pancreas.

pancreatography (păn″krē-ă-tŏg′ră-fē) [″ + ″ + *graphein,* to write] Endoscopic and radiological examination of the pancreas after injection of a radiopaque contrast medium through the duct of Wirsung.

pancreatolith (păn″krē-ăt′ō-lĭth) [″ + ″ + *lithos,* stone] A stone in the pancreatic ducts.

pancreatolithectomy (păn″krē-ăt-ō-lĭth-ĕk′tō-mē) [″ + ″ + ″ + *ektome,* excision] Removal of a calculus from the pancreas.

pancreatolithiasis (păn″krē-ă-tō-lĭ-thī′ă-sĭs) [″ + ″ + ″ + *-iasis,* condition] Stones in the duct system of the pancreas.

pancreatolithotomy (păn″krē-ăt-ō-lĭ-thŏt′ō-mē) [″ + ″ + ″ + *tome,* incision] Incision of the pancreas for removal of a calculus. SYN: *pancreolithotomy.*

pancreatolysis (păn″krē-ă-tŏl′ĭ-sĭs) [″ + ″ + *lysis,* dissolution] Destruction of the pancreatic substance by pancreatic enzymes.

pancreatolytic (păn″krē-ăt-ō-lĭt′ĭk) Destructive to pancreatic tissues.

pancreatomy (păn-krē-ăt′ō-mē) [″ + ″ + *tome,* incision] Pancreatotomy.

pancreatoncus (păn-krē-ăt-ŏng′kŭs) [″ + ″ + *onkos,* tumor] A pancreatic tumor.

pancreatopathy (păn″krē-ă-tŏp′ă-thē) [″ + ″ + *pathos,* disease, suffering] Any pathologic state of the pancreas. SYN: *pancreopathy.*

pancreatotomy (păn″krē-ă-tŏt′ō-mē) [″ + ″ + *tome,* incision] Surgical incision into the pancreas. SYN: *pancreatomy.*

pancreatotropic (păn-krē″ă-tō-trŏp′ĭk) [″ + ″ + *tropikos,* turning] Having an affinity for or action on the pancreas.

pancreectomy (păn″krē-ĕk′tō-mē) [″ + ″ + *ektome,* excision] Partial or total excision of the pancreas.

pancrelipase (păn″krē-lī′pās) A standardized preparation of enzymes, principally lipase, with amylase and protease, obtained from the pancreas of the hog. It is used in treating conditions associated with deficient secretion from the pancreas.

pancreolithotomy (păn″krē-ō-lĭ-thŏt′ō-mē) [″ + *kreas,* flesh, + *lithos,* stone, + *tome,* incision] Pancreatolithotomy.

pancreolysis (păn″krē-ŏl′ĭ-sĭs) [″ + ″ + *lysis,* dissolution] Enzymatic destruction of the pancreas.

pancreopathy (păn″krē-ŏp′ă-thē) [″ + ″ + *pathos,* disease, suffering] Pancreatopathy.

pancreoprivic (păn″krē-ō-prĭv′ĭk) Having no pancreas.

pancuronium bromide (păn″kū-rō′nē-ŭm) A neuromuscular blocking agent.

pancytopenia (păn″sī-tō-pē′nē-ă) [″ + *kytos,* cell, + *penia,* poverty] A reduction in all cellular elements of the blood.

pandemic (păn-dĕm′ĭk) A disease affecting the majority of the population of a large region, such as dental caries or periodontal disease, or one that is epidemic at the same time in many different parts of the world.

pandiculation (păn″dĭk-ū-lā′shŭn) [L. *pandiculari,* to stretch one's self] Stretching of the limbs and yawning, as on awakening from normal sleep.

panel **1.** A number of patients or normal subjects who participate in medical investigations, esp. studies in which new drugs, devices, or procedures are tested. SEE: *informed consent; institutional review board.* **2.** The list of patients who obtain their primary medical care from the physician to whom they are assigned. This system is used in some health care plans.

panencephalitis (păn″ĕn-sĕf″ă-lī′tĭs) [Gr. *pan,* all, + *enkephalos,* brain, + *itis,* inflammation] A diffuse inflammation of the brain.

subacute sclerosing p. ABBR: SSPE. A disease of childhood and adolescence marked by gradual and progressive intellectual and behavioral deterioration followed by seizures, muscle jerking, gait disturbances, and eventually coma. The illness is a late complication of measles infection (usually developing about 5 years after the child had measles). It has been almost completely eradicated in the U.S. as a result of universal measles vaccination.

panendoscope (păn-ĕn′dō-skōp) [″ + *endon,* within, + *skopein,* to view] A cystoscope that gives a wide view of the bladder.

Paneth cells (pă′nāt) [Josef Paneth, Ger. physician, 1857–1890] Large secretory cells containing coarse granules, found at the blind end of the crypts of Lieberkühn (the intestinal glands). They secrete lysozyme.

pang **1.** A paroxysm of extreme agony. **2.** A sudden attack of any emotion.

pangenesis (păn″jĕn′ĕ-sĭs) [Gr. *pan,* all, + *genesis,* generation, birth] The discredited hypothesis that each cell of the parent is represented by a particle in the reproductive cell, and thus each part of the organism reproduces itself in the progeny.

panhypopituitarism (păn-hī″pō-pĭ-tū′ĭ-tăr-ĭzm) [″ + *hypo,* under, + L. *pituita,* mucus, + Gr. *-ismos,* condition] Defective or absent function of the entire pituitary gland. SEE: *Simmonds' disease.*

panhysterectomy (păn″hĭs-tĕr-ĕk′tō-mē) [″ + *hystera,* womb, + *ektome,* excision] Excision of the entire uterus including the cervix uteri. SEE: *hysterectomy.*

panhysterocolpectomy (păn-hĭs″tĕr-ō-kŏl-pĕk′tō-mē) [″ + ″ + *kolpos,* vagina, + *ektome,* excision] Total excision of the uterus and vagina.

panhystero-oophorectomy (păn-hĭs″tĕr-ō-ō-ŏf-ō-rĕk′tō-mē) [″ + ″ + *oophoros,* bearing eggs, + *ektome,* excision] Excision of the uterus, cervix, and one or both ovaries.

panhysterosalpingectomy (păn-hĭs″tĕr-ō-săl″pĭn-jĕk′tō-mē) [″ + ″ + *salpinx,* tube, + *ektome,* excision] Surgical removal of the uterus, cervix, and fallopian tubes.

panhysterosalpingo-oophorectomy (păn-hĭs″tĕr-ō-săl″pĭng-gō-ō-ŏf-ō-rĕk′tō-mē) [″ + ″ + ″ + *oophoros,* bearing eggs, + *ektome,* excision] Excision of the entire uterus, including the cervix, ovaries, and uterine tubes.

panic (păn′ĭk) Acute anxiety, terror, or fright that is usually of sudden onset and may be uncontrollable. SEE: *panic attack.*

p. attack A discrete period of intense fear or discomfort that is accompanied by at least 4 of the following symptoms: palpitations, sweating, trembling or shaking, sensations of shortness of breath or smothering, feeling of choking, chest pain or discomfort, nausea or abdominal distress, dizziness or lightheadedness, feeling of unreality or being detached from oneself, feeling of losing control or going crazy, fear of dying, paresthesias (numbness or tingling sensations), and chills or hot flushes. The onset is sudden and builds to a peak usually in 10 min or less and may include a sense of imminent danger or impending doom and an urge to escape.

PATIENT CARE: The caregivers allow the patient to release energy and express feelings of anxiety. Precautions are taken to ensure the patient's safety. A calm, quiet, and reassuring environment helps the patient to overcome feelings of anxiety.

p. disorder An anxiety disorder characterized by panic attacks (e.g., agoraphobia with panic attacks).

homosexual p. **1.** In classic freudian psychiatry, fear, anxiety, aggression, or psychosis that originates in conflicts that arise from an attraction to members of one's own gender. **2.** An irrational fear of contracting illnesses from casual contact with people who have sex with members of their own gender.

panmyeloid (păn-mī′ĕ-loyd) [Gr. *pan,* all, + *myelos,* marrow, + *eidos,* form, shape] Concerning all of the elements of the bone marrow.

panneuritis (păn″ū-rī′tĭs) [″ + *neuron,* sinew, + *itis,* inflammation] Generalized neuritis.

p. epidemica Beriberi.

panniculectomy The excision of an apron of abdominal subcutaneous fat that lacks adequate supportive tissue from people who are morbidly obese. Cosmesis can be achieved by panniculectomy and concomitant abdominoplasty.

panniculitis (păn-ĭk″ū-lī′tĭs) [L. *panniculus,* a small piece of cloth, + *itis,* inflammation] Inflammation of a layer of fatty connective tissue in the anterior wall of the abdomen. Patients experience pain, tenderness, and hypertrophy of tissue in parts where fat is the thickest.

nodular nonsuppurative p. Weber-Christian disease.

panniculus (păn-ĭk′ū-lŭs) [L., a small piece of cloth] Any clothlike sheet or layer of tissue.

p. adiposus The subcutaneous layer of fat, esp. where fat is abundant; the superficial fascia that is heavily laden with fat cells.

p. carnosus The thin layer of muscular tissue in the superficial fascia. SEE: *platysma myoides*.

pannus (păn′ŭs) [L., cloth] **1.** Superficial vascular inflammation of the cornea. The area is cloudy, and its surface is uneven because it is infiltrated with a film of new capillary blood vessels. This condition may be seen in trachoma, acne rosacea, eczema, and as a result of irritation in granular conjunctivitis. SEE: *micropannus*. **2.** Inflamed synovial granulation tissue seen in chronic rheumatoid arthritis.

corneal p. An overgrowth of vascular tissue in the periphery of the cornea, occurring in response to inflammation of the cornea, esp. in trachoma.

p. crassus Pannus that is highly vascularized, thick, and opaque.

phlyctenular p. Pannus that occurs in conjunction with phlyctenular conjunctivitis.

p. siccus Pannus accompanying xerophthalmia. It is composed principally of connective tissue that is dry and poorly vascularized.

p. tenuis Pannus that is thin, poorly vascularized, and slightly opaque.

panodic (pă-nŏd′ĭk) Radiating in all directions, esp. said of a nerve impulse.

panography (păn-nŏg′ră-fē) A radiographic procedure that produces a panoramic view of an entire dental arch on a single film.

panophobia (păn-ō-fō′bē-ă) [Gr. *pan,* all, + *phobos,* fear] Morbid groundless fear of some unknown evil or of everything in general; general apprehension. SYN: *pantophobia*.

panophthalmia, panophthalmitis (păn-ŏf-thăl′mē-ă, -thăl-mī′tĭs) [″ + *ophthalmos,* eye, + *itis,* inflammation] Inflammation of the entire eye.

panoptic (păn-ŏp′tĭk) [″ + *optikos,* vision] Making every part visible.

panoptosis (păn-ŏp-tō′sĭs) [″ + *ptosis,* a dropping] General prolapse of the abdominal organs.

panphobia (păn-fō′bē-ă) [″ + *phobos,* fear] Panophobia.

panplegia (păn-plē′jē-ă) [″ + *plege,* stroke] Total paralysis.

pansclerosis (păn″sklē-rō′sĭs) [″ + *sklerosis,* hardening] Hardening of an entire organ.

pansinusitis (păn″sī-nŭs-ī′tĭs) [″ + L. *sinus,* curve, hollow, + *itis,* inflammation] Inflammation of all of the paranasal sinuses.

pansphygmograph (păn-sfĭg′mō-grăf) [″ + *sphygmos,* pulse, + *graphein,* to write] An apparatus for registering cardiac movements, the pulse wave, and chest movements at the same time.

Panstrongylus (păn-strŏn′jĭ-lŭs) A genus of insects belonging to the order Hemiptera, family Reduviidae. This genus may be the vector for *Trypanosoma cruzi,* the causative agent of Chagas' disease.

pansystolic Throughout systole; used to describe the murmur of mitral regurgitation. SYN: *holosystolic*.

pant [ME. *panten*] **1.** To gasp for breath. **2.** A short and shallow breath. Panting is produced by physical overexertion, as in running, or from fear.

pant-, panto- [Gr. *pantos,* all] Combining form indicating *all, whole*.

pantanencephaly (păn″tăn-ĕn-sĕf′ă-lē) [″ + *an-,* not, + *enkephalos,* brain] Complete absence of the brain in the fetus.

pantankyloblepharon (păn-tăng″kĭ-lō-blĕf′ă-rŏn) [″ + *ankyle,* noose, + *blepharon,* lid] Generalized adhesion of the eyelids to the eyeball.

pantetheine (păn-tĕ-thē′ĭn) The naturally occurring amide of pantothenic acid. It is a growth factor for *Lactobacillus bulgaricus*.

panting (pănt′ĭng) [ME. *panten*] Short, shallow, rapid respirations. SYN: *polypnea*.

pantograph (păn′tō-grăf) [Gr. *pantos,* all, + *graphein,* to write] A device that will reproduce, through a system of levers connected to a stylus, a duplicate of whatever figure or drawing is being copied by the device.

pantomography (păn″tō-mŏg′ră-fē) SEE: *panoramic radiograph*.

pantomorphia (păn″tō-mor′fē-ă) [″ + *morphe,* form] **1.** The state of being symmetrical. **2.** Able to assume any shape.

pantopaque (păn-tō′păk) An oil-based, iodine-containing contrast medium used to outline body structures during radiographic or fluoroscopic examinations, such as myelograms.

pantophobia (păn-tō-fō′bē-ă) [″ + *phobos,* fear] Panophobia.

pantothenate (păn-tō′thĕn-āt) A salt of pantothenic acid.

pantothenic acid (păn-tō-thĕn′ĭk) $C_9H_{17}NO_5$; a vitamin of the B-complex group widely distributed in nature, occurring naturally in yeast, liver, heart, salmon, eggs, and various grains. It was synthesized in 1940. It is part of coenzyme A, which is necessary for the Krebs cycle and for conversion of amino acids and lipids to carbohydrates.

pan troglodytes troglodytes A subspecies of chimpanzee believed to be the primary host of human immunodeficiency virus (HIV) before the illness became epidemic in humans.

panturbinate (păn-tŭr′bĭ-nāt) [″ + L. *turbinatus,* shaped like a top] All of the turbinate structures of the nose; the nasal conchae.

panzootic (păn″zō-ŏt′ĭk) [″ + *zoon,* animal] Any animal disease that is widespread.

PaO₂ The partial pressure of oxygen in arterial blood; arterial oxygen concentration, or tension; usually expressed in millimeters of mercury (mm Hg).

pap (păp) [L. *pappa,* infant's sound for food] Any soft, semiliquid food.

papain (pă-pā′ĭn) Proteolytic enzyme obtained from the fruit of the papaya, *Carica papaya;* used to tenderize meat.

Papanicolaou test [George Nicholas Papanicolaou, Gr.-born U.S. scientist, 1883–1962] ABBR: Pap test. A cytological study used to detect cancer in cells that an organ has shed. The Pap test has been used most often in the diagnosis and prevention of cervical cancers, but it also is valuable in the detection of pleural or peritoneal malignancies, and in the evaluation of cellular changes caused by radiation, infection, or atrophy.

In the detection of cervical cancer cellular material is collected, first from outside the cervix with a wooden spatula and next from the endocervix with a specially formed brush. Samples taken with these tools are smeared onto glass slides and rapidly fixed to avoid artifacts caused by drying. When suspicious cells are identified (e.g., cells with large nuclei or high nuclear-to-cytoplasmic ratios), the patient will need follow-up testing, such as repeat Pap screening or colposcopy. SEE: illus.

Since the introduction of the Pap test, death from cervical cancer has declined by 70%. Although interpretation of the test is subject to human error, a variety of developments have improved test accuracy, including use of computer-generated procedures for detection and examination of abnormal cells and mandated reexamination of sample batches to test quality control. A woman may augment the accuracy and value of the Pap test by following these guidelines: Asking her physician about the quality of the laboratory evaluating the results; having an annual Pap test beginning at age 18; scheduling the test 2 weeks after the end of a menstrual period; abstaining from sexual intercourse and douching for 48 hr before the test; providing a detailed medical history, including use of birth control pills or hormones and results of past Pap tests; and requesting a second opinion on the Pap test if she is at risk for cancer of the reproductive tract.

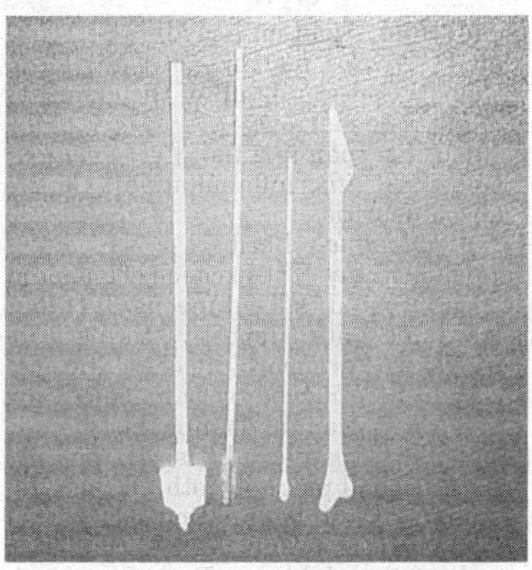

TOOLS FOR PAP TEST

(L to R) cervical broom, Cytobrush, cotton-tipped applicator, and wooden paddle

CAUTION: As with any test, it is possible that human errors may cause an incorrect interpretation of the slides. It is important that the quality of performance of the technicians and physicians be periodically reviewed by persons not employed by the laboratory or hospital.

SCREENING RECOMMENDATIONS: Most authorities recommend that women over age 18, and all sexually active women, have three consecutive annual Pap tests; if the results of these are all negative for dysplasia, subsequent screening may continue less frequently, at the clinician's discretion. Screening for women over age 69 who have never before had abnormal findings on repeated Pap smears is not considered cost effective.

Certain women are at high risk for cervical cancer and may need more frequent testing than the general population. These include women with HIV infection and those who are immunosuppressed as a result of other illnesses. Additional risk factors for cervical cancer include early age at first intercourse, a history of sexually transmitted illnesses, cigarette smoking or substance abuse, a previous history of cervical dysplasia, a history of multiple sexual partners, or having a sexual partner who has other partners with cervical cancer.

PATIENT CARE: Because Pap testing has been effective in detecting the early stages of cervical cancer, health care professionals should advocate this procedure for their female patients and participate in health promotion efforts to increase the number of women who have the test done regularly.

papaverine hydrochloride (pă-păv′ĕr-ēn) [L., poppy] The salt of an alkaloid obtained from opium; used as a smooth muscle relaxant, esp. in gastric and intestinal distress and in bronchial spasm.

papaya (pă-pā′yă) [Sp. Amerind.] **1.** *Carica papaya,* a large herb of the family Caricaceae, native to the American tropics and cultivated for its edible fruit and latex-bearing leaves and stem, which contain digestive enzymes. **2.** Large, oblong, edible fruit of the *Carica papaya* plant; the source of the digestive enzyme papain.

paper [L. *papyrus,* paper] **1.** Cellulose pulp prepared in thin sheets from fibers of wood, rags, and other substances. **2.** Charta. **3.** A thin sheet of cellulosic material impregnated with specific chemicals that react in a definite manner when exposed to certain solutions. This permits use of these papers for testing purposes.

articulating p. Paper coated on one or both sides with a pigment that marks the teeth when their occlusal surfaces contact the paper. This allows the contact points of the teeth to be demonstrated.

bibulous p. Paper that absorbs water readily.

filter p. A porous, unglazed paper used for filtration.

indicator p. Paper saturated with a solution of known strength and then dried; used for testing the pH (acidity or alkalinity) of a solution.

litmus p. An indicator paper impregnated with litmus, which turns blue in alkaline solutions and red in acidic solutions.

test p. Paper impregnated with a substance that will change color when exposed to solutions of a certain pH or to specific chemicals.

papilla (pă-pĭl′ă) *pl.* **papillae** [L.] A small, nipple-like protuberance or elevation.

acoustic p. The spiral organ of the ear.

Bergmeister's p. A veil in front of the retina of the eye. It is made of a conical mass of glial remnants that are the developmental tissue of the eye that has not been reabsorbed.

circumvallate p. One of the large papillae near the base on the dorsal aspect of the tongue, arranged in a V-shape. The taste buds are located in the epithelium of the trench surrounding the papilla.

clavate p. Fungiform p.

conical p. **1.** Papillae on the dorsum of the tongue. **2.** Papillae in the ridge-like projections of the dermis. SYN: *p. of corium.*

p. of corium Conical p. (2).

dental p. A mass of connective tissue that becomes enclosed by the developing enamel organ. It gives rise to dentin and dental pulp.

dermal p. Small elevations of the corium that indent the inner surface of the epidermis.

duodenal p. P. of Vater.

filiform p. One of the very slender papillae at the tip of the tongue.

foliate p. Folds, which are rudimentary papillae, in the sides of the tongue.

fungiform p. One of the broad flat papillae resembling a mushroom, chiefly found on the dorsal central area of the tongue. SYN: *clavate p.*

gingival p. The gingiva that fills the space between adjacent teeth.

gustatory p. Taste papilla of tongue; one of those possessing a taste bud. SYN: *taste p.*

p. of hair A conical process of the corium that projects into the undersurface of a hair bulb. It contains capillaries through which a hair receives its nourishment. SYN: *p. pili.*

incisive p. Projection on the anterior portion of the raphe of the palate. SYN: *palatine p.*

interdental p. The triangular part of the gingivae that fills the area between adjacent teeth. The papilla includes free gingiva and attached gingiva and projections seen from the lingual, buccal, or labial sides of the tooth. SYN: *interproximal p.*

interproximal p. Interdental p.

lacrimal p. An elevation in the medial edge of each eyelid, in the center of which is the opening of the lacrimal duct.

lenticular p. A small rounded elevation underlying lymphatic nodules in the mucosa of the root of the tongue.

lingual p. Any one of the tiny eminences covering the anterior two thirds of the tongue, including circumvallate, filiform, fungiform, and conical papillae.

p. mammae The nipple of the mammary gland.

optic p. Blind spot (1).

palatine p. Incisive p.

parotid p. The projections around the opening of the parotid duct into the mouth.

p. pili P. of hair.

renal p. The apex of a renal pyramid in the kidney.

tactile p. A dermal papilla that contains a sensory end organ for touch.

taste p. Gustatory p.

urethral p. The small projection in the vestibule of the vagina at the entrance of the urethra.

vallate p. Circumvallate p.

p. of Vater The duodenal end of the drainage systems of the pancreatic and common bile ducts; commonly, but inaccurately, called the ampulla of Vater. SYN: *duodenal p.; hepatopancreatic ampulla.*

papillary (păp′ĭ-lăr-ē) [L. *papilla,* nipple] **1.** Concerning a nipple or papilla. **2.** Resembling or composed of papillae.

p. cystadenoma lymphomatosum Warthin's tumor.

p. ducts of Bellini Short ducts that open on the tip of the renal papillae. They are formed by the union of the straight collecting tubules.

p. layer The layer of the corium that adjoins the epidermis. SYN: *stratum papillare.*

p. tumor Neoplasm composed of or resembling enlarged papillae. SEE: *papilloma.*

papillate (păp′ĭ-lāt) [L. *papilla,* nipple] Having nipple-like growths on the surface, as a culture in bacteriology.

papillectomy (păp″ĭ-lĕk′tō-mē) [″ + Gr. *ektome,* excision] Excision of any papilla or papillae.

papilledema (păp″ĭl-ĕ-dē′mă) [″ + Gr. *oidema,* swelling] Edema and inflammation of the optic nerve at its point of entrance into the retina. It is caused by increased intracranial pressure, often due to a tumor of the brain pressing on the optic nerve. Blindness may result very rapidly unless relieved. SYN: *choked disk; papillitis.*

papilliferous (păp″ĭ-lĭf′ĕr-ŭs) [″ + *ferre,* to carry] Having or containing papillae.

papilliform (pă-pĭl′ĭ-form) [″ + *forma,* shape] Having the characteristics or appearance of papillae.

papillitis (păp-ĭ-lī′tĭs) [″ + Gr. *itis,* inflammation] Papilledema.

papilloadenocystoma (păp″ĭl-ō-ăd″ē-nō-sĭs-tō′mă) [″ + Gr. *aden,* gland, + *kystis,* a cyst, + *oma,* tumor] A tumor composed of elements of papilloma, adenoma, and cystoma.

papillocarcinoma (păp″ĭl-ō-kăr-sĭ-nō′mă) [″ + Gr. *karkinos,* crab, + *oma,* tumor] **1.** A malignant tumor of hypertrophied papillae. **2.** Carcinoma with papillary growths.

papilloma (păp-ĭ-lō′mă) [″ + Gr. *oma,* tumor] **1.** A benign epithelial tumor. **2.** Epithelial tumor of skin or mucous membrane consisting of hypertrophied papillae covered by a layer of epithelium. Included in this group are warts, condylomas, and polyps. SEE: *acanthoma; papillomavirus.*

p. durum A hardened papilloma, as a wart or corn.

fibroepithelial p. A skin tag containing fibrous tissue.

hard p. Papilloma that develops from squamous epithelium.

Hopmann's p. [Carl Melchior Hopmann, Ger. physician, 1849–1925] Papillomatous overgrowth of the nasal mucosa.

intracystic p. Papilloma within a cystic adenoma.

intraductal p. A solitary neoplasm of the breast that occurs in the large, lactiferous ducts. A distinct neoplasm that displays a papillary histological pattern.

p. molle Condyloma.

soft p. Papilloma formed from columnar epithelium; applies to any small, soft growth.

villous p. Papilloma with thin, long excrescences present in the urinary bladder, breast, intestinal tract, or choroid plexus of the cerebral ventricles.

papillomatosis (păp″ĭ-lō-mă-tō′sĭs) [″ + Gr. *oma,* tumor, + *osis,* condition] **1.** Widespread formation of papillomas. **2.** The condition of being afflicted with many papillomas.

papillomavirus Any of a group of viruses that cause papillomas or warts in humans and animals. They belong to the papovavirus family or group. SEE: *wart, genital.*

human p. ABBR: HPV. A papillomavirus that is specific to humans. HPVs cause three types of cutaneous infections: common warts, plantar warts, and juvenile or flat warts. A fourth type of infection, condyloma acuminata or genital warts, is a common viral sexually transmitted disease in the U.S. A number of HPV types, esp. numbers 16 and 18, are believed to be important in the pathogenisis of cancer of the uterine cervix and development of some vaginal, vulvar, anal, and penile squamous cell cancers. SEE: *wart, genital.*

TREATMENT: Imiquimod is used to treat warts of the genitals or anus. An alternative drug treatment is podophyllin. Cervical HPV lesions may be removed by loop electrosurgical excision procedure. Cryotherapy and laser surgery also may be used in treatment.

papilloretinitis (păp″ĭ-lō-rĕt-ĭn-ī′tĭs) [″ + *rete,* net, + Gr. *itis,* inflammation] Inflammation of the papilla and retina, extending to the optic disk. SYN: *retinopapillitis.*

papovavirus (păp″ō-vă-vī′rŭs) [*pap*illoma, + *po*lyoma, + *va*cuolating agent + *virus*] Any of a group of viruses important in investigating viral carcinogenesis; including polyoma virus, simian virus 40 (SV 40), and papillomaviruses.

pappataci fever Sandfly fever.

pappose (păp′pōs) [L. *pappus,* down] Covered with fine, downy hair.

pappus [L.] The first growth of beard hair appearing on the cheeks and chin as fine, downy hair.

Pap smear, Pap test Papanicolaou test.

papular mucinosis A rare rash of unknown etiology, in which mucin deposits are found in the dermis, creating a bumpy (papular) eruption often found on the face or arms. The condition often is associated with lesions of the internal organs and the presence of paraproteins in the bloodstream.

papule (păp′ūl) [L. *papula,* pimple] A small bump or pimple, typically larger than a grain of salt but smaller than a peppercorn, that rises above the surface of the neighboring skin. Papules may appear in numerous skin diseases, including prickly heat, psoriasis, xanthomatosis, eczema, and skin cancers. Their color may range from pale, to yellow, red, brown, or black. SEE: illus. **papular,** *adj.*

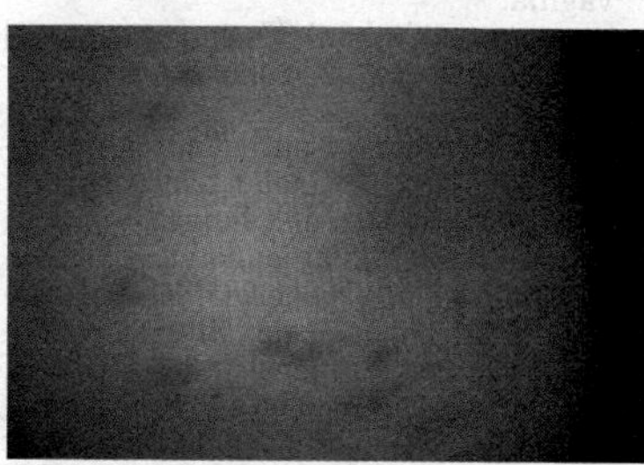

PAPULES

dry p. Chancre.

moist p. Condyloma latum.

pearly penile p. An asymptomatic white papule with a pink, white, or pearly surface on the dorsum of the penis of blacks and uncircumcised men. No treatment is indicated, just reassurance.

piezogenic pedal p. A soft painful skin-colored papule present on the non–weight-bearing portion of the heel. It disappears when weight is taken off the foot and heel. This papule is caused by herniation of fat through connective tissue defects.

split p. Fissures at the corners of the mouth; seen in some cases of secondary syphilis.

papulo- [L. *papula,* pimple] Combining form indicating *pimple, papule.*

papuloerythematous (păp″ū-lō-ĕr″ĕ-thĕm′ă-tŭs) [″ + Gr. *erythema,* redness] Denoting the occurrence of papules on reddened skin.

papulopustular (păp″ū-lō-pŭs′tū-lăr) [″ + *pustula,* blister] Denoting the presence of both pustules and papules.

papulosis (păp-ū-lō′sĭs) [″ + Gr. *osis,* condition] The presence of numerous and generalized papules.

papulosquamous (păp″ū-lō-skwā′mŭs) [″ + *squamosus,* scalelike] Denoting the presence of both papules and scales.

papulovesicular (păp″ū-lō-vē-sĭk′ū-lăr) [″ + *vesicula,* tiny bladder] Denoting the presence of both papules and vesicles.

papyraceous (păp-ĭ-rā′shŭs) [L.] Parchment-like; in obstetrics, denoting a fetus that is retained in the uterus beyond natural term and appears mummified.

par [L., equal] A pair, esp. a pair of cranial nerves.

para (păr′ă) [L. *parere,* to bring forth, to bear] A woman who has produced a viable infant (weighing at least 500 g or of more than 20 weeks' gestation) regardless of whether the infant is alive at birth. A multiple birth is considered to be a single parous experience. SEE: *gravida; multipara.*

para- [Gr. *para,* beyond; L. *par,* equal, pair] Prefix meaning *near, beside, past, beyond, opposite, abnormal, irregular, two like parts.*

-para Suffix meaning *to bear forth* (offspring).

para-aminobenzoic acid (păr″ă-ăm″ĭ-nō-bĕn-zō′ĭk) ABBR: PABA. Previously used name for aminobenzoic acid.

para-aminohippuric acid ABBR: PAHA. A derivative of aminobenzoic acid. The salt, para-aminohippurate, is used to test the excretory capacity of the renal tubules.

para-aminosalicylic acid (păr″ă-ăm″ĭ-nō-săl″ĭ-sĭl′ĭk) ABBR: PAS. $C_7H_7NO_3$; a white or nearly white and practically odorless powder that darkens when exposed to air or light. It is a second-line drug used to treat tuberculosis that is resistant to multiple first-line agents. SYN: *aminosalicylic acid.*

para-aortic body One of the small masses of chromaffin tissue along the abdominal aorta that secrete epinephrine.

parabionts (păr-ăb′ē-ŏnts) [″ + *bioun,* to live] Two individuals living in the condition of parabiosis.

parabiosis (păr″ă-bī-ō′sĭs) [″ + *biosis,* living] **1.** The joining together of two individuals. It may occur congenitally as with conjoined twins or may be produced surgically for experimentation in animals. **2.** The temporary suppression of the excitability of a nerve. **parabiotic** (-ŏt′ĭk), *adj.*

parablepsia, parablepsis (păr″ă-blĕp′sē-ă, -sĭs) [Gr. *para,* beside, + *blepsis,* vision] Abnormality of vision (e.g., visual hallucinations).

paracanthoma (păr″ă-kăn-thō′mă) [Gr.

para, beside, + *akantha,* thorn, + *oma,* tumor] A tumor involving the prickle-cell layer of the epidermis.

paracasein (păr-ă-kā′sē-ĭn) An insoluble protein formed when rennin or pepsin acts on the casein in milk; this reaction, which results in the curdling of milk, occurs only in the presence of calcium ions.

Paracelsus (păr-ă-sĕl′sŭs) [Philippus Aureolus Theophrastus Bombastus von Hohenheim, 1493–1541] Swiss alchemist and physician who introduced several chemicals (lead, sulfur, iron, and arsenic) into pharmaceutical chemistry.

paracentesis (păr″ă-sĕn-tē′sĭs) [Gr. *para,* beside, + *kentesis,* a puncture] The puncture of a cavity with removal of fluid, as in pleural effusion or ascites. **paracentetic** (-tĕt′ĭk), *adj.*

PATIENT CARE: The procedure is explained to the patient, who may choose to void before treatment. Emotional support is offered during the procedure, and the patient is encouraged to express feelings. The patient is positioned as directed by the physician. Vital signs are monitored, especially for changes in respiratory rate, pulse, and blood pressure. The amount of fluid removed is measured and recorded, and its appearance, color, odor, specific gravity, and tendency to clot when the patient stands are described. The puncture site is observed and redressed as necessary. Specimens are sent to laboratories as directed. The procedure and the patient's response are documented, and the patient is monitored for several hours after the procedure.

abdominal p. Paracentesis of the abdominal cavity.

p. pulmonis Removal of fluid from a lung.

p. thoracis Thoracentesis.

p. tympani Drainage or irrigation through incision of the tympanic membrane.

p. vesicae Puncture of the wall of the urinary bladder.

paracentral (păr″ă-sĕn′trăl) [″ + L. *centralis,* center] Located near the center.

paracentral lobule A cerebral convolution on the medial surface joining the upper terminations of the ascending parietal and frontal convolutions.

paracephalus (păr″ă-sĕf′ă-lŭs) [″ + *kephale,* head] A parasitic placental twin with a small rudimentary head.

paracholera (păr″ă-kŏl′ĕr-ă) [″ + L. *cholera,* cholera] A disease resembling cholera but caused by vibriones other than true *Vibrio cholerae.*

parachordal (păr-ă-kor′dăl) [Gr. *para,* beside, + *chorde,* cord] Lying alongside the anterior portion of the notochord in the embryo.

parachordal cartilage One of a pair of cartilages in the cephalic portion of the notochord of the embryo that unite in humans to form a single basal plate that is the forerunner of the occipital bone.

parachromatism (păr″ă-krō′mă-tĭzm) [″ + *chroma,* color, + *-ismos,* condition] Incorrect perception of colors but not true color blindness.

parachromatopsia (păr″ă-krō-mă-tŏp′sē-ă) [″ + ″ + *opsis,* vision] Color blindness.

paracinesia, paracinesis (păr″ă-sī-nē′zē-ă, -sĭs) [″ + *kinesis,* movement] A condition in which movement is abnormal.

Paracoccidioides (păr″ă-kŏk-sĭd″ē-oy′dēz) A genus of yeastlike fungi.

P. brasiliensis Blastomyces brasiliensis.

paracoccidioidomycosis (păr″ă-kŏk-sĭd″ē-ŏy″dō-mī-kō′sĭs) A chronic granulomatous disease of the skin caused by *Paracoccidioides brasiliensis.* SYN: *South American blastomycosis.*

paracolitis (păr″ă-kō-lī′tĭs) Inflammation of the tissue surrounding the colon.

paracolpitis (păr″ă-kŏl-pī′tĭs) [″ + *kolpos,* vagina, + *itis,* inflammation] Inflammation of tissues surrounding the vagina.

paracone (păr′ă-kōn) [″ + *konos,* cone] The mesiobuccal cusp of an upper molar tooth.

paraconid (păr″ă-kō′nĭd) The mesiobuccal cusp of a lower molar tooth.

paracrine Secretion of a hormone from a source other than an endocrine gland.

p. control A general form of bioregulation in which one cell type in a tissue selectively influences the activity of an adjacent cell type by secreting chemicals that diffuse into the tissue and act specifically on cells in that area. SEE: *autocrine factor.*

paracusia, paracusis (păr″ă-kū′sē-ă, -kŭ′sĭs) [″ + *akousis,* hearing] Any abnormality or disorder of the sense of hearing.

p. loci Difficulty in locating the direction of sound.

p. willisiana An apparent ability to hear better in a noisy place, found in deafness due to stapes fixation and adhesive processes. SEE: *otosclerosis.*

paracystitis (păr″ă-sĭs-tī′tĭs) [″ + ″ + *itis,* inflammation] Inflammation of connective tissues and other structures around the urinary bladder.

paracytic (păr″ă-sĭt′ĭk) [″ + *kytos,* cell] Concerning cells other than those normally present in a specific location.

paradenitis (păr″ăd-ĕn-ī′tĭs) [″ + *aden,* gland, + *itis,* inflammation] Inflammation of tissues around a gland.

paradental (păr″ă-dĕn′tăl) [″ + L. *dens,* tooth] **1.** Concerning the practice of dentistry. **2.** Periodontal.

paradentium (păr″ă-dĕn′shē-ŭm) Periodontium.

paradidymal (păr″ă-dĭd′ĭ-măl) [″ + *didymos,* testicle] **1.** Concerning the paradidymis. **2.** Adjacent to the testis.

paradidymis (păr-ă-dĭd′ĭ-mĭs) [″ + *didymos,* testicle] The atrophic remnants of the tubules of the wolffian body, situated on the spermatic cord above the epididymis.

paradigm **1.** An example that serves as a model. **2.** Conceptual model.

paradox [Gr. *paradoxos,* conflicting with expectation] Something that seems untrue or illogical, but is in fact actually true.

Weber's p. Paradox that states that a muscle loaded beyond its ability to contract may elongate.

paradoxic, paradoxical (păr″ă-dŏk′sĭk, -sĭ-kăl) Seemingly contradictory but demonstrably true.

paraffin (păr′ă-fĭn) [L. *parum,* too little, + *affinis,* neighboring] **1.** A waxy, white, tasteless, odorless mixture of solid hydrocarbons obtained from petroleum; used as an ointment base or wound dressing. SEE: *petrolatum.* **2.** One of a series of saturated aliphatic hydrocarbons having the formula C_nH_{2n+2}. Paraffins constitute the methane or paraffin series. **3.** A series of solid waxes prepared according to their melting point, to be used to infiltrate and embed tissues for sectioning in the preparation of microscope slides.

hard p. Solid paraffin with a melting point between 45°C and 60°C.

liquid p. Liquid petrolatum.

soft p. Petrolatum.

white soft p. White petrolatum.

yellow soft p. Petrolatum.

paraffinoma (păr″ă-fĭn-ō′mă) [″ + ″ + Gr. *oma,* tumor] A tumor that arises at the site of an injection of paraffin.

paraformaldehyde (păr″ă-for-măl′dĕ-hīd) A white, powdered antiseptic and disinfectant, a polymer of formaldehyde.

paragammacism (păr″ă-găm′mă-sĭzm) [Gr. *para,* beside, + *gamma,* Gr. letter G, + *-ismos,* condition] An inability to pronounce "g," "k," and "ch" sounds, with substitution of other consonants such as "d" or "t."

paraganglia (păr″ă-găng′lē-ă) *sing.,* **paraganglion** [″ + *ganglion,* knot] Groups of chromaffin cells, similar in staining reaction to cells of the adrenal medulla, associated anatomically and embryologically with the sympathetic system. They are located in various organs and parts of the body.

paraganglioma (păr″ă-găng-lē-ō′mă) [″ + ″ + *oma,* tumor] An extra-adrenal tumor composed of neural crest cells, which may release catecholamines into the systemic circulation and cause symptoms of sustained or episodic hypertension, with sweating, palpitations, and headache. Paragangliomas usually are found in the paravertebral ganglia or the carotid bodies.

paraganglion (păr″ă-găng′lē-ŏn) [″ + *ganglion,* knot] Sing. of paraganglia.

parageusia, parageusis (păr-ă-gū′sē-ă, -sĭs) [″ + *geusis,* taste] Disorder or abnormality of the sense of taste. Intravenous fluid therapy, esp. postoperatively, may create temporary parageusia and parosmia.

paragnathus (păr-ăg′nă-thŭs) [″ + *gnathos,* jaw] **1.** A congenital deformity in which there is an accessory jaw. **2.** A parasitic fetus attached to the outer part of the jaw of the autosite.

paragonimiasis (păr″ă-gŏn″ĭ-mī′ă-sĭs) [*Paragonimus* + *-iasis,* condition] Infection with worms of the genus *Paragonimus.* The clinical signs depend on the path the worm takes in migrating through the body, after the larvae contained in partially cooked freshwater crabs or crayfish are eaten. The larvae migrate from the duodenum to various organs, including the lungs, intestinal wall, lymph nodes, brain, subcutaneous tissues, and genitourinary tract. When the lungs are involved, the symptoms are cough and hemoptysis. In peritoneal infections, there may be an abdominal mass, pain, and dysentery. When the larvae invade the brain, paralysis, epilepsy, homonymous hemianopsia, optic atrophy, and papilledema are common. In some cases, the infected person may appear to be well. This infection is treated by administration of praziquantel.

Paragonimus (păr″ă-gŏn′ĭ-mŭs) A genus of trematode worms.

P. westermani The lung fluke, a common parasite of certain mammals including humans, dogs, cats, pigs, and minks. Human infestation occurs through eating partially cooked crabs or crayfish, the second intermediate host. This infestation is endemic in certain parts of Asia. SEE: illus.

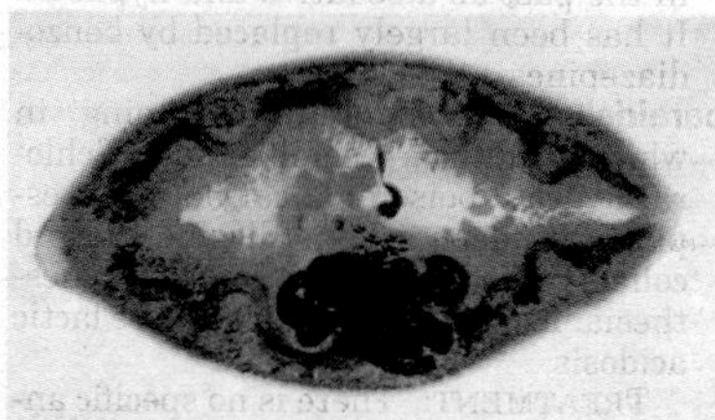

PARAGONIMUS WESTERMANI (X4)

paragrammatism A speech defect characterized by improper use of words and inability to arrange them grammatically.

paragranuloma (păr″ă-grăn″ū-lō′mă) [Gr. *para,* beside, + L. *granulum,* little grain, + Gr. *oma,* tumor] A benign form of Hodgkin's disease usually limited to lymph nodes.

paragraphia (păr-ă-grăf′ē-ă) [″ + *graphein,* to write] The writing of letters or words other than those intended.

parahepatic (păr″ă-hē-păt′ĭk) [″ + *hepar,* liver] Adjacent to the liver.

parahypnosis [″ + *hypnos,* sleep] Abnormal or disordered sleep.

parahypophysis (păr″ă-hī-pŏf′ĭ-sĭs) [″ + *hypophysis,* an undergrowth] Accessory to the pituitary tissue.

parainfluenza viruses A group of viruses that cause acute respiratory infections in humans, esp. in children. Virtually all children in the U.S. have been infected by age 6.

parakeratosis (păr″ă-kĕr″ă-tō′sĭs) [″ + *keras,* horn, + *osis,* condition] The persistence of nuclei within the keratinocytes of the stratum corneum of epidermis or mucosal layers, which indicates a partial keratinization process; a general term applied to disorders of the keratinized layer of the skin.

p. ostracea P. scutularis.

p. psoriasiformis Scab formation resembling that of psoriasis.

p. scutularis A scalp disease with hairs encircled by epidermic crust formation.

paralalia (păr″ă-lā′lē-ă) [″ + *lalein,* to babble] Any speech defect characterized by sound distortion.

p. literalis Stammering.

paralambdacism (păr″ă-lăm′dă-sĭzm) [″ + *lambda,* Gr. letter L, + *-ismos,* condition] An inability to sound the letter "l" correctly, substituting some other letter for it.

paraldehyde (păr-ăl′dĕ-hīd) $C_6H_{12}O_3$; a liquid polymer of acetaldehyde that is colorless, has an unpleasant taste, and has a characteristic odor. It is made by the action of hydrochloric acid on acetic aldehyde.

ACTION/USES: The agent was used in the past as a sedative and hypnotic. It has been largely replaced by benzodiazepines.

paraldehyde poisoning Poisoning in which symptoms resemble those of chloral hydrate poisoning: cardiac and respiratory depression, dizziness, and collapse with partial or complete anesthesia. It may also produce severe lactic acidosis.

TREATMENT: There is no specific antidote. Supportive care includes (when appropriate) airway management, ventilation, and hemodialysis.

paralepsy (păr′ă-lĕp″sē) [″ + *lepsis,* seizure] A temporary attack of mental inertia and hopelessness, or sudden alteration in mood or mental tension.

paralexia (păr″ă-lĕk′sē-ă) [″ + *lexis,* speech] An inability to comprehend printed words or sentences, together with substitution of meaningless combinations of words.

paralgia (păr-ăl′jē-ă) [″ + *algos,* pain] An abnormal sensation that is painful.

paralipophobia Fear of omitting or neglecting a duty.

parallagma (păr″ăl-ăg′mă) [Gr., alternation] Overlapping or displacement of the fragments of a fractured bone.

parallax (păr′ă-lăks) [Gr. *parallaxis,* change of position] The apparent movement or displacement of objects caused by change in the observer's position or by movement of the head or eyes.

binocular p. The basis of stereoscopic vision; the difference in the angles formed by the lines of sight to two objects at different distances from the eyes. This is important in depth perception.

heteronymous p. Parallax in which, when one eye is closed, the object viewed appears to move closer to the closed eye.

homonymous p. Parallax in which, when one eye is covered, the object viewed appears to move closer to the uncovered eye.

parallelometer (păr″ă-lĕl-ŏm′ĕ-tĕr) A device used in dentistry to determine whether or not lines and tooth surfaces are parallel to each other.

parallel play The stage in social development in which a child plays alongside, but not with, other children; characteristic of toddlers.

parallergy (păr-ăl′ĕr-jē) The condition of being allergic to nonspecific stimuli after having been sensitized with a specific allergen. **parallergic** (păr″ă-lĕr′jĭk), *adj.*

paralogia (păr″ă-lō′jē-ă) [Gr. *para,* beside, + *logos,* word, reason] A disorder of reasoning.

benign p. Disordered thinking and communication of thought in which delusions, bizarre thoughts, hallucinations, and regressive behavior are absent. The patient is not severely incapacitated and should not be considered to have schizophrenia.

paralogism (păr″ă-lō′jĭz-ĕm) An incorrectly chosen word inserted into speech, esp. in patients with fluent aphasias. SEE: *neologism; paraphasia.*

paralysis (pă-răl′ĭ-sĭs) *pl.* **paralyses** [Gr. *paralyein,* to disable] **1.** Loss of sensation; anesthesia. **2.** Loss of purposeful movement, usually as a result of neurological disease (e.g., strokes and spinal cord injuries), drugs, or toxins. Loss of motor function may be complete (paralysis) or partial (paresis); unilateral (hemiplegic) or bilateral (diplegic); confined to the lower extremities (paraplegic) or present in all four extremities (tetraplegic); accompanied by increased muscular tension and hyperactive reflexes (spastic) or by loss of reflexes and tone (flaccid). SYN: *palsy.*

PATIENT CARE: Referral is made to the rehabilitation therapists for evaluation of the patient's motor and sensory capabilities (muscle size, tone and strength, reflex or involuntary movement, response to touch or to painful stimuli). The patient is positioned to prevent deformities. Passive range of motion is performed on the involved extremities to prevent contractures. The patient is repositioned frequently to prevent pressure sores. Local and systemic responses, including fatigue, are evaluated. The rehabilitation team assesses and attends to any self-care deficits the patient may have. Support is offered to the patient and family to assist them in dealing with psychological concerns and the grief and loss response. Assistance is provided to help the patient in achieving optimal level of function and in adapting to the disability.

Key concerns include functional positioning, the prevention of deformities secondary to spasticity, and the prevention of injury when sensation is absent. A plan involving muscle reeducation and compensatory training may be prescribed. Functional orthoses and assistive technology devices may be necessary to assist the patient in performing self-care and other tasks of daily living. Support is offered to the patient and family to assist them in dealing with psychological concerns.

p. of accommodation Inability of the eye to adjust itself to various distances owing to paralysis of ciliary muscles.

acoustic p. Deafness.

p. agitans Parkinson's disease.

alcoholic p. Paralysis caused by the toxic effect of alcohol on nerve tissue.

anesthesia p. Paralysis that develops following administration of anesthesia.

arsenical p. Paralysis caused by the toxic effect of arsenic.

Bell's p. Bell's palsy.

birth p. Loss of function related to nerve injury during delivery. Trauma to the baby during delivery may result, for example, in damage to the brachial nerves, facial nerves, or diaphragm. Asymmetrical movements or reflexes of the affected part are present. Prognosis depends on the amount of nerve damage sustained; however, permanent damage is rare. Most newborn paralyses resolve without sequelae within a few weeks to a few months of birth. SYN: *obstetrical p.*

brachial p. Paralysis of one or both arms.

brachiofacial p. Paralysis of the face and an arm.

bulbar p. Paralysis caused by changes in the motor centers of the medulla oblongata. SYN: *progressive bulbar p.*

complete p. Paralysis in which there is total loss of function and sensation.

compression p. Paralysis due to prolonged pressure on a nerve, as by improper use of a crutch or during sleep.

conjugate p. Paralysis of the conjugate movement of the eyes in all directions even though the fixation axis remains parallel.

crossed p. Paralysis affecting one side of the face and limbs of the opposite side of the body.

crutch p. Paralysis due to pressure on nerves in the axilla caused by improper use of a crutch.

decubitus p. Paralysis due to pressure on a nerve from lying in one position for a long time, as in sleep or while in a coma.

diphtheritic p. Paralysis of the muscles of the palate, eyes, limbs, diaphragm, and intercostal muscles that occurs as a complication of diphtheria. It is caused by a toxin produced by the diphtheria bacillus. SYN: *postdiphtheritic p.*

diver's p. Decompression illness.

Duchenne-Erb p. Paralysis of the muscles of the upper arm due to injury of the upper nerves, the fifth and sixth cervical roots, of the brachial plexus. The hand muscles are unaffected.

facial p. Bell's palsy.

flaccid p. Paralysis in which there is loss of muscle tone, loss or reduction of tendon reflexes, atrophy and degeneration of muscles, and reaction of degeneration; caused by lesions of lower motor neurons of the spinal cord.

general p. Paresis.

ginger p. Jamaica ginger p.

glossolabial p. Paralysis of the tongue and lips; occurs in bulbar paralysis.

Gubler's p. A form of alternate hemiplegia in which a brainstem lesion causes paralysis of the cranial nerves on one side and of the body on the opposite side.

hyperkalemic p. A rare form of periodic paralysis characterized by brief, 1- to 2-hr attacks of limb weakness. In some cases, respiratory muscles are involved. The term "hyperkalemic" is misleading in that the potassium levels may be normal. However, because an attack is precipitated by the administration of potassium, this form of paralysis should be termed "potassium-sensitive periodic paralysis."

TREATMENT: Emergency treatment is seldom necessary. Oral glucose hastens recovery. In addition, attacks may be prevented by use of acetazolamide or thiazide diuretics.

hypokalemic periodic p. A form of periodic paralysis with onset usually prior to adulthood. An attack typically comes on during sleep, after strenuous exercise during the day. The weakness may be so pronounced as to prevent the patient from being able to call for help. The attack may last from several hours to a day or more. The diagnosis is established by determining that the serum potassium level is decreased during an attack.

TREATMENT: Administration of oral potassium salts improves the paralysis. If the patient is too weak to swallow, intravenous potassium salts are required. Attacks may be prevented by oral administration of 5 to 10 g of potassium chloride daily.

hysterical p. Loss of movement without a demonstrable organic cause. Typically the patient's reflexes are preserved in the affected body part despite its apparent immobility, and bowel and bladder function are preserved. In Western medicine, functional disorders such as this are treated with occupational therapy or supportive psychotherapy; in traditional Chinese medicine, acupuncture is used. SEE: *Hoover sign*.

immunological p. The inability to form antibodies after exposure to large doses of an antigen.

incomplete p. Partial paralysis of the body or a part.

infantile p. Poliomyelitis.

infantile cerebral ataxic p. Cerebral palsy.

ischemic p. Volkmann's contracture.

Jamaica ginger p. Paralysis due to polyneuropathy that affects the muscles of the distal portions of the limbs. It is caused by drinking an alcoholic beverage called Jamaica ginger that contains the toxic substance triorthocresylphosphate.

Klumpke's p. Wasting paralysis of the arms and hands, often resulting from birth injury.

Landry's p. Flaccid paralysis that begins in the lower extremities and rapidly ascends to the trunk.

laryngeal p. Loss of vocal fold mobility. Common causes include surgical trauma to the recurrent laryngeal nerve or invasion of the nerve by tumor. SYN: *vocal paralysis*.

lead p. Paralysis due to lead poisoning.

local p. Paralysis of a single muscle or one group of muscles.

mimetic p. Paralysis of the facial muscles.

mixed p. Paralysis of motor and sensory nerves.

muscular p. Loss of the capacity of muscles to contract; may be due to a structural or functional disorder in the muscle at the myoneural junction, in efferent nerve fibers, in cell bodies of nuclei of origin of brain or gray matter of spinal cord, in conducting pathways of brain or spinal cord, or in motor centers of the brain.

musculospiral p. Paralysis due to prolonged ischemia of the musculospiral nerve incident to compressing an arm against a hard edge. It occurs if the patient has been comatose or in a stupor or has fallen asleep with the arm hanging over the edge of a bed or chair. Sometimes called "Saturday night paralysis" because in some cultures individuals traditionally become intoxicated on Saturday night; while stuporous, they may remain in a position that allows nerve compression. SYN: *radial p.; Saturday night p.*

nuclear p. Paralysis caused by lesion of nuclei in the central nervous system.

obstetrical p. Birth p.

ocular p. Paralysis of the extraocular and intraocular muscles.

postdiphtheritic p. Diphtheritic p.

posticus p. Paralysis of the posterior cricothyroid muscles.

Pott's p. Paralysis of the lower part of the body owing to tuberculosis of the spine (Pott's disease).

pressure p. Paralysis due to pressure on the spinal cord or a nerve. This may be caused by injury, tumor, or gummata.

primary periodic p. The occurrence of intermittent weakness, usually following rest or sleep, and almost never during vigorous activity. The condition usually begins in early life and rarely has its onset after age 25. The attacks may last from a few hours to a day or more. The patient is alert during an attack.

The causes include hypokalemia, hyperkalemia, thyrotoxicosis, and a form of paramyotonia. Both forms of the disease in which potassium regulation is a factor respond to acetazolamide; the thyrotoxicosis-related disorder is treated by correcting the underlying thyrotoxicosis. In cases of paramyotonia congenita with periodic paralysis, the treatment is spironolactone.

progressive bulbar p. Bulbar p.

pseudobulbar p. Paralysis caused by cerebral center lesions, simulating the bulbar types of paralysis.

pseudohypertrophic muscular p. SEE: *dystrophy, pseudohypertrophic muscular*.

radial p. Musculospiral p.

Saturday night p. Musculospiral p.

sensory p. Loss of sensation; may be due to a structural or functional disorder of the sensory end organs, sensory nerves, conducting pathways of spinal cord or brain, or sensory centers in the brain.

sleep p. Brief, temporary inability to move or speak that occurs when falling asleep or awakening.

spastic p. Paralysis usually involving groups of muscles; characterized by excessive tone and spasticity of muscles, exaggeration of tendon reflexes but loss of superficial reflexes, positive Babinski's reflex, no atrophy or wasting except from prolonged disuse, and absence of reaction of degeneration. This form of paralysis is due to lesions of the upper motor neurons.

spinal p. Paralysis due to injury or disease of the spinal cord.

supranuclear p. Paralysis resulting from disorders in pathways or centers above the nuclei of origin.

tick-bite p. Paralysis resulting from bites of certain species of ticks, esp. of the genera *Ixodes* and *Dermacentor,* due to a toxin in tick saliva. It affects domestic animals and humans, esp. children, and causes a progressive ascending, flaccid motor paralysis. Recovery usually occurs after removal of the ticks.

tourniquet p. Paralysis, esp. of the arm, resulting from a tourniquet being applied for too long a time.

vasomotor p. Paralysis of the vasomotor centers, resulting in lack of tone and dilation of the blood vessels.

vocal p. Laryngeal p.

Volkmann's p. Volkmann's contracture.

wasting p. Progressive muscular atrophy.

paralytic (păr″ă-lĭt′ĭk) [Gr. *paralyein,* to disable] **1.** Concerning paralysis. **2.** One afflicted with paralysis.

paralytic dementia Paresis.

paralytic ileus Paralysis of the movement of the smooth muscles of the intestines, usually temporary, with distention and symptoms of acute obstruction; may occur after any abdominal surgery. It can also be a side effect of many drugs.

paralyzant (păr′ă-līz″ănt) [Fr. *paralyser,* paralyze] **1.** Causing paralysis. **2.** A drug or other agent that induces paralysis.

paralyze (păr′ă-līz) [Fr. *paralyse*] **1.** To cause temporary or permanent loss of muscular power or sensation. **2.** To render ineffective.

paralyzer (păr′ă-līz″ĕr) **1.** That which causes paralysis. **2.** A substance that inhibits a chemical reaction.

paramagnetic (păr″ă-măg-nĕt′ĭk) Anything that is attracted by the poles of a magnet and becomes parallel to the lines of magnetic force.

paramania (păr″ă-mā′nē-ă) [Gr. *para,* beside, + *mania,* madness] A type of emotional disturbance in which the individual derives pleasure from complaining.

paramastigote (păr″ă-măs′tĭ-gōt) [″ + *mastix,* lash] Having a small supernumerary flagellum next to a larger one.

paramastitis (păr″ă-măs-tī′tĭs) [″ + *mastos,* breast, + *itis,* inflammation] Inflammation around the breast.

paramastoid (păr″ă-măs′toyd) [″ + ″ + *eidos,* form, shape] Next to the mastoid.

paramedian (păr″ă-mē′dē-ăn) [″ + L. *medianus,* median] Close to the midline. SYN: *paramesial.*

paramedian incision A surgical incision, esp. of the abdominal wall, close to the midline.

paramedic (păr″ă-mĕd′ĭk) [Gr. *para,* beside, + L. *medicus,* doctor] A health care professional trained in the emergency care of patients who suffer from sudden illnesses or injuries. Paramedics typically function in the prehospital environment, under the medical direction of a physician. SEE: *emergency medical technician.*

paramedical Supplementing the work of medical personnel in related fields: social work; physical, occupational, and speech therapy.

paramedical personnel Health care workers who are not physicians or nurses. These include medical technicians, emergency medical technicians, and physician's assistants. SEE: *allied health professional.*

paramesial (păr″ă-mē′sē-ăl) [″ + *mesos,* middle] Paramedian.

parameter (păr-ăm′ĕ-tĕr) [″ + *metron,* measure] **1.** In mathematics, an arbitrary constant, each value of which determines the specific form of the equation in which it appears; often misused to indicate a variable. **2.** In biostatistics, a measurement taken on a population, which consists of all the subjects in a defined group.

paramethasone acetate (păr″ă-mĕth′ă-sōn) A glucocorticosteroid drug.

parametric (păr″ă-mĕt′rĭk) [Gr. *para,* beside, + *metra,* uterus] **1.** Concerning the area near the uterus. **2.** Rel. to the parametrium, the tissue surrounding the uterus.

parametric (păr″ă-mĕt′rĭk) [Gr. *para,* beside, + *metron,* measure] Adjectival form of parameter.

parametric statistics The class of statistics based on the assumption that the samples measured are from normally distributed populations.

parametritic (păr″ă-mē-trĭt′ĭk) Concerning parametritis.

parametritis (păr″ă-mē-trī′tĭs) [″ + *metra,* uterus, + *itis,* inflammation] An inflammation of the parametrium, the cellular tissue adjacent to the uterus. It may occur in puerperal fever or septic conditions of the uterus and appendages. SYN: *pelvic cellulitis.*

parametrium (păr-ă-mē′trē-ŭm) [″ + *metra,* uterus] Loose connective tissue around the uterus.

paramimia (păr″ă-mĭm′ē-ă) [″ + *mimeisthai,* to imitate] The use of gestures that are inappropriate to the spoken words that they accompany.

paramnesia (păr″ăm-nē′zē-ă) [″ + *amnesia,* loss of memory] **1.** Use of words without meaning. **2.** Distortion of memory in which there is inability to distinguish imaginary or suggested experiences from those that have actually occurred. **3.** Seeming recall of events that never have occurred.

paramolar (păr″ă-mō′lăr) A supernumerary tooth close to a molar.

paramucin (păr″ă-mū′sĭn) A glycoprotein found in ovarian and some other cysts.

paramusia (păr″ă-mū′zē-ă) [″ + *mousa,* music] A form of aphasia in which the ability to render music correctly is lost.

paramyloidosis (păr-ăm″ĭ-loy-dō′sĭs) [″ + L. *amylum,* starch, + Gr. *eidos,* form, shape, + *osis,* condition] The presence and build-up of atypical amyloid in tissues.

paramyoclonus multiplex (păr-ă-mī-ŏk′lō-nŭs mŭl′tĭ-plĕks) [″ + *mys,* muscle, + *klonos,* tumult] Sudden and frequent shocklike contractions usually affecting the muscles of both legs, and particularly the trunk muscles. The contractions, which disappear during sleep and motion, may occur 10 to 50 times each minute. Usually the condition develops spontaneously, but it has been known to follow fright, trauma, infectious diseases, and poliomyelitis. SYN: *polymyoclonus.*

paramyosinogen (păr″ă-mī″ō-sĭn′ō-jĕn) [Gr. *para,* beside, + *myosin,* protein globin of muscle, + *gennan,* to produce] Protein derived from muscle tissue.

paramyotonia (păr″ă-mī″ō-tō′nē-ă) [″ + *mys,* muscle, + *tonos,* tone] A disorder marked by muscular spasms and abnormal muscular tonicity.

ataxic p. Tonic muscular spasm with slight ataxia or paresis during any attempt at movement.

p. congenita A congenital condition of tonic muscular spasms when the body is exposed to cold. SYN: *Eulenburg's disease.*

symptomatic p. Temporary muscular rigidity when one first tries to walk, as in Parkinson's disease.

paramyxovirus Any virus of a subgroup of the myxoviruses that are similar in physical, chemical, and biological characteristics, even though they are quite different pathogenetically. The group includes parainfluenza, measles, mumps, Newcastle disease, and respiratory syncytial viruses.

paranasal (păr″ă-nā′săl) [″ + L. *nasalis,* pert. to the nose] Situated near or along the nasal cavities.

paraneoplastic syndromes Indirect effects of cancers, such as metabolic disturbances or hormonal excesses produced by chemicals released by tumor cells. Tumors such as small cell carcinoma of the lung, hypernephroma, and neuroendocrine cancers are often responsible.

paranephric (păr″ă-nĕf′rĭk) [″ + *nephros,* kidney] **1.** Close to the kidney. **2.** Concerning the adrenal glands.

paranephros (păr-ă-nĕf′rŏs) A suprarenal or adrenal capsule.

paranesthesia (păr″ăn-ĕs-thē′zē-ă) [″ + *an-,* not, + *aisthesis,* sensation] Anesthesia of the lower body.

paraneural (păr″ă-nū′răl) [″ + *neuron,* nerve] Adjacent to a nerve.

paranoia (păr″ă-noy′ă) [Gr. *para,* beside, + *nous,* mind] A condition in which patients show persistent persecutory delusions or delusional jealousy. The disorder must be persistent, lasting at least 1 week. The condition may be accompanied by symptoms of schizophrenia such as bizarre delusions or incoherence. There are no prominent hallucinations and a full depressive or manic syndrome is either not present or is of brief duration. The illness is not due to organic disease of the brain.

This disorder, which usually occurs in middle or late adult life and may be chronic, often includes resentment and anger that may lead to violence. Paranoid people rarely seek medical attention but are brought for care by associates or relatives.

erotomanic type p. A form of paranoid delusion that one is loved by another. The delusion is more nearly one of romantic or spiritual love, rather than physical. The object is usually someone who is of a higher status or who is famous, but may be a complete stranger.

jealous type p. The unfounded conviction that the patient's spouse or lover is unfaithful.

litigious p. Paranoia in which the patient institutes or threatens to institute legal action because of the imagined persecution.

somatic p. The delusion that one's body is malodorous, or is infested with an internal or external parasite, or that the body is physically misshapen or unduly ugly.

paranoiac (păr-ă-noy′ăk) **1.** Concerning or afflicted with paranoia. **2.** One suffering from paranoia.

paranoid (păr′ă-noyd) [″ + *nous,* mind, + *eidos,* form, shape] **1.** Resembling paranoia. **2.** A person afflicted with paranoia.

paranoid disorder Paranoia. SEE: *Nursing Diagnoses Appendix; personality disorder, paranoid.*

paranoid ideation Suspicious thinking that is persecutory, accompanied by feelings that one is being harassed, treated wrongly, or being judged critically.

paranoid reaction type An individual who has fixed systematized delusions, is suspicious, has a persecution complex, is resentful and bitter, and is a megalomaniac. Many states approach true paranoia and resemble it but lack one or more of its distinguishing features. Some of these are transitory paranoid states caused by toxic conditions, a paranoid type of schizophrenia, and paranoid states due to alcoholism.

paranomia (păr″ă-nō′mē-ă) [″ + *onoma,* name] Form of aphasia in which there is an inability to remember correct names of objects shortly after seeing or using them.

paranormal **1.** Pert. to claimed experiences that are not within the range of normal experiences or are not scientifically explainable. SEE: *extrasensory perception; psychokinesis.* **2.** Moderately abnormal.

paranuclear (păr″ă-nū′klē-ăr) Adjacent to the nucleus of a cell.

paranucleolus (păr″ă-nū-klē′ō-lŭs) A small basophil body in the sac enclosing the nucleus.

paranucleus (păr″ă-nū′klē-ŭs) [Gr. *para,* beside, + L. *nucleus,* a kernel] A small body lying close to a cell nucleus.

paraoperative (păr″ă-ŏp′ĕr-ă-tĭv) [″ + L. *operari,* to work] Perioperative.

parapancreatic (păr″ă-păn″krē-ăt′ĭk) [″ + *pan,* all, + *kreas,* flesh] Located close to the pancreas.

paraparesis (păr″ă-păr-ē′sĭs, -păr′ĕ-sĭs) [″ + *parienai,* to let fall] Partial paralysis affecting the lower limbs.

parapeptone (păr″ă-pĕp′tōn) [″ + *peptein,* to digest] Intermediate digestion product of albumin. SEE: *peptone.*

paraperitoneal (păr″ă-pĕr″ĭ-tō-nē′ăl) [″ + *peritonaion,* peritoneum] Near the peritoneum.

paraphasia (păr-ă-fā′zē-ă) [″ + *aphasis,* speech loss] The misuse of spoken words or word combinations, in which a meaningless or inappropriate word or syllable is substituted for the correct word; a form of aphasia. SEE: *paraphrasia.*

paraphemia (păr″ă-fē′mē-ă) [″ + *pheme,* speech] A disorder marked by consistent use of the wrong words or by mispronunciation of words.

paraphilia [″ + *philein,* to love] A psychosexual disorder in which unusual or bizarre imagery or acts are necessary for realization of sexual excitement. Included in this disorder are bestiality, fetishism, transvestism, zoophilia, pedophilia, exhibitionism, voyeurism, sexual masochism, and sexual sadism.

paraphimosis (păr″ă-fī-mō′sĭs) [″ + *phimoun,* to muzzle, + *osis,* condition] Strangulation of the glans penis due to retraction of a narrowed or inflamed foreskin.

p. oculi Retraction of the eyelid behind a protruding eyeball.

paraphobia (păr″ă-fō′bē-ă) [″ + *phobos,* fear] A mild form of phobia.

paraphrasia (păr-ă-frā′zē-ă) [Gr. *para,* beside, + *phrasis,* speech] A condition characterized by loss of ability to use words correctly and coherently. The words spoken are so jumbled and misused as to make speech unintelligible.

paraphrenitis (păr″ă-frē-nī′tĭs) [″ + *phren,* diaphragm, + *itis,* inflammation] Inflammation of the tissues around the diaphragm.

paraphysis (pă-răf′ĭ-sĭs) [Gr., offshoot] The vestigial structure that originates from the roof plate of the telencephalon. Presumably the colloid cyst of the third ventricle arises from it. It is also a midline organ that develops from the roof plate of the diencephalon of some lower vertebrates.

paraplasm (păr′ă-plăzm) [Gr. *para,* beside, + LL. *plasma,* form, mold] **1.** Any abnormal new formation or malformation. **2.** Cytoplasm.

paraplastic (păr″ă-plăs′tĭk) [″ + *plastikos,* formed] **1.** Misshapen; deformed. **2.** Pert. to the fluid portion of the protoplasm.

paraplegia (păr-ă-plē′jē-ă) [Gr. *paraplegia,* stroke on one side] Paralysis of the lower portion of the body and of both legs. It is caused by a lesion involving the spinal cord that may be due to maldevelopment, epidural abscess, hematomyelia, acute transverse myelitis, spinal neoplasms, multiple sclerosis, syringomyelia, or trauma. SEE: *Nursing Diagnoses Appendix.*

PATIENT CARE: Patient care during the acute period, immediately following traumatic injury, aims at stabilizing the patient and preventing further injury or deterioration. Initial and ongoing neurological assessment by nurses, the neurologist, and the neurosurgeon helps to determine the level and degree of paralysis and the patient's potential for recovery. Supportive medical therapy, based on assessment results, is provided. Specific medical, neurological, and neurosurgical interventions depend on the etiology of the paraplegia. Prescribed therapies are administered, and desired and adverse effects assessed for.

The patient should have early consultations with physical and occupational therapy staff, because correct body alignment, positioning, and exercise can prevent complications, encouraging the patient to think about rehabilitation from the beginning. The respiratory therapist also is involved early on to monitor ventilatory activity and help prevent respiratory complications. If intensive care is required, the health care provider recognizes the need to limit sensory overload by controlling and moderating environmental stimuli and to avoid sleep deprivation by planning an uninterrupted sleep time. Because immobility affects all body systems, they must each be monitored for expected and complicating changes. Medical consultations (e.g., with a pulmonologist, urologist) are made as necessary and treatment regimens are developed based on each patient's needs.

The patient experiences paraplegia as a profound loss, affecting not only independent mobility but also self-image and self-esteem. Although the loss may be sudden or gradual, predictable or unexpected, and temporary or permanent, depending on the cause of the patient's paraplegia, it is present nevertheless. Because family members also are affected, the health care provider includes them when helping the patient with grief-work and mourning, recognizing that anger and despondency are expected responses. Referral to a mental health care provider can help patients cope with their loss.

Patients with paraplegia are usually transferred to a rehabilitation facility once the acute period has passed. This move often engenders transfer anxiety, as the patient and family fear a lesser level of care as a threat to security and well-being. Behavioral and psychosomatic manifestations may occur. A liaison nurse from the new facility can help the patient bridge the transition by providing information about the facility and the vigorous program the patient will encounter. The family should be encouraged to visit the facility and to bring any questions or concerns to their liaison, while giving the patient positive input.

Rehabilitation requires the patient's active participation to achieve his or her highest potential, and this participation begins with planning. The patient's individualized plan of care should be developed by the entire rehabilitation team, which includes the patient and significant others who make up the support system, as well as the primary physician, nurse, physiatrist, physical therapist, occupational therapist, vocational counselor, dietitian, social worker, psychologist, and neuropsychologist. The goals of the plan include learning to manage neuromuscular deficits and being able to perform activities of daily living (ADLs) with enough independence to function successfully in the home, workplace, and social situations. Activities include proper positioning, range-of-motion exercises, balancing and sitting, transfer activities, ambulation, and use of equipment to aid ambulation (if the patient will be able to walk with the aid of braces, canes, or crutches) or adjustment to being in a wheelchair. Skin care is of great importance, as persons with paraplegia are at risk for pressure sore development because of their motor, sensory, and vasomotor deficits. Poor nutrition, infection, debilitation, edema, and prolonged immobility are contributing factors. Assessment and prevention of breakdown, as well as treatment of most areas of broken skin, fall within the purview of nursing, although severe pressure sores may require surgical débridement and plastic surgery.

Cystometric studies help to assess bladder function and determine the patient's ability to participate in a bladder-retraining program, as opposed to requiring catheter or condom-catheter drainage methods. Bowel incontinence also demands assessment of cause and contributing factors (autonomic dysfunction, sacral injury, immobility, decreased food intake, esp. roughage). Incontinence is managed matter-of-factly, getting the patient involved, observing behavioral cues related to the need for defecation, noting defecation habits and using them for appropriate toileting, and supporting the patient's self-esteem. Bowel retraining involves establishing and maintaining a defecation routine. All members of the rehabilitation team, but esp. mental health care providers, are involved in helping the patient and family cope with the lifestyle changes necessitated by the illness or injury. Psychosocial care begins with hearing the patient's and family's perceptions of the impact of the disability and their expectations for the future, and learning about their personalities, previous coping abilities, and previous adjustment patterns.

The adjustment to discharge to home or group living adds its own set of transfer anxieties. The team teaches the patient and family any special procedures they will need, and determines home and vehicle modifications needed to provide access for wheelchair or other necessary equipment. Group sessions with others who have faced similar situations often help both the patient and family. Initiating the move with a "weekend pass," followed by a return to process feelings and activities, can also help. It is important to note that rehabilitation, instead of ending with discharge, is an ongoing process central to living a worthwhile life.

alcoholic p. Paraplegia of spinal origin due to excessive use of alcohol.

ataxic p. Lateral and posterior sclerosis of the spinal cord characterized by slowly progressing ataxia and paresis.

cerebral p. Paraplegia from a bilateral cerebral lesion.

congenital spastic p. Infantile spastic p.

p. dolorosa Paraplegia due to pressure of a neoplasm on the posterior spinal cord and nerve roots; extremely painful despite paralysis.

infantile spastic p. Spastic paraplegia that occurs in infants, usually due to birth injury. SYN: *congenital spastic p.* SEE: *spastic p.*

peripheral p. Paraplegia due to pressure on, injury to, or disease of peripheral nerves.

Pott's p. Paraplegia associated with tuberculosis of the spine.

primary spastic p. Paraplegia from degeneration in corticospinal tracts.

senile p. Paraplegia resulting from sclerosis of arteries supplying the spinal cord.

spastic p. Paraplegia characterized by increased muscular tone and accentuated tendon reflexes; seen in upper motor neuron diseases. SYN: *tetanoid p.*

superior p. Paralysis of both arms.

tetanoid p. Spastic p.

paraplegic (păr-ă-plē′jĭk) [Gr. *paraplegia,* stroke on one side] Pert. to, or afflicted with, paraplegia.

paraplegiform (păr″ă-plĕj′ĭ-form) [″ + L. *forma,* form] Similar to paraplegia.

parapleuritis (păr″ă-plū-rī′tĭs) [Gr. *para,* beside, + *pleura,* side, + *itis,* inflammation] **1.** Inflammation in the thoracic wall. **2.** Mild inflammation of the pleura. **3.** Pleurodynia.

parapoplexy (păr-ăp′ō-plĕk″sē) [″ + *apoplessein,* to cripple by a stroke] A mild or slight apoplexy with partial stupor; a stupor resembling apoplexy. SYN: *pseudoapoplexy.*

parapraxia (păr-ă-prăk′sē-ă) [″ + *praxis,* doing] Disturbed mental processes producing inaccuracy, forgetfulness, and tendency to misplace things and make slips of speech or pen.

paraproctitis (păr″ă-prŏk-tī′tĭs) [Gr. *para,* beside, + *proktos,* anus, + *itis,* inflammation] Inflammation of the tissues near the rectum.

paraproctium (păr″ă-prŏk′shē-ŭm) [″ + *proktos,* anus] The connective tissue around the anus and rectum.

paraprofessional (păr″ă-prō-fĕsh′ŭn-ăl) A person with education and training in a specific area of one of the professions (e.g., medicine or law), who provides services in that profession as an extension of an individual licensed to practice independently.

paraprostatitis (păr″ă-prŏs″tă-tī′tĭs) [″ + *prostates,* prostate, + *itis,* inflammation] Inflammation of the tissues around the prostate.

paraprotein (păr″ă-prō′tē-ĭn) An abnormal plasma protein, such as a macroglobulin, cryoglobulin, or immunoglobulin. SEE: *paraproteinemia.*

paraproteinemia The presence of abnormal or excessive amounts of proteins, such as immunoglobulins or cryoglobulins, in the blood. Paraproteinemias include amyloidosis, cryoglobulinemia, cryofibrinogenemia, cold IgM antibody disease, light chain disease, monoclonal gammopathy, multiple myeloma, and Waldenström's macroglobulinemia. Plasma exchange therapy, immunomodulating drugs, or specific chemotherapeutic agents are used to treat these disorders. SEE: *Bence Jones protein.*

parapsoriasis (păr″ă-sō-rī′ă-sĭs) [″ + *psoriasis,* an itching] A chronic disorder of the skin marked by scaly red lesions.

p. en plaque A form of parapsoriasis that is often the precursor of mycosis fungoides.

p. lichenoides chronica A form of parapsoriasis that forms a widespread network over the extremities and trunk that is red to blue, sometimes resembling psoriasis or lichen planus.

parapsychology (păr″ă-sī-kŏl′ō-jē) The division of psychology that deals with alleged instances of extrasensory perception, telepathy, psychokinesis, clairvoyance, and associated phenomena.

paraquat (păr′ă-kwăt) A toxic chemical used in agriculture to kill certain weeds. It damages the skin on contact and if ingested may cause vomiting, diarrhea, liver, renal, and pulmonary disease. This chemical is sometimes present as a contaminant in marijuana.

p. poisoning Poisoning due to ingestion of paraquat. Persons who have consumed paraquat may be treated with oral activated charcoal and, if kidney failure is present, hemodialysis.

pararectal (păr″ă-rĕk′tăl) [″ + L. *rectum,* straight] Close to the rectum.

parareflexia (păr″ă-rē-flĕk′sē-ă) An abnormal condition of the reflexes.

pararenal (păr″ă-rē′năl) [″ + L. *ren,* kidney] Near the kidneys.

pararhotacism (păr″ă-rō′tă-sĭzm) [″ + *rho,* Gr. letter R, + *-ismos,* condition] Constant erroneous use of the letter "r" or the placing of undue emphasis on the letter "r."

pararthria (păr-ăr′thrē-ă) [″ + *arthron,* articulation] A speech disorder characterized by difficulty in uttering sounds.

parasacral (păr″ă-sā′krăl) [″ + L. *sacrum,* sacred] Close to the sacrum.

parasalpingitis (păr″ă-săl-pĭn-jī′tĭs) [″ + *salpinx,* tube, + *itis,* inflammation] Inflammation of the tissues around an oviduct or a eustachian tube.

parasecretion (păr″ă-sē-krē′shŭn) [″ + L. *secretio,* secretion] **1.** An abnormality in secretion. **2.** A substance abnormally secreted.

parasexuality (păr″ă-sĕks″ū-ăl′ĭ-tē) [″ + L. *sexus,* sex] Any sexually deviant act.

parasigmatism (păr″ă-sĭg′mă-tĭzm) [″ + *sigma,* Gr. letter S, + *-ismos,* condition] Lisping.

parasinoidal (păr″ă-sī-noy′dăl) [″ + L. *sinus,* a curve] Close to a sinus.

parasite (păr′ă-sīt) [″ + *sitos,* food] **1.** An organism that lives within, upon, or at the expense of another organism (host) without contributing to its survival. **2.** The smaller or incomplete element of conjoined twins that is attached to and dependent on the more nearly normal twin (autosite).

accidental p. A parasite infesting a host that is not its normal host. SYN: *incidental p.*

external p. A parasite that lives on the outer surface of its hosts, such as fleas, lice, mites, or ticks. SYN: *ectoparasite.*

facultative p. A parasite capable of living independently of its host at times; the opposite of an obligate parasite.

incidental p. Accidental p.

intermittent p. A parasite that visits its host at intervals for nourishment. SYN: *occasional p.*

internal p. A parasite such as a protozoon or worm that lives within the body of the host, occupying the digestive tract or body cavities, or living within body organs, blood, tissues, or cells.

malarial p. Any one of the four species of *Plasmodium* that can cause malaria. SEE: *malaria.*

obligate p. A parasite completely dependent on its host; the opposite of a facultative parasite.

occasional p. Intermittent p.

periodic p. A parasite that lives on the host for short periods of time.

permanent p. A parasite, such as a fluke or an itch mite, that lives on its host until maturity or spends its entire life on its host.

specific p. A parasite that requires a specific host in order to complete its life cycle.

temporary p. A parasite that is free-living during a part of its life cycle.

parasitemia (păr″ă-sī-tē′mē-ă) [″ + ″ + *haima,* blood] The presence of parasites in the blood.

parasitic (păr″ă-sĭt′ĭk) [Gr. *para,* beside, + *sitos,* food] Resembling, caused by, or concerning a parasite.

parasiticide (păr″ă-sĭt′ĭ-sīd) [″ + ″ + L. *caedere,* to kill] **1.** Destructive to parasites. **2.** An agent that kills parasites.

parasitism (păr′ă-sīt″ĭzm) [″ + ″ + *-ismos,* condition] **1.** The state or condition of being infected or infested with parasites. **2.** The behavior of a parasite.

parasitize (păr′ă-sĭt-īz″, -sīt-īz″) To infest or infect with a parasite.

parasitogenic (păr″ă-sī″tō-jĕn′ĭk) [″ + ″ + *gennan,* to produce] **1.** Caused by parasites. **2.** Favoring parasitic development.

parasitologist (păr″ă-sī-tŏl′ō-jĭst) [″ + ″ + *logos,* word, reason] One who specializes in the science of parasitology.

parasitology (păr″ă-sī-tŏl′ō-jē) [″ + ″ + *logos,* word, reason] The study of parasites and parasitism.

parasitophobia (păr″ă-sī″tō-fō′bē-ă) [″ + ″ + *phobos,* fear] An unusual fear of parasites.

parasitosis (păr″ă-sī-tō′sĭs) [″ + ″ + *osis,* condition] A disease or condition resulting from parasitism.

parasitotropic (păr″ă-sī″tō-trŏp′ĭk) [″ + ″ + *tropos,* turning] Having an attraction for parasites, esp. certain drugs that act chiefly on parasites in the body.

parasitotropism (păr″ă-sī-tŏt′rō-pĭzm) [″ + ″ + ″ + *-ismos,* condition] The special affinity of drugs or other agents for parasites.

parasitotropy (păr″ă-sī-tŏt′rō-pē) Parasitotropism.

parasomnias (păr″ă-sŏm′nē-ăz) [″ + L. *somnus,* sleep] An abnormal event that occurs during sleep. SEE: *sleep disorder.*

paraspadia (păr-ă-spā′dē-ă) [Gr. *paraspadein,* to draw aside] A condition in which the urethra has an opening through one side of the penis.

paraspasm (păr′ă-spăzm) [L. *paraspasmus*] **1.** Muscular spasm of the lower extremities. **2.** Spastic paralysis of the lower extremities.

parasteatosis (păr″ă-stē″ă-tō′sĭs) [Gr. *para,* beside, + *steatos,* fat, + *osis,* condition] Any disordered condition of the sebaceous glands.

parasternal (păr-ă-stĕrn′ăl) [″ + *sternon,* chest] Beside the sternum.

p. region The area between the sternal margin and parasternal line.

parasympathetic (păr″ă-sĭm″pă-thĕt′ĭk) [″ + *sympathetikos,* sympathetic nerve] Of or pert. to the craniosacral division of the autonomic nervous system.

p. nervous system The craniosacral division of the autonomic nervous system. Preganglionic fibers originate from nuclei in the midbrain, medulla, and sacral portion of the spinal cord. They pass through the third, seventh, ninth, and tenth cranial nerves and the second, third, and fourth sacral nerves, and synapse with postganglionic neurons located in autonomic (terminal) ganglia that lie in the walls of or near the organ innervated.

Some effects of parasympathetic stimulation are constriction of the pupil, contraction of the smooth muscle of the alimentary canal, constriction of the bronchioles, slowing of the heart rate, and increased secretion by the glands, except the sweat glands.

parasympathicotonia (păr″ă-sĭm-păth″ĭk-ō-tō′nē-ă) [″ + *sympathetikos,* sympathetic nerve, + *tonos,* tension] A condition in which there is an imbalance in functioning of the autonomic nervous system, the parasympathetic division dominating over the sympathetic. SYN: *vagotonia.*

parasympatholytic (păr″ă-sĭm″pă-thō-lĭt′ĭk) [″ + ″ + *lytikos,* dissolving]

Having a destructive effect on or blocking parasympathetic nerve fibers.

parasympathomimetic (păr″ă-sĭm″pă-thō-mĭm-ĕt′ĭk) [″ + ″ + *mimetikos,* imitative] Producing effects similar to those resulting from stimulation of the parasympathetic nervous system.

parasynovitis (păr″ă-sĭn″ō-vī′tĭs) [″ + *syn,* with, + *oon,* egg, + *itis,* inflammation] Inflammation of tissues around a synovial sac.

parasystole (păr-ă-sĭs′tō-lē) [″ + *systole,* contraction] An ectopically originating cardiac rhythm independent of the normal sinus rhythm.

paratarsium (păr-ă-tăr′sē-ŭm) [″ + *tarsos,* tarsus] The covering and connective tissues of the tarsus of the feet.

paratenon (păr″ă-tĕn′ŏn) [″ + *tenon,* tendon] Fatty and areolar tissue that fills the spaces within the facscia around a tendon.

paratereseomania (păr″ă-tĕr-ē″sē-ō-mā′nē-ă) [Gr. *parateresis,* observation, + *mania,* madness] The insane desire to investigate new scenes and subjects.

parathion (păr″ă-thī′ŏn) An agricultural insecticide that is highly toxic to humans and animals.

p. poisoning Poisoning contracted by accidental inhalation or ingestion while working with the pesticide or because of the inadvertent contamination of food products eaten. Shortly after exposure, headache, sweating, salivation, lacrimation, vomiting, diarrhea, muscular twitching, convulsions, dyspnea, and blurred vision occur. SEE: *Poisons and Poisoning Appendix.*

parathormone (păr″ă-thor′mōn) [Gr. *para,* beside, + *thyreos,* shield, + *eidos,* form, shape, + *hormaein,* to excite] Parathyroid hormone.

parathyroid (păr-ă-thī′royd) [″ + *thyreos,* shield, + *eidos,* form, shape] **1.** Located close to the thyroid gland. **2.** One of four small endocrine glands about 6 mm long by 3 to 4 mm broad on the back of and at the lower edge of the thyroid gland, or embedded within it. These glands secrete a hormone, parathyroid hormone (parathormone), that regulates calcium and phosphorus metabolism. SEE: *calcitonin* for illus.

ABNORMALITIES: Hypoparathyroidism or hyposecretion results in neuromuscular hyperexcitability manifested by convulsions and tetany, carpopedal spasm, wheezing, muscle cramps, urinary frequency, mood changes, and lassitude. Blood calcium falls and blood phosphorus rises. Other symptoms include blurring of vision caused by cataracts, poorly formed teeth if onset was in childhood, maldevelopment of hair and nails, and dry and scaly skin. Hyperparathyroidism or hypersecretion results in a rise in blood calcium and fall in blood phosphorus. Calcium is removed from bones, resulting in increased fragility. Muscular weakness, reduced muscular tone, and general neuromuscular hypoexcitability occur. Generalized osteitis fibrosa, or osteitis fibrosa cystica, is a clinical entity associated with hyperplasia and resulting hypersecretion of the parathyroids.

p. injection A standard preparation of the water-soluble parathyroid hormone. It increases the calcium content of the blood.

parathyroidectomy (păr″ă-thī-roydĕk′tō-mē) [″ + ″ + ″ + *ektome,* excision] Surgical removal of one or more of the parathyroid glands; used as a treatment for hyperparathyroidism or neoplasm. Because the parathyroid glands maintain serum calcium levels, removal of the parathyroid glands may produce profound hypocalcemia. SEE: *Nursing Diagnoses Appendix.*

PATIENT CARE: The patient's understanding of the procedure and postoperative care is assessed. The health care provider gives additional information and answers questions. The patient's bed should be slightly elevated, and vital signs monitored regularly. The patient is observed for signs of calcium deficiency, and serum electrolyte levels are monitored. The patient is instructed to report immediately hoarseness or loss of voice. Pain is monitored, and pain relief is provided. Before discharge, the patient is taught the importance of recognizing and seeking medical attention for signs of calcium deficiency. Instruction is provided in incisional care. The importance of early ambulation and activity is emphasized.

parathyroprivia (păr″ă-thī″rō-prĭ′vē-ă) [″ + ″ + L. *privus,* deprived of] A condition that results when the parathyroids are removed or cease functioning.

parathyrotropic (păr″ă-thī-rō-trŏp′ĭk) [″ + ″ + *tropikos,* turning] Having an affinity for the parathyroid gland.

paratonsillar (păr″ă-tŏn′sĭl-ăr) [″ + L. *tonsillaris,* pert. to tonsil] Near or about the tonsil.

paratope (păr′ă-tōp) [″ + *topos,* a place] The site on an antibody to which an antigen attaches. SEE: *epitope.*

paratrichosis (păr″ă-trĭ-kō′sĭs) [″ + *trichosis,* being hairy] An abnormality of the hair or of its location.

paratripsis (păr″ă-trĭp′sĭs) [″ + *tribein,* to rub] Rubbing, chafing.

paratrophic (păr″ă-trō′fĭk) [″ + *trophe,* nourishment] **1.** Requiring living substances for food; parasitic. **2.** Pert. to abnormal nutrition.

paratyphlitis (păr″ă-tĭf-lī′tĭs) [″ + *typhlos,* blind, + *itis,* inflammation] An inflammation of the connective tissue close to the cecum.

paratyphoid fever A rare form of febrile gastroenteritis in Western societies, marked by fevers, abdominal pain, diarrhea, headache, and occasionally intestinal perforation. It is caused by *Salmonella paratyphi* (A and B strains) and related *Salmonella* species, typically contracted by travelers who have visited tropical countries. Antibiotic treatments include ciprofloxacin or chloramphenicol.

paratypic (păr″ă-tĭp′ĭk) [″ + *typos,* type] Diverging from a type.

paraumbilical (păr″ă-ŭm-bĭl′ĭk-ăl) [″ + L. *umbilicus,* navel] Located close to the navel.

paraurethral (păr″ă-ū-rē′thrăl) [″ + *ourethra,* urethra] Located close to the urethra.

parauterine (păr″ă-ū′tĕr-ĭn) [″ + L. *uterus,* womb] Located close to or around the uterus.

paravaccinia (păr″ă-văk-sĭn′ē-ă) A viral disease that affects the udders of cows and may be transmitted to humans. In humans, the virus produces painless smooth or warty lesions, called "milker's nodules," on the hands and arms. SEE: *milker's nodules*.

paravaginal (păr″ă-văj′ĭn-ăl) [″ + *vagina,* sheath] Located close to or around the vagina.

paravaginitis (păr″ă-văj-ĭn-ī′tĭs) [″ + ″ + *itis,* inflammation] Inflammation of the tissue surrounding the vagina.

paravenous (păr″ă-vē′nŭs) [″ + L. *vena,* vein] Located close to a vein.

paravertebral (păr″ă-vĕr′tĕ-brăl) [″ + L. *vertebralis,* pert. to vertebrae] Alongside or near the vertebral column.

paravertebral anesthesia Injection of a local anesthetic at the roots of spinal nerves.

paravesical (păr″ă-vĕs′ĭk-ăl) [″ + L. *vesica,* bladder] Near the urinary bladder.

paraxial (păr-ăk′sē-ăl) [″ + L. *axis,* axis] On either side of the axis of the body or one of its parts.

paraxon (păr-ăk′sŏn) [″ + *axon,* axis] A collateral branch of an axon.

parazoon (păr″ă-zō′ŏn) [″ + *zoon,* animal] An animal that lives as a parasite on another animal.

parched [ME. *parchen*] Extremely dry.

Paré, Ambroise (păr-ā′) French surgeon, 1510–1590, who instituted certain refined techniques into surgery, obstetrics, and wound care.

parectasia, parectasis (păr″ĕk-tā′sē-ă, -tă-sĭs) [Gr. *para,* beside, + *ektasis,* stretching] Excessive dilatation or stretching of a structure.

parectropia (păr″ĕk-trō′pē-ă) [″ + *ek,* out, + *trope,* a turn] Apraxia.

paregoric (păr-ĕ-gor′ĭk) [L. *paregoricus,* soothing] **1.** Camphorated tincture of opium, a narcotic-containing drug that in large doses is poisonous; used in the symptomatic treatment of diarrhea. **2.** Soothing.

p. poisoning SEE: *opiate poisoning*.

parelectronomic (păr″ē-lĕk″trō-nŏm′ĭk) [Gr. *para,* beside, + *elektron,* amber, + *nomos,* law] Not subject to electric stimulus.

parencephalia (păr″ĕn-sĕ-fā′lē-ă) [″ + *enkephalos,* brain] A congenital defect of the brain.

parencephalocele (păr″ĕn-sĕf′ă-lō-sēl) [″ + ″ + *kele,* tumor, swelling] Herniation of the cerebellum through a defect in the cranium.

parencephalous (păr″ĕn-sĕf′ă-lŭs) [″ + *enkephalos,* brain] A fetus with imperfect development of the cranium.

parenchyma (păr-ĕn′kĭ-mă) [Gr. *parenkheim,* to pour in beside] The essential parts of an organ that are concerned with its function in contradistinction to its framework.

p. testis The functional portion of the testis, including the seminiferous tubules within the lobules.

parenchymatitis (păr″ĕn-kĭm″ă-tī′tĭs) [″ + *itis,* inflammation] Inflammation of the parenchyma or substance of a gland.

parenchymatous (păr″ĕn-kĭm′ă-tŭs) Concerning the essential tissues of an organ.

parent [L. *parens*] A father or a mother; one who begets offspring.

parentage, determination of SEE: *paternity test*.

parental leave The policy of allowing one or both parents to have leave from work following the birth of their child.

parental role conflict The state in which a parent experiences role confusion and conflict in response to crisis. SEE: *Nursing Diagnoses Appendix*.

parenteral (păr-ĕn′tĕr-ăl) [Gr. *para,* beside, + *enteron,* intestine] Denoting any medication route other than the alimentary canal, such as intravenous, subcutaneous, intramuscular, or mucosal. SEE: *medication route*.

p. digestion The digestion of foreign substances by body cells as opposed to enteral digestion, which occurs in the alimentary canal.

p. nutrition SEE: *total parenteral nutrition*.

parent/infant/child attachment, altered, risk for Disruption of the interactive process between parent/significant other and infant that fosters the development of a protective and nurturing reciprocal relationship. SEE: *Nursing Diagnoses Appendix*.

parenting **1.** Caring for and raising a child or children. **2.** Producing offspring.

altered p. Inability of the primary caretaker to create an environment that promotes the optimum growth and development of the child. SEE: *Nursing Diagnoses Appendix*.

altered p., risk for Risk for inability of the primary caretaker to create, maintain, or regain an environment that promotes the optimum growth and development of the child. SEE: *Nursing Diagnoses Appendix.*

surrogate p. An alternative method of childbearing for an infertile couple in which the wife is unable to bear a child. The surrogate mother agrees to be artificially inseminated by the husband's sperm and to relinquish the baby to the couple. Another approach is to retrieve eggs from the infertile wife and have them impregnated in vitro by her husband. The fertilized ovum is then implanted in the surrogate mother. SEE: *fertilization, in vitro; GIFT; surrogate parenting.*

parepithymia (păr″ĕp-ĭ-thī′mē-ă) [″ + *epithymia,* desire] An abnormal desire or craving.

paresis (păr′ĕ-sĭs, pă-rē′sĭs) [Gr. *parienai,* to let fall] **1.** Partial or incomplete paralysis. SEE: *paralysis.* **2.** An organic mental disease with somatic, irritative, and paralytic focal symptoms and signs running a slow, chronic, progressive course. SYN: *dementia paralytica; paralytic dementia.*

juvenile p. General paresis due to congenital syphilis; seen in children.

paresthesia (păr″ĕs-thē′zē-ă) [Gr. *para,* beside, + *aisthesis,* sensation] An abnormal or unpleasant sensation that results from injury to one or more nerves, often described by patients as numbness or as a prickly, stinging, or burning feeling.

Berger's p. Paresthesia of the legs that occurs in young people.

paretic (pă-rĕt′ĭk, pă-rē′tĭk) [Gr. *parienai,* to let fall] Afflicted with or concerning paresis.

pareunia [Gr. *pareunos,* lying beside] Sexual intercourse. SEE: *dyspareunia.*

pargyline hydrochloride (păr′gĭ-lēn) An antihypertensive drug.

parhidrosis (păr″hī-drō′sĭs) [Gr. *para,* beside, + *hidrosis,* sweat] Any disordered secretion of perspiration.

paries (pā′rē-ēs) *pl.* **parietes** [L., a wall] The enveloping wall of any structure; applied esp. to hollow organs.

parietal (pă-rī′ĕ-tăl) [L. *parietalis*] **1.** Pert. to, or forming, the wall of a cavity. **2.** Pert. to the parietal bone.

p. bone One of two bones that together form the posterior roof and sides of the skull.

p. cell A large cell on the margin of the gastric glands of the stomach that secretes hydrochloric acid and intrinsic factor. SYN: *oxyntic cell.* SEE: *achlorhydria; anemia, pernicious; intrinsic factor.*

parietofrontal (pă-rī″ĕ-tō-frŏn′tăl) Concerning the parietal or frontal bones or lobes.

parietography (pă-rī″ĕ-tŏg′ră-fē) [″ + Gr. *graphein,* to write] A radiographical study of the walls of an organ.

parieto-occipital (pă-rī″ĕ-tō-ŏk-sĭp′ĭ-tăl) Concerning the parietal and occipital bones or lobes.

parietosquamosal (pă-rī″ĕ-tō-skwă-mō′săl) Concerning the parietal bone and squamous part of the temporal bone.

parietotemporal (pă-rī″ĕ-tō-tĕm′pō-răl) Concerning the parietal and temporal bones or lobes.

parietovisceral (pă-rī″ĕ-tō-vĭs′ĕr-ăl) Concerning the wall of a body cavity and the viscera within.

Parinaud, Henri (pă-rĭ-nō′) French ophthalmologist, 1844–1905.

P.'s oculoglandular syndrome Conjunctivitis with palpable preauricular lymph nodes.

P.'s ophthalmoplegia syndrome Palsy of vertical gaze that may or may not be associated with pupillary or oculomotor nerve paresis. It is caused by a lesion at the level of the anterior corpora quadrigemina of the brain.

pari passu (păr′ē-păs′ū) [L., with equal speed] Occurring at the same time or at the same rate; side by side.

parity (păr′ĭ-tē) [L. *par,* equal] Equality, similarity.

parity (păr′ĭ-tē) [L. *parere,* to bring forth, to bear] The condition of having carried a pregnancy to a point of viability (500 g birth weight or 20 weeks' gestation), regardless of the outcome. SEE: *multiparity; nulliparity.*

Parkinson, James British physician, 1755–1824.

P.'s disease A common, chronic degenerative disease of the central nervous system that produces movement disorders and changes in cognition and mood. Its hallmarks include a pill-rolling tremor of the hands, muscular rigidity, a loss of facial expression, and gait disturbances (esp. shuffling gait, festination, and, sometimes, difficulty initiating forward movements). The disease is usually found among the elderly (its prevalence is highest in persons age 75 to 85). Its underlying cause is unknown, although the disease often is found in families; whether this is the result of genetics or common exposure to toxins (e.g., pesticides, aluminum) is uncertain. SYN: *paralysis agitans; parkinsonism;.* SEE: *Nursing Diagnoses Appendix.*

SYMPTOMS: The onset may be abrupt, but is usually insidious. Early changes may include aching, fatigue, and malaise. However, in over half the cases, the first symptoms are rigidity and immobility of the hands, followed by a fine tremor (pill-rolling tremor) beginning in the hand or the foot that may spread until it involves all the members. At first the tremor is paroxysmal but becomes almost continuous. The face becomes expressionless and fixed. Infrequent eye blinking is often an early sign.

The speech becomes slow and measured, and later generalized muscular rigidity occurs. The head becomes bowed, the body bent forward, the arms flexed, the thumbs turned in toward the palms, the knees slightly bent. The patient often has difficulty rising from a seated position, and when he or she begins to walk, the gait appears to have a shuffling quality; after several steps the walking pace often grows faster and faster (festination) until the patient may lose balance or fall. Occasionally, a tendency to fall backward (retropulsion) replaces festination. Numbness, tingling, and a sensation of heat may be present. Drooling, due to failure to swallow rather than increased saliva production, may become troublesome.

TREATMENT: Medical therapies include levodopa/carbidopa; dopamine agonists (e.g., bromocriptine or pergolide); and monoamine oxidase-B inhibitors (e.g., deprenyl). Surgical therapy, which is performed at very few hospitals, may involve transplantation of dopamine-secreting cells into affected areas of the brain or insertion of electrical brain stimulators into the subthalamic nucleus, globus pallidus internus, or ventral intermediate nucleus.

PATIENT CARE: Prescribed drugs are administered and evaluated for desired effects and any adverse reactions, and the patient is instructed in their use and potential side effects so that the dosage can be adjusted to minimize these effects. The nurse, physician, or occupational or physical therapist teaches the patient and family about safety measures to prevent injury; about drug-related dietary restrictions; and about the need for frequent small feedings, to provide needed fluids, calories, and dietary bulk. The patient should plan daily activities to occur when he or she feels rested, to prevent fatigue. The patient is also referred to national organizations (e.g., the National Parkinson Foundation, Inc.; www.parkinson.org) for additional information.

P.'s facies The immobile, or masklike, facial expression that is a hallmark of Parkinson's disease and postencephalitic states. SYN: *Parkinson's mask*.

parkinsonian (păr″kĭn-sōn′ē-ăn) Concerning parkinsonism.

parkinsonism (păr′kĭn-sŏn-ĭzm″) Parkinson's disease.

PAR nurse *Postanesthesia recovery room nurse.*

paroccipital (păr-ŏk-sĭp′ĭt-ăl) [Gr. *para,* beside, + L. *occiput,* occiput] **1.** Close to the occipital bone. **2.** The paramastoid process.

parodontitis (păr″ō-dŏn-tī′tĭs) [″ + *odous,* tooth, + *itis,* inflammation] Inflammation of the tissues around a tooth.

parodontium (păr″ō-dŏn′shē-ŭm) Periodontium.

parole [Fr. *parole,* short for *parole d'honneur,* word of honor] In psychiatry, the release of a patient from the hospital on a trial basis.

parolivary (păr-ŏl′ĭ-vă″rē) [Gr. *para,* beside, + L. *oliva,* olive] Situated close to the olivary body.

p. bodies Nuclei in the medulla oblongata, lying close to the olivary bodies.

paromomycin sulfate (păr′ō-mō-mī″sĭn) An aminoglycoside antibiotic used in treating intestinal amebiasis and various tapeworms. It is not effective against extraintestinal infections with amebae.

paromphalocele (păr″ŏm-făl′ō-sēl″) [″ + *omphalos,* navel, + *kele,* tumor, swelling] A hernia or tumor close to the umbilicus.

paroniria (păr-ō-nī′rē-ă) [″ + *oneiros,* dream] Abnormal or terrifying dreams.

paronychia (păr-ō-nĭk′ē-ă) [″ + *onyx,* nail] An acute or chronic infection of the marginal structures about the nail. SYN: *felon; panaris; runaround; whitlow*. SEE: illus.

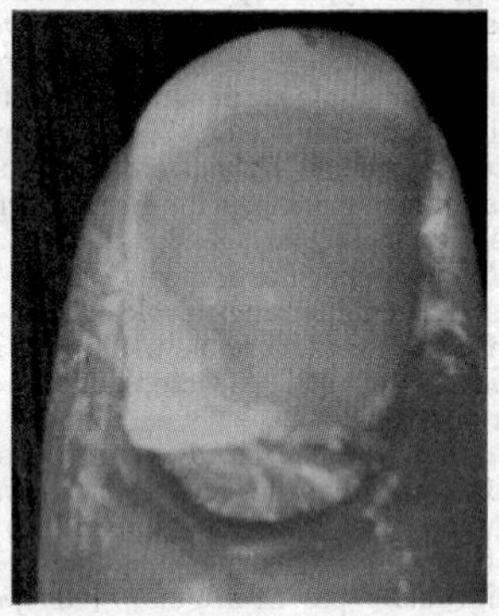

PARONYCHIA

SYMPTOMS: Redness, swelling, and suppuration around the nail edge occur.

TREATMENT: Therapy may involve moist heat application, oral antibiotics, or surgical drainage.

p. tendinosa Inflammation of the sheath of a digital tendon owing to sepsis.

paronychomycosis (păr″ō-nĭk″ō-mī-kō′sĭs) [″ + ″ + *mykes,* fungus, + *osis,* condition] A fungus infection about the nails.

paronychosis (păr-ō-nĭ-kō′sĭs) Growth of a nail in an abnormal position.

paroophoritis (păr″ō-ŏf-ō-rī′tĭs) [″ + *oophoros,* bearing eggs, + *itis,* inflammation] Inflammation of the tissues around the ovary.

paroophoron (păr-ō-ŏf′ō-rŏn) [″ + *oophoros,* bearing eggs] A group of minute tubules located in the mesosalpinx between the uterus and ovary. It is a vestigial structure consisting of the remains of the caudal group of mesonephric tubules and is a homologue of the paradidymis of the male.

parophthalmia (păr-ŏf-thăl′mē-ă) [″ + *ophthalmos,* eye] Inflammation of the tissue around the eye.

parophthalmoncus (păr″ŏf-thăl-mŏn′kŭs) [″ + ″ + *onkos,* mass] A tumor located near the eye.

parorchidium (păr-or-kĭd′ē-ŭm) [″ + *orchis,* testicle] Abnormal position, or nondescent, of a testicle. SYN: *ectopia testis.*

parorexia (păr-ō-rĕk′sē-ă) [″ + *orexis,* appetite] An abnormal or perverted craving for special or strange foods. SEE: *pica; taste.*

parosmia (păr-ŏz′mē-ă) [″ + *osme,* odor] Any disorder or perversion of the sense of smell; a false sense of odors or perception of those that do not exist. Agreeable odors are considered offensive, and disagreeable ones pleasant. Intravenous fluid therapy, esp. postoperatively, may create temporary parageusia and parosmia. SYN: *parosphresia.* SEE: *cacosmia.*

parosphresia, parosphresis (păr″ŏs-frē′zē-ă, -sĭs) [″ + *osphresis,* smell] Parosmia.

parosteal (păr-ŏs′tē-ăl) Concerning the outermost layer of the periosteum.

parosteitis, parostitis (păr-ŏs-tē-ī′tĭs, -tī′tĭs) [Gr. *para,* beside, + *osteon,* bone, + *itis,* inflammation] Inflammation of tissues next to the bone.

parosteosis, parostosis (păr″ŏs-tē-ō′sĭs, -tō′sĭs) [″ + *osteon,* bone, + *osis,* condition] **1.** Bone formation outside of the periosteum. **2.** Bone development in an unusual location.

parotic (pă-rŏt′ĭk) [″ + *ous,* ear] Near the ear.

parotid (pă-rŏt′ĭd) Located near the ear; esp. the parotid gland.

granulomatous p. Granulomatous inflammation of the parotid gland, usually due to tuberculosis or sarcoidosis.

suppurative p. Bacterial infection of the parotid gland, usually in patients with decreased salivary flow. It is often caused by *Staphylococcus aureus.*

parotidectomy (pă-rŏt″ĭ-dĕk′tō-mē) [″ + *ous,* ear, + *ektome,* excision] Excision of the parotid gland. This procedure is most often performed to excise a malignancy and less often to remove a calculus that cannot be extracted from the duct in the mouth.

PATIENT CARE: The patient's understanding of the procedure and postoperative care is assessed, including suctioning and nasogastric tube for drainage. The patient is encouraged to express feelings and anxiety about the surgery and alterations in body image. After surgery, the patient is asked to perform facial movements such as smiling, frowning, and exposing teeth to observe for possible damage to the facial nerve. Drainage should be observed for excessive bleeding. A patent airway is maintained, and good oral hygiene and nutrition are encouraged.

parotidoscirrhus (pă-rŏt″ĭd-ō-skĭr′ŭs) [″ + ″ + *skirrhos,* hardness] **1.** Hardening of the parotid gland. **2.** A scirrhous cancer of the parotid area.

parotitis (pă″rō-tī′tĭs) [″ + *ous,* ear, + *itis,* inflammation] Inflammation of the parotid gland.

parous (păr′ŭs) [L. *pario,* to bear] Parturient; fruitful; having borne at least one child.

parovarian (păr-ō-vā′rē-ăn) [Gr. *para,* beside, + LL. *ovarium,* ovary] **1.** Situated near or beside the ovary. **2.** Pert. to the parovarium, a residual structure in the broad ligament.

parovariotomy (păr″ō-vā″rē-ŏt′ō-mē) [″ + ″ + Gr. *tome,* incision] Removal of a parovarian cyst.

parovaritis (păr″ō-vă-rī′tĭs) [″ + LL. *ovarium,* ovary, + Gr. *itis,* inflammation] Inflammation of the epoophoron.

parovarium (păr″ō-vā′rē-ŭm) Epoophoron.

paroxysm (păr′ŏk-sĭzm) [Gr. *paroxysmos,* irritation] **1.** A sudden, periodic attack or recurrence of symptoms of a disease; an exacerbation of the symptoms of a disease. **2.** A sudden spasm or convulsion of any kind. **3.** A sudden emotional state, as of fear, grief, or joy.

paroxysmal (păr″ŏk-sĭz′măl) Occurring repeatedly and without warning.

p. nocturnal hemoglobinuria ABBR: PNH. A rare form of an acquired hemolytic anemia that results from a defect in membrane-anchored proteins of red blood cells.

SYMPTOMS: The syndrome is characterized by acute onset of fevers and chills, back and extremity pain, and abdominal cramps. Hemoglobinuria occurs if enough red blood cells have been destroyed.

TREATMENT: Erythropoietin may be used to treat the anemia of PNH.

paroxysmal nocturnal dyspnea SEE: *dyspnea, paroxysmal nocturnal.*

Parrot, Joseph Marie Jules (păr-ō′) French physician, 1829–1883.

P.'s disease **1.** Osteochondritis that occurs in infants with congenital syphilis. **2.** A form of dwarfism that is transmitted as an autosomal dominant.

P.'s nodes Bony nodules on the skull of infants with congenital syphilis. Also called *Parrot's sign.*

P.'s pseudoparalysis Pseudoparalysis caused by syphilitic osteochondritis.

P.'s sign P.'s nodes.

P.'s ulcer Lesions seen in thrush or stomatitis.

parrot fever Psittacosis.

Parry's disease (păr′ēz) [Caleb H. Parry, Brit. physician, 1755–1822] Hyperthyroidism.

pars (părz) *pl.* **partes** [L.] A part; portion of a larger structure.

p. basilaris ossis occipitalis The basilar process of the occipital bone.

p. buccalis hypophyseos A developmental protrusion in the primitive buccal cavity of the anterior lobe of the hypophysis.

p. caeca oculi Optic disk.

p. caeca retinae The parts of the retina not sensitive to light (pars ciliaris retinae and pars iridica retinae).

p. cephalica et cervicalis systematis autonomici The cranial and cervical portions of the autonomic nervous system.

p. ciliaris retinae The portion of the retina situated in front of the ora serrata and covering the ciliary body.

p. distalis adenohypophyseos The part of the hypophysis forming the major portion of the anterior lobe. SEE: *pituitary gland.*

p. flaccida membranae tympani The portion of the membrane of the eardrum that fills the notch of Rivinus. This portion of the drum is not taut. SYN: *Shrapnell's membrane.*

p. interarticularis The region between the superior and inferior articulating facets of a vertebra; the region where fracture frequently occurs with spondylolysis.

p. intermedia adenohypophyseos The intermediate lobe of the hypophysis cerebri. SEE: *pituitary gland.*

p. iridica retinae The portion of the retina on the posterior surface of the iris.

p. mastoidea ossis temporalis The mastoid portion of the temporal bone.

p. membranacea urethrae masculinae The membranous portion of the urethra. It extends from the prostate to the bulb of the penis. SEE: *p. spongiosa urethrae masculinae.*

p. nervosa hypophyseos The posterior lobe of the pituitary gland.

p. optica hypothalami Optic chiasm.

p. optica retinae The sensory portion of the retina, extending from the optic disk to the ora serrata.

p. petrosa ossis temporalis The petrous portion of the temporal bone.

p. plana corporis ciliaris The ciliary ring of the eye.

p. radiata lobuli corticalis renis SEE: *ray, medullary.*

p. spongiosa urethrae masculinae The portion of the male urethra included from the point of entrance to the bulb of the penis to its termination at the end of the penis. The bulbourethral glands empty into it via their ducts just after the urethra passes the perineal membrane.

p. squamosa ossis temporalis The flat portion of the temporal bone that forms part of the lateral wall of the skull.

p. tensa membranae tympani The larger portion of the tympanic membrane, a tightly stretched membrane lying inferior to the malleolar folds. SEE: *p. flaccida membranae tympani.*

p. tuberalis adenohypophyseos The portion of the anterior lobe of the hypophysis cerebri that invests the infundibular stalk.

p. tympanica ossis temporalis The tympanic portion of the temporal bone.

Parse, Rosemarie A nursing educator who developed the Theory of Human Becoming. SEE: *Nursing Theory Appendix.*

pars planitis (părs plā-nī′tĭs) Inflammation of the peripheral retina characterized by aggregations of inflammatory cells on the anterior inferior retina. These are called "snowbanks." This chronic condition, which occurs mostly in the young, is sometimes caused by tuberculosis or sarcoidosis, but usually is of unknown etiology. It may cause loss of vision. Corticosteroids are used to treat this condition.

part, presenting Before delivery, the fetal anatomical structure nearest the internal cervical os, identified by sonogram or palpation during vaginal examination. SEE: *presentation* for illus.

part. aeq. *partes aequales,* in equal parts.

partes (păr′tēs) Pl. of pars.

parthenogenesis (păr″thĕn-ō-jĕn′ĕ-sĭs) [Gr. *parthenos,* virgin, + *genesis,* generation, birth] Reproduction arising from a female egg that has not been fertilized by the male; unisexual reproduction.

parthenophobia (păr″thĕ-nō-fō′bē-ă) [″ + *phobos,* fear] Fear of virgins or girls.

participant observation A method of field research whereby the investigator observes and records information about the characteristics of a setting through his or her experiences as a participant in that setting.

particle [L. *particula*] **1.** A very small piece or part of matter; a tiny fragment or trace. **2.** One of several subatomic components of the nuclei of radioactive elements, such as alpha and beta particles. **3.** Attraction particle or centriole of the nucleus of a cell. **4.** Virion.

alpha p. A charged particle emitted from a radioactive substance made up of a helium nucleus consisting of two protons and two electrons. The particle has very low penetrability, but an extremely high linear energy transfer.

beta p. Beta ray.

Dane p. The virion of hepatitis B.

elementary p. The subatomic parts of the atomic nucleus.

particulate (păr-tĭk′ū-lāt) Made up of particles.

parts per million ABBR: PPM; ppm. The concentration of a solute in a liquid gas. For example, a pollutant such as soot may be said to be present in air at a level of 50 parts per million (parts of air). The units also may be expressed as weight of one substance to the weight of another or the volume of a fluid in the volume of another.

parturient (păr-tū′rē-ĕnt) [L. *parturiens,* in labor] Concerning childbirth or parturition; giving birth.

parturifacient (păr-tū-rĭ-fā′shĕnt) [″ + *facere,* to make] **1.** Inducing or accelerating labor. **2.** A drug used to cause or hasten delivery of the fetus.

parturiphobia [″ + Gr. *phobos,* fear] Fear of childbirth.

parturition (păr-tū-rĭsh′ŭn) [L. *parturitio*] The act of giving birth to young. SYN: *childbirth*. SEE: *delivery; labor*.

part. vic. *partitis vicibus,* in divided doses.

party (păr′tē) A person or entity who acts as petitioner, plaintiff, or defendant in a legal action.

parulis (păr-ū′lĭs) [Gr. *para,* beside, + *oulon,* gum] Gumboil.

parumbilical (păr″ŭm-bĭl′ĭ-kăl) [″ + L. *umbilicus,* navel] Close to the navel.

parvovirus (păr″vō-vī′rŭs) [″ + *virus,* poison] A group of viruses similar to adeno-associated viruses. They are pathogenic in animals and humans.

p. B-19 A type of parvovirus that causes erythema infectiosum (fifth disease), a usually benign, nonfebrile disease. However, intrauterine infection may produce fetal anemia with hydrops fetalis and death. Infection of immunocompromised patients or patients with sickle cell anemia may cause aplastic anemia, and complications may lead to death.

parvule (păr′vūl) [L. *parvulus,* very small] A small pill, pellet, or granule.

PAS, PASA *para-aminosalicylic acid.*

pascal A unit of pressure equal to the force of one newton acting uniformly over 1 m^2. SEE: *newton; SI Units Appendix.*

Paschen bodies (pă′shĕn) [Enrique Paschen, Ger. pathologist, 1860–1936] Particles thought to be the pathogenic virus of vaccinia and variola found in great numbers in skin exanthemas.

PASG *pneumatic anti-shock garment.* SEE: *MAST*.

passage (păs′ăj) [ME., to pass] **1.** A channel between cavities and body structures or with the external surface of an organ. **2.** The act of passing. **3.** An evacuation of the bowels. **4.** Introduction of a probe or catheter. **5.** Incubation of a pathogenic organism, esp. a virus, in one or a series of tissue cultures or living organisms.

passion (păsh′ŭn) [L. *passio,* suffering] **1.** Suffering. **2.** Great emotion or zeal; frequently associated with sexual excitement.

heat of p. In forensic medicine, a state of mind that might influence one's propensity to commit violent or aggressive acts.

passive (păs′ĭv) [L. *passivus,* capable of suffering] Submissive; not active.

passivism (păs′ĭ-vĭzm) [″ + Gr. *-ismos,* condition] **1.** Passive behavior or character. **2.** Sexual perversion with subjugation of the will to another.

passivity (păs-sĭv′ĭ-tē) [L. *passivus,* capable of suffering] In psychiatry, the condition of being dependent on others and a reluctance to be assertive or responsible.

Pasteur, Louis (păs-stĕr′) French chemist and bacteriologist, 1822–1895, who founded the science of microbiology. His greatest accomplishments were in the fields of bacteriology and immunology. He developed the technique of immunization and produced vaccines.

P.'s effect The inhibition of fermentation by bacteria when oxygen is abundant.

P.'s treatment An obsolete method of preventing rabies, consisting of a daily injection of increasingly virulent suspensions prepared from the brains or spinal cords of rabbits that have died of rabies. SEE: *rabies*.

Pasteurella (pās-tĕr-ĕl′ă) [Louis Pasteur] A genus of bacteria that at one time included the species *P. pestis, P. tularensis, P. multocida,* and *P. pseudotuberculosis*. *P. pestis,* the organism that causes plague, is now classed as *Yersinia pestis. P. tularensis,* the causative organism of tularemia, is now classed as *Francisella tularensis. P. pseudotuberculosis,* which can cause acute mesenteric lymphadenitis or enterocolitis, is now classed as *Yersinia pseudotuberculosis.*

P. canis Previous name for *P. multocida.*

P. multocida A small nonmotile gram-negative coccobacillus that can cause disease in animals and humans. The infection may be transmitted to humans by animal bites. In other cases the organism can cause cellulitis, abscesses, osteomyelitis, pneumonia, peritonitis, or meningitis. Penicillins, doxycycline, or cephalosporins are used to treat the infection.

pasteurellosis (păs″tĕr-ĕ-lō′sĭs) A disease caused by infection with bacteria of the genus *Pasteurella.*

pasteurization (păs″tūr-ī-zā′shŭn) [Louis Pasteur] The process of heating a fluid at a moderate temperature for a definite period of time to destroy undesirable bacteria without changing to any extent the chemical composition of the fluid. In pasteurization of milk, pathogenic bacteria are destroyed by heating at 62°C for 30 min, or by "flash" heating to higher temperatures for less than 1 min. The pasteurization process, reducing total bacterial count of the milk by 97% to 99%, is effective because the common milk-borne pathogens (tubercle bacillus, and *Salmonella, Streptococcus,* and *Brucella* organisms) do not form spores and are quite sensitive to heat. However, pasteurization should not be considered a substitute for hygienic practices in milk production. SEE: *flash method; milk.*

pastille (păs-tēl′, -tĭl′) [L. *pastillus,* a little roll] **1.** A medicated disk used for local action on the mucosa of the throat and mouth. SYN: *lozenge; troche.* **2.** A small cone used to fumigate or scent the air of a room.

past-pointing The inability to place a finger or some other part of the body accurately on a selected point; seen esp. in cerebellar disorders.

PAT *Paroxysmal atrial tachycardia.* The contemporary, and more accurate, term is paroxysmal supraventricular tachycardia (PSVT).

patagia (pă-tā′jē-ă) [L.] Pl. of patagium.

patagium (pă-tā′jē-ŭm) *pl.* **patagia** [L.] A weblike membrane. SEE: *pterygium.*

patch (păch) [ME. *pacche*] **1.** A small circumscribed area distinct from the surrounding surface in character and appearance. **2.** A drug delivery system that enhances the uptake of a medicine through the skin.

blood p. The injection of a small amount of a patient's blood into the subarachnoid space to heal a headache that occurs after lumbar puncture.

cotton-wool p., cotton-wool spot The appearance of exudative areas in the retina; usually seen in connection with hypertensive retinopathy.

herald p. A solitary oval patch of scaly skin that appears several days before the general eruption of pityriasis rosea.

Hutchinson's p. Salmon patch.

mucous p. A syphilitic eruption having an eroded, moist surface; usually on the mucous membrane of the mouth or external genitals, or on a surface subject to moisture and heat.

nicotine p. A drug delivery device applied to the skin as a form of nicotine replacement. It is most effective in helping smokers to quit using tobacco products when it is used by motivated people who are actively participating in a tobacco cessation program.

Peyer's p. SEE: *Peyer's patch.*

salmon p. A salmon-colored area of the cornea seen in interstitial keratitis caused by syphilis.

smoker's p. Leukoplakia of the oral mucosa.

white p. A white, thickened area of oral mucosa that will not rub off and represents a benign hyperkeratosis. SEE: *leukoplakia.*

patella (pă-tĕl′ă) *pl.* **patellae** [L., a small pan] A lens-shaped sesamoid bone situated in front of the knee in the tendon of the quadriceps femoris muscle. SYN: *kneecap.* SEE: *osteochondritis dissecans.*

p. alta A high-riding patella (high positioning of patella). When a person is standing, the patella rests in a more superior position than normal.

p. baja A low-riding patella (low positioning of patella). When a person is standing, the patella rests in a more inferior position than normal.

bipartite p. The developing patella that matures from two centers rather than one. This usually congenital condition causes no symptoms but may be mistaken for a fracture.

floating p. A patella that rides up from the condyles owing to a large effusion in the knee.

fracture of p. A break in the continuity of the kneecap. Treatment consists of suturing the bone fragments. A cast is applied from the toes to the groin, remaining on for 6 to 8 weeks. Following removal of the cast, gradual exercise may be started and weight placed on the leg for a few weeks, after which the patient may walk.

hypermobile p. Excessive medial and/or lateral motion of the patella. A medially hypermobile patella can be moved greater than 75% of its width medially. A laterally hypermobile patella can be moved greater than 75% of its width laterally. SEE: *hypomobile p.; apprehension test.*

ETIOLOGY: Increased medial patellar hypermobility can result from laxity of the lateral patellar retinaculum. Lateral patellar hypermobility indicates laxity of the medial patellar retinaculum and/or weakness of the oblique fibers of the vastus medialis.

SYMPTOMS: Increased motion of the patella within the femur's trochlea can lead to chondromalacia patellae, producing pain in weight-bearing activities, esp. squatting or climbing or descending stairs. Lateral patellar hypermobility is a predisposition to patellar dislocation or subluxation.

TREATMENT: Treatment and rehabilitation consists of strengthening the muscles on the side opposite the hypermobility. Neuromuscular re-education may be needed to restore the normal recruitment sequence of the oblique fibers of the vastus medialis and the vastus lateralis.

hypomobile p. Lack of normal medial and/or lateral motion of the patella. A medially hypomobile patella cannot be moved more than 25% of its width medially. A laterally hypomobile patella cannot be moved more than 15% of its width laterally. SEE: *hypermobile p.*

ETIOLOGY: Medial hypomobility often results from adhesions of the lateral patellar retinaculum or tightness of the iliotibial band. Lateral hypomobility can result from tightness of the medial patellar retinaculum or hypertrophy or spasm of the oblique fibers of the vastus medialis.

SYMPTOMS: The patient will complain of pain and demonstrate decreased strength during weight-bearing activities. Improper tracking of the patella as the result of hypomobility can lead to chondromalacia patellae.

TREATMENT: Physical agents such as moist heat and/or ultrasound and manual therapy techniques can be used to encourage the elasticity of the offending tissues. A surgical release of the patellar retinaculum may be required.

rider's painful p. Tenderness and pain in the patella from horseback riding.

squinting p. A disorder in which the patella appears to be pointing inward when the patient is standing; caused by excessive femoral anteversion.

patellapexy (pă-tĕl″ă-pĕk″sē) [L. *patella,* small pan, + Gr. *pexis,* fixation] Fixation of the patella to the lower end of the femur to stabilize the joint.

patellar (pă-tĕl′ăr) Concerning the patella.

patellectomy (păt″ĕ-lĕk′tō-mē) [″ + Gr. *ektome,* excision] Surgical removal of the patella.

patelliform (pă-tĕl′ĭ-form) [″ + *forma,* shape] Shaped like the patella.

patellofemoral (pă-tĕl″ō-fĕm′ō-răl) Concerning the patella and femur.

patency (pā′tĕn-sē) [L. *patens,* open] The state of being freely open.

p. of tear duct The open and functional state of a lacrimal duct. The patency of a tear duct can be tested by placing several drops of a weak solution of sugar in the eye. If the person detects a sweet taste in the mouth, then the duct is patent.

patent (păt′ĕnt, pā′tĕnt) Wide open; evident; accessible.

patent ductus arteriosus Persistence, after birth, of a communication between the main pulmonary artery and the aorta. This condition in preterm infants has been treated successfully with drugs, such as indomethacin, that inhibit prostaglandin synthesis. SEE: *prostaglandin.*

paternal (pă-tĕr′năl) [L. *paternis,* fatherly] Of, pert. to, or inherited from the father.

paternalism A type of medical decision making in which health care professionals exercise unilateral authority over patients. When patients are competent to make their own choices and health care professionals seek to act in the patients' best interests, shared decision making is preferable, because it encourages dialogue, preserves autonomy, fosters responsibility, and allows for adaptation.

paternity test A test to determine the father of a child. Because paternity is a clinical estimate, there is the need to have tests to determine whether it would be possible for an individual to have fathered a specific child. At one time, the tests used to prove or exclude the possibility of paternity used blood type data from the child and the suspected father. Tests involving the technique of molecular genetic fingerprinting and of determining genetic markers are available and have the ability to exclude almost all except the father. Use of these techniques makes it possible to distinguish differences between the genotype of all individuals except identical twins.

path A particular course that is followed or traversed. SEE: *pathway.*

p. of closure The path traversed by the mandible as it closes when its neuromuscular mechanisms are in a balanced functional state.

condyle p. The path traversed by the condyle during various mandibular movements.

incisor p. An arc described by the incisal edge of the lower incisors when the mandible closes to normal occlusion.

p. of instantaneous center of rotation ABBR: PICR. The plotted trajectory of the axis of rotation of a joint through its entire range of movement.

PATIENT CARE: Deviation from the ideal PICR may result from muscle strength or length imbalance, internal joint derangement, or joint capsule restriction. These conditions may affect the quality, quantity, efficiency, or pain of joint movement.

path- SEE: *patho-.*

pathetic (pă-thĕt′ĭk) [L. *patheticus*] **1.** Pert. to, or arousing, the emotions of pity, sympathy, or tenderness. **2.** Pert. to the trochlear nerve.

pathfinder [AS. *paeth,* road, + *findan,* to locate] **1.** An instrument for locating stricture of the urethra. **2.** A dental instrument for tracing the course of root canals.

patho-, path- [Gr. *pathos,* disease, suffering] Combining form meaning *disease.* SEE: *-pathy.*

pathoanatomy (păth″ŏ-ă-năt′ō-mē) Anatomic pathology.

pathobiology (păth″ō-bī-ŏl′ō-jē) Pathology.

pathodontia (păth″ō-dŏn′shē-ă) [″ + *odous* tooth] The science of dental pathology.

pathogen (păth′ō-jĕn) [″ + *gennan,* to produce] A microorganism capable of producing a disease.

bloodborne p. A pathogen present in blood that can be transmitted to an individual who is exposed to the blood or body fluids of an infected individual. Three common bloodborne pathogens are hepatitis C, hepatitis B, and human immunodeficiency virus 1 (HIV-1). SEE: *hepatitis B; human immunodeficiency virus; Standard and Universal Precautions Appendix.*

opportunistic p. Opportunistic infection.

pathogenesis (păth″ō-jĕn′ĕ-sĭs) The origin and development of a disease. SYN: *pathogeny.*

bacterial p. The development of a bacterial disease. There are three stages: entry and colonization in the host, bacterial invasion and growth with the production of toxic substances, and the response of the host. The mere presence of an organism in the body does not necessarily mean that disease will follow. This progression of the infection will depend upon a number of interacting factors, including the virulence and number of invading organisms and the ability of the host to respond.

pathogenetic, pathogenic (păth″ō-jĕn-ĕt′ĭk, -jĕn′ĭk) Productive of disease. SYN: *morbific.*

pathogenicity (păth″ō-jĕ-nĭs′ĭ-tē) [″ + *gennan,* to produce] The state of producing or being able to produce pathological changes and disease.

pathogeny (păth-ŏj′ĕn-ē) Pathogenesis.

pathognomonic (păth″ŏg-nō-mŏn′ĭk) [Gr. *pathognomonikos,* skilled in diagnosing] Indicative of a disease, esp. its characteristic symptoms.

pathognomy (păth-ŏg′nō-mē) [Gr. *pathos,* disease, suffering, + *gnome,* a means of knowing] Diagnosing the cause of an illness after careful study of the signs and symptoms of a disease.

pathologic, pathological (păth-ō-lŏj′ĭk, -ĭ-kăl) [Gr. *pathos,* disease, suffering, + *logos,* word, reason] **1.** Concerning pathology. **2.** Diseased; due to a disease. SYN: *morbid.*

pathologist (pă-thŏl′ō-jĭst) [″ + *logos,* word, reason] A medical professional trained to examine tissues, cells, and specimens of body fluids for evidence of disease.

pathology (pă-thŏl′ō-jē) [Gr. *pathos,* disease, suffering, + *logos,* word, reason] **1.** The study of the nature and cause of disease, which involves changes in structure and function. **2.** A condition produced by disease.

anatomic p. The field of pathology that deals with structural changes in disease.

cellular p. Pathology based on microscopic changes in body cells produced by disease.

chemical p. The study of chemical changes that occur in disease.

clinical p. Pathology that uses clinical analysis and other laboratory procedures in the diagnosis and treatment of disease.

comparative p. The observation of pathological condition, spontaneous or artificial, in the lower animals or in vegetable organisms as compared with those of the human body.

dental p. The science of diseases of the mouth. SYN: *oral p.*

experimental p. The study of diseases induced artificially and intentionally, esp. in animals.

functional p. The study of alterations of functions that occur in disease processes without associated structural changes.

geographical p. Pathology in its relationship to climate and geography.

humoral p. Pathology of the fluids of the body.

medical p. Pathology of disorders that are not accessible for surgical procedures.

molecular p. The study of the pathological effects of specific molecules.

oral p. Dental p.

special p. Pathology of particular diseases or organs.

surgical p. The application of pathological procedures and techniques for investigating tissues removed surgically.

pathomimesis (păth″ō-mĭm-ē′sĭs) [Gr. *pathos,* disease, suffering, + *mimesis,* imitation] Intentional (conscious or unconscious) imitation of a disease. SYN: *pathomimicry.*

pathomimicry (păth″ō-mĭm′ĭ-krē) Pathomimesis.

pathophobia (păth-ō-fō′bē-ă) [″ + *phobos,* fear] Morbid fear of disease.

pathophysiology (păth″ō-fĭz″ē-ŏl′ō-jē) [″ + *physis,* nature, + *logos,* word, reason] The study of how normal physiological processes are altered by disease.

pathopsychology (păth″ō-sī-kŏl′ō-jē) [″ + *psyche,* soul, + *logos,* word, reason] The branch of psychology dealing with mental processes during disease.

pathway **1.** A path or a course; e.g., a pathway formed by neurons (cell bodies and their processes) over which impulses pass from their point of origin to their destination. **2.** A chemical or metabolic pathway; the various chemical reactions that occur in metabolism as specific substances are absorbed, metabolized, and altered as they undergo biotransformation in the body. **3.** A course of study or a means to attain professional certification.

afferent p. The pathway leading from a receptor to the spinal cord, the brain, or both.

biosynthetic p. The chemical and metabolic events that lead to the formation of substances in the body.

central p. A pathway within the brain or spinal cord.

clinical p. A method used in health care as a way of organizing, evaluating, and limiting variations in patient care. This method integrates the components of the care plan into one that addresses the needs and services provided to the whole patient. Development of a clinical pathway usually begins with establishment of a multidisciplinary steering committee that examines data to determine which patients will benefit most. Usually, diagnoses that involve costly or complex care (e.g., multidisciplinary care) or common illnesses are selected for study. The following aspects of care are evaluated: consultations and assessments, tests and treatments, nutrition and medications, activity and safety, and teaching and discharge planning. Clinical pathways address timelines, actions, and outcomes, and ensure that essential components of care are provided on time.

Agencies using clinical pathways report the following advantages: reduced length of stay for patients in given DRGs; greater accountability for patient care; greater patient and family satisfaction; enhanced staff and physician satisfaction and communication; an improved and integrated process for care delivery; minimal prejudices and elitism between departments; lower patient charges and costs; and 20% to 40% less time spent on documentation.

complement alternative p. A complement cascade initiated by a foreign protein, usually a bacterium. SEE: *complement.*

complement classic p. A first complement cascade initiated by an antibody-antigen reaction that activates complement factor 1 (C1). SEE: *complement.*

conduction p. A group of fibers in the heart, nerves, spinal cord, or brain that conduct impulses that trigger responses in the same or other tissues.

critical p. Clinical p.

efferent p. A pathway from the central nervous system to an effector.

Embden-Meyerhof p. The anaerobic series of enzymatic reactions involved in glucose metabolism to form pyruvic acid or lactic acid, and to produce adenosine triphosphate, which releases energy for muscular and other cellular activity.

fifth p. A form of postgraduate medical education, in which graduates of international medical training programs undergo supervised clinical clerkships in the U.S. to complete their residency training.

metabolic p. The sequence of chemical reactions that occur as a substance is metabolized.

motor p. A pathway over which motor impulses are conveyed from a motor center to muscles.

p. of incidence The path of a penetrating foreign object from the point of entry into the body to the point where it stops (e.g., the path of a bullet from where it enters the body to where it lodges).

pentose phosphate p. The pathway of glucose metabolism in tissues during which five-carbon sugars are formed.

sensory p. A pathway over which sensory impulses are conveyed from sense organs or receptors to sensory or reflex centers of the spinal cord or brain.

-pathy Combining form indicating *disease.*

patient (pā′shĕnt) [L. *patiens*] **1.** One who is sick with, or being treated for, an illness or injury. **2.** An individual receiving medical care.

p. advocate A person who ensures that a patient is served adequately by the health care system.

p. autonomy The right of an informed patient to choose to accept or to refuse therapy. SEE: *advance directive; informed consent; living will; quality of life.*

p. day The basic time unit for calculating the cost of keeping a patient in a hospital for one day.

p. delay Delay on the part of the patient in seeking medical attention or in taking prescribed medicines or advice.

p. mix The numbers and types of patients served by a hospital or other health program.

surrogate p. A normal, healthy individual who is employed to be examined and perhaps interviewed by health-care students. The purpose is to provide students with the opportunity to examine an individual in a less stressful setting than would be the case if the person being examined were indeed sick. This also prevents persons who are ill from being subjected to multiple examinations by students. In some cases, the surrogate patient is an actor who has been instructed to pretend to be sick, injured, disabled, or hostile.

Patient Advise and Consent Encounter ABBR: PACE. An interactive computer program to assist a patient to understand certain medical and surgical procedures and their risks. The program uses touch-screen technology, animation, and an actor-doctor narrator to communicate with the patient. At the end of each program, the patient may take an interactive quiz that evaluates understanding of the presentation. A printout of the entire session is available for the patient and the physician.

patient education Health information

and instruction to help patients learn about specific or general medical topics, such as the need for preventive services, the adoption of healthy lifestyles, or the care of diseases or injuries at home.

patient management A description of the interaction, from intake to discharge, between the patient and the health care team. It includes communication, empathy, examination, evaluation, diagnosis, prognosis, and intervention. The last element, intervention (or treatment), depends on the others.

patient outcomes research team ABBR: PORT. Those involved in investigating the results of disease interventions and comparing the benefit or lack of benefit of various therapeutic measures.

Patient's Bill of Rights A declaration of the entitlements of hospital patients, compiled by the American Hospital Association. First published in 1973, it emphasizes the responsibilities of hospitals and patients and the need for communication and collaboration between them. The patient is entitled to consideration and respect while receiving care; accurate, understandable information about the condition and treatment; privacy and confidentiality; an appropriate response to the request for treatment; and continued care as necessary after leaving the hospital. The patient may also have an advance directive regarding treatment; designate a surrogate to make decisions; review his or her medical records; be informed of hospital policies or business relationships that may affect care; and agree or refuse to participate in treatments or research studies. Patient responsibilities include providing any information (e.g., an advance directive) that may influence treatment; providing the needed information for insurance claims; and understanding how lifestyle affects health. The full text of the Patient's Bill of Rights is available from the American Hospital Association, One North Franklin, Chicago, IL 60606. SEE: *ombudsman.*

Patient Self-Determination Act ABBR: PSDA. A 1991 act of the U.S. Congress that preserves individual rights to decisions related to personal survival. There are several methods for preserving autonomy: filing appropriate forms for durable power of attorney for health care, making a living will, or giving a directive to the physician.

patricide (păt′rĭ-sīd) [L. *patricida*] The murdering of one's own father or a close relative.

Patrick's test (păt′rĭks) [Hugh Talbot Patrick, U.S. neurologist, 1860–1939] A test for arthritis of the hip. The thigh and knee of the supine patient are flexed, and the external malleolus of the ankle is placed over the patella of the opposite leg. The test result is positive if depression of the knee produces pain. This test is also called the fabere test. "Fabere" is a mnemonic for the position the hip assumes during this test: *F*lexion, *AB*duction, *E*xternal *R*otation, and *E*xtension.

patrilineal (păt-rĕ-lĭn′ē-ăl) [L. *pater,* father, + *linea,* line] Tracing descent through the father.

patten (păt′ĕn) [Fr. *patin,* wooden shoe] A support applied under one shoe as part of the treatment for hip disease or unequal length of the legs. The device may be attached to a leg caliper.

pattern **1.** A design, figure, model, or example. **2.** In psychology, a set or arrangement of ideas or behavior reactions.

capsular p. In a joint, the proportional loss or limitation of passive range of motion that suggests arthritis in that joint (e.g., the capsular pattern of the glenohumeral joint, in order of most restriction, is lateral rotation, abduction, and medial rotation).

cephalocaudal p. of development The principle of maturation that states motor development, control, and coordination progress from the head to the feet.

functional health p. Collective features of an individual's health history used to assess, plan, diagnose, intervene, and evaluate appropriate nursing care. The term is associated with Margery Gordon. SEE: *Nursing Diagnoses Appendix.*

occlusal p. The appearance and anatomical location of the occluding surfaces of teeth.

sinusoidal p. An abnormal fetal heart rate finding in which the monitor records a consistent rhythmic, uniform, undulating wave. Although the number of beats per minute is within normal limits and the recording shows long-term variability, beat-to-beat variability is absent and no accelerations in heart rate occur with fetal movement.

synergy p. Primitive movements that dominate reflex and voluntary effort when spasticity is present following a cerebrovascular accident. They interfere with coordinated volitional movement such as eating, dressing, walking, and isolated movement. *Flexion synergy patterns* include scapular retraction, shoulder abduction and external rotation, elbow flexion, forearm supination, and wrist and finger flexion in the upper extremity; and hip flexion, abduction and external rotation, knee flexion, and ankle dorsiflexion in the lower extremity. *Extension synergy patterns* include scapular protraction, shoulder adduction and internal rotation, elbow extension, forearm pronation, and wrist and finger flexion in the upper extremity;

and hip extension, adduction and internal rotation, knee extension, ankle plantar flexion and inversion, and toe flexion in the lower extremity.

trabecular p. The arrangement of the trabeculae of bone in relation to marrow spaces.

wax p. A molded or carved pattern in wax used extensively in dentistry and jewelry-making whereby casts are made using the lost wax technique.

wear p. The location of tooth erosion as determined by the characteristics of the facets of the teeth.

patterning A therapeutic method used in treating children and adults with brain damage. The patient is guided through movements such as creeping or crawling, based on the theory that undamaged sections of the brain will develop the ability to perform these functions.

patulous (păt′ū-lŭs) [L. *patulus*] Patent.

pauciarticular A classification of juvenile rheumatoid arthritis that indicates that four or fewer joints are affected at the time of onset of the disease.

Paul-Bunnell test [John R. Paul, U.S. physician, 1893–1971; Walls W. Bunnell, U.S. physician, b. 1902] A test for heterophil antibodies in the serum of patients thought to have infectious mononucleosis.

pause [ME.] An interruption; a temporary cessation of activity.

compensatory p. The long interval following a premature ventricular contraction, so called because it does not disturb the normal sinus pacing of the heart.

noncompensatory p. The interval on the electrocardiogram that follows a premature atrial contraction (PAC). Because PACs reset the sinus pacemaker, the next sinus beat does not appear when it would have if there had been no extra beat.

Pautrier microabscess A local collection of malignant lymphocytes, found on microscopic examination of biopsies taken from patients with cutaneous T cell lymphoma.

pavementing A condition occurring during inflammation in which leukocytes adhere to the linings of capillaries.

Pavlik harness A device used to stabilize the hip in neonates with congenital hip dislocation.

Pavlov, Ivan Petrovich (păv′lŏv) Russian physiologist, 1849–1936; winner of Nobel prize in medicine in 1904. He is remembered particularly for his work on conditioned response. SEE: *reflex, conditioned.*

pavor (pā′vor) [L.] Anxiety, dread.

p. diurnus Attacks of terror or fright during the day, esp. in children.

p. nocturnus Night terror during sleep in children and the aged.

PAWP *pulmonary artery wedge pressure.*

P.B. *Pharmacopoeia Britannica,* British pharmacopeia.

Pb [L. *plumbum*] Symbol for the element lead.

PBI *protein-bound iodine.*

P.B.W. *posterior bitewing* in dentistry.

PBZ *pyribenzamine.*

p.c. L. *post cibum,* after a meal.

PCG *phonocardiogram.*

pCi *picocurie.*

P_{CO_2} Symbol for *partial pressure of carbon dioxide.*

PCP *Pneumocystis carinii pneumonia.*

PCR **1.** *polymerase chain reaction.* **2.** *prehospital care report.*

PC-SPES (pē-sē-spēs′) A mixture of herbs (chrysanthemum, *Ganoderma lucidum,* isatis, licorice, *Panax pseudoginseng, Rabdosia rubescens,* saw palmetto, and scutellaria) with estrogen-like effects. The mixture is used by alternative medicine practitioners as a treatment for prostate cancer.

PCV *packed cell volume.*

PCWP *pulmonary capillary wedge pressure.*

Pd Symbol for the element palladium.

p.d. *prism diopter; pupilla diameter; pupillary distance.*

PDA *patent ductus arteriosus.*

PDR *Physicians' Desk Reference.*

PEA *Pulseless electrical activity.*

pearl [ME. *perle*] **1.** A small, tough mass in the sputum in asthma. **2.** A small capsule containing a medicinal fluid for inhalation. The capsule is crushed in a handkerchief and inhaled. **3.** A small mass of cells.

enamel p. Small rounded globules of highly mineralized material seen near or attached to the enamel margin or furcation of the tooth roots. These are formed by aberrant ameloblasts and hypermineralization.

epithelial p. Concentric squamous epithelial cells in carcinoma.

gouty p. Tophus (1).

peau d'orange (pō″dō-rănj′) [Fr., orange skin] Dimpling, pitting, and swelling, seen in skin that is considerably inflamed (e.g., in acne rosacea) or that overlies inflammatory carcinoma of the breast.

peccant (pĕk′ănt) [L. *peccans,* sinning] **1.** Corrupt; producing disease. **2.** Sinning, or violating a law.

peccatiphobia (pĕk″ăt-ĭ-fō′bē-ă) [″ + Gr. *phobos,* fear] Abnormal fear of sinning.

pecilo- words beginning with *poikilo-*.

pecten (pĕk′tĕn) *pl.* **pectines** [L., comb] **1.** A comblike organ. **2.** Pubic bone. **3.** The middle portion of the anal canal.

p. ossis pubis A sharp ridge on the superior ramus of the pubis that forms the pubic portion of the terminal (iliopectineal) line.

pectic acid (pĕk′tĭk) [Gr. *pektos,* congealed] An acid derived from pectin by hydrolyzing the methyl ester group and found in many fruits.

pectin (pĕk'tĭn) [Gr. *pektos,* congealed] Water-soluble polymers of galacturonic acid, found in the skins of grapes, apples, and citrus fruits, which bind in water, cations, and bile acids in the small bowel. SEE: *pectose.*

pectinase (pĕk'tĭ-nās) An enzyme that catalyzes the formation of sugars and galacturonic acid from pectin.

pectinate (pĕk'tĭ-nāt) [L. *pecten,* comb] Having teeth like a comb. SYN: *pectiniform.*

pectineal (pĕk-tĭn'ē-ăl) Relating to the os pubis or the pectineal muscle.

pectineus (pĕk-tĭn-ē'ŭs) [L. *pecten,* comb] A flat quadrangular muscle at the upper and inner part of the thigh, arising from the superior ramus of pubis and inserted between the lesser trochanter and linea aspera of the femur, which flexes and adducts the thigh.

pectiniform (pĕk-tĭn'ĭ-form) [" + *forma,* shape] Pectinate.

pectization (pĕk-tĭ-zā'shŭn) [Gr. *pektos,* congealed] In colloidal chemistry, the conversion of a substance from sol to gel state.

pectora (pĕk'tor-ă) [L.] Pl. of pectus.

pectoral (pĕk'tō-răl) [L. *pectoralis*] **1.** Concerning the chest. **2.** Efficacious in relieving chest conditions, as a cough.

pectoralgia (pĕk"tō-răl'jē-ă) [L. *pectoralis,* chest, + Gr. *algos,* pain] Pain in the chest.

pectoralis (pĕk"tō-rā'lĭs) [L.] **1.** Pert. to the breast or chest. **2.** One of the four muscles of the anterior upper portion of the chest.

p. major A large triangular muscle that extends from the sternum to the humerus and functions to flex, horizontally adduct, and internally rotate the arm, and aids in chest expansion when the upper extremities are stabilized.

p. minor A muscle beneath the pectoralis major, attached to the coracoid process of the scapula that depresses as well as causes anterior tipping of the scapula.

pectoriloquy (pĕk"tō-rĭl'ō-kwē) [L. *pectoralis,* chest, + *loqui,* to speak] The distinct transmission of vocal sounds to the ear through the chest wall in auscultation. The words seem to emanate from the spot that is auscultated. This is heard over cavities that communicate with a bronchus and areas of consolidation near a large bronchus, over pneumothorax when the opening in the lung is patulous, and over some pleural effusions. SYN: *pectorophony.* SEE: *chest.*

aphonic p. In auscultation, a whispered sound heard over a lung with a cavity or pleural effusion.

whispered p. A sound heard in auscultation of the chest over a lung with a cavity of limited extent when the patient whispers.

pectorophony (pĕk"tō-rŏf'ō-nē) [" + Gr. *phone,* voice] Pectoriloquy.

pectose (pĕk'tōs) [Gr. *pektos,* congealed] A substance found in some fruits and vegetables. It yields pectin when boiled.

pectunculus (pĕk-tŭn'kū-lŭs) [L., little comb] One of the tiny longitudinal ridges on the sylvian aqueduct of the brain.

pectus (pĕk'tŭs) *pl.* **pectora** [L.] The chest, breast, or thorax.

p. carinatum Pigeon breast.

p. excavatum A congenital condition in which the sternum is abnormally depressed. SYN: *funnel breast; p. recurvatum.*

p. recurvatum P. excavatum.

ped- SEE: *pedo-.*

pedal (pĕd'l) [L. *pedalis*] Concerning the foot.

pedal spasm Involuntary contractions of the muscles of the feet.

pedarthrocace (pē"dăr-thrŏk'ă-sē) [Gr. *paidos,* child, + *arthron,* joint, + *kakos,* bad] A carious condition of the joints of children.

pedatrophy (pē-dăt'rō-fē) [Gr. *pais,* child, + *atrophia,* want of nourishment] **1.** Marasmus. **2.** Any wasting disease in children. **3.** Tabes mesenterica.

pederast (pĕd'ĕr-ăst) [Gr. *paiderastes,* a lover of boys] A man who indulges in anal intercourse with young boys.

pederasty (pĕd'ĕr-ăs"tē) Anal intercourse between a man and a young boy.

pedesis (pē-dē'sĭs) [Gr., leaping] Brownian movement.

pedi- SEE: *pedo-.*

pedia- [Gr. *pais,* child] Combining form denoting *child.*

pedialgia (pĕd-ē-ăl'jē-ă, pē-dē-) [Gr. *pedion,* foot, + *algos,* pain] Pain of the foot.

Pediamycin Trade name for erythromycin ethylsuccinate.

pediatric (pē-dē-ăt'rĭk) [Gr. *pais,* child, + *iatreia,* treatment] Concerning the treatment of children.

pediatric advanced life support ABBR: PALS. The treatment measures, including basic and advanced life support, needed to stabilize a critically ill or injured child.

pediatric autoimmune neuropsychiatric disorders associated with streptococci ABBR: PANDAS. Childhood behavioral disorders (esp. tic disorders, Tourette's syndrome, and obsessive-compulsive disorder) that begin before puberty and are associated with group A beta-hemolytic streptococcal infections. Affected children become emotionally labile, hyperactive, oppositional, and anxious when infected with *Streptococcus pyogenes.* About 85% of such children have a B-lymphocyte marker for susceptibility to rheumatic fever, called D8/17. Some researchers suspect that an autoimmune response to the infection is responsible for the syndrome.

pediatrician (pē-dē-ă-trĭsh'ăn) [" + *iatrikos,* healing] A specialist in the treatment of children's diseases.

pediatrics (pē-dē-ăt'rĭks) [Gr. *pais,* child, + *iatreia,* treatment] The medical science relating to the care of children and treatment of their diseases.

pediatric trauma score ABBR: PTS. A method for scoring and quantifying the severity of trauma in pediatric patients. SYN: *revised trauma score.*

pedicel (pĕd'ĭ-sĕl) **1.** Foot process or footplate. **2.** A secondary process of a podocyte that in conjunction with other podocytes forms the inner layer of Bowman's capsule of a renal corpuscle.

pedicellation (pĕd"ĭ-sĕl-ā'shŭn) [L. *pediculus,* a little foot; stalk] The formation and development of a pedicle.

pedicle (pĕd'ĭ-k'l) **1.** The stem that attaches a new growth. SYN: *peduncle* (1). **2.** The bony process that projects backward from the body of a vertebra, connecting with the lamina on each side. It forms the root of the vertebral arch.

pedicle flap SEE: *pedicle flap.*

pedicular (pē-dĭk'ū-lar) [L. *pediculus,* a louse] Infested with or concerning lice.

pedicular (pē-dĭk'ū-lar) [L. *pediculus,* a little foot] Concerning a stalk or stem.

pediculate (pē-dĭk'ū-lāt) [L. *pediculus,* a little foot] Pedunculate.

pediculation (pē-dĭk"ū-lā'shŭn) [L. *pediculatio*] **1.** Infestation with lice. **2.** Development of a pedicle.

pediculicide (pē-dĭk'ū-lĭ-sīd) [L. *pediculus,* a louse, + *caedere,* to kill] Destroying, or that which destroys, lice.

Pediculidae A family of lice belonging to the order Anoplura. It includes the species parasitic on primates including humans. SEE: *Pediculus.*

pediculophobia (pē-dĭk"ū-lō-fō'bē-ă) [" + Gr. *phobein,* to fear] Abnormal dread of lice.

pediculosis (pē-dĭk"ū-lō'sĭs) [" + Gr. *osis,* condition] Infestation with lice. SEE: *Pediculus.*

p. capitis A scalp infection caused by *Pediculus humanus capitis,* a common parasite in children; outbreaks are common in schools. The infection is transmitted through use of personal items such as hair ornaments, combs, hairbrushes, hats, scarves, or coats. Lice cause itching, esp. around the ears, in the occipital area, and at the nape of the neck. Long-standing cases may produce chronic inflammation. The adult louse is seen rarely; diagnosis usually is made through the presence of eggs (nits), which appear as whitish sacs attached to the hair. SEE: illus.

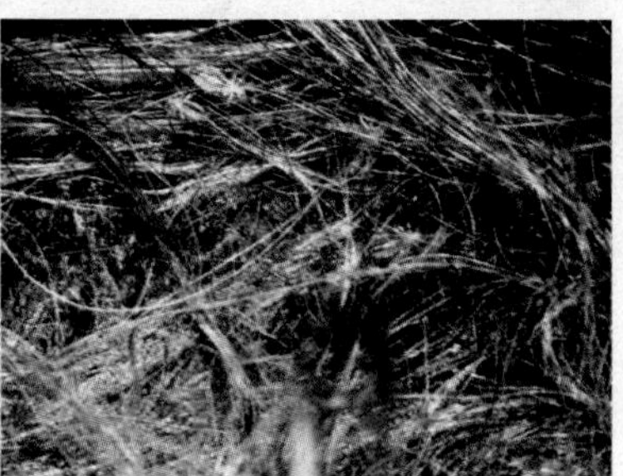

PEDICULOSIS CAPITIS

SYMPTOMS: Itching and eczematous dermatitis. In long-standing, neglected cases, scratching may result in marked inflammation. Secondary infection by bacteria may occur, with formation of pustules, crusts, and suppuration. Hair may become matted and malodorous.

TREATMENT: Therapies for lice infestations are modified frequently, to match the resistance of lice to current therapies and to minimize the toxicities of medications. Manual removal of lice always is appropriate, and is strongly recommended by the National Pediculosis Association (www.headlice.org), an organization that posts regular updates on optimal treatment protocols.

PATIENT CARE: The patient and family are taught how to apply medication to dry hair for lice and are warned that the eyes should be immediately flushed with copious amounts of water if the medication accidentally contacts them. They are informed about minimizing the spread of infection by washing or dry cleaning all clothing and linen used in the home, keeping combs and brushes separate, and using the medicinal shampoo if there has been contact with the patient.

p. corporis Pediculosis caused by the body louse, *Pediculus humanus corporis.* It is transmitted by direct contact or by wearing infested clothing and often is transmitted in crowded or unhygienic conditions. The body louse occasionally is the vector for several important transmissible illnesses, including epidemic typhus, trench fever, and relapsing fever.

SYMPTOMS: Infestation with body lice is marked by intense itching, esp. on the neck, trunk, and thighs. Tiny hemorrhagic points identify the bites. Generalized excoriation, mild fever, and fatigue characterize heavy infestations. In severe cases, pustules may develop.

TREATMENT: The patient first bathes with hot soap and water and then applies prescribed creams containing approved pesticides to affected areas.

PATIENT CARE: The patient should

be assessed for diseases that body lice may transmit. If the patient is homeless or impoverished, social services agencies should be contacted to assist him or her to find shelter and clean clothing. If the patient lives with others, close personal contacts or family members should be screened for lice. All clothing and bedding must be washed with hot water or dry cleaned.

p. palpebrarum Infestation by lice of the eyebrows and eyelashes.

p. pubis Pediculosis caused by the crab louse, *Phthirus pubis,* which usually is confined to pubic hair but also can involve axillary hair; the lice are transmitted by sexual contact. Pubic lice cause intense itching, esp. at night. Brown-red "dust" (lice excreta) can be seen in underwear, and a blue-gray flat rash may appear on the trunk, thighs, or axilla. Treatment may include pesticides such as permethrins or other drugs. SEE: *p. capitis* for treatment.

SYMPTOMS: This condition is characterized by itching and irritation of the external genital area (not introital), esp. the mons. The pubic louse bite produces in light-skinned individuals blue- or slate-colored macules that do not blanch when pressure is applied.

pediculous (pĕ-dĭk′ū-lŭs) Infested with lice.

Pediculus (pē-dĭk′ū-lŭs) A genus of parasitic insects commonly called lice that infest humans and other primates. Lice are sucking insects belonging to the family Pediculidae, order Anoplura. They are of medical importance in that they are the vectors of the causative organisms of epidemic typhus, trench fever, and relapsing fever.

P. humanus capitis The head louse that lives in the fine hair of the head, including the beard and eyebrows. Its eggs, commonly called nits, may be found glued to hairs. They form nests in the vicinity of the ears. This organism is the cause of pediculosis capitis.

P. humanus corporis The body louse that inhabits the seams of clothing worn next to the body and feeds on regions of the body covered by that clothing. Eggs are attached to fibers of the clothing. This organism is the cause of pediculosis corporis.

pediculus (pē-dĭk′ū-lŭs) *pl.* **pediculi** [L.] **1.** A little foot. **2.** Louse. SEE: *Pediculus.*

pedicure (pĕd′ĭ-kūr) [L. *pes,* foot, + *cura,* care] **1.** Care of the feet. **2.** Cosmetic care of the feet and toenails. **3.** Podiatrist.

pediform (pĕd′ĭ-form) [″ + *forma,* shape] Having the shape of a foot.

pedigree A chart, diagram, or table of an individual's ancestors used in human genetics in the analysis of inherited traits and illnesses.

pedionalgia (pē″dē-ō-năl′jē-ă) [Gr. *pedion,* metatarsus, + *algos,* pain] Neuralgic pain in the sole of the foot.

pediophobia (pē″dē-ō-fō′bē-ă) [Gr. *pais,* child, + *phobos,* fear] An unnatural dread of young children or of dolls.

pediphalanx (pĕd″ĭ-fā′lănks) [L. *pes,* foot, + Gr. *phalanx,* closely knit row] A phalanx of the foot. SEE: *maniphalanx.*

pedo-, pedi-, ped- [L. *pes,* foot] Combining form meaning *foot.*

pedobaromacrometer (pē″dō-băr″ō-mă-krŏm′ĕ-tĕr) [Gr. *pais,* child, + *baros,* weight, + *makros,* long, + *metron,* measure] An apparatus for determining the measurement and weight of infants.

pedodontia, pedodontics (pē″dō-dŏn′shē-ă, -tĭks) [Gr. *pais,* child, + *odous,* tooth] Dentistry for children.

pedodontist (pē″dō-dŏn′tĭst) A dentist who specializes in care of children's teeth.

pedodynamometer (pĕd″ō-dī-nă-mŏm′ĕ-tĕr) [L. *pes,* foot, + Gr. *dynamis,* power, + *metron,* measure] A device for measuring the strength of the leg muscles.

pedograph (pĕd′ō-grăf) [″ + Gr. *graphein,* to write] An imprint of the foot on paper.

pedometer (pē-dŏm′ĕ-tĕr) [Gr. *pais,* child, + *metron,* measure] A device for the measurement of infants.

pedometer (pĕd-ŏm′ĕ-tĕr) [L. *pes,* foot, + Gr. *metron,* measurement] An instrument that indicates the number of steps taken while walking.

pedomorphism (pē″dō-mor′fĭzm) [Gr. *pais,* child, + *morphe,* form, + *-ismos,* condition] The retention of juvenile characteristics in the adult.

pedophilia (pē″dō-fĭl′ē-ă) [″ + *philein,* to love] **1.** Fondness for children. **2.** In psychology, an unnatural desire for sexual relations with children.

pedorthics (pĕd′ŏr-thĭks) The making and fitting of shoes and other foot support products to alleviate and prevent foot injury and disease.

pedorthist (pĕd′ŏr-thĭst) A footwear specialist. Pedorthists design and produce individually fitted shoes and foot support products to alleviate and prevent foot injury and disease.

peduncle (pĕ-dŭn′kl) [L. *pedunculus,* a little foot] **1.** Pedicle (1). **2.** A brachium of the brain; a band connecting parts of the brain. SEE: *cimbia; crus; sessile.*

cerebral p. A pair of white bundles from the upper part of the pons to the cerebrum. It constitutes the ventral portion of the midbrain. SYN: *crus cerebri.*

p. of flocculus A band of fibers connecting the flocculus of the cerebellum with the vermis.

inferior cerebellar p. A band of fibers running along the lateral border of the fourth ventricle, connecting the spinal cord and medulla with the cerebellum. SYN: *restiform body*.

mamillary p. A band of fibers extending from the tegmentum of the midbrain to the mamillary body.

middle cerebellar p. A band of fibers connecting the cerebellum with the basilar portion of the pons. SYN: *brachium pontis*.

olfactory p. The long stalk of the olfactory bulb.

pineal p. A band from either side of the pineal gland to the anterior pillars of the fornix.

superior cerebellar p. A band of fibers connecting the cerebellum with the midbrain. SYN: *brachium conjunctivum*.

p. of superior olive A slender band of fibers extending from the superior olivary nucleus in the medulla to the nucleus of the abducens nerve.

thalamic p. One of four groups of fibers known as thalamic radiations that connect the thalamus with the cerebral cortex. SEE: *radiation, thalamic*.

peduncular (pĕ-dŭn′kū-lăr) [L. *pedunculus,* a little foot] Concerning a peduncle.

pedunculate, pedunculated (pĕ-dŭn′kū-lāt, -ĕd) Possessing a stalk or peduncle. SYN: *pediculate*.

pedunculotomy (pĕ-dŭng″kū-lŏt′ō-mē) [″ + Gr. *tome,* incision] Surgical section of a cerebral peduncle. This is done in treating involuntary movement disorders.

peeling [ME. *pelen,* to peel] Shedding of the surface layer of the skin. SYN: *desquamation*.

chemical p. Chemicals applied to skin to produce a mild, superficial burn; done to remove wrinkles.

PEEP *positive end-expiratory pressure.*

peer (pēr) [ME.] One who has an equal standing with another in age, class, or rank.

p. review The evaluation of the quality of the work effort of an individual by his or her peers. It could involve evaluation of articles submitted for publication or the quality of medical care administered by an individual, group, or hospital.

PEG *percutaneous endoscopic gastrostomy.*

peg, rete Rete ridge.

peg tooth An abnormally shaped tooth of genetic origin. Usually noted as a maxillary lateral incisor with a smaller cone-shaped crown.

PEJ *percutaneous endoscopic jejunostomy.*

pejorative (pĭ-jor′ă-tĭv, pē″jă-rā′tĭv) [L. *pejor,* worse] **1.** Tending to become or make worse. **2.** Being disparaging or belittling (e.g., in making a less than flattering remark about something or someone). SEE: *honorific*.

PEL *permissible exposure limits.*

pelade (pĕl-ăd′) [Fr., to remove hair] Alopecia areata.

pelage (pĕl′ĭj) [Fr.] The collective hair of the body.

Pel-Ebstein fever [Pieter K. Pel, Dutch physician, 1852–1919; Wilhelm Ebstein, Ger. physician, 1836–1912] Cyclic fever occurring in Hodgkin's disease in which periods of fever lasting from 3 to 10 days are separated by an afebrile period of about the same length.

Pelger-Huët anomaly (pĕl″jĕr hū′ĕt) [Karel Pelger, Dutch physician, 1885–1931; Gauthier Jean Huët, Dutch physician, 1879–1970] Granulocytes with rodlike, dumbbell, peanut-shaped, and spectacle-like nuclei. The chromatin of the nuclei is unusually coarse. The condition is inherited as an autosomal dominant. The cells function normally and carriers have no demonstrably lowered resistance to infection.

pelioma (pē-lē-ō′mă) [Gr.] Ecchymosis.

peliosis (pē-lē-ō′sĭs) [Gr.] Purpura.

bacillary p. A complication of an infection due to *Bartonella henselae* and *B. quintana,* esp. in immunocompromised patients. The lesions are in the viscera, liver, and spleen, and cause nonspecific symptoms. The prognosis in immunocompromised patients who are not treated is gradual decline and death. If bacteremia is present, the treatment consists of oral doxycycline or erythromycin for 4 weeks. SEE: *Bartonella quintana*.

p. hepatis Multiple, cystic, blood-filled spaces in the liver associated with dilatation of the sinusoids. These cause enlargement of and pain in the liver. These lesions are associated with use of oral contraceptives, certain types of anabolic steroids, and infections with *Bartonella* organisms. If the condition is due to infection, treatment consists of parenteral doxycycline for several weeks followed by several months of oral therapy. SEE: *bacillary angiomatosis; cat scratch disease*.

pellagra (pĕl-ă′gră, pĕ-lăg′ră) [L. *pellis,* skin, + Gr. *agra,* rough] The clinical consequences of profound niacin deficiency characterized by cutaneous, gastrointestinal, mucosal, and neurological symptoms. It is found in regions of the world where malnutrition is endemic.

SYMPTOMS: In advanced cases, stomatitis and glossitis, diarrhea, dermatitis, and central nervous system involvement occur. Cutaneous lesions include erythema followed by vesiculation, crusting, and desquamation. The skin may become dry, scaly, and atrophic. The mucous membranes of the mouth, esophagus, and vagina may atrophy; ulcers and cysts may develop. Anemia is common. Nausea, vomiting, and diarrhea occur, the last being characteristic. Involvement of the central nervous system is first manifested by neurasthenia, followed by organic psychosis characterized by disorientation, memory impairment, and confusion. Later, delirium and clouding of consciousness may occur.

ETIOLOGY: This condition is due to inadequate intake or absorption of niacin (nicotinic acid) or its amide (niacinamide, nicotinamide). It is commonly associated with restricted or limited diets in which a single cereal grain, esp. corn, is consumed without adequate consumption of wheat, eggs, beef, poultry, or other niacin- or tryptophan-rich foods. The condition is often found in chronic alcoholism.

TREATMENT: The disease is treated by following a diet adequate in all vitamins, minerals, and amino acids supplemented by 500 to 1000 mg of niacinamide given orally three times daily. If there is any doubt about the ability of the intestinal tract to absorb vitamins, the vitamins should be given parenterally.

pellagrazein (pĕl-ă-grā′zē-ĭn) A poisonous substance in decomposed cornmeal. At one time it was regarded erroneously as the cause of pellagra.

pellagrin (pĕ-lā′grĭn, -lăg′rĭn) A person afflicted with pellagra.

pellagroid (pĕ-lăg′royd, -lăg′royd) [L. *pellis,* skin, + Gr. *agra,* rough, + *eidos,* form, shape] Resembling pellagra.

Pellegrini's disease, Pellegrini-Stieda disease (pĕl″ā-grē′nē-stē′dă) [Augusto Pellegrini, It. surgeon, b. 1877; Alfred Stieda, Ger. surgeon, 1869–1945] Following trauma, ossification of the superior portion of the medial collateral ligament of the knee.

pellet (pĕl′ĕt) [Fr. *pelote,* a ball] A tiny pill or small ball of medicine or food.

cotton p. A small rolled cottonball, less than ⅜ in. (about 1 cm) in diameter, used for desiccation or topical application of medicaments, particularly in dentistry; also called pledgets.

foil p. Loosely rolled gold foil used for direct filling in dental restoration. SEE: *foil.*

pellicle (pĕl′ĭ-k′l) [L. *pellicula,* a little skin] **1.** A thin piece of cuticle or skin. **2.** Film or surface on a liquid. **3.** Scum.

salivary p. The thin layer of salivary proteins and glycoproteins that quickly adhere to the tooth surface after the tooth has been cleaned; this amorphous, bacteria-free layer may serve as an attachment medium for bacteria, which in turn form plaque.

pellucid (pĕl-lū′sĭd) [L. *pellucidus*] Clear.

pellucid zone Zona pellucida.

pelotherapy (pĕ″lō-thĕr′ă-pē) [Gr. *pelos,* mud, + *therapeia,* treatment] The therapeutic use of mud, peat, moss, or clay applied to all or part of the body.

pelvic (pĕl′vĭk) [L. *pelvis,* basin] Pert. to a pelvis, usually the bony pelvis.

pelvicephalography (pĕl″vē-sĕf″ă-lŏg′ră-fē) [″ + Gr. *kephale,* head, + *graphein,* to write] Radiographical study and measurement of the fetal head and the maternal pelvic outlet.

pelvicephalometry (pĕl″vē-sĕf″ă-lŏm′ĕ-trē) [″ + ″ + *metron,* measure] Measurement of the diameters of the fetal head and comparison of these with the diameters of the maternal pelvis.

pelvic inflammatory disease ABBR: PID. Infection of the uterus, fallopian tubes, and adjacent pelvic structures that is not associated with surgery or pregnancy. PID usually is caused by an ascending infection in which disease-producing germs spread from the vagina and cervix to the upper portions of the female reproductive tract. SEE: *chlamydia; gonorrhea; Nursing Diagnoses Appendix.*

ETIOLOGY: *Chlamydia trachomatis* and *Neisseria gonorrhoeae* are the most frequent causes of PID, although anaerobic microorganisms, *Escherichia coli,* and other microorganisms also are often involved.

SYMPTOMS: The most common symptom is lower abdominal or pelvic pain, typically beginning after the start of a menstrual period. Exquisite tenderness during physical examination of the cervix, fallopian tubes, or ovaries is a common sign. Clear, white, or purulent vaginal discharge is sometimes present. Fevers, chills, nausea, vomiting, vaginal bleeding, dysuria, dyspareunia, or anorectal pain are seen in smaller numbers of patients.

DIAGNOSIS: Distinguishing PID from other causes of lower abdominal or pelvic pain can be difficult. The disease may be confused with appendicitis, diverticulitis, tubo-ovarian abscess, endometritis, ectopic pregnancy, and other serious illnesses. PID is most likely to be found in young, sexually active patients with multiple sexual partners, esp. if there is a history of previous sexually transmitted illnesses or of substance abuse. Leukocytosis and an elevated sedimentation rate are commonly found, and a mucopurulent discharge is often present on pelvic examination. Cultures from the vagina or cervix may be helpful in identifying the causative organism. In patients for whom the diagnosis is unclear, laparoscopy, ultrasonography, or computed tomography may be needed.

COMPLICATIONS: PID may result in adhesions or scarring of the fallopian tubes and pelvis, and is a common cause of pelvic pain and ectopic pregnancy. About a third of all women who are infertile have lost the ability to conceive because of PID. Occasionally, PID causes intraperitoneal abscesses.

TREATMENT: Antibiotics effective against gonococci, chlamydiae, anaerobes, and gram-negative rods usually are used to treat PID. Typical therapy includes a tetracycline derivative, like doxycycline, and a cephalosporin. Early therapy prevents infertility caused by fallopian tube adhesions or scarring. In patients with tubal or pelvic abscesses, drainage is required. Sexual partners should be examined for evidence of sexually transmitted diseases and treated if culture results are positive. SEE: *safe sex*.

pelvic pain, chronic idiopathic ABBR: CIPP. Unexplained pelvic pain in a woman, that has lasted 6 months or longer. A complete medical, social, and sexual history must be obtained. In an experimental study, women with this illness reported more sexual partners, significantly more spontaneous abortions, and previous nongynecological surgery. These women were more likely to have experienced previous significant psychosexual trauma.

TREATMENT: The pain associated with CIPP should be treated symptomatically and sympathetically. The participation of pain management specialists, complementary medical providers, and the primary health care provider should be integrated. Realistic goals (e.g., the reduction of pain rather than its elimination) should be set. Medroxyprogesterone acetate, oral contraceptives, presacral neurectomy, hypnosis, and hysterectomy have been tried with varying degrees of success.

pelvic rock An exercise to strengthen the abdominal muscles and reduce the risk of backache or back stiffness (e.g., during pregnancy). The patient kneels on her hands and knees, hollows her back and pushes out her abdomen while inhaling, and arches her back like a cat and contracts the abdominal, gluteal, and levator muscles while exhaling. The exercise can be done while standing with the hands on the knees. The effects are maximized by concurrent abdominal breathing. SEE: *pelvic tilt*.

pelvic tilt An exercise to strengthen the abdominal muscles and reduce the risk of backache or back stiffness (e.g., during pregnancy). The patient assumes a supine position and flattens the hollow of her back against the floor. The abdominal, gluteal, and levator muscles are contracted with each exhalation and relaxed with each inhalation. The effects are maximized by concurrent abdominal breathing. SEE: *pelvic rock*.

pelvilithotomy (pĕl″vĭ-lĭ-thŏt′ō-mē) [″ + Gr. *lithos,* stone, + *tome,* incision] Pyelolithotomy.

pelvimeter (pĕl-vĭm′ĕ-tĕr) [″ + Gr. *metron,* measure] A device for measuring the pelvis.

pelvimetry (pĕl-vĭm′ĕ-trē) Measurement of the pelvic dimensions or proportions, which helps determine whether or not it will be possible to deliver a fetus through the normal route. This is done by various methods including manual or x-ray. SEE: *pelvis*.

pelviolithotomy (pĕl″vē-ō-lĭ-thŏt′ō-mē) [L. *pelvis,* basin, + Gr. *lithos,* stone, + *tome,* incision] Pyelolithotomy.

pelvioplasty (pĕl′vē-ō-plăs″tē) [″ + Gr. *plassein,* to form] **1.** Enlargement of the pelvic outlet to facilitate childbirth. SYN: *pelviotomy* (1); *pubiotomy; symphysiotomy*. **2.** Plastic surgical procedure on the pelvis of the kidney.

pelvioscopy (pĕl″vē-ŏs′kō-pē) [L. *pelvis,* basin, + Gr. *skopein,* to examine] Inspection of the pelvis.

pelviotomy (pĕl-vē-ŏt′ō-mē) [″ + Gr. *tome,* incision] **1.** Enlargement of the pelvic outlet to facilitate childbirth. **2.** Incision of the renal pelvis; usually done in order to remove a calculus.

pelviperitonitis (pĕl″vĭ-pĕr-ĭ-tō-nī′tĭs) [″ + Gr. *peritonaion,* peritoneum, + *itis,* inflammation] Inflammation of the peritoneum lining the pelvic cavity.

pelvirectal (pĕl″vē-rĕk′tăl) [″ + *rectum,* straight] Concerning the pelvis and rectum.

pelvis (pĕl′vĭs) *pl.* **pelves** [L., basin] **1.** Any basin-shaped structure or cavity. **2.** The bony compartment comprising the innominate bones, the sacrum, and the coccyx, joined at the symphysis pubis, sacroiliac, and sacrococcygeal articulations by a network of cartilage and ligaments. The structure supports the vertebral column and articulates with the lower limbs. SEE: illus. **3.** The cavity encompassed by the innominate bones, the sacrum, and the coccyx.

ANATOMY: The pelvis is separated into a false or superior pelvis and a true or inferior pelvis by the iliopectineal line and the upper margin of the symphysis pubis. The circumference of this area constitutes the inlet of the true pelvis. The lower border of the true pelvis, termed the outlet, is formed by the coccyx, the protuberances of the ischia, the ascending rami of the ischia, and the descending rami of the ossa pubis and the sacrosciatic ligaments. The floor of the pelvis is formed by the perineal fascia, the levator ani, and the coccygeus muscles. All diameters normally are larger in the female than in the male.

EXTERNAL DIAMETERS: *Interspinous:* The distance between the outer edges of the anterosuperior iliac spines, the diameter normally measuring 26 cm (10¼ in.). *Intercristal:* The distance between the outer edges of the most prominent portion of the iliac crests, the diameter normally being 28 cm (11 in.). *Intertrochanteric:* The distance between the most prominent points of the femo-

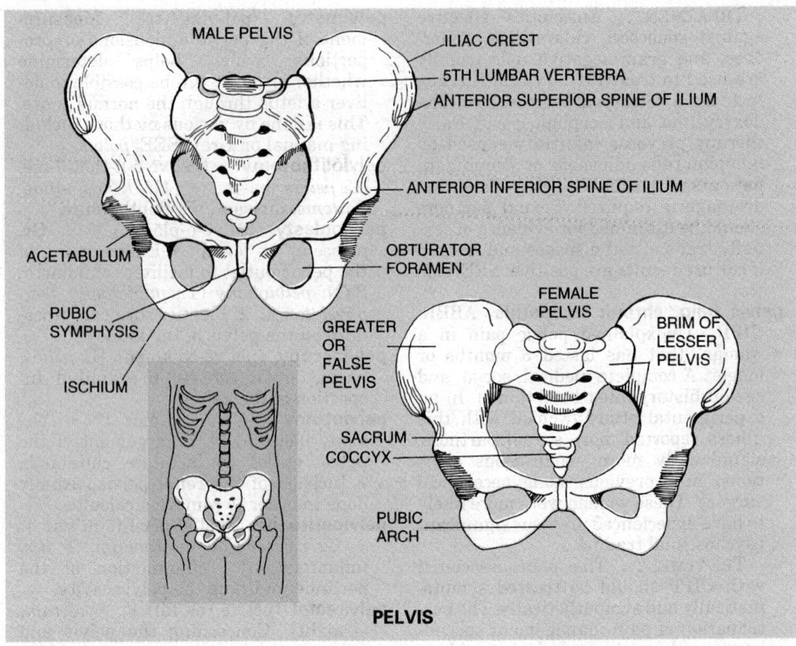

PELVIS

ral trochanters, 32 cm (12½ in.). *Oblique* (right and left): The distance from one posterosuperior iliac spine to the opposite anterosuperior iliac spine, 22 cm (8½ in.), the right being slightly greater than the left. *External conjugate:* The distance from the undersurface of the spinous process of the last lumbar vertebra to the upper margin of the anterior surface of the symphysis pubis, 20 cm (7⅞ in.). SYN: *Baudelocque's diameter.*

INTERNAL DIAMETERS: *True conjugate:* The anteroposterior diameter of the pelvic inlet, 11 cm (4¼ in.), the most important single diameter of the pelvis. *Diagonal conjugate:* The distance between the promontory of the sacrum to the undersurface of the symphysis pubis, 13 cm (5⅛ in.). Two cm (¾ in.) are deducted for the height and inclination of the symphysis pubis to obtain the diameter of the conjugate. *Transverse:* The distance between the ischial tuberosities, 11 cm (4¼ in.). *Anteroposterior* (of outlet): The distance between the lower border of the symphysis pubis and the tip of the sacrum, 11 cm (4¼ in.). *Anterior sagittal:* The distance from the undersurface of the symphysis pubis to the center of the line between the ischial tuberosities, 7 cm (2¾ in.). *Posterior sagittal:* The distance from the center of line between the ischial tuberosities to the tip of the sacrum, 10 cm (4 in.).

p. aequabiliter justo major A pelvis that is symmetrically larger than the standard in all its dimensions. SYN: *giant p.*

p. aequabiliter justo minor A pelvis with all its dimensions uniformly smaller than the standard. SYN: *reduced p.*

android p. The normal shape of the male pelvis. About 30% of women share this bony configuration; however, the heart-shaped inlet convergent sidewalls, slanted sacrum, and narrow sacrosciatic notch pose problems for childbearing. The narrowed dimensions increase the risk of fetopelvic disproportion, obstructed labor, and cesarean delivery. SYN: *masculine p.*

anthropoid p. A structural abnormality that occurs in about 20% of women. Deviations from the normal gynecoid configuration include a long, oval, narrow inlet and narrow sacrum, straight sidewalls, and a wide sacrosciatic notch. The shape increases the potential for fetal posterior positions during childbearing.

assimilation p. A structural abnormality that results from a developmental lumbosacral fusion or from a sacrococcygeal fusion.

beaked p. A pelvis with the pelvic bones laterally compressed and pushed forward so that the outlet is narrow and long. SYN: *rostrate p.; triradiate p.*

brachypellic p. An oval pelvis in which the transverse diameter is at least 1 cm longer, but no more than 3 cm longer, than the anteroposterior diameter of the pelvis.

brim of the p. Inlet of the pelvis. SEE: *brim* (2).

contracted p. A pelvis in which one or more of the principal diameters is reduced to a degree that parturition is impeded.

cordate p. A pelvis possessing a heart-shaped inlet.

coxalgic p. A pelvis deformed subsequent to hip joint disease.

dolichopellic p. An abnormal pelvis in which the anteroposterior diameter is greater than the transverse diameter.

dwarf p. An aequabiliter justo minor pelvis in which all diameters are symmetrically reduced; resembles an infant pelvis. Usually united by cartilage.

elastic p. Osteomalacic p.

extrarenal p. A renal pelvis located outside the kidney. This occurs when there is obstruction of the uteropelvic junction of the ureter.

false p. The portion of the pelvic cavity that lies above the pelvic brim, bounded by the linea terminalis and the iliac fossae. It supports the weight of the growing uterus during the middle and last trimesters of pregnancy. SYN: *p. major*.

fissured p. A structural malformation in which the ilia are pushed forward to an almost parallel position; caused by rickets.

flat p. A pelvis in which the anteroposterior diameters are shortened.

frozen p. Fixation of the pelvic organs in the pelvis caused by infection or neoplastic infiltration.

funnel-shaped p. A pelvis in which the outlet is considerably contracted but the inlet dimensions are normal.

giant p. P. aequabiliter justo major.

gynecoid p. The normal shape of the birth canal. The configuration is nearly circular, and the angle of the pubic arch usually exceeds 90°, allowing exit of the average fetus.

halisteretic p. A deformed pelvis resulting from softening of bones.

infantile p. An adult pelvis that retains its infantile characteristics. SYN: *juvenile p.*

p. justo major An unusually large pelvis.

p. justo minor An unusually small pelvis.

juvenile p. Infantile p.

kyphoscoliotic p. A deformed pelvis caused by rickets.

kyphotic p. A deformed pelvis characterized by an increase of the conjugate diameter at the brim with reduction of the transverse diameter at the outlet.

large p. P. justo major.

lordotic p. A deformed pelvis in which the spinal column has an anterior curvature in the lumbar region.

p. major False p.

malacosteon p. Rachitic p.

masculine p. A female pelvis that resembles a male pelvis, esp. in that it is narrower, more conical, and heavier-boned and has a heart-shaped inlet. SYN: *android p.*

p. minor P. justo minor.

p. obtecta A deformed pelvis in which the vertebral column extends across the pelvic inlet.

osteomalacic p. A pelvis distorted because of osteomalacia. SYN: *elastic p.*

Otto p. SEE: *Otto pelvis*.

platypellic p. A rare structural malformation that resembles a flattened gynecoid pelvis with shortened anteroposterior and wide transverse diameters.

pseudo-osteomalacic p. A rachitic pelvis similar to that of a person with osteomalacia.

rachitic p. A pelvis deformed from rickets. SYN: *malacosteon p.*

reduced p. P. aequabiliter justo minor.

renal p. The expanded proximal end of the ureter. It is within the renal sinus of the kidney and receives the urine through the major calyces.

reniform p. A pelvis shaped like a kidney.

Robert's p. SEE: *Robert's pelvis*.

rostrate p. Beaked p.

p. rotunda A tympanic depression in the inner wall, at the bottom of which is the fenestra rotunda.

round p. A pelvis with a circular inlet.

scoliotic p. A deformed pelvis resulting from spinal curvature.

simple flat p. A pelvis with a shortened anteroposterior diameter.

small p. P. justo minor.

p. spinosa A rachitic pelvis with a pointed pubic crest.

split p. A pelvis with a congenital division at the symphysis pubis.

spondylolisthetic p. A pelvis in which the last lumbar vertebra is dislocated in front of the sacrum, causing occlusion of the brim.

triangular p. A pelvis whose inlet is triangular.

triradiate p. Beaked p.

true p. The portion of the pelvis lying below the iliopectineal line. The dimensions of the true pelvis are of obstetrical significance in determining the success of fetal descent.

pelvitherm (pĕl′vĭ-thĕrm) [L. *pelvis,* basin, + Gr. *therme,* heat] A device for applying heat to the pelvis through the vagina.

pelvoscopy (pĕl-vŏs′kō-pē) [″ + Gr. *skopein,* to examine] Inspection of the pelvis.

pelvospondylitis (pĕl″vō-spŏn″dĭ-lī′tĭs) [″ + Gr. *spondylos,* vertebra, + *itis,* inflammation] Inflammation of the pelvic portion of the spine.

p. ossificans Any inflammatory spondylitis.

pemoline (pĕm′ō-lĕn) A central nervous system–stimulating drug that is used in treating children with hyperkinesis and minimal brain damage. Trade name is Cylert.

pemphigoid (pĕm′fĭ-goyd) [Gr. *pemphigodes,* breaking out in blisters] A skin condition similar to pemphigus.

bullous p. A blistering disease found almost exclusively in the elderly. Large, tense bullae filled with clear serum form on normal and urticarial skin. Lesions predominate in the flexural aspects of the limbs and abdomen. This condition is treated with corticosteroids and immunosuppressive agents, such as azathioprine or cyclophosphamide.

pemphigus (pĕm′fĭ-gŭs) [Gr. *pemphix,* a blister] An acute or chronic autoimmune disease principally of adults but sometimes found in children, characterized by occurrence of successive crops of bullae that appear suddenly on apparently normal skin and disappear, leaving pigmented spots. A characteristic sign is a positive Nikolsky's sign: when pressure is applied to an area as if trying to push the skin parallel to the surface, the skin will detach from the lower layers.

erythematous p. Scaling, erythematous macules and blebs of the scalp, face, and trunk. The lesions have a "butterfly" distribution over the face. The disease resembles pemphigus foliaceus.

p. foliaceus Pemphigus with a chronic course and in which bullous lesions may be absent. Once lesions develop, they may spread to the entire body and mimic generalized exfoliative dermatitis. The positive Nikolsky's sign helps to make the correct diagnosis. The condition is treated with systemic corticosteroids.

p. vegetans A form of pemphigus vulgaris characterized by pustules instead of bullae. Pustules are followed by warty vegetations. Prognosis is good, even prior to therapy with corticosteroids.

p. vulgaris The most common form of pemphigus. Lesions develop suddenly and are round or oval, thin-walled, tense, and translucent with contents bilateral in distribution. The lesions have little tendency to heal, and bleed easily when they burst. Since the introduction of corticosteroids, the prognosis is favorable, but the mortality rate is still high. Immunosuppressive agents, such as azathioprine or cyclophosphamide, are used with corticosteroid therapy. SEE: *photochemotherapy.*

pencil A material rolled into cylindrical form; may contain a caustic substance or a therapeutic paste or ointment.

pendular (pĕn′dū-lĕr) [L. *pendulus*] Hanging so as to swing by an attached part; oscillating like a pendulum.

pendulous (pĕn′dū-lŭs) Swinging freely like a pendulum; hanging.

penectomy Surgical or traumatic removal of the penis.

penetrance 1. The frequency of manifestation of a hereditary condition in individuals. In theory, if the genotype is present, penetrance should be 100%. That is not usually the case, as a result of the modifying effects of other genes. **2.** The extent to which something enters an object.

penetrate (pĕn′ĕ-trāt) [L. *penetrare*] To enter or force into the interior; pierce.

penetrating (pĕn′ĕ-trāt-ĭng) Entering beyond the exterior.

p. power The penetrating capacity of a lens.

p. wound A wound entering the interior of an organ or cavity.

penetration (pĕn″ĕ-trā′shŭn) [L. *penetrare,* to go within] **1.** The process of entering within a part. **2.** The capacity to enter within a part. **3.** The power of a lens to give a clear focus at varying depths. **4.** The ability of radiation to pass through a substance.

penetrometer (pĕn″ĕ-trŏm′ĕ-tĕr) [″ + Gr. *metron,* measure] An instrument that compares roughly the comparative absorption of x-rays in various metals, esp. silver, lead, and aluminum; hence, it gives a rough estimation of the ability of x-rays to penetrate tissues. SYN: *qualimeter.*

-penia (pē′nē-ă) [Gr. *penia,* lack] Combining form indicating *decrease, deficiency.*

penicillamine (pĕn″ĭ-sĭl′ă-mēn) A metal-chelating drug used to treat copper, mercury, zinc, and lead poisoning, and occasionally, rheumatoid arthritis. When taken for a long time, it often causes side effects such as rashes, autoimmune phenomena, renal dysfunction, or bone marrow suppression.

penicillic acid An antibiotic, $C_8H_{10}O_4$, produced by some species of *Penicillium.*

penicillin (pĕn-ĭ-sĭl′ĭn) One of a group of antibiotics biosynthesized by several species of molds, esp. *Penicillium notatum* and *P. chrysogenum.* Penicillin is bactericidal, inhibiting the growth of some gram-positive bacteria and some spirochetes. There are many different penicillins, including synthetic ones, and their effectiveness varies for different organisms. SEE: *penicillin allergy.*

beta-lactamase resistant p. Synthetic penicillins that resist the action of the enzyme beta-lactamase, produced by some microorganisms. Bacteria that produce the enzyme are not susceptible to the action of non–beta-lactamase resistant penicillins.

p. G benzathine An antibiotic of the

penicillin class available in a variety of dosage forms, used orally and parenterally.

penicillinase-resistant p. Any of a group of penicillins that are not inactivated by the enzyme penicillinase. These penicillins retain their effectiveness as antibiotics used for infections caused by bacteria that produce penicillinase. SEE: *bacterial resistance; beta-lactamase resistance; Staphylococcus aureus, methicillin-resistant.*

p. V potassium An antibiotic of the penicillin class. It is relatively stable in an acid medium and is therefore not inactivated by gastric acid when taken orally.

penicillin allergy A hypersensitivity reaction to penicillin, present in about 0.5% to 8% of the population. Although different types of hypersensitivity reactions may occur, the most common and potentially dangerous are the type I (immediate) reactions mediated by immunoglobulin E. If a patient reports a history of signs of local anaphylaxis (e.g., urticaria) or systemic anaphylaxis (e.g., bronchoconstriction, vasodilation) after taking penicillin, no penicillin or other beta-lactam antibiotics (e.g., cephalosporins) should be given to that patient ever again. In those very rare situations in which an infection is susceptible to no other antibiotic and the infection is serious enough to risk the danger of anaphylaxis, the patient may be desensitized with gradually increasing doses of penicillin.

penicillinase (pĕn-ĭ-sĭl′ĭ-nās) A bacterial enzyme that inactivates most but not all penicillins.

penicillinase-producing Neisseria gonorrhoeae ABBR: PPNG. Penicillin-resistant strains of *Neisseria gonorrhoeae.*

penicilliosis (pĕn″ĭ-sĭl″ē-ō′sĭs) [L. *penicillum,* brush, + *osis,* condition] Infection with the fungi of the genus *Penicillium.*

Penicillium (pĕn″ĭ-sĭl′ē-ŭm) [L. *penicillum,* brush] A genus of molds belonging to the Ascomycetes (sac fungi). They form the blue molds that grow on fruits, bread, and cheese. A number of species *(P. chrysogenum, P. notatum)* are the source of penicillin. Occasionally in humans they produce infections of the external ear, skin, or respiratory passageways. They are common allergens. SEE: illus.

P. marneffei A fungus that may cause systemic infections, esp. in immunocompromised patients. It is found most often in Southeast Asia, where it frequently infects patients with acquired immunodeficiency syndrome.

penicilloyl-polylysine (pĕn″ĭ-sĭl′oyl-pŏl″ē-lī′sēn) A substance used to determine sensitivity to some forms of penicillin. When it is injected intradermally into a sensitive individual, a wheal appears within 20 minutes.

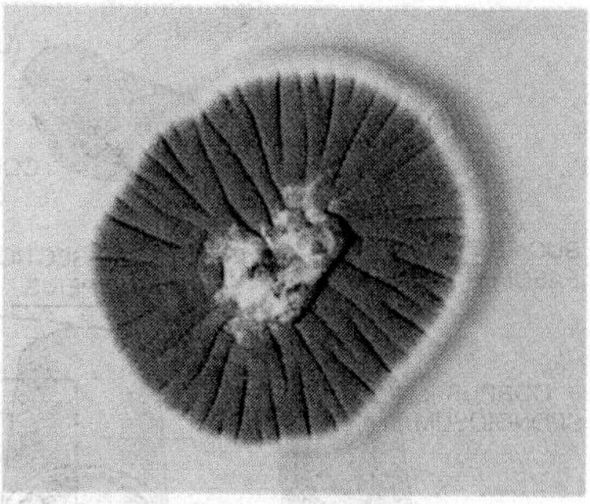

PENICILLIUM IN CULTURE

penicillus (pĕn″ĭ-sĭl′ŭs) *pl.* **penicilli** [L., paint brush] A group of the branches of arteries in the spleen that are arranged like the bristles of a brush. Each consists of successive portions: the pulp arteries, sheathed arteries, and terminal arteries.

penile (pē′nĭl, -nīl) [L. *penis,* penis] Pert. to the penis. SEE: *penile prosthesis.*

penile ring A ring made of metal, plastic, or leather. When placed around the flaccid penis, it is small enough to prevent venous return. Use of the device assists in maintaining erection of the penis and in delaying orgasm.

penis (pē′nĭs) *pl.* **penises, penes** [L.] The male organ of copulation and, in mammals, of urination. It is a cylindrical pendulous organ suspended from the front and sides of the pubic arch. It is homologous to the clitoris in the female. Contrary to popular misconceptions, the size of the normal penis has no physical bearing on the male's or female's enjoyment of sexual intercourse. SEE: illus.; *circumcision; penile prosthesis; Peyronie's disease; priapism.*

ANATOMY: The penis is composed mainly of erectile tissue arranged in three columns, the whole being covered with skin. The two lateral columns are the corpora cavernosa penis. The third or median column, known as the corpus spongiosum, contains the urethra. The body is attached to the descending portion of the pubic bone by the crura of the penis. The cone-shaped head of the penis, the glans penis, contains the urethral orifice. It is covered with a movable hood known as the foreskin or prepuce, under which is secreted the substance called smegma.

Hyperemia of the genitals fills the corpora cavernosa with blood as the result of sexual excitement or stimulation, thus causing an erection. The hyperemia subsides following orgasm and ejaculation of the seminal fluid. The or-

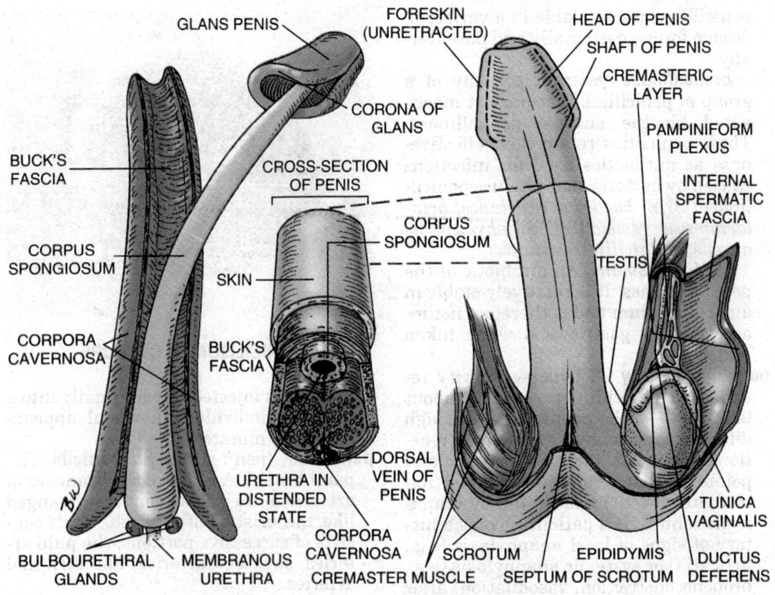

PENIS, INCLUDING TESTICLES AND SCROTUM

gan then returns to its flaccid condition. The size of the flaccid penis does not necessarily correlate with that of the erect penis.

p. captivus During sexual intercourse, the locking of a couple together owing to the penis being entrapped in the vagina. Even though this is quite common in dogs, the evidence that it occurs in human beings for more than a few moments, if ever, is lacking.

clubbed p. The condition in which the penis is curved during erection.

double p. A congenital deformity in which the penis in the embryo is completely divided by the urethral groove.

p. envy In psychoanalysis, the female's desire to have a penis.

p. lunatus Chordee.

p. palmatus A penis enclosed by the scrotum. SYN: *webbed p.*

webbed p. P. palmatus.

penischisis (pĕ-nĭs′kĭ-sĭs) [L. *penis,* penis, + Gr. *schisis,* a splitting] Epispadias, hypospadias, paraspadias, or any fissured condition of the penis.

penitis (pĕ-nī′tĭs) [″ + Gr. *itis,* inflammation] Inflammation of the penis.

pennate (pĕn′āt) [L. *penna,* feather] An object in which parts extend at an angle from a central portion, as do the barbs from a feather.

penniform (pĕn′ĭ-form) [″ + *forma,* shape] Feather-shaped.

pennyroyal (pĕn″ĭ-roy′ăl) Name for various plants, esp. those of the genera *Hedeoma* and *Mentha,* that yield commercial oil used as a carminative and stimulant.

pennyweight Troy weight containing 24 gr or 1/20 of a troy ounce; equal to 1.555 g. This unit of measure was previously used for describing the quantities of precious metals, as the amount of gold needed for dental restorations.

penoscrotal (pē″nō-skrō′tăl) Concerning the penis and scrotum.

pent-, penta- [Gr. *pente,* five] Combining form meaning *five.*

pentabasic (pĕn″tă-bā′sĭk) **1.** A compound that contains five replaceable hydrogen atoms. **2.** An alcohol that contains five hydroxyl groups.

pentachlorophenol C_6HCl_5O; a chemical previously used as a wood preservative for termite control and as a defoliant. It is extremely toxic on its own, but some grades are additionally contaminated with dioxin.

pentad (pĕn′tăd) [Gr. *pente,* five] **1.** A radical or element with a valence of five. **2.** A group of five.

pentadactyl (pĕn″tă-dăk′tĭl) [″ + *daktylos,* finger] Having five digits on each hand and foot.

pentaerythritol tetranitrate (pĕn″tă-ĕ-rĭth′rĭ-tŏl) An organic nitrate drug used in treating angina pectoris.

pentagastrin (pĕn″tă-găs′trĭn) A synthetic gastrin that may be administered to test the ability of the stomach to secrete hydrochloric acid.

pentamethylenediamine (pĕn″tă-mĕth″ĭl-ĕn-dī′ă-mĕn) A ptomaine occurring in tissue decomposed by certain bacteria.

pentamidine (pĕn-tăm′ĭ-dĕn) A drug used by injection or inhalation to treat *Pneumocystis carinii* pneumonia (PCP), leishmaniasis, and early cases of Gambian and Rhodesian trypanosomiasis. Its potential adverse effects include cardiac arrhythmias, kidney failure, and alterations of serum potassium, glucose, magnesium, and calcium levels. When the drug is given by inhalation, PCP may be eliminated from the lungs but may spread to other organs.

pentane (pĕn′tān) C_5H_{12}; one of the hydrocarbons of the methane series. It is a product of petroleum distillation.

pentapeptide (pĕn″tă-pĕp′tĭd) A polypeptide with five amino acid groups.

pentaploid (pĕn′tă-ployd) [″ + *ploos,* a fold, + *eidos,* form, shape] Having five sets of chromosomes.

pentastomiasis (pĕn″tă-stō-mī′ă-sĭs) Infection with certain genera of Pentastomida, the tongue worms. The larval forms usually live in the bodies of animals but have been reported in humans.

pentatomic (pĕn″tă-tŏm′ĭk) [″ + *atomos,* indivisible] **1.** Containing five atoms in the molecule. **2.** An alcohol with five hydroxyl groups.

pentavalent (pĕn″tă-vā′lĕnt, -tăv′ă-lĕnt) [Gr. *pente,* five, + L. *valens,* having power] Having a chemical valence of five.

pentazocine (pĕn-tăz′ō-sēn) An opioid analgesic drug that is effective orally and parenterally. Although originally thought to be nonaddicting, it is potentially addicting. Prolonged injection of the drug may cause a woody sclerosis of the skin and subcutaneous tissues around injection sites. The lesions may also appear on other areas of the skin. Ulcers surrounded by areas of hyperpigmentation may develop. Skin changes do not develop in short-term users of the drug.

pentobarbital (pĕn″tō-băr′bĭ-tăl) A hypnotic sedative drug of the barbiturate class.

p. sodium A barbituric acid derivative used as an oral or intravenous hypnotic agent in preanesthetic medication; used in labor with or without scopolamine.

pentosazon (pĕn″tō-sā′zŏn) A crystalline compound formed when a pentose is treated with phenylhydrazine. It is not normally present in urine.

pentose (pĕn′tōs) [Gr. *pente,* five] $C_5H_{10}O_5$; a monosaccharide containing five carbon atoms, such as ribose in RNA and deoxyribose in DNA.

pentosemia (pĕn″tō-sē′mē-ă) Pentose in the blood.

pentoside (pĕn′tō-sīd) Pentose combined with some other substance. Pentoses combined with purine or pyrimidine bases are present in nucleic acids, DNA, and RNA.

pentostam A drug used in leishmaniasis and available in the U.S. only from the Center for Infectious Disease Control, Drug Service, Atlanta, GA 30333, (404) 639-2888.

pentosuria (pĕn″tō-sū′rē-ă) A condition in which pentose is found in the urine.

pentoxide (pĕn-tŏk′sīd) A chemical molecule containing five atoms of oxygen.

pentoxifylline A drug used in peripheral vascular disease to improve claudication symptoms.

penumbra (pĕ-nŭm′bră) Healthy tissue that surrounds an ischemic or infarcted part.

peotillomania (pē″ō-tĭl″ō-mā′nē-ă) [Gr. *peos,* penis, + *tillein,* to pull, + *mania,* madness] A nervous habit or tic consisting of constant pulling at the penis.

peotomy (pē-ŏt′ō-mē) [″ + *tome,* incision] Surgical removal of the penis.

Peplau, Hildegard A nursing educator (1909–1999) who developed the Theory of Interpersonal Relations in Nursing. SEE: *Nursing Theory Appendix.*

pepper (pĕp′ĕr) [ME. *peper*] A spice that is used as a condiment, stimulant, carminative, and counterirritant. The dried berries of the fruit of plants of the genus *Piper.* These are ground or used whole to season foods. Although pepper irritates the oral mucosa, it does not produce peptic ulcers.

The Scoville scale is used for judging the level of "heat" or spiciness of peppers. Using this scale, the hottest peppers have a rating of 250,000 to 400,000 units. The active ingredient in chile peppers, capsaicin, may cause nasal or ocular irritation; it is wise to wear gloves, or to wash one's hands frequently when handling especially spicy peppers.

peppermint (pĕp′ĕr-mĭnt) A perennial herb, *Mentha piperita,* cultivated for its aromatic leaves and used as a flavoring agent, carminative, and antiemetic.

peppermint spirit The leaves and tops of the plant *Mentha piperita,* from which oil of peppermint is derived. It is used as an aromatic stimulant, carminative, and flavoring agent.

pepsic (pĕp′sĭk) [Gr. *peptein,* to digest] Peptic.

pepsin (pĕp′sĭn) [Gr. *pepsis,* digestion] The chief enzyme of gastric juice, which converts proteins into proteoses and peptones. It is formed by the chief cells of gastric glands and produces its maximum activity at a pH of 1.5 to 2. It is obtainable in granular form. In the presence of hydrochloric acid, it digests proteins in vitro.

pepsinogen (pĕp-sĭn′ō-jĕn) [″ + *gennan,* to produce] The antecedent of pepsin existing in the form of granules in the chief cells of gastric glands.

pepsinuria (pĕp″sĭ-nū′rē-ă) [″ + *ouron,* urine] Excretion of pepsin in the urine.

peptic (pĕp′tĭk) [Gr. *peptikos*] **1.** Concerning digestion. **2.** Concerning pepsin. SYN: *pepsic.*

peptic ulcer An ulcer occurring in the lower end of the esophagus; in the stomach usually along the lesser curvature; in the duodenum; or on the jejunal side of a gastrojejunostomy. Peptic ulcer disease is a common illness, affecting about 10% of men and 5% of women during their lifetimes. SEE: *Curling's ulcer; Helicobacter pylori; stress ulcer; Zollinger-Ellison syndrome; Nursing Diagnoses Appendix.*

ETIOLOGY: Common causes of peptic ulcer include use of nonsteroidal anti-inflammatory drugs (NSAIDs), tobacco smoking, *H. pylori* infection of the upper gastrointestinal tract, and severe physiological stressors. Ulcers are more common in men than in women and occur most frequently in patients over age 65. The relationship between peptic ulcer and emotional stress is not completely understood.

SYMPTOMS: Patients with peptic ulcers may be asymptomatic or have gnawing epigastric pain, esp. in the middle of the night, or when no food has been eaten for several hours. At times, heartburn, nausea, vomiting, hematemesis, melena, or unexplained weight loss may signify peptic disease. Peptic ulcers that perforate the upper gastrointestinal tract may cause symptoms of pancreatitis or an acute abdomen.

DIAGNOSIS: Endoscopy provides the single best test to diagnose peptic ulcers because it allows direct visualization of the mucosa. During endoscopy, tissue can be excised, vessels ligated, or sclerosants injected. Upper gastrointestinal x-ray series may also be used to provide images for diagnosis or follow-up, but biopsy, breath testing for *H. pylori,* and injection therapies (which can all take place during endoscopy) are not part of this procedure.

TREATMENT: *Helicobacter pylori* causes most peptic ulcers in the duodenum; antibiotics and antisecretory drugs like lansoprazole or omeprazole should be given to all patients with duodenal ulcers. Peptic ulceration of the stomach may be treated with the same medications if biopsies or breath tests reveal *H. pylori*. When patients have ulcers caused by the use of NSAIDs or tobacco, withholding these agents and treating with an H_2 blocker (e.g., ranitidine) provides an effective cure. Misoprostol may also be used to prevent peptic ulcer caused by NSAID use. Surgical therapy (including subtotal gastric resection) may be needed in rare instances of uncontrollable hemorrhage or perforation occurring as a result of peptic ulcer disease.

PATIENT CARE: The ambulatory patient is educated about agents that increase the risk for peptic ulceration (e.g., NSAIDs, tobacco products) and given specific instructions to avoid them. Patient teaching should include the importance of adherence to prescription drug therapies and the need for follow-up examination.

In the hospitalized patient with ulcer-related bleeding, careful monitoring of vital signs, fluid balance, hemoglobin levels, and blood losses may enhance early recognition of worsening disease. Endoscopic or other diagnostic procedures are explained to the patient, and the effects of prescribed therapies or transfusions are carefully assessed. Health care professionals should help the patient to develop coping mechanisms to relieve anxiety. Patients are taught to recognize signs and symptoms of disease recurrence (e.g., coffee-ground emesis, the passage of black or tarry stools, or epigastric pain).

peptidase An enzyme that converts peptides to amino acids.

peptide (pĕp'tīd) [Gr. *peptein,* to digest] A compound containing two or more linked amino acids.

peptidoglycan A large, complex carbohydrate that forms layers in the cell walls of bacteria. Gram-positive cell walls have many peptide-linked layers; gram-negative cell walls have few layers.

peptidolytic (pĕp"tĭ-dō-lĭt'ĭk) [" + *lytikos,* dissolving] Causing the splitting up or digestion of peptides.

peptinotoxin (pĕp"tĭn-ō-tŏk'sĭn) [" + *toxikon,* poison] Poisonous ptomaine found in the body as a result of disordered or defective digestion.

peptization (pĕp"tĭ-zā'shŭn) [Gr. *peptein,* to digest] In the chemistry of colloids, the process of making a colloidal solution more stable; conversion of a gel to a sol.

Peptococcaceae A family of bacteria that includes the genus *Peptococcus.* These gram-positive anaerobic cocci may be normal or pathologic inhabitants of the respiratory and intestinal tracts.

Peptococcus (pĕp"tō-kŏk'ŭs) Strictly anaerobic gram-positive cocci that are normally present in the oral cavity, on the skin, and in the intestinal tract. When associated with infection, they usually act synergistically with other organisms.

peptogenic, peptogenous (pĕp-tō-jĕn'ĭk, -tŏj'ĕn-ŭs) [" + *gennan,* to produce] **1.** Producing peptones and pepsin. **2.** Promoting digestion.

peptone (pĕp'tōn) [Gr. *pepton,* digesting] A secondary protein formed by the action of proteolytic enzymes, acids, or alkalies on certain proteins.

peptonization (pĕp"tō-nĭ-zā'shŭn) [Gr. *pepton,* digesting] The action by which proteolytic enzymes break proteins into peptones.

peptonize To convert into peptones; to predigest with pepsin.

peptonuria (pĕp″tō-nū′rē-ă) [″ + *ouron,* urine] Excretion of peptones in the urine.

Peptostreptococcus (pĕp″tō-strĕp″tō-kŏk′ŭs) A genus of gram-positive anaerobic cocci of the Peptococcaceae family. They may be normal or pathogenic inhabitants of the intestinal and respiratory tracts. They are also important as opportunistic pathogens.

peptotoxin (pĕp″tō-tŏk′sĭn) [″+ *toxikon,* poison] Any toxin produced from a peptone.

per [L. *per,* through] **1.** Through, by, by means of. **2.** In chemistry, the highest valence of an element. **3.** For each unit or entity (e.g., milligrams per kilogram, usually written as *mg/kg).*

per- A prefix indicating *throughout, through, utterly, intense.*

peracephalus (pĕr″ă-sĕf′ă-lŭs) [″ + Gr. *a-,* not, + *kephale,* head] A parasitic placental twin. It does not contain a head or arms, and the thorax is malformed.

peracid (pĕr-ăs′ĭd) **1.** An acid that contains the highest valence possible. **2.** An acid containing the peroxide group, O—OH.

peracidity (pĕr″ă-sĭd′ĭ-tē) [L. *per,* through, + *acidus,* sour] Abnormal acidity.

peracute (pĕr″ă-kūt′) [″ + *acutus,* keen] Very acute or violent.

per anum (pĕr ā′nŭm) [L.] Through or by way of the anus.

perarticulation (pĕr″ăr-tĭk″ū-lā′shŭn) [L. *per,* through, + *articulatio,* joint] Diarthrosis.

percent Per hundred; one of each hundred. The symbol, %, is used to indicate that the preceding number is a percentage rather than an absolute number. Thus, 8% of 50 is 4; whereas 8% of 500 is 40.

percentile (pĕr-sĕn′tīl) One of 100 equal divisions of a series of items or data. Thus if a value such as a test score is higher than 92% of all the other test scores, that result is above the 92nd percentile of the range of scores.

percept (pĕr′sĕpt) The mental image of an object seen.

perception (pĕr-sĕp′shŭn) [L. *percepitio,* perceive] **1.** The process of being aware of objects; consciousness. **2.** The process of receiving sensory impressions. **3.** The elaboration of a sensory impression; the ideational association modifying, defining, and usually completing the primary impression or stimulus. Vague or inadequate association occurs in confused and depressed states.

auditory p. **1.** Hearing. **2.** Ability to identify, interpret, and attach meaning to sound.

depth p. The perception of spatial relationships; three-dimensional perception.

extrasensory p. ABBR: ESP. The alleged perception of external events by other than the five senses.

gustatory p. Taste.

olfactory p. Smell.

stereognostic p. The recognition of objects by touch.

tactile p. Touch.

visual p. Sight.

perceptivity (pĕr-sĕp-tĭv′ĭ-tē) The power to receive sense impressions.

perceptual completion An optical illusion in which a boundary, color, texture, light, or object is seen where one does not actually exist. This defect in visual perception, also known as "filling-in," commonly is experienced by people with visual field cuts or defects (scotoma).

percolate (pĕr′kō-lāt) [L. *percolare,* to strain through] **1.** To allow a liquid to seep through a powdered substance. **2.** Any fluid that has been filtered or percolated. **3.** To strain a fluid through powdered substances in order to impregnate it with dissolved chemicals.

percolation (pĕr″kō-lā′shŭn) [L. *percolatio*] **1.** Filtration. **2.** The process of extracting soluble portions of a drug of powdered composition by filtering a liquid solvent through it.

percolator (pĕr′kō-lā″tor) An apparatus used for extraction of a drug with a liquid solvent.

per contiguum (pĕr kŏn-tĭg′ū-ŭm) [L.] Touching, as in the spread of an inflammation from one part to an adjacent structure.

per continuum (pĕr kŏn-tĭn′ū-ŭm) [L.] Continuous, as in the spread of an inflammation from part to part.

percuss (pĕr-kŭs′) [L. *percutere*] To tap parts of the body to aid diagnosis by listening carefully to the sounds they emit.

percussion (pĕr-kŭsh′ŭn) [L. *percussio,* a striking] **1.** Striking the body surface (usually with the fingers or a small hammer) to determine the position, size, or density of underlying structures. **2.** A technique for mobilizing secretions from the lungs by massaging or striking the chest wall with cupped hands. SEE: *cystic fibrosis.*

auscultatory p. Percussion combined with auscultation.

bimanual p. Mediate p.

deep p. Forceful percussion used to elicit a note from a deeply seated tissue or organ.

direct p. Immediate p.

finger p. Striking of the examiner's finger as it rests upon the patient's body with a finger of the examiner's other hand.

immediate p. Percussion performed by striking the surface directly with the fingers. SYN: *direct p.*

indirect p. Mediate p.

mediate p. Percussion performed by using the fingers of one hand as a plexor and those of the opposite hand as a pleximeter. SYN: *bimanual p.; indirect p.*

palpation p. Percussion in which the examiner uses his or her fingers to feel vibrations that are produced within the body, instead of listening for the sounds produced by striking the body.

threshold p. Percussing lightly with the fingers on a glass-rod pleximeter, the far end of which is covered with a rubber cap. The cap is usually placed on an intercostal space. This technique is used to confine the percussion to a very small area.

percussor (pĕr-kŭs′or) [L., striker] A device used for diagnosis by percussion, consisting of a hammer with a rubber or metal head.

percutaneous (pĕr″kū-tā′nē-ŭs) [L. *per,* through, + *cutis,* skin] Effected through the skin; describes the application of a medicated ointment by friction, or the removal or injection of a fluid by needle.

per diem cost Hospital or other inpatient institutional cost per day.

perencephaly (pĕr″ĕn-sĕf′ă-lē) [Gr. *pera,* pouch, + *enkephalos,* brain] Porencephalia.

perfectionism (pĕr-fĕk′shŭn-ĭzm) A type of neurosis in which the individual attempts to achieve goals of behavior or performance that are unrealistic or unnecessary.

perflation (pĕr-flā′shŭn) [L. *perflatio*] The process of blowing air into a cavity to expand its walls or to force out secretions or other matter.

perfluorocarbons A class of solvent molecules that can carry nonpolar gases, such as oxygen, nitrogen, and carbon dioxide. They have been used experimentally in transfusion medicine and in some ophthalmic surgeries. Perfluorocarbons are also used as blood gas controls when prepared in buffered solutions equilibrated with CO_2 and O_2.

perforans (pĕr′fō-răns) [L.] Perforating or penetrating, as a nerve or muscle.

perforate (pĕr′fō-rāt) [L. *perforatus,* pierced with holes] **1.** To puncture or to make holes. **2.** Pierced with holes.

perforation (pĕr″fō-rā′shŭn) **1.** The act or process of making a hole, such as that caused by ulceration. **2.** The hole made through a substance or part.

Bezold's p. [Friedrich Bezold, Ger. physician, 1842–1908] A perforation on the inner surface of the mastoid bone.

p. of stomach or intestine Abdominal crisis due to escape of contents of the perforated viscus into the peritoneal cavity. Peritonitis is certain to develop unless there is immediate surgical intervention. SEE: *intestinal perforation; peritonitis.*

SYMPTOMS: The onset is accompanied by acute pain, beginning over the perforated area and spreading all over the abdomen, which may become rigid. Nausea and vomiting, tachycardia, fevers, chills, sweats, confusion, and decreased urinary output are common.

TREATMENT: Surgical treatment is necessary. Pending operation, the patient is given no oral fluids; parenteral fluids, antibiotics, and other medications are administered.

tooth p. An opening through the wall of a tooth, produced by pathologic processes or accidentally, thereby exposing the dental pulp. It is also called pulp exposure.

perforator (pĕr′fō-rā-tor) [L., a piercing device] An instrument for piercing the skull and other bones.

tympanum p. An instrument for perforating the tympanum.

perforatorium (pĕr″fō-ră-tō′rē-ŭm) The pointed tip of the acrosome of the spermatozoa.

performance **1.** The undertaking and completion of mental or physical work. In rehabilitation, a person's performance is observed and measured to determine functional capability. **2.** An accomplishment; the fulfillment of a task.

perfusate (pĕr-fū′zāt) The fluid used to perfuse a tissue or organ.

perfusion (pĕr-fū′zhŭn) [L. *perfundere,* to pour through] **1.** The circulation of blood through tissues. **2.** Passing of a fluid through spaces. **3.** Pouring of a fluid. **4.** Supplying of an organ or tissue with nutrients and oxygen by injecting blood or a suitable fluid into an artery.

coronary p. The passage of blood through the arteries of the heart. When the heart is unable to do this naturally, an external device may be used to keep blood flowing through these vessels.

perfusionist An individual who assists the physician in all aspects of managing the equipment and techniques used during extracorporeal circulation. A perfusionist may also be involved in inducing hypothermia and the addition of medications on the instruction of the physician.

perhydrocyclopentanophenanthrene (pĕr-hī″drō-sī″klō-pĕn-tăn″ō-phĕn-ăn′thrēn) The name of the ring structure of the chemical nucleus of the steroids. SEE: *steroid hormone* for illus.

peri- [Gr.] Prefix meaning *around, about.*

periadenitis (pĕr″ē-ă″dĕ-nī′tĭs) [″ + *aden,* gland, + *itis,* inflammation] Inflammation of the tissues surrounding a gland.

p. mucosa necrotica recurrens Recurring necrotic or ulcerative lesions on the buccal and pharyngeal mucosa. These start as small hard nodules that ulcerate and leave a deep crater. These may be associated with Behçet's syndrome.

perianal (pĕr″ē-ā′năl) [″ + L. *anus,* anus] Around or close to the anus.
periangiitis (pĕr″ē-ăn″jē-ī′tĭs) [″ + *angeion,* vessel, + *itis,* inflammation] Inflammation of tissue around a blood or lymphatic vessel.
periangiocholitis (pĕr″ē-ăn″jē-ō-kō-lī′tĭs) [″ + ″ + *chole,* bile, + *itis,* inflammation] Pericholangitis.
periaortic (pĕr″ē-ā-or′tĭk) [″ + *aorte,* aorta] Around the aorta.
periaortitis (pĕr″ē-ā-or-tī′tĭs) [″ + *aorte,* aorta, + *itis,* inflammation] Inflammation of adventitia and tissues around the aorta.
periapex (pĕr″ē-ā′pĕks) [″ + L. *apex,* tip] The area around the apex of a tooth.
periapical (pĕr″ē-ăp′ĭ-kăl) [″ + L. *apex,* tip] Around the apex of the root of a tooth.
periappendicitis (pĕr″ē-ă-pĕn″dĭ-sī′tĭs) [″ + L. *appendix,* appendage, + Gr. *itis,* inflammation] Inflammation of the tissues surrounding the appendix secondary to either appendicitis or other intraperitoneal inflammatory process.

p. decidualis A condition in which decidual cells exist in the peritoneum of the appendix vermiformis in cases of tubal pregnancy owing to adhesions between fallopian tubes and the appendix.

periappendicular (pĕr″ē-ăp″ĕn-dĭk′ū-lăr) [″ + L. *appendix,* appendage] Surrounding an appendix.
periarterial (pĕr″ē-ăr-tē′rē-ăl) [″ + *arteria,* artery] Placed around an artery.
periarteritis (pĕr″ē-ăr-tĕr-ī′tĭs) [″ + ″ + *itis,* inflammation] Inflammation of the external coat of an artery.

p. gummosa Gummas in the blood vessels in syphilis.

p. nodosa Polyarteritis nodosa. SEE: *Nursing Diagnoses Appendix.*

periarthric (pĕr″ē-ăr′thrĭk) Circumarticular.
periarthritis (pĕr″ē-ăr-thrī′tĭs) [″ + ″ + *itis,* inflammation] Inflammation of the area around a joint.
periarticular (pĕr″ē-ăr-tĭk′ū-lăr) Circumarticular.
periatrial (pĕr″ē-ā′trē-ăl) [″ + L. *atrium,* corridor] Around the atria of the heart.
periauricular Around the ear.
periaxial (pĕr-ē-ăk′sē-ăl) [″ + *axon,* axis] Located around an axis.
periaxillary (pĕr″ē-ăk′sĭl-ĕ″rē) [″ + L. *axilla,* armpit] Occurring around the axilla.
periaxonal (pĕr″ē-ăk′sō-năl) [″ + *axon,* axis] Around an axon.
peribronchial (pĕr″ĭ-brŏng′kē-ăl) [″ + *bronchos,* windpipe] Surrounding a bronchus.
peribronchiolar (pĕr″ĭ-brŏng-kī′ō-lăr) [″ + L. *bronchiolus,* bronchiole] Surrounding a bronchiole.
peribronchiolitis (pĕr″ĭ-brŏng″kē-ō-lī′tĭs) [″ + ″ + Gr. *itis,* inflammation] Inflammation of the area around the bronchioles.
peribulbar (pĕr″ĭ-bŭl′băr) [″ + L. *bulbus,* bulbous root] Surrounding a bulb, such as the olfactory bulb or the eyeball (previously called the bulb of the eye).
peribursal (pĕr″ĭ-bĕr′săl) [″ + *bursa,* leather sack] Around a bursa.
pericanalicular (pĕr″ĭ-kăn″ă-lĭk′ū-lăr) [″ + L. *canaliculus,* small canal] Around a canaliculus.
pericapsulitis (pĕr″ĭ-kăp″sū-lī′tĭs) Adhesive capsulitis of shoulder.
pericardiac, pericardial (pĕr-ĭ-kăr′dē-ăk, -ăl) [″ + *kardia,* heart] Concerning the pericardium.
pericardicentesis, pericardiocentesis (pĕr″ĭ-kăr″dĭ-sĕn-tē′sĭs, -kăr″dē-ō-sĕn-tē′sĭs) [″ + ″ + *kentesis,* puncture] Surgical perforation of the pericardium. SEE: illus.
pericardiectomy (pĕr″ĭ-kăr-dē-ĕk′tō-mē) [″ + ″ + *ektome,* excision] Puncturing or perforation of the pericardium or creation of a pericardial window, for example, to relieve a pericardial effusion responsible for cardiac tamponade.
pericardiolysis (pĕr″ĭ-kăr″dē-ŏl′ĭ-sĭs) [″ + ″ + *lysis,* dissolution] Separation of adhesions between the visceral and parietal pericardium.
pericardiomediastinitis (pĕr″ĭ-kăr″dē-ō-mē-dē-ăs″tĭ-nī′tĭs) [″ + ″ + L. *mediastinum,* + Gr. *itis,* inflammation] Inflammation of the pericardium and mediastinum.
pericardiopexy [″ + ″ + *pexis,* fixation] A surgical procedure designed to increase the blood supply to the heart by joining the pericardium to an adjacent tissue.
pericardiophrenic (pĕr-ĭ-kăr″dē-ō-frĕn′ĭk) [″ + *kardia,* heart, + *phren,* diaphragm] Concerning the pericardium and diaphragm.
pericardiopleural (pĕr″ĭ-kăr″dē-ō-ploo′răl) [″ + ″ + *pleura,* rib] Concerning the pericardium and pleura.
pericardiorrhaphy (pĕr″ĭ-kăr″dē-or′ă-fē) [″ + ″ + *rhaphe,* seam, ridge] Suture of a wound in the pericardium.
pericardiostomy (pĕr″ĭ-kăr″dē-ŏs′tō-mē) [″ + *kardia,* heart, + *stoma,* mouth] Formation of an opening into the pericardium for drainage.
pericardiosymphysis (pĕr″ĭ-kăr″dē-ō-sĭm′fĭ-sĭs) [″ + ″ + *symphysis,* a joining] Adhesion between the layers of the pericardium.
pericardiotomy (pĕr″ĭ-kăr-dē-ŏt′ō-mē) [″ + ″ + *tome,* incision] Incision of the pericardial sac.
pericarditic (pĕr″ĭ-kăr-dĭt′ĭk) Concerning the pericardium.
pericarditis (pĕr-ĭ-kăr-dī′tĭs) [″ + *kardia,* heart, + *itis,* inflammation] Inflammation of the pericardium, marked by chest pain, fever, and an audible fric-

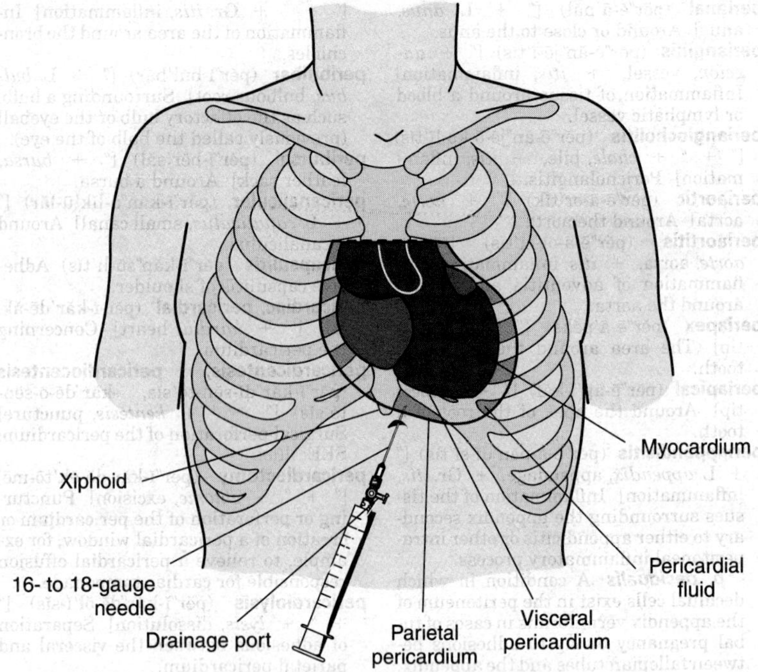

PERICARDIOCENTESIS

tion rub. SEE: *Dressler's syndrome; Nursing Diagnoses Appendix.*

ETIOLOGY: Many diseases and conditions can inflame the membranous covering of the heart, including infections (bacterial, tubercular, viral, fungal); collagen-vascular diseases (e.g., rheumatoid arthritis or systemic lupus erythematosus); myocardial infarction; cancer; renal failure; cardiac surgery; or trauma. In many instances, the precise cause is unknown (idiopathic).

SYMPTOMS: Chest pain that varies with respiration is a hallmark of the disease. The pain often worsens when the patient lies down and improves when the patient sits up. Fever, cough, dyspnea, and palpitations also are characteristic. The classic sign of pericarditis is a friction rub, a multicomponent abnormal heart sound that some observers describe as being scratchy, raspy, or leathery.

TREATMENT: Therapy depends on the cause of the syndrome. Uremic pericarditis, for example, is treated with dialysis, whereas pyogenic pericarditis requires antibiotic therapy and drainage. Prednisone or other anti-inflammatory drugs improve pericardial pain in patients with idiopathic disease.

PATIENT CARE: The patient is observed for symptoms of cardiac tamponade, such as weak or absent peripheral pulses, distended neck veins, decreased blood pressure, and narrowing pulse pressure. Medications are administered as prescribed. In the convalescent phase, the patient is taught about the importance of taking prescribed medications, their purposes, and any potentially recurring symptoms to report.

adhesive p. An old term for constrictive pericarditis.

constrictive p. Scarring of the pericardium after one or more episodes of pericarditis. This limits normal cardiac filling during diastole. Impaired fillling of the heart chambers reduces the volume of blood ejected by the heart with each contraction. The patient often complains of shortness of breath. On physical examination, elevated neck veins, ascites, hepatic enlargement, and lower extremity edema often are found. Surgical stripping of the pericardium (pericardiectomy) is used to relieve the constriction.

external p. Inflammation of the exterior surface of the pericardium.

fibrinous p. Pericarditis in which the membrane is covered with a butter-like exudate that organizes and unites the pericardial surfaces.

SYMPTOMS: The condition is characterized by symptoms of heart failure (e.g., dyspnea, generalized edema, cyanosis).

hemorrhagic p. Pericarditis in which the exudate contains blood.

idiopathic p. Acute nonspecific p.

ischemic p. Pericarditis resulting from myocardial infarction.

neoplastic p. Pericarditis due to invasion of the pericardium by cancer.

p. obliterans Pericardial inflammation causing adhesions and obliteration of the pericardial cavity.

serofibrinous p. Pericarditis in which there is a considerable quantity of serous exudate but little fibrin.

uremic p. Pericarditis associated with end-stage renal failure or hemodialysis. It indicates the need for more frequent or more intensive dialysis.

pericardium (pěr″ĭ-kăr′dē-ŭm) [Gr. *peri,* around, + *kardia,* heart] The membranous fibroserous sac enclosing the heart and the bases of the great vessels. The three layers are the fibrous pericardium (the outer layer); the parietal pericardium, a serous membrane that lines the fibrous pericardium; and the visceral pericardium (epicardium), a serous membrane on the surface of the myocardium. The space between the two serous layers is the pericardial cavity, a potential space filled with serous fluid that reduces friction as the heart beats. Its base is attached to the diaphragm, its apex extending upward as far as the first subdivision of the great blood vessels. It is attached in front to the sternum, laterally to the mediastinal pleura, and posteriorly to the esophagus, trachea, and principal bronchi. SEE: illus.

adherent p. A condition in which fibrous bands form between the two serous layers of the pericardium, obliterating the pericardial cavity. SEE: *pericarditis, constrictive.*

bread-and-butter p. A pathological appearance seen in fibrinous pericarditis, in which the pericardium has a peculiar appearance as a result of fibrinous deposits on the two opposing surfaces.

p. externum Fibrous pericardium. The outer fibrous layer of the pericardium; it extends over the bases of the great vessels and the upper surface of the diaphragm.

fibrous p. The outer fibrous layer of the pericardium; it extends over the bases of the great vessels and the upper surface of the diaphragm.

p. internum Visceral p.

parietal p. The middle layer of the pericardial sac, a serous membrane lining the fibrous pericardium.

serous p. The parietal and visceral pericardial membranes.

shaggy p. A condition occurring in fibrinous pericarditis in which loose shaggy deposits of fibrin are seen on the surfaces of the pericardium.

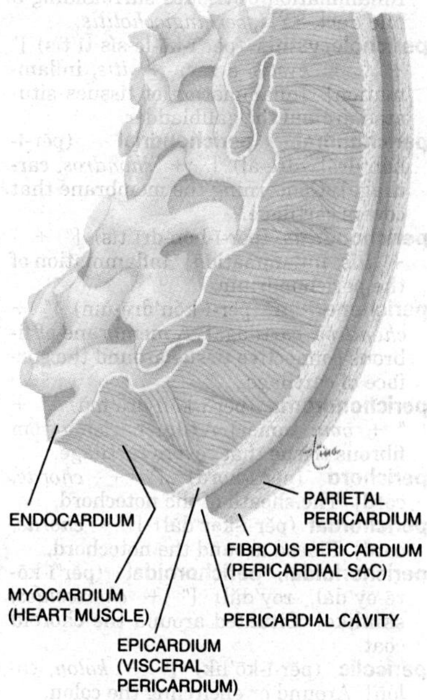

PERICARDIUM

Layers of the heart wall

visceral p. The inner serous layer of the pericardium, on the surface of the myocardium. SYN: *epicardium; P. internum.*

pericardotomy (pěr″ĭ-kăr-dŏt′ō-mē) [Gr. *peri,* around, + *kardia,* heart, + *tome,* incision] Incision of the pericardium.

pericecal (pěr″ĭ-sē′kăl) [″ + L. *caecum,* blind] Situated around the cecum.

pericecitis (pěr″ĭ-sē-sī′tĭs) [″ + ″ + Gr. *itis,* inflammation] Inflammation of the area around the cecum.

pericellular (pěr″ĭ-sĕl′ū-lăr) [″ + L. *cellula, cell*] Around a cell.

pericemental (pěr″ĭ-sē-mĕn′tăl) [″ + L. *caementum,* cement] Concerning the pericementum (i.e., the periodontal ligament).

pericementitis (pěr″ĭ-sē-mĕn-tī′tĭs) [″ + ″ + Gr. *itis,* inflammation] Periodontitis.

apical p. Apical abscess of the tooth.

pericementoclasia (pěr″ĭ-sē-mĕn″tō-klā′zē-ă) [″ + ″ + Gr. *klasis,* a breaking] Dissolution of the pericementum with alveolar absorption.

pericementum (pěr″ĭ-sē-mĕn′tŭm) Periodontal ligament.

pericentral (pěr″ĭ-sĕn′trăl) [″ + *kentron,* center] Around the center.

pericholangitis (pěr″ĭ-kō-lăn-jī′tĭs) [Gr. *peri,* around, + *chole,* bile, + *angeion,* vessel, + *itis,* inflammation]

Inflammation of tissues surrounding a bile duct. SYN: *periangiocholitis.*

pericholecystitis (pĕr″ĭ-kō-lē-sĭs-tī′tĭs) [″ + ″ + *kystis,* a sac, + *itis,* inflammation] Inflammation of tissues situated around the gallbladder.

perichondral, perichondrial (pĕr-ĭ-kŏn′drăl, -drē-ăl) [″ + *chondros,* cartilage] Concerning the membrane that covers cartilage.

perichondritis (pĕr-ĭ-kŏn-drī′tĭs) [″ + ″ + *itis,* inflammation] Inflammation of the perichondrium.

perichondrium (pĕr-ĭ-kŏn′drē-ŭm) [″ + *chondros,* cartilage] A membrane of fibrous connective tissue around the surface of cartilage.

perichondroma (pĕr″ĭ-kŏn-drō′mă) [″ + ″ + *oma,* tumor] A tumor arising from fibrous tissue that covers cartilage.

perichord (pĕr′ĭ-kord) [″ + *chorde,* cord] The sheath of the notochord.

perichordal (pĕr-ĭ-kor′dăl) [″ + *chorde,* cord] Placed around the notochord.

perichorioidal, perichoroidal (pĕr″ĭ-kō-rē-oy′dăl, -roy′dăl) [″ + *chorioeides,* skinlike] Situated around the choroid coat.

pericolic (pĕr-ĭ-kō′lĭk) [″ + *kolon,* colon] Around or encircling the colon.

pericolitis (pĕr″ĭ-kō-lī′tĭs) [″ + ″ + *itis,* inflammation] Inflammation of an area around the colon.

pericolpitis (pĕr″ĭ-kŏl-pī′tĭs) [Gr. *peri,* around, + *kolpos,* vagina, + *itis,* inflammation] Inflammation of connective tissues surrounding the vagina.

periconchal (pĕr-ĭ-kŏng′kăl) [″ + *konche,* concha] Around a concha.

pericorneal (pĕr″ĭ-kor′nē-ăl) [″ + L. *cornu,* horn] Placed around the cornea.

pericoronal (pĕr″ĭ-kor′ō-năl) [″ + *korone,* crown] Around the crown of a tooth.

pericoronitis (pĕr″ĭ-kor″ō-nī′tĭs) [″ + ″ + *itis,* inflammation] Inflammation around the crown of a tooth.

pericranial (pĕr″ĭ-krā′nē-ăl) [″ + *kranion,* skull] Pert. to the periosteum of the skull.

pericranitis (pĕr″ĭ-krā-nī′tĭs) [″ + ″ + *itis,* inflammation] Inflammation of the pericranium.

pericranium (pĕr″ĭ-krā′nē-ŭm) The fibrous membrane surrounding the cranium; periosteum of the skull.

p. internum The lining surface of the cranium. SYN: *endocranium.*

pericystic (pĕr″ĭ-sĭs′tĭk) [″ + *kystis,* bladder] Surrounding a cyst.

pericystitis (pĕr″ĭ-sĭs-tī′tĭs) [″ + ″ + *itis,* inflammation] Inflammation of the tissues about the bladder.

pericystium (pĕr″ĭ-sĭs′tē-ŭm) [″ + *kystis,* bladder] **1.** The vascular wall surrounding a cyst. **2.** The tissues around the urinary bladder or gallbladder.

pericyte (pĕr′ĭ-sīt) [″ + *kytos,* cell] A stem cell that may give rise to smooth muscle cells; often found around capillaries.

pericytial (pĕr-ĭ-sĭsh′ăl) [″ + *kytos,* cell] Placed around a cell.

peridendritic (pĕr″ĭ-dĕn-drĭt′ĭk) [″ + *dendron,* a tree] Surrounding a dendrite of a nerve cell.

peridens (pĕr′ĭ-dĕns) [″ + L. *dens,* tooth] A supernumerary tooth not situated in the dental arch.

peridental (pĕr″ĭ-dĕn′tăl) [″ + L. *dens,* tooth] Surrounding a tooth or part of one. SYN: *periodontal.*

peridentitis [″ + ″ + *itis,* inflammation] Inflammation of tissues surrounding a tooth. SYN: *periodontoclasia.*

peridentium (pĕr″ĭ-dĕn′tē-ŭm) [″ + L. *dens,* tooth] Periodontium.

periderm [″ + *derma,* skin] A thin layer of flattened cells forming a transient layer of embryonic epidermis. SYN: *epitrichial layer; epitrichium.*

peridesmitis (pĕr″ĭ-dĕz-mī′tĭs) [″ + *desmion,* band, + *itis,* inflammation] Inflammation of the areolar tissue around a ligament.

peridesmium (pĕr″ĭ-dĕz′mē-ŭm) The connective tissue membrane sheathing a ligament.

peridiaphragmatic (pĕr-ē-dī′ă-frăg-mă″tĭk) Relating to body areas near the diaphragm.

perididymis (pĕr″ĭ-dĭd′ĭ-mĭs) [″ + *didymos,* testicle] The tunica vaginalis of the testicle.

perididymitis (pĕr″ĭ-dĭd″ĭ-mī′tĭs) [″ + ″ + *itis,* inflammation] Inflammation of the perididymis.

peridiverticulitis (pĕr″ĭ-dī″vĕr-tĭk″ū-lī′tĭs) [″ + L. *diverticulare,* to turn aside, + Gr. *itis,* inflammation] Inflammation of tissues situated around an intestinal diverticulum.

periductal (pĕr-ĭ-dŭk′tăl) [″ + L. *ductus,* a passage] Situated around a duct.

periduodenitis (pĕr″ĭ-dū″ō-dĕ-nī′tĭs) [″ + L. *duodeni,* twelve, + Gr. *itis,* inflammation] Inflammation around the duodenum, often causing adhesions attaching it to the peritoneum.

peridural (pĕr″ĭ-dū′răl) [″ + L. *durus,* hard] Outside the dura mater of the spinal cord.

periencephalitis (pĕr″ē-ĕn-sĕf″ă-lī′tĭs) [″ + *enkephalos,* brain, + *itis,* inflammation] Inflammation of the surface of the brain.

periencephalomeningitis (pĕr″ē-ĕn-sĕf″ă-lō-mĕn″ĭn-jī′tĭs) [″ + ″ + *meninx,* membrane, + *itis,* inflammation] Inflammation of the cerebral cortex and meninges.

periendothelioma (pĕr″ē-ĕn″dō-thē″lē-ō′mă) [″ + *endon,* within, + *thele,* nipple, + *oma,* tumor] A tumor arising from the endothelium of the lymphatics and the perithelium of blood vessels.

perienteric (pĕr″ē-ĕn-tĕr′ĭk) [Gr. *peri,* around, + *enteron,* intestine] Around the intestines.

perienteritis (pĕr″ē-ĕn″tĕr-ī′tĭs) [″ + ″ + *itis,* inflammation] Inflammation of the intestinal peritoneum.

perienteron (pĕr″ē-ĕn′tĕr-ŏn) [″ + *enteron,* intestine] The peritoneal cavity of the embryo.

periependymal (pĕr″ē-ĕp-ĕn′dĭ-măl) [″ + *ependyma,* an upper garment] Around the ependyma.

periesophagitis (pĕr″ē-ĕ-sŏf″ă-jī′tĭs) [″ + *oisophagos,* esophagus, + *itis,* inflammation] Inflammation of the tissues around the esophagus.

perifistular (pĕr-ĭ-fĭs′tū-lĕr) [″ + L. *fistula,* pipe] Located around a fistula.

perifocal (pĕr″ĭ-fō′kăl) [″ + L. *focus,* hearth] Around a focus, esp. around an infected focus.

perifollicular (pĕr″ĭ-fŏl-lĭk′ū-lăr) [″ + L. *folliculus,* a little sac] Around a follicle.

perifolliculitis (pĕr″ĭ-fō-lĭk″ū-lī′tĭs) [″ + ″ + Gr. *itis,* inflammation] Inflammation of an area around the hair follicles.

perigangliitis (pĕr″ĭ-găng″lē-ī′tĭs) [″ + *ganglion,* knot, + *itis,* inflammation] Inflammation of the region around a ganglion.

periganglionic (pĕr″ĭ-găng″glē-ŏn′ĭk) [″ + *ganglion,* knot] Around a ganglion.

perigastric (pĕr″ĭ-găs′trĭk) [″ + *gaster,* belly] Around the stomach.

perigastritis (pĕr″ĭ-găs-trī′tĭs) [″ + ″ + *itis,* inflammation] Inflammation of the peritoneal covering of the stomach.

perigemmal (pĕr″ĭ-jĕm′ăl) [″ + L. *gemma,* bud] Around any bud, esp. a taste bud.

periglandulitis (pĕr″ĭ-glăn″dū-lī′tĭs) [″ + L. *glandula,* small gland, + Gr. *itis,* inflammation] Inflammation of tissues around a gland.

periglottic (pĕr″ĭ-glŏt′ĭk) [″ + *glotta,* tongue] Around the base of the tongue and epiglottis.

perihepatic (pĕr″ĭ-hē-păt′ĭk) [Gr. *peri,* around, + *hepar,* liver] Around the liver.

perihepatitis (pĕr″ĭ-hĕp-ă-tī′tĭs) [″ + ″ + *itis,* inflammation] Inflammation of the peritoneal covering of the liver, usually occurring in circumscribed areas.

perihernial (pĕr″ĭ-hĕr′nē-ăl) [″ + L. *hernia,* rupture] Around a hernia.

perijejunitis (pĕr″ĭ-jē-jū-nī′tĭs) [″ + L. *jejunum,* empty, + Gr. *itis,* inflammation] Inflammation of tissues around the jejunum.

perikaryon (pĕr″ĭ-kăr′ē-ŏn) [″ + *karyon,* nucleus] The cell body of a neuron.

perikeratic (pĕr″ĭ-kĕr-ă′tĭk) [″ + *keras,* horn] About the cornea. SYN: *pericorneal.*

perikymata (pĕr″ĭ-kī′mă-tă) [″ + *kyma,* wave] The transverse wavelike grooves most apparent in the surface enamel of newly erupted anterior teeth; they are more pronounced at eruption and are reduced in depth with wear in advancing age.

perilabyrinthitis (pĕr″ĭ-lăb″ĭr-ĭn-thī′tĭs) [″ + *labyrinthos,* a maze of canals, + *itis,* inflammation] Inflammation of tissues around the labyrinth.

perilaryngeal (pĕr″ĭ-lă-rĭn′jē-ăl) [″ + *larynx,* larynx] Around the larynx.

perilaryngitis (pĕr″ĭ-lăr″ĭn-jī′tĭs) [″ + ″ + *itis,* inflammation] Inflammation of tissues around the larynx.

perilenticular (pĕr″ĭ-lĕn-tĭk′ū-lăr) [″ + L. *lenticularis,* pert. to a lens] Around the lens of the eye.

periligamentous (pĕr″ĭ-lĭg″ă-mĕn′tŭs) [″ + L. *ligamentum,* a band] Around a ligament.

perilymph, perilympha (pĕr′ĭ-lĭmf, pĕr″ĭ-lĭm′fă) [″ + L. *lympha,* serum] The pale, transparent fluid within the bony (not the membranous) labyrinth of the inner ear.

perilymphangeal (pĕr″ĭ-lĭm-făn′jē-ăl) [″ + ″ + Gr. *angeion,* vessel] Around a lymphatic vessel.

perilymphangitis (pĕr″ĭ-lĭmf-ăn-jī′tĭs) [″ + ″ + ″ + *itis,* inflammation] Inflammation of tissues around a lymphatic vessel.

perimastitis (pĕr″ĭ-măs-tī′tĭs) [″ + *mastos,* breast, + *itis,* inflammation] Inflammation of the fibrous tissue around a breast.

perimeningitis (pĕr″ĭ-mĕn″ĭn-jī′tĭs) [Gr. *peri,* around, + *meninx,* membrane, + *itis,* inflammation] Pachymeningitis.

perimenopause The phase prior to the onset of menopause, during which the woman with regular menses changes, perhaps abruptly, to a pattern of irregular cycles and increased periods of amenorrhea. For epidemiological investigations, the inception of perimenopause is characterized by 3 to 11 months of amenorrhea or, for those without amenorrhea, increased menstrual irregularity. While menopause has a clear and accepted definition, perimenopause does not.

perimeter (pĕr-ĭm′ĕ-tĕr) [″ + *metron,* measure] **1.** The outer edge or periphery of a body or measure of the same. **2.** A device for determining the extent of the field of vision. SEE: *perimetry.*

perimetric (pĕr″ĭ-mĕt′rĭk) [″ + *metron,* measure] Concerning perimetry.

perimetric (pĕr″ĭ-mĕt′rĭk) [″ + *metra,* uterus] Around the uterus.

perimetritic (pĕr″ĭ-mē-trĭt′ĭk) [″ + *metra,* uterus, + *itis,* inflammation] Concerning perimetritis.

perimetritis (pĕr″ĭ-mē-trī′tĭs) [″ + ″ + *itis,* inflammation] Inflammation of the peritoneal covering of the uterus; may be associated with parametritis.

perimetrium (pĕr-ĭ-mē′trē-ŭm) The serous layer of the uterus.

perimetry (pĕr-ĭm′ĕ-trē) [″ + *metron,* measure] **1.** Circumference; edge; border of a body. **2.** Measurement of the scope of the field of vision with a perimeter.

perimyelitis (pĕr″ĭ-mī″ĕ-lī′tĭs) [″ + ″ + *itis,* inflammation] **1.** Inflammation of the pia mater and arachnoid of the brain or spinal cord. SYN: *leptomeningitis.* **2.** Inflammation of the endosteum or membrane around medullary cavity of a bone.

perimyelography (pĕr″ĭ-mī″ĕ-lŏg′ră-fē) [″ + ″ + *graphein,* to write] Radiological examination of the area around the spinal cord.

perimyoendocarditis (pĕr″ĭ-mī″ō-ĕn″dō-kăr-dī′tĭs) [″ + *mys,* muscle, + *endon,* within, + *kardia,* heart, + *itis,* inflammation] Inflammation of the muscular wall of the heart, its endothelial lining, and the pericardium.

perimyositis (pĕr″ĭ-mī″ō-sī′tĭs) [″ + ″ + *itis,* inflammation] Inflammation of the connective tissue around a muscle.

perimysia (pĕr″ĭ-mĭs′ē-ă) Pl. of perimysium.

perimysial (pĕr-ĭ-mĭs′ē-ăl) Concerning, or of the nature of, the fibrous sheath of a muscle.

perimysiitis (pĕr″ĭ-mĭs″ē-ī′tĭs) [″ + *mys,* muscle, + *itis,* inflammation] Inflammation of the sheath surrounding a muscle.

perimysium (pĕr″ĭ-mĭs′ē-ŭm) *pl.* **perimysia** A connective tissue sheath that envelops each primary bundle of muscle fibers; sometimes called perimysium internum.

p. externum Epimysium.

perinatal (pĕr″ĭ-nā′tăl) [Gr. *peri,* around, + L. *natalis,* birth] Concerning the period beginning after the 28th week of pregnancy and ending 28 days after birth.

perinatology The study of the fetus and infant during the perinatal period. SEE: *perinatal.*

perineal (pĕr″ĭ-nē′ăl) [Gr. *perinaion,* perineum] Concerning, or situated on, the perineum.

perineo- [Gr. *perinaion*] Combining form meaning *perineum.*

perineocele (pĕr″ĭ-nē′ō-sēl) [Gr. *perinaion,* perineum, + *kele,* tumor, swelling] A hernia in the region of the perineum, between the rectum and vagina or between the rectum and prostate. SYN: *perineal hernia.*

perineocolporectomyomectomy (pĕr″ĭ-nē-ō-kŏl″pō-rĕk″tō-mī″ō-mĕk′tō-mē) [″ + *kolpos,* vagina, + L. *rectus,* straight, + Gr. *mys,* muscle, + *oma,* tumor, + *ektome,* excision] Excision of a myoma by incising the perineum, vagina, and rectum.

perineometer (pĕr″ĭ-nē-ŏm′ĕ-ter) [Gr. *perinaion,* perineum, + *metron,* measure] An apparatus for measuring the pressure or force that is produced in the vagina when the pubococcygeus and levator ani muscles are contracted voluntarily. SEE: *Kegel exercise.*

perineoplasty (pĕr″ĭ-nē′ō-plăs″tē) [″ + *plassein,* to form] Reparative surgery on the perineum.

perineorrhaphy (pĕr″ĭ-nē-or′ă-fē) [″ + *rhaphe,* a sewing] Suture of the perineum to repair a laceration that occurs or is made surgically during the delivery of the fetus.

Patient Care: Caregivers should implement universal precautions, wearing disposable gloves throughout perineal assessment, patient care, and disposal of biohazardous wastes, and performing thorough hand washing before and after procedures. Assessments focus on diet and fluid intake, bowel elimination, and the status of the suture line. To minimize potential for autoinfection, patient care and teaching should emphasize cleansing the perineum from front to rear after urination or defecation with a cascade of warm water, other ordered solution, or an antiseptic towelette. Perineal pads also should be applied from front to rear. Application of an ice pack immediately after delivery and intermittently during the first 24 hr postpartum aids in reducing edema and relieving discomfort. To maximize effects, the ice pack should be removed 20 minutes after its placement and reapplied 10 minutes later. The use of warm Sitz baths or a heat lamp for 20 minutes several times daily is encouraged. Personal portable Sitz baths avoid the possibility of cross-contamination and may be sent home with the mother. Ambulation also is encouraged. Gluteal splinting (i.e., tensing the buttocks while sitting or rising from a seated position) reduces discomfort. Health care professionals should provide support and reassurance because the patient may experience anxiety about the ability to resume normal physical functions and sexual activity and should provide opportunities for the patient to express feelings and to ask questions.

anterior p. Surgical repair of anterior perineum and vaginal wall to correct a cystocele.

posterior p. The removal and repair of a rectocele.

perineoscrotal (pĕr″ĭ-nē-ō-skrō′tăl) [″ + L. *scrotum,* a bag] Concerning the perineum and scrotum.

perineotomy (pĕr″ĭ-nē-ŏt′ō-mē) [″ + *tome,* incision] Surgical incision into the perineum. SYN: *perineal section.*

perineovaginal (pĕr″ĭ-nē″ō-văj′ĭn-ăl) [″ + L. *vagina,* sheath] Concerning the perineum and vagina.

perinephrial (pĕr″ĭ-nĕf′rē-ăl) Concerning the perinephrium.

perinephric (pĕr″ĭ-nĕf′rĭk) [Gr. *peri,* around, + *nephros,* kidney] Located or occurring around the kidney.

perinephritis (pĕr″ĭ-nĕ-frī′tĭs) [″ + ″ + *itis,* inflammation] Inflammation of peritoneal tissues around the kidney.

perinephrium (pĕr″ĭ-nĕf′rē-ŭm) The connective and fatty tissue surrounding the kidney.

perineum (pĕr″ĭ-nē′ŭm) [Gr. *perinaion*] **1.** The structures occupying the pelvic outlet and constituting the pelvic floor. **2.** The external region between the vulva and anus in a female or between the scrotum and anus in a male. It is made up of skin, muscle, and fasciae. The muscles of the perineum are the anterior portion of the intact levator ani muscle, the transverse perineal muscle, and the pubococcygeus muscle. SEE: illus.; *body, perineal.*

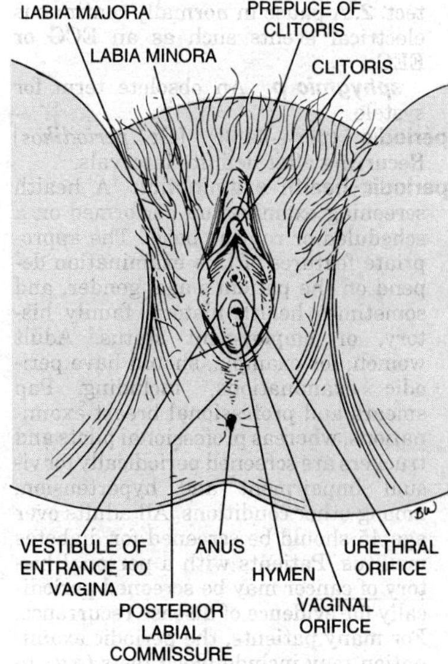

PERINEUM

tears of the p. Laceration of the perineum during delivery. There are four degrees of severity caused by overstretching of the vagina and perineum during delivery. Fetal malposition increases the chance of tears occurring.

A first-degree tear involves superficial tissues of the perineum and vaginal mucosa but does not injure muscular tissue. A second-degree tear involves those tissues included in a first-degree tear and the muscles of the perineum but not the muscles of the anal sphincter. A third-degree tear involves all of the tissues of the second-degree tear and the muscles of the anal sphincter. A fourth-degree tear extends completely through the perineal skin, vaginal mucosa, perineal body, anal sphincter muscles, and the rectal mucosa.

Complications include hemorrhage, infection, cystocele, rectocele, descent of uterus, and perhaps loss of bowel control. Surgery is necessary to treat this condition.

perineural (pĕr″ĭ-nū′răl) [Gr. *peri,* around, + *neuron,* nerve] Around a nerve.

perineurial (pĕr″ĭ-nū′rē-ăl) [″ + *neuron,* sinew] Concerning the perineurium, the sheath around a bundle of nerve fibers.

perineuritis (pĕr″ĭ-nū-rī′tĭs) [″ + ″ + *itis,* inflammation] Inflammation of the sheath enveloping nerve fibers.

perineurium (pĕr″ĭ-nū′rē-ŭm) [″ + *neuron,* sinew] A connective tissue sheath investing a fasciculus or bundle of nerve fibers.

perinuclear (pĕr″ĭ-nū′klē-ăr) [″ + L. *nucleus,* a kernel] Around a nucleus.

periocular (pĕr″ē-ŏk′ū-lăr) [″ + L. *oculus,* eye] Located around the eye. SYN: *circumocular.*

period [L. *periodus*] **1.** The interval between two successive occurrences of any regularly recurring phenomenon or event; a cycle. **2.** Colloquial expression for the menstrual flow. **3.** Time occupied by a disease in running its course, or by a stage of a disease, such as an incubation period.

absolute refractory p. Following contraction of a muscle fiber or transmission of a nerve impulse by a neuron, the period in which a stimulus, no matter how strong, will not elicit a response.

childbearing p. The period in the female during which she is capable of procreation; puberty to the menopause.

communicable p. In epidemiology and infectious diseases, the time during which an infectious agent is transmissible, directly or indirectly, from an infected person or animal to a susceptible person.

critical p. **1.** The phase of the life cycle during which cells are responsive to certain regulators. **2.** The first trimester of pregnancy when organ systems are being formed and the fetus is most vulnerable to environmental factors that may cause deformities.

effective refractory p. In electrocardiography, the interval during which a second action potential cannot occur in an excitable fiber unless the stimulus is much stronger than usual; the membrane is still in the repolarization phase of the previous action potential.

ejection p. Systole.

fertile p. The time during the menstrual cycle when the ovum can be fertilized.

gestation p. The period of pregnancy from conception to parturition. Average length is 10 lunar months or 280 days, measured from the onset of the last menstrual period, but length varies from 250 to 310 days. SEE: *gestation; pregnancy* for table.

incubation p. The time from the moment of infection to the appearance of the first symptom.

isoelectric p. **1.** In an occurrence that normally produces an electric force, such as a muscle contraction, the time or point when no electric energy is produced. **2.** In an electrocardiogram, the period when the electrical tracing is neither positive nor negative.

isometric p. Postsphygmic p.

last menstrual p. ABBR: LMP. The date of the first day of menstruation before the presenting illness or the advent of pregnancy-related amenorrhea; used in estimating the expected date of delivery. SEE: *Naegele's rule.*

latency p. The time from the stimulus to the response of the tissue stimulated.

latent p. **1.** The time between stimulation and the resulting response. SYN: *lag phase.* **2.** The time during which a disease is supposed to be existent without manifesting itself; period of incubation. **3.** The time from exposure to ionizing radiation to the first visible sign of the effects.

menstrual p. Menstruation.

missed p. Menstruation not occurring at the time it was expected.

monthly p. The time of menstrual flow.

neonatal p. The first 30 days of infant life.

patent p. The time in a parasitic disease during which organisms are demonstrable in the body.

postsphygmic p. The short period in diastole when the ventricles are relaxed and no blood is entering. This lasts until the atrioventricular valves open. SYN: *isometric p.*

presphygmic p. The short period in systole beginning with closing of the atrioventricular valves and ending with opening of the valves connecting the right and left ventricles to the pulmonary artery and aorta, respectively.

puerperal p. The interval of time from the birth of a child to approx. 6 weeks later, at which time complete involution of the uterus has occurred.

p. of reactivity In obstetrics, an initial episode of activity, alertness, and responsiveness to interaction, characteristic of newborn physiological and social response to stimuli. The first period of reactivity begins with birth, lasts approx. 30 min, and ends when the infant falls into a deep sleep. Common assessment findings include transient tachypnea, nasal flaring, sternal retraction, crackles, tachycardia, and irregular heart rhythms. The second period of reactivity begins when the infant awakens and usually lasts 4 to 6 hr. Common assessment findings include signs of excessive respiratory and gastric mucus, hunger, apneic episodes, and the passing of a meconium stool.

relative refractory p. The period after activation of a nerve or muscle, during recovery, when it can be excited only by a stronger-than-normal stimulus.

safe p. The time during the menstrual cycle when conception is allegedly not possible. Because of the great variability of the menstrual cycle, it is either extremely difficult or impossible to predict the portion of the cycle in which intercourse may take place and be "safe" from conception.

silent p. **1.** The time in the course of a disease in which the signs and symptoms are so mild as to be difficult to detect. **2.** A pause in normally continuous electrical events such as an ECG or EEG.

sphygmic p. An obsolete term for systole.

periodic (pēr-ē-ŏd′ĭk) [Gr. *periodikos*] Recurring after definite intervals.

periodic health examination A health screening examination performed on a scheduled or routine basis. The appropriate features of this examination depend on the patient's age, gender, and sometimes health history, family history, or employment status. Adult women, for example, should have periodic examinations, including Pap smears and professional breast examinations, whereas professional pilots and truckers are screened periodically for visual impairment and hypertension, among other conditions. All adults over age 45 should be screened for diabetes mellitus. Patients with a personal history of cancer may be screened periodically for evidence of disease recurrence. For many patients, the periodic examination may include blood tests (e.g., to check levels of cholesterol and other lipids), immunological tests (e.g., health care workers are periodically screened for tuberculosis), or invasive examinations (e.g., sigmoidoscopy or colonoscopy to look for colon cancer). SEE: *mammography; Papanicolaou test;* table under *cancer screening.*

periodicity (pēr″ē-ō-dĭs′ĭ-tē) **1.** The state of being regularly recurrent. **2.** The rate of rise and fall or interruption of a unidirectional current in physical therapy.

periodic leg movements Leg movements, originally called nocturnal myoclonus, that consist of repetitive movements occurring every 20 to 40 sec during sleep. Movements usually include extension of the great toe, sometimes followed by flexion of the hip, knee, or ankle. These movements may not be apparent to the patient, yet they are associated with a variety of sleep disturbances. They are not the same as the gross jerks that occur in some normal patients at the time they are falling asleep. Many patients with the restless legs syndrome also have periodic leg movements.

periodic table A chart with the chemical elements arranged by their atomic numbers, that is, by their number of protons, and by the number of electrons in their outermost orbitals. SEE: *law, periodic*.

periodontal (pĕr″ē-ō-dŏn′tăl) [Gr. *peri,* around, + *odous,* tooth] Located around a tooth. SYN: *peridental*.

p. disease A disease of the supporting structures of the teeth, the periodontium, including alveolar bone to which the teeth are anchored. The most common initial symptom is bleeding gums, but loosening of the teeth, receding gums, abscesses in pockets between the gums and the teeth, and necrotizing ulcerative gingivitis may be present as the disease process worsens. Proper dental hygiene, including proper brushing of the teeth, use of dental floss, and periodic removal of plaque by a dentist or dental hygienist, will help to prevent periodontal disease.

TREATMENT: In the early stages of the disease, curettage of the irritating material—plaque and calculus (tartar)—from the crown and root surfaces of the teeth may be the only treatment required. In more advanced stages, procedures such as gingivectomy, gingivoplasty, and correction of the bony architecture of the teeth may be required. Adjustment of the occlusion of the teeth and orthodontic treatment may be used in order to help prevent recurrences. SEE: *plaque; teeth; tooth; toothbrushing*.

PATIENT CARE: Dental professionals teach the patient about the importance of proper dental care, including brushing for two minutes twice a day, flossing, and regular dental examinations and prophylaxis. Patients should consult a dentist if recession of teeth from gums, any drainage from gums, or bleeding gums occur, because these symptoms may indicate periodontal disease.

periodontia (pĕr″ē-ō-dŏn′shē-ă) [Gr. *peri,* around, + *odous,* tooth] **1.** Plural of periodontium. **2.** Periodontics.

periodontics (pĕr″ē-ō-dŏn′tĭks) [″ + *odous,* tooth] The branch of dentistry dealing with treatment of diseases of the tissues around the teeth. SYN: *periodontia* (2); *periodontology*.

periodontitis (pĕr″ē-ō-dŏn-tī′tĭs) [″ + ″ + *itis,* inflammation] Inflammation or degeneration, or both, of the dental periosteum, alveolar bone, cementum, and adjacent gingiva. Suppuration usually occurs, supporting bone is resorbed, teeth become loose, and recession of gingivae occurs. This condition usually follows chronic gingivitis, Vincent's infection, or poor dental hygiene. Systemic factors may predispose one to this condition. SYN: *Riggs' disease*.

apical p. Periodontitis of the periapical region usually leading to formation of periapical abscess.

periodontium (pĕr-ē-ō-dŏn′shē-ŭm) The structures that support the teeth, cushion the shock of chewing, and keep the teeth firmly anchored in the bone. These structures are the gingivae, periodontal membrane or ligament, cementum, and alveolar bone.

periodontoclasia (pĕr″ē-ō-dŏn″tō-klā′zē-ă) [″ + *odous,* tooth, + *klasis,* breaking] A condition characterized by inflammation accompanied by degenerative and retrogressive changes in the periodontium. SYN: *peridentitis*.

periodontology (pĕr″ē-ō-dŏn-tŏl′ō-jē) [″ + ″ + *logos,* word, reason] Periodontics.

periodontosis (pĕr″ē-ō-dŏn-tō′sĭs) [″ + ″ + *osis,* condition] Any degenerative disease of the periodontal tissues.

periodoscope (pĕr″ē-ŏd′ō-skōp) [LL. *periodus,* interval of time, + *skopein,* to examine] A table or dial for the calculation of the expected date of delivery. SEE: *pregnancy* for table.

periomphalic (pĕr″ē-ŏm-făl′ĭk) [Gr. *peri,* around, + *omphalos,* navel] Located around or near the umbilicus.

perionychia (pĕr″ē-ō-nĭk′ē-ă) [″ + *onyx,* nail] Inflammation around a nail.

perionychium (pĕr″ē-ō-nĭk′ē-ŭm) The epidermis surrounding a nail.

perionyx (pĕr″ē-ō′nĭks) [″ + *onyx,* nail] The remnant of the eponychium that persists as a band across the root of the nail.

perionyxis (pĕr″ē-ō-nĭk′sĭs) Inflammation of the epidermis surrounding a nail.

perioophoritis (pĕr″ē-ō-ŏf″ō-rī′tĭs) [″ + *oophoron,* ovary, + *itis,* inflammation] Inflammation of the surface membrane of the ovary. SYN: *perioothecitis; periovaritis*.

perioophorosalpingitis (pĕr″ē-ō-ŏf″ō-rō-săl″pĭn-jī′tĭs) [″ + ″ + *salpinx,* tube, + *itis,* inflammation] Inflammation of the tissues around an ovary and oviduct. SYN: *perioothecosalpingitis; perisalpingoovaritis*.

perioothecitis (pĕr″ē-ō″ō-thē-sī′tĭs) [″ + *oon,* egg, + *theke,* box, + *itis,* inflammation] Perioophoritis.

perioothecosalpingitis (pĕr″ē-ō″ō-thē″kō-săl-pĭn-jī′tĭs) [″ + ″ + ″ + *salpinx,* tube, + *itis,* inflammation] Perioophorosalpingitis.

perioperative Occurring in the period immediately before, during, and/or after surgery.

perioperative positioning injury, risk for A state in which the client is at risk for injury as a result of the environmental conditions found in the perioperative setting. SEE: *Nursing Diagnoses Appendix.*

periophthalmic (pĕr″ē-ŏf-thăl′mĭk) [″ + *ophthalmos,* eye] Around the eye.

perioral (pĕr″ē-or′ăl) [″ + L. *oralis,* mouth] Surrounding the mouth. SYN: *circumoral.*

periorbita (pĕr″ē-or′bĭ-tă) [″ + L. *orbita,* orbit] Connective tissue lining the socket of the eye.

periorbital (pĕr″ē-or′bĭ-tăl) Surrounding the socket of the eye. SYN: *circumorbital.*

periportal tracking In the evaluation of patients with abdominal injuries, the finding of decreased computerized tomographic attenuation around the portal region of the liver. This should be presumed to represent bleeding, and may require operative intervention.

periorbititis (pĕr″ē-or″bĭ-tī′tĭs) [″ + L. *orbita,* orbit, + Gr. *itis,* inflammation] Inflammation of the periorbita.

periorchitis (pĕr″ē-or-kī′tĭs) [″ + *orchis,* testicle, + *itis,* inflammation] Inflammation of the tissues investing a testicle.

p. hemorrhagica A chronic hematocele of the tunica vaginalis of the testis.

periosteal (pĕr-ē-ŏs′tē-ăl) [″ + *osteon,* bone] Concerning the periosteum. SYN: *periosteous.*

periosteitis (pĕr″ē-ŏs″tē-ī′tĭs) [″ + ″ + *itis,* inflammation] Periostitis.

periosteoedema (pĕr″ē-ŏs″tē-ō-ĕ-dē′mă) [Gr. *peri,* around, + *osteon,* bone, + *oidema,* swelling] Edema of the periosteum, the membrane surrounding a bone.

periosteoma (pĕr″ē-ŏs-tē-ō′mă) [″ + ″ + *oma,* tumor] **1.** An abnormal growth surrounding a bone. **2.** A tumor of the periosteum, the tissue surrounding a bone.

periosteomyelitis (pĕr″ē-ŏs″tē-ō-mī″ĕ-lī′tĭs) [″ + ″, + *myelos,* marrow, + *itis,* inflammation] Inflammation of bone, including the periosteum and marrow. SYN: *periostomedullitis.*

periosteophyte (pĕr″ē-ŏs′tē-ō-fīt) [″ + *osteon,* bone, + *phyton,* growth] An abnormal bony growth on the periosteum, or arising from it.

periosteorrhaphy (pĕr″ē-ŏs″tē-or′ă-fē) [″ + ″ + *rhaphe,* seam, ridge] Joining by suture the margins of a severed periosteum.

periosteotome (pĕr″ē-ŏs′tē-ō-tōm) [″ + *osteon,* bone, + *tome,* incision] An instrument for cutting the periosteum or removing it from the bone.

periosteotomy (pĕr″ē-ŏs-tē-ŏt′ō-mē) Incision into the periosteum.

periosteous (pĕr″ē-ŏs′tē-ŭs) [″ + *osteon,* bone] Periosteal.

periosteum (pĕr-ē-ŏs′tē-ŭm) [Gr. *periosteon*] The fibrous membrane that forms the covering of bones except at their articular surfaces; consists of a dense external layer containing numerous blood vessels and an inner layer of connective tissue cells that function as osteoblasts when the bone is injured and then participate in new bone formation. Periosteum serves as a supporting structure for blood vessels nourishing bone and for attachment of tendons and ligaments.

alveolar p. Periodontal ligament.

p. externum Periosteum covering external surfaces of bones.

p. internum Interior periosteum lining the marrow canal of a bone.

periostitis (pĕr″ē-ŏs-tī′tĭs) [″ + *itis,* inflammation] Inflammation of the periosteum, the membrane covering a bone. Findings include pain over the affected part, esp. under pressure; fever; sweats; leukocytosis; skin inflammation, and rigidity of overlying muscles. Infectious diseases, esp. syphilis, and trauma cause this condition. SYN: *periosteitis.*

albuminous p. Periostitis with albuminous serous fluid exudate beneath the membrane affected.

alveolar p. Periodontitis.

diffuse p. Periostitis of the long bones.

hemorrhagic p. Periostitis with extravasation of blood under the periosteum.

periostoma (pĕr″ē-ŏs-tō′mă) [Gr. *peri,* around, + *osteon,* bone, + *oma,* tumor] A bony neoplasm around a bone or arising from its membranous sheath.

periostomedullitis (pĕr″ē-ŏs″tō-mĕd-ū-lī′tĭs) [″ + ″ + L. *medulla,* marrow, + Gr. *itis,* inflammation] Periosteomyelitis.

periostosis (pĕr″ē-ŏs-tō′sĭs) [″ + ″ + *osis,* condition] A bony neoplasm around a bone or arising from it.

periostosteitis (pĕr″ē-ŏs-tŏs″tē-ī′tĭs) [″ + ″ + *osteon,* bone, + *itis,* inflammation] Osteoperiostitis.

periostotome (pĕr″ē-ŏs′tō-tōm) [″ + ″ + *tome,* incision] Periosteotome.

periostotomy (pĕr″ē-ŏs-tŏt′ō-mē) [″ + ″ + *tome,* incision] Periosteotomy.

periotic (pĕr-ē-ō′tĭk) [″ + *ous,* ear] Situated around the ear, esp. the internal ear.

p. bone The mastoid and petrous portions of the temporal bone.

periovaritis (pĕr″ē-ō″vă-rī′tĭs) [″ + L. *ovarium,* ovary, + Gr. *itis,* inflammation] Perioophoritis.

periovular (pĕr″ē-ō′vū-lăr) [″ + L. *ovulum,* little egg] Around an ovum.

peripachymeningitis (pĕr″ĭ-pak″ē-mĕn″ĭn-jī′tĭs) [″ + *pachys,* thick, + *meninx,* membrane, + *itis,* inflammation] Inflammation of the connective tissue between the dura mater and the bone that encloses the central nervous system.

peripancreatitis (pĕr″ĭ-păn″krē-ă-tī′tĭs)

[″ + *pankreas,* pancreas, + *itis,* inflammation] Inflammation of the tissues around the pancreas.

peripapillary (pĕr″ĭ-păp′ĭ-lĕr″ē) [″ + L. *papilla,* nipple] Around a papilla.

peripatetic (pĕr″ĭ-pă-tĕt′ĭk) [L. *peripateticus,* to walk about while teaching] Moving from place to place.

peripenial (pĕr″ĭ-pē′nē-ăl) [Gr. *peri,* around, + L. *penis,* penis] Around the penis.

periphacitis (pĕr-ĭ-fă-sī′tĭs) [″ + *phakos,* lens, + *itis,* inflammation] Inflammation of the capsule of the lens of the eye.

periphakus (pĕr″ĭ-fā′kŭs) The elastic capsule surrounding the lens of the eye.

peripharyngeal (pĕr″ĭ-fă-rĭn′jē-ăl) [″ + *pharynx,* throat] Around the pharynx.

peripherad (pĕr-ĭf′ĕr-ăd) [″ + *pherein,* to bear, + L. *ad,* to] In the direction of the periphery.

peripheral (pĕr-ĭf′ĕr-ăl) Located at, or pert. to, the periphery; occurring away from the center.

peripheral nervous system ABBR: PNS. The portion of the nervous system outside the central nervous system: the 12 pairs of cranial nerves and 31 pairs of spinal nerves. These nerves contain sensory and somatic motor fibers and the motor fibers of the autonomic nervous system.

peripheral neurovascular dysfunction, risk for A state for which an individual is at risk of experiencing a disruption in circulation, sensation, or motion of an extremity. SEE: *Nursing Diagnoses Appendix.*

peripheral vascular disease ABBR: PVD. Any condition that causes partial or complete obstruction of the flow of blood to or from the arteries or veins outside the chest. Peripheral vascular disease includes atherosclerosis of the carotid, aortoiliac, femoral, and axillary arteries, as well as deep venous thromboses of the limbs, pelvis, and vena cava. SEE: *atherosclerosis; claudication; deep venous thrombosis; Nursing Diagnoses Appendix.*

peripheraphose (pĕr-ĭf′ĕr-ă-fōs) A subjective sensation of darkness or shadow that originates in the peripheral optic structures (optic nerve or eyeball).

peripherocentral (pĕ-rĭf″ĕr-ō-sĕn′trăl) [″ + *pherein,* to bear, + *kentron,* center] Concerning both the periphery and central part of an organ.

peripherophose (per-ĭf′ĕr-ō-fōs) A subjective sensation of light or color that originates in the peripheral optic structures (optic nerve or eyeball).

periphery (pĕr-ĭf′ĕ-rē) [Gr. *periphereia*] The outer part or surface of a body; the part away from the center.

periphlebitis (pĕr″ĭ-flĕ-bī′tĭs) [Gr. *peri,* around, + *phleps,* vein, + *itis,* inflammation] Inflammation of the external coat of a vein or tissues around it.

periphoria (pĕr-ĭ-fō′rē-ă) [″ + *phoros,* bearing] The tendency of the axis of the eye to deviate from the normal owing to weakness of oblique muscles. SYN: *cyclophoria.*

periphrastic (pĕr″ĭ-frăs′tĭk) [Gr. *periphrastikos*] Relating to the use of superfluous words in expressing a thought, which appears in the writings and speech of some schizophrenics.

periphrenitis (pĕr″ĭ-frē-nī′tĭs) [Gr. *peri,* around, + *phren,* diaphragm, + *itis,* inflammation] Inflammation of the structures around the diaphragm.

Periplaneta (pĕr″ĭ-plă-nē′tă) A genus of cockroaches belonging to the order Orthoptera. Roaches contaminate food by mechanically transporting disease-producing bacteria, ova, and protozoa to the food.

P. americana The American cockroach.

P. australasiae The Australian cockroach.

periplast (pĕr′ĭ-plăst) [″ + *plassein,* to form] The peripheral protoplasm of a cell exclusive of the nucleus.

peripleural (pĕr″ĭ-plū′răl) [″ + *pleura,* rib] Encircling the pleura.

peripleuritis (pĕr-ĭ-plū-rī′tĭs) [″ + ″ + *itis,* inflammation] Inflammation of the connective tissues between the pleura and wall of the chest.

peripolar (pĕr″ĭ-pō′lăr) [″ + L. *polus,* pole] Around a pole.

peripolesis (pĕr″ĭ-pō-lē′sĭs) [Gr., a going about] In tissue culture, the collecting of lymphocytes around macrophages.

periporitis (pĕr″ĭ-por-ī′tĭs) [Gr. *peri,* around, + L. *porus,* pore, + Gr. *itis*] Multiple abscesses around sweat glands, esp. as a complication of malaria in children.

periportal (pĕr″ĭ-por′tăl) [″ + L. *porta,* gate] Around the portal vein and its branches.

periproctic (pĕr″ĭ-prŏk′tĭk) [″ + *proktos,* anus] Around the anus.

periproctitis (pĕr″ĭ-prŏk-tī′tĭs) [″ + ″ + *itis,* inflammation] Inflammation of the areolar tissues in the region of the rectum and anus. SYN: *perirectitis.*

periprostatic (pĕr″ĭ-prŏs-tăt′ĭk) [″ + *prostates,* prostate] Surrounding or occurring about the prostate.

periprostatitis (pĕr″ĭ-prŏs-tă-tī′tĭs) [″ + ″ + *itis,* inflammation] Inflammation of the tissues surrounding the prostate.

peripylephlebitis (pĕr″ĭ-pī″lē-flĕ-bī′tĭs) [″ + *pyle,* gate, + *phlebos,* vein, + *itis,* inflammation] Inflammation of tissues about the portal vein.

peripyloric (pĕr″ĭ-pī-lor′ĭk) [″ + *pyloros,* pylorus] Extending around the pylorus.

periradicular Around a root or a rootlike process, esp. relating to a tooth.

perirectal (pĕr″ĭ-rĕk′tăl) [″ + L. *rectus,* straight] Extending around the rectum.

perirectitis (pĕr″ĭ-rĕk-tī′tĭs) [″ + ″ + Gr. *itis,* inflammation] Periproctitis.

perirenal (pĕr″ĭ-rē′năl) [″ + L. *ren,* kidney] Extending around the kidney. SYN: *circumrenal; perinephric.*

perirhinal (pĕr″ĭ-rī′năl) [″ + *rhis,* nose] Located about the nose or nasal fossae.

perirhizoclasia (pĕr″ĭ-rī″zō-klā′zē-ă) [″ + *rhiza,* root, + *klasis,* destruction] Inflammation and destruction of tissues extending around the roots of a tooth.

perisalpingitis (pĕr″ĭ-săl″pĭn-jī′tĭs) [″ + *salpinx,* tube, + *itis,* inflammation] Inflammation of the peritoneum on the surface of the fallopian tube, usually as a result of a sexually transmitted infection or endometriosis.

perisalpingoovaritis (pĕr″ĭ-săl-pĭn″gō-ō″văr-ī′tĭs) [″ + ″ + L. *ovarium,* ovary, + Gr. *itis,* inflammation] Perioophorosalpingitis.

perisalpinx (pĕr″ĭ-săl′pĭnks) [″ + *salpinx,* tube] The peritoneum covering the upper borders of the uterine tubes.

perisclerium (pĕr″ĭ-sklē′rē-ŭm) [″ + *skleros,* hard] Fibrous tissue encircling ossifying cartilage.

periscopic (pĕr″ĭ-skŏp′ĭk) [″ + *skopein,* to examine] Viewing on all sides; providing a wide range of vision.

perisigmoiditis (pĕr″ĭ-sĭg″moy-dī′tĭs) [Gr. *peri,* around, + *sigma,* Gr. letter S, + *eidos,* form, shape, + *itis,* inflammation] Inflammation of peritoneal tissues around the sigmoid colon.

perisinuous Adjacent to or around a sinus.

perisinusitis (pĕr″ĭ-sī″nŭ-sī′tĭs) [″ + L. *sinus,* cavity, + Gr. *itis,* inflammation] Inflammation of membranes about a sinus, esp. a venous sinus of the dura mater.

perispermatitis (pĕr″ĭ-spĕr″mă-tī′tĭs) [″ + *sperma,* seed, + *itis,* inflammation] Inflammation of tissues about the spermatic cord.

p. serosa Hydrocele of the spermatic cord.

perisplanchnic (pĕr″ĭ-splănk′nĭk) [″ + *splanchnon,* viscus] Extending around a viscus or the viscera.

perisplanchnitis (pĕr″ĭ-splănk-nī′tĭs) [″ + ″ + *itis,* inflammation] Perivisceritis.

perisplenic (pĕr″ĭ-splĕn′ĭk) [″ + *splen,* spleen] Near or around the spleen.

perisplenitis (pĕr″ĭ-splē-nī′tĭs) [″ + ″ + *itis,* inflammation] Inflammation of the peritoneal coat of the spleen, the splenic capsule.

p. cartilaginea Inflammation of the capsule of the spleen resulting in thickening and hardening.

perispondylic (pĕr″ĭ-spŏn-dĭl′ĭk) [Gr. *peri,* around, + *spondylos,* vertebra] Around a vertebra.

perispondylitis (pĕr″ĭ-spŏn-dĭl-ī′tĭs) [″ + ″ + *itis,* inflammation] Inflammation of the parts around a vertebra.

perissodactylous (pĕr-ĭs″sō-dăk′tĭ-lŭs) [Gr. *perissos,* odd, + *daktylos,* digit] Having an odd number of digits on a hand or foot. SYN: *imparidigitate.*

peristalsis (pĕr-ĭ-stăl′sĭs) [Gr. *peri,* around, + *stalsis,* contraction] A progressive wavelike movement that occurs involuntarily in hollow tubes of the body, esp. the alimentary canal. It is characteristic of tubes possessing longitudinal and circular layers of smooth muscle fibers.

Peristalsis is induced reflexly by distention of the walls of the tube. The wave consists of contraction of the circular muscle above the distention with relaxation of the region immediately distal to the distended portion. The simultaneous contraction and relaxation progresses slowly for a short distance as a wave that causes the contents of the tube to be forced onward.

mass p. Forceful peristaltic movements of short duration in which contents are moved from one section of the colon to another, occurring three or four times daily.

reverse p. Peristalsis in a direction opposite to the normal direction. SYN: *antiperistalsis.*

peristaltic (pĕr″ĭ-stăl′tĭk) Concerning, or of the nature of, peristalsis.

peristaphyline (pĕr″ĭ-stăf′ĭ-lĭn) [″ + *staphyle,* uvula] About the uvula.

peristasis (pĕr-rĭs′tă-sĭs) [″ + *stasis,* standing] **1.** In the early stage of inflammation, the decrease in blood flow in the affected area. **2.** Environment.

peristomatous (pĕr″ĭ-stŏm′ă-tŭs) [″ + *stoma,* mouth] Around the mouth.

peristome (pĕr′ĭ-stōm) [″ + *stoma,* mouth] The channel leading to the cytosome or mouth in certain types of protozoa.

peristrumitis (pĕr″ĭ-stroo-mī′tĭs) [″ + L. *struma,* goiter, + *itis,* inflammation] Perithyroiditis.

peristrumous (pĕr″ĭ-stroo′mŭs) [″ + L. *struma,* goiter] Around a goiter.

perisynovial (pĕr″ĭ-sĭ-nō′vē-ăl) [Gr. *peri,* around, + L. *synovia,* joint fluid] Extending around a synovial structure.

perisystole (pĕr″ĭ-sĭs′tō-lē) [″ + *systole,* contraction] Presystole.

peritectomy (pĕr″ĭ-tĕk′tō-mē) [″ + *ektome,* excision] Surgical removal of a ring of conjunctiva around the cornea.

peritendineum (pĕr″ĭ-tĕn-dĭn′ē-ŭm) [″ + L. *tendo,* tendon] A sheath of fibrous connective tissue investing a fiber bundle of a tendon.

peritendinitis, peritenonitis (pĕr″ĭ-tĕn″dĭ-nī′tĭs, -tĕn″ō-nī′tĭs) [″ + ″ + Gr. *itis,* inflammation] Tenosynovitis.

p. calcarea Calcific tendinitis.

p. serosa Peritendinitis with effusion into the sheath.

peritenon (pĕr″ĭ-tē′nŏn) [″ + *tenon,* tendon] **1.** The sheath of a tendon. **2.** Peritendineum.

perithelioma (pĕr″ĭ-thē-lē-ō′mă) [″ + *thele,* nipple, + *oma,* tumor] A tumor derived from the perithelial layer of the blood vessels.

perithelium (pĕr″ĭ-thē′lē-ŭm) The fibrous outer layer of the smaller blood vessels.

Eberth's p. An incomplete layer of cells covering capillaries.

perithoracic (pĕr″ĭ-thō-răs′ĭk) [″ + *thorax,* chest] Around the thorax.

perithyroiditis (pĕr″ĭ-thī-roy-dī′tĭs) [″ + *thyreos,* shield, + *eidos,* form, shape, + *itis,* inflammation] Inflammation of capsule or tissues sheathing the thyroid gland. SYN: *peristrumitis.*

peritomy (pĕr-ĭt′ō-mē) [″ + *tome,* incision] **1.** Excision of a narrow strip of conjunctiva around the cornea in the treatment of pannus. SYN: *syndectomy.* **2.** Circumcision.

peritoneal (pĕr″ĭ-tō-nē′ăl) [Gr. *peritonaion,* peritoneum] Concerning the peritoneum.

p. fluid The clear straw-colored serous fluid secreted by the cells of the peritoneum. The few milliliters present in the peritoneal cavity moisten the surfaces of the two peritoneal layers and allow them to glide over each other as the intestinal tract changes shape during the process of digestion and absorption. In certain disease states (such as right-sided heart failure, cirrhosis, or ovarian malignancy) the amount of peritoneal fluid is increased. SEE: illus.; *ascites.*

peritonealize During abdominal surgery, to cover a tissue with peritoneum.

peritoneo- Combining form meaning *peritoneum.*

peritoneocentesis (pĕr″ĭ-tō″nē-ō-sĕn-tē′sĭs) [Gr. *peritonaion,* peritoneum, + *kentesis,* puncture] Piercing of the peritoneal cavity to obtain fluid. SEE: *paracentesis.*

peritoneoclysis (pĕr″ĭ-tō″nē-ō-klī′sĭs) [″ + *klysis,* a washing out] Introduction of fluid into the peritoneal cavity.

peritoneopericardial (pĕr″ĭ-tō-nē″ō-pĕr″ĭ-kăr′dē-ăl) [″ + *peri,* around, + *kardia,* heart] Concerning the peritoneum and pericardium.

peritoneopexy (pĕr″ĭ-tō′nē-ō-pĕks″ē) [Gr. *peritonaion,* peritoneum, + *pexis,* fixation] Fixation of the uterus via the vagina.

peritoneoplasty (per″ĭ-tō′nē-ō-plăs″tē) [″ + *plassein,* to form] Surgery to repair separated or denuded segments of the peritoneum.

peritoneoscope (pĕr″ĭ-tō′nē-ō-skōp″) [Gr. *peritonaion,* peritoneum, + *skopein,* to examine] A long, slender periscope or telescope device with a light at one end and an eyepiece at the other; used to inspect the peritoneal and abdominal cavities through a small incision in the abdominal wall. SYN: *laparoscope.*

peritoneoscopy (pĕr″ĭ-tō″nē-ŏs′kō-pē) Examination of the peritoneal cavity with a laparoscope.

peritoneotomy (pĕr″ĭ-tō″nē-ŏt′ō-mē) The process of incising the peritoneum.

peritoneum (pĕr″ĭ-tō-nē′ŭm) [LL., Gr. *peritonaion*] The serous membrane lining the abdominal cavity and reflected over the viscera.

EXAMINATION: Diseases that affect the peritoneum can be assessed with gentle and careful percussion and palpation of the abdomen. Localized or diffuse pertitonitis, for example, may be evident when the abdomen is tapped with a percussing finger (the patient will wince, guard the abdomen, and complain that the percussion is very painful); it may also be evident when the abdominal wall is gently depressed and then released (release of the examining hand causes guarding and discomfort). Fluid within the peritoneum (ascites) may be suggested by shifting dullness on percussion of the abdominal wall, or by the detection of a fluid wave when one hand depresses and releases on one side of the abdomen, while the other hand gently holds the opposite side.

parietal p. Peritoneum lining the abdominal walls and the undersurface of the diaphragm.

visceral p. Peritoneum that invests the abdominal organs. The peritoneum holds the viscera in place by its folds, which are called the *mesentery.*

peritonism (pĕr′ĭ-tō-nĭzm) [Gr. *peritonaion,* peritoneum, + *-ismos,* condi-

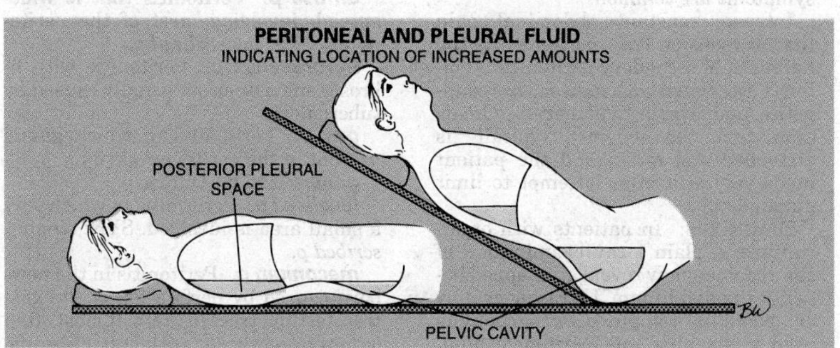

tion] **1.** A condition having the clinical signs of shock and peritonitis. **2.** Symptoms similar to peritonitis, but without actual inflammatory process, due instead to functional disease.

peritonitic (pĕr″ĭ-tō-nĭt′ĭk) [″ + *itis,* inflammation] Affected with or concerning peritonitis.

peritonitis (pĕr″ĭ-tō-nī′tĭs) [″ + *itis,* inflammation] Inflammation of the serous membrane that lines the abdominal cavity and its viscera.

ETIOLOGY: Peritonitis is caused by infection of the abdominal cavity without obvious organ rupture (primary peritonitis); by perforation (rupture) of one of the internal organs (secondary peritonitis); or by instillation of an irritating chemical into the abdominal cavity (chemical peritonitis).

Primary peritonitis occurs in patients with cirrhosis and ascites, in some patients with tuberculosis (esp. those with AIDS), and in patients who use the peritoneum for dialysis. Cirrhotic patients develop peritonitis due to infection of the peritoneal contents by microorganisms such as *Streptococcus pneumoniae,* enterococci, or *Escherichia coli.* Patients who use the peritoneum for dialysis (chronic ambulatory peritoneal dialysis patients) sometimes contaminate their dialysate with microbes such as staphylococci or streptococci, carried on their hands. Dialysis patients also may develop peritonitis after the infusion of irritating substances, such as antibiotics like vancomycin, into the peritoneal cavity during treatment for these infections.

Common causes of secondary peritonitis are ruptured appendix, perforated ulcer, abdominal trauma, and Crohn's disease. The air, acids, fecal material, and bacteria in the ruptured organs spill into and inflame the peritoneum.

SYMPTOMS: Primary peritonitis is marked by moderate or mild abdominal pain, fever, change in bowel habits, and malaise. Dialysis patients may notice clouding of their discharged dialysate. In tuberculous peritonitis, fever, weight loss, inanition, and other systemic symptoms are common.

Intense, constant abdominal pain that worsens on body movement is the hallmark of secondary peritonitis. It often is associated with nausea, loss of appetite, and fever or hypothermia. On examination, the abdomen typically is distended and quiet, and the patient holds very still in an attempt to limit discomfort.

DIAGNOSIS: In patients with organ rupture, a plain x-ray examination of the abdomen may reveal air trapped beneath the diaphragm. Ultrasonography or abdominal computed tomography is used to visualize intraperitoneal fluid, abscesses, and diseased organs. Paracentesis (needle aspiration through the abdominal wall) or peritoneal lavage also is helpful in diagnosis of some cases.

TREATMENT: Primary peritonitis may respond to the administration of antibiotics or antitubercular drugs, but the prognosis is guarded. As many as 50% of affected patients may die of sepsis. Secondary peritonitis is treated with surgical drainage, and repair or removal of the ruptured viscus; fluid resuscitation; and antibiotics. The prognosis depends on the patient's underlying condition, the rapidity of the diagnosis and of subsequent medical intervention, the skill of the surgeon, and other factors.

acute diffuse p. Generalized peritonitis.

adhesive p. Peritonitis in which the visceral and parietal layers stick together by means of adhesions.

aseptic p. Peritonitis due to causes other than bacterial, fungal, or viral infection, such as trauma, presence of chemicals produced naturally or introduced from without, or irradiation.

benign paroxysmal p. Familial paroxysmal polyserositis. SEE: *familial Mediterranean fever.*

bile p. Peritonitis caused by the escape of bile into the peritoneal cavity.

chemical p. Peritonitis due to presence of chemicals such as intestinal juices, pancreatic secretions, or bile in the peritoneal cavity.

chronic p. Peritonitis that is usually due to tuberculosis or cancer. Findings include slight or absent fever, pain, diffuse tenderness, anemia, and emaciation. Rest, paracentesis, and laparotomy are involved in the treatment. The prognosis is guarded.

circumscribed p. Localized p.

p. deformans Chronic peritonitis with a thickened membrane and adhesions contracting and causing retraction of the intestines.

diaphragmatic p. Peritonitis in which the peritoneal surface of the diaphragm is mainly affected.

diffuse p. Peritonitis that is widespread, involving most of the peritoneum. SYN: *generalized p.*

fibrocaseous p. Peritonitis with fibrosis and caseation; usually caused by tuberculosis.

gas p. Peritonitis in which gas is present in the peritoneal cavity.

generalized p. Diffuse p.

localized p. Peritonitis in which only a small area is involved. SYN: *circumscribed p.*

meconium p. Peritonitis in the newborn caused by perforation of the gastrointestinal tract in utero. It most often occurs in newborns with cystic fibrosis.

Neonatal intestinal obstruction is usually present as well. In boys a soft hydrocele or scrotal mass may be found.

pelvic p. Peritonitis involving the peritoneum of the pelvic region, usually the sequela of uterine tube infection in women.

periodic p. Familial Mediterranean fever.

primary p. Peritonitis resulting from infectious organisms transmitted through blood or lymph.

puerperal p. Peritonitis that develops following childbirth.

secondary p. Peritonitis resulting from extension of infection from adjoining structures, rupture of a viscus, abscess, or trauma.

septic p. Peritonitis caused by a pyogenic bacterium.

serous p. Peritonitis in which there is copious liquid exudation.

silent p. Peritonitis in which there are no signs or symptoms.

talc p. Peritonitis due to particles of talcum powder in the peritoneal cavity.

traumatic p. Acute peritonitis due to injury or wound infection.

tuberculous p. Peritonitis caused by tuberculosis.

peritonsillar (pĕr″ĭ-tŏn′sĭ-lăr) [Gr. *peri*, around, + L. *tonsilla*, tonsil] Extending around a tonsil.

peritonsillitis (pĕr″ĭ-tŏn″sĭ-lī′tĭs) [″ + ″ + Gr. *itis*, inflammation] Inflammation of tissues around the tonsils.

peritracheal (pĕr″ĭ-trā′kē-ăl) [″ + *tracheia*, trachea] Around the trachea.

Peritricha (pĕr-ĭt′rĭ-kă) [Gr. *peri*, around, + *thrix*, hair] A group of protozoa having flagella over the entire surface.

peritrichal, peritrichic (pĕ-rĭt′rĭ-kăl, pĕr″ē-trĭk′ĭk) [″ + *thrix*, hair] Peritrichous.

peritrichous (pĕ-rĭt′rĭk-ŭs) [″+ *thrix*, hair] Indicating microorganisms that have cilia or flagella covering the entire surface of the cell. SYN: *peritrichal*.

peritrochanteric (pĕr″ĭ-trō″kăn-tĕr′ĭk) [″ + *trokhanter*, runner] Around a trochanter.

perityphlic (pĕr″ĭ-tĭf′lĭk) [″ + *typhlon*, cecum] Around the cecum.

perityphlitis (pĕr″ĭ-tĭf-lī′tĭs) [″ + ″ + *itis*, inflammation] Appendicitis.

periumbilical (pĕr″ē-ŭm-bĭl′ĭ-kăl) [″ + L. *umbilicus*, a pit] Around the navel (i.e., umbilicus).

periungual (pĕr″ē-ŭng′gwăl) [″ + L. *unguis*, nail] Around a nail.

periureteral (pĕr″ē-ū-rē′tĕr-ăl) [″ + *oureter*, ureter] Around a ureter.

periureteritis (pĕr″ē-ū-rē″tĕr-ī′tĭs) [″ + ″ + *itis*, inflammation] Inflammation of parts about the ureter.

periurethral (pĕr″ē-ū-rē′thrăl) [″ + *ourethra*, urethra] Located about the urethra.

periurethritis (pĕr″ē-ū″rē-thrī′tĭs) [″ + ″ + *itis*, inflammation] Inflammation of the tissues around the urethra.

periuterine (pĕr″ē-ū′tĕr-ĭn) [″ + L. *uterus*, womb] Around the uterus. SYN: *perimetric*.

periuvular (pĕr″ē-ū′vū-lăr) [″ + L. *uvula*, little grape] Around the uvula.

perivaginal (pĕr″ĭ-văj′ĭ-năl) [″ + L. *vagina*, sheath] Around the vagina.

perivaginitis (pĕr″ĭ-văj″ĭ-nī′tĭs) [″ + ″ + Gr. *itis*, inflammation] Inflammation of the region around the vagina. SYN: *pericolpitis*.

perivascular (pĕr″ĭ-văs′kū-lăr) [″ + L. *vasculus*, a little vessel] Around a vessel, esp. a blood vessel.

perivasculitis (pĕr″ĭ-văs″kū-lī′tĭs) [″ + ″ + Gr. *itis*, inflammation] Inflammation of the tissues surrounding a blood vessel. SYN: *periangiitis*.

perivenous (pĕr″ĭ-vē′nŭs) [″ + L. *vena*, vein] Around a vein.

perivertebral (pĕr″ĭ-vĕr′tĕ-brăl) [″ + L. *vertebra*, vertebra] Around a vertebra.

perivesical (pĕr″ĭ-vĕs′ĭ-kăl) [″ + L. *vesicula*, little bladder] Around the urinary bladder.

perivesiculitis (pĕr″ĭ-vĕ-sĭk″ū-lī′tĭs) [″ + ″ + Gr. *itis*, inflammation] Inflammation of tissues around a seminal vesicle.

perivisceral (pĕr″ĭ-vĭs′ĕr-ăl) [″ + L. *viscera*, internal organs] Around the viscera or a seminal vesicle.

perivisceritis (pĕr″ĭ-vĭs″ĕr-ī′tĭs) [″ + ″ + Gr. *itis*, inflammation] Inflammation of the tissues surrounding the viscera. SYN: *perisplanchnitis*.

perivitelline (pĕr″ĭ-vī-tĕl′ēn) [″ + L. *vitellus*, yolk] Around a vitellus or yolk.

perixenitis (pĕr″ĭ-zĕ-nī′tĭs) [″ + *xenos*, strange, + *itis*, inflammation] Noninfection inflammation occurring around a foreign body in a tissue or organ.

perle (pĕrl) [Fr., pearl] A soft capsule containing medicine.

perlèche (pĕr-lĕsh′) [Fr.] A disorder marked by fissures and epithelial desquamation at the corners of the mouth, esp. seen in children. The condition may be due to oral candidiasis or may be a symptom of dietary deficiency, esp. riboflavin deficiency.

perlingual (pĕr-lĭng′gwăl) [L. *per*, through, + *lingua*, tongue] By way of the tongue; a method of administering medicines.

Perl's stain A histochemical stain that demonstrates iron when it is present in body tissues.

permanent (pĕr′mă-nĕnt) [″ + *manere*, to remain] Enduring; without change.

permanganate (pĕr-măn′gă-nāt) Any one of the salts of permanganic acid.

permeability (pĕr″mē-ă-bĭl′ĭ-tē) [LL. *permeabilis*] The quality of being permeable; that which may be traversed.

capillary p. The condition of the capillary wall that enables substances in the blood to pass into tissue spaces or into cells, or vice versa.

permeable (pĕr′mē-ă-b′l) Capable of allowing the passage of fluids or substances in solution. SYN: *pervious* (1).

permeation (pĕr″mē-ā′shŭn) [L. *permeare,* permeate] Penetration of and spreading throughout an organ, tissue, or space.

permethrin An insecticide and insect repellent that has been used to treat scabies and lice infestations, and to protect people from tick exposure while working or playing outdoors.

permissible exposure limits The limits, usually expressed as a combination of time and concentration, to which humans may be safely exposed to physical agents, ionizing radiation, or chemical substances in the environment in general and in work areas specifically. SEE: *hazardous material; health hazard; maximum allowable concentration; right-to-know law; toxic substance.*

permucosal (pĕr-mū-kō′săl, Across mucous membranes.

permutation (pĕr″mū-tā′shŭn) [L. *per,* completely, + *mutare,* to change] Transformation; complete change; act of altering objects in a group.

pernicious (pĕr-nĭsh′ŭs) [L. *perniciosus,* destructive] Destructive; fatal; harmful.

p. trend In psychology, an abnormal departure from conventional ideas and social interests.

pernio (pĕr′nē-ō) [L.] Chilblain.

pero- [Gr. *peros,* maimed] Combining form meaning *deformed.*

perobrachius (pē″rō-brā′kē-ŭs) [″ + *brachion,* arm] An individual with congenitally deformed forearms and hands.

perocephalus (pē″rō-sĕf′ă-lŭs) [″ + *kephale,* head] An individual with a congenitally deformed head.

perochirus (pē″rō-kī′rŭs) [″ + *cheir,* hand] An individual with congenitally deformed hands.

perocormus (pē″rō-kor′mŭs) [″ + *kormos,* trunk] An individual with a congenitally deformed trunk.

perodactylus (pē″rō-dăk′tĭ-lŭs) [″ + *daktylos,* finger] An individual with congenitally deformed fingers or toes.

peromelia (pē″rō-mē′lē-ă) [″ + *melos,* limb] A birth defect with absence or deformity of the terminal part of a limb or limbs.

peromelus (pē-rŏm′ĕ-lŭs) [″+ *melos,* limb] An individual with congenital malformation of the extremities, including absence of a hand or foot.

perone (pĕr-ō′nē) [Gr. *perone,* pin] Fibula.

peroneal (pĕr″ō-nē′ăl) [Gr. *perone,* pin] Concerning the fibula.

p. sign In patients with tetany, eversion and dorsiflexion of the foot caused by tapping on the fibular side over the peroneal nerve.

peroneo- [Gr. *perone,* pin] Combining form meaning *fibula.*

peroneotibial (pĕr″ō-nē″ō-tĭb′ē-ăl) [″ + L. *tibia,* shinbone] Concerning the fibula and tibia.

peroneus (pĕr″ō-nē′ŭs) [Gr. *perone,* pin] One of several muscles of the leg that act to move the foot.

peropus (pē′rō-pŭs) [″ + *pous,* foot] An individual with congenitally deformed feet.

peroral (pĕr-or′ăl) [L. *per,* through, + *oris,* mouth] Administered through the mouth.

per os [L.] By mouth.

perosomus (pē″rō-sō′mŭs) [Gr. *peros,* maimed, + *soma,* body] An individual with a congenitally defective body.

perosplanchnia (pē″rō-splănk′nē-ă) [″ + *splanchnon,* viscus] Congenital malformation of the viscera.

perosseous (pĕr-ŏs′ē-ŭs) [L. *per,* through, + *os,* bone] Through bone.

peroxidase (pĕr-ŏk′sĭ-dās) [″ + Gr. *oxys,* acid, + *-ase,* enzyme] An enzyme that hastens the transfer of oxygen from peroxide to a tissue that requires oxygen. This process is essential to intracellular respiration.

peroxide (pĕr-ŏk′sīd) In chemistry, a compound containing more oxygen than the other oxides of the element in question.

peroxisome (pĕ-rŏks′ĭ-sōm) A class of single-membrane-bound vesicles that contain a variety of enzymes including catalase. They are present in most human cells but are concentrated in the liver. The absence of functional peroxisomes is involved in a number of diseases; the most severe is Zellweger's syndrome, which affects newborns and is usually fatal before one year of age. This syndrome consists of cirrhosis of the liver and congenital malformations of the central nervous system and skeleton.

perphenazine (pĕr-fĕn′ă-zēn) An antipsychotic drug that is also used as an antiemetic and in treating intractable hiccoughs.

per primam intentionem (pĕr prī′măm ĭn-tĕn-shē-ō′nĕm) [L.] By first intention. SEE: *healing.*

per rectum (pĕr rĕk′tŭm) [L.] By the rectum; through the rectum.

PERRLA *pupils equal, round, reactive to light and accommodation.*

persalt (pĕr′sawlt) In chemistry, a salt containing the largest possible amount of an acid radical.

per secundam intentionem (pĕr sē-kŭn′dăm) [L.] By second intention. SEE: *healing.*

perseveration (pĕr-sĕv″ĕr-ā′shŭn) [L. *perseverare,* to persist] **1.** Abnormal, compulsive, and inappropriate repetition of words or behaviors, a symptom observed, for example, in patients with schizophrenia or diseases of the frontal lobes of the brain. **2.** The repetition of rhythmic but meaningless actions, behaviors, or movements.

person A human being.

persona (pěr-sō′nă) [L., mask] The outer attitude or appearance a person presents to others.

personal emergency alert system A device consisting of a portable battery-powered help button and a machine that automatically dials a monitoring station. The device is connected to the individual's telephone or to a phone jack. When the system is activated, it either allows a two-way communication between the monitoring station and the individual or alerts the station personnel to phone the individual. In the latter case, if there is no response the station may call a neighbor or family member or dispatch emergency medical technicians to the person's home.

personal equation A personal bias or peculiarity that may explain a difference in approach or interpretation.

personal identity disturbance Inability to distinguish between self and nonself. SEE: *Nursing Diagnoses Appendix.*

personality [LL. *personalitas*] The unique organization of traits, characteristics, and modes of behavior of an individual, setting the individual apart from others and at the same time determining how others react to the individual. SEE: *personality testing.*

alternating p. Multiple p.

borderline p. SEE: *borderline personality disorder.*

compulsive p. Obsessive-compulsive personality disorder.

extroverted p. A personality type in which activities or libido is directed to other individuals or the environment.

inadequate p. A personality type in which the individual is ineffective and is physically and emotionally unstable to the extent of being unable to cope with the normal stress of living.

introverted p. A personality type in which activities or libido are directed to the individual himself or herself.

multiple p. A state in which two or more personalities alternate in the same individual, usually with each personality unaware of the others. SEE: *dissociation of personality; Nursing Diagnoses Appendix.*

obsessive-compulsive p. Obsessive-compulsive personality disorder.

paranoid p. Paranoid personality disorder.

psychopathic p. Antisocial personality disorder.

type A p. SEE: under *behavior.*

type B p. SEE: under *behavior.*

personality disorder A pathological disturbance of the patterns of perception, communication, and thinking. Personality disorders are manifested in at least two of the following areas: cognition, affect, interpersonal functioning, or impulse control. Generally, the disorder is of long duration and its onset can be traced to early adolescence.

TREATMENT: Psychotherapy, psychopharmacological drugs, or some combination of these approaches, are used in treating these disorders although many personality disorders resist treatment.

antisocial p.d. A type of personality disorder characterized by disregard of the rights of others. It usually begins prior to age 15. In early childhood, lying, stealing, fighting, truancy, and disregard of authority are common. In adolescence, aggressive sexual behavior, excessive use of alcohol, and use of drugs of abuse may be characteristic. In adulthood these behavior patterns continue with the addition of poor work performance, inability to function responsibly as a parent, and inability to accept normal restrictions imposed by laws. Affected persons may repeatedly perform illegal acts (e.g., destroying property, harassing others, or stealing) or pursue illegal occupations. They disregard the safety, wishes, rights, and feelings of others. This type of personality disorder is not due to mental retardation, schizophrenia, or manic episodes. It is much more common in males than females. This condition has been referred to as psychopathy, sociopathy, or dyssocial personality disorder.

avoidant p.d. A personality disorder marked by a pervasive pattern of social inhibition, feelings of inadequacy, and hypersensitivity to criticism. This begins by early adulthood and is present in various situations such as school, work, or activities involving contact with others. Individuals with this disorder desire affection, security, certainty, and acceptance and may fantasize about idealized relationships with others.

borderline p.d. A personality disorder in which there is difficulty in maintaining stable interpersonal relationships and self-image. This manifests as unpredictable and impulsive behavior, outbursts of anger, irritability, sadness, and fear. Self-mutilation or suicidal behavior may be present. Sometimes there is a chronic feeling of emptiness or boredom. SEE: *Nursing Diagnoses Appendix.*

Cluster A p.d. A grouping of personality disorders that share traits of odd behaviors and social isolation. This group of diagnoses includes paranoid, schizoid, and schizotypal personality disorders.

Cluster B p.d. A grouping of personality disorders that share traits of attention seeking, highly excitable emotional states, and unpredictable behavior. This group includes antisocial, borderline, narcissistic, and histrionic personality disorders.

Cluster C p.d. A group of personality disorders that have anxious and fearful behaviors as prominent features. This group includes dependent, avoidant, and obsessive-compulsive personality disorders.

histrionic p.d. A personality disorder marked by excessive emotionalism and attention-seeking. The individual is active, dramatic, prone to exaggerate, and subject to irrational, angry outbursts or tantrums. He or she expresses boredom with normal routines and craves novelty and excitement. Behavior in interpersonal relationships is shallow, vain, demanding, and dependent.

obsessive-compulsive p.d. A disorder characterized by a pervasive pattern of preoccupation with orderliness, perfectionism, and mental and interpersonal control at the expense of flexibility, openness, and efficiency. These symptoms begin by early adulthood and are manifested in various contexts. Four or more of the following criteria must be present: preoccupation with details, rules, lists, order, organization, or schedules to the extent that the major point of the activity is lost; perfectionism interfering with task completion because the person's own overly strict standards are not met; excessive devotion to work and productivity to the exclusion of leisure activities and friendships (not accounted for by obvious economic necessity); overconscientiousness, scrupulousness, and inflexibility about matters of morality, ethics, or values (not accounted for by cultural or religious identification); inability to discard worn-out or worthless objects even when they have no sentimental value; reluctance to delegate tasks or to work with others unless they submit to exactly the person's way of doing things; adoption of a miserly spending style toward both self and others, and a view of money as something to be hoarded for future catastrophes; and showing rigidity and stubbornness.

Even though obsessive-compulsive disorder and obsessive-compulsive personality disorder have similar names, they are usually easily distinguished by the presence of true obsessions and compulsions in the former. Obsessive-compulsive disorder should be considered esp. when hoarding is extreme. When the diagnostic criteria for both disorders are met, both diagnoses should be recorded.

narcissistic p.d. A personality disorder marked by a grandiose sense of self-importance and preoccupation with fantasies of unlimited success, power, brilliance, or beauty. The individual believes that his or her problems are unique and can only be understood by other "special" people. There is an exhibitionistic need for admiration and attention, a lack of empathy, and an inability to understand how others feel.

paranoid p.d. A personality disorder characterized by unwarranted suspiciousness and mistrust of others, hypervigilance directed at hidden motives or intent to harm, hypersensitivity to criticism, tendency to hold grudges and to be easily offended, and reluctance to confide in others. SEE: *paranoid disorder* in *Nursing Diagnoses Appendix.*

passive-aggressive p.d. A personality disorder marked by indirect resistance to demands for adequate occupational or social performance through procrastination, dawdling, stubbornness, inefficiency, or forgetfulness. The disorder begins in early childhood and may manifest as refusal to complete routine tasks, complaints of being misunderstood or unappreciated, sullen or argumentative attitude, pronounced envy of others, and behavior that alternates between hostile defiance and contrition.

schizoid p.d. A personality disorder characterized by shyness, oversensitivity, seclusiveness, dissociation from close interpersonal or competitive relationships, eccentricity, daydreaming, preference for solitary activities, and inability to express anger or joy in situations that would call for such a reaction. In most social interactions these individuals appear cold or aloof.

personality testing Testing that attempts to evaluate an individual's personality dysfunction and stress. A test that has been found to be useful in the fields of mental health, medicine, education, job placement, and counseling is the copyrighted Minnesota Multiphasic Personality Inventory (MMPI). It contains 550 statements that describe a wide variety of thoughts, feelings, attributes, and life experiences. The test requires the individual to answer "true" or "false" to each statement. The responses are measured against those of "normal" adults or adolescents.

personal protective equipment Clothing, masks, gloves, or other gear that protects a person from exposure to noxious chemicals or transmissible diseases.

personnel, unlicensed assistive ABBR: UAP. Any unlicensed health care personnel who work under the direction of a registered nurse. In addition to delivering direct patient care, they may take blood samples, provide respiratory treatments, or keep track of medical records. Some UAPs are multiskilled—they can perform a variety of tasks. Each state regulates UAP practice independently.

persons in need of supervision ABBR: PINS. A legal term for children who, because of behavioral problems, require supervision, usually in an institution.

person-years of life lost A calculation of the impact of a disease on society owing to premature death from the specific disease; that is, the number of years the person would have been alive if the disease had not occurred.

perspiration (pĕr″spĭr-ā′shŭn) [L. *perspirare,* breathe through] **1.** The secretion of the sweat (sudoriferous) glands of the skin; sweating. **2.** The salty fluid secreted through the sweat glands of the skin; sweat. Essentially, the fluid is a weak solution of sodium chloride, but it also contains potassium, lactate, and urea.

Perspiration is a means of removing heat from the body. Evaporation of 1 L of sweat removes 580 kcal of heat from the body. Sweat loss varies from 100 to 1000 ml/hr but may exceed those amounts in a hot climate.

Perspiration is increased by temperature and humidity of the atmosphere, exercise, pain, nausea, nervousness, mental excitement, dyspnea, diaphoretics, and shock. It is decreased by cold, diarrhea, other causes of profound dehydration, and using certain drugs.

insensible p. Evaporation of water vapor from the body without appearing as moisture on the skin.

sensible p. Perspiration that forms moisture on the skin.

perspire (pĕr-spīr′) [L. *perspirare,* breathe through] To secrete fluid through the pores of the skin. SYN: *sweat* (3).

persuasion (pĕr-swā′zhŭn) The act of influencing the thinking or behavior of others.

persulfate (pĕr-sŭl′fāt) One of a series of sulfates containing more sulfuric acid than the others in the same series.

per tertian (pĕr tĕr′shŭn) [L.] By third intention. SEE: *healing.*

Perthes' disease (pĕr′tēz) [Georg C. Perthes, Ger. surgeon, 1869–1927] Osteochondritis deformans juvenilis.

per tubam (pĕr tū′băm) [L.] Through a tube.

perturbation (pĕr″tĕr-bā′shŭn) [L. *perturbare,* thoroughly disordered] The state of being greatly disturbed or agitated; uneasiness of mind.

pertussis (pĕr-tŭs′ĭs) [L. *per,* through, + *tussis,* cough] An acute, infectious disease characterized by a catarrhal stage, followed by a peculiar paroxysmal cough, ending in a whooping inspiration. The disease is caused by a small, nonmotile, gram-negative bacillus, *Bordetella pertussis.* The incubation period is 7 to 10 days. Treatment is symptomatic and supportive. Antibiotics (e.g., erythromycin) are given to treat bacterial pneumonia, otitis media, esp. in infants and young children, early in the course of the infection. SYN: *whooping cough.*

PREVENTION: Pertussis may be prevented by immunization of infants beginning at 3 months of age.

SYMPTOMS: The signs of this disease include elevated white blood count with marked lymphocytosis, possibly in excess of 30,000/mm³. Pertussis is often divided into the following three stages:

Catarrhal: At this stage the symptoms are chiefly suggestive of the common cold—slight elevation of fever, sneezing, rhinitis, dry cough, irritability, and loss of appetite.

Paroxysmal: This stage sets in after approx. 2 weeks. The cough is more violent and consists of a series of several short coughs, followed by a long drawn inspiration during which the typical whoop is heard, this being occasioned by the spasmodic contraction of the glottis. Often with the beginning of each paroxysm, the patient assumes a worried expression, sometimes even one of terror. The face becomes cyanosed, eyes injected, veins distended. With the conclusion of the paroxysm, vomiting is common. Also at this time there may be epistaxis, subconjunctival hemorrhages, or hemorrhages in other portions of the body. The number of paroxysms in 24 hr may vary from 3 or 4 to 40 or 50. The cough is precipitated by eating, drinking, or pressing on the trachea, and may be followed by vomiting.

Decline: This stage begins after an indefinite period of several weeks. Paroxysms grow less frequent and less violent. The child's nutrition improves, and after a period that may be prolonged for several months, the cough finally ceases.

PATIENT CARE: Parents are advised that immunization prevents pertussis in children younger than 7 years, except for those children with a history of known allergy. For those children who contract the disease (mainly nonimmunized children), precautions are taken to prevent spread after the onset of symptoms. Bedrest, isolation, and a quiet environment are provided. Because cough may be severe and debilitating, cough remedies such as guiafenesin or benzonatate may be given. Comfort measures are provided as indicated.

pertussis immune globulin A sterile solution of antibodies derived from the blood of adults who have been immunized with pertussis vaccine; used to produce passive immunity to pertussis.

pertussis vaccine Sterile bacterial fraction of killed pertussis bacilli; used for active immunization against pertussis.

pertussoid (pĕr-tŭs′oyd) [L. *per,* through, + *tussis,* cough, + Gr. *eidos,* form, shape] **1.** Of the nature of whooping cough. **2.** A cough generally similar to that of whooping cough.

per vaginam (pĕr vă-jī′năm) [L.] Through the vagina.

perversion (pĕr-vĕr′zhŭn) [L. *perversus,* perverted] Deviation from the normal path, whether it be in the area of one's intellect, emotions, actions, or reactions.

sexual p. Maladjustment of sexual life in which satisfaction is sought in ways deviating from the accepted norm. In judging the sexual actions of individuals, it is important to remember that what is normal behavior in one society may be regarded as grossly abnormal in another.

pervert (pĕr-vĕrt′) [L. *pervetere,* to turn the wrong way] To turn from the normal; to misuse.

pervert (pĕr′vĕrt) [L. *pervetere,* to turn the wrong way] One who has turned from the normal or socially acceptable path, esp. sexually.

pervious (pĕr′vē-ŭs) [L. *pervius*] **1.** Permeable. **2.** Penetrating.

pes (pĕs) *pl.* **pedes** [L.] The foot or a footlike structure.

p. abductus Talipes valgus.

p. adductus Talipes varus.

p. anserinus **1.** The three primary branches of the facial nerve after leaving the stylomastoid foramen. **2.** The tendinous expansions of the sartorius, gracilis, and semitendinosus muscles at the medial border of the tibial tuberosity.

p. cavus An abnormal hollowness or concavity of the sole of the foot; an excessively high longitudinal arch in the foot.

p. contortus Talipes equinovarus.

p. equinovalgus A condition in which the heel is elevated and turned laterally.

p. equinovarus A condition in which the heel is turned inward and the foot is plantar flexed.

p. equinus A deformity marked by walking without touching the heel to the ground. SYN: *talipes equinus.*

p. gigas Macropodia.

p. hippocampi The lower portion of the hippocampus major.

infraorbital p. Terminal radiating branches of the infraorbital nerve after exit from the infraorbital canal.

p. planus Flatfoot.

p. valgus Talipes valgus.

p. varus Talipes varus.

pessary (pĕs′ă-rē) [L. *pessarium*] A device inserted into the vagina to function as a supportive structure for the uterus. A pessary may be inserted to treat symptomatic uterine displacements. After manually repositioning the uterus, the physician inserts the appropriate-size device; a woman should not feel a well-fitted pessary. The woman is instructed to use a mild acetic acid douche (1 tbs. vinegar to 1 pint warm water) twice weekly to minimize irritation of the vaginal mucosa. Unless discomfort arises, the device is removed about 6 weeks later. If relief and anteversion occur, no further treatment is necessary. If not, the pessary is reinserted for another 6 weeks.

cup p. Pessary that has a cup-shaped hollow that fits over the os uteri.

diaphragm p. A cup-shaped rubber pessary used as a contraceptive device.

Hodge's p. A pessary used to correct retrodeviations of the uterus.

ring p. A round pessary.

pessimism A frame of mind marked by loss of hope, confidence, or trust in a good outcome, even when such an outcome is likely. SEE: *optimism.*

therapeutic p. The tendency not to believe in the effectiveness of therapeutic measures, esp. of drugs.

pest (pĕst) [L. *pestis,* plague] **1.** A noxious, destructive insect. **2.** A fatal epidemic disease, esp. plague.

pesticemia (pĕs″tĭ-sē′mē-ă) [″ + Gr. *haima,* blood] The presence of plague organisms in the blood.

pesticide (pĕs′tĭ-sīd) [″ + *cida,* killer] Any chemical used to kill pests, esp. rodents and insects.

p. residue The amount of any pesticide remaining on or in food or beverages intended for human consumption.

restricted-use p. In the U.S., a pesticide known to have adverse effects on the environment or on people; only individuals who have been specially trained and certified as pesticide applicators may use it.

pestiferous (pĕs-tĭf′ĕr-ŭs) [L. *pestiferus*] Producing a pestilence; carrying infection. SYN: *pestilential.*

pestilence (pĕs′tĭl-ĕns) [L. *pestilentia*] **1.** An epidemic contagious disease. **2.** An epidemic caused by such a disease.

pestilential (pĕs-tĭ-lĕn′shăl) Pestiferous.

pestis (pĕs′tĭs) [L.] Plague.

p. ambulans Ambulatory plague.

p. fulminans The most severe form of plague.

pestle (pĕs′l) [L. *pistillum*] A device for macerating drugs in a mortar.

PET *positron emission tomography.*

petechiae (pē-tē′kē-ē) *sing.,* **petechia** [It. *petecchia,* skin spot] **1.** Small, purplish, hemorrhagic spots on the skin that appear in patients with platelet deficiencies (thrombocytopenias) and in many febrile illnesses. **2.** Red spots from the bite of a flea.

petechial (pē-tē′kē-ăl) Marked by the presence of petechiae.

Peter Pan syndrome The reluctance of an adult to adopt traditional male adult behavior.

petiole (pĕt′ē-ōl) [LL. *petiolus*] A slender stalk or stem, as petiole of the epiglottic cartilage.

petiolus (pē-tī′ō-lŭs) [LL.] The stalk or stem of a fruit; a pedicle.

p. epiglottidis The pedicle of the cartilage of the epiglottis. It is attached to the superior notch of the thyroid cartilage.

Petit, François Pourfour du (pĕt-ē′) French anatomist and surgeon, 1664–1741.

P.'s canal A space or cleft encircling the lens between the points of attachment of fibers of suspensory ligament. SYN: *zonular spaces.*

P.'s sinuses Hollows in the aortic and pulmonary arteries behind the semilunar valves.

Petit, Jean Louis (pĕt-ē′) French surgeon, 1674–1750.

P.'s ligament A thickened portion of the pelvic fascia between the cervix and vagina. It passes posteriorly in the rectouterine fold to attach to the anterior surface of the sacrum.

P.'s triangle The area on the lateral abdominal wall bounded by the crest of the ilium, the posterior margin of the external oblique muscle, and the lateral margin of the latissimus dorsi muscle. SYN: *trigonum lumbale.*

petition Complaint (2).

petit mal SEE: *epilepsy.*

Petri dish (pā′trē) [Julius Petri, Ger. bacteriologist, 1852–1921] A shallow covered dish made of plastic or glass, used to hold solid media for culturing bacteria.

petrifaction (pĕt-rĭ-făk′shŭn) [L. *petra,* stone, + *facere,* to make] The process of changing into stone or hard substance.

petrified (pĕt′rĭ-fīd) Changed into stone; rigid.

petrify (pĕt′rĭ-fī) To convert into stone; make rigid.

pétrissage (pā″trē-săzh′) [Fr.] A massage technique that uses kneading or squeezing of muscle groups across muscle fibers and is performed generally by the tips of the thumbs, with the index finger and thumb, or with the palm of the hand. It is used principally on the extremities. The operator picks up a special muscle or tendon and, placing one finger on each side of the part, proceeds in centripetal motion with a firm pressure. SYN: *kneading.*

petro- [L. *petra,* stone] Combining form meaning *stone;* pert. to the petrous portion of the temporal bone.

petrolatoma (pĕt″rō-lă-tō′mă) [L. *petrolatum,* petroleum] A tumor or swelling caused by the introduction of liquid petrolatum under the skin.

petrolatum (pĕt″rō-lā′tŭm) [L.] A purified semisolid mixture of hydrocarbons obtained from petroleum. This occlusive substance is used as a base for ointments. It is not suitable for use as a vaginal lubricant because it is not miscible in body secretions. SYN: *soft paraffin.*

liquid p. A mixture of liquid hydrocarbons obtained from petroleum. This mixture is used as a vehicle for medicinal substances for local applications. Light petrolatum is employed as a topical spray, whereas heavy petrolatum was once used internally to treat constipation. SYN: *mineral oil.*

white p. A purified mixture of semisolid hydrocarbons obtained from petroleum.

petroleum (pĕ-trō′lē-ŭm) [L. *petra,* stone, + *oleum,* oil] An oily inflammable liquid found in the upper strata of the earth; a hydrocarbon mixture.

petromastoid (pĕt″rō-măs′toyd) Pert. to the petrous and mastoid portions of the temporal and occipital bones.

petro-occipital (pĕt″rō-ŏk-sĭp′ĭ-tăl) [″ + *occipitalis,* occipital] Concerning the petrous portion of the temporal bone and the occipital bone.

petropharyngeus (pĕt″rō-făr-rĭn′jē-ŭs) [″ + Gr. *pharynx,* throat] A small muscle joining the lower surface of the petrous portion of the temporal bone and the pharynx. It helps to constrict the pharynx.

petrosa (pē-trō′să) [L. *petrosus,* stony] The petrous part of the temporal bone.

petrosal (pĕt-rō′săl) [L. *petrosus,* stony] Of, pert. to, or situated near the petrous portion of the temporal bone.

petrosalpingostaphylinus (pĕt″rō-săl-pĭng″gō-stăf″ĭ-lī′nŭs) [L. *petra,* stone, + Gr. *salpinx,* tube, + *staphyle,* uvula] Musculus levator veli palatini.

petrositis (pĕt″rō-sī′tĭs) [″ + Gr. *itis,* inflammation] Inflammation of the petrous region of the temporal bone.

petrosomastoid (pē-trō″sō-măs′toyd) [″ + Gr. *mastos,* breast, + *eidos,* form, shape] Concerning the petrous portion of the temporal bone and its mastoid process.

petrosphenoid (pĕt″rō-sfē′noyd) [″ + Gr. *sphen,* wedge, + *eidos,* form, shape] Pert. to the petrous portion of the temporal bone and sphenoid bone.

petrosquamous (pĕt″rō-skwā′mŭs) [″ + *squamosus,* scaly] Pert. to the petrous and squamous portions of the temporal bone.

petrostaphylinus (pĕt″rō-stăf″ĭ-lī′nŭs) [″ + Gr. *staphyle,* uvula] Musculus levator veli palatini.

petrous (pĕt′rŭs) [L. *petrosus*] **1.** Resembling stone. **2.** Relating to the petrous portion of the temporal bone. SYN: *petrosal.*

Peutz-Jeghers syndrome (pūtz-jā′kĕrs) [Johannes Laurentius Augustinus Peutz, Dutch physician, 1886–1957; Harold J. Jeghers, U.S. physician, b. 1904] An inherited disorder characterized by the presence of polyps of the small intestine and melanin pigmentation of the lips, mucosa, fingers, and toes. Anemia due to bleeding from the intestinal polyps is a common finding.

pexin (pĕk′sĭn) Rennet.

pexis [Gr., fixation] Fixation of material to the tissue.

-pexy [Gr. *pexis,* fixation] A combining form used as a suffix meaning *fixation,* usually surgical.

Peyer's patch (pī′ĕrz) [Johann Conrad Peyer, Swiss anatomist, 1653–1712] A group of diffuse lymphoid nodules in the submucosa of the small bowel. Part of the mucosa-associated lymphoid tissue (MALT), Peyer's patches detect and respond to foreign antigens in the gastrointestinal tract. Antibodies secreted by B cells in Peyer's patches provide a significant defense against ingested pathogens.

peyote (pā-ō′tē) **1.** The cactus plant, *Lophophora williamsii,* from which the hallucinogen mescaline is obtained. **2.** The drug from the flowering heads, buttons, of *L. williamsii,* used by some Native Americans to produce altered states of consciousness. In certain tribes the buttons are used in religious ceremonies. For that reason, members of that tribe are permitted to use this substance even though the drug is classed as a narcotic and its use is otherwise restricted to research.

Peyronie's disease (pā-rō-nēz′) [François de la Peyronie, Fr. surgeon, 1678–1747] A dorsal deformity or curvature of the penis caused by fibrous tissue within the tunica albuginea. When the distortion of the penis is severe, the affected individual may experience erectile dysfunction or pain during sexual intercourse.

TREATMENT: In many cases the contracture is mild, and those patients do not require treatment. When pain is present for more than 12 months, however, or when the deformity is severe or interferes with erectile function, surgical repair of the defect may prove helpful.

Pfannenstiel incision A transverse curvilinear incision immediately above the pubic symphysis extending from the skin into the peritoneum. The skin incision is continued transversely to include the anterior rectus sheath, which is then reflected superiorly; the bellies of the rectus muscle are separated longitudinally and the peritoneum is incised vertically. This surgical approach is used most often in gynecological procedures.

PFD *personal flotation device.*

Pfeiffer, Emil (fī′fĕr) German physician, 1846–1921.

P.'s disease Infectious mononucleosis.

Pfeiffer, Richard F. (fī′fĕr) German bacteriologist, 1858–1945.

P.'s bacillus Haemophilus influenzae.

P.'s phenomenon A discovery made in 1894 stating that the serum of guinea pigs immunized with cholera vibrios destroyed cholera organisms in the peritoneal cavity of immune and nonimmune guinea pigs and that the same reaction occurred in vitro. That same lytic reaction occurred with typhoid and *Escherichia coli.*

Pfiesteria piscicida [L. fish killer] A unicellular marine organism, which may or may not produce a toxin, depending on environmental conditions. When toxic, it has been implicated in the death of millions of fish in the estuaries of North Carolina, Delaware, and Maryland. The toxin can become aerosolized, and if humans are exposed to it severe neurological, mental, and physical illness may occur. Specific therapy to combat the toxin is not available, but concomitant infections can be treated with tetracyclines.

PFT *pulmonary function test.*

PG *prostaglandin.*

pg *picogram.*

PGA *pteroylglutamic acid.*

Ph **1.** *Pharmacopoeia.* **2.** Symbol for phenyl.

pH *potential of hydrogen.* A measure of the hydrogen ion concentration of a solution. In chemistry, the degrees of acidity or alkalinity of a substance are expressed in pH values. A solution that is neither acid nor alkaline, is assigned a pH of 7. Increasing acidity is expressed as a number less than 7, and increasing alkalinity as a number greater than 7. Maximum acidity is pH 0 and maximum alkalinity is pH 14. Because the pH scale is logarithmic, there is a 10-fold difference between each unit. For example, pH 5 is 10 times as acid as pH 6 and pH 4 is 100 times as acid as pH 6. The pH of a solution may be determined electrically by a pH meter or colorimetrically by the use of indicators. A list of indicators and the pH range registered by each is given under the indicator. SEE: illus.; table; *indicator.*

PHA *phytohemagglutinin.*

phacitis (fă-sī′tĭs) [Gr. *phakos,* lens, + *itis,* inflammation] Phakitis.

phaco- [Gr. *phakos*] Combining form denoting *lens.*

phacoanaphylaxis (făk″ō-ăn″ă-fĭ-lăk′sĭs) [Gr. *phakos,* lens, + *ana,* excessive, + *phylaxis,* protection] Hypersensitivity to protein of the crystalline lens.

phacocele (făk′ō-sēl) [″ + *kele,* tumor, swelling] Displacement of the crystalline lens into the interior chamber of the eye. SYN: *phacometachoresis.*

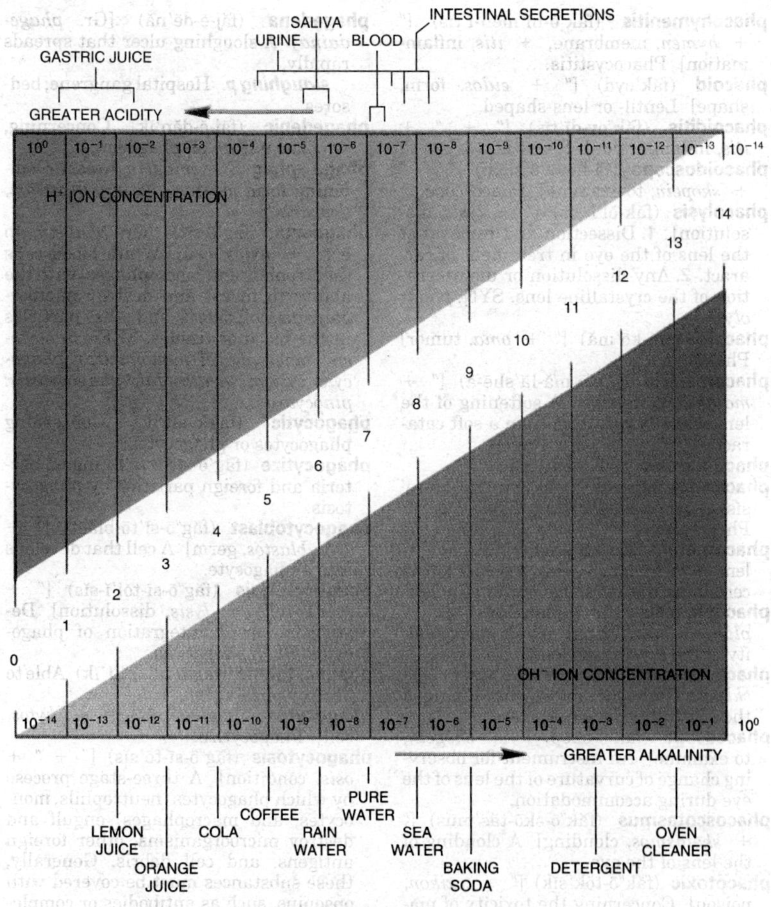

pH SCALE

Values of body fluids and some familiar solutions

phacocyst (făk′ō-sĭst) [Gr. *phakos,* lens, + *kystis,* a sac] The capsule of the crystalline lens.

phacocystectomy (făk″ō-sĭs-tĕk′tō-mē) [″ + ″ + *ektome,* excision] Surgical excision of part of the crystalline lens capsule for treatment of cataract.

phacocystitis (făk″ō-sĭs-tī′tĭs) [″ + ″ + *itis,* inflammation] Inflammation of the capsule of the lens of the eye. SYN: *phacohymenitis*.

phacoemulsification (făk″ō-ē-mŭl′sĭ-fĭ-kā″shŭn) A method of treating cataracts of the lens of the eye. An ultrasonic device is used to disintegrate the cataract, which is then aspirated and removed. SYN: *phacogragmentation*.

phacoerysis (făk″ō-ĕr-ē′sĭs) [″ + *eresis,* removal] Removal of the lens of the eye by attaching a suction device, an erysiphake, to it. SEE: *erysiphake*.

phacogragmentation Phacoemulsification.

phacoglaucoma (făk″ō-glaw-kō′mă) [″ + *glaukos,* green, + *oma,* tumor] Glaucoma and the changes it induces in the crystalline lens. SEE: *glaucoma*.

pH of Some Fluids

Material	pH
Decinormal HCl	1.0
Gastric juice	1.0–5.0
Thousandth-normal HCl	3.0
Pure water (neutral) at 25°C	7.0
Blood plasma	7.35–7.45
Pancreatic juice	8.4–8.9
Thousandth-normal NaOH	11.0
Decinormal NaOH	13.0

HCl—hydrochloric acid; NaOH—sodium hydroxide

phacohymenitis (făk″ō-hī″mĕn-ī′tĭs) [″ + *hymen,* membrane, + *itis,* inflammation] Phacocystitis.

phacoid (făk′oyd) [″ + *eidos,* form, shape] Lentil- or lens-shaped.

phacoiditis (făk″oy-dī′tĭs) [″ + ″ + *itis,* inflammation] Phakitis.

phacoidoscope (fă-koyd′ō-skōp) [″ + ″ + *skopein,* to examine] Phacoscope.

phacolysis (făk-ŏl′ĭ-sĭs) [″ + *lysis,* dissolution] **1.** Dissection and removal of the lens of the eye in treatment of cataract. **2.** Any dissolution or disintegration of the crystalline lens. SYN: *phakolysis.*

phacoma (fă-kō′mă) [″ + *oma,* tumor] Phakoma.

phacomalacia (făk″ō-mă-lā′shē-ă) [″ + *malakia,* softening] A softening of the lens, usually resulting from a soft cataract.

phacomatosis Phakomatosis.

phacometachoresis (făk″ō-mĕt″ă-kō-rē′sĭs) [″ + *metachoresis,* displacement] Phacocele.

phacometer (făk-ŏm′ĕ-tĕr) [Gr. *phakos,* lens, + *metron,* measure] A device for ascertaining the refractive power of a lens.

phacoplanesis (făk″ō-plăn-ē′sĭs) [″ + *planesis,* wandering] Abnormal mobility of the crystalline lens.

phacosclerosis (făk″ō-sklĕr-ō′sĭs) [″ + *sklerosis,* a hardening] A hardening of the crystalline lens of the eye.

phacoscope (făk′ō-skōp) [″ + *skopein,* to examine] An instrument for observing change of curvature of the lens of the eye during accommodation.

phacoscotasmus (făk″ō-skō-tăs′mŭs) [″ + *skotasmos,* clouding] A clouding of the lens of the eye.

phacotoxic (făk″ō-tŏk′sĭk) [″ + *toxikon,* poison] Concerning the toxicity of material in the lens of the eye.

Phaedra complex [Wife of King Theseus of Athens] The love and attraction between a stepparent and a stepchild; so named because of Phaedra's tragic love for the son (Hippolytus) of her husband by a previous marriage.

phag- SEE: *phago-.*

phage (fāj) [Gr. *phagein,* to eat] Bacteriophage.

phagedena (făj-ĕ-dē′nă) [Gr. *phagedaina*] A sloughing ulcer that spreads rapidly.

sloughing p. Hospital gangrene; bedsores.

phagedenic (făj-ĕ-dĕn′ĭk) Concerning, or of the nature of, phagedena.

phago-, phag- [Gr. *phagein,* to eat] Combining form meaning *eating, ingestion, devouring.*

phagocyte (făg′ō-sīt) [Gr. *phagein,* to eat, + *kytos,* cell] White blood cells (neutrophils and macrophages) with the ability to ingest and destroy microorganisms, cell debris, and other particles in the blood or tissues. SEE: *endocytosis; macrophage; mononuclear phagocyte system; neutrophil; phagocytosis; pinocytosis.*

phagocytic (făg″ō-sĭt′ĭk) Concerning phagocytes or phagocytosis.

phagocytize (făg′ō-sīt″īz) To ingest bacteria and foreign particles by phagocytosis.

phagocytoblast (făg″ō-sī′tō-blăst) [″ + ″ + *blastos,* germ] A cell that develops into a phagocyte.

phagocytolysis (făg″ō-sī-tŏl′ĭ-sĭs) [″ + *kytos,* cell, + *lysis,* dissolution] Destruction or disintegration of phagocytes. SYN: *phagolysis.*

phagocytolytic (făg″ō-sī″tō-lĭt′ĭk) Able to destroy phagocytes.

phagocytose (făg″ō-sī′tōs) [″ + *kytos,* cell] Phagocytize.

phagocytosis (făg″ō-sī-tō′sĭs) [″ + ″ + *osis,* condition] A three-stage process by which phagocytes (neutrophils, monocytes, and macrophages) engulf and destroy microorganisms, other foreign antigens, and cell debris. Generally, these substances must be covered with opsonins, such as antibodies or complement, to initiate binding with cell receptors on the phagocytes, the first stage in phagocytosis. In the second stage, the particle is engulfed and enclosed in a vacuole (phagosome). During the third stage, the phagosome merges with lysosomes whose enzymes destroy the engulfed particle. SEE: illus.; *defensin; lysozyme; macrophage; neutrophil; oxygen radical.*

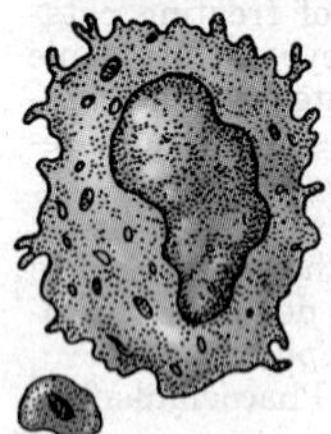

PARTICLE TO BE INGESTED BY CELL

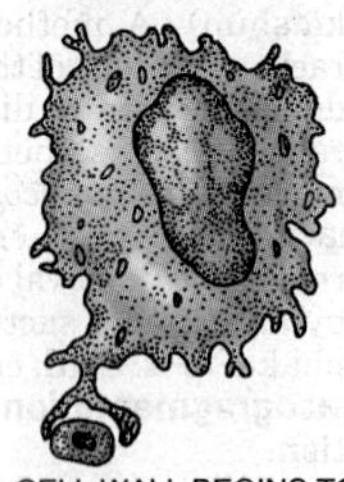

CELL WALL BEGINS TO SURROUND FOREIGN BODY

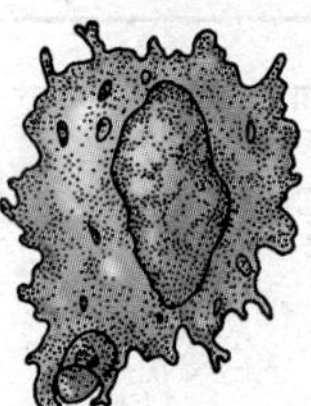

PARTICLE ENCLOSED IN PHAGOLYSOSOME

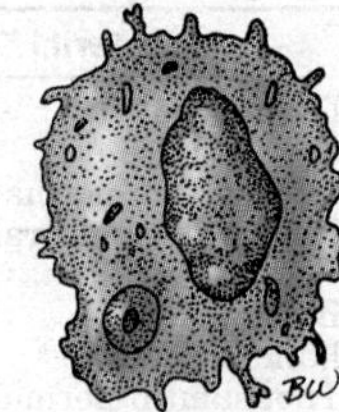

ENZYMATIC DEGRADATION OF PARTICLE BEGINS

PHAGOCYTOSIS

Most bacteria are killed during phagocytosis by oxygen radicals, which are formed during the respiratory burst when phagosomes and lysosomes merge. When oxygen radical production is excessive, tissue damage occurs. Lysozymes, defensins, and bacteriocidal permeability-increasing (BPI) protein also destroy bacteria and other organisms; their actions do not depend on the generation of oxygen radicals.

induced p. Phagocytosis that is aided or stimulated by the effect of serum opsonins or bacteria.

spontaneous p. Phagocytosis occurring in an indifferent medium such as physiological salt solution.

phagodynamometer (făg″ō-dī″nă-mŏm′ĕ-tĕr) [″ + *dynamis,* power, + *metron,* measure] A device that measures energy expended in chewing food.

phagokaryosis (făg″ō-kăr″ē-ō′sĭs) [″ + *karyon,* nucleus, + *osis,* condition] Phagocytic action that is performed by a cell nucleus.

phagolysis (făg-ŏl′ĭ-sĭs) [″ + *lysis,* dissolution] Phagocytolysis.

phagolysosome (făg″ō-lī′sō-sōm) [″ + *lysis,* dissolution, + *soma,* body] The vacuole formed when the membrane-bound phagosome inside a macrophage fuses with a lysosome. SEE: *phagosome.*

phagophobia (făg″ō-fō′bē-ă) [″ + *phobos,* fear] Fear of eating.

phagosome (făg′ō-sōm) [″ + *soma,* body] A membrane-bound vacuole inside a phagocyte that contains material waiting to be digested. Digestion is facilitated by the fusion of the vacuole with the lysosome. The phagosome is then called a phagolysosome or a secondary lysosome. SEE: *phagocytosis.*

phagotype (făg′ō-tīp) [″ + *typos,* mark] The classification of bacteria by their sensitivity to phage types.

phakitis (făk-ī′tĭs) [Gr. *phakos,* lens, + *itis,* inflammation] Inflammation of the crystalline lens of the eye. SYN: *phacitis; lentitis.*

phakolysis (făk-ŏl′ĭ-sĭs) [″ + *lysis,* dissolution] Disintegration or removal of the crystalline lens of the eye. SYN: *phacolysis* (2).

phakoma (fă-kō′mă) [″ + *oma,* tumor] **1.** A microscopic gray white tumor present in the retina in tuberous sclerosis. **2.** An area of myelinated nerve fibers rarely seen in the retina in association with neurofibromatosis. SYN: *phacoma.*

phakomatosis (fă″kō-mă-tō′sĭs) [Gr. *phakos,* lens, + *oma,* tumor, + *osis,* condition] Any genetic neurocutaneous disorders, in which anomalies are spread unevenly through the body. SYN: *phacomatosis.* SEE: *Hippel's disease; neurofibromatosis; sclerosis, tuberous; Sturge-Weber syndrome.*

phalang- SEE: *phalango-.*

phalangeal (fă-lăn′jē-ăl) [Gr. *phalanx,* closely knit row] Concerning a phalanx.

phalangectomy (făl-ăn-jĕk′tō-mē) [″ + *ektome,* excision] Excision of one or more phalanges.

phalanges (fă-lăn′jēz) Pl. of phalanx.

phalangette (făl″ăn-jĕt′) The distal phalanx of a digit.

drop p. Falling of the distal phalanx of a digit with loss of power to extend it when the hand is prone. This is due to trauma or overstretching of the extensor tendon.

phalangitis (făl″ăn-jī′tĭs) [Gr. *phalanx,* closely knit row, + *itis,* inflammation] Inflammation of one or more phalanges.

phalango-, phalang- [Gr. *phalanx,* closely knit row] Combining form meaning *phalanges* (bones of fingers and toes).

phalanx (făl′ănks) *pl.* **phalanges** [Gr., closely knit row] **1.** Any one of the bones of the fingers or toes. SEE: *skeleton.* **2.** One of a set of plates formed of phalangeal cells (inner and outer) forming the reticular membrane of the organ of Corti.

distal p. The phalanx most remote from the metacarpus or metatarsus. SYN: *terminal p.; ungual p.*

metacarpal p. Any phalanx that articulates with a metacarpal bone. SEE: *proximal p.*

metatarsal p. Any phalanx that articulates with a metatarsal bone. SEE: *proximal p.*

middle p. When there are three phalanges, the phalanx intermediate between distal and proximal phalanges.

proximal p. Any phalanx that articulates with a metacarpal or metatarsal bone.

terminal p. Distal p.

ungual p. Distal p.

Phalen's test A physical test involving flexion of the fully extended hand at the wrist to aid in the diagnosis of carpal tunnel syndrome. The test is positive (suggestive of carpal tunnel syndrome) when flexion of the wrist produces numbness in the distribution of the median nerve.

phall- [Gr. *phallos,* penis] Combining form indicating *penis.*

phallalgia (făl-ăl′jē-ă) [Gr. *phallos,* penis, + *algos,* pain] Pain in the penis.

phallectomy (făl-ĕk′tō-mē) [″ + *ektome,* excision] Surgical removal of the penis.

phallic (făl′ĭk) Concerning the penis.

phalliform (făl′ĭ-form) [″ + L. *forma,* form] Shaped like a penis.

phallitis (făl-ī′tĭs) [″ + *itis,* inflammation] Inflammation of the penis.

phallocampsis (făl-ō-kămp′sĭs) [″ + *kampsis,* a bending] Painful downward curvature of the penis when erect.

phallocrypsis (făl″ō-krĭp′sĭs) [″ + *kryp-*

sis, hiding] Contraction of the penis so that it is almost invisible.

phallodynia (făl-ō-dĭn′ē-ă) [″ + *odyne,* pain] Pain in the penis. SYN: *phallalgia.*

phalloid (făl′oyd) [″ + *eidos,* form, shape] Similar to a penis.

phalloidin (fă-loyd′ĭn) A poisonous peptide from the mushroom *Amanita phalloides.* Ingestion of this material can cause death as a result of fulminant hepatic failure.

phalloncus (făl-ŏn′kŭs) [″ + *onkos,* mass] A tumor or swelling on the penis.

phalloplasty (făl′ō-plăs″tē) [″ + *plassein,* to form] Reparative or plastic surgery on the penis.

phallorrhagia (făl-ō-rā′jē-ă) [″ + *rhegnynai,* to burst forth] Hemorrhage from the penis.

phallus (făl′ŭs) [Gr. *phallos,* penis] **1.** The penis. **2.** An artificial penis, used as a symbol. **3.** Embryonic structure developing at the tip of the genital tubercle that in the male develops into the penis and in the female, the clitoris.

phanero-, phaner- [Gr. *phaneros,* visible] Combining form meaning *evident, visible.*

phanerogenic (făn″ĕr-ō-jĕn′ĭk) [″ + *gennan,* to produce] Indicating a disease with a known cause.

phaneromania (făn″ĕr-ō-mā′nē-ă) [″ + *mania,* madness] An abnormal tendency to bite the nails or pick, scratch, or pull a pimple, wart, hair, beard, or mustache.

phanerosis (făn″ĕr-ō′sĭs) [Gr.] The process of becoming visible.

phanic (făn′ĭk) [Gr. *phainein,* to show] Manifest; apparent.

phantasia (făn-tā′zē-ă) [Gr.] An appearance that is imaginary.

phantasm (făn′tăzm) [Gr. *phantasma*] An optical illusion; an apparition, or illusion of something that does not exist.

phantasmagoria [Gr. *phantasma,* an appearance, + *agora,* assembly, gathering] A series of phantasms, deceptive illusions, either imagined or remembered from a dream.

phantasmology (făn″tăz-mŏl′ō-jē) [″ + *logos,* word, reason] The study of dreams, phantoms, and spiritually derived apparitions.

phantasy (făn′tă-sē) [Gr. *phantasia,* imagination] Fantasy.

phantogeusia (făn-tō-gū′sē-ă) [″ + *geusis,* taste] An intermittent or persistent taste sensation not produced by an external stimulus.

phantom (făn′tŭm) [Gr. *phantasma,* an appearance] **1.** An apparition. **2.** A model of the body or of one of its parts.

phantosmia (făn-tŏs′mē-ă) [″ + *osme,* smell] An intermittent or persistent perception of odor when no odor is inhaled.

pharmacal (făr′mă-kăl) [Gr. *pharmakon,* drug] Concerning pharmacy.

pharmaceutical (făr-mă-sū′tĭ-kăl) [Gr. *pharmakeutikos*] Concerning drugs or pharmacy.

pharmaceutics (făr-mă-sū′tĭks) Pharmacy (1).

pharmacist (făr′mă-sĭst) [Gr. *pharmakon,* drug] A druggist; one licensed to prepare and dispense drugs. SYN: *apothecary.*

pharmaco- [Gr. *pharmakon,* drug] Combining form meaning *drug, medicine.*

pharmacochemistry (făr″mă-kō-kĕm′ĭs-trē) [″ + *chemeia,* chemistry] Pharmaceutical chemistry.

pharmacodiagnosis (făr″mă-kō-dī″ăg-nō′sĭs) [″ + *dia,* through, + *gnosis,* knowledge] The use of drugs in making a diagnosis.

pharmacodynamics (făr″mă-kō-dī-năm′ĭks) [″ + *dynamis,* power] The study of drugs and their actions on living organisms.

pharmacoendocrinology (făr″mă-kō-ĕn″dō-krĭ-nŏl′ō-jē) [″ + *endon,* within, + *krinein,* to secrete, + *logos,* word, reason] The pharmacology of the function of endocrine glands.

pharmacoepidemiology The application of the science of epidemiology to the study of the effects of drugs, desired and undesired, and uses of drugs in human populations.

pharmacogenetics (făr″mă-kō-jĕn-ĕt′ĭks) [″ + *genesis,* generation, birth] The study of the influence of hereditary factors on the response of individual organisms to drugs.

pharmacogenomics The study of the effects of genetic differences among people and the impact that these differences have on the uptake, effectiveness, toxicity, and metabolism of drugs.

pharmacogeriatrics The study of the dynamics of medication use in the elderly.

pharmacokinetics (făr″mă-kō-kī-nĕt′ĭks) The study of the metabolism and action of drugs with particular emphasis on the time required for absorption, duration of action, distribution in the body, and method of excretion.

pharmacologist (făr″mă-kŏl′ō-jĭst) An individual who by training and experience is a specialist in pharmacology.

pharmacology (făr″mă-kŏl′ō-jē) [″ + *logos,* word, reason] The study of drugs and their origin, nature, properties, and effects upon living organisms.

pharmacomania (făr″mă-kō-mā′nē-ă) [″ + *mania,* madness] An abnormal desire to give or take medicines.

pharmacopedia (făr″mă-kō-pē′dē-ă) [″ + *paideia,* education] Information concerning drugs and their preparation.

pharmacopeia (făr″mă-kō-pē′ă) [Gr. *pharmakopoeia,* preparation of drugs] An authorized treatise on drugs and their preparation, esp. a book containing formulas and information that provide a standard for preparation and dispensation of drugs.

Pharmacopeia, United States ABBR: USP. A pharmacopeia issued every 5 years, but with periodic supplements, prepared under the supervision of a national committee of pharmacists, pharmacologists, physicians, chemists, biologists, and other scientific and allied personnel. The U.S. Pharmacopeia was adopted as standard in 1906. Beginning with the U.S. Pharmacopeia XIX, 1975, the National Formulary has been included in that publication.

pharmacophobia (făr″mă-kō-fō′bē-ă) [″ + *phobos,* fear] An abnormal fear of taking medicines.

pharmacophore (făr′mă-kō-for) [″ + *phoros,* bearing] The particular group or arrangement of atoms in a molecule that gives the material its medicinal activity.

pharmacotherapy (făr″mă-kō-thĕr′ă-pē) [″ + *therapeia,* treatment] The use of medicine in treatment of disease.

pharmacy (făr′mă-sē) [Gr. *pharmakon,* drug] **1.** The practice of compounding and dispensing medicinal preparations. **2.** A drugstore.

Pharm. D. *Doctor of Pharmacy.*

pharyng- SEE: *pharyngo-*.

pharyngalgia (făr″ĭn-găl′jē-ă) [Gr. *pharynx,* throat, + *algos,* pain] Pain in the pharynx.

pharyngeal (făr-ĭn′jē-ăl) [L. *pharyngeus*] Concerning the pharynx.

pharyngectomy (făr-ĭn-jĕk′tō-mē) [Gr. *pharynx,* throat, + *ektome,* excision] Partial excision of the pharynx to remove growths or abscesses.

pharyngismus (făr″ĭn-jĭz′mŭs) [″ + *-ismos,* condition] Spasm of the muscles in the pharynx. SYN: *pharyngospasm*.

pharyngitis (făr″ĭn-jī′tĭs) [″ + *itis,* inflammation] Inflammation of the mucous membranes and lymphoid tissues of the pharynx, usually as a result of infection.

ETIOLOGY: The disease typically is caused by viral or bacterial infections, including influenza virus, *Streptococcus pyogenes,* or *Mycoplasma pneumoniae*. Occasionally, diphtheria or *Candida albicans* is responsible.

SYMPTOMS: The predominant symptom is throat pain. Fever, malaise, muscle aches, and painful swallowing also are present.

TREATMENT: Gargling with warm salty water provides topical relief. Analgesic drugs, fluids, throat lozenges, or topical anesthetics also are helpful. If rapid tests or culture results identify streptococci, then penicillin or erythromycin usually is curative.

acute p. Inflammation of the pharynx with pain in the throat.

SYMPTOMS: Symptoms include malaise, fever, dysphagia, throat pain, and difficulty swallowing.

TREATMENT: Local treatment includes gargles, lozenges, and topical application to the oral pharynx. General treatment involves bedrest, adequate fluids, and analgesics. An appropriate antibiotic should be given if there is evidence of bacterial infection.

atrophic p. A chronic form of pharyngitis with some atrophy of mucous glands and abnormal secretion.

chronic p. Pharyngitis associated with pathology in the nose and sinuses, mouth breathing, excessive smoking, and chronic tonsillitis. Dryness and irritation of the throat and a cough characterize this condition. Intranasal medication and removal of pathological factors in sinuses and tonsillectomy are the treatment choices.

diphtheritic p. Sore throat with general symptoms of diphtheria and formation of a true membrane.

gangrenous p. Gangrenous inflammation of the mucous membrane of the pharynx.

granular p. Chronic pharyngitis with granulations seen on the pharynx.

p. herpetica Pharyngitis characterized by formation of vesicles and ulcers.

hypertrophic p. Chronic pharyngitis with thickened red mucous membrane on each side with a glazed central portion.

membranous p. Pharyngitis in which a membranous exudate forms a false membrane.

p. ulcerosa Pharyngitis with fever, pain, and the formation of ulcerations.

pharyngo-, pharyng- [Gr. *pharynx,* throat] Combining form meaning *throat.*

pharyngoamygdalitis (fă-rĭn″gō-ă-mĭg″dăl-ī′tĭs) [″ + *amygdale,* tonsil, + *itis,* inflammation] Inflammation of the pharynx and tonsil.

pharyngocele (făr-ĭn′gō-sēl) [″ + *kele,* tumor, swelling] Hernia through the pharyngeal wall.

pharyngoconjunctival fever, acute ABBR: APC. An acute disease consisting of fever, pharyngitis, and conjunctivitis. This disease is caused by adenovirus type 3. It is particularly likely to occur in children in summer camp and may temporarily disable more than half of the campers in a few weeks. Treatment is symptomatic.

pharyngoepiglottic, pharyngoepiglottidean (fă-rĭng″gō-ĕp″ĭ-glŏt′ĭk, -glŏ-tĭd′ē-ăn) [″ + *epi,* upon, + *glottis,* glottis] Concerning the pharynx and glottis.

pharyngoesophageal (fă-rĭng″gō-ē-sŏf′ă-jē″ăl) [″ + *oisophagos,* esophagus] Concerning the pharynx and esophagus.

pharyngoglossal (fă-rĭng″gō-glŏs′ăl) [″ + *glossa,* tongue] Concerning the pharynx and tongue.

pharyngography Radiographical examination of the pharynx after ingestion of a contrast medium.

pharyngokeratosis (făr-ĭn″gō-kĕr″ă-tō′sĭs) [″ + *keras,* horn, + *osis,* condition] Thickening and hardening of the mucous lining of the pharynx.

pharyngolaryngeal (fă-rĭng″gō-lă-rĭn′jē-ăl) [″ + *larynx,* larynx] Concerning the pharynx and larynx.

pharyngolith (făr-ĭn′gō-lĭth) [″ + *lithos,* stone] A stone in pharyngeal walls.

pharyngology (făr″ĭn-gŏl′ō-jē) [″ + *logos,* word, reason] The branch of medicine dealing with the pharynx.

pharyngomaxillary (fă-rĭng″gō-măk′sĭ-lĕr″ē) [″ + L. *maxilla,* jawbone] Concerning the pharynx and maxillae.

pharyngomycosis (făr-ĭn″gō-mī-kō′sĭs) [″ + *mykes,* fungus, + *osis,* condition] Disease of the pharynx caused by fungi.

pharyngonasal (fă-rĭng″gō-nā′săl) [″ + L. *nasus,* nose] Concerning the pharynx and nose.

pharyngo-oral (fă-rĭng″gō-or′ăl) [″ + L. *os,* mouth] Concerning the pharynx and mouth.

pharyngopalatine (fă-rĭng″gō-păl′ă-tīn) [″ + L. *palatum,* palate] Concerning the pharynx and palate.

pharyngoparalysis (făr-ĭn″gō-păr-ăl′ĭ-sĭs) [″ + *paralysis,* a loosening at the side] Paralysis of the muscles of the pharynx.

pharyngopathy (făr″ĭn-gŏp′ă-thē) [″ + *pathos,* disease, suffering] Any disorder of the pharynx.

pharyngoperistole (făr-ĭn″gō-pĕr-ĭs′tō-lē) [″ + *peristole,* contracture] Narrowing or stricture of the lumen of the pharynx.

pharyngoplasty (făr-ĭn′gō-plăs″tē) [″ + *plassein,* to form] Reparative surgery of the pharynx.

pharyngorhinitis (făr-ĭn″gō-rī-nī′tĭs) [″ + *rhis,* nose, + *itis,* inflammation] Inflammation of the nasopharynx.

pharyngorhinoscopy (făr-ĭn″gō-rī-nŏs′kō-pē) [″ + ″ + *skopein,* to examine] Inspection of the nasopharynx and posterior nares.

pharyngorrhea (făr″ĭn-gō-rē′ă) [″ + *rhoia,* flow] Discharge of mucus from the pharynx.

pharyngoscleroma (făr-rĭng″gō-sklē-rō′mă) [″ + *skleroma,* induration] An indurated patch, or scleroma, in the pharynx.

pharyngoscope (făr-ĭn′gō-skōp) [″ + *skopein,* to examine] An instrument for visual examination of the pharynx.

pharyngoscopy (făr″ĭn-gŏs′kō-pē) Visual examination of the pharynx.

pharyngospasm (făr-ĭn′gō-spăzm) [″ + *spasmos,* a convulsion] Pharyngismus.

pharyngostenosis (fă-rĭng″gō-stē-nō′sĭs) [″ + *stenosis,* narrowing] Narrowing or stricture of the pharynx.

pharyngotherapy (făr-ĭn″gō-thĕr′ă-pē) [″ + *therapeia,* treatment] Treatment of pharyngeal disturbances or diseases.

pharyngotome (făr-ĭn′gō-tōm) [″ + *tome,* incision] An instrument for incision of the pharynx.

pharyngotomy (făr-ĭn-gŏt′ō-mē) Incision of the pharynx.

pharyngotonsillitis (fă-rĭng″gō-tŏn″sĭ-lī′tĭs) [″ + L. *tonsilla,* almond, + Gr. *itis,* inflammation] Inflammation of the pharynx and tonsils.

pharyngoxerosis (fă-rĭng″gō-zē-rō′sĭs) [″ + *xerosis,* dryness] Dryness of the pharynx.

pharynx (făr′ĭnks) *pl.* **pharynges** [Gr.] The passageway for air from the nasal cavity to the larynx and for food from the mouth to the esophagus. The pharynx participates in speech as a resonating cavity. SEE: *pharyngitis; mouth* for illus.

ANATOMY: The pharynx is a musculomembranous tube extending from the base of skull to the level of the sixth cervical vertebra, where it becomes continuous with the esophagus. The upper portion, the nasopharynx, is above the soft palate, lined with pseudostratified ciliated epithelium, and has openings to the posterior nares and eustachian tubes. The middle part, the oropharynx, is lined with stratified squamous epithelium and has an opening to the oral cavity. The lowest part, the laryngopharynx, is also lined with stratified squamous epithelium and opens inferiorly to the larynx anteriorly and the esophagus posteriorly.

The pharynx communicates with the posterior nares, eustachian tube, mouth, esophagus, and larynx. The nasopharynx is the section above the palate; the oropharynx lies between the palate and the hyoid bone; and the laryngopharynx is below the hyoid bone.

The nerve supply is from the autonomic nervous system and from the vagus and glossopharyngeal nerves. Blood vessels branch from the exterior carotid artery. Veins form an extensive pharyngeal plexus and drain into the interior jugular vein.

phase (fāz) [Gr. *phasis,* an appearance] **1.** A stage of development. **2.** A transitory appearance. **3.** In chemistry, a distinct component of a larger, heterogeneous system, as oil or water when the two are mixed.

aqueous p. The water portion of a mixture of liquids and solids.

continuous p. The state of a substance in a heterogeneous system in which particles are continuous (e.g., the water particles in which oil has been dispersed).

disperse p. The state of a substance in a heterogeneous system in which particles are separated from each other (e.g., oil particles in water).

lag p. Lag (2).

phasic (fā′sĭk) Of, or pert. to, a phase.

phatnorrhagia (făt″nō-rā′jē-ă) [Gr., socket of a tooth, + *rhegnynai,* to burst forth] Hemorrhage from the socket of a tooth.

Ph.D. *Doctor of Philosophy.*

phenanthrene (fē-năn′thrēn) $C_{14}H_{10}$, a coal tar derivative that is carcinogenic.

phenate (fē′nāt) A salt of phenic acid (phenol).

phenazopyridine hydrochloride (fĕn″ă-zō-pēr′ĭ-dēn) A drug that relieves urinary tract discomfort. It is often given (along with an antibiotic) for urinary tract infections. It causes body fluids to turn red or orange. Trade name is Pyridium.

phencyclidine hydrochloride An anesthetic used in veterinary medicine. It is also used illegally as a hallucinogen, and referred to in slang as "PCP" or "angel dust." The drug is potent; intoxication can occur from passive smoking, and even small doses can produce excitement, hallucinations, and psychotic or extremely violent behavior. Moderate doses also cause elevated blood pressure, rapid pulse, increased skeletal muscle tone, and sometimes, myoclonic jerking. Large doses can cause seizures, ataxia, nystagmus, respiratory depression, and death. The pupils of patients intoxicated with PCP are usually of normal size or small but not the pinpoint size seen in opiate use. This, together with the other physical findings, may help clinicians diagnose overdosed patients.

TREATMENT: For agitation caused by acute intoxication, diazepam is indicated. Because PCP abusers are often hostile, aggressive, and dangerous, efforts to "talk down" these patients are contraindicated. Instead, the patient should be isolated in a quiet room and protective measures taken to avoid injury to self or others.

PROGNOSIS: Despite medication and psychotherapy, the psychotic symptoms produced by PCP may persist for weeks or months.

phenelzine sulfate (fĕn′ĕl-zēn) An antidepressant drug.

phenobarbital (fē″nō-băr′bĭ-tăl) Phenylbarbituric acid, a sedative, hypnotic, and anticonvulsant drug.

sodium p. Soluble phenobarbital; more rapidly absorbed than phenobarbital but with the same uses.

phenocopy (fē′nō-kŏp″ē) [Gr. *phainein,* to show, + *copy*] An individual with a biochemical or physical characteristic that resembles that produced by a genetic mutation but is instead due to an environmental condition.

phenol (fē′nōl) **1.** C_6H_5OH; a crystalline, colorless or light pink solid, melting at 43°C, obtained from the distillation of coal tar. It has a characteristic odor and is dangerous because of its rapid corrosive action on tissues. SYN: *carbolic acid.* **2.** Any of the aromatic derivatives of benzene with one or more hydroxyl groups attached.

p. poisoning Intoxication or chemical burns of the skin, caused by exposure to carbolic acid–containing compounds, such as those found in some dyes, deodorizers, and disinfectants. These substances are corrosive to the skin and mucous membranes. SEE: *Poisons and Poisoning Appendix.*

SYMPTOMS: The patient may present with coagulative necrosis of affected skin or mucous membranes or with evidence of internal organ damage.

TREATMENT: Contaminated clothing should be removed immediately. The skin should then be irrigated with copious amounts of water and either isopropyl alcohol or a polyethylene glycol–containing solution. Patients who have ingested phenols should be treated with activated charcoal, to absorb as much toxin as possible, and general supportive care. Consultation with specialists in toxicology, otorhinolaryngology, and critical care medicine, among others, may be necessary in cases of massive or severe exposure.

p. red An indicator used in determining hydrogen ion concentration.

phenolemia (fē″nō-lē′mē-ă) [*phenol* + Gr. *haima,* blood] The presence of phenol in the blood.

phenology (fē-nŏl′ō-jē) [Gr. *phainesthai,* to appear, + *logos,* word, reason] The study of the effects of climate on living things.

phenolphthalein (fē″nŏl-thăl′ē-ĭn, fē″nōl-thăl′ēn) A white or yellow crystallized powder, produced by the interaction of phenol and phthalic anhydride. It is used as a laxative.

phenolsulfonphthalein (fē″nŏl-sŭl″fōn-thăl′ē-ĭn) ABBR: P.S.P. A substance used to test kidney function.

phenoluria (fē″nŏl-ū′rē-ă) Presence of phenols in the urine.

phenomenology (fĕ-nŏm″ĕ-nŏl′ō-jē) [Gr. *phainomenon,* appearing, + *logos,* word, reason] **1.** The study and classification of phenomena. **2.** The science of the subjective processes by which phenomena are presented, with emphasis on mental processes and essential elements of experiences. A phenomenological study emphasizes a person's descriptions of and feelings about experienced events.

phenomenon (fĕ-nŏm′ĕ-nŏn) *pl.* **phenomena** [Gr. *phainomenon,* appearing] Any observable or objective symptom, sign, event, or fact.

breakaway p. Persons flying in outer space may experience the sensation of losing contact with all other human beings. SYN: *breakoff p.*

breakoff p. Breakaway p.

déjà vu p. SEE: *déjà vu.*

phenothiazines (fē″nō-thī′ă-zēnz) A class of major tranquilizers used to treat psychotic illnesses such as schizophrenia. They have neuroleptic and antiemetic effects. Among the most commonly used agents in this class are chlorpromazine, haloperidol, prochlorperazine, and thioridazine. Side effects of these drugs include dystonic reactions, tardive dyskinesia, seizures, and sedation. Patients who overdose on these medications are treated with airway management, drugs, and fluids to maintain normal blood pressure. Gastric lavage, oral administration of activated charcoal, or both are performed. SEE: *neuroleptic*.

phenotype (fē′nō-tīp) [Gr. *phainein*, to show, + *typos*, type] The expression of the genes present in an individual. This may be directly observable (e.g., eye color) or apparent only with specific tests (e.g., blood type). Some phenotypes, such as the blood groups, are completely determined by heredity, while others are readily altered by environmental agents. SEE: *genotype*.

phenoxybenzamine hydrochloride (fē-nŏk″sē-bĕn′ză-mēn) An alpha-adrenergic blocking agent used to produce peripheral vasodilation.

phenozygous (fē-nŏz′ĭ-gŭs) [″ + *zygon*, yoke] Possessing a cranium much narrower than the face.

phensuximide (fĕn-sŭk′sĭ-mīd) An anticonvulsant drug used in treating absence seizures.

phentermine (fĕn′tĕr-mēn) An amphetamine-like substance that enhances weight loss. When used with fenfluramine hydrochloride, a similar drug, it has been implicated in the destruction of the pulmonary valve of a small percentage of patients.

phentolamine hydrochloride (fĕn-tŏl′ă-mēn) An α-adrenergic blocking agent used in diagnosing pheochromocytoma.

phenyl (fĕn′ĭl, fē′nĭl) The univalent radical of phenol, C_6H_5.

phenylalanine (fĕn″ĭl-ăl′ă-nīn) An essential amino acid; it is one of the two linked amino acids in the sugar substitute Aspartame. The genetically determined inability to dispose of excess phenylalanine is known as phenylketonuria or PKU. SEE: *phenylketonuria*.

phenylamine C_6H_7N; the simplest aromatic amine, an oily liquid derived from benzene. It is used in manufacture of dyes for medical and industrial purposes. SYN: *aminobenzene*.

phenylbutazone (fĕn″ĭl-bū′tă-zōn) A nonsteroidal anti-inflammatory drug used primarily in veterinary medicine. It causes severe bone marrow suppression in humans and is no longer marketed in the U.S.

phenylephrine hydrochloride An adrenergic compound used in a suitably weak concentration to produce nasal decongestion; may also be used in ophthalmic solutions.

phenylethyl alcohol An antibacterial agent that has been used as a preservative in ophthalmic solutions.

phenylhydrazine (fĕn″ĭl-hī′dră-zēn) An oily nitrogenous base used as a test for the presence of sugar in the urine.

phenylketonuria (fĕn″ĭl-kē″tō-nū′rē-ă) ABBR: PKU. A congenital, autosomal recessive disease marked by failure to metabolize the amino acid phenylalanine to tyrosine. It results in severe neurological deficits in infancy if it is unrecognized or left untreated. PKU is present in about 1 in 12,000 newborns in the U.S. In this disease, phenylalanine and its byproducts accumulate in the body, esp. in the nervous system, where they cause severe mental retardation (IQ test results often below 40), seizure disorders, tremors, gait disturbances, coordination deficits, and psychotic or autistic behaviors. Eczema and an abnormal skin odor also are characteristic. The consequences of PKU can be prevented if it is recognized in the first weeks of life and a phenylalanine-restricted (very low protein) diet is maintained throughout infancy, childhood, and young adulthood.

PREVENTION: The U.S. Preventive Services Task Force recommends that all newborns be screened for PKU before discharge from the nursery, or in the first 2 weeks of life. The test's accuracy is highest if it is performed no sooner than 24 hr after birth. Mass screening for the disease began in the 1960s. Some women with PKU are now of childbearing age. During their pregnancies, strict adherence to a low-phenylalanine diet will prevent fetal malformations.

PATIENT CARE: Testing newborns for PKU typically is performed with a heel-stick specimen of blood, which is allowed to dry on blotting paper before being sent to the lab (Guthrie test). If elevated levels of phenylalanine are found, additional tests are performed to confirm the diagnosis.

phenylmercuric acetate (fĕn″ĭl-mĕr-kū′rĭk) A bacteriostatic agent that also acts as a fungicide and herbicide.

phenylpropanolamine hydrochloride (fĕn″ĭl-prō″pă-nŏl′ă-mēn) A sympathomimetic drug used to produce bronchodilation.

phenylpyruvic acid (fĕn″ĭl-pī-roo′vĭk) A metabolic derivative of phenylalanine.

phenylpyruvic acid oligophrenia A form of inherited mental retardation resulting from phenylketonuria.

phenylthiocarbamide (fĕn″ĭl-thī″ō-kăr′bă-mīd) ABBR: PTC. A chemical used in studying medical genetics to detect the presence of a marker gene. About 70% of the population inherit the ability to note the taste of phenylthiocarbamide to be extremely bitter. To the remainder of the population, it is tasteless. The gene for tasting is dominant and is expressed in both homozygous and heterozygous individuals. SYN: *phenylthiourea*.

phenylthiourea (fĕn″ĭl-thī″ō-ū-rē′ă) Phenylthiocarbamide.

phenytoin (fĕn′ĭ-tō-ĭn) An anticonvulsant drug used primarily to treat patients with seizure disorders, including tonic-clonic and partial complex seizures and status epilepticus. It also can be used as an antiarrhythmic drug. Side effects of phenytoin include hyperplasia of the gums, ataxia, nystagmus, and neurological depression. Its use alters the metabolism of many other drugs that the liver degrades.

CAUTION: Because of the drug's effects on heart rhythm, cardiac monitoring is required during intravenous infusions.

pheochrome (fē′ō-krōm) [Gr. *phaios,* dusky, + *chroma,* color] Staining darkly with chrome salts.

pheochromoblast (fē″ō-krō′mō-blăst) [″ + ″ + *blastos,* germ] Embryonic cells that develop into pheochromocytes.

pheochromoblastoma (fē″ō-krō″mō-blăs-tō′mă) [″ + ″ + ″ + *oma,* tumor] A rarely used synonym for pheochromocytoma.

pheochromocyte (fē″ō-krō′mō-sīt) [″ + ″ + *kytos,* cell] A chromaffin cell, such as one of those in the adrenal medulla, that gives a positive chromaffin reaction, that is, it yields a yellowish reaction with chrome salts.

pheochromocytoma (fē-ō-krō″mō-sī-tō′mă) [″ + ″ + ″ + *oma,* tumor] A tumor derived from neural crest cells of the sympathetic nervous system that is responsible for about 0.1% to 2% of all cases of hypertension. The tumor releases catecholamines (e.g., norepinephrine and epinephrine), which cause episodic or sustained signs and symptoms, such as palpitations, sweating, headaches, fainting spells, and hypertensive emergencies. SEE: *catecholamine; multiple endocrine neoplasia; paraganglioma; Nursing Diagnoses Appendix.*

This neuroendocrine tumor is one of the surgically correctable forms of hypertension. It may be difficult to diagnose because the symptoms it causes are found in other, more common conditions, such as anxiety disorders, alcohol withdrawal, and hyperthyroidism, to name just a few.

The tumor is located in the adrenal gland itself in about 85% of cases, but sympathetic tissues are distributed widely throughout the body. As a result, catecholamine-releasing tumors may be found in the urinary bladder, carotid bodies, paravertebral tissues, and other sites in the neck, thorax, abdomen, or pelvis. Neuroendocrine tumors found outside the adrenal glands are called paragangliomas. Some patients have multiple tumors. About 10% of patients with pheochromocytoma also have multiple endocrine neoplasias, one of several genetic syndromes in which pheochromocytomas are associated with adenomas or tumors of other glands.

DIAGNOSIS: The patient's urine or blood is tested to determine whether it contains excessive levels of catecholamines or their metabolites. If so, then imaging studies, such as computed tomography, magnetic resonance imaging, or radioisotope scanning, are used to localize the tumor before surgery.

PATIENT CARE: To collect diagnostic specimens from stress-free subjects, the patient is often placed at bedrest. Drugs are withheld that may block or augment test results for catecholamines or metanephrines. If a tumor is identified and surgery is planned, preoperative hydration of the patient prevents hypotension during anesthetic induction. Medications to blunt the effect of catecholamines (e.g., alpha-adrenergic blocking agents and then beta-adrenergic blocking agents) are administered. Postoperatively, vital signs, cardiac rhythms, fluid balance, and electrolytes are monitored closely. The care team reassures the patient and family throughout diagnosis and management because the symptoms of this condition often fluctuate dramatically.

pheomelanins (fē-ō-mĕl′ă-nĭnz) [″ + Gr. *melas,* black] Yellow-brown, sulfur-containing pigments present as the pigment in human red hair.

pheresis The removal of blood or other body fluids from a patient, separating certain elements (e.g., immunoglobulins, platelets, or red blood cells) and reinfusing the remaining elements into the patient. SEE: *leukapheresis; plateletpheresis; plasmapheresis.*

pheromone (fĕr′ō-mōn) A substance that provides chemical means of communication between animals of the same species. It is probably detected by smell and may affect the development, reproduction, or behavior of other individuals.

Ph.G. *German Pharmacopeia; Graduate in Pharmacy.*

phial (fī′ăl) [Gr. *phiale,* a bowl] A small vessel for medicine; a vial.

Philadelphia collar A lightweight orthosis for the head and neck used to restrict cervical movement.

-philia, -phil, -philic (fĭl′ē-ă) [Gr. *philein,* to love] Combining form used as a suffix meaning *love for, tendency toward, craving for.*

philosophy (fĭ-lŏs′ō-fē) **1.** The love or pursuit of knowledge. **2.** A culturally determined system of beliefs, concepts, theories, or convictions.

philtrum The median groove on the external surface of the upper lip.

phimosis (fī-mō′sĭs) [Gr., a muzzling] Stenosis or narrowness of the preputial orifice so that the foreskin cannot be pushed back over the glans penis. The condition is treated by circumcision.

p. vaginalis Narrowness or closure of the vaginal orifice.

pHisoHex (fī′sō-hĕks) Trade name for an antibacterial skin cleanser containing hexachlorophene as the main ingredient.

phlebalgia (flĕ-băl′jē-ă) [Gr. *phlebos,* vein, + *algos,* pain] Pain arising from a vein.

phlebangioma (flĕb″ăn-jē-ō′mă) [″ + *angeion,* vessel, + *oma,* tumor] An aneurysm occurring in a vein.

phlebarteriectasia (flĕb″ăr-tē″rē-ĕk-tā′zē-ă) [″ + *arteria,* artery, + *ektasis,* dilatation] Dilatation of blood vessels.

phlebectasia, phlebectasis (flĕb-ĕk-tā′zē-ă, -ĕk′tă-sĭs) [″ + *ektasis,* dilatation] Varicosity.

phlebectomy (flĕb-ĕk′tō-mē) [″ + *ektome,* excision] Surgical removal of a vein or part of a vein.

phlebectopia (flĕb″ĕk-tō′pē-ă) [″ + *ek,* out, + *topos,* place] Abnormal position of a vein.

phlebitis (flĕ-bī′tĭs) [″ + *itis,* inflammation] Inflammation of a vein. SYN: *thrombophlebitis*. SEE: *Nursing Diagnoses Appendix.*

ETIOLOGY: Common causes include chemical or mechanical irritation of veins by sclerosing intravenous fluids or indwelling catheters, thrombosis, or venous infections.

SYMPTOMS: The affected vein often is painful, tender, red, or swollen. Inflammation or occlusion of large or deep veins may produce edema distal to the lesion.

PREVENTION: Highly concentrated or irritating infusions should be given through central venous catheters when possible. Irritated or reddened intravenous sites should be changed. Patients with a history of deep venous thrombosis should adhere closely to anticoagulant drug regimens and avoid prolonged sitting or bedrest. They should avoid medications that increase the risk of thrombosis, such as estrogen-containing compounds.

PATIENT CARE: Superficial phlebitis is treated by elevating the extremity and applying warm, moist heat. Any offending solution or catheter is removed from the vein. Phlebitis caused by clots may be treated with antiplatelet or anticoagulant drugs, thrombolytic agents, or, in rare cases, surgery. Antibiotics, surgery, or both, may be required for venous infections.

adhesive p. Phlebitis in which the vein tends to become obliterated.

chemical p. Inflammatory damage to the lining of blood vessels, caused by infusions of highly acidic, highly basic, hypertonic, or sclerosing fluids.

migrating p. A transitory phlebitis that appears in a portion of a vein and then clears up, only to reappear later in another location.

p. nodularis necrotisans Circumscribed inflammation of cutaneous veins resulting in nodules that ulcerate.

obliterative p. Phlebitis in which the lumen of a vein becomes permanently closed.

puerperal p. Venous inflammation following childbirth.

sclerosing p. Phlebitis in which the veins become obstructed and hardened.

sinus p. Inflammation of a sinus of the cerebrum.

suppurative p. Phlebitis characterized by the formation of pus.

phlebo- [Gr. *phleps, phlebos*] Combining form meaning *vein.*

phlebogram (flĕb′ō-grăm) [Gr. *phlebos,* vein, + *gramma,* something written] An infrequently used term for venogram.

phlebography (flĕ-bŏg′ră-fē) [″ + *graphein,* to write] An infrequently used term for venography.

phlebolith, phlebolite (flĕb′ō-lĭth, -līt) [″ + *lithos,* a stone] A stone within a vein.

phlebolithiasis (flĕb″ō-lĭ-thī′ă-sĭs) [″ + *lithiasis,* forming stones] The formation of phleboliths in veins.

phlebology (flĕb-ŏl′ō-jē) [″ + *logos,* word, reason] The science of veins and their diseases.

phlebomanometer (flĕb″ō-mă-nŏm′ĕ-tĕr) [″ + *manos,* thin, + *metron,* measure] A device for the direct measurement of venous pressure.

phlebometritis (flĕb″ō-mĕ-trī′tĭs) [″ + *metra,* uterus, + *itis,* inflammation] Inflammation of uterine veins.

phlebomyomatosis (flĕb″ō-mī″ō-mă-tō′sĭs) [″ + *mys,* muscle, + *oma,* tumor, + *osis,* condition] Thickening of the tissue of a vein from an overgrowth of muscular fibers.

phlebopexy (flĕb′ō-pĕk″sē) [″ + *peksis,* fixation] Extraserous transplantation of the testes for varicocele, with preservation of the venous network.

phlebophlebostomy (flĕb″ō-flĕ-bŏs′tō-mē) [″ + *phlebos,* vein, + *stoma,* mouth] Surgical anastomosis of veins.

phleboplasty (flĕb′ō-plăs″tē) [″ + *plassein,* to form] Plastic repair of an injured vein.

phleborrhagia (flĕb″ō-rā′jē-ă) [″ + *rhegnynai,* to burst forth] Bleeding from a vein.

phleborrhaphy (flĕb-or′ă-fē) [″ + *rhaphe,* seam, ridge] Suturing of a vein.

phleborrhexis (flĕb″ō-rĕk′sĭs) [″ + *rhexis,* rupture] Rupture of a vein.

phlebosclerosis (flĕb″ō-sklē-rō′sĭs) [″ + *sklerosis,* hardening] Fibrous hardening of a vein's walls.

phlebostasia, phlebostasis (flĕb-ō-stā′zē-ă, -ŏs′tă-sĭs) [″ + *stasis,* stoppage] Compression of veins temporarily to restrict an amount of blood from the general circulation. SYN: *bloodless phlebotomy.*

phlebostenosis (flĕb″ō-stĕ-nō′sĭs) [″ + *stenosis,* narrowing] Constriction of a vein.

phlebothrombosis (flĕb″ō-thrŏm-bō′sĭs) [″ + *thrombos,* a clot] Clotting in a vein; phlebitis with secondary thrombosis.

phlebotomist (flĕ-bŏt′ō-mĭst) [″ + *tome,* incision] One who draws blood.

phlebotomize (flĕ-bŏt′ō-mīz) To take blood from a person.

Phlebotomus (flĕ-bŏt′ō-mŭs) [″ + *tome,* incision] A genus of insects, the sandflies, belonging to the family Psychodidae, order Diptera. These blood-sucking insects transmit various forms of leishmaniasis, sandfly (pappataci) fever, and Oroya fever.

P. argentipes In India, the transmitter of *Leishmania donovani,* causative agent of kala-azar.

P. chinensis Transmitter of kala-azar in China.

P. papatasii Transmitter of the causative agent of sandfly fever. The virus is capable of being transmitted through the offspring of flies.

P. sergenti Transmitter of kala-azar in the Middle East and India.

P. verrucarum The transmitter of *Bartonella bacilliformis,* causative agent of Oroya fever (Carrion's disease), in South America.

phlebotomy (flĕ-bŏt′ō-mē) [″ + *tome,* incision] The surgical opening of a vein to withdraw blood. SYN: *venesection.*

bloodless p. Phlebostasia.

phlebovirus (flē′bō-vī-rŭs) Sandfly fever virus.

phlegm (flĕm) [Gr. *phlegma*] **1.** Thick mucus, esp. that from the respiratory passages. **2.** One of the four "humors" of early physiology.

phlegmasia (flĕg-mā′zē-ă) [Gr. *phlegmasia*] Inflammation.

p. alba dolens A complication of deep venous thrombosis of the iliofemoral veins in which the affected leg becomes extremely pale, swollen, and tender. SYN: *milk leg; white leg.* SEE: *deep venous thrombosis.*

cellulitic p. Septic inflammation of the connective tissue of the leg following childbirth.

p. cerulea dolens A complication of deep venous thrombosis of the iliofemoral veins, in which the entire limb distal to the clot becomes swollen, purple, and painful.

phlegmatic (flĕg-măt′ĭk) [Gr. *phlegmatikos*] Of sluggish or dull temperament; apathetic.

phlegmon (flĕg′mŏn) [Gr. *phlegmone,* inflammation] Acute suppurative inflammation of subcutaneous connective tissue, esp. a pyogenic inflammation that spreads along fascial planes or other natural barriers.

diffuse p. Diffuse inflammation of subcutaneous tissues with sepsis.

gas p. Gas gangrene.

phlegmonous (flĕg′mŏn-ŭs) Pert. to inflammation of subcutaneous tissues.

phlogogenic, phlogogenous (flō-gō-jĕn′ĭk, -gŏj′ĕn-ŭs) [Gr. *phlogosis,* inflammation, + *gennan,* to produce] Producing inflammation.

phlorhizin (flō-rī′zĭn) A glycoside present in the bark of some fruit trees. It is a powerful inhibitor of sugar transport in some animals.

phlyctena (flĭk-tē′nă) *pl.* **phlyctenae** [Gr. *phlyktaina*] A vesicle, esp. one of many after a first-degree burn.

phlyctenar (flĭk′tĕ-năr) Concerning a vesicle.

phlyctenular (flĭk-tĕn′ū-lăr) Resembling or pert. to vesicles or pustules.

phlyctenule, phlyctenula (flĭk′tĕn-ūl) [Gr. *phlyktaina,* a blister; L. *phlyctenula*] A small vesicle or blister infiltrated by lymphocytes, as on the cornea or conjunctiva.

phobia (fō′bē-ă) [Gr. *phobos,* fear] Any persistent and irrational fear of a specific object, activity, or situation that results in a compelling desire to avoid the feared stimulus. SEE: *Nursing Diagnoses Appendix; Phobias Appendix.*

social p. Persistent irrational fear of, and the need to avoid, any situation in which one might be exposed to potentially embarrassing or humiliating scrutiny by others. Even the anticipation of a phobia-producing situation, such as speaking or eating in public, socializing, or using a public toilet may cause anxiety or terror. Cognitive therapies, desensitization, relaxation therapy, selective serotonin-reuptake inhibitors, and beta-blocking drugs such as atenolol are used to treat this condition.

-phobia [Gr.] Combining form used as a suffix indicating *fear, aversion.*

phobic (fō′bĭk) [Gr. *phobos,* fear] Concerning a phobia.

phobophobia (fō″bō-fō′bē-ă) [″ + *phobos,* fear] The morbid fear of acquiring a phobia.

phocomelia (fō″kō-mē′lē-ă) [Gr. *phoke,* seal, + *melos,* limb] A congenital malformation in which the proximal portions of the extremities are poorly developed or absent. Thus the hands and feet are attached to the trunk directly or by means of a poorly formed bone. In some cases this condition was due to the pregnant woman taking thalidomide, a sleeping pill, during early pregnancy. That drug is no longer approved for such use. SYN: *amelia*.

phocomelus (fō-kŏm′ĕ-lŭs) A person with phocomelia.

phon- SEE: *phono-*.

phonacoscope (fō-năk′ō-skōp) [Gr. *phone,* voice, + *skopein,* to examine] A device for amplifying the percussion note or voice sounds.

phonacoscopy (fō-nă-kŏs′kō-pē) Examination of the chest with a phonacoscope.

phonal (fō′năl) [Gr. *phone,* voice] Concerning the voice.

phonasthenia (fōn-ăs-thē′nē-ă) [″ + *asthenia,* weakness] Vocal weakness or hoarseness caused by straining the voice.

phonation (fō-nā′shŭn) The process of uttering vocal sounds.

phone (fōn) [Gr. *phone,* voice] A single speech sound.

cell p. A portable telephone, used, for example, in ambulance-to-hospital communications and in 12-lead electrocardiogram transmission in some emergency medical systems.

phoneme (fō′nēm) [Gr. *phonema,* an utterance] In linguistics, the smallest unit of speech that distinguishes one sound from another.

phonendoscope (fō-nĕn′dō-skōp) [Gr. *phone,* voice, + *endon,* within, + *skopein,* to examine] A stethoscope that intensifies sounds.

phonetics (fō-nĕt′ĭks) [Gr. *phonetikos,* spoken] The science of speech and pronunciation. SYN: *phonology*.

phoniatrics (fō″nē-ăt′rĭks) [Gr. *phone,* voice, + *iatrikos,* treatment] The study of the voice and treatment of its disorders.

phonic (fŏ′nĭk) Concerning the voice or sound.

phonism (fō′nĭzm) [″ + *-ismos,* condition] An auditory sensation occurring when another sense is stimulated. SEE: *synesthesia*.

phono- [Gr. *phone,* voice] Combining form indicating *sound, voice.*

phonocardiogram (fō″nō-kăr′dē-ō-grăm) [″ + *kardia,* heart, + *gramma,* something written] A graphic recording of the heart sounds.

phonocardiography (fō″nō-kăr″dē-ŏg′ră-fē) [″ + ″ + *graphein,* to write] The mechanical or electronic registration of heart sounds.

phonocatheter (fō″nō-kăth′ĕ-tĕr) [″ + *katheter,* something inserted] A catheter with a microphone at its end.

phonogram (fō′nō-grăm) [″ + *gramma,* something written] A graphic curve indicating the intensity and duration of a sound.

phonograph (fō′nō-grăf) [″ + *graphein,* to write] An instrument used for the reproduction of recorded sounds.

phonology (fō-nŏl′ō-jē) [″ + *logos,* word, reason] Phonetics.

phonomassage (fō″nō-mă-sahzh′) [Gr. *phone,* voice, + *massein,* to knead] Exciting movements of the ossicles of the ear by means of noise or alternating suction and pressure directed through the external auditory meatus.

phonometer (fō-nŏm′ĕ-tĕr) [″ + *metron,* measure] A device for determining the intensity of vocal sounds.

phonomyoclonus (fō″nō-mī-ŏk′lō-nŭs) [″ + *mys,* muscle, + *klonos,* a contraction] Invisible fibrillary muscular contractions revealed by auscultation.

phonomyogram (fō″nō-mī′ō-grăm) [″ + ″ + *gramma,* something written] A recording of sound produced by the action of a muscle.

phonomyography (fō″nō-mī-ŏg′ră-fē) [″ + ″ + *graphein,* to write] The recording of sounds made by contracting muscular tissue.

phonopathy (fō-nŏp′ă-thē) [″ + *pathos,* disease, suffering] Any disease of organs affecting speech.

phonophobia (fō″nō-fō′bē-ă) [″ + *phobos,* fear] **1.** A morbid fear of sound or noise. **2.** A fear of speaking or hearing one's own voice.

phonophoresis The use of ultrasound to introduce medication into a tissue. This has been used in treating injuries to soft tissues. Not all medicines are suitable for application using this technique.

CAUTION: The use of phonophoresis should be supervised by persons skilled in using the technique.

---

phonopsia (fō-nŏp′sē-ă) [″ + *opsis,* vision] The subjective perception of sensations upon hearing certain sounds.

phonoreceptor A receptor for sound waves.

phonorenogram (fō″nō-rē′nō-grăm) [″ + L. *ren,* kidney, + Gr. *gramma,* something written] A recording of the pulse in the renal artery.

phonoscope (fō′nō-skōp) [″ + *skopein,* to examine] A device for recording heart sounds.

phonoscopy (fō-nŏs′kō-pē) A recording made by use of a phonoscope.

-phoresis (fō-rē′sĭs) [Gr. *phoresis,* being borne] Suffix indicating transmission, as *electrophoresis, cataphoresis, anaphoresis.*

-phoria [Gr. *phoresis,* being borne] In ophthalmology, a combining form meaning *a turning,* with reference to the visual axis, such as cyclophoria.

Phormia (for′mē-ă) A genus of blowflies belonging to the family Calliphoridae. Their larvae normally live in decaying flesh of dead animals, but they may infest neglected wounds or sores, giving rise to myiasis.

phorozoon (fŏ″rō-zō′ŏn) [Gr. *phoros,* fruitful, + *zoon,* animal] The nonsexual stage of an animal that in its life cycle passes through several stages.

phose (fōz) [Gr. *phos,* light] A subjective sensation of light or color. SEE: *chromophose; erythrophose.*

phosgene (fŏs′jēn) [″ + *genes,* born] Carbonyl chloride, $COCl_2$, a poisonous gas that causes nausea and suffocation when inhaled; used in chemical warfare.

phosphagen (fŏs′fă-jĕn) Several chemicals, including phosphocreatine, that release energy when split. They are high-energy phosphate compounds.

phosphatase (fŏs′fă-tās) One of a group of enzymes that catalyze the hydrolysis of phosphoric acid esters. They are of importance in absorption and metabolism of carbohydrates, nucleotides, and phospholipids and are essential in the calcification of bone.

acid p. A phosphatase whose optimum pH is between 4.0 and 5.4. It is present in kidney, semen, serum, and prostate gland, and particularly in osteoclasts or odontoclasts in which it is associated with demineralization or resorption of bone and teeth.

alkaline p. An enzyme, present in the liver, kidneys, intestines, teeth, plasma, and developing bone. Alkaline phosphatase levels greater than 300% of normal usually signify cholestatic disorders like obstructive jaundice or intrahepatic biliary disease.

phosphate (fŏs′fāt) [Gr. *phosphas*] Any salt of phosphoric acid containing the radical PO_4. Phosphates are important in the maintenance of the acid-base balance of the blood, the principal ones being monosodium and disodium phosphate. The former is acid, the latter alkaline. In the blood, because of their low concentration, they exert a minor buffering action.

acid p. A phosphate in which only one or two hydrogen atoms of phosphoric acid have been replaced by a metal.

calcium p. Any one of three salts of calcium and phosphate; used as an antacid and dietary supplement.

creatine p. Phosphocreatine.

normal p. A phosphate in which all three hydrogen atoms of phosphoric acid have been replaced by metals.

triple p. Calcium, ammonium, and magnesium phosphate.

phosphate-bond energy Energy derived from phosphorylated compounds such as adenosine triphosphate (ATP) and creatine phosphate.

phosphatemia (fŏs″fă-tē′mē-ă) [Gr. *phosphas,* phosphate, + *haima,* blood] Phosphates in the blood.

phosphatide (fŏs′fă-tīd) Phospholipid.

phosphatidyl glycerol ABBR: PG. A phospholipid found in amniotic fluid, pulmonary effluent, and semen. It first appears in amniotic fluid during week 36 of pregnancy, confirms fetal gestational age, and is an accurate predictor of fetal lung maturity.

phosphaturia (fŏs″fă-tū′rē-ă) [″ + *ouron,* urine] An excessive amount of phosphates in the urine; often causing renal stones. SYN: *phosphoruria; phosphuria.*

SYMPTOMS: This condition is characterized by cloudy, opaque, alkaline, and pale urine; and pearly or pink-white deposits of phosphates in standing urine.

phosphene (fŏs′fēn) [Gr. *phos,* light, + *phainein,* to show] A subjective sensation of light caused by pressure on the eyeball.

accommodation p. Phosphene resulting from contraction of the ciliary muscles in accommodation. This is seen esp. in the dark.

phosphide (fŏs′fīd) [″ + *phorein,* to carry] A binary compound of phosphorus with an element or radical.

aluminum p. A pesticide used to protect stored grains from insects and rodents; after exposure to water it is converted to hydrogen phosphide, a poison that inhibits cellular oxidative metabolism, esp. in metabolically active organs. It may be toxic or deadly to humans if ingested or inhaled. Its chemical formula is AlP.

TREATMENT: There is no specific antidote. Cardiopulmonary support is given to intoxicated patients.

hydrogen p. A poison that is released when phosphide pesticides react with water. It inhibits oxidative metabolism in cells and may be deadly if eaten or inhaled. Chemical formula is PH_3. SYN: *phosphine.*

zinc p. A toxic pesticide that releases hydrogen phosphide after exposure to water. Its chemical formula is $Z_{n3}P_2$.

phosphine Hydrogen p.

phosphite (fŏs′fīt) A salt of phosphoric acid.

phosphoamidase (fŏs″fō-ăm′ĭ-dās) An enzyme that catalyzes the conversion of phosphocreatine to creatine and orthophosphate.

phosphocreatine (fŏs″fō-krē′ă-tĭn) A compound found in muscle. It is important as an energy source, yielding phosphate and creatine in this process, and releasing energy that is used to synthesize adenosine triphosphate. SYN: *creatine phosphate.*

phosphodiesterase An enzyme critical for the breakdown of cyclic adenosine monophosphate.

phosphofructokinase (fŏs″fō-frŭk″tō-kī′nās) A glycolytic enzyme that catalyzes phosphorylation of fructose-6-phosphate by adenosine triphosphate.

phospholipase (fŏs″fō-lĭp′ās) An enzyme

that catalyzes hydrolysis of a phospholipid.

phospholipid (fŏs″fō-lĭp′ĭd) [Gr. *phos,* light, + *phorein,* to carry, + *lipos,* fat] A diglyceride containing phosphorus, such as lecithin. The lipid portion of cell membranes is primarily phospholipids. SYN: *phosphatide; phospholipin.*

phospholipin (fŏs″fō-lĭp′ĭn) Phospholipid.

phosphonecrosis (fŏs″fō-nĕ-krō′sĭs) [″ + *phorein,* to carry, + *nekros,* dead, + *osis,* condition] Necrosis of the alveolar process in persons working with phosphorus.

phosphonuclease (fŏs″fō-nū′klē-ās) An enzyme that catalyzes the hydrolysis of nucleotides to nucleosides and phosphoric acid.

phosphopenia (fŏs″fō-pē′nē-ă) [″ + *phorein,* to carry, + *penia,* lack] A deficiency of phosphorus in the body.

phosphoprotein (fŏs″fō-prō′tē-ĭn) [″ + ″ + *protos,* first] One of a group of proteins in which the protein is combined with a phosphorus-containing compound. Caseinogen and vitellin are examples. Phosphoprotein was formerly called nucleoalbumin.

phosphor A substance in radiographic intensifying screens, fluoroscopic image intensifiers or other image receptors that convert photons of energy into light, thereby amplifying the image.

rare earth p. An element such as yttrium, gadolinium, or lanthanum, that is used for ultra-high-speed radiographic intensification screens.

phosphorated (fŏs′fō-rā″tĕd) [″ + *phorein,* to carry] Impregnated with phosphorus.

phosphorescence (fŏs-fō-rĕs′ĕns) The induced luminescence that persists after cessation of the irradiation that caused it; the emission of light without appreciable heat.

phosphoribosyltransferase (fŏs″fō-rī″bō-sĭl-trăns′fĕr-ās) An enzyme that catalyzes reconversion to the ribonucleotide stage of the purine bases, hypoxanthine and guanine. The deficiency of this enzyme is inherited as an X–linked trait.

phosphorism (fŏs′for-ĭzm) [″ + ″ + *-ismos,* condition] Chronic poisoning from phosphorus.

phosphorolysis (fŏs″fō-rŏl′ĭ-sĭs) The chemical reaction of incorporating phosphoric acid into a molecule.

phosphorous acid (fŏs-fō′rŭs, fŏs′for-ŭs) [″ + *phoros,* carrying] H_3PO_3; a crystalline acid formed when phosphorus is oxidized in moist air.

phosphoruria (fŏs″for-ū′rē-ă) [″ + *phorein,* to carry, + *ouron,* urine] Phosphaturia.

phosphorus (fŏs′fō-rŭs) [Gr. *phos,* light, + *phoros,* carrying] SYMB: P. A nonmetallic element not found in a free state but in combination with alkalies; atomic weight 30.9738; atomic number 15. The normal serum value of phosphorus is 2.5 to 4.5 mg/dL. Normally, plasma concentrations of phosphorus and calcium have a reciprocal relationship; as one increases, the other decreases.

The adult body contains from 600 to 900 g of phosphorus in various forms: 70% to 80% in bones and teeth, principally combined with calcium; 10% in muscle; and 1% in nerve tissue. Minimum daily requirement is approx. 800 mg. This amount should be increased during pregnancy and lactation. Vitamin D is important in the absorption and metabolism of phosphorus. Excess phosphorus is excreted by the kidneys and intestines, about 60% being excreted in urine principally as phosphates. Abnormal appetite, retarded growth, loss of weight, weakness, rickets, and imperfect bone and teeth development characterize the deficiency of this element.

Phosphorus compounds are found in the nucleic acids DNA and RNA; in adenosine triphosphate, the principal energy source in cells; and in phosphocreatine, a secondary energy source for muscle contraction.

ETIOLOGY: An excess of phosphorus is caused most often by renal disease.

SOURCES: Phosphorus is found in many foods. Excellent sources are almonds, beans, barley, bran, cheese, cocoa, chocolate, eggs, lentils, liver, milk, oatmeal, peanuts, peas, rye, walnuts, and whole wheat. Good sources are asparagus, beef, cabbage, carrots, celery, cauliflower, chard, chicken, clams, corn, cream, cucumbers, eggplant, fish, figs, meat, prunes, pineapples, pumpkin, raisins, and string beans.

p. poisoning Poisoning caused by the ingestion of substances containing yellow phosphorus, such as rat and roach poison. Before the introduction of safety matches (which contain no yellow phosphorus), phosphorus poisoning was quite common. Yellow phosphorus is also used in manufacturing fireworks and fertilizers. SEE: *Poisons and Poisoning Appendix.*

SYMPTOMS: In this type of poisoning acute irritation of the gastrointestinal tract may be followed by liver failure. Kidney damage also may occur. Other symptoms include profound weakness, hemorrhage, and heart failure. Occasionally nervous system symptoms predominate.

PATIENT CARE: Gastric lavage is performed if phosphorus was swallowed. The airway is protected by cuffed endotracheal intubation. Charcoal and a cathartic drug are administered. The patient requires close monitoring for delayed effects for at least 24 hr.

phosphoryl (fŏs′for-ĭl) The radical [PO]≡.

phosphorylase (fŏs-for′ĭ-lās) An enzyme that catalyzes the formation of glucose-1-phosphate from glycogen.

phosphorylation (fŏs″for-ĭ-lā′shŭn) The combining of a phosphate with an organic compound.

phosphuria (fŏs-fū′rē-ă) [Gr. *phos,* light, + *phoros,* a bearer, + *ouron,* urine] Phosphaturia.

phot (fōt) [Gr. *photos,* light] ABBR: ph. The unit of photochemical energy equal to 1 lumen/cm² or about 929 foot-candles.

phot- words beginning with *photo-*.

photalgia (fō-tăl′jē-ă) [Gr. *photos,* light, + *algos,* pain] Pain produced by light.

photaugiaphobia (fō-taw″jē-ă-fō′bē-ă) [Gr. *photaugeia,* glare, + *phobos,* fear] Intolerance of bright light.

photic (fō′tĭk) **1.** Concerning light. **2.** In biology, pert. to the production of light by certain organisms.

p. driving In neurology, altering the electroencephalogram by intermittently flashing light into the eyes.

p. sneezing Sneezing initiated or hastened in its onset by light stimulus. It is sometimes due to light causing tears, which, upon draining into the nasal area, cause sneezing. SYN: *photoptarmosis*.

photism (fō′tĭzm) [″ + *-ismos,* condition] A subjective sensation of color or light produced by a stimulus of another sense, such as smell, hearing, taste, or touch. SEE: *synesthesia.*

photo- [Gr. *photos*] Combining form indicating *light.*

photoactinic (fō″tō-ăk-tĭn′ĭk) Emitting both luminous and actinic rays.

photoaging Skin damage as a result of exposure to ultraviolet rays.

photoallergy (fō″tō-ăl′ĕr-jē) [Gr. *photos,* light, + *allos,* other, + *ergon,* work] A contact dermatitis produced by the interaction between ultraviolet light rays and topically applied chemicals such as sunscreens, perfumes, phenothiazines, sulfonamides, and some components in soaps. Sunlight changes the structure of these chemicals, causing them to become allergens. An eczematous rash results. Avoiding the inciting agent is preventive; topical corticosteroid drugs provide relief from the rash. SEE: *persistent light reaction; photosensitivity; phototoxic.*

photobiology (fō″tō-bī-ŏl′ō-jē) [″ + *bios,* life, + *logos,* word, reason] The study of the effect of light on living things.

photobiotic (fō″tō-bī-ŏt′ĭk) [″ + *bios,* life] Capable of living only in the light.

photocarcinogenesis (fō-tō-căr-sĭn-ō-jĕn′ĕ-sĭs) Malignant skin damage caused by exposure to ultraviolet rays.

photochemistry (fō″tō-kĕm′ĭs-trē) [″ + *chemeia,* chemistry] The branch of chemistry concerned with the effects of light rays.

photochemotherapy The use of light and chemicals together to treat certain conditions, such as psoriasis or cutaneous T cell lymphoma.

extracorporeal p. The exposure of blood that is temporarily removed from the body to ultraviolet A radiation. This is used to treat several diseases, including pemphigus vulgaris and cutaneous T cell lymphoma.

photochromogen [″ + *chroma,* color, + *gennan,* to produce] Certain microorganisms in which a pigment develops when it is grown in the presence of light, such as *Mycobacterium kansasii.*

photocoagulation Thermal alteration of proteins in tissue by the use of light energy in the form of ordinary light rays or a laser beam; used esp. in treating retinal detachments or bleeding from the retina.

photodermatitis (fō″tō-dĕr-mă-tī′tĭs) [″ + *dermatos,* skin, + *itis,* inflammation] Sensitivity of the skin to light; may be due to photoallergy or to phototoxic reaction.

photodynamic (fō″tō-dī-năm′ĭk) [″ + *dynamis,* force] Pert. to the effects of light on biological, chemical, or physical systems.

p. therapy In ophthalmology, the use of laser-activated photosensitizing drugs to treat a variety of tumors and nonmalignant conditions such as age-related macular degeneration.

photodysphoria (fō″tō-dĭs-for′ē-ă) [″ + *dysphoria,* distress] Photophobia.

photoelectricity (fō″tō-ē-lĕk-trĭ′sĭ-tē) [″ + *elektron,* amber] Electricity formed by the action of light.

photoelectron (fō″tō-ē-lĕk′trŏn) [″ + *elektron,* amber] An electron that is ejected from its orbit around the nucleus of an atom by interaction with a photon of energy (light, x-radiation, and so on).

photoerythema (fō″tō-ĕr″ĭ-thē′mă) [″ + *erythema,* redness] Reddening of the skin caused by light.

photofluorography (fō″tō-flū″ĕr-ŏg′ră-fē) Photographing the images seen during fluoroscopic examination.

photogenic, photogenous (fō″tō-jĕn′ĭk, -tŏj′ĕn-ŭs) Induced by, or inducing, light.

photokinetic (fō″tō-kĭn-ĕt′ĭk) [″ + *kinetikos,* motion] Reacting with motion to stimulation by light.

photokymograph (fō″tō-kī′mō-grăf) [″ + *kyma,* wave, + *graphein,* to write] A device for making continuous photographs of a physiological event.

photolabile The characteristic of being destroyed or inactivated by light.

photoluminescence (fō″tō-lū-mĭ-nĕs′ĕns) [″ + L. *lumen,* light] The power of an object to become luminescent when acted on by light.

photolysis (fō-tŏl′ĭ-sĭs) [″ + *lysis,* dissolution] Dissolution or disintegration under stimulus of light rays.

photolytic (fō″tō-lĭt′ĭk) Dissolved by stimulus of light rays.

photomania (fō″tō-mā′nē-ă) [″ + *mania,* madness] **1.** A psychosis produced by prolonged exposure to intense light. **2.** A psychotic desire for light.

photomedicine The use of light to treat certain conditions. SEE: *hemolytic disease of the newborn; phototherapy; psoriasis.*

photometer (fō-tŏm′ĕ-tĕr) [″ + *metron,* measure] A device for measuring the intensity of light.

photometry (fō-tŏm′ĕ-trē) Measurement of light rays.

photomicrograph (fō″tō-mī′krō-grăf) [″ + *mikros,* small, + *graphein,* to write] A photograph of an object under a microscope.

photon (fō′tŏn) [Gr. *photos,* light] A light quantum or unit of energy of a light ray or other form of radiant energy. It is generally considered to be a discrete particle having zero mass, no electric charge, and indefinitely long life.

photo-onycholysis Separation of the nail from the distal nailbed in conjunction with sun exposure and simultaneous use of drugs such as antibiotics.

photo-ophthalmia, photophthalmia (fō″tō-ŏf-thăl′mē-ă, fō″tŏf-thăl′mē-ă) [″ + *ophthalmos,* eye] Keratoconjunctivitis produced by excess exposure to intense light rays.

photoperceptive (fō″tō-pĕr-sĕp′tĭv) [″ + L. *percipere,* to receive] Capable of perceiving light.

photoperiod (fō″tō-pĕr′ē-ŏd) [″ + L. *periodus,* period] The daily duration of exposure to light of a living thing.

photoperiodism (fō″tō-pĕr′ē-ō-dĭzm) [″ + ″ + Gr. *-ismos,* condition] The periodic occurrence of biological phenomena in relationship to the presence or absence of light. In most animals, the sleep-wake cycle is a form of photoperiodism.

photophilic (fō-tō-fĭl′ĭk) [″ + *philein,* to love] Seeking, or fond of, light.

photophobia (fō″tō-fō′bē-ă) [″ + *phobos,* fear] Unusual intolerance of light, occurring in measles, rubella, meningitis, and inflammation of the eyes. SYN: *photodysphoria.*

photophoresis A technique used in treating cutaneous T-cell lymphoma. It incorporates exposure of a lymphocyte-enriched blood fraction, obtained by use of apheresis to ultraviolet A light after the patient has ingested the cytotoxic agent 8-methoxypsoralen. SYN: *extracorporeal photochemotherapy.*

photopia Adjustment of the eye for vision in bright light; the opposite of scotopia.

photopsia, photopsy (fō-tŏp′sē-ă, fō-tŏp′sē) [Gr. *photos,* light, + *opsis,* vision] The subjective sensation of sparks or flashes of light in retinal, optic, or brain diseases.

photopsin (fō-tŏp′sĭn) The protein portion (opsin) of the photopigments in the cones of the retina.

photoptarmosis (fō″tō-tăr-mō′sĭs) [″ + *ptarmosis,* sneezing] Photic sneezing.

photoptometer (fō-tŏp-tŏm′ĕ-tĕr) [″ + *opsis,* vision, + *metron,* measure] A device for determining the smallest amount of light that will make an object visible.

photoradiometer (fō″tō-rā″dē-ŏm′ĕ-tĕr) [″ + L. *radius,* ray, + Gr. *metron,* measure] A device for determining the ability of ionizing radiation to penetrate substances.

photoradiotherapy Photodynamic therapy.

photoreaction (fō″tō-rē-ăk′shŭn) [″ + LL. *reactus,* reacted] A chemical reaction produced or influenced by light.

photoreactivation (fō″tō-rē-ăk″tĭ-vā′shŭn) Enzymatic repair of lesions such as can be produced in DNA by ultraviolet light.

photoreception (fō″tō-rē-sĕp′shŭn) [″ + L. *recipere,* to receive] The perception of light rays in the visible light spectrum.

photoreceptor (fō″tō-rē-sĕp′tor) Sensory nerve endings or cells that are capable of being stimulated by light. In humans, these include the rods and cones of the retina.

photoretinitis (fō″tō-rĕt″ĭ-nī′tĭs) [Gr. *photos,* light, + L. *retina,* retina, + Gr. *itis,* inflammation] Damage to the macula of the eye owing to exposure to intense light. SEE: *blindness, eclipse.*

photoscan A representation of the concentration of a radioisotope outlining an organ in the body. The map is printed on photographic paper. SEE: *scintiscan.*

photosensitivity [″ + L. *sensitivus,* feeling] Sensitivity to light either because of an autoimmune illness, such as systemic lupus erythematosus, or because of the use or application of sensitizing drugs or chemicals.

DRUG-INDUCED PHOTOSENSITIVITY: Individuals using certain drugs or other chemicals may develop dermatitis or sunburn after exposure to light of an intensity or duration that normally would not have affected them. These phototoxic reactions result from interaction between ultraviolet light and chemicals contained in the drug, but are not mediated by the immune system. Agents associated with photosensitizing reactions include coal tar derivatives found in perfumes and dyes, antiemetics, estrogens and progestins, psoralens, sulfonamides, sulfonylureas (oral hypoglycemic agents), thiazide diuretics, and tetracyclines. Persons known to have increased sensitivity to light caused by the medications they are taking should avoid exposure to sunlight or, when in the sun, should use sunscreens or clothing to cover exposed areas of the skin. SEE: *photoallergy*.

photosensitization (fō″tō-sĕn″sĭ-tĭ-zā′shŭn) A condition in which the skin reacts abnormally to light, esp. ultraviolet radiations or sunlight. It is due to the presence of drugs, hormones, or heavy metals in the system. SEE: *photoallergy*.

photosensitizer (fō″tō-sĕn′sĭ-tī″zĕr) A substance that, in combination with light, will cause a sensitivity reaction in the substance or organism.

photosensor A device that detects light.

photostable (fō′tō-stā″b′l) [″ + L. *stabilis*, stable] Uninfluenced by exposure to light.

photosynthesis (fō″tō-sĭn′thĕ-sĭs) [″ + *synthesis*, placing together] The process by which plants manufacture carbohydrates and oxygen by combining carbon dioxide and water, using light energy in the presence of chlorophyll.

phototaxis (fō″tō-tăk′sĭs) [Gr. *photos*, light, + *taxis*, arrangement] The reaction and movement of cells and microorganisms under the stimulus of light.

phototherapy (fō″tō-thĕr′ă-pē) [″ + *therapeia*, treatment] Exposure to sunlight or to ultraviolet (UV) light for therapeutic purposes. One example of phototherapy is the treatment of neonatal jaundice, in which the jaundiced infant is exposed to UV light to decrease bilirubin levels in the bloodstream, thereby reducing the risk of bilirubin deposition in the brain. Phototherapy also is used to treat some skin diseases, including cutaneous T-cell lymphoma and psoriasis, and to relieve the symptoms of seasonal affective disorder. SEE: *photodynamic therapy; seasonal affective disorder*.

CAUTION: The eyes and often the gonads of treated patients are shielded from the light source to prevent them from being damaged.

phototthermal (fō″tō-thĕr′măl) [″ + *therme*, heat] Concerning heat produced by light.

photothermolysis, selective The use of short pulses of light to treat skin conditions. This method causes less damage to normal tissue than do continuous beam lasers. SEE: *laser*.

phototimer SEE: *control, automatic exposure*.

phototoxic (fō″tō-tŏk′sĭk) [″+ *toxikon*, poison] Pert. to the harmful reaction produced by light energy, esp. that produced in the skin. Simple sunburn of the skin is an example of phototoxicity.

phototrophic (fō″tō-trŏf′ĭk) [″ + *trophe*, nutrition] Concerning the ability to use light in metabolism.

phototropism (fō-tŏt′rō-pĭzm) [″+ *tropos*, turning, + *-ismos*, condition] A tendency exhibited by green plants and some microorganisms to turn toward or grow toward light.

photuria (fō-tū′rē-ă) [″ + *ouron*, urine] Excretion of phosphorescent urine.

phren- SEE: *phreno-*.

phrenalgia (frĕ-năl′jē-ă) [Gr. *phren*, mind, diaphragm + *algos*, pain] **1.** Pain of functional origin. **2.** Pain in the diaphragm.

phrenectomy (frĕ-nĕk′tō-mē) [Gr. *phren*, diaphragm, + *ektome*, excision] **1.** Surgical excision of all or part of the diaphragm. **2.** Surgical resection of part of the phrenic nerve.

phrenemphraxis (frĕn″ĕm-frăk′sĭs) [″ + *emphraxis*, stoppage] Crushing of the phrenic nerve in order to induce temporary paralysis of the diaphragm, a therapeutic measure that was previously employed in treatment of pulmonary tuberculosis.

phrenetic (frĕn-ĕt′ĭk) [Gr. *phren*, mind] **1.** Maniacal; frenzied. **2.** A maniac.

-phrenia Combining form indicating *mental disorder*.

phrenic (frĕn′ĭk) [Gr. *phren*, diaphragm] Concerning the diaphragm, as the phrenic nerve.

phrenic (frĕn′ĭk) [Gr. *phren*, mind] Concerning the mind.

phrenicectomy (frĕn-ĭ-sĕk′tō-mē) [Gr. *phren*, diaphragm, + *ektome*, excision] Phreniconeurectomy.

phreniconeurectomy (frĕn″ĭ-kō-nū-rĕk′tō-mē) [″ + *neuron*, nerve, + *ektome*, excision] Excision of part of the phrenic nerve.

phrenicotomy (frĕn″ĭ-kŏt′ō-mē) [″ + *tome*, incision] Cutting of the phrenic nerve to immobilize a lung by inducing paralysis of one side. This causes the diaphragm to rise, compressing the lung and diminishing respiratory movement, thus resting the lung on that side.

phreno-, phren- [Gr. *phren*, mind; L. *phrenicus*, diaphragm] **1.** Combining form meaning *mind*. **2.** Combining form meaning *diaphragm*.

phrenodynia (frĕn″ō-dĭn′ē-ă) [″ + *odyne*, pain] Pain in the diaphragm.

phrenogastric (frĕn″ō-găs′trĭk) [″ + *gaster*, belly] Concerning the diaphragm and stomach.

phrenohepatic (frĕn″ō-hĕ-păt′ĭk) [″ + *hepar*, liver] Concerning the diaphragm and liver.

phrenopericarditis (frē″nō-pĕr″ĭ-kăr-dī′tĭs) [Gr. *phren*, diaphragm, + *peri*, around, + *kardia*, heart, + *itis*, inflammation] Attachment of the heart by adhesions to the diaphragm.

phrenoplegia (frĕn-ō-plē′jē-ă) [Gr. *phren*, mind, diaphragm + *plege*, stroke] **1.** A sudden attack of mental illness. **2.** Paralysis of the diaphragm.

phrenoptosis (frĕn″ŏp-tō′sĭs) [Gr. *phren,* diaphragm, + *ptosis,* a dropping] Downward displacement of the diaphragm.

phrenospasm (frĕn′ō-spăzm) [″ + *spasmos,* a convulsion] Spasm of the diaphragm.

phrenosplenic (frĕn″ō-splĕn′ĭk) [″ + *splen,* spleen] Concerning the diaphragm and spleen.

phthalates (thăl′ātes) Chemical compounds used to improve the flexibility of plastics used in health care (e.g., in intravenous tubing). Some controversial evidence suggests these compounds may have toxic or possibly carcinogenic effects.

Phthirus (thĭr′ŭs) [Gr. *phtheir,* louse] A genus of sucking lice belonging to the order Anoplura.

P. pubis The crab louse. It infests primarily the pubic region but it may also be found in armpits, beard, eyebrows, and eyelashes. SEE: *pediculosis pubis.*

phthisis A wasting illness.

p. bulbi The wasting of ocular tissue.

phyco- [Gr. *phykos,* seaweed] Combining form meaning *seaweed.*

phycology (fī-kŏl′ō-jē) [Gr. *phykos,* seaweed, + *logos,* word, reason] The study of algae.

Phycomycetes (fī″kō-mī-sē′tēz) [″ + *mykes,* fungus] A class of fungi, several genera of which consist of organisms that occasionally cause disease in humans.

phylactic (fī-lăk′tĭk) [Gr. *phylaktikos,* preservative] Concerning or producing phylaxis.

phylaxis (fī-lăk′sĭs) [Gr., protection] The active defense of the body against infection.

phyletic (fī-lĕt′ĭk) [Gr. *phyletikos*] Phylogenetic.

phylloquinone (fĭl″ō-kwĭn′ōn) Phytonadione.

phylogenesis (fī″lō-jĕn′ĕ-sĭs) [Gr. *phyle,* tribe, + *genesis,* generation, birth] The evolutionary development of a group, race, or species. SEE: *phylogeny.*

phylogenetic (fī″lō-jĕ-nĕt′ĭk) Concerning the development of a race or phylum. SYN: *phyletic.*

phylogeny (fī-lŏj′ĕ-nē) Development and growth of a race or group of animals. SEE: *ontogeny.*

phylum (fī′lŭm) *pl.* **phyla** [Gr. *phylon,* tribe] In taxonomy, one of the primary divisions of a kingdom, one division higher than a class.

physaliform, physalliform (fī-săl′ĭ-form) [Gr. *physallis,* bubble, + L. *forma,* shape] Resembling a bleb or bubble.

physaliphorous (fĭs″ă-lĭf′ō-rŭs) Pert. to a highly vacuolated cell present in a chordoma.

physalis (fĭs′ă-lĭs) [Gr. *physallis,* bubble] A large vacuole present in the cell of certain malignancies such as a chondroma.

Physaloptera (fĭs″ă-lŏp′tĕr-ă) [″ + *pteron,* wing] A genus of nematode worms belonging to the suborder Spiruata.

P. caucasica A species that occurs in and damages the upper gastrointestinal tract.

physiatrics (fĭz″ē-ăt′rĭks) [Gr. *physis,* nature, + *iatrikos,* treatment] The curing of disease by natural methods, esp. physical therapy.

physiatrist (fĭz″ē-ăt′rĭst) A physician who specializes in physical medicine.

physic (fĭz′ĭk) [Gr. *physikos,* natural] **1.** The art of medicine and healing. **2.** A medicine, esp. a cathartic.

physical (fĭz′ĭ-kăl) **1.** Of or pert. to nature or material things. **2.** Concerning or pert. to the body; bodily.

p. activity and exercise A general term for any sort of muscular effort but esp. the kind intended to train, condition, or increase flexibility of the muscular and skeletal systems of the body.

p. examination Examination of the body by auscultation, palpation, percussion, inspection, and olfaction.

p. fitness The ability to carry out daily tasks with vigor and alertness, without undue fatigue, and with ample energy to enjoy leisure-time pursuits and meet unforeseen emergencies. It is the ability to withstand stress and persevere under difficult circumstances in which an unfit person would quit. Implied in this is more than lack of illness; it is a positive quality that everyone has to some degree. Physical fitness is minimal in the severely ill and maximal in the highly trained athlete. Persons who maintain a high level of fitness may have increased longevity as compared to those who are sedentary. In addition, the quality of life is enhanced in those who are fit.

physical mobility, impaired A limitation in independent, purposeful physical movement of the body or of one or more extremities. SEE: *Nursing Diagnoses Appendix.*

physical therapy A profession that is responsible for management of the patient's movement system. This includes conducting an examination; alleviating impairments and functional limitation; preventing injury, impairment, functional limitation, and disability; and engaging in consultation, education, and research. Direct interventions include the appropriate use of patient education, therapeutic exercise, and physical agents such massage, thermal modalities, hydrotherapy, and electricity. SYN: *physiotherapy.*

physical therapist assistant ABBR: PTA. A graduate of an accredited physical therapist assistant education program. The physical therapist assistant is a paraprofessional who assists the physical therapist, providing selected interventions under the direction and supervision of the physical therapist.

physical therapy diagnosis **1.** A clinical classification of a patient's impairments, functional limitations, and disabilities by a physical therapist. **2.** The use of data obtained by physical therapy examination and other relevant information to determine the cause and nature of a patient's impairments, functional limitations, and disabilities.

physician (fĭ-zĭsh′ŭn) [O.Fr. *physicien*] A person who has successfully completed the prescribed course of studies in medicine in a medical school officially recognized by the country in which it is located, and who has acquired the requisite qualifications for licensure in the practice of medicine.

attending p. A physician who is on the staff of a hospital and regularly cares for patients therein.

family p. SEE: *primary care p.*

primary care p. A physician to whom a family or individual goes initially when ill or for a periodic health check. This physician assumes medical coordination of care with other physicians for the patient with multiple health concerns.

resident p. A physician who works full or part time in a hospital to continue training after internship; commonly called a resident.

Physicians' Desk Reference ABBR: PDR. An annual compendium of information concerning drugs, primarily prescription and diagnostic products. The information is largely that included by the manufacturer in the labeling or package insert as required by the Food and Drug Administration: indications for use, effects, dosages, administration, warnings, hazards, contraindications, drug interactions, side effects, and precautions.

physician shortage area An area with an inadequate supply of physicians, usually with a physician-to-population ratio less than 1:400.

physicist (fĭz′ĭ-sĭst) [L. *physics,* natural sciences] A specialist in the science of physics.

physico- [Gr. *physikos*] Combining form meaning *physical, natural.*

physicochemical (fĭz″ĭ-kō-kĕm′ĭ-kăl) [″ + *chemeia,* chemistry] Concerning the application of the laws of physics to chemical reactions.

physics (fĭz′ĭks) [Gr. *physis,* nature] The study of the laws of matter and their interactions with energy. Included are the fields of acoustics, optics, mechanics, electricity, and thermodynamics, and ionizing radiation.

physio- [Gr. *physis*] Combining form denoting *nature.*

physiochemical (fĭz″ē-ō-kĕm′ĭ-kăl) [Gr. *physis,* nature, + *chemeia,* chemistry] Concerning clinical chemistry.

physiocogenic (fĭz″ē-ō-kō-jĕn′ĭk) [″ + *gennan,* to produce] Originating from physical causes.

physiocopyrexia (fĭz″ē-ō-kō″pī-rĕk′sē-ă) [″ + *pyressein,* feverish] Fever produced artificially by physical means.

physiognomy (fĭz″ē-ŏg′nō-mē) [Gr. *physis,* nature, + *gnomon,* a judge] **1.** The countenance. **2.** Assumed ability to diagnose a disease or illness based on the appearance and expression(s) on the face.

physiognosis (fĭz″ē-ŏg-nō′sĭs) [″ + *gnosis,* knowledge] Diagnosis determined from one's facial expression and appearance.

physiological (fĭz″ē-ō-lŏj′ĭ-kăl) [Gr. *physis,* nature, + *logos,* word, reason] Concerning body function.

physiologicoanatomical (fĭz″ē-ō-lŏj″ĭ-kō-ăn″ă-tŏm′ĭ-kăl) [″ + ″ + *anatome,* dissection] Concerning physiology and anatomy.

physiologist (fĭz″ē-ŏl′ō-jĭst) A person trained in and capable in the field of physiology.

physiology (fĭz″ē-ŏl′ō-jē) [Gr. *physis,* nature, + *logos,* study] The science of the functions of the living organism and its components and of the chemical and physical processes involved.

cell p. The physiology of cells.

comparative p. The study and comparison of the physiology of different species.

general p. The broad scientific basis of physiology.

pathologic p. The physiological explanation of pathologic events.

special p. The physiology of special organs or systems.

physiopathologic (fĭz″ē-ō-păth″ō-lŏj′ĭk) [″ + *pathos,* disease, suffering, + *logos,* word, reason] **1.** Concerning physiology and pathology. **2.** Pert. to a pathologic alteration in a normal function.

physiotherapy (fĭz″ē-ō-thĕr′ă-pē) [″ + *therapeia,* treatment] Physical therapy.

physique (fĭ-zēk′) [Fr.] Body build; the structure and organization of the body.

physo- [Gr. *physa,* air] Combining form indicating *air, gas.*

physometra (fī″sō-mē′tră) [″ + *metra,* uterus] Air or gas in the uterine cavity.

physopyosalpinx (fī″sō-pī″ō-săl′pĭnks) [″ + *pyon,* pus, + *salpinx,* tube] Pus and gas in a fallopian tube.

physostigmine salicylate (fī″sō-stĭg′mēn săl-ĭs′ĭl-āt) The salicylate of an alkaloid usually obtained from the dried ripe seed of *Physostigma venenosum.*

ACTION/USES: This substance is a cholinergic. It inactivates cholinesterase, thus prolonging and intensifying the action of acetylcholine. It improves the tone and action of skeletal muscle; increases intestinal peristalsis through its effects on the parasympathetic nervous system; and acts as a miotic in the eye. It is used in tetanus and strychnine poisoning and in the treatment of myasthenia gravis.

phytalbumose (fī-tăl′bū-mōs) [Gr. *phyton,* plant, + L. *albumen,* white of egg] An albumose found in plants and vegetables.

phytase (fī′tās) [″ + *ase,* enzyme] An enzyme found in grains and present in the kidneys; important in splitting phytin or phytic acid into inositol and phosphoric acid.

phytin (fī′tĭn) A calcium or magnesium salt of inositol and hexaphosphoric acid, present in cereals. SEE: *inositol.*

phyto-, phyt- [Gr. *phyton*] Combining form indicating *plant, that which grows.*

phytoagglutinin (fī″tō-ă-gloo′tĭ-nĭn) [Gr. *phyton,* plant, + L. *agglutinans,* gluing] A lectin that agglutinates red blood cells and leukocytes.

phytobezoar (fī″tō-bē′zor) [″ + Arabic *bazahr,* protecting against poison] A mass composed of vegetable matter found in the stomach. SYN: *food ball.* SEE: *bezoar.*

phytochemical Any of the hundreds of natural chemicals present in plants. Many have nutritional value; others are protective (e.g., antioxidants) or cause cell damage (e.g., free radicals). Important phytochemicals include indole, phytosterol, polyphenol, saponin, phenolic acids, protease inhibitors, carotenoids, capsaicin, and lignans.

phytochemistry (fī″tō-kĕm′ĭs-trē) [″ + *chemeia,* chemistry] The study of plant chemistry.

phytoestrogen (fī′tō-ĕs′trō-jĕn) Estrogen-like steroid compound found in beans, sprouts, fruits, vegetables, cereals, and some nuts. Phytoestrogens are being examined for their potential role in the management of hormone-sensitive cancers, cardiovascular disease, lipid disorders, and menopause.

phytogenous (fī-tŏj′ĕ-nŭs) [″ + *gennan,* to produce] Arising in or caused by plants.

phytohemagglutinin (fī″tō-hĕm-ă-glū′tĭ-nĭn) [″ + *haima,* blood, + L. *agglutinare,* to glue to] ABBR: PHA. A chemical derived from red kidney beans, used in the laboratory as a mitogen, stimulating T-lymphocyte growth in cultures.

phytoid (fī′toyd) [″ + *eidos,* form, shape] Plantlike.

phytomenadione (fī″tō-mĕn″ă-dī′ōn) Phytonadione.

phytonadione (fī″tō-nă-dī′ōn) **1.** Synthetic vitamin K_1; used as a prothrombogenic agent. **2.** An anticoagulant drug that is little used because of its toxicity. SYN: *phytomenadione.*

phytonutrient (fī″tō-nūt′rē-ĕnt) A metabolically active or nourishing substance derived from plants.

phytopharmacology (fī″tō-făr″mă-kŏl′ō-jē) [″ + *pharmakon,* drug, + *logos,* word, reason] The study of drugs obtained from plants.

phytophotodermatitis (fī″tō-fō″tō-dĕr″mă-tī′tĭs) [″ + *photos,* light, + *derma,* skin, + *itis,* inflammation] A dermatitis produced by exposure to certain plants and then sunlight.

phytoplankton (fī″tō-plănk′tŏn) [″ + *planktos,* wandering] Plant life consisting of the millions of microscopic organisms present in each cubic meter of sea water near the surface.

phytoprecipitin (fī″tō-prē-sĭp′ĭ-tĭn) A precipitin produced by immunization with a plant protein.

phytosis (fī-tō′sĭs) [″ + *osis,* condition] **1.** A disease caused by a vegetable parasite. **2.** The presence of vegetable parasites.

phytosterol (fī″tō-stē′rŏl) Any sterol present in vegetable oil or fat.

phytoremediation The use of trees and plants to remove pollutants from the environment.

phytotherapy (fī′tō-thĕr″ă-pē) The use of plant extracts in the maintenance of health or the treatment of disease.

phytotoxin (fī″tō-tŏk′sĭn) [Gr. *phyton,* plant, + *toxikon,* a poison] A toxin produced by or derived from a plant. SEE: *ricin.*

pI The pH of the isoelectric point of a substance in solution.

pia (pē′ă) [L.] Tender, soft.

pia-arachnitis (pē″ă-ăr″ăk-nī′tĭs) Piarachnitis.

pia-arachnoid Piarachnoid.

Piaget, Jean Swiss philosopher and psychologist, 1896–1980, whose work provided understanding of how children's thinking differs from adults' and of how children learn. Concerning education, he explained, "The goal of education is not to increase the amount of knowledge but to create the possibilities for a child to invent and discover, to create men who are capable of doing new things."

pial (pī′ăl) Concerning the pia mater.

pia mater (pē′ă mā′tĕr) [L. *pia,* soft, + *mater,* mother] A thin vascular membrane closely investing the brain and spinal cord and proximal portions of the nerves. It is the innermost of the three meninges. The other portions of the covering are the dura mater and the arachnoid. SEE: *meninges.*

pian (pē-ăn′) [Fr.] A contagious skin disease of the tropics. SYN: *yaws.*

piarachnitis (pī″ăr-ăk-nī′tĭs) [L. *pia,* tender, + Gr. *arachne,* spider, + *itis,* inflammation] Inflammation of the arachnoid and pia mater. SYN: *leptomeningitis; pia-arachnitis.*

piarachnoid (pī″ăr-ăk′noyd) [″ + ″ + *eidos,* form, shape] The pia mater and arachnoid membranes when regarded as one structure. SYN: *leptomeninges; pia-arachnoid.*

piblokto, pibloktog [Inuit] A syndrome, apparently culturally specific for Eskimo women, in which the individual screams, removes or tears off her clothes, and runs naked in the snow. She then has no recollection of these events.

pica (pī′kă) [L., magpie] An eating disorder manifested by a craving to ingest any material not normally considered as food, including starch, clay, ashes, toy balloons, crayons, cotton, grass, cigarette butts, soap, twigs, wood, paper, metal, or plaster. This condition is seen in pregnancy, chlorosis, hysteria, helminthiasis, and certain psychoses. It may also be associated with iron-deficiency anemia. The importance of this condition, the etiology of which is unknown, stems from the toxicity of ingested material (e.g., paint that contains lead) or from ingesting materials in place of essential nutrients. The inclusion of compulsive ingestion of nonfood and food items such as licorice, croutons, chewing gum, coffee grounds, or oyster shells as examples of pica is controversial. SEE: *appetite; geophagia; taste.*

PICC *Peripherally inserted central catheter.*

pick 1. A sharp, pointed, curved dental instrument used to explore tooth surfaces and restorations for defects. **2.** To remove bits of food from teeth.

Pick, Arnold Czechoslovakian physician, 1851–1924.

P.'s disease A form of presenile dementia due to atrophy of the frontal and temporal lobes. It usually occurs between the ages of 40 and 60, more often in women than in men. The disease involves progressive, irreversible loss of memory, deterioration of intellectual functions, disordered emotions, apathy, speech disturbances, and disorientation. The course may take from a few months to 4 or 5 years to progress to complete loss of intellectual function. SEE: *Alzheimer's disease.*

Pick, Friedel Czechoslovakian physician, 1867–1926.

P.'s disease A form of dementia in which the frontal and temporal lobes of the cerebral cortex atrophy. The disease is sometimes familial.

Pick, Ludwig German physician, 1868–1944.

P.'s cell A foamy, lipid-filled cell present in the spleen and bone marrow in Niemann-Pick disease. SYN: *Niemann-Pick cell.*

P.'s disease Niemann-Pick disease.

pickling 1. A method of preserving and flavoring food in which the food is soaked in a solution of salt and vinegar. **2.** The use of a chemical solution to remove scales and oxides from metals after casting or before plating them.

pickwickian syndrome [Inspired by Joe, an obese character in Pickwick Papers by Charles Dickens.] Obesity, decreased pulmonary function, and polycythemia.

pico- Combining form used to indicate a unit of measurement that is one trillionth of the basic unit.

picocurie ABBR: pCi. An amount of radiation equal to 10^{-12} curies. SEE: *becquerel.*

picogram ABBR: pg. 1×10^{-12} g or 1 trillionth of a gram.

picornavirus (pī-kor″nă-vī′rŭs) [″ + *RNA,* ribonucleic acid, + L. *virus,* virus] Any of a group of very small ether-resistant viruses that includes enteroviruses and rhinoviruses.

picrate (pĭk′răt) A salt of picric acid.

picro-, picr- [Gr. *pikros,* bitter] Combining form meaning *bitter.*

picrotoxin (pĭk″rō-tŏk′sĭn) [″ + *toxikon,* poison] A stimulant to the central nervous system, no longer used as such, obtained from the seed of *Anamirta cocculus,* a shrub.

pictograph (pĭk′tō-grăf) A set of test pictures used for testing vision in children and illiterate adults.

PID *pelvic inflammatory disease.*

piedra (pē-ā′dră) [Sp., stone] Sheath-like nodular masses in the hair of the beard and mustache from growth of either *Piedraia hortai,* which causes black piedra, or *Trichosporon beigelii,* which causes white piedra. The masses surround the hairs, which become brittle; hairs may be penetrated by fungus and thus split. SYN: *tinea nodosa.* SEE: illus.

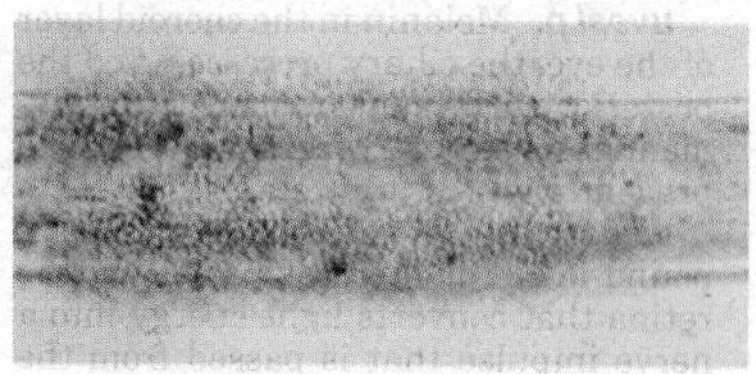

WHITE PIEDRA ON HAIR (X200)

pierce To penetrate body tissue, usually in order to place an ornamental ring or stud on the surface of the skin.

Pierre Robin syndrome [Pierre Robin, French physician, 1867–1950] Unusual smallness of the jaw combined with cleft palate, downward displacement of the tongue, and an absent gag reflex.

piesesthesia (pī-ē″zĕs-thē′zē-ă) [Gr. *piesis,* pressure, + *aisthesis,* sensation] Sensitivity to pressure.

piesimeter, piesometer (pī″ĕ-sĭm′ĕ-tĕr, -sŏm′ĕ-tĕr) [″ + *metron,* measure] A device for measurement of the skin's sensitivity to pressure.

-piesis Combining form used as a suffix meaning *pressure.*

piezoelectricity [″ + *elektron,* amber] Production of an electric current by application of pressure to certain crystals such as mica, quartz, or Rochelle salt. SEE: *triboluminescence.*

PIF *proliferation inhibiting factor.*

pigeon breeder's disease Bird breeder's lung.

pigeon-toed With feet turned inward.

pigment (pĭg′mĕnt) [L. *pigmentum,* paint] Any organic coloring matter in the body. SEE: *albino; carotene; carotenoid;* words beginning with *chrom-.*

bile p. The waste product of the hemoglobin of old red blood cells, found in the bile. Included are bilirubin (orange), biliverdin (green), their derivatives (urobilinogen, urobilin, bilicyanin, and bilifuscin), and stercobilin, which gives brown color to the feces. SYN: *hepatogenous p.*

blood p. A pigment in blood (hemoglobin) or a derivative of it (hematin, hemin, methemoglobin, hemosiderin).

endogenous p. A pigment produced within the human body, as melanin.

exogenous p. A pigment produced outside the human body.

hematogenous p. A pigment from hemoglobin of the erythrocytes.

hepatogenous p. Bile p.

respiratory p. Any pigment such as hemoglobin, myoglobin, or cytochrome that has a part in the metabolism of oxygen within the body.

skin p. Melanin, melanoid, and carotene.

urinary p. Urochrome and sometimes urobilin.

uveal p. Melanin in the choroid layer of the eye, the ciliary processes, and the posterior surface of the iris. Uveal pigment absorbs light within the eyeball to prevent glare.

visual p. A light-absorbing compound in the photoreceptor cells of the retina that converts light energy into a nerve impulse that is passed from the receptor cells to the optic nerve.

pigmentary (pĭg′mĕn-tĕr″ē) [L. *pigmentum,* paint] Concerning, or like, a pigment.

pigmentation (pĭg″mĕn-tā′shŭn) Coloration caused by deposition of pigments. SEE: *albinism; carotenemia;* words beginning with *chrom-.*

hematogenous p. Pigmentation produced by the collection of hemoglobin, or pigment carried to a site through the blood.

pigmented (pĭg′mĕnt-ĕd) Colored by a pigment.

pigmentolysin (pĭg″mĕn-tŏl′ĭ-sĭn) [″ + Gr. *lysis,* dissolution] A substance that destroys a pigment.

pigmentophore (pĭg-mĕn′tō-for) [″ + Gr. *phorein,* to carry] A cell that carries pigment.

pigmentum nigrum (pĭg-mĕn′tŭm nī′grŭm) [L., black paint] The black pigment of the lamina vitrea of the choroid of the eye.

piitis (pī-ī′tĭs) [L. *pia,* tender, + Gr. *itis,* inflammation] Inflammation of the pia mater.

pil L. *pilula,* pill, or *pilulae,* pills.

pila (pī′lă) *pl.* **pilae** [L., pillar] A pillar-like structure in spongy bone.

pilar, pilary (pī′lăr, pĭl′ă-rē) [L. *pilaris*] Concerning, or covered with, hair.

pile [L. *pila,* a ball, a pillar] **1.** A single hemorrhoid. SEE: *hemorrhoid.* **2.** The hair. **3.** A battery for production of electricity. **4.** An apparatus for producing and regulating a nuclear chain-reaction fission process.

sentinel p. A localized thickening of the skin at the distal end of an anal fissure.

pileous (pī′lē-ŭs) [L. *pilus,* hair] Hirsute.

piles (pīls) [L. *pila,* a mass] Hemorrhoids. SEE: *hemorrhoid.*

pileum (pī′lē-ŭm) [L., a cap] Caul.

pileus (pī′lē-ŭs) [L., a cap] Caul.

pili (pī′lē) *sing.,* **pilus** Hairs; in bacteria, filamentous appendages of which there may be hundreds on a single cell. One function of pili is to attach the bacterium to cells of the host; another is to propel the bacterial cell.

p. incarnati The condition of ingrowing hair, esp. in the beard area.

p. tactiles Sensitive or tactile hairs.

p. torti A condition in which hairs are broken and twisted.

piliation (pī-lē-ā′shŭn) [L. *pilus,* hair] The formation and development of hair.

piliform (pī′lĭ-form) [″ + *forma,* shape] Hairlike.

pill (pĭl) [L. *pilula,* small mass] **1.** Medicine in the form of a tiny solid mass or pellet to be swallowed or chewed; may be coated. **2.** Birth control pill.

morning-after p. A pill containing an estrogen or synthetic estrogen that can be taken after intercourse to prevent pregnancy.

pillar (pĭl′ĕr) [L. *pila,* a column] An upright support, column, or structure resembling a column.

anterior p. of the fornix One of two diverging columns extending downward from the anterior extremity of body of the fornix of the cerebrum.

p. cell One of two groups of cells (inner and outer) resting on the basement membrane of the organ of Corti in which elongated bodies (pillars) develop. These enclose the inner tunnel (Corti's tunnel).

p. of Corti Pillar cell.

p. of the diaphragm Crura of the diaphragm, two bundles of muscle fibers extending from the lumbar vertebrae to the central tendon and forming the sides of the hiatus aorticus.

p. of the fauces Folds of mucous membrane, one on each side of the fauces and between which is situated the tonsil. SYN: *glossopalatine arch; pharyngopalatine arch.*

pillion (pĭl′yŭn) [L. *pellis,* skin] A temporary form of artificial leg, esp. a peg-leg type of stump.

pilo- [L. *pilus*] Combining form indicating *hair.*

pilobezoar (pī″lō-bē′zor) [″ + Arabic *bazahr,* protecting against poison] Trichobezoar.

pilocarpine hydrochloride (pī″lō-kăr′pĭn) $C_{11}H_{16}N_2O_2 \cdot HCl$; the hydrochloride of an alkaloid obtained from leaflets of *Pilocarpus jaborandi* and *P. microphyllus.*

ACTION/USES: It is used as a cholinergic. Because it causes contraction of the pupil, it is used topically as a miotic, esp. in glaucoma.

pilocarpine nitrate A nitrate of the alkaloid obtained from leaves of the jaborandi tree. Uses are the same as for pilocarpine hydrochloride.

pilocystic (pī″lō-sĭs′tĭk) [L. *pilus,* hair, + Gr. *kystis,* bladder] Encysted and containing hair, said of a dermoid cyst.

piloerection Elevation of the hair above the skin as a result of contraction of the arrector pili muscles. This may occur after exposure to the cold or during adrenergic stimulation. SYN: *cutis anserina; goose flesh; horripilation.*

pilojection [″ + *jacere,* to throw] Introduction of hairs, by use of a pneumatic gun, into an aneurysm to induce clotting in the aneurysmal sac. It has been used in treating intracranial aneurysms.

pilomotor (pī″lō-mō′tor) [″ + *motor,* mover] Causing movements of hairs, as the arrectores pilorum.

pilonidal (pī″lō-nī′dăl) [″ + *nidus,* nest] Containing hairs most often seen in a dermoid cyst, esp. in the saccrococcygeal region.

pilosebaceous (pī″lō-sē-bā′shŭs) [″ + *sebaceus,* fatty] Concerning the hair and sebaceous glands.

Piltz's reflex (pĭlts′ĕz) [Jan Piltz, Polish neurologist, 1870–1931] Change in the size of the pupil on sudden fixation of attention. SYN: *pupillary reflex.*

pilus (pī′lŭs) *pl.* **pili** [L.] A hair.

p. cuniculatus A hair that burrows into the skin.

p. incarnatus An ingrown hair.

p. tortus A twisted hair.

PImax *maximum inspiratory pressure.* SEE: *force, maximum inspiratory.*

pimel-, pimelo [Gr. *pimele,* fat] Combining form meaning *fat* or *fatty.*

pimelopterygium (pĭm″ĕ-lō-tĕ-rĭj′ē-ŭm) [″ + *pterygion,* wing] A fatty outgrowth of the conjunctiva.

pimelorthopnea (pĭm″ĕl-or″thŏp′nē-ă) [″ + *orthos,* straight, + *pnoia,* breath] Difficulty in breathing when lying down, due to obesity.

pimelosis (pĭm″ĕ-lō′sĭs) [″ + *osis,* condition] **1.** Conversion into fat. **2.** Fatty degeneration of any tissue. **3.** Obesity.

pimple (pĭm′pl) [ME. *pinple*] A papule or pustule of the skin often seen in clusters on skin of the adolescent with acne.

pin A short, slim piece of wire, plastic, or metal. It may have one end blunt and the other sharp.

endodontic p. A straight or threaded pin that is passed through the root canal to the alveolar bone beyond the apex of the tooth root.

self-threading p. A pin screwed through a small hole into dentin.

sprue p. In dentistry, a wax, plastic, or metal pattern used to make the channel or channels through which molten metal flows into a mold to make a casting. Also called *sprue former.*

pincement (păns-mŏn′) [Fr.] Pinching or nipping of the flesh in massage.

pinch A type of hand prehension. The pinch of the human hand is achieved principally through holding objects between the thumb and index finger or the index and long fingers.

Hand pinch is classified according to the anatomical parts involved, as follows:

Pinch, fingertip—pinch using the tips of strongly arched digits, primarily the thumb and index finger; used to pick up very small objects such as pins and needles.

Pinch, palmar tripod or three-jaw chuck—pinch using the palmar pads of the thumb and index and long fingers.

Pinch, lateral—pinch accomplished by clamping the palmar surface of the distal portion of the thumb against the side of the index finger.

pinch meter A device for objectively measuring the strength of hand pinch in grams or pounds.

pindolol (pĭn′dō-lōl) A β-adrenergic blocking agent.

pineal (pĭn′ē-ăl) [Fr., pine cone] **1.** Shaped like a pine cone. **2.** Pert. to the pineal gland.

pinealectomy (pĭn″ē-ăl-ĕk′tō-mē) [L. *pineus,* of the pine, + Gr. *ektome,* excision] Removal of the pineal gland.

pinealoblastoma (pĭn″ē-ă-lō-blăs-tō′mă) [″ + Gr. *blastos,* germ, + *oma,* tumor] Pineoblastoma.

pinealocyte (pĭn′ē-ă-lō-sīt″) [″ + Gr. *kytos,* cell] The principal cell of the pineal gland. It contains pale-staining cytoplasm and has long processes that terminate in bulbous expansions.

pinealoma (pĭn″ē-ă-lō′mă) [″ + Gr. *oma,* tumor] A tumor of the pineal gland, usually encapsulated; often associated with precocious puberty.

pinealopathy (pĭn″ē-ă-lŏp′ă-thē) [″ + Gr. *pathos,* disease, suffering] Any disorder of the pineal gland.

Pinel, Philippe (pē-nĕl′) French psychologist, 1745–1826, who developed a method or system of treating the mentally ill without the use of restraint, at a time when use of restraint was the accepted form of therapy.

pineoblastoma (pĭn″ē-ō-blăs-tō′mă) [L. *pineus,* of the pine, + Gr. *blastos,* germ, + *oma,* tumor] A malignant tumor of the pineal gland that may occur in childhood and early adulthood. SYN: *pinealoblastoma.*

pineocytoma A malignant tumor of the pineal gland of the brain.

ping-ponging [Ping Pong, trademark for table tennis] The transmission of an infectious disease, esp. a sexually transmitted one, between two people. After the first person has been cured, the second person reinfects the first.

pinguecula (pĭn-gwĕk′ū-lă) [L. *pinguiculus,* fatty] A yellow triangular thickening of the bulbar conjunctiva on the inner and outer margins of the cornea. The base of the triangle is toward the limbus. The yellow color is due to an increase in elastic fibers.

pinhole (pĭn′hōl) [AS. *pinn,* pin, + *hol,* hole] A small perforation made by, or size of that made by, a pin.

p. os A very small opening to the uterus from the vagina. It may be present in very young women.

piniform (pĭn′ĭ-form) [L. *pinea,* pine cone, + *forma,* shape] Conical; shaped like a pine cone.

pink disease Acrodynia.

pinkeye [D. *pinck oog*] Acute conjunctivitis. Depending on the cause, this may be treated conservatively (e.g., with warm, moist compresses) or with antibiotics when bacteria are the cause.

pinna (pĭn′ă) *pl.* **pinnae** [L., feather] **1.** The auricle or projected part of the external ear. It directs sound waves into the external acoustic meatus toward the tympanic membrane. **2.** A feather, fin, wing, or similar appendage.

p. nasi A protruding cartilaginous extension on each nostril. SYN: *ala nasi.*

pinnal (pĭn′ăl) Concerning pinna.

pinocyte (pī′nō-sīt) [Gr. *pinein,* to drink, + *kytos,* cell] A cell that exhibits pinocytosis.

pinocytosis (pī″nō-sī-tō′sĭs) [″ + ″ + *osis,* condition] The process by which cells absorb or ingest nutrients and fluid. An invaginating portion of the cell membrane encircles the nutrient, enclosing it in a membrane-bound sac. The sac is brought into the cell and its contents are digested. SEE: illus.

pinosome (pī′nō-, pĭn′ō-sōm) [″ + *soma,* body] The fluid-filled vacuole formed during pinocytosis.

PINS *persons in need of supervision.*

Pins' sign [Emil Pins, Aust. physician, 1845–1913] In pericarditis, disappearance of symptoms of pleurisy when the patient assumes knee-chest position.

PINOCYTOSIS

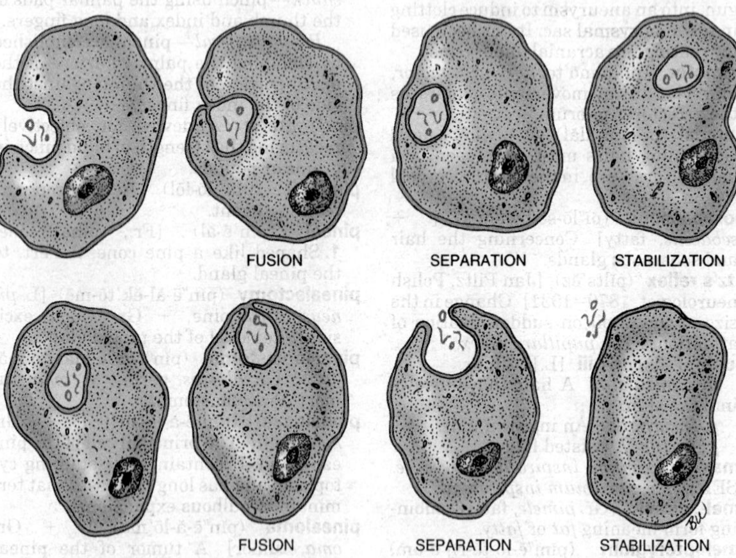

EXOCYTOSIS

pint (pīnt) [ME. *pinte*] ABBR: pt. In the U.S. a measure of capacity equal to ½ qt.; 16 fl. oz; 473.2 ml. SEE: *Weights and Measures Appendix.*

pinta (pēn′tă) [Sp., paint] A nonvenereal disease spread by body contact, caused by the spirochete *Treponema carateum.* It is manifested by depigmented spots or patches. The treatment is administration of penicillin.

pintid (pĭn′tĭd) A flat red skin lesion present in the second stage of pinta.

pinus (pī′nŭs) [L., pine] Pert. to the pineal gland.

pinworm *Enterobius vermicularis.*

pioepithelium (pī″ō-ĕp″ĭ-thē′lē-ŭm) [Gr. *pion,* fat, + *epi,* upon, + *thele,* nipple] Epithelium that contains fat globules.

pion therapy The use of subatomic particles, called pions, to treat brain cancers and some sarcomas.

Piper (pī′pĕr) [L.] Genus of plants that produce pepper.

Piper forceps Forceps designed to deliver the infant's head during a breech delivery, after other maneuvers to deliver the head have failed.

piperazine (pī-pĕr′ă-zēn) A white crystalline powder used in the treatment of ascariasis and enterobiasis.

piperoxan (pī″pĕr-ŏks′ăn) An alpha-adrenergic blocking agent effective in inhibiting the response to catecholamines.

pipet, pipette (pī-pĕt′) [Fr. *pipette,* tiny pipe] Narrow glass tube with both ends open for transferring and measuring liquids by suctioning them into the tube.

pipobroman (pī″pō-brō′măn) A cytotoxic drug used principally to treat polycythemia rubra vera.

piriform, pyriform (pĭr′ĭ-form) [L. *pirum,* pear, + *forma,* shape] Pear-shaped.

piriformis syndrome A condition marked by pain in the hip and buttock that radiates up into the lower back and down the leg. In women, the pain may occur during sexual intercourse. This is caused by entrapment of the sciatic nerve as it passes through the piriformis muscle in the buttock. Because the symptoms mimic those caused by a herniated lumbar disk, the syndrome may be confused with that disease. Treatment includes physical therapy to relieve pressure, ultrasound to reduce muscle spasm, and anti-inflammatory medicines. Surgical therapy to free the entrapped nerve may be necessary. SEE: *sciatica.*

Pirogoff's amputation (pĭr″ō-gŏfs′) [Nikolai Ivanovich Pirogoff, Russ. surgeon, 1810–1881] Foot amputation at the ankle, removing a portion of the os calcis.

piroplasm (pī′rō-plăzm) A member of a class of parasitic protozoa that can cause both human and animal diseases. SEE: *babesia.*

Pirquet's test (pĕr-kāz′) [Clemens Peter Johann von Pirquet, Austrian pediatrician, 1874–1929] A test for tuberculosis by means of a skin reaction, used esp. in children.

piscicide (pĭs′ĭ-sīd) [L. *piscis,* fish, + *caedere,* to kill] An agent that kills fish.

pisiform (pī′sĭ-form) [L. *pisum,* pea, + *forma,* shape] **1.** Pea-shaped. **2.** The smallest carpal bone, located in the flexor carpi ulnaris tendon as a sesamoid bone, on the ulnar side in the proximal row of carpals.

pit (pĭt) [ME. *pitt,* hole] **1.** A tiny hollow or pocket. SYN: *depression; fossa.* **2.** To be or become marked with a shallow depression; to cause a depression on pressure in edema. **3.** A small depression in the enamel surface of a tooth often connected with one or more developmental grooves. It contributes to pit and fissure caries. SYN: *occlusal p.*

anal p. Proctodeum.

auditory p. A pit that develops in the auditory placode.

costal p. The inferior facet on the body of a thoracic vertebra. It articulates with the head of a rib.

gastric p. One of many minute depressions (foveolae) in the gastric mucosa into which the gastric glands open.

lens p. The depression on the skin of the embryonic head where the lens of the eye will develop.

nasal p. In the embryo, one of two horseshoe-shaped depressions on the ventrolateral surface of the head bounded by lateral and median nasal processes. It gives rise to nostrils and a portion of the nasal fossa. SYN: *olfactory p.*

occlusal p. Pit (3).

olfactory p. Nasal p.

primitive p. A minute depression at the anterior end of the primitive groove or streak and immediately posterior to the primitive knot.

p. of the stomach **1.** The depression at the end of the xiphoid process. **2.** The center of the abdominal region above the navel.

pitch (pĭch) [ME. *picchen,* to fix] **1.** That quality of the sensation of sound that enables one to classify it in a scale from high to low. It is dependent principally on frequency of vibrations. **2.** Residue obtained from distillation of coal or wood tar.

pitchblende (pĭch′blĕnd) Uraninite, the principal source of uranium. It is a mineral that resembles pitch.

pith (pĭth) **1.** The center of a hair or the soft material in the stalk of a plant. **2.** Destruction of a part of the central nervous system of an animal being prepared for certain experiments. A blunt probe is inserted in the brain or spinal cord through a foramen.

pithing (pĭth'ĭng) [ME. *pithe*] Destruction of the central nervous system by the piercing of brain or spinal cord, as in vivisection. This is done on experimental animals to render them insensible to pain and to inhibit controlling effects of the central nervous system during research and experimentation. SEE: *decerebration*.

pithode (pī'thōd) [Gr. *pithose,* wine cask, + *eidos,* form, shape] The barrel-shaped spindle formed during karyokinesis.

Pitres' section (pē-trēs') [Jean A. Pitres, Fr. physician, 1848–1927] Any of the series of six coronal vertical sections of the brain for study. The sections are prefrontal, pediculofrontal, frontal, parietal, pediculoparietal, and occipital.

pitting (pĭt'ĭng) [ME. *pitt,* hole] **1.** The formation of pits, depressions, or scars, as in smallpox. **2.** In the spleen, removal of the remains of red blood cells that have completed their lifespan or have been injured. Nucleated red blood cells are also removed from circulating blood in this pitting function. SEE: *culling*. **3.** In dentistry, the formation of depressions in the materials used in restoring teeth. **4.** In radiography, the imperfections created on the face of the x-ray tube anode by overloading current limits.

pituicyte (pĭ-tū'ĭ-sīt) [L. *pituita,* phlegm, + Gr. *kytos,* cell] A modified branched neuroglia cell characteristic of pars nervosa of the posterior lobe of the pituitary gland; also present in the infundibular stalk.

pituitary (pĭ-tū'ĭ-tăr"ē) [L. *pituitarius,* phlegm] The pituitary body or gland. SYN: *hypophysis*. SEE: *releasing hormone; inhibitory hormone; pituitary gland*.

anterior p. A preparation consisting of dried, defatted, powdered anterior lobe of the pituitary gland of domestic animals.

posterior p. The dried, powdered posterior lobe of the pituitary gland of animals used as food by humans.

whole p. The dried, defatted, powdered entire pituitary gland of domestic animals.

pituitary gland A small, gray, rounded gland that develops from ingrown oral epithelium (Rathke's pouch) and is attached to the lower surface of the hypothalamus by the infundibular stalk. The Rathke's pouch portion forms the anterior lobe and an intermediate area; the neural tissue of the infundibular stalk forms the posterior lobe. The pituitary gland averages 1.3 × 1.0 × 0.5 cm in size and weighs 0.55 to 0.6 g. SYN: *hypophysis cerebri*. SEE: illus. (Pituitary Gland and Hypothalamus).

FUNCTION: The pituitary is an endocrine gland secreting a number of hormones that regulate many bodily processes including growth, reproduction, and various metabolic activities. It is often referred to as the "master gland of the body." SEE: illus. (Pituitary Hormones and Target Organs).

Hormones are secreted in the following lobes: *Intermediate lobe:* In cold-blooded animals, intermedin is secreted, influencing the activity of pigment cells (chromatophores) of fishes, amphibians, and reptiles. In warm-blooded animals, no effects are known.

Anterior lobe: Secretions here are the somatotropic, or growth hormone (STH or GH), which regulates cell division and protein synthesis for growth; adrenocorticotropic hormone (ACTH), which regulates functional activity of the adrenal cortex; thyrotropic hormone (TTH or TSH), which regulates functional activity of the thyroid gland; and the following gonadotropic hormones: In women, follicle-stimulating hormone (FSH) stimulates development of ovarian follicles and their secretion of estrogen; in men, it stimulates spermatogenesis in the testes. In women, luteinizing hormone stimulates ovulation and formation of the corpus luteum and its secretion of estrogen and progesterone. In men LH, also called interstitial cell-stimulation hormone (ICSH), stimulates testoterone secretion. Prolactin, also called lactogenic hormone, induces secretion of milk in the adult female.

Posterior lobe: Hormones are secreted by the neurosecretory cells of the hypothalamus and pass through fibers of the supraopticohypophyseal tracts in the infundibular stalk to the neurohypophysis, where they are stored. Secretions here are oxytocin, which acts specifically on smooth muscle of the uterus, increasing tone and contractility; and antidiuretic hormone (ADH), which increases reabsorption of water by the kidney tubules. ADH also has a vasopressor effect and may be called vasopressin.

DISORDERS: *Hypersecretion of anterior lobe* causes gigantism, acromegaly, and pituitary basophilism (Cushing's disease). *Hyposecretion of anterior lobe* causes dwarfism, pituitary cachexia (Simmonds' disease), Sheehan's syndrome, acromicria, eunuchoidism or hypogonadism. *Posterior lobe deficiency* or *hypothalamic lesion* causes diabetes insipidus. *Anterior and posterior lobe deficiency* and *hypothalamic lesion* cause Fröhlich's syndrome (adiposogenital dystrophy) and pituitary obesity.

pituitary (injection), posterior Antidiuretic hormone.

pityriasis (pĭt"ĭ-rī'ă-sĭs) [Gr. *pityron,*

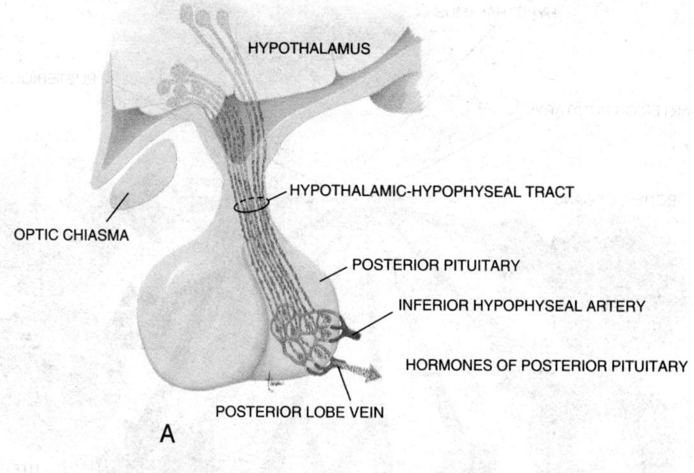

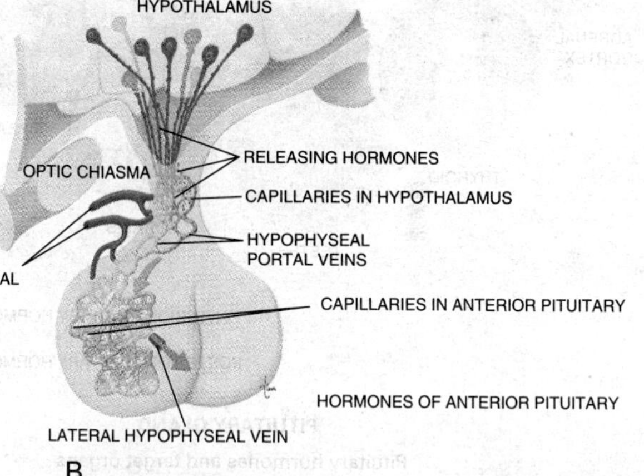

PITUITARY GLAND AND HYPOTHALAMUS

(A) posterior, (B) anterior

bran, + *-iasis,* disease] A skin disease characterized by branny scales.

p. alba A form of decreased melanin in the skin marked by patches of round or oval macular skin lesions with fine adherent scales. The lesions are commonly seen in the facial areas of children. They are virtually painless and usually require no therapy. They may disappear spontaneously. The etiology is unknown, but the disease is regarded as a mild form of eczema.

p. capitis Dandruff.

p. lichenoides, acute A skin disorder characterized by development of an edematous pink papule that undergoes central vesiculation and hemorrhagic necrosis. The lesions clear spontaneously after weeks or months but leave scars.

p. linguae Transitory benign plaques of the tongue. SYN: *geographic tongue.*

p. nigra Tinea nigra.

p. rosea An acute inflammatory skin disease of unknown etiology, marked by a macular eruption on the trunk, obliquely to the ribs, and on the upper extremities. The initial (herald) patch appears in more than half of the cases. In a few days it enlarges to several centimeters. Then, within 2 to 21 days, secondary eruptions occur. They are rose-red and somewhat scaly with a clearing in the center, or reddish ring-shaped patches symmetrically distributed over the limbs. The symptoms disappear spontaneously within 2 to 10 weeks. Treatment consists of the local application of antipruritics.

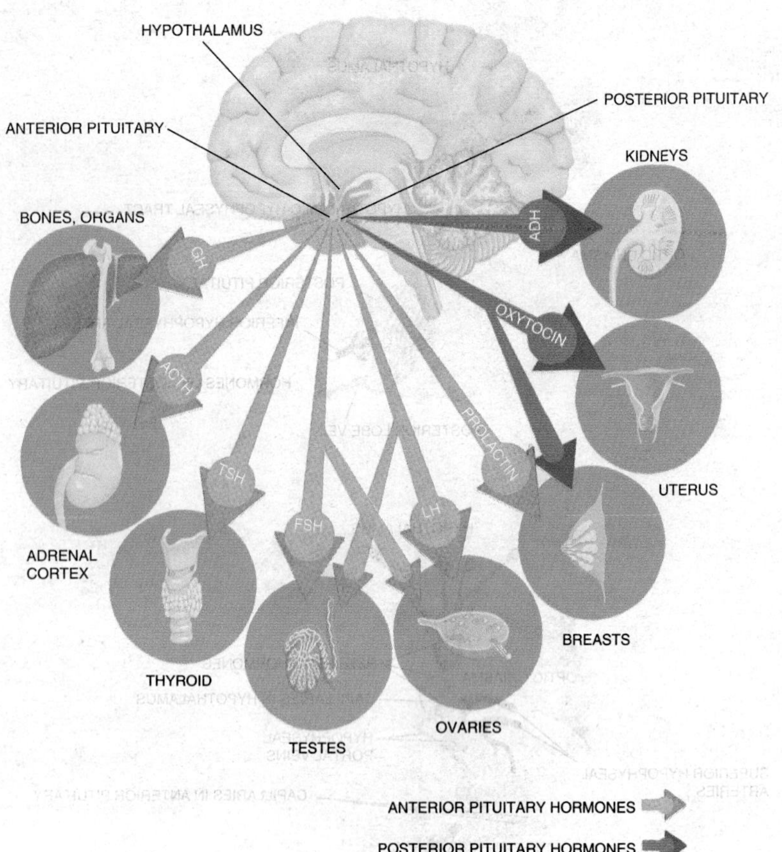

PITUITARY GLAND

Pituitary hormones and target organs

p. rubra pilaris Persistent general exfoliative dermatitis of unknown etiology. SEE: *exfoliative dermatitis*.

p. versicolor Tinea versicolor.

pivot (pĭv′ŭt) In dentistry, a part used for attaching an artificial crown to the base of a natural tooth.

pix (pĭks) [L.] Tar.

PJC *premature junctional contraction.*

PK *psychokinesis.*

pK Abbreviation for the negative logarithm of the ionization constant, called K, of an acid. The closer the pK to the pH, the greater the buffering power of the system.

PKU *phenylketonuria.*

placebo (plă-sē′bō) [L., I shall please] **1.** An inactive substance given to satisfy a patient's demand for medicine. **2.** A drug or treatment used as a nonspecific or inactive control in a test of a therapy that is suspected of being useful for a particular disease or condition. The placebo is given to one group of patients and the drug being tested is given to a similar group; then the results obtained in the two groups are compared. Although a placebo is believed to lack a specific effect, it is often found that administering a placebo elicits a positive patient response. It has been hypothesized that the psychological effects of the patient's expectations of benefit are responsible for the result. SEE: *double-blind technique*.

placenta (plă-sĕn′tă) *pl.* **placentae, placentas** [L., a flat cake] The oval or discoid spongy structure in the uterus of eutherian mammals from which the fetus derives its nourishment and oxygen. SEE: illus. **placental,** *adj.*

ANATOMY: The placenta consists of a fetal portion, the chorion frondosum, bearing many chorionic villi that interlock with the decidua basalis of the uterus, which constitutes the maternal

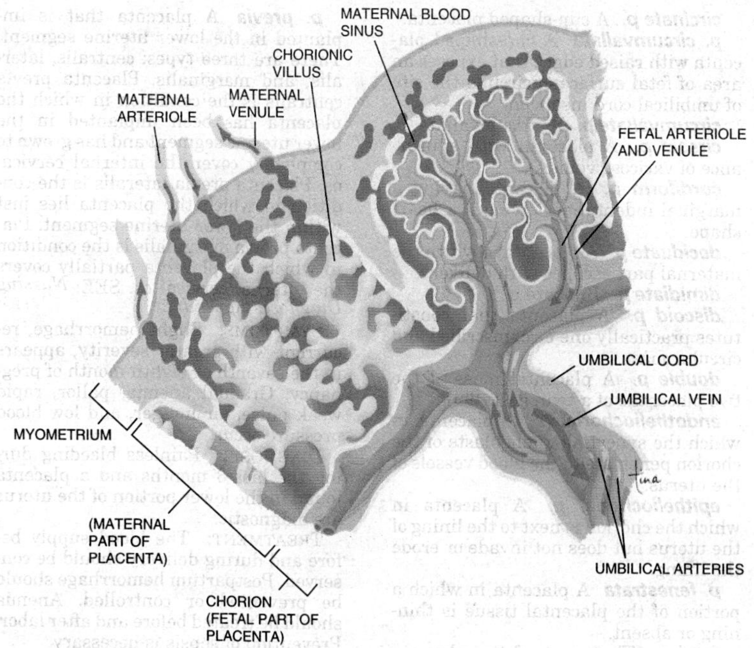

PLACENTA

Maternal and fetal portions

portion. The chorionic villi lie in spaces in the uterine endometrium, where they are bathed in maternal blood and lymph. Groups of villi are separated by placental septa forming about 20 distinct lobules called cotyledons.

Attached to the margin of the placenta is a membrane that encloses the embryo. It is a composite of several structures (decidua parietalis, decidua capsularis, chorion laeve, and amnion). At the center of the concave side is attached the umbilical cord through which the umbilical vessels (two arteries and one vein) pass to the fetus. The cord is approx. 50 cm (20 in.) long at full term.

The mature placenta is 15 to 18 cm (6 to 7 in.) in diameter and weighs about 450 gm (approx. 1 lb). When expelled following parturition, it is known as the afterbirth.

Maternal blood enters the intervillous spaces of the placenta through spiral arteries, branches of the uterine arteries. It bathes the chorionic villi and flows peripherally to the marginal sinus, which leads to uterine veins. Food molecules, oxygen, and antibodies pass into fetal blood of the villi; metabolic waste products pass from fetal blood into the mother's blood. Normally, there is no admixture of fetal and maternal blood. The placenta is also an endocrine organ. It produces chorionic gonadotropins, the presence of which in urine is the basis of one type of pregnancy test. Estrogen and progesterone are also secreted by the placenta.

abruption of p. Abruptio placentae.

accessory p. A placenta separate from the main placenta.

p. accreta A placenta in which the cotyledons have invaded the uterine musculature, resulting in difficult or impossible separation of the placenta.

adherent p. A placenta that remains adherent to the uterine wall after the normal period following childbirth.

annular p. A placenta that extends like a belt around the interior of the uterus. SYN: *zonary p.*

battledore p. A form of insertion of the umbilical cord into the margin of the placenta in which it spreads out to resemble a paddle or battledore.

bidiscoidal p. The presence of two discoidal masses. This is normal in some primates.

bilobate p. A placenta consisting of two lobes. SYN: *dimidiate p.*

bipartite p. A placenta divided into two separate parts.

chorioallantoic p. A placenta in which the allantoic mesoderm and vessels fuse with the inner face of the serosa to form the chorion.

circinate p. A cup-shaped placenta.

p. circumvallata A cup-shaped placenta with raised edges that exposes an area of fetal surface encircling the site of umbilical cord insertion.

circumvallate p. P. circumvallata.

cirsoid p. A placenta with appearance of varicose veins.

cordiform p. A placenta having a marginal indentation, giving it a heart shape.

deciduate p. A placenta of which the maternal part escapes with delivery.

dimidiate p. Bilobate p.

discoid p. A placenta that constitutes practically one circumscribed and circular mass.

double p. A placental mass of the two placentae of a twin gestation.

endotheliochorial p. A placenta in which the syncytial trophoblasts of the chorion penetrate to the blood vessels of the uterus.

epitheliochorial p. A placenta in which the chorion is next to the lining of the uterus but does not invade or erode the lining.

p. fenestrata A placenta in which a portion of the placental tissue is thinning or absent.

fetal p. That part of the placenta formed by aggregation of chorionic villi in which the umbilical vein and arteries ramify.

fundal p. A placenta attached to the uterine wall within the fundal zone.

hemochorial p. A placenta in which the maternal blood is in direct contact with the chorion. The human placenta is of this type.

hemoendothelial p. A placenta in which the maternal blood is in contact with the endothelium of the chorionic vessels.

horseshoe p. A formation in which the two placentae of a twin gestation are united.

incarcerated p. A placenta retained in the uterus by irregular uterine contractions after delivery.

p. increta A form of placenta accreta in which the chorionic villi invade the myometrium.

lateral p. A placenta attached to the lateral wall of the uterus.

maternal p. A portion of the placenta that develops from the decidua basalis of the uterus.

membranous p. Thinning of the placenta from atrophy.

multilobate p. A placenta with more than three lobes.

nondeciduate p. A placenta that does not shed the maternal portion.

p. percreta A type of placenta accreta in which the myometrium is invaded to the serosa of the peritoneum covering the uterus. This may cause rupture of the uterus.

p. previa A placenta that is implanted in the lower uterine segment. There are three types: centralis, lateralis, and marginalis. Placenta previa centralis is the condition in which the placenta has been implanted in the lower uterine segment and has grown to completely cover the internal cervical os. Placenta previa lateralis is the condition in which the placenta lies just within the lower uterine segment. Placenta previa marginalis is the condition in which the placenta partially covers the internal cervical os. SEE: *Nursing Diagnoses Appendix.*

SYMPTOMS: Slight hemorrhage, recurrent with greater severity, appears in the seventh or eighth month of pregnancy. Gradual anemia, pallor, rapid weak pulse, air hunger, and low blood pressure occur.

DIAGNOSIS: Painless bleeding during the last 3 months and a placenta found in the lower portion of the uterus are diagnostic.

TREATMENT: The blood supply before and during delivery should be conserved. Postpartum hemorrhage should be prevented or controlled. Anemia should be treated before and after labor. Prevention of sepsis is necessary.

PROGNOSIS: The prognosis depends on the control of hemorrhage and prevention of sepsis.

PATIENT CARE: In a calm environment, the patient is told what is happening; then the procedure of obstetric ultrasound is explained. The patient is told that if the ultrasound examination reveals a placenta previa, sterile vaginal examination will be delayed if possible until after 34 weeks' (preferably 36 weeks') gestation (to enhance the chances for fetal survival) and then will be carried out only as a "double-setup" procedure, with all preparations needed for immediate vaginal or cesarean delivery. (If, however, the ultrasound examination reveals a normally implanted placenta, a sterile vaginal speculum examination is performed to rule out local bleeding causes and a laboratory study is ordered to rule out coagulation problems.)

The patient is maintained on absolute bedrest and under close supervision in the hospital to extend the period of gestation until 36 weeks, when fetal lung maturity is likely (or can be stimulated to mature 48 hr before delivery). The laboratory types and cross-matches blood for emergency use the number of units based on the assessment of the particular patient's possible requirements. The patient's hematocrit level is kept at 30% or greater. The patient is prepared physically and emotionally for cesarean delivery; vaginal delivery may be attempted, but only if the previa is marginal or partial.

After delivery, the patient is monitored closely for continued bleeding, which may occur from the large vascular channels in the lower uterine segment, even if the fundus is firmly contracted. Prophylactic antibiotic therapy may be prescribed because of the patient's propensity for infection. Oxytocic drugs are given to control bleeding; packed cells or whole blood also are given. The obstetrical surgery team remains available, in case further intervention is required. The patient's hemodynamic status is monitored continuously, to provide blood and fluid replacement needed to prevent and treat hypovolemia while avoiding hypervolemia.

Although maternal mortality remains a concern, the patient and her family should be assured that this is unlikely, but not impossible in most large treatment centers because of the conservative regimen that is followed. In the event of fetal distress or death, the family is informed that these are related to detachment of a significant portion of the placenta or to maternal hypovolemic shock, or both. The patient and family require the health care providers' empathetic concern and support. A social service consultation is set up if financial or home and family care concerns require agency referrals; spiritual counseling is supplied according to the patient's wishes. Reducing maternal anxiety helps reduce uterine irritability, so a mental health practitioner should be consulted if the patient does not respond to nursing interventions (e.g., relaxation techniques, guided imagery) or if the patient's previous coping skills are known to be ineffective.

p. previa partialis A placenta that only partially covers the internal os of the uterus.

p. reflexa An abnormal placenta in which the margin is thickened and appears to turn back on itself.

reniform p. A kidney-shaped placenta.

retained p. A placenta not expelled within 30 minutes after completion of the second stage of labor.

p. spuria An outlying portion of the placenta that has not maintained its vascular connection with the decidua vera.

succenturiate p. An accessory placenta that has a vascular connection to the main part of the placenta.

trilobate p. A placenta with three lobes.

tripartite p. A three-lobed placenta attached to a single fetus.

triple p. A placental mass of three lobes in a triple gestation.

p. uterina The uterine part of the placenta.

velamentous p. A placenta with the umbilical cord attached to the membrane a short distance from the placenta, the vessels entering the placenta at its margin.

villous p. A placenta in which the chorion forms villi.

zonary p. Annular p.

placental (plă-sĕn′tăl) [L. *placenta,* a flat cake] Rel. to the placenta.

p. blood banking The use of human placental tissue as a source of fetal blood and hematopoietic stem cells.

placentation (plă″sĕn-tā′shŭn) The process of formation and attachment of the placenta.

placentitis (plă″sĕn-tī′tĭs) [″ + Gr. *itis,* inflammation] Inflammation of the placenta.

placentography (plă″sĕn-tŏg′ră-fē) [″ + Gr. *graphein,* to write] Examination of the placenta by radiography.

indirect p. Measurement of the space between the placenta and the head of the fetus by means of radiographical examination. It is done to diagnose placenta previa.

Placido's disk (plă-sē′dōz) [Antonio Placido, Portuguese ophthalmologist, 1848–1916] A disk marked with concentric black and white circles used in determining the amount and character of corneal irregularity.

placode (plăk′ōd) [Gr. *plax,* plate, + *eidos,* form, shape] In embryology, a platelike thickening of epithelium, usually the ectoderm, that serves as the precursor of an organ or structure.

auditory p. A dorsolateral placode located alongside the hindbrain that gives rise to the otocyst, which in turn develops into the internal ear.

lens p. A placode developing in the ectoderm directly overlying the optic vesicle. It forms the lens vesicle, which becomes enclosed in the optic cup and eventually becomes the lens of the eye.

olfactory p. A placode that gives rise to the olfactory pit and finally the major portion of the nasal cavity.

placoid (plăk′oyd) [″ + *eidos,* form, shape] Platelike.

pladaroma (plăd-ă-rō′mă) [Gr. *pladaros,* damp, + *oma,* tumor] A soft growth like a wart on the eyelid.

pladarosis (plăd-ă-rō′sĭs) [″ + *osis,* condition] The condition of pladaroma.

plagio- [Gr. *plagios,* slanting or sideways] Combining form meaning *slanting, oblique.*

plagiocephaly (plā″jē-ō-sĕf′ă-lē) A malformation of the skull producing the appearance of a twisted and lopsided head; caused by irregular closure of the cranial sutures.

plague (plāg) [ME., calamity] **1.** Any widespread contagious disease associated with a high death rate. **2.** A highly fatal disease caused by *Yersinia pestis* (previously classed as *Pasteurella pestis*) infection. This disease is characterized by high fever, restlessness, confusion, prostration, delirium, shock, and coma. Streptomycin, gentamicin, tetracyclines, fluoroquinolones, and chloramphenicol are effective in treating plague. In the U.S., about 15 cases of plague are reported annually.

ambulatory p. A mild form of bubonic plague.

black p. Plague.

bubonic p. Plague.

hemorrhagic p. A severe form of bubonic plague in which there is hemorrhage into the skin.

murine p. A plague infecting rats.

pneumonic p. A highly virulent form of plague spread from person to person by respiratory secretions. It occurs as a sequela of bubonic plague or as a primary infection.

septicemic p. A plague characterized by septicemia before the formation of buboes.

sylvatic p. Bubonic plague that is endemic among wild rodents. The causative organism, *Yersinia pestis,* is transmitted to people by fleas. SEE: *plague*.

white p. A historical term for tuberculosis.

plaintiff The person or party who sues or brings a legal action against another and seeks damages or other legal relief. SEE: *defendant*.

plait (plāt) To braid; to make separate strands of tissue into a rope-like structure (e.g., during tendon repair).

plan The conscious design of desired future states and of the goals, objectives, and activities required.

birth p. Written specifications for the management of labor, delivery, and recovery as desired by the expectant mother or couple and approved by the physician or midwife. Components usually include pain management techniques, method of delivery, and family participation. SEE: *Lamaze technique; Leboyer method*.

dental care p. **1.** The statement of the goals, objectives, and procedures related to the dentist's care for the patient, based on the medical history, oral examination, and oral radiographs. **2.** Third-party insurance that covers part or all of the cost for regular dental care.

health p. A corporation that provides medical insurance.

Individual Education P. ABBR: IEP. A federally required, individual program of goals and methods for addressing needs of students receiving special education and related services in public schools. IEPs are required under the provisions of federal legislation providing for a free and appropriate education for individuals with disabilities, as amended (Individuals with Disabilities Education Act [IDEA]-PL 104-134, Amended in 1997). The law mandates that for each child receiving special education services under the act, a written plan, involving input from teachers, service providers, and parents, will document the needs of the child, how those special needs will be addressed, and when and how the effectiveness of the services will be evaluated.

Individualized Family Service p. ABBR: IFSP. A written document, developed collaboratively by parents of young children with disabilities and related service personnel, that describes plans for intervention and educational placement. Twenty-five percent of occupational therapists now practice in school settings with the purpose of meeting the legislated mandate for public schools to provide related services for children with disabilities.

medical care p. The goals and objectives of the physician's care and the treatment instituted to accomplish them.

nursing care p. The statement of the goals and objectives of the nursing care provided for the patient and the activities or tasks required to accomplish the plan, including the criteria to be used to evaluate the effectiveness and appropriateness of the plan.

treatment p. A therapeutic strategy that may incorporate patient education, dietary adjustment, an exercise program, drug therapy, and the participation of nursing and allied health professionals. Treatment plans are esp. important in the optimal management of complex or chronic illnesses.

plan of care, care plan A description of the goals and outcomes, prognosis, and proposed interventions for a particular patient, including criteria for discharge and the optimal duration and frequency of therapeutic interventions.

planaria (plă-năr′ē-ă) Free-living flatworms of the Turbellaria class.

planchet (plăn′chĕt) A small flat container or dish on which a radioactive sample is placed.

plane (plān) [L. *planus*] **1.** A flat or relatively smooth surface. SYN: *planum*. **2.** A flat surface formed by making a cut, imaginary or real, through the body or a part of it. Planes are used as points of reference by which positions of parts of the body are indicated. In the human subject, all planes are based on the body being in an upright anatomical position. SEE: illus.; *anatomical position*. **3.** A certain stage, as in levels of anesthesia. **4.** To smooth a surface or rub away.

Addison's p. [Christopher Addison, Brit. anatomist, 1869–1951] One of the planes used as landmarks in thoracoabdominal topography.

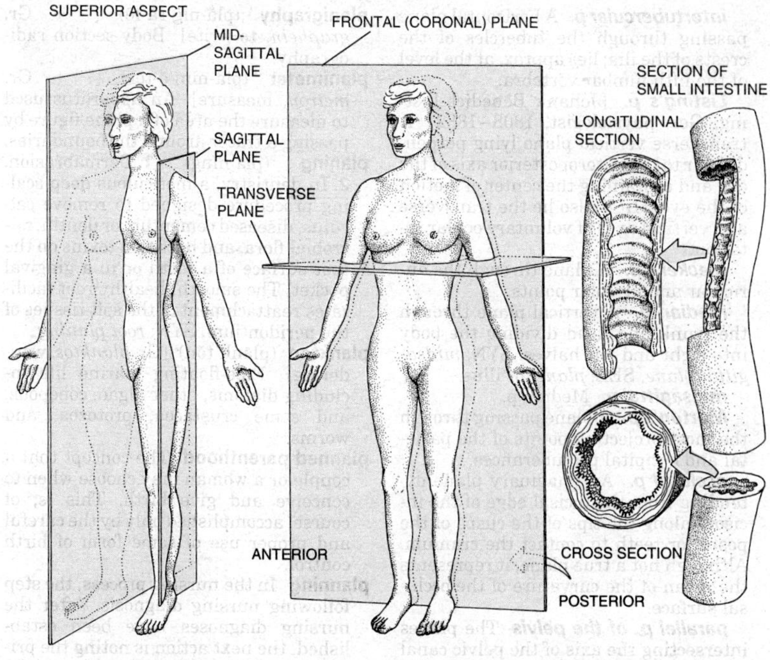

BODY PLANES AND SECTIONS

Aeby's p. [Christopher T. Aeby, Swiss anatomist, 1835–1885] A plane perpendicular to the median plane of the cranium through the basion and nasion.

alveolocondylar p. A plane tangent to the alveolar point with most prominent points on lower aspects of condyles of the occipital bone.

axiolabiolingual p. A plane that passes through an incisor or canine tooth parallel to the long axis of the tooth and in a labiolingual direction.

axiomesiodistal p. A plane that passes through a tooth parallel to the axis and in a mesiodistal direction.

Baer's p. A plane through the upper border of the zygomatic arches.

bite p. A plae formed by the biting surfaces of the teeth.

coccygeal p. The fourth parallel plane of the pelvis.

coronal p. A vertical plane at right angles to a sagittal plane. It divides the body into anterior and posterior portions. SYN: *frontal p.*

datum p. An assumed horizontal plane from which craniometric measurements are taken.

Daubenton's p. [Louis Jean Marie Daubenton, Fr. physician, 1716–1800] A plane passing through the opisthion and inferior bones of the orbits.

focal p. One of two planes through the anterior and posterior principal foci of a dioptric system and perpendicular to the line connecting the two.

Frankfort horizontal p. The cephalometric plane joining the porion and orbitale, the upper part of the ear openings and the lowest margin of the orbit, to establish a reproducible position of the head for radiographical and cephalometric studies.

frontal p. Coronal p.

Hodge's p. [Hugh Lennox Hodge, U.S. physician, 1796–1873] A plane running parallel to the pelvic inlet and passing through the second sacral vertebra and the upper border of the os pubis.

horizontal p. A transverse plane at right angles to the vertical axis of the body. SYN: *transverse p.*

inclined p. of the pelvis Anterior and posterior inclined planes of the pelvic cavity, two unequal sections divided by the sciatic spines. In the larger, anterior section, the lateral walls slope toward the symphysis and arch of the pubes; and the posterior walls slope in the direction of the sacrum and coccyx. The anterior inclined planes are the declivities over which rotation of the occiput takes place in the mechanism of normal labor.

inclined p. of a tooth Any sloping surface of the cusp of a tooth.

intertubercular p. A horizontal plane passing through the tubercles of the crests of the ilia; lies approx. at the level of the fifth lumbar vertebra.

Listing's p. [Johann Benedict Listing, Ger. physiologist, 1808–1882] A transverse vertical plane lying perpendicular to the anteroposterior axis of the eye and containing the center of motion of the eyes. In it also lie the transverse and vertical axes of voluntary ocular rotation.

Meckel's p. A plane through the auricular and alveolar points.

median p. A vertical plane through the trunk and head dividing the body into right and left halves. SYN: *midsagittal plane*. SEE: *plane* for illus.

midsagittal p. Median p.

Morton's p. A plane passing through the most projecting points of the parietal and occipital protuberances.

occlusal p. An imaginary plane extending from the incisal edge of the incisors along the tips of the cusps of the posterior teeth to contact the cranium. Although not a true plane, it represents the mean of the curvature of the occlusal surface.

parallel p. of the pelvis The planes intersecting the axis of the pelvic canal at right angles. The first plane is that of the superior strait; the second that extending from the middle of the sacral vertebra to the level of the subpubic ligament. The third plane is at the level of the spines of the ischia, and the fourth plane is at the outlet.

p. of the pelvis Imaginary planes touching the same parts of the pelvic canal on both sides.

p. of refraction A plane passing through a refracted ray of light and drawn perpendicular to the surface at which refraction takes place.

p. of regard A plane through the fovea of the eye; fixation point.

sagittal p. A vertical plane parallel to the midsagittal plane. It divides the body into right and left portions.

subcostal p. A horizontal plane passing through the lowest points of the 10th costal cartilages. It lies approx. at the level of third lumbar vertebra.

transverse p. Horizontal p.

treatment p. A plane in the concave joint surface that defines the direction of joint mobilization techniques. The plane is perpendicular to a line drawn from the axis of rotation in the convex joint surface to the center of the concave surface. Joint distraction techniques are applied perpendicular to, and gliding techniques parallel to, the treatment plane.

vertical p. Any body plane perpendicular to a horizontal plane.

visual p. A plane passing the visual axis of the eye.

planigraphy (plă-nĭg′ră-fē) [″ + Gr. *graphein,* to write] Body section radiography.

planimeter (plā-nĭm′ĕ-tĕr) [″ + Gr. *metron,* measure] An apparatus used to measure the area of a plane figure by passing a tracer around the boundaries.

planing (plā′nĭng) **1.** Dermabrasion. **2.** In dentistry, a meticulous deep scaling procedure designed to remove calculus, diseased cementum or dentin, microbial flora, and bacterial toxins on the root surface of a tooth or in a gingival pocket. The smooth, healthy root facilitates reattachment of the soft tissues of the peridontium. SYN: *root planing*.

plankton (plănk′tŏn) [Gr. *planktos,* wandering] Free-floating marine life including diatoms, other algae, copepods, and some crustacea, protozoa, and worms.

planned parenthood The concept that a couple or a woman may choose when to conceive and give birth. This is, of course, accomplished only by the careful and proper use of some form of birth control.

planning In the nursing process, the step following nursing diagnosis. After the nursing diagnoses have been established, the next action is noting the priority of the diagnoses and indicating the actions that will accomplish the immediate and long-range goals of the nursing process. Specific nursing interventions are indicated, and the expected outcomes of these actions are recorded on the chart. This portion of the nursing process is dynamic and will need to be altered as the patient's course evolves. The evaluation of the effectiveness of the nursing process will be essential to restating the plan for administering nursing care. SEE: *nursing process; nursing assessment; evaluation; nursing intervention; problem-oriented medical record*.

planocellular (plā″nō-sĕl′ū-lăr) [L. *planus,* plane, + *cellula,* cell] Composed of flat cells.

planoconcave (plā″nō-kŏn′kāv) [″ + *concavus,* hollow] An optical lens that is flat on one side and concave on the other.

planoconvex (plā″nō-kŏn′vĕks) [″ + L. *convexus,* arched] An optical lens that is flat on one side and convex on the other.

planomania (plā″nō-mā′nē-ă) [Gr. *plane,* wandering, + Gr. *mania,* madness] The morbid desire to wander and be free of social restraints.

Planorbis (plăn-or′bĭs) A genus of freshwater snails serving as intermediate hosts for certain species of blood flukes *(Schistosoma)*.

planotopokinesia (plā″nō-tŏp″ō-kī-nē′zē-ă) [″ + *topos,* place, + *kinesis,* movement] Loss of orientation in space.

plant (plănt) [L. *planta,* a sprout] An organism that contains chlorophyll and synthesizes carbohydrates and oxygen from carbon dioxide and water. Plants make up one of the five kingdoms of living things. SEE: *chlorophyll.*

planta pedis (plăn′tă pē′dŭs) *pl.* **plantae** [L.] The sole of the foot.

plantago seed (plăn-tā′gō) The cleaned, dried, ripe seed of *Plantago psyllium* or *P. indica.* It is used as a cathartic, but usually in a powdered form rather than in the form of whole seeds.

plantalgia (plăn-tăl′jē-ă) [L. *planta,* sole of the foot, + Gr. *algos,* pain] Pain in the sole of the foot.

plantar (plăn′tăr) Concerning the sole of the foot.

plantar flexion Extension of the foot so that the forepart is depressed with respect to the position of the ankle. SEE: *dorsiflexion.*

plantaris (plăn-tăr′ĭs) [L.] A long slim muscle of the calf between the gastrocnemius and soleus. It is sometimes double and at other times missing.

plantation (plăn-tā′shŭn) [L. *plantare,* to plant] Insertion of a tooth into the bony socket from which it may have been removed by accident; or transplantation of a tooth into the socket from which a tooth has just been removed. The transplanted tooth may come from the patient or a donor.

plantigrade [L. *planta,* sole of the foot, + *gradi,* to walk] A type of foot posture in which the entire sole of the foot is placed on the ground in walking, as in the bear, rabbit, or human.

planula (plăn′ū-lă) The larval stage of a coelenterate.

planum (plā′nŭm) *pl.* **plana** [L.] A flat or relatively smooth surface; a plane.

nuchal p. The outer surface of the occipital bone between the foramen magnum and superior nuchal line.

occipital p. The outer surface of the occipital bone lying above the superior nuchal line.

orbital p. The portion of the maxilla that forms the greater part of the floor of the orbit.

popliteal p. A smooth triangular area on the posterior surface of distal end of femur. It is bordered by the medial and lateral supracondylar lines and forms the floor of the popliteal fossa.

sternal p. The anterior or ventral surface of the sternum.

temporal p. The depressed area on the side of the skull below the inferior temporal line; underlies the temporal fossa.

planuria (plā-nū′rē-ă) [Gr. *plane,* wandering, + *ouron,* urine] The voiding of urine from an abnormal passage of the body.

plaque (plăk) [Fr., a plate] A patch on the skin or on a mucous surface.

atheromatous p. An obstruction in the lining of an artery, formed by the abnormal accumulation of lipids (fats) and sometimes calcium.

bacterial p. Dental p.

dental p. A tenacious mass of microorganisms that accumulates and grows on the crowns of teeth. Plaque is colorless, transparent, and the forerunner of dental caries and periodontal disease. Measures to prevent plaque build-up include daily self-care of the teeth, careful use of dental floss, and periodic prophylaxis by a dentist or dental hygienist.

TREATMENT: Treatment should include removal on a daily basis. Brushing and flossing are typical methods of plaque removal. Additional techniques may include water irrigation, chemical plaque control, and auxiliary oral hygiene aids. SEE: *calculus; caries; periodontal disease; periodontitis.*

mucous p. Condyloma latum.

senile p. Accumulations of bundled amyloid fibrils surrounding normal and damaged neurons in the brain, a finding on pathological inspection of brain tissue from patients with Alzheimer's dementia.

-plasia [Gr. *plasis,* molding] Combining form used as a suffix indicating *formation, growth, proliferation.*

plasm (plăzm) [LL. *plasma,* form, mold] Plasma.

plasm- [Gr. *plasma,* anything formed] Combining form meaning *living substance, tissue.*

plasma (plăz′mă) [LL. *plasma,* form, mold] **1.** An obsolete term for cytoplasm. **2.** An ointment base of glycerol and starch. **3.** The liquid part of the lymph and of the blood. SYN: *blood p.*

In the blood, cells and platelets are suspended in plasma. The plasma consists of serum, protein, and chemical substances in aqueous solution. The aqueous solution also contains solids and dissolved gases. Among the chemical materials are electrolytes, glucose, proteins including enzymes and hormones, fats, bile pigments, and bilirubin.

Plasma serves as the medium for transporting the substances previously mentioned to various structures and, at the same time, transports waste products to various sites of clearance (i.e., lungs, liver, kidneys, and spleen).

Different constituents of plasma have specific functions within the blood. Proteins, bicarbonates, carbon dioxide, chlorides, phosphates, and ammonia serve to keep the acid-base equilibrium of the blood constant when acid or base substances are added to it. Proteins, esp. albumin, by virtue of their osmotic pressure, tend to prevent undue leakage of fluids out of the capillaries and to maintain a proper exchange of fluid between capillaries and tissues.

Normal plasma is thin and colorless when free of blood cells; it may have a faint yellow tinge when seen in thick layers.

After clotting of the blood, the liquid squeezed out by the clot is called serum. If whole blood is prevented from clotting either by chilling it or by adding anticoagulants, such as sodium citrate, it can be centrifuged. The clear fluid that then occupies the upper half of the centrifuge tube is called plasma.

antihemophilic factor p. Human plasma in which factor VIII, the antihemophilic globulin, has been preserved; used to correct temporarily the bleeding tendency in some forms of hemophilia. SEE: *hemophilia.*

blood p. Plasma 3.

fresh frozen p. ABBR: FFP. The fluid portion of one unit of human blood that has been centrifuged, separated, and frozen solid within 6 hours of collection. SEE: *blood component therapy.*

hyperimmune p. Plasma with a high titer of a specific antibody, administered to create passive immunity to the antigen.

normal human p. Pooled plasma from a number of human donors. The plasma is sterile and the donors are free from diseases that could be transmitted by transfusion.

p. skimming The natural separation of red blood cells from plasma at bifurcations in the vascular tree, thereby allowing the blood to be divided into relatively concentrated and relatively dilute streams.

plasmablast (plăz′mă-blăst) [LL. *plasma,* form, mold, + Gr. *blastos,* germ] The undifferentiated cell that will mature into a B lymphocyte and ultimately into a plasma cell.

plasmacyte (plăz′mă-sīt) [″ + Gr. *kytos,* cell] A plasma cell.

plasmacytoma (plăz″mă-sī′tō′mă) [″ + ″ + *oma,* tumor] A plasma cell myeloma occurring in bone marrow. SEE: *multiple myeloma.*

plasmacytosis (plăz″mă-sī-tō′sĭs) [″ + ″ + *osis,* condition] An excess of plasma cells in the blood.

plasma exchange therapy The removal of plasma from a patient (usually to treat an immmunologically mediated illness such as thrombotic thrombocytopenic purpura or myasthenia gravis) and its replacement with normal plasma. Plasma exchange therapy can also be used to replace excessively viscous plasma in patients with Waldenström's macroglobulinemia. Pathological (disease-causing) antibodies, immune complexes, and protein-bound toxins are removed from the plasma by plasma exchange.

Immunoglobulin infusions are an alternative to plasma exchange when treating some immunological illnesses, including Guillain-Barré syndrome and chronic inflammatory demyelinating polyneuropathy. SYN: *plasmapheresis.*

plasmagel (plăz′mă-jĕl″) [″ + L. *gelare,* to congeal] The peripheral portion of the endoplasm of a cell, such as in an ameba. It is immobile and has the consistency of a gel.

plasmagene (plăz′mă-jēn″) [″ + Gr. *gennan,* to produce] A cytoplasmic hereditary determiner.

plasmalemma (plăz″mă-lĕm′ă) [″ + Gr. *lemma,* husk] Plasma, or cell, membrane.

plasmapheresis (plăz″mă-fĕr-ē′sĭs) [″ + Gr. *aphairesis,* separation] Plasma exchange therapy.

plasma protein fraction A standard sterile preparation of serum albumin and globulin obtained by fractionating blood, serum, or plasma from healthy human donors and testing for absence of hepatitis B surface antigen. It is used as a blood volume expander.

plasmatherapy (plăz″mă-thĕr′ă-pē) [″ + Gr. *therapeia,* service] Plasma exchange therapy.

plasmatic (plăz-măt′ĭk) **1.** Relating to plasma. **2.** Formative or plastic.

plasmatogamy (plăz″mă-tŏg′ă-mē) [″ + Gr. *gamos,* marriage] The union of the cytoplasm of two or more cells without joining of the nuclei.

plasmatorrhexis (plăz″mă-tō-rĕk′sĭs) [″ + Gr. *rhexis,* rupture] The rupture of a cell with loss of its contents, resulting from internal pressure caused by swelling.

plasma volume extender A high-molecular-weight compound in a solution suitable for intravenous use. The materials, such as dextran or certain proteins, are used in treating shock caused by loss of blood volume.

plasmid A diverse group of extrachromosomal genetic elements. They are circular double-stringed DNA molecules present intracellularly and symbiotically in most bacteria. They reproduce inside the bacterial cell but are not essential to its viability. Plasmids can influence a great number of bacterial functions, including resistance to antibiotics, production of enzymes that produce some antibiotics, the ability of the cell to detoxify harmful materials, and production of bacteriocins. Plasmids are gained or lost depending on their value to the bacterial cell in a specific circumstance. SYN: *episome.* SEE: *bacteriocin; transposon.*

plasmin (plăz′mĭn) A fibrinolytic enzyme derived from its precursor plasminogen.

plasminogen (plăz-mĭn′ō-jĕn) A protein found in many tissues and body fluids; important in preventing fibrin clot formation.

plasmocyte (plăz′mō-sīt) [″ + Gr. *kytos,* cell] The malignant cells found in the bone marrow, and occasionally the blood of persons with multiple myeloma.

plasmodesmata (plăz″mō-dĕz′mă-tă) *sing.*, **plasmodesma** [″ + Gr. *desmos,* bond] Tunnels in plant cell walls. These facilitate communication between cells.

plasmodial (plăz-mō′dē-ăl) Concerning *Plasmodia.*

plasmodicidal (plăz″mō-dĭ-sī′dăl) [″ + Gr. *eidos,* form, shape, + L. *caedere,* to kill] Lethal to plasmodia.

Plasmodium (plăz-mō′dē-ŭm) A genus of protozoa belonging to subphylum Sporozoa, class Telosporidia; includes causative agents of malaria in humans and lower animals. SEE: *malaria; mosquito.*

P. falciparum The causative agent of malignant (falciparum) malaria. SEE: illus.

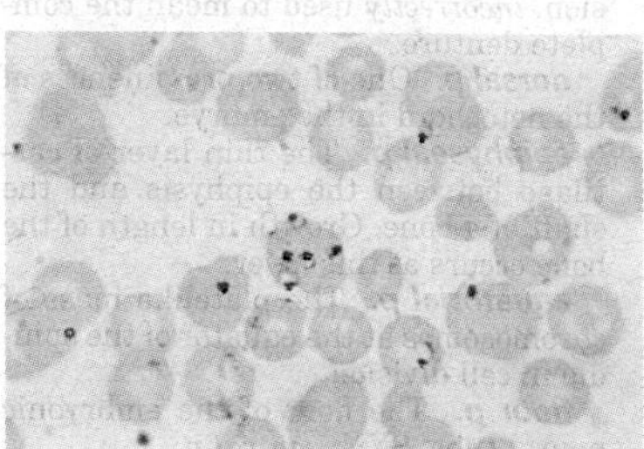

10μm

PLASMODIUM FALCIPARUM

Sporozoite ring forms in red blood cells (×1000)

P. malariae The causative agent of quartan malaria.

P. ovale The causative agent of benign tertian or ovale malaria.

P. vivax The causative agent of benign tertian or vivax malaria.

plasmodium (plăz-mō′dē-ŭm) *pl.* **plasmodia** [LL. *plasma,* form, mold, + Gr. *eidos,* form, shape] **1.** A multinucleate mass of naked protoplasm, occurring commonly among slime molds. **2.** An organism in the genus *Plasmodium.*

plasmogamy (plăs-mŏg′ă-mē) [″ + Gr. *gamos,* marriage] The fusion of cells.

plasmolysis (plăz-mŏl′ĭ-sĭs) [″ + Gr. *lysis,* dissolution] Shrinking of cytoplasm in a living cell caused by loss of water by osmosis.

plasmoma (plăz-mō′mă) [″ + Gr. *oma,* tumor] **1.** A collection of plasma cells. **2.** Plasmacytoma.

plasmoptysis (plăz-mŏp′tĭ-sĭs) [″ + Gr. *ptyein,* to spit] Escape of cytoplasm from a cell.

plasmorrhexis (plăz″mō-rĕk′sĭs) [″ + Gr. *rhexis,* rupture] The rupture of a cell with loss of its contents. SYN: *erythrocytorrhexis; plasmatorrhexis.*

plasmotomy (plăz-mŏt′ō-mē) [″ + Gr. *tome,* incision] Mitosis in which the cytoplasm divides into two or more masses.

plastein (plăs′tē-ĭn) A massive polypeptide formed by the hydrolysis of proteins and the subsequent recombination of amino acid esters. Plasteins can be derived from nonconventional sources of protein (e.g., cassava leaves or other plants) and used to make protein-rich foods.

plaster [Gr. *emplastron*] **1.** A material, usually plaster of Paris, that is applied to a part and allowed to harden in order to immobilize the part or to make an impression. **2.** A topical preparation in which the constituents are formed into a tenacious mass of substance harder than an ointment and spread upon muslin, linen, skin, or paper.

adhesive p. Plaster made of a strong cloth coated on one side with an adhesive substance; used to immobilize a part, to relieve pressure upon sutures, to protect wounds, to secure traction in fractures, to exert pressure, or to hold dressings in place. Hair on the area should be removed before applying any plaster. Plaster should never be applied to abraded or raw surfaces. In reapplying, dead skin should be removed. The surface should be dry and clean.

dental p. A powder, when mixed with water, that hardens to form a stonelike investment or model material. It is composed of a hemihydrate of gypsum ($CaSO_4 \cdot 2H_2O$), which differs in compression strength and expansion coefficient according to how it is treated and rehydrated. There are four classes of dental plaster, with differing uses as materials for casts, impressions, or stone models, based on the differences of characteristics.

mustard p. Sinapism.

p. of Paris Gypsum cement, hemihydrated calcium sulfate ($CaSO_4 \cdot 2H_2O$), mixed with water to form a paste that sets rapidly; used to make casts and stiff bandages.

salicylic acid p. A uniform mixture of salicylic acid spread on an appropriate base such as paper, cotton, or fabric. It is applied topically for use as a keratolytic agent.

plaster cast Rigid dressing made of gauze impregnated with plaster of Paris, used to immobilize an injured part, esp. in bone fractures.

PATIENT CARE: Neurovascular status of the casted part is monitored hourly for 24 hr, then every 4 hr. If the patient is sent home with a cast, the importance of either returning to the hospital or of calling the physician to report any pain is emphasized, particularly in the 24 to 48 hr after cast application. The patient is assessed for pressure areas and skin irritation at least daily and for indications of infection. Once the cast is dry, unfinished edges may be covered with adhesive tape or moleskin strips to prevent irritation. If the patient complains of discomfort not relieved by repositioning or comfort measures, this should be reported immediately; cast removal, bivalving, or windowing may be necessary. Physical mobility is encouraged as permitted or prescribed, and preventive measures pertaining to immobility hazards and safety measures are taught to prevent further injury. The patient should never insert anything under the cast to relieve itching, because further irritation or infection may result. The patient is given instruction regarding self-care and is taught measures to prevent wetting or soiling the cast. Respiratory, nutritional, and elimination statuses are monitored, and respiratory toilet is provided. The patient is prepared for cast removal and advised about the visual appearance of the casted area.

plastic (plăs′tĭk) [Gr. *plastikos,* fit for molding] **1.** Capable of being molded. **2.** Contributing to building tissues.

plasticity (plăs-tĭs′ĭ-tē) **1.** The ability to be molded. **2.** The ability of tissues to grow or integrate with others during development, after trauma, or after an illness.

plastid (plăs′tĭd) [Gr. *plastos,* formed] An organelle in plant cells. It includes chloroplasts (which contain chlorophyll), leukoplasts (colorless), chromoplasts (which contain pigment), and amyloplasts (which store starch). Chloroplasts are the site of photosynthesis.

plastron [Fr., breastplate] The sternum and attached cartilages.

-plasty [Gr. *plastos,* formed] A word ending meaning *molding, surgically forming.*

plate (plāt) [Gr. *plate,* flat] **1.** A thin flattened part or portion, such as a flattened process of a bone. SYN: *lamella; lamina.* **2.** An incorrect reference to a full denture. **3.** A shallow covered dish for culturing microorganisms. **4.** To inoculate and culture microorganisms in a culture plate.

auditory p. The bony roof of the external auditory meatus.

axial p. The primitive streak of the embryo.

belay p. A metal, steel, or aluminum plate that has one or more slots in it, designed to weave a rope through, to create friction with a carabiner.

bite p. In dentistry, a plate made of some suitable plastic material into which the patient bites in order to have a record of the relationship between the upper and lower jaws. The device may be reinforced with wire and used as a splint in the mouth or to treat temporomandibular joint difficulties.

bone p. A flat, round or oval, decalcified bone or metal disk, employed in pairs, used in approximation.

cortical p. The compact layers of bone forming the surfaces of the alveolar processes of the mandible and maxilla.

cribriform p. The thin, perforated, medial portion of the horizontal plate of the ethmoid bone; also, a synonym for alveolar bone proper, the sievelike layer of bone that makes up the wall of the socket and supports the tooth.

deck p. The roof plate of the embryonic neural tube.

dental p. An old term for the denture base of metal or acrylic material that rests on the oral mucosa and to which artificial teeth are attached; by extension, *incorrectly* used to mean the complete denture.

dorsal p. One of two prominences of the notochord in the embryo.

epiphyseal p. The thin layer of cartilage between the epiphysis and the shaft of a bone. Growth in length of the bone occurs at this layer.

equatorial p. The platelike mass of chromosomes at the equator of the spindle in cell division.

floor p. The floor of the embryonic neural tube. SYN: *ventral p.*

medullary p. The central portion of the ectoderm in the embryo developing into the neural canal. SYN: *neural p.*

muscle p. In the somite, the myotome from which the striated muscles are formed.

neural p. Medullary p.

palate p. The part of the palatine bone forming the dorsal half of the roof of the mouth.

polar p. In some cells, the flattened platelike bodies seen at the end of the spindle during mitosis.

pterygoid p. Either of a pair of thin, bony processes that arise from the sphenoid bone. They are termed medial and lateral pterygoid plates on each side and serve to bound the infratemporal fossa and give origin to muscles of mastication.

tarsal p. The dense connective tissue structure that supports the eyelid. It was formerly called *tarsal cartilage;* however, it is not true cartilage.

tympanic p. The bony plate between the anterior wall of the external auditory meatus and the tympanum.

ventral p. Floor p.

plateau **1.** An elevated and usually flat area; a steady and consistent fever appears as a plateau on the patient's chart of vital signs. **2.** The stage in training or skill acquisition when progress occurs at a very slow or flat rate in comparison with earlier phases.

ventricular p. The flat portion of the record of intraventricular pressure during the end of the ejection phase of ventricular systole.

platelet (plāt′lĕt) [Gr. *plate,* flat] A round or oval disk, 2 to 4 μm in diameter, found in the blood of vertebrates. Platelets number 130,000 to 400,000/mm^3. They are fragments of megakaryocytes, large cells found in the bone marrow. SYN: *thrombocyte*. SEE: illus.; *blood* for illus.; *megakaryocyte* for illus.; *thrombopoietin*.

FUNCTION: Platelets play an important role in blood coagulation, hemostasis, and blood thrombus formation. When a small vessel is injured, platelets adhere to each other and the edges of the injury and form a plug that covers the area. This leads to enhancement of the coagulation mechanism and deposition of fibrin. The plug or blood clot formed soon retracts and stops the loss of blood. The actions of platelets, though quite beneficial in initiating the reaction to injury, may actually be harmful in conditions such as coronary occlusion. In that case, platelet function may delay reperfusion and help to cause reocclusion of the vessel.

DISORDERS: Thrombocytopenia (reduced platelet count) occurs in acute infections, anaphylactic shock, and certain hemorrhagic diseases and anemias. Thrombocytosis (increased platelet count) occurs after operations, esp. splenectomy, and after violent exercise and tissue injury.

platelet concentrate Platelets prepared from a single unit of whole blood or plasma and suspended in a specific volume of the original plasma. This blood fraction must be used before the expiration date shown on its label. Platelets are stored at room temperature (22°C) either in plasma or in a concentrated form as platelet-rich plasma.

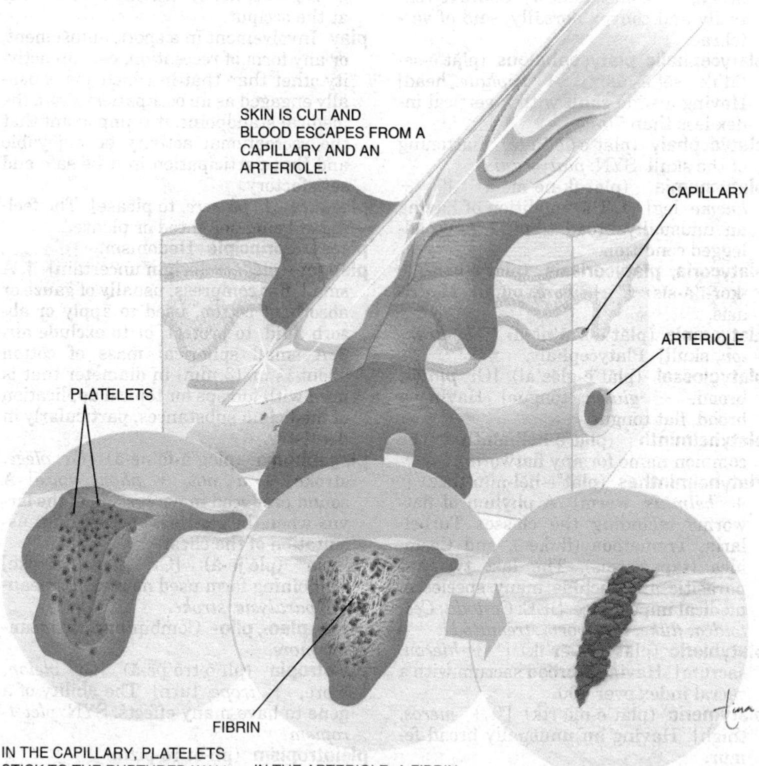
SKIN IS CUT AND BLOOD ESCAPES FROM A CAPILLARY AND AN ARTERIOLE.
CAPILLARY
ARTERIOLE
PLATELETS
FIBRIN
IN THE CAPILLARY, PLATELETS STICK TO THE RUPTURED WALL AND FORM A PLATELET PLUG.
IN THE ARTERIOLE, A FIBRIN CLOT FORMS.
CLOT RETRACTION PULLS THE EDGES OF THE WOUND TOGETHER.

PLATELET PLUG FORMATION AND CLOTTING

plateletpheresis The process of treating donor blood to remove platelets and then returning the remaining blood to the donor.

plating In bacteriology, inoculation of liquefiable, solid media (gelatin or agar) with microorganisms and pouring of medium into a shallow flat dish.

platinic (plă-tĭn′ĭk) Pert. to a compound containing quadrivalent platinum.

platinosis Cutaneous and respiratory allergic reactions to exposure to complex salts of platinum.

platinous (plăt′ĭ-nŭs) A compound containing divalent platinum.

platinum (plăt′ĭ-nŭm) [Sp. *platina*] SYMB: Pt. A heavy silver-white metal; atomic weight 195.09; atomic number 78; specific gravity 21.45.

platy- [Gr. *platys,* broad] Combining form meaning *broad.*

platybasia (plăt″ē-bā′sē-ă) A developmental defect of the skull in which the floor of the posterior fossa of the skull around the foramen magnum protrudes upward.

platycelous (plăt-ē-sē′lŭs) [Gr. *platys,* broad, + *koilos,* hollow] Concave ventrally and convex dorsally, said of vertebrae.

platycephalic, platycephalous (plăt″ē-sē-făl′ĭk, -sĕf′ă-lŭs) [″ + *kephale,* head] Having a wide skull with a vertical index less than 70.

platycephaly (plăt″ē-sĕf′ă-lē) Flattening of the skull. SYN: *platycrania.*

platycnemia (plăt-ĭk-nē′mē-ă) [″ + *kneme,* leg] **1.** The condition of having an unusually broad tibia. **2.** A broad-legged condition.

platycoria, platycoriasis (plăt″ē-kor-ē′ă, -kor-ī′ă-sĭs) [″ + *kore,* pupil] Mydriasis.

platycrania (plăt″ē-krā′nē-ă) [″ + *kranion,* skull] Platycephaly.

platyglossal (plăt″ē-glŏs′ăl) [Gr. *platys,* broad, + *glossa,* tongue] Having a broad, flat tongue.

platyhelminth (plăt″ē-hĕl′mĭnth) The common name for any flatworm.

Platyhelminthes (plăt″ē-hĕl-mĭn′thēz) [″ + *helmins,* worm] A phylum of flatworms including the classes Turbellaria, Trematoda (flukes), and Cestoidea (tapeworms). The last two are parasitic and include many species of medical importance. SEE: *Cestoda; Cestoidea; fluke; tapeworm; trematode.*

platyhieric (plăt″ē-hī-ĕr′ĭk) [″ + *hieron,* sacrum] Having a broad sacrum with a sacral index over 100.

platymeric (plăt″ē-mē′rĭk) [″ + *meros,* thigh] Having an unusually broad femur.

platymorphia (plăt″ē-mor′fē-ă) [″ + *morphe,* form] Having an eye with a shortened anteroposterior diameter, which results in hyperopia.

platyopia (plăt″ē-ō′pē-ă) [″ + *ops,* face] Having a very broad face, with a nasomalar index of less than 107.5.

platyopic (plăt″ē-ŏp′ĭk) Having a broad, flattened face.

platypellic, platypelvic, platypelloid (plăt″ē-pĕl′ĭk, -vĭk, -oyd) [″ + *pella,* a basin] Having a broad pelvis. SEE: under *pelvis.*

platypnea (plă″tĭp′nē-ă) [″ + *pnoia,* breath] Shortness of breath, dyspnea, only when the patient is upright or seated. SEE: *orthopnea.*

platyrrhine (plăt′ĭr-īn) [″ + *rhis,* nose] **1.** Having a very wide nose in proportion to length. **2.** Pert. to a skull with a nasal index between 51.1 and 58.

platysma myoides (plă-tĭz′mă mī-oy′dēz) [Gr. *platysma,* plate, + *mys,* muscle, + *eidos,* form, shape] A broad, thin, platelike layer of muscle that extends from the fascia of both sides of the neck to the jaw and muscles around the mouth. It acts to wrinkle the skin of the neck and depress the jaw.

platyspondylia (plăt″ē-spŏn-dĭl′ē-ă) Flatness of the vertebral bodies.

platystencephaly (plăt″ĭ-stĕn-sĕf′ă-lē) [″ + *kephale,* head] Having a skull wide at the occiput.

play Involvement in a sport, amusement, or any form of recreation, esp. an activity other than that in which one is usually engaged as an occupation. From the medical standpoint, it is important that the recreational activity be enjoyable and that participation in it be safe and satisfactory.

pleasure [L. *placere,* to please] The feeling of being delighted or pleased.

pleasure principle Hedonism.

pledget (plĕj′ĕt) [origin uncertain] **1.** A small, flat compress, usually of gauze or absorbent cotton, used to apply or absorb fluid, to protect, or to exclude air. **2.** A small spherical mass of cotton about ⅛ in. (3 mm) in diameter that is used with forceps for topical application of medicinal substances, particularly in dentistry.

plegaphonia (plĕg″ă-fō′nē-ă) [Gr. *plege,* stroke, + *a-,* not, + *phone,* voice] A sound produced in percussion of the larynx when the glottis is open during auscultation of the chest.

-plegia (plē′jē-ă) [Gr. *plege,* stroke] Combining form used as a suffix meaning *paralysis, stroke.*

pleio-, pleo-, plio- Combining form meaning *more.*

pleiotropia (plī″ō-trō′pē-ă) [Gr. *pleion,* more, + *trope,* turn] The ability of a gene to have many effects. SYN: *pleiotropism.*

pleiotropism (plī-ŏt′rō-pĭzm) [″ + ″ + *-ismos,* condition] Pleiotropia.

Pleistophora A genus of microsporidia. SEE: *microsporidiosis.*

pleochroic (plē″ō-krō′ĭk) [Gr. *pleon,* more, + *chroia,* color] Pleochromatic.

pleochroism (plē-ŏk′rō-ĭzm) [″ + ″ + *-ismos,* condition] The property of a crystal that produces different colors when light passes through it at different angles.

pleochromatic (plē″ō-krō-măt′ĭk) [″ + *chroma,* color] Pert. to the property of crystals and some other bodies that show different colors when seen from different axes. SYN: *pleochroic.*

pleocytosis (plē″ō-sī-tō′sĭs) [″ + *kytos,* cell, + *osis,* condition] An increased number of lymphocytes in the cerebrospinal fluid.

pleomorphic (plē-ō-mor′fĭk) [″ + *morphe,* form] Having many shapes.

pleomorphism (plē-ō-mor′fĭzm) [″ + ″ + *-ismos,* condition] Polymorphism.

pleomorphous (plē-ō-mor′fŭs) Having many shapes or crystallizing into several forms.

pleonasm (plē′ō-năzm) [Gr. *pleonasmos,* exaggeration] **1.** The state of having more than the normal number of organs or parts. **2.** The use of more words than necessary to express an idea.

pleonexia (plē″ō-nĕk′sē-ă) [Gr.] Having a morbid desire for possession of material things; greediness.

pleonosteosis (plē″ŏn-ŏs″tē-ō′sĭs) [Gr. *pleon,* more, + *osteon,* bone, + *osis,* condition] Premature and excessive ossification of bones.

pleoptics (plē-ŏp′tĭks) [″ + *optikos,* sight] An obsolete method of eye exercises created to stimulate and train an amblyopic eye.

plerocercoid The solid wormlike larva of certain tapeworms. Plerocercoids develop in secondary hosts.

plesiomorphism (plē″sē-ō-mor′fĭzm) [Gr. *plesios,* close, + *morphe,* form, + *-ismos,* condition] Similarity of form.

plesiopia (plē″sē-ō′pē-ă) [″ + *ops,* eye] An increase in the convexity of the lens of the eye.

plessesthesia (plĕs″ĕs-thē′zē-ă) [Gr. *plessein,* to strike, + *aisthesis,* sensation] Palpatory percussion with the left middle finger pressed against the body and the right index finger percussing in contact with the left finger.

plessimeter (plĕs-sĭm′ĕ-tĕr) [″ + *metron,* measure] Pleximeter.

plessor (plĕs′or) [Gr. *plessein,* to strike] Plexor.

plethora (plĕth′ō-ră) [Gr. *plethore,* fullness] **1.** Overfullness of blood vessels or of the total quantity of any fluid in the body. SEE: *sanguine.* **2.** Congestion causing distention of the blood vessels.

plethoric (plĕ-thor′ĭk, plĕth′ō-rĭk) Pert. to, or characterized by, plethora; overfull.

plethysmograph (plē-thĭz′mō-grăf) [Gr. *plethysmos,* to increase, + *graphein,* to write] A device for finding variations in the size of a part owing to variations in the amount of blood passing through or contained in the part.

body p. A body box used to measure lung volume and pressure.

impedance p. A device that uses gas-to-tissue ratio to set an alarm or measure a volume.

plethysmography (plĕth″ĭz-mŏg′ră-fē) The use of a plethysmograph to record the changes in volume of an organ or extremity.

pleur-, pleuro- [Gr. *pleura,* rib, side] Combining form meaning *pleura, side, rib.*

pleura (ploo′ră) *pl.* **pleurae** [Gr., side] A serous membrane that enfolds both lungs and is reflected upon the walls of the thorax and diaphragm. The pleurae are moistened with a serous secretion that reduces friction during respiratory movements of the lungs. SEE: *effusion, pleural; mediastinum; thorax.*

costal p. Parietal p.

p. diaphragmatica The part of the pleura covering the upper surface of the diaphragm.

mediastinal p. The portion of the parietal pleura that extends to cover the mediastinum.

parietal p. The serous membrane that lines the chest cavity; it extends from the mediastinal roots of the lungs and covers the sides of the pericardium to the chest wall and backward to the spine. The visceral and parietal pleural layers are separated only by a lubricating secretion. These layers may become adherent or separated by air or by blood, pus, or other fluids, when the lungs or chest wall are injured or inflamed. SYN: *costal p.*

p. pericardiaca The portion of the pleura covering the pericardium.

p. pulmonalis Visceral p.

visceral p. The pleura that covers the lungs and enters into and lines the interlobar fissures. It is loose at the base and at the sternal and vertebral borders to allow for lung expansion.

pleuracotomy (ploor″ă-kŏt′ō-mē) [″ + *tome,* incision] Incision into the pleura through the chest wall.

pleural (ploo′răl) [Gr. *pleura,* side] Concerning the pleura.

p. fibrosis A condition occurring in pulmonary tuberculosis, asbestosis, and other lung diseases in which the pleura becomes thickened and the pleural space may be obliterated.

pleuralgia (ploo-răl′jē-ă) [″ + *algos,* pain] Pain in the pleura, or in the side. SYN: *intercostal neuralgia.*

pleurapophysis (ploo-ră-pŏf′ĭ-sĭs) [″ + *apo,* from, + *physis,* a growth] A rib or a vertebral lateral process.

pleurectomy (ploo-rĕk′tō-mē) [″ + *ektome,* excision] Excision of part of the pleura.

pleurisy (ploo′rĭs-ē) [Gr. *pleuritis*] Inflammation of the pleura. It may be primary or secondary; unilateral, bilateral, or local; acute or chronic; fibrinous, serofibrinous, or purulent. SYN: *pleuritis.* SEE: *Nursing Diagnoses Appendix.*

PATIENT CARE: Respiratory function is monitored by auscultation, observation of breathing pattern, and oximetry. The patient is positioned in the high Fowler position to facilitate chest expansion. Deep breathing and coughing are encouraged every 1 to 2 hr to prevent atelectasis. During coughing, the nurse or respiratory therapist should splint the chest with a pillow as necessary and administer analgesic drugs and use noninvasive measures, such as local application of warm or cool compresses, to reduce pain. Respiratory toilet is provided if secretions are present. Rest is recommended. Prescribed medical regimens are carried out, and the patient's responses evaluated.

adhesive p. Pleurisy in which the exudate causes the parietal pleura to adhere to the visceral. If this is extensive, the pleural space is obliterated.

diaphragmatic p. Inflammation of the diaphragmatic pleura. Symptoms include intense pain under the margin of the ribs, sometimes referred into the abdomen, with tenderness upon pressure; thoracic breathing; tenderness over the phrenic nerve referred to the supraclavicular region in the neck on the same side; hiccough; and extreme dyspnea.

dry p. A condition in which the pleural membrane is covered with a fibrinous exudate.

p. with effusion Pleural effusion.

encysted p. Pleurisy with effusion limited by adhesions.

fibrinous p. Pleurisy with severe and continuous pain. Aspiration gives negative results, and later much retraction of the affected side.

hemorrhagic p. Pleurisy with hemorrhage.

interlobar p. Pleurisy in interlobar spaces.

pulmonary p. Inflammation of the pleura covering the lung.

purulent p. Empyema.

sacculated p. Pleurisy in which inflammatory areas are sealed off and filled with fluid, that is, loculated.

serofibrinous p. Pleurisy with fibrinous exudate and serous effusion.

serous p. Pleural effusion.

tuberculous p. Inflammation of the pleura as a result of tuberculosis. The effusion may be bloody.

typhoid p. Pleurisy with symptoms of typhoid.

wet p. An obsolete term for pleural effusion.

pleuritic (ploo-rĭt′ĭk) [Gr. *pleuritis,* pleurisy] Relating to, or resembling, pleurisy.

pleuritis (ploo-rī′tĭs) [Gr.] Pleurisy.

pleuritogenous (ploor″ĭ-tŏj′ĕ-nŭs) [″ + *gennan,* to produce] Causing pleurisy.

pleurocele (ploo′rō-sēl) [Gr. *pleura,* side, + *kele,* tumor, swelling] **1.** Hernia of the lungs or pleura. **2.** A serous pleural effusion.

pleurocentesis (ploo″rō-sĕn-tē′sĭs) [″ + *kentesis,* a piercing] Thoracentesis.

pleurocentrum (ploo″rō-sĕn′trŭm) *pl.* **pleurocentra** [″ + *kentron,* center] The lateral half of the body of a vertebra.

pleurocholecystitis (ploo″rō-kō″lē-sĭst-ī′tĭs) [″ + *chole,* bile, + *kystis,* bladder, + *itis,* inflammation] Inflammation of the pleura and gallbladder.

pleuroclysis (ploo-rŏk′lĭ-sĭs) [″ + *klysis,* a washing] Injection and removal of fluid into the pleural cavity to wash it out.

pleurodesis (ploo″rō-dē′sĭs) [″ + *desis,* binding] Production of adhesions between the parietal and visceral pleura; it is usually done surgically or by instillation of drugs or chemicals. This method is used to treat recurrent pneumothorax and malignant pleural effusions.

pleurodynia (ploo″rō-dĭn′ē-ă) [″ + *odyne,* pain] Pain of sharp intensity in the intercostal muscles due to chronic inflammatory changes in the chest fasciae; pain of the pleural nerves.

epidemic p. Bornholm disease.

pleurogenic, pleurogenous (ploo-rŏj′ĕn-ŭs) Arising in the pleura.

pleurography (ploo-rŏg′ră-fē) [″ + *graphein,* to write] Radiographical examination of the lungs and pleura.

pleurohepatitis (ploo″rō-hĕp″ă-tī′tĭs) [″ + *hepatos,* liver, + *itis,* inflammation] Inflammation of the pleura and liver.

pleurolith (ploo′rō-lĭth) [″ + *lithos,* stone] A stone between the pleura.

pleurolysis (ploo-rŏl′ĭ-sĭs) [″ + *lysis,* dissolution] Loosening of parietal pleura from intrathoracic fascia to facilitate contraction of the lung or artificial pneumothorax.

pleuromelus (ploor″ō-mē′lŭs) [″ + *melos,* limb] A congenital anomaly in which an accessory limb arises from the thorax or flank.

pleuropericardial (ploor″ō-pĕr-ĭ-kăr′dē-l) [″ + *peri,* around, + *kardia,* heart] Concerning the pleura and pericardium.

pleuropericarditis (ploo″rō-pĕr″ĭ-kăr-dī′tĭs) [″ + ″ + ″ + *itis,* inflammation] Pleuritis accompanied by pericarditis.

pleuroperitoneal (ploo″rō-pĕr″ĭ-tō-nē′ăl) [″ + *peritonaion,* peritoneum] Concerning the pleura and peritoneum.

p. cavity The ventral body cavity. SEE: under *body cavity* for illus.; *coelom.*

pleuropneumonia (ploo″rō-nū-mō′nē-ă) [″ + *pneumon,* lung] Pleurisy accompanied by pneumonia.

pleuropneumonia-like organisms ABBR: PPLO. The name once given organisms that are now called mycoplasmas.

pleuropulmonary (ploor″ō-pŭl′mō-nĕr″ē) [″ + L. *pulmo,* lung] Concerning the pleura and lung.

pleurorrhea (ploor″ō-rē′ă) [″ + *rhoia,* flow] Effusion of fluid into the pleura.

pleuroscopy (ploo-rŏs′kō-pē) [″ + *skopein,* to examine] Inspection of the pleural cavity with an endoscope inserted through an incision into the thorax.

pleurosoma (ploor″ō-sō′mă) [″ + *soma,* body] A fetus with a cleft in the abdominal wall and thorax with protrusion of the contents of the thoracic and abdominal cavities.

pleurothotonos (ploo″rō-thŏt′ō-nŏs) [Gr. *pleurothen,* from the side, + *tonos,* tension] A tetanic spasm in which the body is arched to one side.

pleurotomy (ploo-rŏt′ō-mē) [Gr. *pleura,* side, + *tome,* incision] Incision of the pleura.

pleurotyphoid (ploo″rō-tī′foyd) [″ + *typhos,* fever, + *eidos,* form, shape] Typhoid fever with pleural involvement.

pleurovisceral (ploo″rō-vĭs′ĕr-ăl) [″ + L. *viscera,* viscera] Concerning the pleura and viscera.

plexal (plĕk′săl) [L. *plexus,* a braid] Pert. to, or of the nature of, a plexus.

plexectomy (plĕk-sĕk′tō-mē) [″ + Gr. *ektome,* excision] Surgical removal of a plexus.

plexiform (plĕk′sĭ-form) [″ + *forma,* shape] Resembling a network or plexus.

pleximeter (plĕks-ĭm′ĕ-tĕr) [Gr. *plexis,* stroke, + *metron,* measure] A device for receiving the blow of the percussion hammer, consisting of a disk that is struck in mediate percussion while being held over the surface of the body. SYN: *plessimeter; plexometer*.

plexitis (plĕk-sī′tĭs) [L. *plexus,* a braid, + Gr. *itis,* inflammation] Inflammation of a nerve plexus.

plexometer (plĕk-sŏm′ĕ-tĕr) Pleximeter.

plexopathy A peripheral neuropathy. Any disease of a (peripheral) nerve plexus.

plexor (plĕks′or) A hammer or other device for striking on the pleximeter in percussion. SYN: *plessor*.

plexus (plĕks′ŭs) *pl.* **plexus, plexuses** [L., a braid] A network of nerves or of blood or lymphatic vessels. SEE: *rete*.

autonomic p. An extensive network of nerve fibers and neuron cell bodies belonging to the sympathetic or parasympathetic nervous system.

cavernous p. Plexus of a cavernous part of the body. The following are included: Of the nose: a venous plexus in the mucosa covering the superior and middle conchae. Of the penis: a nerve plexus at the base of the penis giving rise to large and small cavernous nerves. Of the clitoris: nerve plexus at the base of the clitoris, formed of fibers from the uterovaginal plexus. Of the cavernous sinus: a sympathetic plexus that supplies fibers to the internal carotid artery and its branches within the cranium.

celiac p. A sympathetic plexus lying near the origin of the celiac artery.

choroid p. A capillary network located in each of the four ventricles of the brain (two lateral, the third, and the fourth) that produces cerebrospinal fluid by filtration and secretion.

dental p. A network of sensory nerve fibers that are distributed to the teeth. The inferior alveolar nerve is distributed to the mandibular teeth; the anterior, middle, and posterior superior alveolar nerves contribute fibers to innervate the maxillary teeth.

enteric p. One of two plexuses of nerve fibers and ganglion cells that lie in the wall of the alimentary canal. These are the myenteric (Auerbach's) and submucosal (Meissner's) plexuses.

lumbar p. A nerve plexus formed by the ventral branches of the first four lumbar nerves.

lumbosacral p. The lumbar plexus and sacral plexus, considered as one.

myenteric p. Auerbach's plexus.

nerve p. Plexus made of nerve fibers.

pampiniform p. In the male, a complicated network of veins lying in the spermatic cord and draining the testis. In the female, a network of veins lying in the mesovarium and draining the ovary.

prevertebral p. One of three plexuses of autonomic nerve division that lie in body cavities. These are the cardiac, celiac, and hypogastric (pelvic) plexuses.

pliability (plī″ă-bĭl′ĭ-tē) [O.Fr. *pliant,* bend, + L. *abilis,* able] Capacity of being bent or twisted easily.

plica (plī′kă) *pl.* **plicae** [L.] A fold. SEE: *fold*.

circular p. One of the transverse folds of the mucosa and submucosa of the small intestine. Collectively they resemble accordion pleats, do not disappear with distention of the intestine, and increase the surface area for absorption. SYN: *Kerckring's folds; valvulae conniventes*.

epiglottic p. One of three folds of mucosa between the tongue and the epiglottis.

lacrimal p. A mucosal fold at the lower orifice of the nasolacrimal duct.

palmate p. A radiating fold in the uterine mucosa on the anterior and posterior walls of the cervical canal.

semilunar p. of the colon The transverse fold of mucosa of the large intestine lying between sacculations.

semilunar p. of the conjunctiva The mucosal fold at the inner canthus of the eye.

synovial p. A fold of synovial membrane that projects into a joint cavity.

transverse p. of the rectum One of the mucosal folds in the rectum.

plicamycin An antineoplastic agent that has been used in treating Paget's disease of the bone.

plicate (plī'kāt) [L. *plicatus*] Braided or folded.

plication (plī-kā'shŭn) [L. *plicare,* to fold] The stitching of folds or tucks in tissue at an organ's walls to reduce its size.

p. of the stomach A surgical procedure for obesity supplanted by partial gastric bypass. SEE: *fundoplication.*

plicotomy (plī-kŏt'ō-mē) [" + Gr. *tome,* incision] Section of the posterior fold of the tympanic membrane.

pliers **1.** Commonly, a scissor-action, pointed-jawed tool for bending or cutting metal wires or grasping small objects. **2.** In dentistry, a variety of instruments that have been shaped or adapted for special uses such as cutting arch wires or metal clasps, shaping metal crown details, applying cotton pledgets or rolls, carrying metal foils, tying ligatures, and placing or removing matrix bands.

plinth [Gr. *plinthos,* tile] A table, seat, or apparatus on which a patient lies or sits while doing remedial exercise.

-ploid [Gr. *ploos,* fold] Combining form used as a suffix indicating the number of chromosome pairs of the root word to which it is added.

ploidy (ploy'dē) [Gr. *ploos,* a fold, + *eidos,* form, shape] The number of chromosome sets in a cell (e.g., haploidy, diploidy, and triploidy for one, two, and three sets, respectively, of chromosomes).

plombage (plŏm-băzh') [Fr. *plomber,* to plug] A method of collapsing the apex of the lung by stripping the parietal pleura from the chest wall at the site of desired collapse and packing the space between the lung and the chest wall with an inert substance such as small balls made of certain plastic materials.

plototoxin (plō″tō-tŏk'sĭn) A toxic substance present in catfish, *Plotosus lineatus.*

plug (plŭg) [MD. *plugge*] **1.** A mass obstructing a hole or intended to close a hole. **2.** A plastic or metallic device for closing the end of an instrument or tube.

epithelial p. A mass of epithelial cells temporarily plugging an orifice in the embryo, esp. the nasal openings.

mucous p. A mass of cells and mucus that closes the cervical canal of the uterus during pregnancy and between menstrual periods.

vaginal p. A closed tube for maintaining patency of the vagina following operation for fistula.

plugger A hand- or machine-operated device for condensing amalgam, or gold foil, in the cavity preparation of a tooth.

automatic p. A plugger that is run by a machine rather than by hand.

back-action p. A plugger with a bent shank so that the pressure applied is back toward the operator.

foot p. A plugger having a broad, foot-shaped tip.

plumbic (plŭm'bĭk) [L. *plumbicus,* leaden] Pert. to, or containing, lead.

plumbism (plŭm'bĭzm) [L. *plumbum,* lead, + Gr. *-ismos,* condition] Poisoning from lead.

plumbum (plŭm'bŭm) [L.] Lead; a bluish-white metal. SEE: *lead.*

Plummer-Vinson syndrome (plŭm'ĕr-vĭn'sŏn) [Henry S. Plummer, U.S. physician, 1874–1937; Porter P. Vinson, U.S. surgeon, 1890–1959] Iron-deficiency anemia, associated with dysphagia, gastric achlorhydria, splenomegaly, and spooning of the nails due to an esophageal web. It occurs most commonly in premenopausal women. Treatment consists of disrupting the web. SEE: *esophageal web.*

plumose (plū'mōs) [L. *plumosus*] Having a delicate, feathery growth.

plumper (plŭm'pĕr) [Middle Low Ger. *plump,* to fill] A pad for filling out sunken cheeks, sometimes in the form of a flange or extension from artificial dentures.

pluri- [L. *plus,* more] Prefix meaning *several, more.*

pluriceptor (ploo″rĭ-sĕp'tor) [L. *plus,* more, + *ceptor,* a receiver] A receptor that has more than two groups uniting with the complement.

pluriglandular (ploo″rĭ-glănd'ū-lăr) [" + *glandula,* gland] Polyglandular.

plurigravida (ploo″rĭ-grăv'ĭ-dă) [" + *gravida,* pregnant] A pregnant woman who has had three or more pregnancies.

plurilocular (ploo″rĭ-lŏk'ū-lăr) [" + *loculus,* a cell] Multilocular.

plurinuclear (ploor″ĭ-nū'klē-ăr) [" + *nucleus,* kernel] Having a number of nuclei.

pluripara (ploo-rĭp'ă-ră) [" + *parere,* to bring forth, to bear] A woman who has given birth three or more times.

pluriparity (ploo″rĭ-păr'ĭ-tē) The condition of having three or more pregnancies that have reached a point of viability regardless of the outcome.

pluripotent, pluripotential (ploo-rĭp'ō-tĕnt, ploor″ĭ-pō-tĕn'shăl) [" + *potentia,* power] **1.** Concerning an embryonic cell that can form different kinds of cells. **2.** Having a number of different actions.

pluriresistant (ploor″ĭ-rē-zĭs'tănt) [" + *resistens,* standing back] Resistant to several drugs, esp. antibiotics.

plutonium (ploo-tō'nē-ŭm) [Named after the planet Pluto] SYMB: Pu. A radioactive element obtained from neptunium, which in turn is obtained from uranium; atomic weight of the most stable isotope is 244; atomic number 94.

plyometrics A stretching and shortening exercise technique that combines strength with speed to achieve maximum power in functional movements. This regimen combines eccentric training of muscles with concentric contraction.

Pm Symbol for the element promethium.

PML *progressive multifocal leukoencephalopathy.*

PMS *premenstrual syndrome.*

PMSG *pregnant mare serum gonadotropin.* SEE: *gonadotropin, human chorionic.*

PMT *photomultiplier tube; premenstrual tension.*

PNC *premature nodal contraction* or *complex.*

pneo- (nē'ō) [Gr. *pnein,* to breathe] Combining form meaning *breath, breathing.* SEE: *pneumo-.*

pneum-, pneuma-, pneumato- [Gr. *pneuma, pneumatos,* air, breath] Combining form meaning *air, gas, respiration.*

pneumarthrogram (nū-măr'thrō-grăm) [Gr. *pneuma,* air, + *arthron,* joint, + *gramma,* something written] A radiograph of a synovial joint after injection of a radiolucent contrast medium, usually air; an obsolete technique.

pneumarthrography (nū"măr-thrŏg'ră-fē) [" + " + *graphein,* to write] Radiography of a synovial joint after injection of a radiolucent contrast medium, usually air. SYN: *pneumoarthrography.*

pneumarthrosis (nū-măr-thrō'sĭs) [" + " + *osis,* condition] Accumulation of gas or air in a joint.

pneumatic (nū-măt'ĭk) [Gr. *pneumatikos,* pert. to air] **1.** Concerning gas or air. **2.** Relating to respiration. **3.** Relating to rarefied or compressed air.

pneumatics (nū-măt'ĭks) The branch of physics that is concerned with the physical and mechanical properties of gases and air.

pneumatinuria (nū"măt-ĭn-ū'rē-ă) [" + *ouron,* urine] Pneumaturia.

pneumatization (nū"mă-tī-zā'shŭn) The formation of air-filled cavities, usually in bone (e.g., the paranasal sinuses and mastoid sinuses).

pneumatocardia (nū"măt-ō-kăr'dē-ă) [" + *kardia,* heart] Air or gas in the heart chambers.

pneumatocele (nū-măt'ō-sēl) [" + *kele,* tumor, swelling] **1.** A hernia of the lung tissue. **2.** A swelling containing gas or air, esp. a swelling of the scrotum. SYN: *pneumonocele.*

extracranial p. A collection of gas under the scalp, caused by a fracture of the skull that communicates with a paranasal sinus.

intracranial p. A collection of gas within the skull.

pneumatodyspnea (nū"măt-ō-dĭsp'nē-ă) [" + *dys,* bad, + *pneia,* breath] Dyspnea caused by pulmonary emphysema.

pneumatology (nū"mă-tŏl'ō-jē) [" + *logos,* word, reason] The science of gases and air and their chemical properties and use in treatment.

pneumatosis (nū"mă-tō'sĭs) [Gr. *pneumatosis*] The presence of air or gas in an abnormal location in the body.

p. cystoides intestinalis The presence of thin-walled gas-filled cysts in the intestines. The cause is unknown. The cysts usually disappear but occasionally rupture and cause pneumoperitoneum.

pneumatotherapy (nū"măt-ō-thĕr'ă-pē) [Gr. *pneumatos,* air, + *therapeia,* treatment] Pneumotherapy.

pneumaturia (nū"măt-ū'rē-ă) [Gr. *pneuma,* air, + *ouron,* urine] Excretion of urine containing free gas. SYN: *pneumatinuria.*

pneumatype (nū'mă-tīp) [" + *typos,* type] The deposit of moisture on glass from the breath exhaled through the nostrils with the mouth closed for purpose of comparing the airflow through the nostrils.

pneumectomy (nū-mĕk'tō-mē) [Gr. *pneumon,* lung, + *ektome,* excision] Excision of all or part of a lung.

pneumo-, pneumono- [Gr. *pneumon,* lung] Combining form meaning *air, lung.*

pneumoangiography (nū"mō-ăn"jē-g'ră-fē) [Gr. *pneumon,* lung, + *angeion,* vessel, + *graphein,* to write] A radiographical study of the vessels of the lungs; usually performed using a contrast medium.

pneumoarthrography (nū"mō-ăr-thrŏg'ră-fē) [" + *arthron,* joint, + *graphein,* to write] Pneumarthrography.

pneumobilia (nū"mō-bĭll'ē-ah) Air or gas within the biliary ducts, a finding associated primarily with cholecystitis that is caused by gas-forming organisms.

pneumobulbar (nū"mō-bŭl'băr) [" + L. *bulbus,* bulbous root] Concerning the lungs and respiratory center in the medulla oblongata of the brain.

pneumocentesis (nū"mō-sĕn-tē'sĭs) [" + *kentesis,* a piercing] Paracentesis or surgical puncture of a lung to evacuate a cavity. SYN: *pneumonocentesis.*

pneumocephalus (nū"mō-sĕf'ă-lŭs) [Gr. *pneuma,* air, + *kephale,* head] Gas or air in the cavity of the cranium. SYN: *pneumocranium.*

pneumocholecystitis (nū"mō-kō"lē-sĭs-tī'tĭs) [" + *chole,* bile, + *kystis,* bladder, + *itis,* inflammation] Cholecystitis with gas in the gallbladder.

pneumococcal (nū″mō-kŏk′ăl) [″ + *kokkos,* berry] Concerning or caused by pneumococci.

pneumococcemia (nū″mō-kŏk-sē′mē-ă) The presence of pneumococci in the blood.

pneumococcidal (nū″mō-kŏk-sī′dăl) [″ + ″ + L. *cidus,* killing] Killing pneumococci.

pneumococcolysis (nū″mō-kŏk-ŏl′ĭ-sĭs) [″ + *kokkos,* berry, + *lysis,* dissolution] Destruction or lysis of pneumococci.

pneumococcus (nū″mō-kŏk′ŭs) *pl.* **pneumococci** [″ + *kokkos,* berry] An oval-shaped, encapsulated, non–spore-forming, gram-positive bacterium of the genus *Streptococcus,* occurring usually in pairs (diplococcus), with lancet-shaped ends. There are more than 80 serological types of pneumococci. Besides causing pneumonia, pneumococci cause otitis media, mastoiditis, meningitis, bronchitis, bloodstream infections, keratitis, and conjunctivitis. The risk of infection is greatest in children, elderly people, asplenic persons, and those with acquired immunodeficiency syndrome. About half of all pneumonias acquired by outpatients are caused by pneumococcus; many of these are preventable with pneumococcal vaccination. Although the pneumococcus used to be uniformly sensitive to treatment with penicillins, drug-resistant strains are exceptionally common, making the choice of antibiotic therapy increasingly difficult. SYN: *Streptococcus pneumoniae*. SEE: *pneumonia; polyvalent pneumococcal vaccine.*

pneumocolon (nū″mō-kō′lŏn) [″ + *kolon,* colon] Air in the colon. This may be introduced as an aid in radiological diagnosis.

pneumoconiosis (nū″mō-kō″nē-ō′sĭs) [″ + *konis,* dust, + *osis,* condition] Any disease of the respiratory tract owing to inhalation of dust particles; an occupational disorder such as that caused by mining or stonecutting. SYN: *pneumonoconiosis*.

pneumocranium (nū″mō-krā′nē-ŭm) [″ + *kranion,* skull] Pneumocephalus.

Pneumocystis carinii (nū″mō-sĭs′tĭs kă-rī′nē-ī) The causative organism of *Pneumocystis carinii* pneumonia. SEE: illus.; *AIDS*.

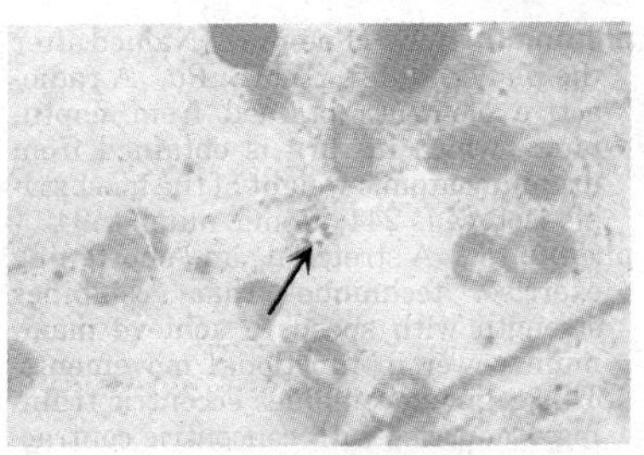

PNEUMOCYSTIS CARINII (X1000)

pneumocystography (nū″mō-sĭs-tŏg′ră-fē) [Gr. *pneuma,* air, + *kystis,* bladder, + *graphein,* to write] A cystogram done after air has been introduced into the urinary bladder.

pneumocystosis (nū″mō-sĭs-tō′sĭs) *Pneumocystis carinii* pneumonia.

pneumocyte Either of the two types of cells that form the alveoli of the lung. Type I cells are simple squamous epithelium that permit gas exchange. Type II cells are rounded and produce surfactant.

pneumoderma (nū″mō-dĕr′mă) [″ + *derma,* skin] Subcutaneous emphysema.

pneumodynamics (nū″mō-dī-năm′ĭks) [″ + *dynamis,* force] The branch of science dealing with force employed in respiration.

pneumoempyema (nū″mō-ĕm-pī-ē′mă) [″ + *en,* in + *pyon,* pus] Empyema accompanied by an accumulation of gas.

pneumoencephalitis (nū″mō-ĕn-sĕf″ă-lī′tĭs) [″ + *enkephalos,* brain, + *itis,* inflammation] Newcastle disease.

pneumoencephalogram (nū″mō-ĕn-sĕf′ă-lō-grăm) [″ + ″ + *gramma,* something written] An obsolete term for a radiograph of the subarachnoid space and ventricular system of the brain during pneumoencephalography.

pneumoencephalography (nū″mō-ĕn-sĕf″ă-lŏg′ră-fē) [″ + ″ + *graphein,* to write] An obsolete term for radiography of the ventricles and subarachnoid spaces of the brain following withdrawal of cerebrospinal fluid and injection of air or gas via lumbar puncture. This technique has been replaced by computed tomography and magnetic resonance imaging.

pneumofasciogram (nū″mō-făs′ē-ō-grăm) [″ + L. *fascia,* a band, + Gr. *gramma,* something written] An obsolete term for radiograph of fascial tissues and spaces after air has been injected in the fascia.

pneumogalactocele (nū″mō-găl-ăk′tō-sēl) [″ + *gala,* milk, + *kele,* tumor, swelling] A breast tumor containing milk and gas.

pneumogastric (nū″mō-găs′trĭk) [Gr. *pneumon,* lung, + *gaster,* stomach] Pert. to the lungs and stomach.

pneumogastric nerve Term formerly used for the vagus nerve.

pneumogastrography (nū″mō-găs-trŏg′ră-fē) [Gr. *pneuma,* air, + *gaster,* stomach, + *graphein,* to write] A radiographical study of the stomach after air has been introduced into it.

pneumogram (nū′mō-grăm) [″ + *gramma,* something written] **1.** A record of respiratory movements. **2.** A radiograph following injection of air.

pneumograph (nū′mō-grăf) [″ + *graphein,* to write] A device for recording the frequency and intensity of respiration.

pneumography (nū-mŏg′ră-fē) **1.** An anatomical description or illustration of the lung. **2.** The recording of respiratory movements on a graph. **3.** Radiography of a part or organ after injection of air.

pelvic p. An obsolete term for radiography of the pelvis after injection of carbon dioxide into the peritoneal cavity.

pneumohemopericardium (nū″mō-hēm″ō-pĕr-ĭ-kăr′dē-ŭm) [Gr. *pneumon,* lung, + *haima,* blood, + *peri,* around, + *kardia,* heart] The accumulation of air and blood in the pericardium.

pneumohemothorax (nū″mō-hēm″ō-thō′răks) [″ + ″ + *thorax,* chest] Gas or air and blood collected in the pleural cavity.

pneumohydrometra (nū″mō-hī″drō-mē′tră) [″ + *hydor,* water, + *metra,* uterus] The accumulation of gas and fluid in the uterus.

pneumohydropericardium (nū″mō-hī″drō-pĕr-ĭ-kăr′dē-ŭm) [″ + *hydor,* water, + *peri,* around, + *kardia,* heart] Air and fluid accumulated in the pericardium.

pneumohydrothorax (nū″mō-hī″drō-thō′răks) [″ + ″ + *thorax,* chest] Gas or air and fluid in the pleural cavity.

pneumohypoderma (nū″mō-hī″pō-dĕr′mă) [″ + *hypo,* under, + *derma,* skin] Subcutaneous emphysema.

pneumokidney (nū″mō-kĭd′nē) [″ + ME. *kidenei,* kidney] Air in the pelvis of the kidney.

pneumolith (nū′mō-lĭth) [″ + *lithos,* stone] A pulmonary stone.

pneumolithiasis (nū″mō-lĭth-ī′ăs-ĭs) [″ + ″ + *-iasis,* condition] Formation of stones in the lungs.

pneumolysin (nū-mŏl′ĭ-sĭn) A hemolytic toxin produced by pneumococci.

pneumomalacia (nū″mō-mă-lā′shē-ă) [″ + *malakia,* a softening] Abnormal softening of the lung.

pneumomassage (nū″mō-mă-săzh′) [Gr. *pneuma,* air, + *massein,* to knead] Massage of the tympanum with air to cause movement of the ossicles of the inner ear.

pneumomediastinum (nū″mō-mē″dē-ăs-tī′nŭm) [″ + L. *mediastinum,* in the middle] The presence of air or gas in the mediastinal tissues, either owing to disease or following injection of air into the area. It is a cause of intense chest pain that worsens with movement.

pneumomelanosis (nū″mō-mĕl-ăn-ō′sĭs) [Gr. *pneumon,* lung, + *melano,* black, + *osis,* condition] Pigmentation of the lung seen in pneumoconiosis. SYN: *pneumonomelanosis.*

pneumometer (nū-mŏm′ĕt-ĕr) [Gr. *pneuma,* air, + *metron,* measure] Spirometer.

pneumomycosis (nū″mō-mī-kō′sĭs) [Gr. *pneumon,* lung, + *mykes,* fungus, + *osis,* condition] A fungal pulmonary disease. SYN: *pneumonomycosis.*

pneumomyelography (nū″mō-mī-ĕl-g′ră-fē) [Gr. *pneuma,* air + *myelos,* marrow, + *graphein,* to write] An obsolete term for a radiographical study of the spinal canal following injection of air or other gas.

pneumonectasia, pneumonectasis (nū″mŏn-ĕk-tā′zē-ă, -ĕk′tă-sĭs) [″ + *ektasis,* dilatation] Distention of the lungs with air.

pneumonectomy (nū″mŏn-ĕk′tō-mē) [Gr. *pneumon,* lung, + *ektome,* excision] Pneumectomy.

pneumonia (nū-mō′nē-ă) [Gr.] Inflammation of the lungs, usually due to infection with bacteria, viruses, or other pathogenic organisms. Clinically, the term “pneumonia” is used to indicate an infectious disease. Pulmonary inflammation due to other causes is generally called “pneumonitis.” In the U.S., about 4,500,000 persons contract pneumonia each year. The disease is the sixth most common cause of death in the U.S. and the most common cause of death due to infectious disease. Pneumonia occurs most commonly in weakened individuals, such as those with cancer, heart or lung disease, immunosuppressive illnesses, diabetes mellitus, cirrhosis, malnutrition, and renal failure, but virulent pathogens can cause pneumonia in healthy persons as well. Smoking, general anesthesia, and endotracheal intubation each increase the risk for developing pneumonia by inhibiting airway defenses and helping disease-causing germs reach the alveoli of the lungs. SEE: *aspiration; pleural effusion; empyema; pleurisy; pneumonitis; tuberculosis* (and names of lung pathogens); *Nursing Diagnoses Appendix.*

ETIOLOGY: Pneumonias are categorized by site and by causative agent. Lobar pneumonia affects most of a single lobe; bronchopneumonia involves smaller lung areas in several lobes; interstitial pneumonia affects tissues surrounding the alveoli and bronchi of the lung. Atypical pneumonias diffusely affect lung tissues rather than anatomical lobes or lobules. Community-acquired pneumonia implies lung infection that develops in noninstitutionalized patients, typically involving organisms such as *Klebsiella pneumoniae, Mycoplasma pneumoniae, Legionella pneumophila, Chlamydia pneumoniae, Moraxella,* or *Pneumocystis carinii.* Nosocomial pneumonia develops in patients in the hospital or nursing home; this type is most likely to be caused by gram-negative rods or staphylococcal species. Aspiration pneumonias result from the inhalation of oropharyngeal microorganisms and often involve anaerobic organisms. Pneumonias in immunocompromised patients sometimes are caused by *Pneumocystis carinii* or by fungal species such as *Aspergillus* or *Candida*. Some fungal pneumonias occur in specific geographical regions of the U.S. For example, histoplasmosis is common in the Ohio River Valley, and coccidioidomycosis is found in the San Joaquin River Valley of southern California. Viral pneumonias may be caused by influenza, varicella-zoster, herpes, or adenoviruses, among others.

SYMPTOMS: Most patients with pneumonia have cough, shortness of breath, and fever, although these symptoms are not universal. Bacterial pneumonias are marked by abrupt onset, with high fevers, shaking chills, pleuritic chest pain, and prostration. Patients with atypical pneumonias usually have lower temperatures and nonproductive coughs and appear less ill.

PREVENTION: Pneumococcal vaccine effectively prevents many forms of streptococcal pneumonia; this vaccine is recommended for persons over age 65; those with chronic respiratory, cardiac, or neuromuscular diseases; and patients with diabetes mellitus or renal failure, among others.

TREATMENT: Treatment is based on the clinical presentation (e.g., community-acquired versus nosocomial), results of the Gram stain of sputum specimens, the radiographic appearance of the pneumonia, the degree of respiratory impairment, and the results of cultures. Many patients hospitalized with pneumonia require supplemental oxygen and analgesics. Erythromycin and cephalosporins, for example, are empirical treatments for community-acquired pneumonias.

PATIENT CARE: Supportive care is provided for the patient with pneumonia to remove secretions and to improve gas exchange. Such care includes position changes, deep-breathing and coughing exercises and respiratory toilet, active and passive limb exercises, and assistance with self-care. Oxygen therapy may be needed in more severe cases, esp. if the patient has a preexisting lung disease. Respiratory status is monitored by chest assessment, oximetry, and arterial blood gas studies. The patient is assessed for signs and symptoms of respiratory failure, sepsis, and shock. Prescribed analgesics are administered. The prescribed medical regimen is carried out, and the patient's response is evaluated. The patient is encouraged to verbalize concerns; diagnostic studies and therapeutic measures are explained, and the patient is taught about the importance of follow-up care.

abortive p. Mild pneumonia with a brief course.

acute lobar p. Lobar p.

p. alba A pneumonia seen in stillborn infants; it is caused by congenital syphilis.

aspiration p. Pneumonia caused by inhalation of gastric contents, food, or other substances. A frequent cause is loss of the gag reflex in patients with central nervous system depression or damage or alcoholic intoxication with stupor and vomiting. This condition also occurs in newborns who inhale infected amniotic fluid, meconium, or vaginal secretions during delivery.

atypical p. Pneumonia caused by a virus or *Mycoplasma pneumoniae*. The symptoms are low-grade fever, nonproductive cough, pharyngitis, myalgia, and minimal adventitious lung sounds.

community-acquired p. Pneumonia occurring in outpatients, often caused by infection with streptococcus, *Haemophilus influenzae, Staphylococcus aureus,* and atypical organisms. Mortality is approximately 15% but depends on many host and pathogen features.

desquamative interstitial p. Pneumonia of unknown etiology accompanied by cellular infiltration or fibrosis in the pulmonary interstitium. Progressive dyspnea and a nonproductive cough are symptoms characterizing this disease. Clubbing of the fingers is a common finding. Diffusion of oxygen and carbon dioxide is abnormal. Diagnosis is made by lung biopsy. The condition is treated by corticosteroids.

double p. Pneumonia that involves both lungs or two lobes.

embolic p. Pneumonia following embolization of a pulmonary blood vessel.

eosinophilic p. Infiltration of the lung by eosinophils, typically found in patients with peripheral eosinophilia. The etiology usually is unknown; occasionally, the condition responds to the administration of corticosteroids. In some cases, a specific underlying cause is found, such as the recent initiation of cigarette smoking or an allergic drug reaction. Infection with some parasites or fungi also can trigger the disease.

fibrous p. Pneumonia followed by formation of scar tissue.

Friedländer's p. A form of lobar pneumonia caused by the specific organism *Klebsiella pneumoniae*.

gangrenous p. Pulmonary gangrene.

giant cell p. An interstitial pneumonitis of infancy and childhood. The lung tissue contains multinucleated giant cells. The disease often occurs in connection with measles.

hypostatic p. Pneumonia occurring in elderly or bed-ridden patients who re-

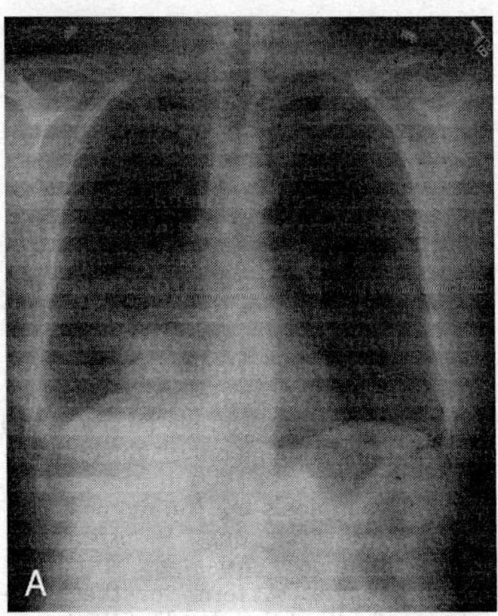

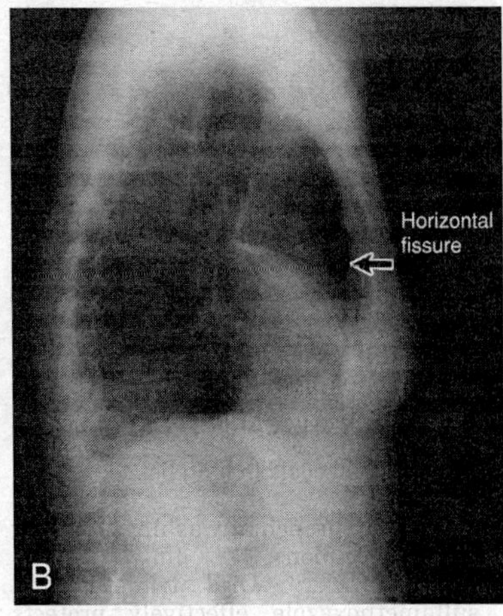

LOBAR PNEUMONIA

(A) The right heart border is obscured by the infection, (B) Lateral view shows dense (white) infiltrate sharply defined by horizontal fissure (Courtesy of Harvey Hatch, MD, Curry General Hospital)

main constantly in the same position. Ventilation is greatest in dependent areas; remaining in one position causes hypoventilation in many areas, causing alveolar collapse (atelectasis) and creating a pulmonary environment that supports the growth of bacteria or other organisms. Development of this condition is prevented by having the patient change positions and take deep breaths to inflate peripheral alveoli. SEE: *pneumonia*.

PATIENT CARE: Prevention is the most important factor, esp. in elderly and immobile persons. Patients should be moved and turned frequently at least every 1 to 2 hr. The nurse and respiratory therapist should encourage the patient to engage in active movement and to perform deep-breathing coughing exercises frequently and regularly. Incentive spirometry may prove useful in patients who need added encouragement to deep breathe periodically.

intrauterine p. Pneumonia contracted in utero.

Legionella p. SEE: *Legionnaires' disease*.

lipoid p. Damage to lung tissue that results from aspiration of oils. It may occur repeatedly in patients with impaired swallowing mechanisms or in persons affected by esophageal disorders, such as esophageal carcinoma, achalasia, or scleroderma. Mineral oils and cooking oils often are responsible. Most cases resolve spontaneously, but corticosteroids sometimes are used as treatment to reduce inflammatory changes. Distinguishing lipoid pneumonia from bacterial pneumonia may require endoscopy.

lobar p. Pneumonia infecting one or more lobes of the lung, usually caused by *Streptococcus pneumoniae*. The pathologic changes are, in order, congestion; redness and firmness due to exudate and red blood cells in the alveoli; and, finally, gray hepatization as the exudate degenerates and is absorbed. SYN: *acute lobar p.* SEE: illus.

nosocomial p. Pneumonia occurring after 48 hours of hospitalization. It is often the result of infection with gram-negative pathogens or multiply drug-resistant bacteria. Mortality is approximately 50%.

Pneumocystis carinii p. ABBR: PCP. A subacute opportunistic infection marked by fever, nonproductive cough, tachypnea, dyspnea, and hypoxemia. It is caused by *Pneumocystis carinii,* an organism formerly thought to be a protozoan but now generally accepted as a fungus. The disease is seen principally in immunosuppressed patients, such as persons with the acquired immunodeficiency syndrome (AIDS) or who have received an organ transplant and immunosuppressant drugs. Without treatment, the progressive respiratory failure that the infection causes is ultimately fatal.

DIAGNOSIS: The disease should be suspected in patients with human immunodeficiency virus (HIV) infection or other risk factors for the disease who present with cough and shortness of breath. Chest x-ray examination may reveal diffuse interstitial infiltrates, upper lobe disease, spontaneous pneumothorax, or cystic lung disease. The diagnosis is confirmed with special stains

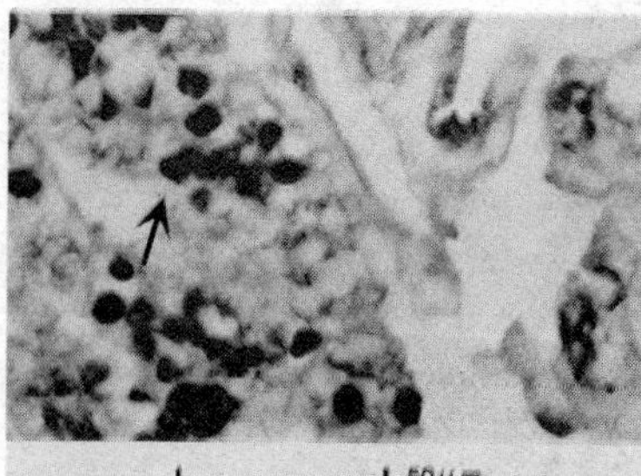

PNEUMOCYSTIS CARINII PNEUMONIA

Silver-stained cysts in lung tissue (×400)

of sputum, bronchial washings, or lung biopsy specimens. SEE: illus.

TREATMENT: Oral trimethoprim-sulfamethoxazole effectively protects against PCP, and is also the drug of choice for active infection. Other drugs that are active against PCP include pentamidine, trimethoprim in combination with dapsone, and atovaquone. Corticosteroids are used as adjunctive therapy when treating markedly hypoxic patients (e.g., those who present with an alveolar-arterial oxygen gradient of more than 35 mm Hg). The introduction of highly active antiretroviral drug cocktails for AIDS patients has restored immune function to many patients and markedly reduced the incidence of PCP.

secondary p. Pneumonia that occurs in connection with a specific systemic disease such as typhoid, diphtheria, or plague.

tuberculous p. Pneumonia caused by *Mycobacterium tuberculosis*. SEE: *tuberculosis*.

tularemic p. Pneumonia caused by *Francisella tularensis*. It may be primary or associated with tularemia.

woolsorter's p. Pulmonary anthrax.

pneumonic (nū-mŏn'ĭk) [Gr. *pneumon,* lung] Concerning the lungs or pneumonia.

pneumonitis (nū"mō-nī'tĭs) [" + *itis,* inflammation] Inflammation of the lung, usually due to hypersensitivity (allergy), radiation exposure, aspiration, viral infection, or autoimmune illnesses, such as systemic lupus erythematosus.

hypersensitivity p. Immunologically induced inflammation of the lungs of a susceptible host caused by repeated inhalation of a variety of substances including organic dusts. Included are molds and other fungi from sources such as cheese, vegetables, mushrooms, flour, mushroom compost, bark of trees, detergents, and contaminated humidification systems. In the acute stage, patients may present with cough, fever, chills, malaise, and shortness of breath. In the subacute and chronic forms, the onset of symptoms is gradual and prolonged. Treatment includes identifying and avoiding causative agents.

mycoplasma p. A form of atypical pneumonia caused by *Mycoplasma pneumoniae*.

pneumococcal p. Pneumonia in which the causative agent is pneumococci. SEE: *Streptococcus pneumoniae*.

pneumono- [Gr. *pneumon,* lung] SEE: *pneumo-*.

pneumonocele (nū-mŏn'ō-sēl) [" + *kele,* tumor, swelling] Pneumatocele.

pneumonocentesis (nū-mō"nō-sĕn-tē'sĭs) [" + *kentesis,* a piercing] Pneumocentesis.

pneumonoconiosis (nū-mō"nō-kō"nē-'sĭs) [" + *konis,* dust, + *osis,* condition] Pneumoconiosis.

pneumonocyte A term for the three types of cells of the alveoli of the lungs: type I and II alveolar cells and alveolar macrophages.

pneumonolysis (nū"mŏ-nŏl'ĭ-sĭs) [" + *lysis,* dissolution] The loosening and separation of an adherent lung from the costal pleura.

extrapleural p. Separation of the parietal pleura from the chest wall. SEE: *apicolysis*.

intrapleural p. Separation of adhering visceral and parietal layers of pleura.

pneumonomelanosis (nū"mō-nō-mĕl"ăn-'sĭs) [" + *melano,* black, + *osis,* condition] Pneumomelanosis.

pneumonomycosis (nū-mōn"ō-mī-kō'sĭs) [" + *mykes,* fungus, + *osis,* condition] Pneumomycosis.

pneumonopathy (nū"mō-nŏp'ăth-ē) [" + *pathos,* disease, suffering] Any diseased condition of the lung.

pneumonoperitonitis (nū"mō-nō-pĕr"ĭ-tō-nī'tĭs) [" + *peritonaion,* peritoneum, + *itis,* inflammation] Pneumoperitonitis.

pneumonopleuritis (nū-mō"nō-ploo-rī'tĭs) [Gr. *pneumon,* lung, + *pleura,* side, + *itis,* inflammation] Pneumopleuritis.

pneumonorrhapy (nū"mō-nor'ă-fē) [" + *rhaphe,* seam, ridge] Suture of a lung.

pneumonotherapy Pneumotherapy.

pneumonotomy (nū-mō-nŏt'ō-mē) [" + *tome,* incision] Incision into the lung. SYN: *pneumotomy*.

pneumopericardium (nū"mō-pĕr-ĭ-kăr'dē-ŭm) [Gr. *pneuma,* air, + *peri,* around, + *kardia,* heart] Air or gas in the pericardial sac; caused by trauma or pathological communication between the esophagus, stomach, or lungs and the pericardium. On examination one finds unusual metallic heart sounds and tympany over the precordial area.

pneumoperitoneography An obsolete term for radiographical examination of the peritoneum and internal organs after introduction of sterile air into the peritoneal cavity.

pneumoperitoneum (nū″mō-pĕr-ĭ-tō-nē′ŭm) [″ + *peritonaion,* peritoneum] **1.** A condition in which air or gas collects in the peritoneal cavity. This may occur catastrophically when internal organs rupture. **2.** Air or gas that has been injected into the peritoneal cavity to facilitate laparoscopy.

pneumoperitonitis (nū″mō-pĕr-ĭ-tō-nī′tĭs) [″ + *peritonaion,* peritoneum, + *itis,* inflammation] Peritonitis with gas accumulation.

pneumopexy (nū′mō-pĕks″ē) [Gr. *pneumon,* lung, + *pexis,* fixation] Pneumonopexy.

pneumopleuritis (nū″mō-ploo-rī′tĭs) [″ + *pleura,* a side, + *itis,* inflammation] Inflammation of the lungs and pleura.

pneumopyelography (nū″mō-pī-ĕ-lŏg′ră-fē) [Gr. *pneuma,* air, + *pyelos,* pelvis, + *graphein,* to write] An obsolete term for a radiographical examination of the renal pelvis and ureters after they are injected with oxygen.

pneumopyopericardium (nū″mō-pī″ō-pĕr-ĭ-kar′dē-ŭm) [″ + *pyon,* pus, + *peri,* around, + *kardia,* heart] Air, gas, and pus collected in the pericardium.

pneumopyothorax (nū″mō-pī″ō-thō′răks) [″ + ″ + *thorax,* chest] Air and pus collected in the pleural cavity.

pneumoradiography (nū″mō-rā-dē-g′ră-fē) [″ + L. *radius,* ray, + Gr. *graphein,* to write] Injection of air into a part for the purpose of x-ray examination. This procedure has been replaced by computed tomography and magnetic resonance imaging.

pneumoretroperitoneum (nū″mō-rĕt″rō-pĕr″ĭ-tō-nē′ŭm) [″ + L. *retro,* backwards, + Gr. *peritonaion,* peritoneum] Air or gas in the retroperitoneal space.

pneumorrhachis (nū″mō-rā′kĭs) [Gr. *pneumon,* lung, + *rhachis,* spine] Gas accumulation in the spinal canal.

pneumorrhagia (nū″mō-rā′jē-ă) [Gr. *pneumon,* lung, + *rhegnynai,* to burst forth] Lung hemorrhage. SEE: *hemoptysis.*

pneumoserothorax (nū″mō-sē-rō-thō′răks) [Gr. *pneuma,* air, + L. *serum,* whey, + Gr. *thorax,* chest] Air or gas and serum collected in the pleural cavity.

pneumosilicosis (nū″mō-sĭl″ĭ-kō′sĭs) [Gr. *pneumon,* lung, + L. *silex,* flint, + Gr. *osis,* condition] Silicosis.

pneumotaxic (nū″mō-tăk′sĭk) [″ + *taxis,* arrangement] Concerning the regulation of breathing.

pneumotherapy (nū-mō-thĕr′ă-pē) [Gr. *pneumon,* lung, + *therapeia,* treatment] The treatment of diseases of the lungs.

pneumotherapy (nū-mō-thĕr′ă-pē) [Gr. *pneuma,* air, + *therapeia,* treatment] The treatment of diseases by the use of rarefied or condensed gases. SYN: *pneumatotherapy; pneumonotherapy.*

pneumothorax (nū-mō-thō′răks) [″ + *thorax,* chest] A collection of air or gas in the pleural cavity. The gas enters as the result of a perforation through the chest wall or the pleura covering the lung (visceral pleura). This perforation may be the result of an injury or of the rupture of an emphysematous bleb or superficial lung abscess. Some tall slender young men and women suffer repeated episodes of spontaneous pneumothorax. SEE: illus.; *Nursing Diagnoses Appendix.*

SYMPTOMS: The onset is sudden, usually with a severe sharp pain in the side and marked dyspnea. The physical signs are those of a distended unilateral chest, tympanitic resonance, absence of breath sounds, and, if fluid is present, a splashing sound on succussion (or shaking) of the patient.

TREATMENT: The affected lung may need to be reinflated with chest tube thoracostomy.

PATIENT CARE: The nurse or respiratory therapist explains the procedure for chest tube insertion and assists the physician as necessary. Vital signs, breath sounds, chest expansion, chest tube site, drainage, and blood gas analysis are assessed. The skin around the thorax is palpated for subcutaneous emphysema, which indicates air leak into the soft tissues. Oxygen is administered as prescribed. The patient is placed in the semi-Fowler position to promote drainage, comfort, and ease of breathing. Adequate rest periods are provided. Medications are administered as prescribed (analgesics, antibiotics, expectorants). Intake and output are monitored. The patient should maintain adequate nutrition and fluid intake to promote tissue healing and repair and to maintain proper hydration. The catheter site is observed daily and redressed as necessary. The patient should avoid excessive exercise and smoking. The importance of follow-up examination is stressed to the patient and care of the chest tube insertion site is taught.

artificial p. A pneumothorax induced intentionally by artificial means, used to treat pulmonary tuberculosis or pneumonia. Pneumothorax allows the diseased lung to rest temporarily. The lung collapses when the air enters the pleural space.

Scattered adhesions may afford only a partial collapse. Effusion may occur in about one third of the cases. Hazards include pain, infection, and respiratory distress.

extrapleural p. The formation of a pneumothorax by introducing air into

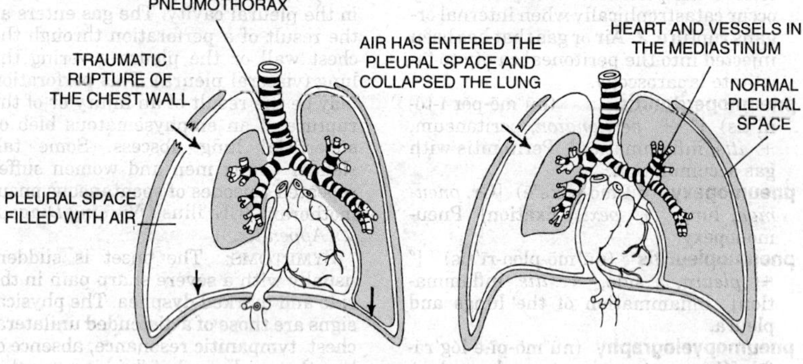
(CHEST WALL INJURY PERMITS
AIR TO FLOW IN AND OUT OF THE PLEURAL
SPACE ON THE AFFECTED SIDE)
TRACHEA AND MEDIASTINUM
SHIFTED AWAY FROM
PNEUMOTHORAX
HEART AND VESSELS IN
THE MEDIASTINUM
AIR HAS ENTERED THE
PLEURAL SPACE AND
COLLAPSED THE LUNG
TRAUMATIC
RUPTURE OF
THE CHEST WALL
NORMAL
PLEURAL
SPACE
PLEURAL SPACE
FILLED WITH AIR
INHALATION: AIR ENTERS THE INJURED
SIDE, CAUSING COLLAPSE OF THE LUNG
AND SHIFT OF THE MEDIASTINUM AND
HEART TOWARD THE UNAFFECTED SIDE
EXHALATION: THE AIR IS PARTIALLY
FORCED FROM THE AFFECTED SIDE
PLEURAL SPACE AND THE MEDIASTINUM
SHIFTS TOWARD THE AFFECTED SIDE

OPEN PNEUMOTHORAX

the space between the pleura and the inside of the rib cage.

open p. A pneumothorax in which the pleural cavity is exposed to the atmosphere through an open wound in the chest wall.

spontaneous p. The spontaneous entrance of air into the pleural cavity. The pressure may collapse the lung and displace the mediastinum away from the side of the lesion.

SYMPTOMS: Sudden sharp pain, dyspnea, and cough characterize this condition although it may be asymptomatic (silent). Pain may be referred to the shoulder. The majority of cases are mild and require only rest. Rarely shock and collapse occur.

tension p. A type of pneumothorax in which air can enter the pleural space but cannot escape via the route of entry. This leads to increased pressure in the pleural space, resulting in lung collapse. The increase in pressure also compresses the heart and vena cavae, which impairs circulation.

PATIENT CARE: The patient is assessed for respiratory failure. The chest is auscultated for decreased breath sounds over the collapsed lung and inspected for signs of mediastinal shift (deviation of the trachea away from the affected side). Vital signs are assessed for evidence of hypotension, tachypnea, and tachycardia, ominous signs indicating need for immediate water-seal chest tube drainage or needle chest decompression.

pneumotomy (nū-mŏt′ō-mē) [Gr. *pneumon,* lung, + *tome,* incision] Pneumonotomy.

pneumotoxin (nū″mō-tŏks′ĭn) [″ + *toxikon,* poison] A toxin produced by pneumococcus.

pneumotyphus (nū″mō-tī′fŭs) [″ + *typhos,* fever] **1.** Typhoid fever with pneumonia at onset. **2.** The development of pneumonia during typhoid fever.

pneumoventricle (nū″mō-vĕn′trĭ-k′l) [″ + L. *ventriculus,* little belly] Air accumulation in the cerebral ventricles.

pneumoventriculography (nū″mō-vĕn-trĭk″ū-lŏg′ră-fē) [″ + ″ + Gr. *graphein,* to write] An obsolete term for radiography of the ventricles of the brain after the injection of air.

pnigophobia (nī″gō-fō′bē-ă) [Gr. *pnigos,* choking, + *phobos,* fear] Morbid fear of choking; sometimes experienced in angina pectoris.

Po Symbol for the element polonium.

PO_2 Abbr. for *partial pressure of oxygen.*

p.o. L. *per os,* by mouth.

pock (pŏk) [AS. *poc,* pustule] A pustule of an eruptive fever, esp. of smallpox.

pocket (pŏk′ĕt) [ME. *poket,* pouch] A saclike cavity.

gingival p. Periodontal p.

periodontal p. A gingival sulcus enlarged beyond normal limits as a result of poor oral hygiene; the space bordered on one side by the tooth and the other side by ulcerated sulcular epithelium. It will be several millimeters deep when probed and limited at its apex by attachment epithelium.

pocketing A method of treating the pedicle in ovariotomy by enclosing it within the edges of the wound.

pockmarked Pitted or marked with scars from healed pustules, esp. those due to smallpox.

poculum diogenis (pŏk′ū-lŭm dī-ŏj′ē-nĭs) [L. *poculum,* cup, + Diogenes, Gr. philosopher, 4th century B.C.] The concavity formed by contracting the muscles of the hand so the palm becomes cupped instead of flat.

podagra (pō-dăg′ră) [Gr. *podos,* foot, + *agra,* seizure] Gout, esp. of the joints of the great toe.

podalgia (pō-dăl′jē-ă) [″ + *algos,* pain] Pain in the feet.

podalic (pō-dăl′ĭk) [Gr. *podos,* foot] Pert. to the feet.

podencephalus (pŏd″ĕn-sĕf′ă-lŭs) [″ + *enkephalos,* brain] A deformed fetus in whom most of the brain is outside the skull and is attached by a thin pedicle.

podiatrist (pō-dī′ă-trĭst″) [″ + *iatreia,* treatment] A health professional responsible for the examination, diagnosis, prevention, treatment, and care of conditions and functions of the human foot. A podiatrist performs surgical procedures and prescribes corrective devices, drugs, and physical therapy as legally authorized in the state in which he or she is practicing. SYN: *chiropodist.*

podiatry (pō-dī′ă-trē) The diagnosis, treatment, and prevention of conditions of human feet. SYN: *chiropody.*

podium (pō′dē-ŭm) [Gr. *podos,* foot] A footlike projection.

podo-, pod- [Gr. *pous, podos,* foot] Combining form meaning *foot.*

podobromidrosis (pŏd″ō-brō″mĭ-drō′sĭs) [″ + *bromos,* stench, + *hidros,* sweat] Offensive perspiration of the feet.

podocyte (pŏd′ō-sīt) [″ + *kytos,* cell] A special epithelial cell with numerous footplates (pedicels). These form the inner layer of Bowman's capsule of the renal corpuscle and have spaces for the passage of renal filtrate from the glomerulus.

pododynamometer (pŏd″ō-dī″nă-mŏm′ĕ-tĕr) [″ + *dynamis,* force, + *metron,* measure] A device for testing the strength of the leg and foot muscles.

podophyllum (pŏd-ō-fĭl′ŭm) [″ + *phyllon,* leaf] The dried rhizome and roots of *Podophyllum peltatum;* used for treating, by direct application, certain papillomas such as condyloma acuminata.

podophyllum resin (pŏd″ō-fĭl′ŭm) The resinous extract from podophyllum.

POEMS An acronym for *p*olyneuropathy, *o*rganomegaly, *e*ndocrinopathy, *m*onoclonal gammopathy, and *s*kin changes.

pogoniasis (pō″gō-nī′ă-sĭs) [Gr. *pogon,* beard, + *-iasis,* disorder] **1.** Excessive growth of the beard. **2.** Growth of a beard in a woman.

pogonion (pō-gō′nē-ŏn) Mental point.

-poiesis [Gr.] Combining form used as a suffix meaning *formation, production.*

poikilo- Combining form meaning *irregular, varied.*

poikilocyte A teardrop or pear-shaped red blood cell, seen in myelofibrosis and certain anemias. SEE: illus.

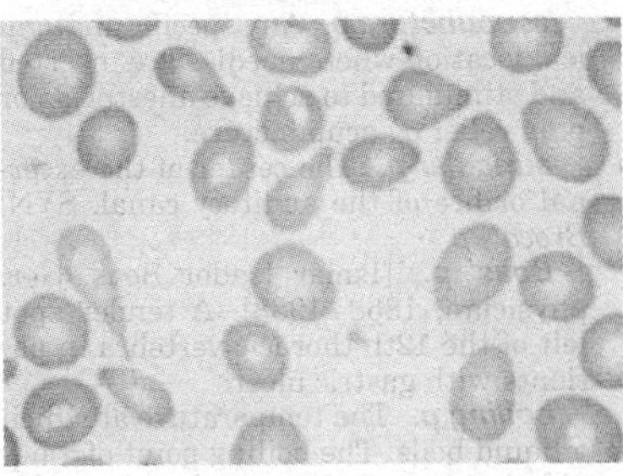

POIKILOCYTES (X640)

poikilocytosis (poy″kĭl-ō-sī-tō′sĭs) [″ + ″ + *osis,* condition] A term used to describe variations in shape of red blood cells (e.g., elliptocytes, spherocytes, dacryocytes, sickle cells, schizocytes, echinocytes, and acanthocytes).

poikilodentosis (poy″kĭ-lō-dĕn-tō′sĭs) [″ + L. *dens,* tooth, + Gr. *osis,* condition] Mottling of the teeth usually caused by an excess of fluoride in the drinking water.

poikiloderma (poy-kĭl-ō-dĕr′mă) [″ + *derma,* skin] A skin disorder characterized by pigmentation, telangiectasia, purpura, pruritus, and atrophy.

p. atrophicans vasculare A generalized dermatitis of unknown cause. It is symmetrical and occurs almost exclusively in adults. There is widespread telangiectasia, pigmentation, and atrophy of the skin.

p. of Civatte Reticulated pigmentation and telangiectasia of the sides of the face and neck; seen quite commonly in middle-aged women.

poikilonymy (poy″kĭ-lŏn′ĭ-mē) [″ + *onoma,* name] The use of terms from several nomenclature systems.

poikilotherm (poy-kĭl′ō-thĕrm) [″ + *therme,* heat] An animal whose body temperature varies according to the temperature of the environment. A cold blooded animal. SYN: *allotherm.* SEE: *homotherm.*

poikilothermal, poikilothermic (poy″kĭ-lō-thĕr′măl, -mĭk) Concerning poikilothermy.

poikilothermy (poy″kĭ-lō-thĕr′mē) The condition of having the temperature of the organism or animal match the temperature of the environment. Reptiles have this property. SEE: *homoiotherm.*

poikilothrombocyte (poy-kĭl″ō-thrŏm′bō-sīt) [″ + *thrombos,* clot, + *kytos,* cell] An abnormally shaped platelet.

point (poynt) [O.Fr., a prick, a dot] **1.** The sharp end of any object. **2.** The stage at which the surface of an abscess is about to rupture. **3.** A minute spot. **4.** A position in space, time, or degree.

absorbent p. A cone of paper used in drying or in keeping liquid medicines in a root canal of a tooth.

acupuncture p. Any specific anatomical location where needles are inserted and stimulated to achieve anesthesia or pain relief by acupuncture.

auricular p. The center of the external orifice of the auditory canal. SYN: *Broca's p.*

Boas' p. [Ismar Isador Boas, Ger. physician, 1858–1938] A tender spot left of the 12th thoracic vertebra in patients with gastric ulcer.

boiling p. The temperature at which a liquid boils. The boiling point of a liquid varies according to the chemicals present in it. Under ordinary conditions water boils at 212°F (100°C) at sea level. To kill most vegetative forms of microorganisms, water should be boiled for 30 min.

Broca's p. Auricular p.

Capuron's p. One of four fixed points in the pelvic inlet, the two iliopectineal eminences and the two sacroiliac joints. SYN: *cardinal p.* (2).

cardinal p. **1.** One of six points determining the direction of light rays emerging from and entering the eye. SEE: *nodal p.; principal p.* **2.** Capuron's p.

cold rigor p. The temperature at which cell activity ceases.

contact p. The point on a tooth that touches an opposed tooth.

convergence p. **1.** The point to which rays of light converge. **2.** The closest point to the patient on which the eyes can converge as the object is moved closer and closer.

corresponding p. The point in the retina of each eye that, when stimulated simultaneously, results in a single visual sensation.

craniometric p. One of the fixed points of the skull used in craniometry.

critical p. of gases The temperature at or above which a gas is no longer liquefied by pressure.

critical p. of liquids The temperature above which no pressure may retain a substance in a liquid form.

deaf p. of the ear One of several points or areas close to the external auditory meatus where a vibrating tuning fork is not heard.

disparate p. Points on the retinas that are unequally paired.

end p. The point or time at which a reaction or activity is completed.

external orbital p. The prominent point at the outer edge of the orbit above the frontomalar suture.

far p. Point (normally 20 ft [6.1 m] or more) at which distinct vision is possible without aid of the muscles of accommodation. It may be nearer than 20 ft (6.1 m) according to the degree of myopia. There is no far point in the hypermetropic eye.

fixation p. The fovea or point on the retina where the visual axes (lines) meet the point of clearest vision.

flash p. The temperature at which a substance bursts into flame spontaneously.

focal p. The point at which a group of light rays converge.

freezing p. The temperature at which liquids become solid.

fusion p. Melting p.

Guéneau de Mussy's p. The point located at the junction of a line extending down from the left border of the sternum with a horizontal line at the level of the bony part of the anterior portion of the tenth rib. Pressure on this point causes pain in cases of diaphragmatic pleurisy.

gutta-percha p. A cone made of gutta-percha combined with other material that is used in filling root canals of teeth.

Halle's p. [Adrien Joseph Marie Nöel Halle, Fr. physician, 1859–1947] The point at the intersection of a horizontal line drawn from the anterior superior iliac spines and an angled line extending up from the pubic spine. At that point, the ureter is palpable as it crosses the pelvic brim.

hot p. A spot on the skin that perceives hot but not cold stimuli.

hysterogenic p. One of the circumscribed areas of the body that produce symptoms of a hysterical aura, and eventually a hysterical attack, when rubbed or pressed.

ice p. The temperature at which there is equilibrium between ice and air-saturated water at one atmosphere of pressure.

identical retinal p. The points in the two retinas upon which the images are seen as one.

isoelectric p. The particular pH of a solution of an amphoteric electrolyte such as an amino acid or protein in which the charged molecules do not migrate to either electrode. Proteins are least soluble at this point. Thus at the appropriate pH, proteins may be precipitated.

isoionic p. The pH at which a solution of ionized material has as many negative as positive ions.

J p. On the electrocardiogram, the juncture between the end of the QRS complex and the beginning of the T wave; that is, between the representations of ventricular depolarization and repolarization.

jugal p. The posterior border of the

frontal process of the malar bone where bisected by a line tangent to the upper border of the zygoma.

lacrimal p. The outlet of the lacrimal canaliculus. SYN: *punctum lacrimale*.

Lanz's p. [Otto Lanz, Swiss surgeon in the Netherlands, 1865–1935] The point on the line between the two anterior superior iliac spines, one third of the distance from the right spine, indicating the origin of the vermiform appendix.

Lian's p. The point at the junction of the outer and middle thirds of a line from the umbilicus to the anterior superior spine of the ilium where a trocar may be introduced safely for paracentesis.

malar p. The most prominent point on the external tubercle of the malar bone.

p. of maximal impulse ABBR: P.M.I. The point on the chest wall over the heart at which the contraction of the heart is best seen or felt; normally at the fourth to fifth intercostal space in the midclavicular line.

maximum occipital p. The point on the occipital bone farthest from the glabella.

median mandibular p. The point on the anteroposterior center of the mandibular ridge in the median sagittal plane.

melting p. The temperature at which a solid becomes a liquid. This is a constant for each material.

mental p. The most anterior point of the midline of the chin. SYN: *pogonion*.

metopic p. Glabella.

motor p. The point usually about the middle of a muscle where a motor nerve enters the muscle at which a minimal electrical stimulus to the overlying skin will elicit a visible contraction.

Munro's p. [John Cummings Munro, U.S. surgeon, 1858–1910] The point halfway between the left anterior iliac spine and the umbilicus.

nasal p. Nasion.

near p. The nearest point at which the eye can accommodate for distinct vision.

p. of no return An unofficial term describing a critical biochemical event that indicates lethal, irreversible changes in cells following ischemic cell injury.

nodal p. Either of a pair of points situated on the axis of an optical system so that any incident ray sent through one will produce a parallel emergent ray sent through the other.

occipital p. The most posterior point on the occipital bone.

painful p. Valleix's p.

preauricular p. The point immediately in front of the auricular point.

pressure p. **1.** A point on the skin that, when stimulated, gives rise to a sensation of pressure. **2.** A point where an artery comes near the surface and at which pressure may be applied to stop arterial bleeding.

principal p. One of two points so situated that the optical axis is cut by the two principal planes.

p. of regard The point at which the eye is looking.

silver p. An elongated, tapered silver plug used to fill the root canal in the endodontic treatment of teeth.

spinal p. Subnasal p.

subnasal p. The center of the root of the anterior nasal spine. SYN: *spinal p.*

supra-auricular p. The point on the skull on the posterior root of the zygomatic process of the temporal bone, directly above the auricular point.

supranasal p. Supraorbital p.

supraorbital p. **1.** The point on the skull in the midline of the forehead, just above the glabella. SYN: *ophryon*. **2.** A neuralgic point just above the supraorbital notch.

tender p. One of the anatomic locations used to identify fibromyalgia. The deep diffuse muscular pain is localized to a number of reproducible (from patient to patient) areas that are tender when palpated. Tender points differ from trigger points in that pain does not radiate to referred areas. SEE: *fibromyalgia* for table.

thermal death p. The temperature required to kill all of the organisms in a culture in a specified time.

trigger p. SEE: *trigger point*.

triple p. The temperature and pressure that allow the solid, liquid, and vapor forms of a substance to exist in equilibrium.

Trousseau's apophysiary p. Sensitive points over the dorsal and lumbar vertebrae in neuralgia.

Valleix's p. Tender spots upon pressure over the course of a nerve in neuralgia. SYN: *painful p.*

vital p. The point in the medulla oblongata close to the floor of the fourth ventricle, the puncture of which causes instant death owing to destruction of the respiratory center.

Voillemier's p. The point on the linea alba of the abdominal wall about 6 to 7 cm below a line connecting the anterior superior iliac spines. Suprapubic puncture of the bladder may be made at this point in obese or edematous individuals.

pointer, light A head-mounted input device to enable computer use by persons with paralysis or limited movement. These devices typically operate through visible or invisible light sources at the tip of the pointer, which transmits a signal to a computer-mounted light sensor or receiver.

pointillage (pwăn″tĭ-yăzh′) [Fr.] Massage with the fingertips.

pointing 1. Reaching a point. 2. Forming a localized collection of pus near the body surface.

point of service A form of extended health-care coverage granted to members of managed-care plans who opt to pay additional premiums for medical services provided by special panels of providers.

poise (poyz) [J. M. Poiseuille] The unit of viscosity; the tangential shearing force required to be applied to an area of 1 cm^2 between two parallel planes of 1 cm^2 in area and 1 cm apart in order to produce a velocity of flow of the liquid of 1 cm/sec.

Poiseuille's law (pwă-zŭ'yĕz) [Jean Marie Poiseuille, Fr. physiologist, 1799–1869] A law that states that the rapidity of the capillary current is directly proportional to the fourth power of the radius of the capillary tube, the pressure on the fluid, and inversely proportional to the viscosity of the liquid and the length of the tube.

Poiseuille's space The inert capillary current in which leukocytes close to the wall of the vessel move slowly; the erythrocytes travel more rapidly in the middle current.

POISINDEX® A computerized database, revised quarterly, on over 300,000 commercial compounds. For information, contact Micromedex, Inc., 600 Grant St., Denver, CO 80203; (800) 525-9083.

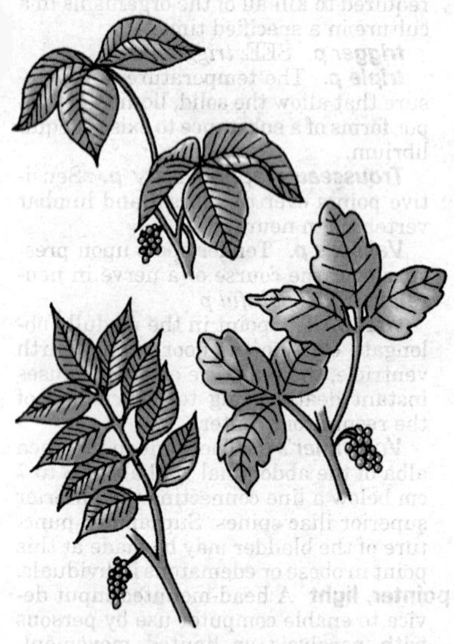

POISON IVY - POISON OAK
POISON SUMAC
(FROM TOP TO BOTTOM)

poison (poy'zn) [L. *potio*, a poisonous draft] Any substance taken into the body by ingestion, inhalation, injection, or absorption that interferes with normal physiological functions. Virtually any substance can be poisonous if consumed in sufficient quantity; therefore the term poison more often implies an excessive degree of dosage rather than a specific group of substances. Aspirin is not usually thought of as a poison, but overdoses of this drug kill more children accidentally each year than any of the traditional poisons. SEE: *poisoning; Poisons and Poisoning Appendix.*

cellular p. Anything that damages or kills cells.

p. ivy A climbing vine, *Rhus toxicodendron,* which on contact may produce a severe form of pruritic dermatitis. *Rhus* species contain urushiol, an extremely irritating oily resin, and pentadecylcatechol, a common allergen, which stimulates a type IV hypersensitivity reaction. First contact produces sensitization; later contacts cause severe blistering, eczema, and itching. SEE: illus (Poison Ivy-Poison Oak-Poison Sumac; Poison Ivy Dermatitis).

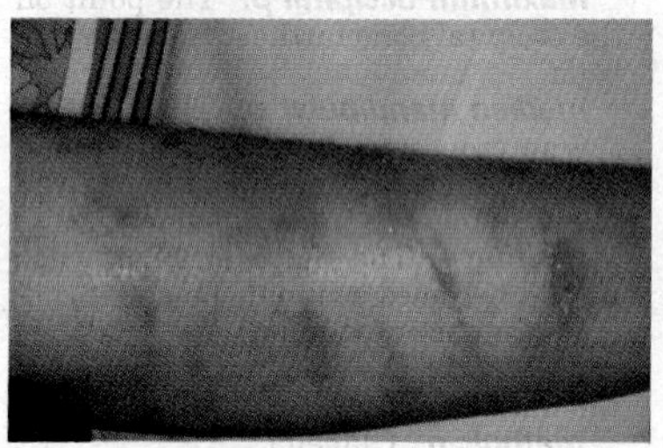

POISION IVY DERMATITIS

p. oak A climbing vine, *Rhus radicans* or *R. diversiloba,* closely related to poison ivy and having the same active substances. SEE: *poison ivy* for illus.

pesticidal p. Chemicals whose toxic properties are commercially exploited in agriculture, industry, or commerce to increase quantity, improve quality, or generally promote consumer acceptability of a variety of products. Common types include insecticides, rodenticides, herbicides, defoliants, fungicides, insect repellents, molluscicides, and some kinds of food additives. The wide variety of poisons commonly found in and around the home constitutes an important source of accidental poisonings. SEE: *Poisons and Poisoning Appendix.*

p. sumac A shrublike plant, *Toxicodendron vernix,* widely distributed in the U.S. Because it contains the same active substances as poison ivy, the symptoms and treatment of poison sumac dermatitis are the same as for poison ivy dermatitis. SEE: *poison ivy* for illus.

poison control center A facility meeting the staffing and equipment standards of the American Association of Poison Control Centers and recognized to be able to give information on, or treatment to patients suffering from, poisoning. A poison information center consists of specially trained staff and a reference library but does not have treatment facilities. More than 400 poison centers are scattered throughout the U.S. They offer 24-hr service. They are commonly associated with or are part of large hospitals or medical schools. A government agency—the Bureau of Drugs Division of the Poison Control Branch of the Food and Drug Administration, U.S. Department of Health and Human Services—is also active in poison control programs and in coordinating the efforts of individual centers. For the address and telephone number of state or province poison control centers, SEE: *Health Care Resources Appendix.*

poisoning [L. *potio,* a poisonous draft] **1.** The illness produced by the introduction of a toxic substance into the body. **2.** Administration of a noxious substance. SEE: *intoxication; Poisons and Poisoning Appendix.*

PATIENT CARE: The standard care of the poisoned patient begins with immediate stabilization of the patient's airway, breathing, circulation, and neurological status if these are compromised. This may require oximetry, blood gas analysis, electrocardiographic monitoring, airway placement, endotracheal intubation, fluid resuscitation, the giving of naloxone and dextrose, or the use of pressors in some severely intoxicated patients. If the intoxicating substance can be identified, reference texts or local poison control centers should be contacted to determine specific antidotes or treatments. When the poison is not identified or when rescuers are uncertain about the underlying cause, it is safest to test blood and urine for acetaminophen, aspirin, and commonly abused drugs, as well as performing standard blood chemistries. Women of childbearing age also should be screened routinely for pregnancy.

Decontamination of the gastrointestinal tract may include the use of activated charcoal, if the patient has ingested a drug or chemical that it can bind; or whole bowel irrigation, which sweeps toxins from the bowel before they are absorbed. Inducing vomiting, a practice formerly relied on in poisonings, is now used rarely because it has not been shown to improve outcome and may cause complications such as aspiration pneumonia. After decontamination procedures, specific antidotes, if available, should be administered.

The elimination of many drugs from the body can be enhanced by other means, including, in some instances, the administration of alkaline fluids, hemodialysis, or hemoperfusion.

Once the patient is physically stabilized, the underlying reason for the intoxication should be addressed. Patients with substance abuse problems, for example, should be referred for detoxification, support, and counseling; suicidal and depressed patients may benefit from counseling or drug therapy. Demented patients who have poisoned themselves because of confusion about their medications should have the administration of their medications supervised. In some cases, poisonings are iatrogenic; that is, they occur because of unintended consequences of prescribed drugs or drug-drug interactions. Careful prescribing may prevent future intoxications.

CAUTION: Many illnesses (e.g., massive strokes, postictal states, insulin reactions, sepsis, meningitis, uremia) mimic the symptoms of poisoning, especially when the patient presents with altered mental status.

---

aluminum p. Nausea, vomiting, renal dysfunction, and cognitive disorders that result from excessive exposure to aluminum. Aluminum toxicity–impaired cognition ("dialysis dementia") in patients with end-stage renal disease has been practically eliminated now that dialysates no longer contain aluminum.

arsenic p. Illness produced by ingestion of arsenic.

SYMPTOMS: Symptoms include a burning pain throughout the gastrointestinal tract, vomiting, dehydration, shock, dysrhythmias, coma, convulsions, paralysis, and death.

FIRST AID: The stomach should be lavaged with copious amounts of water. Dimercaprol (British antilewisite) or other chelators (e.g., penicillamine) should be given immediately.

TREATMENT: After first aid, fluid and electrolyte balance must be maintained. Morphine should be given for pain. The patient is treated for shock and pulmonary edema. Blood transfusion may be required. SEE: *arsenic in Poisons and Poisoning Appendix.*

barbiturate p. Excessive sedation, sometimes accompanied by an inability to protect the airway; coma; shock; and hypothermia as a result of overdose with barbiturates. Agents that are commonly taken in overdose include secobarbital, phenobarbital, or butalbital.

TREATMENT: When oxygenation and ventilation are compromised, intubation and mechanical ventilation may be needed. Other supportive treatments include the administration of activated charcoal, bicarbonate-containing fluids (to make the urine alkaline and increase barbiturate excretion), rewarming techniques, and fluids or drugs to support blood pressure.

blood p. An outdated term for septicemia.

buckthorn p. Motor paralysis that results from consumption of the fruit of the buckthorn (a species of *Bumelia*) that grows in the southeastern U.S.

corrosive p. Poisoning by strong acids, alkalies, strong antiseptics including bichloride of mercury, carbolic acid (phenol), Lysol, cresol compounds, tincture of iodine, and arsenic compounds. These are destructive and cause tissue damage similar to that caused by burns. If the substances have been swallowed, any part of the alimentary canal may be affected. Tissues involved are easily perforated. Death may result from shock or from swelling of the throat and pharynx, which causes asphyxiation. Esophageal injury and stricture may be a late complication. SEE: *individual poisons in Poisons and Poisoning Appendix.*

SYMPTOMS: This type of poisoning is marked by intense burning of the mouth, throat, pharynx, and abdomen; abdominal cramping, retching, nausea, and vomiting, and often collapse. There may be bloody vomit (hematemesis) and diarrhea; the stools are watery, mucoid, bloody, and possibly stained with the poison or its products, resulting from its action on the contents of the alimentary tract. Stains of the lips, cheeks, tongue, mouth, or pharynx are often a characteristic brown; stains on the mucous membranes may be violet or black. Carbolic acid (phenol) leaves white or gray stains resembling boiled meat, hydrochloric acid stains are grayish, nitric acid leaves yellow stains, and sulfuric acid leaves tan or dark burns.

TREATMENT: Immediate treatment in a hospital is mandatory. It is also important to attempt to discover the chemical substance ingested. For this reason, all materials such as food, bottles, jars, or containers that may help to answer this question should be saved. This is essential if the patient is either comatose or an infant.

CAUTION: In treating corrosive poisoning, vomiting must NOT be induced; gastric lavage must not be attempted; and no attempt should be made to neutralize the corrosive substance.

Vomiting will increase the severity of damage to the esophagus by renewing contact with the corrosive substance. Gastric lavage may cause the esophagus or stomach to perforate. If the trachea has been damaged, tracheostomy may be needed. Emergency surgery must be considered if there are signs of possible esophageal perforation or perforation of abdominal viscera. Opiates will be needed to control pain. For esophageal burns, broad-spectrum antibiotic and corticosteroid therapy should be started. Intravenous fluids will be required if esophageal or gastric damage prevents ingestion of liquids. Long-range therapy will be directed toward preventing or treating esophageal scars and strictures.

fish p. A form of food poisoning caused by eating fish that are inherently poisonous or that are poisonous because they had decomposed, become infected, or been feeding on other poisonous life forms.

Ciguatera poisoning: Poisoning due to eating certain types of bottom-dwelling shore fish. These include grouper, red snapper, and barracuda. The toxin, ciguatoxin, is present in fish that feed on dinoflagellates. It acts within 5 hr of ingestion, and symptoms may persist for 8 days or longer. Symptoms include abdominal cramps, nausea, vomiting, diarrhea, paresthesia, hypotension, and respiratory paralysis. Treatment is supportive.

Scromboid fish poisoning: Poisoning due to eating fish that have spoiled and are infested with bacteria, usually *Proteus morganii,* that degrade the protein in fish to produce scrombotoxin.

SYMPTOMS: About 30 min to 2 hr after eating the fish, a peppery sensation of the tongue develops, followed by a rash, pruritus, headache, dizziness, periorbital edema, thirst, nausea, vomiting, diarrhea, and abdominal cramps. These symptoms last about 12 to 24 hr.

TREATMENT: Treatment is symptomatic, but antihistamines may be of benefit. If the stomach has not been emptied by vomiting, gastric lavage should be used. SEE: *shellfish p.*

food p. Illness resulting from ingestion of foods containing poisonous substances. These include mushrooms; shellfish; foods contaminated with pesticides, lead, or mercury; milk from cows that have fed on poisonous plants; or foods that have putrefied or decomposed due to bacterial action.

heavy metal p. Toxicity caused by ingestion, inhalation, or absorption of any heavy metal, esp. lead or mercury. Symptoms are determined by the type and duration of exposure and may include pulmonary, neurological, integumentary, or gastrointestinal disorders.

ink p. Poisonings caused by contact with ink. Many are forms of dermatitis caused by several types of materials. Ordinary ink may cause irritation because of its composition or because of a person's sensitivity to certain ingredients in the ink. Sometimes cleaning materials used to remove ink stains are toxic. Symptoms of ink poisoning include redness, pustule formation, and cracking of the skin.

FIRST AID: The area should be washed with alcohol, soap, and water. It then should be rinsed carefully and covered with a bland dressing such as cold cream.

iodine p. An acute condition caused by the accidental ingestion of iodine or its compounds. This condition is marked by brown stains on the lips and mouth; burning pain in the mouth, throat, and stomach; vomiting (blue vomit if the stomach contained starches, otherwise yellow vomit); bloody diarrhea. SEE: *Poisons and Poisoning Appendix.*

FIRST AID: The patient should be given immediately by mouth a cornstarch or flour solution, 15 g in 500 ml (2 cups) of water. Lavage should be performed, with starch solution or 2% sodium thiosulfate solution. Morphine may be given for pain, as well as mild stimulants as indicated. After this therapy, catharsis should be promoted.

iron p. Acute poisoning usually caused by the accidental ingestion (usually by infants or small children) of iron-containing medications intended for use by adults. In the U.S., about 20,000 accidental iron exposures are reported each year.

SYMPTOMS: The victim vomits, usually within an hour of taking the iron. Vomiting of blood and melena may occur. If untreated, restlessness, hypotension, rapid respirations, and cyanosis may develop, followed within a few hours by coma and death.

TREATMENT: Whole bowel irrigation should be used to force ingested iron out of the gastrointestinal tract. Chelation of iron can be performed with deferoxamine, which binds circulating iron from the bloodstream.

lead p. Ingestion or inhalation of substances containing lead. Symptoms of acute poisoning include a metallic taste in the mouth, burns in the throat and pharynx, and later abdominal cramps and prostration. Chronic lead poisoning is characterized by anorexia, nausea, vomiting, excess salivation, anemia, a lead line on the gums, abdominal pains, muscle cramps, kidney failure, encephalopathy, seizures, learning disabilities, and pains in the joints.

TREATMENT: Seizures are treated with diazepam. Fluid and electrolyte balance is maintained. Cerebral edema is treated with mannitol and dexamethasone. The blood lead level is determined. If it is above 50 to 60 μg/dl, the lead is removed from the body with a chelator (e.g., edetate calcium disodium, dimercaprol, D-penicillamine, or succimer). Succimer has the advantage of being orally active and is esp. helpful in treating children. The effect of treatment is monitored closely and may have to be continued for a week or longer or repeated if the lead level rebounds.

mercury p. The acute or chronic consequences of the ingestion or inhalation of mercury. These include nausea, vomiting, abdominal pain, renal failure, gingivitis, behavioral and cognitive deficits, seizures, paralysis, pneumonitis, and/or death.

TREATMENT: Gastric lavage or whole bowel irrigation may be used to empty the gastrointestinal tract. Hemodialysis or chelation therapy (e.g., with succimer or penicillamine) may also be helpful. SEE: *mercuric chloride in Poisons and Poisoning Appendix.*

mushroom p. Poisoning caused by ingestion of mushrooms such as *Amanita muscaria,* which contains muscarine, or species that contain phalloidin, a component of the amanita toxin. The nearest poison control center should be called for emergency treatment. SEE: *amanita in Poisons and Poisoning Appendix.*

oxalic acid p. Acute poisoning occurring when oxalic acid is accidentally ingested or when large quantities of foods rich in oxalic acid are eaten. Ingestion of 5 g of oxalic acid may be fatal. Chronic poisoning may result from inhalation of vapors. SEE: *Poisons and Poisoning Appendix.*

SYMPTOMS: Signs and symptoms include a corrosive action on the mucosa of the mouth, esophagus, and stomach; a sour taste; burning in the mouth, throat, and stomach; great thirst; bloody vomitus; collapse; and sometimes convulsions and coma.

TREATMENT: Gastric lavage should be used to empty the gastrointestinal tract. Activated charcoal can be given to bind the acid. Vomiting should not be induced.

pokeroot p. Poisoning resulting from ingestion of pokeroot. Nausea, vomiting, drowsiness, vertigo, and possibly convulsions and respiratory paralysis characterize this type of poisoning. Treatment includes administration of whole bowel irrigation or gastric lavage.

potato p. Poisoning due to ingestion of potatoes that contain excess amounts of solanine. This toxic substance is present in the potato peel and in the green sprouts. Potatoes usually contain about 7 mg of solanine per 100 g; the toxic dose of solanine is about 20 to 25 g. Boiling but not baking removes most of the solanine from the potato. Symptoms of poisoning include headache, vomiting, abdominal pain, diarrhea, and fever. Neurological disturbances include apathy, restlessness, drowsiness, confusion, stupor, hallucinations, and visual disturbances. There is no specific therapy. With appropriate supportive and symptomatic therapy, prognosis is good.

risk for p. Accentuated risk of accidental exposure to or ingestion of drugs or dangerous products in doses sufficient to cause poisoning. SEE: *Nursing Diagnoses Appendix.*

shellfish p. Poisoning produced when humans ingest shellfish that have themselves ingested toxic phytoplankton. Symptoms of shellfish poisoning include muscular weakness, dysphonia, paresthesias of the face and extremities, nausea and vomiting, and occasionally paralysis and respiratory distress. Treatment is symptomatic. Spontaneous recovery usually takes place in 24 hr. SEE: *fish p.*

theophylline p. Nausea, vomiting, agitation, cardiac arrhythmias, and, in some instances, seizures or death that result from excessive levels of theophylline-containing compounds in the blood. For young patients with asthma, theophylline levels exceeding 20 mg/dl are typically toxic; even lower levels (e.g., 15 mg/dl) may produce toxic effects in people over age 60. Theophylline levels above 30 mg/dl have a high likelihood of adverse effects at any age.

PATIENT CARE: Theophylline toxicity may occur if the patient's symptoms and drug levels while using theophylline-containing compounds are not monitored regularly. Many commonly used drugs such as cimetidine, ciprofloxacin, erythromycin, and rifampin alter the metabolism of theophylline and may produce toxic reactions if they are taken during theophylline therapy. They should be avoided. Because of the risk of theophylline poisoning, most patients with reactive airway diseases such as asthma or asthmatic bronchitis are treated with inhaled bronchodilators instead of theophylline.

The theophylline-poisoned patient may require monitoring in a critical care unit, where blood pressure and cardiac rhythm can be observed closely, and early interventions taken in the case of seizures or potentially fatal arrhythmias. Anticonvulsants are given for seizures (or to prevent seizures when theophylline levels exceed 100 mg/dl); the gastrointestinal tract should be decontaminated with activated charcoal, and antiarrhythmic drugs are administered, as indicated, for cardiac rhythm disturbances. Severe overdoses or ones with refractory symptoms should be treated with charcoal hemoperfusion.

p. by unknown substances Cases in which there is no information concerning the nature of the poison taken, and the signs and symptoms are not recognized as being due to any particular substance. Specific antidotes cannot be given in this situation. There are, however, certain agents that act in a general manner and may be efficacious.

One of these is activated charcoal, which binds most organic toxins. Whole bowel irrigation can be used to flush ingested substances from the gastrointestinal tract when dermal exposures are suspected. The patient should be showered to remove chemicals from the skin.

poisonous (poy'zŏn-ŭs) [L. *potio,* a poisonous draft] Having the properties or qualities of a poison. SYN: *toxic; venomous.*

poisonous plants Plants containing a poisonous substance that may be fatal if ingested, including azalea, castor bean, chinaberry, European bittersweet, wild or black cherry, oleander, berries of holly and mistletoe, dieffenbachia, horse chestnuts, poison hemlock, laurel, death cup, black nightshade or deadly nightshade, rhododendron, choke cherry, Japanese yew, unripe fruit of akee, cassava roots, betel nut, seeds and pods of bird-of-paradise, belladonna, angels trumpet, fava bean (if eaten by a person with glucose-6-phosphate deficiency), foxglove, bulb of hyacinth, Indian tobacco, iris root, poinsettia, pokeroot, apricot kernels, apple seeds, green tubers and new sprouts of potatoes, privet, rhubarb leaves, wild tomatoes, skunk cabbage, and jimsonweed; and plants containing irritating substances, such as poison ivy, poison oak, and poison sumac.

poker back Stiffness of the spine that may result from ankylosing spondylitis or related conditions.

pokeroot (pōk'root) An herb, *Phytolacca americana,* with white flowers and purple berries. The root is poisonous. Also called *pokeweed.*

polar [L. *polaris*] Concerning a pole.

polarimeter (pō″lăr-ĭm'ĕ-tĕr) [″ + Gr. *metron,* measure] An instrument for measuring amount of polarization of light or rotation of polarized light.

polarimetry (pō″lăr-ĭm'ĕ-trē) The measurement of the amount and rotation of polarized light.

polariscope (pō-lăr'ĭ-skōp) [L. *polaris,* pole, + Gr. *skopein,* to examine] An apparatus used in the measurement of polarized light.

polariscopy (pō″lăr-ĭs'kō-pē) The study of polarized light by the use of a polariscope.

polarity (pō-lăr'ĭ-tē) **1.** The quality of having poles. **2.** The exhibition of opposite effects at the two extremities in physical therapy. **3.** The positive or negative state of an electrical battery. **4.** In cell division, the relation of cell constituents to the poles of the cell.

polarization (pō″lăr-ī-zā′shŭn) [L. *polaris,* pole] **1.** A condition in a ray of light in which vibrations occur in only one plane. **2.** In a galvanic battery, collection of hydrogen bubbles on the negative plate and oxygen on the positive plate, whereby generation of current is impeded. **3.** The electrical state that exists at the cell membrane of an excitable cell at rest; the inside is negatively charged in relation to the outside. The difference is created by the distribution of ions within the cell and in the extracellular fluid. SYN: *potential, resting.* SEE: *depolarization* for illus.

polarizer (pō′lă-rīz″ĕr) The part of a polariscope that polarizes light.

pole (pōl) [L. *polus*] **1.** The extremity of any axis about which forces acting on it are symmetrically disposed. SYN: *polus.* **2.** One of two points in a magnet, cell, or battery having opposite physical qualities.

animal p. The pole opposite the yolk in an ovum. At this point, polar bodies are formed and pinched off and protoplasm is concentrated and has its greatest activity.

p. of the eye The anterior and posterior extremities of the optic axis.

frontal p. The farthest projecting part of the anterior extremity of both cerebral hemispheres.

germinal p. The pole of an ovum at which the development begins.

p. of the kidney The upper and lower extremities of the kidney.

occipital p. The posterior extremity of the occipital lobe.

pelvic p. The breech of a fetus.

placental p. of the chorion The spot at which the domelike placenta is situated.

temporal p. The anterior extremity of the temporal lobe.

p. of the testicle The upper and lower extremities of a testicle.

vegetal p. The part of the egg containing the yolk.

polio *acute anterior poliomyelitis.*

polio- Combining form indicating *gray.*

polioclastic (pŏl″ē-ō-klăs′tĭk) [Gr. *polios,* gray, + *klastos,* breaking] Destructive to the gray matter of the nervous system.

polioencephalitis (pŏl″ē-ō-ĕn-sĕf″ă-lī′tĭs) [″ + *enkephalos,* brain, + *itis,* inflammation] A condition characterized by inflammatory lesions of the gray matter of the brain.

anterior superior p. Inflammatory changes in the gray matter around the third ventricle, the anterior portion of the fourth ventricle, and the aqueduct of Sylvius. It is characterized by ocular abnormalities, mental disturbances, and ataxia. The origin of the disease is thiamine (vitamin B_1) deficiency. SYN: *Korsakoff's syndrome.*

p. hemorrhagica Polioencephalitis accompanied by hemorrhagic lesions.

posterior p. Polioencephalitis involving the gray matter around the fourth ventricle.

polioencephalomeningomyelitis (pŏl″ē-ō-ĕn-sĕf″ăl-ō-mĕn-ĭn″gō-mī-ĕl-ī′tĭs) [″ + ″ + *meninx,* membrane, + *myelos,* marrow, + *itis,* inflammation] Inflammation of the gray matter of the brain and spinal cord and their meninges.

polioencephalomyelitis (pŏl″ē-ō-ĕn-sĕf″ăl-ō-mī″ĕl-ī′tĭs) Inflammation of the gray matter of the brain and spinal cord.

polioencephalopathy (pŏl″ē-ō-ĕn-sĕf″ăl-ŏp′ă-thē) [Gr. *polios,* gray, + *enkephalos,* brain, + *pathos,* disease, suffering] Disease of the gray matter of the brain.

poliomyelencephalitis (pŏl″ē-ō-mī″ĕl-ĕn-sĕf″ăl-ī′tĭs) [″ + *myelos,* marrow, + *enkephalos,* brain, + *itis,* inflammation] Poliomyelitis with polioencephalitis.

poliomyelitis (pŏl″ē-ō-mī″ĕl-ī′tĭs) [″ + ″ + *itis,* inflammation] Inflammation of the gray matter of the spinal cord. It is an acute viral disease characterized by fever, sore throat, headache, vomiting, and often stiffness of the neck and back. Late consequences of the infection include atrophy of groups of muscles ending in contraction and permanent deformity. Polio is preventable with standard vaccinations given to children.

abortive p. Poliomyelitis in which the illness is mild with no involvement of the central nervous system.

acute anterior p. An acute infectious inflammation of the anterior horns of the gray matter of the spinal cord, a rare illness in the U.S. since the introduction of effective polio vaccines. In this disease, paralysis may or may not occur. In the majority of patients, the disease is mild, being limited to respiratory and gastrointestinal symptoms, such constituting the minor illness or the abortive type, which lasts only a few days. In the major illness, muscle paralysis or weakness occurs with loss of superficial and deep reflexes. In such cases characteristic lesions are found in the gray matter of the spinal cord, medulla, motor area of cerebral cortex, and cerebellum.

ETIOLOGY: The causative agent is the polio virus. The virus that is excreted in the feces is resistant and stable, remaining viable for months outside the body. Three immunological types exist. The incubation period ranges from 5 to 35 days but is usually 7 to 12 days.

SYMPTOMS: The onset often is abrupt, although the ordinary manifestations of a severe cold or some gastrointestinal disturbances may come on gradually, accompanied by slight elevation of temperature, frequently enduring for not more than 3 days. At the end of this period, paralysis may or may not develop. The extent of any paralysis necessarily depends on the degree of nerve involvement. Consequently, paralysis may be confined to one small group of muscles or affect one or all extremities. When the respiratory muscles also are involved, death is likely to ensue. In the average paralytic case it is the extensor muscles in particular that are affected.

DIFFERENTIAL DIAGNOSIS: Among the diseases confused with this infection are the various types of meningitis, postinfection encephalomyelitis, and conversion disorders.

PROPHYLAXIS: Active immunization with inactivated poliovirus vaccine has greatly reduced the incidence of paralytic poliomyelitis. SEE: *inactivated poliovirus vaccine.*

COMPLICATIONS: Paralysis, atrophy of muscles, and ultimate deformities constitute the complications of this disease. Aside from bronchopneumonia, which may develop in very severe cases, other complications are surprisingly few.

PROGNOSIS: Ordinarily the outcome is good (mortality from polio is less than 10%). When paralysis develops, 50% of the patients make a full recovery and about 25% have mild permanent paralysis.

Progressive paralysis may occur years after the acute attack. This syndrome (postpolio syndrome) often first appears many decades after the initial infection. SEE: *postpoliomyelitis muscular atrophy; postpolio syndrome.*

INCIDENCE: Poliomyelitis is endemic throughout the world but occurs in epidemics in certain countries. Polio no longer occurs in epidemics in the U.S. Virtually all cases for the last several years have been vaccine-associated. In countries where polio vaccine has not been used extensively, epidemics are seasonal, occurring in summer and fall. Children are more susceptible than adults. Infection is spread by direct contact, the virus probably entering the body via the mouth. It reaches the central nervous system through the blood.

TREATMENT: Treatment is supportive. A respirator is used for patients whose respiratory muscles are paralyzed. Physical therapy is used to attain maximum function and prevent deformities that are late manifestations of the disease.

PATIENT CARE: Strict isolation with concurrent disinfection of throat discharge and feces is enforced to prevent transmission of polio virus. A patent airway is maintained, the patient is observed closely for signs of respiratory distress, oxygen is administered as necessary, and a tracheostomy tray is kept at bedside.

The patient should maintain strict bedrest during the acute phase. Gentle passive range-of-motion exercises and application of hot moist packs at 20-min intervals, or tub baths for children, help to alleviate muscle pain. Proper body alignment is maintained, and the patient turned frequently to prevent deformity and decubiti. A mild sedative or analgesic is administered to decrease pain and anxiety and to promote rest. The patient is observed for distended bladder due to transitory paralysis. Personal hygiene is provided, and oral hygiene is promoted. Appetizing food is offered because anorexia is common. Antipyretics are administered to reduce fever. Fluid and electrolyte balance and elimination are monitored closely. A foot board is used to prevent footdrop. Emotional support is provided to assist the patient to cope with loss of body function and paralysis.

anterior p. Inflammation of the anterior horns of the spinal cord.

ascending p. Poliomyelitis in which paralysis begins in the lower extremities and progresses up the legs, thighs, and trunk, and finally involves the respiratory muscles.

bulbar p. Poliomyelitis in which the gray matter of the medulla oblongata is involved, resulting in paralysis and usually respiratory failure.

chronic anterior p. Progressive wasting of the muscles; myelopathic progressive muscular atrophy.

nonparalytic p. Pain and stiffness in the muscles of the axial skeleton, esp. of the neck and back; mild fever; increased proteins and leukocytes in the cerebrospinal fluid. Diagnosis depends on the isolation of the virus and serological reactions.

paralytic p. Poliomyelitis with a variable combination of signs of damage of the central nervous system. These include weakness, incoordination, muscle tenderness and spasms, flaccid paralysis, and disturbance of consciousness.

provocative p. During an epidemic of poliomyelitis, the onset of paralysis in the area close to the site of an invasive procedure. Thus an injection in muscle increases the risk of paralysis of the side of the body injected; and tonsillectomy and adenoidectomy increases the risk that poliomyelitis will affect the brain stem.

poliosis (pŏl″ē-ō′sĭs) [Gr. *polios,* gray, + *osis,* condition] Whiteness of the hair, esp. when due to a hereditary condition or as a result of infection. SYN: *canities.*

poliovirus (pō″lē-ō-vī′rŭs) The etiological agent of poliomyelitis, separable into three serotypes based on the specificity of the neutralizing antibody. The three serotypes are types I, II, and III. A virus found worldwide, it spreads directly or indirectly from infected persons or convalescent carriers. Epidemics of poliomyelitis that were characteristic of infections with this virus have been virtually eliminated by the poliovirus vaccine. SEE: *poliovirus vaccine, inactivated.*

poliovirus vaccine, inactivated ABBR: IPV. A poliovirus vaccine recommended for the prevention of paralytic poliomyelitis. The vaccine, which contains inactivated types I, II, and III polioviruses, is suitable for parenteral administration to all infants and children.

Infants should be given three doses, the first at 2 months of age, followed by two more doses at 8-week intervals. A fourth dose should be given at age 18 months unless poliomyelitis is endemic in the area, in which case the fourth dose is given 6 to 12 months after the third. Additional doses are recommended prior to school entry and then every 5 years until age 18.

poliovirus vaccine, live oral ABBR: OPV. A standard preparation of one type or a combination of the three types of live, attenuated polioviruses. In 1999, an advisory panel to the Centers for Disease Control and Prevention (CDC) recommended that live oral poliovirus no longer be used routinely because it has caused 8-10 cases of polio each year. This risk is no longer acceptable now that the polio epidemic has been eliminated in the U.S. SEE: *vaccine.*

polishing (pŏl′ĭsh-ĭng) Producing a smooth, glossy finish on a denture or a dental restoration.

Politzer bag (pŏl′ĭt-zĕr) [Adam Politzer, Hungarian otologist, 1835–1920] A soft rubber bag with a rubber tip for inflating the middle ear by increasing the pressure in the nasopharynx. SEE: *aerotitis.*

politzerization (pŏl″ĭt-sĕr-ĭ-zā′shŭn) The inflation of the middle ear by means of a Politzer bag.

pollen (pŏl′ĕn) [L., dust] The microspores of a seed plant that develop in the anther at the tip of the stamen. Each pollen grain develops a pollen tube and constitutes the male gametophyte. Within it develops a tube nucleus and two sperm nuclei, which are the male reproductive cells. Many airborne pollens are allergens. SEE: *hay fever.*

pollenogenic (pŏl″ĕn-ō-jĕn′ĭk) [″ + Gr. *gennan,* to produce] Caused by the pollen of plants, or producing plant pollen.

pollex (pŏl′ĕks) *pl.* **pollices** [L.] The thumb.

p. extensus Backward deviation of the thumb.

p. flexus Permanent flexion of the thumb.

p. valgus Abnormal deviation of the thumb toward the ulnar side.

p. varus Abnormal deviation of the thumb toward the radial side.

pollicization (pŏl″ĭs-ĭ-zā′shŭn) [L. *pollex,* thumb] The plastic surgical procedure of constructing a thumb from adjacent tissues.

pollinosis (pŏl-ĭn-ō′sĭs) [L. *pollen,* dust, + Gr. *osis,* disease] Hay fever.

pollute (pŭ-loot′) To ruin, contaminate, or spoil; to make something, such as water, food, or the environment, unfit for use or unsafe for living things.

pollution (pŭ-loo′shŭn) [ME. *polluten*] The state of making impure or defiling.

polocyte (pō′lō-sīt) [Gr. *polos,* pole, + *kytos,* cell] Polar body.

polonium (pō-lō′nē-ŭm) [L. *Polonia,* Poland, native country of its discoverers, the Curies] SYMB: Po. A radioactive element isolated from pitchblende; atomic weight 210; atomic number 84.

polus (pō′lŭs) *pl.* **poli** [L.] Pole (1).

poly (pŏl′ē) *polymorphonuclear leukocyte.*

poly- [Gr. *polys,* many] Combining form indicating *many, much.*

polyacid (pŏl″ē-ăs′ĭd) An alcohol or a base with two or more hydroxyl groups that will combine with an acid.

polyacrylonitrile A synthetic polymer used in the fabrication of dialysis membranes with high biocompatibility.

polyadenitis (pŏl″ē-ăd″ĕ-nī′tĭs) [″ + Gr. *aden,* gland, + *itis,* inflammation] Inflammation of the lymph nodes, esp. the cervical lymph nodes.

polyadenomatosis (pŏl″ē-ăd″ĕ-nō-mă-tō′sĭs) [″ + ″ + *oma,* tumor, + *osis,* condition] Adenomas in many glands.

polyadenopathy (pŏl″ē-ăd″ĕ-nŏp′ă-thē) [″ + ″ + *pathos,* disease, suffering] Any disease in which many glands are involved.

polyadenous (pŏl″ē-ăd′ĕ-nŭs) Involving or relating to many glands.

polyagglutination Red cells that are agglutinated by a large proportion of adult human sera regardless of blood group.

polyalgesia (pŏl″ē-ăl-jē′zē-ă) [″ + *algesis,* sense of pain] A single stimulus of a part, producing sensation in many parts.

polyandry (pŏl″ē-ăn′drē) [Gr. *polyandria*] The practice of having more than one husband at the same time. SEE: *polygamy.*

polyangiitis (pŏl″ē-ăn″jē-ī′tĭs) [Gr. *polys,* many, + *angeion,* vessel, + *itis,* inflammation] Inflammation of a number of blood vessels.

polyarteritis nodosa (pŏl″ē-ăr″tĕr-ī′tĭs) [″ + *arteria,* artery, + *itis,* inflammation] ABBR: PAN. A form of vasculitis affecting medium and small arteries, particularly at the point of bifurcation and branching. Segmental inflammation and fibrinoid necrosis of blood vessels lead to diminished blood flow (ischemia) to the areas normally supplied by these arteries. Although signs and symptoms depend on the location of the affected vessels and organs, patients usually present with symptoms of multisystem disease, including fever, malaise, weight loss, hypertension, renal failure, myalgia, peripheral neuritis, and gastrointestinal bleeding; these may occur episodically. Unlike most types of vasculitis, polyarteritis nodosa does not affect glomerular capillaries, although other renal vessels are involved. SYN: *periarteritis nodosa*. SEE: *Nursing Diagnoses Appendix*.

ETIOLOGY: The cause is unknown, but the disease is associated with immunological disorders. Hepatitis B antigens are present in the blood of approx. 30% of patients.

polyarthritis (pŏl-ē-ăr-thrī′tĭs) [″ +*arthron,* joint + *itis,* inflammation] Inflammation of more than one joint seen in rheumatoid arthritis, juvenile rheumatoid arthritis, and psoriatic arthritis. It usually refers to involvement of more than four joints. **polyarthritic** (pŏl″ē-ăr-thrĭt′ĭk), *adj.*

acute p. rheumatica An obsolete term for acute rheumatic fever.

chronic villous p. Chronic inflammation of the synovial membrane of multiple joints.

polyarticular (pŏl″ē-ăr-tĭk′ū-lăr) [″ + L. *articulus,* a joint] Concerning, having, or affecting many joints. SYN: *multiarticular*.

polyatomic (pŏl″ē-ă-tŏm′ĭk) [″ + *atomon,* atom] **1.** Having several atoms. **2.** Having more than two replaceable hydrogen atoms.

polyavitaminosis (pŏl″ē-ā-vī″tă-mĭn-ō′sĭs) [″ + *a-,* not, + L. *vita,* life, + *amine* + Gr. *osis,* condition] A deficiency of more than one vitamin.

polybasic (pŏl″ē-bā′sĭk) [Gr. *polys,* many, + *basis,* base] Pert. to an acid with two or more hydrogen ions that will combine with a base.

polyblennia (pŏl″ē-blĕ′nē-ă) [″ + *blennos,* mucus] Secretion of an abnormal amount of mucus.

polycarbophil (pŏl″ē-kăr′bō-fĭl) A hydrophilic substance that is used as a bulk-forming laxative.

polycentric (pŏl″ē-sĕn′trĭk) [″ + *kentron,* center] The condition of having many centers.

polycheiria (pŏl″ē-kī′rē-ă) [″ + *cheir,* hand] Having more than two hands.

polychemotherapy (pŏl″ē-kē″mō-thĕr′ă-pē) [″ + *chemeia,* chemistry, + *therapeia,* treatment] Treatment with several chemotherapeutic agents at once.

polychlorinated biphenyls ABBR: PCBs. A group of complex chemicals classed as chlorinated aromatic hydrocarbons. They were widely used in industry as a component of transformers and capacitors; in paints and hydraulic systems; and in carbonless NCR paper. Because of their extremely low rate of biodegradation, accumulation in animal tissues (particularly in adipose tissue), and their potential for chronic or delayed toxic effects, the manufacture of PCBs was discontinued in the U.S. in 1977. PCBs were sold in the U.S. under the trade name Aroclor.

polychondritis (pŏl″ē-kŏn-drī′tĭs) [″ + *chondros,* cartilage, + *itis,* inflammation] Inflammation of several cartilaginous areas.

relapsing p. A rare inflammatory disease of cartilage associated with polyarthritis and involvement of the cartilage of the nose, ears, joints, bronchi, and trachea. It is most common between the ages of 40 and 60 years but may occur at any time. The cause is unknown. Because of the collapse of the bronchial walls, repeated infections of the lungs may occur, and death may result from respiratory compromise.

TREATMENT: Prednisone is the treatment of choice. Immunosuppressive drugs such as cyclophosphamide or azathioprine are used if patients fail to respond to prednisone. Heart valve replacement or repair of aortic aneurysm may be necessary.

polychromasia (pŏl″ē-krō-mā′zē-ă) [″ + *chroma,* color] The quality of having many colors.

polychromatic (pŏl″ē-krō-măt′ĭk) Multicolored.

polychromatocyte (pŏl″ē-krō-măt′ō-sīt) [″ + ″ + *kytos,* cell] A cell that has an affinity for various stains. SEE: *polychromatophilia* (1).

polychromatophil(e) (pŏl″ē-krō-măt′ō-fĭl) [Gr. *polys,* many, + *chroma,* color, + *philein,* to love] A cell, esp. a red blood cell, that is stainable with more than one kind of stain.

polychromatophilia (pŏl″ē-krō-măt″ō-fĭl′ē-ă) **1.** The quality of being stainable with more than one stain. **2.** An excess of polychromatophils in the blood.

polychylia (pŏl″ē-kī′lē-ă) [″ + *chylos,* juice] Excessive secretion of chyle.

polyclinic (pŏl″ē-klĭn′ĭk) [″ + *kline,* bed] A hospital or clinic treating patients with various medical and surgical conditions; a general hospital.

polyclonal (pŏl″ē-klōn′ăl) Arising from different cell lines.

polycoria (pŏl″ē-kō′rē-ă) [″ + *kore,* pupil] The state of having more than one pupil in one eye.

polycrotic (pŏl″ē-krŏt′ĭk) [″ + *krotos,* beat] Having several pulse waves for each heartbeat.

polycrotism (pŏl-ĭk′rō-tĭzm) [″ + ″ + *-ismos,* condition] The condition of having several pulse waves for each heartbeat.

polycystic (pŏl″ē-sĭs′tĭk) [″ + *kystis,* cyst] Composed of many cysts.

polycystic ovary syndrome Stein-Leventhal syndrome.

polycythemia (pŏl″ē-sī-thē′mē-ă) [″ + *kytos,* cell, + *haima,* blood] An excess of red blood cells. In a newborn, it may reflect hemoconcentration due to hypovolcmia or prolonged intrauterine hypoxia, or hypervolemia due to intrauterine twin-to-twin transfusion or placental transfusion resulting in delayed clamping of the umbilical cord. SYN: *erythrocytosis.*

relative p. A relative increase in the number of erythrocytes that occurs in hemoconcentration.

secondary p. Polycythemia resulting from some physiological condition that stimulates erythropoiesis, such as lowered oxygen tension in blood.

spurious p. Stress erythrocytosis.

p. vera A chronic, life-shortening myeloproliferative disorder resulting from the reproduction of a single cell clone; characterized by an increase in red blood cell mass and hemoglobin concentration that occurs independently of erythropoietin stimulation. SYN: *erythremia.* SEE: illus; *Nursing Diagnoses Appendix.*

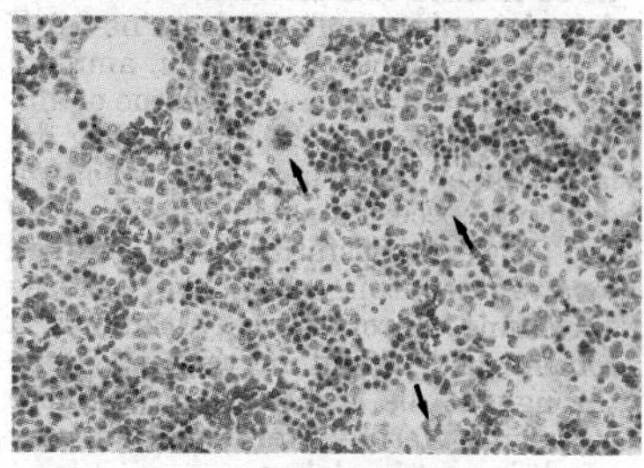

POLYCYTHEMIA VERA

Bone marrow showing hypercellularity and increased megakaryocytes (arrows)

SYMPTOMS: Weakness, fatigue, blood clotting, vertigo, tinnitus, irritability, flushing of face, redness, and pain of extremities occur commonly. The bone marrow shows increased cellularity. Peptic ulcers are often reported.

TREATMENT: Permanent cure cannot be achieved today, but remissions of many years can be produced. Phlebotomy, radioactive phosphorus (^{32}P), cyclophosphamide, hydroxyurea, or melphalan is used.

PATIENT CARE: The symptoms and the need to seek medical attention when signs and symptoms of bleeding and thrombus formation occur are explained to the patient. Rest should be balanced with exercise. Limbs should be protected from injury due to heat, cold, and pressure, and safety precautions, including use of a soft toothbrush, should be instituted to prevent injury. Reassurance and support are provided to the patient and family, and opportunities are provided for questions and discussion of concerns.

polydactylism (pŏl″ē-dăk′tĭ-lĭzm) [Gr. *polys,* many, + *daktylos,* digit, + *-ismos,* condition] The state of having supernumerary fingers or toes.

polydactyly (pŏl″ē-dăk′tĭ-lē) [″ + *daktylos,* finger] The condition of having more than the normal number of fingers and toes.

polydipsia (pŏl″ē-dĭp′sē-ă) [″ + *dipsa,* thirst] Excessive thirst.

polydrug use In drug abusers, the practice of concurrent use of several dissimilar drugs, such as alcohol, cocaine, opiates, and other drugs. The toxic potential of multiple drug use is increased as compared with use of a single drug.

polydysplasia (pŏl″ē-dĭs-plā′zē-ă) [″ + *dys,* bad, + *plassein,* to form] The condition of having multiple developmental abnormalities.

polydystrophic (pŏl″ē-dĭs-trō′fĭk) Concerning or having polydystrophy.

polydystrophy (pŏl″ē-dĭs′trō-fē) [″ + ″ + *trophe,* nourishment] The condition of having multiple congenital anomalies of the connective tissues.

polyendocrine deficiency syndromes *Type I:* A disease that begins at about age 12, characterized by hypoparathyroidism, primary adrenal insufficiency, and mucocutaneous candidiasis. Alopecia, pernicious anemia, malabsorption, and chronic hepatitis may also be present. *Type II:* A disease for which the average age of onset is about 30 years and which is characterized by primary adrenal insufficiency, autoimmune thyroid disease, and insulin-dependent diabetes mellitus. SYN: *autoimmune endrocrine failure syndrome.*

polyene (pŏl-ē′ēn) An organic compound containing alternating, or conjugate, double bonds. An example is butadiene, $CH_2{=}CHCH{=}CH_2$.

polyesthesia (pŏl″ē-ĕs-thē′zē-ă) [″ + *aisthesis,* sensation] An abnormal sensation of touch in which a single stimulus is felt at two or more places.

polyesthetic (pŏl″ē-ĕs-thĕt′ĭk) **1.** Pert. to polyesthesia. **2.** Pert. to several senses or sensations.

polyestrous (pŏl″ē-ĕs′trŭs) [″ + *oistros,* mad desire] Having two or more estrous cycles in each mating season.

polyethylene (pŏl″ē-ĕth′ĭ-lēn) A polymerized resin of ethylene; used to make a wide variety of products, including tubing used in intravenous sets.

p. glycol 400 A polymer consisting of

ethylene oxide and water. The formula is $H(OCH_2CH_2)_nOH$, in which the value of *n* is from 8.2 to 9.1. It is used as a water-soluble ointment base.

p. glycol 4000 A polymer consisting of ethylene oxide and water. The formula is $H(OCH_2CH_2)_nOH$, in which the value of *n* is from 68 to 84. It is used as a water-soluble ointment base.

p. glycol electrolyte for gastrointestinal lavage solution A white powder added to water to make a volume of 4 L. An isosmotic solution for oral administration, it contains 236 g of polyethylene glycol 3350; 23.74 g of sodium sulfate; 6.74 g of sodium bicarbonate; 5.86 g of sodium chloride; and 2.97 g of potassium chloride. For adults the 4 L are given at the rate of 8 oz (240 ml) every 10 min until completed. This solution is given before colonoscopy and barium enema examinations. The bowel will be cleansed within 3 to 4 hr. Trade name is Golytely.

polygalactia (pŏl″ē-gă-lăk′shē-ă) [Gr. *polys,* many, + *gala,* milk] Excessive secretion or flow of milk.

polygamy (pō-lĭg′ă-mē) [″ + *gamos,* marriage] The practice of having several wives, husbands, or mates at the same time. SEE: *polyandry; polygyny.*

polyganglionic (pŏl″ē-găng″glē-ŏn′ĭk) [″ + *ganglion,* ganglion] Concerning many ganglia.

polygastria (pŏl″ē-găs′trē-ă) [″ + *gaster,* stomach] Excessive secretion or flow of gastric juice.

polygen (pŏl′ĕ-jĕn) **1.** An element that has more than one valency and that can form more than one series of compounds. **2.** An antigen that will cause the formation of two or more specific antibodies.

polygenic (pŏl″ē-jĕn′ĭk) [″ + *gennan,* to produce] Pert. to or caused by several genes.

polyglactin An absorbable polymer used to manufacture sutures and surgical mesh. Trade name is Vicryl.

polyglandular (pŏl″ē-glăn′dū-lăr) [″ + L. *glandula,* a little kernel] Pert. to or affecting many glands. SYN: *pluriglandular.*

polyglycolic acid A polymer of glycolic acid anhydride units. It is used to manufacture surgical sutures, clips, and mesh.

polygnathus (pō-lĭg′nă-thŭs) [″ + *gnathos,* jaw] Conjoined twins of unequal size in which the smaller is attached to the jaw of the larger.

polygram (pŏl′ē-grăm) [″ + *gramma,* something written] A tracing or record made by a polygraph.

polygraph (pŏl′ē-grăf) [″ + *graphein,* to write] An instrument for determining minor physiological changes assumed to occur under the stress of lying (or any other emotion). Variations in respiratory rhythm, pulse rate, blood pressure, and sweating of the hands are among the functions that are monitored. Increased perspiration lessens resistance to passage of electrical current. The test has popular appeal among law enforcement departments, but results obtained are presumptive and not absolute; nevertheless, interpretations of polygraph data have been admitted as evidence in some legal proceedings. The advisability of accepting the results of polygraph tests is controversial. SYN: *sphygmograph.*

polygyny (pŏ-lĭj′ŏ-nē) The practice of having more than one female mate at a time. SEE: *polygamy.*

polygyria (pŏl″ē-jī′rē-ă) [″ + *gyros,* circle] Excess of the normal number of convolutions in the brain.

polyhedral (pŏl″ē-hē′drăl) [Gr. *polys,* many, + *hedra,* base] Having many surfaces.

polyhistor (pŏl″ē-hĭs′tŭr) [″ + *histor,* learned] A scholar or physician who has great and varied abilities and knowledge (e.g., Hippocrates, Galen, Paracelsus, Leonardo da Vinci, Boerhaave, Sir William Osler, Richard Mead, and Thomas Jefferson).

polyhybrid (pŏl″ē-hī′brĭd) [″ + L. *hybrida,* mongrel] The offspring of parents that are different with respect to three or more characteristics.

polyhydramnios (pŏl″ē-hī-drăm′nē-ŏs) [″ + *hydor,* water, + *amnion,* amnion] A condition in which the volume of amniotic fluid exceeds 2000 ml during the last half of pregnancy. Acute polyhydramnios occurs suddenly between 20 and 24 weeks' gestation and is marked by a rapid (within a few days) increase in volume. Chronic polyhydramnios, a continuous, gradual increase in volume throughout the last trimester, is more common. Uterine overdistention may result in preterm labor.

ETIOLOGY: The cause is unknown; however, the condition occurs more frequently in association with congenital fetal anomalies that interfere with swallowing, in anencephaly, in monozygotic multiple gestation, and in 10% of pregnancies in diabetic women.

SYMPTOMS: Suspicious clinical signs include a taut abdomen, a fundal height increased out of proportion to gestation, and difficulty in auscultating the fetal heart rate. When the amniotic fluid volume exceeds 3000 ml, interference with diaphragmatic excursion and vena caval compression are reflected in maternal shortness of breath and increased dependent edema.

DIAGNOSIS: Ultrasonography confirms the presence of polyhydramnios and will identify fetal anomalies such as anencephaly or exposed fetal meninges.

TREATMENT: Amniocentesis is performed to reduce the amniotic volume in women who are experiencing severe discomfort and/or respiratory embarrassment. In most cases, however, conservative management includes bedrest in the left lateral position to encourage placental perfusion and diuresis.

polyhydric (pŏl″ē-hī′drĭk) Containing more than two hydroxyl groups.

polyhydruria (pŏl″ē-hī-droo′rē-ă) [″ + ″ + *ouron,* urine] An excessive amount of water in the urine.

polyhypermenorrhea (pŏl″ē-hī″pĕr-mĕn″ō-rē′ă) [″ + *hyper,* over, + *men,* month, + *rhoia,* flow] Frequent menstruation with excessive discharge.

polyhypomenorrhea (pŏl″ē-hī″pō-mĕn″ō-rē′ă) [″ + *hypo,* under, + *men,* month, + *rhoia,* flow] Frequent menstruation with scanty discharge.

polyidrosis (pŏl″ē-ĭd-rō′sĭs) [″ + *hidrosis,* sweat] Hyperhidrosis.

polyinfection (pŏl″ē-ĭn-fĕk′shŭn) [″ + ME. *infecten,* infect] Infection with two or more microorganisms. SYN: *multiinfection.*

polykaryocyte (pŏl″ē-kăr′ē-ō-sīt) [″ + *karyon,* nucleus, + *kytos,* cell] A cell possessing several nuclei.

polylysine (pŏl″ē-lī′sĭn) A polypeptide in which two lysine molecules are joined by a peptide linkage.

polymastia (pŏl″ē-măs′tē-ă) [Gr. *polys,* many, + *mastos,* breast] The condition of having more than two breasts. SYN: *multimammae; polymazia.*

polymastigote (pŏl″ē-măs′tĭ-gōt) [″ + *mastix,* whip] Possessing several flagella.

polymazia [″ + *mazos,* breast] Polymastia.

polymelia (pŏl″ē-mē′lē-ă) [″ + *melos,* limb] A congenital abnormality in which there are supernumerary limbs.

polymelus (pō-lĭm′ĕ-lŭs) [″ + *melos,* limb] One having polymelia.

polymenorrhea (pŏl″ē-mĕn-ō-rē′ă) [″ + ″ + *rhoia,* to flow] Menstrual periods occurring with abnormal frequency.

polymer (pŏl′ĭ-mĕr) [″ + *meros,* a part] A natural or synthetic substance formed by a combination of two or more molecules (and up to millions) of the same substance.

polymerase (pŏl-ĭm′ĕr-ās) An enzyme that catalyzes polymerization of nucleotides to form DNA molecules before cell division, or RNA molecules before protein synthesis.

p. chain reaction ABBR: PCR. A process that permits making, in the laboratory, unlimited numbers of copies of genes. This is done beginning with a single molecule of the genetic material DNA. The technique can be used in investigating and diagnosing numerous bacterial diseases, viruses associated with cancer, genetic diseases such as diabetes mellitus, human immunodeficiency virus (HIV), pemphigus vulgaris, and various diseases of the blood (e.g., sickle cell anemia) and of muscles.

RNA p. Transcriptase.

polymer fume fever Condition resulting from breathing fumes produced by certain polymers when they are heated to 300° to 700°C or higher. Symptoms include a tight gripping sensation of the chest associated with shivering, sore throat, fever, and weakness. Treatment consists of discontinuance of exposure to fumes. SEE: *metal fume fever.*

polymeria (pŏl-ĭ-mē′rē-ă) The condition of having more than normal number of parts. SYN: *polymerism.*

polymeric (pŏl″ĭ-mĕr′ĭk) **1.** Having the characteristics of a polymer. **2.** Muscles derived from more than one myotome.

polymerid (pō-lĭm′ĕr-ĭd) Polymer.

polymerism (pŏl′ĭ-mĕr″ĭzm, pō-lĭm′ĕr-ĭzm) [″ + *meros,* part, + *-ismos,* condition] Polymeria.

polymerization (pŏl″ĭ-mĕr″ĭ-zā′shŭn) The process of changing a simple chemical substance or substances into another compound having the same elements usually in the same proportions but with a higher molecular weight.

polymerize (pŏl′ĭ-mĕr-īz) To cause polymerization.

polymethylmacrylate A synthetic polymer used in the fabrication of dialysis membranes with high biocompatibility.

polymicrobial (pŏl″ē-mī-krō′bē-ăl) [Gr. *polys,* many, + *mikros,* small, + *bios,* life] Concerning a number of species of microorganisms.

polymicrobic infections Bacterial infections caused by two or more different microorganisms.

polymicrogyria (pŏl″ē-mī″krō-jī′rē-ă) [″ + ″ + *gyros,* convolution] A malformed brain in which multiple small convolutions have developed.

polymorph (pŏl′ē-morf) [″ + *morphe,* form] A polymorphonuclear leukocyte.

polymorphic Occurring in more than one form. SYN: *multiform; polymorphous.*

polymorphism [″ + *morphe,* form, + *-ismos,* condition] **1.** The property of crystallizing into two or more different forms. **2.** The occurrence of more than one form in a life cycle. **3.** An allelic variation within a species. SYN: *pleomorphism.*

restriction fragment length p. DNA fingerprinting with a specific nucleotide insertion sequence.

polymorphocellular (pŏl″ē-mor″fō-sĕl′ū-lăr) [″ + ″ + L. *cellula,* a small chamber] Composed of cells of many forms.

polymorphonuclear (pŏl″ē-mor″fō-nū′klē-ăr) [″ + ″ + L. *nucleus,* a kernel] Possessing a nucleus consisting of several parts or lobes connected by fine strands.

polymorphous (pŏl″ē-mor′fŭs) Polymorphic.

polymyalgia arteritica (pŏl″ē-mī-ăl′jē-ă) [″ + *mys,* muscle, + *algos,* pain] Polymyalgia rheumatica.

polymyalgia rheumatica ABBR: PMR. A rheumatologic illness marked by fevers, malaise, weight loss, muscle pain and stiffness (esp. of the shoulders and pelvis), and morning stiffness. It occurs primarily, but not exclusively, in white individuals over age 60. The cause of the syndrome is unknown. Although there is no single diagnostic test for this condition, patients typically have a markedly elevated erythrocyte sedimentation rate (>50 mm/hr) and no evidence of another disease (e.g., infection, cancer, rheumatoid arthritis, or lupus) as the underlying cause. Patients with the syndrome obtain rapid and durable relief from corticosteroids but usually require a course of treatment lasting 6 to 18 months. Pathologically, the syndrome is related to giant cell arteritis. SYN: *polymyalgia arteritica*.

polymyoclonus (pŏl″ē-mī-ŏk′lō-nŭs) [″ + ″ + *klonos,* tumult] Paramyoclonus multiplex.

polymyositis (pŏl″ē-mī″ō-sī′tĭs) [″ + ″ + *itis,* inflammation] A relatively uncommon inflammatory disease of skeletal muscles, marked by symmetrical weakness of the proximal muscles of the limbs, elevated serum muscle enzymes, evidence of muscle necrosis on biopsy, and electromyographic abnormalities when the characteristic heliotrope rash of the eyelids or papules over the dorsal surfaces of the knuckles occur. The condition is called dermatomyositis.

TREATMENT: Physical therapy and corticosteroids are used initially. In patients who fail to respond, methotrexate, azathioprine, or other immunosuppressant drugs are used.

polymyxin (pŏl″ē-mĭks′ĭn) One of several closely related antibiotics isolated from various strains of *Bacillus polymyxa* and designated polymyxins A, B, C, D, and E. Most polymyxins cause renal toxicity.

p. B sulfate The least toxic of the antibiotic fractions of polymyxin, and the only one used therapeutically for treating infection.

polyneural (pŏl″ē-nū′răl) [″ + *neuron,* nerve, sinew] Pert. to, innervated, or supplied by many nerves.

polyneuralgia (pŏl″ē-nū-răl′jē-ă) [″ + ″ + *algos,* pain] Neuralgia in several nerves.

polyneuritic (pŏl″ē-nū-rĭt′ĭk) [″ + ″ + *itis,* inflammation] Inflammation of several nerves at once.

polyneuritis (pŏl″ē-nū-rī′tĭs) [″ + ″ + *itis,* inflammation] Multiple neuritis.

acute idiopathic p. Guillain-Barré syndrome.

diabetic p. Diabetic polyneuropathy.

Jamaica ginger p. Jamaica ginger paralysis.

metabolic p. Polyneuritis resulting from metabolic disorders such as nutritional deficiency, esp. the lack of thiamine; gastrointestinal disorders; or pathologic conditions such as diabetes, pernicious anemia, and toxemias of pregnancy.

toxic p. Polyneuritis resulting from poisons such as heavy metals, alcohol, carbon monoxide, or various organic compounds.

polyneuromyositis (pŏl″ē-nū″rō-mī″ō-sī′tĭs) [″ + ″ + *mys,* muscle, + *itis,* inflammation] A disease in which polyneuritis and polymyositis occur together.

polyneuropathy (pŏl″ē-nū-rŏp′ă-thē) [Gr. *polys,* many, + *neuron,* nerve, sinew, + *pathos,* disease, suffering] Any disease that affects multiple peripheral nerves.

acute inflammatory p. Guillain-Barré syndrome.

amyloid p. Polyneuropathy characterized by deposition of amyloid in nerves.

chronic inflammatory demyelinating p. ABBR: CIDP. A gradually progressing autoimmune muscle weakness in arms and legs caused by inflammation of the myelin sheath covering peripheral nerve axons. Myelin destruction (demyelination) slows or blocks conduction of impulses to muscles. Numbness and paresthesia may accompany or precede loss of motor function, which varies from mild to severe. Laboratory findings include elevated protein levels in the cerebrospinal fluid. The disorder is marked by remissions and exacerbations. The inflammatory damage involves not only phagocytes (neutrophils and macrophages), but also immune complexes and complement activation by myelin autoantigens. Immunosuppressive drugs are used to treat this illness. Plasma exchange therapy or infusions of immunoglobulins often are used first, to produce a remission.

diabetic p. A common disabling chronic complication of diabetes mellitus, affecting up to 50% of patients with either type of diabetes. The neuropathy may be symmetrical or asymmetrical and affects peripheral nerves as well as the autonomic nervous system and cranial nerves. Clinically, neuropathic ulcers may develop, esp. on the feet. If these are not appropriately treated, they may result in serious infections that may only resolve with amputation. Thus, patients should be instructed to examine their feet daily for evidence of trauma, callous formation, and blisters. Treatment is supportive, with emphasis on preventing tissue damage. SYN: *diabetic polyneuritis*.

paraproteinemic p. Nerve damage caused by excessive levels of immunoglobulin in the blood.

porphyric p. Polyneuropathy resulting from acute porphyria, characterized by pains and paresthesias in the extremities and by flaccid paralysis.

progressive hypertrophic p. A rare familial disease beginning in childhood and characterized by increased size of peripheral nerves owing to multiplication and hypertrophy of cells of the sheath of Schwann.

polyneuroradiculitis (pŏl″ē-nū″rō-ră-dĭk″ū-lī′tĭs) [″ + ″ + *radix,* root, + *itis,* inflammation] Inflammation of the nerve roots, the peripheral nerves, and spinal ganglia.

polynuclear, polynucleate (pŏl″ē-nū′klē-ăr, -āt) [″ + L. *nucleus,* a kernel] Possessing more than one nucleus. SYN: *multinuclear; multinucleate.*

polynucleotidase (pŏl″ē-nū″klē-ō′tĭ-dās) An enzyme present in intestinal mucosa and intestinal juice that catalyzes the breakdown of nucleic acid to nucleotides.

polynucleotide (pŏl″ē-nū′klē-ō-tīd) Nucleic acid composed of two or more nucleotides.

polyodontia (pŏl″ē-ō-dŏn′shē-ă) [″ + *odous,* tooth] The state of having supernumerary teeth.

polyomavirus (pŏl″ē-ō-mă-vī′rŭs) A DNA tumor virus of the papovavirus family that produces kidney, neurological, and lymphoid diseases in humans.

polyonychia (pŏl″ē-ō-nĭk′ē-ă) [″ + *onyx,* nail] Having an excessive number of nails.

polyopia, polyopsia (pŏl″ē-ō′pē-ă, -ŏp′sē-ă) [″ + *opsis,* vision] Multiple vision; perception of more than one image of the same object.

polyorchidism (pŏl″ē-or′kĭ-dĭzm) [″ + *orchis,* testicle, + *-ismos,* condition] The condition of having more than two testicles.

polyorchis (pŏl″ē-or′kĭs) An individual with more than two testicles.

polyostotic (pŏl″ē-ŏs-tŏt′ĭk) [″ + *osteon,* bone] Concerning many bones.

polyotia (pŏl″ē-ō′shē-ă) [″ + *ous,* ear] The state of having more than two ears.

polyovulatory (pŏl″ē-ŏv′ū-lă-tō″rē) [″ + L. *ovulum,* little egg] Releasing several ova in a single ovulatory cycle.

polyoxyl stearate (pŏl″ē-ŏks′ĭl) Any of several polyoxyethylene stearates. They have varying lengths of the polymer chain (e.g., polyoxyl 8 stearate and polyoxyl 40 stearate [trade name Myrj 52] have polymer lengths of 8 and 40, respectively). They are nonionic surface-active agents that are useful emulsifiers.

polyp (pŏl′ĭp) [Gr. *polypous,* many-footed] A tumor with a pedicle; commonly found in vascular organs such as the nose, uterus, colon, and rectum. Polyps bleed easily; if there is a possibility that they will become malignant, they should be removed surgically. SYN: *polypus.*

adenomatous p. Benign neoplastic tissue originating in the glandular epithelium.

antrochoanal p. A nasal polyp found near the posterior wall of the maxillary sinus.

aural p. Polypoid granulation tissue in the external canal of the ear attached to the tympanic membrane or middle ear structures.

bleeding p. An angioma of the nasal mucous membrane.

cardiac p. A pedunculated tumor attached to the inside of the heart. If situated close to a valve, it may cause blockage of the valve intermittently.

cervical p. A fibrous or mucous polyp of the cervical mucosa.

choanal p. A nasal polyp that extends into the pharynx.

colonic p. An abnormal tissue growth within the lumen of the colon. It may be benign or malignant.

fibrinous p. A polyp containing fibrin and blood, located in the uterine cavity.

fibroepithelial p. A smooth-surfaced polyp of the oral mucosa, usually developing after trauma to the area. SEE: *acrochordon.*

fleshy p. A submucous myoma in the uterus.

gelatinous p. **1.** A polyp made up of loose swollen edematous tissue. **2.** A myxoma.

Hopmann's p. A papillary growth of the nasal mucosa.

hydatid p. A cystic polyp.

juvenile p. A benign rounded mucosal hamartoma of the large bowel. This type of polyp may be present in large numbers in infants and are commonly associated with rectal bleeding. SYN: *retention p.*

laryngeal p. A polyp attached to the vocal cords and extending to the air passageway.

lymphoid p. A benign lymphoma of the rectum.

mucous p. A polyp of soft or jelly-like consistency and exhibiting mucoid degeneration.

placental p. A polyp composed of retained placental tissue.

retention p. Juvenile p.

vascular p. A pedunculated angioma.

polypapilloma (pŏl″ē-păp″ĭ-lō′mă) [Gr. *polys,* many, + L. *papilla,* nipple, + Gr. *oma,* tumor] Yaws.

polypectomy (pŏl″ĭ-pĕk′tō-mē) [″ + *pous,* foot, + *ektome,* excision] The surgical removal of a polyp. In the U.S., about 1 million colonic polypectomies are performed each year.

polypeptidase (pŏl″ē-pĕp′tĭ-dās) An enzyme that catalyzes the hydrolysis of peptides.

polypeptide (pŏl″ē-pĕp′tīd) [″ + *pep-*

tein, to digest] A union of two or more amino acids. SEE: *peptide.*

polypeptidorrhachia (pŏl″ē-pĕp″tĭ-dō-ră′kē-ă) [″ + ″ + *rhachis,* spine] The presence of polypeptides in the cerebrospinal fluid.

polyphagia (pŏl″ē-fā′jē-ă) [Gr. *polys,* many, + *phagein,* to eat] Eating abnormally large amounts of food; gluttony.

polyphalangism (pŏl″ē-fă-lăn′jĭzm) [″ + *phalanx,* closely knit row, + *-ismos,* condition] Hyperphalangism.

polypharmacy (pŏl″ē-făr′mă-sē) [″ + *pharmakon,* drug] **1.** Concurrent use of a large number of drugs, a condition that increases the likelihood of unwanted side effects and adverse drug-to-drug interactions. This situation is esp. liable to occur when the elderly with multiple diseases and complaints are treated by several physicians. Any person taking more than one drug should keep a careful record of all of the drugs being taken, how often they are taken, and by whom they were prescribed, and share that information with all health care providers. The information on the patient's chart should be shown at each office visit to all of those involved in administering medicines to the patient. **2.** Excessive use of drugs.

polyphenoloxidase (pŏl″ē-fē″nŏl-ŏk′sĭ-dās) An enzyme present in bacteria, fungi, and some plants that catalyzes the oxidation of polyphenols, but not monophenols such as tyrosine, to quinones.

polyphobia (pŏl″ē-fō′bē-ă) [Gr. *polys,* many, + *phobos,* fear] Excessive or abnormal fear of a number of things.

polyphrasia (pŏl″ē-frā′zē-ă) [″ + *phrasis,* speech] Excessive talkativeness.

polyphyletic (pŏl″ē-fī-lĕt′ĭk) [″ + *phyle,* tribe] Having more than one origin; opposite of monophyletic.

polyphyodont (pŏl″ē-fī′ō-dŏnt) [″ + *phyein,* to produce, + *odous,* tooth] Developing more than two sets of teeth at intervals during a lifetime.

polypiform (pō-lĭp′ĭ-form) [″ + *pous,* foot, + L. *forma,* form] Resembling a polyp.

polyplastic (pŏl″ē-plăs′tĭk) [″ + *plastos,* formed] **1.** Having had many evolutionary modifications. **2.** Having many substances in the cellular composition.

polyplegia (pŏl″ē-plē′jē-ă) [″ + *plege,* stroke] Paralysis affecting several muscles.

polyploid (pŏl′ē-ployd) **1.** Characterized by polyploidy. **2.** An individual in which the chromosome number is two or more times the normal haploid number.

polyploidy (pŏl′ē-ploy″dē) A condition in which the chromosome number is two or more times the normal haploid number found in gametes.

polypnea (pŏl″ĭp-nē′ă) [″ + *pnoia,* breath] Panting.

polypodia (pŏl″ē-pō′dē-ă) [″ + *pous,* foot] Possession of more than the normal number of feet.

polypoid (pŏl′ē-poyd) [″ + ″ + *eidos,* form, shape] Like a polyp.

polyporous (pŏl-ĭp′ō-rŭs) [″ + *poros,* pore] Possessing many small openings or pores.

polyposia (pŏl″ē-pō′zē-ă) [″ + *posis,* drinking] The sustained ingestion of large amounts of fluid.

polyposis (pŏl″ē-pō′sĭs) [″ + *pous,* foot, + *osis,* condition] The presence of numerous polyps.

p. coli Polyposis of the large intestine.

familial p. A rare familial condition transmitted by a dominant gene in which thousands of polyps develop in the mucosa of the colon and often other organs. They may produce intestinal bleeding, anemia, or pain, but most importantly affected persons nearly always develop colon cancer. They are treated with prophylactic colectomy. SYN: *multiple intestinal p.* SEE: *Gardner's syndrome.*

multiple intestinal p. Familial polyposis.

p. ventriculi The presence of numerous polyps in the stomach, sometimes involving the entire mucosa, accompanied by chronic atrophic gastritis.

polyptychial (pŏl″ē-tī′kē-ăl) [″ + *ptyche,* fold] Arranged in several layers, as is the case in some glands.

polypus (pŏl′ĭ-pŭs) *pl.* **polypi** [L.] Polyp.

polyradiculitis (pŏl″ē-ră-dĭk′ū-lī′tĭs) [″ + L. *radix,* root, + Gr. *itis,* inflammation] Inflammation of nerve roots, esp. the roots of spinal nerves. SEE: *Nursing Diagnoses Appendix.*

polyradiculoneuritis (pŏl″ē-ră-dĭk″ū-lō-nū-rī′tĭs) [″ + ″ + Gr. *neuron,* nerve, + *itis,* inflammation] Inflammation of the peripheral nerves and spinal ganglia.

polyradiculopathy, acute inflammatory Guillain-Barré syndrome.

polyribosome (pŏl″ē-rī′bō-sōm) A cluster or group of ribosomes. They are the site of attachment for mRNA in the cytoplasm and the translation of genetic information into the synthesis of specific proteins. SYN: *polysome.*

polyrrhea, polyrrhoea (pŏl″ē-rē′ă) [″ + *rhoia,* flow] The excessive secretion of fluid.

polysaccharide (pŏl″ē-săk′ă-rīd) [″ + Sanskrit *sarkara,* sugar] One of a group of carbohydrates that, upon hydrolysis, yield more than 20 monosaccharide molecules. They are complex carbohydrates of high molecular weight, usually insoluble in water, but when soluble, they form colloidal solutions. Their basic formula is $(C_6H_{12}O_6)_n$. They include two groups: starch (e.g., starch, inulin, glycogen, dextrin) and cellulose (e.g., cellulose and hemicelluloses). The hemicelluloses include the pentosans (e.g., gum arabic), hexosans (e.g., agar-agar), and hexopentosans (e.g., pectin). SEE: *carbohydrate; disaccharide; monosaccharide.*

immune p. Polysaccharides in bacteria, esp. in the cell wall, that are antigenic.

polysaccharose (pŏl″ē-săk′ă-rōs) A polysaccharide.

polyscelia (pŏl″ē-sē′lē-ă) [″ + *skelos,* leg] The condition of having more than the normal number of legs.

polyscelus (pŏ-lĭs′ĕ-lŭs) One having polyscelia.

polyserositis (pŏl″ē-sē-rō-sī′tĭs) [″ + L. *serum,* whey, + *itis,* inflammation] Inflammation of several serous membranes simultaneously. SYN: *Concato's disease.*

recurrent p. Familial Mediterranean fever.

polysinusitis, polysinuitis (pŏl″ē-sī″nŭs-ī′tĭs, -nū-ī′tĭs) [″ + L. *sinus,* a hollow, + Gr. *itis,* inflammation] Inflammation of several sinuses simultaneously.

polysomaty (pŏl″ē-sō′mă-tē) [″ + *soma,* body] Having reduplicated chromatin in the nucleus.

polysome Polyribosome.

polysomia (pŏl″ē-sō′mē-ă) [″ + *soma,* body] Having more than one body, as in the doubling of the body of a fetus.

polysomnography The simultaneous monitoring of respiratory, cardiac, muscle, brain, and ocular function during sleep. It is used most often to diagnose sleep apnea.

polysorbates (pŏl″ē-sor′bāts) Nonionic surface-active agents composed of polyoxyethylene esters of sorbitol. They usually contain associated fatty acids. The series includes polysorbates 20, 40, 60, and 80, which are used in preparing pharmaceuticals. These polysorbates have the trade names of Tween 20, Tween 40, and so forth.

polyspermia (pŏl″ē-spĕr′mē-ă) [Gr. *polys,* many, + *sperma,* seed] **1.** The excessive secretion of seminal fluid. **2.** The entrance of several spermatozoa into one ovum. SYN: *polyspermism.*

polyspermism (pŏl″ē-spĕrm′ĭzm) Polyspermia.

polyspermy (pŏl″ē-spĕr′mē) The fertilization of an ovum by multiple spermatozoa.

polystichia (pŏl″ē-stĭk′ē-ă) [″ + *stichos,* a row] A condition in which there are two or more rows of eyelashes.

polystomatous (pŏl″ē-stō′mă-tŭs) [″ + *stoma,* mouth] Possessing many mouths or openings.

polystyrene (pŏl″ē-stī′rēn) A synthetic resin produced by the polymerization of styrene from ethylene and benzene. The formula is $(CH_2CHC_6H_5)_n$. It is used in the plastics industry.

polysulfone A synthetic polymer used in the fabrication of dialysis membranes with high biocompatibility.

polysynaptic (pŏl″ē-sĭ-năp′tĭk) [″ + *synapsis,* point of contact] Pert. to nerve pathways involving multiple synapses.

polysyndactyly (pŏl″ē-sĭn-dăk′tĭl-ē) [″ + *syn,* together, + *daktylos,* finger] Multiple syndactyly.

polytendinitis (pŏl″ē-tĕn″dĭ-nī′tĭs) [″ + L. *tendo,* tendon, + Gr. *itis,* inflammation] Inflammation of several tendons.

polytene (pŏl′ĕ-tēn) [″ + *tainia,* band] Composed of many filaments of chromatin.

polyteny (pŏl″ē-tē′nē) [″ + *tainia,* band] Multiple lateral duplication of the chromosome. This produces a giant chromosome.

polytetrafluoroethylene ABBR: PTFE. A synthetic polymer that has slippery, nonsticking properties. It is used in a variety of products, including vascular grafts used to bypass obstructed blood vessels and grafts used for dialysis access.

polythelia (pŏl″ē-thē′lē-ă) [″ + *thele,* nipple, + *-ismos,* condition] The presence of more than one nipple on a mamma.

polythiazide (pŏl″ē-thī′ă-zīd) A diuretic drug.

polytrichia (pŏl″ē-trĭk′ē-ă) [″ + *thrix,* hair] Hypertrichosis.

polytrichosis (pŏl″ē-trĭ-kō′sĭs) [″ + ″ + *osis,* condition] Hypertrichosis.

polytropic (pŏl″ē-trŏp′ĭk) [″ + *trope,* a turning] Affecting more than one type of cell, said of viruses, or affecting more than one type of tissue, said of certain poisons.

polyunguia (pŏl″ē-ŭng′gwē-ă) [″ + L. *unguis,* nail] Polyonychia.

polyunsaturated In chemistry, relating to long-chain carbon compounds, esp. fats that have many carbon atoms joined by double or triple bonds.

polyuria (pŏl″ē-ū′rē-ă) [″ + *ouron,* urine] Excessive secretion and discharge of urine. The urine does not, as a rule, contain abnormal constituents. Several liters in excess of normal may be voided each day. The urine is virtually colorless. Specific gravity is 1.000 to 1.002 (higher in diabetes mellitus). Polyuria occurs in diabetes insipidus; diabetes mellitus; chronic nephritis; nephrosclerosis; hyperthyroidism; following edematous states, esp. those induced by heart failure treated with diuretics; and following excessive intake of liquids.

polyvalent (pŏl″ē-vā′lĕnt, pō-lĭv′ă-lĕnt) [″ + L. *valere,* to be strong] Multivalent; having a combining power of more than two atoms of hydrogen.

polyvinyl alcohol (pŏl″ē-vī′nĭl) A water-soluble synthetic resin used in preparing medicines, esp. ophthalmic solutions.

polyvinyl chloride ABBR: PVC. A thermoplastic polymer formed from vinyl chloride, used in the manufacture of many products such as rainwear, garden hoses, and floor tiles.

CAUTION: Exposure to toxic fumes of PVC can cause respiratory irritation, asthma, or decompensation. Some evidence suggests PVCs can cause cancer.

---

polyvinylpyrrolidone (pŏl″ē-vī″nĭl-pĕr-rŏl′ĭ-dōn) ABBR: PVP. Previously used name for povidone.

pomatum (pō-mā′tŭm) A medicinal ointment, esp. one used on the hair.

Pompe's disease Glycogen storage disease type II.

pompholyx A blistering itchy rash of the hands and feet, marked by episodic and recurring deep-seated vesicles or bullae. The rash is most often found in adolescents and young adults, esp. during spring and summer. SYN: *dyshidrosis; dyshidrotic eczema*. SEE: illus.

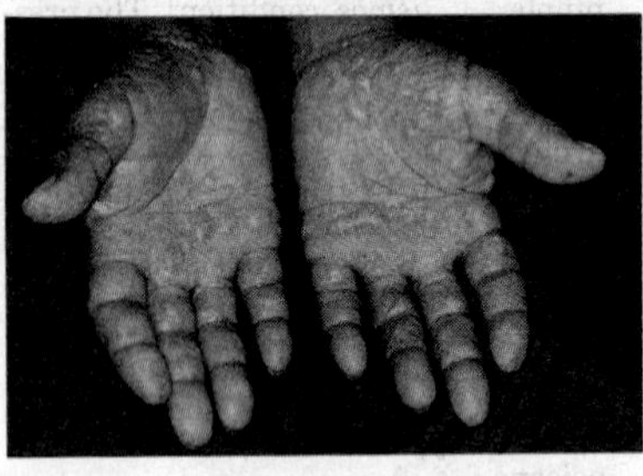

POMPHOLYX

ETIOLOGY: Although the cause is unknown, emotional stress, an allergic predisposition, and fungal infections have each been associated with episodes of the rash.

TREATMENT: Burow's or permanganate solution and potent topical steroids sometimes are effective. The rash tends to appear less often as patients reach middle age.

pomphus (pŏm′fŭs) *pl.* **pomphi** [L.] A blister or a circumscribed elevation on the skin; a wheal.

POMR *problem-oriented medical record.*

pomum (pō′mŭm) [L.] An apple.

p. adami A prominence in the middle line of the throat, caused by junction of two lateral wings of the thyroid cartilage. SYN: *Adam's apple*.

ponderal (pŏn′dĕr-ăl) [L. *pondus*, weight] Relating to weight.

ponderal index The ratio of an individual's height to the cube root of his or her weight; used to determine body mass. SEE: *Quatelet index*.

ponophobia (pŏ″nō-fō′bē-ă) [Gr. *ponos*, pain, + *phobos*, fear] **1.** An abnormal distaste for exerting oneself. **2.** A dread of pain.

pons (pŏnz) *pl.* **pontes** [L., bridge] **1.** A process of tissue connecting two or more parts. **2.** P. varolii.

p. cerebelli P. varolii.

p. hepatis The part of the liver sometimes present that extends from the quadrate lobe to the left lobe across the umbilical fissure.

p. varolii A rounded eminence on the ventral surface of the brain stem. It lies between the medulla and cerebral peduncles, and appears externally as a broad band of transverse fibers. It is connected to the cerebellum by the midcerebellar peduncle, or brachium pontis. It contains fiber tracts connecting the medulla oblongata and cerebellum with the upper portions of the brain, and contains two respiratory centers that work with those in the medulla. The origins of the abducens, facial, trigeminal, and cochlear divisions of the eighth (vestibulocochlear) nerve are at the borders of the pons. SYN: *pons* (2); *p. cerebelli*.

pontic (pŏn′tĭk) [L. *pons, pontis*, bridge] An artificial tooth set in a bridge.

pontile (pŏn′tēl) Pert. to the pons varolii.

pontile nuclei The gray matter in the pons.

pontine (pŏn′tēn) Pert. to the pons varolii.

pontobulbar (pŏn″tō-bŭl′bar) Pert. to the pons and medulla oblongata.

pool **1.** To mix blood from several donors. **2.** The accumulation of blood in a body site. **3.** A source of similar substances or cells.

abdominal p. The accumulation of blood in the visceral organs of the abdominal cavity. This may occur as a result of abdominal trauma.

amino acid p. The amino acids available for protein synthesis at any given time; the liver regulates the blood level of amino acids based on tissue needs and converts excess amino acids to carbohydrates for energy production.

gene p. The sum of the genetic material in the members of a specified population.

metabolic p. All of the chemical compounds included in metabolic processes in the body.

vaginal p. The mucus and cells that are present in the posterior fornix of the vagina when the patient is in a supine position. Material obtained from this site is used in cancer detection and in evaluating the character of the vaginal fluid in investigating infertility problems.

poples (pŏp′lēz) [L., ham of the knee]

The popliteal or posterior region of the knee.

popliteus (pŏp-lĭt′ē-ŭs, -lĭt-ē′ŭs) [L. *poples,* ham of the knee] Muscle located in the hind part of the knee joint that flexes the leg and aids it in rotating. **popliteal** (pŏp″lĭt-ē′ăl, pŏp-lĭt′ē-ăl), *adj.*

poppy Any of the several plants of the genus *Papaver.* Opium is obtained from the juice of the unripe pods of *Papaver somniferum.*

population **1.** All persons, plants, or animals inhabiting a specified area. **2.** The group of persons from which a research sample is drawn.

POR *problem-oriented record.*

poradenitis (por″ăd-ĕ-nī′tĭs) [Gr. *poros,* passage, + *aden,* gland, + *itis,* inflammation] The formation of small abscesses in the iliac lymph nodes.

porcelain (por′sĕ-lĭn) A hard, translucent ceramic made by fusing clay and colored by glazing with fusible pigments. It is used in dentistry.

porcelaneous, porcelanous (por″sĕ-lā′nē-ŭs, -sĕl′ăn-ŭs) [Fr. *porcelaine*] Translucent or white like porcelain, as the skin.

porcine (por′sīn) [L. *porcus,* pig] Relating to or concerning swine.

pore (por) [Gr. *poros,* passage.] **1.** A minute opening, esp. one on an epithelial surface. SYN: *porus.* **2.** The opening of the secretory duct of a sweat gland. SEE: *skin; stoma; sweat glands.*

alveolar p. A minute opening that is thought to exist between adjacent alveoli of the lung.

gustatory p. Taste p.

taste p. The external opening of a taste bud. SYN: *gustatory p.* SEE: *taste.*

porencephalia, porencephaly (por″ĕn-sĕf-ā′lē-ă, por″ĕn-sĕf′ă-lē) [″ + *enkephalos,* brain] An anomalous condition in which the ventricles of the brain are connected with the subarachnoid space.

porencephalitis (por″ĕn-sĕf″ă-lī′tĭs) [″ + ″ + *itis,* inflammation] Inflammation of the brain with development of cavities communicating with the subarachnoid space.

pores of Kohn [Hans Kohn, Ger. pathologist, b. 1866] A passageway for gas from one alveolus of the lung to an adjacent one. These may be of assistance in preventing atelectasis.

pori Pl. of porus.

poriomania [Gr. *poreia,* walking, + *mania,* madness] The morbid desire to wander from home.

porion (pō′rē-ŏn) [Gr. *poros,* passage] The midpoint of the upper margin of the auditory meatus.

porocele (pō′rō-sēl) [Gr. *poros,* passage, + *kele,* tumor, swelling] A herniation into the scrotal sac. This causes hardening and thickening of the scrotum.

porocephaliasis, porocephalosis (pō″rō-sĕf″ă-lī′ă-sĭs, -lō′sĭs) [″ + *kephale,* head, + *-iasis,* state or condition of] Infection with a species of *Porocephalus.*

Porocephalus (pō″rō-sĕf′ă-lŭs) A genus of wormlike arthropods found commonly in snakes. The young sometimes infest mammals, including humans.

porokeratosis (pō″rō-kĕr″ă-tō′sĭs) [″ + *keras,* horn, + *osis,* condition] A rare skin disease marked by thickening of the stratum corneum in a linear arrangement, followed by its atrophy. Porokeratosis appears on smooth areas. It is irregular in form and size with a circumscribed outline and affects the hands and feet, forearms and legs, the face, neck, and scalp.

poroma (pō-rō′mă) [Gr.] **1.** Callosity. **2.** A tumor of cells lining the opening of the sweat glands.

cerebral p. At postmortem examination, the presence of cavities in the brain substance caused by gas-forming bacteria.

eccrine p. A tumor arising from the duct of an eccrine gland; usually occurring on the palm or sole.

porosis (pō-rō′sĭs) [Gr. *poros,* passage, + *osis,* condition] Callus formation in repair of fractured bone. SEE: *callus.*

porosity (pō-rŏs′ĭ-tē) [Gr. *poros,* passage] The state of being porous.

porous (pō′rŭs) Full of pores; able to admit passage of a liquid.

porphin (por′fĭn) The basic ring structure forming the framework of all porphyrins. Consisting of four pyrrole rings united by methene couplings.

porphobilinogen (por″fō-bī-lĭn′ō-jĕn) An intermediate product in heme synthesis sometimes found in the urine of patients with acute porphyria. The urine may appear normal when fresh but will change to a burgundy wine color or even to black when heated with dilute hydrochloric acid to 100°C.

porphyria (por-fī′rē-ă, por-fĭr′ē-ă) [Gr. *porphyra,* purple] A group of disorders that result from a disturbance in porphyrin metabolism, causing increased formation and excretion of porphyrin or its precursors.

acute intermittent p. A rare metabolic disorder inherited as an autosomal dominant trait. It is characterized by excessive excretion of porphyrins, episodes of acute abdominal pain, sensitivity to light, and neurological disturbances. The disorder is sometimes precipitated by the excessive use of sulfonamides, barbiturates, or other drugs.

congenital erythropoietic p. A rare condition inherited as an autosomal recessive trait. It is characterized by severe skin lesions, hemolytic anemia, and splenomegaly.

p. cutanea tarda A form of porphyria in which patients develop liver disease and rashes on sun-exposed parts of their bodies (e.g., knuckles or face). The use of alcohol or estrogens may worsen the condition. The cause is a deficiency of uroporphylinogen decarboxylase.

p. erythropoietica A mild form of porphyria characterized by cutaneous lesions and excess protoporphyrin in the erythrocytes and feces.

p. hepatica Porphyria caused by a disturbance in liver metabolism such as occurs following hepatitis, poisoning by heavy metals, certain anemias, and other conditions.

South African genetic p. Variegate p.

variegate p. A form of hepatic porphyria in which there are recurrent episodes of abdominal pain and neuropathy. The skin is esp. fragile. SYN: *South African genetic p.*

porphyrin (por′fĭ-rĭn) [Gr. *porphyra,* purple] Any of a group of nitrogen-containing organic compounds that occur in protoplasm and form the basis of animal and plant respiratory pigments; obtained from hemoglobin and chlorophyll.

porphyrinuria (por″fĭ-rĭ-nū′rē-ă) [″ + *ouron,* urine] Excretion of an increased amount of porphyrin in the urine. SYN: *porphyruria.*

porphyruria (por″fĭr-ū′rē-ă) [″ + *ouron,* urine] Porphyrinuria.

Porro's operation (por′ōz) [Eduardo Porro, It. obstetrician, 1842–1902] Cesarean section followed by removal of the uterus, the ovaries, and fallopian tubes. SYN: *cesarean hysterectomy.*

PORT *patient outcomes research team.*

porta [L., gate] The point of entry of nerves and vessels into an organ or part.

p. hepatis The fissure of the liver where the portal vein and hepatic artery enter and the hepatic duct leaves.

p. lienis The hilus of the spleen where vessels enter and leave.

p. pulmonis A pulmonary hilus for the entry and exit of the bronchi, nerves, and vessels.

p. renis The hilus of the kidney; the site of entry and exit of vessels and the ureter.

portacaval (por″tă-kā′văl) Concerning the portal vein and the vena cava.

portal [L. *porta,* gate] **1.** An entryway. **2.** Concerning a porta or entrance to an organ, esp. that through which the blood is carried to the liver.

p. of entry The pathway by which infectious organisms gain access to the body (e.g., respiratory tract, breaks in skin).

p. of exit The pathway by which pathogens leave the body of a host (e.g., respiratory droplets, feces, urine, blood).

intestinal p. The opening of the midgut or yolk sac into the foregut or hindgut of an embryo.

p. vein Vein formed by the veins of the splanchnic area that conveys its blood into the liver. It is made of the combined superior and inferior mesenteric, splenic, gastric, and cystic veins.

portio (por′shē-ō) *pl.* **portiones** [L.] A part. In anatomy, it designates a certain portion of a structure or organ.

p. dura Facial nerve.

p. intermedia Nervus intermedius.

p. vaginalis The part of the cervix within the vagina.

portoenterostomy, hepatic A surgical procedure performed to establish bile flow in an infant who has external biliary atresia associated with absence of the extrahepatic biliary system. A section of the jejunum is attached to the liver at the normal exit site of the hepatic duct to allow bile drainage into the small intestine. The jejunal segment may be looped to form a cutaneous double-barreled ostomy. Postoperatively, liver function continues to deteriorate in most children, and liver transplantation is often needed. SYN: *Kasai procedure.*

portogram (por′tō-grăm) [L. *porta,* gate, + Gr. *gramma,* something written] A radiograph of the portal vein after injection of a contrast medium.

portography (por-tŏg′ră-fē) [″ + Gr. *graphein,* to write] Radiography of the portal vein after injection of a radiopaque contrast medium.

portal p. Portography after injection of opaque material into the superior mesenteric vein. This is usually done during laparotomy.

splenic p. Radiography of the splenic and portal veins after injection of a contrast medium into the splenic artery.

portosystemic (por″tō-sĭs-tĕm′ĭk) Joining the portal and systemic venous circulation.

Portuguese man-of-war A type of jellyfish, *Physalia physalis,* whose tentacles contain a neurotoxin that produces a burning sensation on contact. SEE: *bite.*

port-wine stain Nevus flammeus.

porus (pō′rŭs) *pl.* **pori** [L.] A meatus or foramen; a tiny aperture in a structure; a pore.

p. acusticus externus The outer opening of the external acoustic meatus.

p. acusticus internus The opening of the internal acoustic meatus into the cranial cavity.

p. gustatorius The small taste pore openings in the taste buds of the tongue.

p. lactiferous The opening of a lactiferous duct on the tip of the nipple of the mammary gland.

p. opticus The opening in the center of the optic disk through which retinal vessels (central artery and vein) reach the retina through the lamina cribrosa of the sclera.

p. sudoriferus The opening of a sweat gland.

position (pō-zĭsh′ŭn) [L. *positio*] **1.** The place or arrangement in which a thing is put. **2.** The manner in which a body is arranged, as by the nurse or physician for examination. **3.** In obstetrics, the relationship of a selected fetal landmark to the maternal front or back, and on the right or left side. SEE: table; *presentation* for illus.

anatomical p. The position assumed when a person is standing erect with arms at the sides, palms forward. SYN: *orthograde p.*

anteroposterior p. A radiographical examination position in which the central ray enters the front of the body and exits from the back.

axial p. A radiographical examination position in which an image is obtained with the central ray entering the body at an angle.

Bonnet's p. In inflammation of the hip joint, the flexion, abduction, and outward rotation of the thigh, which produces relief.

Positions of Fetus in Utero

Vertex Presentation (point of designation—occiput)	
Left occiput anterior	LOA
Right occiput posterior	ROP
Right occiput anterior	ROA
Left occiput posterior	LOP
Right occiput transverse	ROT
Occiput anterior	OA
Occiput posterior	OP
Breech Presentation (point of designation—sacrum)	
Left sacroanterior	LSA
Right sacroposterior	RSP
Right sacroanterior	RSA
Left sacroposterior	LSP
Sacroanterior	SA
Sacroposterior	SP
Left sacrotransverse	LST
Right sacrotransverse	RST
Face Presentation (point of designation—mentum)	
Left mentoanterior	LMA
Right mentoposterior	RMP
Right mentoanterior	RMA
Left mentoposterior	LMP
Mentoposterior	MP
Mentoanterior	MA
Left mentotransverse	LMT
Right mentotransverse	RMT
Transverse Presentation (point of designation—scapula of presenting shoulder)	
Left acromiodorso-anterior	LADA
Right acromiodorso-posterior	RADP
Right acromiodorso-anterior	RADA
Left acromiodorso-posterior	LADP

Brickner p. A method of obtaining traction, abduction, and external rotation of the shoulder by tying the patient's wrists to the head of the bed.

centric p. The most posterior position of the mandible in relation to the maxilla.

decubitus p. The position of the patient on a flat surface. The exact position is indicated by which surface of the body is closest to the flat surface (i.e., in left or right lateral decubitus, the patient is flat on the left or right side, respectively; in dorsal or ventral decubitus, the patient is on the back or abdomen, respectively).

dorsal p. A position in which the patient lies on the back. SYN: *supine.*

dorsal elevated p. A position in which the patient lies on the back with the head and shoulders elevated at an angle of 30° or more. It is employed in digital examination of genitalia and in bimanual examination of the vagina.

dorsal recumbent p. A position in which the patient lies on the back with the lower extremities moderately flexed and rotated outward. It is employed in the application of obstetrical forceps, repair of lesions following parturition, vaginal examination, and bimanual palpation. SEE: illus.

dorsosacral p. Lithotomy p. SEE: *dorsal recumbent p.* for illus.

Edebohls' p. Simon's position.

Elliot's p. A position in which supports are placed under the small of the patient's back so that the patient is in a posture resembling a double inclined plane.

en face p. In obstetrics, a position in which the mother and infant are face to face. This position encourages eye contact and is conducive to attachment.

English p. Left lateral recumbent p.

fetal p. The relationship of a specified bony landmark on the fetal presenting part to the quadrants of the maternal pelvis.

Fowler's p. SEE: *dorsal recumbent p.* for illus.; *Fowler's position.*

genucubital p. A position with the patient on the knees, thighs upright, body resting on elbows, head down on hands. Employed when it is not possible to use the classic knee-chest position. SYN: *knee-elbow position.*

genupectoral p. A position with the patient on the knees, thighs upright, the head and upper part of the chest resting on the table, arms crossed above the head. It is employed in displacement of a prolapsed fundus, dislodgment of the impacted head of a fetus, management of transverse presentation, replacement of a retroverted uterus or displaced ovary, or flushing of the intestinal canal. SYN: *knee-chest p.* SEE: *dorsal recumbent p.* for illus.

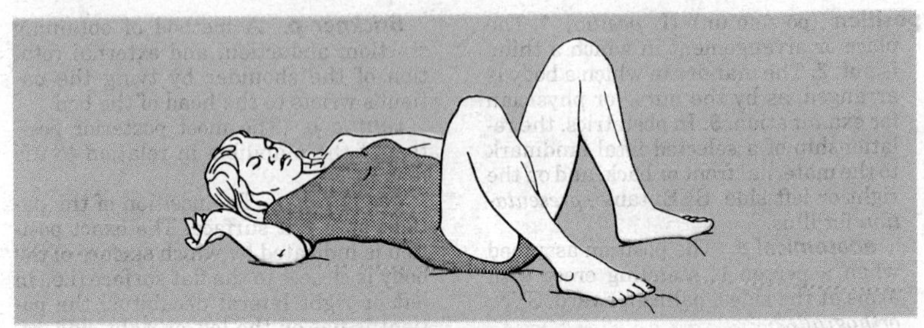
DORSAL RECUMBENT POSITION

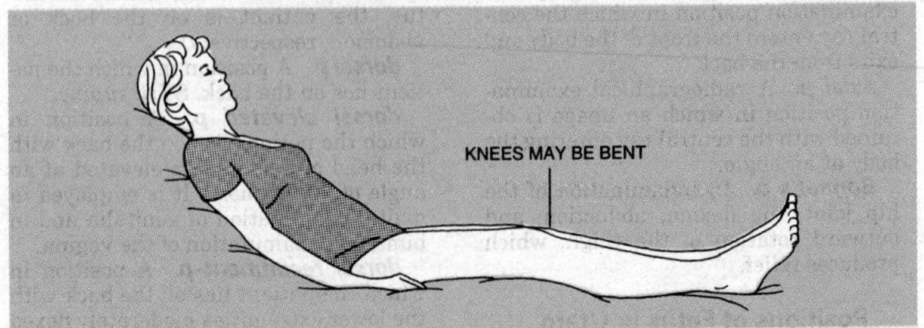

FOWLER'S POSITION

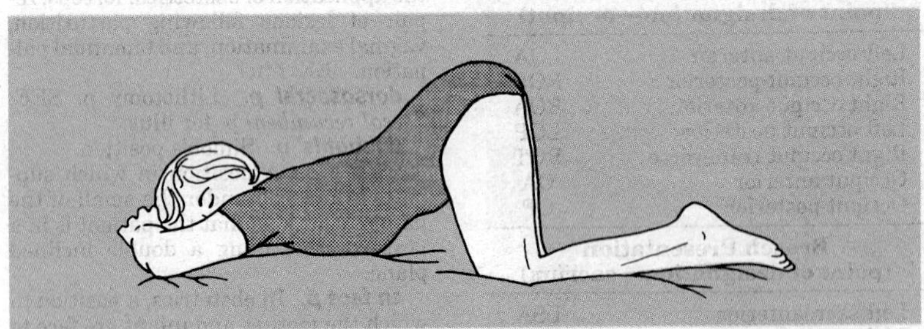
KNEE-CHEST OR GENUPECTORAL POSITION

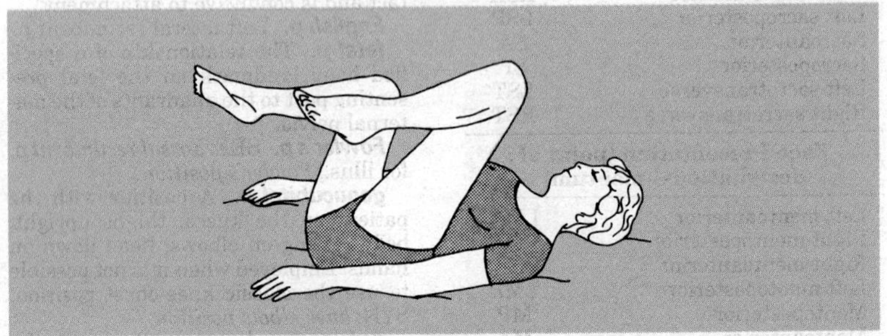
LITHOTOMY OR DORSOSACRAL POSITION

POSITIONS (CONTINUED)

gravity-dependent p. Placing a limb so that its distal end is lower than the level of the heart. Gravity affects the fluids within the limb, drawing or retaining them to the distal aspect. When limbs, esp. injured limbs, are placed below the level of the heart, interstitial pressure is increased, encouraging the formation and retention of edema within the extremity.

horizontal p. A position in which the patient lies supine with feet extended. It is used in palpation, in auscultation of fetal heart, and in operative procedures.

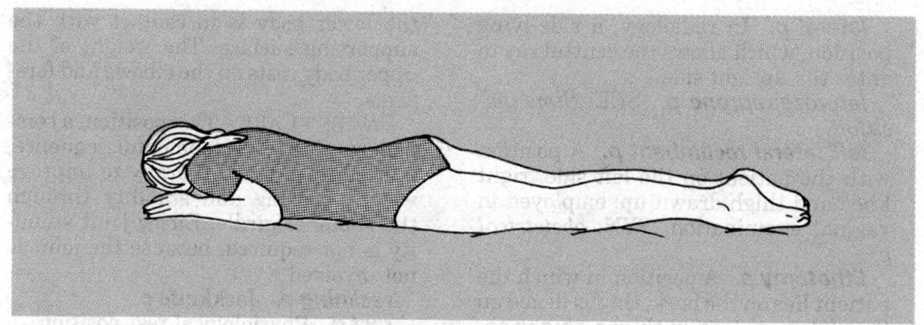

PRONE POSITION

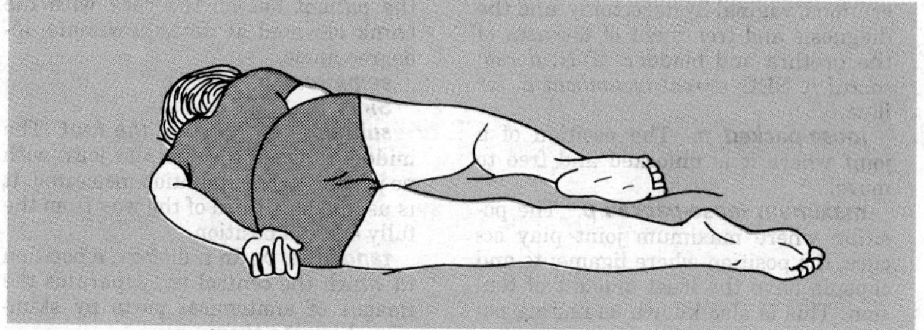

SIMS' POSITION

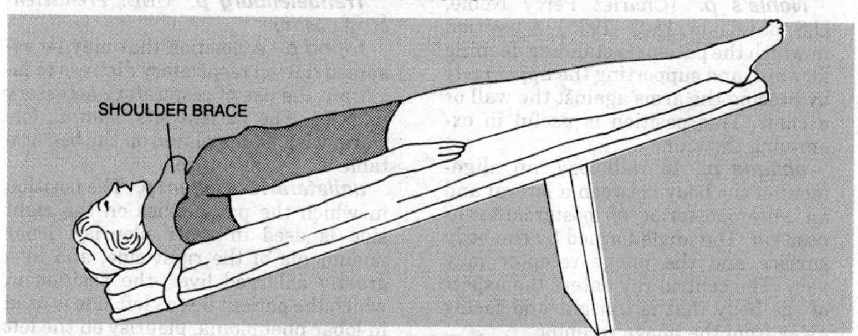

TRENDELENBURG POSITION

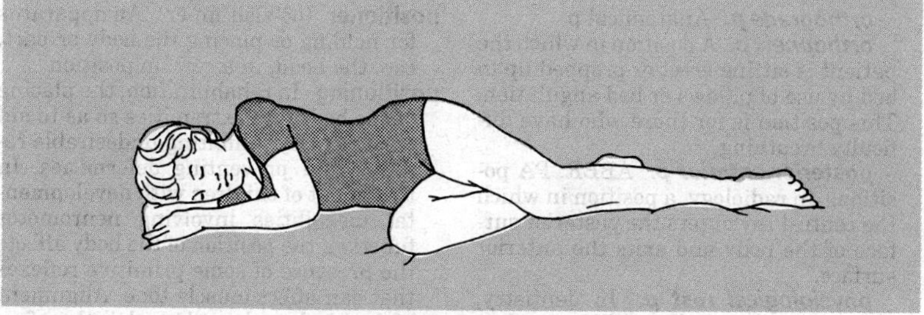

RIGHT LATERAL RECUMBENT POSITION

POSITIONS

horizontal abdominal p. A position in which the patient lies flat on the abdomen, feet extended; employed in examination of the back and spinal column.

jackknife p. A position in which the patient lies on the back, shoulders elevated, legs flexed on thighs, thighs at right angles to the abdomen. It is employed when introducing a urethral sound. SYN: *reclining p.*

knee-chest p. Genupectoral p. SEE: *dorsal recumbent p.* for illus.

knee-elbow p. Genucubital p.

lateral p. In radiology, a side-lying position, which allows the central ray to enter the upright side.

laterosemiprone p. SEE: *Sims' position.*

left lateral recumbent p. A position with the patient on the left side, right knee and thigh drawn up; employed in vaginal examination. SYN: *obstetrical p.*

lithotomy p. A position in which the patient lies on the back, thighs flexed on the abdomen, legs on thighs, thighs abducted. This is used in genital tract operations, vaginal hysterectomy, and the diagnosis and treatment of diseases of the urethra and bladder. SYN: *dorsosacral p.* SEE: *dorsal recumbent p.* for illus.

loose-packed p. The position of a joint where it is unlocked and free to move.

maximum loose-packed p. The position where maximum joint play occurs; the position where ligaments and capsule have the least amount of tension. This is also known as resting position.

Noble's p. [Charles Percy Noble, U.S. physician, 1863–1935] A position in which the patient is standing, leaning forward, and supporting the upper body by bracing the arms against the wall or a chair. This position is useful in examining the kidney.

oblique p. In radiology, an alignment of the body between a lateral and an anteroposterior or posteroanterior position. The angle formed by the body surface and the image receptor may vary. The central ray enters the aspect of the body that is upright and facing away from the image receptor.

obstetrical p. Left lateral recumbent p.

orthograde p. Anatomical p.

orthopneic p. A position in which the patient is sitting erect or propped up in bed by use of pillows or bed angulation. This position is for those who have difficulty breathing.

posterior-anterior p. ABBR: PA position. In radiology, a position in which the central ray enters the posterior surface of the body and exits the anterior surface.

physiological rest p. In dentistry, the position of the mandible at rest when the patient is sitting upright and the condyles are in an unstrained position. The jaw muscles are relaxed. SYN: *rest p.*

prone p. A position in which the patient is lying face downward. SEE: *dorsal recumbent p.* for illus.

prone on elbows p. ABBR: POE. A position in which the body is lying face down with the upper trunk and head elevated, propped up by the arms, while the lower body is in contact with the supporting surface. The weight of the upper body rests on the elbows and forearms.

PATIENT CARE: This position, a component of the developmental sequence, is used in physical therapy to improve weight bearing and stability through the shoulder girdle. Elbow joint stability is not required, because the joint is not involved.

reclining p. Jackknife p.

rest p. Physiological rest position.

semi-Fowler's p. A position in which the patient lies on the back with the trunk elevated at an approximate 45-degree angle.

semiprone p. Sims' p.

Sims' p. Sims' position.

subtalar neutral p. of the foot The middle range of the subtalar joint with no pronation or supination measured. It is usually one third of the way from the fully everted position.

tangential p. In radiology, a position in which the central ray separates the images of anatomical parts by skimming between them.

Trendelenburg p. SEE: *Trendelenburg position.*

tripod p. A position that may be assumed during respiratory distress to facilitate the use of respiratory accessory muscles. The patient sits, leaning forward, with hands placed on the bed or a table with arms braced.

unilateral recumbent p. The position in which the patient lies on the right side is used in acute pleurisy, lobar pneumonia of the right side, and in a greatly enlarged liver; the position in which the patient lies on left side is used in lobar pneumonia, pleurisy on the left side, and in large pericardial effusions. SEE: *dorsal recumbent p.* for illus.

positioner (pō-zĭsh'ŭn-ĕr) An apparatus for holding or placing the body or part, esp. the head, in a certain position.

positioning In rehabilitation, the placing of the body and extremities so as to aid treatment by inhibiting undesirable reflexes and preventing deformities. In treatment of children with developmental disabilities involving neuromotor function, the position of the body affects the presence of some primitive reflexes that can affect muscle tone. Alignment of the head, neck, and trunk is therefore thought to be important to reduce unnecessary influences on muscle tone, and the careful placement of the limbs is important to reduce or prevent contractions and deformities.

positive (pŏz'ĭ-tĭv) [L. *positivus,* ruling] **1.** Definite; affirmative; opposite of negative. **2.** Indicating an abnormal condition in examination and diagnosis. **3.** Having a value greater than zero. In laboratory findings and mathematical expressions, positive is indicated by a plus (+) sign.

positron (pŏz′ĭ-trŏn) A particle having the same mass as a negative electron but possessing a positive charge.

Possum (pŏs′ŭm) [*p*atient *o*perated *s*elector *m*echanism] A device that permits a disabled individual to control and operate various machines such as switches, telephones, and typewriters by breathing into the master control of the apparatus.

post In dentistry, a dowel or pin anchored in an upright position in a tooth or bone for the attachment of a dental crown or prosthesis.

post- [L.] A prefix meaning *behind, after, posterior.*

postabortal (pōst″ă-bor′tăl) [L. *post,* behind, after, + *abortus,* abortion] Happening subsequent to abortion.

postacetabular (pōst″ăs-ĕ-tăb′ū-lăr) [″ + *acetabulum,* a little saucer for vinegar] Behind the acetabulum.

postadolescent (pōst″ăd-ō-lĕs′ĕnt) [″ + *adolescens,* to grow up] An individual who has passed adolescence.

postanal (pōst-ā′năl) [″ + *anus,* anus] Located behind the anus.

postanesthesia recovery room nurse ABBR: PAR nurse. A nurse who has received special training in caring for patients who have come from surgery and are recovering from the effects of anesthesia.

postanesthetic (pōst″ăn-ĕs-thĕt′ĭk) [″ + Gr. *an-,* not, + *aisthesis,* sensation] Pert. to the period following anesthesia.

postapoplectic (pōst″ăp-ō-plĕk′tĭk) [″ + Gr. *apoplessein,* to cripple by a stroke] Pert. to the period immediately following a stroke or apoplexy.

postaxial (pōst-ăk′sē-ăl) [″ + Gr. *axon,* axis] Situated or happening behind an axis.

postbrachial (pōst-brā′kē-ăl) [″ + *brachiolis,* arm] Pert. to the posterior portion of the upper arm.

postcapillary (pōst-kăp′ĭl-lā-rē) Venous capillary.

postcardial (pōst-kăr′dē-ăl) [″ + Gr. *kardia,* heart] Behind the heart.

postcardiotomy (pōst-kăr″dē-ŏt′ō-mē) [″ + ″ + *tome,* incision] The period after open-heart surgery.

postcaval Concerning the postcava, the ascending or inferior vena cava.

postcentral (pōst-sĕn′trăl) [″ + Gr. *kentron,* center] **1.** Situated or happening behind a center. **2.** Located behind the fissure of Rolando.

postcibal (pōst-sī′băl) [″ + *cibum,* food] ABBR: pc. Occurring after meals.

postclavicular (pōst″klă-vĭk′ū-lăr) [″ + *clavicula,* a little key] Located or occurring behind the clavicle.

postclimacteric (pōst″klī-măk-tĕr′ĭk, -măk′tĕr-ĭk) [″ + Gr. *klimakter,* rung of a ladder] Occurring after menopause.

postcoital (pōst-kō′ĭt-ăl) [″ + *coitio,* a coming together] Subsequent to sexual intercourse.

postconnubial (pōst″kŏn-ū′bē-ăl) [″ + *connubium,* marriage] Occurring after marriage.

postconvulsive (pōst″kŏn-vŭl′sĭv) [″ + *convulsus,* pull violently] Occurring after a convulsion.

postdiastolic (pōst″dī-ăs-tŏl′ĭk) [″ + Gr. *diastole,* expansion] Occurring after the cardiac diastole.

postdicrotic (pōst″dī-krŏt′ĭk) [″ + Gr. *dikrotos,* beating double] Occurring after the dicrotic pulse wave.

p. wave A recoil or second wave (not always present) in a blood pressure tracing.

postdiphtheritic (pōst″dĭf-thĕr-ĭt′ĭk) Following diphtheria.

postencephalitis (pōst″ĕn-sĕf-ă-lī′tĭs) [″ + Gr. *enkephalos,* brain, + *itis,* inflammation] Occurring after encephalitis; an abnormal state remaining after the acute stage of encephalitis has passed.

postepileptic (pōst″ĕp-ĭ-lĕp′tĭk) [″ + Gr. *epi,* upon, + *lepsis,* a seizure] Following an epileptic seizure. SEE: *postictal.*

posterior (pŏs-tē′rē-or) [L. *posterus,* behind] **1.** Toward the rear or caudal end; opposite of anterior. **2.** In humans, toward the back; dorsal. **3.** Situated behind; coming after.

posterior pituitary injection A standard preparation of the polypeptide hormones obtained from the posterior lobe of the pituitary body of healthy domestic animals.

postero- (pŏs′tĕr-ō) [L.] Prefix indicating *posterior, situated behind, toward the back.*

posteroanterior (pŏs″tĕr-ō-ăn-tĕr′ē-or) [L. *posterus,* behind, + *anterior,* anterior] Indicating the flow or movement from back to front.

posteroexternal (pŏs″tĕr-ō-ĕks-tĕr′năl) [″ + *externus,* outer] Toward the back and outer side.

posteroinferior (pŏs″tĕr-ō-ĭn-fĕr′ē-or) [″ + *inferus,* below] Located behind and below a part.

posterointernal [″ + *internus,* inner] Toward the back and inner side.

posterolateral [″ + *lateralis,* side] Located behind and at the side of a part.

posteromedial (pŏs″tĕr-ō-mē′dē-ăl) [″ + *medius,* middle] Toward the back and toward the median plane.

posteromedian Situated posteriorly and in the median plane.

posteroparietal (pŏs″tĕr-ō-pă-rī′ĕ-tăl) [″ + *paries,* a wall] Located at the back of the parietal bone.

posterosuperior (pŏs″tĕr-ō-sū-pē′rē-or) [″ + *superior,* upper] Located behind and above a part.

posterotemporal (pŏs″tĕr-ō-tĕm′pō-răl) [″ + *temporalis,* temporal] Located at the back of the temporal bone.

posteruption Referring to the stage of tooth eruption in which the tooth has reached the occlusal plane and is functional, but continues to erupt to compensate for loss of tooth substance because of wear. SEE: *eruption; preeruption.*

postesophageal (pōst″ē-sŏf″ă-jē′ăl) [L. *post,* behind, after, + Gr. *oisophagos,* gullet] Located behind the esophagus.

postethmoid (pōst-ĕth′moyd) [″ + Gr. *ethmos,* sieve, + *eidos,* form, shape] Located behind the ethmoid bone.

postfebrile (pōst-fē′brĭl) [″ + *febris,* fever] Occurring after a fever.

postganglionic (pōst″găn-glē-ŏn′ĭk) [″ + Gr. *ganglion,* knot] Situated posterior or distal to a ganglion.

postgraduate year one ABBR: PGY-1. The first year of graduate training after completion of the formal 4 yr of medical school. Previously, this year was known as the internship year. Similarly, PGY-2 and PGY-3 are the abbreviations for postgraduate year two and three.

posthemiplegic (pōst″hĕm-ĭ-plē′jĭk) [″ + Gr. *hemi,* half, + *plege,* a stroke] Occurring after hemiplegia.

posthemorrhagic (pōst-hĕm″ō-răj′ĭk) [″ + Gr. *haima,* blood, + *rhegnynai,* to burst forth] Occurring after hemorrhage.

posthepatic Originating after bile leaves the liver, as in posthepatic jaundice, in which obstruction of bile ducts causes the jaundice.

posthepatitic (pōst″hĕp-ă-tĭt′ĭk) [″ + Gr. *hepar,* liver, + *itis,* inflammation] Occurring after hepatitis.

posthioplasty (pŏs′thē-ō-plăs″tē) [″ + *plastos,* formed] Plastic surgery of the prepuce or foreskin.

posthitis (pŏs-thī′tĭs) [″ + *itis,* inflammation] Inflammation of the foreskin. SYN: *acroposthitis.*

posthumous (pŏs′tū-mŭs) [L. *postumus,* last] **1.** Occurring after death. **2.** Born after the death of the father. **3.** Said of a child taken by cesarean section after the death of the mother.

posthypnotic (pōst″hĭp-nŏt′ĭk) [L. *post,* behind, after, + Gr. *hypnos,* sleep] Occurring or performed subsequent to the hypnotic state.

p. suggestion A suggestion given during the hypnotic state influencing a later action when an individual is awake and alert.

posthypoxia syndrome One of several syndromes occurring after an individual has experienced severe hypoxia including persistent coma or stupor, dementia, visual agnosia, parkinsonism, choreoathetosis, cerebral ataxia, inattention or action myoclonus, and amnesic state. SEE: *hypoxia.*

postictal (pōst-ĭk′tăl) [″ + *ictus,* a blow or stroke] Occurring after a sudden attack or stroke, as an epileptic seizure or apoplexy.

p. confusion Confusion that follows a seizure. It usually resolves in an hour unless complicated by head injury, hypoxia, or status epilepticus. SEE: *epilepsy.*

posticteric (pōst″ĭk-tĕr′ĭk) [″ + Gr. *ikteros,* jaundice] Occurring after jaundice.

postmalarial (pōst″mă-lā′rē-ăl) [″ + It. *malaria,* bad air] Occurring after malaria.

postmature (pōst″mă-tūr′) [″ + *maturus,* ripe] Pert. to an infant born after an estimated 42 weeks' gestation, who exhibits findings consistent with postmaturity syndrome.

postmaturity SEE: *syndrome, postmaturity.*

postmediastinal (pōst″mē-dē-ăs′tĭ-năl) [″ + *mediastinum,* in the middle] Behind the mediastinum.

postmenopausal (pōst″mĕn-ō-paw′zăl) [″ + Gr. *men,* month, + *pausis,* cessation] Occurring after permanent cessation of menstruation.

postmortem [L.] **1.** Occurring or performed after death. **2.** Autopsy.

postmyocardial infarction syndrome Pericardial chest pain occurring as a result of myocardial infarction. The pain is aggravated by deep breathing, swallowing, and change in body position. Fever and a pericardial friction rub are usually present. The white blood cell count and sedimentation rate may be elevated. SYN: *Dressler's syndrome.*

ETIOLOGY: The cause is unknown but thought to be due to an autoimmune response.

TREATMENT: This syndrome usually responds to salicylates or other anti-inflammatory drugs.

postnasal (pōst-nā′zăl) [L. *post,* behind, after, + *nasus,* nose] Located behind the nose.

postnatal [″ + *natus,* birth] Occurring after birth.

postnecrotic (pōst″nĕ-krŏt′ĭk) [″ + Gr. *nekros,* corpse] Occurring after the death of a tissue or a part.

postneuritic (pōst″nū-rĭt′ĭk) [″ + Gr. *neuron,* nerve, + *itis,* inflammation] Occurring after neuritis.

postocular (pōst-ŏk′ū-lar) [″ + *oculus,* eye] Behind the eye.

postocular neuritis Inflammation of the optic nerve behind the retina.

postolivary (pōst-ŏl′ĭ-vā-rē) [″ + *oliva,* olive] Behind the olivary body; the back of the anterior pyramid of the medulla.

postoperculum (pōst-ō-pŭr′kū-lŭm) [″ + *operculum,* a covering] The fold covering the insula that is formed of part of the superior temporal gyrus of the brain.

postoral (pōst-or'ăl) [" + *os,* mouth] Behind, or in the posterior part of, the mouth.

postorbital (pōst-or'bĭ-tăl) [" + *orbita,* track] Behind the orbit of the eye.

postpalatine (pōst-păl'ă-tĭn) [" + *palatum,* palate] Behind the palate.

postpallium (pōst-păl'ē-ŭm) [" + *pallium,* cloak] That part of the cerebral cortex behind the fissure of Rolando.

postpaludal (pōst-păl'ū-dăl) [" + *palus,* swamp] Occurring after a malarial attack.

postparalytic (pōst"păr-ă-lĭt'ĭk) [" + *para,* beside, + *lyein,* to loosen] Subsequent to an attack of paralysis.

postpartal period, postpartum period Pert. to the 6-week period after childbirth, during which progressive physiological changes restore uterine size and system functions to nonpregnant status. SEE: *Nursing Diagnoses Appendix.*

postpartum (pōst-păr'tŭm) [L. *post,* after, + *partus,* birth] Occurring after childbirth.

p. blues A colloquial term for postpartum depression.

p. pituitary necrosis Sheehan's syndrome.

postpharyngeal (pōst-fă-rĭn'jē-ăl) [L. *post,* after, + Gr. *pharynx,* throat] Behind the pharynx.

postpneumonic (pōst"nū-mŏn'ĭk) [" + Gr. *pneumon,* lung] Occurring after pneumonia.

postpoliomyelitis muscular atrophy ABBR: PPMA. The development of new neuromuscular symptoms, including muscle weakness, many years after recovery from acute paralytic poliomyelitis. This may occur in muscles that were previously affected by polio and recovered or in muscles that were clinically unaffected by the acute disease. There is no treatment for this slowly progressing atrophy, but the unaffected muscles remain strong. SEE: *poliomyelitis, acute anterior.*

postpolio syndrome A variety of musculoskeletal symptoms and muscular atrophy that create new difficulties with activities of daily living 25 to 30 years after the original attack of acute paralytic poliomyelitis.

postpontile (pōst-pŏn'tĭl) [" + *pons,* bridge] Situated behind the pons varolii.

postprandial (pōst-prăn'dē-ăl) Following a meal.

p. dumping syndrome Dumping syndrome.

postpuberty (pōst-pū'bĕr-tē) [" + *pubertas,* puberty] The period after puberty. **postpubertal** (-tăl), *adj.*

postpubescent (pōst"pū-bĕs'ĕnt) [" + *pubescens,* becoming hairy] Following puberty.

postpyramidal (pōst-pĭ-răm'ĭd-ăl) Behind a pyramidal tract.

postradiation (pōst"rā-dē-ā'shŭn) Occurring after exposure to ionizing radiation.

postsacral (pōst-sā'krăl) [" + *sacrum,* sacred] Below the sacrum.

postscapular (pōst-skăp'ū-lăr) [" + *scapula,* shoulder blade] Below or behind the scapula.

postscarlatinal (pōst"skăr-lă-tī'năl) [" + *scarlatina,* scarlet fever] Following scarlet fever.

postsphygmic (pōst-sfĭg'mĭk) [" + Gr. *sphygmos,* pulse] Following the pulse wave.

postsplenic (pōst-splĕn'ĭk) [" + Gr. *splen,* spleen] Behind the spleen.

poststenotic (pōst"stĕ-nŏt'ĭk) [" + Gr. *stenosis,* act of narrowing] Distal to a stenosed or constricted area, esp. of an artery.

postsynaptic (pōst"sĭ-năp'tĭk) [" + Gr. *synapsis,* point of contact] Located distal to a synapse.

post-tarsal (pōst-tăr'săl) [" + Gr. *tarsos,* a broad, flat surface] Behind the tarsus.

post-term pregnancy Pregnancy continuing beyond the beginning of the 42nd week (294 days) of gestation, as counted from the first day of the last normal menstrual period. This occurs in an estimated 3% to 12% of pregnancies. Complications include oligohydramnios, meconium passage, macrosomatia, and dysmaturity, all of which may lead to poor pregnancy outcome. The fetus should be delivered if any sign of fetal distress is detected. SEE: *syndrome, postmaturity.*

post-tibial (pōst-tĭb'ē-ăl) [" + *tibia,* shinbone] Behind the tibia.

post-transfusion syndrome A condition consisting of fever, splenomegaly, atypical lymphocytes, abnormal liver function tests, and occasionally a skin rash that develops following blood transfusion or perfusion of an organ during surgery. The syndrome appears 3 to 5 weeks after transfusion or perfusion with fresh (less than 24 hr old) blood, usually in large quantities. The causative agent is thought to be cytomegalovirus.

post-traumatic (pōst"traw-măt'ĭk) [" + Gr. *traumatikos,* traumatic] Following an injury or traumatic event.

post-traumatic stress disorder ABBR: PTSD. Intense psychological distress, marked by horrifying memories, recurring fears, and feelings of helplessness that develop after a psychologically traumatic event, such as the experience of combat, criminal assault, life-threatening accidents, natural disasters, or rape. The symptoms of PTSD may include re-experiencing the traumatic event (a phenomenon called "flashback"); avoiding stimuli associated with the trauma; memory disturbances; psychological or social withdrawal; or increased aggressiveness, irritability, insomnia, startle responses, and vigilance. The symptoms may last for years after the event, but often can be managed with supportive psychotherapy or medications such as antidepressants.

postulate (pŏs′tū-lāt) [L. *postulare,* to request] A supposition or view, usually self-evident, that is assumed without proof. SEE: *Koch's law.*

postural (pŏs′tū-răl) [L. *postura,* position] Pert. to or affected by posture.

postural drainage A passive airway clearance technique in which patients are positioned so that gravity will assist the removal of secretions from specific lobes of the lung, bronchi, or lung cavities. It can be used for patients with pneumonias, chronic bronchitis, cystic fibrosis, bronchiectasis, inhaled foreign bodies, before operation for lobectomy, or in any patient having difficulty with retained secretions. A side effect of the treatment in some patients is gastroesophageal reflux. SEE: illus.

PATIENT CARE: Physical tolerance to the procedure is evaluated. The respiratory therapist teaches and assists the patient in the procedure, as ordered, by positioning the patient for effective drainage of the affected lung region(s). The patient is encouraged to remove secretions with an effective cough. To decrease the risk of aspiration, the patient should not perform the procedure after meals. Percussion is often done at the same time to assist movement of retained secretions in the lung.

postural hypotension Orthostatic hypotension.

posture (pŏs′tŭr) [L. *postura*] Attitude or position of the body.

coiled p. Posture in which the body is on one side with legs drawn up to meet the trunk. It is used sometimes during lumbar punctures.

dorsal rigid p. Posture in which the patient lies on the back with both legs drawn up. This is a position that is maintained by some patients suffering the pain of peritonitis.

kyphosis-lordosis p. A stance in which the pelvis is tilted forward, causing hip flexion, increased lumbar lordosis, and thoracic kyphosis.

modified plantigrade p. A standing position with the lower extremities on the ground and the upper extremities bearing weight on a table or other surface. The body weight is stabilized on all four extremities. This posture is used developmentally and in physical therapy to prepare for independent standing and gait.

orthopnea p. Posture in which the patient sits upright, hands or elbows resting upon some support; seen in asthma, emphysema, dyspnea, ascites, effusions into the pleural and pericardial cavities, congestive heart failure.

orthotonos p. Posture in which the neck and trunk are extended rigidly in a straight line; seen in tetanus, strychnine poisoning, rabies, and meningitis.

prone p. Prone.

semireclining p. Posture used instead of lying supine, by patients who are short of breath, e.g., because of heart failure.

standard p. The skeletal alignment accepted as normal; used for evaluating posture. There is equilibrium around the line of gravity and the least amount of stress and strain on supporting muscles, joints, and ligaments. From either the front or the back, a plumb bob would bisect the body equally. From the side, a plumb bob would be anterior to the lateral malleolus and the axis of the knee, posterior to the axis of the hip and the apex of the coronal suture, and through the bodies of the lumbar vertebrae, the tip of the shoulder, the bodies of the cervical vertebrae, and the external auditory meatus.

swayback p. A relaxed stance in which the pelvis is shifted forward, resulting in hip extension, and the thorax is shifted backward, resulting in an increased thoracic kyphosis and forward head. Also called *slouched posture.*

postuterine (pōst-ū′tĕr-ĭn) [L. *post,* behind, after, + *uterus,* womb] Referring to the anatomical area behind the uterus. SEE: *retrouterine.*

postvaccinal (pōst-văk′sĭ-năl) [″ + *vaccinus,* pert. to cows] Following vaccination; used esp. with reference to safety issues or immune responses that result from immunization.

postviral fatigue syndrome Chronic disability following a presumed viral infection. The most characteristic and persistent feature of the disease is muscle fatigability unrelieved by rest. Other symptoms and signs include low-grade fever, headache, blurred vision or diplopia, stiff neck, vertigo, nausea and vomiting, lymphadenopathy, emotional lability, insomnia, urinary frequency, and either deafness or hyperacusis. In addition, psychological disturbances are usually present. These include mild depression, anxiety, or severe behavioral abnormalities. There is no effective treatment, but the usual course is slow recovery. SYN: *Royal Free disease.*

post-void residual Residual urine.

potable (pō′tă-bl) [LL. *potabilis*] Suitable for drinking, esp. pert. to water free of harmful organic or inorganic ingredients.

Potain's apparatus (pō-tānz′) [Pierre C. E. Potain, Fr. physician, 1825–1901] A form of aspirator.

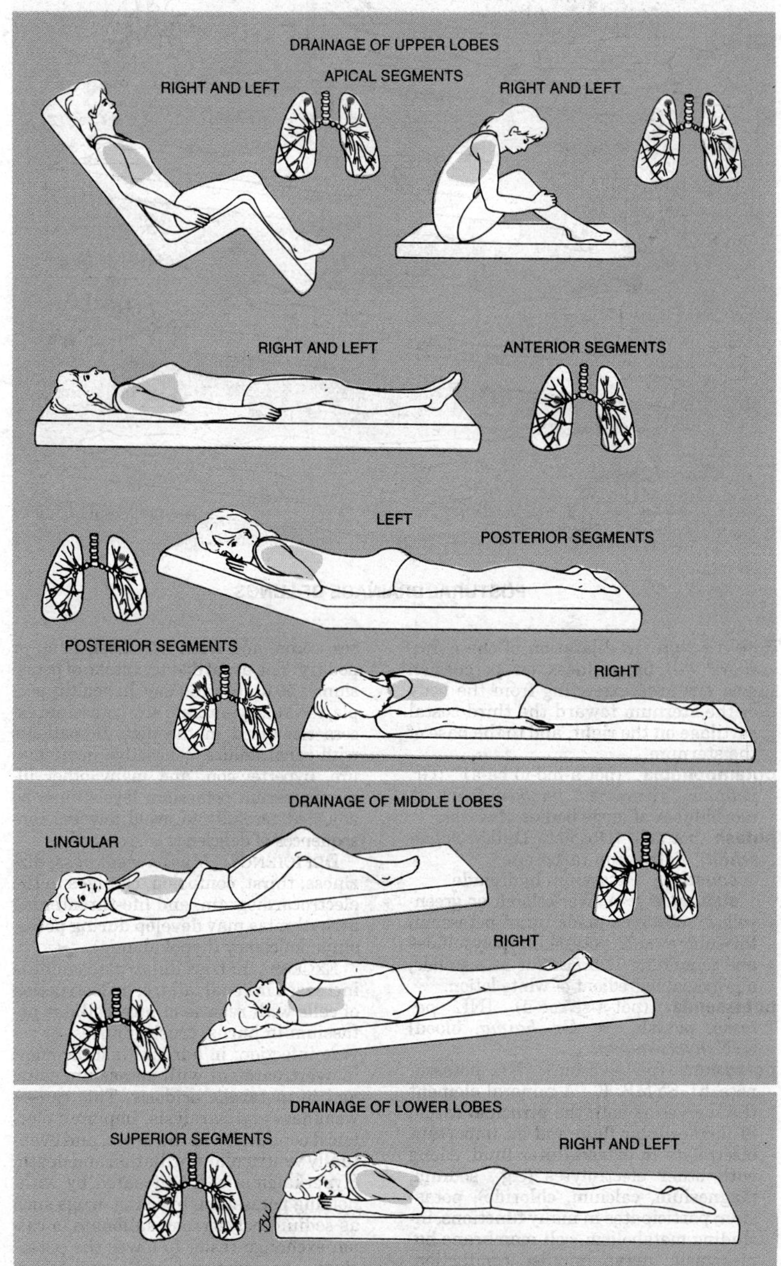

POSTURAL DRAINAGE OF LUNGS (CONTINUED)

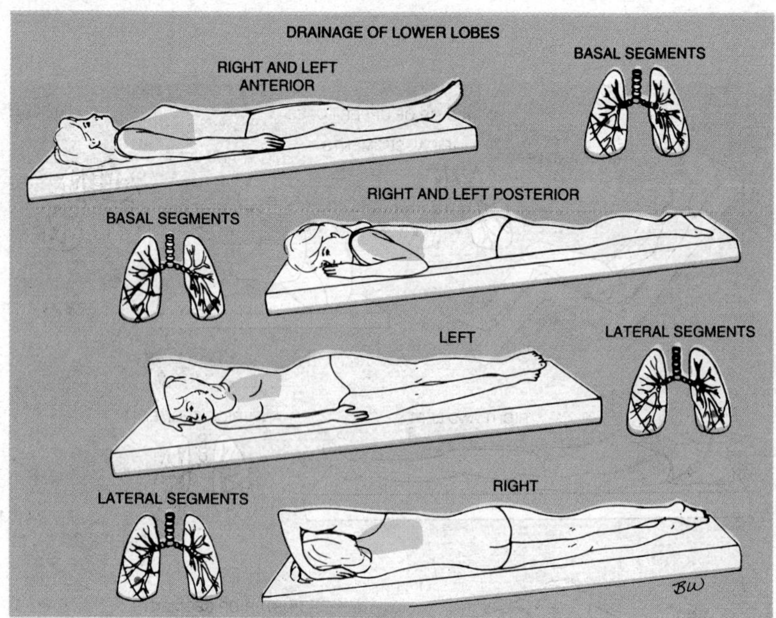

POSTURAL DRAINAGE OF LUNGS

Potain's sign In dilatation of the aorta, there will be dullness on percussion over the area extending from the body of the sternum toward the third costal cartilage on the right, and to the base of the sternum.

potamophobia (pŏt″ă-mō-fō′bē-ă) [Gr. *potamos,* river, + *phobos,* fear] A morbid fear of large bodies of water.

potash (pŏt′ăsh) [Obsolete Dutch, *potasschan*] Potassium carbonate.

caustic p. Potassium hydroxide.

sulfurated p. A liver-colored or green-yellow substance made up of potassium thiosulfate and potassium polysulfides and containing 12.8% sulfur as a sulfide; a principal ingredient of white lotion.

potassemia (pŏt-ă-sē′mē-ă) [NL. *potassa,* potash, + Gr. *haima,* blood] SYN: *hyperkalemia.*

potassium (pō-tăs′ē-ŭm) [NL. *potassa,* potash] SYMB: K. A mineral element that serves as both the principal cation in intracellular fluid and an important electrolyte in extracellular fluid. Along with other electrolytes (e.g., sodium, magnesium, calcium, chloride), potassium participates in many functions, including metabolism, cell membrane homeostasis, nerve impulse conduction, and muscle contraction.

Potassium, which constitutes 0.35% of body weight, is found in most foods, including cereals, dried peas and beans, fresh vegetables, fresh or dried fruits, fruit juices, sunflower seeds, nuts, molasses, cocoa, and fresh fish, beef, ham, or poultry. The usual dietary intake of potassium is 50 to 150 mEq/day. In healthy people, the kidneys excrete any potassium excess consumed in the diet. In patients with renal failure, congestive heart failure, hypertension, and many other illnesses, serum potassium levels must be adjusted carefully to avoid adverse consequences of deficiency or excess.

DEFICIENCY: Muscle weakness, dizziness, thirst, confusion, changes in the electrocardiogram, and life-threatening arrhythmias may develop during potassium deficiency (hypokalemia).

EXCESS: Extracellular potassium is increased in renal failure; in destruction of cells with release of intracellular potassium in burns, crush injuries, or severe infection; in adrenal insufficiency; in overtreatment with potassium salts; and in metabolic acidosis. This causes weakness and paralysis, impaired electrical conduction in the heart, and eventually ventricular fibrillation and death. Hyperkalemia can be treated by withholding potassium, by using drugs such as sodium polystyrene sulfonate, a cation exchange resin, to lower the potassium concentration in cells, and by using calcium gluconate to counteract the effects on the heart.

CAUTION: Rapid infusion of potassium is painful and may cause severe hyperkalemia, complicated by cardiac arrhythmias. Institutional protocols for the use of intravenous potassium should be followed carefully.

---

p. alum Aluminum potassium sulfate; strongly astringent, used topically as a styptic. SEE: *alum*.

p. aminosalicylate Para-aminosalicylic acid.

p. arsenite solution An arsenical solution containing 0.95 to 1.5 g of arsenic trioxide for each 100 ml of solution.

p. bicarbonate $KHCO_3$; white crystals or powder used to neutralize acid of the stomach and to treat acid-base imbalance.

p. carbonate K_2CO_3; a white crystalline powder used in pharmaceutical and chemical preparations. SYN: *potash*.

p. chloride A white crystalline salt, KCl, that is soluble in water; one of the three chlorides used in preparation of Ringer's solution. It is used in the treatment of potassium deficiencies (hypokalemia).

p. chromate K_2CrO_4; lemon-yellow crystals used as a dye and furniture stain, in manufacture of batteries, in photography, and in laboratories to preserve tissue.

p. citrate $C_6H_5K_3O_7 \cdot H_2O$; transparent prismatic crystals used as an alkalizer.

p. cyanide KCN; a highly poisonous compound used as a fumigant.

dibasic p. phosphate K_2HPO_4; a drug used to treat calcium imbalance.

p. gluconate $C_6H_{11}KO_7$; a drug used orally to replenish loss of potassium ion.

p. guaiacolsulfonate An expectorant.

p. hydroxide KOH; a gray-white compound used in the preparation of soap and as a chemical reagent. SYN: *caustic potash*.

p. iodide KI; colorless or white crystals having a faint odor of iodine, used as an expectorant. This form of potassium is recommended for use following exposure to radioactive iodides downwind from a nuclear reactor accident. The rationale is that it blocks the uptake of radioactive iodides by the thyroid gland, thus preventing or decreasing the chance of developing cancer of the thyroid many years later.

p. permanganate $KMnO_4$; crystals of dark purple prisms that are sweet and odorless. It is used as a topical astringent and antiseptic, as an oxidizing agent, and as an antidote in phosphorus poisoning. Concentrated solutions irritate and even corrode the skin and, when swallowed, induce gastroenteritis. The solutions have considerable power as disinfectants because their oxidizing ability destroys bacteria. They fail to penetrate deeply in an active form, which renders them of less value than many other disinfectants, except for use in very superficial infections.

p. sodium tartrate $C_4H_4KNaO_6 \cdot 4H_2O$; a saline cathartic.

p. tartrate $C_4H_4K_2O_6$; a medicine used as a cathartic.

potassium chlorate poisoning Poisoning by potassium chlorate, large doses of which cause abdominal discomfort, vomiting, diarrhea, hematuria with nephritis, and disturbances of the blood. Gastric lavage should be used to empty the stomach. Other treatment is symptomatic.

CAUTION: Vomiting should not be induced.

---

potassium chromate poisoning Poisoning by potassium chromate, possibly contracted by inhalation or from touching the nose with contaminated fingers, causing deep indolent ulcers.

SYMPTOMS: When taken by mouth potassium chromate has a disagreeable taste; causes cramping, pain, vomiting, diarrhea, slow respiration; and may affect the liver and kidneys.

CAUTION: Vomiting should not be induced.

PATIENT CARE: For ingestion, the patient is treated as if poisoned with a strong acid. Gastric lavage is administered through a nasogastric tube. Bronchoalveolar lavage or penicillamine may be used.

potassium hydroxide poisoning Poisoning by potassium hydroxide, characterized by nausea, soapy taste, and burning pain in the mouth; bloody, slimy vomitus; abdominal cramping; bloody purging and prostration.

CAUTION: Vomiting should not be induced.

PATIENT CARE: The patient requires hospitalization, morphine for pain, and most probably treatment for shock. If the patient's airway has been burned, tracheostomy may be required. Corticosterioids and antibiotics may be given.

potbelly Slang term for the selective deposition of adipose tissue in the abdominal subcutaneous tissue. This condition usually occurs in middle-aged persons who have sedentary occupations. It is accentuated by weakening of the anterior abdominal musculature and lumbar lordosis. Weight reduction, exercises to strengthen the abdominal muscles, and therapy for lordosis are the treatment for this condition.

potency (pō′tĕn-sē) [L. *potentia,* power] **1.** Strength; force; power. **2.** Strength of a medicine. **3.** The ability of a man to perform coitus.

potent (pō′tĕnt) [L. *potens,* powerful] **1.** Powerful. **2.** Highly effective medicinally. **3.** Having the power of procreation.

potentia coeundi (pō-tĕn′shē-ă kō-ē-ŭn′dī) [L.] The ability to perform sexual intercourse in a normal manner.

potential 1. Latent; existing in possibility. **2.** In electricity, voltage or electrical pressure; a condition in which a state of tension or pressure, capable of doing work, exists. When two electrically charged bodies of different potentials are brought together, an electric current passes from the body of high potential to that of low.

action p. ABBR: A.P. The change in electrical potential of nerve or muscle fiber when it is stimulated; depolarization followed by repolarization.

after p. The period occurring subsequent to the spike potential.

demarcation p. The difference in potential between an intact longitudinal surface and the injured end of a muscle or nerve. SYN: *injury p.*

injury p. Demarcation p.

late p. Deflections found on signal-averaged electrocardiograms that follow the QRS complex, and point to an increased likelihood of ventricular dysrhythmias. These deflections represent delays in electrical conduction through the ventricles.

liquid junction p. The potential voltage developed in an electrode measurement system at the point where two solutions are in contact. Most often the solutions are the test solution and a liquid bridging solution such as saturated KCl, although any liquid-liquid interface may be involved. An example is the pH reference electrode.

membrane p. The electrical charge or potential difference between the inside and outside of a cell membrane.

resting p. Polarization (3).

spike p. A change in potential that occurs when a cell membrane is stimulated.

potentiate (pō-tĕn′shē-āt) To increase the potency or action.

potentiation (pō-tĕn″shē-ā′shŭn) The synergistic action of two substances, such as hormones or drugs, in which the total effects are greater than the sum of the independent effects of the two substances.

potentiometer (pō-tĕn″shē-ŏm′ĕ-tĕr) A voltmeter.

calibration p. A mechanically adjusted resistance used as a calibration control on many instruments. It adjusts a voltage or current within the device.

potion (pō′shŭn) [L. *potio,* draft] A drink or draft; a dose of poison or liquid medicine.

Pott, Sir Percivall British surgeon, 1714–1788. He pioneered research into chemical carcinogenesis by describing scrotal cancer in chimney sweeps.

Pott's disease Infection of the vertebrae of the spine caused by miliary (disseminated) tuberculosis. About 1% to 3% of patients with tuberculosis have infections in the bone; the spine is the most common site. Organisms spread from the site of primary infection through the blood. Once established in the spine, the infection moves through the intervertebral disks to multiple vertebrae. When it extends into the surrounding soft tissue, abscesses may be created. SYN: *tuberculous spondylitis*. SEE: *kyphosis*.

SYMPTOMS: Patients report pain when they move their back. Signs include a low-grade fever, weight loss, and local tenderness. When several upper vertebrae are involved, compression fractures, curvature of the spine (kyphosis), or nerve injury may occur.

TREATMENT: See Treatment section under tuberculosis.

Pott's fracture Fracture of the lower end of the fibula and medial malleolus of the tibia, with dislocation of the foot outward and backward. After reduction, foot and leg are put in a cast in which a walking iron is incorporated. The patient is able to walk, and the cast is removed in about 6 weeks.

pouch (powch) [ME. *pouche*] Any pocket or sac.

branchial p. Pharyngeal p.

Broca's p. A sac in the tissues of the labia majora.

p. of Douglas Rectouterine p.

Heidenhain p. A small, surgically constructed pouch of the stomach that is denervated and separated from the stomach and drained to the outside of the body. It is used to study the physiology of the stomach.

laryngeal p. A blind pouch of mucosa entering the ventral portion of the ventricle of the larynx.

Pavlov p. A stomach pouch formed surgically for the experimental study of gastric secretion. A section of the stomach is separated from the main stomach except for the vagus nerves. This pouch is named after I. P. Pavlov, who devised it to investigate gastric function and conditioned reflexes.

pharyngeal p. One of a series of five pairs of entodermal outpocketings that develop in lateral walls of the pharynx of the embryo. SYN: *branchial p.*

Prussak's p. The anterior recess of the tympanic membrane.

Rathke's p. An outpocketing of the roof of embryonic stomodeum. It gives rise to the anterior lobe of the hypophysis cerebri.

rectouterine p. The pouch between the anterior rectal wall and the posterior uterine wall. SYN: *p. of Douglas; cul-de-sac.*

rectovesical p. A fold of peritoneum that in men extends downward between the bladder and rectum.

pouchitis Acute or chronic inflammation of the surgically produced pouch used in restorative proctocolectomy.

poudrage (pū-drăzh′) [Fr.] Application of an irritating, but otherwise nontoxic, powder to the pleural space of the lung in order to produce pleural adhesions.

poultice (pōl′tĭs) [L. *pultes,* thick paste] A hot, moist, usually medicated mass that is placed between cloth sheets and applied to the skin to relieve pain, soothe injured tissues, stimulate the circulation, or act as a counterirritant. SEE: *plaster.*

pound (pownd) [L. *pondus,* weight] SYMB: lb. A measure of weight of the avoirdupois and the apothecaries' systems that is equal to 16 oz. SEE: *Weights and Measures Appendix.*

avoirdupois p. Sixteen ounces, equal to 453.59 g.

troy p. Twelve ounces, 5760 gr, equal to 373.242 g.

Poupart's ligament (pū-părz′) [François Poupart, Fr. anatomist, 1661–1708] The ligament forming the lower border of aponeurosis of the external oblique muscle between the anterosuperior spine of the ilium and spine of the pubis. SYN: *inguinal ligament.*

poverty The condition of having an inadequate supply of money, resources, or means of subsistence.

p. of thought The mental state of being devoid of thought and having a feeling of emptiness.

poverty level The relative standard of living of individuals or families who have inadequate funds to afford basic needs, such as shelter, food, clothing, or health care.

povidone (pō′vĭ-dōn) A synthetic polymer used as a dispersing and suspending agent in manufacturing drugs.

povidone-iodine A complex of iodine with povidone. It contains not less than 9% and not more than 12% available iodine. This iodophor is used in dilute concentration as a surgical scrub, in aerosol spray, in vaginal douche solutions, and in ointments and gels.

powder [ME. *poudre*] **1.** An aggregation of fine particles of one or more substances that may be passed through fine meshes. **2.** A dose of such a powder, contained in a paper.

power [ME. *power*] **1.** The rate at which work is done. Power may be calculated by multiplying force times velocity. The metric unit for power is the watt. One watt equals one newton meter per second, or 0.7376 foot pound per second. Sometimes power is measured in horsepower. A horsepower unit equals 745.7 watts or 550 foot pounds per second. **2.** The capacity for action. **3.** In optics, the degree to which a lens or optical instrument magnifies. **4.** In microscopy, the number of times the diameter of an object is magnified, indicated by placing an × after the number (e.g., 10× indicates magnification of 10 times). **5.** In mathematics and in scientific nomenclature, the number of times a value is to be multiplied by itself, the exponent (i.e., $10^2 = 10 \times 10 = 100$; $10^3 = 10 \times 10 \times 10 = 1000$). **6.** In statistics, the probability that a planned investigation will yield a statistically significant result. This is estimated by calculating how many individuals need to be randomly assigned to each group studied and how many would have to demonstrate improvement after receiving therapy in order to be able to conclude that one result meaningfully differs from another.

power of attorney ABBR: POA. A legal document by which a person identifies someone to make financial decisions if he or she is unable to perform this task independently. SEE: *power of attorney, durable, for health care.*

power of attorney, durable, for health care An advance directive that designates another person to make health care decisions regarding how aggressive treatment should be if the patient becomes incompetent or unable to make decisions in the future, for example, in the case of coma or a persistent vegetative state. The document also lists medical treatments that the person would not want to have. Durable power of attorney goes into effect when the document is signed. The Patient Self-Determination Act, enacted in 1991, mandates the responsibility of health care providers to develop written materials concerning advance directives. Also called *health care proxy.* SEE: *advance directive; living will.*

powerlessness Perception that one's own action will not significantly affect an outcome; a perceived lack of control over a current situation or immediate happening. SEE: *Nursing Diagnoses Appendix.*

pox (pŏks) [ME. *pokkes,* pits] **1.** An eruptive, contagious disease. **2.** A papular eruption that becomes pustular. SEE: *chickenpox; smallpox.*

poxvirus (pŏks′vī-rŭs) One of a group of DNA viruses that produce characteristic spreading vesicular lesions, often called pocks. It is the largest of the true viruses and includes viruses responsible for smallpox, vaccinia, molluscum contagiosum, and orf.

p.p. *punctum proximum,* the near point of accommodation (in vision).

ppb *parts per billion.*

P.P.D. *purified protein derivative,* the substance used in an intradermal test for tuberculosis. SEE: *tuberculin skin test.*

PPE *personal protective equipment.*

PPLO *pleuropneumonia-like organisms,* now called mycoplasmas.

ppm *parts per million.*

ppt *parts per trillion; precipitate; prepared.*

Pr **1.** *presbyopia.* **2.** Symbol for the element praseodymium.

p.r. L. *punctum remotum,* the far point of visual accommodation.

practice (prăk'tĭs) [Gr. *praxis,* practice] **1.** The use, by a health care professional, of knowledge and skill to provide a service in the prevention, diagnosis, and treatment of illness and in the maintenance of health. **2.** The continuing and repetitive effort to become proficient and to improve one's skill in the practice of medicine.

scope of p. The extent and limits of the medical interventions that a health care provider may perform.

practice guidelines Consensus statements by professional societies or agents suggesting appropriate diagnostic and therapeutic options for patients with a specified diagnosis.

practitioner (prăk-tĭsh'ŭn-ĕr) One who has met the professional and legal requirements necessary to provide a health care service, such as a physician, nurse, dentist, dental hygientist, or physical therapist.

acute care nurse p. A nurse who is licensed to manage the care of select patient groups that have acute and specialized health care needs. The practice of the acute care nurse practitioner may be within a hospital setting or may extend into other areas of the community.

adult nurse p. ABBR: ANP. A nurse practitioner who is licensed to treat people over 18 years of age.

advanced nurse p. An umbrella term that includes the following health care workers: Certified Midwife, Certified Registered Nurse Anesthetist, Clinical Nurse Specialist, and Nurse Practitioner.

emergency room p. A nurse certified in the area of urgent care, who possesses skills in triage and the knowledge to meet the emergent needs of clients.

family nurse p. ABBR: FNP. A nurse practitioner who is licensed to treat people of any age. SEE: *adult nurse p.*

geriatric nurse p. A certified nurse who practices multilevel health care with elderly people. Duties of the GNP include examining, diagnosing, and managing acute and chronic illnesses. The GNP also may supervise routine foot care clinics, allergy shots, and immunizations for elderly persons.

mid-level p. Mid-level provider.

nurse p. SEE: *nurse practitioner.*

pediatric nurse p. A certified nurse who focuses on the common acute and chronic illnesses experienced by children and adolescents. The pediatric nurse practitioner integrates concepts of growth and development in assessing health care needs.

Practitioners' Reporting Network, USP ABBR: USP-PRN. Three separate programs designed to collect practitioners' experience with unreliable drug products, defective medical devices, drug problems with radiopharmaceuticals, and medication errors. Practitioners and pharmacists report their experience to the United States Pharmacopeia, 12601 Twinbrook Parkway, Rockville, MD 20852. The USP receives the reports and publishes the results. Drug problem reports and medical device and laboratory product problem reports may be made by calling (800) 638-6725; medication errors may be reported by calling (800) 23ERROR.

prae- SEE: *pre-.*

praecox (prē'kŏks) [L.] Early.

praevia, praevius (prē'vē-ă, prē'vē-ŭs) [L.] Going before in time or place.

pragmatagnosia (prăg"măt-ăg-nō'zē-ă) [Gr. *pragma,* object, + *agnosia,* lack of recognition] Inability to recognize once familiar objects.

pragmatamnesia (prăg"măt-ăm-nē'zē-ă) [" + *amnesia,* forgetfulness] The inability to recall the appearance of an object.

visual p. The mental condition making possible pragmatamnesia.

pragmatism (prăg'mă-tĭzm) [Gr. *pragma,* a thing done, + *-ismos,* condition] The belief that the practical application of a principle should be the determining factor. **pragmatic** (prăg-măt'ĭk), *adj.*

pragmatist (prăg'mă-tĭst) A person whose goals are achieved or attempted from a practical concept, action, or approach; a practical person.

pralidoxime chloride (prăl"ĭ-dŏks'ēm) A cholinesterase reactivator used in treating poisoning due to certain pesticides or drugs with anticholinesterase activity.

pramoxine hydrochloride (prăm-ŏk'sēn) A topical anesthetic. It should not be used on mucous membranes.

prandial (prăn'dē-ăl) [L. *prandium,* breakfast] Relating to a meal.

praseodymium (prā"sē-ō-dĭm'ē-ŭm) [Gr. *prasios,* leek-green, + *didymium*] SYMB: Pr. A metallic element in the rare earth series; atomic weight 140.907; atomic number 59.

Prausnitz-Küstner reaction (prows'nĭts-kĭst'nĕr) [Carl Willi Prausnitz, Ger.

bacteriologist, b. 1876; Heinz Küstner, Ger. gynecologist, b. 1897] The intracutaneous injection of a hypersensitive patient's serum into a nonallergic person followed, 24 to 48 hr later, by the application of the suspected antigen to the injection site. If a wheal and flare occur, there is evidence that the suspected antigen is causing the hypersensitivity. Because of the danger of transmitting viral hepatitis and AIDS, this test is no longer used.

praxinoscope (prăk-sĭn′ō-skōp) [Gr. *praxis,* action, + *skopein,* to examine] A device for studying the larynx.

praxiology (prăk″sē-ŏl′ō-jē) [″ + *logos,* word, reason] The study of behavior.

praxis (prăk′sĭs) [Gr., action] The ability to plan and execute coordinated movement.

-praxis [Gr., action] Combining form indicating *act, activity, practice, use.*

Prayer of Maimonides [Rabbi Moses ben Maimon, Jewish philosopher and physician in Egypt, 1135–1204] A prayer used at graduation ceremonies by some medical schools. SEE: *Declaration of Geneva; Declaration of Hawaii; Hippocratic Oath; Nightingale Pledge.*

"Thy eternal providence has appointed me to watch over the life and health of Thy creatures. May the love for my art actuate me at all times; may neither avarice nor miserliness, nor thirst for glory, or for a great reputation engage my mind; for the enemies of truth and philanthropy could easily deceive me and make me forgetful of my lofty aim of doing good to Thy children.

"May I never see in the patient anything but a fellow creature in pain.

"Grant me strength, time, opportunity always to correct what I have acquired, always to extend its domain; for knowledge is immense and the spirit of man can extend indefinitely to enrich itself daily with new requirements.

"Today he can discover his errors of yesterday and tomorrow he can obtain a new light on what he thinks himself sure of today. Oh, God, Thou has appointed me to watch over the life and death of Thy creatures; here am I ready for my vocation and now I turn unto my calling."

praziquantel A broad-spectrum drug that is useful in treating infections with helminths such as *Schistosoma* species, *Hymenolepis nana,* and *Taenia saginata.* It is also effective in treating infections with *Diphyllobothrium latum.*

prazosin hydrochloride A drug used in treating hypertension. It acts as an alpha-adrenergic receptor blocker.

pre- [L. *prae,* before] Prefix indicating *before, in front of.* SEE: *anti-; pro-.*

preadmission certification Authorization granted to the patient for hospital admission, after a review of the patient's proposed need for inpatient services. In some settings, if predetermined criteria are not met, then the admission is not allowed.

preagonal (prē-ăg′ō-năl) [L. *prae,* before, in front of, + Gr. *agonia,* agony] Pert. to the condition immediately before death.

preanal (prē-ā′năl) [″ + *anus,* anus] In front of the anus.

preanesthesia (prē″ăn-ĕs-thē′zē-ă) A light anesthesia produced by a medication given before the anesthesia.

preanesthetic (prē″ăn-ĕs-thĕt′ĭk) [″ + Gr. *anaisthesia,* lack of sensation] A preliminary drug given to facilitate induction of general anesthesia.

preaortic (prē″ā-or′tĭk) [″ + Gr. *aorte,* aorta] Located in front of the aorta.

preataxic (prē-ă-tăk′sĭk) [″ + Gr. *ataxia,* lack of order] Before the onset of ataxia.

preauricular (prē″aw-rĭk′ū-lăr) [″ + *auricula,* little ear] Located in front of the ear.

preaxial (prē-ăk′sē-ăl) [″ + Gr. *axon,* axis] In front of the axis of a limb or of the body.

precancer (prē′kăn-sĕr) [″ + *cancer,* crab] A condition that tends to become malignant.

precancerous (prē-kăn′sĕr-ŭs) [″ + *cancer,* crab] Said of a growth that is not yet, but probably will become, cancerous.

precapillary [″ + *capillaris,* hairlike] Before or at the beginning of a capillary network, such as a precapillary sphincter.

precaution An action taken in advance to protect against danger, harm, or possible failure.

precautionary principle, principle of precaution A risk management principle, originally developed in the environmental movement, based on the concept of avoiding any new action (e.g., introducing a new technology or a new drug) that carries a hypothetical risk for human or planetary health, regardless of whether the hypothesis has been subjected to formal testing.

precautions, blood and body fluid Universal precautions. SEE: *Standard and Universal Precautions Appendix.*

precautions, standard Guidelines recommended by the Centers for Disease Control and Prevention to reduce the risk of the spread of infection in hospitals. These precautions (e.g., handwashing and wearing personal protective equipment such as gloves, mask, eye protection, gown) apply to blood, all body fluids, secretions, excretions (except sweat), nonintact skin, and mucous membranes of all patients and are the primary strategy for successful nosocomial infection control. SEE: *Standard and Universal Precautions Appendix.*

precautions, universal SEE: under *universal*; *Standard and Universal Precautions Appendix.*

precava (prē-kā'vă) [" + *cavus,* hollow] The descending or superior vena cava. SEE: *vena cava superior.*

precedent In law, an action, ruling, or verdict that may be used as an example to be followed in the future.

precentral (prē-sĕn'trăl) [" + Gr. *kentron,* center] In front of a center, as the central fissure of the brain.

precentral convolution The ascending frontal convolution of the brain.

prechordal (prē-kor'dăl) [" + Gr. *chorde,* cord] In front of the notochord.

precipitable (prē-sĭp'ĭ-tă-b'l) Capable of being precipitated.

precipitant (prē-sĭp'ĭ-tănt) [L. *praecipitare,* to cast down] A substance bringing about precipitation.

precipitate (prē-sĭp'ĭ-tāt) **1.** A deposit separated from a suspension or solution by precipitation, the reaction of a reagent that causes the deposit to fall to the bottom or float near the top. **2.** To separate as a precipitate. **3.** Occurring suddenly or unexpectedly.

precipitation (prē-sĭp"ĭ-tā'shŭn) [L. *praecipitatio*] **1.** The process of a substance being separated from a solution by the action of a reagent so that a precipitate forms. **2.** The sudden and unprepared-for delivery of an infant. SEE: *precipitous delivery.*

precipitation test A test in which a positive reaction is indicated by formation of a precipitate in the solution being tested.

precipitin (prē-sĭp'ĭ-tĭn) An antibody formed in the blood serum of an animal owing to the presence of a soluble antigen, usually a protein. When added to a solution of the antigen, it brings about precipitation. The injected protein is called the antigen, and the antibody produced is the precipitin. It was originally thought that these antibodies were members of a unique class, but most antibodies are capable of precipitating when combined with their antigens. SEE: *autoprecipitin; precipitinogen.*

precipitinogen (prē-sĭp"ĭ-tĭn'ō-jĕn) Any protein that, acting as an antigen, stimulates the production of a specific precipitin.

precipitinoid (prĕ-sĭp'ĭt-ĭn-oyd) A precipitin that can no longer cause precipitation when mixed with its antigen but that retains its affinity to the antigen.

precipitin test A laboratory test in which an insoluble precipitate forms when relatively equal concentrations of soluble antigen and soluble antibody, each with multiple binding sites for each other, are mixed. The results depend on the strength of the attraction between the Fab fragment on the antibody and the corresponding epitope on the antigen (affinity) and on the stability of the complex (antibody avidity). The test demonstrates how immune complexes form in the circulation and are deposited in blood vessel walls. SEE: *precipitation test.*

precipitophore (prē-sĭp'ĭt-ō-for") The part of a precipitin that produces the actual precipitation.

precipitum (prē-sĭp'ĭ-tŭm) The precipitate produced by action of a precipitin.

preclinical (prē-klĭn'ĭ-kăl) [L. *prae,* before, in front of, + Gr. *klinike,* medical treatment in bed] **1.** Occurring before diagnosis of a definite disease is possible. **2.** Classroom training and education that occurs before actual observation and treatment of patients.

preclinical dental training Study and mastery of the theory and techniques related to the various dental procedures required prior to treating human patients.

preclinical technique In dentistry, the use of manikins, mechanical articulator, artificial or extracted teeth, and the variety of dental instruments and materials to study and master the techniques necessary to do clinical dentistry.

preclival (prē-klī'văl) [" + *clivus,* slope] In front of the cerebellar clivus.

precocious (prē-kō'shŭs) [L. *praecox,* ripening early] Mental or physical development earlier than would be expected.

precocity (prē-kŏs'ĭ-tē) Premature development of physical or mental traits.

sexual p. Evidence of the development of secondary sex characteristics before age 8 in girls and age 9 in boys. SYN: *precocious p.*

precognition (prē"kŏg-nĭsh'ŭn) [L. *prae,* before, in front of, + *cognoscere,* to know] Prior knowledge that an event will occur acquired pre-rationally.

precoital (prē-kō'ĭ-tăl) [" + *coitio,* a going together] Prior to sexual intercourse.

precoma (prē-kō'mă) [" + Gr. *koma,* a deep sleep] Stupor.

preconscious (prē-kŏn'shŭs) [" + *conscius,* aware] Not present in consciousness but able to be recalled as desired.

preconvulsive (prē"kŏn-vŭl'sĭv) [" + *convulsio,* pulling together] Before a convulsion.

precordia (prē-kor'dē-ă) [L. *praecordia*] The precordium.

precordial (prē-kor'dē-ăl) Pert. to the precordium or epigastrium.

precordium (prē-kor'dē-ŭm) The area on the anterior surface of the body overlying the heart and lower part of the thorax. SYN: *antecardium; precordia.*

precornu (prē-kor'nū) [L. *prae,* before, in front of, + *cornu,* horn] The anterior horn of the lateral ventricle of the brain.

precostal (prē-kŏs′tăl) [″ + Gr. *costa,* rib] In front of the ribs.

precuneus (prē-kū′nē-ŭs) [″ + *cuneus,* wedge] The division of the mesial surface of a cerebral hemisphere between the cuneus and the paracentral lobule.

precursor A substance that precedes another substance, or a substance from which another is synthesized.

predentin Uncalcified dentinal matrix.

prediabetes (prē-dī″ă-bē′tēz) [″ + Gr. *diabetes,* passing through] Early evidence of autoimmune disease or impaired carbohydrate metabolism in patients who later develop overt diabetes mellitus.

prediastole (prē″dī-ăs′tō-lē) [″ + Gr. *diastellein,* to expand] The period in the cardiac cycle just before diastole.

prediastolic (prē″dī-ă-stŏl′ĭk) [″ + Gr. *diastole,* expansion] Before the diastole, or interval in the cardiac cycle that precedes it.

predicrotic (prē″dī-krŏt′ĭk) [″ + Gr. *dikrotos,* beating double] Preceding the dicrotic wave of the sphygmographic tracing.

prediction rules Identifying and giving weight to the factors important in formulating a diagnosis, in order to establish the probability that a disease is present.

predigestion (prē″dĭ-jĕs′chŭn) [″ + *digestio,* carrying apart] Artificial proteolysis or digestion of proteins and amylolysis of starches before ingestion.

predisposing (prē″dĭs-pōz′ĭng) [″ + *disponere,* to dispose] Indicating a tendency to, or susceptibility to, disease.

predisposition (prē″dĭs-pō-zĭsh′ŭn) The potential to develop a certain disease or condition in the presence of specific environmental stimuli.

prednisolone (prĕd-nĭs′ō-lōn) A glucocorticosteroid drug, available in a variety of dosage forms. It is similar in action to cortisone.

prednisone (prĕd′nĭ-sōn) A glucocorticosteroid with the same effects as cortisone.

pre-eclampsia (prē″ē-klămp′sē-ă) [″ + Gr. *ek,* out, + *lampein,* to flash] A complication of pregnancy characterized by increasing hypertension, proteinuria, and edema. The condition may progress rapidly from mild to severe and, if untreated, to eclampsia. It is the leading cause of fetal and maternal morbidity and death, esp. in underdeveloped countries. SYN: *pregnancy-induced hypertension*. SEE: *eclampsia; HELLP syndrome; Nursing Diagnoses Appendix.*

ETIOLOGY: The cause is unknown; however, the incidence is higher among adolescent and older primigravidas, diabetic patients, and in multiple pregnancy. Pathophysiology associated with pre-eclampsia includes generalized vasospasm, damage to the glomerular membranes, and hypovolemia and hemoconcentration due to a fluid shift from intravascular to interstitial compartments.

SYMPTOMS: The condition develops between the 20th week of gestation and the end of the first postpartum week; however, most commonly it occurs during the last trimester. Characteristic complaints include sudden weight gain, severe headaches, and visual disturbances. Indications of increasing severity include complaints of epigastric or abdominal pain; generalized, presacral, and facial edema; oliguria; and hyperreflexia. Objective findings include hypertension, edema, proteinuria, and hyperreflexia. SEE: *deep tendon reflex*.

TREATMENT: Treatment includes bedrest; high-protein diet; and medications including mild sedatives, antihypertensives, and, if indicated, intravenous anticonvulsants. Magnesium sulfate is the drug of choice.

pre-embryo The morula and blastocyst stages produced by the division of the zygote until the formation of the embryo proper at the appearance of the primitive streak about 14 days after fertilization.

pre-eruption (prē″ē-rŭp′shŭn) [″ + *eruptio,* a breaking out] **1.** Before an eruption. **2.** The stage of tooth eruption when the tooth bud is in the bony socket prior to root formation. SEE: *eruptive stage* (2).

pre-excitation, ventricular (prē-ĕk″sī-tā′shŭn) [″ + *excitare,* to arouse] Premature excitation of the ventricle by an impulse that traveled a path other than through the atrioventricular node. This produces a short P-R interval. SEE: *Wolff-Parkinson-White syndrome*.

pre-existing condition Any injury, disease, or physical condition occurring prior to an arbitrary date; usually used in reference to the date of issuance of a health insurance policy. In some cases, a pre-existing condition results in an exclusion from coverage for costs resulting from the injury, disease, or condition.

preferred provider organization ABBR: PPO. An incorporated group of physicians, hospital(s), nurses, and other health care workers, who jointly assume the clinical and financial responsibilities for delivering health care to enrolled groups of insured patients. The providers are semi-independent agents who agree to provide care at reduced rates.

prefrontal (prē-frŏn′tăl) [″ + *frons,* front] **1.** The middle portion of the ethmoid bone. **2.** In the anterior part of the frontal lobe of the brain.

preganglionic (prē″găng-lē-ŏn′ĭk) [″ + Gr. *ganglion,* knot] **1.** Situated in front of or anterior to a ganglion. **2.** Situated before a ganglion, such as a preganglionic neuron.

preganglionic fiber The axon of a preganglionic neuron.

preganglionic neuron The first of a series of two efferent neurons that transmit impulses to visceral effectors. Its cell body lies in the central nervous system. Its axon terminates in an autonomic ganglion.

pregenital (prē-jĕn′ĭ-tăl) [″ + *genitalia*, genitals] In psychology, relating to that period when erotic interest in the reproductive organs and functions is not yet organized.

pregnancy (prĕg′năn-sē) [L. *praegnans*] The condition of having a developing embryo or fetus in the body after successful conception. The average duration of pregnancy is about 280 days. Estimation of the date on which delivery should occur is based on the first day of the last menstrual period. SEE: *Naegeli's rule;* table; *prenatal care; prenatal diagnosis; Nursing Diagnoses Appendix.*

DEMOGRAPHICS: About 7 million Americans become pregnant each year, and about two-thirds of these pregnancies result in live births. In 1998 there were 3.94 million live births in the U.S.

SIGNS AND SYMPTOMS: Presumptive and probable signs are those commonly associated with pregnancy but may be due to other causes, such as oral contraceptive therapy. *Presumptive symptoms* include amenorrhea, nausea and vomiting, breast tenderness, urinary frequency, fatigue, chloasma, vaginal hyperemia (Chadwick's sign), and "quickening." *Probable signs* include increased abdominal girth, palpable fetal outline, softening of the lower uterine segment (Hegar's sign), softening of the cervix (Goodell's sign), and immunodiagnostic pregnancy tests. *Positive signs and symptoms* of pregnancy are auscultation of fetal heart sounds, fetal movements felt by the examiner, and an identifiable embryonic outline on ultrasound.

PHYSICAL CHANGES: The pregnant woman experiences many physiological alterations related to the increased levels of estrogen and progesterone and to the demands of the growing fetus; every system in the woman's body responds to these changes.

Reproductive tract changes: Alterations in uterine size, shape, and consistency include an increase in uterine muscle mass over the months of pregnancy. In response to elevated estrogen and progesterone levels, the cervix and lower uterine segment soften. Vaginal secretions increase, and vaginal pH is more acidic (pH = 3.5 to 6.0). Change in vaginal pH discourages the survival and multiplication of bacteria; however, it also encourages infection by *Candida albicans*. The vagina elongates as the uterus rises in the pelvis; the mucosa thickens, with increases in secretions, vascularity, and elasticity. SEE: *Chadwick's sign; Goodell's sign; Hegar's sign.*

Breast changes: The breasts become enlarged, tender, and more nodular. The areolae darken; the nipples become more sensitive and erectile; and Montgomery's tubercles enlarge. Colostrum may leak out during the last trimester, as the breasts prepare for lactation.

Endocrine glands: The size and activity of the thyroid gland increase markedly. Thyroid-binding globulin and triiodothyronine levels rise, while thyroid stimulating hormone levels drop slightly. These changes allow the pregnant woman to meet the endocrine needs imposed by the developing fetus, and other body changes that occur during pregnancy. Pituitary activity increases; placental hormones prevent ovulation and encourage development of the corpus luteum.

Cardiovascular alterations: Circulating blood volume increases progressively throughout pregnancy, peaking in the middle of the third trimester. Although the red blood cell count rises by about 30%, the 50% increase in blood volume creates a false impression of anemia. Rising levels of clotting factors VII, VIII, IX, and X increase coagulability. The pulse rate increases, along with cardiac stroke volume. Mid-trimester blood pressure may be slightly lower than normal but remains essentially unchanged.

Skeletal system: Softening and increased mobility of the pelvic articulations is reflected in the waddling gait of pregnancy. As pregnancy progresses, the woman's center of gravity shifts, and the lumbar curve increases to compensate for the growing anterior weight of the gravid uterus. Problems with dental caries may become more prominent during pregnancy, but can be prevented with oral rinses (such as chlorhexidine) and regular brushing and flossing.

Respiratory system: The effects of progesterone on smooth muscle include a decreased airway resistance, which enables the woman to meet her increased needs for oxygen by permitting a 30% to 40% increase in tidal volume and a 15% to 20% rise in oxygen consumption. The effects of estrogen include edema and congestion of the nasal mucosa, reflected in nosebleeds and nasal stuffiness.

Gastrointestinal system: Nausea and vomiting is the single most common complaint during the first trimester. Progesterone-related diminished motility contributes to common complaints of heartburn and constipation.

Pregnancy Table for Expected Date of Delivery

Jan.	1	2	3	4	5	6	7	8	9	10	11	12	13	14	15	16	17	18	19	20	21	22	23	24	25	26	27	28	29	30	31	
Oct.	**8**	**9**	**10**	**11**	**12**	**13**	**14**	**15**	**16**	**17**	**18**	**19**	**20**	**21**	**22**	**23**	**24**	**25**	**26**	**27**	**28**	**29**	**30**	**31**	**1**	**2**	**3**	**4**	**5**	**6**	**7**	**Nov.**
Feb.	1	2	3	4	5	6	7	8	9	10	11	12	13	14	15	16	17	18	19	20	21	22	23	24	25	26	27	28				
Nov.	**8**	**9**	**10**	**11**	**12**	**13**	**14**	**15**	**16**	**17**	**18**	**19**	**20**	**21**	**22**	**23**	**24**	**25**	**26**	**27**	**28**	**29**	**30**	**1**	**2**	**3**	**4**	**5**				**Dec.**
Mar.	1	2	3	4	5	6	7	8	9	10	11	12	13	14	15	16	17	18	19	20	21	22	23	24	25	26	27	28	29	30	31	
Dec.	**6**	**7**	**8**	**9**	**10**	**11**	**12**	**13**	**14**	**15**	**16**	**17**	**18**	**19**	**20**	**21**	**22**	**23**	**24**	**25**	**26**	**27**	**28**	**29**	**30**	**31**	**1**	**2**	**3**	**4**	**5**	**Jan.**
April	1	2	3	4	5	6	7	8	9	10	11	12	13	14	15	16	17	18	19	20	21	22	23	24	25	26	27	28	29	30		
Jan.	**6**	**7**	**8**	**9**	**10**	**11**	**12**	**13**	**14**	**15**	**16**	**17**	**18**	**19**	**20**	**21**	**22**	**23**	**24**	**25**	**26**	**27**	**28**	**29**	**30**	**31**	**1**	**2**	**3**	**4**		**Feb.**
May	1	2	3	4	5	6	7	8	9	10	11	12	13	14	15	16	17	18	19	20	21	22	23	24	25	26	27	28	29	30	31	
Feb.	**5**	**6**	**7**	**8**	**9**	**10**	**11**	**12**	**13**	**14**	**15**	**16**	**17**	**18**	**19**	**20**	**21**	**22**	**23**	**24**	**25**	**26**	**27**	**28**	**1**	**2**	**3**	**4**	**5**	**6**	**7**	**Mar.**
June	1	2	3	4	5	6	7	8	9	10	11	12	13	14	15	16	17	18	19	20	21	22	23	24	25	26	27	28	29	30		
Mar.	**8**	**9**	**10**	**11**	**12**	**13**	**14**	**15**	**16**	**17**	**18**	**19**	**20**	**21**	**22**	**23**	**24**	**25**	**26**	**27**	**28**	**29**	**30**	**31**	**1**	**2**	**3**	**4**	**5**	**6**		**April**
July	1	2	3	4	5	6	7	8	9	10	11	12	13	14	15	16	17	18	19	20	21	22	23	24	25	26	27	28	29	30	31	
April	**7**	**8**	**9**	**10**	**11**	**12**	**13**	**14**	**15**	**16**	**17**	**18**	**19**	**20**	**21**	**22**	**23**	**24**	**25**	**26**	**27**	**28**	**29**	**30**	**1**	**2**	**3**	**4**	**5**	**6**	**7**	**May**
Aug.	1	2	3	4	5	6	7	8	9	10	11	12	13	14	15	16	17	18	19	20	21	22	23	24	25	26	27	28	29	30	31	
May	**8**	**9**	**10**	**11**	**12**	**13**	**14**	**15**	**16**	**17**	**18**	**19**	**20**	**21**	**22**	**23**	**24**	**25**	**26**	**27**	**28**	**29**	**30**	**31**	**1**	**2**	**3**	**4**	**5**	**6**	**7**	**June**
Sept.	1	2	3	4	5	6	7	8	9	10	11	12	13	14	15	16	17	18	19	20	21	22	23	24	25	26	27	28	29	30		
June	**8**	**9**	**10**	**11**	**12**	**13**	**14**	**15**	**16**	**17**	**18**	**19**	**20**	**21**	**22**	**23**	**24**	**25**	**26**	**27**	**28**	**29**	**30**	**1**	**2**	**3**	**4**	**5**	**6**	**7**		**July**
Oct.	1	2	3	4	5	6	7	8	9	10	11	12	13	14	15	16	17	18	19	20	21	22	23	24	25	26	27	28	29	30	31	
July	**8**	**9**	**10**	**11**	**12**	**13**	**14**	**15**	**16**	**17**	**18**	**19**	**20**	**21**	**22**	**23**	**24**	**25**	**26**	**27**	**28**	**29**	**30**	**31**	**1**	**2**	**3**	**4**	**5**	**6**	**7**	**Aug.**
Nov.	1	2	3	4	5	6	7	8	9	10	11	12	13	14	15	16	17	18	19	20	21	22	23	24	25	26	27	28	29	30		
Aug.	**8**	**9**	**10**	**11**	**12**	**13**	**14**	**15**	**16**	**17**	**18**	**19**	**20**	**21**	**22**	**23**	**24**	**25**	**26**	**27**	**28**	**29**	**30**	**31**	**1**	**2**	**3**	**4**	**5**	**6**		**Sept.**
Dec.	1	2	3	4	5	6	7	8	9	10	11	12	13	14	15	16	17	18	19	20	21	22	23	24	25	26	27	28	29	30	31	
Sept.	**7**	**8**	**9**	**10**	**11**	**12**	**13**	**14**	**15**	**16**	**17**	**18**	**19**	**20**	**21**	**22**	**23**	**24**	**25**	**26**	**27**	**28**	**29**	**30**	**1**	**2**	**3**	**4**	**5**	**6**	**7**	**Oct.**

The date of the last menstrual period is in the top line (light-face type) of the pair of lines. The dark number (bold-face type) in the line below will be the expected day of delivery.

Skin: Pigmentation changes in pregnancy include chloasma (the so-called mask of pregnancy), areolar darkening, and linea nigra (a pigmented line that vertically bisects the abdomen). They reflect estrogen-related stimulation of skin melanocytes.

Urinary system: By middle of the first trimester, the glomerular filtration rate (GFR) has risen by about 50%; in compensation, tubular reabsorption also increases. Although urinary frequency is common in the first and last trimesters, bladder capacity actually increases; however, pressure from the growing uterus reduces the volume required to stimulate voiding. During the second trimester, the uterus rises out of the pelvis, becoming an abdominal organ and relieving bladder compression.

Weight: In average-sized individuals, expected first trimester weight gain is 2 to 5 lb. Total weight gain and the pattern by which it increases should be monitored to enable early signs of pregnancy-related problems common to the particular point in gestation. The Institute of Medicine recommends the following weight gains during singleton pregnancies: a woman with a prepregnancy body mass index less than 19.8 should gain 25 to 39 lb (11.4 to 17.7 kg); a woman with a prepregnancy body mass index from 19.8 to 26 should gain 25 to 34 lb (11.4 to 15.5 kg); and a woman with a prepregnancy body mass index from 26 to 29 should gain 15 to 24 lb (6.8 to 10.9 kg). The recommended weight gains during pregnancy are different for multiple gestations (e.g., a woman carrying triplets should gain about 50 lb (22.7 kg) during the course of her pregnancy).

PATIENT CARE: An essential component to anticipatory guidance and patient teaching is to encourage the woman's active participation in her own health maintenance and pregnancy progress. Health care providers describe to pregnant women common complaints related to normal physiological changes of pregnancy and suggest actions to minimize discomfort.

DISORDERS: *Nausea and vomiting* SEE: *morning sickness*.

Heartburn: Hormone-related delayed gastric emptying, cardiac sphincter relaxation, and stomach displacement by the growing uterus contribute to reflux. The use of low-sodium or combination aluminum hydroxide/magnesium hydroxide preparations is recommended for symptomatic relief. For severe, unresponsive heartburn, over-the-counter H2 blockers, such as ranitidine (Zantac) or famotidine (Pepcid), may be recommended.

Constipation: The woman should increase fiber and fluid intake. She also may use stool softeners.

Muscle cramps: The woman may relieve the so-called "charleyhorse" that occurs during sleep by dorsiflexing the foot of the affected leg. A calcium-phosphorus imbalance may contribute to increased frequency of this problem. The woman can increase calcium intake by drinking the recommended daily quart of milk or by drinking a pint of milk daily and taking a calcium supplement.

Back pain: Growing anterior mass, shift in center of gravity, and increased lumbar curve contribute to backaches. To relieve discomfort, the pregnant woman should wear well-fitting, low-heeled shoes and perform exercises that increase abdominal muscle tone. SEE: *pelvic rock; pelvic tilt*.

Dependent edema: Pedal edema is a common third-trimester complaint related to decreased venous return from the extremities. The woman is advised to rest frequently and to elevate her feet. She should report promptly any edema of the face, hands, or sacral area to facilitate early diagnosis and management of pregnancy-induced hypertension.

Varicose veins: Decreased venous return from the extremities and compression of vascular structures by the growing uterus aggravate any weakness in the vascular wall. Varicosities often occur in the legs, vulva, and pelvis. The woman should avoid tight clothing and prolonged standing. Other preventive and therapeutic measures include wearing support stockings, resting in left Sims' position, and elevating the lower limbs during sleep.

Hemorrhoids: Temporary symptomatic relief may be obtained by Sitz baths and analgesic ointments. The woman also should be instructed in how to reinsert the hemorrhoid with a well-lubricated finger, holding it in place for 1 to 2 min before releasing the pressure. SEE: *constipation*.

Vaginal discharge: A normal increase in vaginal discharge occurs during pregnancy. Common perineal hygiene usually is effective as a comfort measure; douching is contraindicated during pregnancy. The woman should contact her primary caregiver promptly if profuse, malodorous, or blood-tinged discharge occurs. SEE: *vaginitis*.

Dyspnea: Shortness of breath occurs as the growing uterus presses on the woman's diaphragm. Elevation of the head and shoulders may provide some relief. The dyspnea disappears when lightening occurs.

Pruritus: The normal stretching of the skin may generate itching on the breasts, abdomen, and vulva. Use of an emollient lotion may be suggested; the patient is instructed to inform her primary caregiver if vulvovaginal itching occurs in conjunction with an increase or alteration in vaginal discharge. SEE: *vaginitis*.

NUTRITION: A woman's nutritional status before and during pregnancy is an important factor that affects both her health and that of her unborn child. Nutritional assessment is an essential part of antepartal care. In addition, the presence of pre-existing and coexisting disorders, such as anemia, diabetes mellitus, chronic renal disease, and phenylketonuria, may affect dietary recommendations. Substance abuse increases the risk of inadequate nutrition, low maternal weight gain, low-birth-weight infants, and perinatal mortality.

Dietary recommendations emphasize a high-quality, well-balanced diet. Increased amounts of essential nutrients (i.e., protein, calcium, magnesium, zinc, and selenium, B vitamins, vitamin C, folate, and iron) are necessary to meet nutritional needs of both mother and fetus. Most nutritional and metabolic needs can be met by eating a balanced daily diet containing approximately 35 kcal for each kilogram of optimal body weight plus an additional 300 kcal/day during the second and third trimesters. Vitamin supplements are not required if the woman adheres to the dietary recommendations; however, daily iron supplements are recommended.

CONSIDERATIONS: *Travel during pregnancy:* Preparing for travel during pregnancy will depend upon the number of weeks gestation, the duration of the travel, and the method (i.e., auto, boat, bus, train, airplane).

Safety belts, preferably the combined lap and shoulder type, should be worn. If nausea and vomiting of pregnancy is a factor, travel by sea isn't advisable. If antimotion medication is used, it should be approved for use during pregnancy. Travel during the last part of pregnancy isn't advised unless obstetrical care is available at the destination(s). It is important to have a copy of current medical records along when traveling. Travel abroad should be discussed with the obstetrician so that appropriate immunizations can be given. For travel in an area known to be endemic for malaria, certain drugs will be needed for prophylaxis.

CAUTION: Not all antimalarials are safe for use during pregnancy. Live virus immunization should not be administered during pregnancy.

Working during pregnancy: Healthy pregnant women who are employed in jobs that present no more risk than those in daily life are encouraged to continue working if they desire until shortly before delivery.

Exercise during pregnancy: If the pregnancy is progressing normally, exercise may and should be continued. The amount and type of exercise is an individual matter. A woman who has exercised regularly before her pregnancy should experience no difficulty with continuing; however, a previously sedentary woman should not attempt to institute a vigorous exercise program such as long-distance running or jogging during her pregnancy. No matter what the type of exercise, it is important to remember that, with the progress of pregnancy, the center of gravity will change and probably prevent participation at the same level and skill as before pregnancy. Sports to avoid include water skiing, horseback riding, and scuba diving. In water skiing, high-speed falls could cause miscarriage due to an inadvertent, forceful vaginal douche. In horseback riding, in addition to the possibility of falling from the horse, the repeated bouncing may lead to bruising of the perianal area. Scuba diving may lead to decompression sickness and bends and to intravascular air embolism in the fetus. Women who breast-feed their children can continue exercising if they maintain hydration and adequate breast support.

Sexual intercourse during pregnancy: Women who are experiencing normally progressing pregnancies need not avoid intercourse. Pregnant women should refrain from coitus if they have a history of preterm labor or premature rupture of membranes and if they are bleeding or have ruptured membranes.

Tests during pregnancy: Common tests include blood tests for nutritional or sickle cell anemia, blood type and Rh factor, rubella titers, syphilis, and serum alpha-fetoprotein for the presence of neural tube defects such as spina bifida. Ultrasound may be used to determine age, rate of growth, position, some birth defects, and fetal sex. Chorionic villus sampling is done early in pregnancy if the family history indicates potential for genetic diseases. Second trimester amniocentesis may be used to detect chromosomal abnormalities, genetic disorders, and fetal sex. Additional testing may include determining HIV status and hepatitis immunity. In late pregnancy, nonstress tests, contraction stress tests, and fetal biophysical profiles may be done; amniocentesis may be done to evaluate fetal lung maturity.

Pregnancy in adolescence: Although pregnancy among teenagers is decreasing in the United States, about 7% of all American teenage girls still become pregnant in any given year—this is one of the highest rates of teen pregnancy in developed cultures. Sociocultural factors are believed to contribute to the high incidence of pregnancies among this population. Demographic data indicate that teen pregnancy is more likely to be associated with being single, having low socioeconomic status, and lacking social support systems. Pregnant teenagers are believed to be at high risk for some complications of pregnancy; if, however, they seek prenatal care early and consistently cooperate with recommendations, the risk is comparable to that for other age groups. Clinical data identify a common pattern of late entry to the prenatal care system, failure to return for scheduled appointments, and noncompliance with medical and nursing recommendations. As a result of these behaviors, adolescents are at higher risk for pregnancy-related complications, such as iron-deficiency anemia, pregnancy-induced hypertension, preterm labor and delivery, low birthweight newborns, and cephalopelvic disproportion. Other health problems seen more commonly in pregnant adolescents include sexually transmitted diseases and substance abuse. SEE: *high-risk pregnancy; Nursing Diagnoses Appendix.*

Mature pregnancy: A growing number of women are experiencing their first pregnancies after age 35. The incidence of fetal demise among this population is 6:1000 births, double the rate for women under 35. Many factors may contribute to the increased risk, including pre-existing and coexisting conditions, such as diabetes mellitus, hypertension, and uterine fibroids. Mature women are identified as being at higher risk for spontaneous abortion, pre-eclampsia, abruptio placentae, placenta previa, gestational diabetes, cesarean birth, and chromosomal abnormalities such as Down syndrome. Multiple gestation secondary to the use of fertility drugs also may be a factor in fetal loss.

Pregnancy after menopause: Very rarely, postmenopausal women have become pregnant through embryo donation and have successfully carried the pregnancy to term delivery. Prior to undergoing this procedure, the women had been taking hormone replacement therapy. Previously, it had been assumed that the postmenopausal uterus would not be capable of supporting the growth and development of an embryo. Pregnancies in older women are considered high risk for reasons similar to those related to mature pregnancy. Late in the third trimester, the woman may be instructed to keep a fetal activity record and undergo regularly scheduled nonstress tests.

abdominal p. Ectopic gestation in which the embryo develops in the peritoneal cavity. SYN: *abdominocyesis.* SEE: *ectopic pregnancy.*

ampullar p. Ectopic implantation of the zygote in the ampulla of a fallopian tube; 78% of all ectopic pregnancies occur in this site.

bigeminal p. Intrauterine twin gestation.

cervical p. Pregnancy with implantation of the embryo in the cervical canal.

coitus during p. Sexual intercourse during pregnancy. There is no evidence that this has adverse effects on the pregnancy or the embryo (i.e., perinatal mortality). Also, sexual intercourse does not initiate labor.

cornual p. A rare type of ectopic pregnancy (found in about 2% to 4% of all ectopic pregnancies) in which implantation takes place in one of the horns of the uterus. The uterine horn may rupture between the 12 and 16 weeks' gestation, causing life-threatening shock. Traditionally, cornual pregnancies have been managed with laparotomy and hysterectomy, although conservative management strategies are employed occasionally.

ectopic p. Extrauterine implantation of a fertilized ovum, usually in the fallopian tubes, but occasionally in the peritoneum, ovary, or other locations. Ectopic implantation occurs in about 1 of every 150 pregnancies; it is responsible for approximately 10% of maternal deaths. Symptoms usually occur between 6 and 12 weeks after conception. SEE: illus.; *pregnancy.*

SYMPTOMS: Early complaints are consistent with those of a normal pregnancy (i.e., amenorrhea, breast tenderness, nausea). Pregnancy test results are positive owing to the presence of human chorionic gonadotropin (hCG) in blood and urine. Signs and symptoms arise as the growing embryo distends the fallopian tube; associated complaints include intermittent, unilateral, colicky abdominal pain. Complaints associated with tubal rupture include sharp unilateral pelvic or lower abdominal pain; orthostatic dizziness and vertigo or syncope; and referred shoulder pain related to peritoneal irritation from abdominal bleeding (hemoperitoneum). Signs of hypovolemic shock may indicate extensive abdominal bleeding. Vaginal bleeding, typically occurring after the onset of pain, is the result of decidual sloughing.

LOCATIONS: *Abdominal:* The incidence of pregnancy in the abdominal cavity with the conceptus attached to an abdominal organ is between 1:3000 and 1:4000 births. *Ovarian:* Conception and implantation within the ovary itself occurs in approximately 1 in 7,000 to 1 in

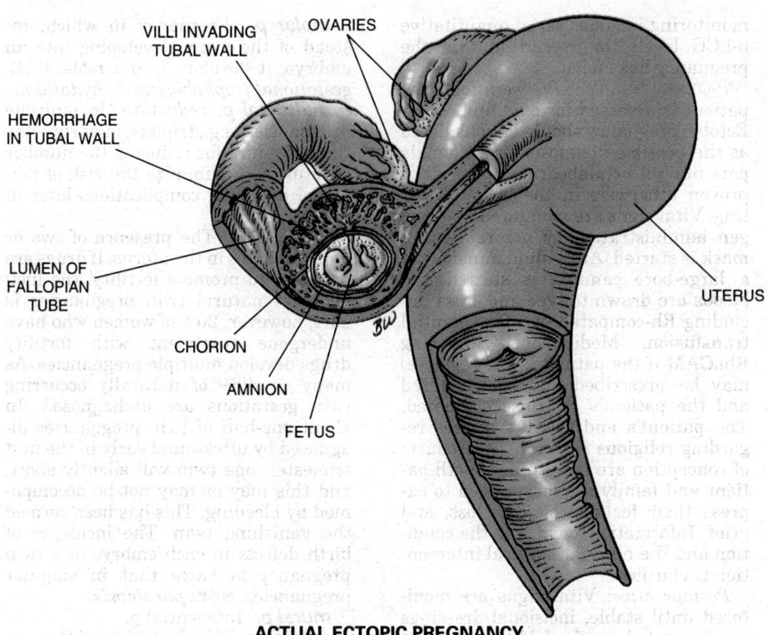

ACTUAL ECTOPIC PREGNANCY

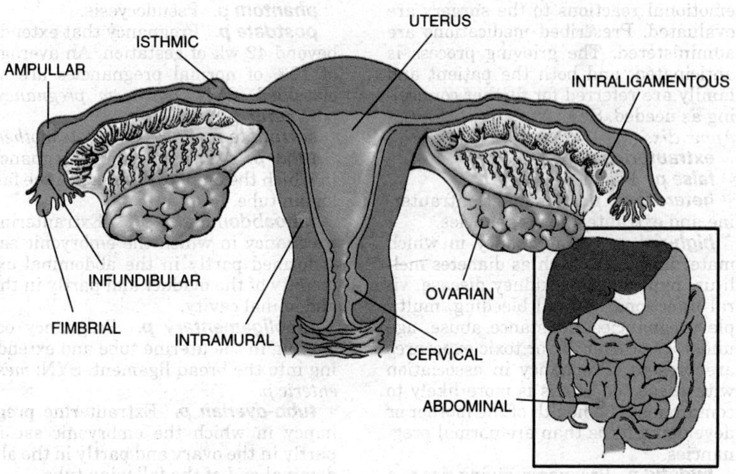

VARIOUS SITES OF ECTOPIC PREGNANCY

50,000 pregnancies. *Tubal:* Ninety to 95% of ectopic pregnancies occur in the fallopian tube; of these, 78% become implanted in the uterine ampulla, 12% in the isthmus, and 2% to 3% in the interstices.

DIAGNOSIS: Transabdominal pelvic ultrasonography is used to identify the location of the pregnancy. It has also largely replaced culdocentesis for confirmation of hemoperitoneum.

TREATMENT: An operative approach is most common. Laparoscopy and linear laser salpingostomy can be used to excise early ectopic implantations; healing is by secondary intention. Segmental resection allows salvage and later reconstruction of the affected tube. Salpingectomy is reserved for cases in which tubal damage is so extensive that reanastomosis is not possible. Methotrexate has been used successfully to induce dissolution of unruptured tubal masses less than 3.5 cm. Posttreatment monitoring includes serial quantitative b-hCG levels, to be certain that the pregnancy has ended.

PATIENT CARE: *Preoperative:* The patient is assessed for pain and shock. Ectopic pregnancy should be considered as the possible diagnosis for all female patients of childbearing age until proven otherwise in the hospital setting. Vital signs are monitored and oxygen administration by non-rebreather mask is started. An IV fluid infusion via a large-bore cannula is started and bloods are drawn to type and cross (including Rh-compatability) for potential transfusion. Medications (including RhoGAM if the patient is Rh negative) may be prescribed and administered and the patient's response evaluated. The patient's and family's wishes regarding religious rites for the products of conception are determined. Both patient and family are encouraged to express their feelings of fear, loss, and grief. Information regarding the condition and the need for surgical intervention is clarified.

Postoperative: Vital signs are monitored until stable, incisional dressings are inspected, vaginal bleeding is assessed, and the patient's physical and emotional reactions to the surgery are evaluated. Prescribed medications are administered. The grieving process is anticipated, and both the patient and family are referred for further counseling as needed. SEE: *Nursing Diagnoses Appendix.*

extrauterine p. Ectopic p.

false p. Pseudocyesis.

heterotopic p. Combined intrauterine and extrauterine pregnancies.

high-risk p. A pregnancy in which maternal factors such as diabetes mellitus, hypertension, kidney disease, viral infections, vaginal bleeding, multiple pregnancies, substance abuse, age under 17 or over 35, or toxic exposures are present. Pregnancy in association with these conditions is more likely to compromise the health of the mother or developing fetus than are normal pregnancies.

hydatid p. Pregnancy giving rise to a hydatidiform mole. SEE: *gestational trophoblastic d. hydatid mole.*

interstitial p. Rare condition in which the zygote implants in the portion of the fallopian tube that traverses the wall of the uterus. SYN: *mural p.*

intraligamentary p. Pregnancy that occurs within the broad ligament.

mask of p. Chloasma gravidarum. SEE: *chloasma.*

membranous p. Pregnancy in which the amniotic sac ruptures and the embryo comes to lie in direct contact with the uterine wall.

mesenteric p. Tuboligamentary p.

molar p. Pregnancy in which, instead of the ovum developing into an embryo, it develops into a mole. SEE: *gestational trophoblastic d.; hydatid m.*

multifetal p. reduction In multiple pregnancies (e.g., triplets, quadruplets), the procedure for reducing the number of fetuses, to minimize the risk of maternal and fetal complications later in the pregnancy.

multiple p. The presence of two or more embryos in the uterus. If drugs are not used to promote fertility, the incidence of natural twin pregnancies is 1:94; however, 20% of women who have undergone treatment with fertility drugs develop multiple pregnancies. As many as 40% of naturally occurring twin gestations are undiagnosed. In about one-half of twin pregnancies diagnosed by ultrasound early in the first trimester, one twin will silently abort, and this may or may not be accompanied by bleeding. This has been termed the vanishing twin. The incidence of birth defects in each embryo of a twin pregnancy is twice that in singular pregnancies. SEE: *parabiosis.*

mural p. Interstitial p.

ovarian p. Implantation of the embryo in the substance of the ovary.

phantom p. Pseudocyesis.

postdate p. Pregnancy that extends beyond 42 wk of gestation. An average of 10% of normal pregnancies are so classified. SYN: *post-term pregnancy; postmaturity s.*

surrogate p. SEE: *surrogate mother.*

tubal p. A form of ectopic pregnancy in which the embryo develops in the fallopian tube.

tuboabdominal p. Extrauterine pregnancy in which the embryonic sac is formed partly in the abdominal extremity of the oviduct and partly in the abdominal cavity.

tuboligamentary p. Pregnancy occurring in the uterine tube and extending into the broad ligament. SYN: *mesenteric p.*

tubo-ovarian p. Extrauterine pregnancy in which the embryonic sac is partly in the ovary and partly in the abdominal end of the fallopian tube.

uteroabdominal p. Twin pregnancy with one embryo in the uterus and the other in the abdominal cavity.

pregnancy-specific β_1 glycoprotein A protein found in 97% of women who have been pregnant for 6 to 8 weeks and in 100% of those at later stages of pregnancy. The function of this protein is not known, but it may be useful in estimating the quality of placental function.

pregnancy test A test used to determine whether conception has occurred. In addition to the clinical signs and symptoms of pregnancy, almost none of which are reliable within the first several weeks of pregnancy, chemical tests done in the physician's office are quite accurate by as early as the time the first menstrual period is missed. There are also test kits available for purchase without a prescription. If that type of test is used, it is very important to follow the directions carefully.

A major class of pregnancy tests is those using immunodiagnostic procedures. They are the hemagglutination inhibition test, which requires a sample of urine; radioreceptor assay, which requires blood from the patient; radioimmunoassay, which requires a blood sample; and monoclonal antibody determination, which requires a sample of urine. In general, these tests are accurate beginning the 40th day following the first day of the last menstrual period; the monoclonal antibody test is somewhat more sensitive. The reliability of the test methods increases as pregnancy continues.

pregnane (prĕg′nān) $C_{21}H_{36}$ The organic compound that is a precursor of two series of steroid hormones: the progesterones and several adrenal cortical hormones.

pregnanediol (prĕg″nān-dī′ŏl) $C_{21}H_{36}O_2$; the inactive end product of metabolism of progesterone present in the urine. The amount in the urine increases during the premenstrual or luteal phase of the menstrual cycle and during pregnancy.

pregnanetriol (prĕg″nān-trī′ŏl) A metabolite of progesterone. Its presence in the urine is increased in those who have congenital adrenal hyperplasia.

pregnant (prĕg′nănt) [L. *praegnans*] Having conceived; with child. SYN: *gravid*.

pregnene (prĕg′nēn) A steroid that forms the nucleus of progesterone.

pregneninolone (prĕg″nēn-ĭn′ō-lōn) A progestin, ethisterone.

pregnenolone (prĕg-nĕn′ō-lōn) A synthetic corticosteroid hormone produced from progesterone.

pregravidic (prē-gră-vĭd′ĭk) [L. *prae,* before, in front of, + *gravida,* pregnant] Before pregnancy.

prehallux (prē-hăl′ŭks) [″ + *hallux,* the great toe] A supernumerary bone, accessory naviculare pedis, or sometimes a prolongation inward of it on the foot.

prehemiplegic (prē″hĕm-ĭ-plē′jĭk) [″ + Gr. *hemi,* half, + *plege,* a stroke] Occurring before an attack of hemiplegia.

prehensile (prē-hĕn′sĭl) [L. *prehendere,* to seize] Adapted for grasping or holding, esp. by encircling an object.

prehension (prē-hĕn′shŭn) [L. *prehensio*] The primary function of the hand; includes pinching, grasping, and seizing.

prehormone A precursor of a hormone.

prehospital care The care a patient receives from emergency medical service before arriving at the hospital. This is usually done by emergency medical technicians and paramedics.

prehospital care report ABBR: PCR. The standardized form used by all emergency medical service agencies within an EMS system, to document patient care and assessments conducted in the field.

prehospital provider A medical technician who provides care to emergency patients before they arrive at a hospital.

prehyoid (prē-hī′oyd) [L. *prae,* before, in front of, + Gr. *hyoeides,* U-shaped] In front of the hyoid bone.

prehypophysis (prē″hī-pŏf′ĭ-sĭs) [″ + Gr. *hypophysis,* an undergrowth] The anterior lobe of the pituitary gland.

preictal (prē-ĭk′tăl) [″ + *ictus,* stroke] The period just prior to a stroke or convulsion.

preicteric (prē-ĭk-tĕr′ĭk) [″ + *ikteros,* jaundice] In liver disease, the period prior to the appearance of jaundice.

preimmunization (prē-ĭm″ū-nĭ-zā′shŭn) [″ + *immunis,* safe] Immunization produced artificially in very young infants.

preinvasive (prē″ĭn-vā′sĭv) [″ + *in,* into, + *vadere,* to go] Referring to a stage of development of a malignancy in which the neoplastic cells have not metastasized.

Preiser's disease (prī′zĕrz) [Georg K.F. Preiser, Ger. orthopedic surgeon, 1879–1913] Osteoporosis caused by trauma and affecting the scaphoid bone of the wrist.

prejudice **1.** A preconceived judgment or opinion formed without factual knowledge. **2.** Irrational hostility, hatred, or suspicion of a particular group, race, or religion.

prekallikrein A cofactor in blood coagulation. SEE: *coagulation, blood.*

preleukemia Myelodysplasia (1).

preload In cardiac physiology, the end-diastolic stretch of a heart muscle fiber. In the intact ventricle, this is approx. equal to the end-diastolic volume or pressure. At the bedside, preload is estimated by measuring the central venous pressure or the pulmonary capillary wedge pressure. SEE: *afterload.*

premaniacal (prē″mā-nī′ă-kăl) [L. *prae,* before, in front of, + Gr. *mania,* madness] Prior to an attack of mania.

premature (prē-mă-chūr′) [L. *praematurus,* ripening early] Born or manifest before full development has been achieved.

premature rupture of membranes ABBR: PROM. In pregnancy, rupture of the amniotic membrane prior to the time labor was expected. This occurs in about 10% of patients. PROM is the single most common diagnosis leading to admission of the newborn to intensive care nursing.

PROM is more common in women of poor socioeconomic groups, teenagers, single women, smokers, and women who have a sexually transmitted organism cultured from the cervix or vagina in the first half of pregnancy. PROM increases the risk of intrauterine infection.

preterm p.r.o.m. ABBR: PPROM. Rupture of the fetal membranes before completion of week 37 of pregnancy. SEE: *prematurity*.

premature ventricular contraction ABBR: PVC. The contraction of the cardiac ventricle prior to the normal time, caused by an electrical impulse to the ventricle arising from a site other than the sinoatrial node. The PVC may be a single event or occur several times in a minute or in pairs or strings. Three or more PVCs in a row constitute ventricular tachycardia.

prematurity The state of an infant born any time prior to completion of the 37th week of gestation. The normal gestation period for the human being is 40 weeks. Because of the difficulty of obtaining accurate and objective data on the exact length of gestation, a birth weight of 2500 g (5.5 lb) or less has been accepted internationally as the clinical criterion of prematurity regardless of the period of gestation. Other measures suggestive of prematurity are crown-heel length (47 cm or less), crown-rump length (32 cm or less), occipitofrontal circumference (33 cm or less), occipitofrontal diameter (11.5 cm or less), and ratio of the thorax circumference to the head circumference (less than 93%).

The use of a single-criterion measure (birth weight) imposes limitations in accurately identifying those infants born before adequate development of body organs and systems has been achieved. It can easily include mature infants who are of low birth weight for reasons other than a shortened gestation period. The Expert Committee on Prematurity of the World Health Organization (1961) recommended that the concept of prematurity in the international definition be replaced by that of low birth weight. The term *low birth weight* more accurately describes infants weighing less than 2500 g at birth than does the term *prematurity*. The latter term should be reserved for those neonates within the low birth weight group with evidence of incomplete development.

In the United States approx. 7.1% white liveborn and 13.4% nonwhite liveborn infants weigh 2500 g or less. Chances of survival depend on the degree of maturity achieved, general medical condition, and quality of care received.

Prematurity is the leading cause of death in the neonatal period. Mortality among infants weighing less than 2500 g at birth is 17 times greater than among infants with birth weight above 2500 g. Chief causes of mortality are abnormal pulmonary ventilation, infection, intracranial hemorrhage, abnormal blood conditions, and congenital anomalies.

ETIOLOGY: The incidence of neonates of low birth weight is more frequent among the female sex, nonwhite races, plural births, and the first- and fifth- (and over) born infants. Delivery of infants of low birth weight is reported to be more frequent among women with one or more of the following characteristics: having their children at either a very young age or between ages 45 and 49; being unmarried; having children closely spaced (i.e., less than 2 to 4 years between births); and living in a large urban area.

Another factor associated with low birth weight is the socioeconomic status of the family as measured by the mother's educational attainment. The proportion of infants of low birth weight born to mothers with 16 years or more of education was half of that of infants born to mothers with less than 9 years of education. Low birth weight is also associated with generally elevated risk of infant mortality, congenital malformations, mental retardation, and various other physical and neurological impairments.

COMPLICATIONS: Frequently, premature infants are handicapped by a number of anatomical and physiological limitations. These limitations vary in direct proportion to the degree of immaturity present. Limitations include weakness of the sucking and swallowing reflexes, small capacity of stomach, impairment of renal function, incomplete development of capillaries of the lungs, immature alveoli of the lungs, weakness of the cough and gag reflexes, weakness of the thoracic cage muscles and other muscles used in respiration, inadequate regulation of body temperature, incomplete or poorly developed enzyme systems, hepatic immaturity, and deficient placental transfer and antenatal storage of minerals, vitamins, and immune substances. SEE: *intrauterine growth retardation; premature rupture of membranes*.

PATIENT CARE: A physical assessment correlated with the expected maturation for fetal age is performed. Health care providers perform a neurological evaluation, obtain an Apgar score, ensure proper environmental temperature, provide proper fluid and caloric intake, ensure parental bonding and support, assess laboratory reports, monitor intake and output, notify the nursery of the premature birth, weigh the infant daily at the same time without clothing and on the same scale, monitor oxygen concentration at frequent intervals, hold and cuddle the infant during feedings, cover the infant when removing from isolette, and provide adequate time for feeding.

Care of low-birth-weight infants: Care of low-birth-weight infants should be individualized and reflect the needs of the developing infant with regard to anatomical and physiological handicaps. Evaluation for degree of immaturity and identification of special problems after birth dictates care required by these infants. In general, care centers on prevention of infection, stabilization of body temperature, maintenance of respiration, and provision of adequate nutrition and hydration.

Aseptic technique is required. An incubator or heated bed provides a suitable environment for maintenance of body temperature. A high-humidity environment may be of value for infants with respiratory difficulties. Gentle nasal and pharyngeal suctioning aids in keeping airways clear. Use of oxygen should be restricted to the minimal amounts required for survival of the infant. Because of the danger of retrolental fibroplasia, the oxygen concentration should not exceed 30%.

Depending on the infant's sucking and swallowing abilities, gavage feeding may be necessary. Some of these infants may not be given anything by mouth for as long as 72 hr after birth. Caloric and fluid intakes are increased gradually until 100 to 120 cal/kg and 140 to 150 ml/kg, respectively, in 24 hr are reached. The time required to achieve these intake levels depends on the newborn's condition. The infant may require small, frequent feedings to cope with the small capacity of the stomach, to prevent vomiting and distention, and to meet the body's caloric and fluid requirements. Overfeeding should be avoided. During the early days of life, clyses are sometimes administered to maintain adequate hydration.

The infant should not be allowed to become fatigued from excessive handling, prolonged feeding procedures, or too much crying. Body position should be changed every 2 to 4 hr. Gentle handling should be practiced. The newborn and infant should receive cuddling several times a day.

Because of the possibility of retinal damage, premature infants should not be exposed to bright light.

premaxilla (prē″măk-sĭl′ă) [L. *prae,* before, in front of, + *maxilla,* jawbone] A separate bone, derived from the median nasal process embryologically, that fuses with the maxilla in humans; formerly called the incisive bone.

premaxillary (prē-măk′sĭ-lĕr″ē) Located before the maxilla.

premedication (prē″mĕd-ĭ-kā′shŭn) [″ + *medicari,* to heal] **1.** Administration of drugs before treatment to enhance the therapeutic effect and safety of a given procedure. **2.** SYN: *preanesthetic.*

premenarchal (prē″mĕ-năr′kăl) [″ + Gr. *men,* mouth, + *arche,* beginning] The time prior to the first menstrual period (i.e., prior to menarche).

premenstrual (prē-mĕn′stroo-ăl) [″ + *menstruare,* to discharge the menses] Before menstruation.

premenstrual dysphoric disorder A disorder characterized by symptoms such as markedly depressed mood, marked anxiety, marked affective lability, and decreased interest in activities. It is the current term, according to *DSM-IV,* for what was previously known as premenstrual tension syndrome.

SYMPTOMS: In patients with this disease, the symptoms occur regularly during the last week of the luteal phase in most menstrual cycles during the year preceding diagnosis. These symptoms begin to remit within a few days of the onset of the menses (the follicular phase) and are always absent the week following menses.

DIAGNOSIS: For diagnosis, five or more of the following must be present most of the time during the last week of the luteal phase, with at least one of the symptoms being one of the first four: feeling sad, hopeless, or self-deprecating; feeling tense, anxious, or "on edge"; marked lability of mood interspersed with frequent tearfulness; persistent irritability, anger, and increased interpersonal conflicts; decreased interest in usual activities, which may be associated with withdrawal from social relationships; difficulty concentrating; feeling fatigued, lethargic, or lacking in energy; marked changes in appetite, which may be associated with binge eating or craving certain foods; hypersomnia or insomnia; a subjective feeling of being overwhelmed or out of control; and physical symptoms such as breast tenderness or swelling, headaches, or sensation of "bloating" or weight gain, with tightness of fit of clothing, shoes, or rings. There may also be joint or muscle pain. The symptoms may be accompanied by suicidal thoughts.

The pattern of symptoms must have occurred most months for the previous 12 months. The symptoms disappear completely shortly after the onset of menstruation. In atypical cases, some women also have symptoms for a few days around ovulation; and a few women with short cycles might, therefore, be symptom-free for only 1 week per cycle. Women commonly report that their symptoms worsen with age until relieved by the onset of menopause.

TREATMENT: The selective serotonin reuptake inhibitors, such as fluoxetine and sertraline, but not tricyclic antidepressants, help improve symptoms of the disorder for many patients. Some people believe that symptoms are diminished by limiting one's intake of salt, refined sugars, caffeine (e.g., in chocolate, colas, and coffee), nicotine, alcohol, red meat, and animal fat, and increasing consumption of leafy green vegetables, whole-grain cereals, vitamins B_6 and E, and complex carbohydrates. The hypothesis that dietary changes influence PDD, however, has not been rigorously tested.

PATIENT CARE: Support and reassurance are offered, and the woman is encouraged to develop her own resources to help her cope with the syndrome.

premenstrual tension syndrome ABBR: PMS. Premenstrual dysphoric disorder. SEE: *Nursing Diagnoses Appendix.*

premenstruum (prē-mĕn'stroo-ŭm) [" + *menstruus,* menstrual fluid] The period of time prior to menstruation.

premise (prĕm'ĭs) A proposition or starting point that is taken as a given. SEE: *assumption.*

premium (prē'mē-uhm) A payment made periodically to a health care insurer in exchange for benefits coverage (indemnity against future expenses).

premolar (prē-mō'lĕr) [" + *moles,* a mass] One of the permanent teeth that erupt to replace the deciduous molars. They are often called bicuspid teeth, for the maxillary premolars have two cusps, whereas the mandibular premolars may have from one to three cusps. They are located between the canine and first molar of each quadrant of the dental arches. SEE: *dentition.*

premonition (prĕm"ĕ-, prē-mĕ-nĭsh'ŭn) [L. *praemonere,* to warn beforehand] A feeling of an impending event.

premonitory (prē-mŏn'ĭ-tō-rē) [LL. *praemonitorius*] Giving a warning, as an early symptom.

premonocyte (prē-mŏn'ō-sīt) [L. *prae,* before, in front of, + Gr. *monos,* alone, + *kytos,* cell] An embryonic cell transitional in development prior to a monocyte.

premorbid (prē-mor'bĭd) [" + *morbidus,* sick] Prior to the development of disease.

premyeloblast (prē-mī'ĕ-lō-blăst) [" + Gr. *myelos,* marrow, + *blastos,* germ] A precursor of the mature myeloblast.

premyelocyte (prē-mī'ĕl-ō-sīt) [" + " + *kytos,* cell] The cell that is the immediate precursor of a myelocyte.

prenarcosis (prē-năr-kō'sĭs) [" + Gr. *narkosis,* a benumbing] Preanesthetic.

prenatal (prē-nā'tl) [" + *natalis,* birth] Before birth.

prenatal care The regular monitoring and management of the health status of the pregnant woman and her fetus during the period of gestation. Comprehensive care is based on a thorough review of the woman's medical, surgical, obstetrical and gynecological, nutritional, and social history, and that of the family for indications of genetic or other risk factors. Laboratory analyses provide important data describing the woman's current health status and indications for treatment and anticipatory guidance. Periodic visits are scheduled to evaluate changes in blood pressure, weight, fundal height, fetal heart rate, and fetal activity, and to assess for any signs of emerging health problems. To enable the patient's active participation in care and to facilitate early diagnosis and prompt treatment of emerging problems, emphasis is placed on anticipatory guidance and patient teaching. The health care professional describes and discusses nutrition and diet (including the importance of folate supplementation), self-management of common minor complaints, and signs to report promptly to the primary caregiver; helps patients gain access to resources available for preparation for childbirth, breastfeeding, newborn care, and parenting; and provides support and counseling. SEE: *pregnancy; prenatal diagnosis.*

prenatal surgery Intrauterine surgical procedures. These techniques have been used to repair heart defects and anatomical defects of other organs. SEE: *prenatal diagnosis.*

preobese (prē-ō-bēs') The term used by the World Health Organization for "overweight."

preoperative care (prē-ŏp'ĕr-ă-tĭv) [" + *operatus,* work] Care preceding an operation, including the medical evaluation of the risks of surgery, and the psychological adjustment of the patient.

PATIENT CARE: Time to discuss the meaning of the procedure with the patient and to allow the patient to express concerns and fears is essential. The patient should be instructed to cough, breathe deeply (splinting incision as necessary), turn, and exercise the extremities at frequent intervals. The operative site is prepared as prescribed; the gastrointestinal tract is prepared as indicated (restrict food and fluids as ordered). Rest and sleep are promoted; laboratory results are reviewed; and preoperative medications are administered as prescribed after the patient has voided. The patient should perform oral hygiene; remove dentures, if present, as well as jewelry and make-up; and dress in a hospital gown. Proper identification on the patient identification bracelet is verified. If the patient is menstruating, the type of menstrual protection used should be noted on the chart. The patient's tampons or pads should be changed, at least every 4 to 6 hr in the case of tampons.

The patient requires guidance concerning the timing of prescribed activities, including when to return to work and athletic endeavors, when sexual activity may be resumed, and whether there will be postoperative restriction on driving automobiles.

preoptic area The anterior portion of the hypothalamus. It is above the optic chiasma and on the sides of the third ventricle.

preoral (prē-ō'răl) [L. *prae,* before, in front of, + *os,* mouth] In front of the mouth.

preoxygenation Breathing of 100% oxygen via a face mask by the fully conscious patient prior to induction of anesthesia. Duration is 2 to 7 min. In that time, the nitrogen is washed out of the lungs and oxygen replaces it.

This same procedure is used for a longer period of time in persons prior to exposure to very low atmospheric pressure (e.g., aviators prior to flying to high altitudes) or to very high atmospheric pressure (e.g., divers descending to a great depth in water). In both cases, the goal is to rid the body of nitrogen to prevent bends.

prep (prĕp) [*prepare; preparation*] Used esp. when referring to preparation for surgery. SEE: *preoperative care.*

bowel p. The administration of a clear liquid diet with laxatives, enemas, or both, in anticipation of endoscopy of the lower gastrointestinal tract to provide an optimal view of the bowel wall.

prepaid care Managed care in which a patient or group contracts for all its health care services in advance, instead of paying for each service when it is delivered.

prepalatal (prē-păl'ă-tăl) [L. *prae,* before, in front of, + *palatum,* plate] Located in front of the teeth.

preparalytic (prē"păr-ă-lĭt'ĭk) [" + Gr. *para,* at the side, + *lyein,* to loosen] Before the appearance of paralysis.

preparation (prĕp-ă-rā'shŭn) [L. *praeparatio*] **1.** The making ready, esp. of a medicine for use. **2.** A specimen set up for demonstration in anatomy, pathology, or histology. **3.** A medicine made ready for use.

cavity p. The preparation of an artificial hole in a tooth so that the tooth can be restored by use of appropriate dental materials.

chlorine p. A disinfectant solution such as Dakin's solution or Javelle water, made from hypochlorites in water.

corrosion p. In anatomical and pathology investigations, hollow organs and structures such as vessels are filled with a liquid substance that hardens. Then the surrounding tissues are dissolved by use of suitable chemicals. This leaves a cast of the structures.

heart-lung p. In animal studies and in open-heart surgery, the use of devices that take over the function of the heart and lungs while those organs are being treated or possibly replaced.

prepatellar (prē"pă-tĕl'ăr) [L. *prae,* before, in front of, + *patella,* pan] In front of the patella.

prepatellar bursitis Inflammation of the bursa in front of the patella. SYN: *housemaid's knee.* SEE: *bursitis.*

prepatent Before becoming evident or manifest.

prepatent period The period between the time of introduction of parasitic organisms into the body and their appearance in the blood or tissues.

preperception (prē"pĕr-sĕp'shŭn) [" + *percepitio,* to perceive] The anticipation of a perception. This intensifies the response to the perception.

preperitoneal (prē"pĕr-ĭ-tō-nē'ăl) [" + Gr. *peritonaion,* peritoneum] Located in front of the peritoneum.

preplacental (prē"plă-sĕn'tăl) [" + *placenta,* a flat cake] Occurring prior to formation of the placenta.

prepotent (prē-pō'tĕnt) [" + *potentia,* power] Pert. to the greater power of one parent to transmit inherited characteristics to the offspring.

preprandial (prē-prăn'dē-ăl) [" + *prandium,* breakfast] Before a meal.

prepuberal, prepubertal (prē-pū'bĕr-ăl, -tăl) [" + *pubertas,* puberty] Before puberty.

prepubescent (prē"pū-bĕs'ĕnt) [" + *pubescens,* becoming hairy] Pert. to the period just before puberty.

prepuce (prē'pūs) [L. *praeputium,* prepuce] Foreskin.

p. of the clitoris A fold of the labia minora that covers the clitoris. SEE: *clitoris.*

preputial (prē-pū'shăl) Concerning the prepuce.

preputial gland Tyson's gland.

preputiotomy (prē-pū"shē-ŏt'ō-mē) [" + Gr. *tome,* incision] Incision of the prepuce of the penis to relieve phimosis.

preputium (prē-pū'shē-ŭm) *pl.* **preputia** Prepuce.

p. clitoridis The prepuce of the clitoris.

p. penis Foreskin.

prepyloric (prē"pī-lor'ĭk) Anterior to, or preceding, the pylorus of the stomach.

prerectal (prē-rĕk'tăl) [L. *prae,* before, + *rectus,* straight] Located in front of the rectum.

prerenal (prē-rē'năl) [" + *ren,* kidney] **1.** Located in front of the kidney. **2.** Occurring prior to reaching the kidney, such as changes in consistency of the blood prior to its flow to the kidney.

preretinal (prē-rĕt'ĭ-năl) [" + *retina,* retina] In front of the retina of the eye.

presacral (prē-sā′krăl) [″ + *sacrum,* sacred] In front of the sacrum.

presby- Combining form meaning *old.*

presbyacusia, presbyacousia (prĕz″bē-ă-kū′sē-ă) [Gr. *presbys,* old, + *akousis,* hearing] Presbycusis.

presbyatrics, presbyatry (prĕz-bē-ăt′rĭks, prĕz′bē-ăt-rē) [″ + *iatrikos,* healing] An infrequently used synonym for geriatrics.

presbycardia (prĕz-bĭ-kăr′dē-ă) [″ + *kardia,* heart] Decreased functional capacity of the heart, as a result of age-related muscular hypertrophy, loss of myocytes, and decreased cardiac elasticity and compliance.

presbycusis, presbykousis (prĕz-bĭ-kū′sĭs) [″ + *akousis,* hearing] The progressive loss of hearing due to the normal aging process, especially for high-pitched sounds. The use of amplifiers (hearing aids) may help affected patients maintain active social interactions with others. SYN: *presbyacusia.*

presbyope (prĕs′bē-ōp) [″ + *ops,* eye] A person who is presbyopic.

presbyopia (prĕz-bē-ō′pē-ă) [″ + *ops,* eye] The permanent loss of accommodation of the crystalline lens of the eye that occurs when people are in their mid-40s, marked by the inability to maintain focus on objects held near to the eye (i.e., at reading distance). SEE: *farsightedness.*

presbyopic (prĕs″bē-ŏp′ĭk) Concerning presbyopia.

presbytiatrics (prĕz″bĭ-tē-ăt′rĭks) [″ + *iatrikos,* healing] Geriatrics.

prescribe (prē-skrīb′) [L. *praescriptio,* prescription] To indicate the medicine to be administered. This can be done orally but is usually done by writing a prescription or an order in the patient's hospital chart.

prescribing error An error in the choice or administration of drugs for patients. Included are incorrect dose or medicine, duplicate therapy, incorrect route of administration, or wrong patient. In one extensive study of prescriptions written by physicians in a tertiary-care teaching hospital, 0.3% were erroneous and more than half of these were rated as having the potential for adverse consequences. Monitoring of medications and patients is thought to be helpful in limiting these errors.

prescription (prē-skrĭp′shŭn) [L. *praescriptio*] A written direction or order for dispensing and administering drugs. It is signed by a physician, dentist, or other practitioner licensed by law to prescribe such a drug. Historically, a prescription consists of four main parts.

Superscription: Represented by the symbol ℞, which signifies Recipe, meaning to take.

Inscription: Containing the ingredients.

Subscription: Directions to the dispenser as to the manner of preparation of the drugs.

Signature: Directions to the patient with regard to the manner of taking dosage and the physician's signature, address, telephone number, date, and whether or not the prescription may be refilled. When applicable, the physician's Drug Enforcement Administration (DEA) number must be included. Also, some states require that the prescriber indicate on the prescription whether or not a generic drug may be substituted for the trade name equivalent.

CAUTION: Unused prescription pads should be kept in a secure place in order to prevent their being misused or stolen. Each prescription should be numbered consecutively. One should never sign a prescription blank in advance. The prescriber should use ink to prevent changes being made and not use prescription pads for writing notes or memos.

---

p. drug A drug available to the public only upon prescription written by a physician, dentist, or other practitioner licensed to do so.

shotgun p. A prescription containing many drugs, given with the hope that one of them may prove effective; it is not a recommended approach to the treatment of disease.

prescriptive authority The limited authority to prescribe certain medications according to established protocol.

presenile (prē-sē′nīl) [L. *prae,* before, in front of, + *senilis,* old] Occurring before the expected onset of age-related changes, that is, in middle age. The word is usually used to describe dementia that occurs relatively early in life.

presenium (prē-sē′nē-ŭm) [″ + *senium,* old age] Prior to the onset of senility.

present [L. *praesent,* to be present before others] The presence of the patient for examination.

presentation (prē″zĕn-tā′shŭn) [L. *praesentatio*] **1.** In obstetrics, the position of the fetus presenting itself to the examining finger in the vagina or rectum (e.g., longitudinal or normal and transverse or pathologic presentation). **2.** The relationship of the long axis of fetus to that of the mother; also called *lie.* SEE: illus.; *position* for table. **3.** The fetal body part that first enters the maternal pelvis. SEE: *position* for table.

breech p. Fetal position in which the buttocks comes first. Breech presentation is of three types: complete breech, when the thighs of the fetus are flexed on the abdomen and the legs flexed upon the thighs; frank breech, when the legs of the fetus are extended over the

ATTITUDES OF THE FETUS

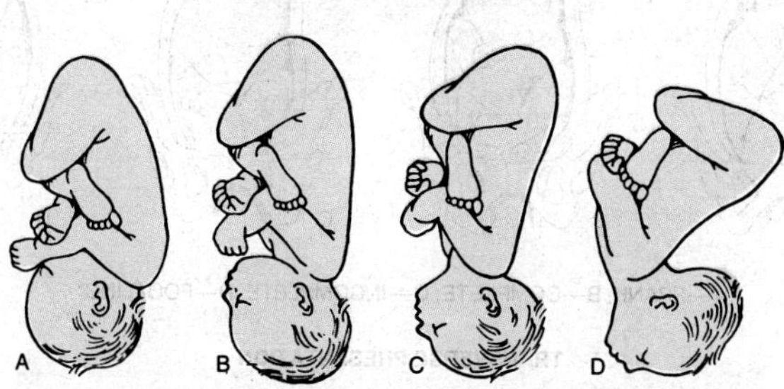

A—VERTEX PRESENTATION; B—SINCIPUT PRESENTATION; C—BROW PRESENTATION; D—FACE PRESENTATION*

BROW PRESENTATION

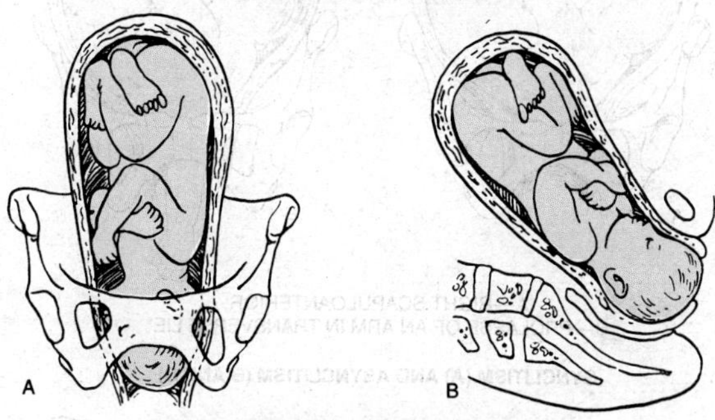

A—ANTERIOR VIEW; B—SAGITTAL VIEW*

FACE PRESENTATIONS

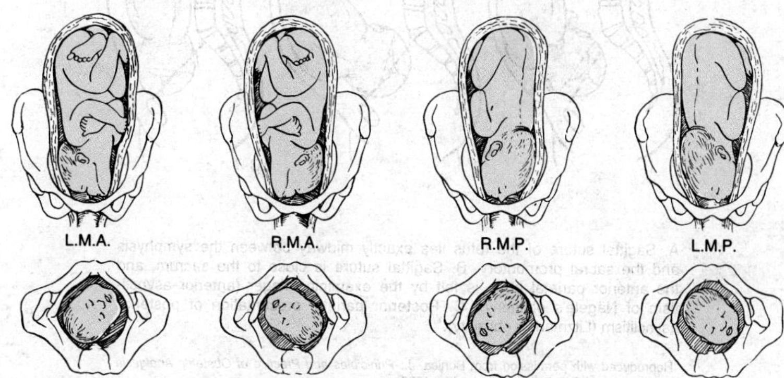

LEFT MENTOANTERIOR (L.M.A.); RIGHT MENTOANTERIOR (R.M.A.); RIGHT MENTOPOSTERIOR (R.M.P.); LEFT MENTOPOSTERIOR (L.M.P.)*

*Reproduced with permission from Bonica, J.: *Principles and Practice of Obstetric Analgesia and Anesthesia*. F.A. Davis, Philadelphia, 1972.

PRESENTATIONS OF FETUS (CONTINUED)

TYPES OF BREECH PRESENTATIONS

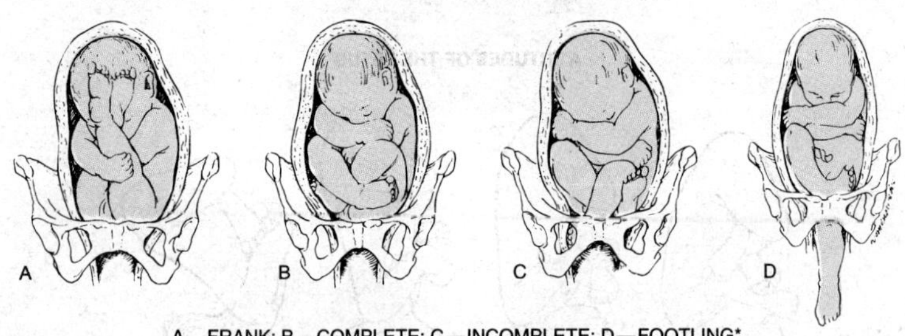

A—FRANK; B—COMPLETE; C—INCOMPLETE; D—FOOTLING*

TRANSVERSE PRESENTATION

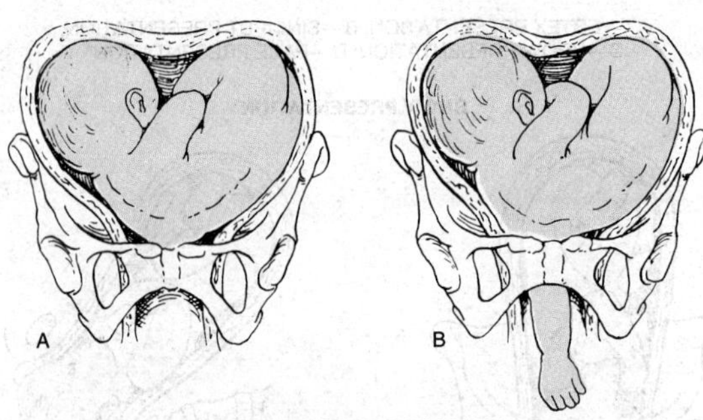

A—RIGHT SCAPULOANTERIOR;
B—PROLAPSE OF AN ARM IN TRANSVERSE LIE*

SYNCLITISM (A) AND ASYNCLITISM (B AND C)

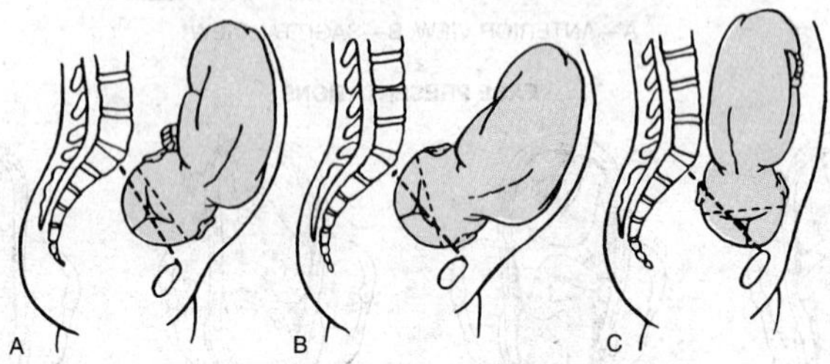

A. Sagittal suture of the fetus lies exactly midway between the symphysis and the sacral promontory. B. Sagittal suture is close to the sacrum, and the anterior parietal bone is felt by the examining finger (anterior asynclitism of Nägele's obliquity). C. Posterior parietal presentation of posterior asynclitism (Litzmann's obliquity).*

*Reproduced with permission from Bonica, J.: *Prinicíples and Practice of Obstetric Analgesia and Anesthesia*. F.A. Davis, Philadelphia, 1972.

PRESENTATIONS OF FETUS

anterior surface of the body; and footling, when a foot or feet present. Footling can be single, double, or, if the leg remains flexed, knee presentation. SYN: *pelvic p.*

brow p. Fetal position in which the brow or face of the infant comes first during labor, making vaginal delivery almost impossible. Cesarean section may be needed if the presentation cannot be altered.

cephalic p. Presentation of the head of the fetus in any position.

compound p. Fetal position in which

a prolapsed limb is alongside the main presenting part.

face p. Fetal position in which the head of the fetus is sharply extended so that the face comes first.

footling p. Fetal position in which the feet come first. SEE: *breech p.*

funic p. Appearance of the umbilical cord during labor.

longitudinal p. Presentation in which the long axis of the fetus is parallel to the long axis of the mother.

oblique p. Presentation in which the long axis of the fetus is oblique to that of the mother.

pelvic p. Breech p.

placental p. Placenta previa.

shoulder p. Presentation in which the shoulder of the fetus is the presenting part.

transverse p. Presentation with the fetus lying crosswise.

vertex p. Presentation of the upper and back part of the fetal head.

preservative (prē-zĕr′vă-tĭv) [L. *prae,* before, in front of, + *servare,* to keep] A substance added to medicines or foods to prevent them from spoiling. It may act by interfering with certain chemical reactions or with the growth of molds, fungi, bacteria, or parasites. Some common preservatives are sugar, salt, vinegar, ethyl alcohol, sulfur dioxide, and benzoic acid.

presomite (prē-sō′mīt) [″ + Gr. *soma,* body] The embryonic stage prior to the formation of somites.

presphenoid (prē-sfē′noyd) [″ + Gr. *sphen,* wedge, + *eidos,* form, shape] The anterior region of the body on the sphenoid bone.

presphygmic (prē-sfĭg′mĭk) [″ + Gr. *sphygmos,* pulse] Pert. to the period preceding the pulse wave.

prespinal (prē-spī′năl) [″ + *spina,* thorn] In front of the spine, or ventral to it.

prespondylolisthesis (prē-spŏn″dĭl-ō-lĭs-thē′sĭs) [″ + Gr. *spondylos,* vertebra, + *olisthanein,* to slip] A congenital defect of both pedicles of the fifth lumbar vertebra without displacement, predisposing the individual to spondylolisthesis.

pressor (prĕs′or) [O.Fr. *presser,* to press] **1.** Stimulating, increasing the activity of a function, esp. of vasomotor activity, as a nerve. **2.** Inducing an elevation in blood pressure. **3.** One of several drugs, such as dopamine, epinephrine, and norepinephrine, that are used to increase the blood pressure of patients in shock.

pressoreceptive (prĕs″ō-rē-sĕp′tĭv) Sensitive to pressure stimuli. SYN: *pressosensitive.*

pressoreceptor (prĕs″ō-rē-sĕp′tor) A sensory nerve ending, such as those in the aorta and carotid sinus, that is stimulated by changes in blood pressure. SYN: *baroreceptor.*

pressosensitive (prĕs″ō-sĕn′sĭ-tĭv) Pressoreceptive.

pressure (prĕsh′ŭr) [L. *pressura*] **1.** A compression. **2.** Stress or force exerted on a body, as by tension, weight, or pulling. **3.** In psychology, the quality of sensation aroused by moderate compression of the skin. **4.** In physics, the quotient obtained by dividing a force by the area of the surface on which it acts.

alveolar p. Air pressure in the alveoli and bronchial tree. It fluctuates below and above atmospheric pressure during breathing; this causes air to enter or leave the lungs. SYN: *intrapulmonic p.*

arterial p. The pressure of the blood in the arteries. For a normal young person at physical and mental rest and in sitting position, systolic blood pressure averages about 120 mm Hg; diastolic pressure about 80 mm Hg. A wide range of normal variation is due to constitutional, physical, and psychic factors. For women, the figures are slightly lower. For older people, they are higher. Normally there is little difference in the blood pressure recorded in the two arms. SEE: *blood pressure.*

atmospheric p. The pressure of the weight of the atmosphere; at sea level it averages about 760 mm Hg.

bilevel positive airway p. ABBR: BiPAP. A type of continuous positive airway pressure in which both inspiratory and expiratory pressure are set.

biting p. The pressure exerted on the teeth during biting. SYN: *occlusal p.*

blood p. SEE: *blood pressure.*

capillary p. The blood pressure in the capillaries.

central venous p. ABBR: CVP. The pressure within the superior vena cava. It reflects the pressure under which the blood is returned to the right atrium. The normal range is between 5 and 10 cm H_2O. A high CVP indicates circulatory overload (as in congestive heart failure), whereas a low CVP indicates reduced blood volume (as in hemorrhage or fluid loss). CVP can be estimated by examining the cervical veins or the dorsal veins of the hand if the neck and hand are at the level of the heart. Those veins are well filled if CVP is normal or high, and tend to collapse if it is low.

cerebrospinal p. The pressure of the cerebrospinal fluid. This varies with body position but is normally about 100 to 180 mm H_2O when the spinal canal is initially entered during lumbar puncture with the patient lying on his or her side.

continuous positive airway p. ABBR: CPAP. A method of ventilatory support applied to the spontaneously breathing patient in which airway pressure is maintained above atmospheric pressure throughout the respiratory cycle. CPAP can be applied by way of a nasal mask, a face mask, or an endotracheal tube. It can be used to treat congestive heart failure, acute pulmonary edema, obstructive sleep apnea syndrome, and other conditions. A potential adverse effect of CPAP is barotrauma to the lungs.

cricoid p. The application of manual pressure onto the cricoid cartilage during intubation and mechanical ventilation. This technique helps to occlude the esophagus and prevent the entry of air into the gastrointestinal tract during ventilation. It also diminishes the chances for regurgitation from the stomach and aspiration of gastric contents.

critical p. The pressure exerted by a vapor at its critical temperature in an evacuated container.

effective osmotic p. That portion of the total osmotic pressure of a solution that determines the tendency of the solvent to pass through a membrane, usually one that is semipermeable. The tendency is for the solvent to pass from a solution containing a high concentration of the solute to the side of the membrane with the low concentration.

end-diastolic p. Blood pressure in a ventricle of the heart at the end of diastole.

filling p. The average pressure in the atria or the ventricles at the end of diastole.

hydrostatic p. The pressure exerted by a fluid within a closed system.

intra-abdominal p. Pressure within the abdominal cavity, such as that caused by descent of the diaphragm.

intracranial p. The pressure of the cerebrospinal fluid in the subarachnoid space between the skull and the brain. The pressure is normally the same as that found during lumbar puncture.

intraocular p. Normal tension within the eyeball, equal to approx. 12 to 20 mm Hg.

intrapleural p. The pressure between the two pleural membranes. It is normally always lower than atmospheric pressure and therefore sometimes called a negative pressure. SYN: *intrathoracic p.*

intrapulmonic p. Alveolar p.

intrathoracic p. Intrapleural p.

intraventricular p. The pressure within the ventricles of the heart during different phases of diastole and systole.

negative p. Any pressure less than that of the atmosphere, or less than that pressure to which the initial pressure is being compared.

occlusal p. Biting p.

oncotic p. Osmotic pressure exerted by colloids in a solution.

opening p. ABBR: OP. The pressure of the cerebrospinal fluid that is detected just after a needle is placed into the spinal canal. It is normally 100 to 180 mm H_2O.

osmotic p. The force with which a solvent, usually water, passes through a semipermeable membrane separating solutions of different concentrations. It is measured by determining the hydrostatic (mechanical) pressure that must be opposed to the osmotic force to bring the passage to a standstill.

partial p. In a gas containing several different components, the pressure exerted by each component.

positive p. Pressure greater than atmospheric or greater than the pressure to which the initial pressure is being compared.

positive end-expiratory p. ABBR: PEEP. In respiratory medicine, a method of holding alveoli open during expiration. This is done by gradually increasing the expiratory pressure during mechanical ventilation. When PEEP is used, it is important to monitor the hemodynamic status of the patient because PEEP reduces venous return to the heart and cardiac output. The goal is to achieve adequate arterial oxygenation, without using toxic levels of oxygen and without compromising cardiac output.

CAUTION: The patient must be carefully monitored during the therapy to ensure compliance and to allow observation for undesired side effects such as pneumomediastinum, subcutaneous emphysema, and pneumothorax.

---

positive end-expiratory p., auto ABBR: auto-PEEP. A complication of mechanical ventilation in which the device does not permit the patient sufficient time to exhale. This causes air to be trapped in the lungs, particularly the alveoli. If continued, auto-PEEP causes respiratory muscle fatigue and can cause rupture of the lung (i.e., pneumothorax). Auto-PEEP may be corrected by increasing exhalation time, decreasing the ventilator rate, or switching the ventilation mode so that the patient's spontaneous respiratory pattern governs the inspiratory and expiratory times.

posterior cricoid p. Pressure applied by firmly placing the thumb and index finger on the lateral aspects of a patient's cricoid ring to occlude the esophagus. SYN: *Sellick's maneuver.*

pulse p. The difference between systolic and diastolic pressures. The systolic pressure is normally about 40 points greater than the diastolic. A pulse pressure over 50 points or under 30 points is considered abnormal.

solution p. Pressure that tends to dissolve a solid present in a solution.

static p. The pressure existing in all points in the circulation when the heart is stopped. It provides a measure of how well the circulatory bed is filled with blood.

systolic p. Arterial pressure at the time of the contraction of the ventricles.

transpulmonary p. Alveolar pressure minus pleural pressure. When normal transpulmonary pressures are exceeded, air leaks may develop.

venous p. The pressure of the blood within the veins. It is highest near the periphery, diminishing progressively from capillaries to the heart. Near the heart the venous pressure may be below zero (negative pressure) owing to negative intrathoracic pressure.

wedge p. Pressure determined by use of a fluid-filled catheter wedged in a branch of the pulmonary artery. This provides an indirect measurement of the pressure in the left atrium of the heart.

pressure of speech Loud and emphatic speech that is increased in amount, accelerated, and usually difficult or impossible to interrupt. The speech is not in response to a stimulus and may continue even though no one is listening. It may be present in manic episodes, organic brain disease, depression with agitation, psychotic disorders, and sometimes as an acute reaction to stress.

pressure point **1.** A cutaneous area that can be used for exerting pressure to control bleeding. For control of hemorrhage, pressure above the bleeding point when an artery passes over a bone may be sufficient. SEE: *bleeding* for table. **2.** An anatomical location used in shiatsu (acupressure) to relieve pain or improve the health of organs or tissues.

equal p. p. During forced exhalation, the point at an airway where the pressure inside the wall equals the intrapleural pressure. The pleural pressure is greater than the pressure inside the airway, tending to cause bronchiolar collapse.

pressure sore Damage to the skin or underlying structures as a result of tissue compression and inadequate perfusion. Pressure ulcers typically occur in patients who are bed or chair bound. Patients with sensory and mobility deficits (e.g., individuals with spinal cord injury, stroke, or coma); malnourished patients; patients with peripheral vascular disease; hospitalized elderly patients; and nursing home residents are all at risk. Some evidence also suggests that incontinence is a risk factor.

The most common sites of skin breakdown are over bony prominences (i.e., the sacrum and the trochanters, the heels, the lateral malleoli). The combination of pressure, shearing forces, friction, and moisture leads to tissue injury and occasionally necrosis. If not treated vigorously, the ulcer will progress from a simple red patch of skin to erosion into the subcutaneous tissues, eventually extending to muscle or bone. Deep ulcers often become infected with bacteria and develop gangrene. SEE: illus.

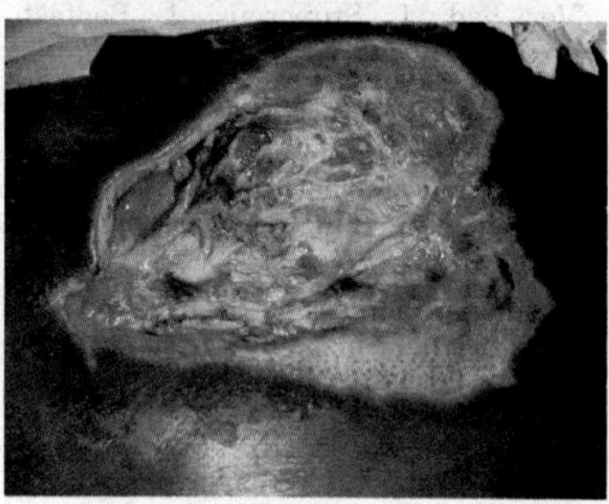

PRESSURE SORE

TREATMENT AND PREVENTION: The most important principle of therapy is to prevent the initial skin damage that promotes ulceration. In patients at risk, aggressive nursing practices, such as frequent turning of immobile patients and the application of skin protection to bony body parts, frequently are effective. Specialized air-fluid beds, waterbeds, or beds with polystyrene beads provide expensive but effective prophylaxis as well. Once ulcers have formed, topical treatments with occlusive hydrocolloid dressings, polyurethane films, and antibiotic ointments aid the healing of partial-thickness sores. Deeper lesions may need surgical débridement.

PATIENT CARE: In at-risk patients (one method of determining patient risk is with simple assessment tools, such as the Norton scale), decubiti can be prevented by inspecting the skin regularly for redness and signs of breakdown, documenting findings, and instituting any preventive measures or treatment. Reddened areas should not be massaged because this can damage ischemic deep layers of tissue. The skin is thoroughly cleansed, rinsed, and dried, and emollients are gently applied by minimizing the force and friction used, esp. over bony prominences. The patient is repositioned every 1 to 2 hr with a turning sheet or pad and by lifting rather than sliding to relieve pressure. Raising the head higher than 30 degrees except for short periods should be avoided to decrease shearing forces. Range-of-motion exercises are provided, early ambulation is encouraged, and nutritious high-protein meals are offered. Low-pressure mattresses and special beds are kept in proper working order. Doughnut-type

The Norton Scale*

Physical Condition		Mental State		Activity		Mobility		Incontinence	
Good	4	Alert	4	Ambulatory	4	Full	4	Not	4
Fair	3	Apathetic	3	Walks with help	3	Slightly limited	3	Occasionally	3
Poor	2	Confused	2	Chairbound	2	Very limited	2	Usually urinary	2
Very bad	1	Stuporous	1	Bedfast	1	Immobile	1	Double	1

* The patient is rated from 1 to 4 on the five risk factors listed. A score ≤14 indicates risk for decubitus ulcers, or pressure sores.

SOURCE: Doreen Norton, Rhoda McLaren, and A.N. Exton-Smith. An investigation of geriatric nursing problems in the hospital. London: National Corporation for the Care of Old People (now the Centre for Policy on Ageing), 1962.

cushions should not be used because they decrease blood flow to tissues resting in the center of the doughnut. SEE: table.

Ulcers are cleansed and débrided, and other therapeutic measures are instituted according to institutional protocol or prescription. Topical agents include absorbable gelatin sponges, karaya gum patches, antiseptic irrigations, air-permeable occlusive clear dressings that allow aspiration of collected fluid, supportive adhesive-backed foam padding, surgical débridement, proteolytic enzyme débriding agents, and absorptive dextranomer beads. Continuity of care is probably more important than the agent used; the nurse's main efforts are directed at relieving pressure and preventing further damage. SYN: *decubitus ulcer*. SEE: *Nursing Diagnoses Appendix*.

presternum (prē-stĕr′nŭm) [L. *prae,* before, in front of, + Gr. *sternon,* chest] The upper part of the sternum. SYN: *manubrium sterni*.

presuppurative (prē-sŭp′ū-rā″tĭv) [″ + *sub,* under, + *puris,* pus] Relating to the period of inflammation before suppuration.

presylvian fissure (prē-sĭl′vē-ăn) The anterior division of the sylvian fissure.

presymptomatic (prē″sĭmp-tō-măt′ĭk) The state of health prior to the clinical appearance of the signs and symptoms of a disease.

presynaptic (prē″sĭ-năp′tĭk) [″ + Gr. *synapsis,* point of contact] Located before the nerve synapse.

presyncope Near fainting; the sensation that one is about to pass out.

presystole (prē-sĭs′tō-lē) [L. *prae,* before, in front of, + Gr. *systole,* contraction] The period in the heart's cycle just before the systole. SYN: *perisystole*.

presystolic (prē-sĭs-tŏl′ĭk) Before the systole of the heart.

pretarsal (prē-tăr′săl) [″ + Gr. *tarsos,* a broad flat surface] In front of the tarsus.

preterm In obstetrics, occurring prior to the 37th week of gestation. SYN: *premature*.

preterm birth Delivery occurring between 20 and 38 weeks' gestation. Neonatal morbidity and mortality are high because of physiological immaturity. Preterm neonates are at high risk for developing respiratory distress syndrome; intraventricular hemorrhage; sepsis; patent ductus arteriosus; retinopathy of prematurity; and necrotizing enterocolitis. SEE: *prematurity; preterm labor*.

TREATMENT: When there is a risk of birth occurring between 24 and 34 weeks' gestation, corticosteroid therapy to stimulate fetal lung maturation and production of pulmonary surfactant should be considered; however, birth must occur in no less than 24 hr after administration. Therapy should be repeated weekly until 34 weeks' gestation. There is no evidence that this treatment is harmful to fetuses of either gender.

CONTRAINDICATIONS: Corticosteroid therapy should not be administered if the mother has chorioamnionitis or if there is evidence that the drug will have an adverse effect on the mother. Caution is recommended in women who have diabetes mellitus and/or hypertension.

preterm labor SEE: under *labor*.

pretibial (prē-tĭb′ē-ăl) [″ + *tibia,* shinbone] In front of the tibia.

pretibial fever A form of leptospirosis caused by one of the several serotypes of the autumnalis serogroup. It is characterized by fever, a rash on the legs, prostration, splenomegaly, and respiratory disturbances. SYN: *Fort Bragg fever*.

pretreatment **1.** A priming treatment given before the main course of therapy or the main chemical modification of a substance. **2.** Before therapy.

wastewater p. In environmental practice, acting to attempt to eliminate, reduce, or alter polluted water after it enters the water treatment works.

pretympanic (prē″tĭm-păn′ĭk) [″ + *tympanon,* drum] Located in front of the tympanic membrane.

preurethritis (prē″ū-rē-thrī′tĭs) [″ + Gr. *ourethra,* urethra, + *itis,* inflammation] Inflammation around the urethral orifice of the vaginal vestibule.

prevalence (prĕv′ă-lĕns) [L. *praevalens,* prevail] The number of cases of a disease present in a specified population at a given time. SEE: *incidence*.

prevention (prē-vĕn′shŭn) The anticipation and forestallment of harm, disease, or injury. SEE: *p. medicine; p. nursing*. **preventive,** *adj.*

primary p. Limiting the spread of illness to previously unaffected patients or populations.

p. paradox A preventive measure that brings benefits to the community at large but affords little benefit to each participating individual.

secondary p. Limiting the impact or the recurrence of an illness in patients already afflicted by it.

preventive (prē-vĕn′tĭv) [ME. *preventen,* to anticipate] Hindering the occurrence of something, esp. disease. SYN: *prophylactic* (1).

preventive medicine The anticipation and thwarting of disease in individuals and populations. SEE: *prevention; preventive nursing*.

preventive nursing The branch of nursing concerned with preventing the occurrence of both mental and physical illness and disease. The nurse is an essential part of the health care team and has the opportunity to emphasize and indeed implement health care services to promote health and prevent disease. Nursing expertise and general professional competence can also be used in supporting community action at all levels for promoting public health measures. There are three levels of preventive nursing:

A. Primary. Nursing care aimed at general health promotion. This includes whatever intervention is required to provide a health-promoting environment at home, in the schools, in public places, and in the workplace by ensuring good nutrition, adequate clothing and shelter, rest and recreation, and health education (including sex education and, for the aging, realistic plans for retirement). Areas of emphasis are specific protective measures such as immunizations, environmental sanitation, accident prevention, and protection from occupational hazards. Changes in lifestyle through behavior therapy, though difficult, must be attempted with respect to those areas known to represent major health risk factors (i.e., smoking, obesity, sedentary lifestyle, improper diet, alcohol and drug abuse, sexual promiscuity and not practicing safe sex, and falls). Major efforts must be made to prevent automobile accidents.

B. Secondary. Nursing care aimed at early recognition and treatment of disease. It includes general nursing interventions and teaching of early signs of disease conditions. Infectious diseases, glaucoma, obesity, and cancer fall into this category.

C. Tertiary. Nursing care for patients with incurable diseases, and patient instruction concerning how to manage those conditions and diseases. Parkinson's disease, multiple sclerosis, and cancer are conditions that lend themselves to tertiary prevention. The goal is to prevent further deterioration of physical and mental function, and to have the patient use whatever residual function is available for maximum enjoyment of and participation in life's activities. Rehabilitation is an essential part of tertiary prevention. SEE: *preventive medicine; public health*.

prevertebral (prē-vĕr′tē-brăl) [L. *prae,* before, in front of, + *vertebra,* vertebra] In front of a vertebra.

prevertebral ganglion Any of the ganglia of the sympathetic division of the autonomic nervous system, located near origins of the celiac and mesenteric arteries. These include the celiac and mesenteric ganglia. SYN: *ganglion, collateral*.

prevertiginous (prē-vĕr-tĭj′ĭ-nŭs) [″ + *vertigo,* a turning round] Giddiness or dizziness rather than true vertigo.

prevesical (prē-vĕs′ĭ-kl) [″ + *vesica,* bladder] Located in front of the bladder.

previa, praevia (prē′vē-ă) [L.] Appearing before or in front of.

previable Pert. to a fetus not sufficiently mature to survive outside the uterus.

prevocational evaluation In rehabilitation, the assessment of those interests, aptitudes, abilities, and behavioral traits that are necessary for developing or performing specific job skills.

prezonular Pert. to the posterior chamber of the eye, the space between the iris and ciliary zonule (suspensory ligament).

prezygotic (prē-zī-gŏt′ĭk) [″ + *zygotos,* yoked] Happening prior to fertilization of the ovum.

priapism (prī′ă-pĭzm) [LL. *priapismus*] Abnormal, painful, and continued erection of the penis caused by disease, occurring usually without sexual desire. SEE: *erection; gonorrhea*.

ETIOLOGY: It may be due to lesions of the cord above the lumbar region; turgescence of the corpora cavernosa without erection may exist. It may be reflex from peripheral sensory irritants, from organic irritation of nerve tracts or nerve centers when libido may be lacking. It is sometimes seen in patients as a complication of sickle cell disease or acute leukemia. It can also be due to medicines injected into the penis to promote erection.

stuttering p. Painful, recurrent attacks of priapism that last 2 to 6 hr. The condition is seen in some patients with homozygous sickle cell disease.

priapitis (prī-ă-pī′tĭs) [Gr. *priapos,* phallus, + *itis,* inflammation] Inflammation of the penis.

priapus (prī′ă-pŭs) [Gr. *priapos*] Penis.

prickly heat Miliaria rubra; an inflamed papular or vesicular rash that results when the flow of sweat from sweat glands is blocked.

prilocaine hydrochloride (prĭl′ō-kān) A local anesthetic. It may cause methemoglobinemia.

primal scene In psychiatry, the term for a child's first observation of sexual intercourse, real or imagined.

primary (prī′mă-rē) [L. *primarius,* principal] First in time or order. SYN: *principal.*

primary bubo An inflamed lymph node that represents the initial lesion following exposure to a venereal disease, esp. to syphilis. Also called *bubon d'emblée.*

primary care, primary health care Integrated, accessible health care, provided where the patient first seeks medical assistance, by clinicians who are responsible for most of a patient's personal health care, including health maintenance, therapy during illnesses, and consultation with specialists.

primary cell In physical therapy, a device consisting of a container, two solid conducting elements, and an electrolyte for the production of electric current by chemical energy.

primary health care Primary care.

primary nursing The nursing practice system in which the entire nursing care of a patient is managed and coordinated by one nurse for a 24-hr period. The nurse is involved in, manages, and coordinates all aspects of the patient's care in that period. This includes scheduling of activities, tests, and procedures.

primary radiation That radiation being emitted directly to the patient from the x-ray source.

primary sore The initial sore or hard chancre of syphilis.

primate (prī′māt) [L. *primus,* first] A member of the order Primates.

Primates (prī-mā′tēz) An order of vertebrates belonging to the class Mammalia, subclass Theria, including the lemurs, tarsiers, monkeys, apes, and humans. This order is most highly developed with respect to the brain and nervous system.

prime (prīm) [L. *primus,* first] **1.** The period of greatest health and strength. **2.** To give an initial treatment in preparation for either a larger dose of the same medicine, or a different medicine.

primidone (prĭm′ĭ-dōn) An anticonvulsive drug used in treating epilepsy.

primigravida (prī-mĭ-grăv′ĭ-dă) [″ + *gravida,* pregnant] A woman during her first pregnancy.

elderly p. A woman who is 35 years of age or older and pregnant for the first time. In the past, women were informed that delaying childbearing until age 35 or more would greatly increase the chance of an adverse outcome of pregnancy. A well-controlled study of the outcome of first pregnancy in this age group indicates little, if any, increased risk of adverse fetal outcome. The women themselves had significantly more antepartum and intrapartum complications than younger women. The women studied were private patients who were predominantly white, college educated, married, nonsmoking, and had had excellent prenatal care.

primipara (prī-mĭp′ă-ră) [″ + *parere,* to bring forth, to bear] A woman who has been delivered of one infant of 500 g (or of 20 weeks' gestation), regardless of its viability.

primiparous (prī-mĭp′ă-rŭs) Pert. to a primipara.

primitiae (prī-mĭsh′ē-ē) [L. *primus,* first] Liquor amnii appearing just before the birth of the fetus. SEE: *amnion; bag of waters; labor; liquor amnii.*

primitive (prĭm′ĭ-tĭv) [L. *primitivus*] Original; early in point of time; embryonic.

primitive streak In embryology, the initial band of cells from which the embryo begins to develop. These cells are at the caudal end of the embryonic disk. It is present at about 15 days after fertilization.

primordial (prī-mor′dē-ăl) [L. *primordialis*] **1.** Existing first. **2.** Existing in an undeveloped, primitive, or early form.

primordium (prī-mor′dē-ŭm) *pl.* **primordia** [L., origin] The first accumulation of cells in an embryo that constitutes the beginning of a future tissue, organ, or part. SYN: *anlage.*

primum non nocere (prī″mŭm nōn nō′sĕ-rā) [L.] "First do no harm," the goal in health care, of avoiding actions that may worsen a patient's disease or suffering. SEE: *risk-benefit analysis.*

princeps (prĭn′sĕps) [L., chief] **1.** Original; first. **2.** The name of certain arteries (e.g., princeps cervicis). **3.** Chief, principal.

principal (prĭn′sĭ-păl) **1.** Chief. **2.** Outstanding.

principal fibers of the periodontal ligament ABBR: PDL. The oriented bundles of collagen fibers that, by their attachments and position within the periodontal ligament space, are recognized as specific parts of the alveolodental ligament. Bundles of PDL fibers are named according to orientation and attachment.

principle (prĭn′sĭ-pl) [L. *principium,*

foundation] **1.** A constituent of a compound representing its essential properties. **2.** A fundamental truth. **3.** An established rule of action.

active p. The portion of a pharmaceutical preparation that produces the therapeutic action.

antidiuretic p. A term formerly used to indicate "antidiuretic hormone." SEE: *antidiuretic hormone.*

gastrointestinal p. An archaic term used to denote hormones, such as cholecystokinin, gastrin, and secretin, which are secreted by mucosal cells of the gastrointestinal tract and absorbed into the blood.

oxytocic p. An obsolete term for oxytoxin.

pleasure p. In psychoanalysis, the idea that unconsciously the individual is striving to attain pleasure and avoid painful situations.

proximate p. An obsolete term for a substance that may be extracted from its complex form without destroying or altering its chemical properties.

reality p. In psychoanalysis, the idea that the striving for pleasure is balanced by the situations produced by the real world.

Prinzmetal's angina [Myron Prinzmetal, U.S. cardiologist, b. 1908] Chest pain caused by vasospasm of the coronary arteries. It typically occurs while the patient is at rest rather than during exertion and may occur in patients with anatomically normal-appearing coronary arteries. An electrocardiogram taken during an attack will show ST-segment elevation, rather than the ST-segment depression seen in typical angina pectoris. Nitroglycerin and calcium channel blocking agents relieve the spasm of the arteries and the associated symptoms. SYN: *variant angina.*

prion (prē'ŏn) A small proteinaceous infection particle that is believed to be responsible for central nervous system diseases (*spongiform encephalopathies*) in humans.

prion disease Any transmissible neurodegenerative disease believed to be caused by a proteinaceous infectious particle (also known as prion proteins, or PrPs). PrPs change other cellular proteins, producing intracellular vacuoles ("spongiform change") that disrupt the functioning of neurons. Included in this group are Creutzfeldt-Jacob disease, Gerstmann-Strüssler-Scheinker syndrome, kuru, and fatal familial insomnia in humans, mad cow disease (bovine spongiform encephalopathy), and scrapie in sheep and goats. Prion diseases may be transmitted by hereditary changes in the gene coding PrP; by contaminated biological agents such as plasma or serum, human growth hormone, and organ transplants; and possibly, by eating the flesh of infected animals. All prion diseases are characterized by a long incubation period, followed by a rapidly progressive dementia. SYN: *transmissible spongiform encephalopathy.* SEE: *Creutzfeldt-Jakob disease; fatal familial insomnia; Gerstmann-Sträussler-Scheinker syndrome; kuru.*

prior authorization The approval by an insurer or other third-party payor of a health care service before the service is rendered. This approval is required in order for the insurer to pay the provider for the service.

prism (prĭzm) [Gr. *prisma*] A transparent solid, three sides of which are parallelograms. The bases, perpendicular to the three sides, are triangles, and a transverse section of the solid is a triangle. Light rays going through a prism are deflected toward the base of the triangle and at the same time are split into the primary colors.

enamel p. A minute rod of calcareous material deposited at the end of an ameloblast in the formation of the enamel of a tooth.

Maddox p. Two base-together prisms used in testing for cyclophoria or torsion of the eyeball.

Nicol p. A prism made by splitting a prism of Icelandic spar and rejoining the cut surfaces. This causes the light passing through to be split. Ordinary light rays are reflected by the joined surfaces, and polarized light is transmitted.

Risley's rotary p. A prism mounted in a device that allows it to be rotated. This is used in testing eye muscle imbalance.

prismatic (prĭz-măt'ĭk) **1.** Shaped like a prism. **2.** Produced by a prism.

prismoid (prĭz'moyd) [" + *eidos,* form, shape] Resembling a prism.

prismoptometer (prĭz-mŏp-tŏm'ĕ-tĕr) [" + *opsis,* vision, + *metron,* measure] A device for estimating abnormal refraction of the eye by using prisms.

privacy In the medical context, the rights of a patient to control the distribution and release of data concerning his or her illness. This includes information the patient has provided to the health care professionals and all additional information contained in the chart, medical records, and laboratory data. Failure to observe this aspect of a patient's rights is classed as an invasion of privacy.

private patient A patient whose care is the responsibility of one identifiable health care professional, usually a physician or dentist. The health care professional is paid directly, either by the patient or by the patient's insurer.

private practice The practice by a health care professional, usually a physician or dentist, in a setting in which the practice and the practitioner are independent of external policy control other than ethics of the professional and state licensing laws.

privileged communication Confidential information furnished (to facilitate diagnosis and treatment) by the patient to a professional authorized by law to provide care and treatment. In some states, the person who has received this communication cannot be made to divulge it. When this is the case, communication between the patient and the recipient is classed as privileged.

Information given by the patient with the family present may not be considered privileged.

p.r.n. L. *pro re nata,;* according to circumstances; as necessary. Frequently used in prescription and order writing.

pro- [L., Gr. *pro,* before] Prefix indicating *for, in front of, before, from, in behalf of, on account of.* SEE: also *ante-; pre-*.

proaccelerin The fifth factor (factor V) in blood coagulation. SEE: *coagulation factor*.

proagglutinoid (prō″ă-gloo′tĭ-noyd) An agglutinoid having a greater affinity for the agglutinogen than that possessed by the agglutinin.

proal (prō′ăl) [Gr. *pro,* before] Concerning forward movement.

proamnion (prō-ăm′nē-ŏn) [Gr. *pro,* before, + *amnion,* amnion] A region anterior to the head in a vertebrate embryo in which mesoderm is lacking.

proarrhythmia An arrhythmia that is stimulated, provoked, or worsened by drug therapy. **proarrhythmic,** *adj.*

proatlas (prō-ăt′lăs) [″ + *atlas,* a support] A rudimentary vertebra in front of the atlas of small animals. It may be present as an anomaly in the understructure of the occipital bone in humans.

probability The ratio that expresses the likelihood of the occurrence of a specific event. The probability of a tossed coin landing head side up is one-half or 50%, as is the probability of the tail side landing up. This 50% probability remains the same each time a coin is tossed. Probability ratios based on sophisticated techniques are used for estimating the chance of occurrence of diseases in a population and in projecting vital statistics such as birth and death rates.

proband [L. *probare,* to test] The initial subject presenting a mental or physical disorder, who causes a study of his or her heredity in order to determine if other members of the family have had the same disease or carry it. SYN: *index case; propositus*.

probang (prō′băng) A slim, flexible rod with a sponge or similar material attached to the end; used for determining the location of strictures in the larynx or esophagus and for removing objects from the trachea. Medicines may also be applied to these areas by use of this device.

probationer (prō-bā′shŭn-ĕr) A person working during a trial period, as a student nurse just after entering training.

probe (prōb) [L. *probare,* to test] An instrument, usually flexible, for exploring the depth and direction of a wound or sinus.

dental p. A sharp, pointed hand instrument used to examine the surface features of teeth and dental restorations for irregularities, cracks, and soft or carious enamel. SYN: *dental explorer*.

Florida p. A periodontal probe connected to a computer that measures the depth of periodontal pockets automatically.

heater p. A surgical instrument that is advanced through an endoscope and used to cauterize bleeding peptic ulcers. The probe applies thermal energy directly to the bleeding vessel, and works best when it is pressed forcefully onto the lesion.

periodontal p. A fine-caliber probe, calibrated in millimeters, designed and used to measure the depth and extent of the gingival sulcus and periodontal pockets present.

probenecid A drug used occasionally to treat gout. It prevents the reabsorption of many chemicals by the kidney, including uric acid and penicillin.

probity Rectitude, integrity, or honesty; a characteristic expected of professionals.

problem-oriented medical record ABBR: POMR. Method of establishing and maintaining the patient's medical record so that problems are clearly listed, usually in order of importance, and a rational plan for dealing with them is stated. These data are kept at the front of the chart and are evaluated as frequently as indicated with respect to recording changes in the patient's status as well as progress made in solving the problems. Use of this system may bring a degree of comprehensiveness to total patient care that might not be possible with conventional medical records.

problem-oriented record ABBR: POR. SEE: *problem-oriented medical record.*

pro bono publico Rendered for the public good (i.e., without financial reward).

probucol (prō′bū-kōl) An antihypercholesteremic drug.

procainamide hydrochloride An antiarrhythmic drug used to treat atrial and ventricular cardiac rhythm disturbances; its adverse effects may include proarrhythmia and lupus-like syndromes, among others.

procaine hydrochloride (prō′kān) A local anesthetic agent.

procarbazine hydrochloride (prō-kăr′bă-zēn) A cytotoxic drug used in treating Hodgkin's disease and certain other neoplastic diseases.

procarboxypeptidase (prō″kăr-bŏk″sē-pĕp′tĭ-dās) The inactive precursor of carboxypeptidase, which is activated by trypsin.

procaryote (prō-kăr′ē-ōt) [Gr. *pro,* before, + *karyon,* nucleus] Prokaryote.

procedure (prō-sē′dūr) [L. *procedere,* to proceed] A particular way of accomplishing a desired result.

staged p. Any operation undertaken in two or more separate parts, with a lull between the two stages to facilitate tissue healing or clearance of infection.

procentriole (prō-sĕn′trē-ōl) The early form of the centrioles and ciliary basal bodies in the cell. SEE: *centriole.*

procephalic (prō″sē-făl′ĭk) [″ + *kephale,* head] Of, or relating to, the anterior part of the head.

procercoid (prō-sĕr′koyd) The first larval stage in the development of certain cestodes belonging to the order Pseudophyllidea. It is an elongated structure that develops in crustaceans.

procerus muscle A muscle that arises in the skin over the nose and is connected to the forehead. It acts to draw the eyebrows down.

process (prŏs′ĕs) [L. *processus,* going before] **1.** A method of action. **2.** The state of progress of a disease. **3.** A projection or outgrowth of bone or tissue. SYN: *processus.* **4.** A series of steps or events that lead to achievement of specific results.

acromion p. Acromion.

alar p. The process of the cribriform plate of the ethmoid bone that articulates with the frontal bone.

alveolar p. The portion of the mandible and maxilla containing the tooth sockets. SYN: *alveolar bone.*

articular p. of vertebra One of four processes (two superior and two inferior) by which vertebrae articulate with each other.

basilar p. The narrow part of the base of the occipital bone, in front of the foramen magnum, articulating with the sphenoid bone. SYN: *pars basilaris ossis occipitalis.*

caudate p. The process of the caudate lobe of the liver extending under the right lobe.

ciliary p. One of about 70 prominent meridional ridges projecting from the corona ciliaris of the choroid coat of the eye to which the suspensory ligament of the lens is attached. These have the same structure as the rest of the choroid and secrete nutrient fluids that nourish neighboring parts, the cornea, and lens.

clinoid p. One of the three processes of the sphenoid bone: anterior, middle, and posterior clinoid.

condyloid p. A posterior process on the superior border of the ramus of the mandible consisting of a capitulum and neck. It articulates with the mandibular fossa of the temporal bone.

coracoid p. A beak-shaped process extending upward and laterally from the neck of the scapula.

coronoid p. **1.** The process on the proximal end of the ulna that forms the anterior portion of the semilunar notch. **2.** The process on the anterior upper end of the ramus of the mandible that serves for attachment of the temporalis muscle.

ensiform p. Xiphoid p.

ethmoidal p. A small process on the superior border of the inferior concha that articulates with the uncinate process of the ethmoid.

falciform p. An extension of the posterior edge of the sacrotuberous ligament to the ramus of the ischium.

frontal p. An upward projection of the maxilla that articulates with the frontal bone; forms part of the orbit and nasal fossa.

frontonasal p. In the area of the primitive mouth of the embryo, a median swelling that is the precursor of the nose, upper lip, and front part of the palate.

frontosphenoidal p. The upward-projecting process of the zygomatic bone.

head p. An axial strand of cells in vertebrate embryos extending forward from the primitive knot. It forms a primitive axis about which the embryo differentiates.

horizontal p. The part of the palatine bone that fuses with its counterpart at the midline to form the dorsal extension of the hard palate.

infraorbital p. The medially projecting process of the zygomatic bone that articulates with the maxilla. It forms the inferior lateral margin of orbit.

jugal p. A temporal bone process forming the zygomatic arch. SYN: *zygomatic p.*

jugular p. A process of the occipital bone lying lateral to the occipital condyle.

lacrimal p. A short process of the inferior concha that articulates with the lacrimal bone.

lenticular p. A knob on the incus in the middle ear that articulates with the stapes.

malar p. A projection from the maxilla that articulates with the zygomatic bone.

mandibular p. The posterior portion of the first branchial arch from which the lower jaw develops.

mastoid p. A projection of the mastoid portion of the temporal bone.

maxillary p. **1.** The anterior portion of the first branchial arch, which, with medial nasal processes, forms the upper jaw. **2.** The process of the inferior nasal concha extending laterally and covering the orifice of the antrum. **3.** A process on the anterior border of the perpendicular portion of the palatine bone.

nursing p. SEE: *nursing process.*

odontoid p. A toothlike process extending upward from the axis and about which the atlas rotates. SYN: *dens.*

olecranon p. The olecranon, an extension at the proximal end of the ulna.

orbital p. **1.** The process at the tip of the perpendicular portion of the palatine bone directed upward and backward. **2.** The process of the zygomatic bone that forms the anterior boundary of the temporal fossa.

palatine p. A process extending transversely from the medial surface of the maxilla. With the corresponding process from the other side, it forms the major portion of the hard palate.

postglenoid p. The process of the temporal bone separating the mandibular fossa from the external acoustic meatus.

pterygoid p. The process of the sphenoid bone extending downward from the junction of the body and great wing. It consists of the lateral and medial pterygoid plates.

spinous p. of vertebrae The posteriormost part of a vertebra. This spine projects back and serves as a point of attachment for muscles of the back.

styloid p. **1.** A pointed process of the temporal bone, projecting downward, and to which some of the muscles of the tongue are attached. **2.** A pointed projection behind the head of the fibula. **3.** A protuberance on the outer portion of the distal end of the radius. **4.** An ulnar projection on the inner side of the distal end.

transverse p. The process extending laterally and dorsally from the arch of a vertebra.

uncinate p. of the ethmoid bone A sickle-shaped bony process on the medial wall of the ethmoidal labyrinth below the concha.

vermiform p. Vermiform appendix.

vocal p. The process of the arytenoid cartilage that serves for attachment of the vocal ligament.

xiphoid p. A thin, elongated process extending caudally from the body of the sternum. SYN: *ensiform p.*

zygomatic p. **1.** A thin projection from the temporal bone bounding its squamous portion. **2.** A part of the malar bone helping to form the zygoma.

processing In radiology, the use of a developer, fixer, washer, and dryer to change a latent film image or electrical impulses to a visible image for interpretation.

daylight p. The use of an automatic system that accepts radiographic film, inserts it into the processor, and refills the cassette without the need for a darkroom.

extended p. In mammography, extension of the development time or developer temperature to enhance image contrast and lower the patient dose.

processor In radiology, an automatic machine that helps to convert the latent image to a visible image. It consists of a transporter, electrical system, temperature control, circulation system, and dryer.

processus (prō-sĕs′ŭs) *pl.* **processus** [L.] Process (3).

p. cochleariformis The curved portion of a thin plate of bone separating the eustachian tube from the canal for the tensor tympani muscle over which the tendon of the muscle passes before insertion into the manubrium of the malleus.

p. retromandibularis The wedge-shaped portion of the parotid gland that projects medially toward the pharynx.

p. uncinatus **1.** The curved process of the ethmoid labyrinth projecting from the lateral wall of the middle meatus that forms the inferior border of hiatus semilunaris. **2.** A hooklike portion of the head of the pancreas that curves around the superior mesenteric vessels.

procheilon (prō-kī′lŏn) [Gr. *pro,* before, + *cheilon,* lip] A prominence in the central portion of the upper lip.

prochlorperazine (prō″klor-pĕr′ă-zēn) A phenothiazine-type drug used to treat nausea and vomiting.

prochondral (prō-kŏn′drăl) [″ + *chondros,* cartilage] Preceding the formation of cartilage.

prochordal (prō-kor′dăl) [″ + *chorde,* cord] In front of the notochord.

procidentia (prō″sĭ-dĕn′shē-ă) [L.] A complete prolapse, esp. of the uterus, to such an extent that the uterus lies outside of the vulva with everted vaginal walls. This is generally due to relaxation of the tissues that provide support for the pelvic organs. SYN: *hysteroptosia.*

procoagulant factor A lymphokine that can assume the role of factor VIII, antihemophilic factor, in coagulation cascade.

procollagen (prō-kŏl′ă-jĕn) [″ + *kolla,* glue, + *gennan,* to produce] Precursor of collagen.

proconvertin (prō″kŏn-vĕr′tĭn) Coagulation factor VII.

proconvulsive (prō-kŏn-vŭl′sĭv) Able or likely to provoke seizures.

procreate [L. *procreare*] To beget; to be the parents of an infant.

procreation (prō″krē-ā′shŭn) The act or state of conceiving and giving birth to an infant. SYN: *reproduction.*

proct- SEE: *procto-.*

proctalgia (prŏk-tăl′jē-ă) [″ + *algos,* pain] Pain in or around the anus and rectum.

p. fugax Severe rectal or anal pain, usually occurring in young men, possibly as a result of muscular spasms.

proctatresia (prŏk″tă-trē′zē-ă) [″ + *atresis,* imperforation] Imperforation of the anus.

proctectasia (prŏk″tĕk-tā′sē-ă) [″ + *ektasis,* dilatation] Dilatation of the anus or rectum.

proctectomy (prŏk-tĕk′tō-mē) [″ + *ektome,* excision] Excision of the rectum or anus.

proctitis [″ + *itis,* inflammation] Inflammation of the rectum and anus that may be caused by sexually transmitted diseases (e.g., infections with herpes simplex virus, *Neisseria gonorrhoeae, Chlamydia trachomatis,* and others); radiation injury (e.g., after treatment of pelvic cancers); inflammatory bowel disease (e.g., ulcerative colitis); allergy; trauma; or ischemia.

diphtheritic p. Proctitis caused by diphtheria; a rare condition in a time when vaccination against diphtheria is routine.

dysenteric p. Proctitis resulting from infectious diarrhea. It may produce ulcers and scarring of the rectum and anus.

gonococcal p. Gonorrheal infection around the rectum and anus.

traumatic p. Proctitis that results from anal or rectal injury.

procto-, proct- Combining form meaning *anus, rectum.*

proctocele (prŏk′tō-sēl) [Gr. *proktos,* anus, + *kele,* tumor, swelling] A protrusion of the rectal mucosa into the vagina. SYN: *rectocele.*

proctoclysis (prŏk-tŏk′lĭ-sĭs) [″ + *klysis,* a washing] Hydration of patients using a continuous infusion of fluids into the rectum and colon. The treatment sometimes is used for palliation of thirst in terminally ill patients who cannot receive fluids by other means. SEE: *enteroclysis.*

THERAPEUTIC EFFECT: This procedure has the following therapeutic effects: to supply fluid in postoperative cases when fluids cannot be taken otherwise; to supply the body with fluid as in hemorrhage, vomiting, or diarrhea; to relieve thirst as in persistent vomiting; and to lower body temperature by giving ice water enemas.

PATIENT CARE: Any hydrating solution may be used (saline, free water, dextrose in water, etc.) depending on the patient's fluid or electrolyte needs. After the bowel is evacuated, a catheter is inserted approx. 40 cm into the bowel, and fluids are given at 250 to 300 cc/hr or less, depending on tolerance. If pain or distention develop, treatment should be discontinued.

proctococcypexia, proctococcypexy (prŏk″tō-kŏk-sĭ-pĕk′sē-ă, -kŏk′sĭ-pĕk″sē) [″ + *kokkyx,* coccyx, + *pexis,* fixation] Suture of the rectum to the coccyx.

proctocolitis (prŏk″tō-kō-lī′tĭs) [″ + *kolon,* colon, + *itis,* inflammation] Inflammation of the colon and rectum.

proctocolonoscopy (prŏk″tō-kō″lŏn-ŏs′kō-pē) [″ + ″ + *skopein,* to examine] Examination of the interior of the rectum and lower colon.

proctocystoplasty (prŏk″tō-sĭs′tō-plăs″tē) [Gr. *proktos,* anus, + *kystis,* bladder, + *plastos,* formed] Plastic surgery involving the rectum and bladder.

proctocystotomy (prŏk″tō-sĭs-tŏt′ō-mē) [″ + *kystis,* bladder, + *tome,* incision] Incision into the bladder through the rectum.

proctodeum (prŏk-tō-dē′ŭm) [″ + *hodaios,* a way] An ectodermal depression located caudally that, upon rupture of the cloacal membrane, forms the anal canal.

proctodynia (prŏk″tō-dĭn′ē-ă) [″ + *odyne,* pain] Pain in the rectum or around the anus.

proctologic (prŏk″tō-lŏj′ĭk) [″ + *logos,* word, reason] Concerning proctology.

proctologist (prŏk-tŏl′ō-jĭst) [″ + *logos,* word, reason] One who specializes in diseases of the colon, rectum, and anus.

proctology (prŏk-tŏl′ō-jē) The phase of medicine dealing with treatment of diseases of the colon, rectum, and anus.

proctoparalysis (prŏk″tō-păr-ăl′ĭ-sĭs) [″ + *para,* at the side, + *lyein,* to loosen] Paralysis of the anal sphincter muscle.

proctoperineoplasty (prŏk″tō-pĕr″ĭ-nē′ō-plăs″tē) [″ + *perinaion,* perineum, + *plassein,* to form] Plastic surgery of the anus and rectum.

proctopexia, proctopexy (prŏk-tō-pĕk′sē-ă, prŏk′tō-pĕk″sē) [″ + *pexis,* fixation] Suture of the rectum to some other part, for example, presacral fascia.

proctophobia (prŏk″tō-fō′bē-ă) [″ + *phobos,* fear] Abnormal apprehension in those suffering from rectal disease.

proctoplasty (prŏk′tō-plăs″tē) [″ + *plastos,* formed] Plastic surgery of the anus or rectum.

proctopolypus (prŏk″tō-pŏl′ĭ-pŭs) [″ + *polys,* many, + *pous,* foot] Polyp of the rectum.

proctoptosis (prŏk″tŏp-tō′sĭs) [″ + *ptosis,* a dropping] Prolapse of the anus and rectum. SEE: *procidentia.*

proctorrhagia (prŏk″tō-rā′jē-ă) [″ + *rhegnynai,* to burst forth] Bleeding from the rectum.

proctorrhaphy (prŏk-tor′ă-fē) [″ + *rhaphe,* seam, ridge] Suturing of the rectum or anus.

proctorrhea (prŏk-tōr-ē′ă) [″ + *rhoia,* flow] Mucous discharge from the anus.

proctoscope [″ + *skopein,* to examine]

An instrument for inspection of the rectum.

proctoscopy (prŏk-tŏs′kō-pē) Inspection of the rectum with a proctoscope.

proctosigmoidectomy (prŏk″tō-sĭg″moy-dĕk′tō-mē) [″ + *sigma,* Gr. letter S, + *eidos,* form, shape, + *ektome,* excision] Surgical removal of the anus, rectum, and sigmoid flexure of the colon.

proctosigmoiditis (prŏk″tō-sĭg″moyd-ī′tĭs) [″ + ″ + *eidos,* form, shape, + *itis,* inflammation] Inflammation of the rectum and sigmoid.

proctosigmoidoscopy (prŏk″tō-sĭg-moyd-ŏs′kō-pē) Visual examination of the rectum and sigmoid colon by use of a sigmoidoscope.

proctospasm (prŏk′tō-spăzm) [″ + *spasmos,* a convulsion] Rectal spasm.

proctostasis (prŏk″tō-stā′sĭs) [″ + *stasis,* stoppage] Constipation resulting from failure of the rectum to respond to defecation stimulus.

proctostenosis (prŏk″tō-stĕn-ō′sĭs) [″ + *stenosis,* act of narrowing] Stricture of the anus or rectum.

proctostomy (prŏk-tŏs′tō-mē) [″ + *stoma,* mouth] Surgical creation of a permanent opening into the rectum.

proctotome (prŏk′tō-tōm) [″ + *tome,* incision] A knife for incision into the rectum.

proctotomy (prŏk-tŏt′ō-mē) Incision of the rectum or anus.

PATIENT CARE: The dressing is assessed frequently and the presence and amount of bleeding and drainage are recorded. Dressings should be changed or reinforced as prescribed by the physician. A T binder (female patients) or split T binder (male patients) is advantageous to ensure proper placement of the dressing.

proctovalvotomy (prŏk″tō-văl-vŏt′ō-mē) [″ + L. *valva,* leaf of a folding door, + Gr. *tome,* incision] Incision of the rectal valves.

procumbent [L. *procumbens,* lying down] Prone.

procursive (prō-kŭr′sĭv) [L. *procursivus*] Having an involuntary tendency to run forward.

procurvation (prō″kŭr-vā′shŭn) [L. *procurvare,* to bend forward] A bending forward.

procyclidine hydrochloride (prō-sī′klĭ-dēn) An antiparkinsonism drug.

prodromal (prō-drō′măl) [Gr. *prodromos,* running before] Pert. to the initial stage of a disease; the interval between the earliest symptoms and the appearance of a rash or fever.

prodromal rash A rash that precedes the true rash of an infectious disease.

prodrome *pl.* **prodromes, prodromata** A symptom indicative of an approaching disease.

prodrug An inert drug that becomes active only after it is transformed or metabolized by the body.

product (prŏd′ŭkt) [L. *productum*] Anything that is made; also, the resulting compound after the reaction of two chemical substances.

product liability The debt that manufacturers and sellers owe the public for any damages their products cause. In health care, the U.S. Food and Drug Administration and applicable tort law regulate the responsibility for consumer product safety of medical devices, new technologies, prostheses and implants, telecommunications machinery, office equipment, supplies, and drugs.

production (prō-dŭk′shŭn) Development or formation of a substance.

productive (prō-dŭk′tĭv) Forming, esp. new tissue.

productive inflammation An infrequently used term for any inflammatory process in which there is marked cellular proliferation (e.g., in proliferative retinopathy).

proencephalus (prō″ĕn-sĕf′ă-lŭs) [Gr. *pro,* before, + *enkephalos,* brain] A deformed fetus in which the brain protrudes through a fissure in the frontal area of the skull.

proenzyme (prō-ĕn′zīm) [″ + *en,* in, + *zyme,* a leaven] The inactive form of an enzyme found within a cell, which, upon leaving the cell, is converted into the active form, such as pepsinogen, which is cleaved to pepsin by hydrochloric acid in gastric juice.

proerythroblast (prō″ĕ-rĭth′rō-blăst) [″ + *erythros,* red, + *blastos,* germ] An old term for a pronormoblast.

proestrus (prō-ĕs′trŭs) The period preceding estrus in females, characterized by development of ovarian follicles and uterine endometrium.

professional (prō-fĕsh′ŭn-ăl) [ME. *profession,* sacred vow] Pert. to a profession.

p. misconduct Behavior that is professionally unsuitable, potentially dangerous to patients, incompetent, disruptive, abusive, or illegal.

professional liability The obligation of health care providers or their insurers to pay for damages resulting from the providers' acts of omission or commission in treating patients.

professional liability insurance A type of insurance contract that provides compensation for a person or party injured by a professional's acts or omissions. Two common types of policies are as follows: (1) *Claims made.* The claim for damages by the injured party must be made during the policy coverage period in order for the professional to be covered and represented by the insurance company. (2) *Occurrence basis.* The claim for damages by the injured party is covered by the insurance company as long as the act of professional liability occurs during the policy coverage period, even though the claim is filed after the coverage period ends.

Professional Standards Review Organization ABBR: PSRO. Peer review at the local level required by Public Law 92-603 of the U.S. for the services provided under the Medicare, Medicaid, and maternal and child health programs funded by the federal government. The major goals of the PSRO program are as follows: to ensure that health care services are of acceptable professional quality; to ensure appropriate use of health care facilities at the most economical level consistent with professional standards; to identify lack of quality and overuse problems in health care and improve those conditions; to attempt to obtain voluntary correction of inappropriate or unnecessary practitioner and facility practices, and, if unable to do so, recommend sanctions against violators.

profibrinolysin (prō″fī-brĭ-nō-lī′sĭn) [Gr. *pro,* before, + L. *fibra,* fiber, + Gr. *lysis,* dissolution] The inactive precursor of the proteolytic enzyme fibrinolysin.

profile (prō′fīl) [L. *pro,* forward, + *filare,* to draw a line] **1.** An outline of the lateral view of an object, esp. the human head. **2.** A summary, graph, or table presenting a subject's most notable characteristics. **3.** A comprehensive history of the use of health care services. SEE: *practice p.*

biophysical p. ABBR: BPP. A system of estimating current fetal status, determined by analyzing five variables via ultrasonography and nonstress testing. Fetal breathing movements, gross body movement, fetal tone, amniotic fluid volume, and fetal heart rate reactivity are each assigned specific values. Each expected normal finding is rated as 2; each abnormal finding is rated as 0. Scores of 8 to 10 with normal amniotic fluid volume indicate satisfactory fetal status. A score of 6 with normal amniotic fluid volume requires reassessment of a preterm fetus within 24 hr of delivery. Scores less than 6 indicate fetal compromise and require prompt delivery. SEE: *Apgar score.*

drug p. The unique characteristics of a drug or class of drugs, including their administration, absorption, metabolism, duration of action, toxicity, and interactions with foods or other medications.

iceberg p. Profile of a person with a psychological outlook characterized by more vigor and less tension, depression, anger, fatigue, and confusion than is found in others. This type of affect often is found in elite athletes and others with physically active lifestyles.

practice p. A performance-based method of assessing the professional behaviors of individual practitioners. A typical profile may include data about a practioner's patients, their known illnesses, their drug therapies, their immunization history, hospitalization rate, use of other services, and the cost of specific aspects of their care. The profile of an individual practitioner's performance could provide information such as the number of his or her patients who are screened for cancer or diabetes mellitus, or the number of patients treated for a particular condition who survive. The profile could be used to further a practitioner's education, to influence future care patterns, to certify or recertify health care providers, or to assist decisions about the hiring, retention, or dismissal of professionals who provide health care services. The outcome of establishing practice profiles could help to increase the quality of medical care and to provide patients the opportunity of evaluating physicians. The methods used to profile practice are constantly evolving.

PULSES p. One of the first formal, widely used scales to assess daily living skills. PULSES is an acronym formed by the domains measured: *P*hysical condition, *U*pper extremity function, *L*ower extremity function, *S*ensory, *E*xcretory, and psychosocial *S*tatus. SEE: *activities of daily living.*

safety p. The chemistry, pharmacology, therapeutic effects, and adverse effects of an administered drug or other substance.

profluvium (prō-floo′vē-ŭm) [L.] An excessive flow or discharge; a flux.

p. seminis The flow from the vagina of semen deposited during coition.

profunda [L.] Deep seated; term applied to certain deeply located blood vessels.

profundaplasty An operation to repair an obstructing lesion in a deep blood vessel, for example, of the deep femoral artery.

profundus (prō-fŭn′dŭs) [L.] Located deeper than the indicated reference point.

progastrin (prō-găs′trĭn) The inactive precursor of gastrin.

progenitor (prō-jĕn′ĭ-tor) [L.] An ancestor.

progeny (prŏj′ĕ-nē) [ME. *progenie*] Offspring.

progeria (prō-jē′rē-ă) [Gr. *pro,* before, + *geras,* old age] The syndrome of premature aging, which may be an inherited disorder that is transmitted as an autosomal dominant trait. The incidence appears higher in children of older fathers. Onset is from birth to 18 months of age and the average age at death is 12 to 13 years.

FINDINGS: The child has an aged and wizened appearance. In addition there is small stature, slightness of build, alopecia, thick and inelastic skin that has brownish spots on it, delayed dentition, high-pitched voice, prominent eyes, and infantile sex organs.

progestational (prō″jĕs-tā′shŭn-ăl) Concerned with the luteal phase of the menstrual cycle, at which time, by the action of the hormone progesterone, the endometrium is further prepared for implantation of the fertilized ovum.

progestational agent Progestin (1).

progesterone (prō-jĕs′tĕr-ōn) A steroid hormone, $C_{21}H_{30}O_2$, obtained from the corpus luteum and placenta. It is responsible for changes in the endometrium in the second half of the menstrual cycle preparatory to implantation of the blastocyst. It facilitates implantation by inhibiting uterine motility and stimulates the development of the mammary glands. Progesterone is used to treat patients with menstrual disorders (secondary amenorrhea, abnormal uterine bleeding, luteal phase deficiency) and to manage renal or endometrial carcinoma. In combination with estrogen, it is used for contraception and postmenopausal hormone replacement therapy. SYN: *progestin* (1).

progestin (prō-jĕs′tĭn) **1.** A corpus luteum hormone that prepares the endometrium for implantation of the fertilized ovum. SYN: *progesterone*. **2.** A term used to cover a large group of synthetic drugs that have a progesterone-like effect on the uterus.

progestogen (prō-jĕs′tō-jĕn) Any natural or synthetic hormonal substance that produces effects similar to those due to progesterone.

proglossis (prō-glŏs′ĭs) [Gr.] The tip of the tongue.

proglottid (prō-glŏt′tĭd) *pl.* **proglottides** [Gr. *pro,* before, + *glossa,* tongue] A segment of a tapeworm, containing both male and female reproductive organs. SEE: *Cestoda; tapeworm*.

proglottis SEE: *proglottid*.

prognathic (prŏg-nā′thĭk) [″ + *gnathos,* jaw] Prognathous.

prognathism (prŏg′nă-thĭzm) [″ + *gnathos,* jaw + *-ismos,* condition] Projection of the jaws beyond projection of the forehead.

prognathous (prŏg′nă-thŭs) Having jaws projecting forward beyond the rest of the face.

prognose (prŏg-nōs′) To predict the course of a disease.

prognosis (prŏg-nō′sĭs) [Gr., foreknowledge] Prediction of the course and end of a disease, and the estimate of chance for recovery.

prognosticate (prŏg-nŏs′tĭ-kāt) [Gr. *prognostikon,* knowing before] To make a statement on the probable outcome of an illness.

program A plan or system, usually printed, outlining procedures or actions to be followed.

employee benefit p. A group of economically useful goods or services workers receive from their employer in addition to salary. These often provide protection against unpleasant or catastrophic events. Examples include medical and dental insurance, disability income, retirement income, and life insurance.

Individualized Education P. ABBR: IEP. A documented program of intervention mandated for each child provided education-related rehabilitation services under federal legislation. The program guarantees a free and appropriate public education for children with disabilities. Decisions relating to Individual Educational Programs must be approved in Admission, Review and Discharge (ARD) conferences mandated by federal legislation. Participants in these conferences should include parents or guardians, special educators, rehabilitation providers, and others as appropriate.

needle exchange p. Syringe exchange p.

preprosthetic p. Postsurgical intervention following amputation during which the patient is taught stump care, positioning, sitting tolerance, transfer techniques, and other skills that are necessary before prosthetic training can begin.

prosthetic training p. Systematic education and training provided to persons with amputations following fitting of a prosthetic device.

syringe exchange p. A public health program responsible for collecting used hypodermic syringes and exchanging them for sterile ones. Such programs are designed to decrease the spread of diseases (like AIDS and hepatitis C) that are transmitted by the sharing of contaminated needles. SYN: *needle exchange p.*

12-step p. A form of treatment, used primarily by persons who abuse alcohol or other substances, that relies on social support, interpersonal motivation, abstinence from the addictive substance, and spirituality.

progranulocyte (prō-grăn′ū-lō-sīt) [″ + L. *granula,* granule, + Gr. *kytos,* cell] Promyelocyte.

progravid (prō-grăv′ĭd) [″ + L. *gravidus,* pregnant] Preceding pregnancy.

progress [L. *progressus,* a going forward] The ongoing sequence of events of an illness.

progression (prō-grĕsh′ŭn) [L. *progressus*] An advancing or moving forward.

progressive (prō-grĕs′ĭv) Advancing, as a disease from bad to worse.

progressive lens An eyeglass lens that gradually changes prescription strength from the top of the lens, which is used for viewing distance, to the bottom of the lens, which is used for seeing objects that are nearby. Progressive lenses enable the eyes to adjust from one distance to another (e.g., when looking up from a book) without the "image jump" associated with bifocals, lenses that require the eye to shift between two separate prescriptions.

progressive ossifying myositis A tendency to bony deposits in the muscles with chronic inflammation.

progressive resistive exercise ABBR: PRE. A form of active resistive exercise based on a principle of gradual increase in the amount of resistance in order to achieve maximum strength.

progress notes Notes made on the chart by those involved in caring for a patient. Physicians, nurses, consultants, and therapists may record their notes concerning the progress or lack of progress made by the patient in the interim between the previous note and the time of the most recent note. In patients who are not critically ill, a note concerning progress might be made daily or less frequently; in critical care situations, notes could be made hourly. It is important that each note be signed and written clearly, and the date and time recorded.

progress report The written or verbal account of a patient's present condition, esp. as compared with the previous state.

prohormone (prō-hor′mōn) Precursor of a hormone.

proinsulin Precursor of insulin produced in the beta cells of the pancreas.

projection (prō″jĕk′shŭn) [Gr. *pro,* before, + *jacere,* to throw] **1.** The act of throwing forward. **2.** A part extending beyond the level of its surroundings. **3.** The mental process by which sensations are referred to the sense organs or receptors stimulated, or outside the body to the object that is the stimulus. **4.** The distortion of a perception as a result of its repression, resulting in such a phenomenon as hating without cause one who has been dearly loved, or attributing to others one's own undesirable traits. These are characteristics of the paranoid reaction. **5.** In radiology, the path of the x-ray photon beam. In an anteroposterior projection, for example, the beam enters the anterior surface of the body and exits the posterior surface.

isometric p. A projection of an x-ray photon beam that yields an image having the same dimensions as the object being examined.

projective technique Any one of several forms of psychological assessment or evaluation. Using ambiguous activities and tasks which encourage self-expression, the products or results and the individual's verbalizations about them are evaluated and interpreted to determine indications of unconscious needs, thoughts, or concerns.

prokaryon (prō-kăr′ē-ŏn) [″ + *karyon,* nucleus] **1.** Nuclear material that is spread throughout the cell cytoplasm and is not bounded by a membrane. **2.** Prokaryote.

Prokaryotae In taxonomy, the kingdom of organisms with prokaryotic cell structure, that is, they lack membrane-bound cell organelles and a nuclear membrane around the chromosome. Included are the bacteria and cyanobacteria (formerly the blue-green algae). SYN: *Monera.*

prokaryote (prō-kăr′ē-ōt) [″ + *karyon,* nucleus] An organism of the kingdom Monera with a single, circular chromosome, without a nuclear membrane, or membrane-bound organelles (i.e., mitochondria and lysosomes). Included in this classification are bacteria and cyanobacteria (formerly the blue-green algae). SYN: *procaryote; prokaryon* (2). SEE: *eukaryote.*

prokinetic Stimulating aboral gastrointestinal activity.

prolabium (prō-lā′bē-ŭm) [″ + *labium,* lip] The entire central portion of the upper lip.

prolactin (prō-lăk′tĭn) [″ + *lac,* milk] A hormone produced by the anterior pituitary gland. In humans, prolactin in association with estrogen and progesterone stimulates breast development and the formation of milk during pregnancy. The act of sucking is an important stimulus for the production of prolactin in the postpartum period. Some of the metabolic effects of prolactin resemble those of growth hormone. In the female this includes amenorrhea, galactorrhea, and infertility. In the male it may cause erectile dysfunction. Hyperprolactinemia may be associated with amenorrhea in women and reduced sexual potency in men. Thyrotropin-releasing hormone and stress of all kinds can stimulate prolactin release.

prolactinoma An adenoma of the pituitary gland (found more often in women than in men) that produces excessive amounts of prolactin and, in some cases, endocrine effects such as galactorrhea or amenorrhea, or visual effects due to compression of the optic chiasm. Treatments may include surgical removal of the tumor or suppression of the gland with drugs such as bromocriptine.

prolapse (prō-lăps′) [L. *prolapsus*] A falling or dropping down of an organ or internal part, such as the uterus or rectum. SEE: *mitral valve prolapse; procidentia; ptosis.*

p. of the iris Protrusion of the iris through an injury in the cornea.

lumbar disk p. Herniated intervertebral disk.

pelvic organ p. Protrusion of the pelvic organs into or through the vaginal canal. This condition is usually due to direct or indirect damage to the vagina and its pelvic support system. The damage may be related to stretching or laceration of the vaginal wall, hypoestrogenic atrophy, or injury to the nerves of the pelvic support structures.

SYMPTOMS: Symptoms include a sensation of pelvic pressure, groin pain, coital difficulty, sacral backache, bloody vaginal discharge, difficult bowel movements, and urinary frequency, urgency, or incontinence.

PROPHYLAXIS: Preventive measures include treatment of chronic respiratory disorders or constipation, estrogen replacement for menopausal women, weight control, smoking cessation, avoidance of strenuous occupational or recreational stresses to the pelvic support system, and pelvic muscle exercise to strengthen the pelvic diaphragm.

TREATMENT: Treatment may be nonsurgical (e.g., use of a vaginal pessary) or surgical, including reconstructive operations, vaginal hysterectomy, and cystocele or rectocele repair.

p. of the rectum Protrusion of the rectal mucosa or full thickness of the rectum (procidentia). Internal or complete rectal prolapse can be identified radiographically or endoscopically without transanal protrusion.

p. of the umbilical cord Premature expulsion of a loop of umbilical cord into the cervical or vaginal canal during labor before engagement of the presenting part, a potentially life-threatening event that occurs in about 2 of 1000 births. The greatest danger of cord prolapse is neonatal asphyxia and death. SEE: *deceleration*.

p. of the uterus Downward displacement of the uterus, the cervix sometimes protruding from the vaginal orifice. The causes include age with weakening of pelvic musculature, traumatic vaginal delivery, chronic straining in association with coughing or difficult bowel movements, and pelvic tumors that push the uterus down.

prolapsus [L.] Prolapse.

prolepsis [Gr. *pro*, before, + *lepsis*, a seizure] The return of paroxysmal attacks at successively shorter intervals.

proleptic Recurring before the time expected, said of paroxysms.

proleukocyte (prō-lū′kō-sīt) [″ + *leukos*, white, + *kytos*, cell] An undeveloped leukocyte.

proliferate (prō-lĭf′ĕr-āt) [L. *proles*, offspring, + *ferre*, to bear] To increase by reproduction of similar forms.

proliferation (prō-lĭf″ĕr-ā′shŭn) **1.** Rapid and repeated reproduction of new parts, as by cell division. **2.** The process or result of rapid reproduction.

proliferous **1.** Multiplying, as by formation of new tissue cells. **2.** Bearing offspring.

prolific [L. *prolificus*] Fruitful; reproductive. SYN: *fertile*.

prolinase An enzyme that is found in animal tissues and yeast and that hydrolyzes proline peptides to simpler peptide and proline.

proline (prō′lēn) C_4H_8NCOOH; an amino acid formed by digestion of protein. Proline is a significant constituent of collagens.

prolotherapy The injection of sclerosing solutions into the ligaments of the back as a treatment for back pain. Objective validation of the efficacy of this technique is lacking.

prolymphocyte (prō″lĭmf′ō-sīt) [″ + L. *lympha*, lymph, + Gr. *kytos*, cell] A cell intermediate between a lymphoblast and lymphocyte.

PROM *premature rupture of membranes.*

promegakaryocyte (prō-mĕg″ă-kăr′ē-ō-sīt) [″ + *megas*, big, + *karyon*, nucleus, + *kytos*, cell] A cell from which a megakaryocyte develops.

promegaloblast (prō-mĕg′ă-lō-blast″) [″ + ″ + *blastos*, germ] A cell of the erythrocyte series preceding the megaloblast.

prometaphase (prō-mĕt′ă-fāz) [″ + *meta*, change, + *phasis*, to appear] The stage of mitosis in which the nuclear membrane disintegrates, and the chromosomes move toward the equatorial plate.

promethazine hydrochloride (prō-mĕth′ă-zēn) An antihistamine drug used as an antiemetic and anticough medicine.

promethium (prō-mē′thē-ŭm) SYMB: Pm. A radioactive element of the rare earth series; atomic weight 144.9128; atomic number 61.

prominence (prŏm′ĭ-nĕns) [L. *prominens*, project] A projection or protrusion.

prominentia (prŏm″ĭ-nĕn′shē-ă) *pl.* **prominentiae** [L.] A projection.

p. laryngea The laryngeal prominence; Adam's apple.

p. spiralis A small ridge extending the entire length of the cochlea located on the inner surface of the spiral ligament. It projects slightly into the cochlear canal and contains blood vessels, including the vas prominens.

promonocyte (prō-mŏn′ō-sīt) [Gr. *pro*, before, + *monos*, single, + *kytos*, cell] In the development of white blood cells, the precursor of the monocyte. It is between the monoblast and monocyte.

promontory (prŏm′ŏn-tor″ē) [L. *promontorium*] A projecting process or part.

p. of the sacrum The anterior projecting portion of the pelvic surface of the base of the sacrum. With the fifth lumbar vertebra, it forms the sacrovertebral angle.

p. of the tympanic cavity The projection on the medial wall of the tympanic cavity produced by the first turn of the cochlea.

promoter (prō-mō′tĕr) A substance that assists a catalyst to act. SEE: *coenzyme*.

prompt Assistance, reinforcement, or feedback given during the acquisition or relearning of skills necessary for task completion.

promyelocyte (prō-mī′ĕl-ō-sīt) [Gr. *pro,* before, + *myelos,* marrow, + *kytos,* cell] **1.** A large mononuclear myeloid cell seen in the blood in leukemia. **2.** Cell development between a myeloblast and a myelocyte, resembling a myeloblast. SEE: illus.

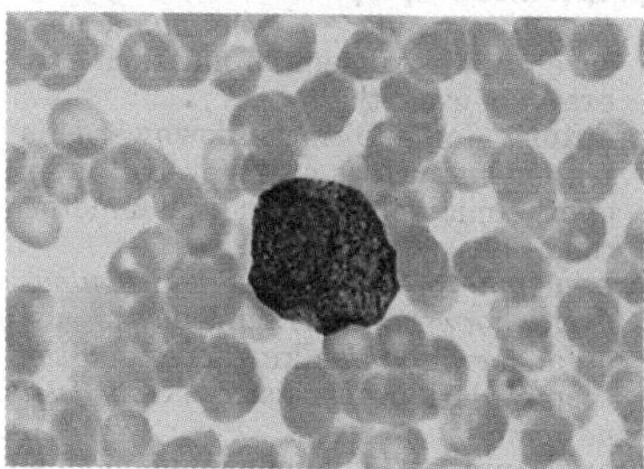

PROMYELOCYTE (X600)

pronate (prō′nāt) To place in a prone position. SEE: *supinate*.

pronation (prō-nā′shŭn) [L. *pronus,* prone] **1.** The act of lying prone or face downward. **2.** The act of turning the hand so that the palm faces downward or backward. SEE: *supination*.

pronator A muscle that pronates.

pronator syndrome A neurological disorder caused by entrapment of the median nerve at the elbow. Symptoms and signs include aching in the wrist with a subjective feeling of poor coordination; paresthesias extending into the hand; paresis of the thumb muscles; pain on pronation of the forearm and flexion of the wrist against resistance; and tenderness in the proximal thenar muscles. A positive Tinel's sign over the pronator teres muscles may be present. The disease usually affects the dominant arm in men. The condition may be treated with corticosteroid injections or orthopedic surgery.

pronaus, pronaeus (prō-nā′ŭs) [Gr. *pro,* before, + *naos,* temple] The vagina or vestibule of the vagina.

prone (prōn) [ME.] **1.** Horizontal with the face downward. **2.** Denoting the hand with the palm turned downward. It is the opposite of supine. SYN: *prone posture*.

pronephros, pronephron (prō-nĕf′rŏs, -rŏn) The earliest and simplest type of excretory organ of vertebrates, functional in simpler forms (cyclostomes), and serving as a provisional kidney in some fishes and amphibians. In reptiles, birds, and mammals, it appears in the embryo as a temporary, functionless structure.

prong (prŏng) A cone-shaped body such as the root of a tooth.

pronograde (prō′nō-grād) [L. *pronus,* prone, + *gradus,* a step] In animals, walking on the hands and feet or resting with the body in a horizontal position. It is the opposite of orthograde.

pronometer (prō-nŏm′ĕ-tĕr) [″ + Gr. *metron,* measure] A device for showing the amount of pronation or supination of the forearm.

pronormoblast (prō-nor′mō-blăst) [Gr. *pro,* before, + L. *norma,* rule, + Gr. *blastos,* germ] An early precursor of the red blood cell.

pronucleus (prō-nū′klē-ŭs) [Gr. *pro,* before, + *nucleus,* little kernel] The nucleus of the ovum (the female pronucleus) or of the spermatozoon (the male pronucleus) after fertilization of the ovum.

prootic (prō-ŏt′ĭk, -ō′tĭk) [″ + *ous,* ear] In front of the ear.

prop A device of sturdy material used to support or hold something in place.

mouth p. A metal or rubber device inserted between the jaws to maintain the mouth in an open position. SYN: *bite block*.

propagation (prŏp-ă-gā′shŭn) [L.] The act of reproducing or giving birth. SYN: *generation; reproduction*.

propagative (prŏp′ă-gā″tĭv) Pert. to or taking part in reproduction.

propalinal (prō-păl′ĭ-năl) [Gr. *pro,* before, + *palin,* back] Applied to a backward and forward movement, as of the jaws.

propane (prō′pān) An inflammable odorless, colorless hydrocarbon, C_3H_8, that is present in natural gas.

propantheline bromide (prō-păn′thĕ-lēn) A anticholinergic drug that acts like belladonna.

proparacaine hydrochloride (prō-păr′ă-kān) A topical anesthetic drug used in ophthalmology.

propepsin (prō-pĕp′sĭn) Pepsinogen.

propeptone (prō-pĕp′tōn) [″ + *peptein,* to digest] An intermediate product in the digestive conversion of protein into peptone. SYN: *hemialbumose*.

propeptonuria (prō″pĕp-tō-nū′rē-ă) [″ + ″ + *ouron,* urine] Excretion of propeptone in the urine. SYN: *hemialbumosuria*.

properdin (prō-pĕrd′ĭn) A plasma protein that stabilizes the enzyme C3 convertase, and helps to activate the alternative pathway of the complement cascade. SEE: *complement*.

prophase (prō′fāz) [″ + *phasis,* an appearance] The first stage of cell division. SEE: *mitosis* for illustration.

prophylactic (prō-fĭ-lăk′tĭk) [Gr. *prophy-*

laktikos, guarding] **1.** Any agent or regimen that contributes to the prevention of infection and disease. **2.** A popular term for a condom.

prophylaxis (prō-fĭ-lăk′sĭs, prō-fĭl-ăks′ĭs) [Gr. *prophylassein,* to guard against] Observance of rules necessary to prevent disease.

oral p. The removal of plaque, calculus, stains, and necrotic cementum from the exposed and unexposed surfaces of the teeth by scaling and polishing. A preventive measure for the control of caries and periodontal disease.

propiolactone (prō″pē-ō-lăk′tōn) A disinfectant used in preparing certain viral and bacterial vaccines.

propionic acid C_2H_5COOH, methylacetic acid, which is present in sweat.

Propionibacterium acnes A gram-positive rod bacterium that may be part of the normal skin flora, but can also be pathogenic in wounds and infected prosthetic devices. It was formerly called *Corynebacterium acnes.*

proplasmacyte (prō-plăz′mă-sīt) [Gr. *pro,* before, + LL. *plasma,* form, mold, + Gr. *kytos,* cell] The precursor of the plasma cell.

proplastid (prō-plăs′tĭd) The cytoplasmic body from which a plastid is formed.

propofol (prŏ′pō-fŏl) A nonbarbiturate sedative used to induce anesthesia. It has a short duration of action and a rapid recovery time. Common side effects of its use include pain during injection and bradycardia.

propolis [Gr. *pro,* before, + *polis,* city] A sticky resin present in the buds and bark of certain trees and plants. It is collected by bees for the purpose of repairing combs, filling cracks, and making the entrance to the hive waterproof.

proposition (prŏp-uh-zĭsh′ĕn) A statement about a concept or about the relationship between concepts. A proposition may be an assumption, a premise, a theorem, or a hypothesis. SEE: *assumption; hypothesis; premise; theorem.*

propositus (prō-pŏz′ĭ-tŭs) [L. *proponere,* to put on view] Proband.

propoxycaine hydrochloride (prō-pŏk′sē-kān) A local anesthetic drug.

propoxyphene hydrochloride (prō-pŏk′sē-fēn) A mild opioid pain reliever.

propranolol hydrochloride A beta-adrenergic blocking agent used primarily to treat hypertension, angina pectoris, and many cardiac rhythm disturbances. It also may be used to prevent migraine headaches and to treat drug-induced akathesia.

CAUTION: Persons with asthma, heart block, or decompensated heart failure should not be treated with this drug.

proprioception (prō″prē-ō-sĕp′shŭn) [L. *proprius,* one's own, + *capio,* to take] The awareness of posture, movement, and changes in equilibrium and the knowledge of position, weight, and resistance of objects in relation to the body. **proprioceptive** (-tĭv), *adj.*

proprioceptor (prō″prē-ō-sĕp′tor) [″ + *ceptor,* a receiver] A receptor that responds to stimuli originating within the body itself, esp. one that responds to pressure, position, or stretch (e.g., muscle spindles, pacinian corpuscles, and labyrinthine receptors).

propriospinal (prō″prē-ō-spī′năl) [″ + *spina,* thorn] Concerned exclusively with the spinal cord.

proptometer (prŏp-tŏm′ĕ-tĕr) [Gr. *proptosis,* protrusion, + *metron,* a measure] An instrument for measuring the extent of exophthalmos.

proptosis (prŏp-tō′sĭs) A downward displacement such as of the eyeball in exophthalmic goiter or in inflammatory conditions of the orbit.

propulsion (prō-pŭl′shŭn) [L. *propulsus,* driven forward] **1.** A tendency to push or fall forward in walking. **2.** A condition seen in Parkinson's disease. SEE: *festination.*

propyl (prō′pĭl) The radical of propyl alcohol or propane, $CH_3—CH_2—CH_2—$.

propylene glycol (prŏp′ĭ-lēn) A demulcent agent used as a solvent for medicines, and in cosmetics.

propyliodone (prō″pĭl-ī′ō-dōn) A radiopaque dye used formerly in radiographical studies of the bronchi.

propylparaben (prō″pĭl-păr′ă-bĕn) Propyl *p*-hydroxybenzoate, $C_{10}H_{12}O_3$, a chemical used as an antifungal agent and as a preservative in pharmaceuticals.

propylthiouracil (prō″pĭl-thī″ō-ū′ră-sĭl) An antithyroid drug used to treat hyperthyroidism. One of its most important, but rare, adverse effects is suppression of white blood cell production by the bone marrow.

pro re nata (prō rē nā′tă) [L.] ABBR: p.r.n. According to the circumstances; as necessary.

prorrhaphy (prō′ră-fē) [Gr. *pro,* before, + *rhaphe,* seam, ridge] Surgical movement of a muscle or tendon insertion to a point farther away; done to change the action of a muscle. SYN: *advancement.*

prorsad (pror′săd) In a forward direction.

prorubricyte (prō-roo′brĭ-sīt) A basophilic normoblast.

proscription Behavior that is forbidden by religious or cultural tenet or belief. SEE: *taboo.*

prosecretin (prō″sē-krē′tĭn) [″ + *secretio,* separation] A substance present in the duodenal mucosa that, when acted on by hydrochloric acid in chyme, is converted into secretin. SEE: *secretin.*

prosection (prō-sĕk′shŭn) [″ + L. *sectio,* a cutting] Dissection for the purpose of demonstrating anatomical structure.

prosector (prō-sĕk′tor) [L.] One who prepares cadavers for dissection or dissects for demonstration.

prosencephalon (prŏs″ĕn-sĕf′ă-lŏn) [Gr. *proso,* before, + *enkephalos,* brain] The embryonic forebrain, which gives rise to the telencephalon and diencephalon.

proso- [Gr. *proso,* forward] Combining form indicating *forward, anterior.*

prosodemic (prŏs″ō-dĕm′ĭk) [″ + *demos,* people] Spread by individual contact; said of a disease. SEE: *epidemic.*

prosody (prŏs′ă-dē) [L. *prosodia,* accent of a syllable] The normal rhythm, melody, and articulation of speech.

prosopagnosia (prŏs″ō-păg-nō′sē-ă) [Gr. *prosopon,* face, + *a-,* not, + *gnosis,* recognition] An inability to recognize faces, even one's own face.

prosopalgia (prŏs″ō-păl′jē-ă) [″ + *algos,* pain] Trigeminal neuralgia.

prosopectasia (prŏs″ō-pĕk-tā′zē-ă) [″ + *ektasis,* dilatation] Abnormal enlargement of the face.

prosopic (prō″sŏp′ĭk) Pert. to a face or facial skeleton that is convex anteriorly.

prosoplasia (prŏs″ō-plā′sē-ă) [Gr. *proso,* forward, + *plassein,* to form] Progressive transformation of cells until they develop into cells with a higher degree of function.

prosopoanoschisis (prŏs″ō-pō″ă-nŏs′kĭ-sĭs) [Gr. *prosopon,* face, + *ana,* up, + *schisis,* a splitting] An oblique facial cleft, a slanting furrow extending from mouth to eye.

prosopodiplegia (prŏs″ō-pō-dī-plē′jē-ă) [″ + *dis,* twice, + *plege,* a stroke] Paralysis on both sides of the face.

prosopodynia (prŏs″ō-pō-dĭn′ē-ă) [″ + *odyne,* pain] Tic douloureux.

prosoponeuralgia (prŏs″ō-pō-nū-răl′jē-ă) [″ + *neuron,* sinew, + *algos,* pain] Trigeminal neuralgia.

prosopopagus (prŏs″ō-pŏp′ă-gŭs) [″ + *pagos,* a thing fixed] Unequal conjoined twins in which the parasite is attached to some part of the face other than the jaw.

prosopoplegia (prŏs″ō-pō-plē′jē-ă) [″ + *plege,* stroke] Facial paralysis.

prosoposchisis (prŏs-ō-pŏs′kĭ-sĭs) [Gr. *prosopon,* face, + *schisis,* a splitting] A congenital cleft of the face.

prosopospasm (prŏs′ō-pō-spăzm) [″ + *spasmos,* a convulsion] Facial spasm.

prosopothoracopagus (prŏs″ō-pō-thō″ră-kŏp′ă-gŭs) [″ + *thorax,* chest, + *pagos,* a thing fixed] Conjoined twins joined in the frontal area between the face and the chest.

prosopotocia (prŏs″ō-pō-tō′shē-ă) [″ + *tokos,* birth] Presentation of the face in parturition.

prosopus varus (prŏs′ō-pŭs vā′rŭs) [Gr. *prosopon,* face, + L. *varus,* crooked] Congenital obliquity of the face caused by atrophy of one side of the head.

prospective payment system A reimbursement method used in which a fixed, predetermined amount is allocated for treating patients with a specific diagnosis when an individual is hospitalized. It was originally developed for use with Medicare recipients. It is also referred to as payment-by-diagnosis.

prospective study A clinical or epidemiological investigation of patients or health subjects with respect to the medical, social, and environmental factors encountered from the time of the beginning of the study until the investigation is terminated. SEE: *retrospective study.*

prostacyclin Prostaglandin GI_2.

prostaglandin (prŏs′tă-glănd-ĭn) ABBR: PG. Any of a large group of biologically active, carbon-20, unsaturated fatty acids that are produced by the metabolism of arachidonic acid through the cyclo-oxygenase pathway. They are autacoids: local short-range hormones that are formed rapidly, act in the immediate area, and then decay or are destroyed by enzymes. PGD_2, PGE_2, $PGF_{2\alpha}$, and PGI_1PGI_2 (prostacyclin), and TXA_2 (thromboxane) are important mediators of inflammation. Nonsteroidal anti-inflammatory drugs block the production of prostaglandins.

PGs influence a broad range of biological effects, including vasodilation, vascular permeability, bronchoconstriction, platelet aggregation, dysmenorrhea, inhibition of gastric acid secretion, stimulation of neural receptors for pain during tissue damage, sleep inhibition, and maintenance of patent ductus arteriosus. Exogenous PGE_2 gel may be used to soften the cervix before induction of labor. SEE: *arachidonic acid; nonsteroidal anti-inflammatory drug; patent ductus arteriosus.*

prostaglandin GI_2 ABBR: PGI_2. A compound formed from the metabolism of arachidonic acid. It is a potent vasodilator and inhibitor of platelet aggregation.

prostaglandin inhibitor A substance that inhibits the production of prostaglandins. Nonsteroidal and steroid anti-inflammatory agents are two major categories that inhibit prostaglandins.

prostanoids The name of the end products of the cyclo-oxygenase pathway of the metabolism of arachidonic acid. These are prostaglandins and thromboxanes. SEE: *eicosanoid; prostaglandin; thromboxane A_2.*

prostat- SEE: *prostato-.*

prostatalgia (prŏs-tă-tăl′jē-ă) [Gr. *prostates,* prostate, + *algos,* pain] Prostatodynia.

prostate (prŏs′tāt) [Gr. *prostates*] A gland, consisting of a median lobe and two lateral lobes, that surrounds the neck of the bladder and the urethra in the male. It is partly muscular and partly glandular, with ducts opening into the prostatic portion of the urethra. About 2 × 4 × 3 cm, and weighing about 20 g, it is enclosed in a fibrous capsule containing smooth muscle fibers in its inner layer. Muscle fibers also separate the glandular tissue and encircle the urethra. The gland secretes a thin, opalescent, slightly alkaline fluid that forms part of the seminal fluid.

PATHOLOGY: Inflammation of the prostate may occur, often the result of gonorrheal urethritis. Enlargement of the prostate is common, esp. after middle age. This results in urethral obstruction, impeding urination and sometimes leading to retention. Benign and malignant tumors, calculi, and nodular hyperplasia are common, particularly in men past 60. SEE: *benign prostatic hypertrophy; prostate cancer*.

balloon dilatation of the p. A treatment for prostatic hyperplasia.

transrectal ultrasonography of the p. The use of an ultrasonic detection device placed in the rectum in order to guide biopsy of the prostate.

prostate cancer A malignant tumor (almost always an adenocarcinoma) of the prostate gland. Other than skin cancers, it is the most common neoplasm in men; in 2000 the American Cancer Society estimated that there would be 180,400 cases of the disease and 31,900 fatalities. The incidence of the disease rose sharply in the 1990s after the introduction of simple screening techniques for this cancer, esp. the prostate specific antigen blood test. The disease is more common in African-American than European-American men. SEE: *benign prostatic hypertrophy; brachytherapy; prostatectomy*.

ETIOLOGY: Although the cancer may have many causes, it is a hormone (i.e. testosterone) sensitive tumor.

SYMPTOMS: The disease often is asymptomatic, or it may present with symptoms such as difficulty urinating, urinary hesitancy, nocturia, symptoms of urinary tract infection, or in cases in which the cancer has spread to bone, localized or generalized bone pain.

TREATMENT: Therapeutic options include conservative management (for patients with localized disease), orchiectomy, drug therapies to reduce testosterone concentrations, surgical resection, or radiation therapy. The procedure(s) chosen depend on the patient's expected lifespan (the disease often is diagnosed in elderly or infirm patients), the aggressiveness of the tumor, and the patient's decision after consultation with his health care team.

PATIENT CARE: Whether to screen for prostate cancer and, if so, how are topics of active research. The available options include blood tests to assess levels of prostate specific antigen (PSA), digital rectal examinations, or assessment of the gland with ultrasonography. Most experts recommend screening for men over the age of 50 who have a close relative with the disease, or who are African-American. Many urologists are convinced that screening for all men over the age of 50 increases the detection of the cancer and allows the disease to be detected at early stages when it is most likely to respond to therapy. Mass screening is controversial, however, because it detects many prostate cancers that may never damage a patient (the tumor may develop extremely slowly in a large number of men), and because some therapies used to treat the disease may themselves cause considerable morbidity and mortality. In general, when most men are given the option to screen for the disease or not they opt for a PSA test or one of its enhancements (e.g., a "free PSA" test, which measures unbound PSA in the serum).

prostatectomy (prŏs″tă-tĕk′tō-mē) [Gr. *prostates,* prostate, + *ektome,* excision] Excision of part or all of the prostate gland. The operation may be performed through an incision in the perineum (perineal prostatectomy), into the bladder (suprapubic prostatectomy), or through the urethra (transurethral prostatectomy, TURP). After prostatectomy the libido is unaffected, but during ejaculation sperm enters the bladder rather than the urethra. In the past, about 90% of patients who had prostatectomy became impotent. New surgical techniques, however, have made it possible to preserve the autonomic nerves to the corpora cavernosa of the penis. Radical prostatectomy in which the nerves important to potency are not removed or traumatized (nerve-sparing technique) has improved the chances that impotency or incontinence will not persist after the initial recovery period. Up to 70% of men having surgery done by urologists who do not use the nerve-sparing procedure will have impotency and up to 30% will have incontinence. Of patients whose surgeons use the nerve-sparing technique, 20% to 30% will be impotent and 4% to 7% or less will have mild incontinence. Complications include retention or incontinence of urine, impotence, hematuria, cystitis, infection of kidney, pyelitis, infective nephritis, and renal failure. SEE: *Nursing Diagnoses Appendix*.

PATIENT CARE: *Preoperative:* To prepare the patient for surgery and postoperative recovery, the type of procedure planned and expected results are explained, as well as the process of retrograde ejaculation. The patient is encouraged to verbalize feelings and concerns (the patient may fear loss of erectile function more than he fears cancer). The patient is prepared physically for the procedure according to the urologist's protocol.

Postoperative: Vital signs are monitored closely for indications of hemorrhage or shock. Any dressings and drainage tubes are managed, skin is protected from excoriation, and incisions or tube insertion wounds are inspected for signs of infection. If a suprapubic tube is present, patency and drainage are monitored; drainage fluid should be amber to pink tinged. Urinary catheter patency is monitored, and intermittent or continuous bladder irrigation is maintained as prescribed, usually via a three-channel indwelling catheter. Irrigation rate should be fast enough to limit drainage color change to amber to pink tinged, rather than red; rate should be increased if color deepens or clots appear. Volume of irrigant and amount of drainage are carefully tracked, and the former is subtracted from the latter to determine urinary output. This figure is then compared with intake to assess fluid balance. Findings are documented, and any abnormalities in drainage color, output volume, or patient's response to surgery are reported. If bleeding increases, traction may be applied to the catheter as directed to provide tamponade. Medicines are administered as prescribed to reduce bladder spasms and pain. Sitz baths also may be used to relieve pain and discomfort.

When the catheter is removed, the patient should void every 2 hr, and serial urines are monitored for color, time, and amount of each voiding. Fluid intake of 2 to 3 L/day (unless restricted by cardiac or renal deficits), mainly as water, is encouraged; caffeine is avoided. The patient may experience urinary frequency temporarily and dribbling, but he can regain control of urinary function with Kegel exercises. Urine may be blood tinged for a few weeks, but any bright red bleeding and fever, chills, or other signs of infection should be reported. The patient should avoid straining at stool (stool softeners are often prescribed) and lifting objects of more than 10 lb, long automobile trips, and strenuous exercise for several weeks. Walking usually is considered acceptable exercise. Sexual intercourse should be delayed until the patient has been evaluated by the physician at the follow-up visit and has the physician's permission to begin such activity. The patient also should continue prescribed medications at least until the follow-up visit and should have an annual prostatic examination if prostate removal was partial.

prostatic (prŏs-tăt′ĭk) [Gr. *prostates,* prostate] Concerning the prostate gland.

prostatic calculus A stone in the prostate.

prostatic plexus **1.** The veins around the base and neck of the bladder and prostate gland. **2.** The nerves from the pelvic plexus to the prostate gland, erectile tissue of the penis, and the seminal vesicles.

prostatic syncope Fainting during examination of the prostate. It is a rare occurrence that usually can be avoided by examining the patient in the lateral recumbent position.

prostatic urethra That part of the urethra surrounded by the prostate gland.

prostatism (prŏs′tă-tĭzm) [″ + *-ismos,* condition] Any condition of the prostate gland that interferes with the flow of urine from the bladder. The condition is characterized by frequent uncomfortable urination and nocturia. Retention of urine may occur with development of uremia. Causes include benign hypertrophy, carcinoma, prostatitis, and nodular hyperplasia.

prostatitis (prŏs″tă-tī′tĭs) [″ + *itis,* inflammation] Inflammation of the prostate gland, usually as a result of infection.

acute bacterial p. Inflammation of the prostate, commonly associated with urinary tract infections caused by enterococci, staphylococci, or gram-negative bacteria such as *Escherichia coli*. It often is caused by reflux of urine resulting from an anatomical abnormality. Patients present with fever, chills, urethral discharge, pain on urination, difficulty voiding, malaise, myalgias, and discomfort in the perineal area; the prostate is soft, swollen, and tender on examination.

The causative organism is identified through a culture of prostatic secretions and is treated with an extended course of antibiotics. Narcotics and antispasmodics may be needed to relieve pain.

chronic abacterial p. Inflammation of the prostate gland, marked by dull, aching pain in the perineum, usually of long duration. Although this is the most common type of chronic prostatitis, its cause is unknown.

chronic bacterial p. ABBR: CBP. Inflammation of the prostate caused by a long-standing bacterial infection that often develops insidiously; causative organisms include gram-negative bacteria and enterococci. Clinically, the patient may have mild to moderate low back pain, pain with urination, and perineal discomfort, or he may be asymptomatic. Patients may have a history of multiple urinary tract infections; bacteria can hide in the prostate, which resists penetration by antibiotics, and reinfect the urinary tract. Causal bacteria are identified by culture of prostatic secretions and urine. Treatment consists of ciprofloxacin or another fluoroquinolone antibiotic for 4 to 6 weeks. The long course is needed because of poor penetration into the prostate.

prostato-, prostat- [Gr. *prostrates,* prostate] Combining form meaning prostate gland.

prostatocystitis (prŏs″tă-tō-sĭs-tī′tĭs) [Gr. *prostates,* prostate, + *kystis,* bladder, + *itis,* inflammation] Inflammation of the prostatic urethra involving the bladder.

prostatocystotomy (prŏs″tă-tō-sĭs-tŏt′ō-mē) [″ + ″ + *tome,* incision] Surgical incision of the prostate and bladder.

prostatodynia (prŏs″tă-tō-dĭn′ē-ă) [″ + *odyne,* pain] The condition of having the symptoms and signs of prostatitis but no evidence of inflammation of the prostate, with negative urine culture. Use of antibiotics in patients with prostatodynia is unnecessary. SYN: *proctalgia fugax; prostatalgia.*

prostatolith (prŏs-tăt′ō-lĭth) [″ + *lithos,* stone] A calculus of the prostate gland.

prostatolithotomy (prŏs-tăt″ō-lĭ-thŏt′ō-mē) [″ + ″ + *tome,* incision] Incision of the prostate in order to remove a calculus.

prostatomegaly (prŏs″tă-tō-mĕg′ă-lē) [″ + *megas,* large] Enlargement of the prostate gland.

prostatomy, prostatotomy (prŏs-tăt′ō-mē, prŏs″tă-tŏt′ō-mē) [″ + *tome,* incision] Incision into the prostate.

prostatomyomectomy (prŏs″tă-tō-mī″ō-mĕk′tō-mē) [″ + *mys,* muscle, + *ektome,* excision] Surgical excision of a prostatic myoma.

prostatorrhea (prŏs″tă-tō-rē′ă) [″ + *rhoia,* flow] Abnormal discharge from the prostate gland.

prostatovesiculectomy (prŏs″tă-tō-vē-sĭk″ū-lĕk′tō-mē) [Gr. *prostates,* prostate, + L. *vesiculus,* a little sac, + Gr. *ektome,* excision] Removal of the prostate gland and seminal vesicles.

prostatovesiculitis (prŏs″tă-tō-vē-sĭk″ū-lī′tĭs) [″ + ″ + Gr. *itis,* inflammation] Inflammation of the seminal vesicles and prostate gland.

prosternation (prō″stĕr-nā′shŭn) [Gr. *pro,* before, + *sternon,* chest] Camptocormia.

prostheon (prŏs′thē-ŏn) [Gr. *prosthios,* foremost] The alveolar point; the midpoint of the lower border of the upper alveolar arch of the jaw.

prosthesis (prŏs′thē-sĭs) *pl.* **prostheses** [Gr. *prosthesis,* an addition] **1.** Replacement of a missing part by an artificial substitute, such as an artificial extremity. **2.** An artificial organ or part, including arms, hands, joints, heart valves, teeth, and others. SEE: *Boston arm.* **3.** A device to augment performance of a natural function, such as a hearing aid.

dental p. A dental appliance used to restore soft and hard oral tissue. The prosthesis may be internal or external to the oral cavity. Examples include dentures, partial dentures, orthodontic retainers, obturators, fixed bridges, and removable bridges.

PATIENT CARE: Care should be taken to remove, maintain, and clean dental prostheses regularly.

expansion p. A prosthesis that expands the lateral segment of the maxilla; used in clefts of the soft and hard palates and alveolar processes.

externally powered p. Any prosthesis in which a small electric motor has been incorporated for the purpose of providing force to control various functions.

hair p. Wig.

maxillofacial p. The repair and artificial replacement of the face and jaw missing because of disease or injury.

myoelectric p. An advanced prosthetic device operated by battery-powered electric motors that are activated through electrodes by the myoelectric potentials provided by muscles.

neural p. Any device or electrode that improves function by substituting for an injured or diseased part of the nervous system.

penile p. A device implanted in the penis that assists it to become erect. The device is used in patients with erectile dysfunction due to such organic causes as trauma, prostatectomy, or diabetes. It is usually in the form of inflatable plastic cylinders implanted in each corpus cavernosum of the penis. These cylinders are attached to a pump embedded in the scrotal pouch. A reservoir for the fluid used to fill the cylinders is implanted behind the rectus muscle. This system allows the cylinders to be filled when an erection is desired and the fluid to be drained back into the reservoir when the need for the erection has passed. In most patients, this device permits the attaining of a nearly physiological erection. SEE: *Peyronie's disease.*

porcine valvular p. A biological prosthesis made from the heart valve of a pig, used to replace a diseased cardiac valve.

voice p. A device that synthesizes the human voice. It is used in patients who have undergone laryngeal surgery.

prosthetic group (prŏs-thĕt′ĭk) The non–amino acid component of a conjugated protein; usually the portion of an enzyme that is not an amino acid. SEE: *apoenzyme; holoenzyme.*

prosthetics (prŏs-thĕt′ĭks) The branch of surgery or physiatry (physical medicine) dealing with construction, replacement, and adaptation of missing or damaged parts.

prosthetist (prŏs′thĕ-tĭst) **1.** A specialist in artificial dentures. **2.** A maker of artificial limbs.

prosthetosclerokeratoplasty (prŏs″thĕ-tō-sklē″rō-kĕr′ă-tō-plăs″tē) The surgical procedure for replacement of diseased scleral and corneal tissue with a transparent prosthesis.

prosthion (prŏs′thē-ŏn) [Gr. *prosthios,* foremost] The lowest point on the alveolar process of the maxilla.

prosthodontics (prŏs″thō-dŏn′tĭks) [″ + *odous,* tooth] The branch of dentistry dealing with construction of artificial appliances for the mouth.

prosthodontist (prŏs″thō-dŏn′tĭst) A dentist who specializes in the mechanics of making and fitting artificial teeth, dental appliances, and other prostheses that replace structures of the maxillofacial region.

prosthokeratoplasty (prŏs″thō-kĕr′ă-tō-plăs″tē) [″ + *keras,* horn, + *plassein,* to form] Surgical replacement of diseased or scarred corneal tissue with a transparent prosthesis.

prostitution (prŏs″tĭ-tū′shŭn) [L. *prostituere,* to prostitute] The act of exchanging sexual favors for money. It is a risk factor for the spread of sexually transmitted diseases, including chlamydia, gonorrhea, trichomoniasis, syphilis, hepatitis, and acquired immunodeficiency syndrome.

prostrate (prŏs′trāt) [Gr. *pro,* before, + L. *sternere,* stretch out] **1.** Lying with the body extended, usually face down. **2.** To deprive of strength or to exhaust.

prostrated Depleted of strength; exhausted.

prostration (prŏs-trā′shŭn) Absolute exhaustion.

heat p. Exhaustion resulting from exposure to excessive heat.

nervous p. General physical and nervous exhaustion. SYN: *neurasthenia.*

protactinium (prō″tăk-tĭn′ē-ŭm) SYMB: Pa. A radioactive element; atomic weight 231; atomic number 91.

protal (prō′tăl) [Gr. *protos,* first] Congenital.

protamine (prō′tă-mĭn) **1.** One of a class of simple proteins that are strongly basic, noncoagulable in heat, and yield diamino acids when hydrolyzed. **2.** An amine isolated from spermatozoa and the spawn of fish, and named for the fish from which it is derived. SEE: *salmin(e).*

p. insulin Preparations of insulin that are more slowly dissolved and absorbed by body tissues than ordinary insulin. They are longer-acting than ordinary insulin and lower the blood sugar for 20 to 24 hr. Examples are NPH (isophane) insulin and protamine zinc insulin.

p. sulfate A purified form of protamine used to neutralize the anticoagulant action of heparin.

protanope (prō′tă-nōp) [Gr. *protos,* first, + *an-,* not, + *opsis,* vision] A person with protanopia.

protanopia (prō-tăn-ō′pē-ă) [″ + ″ + *opsis,* vision] Red blindness; color blindness in which there is a defect in the perception of red. SEE: *color blindness.*

protean (prō′tē-ăn) [Gr. *Proteus,* a god who could change his form] Having the ability to change form, as the ameba; variable.

protease inhibitor **1.** A substance that inhibits the action of enzymes. **2.** One of a class of medications that prevent immature virions of the human immunodeficiency virus (HIV) from assembling into structures capable of replication.

proteases (prō′tē-ās-ĕs) [Gr. *protos,* first, + *-ase,* enzyme] A class of enzymes that break down, or hydrolyze, the peptide bonds that join the amino acids in a protein. The protein is broken down into its basic building blocks (i.e., amino acids). SEE: *digestion.*

protection, altered The state in which an individual experiences a decrease in the ability to guard the self from internal or external threats such as illness or injury. SEE: *Nursing Diagnoses Appendix.*

protective (prō-tĕk′tĭv) [L. *protectus,* shielding] **1.** Covering, preventing infection, providing immunity. **2.** Dressing.

proteidogenous (prō″tē-ĭd-ŏj′ĕn-ŭs) Producing proteins.

protein (prō′tēn, prō′tē-ĭn) [Gr. *protos,* first] One of a class of complex nitrogenous compounds that are synthesized by all living organisms and yield amino acids when hydrolyzed. Proteins in the diet provide the amino acids necessary for the growth and repair of animal tissue.

COMPOSITION: All amino acids contain carbon, hydrogen, oxygen, and nitrogen; some also contain sulfur. About 20 different amino acids make up human proteins, which may contain other minerals such as iron or copper. A protein consists of from 50 to thousands of amino acids arranged in a very specific sequence. The essential amino acids are those the liver cannot synthesize (tryptophan, lysine, methionine, valine, leucine, isoleucine, phenylalanine, threonine, arginine, and histidine); they are essential in the diet, and a protein containing all of them is called a complete protein. An incomplete protein lacks one or more of the essential amino acids. The nonessential amino acids are synthesized by the liver.

SOURCES: Milk, eggs, cheese, meat, fish, and some vegetables such as soybeans are the best sources. Proteins are found in both vegetable and animal sources of food. Many incomplete proteins are found in vegetables; they contain some of the essential amino acids. A vegetarian diet can make up for this by combining vegetable groups that complement each other in their basic amino acid groups. This provides the body with complete protein.

Principal animal proteins are lactalbumin and lactoglobulin in milk; ovalbumin and ovoglobulin in eggs; serum albumin in serum; myosin and actin in striated muscle tissue; fibrinogen in blood; serum globulin in serum; thyroglobulin in thyroid; globin in blood; thymus histones in thymus; collagen and gelatin in connective tissue; collagen and elastin in connective tissue; and keratin in the epidermis. Chondroprotein is found in tendons and cartilage; mucin and mucoids are found in various secreting glands and animal mucilaginous substances; caseinogen in milk; vitellin in egg yolk; hemoglobin in red blood cells; and lecithoprotein in the blood, brain, and bile.

FUNCTION: Ingested proteins are a source of amino acids needed to synthesize the body's own proteins, which are essential for the growth of new tissue or the repair of damaged tissue; proteins are part of all cell membranes. Excess amino acids in the diet may be changed to simple carbohydrates and oxidized to produce adenosine triphosphate and heat; 1 g supplies 4 kcal of heat.

Infants and children require from 2 to 2.2 g of protein per kilogram of body weight per day. This should be calculated on the basis of the ideal, rather than the actual, weight of the child. Age also is a factor in determining protein requirements, the amount decreasing with age. Physical work, menstruation, pregnancy, lactation, and convalescence require increased protein intake. Excess protein in the diet results in increased nitrogen excretion in the urine.

activator p. A protein that stimulates the expression of a gene.

acute phase p. Any of the plasma proteins whose concentration increases or decreases by at least 25% during inflammation. Acute-phase proteins include C-reactive protein, several complement and coagulation factors, transport proteins, amyloid, and antiprotease enzymes. They help mediate both positive and negative effects of acute and chronic inflammation, including chemotaxis, phagocytosis, protection against oxygen radicals, and tissue repair. In clinical medicine, the erythrocyte sedimentation rate or serum C-reactive protein level sometimes is used as a marker of increased amounts of acute-phase proteins. SEE: *inflammation.*

amyloid precursor p. ABBR: APP. A brain peptide that is cleaved biochemically into components, one of which is the Alzheimer's disease–associated amyloid. Mutations in the gene for APP on chromosome 21 account for less than 5% of early-onset familial Alzheimer's disease.

blood p. A broad term encompassing numerous proteins, including hemoglobin, albumin, globulins, the acute-phase reactants, transporter molecules, and many others. Normal values are hemoglobin, 13 to 18 g/dl in men and 12 to 16 g/dl in women; albumin, 3.5 to 5.0 g/dl of serum; globulin, 2.3 to 3.5 g/dl of serum. The amount of albumin in relation to the amount of globulin is referred to as the albumin-globulin (A/G) ratio, which is normally 1.5:1 to 2.5:1.

carrier p. A protein that elicits an immune response when coupled with a hapten.

coagulated p. One of the derived (insoluble) proteins resulting from the action of alcohol, heat, or other physicochemical entities on protein solutions.

complete p. A protein containing all the essential amino acids.

conjugated p. A protein that is chemically linked with a non-protein molecule. Included are chromoproteins (e.g., hemoglobin); glycoproteins (e.g., mucin); lecithoproteins, nucleoproteins, and phosphoproteins (e.g., casein).

C reactive p. The first acute phase protein identified. It binds with phospholipids on foreign substances, activates the complement system, stimulates the production of cytokines, and inhibits the production of oxygen radicals by neutrophils. Increased blood levels of C-reactive protein are present in many infectious and inflammatory diseases. SEE: *acute phase p.*

denatured p. A protein in which the amino acid composition and stereochemical structure (shape) have been altered by physical or chemical means. SEE: *coagulated p.*

derived p. A protein altered chemically or physically.

G p. A cellular protein activated by the binding of an intercellular signal to its receptor on the cell membrane; the G-protein then activates the enzyme adenyl cyclase within the cell, triggering the formation of cyclic AMP and a stereotyped response.

immune p. An antibody or immunoglobulin produced by plasma cells that identifies foreign antigens and initiates their destruction.

incomplete p. A protein lacking one or more of the essential amino acids. SEE: *amino acid, essential.*

lipopolysaccharide-binding p. One of many acute-phase proteins released into the serum in patients with a gram-negative bacterial infection; it helps to defend the body against sepsis by binding and transferring bacterial endotoxin.

membrane-bound p. A protein that is part of a cell membrane and acts as a receptor for substances transported in extracellular fluid or as an agent that mediates the transport of chemicals into or out of the cell.

native p. A protein in its natural state; one that has not been denatured.

oncofetal p. A cell surface marker, such as carcinoembryonic antigen or alpha-fetoprotein, that is expressed on some malignant cells. The detection of such proteins may be used to monitor the clinical course of some cancers (e.g., cancer of the colon or liver).

plasma p. A protein present in blood plasma, such as albumin or globulin.

pregnancy-associated p. A A serum protein that is diminished in pregnancies in which the fetus suffers from Down syndrome. It may be used as a screening test for this condition.

serum p. Any protein in the blood serum. The two main fractions are albumin and the globulins. Serum protein forms weak acids mixed with alkali salts; this increases the buffer effects of the blood but to a lesser extent than does cellular protein.

simple p. Any of the proteins that produce alpha amino acids on hydrolysis (e.g., albumins, albuminoids, globulins, glutelins, histones, prolamines, and protamines).

steroidogenic acute regulatory p. ABBR: StAR protein. A protein found within cells of the adrenal glands and gonads that stimulates the conversion of cholesterol into sex hormones, corticosteroids, and mineralocorticoids.

proteinaceous (prō″tē-ĭn-ā′shŭs) Concerning, derived from, or resembling proteins.

proteinase (prō′tē-ĭn-ās) [Gr. *protos,* first, + *lase,* enzyme] A proteolytic enzyme; an enzyme that catalyzes the breakdown of native proteins.

protein balance Equilibrium between protein intake and anabolism, and protein catabolism and elimination of nitrogenous products. SEE: *nitrogen equilibrium.*

protein C A plasma protein that inhibits coagulation factors V and XIII, preventing excessive clotting. Deficiency of this protein causes thrombosis.

protein-calorie malnutrition Malnutrition usually seen in infants and young children whose diets are deficient in both proteins and calories. Clinically the condition may be precipitated by other factors such as infection or intestinal parasites. SEE: *kwashiorkor.*

protein hydrolysate injection A sterile solution of amino acids and short-chain peptides. They represent the approximate nutritive equivalent of casein, lactalbumin, plasma, fibrin, or other suitable proteins from which the hydrolysate is derived by acid, enzymatic, or other method of hydrolysis. It may contain dextrose or other carbohydrates suitable for intravenous infusion. It is used intravenously in the treatment of hypoproteinemia in patients who are unable to eat or absorb food.

protein kinase An enzyme that activates or inactivates cell proteins or enzymes by adding a phosphate moiety, thereby changing cell functions.

protein-losing enteropathy The abnormal loss of protein into the gastrointestinal tract. It may be due to any disease that causes extensive ulceration of the intestinal mucosa.

proteinogenous (prō″tē-ĭn-ŏj′ĕn-ŭs) [″ + *gennan,* to produce] Developing from a protein.

proteinophobia (prō″tē-ĭn-ō-fō′bē-ă) [″ + *phobos,* fear] An aversion to foods containing protein.

proteinosis (prō″tē-ĭn-ō′sĭs) [″ + *osis,* condition] Accumulation of excess proteins in the tissues.

lipoid p. A rare autosomal recessive condition resulting from an undefined metabolic defect. Yellow deposits of a mixture of protein and lipoid occur, esp. on the mucous surface of the mouth and tongue. Nodules may appear on the face, extremities, and on the epiglottis and vocal cords, the latter producing hoarseness.

pulmonary alveolar p. A disease of unknown cause in which eosinophilic material is deposited in the alveoli. The principal symptom is dyspnea. Death from pulmonary insufficiency may occur, but complete recovery has been observed. There is no specific treatment, but general supportive measures including antibiotics and bronchopulmonary lavage have helped. In about 25% of cases, the disease clears spontaneously, but in most untreated cases the disease is progressive and leads to respiratory failure. SEE: *bronchoalveolar lavage.*

protein sparer A substance in the diet such as carbohydrate or fat that prevents the use of protein for energy needs.

proteinuria (prō″tē-ĭn-ū′rē-ă) [″ + *ouron,* urine] Protein, usually albumin, in the urine. This finding may be transient and entirely benign or a sign of severe renal disease. SYN: *albuminuria.* SEE: *microalbuminuria; nephrotic syndrome.*

nephrotic range p. Loss of massive amounts of protein in the urine (more than 3 g/day).

orthostatic p. Protein in the urine when the patient has been standing but not while reclining.

postural p. Protein in the urine in relation to bodily position.
proteoglycans (prō″tē-ō-glī′kăns) A family of molecules that are fundamental components of mucus and connective tissues. They are composed of sugars linked to polypeptides and are found in organs and tissues throughout the body.
proteolipid (prō″tē-ō-lĭp′ĭd) A lipid-protein complex that is insoluble in water. It is found principally in the brain.
proteolysin (prō″tē-ŏl′ĭ-sĭn) [″ + *lysis,* dissolution] A specific substance causing decomposition of proteins.
proteolysis (prō″tē-ŏl′ĭ-sĭs) The hydrolysis of proteins, usually by enzyme action, into simpler substances.
proteolytic (prō″tē-ō-lĭt′ĭk) Hastening the hydrolysis of proteins.
proteometabolism (prō″tē-ō-mĕ-tăb′ō-lĭzm) [″ + *metabole,* change, + *-ismos,* condition] Digestion, absorption, and assimilation of proteins.
proteopepsis (prō″tē-ō-pĕp′sĭs) [″ + *peptein,* to digest] The digestion of proteins.
proteopeptic (prō″tē-ō-pĕp′tĭk) [″ + *peptein,* to digest] Pert. to the digestion of protein.
proteopexy (prō″tē-ō-pĕks′ē) [″ + *pexis,* fixation] The fixation of proteins within the body. **proteopexic** (prō-tē-ō-pĕks′ĭk), *adj.*
proteose (prō′tē-ōs) [Gr. *protos,* first] One of the class of intermediate products of proteolysis between protein and peptone.
primary p. The first products formed during proteolysis of proteins.
secondary p. The protein resulting from further hydrolysis of primary proteoses.
proteosuria (prō″tē-ōs-ū′rē-ă) [″ + *ouron,* urine] Proteose in urine.
Proteus (prō′tē-ŭs) [Gr. *Proteus,* a god who could change his form] A genus of gram-negative enteric bacilli, found in intestines and decaying material, causing protein decomposition.
P. mirabilis A species abundant in nature and an occasional human pathogen (e.g., of the urinary tract).
P. morganii Previous name of *Morganella morganii.*
P. vulgaris An essentially saprophytic species that may produce urinary tract infections.
prothrombin A plasma protein coagulation factor synthesized by the liver (vitamin K is necessary) that is converted to thrombin by prothrombinase and thrombokinase (activated factor X) in the presence of calcium ions. SEE: *coagulation factor*.
prothrombinase An enzyme important in blood coagulation. In a reaction with activated factors X (Xa) and V (Va) in the presence of calcium and platelets, prothrombinase catalyzes the conversion of prothrombin to thrombin.
prothrombinemia (prō-thrŏm″bĭn-ē′mē-ă) [Gr. *pro,* before, + *thrombos,* clot, + *haima,* blood] The presence of prothrombin in the blood.
prothrombinogenic (prō-thrŏm″bĭ-nō-jĕn′ĭk) [″ + ″ + *gennan,* to produce] Promoting the formation of prothrombin.
prothrombinopenia (prō-thrŏm″bĭ-nō-pē′nē-ă) [″ + ″ + *penia,* lack] A deficiency of prothrombin in the blood. SYN: *hypoprothrombinemia*.
prothrombin time The time it takes for clotting to occur after thromboplastin and calcium are added to decalcified plasma. The test is used to assess levels of anticoagulation in patients taking warfarin, to determine the cause of unexplained bleeding (e.g., in patients with hemophilia), or to assess the ability of the liver to synthesize blood-clotting proteins.
prothymocyte A precursor cell that matures and differentiates into a functioning T cell in the thymus gland. SEE: *T cell*.
protide (prō′tīd) Protein.
protist (prō′tĭst) Any member of the Protista kingdom.
Protista (prō-tĭs′tă) [LL., simplest organisms] In taxonomy, a kingdom of organisms that includes the protozoa, unicellular and multicellular algae, and the slime molds. The cells are eukaryotic. SEE: *Protozoa* for illus.; *eukaryote; prokaryote*.
protistologist (prō-tĭs-tŏl′ō-jĭst) [″ + *logos,* word, reason] One who studies the Protista, the unicellular organisms.
protium (prō-tē-ŭm) Hydrogen with an atomic weight of one.
proto- **1.** Combining form meaning *first.* **2.** Prefix indicating the lowest of a series of compounds having the same elements.
protobiology (prō″tō-bī-ŏl′ō-jē) [Gr. *protos,* first, + *bios,* life, + *logos,* word, reason] The phase of science dealing with life forms more minute than bacteria (i.e., the ultraviruses and bacteriophages).
protocol (prō′tō-kŏl) [Gr. *protokollon,* first notes glued to manuscript] **1.** Formal ideas, plans, or expectations concerning the actions of those involved in patient care, bench work, administration, or research. **2.** In computer science, the rules or conventions governing the formats and timing of information exchange between communicating devices or processes. SEE: *algorithm*. **3.** A description of the steps to be taken in an experiment.
therapist-driven p. A patient care plan initiated and carried out by a respiratory care practitioner with the approval of the hospital medical staff.
treatment p. An algorithm or recipe for managing a disease or condition.

protodiastole (prō″tō-dī-ăs′tō-lē) [Gr. *protos,* first, + *diastole,* expansion] The first of four phases of ventricular diastole characterized by a drop in intraventricular pressure. This occurs immediately after the second heart sound.

protoduodenum (prō″tō-dū-ō-dē′nŭm) [″ + L. *duodeni,* twelve] The upper half of the duodenum. It is derived from the embryonic foregut.

protogaster (prō″tō-găs′tĕr) [″ + *gaster,* belly] The archenteron or gastrocele; the cavity in a gastrula or developing embryo from which the digestive tract develops.

protoleukocyte (prō″tō-lū′kō-sīt) [″ + *leukos,* white, + *kytos,* cell] A minute lymphoid cell in the red bone marrow and spleen.

Protomastigida (prō″tō-măst-ĭj′ĭ-dă) [″ + *mastix,* whip, + *eidos,* form, shape] An order of flagellate protozoa. It contains several pathogenic genera including *Leishmania* and *Trypanosoma.*

proton (prō′tŏn) [Gr. *protos,* first] A positively charged particle forming the nucleus of hydrogen and present in the nuclei of all elements, the atomic number of the element indicating the number of protons present. Its mass is 1836 times that of an electron. SEE: *atom; atomic theory; electron; element.*

protoneuron (prō″tō-nū′rŏn) [″ + *neuron,* nerve] The initial neuron in a reflex arc.

protopathic [″ + *pathos,* disease, suffering] Primitive, undiscriminating, esp. with respect to sensing and localizing pain stimuli. SEE: *sensibility.*

protoplasia (prō-tō-plā′zē-ă) [″ + *plassein,* to form] The primary formation of tissue.

protoplasm (prō′tō-plăzm) [″ + LL. *plasma,* form, mold] A thick, viscous colloidal substance that constitutes the physical basis of all living activities, exhibiting the properties of assimilation, growth, motility, secretion, irritability, and reproduction. It is a complex mixture of heterogeneous substances surrounded by a chemically active membrane that regulates the interchange of substances with the surrounding medium. It possesses the physical properties of a colloidal mass, the medium of dispersion being water.

Protoplasm consists of inorganic substances (water, mineral compounds) and organic substances (proteins, carbohydrates, and lipids). The principal elements present are oxygen, carbon, hydrogen, nitrogen, calcium, sulfur, and phosphorus, which constitute about 99% of protoplasm. Others present in small amounts are potassium, chlorine, sodium, magnesium, and iron, together with trace elements (copper, cobalt, manganese, zinc, and others). SEE: *cell; cytoplasm; nucleus.* **protoplasmic** (prō-tō-plăz′mĭk), *adj.*

protoplast (prō′tō-plăst) [″ + *plassein,* to form] In bacteriology, the sphere remaining after gram-positive bacteria have had their cell contents lysed. The bacterial cell wall constituents are absent. In gram-negative organisms these spheres retain an outer wall layer and are called spheroplasts.

protoporphyria (prō″tō-por-fĭr′ē-ă) Porphyria erythropoietica.

protoporphyrin (prō″tō-por′fĭ-rĭn) A derivative of hemoglobin containing four pyrrole nuclei; $C_{34}H_{34}N_4O_4$. It occurs naturally and is formed from heme (ferriprotoporphyrin) by deletion of an atom of iron.

protoporphyrinuria (prō″tō-por″fĭ-rĭn-ū′rē-ă) Protoporphyrin in the urine.

protoproteose (prō″tō-prō′tē-ōz) A primary proteose that, upon further digestion, is converted to deuteroproteose.

protospasm (prō′tō-spăzm) [Gr. *protos,* first, + *spasmos,* a convulsion] A spasm beginning in one area and extending to other parts.

prototype (prō″tō-tīp) An original or initial model or type from which subsequent types arise.

protovertebra (prō″tō-vĕr′tĕ-bră) [″ + L. *vertebra,* vertebra] Primitive vertebra in the notochord. SYN: *provertebra.*

Protozoa [″ + *zoon,* animal] The phylum of the kingdom Protista that includes unicellular, animal-like microorganisms. Most protozoa are saprophytes, living in the soil and obtaining nourishment from dead or decaying organic material. Most protozoa infect only humans without adequate immunological defenses, although a few infect immunocompetent persons. Infections are spread by the fecal-oral route, through ingestion of food or water contaminated with cysts or spores, or by the bite of a mosquito or other insect that has previously bitten an infected person. Common protozoan infections include malaria (*Plasmodium vivax, P. malariae*); gastroenteritis (*Entamoeba histolytica, Giardia lamblia*); leishmaniasis, an inflammatory skin or visceral disease (*Leishmania* species); sleeping sickness (*Trypanosoma gambiense*); and vaginal infections (*Trichomonas vaginalis*). *Pneumocystis carinii,* previously classified as a protozoon, is now categorized as a fungus. Opportunistic protozoan infections caused by *Cryptosporidium parvum* and *Toxoplasma gondii* are seen in patients who are immunosuppressed by disease or drug therapy. SEE: illus.; table.

protozoa Pl. of protozoon.

protozoacide (prō-tō-zō′ă-sīd) [″ + *zoon,* animal, + L. *cidus,* kill] Destructive to, or that which kills, protozoa.

protozoal (prō″tō-zō′ăl) Pert. to protozoa, unicellular organisms.

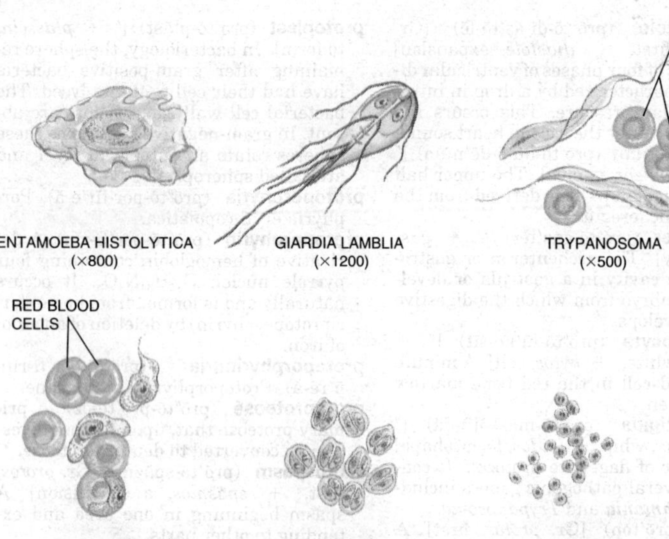

PROTOZOA

Table of Pathogenic Protozoa

Subphylum	Genus and Species	Disease Caused
Zoomastigophora (Mastigophora) Locomotion by flagella	*Giardia lamblia*	Gastroenteritis
	Leishmania donovani	Kala azar
	Leishmania braziliensis	American leishmaniasis
	Leishmania tropica	Oriental sore
	Trichomonas vaginalis	Trichomoniasis
	Trypanosoma gambiense	Sleeping sickness
	Trypanosoma rhodesiense	Sleeping sickness
	Trypanosoma cruzi	Chagas' disease
Rhizopoda (Sarcodinae) Locomotion by pseudopodia	*Acanthamoeba castellani*	Amebic meningoencephalitis
	A. culbertsonii	
	A. astromyxis	
	Dientamoeba fragilis	Diarrhea, fever
	Entamoeba histolytica	Amebic dysentery
	Naegleria fowleri	Amebic meningoencephalitis
Apicomplexa (Sporozoa) No locomotion in adult stage	*Babesia microti*	Babesiosis
	B. divergens	
	Cryptosporidium parvum	Cryptosporidiosis
	Cyclospora cayetanensis	Diarrhea, gastroenteritis
	Isospora belli	Diarrhea
	Microspora (multiple spp.)	Diarrhea, chronic
	Plasmodium malariae	Quartan malaria
	Plasmodium falciparum	Malignant tertian malaria
	Plasmodium vivax	Tertian malaria
	Plasmodium ovale	Tertian malaria
	Toxoplasma gondii	Toxoplasmosis
Ciliophora Possession of cilia in some stage of life cycle	*Balantidium coli*	Balantidiasis

protozoal disease A disease produced by parasitic protozoa. Examples are amebic dysentery, sleeping sickness, and malaria.

protozoan (prō″tō-zō′ăn) [″ + *zoon,* animal] Concerning protozoa.

protozoology (prō″tō-zō-ŏl′ō-jē) [Gr. *protos,* first, + *zoon,* animal, + *logos,* word, reason] The branch of science dealing with the study of protozoa.

protozoon *pl.* **protozoa** Unicellular organism. SEE: *Protozoa.*

protozoophage (prō″tō-zō′ō-fāj) [″ + *zoon,* animal, + *phagein,* to eat] A phagocyte that ingests protozoa.

protraction (prō-trăk′shŭn) [″ + L. *protractus,* dragged out] The extension forward or drawing forward of a part of the body such as the mandible.

protractor (prō-trăk′tor) [L. *protractus,* dragged out] **1.** An instrument formerly used to remove foreign bodies from wounds. **2.** A muscle that draws a part forward; the opposite of retractor. **3.** Semicircular device for drawing angles.

protriptyline hydrochloride (prō-trĭp′tĭ-lēn) A tricyclic antidepressant drug. Its side effects may include dry mouth, sedation, constipation, and urinary retention, among others.

protrude [L. *protrudere*] To project; to extend beyond a border or limit.

protrusion (prō-troo′zhŭn) The state or condition of being thrust forward or projecting. In dentistry, particularly related to the position of the mandible, as opposed to retrusion.

protuberance (prō-tū′bĕr-ăns) [Gr. *pro,* before, + L. *tuber,* bulge] A part that is prominent beyond a surface, like a knob.

protuberantia (prō-tū″bĕr-ăn′shē-ă) A protuberance, eminence, or projection.

proud flesh A mass of excessive granulation formed when a wound shows no other sign of healing or tendency to cicatrization.

provertebra (prō-vĕr′tĕ-bră) Protovertebra.

provider A professional who gives health care services, or an institution that supervises the rendering of such services.

mid-level p. A category of health care professionals that includes physician assistants, nurse midwives, nurse anesthetists, and nurse practitioners. SYN: *mid-level practitioner.*

provirus (prō-vī′rŭs) The precursor of a virus.

provisional (prō-vĭzh′ŭn-ăl) [L. *provisio,* provision] Serving a temporary use pending permanent arrangements.

provitamin (prō-vī′tă-mĭn) [L. *pro,* before, + *vita,* life, + *amine*] An inactive substance that can be transformed in the body to a corresponding active vitamin and thus function as a vitamin.

p. A Carotene, the precursor of vitamin A.

proximad (prŏk′sĭm-ăd) [L. *proximus,* next, + *ad,* toward] Toward the proximal or central point.

proximal (prŏk′sĭm-ăl) Nearest the point of attachment, center of the body, or point of reference; the opposite of distal.

proximate (prŏk′sĭm-āt) Closely related with respect to space, time, or sequence. Next to, or nearest.

proximate cause An event that immediately precedes another and is felt to be responsible for its occurrence.

proximoataxia (prŏk″sĭ-mō-ă-tăk′sē-ă) [″ + Gr. *ataxia,* lack of order] A lack of coordination in the muscles of the proximal area of an extremity, as the arm, forearm, thigh, or leg.

proximobuccal (prŏk″sĭ-mō-bŭk′ăl) [″ + *bucca,* cheek] Concerning the proximal and buccal surfaces of a tooth.

proximolabial (prŏk″sĭ-mō-lā′bē-ăl) [″ + *labialis,* pert. to the lips] Concerning the proximal and labial surfaces of a tooth.

proximolingual (prŏk″sĭ-mō-lĭng′gwăl) [″ + *lingua,* tongue] Concerning the proximal and lingual surfaces of a tooth.

prozone That portion of the low dilution range of a homologous serum that fails to agglutinate bacteria that are agglutinated by the same serum in a higher dilution.

prozymogen (prō-zī′mō-jĕn) [Gr. *pro,* before, + *zyme,* leaven, + *gennan,* to produce] An intranuclear substance that is a precursor of zymogen.

prune (proon) [L. *pruna*] A dried plum, rich in carbohydrate, that contains dihydroxyphenyl isatin, a laxative. Regular consumption may lead to dependence on its laxative properties.

prune-belly defect A nonstandard, but descriptive, term for children with congenital absence of one or more layers of abdominal muscles.

pruriginous (proo-rĭj′ĭ-nŭs) [L. *prurigo,* itch] Pert. to, or of the nature of, prurigo.

prurigo (proo-rī′gō) [L., the itch] A chronic skin disease of unknown etiology, marked by constantly recurring, discrete, pale, deep-seated, intensely itchy papules on extensor surfaces of limbs. Superimposed exanthematous manifestations may mask the true nature. This term is used by dermatologists throughout the world, but it has not received a universally acceptable definition. Treatment is constitutional and local, with antipruritics given locally. Prurigo begins in childhood and may last a lifetime.

p. agria A severe type of prurigo that starts in childhood and persists. The skin becomes thickened and pigmented. Because of the severe itching and scratching, secondary pustules, boils, and abscesses may develop.

p. estivalis A form of polymorphic light eruption characterized by prurigo and photodermatitis. It recurs every summer and continues during hot weather.

p. mitis Mild prurigo.

pregnancy p. A form of prurigo that usually has its onset in the middle trimester of pregnancy or later. The lesions occur on the proximal portion of the limbs and upper part of the trunk and usually improves spontaneously before term or rapidly after delivery.

simple acute p. A simple form of prurigo with recurring tendency. It is thought to be caused by a reaction to bites in sensitive subjects.

p. simplex Urticaria papulosa.

pruritogenic (proo″rĭ-tō-jĕn′ĭk) [L. *pruritus,* itching, + *gennan,* to produce] Causing pruritus.

pruritus (proo-rī′tŭs) [L., itching] Itch; a tingling or faintly burning skin sensation that prompts a person to rub or scratch. It may be a symptom of a disease process, such as an allergic response or hyperbilirubinemia, or it may be due to emotional factors. SEE: *Nursing Diagnoses Appendix.* **pruritic,** *adj.*

TREATMENT: Any inciting or contributory cause should be identified and removed if possible.

p. ani Itching around the anus. This may be due to poor perineal hygiene; perianal skin damage caused by scratching, or abrasion due to use of harsh, dry paper; excess moisture caused by wearing tight, nonporous clothing; decreased resistance to fungi and yeasts during steroid therapy; ingestion of dietary irritants; pinworms; anal fistula or hemorrhoids; or contact with soap or detergents that remain in underclothing following improper washing.

TREATMENT: The primary cause should be removed or avoided. The anus should be kept scrupulously clean by use of a mild soap, and applications of drugs that produce sensitivity and irritation should be avoided.

aquagenic p. Pruritus produced by contact with water.

emperor of p. SEE: *emperor of pruritus.*

essential p. Pruritus without apparent skin lesion.

p. estivalis Pruritus with prickly heat occurring in hot weather.

p. hiemalis Winter itch.

p. senilis Pruritus in the aged with degenerative skin changes sometimes caused by loss of epidermal hydration.

vulvar p. Lichen sclerosis et atrophicus.

Prussak's space (proo′săks) [Alexander Prussak, Russ. otologist, 1839–1897] The tiny space in the middle ear between Shrapnell's membrane laterally and the neck of the malleus medially.

PSA *prostate-specific antigen.*

psalterium (săl-tē′rē-ŭm) [Gr. *psalterion,* harp] **1.** The third division of a ruminant's stomach. **2.** Commissure of the fornix of the brain.

psammoma (săm-ō′mă) [Gr. *psammos,* sand, + *oma,* tumor] A small tumor of the brain, the choroid plexus, and other areas, containing calcareous particles.

psammosarcoma (săm″o-săr-kō′mă) [″ + *sarx,* flesh, + *oma,* tumor] A sarcoma in which psammoma bodies are present.

psammotherapy (săm″ō-thĕr′ă-pē) [″ + *therapeia,* treatment] The application of sand baths in treatment.

psammous (săm′ŭs) Sandy, gritty.

PSDE *painful swollen deformed extremity.*

psellism, psellismus (sĕl′ĭzm, sĕl-ĭz′mŭs) [Gr. *psellisma,* stammer] Defective pronunciation, stuttering, or stammering.

p. mercurialis Jerking, hurried, unintelligible speech present as part of the tremor that accompanies mercury poisoning.

pseudacousma (soo″dă-kooz′mă) [Gr. *pseudes,* false, + *akousma,* a thing heard] A condition in which all sounds are heard falsely, seeming to be altered in quality of pitch, or imaginary sounds are heard. SYN: *pseudacusis.*

pseudacusis (soo″dă-kū′sĭs) Pseudacousma.

pseudagraphia (soo″dă-grăf′ē-ă) [″ + *a-,* not, + *graphein,* to write] A form of agraphia in which a person is unable to write independently, but is able to copy words or letters. SYN: *pseudoagraphia.*

pseudarthritis (soo″dăr-thrī′tĭs) [″ + *arthron,* joint, + *itis,* inflammation] A condition that imitates arthritis. Also known as pseudoarteritis.

pseudarthrosis, pseudoarthrosis (soo″dăr-thrō′sĭs) [″ + *arthron,* joint, + *osis,* condition] A false joint or abnormal articulation, as one developing after a fracture that has not united. SYN: *nearthrosis.*

pseudencephalus (soo″dĕn-sĕf′ă-lŭs) [″ + *enkephalos,* brain] A congenital deformity in which the cranium is open and contains poorly organized vascular tissue.

pseudesthesia (soo″dĕs-thē′zē-ă) [″ + *aisthesis,* sensation] **1.** An imaginary or false sensation, as that felt in the lost part after amputation. **2.** A sense of feeling not caused by external stimulation. SYN: *pseudoesthesia.*

pseudo- (soo′dō) [Gr. *pseudes,* false] Combining form meaning *false.*

pseudoacanthosis nigricans (soo″dō-ăk″ăn-thō′sĭs) [″ + *akantha,* thorn, + *osis,* condition] A velvety, pigmented thickening of the flexural surfaces, occurring in dark-skinned obese persons.

pseudoacephalus (soo″dō-ā-sĕf′ă-lŭs) [″ + *a-,* not, + *kephale,* head] A parasitic twin that has a rudimentary cranium.

pseudoagglutination (soo″dō-ă-glū″tĭ-nā′shŭn) The clumping together of red blood cells as in the formation of rouleaux, but differing from true agglutination in that the cells can be dispersed by shaking.

pseudoagraphia Pseudagraphia.

pseudoalbinism (soo″dō-ăl′bĭ-nĭzm) [″ + L. *albus,* white, + Gr. *-ismos,* condition] Loss of pigment of the skin, as occurs in leukopathia or vitiligo.

pseudoalleles (soo″dō-ă-lēlz′) [″ + *allelon,* of one another] A set of genes that seem to be present in the same locus in certain conditions and in closely situated loci in other conditions.

pseudoanemia (soo″dō-ă-nē′mē-ă) [″ + *an-,* not, + *haima,* blood] Pallor of mucous membranes and skin without other signs of true anemia.

p. of pregnancy A drop in hematocrit during pregnancy. The increase in circulating blood volume reflects an altered ratio of serum to red blood cells; plasma volume increases by 50%, whereas the red blood cell count increases by 30%.

pseudoaneurysm (soo″dō-ăn′ū-rĭzm) [″ + *aneurysma,* a widening] A dilation or tortuosity in a vessel that gives the impression of an aneurysm.

pseudoangina (soo″dō-ăn′jĭ-nă, -ăn-jī′nă) [″ + L. *angina,* a choking] Chest pain in patients who have healthy coronary arteries. The syndrome may be caused by esophageal, peptic, gallbladder, musculoskeletal, pulmonary, pleural, or psychogenic illnesses.

pseudoankylosis (soo″dō-ăng″kĭ-lō′sĭs) [″ + *ankyle,* stiff joint, + *osis,* condition] A false joint.

pseudoapoplexy (soo″dō-ăp′ŏ-plĕk″sē) A mild condition simulating a stroke but not accompanied by cerebral hemorrhage. SYN: *parapoplexy.* SEE: *transient ischemic attack.*

pseudoataxia (soo″dō-ă-tăk′sē-ă) [″ + *ataxia,* lack of order] A condition resembling ataxia but not due to tabes dorsalis.

pseudoblepsia, pseudoblepsis (soo″dō-blĕp′sē-ă, -sĭs) [″ + *blepsis,* sight] False or imaginary vision. SYN: *parablepsia; pseudopsia.*

pseudocartilaginous (soo″dō-kăr″tĭ-lăj′ĭ-nŭs) [″ + L. *cartilago,* gristle] Pert. to, or formed of, a substance resembling cartilage.

pseudocast (soo′dō-kăst) [″ + ME. *casten,* to carry] A sediment in urine composed of epithelial cells and resembling a true cast; a false cast. Alkaline urine tends to dissolve pseudocasts.

pseudocele (soo′dō-sēl) [″ + *koilos,* hollow] The cavity of the septum pellucidum, the so-called fifth ventricle. SYN: *pseudocoele.* SEE: *cavum septi pellucidi.*

pseudocholesteatoma (soo″dō-kō″lĕs-tē-ă-tō′mă) [″ + *chole,* bile, + *steatos,* fat, + *oma,* tumor] Hard epithelium present as a mass in the tympanic cavity in association with chronic inflammation of the middle ear.

pseudocholinesterase (soo″dō-kō″lĭn-ĕs′tĕr-ās) A nonspecific cholinesterase that hydrolyzes noncholine esters as well as acetylcholine. It is found in serum and pancreatic tissue.

pseudochorea (soo″dō-kō-rē′ă) [″ + *choreia,* dance] A somatoform disorder resembling chorea.

pseudochromesthesia (soo″dō-krō″mĕs-thē′zē-ă) [″ + *chroma,* color, + *aisthesis,* sensation] A condition in which sounds, esp. of the vowels, seem to induce a sensation of a distinct visual color. SEE: *phonism; photism; synesthesia.*

pseudochromidrosis (soo″dō-krō″mĭd-rō′sĭs) [″ + ″ + *hidros,* sweat, + *osis,* condition] The appearance of colored sweat, in which the sweat acquires its color after it is excreted.

pseudocirrhosis (soo″dō-sĭr-ō′sĭs) [″ + *kirrhos,* orange yellow, + *osis,* disease] A condition with symptoms of cirrhosis of the liver, caused by any process that causes obstruction of venous flow from the liver. Constrictive pericarditis can cause this condition. Cyanosis, ascites, and dyspnea characterize this condition.

pseudocoele (soo′dō-sēl) [″ + *koilos,* hollow] Pseudocele.

pseudocolloid (soo″dō-kŏl′oyd) [″ + *kollodes,* glutinous] A mucoid substance present in various locations and in ovarian cysts.

pseudocoloboma (soo″dō-kŏl-ō-bō′mă) [″ + *koloboma,* a mutilation] A scarcely noticeable scar on the iris from an embryonic fissure.

pseudocoma Locked-in syndrome.

pseudocoxalgia (soo″dō-kŏk-săl′jē-ă) [″ + L. *coxa,* hip, + Gr. *algos,* pain] Legg-Calvé-Perthes disease.

pseudocrisis (soo-dō-krī′sĭs) [″ + *krisis,* turning point] A false crisis; a temporary fall of body temperature, which may be followed by a rise.

pseudocroup (soo-dō-kroop′) False croup.

pseudocyesis (soo″dō-sī-ē′sĭs) [″ + *kyesis,* pregnancy] A condition in which a patient has nearly all of the usual signs and symptoms of pregnancy, such as enlargement of the abdomen, weight gain, cessation of menses, and morning sickness, but is not pregnant. It is usually seen in women who either are very desirous of having children or wish to avoid pregnancy. Treatment usually is done by psychiatric means. Pseudocyesis also occurs in men. SYN: *phantom pregnancy; pseudopregnancy* (2).

pseudocylindroid (soo″dō-sĭ-lĭn′droyd) [″ + *kylindros,* cylinder, + *eidos,* form, shape] A shred of mucus in the urine that resembles a cast.

pseudocyst (soo′dō-sĭst) [″ + *kystis,* bladder] A dilatation resembling a cyst.

pseudodementia (soo″dō-dē-mĕn′shē-ă) [″ + L. *dementare,* to make insane] An impairment in thinking accompanied by a withdrawal from social interactions that resembles dementia but instead is the result of depression, esp. in the elderly.

pseudodiphtheria (soo″dō-dĭf-thē′rē-ă) [″ + *diphthera,* membrane] A condition resembling diphtheria but not due to *Corynebacterium diphtheriae.*

pseudoedema (soo″dō-ē-dē′mă) [″ + *oidema,* a swelling] A puffy condition of the skin simulating edema.

pseudoemphysema (soo″dō-ĕm-fĭ-zē′mă) [″ + *emphysema,* an inflation] A bronchial condition simulating emphysema, caused by temporary blockage of the bronchi.

pseudoencephalitis (soo″dō-ĕn-sĕf″ă-lī′tĭs) [″ + *enkephalos,* brain, + *itis,* inflammation] A false encephalitis due to profuse diarrhea.

pseudoephedrine hydrochloride (soo″dō-ĕ-fĕd′rĭn) A sympathomimetic drug, an isomer of ephedrine, that has actions similar to those of ephedrine. Trade names is Sudafed.

pseudoerysipelas (soo″dō-ĕr-ĭ-sĭp′ĕ-lăs) [″ + *erythros,* red, + *pella,* skin] An inflammation of subcutaneous cellular tissue simulating erysipelas.

pseudoesthesia (soo″dō-ĕs-thē′zē-ă) [″ + *aisthesis,* sensation] Pseudesthesia.

pseudofolliculitis barbae Inflammation of beard follicles when tightly coiled hairs become ingrown. The only sure prevention is not shaving. SEE: illus.

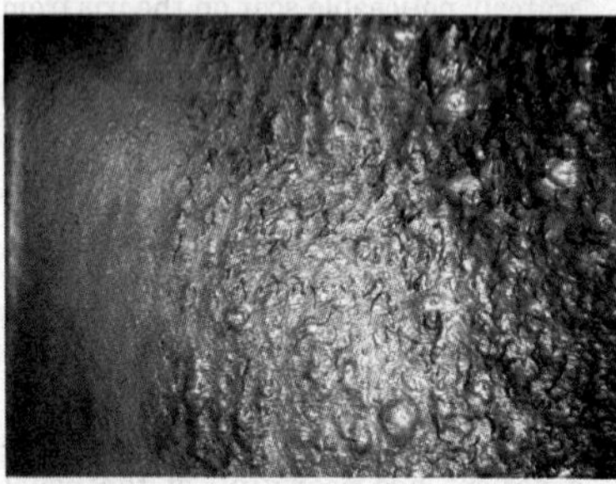

PSEUDOFOLLICULITIS BARBAE

pseudofracture (soo″dō-frăk′chūr) A ribbon-like zone of decalcification seen in certain types of osteomalacia.

pseudoganglion (soo″dō-găn′glē-ŏn) [″ + *ganglion,* knot] A slight thickening of a nerve, resembling a ganglion.

pseudogeusesthesia (soo″dō-gūs″ĕs-thē′zē-ă) [″ + *geusis,* taste, + *aisthesis,* sensation] A sense of taste stimulated by one of the other senses.

pseudogeusia (soo″dō-gū′sē-ă) A subjective sensation of taste not produced by external stimulus.

pseudoglioma (soo″dō-glī-ō′mă) [″ + *glia,* glue, + *oma,* tumor] Inflammatory changes occurring in the vitreous body that simulate glioma of retina but are due to iridochoroiditis.

pseudoglobulin (soo″dō-glŏb′ū-lĭn) [″ + L. *globulus,* little globe] Onc of a class of globulins characterized by being soluble in salt-free water. SEE: *euglobulin.*

pseudoglottis (soo″dō-glŏt′ĭs) [″ + *glottis,* back of tongue] The area between the false vocal cords.

pseudogout (soo′dō-gowt″) Chronic recurrent arthritis that may be clinically similar to gout. The crystals found in synovial fluid are composed of calcium pyrophosphate dihydrate (CPPD), instead of urate (urate crystals accumulate in the synovial fluid in gout). CPPD crystals deposit in fibrocartilage (e.g., meniscus of knee, triangular fibrocartilage of wrist), and these deposits can be identified on radiographs as chondrocalcinosis. The most commonly involved joint is the knee. Multiple joints are involved in two thirds of patients. This condition is treated by joint aspiration, nonsteroidal anti-inflammatory agents, and intra-articular injection of glucocorticoids. SEE: *chondrocalcinosis.*

pseudogynecomastia (soo″dō-jĭn″ĕ-kō-măs′tē-ă) [Gr. *pseudes,* false, + *gyne,* woman, + *mastos,* breast] Excess adipose tissue in the male breast but with no increase in glandular tissue.

pseudohematuria (soo″dō-hē″mă-tū′rē-ă) [″ + *haima,* blood, + *ouron,* urine] A red pigment in the urine that makes the urine appear to have blood in it.

pseudohemophilia (soo″dō-hē″mō-fĭl′ē-ă) [″ + ″ + *philos,* to love] Von Willebrand's disease.

pseudohemoptysis (soo″dō-hē-mŏp′tĭ-sĭs) [″ + *haima,* blood, + *ptyein,* to spit] Spitting of blood that does not arise from the bronchi or the lungs.

pseudohermaphrodite (soo″dō-hĕr-măf′rō-dīt) An individual having the sex glands of only one sex but having some of the physical appearances of an individual of the opposite sex.

pseudohermaphroditism (soo″dō-hĕr-măf′rō-dīt″ĭzm) [″ + *Hermaphroditos,* mythical two-sexed god, + *-ismos,* condition] A condition in which an individual has both male and female external genitalia but the internal reproductive organs of only one gender. SYN: *false hermaphroditism.* SEE: *intersex; macrogenitosomia praecox.*

female p. A condition in a female marked by a large clitoris, resembling the penis, and hypertrophied labia majora, resembling the scrotum, thus producing a resemblance to male genitalia. This condition can be caused by disease of the adrenal gland.

male p. A condition in a male

marked by a small penis, perineal hypospadias, and scrotum without testes, thereby resembling the vulva. This condition can be due to disease of the adrenal gland or a feminizing tumor of the undescended testis.

pseudohernia (soo″dō-hĕr′nē-ă) [″ + L. *hernia,* rupture] Inflammation in the scrotal area resembling a hernia.

pseudohypertension The observation of elevated blood pressure when taken by conventional means (i.e., sphygmomanometer), that is in reality not elevated when compared with the actual pressure in the artery when determined by more accurate methods. Accurate blood pressure may be obtained with an intra-arterial catheter or an infrasonic recorder. Pseudohypertension usually is found in elderly persons, who may have arterial calcifications that interfere with blood pressure measurements obtained with a cuff. SEE: *indirect measurement of blood pressure; hypertension; infrasonic recorder.*

pseudohypertrophy (soo″dō-hī-pĕr′trō-fē) [″ + *hyper,* above, + *trophe,* nourishment] The increase in size of an organ or structure owing to hypertrophy or hyperplasia of tissue other than parenchyma. It often is accompanied by diminution of function. **pseudohypertrophic** (-trō′fĭk), *adj.*

pseudohypoparathyroidism (soo″dō-hī″pō-păr″ă-thī′royd-ĭzm) A group of hereditary diseases resembling hypoparathyroidism but caused by an inadequate response to parathyroid hormone rather than a deficiency of the hormone. Some of these patients are obese with short, stocky build and a moonface.

pseudoicterus (soo″dō-ĭk′tĕr-ŭs) [″ + *ikteros,* jaundice] Pseudojaundice.

pseudoisochromatic (soo″dō-ī″sō-krō-măt′ĭk) [″ + *isos,* equal, + *chroma,* color] Seemingly of the same color; colors used in charts testing for color blindness.

pseudojaundice (soo″dō-jawn′dĭs) [″ + Fr. *jaune,* yellow] Pigment in the skin, such as in carotenemia, that resembles jaundice, but is not due to elevated serum bilirubin levels. SYN: *pseudoicterus.* SEE: *carotenemia.*

pseudologia (soo-dō-lō′jē-ă) [″ + *logos,* word, reason] Falsification in writing or in speech, a form of pathological lying.

p. fantastica Pathological lying, usually for psychological reasons rather than for personal gain. The condition is considered to be a type of factitious disorder.

pseudomania (soo-dō-mā′nē-ă) [″ + *mania,* madness] **1.** A psychosis in which patients falsely accuse themselves of crimes that they think they have committed. **2.** Pathological lying.

pseudomasturbation (soo″dō-măs-tŭr-bā′shŭn) [″ + L. *manus,* hand, + *stuprare,* to rape] Peotillomania.

pseudomelanosis (soo″dō-mĕl-ă-nō′sĭs) [″ + *melas,* black, + *osis,* condition] Discoloration of the tissues after death.

pseudomembrane (soo″dō-mĕm′brān) [″ + L. *membrana,* membrane] A leaf- or shelf-like exudate made of inflammatory debris and fibrin that may form on epithelial surfaces (e.g., in the colitis caused by *Clostridium difficile,* or the pharyngitis caused by *Corynebacterium diphtheriae*. **pseudomembranous,** *adj.*

pseudomeningitis (soo″dō-mĕn-ĭn-jī′tĭs) [″ + *meninx,* membrane, + *itis,* inflammation] A condition resembling the symptoms of meningitis without the meningeal inflammation.

pseudomenstruation (soo″dō-mĕn″strū-ā′ shŭn) [″ + L. *menstruare,* menstruate] Bleeding from the uterus not accompanied by the usual changes in the endometrium.

p. of the newborn Withdrawal bleeding after birth, a scant vaginal discharge that reflects the physiological response of some female infants to an exposure to high levels of maternal hormones in utero.

pseudomnesia (soo″dŏm-nē′zē-ă) [″ + *mnesis,* memory] A memory disturbance in which the patient remembers that which never occurred.

Pseudomonas (soo-dō-mō′năs) [″ + *monas,* single] A genus of small, motile, gram-negative bacilli with polar flagella. Most are saprophytic, living in soil and decomposing organic matter. Some produce blue and yellow pigments.

P. aeruginosa A species that grows easily in water and sometimes causes life-threatening infections in humans, including nosocomial pneumonia, urinary tract infections, and sepsis. It may also cause folliculitis, malignant otitis externa, and skin infections in patients who have suffered burns.

P. cepacia Burkholderia cepacia.

P. mallei A species that causes glanders in horses.

P. maltophilia Former name for *Stenotrophomonas maltophilia.*

P. pseudomallei A species that causes melioidosis in humans and animals.

pseudomucin (soo-dō-mū′sĭn) [″ + L. *mucus,* mucus] A variety of mucin found in ovarian cysts.

pseudomyopia (soo″dō-mī-ō′pē-ă) [″ + *myein,* to shut, + *ops,* eye] A condition in which defective vision causes persons to hold objects close in order to see them, even though myopia is not present.

pseudomyxoma (soo″dō-mĭk-sō′mă) [″ + *myxa,* mucus, + *oma,* tumor] A peritoneal tumor resembling a myxoma and containing a thick viscid fluid.

p. peritonei A type of tumor that develops in the peritoneum from implantation metastases resulting from rupture of ovarian cystadenoma or cells escaping during surgical removal. Numerous papillomas develop, attached to the abdominal wall and intestine, and the peritoneal cavity becomes filled with mucus-like fluid.

pseudoneoplasm (soo-dō-nē′ō-plăsm) [″ + *neos,* new, + LL. *plasma,* form, mold] A false or phantom tumor; a temporary swelling, usually of an inflammatory nature, that simulates a tumor.

pseudoneuritis (soo″dō-nū-rī′tĭs) [″ + *neuron,* nerve, + *itis,* inflammation] Reddening and blurring of the optic disk, which resembles optic neuritis.

pseudoneuroma (soo″dō-nū-rō′mă) [″ + ″ + *oma,* tumor] A mass of interlacing, coiled fibers, cells of Schwann, and fibrous tissue forming a mass at the end of an amputation stump. Also called amputation or traumatic neuroma, this is not a true neuroma.

pseudonucleolus (soo″dō-nū″klē-ōl′ŭs) [″ + L. *nucleus,* a nut] The false nucleolus or karyosome.

pseudopapilledema (soo″dō-păp″ĭ-lĕ-dē′mă) [″ + *papilla,* nipple, + *oidema,* swelling] A swelling of the optic nerve head that is not caused by optic neuritis.

pseudoparalysis (soo″dō-pă-răl′ĭ-sĭs) [″ + *para,* at the side, + *lyein,* to loosen] A loss of movement caused by the pain and inflammation of a localized injury, an infection, or a factitious disorder, rather than caused by a nerve injury or stroke.

pseudoparaplegia (soo″dō-păr-ă-plē′jē-ă) [″ + ″ + *plege,* a stroke] A seeming paralysis of the lower extremities without impairment of the reflexes.

pseudoparasite (soo″dō-păr′ă-sīt) [″ + ″ + *sitos,* food] **1.** Anything resembling a parasite. **2.** An organism that can live as a parasite, although it is normally not one. SEE: *parasite, facultative.*

Pseudophyllidea (soo″dō-fĭ-lĭd′ē-ă) An order belonging to the class Cestoidea, subclass Cestoda. It includes tapeworms with scolices bearing two lateral (or one terminal) sucking grooves (bothria) and includes *Diphyllobothrium latum,* the fish tapeworm of humans.

pseudopocket A pocket that results from gingival inflammation with edema that produces an apparent abnormal depth of the gingival sulcus without apical movement of the bottom of the sulcus; a false pocket. SEE: *gingivitis.*

pseudopod (soo′dō-pŏd) [″ + *pous,* foot] Pseudopodium (1).

pseudopodium (soo″dō-pō′dē-ŭm) *pl.* **pseudopodia 1.** A temporary protruding process of a protozoan or ameboid cell, such as a leukocyte, into which the cell flows, for locomotion and the engulfing of food particles or foreign substances, as in phagocytosis. SYN: *pseudopod.* **2.** An irregular projection at the edge of a wheal.

pseudopolyp (soo″dō-pŏl′ĭp) [″ + *polys,* many, + *pous,* foot] A hypertrophied area of mucous membrane resembling a polyp.

pseudopolyposis (soo″dō-pŏl″ĭ-pō′sĭs) [″ + ″ + ″ + *osis,* condition] A large number of pseudopolyps in the colon due to chronic inflammation.

pseudopregnancy (soo″dō-prĕg′năn-sē) [Gr. *pseudes,* false, + L. *praegnans,* with child] **1.** A condition in animals following sterile matings in which anatomical and physiological changes occur, similar to those of pregnancy. **2.** Pseudocyesis.

pseudopuberty, precocious Feminization of a young girl due to enhanced estrogen production, but ovulation and cyclic menstruation are absent. Estrogen-secreting tumors of the ovary are the usual cause. Treatment is removal of the tumor.

pseudo-pseudohypoparathyroidism (soo″dō-soo″dō-hī″pō-păr″ă-thī′royd-ĭzm) [″ + *pseudes,* false, + *hypo,* under, + *para,* beside, + *thyreos,* shield, + *eidos,* form, shape + *-ismos,* condition] Pseudohypoparathyroidism in which most of the clinical but none of the biochemical changes are present.

pseudopsia (soo-dŏp′sē-ă) [″ + *opsis,* vision] Visual hallucinations or false perceptions. SYN: *parablepsia; pseudoblepsia.*

pseudopterygium (soo″dō-tĕr-ĭj′ē-ŭm) [″ + *pterygion,* wing] A scar on the conjunctiva of the eye that is firmly attached to the underlying tissue.

pseudoptosis (soo-dō-tō′sĭs) [″ + *ptosis,* a dropping] Apparent ptosis of the eyelid, resulting from a fold of skin or fat projecting below the edge of the eyelid.

pseudorabies (soo″dō-rā′bēz) [″ + L. *rabere,* to rage] A rabies-like disease in animals that is due to a type of herpesvirus. It causes death within several days.

pseudoreaction (soo″dō-rē-ăk′shŭn) A false reaction; a response to injection of a test substance into the tissues owing to the presence of an allergen other than one for which the test is made.

pseudorickets (soo″dō-rĭk′ĕts) Renal rickets.

pseudoscarlatina (soo″dō-skăr-lă-tē′nă) A septic febrile condition with a rash resembling scarlatina.

pseudosclerosis (soo″dō-sklē-rō′sĭs) [″ + *sklerosis,* a hardening] A condition with the symptoms, but without the lesions, of multiple sclerosis of the nervous system.

pseudosmia (soo-dŏz′mē-ă) [″ + *osme,* smell] An olfactory hallucination or perversion of the sense of smell.

pseudostoma (soo-dŏs′tō-mă) [″ + *stoma,* mouth] An apparent opening or window between endothelial cells that have been stained.

pseudostratified (soo-dō-străt′ĭ-fīd) [″ + L. *stratificare,* to arrange in layers] Apparently composed of layers.

pseudosyphilis (soo″dō-sĭf′ĭ-lĭs) A nonspecific condition resembling syphilis.

pseudotabes (soo″dō-tā′bēz) [Gr. *pseudes,* false, + L. *tabes,* wasting away] A neural disease simulating tabes dorsalis.

pseudotetanus (soo″dō-tĕt′ă-nŭs) [″ + *tetanos,* stretched] Persistent muscular contractions resembling tetanus.

pseudotruncus arteriosus (soo″dō-trŭnk′ŭs ăr-tē″rē-ō′sŭs) The severest form of tetralogy of Fallot.

pseudotuberculosis (soo″dō-tū-ber″kū-lō′sĭs) [″ + L. *tuberculus,* tubercle, + Gr. *osis,* condition] A group of diseases that resemble tuberculosis but are due to an organism other than the tubercle bacillus. In humans the most common cause is *Yersinia pseudotuberculosis,* a gram-negative organism.

pseudotumor cerebri (soo″dō-tū′mor sĕr′ĕ-brī) Benign intracranial hypertension. A relatively uncommon neurological condition—found in young overweight women more than other groups of the population—whose hallmarks are moderately severe headaches associated with papilledema on physical examination. Imaging studies do not reveal a mass lesion in the brain. Cerebrospinal fluid pressures are markedly elevated when measured by lumbar puncture. Treatment may include diuretics, or the surgical construction of a shunt to relieve intracranial hypertension.

pseudoxanthoma (soo″dō-zăn-thō′mă) [″ + *xanthos,* yellow, + *oma,* tumor] A condition resembling xanthoma.

p. elasticum A chronic degenerative cutaneous disease marked by yellow patches and stretching of the skin. It is associated with hypertension and degeneration of the elastic coat of the arteries. Angioid streaks in the retina are common.

p.s.i. *pounds per square inch.*

psilocin (sī′lō-sĭn) A hallucinogen similar to psilocybin.

psilocybin (sī″lō-sī′bĭn) A rapidly acting visual hallucinogen derived from the mushroom *Psilocybe mexicana* and related species, sometimes used by recreational substance abusers.

psi phenomena Occurrences, events, or actions that have no logical explanation (e.g., extrasensory perception, clairvoyance, precognition, psychokinesis, and telepathy).

psittacosis (sĭt-ă-kō′sĭs) [Gr. *psittakos,* parrot, + *osis,* condition] A relatively uncommon flulike illness caused by *Chlamydia psittaci,* a microbe that is transmitted to humans from infected birds. It causes an atypical pneumonia with headache, sore throat, fevers and chills, cough, anorexia, muscle aches, and other nonspecific symptoms. It is treated with tetracyclines. SYN: *ornithosis; parrot fever.* SEE: *Chlamydia.*

psoas (sō′ăs) [Gr. *psoa*] One of two muscles of the loins.

psoitis (sō-ī′tĭs) [Gr. *psoa,* muscle of the loin, + *itis,* inflammation] Inflammation of the psoas muscles or of the area of the loins.

psomophagia (sō″mō-fā′jē-ă) [Gr. *psomos,* morsel, + *phagein,* to eat] The habit of swallowing food without thoroughly chewing it. SEE: *fletcherism.*

psoralen One of a group of plant-derived chemicals that sensitize the skin to damage by ultraviolet light. Drugs derived from psoralens, such as methoxsalen and trioxsalen, are used to treat vitiligo, psoriasis, and cutaneous T-cell lymphoma. Side effects from the use of psoralens may include drying and chapping of the skin and an increased risk of developing skin cancer. SEE: *psoriasis; PUVA therapy; vitiligo.*

psorelcosis (sō″rĕl-kō′sĭs) [″ + *helkosis,* ulceration] Ulceration occurring as a result of scabies.

psoriasiform (sō-rī′ă-sĭ-form) Resembling psoriasis; psoriasis-like. Applies to a rash that resembles the plaquelike erythematous lesions of psoriasis; also used in reference to joint conditions resembling those of psoriatic arthritis. SEE: *psoriasis; psoriatic arthritis.*

psoriasis (sō-rī′ă-sĭs) [Gr., an itching] A chronic skin disorder affecting 1% to 2% of the population, in which red, scaly plaques with sharply defined borders appear on the body surface. The rash commonly is found on the knees, shins, elbows, umbilicus, lower back, buttocks, ears, and along the hairline. Pitting of the nails also occurs frequently. The severity of the disease may range from a minimal cosmetic problem to total body surface involvement. About a third of all affected patients have a family history of the disease. SEE: illus.

Although psoriasis may begin at any time of life, the most common age of on-

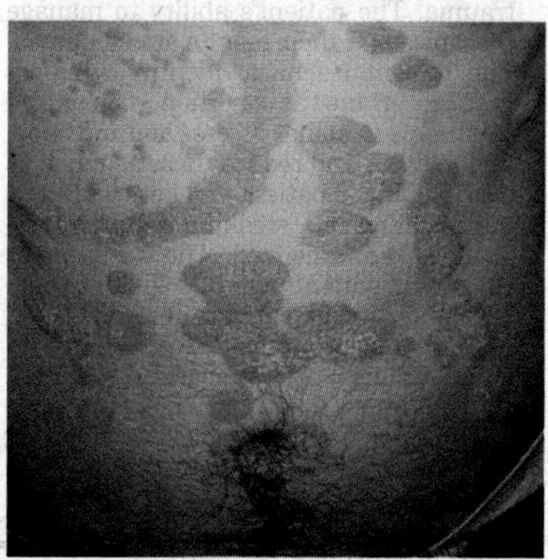

PSORIASIS

set is between 10 and 40 years. The condition has relapses and remissions, but established lesions often persist for many months or years. About 5% of patients with psoriasis also develop an inflammatory arthritis, and patients with psoriasis have an increased rate of inflammatory bowel disease. SEE: *Nursing Diagnoses Appendix.*

ETIOLOGY: Although the cause of psoriasis is unknown, emotional stress, skin trauma, cold weather, infections, and some drugs may trigger attacks.

TREATMENT: Topical corticosteroids, coal tar derivatives, vitamin D_3 analogs (e.g., calcipotriene), retinoids (e.g., etretinate), ultraviolet light exposure, and saltwater immersion are among the many methods that have been used effectively to treat this condition. For severe disease, immune-modulating drugs like methotrexate or cyclosporine sometimes are used, with close monitoring to prevent side effects.

CAUTION: Many treatments for psoriasis carry some risk for the patient. Etretinate, for example, produces fetal abnormalities and should never be used by women of childbearing age. Phototherapy with ultraviolet light increases the risk of developing many types of skin cancer. Methotrexate use requires regular monitoring of liver function, renal function, complete blood counts, and lung function.

PATIENT CARE: The nurse teaches the patient about the prescribed therapy, to soften and remove scales, to relieve pruritus, to reduce pain and discomfort, to retard rapid cell proliferation, and to help induce remission and monitors for adverse reactions. Assistance is provided to help the patient gain confidence in managing these largely palliative treatments, many of which require special instructions for application and removal. The patient should protect against and minimize trauma. The patient's ability to manage therapies and their results are evaluated. The patient learns to identify stressors that exacerbate the condition, such as cold weather, emotional stress, and infection, and to avoid and reduce these as much as possible. If the patient smokes cigarettes, participation in a smoking cessation program is recommended. The nurse helps the young patient (aged 20 to 30) to deal with body image changes and effects on self-esteem, encourages the patient to verbalize feelings, and supports the patient through loss of body image and associated grief. Referral for psychological counseling or cosmetic concealment therapy may be necessary.

p. annularis Circular or ringlike lesions of psoriasis.

p. buccalis Leukoplakia of the oral mucosa.

elephantine p. A rare but persistent psoriasis that occurs on the back, thighs, and hips in thick scaling plaques.

guttate p. Psoriasis characterized by small distinct lesions that generally occur over the body. The lesions appear particularly in the young after acute streptococcal infections. SEE: illus.

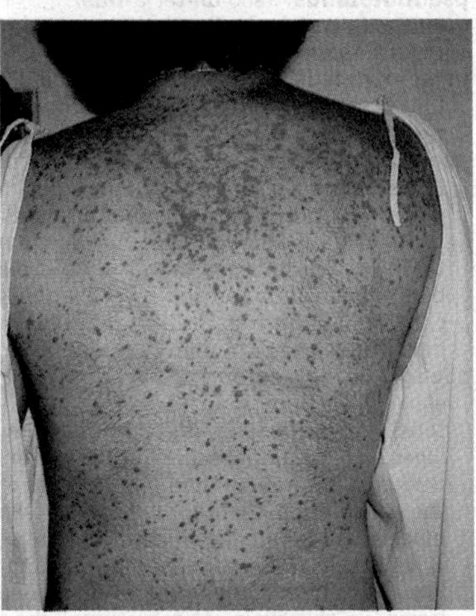

GUTTATE PSORIASIS

nummular p. The most common form of psoriasis with disks and plaques of varying sizes on the extremities and trunk. There may be a great number of lesions or a solitary lesion.

pustular p. Psoriasis in which small sterile pustules form, dry up, and then form a scab.

rupioid p. Psoriasis with hyperkeratotic lesions on the feet.

p. universalis Severe generalized psoriasis.

psorophthalmia (sō″rŏf-thăl′mē-ă) [Gr.] Marginal inflammation of the eyelids with ulceration.

psorous (sō′rŭs) [Gr. *psoros*] Relating to, or affected with, itch.

P.S.P. *phenolsulfonphthalein.*

PSRO *Professional Standards Review Organization.*

PSV *pressure support ventilation.*

PSVT *paroxysmal supraventricular tachycardia.*

psych-, psycho- Combining form meaning *mind, mental processes.*

psychalgia (sī-kăl′jē-ă) [″ + *algos,* pain] **1.** Pain of somatoform origin. **2.** Mental distress marked by auditory and visual hallucinations, often associated with melancholia.

psychataxia (sī″kă-tăk′sē-ă) [″ + *ataxia,* lack of order] Disordered power of concentration.

psychauditory (sīk-aw′dĭ-tor-ē) [″ + L.

auditorius, hearing] Pert. to the perception and interpretation of sounds.

psyche (sī'kē) [Gr. *psyche,* soul, mind] All that constitutes the mind and its processes.

psychedelic (sī"kĕ-dĕl'ĭk) [" + *delos,* manifest] Mind-altering; hallucinogenic; capable of producing an altered state of awareness or consciousness. It is said of drugs such as lysergic acid diethylamide (LSD).

psychiatric (sī-kē-ă'trĭk) [" + *iatrikos,* healing] Pert. to psychiatry, the science concerned with the study, diagnosis, and prevention of mental illness.

psychiatrist (sī-kī'ă-trĭst) A physician who specializes in the study, treatment, and prevention of mental disorders.

psychiatry (sī-kī'ă-trē) The branch of medicine that deals with the diagnosis, treatment, and prevention of mental illness.

descriptive p. A system of psychiatry concerned with readily observable external factors that influence the mental state of an individual. SEE: *dynamic p.*

dynamic p. The study of the origin, influence, and control of emotions. This involves investigating the factors both from within and without that alter emotions and motivation. Such analysis provides a basis for judging regression or progression.

emergency p. The emergency therapy and intervention in patients who are suicidal, homicidal, or perpetrators or victims of child abuse, spouse abuse, or incest. Most of these individuals see a physician within hours or days of their violent or abusive act. Many physician training programs fail to prepare a student for managing patients who need this emergency service.

forensic p. The use of psychiatry in legal matters, esp. in determining social adaptability of an individual suspected of insanity; or the presence or absence of insanity, esp. at the time the individual committed a crime.

orthomolecular p. The concept that mental illness is due to biochemical abnormalities resulting in increased requirements for specific substances, such as vitamins and minerals.

psychic (sī'kĭk) [Gr. *psychikos*] **1.** Concerning the mind or psyche. **2.** An individual said to be endowed with supernatural powers, such as the ability to read the minds of others or to foresee coming events; one who claims to be sensitive to nonphysical forces.

p. determinism The theory that mental processes are determined by conscious or unconscious motives and are never irrelevant.

p. force Force generated apart from physical energy.

psychoactive (sī"kō-ăk'tĭv) [" + L. *actio,* action] Having an impact on thinking, mood, or behavior. The term typically is used to describe the effects of drugs or toxins.

psychoanaleptic (sī"kō-ăn"ă-lĕp'tĭk) [" + *analepsis,* a taking up] Having a stimulating effect on the mind.

psychoanalysis (sī"kō-ă-năl'ĭ-sĭs) [" + *analysis,* a dissolving] A method of obtaining a detailed account of past and present mental and emotional experiences and repressions in order to determine the source and to eliminate or diminish the undesirable effects of unconscious conflicts by making patients aware of their existence, origin, and inappropriate expression in emotions and behavior. It is largely a system created by Sigmund Freud that was originally the outgrowth of his observations of neurotics. Frequently the term is used synonymously with freudianism, but more commonly it is used for a more extensive system of psychological fact and theory applying both to normal and abnormal groups.

Psychoanalysis is based on the theory that abnormal phenomena are caused by repression of painful or undesirable past experiences that, although forgotten, later manifest themselves in various abnormal ways. Psychoanalysis includes a study of the ego in relationship to reality and the conflicting goals so created. This conflict is solved by repressing one component. This repressed or censored emotion-laden complex of ideas exists in the subconscious, manifesting itself in the hidden content of dreams, neuroses, and tension states. Angry outbursts, rationalization of unfair attitudes, or slips of the tongue occur because the patient is unaware of the influence of the subconscious.

Repressed material is, in Freudian analysis, sexual. The peculiar conditioning of the patient is determined chiefly by emotional experiences of earlier years. Reactions of inferiority may result in a compensatory reaction of goodness or ambition. Sublimation is the escape of creative interest on levels not socially taboo. Therefore, psychoanalysis makes an effort to bring forgotten memories into the conscious mind. The patient thus is enabled to view the occurrence in its true perspective and to minimize its harm.

In addition to the freudian method, other schools of thought used in psychoanalysis include analytical psychology (Jung), psychobiology (Meyer), and individual psychology (Adler).

psychoanalyst (sī"kō-ăn'ă-lĭst) [Gr. *psyche,* mind, + *analysis,* a dissolving] One who practices psychoanalysis.

psychobiology (sī"kō-bī-ŏl'ō-jē) [" + *bios,* life, + *logos,* word, reason] **1.** The study of the biology of the psyche, including the anatomy, physiology, and pathology of the mind. **2.** A method of psychoanalysis employing distributive analysis, which includes a study of all mental and physical factors involved in an individual's growth and development.

objective p. Psychobiology in which special emphasis is placed on the relationship of the individual to his or her environment.

psychocatharsis (sī″kō-kă-thăr′sĭs) [″ + *katharsis,* purification] The bringing of so-called traumatic experiences and their affective associations into consciousness by interview, hypnosis, or in the past, drugs such as sodium amytal. SEE: *catharsis.*

psychochrome (sī′kō-krōm) [″ + *chroma,* color] Color impression resulting from sensory stimulation of a part other than the visual organ.

psychochromesthesia (sī″kō-krōm″ĕs-thē′zē-ă) [″ + ″ + *aisthesis* , sensation] Color sensation produced by the stimulus of a sense organ other than that of vision. SEE: *pseudochromesthesia.*

psychocortical (sī″kō-kor′tĭ-kăl) [″ + L. *cortex,* rind] Pert. to the cerebral cortex as the seat of sensory, motor, and psychic functions.

psychodiagnosis (sī″kō-dī″ăg-nō′sĭs) [″ + *diagignoskein,* to discern] The use of psychological tests to assist in diagnosing diseases, esp. mental illness.

psychodiagnostics (sī″kō-dī″ăg-nŏs′tĭks) The use of psychological testing as an aid in diagnosing mental disorders.

Psychodidae (sī″kŏd′ĭ-dē) A family of the order Diptera, characterized by minute size, long legs, and hairy bodies and wings. It includes moth flies, owl midges, and sandflies. SEE: *Phlebotomus.*

psychodrama (sī″kō-drăm′ă) [″ + L. *drama,* drama] A form of group psychotherapy. Patients act out assigned roles and, in so doing, are able to gain insight into their own mental disturbances.

psychodynamics (sī″kō-dī-năm′ĭks) [″ + *dynamis,* power] The scientific study of mental action or force.

psychogalvanometer (sī″kō-găl″vă-nŏm′ĕ-tĕr) [″ + *galvanism* + Gr. *metron,* measure] A device for determining the changes in the electrical resistance of the skin in response to emotional stimuli.

psychogenesis (sī″kō-jĕn′ĕ-sĭs) [″ + *genesis,* generation, birth] **1.** The origin and development of mind; the formation of mental traits. **2.** Origin within the mind or psyche.

psychogenetic (sī″kō-jĕn-ĕt′ĭk) **1.** Originating in the mind, as a disease. **2.** Concerning formation of mental traits.

psychogenic (sī-kō-jĕn′ĭk) [″ + *gennan,* to produce] **1.** Of mental origin. **2.** Concerning the development of the mind. SYN: *psychogenetic.*

psychogeriatric Concerning the psychiatric disorders that may affect elderly persons.

psychogeusic (sī″kō-gū′sĭk) [″ + *geusis,* taste] Pert. to perception of taste.

psychograph (sī′kō-grăf) [″ + *graphein,* to write] **1.** A chart that lists personality traits. **2.** A history of the personality of an individual.

psychokinesis (sī″kō-kĭ-nē′sĭs) [″ + *kinesis,* movement] **1.** Explosive or impulsive maniacal action caused by defective inhibition. **2.** In parapsychology, claimed or alleged influence exerted on a physical object by a subject without any intermediate physical energy or instrumentation. SEE: *paranormal; psi phenomena.*

psycholagny (sī″kō-lăg′nē) [″ + *lagneia,* lust] Sexual excitation brought about by mental imagery; psychic or mental masturbation.

psycholinguistics (sī″kō-lĭng-gwĭs′tĭks) The study of linguistics as it relates to human behavior.

psychological (sī″kō-lŏj′ĭ-kăl) [″ + *logos,* word, reason] Pert. to the study of the mind in all of its relationships, normal and abnormal.

psychologist (sī-kŏl′ō-jĭst) One who is trained in methods of psychological analysis, therapy, and research.

psychology (sī-kŏl′ō-jē) [″ + *logos,* word, reason] The science dealing with mental processes, both normal and abnormal, and their effects upon behavior. There are two main approaches to the study: introspective, looking inward or self-examination of one's own mental processes; and objective studying of the minds of others.

abnormal p. The study of deviant behavior and the associated mental phenomena.

analytic p. Psychoanalysis based on the concepts of Carl Jung, de-emphasizing sexual factors in motivation and emphasizing the "collective unconscious" and "psychological types" (introvert and extrovert).

animal p. The study of animal behavior.

applied p. The application of the principles of psychology to special fields, such as clinical, industrial, educational, nursing, or pastoral applications.

clinical p. The branch of psychology concerned with diagnosing and treating mental disorders.

criminal p. The branch of psychology concerned with the behavior and therapy of criminals.

dynamic p. Psychology of motivation; that which seeks the causes of mental phenomena.

experimental p. The study of mental acts by tests and experiments.

genetic p. The branch of psychology concerned with the evolution of and inheritance of psychological characteristics.

gestalt p. Psychology that emphasizes the wholeness of psychological processes and behavior, maintaining that such cannot be adequately explained by breaking down into constituent parts.

individual p. A system of psychological thinking developed by Alfred Adler in which an individual is regarded as having three life goals: physical security, sexual satisfaction, and social integration. Self-evaluations lead to feelings of inferiority and inadequacy, which often lead to overcompensation or a striving for superiority.

physiological p. Psychology that deals with the structure and function of the nervous system and other bodily organs and their relationship to behavior.

social p. The branch of psychology concerned with the study of groups and their influence on the individual's actions and mental processes.

psychometrician (sī″kō-mĕ-trĭsh′ăn) [Gr. *psyche,* mind, + *metron,* measure] **1.** A person skilled in psychometry. **2.** A person skilled in the application of statistical analysis to psychological data.

psychometry (sī-kŏm′ĕ-trē) [″ + *metron,* measure] The measurement of psychological variables, such as intelligence, aptitude, behavior, and emotional reactions.

psychomotor (sī″kō-mō′tor) [″ + L. *motor,* a mover] Concerning or causing physical activity associated with mental processes.

psychomotor and physical development of infant The physical growth of an infant and the effect of mental activity on motor skills. It is important that all concerned with the care of the newborn through infancy have guidelines for comparing the growth and development of an individual with normal standards. Certain activities of infants serve as general indicators of normal psychomotor development. The average ages for certain of these activities are shown in the accompanying table. SEE: table; *arousal level.*

Appearance and loss of certain reflexes and reactions: The Moro reflex is present at birth and disappears by 3 months; the stepping and placing reflexes are present at birth and are no longer obtainable by 6 weeks; the tonic neck reflex is usually present at 2 months and is gone by 6 months; neck righting appears at 4 to 6 months and is gone by 24 months; the parachute reaction is present at 9 months and persists; sucking and rooting are present at birth and are usually gone by 4 months if tested while awake and by 7 months if tested while the infant is asleep; palmar grasp is present from birth to 6 months; plantar grasp is present from birth to 10 months.

psychomotor epilepsy Temporal lobe epilepsy.

psychomotor retardation A generalized slowing of physical and mental reactions; seen frequently in depression, intoxications, and other conditions.

psychoneuroimmunology The study of the relationships that exist among the central nervous system, autonomic nervous system, endocrine system, and immune system. Social scientists use the data gathered from studies as they examine the impact of psychosocial stressors and the psychophysiological stress response on the development of disease.

psychoneurosis (sī″kō-nū-rō′sĭs) [″ + *neuron,* sinew, + *osis,* condition] Neurosis.

psychoneurotic (sī″kō-nū-rŏt′ĭk) [Gr. *psyche,* mind, + *neuron,* sinew] **1.** Pert. to a functional disorder of mental origin. **2.** A person suffering from a psychoneurosis.

psychopath (sī′kō-păth) [″ + *pathos,* disease, suffering] A person who consistently and repeatedly treads on, abuses, or violates the rights of others, often causing considerable harm. SEE: *antisocial personality disorder.*

psychopathic (sī″kō-păth′ĭk) **1.** Concerning or characterized by a mental disorder. **2.** Concerning the treatment of mental disorders. **3.** Abnormal.

psychopathology (sī″kō-păth-ŏl′ō-jē) [″ + *pathos,* disease, suffering + *logos,* word, reason] The study of the causes and nature of mental disease or abnormal behavior.

psychopathy (sī-kŏp′ă-thē) Any mental disease, esp. one associated with defective character or personality. SEE: *antisocial personality disorder.*

psychopharmacology (sī″kō-făr″mă-kŏl′ō-jē) The science of drugs having an effect on psychomotor behavior and emotional states.

psychophysical (sī″kō-fĭz′ĭ-kăl) [″ + *physikos,* natural] Concerning the relationship of the physical and the mental.

psychophysics (sī″kō-fĭz′ĭks) **1.** The study of mental processes in relationship to physical processes. **2.** The study of stimuli in relationship to the effects they produce.

psychophysiological (sī″kō-fĭz-ē-ō-lŏj′ĭ-kăl) Pert. to psychophysiology.

psychophysiological disorder An outdated term for *somatization disorder.*

psychophysiology (sī″kō-fĭz″ē-ŏl′ō-jē) Physiology of the mind; science of the correlation of body and mind.

psychoplegic (sī″kō-plē′jĭk) [″ + *plege,* a stroke] An agent reducing excitability of the mental processes; a sedative.

psychoprophylactic preparation for childbirth Mental and physical training of the mother in preparation for delivery. The goals of the preparation are the dispelling of the fear of pain and the delivery of a healthy child. SEE: *natural childbirth; prepared childbirth; Lamaze technique.*

psychoprophylaxis (sī″kō-prō″fĭ-lăk′sĭs)

Psychomotor and Physical Development: Birth to 1 Year

Physical Development						
		Length Range		Weight Range		
		In.	Cm	Lb	Kg	
Birth	boys	18¼–21½	46.4–54.4	5½–9¼	2.54–4.15
	girls	17¾–20¾	45.4–52.9	5¼–8½	2.36–3.81
1 Month	boys	19¾–23	50.4–58.6	7–11¾	3.16–5.38
	girls	19¼–22½	49.2–56.9	6½–10¾	2.97–4.92
3 Months	boys	22¼–25¾	56.7–65.4	9¾–16¼	4.43–7.37
	girls	21¾–25	55.4–63.4	9¼–14¾	4.18–6.74
6 Months	boys	25–28½	63.4–72.3	13¾–20¾	6.20–9.46
	girls	24¼–27¾	61.8–70.2	12¾–19¼	5.79–8.73
9 Months	boys	26¾–30¼	68.0–77.1	16½–24	7.52–10.93
	girls	26–29½	66.1–75.0	15½–22½	7.0–10.17
12 Months	boys	28¼–32	71.7–81.2	18½–26½	8.43–11.99
	girls	27½–31¼	69.8–79.1	17¼–24¾	7.84–11.24

Psychomotor Development	
Birth through 1st Month	Ability to suck, swallow, gag, cry, and maintain eye contact with a person. Head needs to be supported. Loud noises may cause a startle reflex.
2nd Month	May turn to either side when on their backs; will follow moving objects; able to lift head but not for a sustained period; begin to smile, frown, and turn away.
3rd Month	Greater movement and vocal response to stimuli; notice own hands and suck on them; head steady while supported.
4th and 5th Months	Able to lift head higher when lying on stomach; will reach for objects and may be able to encircle a bottle with both hands; may drool a lot; attempt to put all kinds of objects in mouth.
6th–9th Month	Develop ability to grasp and pick up food; are able to pull up to a sitting position and eventually will crawl; begin to make noises that sound like words and to recognize certain words; will play peek-a-boo.
9th–11th Month	Develop ability to handle food and to drink from a cup; may imitate sounds and say certain words; crawl by pulling body along with arms, and pull themselves to a standing position; they will point at objects and throw things; they want to feed themselves and to help with dressing and undressing; they will walk while holding a person's hand.
12th Month	Can eat food alone and drink from a cup with assistance; able to move around easily and crawl up stairs and out of crib.

In obstetrics, a method of mental and physical preparation for natural childbirth. SEE: *natural childbirth; Lamaze technique.*

psychosensory (sī″kō-sĕn′sō-rē) [″ + L. *sensorius,* organ of sensation] **1.** Understanding and interpreting sensory stimuli. **2.** Concerning perceptions not arising in sensory organs, as hallucinations.

psychosexual (sī″kō-sĕks′ū-ăl) [Gr. *psyche,* soul, mind, + L. *sexus,* sex] Concerning the emotional components of sexual instinct.

psychosexual development Evolution of personality through infantile and pregenital periods to sexual maturity.

psychosexual disorder A disorder of sexual function not due to organic causes. Included are gender identity disorders, transsexualism, paraphilias, transvestism, zoophilia, pedophilia, exhibitionism, voyeurism, and sexual sadism.

psychosis (sī-kō′sĭs) *pl.* **psychoses** [″ + *osis,* condition] A mental disorder in which there is severe loss of contact with reality, evidenced by delusions, hallucinations, disorganized speech patterns, and bizarre or catatonic behaviors. Psychotic disorders are common features of schizophrenia, mania, and some affective disorders. They can also result from substance abuse (e.g., the use of hallucinogens), substance withdrawal (e.g., delirium tremens), or side effects of some prescription drugs.

SYMPTOMS: In psychotic states patients may express unusual ideas (e.g., that they can read the minds of others, send radio messages directly to God or inanimate objects, travel to distant galaxies). These ideas are called delusions. Psychosis also is marked by patient reports of hearing voices (auditory hallucinations) or seeing objects or persons not visible to others (visual hallucinations). Auditory hallucinations are hallmarks of schizophrenic and manic states, while visual hallucinations are characteristic of drug intoxication or withdrawal.

TREATMENT: Patients with psychosis are treated effectively with neuroleptic drugs, such as haloperidol, risperidone, or chlorpromazine. Side effects of some of these medications include dystonic reactions and tardive dyskinesia.

PATIENT CARE: The psychotic patient should be treated gently and with respect. Attempts to correct delusional thinking should be avoided because delusions are resistant to logical argument, and discussion about them may be misinterpreted. Because psychotic patients behave violently on occasion, careful practitioners eschew confrontation with them.

CAUTION: 1. Unfamiliar religious experiences and rituals may have all the hallmarks of psychosis when viewed by individuals from different cultures. What constitutes an especially meaningful experience in one society may be recognized as psychosis by another. 2. When assisting a psychotic patient, most clinicians sit close to a door, so that if they feel the need to leave the room quickly, they can do so unimpeded.

---

alcoholic p. Loss of contact with reality that results from acute or chronic alcohol use. Included are pathological intoxication, delirium tremens, Korsakoff's psychosis, and acute hallucinosis. SEE: *acute alcoholism; acute alcoholic hallucinosis; delirium tremens; intoxication; Korsakoff's syndrome.*

depressive p. Psychosis characterized by extreme depression, melancholia, and feelings of unworthiness.

drug p. Psychosis caused by ingestion of a drug.

exhaustion p. An acute state of confusion and delirium that occurs in relation to extreme fatigue, chronic illness, prolonged sleeplessness, or tension.

functional p. A psychosis in which there is no apparent pathology of the central nervous system.

gestational p. Psychosis that occurs during pregnancy.

involutional p. Psychosis occurring during the period of bodily and intellectual decline.

manic-depressive p. SYN: *bipolar disorder.*

organic p. Psychosis induced by structural brain changes. Emotional instability, irritability, angry outbursts, and inattention are typical symptoms. At any time in the course of the disease, memory, comprehension, ideation, and orientation may become defective. Possible causes include alcohol, narcotics, trauma, syphilis, drugs, poisons, chronic infections, encephalitis, and brain tumors, among many others.

polyneuritic p. Korsakoff's syndrome.

postinfectious p. A psychosis following an infectious disease such as meningitis, pneumonia, or typhoid fever.

postpartum p. A psychosis that develops during the 6 months following childbirth, the highest incidence being in the third to sixth day after delivery through the first month postpartum. The symptoms and signs include hallucinations, delusions, preoccupation with death, self-mutilation, infanticide, distorted reality, and extreme dependency. This psychosis may become a chronic condition, but for most women it is an isolated event in their lives. SYN: *puerperal p.* SEE: *postpartum blues.*

puerperal p. Postpartum p.

senile p. Psychosis in which onset occurs in an aged individual. This term is rarely used in the English-language health care literature but remains in use in non–English-speaking countries.

situational p. Psychosis due to excessive stress in an unbearable environmental situation.

toxic p. Psychosis resulting from toxic agents.

traumatic p. Psychosis resulting from head injuries and belonging to the organic group.

psychosocial (sī″kō-sō′shăl) Related to both psychological and social factors.

psychosomatic (sī″kō-sō-măt′ĭk) [Gr. *psyche,* mind, + *soma,* body] Pertaining to the relationship of the brain and body; pert. to disorders that have a physiological component but are thought to originate in the emotional state of the patient. When so used, the impression is created that the brain and body are separate entities and that a disease may be purely somatic in its effect or entirely emotional. This partitioning of the human being is not possible; thus no disease is limited to only the brain or the body. A complex interaction is always present even though in specific instances a disease might on superficial examination appear to involve only the body or the mind.

psychosurgery (sī″kō-sur′jĕr-ē) [″ + L. *chirurgia,* surgery] Surgical intervention for mental disorders, e.g., frontal lobotomy.

psychotechnics (sī″kō-tĕk′nĭks) [″ + *techne,* art] The use of psychological methods in the study of economic and social problems.

psychotherapeutic drug A drug that is

used because of its effects in ameliorating the principal symptoms that occur in mentally disturbed persons, such as anxiety, depression, and psychosis.

psychotherapy (sī-kō-thĕr′ă-pē) [Gr. *psyche,* mind, + *therapeia,* treatment] A method of treating disease, esp. psychic disorders, by mental rather than pharmacological means (e.g., suggestion, re-education, hypnotism, and psychoanalysis).

psychotherapist (sī″kō-thĕr′ă-pĭst) An individual trained or skilled in the management of psychological disorders.

psychotic (sī-kŏt′ĭk) Pert. to or affected by psychosis.

psychotogenic (sī-kŏt″ō-jĕn′ĭk) [″ + *gennan,* to produce] Producing a psychosis, usually temporary and due to certain powerful drugs.

psychotomimetic (sī-kŏt″ō-mĭ-mĕ′tĭk) [″ + *mimetikos,* imitative] Relating to or producing a state resembling psychosis.

psychotropic drug [″ + *trope,* a turning] A drug that affects psychic function, behavior, or experience. Many drugs can be classed as being intentionally psychotropic, but many other drugs also occasionally may produce undesired psychotropic side effects.

psychro- Combining form meaning *cold.* SEE: also *cryo-*.

psychroalgia (sī″krō-ăl′jē-ă) [Gr. *psychros,* cold, + *algos,* pain] A painful sensation of cold.

psychroesthesia (sī″krō-ĕs-thē′zē-ă) [″ + *aisthesis,* sensation] A sensation of cold in a part of the body, even though it is warm.

psychrometer (sī-krŏm′ĕ-tĕr) [″ + *metron,* measure] A device for measuring relative humidity of the atmosphere. Calculations are made using the readings of two thermometers, one with a dry bulb and one with a wet bulb.

psychrophilic (sī-krō-fĭl′ĭk) [″ + *philein,* to love] Preferring cold, as bacteria that thrive at low temperatures, between 0° and 30°C (32° and 86°F).

psychrophobia (sī-krō-fō′bē-ă) [″ + *phobos,* fear] Abnormal aversion or sensitiveness to cold.

psychrophore (sī′krō-for) [″ + *phorein,* to carry] A double-lumen catheter for applying cold to the urethra or any canal.

psychrotherapy (sī″krō-thĕr′ă-pē) [″ + *therapeia,* treatment] The treatment of disease by the use of cold.

psyllium seed (sĭl′ē-ŭm) The dried ripe seed of the psyllium plant (*Plantago afra*), grown in France, Spain, and India; used as a mild laxative. It is also used in symptomatic treatment of diarrhea. It enhances stool consistency by absorbing water from the bowel contents.

PT *prothrombin time; physical therapist.*

Pt Symbol for the element platinum.

pt *pint; patient.*

PTA *plasma thromboplastin antecedent; physical therapy assistant.*

ptarmic (tăr′mĭk) [Gr. *ptarmikos,* causing to sneeze] **1.** Causing sneezing. **2.** An agent that causes sneezing. SYN: *sternutatory.*

ptarmus (tar′mŭs) Spasmodic sneezing.

PTC *percutaneous transhepatic cholangiography; phenylthiocarbamide; plasma thromboplastin component.*

PTCA *percutaneous transluminal coronary angioplasty.*

pterion (tē′rē-ŏn) [Gr. *pteron,* wing] Point of suture of frontal, parietal, temporal, and sphenoid bones.

pternalgia (tĕr-năl′jē-ă) [Gr. *pterna,* heel, + *algos,* pain] Pain in the heel.

pterygium (tĕr-ĭj′ē-ŭm) [Gr. *pterygion,* wing] Triangular thickening of the bulbar conjunctiva extending from the inner canthus to the border of the cornea with the apex toward the pupil.

p. colli A congenital band of fascia extending from the mastoid process of the temporal bone to the clavicle.

progressive p. A stage in which the growth extends toward the center of the cornea.

pterygoid (tĕr′ĭ-goyd) [Gr. *pterygoeides*] Wing-shaped.

p. hamulus A small bony projection, just medial to the pterygoid process, that serves as an attachment for the tensor veli palatini muscle.

pterygomandibular (tĕr″ĭ-gō-măn-dĭb′ū-lăr) [″ + L. *mandibula,* lower jawbone] Concerning the pterygoid process of the sphenoid bone and mandible.

pterygomaxillary (tĕr″ĭ-gō-măk′sĭ-lĕr″ē) [″ + L. *maxillaris,* upper jaw] Concerning the pterygoid process and upper jaw.

pterygopalatine (tĕr″ĭ-gō-păl′ă-tĭn) [″ + L. *palatinus,* palate] Relating to the pterygoid process and the palate bone.

PTFE *polytetrafluoroethylene* (Teflon).

PTH *parathyroid hormone.*

ptilosis (tī-lō′sĭs) [Gr.] Loss of eyelashes.

ptomaine (tō′mān, tō-mān′) [Gr. *ptoma,* dead body] One of a class of nitrogenous organic bases formed in the action of putrefactive bacteria on proteins and amino acids.

ptosed (tōst) Having ptosis.

ptosis (tō′sĭs) [Gr. *ptosis,* a dropping] Dropping or drooping of an organ or part, as the upper eyelid from paralysis, or the visceral organs from weakness of the abdominal muscles. **ptotic** (tŏt′ĭk), *adj.* SEE: illus.

morning p. Difficulty in raising the eyelids upon awakening.

waking p. Morning p.

PTT *partial thromboplastin time.*

ptyalagogue (tī-ăl′ă-gŏg) [Gr. *ptyalon,* saliva, + *agogos,* leading] Causing, or something that causes, a flow of saliva. SYN: *sialagogue.*

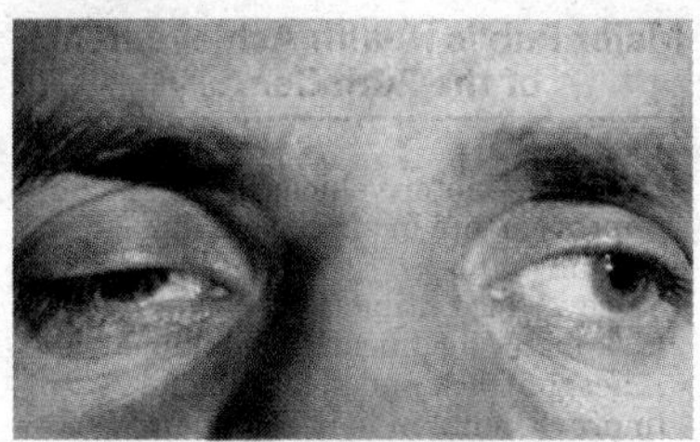

PTOSIS

ptyalectasis (tī″ă-lĕk′tă-sĭs) [″ + *ektasis,* dilation] Surgical dilation of a salivary duct.

ptyalin (tī′ă-lĭn) A salivary enzyme that hydrolyzes starch and glycogen to maltose and a small amount of glucose. The optimum pH for ptyalin activity is 6.9. SYN: *amylase, salivary.* SEE: *enzyme; ptyalism; saliva.*

ptyalism (tī′ă-lĭzm) [″ + *-ismos,* condition] Excessive secretion of saliva. This may be due to pregnancy, stomatitis, rabies, exophthalmic goiter, menstruation, epilepsy, hysteria, nervous conditions, and gastrointestinal disorders and may be induced by mercury, iodides, pilocarpine, and other drugs. SYN: *hyperptyalism; hypersalivation; salivation.* SEE: *xerostomia.*

ptyalith (tī′ă-lĭth) [″ + *lithos,* stone] A salivary gland stone.

ptyalocele (tī-ăl′ō-sēl) [″ + *kele,* tumor, swelling] A salivary cystic tumor or cystic dilatation of a salivary duct.

ptyalogenic (tī″ăl-ō-jĕn′ĭk) [Gr. *ptyalon;* saliva, + *gennan,* to produce] Of salivary origin.

ptyalogogue (tī″ăl′ō-gŏg) [″ + *agogos,* leading] An agent that causes the flow of saliva. SYN: *sialogogue.*

ptyalography (tī-ăl-ŏg′ră-fē) [″ + *graphein,* to write] SEE: *sialography.*

ptyalolith (tī′ă-lō-lĭth) [″ + *lithos,* stone] A salivary concretion.

ptyalolithiasis (tī″ă-lō-lĭ-thī′ă-sĭs) The presence of a stone in a salivary gland or duct.

ptyalolithotomy (tī″ăl-ō-lĭ-thŏt′ō-mē) [Gr. *ptyalon,* saliva, + *lithos,* stone, + *tome,* incision] The surgical removal of a stone from a salivary duct or gland.

ptyaloreaction (tī″ă-lō-rē-ăk′shŭn) A reaction occurring in saliva.

ptyalorrhea (tī″ă-lō-rē′ă) [″ + *rhoia,* flow] An excessive flow of saliva.

ptyocrinous (tī-ŏk′rĭ-nŭs) A type of glandular secretion in which the contents of the cell are discharged.

ptysis (tī′sĭs) [Gr.] Spitting; the ejection of saliva from the mouth.

Pu Symbol for the element plutonium.

pubalgia (pyū′bal-ja) Pain arising from the groin or pubic symphysis. Diagnosis is made after ruling out the presence of an inguinal hernia.

ETIOLOGY: Symptoms are often secondary to strain of the muscles that attach in the area (e.g., rectus abdominis, iliopsoas, adductor longus, or rectus femoris), inflammation in the urogenital system (e.g., urethritis, epididymitis), inflammation of the hip (e.g., bursitis, arthritis), or weaknesses in the abdominal wall.

pubarche (pū-băr′kē) [L. *puber,* grown up, + Gr. *arche,* beginning] **1.** The beginning of puberty. **2.** Beginning development of pubic hair. SEE: *semenarche; thelarche.*

puber (pū′bĕr) [L., grown up] One at the onset of puberty.

puberal (pū′bĕr-ăl) [L. *pubertas,* puberty] Pubertal.

pubertal Pert. to puberty.

pubertas (pū′bĕr-tăs) [L.] Puberty.

p. praecox Precocious puberty or puberty at an early age.

puberty (pū′bĕr-tē) The stage in life at which members of both sexes become functionally capable of reproduction. A period of rapid change occurs between the ages of 13 and 15 in boys and 9 to 16 in girls, ending in the attainment of sexual maturity. There is evidence that the onset of puberty is related to a decrease in secretion of the pineal gland.

onset of p. *Boys:* Between the ages of 13 and 15, a relatively rapid increase in height and weight occurs, with broadening of the shoulders and increase in size of the penis and testicles. Pubic and facial hair begin to grow. Endocrine and sebaceous gland activity is increased. Nocturnal emissions usually occur.

Girls: Between the ages of 9 and 16, a marked increase in growth is accompanied by breast enlargement and appearance of pubic hair. Within 1 to 2 years after these changes, underarm hair grows and the normal whitish vaginal secretion (physiological leukorrhea) characteristic of the adult female is noticed. Several months later the first menstrual period (menarche) occurs. Each individual will vary somewhat from this schedule.

PATIENT CARE: Before puberty, young girls should be told about menstruation and the techniques of menstrual protection through use of perineal pads or tampons. In addition, she should be told that a certain amount of intermenstrual vaginal discharge (leukorrhea) is normal but if the secretion is malodorous or causes irritation of the vulva, a physician should be consulted. SEE: *menstruation.*

Young boys should be assured that the size of the penis is not related to the degree of masculinity and is not an important factor in experiencing or providing sexual gratification.

precocious p. The appearance of secondary sex characteristics before 8 years of age in girls and 9 years of age in boys. The pituitary and hypothalamus glands may be involved, or the condition may result from premature secretion of sex hormones not caused by pituitary or hypothalamic action. Gonadotropin-releasing hormone (GnRH) has been used to treat this condition.

pubes (pū′bēz) *sing.*, **pubis** [L., grown up] **1.** The anterior part of the innominate bone. SYN: *os pubis*. **2.** The pubic region. **3.** The pubic hair.

pubescence (pū-bĕs′ĕns) [L. *pubescens,* becoming hairy] **1.** Puberty or its approach. **2.** A covering of fine, soft hairs on the body. SYN: *lanugo*. **pubescent,** *adj.*

pubetrotomy (pū″bĕ-trŏt′ō-mē) [NL. *(os) pubis,* bone of the groin, + Gr. *etron,* belly, + *tome,* incision] Section through the os pubis and lower abdominal wall.

pubic (pū′bĭk) [L. *pubes,* pubic hair] Concerning the pubes.

pubic bone The lower anterior part of the innominate bone. SYN: *os pubis*.

pubic hair Hair over the pubes, which appears at onset of sexual maturity. The distribution is somewhat different in men than in women. SEE: *m. pubis; m. veneris*.

pubio-, pubo- Combining form meaning *pubic bone, pubic region.*

pubiotomy (pū-bē-ŏt′ō-mē) [L. *pubes,* pubic region, + *tome,* incision] Incision across the pubis in order to enlarge the pelvic passage, facilitating the delivery of the fetus when the pelvis is malformed. SYN: *hebotomy*.

pubis (pū′bĭs) *pl.* **pubes** [NL. *(os) pubis,* bone of the groin] Pubic bone.

public health The discipline concerned with preventive measures intended to improve the health of communities. It includes the study and practice of techniques that protect communities from epidemics or toxic exposures, predict environmental disasters, and enforce the laws that provide a safe supply of water and food. Various government agencies such as the Centers for Disease Control and Prevention, Food and Drug Administration, and National Institutes of Health are active in maintaining the public health. Each of the 50 states has a health department in which at least one physician is the public health official. SEE: table; *preventive medicine; preventive nursing*.

Public Health Service Act One of the principal laws of Congress giving the authority for federal health activities. First enacted July 1, 1944, it provided a complete codification of all the federal public health laws. Many of the health laws since 1944 have actually been amendments to the Public Health Service Act that have revised, extended, or given new authority to the act.

pubococcygeal (pū″bō-kŏk-sĭj′ē-ăl) [″ + Gr. *kokkyx,* coccyx] Concerning the pubis and coccyx.

Major Public Health Achievements of the 20th Century

Vaccination
Enhanced motor vehicle safety
Improvements in sanitation and clean water
Discovery of antibiotics
Risk factor modification to reduce heart attack and stroke
Improvements in food safety and nutrition
Maternal/child care innovations
Family planning
Fluoridation of drinking water
Antismoking campaigns

SOURCE: Adapted from the Centers for Disease Control and Prevention. *MMWR* 1999; 48:241–243.

pubofemoral (pū″bō-fĕm′or-ăl) [″ + *femur,* thigh bone] Pert. to the os pubis and femur.

pubomadesis [L. *pubes,* pubic hair, + Gr. *madesis,* baldness] Loss of or absent pubic hair.

puboprostatic (pū″bō-prŏs-tăt′ĭk) [″ + Gr. *prostates,* prostate] Relating to the os pubis and prostate gland.

puborectal (pū″bō-rĕk′tăl) [″ + *rectus,* straight] Concerning the pubis and rectum.

pubovaginal device An apparatus that is fitted for use in the vagina to help prevent urinary incontinence. *SEE: pessary*.

pubovesical (pū″bō-vĕs′ĭ-kl) [″ + *vesiculus,* a little sac] Pert. to the os pubis and bladder.

pudenda (pū-dĕn′dă) *sing.*, **pudendum** [L.] Vulva.

pudendagra (pū″dĕn-dăg′ră) [″ + Gr. *agra,* seizure] Pain in the external genitals.

pudendal (pū-dĕn′dăl) [L. *pudenda,* external genitals] Relating to the external genitals of the female.

pudendum (pū-dĕn′dŭm) *pl.* **pudenda** [L.] Vulva.

p. femininum Vulva.

p. muliebre External genitals of the female.

puerile (pū′ĕ-rĭl) [L. *puerilis*] Concerning a child; childlike.

puerilism (pū′ĕr-ĭl-ĭzm) [″ + Gr. *-ismos,* condition] Childishness; second childhood.

puerperal eclampsia Convulsions occurring immediately after childbirth.

puerperal fever Septicemia following childbirth. SYN: *childbed fever; puerperal sepsis*.

puerperalism (pū-ĕr′pĕr-ăl-ĭzm) [L. *puer,* child, + *parere,* to bring forth, to bear, + Gr. *-ismos,* condition] A pathologic condition accompanying childbirth.

puerperant (pū-ĕr′pĕr-ănt) A woman in labor, or one who has recently given birth.

puerperium (pū″ĕr-pē′rē-ŭm) [L.] The period of 42 days following childbirth and expulsion of the placenta and membranes. The generative organs usually return to normal during this time. SYN: *postpartum*. **puerperal,** *adj.*

PUFA *polyunsaturated fatty acids*. SEE: *fatty acid*.

puff A soft, short, blowing sound heard on auscultation.

Pulex (pū′lĕks) [L., flea] A genus of fleas belonging to the order Siphonaptera.

P. irritans The human flea, which also infests dogs, hogs, and other mammals. It is an intermediate host of the tapeworms *Dipylidium caninum* and *Hymenolepis diminuta*. SEE: *flea*.

pulicatio (pū″lĭ-kā′tē-ō) Infested with fleas.

Pulicidae (pū-lĭs′ĭ-dē) A family of fleas belonging to the order Siphonaptera. Pulicidae includes the genera *Pulex, Echidnophaga, Ctenocephalides,* and *Xenopsylla*. SEE: *flea*.

pulicide (pū′lĭ-sīd) [L. *pulex,* flea, + *caedere,* to kill] An agent that kills fleas.

pullulate (pŭl″ū-lāt) [L. *pullulare,* to sprout] To bud or germinate.

pullulation (pŭl″ū-lā′shŭn) The act of budding or germinating, as seen in yeast.

pulmo- (pŭl′mō-, pool′mō-) Combining form meaning *lung*.

pulmoaortic (pŭl″mō-ā-or′tĭk) [L. *pulmo,* lung, + Gr. *aorte,* aorta] **1.** Concerning the lungs and the aorta. **2.** Relating to the pulmonary artery and aorta.

pulmometry (pūl-mŏm′ĕ-trē) Determination of capacity of the lungs.

pulmonary (pŭl′mō-nĕ-rē) [L. *pulmonarius*] Concerning or involving the lungs.

pulmonary arterial web A weblike deformity seen in pulmonary angiograms at the site of previous pulmonary thromboembolism.

pulmonary artery The artery leading from the right ventricle of the heart to the lungs.

pulmonary artery wedge pressure, pulmonary artery occlusive pressure ABBR: PAWP. Pressure measured in the pulmonary artery after catheterization. The catheter is positioned in the pulmonary artery, and the distal portion of the catheter is isolated from pressure behind it in the artery by inflating a balloon with air. This allows the catheter to float into a wedged position, and permits sensing of transmission of pressures ahead of the catheter (in the pulmonary capillary bed) by the transducer. Because no valve is present between this location and the left atrium, the measurement reflects left atrial pressure, and, in the presence of a competent mitral valve, the measurement provides an indication of left ventricular end-diastolic pressure. The balloon is then passively deflated after measurements of wedge pressure are completed. Elevated wedge pressures are found characteristically in patients with congestive heart failure or fluid overload. SYN: *wedge pressure*. SEE: *Swan-Ganz catheter*.

PATIENT CARE: The nurse prepares and sets up the transducer equipment to monitor pulmonary artery pressure and PAWP alternately according to institutional protocol and manufacturer's instructions. The transducer is balanced and calibrated as required (every 4 to 8 hr). Hemodynamic status is monitored, and findings are documented, including pulmonary artery pressure (normally 20 to 30 mm Hg systolic and 8 to 12 mm Hg diastolic) every hour as directed. To measure PAWP every 1 to 4 hr as directed, the nurse inflates the balloon with 0.75 to 1.5 cc of air depending on balloon size (balloon with fluid is never inflated) while watching for change in waveform indicating wedging and assessing for balloon rupture (lack of resistance on inflation, with absence of wedging). If this occurs, the wedging procedure is discontinued (because of concern for air embolism), and therapy is managed based on pulmonary artery diastolic pressures. Pulmonary artery wedge pressure is read, documented (normally 4 to 12 mm Hg), and correlated to clinical findings and other hemodynamic values, and any abnormal findings are reported. The nurse then removes the syringe and permits passive deflation of the balloon while observing for reappearance of pulmonary artery pressure waveform. If the balloon remains inflated, the patient is at risk for pulmonary artery necrosis. The patient should be positioned on the right side and encouraged to take deep breaths and to cough as the nurse mobilizes the right arm. If balloon remains wedged, the physician should be notified. Fluid and diuretic therapy are adjusted based on PAWP and other values as prescribed.

pulmonary function test One of several different tests used to evaluate the condition of the respiratory system. Measures of expiratory flow and lung volumes and capacities are obtained. The forced vital capacity is one of the more important pulmonary function tests; it provides a measure of the amount of air that can be maximally exhaled after a maximum inspiration and the time required for that expiration. Pulmonary function tests can also determine the diffusion ability of the alveolar-capillary membrane. SEE: illus.

pulmonary mucociliary clearance The removal of inhaled particles, endogenous cellular debris, and excessive secretions from the tracheobronchial tree by the action of the ciliated cells that live in the respiratory tract. The cilia of

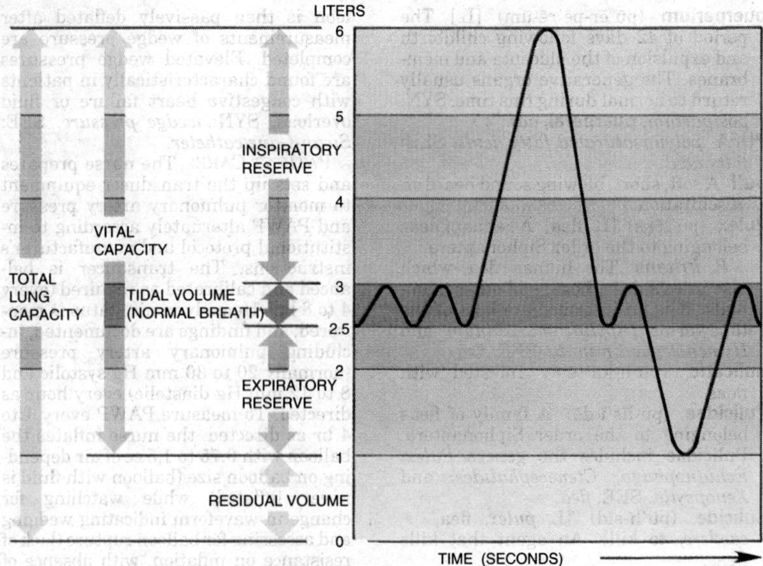

PULMONARY FUNCTION TEST

Pulmonary volumes

these cells beat and are therefore able to propel mucus and debris upward and out of the tracheobronchial tree. This action is one of the most important defenses of the respiratory tract.

pulmonary vein One of the four veins draining the lungs and returning the blood to the left atrium of the heart.

pulmonectomy (pŭl″mō-nĕk′tō-mē) [L. *pulmonis,* lung, + Gr. *ektome,* excision] Pneumectomy.

pulmonic (pŭl-mŏn′ĭk) **1.** Concerning the lungs. **2.** Concerning the pulmonary artery.

pulmonitis (pŭl-mō-nī′tĭs) [″ + Gr. *itis,* inflammation] Pneumonia.

pulmonologist A physician trained and certified to treat pulmonary diseases.

pulmotor (pŭl′mō-tor) [″ + *motor,* mover] An apparatus for inducing artificial respiration by forcing air or oxygen into the lungs.

pulp, pulpa [L. *pulpa,* flesh] **1.** The soft part of fruit. **2.** The soft part of an organ. **3.** A mass of partly digested food passed from stomach to duodenum. SYN: *chyme*. **4.** The soft vascular portion of the center of a tooth.

p. amputation The technique of removing the coronal portion of an exposed or involved vital pulp in an effort to retain the radicular pulp in a healthy, vital condition. SYN: *pulpotomy*.

p. capping The technique and material for covering and protecting from external conditions a vital, exposed pulp while the pulp heals and secondary or tertiary dentin forms to cover it.

coronal p. The portion of dental pulp in the crown of the pulp cavity.

dead p. Devitalized or necrotic dental pulp that will result in an abscess.

TREATMENT: Recommended treatment includes endodontic therapy.

dental p. The connective tissues that fill the pulp cavity enclosed by dentin of the tooth; it includes a vascular and nerve network, a peripheral layer of odontoblasts involved with dentin formation, and other cellular and fibrous components.

devitalized p. A dead or necrotic dental pulp as indicated by a vitalometer used for pulp testing.

digital p. The elastic, soft prominence on the palmar or plantar surface of the last phalanx of a finger or toe.

enamel p. Cells forming a stellate reticulum lying between outer and inner layers of the enamel organ of a tooth.

exposed p. Pulp that, due to disease, is exposed to the air and saliva in the mouth.

p. extirpation The complete removal of the pulp tissue from the pulp chamber and root canal, irrespective of the state of health of the pulp. SYN: *pulpectomy*.

putrescent p. Dead pulp that has a foul odor because of the action of anaerobic bacteria.

radicular p. Pulp that is in the root canal of a tooth.

red p. The portion of splenic pulp consisting of vascular sinuses through which blood flows. The sinuses are separated by pulp cords, made up of loosely connected macrophages that phagocytize foreign antigens and red blood cells. SEE: *spleen*.

splenic p. The soft spongelike tissue-forming substance of the spleen.

tooth p. SEE: *tooth*.

vertebral p. Nucleus pulposus of the intervertebral disk.

vital p. Dental pulp that is alive and thus normal.

white p. The portion of splenic pulp, consisting of T and B lymphocytes, that forms sheaths around arteries. The sheaths are thickest around the large arteries and grow progressively thinner as the arteries progress into the spleen. SEE: *spleen*.

wood p. A soft form of cellulose, derived from wood or cotton, used as a food additive.

pulpalgia (pŭl-păl′jē-ă) [″ + Gr. *algos,* pain] Pain in the pulp of a tooth.

pulpectomy (pŭl-pĕk′tō-mē) [″ + Gr. *ektome,* excision] Pulp extirpation.

pulpefaction (pŭl-pĭ-făk′shŭn) [L. *pulpa,* pulp, + *facere,* to make] Conversion into a pulpy substance.

pulpitis (pŭl-pī′tĭs) *pl.* **pulpitides** [″ + *itis,* inflammation] Inflammation of the pulp of a tooth.

pulpotomy (pŭl-pŏt′ō-mē) [″ + Gr. *tome,* incision] Pulp amputation.

pulpy (pŭl′pē) Resembling pulp; flabby.

pulsate (pŭl′sāt) [L. *pulsare*] To throb or beat in rhythm.

pulsatile (pŭl′să-tĭl) Pulsating; characterized by a rhythmic beat. SYN: *throbbing*.

pulsation (pŭl-sā′shŭn) [L. *pulsatio,* a beating] The rhythmic beat, as of the heart and blood vessels; a throbbing. SEE: *pulse*.

pulse (pŭls) [L. *pulsus,* beating] **1.** Rate, rhythm, condition of arterial walls, compressibility and tension, and size and shape of the fluid wave of blood traveling through the arteries as a result of each heartbeat. **2.** Rhythmical throbbing. **3.** Throbbing caused by the regular contraction and alternate expansion of an artery as the wave of blood passes through the vessel; the periodic thrust felt over arteries in time with the heartbeat.

A tracing of this is called a sphygmogram and consists of a series of waves in which the upstroke is called the anacrotic limb, and the downstroke (on which is normally seen the dicrotic notch), the catacrotic limb.

The normal resting pulse in adults is between 60 and 100 beats per minute. The resting pulse is faster, for example, in febrile patients, anemic or hypovolemic persons, persons in shock, and patients who have taken drugs that stimulate the heart, such as theophylline, caffeine, nicotine, or cocaine. It may be slower in well-trained athletes; in patients using beta blockers, calcium channel blockers, or other agents; and during sleep or deep relaxation.

PATIENT CARE: In patients complaining of chest pain, pulses should be assessed in at least two extremities (e.g., both radial arteries). A strong pulse on the right side with a weak one on the left may suggest an aortic dissection or a stenosis of the left subclavian artery. Young patients with high blood pressure should have pulses assessed simultaneously at the radial and femoral artery because a significant delay in the femoral pulse may suggest coarctation of the aorta. Patients with recent symptoms of stroke or claudication should have pulses checked at the carotid, radial, femoral, popliteal, and posterior tibial arteries, to see whether any palpable evidence of arterial insufficiency exists at any of these locations. If a decreased pulse is detected, further evaluation might include ultrasonography or assessments of the ankle brachial index. Patients who are lightheaded or dizzy or who notice palpitations may have detectable premature beats or other pulse irregularities (e.g., the irregularly irregular pulse of atrial fibrillation).

abdominal p. A palpable pulse felt between the xiphoid process and the navel. This is produced by the pulse of the abdominal aorta.

accelerated p. Tachycardia.

alternating p. A pulse with alternating weak and strong pulsations.

anacrotic p. A pulse showing a secondary wave on the ascending limb of the main wave.

anadicrotic p. A pulse wave with two small notches on the ascending portion.

apical p. A pulse felt or heard over the apex of the heart.

asymmetrical radial p. Unequal p.

basal p. Resting p.

bigeminal p. A pulse in which two regular beats are followed by a longer pause. SYN: *coupled p.*

bisferiens p. A pulse marked by two systolic peaks on the pulse waveform. It is characteristic of aortic regurgitation (with or without aortic stenosis) and hypertrophic cardiomyopathy.

bounding p. A pulse that reaches a higher intensity than normal, then disappears quickly. Best detected when the arm is held aloft. SYN: *collapsing p.*

brachial p. A pulse felt in the brachial artery.

capillary p. Alternating redness and pallor of a capillary region, as in the matrices beneath the nails, occurring chiefly in aortic insufficiency. SYN: *Quincke's pulse*.

carotid p. A pulse felt in the carotid artery.

catacrotic p. A pulse showing one or more secondary waves on the descending limb of the main wave.

***catadicrotic* p.** A pulse wave with two small notches on the descending portion.

***central* p.** A pulse recorded near the origin of the carotid or subclavian arteries.

***collapsing* p.** Bounding p.

***coupled* p.** Bigeminal p.

p. deficit A condition in which the number of pulse beats counted at the wrist is less than those counted in the same period of time at the heart. This is seen in atrial fibrillation.

***dicrotic* p.** A pulse with a double beat, one heartbeat for two arterial pulsations, or a seemingly weak wave between the usual heartbeats. This weak wave should not be counted as a regular beat. It is indicative of low arterial tension and is noted in fevers.

***dorsalis pedis* p.** A pulse felt over the dorsalis pedis artery of the foot.

***entoptic* p.** Intermittent subjective sensations of light that accompany the heartbeat.

***femoral* p.** A pulse felt over the femoral artery.

***filiform* p.** Thready p.

***hepatic* p.** A pulse due to expansion of veins of the liver at each ventricular contraction.

***intermediate* p.** A pulse recorded in the proximal portions of the carotid, femoral, and brachial arteries.

***intermittent* p.** A pulse in which occasional beats are skipped, caused by conditions such as premature atrial contractions, premature ventricular contractions, and atrial fibrillation. SYN: *irregular p.*

***irregular* p.** Intermittent pulse.

***irregularly irregular* p.** The erratic, unpredictable pulse that is present in atrial fibrillation.

***jugular* p.** A venous pulse felt in the jugular vein.

***Kussmaul's* p.** Paradoxical p.

***monocrotic* p.** A pulse in which the sphygmogram shows a simple ascending and descending uninterrupted line and no dicrotism.

***nail* p.** A visible pulsation in the capillaries under the nails.

***paradoxical* p.** A decrease in the strength of the pulse (and of systolic blood pressure) during inspiration, a condition that may be esp. prominent in severe asthma, cardiac tamponade, obstructive sleep apnea, croup, and other conditions that alter pressure relationships within the chest. SYN: *Kussmaul's p.; p. paradoxus.*

p. parvus Pulsus parvus et tardus.

***peripheral* p.** A pulse recorded in the arteries (radial or pedal) in the distal portion of the limbs.

***pistol-shot* p.** A pulse resulting from rapid distention and collapse of an artery as occurs in aortic regurgitation.

***plateau* p.** A pulse associated with an increase in pressure that slowly rises but is maintained.

***popliteal* p.** A pulse felt over the popliteal artery.

***radial* p.** A pulse felt over the radial artery.

***rapid* p.** Tachycardia.

***regular* p.** A pulse felt when the force and frequency are the same (i.e., when the length of beat and number of beats per minute and the strength are the same).

***respiratory* p.** Alternate dilatation and contraction of the large veins of the neck occurring simultaneously with inspiration and expiration.

***resting* p.** A pulse rate obtained while an individual is at rest and calm.

***Riegel's* p.** A diminution of the pulse during expiration.

***running* p.** A weak, rapid pulse with one wave continuing into the next.

***short* p.** A pulse with a short, quick systolic wave.

***slow* p.** A pulse rate that is less than 60 beats per minute.

***small* p.** SEE: *pulsus parvus et tardus.*

***soft* p.** A pulse that may be stopped by moderate digital compression.

***tense* p.** A full but not bounding pulse.

***thready* p.** A fine, scarcely perceptible pulse. SYN: *filiform p.*

***tremulous* p.** A pulse in which a series of oscillations is felt with each beat.

***tricrotic* p.** A pulse with three separate expansions during each heartbeat.

***trigeminal* p.** A pulse in which a pause follows three regular beats.

***triphammer* p.** Waterhammer p.

***undulating* p.** A pulse that seems to have several successive waves.

***unequal* p.** A pulse in which beats vary in force. SYN: *asymmetrical radial p.*

***vagus* p.** A slow pulse resulting from vagal inhibition of the heart.

***venous* p.** A pulse in a vein, esp. one of the large veins near the heart, such as the internal or external jugular. Normally it is undulating and scarcely palpable. In conditions such as tricuspid regurgitation, it is pronounced.

***vermicular* p.** A small, frequent pulse with a wormlike feeling.

***waterhammer* p.** A pulse with a powerful upstroke and then sudden disappearance; a hallmark of aortic regurgitation. SYN: *triphammer p.; Corrigan's pulse.*

***wiry* p.** A tense pulse that feels like a wire or firm cord.

pulseless disease Takayasu's arteritis.

pulseless electrical activity A form of cardiac arrest in which the continuation of organized electrical activity in the heart is not accompanied by a palpable pulse or effective circulation of blood. SEE: *cardiopulmonary resuscitation.*

ETIOLOGY: PEA may be caused by severe acidosis; cardiac ischemia or infarction; hyperkalemia; hypothermia; hypoxia; hypovolemia (e.g., bleeding or dehydration); massive pulmonary embolism (which blocks the return of blood from the body to the heart); cardiac tamponade; and tension pneumothorax.

SYMPTOMS: The patient is unresponsive, pulseless, and apneic.

TREATMENT: Intravenous fluids are given, and potentially correctable conditions are addressed (e.g., when cardiac tamponade is suspected, pericardiocentesis is performed; for tension pneumothorax, needle decompression of the chest is performed).

pulsing electromagnetic field ABBR: PEMF. An alternating electrical current used to produce an electromagnetic field. This may induce healing when applied to a fractured bone. The field is applied noninvasively to the affected limb. It may be moderately helpful in treating bony nonunion. SEE: *diathermy*.

pulsion (pŭl′shŭn) Driving or propelling in any direction.

lateral p. Movement, particularly walking as if pulled to one side.

pulsus (pŭl′sŭs) [L.] Pulse.

p. alternans A weak pulse alternating with a strong one.

p. bigeminus Bigeminal pulse.

p. celer A quick pulse that rises and falls suddenly.

p. differens A condition in which the pulses on either side of the body are of unequal intensity. It is seen sometimes in aortic dissection, or in atherosclerotic obstruction of one of the subclavian arteries.

p. paradoxus Paradoxical pulse.

p. parvus et tardus A pulse that is small and rises and falls slowly, indicative of severe aortic stenosis. SYN: *p. parvus*.

p. tardus An abnormally slow pulse.

pulv L. *pulvis,* powder.

pulverization (pŭl″vĕr-ī-zā′shŭn) [L. *pulvis,* powder] The crushing of any substance to powder or tiny particles.

pulverulent (pŭl-vĕr′ū-lĕnt) Of the nature of, or resembling, powder.

pulvinar (pŭl-vī′năr) [L., cushioned seat] The part of the thalamus comprising a portion of the posterior nuclei. It projects posteriorly and medially, partially overlying the midbrain.

pulvinate (pŭl′vĭ-nāt) [L. *pulvinus,* cushion] Convex; shaped like a cushion.

pulvis [L.] Powder.

pumice (pŭm′ĭs) An abrasive polishing agent derived from volcanic material. Pumice consists chiefly of complex silicates of aluminum, potassium, and sodium.

pump [ME. *pumpe*] **1.** An apparatus that transfers fluids or gases by pressure or suction. **2.** To force air or fluid along a certain pathway, as when the heart pumps blood.

air p. A device for forcing air in or out of a chamber.

blood p. **1.** A device for pumping blood. It is attached to an extracorporeal circulation system. **2.** A compression sleeve placed about a plastic transfusion bag.

breast p. An apparatus for removing milk from the breasts.

dental p. An apparatus for removing saliva from the mouth during operation on teeth or jaws.

insulin p. SEE: under *insulin*.

lymphedema p. A pneumatic compression device for application to an edematous limb. It works best when combined with elevation of the limb and manual massage. The device, which may be single-chambered or multichambered, is designed to provide calibrated, sequential pressure to the extremity. This action "milks" edema fluid from the extremity. It is essential that the device be used in the early phase of the development of lymphedema. If the affected lymph vessels develop fibrotic changes (i.e., scar tissue), then pneumatic compression devices are of questionable benefit.

sodium p. The active transport mechanism that moves sodium ions across a membrane to their area of greater concentration. In neurons and muscle cells, this is outside the cell. In many cells, the sodium pump is linked with the potassium pump that transports potassium ions into the cell, also against a concentration gradient, and may be called the *sodium-potassium pump*. In neurons and muscle fibers, this pump maintains the polarization of the membrane.

stomach p. An apparatus consisting of tubing and suction for removing contents from the stomach, e.g., after oral overdose.

pumping (pŭm′pēng) Draining or emptying of fluids by hydraulic suction.

lymphatic p. In osteopathic practice, manipulation of the thoracic cavity to facilitate lymphatic circulation.

pump-oxygenator A device that pumps and oxygenates blood.

punch An instrument for making a small circular hole in material or tissue, esp. the skin.

punchdrunk **1.** An imprecise term for the behavioral consequences of traumatic brain injury, present in persons who have boxed and experienced multiple episodes of trauma to the head. If severe, both the cognitive and memory functions of the brain are affected. Symptoms may resemble those of Parkinson's disease. SYN: *dementia pugilistica*. **2.** One who is punchdrunk.

punched out Appearing as if holes have been made; used to describe appearance of bones (as seen on x-ray film) in diseases like multiple myeloma.

puncta (pŭnk′tă) *sing.,* **punctum** [L.] Points.

punctate (pŭnk′tāt) [L. *punctum,* point] Having pinpoint punctures or depressions on the surface; marked with dots.

p. keratoses Discrete yellow-to-brown firm papules of the palms and soles that appear after skin trauma, e.g., in walking or regular use of the hands or feet at work. The lesions are found in patients with a genetic predisposition to keratoderma.

p. pits Depressed areas of the skin, esp. of the palmar creases of the hands and soles.

p. rash A rash with minute red points.

punctiform (pŭnk′tĭ-form) [″ + *forma,* shape] **1.** Formed like a point. **2.** In bacteriology, referring to pinpoint colonies of less than 1 mm in diameter.

punctio (pŭnk′shē-ō) [L. *punctura,* a point] The act of puncturing or pricking.

punctum (pŭnk′tŭm) *pl.* **puncta** [L.] Point.

p. caecum Blind spot (1).

p. dolorosa Painful points in the course of, or at the exit of, nerves affected by neuralgia.

p. lacrimale The outlet of a lacrimal canaliculus.

p. nasale inferius Rhinion.

p. proximum ABBR: P.P. Visual accommodation near-point.

p. remotum ABBR: P.R. Visual accommodation far-point.

p. saliens The first trace of the embryonic heart.

p. vasculosa Minute red areas that mark the cut surface of white central substance of the brain, caused by blood escaping from divided blood vessels.

puncture (pŭnk′chūr) [L. *punctura,* prick] **1.** A hole or wound made by a sharp pointed instrument. **2.** To make a hole with such an instrument.

cisternal p. A spinal puncture with a hollow needle between the cervical vertebrae, through the dura mater, and into the cisterna at the base of the brain. This is done to inject a drug as in meningitis or cerebral syphilis, to remove spinal fluid for diagnostic purposes, or to reduce intracranial pressure. It should be used as a source of spinal fluid only if fluid cannot be obtained by lumbar puncture. SEE: *cerebrospinal fluid; lumbar puncture.*

CAUTION: This procedure may be lethal if not done by one skilled in this technique.

---

diabetic p. Puncture in the floor of the fourth ventricle, which results in glycosuria. This lesion was produced experimentally by the French physiologist Claude Bernard.

exploratory p. Piercing of a cavity or cyst for the purpose of examining the fluid or pus removed.

lumbar p. SEE: *lumbar puncture.*

Quincke's p. Lumbar puncture.

spinal p. Lumbar puncture.

sternal p. Puncture of the sternum to obtain a bone marrow specimen.

tracheoesophageal p. The surgical creation of a passage between the trachea and esophagus. It is used for vocal restoration in patients who have undergone laryngectomy. The technique provides air to the esophagus. The patient is trained to use that air to make vibrations that recreate speech.

ventricular p. Puncture of a ventricle of the brain for purpose of withdrawing fluid or introducing air for ventriculography.

pungency (pŭn′jĕn-sē) [L. *pungens,* prick] The quality of being sharp, strong, or bitter, as an odor or taste.

pungent (pŭn′jĕnt) Acrid or sharp, as applied to an odor or taste.

punitive damages Compensation awarded in an amount intended to punish the defendant (the person committing the tort) for the obvious and preventable harmful act. The defendant's actions must be willful and wanton, and the damages are not based on the plaintiff's actual monetary loss. SEE: *tort.*

P.U.O. *pyrexia of unknown origin.*

pupa (pū′pă) [L., girl] The stage in complete metamorphosis of an insect that follows the larva and precedes the adult or imago. The insect does not feed during this stage and usually is inactive.

pupil (pū′pĭl) [L. *pupilla*] The contractile opening at the center of the iris of the eye. It is constricted when exposed to strong light and when the focus is on a near object; is dilated in the dark and when the focus is on a distant object. Average diameter is 4 to 5 mm. The pupils should be equal. SYN: *pupilla.*

DIFFERENTIAL DIAGNOSIS: Constriction of the pupil occurs, for example, in bright light and after exposure to drugs such as morphine, pilocarpin, physostigmine, eserine, and other miotics.

Dilation of the pupil is most often observed after treatment with mydriatic drugs (such as atropine, scopolamine, or homatropine), but may also be caused by paralysis of cranial nerve III, intracranial masses or trauma, sympathetic nervous system stimulation, and other pupillary stimuli.

Adie's p. Tonic p. SEE: *Adie's syndrome.*

artificial p. A pupil made by iridectomy when the normal pupil is occluded.

bounding p. Rapid dilatation of a pupil, alternating with contraction.

Bumke's p. Dilatation of the pupil owing to psychic stimulus.

cat's-eye p. A pupil that is narrow and slitlike.

cornpicker's p. Dilated pupils found in agricultural workers who are exposed to dust from jimsonweed. The dust contains stramonium, a mydriatic.

fixed p. A pupil that does not react to stimuli.

keyhole p. A pupil with an artificial coloboma at the pupillary margin.

luetic p. Argyll Robertson pupil.

occlusion of the p. A pupil with an opaque membrane shutting off the pupillary area.

pinhole p. A pupil of minute size; one excessively constricted; seen after use of miotics, in opium poisoning, and in certain brain disorders.

stiff p. Argyll Robertson pupil.

tonic p. A pupil that reacts slowly in accommodation-convergence reflexes.

pupilla (pū-pĭl′ă) [L., pupil] The pupil of the eye.

pupillary (pū′pĭ-lĕr-ē) [L. *pupilla,* pupil] Concerning the pupil.

pupillography Recording movements of the pupil of the eye.

pupillometer (pū-pĭl-ŏm′ĕ-tĕr) [″ + Gr. *metron,* measure] A device for measuring the diameter of a pupil.

pupillometry (pū-pĭl-lŏm′ĕ-trē) [″ + *metron,* measure] Measurement of the diameter of the pupil.

pupillomotor reflex Purkinje phenomenon.

pupilloplegia (pū″pĭ-lō-plē′jē-ă) [″ + *plege,* stroke] Slow reaction of the pupil of the eye.

pupilloscopy (pū-pĭl-ŏs′kō-pē) [″ + Gr. *skopein,* to examine] **1.** Retinoscopy. **2.** Examination of the pupil.

pupillostatometer (pū″pĭl-ō-stă-tŏm′ĕ-tĕr) [″ + Gr. *statos,* placed, + *metron,* measure] A device for measuring the distance between the centers of the pupils.

Purdue Pegboard Test A standardized test of manual dexterity for adults and children.

pure (pūr) [ME.] Free from pollution; uncontaminated.

pure line **1.** The progeny of a single homozygous individual obtained by self-fertilization. **2.** The progeny of an individual reproducing asexually by simple fission, or by buds, runners, stolons, and so on. **3.** The progeny of two homozygous individuals reproducing sexually.

purgation (pŭr-gā′shŭn) [L. *purgatio*] **1.** Cleansing. **2.** Evacuation of the bowels by the action of a purgative medicine. SYN: *catharsis.*

purgative (pŭr′gă-tĭv) [L. *purgativus*] **1.** Cleansing. **2.** An agent that will stimulate the production of bowel movements. SEE: *catharsis; cathartic.*

cholagogue p. A purgative that stimulates the flow of bile, producing green stools.

drastic p. A purgative that produces violent bowel movements.

saline p. A purgative that produces copious watery diarrhea.

purgative enema A strong, high colonic purgative that is used when other enemas fail. SEE: *enema.*

purge (pŭrj) [L. *purgare,* to cleanse] **1.** To evacuate the bowels by means of a cathartic. **2.** A drug that causes evacuation of the bowels. **3.** Removal of malignant or other pathologic cells from bone marrow.

purging (pŭr′jĭng) In eating disorders, the act of eliminating ingested calories, either by vomiting or by evacuation of the bowels. Purging behaviors may include misuse of emetics, diuretics, laxatives, or enemas.

puriform (pū′rĭ-form) [L. *pus,* pus, + *forma,* shape] Resembling pus. SYN: *puruloid.*

purinase (pū′rĭ-nās) An enzyme that catalyzes purine metabolism.

purine (pū′rēn″) [L. *purum,* pure, + *uricus,* uric acid] Parent compound of nitrogenous bases, as adenine, guanine, xanthine, caffeine, and uric acid. Purines are the end products of nucleoprotein digestion, and are catabolized to uric acid, which is excreted by the kidneys. Adenine and guanine are synthesized within cells for incorporation into the genetic code of DNA and RNA. SEE: *aminopurine; oxypurine; methyl purine.*

endogenous p. Purine originating from nucleoproteins within the tissues.

exogenous p. Purine present in, or derived from, foods. SEE: table.

purine base Xanthine base.

purinemia (pū″rĭ-nē′mē-ă) [*purine,* + Gr. *haima,* blood] Purine in the blood.

purity [L. *puris,* clean, pure, unmixed] The state of being free of contamination.

Purkinje, Johannes E. von (pŭr-kĭn′jē) Bohemian anatomist and physiologist, 1787–1869.

P. cell A large neuron that has dendrites extending to the molecular layer of the cerebellar cortex and into the white matter of the cerebellum.

P. fiber A cardiac muscle cell beneath the endocardium of the ventricles of the heart. These extend from the bundle branches to the ventricular myocardium and form the last part of the cardiac conduction system.

P. figures Shadows of blood vessels perceived when light is projected out of focus or obliquely onto the retina.

P. layer A single row of large flask-shaped cells (Purkinje cells) lying between molecular and granular layers of the cerebellar cortex.

P. network A network of Purkinje fibers found in cardiac muscle.

P. phenomenon The adjustment of the pupil of the eye to light intensity. When the eye adapts from light to dark conditions, the maximum pupillary movement is caused by green instead of yellow light. SYN: *pupillomotor reflex.*

P.-Sanson images Three images of the same object, produced by reflections from the surface of the cornea and the anterior and posterior surfaces of the lens of the eye. For the most part, the viewer adapts to this phenomenon and ignores these "extra" images.

P. vesicle The nuclear portion of an ovum. SYN: *germinal vesicle*.

purohepatitis (pū″rō-hĕp″ă-tī′tĭs) [L. *pus*, pus + Gr. *hepar*, liver, + *itis*, inflammation] Purulent inflammation of the liver.

puromucous (pū″rō-mū′kŭs) [″ + *mucus*, mucus] Mucopurulent, containing both mucus and pus.

purple A color formed by mixing red with blue.

visual p. Rhodopsin.

purposeful movement Motor activity requiring the planned and consciously directed involvement of the patient. It is hypothesized that evoking cortical involvement in movement patterns during sensorimotor rehabilitation will enhance the development of coordination and voluntary control.

purpura (pŭr′pū-ră) [L., purple] Any rash in which blood cells leak into the skin or mucous membranes, usually at multiple sites. Purpuric rashes often are associated with disorders of coagulation or thrombosis. Pinpoint purpuric lesions are called petechiae; larger hemorrhages into the skin are called ecchymoses. SEE: illus.

Purines in Food

Group A: High Concentration (150–1000 mg/100 g)	
Liver	Sardines (in oil)
Kidney	Meat extracts
Sweetbreads	Consommé
Brains	Gravies
Heart	Fish roes
Anchovies	Herring
Group B: Moderate Amounts (50–150 mg/100 g)	
Meat, game, and fish other than those mentioned in Group A	
Fowl	Asparagus
Lentils	Cauliflower
Whole-grain cereals	Mushrooms
Beans	Spinach
Peas	
Group C: Very Small Amounts: Need Not be Restricted in Diet of Persons with Gout	
Vegetables other than those mentioned above	
Fruits of all kinds	Coffee
Milk	Tea
Cheese	Chocolate
Eggs	Carbonated beverages
Refined cereals, spaghetti, macaroni	Tapioca
	Yeast
Butter, fats, nuts, peanut butter*	
Sugars and sweets	
Vegetable soups	

* Fats interfere with the urinary excretion of urates and thus should be limited if the objective is to promote excretion of uric acid.

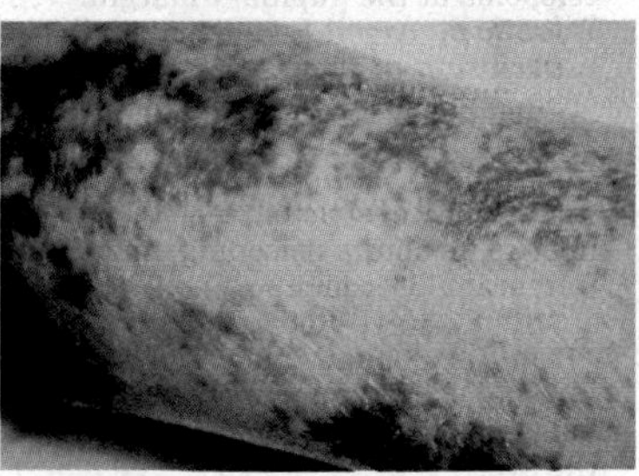

PURPURA

allergic p. Any of a group of purpuras caused by a variety of agents, including bacteria, drugs, and food. The immune complexes associated with type III hypersensitivity reaction damage the walls of small blood vessels, leading to bleeding. SYN: *nonthrombocytopenic p.*

anaphylactoid p. Henoch-Schönlein p.

p. annularis telangiectodes Majocchi's disease.

fibrinolytic p. Purpura resulting from excess fibrinolytic activity of the blood.

p. fulminans A rapidly progressing form of purpura occurring principally in children; of short duration and frequently fatal.

hemorrhagic p. Idiopathic thrombocytopenic p.

Henoch-Schönlein p. A form of small vessel vasculitis that affects children more commonly than adults. It is marked by abdominal pain, polyarticular joint disease, and purpuric lesions of the lower extremities. The illness usually lasts about 2 weeks before resolving spontaneously. In some instances, renal failure or gastrointestinal bleeding can complicate the course. SYN: *anaphylactoid p.* SEE: illus.

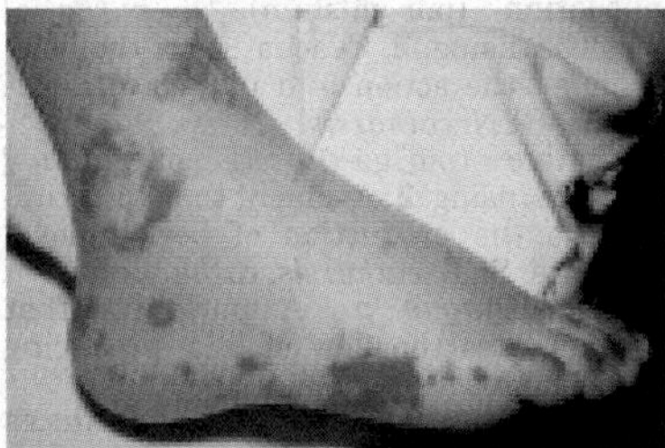

HENOCH–SCHÖNLEIN PURPURA

TREATMENT: Joint symptoms respond to rest and administration of nonsteroidal anti-inflammatory drugs. Corticosteroid drugs, such as prednisone, are used to treat patients with severe gastrointestinal or renal involvement.

idiopathic thrombocytopenic p. ABBR: ITP. Hemorrhagic autoimmune disease in which there is destruction of circulating platelets, caused by autoantibodies that bind with antigens on the platelet membrane. It occurs as a chronic disease in children and often follows a viral infection. Opsonization of platelets by autoantibodies stimulates their lysis by macrophages, esp. in the spleen. SYN: *thrombocytopenic p.; thrombopenic p.; Schönlein's disease.* SEE: illus.; *Nursing Diagnoses Appendix.*

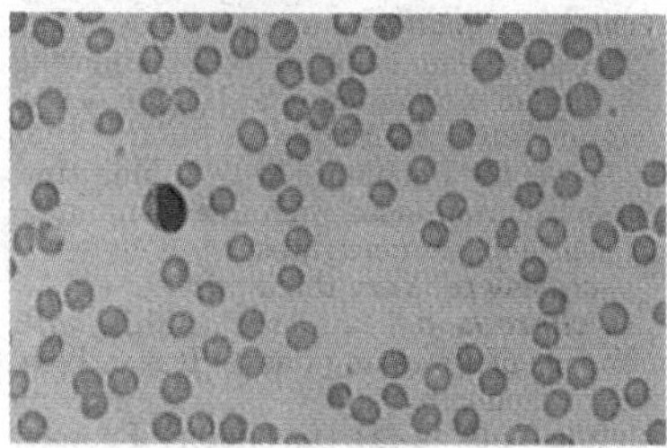

IDIOPATHIC THROMBOCYTOPENIC PURPURA

Virtual absence of platelets in peripheral blood (×400)

SYMPTOMS: Symptoms may include bleeding from the nose, the gums, or the gastrointestinal tract. Physical findings include petechiae, esp on the lower extremities, and ecchymoses. Laboratory findings: The platelet count is usually less than 100,000/mm³ and may be associated with mild anemia as a result of bleeding.

TREATMENT: If patients are aysmptomatic and the platelet count is about 40,000/mm³, treatment is unnecessary. Treatment regimens for symptomatic patients may include high-dose corticosteroids, intravenous immune globulin (IVIG), splenectomy, or chemotherapeutic drugs such as vincristine or cyclophosphamide.

PATIENT CARE: Platelet count is monitored daily. The patient is observed for bleeding (petechiae, ecchymoses, epistaxis, oral mucous membrane or G.I. bleeding, hematuria, menorrhagia) and stools, urine, and vomitus are tested for occult blood. The amount of bleeding or size of ecchymoses is measured at least every 24 hr. Any complications of ITP are monitored. The patient is educated about the disorder, prescribed treatments, and importance of reporting bleeding (such as epistaxis, gingival, urinary tract, or uterine or rectal bleeding) and signs of internal bleeding (such as tarry stools or coffee-ground vomitus). The patient should avoid straining during defecation or coughing because both can lead to increased intracranial pressure, possibly causing cerebral hemorrhage. Stool softeners are provided as necessary to prevent tearing of the rectal mucosa and bleeding due to passage of constipated or hard stools. The purpose, procedure, and expected sensations of each diagnostic test are explained. The role of platelets and the way in which the results of platelet counts can help to identify symptoms of abnormal bleeding are also explained. The lower the platelet count falls, the more precautions the patient will need to take; in severe thrombocytopenia, even minor bumps or scrapes can result in bleeding. The nurse guards against bleeding by taking the following precautions to protect the patient from trauma: keeping the side rails of the bed raised and padded, promoting use of a soft toothbrush or sponge-stick and an electric razor, and avoiding invasive procedures if possible. When venipuncture is unavoidable, pressure is exerted on the puncture site for at least 20 min or until the bleeding stops. During active bleeding, the patient maintains strict bedrest, with the head of the bed elevated to prevent gravity-related intracranial pressure increases, possibly leading to intracranial bleeding. All areas of petechiae and ecchymoses are protected from further injury. Rest periods are provided between activities if the patient tires easily. Both patient and family are encouraged to discuss their concerns about the disease and its treatment, and emotional support is provided and questions answered honestly. The nurse reassures the patient that areas of petechiae and ecchymoses will heal as the disease resolves. The patient should avoid taking aspirin in any form as well as any other drugs that impair coagulation including nonsteroidal anti-inflammatory drugs listed on the labels of nonprescription remedies. If the patient experiences frequent nosebleeds, the patient should use a humidifier at night and should moisten the inner nostrils twice a day with an anti-infective ointment. The nurse teaches the patient to monitor the condition by examining the skin for petechiae and ecchymoses and demonstrates the correct method to test stools for occult blood. If the patient is receiving corticosteroid therapy, fluid and electrolyte balance is monitored and the patient is assessed for signs of infection, pathological fractures, and mood changes. If the patient is receiving blood or blood components, they are administered according to protocol; vital signs are monitored before, during, and after the transfusion, and the patient is observed closely for adverse reactions. If the patient is receiving immunosuppressants, the patient is monitored closely for signs of bone marrow depression, opportunistic infections, mucositis, G.I. tract ulceration, and severe diarrhea or vomiting. If the patient is scheduled for a splenectomy, the nurse determines the patient's understanding of the procedure, corrects misinformation, administers prescribed blood transfusions, explains postoperative care and expected activities and sensations, ensures that a signed informed consent has been obtained, and prepares the patient physically (according to institutional or surgeon's protocol) and emotionally for the surgery. The patient with chronic ITP should wear or carry a medical identification device.

p. nervosa An obsolete term for Henoch-Schönlein p.

nonthrombocytopenic p. Allergic p.

p. rheumatica Purpura with joint pain, colic, bloody stools, and vomiting of blood.

senile p. Purpura occurring in debilitated and aged persons with ecchymoses and petechiae on the legs.

p. simplex Purpura that is not associated with systemic illness.

thrombocytopenic p. Idiopathic thrombocytopenic p.

thrombopenic p. Idiopathic thrombocytopenic p.

thrombotic thrombocytopenic p. ABBR: TTP. A rare life-threatening disease marked by widespread aggregation of platelets throughout the body, neurological dysfunction, and renal insufficiency. The disease is triggered by a deficiency of an enzyme that cleaves von Willebrand factor (a blood clotting protein). This deficiency results in blood clots in small blood vessels throughout the body. Shifting neurological signs such as aphasia, blindness, and convulsions are often present. SEE: *hemolytic uremic syndrome*.

ETIOLOGY: The disease has occurred in patients taking certain drugs (e.g., ticlopidine); in some patients with cancer or HIV-1 infection; and in some pregnant women.

TREATMENT: Plasmapheresis or infusions of fresh frozen plasma are effective in treating the disease.

purpureaglycosides A and B (pŭr-pū″rē-ă-glī′kō-sīds) True cardiac glycosides present in the leaves of *Digitalis purpurea*, foxglove.

purpuric (pŭr-pū′rĭk) [L. *purpura*, purple] Pert. to, resembling, or suffering from purpura.

purring thrill A vibration, like a cat's purring, due to mitral stenosis, aneurysm, or valvular disease of the heart; felt by palpation over the precordium.

purulence (pūr′ū-lĕns) [L. *purulentus*, full of pus] The state of containing pus. SEE: *pus*.

purulency (pūr′ū-lĕn″sē) Purulence.

purulent (pūr′ū-lĕnt) [L. *purulentus*, full of pus] Suppurative; forming or containing pus. SEE: *sputum*.

puruloid (pūr′ū-loyd) [L. *pus*, pus, + Gr. *eidos*, form, shape] Like pus. SYN: *puriform*.

pus (pŭs) [L.] Protein-rich fluid (exudate) containing white blood cells, esp. neutrophils, and cell debris produced during inflammation. It commonly is caused by infection with pyogenic (pus-forming) bacteria such as streptococci, staphylococci, gonococci, and pneumococci. Normally, pus is yellow; red pus may contain blood from the rupture of small vessels, and bluish-green pus may contain *Pseudomonas aeruginosa*. Pus that has been walled off by a membrane is called an abscess. SYN: *purulence; suppuration*. SEE: *abscess*.

blue p. Purulence with a blue tint; usually associated with infection due to *Pseudomonas aeruginosa*.

cheesy p. Very thick pus.

ichorous p. Pus that is thin with shreds of sloughing tissue. It may have a fetid odor.

pustula (pŭs′tū-lă) [L., blister] Pustule.

pustulant (pŭs′tū-lănt) [L. *pustula*, blister] **1.** Causing pustules. **2.** An agent that produces the formation of pustules.

pustular (pŭs′tū-lĕr) Pert. to, or characterized by, pustules.

pustulation (pŭs″tū-lā′shŭn) The development of pustules.

pustule (pŭs′tūl) [L. *pustula*, blister] A small, elevated skin lesion filled with white blood cells and, sometimes, bacteria or the products of broken-down cells. Pustules are found in many common skin disorders, including acne vulgaris, some drug rashes, many viral exanthems (e.g., herpes simplex or varicella-zoster viruses), and pustular psoriasis.

pustulocrustaceous (pŭs″tū-lō-krŭs-tā′shŭs) [″ + *crusta*, shell] Characterized by formation of pustules and crusts.

pustulosis (pŭs″tū-lō′sĭs) [″ + Gr. *osis*, condition] A generalized eruption of pustules.

putamen (pū-tā′mĕn) [L., shell] The darker outer layer of the lenticular nucleus.

Putnam-Dana syndrome (pŭt′năm-dā′nă) [James J. Putnam, U.S. neurologist, 1846–1918; Charles L. Dana, U.S. neurologist, 1852–1935] Subacute combined degeneration of the spinal cord that may be present in patients with untreated pernicious anemia.

putrefaction (pū″trĕ-făk′shŭn) [L. *putrefactio*] Decomposition of animal matter, esp. protein associated with malodorous and poisonous products such as the ptomaines, mercaptans, and hydrogen sulfide, caused by certain kinds of bacteria and fungi. Decomposition occurring spontaneously in sterile tissue after death is called autolysis. SEE: *sepsis.*

intestinal p. The chemical changes by bacteria in the intestine, forming indole, skatole, paracresol, phenol, phenylpropionic acid, phenylacetic acid, paraoxyphenylacetic acid, hydroparacumaric acid, fatty acids, carbon dioxide, hydrogen, methane, methylmercaptan, and sulfurated hydrogen.

putrefactive (pū″trĕ-făk′tĭv) [L. *putrefacere,* to putrefy] **1.** Causing, or pert. to, putrefaction. **2.** Agent promoting putrefaction.

putrefy (pū′trĕ-fī) [L. *putrefacere,* to putrefy] To undergo putrefaction.

putrescence (pū-trĕs′ĕns) [L. *putrescens,* grow rotten] Decay; rottenness.

putrescine (pū-trĕs′ĭn) A poisonous polyamine formed by bacterial action on the amino acid arginine.

putrid (pū′trĭd) [L. *putridus*] Decayed; rotten; foul.

PUVA therapy [*p*soralen + *u*ltra*v*iolet *A*] The treatment of skin conditions (e.g., psoriasis or cutaneous T-cell lymphoma) with a photosensitizing drug, psoralens, and gradually increasing doses of long-wave ultraviolet light. SEE: *psoralen; psoriasis.*

PVC *polyvinyl chloride; premature ventricular contraction.*

P$\bar{v}$O$_2$ Symbol for partial pressure of oxygen in mixed venous blood.

PVP *polyvinylpyrrolidone.*

PVP-iodine *povidone-iodine.*

PWA *person with AIDS.*

PWB *partial weight bearing.*

pyarthrosis (pī″ăr-thrō′sĭs) [Gr. *pyon,* pus, + *arthron,* joint, + *osis,* condition] Pus in the cavity of a joint.

pycno-, pycn- (pĭk′nō) [Gr. *pyknos,* thick] Combining form meaning *dense, thick, compact, frequent.* SEE: also *pykno-.*

pyecchysis (pī-ĕk′ĭ-sĭs) [Gr. *pyon,* pus, + *ek,* out, + *chein,* to pour] An effusion of pus.

pyelectasia, pyelectasis (pī″ĕ-lĕk-tā′zē-ă, -lĕk′tăs-ĭs) [Gr. *pyelos,* pelvis, + *ektasis,* dilatation] Dilatation of the renal pelvis.

pyelitis (pī″ĕ-lī′tĭs) [Gr. *pyelos,* pelvis, + *itis,* inflammation] Inflammation of the pelvis of the kidney and its calices. **pyelitic,** *adj.*

calculous p. Pyelitis resulting from a kidney stone.

p. cystica Pyelitis associated with multiple small cysts in the mucosa of the renal pelvis.

pyelo- [Gr. *pyelos,* pelvis] Combining form meaning *pelvis.*

pyelocaliectasis (pī″ĕ-lō-kăl″ē-ĕk′tă-sĭs) [″ + *kalyx,* cup, + *ektasis,* dilation] Dilation of the pelvis and calices of the kidney.

pyelocystitis (pī″ĕ-lō-sĭs-tī′tĭs) [″ + *kystis,* bladder, + *itis,* inflammation] Inflammation of the renal pelvis and bladder.

pyelocystostomosis (pī″ĕ-lō-sĭs″tō-stō-mō′sĭs) [″ + ″ + *stoma,* mouth, + *osis,* condition] The surgical establishment of communication between the kidney and bladder.

pyelogram (pī′ĕ-lō-grăm) [Gr. *pyelos,* pelvis, + *gramma,* something written] A radiograph of the ureter and renal pelvis.

intravenous p. ABBR: I.V.P. A pyelogram in which a radiopaque material is given intravenously. Multiple radiographs of the urinary tract taken while the material is excreted provide important information about the structure and function of the kidney, ureter, and bladder. This examination may be used to detect kidney stones and other lesions that may block or irritate the urinary tract.

pyelography (pī″ĕ-lŏg′ră-fē) [″ + *graphein,* to write] Radiography of the renal pelvis and ureter after injection of a radiopaque contrast medium.

pyelolithotomy (pī″ĕ-lō-lĭth-ŏt′ō-mē) [″ + *lithos,* stone, + *tome,* incision] The removal of a stone from the pelvis of a kidney through an incision.

pyelonephritis (pī″ĕ-lō-nĕ-frī′tĭs) [″ + *nephros,* kidney, + *itis,* inflammation] Inflammation of the kidney and renal pelvis, usually as a result of a bacterial infection that has ascended from the urinary bladder. SEE: *Nursing Diagnoses Appendix.*

ETIOLOGY: *Escherichia coli* is the responsible microbe in most cases. Cultures of urine and blood are obtained to guide therapy.

SYMPTOMS: This condition is characterized by the sudden onset of chills and fever with dull pain in the flank over either or both kidneys. There is tenderness when the kidney is palpated. Usually there are signs of cystitis (i.e., pyuria, urgency with burning, and frequency of urination).

TREATMENT: Antibiotics (e.g., fluoroquinolones, sulfa drugs, cephalosporins, or aminoglycosides) that effectively treat common urinary tract pathogens are administered, pending the results of cultures. Antiemetics are given to control nausea and vomiting. If patients are unable to take medications by mouth or if they have predisposing conditions (e.g., pregnancy or diabetes) that increase the likelihood of a bad outcome, they may be admitted to the hospital for observation, monitoring, and hydration.

PROGNOSIS: The outcome depends on the character and virulence of the infection, accessory etiological factors, drainage of the kidney, presence or absence of complications, and general physical condition of the patient.

PATIENT CARE: Antibiotics and antipyretics are administered as prescribed. The patient is encouraged to complete the full course of antibiotics and drink 2 to 3 L of fluids per day to prevent urinary stasis and to flush byproducts of the inflammatory process. After the completion of therapy, the patient should report any signs of infection during scheduled follow-up care.

pyelonephrosis (pī″ĕ-lō-nĕ-frō′sĭs) [″ + ″ + *osis,* condition] Any disease of the pelvis of the kidney. SYN: *pyelopathy.*

pyelopathy (pī″ĕ-lŏp′ăth-ē) [″ + *pathos,* disease, suffering] Pyelonephrosis.

pyeloplasty (pī′ĕ-lō-plăs″tē) [″ + *plastos,* formed] Reparative surgery on the pelvis of the kidney.

pyeloplication (pī″ĕ-lō-plĭ-kā′shŭn) [″ + L. *plicare,* to fold] Shortening of the wall of a dilated renal pelvis by taking tucks in it.

pyelostomy (pī″ĕ-lŏs′tō-mē) [″ + *stoma,* mouth] Creation of an opening into the renal pelvis.

pyelotomy (pī″ĕ-lŏt′ō-mē) [″ + *tome,* incision] Incision of the renal pelvis.

PATIENT CARE: All catheters should be secured to the patient to prevent dislodgement. The nurse should assess and record the appearance of the urine, including color, consistency, and amount. Catheter drainage tubing must be kept free of kinks. Catheters should never be clamped. The nurse should monitor and record intake and output. After removal of the catheter, a stoma-bag collection device should be used to collect any drainage and maintain skin integrity while the wound heals.

pyeloureterectasis Dilatation of the pelvis of the kidney and ureter.

pyemia (pī-ē′mē-ă) [″ + *haima,* blood] A form of septicemia due to the presence of pus-forming organisms in the blood, manifested by formation of multiple abscesses of a metastatic nature.

SYMPTOMS: The disease is characterized by intermittent high temperature with recurrent chills; metastatic processes in various parts of the body, esp. in lungs; septic pneumonia; empyema. It may be fatal.

TREATMENT: Antibiotics are effective. Prophylactic treatment consists in prevention of suppuration.

arterial p. Pyemia resulting from dissemination of emboli from a thrombus in cardiac vessels.

cryptogenic p. Pyemia of an origin that is hidden in the deeper tissues.

metastatic p. Multiple abscesses resulting from infected pyemic thrombi.

portal p. Suppurative inflammation of the portal vein.

pyemic (pī-ē′mĭk) [Gr. *pyon,* pus, + *haima,* blood] Relating to, or affected with, septicemia.

Pyemotes (pī-ĕ-mō′tēz) A genus of mites parasitic on the larvae of insects.

P. ventricosus A mite present in the straw of some cereals, contact with which causes a vesiculopapular dermatitis in humans. This is called grain itch.

pyencephalus (pī″ĕn-sĕf′ă-lŭs) [″ + *enkephalos,* brain] A brain abscess with suppuration within the cranium. SYN: *pyocephalus.*

pyg- SEE: *pygo-.*

pygal (pī′găl) [Gr. *pyge,* rump] Concerning the buttocks. SEE: *steatopygia.*

pygalgia (pī-găl′jē-ă) [″ + *algos,* pain] Pain in the buttocks.

pygmalionism (pĭg-mā′lē-ŏn-ĭzm) [named for Pygmalion, a sculptor and king in Gr. mythology, who fell in love with a figure he carved] The psychopathic condition of falling in love with one's own creation.

pygmy (pĭg′mē) A very small person, a dwarf.

pygo-, pyg- Combining form meaning *buttocks.*

pygoamorphus (pī″gō-ă-mor′fŭs) [Gr. *pyge,* rump, + *a-,* not, + *morphe,* form] Conjoined twins in which the parasite, joined to the buttocks, is an amorphous mass of tissue, or a teratoma.

pygodidymus (pī″gō-dĭd′ĭ-mŭs) [″ + *didymos,* twin] Conjoined twins with fusion of the cephalothoracic area, but with doubling of the pelvis and extremities.

pygomelus (pī-gŏm′ĕ-lŭs) [″ + *melos,* limb] Unequal conjoined twins with the parasite represented by an accessory limb attached to the pelvic area.

pykn- SEE: *pykno-.*

pyknic (pĭk′nĭk) [Gr. *pyknos,* thick] Pert. to a body type characterized by roundness of the extremities, stockiness, large chest and abdomen, and tendency to obesity.

pykno-, pykn- [Gr. *pyknos,* thick] Combining form meaning *thick, compact, dense, frequent.* SEE: also *pycno-.*

pyknocyte (pĭk′nō-sīt) [″ + *kytos,* cell] A form of spiculed red cell. SEE: *spiculed red cell.*

pyknodysostosis (pĭk″nō-dĭs″ŏs-tō′sĭs) [″ + *dys,* bad, + *osteon,* bone, + *osis,* condition] An autosomal recessive disease that affects bones and resembles osteopetrosis, but the disease is mild and not associated with hematological or neurological abnormalities. Affected children have short stature, open fontanels, frontal bossing, hypoplastic facial bones, blue sclerae, and dental abnormalities. There may be double rows of malformed teeth. Despite the multiple abnormalities, life span is unaffected. The patient usually seeks medical care because of frequent fractures. The only treatment is surgical correction of deformities and fractures.

pyknomorphous (pĭk″nō-morf′ŭs) [″ + *morphe,* form] Characterized by compact arrangement of the stainable portions, said esp. of certain nerve cells.

pyknophrasia (pĭk″nō-frā′zē-ă) [″ + *phrasis,* speech] Thickness of words uttered in speech.

pyknosis (pĭk-nō′sĭs) [″ + *osis,* condition] Thickness, esp. shrinking of cells through degeneration. SYN: *inspissation.*

pyle- [Gr. *pyle,* gate] Combining form meaning *orifice,* esp. that of the portal vein.

pylemphraxis (pī″lĕm-frăk′sĭs) [″ + *emphraxis,* stoppage] Occlusion of the portal vein.

pylephlebectasia, pylephlebectasis (pī″lē-flē-bĕk-tā′zē-ă, -bĕk′tă-sĭs) [″ + *phleps,* vein, + *ektasis,* dilatation] Distention of the portal vein.

pylephlebitis (pī″lē-flē-bī′tĭs) [″ + ″ + *itis,* inflammation] Inflammation of the portal vein, generally suppurative.

adhesive p. Thrombosis of the portal vein.

p. obturans Pylephlebitis with obstructed flow in the portal vein.

pylethrombophlebitis (pī″lē-thrŏm″bō-flē-bī′tĭs) [″ + *thrombos,* clot, + *phleps,* vein, + *itis,* inflammation] Thrombosis and inflammation of the portal vein.

pylethrombosis (pī″lē-thrŏm-bō′sĭs) [Gr. *pyle,* gate, + *thrombos,* clot, + *osis,* condition] Occlusion of the portal vein by a thrombus.

pylon (pī′lŏn) A temporary artificial leg.

pylorectomy (pī″lō-rĕk′tō-mē) [″ + *ektome,* excision] Surgical removal of the pylorus.

pyloric (pī-lor′ĭk) [Gr. *pyloros,* gatekeeper] Pert. to the distal portion of the stomach or to the opening between the stomach and duodenum.

pyloric canal The narrow constricted region of the pyloric portion of the stomach that opens through the pylorus into the duodenum.

pyloric cap An outdated term for the duodenal bulb.

pyloric obstruction and dilatation Blockage of the lower orifice of the stomach with consequent hypertrophy and dilatation. Pyloric obstruction increases the resistance offered to the expulsion of food from the stomach. The causes of dilatation are pyloric obstruction, laxness of walls from simple atony, or excessive ingestion of food or drink.

SYMPTOMS: The typical findings are dyspepsia, vomiting (occasionally projectile vomiting), wasting, and dehydration. Vomiting may occur long after eating, sometimes several hours or days. Constipation is present. There is bulging over the epigastrium. In thin subjects, the outline of the stomach may be visible. Palpation gives a splashing fremitus. In percussion there is an increased area of gastric tympany. In auscultation, splashing sounds often are audible at some distance.

TREATMENT: In acute obstruction, treatment includes nasogastric decompression of the stomach with parenteral fluid administration and gradual resumption of oral feeding. In chronic obstruction (congenital, neoplastic, inflammatory), surgery is indicated.

PROGNOSIS: Outcome relates to cause and promptness of treatment. It is generally favorable in cases of acute dilatation without obstruction.

pyloric sphincter The thickened circular smooth muscle around the pyloric orifice at the junction of the stomach and duodenum. The sphincter is usually contracted but relaxes at intervals (when gastric pressure exceeds duodenal pressure) to permit acid chyme to enter the duodenum. It then contracts to prevent backup of chyme to the stomach.

pyloric stenosis Narrowing of the pyloric orifice. In children, excessive thickening of the pyloric sphincter or hypertrophy and hyperplasia of the mucosa and submucosa of the pylorus typically are responsible. In adults, obstruction of the pylorus typically results from peptic ulcer disease, malignant compression of the gastric outlet, or pneumatosis intestinalis.

TREATMENT: In infants, treatment may involve open or laparoscopic division of the muscles of the pylorus. In adults, endoscopic stents may be placed to open malignant obstructions.

pyloristenosis (pī-lor″ĭ-stĕn-ō′sĭs) [Gr. *pyloros,* gatekeeper, + *stenos,* narrow] SEE: *pyloric stenosis.*

pyloritis (pī″lō-rī′tĭs) [″ + *itis,* inflammation] Inflammation of the pylorus.

pyloro- Combining form meaning *gatekeeper,* applied to the pylorus.

pylorodiosis (pī-lō″rō-dī-ō′sĭs) [Gr. *pyloros,* gatekeeper, + *diosis,* pushing under] Dilation of the pylorus of the stomach.

pyloroduodenitis (pī-lor″ō-dū″ō-dē-nī′tĭs) [″ + L. *duodeni,* twelve, + Gr. *itis,* inflammation] Inflammation of the mucosa of the pyloric outlet of the stomach and duodenum.

pylorogastrectomy (pī-lor″ō-găs-trĕk′tō-mē) [″ + *gaster,* belly, + *ektome,* excision] Excision of the pyloric portion of the stomach.

pyloromyotomy (pī-lor″ō-mī-ŏt′ō-mē) [″ + *mys,* muscle, + *tome,* incision] Incision (and suture) of the pyloric sphincter.

pyloroplasty (pī-lor′ō-plăs″tē) [″ + *plassein,* to form] Operation to repair the pylorus, esp. one to increase the caliber of the pyloric opening by stretching.

Finney p. Surgical procedure for enlarging the opening from the stomach to the duodenum.

pyloroscopy (pī-lō-rŏs′kō-pē) [Gr. *pyloros,* gatekeeper, + *skopein,* to examine] Fluoroscopic examination of the pylorus.

pylorospasm (pī-lor′ō-spăzm) [″ + *spasmos,* a convulsion] Spasmodic contraction of the pyloric orifice. The usual cause is a disturbance in the motor innervation of the pyloric sphincter. It may occur secondary to lesions of the stomach or duodenum near the pyloric orifice.

pylorostenosis (pī-lor″ō-stĕn-ō′sĭs) [″ + *stenos,* narrow] Abnormal narrowing or stricture of the pyloric orifice. SEE: *pyloric stenosis.*

pylorotomy (pī-lor-ŏt′ō-mē) [″ + *tome,* incision] Incision of the pylorus through its muscular layers to the level of the submucosa to relieve hypertrophic stenosis.

pylorus (pī-lor′ŭs) [Gr. *pyloros,* gatekeeper] **1.** The lower portion of the stomach that opens into the duodenum, consisting of the pyloric antrum and pyloric canal. **2.** In older texts, a term that may be used for the pyloric orifice or the pyloric sphincter. **pyloric,** *adj.*

pyo-, py- [Gr. *pyon,* pus] Combining form meaning *pus.*

pyocele (pī′ō-sēl) [Gr. *pyon,* pus, + *kele,* tumor, swelling] A hernia or distended cavity containing pus.

pyocephalus (pī″ō-sĕf′ă-lŭs) [″ + *kephale,* head] Effusion of purulent nature within the cranium.

pyococcus (pī″ō-kŏk′ŭs) [″ + *kokkos,* berry] A micrococcus that causes pus formation, such as *Staphylococcus aureus.*

pyocolpocele (pī″ō-kŏl′pō-sēl) [″ + *kolpos,* vagina, + *kele,* tumor, swelling] A vaginal tumor containing pus. SEE: *pyocolpos.*

pyocolpos (pī″ō-kŏl′pōs) Accumulation of pus in the vagina.

pyocyanic (pī″ō-sī-ăn′ĭk) [″ + *kyanos,* dark blue] Pert. to pyocyanin or blue pus.

pyocyst (pī′ō-sĭst) [″ + *kystis,* sac] A cyst containing pus.

pyoderma (pī-ō-dĕr′mă) [″ + *derma,* skin] Any acute, inflammatory, purulent bacterial dermatitis.

p. gangrenosum Pyoderma usually associated with ulcerative colitis or any severe chronic disease that leads to wasting; occurs principally on the trunk.

pyodermatitis (pī″ō-dĕr″mă-tī′tĭs) [″ + ″ + *itis,* inflammation] Pyogenic infection of the skin causing a dermatitis.

pyodermia (pī″ō-dĕr′mē-ă) Any suppurative skin disease.

pyogenesis (pī″ō-jĕn′ĕ-sĭs) [″ + *genesis,* generation, birth] The formation of pus. SEE: *pus.*

pyogenic (pī-ō-jĕn′ĭk) [″ + *gennan,* to produce] Producing pus.

pyogenic microorganism A microorganism that forms pus. The principal ones are *Staphylococcus aureus, Staphylococcus epidermidis, Streptococcus hemolyticus, Bacillus anthracis, Bacillus subtilis, Clostridium perfringens, Pseudomonas aeruginosa,* and *Neisseria gonorrhoeae.* These pathogens stimulate a huge influx of neutrophils to the site. The pus is formed from dead organisms, white blood cells, and other cells destroyed during the immune response.

pyohemothorax (pī″ō-hē″mō-thō′răks) [″ + *haima,* blood, + *thorax,* chest] Pus and blood in the pleural cavity.

pyoid (pī′oyd) [″ + *eidos,* form, shape] Resembling pus.

pyolabyrinthitis (pī″ō-lăb″ĭ-rĭn-thī′tĭs) [″ + *labyrinthos,* maze, + *itis,* inflammation] Inflammation with suppuration of the labyrinth of the ear.

pyometra (pī″ō-mē′tră) [″ + *metra,* uterus] Retained pus accumulation in the uterine cavity.

pyometritis (pī″ō-mē-trī′tĭs) [″ + ″ + *itis,* inflammation] Inflammation of the uterus with purulent exudate.

pyonephritis (pī″ō-nĕf-rī′tĭs) [″ + *nephros,* kidney, + *itis,* inflammation] Inflammation of the kidney, suppurative in character.

pyonephrolithiasis (pī″ō-nĕf″rō-lĭth-ī′ă-sĭs) [″ + ″ + *lithos,* stone, + *-iasis,* condition] Pus and stones in the kidney.

pyonephrosis (pī″ō-nĕf-rō′sĭs) [″ + ″ + *osis,* condition] Pus accumulation in the pelvis of the kidney.

pyoovarium (pī″ō-ō-vā′rē-ŭm) [″ + LL. *ovarium,* ovary] Abscess formation in an ovary.

pyopericarditis (pī″ō-pĕr″ĭ-kăr-dī′tĭs) [″ + *peri,* around, + *kardia,* heart, + *itis,* inflammation] Pericarditis with suppuration.

pyopericardium (pī″ō-pĕr″ĭ-kăr′dē-ŭm) Pus formation in the pericardium.

pyoperitoneum (pī″ō-pĕr″ĭ-tō-nē′ŭm) [Gr. *pyon,* pus, + *peritonaion,* peritoneum] Pus formation in the peritoneal cavity.

pyoperitonitis (pī″ō-pĕr″ĭ-tō-nī′tĭs) [″ + ″ + *itis,* inflammation] Purulent inflammation of the lining of peritoneum.

pyophthalmia (pī″ŏf-thăl′mē-ă) [″ + *ophthalmos,* eye] Pyophthalmitis.

pyophthalmitis (pī″ŏf-thăl-mī′tĭs) [″ + ″ + *itis,* inflammation] Suppurative inflammation of the eye. SYN: *pyophthalmia.*

pyophysometra (pī″ō-fī″sō-mē′tră) [″ + *physa,* air, + *metra,* uterus] Pus and gas accumulation in the uterus.

pyopneumocholecystitis (pī″ō-nū″mō-kō-lē-sĭs-tī′tĭs) [″ + *pneuma,* air, + *chole,* bile, + *kystis,* sac, + *itis,* inflammation] Distention of the gallbladder with air and pus.

pyopneumocyst (pī″ō-nū′mō-sĭst) [″ + ″ + *kystis,* bladder] A cyst enclosing pus and gas.

pyopneumohepatitis (pī″ō-nū″mō-hĕp″ă-tī′tĭs) [″ + *pneuma,* air, + *hepar,* liver, + *itis,* inflammation] A liver abscess with gas in the abscess cavity.

pyopneumopericardium (pī″ō-nū″mō-pĕr″ĭ-kăr′dē-ŭm) [″ + ″ + *peri,* around, + *kardia,* heart] Pus and air or gas in the pericardium.

pyopneumoperitoneum (pī″ō-nū″mō-pĕr″ĭ-tō-nē′ŭm) [″ + ″ + *peritonaion,* peritoneum] Peritonitis with gas and pus in the peritoneal cavity.

pyopneumoperitonitis (pī″ō-nū″mō-pĕr″ĭ-tō-nī′tĭs) [″ + ″ + ″ + *itis,* inflammation] Pus and air in the peritoneal cavity complicating peritonitis.

pyopneumothorax (pī″ō-nū″mō-thō′răks) [″ + ″ + *thorax,* chest] The presence of pus and gas in the pleural cavity.

pyoptysis (pī-ŏp′tĭ-sĭs) [″ + *ptysis,* spitting] Spitting of pus.

pyopyelectasis (pī″ō-pī″ĕ-lĕk′tă-sĭs) [″ + *pyelos,* pelvis, + *ektasis,* dilation] Purulent fluid in the dilated renal pelvis.

pyorrhea (pī″ō-rē′ă) [″ + *rhoia,* flow] A discharge of purulent matter.

pyosalpingitis (pī″ō-săl″pĭn-jī′tĭs) [Gr. *pyon,* pus, + *salpinx,* tube, + *itis,* inflammation] Retained pus in the oviduct with inflammation.

pyosalpingo-oophoritis (pī″ō-săl-pĭn″gō-ō″ŏf-ō-rī′tĭs) [″ + ″ + *oon,* ovum, + *phoros,* a bearer, + *itis,* inflammation] Inflammation of the ovary and oviduct, with suppuration.

pyosalpinx (pī″ō-săl′pĭnks) Pus in the fallopian tube.

pyosemia (pī″ō-sē′mē-ă) [Gr. *pyon,* pus, + L. *semen,* seed] Pus in the semen.

pyostatic (pī″ō-stăt′ĭk) [″ + *statikos,* standing] **1.** Preventing pus formation. **2.** An agent preventing the development of pus.

pyothorax (pī″ō-thō′răks) [″ + *thorax,* chest] Empyema.

pyotorrhea (pī″ō-tō-rē′ă) [″ + *ous,* ear, + *rhoia,* flow] Purulent discharge from the ear.

pyourachus (pī″ō-ū′ră-kŭs) [″ + *ourachos,* fetal urinary canal] Accumulation of pus in the urachus.

pyoureter (pī″ō-ū-rē′tĕr) [″ + *oureter,* ureter] Pus collection in the ureter.

pyovesiculosis (pī″ō-vĕ-sĭk″ū-lō′sĭs) [″ + L. *vesiculus,* a small vessel, + Gr. *osis,* condition] Pus collection in the seminal vesicles.

pyoxanthin(e) (pī″ō-zăn′thĭn) [″ + *xanthos,* yellow] A yellow pigment resulting from oxidation of pyocyanin, sometimes present in pus.

pyramid (pĭr′ă-mĭd) [Gr. *pyramis,* a pyramid] **1.** A solid on the base with three or more triangular sides that meet at an apex. **2.** Any part of the body resembling a pyramid. **3.** A compact bundle of nerve fibers in the medulla oblongata. **4.** The petrous portion of the temporal bone.

p. of the cerebellum A median ventral projection of the vermis of the cerebellum lying between the tuber and uvula.

p. of light The triangular light reflex from the typanic membrane of the ear.

malpighian p. Renal p.

p. of the medulla One of a pair of elongated tapering prominences on the anterior surface of the medulla oblongata, composed of descending corticospinal fibers.

renal p. One of a number of cone-shaped structures making up the medulla of the kidney along with renal columns. Each pyramid has its base adjacent to the renal cortex, with the apex projecting as a renal papilla into a calyx of the renal pelvis. Parts of the nephron found in a pyramid are the loops of Henle and collecting tubules; a papillary duct terminates at the apex and empties urine into the renal pelvis. The pyramids converge. SYN: *malpighian p.*

p. of the temporal bone The pyramis or petrous portion of the temporal bone.

p. of the thyroid A conical process sometimes present, extending cephalad from the isthmus of the thyroid gland.

p. of the tympanum A hollow projection on the inner wall of the middle ear through which passes the stapedius muscle.

pyramidal (pĭ-răm′ĭ-dăl) [L. *pyramidalis*] In the shape of a pyramid.

pyramidalis (pĭ-răm″ĭ-dăl′ĭs) [L.] The muscle that arises from the crest of the pubis and is inserted into the linea alba upward about halfway to the navel.

p. auriculae A small muscle inserted into the auricle of the ear. It is often absent.

pyramidotomy (pĭ-răm-ĭ-dŏt′ō-mē) [Gr. *pyramis,* a pyramid, + *tome,* incision] Excision of the pyramidal tracts of the spinal cord in order to alleviate involuntary muscular movements.

pyran (pī′răn) The compound C_5H_6O, the ring structure of which consists of five carbon atoms and one oxygen atom.

pyranose (pī′ră-nōs) A cyclic sugar or glycoside with a structure similar to a pyran.

pyrantel pamoate (pĭ-răn′tĕl) A drug used in treating the parasitic diseases ascariasis and enterobiasis, as well as those caused by *Ancylostoma, Necator americanus,* and *Trichostrongylus.*

pyrazinamide (pī″ră-zĭn′ă-mīd) A drug used in treating tuberculosis that is given typically with isoniazid, rifampin, or other agents.

pyrectic (pī-rĕk′tĭk) Concerning fever.

pyrenemia (pī″rĕ-nē′mē-ă) [Gr. *pyren,* fruit stone, + *haima,* blood] A condition in which there are nucleated red cells in the blood.

pyretherapy (pī″rĕ-thĕr′ă-pē) [Gr. *pyr,* fever, + *therapeia,* treatment] Treatment by artificially raising the patient's temperature.

pyrethrins (pī-rē′thrĭnz) The general name given to substances derived from pyrethrum flowers (chrysanthemums); used as insecticides.

pyretic (pī-rĕt′ĭk) [Gr. *pyretos,* fever] Concerning fever.

pyreto- (pī-rĕt′ō) Prefix indicating *fever.*

pyretogenesia, pyretogenesis (pī″rĕ-tō-jĕn-ē′zē-ă, -jĕn′ĕ-sĭs) [″ + *genesis,* generation, birth] Origin and production of fever.

pyretogenic bacteria Pathogenic bacteria causing fever.

pyretolysis (pī″rĕ-tŏl′ĭ-sĭs) [″ + *lysis,* dissolution] **1.** Reduction of fever. **2.** Lysis of symptoms of a disease process that is accelerated by fever.

pyretotyphosis (pī″rĕ-tō-tī-fō′sĭs) [″ + *typhosis,* delirium] The delirious or stuporous condition characteristic of high fever.

pyrexia (pī-rĕk′sē-ă) [Gr. *pyressein,* to be feverish] Fever.

pyrexin (pī′rĕks′ĭn) Pyrogen.

pyridine (pēr′ĭ-dēn) A colorless, volatile liquid with a charred odor. It is obtained by dry distillation of nitrogen-containing organic matter. It is used as an industrial solvent.

pyridostigmine bromide (pēr″ĭ-dō-stĭg′mēn) An anticholinesterase drug used in treating myasthenia gravis.

pyridoxal 5-phosphate A derivative of pyridoxine. It serves as a coenzyme of certain amino-acid decarboxylases in bacteria, and in animal tissues of 3,4-dihydroxyphenylalanine (dopa) decarboxylase.

pyridoxamine (pĭr″ĭ-dŏks′ă-mīn) One of the vitamin B_6 group; a 4-aminoethyl analog of pyridoxine.

4-pyridoxic acid (pĭr″ĭ-dŏks′ĭk) The principal end product of pyridoxine metabolism, excreted in human urine.

pyridoxine hydrochloride (pĭ-rĭ-dŏks′ēn) One of a group of substances, including pyridoxal and pyridoxamine, that make up vitamin B_6. SEE: vitamin B_6 in *Vitamins Appendix.*

pyriform (pĭr′ĭ-form) [L. *pirum,* pear, + *forma,* shape] Shaped like a pear. Also spelled piriform.

pyrimethamine (pĭr-ĭ-mĕth′ă-mēn) An antimalarial drug used in prophylaxis against malaria rather than in treatment of an acute attack. The drug is also used in the treatment of toxoplasmosis, an opportunistic infection of the central nervous system found in AIDS. Trade name is Daraprim.

pyrimidine (pĭ-rĭm′ĭd-ĭn) The parent of a group of heterocyclic nitrogen compounds, $C_4H_4N_2$. Cytosine and thymine are found in DNA; cytosine and uracil, in RNA.

pyrithiamine (pĭr″ĭ-thī′ă-mĭn) A synthetic analog of thiamine that acts as an antithiamine substance. When administered, it produces many of the symptoms of thiamine deficiency.

pyro- (pī′rō) [Gr. *pyr,* fire] Prefix meaning *heat, fire.*

pyrogallol (pī″rō-găl′ōl) $C_6H_6O_3$; a toxic chemical derived from gallic acid.

pyrogen (pī′rō-jĕn) [Gr. *pyr,* fire, + *gennan,* to produce] Any agent that causes fever. It may be exogenous, such as bacteria or viruses, or endogenous, produced in the body. The latter are usually in response to stimuli accompanying infection or inflammation. SYN: *pyrexin.*

CAUTION: A fluid that has been opened previously and allowed to stand should not be given intravenously, even though the top may have been closed tightly, because pyrogens will have formed within it.

leukocytic p. A substance found in the blood during a fever that acts upon the thermoregulatory centers of the hypothalamus.

pyrogenic (pī″rō-jĕn′ĭk) [Gr. *pyr,* fire, + *gennan,* to produce] Producing fever.

pyroglobulinemia (pī″rō-glŏb″ū-lĭ-nē′mē-ă) [″ + *globulus,* globule, + *haima,* blood] An obsolete term for *paraproteinemia.*

pyrolysis (pī-rŏl′ĭ-sĭs) [″ + *lysis,* dissolution] The decomposition of organic matter when there is a rise in temperature.

pyromania (pī″rō-mā′nē-ă) [″ + *mania,* madness] Fire madness; a mania for setting fires or seeing them.

pyrometer (pī-rŏm′ĕ-tĕr) [″ + *metron,* measure] A device for measuring a very high temperature.

pyronine (pī′rō-nĭn) A histological stain used to demonstrate the presence of RNA and DNA.

pyronyxis (pī″rō-nĭk′sĭs) [″ + *nyxis,* a piercing] Treatment or cauterization by puncturing a part with hot needles.

pyrophobia (pī″rō-fō′bē-ă) [″ + *phobos,* fear] Abnormal fear of fire.

pyrophosphatase (pī″rō-fŏs′fă-tās) An enzyme that catalyzes splitting of phosphoric groups.

pyrophosphate (pī″rō-fŏs′fāt) Any salt of phosphoric acid.

pyroptothymia (pī″rŏp-tō-thī′mē-ă) [″ + *ptoein,* to scare, + *thymos,* mind] A psychosis in which one imagines himself or herself surrounded by flames.

pyropuncture (pī″rō-pŭnk′chūr) [″ + L. *punctura,* piercing] A Treatment by puncture of a part with hot needles. SEE: *counterirritation.*

pyrosis (pī-rō′sĭs) [Gr. *pyrosis,* burning] Heartburn.

PATIENT CARE: The caregivers assess the meaning of this term to the patient and determines the exact location, timing, and duration of discomfort. If position changes exaggerate discomfort, precipitating factors (such as type and amount of food), method of relief, and factors that aggravate the discomfort are determined.

pyrotic (pī-rŏt′ĭk) [Gr. *pyrotikos*] **1.** Caustic; burning. **2.** Pert. to pyrosis.

pyrotoxin (pī″rō-tŏk′sĭn) [Gr. *pyr,* fire, + *toxikon,* poison] A toxin produced during a febrile disease.

pyrrobutamine phosphate (pĕr″rō-bū′tă-mēn) An antihistamine.

pyrrole (pĕr′ŏl) A heterocyclic substance that provides the building blocks for a large number of vital compounds such as hemoglobin, chlorophyll, and bile acids. It is a colorless liquid with the odor of chloroform.

pyrrolidine (pĭ-rŏl′ĭ-dĭn) Tetramethylamine, $(CH_2)_4NH$. It may be obtained from pyrrole or tobacco, which contains pyrrole.

pyruvate (pī′roo-vāt) A salt or ester of pyruvic acid.

pythogenesis (pī″thō-jĕn′ĕ-sĭs) [Gr. *pythein,* to rot, + *genesis,* generation, birth] Originating in decaying matter.

pyuria (pī-ū′rē-ă) [Gr. *pyon,* pus, + *ouron,* urine] Pus in the urine; evidence of renal disease; a condition in which there are more than the normal number of white blood cells in the urine. Freshly passed urine may be cloudy due to the presence of phosphates or pus. If the former are present, the addition of acid will cause it to clear; if the latter, it will not clear but may become gelatinous. The etiology includes lesions or infections of the urethra, ureters, bladder, or kidneys.

PZI *protamine zinc insulin.*

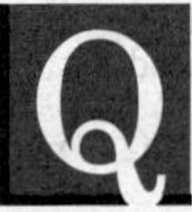

Q **1.** *quantity*. **2.** Symbol for coulomb.

q Symbol for long arm of a chromosome.

Q angle The acute angle formed by a line from the anterior superior iliac spine of the pelvis through the center of the patella and a line from the tibial tubercle through the patella. The angle describes the tracking of the patella in the trochlear groove of the femur. The normal angle is around 15 degrees. It is usually greater in females.

Q_{CO_2} The number of microliters of CO_2 given off per milligram of dry weight of tissue per hour.

q.d. L. *quaque die,* every day.

Q fever [Q is for *query* because its etiology was unknown] An acute infectious disease characterized by headache, fever, severe sweating, malaise, myalgia, and anorexia. Q fever is caused by rickettsia, *Coxiella burnetii,* an intracellular, gram-negative bacterium, and is contracted by inhaling infected dusts, drinking unpasteurized milk from infected animals, or handling infected animals such as goats, cows, or sheep. Transmission by human contact is rare but has occurred. An effective vaccine is available for the prevention of infection in persons who have a good chance of being exposed to the disease. Tetracyclines are used to treat the infection.

q.h. L. *quaque hora,* every hour.

q.l. L. *quantum libet,* as much as one pleases.

q.i.d. L. *quater in die,* four times a day.

qi gong, qigong (chē-gŏng) An ancient Chinese martial art used to develop flexibility, strength, relaxation, and mental concentration.

Q law As temperature decreases, chemical activity decreases.

Q_{O_2} The number of microliters of O_2 taken up per milligram of dry weight of tissue per hour.

q.q.h. L. *quaque quarta hora,* every four hours.

QRS complex The pattern traced on the surface electrocardiogram by depolarization of the ventricles. In the anterior chest leads (e.g., V_1 to V_3) the complex normally consists of a small initial downward deflection (Q wave), a large upward deflection (R wave), and a second downward deflection (S wave). The normal duration of the complex is 0.06 to 0.11 sec. Longer QRS complexes are seen in premature ventricular beats and ventricular arrhythmias.

QRST complex Q-T interval.

q.s. L. *quantum sufficit,* as much as suffices.

qt *quart.*

QTc In electrocardiography, the duration of the QT interval adjusted for the patient's heart rate. Prolonged QTc's are associated with an increased risk of ventricular dysrhythmia and sudden death.

Q-T interval, Q-T segment The representation on the electrocardiogram of ventricular depolarization and repolarization, beginning with the QRS complex and ending with the T wave.

Quaalude The former trade name and the street name for methaqualone hydrochloride, a euphoriant and sedative used as a drug of abuse. The proprietary drug is no longer distributed in the U.S.

quack (kwăk) [D. *kwaksalven,* to peddle salve] One who pretends to have knowledge or skill in medicine. SYN: *charlatan.*

quad Medical "shorthand" for quadriceps, quadrilateral, quadrant, quadriplegia.

quadrangular (kwŏd-răng′ū-lĕr) [L. *quadri,* four, + *angulus,* angle] Having four angles.

quadrangular lobe A region forming the superior portion of each cerebellar hemisphere.

quadrant (kwŏd′rănt) [L. *quadrans,* a fourth] **1.** One quarter or fourth of a circle. **2.** One of four corresponding regions, as of the abdomen, divided for descriptive and diagnostic purposes.

dental q. One quarter of the mouth. Each arch is divided in half so that one can easily describe the location of teeth or soft tissue observations. Quadrants are labeled as maxillary right and left or mandibular right and left and are shown in diagram form for dental records.

quadrantanopia (kwŏd″rănt-ă-nō′pē-ă) [″ + Gr. *an-,* not, + *opsis,* vision] Blindness or diminished visual acuity in one fourth of the visual field.

quadrantanopsia (kwŏd″rănt-ăn-ŏp′sē-ă) [″ + ″ + *opsis,* vision] Loss of sight in approx. one fourth of the visual field.

quadrate (kwŏd′rāt) [L. *quadratus,* squared] Square, or having four equal sides.

quadrate lobe A small lobe of liver located on the visceral surface and lying in contact with the pylorus and duodenum.

quadrate lobule The square lobule of the upper surface of the cerebellum.

quadri-, quadr- Combining form meaning *four.*
quadribasic (kwŏd″rĭ-bā′sĭk) [L. *quattuor,* four + basic] Having four replaceable atoms of hydrogen.
quadriceps (kwŏd′rĭ-sĕps) [″ + *caput,* head] Four-headed, as a quadriceps muscle.
quadriceps femoris A large muscle on the anterior surface of the thigh composed of the rectus femoris, vastus lateralis, vastus medialis, and vastus intermedius muscles. These muscles are inserted by a common tendon on the tuberosity of the tibia. The quadriceps femoris is an extensor of the leg.
quadricepsplasty (kwŏd″rĭ-sĕps′plăs-tē) [″ + ″ + Gr. *plassein,* to form] Plastic surgery to repair adhesions and scars around the quadriceps femoris muscle in order to restore function.
quadricuspid (kwŏd″rĭ-kŭs′pĭd) [″ + *cuspis,* point] Having four cusps, as a tooth.
quadridigitate (kwŏd″rĭ-dĭj′ĭ-tāt) Having only four fingers on a hand or four toes on a foot.
quadrigemina (kwŏd″rĭ-jĕm′ĭn-ă) [″ + *geminus,* twin] The corpora quadrigemina. SEE: *colliculus inferior; colliculus superior.*
quadrigeminal (kwŏd″rĭ-jĕm′ĭn-ăl) Fourfold; having four symmetrical parts; pert. to the corpora quadrigemina.
quadrigeminum (kwŏd″rĭ-jĕm′ĭ-nŭm) One of the four quadrigeminal bodies of the brain.
quadrigeminus (kwŏd″rĭ-jĕm′ĭ-nŭs) Composed of four parts.
quadrilateral (kwŏd″rĭ-lăt′ĕr-ăl) [″ + *latus,* side] Having four sides.
quadrilocular (kwŏd″rĭ-lŏk′ū-lăr) [″ + *loculus,* a small space] Having four chambers, cavities, or spaces.
quadripara (kwŏd-rĭp′ă-ră) [″ + *parere,* to bring forth, to bear] A woman who has had four pregnancies that have continued beyond the 20th week of gestation. SYN: *quartipara.* SEE: *para.*
quadripartite (kwŏd″rĭ-păr′tīt) [″ + *partire,* to divide] Divided into four parts.
quadriplegia (kwŏd″rĭ-plē′jē-ă) [″ + Gr. *plege,* stroke] Paralysis of all four extremities, usually caused by a lesion of the cervical spinal cord. Quadriplegia most often results from trauma to the neck, although it may occasionally result from spinal stenosis, infections, aneurysms, vasculitis, autoimmune diseases, neurosurgery, or mass lesions. The higher the injury, the less function will be present in the arms. Injury above the third cervical vertebra paralyzes the diaphragm; in patients with high cervical lesions, life can be sustained only with mechanical ventilation. SEE: *Nursing Diagnoses Appendix.*

EMERGENCY MEASURES: When a fracture of a cervical vertebra is suspected, the injured patient's head, neck, and torso should be stabilized during transportation.

TREATMENT: Immediately after an acute injury, potent corticosteroids may be given to limit swelling of the spinal cord.

PATIENT CARE: After an injury, the patient's neck is immobilized and in-line traction is maintained according to established procedures. A patent airway is established and maintained, and respiratory status is monitored for signs of insufficiency (hypoxemia, hypercapnia, and acidemia). Bowel sounds are assessed for development of paralytic ileus. Catheterization of the urinary bladder is necessary, and antithrombotic therapies are used to prevent deep venous thrombosis or pulmonary embolism. After the patient's condition has stabilized, physical therapy, occupational therapy, and respiratory care are critical to regaining or attaining optimal functioning. When the patient can be ambulatory, he or she should be monitored for evidence of orthostatic hypotension. Assistance is provided with self-care deficits, including skin and oral care, feeding and nutrition, elimination, respiratory toilet, positioning, and exercise. The patency of the urinary catheter is checked, and a bulk diet is provided to prevent impaction. Both patient and family are encouraged to verbalize their concerns, and support is offered to help them cope with their grief and loss. Assistance is provided to help the family set realistic plans for the future in view of the patient's functional abilities, body image, and self-concept. The patient is urged to participate in a rehabilitation program as soon as stabilized.

quadripolar (kwŏd″rĭ-pō′lăr) Pert. to a cell having four poles.
quadrisect (kwŏd′rĭ-sĕkt) [″ + *sectio,* a cutting] To divide into four parts.
quadrisection (kwŏd″rĭ-sĕk′shŭn) Dividing into four sections or parts.
quadritubercular (kwŏd″rĭ-tū-bĕr′kū-lĕr) [″ + *tuberculum,* a little swelling] Having four tubercles or cusps.
quadrivalent (kwŏd″rĭ-vā′lĕnt) [″ + *valens,* powerful] Having the ability to replace four atoms of hydrogen in a compound (i.e., a chemical valence of four).
quadruped (kwŏd′roo-pĕd″) [″ + *pes,* foot] **1.** A four-footed animal. **2.** Assuming a position with hands and feet on the floor.
quadrupedal reflex (kwŏd-roop′ĕd-ăl) Extension of the flexed arm on assuming a quadrupedal posture.
quadruplet (kwŏd′roo-plĕt, kwŏ-droo′plĕt) [L. *quadruplus,* fourfold]

One of four children born of the same mother in the same confinement. SEE: *Hellin's law*.

quail poisoning Acute myoglobinuria following ingestion of game birds of the species *Coturnix coturnix*. The cause is unknown but is suspected to be toxic rather than genetic (as was once believed).

quale (kwā'lē) [L. *qualis,* of what kind] The quality of anything, esp. of a sensation.

qualimeter (kwŏl-ĭm'ĕt-ĕr) [" + Gr. *metron,* measure] A device for measuring the quality of x-ray photons. SEE: *penetrometer*.

qualitative (kwŏl'ĭ-tā"tĭv) [L. *qualitativus*] Referring to the quality of anything. SEE: *quantitative*.

quality (kwŏl'ĭ-tē) [L. *qualitas,* quality] **1.** That which constitutes or characterizes a thing; the natural character. **2.** In radiology, the energy or penetrating power of the x-ray beam, which is controlled by kilovoltage peak.

quality-adjusted life-years ABBR: QALY. A measure of the health of a population that combines an assessment of both mortality and disability.

quality assurance Activities and programs designed to achieve desired levels of care.

quality of life The worth, meaning, or satisfaction obtained from living. The concept holds varying meanings for different people and may evolve over time. For some individuals it implies autonomy, empowerment, capability, and choice; for others, security, social integration, or freedom from stress or illness.

quanta (kwŏn'tă) [L.] Pl. of quantum.

quantimeter (kwŏn-tĭm'ĕt-ĕr) [L. *quantus,* how great, + Gr. *metron,* measure] A device for measuring the amount of x-ray photons given during an exposure.

quanti-Pirquet (kwŏn"tĭ-pēr-kā') [Clemens Peter Johann von Pirquet, Austrian pediatrician, 1874–1929] A quantitative cutaneous test of sensitivity to tuberculin by the use of graduated dilutions.

quantitative (kwŏn"tĭ-tā'tĭv) [LL. *quantitativus*] **1.** Concerning measurement **2.** Capable of being counted. SEE: *qualitative*.

quantity (kwŏn'tĭ-tē) [L. *quantitas,* quantity] Amount; portion.

quantivalence The number of hydrogen atoms with which an element or radical will combine.

quantum (kwŏn'tŭm) *pl.* **quanta** [L., how much] **1.** A definite amount. **2.** A unit of radiant energy.

quantum libet (kwŏn'tŭm lī'bĕt) [L.] ABBR: q.l. As much as desired.

quantum mottle A phenomena where an insufficient number of x-ray photons strike the radiographic image receptor during an exposure. This phenomenon causes a speckled or snowy appearing nonuniform intensity over the areas of similar densities on the film. In radiography it is corrected by increasing milliampere-seconds (mAS).

quantum sufficit (kwŏn'tŭm sŭf'fĭ-sĭt) [L.] ABBR: q.s. As much as suffices.

quarantine (kwor'ăn-tēn") [It. *quarantina,* 40 days] **1.** The period during which free entry to a country by humans, animals, plants, or agricultural products is prohibited, in order to limit the spread of potentially infectious diseases. **2.** The period of isolation from public contact after contracting a contagious disease, such as rabies. Complete quarantine is the limitation of the freedom of movement of healthy persons or domestic animals that have been exposed to a communicable disease for a period of time equal to the longest incubation period of the disease, in such a manner as to prevent effective contact with those not so exposed. SEE: *contagious; isolation; reportable disease*.

quart (kwort) [L. *quartus,* a fourth] ABBR: qt. A unit of fluid equal to one fourth of a gallon, or 2 pints, or 946 ml; in dry measure, one eighth of a peck.

quartan (kwor'tăn) [L. *quartana,* of the fourth] Occurring every fourth day. SEE: *malaria*.

quartile (kwor'tĭl) [L. *quartus,* a fourth] One of the two middle values of each half of a series of variables.

quartipara (kwor-tĭp'ă-ră) [" + *parere,* to bring forth, to bear] Quadripara.

quartz (kwărts) [Ger. *quarz*] Silicon dioxide, the principal ingredient of sandstone (crystallized silica; rock crystal). When crystal is clear and colorless, it permits the passage of large amounts of ultraviolet rays.

q. applicator A quartz rod containing various shapes and angles used to conduct, by total internal reflection, ultraviolet radiation from a water-cooled mercury arc quartz lamp.

q. glass Crystalline quartz used for prisms and lenses; fused quartz used for windows, through which ultraviolet radiations are freely transmitted.

Quatelet index Body mass index.

quater in die (kwŏ'tĕr ĭn dē'ă) [L.] ABBR: q.i.d. Four times a day.

quaternary (kwŏ-tĕr'nă-rē) [L. *quaternarius,* of four] **1.** The fourth in order. **2.** Composed of four elements.

Queckenstedt's sign (kwĕk'ĕn-stĕts) [Hans Queckenstedt, Ger. physician, 1876–1918] In vertebral canal block, the cerebrospinal fluid pressure is scarcely affected by compression of the veins of the neck, unilaterally or bilaterally. In healthy persons, the pressure rises rapidly on compression, then disappears when the compression is released.

quenching (kwĕnch'ĭng) **1.** Cooling something that is hot; or decreasing the radioactive energy released. **2.** The ability of any material to decrease the toxicity of a poison. **3.** In MRI, the emergency release of cooling cyrogens that maintain the necessary super-cooling condition of the primary magnet in order to turn off the magnetic field as a safety measure.

fluorescence q. A technique for investigating antigen-antibody reactions by measuring the light absorbed by an antigen mixed with a fluorescent-labeled antibody.

querulent (kwĕr'ū-lĕnt) [L. *querulus,* complaining] **1.** Complaining; fretful. **2.** One who is dissatisfied, complaining, and suspicious.

Quervain's disease (kār'vănz) [Fritz de Quervain, Swiss surgeon, 1868–1940] De Quervain's disease.

questionnaire A list of questions submitted to a patient or research subject in order to obtain data for analysis.

quick (kwĭk) [ME. *quicke,* alive] **1.** A part susceptible to keen feeling, esp. the part of a finger or toe to which the nail is attached. **2.** Pregnant and experiencing fetal movements.

quickening (kwĭk'ĕn-ĭng) A woman's initial awareness of the movement of the fetus within her womb (uterus). Most commonly, fetal activity is first reported between 18 and 20 weeks' gestation.

quicklime CaO; calcium oxide (unslaked lime). It forms calcium hydroxide when water is added to it.

Quick Neurological Screening Test ABBR: QNST. A standardized test of neurological function for persons 5 years of age or older. It assesses various areas, including attention, balance, motor planning, coordination, and spatial organization.

quicksilver [ME. *quicke,* alive, + *silver,* silver] The metal mercury.

Quick's test (kwĭks) [Armand James Quick, U.S. physician, 1894–1978] **1.** A liver function test that measures the amount of hippuric acid excreted after a dose of sodium benzoate is given. **2.** A test for the amount of prothrombin present in blood plasma. **3.** Quick Neurological Screening Test.

quiescent The condition of being inactive or at rest. SYN: *dormant; latent.*

quinacrine hydrochloride A drug used to treat protozoan infections, such as malaria or giardiasis.

Quincke's disease (kwĭnk'ēz) [Heinrich I. Quincke, Ger. physician, 1842–1922] Angioedema.

Quincke's pulse Visible inflow and outflow of blood from the nailbed, a physical finding in patients with aortic regurgitation when their fingernails or toenails are gently depressed by the examiner's finger.

Quincke's puncture Lumbar puncture to determine the pressure of the spinal fluid, or to remove some of the spinal fluid.

quinestrol (kwĭn-ĕs'trōl) An estrogen.

quinic acid $C_7H_{12}O_6$; a substance present in some plants, including cinchona bark, and berries.

quinidine sulfate (kwĭn'ĭ-dēn) An antiarrhythmic drug that can be used to control atrial fibrillation. Its use is associated with an increased risk, in some patients, of sudden death.

quinine (kwī'nīn", kwĭ-nēn') [Sp. *quina*] A bitter white crystalline alkaloid derived from cinchona bark and used as an antimalarial. It is usually administered in the form of its salts.

q. sulfate The sulfate of a cinchona alkaloid, used to treat nocturnal leg cramps and malaria. Controlled trials have not shown it to be effective for leg cramps.

quinine and urea hydrochloride The combination used, in dilute solutions, as a sclerosing agent for injection treatment of hemorrhoids and varicose veins.

quininism (kwī'nīn-ĭzm, kwĭ-nēn'ĭzm) Cinchonism.

quinolone Any of a class of antibiotics that inhibit bacterial DNA gyrase. Commonly prescribed agents include ciprofloxacin, levofloxacin, norfloxacin, and ofloxacin.

quinone (kwĭn'ōn) **1.** $C_6H_4O_2$; a yellow crystalline oxidation product of quinic acid. **2.** A class of organic compounds in which two atoms of hydrogen are replaced by two oxygen atoms.

quinqu- Combining form meaning *five.*

Quinquaud's disease (kăn-kōz') [Charles E. Quinquaud, Fr. physician, 1841–1894] Purulent inflammation of the hair follicles of the scalp, resulting in bald patches. SEE: *folliculitis.*

quinquetubercular (kwĭn"kwē-tū-bĕr'kū-lăr) [L. *quinque,* five] Having five cusps or tubercles.

quinquevalent (kwĭng"kwĕ-vā'lĕnt) Pert. to a radical or element with a valence of five.

quinquina (kwĭn-kwī'nă, kĭn-kē'nă) Cinchona.

quintan (kwĭn'tăn) [L. *quintanus,* of a fifth] **1.** Occurring every fifth day. **2.** Trench fever.

quinti- [L. *quintus,* fifth] Combining form meaning *fifth.*

quintipara (kwĭn-tĭp'ă-ră) [" + *parere,* to bear] A woman who has had five pregnancies that have continued beyond the 20th week of gestation. SEE: *para.*

quintuplet (kwĭn'tū-plĕt, kwĭn-tŭp'lĕt)

[LL. *quintuplex,* fivefold] One of five children born of one mother during the same confinement. SEE: *Hellin's law.*

quotidian (kwō-tĭd′ē-ăn) [L. *quotidianus,* daily] Occurring daily.

quotient (kwō′shĕnt) [L. *quotiens,* how many times] The number of times one number is contained in another.

achievement q. A percentile rating of a child's score on a test with respect to age, level of education, and peer performance.

intelligence q. ABBR: IQ. An index of relative intelligence determined through the subject's answers to arbitrarily chosen questions. The IQ test may not be an accurate indicator of an individual's skills or potential in creative, artistic, or motor skills areas. SEE: *intelligence; mental retardation; test, intelligence.*

respiratory q. **1.** The amount of energy derived from carbohydrate, rather than fat, metabolism. **2.** The result of dividing the amount of carbon dioxide exhaled per minute by the amount of oxygen consumed each minute, normally 0.9.

q.v. L. *quantum vis,* as much as you please; *quod vide,* which see.

R

R 1. *respiration; right; roentgen.* 2. In chemistry, a radical. 3. In the ideal gas equation, PV = nRT, R is the gas constant. Its value is 0.082 liter-atmospheres per degree per mole.

R– Abbr. used in organic chemistry to indicate part of a molecule.

R– Rinne negative. SEE: *Rinne test.*

+R+ Rinne positive. SEE: *Rinne test.*

℞ Symbol for L. *recipe,* take. SEE: *prescription.*

RA *rheumatoid arthritis; right atrium.*

Ra Symbol for the element radium.

rabbetting (răb′ĕt-ĭng) [Fr. *raboter,* to plane] Interlocking of the jagged edges of a fractured bone.

rabbit fever Tularemia.

rabbitpox An acute viral disease of laboratory rabbits.

rabiate (rā′bē-āt) [L. *rabies,* rage] Rabid.

rabic (răb′ĭk) Pert. to rabies.

rabicidal (răb-ĭ-sī′dăl) [L. *rabies,* rage, + *cidus,* kill] Destructive to the virus causing rabies.

rabid (răb′ĭd) Pert. to or affected with rabies. SYN: *rabiate.*

rabies (rā′bēez) [L. *rabere,* to rage] A fatal infection of the central nervous system caused by the rabies virus. Human infection occurs as the result of a bite from a wild animal in which the virus is present. Rarely, it may be transmitted by inhalation of infectious aerosol particles or contamination of conjunctiva or other mucous membranes by the saliva of an infected animal. The long incubation period, before signs of rabies appear, is 3 to 12 weeks; this means that wild animals that are displaying no signs of the disease may still be infected, thereby increasing the risk of human infection. SYN: *hydrophobia.* SEE: *immune globulin; rabies vaccine.*

ETIOLOGY: Rabies is found almost exclusively in wild animals (e.g., raccoons, skunks, coyotes, foxes, and bats), which serve as reservoirs for infection. Domestic animal infections have been rare in the U.S. since 1960, but dogs and cats in developing countries may be infected. After infection, the virus replicates in the animal for several days to months; this period stimulates an immune response to viral antigens. The virus then spreads through the cytoplasm of peripheral nerve axons to the central nervous system.

SYMPTOMS: Early symptoms in humans usually are nonspecific and include fever, malaise, and headache. Progressive signs of cerebral infection are those of encephalitis, including anxiety, confusion, insomnia, agitation, delirium, hallucinations, hypersalivation, hyperactive reflexes, and convulsions; periods of stupor alternate cyclically with episodes of extreme agitation. The classic symptom of hydrophobia (fear of water) is probably related to the painful contracture of the pharyngeal muscles that occurs during swallowing. Once clinical signs occur, the disease usually is fatal within days.

DIAGNOSIS: The diagnosis of rabies is made in animals by a direct fluorescent antibody test on brain tissue. In humans, brain biopsies, skin biopsies from the nape of the neck, corneal impression tests, and/or spinal fluid, blood, or salivary antibody tests are conducted.

PREVENTION: Veterinarians, animal handlers, and those who come in frequent contact with wild animals should receive preexposure prophylaxis with rabies vaccine. The vaccine does not prevent infection with rabies but simplifies treatment because it eliminates the need for immune globulin and decreases the amount of rabies vaccine required postexposure.

To decrease the spread of rabies, the Centers for Disease Control and Prevention recommends that all domestic animals be vaccinated routinely (consult local veterinarian and public health department) and that contact between pets and wild animals be minimized. Control of rabies in pets through vaccination and elimination of contact with stray animals significantly reduces the risk of human infection. Garbage containers should be designed to prevent attracting raccoons and skunks. Physical contact with raccoons, skunks, foxes, coyotes, and bats should be reported immediately. SEE: *Standard and Universal Precautions Appendix.*

TREATMENT: Physicians should contact the local or state health department to determine the need for postexposure prophylaxis. All wounds are vigorously cleaned. Intravenous immune globulin containing preformed antibodies and one dose of rabies vaccine are given immediately (day 1); an additional four doses of vaccine are administered on days 3, 7, 14, and 28. No cases of rabies have occurred when this protocol has been followed promptly after exposure. Most fatalities occur when people do not seek medical assistance because they are not aware of the possibility of rabies infection.

rabies immune globulin, human rabies immune globulin ABBR: RIG, HRIG. A standardized preparation of globulins derived from blood plasma or serum from selected human donors who have been immunized with rabies vaccine and have developed high titers of rabies antibody. It is used to produce passive immunity in persons bitten by animals. Trade name is Hyperab. SEE: *rabies.*

rabies virus group A genus of viruses whose official designation is *Lyssavirus.* The virus that causes human rabies is included in this group.

rabiform (rā'bĭ-form) [" + *forma,* shape] Resembling rabies.

raccoon sign [raccoons have distinctive periorbital coloration] Periorbital ecchymosis, which may be present in patients who have a basilar skull fracture.

race (rās) [Fr.] **1.** The descendants of a genetically cohesive ancestral group. **2.** A group of organisms identifiable within a species. **3.** A political or social designation for a group of people thought to share a common ancestry or common ethnicity. In contemporary societies, such designations have limited validity and value, although they are sometimes employed as a means of social, economic, or political discrimination.

racemase (rā'sē-mās) An enzyme that catalyzes racemization (i.e., the production of an optically active compound).

racemate (rā'sē-māt) A racemic compound.

racemic (rā-sē'mĭk) Optically active; used of compounds.

racemization (rā"sē-mī-zā'shŭn) The production of a racemic form of an optically active compound.

racemose (răs'ĕ-mōs) [L. *racemosus,* full of clusters] Resembling a clustered bunch of grapes, as a gland; divided and subdivided; ending in a bunch of follicles.

rachi-, rachio- [Gr. *rhachis,* spine] Combining form meaning *spine.*

rachial (rā'kē-ăl) [Gr. *rhachis,* spine] Spinal.

rachicele (rā'kĭ-sēl) [" + *kele,* tumor, swelling] Protrusion of the contents of the spinal canal in spina bifida cystica.

rachidial (ră-kĭd'ē-ăl) Spinal.

rachidian (ră-kĭd'ē-ăn) Pert. to the spinal column.

rachilysis (rā-kĭl'ĭ-sĭs) [" + *lysis,* dissolution] The mechanical treatment of lateral curvature of the spine through traction and pressure.

rachiometer (rā-kē-ŏm'ĕ-tĕr) [" + *metron,* measure] An instrument for measuring a spinal curvature.

rachiopagus (rā"kē-ŏp'ă-gŭs) [" + *pagos,* thing fixed] A conjoined twin deformity in which the two are joined at the vertebral column.

rachiotome (rā'kē-ō-tōm") [" + *tome,* incision] An instrument for dividing the vertebrae.

rachis (rā'kĭs) *pl.* **rachises** [Gr. *rhachis*] The spinal column.

rachischisis (ră-kĭs'kĭ-sĭs) [" + *schisis,* a splitting] A congenital spinal column fissure (e.g., spina bifida).

posterior r. Spina bifida.

rachitic (ră-kĭt'ĭk) Pert. to or affected with rickets.

rachitis (ră-kī'tĭs) [" + *itis,* inflammatory] **1.** Inflammation of the spine. **2.** Rickets.

r. fetalis annularis Congenital enlargement of the epiphyses of the long bones.

r. fetalis micromelica Congenital shortness of the bones.

rachitome (răk'ĭ-tōm") [" + *tome,* incision] An instrument used to open the spinal canal.

rachitomy (ră-kĭt'ō-mē) [" + *tome,* incision] Surgical cutting of the vertebral column.

raclage (ră-klŏzh') [Fr.] The destruction and removal of a soft growth by scraping or rubbing. SEE: *curettage.*

rad *radiation absorbed dose.*

radectomy (rā-dĕk'tō-mē) [L. *radix,* root, + Gr. *ektome,* excision] Surgical removal of all or a portion of a dental root.

radiability (rā"dē-ă-bĭl'ĭ-tē) [L. *radius,* ray, + *habilitas,* able] The capability of being penetrated readily by ionizing radiation. **radiable** (rā'dē-ă-băl), *adj.*

radiad (rā'dē-ăd) [L. *radialis,* radial, + *ad,* toward] In the direction of the radial side.

radial (rā'dē-ăl) **1.** Radiating out from a given center. **2.** Pert. to the radius.

radialis (rā"dē-ā'lĭs) [L.] Pert. to the radius bone.

radian (rā'dē-ăn) **1.** A unit of angular measurement equivalent to 57.295 degrees. It is subtended at the center of a circle by an arc the length of the radius of the circle. **2.** In ophthalmometry, a lens of 1 radian would have one plane surface equal in length to the radius of curvature of the curved surface.

radiant (rā'dē-ănt) [L. *radians,* radiate] **1.** Emitting beams of light. **2.** Transmitted by radiation. **3.** Emanating from a common center. SEE: *energy; heat; radiation.*

radiate (rā'dē-āt) [L. *radiatre,* to emit rays] To spread from a common center.

radiatio (rā-dē-ā'shē-ō) [L.] An anatomical structure, esp. a neurological one, that forms interconnections between parts by means of radiating fibers.

radiation (rā-dē-ā'shŭn) [L. *radiatio,* to radiate] **1.** The process by which energy is propagated through space or matter. **2.** The emission of rays in all directions from a common center. **3.** Ionizing rays used for diagnostic or therapeutic purposes. Two types of radiation therapy are commonly used for patients with cancer: teletherapy and brachytherapy. SEE: *brachytherapy*. **4.** A general term for any form of radiant energy emission or divergence, as of energy in all directions from luminous bodies, radiographical tubes, particle accelerators, radioactive elements, and fluorescent substances. **5.** In neurology, a group of fibers that diverge from a common origin.

acoustic r. Auditory r.

actinic r. Ionizing, electromagnetic radiation that can produce chemical changes, such as the damage done to skin by ultraviolet sunlight.

auditory r. A band of fibers that connect auditory areas of the cerebral cortex with the medial geniculate body of the thalamus. SYN: *acoustic r.*

Bremsstrahlung r. Diagnostic radiation produced at the target of the anode in an x-ray tube. An electron is accelerated at high speed from the x-ray tube cathode filament. It interacts with the nuclear field of a target atom, changing direction and losing energy that is emitted in the form of an ionizing radiation photon. The result is a heterogeneous beam.

characteristic r. In radiology, the production of radiation in an anode caused by an interaction between an electron from the electron stream and an inner-shell electron of the target material. The result is an ejected electron, a positive atom, and an x-ray photon characteristic of the difference in binding energies between the atomic shells.

r. of corpus callosum All the fibers emanating from the corpus callosum into each cerebral hemisphere.

corpuscular r. Radiation composed of discrete elements or particles such as elements of atomic nuclei (i.e., alpha, beta, neutron, positron, or proton particles).

cosmic r. Ionizing radiation from the sun and other extraterrestrial sources. It has a short wavelength, high velocity, and an exceptional ability to penetrate tissue. It accounts for about one tenth of the yearly total of ionizing radiation exposure for each person. Colloquially, it is known as "cosmic rays."

electromagnetic r. Rays that travel at the speed of light. They exhibit both magnetic and electrical properties. SEE: *electromagnetic spectrum* for table.

heterogeneous r. Radiation containing waves of various wavelengths.

homogeneous r. Radiation containing photons of similar wavelength.

infrared r. Infrared ray.

interstitial r. Radiation treatment accomplished by inserting sealed sources of a particle emitter directly into tissues.

ionizing r. Electromagnetic waves capable of producing ions after interaction with matter. Examples include x-rays, gamma rays, and beta particles. SEE: *radiation injury, ionizing*.

irritative r. An overdose of ultraviolet irradiation resulting in erythema and, in exceptional cases, blister formation.

low-level r. Electromagnetic waves at intensity levels below that known to cause obvious damage to living things. Low-level radiation includes that emitted by power lines, nuclear power plants, and appliances such as electric blankets, television sets, and computer terminals.

nonionizing r. ABBR: NIR. Electromagnetic radiation such as that in visible light, ultraviolet light, infrared light, microwaves, ultrasound, and radiofrequency emissions.

optic r. A system of fibers extending from the lateral geniculate body of the thalamus through the sublenticular portion of the internal capsule to the calcarine occipital cortex (striate area). SYN: *geniculocalcarine tract*.

photochemical r. Light rays that penetrate tissues only fractions of a millimeter, are absorbed by cells, and cause physical and biological changes. This type of radiation causes surface heating.

photothermal r. Radiation of heat by a source of light, as that from an electric bulb.

pyramidal r. The radiation of fibers from the cerebral cortex to the pyramidal tract.

solar r. Radiation from the sun; 60% is infrared and 40% is visible and ultraviolet.

striatomesencephalic r. Fibers originating in the corpus striatum and terminating principally in the substantia nigra of the midbrain.

striatosubthalamic r. A system of fibers consisting of three groups that emerge from the medial aspect of the lentiform nucleus and enter the subthalamic region, most terminating there but some continuing into the midbrain. SYN: *ansa lenticularis*.

striatothalamic r. Groups of fibers connecting the corpus striatum with the thalamus and subthalamus.

thalamic r. Groups of fibers connecting the thalamus with the cerebral hemispheres. These include frontal, centroparietal, occipital, and optic radiations.

ultraviolet r. Radiant energy extending from 3900 to 200 angstrom units (A.U.) Divided into near ultraviolet, which extends from 3900 to 2900 A.U., and far ultraviolet, which extends from 2900 to 200 A.U.

visible r. The radiation of the visible spectrum, which may be broken up into different wavelengths representing different colors:

Violet, 3900–4550 angstrom units (A.U.)

Blue, 4550–4920 A.U.
Green, 4920–5770 A.U.
Yellow, 5770–5970 A.U.
Orange, 5970–6220 A.U.
Red, 6220–7700 A.U.

radiation absorbed dose ABBR: rad. The quantity of ionizing radiation, measured in rad or gray (Gy), absorbed by any material per unit mass of matter. One Gy equals 100 rad.

radiation injury, ionizing Damage to cells and intracellular molecules by x-rays, gamma rays, radionuclides, or other sources of radioactive energy. In sufficient doses, radioactive energy can damage the cytoplasm and the genetic material of the cell, leading to organ dysfunction (esp. in rapidly dividing tissues such as the skin and the lining of the gastrointestinal tract), mutations, inhibition of cell division, cell death, or carcinogenesis. When the developing fetus is exposed to radiation in the womb, developmental malformations may result. SEE: *low-level radiation; radiation syndrome*.

radiation protection Prophylaxis against injury from ionizing radiation. The only effective preventive measures are shielding the source and the operator, handlers, and patients; maintaining appropriate distance from the source; and limiting the time and amount of exposure. In general, the use of drugs to protect against radiation is not practical because of their toxicity. An exception is the use of orally administered potassium iodide to protect the thyroid from radioactive iodine.

radiation sickness Radiation syndrome.

radiation symbol An international symbol used to indicate radioactive sources, containers for radioactive materials, and areas where radioactive materials are stored and used. The presence of this symbol (a magenta or black propeller on a yellow background) on a sign denotes the need for caution to avoid contamination with or undue exposure to atomic radiation. The wording on the sign varies with the level of potential radiation in the area. SEE: illus.

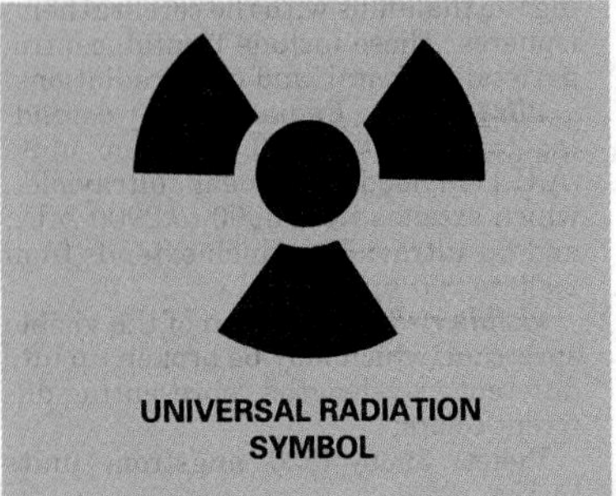
UNIVERSAL RADIATION SYMBOL

radiation syndrome Illness due to overexposure to harmful electromagnetic waves, usually x-rays or gamma rays. Mild acute illness is manifested by anorexia, headache, nausea, vomiting, and diarrhea. Delayed effects resulting from repeated or prolonged exposure may result in skin ulcers, alopecia, proctitis, enteritis, amenorrhea, sterility, disturbances in blood cell formation, cataract formation, premature aging, and cancer. SYN: *radiation sickness.*

radiator (rā′dē-ā″tor) [LL. *radiatus,* radiate] A device for radiating heat or light.

infrared r. A device for transmitting infrared rays.

radical (răd′ĭ-kăl) [LL. *radicalis,* having roots] **1.** In chemistry, a group of atoms acting as a single unit, passing without change from one compound to another, but unable to exist in a free state. **2.** Oriented toward the origin or root. **3.** A foundation or principle.

acid r. The electronegative portion of a molecule when the acid hydrogen is removed.

alcohol r. The portion of an alcohol molecule left when the hydrogen of the OH-group is removed.

free r. A molecule containing an odd number of electrons. These molecules contain an open bond or a half bond and are highly reactive. The odd electron is represented in the chemical formula by a dot. If two radicals react, both are eliminated; if a radical reacts with a nonradical, another free radical is produced. This type of event may become a chain reaction. In ischemic injury to tissues (e.g., myocardial infarction), free radical production may play an important role at certain stages in the progression of the injury.

The body has developed methods of defending against the harmful effects of free radicals. Superoxide dismutases, enzymes in mitochondria, and antioxidants are effective in counteracting the harmful effects of free radicals. SEE: *antioxidant; oxidative stress; superoxide; superoxide dismutase.*

radical treatment An extensive or complete therapy, such as surgical removal of an entire diseased organ and its associated lymphatic drainage. Alternatives to radical treatment may include observation, palliation, modified procedures, lumpectomies, or conservative treatments.

radices (răd′ĭ-sēz) [L.] Pl. of radix.

radiciform Resembling a root.

radicle (răd′ĭ-kl) [L. *radicula,* little root] A structure resembling a rootlet, as a radicle of a nerve or vein. SYN: *radicula.*

radicotomy (răd″ĭ-kŏt′ō-mē) [L. *radix,* root, + Gr. *tome,* incision] Rhizotomy. SEE: *radiculectomy.*

radicula (ră-dĭk′ū-lă) [L.] Radicle.

radiculalgia (ră-dĭk″ū-lăl′jē-ă) [L. *radix,*

root, + Gr. *algos,* pain] Neuralgia of nerve roots.

radicular (ră-dĭk′ū-lăr) [L. *radix,* root] **1.** Pert. to a root or radicle. **2.** Pert. to the tissues on or around a tooth root (e.g., radicular dentin, radicular bone).

radiculectomy (ră-dĭk″ū-lĕk′tō-mē) [″ + Gr. *ektome,* excision] **1.** Excision of a spinal nerve root. **2.** Resection of a posterior spinal nerve root. SEE: *rhizotomy.*

radiculitis (ră-dĭk″ū-lī′tĭs) [L. *radicula,* little root, + Gr. *itis,* inflammation] Inflammation of the spinal nerve roots, accompanied by pain and hyperesthesia.

radiculoganglionitis (ră-dĭk″ū-lō-găng″glē-ō-nī′tĭs) [″ + Gr. *ganglion,* knot, + *itis,* inflammation] Inflammation of the posterior spinal roots and their ganglia.

radiculomedullary (ră-dĭk″ū-lō-mĕd′ū-lĕr″ē) [″ + *medullaris,* marrow] Pert. to the nerve roots and the spinal cord.

radiculomeningomyelitis (ră-dĭk″ū-lō-mĕ-nĭn″gō-mī-ĕl-ī′tĭs) [″ + Gr. *meninx,* membrane, + *myelos,* marrow, + *itis,* inflammation] Inflammation of the nerve roots, meninges, and spinal cord.

radiculoneuritis (ră-dĭk″ū-lō″nū-rī′tĭs) [L. *radicula,* little root, + Gr. *neuron,* sinew, + *itis,* inflammation] Inflammation of the spinal nerve roots.

radiculopathy (ră-dĭk-ū-lŏp′ă-thē) [″ + ″ + *pathos,* disease, suffering] Any disease of a nerve root.

radiectomy (rā″dē-ĕk′tō-mē) [L. *radix,* root, + Gr. *ektome,* excision] Surgical removal of the root of a tooth.

radii (rā′dē-ī) [L.] Pl. of radius.

radio- [L. *radius,* ray] **1.** Combining form indicating *radiant energy, radioactive substances.* **2.** Combining form used as a prefix indicating *radioactive isotope.*

radioactinium (rā″dē-ō-ăk-tĭn′ē-ŭm) A radioactive product formed from disintegration of the element actinium.

radioactive (rā″dē-ō-ăk′tĭv) [L. *radius,* ray, + *activus,* acting] Capable of spontaneous emission of alpha, beta, or gamma rays as a result of the disintegration of the nucleus of an atom.

radioactive patient An individual treated or accidentally contaminated with radioactive materials. The patient should be told how long to avoid close contact with children and pregnant women.

radioactivity (rā″dē-ō-ăk″tĭv′ĭ-tē) Spontaneous disintegration of an atomic nucleus resulting in the emission of alpha, beta, or gamma rays.

artificial r. Radioactivity resulting from bombardment of a substance with high-energy particles in a cyclotron, betatron, or other apparatus.

induced r. Temporary radioactivity of a substance that has been exposed to a radioactive element.

natural r. Radioactivity emitted by elements in the environment, such as radon in soil. It may include alpha particles, beta particles, or gamma rays.

radioallergosorbent test (rā″dē-ō-ăl″ĕr-gō-sor′bĕnt) ABBR: RAST. A blood test for allergy that measures minute quantities of immunoglobulin E in blood. People who have type I hypersensitivity reactions to common allergens (e.g., ragweed, trees, molds, milk, eggs, and animal dander) have elevated levels of IgE. For these individuals and others, RAST is safer than skin testing, because it carries no risk of systemic anaphylaxis. RAST is not as sensitive as skin testing, however.

radioautograph (rā″dē-ō-aw′tō-grăf) [″ + ″ + *graphein,* to write] A photograph of a histologic section of a tissue showing the distribution of radioactive substances in the tissue.

radiobicipital (rā″dē-ō-bī-sĭp′ĭ-tăl) Pert. to the radius and biceps muscle of the arm.

radiobiology (rā″dē-ō-bī-ŏl′ō-jē) The branch of biology that deals with the effects of ionizing radiations on living organisms.

radiocalcium (rā″dē-ō-kăl′sē-ŭm) A radioisotope of calcium; ^{45}Ca and ^{47}Ca are used in medical studies.

radiocarbon (rā″dē-ō-kăr′bŏn) A radioisotope of carbon; ^{11}C and ^{14}C are used in medical studies.

radiocardiogram (rā″dē-ō-kăr′dē-ō-grăm) [L. *radius,* ray, + Gr. *kardia,* heart, + *gramma,* something written] The record or film obtained during radiocardiography.

radiocardiography (rā″dē-ō-kăr″dē-ŏg′ră-fē) [″ + ″ + *graphein,* to write] The investigation of the anatomy and function of the heart by obtaining a record or film of a radioactive substance as it travels through the heart.

radiocarpal (rā″dē-ō-kăr′păl) [″ + Gr. *karpos,* wrist] Pert. to the radius and carpus.

radiochemistry [″ + Gr. *chemeia,* chemistry] The branch of chemistry dealing with radioactive phenomena.

radiocurable (rā″dē-ō-kūr′ă-bl) Curable by radiation therapy.

radiocystitis (rā″dē-ō-sĭs-tī′tĭs) [″ + Gr. *kystis,* bladder, + *itis,* inflammation] Inflammation of the bladder following radiation therapy as a result of cell and tissue damage.

radiodensity The impenetrability of a substance or tissue by x-rays. SYN: *radiopacity.*

radiodermatitis (rā″dē-ō-dĕr″mă-tī′tĭs) [″ + Gr. *derma,* skin, + *osis,* condition] Inflammation of the skin caused by exposure to x-rays or emissions from radioactive particles. SYN: *radioepidermitis.*

radiodiagnosis (rā″dē-ō-dī″ăg-nō′sĭs) [″

+ Gr. *dia,* through, + *gnosis,* knowledge] Diagnosis with radiological imaging.

radiodigital (rā″dē-ō-dĭg′ĭ-tăl) Pert. to the radius and the fingers.

radiodontia (rā″dē-ō-dŏn′shē-ă) [″ + Gr. *odous,* tooth] Radiography of the teeth.

radioecology (rā″dē-ō-ē-kŏl′ō-jē) [″ + Gr. *oikos,* house, + *logos,* word, reason] Investigation of the effect of radiation on the living organisms in the environment.

radioelectrocardiogram (rā″dē-ō-ē-lĕk″trō-kăr′dē-ō-grăm) The record obtained by radioelectrocardiography.

radioelectrocardiography (rā″dē-ō-ē-lĕk″trō-kăr″dē-ŏg′ră-fē) [L. *radius,* ray, + Gr. *elektron,* amber, + *kardia,* heart, + *graphein,* to write] An infrequently used term for telemetry.

radioelement (rā″dē-ō-ĕl′ĕ-mĕnt) [″ + *elementum,* a rudiment] Any of the radioactive elements.

radioencephalogram (rā″dē-ō-ĕn-sĕf′ă-lō-grăm″) [″ + Gr. *enkephalos,* brain, + *gramma,* something written] The record obtained when a radioactive tracer passes through the blood vessels of the brain.

radioencephalography (rā″dē-ō-ĕn-sĕf″ă-lŏg′ră-fē) [″ + ″ + *graphein,* to write] The recording of radio waves transmitted from the brain to a receiver but without electrodes being placed on the scalp.

radioepidermitis (rā″dē-ō-ĕp″ĭ-dĕr-mī′tĭs) [″ + Gr. *epi,* upon, + *derma,* skin, + *itis,* inflammation] Radiodermatitis.

radioepithelitis (rā″dē-ō-ĕp″ĭ-thē-lī′tĭs) [″ + ″ + *thele,* nipple, + *itis,* inflammation] Disintegration of the epithelium due to exposure to radiation.

radiofrequency electrophrenic respiration A method of stimulating respiration in cases of respiratory paralysis from spinal cord injury at the cervical level. Intermittent electrical stimuli to the phrenic nerves are supplied by a radiofrequency transmitter implanted subcutaneously. The diaphragmatic muscles contract in response to these stimuli.

radiogenic (rā″dē-ō-jĕn′ĭk) [″ + *gennan,* to produce] **1.** Producing radiation. **2.** Caused by radiation. SYN: *actinogenic.*

radiogold (rā′dē-ō-gōld) A radioisotope of gold.

radiograph (rā′dē-ō-grăf) [″ + Gr. *graphein,* to write] **1.** The film on which an image is produced through exposure to x-rays. SYN: *roentgenogram.* **2.** To make a radiograph.

bitewing r. A type of radiograph that shows the crowns and upper third of the roots of upper and lower teeth. It is made by using a dental film with a tab (bitewing) or placement device that holds the film in place when the jaws are closed on the tab. The purpose is to detect proximal caries and the interdental bone. SYN: *interproximal radiograph.*

body section r. Tomogram.

bregma-menton r. A radiograph taken in the submental-vertex plane, from below the chin to the top of the skull. It shows the contour of the zygomatic arches and the lateral separation of the mandibular condyles, coronoid processes, or both.

bucket-handle r. A slang term for an x-ray examination taken with the beam aimed from beneath the chin toward the vertex of the skull; used to assess facial and orbital floor injuries.

cephalogram r. A radiograph of the jaws and skull on which anatomical points, planes, and angles may be drawn to assist in measurement.

dental r. An image of dental structures made on x-ray film. Radiographs may be extraoral or intraoral. Three common types of intraoral dental images are periapical, interproximal, and occlusal radiographs.

interproximal r. Bitewing radiograph.

lateral cephalometric r. A film of the entire head, taken from the side with the head in a known, fixed position for the purpose of making definitive observations or measurements.

lateral oblique r. A radiograph used to examine the body of the mandible and the ramus. Projections may be performed with conventional dental radiographical film and cover a broader area than a typical periapical radiograph. Also called *lateral jaw survey.*

lateral skull r. A radiograph of the sinuses and lateral aspects of the cranial skeleton.

maxillary sinus r. A frontal x-ray of the maxillary sinuses and the zygomas that allows direct comparison of both sides.

panoramic r. A type of extraoral curved-surface radiograph that shows the entire upper and lower jaws in a continuous single film.

periapical r. An intraoral film that depicts the tooth and surrounding tissues extending to the apical region. SYN: *dental r.*

posteroanterior r. A frontal radiograph of the skull; used to examine the skull for disease, trauma, and developmental abnormalities.

rotational r. Panoramic r.

transcranial r. A radiograph of the temporomandibular articulation.

radiographer A health care professional who operates radiological equipment. Internationally, the term includes other imaging and radiation therapy technologists, such as those who perform computed tomography, mammography, and nuclear magnetic resonance examinations.

radiography (rā-dē-ŏg′ră-fē) The process of obtaining an image for diagnosis using a radiological modality.
radiohumeral (rā″dē-ō-hū′mĕr-ăl) [″ + *humerus,* upper arm] Pert. to the radius and humerus.
radioimmunity (rā″dē-ō-ĭ-mū′nĭ-tē) [″ + *immunitas,* immunity] Apparent decreased sensitivity to radiation that may follow repeated radiation therapy.
radioimmunoassay (rā″dē-ō-ĭm″ū-nō-ăs′ā) ABBR: RIA. A method of determining the concentration of a substance, esp. hormones, based on the competitive inhibition of binding of a radioactively labeled substance to a specific antibody. Protein concentrations in the picogram (10^{-12} g) range can be measured by this technique.
radioimmunodiffusion (rā″dē-ō-ĭm″ū-nō-dĭf-fū′zhŭn) [″ + ″ + *dis,* apart, + *fundere,* to pour] A method of studying antigen-antibody interaction by use of radioisotope-labeled antigens or antibodies diffused through a gel.
radioimmunoelectrophoresis (rā″dē-ō-ĭm″ū-nō-ē-lĕk″trō-fō-rē′sĭs) [″ + ″ + Gr. *elektron,* amber, + *phoresis,* bearing] Electrophoresis involving the use of a radioisotope-labeled antigen or antibody. An autoradiograph is taken of the electrophoretic pattern produced.
radioiodine (rā″dē-ō-ī′ō-dīn) A radioactive isotope of iodine, used in the diagnosis and treatment of thyroid disorders. The most commonly used isotope is ^{131}I.
radioiron (rā″dē-ō-ī′ĕrn) A radioactive isotope of iron; ^{55}Fe and ^{59}Fe are used in medical studies.
radioisotope (rā″dē-ō-ī′sō-tōp) A radioactive form of an element.
radiolead (rā″dē-ō-lĕd′) A radioactive isotope of lead.
radiolesion (rā″dē-ō-lē′zhŭn) An injury caused by radiation.
radioligand (rā″dē-ō-lī′gănd, răd″dē-ō-lĭg′ ănd) A molecule, esp. an antigen or antibody, with a radioactive tracer attached to it.
radiological emergency assistance Urgent care provided to individuals exposed to ionizing radiation.
radiologist (rā-dē-ŏl′ō-jĭst) [L. *radius,* ray, + Gr. *logos,* word, reason] A physician who uses x-rays or other sources of ionizing radiation, sound, or radiofrequencies for diagnosis and treatment.
 dental r. A dentist whose specialty is the production of radiographs and their use in diagnosing dental and oral diseases.
radiology (rā-dē-ŏl′ō-jē) The branch of medicine concerned with radioactive substances, including x-rays, radioactive isotopes, and ionizing radiation, and the application of this information to prevention, diagnosis, and treatment of disease.
radiolucency (rā″dē-ō-lū′sĕn-sē) [″ + *lucere,* to shine] The property of being partly or wholly penetrable by radiant energy.
radiolucent (rā″dē-ō-lū′sĕnt) [″ + *lucere,* to shine] Penetrable by x-rays.
radiolus (rā-dē′ō-lŭs) [L., a little ray] A sound or probe.
radiometer (rā-dē-ŏm′ĕ-tĕr) [″ + Gr. *metron,* measure] An instrument for measuring the intensity of radiation.
radiomicrometer (rā″dē-ō-mī-krŏm′ĕ-tĕr) [″ + Gr. *mikros,* small, + *metron,* measure] An instrument for measuring small changes in radiation.
radiomimetic (rā″dē-ō-mĭm-ĕt′ĭk) [″ + Gr. *mimetikos,* imitation] Imitating the biological effects of radiation. Alkylating agents are examples of substances with this property. SEE: *alkylating agent.*
radiomuscular (rā″dē-ō-mŭs′kū-lăr) Pert. to the radius or radial artery and the muscles of the arm.
radiomutation The permanent alteration of the genetic material of a cell caused by the effects of ionizing radiation.
radionecrosis (rā″dē-ō-nĕ-krō′sĭs) [″ + Gr. *nekrosis,* state of death] The disintegration of tissue resulting from exposure to ionizing radiation.
radioneuritis (rā″dē-ō-nū-rī′tĭs) [″ + Gr. *neuron,* sinew, + *itis,* inflammation] Inflammation of a nerve caused by exposure to a radioactive substance.
radionitrogen (rā″dē-ō-nī′trō-jĕn) A radioisotope of nitrogen.
radionuclide (rā″dē-ō-nū′klīd) An atom that disintegrates by emitting electromagnetic rays, known as gamma rays.
radiopacity (rā″dē-ō-păs′ĭ-tē) Radiodensity.
radiopaque (rā-dē-ō-pāk′) [″ + *opacus,* dark] Impenetrable to x-rays or other forms of radiation.
radioparency (rā″dē-ō-păr′ĕn-sē) Condition of being radiolucent or radioparent.
radioparent (rā″dē-ō-păr′ĕnt) [″ + *parere,* to appear] Penetrable by x-rays or other forms of radiation.
radiopathology (rā″dē-ō-pă-thŏl′ō-jē) [″ + Gr. *pathos,* disease, suffering, + *logos,* word, reason] The study of radiation injuries.
radiopelvimetry (rā″dē-ō-pĕl-vĭm′ĕt-rē) [″ + *pelvis,* basin, + Gr. *metron,* measure] Measurement of the pelvis by use of x-rays.
radiopharmaceutical (rā″dē-ō-fărm″ă-sū′tĭ-kăl) A radioactive chemical or drug (e.g., an isotope of technetium or iodine) that has a specific affinity for a particular body tissue or organ. It can be used in nuclear medicine to obtain images of structures, or to treat radiation-sensitive diseases.

CAUTION: Radiopharmaceuticals must be handled in accordance with prescribed methods to prevent the patient or those treating the patient from being exposed to unnecessary ionizing radiation.

---

radiophobia (rā″dē-ō-fō′bē-ă) [″ + Gr. *phobos,* fear] An abnormal fear of x-rays and radiation.

radiophosphorus (rā″dē-ō-fŏs′fō-rŭs) A radioactive isotope of phosphorus. ^{32}P is used in medical studies.

radiopotassium (rā″dē-ō-pō-tăs′ē-ŭm) A radioactive isotope of potassium. ^{42}K is used in medical studies.

radiopotentiation (rā″dē-ō-pō-tĕn″shē-ā′shŭn) [″ + *potentia,* power] The augmentation of the effect of radiation. This may be produced by certain drugs and by oxygen.

radioprotective drug A drug that protects humans against the damaging or lethal effects of ionizing radiation. For example, Lugol's solution or a saturated solution of potassium iodide blocks the uptake of inhaled or ingested radioactive iodine by the thyroid.

radiopulmonography (rā″dē-ō-pŭl″mō-nŏg′ră-fē) [″ + *pulmo,* lung, + Gr. *graphein,* to write] The use of radioactive materials to measure the flow, or lack of flow, of gases through the lung during respiration.

radioreaction (rā″dē-ō-rē-ăk′shŭn) The reaction of the body to radiation.

radioreceptor (rā″dē-ō-rē-sĕp′tor) Something that receives radiant energy such as light, heat, or x-rays.

radioresistant Resistant to the action of radiation; used esp. of a tumor that cannot be destroyed by radiation treatment.

radioresponsive (rā″dē-ō-rē-spŏn′sĭv) Radiosensitive.

radioscopy (rā-dē-ŏs′kō-pē) [L. *radius,* ray, + Gr. *skopein,* to examine] Inspection and examination of the internal structures of the body by fluoroscopic procedures. SYN: *fluoroscopy*.

radiosensibility Radiosensitivity.

radiosensitivity (rā″dē-ō-sĕn″sĭ-tĭv′ĭ-tē) Reactiveness or responsiveness of a cell to radiation. SYN: *radiosensibility*. **radiosensitive,** *adj.*

radiosodium (rā″dē-ō-sō′dē-ŭm) A radioisotope of sodium such as ^{24}Na and ^{22}Na.

radiostrontium (rā″dē-ō-strŏn′shē-ŭm) A radioisotope of strontium.

radiosulfur (rā″dē-ō-sŭl′fŭr) A radioisotope of sulfur.

radiosurgery (rā″dē-ō-sŭr′jĕr-ē) [″ + Gr. *cheirurgia,* handwork] The use of ionizing radiation in surgery. SEE: *gamma knife surgery*.

radiotelemetry (rā″dē-ō-tĕl-ĕm′ĕ-trē) [″ + Gr. *tele,* distant, + *metron,* measure] The transmission of data, including biological data, by radio from a patient to a remote monitor or recording device for storage, analysis, and interpretation.

radiotherapeutics (rā″dē-ō-thĕr″ă-pū′tĭks) **1.** Radiotherapy. **2.** The study of radiotherapeutic agents.

radiotherapist (rā″dē-ō-thĕr′ă-pĭst) [″ + Gr. *therapeia,* treatment] Someone trained in use of ionizing radiation for therapeutic purposes.

radiotherapy (rā″dē-ō-thĕr′ă-pē) The treatment of disease with ionizing or nonionizing radiation.

radiothermy (rā″dē-ō-thĕr′mē) [″ + Gr. *therme,* heat] **1.** The use of radiant heat or heat from radioactive substances for therapeutic purposes. **2.** Short-wave diathermy.

radiothorium (rā″dē-ō-thō′rē-ŭm) A radioisotope of thorium.

radiotoxemia (rā″dē-ō-tŏk-sē′mē-ă) [″ + Gr. *toxikon,* poison, + *haima,* blood] A rarely used term for radiation syndrome.

radiotransparent (rā″dē-ō-trăns-păr′ĕnt) [″ + *trans,* across, + *parere,* to appear] Penetrable by radiation.

radioulnar (rā″dē-ō-ŭl′năr) [″ + *ulna,* arm] Concerning the radius and ulna.

radium (rā′dē-ŭm) [L. *radius,* ray] SYMB: Ra. A metallic element found in very small quantities in uranium ores such as pitchblende; atomic number 88, atomic weight 226, half-life 1622 years. It is radioactive and fluorescent. Radon is produced by the breakdown of radium. The most stable isotope, ^{226}Ra, has been used as a source of radioactivity in medical research and therapy.

radium needle A slender tissue implant containing radium that is used to treat internal malignancies.

radium therapy [″ + Gr. *therapeia,* treatment] Radiotherapy.

radius [L., ray] **1.** A line extending from a circle's center point to its circumference. **2.** The outer and shorter bone of the forearm. It revolves partially about the ulna. Its head articulates with the capitulum of the humerus and with the radial notch on the ulna and is encircled by the annular ligament. Its lower portion articulates with the ulna by the ulnar notch, and by another articulation with the navicular (scaphoid) and lunate bones of the wrist. **radial,** *adj.*

fracture of r. A break in the radius. A common fracture of the lower end of the radius is a Colles' fracture, caused by falling on the outstretched hand. Fractures also occur along the shaft or at the upper end frequently involving the radial head. SEE: under *fracture*.

radix (rā′dĭks) *pl.* **radices** [L., root] **1.** The root portion of a cranial or spinal nerve. **2.** The root of a plant.

radon (rā′dŏn) [L. *radius,* ray] SYMB: Rn. A radioactive gaseous element resulting from the disintegration of isotopes of radium; atomic weight 222, atomic number 86. Because radium is present in the earth's crust, radon and its disintegration products accumulate in caves, mines, houses (particularly those that are energy efficient), and any space where no free exchange exists between the air contained in it and the air outside it. Exposure to radon above acceptable limits is believed to be a risk factor for lung cancer.

PATIENT CARE: If the level of radon in a house is measured and exceeds acceptable limits, steps should be taken to reduce it. Methods for removing or decreasing radon exposure in buildings are available.

r. seed A tissue implant containing radon that is used to treat internal malignancies.

raffinose (răf'ĭ-nōs) A trisaccharide, melitose, present in certain plants, cereals, and fungi. Hydrolysis yields fructose and melibiose.

rage (rāj') [ME.] Violent anger.

sham r. A rage reaction produced by stimuli in decorticated animals.

ragsorter's disease A febrile pulmonary disease that may occur in people who sort paper and rags. It is caused by inhalation of anthrax.

ragweed One of several species of the genus *Ambrosia,* whose pollen is an important allergen. The pollen-producing period of grasses in temperate zones is from the middle of August to the first hard frost. SEE: *allergy*.

Raillietina (rī"lē-ĕ-tī'nă) A genus of tapeworms belonging to the family Davaineidae.

R. demerariensis A species that infests humans, reported from several South American countries, esp. Ecuador.

Raimiste's phenomenon, Raimiste's sign An associated reaction in hemiplegia in which resistance to hip abduction or adduction in the noninvolved extremity evokes the same motion in the involved extremity.

raised (rāzd) [ME. *reisen,* to rise] Elevated above a surface.

rale Crackle.

ramal (rā'măl) [L. *ramus,* branch] Pert. to a ramus.

rami (rā'mī) [L.] Pl. of ramus.

ramicotomy (răm"ĭ-kŏt'ō-mē) [L. *ramus,* branch, + Gr. *tome,* incision] Ramisection.

ramification (răm"ĭ-fĭ-kā'shŭn) [L. *ramificare,* to make branches] **1.** The process of branching. **2.** A branch. **3.** Arrangement in branches.

ramify (răm'ĭ-fī) To branch; to spread out in different directions.

ramisection (răm'ĭ-sĕk"shŭn) [L. *ramus,* branch, + *sectio,* a cutting] The surgical division of a ramus communicans between a spinal nerve and a ganglion of the sympathetic trunk.

ramisectomy (răm-ĭs-ĕk'tō-mē) [" + Gr. *ektome,* excision] Excision of a ramus, specifically a ramus communicans. SEE: *ramisection*.

ramitis (răm-ī'tĭs) [" + Gr. *itis,* inflammation] Inflammation of a ramus.

ramose (rā'mōs) [L. *ramus,* branch] Branching; having many branches.

Ramsay Hunt syndrome A condition caused by herpes zoster of the geniculate ganglion of the brain or neuritis of the facial nerve and characterized by severe facial palsy and vesicular eruption in the pharynx, external ear canal, tongue, and occipital area. Deafness, tinnitus, and vertigo may be present.

ramulus [L.] A small branch or ramus.

ramus (rā'mŭs) *pl.* **rami** [L., branch] A branch; one of the divisions of a forked structure. **ramal** (-măl), *adj.*

anterior r. One of the primary branches of a spinal nerve that supplies the lateral and ventral portions of the body wall, limbs, and perineum.

bronchial r. One of the collateral branches of each primary bronchus.

r. communicans One of the primary branches of a spinal nerve that connects with a sympathetic ganglion. Each consists of a white portion (white ramus communicans) composed of myelinated preganglionic sympathetic fibers and a gray portion (gray ramus communicans) composed of unmyelinated postganglionic fibers.

mandibular r. The vertical portion of the mandible.

meningeal r. One of the primary branches of a spinal nerve that reenters the vertebral foramen and supplies the meninges and vertebral column.

posterior r. One of the primary branches of a spinal nerve that supplies the muscles and skin of the back.

Rancho Los Amigos Guide to Cognitive Levels A scale widely used to classify a neurological patient's level of cognitive dysfunction according to behavior. This scale provides eight levels with descriptors, progressing from level I (no response) to level VIII (purposeful and appropriate response), as follows:

1. No response: is unresponsive to any stimuli.

2. Generalized response: exhibits limited, inconsistent, nonpurposeful responses, often to pain only.

3. Localized response: displays purposeful responses; may follow simple commands; may focus on presented object.

4. Confused, agitated: demonstrates heightened state of activity; confusion, disorientation; aggressive behavior; inability to perform self-care; unawareness of present events; agitation, which appears as internal confusion.

5. Confused, inappropriate: is nonagitated; appears alert; responds to commands; is distractible; does not concentrate on task; demonstrates agitated responses to external stimuli; is verbally inappropriate; does not learn new information.

6. Confused, appropriate: demonstrates goal-directed behavior, needs cueing; can relearn old skills, such as activities of daily living; displays serious memory problems; exhibits some awareness of self and others.

7. Automatic, appropriate: appears appropriate, oriented; frequently acts robot-like in daily routine; has minimal or no confusion; demonstrates shallow recall; exhibits increased awareness of self, interaction in environment; lacks insight into condition; shows decreased judgment and problem solving ability; lacks realistic planning for future.

8. Purposeful, appropriate: is alert, oriented; recalls and integrates past events; learns new activities and can continue without supervision; is independent in home and living skills; is capable of driving; demonstrates defects in stress tolerance, judgment, abstract reasoning; possibly functions at reduced levels in society.

rancid (răn′sĭd) [L. *rancidus,* stink] Having a disagreeable odor resulting from the breakdown of double bonds in fatty acids.

rancidity (răn-sĭd′ĭ-tē) The condition of being rancid.

randomization In research, a method used to assign subjects to experimental groups without introducing biases into a study. SEE: *clinical trial; double-blind technique.*

randomized controlled trial ABBR: RCT. An experimental study to assess the effects of a particular variable (e.g., a drug or treatment) in which subjects are assigned randomly to an experimental, placebo, or control group. The experimental group receives the drug or procedure; the placebo group's medication is disguised to resemble the drug being investigated. The control group receives nothing. Laboratory tests or clinical evaluations are performed on the groups (usually using the double-blind technique) to determine the effects of the drug or procedure.

random sample In experimental medicine and epidemiology, a scrupulously unbiased selection of individuals or items from a population or other grouping, such that the study results will have a high probability of reflecting the variables under study, rather than unintentionally reflecting a characteristic of the research subjects.

range [ME., series] The difference between the highest and lowest in a set of variables or in a series of values or observations.

r. of accommodation The difference between the least and the greatest distance of distinct vision. SEE: *accommodation.*

r. of motion ABBR: ROM. **1.** The amount of excursion through which a joint can move, measured in degrees of a circle. SEE: *range-of-motion exercise* for illus.; *goniometer.* **2.** An exercise that moves a joint through the extent of its limitations. This exercise can be active, active assisted, or passive.

continuous passive r. of motion Continuous passive motion.

passive r. of motion ABBR: PROM. **1.** The possible excursion of motion at a joint, accomplished by an examiner, without any muscle contraction by the patient. This can be measured by a goniometer. The excursion is normally slightly greater than active range of motion. The examiner assesses the end point. **2.** An exercise in which an external force moves a joint through its excursion without any effort by the patient. PROM exercise is used when the patient is unable to move or when active motion is prohibited.

ranine (rā′nīn) [L. *rana,* a frog] **1.** Pert. to a ranula, or the region beneath the tip of the tongue. **2.** The branch of the lingual artery supplying that area. **3.** Pert. to frogs.

Ransohoff's sign (răn′zō-hŏfz) [Joseph Ransohoff, American surgeon, 1853–1921] Yellow staining of the skin around the umbilicus. The sign suggests rupture of the biliary ducts.

ranula (răn′ū-lă) [L., little frog] A cystic tumor seen on the underside of the tongue on either side of the frenum; a retention cyst of the submandibular or sublingual ducts. The swelling may be small or large.

SYMPTOMS: The tumor is semitranslucent, with soft, dilated veins coursing over it. The patient experiences fullness and discomfort, but usually no pain. The tumor contains clear fluid owing to dilatation of the salivary glands and obstruction of the sublingual mucous glands.

TREATMENT: Periodic emptying of the sac by careful needle aspiration provides temporary relief. Surgical intervention is required for complete removal.

pancreatic r. Cystic disease of the pancreas caused by obstruction of its ducts.

Ranvier's node (rŏn-vē-āz′) [Louis A. Ranvier, Fr. pathologist, 1835–1922] A space between adjacent Schwann cells along a nerve fiber; no myelin sheath is present. SYN: *neurofibril node.* SEE: *nerve fiber; neuron* for illus.; *Schwann cell.*

RAO *right anterior oblique* position.

rape (rāp) [L. *rapere,* to seize] Sexual assault or sexual violence perpetrated on one person by another against the will of the victim. Rape involves an attempt at or actual penetration of the vagina or another body orifice by a penis, finger, or inanimate object. Complete penetration by the penis or emission of seminal fluid is not necessary to constitute rape. Most rapes include force, intimidation, or violence, but acquiescence because of verbal threats does not indicate consent. Studies, which may have disclosure or reporting biases, indicate that an incident involving rape occurs about every 1.2 minutes, and that 1 out of 3 women will be raped sometime during her life. The peak incidence is among women 16 to 19 years of age in the U.S. Nevertheless, more than 60,000 rapes of women older than 50 years of age are reported annually. SEE: *rape and sexual assault prevention; rape-trauma syndrome; sexual abuse; Nursing Diagnoses Appendix.*

TREATMENT: The medical care of the rape victim must include appropriate antibiotic prophylactic treatment for sexually transmitted diseases, and prophylaxis against hepatitis B, which will require administration of hepatitis B immune globulin (0.06 ml/kg of body weight). This should be given within 24 hr of exposure. The importance of HIV testing while in the treatment center and scheduling of repeat tests at monthly intervals for at least 6 months should be stressed. In cases where semen entered the vagina, medication to prevent pregnancy may be given.

PATIENT CARE: The health care professional provides sensitive care, esp. psychological support, by remaining with the patient and by encouraging verbalization of feelings. If available, a Sexual Assault Nurse Examiner should be summoned. State regulations regarding the reporting of rape should be followed. The health care professional explains and assists with the physical, pelvic, and rectal examinations and diagnostic tests. Directions should be followed exactly in collecting rape evidence such as head and pubic hair combings, nail scrapings, and vaginal, oral, or anal specimens for police investigation. The patient should be allowed as much control as possible throughout examination, treatment, and interview procedures. An assault and sexual history is obtained, including whether the female rape victim was menstruating and, if so, the type of menstrual protection used.

Prescribed treatments of associated injuries are performed. Photographs to document any injuries are taken. Tests for sexually transmitted illnesses may be performed, including tests for human immunodeficiency virus. Crisis intervention services are offered to assist the patient with emotional expression. Information regarding antipregnancy measures is provided. Assistance is offered to help the patient explain the rape to family. Follow-up services and written and verbal instructions for prescribed medications, including drug actions and possible side effects, are provided. Arrangements are made for someone to escort the patient home.

date r. Nonconsensual, unsolicited, and unwelcome sexual relations between individuals who are currently or were previously romantically involved or sexually intimate.

gang r. Forcible sexual intercourse or other sexual activity committed on an individual by several persons. SEE: *rape.*

male r. Sexual assault, usually penetrative, of a man by a man. Estimating the prevalence of male rape is difficult because it often is not reported.

marital r. Forcible sexual assault by a spouse at a time when the sexual encounter was neither solicited nor welcome.

prison r. Rape that occurs when the victim is assaulted by another prisoner or by a prison employee.

statutory r. Sexual intercourse with an individual younger than the legal age of consent.

rape and sexual assault prevention The precautions taken to decrease the chances of one's being forced to engage in unwanted sexual behaviors. In the US., about 700,000–1,000,000 sexual assaults occur each year; 75–85% of all sexual assaults are committed by friends, family members, or sexual partners of the victim; 95% of all sexual assaults are committed against women, the majority of whom are under 18 years old. Because of this, a crucial element in the prevention of sexual assault is the education of young men and adolescent boys about respectful sexual interactions with women. In addition, women who feel threatened, dominated, or controlled by men or boys in their home, school, or work environments should proactively seek help from sexual assault crisis services in their neighborhood.

Personal safety tips. (1) Because alcohol consumption is a related factor in many rapes, it is advisable to keep alcohol intake to a minimum and not allow a companion who is intoxicated into one's home. (2) As much as possible, preventive measures should be directed at remaining in a well-secured area and being close to persons who can be called for assistance day or night. (3) Emergency police and fire department telephone numbers should be kept readily available. Help should be summoned without delay if it is suspected that one's apartment or home is being illegally entered. (4) When preparing to enter a car or home, one should be constantly alert for the presence of strangers. (5) Before leaving a well-lighted and populated area, one should have the car keys in hand and ready for quick use. It is advisable to leave one arm free of packages, handbag, or other items and to carry a noise making device. (6) When driving, it is important to lock the car doors and close any open windows immediately, and stay on well-lit streets. (7) When outdoors at night, one should enlist the assistance of a known neighbor, law enforcement officer, or friend to search the home. Once one is safely inside, the door should be locked securely. (8) If a stranger comes to the door, a security chain should be kept on and a peephole preferably used for communication until proper identification has been presented. If doubt exists about the credentials or demeanor of the stranger, admission should be refused and help summoned immediately. (9) Always walk quickly and with assurance. (10) Avoid automated teller machines at night. (11) If attacked, make as much noise and resist assault vigorously, unless you believe that to do so would increase the likelihood of physical harm or death. (12) Never leave children unattended. (13) Do not allow strangers to enter your car. (14) If you are assaulted, seek immediate help from local medical, social, and policing agencies. Do not wash or bathe. (15) Attempt to remember as many details as possible about the attacker: clothes, size, race, accent, hair color, identifying marks and scars, facial hair, vehicle, and evidence of drug or alcohol use.

rape counseling The provision of advice, comfort, and sources of therapy for victims of sexual assault. The emotional reaction and sequelae of rape may be devastating to the mental well-being of the victim. It is therefore important that the victim be reassured about what to expect from both internal feelings and the potential reactions of society. Historically, law enforcement officers have been less than sympathetic to rape victims, but now most police departments have officers trained in rape investigation who are sensitive to the emotional and physical trauma the victim has experienced. Frequently, specially trained Sexual Assault Nurse Examiners (SANE) are available to provide care and support. Various services are available to the victim, including advocate groups and health care professionals experienced in counseling rape victims.

rapeseed [L. *rapa,* turnip] The seed of *Brassica campestris* and other *Brassica* species, whose oil is used in the manufacture of lubricants and canola oil. The oil made from the seeds of the variety high in erucic acid is used as an industrial lubricant. Oil made from the seeds of the low-erucic-acid variety is relatively low in saturated fat and is commonly known as canola oil.

raphania (ră-fā′nē-ă) [Gr. *rhaphanos,* radish] A spasmodic disease caused by eating seeds of the wild radish; allied to ergotism. SYN: *rhaphania.*

raphe (rā′fē) [Gr. *rhaphe*] A crease, ridge, or seam denoting union of the halves of a part. SYN: *rhaphe.*

abdominal r. Linea alba.

buccal r. In the embryo, a raphe on the cheek indicating the line of fusion of the maxillary and mandibular processes.

lateral r. A ridge along the lateral margin of the erector spinae muscles formed by the aponeurosis of the latissimus dorsi internal oblique and transversus abdominis muscles and the layers of the thoracolumbar fascia.

palatine r. A line or ridge in the median line of the palate.

r. of penis A median ridge on the posterior surface of the penis, a continuation of the raphe of the scrotum.

perineal r. A line or ridge in the midline of the perineum.

pterygomandibular r. A tendinous line of fusion between the buccinator and superior pharyngeal constrictor muscles that passes between the pterygoid process and the mandible, serving as an important landmark in dental anesthesia.

r. of scrotum A ridge in the midline of the scrotum.

r. of tongue A median groove on the dorsum of the tongue.

rapid eye movement ABBR: REM. Cyclic movement of the closed eyes observed or recorded during sleep.

rapid cycling Four or more episodes of depression, mania, hypomania, or other alternating mood disturbances occurring in a single year. Roughly 10% of patients with bipolar illness have this condition; more men than women are affected. Lithium carbonate is less effective in treating rapid cycling than in treating other forms of bipolar disorder.

rappel (ră-pĕl′) To slide down a rope, as in a lifesaving rescue.

rapport (ră-por′) [Fr. *rapporter,* to bring back] A relationship of mutual trust and understanding, esp. between the patient and physician, nurse, or other health care provider.

rapture A state of great joy, delight, or ecstasy.

rarefaction (răr″ĕ-făk′shŭn) [L. *rarefacere,* to make thin] The process of decreasing in density and weight.

r. of bone Loss of bone mineral density. SEE: *osteoporosis; parathyroid.*

rarefy (rār′ĕ-fī) To make less dense; to increase the porosity of something.

RAS *reticular activating system.*

rash (răsh) [O.Fr. *rasche*] A general term for any eruption that appears on the skin transiently (as opposed to durable skin lesions such as scars, tattoos, or moles). SYN: *exanthem.*

PATIENT CARE: Assessments are made of the location and characteristics of the lesion, such as color; size (height and diameter); pattern, whether discrete or coalesced; and any secondary changes (crusting, scaling, lichenification). Associated symptoms such as pruritus or discomfort, temporal elements, history of known allergies, drugs used, and contacts with communicable diseases during prior 2-week period also are assessed. Suspected drugs are discontinued, and the potential communicable disease patient is isolated and assessed. Cool compresses are applied to relieve itching. Topical preparations and dressings are applied and systemic medications administered as prescribed. The patient is instructed to keep hands clean and nails short and even, and to avoid scratching. The patient also is taught about the treatment regimen, its actions, and its side effects and evaluates for desired effects and side effects.

butterfly r. A rash on both cheeks joined by an extension across the bridge of the nose. It is seen in systemic lupus erythematosus, esp. after the patient's face has been exposed to sunlight, and in seborrheic dermatitis, tuberous sclerosis, and dermatomyositis. SEE: *discoid lupus erythematosus*.

diaper r. Irritant contact dermatitis as a reaction to friction, maceration, and prolonged contact with urine, feces, soap retained in diapers, and topical preparations. A persistent diaper rash may be colonized by yeast or bacteria. SYN: *diaper dermatitis*. SEE: illus.

TREATMENT: Treatment is symptomatic. Diapers should be changed frequently. If washable cloth diapers are used, they should be thoroughly washed and rinsed; occlusive plastic pants should not be used over diaper; the perianal and genital areas should be washed with warm water and mild, nonperfumed soap. If these measures and application of a bland protective agent (e.g., zinc oxide paste) do not promote healing, then a small amount of 0.5% to 1% topical hydrocortisone cream should be applied to the area after each diaper change, until the rash has completely resolved.

drug r. Drug eruption.

ecchymotic r. Hemorrhagic r.

gum r. A red, papular eruption of an infant's chin and anterior chest area seen during teething. A form of miliaria due to excess saliva coming in contact with the skin. SYN: *red r.; tooth r.*

heat r. Miliaria.

hemorrhagic r. A rash consisting chiefly of hemorrhages or ecchymoses. SYN: *ecchymotic r.*

macular r. A rash in which the lesions are flat and level with the surrounding skin.

maculopapular r. A rash in which there are discrete macular and papular lesions or a combination of both.

mercurial r. A rash caused by local application of mercurial preparations.

mulberry r. A dusky rash seen in typhus fever.

nettle r. Urticaria.

red r. Gum r.

serum r. A pruritic, hivelike rash (urticaria or angioedema) or a vasculitis (palpable purpura) that accompanies serum sickness, which usually is caused by a hypersensitivity reaction to drugs or immune globulins obtained from animals. Malaise, joint pains, fevers, and other symptoms may accompany the rash. SEE: *serum sickness*.

sunburn-like r. A macular rash resembling the reddened skin character-

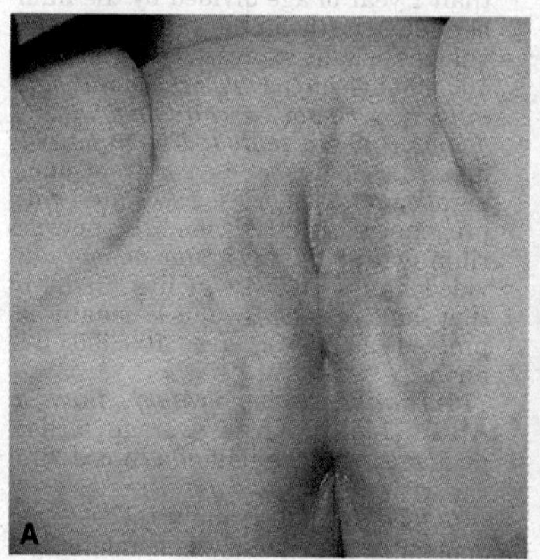

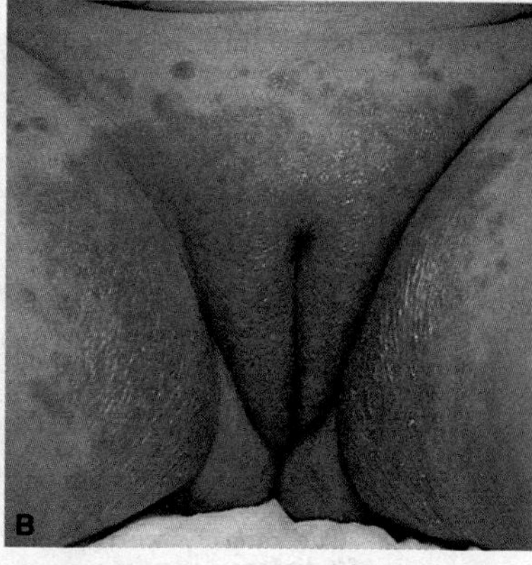

DIAPER RASH

(A) mild diaper rash, (B) severe yeast infection in diaper area

istic of a severe sunburn. SEE: *exfoliative dermatitis; toxic shock syndrome.*

tooth r. Gum r.

wandering r. Geographic tongue.

Rashkind procedure **1.** Balloon atrial septostomy. **2.** The closure of an atrial septal defect, ventricular septal defect, or patent ductus arteriosus with a double disk prosthesis that is placed during cardiac catheterization. It is used as an alternative to septostomy.

rasion (rā'zhŭn) [L. *rasio*] The grating of drugs by use of a file.

raspatory (răs'pă-tō"rē) [L. *raspatorium*] A file used in surgery, esp. for trimming bone surfaces. SYN: *xyster.*

RAST *radioallergosorbent test.*

Rastafarian cult A religious cult that originated in Jamaica in the 1930s and has members in the Caribbean, Europe, Canada, and the U.S. It is of medical importance because cult members' dietary practices may lead to vitamin B_{12} deficiency with subsequent neurological disease, megaloblastic anemia, or both.

rasura (ră-sū'ră) [L. *rasura,* a scraping] **1.** The process of scraping or shaving. **2.** Scrapings or filings.

rat [ME.] A rodent of the genus *Rattus,* found in and around human habitations. In addition to causing economic loss from crop destruction, rats are of primary importance in the spread of human and animal diseases. They are hosts of various protozoans, flukes, tapeworms, and threadworms, and reservoirs of amebiasis, murine and scrub typhus, and bubonic plague. Typhus and plague are transmitted to people mainly by the rat flea. Rats also transmit rat-bite fever.

rat-bite fever Either of two infectious diseases transmitted by the bite of a rat. One is caused by *Streptobacillus moniliformis* and is marked by skin inflammation, fever, chills, headache, vomiting, and back and joint pain. The other is caused by *Spirillum minus* and is associated with ulceration, rash, and recurrent fever. The latter disease is rare in the U.S. SYN: *sodokosis; sodoku.*

TREATMENT: Both diseases are treated with penicillin. Therapy is most effective when penicillin is given intravenously for 1 week, then orally for 1 week. Tetanus prophylaxis is also administered.

rate (rāt) [L. *rata,* calculated] The speed or frequency of occurrence of an event, usually expressed with respect to time or some other known standard.

acquisition r. In radiology, the speed with which medical images are recorded, usually expressed in images per second.

attack r. The rate of occurrence of new cases of a disease.

basal metabolic r. SEE: *basal metabolic rate.*

baseline fetal heart r. ABBR: FHR. Average range of beats per minute recorded within a 10-minute time frame. Normal range is between 120 and 160 beats per minute.

birth r. The number of live births per 1000 in the population in a given year.

case r. Morbidity r.

case fatality r. The percentage of individuals afflicted with an illness who die as a result of it.

death r. The number of deaths in a specified population, usually expressed per 100,000 population, over a given period, usually 1 year. SYN: *mortality r.*

DMF r. An expression pert. to dental caries in school children. It is noted how many teeth are decayed (D), missing or requiring extraction (M), and filled or with restorations (F). SEE: *DMF index.*

dose r. The quantity of medicine administered per unit of time.

erythrocyte sedimentation r. ABBR: ESR. SEE: *sedimentation r.*

false-negative r. The rate of occurrence of negative test results in individuals who actually have the attribute or disease for which they are being tested.

false-positive r. The rate of occurrence of positive test results in individuals who actually do not have the attribute or disease for which they are being tested.

fertility r. The number of births per year per 1000 women between ages 15 and 44 in a given population.

glomerular filtration r. ABBR: GFR. The rate of urine formation as plasma passes through the glomeruli of the kidneys.

growth r. The rate at which an individual, tissue, or organ grows over time.

heart r. The number of heartbeats per unit of time, usually expressed or written as number per minute.

infant mortality r. The number of deaths per year of live-born infants less than 1 year of age divided by the number of live births in the same year. This value is usually expressed as deaths per 100,000 live births. SEE: *neonatal mortality r.; perinatal mortality r.*

maternal mortality r. The number of maternal deaths in 1 year from puerperal causes (i.e., those associated with pregnancy, childbirth, and the puerperium) within 42 days after delivery divided by the number of live births in that same year. This value is usually expressed as deaths per 100,000 live births.

maximum midexpiratory flow r. ABBR: MMFR. The average airflow during the middle half of a forced vital capacity effort.

morbidity r. The number of cases per year of certain diseases in relation to the population in which they occur. SYN: *case r.*

mortality r. Death r.

neonatal mortality r. The number of

deaths in 1 year of infants aged 0 to 28 days divided by the number of live births in that same year. SEE: *maternal mortality r.; perinatal mortality r.*

peak expiratory flow r. The maximum rate of exhalation during a forced expiration, measured in liters per second or liters per minute. It is used as a test of airway obstruction.

perinatal mortality r. The number of stillbirths (in which the gestation period was 28 weeks or more) in the first 7 days of life divided by the number of live births plus stillbirths in the same year. This value is usually expressed as deaths per 100,000 live births plus stillbirths. SEE: *infant mortality r.; neonatal mortality r.*

periodontal disease r. SEE: *periodontal (Ramfjord) index.*

pulse r. The number of heartbeats per unit of time that can be detected by palpating any accessible artery.

respiration r. The number of breaths per unit of time.

sedimentation r. ABBR: ESR (erythrocyte sedimentation rate). A nonspecific laboratory test of the speed at which erythrocytes settle out of unclotted blood. In this test, blood to which an anticoagulant has been added is placed in a long, narrow tube, and the distance the red cells fall in 1 hr is the ESR. Normally, it is less than 10 mm/hr in men and slightly higher in women.

The speed at which the cells settle depends on how many red blood cells clump together. Clumping is increased by the presence of acute-phase proteins, released during inflammation. Therefore, the sedimentation rate indicates the presence of inflammation and is used to track the onset and progress of inflammatory disorders. An elevated ESR helps to differentiate an acute myocardial infarction from angina pectoris because no inflammation is present in the latter state.

ventilation r. ABBR: VR. The number of breaths per minute.

rate of perceived exertion ABBR: RPE. A 15-point grading scale developed by physiologist G. A. Borg, in which a patient reports his or her level of effort during exercise. The corresponding written descriptions range from "very light" to "very, very hard." The scale correlates well with cardiorespiratory and metabolic variables such as minute ventilation, heart rate, and blood lactate levels.

PATIENT CARE: This scale is helpful when patients are unable to take their own pulses during exercise or have abnormal heart rate responses to exercise.

Rathke's pouch (răth'kĕz) [Martin H. Rathke, Ger. anatomist, 1793–1860] A depression in the mouth of the embryo just anterior to the buccopharyngeal membrane. The anterior lobe of the pituitary arises from this structure.

ratio (rā'shē-ō) [L., computation] The relationship in degree or number between two things.

a–A r. The ratio of arterial oxygen partial pressure (PaO_2) to alveolar oxygen partial pressure (PAO_2), a measure of oxygen transfer across the lung. This figure is normally greater than 0.9.

A/G r. Albumin-globulin ratio.

albumin-globulin r. ABBR: A/G r. The ratio of albumin to globulin in blood plasma or serum. Normally this value is 1.3:1 to 3.0:1.

arm r. In chromosomes, the relation of the length of the long arm of the mitotic chromosome to that of the short arm.

beam nonuniformity r. ABBR: BNR. A measure of the homogeneity of a therapeutic ultrasound wave, expressed as a ratio between the ultrasound unit's average intensity (the metered output) and the peak intensity within the output wave. A completely homogeneous wave is represented by a 1:1 BNR.

CAUTION: FDA regulations require that the BNR be clearly labeled on therapeutic ultrasound units. A BNR of greater than 8:1 is considered to be potentially harmful.

---

body weight r. Body weight in grams divided by body height in centimeters.

cardiothoracic r. The relation of the overall diameter of the heart to the widest part of the inside of the thoracic cavity. Usually the heart's diameter is half or less than half that of the thoracic cavity.

common mode rejection r. ABBR: CMRR. The ability of an amplifier to amplify a signal in the presence of electrical noise. The higher the number, the better the amplification.

curative r. Therapeutic r.

dextrose-nitrogen r. The ratio of dextrose to nitrogen in urine.

false-negative r. ABBR: FNR. The ratio of subjects affected by an illness whose test results wrongly suggest they are disease-free to all those subjects who have the disease. The false-negative ratio of a test is useful in determining the test's reliability (i.e., the higher the ratio, the less reliable the test).

A high FNR may be biological or analytical in origin. Biological false-negative test results may occur when a test is performed at the wrong stage of an illness (e.g., before an antibody or antigen is found in the blood). Analytical false negatives may result when a test lacks adequate sensitivity or specificity to detect an agent that is already present.

false-positive r. ABBR: FPR. The ratio of patients who are disease-free but test positive for an illness, as a result of error, to all patients who do not have the disease.

grid r. In a radiographical grid, the ratio of the height of the lead strips to the distance of the interspace. High ratios indicate increased ability of the grid to remove scatter.

I:E r. In respiratory therapy or mechanical ventilation, the ratio of a patient's inspiratory to expiratory time.

international normalized r. ABBR: INR. The standard measurement of oral anticoagulation, introduced by the World Health Organization (WHO) in 1983 to replace the prothrombin time (PT). When a patient's blood is tested to determine its level of anticoagulation, the sample is treated with a thromboplastin, a laboratory reagent that may vary considerably depending on its chemical constituents. As a result, a single sample of blood tested in several different laboratories may give different PT results. To resolve the potential difficulties that this may create for patients who need to achieve a stable level of anticoagulation, the WHO has created the INR to be a rating scale for thromboplastins used around the world that standardizes the PT result. SEE: *International Sensitivity Index.*

PATIENT CARE: The INR is used in managing oral anticoagulant (warfarin) therapy. SEE: table.

lecithin-sphingomyelin r. ABBR: L/S ratio. One of several laboratory tests performed on amniotic fluid to determine the maturity of the fetal lungs. Other tests commonly used for this purpose include the amniotic lamellar body count, phosphatidylglycerol presence, and the shake test.

odds r. In epidemiological case-control studies, a relative measure of disease occurrence. The odds in favor of a particular disease occurring in an exposed group are divided by the odds in favor of its occurring in an unexposed group. If the condition being studied is rare, the odds ratio is a close approximation to the relative risk. SEE: *relative risk.*

P:F r. The ratio of arterial partial pressure of oxygen to inspired fractional concentration of oxygen; used to measure oxygen transfer.

sex r. The ratio of males to females in a given population, usually expressed as the number of males per 100 females. It is used in defining the proportion of births of the two sexes or in the representation by sexual distribution in certain diseases.

therapeutic r. The ratio obtained by dividing the effective therapeutic dose by the minimum lethal dose. SYN: *curative r.*

urea-reduction r. The relative decrease (or clearance) of blood urea nitrogen during hemodialysis. The ratio is a measure of the adequacy of renal replacement. The failure to achieve an adequate ratio leads to increased morbidity and mortality among renal failure patients.

ration (rā′shŭn) A fixed allowance of food and drink for a certain period.

rational (răsh′ŭn-ăl) [L. *rationalis,* reason] **1.** Of sound mind. SYN: *sane.* **2.** Reasonable or logical; employing treatments based on reasoning or general principles; opposed to empiric.

rationale (răsh″ŭn-ăl′) [L.] The logical or fundamental reason for a course of action or procedure.

rationalization (răsh″ŭn-ăl-ĭ-zā′shŭn) In psychology, a justification for an unreasonable or illogical act or idea to make it appear reasonable.

rationing Resource allocation in health care, esp. in managed health care systems.

rattle (răt′l) [ME. *ratelen,* to rattle] A coarse crackle heard during auscultation of the chest. This finding suggests excessive airway secretions are present.

death r. A gurgling sound or subcrepitant crackle heard in the breathing of patients with life-threatening respiratory illnesses.

rattlesnake A poisonous snake of the genus *Crotalus.* Its bite may produce coagulation disorders, anaphylaxis, or injury to local tissues.

raucous (raw′kŭs) [L. *raucus, hoarse*] Hoarse, harsh, as the sound of a voice.

Rauscher leukemia virus [Frank J. Rauscher, U.S. virologist, b. 1931] A virus known to cause leukemia in mice.

rauwolfia serpentina (raw-wŏlf′ē-ă) [Leonhard Rauwolf, Ger. botanist, 1535–1596] The dried roots of a tropical shrub of the family Apocynaceae, whose extracts are potent hypotensive and sedative drugs. Derivatives include reserpine, serpentine, and serpentinine.

Desirable Levels of Anticoagulation

Disease or Condition	Optimal Anticoagulant Range (INR)
Deep venous thrombosis	2.0 – 3.0
Pulmonary embolism	2.0 – 3.0
Stroke prevention in atrial fibrillation	2.0 – 3.0
Prevention of clots in patients with mechanical heart valves	2.5 – 3.5
Hypercoagulable states	Variable, but often 3.0 or higher

rave (rāv) [ME. *raven*, to be delirious] To talk irrationally, as in delirium.

raving **1.** Irrational utterance. **2.** Talking irrationally.

raw data The information obtained during an experiment, before the information has been analyzed or statistically manipulated.

ray (rā) [L. *radius*, ray] **1.** One of several lines diverging from a common center. **2.** A line of propagation of any form of radiant energy, esp. light or heat; loosely, any narrow beam of light.

actinic r. A solar ray capable of producing chemical changes. SYN: *chemical r.*

alpha r. A ray composed of positively charged helium particles derived from atomic disintegration of radioactive elements. Its velocity is one tenth the speed of light. Alpha rays are completely absorbed by a thin sheet of paper and possess powerful fluorescent, photographic, and ionizing properties. They penetrate tissues less than beta rays.

beta r. A ray composed of negatively charged electrons expelled from atoms of disintegrating radioactive elements. SYN: *beta particle.*

border r. Grenz r.

cathode r. A ray composed of negatively charged electrons discharged by a cathode through a vacuum, moving in a straight line and producing x-ray photons on hitting solid matter.

central r. The theoretical center of an x-ray beam. The term designates the direction of the x-ray photons as projected from the focal spot of the x-ray tube to the radiographical film.

characteristic r. A secondary photon produced by an electron giving up energy as it changes location from an outer to a more inner shell in an atom. The wavelengths are characteristic of the difference in binding energies.

chemical r. Actinic r.

cosmic r. Cosmic radiation.

delta r. Highly penetrative waves given off by radioactive substances.

erythema-producing r. Ultraviolet radiation (wavelengths between 2050 and 3100 A.U.) that is capable of reddening skin.

gamma r. Short wavelength, high-energy electromagnetic radiation emitted by disintegrating atomic nuclei.

grenz r. A low-energy x-ray photon with an average wavelength of 2 A.U. (range from 1 to 3 A.U.); obtained with peak voltage of less than 10 kV. Grenz rays lie between ultraviolet and x-rays. SYN: *border r.*

hard r. An x-ray photon of short wavelength and great penetrative power.

heat r. Radiation whose wavelength is between 3,900 and 14,000 A.U. Shorter wavelength heat sources penetrate tissues better than longer (infrared) sources. SEE: *heat.*

infrared r. An invisible heat ray from beyond the red end of the spectrum. Infrared wavelengths range from 7700 angstrom units (A.U.) to 1 mm. Long-wave infrared rays (15,000 to 150,000 A.U.) are emitted by all heated bodies and exclusively by bodies of low temperature such as hot water bottles and electric heating pads; short-wave infrared rays (7,200 to 15,000 A.U.) are emitted by all incandescent heaters. The sun, electric arcs, incandescent globes, and so-called infrared burners are sources of infrared rays.

USES: Infrared ray energy is transformed into heat in a superficial layer of the tissues. It is used therapeutically to stimulate local and general circulation and to relieve pain. The infrared thermograph, a device for detecting and photographing infrared rays, has been useful in studying the heat of tissues. This device has many applications such as in investigation of the rate of blood flow through a part. SEE: *radiation; thermography.*

luminous r. One of the visible rays of the spectrum.

medullary r. In the kidney, one of many slender processes composed of straight tubules that project into the cortex from the bases of renal pyramids. SYN: *pars radiata lobuli corticalis renis.*

monochromatic r. A ray characterized by a definite wavelength, as a secondary ray.

pigment-producing r. A ray between 2540 and 3100 A.U. that is most effective in stimulating pigment production in the skin. This is due to a local response to irritation of cutaneous prickle cells.

positive r. A ray composed of positively charged ions that in a discharge tube moves from the anode toward the cathode.

primary r. A ray discharged directly from a radioactive substance, as the alpha, beta, and gamma rays.

roentgen r. X-ray photon.

scattered r. An x-ray photon or gamma ray that has been deflected in its passage through a substance and changed by an increase in wavelength.

secondary r. X-ray photons produced after the incoming, primary x-ray photons remove an inner-shell electron from the atom. They are of lower energy than the primary radiation and usually are absorbed in matter.

ultraviolet r. An invisible ray of the spectrum beyond the violet rays. The wavelengths of ultraviolet rays vary. They may be refracted, reflected, and polarized, but will not traverse many substances impervious to the rays of the visible spectrum. They rapidly destroy the vitality of bacteria, and are able to produce photochemical and photographic effects.

Raynaud, Maurice (rā-nōz′) French physician, 1834–1881.

R.'s disease [Maurice Raynaud, Fr. physician, 1834–1881] A primary vasospastic disease of small arteries and arterioles; the cause is unknown. There is an exaggerated response of vasomotor controls to cold or emotion.

SYMPTOMS: Patients have intermittent vasospastic attacks of varying severity and frequency that affect the digits of the hands bilaterally; the toes are less commonly involved. Color changes occur in sequence, first white (pallor), then blue (cyanosis), and then red (hyperemia as blood flow returns). Initially, there is numbness and sensation of cold; during the red phase patients may have throbbing and paresthesia. Normal skin color returns after the attack. Patients with long-term disease may develop atrophy of the skin and subcutaneous tissues, brittle nails, and occasionally skin ulcerations or gangrene.

PATIENT CARE: Persons with this disease should maintain warmth in the extremities by wearing wool gloves and socks. They should avoid contact with cold materials and prolonged exposure to cold environments. Use of tobacco is contraindicated because of the vasoconstrictive effects of nicotine. Increasing hydrostatic pressure, and therefore circulation, by vigorous exercise of the arms may be useful. If attacks are prolonged and frequent, vasodilator drugs, including calcium channel blockers, may be helpful. A sympathectomy to prevent vasoconstriction may be tried but is not always successful.

R.'s phenomenon Intermittent attacks of pallor or cyanosis of the small arteries and arterioles of the fingers as the result of inadequate arterial blood flow. This condition is associated with scleroderma, systemic lupus erythematosus, Buerger's disease, nerve entrapment, and anorexia-bulimia. The signs, symptoms, and treatment are identical to those of Raynaud's disease. SEE: illus.; *Nursing Diagnoses Appendix.*

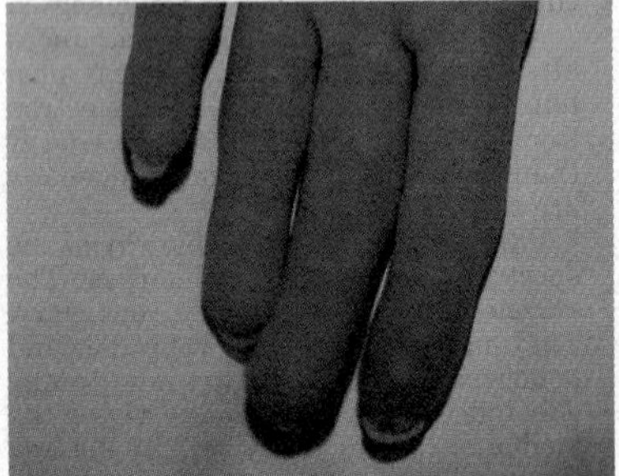

RAYNAUD'S PHENOMENON

rayon, purified A fibrous form of regenerated cellulose manufactured by the viscose process, desulfured, washed, and bleached. Once used in surgical dressings and bandages.

Rb Symbol for the element rubidium.

RBBB *right bundle branch block.*

RBC, rbc *red blood cell; red blood count.*

R.B.E. *relative biological effectiveness.*

RBRVS *resource-based relative value scale.*

R.C.D. *relative cardiac dullness.*

R.C.P. *Royal College of Physicians; Respiratory Care Practitioner.*

R.C.S. *Royal College of Surgeons.*

R.D. *Registered Dietitian.*

R.D.A. *right dorsoanterior,* presentation position of the fetus; *recommended dietary allowance.*

R.D.D.A. *recommended daily dietary allowance.*

R.D.H. *registered dental hygienist.*

RDMS *registered diagnostic medical sonographer.*

R.D.P. *right dorsoposterior,* presentation position of the fetus.

RDS *respiratory distress syndrome.*

R.E. *radium emanation; right eye; reticuloendothelium.*

Re Symbol for the element rhenium.

re- [L.] Prefix meaning *back, again.*

reabsorb (rē″ăb-sorb′) To absorb again.

reabsorption (rē″ăb-sorp′shŭn) The process of absorbing again. It occurs in the kidney when some of the materials filtered out of the blood by the glomerulus are reabsorbed as the filtrate passes through the nephron.

reacher A type of extension device for assisting persons with limited reach to grasp and manipulate objects in the performance of everyday tasks.

react (rē-ăkt′) [L. *re,* again, + *agere,* to act] **1.** To respond to a stimulus. **2.** To participate in a chemical reaction.

reactant (rē-ăk′tănt) A chemical or substance taking part in a chemical reaction.

acute phase r. Any one of several serum proteins that increase or decrease in response to the progress or decline of inflammation.

reaction (rē-ăk′shŭn) [LL. *reactus,* reacted] **1.** The response of an organism, or part of it, to a stimulus. **2.** In chemistry, a chemical process or change; transformation of one substance into another in response to a stimulus. **3.** An opposing action or counteraction. **4.** An emotional and mental response to a stimulus.

acrosomal r. The release of enzymes from the head of the sperm, a complex process that helps sperm to penetrate the zona pellucida of the egg and thus to begin fertilization.

alarm r. The first stage in the general adaptation syndrome, which includes changes occurring in the body when subjected to stressful stimuli. Physiological changes that occur are direct results of damage, shock, or both, or reactions of the body to defend itself against shock.

allergic r. A reaction resulting from hypersensitivity to an antigen. SEE: *allergy; hypersensitivity.*

anamnestic r. The rapid reappearance of antibodies in the blood as a result of a second contact with a foreign antigen, due to the presence of antigen-specific memory B cells, which were created during the first contact with the antigen.

anaphylactic r. Anaphylaxis.

anaphylactoid r. A reaction that resembles anaphylaxis (e.g., characterized by hives, angioedema, laryngeal edema, or shock) but does not involve IgE antibodies or allergens, and therefore is without an allergic basis.

ETIOLOGY: This relatively uncommon type of reaction can be caused by exercise; as the result of the release of histamine when body temperature rises or elevated endorphin levels; by ionic compounds, such as contrast media that contain radiographic iodine, or polymyxin B antibiotic; by solutions containing polysaccharides, such as dextran; by morphine, codeine, or meperidine; and by NSAIDs. The term should not be used as a synonym for mild anaphylaxis produced by IgE-allergen reactions.

SYMPTOMS: Anaphylactoid reactions produce hives and itching identical to those caused by anaphylaxis. Very rarely severe anaphylaxis or anaphylactic shock occurs. Anaphylactoid reactions are treated with the same drugs used to treat anaphylaxis.

antigen-antibody r. The combination of an antigen with its specific antibody. It may result in agglutination, precipitation, neutralization, complement fixation, or increased susceptibility to phagocytosis. The antigen-antibody reaction forms the basis for B-cell–mediated immunity.

anxiety r. Anxiety disorder.

Arias-Stella r. A reaction marked by decidual changes in the endometrial epithelium. These changes consist of hyperchromatic cells with large nuclei; they may be associated with ectopic pregnancy.

automatic movement r. Automatic r.

automatic r. A category of reflexes that includes righting and equilibrium reactions. SYN: *automatic movement r.*

biuret r. Biuret test.

chain r. A self-renewing reaction in which the initial stage triggers a subsequent reaction, which in turn causes the next, and so on.

complement-fixation r. A reaction seen when complement enters into combinations formed between soluble or particulate antigens and antibody. It is used to diagnosis many infectious illnesses, including chlamydia, syphilis, and mycoplasma, among many others. SEE: *complement; complement fixation.*

consensual r. **1.** An involuntary action. **2.** A crossed reflex.

conversion r. A type of neurosis in which loss or alteration of physical functioning suggests a physical disorder but instead expresses a psychological conflict or need. The disturbance is not under voluntary control and cannot be explained by a disease process; it is not limited to pain or sexual dysfunction. SEE: *somatoform disorder.*

cross r. A reaction between an antibody and an antigen that is similar to the specific antigen for which the antibody was created. It enables immunoglobulins to cross-link and activate B cells.

defense r. A mental response whose purpose (according to classical psychoanalysis) is to protect the ego.

r. of degeneration A change in muscle reactivity to electricity, seen in lower motor neuron paralysis.

delayed r. A reaction occurring a considerable time after a stimulus, esp. a reaction such as a skin inflammation occurring hours or days after exposure to the allergen.

delayed hypersensitivity r. A localized skin response mediated by T cells, which occurs 24 to 72 hr after injection of a specific antigen to which the person has been previously sensitized. It is used routinely to screen for tuberculosis infection through injection with purified protein derivative of *Mycobacterium tuberculosis*. In patients with immunodeficiency, common microbial antigens to which most people have been exposed, such as diphtheria, tetanus, measles, or *Candida,* are used to determine the presence of defects in T-cell–mediated immunity (CMI). If patients do not develop induration at the site, indicating a positive response to the antigen, a CMI defect is present. Delayed hypersensitivity is a type IV hypersensitivity reaction mediated by cytokines released by macrophages and T helper cells.

dissociative r. A sudden, temporary alteration in the normal functions of consciousness, identity, or motor behavior. SEE: *dissociation* (3).

false-negative r. A test result that is negative in an individual who nonetheless has the attribute or disease being tested for.

false-positive r. A positive reaction in a test in a person who is actually healthy due to faulty technique or the presence of another disease.

foreign body r. A localized inflammatory response elicited by any material (e.g., a splinter or a suture) that would not normally be found within the body.

hemianopic r. A reaction in which the pupils of both eyes fail to react to a thin pencil of light from the blind side but react normally to light from the normal side. It is seen in some forms of homonymous hemianopia.

hemiopic pupillary r. A reaction in which light from one side causes the iris to contract but light from the other side does not cause the contraction. It is seen in certain cases of hemianopia.

hypersensitivity r. Allergy.

immune-mediated inflammatory r. The process by which the immune system destroys, dilutes, or walls off injurious agents and injured tissue. Small blood vessels dilate and become permeable. This increases blood flow and permits exudation of plasma and leukocytes. The cells arriving from the blood include monocytes, neutrophils, basophils, and lymphocytes; those of local origin include endothelial cells, mast cells, tissue fibroblasts, and macrophages. Other mediators of inflammation include cytokines, interleukins, and neuropathies.

intracutaneous r. A reaction following the injection of a substance into the skin. SYN: *intradermal r.* SEE: *skin test.*

intradermal r. Intracutaneous r.

late-phase r. Inflammation of any part of the body caused by the release of cytokines; leukotrienes B4, C4, and D4; and prostaglandin D2, occurring approx. 6 hours after the body's initial response to an antigen, during a type I hypersensitivity response. Late-phase reactions play a significant role in prolonging illnesses such as asthma after the initial, immediate histamine-based response has subsided. These are treated with and prevented by the use of corticosteroids, such as prednisone, and other drugs.

leukemoid r. An extreme elevation in the white blood cell count (about 50,000 cells/mm^3), which superficially resembles a leukemia but which has another explanation, such as severe infection, trauma, large burn, ketoacidosis, or other stressful illness.

ligase chain r. A technique for amplifying the quantity of specific sequences of nucleic acid in a specimen. The patient's DNA, or specimens thought to contain pathogenic DNA, are mixed with DNA ligase and oligonucleotide probes. Double-stranded DNA is denatured. Probes bind to the complementary strands on any denatured target DNA. Ligase joins the bound probes, and multiple copies of the DNA of interest are made. In clinical practice, ligase chain reactions are used primarily in urinary (noninvasive) assays to detect genital infections with chlamydia or gonorrhea.

local r. A reaction occurring at the point of stimulation or injection of foreign substances.

myasthenic r. A gradual decrease and eventual cessation of muscle contractions when a muscle is stimulated repeatedly.

neutral r. In chemistry, a reaction indicating the absence of acid or alkaline properties; expressed as pH 7.0.

ophthalmic r. SEE: *ophthalmic reaction.*

persistent light r. Photosensitivity.

Prausnitz-Küstner r. SEE: *Prausnitz-Küstner reaction.*

quellung r. The swelling of capsules of bacteria when they are mixed with their specific immune serum.

tuberculin r. Tuberculin test.

wheal and flare r. The response within 10 to 15 min to an antigen injected into the skin. The injected skin elevates and blanches, and becomes surrounded by a red rim of inflamed tissue.

reactivate To make active again, for example, to restore to a physiological response or to awaken a dormant infection.

reactivation (rē-ăk″tĭ-vā′shŭn) The process of making something active again.

reactivity (rē″ăk-tĭv′ĭ-tē) **1.** The ability to respond to a stimulus. **2.** In measurement of function or behavior, the influence that the presence of the examiner and the assessment process may have on performance and therefore on the outcome or finding.

cross r. The ability of an antibody to bind with more than one antigen or of an antigen to bind with more than one antibody.

Read method [Grantley Dick-Read, Brit. physician, 1890–1959] The original psychoprophylactic method of prepared childbirth, based on the premise that fear causes tension, which generates or increases pain during labor. Women are taught to control the response to each uterine contraction with slow abdominal breathing. Each breath is evenly divided between inhalation and exhalation.

reading Interpreting or perusing written or printed characters or material. Reading may or may not include comprehension of the material.

lip r. Interpretation of what is being spoken by watching the movements of the speaker's lips.

pulse r. In traditional Chinese medicine, assessment of the pulse as an aid in diagnosis.

reading disorder A condition that interferes with or prevents comprehension of written or printed material; used esp. in reference to children. In some adults, the condition may have developed from a brain injury or may have persisted from infancy. SEE: *dyslexia*.

reading machine for the blind An electronic device that converts printed matter into speech. Several machines for home use are available. Information may be obtained from the Lighthouse National Center for Vision and Aging at (800) 334-5497 or the American Foundation for the Blind at (800) 232-5463.

reagent (rē-ā′jĕnt) [L. *reagere,* to react] **1.** A substance involved in a chemical reaction. **2.** A substance used to detect the presence or amount of another substance. **3.** A subject of a psychological experiment, esp. one reacting to a stimulus.

reagin (rē′ă-jĭn) A type of immunoglobulin E (IgE) present in the serum of atopic individuals that mediates hypersensitivity reactions.

rapid plasma r. ABBR: RPR. A nonspecific serological test for syphilis. The RPR titer is elevated in most patients with syphilis (and falsely elevated in some patients with other diseases). The titer decreases or returns to normal after successful eradication of the disease.

reaginic (rē-ă-jĭn′ĭk), *adj.*

reality The quality of being genuine or actual.

reality orientation An intervention intended to orient persons with early dementia or delirium. It involves repetition of verbal and nonverbal information. The environment remains constant and the person is reminded and reviewed about names, dates, weather, and other pertinent information.

reality principle (rē-ăl′ĭ-tē) Awareness of external demands and adjustment in a manner that meets these demands, yet assures continued self-gratification.

reality testing The attempt by the individual to evaluate and understand the real world and his or her relation to it.

reality therapy A psychiatric treatment based on the concept that some patients deny the reality of the world around them. Therapy is directed to assist such patients in recognizing and accepting the present situation. The main technique is confrontation; the purpose of the confrontation is to minimize distortion, and improve coping and insight.

reamer (rē′mĕr) A small instrument used in dentistry for enlarging the root canal of a tooth.

reanastomosis, surgical The rejoining of structures, esp. vessels or tubes, that had been previously ligated.

reanimate (rē-ăn′ĭ-māt) [L. *re,* again, + *animare,* fill with life] To reactivate, restore to life, revive, or resuscitate.

reapers' keratitis (rēp′ĕrs kĕr-ă-tī′tĭs) Corneal inflammation caused by grain dust. SEE: *keratitis*.

rearfoot Hindfoot.

reasonable care In law, the degree of care that an ordinarily prudent person or professional would exercise under given circumstances.

reasonable cost The amount a third party (usually the medical insurer) will actually reimburse for health care. This amount is based on the cost to the provider for delivering that service.

reasonable and customary fees In health care finance, the prevailing reimbursement for health services or medical care in a specific region or state.

reattachment (rē″ă-tăch′mĕnt) **1.** Recementing of a dental crown. **2.** Reembedding of periodontal ligament fibers into the cementum of a tooth that has become dislodged. **3.** Rejoining of parts that have been separated, as a finger that has been traumatically detached.

rebase (rē-bās′) To refit a denture by replacing the base material without altering the occlusal characteristics.

rebound [ME. *rebounden,* to leap back] A reflex response in which sudden withdrawal of a stimulus is followed by increased activity, such as an increase in heart rate or blood pressure when beta-blocking drugs or clonidine are withheld.

rebound phenomenon **1.** In pharmacology and physiology, the worsening of a disease or condition (e.g., hypertension or anxiety) when a drug used to treat the condition is suddenly withdrawn. **2.** A symptom indicating a cerebellar lesion. When a limb or part is acting against a resistance and the resistance is suddenly removed, the limb moves forcibly in the direction toward which effort was being directed.

rebreathing The inhalation of gases that had been previously exhaled.

Rebuck skin window test An in vivo method of assessing inflammation. A superficial abrasion is made in the skin and a glass coverslip applied to the area. Leukocytes accumulate at the site and adhere to the coverslip.

recalcification (rē″kăl-sĭ-fĭ-kā′shŭn) [L. *re,* again, + *calx,* lime, + *facere,* to make] The restoration of calcium salts to tissues from which they have been withdrawn.

recall [″ + AS. *ceallian,* to call] The act of bringing back to mind something previously learned or experienced. SEE: *memory*.

24-hr dietary r. One means of obtaining a diet history in which the individual being assessed lists all the foods along with the portion size of everything eaten or drunk in the preceding 24 hr. The information obtained is rarely accurate enough to be valid.

recanalization Re-establishment of an opening through a vessel that had been previously occluded.

receiver (rē-sēv′ĕr) [" + *capere*, to take] **1.** A container for holding a gas or a distillate. **2.** An apparatus for receiving electric waves or current, such as a radio receiver.

receptaculum (rē″sĕp-tăk′ū-lŭm) *pl.* **receptacula** [L.] A vessel or cavity in which a fluid is contained.

r. chyli Inferior, pear-shaped, expanded portion of the lower end of the thoracic duct, near the first and second lumbar vertebrae, into which the right and left lumbar trunks, an intestinal trunk, and some thoracic vessels empty. SYN: *cisterna chyli*.

receptor (rē-sĕp′tor) [L., a receiver] **1.** In cell biology, a structure in the cell membrane that combines with a drug, hormone, infectious particle, or chemical mediator to alter the function of the cell. **2.** A sensory nerve ending. SYN: *ceptor*.

accessory r. Proteins on the surface of T lymphocytes that enhance the response of the T-cell receptor to foreign antigens and stimulate signals from the receptor to the cytoplasm. SEE: *antigen-presenting cell; T-cell receptor*.

adrenergic r. A cell membrane protein that mediates the effects of adrenergic stimulation on target organs by catecholamines.

antigen r. Receptors, primarily on white blood cells, that bind with the epitope on foreign antigens, stimulating an immune response.

auditory r. One of the hair cells in the organ of Corti in the cochlea of the ear.

cell r. Cell membrane proteins or intracellular proteins that react with chemicals (e.g., hormones) circulating in the cell's environment. The reaction triggers the cell's characteristic response to the hormone or other chemical. SEE: *drug r.*

cholinergic r. A site in a nerve synapse or effector cell that responds to the effect of acetylcholine.

complement r. ABBR: CR. A receptor on phagocytes, neutrophils, and macrophages that allows complement factors to bind, thus stimulating inflammation, phagocytosis, and cell destruction.

contact r. A receptor that produces a sensation such as touch, temperature, or pain that can be localized in or on the surface of the body.

cutaneous r. A receptor located in the skin.

distance r. Teleceptor.

drug r. A protein-containing complex on a cell membrane that is capable of being stimulated by drugs in the extracellular fluid and translating that stimulation into an intracellular response. There may be thousands of such receptors on the surface of each cell. SYN: *cell r.*

gravity r. A macular hair cell of the utricle and saccule. It responds to changes in position of the head and linear acceleration.

immunologic r. A receptor on the surface of white blood cells that identifies the type of cell and links with monokines, lymphokines, or other chemical mediators during the immune response.

killer cell inhibitory r. ABBR: KIR. Molecules on the surface of natural killer (NK) cells that bind with major histocompatibility complex (MHC) class I markers and inhibit the ability of NK cells to destroy target cells. Different groups of KIRs may create subsets of NK cells that bind to and destroy different targets.

olfactory r. One of the bipolar nerve cells found in olfactory epithelium whose axons form olfactory nerve fibers.

optic r. A rod or cone cell of the retina.

proprioceptive r. A muscle or tendon spindle. These are the receptors of muscle or kinesthetic stimuli.

rotary r. One of the hair cells in the cristae of the ampulla of the semicircular ducts of the ear. It is stimulated by angular acceleration or rotation.

ryanodine r. ABBR: RyR. The release channel for calcium ions that is found on the membranes of the sarcoplasmic reticulum of skeletal muscles.

sensory r. A sensory nerve ending, a cell or group of cells, or a sense organ that when stimulated produces an afferent or sensory impulse.

CLASSIFICATION: *Exteroreceptors* are receptors located on or near the surface that respond to stimuli from the outside world. They include eye and ear receptors (for remote stimuli) and touch, temperature, and pain receptors (for contact). *Interoceptors* are those in the mucous linings of the respiratory and digestive tracts that respond to internal stimuli; also called visceroceptors. *Proprioceptors* are those responding to stimuli arising within body tissues.

Receptors also are classified according to the nature of stimuli to which they respond. These include *chemoreceptors,* which respond to chemical substances (taste buds, olfactory cells, receptors in aortic and carotid bodies); *pressoreceptors,* which respond to pressure (receptors in the aortic and carotid sinuses); *photoreceptors,* which respond to light (rods and cones); and *tactile receptors,* which respond to touch (Meissner's corpuscle).

stretch r. One of the neuromuscular and neurotendinar spindles and organs of Golgi, which are stimulated by stretch. SEE: *proprioceptor*.

taste r. A gustatory cell of a taste bud.

temperature r. A Krause's end-bulb

(a cold receptor) or a Ruffini's corpuscle (a warmth receptor).

touch r. A Merkel's disk, a Meissner's corpuscle, or a nerve plexus around a hair root.

receptosome Endosome.

recess (rē′sĕs) [L. *recessus,* receded] A small indentation, depression, or cavity. SYN: *recessus.*

cochlear r. A small concavity, lying between the two limbs of the vestibular crest in the vestibule of the ear, that lodges the beginning of the cochlear duct.

elliptical r. A small concavity lying superiorly and posteriorly on the medial wall of the vestibule that lodges the utricle of the ear.

epitympanic r. Attic.

infundibular r. A small projection of the third ventricle that extends into the infundibular stalk of the hypophysis.

lateral r. of fourth ventricle One of two lateral extensions of the fourth ventricle, forming narrow pockets on each side and around the upper portions of the restiform bodies.

nasopalatine r. A small depression on the floor of the nasal cavity near the nasal septum, lying immediately over the incisive foramen.

omental r. One of three pocket-like extensions of the omental bursa. The superior recess extends upward behind the caudate lobe of the liver, the inferior recess extends downward into the great omentum, and the lineal recess extends laterally to the hilus of the spleen.

optic r. A pocket of the third ventricle lying anterior to the infundibular recess. It is bound inferiorly by the optic chiasma.

pharyngeal r. A recess in the lateral wall of the nasopharynx lying above and behind the opening to the auditory tube. SYN: *Rosenmüller's fossa.*

pineal r. Recess of the roof of the third ventricle extending into the stalk of the pineal body.

piriform r. A deep depression in the wall of the laryngeal pharynx lying lateral to the orifice of the larynx. It is bounded laterally by the thyroid cartilage and medially by the cricoid and arytenoid cartilages. It is a common site for lodgment of foreign objects.

sphenoethmoidal r. A small space in the nasal fossa above the superior concha. It lies between the ethmoid bone and the anterior surface of the body of the sphenoid bone and posteriorly receives the opening of the sphenoidal sinus.

spherical r. A recess on the medial wall of the vestibule of the inner ear that accommodates the saccule.

suprapineal r. A posterior extension of the roof of the third ventricle forming a small cavity above the pineal body.

tympanic membrane r. One of two pouches of tympanic mucous membrane (anterior and posterior) lying between the tympanic membrane and anterior and posterior malleolar folds.

umbilical r. A dilatation on the left main branch of the portal vein that marks the position where the umbilical vein was originally attached.

recession (rē-sĕsh′ŭn) [L. *recessus,* recess] The withdrawal of a part from its normal position.

gingival r. Apical migration of the gingiva resulting from faulty toothbrushing technique, tooth malposition, friction from soft tissues, gingival inflammation, and high frenum attachment. The incidence of recession may result in sensitivity, increased susceptibility to caries, and difficulty maintaining clean teeth. SEE: *gingivitis.*

recessive Tending to recede or go back; lacking control; not dominant.

recessus (rē-sĕs′ŭs) [L.] Recess.

recidivation (rē-sĭd″ĭ-vā′shŭn) [L. *recidivus,* falling back] **1.** The relapse of a disease or recurrence of a symptom. **2.** The return to criminal activity.

recidivism Habitual criminality; the repetition of antisocial acts.

recidivist **1.** A confirmed criminal. **2.** A patient, esp. one with mental illness, who has repeated relapses into behavior marked by antisocial acts.

recidivity Tendency to relapse, or to return to a former condition.

recipe (rĕs′ĭ-pē) [L., take] **1.** Take, indicated by the sign ℞. **2.** A prescription or formula for a medicine. SEE: *prescription.*

recipient (rĭ-sĭp′ē-ĕnt) [L. *recipiens,* receiving] One who receives something, esp. blood, tissues, or an organ, provided by a donor, as in a blood transfusion or kidney transplant. SEE: *donor.*

reciprocal (rĭ-sĭp′rō-kăl) [L. *reciprocus,* alternate] Interchangeable.

reciprocal inhibition **1.** The inhibition of muscles antagonistic to those being facilitated; this is essential for coordinated movement. **2.** Inhibition of a complementary nerve center by the one being stimulated (e.g., the inspiration center in the medulla generates impulses to the respiratory muscles to bring about inhalation, and inhibits the expiration center at the same time).

reciprocation (rĭ-sĭp″rō-kā′shŭn) [L. *reciprocare,* to move backward and forward] The countering of a reaction by an action. In dentistry, the action of one part of a dental device to counter the effect of another part.

reciprocity The recognition by one state of the license to practice granted to a health care professional by another state.

Recklinghausen, Friedrich D. von (rĕk′lĭng-how″zĕn) German pathologist, 1833–1910.

R.'s canals Rootlets of the lymphatics, minute spaces in connective tissue. SYN: *von Recklinghausen's canals*.

R.'s disease Type 1 neurofibromatosis.

R.'s tumor An adenoleiomyofibroma on the wall of the fallopian tube or the posterior uterine wall. SYN: *von Recklinghausen's tumor*.

reclination (rĕk″lĭ-nā′shŭn) [L. *reclinatio,* lean back] The turning of a cataract-covered lens over into the vitreous to remove it from the line of vision.

recline (rē-klīn′) [L. *reclinare*] To be in recumbent position; to lie down.

Reclus' disease (rā-klooz′) [Paul Reclus, Fr. surgeon, 1847–1914] Multiple benign cystic growths in the breast.

recombinant In genetics and molecular biology, pert. to genetic material combined from different sources.

recombinant DNA Segments of DNA from one organism artificially manipulated or inserted into the DNA of another organism, using a technique known as gene splicing. When the host's genetic material is reproduced, the transplanted genetic material is also copied. This technique permits isolating and examining the properties and action of specific genes. SEE: *plasmid; gene splicing*.

recombinant TPA Tissue plasminogen activator.

recombination (rē″kŏm-bĭ-nā′shŭn) **1.** Joining again. **2.** In genetics, the joining of gene combinations in the offspring that were not present in the parents.

recomposition [L. *re,* again, + *composer,* to place together] The recombination of constituents or parts.

recompression [″ + LL. *compressare,* press together] The resubjection of a person to increased atmospheric pressure, a procedure used in the treatment of caisson disease (bends).

reconcentration The process of repeated concentration.

reconstitution (rē″kŏn-stĭ-tū′shŭn) The return of a substance previously altered for preservation and storage to its original state, as is done with dried blood plasma.

reconstruction Surgical repair or restoration of a missing part or organ.

r. of the knee Procedures to reestablish knee stability following injury, usually to the anterior or posterior cruciate ligaments or both.

neovaginal r. Construction of an artificial vagina after the vagina has been removed because of cancer, or trauma of the pelvic area. The tissue used may be obtained from muscle and skin tissue from the abdomen. Normal sexual function is possible after the area has healed.

record (rĕk′ord) **1.** A written account of something. SEE: *problem-oriented medical record*. **2.** In dentistry, a registration of jaw relations in a malleable material or on a device.

functional chew-in r. A record of the natural chewing action of the mandible made on an occlusion rim by the teeth or scribing studs.

interocclusal r. A record of the positional relationship of the teeth or jaws to each other. A plastic material that hardens is placed between the teeth, and the patient bites down on it.

medication administration r. ABBR: MAR. A file maintained on hospital wards that documents the schedule and dosing of medications given to patients.

recover (rĭ-kŭv′ĕr) [O.Fr. *recoverer*] **1.** To regain health after illness; to regain a former state of health. **2.** To regain a normal state, as to recover from fright.

recovery (rĭ-kŭv′ĕr-ē) **1.** The process or act of becoming well or returning to a state of health. **2.** Compensation awarded by a court to individuals who prevailed in a lawsuit (e.g., those who had been injured as a result of the health care provider's negligence or malpractice).

delayed surgical r. An extension of the number of postoperative days required for individuals to initiate and perform on their own behalf activities that maintain life, health, and wellbeing. SEE: *Nursing Diagnoses Appendix*.

inversion r. In magnetic resonance imaging, a standard pulse sequence used to produce T1 weighted images.

recovery position The position in which the patient is placed on the left side with the left arm moved aside and supported to allow for lung expansion and the right leg crossed over the left. This position affords the unconscious, breathing patient the best protection from airway occlusion or aspiration of fluids into the lungs.

recreation Participation in any endeavor that is entertaining, relaxing, or refreshing. Recreational activities may be personal or private (e.g., reading, painting), social (e.g., team sports or dance), physical (e.g., hunting), or mental (e.g., meditating or praying); they may be active or passive. Many recreational activities combine more than one of these elements.

recredentialing The process whereby an individual certified in a profession completes the current requirements for certification in that profession.

recrement (rĕk′rē-mĕnt) [L. *recrementum,* sifted again] A secretion, such as saliva or part of the bile, that is reabsorbed by the body.

recrudescence (rē″kroo-dĕs′ĕns) Relapse.

recrudescent (rē″kroo-dĕs′ĕnt) Assuming renewed activity after a dormant or inactive period.

recruitment (rĭ-kroot′mĕnt) [O.Fr. *recrute,* new growth] **1.** An increased response to a reflex when a stimulus is prolonged, even though the strength of the stimulus is unchanged, due to activation of increasingly greater numbers of motor neurons **2.** In audiology, an increase in the perceived intensity of a sound out of proportion to the actual increase in the sound level. **3.** The addition of staff to a hospital or clinic during expansion of employment.

r. of end organs An increase in discharge from sensory end organs, resulting from an increase in the number of end organs discharging and an increase in frequency of discharge from each.

rectal (rĕk′tăl) [L. *rectus,* straight] Pert. to the rectum.

rectal crisis Tenesmus and rectal pain in locomotor ataxia.

rectalgia (rĕk-tăl′jē-ă) [L. *rectus,* straight, + Gr. *algos,* pain] Pain in the rectum.

rectal reflex The normal desire to evacuate feces present in the rectum.

rectification (rĕk″tĭ-fĭ-kā′shŭn) [″ + *facere,* to make] **1.** The process of refining or purifying a substance. **2.** The act of straightening or correcting. **3.** The process of changing an alternating current into a pulsating direct current.

rectified (rĕk′tĭ-fīd) Made pure or straight; set right.

rectifier (rĕk′tĭ-fī″ĕr) [L. *rectum,* straight, + *-ficare,* to make] In electricity, a device for transforming an alternating current into a pulsating direct current.

rectitis (rĕk-tī′tĭs) Proctitis.

recto- Combining form meaning *straight.*

rectoabdominal (rĕk″tō-ăb-dŏm′ĭ-năl) [L. *rectus,* straight, + *abdomen,* belly] Pert. to the rectum and abdomen.

rectocele (rĕk′tō-sēl) [″ + Gr. *kele,* tumor, swelling] Protrusion or herniation of the posterior vaginal wall with the anterior wall of the rectum through the vagina. SEE: *cystocele.*

rectoclysis (rĕk-tŏk′lĭ-sĭs) [″ + Gr. *klysis,* a washing] The slow introduction of fluid into the rectum.

rectococcygeal (rĕk-tō-kŏk-sĭj′ē-ăl) [″ + Gr. *kokkyx,* coccyx] Pert. to the rectum and coccyx.

rectococcypexia (rĕk″tō-kŏk-sĭ-pĕks′sē-ă) [″ + ″ + *pexis,* fixation] Fixation of the rectum by suturing it to the coccyx.

rectocolitis (rĕk″tō-kō-lī′tĭs) Proctocolitis.

rectocystotomy (rĕk″tō-sĭs-tŏt′ō-mē) [″ + Gr. *kystis,* bladder, + *tome,* incision] An incision of the bladder through the rectum, usually to remove a stone.

rectolabial (rĕk″tō-lā′bē-ăl) [″ + *labium,* lip] Pert. to the rectum and a labium of the vulva.

rectoperineorrhaphy (rĕk″tō-pĕr″ĭ-nē-or′ă-fē) Proctoperineoplasty.

rectopexy (rĕk′tō-pĕk-sē) Proctopexia.

rectophobia (rĕk″tō-fō′bē-ă) [″ + Gr. *phobos,* fear] Acute anxiety in patients with rectal disease concerning the possibility of having cancer.

rectoplasty (rĕk′tō-plăs″tē) Proctoplasty.

rectorrhaphy (rĕk-tor′ă-fē) Proctorrhaphy.

rectoscope (rĕk′tō-skōp) [″ + Gr. *skopein,* to examine] Proctoscope.

rectoscopy (rĕk-tŏs′kō-pē) Proctoscopy.

rectosigmoid (rĕk″tō-sĭg′moyd) [″ + Gr. *sigma,* letter S, + *eidos,* form, shape] The upper part of the rectum and the adjoining portion of the sigmoid colon.

rectosigmoidectomy (rĕk″tō-sĭg″moy-dĕk′tō-mē) [″ + ″ + *ektome,* excision] Surgical removal of the rectum and sigmoid colon.

rectostenosis (rĕk″tō-stĕn-ō′sĭs) [″ + Gr. *stenos,* narrow] Stricture of the rectum.

rectostomy (rĕk-tŏs′tō-mē) Proctostomy.

rectotomy (rĕk-tŏt′ō-mē) Proctotomy.

rectourethral (rĕk″tō-ū-rē′thrăl) [″ + Gr. *ourethra,* urethra] Pert. to the rectum and urethra.

rectouterine (rĕk″tō-ū′tĕr-ĭn) [″ + *uterus,* womb] Pert. to the rectum and uterus.

rectovaginal (rĕk″tō-văj′ĭ-năl) [″ + *vagina,* sheath] Pert. to the rectum and vagina.

rectovesical (rĕk″tō-vĕs′ĭ-kăl) [″ + *vesica,* bladder] Pert. to the rectum and bladder.

rectovestibular (rĕk″tō-vĕs-tĭb′ū-lăr) [″ + *vestibulum,* vestibule] Pert. to the rectum and vestibule of the vagina.

rectovulvar (rĕk″tō-vŭl′văr) [″ + *vulva,* covering] Pert. to the rectum and vulva.

rectum (rĕk′tŭm) [L., straight] The lower part of the large intestine, about 5 in. (12.7 cm) long, between the sigmoid colon and the anal canal. The centers for the defecation reflex are in the second, third, and fourth sacral segments of the spinal cord. SEE: *colon* for illus.

rectus (rĕk′tŭs) [L.] Straight; not crooked.

rectus muscle **1.** One of two external abdominal muscles on either side, from the pubic bone to the xiphoid process and the fifth, sixth, and seventh ribs. **2.** One of the four short muscles of the eye: lateral, medial, superior, and inferior.

recumbency (rĭ-kŭm′bĕn-sē) [L. *recumbens,* lying down] The condition of leaning or reclining.

recumbent **1.** Lying down. SEE: *position,*

left lateral recumbent; position, unilateral recumbent; prone. **2.** Inactive, idle.

dorsal r. Lying on one's back. SYN: *supine* (1).

lateral r. Lying on one's side.

ventral r. Lying with one's anterior side down. SYN: *prone* (1).

recuperation (rĭ-kū″pĕr-ā′shŭn) [L. *recuperare,* to recover] The process of returning to normal health following an illness.

recurrence (rĭ-kŭr′ĕns) Relapse. **recurrent** (-ĕnt), *adj.*

recurvation (rĭ″kŭr-vā′shŭn) [L. *recurvus,* bent back] The act of bending backward.

recurvatum Backward bowing. At the knee, it is called genu recurvatum or back knee.

recurve (rē-kŭrv′) To bend backward.

red (rĕd) [AS. *read*] A primary color of the spectrum that, when added to blue, forms green, and when added to yellow, forms orange.

Congo r. An odorless red-brown powder used in testing for amyloid. In polarized light, amyloid treated with Congo red produces a green fluorescence.

cresol r. An indicator of pH. It is yellow below pH 7.4 and red above 9.0.

methyl r. An indicator of pH. It is red at pH 4.4 and yellow at 6.2.

neutral r. An indicator of pH. It is red at pH 6.8 and yellow at 8.0.

phenol r. Phenolsulfonphthalein.

scarlet r. A red azo dye used to stimulate healing of indolent ulcers, burns, wounds, and so on; in histology, used as a stain. SYN: *rubrum scarlatinum.*

vital r. A stain used in preparing tissues for microscopic examination.

red bag waste Medical refuse, including potentially infectious materials and other hazardous products, that is placed in special containers to prevent them from contaminating the environment or spreading disease. SEE: *Standard and Universal Precautions Appendix.*

red blood cell Erythrocyte.

spiculed r.b.c. Spiculed red cell.

redbug Chiggers.

red cross **1.** A red cross on a white background; an internationally recognized sign of a medical installation or of medical personnel. **2.** The emblem of the American Red Cross.

red-green color blindness Inability to see red hues; the most frequent type of color blindness.

redia (rē′dē-ă) *pl.* **rediae** [Francesco Redi, It. naturalist, 1626–1698] The stage in the life cycle of a trematode that follows the sporocyst stage. Rediae are saclike structures possessing an oral sucker and a blind gut. They arise parthenogenetically from germ masses within the sporocyst and in turn produce second- or third-generation rediae or cercaria.

redifferentiation (rē″dĭf-ĕr-ĕn″shē-ā′shŭn) The resumption of the characteristics of mature cells by malignant cells.

red. in pulv. [L., *reductus in pulverum*] Let it be reduced to powder.

redintegration (rĕd-ĭn″tē-grā′shŭn) [L. *redintegratio*] **1.** Restitution of a part. **2.** Restoration to health. **3.** Recall by mental association.

redistribution **1.** The matching of care personnel resources to the population's site of care. The term usually is used in discussing the maldistribution of in-hospital personnel compared with in-community personnel. **2.** The return of blood flow to an ischemic segment of myocardium. During exercise, regions of the heart supplied by partially occluded arteries are deprived of blood, a condition that may foster angina pectoris. With rest, healthy blood flow to the affected areas is restored. Radionuclide agents (e.g., thallium-201 or sestamibi) can be used to demonstrate regions of the coronary circulation where this effect occurs, and aid in the diagnosis and management of ischemic heart disease.

red lead Pb_3O_4; lead tetroxide.

red man (neck) syndrome An adverse anaphylactoid reaction to vancomycin therapy, causing pruritus, flushing, and erythema of the head and upper body. The condition is caused by release of histamine. It can be prevented by slowing the infusion rate.

red-out (rĕd′owt) A term used in aerospace medicine to describe what happens to the vision and central nervous system (i.e., seeing red and perhaps experiencing unconsciousness) when the aircraft is doing part or all of an outside loop at high speed, or any other maneuver that causes the pilot to experience a negative force of gravity. The condition is due to engorgement of the vessels of the head including those of the retina.

redox Combined form indicating oxidation-reduction system or reaction.

red precipitate Red mercuric oxide. Poisoning symptoms are similar to those of mercuric chloride.

red tide Seasonal proliferation of certain dinoflagellates in coastal waters. These blooms change the color of the water to red, green, or brown and produce a potent neurotoxin that kills fish and contaminates shellfish. SEE: *poisoning, shellfish.*

reduce (rĭ-dūs′) [L. *re,* again, + *ducere,* to lead] **1.** To restore to usual relationship, as the ends of a fractured bone. **2.** To weaken, as a solution. **3.** To diminish, as bulk or weight.

reducible (rĭ-dūs′ĭ-bl) Capable of being replaced in a normal position, as a dislocated bone or a hernia.

reducing agent A substance that loses electrons easily and therefore causes other substances to be reduced (e.g., hydrogen sulfide, sulfur dioxide).

reductant (rĭ-dŭk′tănt) The atom that is oxidized in an oxidation-reduction reaction.

reductase (rĭ-dŭk′tās) [″ + *ducere,* to lead, + *ase,* enzyme] An enzyme that accelerates the reduction process of chemical compounds.

reduction (rĭ-dŭk′shŭn) [L. *reductio,* leading back] **1.** Restoration to a normal position, as a fractured bone or a hernia. **2.** In chemistry, a type of reaction in which a substance gains electrons and positive valence is decreased. SEE: *oxidation.*

closed r. of fractures The treatment of bone fractures by placing the bones in their proper position without surgery.

open r. of fractures The treatment of bone fractures by the use of surgery to place the bones in their proper position.

pregnancy r. The intentional elimination of one or more fetuses carried by a woman with a multifetal pregnancy.

risk r. **1.** A decrease in the probability of an adverse outcome. **2.** Any lowering of factors considered hazards for a specified disease, such as wearing a condom to lower the risk for sexually transmitted diseases, ceasing smoking to prevent lung cancer or emphysema, or lowering the intake of dietary cholesterol and fats to prevent heart disease. SEE: *risk-benefit analysis; risk factor; risk management.*

salt r. Limiting the quantity of sodium chloride in the diet, usually as a means of lowering blood pressure or preventing fluid retention.

reduction division Meiosis.

redundant (rĭ-dŭn′dĕnt) [L. *redundare,* to overflow] More than necessary.

reduplicated (rĭ-dū′plĭ-kā″tĕd) [L. *re,* again, + *duplicare,* to double] **1.** Doubled. **2.** Bent backward on itself, as a fold.

reduplication (rĭ-dū″plĭ-kā′shŭn) **1.** A doubling, as of the heart sounds in some morbid conditions. **2.** A fold.

Reduviidae (rē″dū-vī′ĭ-dē) A family of the order Hemiptera, including the assassin bugs.

Reduvius (rē-dū′vē-ŭs) A genus of true bugs belonging to the family Reduviidae.

R. personatus A species that normally feeds on other insects but sometimes preys on humans. In some cases the bite may transmit *Trypanosoma cruzi,* a protozoan responsible for Chagas' disease. SYN: *kissing bug.*

Reed-Sternberg cell [Dorothy Reed, U.S. pathologist, 1874–1964; Karl Sternberg, Aust. pathologist, 1872–1935] A giant, malignant, multinucleated B lymphocyte, the presence of which is the pathologic hallmark of Hodgkin's disease. SEE: illus.

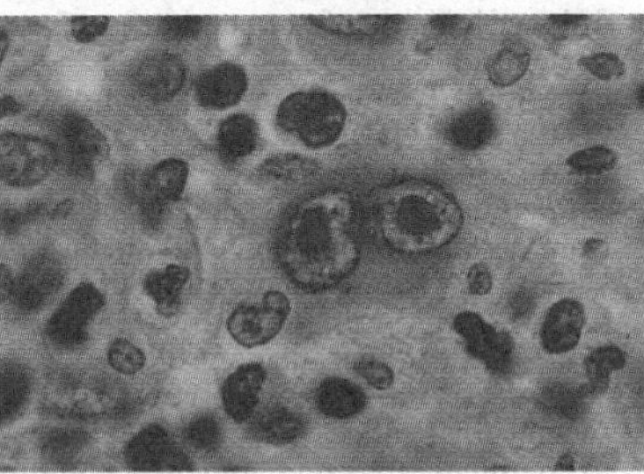

REED-STERNBERG CELL (CENTER)

(Orig. mag. ×600)

re-education (rē″ĕd-ū-kā′shŭn) [L. *re,* again, + *educare,* to educate] **1.** Training to restore competence to a person with functional limitations. **2.** A physical technique to facilitate restoration of motor control.

sensory r. A rehabilitation regimen used after sensation is impaired by peripheral nerve injuries or surgery to the hand. The purpose is to relearn the interpretation of sensory information related to pain, temperature, and object identification.

reef (rēf) A fold or tuck, usually taken in redundant tissue.

re-entry (rē-ĕn′trē) In cardiology, the cycling of an electrical impulse through conductive tissue that has been recently stimulated. This is the cause of many tachycardic heart rhythms (e.g., those originating in the atrioventricular node).

refection (rē-fĕk′shŭn) [L. *reficere,* to refresh] **1.** Restoration after hunger or fatigue, esp. with food or drink. **2.** Recovery by laboratory rats from the symptoms of vitamin B deficiency caused by consuming a diet deficient in vitamin B, due to vitamin synthesis by intestinal flora.

reference man An idealized male, used in models of nutritional, pharmacological, and toxicological research, of 22 years, weighing 70 kg, living in an environment with a mean temperature of 20°C, wearing clothing compatible with thermal comfort, engaged in light physical activity, and with an estimated caloric intake of 2800 kcal/day.

reference woman An idealized female, used in research models, described the same as reference man, except in weight (58 kg) and caloric intake (2000 kcal/day).

referral The practice of sending a patient to another practitioner or specialty program for consultation or service. Such a practice involves a delegation of responsibility for patient care, which should be followed up to ensure satisfactory care.

refine (rē-fīn′) [L. *re,* again, + ME. *fin,*

finished] To purify or render free from foreign material.

reflectance The fraction of total light reflected after it hits a surface, and the angle at which it is reflected.

diffuse r. The reflectance of light from a rough or nonpolished surface in which the radiant energy tends to scatter. The angle of reflectance does not equal the angle of incidence.

r. photometer An instrument used to measure reflectance; used clinically in chemical analyzers, glucometers, and dipstick readers.

spectral r. The reflectance of light from a polished surface in which the angle of reflectance equals the angle of incidence.

reflection (rĭ-flĕk′shŭn) [L. *reflexio,* a bending back] **1.** The condition of being turned back on itself, as when the peritoneum passes from the wall of a body cavity to and around an organ and back to the body wall. **2.** The throwing back of a ray of radiant energy from a surface not penetrated. **3.** Mental consideration of something previously considered.

diffuse r. The reflection of a light ray by a rough surface in which the angle of reflection is NOT equal to the angle of incidence. As opposed to *specular* reflection by a smooth surface in which the angle of reflection equals the angle of incidence. Employed in the analytical technique of reflectometry.

reflectometer An instrument that measures the light reflected by a surface. Reflectometers are used to analyze blood and urine specimens.

reflector (rĭ-flĕk′tor) [L. *re,* again, + *flectere,* to bend] A device or surface that reflects waves, radiant energy, or sound.

reflex (rē′flĕks) [L. *reflexus,* bend back] An involuntary response to a stimulus; an involuntary action. Reflexes are specific and predictable and are usually purposeful and adaptive. They depend on an intact neural pathway between the stimulation point and a responding organ (a muscle or gland). This pathway is called the reflex arc. In a simple reflex this includes a sensory receptor, afferent or sensory neuron, reflex center in the brain or spinal cord, one or more efferent neurons, and an effector organ (a muscle or gland). Most reflexes, however, are more complicated and include internuncial or associative neurons intercalated between afferent and efferent neurons. SEE: *arc, reflex* for illus.

abdominal r. SEE: *abdominal reflexes.*

abdominocardiac r. A change in heart rate, usually a slowing, resulting from mechanical stimulation of abdominal viscera.

accommodation r. One of the changes that take place when the eye adjusts to bring light rays from an object to focus on the retina. This involves a change in the size of the pupil, convergence or divergence of the eyes, and either a decrease or an increase in the convexity of the lens depending on the previous condition of the lens.

Achilles r. SEE: *Achilles tendon reflex.*

acoustic blink r. Involuntary closure of the eyelids after exposure to a sharp, sudden noise. This is a normal startle response that may be exaggerated in patients with anxiety disorders or hyperacusis or blunted in infants or adults with a hearing disorder or facial nerve paralysis.

acquired r. Conditioned r.

allied r. Reflexes initiated by several stimuli originating in widely separated receptors whose impulses follow the final common path to the effector organ and reinforce one another.

anal r. Contraction of the anal sphincter, following irritation or stimulation of the skin around the anus. This reflex is lost if the second to fourth sacral nerves are injured. SYN: *anal wink.*

ankle r. Achilles tendon reflex.

antagonistic r. Two or more reflexes initiated simultaneously in different receptors that involve the same motor center but produce opposite effects.

asymmetrical tonic neck r. In an infant, extension of one or both extremities on the side to which the head is forcibly turned. Flexion of the extremities occurs on the other side.

auditory r. Any reflex produced by stimulation of the auditory nerve, esp. blinking of the eyes at the sudden unexpected production of a sound.

autonomic r. Any reflex involving the response of a visceral effector (cardiac muscle, smooth muscle, or gland). Such reflexes always involve two efferent neurons (preganglionic and postganglionic).

axon r. A reflex that does not involve a complete reflex arc and hence is not a true reflex. Its afferent and efferent limbs are branches of a single nerve fiber, the axon (axon-like dendrite) of a sensory neuron. An example is vasodilation resulting from stimulation of the skin.

Babinski's r. SEE: *Babinski's reflex.*

Bainbridge r. An increase in heart rate caused by an increase in blood pressure or distention of the heart. SYN: *Bainbridge effect.*

biceps r. Flexion of the forearm on percussion of the tendon of the biceps brachii.

brachioradial r. Supinator longus r.

Brain's r. SEE: *Brain's reflex.*

carotid sinus r. A slowing of the heart rate along with a fall in blood pressure when the carotid sinus is massaged. Carotid sinus massage may be used therapeutically as a treatment for paroxysmal supraventricular tachycardia.

cat's eye r. In children, an abnormal pupillary flash or reflection from the eye that may be momentary; may be white, yellow, or pink; and is best seen under diminished natural illumination. This reflex, which may be noticed first by a parent, may be caused by various conditions, the most important of which is retinoblastoma. It is also observed in tuberous sclerosis, inflammatory eye diseases, and certain congenital malformations of the eye. SEE: *retinoblastoma.*

Chaddock's r. SEE: *Chaddock's reflex.*

chain r. A reflex initiated by several separate serial reflexes, each activated by the preceding one.

chin r. A clonic movement resulting from percussion or stroking of the lower jaw.

ciliary r. The normal contraction of the pupil in accommodation of vision from distant to near.

ciliospinal r. Dilation of the pupil following stimulation of the skin of the neck by pinching or scratching.

clasp-knife r. Quick inhibition of the stretch reflex when extensor muscles are forcibly stretched by flexing the limb.

conditioned r. A reflex acquired as a result of training in which the cerebral cortex plays an essential part. Conditioned reflexes are not inborn or inherited; rather, they are learned. SYN: *acquired r.*

conjunctival r. Closure of eyelids when the conjunctiva is touched or threatened.

consensual r. Crossed r.

convulsive r. A reflex induced by a weak stimulus and causing widespread uncoordinated and purposeless muscle contractions; seen in strychnine poisoning.

corneal r. Closure of eyelids resulting from direct corneal irritation.

cough r. SEE: *cough reflex.*

cranial r. Any reflex whose origin is in the brain.

cremasteric r. Retraction of the testis when the skin is stroked on the front inner side of the thigh.

crossed r. A reflex in which stimulation of one side of the body results in response on the opposite side. SYN: *consensual r.; indirect r.*

crossed extension r. An extension of the lower extremity on the opposite side when a painful stimulus is applied to the skin.

deep r. Deep tendon reflex.

deep tendon r. ABBR: DTR. An automatic motor response elicited by stimulating stretch receptors in subcutaneous tissues surrounding joints and tendons. The assessment of DTRs typically is made by striking a tendon (e.g., Achilles, patellar, biceps, triceps, or brachioradialis tendons) with a weighted hammer. Brisk or hyperactive responses are seen in conditions such as hyperthyroidism, stroke, pre-eclampsia, or spastic disorders; diminished responses may be seen in patients with hypothyroidism, drug intoxication, and flaccid neuromuscular disorders, among others. SYN: *deep reflex.* SEE: *clonus; knee-jerk reflex.*

delayed r. A reflex that does not occur until several seconds after the application of a stimulus.

digital r. Sudden flexion of the terminal phalanx of a finger or thumb when the nail is suddenly tapped.

diving r. Slowing of the heart rate when the head is immersed in water. This reflex helps to protect a person from drowning, esp. during immersion in cold water. SEE: *drowning.*

elbow r. An involuntary response in the elbow region to stimulation of the biceps and triceps muscles. SYN: *elbow jerk.* SEE: *biceps reflex; triceps reflex.*

elementary r. A typical reflex common to all vertebrates; includes the postural, flexion, stretch, and extensor thrust reflexes.

embrace r. Moro reflex.

extensor plantar r. Extension of the great toe when the sole of the foot is stimulated. SEE: *Babinski's reflex.*

extensor thrust r. A quick and brief extension of a limb on application of pressure to the plantar surface.

fencing r. Tonic neck r.

flexor withdrawal r. Flexion of a body part in response to a painful stimulus. SYN: *withdrawal r.*

gag r. Gagging and vomiting resulting from irritation of the throat or pharynx.

gastrocolic r. Peristaltic wave in the colon induced by entrance of food into the stomach.

gastroileac r. The physiological relaxation of the ileocecal valve resulting from food in the stomach.

Gault's r. SEE: *Gault's reflex.*

Geigel's r. SEE: *Geigel's reflex.*

gluteal r. Contraction of the gluteal muscles from stimulation of the overlying skin.

grasp r. The grasping reaction of the fingers and toes when stimulated. This reflex is normal in the newborn but disappears as the nervous system matures. It may reappear later in life if an individual suffers an injury to the frontal lobes of the brain.

Grünfelder's r. SEE: *Grünfelder's reflex.*

heart r. Any reflex in which the stimulation of a sensory nerve causes the heart rate to increase or decrease. An example is the Bainbridge reflex, in which stimulation of sensory receptors in the right atrium by increased venous return results in an increase in heart rate.

Hering-Breuer r. SEE: *Hering-Breuer reflex*.

Hoffmann's r. A reflex that occurs when the tip of the nail of the ring, middle, or index finger is flicked, producing flexion of the terminal phalanx of the thumb and the second and third phalanges of another finger. This reflex is evidence of disease in the frontal lobes of the brain.

hung-up r. Slowness of the relaxation phase of deep tendon reflexes; present in hypothyroidism.

hypochondrial r. Sudden inspiration resulting from abrupt pressure below the costal border.

inborn r. An unconditioned reflex; an innate or inherited reflex.

indirect r. Crossed r.

inhibition of r. The prevention of a reflex action, as inhibiting a sneeze by pressure on a facial nerve as it passes just under the upper lip.

interscapular r. A scapular muscular contraction following percussion or stimulus between the scapulae.

intersegmental r. A reflex involving several segments of the spinal cord. SYN: *long r.*

intestinal r. Myenteric r.

intrasegmental r. Reflex that involves only a single segment of the spinal cord.

irradiation of r. The spreading of reflexes through the central nervous system whereby impulses entering the cord in one segment activate motor neurons located in many segments.

jaw r. Chin r.

kinetic r. Labyrinthine righting r.

Kisch's r. SEE: *Kisch's reflex*.

knee-jerk r. Extension of the leg resulting from percussion of the patellar tendon. This is one of the myotatic or stretch reflexes important in maintaining posture. SYN: *patellar r.*

labyrinthine righting r. A reflex, esp. a postural reflex, resulting from stimulation of receptors in the semicircular ducts, utricle, and saccule of the inner ear. This reflex helps orient the head in space and to the rest of the body. SYN: *kinetic r.; optical righting r.*

lacrimal r. Secretion of fluid resulting from irritation of the corneal conjunctiva.

laryngeal r. Coughing as a result of irritation of the larynx or fauces.

letdown r. The movement of breast milk from the alveoli into the lactiferous ducts in response to oxytocin-stimulated contractions. The reflex may be stimulated by suckling or by infant crying. Stimulation of the nipple increases the secretion of oxytocin and this technique may be used to stimulate contraction of the postpartum uterus.

lid r. Closure of eyelids resulting from direct corneal stimulation. This reflex is mediated by the fifth cranial nerve. SYN: *corneal reflex*.

light r. Constriction of the pupil when light is flashed into the eye.

lip r. The reflex movement of the lips when the angle of the mouth is suddenly and lightly tapped during sleep.

local r. A reflex that does not involve the central nervous system (e.g., the myenteric reflex, which occurs even when extrinsic nerves to the intestine have been cut).

long r. Intersegmental r.

lumbar r. An irritation of the skin over the erector spinae muscles, causing contraction of the back muscles.

Magnus-de Kleijn r. In decerebrate rigidity, extension of the limbs on the side to which the chin is turned by rotating the head. There is flexion of the limbs on the opposite side.

mandibular r. Clonic movement resulting from percussing or stroking the lower jaw.

mass r. Autonomic dysfunction that may occur as a late consequence of transection of the spinal cord. It is marked by episodes of sweating, bradycardia, hypotension, urinary incontinence, and muscular spasms of the legs.

Mayer's r. Opposition and adduction of the thumb, flexion at the metacarpophalangeal joint, and extension at the interphalangeal joint in response to downward pressure on the index finger.

Mendel-Bekhterev r. Plantar flexion of the toes in response to percussion of the dorsum of the foot.

monosynaptic r. A reflex involving only two neurons, an afferent and an efferent.

Moro r. SEE: *Moro reflex*.

myenteric r. Reflex caused by distention of the intestine, resulting in contraction above the point of stimulation and relaxation below it. SYN: *intestinal r.*

myotatic r. Stretch r.

near r. Accommodation r.

neck-righting r. In a supine infant, rotation of the trunk in the same direction as that in which the head is turned. This reflex appears at age 4 to 6 months and is no longer obtainable by age 2 years.

nociceptive r. A reflex initiated by a painful stimulus.

obliquus r. Contraction of the entire external obliquus muscle on application of stimulus to the skin of the thigh below Poupart's ligament.

oculocardiac r. SEE: *Aschner's phenomenon*.

oculocephalic r. The deviation of a person's eyes to the opposite side when the head is rapidly rotated. This is a normal finding in neonates; in adults it is indicative of coma. SYN: *doll's eye movement.*

optical blink r. Involuntary closure of the eyelids after exposure to a bright light source. Shining a bright light at an infant's eyes causes the eyes to blink and the head to flex backward. If this reflex is absent, further testing of cranial nerves II, III, IV, and VI is required.

optical righting r. Labyrinthine righting r.

palatal r. Swallowing induced by stimulation of the soft palate.

palmar grasp r. A normal newborn reflex in which the baby's fingers spontaneously curl around any object placed within them and do not spontaneously let go. This reflex usually diminishes by age 3 to 4 months and disappears before age 6 months. The reflex reappears later in life in diseases that affect the brain's frontal lobes.

palmar r. Swallowing induced by stimulation of the soft palate.

palmomental r. A contraction of the superficial muscles of the eye and chin produced on the same side as the palmar area that is stimulated by an examiner. This is an abnormal finding that indicates frontal disease.

parachute r. (response) Extension of the arms, hands, and fingers when the infant is suspended in the prone position and dropped a short distance onto a soft surface. This reaction appears at age 9 months and persists. An asymmetrical response indicates a motor nerve abnormality.

paradoxical r. A response to a stimulus that is unexpected and may be the opposite of what would be considered normal.

patellar r. Knee-jerk r.

pathological r. Any abnormal reflex due to disease.

penile r. **1.** Sudden downward movement of the penis when the prepuce or gland of a completely relaxed penis is pulled upward. **2.** Contraction of the bulbocavernous muscle on percussing the dorsum of the penis. **3.** Contraction of the bulbocavernous muscle resulting from compression of the glans penis.

pharyngeal r. An attempt to swallow following any application of stimulus to the pharynx.

pilomotor r. Piloerection when skin is cooled or as a result of emotional reaction.

placing r. Flexion and then extension of an infant's leg that occurs when an infant is held erect and the dorsum of one foot is dragged along the underedge of a table top. This reflex lasts from birth until age 6 weeks.

plantar r. SEE: *plantar grasp.*

plantar grasp r. A grasp reflex resulting from light stimulation of the sole of the foot. This reflex lasts from birth until age 10 months.

platysmal r. Dilation of the pupil resulting from sharp pinching of the platysma myoides.

pneocardiac r. A change in the rate and rhythm of the heart and blood pressure when an irritant vapor is inhaled.

pneopneic r. A change in respiratory depth and rate, coughing, suffocation, and pulmonary edema when an irritant vapor is inhaled.

postural r. Any reflex that is concerned with maintaining posture.

pressor r. A reflex in which the response to stimulation is an increase in blood pressure brought about by constriction of arterioles.

proprioceptive r. A reflex initiated by body movement to maintain the position of the moved part; any reflex initiated by stimulation of a proprioceptor.

psychogalvanic r. Decreased electric resistance of the skin in response to emotional stress or stimuli.

pupillary r. **1.** Constriction of the pupil upon stimulation of the retina by light. This reflex is mediated by the third cranial nerve. **2.** Constriction of the pupil upon accommodation for near vision, and dilatation upon accommodation for far vision. **3.** Constriction of the pupil of one eye in response to stimulation of the other by light. **4.** Constriction of the pupil upon attempted closure of eyelids that are held apart.

quadriceps r. Knee-jerk r.

quadrupedal extensor r. Brain's reflex.

radial r. Flexion of forearm resulting when the lower end of the radius is percussed.

red r. The red light reflection seen in ophthalmoscopic examination of the eye.

righting r. Any of the reflexes that enable an animal to maintain the body in a definite relationship to the head and thus maintain its body right side up.

rooting r. The turning of an infant's mouth toward the stimulus when the infant's cheek is stroked. This reflex is present at birth; by age 4 months it is gone when the infant is awake; by age 7 months it is gone when the infant is asleep.

Rossolimo's r. SEE: *Rossolimo's reflex.*

scapular r. Muscular contraction following percussion or stimulus between the scapulae.

scapulohumeral r. A reflex in which the upper arm is adducted and rotated outward when the vertebral border of the scapula is percussed.

scrotal r. Slow vermicular contraction of the scrotal muscle when the perineum is stroked or cold is applied.

segmental r. A reflex in which afferent impulses enter the cord in the same segment or segments from which the efferent impulses emerge.

sexual r. A reflex concerned with sexual activities, esp. erection and ejaculation, which results from direct genital stimulation or indirectly from emotion, whether the individual is asleep or awake.

short r. A reflex involving one or a few segments of spinal cord.

simple r. A reflex in which only two or possibly three neurons are interposed between receptor and effector organs.

solar sneeze r. A sneeze that occurs following exposure to bright sunlight. This benign condition may affect a great number of normal persons, and it may also be associated with rhinitis. The mechanism of the cause of this type of sneeze reflex is unknown.

sole r. Plantar reflex.

somatic r. A reflex induced by stimulation of somatic sensory nerve endings.

spinal r. A reflex whose center is in the spinal cord.

startle r. Moro reflex.

static r. A reflex concerned with establishing and maintaining posture when the body is at rest.

statokinetic r. A reflex that occurs when the body is moving (e.g., walking or running).

stepping r. Movements of progression elicited by holding an infant upright, inclined forward, and touching the soles of the feet to a flat surface. This reflex lasts from birth to age 6 weeks.

stretch r. The contraction of a muscle as a result of quickly stretching the same muscle. Stretch reflexes are of primary importance in the maintenance of posture. SYN: *myotatic r.*

sucking r. A sucking movement of an infant's mouth produced by stroking the lips. A primitive form of this reflex is present in the fetus by the 16th week of gestation; it is fully developed by the time of birth. In adults, the presence of a sucking reflex is an indicator of severe dementia, frontal lobe disease, or extrapyramidal diseases.

superficial r. A cutaneous reflex caused by irritation of the skin or of areas that depend on the spinal cord as a motor center (e.g., the scapular, epigastric, abdominal, cremasteric, gluteal, and plantar reflexes) or on centers in the medulla (e.g., the conjunctival, pupillary, and palatal reflexes). This reflex is induced by a very light stimulus, such as stroking the skin lightly with a soft cotton swab.

supinator longus r. Flexion of the forearm caused by tapping of the tendon of the supinator longus. SYN: *brachioradial r.*

supraorbital r. A contraction of the orbicularis oculi muscle with closure of lids resulting from percussion above the supraorbital nerve.

suprapubic r. Deflection of the linea alba toward the stroked side when the abdomen is stroked above Poupart's ligament.

swallowing r. Involuntary muscular activity in the oropharynx and nasopharynx when foods, tongue depressors, or other objects stimulate the back of the throat. In humans, swallowing is mediated by cranial nerves VII, IX, X, and XI.

symmetrical tonic neck r. In an infant, flexion or extension of the arms in response to flexion and extension, respectively, of the neck.

tendon r. A deep reflex obtained by sharply tapping the skin over the tendon of a muscle. It is exaggerated in upper neuron disease and diminished or lost in lower neuron disease.

tonic neck r. The ipsilateral extension and contralateral flexion of the supine infant's extremities when the head is turned to one side. This normal newborn reflex may not be evident immediately after birth; however, once it appears, it persists until about the third postnatal month.

tonic vibration r. ABBR: T.V.R. A polysynaptic reflex believed to depend on spinal and supraspinal pathways.

triceps r. Sharp extension of the forearm resulting from tapping of the triceps tendon while the arm is held loosely in a bent position. SYN: *elbow r.*

triceps surae r. Achilles tendon reflex.

true autonomic r. A visceral response in which afferent impulses do not pass through the central nervous system, but instead enter prevertebral ganglia where connections are made with efferent neurons.

unconditioned r. A natural or inherited reflex action; one not acquired.

urinary r. The spinal cord reflex, initiated by accumulated urine stretching the bladder and the resulting contraction of the bladder to expel urine.

vascular r. Vasomotor r.

vasomotor r. The constriction or dilatation of a blood vessel in response to a stimulus, as in becoming pale from fright. SYN: *vascular r.*

visceral r. Any reflex induced by stimulation of the visceral nerves.

visceromotor r. Contraction or tenseness of the skeletal muscles resulting from painful stimuli originating in visceral organs.

withdrawal r. Flexor withdrawal r.

reflexogenic (rĭ-flĕks″ō-jĕn′ĭk) [L. *re-*

flexus, bend back, + Gr. *gennan,* to produce] Causing a reflex action.

reflexogenous (rĭ″flĕks-ŏj′ĕ-nŭs) Reflexogenic.

reflexograph (rĭ-flĕks′ō-grăf) [″ + Gr. *graphein,* to write] A device for recording and graphing a reflex, esp. one produced by muscular activity.

reflexology (rē″flĕk-sŏl′ō-jē) [″ + Gr. *logos,* word, reason] **1.** The study of the anatomy and physiology of reflexes. **2.** A system of massage in which the feet and sometimes the hands are massaged in an attempt to favorably influence other body functions.

reflexometer (rē″flĕks-ŏm′ĕ-tĕr) [″ + Gr. *metron,* measure] An instrument that measures the force of the tap required to produce a reflex.

reflexophil (rē-flĕks′ō-fĭl) [″ + Gr. *philein,* to love] Marked by reflex activity or by exaggerated reflexes.

reflexotherapy (rē-flĕks″ō-thĕr′ă-pē) [″ + Gr. *therapeia,* treatment] Treatment by manipulating, anesthetizing, or cauterizing an area distant from the location of the disorder. SEE: *spondylotherapy.*

reflex sympathetic dystrophy An abnormal response of the nerves of the face or an extremity, marked by pain, autonomic dysfunction, vasomotor instability, and tissue swelling. Although the precise cause of the syndrome is unknown, it often follows trauma, stroke, neuropathy, or radiculopathy. In about one third of all patients, the onset is insidious. Affected patients often complain of burning pain with any movement of an affected body part, excessive sensitivity to light touch or minor stimulation, temperature changes (heat or cold) in the affected limb, localized sweating, localized changes of skin color, or atrophic changes in the skin, nails, or musculature. SYN: *shoulder-hand syndrome; Sudeck's atrophy.* SEE: *Nursing Diagnoses Appendix.*

TREATMENT: Early mobilization of the body part, with multimodality therapy, may improve the symptoms of RSD. Drug therapies often include prednisone or other corticosteroids and narcotic analgesics; trancutaneous electrical stimulation, physical therapy, or nerve blocks may also prove helpful.

reflux (rē′flŭks) [L. *re,* back, + *fluxus,* flow] A return or backward flow. SEE: *regurgitation.*

hepatojugular r. Distention of the veins of the neck when the liver is compressed during physical examination of the abdomen. Neck vein filling during liver examination commonly is seen in patients with congestive heart failure but also may be a normal finding.

vesicoureteral r. The backward flow of urine up the ureter during urination, instead of downward into the bladder. This condition may cause recurrent urinary tract infections in infants and children and may produce kidney scarring and failure if it is untreated. Depending on the underlying cause, treatment may include endoscopic or open surgical procedures.

reflux disease Gastroesophageal reflux disease.

refract (rĭ-frăkt′) [L. *refractus,* broken off] **1.** To turn back; to deflect. **2.** To detect and correct refractive errors in the eyes.

refracta dosi (rē-frăk′tă dō′sē) [L.] In divided doses, denoting a definite amount of drug taken within a given time in a number of fractional equal parts.

refraction (rĭ-frăk′shŭn) [LL. *refractio,* break back] **1.** Deflection from a straight path, as of light rays as they pass through media of different densities; the change in direction of a ray when it passes from one medium to another of a different density. **2.** Determination of the amount of ocular refractive errors and their correction.

angle of r. The angle formed by a refracted ray of light with a line perpendicular to the surface at the refraction point.

coefficient of r. The quotient of the sine of the angle of incidence divided by the sine of the angle of refraction.

double r. Possession of more than one refractive index, resulting in a double image. SEE: *birefractive; birefringence.*

dynamic r. The static refraction of the eye plus that accomplished by accommodation; the reciprocal of the near-point distance.

error of r. Ametropia.

r. of eye The refraction brought about by the refractive media of the eye (cornea, aqueous humor, crystalline lens, vitreous body). SYN: *ocular r.*

index of r. **1.** The ratio of the angle made by the incident ray with the perpendicular (angle of incidence) to that made by the emergent ray (angle of refraction). **2.** The ratio of the speed of light in a vacuum to its speed in another medium. The refractive index of water is 1.33; that of the crystalline lens of the eye is 1.413.

ocular r. R. of eye.

static r. Refraction of the eye when accommodation is at rest or paralyzed.

refractionist (rĭ-frăk′shŭn-ĭst) [LL. *refractio,* break back] A person skilled in determining and correcting ocular refractive errors.

refractive (rĭ-frăk′tĭv) [L. *refractus,* broken off] Concerning refraction. SYN: *refringent.*

refractive media The structures of the eye that deflect light: the cornea, aqueous, crystalline lens, and vitreous.

refractive power The degree to which a transparent body deflects a ray of light from a straight path. SEE: *diopter*.

refractivity (rē″frăk-tĭv′ĭ-tē) The quality of being refractive; the ability to refract.

refractometer (rē-frăk-tŏm′ĕt-ĕr) [″ + Gr. *metron,* measure] A device for measuring refractive power, as of the eye.

refractometry (rē″frăk-tŏm′ĕ-trē) Measurement of the refractive power of lenses.

refractory (rē-frăk′tō-rē) [L. *refractarius*] **1.** Obstinate; stubborn. **2.** Resistant to ordinary treatment. **3.** Resistant to stimulation; used of muscle or nerve.

refractory period, absolute The brief period during depolarization of a neuron or muscle fiber when the cell does not respond to any stimulus, no matter how strong.

refractory period, relative The brief period during repolarization of a neuron or muscle fiber when excitability is depressed. If stimulated, the cell may respond, but a stronger than usual stimulus is required.

refracture (rē-frăk′chūr) [L. *refractus,* broken off] **1.** To break again, as a bone set wrongly. **2.** Rebreaking of a fracture united in a malaligned or incorrect position.

refrangible (rē-frăn′jĭ-bl) [L. *re,* again, + ME. *frangible,* breakable] Capable of being refracted.

refresh (rĭ-frĕsh′) [O.Fr. *refreschir,* to renew] **1.** To restore strength; to relieve from fatigue; to renew; to revive. **2.** To scrape epithelial covering from two opposing surfaces of a wound to facilitate healing and joining together.

refrigerant (rĭ-frĭj′ĕr-ănt) [L. *refrigerans,* making cold] **1.** Cooling. **2.** An agent that produces coolness or reduces fever. SYN: *algefacient*.

refrigerant gas One of several gases (e.g., Freon, a fluorinated hydrocarbon) used in ordinary household refrigerators. Poisoning may be caused by leaks, faulty connections or breakage, or gas dissipated into the atmosphere.

refrigeration (rĭ-frĭj″ĕr-ā′shŭn) [L. *refrigeratio,* make cold] Cooling; reduction of heat.

refringent Refractive.

Refsum's disease (rĕf′soomz) [Sigvald Bernhard Refsum, Norwegian physician, b. 1907] An autosomal recessive disease caused by the inability to metabolize phytanic acid. Clinical symptoms include visual disturbances, peripheral neuropathy, ataxia, and liver, kidney, and heart disease. Diets low in animal fat and milk products may relieve some of the symptoms.

regainer (rē-gān′ĕr) **1.** A device that ameliorates or restores something that was lost. **2.** A device that applies pressure between teeth on either side of the space left by a missing tooth. This is done to push the teeth toward the edentulous space.

regeneration (rē-jĕn″ĕr-ā′shŭn) [L. *re,* again, + *generare,* to produce] Repair, regrowth, or restoration of a part, such as tissues. Opposite of degeneration.

regimen (rĕj′ĭ-mĕn) [L., rule] A systematic plan of activities, treatments, diet, sleep, and exercise designed to improve, maintain, or restore health.

regio (rē′jē-ō) [L.] Region.

region (rē′jŭn) [L. *regio,* boundary] A portion of the body with natural or arbitrary boundaries. SYN: *regio*. **regional** (-ăl), *adj.*

register [LL. *regesta,* list] **1.** An official recording of vital statistics, including date and place of birth, marriage(s), and death. Recording these data is a legal requirement in the U.S. **2.** The compass or range of a voice. **3.** A series of tones of like quality or character, as low or high register, chest or head register.

registered record administrator ABBR: RRA. A person registered by the American Medical Records Association, who plans, supervises, designs, and develops medical records systems for health care facilities.

registrant (rĕj′ĭs-trănt) [L. *registrans,* registering] A nurse named on the books of a registry as being "on call" or available to be called for duty.

registrar (rĕj′ĭs-trăr) [O.Fr. *registreur*] The official manager of a registry.

registration [L. *registratio*] The recording of information such as births or deaths; the recording of those who are registered or licensed to practice within a state.

registry (rĕj′ĭs-trē) [LL. *regesta,* list] An office or book containing a list of nurses ready for duty; a placement bureau for nurses.

cancer r. A list of patients diagnosed with cancer, kept to facilitate patient follow-up, as well as research about cancer causes, therapies, and outcomes.

regression (rĭ-grĕsh′ŭn) [L. *regressio,* go back] **1.** A turning back or return to a former state. **2.** A return of symptoms. **3.** Retrogression. **4.** In psychology, an abnormal return to an earlier reaction, characterized by a mental state and behavior inappropriate to the situation. Regression may occur as a result of frustration or in states of fatigue, dreams, hypnosis, intoxication, illness, and certain psychoses (e.g., schizophrenia). **5.** In statistics, a procedure used to predict one variable on the basis of data about one or more other variables. **regressive** (-grĕs′ĭv), *adj.*

regressive resistive exercise ABBR: RRE. A form of active resistive exercise that advocates gradual reduction in the amount of resistance as muscles fatigue.

regular (rĕg′ū-lăr) [L. *regula,* rule] **1.** Conforming to a rule or custom. **2.** Methodical, steady in course, as a pulse. SEE: *normal; typical.*

regulation **1.** The condition of being controlled or directed. **2.** The ability of an organism, such as a developing embryo, to develop normally despite experimental modifications. **regulative,** *adj.*

regulation development In embryology, the condition in which a single blastomere or a portion of an embryo can give rise to a whole embryo; the opposite of mosaic development.

regulator **1.** A device for adjusting or controlling the rate of flow or administration of gases (e.g., oxygen) or fluids (including blood). **2.** A gene that alters the expression of other genes.

regurgitant (rē-gŭr′jĭ-tănt) [L. *re,* again, + *gurgitare,* to flood] Throwing back or flowing in a direction opposite to normal.

regurgitation (rē-gŭr″jĭ-tā′shŭn) A backward flowing, as in the return of solids or fluids to the mouth from the stomach or the backflow of blood through a defective heart valve.

aortic r. Aortic insufficiency.

duodenal r. A return flow of chyme from the duodenum to the stomach.

functional r. Regurgitation caused not by valvular disorder but by dilatation of ventricles, the great vessels, or valve rings.

mitral r. ABBR: MR. A backflow of blood from the left ventricle into the left atrium, resulting from imperfect closure of the mitral (bicuspid) valve. It may result from congenital anomalies of the valve, connective tissue disorders (e.g., Marfan's disease), infective endocarditis, ischemic damage to the valve or its supporting chordae, rheumatic valvulitis, or other degenerative conditions.

Congestive heart failure or atrial fibrillation may be complications of severe MR. The degree of regurgitation also can be judged echocardiographically or by other diagnostic modalities (e.g., angiographically). Valve reconstruction or valve replacement surgeries can be used to repair the defect.

pulmonic r. A backflow of blood from the pulmonary artery into the right ventricle.

tricuspid r. A backflow of blood from the right ventricle into the right atrium.

valvular r. A backflow of blood through a valve, esp. a heart valve, that is not completely closed as it would normally be.

REHABDATA A computerized bibliographical database of rehabilitation information supplied by the National Rehabilitation Information Center (NARIC). Topics included in the REHABDATA database include vocational rehabilitation, the cost of rehabilitation and community-based services; medical rehabilitation and policy issues, including health care policy and costs as they relate to people with disabilities; and community integration. For information, contact NARIC, 8455 Colesville Road, Suite 935, Silver Spring, MD 20910-3319; (800) 346-2742; www.naric.com

rehabilitation (rē″hă-bĭl″ĭ-tā′shŭn) [L. *rehabilitare*] **1.** The processes of treatment and education that help disabled individuals to attain maximum function, a sense of well-being, and a personally satisfying level of independence. Rehabilitation may be necessitated by any disease or injury that causes mental or physical impairment serious enough to result in functional limitation or disability. The postmyocardial infarction patient, the posttrauma patient, patients with psychological illnesses, and the postsurgical patient need and can benefit from rehabilitation efforts. The combined efforts of the individual, family, friends, medical, nursing, allied health personnel, and community resources are essential to making rehabilitation possible. **2.** In dentistry, the methods used to restore dentition to its optimal functional condition. It may involve restoration of teeth by fillings, crowns, or bridgework; adjustment of occlusal surfaces by selective grinding; orthodontic realignment of teeth; or surgical correction of diseased or malaligned parts. It may be done to improve chewing, to enhance the aesthetic appearance of the face and teeth, to enhance speech, or to preserve the dentition and supporting tissues. Also called *occlusorehabilitation* and *mouth,* or *oral, rehabilitation.*

cardiac r. A structured, interdisciplinary program of progressive exercise, psychological support, nutritional counseling, and patient education to enable attainment of maximum functional capacity by patients who have experienced a myocardial infarction.

pool r. Aquatic therapy.

aquatic r. Aquatic therapy.

neurological r. A supervised program of formal training to restore function to patients who have neurodegenerative diseases, spinal cord injuries, strokes, or traumatic brain injury.

pulmonary r. A structured program of activity, progressive breathing and conditioning exercises, and patient education designed to return patients with pulmonary disease to maximum function.

rehabilitee (rē″hă-bĭl′ĭ-tē) A person who has been rehabilitated.

rehydration (rē″hī-drā′shŭn) [″ + Gr. *hydor,* water] The restoration of fluid volume to a dehydrated person, either orally or parenterally.

Reichert's cartilage (rī′kĕrts) [Karl Bogislaus Reichert, Ger. anatomist, 1811–1883] The second branchial arch of the embryo, which gives rise to the stapes, styloid process, stylohyoid ligament, and lesser cornua to the hyoid bone.

Reid's base line (rēdz) [Robert William Reid, Scottish anatomist, 1851–1939] The line extending from the lower edge of the orbit to the center of the aperture of the external auditory canal and backward to the center of the occipital bone.

reiki (rī′kē) An alternative medical practice of massage in which the patient is not physically touched.

Reil's island (rīlz) Island of Reil.

reimbursement (rē-ĭm-bŭrs′mĕnt) Payment for health care services.

reimplantation (rē″ĭm-plăn-tā′shŭn) [L. *re,* again, + *in,* into, + *plantare,* to set] Replantation.

reinfection (rē″ĭn-fĕk′shŭn) [″ + ME. *infecten,* infect] A second infection by the same organism. SEE: *superinfection.*

reinforcement (rē″ĭn-fors′mĕnt) [″ + *inforce,* enforce] Strengthening; an augmentation of force; part of the fundamental learning process, along with motivation, stimulation, and action. Reinforcement is the reward for the appropriate response in a learning situation.

reinforcement of reflex Strengthening of the response to one stimulus by concurrent action of another; the exaggeration of a reflex by nerve activity elsewhere. Thus, during the raising of a heavy weight, the knee jerk is stronger. SEE: *Jendrassik's maneuver.*

reinforcer (rē″ĭn-fors′ĕr) Something that produces reinforcement.

reinfusion (rē″ĭn-fū′zhŭn) [″ + *infusio,* to pour in] The reinjection of blood serum or cerebrospinal fluid.

reinnervation (rē″ĭn-ĕr-vā′shŭn) [″ + *in,* into, + *nervus,* nerve] **1.** Anastomosis of a paralyzed part with a living nerve. **2.** Grafting of a fresh nerve for restoration of function in a paralyzed muscle.

reinoculation (rē″ĭn-ŏk″ū-lā′shŭn) [″ + *in,* into, + *oculus,* bud] A second inoculation with the same organism or its antigens. SEE: *reinfection.*

reintegration In psychology, the resumption of normal behavior and mental functioning following disintegration of personality in mental illness.

reinversion (rē″ĭn-vĕr′shŭn) [″ + *in,* into, + *versio,* turning] Correction of an inverted organ.

Reissner's membrane (rĭs′nĕrz) [Ernst Reissner, Ger. anatomist, 1824–1878] A delicate membrane separating the cochlear canal from the scala vestibuli.

Reiter's syndrome (rī′tĕrz) [Hans Conrad Julius Reiter, Ger. physician, 1881–1969] ABBR: RS. A syndrome consisting of urethritis, which usually occurs first; arthritis; and conjunctivitis. It occurs mainly in young men. When an organism is implicated, it is most frequently *Chlamydia.* The prognosis is generally good; however, recurrences are common.

TREATMENT: There is no specific therapy. Tetracyclines or erythromycins are used for urethritis. The sexual partner should be treated if RS was transmitted sexually. Arthritis and conjunctivitis are treated symptomatically.

rejection [L. *rejicere,* to throw back] **1.** Refusal to accept or to show affection. In animals, for example, the young may be ignored or driven away by their mother. **2.** In tissue and organ transplantation, destruction of transplanted material at the cellular level by the host's immune mechanism. Transplant rejection is controlled primarily by T cells, but macrophages and B lymphocytes are also involved. Immunosuppressive therapy with cyclosporine, mycophenolate mofetil, tacrolimus, antilymphocyte immune globulin, and monoclonal antibodies, which inhibit or block T-cell activity, has markedly lowered the risk of transplant organ rejection.

acute r. The early destruction of grafted or transplanted material, usually beginning a week after implantation. Acute rejection is identified clinically by decreased function of the transplanted organ. High-dose corticosteroids are the first treatment of acute rejection; they are typically quite effective. Antilymphocyte globulin (ALG), the monoclonal antibody OKT 3, mycophenolate mofetil, and tacrolimus, among other agents, are used when corticosteroids are not effective. SEE: *suppressive immunotherapy; macrophage processing; major histocompatibility complex; T cell.*

chronic r. Late and ongoing destruction of grafted or transplanted tissue. It most commonly involves vascular changes and interstitial fibrosis. Immunosuppressive therapy with tacrolimus and cyclosporine has significantly reduced this T-cell–mediated rejection process.

hyperacute r. Immediate, intense, and irreversible destruction of grafted material due to preformed antibodies. These antibodies are most common in patients who have rejected a previously transplanted organ or who have received multiple blood transfusions. The risk of hyperacute rejection has been nearly eliminated by testing the recipient's blood for antibodies against donor lymphocytes before surgery.

parental r. The refusal of a parent to accept or show affection for a son or daughter.

rejuvenation (rĭ-jū″vĕ-nā′shŭn) [L. *re,* again, + *juvenis,* young] A return to a youthful condition or to the normal.

rejuvenescence (rĭ-jū″vĕ-nĕs′ĕns) [″ + *juvenescere,* to become young] The renewal of youth; the return to an earlier stage of existence.

relapse (rē-lăps′) [L. *relapsus*] The recurrence of a disease or symptoms after apparent recovery.

relapsing Recurring after apparent recovery.

relation (rĭ-lā′shŭn) [L. *relatio,* a carrying back] The condition, connection, or state of one thing compared with another.

jaw r. Any relation of the position of the maxilla to that of the mandible.

occlusal jaw r. The relation of the mandibular teeth to the maxillary teeth when the teeth are in contact.

unstrained jaw r. The position of the jaw during normal tonus of all the jaw muscles.

relative biological effect The effectiveness of types of radiation compared with that of x-rays or gamma rays.

relax [L. *relaxare,* to loosen] To decrease tension or intensity; to be rid of strain, anxiety, and nervousness.

relaxant (rĭ-lăk′sănt) **1.** Pert. to or producing relaxation. **2.** A drug that reduces tension. **3.** A laxative.

muscle r. A drug or therapeutic treatment that specifically relieves muscular tension.

neuromuscular r. A drug (e.g., succinylcholine) that prevents transmission of stimuli to muscle tissue, esp. striated muscle.

smooth muscle r. A drug that reduces the tension of smooth muscles such as those in the intestinal tract or bronchi.

relaxation (rē-lăk-sā′shŭn) **1.** A lessening of tension or activity in a part. **2.** A phase or period in a single muscle twitch following contraction in which tension decreases, fibers lengthen, and the muscle returns to a resting position. **3.** In magnetic resonance imaging, the return of an excited atom to alignment with the applied magnetic field.

general r. Relaxation of the entire body.

local r. Relaxation limited to a particular muscle group or to a certain part.

pelvic r. Diminished support of the pelvic tissues and organs, esp. in women; usually due to childbirth or aging. The organs affected and the pathological conditions associated with this condition are the bladder (cystocele), rectum (rectocele), uterus (uterine prolapse), small intestine (enterocele), and urethra (protrusion of the urethra into the vagina). Symptoms are related to the organ(s) affected. Treatment is determined by the severity of the relaxation. Medical treatments, including pelvic muscle exercises, pessaries, prompted voiding regimens, and estrogen therapy, may be helpful to patients; however, many patients require surgery.

relaxation response The physiological responses (slower heart rate, decreased blood pressure, lowered cutaneous resistance) produced by sitting quietly with the eyes closed and breathing slowly and methodically. A brief word or phrase (in Hindu cultures, this is called a mantra) may be repeated to oneself to help focus the mind or reduce stray thoughts. This approach to meditation or stress reduction may be undertaken once or twice a day, usually for 10 to 30 minutes. The relaxation response helps reduce anxiety, high blood pressure, pain, postmenopausal symptoms, and medication use.

relaxed movement Passive exercise.

relaxin (rĭ-lăk′sĭn) A polypeptide hormone related to insulin in women secreted in the corpus luteum during pregnancy and by the prostate in men. It has many effects on breast, uterine, cardiac, and other tissues.

relearning Acquiring a skill or ability that had been previously present but was lost or removed as a result of physical damage to the muscles or brain.

release **1.** A document that, if signed by the patient or the patient's legal representative in the case of a minor, permits the treating physician to perform certain procedures (e.g., surgery, anesthesia, blood transfusion, removal of tissues or fluids for analysis). In addition to being signed by the patient, the release should also be signed by a witness. Most releases have a notation indicating the applicable time of the release. **2.** To discharge. **3.** To remove restraints.

myofascial r. ABBR: MFR. The manipulation of soft tissue to facilitate improved posture and range of motion and to decrease pain. SEE: *soft-tissue mobilization.*

sustained r. The delivery of a drug from a tablet or other reservoir over many hours or days (instead of minutes or hours), to provide a durable therapeutic effect.

reliability **1.** The condition of being dependable, accurate, and honest. **2.** In statistics, the ability of the measuring method or device to produce reproducible data or information.

relief (rĭ-lēf′) [ME.] **1.** The alleviation or removal of a distressing or painful symptom. **2.** Assistance given to the poor, homeless, or those whose lives have been changed by mass casualty incidents or other catastrophes. Relief may be provided in the form of food, clothing, shelter, loans, or cash, as well as other goods and services.

relieve [L. *relevare,* to raise] To provide relief.

reline (rē-līn′) To replace or resurface the lining of a denture.

relinquishment, infant The psychological process experienced by a birth mother during adoption of her child by others.

relocation stress syndrome Physiological and/or psychosocial disturbances as a result of transfer from one environment to another. SEE: *Nursing Diagnoses Appendix.*

REM *rapid eye movement.*

rem *roentgen equivalent* (in) *man.*

Remak, Robert (ră′māk) German neurologist, 1815–1865.

R.'s axis cylinder The conducting part of a nerve.

R.'s band The axis cylinder of a neuron.

R.'s fibers The nonmyelinated nerve fibers.

R.'s ganglion A group of nerve cells in the coronary sinus near its entry into the right atrium.

Remak's sign [Ernest Julius Remak, Ger. neurologist, 1849–1911] A sign or symptom pert. to perception of stimuli. It can be one of two types: a single stimulus may be perceived as if it were several stimuli applied in separate locations (polyesthesia), or there may be a delay in perception of stimuli. Both types are seen in tabes dorsalis.

remedial (rĭ-mē′dē-ăl) [L. *remedialis*] Curative; intended as a remedy.

remedy (rĕm′ĕd-ē) [L. *remedium,* medicine] **1.** To cure or relieve a disease. **2.** Anything that relieves or cures a disease.

herbal r. Plant leaves, roots, seeds, or extracts used to prevent or treat human ailments. Many herbs contain small concentrations of chemicals with therapeutic properties, and many cultures rely on plant-derived preparations for cures. A few herbs, however, may produce serious adverse or allergic responses. Problems may arise as a result of the lack of uniformity of the ingredients, misidentification of the ingredients, or variations in their potency. In the U.S., herbal remedies are considered nutrients rather than drugs; the Food and Drug Administration does not regulate their manufacture and sale. SEE: Entries beginning with the prefix "phyto-"; *alternative medicine.*

CAUTION: Herbal remedies of unknown potency should not be taken during pregnancy, while nursing, or in place of other therapies if such therapies are known to be more effective. Patients with complex illnesses should consult licensed health care professionals before initiating, and while undertaking, herbal therapies.

---

local r. An agent used to relieve a local condition such as a sore.

systemic r. An agent used to relieve or cure a disease affecting the entire organism.

remineralization (rē-mĭn″ĕr-ăl-ī-zā′shŭn) Therapeutic replacement of the mineral content of the body after it has been disrupted by disease or improper diet.

reminiscence therapy A form of supportive psychotherapy for elderly patients experiencing depression or loss. Reminiscence therapy assists patients to review and highlight the meaningful components of their past. This is thought to increase self-esteem and life satisfaction. It can be conducted in groups or individually.

remission (rĭ-mĭsh′ŭn) [L. *remissio,* remit] **1.** A lessening in severity or an abatement of symptoms. **2.** The period during which symptoms abate. **3.** The period when no evidence of underlying disease exists.

remittance (rē-mĭt′ĕns) A temporary abatement of symptoms.

remittent (rē-mĭt′ĕnt) [L. *remittere,* to send back] Alternately abating and returning at certain intervals. SEE: *fever.*

remnant Something that remains or is left over.

remnant radiation Ionizing radiation that passes through the part being examined to make the radiographical image.

remodeling **1.** The reshaping or reconstruction of a part of the body, esp. to repair a part that has been injured (e.g., the walls of the heart after myocardial infarction or the airways in patients with asthma). **2.** Bone change or growth that is the net effect of all appositional growth and bone resorption and that continues throughout life to adapt individual bones to the changing forces of growth, muscular activity, gravity, or mechanical pressures.

temporomandibular joint r. The slow changes in the articular surfaces of the temporomandibular joint as it adapts to changing occlusal forces, resulting in shape changes or irregularities of the condyle or articular eminence.

ren (rĕn) *pl.* **renes** [L.] The kidney.

renal (rē′năl) [LL. *renalis,* kidney] **1.** Pert. to the kidney. SYN: *nephric.* SEE: *kidney* for illus. **2.** Shaped like a kidney.

renal biopsy, percutaneous Obtaining renal tissue for analysis with a needle inserted through the skin, usually done after the kidney has been localized by ultrasound, computed tomography, or angiography. The most common complication is urinary bleeding, which tends to clear gradually over several days. This technique is used to establish a diagnosis of renal dysfunction, determine prognosis in patients with renal disease, evaluate the extent of renal injury, and determine appropriate therapy.

renal clearance test One of several kidney function tests based on the kidney's ability to eliminate a given substance in a standard time. Urea, phenolsulfonphthalein (PSP), iodopyracet, and other substances are employed.

renal failure, acute ABBR: ARF. An acute rise in the serum creatinine level of 25% or more. Acute renal failure may be transient (lasting days or weeks before resolving), or it may develop into chronic (end-stage) renal disease. SEE: *dialysis;* table; *Nursing Diagnoses Appendix.*

TREATMENT: Acute renal failure caused by urinary outlet obstruction often completely resolves when urinary flow is restored (i.e., after a urinary catheter is placed or a prostatectomy performed). Renal failure caused by prerenal conditions sometimes improves with fluid and pressor support but may require other therapies, including dialysis. The resolution of ARF caused by intrarenal diseases and kidney toxins depends on the underlying cause and the duration of the exposure. For example, immunosuppressant drugs may reverse the lesions in patients with ARF due to glomerulonephritis or renal vasculitis, whereas forced diuresis is the treatment for those whose disease is caused by rhabdomyolysis.

PATIENT CARE: The specific cause is identified and removed if possible. The nurse instructs the patient regarding dietary and fluid restrictions and implements these restrictions, promotes infection prevention, and advises the patient about activity restrictions due to metabolic alterations.

Neurological status is assessed, and safety measures are instituted. Intake and output and daily weights (measures of fluid status) are monitored. Daily blood tests determine acid-base and electrolyte balance. The patient is assessed for G.I. and cutaneous bleeding and anemia, and blood components are replaced or erythropoietin therapy is administered as prescribed. Blood pressure, pulse, respiratory rate, and heart and lung sounds are regularly assessed (e.g., for evidence of pericarditis or fluid overload).

If ARF is not reversed but progresses to chronic (end-stage) renal failure, follow-up care is arranged, and evaluation and teaching are provided for possible dialysis. Referral is made for vocational, sexual, or other counseling as needed.

renal papillary necrosis Destruction of the papillae of the kidney, usually as a result of pyelonephritis, diabetes mellitus, sickle cell disease, urinary obstruction, or the toxic effects of nonsteroidal anti-inflammatory drugs. If the necrotic tissue sloughs into the ureters, it may cause renal colic similar to the pain caused by a kidney stone.

renal scanning A scintigraphic method of determining renal function, size, and shape. A radioactive substance that concentrates in the kidney is given intravenously. The radiation emitted from the substance as it accumulates in the kidneys is recorded on a suitable photographic film.

renal tubular acidosis ABBR: RTA. A group of non–anion gap metabolic acidoses marked by either loss of bicarbonate or failure to excrete hydrogen ions in the urine. Type I (distal RTA) is marked by low serum potassium, elevated serum chloride, a urinary pH greater than 5.5, nephrocalcinosis, and nephrolithiasis. Alkalis such as sodium bicarbonate or Shohl's solution are effective treatments.

Type II (proximal RTA) is caused by impaired reabsorption of bicarbonate by the proximal tubules. Its hallmarks include preserved glomerular filtration, hypokalemia, excessive bicarbonate excretion in the urine during bicarbonate loading, and a urinary pH less than 5.5. Osteopenia and osteomalacia are common clinical consequences. Treatments may include volume restriction and potassium and bicarbonate supplementation.

Type IV (hyperkalemia RTA) usually is associated with hyporeninemic hypoaldosteronism due to diabetic nephropathy, nephrosclerosis associated with hypertension, or chronic nephropathy. Affected patients have high serum potassium levels and low urine ammonia excretion. They do not have renal cal-

Causes of Acute Renal Failure

Where	What's Responsible	Examples
Prerenal	Inadequate blood flow to the kidney	Severe dehydration; prolonged hypotension; renal ischemia or emboli; septic or cardiogenic shock
Renal	Injury to kidney glomeruli or tubules	Glomerulonephritis; toxic injury to the kidneys (e.g., by drugs or poisons)
Postrenal	Obstruction to urinary outflow	Prostatic hyperplasia; bladder outlet obstruction

culi. The hyperkalemia may be managed by administration of mineralocorticoids in combination with furosemide. Glomerular filtration is reduced in this disorder.

rendering, food The conversion of the waste products of animal butchery into feeds, bone meal, tallows, oils, and fertilizer. Consumption of rendered feed products sometimes results in animal and human infections, such as bovine spongiform encephalopathy (mad cow disease).

Rendu-Osler-Weber syndrome Hereditary hemorrhagic telangiectasia.

reniculus (rĕ-nĭk′ū-lŭs) [L.] A lobule of the kidney.

renifleur (rā-nĭ-flŭr′) [Fr.] One stimulated sexually by certain odors, esp. that of the the urine of others.

reniform (rĕn′ĭ-form) [L. *ren,* kidney, + *forma,* shape] Shaped like a kidney. SYN: *nephroid.*

renin (rĕn′ĭn) An enzyme produced by the kidney that splits angiotensinogen to form angiotensin I, which is then transformed to angiotensin II, which stimulates vasoconstriction and secretion of aldosterone. The blood renin level is elevated in some forms of hypertension.

renin substrate Angiotensinogen.

renipelvic (rĕn″ĭ-pĕl′vĭk) [″ + *pelvis,* basin] Pert. to the renal pelvis.

reniportal (rĕn″ĭ-por′tăl) [″ + *porta,* gate] **1.** Pert. to the "hilum" of the kidney. **2.** Pert. to the renal and portal circulations.

renipuncture (rĕn″ĭ-pŭnk′chūr) [″ + *punctura,* a piercing] Surgical puncture of the renal capsule.

rennet (rĕn′ĕt) [ME.] **1.** The lining of the fourth stomach of a calf. **2.** A fluid containing rennin (chymosin), a coagulating enzyme, used for making junket or cheese.

rennin (rĕn′ĭn) Chymosin.

renninogen (rĕn-ĭn′ō-jĕn) [ME. *rennet,* rennet, + Gr. *gennan,* to produce] The antecedent or zymogen from which rennin is formed; the inactive form of rennin.

reno-, ren- Combining form meaning *kidney.* SEE: *nephro-.*

renocutaneous (rē″nō-kū-tā′nē-ŭs) [″ + *cutis,* skin] Pert. to the kidneys and skin.

renogastric (rē″nō-găs′trĭk) [L. *ren,* kidney, + Gr. *gaster,* belly] Pert. to the kidneys and stomach.

renogram (rē′nō-grăm) [″ + Gr. *gramma,* something written] A record of the rate of removal of an intravenously injected dose of radioactive iodine (^{131}I) from the blood by the kidneys.

renography (rē-nŏg′ră-fē) [″ + Gr. *graphein,* to write] Radiography of the kidney.

renointestinal (rē″nō-ĭn-tĕs′tĭn-ăl) [″ + *intestinum,* intestine] Pert. to the kidneys and intestine.

renoprival (rē″nō-prī′văl) Pert. to loss of kidney function.

renovascular Pert. to the vascular supply of the kidney.

Renshaw cell (rĕn′shaw) [B. Renshaw, U.S. neurophysiologist, 1911–1948] An interneuron of the spinal cord that inhibits motor neurons.

reocclusion (rē′ŏ-kloo″zhŭn) Closure of a structure (e.g., a blood vessel) that had been previously stenosed and then unclogged by mechanical dilation or the use of medications.

reovirus (rē″ō-vī′rŭs) [*re*spiratory *en*teric *o*rphan *virus*] A double-stranded RNA virus found in the respiratory and digestive tracts of apparently healthy persons, and occasionally associated with respiratory, digestive, or neurological diseases.

rep [L., *repetatur*] Let it be repeated.

repair (rĭ-păr′) [L. *reparare,* to prepare again] To remedy, replace, or heal, as in a wound or a lost part.

plastic r. Use of plastic surgery to repair tissue.

tooth r. Recovery from pathological changes, involving the reduction of inflammation and the production of tertiary or reparative cementum. This is usually accompanied by improved health of the gingiva and the periodontal ligament.

repellent [L. *repellere,* to drive back] An agent that repels noxious organisms such as insects, ticks, and mites. Repellents may be applied to the surface of the body as a liquid, spray, or dust, or they may be used to impregnate clothing.

insect r. A commercial preparation effective in repelling insects. Many insect repellents contain diethyltoluamide, a safe and effective agent popularly known as DEET. When applying insect repellent, do not allow it to contact the eyes.

repercolation (rē″pĕr-kō-lā′shŭn) [L. *re,* again, + *percolare,* to filter] Repeated percolation using the same materials.

repercussion (rē-pĕr-kŭsh′ŭn) [L. *repercussio,* rebound] **1.** A reciprocal action. **2.** An action involved in causing the subsidence of a swelling, tumor, or eruption. **3.** Ballottement.

repercussive (rē″pĕr-kŭs′ĭv) **1.** Causing repercussion. **2.** An agent that repels; a repellent.

reperfusion [L. *re,* back, + *perfundere,* to pour through] **1.** The restoration of blood flow to a part of the body previously deprived of adequate circulation, such as the heart muscle (in myocardial infarction) or the brain (in stroke). This may be accomplished through the use of thrombolytic agents, sometimes called "clot busters" (e.g., streptokinase or tissue plasminogen activator), or mechanical interventions (e.g., balloon angioplasty). The use of these interventions has improved patient outcomes in acute coronary syndromes and patients with stroke who come to medical attention in the first few hours of their illness. **2.** The reinstitution of blood flow to tissues that have been traumatized, esp. by a long period of crushing. SEE: *crush syndrome; rhabdomyolysis*.

r. injury Cellular damage that occurs after blood flow is restored to ischemic tissues.

repetitive motion injury Tissue damage caused by repeated trauma, usually associated with writing, painting, typing, or use of vibrating tools or hand tools. Almost any form of activity that produces repeated trauma to a particular area of soft tissue, including tendons and synovial sheaths, may cause this type of injury. Carpal tunnel syndrome, other nerve compression syndromes, and shin splints are examples of repetitive motion injuries. SYN: *cumulative trauma syndrome; repetitive strain injury; overuse syndrome*.

replacement **1.** The restoration of a structure to its original position. **2.** The repletion of lost fluids (e.g., by fluid infusions or blood transfusion).

orthotopic bladder r. Neobladder.

replantation [L. *re*, again, + *planto*, to plant] Surgical reimplantation of something removed from the body, esp. the surgical procedure of rejoining a hand, arm, or leg to the body after its accidental detachment. In dentistry, replantation is the replacement of a tooth that has been removed from its socket.

repletion (rē-plē′shŭn) [L. *repletio*, a filling up] The condition of being full or satisfied.

replication (rĕp″lĭ-kā′shŭn) **1.** A doubling back of tissue. **2.** In medical investigations, the repetition of an experiment. **3.** In genetics, the duplication process of genetic material.

replicon (rĕp′lĭ-kŏn) A segment of DNA that includes the "start" and "stop" nucleotide sequences and can replicate as a unit. In a human chromosome, these are genes.

repolarization Restoration of the polarized state at a cell membrane (negative inside in relation to the outside) following depolarization as in muscle or nerve fibers.

report The account, usually verbal, that the nursing staff going off duty gives to the oncoming staff. The purpose is to provide continuity of care despite the change in staff. The information provided is of the utmost importance in caring for critically ill patients.

reportable disease Notifiable disease.

reposition (rē″pō-zĭsh′ŭn) [L. *repositio*, a replacing] Restoration of an organ or tissue to its correct or original position.

repositioning (rē″pō-zĭsh′ŭn-ĭng) Replacement of a structure to its original site or a new site.

jaw r. Changing of the position of the mandible in relation to the maxilla by altering the occlusion of the teeth.

muscle r. Surgical placement of a muscle to another attachment point to enhance function.

repositor An instrument for restoring a tissue or an organ to its normal position.

inversion r. An instrument for replacing an inverted uterus.

uterine r. A lever for replacing the uterus when it is out of normal position.

repression (rē-prĕsh′ŭn) [L. *repressus*, press back] In psychology, the refusal to entertain distressing or painful ideas. In Freudian theory, the submersion of such thoughts in the unconscious, where they continue to influence the individual. Psychoanalysis seeks to discover and release repressions.

coordinate r. Simultaneous reduction of the enzyme levels of a metabolic pathway.

enzyme r. Interference with enzyme synthesis by a metabolic product.

repressor (rē-prĕs′or) [L. *repressus*, press back] Something, esp. an enzyme, that inhibits or interferes with the initiation of protein synthesis by genetic material.

reprocessing Preparation of a dialysis membrane for reuse with rinses and sterilizing solutions.

reprocessing of endoscopes Preparation of endoscopes for reuse by disinfecting and decontaminating them.

PATIENT CARE: To protect patients from infections transmitted by reused endoscopes, the following procedure is followed: (1) The endoscope is manually cleaned externally; (2) Detergent is drawn through the accessory channel; (3) The accessory channel's chamber and valves are carefully brushed; (4) Reusable forceps are sterilized; (5) The endoscope is treated with a 2.4% solution of glutaraldehyde, heated to 25°C for 45 minutes; (6) The strength of the disinfectant solution is tested daily.

reproducibility **1.** The quality of being provable again by repeated experimentation. SEE: *research*. **2.** A quality control test of radiographical output for multiple exposures using the same exposure factors. These factors must not vary by more than ±5%.

reproduction (rē-prō-dŭk′shŭn) [L. *re*, again, + *productio*, production] **1.** The process by which plants and animals produce offspring. SEE: *ovary* for illus. **2.** The creation of a similar structure or situation; the act of duplicating.

asexual r. Reproduction in which sex cells are not involved, as by fission or budding.

cytogenic r. Reproduction by means of asexual single germ cells.

sexual r. Reproduction by means of sexual or germ cells. Usually a male cell (spermatozoon) fuses with a female cell (egg or ovum). SYN: *syngamy*.

somatic r. Asexual reproduction by budding of somatic cells.

reproductive (rē″prō-dŭk′tĭv) Pert. to or employed in reproduction.

repulsion (rĭ-pŭl′shŭn) [L. *repulsio*, a thrusting back] **1.** The act of driving back. **2.** The force exerted by one body on another to cause separation; the opposite of attraction.

request for production of documents and things A discovery technique in which the plaintiff or defendant requests in a written form that the other party furnish information pertaining to the issues of the lawsuit.

In medical negligence cases, requests can be for: medical records, office records, facility policies and procedures, staffing schedules, personnel records, ambulance run sheets, and autopsy protocols, in addition to other items.

request for proposal ABBR: RFP. Notification by a foundation or government agency that funds are available for research projects and that research sponsors are seeking applicants for those funds.

required service A service that must be included in a health program for it to qualify for federal funds.

RES *reticuloendothelial system;* an old name for mononuclear phagocytic system.

rescinnamine (rē-sĭn′ă-mĭn) An antihypertensive drug derived from species of *Rauwolfia*.

rescue 1. To free a person from a hazardous situation such as entrapment in an automobile, trench, cave, or burning building, or from the site of a hazardous material spill. **2.** To restore an organ to its normal function after an illness or a treatment that has damaged it.

rescue tool A piece of equipment used by rescuers in emergency medical service to free trapped victims. Rescue tools include a come-a-long, a hand-operated winch used to gain forceful entry during a rescue; cutting tools, used to cut open vehicles and metal to gain access to a patient; a hydraulic jack, a hand-operated jack used to lift objects away from patients; pneumatic air bags, used to lift or spread heavy objects; and a power chisel, a pressure-operated device used to cut into sheet metal. The trade name of one familiar rescue tool is Jaws of Life.

research (rĭ-sĕrch′, rē′sĕrch) [O.Fr. *recerche*, research] Scientific study, investigation, or experimentation to establish facts and analyze their significance.

clinical r. Research based mainly on bedside observation of the patient rather than on laboratory work.

laboratory r. Research done principally in the laboratory.

medical r. Research concerned with any phase of medical science.

outcomes r. An analysis of the value of provided health care services. SEE: *outcome criteria*.

preembryo r. Research involving the use of the fertilized egg from its unicellular zygote stage until the embryo stage (i.e., to the 14th day following fertilization), for example, for studies of in vitro fertilization, conception, gene therapy, or studies of cancer.

resect (rē-sĕkt′) [L. *resectus*, cut off] To cut off or cut out a portion of a structure or organ, as to cut off the end of a bone or to remove a segment of the intestine.

resectable (rē-sĕk′tă-bl) Able to be removed surgically; usually used in reference to malignant growths.

resection (rē-sĕk′shŭn) [L. *resectio*, a cutting off] Partial excision of a bone or other structure.

gastric r. Surgical resection of all or a part of the stomach.

transurethral r. Surgical removal of the prostate using an instrument introduced through the urethra.

wedge r. Surgical removal of a triangular-shaped piece of tissue (e.g., from the lung, gastrointestinal tract, uterus, ovary, or other organs). Wedge resection is often used to remove malignant tissue.

window r. Resection of a portion of the nasal septum after reflection of a flap of mucous membrane.

resectoscope (rē-sĕk′tō-skōp) [L. *resectus*, cut off, + Gr. *skopein*, to examine] An instrument for resection of the prostate gland through the urethra.

resectoscopy (rē″sĕk-tŏs′kō-pē) Resection of the prostate through the urethra.

reserpine (rĭ-sĕr′pĭn) A chemically pure derivative of the plant *Rauwolfia serpentina*. It lowers blood pressure and acts as a tranquilizer.

reserve (rē-zĕrv′) [L. *reservare*, to keep back] **1.** Something held back for future use. **2.** Self-control of one's feelings and thoughts.

alkali r. Alkaline r.

alkaline r. The amount of base in the blood, principally bicarbonates, available for neutralization of fixed acids (acetoacetate, β-hydroxybutyrate, and lactate). A fall in alkaline reserve is called acidosis; a rise, alkalosis. SYN: *alkali r.*

cardiac r. The ability of the heart to increase cardiac output to meet the needs of increased energy output.

reservoir (rĕz′ĕr-vwor) [Fr.] A place or cavity for storage of fluids.

cardiotomy r. A device used to salvage autologous blood lost by patients as they undergo cardiovascular surgery.

r. of infectious agents Any person,

animal, arthropod, plant, soil, or substance in which an infectious agent normally lives and multiplies, on which it depends primarily for survival, and where it reproduces itself in a way that allows transmission to a susceptible host.

residency A period of at least 1 year and often 3 to 7 years of on-the-job training, usually postgraduate, that is part of the formal educational program for health care professionals.

resident A physician obtaining further clinical training after internship, usually as a member of the house staff of a hospital.

residual (rĭ-zĭd′ū-ăl) [L. *residuum,* residue] **1.** Pert. to something left as a residue. **2.** In psychology, any aftereffect of experience influencing later behavior.

residual function The functional capacity remaining after an illness or injury.

residue (rĕz′ĭ-dū) The remainder of something after a part is removed.

residue-free diet A diet without cellulose or roughage. Semisolid and bland foods are included. Low-residue diets are used to prepare the colon for barium enemas or colonoscopy and occasionally to help manage Crohn's disease.

residuum (rē-zĭd′ū-ŭm) *pl.* **residua** [L.] Residue.

resilience (rē-zĭl′ē-ĕns) [L. *resiliens,* leaping back] **1.** Elasticity. **2.** The ability to withstand mental or physical stress.

resilient (rē-zĭl′ē-ĕnt) Elastic.

resin (rĕz′ĭn) [L. *resina,* fr. Gr. *rhetine,* resin of the pine] **1.** An amorphous, nonvolatile solid or soft-solid substance, which is a natural exudation from plants. It is practically insoluble in water but dissolves in alcohol. SEE: *rosin.* **2.** Any of a class of solid or soft organic compounds of natural or synthetic origin. They are usually of high molecular weight and most are polymers. Included are polyvinyl, polyethylene, and polystyrene. These are combined with chemicals such as epoxides, plasticizers, pigments, fillers, and stabilizers to form plastics.

acrylic r. Quick-cure r.

anion-exchange r. SEE: *ion-exchange r.*

cation-exchange r. SEE: *ion-exchange r.*

cold-cure r. Quick-cure r.

ion-exchange r. An ionizable synthetic substance, which may be acid or basic, used accordingly to remove either acid or basic ions from solutions. Anion-exchange resins are used to absorb acid in the stomach, and cation-exchange resins are used to remove basic (alkaline) ions from solutions.

quick-cure r. An autopolymer resin, used in many dental procedures, that can be polymerized by an activator and catalyst without applying external heat. SYN: *acrylic r.; cold-cure r.; self-curing r.*

self-curing r. Quick-cure r.

resinoid (rĕz′ĭ-noyd) [″ + Gr. *eidos,* form, shape] Resembling a resin.

resinous (rĕz′ĭ-nŭs) Having the nature of or pert. to resin.

res ipsa loquitur [L.] Literally, "the thing speaks for itself." In malpractice this concept is used for cases in which an injury occurs to the plaintiff in a situation solely under the control of the defendant. The injury would not have occurred had the defendant exercised due care. The defendant must then defend his or her actions. In medicine the classic example of this situation is the leaving of an object such as a sponge or clamp in a patient's body after a surgical procedure, or the inadvertent removal of a healthy organ or extremity.

resistance (rĭ-zĭs′tăns) [L. *resistens,* standing back] **1.** Opposition to a disease, a toxin, or to a physical force. **2.** The force exerted to penetrate the unconscious or to submerge memories in the unconscious. **3.** In psychoanalysis, a condition in which the ego avoids bringing into consciousness conflicts and unpleasant events responsible for neurosis; the reluctance of a patient to give up old patterns of thought and behavior. It may take various forms such as silence, failure to remember dreams, forgetfulness, and undue annoyance with trivial aspects of the treatment situation. **4.** Force applied to a body part by weights, machinery, or another person to load muscles as an exercise to increase muscle strength.

airway r. The impedance to the flow of air into and out of the respiratory tract.

antibiotic r. The evolution of microorganisms that has provided them with mechanisms to block the action of antibiotics. Chance mutations have provided some bacteria with genes for enzymes that destroy antibiotics such as penicillins, cephalosporins, or aminoglycosides. Other mutations have changed the structure of bacterial cell walls previously penetrable by antibiotics or have created new enzymes for cellular functions that were previously blocked by drugs. SYN: *bacterial resistance.* SEE: *vancomycin-resistant enterococci; resistance transfer factor; methicillin-resistant* Staphylococcus aureus.

CAUTION: The indiscriminate use of antibiotics provides the selection pressure that creates ever more resistant strains. The most effective, and frequently ignored, measure to reduce the spread of many organisms is *careful handwashing with antimicrobial soap* after contact with *all* patients.

---

cross r. Multidrug resistance.

drug r. The ability to withstand drug treatment.

expiratory r. The use of a restricted orifice, or flow resistor, during positive-pressure ventilation to retard the flow of exhaled gases.

insulin r. Cellular phenomena that prevent insulin from stimulating the uptake of glucose from the bloodstream and the synthesis of glycogen. Insulin resistance is one of the fundamental metabolic defects found in patients with type 2 diabetes mellitus.

multidrug r. ABBR: MDR. The ability of germs or cancer cells to withstand treatment with more than one drug.

peripheral r. The resistance of the arterial vascular system, esp. the arterioles and capillaries, to the flow of blood.

systemic vascular r. ABBR: SVR. The resistance to the flow of blood through the body's blood vessels. It increases as vessels constrict (e.g., when a drug like norepinephrine is given) and decreases when vessels dilate (e.g., in septic shock). Any change in the diameter, elasticity, or number of vessels recruited can influence the measured amount of resistance to the flow of blood through the body.

threshold r. The amount of pressure necessary in overcoming resistance to flow.

transthoracic r. The amount of resistance to the flow of electrical energy across the chest. This is an important factor to consider when electrical therapies such as defibrillation, cardioversion, and transthoracic pacing are used to treat abnormal cardiac rhythms.

viscous r. Nonelastic opposition of tissue to ventilation due to the energy required to displace the thorax and airways.

resistance exercise Exercise in which a muscle contraction is opposed by an outside force, to increase strength or endurance. If the resistance is applied by using weights, it is called mechanical resistance; if applied by a clinician, it is called manual resistance.

resistance transfer factor ABBR: R factor. A genetic factor in bacteria that controls resistance to certain antibiotic drugs. The factor may be passed from one bacterium to another. This makes it possible for nonpathogenic bacteria to become resistant to antibiotics and to transfer that resistance to pathogens, thereby establishing a potential source for an epidemic. SEE: *plasmid.*

resolution (rĕz-ō-lū′shŭn) [L. *resolutio,* a relaxing] **1.** Decomposition; absorption or breaking down of the products of inflammation. **2.** Cessation of illness; a return to normal. **3.** The ability of the eye or a series of lenses to distinguish fine detail. **4.** In radiology, the ability to record small images placed very close together as separate images.

resolve (rē-zŏlv′) [L. *resolvere,* to release] **1.** To return to normal as after a pathological process. **2.** To separate into components.

resonance (rĕz′ō-năns) [L. *resonantia,* resound] **1.** The quality or act of resounding. **2.** The quality of the sound heard on percussion of a hollow structure such as the chest or abdomen. An absence of resonance is termed *flatness;* diminished resonance, *dullness.* **3.** In physics, the modification of sound caused by vibrations of a body that are set up by waves from another vibrating body. **4.** In electricity, a state in which two electrical circuits are in tune with each other.

amphoric r. A sound similar to that produced by blowing across the mouth of an empty bottle.

bandbox r. The pulmonary resonance heard during chest percussion in patients with emphysema.

bell-metal r. The sound heard in pneumothorax on auscultation when a coin is held against the chest wall and struck by another coin.

cracked-pot r. The peculiar clinking sound sometimes heard on chest percussion in cases of advanced tuberculosis when cavities are present.

electron spin r. ABBR: ESR. A technique used in medical imaging that identifies atoms by their electron spin characteristics.

normal r. Vesicular r.

skodaic r. An increased percussion sound over the upper lung when there is a pleural effusion in the lower part.

tympanic r. A low-pitched, drumlike sound heard on percussion over a large air-containing space.

tympanitic r. The resonance obtained by percussion of a hollow structure, such as the stomach or colon, when it is moderately distended with air.

vesicular r. The resonance obtained by percussion of normal lungs. SYN: *normal r.*

vocal r. In auscultation, the vibrations of the voice transmitted to the examiner's ear, normally more marked over the right apex of the lung. These vibrations are abnormally increased in pneumonic consolidation, in lungs infiltrated with tuberculosis, or in cavities that communicate freely with a bronchus.

Vocal resonance is diminished or absent in pleural effusion (air, pus, serum, lymph, or blood); emphysema; pulmonary collapse; pulmonary edema; and egophony, a modified bronchophony characterized by a trembling, bleating sound usually heard above the upper border of dullness of pleural effusions and occasionally heard in beginning pneumonia.

whispering r. The auscultation sound heard when a patient whispers.

resonant (rĕz′ō-nănt) Producing a vibrating sound on percussion.

resonating [L. *resonantia,* resound] Vibrating sympathetically with a source of sound or electrical oscillations.

resonating cavities The anatomic intensifiers of the human voice, including the upper portion of the larynx, pharynx, nasal cavity, paranasal sinuses, and oral cavity.

resonator (rĕz′ō-nā″tĕr) **1.** A structure that can be set into sympathetic vibration when sound waves of the same frequency from another vibrating body strike it. **2.** In electricity, an apparatus consisting of an electric circuit in which oscillations of a certain frequency are set up by oscillations of the same frequency in another circuit.

resorb (rē-sorb′, rē-zorb′) [L. *resorbere,* to suck in] **1.** To undergo resorption. **2.** To absorb again.

resorbent (rē-sor′bĕnt) [L. *resorbens,* sucking in] An agent that promotes the absorption of abnormal matters, as exudates or blood clots (e.g., potassium iodide, ammonium chloride).

resorcin (rĕ-zor′sĭn) Resorcinol.

resorcinol (rĕ-zor′sĭ-nŏl) An agent with keratolytic, fungicidal, and bactericidal actions, used in treating certain skin diseases. SYN: *resorcin.*

resorcinolphthalein (rē-zor″sĭ-nŏl-thăl′ē-ĭn) Fluorescein sodium.

resorption (rē-sorp′shŭn) [L. *resorbere,* to suck in] **1.** Removal by absorption, as of an exudate or pus. **2.** The removal of enamel and other calcific portions of a tooth as a result of lysis and other pathological processes. It often results from pressure or vascular changes as in root resorption of deciduous teeth prior to shedding, or bone resorption on the pressure side during tooth movement.

bone r. The removal of bone tissue by resorption.

resource allocation **1.** The management of economic and administrative reserves by choosing from among competing claims for assets and services. **2.** Health care rationing.

resource-based relative value scale ABBR: RBRVS. A measuring tool developed to increase payment to nonsurgeons for cognitive services (i.e., evaluation and management of patients). The scale is based on the total work required for a given service and on other considerations, including the cost of the physician's practice, the income lost during training, and the relative cost of liability insurance. This method of calculating medical care services was implemented by law in January 1992. SEE: *managed care; managed competition.*

Resource, Conservation, and Recovery Act ABBR: RCRA. An act passed in 1976 that gave the Environmental Protection Agency the authority to control hazardous waste disposal, including the disposal of infectious and radioactive medical waste products.

resource depletion The dissipation of assets or reserves, esp. (in health care and the environment) those that affect public health.

respirable (rē-spīr′ă-bl, rĕs′pĕr-ă-bl) [L. *respirare,* breathe again] Fit or adapted for respiration.

respiration (rĕs-pĭr-ā′shŭn) [L. *respiratio,* breathing] **1.** The interchange of gases between an organism and the medium in which it lives. **2.** The act of breathing (i.e., inhaling and exhaling) during which the lungs are provided with air through inhaling and the carbon dioxide is removed through exhaling. Normal respiratory exchange of oxygen and carbon dioxide in the lungs is impossible unless the pulmonary tissue is adequately perfused with blood. SEE: table; *diaphragm* for illus.; *lung; ventilation.*

Rate of Respiration (breaths/min)

Premature infant	40–90
Newborn	30–60
1st yr	20–40
2nd yr	20–30
5th yr	20–25
15th yr	15–20
Adult	8–20

abdominal r. Respiration in which chiefly the diaphragm exerts itself while the chest wall muscles are nearly at rest; used in normal, quiet breathing—and in pathological conditions such as pleurisy, pericarditis, and rib fracture. SYN: *diaphragmatic r.*

absent r. Respiration in which respiratory sounds are suppressed.

accelerated r. Respiration occurring at a faster rate than normal, considered accelerated when it exceeds 25 per minute in adults. Increased frequency may result from exercise, physical exertion, excitement, fear, exposure to high altitudes, and many metabolic, hematological, cardiac, and pulmonary diseases.

aerobic r. Cellular respiration in which oxygen is used in the production of energy.

amphoric r. Respiration having amphoric resonance. SEE: *resonance, amphoric.*

anaerobic r. Cellular respiration in which energy is obtained from chemical reactions that do not involve free oxygen.

apneustic r. Breathing marked by prolonged inspiration unrelieved by attempts to exhale. Seen in patients who have had the upper part of the pons of the brain removed or damaged.

artificial r. Maintenance of respiratory movement by artificial means, such as rescue breathing, bag-valve-mask, pocket mask, automatic transport ventilator, manual transport ventilator, or a flow-restricted oxygen-powered ventilation device. SEE: *cardiopulmonary resuscitation.*

Biot's r. Biot's breathing.

cell r. The gradual breakdown of food molecules in the presence of oxygen within cells, resulting in the formation of carbon dioxide and water and the release of energy in the forms of ATP and heat. In many intermediary reactions, substances other than oxygen act as oxidizing agents (i.e., hydrogen or electron acceptors). Reactions are catalyzed by respiratory enzymes, which include the flavoproteins, cytochromes, and other enzymes. Certain vitamins (nicotinamide, riboflavin, thiamine, pyridoxine, and pantothenic acid) are essential in the formation of components of various intracellular enzyme systems.

Cheyne-Stokes r. A common and bizarre breathing pattern marked by a period of apnea lasting 10 to 60 sec, followed by gradually increasing depth and frequency of respirations. It accompanies coma, encephalopathy, and other neurological disorders. This condition may be present as a normal finding in children. SEE: illus.

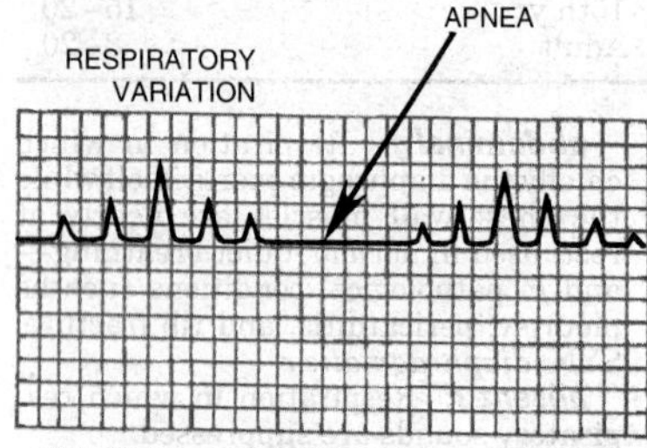

GRAPH OF RESPIRATORY MOVEMENTS IN CHEYNE-STOKES BREATHING

cogwheel r. Interrupted r.

costal r. Respiration in which the chest cavity expands by raising the ribs.

decreased r. Respiration at less than a normal rate for the individual's age. In adults, a respiratory rate of less than 12 breaths per minute. Slower than normal respiratory rates occur after opiate or sedative use, during sleep, in coma, and many other conditions, and may result in respiratory failure or carbon dioxide retention. SYN: *slow r.*

diaphragmatic r. Abdominal r.

direct r. Respiration in which an organism, such as a one-celled ameba, secures its oxygen and gives up carbon dioxide directly to the surrounding medium.

electrophrenic r. Radiofrequency electrophrenic respiration.

external r. Breathing, that is, inspiration and expiration.

fetal r. Gas exchange in the placenta between the fetal and maternal blood. SYN: *placental r.*

forced r. Voluntary hyperpnea (increase in rate and depth of breathing).

internal r. The passage of oxygen from the blood into the cells, its use by the cells, and the passage of carbon dioxide from the cells into the blood. Oxygen is carried in combination with hemoglobin. Oxyhemoglobin gives arterial blood its red color; reduced hemoglobin gives venous blood its dark red color. Carbon dioxide is carried in combination with metallic elements in the blood as bicarbonates and carbonic acid. Normally the partial pressure of oxygen in the blood is 75 to 100 mm Hg, depending on age; for carbon dioxide it is 35 to 45 mm Hg. SYN: *tissue r.*

interrupted r. Respiration in which inspiratory or expiratory sounds are not continuous. SYN: *cogwheel r.*

intrauterine r. Respiration by the fetus before birth. SEE: *fetal respiration.*

Kussmaul's r. Kussmaul's breathing.

labored r. Dyspnea or difficult breathing; respiration that involves active participation of accessory inspiratory and expiratory muscles.

muscles of r. *Inspiration:* diaphragm and external intercostals. *Forced inspiration* (assist in elevating ribs and sternum): scaleni, levatores costorum, sternocleidomastoideus, pectoralis major, platysma myoides, and serratus posterior superior. *Expiration* (voluntary deep breathing or forced expiration): internal intercostals, rectus abdominis, external and internal oblique, transverse abdominis. SEE: *diaphragm; expiration; inspiration.*

The following accessory muscles may assist in depressing the ribs: serratus posterior inferior, quadratus lumborum.

paradoxical r. **1.** Respiration occurring in patients with chest trauma and multiple rib fractures in which a portion of the chest wall sinks inward with each spontaneous inspiratory effort. **2.** A condition seen in paralysis of the diaphragm in which the diaphragm ascends during inspiration.

periodic r. Periodic breathing.

placental r. Fetal r.

slow r. Decreased respiration.

stertorous r. Respiration marked by rattling or bubbling sounds.

stridulous r. Respiration marked by high-pitched crowing or barking sound heard on inspiration, caused by an obstruction near the glottis or in the respiratory passageway.

thoracic r. Respiration performed entirely by expansion of the chest when the abdomen does not move. It is seen when the peritoneum or diaphragm is inflamed, when the abdominal cavity is restricted by tight bandages or clothes, or during abdominal surgery.

tissue r. Internal r.

respirator (rĕs′pĭ-rā″tor) [L. *respirare,* to breathe] A machine used to assist ventilation and/or oxygenation. Mechanical methods of assisting respiration usually include the capability of producing either intermittent or continuous positive pressure in the lungs.

abdominal belt r. An obsolete device used for noninvasive ventilatory assistance by patients with chronic respiratory failure, consisting of an inflatable rubber bladder held over the abdomen that inflates and deflates to assist diaphragm movement and ventilation.

respiratory (rĕs-pīr′ă-tō-rē, rĕs′pĭ-ră-tō″rē) [L. *respiratio,* breathing] Pert. to respiration.

respiratory anemometer An obsolete form of respirometer formerly used in investigating pulmonary function.

respiratory center A region in the medulla oblongata of the brainstem that regulates movements of respiration. This area consists of an inspiratory center, located in the rostral half of the reticular formation overlying the olivary nuclei, and an expiratory center, located dorsal to the inspiratory center. The pons contains the apneustic center, which prolongs inhalation, and the pneumotaxic center, which helps bring about exhalation.

respiratory defense mechanisms Ciliated epithelium, mucus, immunoglobulins, and other devices present in the trachea, bronchi, and lungs, used to defend the respiratory tract against microorganisms and other inhaled particles.

respiratory distress syndrome of the preterm infant ABBR: RDS. Severe impairment of respiratory function in a preterm newborn, caused by immaturity of the lungs. This condition is rarely present in a newborn of more than 37 weeks' gestation or in one weighing at least 2.2 kg (5 lb). RDS is the leading cause of death in prematurely born infants in the U.S. SYN: *hyaline membrane disease*. SEE: *acute respiratory distress syndrome; preterm labor; Nursing Diagnoses Appendix.*

SYMPTOMS: Shortly after birth the preterm infant with RDS has a low Apgar score, and develops signs of acute respiratory distress owing to atelectasis of the lung, impaired perfusion of the lung, and reduced pulmonary compliance. Tachypnea, tachycardia, retraction of the rib cage during inspiration, cyanosis, and grunting during expiration are present. Blood gas studies reflect the impaired ventilatory function. Radiographical examination of the lung reveals atelectasis.

TREATMENT: Preterm infants with RDS require treatment in a specially staffed and equipped neonatal intensive care unit. Therapy is supportive to ensure adequate hydration and electrolyte control. Every attempt should be made to reduce oxygen requirements by reducing any fever and minimizing activity. Supplemental oxygen is given. If necessary, assisted ventilation is used with care to prevent the traumatic formation of pulmonary air leaks that could cause pulmonary emphysema and tension pneumothorax. Instillation of surfactant into the respiratory tract is essential in managing this condition.

PATIENT CARE: *To prevent RDS,* as soon after birth as possible (preferably within 15 min), the health care professional administers neonatal lung surfactant intratracheally. The neonate's response to the medication is monitored carefully, and used to guide changes in ventilation (e.g., inspiratory pressures, tidal volume) and oxygenation.

The skin and mucous membranes are frequently inspected and lubricated with a water-soluble lubricant to prevent irritation, inflammation, and perforation.

The newborn is maintained in a thermoneutral environment to stabilize body temperature at 97.6°F (36.5°C). The newborn requires gentle and minimal handling, with assessment and care procedures separated by rest periods. Caloric intake is provided orally or by gavage feeding in quantity to prevent catabolic breakdown. Ongoing laboratory testing of blood contributes to blood loss, which may then require replacement. Because of hypoxia, low serum albumin, and acidosis, limited binding of albumin to bilirubin occurs, so these newborns are at risk for kernicterus. Phototherapy or exchange transfusions, or both, control resultant increased serum bilirubin levels.

The parents require ongoing support in the face of such serious neonatal illness. The parents are encouraged to ask questions and raise concerns to be addressed. The parents' presence at cribside is encouraged and they are shown ways to approach the infant without adding to his or her stress. The parents may require social services and psychological referrals or the support of family, friends, or clergy to help them deal with familial, financial, and emotional stresses imposed by the illness.

respiratory failure, acute Any impairment in oxygen uptake, carbon dioxide exhalation, and arterial pH in which the arterial oxygen tension falls below 60 mm Hg, the carbon dioxide tension rises above 50, and the pH drops below 7.35.

TREATMENT: In most cases, the patient will need supplemental oxygen therapy. Intubation and mechanical ventilation may be needed if the patient cannot oxygenate and ventilate adequately (i.e., if carbon dioxide retention occurs). Treatment depends on the underlying cause of the respiratory failure (e.g., bronchodilators for asthma, antibiotics for pneumonia, diuretics or vasodilators for congestive heart failure).

PATIENT CARE: Patients with acute respiratory failure are usually admitted to an acute care unit. The patient is positioned for optimal gas exchange, as well as for comfort. Supplemental oxygen is provided, but patients with chronic obstructive lung disease who retain carbon dioxide are closely monitored for adverse effects. A normothermic state is maintained to reduce the patient's oxygen demand. If mechanical ventilation is needed, ventilator settings and inspired oxygen concentrations are adjusted based on arterial blood gas results. The trachea is suctioned after oxygenation as necessary, and humidification is provided to help loosen and liquefy secretions. Secretions are collected as needed for culture and sensitivity testing. Sterile technique during suctioning and change of ventilator tubing helps to prevent infection. Using the minimal leak technique for endotracheal tube cuff inflation helps to prevent tracheal erosion. Positioning the nasoendotracheal tube midline within the nostril, avoiding excessive tube movement, and providing adequate support for ventilator tubing all help to prevent nasal and endotracheal tissue necrosis. Periodically loosening the securing tapes and supports prevents skin irritation and breakdown. The patient is assessed for complications of mechanical ventilation, including reduced cardiac output, pneumothorax or other barotrauma, increased pulmonary vascular resistance, diminished urine output, increased intracranial pressure, and gastrointestinal bleeding.

The patient is monitored closely for signs of respiratory arrest; lung sounds are auscultated and any deterioration in oxygen saturation immediately reported. The patient is also watched for adverse drug effects and treatment complications such as oxygen toxicity and acute respiratory distress syndrome. Vital signs are assessed frequently, and fever, tachycardia, tachypnea or bradypnea, and hypotension are reported. The electrocardiogram is monitored for arrhythmias. Serum electrolyte levels and fluid balance are monitored and steps are taken to correct and prevent imbalances.

All tests, procedures, and treatments should be explained to the patient and family. Rationales for such measures should be presented, and concerns elicited and answered. If the patient is intubated (or has had a tracheostomy), the patient should be told why speech is not possible and should be taught how to use alternative methods to communicate needs, wishes, and concerns to health care staff and family members.

respiratory failure, chronic Chronic inability of the respiratory system to maintain the function of oxygenating blood and remove carbon dioxide from the lungs. Many diseases can cause chronic pulmonary insufficiency, including asthmatic airway obstruction, emphysema, chronic bronchitis, and cystic fibrosis; and chronic pulmonary interstitial tissue diseases such as sarcoidosis, pneumoconiosis, idiopathic pulmonary fibrosis, disseminated carcinoma, radiation injury, and leukemia.

PATIENT CARE: The focus of patient care is on relieving respiratory symptoms, managing hypoxia, conserving energy, and avoiding respiratory irritants and infections. The nurse, respiratory therapist, primary care physician, and pulmonologist carry out the prescribed treatment regimen and teach the patient and family to manage care at home.

Patients may require supplemental oxygen. The patient is taught how to use the equipment and the importance of maintaining an appropriate flow rate. Low flow rates (1–2 L/m) are often best for patients with chronic obstructive lung disease. Drug therapy can include inhaled bronchodilators (if bronchospasm is reversible), oral or inhaled corticosteroids, oral or inhaled sympathomimetics, inhaled mucolytic therapy, and prompt use of oral antibiotics in the presence of respiratory infection. The patient and family are taught the order and spacing for administering these drugs, as well as how to use a metered-dose inhaler (with spacer if necessary). They are taught the desired effects, serious adverse reactions to report, and minor adverse effects and how to deal with them. Patients are taught care of inhalers and other respiratory equipment and are advised to rinse the mouth after using these devices to help limit bad tastes, dryness, and *Candida* infections.

Unless otherwise restricted, the patient will benefit from increased fluid intake (to 3 L/day) to help liquefy secretions and aid in their expectoration. Deep-breathing and coughing techniques are taught to promote ventilation and remove secretions. The patient also may be taught postural drainage and chest physiotherapy to help mobilize secretions and clear airways. Such therapy is to be carried out at least 1 hr before or after meals. Incentive spirometry may help to promote optimal lung expansion. A high-calorie, high-protein diet, offered as small, frequent meals, helps the patient maintain needed nutrition, while conserving energy and reducing fatigue.

Daily activity is encouraged, alternating with rest to prevent fatigue. Patients may benefit from a planned respiratory rehabilitation program to teach breathing techniques, provide conditioning, and help increase exercise tolerance. Diversional activities also should be provided, based on the patient's interests.

The patient is assessed for changes in baseline respiratory function; restlessness, changes in breath sounds, and tachypnea may signal an exacerbation. Any changes in sputum quality or quantity are noted. The patient is taught to be aware of these changes.

Patients need help in adjusting to lifestyle changes necessitated by this chronic illness. Patients and their families are encouraged to ask questions and voice concerns; answers are provided when possible, and support is given throughout. The patient and family should be included in all care planning and related decisions. The patient also is taught to avoid air pollutants such as automobile exhaust fumes and aerosol sprays, as well as crowds and people with respiratory infections. Patients should obtain influenza immunization annually and pneumonia immunization every 6 years. The patient also may benefit from avoiding exposure to cold air and covering the nose and mouth with a scarf or mask when outdoors in cold, windy weather. Patients who smoke tobacco are advised to abstain, using nicotine replacement therapy, hypnotism, support groups, or other methods.

respiratory function monitoring The use of various techniques to provide alarms that alert a patient's attendants to a change in the ability of the lungs to perform their functions. These techniques include noninvasive devices for measuring the oxygen content of the blood (e.g., pulse oximetry); methods of monitoring respiratory muscle function and breathing pattern; or devices for monitoring the carbon dioxide content of expired air (i.e., capnography). SEE: *apnea monitoring*.

respiratory myoclonus Leeuwenhoek's disease.

respiratory therapy Treatment to preserve or improve pulmonary function.

respiratory triggering In radiology, image acquisition that is synchronized to the patient's breathing, used to minimize motion artifact.

respire To breathe and to consume oxygen and release carbon dioxide.

respirometer (rĕs″pĭr-ŏm′ĕt-ĕr) [L. *respirare,* to breathe, + Gr. *metron,* a measure] An instrument to ascertain the character of respirations. Several devices are available for measuring specific respiratory qualities such as minute ventilation and tidal volume. SEE: *respiratory anemometer*.

respite Short-term, intermittent care, often for persons with chronic or debilitating conditions. One of the goals is to provide rest for family members or caregivers from the burden and stress of sustained caregiving.

respondeat superior [L., let the master answer] A Latin term meaning "Let the master answer." The "master," or employer, is held liable for wrongful acts of the "servant," or employee, in causing injury or damage during employed activities.

response [L. *respondere,* to reply] **1.** A reaction, such as contraction of a muscle or secretion of a gland, resulting from a stimulus. SEE: *reaction*. **2.** The sum total of an individual's reactions to specific conditions, such as the response (favorable or unfavorable) of a patient to a certain treatment or to a challenge to the immune system.

acute phase r. Systemic changes that occur as part of both acute and chronic inflammation. The acute phase response involves the production of plasma proteins, as well as other metabolic, hematological, and neuroendocrine events. Cytokines, produced by white blood cells, esp. macrophages, stimulate the liver's production of acute phase proteins: interleukin-6, interleukin-1β, tumor necrosis factor α, interferon-γ, and transforming growth factor β. These proteins, which increase or decrease in the blood by at least 25%, include C-reactive protein, complement, and coagulation factors; they enhance the immune response and tissue repair. Cytokines also stimulate systemic changes, producing diverse beneficial effects including fever, which enhances the immune response and stabilizes cell membranes; increased adrenal cortisol and catecholamine production, which helps maintain hemodynamic stability; thrombocytosis and leukocytosis; and increased gluconeogenesis and lipolysis, which provide nutrients for cells. There are also negative effects, however, including decreased production of erythropoietin, causing anemia; impaired growth; anorexia; lethargy; and, if prolonged, the loss of skeletal muscle and fat (cachexia). SEE: *acute phase protein; cachexia; inflammation*.

complete r. ABBR: CR. In cancer care, the eradication by treatment of all readily identifiable tumor. A complete response differs from a cure in that microscopic amounts of tumor may remain in the patient and later produce a relapse.

conditioned r. SEE: *reflex, conditioned.*

durable r. In cancer care, a long-lasting positive reaction to tumor therapy, usually lasting at least a year.

duration of r. In cancer care, the time between an initial response to therapy and subsequent disease progression or relapse.

galvanic skin r. The measurement of the change in the electrical resistance of the skin in response to stimuli.

inflammatory r. Inflammation.

minor r. In cancer care, a reduction in tumor size by less than 50%, but more than 25%.

partial r. ABBR: PR. In cancer care, a reduction in the size of readily identifiable tumors by 50% or more.

physiological stress r. Stress r.

reticulocyte r. An increase in reticulocyte production in response to the administration of a hematinic agent.

stress r. The predictable physiological response that occurs in humans as a result of injury, surgery, shock, ischemia, or sepsis. SYN: *physiological stress r.*

This response is hormonally mediated and is divided into three distinct phases:

Ebb phase (lag phase): For 12 to 36 hr after the precipitating event, the body attempts to conserve its resources. Vital signs (heart, respiration, temperature) are less than normal. *Flow phase (hypermetabolic phase):* This stage peaks in 3 to 4 days and lasts 9 to 14 days, depending on the extent of the injury or infection and the person's physical and nutritional status. Carbohydrate, protein, and fat are mobilized from tissue stores and catabolized to meet the energy needs of an increased metabolic rate (hypermetabolism). Serum levels of glucose and electrolytes such as potassium can increase dramatically. If this stage is not controlled by removal of the cause or activator, multiple system organ failure or death can result. *Anabolic phase (recovery):* The anabolic, or healing, phase occurs as the catabolism declines, and electrolyte balances are restored. Often, aggressive nutritional support is necessary to promote a positive nitrogen balance.

triple r. The three phases of vasomotor reactions that occur when a sharp object is drawn across the skin. In order of appearance, these are red reaction, flare or spreading flush, and wheal.

unconditioned r. An inherent response rather than one that is learned. SEE: *reflex, conditioned.*

responsible party The individual whose actions or inactions caused injury, harm, or damage to something or someone.

responsibility (rē-spŏn″sĭ-bĭ′lĭ-tē) **1.** Accountability. **2.** Trustworthiness.

rest (rĕst) [AS. *raest*] **1.** Repose of the body caused by sleep. **2.** Freedom from activity, as of mind or body. **3.** To lie down; to cease voluntary motion. **4.** A remnant of embryonic tissue that persists in the adult.

restenosis (rē″stĕ-nō′sĭs) [L. *re,* again, + Gr. *stenos,* narrow] The recurrence of a stenotic condition as in a heart valve or vessel.

restiform (rĕs′tĭ-form) [L. *restis,* rope, + *forma,* shape] Ropelike; rope-shaped.

resting Inactive, motionless, at rest.

resting cell **1.** A cell not in the process of dividing. SEE: *interphase.* **2.** A cell that is not performing its normal function (i.e., a nerve cell that is not conducting an impulse or a muscle cell that is not contracting).

resting pan splint Splint designed to position fingers and stabilize hand in a functional position with the fingers held in opposition. Also called *resting hand splint.*

restitutio ad integrum (rĕs″tĭ-tū′shē-ō ăd ĭn-tĕ′grŭm) [L.] Complete restoration to health.

restitution (rĕs″tĭ-tū′shŭn) [L. *restitutio*] **1.** The return to a former status. **2.** The act of making amends. **3.** The turning of a fetal head to the right or left after it has completely emerged through the vagina.

restless legs syndrome A condition of unknown etiology marked by an intolerable creeping and internal itching sensation occurring in the lower extremities and causing an almost irresistible urge to move the legs. The symptoms are worse at the end of the day when the patient is either seated or in bed and may produce insomnia. SYN: *Ekbom's syndrome.*

TREATMENT: Treatments include levodopa/carbidopa, benzodiazepines, or tricyclic antidepressants.

restoration (rĕs″tō-rā′shŭn) [L. *restaurare,* to fix] **1.** The return of something to its previous state. **2.** In dentistry, any treatment, material, or device that restores a tooth surface, or replaces a tooth or all of the teeth and adjacent tissues.

temporary r. A temporary filling of a tooth cavity made from zinc oxide and eugenol or some plastic material.

restorative (rĭ-stor′ă-tĭv) [L. *restaurare,* to fix] **1.** Pert. to restoration. **2.** An agent that is effective in the regaining of health and strength.

restraint (rĭ-strānt′) [O.Fr. *restrainte*] **1.** The process of refraining from any action, mental or physical. **2.** The condition of being hindered. **3.** In medicine, the use of major tranquilizers or physical means to prevent patients from harming themselves or others. In nursing homes, restraints are used in 36% to 85% of patients; in acute care hospitals, between 7.4% and 17% of patients will be restrained.

The Food and Drug Administration, which regulates medical devices, has defined restraint as "a device, usually a wristlet, anklet, or other type of strap intended for medical purposes and that limits a patient's movements to the extent necessary for treatment, examination, or protection of the patient." Protective devices include safety vests, hand mitts, lap and wheelchair belts, body holders, straitjackets, and protection nets.

Restraints should be fitted properly (i.e., neither too loose nor too tight). They should be applied in a manner that will protect the patient from accidental self-injury, such as strangling or smothering themselves by slipping down in a bed, wheelchair, or chair.

Caregivers are legally and ethically responsible for the safety and well-being of patients in their care; however, when patient protection or achieving the therapeutic goal appears to require physical or pharmacological restraint, health care providers must consider that such action limits the patient's legal rights to autonomy and self-determination. Decisions to institute physical or pharmacological restraint must be based on a clear, identifiable, documented need for their use (i.e., that protecting the patient from harm or achievement of the therapeutic goals cannot be met in any other manner).

With many patients, effective alternatives to physical restraint include providing companionship and close supervision of activities; explaining procedures to reduce anxiety; when possible, removing indwelling tubes, drains, and catheters to reduce discomfort and the potential for displacement; providing good lighting, ensuring that pathways are clear, and that furniture is adequately secured to minimize potential environmental hazards; ensuring that the call button is easily accessible to facilitate patient requests for assistance with ambulation; reducing unwelcome distractions (e.g., background noise) and enabling patient access to diversions such as music and video movies to encourage relaxation; and encouraging ambulation and exercise to meet patient needs for mobility.

CAUTION: Informed consent must be obtained from the patient or guardian prior to use of restraints. Restraints should not be used without a specific order from the treating physician. Almost any type of restraint has the potential for harming the patient; thus it is extremely important to monitor use and be certain that it is applied correctly and removed periodically.

PATIENT CARE: The nurse records and reports patient behaviors that demonstrate a need for restraint to ensure safety and achievement of therapeutic goals; describes nursing actions designed to achieve care objectives without resort to restraint and their effects; suggests the minimum amount of restraint required to achieve the objectives of care (i.e., restriction of mobility only to the degree necessary); secures or reviews physician orders for specific types of restraints; validates informed consent; explains the use of the specific type of restraint to the patient and family members as a "reminder" needed for protection; and encourages verbalization of feelings and concerns and provides emotional support.

The nurse follows these general guidelines for application of restraints: the device that is most appropriate for the purpose is selected (e.g., padded mitts protect against patient removal of intravenous or other invasive tubing by limiting the ability to manipulate equipment with fingers but do not elicit the restlessness and frustration that occurs when the hands are tied down with wrist restraints). The status of tissues is assessed and documented before application. Bony prominences that will be in contact with the restraining devices are padded before application of such restraints. Restraints are applied to maintain a comfortable normal anatomic position, and mobility is limited only as much as is necessary to protect the patient (i.e., the nurse may change the position without defeating the objectives of the restraint). The nurse anchors restraint devices securely and ensures that they do not interfere with blood flow to the limbs or trunk; ensures that the restraints can be released quickly in the event of emergency; documents application and evaluation of current status; assesses and records the effects of the restraint on patient behavior and on the neurovascular status distal to the site of the restraint at frequent intervals (e.g., every 30 min); reports signs of increased agitation promptly; releases restraints (one at a time if the patient is unreliable or combative) and allows or provides range-of-motion exercises two to four times each shift; and evaluates the need for continuing restraint at least once each shift, discontinuing the devices as soon as the patient's status permits.

r. in bed The therapeutic use of physical means to prevent limb or body motion in bed. If a proper bed is not available, the following may provide a makeshift alternative. With the bed against the wall, straight-backed chairs are placed along the open side of the bed. They are tied into place by interlacing them with rope and then tying the rope to the foot and head of the bed. Another method is to place a wide board the length of the bed on either side and to fasten it through three or four holes bored near the ends of the boards. A sheet is folded lengthwise to a 1-ft width, placed under the patient's back, and crossed in front below the armpits. The hem ends are secured at the side to the side bar or the bedsprings. This allows some freedom for turning from side to side. The patient's hands and feet may be restrained by a clove hitch of wide bandage around the wrists and ankles and tied to the side or foot of the bed.

PATIENT CARE: The nurse follows general guidelines for restraint application. The nurse never ties restraints to bed siderails; rather, the restraint is anchored to a part of the bed that moves when the head is lowered or elevated; the nurse uses a clove hitch to secure restraints so they will not tighten if tension is applied and so that they can be released rapidly if an emergency arises. A simple body restraint can be made by folding a sheet lengthwise to a 1-ft width. This restraint is placed under the patient's back and crossed in front below the armpits. The ends are secured to the side bar of the bed. This prevents some freedom in side-to-side movement.

clove hitch r. A device used to restrain a person's arm or leg. Gauze or other soft material is placed on a flat surface in a figure-8 configuration. The loops are then lifted from the underside and the tops brought together. The extremity is placed through both loops at once and the loose ends of the material are tied to an immobile surface. It is important to check circulation regularly in any extremity restrained by this device.

r. of lower extremities The use of physical means to restrict movement of the legs and feet. A sheet is tied across the knees and the feet are tied together with a figure-of-eight bandage. The correct method is to start the loop under the ankles, cross it between the feet, bring the ends around the feet, and tie them on top.

CAUTION: The restraint should not interfere with blood circulation to an extremity.

mechanical r. Restraint by physical devices, esp. restraint of the mentally ill.

medicinal r. Restraint of combative or violent patients through use of narcotics or sedatives.

resurfacing (rē-sŭr′fă-sĭng) Repair of damaged body surfaces, such as articular cartilage or skin. In cosmetic surgery, resurfacing of the skin may involve dermabrasion, chemical peels, cutaneous lasers, and other techniques.

laser r. of skin Use of laser treatments to repair wrinkled or photoaged skin for aesthetic purposes. Carbon dioxide and other lasers are used to remove the damaged dermis and repair underlying connective tissues. Whether these treatments have long-term adverse effects is unknown.

Resusci-Anne™ A mannikin used in cardiopulmonary resuscitation training.

resuscitation (rĭ-sŭs″ĭ-tā′shŭn) [L. *resuscitatio*] Revival after apparent death; also called *anabiosis*. SEE: *cardiopulmonary r.*

cardiopulmonary r. ABBR: CPR. Basic life support. In emergency cardiac care, CPR involves opening the airway, providing artificial breathing, and assisting circulation until definitive treatments can restore spontaneous cardiac, pulmonary, and cerebral function. When trained providers are available, CPR includes defibrillation with automated external defibrillators. In the U.S., the American Heart Association develops and disseminates standard techniques for emergency cardiac care.

The first step in CPR is making certain that an unarousable patient is in need of cardiopulmonary support and not merely asleep or unconscious. If the patient does not respond to a loud voice or a gentle shake, the most important role for the rescuer is to call for skilled assistance, because the likelihood of a successful resuscitation usually depends on the speed with which the patient can be defibrillated.

Before the defibrillator arrives, the rescuer can position the patient and begin rescue breathing. The patient should be placed supine on a firm, flat surface, with care taken to protect his or her cervical spine if traumatic injury is suspected. Kneeling at the level of the patient's shoulder, the rescuer should open the patient's *airway*, either with the jaw-thrust or the head-tilt chin-lift technique. If foreign bodies are present in the airway, they must be removed; dentures are also removed if they interfere with resuscitation. Next *breathing* is assessed by listening for breath sounds at the nose and lips and watching for the rise and fall of the chest. If these signs are not present, the patient is apneic, and rescue breathing must begin.

Rescue breathing can be performed with mouth-to-mouth technique or through a mask with a one-way valve, if one is available. Two deep, slow positive-pressure breaths are given to the patient; the duration of each depends on the patient's age. If supplied breaths meet obvious resistance, an attempt should be made again to reopen the airway, and if this is ineffective, to clear the airway with the Heimlich maneuver in children and adults. Infants should receive chest thrusts and blows to the back instead of the Heimlich maneuver.

After the first two breaths, the American Heart Association formerly suggested checking the victim for a pulse. In guidelines revised in 2000, the pulse check was eliminated. If the patient is not breathing on his own rescue breathing continues. If there is no pulse, external chest compression begins and continues, with periodically interposed ventilations, until a defibrillator arrives or the patient revives. The precise number of ventilations and chest compressions per minute depend on the patient's age and the number of rescuers. For a single rescuer caring for an adult patient, two breaths are given for every 15 chest compressions.

Compressions are given to adults (the most common victims of cardiac arrest) on the inferior half of the sternum, using the heel of one hand below the other hand; the fingers of the two hands are often interlaced for support. The elbows of the rescuer should be locked and straight, and the direction of compression should be exactly perpendicular to the patient's chest.

The chest is depressed 1.5 to 2.0 in. for a normal-sized adult. For a child, the chest is depressed 1.0 to 1.5 in.; for an infant, 0.5. to 1.0 in. The chest should return to its normally inflated position after each compression.

When professional rescuers arrive, the patient should be defibrillated immediately. If a defibrillator is not available, two-person CPR continues; the two rescuers alternate in giving rescue breaths and chest compressions to minimize rescuer fatigue. Ventilation and chest compressions are held for 5 seconds at the end of the first minute, and every few minutes thereafter to determine whether the patient has responded. SEE: illus.; *advanced cardiac life support; defibrillation; emergency cardiac care; Standard and Universal Precautions Appendix.*

cerebral r. The restoration of a patient's normal neurological function due to effective revival from cardiopulmonary arrest.

mouth-to-mouth r. Providing respiratory gases to a patient in cardiopulmonary arrest by exhaling directly into the open mouth of an unconscious victim. SEE: *cardiopulmonary resuscitation.*

oral r. SEE: *artificial respiration.*

resuscitator (rĭ-sŭs'ĭ-tā"tor) [L. *resuscitare,* to revive] A breathing-assist device used to oxygenate and ventilate a patient who can no longer breathe spontaneously. Most resuscitators are portable and capable of delivering high concentrations of oxygen.

manual r. A disposable, hand-held mask, with an attached self-inflating bag, that permits air to be forced into the lungs each time it is squeezed. Manual resuscitators can be difficult to use properly; complications can arise if the mask does not seal the patient's face properly; excessive pressure is used during ventilation; inadequate supplemental oxygen is provided; or the rate or volume of ventilations is insufficient to inflate the lungs and remove carbon dioxide.

resveratrol (rĕs-vĕr'ă-trŏl) A plant-derived polyphenol that is structurally related to diethylstilbestrol. It is found in grapes and wine, and is believed to have antioxidant effects.

ret *roentgen equivalent therapy.* It is analogous to rem, used in describing radiation protection or exposure.

retainer (rĭ-tān'ĕr) **1.** Any device or attachment for keeping something in place. **2.** In dentistry, a device used in orthodontia for maintaining the teeth and jaws in position.

retardate (rĭ-tăr'dāt) [L. *retardare,* to delay] One who is mentally retarded.

retardation (rē"tăr-dā'shŭn) [L. *retardare,* to delay] **1.** A holding back or slowing down; a delay. **2.** Delayed mental or physical response resulting from pathological conditions. SEE: *mental retardation.*

retarder A substance used in dentistry to decrease the setting of a dental material.

retch (rĕch) [AS. *hraecan,* to cough up phlegm] To make an involuntary attempt to vomit.

retching (rĕch'ĭng) Intense rhythmic contraction of the respiratory and abdominal muscles that may precede or accompany vomiting.

rete (rē'tē) *pl.* **retia** [L.] A network; a plexus of nerves or blood vessels.

arterial r. A vascular arterial network just before the point where arteries become capillaries.

articular r. A rete about a joint, esp. a deep anastomosis at the knee joint.

r. cutaneum A network of blood vessels at the junction of the dermis and superficial fascia.

malpighian r. Stratum germinativum.

r. mirabile A plexus formed by the sudden division of a vessel into capillaries that reunite to form one vessel, as in the glomeruli of the kidneys.

r. olecrani A network of vessels at the back of the elbow formed by divisions of the recurrent ulnar arteries.

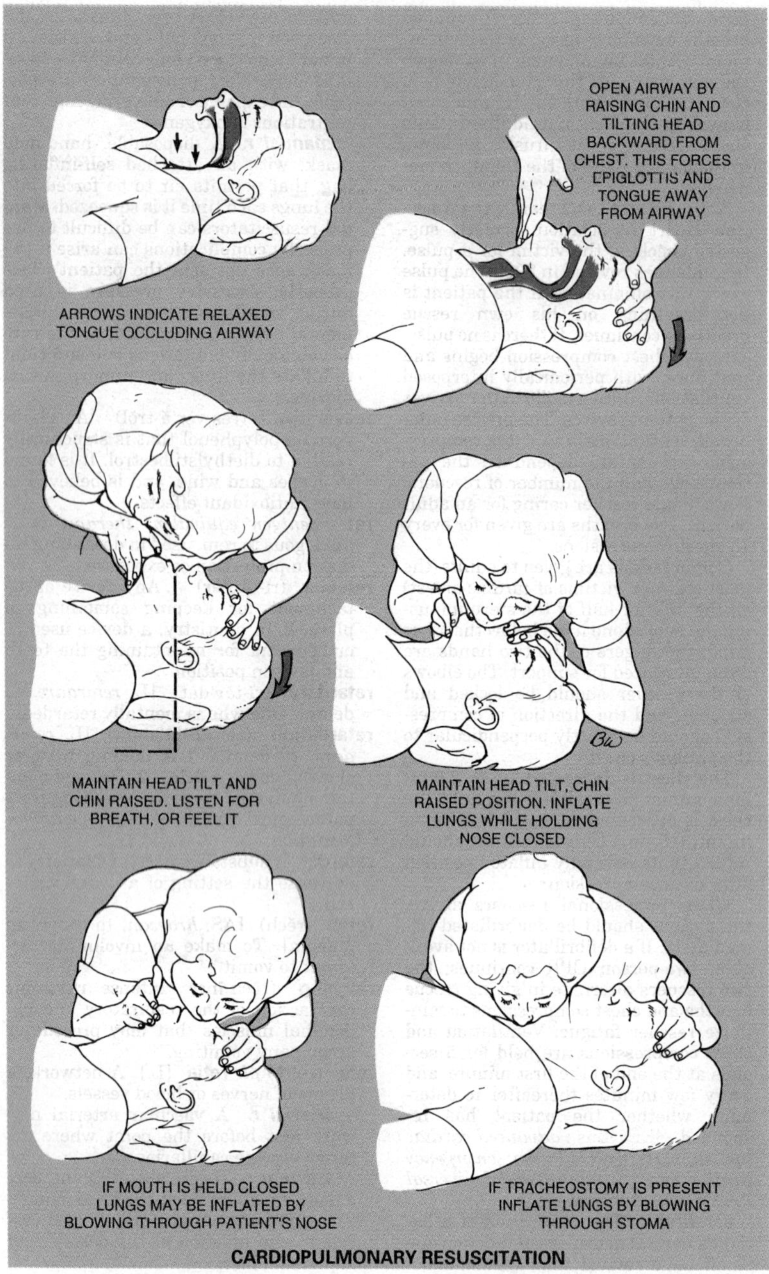
ARROWS INDICATE RELAXED
TONGUE OCCLUDING AIRWAY
OPEN AIRWAY BY
RAISING CHIN AND
TILTING HEAD
BACKWARD FROM
CHEST. THIS FORCES
EPIGLOTTIS AND
TONGUE AWAY
FROM AIRWAY
MAINTAIN HEAD TILT AND
CHIN RAISED. LISTEN FOR
BREATH, OR FEEL IT
MAINTAIN HEAD TILT, CHIN
RAISED POSITION. INFLATE
LUNGS WHILE HOLDING
NOSE CLOSED
IF MOUTH IS HELD CLOSED
LUNGS MAY BE INFLATED BY
BLOWING THROUGH PATIENT'S NOSE
IF TRACHEOSTOMY IS PRESENT
INFLATE LUNGS BY BLOWING
THROUGH STOMA

CARDIOPULMONARY RESUSCITATION

r. ovarii A layer of cells in the broad ligament and mesovarium of the ovary. It is homologous to rete testes in men.

r. patellae A superficial network of vessels around the patella; formed by branches of genicular arteries.

r. subpapillare A network of vessels between the papillary and reticular layers of the dermis.

r. testis A network of tubules in the mediastinum testis that receives sperm through the tubuli recti from the seminiferous tubules. From the rete testis, efferent ducts convey sperm to the epi-

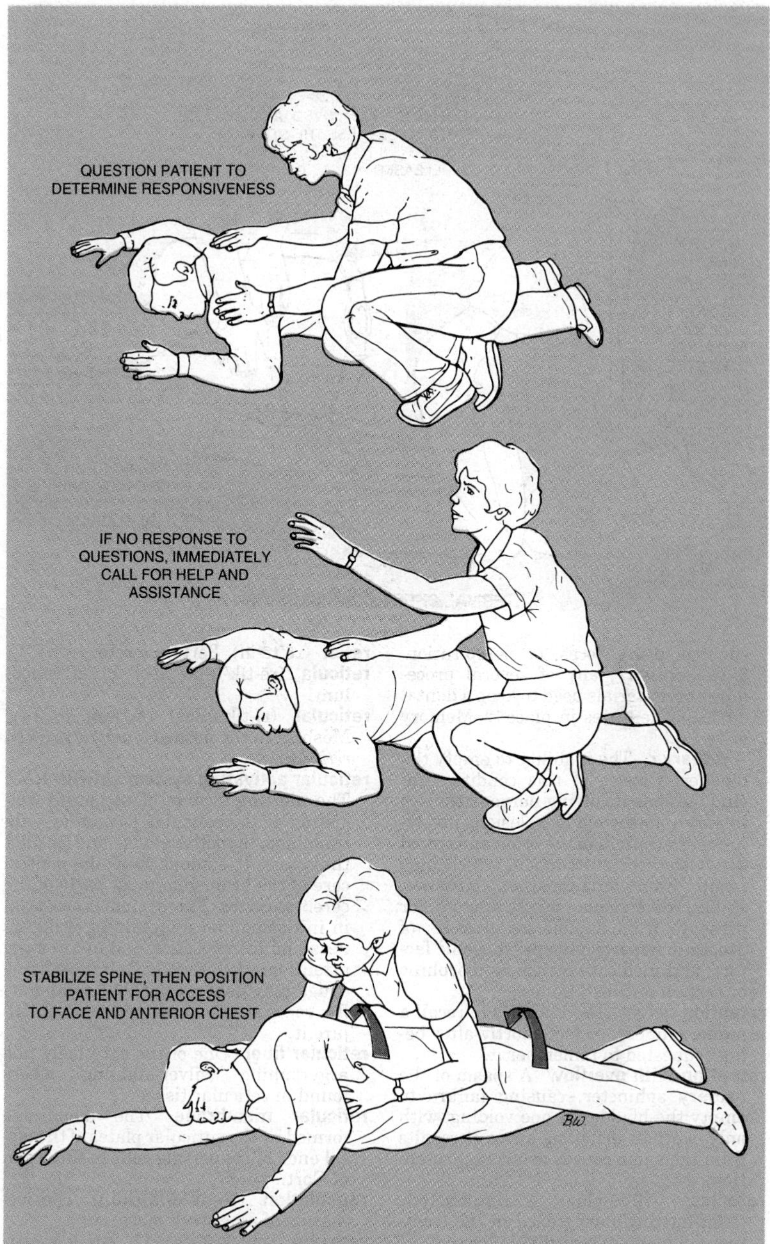
QUESTION PATIENT TO
DETERMINE RESPONSIVENESS
IF NO RESPONSE TO
QUESTIONS, IMMEDIATELY
CALL FOR HELP AND
ASSISTANCE
STABILIZE SPINE, THEN POSITION
PATIENT FOR ACCESS
TO FACE AND ANTERIOR CHEST
BW

INITIAL APPROACH TO PATIENT WHO MAY NEED CARDIOPULMONARY RESUSCITATION

didymis. The rete testis is homologous to the rete ovarii in women.

r. venosum Venous network.

vertebral r. One of two plexuses within the vertebral canal that extends from the foramen magnum to the coccyx. These retia lie posteriorly and laterally to the dura and between the dura and the arches of the vertebrae.

retention (rĭ-tĕn′shŭn) [L. *retentio,* a holding back] **1.** The act or process of keeping in possession or of holding in place. **2.** The persistent keeping within the body of materials normally excreted,

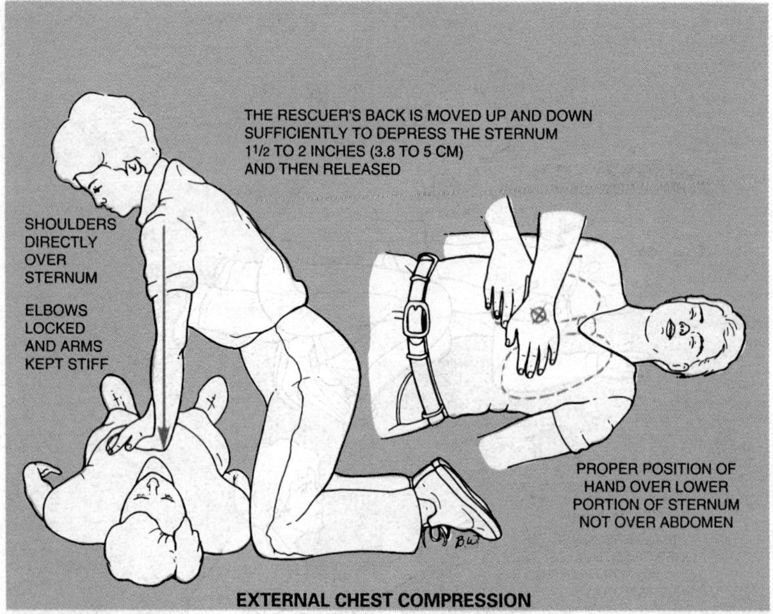
THE RESCUER'S BACK IS MOVED UP AND DOWN SUFFICIENTLY TO DEPRESS THE STERNUM 1 1/2 TO 2 INCHES (3.8 TO 5 CM) AND THEN RELEASED
SHOULDERS DIRECTLY OVER STERNUM
ELBOWS LOCKED AND ARMS KEPT STIFF
PROPER POSITION OF HAND OVER LOWER PORTION OF STERNUM NOT OVER ABDOMEN
EXTERNAL CHEST COMPRESSION

such as urine, feces, or perspiration. **3.** In dentistry, any of several procedures or materials used to keep a dental device or dentures in place. **4.** Memory or recall.

urinary r. The inability to empty the bladder. Causes of this condition include lesions involving nerve pathways to and from the bladder; lesions involving reflex centers in the brain and spinal cord; urethral obstruction, which may result from inflammation, stricture, stones, diverticula, cysts, tumors, or pressure from outside as in cases of prostatic hypertrophy; psychogenic factors; and medication such as morphine or certain antihistamines.

retention defect The inability to recall a name, number, or fact shortly after being requested to remember it.

retention with overflow A spasm of the urinary sphincter, causing failure to empty the bladder at one voiding, with only overflow dribbling away. It results from the same causes as urinary retention.

reteplase (rĕ′tĕ-plāz) A thrombolytic ("clot-busting") drug used in the treatment of acute myocardial infarction.

rete ridge One of the downgrowths of epithelium surrounding the connective tissue papillae in the irregular internal surface of the epidermis. Microscopic sections often appear as single downgrowths when in fact the epithelium is in a series of interconnecting ridges at the dermis-epidermis interface. SYN: *peg, rete.*

retia (rē′tē-ă) [L.] Pl. of rete.

retial (rē′tē-ăl) Pert. to a rete.

reticula (rē-tĭk′ū-lă) [L.] Pl. of reticulum.

reticular (rĭ-tĭk′ū-lăr) [L. *reticula,* net] Meshed; in the form of a network. SYN: *retiform.*

reticular activating system ABBR: RAS. The alerting system of the brain consisting of the reticular formation, subthalamus, hypothalamus, and medial thalamus. It extends from the central core of the brainstem to all parts of the cerebral cortex. This system is essential in initiating and maintaining wakefulness and introspection and in directing attention. Sedative and tranquilizing drugs may depress the RAS temporarily; some strokes may permanently injure it.

reticular fiber One of the extremely fine argyrophilic (silver-staining) fibers found in reticular tissue.

reticular membrane The membrane formed by the cuticular plates of the distal ends of supporting cells in the organ of Corti.

reticulation (rē-tĭk″ū-lā′shŭn) The formation of a network mass.

reticulin (rē-tĭk′ū-lĭn) [L. *reticula,* net] An albuminoid or scleroprotein in the connective tissue framework of reticular tissue.

reticulo- Combining form meaning *network.*

reticulocyte (rĕ-tĭk′ū-lō-sīt) [″ + Gr. *kytos,* cell] The last immature stage of a red blood cell. Its darkly staining granules are fragments of the endoplasmic reticulum. Reticulocytes normally constitute about 1% of the circulating red blood cells. SEE: illus.

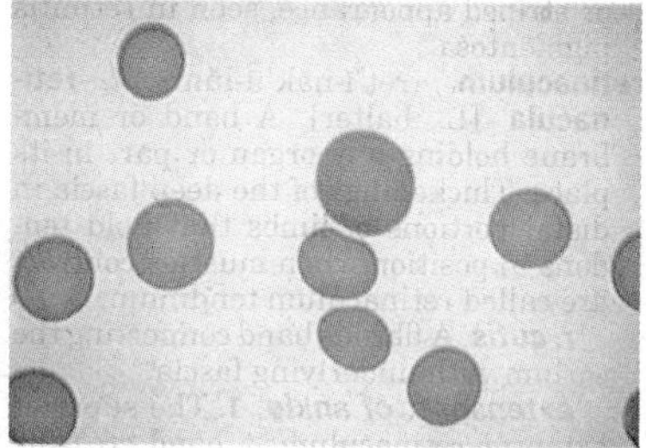

RETICULOCYTE

reticulocytopenia (rē-tĭk″ū-lō-sī″tō-pē′nē-ă) [″ + ″ + *penia,* poverty] A decreased number of the reticulocytes of the blood.

reticulocytosis (rē-tĭk″ū-lō-sī-tō′sĭs) [″ + ″ + *osis,* condition] An increased number of reticulocytes in the circulating blood. This condition indicates active erythropoiesis in the red bone marrow and the need for greater oxygen-carrying capacity of the blood. It occurs after hemorrhage, during acclimatization to high altitude, during any pulmonary disorder that induces hypoxia, and in all types of anemia.

reticuloendothelial (rē-tĭk″ū-lō-ĕn″dō-thē′lē-ăl) [″ + Gr. *endon,* within, + *thele,* nipple] Pert. to the reticuloendothelial system, which is the old name for the mononuclear phagocytic system.

reticuloendothelioma (rĕ-tĭk″ū-lō-ĕn″dō-thē-lē-ō′mă) [″ + ″ + ″ + *oma,* tumor] A neoplasm composed of cells of the mononuclear phagocytic system.

reticuloendotheliosis (rĕ-tĭk″ū-lō-ĕn″dō-thē-lē-ō′sĭs) [″ + ″ + *thele,* nipple, + *osis,* condition] Hyperplasia of reticuloendothelium.

reticuloendothelium (rĕ-tĭk″ū-lō-ĕn″dō-thē′lē-ŭm) The tissue of the reticuloendothelial system, which is the old name for the mononuclear phagocytic system.

reticulohistiocytoma (rĕ-tĭk″ū-lō-hĭs″tē-ō-sī-tō′mă) [L. *reticula,* net, + Gr. *histion,* little web, + *kytos,* cell, + *oma,* tumor] A malignant connective tissue tumor composed of multinucleated giant cells in the skin, mucous membranes, or synovium.

reticulohistiocytosis (rĕ-tĭk″ū-lō-hĭs″tē-ō-sī-tō′sĭs) [″ + ″ + ″ + *osis,* condition] Reticuloendotheliosis.

reticuloid (rĕ-tĭk′ū-loyd) [″ + Gr. *eidos,* form, shape] Resembling reticulosis.

reticuloma (rĕ-tĭk″ū-lō′mă) [″ + Gr. *oma,* tumor] A neoplasm composed of cells of the mononuclear phagocytic system.

reticulopenia (rĕ-tĭk″ū-lō-pē′nē-ă) [″ + Gr. *penia,* lack] A decreased number of reticulocytes in the blood.

reticulopodium (rĕ-tĭk″ū-lō-pō′dē-ŭm) A branching pseudopod.

reticulosarcoma (rĕ-tĭk″ū-lō-săr-kō′mă) [″ + Gr. *sarx,* flesh, + *oma,* tumor] A neoplasm composed of large monocytic cells that originated in the mononuclear phagocyte of the lymph and other glands.

reticulosis (rĕ-tĭk-ū-lō′sĭs) [″ + Gr. *osis,* condition] Reticulocytosis.

histiocytic medullary r. A form of malignant histiocytosis marked by anemia; granulocytopenia; enlargement of the spleen, liver, and lymph nodes; and phagocytosis of red blood cells.

reticulum (rĕ-tĭk′ū-lŭm) *pl.* **reticula** [L., a little net] A network. **reticulate, reticulated** (-lāt, -lāt″ĕd), *adj.*

endoplasmic r. ABBR: ER. A cell organelle that is a complex network of membranous tubules in the cytoplasm between the nuclear and cell membranes; it is visible only with an electron microscope. It is involved in the manufacturing of proteins, fats, and carbohydrates, and in the regulation of intracellular ions. One form with ribosomes attached is called *granular* or *rough ER;* another form that is free of ribosomes is called *agranular* or *smooth ER.* Rough ER transports proteins produced on the ribosomes; smooth ER synthesizes lipids. SEE: *cell* for illus.

r. of nucleus The netlike contents of a nondividing nucleus of a cell; the chromatin, the long, uncoiled chromosomes.

sarcoplasmic r. The endoplasmic reticulum of striated muscle cells, surrounding the sarcomeres. In response to an action potential, it releases calcium ions to induce contraction, then reabsorbs calcium ions to induce relaxation.

stellate r. The enamel pulp of a developing tooth, consisting of stellate cells lying between the inner and outer epithelial layers of the enamel organ.

retiform (rĕt′ĭ-form) [L. *rete,* net, + *forma,* shape] Reticular.

retina (rĕt′ĭ-nă) *pl.* **retinae** [L.] The innermost layer of the eye, which receives images transmitted through the lens and contains the receptors for vision, the rods and cones. SEE: illus. (Retina of Right Eye). **retinal** (-năl), *adj.*

The retina is a light-sensitive membrane on which light rays are focused. It extends from the entrance point of the optic nerve anteriorly to the margin of the pupil, completely lining the interior of the eye. It consists of three parts. The pars optica, the nervous or sensory portion, extends from the optic disk forward to the ora serrata, a wavy line immediately behind the ciliary process; the pars ciliaris lines the inner surface of the ciliary process; and the pars iridica forms the posterior surface of the

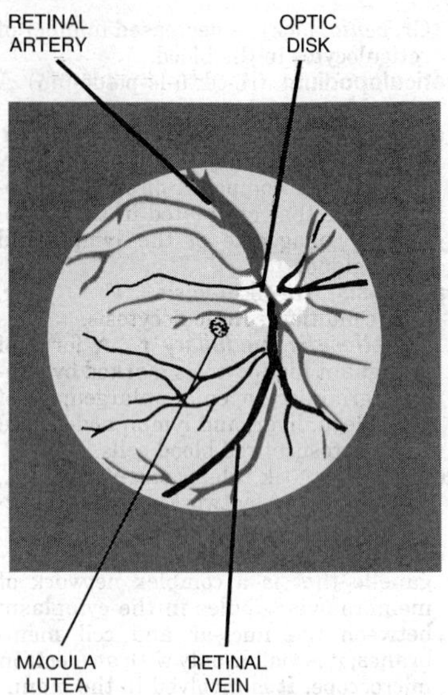

RETINA OF RIGHT EYE

iris. Slightly lateral to the posterior pole of the eye is a small, oval, yellowish spot, the macula lutea, in the center of which is a depression, the fovea centralis. This region contains only cones and is the region of the most acute vision. About 3.5 mm nasally from the fovea is the optic papilla (optic disk), where nerve fibers from the retina make their exit and form the optic nerve. This region is devoid of rods and cones and is insensitive to light; hence it is named the blind spot.

The layers of the retina, in the order light strikes them, are the optic nerve fiber layer, ganglion cell layer, inner synaptic layer, bipolar cell layer, outer synaptic layer, layer of rods and cones, and pigment epithelium. SEE: illus. (Retina).

COLOR: The retina is normally red, reflecting blood flow, and is pale in anemia or ischemia.

VESSELS: The arteries are branches of a single central artery, which is a branch of the ophthalmic artery. The central artery enters at the center of the optic papilla and supplies the inner layers of the retina. The outer layers, including rods and cones, are nourished by capillaries of the choroid layer. The veins lack muscular coats. They parallel the arteries; blood leaves by a central vein that leads to the superior ophthalmic vein.

coarctate r. A condition in which there is an effusion of fluid between the retina and choroid, giving the retina a funnel shape.

shot-silk r. A retina having an opalescent appearance, sometimes seen in young persons.

tigroid r. A retina having a spotted or striped appearance, seen in retinitis pigmentosa.

retinaculum (rĕt″ĭ-năk′ū-lŭm) *pl.* **retinacula** [L., halter] A band or membrane holding any organ or part in its place. Thickenings of the deep fascia in distal portions of limbs that hold tendons in position when muscles contract are called retinaculum tendinum.

r. cutis A fibrous band connecting the corium with underlying fascia.

extensor r. of ankle **1.** The superior extensor retinaculum, a band crossing the extensor tendons of the foot and attached to the lower portion of the tibia and fibula. **2.** The inferior extensor retinaculum, a band located on the dorsum of the foot. It consists of two limbs having a common origin on the lateral surface of the calcaneum. The upper limb is attached to the medial malleolus; the lower limb curves around the instep and is attached to the fascia of the abductor hallucis on the medial side of the foot.

extensor r. of wrist An oblique band attached medially to the styloid process of the ulna, the hammate bone, and the medial ligament of the wrist joint. Laterally it is attached to the anterior border of the radius. It contains six separate compartments for passage of the extensor tendons to the hand.

flexor r. of ankle The retinaculum extending from the medial malleolus to the medial tubercle of the calcaneum.

flexor r. of hand The fascial band that holds down the flexor tendons of the digits.

flexor r. of wrist The retinaculum extending from the trapezium and scaphoid bones laterally to the hammate and pisiform bones medially.

r. of hip joint Any of three flat bands lying along the neck of the femur and continuous with the capsule of the hip joint.

r. mammae Strands of connective tissue in the mammary gland extending from glandular tissue through fat toward the skin, where they are attached to the dermis. Over the cephalic portion of the mammae, they are well developed and are called suspensory ligaments of Cooper.

patellar r. One of two fibrous bands (medial and lateral) lying on either side of the knee joint and forming part of the joint capsule. These bands are extensions of the insertions of the medial and lateral vastus muscles of the thigh.

peroneal r. One of two fibrous bands on the lateral side of the foot that contains the tendons of the peroneus longus and brevis muscles. The superior peroneal retinaculum extends from the lateral malleolus to the lateral surface of

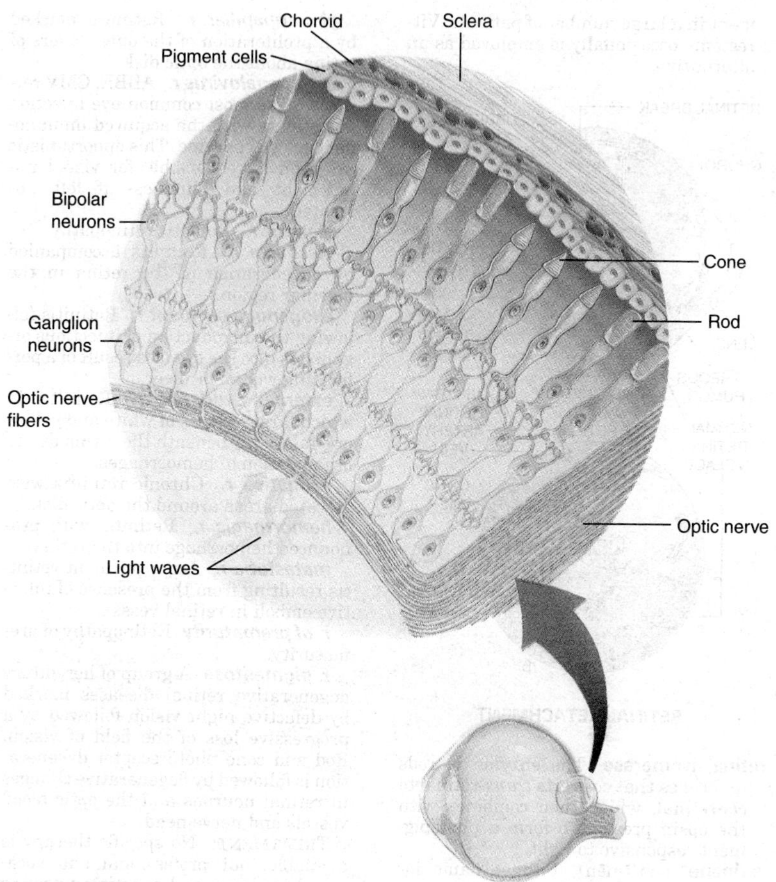

RETINA

Microscopic structure of optic disk area

the calcaneus; the inferior peroneal retinaculum is attached below to the calcaneus and above to the lower border of the inferior extensor retinaculum.

r. tendinum The annular band of the wrist or ankle.

retinal (rĕt′ĭ-năl) **1.** Pertaining to the retina. **2.** The light-absorbing portion of a photopigment, a derivative of vitamin A.

retinal break A break in the continuity of the retina, usually caused by trauma to the eye. Detachment of the retina may follow the appearance of the break.

retinal correspondence A condition in which simultaneous stimulation of points in the retina of each eye results in formation of a single visual sensation. These points, called corresponding points, lie in the foveae of the two retinas, or in the nasal half of one retina and the temporal half of the other. Abnormal correspondence results in double vision (diplopia) and usually is caused by imbalance of the ocular muscles. SEE: *strabismus*.

retinal detachment Separation of the inner sensory layer of the retina from the outer pigment epithelium. It is usually caused by a hole or break in the inner sensory layer that permits fluid from the vitreous to leak under the retina and lift off its innermost layer. Causes include trauma and any disease that causes retinopathy, such as diabetes or sickle cell disease. Symptoms are blurred vision, flashes of light, vitreous floaters, and loss of visual acuity. The location of holes must be determined so that they can be repaired by laser therapy (i.e., photocoagulation). SEE: illus.; *Nursing Diagnoses Appendix*.

TREATMENT: Scleral buckling techniques are used to treat retinal detachment in a large number of patients. Vitrectomy occasionally is employed as an alternative.

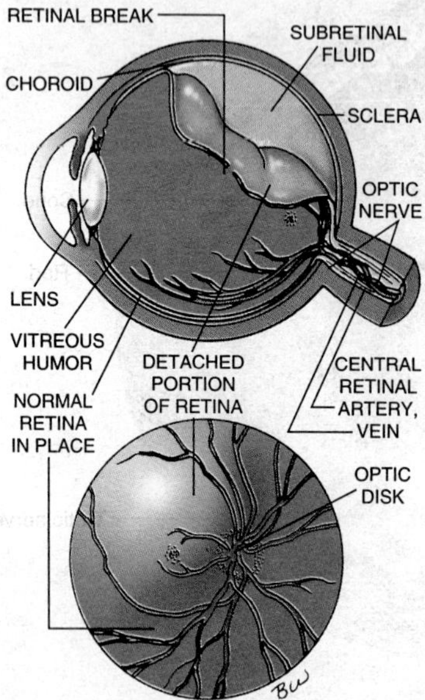

RETINAL DETACHMENT

retinal isomerase The enzyme in rods and cones that converts *trans*-retinal to *cis*-retinal, which then combines with the opsin present to form a photopigment responsive to light.

retinene (rĕt′ĭ-nēn) Former name for retinal.

retinitis (rĕt-ĭ-nī′tĭs) [L. *retina,* retina, + Gr. *itis,* inflammation] Inflammation of the retina. Symptoms include diminished vision, contractions of fields or scotomata, alteration in the apparent size of objects, and photophobia. This condition is treated by absolute rest of the eyes, protection from light, and treatment of the underlying cause. SEE: *retinopathy*.

actinic r. Retinitis caused by exposure to intense light or other forms of radiant energy.

albuminuric r. Retinitis associated with chronic kidney disease and malignant hypertension. Findings on physical examination include a hazy retina, blurred disk margins, distention of retinal arteries, retinal hemorrhages and white patches in the fundus, esp. surrounding the papilla and at the stellate figure at the macula.

apoplectic r. Retinitis associated with hemorrhaging of the retinal vessels.

circinate r. Retinitis marked by a circle of white spots about the macula.

circumpapillar r. Retinitis marked by a proliferation of the outer layers of retina about the optic disk.

cytomegalovirus r. ABBR: CMV retinitis. The most common eye infection in patients with the acquired immunodeficiency syndrome. This opportunistic infection is responsible for visual impairment and blindness if left untreated.

diabetic r. Diabetic retinopathy.

disciform r. Retinitis accompanied by degeneration of the retina in the macular region.

exogenous purulent r. Retinitis following the introduction of infectious organisms into the eye as a result of a perforating wound or ulcer.

external exudative r. Retinitis in which large masses of white and yellow crystals occur beneath the retina due to organization of hemorrhages.

exudative r. Chronic retinitis with elevated areas around the optic disk.

hemorrhagic r. Retinitis with pronounced hemorrhage into the retina.

metastatic r. Acute purulent retinitis resulting from the presence of infective emboli in retinal vessels.

r. of prematurity Retinopathy of prematurity.

r. pigmentosa A group of hereditary degenerative retinal diseases marked by defective night vision followed by a progressive loss of the field of vision. Rod and cone photoreceptor degeneration is followed by degenerative changes in retinal neurons and the optic blood vessels and nerve head.

TREATMENT: No specific therapy is available, but professional and vocational guidance and genetic counseling can be provided. Family members should be examined to determine whether their vision is affected.

r. proliferans Retinitis marked by vascularized masses of connective tissue that project from the retina into the vitreous; the end result of recurrent hemorrhage from the retina into the vitreous.

r. punctata albescens A nonprogressive, degenerative familial disease in which innumerable minute white spots are scattered over entire retina. There are no pigmentary changes. The disease usually starts early in life.

punctate r. Retinitis marked by numerous white or yellow spots in the fundus of the eye.

solar r. Solar retinopathy.

stellate r. Retinitis marked by exudates, hemorrhages, blurring of the optic disk, and formation of a star-shaped figure around the macula.

suppurative r. Retinitis associated with septicemia resulting from pyogenic organisms.

syphilitic r. Retinitis resulting from

or associated with syphilis. It may also involve the optic nerve (syphilitic neuroretinitis).

retinoblastoma (rĕt″ĭ-nō-blăs-tō′mă) [L. *retina,* retina, + Gr. *blastos,* germ, + *oma,* tumor] A malignant glioma of the retina, usually unilateral, that occurs in young children and usually is hereditary. One of hundreds of genetic mutations in a tumor regulatory protein (the retinoblastoma protein) may be responsible. The initial diagnostic finding is usually a yellow or white light reflex seen at the pupil (cat's eye reflex). Several treatment options are available depending on the size and extent of the tumor, whether both eyes are involved, and the general health of the patient. Included are enucleation, radiation, scleral plaque irradiation, cryotherapy, photocoagulation, and chemotherapy.

retinochoroid (rĕt″ĭ-nō-kō′royd) [″ + Gr. *chorioeides,* skinlike] Pert. to the retina and choroid. SYN: *chorioretinal.*

retinochoroiditis (rĕt″ĭ-nō-kō-royd-ī′tĭs) [″ + ″ + *itis,* inflammation] Inflammation of the retina and choroid. SYN: *chorioretinitis; choroidoretinitis.*

r. juxtapapillaris Retinochoroiditis close to the optic nerve.

retinocystoma (rĕt″ĭ-nō-sĭs-tō′mă) [″ + Gr. *kysis,* sac, + *oma,* tumor] Glioma of the retina.

retinodialysis (rĕt″ĭ-nō-dī-ăl′ĭ-sĭs) [″ + Gr. *dialysis,* separation] Detachment of the retina at its periphery. SYN: *disinsertion.*

retinoic acid A metabolite of vitamin A used in the treatment of cystic acne.

retinol (rĕt′ĭ-nŏl) One of the active forms of vitamin A; it is stored in the body primarily in the liver and in adipose tissue. Sources of this 20-carbon alcohol include liver, egg yolk, chicken, whole milk, butter, and fortified breakfast cereal. Vitamin A activity in foods is expressed as retinol equivalents (RE), the resulting amount of retinol after conversion in the body.

CAUTION: Excessive consumption of retinol supplements, esp. by the elderly, can produce vitamin A toxicity.

---

retinopapillitis (rĕt″ĭ-nō-pă″pĭl-ī′tĭs) [L. *retina,* retina, + *papilla,* nipple, + Gr. *itis,* inflammation] Inflammation of the retina and optic papilla extending to the optic disk. SYN: *papilloretinitis.*

retinopathy (rĕt″ĭn-ŏp′ă-thē) [″ + Gr. *pathos,* disease, suffering] Any disorder of the retina.

arteriosclerotic r. Retinopathy accompanying generalized arteriosclerosis and hypertension.

circinate r. A ring of degenerated white exudative area of the retina around the macula.

diabetic r. Retinal damage, marked by aneurysmal dilation of blood vessels, hemorrhage, macular edema or macular ischemia, or retinal exudates in patients with diabetes mellitus. This common complication of long-standing diabetes may result in blindness; it is found in nearly all patients who have had diabetes for more than 15 years. Strict control of blood sugar levels and of high blood pressure reduces the incidence of the disease. Regular ophthalmological screening helps to detect the disease before it causes irreversible visual loss. Treatment includes retinal laser surgery or vitrectomy. SEE: *visual field* for illus.

hypertensive r. Retinopathy associated with hypertension, toxemia of pregnancy, or glomerulonephritis. SEE: *Keith-Wagener-Barker classification.*

r. of prematurity ABBR: ROP. A bilateral disease of the retinal vessels in preterm infants that is the most prominent cause of blindness in this population. Its cause remains uncertain despite much research, but oxygen levels and other environmental factors may contribute.The disease is marked by retinal neovascularization in the first weeks of life. Retinal detachment may occur. Cryotherapy or laser photocoagulation can be curative if instituted early in the course of the illness. SYN: *retrolental fibroplasia.*

In treating preterm infants, it is possible to prevent ROP by using only the lowest possible effective oxygen concentration that will not endanger the life of the infant. Monitoring arterial blood oxygen levels is essential in preventing ROP. Too severe oxygen restriction, however, increases the likelihood of hyaline membrane disease and neurological disorders. All preterm infants treated with supplemental oxygen should be examined carefully by an ophthalmologist before discharge from the hospital. Once blindness develops, there is no effective treatment.

solar r. Pathological changes in the retina after looking directly at the sun. This condition is seen frequently following an eclipse of the sun. SEE: *scotoma, eclipse.*

syphilitic r. Syphilitic retinitis.

retinopexy (rĕt″ĭn-ō-pĕk′sē) [″+ Gr. *pexis,* fixation] In the treatment of retinal detachment, the formation of adhesions between the detached portion and the underlying tissue.

pneumatic r. A treatment for retinal detachment, in which a bubble of gas is instilled into the vitreous. As the bubble attains equilibrium with body gases, it expands and forces the detached area back into place; then, cryotherapy or photocoagulation is used to reattach the retina permanently. SEE: *retinal detachment.*

retinoschisis (rĕt″ĭ-nŏs′kĭ-sĭs) [″ + Gr. *schisis,* a splitting] A splitting of the retina into two layers with cyst formation between the layers.

retinoscope (rĕt′ĭ-nō-skōp) [″ + Gr. *skopein,* to examine] An instrument used in performing retinoscopy.

retinoscopy (rĕt″ĭn-ŏs′kō-pē) An objective method of determining refractive errors of the eye. The examiner projects light into the eyes and judges error of refraction by the movement of reflected light rays. SYN: *skiascopy* (1).

retinosis (rĕt″ĭ-nō′sĭs) [″ + Gr. *osis,* condition] Any degenerative process of the retina not associated with inflammation.

retire **1.** To discontinue formal employment or work at a specific place or task. In the past, in many industries, educational institutions, and public service, retirement was mandated when an employee had attained a specified age. This practice has lost its attractiveness to a large segment of the work force, esp. among those who enjoy work. SEE: *recreation.* **2.** To go to bed.

retisolution (rĕt″ĭ-sō-lū′shŭn) [L. *rete,* net, + *solutio,* dissolution] Dissolution of the Golgi structures.

retispersion (rĕt″ĭ-spĕr′zhŭn) [″ + *spersio,* a scattering] Transference of Golgi structures to the periphery of the cell.

retoperithelium (rē″tō-pĕr″ĭ-thē′lē-ŭm) [L. *rete,* net, + Gr. *peri,* around, + *thele,* nipple] Epithelium covering a reticulum.

retort (rē-tort′) [L. *retortus,* bent back] A flasklike, long-necked vessel used in distillation.

retothelium (rē″tō-thē′lē-ŭm) Reticuloendothelium.

retract (rĭ-trăkt′) [L. *retractus*] To draw back.

retractile (rĭ-trăkt′ĭl) [L. *retractilis*] Capable of being drawn back or in.

retraction (rĭ-trăk′shŭn) A shortening; the act of drawing backward or the condition of being drawn back.

clot r. **1.** The shrinking of the clot that forms when blood is allowed to stand, due to the fibrin network formed in the clot. **2.** The platelet-mediated folding of fibrin threads in a formed clot, which diminishes the size of the damaged area.

genital r. Koro.

uterine r. The process by which the muscular fibers of the uterus remain permanently shortened to a small degree following each contraction or labor pain.

retraction ring A ridge sometimes felt on the uterus above the pubes, marking the line of separation between the upper contractile and lower dilatable segments of the uterus. SEE: *Bandl's ring.*

retractor **1.** An instrument for holding back the margins of a wound or structures within the wound. **2.** A muscle that draws in any organ or part.

retrad (rē′trăd) [L. *retro,* backward] Toward the posterior part of the body.

retrain To instruct a person in a skill or trade different from the person's previous work.

retreat (rĭ-trēt′) [ME. *retret,* draw back] A withdrawal (e.g., in psychology) from difficult life situations. This may be direct, as in physical flight, or indirect, as in malingering, illness, abnormal preoccupation, and self-deception.

retrenchment [Fr. *retrenchier,* to cut back] **1.** A budgetary reduction; a cutback in the amount of funds allocated for a purpose. **2.** A procedure used in plastic surgery to remove excess tissue.

retrieval (rĭ-trē′văl) In psychology, the process of bringing remembered information back to the conscious level.

oocyte r. A procedure to collect eggs contained in the ovarian follicles for use in assisted reproduction.

retro- [L.] Prefix meaning *backward, back, behind.*

retroaction (rĕt″rō-ăk′shŭn) Action in a reverse direction.

retroauricular (rĕt″rō-aw-rĭk′ū-lăr) [L. *retro,* behind, + *auricula,* ear] Behind the auricle or ear.

retrobuccal (rĕt″rō-bŭk′ăl) [L. *retro,* back, + *bucca,* cheek] Pert. to the back part of the mouth or the area behind the mouth.

retrobulbar (rĕt″rō-bŭl′băr) [L. *retro,* behind, + Gr. *bulbus,* bulb] **1.** Behind the eyeball. **2.** Posterior to the medulla oblongata.

retrocecal (rĕt″rō-sē′kăl) [L. *retro,* back, + *caecum,* cecum] Behind or pert. to the area posterior to the cecum.

retrocedent (rĕt″rō-sē′dĕnt) [L. *retrocedere*] Going backward, returning.

retrocervical (rĕt″rō-sĕr′vĭ-kăl) [L. *retro,* back, + *cervix,* neck] Posterior to the cervix uteri.

retrocession (rĕt″rō-sĕsh′ŭn) [L. *retrocessio,* going back] **1.** A going back; a relapse. **2.** Metastasis from the surface to an internal organ. **3.** Backward displacement of the uterus.

retroclusion (rĕt″rō-kloo′zhŭn) [″ + *claudere,* to close] A method of stopping arterial bleeding. A needle is placed through the tissues over a severed artery and then turned around and down so that it is passed back through the tissues under the artery. This compresses the vessel.

retrocolic (rĕt″rō-kŏl′ĭk) [L. *retro,* back, + Gr. *kolon,* colon] Posterior to the colon.

retrocollic (rĕt″rō-kŏl′ĭk) [″ + *collum,* neck] Pert. to the back of the neck.

retrocollic spasm, retrocollis Torticollis with spasms affecting the posterior neck muscles.

retrocursive (rĕt″rō-kŭr′sĭv) [L. *retro,* back, + *curro,* to run] Stepping or turning backward.

retrodeviation (rĕt″rō-dē″vē-ā′shŭn) [″ + *deviare,* to turn aside] Backward displacement, as of an organ.

retrodisplacement (rĕt″rō-dĭs-plās′mĕnt) [″ + Fr. *desplacer,* displace] Backward displacement of a part.

retroesophageal (rĕt″rō-ē-sŏf″ă-jē′ăl) [L. *retro,* behind, + Gr. *oisophagos,* gullet] Behind the esophagus.

retrofilling (rĕt″rō-fĭl′ĭng) The placement of filling material in a root canal through an opening made in the apex of the tooth.

retroflexion (rĕt″rō-flĕk′shŭn) A bending or flexing backward. **retroflexed,** *adj.*

r. of uterus A condition in which the body of the uterus is bent backward at an angle with the cervix, whose position usually remains unchanged.

retrogasserian (rĕt″rō-găs-sē′rē-ăn) Pert. to the posterior root of the gasserian ganglion.

retrognathia (rĕt″rō-năth′ē-ă) [L. *retro,* back, + Gr. *gnathos,* jaw] Location of the mandible behind the frontal plane of the maxilla.

retrognathism (rĕt″rō-năth′ĭzm) [″ + Gr. *gnathos,* jaw] The condition of having retrognathia.

retrograde (rĕt′rō-grād) [L. *retro,* backward, + *gradi,* to step] Moving backward; degenerating from a better to a worse state.

retrograde flow The flow of fluid in a direction opposite to that considered normal.

retrograde pyelography A surgical procedure used to visualize the renal pelvis and ureter in which an endoscope is placed through the urethra into the urinary bladder and a catheter is placed into the ureter to instill a contrast medium.

retrography (rĕt″rŏg′ră-fē) [″ + Gr. *graphein,* to write] Mirror writing, a symptom of certain brain diseases. It also may be present in persons with dyslexia.

retrogression (rĕt″rō-grĕsh′ŭn) [L. *retrogressus,* go backward] A going backward, as in the involution, degeneration, or atrophy of a tissue or structure.

retroinfection (rĕt″rō-ĭn-fĕk′shŭn) [L. *retro,* backward, + *infectio,* infection] An infection communicated by the fetus in utero to the mother.

retroinsular (rĕt″rō-ĭn′sū-lăr) [″ + *insula,* island] Located behind the island of Reil in the brain.

retroiridian (rĕt″rō-ī-rĭd′ē-ăn) [L. *retro,* behind, + Gr. *iridos,* colored circle] Posterior to the iris.

retrojection (rĕt″rō-jĕk′shŭn) [″ + *jacio,* throw] Washing out a cavity from within by injection of a fluid.

retrolabyrinthine (rĕt″rō-lăb″ĭ-rĭn′thĭn) [L. *retro,* behind + Gr. *labyrinthos,* a maze] Located behind the labyrinth of the ear.

retrolental Behind the crystalline lens. SYN: *retrolenticular.*

retrolenticular (rĕt″rō-lĕn-tĭk′ū-lăr) Retrolental.

retrolingual (rĕt″rō-lĭng′gwăl) [L. *retro,* behind, + *lingua,* tongue] Behind the tongue.

retromammary (rĕt″rō-măm′mă-rē) [″ + *mamma,* breast] Behind the mammary gland.

retromandibular (rĕt″rō-măn-dĭb′ū-lăr) [″ + *mandibulum,* jaw] Behind the lower jaw.

retromastoid (rĕt″rō-măs′toyd) [″ + Gr. *mastos,* breast, + *eidos,* form, shape] Behind the mastoid process.

retromorphosis (rĕt″rō-mor′fō-sĭs) [″ + Gr. *morphe,* form, + *osis,* condition] **1.** A change in shape accompanying a transition from a higher to a lower type of structure. **2.** Retrogressive changes within cells or tissues. SYN: *catabolism.*

retronasal (rĕt″rō-nā′zăl) [L. *retro,* back, + *nasus,* nose] Pert. to or situated at the back part of the nose.

retro-ocular (rĕt″rō-ŏk′ū-lar) [L. *retro,* behind, + *oculus,* eye] Behind the eye.

retroparotid (rĕt″ō-pă-rŏt′ĭd) [″ + Gr. *para,* beside, + *ous,* ear] Behind the parotid gland.

retroperitoneal (rĕt″rō-pĕr″ĭ-tō-nē′ăl) [″ + Gr. *peritonaion,* peritoneum] Behind the peritoneum and outside the peritoneal cavity (e.g., the kidneys).

retroperitoneal fibrosis Development of a mass of scar tissue in the retroperitoneal space. This may lead to physical compression of the ureters, vena cava, or aorta. This disease may be associated with taking methysergide for migraine, and with other drugs. SYN: *Ormond's disease.*

retroperitoneum (rĕt″rō-pĕr-ĭ-tō-nē′ŭm) The space behind the peritoneum.

retroperitonitis (rĕt″rō-pĕr″ĭ-tō-nī′tĭs) Inflammation behind the peritoneum.

retropharyngeal (rĕt″rō-făr-ĭn′jē-ăl) [L. *retro,* behind, + Gr. *pharynx,* throat] Behind the pharynx.

retropharyngitis (rĕt″rō-făr″ĭn-jī′tĭs) [″ + ″ + *itis,* inflammation] Inflammation of the retropharyngeal tissue.

retropharynx (rĕt″rō-făr′ĭnks) [″ + Gr. *pharynx,* throat] The posterior portion of the pharynx.

retroplacental (rĕt″rō-plă-sĕn′tăl) [″ + *placenta,* a flat cake] Behind the placenta, or between the placenta and the uterine wall.

retroplasia (rĕt″rō-plā′zē-ă) [″ + Gr. *plassein,* to form] The degenerative change of a cell or tissue into a more primitive form.

retroposed (rĕt-rō-pōsd′) [L. *retro,* backward, + *positus,* placed] Displaced backward.

retroposition (rĕt″rō-pō-zĭsh′ŭn) The backward displacement of a tissue or organ.

retropulsion (rĕt″rō-pŭl′shŭn) [″ + *pulsio,* a thrusting] **1.** The pushing back of any part, as of the fetal head in labor. **2.** A gait disturbance in which patients involuntarily walk backward, seen in some diseases of the central nervous system, including Parkinson's disease. **3.** Movement of intestinal contents backward (i.e., toward the mouth instead of the anus).

retrorunning The act of running backwards, esp. for conditioning of the hamstring muscle groups for sport-specific training. [Because of the risk of falling, retrorunning regimens should be performed with close supervision when dealing with a nonathletic population.]

retrospective Looking backward.

retrospective study A clinical study in which patients or their records are investigated after the patients have experienced the disease, condition, or treatment. SEE: *prospective study*.

retrospondylolisthesis (rĕt″rō-spŏn″dĭ-lō-lĭs-thē′sĭs) [L. *retro,* behind + Gr. *spondylos,* vertebra, + *olisthesis,* a slipping] The posterior displacement of a vertebra.

retrosternal (rĕt″rō-stĕr′năl) [″ + Gr. *sternon,* chest] Behind the sternum.

retrosternal pulse A venous pulse felt over the suprasternal notch.

retrotarsal (rĕt″rō-tăr′săl) [″ + Gr. *tarsos,* a broad, flat surface] Behind the tarsus of the eyelid.

retrouterine (rĕt″rō-ū′tĕr-ĭn) [L. *retro,* backward, + *uterus,* womb] Behind the uterus.

retroversioflexion (rĕt″rō-vĕr″sē-ō-flĕk′shŭn) [″ + *versio,* a turning, + *flexio,* flexion] Retroversion and retroflexion of the uterus.

retroversion (rĕt″rō-vĕr′shŭn) [L. *retro,* back, + *versio,* a turning] A turning, or a state of being turned back; esp., the tipping of an entire organ.

femoral r. A decrease in the head-neck angle of the femur, causing outward rotation of the shaft of the bone when the person is standing.

r. of uterus Backward displacement of the uterus with the cervix pointing forward toward the symphysis pubis. Normally the cervix points toward the lower end of the sacrum with the fundus toward the suprapubic region.

retroviruses (rĕt″rō-vī′rŭs-ĕs) The common name for the family of Retroviridae. Some of these RNA-containing tumor viruses are oncogenic and induce sarcomas, leukemias, lymphomas, and mammary carcinomas in lower animals. These viruses contain reverse transcriptase, an enzyme essential for reverse transcription (i.e., the production of a DNA molecule from an RNA model).

retrude (rĭ-trood′) [L. *re,* back, + *trudere,* to shove] To force inward or backward.

retrusion (rĭ-troo′shŭn) **1.** The process of forcing backward, esp. with reference to the teeth. **2.** A condition in which teeth are retroposed.

Rett's syndrome [Andreas Rett, contemporary Austrian physician] A multiple-deficit X-linked developmental disorder marked by mental retardation, impaired language use, breath holding and hyperventilation, seizures, loss of communication skills, tremors of the trunk, difficulties walking, and abnormally small development of the head. It occurs almost exclusively in girls, after the age of 6 to 18 months, in about one of every 10,000 to 15,000 female children.

Retzius, lines of (rĕt′zē-ŭs) [Gustav Magnus Retzius, Swedish anatomist, 1842–1919] Brownish incremental lines seen in microscopic sections of tooth enamel. They appear as concentric lines in transverse sections through the enamel crown.

Retzius, Anders Adolf Swedish anatomist, 1796–1860.

space of R. An area in the lower portion of the abdomen between the bladder and pubic bones and bounded superiorly by the peritoneum. It contains areolar tissue, fat, and a plexus of veins.

veins of R. The veins that communicate between the mesenteric veins and the inferior vena cava.

reunient (rē-ūn′yĕnt) [L. *re,* again,+ *unire,* to unite] **1.** Connecting or uniting tissue. **2.** Ductus reuniens.

Reuss's color charts (roys) [August R. von Reuss, Austrian ophthalmologist, 1841–1924] Colored letters printed on colored backgrounds to test color vision. A color-blind person sees the letters as being the same color as the background.

revaccination (rē″văk-sĭ-nā′shŭn) An inoculation against a disease to sustain a passive immune response (protective antibodies) against a potentially infectious organism.

revascularization (rē-văs″kū-lăr-ī-zā′shŭn) Restoration of blood flow to a part. This may be done surgically or by removing or dissolving thrombi occluding arteries, esp. coronary or renal arteries.

transmyocardial r. ABBR: TMR. The use of a laser to bore tiny channels directly through the wall of the heart in an attempt to bring oxygen-rich blood from the left ventricular cavity to areas where the heart muscle is oxygen-deprived, or ischemic. TMR is a potential alternative to coronary bypass surgery or angioplasty, esp. in patients with complex plaques that would be difficult to reach with standard interventions or in patients who have already undergone many other procedures without effect. A variant of TMR is percutaneous myocardial revascularization.

reverberation (rĭ″vĕr-bĕr-ā′shŭn) [L. *reverberare,* to cause to rebound] **1.** The process by which closed chains of neurons, when excited by a single impulse, continue to discharge impulses from collaterals of their cells. **2.** The repeated echoing of a sound.

Reverdin's needle (rā-vĕr-dănz′) [Jacques L. Reverdin, Swiss surgeon, 1842–1929] A needle with an eye at the tip that can be opened and closed by a lever.

reversal (rĭ-vĕr′săl) [L. *reversus,* revert] **1.** A change or turning in the opposite direction. **2.** In psychology, a change in an instinct or emotion to its opposite, as from love to hate.

sex r. The changing of an individual's sexual phenotype to that of the opposite sex. SEE: *sexual reassignment.*

reversible (rĭ-vĕr′sĭ-bl) Able to change back and forth.

reversion (rĭ-vĕr′zhŭn) **1.** A return to a previously existing condition. **2.** In genetics, the appearance of traits possessed by a remote ancestor. SEE: *atavism.*

revertant An organism that has reverted to a previous phenotype by mutation.

review, chart A method of quality assurance (and sometimes clinical research) that relies on the systematic analysis of individual patient records. Data may be used to determine the incidence of adverse events, the allocation of resources, the employment of specific therapies, or the degree of compliance with specified standards of care.

review of systems ABBR: ROS. A series of questions concerning each organ system and region of the body, asked of the patient during history taking and physical examination for the purpose of gaining an optimal understanding of the patient's presenting illness and medical history.

An example of ROS follows: *General.* The examiner should determine any history of fatigue, travel to other climates or countries, recent weight change, chills, fever, and lifestyle change in the patient. How many persons occupy the patient's dwelling? What is the patient's relationship to the persons with whom he or she lives? Is it a happy home? What are the patient's hobbies and outside interests? How does the patient usually exercise? Does the patient have pets? Any history of military service? Any job-related illnesses? Any sexual partners? Any use of injected drugs? Any recent hospitalizations or illnesses?

Skin. Is the patient experiencing any rash, itching, sunburn, change in the size of moles, vesicles, or hair loss?

Head, face, and neck. Does the patient have headaches, migraine, vertigo, stiffness, pain, or swelling? Has there been trauma to this area?

Eyes. Are glasses worn and when were the eyes last examined for visual acuity and glaucoma? Is the patient experiencing pain, diplopia, scotomata, itch, discharge, redness, or infection?

Ears. Does the patient have acute or chronic hearing loss, pain, discharge, tinnitus, or vertigo? Is there a history of failure to adjust to descent from a high altitude?

Nose. Is there any dryness, crust formation, bleeding, pain, discharge, obstruction, malodor, or sneezing? How acute is the patient's sense of smell?

Mouth and teeth. The patient should be asked about any soreness, ulcers, pain, dryness, infection, hoarseness, bleeding gums, swallowing difficulty, bruxism, or temporomandibular syndrome. What is the condition of the patient's teeth (real or false)?

Breasts. Has the patient had any pain, swelling, tenderness, lumps, bleeding from the nipple, infection, or change in the ability of the nipples to become erect? Has plastic surgery been done, and if so, were implants used?

Respiratory. Has there been any cough, pain, wheezing, sputum production (including character of sputum), hemoptysis, or exposure to persons with contagious diseases such as tuberculosis? Is there a history of occupational or other exposure to asbestos, silica, chickens, parrots, or a dusty environment? The presence of dyspnea, cyanosis, tuberculosis, pneumonia, and pleurisy should be determined. If pulmonary function tests were done, the date or dates should be recorded. The extent and duration of all forms of tobacco use should be determined.

Cardiac. The following should be determined: angina, dyspnea, orthopnea, palpitations, heart murmur, heart failure, myocardial infarction, surgical procedures on coronary arteries or heart valves, history of stress tests or angiography, hypertension, rheumatic fever, cardiac arrhythmias, exercise tolerance, history of athletic participation (including jogging and running) and if these are current activities, the dates of electrocardiograms if they were ever taken.

Vascular. Has the patient experienced claudication, cold intolerance (esp. of the extremities), frostbite, phlebitis, or ulcers (esp. of the extremities) due to poor blood supply?

Gastrointestinal. The examiner should assess the patient's appetite, history of recent weight gain or loss, and whether the patient has been following a particular diet for gaining or losing weight. Is the patient a vegetarian? Has he or she had any difficulty in swallowing? Anorexia, nausea, vomiting (including the character of the vomitus), diarrhea and its possible explanation (such as foreign travel or food poisoning), belching, constipation, change in bowel habits, melena, hemorrhoids and history of surgery for this condition, use of laxatives or antacids, jaundice, hepatitis, and other liver disease should be determined.

Renal; urinary and genital tract. The examiner should take a history of kidney or bladder stones and date of last occurrence, dysuria, hematuria, pyuria, nocturia, incontinence, urgency, antibiotics used for urinary tract infections, bedwetting, sexually transmitted diseases, libido, sexual partners, penile or urethral discharge, and frequency of sexual activity.

Women should be questioned regarding any vulval pruritus, vaginal discharge, vaginal malodor, history of menarche, frequency and duration of menstrual periods, amount of flow, type of menstrual protection used, type or types of contraception and douches used, and the total number of pregnancies, abortions, miscarriages, and normal deliveries. The number, sex, age, and health status of living children, and the cause of death of children who died, should be determined. Vaginal, cervical, and uterine infections; pelvic inflammatory disease; tubal ligation; dilation and curettement; hysterectomy; and dyspareunia should be recorded. Any history of the mother's use of diethylstilbestrol while pregnant with the patient should be determined.

Men should be asked about vasectomy, scrotal pain or swelling, and urinary hesitancy or double voiding.

Musculoskeletal. The examiner should ask about muscle twitches, pain, heat, tenderness, swelling, loss of range of motion or strength, cramps, sprains, strains, trauma, fractures, stiffness, back pain, osteoporosis, and character regarding time of day of onset and duration (esp. with respect to the effect of exercise, back pain, and osteoporosis).

Hematological. A history of anemia, bleeding, bruising, hemarthrosis, hemophilia, sickle cell disease or trait, recent blood loss, transfusions received, and blood donation should be recorded. Was a transfusion received at a time when blood was not being screened for hepatitis or AIDS? Was the patient ever turned down as a blood donor?

Endocrine. The patient should be questioned about sexual maturation and development, weight change, tolerance to heat or cold (esp. with respect to other persons in the same environment), dryness of hair and skin, hair loss, and voice change. Any change in the rate of beard growth in men, development of facial hair in women, increase in or loss of libido, polyuria, polydipsia, polyphagia, pruritus, diabetes, exophthalmos, goiter, unexplained flushing, and sweating should be noted.

Nervous system. Has the patient experienced any recent change in ability to control muscular activity, or any syncope, stroke ("shock"), seizures, tremor, coordination, sensory disturbance, falls, pain, change in memory, dizziness, or head trauma?

Emotional and psychological status. Has there been a history of psychiatric illness, anxiety, depression, overactivity, mania, lassitude, change in sleep pattern, insomnia, hypersomnia, nightmares, sleepwalking, hallucinations, feeling of unreality, paranoia, phobias, obsessions, compulsions, criminal behavior, increase in or loss of libido, or suicidal thoughts? Is the patient satisfied with his or her occupation and life in general? What is his or her marital and divorce record? Has there been family discord? Does the patient attend church? The patient's employment history and any recent job changes, educational history and achievement, and self-image should be assessed.

Révilliod sign SEE: *wink.*

revised trauma score ABBR: RTS. Pediatric trauma score.

revivification (rē-vĭv″ĭ-fĭ-kā′shŭn) [L. *re,* again, + *vivere,* to live, + *facere,* to make] **1.** An attempt to restore life to those apparently dead; restoration to life or consciousness; also the restoration of life in local parts, as a limb after freezing. **2.** The pairing of surfaces to facilitate healing, as in a wound.

revulsant (rĭ-vŭl′sănt) [L. *revulsio,* pulling back] **1.** Causing transfer of disease or blood from one part of the body to another. **2.** A counterirritant that increases blood flow to an inflamed part.

revulsion (rĭ-vŭl′shŭn) **1.** Repugnance, hostility, or extreme distaste for a person or thing. **2.** The act of driving backward, as diverting disease from one part to another by a quick withdrawal of blood from that part—a treatment that has its origins in ancient medical care. **3.** Circulatory changes obtained by sudden and intense reactions to heat and cold. SEE: *counterirritation.*

revulsive (rĭ-vŭl′sĭv) **1.** Causing revulsion. **2.** A counterirritant.

reward 1. In behavioral science, a positive reinforcement. **2.** Something given to an individual as recognition of a good performance or of having achieved a certain level of competence in a field of endeavor.

rewarming Restoring a hypothermic patient's body temperature to normal. Techniques used include removing wet clothing; wrapping patients in blankets, hotpacks, or foils; infusing intravenous, nasogastric, or intraperitoneal fluids warmed to about 40°C; increasing the temperature of the patient's blood with extracorporeal bypass machines, or, rarely, immersing the patient in warm water.

Reye's syndrome (rīz) [R. D. K. Reye, Australian pathologist, 1912–1977] A syndrome marked by acute encephalopathy and fatty infiltration of the liver and possibly of the pancreas, heart, kidney, spleen, and lymph nodes. It is seen in children under age 15 after an acute viral infection such as chickenpox or influenza. The mortality rate depends on the severity of the central nervous system involvement but may be as high as 80%. The cause of the disease is unknown, but association with increased use of aspirin and other salicylates is evident from epidemiological studies. SEE: *Nursing Diagnoses Appendix.*

SYMPTOMS: The patient experiences a viral upper respiratory infection followed in about 6 days by severe nausea and vomiting, a change in mental status (disorientation, agitation, coma, seizures), and hepatomegaly without jaundice in 40% of cases. The disease should be suspected in any child with acute onset of encephalopathy, nausea and vomiting, or altered liver function, esp. after a recent illness.

CAUTION: Aspirin and other salicylates should not be used for any reason in treating children with viral infections.

TREATMENT: Supportive care includes intravenous administration of fluids and electrolytes. The blood electrolytes should be controlled carefully.

PATIENT CARE: Neurological assessment is performed at frequent intervals. Temperature is monitored, and prescribed measures to alleviate hyperthermia are instituted. Seizure precautions are also instituted. Intake and output are monitored carefully. The patient is observed for evidence of impaired hepatic function, such as signs of bleeding or encephalopathy.

RF, Rf *rheumatoid factor.*

R.F.A. *right frontoanterior* fetal position.

R factor *resistance transfer factor.*

R.F.P. *right frontoposterior* fetal position.

R.F.T. *right frontotransverse* fetal position.

RH *releasing hormone.*

Rh **1.** Symbol for the element rhodium. **2.** *Rhesus,* a monkey (*Macaca rhesus*) in which the Rh factor was first identified.

Rhabditis (răb-dī'tĭs) [Gr. *rhabdos,* rod] A genus of small nematode worms, some of which are parasitic.

rhabdo- Combining form meaning *rod.*

rhabdoid (răb'doyd) [Gr. *rhabdos,* rod, + *eidos,* form, shape] Resembling a rod.

rhabdomyoblastoma (răb"dō-mī"ō-blăs-tō'mă) Rhabdomyosarcoma.

rhabdomyolysis (răb"dō-mī-ŏl'ĭ-sĭs) [" + " + *lysis,* dissolution] An acute, sometimes fatal disease in which the byproducts of skeletal muscle destruction accumulate in the renal tubules and produce acute renal failure. Rhabdomyolysis may result from crush injuries, the toxic effect of drugs or chemicals on skeletal muscle, extremes of exertion, sepsis, shock, and severe hyponatremia, among other diseases and conditions. Life-threatening hyperkalemia and metabolic acidosis may result. Management may include the infusion of bicarbonate-containing fluids (to enhance urinary secretion of myoglobin and iron) or hemodialysis. SEE: *reperfusion.*

traumatic r. SEE: *crush syndrome; reperfusion* (2).

rhabdomyoma (răb"dō-mī-ō'mă) [" + " + *oma,* tumor] A striated muscular tissue tumor. SYN: *myoma striocellulare.*

rhabdomyosarcoma (răb"dō-mī"ō-săr-kō'mă) [" + " + *sarx,* flesh, + *oma,* tumor] A malignant neoplasm originating in skeletal muscle. SYN: *rhabdomyoblastoma.*

rhabdophobia (răb-dō-fō'bē-ă) [" + *phobos,* fear] An abnormal fear of being hit or beaten with a stick or rod.

rhabdosarcoma, embryonal Botryoid sarcoma.

rhabdovirus (răb"dō-vī'rŭs) [" + L. *virus,* poison] Any of a group of rod-shaped RNA viruses with one important member, the rabies virus, being pathogenic to humans. The virus has a predilection for the tissue of mucus-secreting glands and the central nervous system. All warm-blooded animals are susceptible to infection with these viruses.

rhachialgia (rā"kē-ăl'jē-ă) [Gr. *rhachis,* spine, + *algos,* pain] Pain in the spine.

rhachiocampsis (rā"kē-ō-kămp'sĭs) [" + *kampsis,* a bending] Curvature of the spine.

rhachioplegia (rā"kē-ō-plē'jē-ă) [" + *plege,* stroke] Spinal paralysis.

rhachioscoliosis (rā"kē-ō-skō"lē-ō'sĭs) [" + *skoliosis,* curvature] Curvature of the spine laterally.

rhachis (rā'kĭs) [Gr.] The spinal column.

rhachischisis (ră-kĭs'kĭ-sĭs) [" + *schisis,* a splitting] A congenital cleft in the spinal column. SYN: *spondyloschisis.*

rhagades (răg'ă-dēz) [Gr., tears] Linear fissures appearing in the skin, esp. at the corner of the mouth or anus, causing pain. If due to syphilis, they form a radiating scar on healing.

rhagadiform (rā-găd′ĭ-form) [Gr. *rhagas,* tear, + L. *forma,* shape] Fissured; having cracks.

-rhage, -rhagia SEE: *-rrhage; -rrhagia.*

Rh antiserum Human serum that contains antibodies to the Rh factor.

rhaphania (ră-fā′nē-ă) Raphania.

rhaphe (rā′fē) Raphe.

Rh blood group A group of antigens on the surface of red blood cells present to a variable degree in human populations. When the Rh factor (an antigen often called D) is present, an individual's blood type is designated Rh^+ (Rh positive); when the Rh antigen is absent, the blood type is Rh^- (Rh negative). If an individual with Rh^- blood receives a transfusion of Rh^+ blood, anti-Rh antibodies form. Subsequent transfusions of Rh^+ blood may result in serious transfusion reactions (agglutination and hemolysis of red blood cells). A pregnant woman who is Rh^- may become sensitized by entry of red blood cells from an Rh^+ fetus into the maternal circulation after abortion, ectopic pregnancy, or delivery. In subsequent pregnancies, if the fetus is Rh^+, Rh antibodies produced in maternal blood may cross the placenta and destroy fetal cells, causing erythroblastosis fetalis. SEE: *Rh_0(D) immune globulin.*

-rhea SEE: *-rrhea.*

rhenium (rē′nē-ŭm) SYMB: Re. A metallic element similar to manganese; atomic weight 186.2, atomic number 75.

rheo- [Gr. *rheos,* current] Combining form meaning *current, stream, flow.*

rheobase (rē′ō-bās) [″ + *basis,* base] In unipolar testing with the galvanic current using the negative as the active pole, the minimal voltage required to produce a stimulated response. Also called *threshold of excitation.* SEE: *chronaxie.*

rheobasic (rē″ō-bā′sĭk) Concerning the rheobase.

rheology (rē-ŏl′ō-jē) [″ + *logos,* word, reason] The study of the deformation and flow of materials.

rheostat (rē′ō-stăt) [″ + *statos,* standing] A device maintaining fixed or variable resistance for controlling the amount of electric current entering a circuit.

rheostosis (rē-ŏs-tō′sĭs) [″ + *osteon,* bone] A hypertrophying and condensing osteitis occurring in streaks, involving the long bones; also known as melorheostosis.

rheotaxis (rē″ō-tăk′sĭs) [″ + *taxis,* arrangement] A reaction to a current of fluid, in which an organism orients itself with the current.

rheum, rheuma (room, room′ă) [Gr. *rheuma,* discharge] Any catarrhal or watery discharge.

rheumatic (roo-măt′ĭk) [Gr. *rheumatikos*] Pert. to rheumatism.

rheumatic disease, functional class Classifications created by the American Rheumatism Association (now the American College of Rheumatology) that define the capacity level at which a patient with rheumatic disease is capable of functioning. Class I is complete functional capacity with ability to carry on all usual duties without handicaps; class II is functional capacity adequate to conduct normal activities despite handicap or discomfort or limited mobility of one or more joints; class III is functional capacity adequate to perform only a few or none of the duties of usual occupations or of self-care; and class IV indicates a patient who is largely or wholly incapacitated and is bedridden or confined to a wheelchair, permitting little or no self-care.

rheumatic fever A multisystem, febrile inflammatory disease that is a delayed complication of untreated group A streptococcal pharyngitis. It is believed to be caused by an autoimmune response to bacterial antigens in the streptococci, although the precise mechanism responsible for the illness has not been identified. The disease is now uncommon in Western societies because of effective and prompt treatment for strep throat, but it remains a major cause of morbidity in the developing world. SEE: illus.; *Nursing Diagnoses Appendix.*

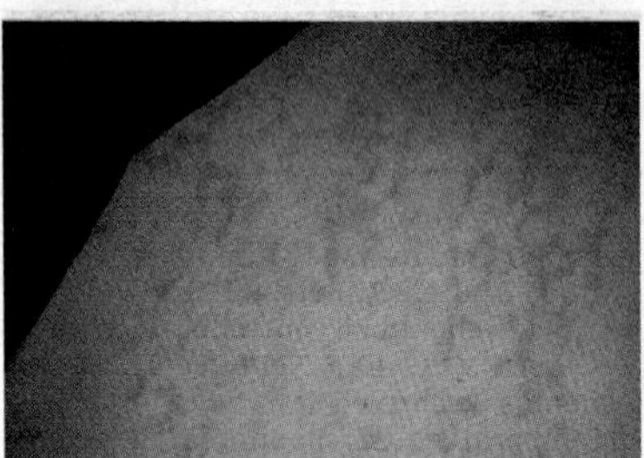

RHEUMATIC FEVER

Erythema marginatum

SYMPTOMS: Following a pharyngeal infection with group A streptococci, some patients experience sudden fever and joint pain; this is the most common type of onset. Other symptoms include fever, migratory polyarthritis, pain on motion, abdominal pain, chorea, and cardiac involvement (pericarditis, myocarditis, and endocarditis). Precordial discomfort and heart murmurs develop suddenly. Skin manifestations include erythema marginatum or circinatum and the development of subcutaneous nodules.

Rheumatic fever may occur without any sign or symptom of joint involvement. Two major manifestations (carditis, polyarthritis, chorea, erythema marginatum, subcutaneous nodules) or one major and two minor criteria (fever, arthralgia, previous rheumatic fever, elevated erythrocyte sedimentation rate or positive C-reactive protein, prolonged P-R interval) are required to establish the diagnosis of acute rheumatic fever.

PROPHYLAXIS: Prompt and adequate treatment of streptococcal infections with oral penicillin or cephalosporin is given for at least 10 days. Erythromycin is substituted in patients with penicillin allergy.

Patients known to have carditis who must undergo dental or surgical procedures (esp. those involving instrumentation of the urinary tract, rectum, or colon) should receive additional antibiotic coverage on the day of the procedure and for several days thereafter.

To prevent recurrence of rheumatic fever in a patient who has already been affected by the disease, penicillin, erythromycin, or sulfa drugs are taken daily for at least 5 years after the initial infection (10 years for patients who have had heart valve involvement).

TREATMENT: The treatment also involves bedrest until the signs of active rheumatic fever have disappeared. Salicylates may be given for symptomatic relief. Diuretics or antiarrhythmics may be given for congestive heart failure or cardiac rhythm disturbances.

PATIENT CARE: Health care professionals advise the patient about lifestyle and activity modifications, as well as the importance of taking prescribed antibiotics for the full course of treatment and prophylaxis. The importance of maintaining a salt-restricted diet and of adhering to treatment with diuretics, digoxin, or afterload-reducing drugs is emphasized for patients with congestive heart failure.

rheumatid (roo'mă-tĭd) A skin lesion associated with rheumatic disease.

rheumatism (roo'mă-tĭzm) [Gr. *rheumatismos*] A general, but somewhat archaic term for acute and chronic conditions marked by inflammation, muscle soreness and stiffness, and pain in joints and associated structures. It includes inflammatory arthritis (infectious, rheumatoid, gouty), arthritis due to rheumatic fever or trauma, degenerative joint disease, neurogenic arthropathy, hydroarthrosis, myositis, bursitis, fibromyalgia, and many other conditions. SEE: *arthritis; rheumatic fever*.

acute articular r. Rheumatic fever.

chronic r. Rheumatism associated with a joint disorder, such as rheumatoid arthritis, gout, or degenerative joint disease, usually resulting in deformity of the joint.

gonorrheal r. Arthritis resulting from gonorrheal infection. SEE: *gonorrhea*.

inflammatory r. Rheumatism caused by rheumatic fever.

muscular r. One of several muscular conditions marked by tenderness, soreness, pain, and local spasm, including fibromyalgia, myositis, polymyalgia, and torticollis.

palindromic r. Intermittent migrating joint pain with tenderness, heat, and swelling that lasts from a few hours to as long as a week. The knee is most often involved, but each recurrence often involves a different joint. Between attacks there is no evidence of joint disease. The cause is unknown, and there is no specific treatment.

psychogenic r. An out-of-date and discredited term for fibromyalgia.

soft tissue r. Any of several localized or generalized conditions that cause pain around joints but are not related to or caused by joint disease (e.g., bursitis, tennis elbow, tendinitis, perichondritis, stiff man syndrome, Tietze's disease).

rheumatoid (roo'mă-toyd) [Gr. *rheuma*, discharge, + *eidos*, form, shape] Of the nature of rheumatism; resembling rheumatism.

rheumatoid factor Antibodies raised by the body against immunoglobulins. They are present in roughly 80% of patients with rheumatoid arthritis and in many patients with other rheumatological and infectious illnesses. This factor is used, with other clinical indicators, in the diagnosis and management of rheumatoid arthritis.

rheumatologist (roo"mă-tŏl'ō-jĭst) A physician who specializes in rheumatic diseases.

rheumatology (roo"mă-tŏl'ō-jē) The division of medicine concerned with rheumatic diseases.

rhexis (rĕk'sĭs) [Gr., rupture] The rupture of any organ, blood vessel, or tissue.

Rh factor Rh antigen. SEE: *Rh blood group*.

Rh gene Any of eight allelic genes that are responsible for the various Rh blood types. They have been designated as R^1, R^2, R^0, R^z, r, r', r", and r_y. Genes represented by small r's are responsible for the Rh-negative (Rh^-) blood type; those by capital R's, for the Rh-positive (Rh^+) blood type.

rhigosis (rī-gō'sĭs) [Gr., shivering] Perception of cold.

rhinal (rī'năl) Nasal.

rhinalgia (rī-năl'jē-ă) [" + *algos*, pain] Pain in the nose; nasal neuralgia.

rhinedema (rī"nĕ-dē'mă) [" + *oidema*, swelling] Edema of the nose.

rhinencephalon (rī-nĕn-sĕf'ă-lŏn) [" + *enkephalos*, brain] The portion of brain concerned with receiving and integrating olfactory impulses. It includes the olfactory bulb, olfactory tract and striae, intermediate olfactory area, pyriform area, paraterminal area, hippocampal formation, and fornix, and constitutes the paleopallium and archipallium.

rhinencephalus (rī″nĕn-sĕf′ă-lŭs) [″ + *enkephalos,* brain] Rhinocephalus.

rhinenchysis [″ + Gr. *enchein,* to pour in] A nasal douche using a medicated or nonmedicated solution.

rhinesthesia (rī-nĕs-thē′zē-ă) [″ + *aisthesis,* sensation] The sense of smell.

rhineurynter (rĭn″ū-rĭn′tĕr) [″ + *eurynein,* to dilate] An elastic bag used for dilating the nostrils.

rhinion (rĭn′ē-ŏn) [Gr.] The lower end of the suture between the nasal bones; a craniometric point. SYN: *punctum nasale inferius.*

rhinism (rī′nĭzm) Rhinolalia.

rhinitis (rī-nī′tĭs) [″ + *itis,* inflammation] A seasonal or year-round IgE-mediated inflammation of the nasal mucosa. SEE: *hay fever.*

acute r. Acute nasal congestion with increased mucus secretion. This condition is the usual manifestation of the common cold. SEE: *coryza.*

TREATMENT: General measures include rest, adequate fluids, and a well-balanced diet. Analgesics and antipyretics may be used to make the patient comfortable. Antibiotics are of no value and should not be administered. Antihistamines may relieve early symptoms but do not abort or alter the course. Inhaled ipratropium lessens secretions. Vasoconstrictors in the form of inhalants, nasal sprays, or drops may give temporary relief. Their use helps prevent the development of middle ear infections by helping to maintain the patency of the eustachian tubes.

allergic r. Hay fever.

atrophic r. Chronic inflammation with marked atrophy of the mucous membrane and disturbance in the sense of smell; usually accompanied by ozena. The throat is dry and usually contains crusts. A husky voice or hoarseness is common.

TREATMENT: The nose should be irrigated using warm alkalinized saline solution twice daily. Surgery is seldom helpful.

r. caseosa Rhinitis characterized by the accumulation of offensive cheeselike masses in the nose and sinuses and accompanied by a seropurulent discharge.

chronic hyperplastic r. Chronic inflammation of the nasal mucous membrane accompanied by polypoid formation and underlying sinus pathology. SEE: *sinus.*

chronic hypertrophic r. Inflammation of the nasal mucous membrane marked by hypertrophy of the mucous membrane of the turbinates and the septum. The symptoms are those of nasal obstruction, postnasal discharge, and recurrent head colds. The treatment is surgical removal of the hypertrophic or mulberry ends of the inferior turbinates and cauterization of the mucosa of the inferior turbinates and septum.

fibrinous r. Rhinitis marked by the formation of a false membrane in the nasal cavities. SYN: *pseudomembranous r.*

hypertrophic r. Rhinitis marked by thickening and swelling of the nasal mucosa.

infectious r. Rhinitis due to infections of the nasal mucosa.

membranous r. Chronic rhinitis accompanied by a fibrinous exudate.

perennial r. Year-round, rather than seasonal, rhinitis.

pseudomembranous r. Fibrinous r.

purulent r. Chronic rhinitis accompanied by pus formation.

vasomotor r. Nonallergic rhinitis.

rhino- [Gr. *rhis*] Combining form meaning *nose.* SEE: *naso-.*

rhinoanemometer (rī″nō-ăn″ĕ-mŏm′ĕ-tĕr) A device that determines the presence of nasal obstruction by measuring the rate of air flow through the nasal passages.

rhinoantritis (rī″nō-ăn-trī′tĭs) [″ + *antron,* cavity, + *itis,* inflammation] Inflammation of the nasal cavities and one or both maxillary sinuses (antra).

rhinocanthectomy (rī″nō-kăn-thĕk′tō-mē) [Gr. *rhis,* nose, + *kanthos,* canthus, + *ektome,* excision] Surgical excision of the inner corner of the eye. SYN: *rhinommectomy.*

rhinocele (rī′nō-sēl) [″ + *koilia,* cavity] The ventricle or hollow of the olfactory lobe or rhinencephalon.

rhinocephalus (rī″nō-sĕf′ă-lŭs) [″ + *kephale,* head] An individual with rhinocephaly. SYN: *rhinencephalus.*

rhinocephaly (rī″nō-sĕf′ă-lē) [″ + *kephale,* head] A congenital deformity in which the eyes are fused and the nose is present as a fleshy protuberance above the eyes.

rhinocheiloplasty (rī″nō-kī′lō-plăs″tē) [″ + *cheilos,* lip, + *plastos,* formed] Plastic surgery of the nose and upper lip.

rhinodacryolith (rī″nō-dăk′rē-ō-lĭth) [″ + *dakryon,* tear, + *lithos,* stone] A stone in the nasolacrimal duct.

Rhinoestrus (rī-nĕs′trŭs) A genus of flies belonging to the family Oestridae. Larvae may be deposited in the eye or in the nasal or buccal cavity of mammals.

R. purpureus The Russian gadfly, whose larvae sometimes cause nasomyiasis and ophthalmomyiasis in humans.

rhinogenous (rī-nŏj′ĕn-ŭs) [″ + *gennan,* to produce] Originating in the nose.

rhinokyphosis (rī″nō-kī-fō′sĭs) [″ + *ky-*

phos, hump, + *osis,* condition] A deformity of the bridge of the nose.
rhinolalia (rī″nō-lā′lē-ă) [″ + *lalia,* speech] A nasal quality of the voice.
r. aperta Rhinolalia caused by undue patency of the posterior nares.
r. clausa Rhinolalia caused by closure of the nasal passages.
rhinolaryngitis (rī″nō-lăr″ĭn-jī′tĭs) [″ + *larynx,* larynx, + *itis,* inflammation] Simultaneous inflammation of the mucosa of the nose and larynx.
rhinolith (rī′nō-lĭth) [″ + *lithos,* stone] A nasal concretion.
rhinolithiasis (rī″nō-lĭth-ī′ă-sĭs) The formation of nasal stones.
rhinologist (rī-nŏl′ō-jĭst) [″ + *logos,* word, reason] A specialist in diseases of the nose.
rhinology (rī-nŏl′ō-jē) The science of the nose and its diseases.
rhinomanometry (rī″nō-mă-nŏm′ĕ-trē) The measurement of air flow through and air pressure in the nose.
rhinometer (rī-nŏm′ĕt-ĕr) A device for measuring the nose or its cavities.
rhinomiosis (rī″nō-mī-ō′sĭs) [″ + *meiosis,* a lessening] Surgical reduction in the size of the nose. SEE: *rhinoplasty.*
rhinommectomy (rī″nŏm-mĕk′tō-mē) [″ + *omma,* eye, + *ektome,* excision] Rhinocanthectomy.
rhinomycosis (rī″nō-mī-kō′sĭs) [″ + *mykes,* fungus, + *osis,* condition] Fungi in the mucous membranes and secretions of the nose.
rhinonecrosis (rī″nō-nē-krō′sĭs) [″ + *nekrosis,* state of death] Necrosis of the nasal bones.
rhinopathy (rī-nŏp′ă-thē) [″ + *pathos,* disease] Any nasal disease.
rhinopharyngeal (rī″nō-fă-rĭn′jē-ăl) Pert. to the nasopharynx.
rhinopharyngitis (rī″nō-făr-ĭn-jī′tĭs) [″ + *pharynx,* throat, + *itis,* inflammation] Inflammation of the nasopharynx.
rhinopharyngocele (rī″nō-făr-ĭn′gō-sēl) [″ + ″ + *kele,* tumor, swelling] A nasopharyngeal tumor.
rhinopharyngolith (rī″nō-făr-ĭn′gō-lĭth) [″ + ″ + *lithos,* stone] A concretion in the nasal pharynx.
rhinopharynx (rī″nō-făr′ĭnks) Nasopharynx.
rhinophonia (rī″nō-fō′nē-ă) Rhinolalia.
rhinophycomycosis (rī″nō-fī″kō-mī-kō′sĭs) [″ + *phykos,* seaweed, + *mykes,* fungus, + *osis,* condition] A fungal infection that may occur in humans or animals. It affects the nasal and paranasal sinuses and may spread to the brain. It is caused by the phycomycete *Entomophthora coronata.*
rhinophyma (rī-nō-fī′mă) [″ + *phyma,* growth] Nodular swelling and congestion of the nose associated with advanced acne rosacea. SEE: illus.; *rosacea.*

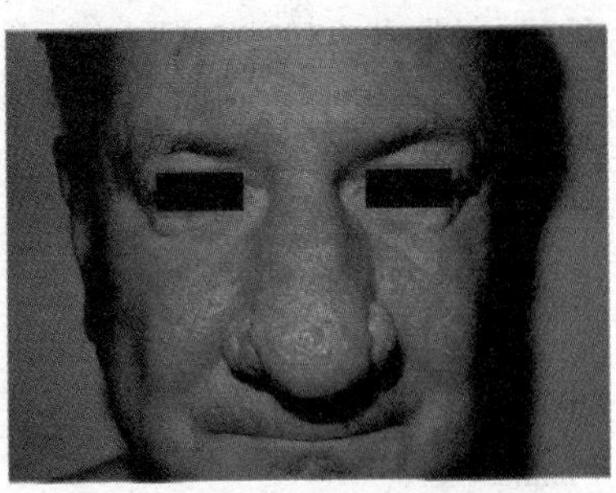

RHINOPHYMA AND ROSACEA

rhinoplasty (rī′nō-plăs″tē) [″ + *plastos,* formed] Plastic surgery of the nose.
rhinopneumonitis (rī″nō-nū″mō-nī′tĭs) [Gr. *rhis,* nose, + *pneumon,* lung, + *itis,* inflammation] Inflammation of the nasal and pulmonary mucous membranes.
rhinopolypus (rī″nō-pŏl′ĭ-pŭs) [″ + *polys,* many, + *pous,* foot] A nasal polyp.
rhinorrhagia (rī″nō-rā′jē-ă) Epistaxis.
rhinorrhea (rī″nō-rē′ă) [″ + *rhoia,* flow] A thin watery discharge from the nose.
cerebrospinal r. A discharge of spinal fluid from the nose caused by a defect in or trauma to the cribriform plate.
gustatory r. A flow of thin watery material from the nose while one is eating.
rhinosalpingitis (rī″nō-săl″pĭn-jī′tĭs) [″ + *salpinx,* tube, + *itis,* inflammation] Inflammation of the mucosa of the nose and eustachian tube.
rhinoscleroma (rī″nō-sklē-rō′mă) [″ + *skleros,* hard, + *oma,* tumor] A chronic, recurring granulomatous infection of the nasal passages and surrounding structures, sometimes leading to marked deformity of the nasal cavity, nasopharynx, paranasal sinuses, or eyes. The disease is caused by *Klebsiella rhinoscleromatis,* a gram-negative encapsulated bacillus.

TREATMENT: Surgical débridement is combined with prolonged antimicrobial therapy.

SYMPTOMS: The disease presents a hard, nodular growth, which usually begins at the anterior end of the nose and spreads to the lower respiratory tract. There usually is no pain and no tendency to ulceration.
rhinoscope (rī′nō-skōp) [″ + *skopein,* to examine] An instrument for examining the nose.
rhinoscopy (rī-nŏs′kō-pē) Examination of nasal passages. **rhinoscopic** (rī″nō-skŏp′ĭk), *adj.*
anterior r. Examination through the anterior nares.
posterior r. Examination through the posterior nares, usually with a small mirror in the nasopharynx.

rhinosporidiosis (rī″nō-spō-rĭd″ē-ō′sĭs) [″ + *sporidion,* little seed, + *osis,* condition] A condition caused by a fungus, *Rhinosporidium seeberi,* and marked by development of pedunculated polyps on the mucous membranes of the nose, larynx, eyes, penis, vagina, and sometimes skin of various parts of the body. The disease is contracted from cattle and is found in India, Sri Lanka, and other parts of the world.

Rhinosporidium (rī″nō-spō-rĭd′ē-ŭm) A genus of fungi that is pathogenic to humans.

R. seeberi The causative agent of rhinosporidiosis.

rhinostenosis (rī″nō-stěn-ō′sĭs) [″ + *stenos,* narrow, + *osis,* condition] Obstruction of the nasal passages.

rhinotomy (rī-nŏt′ō-mē) [″ + *tome,* incision] Incision of the nose for drainage purposes.

rhinotracheitis (rī″nō-trā″kē-ī′tĭs) [″ + *tracheia,* rough, + *itis,* inflammation] Inflammation of the nasal mucous membranes and the trachea.

rhinovirus (rī″nō-vī′rŭs) One of hundreds of species of picornaviruses that are responsible for upper respiratory infections ("common cold") in humans. Rhinoviruses commonly produce runny nose and congestion, postnasal drainage, cough, malaise, and, in some cases, exacerbations of asthma. The symptoms of rhinoviral infection are treatable, through the use of oxymetazoline nasal spray, pseudoephedrine, or inhaled ipratropium bromide.

Rhipicephalus (rī″pĭ-sěf′ă-lŭs) [Gr. *rhipis,* fan, + *kephale,* head] A genus of ticks belonging to the family Ixodidae. Several species, esp. *R. sanguineus,* are vectors for the organisms of spotted fever, boutonneuse fever, and other rickettsial diseases.

rhitidectomy (rĭt″ĭ-děk′tō-mē) Rhytidectomy.

rhitidosis (rĭt-ĭ-dō′sĭs) Rhytidosis.

rhizo- [Gr. *rhiza*] Combining form meaning *root.*

rhizodontropy (rī″zō-dŏn′trō-pē) [Gr. *rhiza,* root, + *odous,* tooth, + *trope,* a turning] The process of attaching an artificial crown onto the root of a tooth.

rhizodontrypy (rī″zō-dŏn′trĭ-pē) [″ + ″ + *trype,* a hole] The puncture of the root of a tooth.

rhizoid (rī′zoyd) [″ + *eidos,* form, shape] **1.** Rootlike. **2.** A rootlike structure, usually one-celled, occurring in lower forms of plant life. **3.** In bacteriology, a colony showing an irregular rootlike system of branching.

rhizome (rī′zōm) [Gr. *rhizoma,* mass of roots] A rootlike stem growing horizontally along or below the ground and sending out roots and shoots.

rhizomelic (rī″zō-měl′ĭk) [Gr. *rhiza,* root, + *melos,* limb] Concerning the hip joint and the shoulder joint.

rhizomeningomyelitis (rī″zō-mě-nĭn″gō-mī″ě-lī′tĭs) Radiculomeningomyelitis.

Rhizopoda (rī-zŏp′ō-dā) [″ + *pous,* foot] A phylum of the kingdom Protista; unicellular amebas with pseudopod locomotion. It includes free-living and pathogenic species such as *Entamoeba histolytica.*

rhizotomy (rī-zŏt′ō-mē) [″ + *tome,* incision] Surgical section of a nerve root (e.g., the root of a spinal or dental nerve) to relieve pain or reduce spasticity.

anterior r. Surgical section of the ventral root of the spinal nerve.

posterior r. Surgical section of the dorsal root of the spinal nerve.

rhodium (rō′dē-ŭm) SYMB: Rh. A rare metallic element; atomic weight 102.905, atomic number 45.

rhodo- (rō′dō) Combining form meaning *red.*

rhodogenesis (rō″dō-jěn′ě-sĭs) [Gr. *rhodon,* rose, + *genesis,* generation, birth] Regeneration of rhodopsin that has been bleached by light.

rhodophylaxis (rō″dō-fī-lăk′sĭs) [″ + *phylaxis,* protection] The ability of the retinal epithelium to regenerate rhodopsin that has been bleached by light.

rhodopsin (rō-dŏp′sĭn) [″ + *opsis,* vision] The glycoprotein opsin of the rods of the retina; combines with retinal to form a functional photopigment responsive to light. Formerly called visual purple.

rhombencephalon (rŏm″běn-sěf′ă-lŏn) Hindbrain.

rhombocele (rŏm′bō-sēl) [″ + *koilos,* a hollow] The cavity of the rhombencephalon.

rhomboid (rŏm′boyd) [″ + *eidos,* form, shape] An oblique parallelogram.

rhomboideus (rŏm-bō-ĭd′ē-ŭs) [L.] One of two muscles beneath the trapezius muscle. SEE: *muscle* for illus.

rhomboid fossa The fourth ventricle of the brain.

rhombomere (rŏm′bō-mēr) Neuromere.

rhoncal, rhonchial (rŏng′kăl, rŏng′kē-ăl) [Gr. *rhonchos,* a snore] Pert. to or produced by a rattle in the throat.

rhonchi Pl. of rhonchus.

rhonchus (rŏng′kŭs) *pl.* **rhonchi** A wheezing, snoring, or squeaking sound heard during auscultation of the chest of a person with partial airway obstruction. Mucus or other secretions in the airway, bronchial hyperreactivity, or tumors that occlude respiratory passages can all cause rhonchi.

rhopheocytosis (rō″fē-ō-sī-tō′sĭs) [Gr. *rhophein,* gulp down, + *kytos,* cell, + *osis,* condition] The mechanism by which ferritin is transferred from macrophages in the bone marrow to normoblasts. SEE: *pinocytosis.*

rhotacism (rō′tă-sĭzm) [Gr. *rhotakizein,* to overuse letter "r"] Overuse or improper utterance of "r" sounds.

rhubarb (roo'bărb) [ME. *rubarbe*] An extract made from the roots and rhizome of *Rheum officinale, R. palmatum,* and other species, used as a cathartic and astringent. It is high in oxalic acid. The stems are used as food.

rHuEPO *recombinant human erythropoietin.*

Rhus (rŭs) [L.] A genus of trees and shrubs, some of which are poisonous and produce a severe dermatitis, such as poison ivy *(R. toxicodendron)* and poison sumac *(R. venenata).*

rhypophobia (rī"pō-fō'bē-ă) [Gr. *rhypos,* filth, + *phobos,* fear] An abnormal disgust at the act of defecation, feces, or filth. SYN: *rupophobia.*

rhythm (rĭth'ŭm) [Gr. *rhythmos,* measured motion] **1.** A measured time or movement; regularity of occurrence of action or function. **2.** In electroencephalography, the regular occurrence of an impulse. **rhythmic** (-mĭk), *adj.*

alpha r. In electroencephalography, oscillations in electric potential occurring at a rate of 8½ to 12 per second.

atrioventricular r. The rhythmic discharges of impulses from the atrioventricular node that occur when the activity of the sinoatrial node is depressed or abolished. SYN: *nodal r.*

beta r. In electroencephalography, waves ranging in frequency from 15 to 30 per second and of lower voltage than alpha waves. This rhythm is more pronounced in the frontomotor leads.

bigeminal r. The coupling of extrasystoles with previously normal beats of the heart. SEE: *bigeminal pulse.*

biological r. The regular occurrence of certain phenomena in living organisms. SEE: *circadian r.; clock, biological.*

cantering r. Gallop.

cardiac r. The predominant electrical activity of the heart. It may be determined by recording an electrocardiogram or by evaluating tracings made by a cardiac monitor. SEE: *cardiac cycle; electrocardiogram; conduction system of the heart.*

circadian r. Diverse yet predictable changes in physiological variables, including sleep, appetite, temperature, and hormone secretion, over a 24-hour period. SYN: *diurnal r.*

coupled r. A rhythm in which every other heartbeat produces no pulse at the wrist.

delta r. In electroencephalography, slow waves with a frequency of 4 or fewer per second and of relatively high voltage (20 to 200 μV). It may be found over the area of a gross lesion such as a tumor or hemorrhage.

diurnal r. Circadian r.

ectopic r. A heart rhythm originating outside the sinoatrial node.

escape r. A heart rhythm that arises from a junctional or ventricular source when impulses from the atria or atrioventricular node are blocked.

gamma r. The 50-per-second rhythm seen in the electroencephalogram.

idioventricular r. A cardiac rhythm that arises from pacemakers in ventricular muscle.

junctional r. An electrocardiographic rhythm arising in the atrioventricular junction. It appears as an electrocardiogram as a narrow QRS complex that lacks an upright P wave preceding it.

nodal r. Atrioventricular r.

normal sinus r. The normal heart rhythm whose pacemaker is in the sinoatrial node and whose conduction through the atria, atrioventricular node, and ventricles in unimpaired. The interval between complexes is regular, the ventricular rate is 60 to 100, there are upright P waves in leads I and II, a negative P wave in lead AVR, a P-R interval of 0.12 to 0.20 sec, and one P wave preceding each QRS complex. SYN: *sinus r.*

nyctohemeral r. Day and night rhythm.

sinus r. Normal sinus rhythm.

theta r. The 4 to 7 per second rhythm seen in the electroencephalogram.

ventricular r. **1.** The pace and synchrony of ventricular depolarization. **2.** An escape rhythm that arises in the ventricles, typically with wide QRS complexes and a rate of 30–40 beats per minute.

rhythmicity (rĭth-mĭs'ĭ-tē) The condition of being rhythmic.

rhythm method of birth control A method preventing pregnancy that uses abstinence from sexual relations around the time of ovulation. SEE: *contraception.*

rhytide (rī'tĭd) Wrinkle.

rhytidectomy (rĭt"ĭ-dĕk'tō-mē) [Gr. *rhytis,* wrinkle, + *ektome,* excision] The excision of wrinkles by plastic surgery; often called a "face-lift." SYN: *rhitidectomy.*

rhytidoplasty (rĭt'ĭ-dō-plăs"tē) [" + *plassein,* to form] The elimination of facial wrinkles by plastic surgery.

rhytidosis (rĭt"ĭ-dō'sĭs) [" + *osis,* condition] Wrinkling of the cornea, which occurs when tension in the eyeball is greatly diminished, particularly after the escape of aqueous or vitreous humor; usually a sign of impending death. SYN: *rhitidosis.*

RIA *radioimmunoassay.*

rib (rĭb) [AS. *ribb*] One of a series of 12 pairs of narrow, curved bones extending laterally and anteriorly from the sides of the thoracic vertebrae and forming a part of the skeletal thorax. With the exception of the floating ribs, they are connected to the sternum by costal cartilages. SEE: illus.

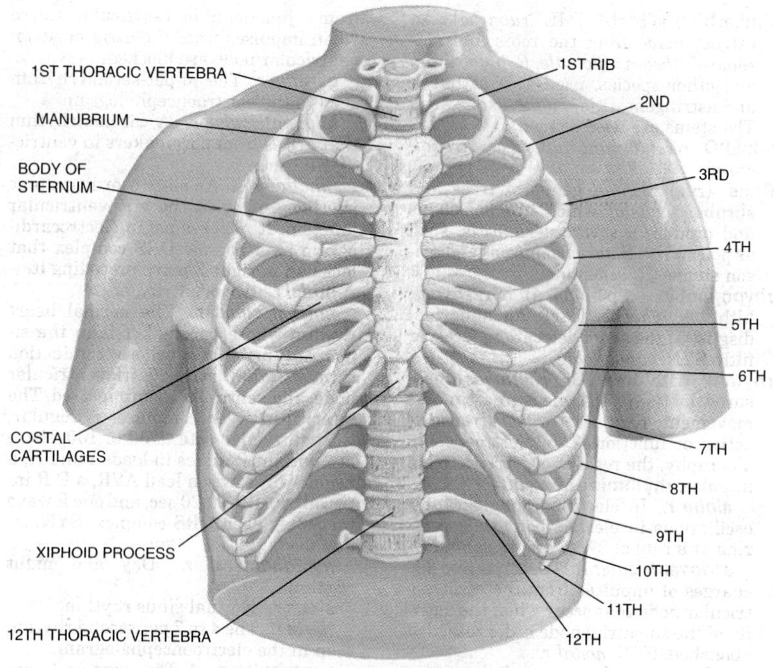

RIB CAGE
Anterior view

abdominal r. False r.

asternal r. False r.

bicipital r. An irregular condition resulting from the fusion of two ribs, usually involving the first rib.

cervical r. A supernumerary rib sometimes developing in connection with a cervical vertebra, usually the lowest.

false r. One of the lower ribs (8, 9, and 10) that do not join the sternum directly. Their cartilage connects to the cartilage of the seventh rib. The variation in the anatomy of the lower ribs may be considerable (i.e., there may be only two false ribs).

floating r. Ribs 11 and 12 on each side, not attached to the sternum. SYN: *vertebral r.*

lumbar r. A rudimentary rib that develops in relation to a lumbar vertebra.

slipping r. A rib in which the costal cartilage dislocates repeatedly.

spring fracture of r. Outward displacement of the end of a broken rib, seen on x-ray examination of ribs that are broken by compression rather than by direct blows to the chest.

sternal r. True r.

true r. Any of the upper seven ribs on each side, which join the sternum by separate cartilages. SYN: *sternal r.; vertebrosternal r.*

vertebral r. Floating r.

vertebrocostal r. Any of the three false ribs on each side.

vertebrosternal r. True r.

ribavirin (rī″bă-vī-rĕn) An antiviral agent used to treat respiratory syncytial viral infection and hepatitis C.

ribbon (rĭb′ŭn) A long, thin, band-shaped structure.

riboflavin (rī″bō-flā′vĭn) $C_{17}H_{20}N_4O_6$; a water-soluble vitamin of the B complex group. It is an orange-yellow crystalline powder. Symptoms of riboflavin deficiency are photophobia, cheilosis, glossitis, and seborrheic dermatitis, esp. of the face and scalp. SYN: *vitamin B_2.*

FUNCTION: Riboflavin is a constituent of certain flavoproteins that function as coenzymes in cellular oxidation. It is essential for tissue repair.

SOURCES: Riboflavin is found in milk and milk products, leafy green vegetables, liver, beef, fish, and dry yeast. It is also synthesized by bacteria in the body.

DAILY REQUIREMENT: Adults require 0.6 mg/1000 kcal of food intake. Infants, children, and pregnant and lactating women require increased amounts.

ribonuclease (rī″bō-nū′klē-ās) ABBR: RNase. An enzyme that catalyzes the depolymerization of ribonucleic acid

(RNA) with formation of mononucleotides.

ribonucleoprotein (rī″bō-nū″klē-ō-prō′tē-ĭn) A compound containing both protein and ribonucleic acid.

ribonucleotide (rī″bō-nū′klē-ō-tīd) A nucleotide in which the sugar ribose is combined with the purine or pyrimidine base.

ribose (rī′bōs) $C_5H_{10}O_5$, a pentose sugar present in ribonucleic acids, riboflavin, and some nucleotides.

ribosome (rī′bō-sōm) A cell organelle made of ribosomal RNA and protein. Ribosomes may exist singly, in clusters called polyribosomes, or on the surface of rough endoplasmic reticulum. In protein synthesis, they are the site of messenger RNA attachment and amino acid assembly in the sequence ordered by the genetic code carried by mRNA.

ribosyl (rī′bō-sĭl) The compound glycosyl, $C_5H_9O_4$, formed from ribose.

ribozyme (rī′bō-zīm) A ribonucleic acid molecule with catalytic properties, used to damage nucleic acid sequences in diseased cells and prevent their gene products from being expressed.

RICE Acronym for *r*est, *i*ce, *c*ompression, and *e*levation, the elements of management of soft tissue stress or trauma, esp. sports injuries.

rice, polished Rice that has been milled to produce the commercially available white product commonly consumed in Western countries. This treatment removes most of the protein and vitamin B_1, thiamine, from the grain. When polished rice is the major source of calories in the diet, it is associated with the deficiency disease beriberi.

rice water, boiled The water remaining after rice has been cooked in it and removed; formerly used as an oral rehydration agent, esp. for children with diarrhea. The use of oral rehydration solutions, however, has provided a better supply of fluids and electrolytes and has replaced the practice of using boiled rice water for rehydration. SEE: *oral rehydration therapy.*

ricin (rī′sĭn) A white, amorphous, highly toxic protein present in the seed of the castor bean, *Ricinus communis.*

ricinine (rĭs′ĭn-ēn, -īn) A poisonous alkaloid present in the leaves and seeds of the castor bean plant, *Ricinus communis.*

ricinoleic acid $C_{19}H_{34}O_3$, 12-hydroxy-9-octadecenoic acid; an unsaturated hydroxy acid comprising about 80% of fatty acids in the glycerides of castor oil. It has a strong laxative action.

rickets (rĭk′ĕts) A disease of bone formation in children, most commonly the result of vitamin D deficiency, marked by inadequate mineralization of developing cartilage and newly formed bone, causing abnormalities in the shape, structure, and strength of the skeleton. This condition may be prevented by exposure to ultraviolet light (sunlight or artificial light) and administration of vitamin D in quantities that provide 400 I.U. of vitamin D activity per day. Vitamin D deficiency disease in adults is known as osteomalacia. SYN: *rachitis* (2). SEE: *osteomalacia; Nursing Diagnoses Appendix.*

ETIOLOGY: Rickets has many causes, including diseases that affect vitamin D or phosphorus intake, absorption, and metabolism; renal tubular disorders; and diseases in which the child is chronically acidotic, among others.

FINDINGS: Affected children are often lethargic, and may have flaccid musculature and decreased muscular strength. On physical examination, multiple bony abnormalities are present, including frontal bossing, bowing of the long bones, flattening of the sides of the thoracic cavity, kyphosis, scoliosis, or lordosis.

TREATMENT: Treatment and prognosis depend on the correction of the underlying cause. Supplemental vitamin D therapy is appropriate for some patients.

CAUTION: Excessive use of vitamin D (in infants, more than 20,000 I.U. daily; in adults, more than 100,000 I.U. daily) should be avoided because of the risk of hypervitaminosis D.

adult r. Osteomalacia.

late r. Rickets that has its onset in older children.

renal r. A disturbance in epiphyseal growth during childhood due to severe chronic renal insufficiency resulting in persistent acidosis. Dwarfism and failure of gonadal development result. The prognosis is poor.

TREATMENT: Renal rickets is treated with a diet low in meat, milk, cheese, and egg yolk. Calcium lactate or calcium gluconate is given in large doses.

vitamin D refractory r. A rare form of rickets that is not caused by vitamin D deficiency and is thus not responsive to vitamin D treatment. It is caused by a defect in renal tubular function that results in excessive loss of phosphorus.

Rickettsia (rĭ-kĕt′sē-ă) [Howard T. Ricketts, U.S. pathologist, 1871–1910] A genus of bacteria of the family Rickettsiaceae, order Rickettsiales. They are obligate intracellular parasites (must be in living cells to reproduce) and are the causative agents of many diseases. Their vectors are arthropods such as fleas, ticks, mites, and lice. SEE: *rickettsial disease; rickettsialpox; rickettsiosis; tick-borne rickettsiosis.*

R. akari The causative agent of rickettsialpox. The animal reservoir is the house mouse and the vector is a mite.

R. prowazekii The causative agent of epidemic typhus, spread by the human body louse. It was once thought to be a strictly human pathogen. Flying squirrels may be animal reservoirs; and humans acquire infection from their lice or fleas.

R. rickettsii The causative agent of Rocky Mountain spotted fever. The animal reservoirs are rodents and dogs and the vectors are ticks of several genera.

R. typhi The agent that causes flea-borne murine (endemic) typhus.

rickettsia (rĭ-kĕt′sē-ă) *pl.* **rickettsiae** Term applied to any of the bacteria belonging to the genus *Rickettsia*.

rickettsial disease A disease caused by an organism of the genus *Rickettsia*. The most common types are the spotted-fever group (Rocky Mountain spotted fever and rickettsialpox), epidemic typhus, endemic typhus, Brill's disease, Q fever, scrub typhus, and trench fever.

rickettsialpox (rĭ-kĕt′sē-ăl-pŏks″) An acute, febrile, self-limited disease caused by *Rickettsia akari*. It is transmitted from the house mouse to humans by a small colorless mite, *Allodermanyssus sanguineus*.

rickettsicidal (rĭ-kĕt″sĭ-sī′dăl) Lethal to rickettsiae.

rickettsiosis (rĭ-kĕt″sē-ō′sĭs) Infection with rickettsiae.

rickettsiostatic (rĭ-kĕt″sē-ō-stăt′ĭk) Preventing or slowing the growth of rickettsiae.

ridge (rĭj) [ME. *rigge*] An elongated projecting structure or crest.

alveolar r. The bony process of the maxilla or mandible that contains the alveoli or tooth sockets; the alveolar process without teeth present.

carotid r. The sharp ridge between the carotid canal and the jugular fossa.

dental r. Any elevation on the crown of a tooth.

dermal r. One of the ridges on the surface of the fingers that make up the fingerprints; also called *crista cutis*.

epicondylic r. One of two ridges for muscular attachments on the humerus.

external oblique r. An anatomical landmark that is a continuation of the anterior border of the mandibular ramus and extends obliquely to the region of the first molar. It serves as an attachment of the buccinator muscle and appears superior to the mylohyoid ridge on a dental radiograph.

gastrocnemial r. A ridge on the posterior femoral surface for attachment of the gastrocnemius muscle.

genital r. A ridge that develops on the ventromedial surface of the urogenital ridge and gives rise to the gonads.

gluteal r. A ridge extending obliquely downward from the greater trochanter of the femur for attachment of the gluteus maximus muscle.

interosseous r. A ridge on the fibula for attachment of the interosseous membrane.

interureteric r. A ridge between the openings of the ureters in the bladder.

mammary r. In mammal embryos, a ridge extending from the axilla to the groin. The breasts arise from this ridge. In humans, only one breast normally remains on each side. SYN: *milk line*.

mesonephric r. A ridge that develops on the lateral surface of the urogenital ridge and gives rise to the mesonephros. SYN: *wolffian r.*

mylohyoid r. The line of attachment on the medial aspect of the body of the mandible for the mylohyoid muscle, which forms the floor of the mouth.

pronator r. An oblique ridge on the anterior surface of the ulna for attachment of the pronator quadratus.

pterygoid r. A ridge at the angle of junction of the temporal and infratemporal surfaces of the greater wing of the sphenoid bone.

superciliary r. A curved ridge of the frontal bone over the supraorbital arch.

supracondylar r. One of two ridges (lateral and medial) on the distal end of the humerus, extending upward from the lateral to the medial epicondyles.

tentorial r. A ridge on the upper inner surface of the cranium to which the tentorium is attached.

trapezoid r. An oblique ridge on the upper surface of the clavicle for attachment of the trapezoid ligament.

urogenital r. A ridge on the dorsal wall of the coelom that gives rise to the genital and mesonephric ridges. SYN: *urogenital fold*. SEE: *genital r.; mesonephric r.*

wolffian r. Mesonephric r.

ridgel (rĭj′ĕl) A male animal, esp. a horse, with only one testicle, or only one descended testicle.

Riedel's lobe (rē′dĕlz) [Bernhard M. C. L. Riedel, Ger. surgeon, 1846–1916] A tongue-shaped process of the liver that often protrudes over the gallbladder in cases of chronic cholecystitis.

Rieder cell A white blood cell with radially segmented nucleus, found in some T cells in patients with lymphoproliferative disorders.

rifampin (rĭf′ăm-pĭn) An antibiotic synthesized from rifamycin B, which in turn is produced by fermentation of *Streptomyces mediterranei*. It is used primarily to treat infections caused by *Mycobacterium tuberculosis*. This agent also has good activity against *Staphylococcus aureus* but must be used in combination with other drugs when treating this microorganism because of the rapid emergence of resistance.

rifamycin (rĭf″ă-mī′sĭn) An antibiotic produced by certain strains of *Streptomyces mediterranei.*

Riga-Fede's disease (rē′gă fā′dāz) [Antonio Riga, It. physician, 1832–1919; Francesco Fede, It. physician, 1832–1913] Ulceration of the frenum of the tongue with membrane formation. It occurs after abrasion by the lower central incisors.

Riggs' disease [John M. Riggs, U.S. dentist, 1810–1885] Periodontitis.

right (rīt) [AS. *riht*] ABBR: R; rt. **1.** Pert. to the dextral side of the body (the side away from the heart), which in most persons is the stronger or preferred. SYN: *dexter*. **2.** Legal authority to supervise and control one's own actions or the actions of others.

right-handedness The condition of greater adeptness in using the right hand. This characteristic is found in about 93% of the population. SYN: *dextrality*. SEE: *sinistrality*.

right to die The freedom to choose one's own end-of-life care by specifying, for example, whether one would permit or want life-prolonging treatments (e.g., intubation and mechanical ventilation); intravenous or enteral feedings; antibiotics (if infected); narcotic analgesics (if in pain); or medications to hasten death (e.g., in assisted suicide or euthanasia). The moral, ethical, or legal authority to make decisions about many of these issues are topics of considerable controversy and confusion. Contemporary health care techniques often permit the prolongation of a patient's life, when, in the natural course of biological events, that life might have ended. The ability to postpone death, and the difficulty that health care providers have in predicting when death will occur, has generated many questions about the meaning of care and well-being at the margins of existence. Who should make decisions for patients when they cannot speak for themselves? How should one's wishes be expressed or codified? Who should carry them out if the patient cannot act on his or her own? When must a person's stated wishes be followed precisely, and when should they be factored in with the wishes of loved ones or of those acting on behalf of the patient? Should they ever be ignored or overruled? When does the aid given to a dying person compromise the moral or professional values of others or jeopardize the legal standing of the patient's caregiver? Many of these challenging questions remain unresolved. SEE: *advance directive; assisted suicide; care, end-of-life; euthanasia; suicide*.

right-to-know law A law that dictates that employers must inform their employees of the health effects and chemical hazards of the toxic substances used in each workplace. The employer must provide information concerning the generic and chemical names of the substances used; the level at which the exposure is hazardous; the effects of exposure at hazardous levels; the symptoms of such effects; the potential for flammability, explosion, and reactivity of the substances; the appropriate emergency treatment; proper conditions for safe use and exposure to the substances; and procedures for cleanup of leaks and spills. The law provides that an employee may refuse to work with a toxic substance until he or she has received information concerning its potential for hazard. SEE: *hazardous material; health hazard; material safety data sheet; permissible exposure limits; toxic substance*.

rigid (rĭ′jĭd) [L. *rigidus*] Stiff, hard, unyielding.

rigidity (rĭ-jĭd′ĭ-tē) **1.** Tenseness; immovability; stiffness; inability to bend or be bent. **2.** In psychiatry, an excessive resistance to change.

cadaveric r. Rigor mortis.

cerebellar r. Stiffness of the body and extremities resulting from a lesion of the middle lobe of the cerebellum.

clasp-knife r. A condition in which passive flexion of the joint causes increased resistance of the extensors. This gives way abruptly if the pressure to produce flexion is continued.

cogwheel r. The condition that occurs when tremor coexists with rigidity as in Parkinson's syndrome. In this condition, manually manipulated body parts may take on the feel of a cogwheel. This can occur also as an extrapyramidal side effect of antipsychotic drug therapy.

decerebrate r. Sustained contraction of the extensor muscles of the limbs resulting from a lesion in the brainstem between the superior colliculi and the vestibular nuclei.

lead-pipe r. The generalized muscular rigidity seen in parkinsonism.

nuchal r. Inflexibility of the neck movement, esp. forward flexion of the neck. It is a sign of meningeal irritation.

rigor (rĭg′or) [L. *rigor,* stiffness] **1.** A sudden paroxysmal shaking chill occurring during a febrile illness. Onset of rigors often corresponds to bacteremia. **2.** A state of hardness and stiffness, as in a muscle.

r. mortis The stiffness that occurs in dead bodies. SYN: *cadaveric rigidity*. SEE: *Nysten's law*.

rim An edge or border.

bite r. Occlusion r.

occlusion r. The biting surfaces built on denture bases to make maxillomandibular relation records and to arrange teeth. SYN: *bite r.*

rima (rī′mă) *pl.* **rimae** [L., a slit] A slit, fissure, or crack.

r. cornealis A groove in the sclera holding edge of the cornea.

r. glottidis An elongated slit between the vocal folds. SYN: *r. vocalis*.

r. oris The aperture of the mouth.

r. palpebrarum The slit between the eyelids.

r. pudendi The space between the labia majora, into which the urethra and vagina open. SYN: *vestibule of vagina*.

r. respiratoria The space behind the arytenoid cartilages.

r. vestibuli The space between the false vocal cords.

r. vocalis R. glottidis.

rimantadine hydrochloride An antiviral drug given orally to treat influenza A.

rimose (rī′mōs, rī-mōs′) [L. *rimosus*] Fissured or marked by cracks.

rimula (rĭm′ū-lă) *pl.* **rimulae** [L.] A minute fissure or slit, esp. of the spinal cord or brain.

rind (rīnd) [AS.] A thick or firm outer coating of an organ, plant, or animal.

ring (rĭng) [AS. *hring*] **1.** Any round area, organ, or band around a circular opening. SEE: *annulus*. **2.** In chemistry, a collection of atoms chemically bound in a circle.

abdominal r. SEE: *abdominal ring*.

abdominal inguinal r. The internal opening of the inguinal canal. SEE: *abdominal ring*.

Albl's r. A curved thin shadow seen on roentgenogram of an intracranial aneurysm.

Bandl's r. SEE: *Bandl's ring*.

benzene r. The closed ring of six carbon atoms.

Cannon's r. A contracted band of muscles in the transverse colon near the hepatic flexure.

ciliary r. Orbiculus ciliaris.

conjunctival r. A narrow ring at the junction of the edge of the cornea with the conjunctiva; also called *anulus conjunctiva*.

constriction r. A stricture of the body of the uterus; a circular area of the uterus that contracts around a part of the fetus.

deep inguinal r. The opening of the inguinal canal deep inside the abdominal wall.

femoral r. The superior aperture of the femoral canal.

lymphoid r. A ringlike arrangement of lymphoid tonsillar tissue around the oronasal region of the pharynx. It consists of the palatine, pharyngeal, and lingual tonsils and provides protection against invading bacteria, viruses, and other foreign antigens. SYN: *Waldeyer's ring*.

pathologic retraction r. During delivery, a prolonged contraction of the ring formed by the junction of the body and isthmus of the uterus. SYN: *Bandl's r.*

physiologic retraction r. A normal contraction of the ring formed by the junction of the body and isthmus of the uterus.

Schatzki r. SEE: *Schatzki ring*.

subcutaneous inguinal r. Superficial inguinal ring.

superficial inguinal r. The opening of the superficial end of the inguinal canal. SYN: *subcutaneous inguinal r.* SEE: *abdominal ring*.

tympanic r. A band of bone formed by three parts (squamous, petromastoid, and tympanic) that develops into the tympanic plate.

umbilical r. The opening in the linea alba of the embryo through which the umbilical vessels pass.

vascular r. An anomalous ring of vascular structures around the trachea and esophagus.

Waldeyer's r. Lymphoid r.

ring, removal from swollen finger A technique for the removal of a ring from an injured or swollen finger. One method is described here: One end of a length of string is passed under the ring. The ring is pushed as far from the swollen area toward the hand as possible; the string is wrapped on the side of the swollen area around the finger for about a dozen turns. The end of the string that extends under the ring is grasped. While being held firmly, the string is unwound from the hand side of the ring. This moves the ring toward the free end of the finger. This procedure should be continued until the ring is free. If this technique fails, the ring must be cut from the finger.

Ringer, Sydney (rĭng′ĕr) British physiologist, 1835–1910.

lactated R.'s solution A crystalloid electrolyte sterile solution of specified amounts of calcium chloride, potassium chloride, sodium chloride, and sodium lactate in water for injection. It is used intravenously to replace electrolytes.

R.'s solution A physiologic solution of distilled water containing 8.6 g sodium chloride, 0.3 g potassium chloride, and 0.33 g calcium chloride per liter; for topical (Ringer's irrigation) or intravenous use.

ringworm (rĭng′wŭrm) The popular term for any contagious skin infection caused by fungi of the genera *Microsporum* or *Trichophyton*. The hallmark of these conditions is a well-defined red rash, with an elevated, wavy, or worm-shaped border. Ringworm of the scalp is called tinea capitis; of the body, tinea corporis; of the groin, tinea cruris; of the hand, tinea manus; of the beard, tinea barbae; of the nails, tinea unguium; and of the feet, tinea pedis or athlete's foot. SEE: illus.; *Nursing Diagnoses Appendix*.

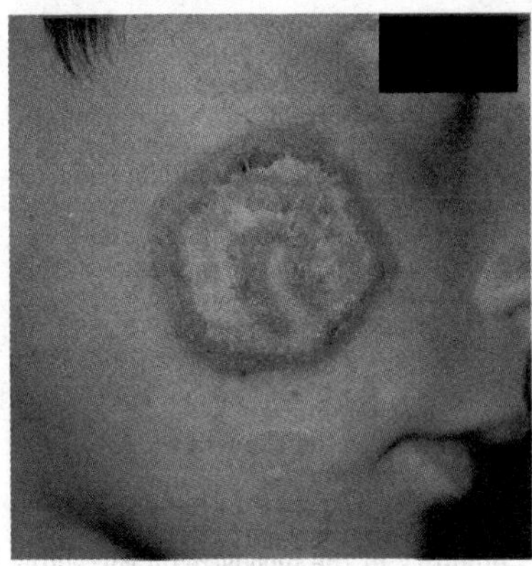

RING WORM

Rinne test (rĭn′nē) [Heinrich Adolf Rinne, Ger. otologist, 1819–1868] The use of a tuning fork to compare bone conduction hearing with air conduction. The vibrating fork is held by its stem on the mastoid process of the ear until the patient no longer hears it. Then it is held close to the external auditory meatus. If the subject still hears the vibrations, air conduction exceeds bone conduction (this is the normal finding). SEE: *Weber test*.

rinse **1.** To wash lightly. **2.** A solution used for irrigation or bathing.

mouth r. A flavored, sometimes mildly antiseptic solution which may improve breath odor and reduce bacteria within the oral cavity.

sodium fluoride r. A 0.05% aqueous solution of sodium fluoride also containing coloring and flavoring agents, used as a mouth rinse to help prevent dental caries.

Riolan (rē″ō-lănz′) Jean, French anatomist, 1577–1657.

R.'s arch The arch formed by the mesentery of the transverse colon.

R.'s bouquet The two ligaments and three muscles attached to the styloid process of the temporal bone.

R.'s muscle The ciliary portion of the orbicularis oculi.

ripa (rī′pă) [L., bank] Any reflection line of the ependyma of the brain from the ventricular wall to the choroid plexus.

Ripault's sign (rē-pōz′) [Louis H. A. Ripault, Fr. physician, 1807–1856] A change in the shape of the pupil produced by unilateral (external) pressure on the eyeball.

ripening **1.** Softening, effacement, and dilation before labor. SEE: *Bishop's score; prostaglandin.* **2.** Maturation of a cataract.

risk [origin obscure] The probability that a loss or something dangerous or harmful will occur.

acceptable r. In toxicology and public health, the concept that a particular exposure or environmental level of an agent (chemical or other) poses a tolerable level of harm to individuals or populations.

r. assessment Quantitation of the risks to which people are exposed by compilation of morbidity and mortality data over specified periods of time.

attributable r. The portion of the risk of developing a condition that can be traced to each known risk factor (e.g., persons exposed to asbestos have a certain risk of developing lung cancer, and if they also smoke tobacco, they are also at risk from that factor). These risks may be estimated from cohort studies.

material r. A significant potential for harm that a reasonable person would want to consider when making a decision about undergoing a medical or surgical treatment.

relative r. In epidemiological studies, a method of measuring the relative amount of disease occurring in different populations; the ratio of incidence rate in the exposed group to that in the unexposed group. SEE: *ratio, odds*.

risk-benefit analysis Examination of the potential positive and negative results of undertaking a specific therapeutic course of action. An example would be the risk of dying from a surgical procedure versus the outcome if the procedure were successful and the course of the disease if the procedure were not done.

risk factor An environmental, chemical, psychological, physiological, or genetic element that predisposes an individual to the development of a disease. For example, risk factors for coronary artery disease include hypertension, high circulating blood lipids and cholesterol, obesity, cigarette smoking, diabetes mellitus, physical inactivity, and a family history of atherosclerosis. SEE: *ratio, odds; risk, relative*.

risk management A subspecialty in health care that addresses the prevention and containment of liability by careful and objective investigation and documentation of critical or unusual patient care incidents. In psychiatry, for example, risk management may be concerned with preventing suicide and patient-related violence and its associated liability.

risk-taker An individual who willfully exposes himself or herself to activities that others regard as hazardous.

risorius (rī-sŏ′rē-ŭs) [L., laughing] The muscular fibrous band arising over the masseter muscle and inserted into the tissues at the corner of the mouth.

RIST *radioimmunosorbent test.*

ristocetin (rĭs″tō-sē′tĭn) An antibiotic obtained from cultures of *Nocardia lurida*.

risus (rī'sŭs) [L.] Laughter; a laugh.

r. sardonicus A peculiar grin, as seen in tetanus, caused by acute facial spasm.

Ritgen's maneuver [A. M. F. von Ritgen, German obstetrician, 1787–1867] A manual method of controlling the delivery of the fetal head. The nondominant hand exerts pressure against the fetal chin through the perineum. At the same time, the dominant hand exerts pressure against the fetal occiput. The maneuver should be performed slowly and between contractions to avoid perineal lacerations.

Ritter's disease (rĭt'ĕrz) [Gottfried Ritter von Rittershain, Ger. physician, 1820–1883] A generalized form of impetigo of the newborn.

ritual (rĭch'ū-ăl) **1.** A routine that the individual feels is essential and must be carried out. **2.** In psychiatry, any activity that is performed compulsively in an attempt to relieve anxiety.

ritualistic surgery Surgical procedures without scientific justification, performed in primitive societies without the purpose of treating or preventing disease. Included are alterations of the skin, ears, lips, teeth, genitalia, and head. In some cases, even in nonprimitive societies, surgical procedures without rational justification are considered ritualistic. SEE: *circumcision*.

rivalry (rī'văl-rē) Competition between two or more individuals, groups, or systems seeking to attain the same goal.

binocular r. The continuous alternation in the conscious perception of visual stimuli to the two eyes.

retinal r. Binocular r.

sibling r. The competition between children for attention and affection from others, esp. their parents.

rivalry strife Alternate sensations of color and shape when the fields of vision of the two eyes cannot combine in one visual image.

Rivinus, August Quirinus (rē-vē'nŭs) German anatomist, 1652–1723.

R.'s canal Any duct of the sublingual glands.

R.'s gland A sublingual gland.

R.'s incisure The tympanic notch in the upper part of the tympanic portion of the temporal bone. It extends from the lesser to the greater tympanic spines and is occupied by the pars flaccida of the tympanic membrane. SYN: *notch of Rivinus*.

R.'s ligament The small portion of the tympanic membrane in Rivinus' incisure. SYN: *Shrapnell's membrane*.

rivus lacrimalis (rī'vŭs) [L. *rivus,* little stream, + *lacrima,* tear] The pathway under the eyelids through which tears travel from their source in the lacrimal glands to the punctum lacrimale.

riziform (rĭz'ĭ-form) [Fr. *riz,* rice, + L. *forma,* form] Resembling rice grains.

R.L.E. *right lower extremity.*

RLF *retrolental fibroplasia.*

R.L.L. *right lower lobe* of the lung.

RLQ *right lower quadrant* (of abdomen).

R.M.A. *registered medical assistant; right mentoanterior presentation* (of the fetal face).

RML *right middle lobe* (of the lung).

R.M.P. *right mentoposterior presentation* (of the fetal face).

RMS *rhabdomyosarcoma.*

R.M.T. *right mentotransverse* (fetal position).

R.N. *registered nurse.*

Rn Symbol for the element radon.

RNA *ribonucleic acid.*

HIV R. The genetic material of the human immunodeficiency virus. Its quantity in the bloodstream correlates with the severity and prognosis of the acquired immunodeficiency syndrome. Drug regimens for AIDS, esp. those that use a combination of protease inhibitors and reverse transcriptase inhibitors, aim to decrease the amount of HIV RNA in the blood to undetectable levels.

RNase *ribonuclease.*

RNC *registered nurse certified.*

R.O.A. *right occipitoanterior* (fetal position).

Robert's pelvis (rō'bārts) [Heinrich L. F. Robert, Ger. gynecologist, 1814–1874] A transverse contraction of the pelvis caused by osteoarthritis of the sacroiliac joints.

Robertson's pupil Argyll Robertson pupil.

Rochalimaea Former name for the genus *Bartonella.*

R. quintana SEE: *Bartonella quintana.*

Rochelle salt (rō-shĕl') Potassium sodium tartrate, a colorless, transparent powder having a cooling and saline taste and formerly used as a saline cathartic.

rocker board A board with rockers or a partial sphere on the undersurface so that a rocking motion occurs when a person stands on it. It is used for proprioception and balance training, esp. in lower-extremity injuries and central nervous system disturbances. Also called *balance board; wobble board.*

rocker knife An assistive device for persons with limited upper-extremity function. It allows one-handed stabilization and cutting of food.

rocking A technique in neurodevelopmental rehabilitation designed to increase muscle tone in hypotonic patients through vestibular stimulation.

Rocky Mountain spotted fever An infectious disease caused by the bacterium *Rickettsia ricketsii* and transmitted by the wood tick *Dermacentor andersoni* or *D. variabilis*. Originally thought to exist only in the western U.S., it can occur anywhere that the tick vector is present. SEE: illus.

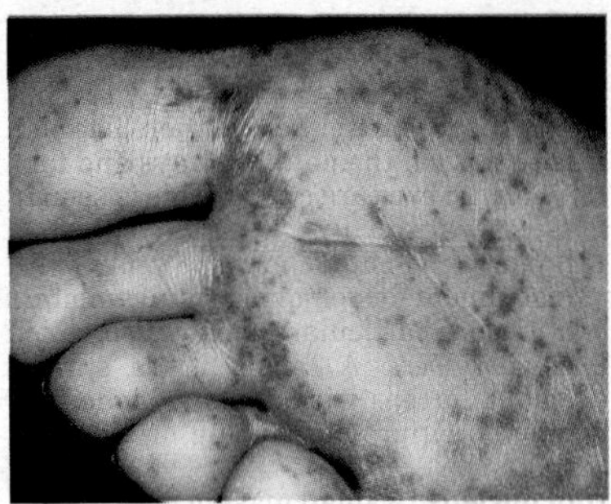

ROCKY MOUNTAIN SPOTTED FEVER

The organism causes fever, headache, myalgia, and a characteristic vasculitic rash. The rash appears several days after the other symptoms, first erupting on the wrists and ankles, then on the palms and soles. It is nonpruritic and macular and spreads to the legs, arms, trunk, and face. Disseminated intravascular coagulation or pneumonia may be serious complications. Tetracyclines are the drug of choice for treating this disease, but their use in pregnant women is not advised. Chloramphenicol may be substituted.

Persons living in areas with wood ticks should wear clothing that covers much of their bodies, including the neck, to prevent ticks carrying the disease from attaching to the skin. People who live in or travel to areas where ticks flourish should examine their scalps, skin, and clothing daily. Ticks should be grasped close to the mouthparts (not on the tick's body), as close to their point of attachment to their human host as possible. Pets should be examined regularly for ticks.

rod (rŏd) [AS. *rodd,* club] **1.** A slender, straight bar. **2.** One of the slender, long sensory bodies in the retina, which respond to faint light. **3.** A bacterium shaped like a rod.

Corti's r. Pillar cell.

enamel r. One of the minute calcium-rich rods or prisms laid down by ameloblasts and forming tooth enamel.

retinal r. A receptor in the retina that responds to dim light. SEE: *retina* for illus.

rodent Any mammal of the Rodentia order, such as mice, rats, and squirrels.

rodenticide (rō-dĕn′tĭ-sīd) [L. *rodens,* gnawing, + *caedere,* to kill] An agent that kills rodents.

rods and cones The photoreceptor cells of the retina. They are between the pigment epithelium and the bipolar layer of neurons. The rods contain rhodopsin, which is stimulated by dim light; the cones contain one of three other photopigments, which are stimulated by various wavelengths of visible light (colors). SEE: *cone (2); night vision; rod (2).*

Roentgen, Wilhelm Konrad (rĕnt′gĕn) German physicist, 1845–1923, who discovered roentgen rays (x-rays) in 1895. He won the Nobel Prize in physics in 1901.

roentgen (rĕnt′gĕn) ABBR: R. A unit for describing the exposure dose of x-rays or gamma rays. One unit can liberate enough electrons and positrons to produce emissions of either charge of one electrostatic unit of electricity per 0.001293 g of air (the weight of 1 cm^3 of dry air at 0°C and at 760 mm Hg).

roentgenocinematography (rĕnt″gĕn-ō-sĭn″ĕ-mă-tŏg′ră-fē) [″ + Gr. *kinema,* motion, + *graphein,* to write] Moving picture photography of x-ray studies.

roentgenogram (rĕnt-gĕn′ō-grăm, rĕnt′gĕn-ō-grăm″) Radiograph.

roentgenography (rĕnt″gĕn-ŏg′ră-fē) Radiography.

body section r. Tomography.

mucosal relief r. An x-ray examination of the intestinal mucosa after ingested barium has been removed and air under slight pressure has been injected. This leaves a light coat of barium on the mucosa and permits x-ray pictures of the fine detail of the mucosa.

serial r. Repeated x-ray pictures taken of an area at defined but arbitrary intervals.

spot-film r. An x-ray picture taken of a small area during fluoroscopy.

roentgenology (rĕnt″gĕn-ŏl′ō-jē) Radiology.

roentgenometer (rĕnt″gĕ-nŏm′ĕ-tĕr) Radiometer.

roentgenotherapy, roentgentherapy (rĕnt″gĕn-ō-thĕr′ăp-ē) Radiotherapy.

roeteln, roetheln (rĕt′ĕln) [Ger.] Rubella.

Roger's disease (rō-zhāz′) [Henri L. Roger, Fr. physician, 1809–1891] Ventricular septal defect.

Rogers, Martha A nursing educator, 1914–1994, who developed the Science of Unitary Human Beings. SEE: *Nursing Theory Appendix.*

Rokitansky's disease (rō″kĭ-tăn′skēz) [Karl Freiherr von Rokitansky, Austrian pathologist, 1804–1878] Fulminant hepatitis.

Rolando's area (rō-lăn′dōz) [Luigi Rolando, It. anatomist, 1773–1831] A motor area in the cerebral cortex, situated in the anterior central convolution in front of Rolando's fissure in each hemisphere.

Rolando's fissure Sulcus centralis.

role (rōl) [O.Fr. *rolle,* roll of paper on which a part is written] The characteristic social behavior of an individual in relationship to the group.

gender r. The characteristic lifestyle and behavior pattern of a person with respect to sexual and social conditions associated with being of a particular sex. Usually this behavior represents how the individual feels about his or her own sexual preference; it may not coincide with the true chromosomal and anatomical sexual differentiation of the person.

sick r. A dependent affect or behavior, or both, associated with physical or mental illness.

role model Someone who serves as an example for others by demonstrating the behavior associated with a particular position or profession.

role performance, altered A change in patterns of behavior and self-expression that do not match the environmental context, norms, and expectations. SEE: *Nursing Diagnoses Appendix.*

role playing The assignment and acting out of a role in a treatment setting to provide individuals an opportunity for people to explore the behaviors and feelings of others, or to see themselves as others see them. It is also used to teach such skills as interviewing, history taking, and doing a physical examination.

Rolfing [Ida P. Rolf, U.S. biochemist, 1897–1979] A therapy designed to realign the body with gravity through fascial manipulation.

roll An usually solid, cylindrical structure.

cotton r. A cylindrical mass of purified and sterilized cotton used as packing or absorbent material in various dental procedures.

ilial r. A sausage-shaped mass in the left iliac fossa. It is due to a collection of feces in or induration of the walls of the sigmoid colon.

scleral r. SEE: *spur, scleral.*

roller (rōl′ĕr) [O.Fr., roll] **1.** A strip of muslin or other cloth rolled up in cylinder form for surgical use. **2.** A roller bandage.

ROM *read-only memory; rupture of membranes.*

R.O.M. *range of motion.*

roman numeral One of the letters used by the ancient Romans for numeration, as distinct from the arabic numerals that we now use. In roman notation, values are changed either by adding one or more symbols to the initial symbol or by subtracting a symbol to the right of it. For example, V is 5, IV is 4, and VI is 6. Hence, because X is 10, IX is 9 and XI is 11. SEE: roman numerals in *Latin and Greek Nomenclature Appendix.*

romanopexy (rō-măn′ō-pĕk″sē) Sigmoidopexy.

romanoscope (rō-măn′ō-skōp) Sigmoidoscope.

rombergism (rŏm′bĕrg-ĭzm) The tendency to fall from a standing position when the eyes are closed and the feet are close together. SEE: *Romberg's sign.*

Romberg's sign (rŏm′bĕrgs) [Moritz Heinrich Romberg, Ger. physician, 1795–1873] The inability to maintain body balance when the eyes are shut and the feet are close together. The sign is positive if the patient sways and falls when the eyes are closed. This is seen in sensory ataxia.

rongeur (rŏn-zhŭr′) [Fr., to gnaw] An instrument for removing small amounts of tissue, particularly bone; also called *bone nippers.* A rongeur is a spring-loaded forceps with a sharp blade that may be either end cutting or side cutting.

roof nucleus A small mass of gray matter in the white matter of the vermis of the cerebellum.

room (rūm) [AS. *rum*] An area or space in a building, partitioned off for occupancy or available for specific procedures.

clean r. A controlled environment facility in which all incoming air passes through a filter capable of removing 99.97% of all particles 0.3 μm and larger. The temperature, pressure, and humidity in the room are controlled. Clean rooms are used in research and in controlling infections, esp. for persons who may not have normally functioning immune systems (e.g., individuals who have been treated with immunosuppressive drugs in preparation for organ transplantation).

In very rare instances a child is born without the ability to develop an immune system. Such children are kept in a clean room while waiting for specific therapy such as bone marrow transplantation.

delivery r. A room to which an obstetrical patient may be taken for childbirth.

dust-free r. A type of room designed to eliminate or reduce circulating particulate matter, including airborne microorganisms. This kind of room is useful for housing burn patients, removing allergens from the air, providing an environment for transplantation surgery, and preparing drugs and solutions for intravenous use.

labor r. A room in which an obstetrical mother may be placed during the first stage of labor.

operating r. A room used and equipped for surgical procedures (e.g., in a hospital, surgicenter, or doctor's office).

recovery r. An area provided with equipment and nurses needed to care for patients who have just come from surgery. Patients remain there until they regain consciousness and are no longer drowsy and stuporous from the effects of the anesthesia.

rooming-in The practice of placing an infant in the same hospital room as the mother, beginning immediately after birth.

root (rūt) [AS. *rot*] **1.** The underground part of a plant. **2.** The proximal end of a nerve. **3.** A portion of an organ implanted in tissues. SYN: *radix*. **4.** The part of the human tooth covered by cementum; designated by location (mesial, distal, buccal, lingual). **5.** A hex or spell, esp. one that relies on herbal rituals to produce or heal disease; sorcery; voodoo. In the coastal regions of the southeastern U.S., esp. among those of Caribbean or African descent, "rootwork" is relied on as a traditional form of healing and hexing.

anterior r. One of the two roots by which a spinal nerve is attached to the spinal cord; contains efferent nerve fibers.

dorsal r. The radix dorsalis or sensory root of each spinal nerve. SYN: *sensory r.*

motor r. The anterior root of a spinal nerve. SYN: *ventral r.*

posterior r. One of the two roots by which a spinal nerve is attached to the spinal cord; contains afferent nerve fibers.

sensory r. Dorsal r.

ventral r. Motor r.

root artery An artery accompanying a nerve root into the spinal cord.

root formation The development of tooth roots by Hertwig's root sheath and the epithelial diaphragm. It involves the formation of root dentin with a covering of cementum essential for the attachment of the tooth to the surrounding bony tissues. Root formation or development continues for months or years after the tooth has erupted into the mouth.

root pick A dental instrument for retrieving root fragments resulting from tooth extraction; also called *apical elevator*.

root planing SEE: *planing* (2).

root resorption of teeth Degeneration of tooth roots caused by endocrine imbalance or excessive pressure of orthodontic appliances. Root resorption may be categorized as internal or external. Internal root resorption, sometimes called internal granuloma, is usually a result of pulpal trauma. Affected teeth demonstrate a radiolucent enlargement within the pulp canal on a dental radiograph. External root resorption has a variety of causes, including eruption pressure, localized infection, and forced orthodontic pressure. Radiographs demonstrate roots that appear to be sawed off or shortened.

ETIOLOGY: Traumatic sources of resorption may include pulpal trauma, eruption pressure, localized infection, previous injury, and forced orthodontic pressure; however, resorption has occurred with no identifiable source of trauma.

SYMPTOMS: Patients may be asymptomatic or they may experience localized sensitivity.

TREATMENT: The treatment includes eliminating the trauma, if possible.

root zone Fasciculus cuneatus.

R.O.P. *right occipitoposterior.* In this fetal presentation, the occiput of the fetus is in relationship to the right sacroiliac joint of the mother.

Rorschach test (ror′shăk) [Hermann Rorschach, Swiss pyschiatrist, 1884–1922] A psychological test consisting of 10 different inkblot designs. The subject is asked to interpret each design individually. The test has been used to reveal personality disturbances.

rosa (rō′ză) [L.] Rose.

rosacea (rō-zā′sē-ă) [L. *rosaceus,* rosy] A chronic eruption, usually localized to the middle of the face (nose, cheeks, forehead, around the eyes, on the chin) in which papules and pustules appear on a flushed or red background. As the condition progresses, small vascular malformations of the skin may appear, and eventually the sebaceous glands of the nose may swell and produce deformities (rhinophyma). The condition is common, esp. in middle-aged persons of Northern European ancestry. Women are affected more often than men. SEE: illus.

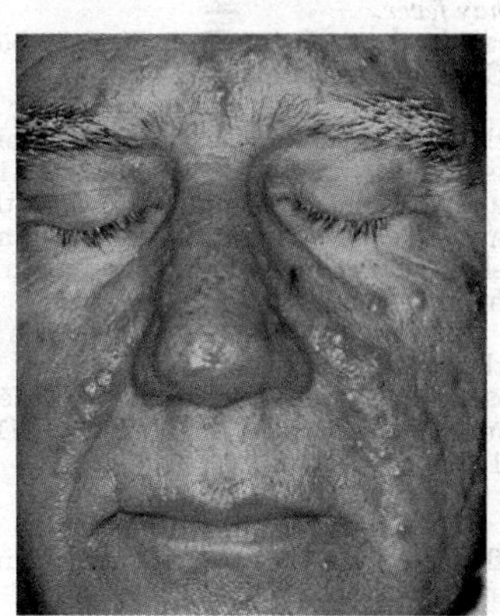

ROSACEA

TREATMENT: Topically applied metronidazole, clindamycin, or erythromycin; oral tetracyclines; and retinoids are all helpful, but the condition is chronic. The disease is managed, not cured.

steroid r. Acne caused by systemic or topical use of corticosteroid drugs. SEE: illus.

rosaniline (rō-zăn′ĭ-lĭn) A basic dye used in preparing other dyes.

rosary (rō′ză-rē) Something that resembles a string of beads.

rachitic r. Palpable areas at the junc-

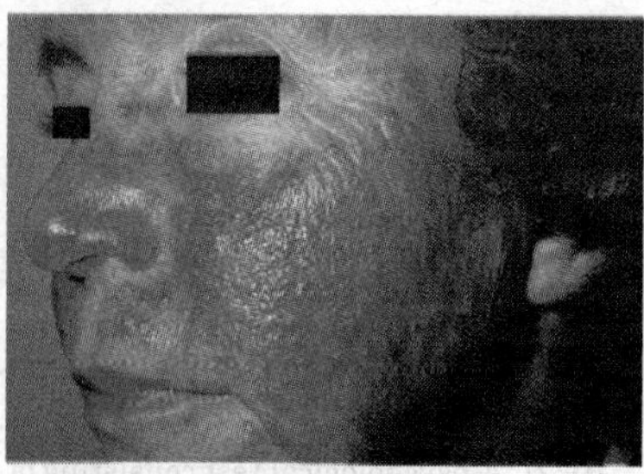

STEROID ROSACEA

ture of the ribs with their cartilages. This is seen in conjunction with rickets. SEE: *rachitic beads*.

Rose's position (rōz) [Frank A. Rose, Brit. surgeon, 1873–1935] A fully extended position in which the patient's head is allowed to hang over the end of the operating room table to prevent aspiration of blood during surgery on the mouth and lips.

rose bengal sodium I 131 A standardized preparation of radioactive iodine and rose bengal used in photoscanning the liver and testing liver function.

rose fever Hay fever of early summer attributed to inhaling rose pollen. SEE: *hay fever*.

Rosenbach, Ottomar (rō'zĕn-bŏk) German physician, 1851–1907.

R.'s sign **1.** A fine, rapid tremor of the closed eyelids, seen in hyperthyroidism. **2.** In functional disorders, the inability to obey a command to close the eyes. **3.** The absence of an abdominal skin reflex in intestinal inflammation or hemiplegia.

R.'s test An obsolete test for bile in the urine.

Rosenmüller, Johann Christian (rō'zĕn-mül"ĕr) German anatomist, 1771–1820.

R.'s body Epoophoron.

R.'s cavity A slitlike depression in the pharyngeal wall behind the opening of the eustachian tube.

roseo- **1.** Combining form meaning *rose-colored*. **2.** A prefix in chemical terms.

roseola (rō-zē'ō-lă, rō"zē-ō'lă) [L. *roseus*, rosy] A skin condition marked by maculae or red spots of varying sizes on the skin; any rose-colored rash.

r. idiopathica A macular eruption not associated with any well-defined symptoms.

r. infantum Exanthem subitum.

roseolous (rō-zē'ō-lŭs) [L. *roseus*, rosy] Resembling or pert. to roseola.

rosette [Fr., small rose] **1.** A structure that has a rose shape, such as an array of phagocytic cells around an object they are consuming. **2.** A spherical group of fine red vacuoles surrounding the centrosome of a monocyte. SEE: illus. **3.** A mature schizont. SYN: *segmenter*.

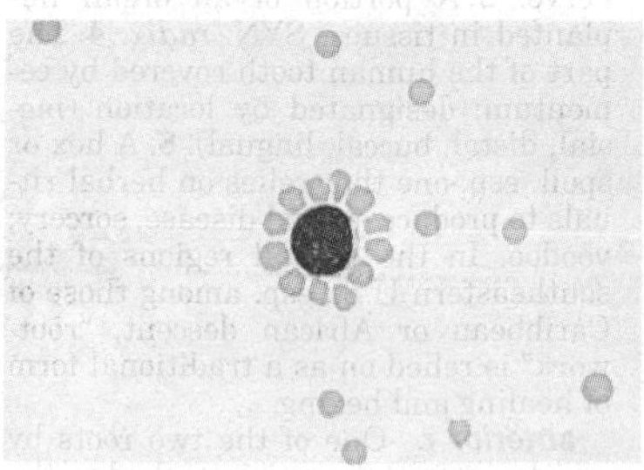

ROSETTE OF RED BLOOD CELLS

rose water A saturated aqueous solution of rose oil, used to impart agreeable odor to lotions.

rose water ointment An emollient used to soften the skin. It contains waxes, almond oil, sodium borate, rose water, rose oil, and purified water.

rosin (rŏz'ĭn) [L. *resina*] A substance distilled from pine trees, sometimes used in adhesives, plastics, or polishes, and occasionally causing allergic contact dermatitis.

Ross' body [Edward Halford Ross, Brit. pathologist, 1875–1928] A copper-colored, round body, showing dark granules, that is found in blood and tissue fluids in syphilis. Sometimes these exhibit ameboid movements.

Rossolimo's reflex (rŏs"ō-lē'mōz) [Gregoriy I. Rossolimo, Russian neurologist, 1860–1928] Plantar flexion of the second to fifth toes in response to percussion of the plantar surface of the toes.

rostellum (rŏs-tĕl'lŭm) *pl.* **rostella** [L., little beak] A fleshy protrusion on the anterior end of the scolex of a tapeworm, bearing one or more rows of spines or hooks.

rostral (rŏs'trăl) [L. *rostralis*] **1.** Resembling a beak. **2.** Toward the front or cephalic end of the body.

rostrate (rŏs'trāt) [L. *rostratus*, beaked] Having a beak or hook formation.

rostriform (rŏs'trĭ-form) [" + *forma*, shape] Shaped like a beak.

rostrum (rŏs'trŭm) *pl.* **rostrums rostra** [L., beak] Any hooked or beaked structure.

rosulate (rŏs'ū-lāt) [L. *rosulatus*, like a rose] Shaped like a rosette.

R.O.T. *right occipito transverse* (fetal position).

rot (rŏt) [ME. *roten*] To decay or decompose.

jungle r. The common term for certain fungal skin diseases that occur in the tropics.

rotameter (rō-tăm'ĕ-tĕr) A device for measuring the flow of a gas or liquid.

rotate (rō-tāt) [L. *rotare*, to turn] To twist or revolve.

rotation (rō-tā′shŭn) [L. *rotatio,* a turning] The process of turning on an axis.

fetal r. Twisting of the fetal head as it follows the curves of the birth canal downward.

optical r. SEE: *optical activity.*

tooth r. The repositioning of a tooth by turning it on its long axis to a more normal occlusal position.

rotator (rō-tā′tor) *pl.* **rotatores** A muscle revolving a part on its axis.

rotaviruses (rō′tă-vī″rŭs-ĕs) [L. *rota,* wheel, + *virus,* poison] A group of viruses that worldwide is the most common cause of dehydrating diarrhea in children. In the U.S. during the peak season (October through May), these viruses account for one third of all hospitalizations for diarrhea in children younger than age 5, and 500 or so rotavirus-associated deaths are reported annually, most in children under age 2. The incubation period of the disease is short (1 to 3 days), and the transmission is via the fecal-oral route. The first effective vaccine was withdrawn when its use in infants was associated with intussusception (a type of bowel obstruction).

röteln, rötheln (rĕt′ĕln) Rubella.

rotenone (rō′tĕn-nōn) A poisonous chemical, $C_{23}H_{22}O_6$, used as an insecticide.

Roth's spots [Moritz Roth, Swiss physician and pathologist, 1839–1914] Small white spots in the retina close to the optic disk, often surrounded by areas of hemorrhage. The condition is caused by a systemic infection, particularly acute infective endocarditis.

Rotor syndrome A benign form of hyperbilirubinemia transmitted as an autosomal recessive trait, in which there is jaundice, but normal aminotransferase levels and normal hepatic synthesis of albumin and clotting factors.

rototome A device for cutting tissue, used in arthroscopic surgery.

rotoxamine (rō-tŏks′ă-mēn) An antihistaminic drug.

Rouget's cells (roo-zhāz′) [Charles M. B. Rouget, Fr. physiologist, 1824–1904] Contractile cells that surround the capillaries, observed in frogs and salamanders.

rough (rŭf) Not smooth.

roughage Food fiber that is largely indigestible. SEE: *cellulose; fiber, dietary.*

rouleau (roo-lō′) *pl.* **rouleaux** [Fr., roll] A group of red blood cells that are stuck together, resembling a roll of coins. SEE: illus.

round (rownd) [O.Fr. *ronde*] **1.** Circular. **2.** Spherical, globular.

rounds, grand A medical education procedure, used esp. in teaching hospitals, in which all aspects of a patient's condition, management, and problems encountered are presented to faculty members, medical students, and health care workers. This provides an opportunity for all concerned to ask questions and provide comments on the patient's diagnosis, care, and clinical program. The patient is usually, but not always, present during the conference. This method of teaching was begun in America by Sir William Osler at Johns Hopkins Hospital, Baltimore, Maryland.

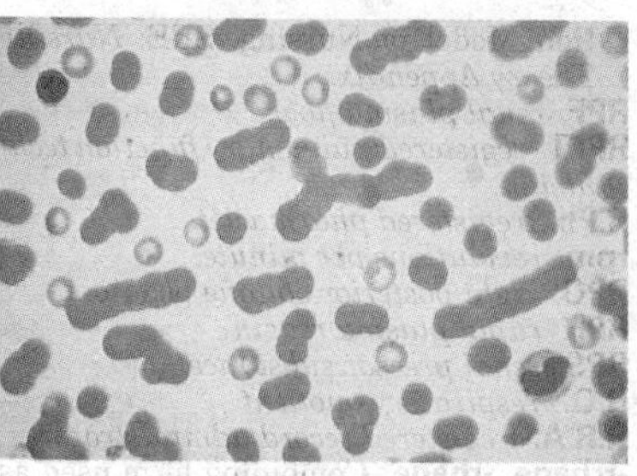

ROULEAUX FORMATION

roundworm Any member of the phylum Nemathelminthes (Aschelminthes), esp. one belonging to the class Nematoda. SEE: *threadworm.*

Roux-en-Y An anastomosis of the distal divided end of the small bowel to another organ such as the stomach, pancreas, or esophagus. The proximal end is anastomosed to the small bowel below the anastomosis.

Roven's IMDC [Milton D. Roven, contemporary U.S. podiatrist] A new procedure for *i*ntramedullary *m*etatarsal *d*ecompression performed through a small dorsal incision. It is less traumatic than previous procedures, allowing immediate ambulation and minimal postoperative pain and edema.

Rovsing's sign (rŏv′zĭngz) [Niels Thorkild Rovsing, Danish surgeon, 1862-1927] Pain referred to McBurney's point on palpation of the left lower abdomen. The sign suggests peritoneal irritation in appendicitis.

Roy Adaptation Model A conceptual model of nursing developed by Callista Roy. Individuals and groups are adaptive systems with physiological, self-concept, role function, and interdependence modes of response to focal, contextual, and residual environmental stimuli. The goal of nursing is promotion of adaptation through increasing, decreasing, maintaining, removing, altering, or changing environmental stimuli. SEE: *Nursing Theory Appendix.*

Royal Free disease [After Royal Free Hospital, London, from which cases were reported in 1955] Postviral fatigue syndrome.

Roy, Callista A nursing educator, born 1939, who developed the Roy Adaptation Model of Nursing. SEE: *Nursing Theory Appendix.*

RPF *renal plasma flow.*

RPFT *registered pulmonary function technician.*

R.Ph. *registered pharmacist.*

rpm *revolutions per minute.*

RPO *right posterior oblique* position.

RPR *rapid plasma reagin.*

RPS *renal pressor substance.*

R.Q. *respiratory quotient.*

R.R.A. *registered record administrator.*

-rrhage, -rhage Combining form used as a suffix meaning *rupture, profuse fluid discharge,* as in hemorrhage.

-rrhagia, -rhagia (rā′jē-ă) [Gr. *rhegnynai,* to burst forth] Combining form used as a suffix meaning *rupture, profuse fluid discharge.*

-rrhaphy [Gr. *raphe,* suture] Combining form used as a suffix meaning *suture, surgical repair.*

-rrhea, -rhea [Gr. *rhoia,* flow] Combining form used as a suffix denoting *flow, discharge.*

-rrhexis, -rhexis [Gr. *rhexis,* a breaking, bursting] Combining form used as a suffix meaning *rupture.*

rRNA *ribosomal RNA.*

RRT *registered respiratory therapist.*

R.S.A. *right sacroanterior* (fetal position).

R.Sc.A. *right scapuloanterior* (fetal position).

R.Sc.P. *right scapuloposterior* (fetal position).

RSI *rapid-sequence induction.*

R.S.P. *right sacroposterior* (fetal position).

R.S.T. *right sacrotransverse* (fetal position).

R.S.V. *respiratory syncytial virus; Rous sarcoma virus.*

R.T. *radiation therapy; reading test; registered technologist.*

R.T.(N.) *registered technologist—nuclear medicine.*

R.T.(R.) *registered technologist radiographer.*

R.T.(T.) *registered technologist—radiation therapy.*

R.U. *rat unit.*

RU 486 Mifepristone.

Ru Symbol for the element ruthenium.

rub Friction of one surface moving over another. In auscultation, a roughened surface moving over another causes a characteristic sound.

pericardial r. The sounds heard during auscultation with each heartbeat when the inflamed pericardial surface moves over the heart.

pleural friction r. The friction rub caused by inflammation of the pleural space.

rubber dam SEE: *dam.*

rubedo [L. *ruber,* red] Redness of the skin that may be temporary.

rubefacient (roo″bĕ-fā′shĕnt) [L. *rubefaciens,* making red] **1.** Causing redness, esp. of the skin. **2.** An agent that reddens the skin by increasing its blood flow (e.g., rubbing alcohol or capsaicin).

rubella (roo-bĕl′lă) [L. *rubellus,* reddish] A mild, febrile, highly infectious viral disease historically common in childhood prior to the advent of an effective vaccine. SYN: *German measles; roeteln; röteln.* SEE: *Nursing Diagnoses Appendix.*

SYMPTOMS: A variable 1- to 5-day prodromal period of drowsiness, mild temperature elevation, slight sore throat, Forschheimer spots (pinpoint reddish areas on the palate), and postauricular, postcervical, and occipital lymphadenopathy commonly precedes the rash eruption. The rash resembles that of measles or scarlet fever, begins on the forehead and face, spreads downward to the trunk and extremities, and lasts about 3 days. The rash appears in only about 50% of infections.

INCUBATION: Infection occurs approx. 14 to 23 days before the advent of symptoms.

COMPLICATIONS: Complications include generalized lymphadenopathy and splenomegaly. A transient polyarthritis (inflammation of the wrist, finger, knee, toe, and ankle joints) may occur within 5 days of the rash, but usually lasts less than 2 weeks. Encephalomyelitis is rare and usually self-limiting. The disease is most important because of its ability to produce defects in the developing fetus. Rubella infection during the first trimester of pregnancy is of concern; transplacental transmission to the fetus may result in several types of congenital anomalies. SEE: *congenital r. syndrome.*

PREVENTION: Prophylaxis consists of childhood immunization with a combination measles, mumps, rubella (MMR) vaccine.

CAUTION: Administration of live virus vaccines is contraindicated during pregnancy.

PATIENT CARE: *Injection Site:* For 30 min after receiving the vaccine, the patient is observed for indications of anaphylaxis, and epinephrine 1:10,000 is kept readily available. Warmth should be applied to the injection site for 24 hr following immunization, to aid absorption. If swelling persists beyond the initial 24 hr, cold should be applied, to promote vasoconstriction and prevent antigenic cyst formation. Acetaminophen (for children) or aspirin (for adults) can be taken for relief of fever.

Confirmed cases of rubella should be reported to local public health officials. Parents need to be taught about respiratory isolation and why it is necessary, emphasizing the need to prevent exposure of pregnant women to this disease.

Children with rubella virus should be made as comfortable as possible, allowed to occupy themselves with age-appropriate books, games, and television. Adolescent or adult patients may experience fever and joint pain. If medication is needed for symptomatic relief, adults may use aspirin, but children and adolescents should use acetaminophen.

If a pregnant unimmunized woman develops rubella in her first trimester, she must be informed of the potential for fetal infection and its serious consequences. Appropriate immunoglobulin laboratory studies determine the presence of fetal infection. Counseling is offered regarding the woman's choice for aborting the pregnancy, and the patient is supported in her decision.

Infants born with congenital rubella require isolation until they are no longer excreting the virus. The duration of the viral excretion is variable. Parents are taught that congenital rubella is a lifelong disease, that many related disorders may not appear until later in life, and that cataract and cardiac surgery may be required. Emotional support is offered to parents of an affected child. A referral to social service helps the parents locate help from appropriate community resources and organizations. A mental health referral may help them deal with their grief, frustration, and anxiety.

congenital r. syndrome ABBR: CRS. Transplacental transmission of the rubella virus to a fetus, resulting in spontaneous abortion, stillbirth, or major birth defects of the heart, eyes, or central nervous system, including deafness. Women who become pregnant and have not received rubella immunization should be advised of the risk of fetal development of CRS. For unimmunized women who develop rubella in the first trimester of pregnancy, the risk of CRS may be as high as 85%. The risk decreases sharply after the eighth week of pregnancy, and is absent after the 20th week of gestation. Fetal infection can be determined by serial studies of the immunoglobulin gamma M and immunoglobulin gamma G rubella antibodies. Prevention of CRS consists of active immunization of all children and of women of childbearing age.

CAUTION: Immunization with live rubella virus is contraindicated during pregnancy. It is recommended that women avoid pregnancy during the 3-month period after immunization. Infants with CRS are considered to be contagious. Only health care workers known to be immune to rubella (seropositive) should be permitted to care for infants with CRS.

---

rubella titer A blood test to determine a person's immune status to rubella.

rubella virus vaccine, live SEE: under *vaccine*.

rubeola (roo-bē′ō-lă, roo″bē-ō′lă) [L. *rubeolus*, reddish] **1.** Measles. **2.** Term occasionally applied to an acute infectious disease with mild symptoms and a rose-colored macular eruption.

rubeosis iridis A condition in which new blood vessels form on the anterior surface of the iris. It is associated with vascular disease that affects the retinal vein of the eye and is seen most frequently in diabetics, although not limited to these patients. It leads to painful, hemorrhagic glaucoma.

ruber (roo′bĕr) [L.] Red.

rubescent (roo-bĕs′ĕnt) [L. *rubescere*, to grow red] Growing red; flushing.

rubidium (roo-bĭd′ē-ŭm) [L. *rubidus*, red] SYMB: Rb. A soft, silvery metal; atomic weight 85.47, atomic number 37. Its salts are used medicinally.

rubiginous (roo-bĭj′ĭ-nŭs) [L. *rubiginosus*] Rusty.

rubigo (roo-bī′gō) [L., rust] Rust; mildew.

Rubin, Reva A nursing educator, 1916–1995, who developed the Theory of Maternal Identity. SEE: *Nursing Theory Appendix*.

Rubin's test (roo′bĭns) [Isidor Clinton Rubin, U.S. physician, 1883–1958] Transuterine insufflation of the fallopian tubes with carbon dioxide to test their patency. SYN: *tubal insufflation*. SEE: *sterility*.

Rubner's test (roob′nĕrz) [Max Rubner, Ger. physiologist, 1854–1932] **1.** A test for lactose or glucose in urine. **2.** A test for carbon monoxide in blood.

rubor (roo′bor) [L.] Discoloration or redness caused by inflammation. It is one of the four classic symptoms of inflammation. The others are calor (heat), dolor (pain), and tumor (swelling).

rubriblast (roo′brĭ-blăst) Pronormoblast.

rubricyte (roo′brĭ-sīt) [L. *ruber*, red, + Gr. *kytos*, cell] A polychromatic normoblast.

rubrospinal (roo″brō-spī′năl) [″ + *spina*, thorn] Pert. to a descending tract that consists of a small bundle of nerve fibers in the lateral funiculus of the spinal cord. Fibers arise in the cells of the red nucleus of the midbrain and terminate in the ventral horn of the gray matter.

rubrothalamic (roo″brō-thăl-lăm′ĭk) [″ + Gr. *thalamos*, chamber] Pert. to the red nucleus of the brain and thalamus.

rubrum (roo′brŭm) [L., red] The red nucleus of the gray matter in the crus cerebri near the optic thalamus.

r. scarlatinum Scarlet red, a substance used as a stain.

rudiment (roo′dĭ-mĕnt) [L. *rudimentum,* beginning] **1.** Something undeveloped. **2.** In biology, a part just beginning to develop. **3.** The remains of a part that was functional at an earlier stage of one's development or in one's ancestors. SYN: *rudimentum.*

rudimentary (roo″dĭ-mĕn′tă-rē) **1.** Elementary. **2.** Undeveloped; not fully formed; remaining from an earlier stage. SYN: *vestigial.*

rudimentum (roo″dĭ-mĕn′tŭm) [L., beginning] Rudiment.

Ruffini's corpuscle (roo-fē′nēz) [Angelo Ruffini, It. anatomist, 1864–1929] One of the encapsulated sensory nerve endings found in the dermis and subcutaneous tissue, once thought to mediate the sense of warmth, now believed to be a pressure receptor. SYN: *organ of Ruffini.*

rufous (roo′fŭs) [L. *rufus,* red] Ruddy; having a ruddy complexion and reddish hair.

ruga (roo′gă) *pl.* **rugae** [L.] A fold or crease, esp. one of the folds of mucous membrane on the internal surface of the stomach. SEE: illus.

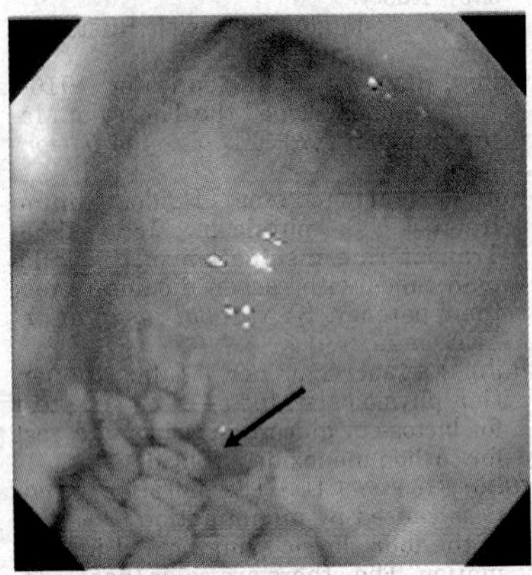

RUGAE

Rugae of stomach as seen through an endoscope

palatal r. One of the folds of the mucous membrane of the roof of the mouth. SYN: *palatine r.*

palatine r. Palatal r.

r. of vagina One of the small ridges on the inner surface of the vagina extending laterally and upward from the columna rugarum (long ridges on the anterior and posterior walls).

Ruggeri's reflex [Ruggero Ruggeri, It. physician, d. 1905] The increase in pulse rate that occurs when the eyes are strongly converged on a near object.

rugine (roo-zhēn′) **1.** Periosteal elevator. **2.** A raspatory.

rugose, rugous (roo′gōs, -gŭs) [L. *rugosus,* wrinkled] Having many wrinkles or creases; used in describing microbiological colonies. SEE: illus.

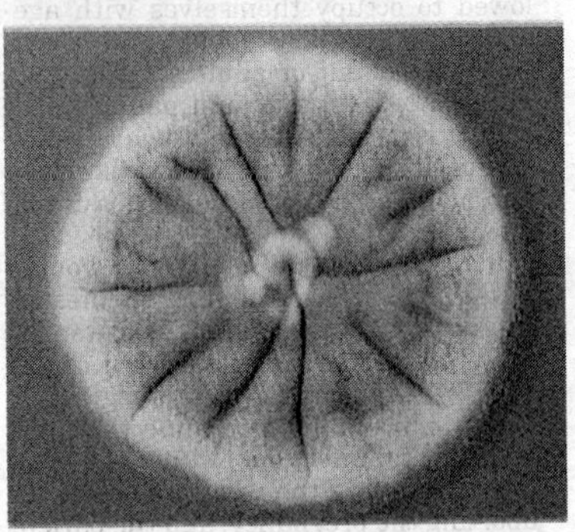

RUGOSE

Rugose appearance of *Aspergillus* culture

rugosity (rū-gŏs′ĭ-tē) [L. *rugositas*] **1.** The condition of being folded or wrinkled. **2.** A ridge or wrinkle.

R.U.L. *right upper lobe* of lung.

rule (rool) [ME. *riule*] A guide or principle based on experience or observation.

buccal object r. A dental radiographical technique used to identify the position of an object within a three-dimensional area. A reference radiograph is taken. The projection angle is changed and the resulting radiograph compared with the reference radiograph. If the image remains in the same position, the object is located buccal to the reference object. If the image changes position, the object is lingual to the reference object. Also called *Clark's rule; Clark's technique; tube shift technique.*

r. of nines A formula for estimating percentage of body surface areas, particularly helpful in judging the portion of skin that has been burned. For the adult, the head represents 9%; each upper extremity 9%; the back of the trunk 18%, and the front 18%; each lower extremity 18%; and the perineum the remaining 1%. SEE: illus.

r. of ten The criteria used to judge the readiness of an infant for surgical repair of a cleft lip. The infant must weigh 10 lb, be 10 weeks old, have a hemoglobin value of 10 g, and have a white blood cell count less than 10,000.

r. of thirds The classification of bone shaft fractures: proximal third, midshaft, and distal third. Midshaft fractures heal more slowly than other fractures because the blood supply in the middle of a bone is less than that at either end.

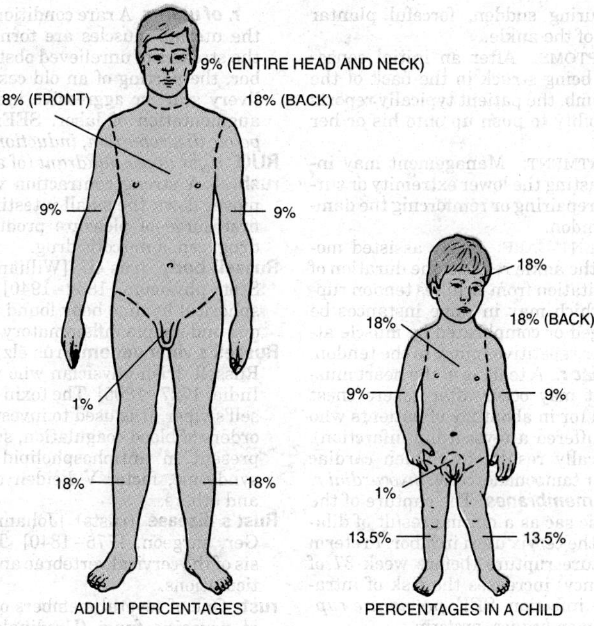

RULE OF NINES

rum [origin obscure] **1.** An alcoholic beverage prepared from fermented sugar cane juice. **2.** Colloquially, any alcoholic beverage.

rum fits A colloquial phrase for alcohol withdrawal seizures. Most occur during the 7- to 48-hr period following abstinence. There may be a single seizure, but most occur in bursts of two to six. These seizures do not represent latent epilepsy.

ruminant (roo′mĭ-nănt) An animal that regurgitates food in order to chew it again. This is called chewing the cud.

rumination (roo″mĭ-nā′shŭn) [L. *ruminatio*] **1.** Regurgitation, esp. with rechewing, of previously swallowed food. This condition may be present in otherwise normal individuals, in emotionally deprived or mentally retarded infants, or in mentally retarded adults. Infants with rumination disorder often have weight loss, malnutrition, and failure to thrive. **2.** In psychiatry, an obsessional preoccupation by a single idea or a set of thoughts, with an inability to dismiss or dislodge them. Also called *merycism.*

rump (rŭmp) [ME. *rumpe*] The posterior end of the back, the gluteal region, or the buttocks.

Rumpf's symptom (roompfs) [Heinrich Theodor Rumpf, Ger. physician, 1851–1923] A quickening of the pulse when pressure is exerted over a painful spot.

run [AS. *rinnan,* run] To exude pus or mucus.

runaround, runround Whitlow.

runners' high Feelings of relaxation experienced by many persons who participate in an intensive aerobic exercise program.

rupia (roo′pē-ă) [Gr. *rhypos,* filth] A rash, usually caused by tertiary syphilis, first manifested by large elevations of the epidermis filled with a clear, bloodstained, turbid, or purulent serum. The bulla bursts and allows some fluid to escape. As it desiccates, it is covered with a crust that dries, accumulates new layers, and becomes covered with greenish-brown scales, sometimes to a depth of ½ in. (13 mm). It is the thickest of all syphilides and presents the most extensive ulcerations. The condition is treated with antisyphilitic antibiotics.

rupioid (roo′pē-oyd) [″ + *eidos,* form, shape] Resembling rupia.

rupophobia (roo″pō-fō′bē-ă) Rhypophobia.

rupture (rŭp′chūr) [L. *ruptura,* breaking] **1.** A breaking apart of an organ or tissue. **2.** Hernia.

r. of the Achilles tendon Disruption of the attachments of the gastrocnemius and soleus muscles to the posterior calcaneus, an injury that typically occurs in middle-aged male athletes participating in basketball or other ball sports, some divers, or patients treated with steroid injections for Achilles tendonitis.

ETIOLOGY: The injury typically occurs during sudden, forceful plantar flexion of the ankle.

SYMPTOMS: After an initial sensation of being struck in the back of the lower limb, the patient typically reports an inability to push up onto his or her tiptoes.

TREATMENT: Management may involve casting the lower extremity or surgically repairing or reinforcing the damaged tendon.

PATIENT CARE: Early assisted motion of the ankle reduces the duration of rehabilitation from Achilles tendon rupture, which may in some instances be prolonged or complicated by muscle atrophy or repetitive injury to the tendon.

cardiac r. A tearing of the heart muscle that may occur after severe chest trauma (or in about 2% of patients who have suffered a myocardial infarction). It typically results in sudden cardiac death or tamponade. SYN: *myocardial r.*

r. of membranes The rupture of the amniotic sac as a normal result of dilation of the cervix uteri in labor. Preterm premature rupture (before week 37 of pregnancy) increases the risk of intrauterine infection. SEE: *premature rupture of membranes, preterm.*

myocardial r. Cardiac r.

r. of perineum Spontaneous laceration of the perineum during the second stage of labor. The event occurs more commonly in primiparas and may be avoided by having an episiotomy.

plaque r. The separation of a lipid-rich lesion from the wall of a blood vessel. The damage this does to the lining of a blood vessel triggers a cascade of events that result in blood clot formation within the vessel and its eventual obstruction. This is the immediate cause of acute myocardial infarction.

splenic r. An abdominal catastrophe marked by severe, often pleuritic pain, hemodynamic instability, blood loss into the peritoneum, and occasionally cardiovascular collapse and death. It may occur as a result of trauma or rarely in patients with infectious mononucleosis. Treatment may be conservative or may involve removal of the spleen. In delayed rupture of the spleen, a catastrophic illness may not present until days or weeks after the causative injury.

r. of tubes A rupture of a fallopian tube, a surgical emergency in ectopic pregnancy. This may occur without the woman's knowledge of her pregnancy.

r. of the tympanic membrane A disruption of the epithelium that separates the external auditory canal from the middle ear. This can occur as a result of trauma, or more often as a consequence of a middle ear infection.

r. of uterus A rare condition in which the uterine muscles are torn apart by the stresses of unrelieved obstructed labor, the parting of an old cesarean delivery scar, or aggressive induction or augmentation of labor. SEE: *cephalopelvic disproportion; induction of labor.*

RUQ *right upper quadrant* (of abdomen).

rush **1.** A strong contraction wave that moves down the small intestine. **2.** The first surge of pleasure produced by a drug, esp. a narcotic drug.

Russell body (rŭs′ĕl) [William Russell, Scot. physician, 1852–1940] A small spherical hyaline body found in cancerous and simple inflammatory growths.

Russell's viper venom (rŭs′ĕlz) [Patrick Russell, Irish physician who worked in India, 1727–1805] The toxin from Russell's viper. It is used to investigate disorders of blood coagulation, such as are present in antiphospholipid antibody syndrome, factor V Leiden deficiency, and others.

Rust's disease (rŭsts) [Johann N. Rust, Ger. surgeon, 1775–1840] Tuberculosis of the cervical vertebrae and their articulations.

rust One of several members of an order of parasitic fungi (Uredinales), all of which are parasitic on plants. Many of these are allergens.

rusty (rŭst′ē) [AS. *rustig*] Reddish; resembling or containing rust. SYN: *rubiginous.*

rut-formation In psychology, a loss of interest in the environment, the fixation on a single object, and the narrowing of concentration of emotional or other interests.

ruthenium (roo-thē′nē-ŭm) SYMB: Ru. A hard, brittle, metallic element of the platinum group; atomic weight 101.07, atomic number 44.

rutherford [Ernest Rutherford, Brit. physicist, 1871–1937] ABBR: rd. A unit of radioactivity representing 10^6 disintegrations per second.

rutidosis (roo″tĭ-dō′sĭs) Rhytidosis.

rutilism (roo′tĭl-ĭzm) [L. *rutilis,* red, + Gr. *-ismos,* condition] Having red or auburn hair.

rutin (roo′tĭn) A flavonoid present in many plants including whole grains and the inner rind of lemons and oranges.

Ruysch's membrane [Frederik Ruysch, Dutch anatomist, 1638–1731] Lamina choriocapillaris.

RV *residual volume; right ventricle.*

rye (rī) [AS. *ryge*] A cereal grass that produces a grain used in food and beverage production. When rye grain is infected with a certain fungus, ergot is produced.

rytidosis (rĭt″ĭ-dō′sĭs) Rhytidosis.

S

σ Sigma, the 18th letter of the Greek alphabet. In statistics, this is the symbol for standard deviation.

Σ The capital of the Greek letter sigma. In statistics, this is the symbol for summation.

S L. *signa,* mark, or let it be written. **1.** Symbol for the element sulfur. **2.** In prescription writing, the symbol indicating the instructions to the patient that the pharmacist will place on the dispensed medicine. **3.** *Smooth,* in reference to bacterial colonies. **4.** *Spherical* or *spherical lens.* **5.** *Subject* (pl. Ss); a participant in an experiment. **6.** Symbol for siemens.

s L. *semis,* half; *sinister,* left.

s̄, s Symbol for [L.] *sine,* without; used as a form of shorthand in hospital charts and clinical records.

S1, S2, etc. *first sacral nerve, second sacral nerve,* and so forth.

S_1, S_2 Normal first and second heart sounds.

S_3 Ventricular gallop heard after S_2, an abnormal heart sound.

S_4 Atrial gallop, heard before S_1, an abnormal heart sound.

S-A, SA, S.A. *sinoatrial.*

SAARD *slow-acting antirheumatic drug.*

Sabiá virus An arenavirus that causes Brazilian hemorrhagic fever, a potentially fatal acute febrile disease. The reservoir for the virus is unknown. Ribavirin, which is effective against Lassa fever, also caused by an arenavirus, may be effective in this illness.

Sabin vaccine [Albert Bruce Sabin, Russ.-born U.S. virologist, 1906–1993] Live oral poliovirus vaccine.

sabulous (săb′ū-lŭs) [L. *sabulosus,* sand] Gritty; sandy.

sac (săk) [L. *saccus,* sack, bag] A baglike part of an organ, a cavity or pouch, sometimes containing fluid. SYN: *saccus.* SEE: *cyst.*

air s. Alveolar sac.

allantoic s. The expanded end of the allantois, well developed in birds and reptiles.

alveolar s. The terminal portion of an air passageway within the lung. Its wall is made of simple squamous epithelium and is surrounded by pulmonary capillaries. This is the site of gas exchange. Each alveolar sac is connected to a respiratory bronchiole by an alveolar duct. SYN: *air s.*

amniotic s. The inner fetal membrane that encloses the developing fetus and produces amniotic fluid. SEE: *chorion.*

chorionic s. The outer fetal membrane that encloses the developing embryo.

conjunctival s. The cavity, lined with conjunctiva, that lies between the eyelids and the anterior surface of the eye.

dental s. The mesenchymal tissue surrounding a developing tooth.

endolymphatic s. The expanded distal end of the endolymphatic duct. SYN: *saccus endolymphaticus.*

heart s. The pericardium.

hernial s. In the peritoneum, a saclike protrusion containing a herniated organ. SEE: *hernia.*

lacrimal s. The upper dilated portion of the nasolacrimal duct situated in the groove of the lacrimal bone. The upper part is behind the internal tarsal ligament. It is 12 to 15 mm long. SYN: *saccus lacrimalis.*

lesser peritoneal s. Omental bursa.

vitelline s. Yolk s.

yolk s. In mammals, the embryonic membrane that is the site of formation of the first red blood cells and the cells that will become oogonia or spermatogonia. SYN: *vitelline s.* SEE: *embryo* for illus.

saccades (să-kāds′) [Fr. *saccade,* jerk] Fast, involuntary movements of the eyes as they change from one point of gaze to another. SEE: *nystagmus; vergence.* **saccadic,** *adj.*

saccate (săk′āt) [NL. *saccatus,* baglike] **1.** Encysted. **2.** In bacteriology, making a sac shape, as in a type of liquefaction.

saccharase (săk′ă-rās) [Sanskrit *sarkara,* sugar] An enzyme such as sucrase that catalyzes the hydrolysis of a disaccharide to monosaccharides.

saccharated (săk′ă-rāt″ĕd) Containing sugar.

saccharide (săk′ă-rīd) A group of carbohydrates including sugars. It is divided into the following classifications: monosaccharides, disaccharides, oligosaccharides, and polysaccharides.

saccharin (săk′ă-rĭn) $C_7H_5NO_3S$; a sweet, white, powdered, synthetic product derived from coal tar, 300 to 500 times sweeter than sugar, used as an artificial sweetener.

saccharine (săk′ă-rĭn, -rīn) [L. *saccharum,* sugar] Of the nature of, or having the quality of, sugar. SYN: *sweet.*

saccharo- Combining form meaning *sugar.*

saccharogalactorrhea (săk″ă-rō-gă-lăk″tō-rē′ă) [Sanskrit *sarkara,* sugar, + Gr. *gala,* milk, + *rhoia,* flow] Excessive lactose secreted in milk.

saccharolytic (săk″ă-rō-lĭt′ĭk) [″ + Gr. *lysis,* dissolution] Able to split up sugar.

Saccharomyces (săk″ă-rō-mī′sēz) [Sanskrit *sarkara,* sugar, + Gr. *mykes,* fungus] SEE: *yeast* (1).

saccharomycosis (săk″ă-rō-mī-kō′sĭs) [″ + ″ + *osis,* condition] Any disease or pathologic condition caused by yeasts (saccharomycetes).

saccharum (săk′ă-rŭm) [L.] Sugar.

sacciform (săk′sĭ-form) [L. *saccus,* sack, bag, + *forma,* shape] Bag-shaped or saclike. SYN: *encysted.*

saccular (săk′ū-lăr) [NL. *sacculus,* small bag] Sac-shaped or saclike.

sacculated (săk′ū-lāt″ĕd) [NL. *sacculus,* small bag] Consisting of small sacs or saccules.

sacculation (săk″ū-lā′shŭn) **1.** Formation into a sac or sacs. **2.** Group of sacs, collectively.

saccule (săk′ūl) [NL. *sacculus,* small bag] **1.** A small sac. SYN: *sacculus.* **2.** The smaller of two sacs of the membranous labyrinth in the vestibule of the inner ear. It communicates with the utricle, cochlear duct, and endolymphatic duct, all of which are filled with endolymph. In its wall is the macula sacculi, a sensory area containing hair cells that respond to gravity or bodily movement. SEE: *labyrinth* for illus.

laryngeal s. A small diverticulum extending ventrally from the laryngeal ventricle lying between the ventricular fold and the thyroarytenoid muscle. SYN: *sacculus laryngis; ventricular appendix.*

sacculocochlear (săk″ū-lō-kŏk′lē-ăr) [″ + Gr. *kokhlos,* land snail] Concerning the saccule and cochlea of the ear.

sacculus (săk′ū-lŭs) *pl.* **sacculi** [NL., small bag] Saccule.

s. laryngis Laryngeal saccule.

saccus (săk′ŭs) *pl.* **sacci** [L., sack, bag] Sac.

s. endolymphaticus Endolymphatic sac.

s. lacrimalis Lacrimal sac.

SACH foot *Solid ankle cushion heel* foot; a prosthetic (artificial) foot that has no definite ankle joint but is designed to absorb shock and allow movement of the shank over the foot during ambulation.

sacrad (sā′krăd) [L. *sacrum,* sacred, + *ad,* toward] Toward the sacrum.

sacral (sā′krăl) [L. *sacralis*] Relating to the sacrum.

sacral bone Sacrum.

sacral flexure Rectal curve in front of the sacrum.

sacralgia (sā-krăl′jē-ă) [L. *sacrum,* sacred, + Gr. *algos,* pain] Pain in the sacrum.

sacral index Sacral breadth multiplied by 100 and divided by sacral length.

sacralization (sā″krăl-ĭ-zā′shŭn) Fusion of the sacrum and the fifth lumbar vertebra.

sacral nerves Five pairs of spinal nerves, the upper four of which emerge through the posterior sacral foramina, the fifth pair through the sacral hiatus (termination of the sacral canal). All are mixed nerves (motor and sensory).

sacral plexus A nerve plexus formed by the ventral branches of the fourth and fifth lumbar nerves and the first four sacral nerves, from which the sciatic nerve originates.

sacrectomy (sā-krĕk′tō-mē) [L. *sacrum,* sacred, + Gr. *ektome,* excision] Excision of part of the sacrum.

sacro- (sā′krō) Combining form meaning *sacrum.*

sacroanterior (sā″krō-ăn-tē′rē-or) [L. *sacrum,* sacred, + *anterior,* before] Denoting intrauterine fetal position in which the fetal sacrum is directed anteriorly.

sacrococcygeal (sā″krō-kŏk-sĭj′ē-ăl) [″ + Gr. *kokkyx,* coccyx] Concerning the sacrum and coccyx.

sacrococcygeus (săk″rō-kŏk-sĭj′ē-ŭs) One of two small muscles (anterior and posterior) extending from the sacrum to the coccyx.

sacrocoxalgia (sā″krō-kŏks-ăl′jē-ă) [″ + *coxa,* hip, + Gr. *algos,* pain] Pain in the sacroiliac joint, usually owing to inflammation. SEE: *sacrocoxitis.*

sacrocoxitis (sā″krō-kŏks-ī′tĭs) [″ + ″ + Gr. *itis,* inflammation] Inflammation of the sacroiliac joint. SEE: *sacrocoxalgia.*

sacrodynia (sā″krō-dĭn′ē-ă) [″ + *odyne,* pain] Pain in the region of the sacrum.

sacroiliac (sā″krō-ĭl′ē-ăk) [″ + *iliacus,* hipbone] Of, or pert. to, the sacrum and ilium.

sacroiliac joint The articulation between the sacrum and the innominate bone of the pelvis. Joint movement is limited because of interlocking of the articular surfaces.

sacroiliitis (sā″krō-ĭl″ē-ī′tĭs) [″ + ″ + Gr. *itis,* inflammation] Inflammation of the sacroiliac joint.

sacrolisthesis (sā″krō-lĭs-thē′sĭs) [″ + Gr. *olisthesis,* a slipping] A deformity in which the sacrum is in front of the last lumbar vertebra. SEE: *spondylolisthesis.*

sacrolumbar (sā″krō-lŭm′băr) [″ + *lumbus,* loin] Of, or concerning, the sacrum and lumbar area.

sacrolumbar angle The angle formed by articulation of the last lumbar vertebra and the sacrum.

sacroposterior (sā″krō-pŏs-tē′rē-or) [″ + *posterus,* behind] Denoting intrauterine fetal position in which the fetal sacrum is directed posteriorly.

sacrosciatic (sā″krō-sī-ăt′ĭk) [″ + *sciaticus,* hip joint] Concerning the sacrum and ischium.

sacrospinal (sā″krō-spī′năl) [″ + *spina,* thorn] Concerning the sacrum and spine.

sacrospinalis [″ + *spina,* thorn] A large muscle group lying on either side of the vertebral column extending from the sacrum to the head. Its two chief components are the iliocostalis and longissimus muscles.

sacrotomy (sā-krŏt′ō-mē) [″ + Gr. *tome,* incision] Surgical excision of the lower part of the sacrum.

sacrouterine (sā″krō-ū′tĕr-ĭn) [″ + *uterus,* womb] Concerning the sacrum and the uterus.

sacrovertebral (sā″krō-vĕr′tĕ-brăl) [″ + *vertebra,* vertebra] Concerning the sacrum and the spinal column.

sacrovertebral angle The angle formed by the base of the sacrum and the fifth lumbar vertebra.

sacrum (sā′krŭm) [L., sacred] The triangular bone situated dorsal and caudal from the two ilia between the fifth lumbar vertebra and the coccyx. It is formed of five united vertebrae and is wedged between the two innominate bones, its articulations forming the sacroiliac joints. It is the base of the vertebral column and, with the coccyx, forms the posterior boundary of the true pelvis. The male sacrum is narrower and more curved than the female sacrum. SYN: *sacral bone; vertebra magnum*. SEE: illus.

sactosalpinx (săk″tō-săl′pĭnks) [Gr. *saktos,* stuffed, + *salpinx,* tube] A dilated fallopian tube owing to retention of secretions, as in pyosalpinx or hydrosalpinx.

SAD *seasonal affective disorder; source-to-axis distance.*

saddle A surface or structure that resembles a seat used to ride a horse. The base of artificial dentures is often referred to as a saddle.

s. area The portion of the buttocks, perineum, and thighs that comes in contact with the seat of the saddle when one rides a horse.

s. back Lordosis.

s. block anesthesia Anesthesia of the buttocks and perineum.

S-adenosylmethionine ABBR: SAM-e. A compound that is synthesized naturally in the central nervous system when folate and vitamin B_{12} levels are adequate. It is involved in the methylation of neurotransmitters, amino acids, proteins, phospholipids, and other neurochemicals. Preliminary studies suggest it may act rapidly and with few side effects in the treatment of depression. The chemical is marketed as a nutritional supplement. Its safety and efficacy have not been formally evaluated by the U.S. Food and Drug Administration.

sadism (sā′dĭzm, săd′ĭzm) [Comte Donatien Alphonse François de Sade, Marquis de Sade, 1740–1814] Conscious or unconscious sexual pleasure derived from inflicting mental or physical pain on others. SEE: *algolagnia; masochism.*

sadist (sā′dĭst, săd′ĭst) One who practices sadism.

sadness A normal emotional feeling of dejection or melancholy that one may experience after an unhappy event.

sadomasochism (sā″dō-măs′ĕ-kĭzm,

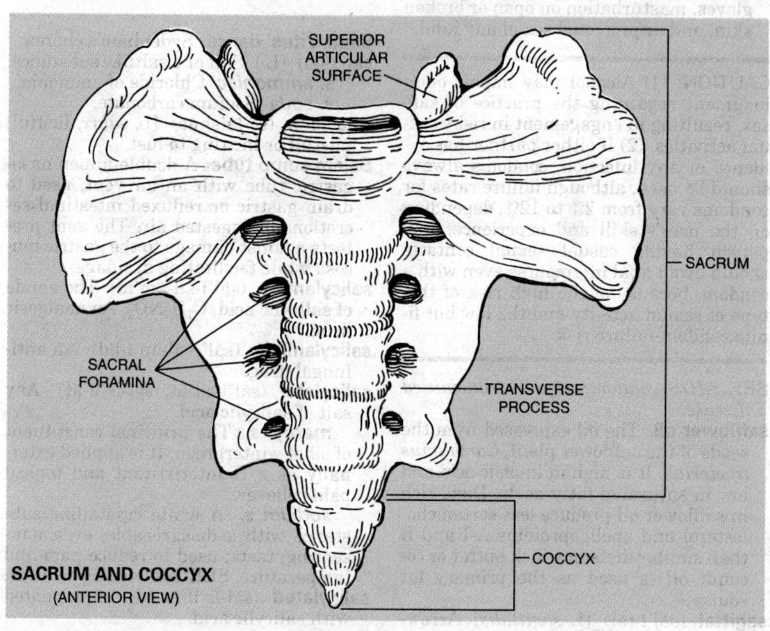

SACRUM AND COCCYX
(ANTERIOR VIEW)

săd″ō-măs′ĕ-kĭzm) Sexual pleasure related to both sadism and masochism.

sadomasochist (sā″dō-măs′ĕ-kĭst) One whose personality includes sadistic and masochistic components.

Saemisch's ulcer (sā′mĭsh-ĕs) [Edwin Theodor Saemisch, Ger. ophthalmologist, 1833–1909] Serpiginous infectious ulcer of the cornea.

Safe Drinking Water Act A federal law that created the infrastructure, standards, and regulations to ensure the quality of drinking water.

safelight A darkroom device that emits a light of a specified wavelength that causes less fogging of undeveloped film than white light does.

safe sex The practice of protecting oneself and one's partner(s) from sexually transmitted diseases (STDs), including chlamydia, gonorrhea, trichomoniasis, syphilis, herpesviruses, hepatitis viruses, and human immunodeficiency virus. Safe sexual practices involve avoiding contact with one's partner's blood or body fluids (e.g., seminal fluid) by wearing condoms during any form of oral, vaginal, or anal intercourse. The risks of transmitting STDs may be further classified as follows: *Safe:* Celibacy; masturbation; dry kissing; masturbation of a partner on healthy, intact skin; oral sex with use of a condom; touching; fantasy. *Possibly Safe:* Condom-protected vaginal or anal intercourse. *Risky:* Wet kissing, oral sex (without a dental dam or latex or plastic barrier or condom), masturbation of a woman without a latex barrier or use of latex gloves, masturbation on open or broken skin, and unprotected sex of any kind.

CAUTION: (1) Alcohol may impair one's judgment regarding the practice of safe sex, resulting in engagement in risky sexual activities. (2) If either partner has evidence of any infection, condoms always should be used, although failure rates for condoms vary from 2% to 12%, depending on the user's skill and experience. Any person having casual sexual contacts should avoid anal intercourse even with a condom, because of the high risk of this type of sexual activity and the low but finite condom-failure risk.

SEE: *AIDS; condom; sexually transmitted disease.*

safflower oil The oil expressed from the seeds of the safflower plant, *Carthamus tinctorius.* It is high in linoleic acid and low in saturated fatty acids. Diets rich in safflower oil produce less serum cholesterol and apolipoproteins A-I and B than similar diets in which butter or coconut oil is used as the primary fat source.

sagittal (săj′ĭ-tăl) [L. *sagittalis*] Arrow-like; in an anteroposterior direction. SYN: *sagittalis.*

sagittalis (săj″ĭ-tā′lĭs) [L.] Sagittal.

sagittal plane A vertical plane through the longitudinal axis of the trunk dividing the body into right and left portions. If it is through the anteroposterior midaxis and divides the body into right and left halves, it is called a *median* or *midsagittal plane.*

sagittal sulcus A groove on the inner surface of the parietal bones, forming a channel for the superior sagittal sinus.

sago (sā′gō) [Malay *sagu*] A substance prepared from various palms, consisting principally of starches; used as a demulcent and as a food with little residue.

Saint John's wort An herbal remedy recommended by alternative medical practitioners for the treatment of mood disorders. SEE: illus.

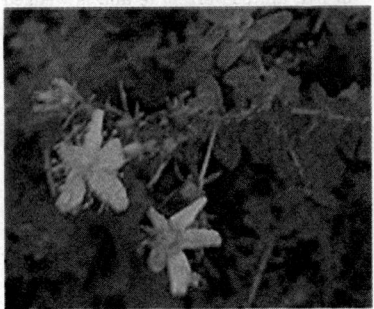

SAINT JOHN'S WORT

Saint Vitus' dance Sydenham's chorea.

sal (săl) [L.] Salt or a saltlike substance.

s. ammoniac Chloride of ammonia.

s. soda Sodium carbonate.

salacious (sĕ-lā′shŭs) [L. *salax,* lustful] Lustful or inciting to lust.

Salem sump tube A double-lumen nasogastric tube with an air vent, used to drain gastric or refluxed intestinal secretions or ingested air. The vent protects against damage to the gastric mucosa while facilitating drainage.

salicylamide (săl″ĭ-sĭl-ăm′ĭd) The amide of salicylic acid, $C_7H_7NO_2$. An analgesic drug.

salicylanilide (săl″ĭ-sĭl-ăn′ĭ-lĭd) An antifungal drug.

salicylate (săl″ĭ-sĭl′āt, săl-ĭs′ĭl-āt) Any salt of salicylic acid.

methyl s. The principal constituent of oil of wintergreen. It is applied externally as a counterirritant and topical pain reliever.

sodium s. A white crystalline substance with a disagreeable, even nauseating, taste; used to reduce pain and temperature. SEE: *acetylsalicylic acid.*

salicylated (săl-ĭs′ĭl-āt-ĕd) Impregnated with salicylic acid.

salicylate poisoning Intoxication with aspirin or one of its derivatives. SEE: *aspirin poisoning*.

salicylic acid (săl″ĭ-sĭl′ĭk) $C_7H_6O_3$; a white crystalline acid derived from phenol used to make aspirin, as a preservative and flavoring agent, and in the topical treatment of some skin conditions, such as warts and wrinkles. SEE: *chemical peeling*.

salicylism (săl′ĭ-sĭl″ĭzm) Intoxication caused by an overdose of salicylic acid or its derivatives.

salicyluric acid (săl″ĭ-sĭ-lū′rĭk) Acid found in the urine after an individual takes salicylic acid or its derivatives.

salient [L. *salio*, to spring, jump] Prominent, conspicuous.

saline (sā′līn, sā′lēn) [L. *salinus*, of salt] Containing or pert. to salt; salty.

s. cathartic A salt, such as epsom salts, used to produce evacuation of the bowel.

hypertonic s. An aqueous solution of sodium chloride of greater than 0.85%.

hypotonic s. An aqueous solution of sodium chloride of less than 0.85%.

salinometer (săl″ĭ-nŏm′ĕ-tĕr) [L. *salinus*, of salt, + *metron*, measure] An instrument for determining the salt content of a solution.

saliva (să-lī′vă) [L., spittle] Salivary gland and oral mucous gland fluid; the secretion that begins the process of digesting food. Saliva moistens food for tasting, chewing, and swallowing; initiates digestion of starches; moistens and lubricates the mouth; and acts as a solvent for excretion of waste products. SYN: *spit* (1); *spittle*.

CHARACTERISTICS: It is normally tasteless, clear, odorless, viscid, and weakly alkaline, being neutralized after being acted on by gastric acid in the stomach. Its specific gravity is 1.002 to 1.006. The amount secreted in 24 hr is estimated to be 1500 ml. The flow varies from 0.2 ml/min from resting glands to 4.0 ml/min with maximum secretion.

COMPOSITION: Saliva is 99.5% water. Inorganic constituents include salts (chlorides, carbonates, phosphates, sulfates) and dissolved gases. Organic constituents include enzymes (amylase and lysozyme), proteins (mucin, albumin, and globulins), small amounts of urea, and unusual waste products (e.g., acetone). Epithelial cells and leukocytes are also present.

DIAGNOSTIC TESTING: Like urine and blood, saliva is readily accessible and easy to transport and store. As a result it has become a target for clinical laboratory testing. In the year 2000, U.S. Food and Drug Administration-approved diagnostic tests on saliva include assays for antibodies to human immunodeficiency virus, estrogen levels, drugs of abuse, and alcohol levels. Other tests that are readily available, but not FDA-approved, include assays for hepatitis virus infections, prostate-specific antigen, and cholesterol.

artificial s. A solution that is useful in treating excessive dryness of the mouth (xerostomia). One such formula is 20 ml of a 4% solution of methylcellulose, 10 ml of glycerin, sufficient normal saline to make 90 ml, and one drop of lemon oil.

saliva ejector A device used during dental procedures to remove saliva.

salivant (săl′ĭ-vănt) [L. *saliva*, spittle] Something that stimulates the flow of saliva.

salivary (săl′ĭ-vĕr-ē) [L. *salivarius*, slimy] Pert. to, producing, or formed from saliva.

salivary corpuscle A white blood cell found in saliva.

salivary gland Any of the glands near the oral cavity that secrete saliva. The major glands are paired and include the parotid, below the ear and inside the ramus of the mandible; the sublingual, below the tongue in the anterior floor of the mouth; and the submandibular, below the posterior floor of the mouth, medial to the body of the mandible. Minor salivary glands are numerous in the oral cavity and are named according to their locations: lingual, sublingual, palatal, buccal, labial, and glossopharyngeal. SEE: illus.

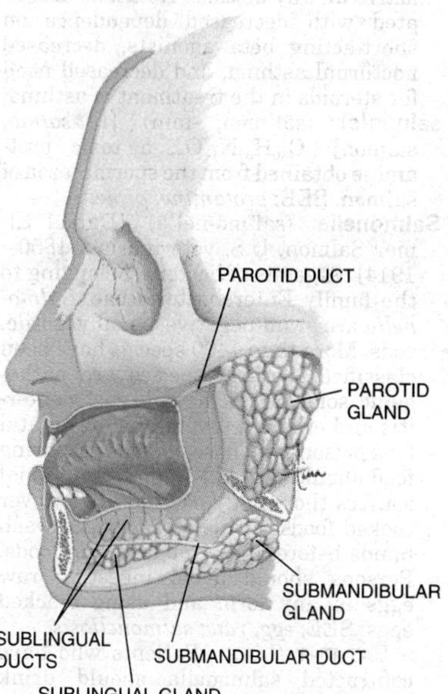

SALIVARY GLANDS

Salivary secretion is under nervous control, reflexly initiated by mechanical, chemical, or radiant stimuli acting on gustatory receptors (taste buds) in the mouth, olfactory receptors, visual receptors (eyes), or other sense organs. Secretion may also occur as a result of conditioned reflexes, as when one thinks about food or hears a dinner bell. The nerve supply of the salivary glands is from the facial and glossopharyngeal nerves, which are parasympathetic and increase secretion, and from the sympathetic nerves, which decrease secretion. The blood supply is from branches of the external carotid artery.

salivation (săl″ĭ-vā′shŭn) [LL. *salivatio,* to spit out] **1.** The act of secreting saliva. **2.** Excessive secretion of saliva. SYN: *ptyalism.*

salivatory (săl′ĭ-vă-tor″ē) Producing the secretion of saliva.

salivolithiasis (să-lī″vō-lĭ-thī′ă-sĭs) [L. *saliva,* spittle, + Gr. *lithos,* stone, + *-iasis,* condition] Sialolithiasis.

Salk vaccine (sŏlk) [Jonas E. Salk, U.S. microbiologist, 1914–1995] The first successful poliomyelitis vaccine. It contains three types of formalin-inactivated poliomyelitis viruses and induces immunity against the disease. SEE: *poliomyelitis.*

sallow (săl′ō) [AS. *salo*] A sickly yellow color, usually describing complexion or skin color.

salmeterol (săl-mē-tĕr′al) A long-acting β_2 agonist used to treat patients with reactive airway disease. Its use is associated with decreased dependence on short-acting beta agonists, decreased nocturnal asthma, and decreased need for steroids in the treatment of asthma.

salmin(e) (săl′mēn, -mĭn) [L. *salmo,* salmon] $C_{30}H_{57}N_{14}O_6$; a toxic protamine obtained from the spermatozoa of salmon. SEE: *protamine; protein.*

Salmonella (săl″mō-nĕl′ă) [Daniel Elmer Salmon, U.S. veterinarian, 1850–1914] A genus of bacteria belonging to the family Enterobacteriaceae. *Salmonella* are gram-negative, usually motile, rods. More than 1400 species have been classified. Several species are pathogenic, some producing mild gastroenteritis and others a severe and often fatal food poisoning. Those persons preparing food should cook all foods from animal sources thoroughly, refrigerate leftover cooked foods during storage, and wash hands before and after handling foods. Persons should avoid ingesting raw eggs in any form and using cracked eggs. SEE: *egg, raw; salmonellosis.*

PATIENT CARE: Patients who have contracted salmonella should drink clear fluids until abdominal pain has subsided. Fluid and electrolyte balance is monitored, and supportive therapy is maintained as indicated. Enteric precautions are used until infection has subsided.

S. arizonae A species that may infect animals and humans and cause gastroenteritis, urinary tract infection, bacteremia, meningitis, osteomyelitis, and brain abscess.

S. choleraesuis A species often found to be the cause of septicemia.

S. enteritidis An organism that commonly causes gastrointestinal infections. Approx. 10% to 20% of food poisoning cases are caused by *S. enteritidis.* The organism lives in the ovaries of chickens and contaminates eggs before the shells are formed. The infection is passed to humans when they eat raw eggs (e.g., in homemade ice cream, salad dressings, eggnog) or cooked eggs in which the yolk is still runny. It also lives in the intestinal tracts of animals and may be found in water or meat that is contaminated with feces and is inadequately washed and cooked. Infants, elderly persons, and immunocompromised patients are at greatest risk. SEE: *diarrhea; raw egg; enterocolitis.*

S. paratyphi A group of organisms of *Salmonella,* types A, B, and C, that cause paratyphoid fever.

S. typhi A species causing typhoid fever in humans.

S. typhimurium A species frequently isolated from persons having acute gastroenteritis.

salmonellosis (săl-mō-nĕ-lō′sĭs) Infection with gram-negative bacteria of the genus *Salmonella.* In the U.S., the most common infection is acute gastroenteritis caused by *S. enteritidis, S. typhimurium,* or other strains. Typhoid fever, found in developing countries with inadequate sanitation, is caused by *S. typhi.*

SYMPTOMS: Salmonella gastroenteritis is characterized by fever, nausea and vomiting, watery diarrhea, and abdominal cramps 12 to 72 hr after consuming contaminated food or water. The illness usually is self-limiting and lasts from 4 to 7 days.

TREATMENT: Unless severe, salmonella gastroenteritis is treated with fluid replacement and antimotility drugs; antibiotics are not used. For immunocompromised patients, those with severe diarrhea and fever greater than 101°F, and elderly persons or infants, ciprofloxacin or trimethoprim-sulfamethoxazole may be prescribed for 3 to 7 days.

PREVENTION: To reduce the risk of *S. enteritidis* infection, eggs should be kept refrigerated at all times to prevent increased bacterial growth; cracked or dirty eggs should be discarded. Hands and equipment in contact with raw eggs should be washed thoroughly in soap and hot water before other foods are touched. Eggs should be cooked until the yolk is solid, and eaten promptly;

food containing cooked eggs should not be kept warm for more than 2 hr.

salpingectomy (săl″pĭn-jĕk′tō-mē) [Gr. *salpinx,* tube, + *ektome,* excision] The surgical removal of a fallopian tube.

salpingemphraxis (săl″pĭn-jĕm-frăk′sĭs) [″ + *emphraxis,* a stoppage] An obstruction of the eustachian tube.

salpingian (săl-pĭn′jē-ăn) Concerning the eustachian tube or a fallopian tube.

salpingion (săl-pĭn′jē-ŏn) A point at the inferior surface of the apex of the petrous portion of the temporal bone.

salpingitis (săl″pĭn-jī′tĭs) [Gr. *salpinx,* tube, + *itis,* inflammation] Inflammation of a fallopian tube, usually as a result of a sexually transmitted infection. The prognosis is affected by the virulence of the organism, degree of inflammation, and promptness of treatment. The long-term consequences of the infection may include scarring of the fallopian tubes and infertility.

ETIOLOGY: The most common causative organisms are *Neisseria gonorrhoeae* and *Chlamydia trachomatis.* Additional microbes include *Staphylococcus aureus, Escherichia coli,* and other aerobic and anaerobic bacilli and cocci. Although common among other cultures, tubercular salpingitis is rare in the U.S.; it is most likely to be present in immunosuppressed women and some immigrant populations. Postpartum salpingitis often results from the upward migration of commensal vaginal streptococci.

SYMPTOMS: Although the disease may be asymptomatic, the patient often presents with signs of an acute pelvic infection. Complaints include unilateral or bilateral pelvic or lower abdominal pain; fever; and chills.

EXAMINATION: If an abscess has formed, bimanual palpation or ultrasonography may reveal a tender adnexal mass.

TREATMENT: Empirical antibiotic therapies may include fluoroquinolones or combination therapies using tetracycline derivatives and cephalosporins. Care must be taken to avoid using fluoroquinolones or tetracyclines in pregnancy. Bedrest and analgesics assist in pain management.

eustachian s. Eustachitis.

gonococcal s. Salpingitis due to gonococci.

salpingo- Combining form indicating *tube.*

salpingocatheterism (săl-pĭng″gō-kăth′ĕt-ĕr-ĭzm) [Gr. *salpinx,* tube, + *katheter,* something inserted, + *-ismos,* condition] Catheterization of the eustachian tube.

salpingocele (săl-pĭng′gō-sēl) [″ + *kele,* tumor, swelling] The hernial protrusion of a fallopian tube.

salpingocyesis (săl-pĭng″ō-sī-ē′sĭs) [″ + *kyesis,* pregnancy] Tubal pregnancy.

salpingography (săl″pĭng-gŏg′ră-fē) [″ + *graphein,* to write] Radiography of the fallopian tubes after the introduction of a radiopaque contrast medium; used in testing for patency of the tubes in investigating infertility.

salpingolithiasis (săl-pĭng″gō-lĭ-thī′ă-sĭs) [″ + *lithos,* stone, + *iasis,* condition] The presence of stones in a fallopian tube.

salpingolysis (săl″pĭng-gŏl′ĭ-sĭs) [″ + *lysis,* dissolution] The surgical disruption of adhesions in a fallopian tube.

salpingo-oophorectomy (săl-pĭng″gō-ō″ŏf-ō-rĕk′tō-mē) [″ + *oon,* egg, + *phoros,* a bearer, + *ektome,* excision] Excision of an ovary and a fallopian tube. SYN: *oophorosalpingectomy; ovariosalpingectomy; salpingo-ovariectomy.*

salpingo-oophoritis (săl-pĭng″ō-ō″ŏf-ō-rī′tĭs) [″ + ″ + ″ + *itis,* inflammation] Inflammation of a fallopian tube and an ovary. SYN: *salpingo-oothecitis.* SEE: *pelvic inflammatory disease; salpingitis.*

salpingo-oophorocele (săl-pĭng″gō-ō-ŏf′or-ō-sēl) [Gr. *salpinx,* tube, + *oon,* egg, + *phoros,* a bearer, + *kele,* tumor, swelling] A hernia enclosing an ovary and a fallopian tube.

salpingo-oothecitis (săl-pĭng″gō-ō″ō-thē-sī′tĭs) [″ + *ootheke,* ovary, + *itis,* inflammation] Salpingo-oophoritis.

salpingo-oothecocele (săl-pĭng″gō-ō″ō-thē′kō-sēl) [″ + ″ + *kele,* tumor, swelling] A hernia of an ovary and a fallopian tube.

salpingo-ovariectomy (săl-pĭng″gō-ō″văr-ē-ĕk′tō-mē) [″ + LL. *ovarium,* ovary, + Gr. *ektome,* excision] Salpingo-oophorectomy.

salpingoperitonitis (săl-pĭng″gō-pĕr″ĭ-tō-nī′tĭs) [″ + *peritonaion,* peritoneum, + *itis,* inflammation] Inflammation of the serosal covering of the fallopian tubes.

salpingopexy (săl-pĭng′ō-pĕk″sē) [″ + *pexis,* fixation] Fixation of a fallopian tube.

salpingopharyngeal (săl-pĭng″gō-fă-rĭn′jē-ăl) [″ + *pharynx,* throat] Concerning the eustachian tube and the pharynx.

salpingopharyngeus (săl-pĭng″gō-făr-ĭn′jē-ŭs) [″ + *pharynx,* throat] The muscle near the opening of the eustachian tube that raises the nasopharynx and also may help open the eustachian tube.

salpingoplasty (săl-pĭng′gō-plăs″tē) [″ + *plassein,* to form] Plastic surgery of a fallopian tube; used in treating female infertility. SYN: *tuboplasty.*

salpingorrhaphy (săl″pĭng-gor′ă-fē) [″ + *rhaphe,* seam, ridge] Suture of a fallopian tube.

salpingosalpingostomy (săl-pĭng″gō-săl″pĭng-gŏs′tō-mē) [″ + *salpinx,* tube, + *stoma,* mouth] The operation of attaching one fallopian tube to the other.

salpingoscope (săl-pĭng′gō-skōp″) [″ + *skopein,* to examine] A device for examining the nasopharynx and the eustachian tube.

salpingostenochoria (săl-pĭng″gō-stĕn″ō-kor′ē-ă) [″ + *stenos,* narrow, + *choreia,* dance] A stenosis or stricture of the eustachian tube.

salpingostomatomy (săl-pĭng″gō-stō-măt′ō-mē) [″ + *stoma,* mouth, + *tome,* incision] The creation of an artificial opening in a fallopian tube after it has been occluded as a result of inflammation and scarring.

salpingostomy (săl-pĭng-ŏs′tō-mē) The surgical opening of a fallopian tube that has been occluded, or for drainage purposes.

salpingotomy (săl-pĭng-ŏt′ō-mē) [″ + *tome,* incision] Incision of a fallopian tube.

salpingo-ureterostomy (săl-pĭng″gō-ūr-ēt″ĕr-ŏs′tō-mē) [″ + *oureter,* ureter, + *stoma,* mouth] A surgical connection of the ureter and a fallopian tube.

salpinx (săl′pĭnks) *pl.* **salpinges** [Gr., tube] A fallopian tube or the eustachian tube.

salt [AS. *sealt*] **1.** White crystalline compound occurring in nature, known chemically as sodium chloride, NaCl. **2.** Containing or treated with salt. **3.** To treat with salt. **4.** In the plural, any mineral salt or saline mixture used as an aperient or cathartic, esp. epsom salts or Glauber's salt. **5.** In chemistry, a compound consisting of a positive ion other than hydrogen and a negative ion other than hydroxyl. **6.** A chemical compound resulting from the interaction of an acid and a base.

Salts and water are the inorganic or mineral constituents of the body. They play specific roles in the functions of cells and are indispensable for life. The principal salts are chlorides, carbonates, bicarbonates, sulfates, and phosphates, combined with sodium, potassium, calcium, or magnesium.

In general, salts serve the following roles in the body: maintenance of proper osmotic conditions; maintenance of water balance and regulation of blood volume; maintenance of proper acid-base balance; provision for essential constituents of tissue, esp. bones and teeth; maintenance of normal irritability of muscle and nerve cells; maintenance of condition for coagulation of the blood; provision for essential components of certain enzyme systems, respiratory pigments, and hormones; and regulation of cell membrane and capillary permeability. SEE: *sodium chloride*.

acid s. A salt in which one or more hydrogen atoms remain unreplaced by the hydroxyl (OH) radical.

basic s. A salt retaining the ability to react with an acid radical.

bile s. A salt of glycocholic and taurocholic acid present in bile.

buffer s. A salt that fixes excess amounts of acid or alkali without a change in hydrogen ion concentration.

double s. Any salt formed from two other salts.

epsom s. Magnesium sulfate.

Glauber's s. Sodium sulfate.

glow s. Rubbing of the entire body with moist salt for stimulation.

haloid s. A salt made up of a base and a halogen (i.e., chloride, iodide, bromide, fluorine, or astatine).

hypochlorite s. A salt of hypochlorous acid used in household bleach and as an oxidizer, deodorant, and disinfectant.

iodized s. A salt containing 1 part sodium or potassium iodide to 10,000 parts of sodium chloride. It is an important source of iodine in the diet. Its use prevents goiter due to iodine deficiency.

neutral s. Normal s.

normal s. An ionic compound containing no replaceable hydrogen or hydroxyl ions. SYN: *neutral salt.*

Rochelle s. SEE: *Rochelle salt*.

rock s. Natural sodium chloride.

sea s. Sodium chloride obtained from sea water.

smelling s. Aromatized ammonium carbonate.

substitute s. A chemical, such as potassium chloride, that has a flavor similar to that of salt but has negligible sodium content. It is used by individuals whose medical condition requires limited sodium intake.

saltation (săl-tā′shŭn) [L. *saltatio,* leaping] Act of leaping or dancing, as in chorea.

saltatory (săl′tă-tō″rē) Marked by dancing or leaping.

saltatory conduction The transmission of a nerve impulse along a myelinated nerve fiber. The action potential occurs only at the nodes of Ranvier, making velocity faster than along unmyelinated fibers.

salt-free diet A low-sodium diet containing about 500 mg (approx. 10 mmol) of sodium daily. It is used occasionally to help manage hypertension, congestive heart failure, or renal failure. On this diet, table salt should not be added to food, and the salt content of commonly used beverages such as beer or soft drinks should be noted. To help regulate sodium consumption, sodium-containing medicines should be avoided. SEE: *salt.*

salting out A method of separating a specific protein from a mixture of proteins by the addition of a salt (e.g., ammonium sulfate).

salt-losing syndrome The condition of greatly increased sodium loss from the body as a result of renal disease, adrenocortical insufficiency, or gastrointestinal disease.

saltpeter, saltpetre (sawlt-pē′tĕr) [L. *sal,* salt, + *petra,* rock] A common name for *potassium nitrate.*

Chile s. A common name for sodium nitrate, $NaNO_3$; a crystalline powder, saline in taste and soluble in water.

salubrious (să-lū′brē-ŭs) [L. *salubris,* healthful] Promoting or favorable to health; wholesome.

salutary (săl′ū-tā″rē) [L. *salutaris,* health] Healthful; promoting health; curative.

Salvarsan (săl′văr-săn) [L. *salvus,* safe, + Gr. *arsen,* arsenic] An arsenical, yellow powder preparation developed by Paul Ehrlich for treatment of syphilis. Since the development of penicillin, there has been little need for Salvarsan. SYN: *arsphenamine.*

salve (săv) [AS. *sealf*] Ointment.

samaritanism Compassion.

samarium (să-mā′rē-ŭm) SYMB: Sm. A very rare metallic element. Atomic weight 150.35; atomic number 62; specific gravity approx. 7.50.

SAM-e *S-adenosylmethionine.*

SAMPLE An acronym designed to remind the emergency medical service provider of the appropriate questions to ask about the patient's pertinent past medical history. It stands for symptoms, allergies, medications, past medical history, last oral intake, and events leading up to today's complaint. The SAMPLE history is a part of the focused history and physical examination of a patient.

sample **1.** A piece or portion of a whole that demonstrates the characteristics or quality of the whole, such as a specimen of blood. **2.** In research, a portion of a population selected to represent the entire population.

biased s. In epidemiology or medical research, a sample of a group that does not equally represent the members of the group.

fetal blood s. A small amount of blood drawn from a fetal scalp vein to assess acid-base status. The normal fetal blood pH level is 7.25. Levels between 7.20 and 7.24 reflect a preacidotic state; levels below 7.20 indicate acidosis and fetal jeopardy.

grab s. In public health and medical statistics, a chaotic set of data from which conclusions are injudiciously drawn. Because the sample is not carefully randomized or scientifically selected, the conclusions derived from such sample groups may be inaccurate.

sampling The process of selecting a portion or part to represent the whole.

random s. A method of selecting a sample population using a table of random numbers to select the sample from a listing of the population.

sanatorium (săn″ă-tō′rē-ŭm) [L. *sanatorius,* healing] Sanitarium.

sand (sănd) [AS.] Fine grains of disintegrated rock.

auditory s. An out-of-date term for otolith or statoconia.

brain s. Concretion of matter near the base of the pineal gland. SYN: *corpora arenacea.*

sandflies Flies of the order Diptera belonging to the genus *Phlebotomus.* They transmit sandfly fever, Oroya fever, and various types of leishmaniasis.

sandfly fever A mild viral disease that clinically resembles influenza, with headache, sore throat, muscle aches, and malaise. The causative organism, any one of several species of *Bunyaviridae* viruses, is transmitted by the common sandfly *Phlebotomus papatasi,* a small, hairy, blood-sucking midge that bites at night. The disease occurs in tropical and subtropical areas that experience long periods of hot, dry weather. Several antiviral drugs (e.g., interferon alpha and ribavirin) have some activity against the disease. SYN: *pappataci fever; phlebotomus fever.*

Sandhoff's disease A rare form of Tay-Sachs disease in which two essential enzymes (hexosaminidase A and B) for metabolizing gangliosides are absent. In Tay-Sachs disease only one enzyme, hexosaminidase A, is absent.

Sandwith's bald tongue (sănd′wĭths) [Fleming M. Sandwith, Brit. physician, 1777–1843] An abnormally clean tongue seen in the late stages of pellagra.

SANE *Sexual Assault Nurse Examiner.*

sane (sān) [L. *sanus,* healthy] Sound of mind; mentally normal.

Sanfilippo's disease [S. J. Sanfilippo, contemporary U.S. pediatrician] Mucopolysaccharidosis III.

sanguicolous (săng-gwĭk′ō-lŭs) [L. *sanguis,* blood, + *colere,* to dwell] Inhabiting the blood, as a parasite.

sanguiferous (săng-gwĭf′ĕr-ŭs) [″ + *ferre,* to carry] Conducting or containing blood, as the circulatory organs.

sanguinarine (săng′gwĭn-ă-rĭn) A benzophenanthridine alkaloid available as an oral rinse and toothpaste. It is used to treat dental plaque and gingivitis.

sanguine (săng′gwĭn) [L. *sanguineus,* bloody] **1.** Optimistic; cheerful. **2.** Plethoric, bloody; marked by abundant and active blood circulation, particularly a ruddy complexion. **3.** Pert. to, or consisting of, blood.

sanguineous (săng-gwĭn′ē-ŭs) [L. *sanguineus,* bloody] **1.** Bloody; relating to blood. **2.** Having an abundance of blood. SYN: *plethoric.*

sanguinopurulent (săng″gwĭ-nō-pū′rū-lĕnt) [″ + *purulentus,* full of pus] Concerning or containing blood and pus.

sanguirenal (săng″gwĭ-rē′năl) [L. *sanguis,* blood, + *ren,* kidney] Pert. to the blood supply of the kidneys.

sanguis (săng′gwĭs) [L.] Blood.

sanguisuga (săng-gwĭ-sū′gă) [″ + *sugere,* to suck] A leech or bloodsucker. SEE: *Hirudo*.

sanies (sā′nē-ēz) [L., thin, fetid pus] A thin, fetid, greenish discharge from a wound or ulcer, appearing as pus tinged with blood.

saniopurulent (sā″nē-ō-pū′roo-lĕnt) [L. *sanies,* thin, fetid pus, + *purulentus,* full of pus] Having characteristics of sanies and pus; pert. to a fetid, serous, blood-tinged discharge containing pus.

sanitarian (săn″ĭ-tā′rē-ăn) [L. *sanitas,* health] A person who by training and experience is skilled in sanitation and public health.

sanitarium (săn-ĭ-tā′rē-ŭm) [L. *sanitas,* health] An institution for the treatment and recuperation of persons having physical or mental disorders. SYN: *sanatorium*.

sanitary (săn′ĭ-tā″rē) [L. *sanitas,* health] **1.** Promoting or pert. to conditions that are conducive to good health. **2.** Clean, free of dirt.

sanitary napkin Perineal pad, esp. one used for absorbing menstrual fluid. SEE: *menstrual tampon; menstruation*.

sanitation (săn″ĭ-tā′shŭn) [L. *sanitas,* health] The formulation and application of measures to promote and establish conditions favorable to health, esp. public health. SEE: *hygiene*.

sanitization (săn″ĭ-tĭ-zā′shŭn) [L. *sanitas,* health] The act of making sanitary.

sanitize (săn′ĭ-tīz) **1.** To make sanitary. **2.** To inactivate or remove microorganisms from equipment and surfaces. Chemicals, heat, and ionizing radiation can be used for this purpose.

sanitizer An agent that reduces the number of bacterial contaminants to safe levels as judged by public health requirements. Usually used to describe agents applied to eating and drinking utensils and dairy equipment. All chemicals are removed from equipment and surfaces before food preparation or processing.

sanity (săn′ĭ-tē) **1.** Soundness of health or mind; mentally normal. **2.** The ability to think logically or rationally.

San Joaquin valley fever Coccidioidomycosis.

SA node Sinoatrial node of the heart.

SaO_2 Saturation, oxygen.

sap (săp) [AS. *saep*] **1.** Any fluid essential to the life of plants. **2.** To cause gradual exhaustion or weakness, as to sap one's strength.

cell s. Cytoplasm.

nuclear s. An old term for the contents of a cell's nucleus.

saphena (să-fē′nă) *pl.* **saphenae** [Gr. *saphenes,* manifest] A saphenous vein.

saphenectomy (săf″ĕ-nĕk′tō-mē) [″ + *ektome,* excision] The surgical removal of a saphenous vein.

saphenous (să-fē′nŭs) Pert. to, or associated with, a saphenous vein or nerve in the leg.

saphenous nerve A deep branch of the femoral nerve. In the lower leg, it follows the great saphenous vein and supplies the medial side of the leg, ankle, and foot.

saphenous opening An oval aperture in the fascia in the inner and upper part of the thigh, transmitting the saphenous vein below Poupart's ligament. SYN: *fossa ovalis*.

saphenous vein One of two superficial veins, the great and small, passing up the leg. The great saphenous vein extends from the foot to the saphenous opening; the small vein runs behind the outer malleolus up the back of the leg, joining the popliteal vein. SYN: *saphena*.

saponification (să-pŏn″ĭ-fĭ-kā′shŭn) [L. *sapo,* soap, + *facere,* to make] **1.** Conversion into soap; chemically, the hydrolysis or the splitting of fat by an alkali yielding glycerol and three molecules of alkali salt of the fatty acid, the soap. **2.** In chemistry, hydrolysis of an ester into its corresponding alcohol and acid (free or in the form of a salt).

s. number In analysis of fats, the number of milligrams of potassium hydroxide needed to saponify 1 g of oil or fat.

saponify (să-pŏn′ĭ-fī) To convert into a soap, as when fats are treated with an alkali to produce a free alcohol plus the salt of the fatty acid. Thus, stearin, saponified with sodium hydroxide, yields the alcohol glycerol plus the soap sodium stearate.

saponin (săp′ō-nĭn) [Fr. *saponine,* soap] An unabsorbable glucoside contained in the roots of some plants that forms a lather in an aqueous solution. Saponins cause hemolysis of red blood cells even in high dilutions. When taken orally, they may cause diarrhea and vomiting. Mixtures of saponins are used as laboratory reagents to hemolyze specimens before analysis.

sapophore (săp′ō-for) [L. *sapor,* taste, + Gr. *phoros,* bearing] The component of a molecule that gives a substance its taste.

saporific (săp″ō-rĭf′ĭk) [NL. *saporificus,* producing taste] Imparting or affecting a taste or flavor.

sapphism (săf′ĭzm) [Sappho, Gr. poetess, 7th-century B.C.] Lesbianism.

sapro- Combining form meaning *putrid, rotten*.

saprobe (să′prōb) [Gr. *sapros,* putrid, + *bios,* life] Saprophyte. **saprobic,** *adj.*

saprogenic (săp″rō-jĕn′ĭk) Causing putrefaction, or resulting from it.

saprophilous (săp-rŏf′ĭl-ŭs) [Gr. *sapros,* putrid, + *philein,* to love] Living on decaying or dead substances, as a microorganism.

saprophyte (săp′rō-fīt) [″ + *phyton,* plant] Any organism living on decaying or dead organic matter. Most of the higher fungi are saprophytes. SYN: *saprobe.* SEE: *parasite.* **saprophytic** (fĭt′ĭk), *adj.*

saquinavir A protease inhibitor that, in combination with other antiretroviral drugs (e.g., zidovudine), is used to treat HIV infection.

Sarcina (săr′sĭ-nă) [L., bundle] A genus of spherical saprophytic bacteria of the family Micrococcaceae. The individual organisms remain adherent to each other after splitting in three planes.

sarcina (săr′sĭ-nă) *pl.* **sarcinas sarcinae** Any organism of the genus *Sarcina.* SEE: *bacteria* for illus.

sarcitis (săr-sī′tĭs) [Gr. *sarx,* flesh, + *itis,* inflammation] Inflammation of muscle tissue. SYN: *myositis.*

sarco- Combining form meaning *flesh.*

sarcoadenoma (săr″kō-ăd″ĕn-ō′mă) [Gr. *sarx,* flesh, + *aden,* gland, + *oma,* tumor] A fleshy tumor of a gland. SYN: *adenosarcoma.*

sarcocarcinoma (săr″kō-kăr″sĭn-ō′mă) [″ + *karkinos,* crab, + *oma,* tumor] A malignant tumor of sarcomatous and carcinomatous types.

sarcocele (săr′kō-sēl) [″ + *kele,* tumor, swelling] A fleshy tumor of the testicle.

sarcocyst (săr′kō-sĭst) [″ + *kystis,* bladder] An elongated tubular body produced by *Sarcocystis.*

Sarcocystis (săr″kō-sĭs′tĭs) [″ + *kystis,* bladder] A genus of sporozoa found in the muscles of higher vertebrates (reptiles, birds, and mammals).

S. lindemanni A species infesting the muscles of humans, causing myositis, eosinophilia, and fever.

Sarcodina (săr-kō-dī′nă) [″ + *eidos,* form, shape] A subphylum of protozoa that includes the order Amoebida. It is characterized by pseudopod locomotion.

sarcoid (săr′koyd) [″ + *eidos,* form, shape] **1.** Resembling flesh. **2.** A small epithelioid tubercle-like lesion characteristic of sarcoidosis.

sarcoidosis (săr″koyd-ō′sĭs) [″ + ″ + *osis,* condition] A chronic multisystem disease of unknown etiology, characterized by noncaseating (hard) granulomas and lymphocytic alveolitis. Sarcoidosis occurs most often in the southeastern U.S., is 10 times more common in blacks than whites, and is more common in women than men. SEE: illus.

SYMPTOMS: The lungs are involved in 90% of cases of sarcoidosis, and are the basis for the initial symptoms of fatigue, weight loss, anorexia, night sweats, shortness of breath, and a nonproductive cough. Hilar lymphadenopathy may precede the development of respiratory symptoms from alveolitis. Peripheral lymphadenopathy, iritis, skin lesions, splenomegaly, hepatomegaly, interstitial nephritis, peritoneal disease, involvement of other visceral organs, and skeletal changes are seen in patients with widespread disease. Immunological abnormalities include T-cell lymphocytopenia, increased blood monocyte count, and anergic reactions to skin tests for common allergens. In approx. 60% to 70% of patients, no permanent damage to the lungs or other organs occurs. Approx. 20% develop residual lung or eye damage, and 10% die of progressive pulmonary fibrosis or associated right-sided heart failure (cor pulmonale).

DIAGNOSIS: Diagnosis is made through a combination of clinical, radiographical, and histological findings. Sarcoidosis must be differentiated from other diseases that cause granulomas, such as tuberculosis, histoplasmosis, and some other fungal infections.

TREATMENT: Sarcoidosis may progress insidiously or rapidly or may remit as the result of treatment with corticosteroids.

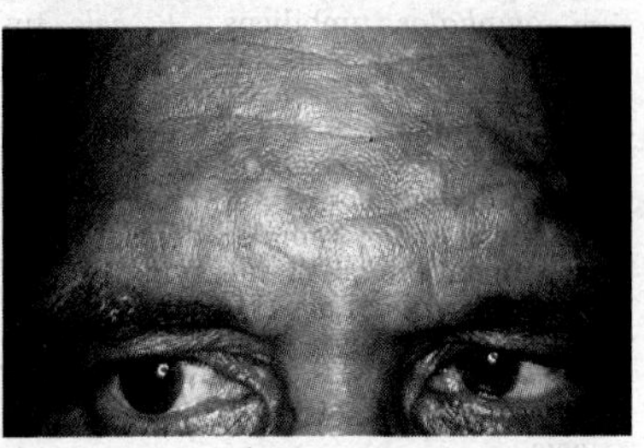

SARCOIDOSIS

sarcolemma (săr″kō-lĕm′ă) [″ + *lemma,* husk] The cell membrane of a muscle cell. Invaginations called transverse tubules (T-tubules) penetrate the cytoplasm adjacent to the myofibrils and carry the action potential to the interior of the muscle cell.

sarcology (săr-kŏl′ō-jē) [″ + *logos,* word, reason] The branch of medicine dealing with study of the soft tissues of the body.

sarcolysis (săr-kŏl′ĭ-sĭs) [″ + *lysis,* dissolution] Decomposition of the soft tissues or flesh.

sarcoma (săr-kō′mă) *pl.* **sarcomata** [″ + *oma,* tumor] A cancer arising from mesenchymal tissue such as muscle or bone, which may affect the bones, bladder, kidneys, liver, lungs, parotids, and spleen. SEE: *Kaposi's sarcoma.*

alveolar soft part s. A malignant neoplasm that usually affects teen-agers, composed of a reticular stroma of connective tissue surrounding clumps of large round cells.

botryoid s. A rare malignant connective tissue tumor occurring in the uterus, bladder, vagina, liver, or biliary tree. SYN: *rhabdosarcoma, embryonal.*

endometrial s. A malignant neoplasm of the endometrial stroma.

giant-cell s. Giant cell tumor.

osteogenic s. A sarcoma composed of bony tissue. It is the most common bony cancer and typically afflicts adolescents.

reticulum cell s. A rare form of malignant large cell lymphoma.

spindle cell s. A sarcoma consisting of small and large spindle-shaped cells.

sarcomatoid (sar-kō′mă-toyd) [Gr. *sarx,* flesh, + *oma,* tumor, + *eidos,* form, shape] Resembling a sarcoma.

sarcomatosis (săr″kō-mă-tō′sĭs) [″ + ″ + *osis,* condition] A condition marked by the presence and spread of a sarcoma; sarcomatous degeneration.

sarcomatous (săr-kō′mă-tŭs) Of the nature of, or like, a sarcoma.

sarcomere (săr′kō-mēr) [″ + *meros,* a part] The contraction unit of the myofibrils of muscle tissue, made of myosin and actin filaments arranged between two Z disks.

sarcomphalocele (săr″kŏm-făl′ō-sēl) [″ + *omphalos,* umbilicus, + *kele,* tumor, swelling] A fleshy tumor of the umbilicus.

Sarcophagidae (săr″kō-făj′ĭ-dē) [Gr. *sarx,* flesh, + *phagein,* to eat] The family of the order Diptera that includes the flesh flies. Females deposit their eggs or larvae on the decaying flesh of dead animals. Larvae of two genera, *Sarcophaga* and *Wohlfahrtia,* frequently infest open sores and wounds of humans, giving rise to cutaneous myiasis.

sarcoplasm (săr′kō-plăzm) [″ + LL. *plasma,* form, mold] The cytoplasm of muscle cells, esp. striated muscle cells.

sarcoplasmic (săr″kō-plăz′mĭk) Concerning or containing sarcoplasm.

Sarcoptes (săr-kŏp′tēz) A genus of Acarina that includes the mites that infest humans and animals. *Sarcoptes scabiei* causes scabies in humans. SEE: illus.

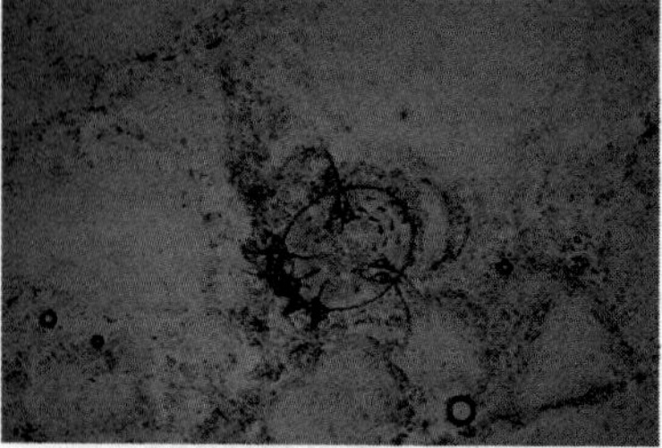

SARCOPTES SCABIEI

Sarcoptidae (săr-kŏp′tĭ-dē) A family of mites of the order Acarina, class Arachnida, that includes *Sarcoptes scabiei,* the causative agent of scabies or itch in humans and of mange and scab in other animals.

sarcosis (săr-kō′sĭs) [″ + *osis,* condition] Abnormal formation of flesh.

sarcosome (săr′kō-sōm) [″ + *soma,* body] Former term for *mitochondria,* particularly of muscle cells.

Sarcosporidia (săr″kō-spō-rĭd′ē-ă) [″ + *sporos,* a seed] An order of protozoa that belong to the class Sporozoa and are parasitic in the muscles of higher vertebrates. It includes the genus *Sarcocystis.*

sarcosporidiosis (săr″kō-spō-rĭd″ē-ō′sĭs) [″ + ″ + *osis,* condition] Infestation with organisms of the order Sarcosporidia or the condition produced by them.

sarcostosis (săr″kŏs-tō′sĭs) [″ + *osteon,* bone, + *osis,* condition] Ossification of fleshy or muscular tissue.

sarcostyle (săr′kō-stīl) [″ + *stylos,* a column] Former term for myofibril.

sarcotubule (săr″kō-tū′būl) Term previously used for the sarcoplasmic reticulum of striated muscle cells.

sarcous (săr′kŭs) [Gr. *sarko,* flesh] Concerning flesh or muscle.

sarin (GB) Isopropylmethylphosphonofluoridate; an extremely toxic nerve gas.

SART *Sexual Assault Response Team.*

sartorius (săr-tō′rē-ŭs) [L. *sartor,* tailor] A long, ribbon-shaped muscle in the leg that flexes, abducts, laterally rotates the thigh, and flexes the lower leg. This muscle, the longest in the body, enables the crossing of the legs in the tailor's position, the function for which it is named.

sashimi A traditional Japanese food made of raw fish usually served as an appetizer. It can occasionally be a source of food-borne toxins or infections.

sat *saturated.*

satellite (săt′l-īt) [L. *satelles,* attendant] A small structure attached to a larger one, esp. a minute body attached to a chromosome by a slender chromatin filament.

bacterial s. A bacterial colony that grows best when close to a colony of another microorganism.

satellitosis (săt″l-ī-tō′sĭs) [″ + Gr. *osis,* condition] The accumulation of neuroglial cells about neurons of the central nervous system. This condition is seen in certain degenerative and inflammatory conditions.

satiety (sā-tī′ĕt-ē) [L. *satietas,* enough] Being full to satisfaction, esp. with food.

saturated (săt′ū-rā″tĕd) [L. *saturare,* to fill] Holding all that can be absorbed, received, or combined, as a solution in which no more of a substance can be dissolved. This term is applied to hydrocarbons in which the maximum number of hydrogen atoms is present and there are no double or triple bonds between the carbon atoms. It is also applied to the hemoglobin-oxygen complex found in red blood cells when no more oxygen can reversibly bind to the hemoglobin.

saturated compound An organic compound with all carbon bonds filled. It does not contain double or triple bonds. SEE: *unsaturated compound*.

saturated hydrocarbon A carbon-hydrogen compound with all carbon bonds filled so there are no double or triple bonds. SEE: *polyunsaturated*.

saturation (săt″ū-rā′shŭn) **1.** State in which all of a substance that can be dissolved in a solution is dissolved. Adding more of the substance will not increase the concentration. **2.** In organic chemistry, to have all available carbon atom valences satisfied so that there are no double or triple bonds between the carbon atoms.

saturation index In hematology, the amount of hemoglobin present in a known volume of blood compared with the normal.

saturation, oxygen The saturation of the arterial blood with oxygen, expressed as a percentage. SaO_2 can be monitored noninvasively with a pulse oximeter. It is normally greater than 96%.

saturation time The time required for the arterial blood of a person inhaling pure oxygen to become saturated.

saturnine (săt′ŭr-nīn) [L. *saturnus*, lead] Concerning or produced by lead.

saturnine breath Sweet breath produced by lead poisoning.

saturnism (săt′ŭr-nĭzm) [″ + Gr. *-ismos*, condition] Lead poisoning. SYN: *plumbism*.

satyriasis (săt-ĭ-rī′ă-sĭs) [LL.] An excessive, and often uncontrollable, sexual drive in men. SYN: *satyromania*. SEE: *nymphomania*.

satyromania (săt″ĭ-rō-mā′nē-ă) Satyriasis.

saucerization (saw″sĕr-ĭ-zā′shŭn) The creation of a shallow area in tissue surgically to remove devitalized tissue and to facilitate drainage.

sauna An enclosure in which a person is exposed to moderate to very high temperatures and often high humidity, produced by water poured on heated stones. A stay in the sauna may be followed by a cool bath or shower. Sauna water is not sterile and may contain harmful microorganisms, including yeasts and molds. Even though the sauna has no proven benefits in preventing illnesses or promoting fitness, the regimen does help to promote relaxation, relieve aches and pains, and loosen stiff joints.

CAUTION: Saunas are not advised for those with fever, those who are dehydrated, or those who are unable to sweat. Those who have recently used alcohol or have participated in strenuous exercise should not use a sauna. If soft tissue has been traumatized in the past 24 to 48 hr, the sauna should not be used. Prolonged exposure to the sauna may be dangerous due to induced hyperpyrexia, dehydration, and renal failure.

---

savings account, medical A form of savings account in which deposits may accumulate tax-free and be used as a form of self-financed health insurance to pay incurred or anticipated medical expenses.

saw [AS. *sagu*] A cutting instrument with an edge of sharp toothlike projections; used esp. for cutting bone in surgery.

saw palmetto A low-growing, spreading palm (*Serenoa repens*) native to Florida and the coastal southeastern U.S. whose extract is used by alternative and complementary medicine practitioners to treat benign prostatic hyperplasia.

saxifragant (săks-ĭf′ră-gănt) [L. *saxum*, rock, + *frangere*, to break] Dissolving or breaking stones, esp. in the bladder.

saxitoxin (săk″sĭ-tŏk′sĭn) A paralytic shellfish toxin obtained from some forms of marine life, including mussels, clams, and plankton. It is the active ingredient in paralytic shellfish poisoning. If ingested, saxitoxin can produce death in hours; if inhaled, it can be lethal in minutes.

Sayre's jacket (sārz) [Lewis Albert Sayre, U.S. surgeon, 1820–1900] A jacket of plaster of Paris formerly used to support the spine in vertebral diseases.

Sb Symbol for the element antimony.

$SbCl_3$ Antimony trichloride.

SBE *subacute bacterial endocarditis*.

Sb_2O_5 Antimonic oxide; antimony pentoxide.

Sb_4O_6 Antimonious oxide.

Sc Symbol for the element scandium.

s.c. *subcutaneously*.

scab (skăb) [ME. *scabbe*] **1.** Crust of a cutaneous sore, wound, ulcer, or pustule formed by drying of the discharge. **2.** To become covered with a crust.

scabicide (skā′bĭ-sīd) An agent that kills mites, esp. the causative agent of scabies. SYN: *scabieticide*.

scabies (skā′bēz) [L. *scabies*, itch] A contagious infestation of the skin with the itch mite, *Sarcoptes scabiei*. It typically presents as an intensely pruritic rash, composed of scaly papules, insect burrows, and secondarily infected lesions distributed in the webs between the fingers and on the waistline, trunk (esp. the axillae), penis, and arms. It readily spreads in households, among playmates, and between sexual partners—that is, among people having close physical contact. SEE: illus.; *Nursing Diagnoses Appendix*. **scabietic** (-ĕt′ĭk), *adj*.

SYMPTOMS: An itchy rash that worsens at night and that involves multiple members of the same household is a common presentation.

DIAGNOSIS: Because the disease is often missed and occasionally overdiagnosed, scrapings from suspect lesions are examined microscopically to confirm the presence of the mite, its eggs, or its excretions.

TREATMENT: For children 2 months and older and nonpregnant adults, permethrin 5% cream is applied to the entire body surface, avoiding the eyes and the mouth. The cream is thoroughly washed off after about 8 to 14 hr. Retreatment is sometimes required in 14 days. Pregnant women and infants under 2 months of age should be treated with 6% precipitated sulfur in petrolatum, daily for 3 days.

Norwegian s. A rare form of scabies in which the mites are present in great number. It often is found in patients with human immunodeficiency virus infection. Ivermectin is used to treat the infestation.

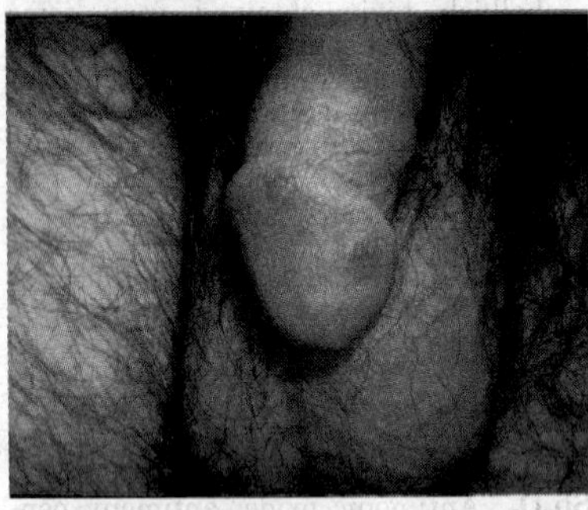

SCABIES

scabieticide (skā″bē-ĕt′ĭ-sīd) [″ + *cidus,* killing] Scabicide.

scabiphobia (skă″bĭ-fō′bē-ă) [″ + Gr. *phobos,* fear] An abnormal fear of acquiring scabies.

scabrities (skā-brĭsh′ē-ēz) [L. *scaber,* rough] A scaly, roughened condition of the skin.

s. unguium Morbid degeneration of the nails, making them rough, thick, distorted, and separated from the flesh at the root; symptomatic of syphilis and leprosy.

scala (skā′lă) [L. *scala,* staircase] Any one of the three spiral passages of the cochlea of the inner ear.

s. media The cochlear duct, the duct that contains the spiral organ of Corti. It is between the scala tympani below and the scala vestibuli above, contains endolymph, and extends from the saccule to the tip of the cochlea.

s. tympani The duct filled with perilymph that is below the organ of Corti. It extends from the round window to the tip of the cochlea.

s. vestibuli The duct filled with perilymph that is above the organ of Corti. It extends from the oval window to the tip of the cochlea, where it communicates with the scala tympani through an aperture, the helicotrema.

scald (skŏld) [ME. *scalden,* to burn with hot liquid] **1.** A burn of the skin or flesh caused by moist heat and hot vapors, as steam. **2.** To cause a burn with hot liquid or steam.

When the heat applied is approx. equivalent, a scald is deeper than a burn from dry heat. Healing is slower and scar formation greater in scalds. Emergency treatment of a scalded area should include immediate application of cold in the most readily available form, (i.e., ice packs or immersion of the part in very cold water). This should be continued for at least 1 hr.

scalded skin syndrome, staphylococcal Infection and inflammation of the outer layers of skin, predominantly but not exclusively found in children, elderly persons, and immunosuppressed patients. It is caused by exotoxins produced by *Staphylococcus aureus*. Initially, the skin in the affected areas is rough, with a bright red, flat rash; it then becomes wrinkled, and blisters form. The syndrome is treated with antistaphylococcal antibiotics (e.g., nafcillin), and supportive care is provided to minimize the risk of cellulitis or pneumonia. About 2% to 3% of affected patients die of the disease. In survivors, the blisters heal without scarring.

TREATMENT: Beta-lactamase–resistant synthetic penicillin is given. The bullae and denuded skin should be treated symptomatically. Uncomplicated lesions heal without scarring.

scale (skāl) [O.Fr. *escale,* husk] **1.** A small dry flake, shed from the upper layers of skin. Some shedding of skin is normal; scale increases in diseases like pityriasis rosea, psoriasis, and tinea pedis, and after scratching the skin. **2.** A film of tartar encrusting the teeth. **3.** To remove a film of tartar from the teeth. **4.** To form a scale on. **5.** To shed scales.

scale (skāl) [ME. *scole,* balance] An instrument for weighing. SEE: illus.

scale (skāl) [L. *scala,* staircase] A graduated or proportioned measure, a series of tests, or an instrument for measuring quantities or for rating some individual intelligence characteristics.

absolute s. Scale used for indicating low temperatures based on absolute zero. SYN: *Kelvin scale*. SEE: *absolute temperature; absolute zero.*

Borg's dyspnea s. SEE: *Borg's dyspnea scale.*

Braden s. SEE: *Braden scale.*

centigrade s. Celsius scale.

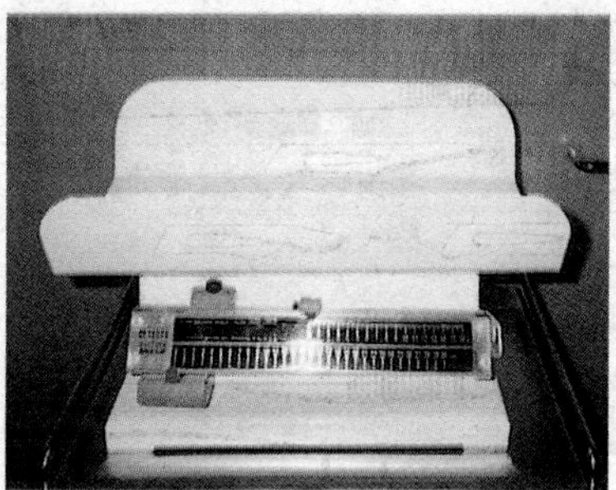

SCALE FOR INFANTS

s. of contrast The range of densities on a radiograph; the number of tonal grays that are visible.

hydrogen ion s. A scale used to express the degree of acidity or alkalinity of a solution. It extends from 0.00 (total acidity) to 14 (total alkalinity), the numbers running in inverse order of hydrogen ion concentration. The pH value is the negative logarithm of the hydrogen ion concentration of a solution, expressed in moles per liter.

As the hydrogen ion concentration decreases, a change of 1 pH unit means a 10-fold decrease in hydrogen ion concentration. Thus a solution with a pH of 1.0 is 10 times more acid than one with a pH of 2.0 and 100 times more acid than one with a pH of 3.0. A pH of 7.0 indicates neutrality.

As the hydrogen ion concentration varies in a definite reciprocal manner with the hydroxyl ion (OH^-) concentration, a pH reading above 7.0 indicates alkalinity. In the human body, arterial blood is slightly alkaline, having a normal pH range of 7.35 to 7.45. SEE: *pH.*

Norton s. SEE: *Norton scale.*

Numerical Rating S. ABBR: NRS. Visual analog scale.

visual analog s. An instrument used to quantify a subjective experience, such as the intensity of pain. A commonly used visual analog scale is a 10-cm line labeled with "worst pain imaginable" on the left border and "no pain" on the right border. The patient is instructed to make a mark along the line to represent the intensity of pain currently being experienced. The clinician records the distance of the mark in centimeters from the right end of the scale.

scalene (skā-lēn′) [Gr. *skalenos,* uneven] **1.** Having unequal sides and angles, said of a triangle. **2.** Designating a scalenus muscle.

s. tubercle Lisfranc's tubercle.

scalenectomy (skā″lĕ-nĕk′tō-mē) [″ + *ektome,* excision] Resection of any of the scalenus muscles.

scaleniotomy (skā-lēn″ē-ŏt′ō-mē) [″ + *tome,* incision] Incision of scalenus muscles near their insertion to check expansive movements in tuberculosis of the apex of the lung.

scalenotomy (skā″lĕ-nŏt′ō-mē) [″ + *tome,* incision] Surgical division of one or more of the scalenus muscles.

scalenus (skā-lē′nŭs) [L., uneven] One of three deeply situated muscles on each side of the neck, extending from the tubercles of the transverse processes of the third through sixth cervical vertebrae to the first or second rib. The three muscles are the scalenus anterior (anticus), medius, and posterior.

scalenus syndrome A symptom complex characterized by brachial neuritis with or without vascular or vasomotor disturbance in the upper extremities. Also called *scalenus anticus syndrome.*

SYMPTOMS: The symptoms include pain, tingling, and numbness anywhere from the shoulder to the fingers. Small muscles of the hand or even the deltoid or other muscles of the arm atrophy.

TREATMENT: The posture should be corrected, and sometimes the arm and shoulder are immobilized. When relief is not obtained, surgical correction may be required.

scaler (skā′lĕr) [O.Fr. *escale,* husk] **1.** A dental instrument used to remove calculus from teeth. **2.** A device for counting pulses detected by a radiation detector.

ultrasonic s. A device that uses high-frequency vibration to remove stains and adherent deposits on the teeth.

scaling (skāl′ĭng) [O.Fr. *escale,* husk] The removal of calculus from the teeth.

scall (skawl) [Norse *skalli,* baldhead] Dermatitis of the scalp producing a crusted scabby eruption.

scalp (skălp) [ME., sheath] The hairy integument of the head. In anatomy, this includes the skin, dense subcutaneous tissue, occipitofrontalis muscle with the galea aponeurotica, loose subaponeurotic tissue, and cranial periosteum.

scalpel (skăl′pĕl) [L. *scalpellum,* knife] A small, straight surgical knife with a convex edge and thin keen blade. SEE: illus.

harmonic s. A tool for excising and coagulating tissue, using a higher frequency (55,000 Hz) than that of the ultrasonic scalpel; this energy breaks hydrogen bonds in tissue, resulting in the dissection or coaptation of blood vessels. The harmonic scalpel facilitates many surgeries (e.g., thorascopic internal mammary artery harvesting). In most surgical applications, tissue destruction is minimal, but when coagulating larger vessels hemostasis is not as effective as with other modalities, even at maximal power. When a blade-extender sheath is used with the scalpel, there is an increased possibility of damage to tissue that extends beyond the sheath.

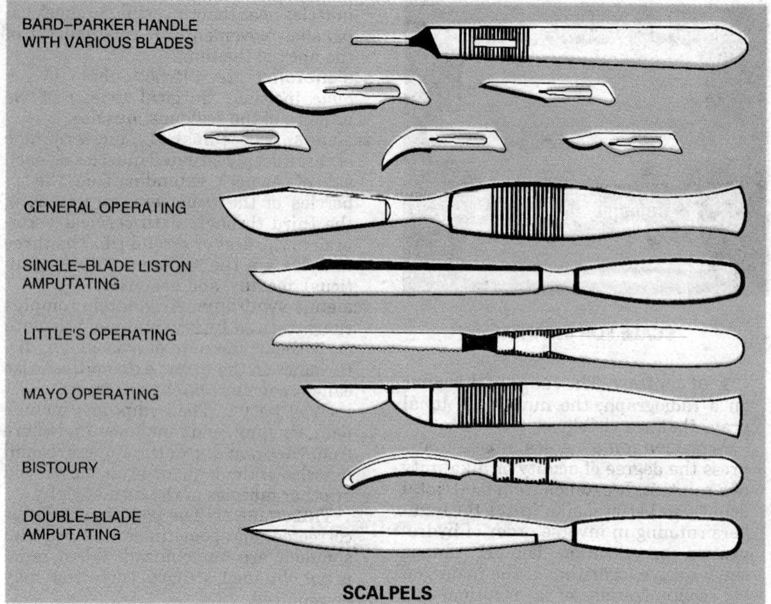

SCALPELS

scalpriform (skăl′prĭ-form) [L. *scalprum,* knife, + *forma,* shape] Shaped like a chisel.

scalprum (skăl′prŭm) *pl.* **scalpra** [L., knife] **1.** A toothed instrument for removal of carious bone or for trephining. **2.** A large scalpel. **3.** The cutting edge of an incisor tooth.

scalp tourniquet A tourniquet applied to the scalp during I.V. administration of antineoplastic drugs to restrict blood flow to the hair-bearing portion of the scalp. This procedure helps prevent the cranial alopecia that may accompany the chemotherapy used to treat certain types of cancer.

scaly (skā′lē) [O.Fr. *escale,* husk] Resembling or characterized by scales.

scan 1. An image obtained from a system that compiles information in a sequence pattern, such as computed tomography, ultrasound, or magnetic resonance imaging. **2.** Scintiscan.

DEXA s. *Dual-energy x-ray absorptiometry scan.*

dual-energy x-ray absorptiometry s. ABBR: DEXA scan. An imaging procedure used to quantify bone density in the diagnosis and management of osteoporosis.

ventilation/perfusion s. V/Q s.

V/Q s. An imaging procedure used in the diagnosis of pulmonary embolism. The procedure has two parts: (1) the injection of microscopic spheres into the bloodstream to evaluate perfusion of the lung, then (2) the inhalation of xenon gas to assess pulmonary aeration. Certain patterns of mismatching between ventilation and perfusion of the lung are considered diagnostic of pulmonary embolism. SYN: *ventilation/perfusion s.*

scandium [L. *Scandia,* Scandinavia] SYMB: Sc. A rare metal belonging to the aluminum group; atomic weight 44.956; atomic number 21.

scanning 1. Recording on an image receptor the emission of radioactive waves from a specific substance injected into the body. The radioactive agent selected is concentrated in a specific tissue, such as thyroid, brain, or liver. **2.** The process of obtaining different images of a specified anatomical part through a system that compiles information in a sequential pattern, such as computed tomography, ultrasound, or magnetic resonance imaging.

radioisotope s. Recording of gamma ray photons from radioisotopes that have been introduced into tissue, usually by chemical bonding with a drug that targets the tissue or organ of interest. The scanner can be moved around the site and a multiview image obtained.

scanty (skăn′tē) [ME. from O. Norse, *skamt,* short] Not abundant; insufficient, as a secretion.

scapha (skā′fă) [NL., skiff] An elongated depression of the ear between the helix and antihelix. SYN: *scaphoid fossa.*

scapho- Combining form meaning *boat-shaped.*

scaphocephalism (skăf″ō-sĕf′ăl-ĭzm) [″ + ″ + *-ismos,* condition] Condition of having a deformed head, projecting like

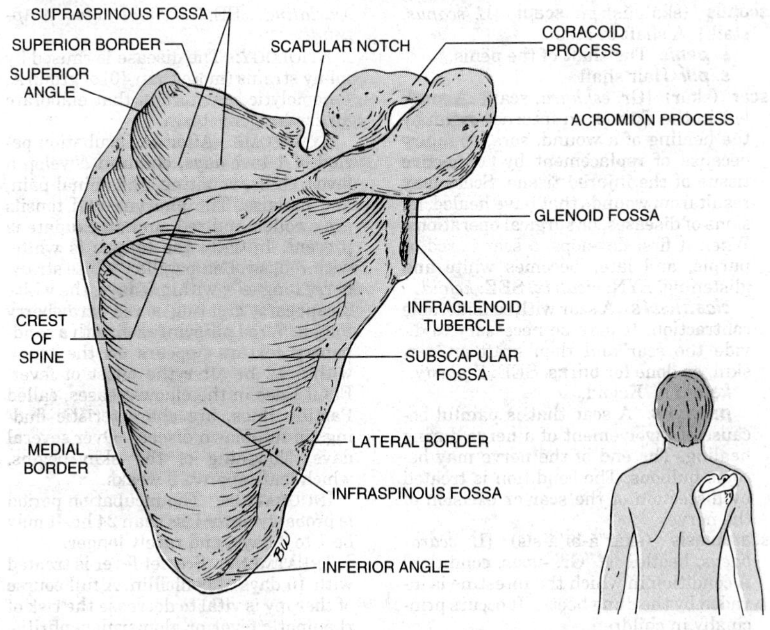

SCAPULA

the keel of a boat. SYN: *scaphocephaly*.
scaphocephalic (-ăl′ĭk), *adj.*

scaphocephalous (skăf″ō-sĕf′ă-lŭs) [″ + *kephale,* head] SEE: *scaphocephalism*.

scaphocephaly (skăf″ō-sĕf′ă-lē) [″ + *kephale,* head] Scaphocephalism.

scaphohydrocephaly (skăf″ō-hī″drō-sĕf′ă-lē) [″ + *hydor,* water, + *kephale,* head] Hydrocephalus combined with scaphocephalism.

scaphoid (skăf′oyd) [″ + *eidos,* form, shape] **1.** Boat-shaped, navicular, hollowed. **2.** A proximal boat-shaped bone of the carpus. SYN: *os scaphoideum*.

scaphoid fossa Scapha.

scaphoiditis (skăf″oyd-ī′tĭs) [″ + ″ + *itis,* inflammation] Inflammation of the scaphoid bone.

scapula [L., shoulder blade] The large, flat, triangular bone that forms the posterior part of the shoulder. It articulates with the clavicle and the humerus. SYN: *shoulder blade*. SEE: illus.; *triceps*.

plane of s. The angle of the scapula in its resting position, normally 30° to 45° forward from the frontal plane toward the sagittal plane. Movement of the humerus in this plane is less restricted than in the frontal or sagittal planes because the capsule is not twisted.

tipped s. A condition in which the inferior angle of the scapula is prominent, usually the result of faulty posture and a tight pectoralis minor muscle. Tipping is a normal motion when a person reaches with the hand behind the back.

winged s. Condition in which the medial border of the scapula is prominent, usually the result of paralysis of the serratus anterior or trapezius muscles. SYN: *angel's wing*.

scapular (skăp′ū-lăr) Of, or pert. to, the shoulder blade.

scapulary (skăp′ū-lā-rē) A shoulder bandage for keeping a body bandage in place. A broad roller bandage is split in half. The undivided section of the roller bandage is fastened in front with the two ends passing over the shoulders and attached to the back of the body bandage.

scapulectomy (skăp″ū-lĕk′tō-mē) [L. *scapula,* shoulder blade, + Gr. *ektome,* excision] Surgical excision of the scapula.

scapulo- Combining form meaning *shoulder*.

scapuloclavicular (skăp″ū-lō-klă-vĭk′ū-lar) [L. *scapula,* shoulder blade, + *clavicula,* little key] Concerning the scapula and clavicle.

scapulodynia (skăp″ū-lō-dĭn′ē-ă) [″ + *odyne,* pain] Inflammation and pain in the shoulder muscles.

scapulohumeral (skăp″ū-lō-hū′mĕr-ăl) [″ + *humerus,* upper arm] Concerning the scapula and humerus.

scapulopexy (skăp″ū-lō-pĕk′sē) [″ + Gr. *pexis,* fixation] Fixation of the scapula to the ribs.

scapulothoracic (skăp″ū-lō-thō-răs′ĭk) [″ + Gr. *thorax,* chest] Concerning the scapula and thorax.

scapus (skā'pŭs) *pl.* **scapi** [L. *scapus,* stalk] A shaft or stem.

s. penis The shaft of the penis.

s. pili Hair shaft.

scar (skăr) [Gr. *eskhara,* scab] A mark left in the skin or an internal organ by the healing of a wound, sore, or injury because of replacement by connective tissue of the injured tissue. Scars may result from wounds that have healed, lesions of diseases, or surgical operations. When it first develops, a scar is red or purple, and later becomes white and glistening. SYN: *cicatrix*. SEE: *keloid*.

cicatricial s. A scar with considerable contraction. It may be necessary to divide the scar and then graft on new skin, as done for burns. SEE: *Z-plasty*.

keloid s. Keloid.

painful s. A scar that is painful because of involvement of a nerve during healing. The end of the nerve may become bulbous. The condition is treated by dissection of the scar or excision of the nerve.

scarabiasis (skăr"ă-bī'ă-sĭs) [L. *scarabaeus,* beetle, + Gr. *-iasis,* condition] A condition in which the intestine is invaded by the dung beetle. It occurs principally in children.

Scarf sign A newborn assessment finding in which the infant's elbow crosses the body midline without resistance as the examiner draws the arm across the chest to the opposite shoulder. This is characteristic of preterm infants born before 30 weeks gestation.

scarification (skăr"ĭ-fĭ-kā'shŭn) [Gr. *skariphismos,* scratching up] The making of numerous superficial incisions in the skin.

scarificator (skăr'ĭf-ĭ-kā"tor) An instrument used for making small incisions in the skin. SYN: *scarifier*.

scarifier Scarificator.

scarlatina (skăr"lă-tē'nă) [NL., red] Scarlet fever.

s. anginosa A severe form of scarlatina with extensive necrosis and ulceration of the pharynx, and in some cases peritonsillar abscess.

s. hemorrhagica Scarlatina with hemorrhage into the skin and mucous membranes.

s. maligna A fulminant and usually lethal form of scarlatina. **scarlatinal** (-năl), *adj.*

scarlatiniform (skăr-lă-tĭn'ĭ-form) [L. *scarlatina,* red, + *forma,* shape] Resembling scarlatina or its rash.

scarlatinoid (skăr-lăt'ĭ-noyd) [" + Gr. *eidos,* form, shape] Resembling scarlet fever.

scarlet fever [L. *scarlatum,* red] An acute, contagious disease characterized by pharyngitis and a pimply red rash. It is caused by group A beta-hemolytic streptococcus and usually affects children between the ages of 3 and 15. SYN: *scarlatina*. SEE: *Nursing Diagnoses Appendix*.

ETIOLOGY: The disease is caused by many strains (more than 40) of group A, β-hemolytic streptococci that elaborate an erythrogenic toxin.

SYMPTOMS: After an incubation period of 1 to 7 days, children develop a fever, chills, vomiting, abdominal pain, and malaise. The pharynx and tonsils are swollen and red, and an exudate is present. Initially the tongue is white, with red, swollen papilla ("white strawberry tongue"); within 5 days, the white disappears, creating a red strawberry tongue. A red pinpoint rash with a sandpapery texture appears on the trunk within 12 hr after the onset of fever. Faint lines in the elbow creases, called Pastia's lines, are characteristic findings in full-blown disease. Over several days, sloughing of the skin begins, which lasts approx. 3 weeks.

INCUBATION: The incubation period is probably never less than 24 hr. It may be 1 to 3 days, and rarely longer.

TREATMENT: Scarlet fever is treated with 10 days of penicillin. A full course of therapy is vital to decrease the risk of rheumatic fever or glomerulonephritis. Generally, children are isolated from siblings until they have received penicillin for 24 hr.

PATIENT CARE: Parents of children with scarlet fever are taught about the importance of isolating the patient for at least 24 hr after antibiotic therapy. Good handwashing techniques are emphasized. The parents also are advised about the importance of administering the prescribed antibiotic as directed for the entire course of treatment, even if the child looks and feels better. Because the child may be irritable and restless, the parents are taught methods to encourage bedrest and relaxation. The child should be kept occupied with age-appropriate books, games, toys, and television.

scarlet rash A rose-colored rash, specifically that of German measles.

Scarpa, Antonio (skăr'pă) Italian anatomist, 1752–1832.

S.'s fascia The deep layer of superficial abdominal fascia around the edge of the subcutaneous inguinal ring.

S.'s fluid Fluid in the membranous labyrinth of the ear. SYN: *endolymph*.

S.'s foramen One of the two bony passages opening into the incisor canal for passage of the nasopalatine nerves.

S.'s ganglion The vestibular ganglion.

S.'s membrane The membrane that closes the fenestra rotunda of the tympanic cavity.

S.'s triangle Triangular space bounded laterally by the inner edge of the sartorius, above by Poupart's ligament, and medially by the adductor longus.

SCAT *sheep cell agglutination test.*

scato- Combining form denoting *excrement, fecal matter.* SEE: *sterco-.*

scatologic (skăt″ō-lŏj′ĭk) Concerning fecal matter.

scatology (skă-tŏl′ō-jē) [Gr. *skato-,* dung, + *logos,* word, reason] **1.** Scientific study and analysis of the feces. SYN: *coprology.* **2.** Interest in obscene things, esp. obscene literature.

scatoma (skă-tō′mă) [″ + *oma,* tumor] A mass of inspissated feces in the colon or rectum, resembling an abdominal tumor. SYN: *fecaloma.*

scatophagy (skă-tŏf′ă-jē) Coprophagy.

scatoscopy (skă-tŏs′kō-pē) [″ + *skopein,* to examine] The examination of feces for diagnostic purposes.

scatter (skăt′ĕr) The diffusion of x-rays when they strike an object.

coherent s. An interaction between x-rays and matter in which the incoming photon is absorbed by the atom and leaves with the same energy in a different direction. Fewer than 5% of the interactions between x-rays and matter in tissue are of this type.

scattered radiation X-rays that have changed direction because of a collision with matter.

scattergram (skăt′ĕr-grăm) **1.** A graphical means of displaying information, in which multiple data points, representing the relation between two variables, are clustered. **2.** A graphic interpretation of blood cell populations generated by some types of blood cell analyzers.

scavenger cell (skăv′ĕn-jĕr) [ME. *skawager,* toll collector] A phagocytic cell, such as a macrophage or a neutrophil, that cleans up disintegrating tissues or cells.

SCBA *self-contained breathing apparatus.*

Sc.D. *Doctor of Science* (degree).

SCE *saturated calomel electrode.*

scent (sĕnt) Odor.

Schäffer's reflex (shā′fĕrs) [Max Schäffer, Ger. neurologist, 1852–1923] Dorsiflexion of the toes and flexion of the foot resulting when the middle portion of the Achilles tendon is pinched.

Schatzki ring [Richard Schatzki, U.S. radiologist, 1901–1992] A lower esophageal mucosal ring composed of an annular, thin, weblike tissue located at the squamocolumnar junction at or near the border of the lower esophageal sphincter. When the diameter of the ring is less than 1.3 cm, dysphagia is present. The treatment involves stretching the ring with dilators.

schedule A timetable, usually written; a plan for action to achieve a certain goal.

s. of controlled substances The list of medications whose prescription is limited to and regulated by the controlled substance act.

fee s., fee sheet A list of charges for health care services. Health care providers keep fee schedules in their offices to specify the amount of compensation they want for providing selected services. Managed care organizations and other medical insurance providers publish lists representing the maximum charges they will reimburse for the same services. In many instances, the reimbursement offered by insurers is less than that charged by health care providers.

Scheie's syndrome [Harold Glendon Scheie, U.S. ophthalmologist, 1909–1990] Mucopolysaccharidosis IS.

schema (skē′mă) [Gr., shape] Shape, plan, or outline.

schematic (skē-măt′ĭk) [NL. *schematicus,* shape, figure] Pert. to a diagram or model; showing part for part in a diagram.

scheroma (shē-rō′mă) Xerophthalmia.

Scheuermann's disease [Holger W. Scheuermann, Danish physician, 1877–1960] A spinal deformity with an autosomal dominant inheritance, occurring most commonly in early adolescence, and characterized by a marked thoracolumbar kyphosis (an increased convexity of the back in the thoracic area, sometimes referred to as "roundback"). The incidence is about 0.4%, with no gender preference.

SYMPTOMS: About 50% of patients complain of back pain in the affected area; others complain of poor posture or fatigue. There are usually no neurological symptoms unless cord compression occurs.

DIAGNOSIS: The diagnosis is usually made from clinical presentation and the results of a standing x-ray examination of the spine.

TREATMENT: Symptomatic treatment may include nonsteroidal anti-inflammatory drugs, rest, and activity modification. Plaster casts and braces (including the Milwaukee brace) are used to correct the deformity and are usually successful if the child has not stopped growing. Operative treatment is reserved for those with a significant deformity and those who have stopped growing.

Schick test (shĭk) [Béla Schick, Hungarian-born U.S. pediatrician, 1877–1967] A test to determine the degree of immunity to diphtheria, involving the injection intradermally of 0.1 ml of dilute diphtheria toxin, 1/50 MLD. (MLD: minimum lethal dose, the amount of diphtheria toxin that would kill a small guinea pig in 4 days.) Results are obtained 3 to 4 days later. Susceptibility (positive test result) is indicated by the development of a red inflamed area at the point of injection, which slowly disappears after a few days. A negative test result (little or no reaction) indicates the presence of antibodies sufficient to neutralize the toxin; hence, the person is immune. SEE: *diphtheria*.

Schick test control Inactivated diphtheria toxin for the Schick test. It is used in the Schick test as a control.

Schilder's disease (shĭl′dĕrs) [Paul Ferdinand Schilder, Austrian-U.S. neurologist, 1886–1940] A rare demyelinating disease of the pediatric central nervous system that produces brain lesions that may be confused with intracranial tumors. The lesions may respond to treatment with immunosuppressant drugs.

Schiller's test (shĭl′ĕrs) [Walter Schiller, Austrian-U.S. pathologist, 1887–1960] A test for superficial cancer, esp. of the uterine cervix. The tissue is painted with an iodine solution. Cells lacking glycogen fail to stain, and their presence may indicate a malignant change.

Schilling's classification [Victor Schilling, Ger. hematologist, 1883–1960] A method of classifying polymorphonuclear neutrophils into four categories according to the number and arrangement of the nuclei in the cells.

Schilling test [Robert F. Schilling, U.S. hematologist, b. 1919] A test, using radioactive vitamin B_{12}, that assesses the gastrointestinal absorption of vitamin B_{12} in order to diagnose primary pernicious anemia.

schindylesis (skĭn″dĭ-lē′sĭs) [Gr. *schindylesis,* a splitting] A form of wedge and groove suture in which a crest of one bone fits into a groove of another.

Schiötz tonometer [Hjalamar Schiötz, Norwegian physician, 1850–1927] An instrument for measuring intraocular pressure by the degree of indentation produced by pressure on the cornea.

Schirmer's test [Rudolph Schirmer, Ger. ophthalmologist, 1831–1896] The use of an absorbent paper placed in the conjunctival sac, as a test for patients with ocular irritation and dry eye (e.g., keratoconjunctivitis sicca). The rate and amount of wetting of the paper provide an estimate of tear production.

schisto- (skĭs′tō) Combining form meaning *split, cleft.*

schistocelia (skĭs″tō-sē′lē-ă) [Gr. *schistos,* divided, + *koilia,* belly] A congenital abdominal fissure.

schistocephalus (skĭs″tō-sĕf′ă-lŭs) [″ + *kephale,* head] A fetus with a cleft head.

schistocormia (skĭs″tō-kor′mē-ă) [″ + *kormos,* trunk] A fetus with a cleft trunk.

schistocystis (skĭs″tō-sĭs′tĭs) [″ + *kystis,* bladder] A fissure of the bladder.

schistocyte (skĭs′tō-sīt) [″ + *kytos,* cell] Fragmented red blood cells that appear in a variety of shapes, from small triangular forms to round cells with irregular surfaces. Schistocytes appear in the blood of patients with hemolytic anemias, severe burns, and several other conditions. SYN: *schizocyte.* SEE: illus.

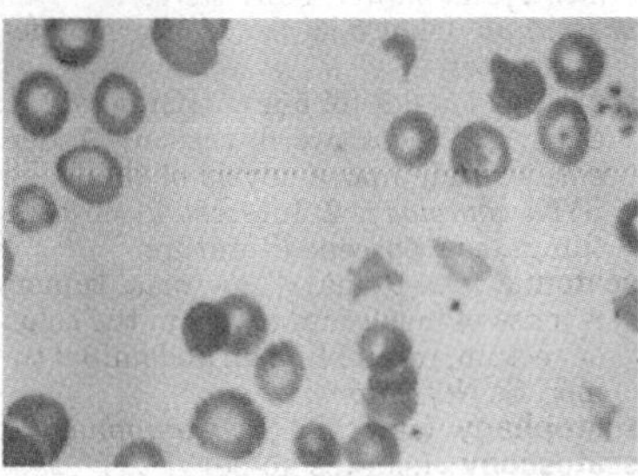

SCHISTOCYTES

In peripheral blood (×600)

schistocytosis (skĭs″tō-sī-tō′sĭs) [″ + ″ + *osis,* condition] Schistocytes in the blood. SYN: *schizocytosis.*

schistoglossia (skĭs″tō-glŏs′ē-ă) [″ + *glossa,* tongue] A cleft tongue.

schistomelus (skĭs-tŏm′ĕ-lŭs) [″ + *melos,* limb] A fetus with a cleft in a limb.

schistoprosopia (skĭs″tō-prō-sō′pē-ă) [″ + *prosopon,* face] A congenital fissure of the face.

schistorachis (skĭs-tor′ă-kĭs) [″ + *rhachis,* spine] Protrusion of membranes through a congenital cleft in the lower vertebral column. SYN: *spina bifida cystica; rachischisis.*

Schistosoma (skĭs″tō-sō′mă) [″ + *soma,* body] A genus of parasitic blood flukes belonging to the family Schistosomatidae, class Trematoda. Adults live in blood vessels of visceral organs. Eggs make their way into the bladder or intestine of the host and are discharged in the urine or feces. Eggs hatch into miracidia, which enter snails and transform into sporocysts. These develop daughter sporocysts, which give rise to fork-tailed cercariae. These leave the snail and enter the final host directly through the skin or mucous membrane. SEE: illus.

S. haematobium A species common in Africa and southwestern Asia. Adults infest the pelvic veins of the vesical plexus. Eggs work their way through the bladder wall of the host and are discharged in the urine. Urinary schistosomiasis is caused by this organism.

S. japonicum A species common in many parts of Asia. Adults live principally in branches of the superior mesenteric vein. Eggs work their way through the intestinal wall of the host into the lumen and are discharged with feces. Oriental schistosomiasis is caused by this species.

S. mansoni A species occurring in many parts of Africa and tropical Amer-

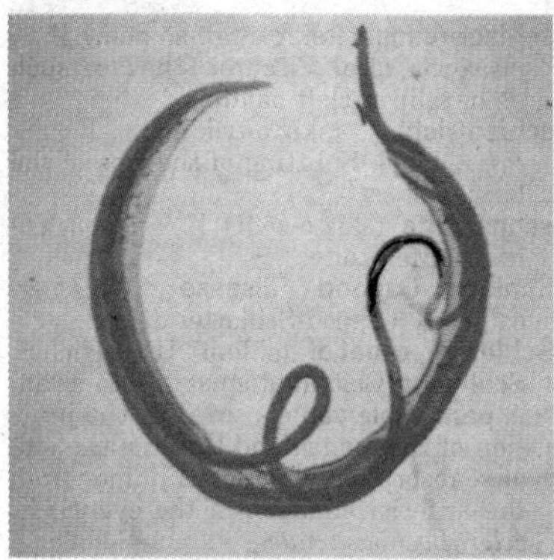

SCHISTOSOMA

Female (larger) and male (×5)

ica, including the West Indies. Adults live in branches of the inferior mesenteric veins. Eggs are discharged through either the host's intestine or bladder. This species causes bilharzial dysentery or Manson's intestinal schistosomiasis.

schistosomia (skĭs″tō-sō′mē-ă) [″ + *soma,* body] A deformed fetus with a fissure in the abdomen. The limbs are rudimentary if present.

schistosomiasis (skĭs″tō-sō-mī′ăs-ĭs) [Gr. *schistos,* divided, + *soma,* body, + *-iasis,* infection] One of several parasitic diseases due to infestation with blood flukes belonging to the genus *Schistosoma*. The flukes may colonize the urinary tract, mesenteries, liver, spleen, or biliary tree, causing symptoms from these organs. Although schistosomiasis rarely is encountered in the U.S., it is endemic throughout Asia, Africa, and South America, as well as some Caribbean islands. An estimated 200 million people are affected worldwide. Infestation occurs by wading or bathing in water contaminated by immature forms of the fluke called cercariae. SYN: *bilharziasis*.

TREATMENT: The drug of choice is praziquantel.

schistosomicide (skĭs″tō-sō′mĭ-sīd) [″ + ″ + L. *cidus,* killing] A drug or toxin that kills parasites of the genus *Schistosoma*.

schistosternia (skĭs″tō-stĕr′nē-ă) [″ + *sternon,* chest] Schistothorax.

schistothorax (skĭs″tō-thō′răks) [″ + *thorax,* chest] A fissure of the thorax. SYN: *schistosternia*.

schistotrachelus (skĭs″tō-tră-kē′lŭs) A fetus with a cleft in the neck.

schizamnion (skĭz-ăm′nē-ŏn) [Gr. *schizein,* to divide, + *amnion,* lamb] An amnion formed by development of a cavity in the inner cell mass.

schizaxon (skĭz-ăk′sŏn) [″ + *axon,* axle] An axon that divides in two equal, or nearly equal, branches.

schizencephaly (skĭz″ĕn-sĕf′ă-lē) [″ + *enkephalos,* brain] A deformed fetus with a longitudinal cleft in the skull.

schizo- (skĭz′ō) Combining form indicating *division*.

schizoblepharia (skĭz″ō-blĕf′ă-rē″ă) [Gr. *schizein,* to split, + *blepharon,* eyelid] A fissure of an eyelid.

schizocyte (skĭz′ō-sīt) [″ + *kytos,* cell] Schistocyte.

schizocytosis (skĭz″ō-sī-tō′sĭs) [″ + ″ + *osis,* condition] Schistocytosis.

schizogenesis (skĭz″ō-jĕn′ĕs-ĭs) [″ + *genesis,* generation, birth] Reproduction by fission.

schizogony (skĭz-ŏg′ō-nē) [″ + *gone,* seed] Reproduction by multiple asexual fission characteristic of sporozoa, esp. the life cycle of the malarial parasite.

schizogyria (skĭz″ō-jī′rē-ă) [″ + *gyros,* a circle] A cleft in the cerebral convolutions.

schizoid (skĭz′oyd) [″ + *eidos,* form, shape] **1.** Severely introverted; socially isolated; lacking close personal relationships or the ability to form them. **2.** Resembling schizophrenia.

schizomycete (skĭz″ō-mī-sēt′) [″ + *mykes,* fungus] Any organism belonging to the class Schizomycetes.

Schizomycetes (skĭz″ō-mī-sē′tēz) [″ + *mykes,* fungus] An obsolete classification, formerly used to denote bacteria.

schizont (skĭz′ŏnt) [″ + *ontos,* being] **1.** A stage appearing in the life cycle of a sporozoan protozoon resulting from multiple division or schizogony. **2.** A stage in the asexual phase of the life cycle of *Plasmodium* organisms found in red blood cells. By schizogony, each gives rise to 12 to 24 or more merozoites. An early schizont is called a *presegmenter;* a mature schizont is called a *rosette* or *segmenter*.

schizonticide (skĭ-zŏn′tĭ-sīd) [″ + ″ + L. *cidus,* killing] Something that destroys schizonts.

schizonychia (skĭz″ō-nĭk′ē-ă) [″ + *onyx,* nail] A split condition of the nails.

schizophasia (skĭz″ō-fā′zē-ă) [″ + *phasis,* speech] Speech marked by looseness of associations and flights of ideas.

schizophrenia (skĭz″ō-frĕn′ē-ă) [Gr. *schizein,* to divide, + *phren,* mind] A common thought disorder affecting about 1% of the population, marked by delusions, hallucinations, and disorganized speech and behavior (the "positive" symptoms) and by flat affect, social withdrawal, and absence of volition (the "negative" symptoms). Schizophrenia involves dysfunction in one or more areas such as interpersonal relations, work or education, or self-care. Associated features include inappropriate affect, anhedonia, dysphoric mood, abnormal psychomotor activity, cognitive dysfunction, confusion, lack of insight, and depersonalization. Abnormal neurological findings may show a broad range of dysfunction including slow reaction time, poor coordination, abnormalities in eye tracking, and impaired sensory gating. Some individuals drink excessive amounts of water (water intoxication) and develop abnormalities in urine specific gravity or electrolyte imbalance. Because none of its clinical features are diagnostic, schizophrenia remains a diagnosis of exclusion. It is important to exclude psychoses with known organic causes such as temporal lobe epilepsy, metabolic disturbances, toxic substances, or psychoactive drugs.

The onset of schizophrenia typically occurs between the late teens and the mid-30s; onset prior to adolescence is rare. Gender differences suggest that women are more likely to have a later onset, more prominent mood symptoms, and a better prognosis. Hospital-based studies show a higher rate of schizophrenia in men, whereas community-based studies suggest an equal sex ratio. The onset of symptoms usually occurs between the ages of 17 and 30 years in men and between 20 and 40 in women. Although complete remission is not common, the prognosis is variable.

schizophrenic (-ĭk), *adj.* SEE: *Nursing Diagnoses Appendix.*

ETIOLOGY: The cause of schizophrenia is unknown. However, some research suggests the illness may be familial, and other evidence links the illness to infection with Borna disease virus.

TREATMENT: Medications used to control schizophrenia include antipsychotic drugs that act on dopamine receptors in the brain, such as chlorpromazine, fluphenazine, haloperidol, clozapine, and risperidone. Each of these may be associated with significant side effects; as a result, drug treatment with any of them requires careful monitoring. Supportive psychotherapy may be helpful for the patient and family.

catatonic s. A schizophrenic disorder marked by motor immobility or stupor; excessive, purposeless motor activity; extreme negativism or mutism; echolalia or echopraxia; and peculiar voluntary movements such as posturing.

paranoid s. A type of schizophrenic disorder characterized by delusions of persecution, grandiosity, jealousy, or hallucinations with persecutory or grandiose content.

residual s. A schizophrenic disorder marked by continuing evidence of flat affect, impoverished or disorganized speech, and eccentric or odd behavior, but showing no evidence of delusions, hallucinations, or disorganized speech.

schizoprosopia (skĭz″ō-prō-sō′pē-ă) [″ + *prosopon,* face] Fissure of the face, such as harelip or cleft palate.

schizotrichia (skĭz″ō-trĭk′ē-ă) [″ + *thrix,* hair] Splitting of the tips of the hair.

schizozoite (skĭz″ō-zō′īt) [″ + *zoon,* animal] Merozoite.

Schlatter-Osgood disease (shlăt′ĕr-ŏz′good) Osgood-Schlatter disease.

Schlemm, canal of (shlĕm) [Friedrich S. Schlemm, Ger. anatomist, 1795–1858] A permeable venous sinus at the junction of the cornea and the iris; the site of reabsorption of aqueous humor from the anterior chamber of the eye. SYN: *scleral venous sinus.*

Schmorl's disease [Christian G. Schmorl, Ger. pathologist, 1861–1932] Herniation of the nucleus pulposus through a cracked vertebral end plate into the vertebral body. The resulting bone necrosis is detectable on radiograph and is called *Schmorl's nodes.*

Schmorl's nodes SEE: *Schmorl's disease.*

schneiderian membrane (shnī-dē′rē-ăn) [Conrad Viktor Schneider, Ger. anatomist, 1614–1680] The nasal mucosa.

Schober's maneuver (shō′bĕrz) A test for flexibility of the lumbar spine; used to determine the presence of ankylosis spondylitis (AS) in patients with low back pain.

PATIENT CARE: The patient is asked to stand erect and a mark is placed on the skin overlying the second sacral vertebra. A second mark is placed on the skin 10 cm above the first. The patient then is asked to bend forward. A repeat measurement of the distance between the two marks should equal or exceed 15 cm. If it does not, the patient may have an inflexible or "bamboo" spine, characteristic of AS.

Schönlein's disease (shān′līnz) [Johann Lukas Schönlein, Ger. physician, 1793–1864] Idiopathic thrombocytopenic purpura.

Schönlein-Henoch purpura SEE: *Henoch-Schönlein purpura.*

school phobia A child's avoidance of school because of fear.

Schüffner's dots (shĭf′nĕrz) [Wilhelm P. A. Schüffner, Ger. pathologist, 1867–1949] Minute granules present in the red blood cells when they are infected by *Plasmodium vivax.*

Schüller's disease Histiocytosis.

Schultze's bundle, Schultze's tract (shooltz′ĕs) [Max Johann Schultze, Ger. biologist, 1825–1874] A longitudinal, comma-shaped mass of descending fibers in the fasciculus cuneatus of the spinal cord.

Schultze's cell Olfactory cell.

Schultz reaction [Werner Schultz, Ger. physician, 1878–1947] A test that demonstrates the ability of muscle tissues from an animal that has been made anaphylactic to contract when reexposed to the antigen. SYN: *Dale reaction.*

Schulze mechanism Placental expulsion with the fetal surface presenting. This indicates placental separation progressed from the inside to the outer margins. SEE: *mechanism, Duncan's.*

Schwabach test (shvă′băk) [Dagobert Schwabach, Ger. otologist, 1846–1920] An obsolete test for hearing, using five tuning forks, each of a different tone. Hearing tests are now performed with more precise audiological devices. SEE: *audiometry.*

Schwalbe's ring (shvăl′bĕz) [Gustav Albert Schwalbe, Ger. anatomist, 1844–1916] The thickened peripheral margin of the Descemet's membrane of the cornea of the eye; it is formed by a circular bundle of connective tissue. Also called *Schwalbe's line.*

Schwann cell (shvŏn) [Theodor Schwann, Ger. anatomist, 1810–1882] One of the cells of the peripheral nervous system that form the myelin sheath and neurilemma of peripheral nerve fibers. In the embryo, the Schwann cells grow around the nerve fiber, forming concentric layers of cell membrane (the myelin sheath). The cytoplasm and nuclei of the Schwann cells, external to the myelin sheath, form the neurilemma. SEE: *neuron* for illus.

schwannoma (shwŏn-nō′mă) A benign tumor of the neurilemma of a nerve.

schwannosis (shwŏn-nō′sĭs) Hypertrophy of the neurilemma of a nerve.

Schwann's sheath Neurilemma.

Schwann's white substance Myelin of a medullated nerve fiber.

sciage (sē-ăzh′) [Fr., a sawing] A movement of the hand used in massage resembling that used in sawing.

sciatic (sī-ăt′ĭk) [L. *sciaticus*] **1.** Pert. to the hip or ischium. **2.** Pert. to, due to, or afflicted with sciatica. SYN: *ischiac; ischiatic.* SEE: *sciatica.*

sciatica (sī-ăt′ĭ-kă) [L.] Pain emanating from the lower back that is felt along the distribution of the sciatic nerve in the lower extremity. It typically occurs as a result of lumbar disk disease and is felt in the back of the thigh and sometimes the rest of the lower extremity. In Western countries like the U.S., about 40% to 50% of the population will experience sciatica at some time during their lives. Recovery follows conservative treatment in 3 to 4 weeks in the vast majority of patients. SEE: *meralgia; piriformis syndrome; sciatic nerve; Nursing Diagnoses Appendix.*

ETIOLOGY: The condition may be caused by compression or trauma of the sciatic nerve or its roots, esp. that resulting from a ruptured intervertebral disk or osteoarthrosis of the lumbosacral vertebrae; inflammation of the sciatic nerve resulting from metabolic, toxic, or infectious disorders; or pain referred to the distribution of the sciatic nerve from other sources.

SYMPTOMS: This condition may begin abruptly or gradually and is characterized by a sharp shooting pain running down the back of the thigh. Movement of the limb or lower back generally intensifies the suffering. Pain may be uniformly distributed along the limb, but frequently there are certain spots where it is more intense. Numbness and tingling may be present, and the skin innervated by the nerve may occasionally be hypersensitive to light touch.

DIAGNOSIS: Physical examination of the patient with sciatica may reveal pain in the lower back during straight leg raising or changes in lower extremity reflexes.

TREATMENT: Although sciatica may be extremely painful and temporarily disabling, in more than 80% of patients it gradually resolves with mild activity restrictions and nonsteroidal antiinflammatories, narcotic analgesic drugs, or muscle relaxers. Patients whose symptoms do not improve with these therapies should be re-evaluated professionally. Occasionally surgery of the lower back (e.g., to remove a herniated disk) is needed, although this intervention is now used much less often than in the past.

PATIENT CARE: Patients with sciatica who have had a history of cancer, inject drugs, have fevers associated with sciatica, or lose control of bowel or bladder function in association with the illness should be evaluated immediately with radiographic studies of the lower back (e.g., computerized tomographic or magnetic resonance scans). Elderly patients also may require earlier and closer follow-up care than younger patients. Patients for whom sciatic pain is disabling, but in whom objective pathology is not easily demonstrated, may benefit from multidisciplinary approaches to their symptoms (e.g., with referrals to chronic pain clinics, physical and occupational therapists, physiatrists, or other specialists).

sciatic nerve The largest nerve in the body, arising from the sacral plexus on either side, passing from the pelvis through the greater sciatic foramen, and down the back of the thigh, where it divides into the tibial and peroneal nerves. Lesions cause paralysis of flexion and extension of the toes, abduction and adduction of the toes, rotation inward and adduction of the foot, plantar flexion and lowering of the ball of the foot; paralysis of dorsiflexion and adduction of the foot; and paralysis of the rotation of the ball of the foot outward and of raising the external border of the foot. Lesions also cause anesthesia in cutaneous distribution.

sciatic nerve, small The posterior femoral cutaneous nerve, a cutaneous nerve supplying the skin of the buttocks, perineum, popliteal region, and the back of the thigh and the leg.

science (sī′ĕns) [L. *scientia,* knowledge] The intellectual process using all available mental and physical resources to better understand, explain, quantitate, and predict normal as well as unusual natural phenomena. The scientific approach involves observation, measurement, and the accumulation and analysis of verifiable data.

life s. The scientific disciplines concerned with living things; included are biology, zoology, medicine, dentistry, surgery, nursing, and psychology.

Science of Unitary Human Beings A conceptual model of nursing developed by Martha Rogers. The human being and the environment are conceived of as being unitary, patterned, open, and pandimensional energy fields. The goal of nursing is to promote human betterment wherever people are, on planet earth or in outer space. SEE: *homeodynamics; Nursing Theory Appendix.*

scieropia (sī-ĕr-ō′pē-ă) [Gr. *skieros,* shadow, + *opsis,* vision] Abnormal vision in which things appear to be in a shadow.

scintigram (sĭn′tĭ-grăm) The record produced by a scintiscan.

scintigraphy (sĭn-tĭg′ră-fē) The injection and subsequent detection of radioactive isotopes to create images of body parts, and identify body functions and diseases.

scintillascope (sĭn-tĭl′ă-skōp) [L. *scintilla,* spark, + Gr. *skopein,* to examine] An obsolete device for viewing the effect of ionizing radiation, alpha particles, on a fluorescent screen.

scintillation (sĭn″tĭ-lā′shŭn) [L. *scintillatio*] **1.** Sparkling; a subjective sensation, as of seeing sparks. **2.** The response of specific crystals to electromagnetic radiation, such as the emissions that come from radioactive substances.

scintiphotography (sĭn″tĭ-fō-tŏg′ră-fē) Making images from radioactive emissions, for example, from radioisotopes injected into the body to determine the health or disease of body structures and functions. SEE: *scintigraphy.*

scintiscan (sĭn′tĭ-skăn) The use of scintiphotography to create a map of scintillations produced when a radioactive substance is introduced into the body. The intensity of the record indicates the differential accumulation of a substance in the various parts of the body.

scintiscanner (sĭn″tĭ-skăn′ĕr) The device used in doing a scintiscan.

scirrho- A combining form meaning *hard.*

scirrhoid (skĭr′oyd) [Gr. *skirrhos,* hard, + *eidos,* form, shape] Pert. to, or like, a hard carcinoma.

scirrhoma (skĭr-ō′mă) [″ + *oma,* tumor] A hard carcinoma.

scirrhosarca (skĭr″ō-săr′kă) [″ + *sarx,* flesh] Scleroderma neonatorum.

scirrhous (skĭr′rŭs) [NL. *scirrhosus,* hard] Hard, like a scirrhus.

scirrhus (skĭr′ŭs) [Gr. *skirrhos,* hard tumor] A hard, cancerous tumor caused by an overgrowth of fibrous tissue.

scission (sĭzh′ŭn) [L. *scindere,* to split] Dividing, cutting, or splitting.

scissors (sĭz′ors) [LL. *cisorium*] A cutting instrument composed of two opposed cutting blades with handles, held together by a central pin. This allows the cutting edge to be opened and closed.

scissura (sĭ-sū′ră) *pl.* **scissurae** [L., to split] A fissure or cleft; a splitting.

sclera (sklĕr′ă) *pl.* **sclerae** [Gr. *skleros,* hard] The outer layer of the eyeball made of fibrous connective tissue. At the front of the eye, it is visible as the white of the eye and ends at the cornea, which is transparent. SYN: *sclerotica.* **scleral,** *adj.*

blue s. An abnormal thinning of the sclera through which a blue uveal pigment is seen. This may be found in persons with disorders of collagen formation such as osteogenesis imperfecta.

scleradenitis (sklĕ″răd-ĕn-ī′tĭs) [″ + *aden,* gland, + *itis,* inflammation] Inflammation and induration of a gland.

scleratogenous (sklĕ″ră-tŏj′ĕ-nŭs) Sclerogenous.

sclerectasia (sklĕ″rĕk-tā′zē-ă) [″ + *ektasis,* dilatation] Protrusion of the sclera.

sclerectoiridectomy (sklĕ-rĕk″tō-ĭr″ĭ-dĕk′tō-mē) [″ + *iris,* colored circle, + *ektome,* excision] Formation of a filtering scar in glaucoma by combined sclerectomy and iridectomy.

sclerectoiridodialysis (sklĕ-rĕk″tō-ĭr″ĭd-ō-dī-ăl′ĭ-sĭs) [″ + ″ + *dialysis,* loosening] Sclerectomy and iridodialysis for the relief of glaucoma.

sclerectomy (sklĕ-rĕk′tō-mē) [″ + *ektome,* excision] **1.** Excision of a portion of the sclera. SYN: *scleroticectomy.* **2.** Removal of adhesions in chronic otitis media.

scleredema (sklĕr″ĕ-dē′mă) [″ + *oidema,* swelling] A condition marked by edema and induration of the skin usually followed by an acute infection. It is a benign self-limited disease occurring more often in women than in men. It is often confused with scleroderma. SEE: illus.

s. adultorum Buschke's scleredema.

s. neonatorum Scleroderma neonatorum.

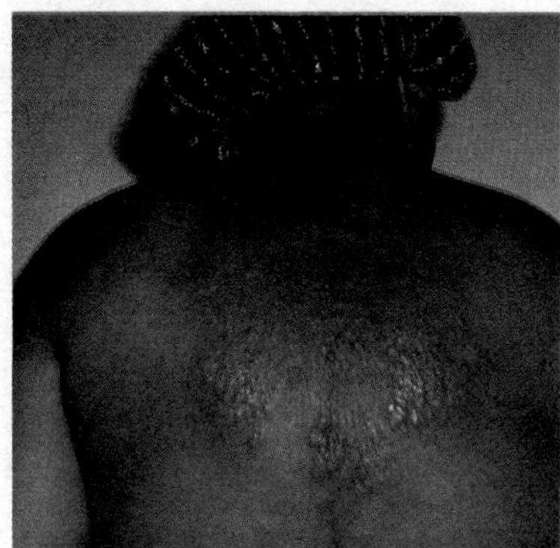

SCLEREDEMA

sclerema (sklĕ-rē′mă) [Gr. *skleros,* hard] Scleroderma.

s. adiposum Sclerema neonatorum.

s. adultorum Scleroderma.

s. neonatorum Hardening and tightening of the skin and subcutaneous tissue of the newborn. This is a rare disease, sometimes associated with premature birth, neonatal sepsis, and dehydration. SYN: *s. adiposum; scleroderma neonatorum.*

sclerencephalia (sklĕ″rĕn-sĕ-fā′lē-ă) [″ + *enkephalos,* brain] Sclerosis of the brain.

scleriasis (sklĕ-rī′ă-sĭs) [Gr. *skleriasis*] **1.** Progressive hardening of the skin. **2.** Hardening of the eyelid.

scleriritomy (sklĕ-rĭ-rĭt′ō-mē) [″ + *iris,* colored circle, + *tome,* incision] Incision of the iris and sclera.

scleritis (sklĕ-rī′tĭs) [″ + *itis,* inflammation] Superficial and deep inflammation of the sclera. SYN: *sclerotitis.* SEE: *episcleritis.*

annular s. Inflammation limited to the area surrounding the limbus of the cornea. A complete ring is formed.

anterior s. Scleritis of the area adjacent to the limbus of the cornea.

posterior s. Scleritis limited to the posterior half of the globe of the eye with loss of vision and ocular pain.

scleroblastema (sklĕ″rō-blăs-tē′mă) [Gr. *skleros,* hard, + *blastema,* sprout] The embryonic tissue from which formation of bone takes place.

scleroblastemic (sklĕ″rō-blăs-tĕm′ĭk) Relating to or derived from scleroblastema.

sclerochoroiditis (sklĕ″rō-kō″royd-ī′tĭs) [″ + *chorioeides,* skinlike, + *itis,* inflammation] Inflammation of the sclera and choroid coat of the eye. SYN: *scleroticochoroiditis.*

posterior s. Posterior staphyloma.

scleroconjunctival (sklĕ″rō-kŏn″jŭnk-tī′văl) [″ + L. *conjunctivus,* to bind together] Pert. to the sclera and conjunctiva.

sclerocornea (sklĕ″rō-kor′nē-ă) [″ + L. *corneus,* horny] The sclera and cornea together considered as one coat.

sclerodactylia (sklĕr″ō-dăk-tĭl′ē-ă) [″ + *daktylos,* a finger] Induration of the skin of the fingers and toes. SYN: *acroscleroderma.*

scleroderma (sklĕr″ă-dĕr′mă) [Gr. *skleros,* hard, + *derma,* skin] A chronic manifestation of progressive systemic sclerosis in which the skin is taut, firm, and edematous, limiting movement. SEE: illus; *sclerosis, progressive systemic; Nursing Diagnoses Appendix.* **sclerodermatous,** *adj.*

circumscribed s. Localized patches of linear sclerosis of the skin. There is no systemic involvement, and the course of the disease is usually benign.

s. neonatorum Sclerema neonatorum.

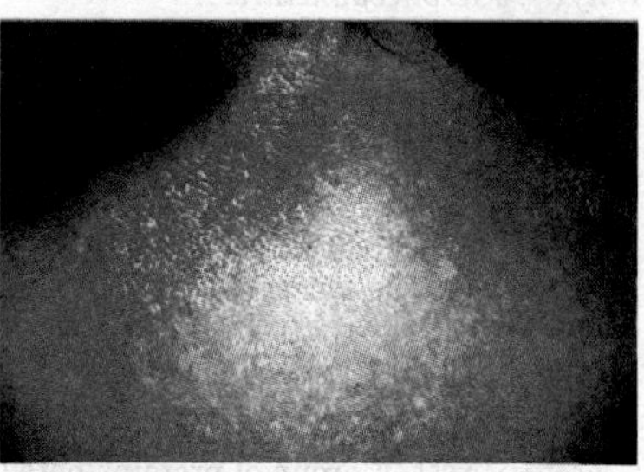

SCLERODERMA

sclerodermatitis (sklĕ″rō-dĕr-mă-tī′tĭs) [Gr. *skleros,* hard, + *derma,* skin, + *itis,* inflammation] Inflammation of the skin accompanied by thickening and hardening.

sclerogenic (sklĕ″rō-jĕn′ĭk) [″ + *gennan,* to produce] Sclerogenous.

sclerogenous (sklĕ-rŏj′ĕ-nŭs) [″ + *gennan,* to produce] Causing sclerosis or hardening of tissue. SYN: *sclerogenic.*

scleroid (sklĕ′rŏyd) [″ + *eidos,* form, shape] Having a hard or firm texture.

scleroiritis (sklĕ″rō-ī-rī′tĭs) [″ + *iris,* colored circle + *itis,* inflammation] Inflammation of both the sclera and iris.

sclerokeratitis (sklĕr″ō-kĕr-ă-tī′tĭs) [″ + *keras,* horn, + *itis,* inflammation] Cellular infiltration with inflammation of the sclera and cornea. SYN: *sclerokeratosis.*

sclerokeratoiritis (sklĕ″rō-kĕr″ă-tō-ī-rī′tĭs) [″ + ″ + *iris,* colored circle, + *itis,* inflammation] Inflammation of the sclera, cornea, and iris.

sclerokeratosis (sklĕr″ō-kĕr″ă-tō′sĭs) [″ + ″ + *osis,* condition] Sclerokeratitis.

scleroma (sklĕ-rō′mă) [″ + *oma,* tumor] Indurated, circumscribed area of granulation tissue in the mucous membrane or skin. SEE: *sclerosis.*

scleromalacia (sklĕ″rō-mā-lā′sē-ă) [Gr.

skleros, hard, + *malakia,* softening] A softening of the sclera.

s. perforans Scleromalacia accompanied by perforation.

scleromere (sklĕr′ō-mēr) [″ + *meros,* a part] **1.** Any segment of the metamere of the skeleton. **2.** The caudal half of a sclerotome.

scleromyxedema (sklĕr″ō-mĭk″sē-dē′mă) [″ + *myxa,* mucus, + *oidema,* swelling] A systemic form of papular mucinosis (also known as lichen myxedematosus), in which a scleroderma-like rash is accompanied by lesions of visceral organs and often paraproteinemia.

scleronychia (sklĕ″rō-nĭk′ē-ă) [″ + *onyx,* nail] Thickening and hardening of the nails.

scleronyxis (sklĕ-rō-nĭk′sĭs) [Gr. *skleros,* hard, + *nyxis,* a piercing] Surgical puncture of the sclera. SYN: *scleroticonyxis; scleroticopuncture.*

sclero-oophoritis (sklĕ″rō-ō-ŏf″ō-rī′tĭs) [″ + *oophoros,* bearing eggs, + *itis,* inflammation] Induration and inflammation of the ovary.

sclerophthalmia (sklĕ″rŏf-thăl′mē-ă) [″ + *ophthalmos,* eye] A congenital condition in which opacity of the sclera advances over the cornea.

scleroplasty (sklĕ′rō-plăs″tē) [″ + *plassein,* to form] Plastic surgery of the sclera.

scleroprotein (sklĕ″rō-prō′tē-ĭn) [″ + *protos,* first] A group of proteins noted for their insolubility in most chemicals; found in skeletal tissue, cartilage, hair, and nails, and in animal claws and horns.

sclerosal (sklĕ-rō′săl) Sclerous.

sclerosant (sklĕ-rō′sănt) [Gr. *skleros,* hard] Something that produces sclerosis.

sclerose (sklĕ-rōs′) [Gr. *skleros,* hard] To become hardened. **sclerosing, sclerosed,** *adj.*

sclerosis (sklĕ-rō′sĭs) [Gr. *sklerosis,* to harden] A hardening or induration of an organ or tissue, esp. that due to excessive growth of fibrous tissue. SEE: *arteriosclerosis; cerebrosclerosis.* **sclerotic,** *adj.*

amyotrophic lateral s. ABBR: ALS. motor neuron disease. SEE: *Nursing Diagnoses Appendix.*

annular s. Sclerosis in which a hardened substance forms a band about the spinal cord.

arterial s. Arteriosclerosis.

arteriolar s. Sclerosis of the arterioles.

diffuse s. Sclerosis affecting large areas of the brain and spinal cord.

hyperplastic s. Medial s.

insular s. Multiple s.

intimal s. Atherosclerosis.

lateral s. Sclerosis of the lateral column of the spinal cord. SEE: *amyotrophic lateral sclerosis.*

lobar s. Sclerosis of the cerebrum resulting in mental disturbances.

medial s. Sclerosis involving the tunica media of arteries, usually the result of involutional changes accompanying aging. SYN: *hyperplastic s.*

multiple s. ABBR: MS. A chronic disease of the central nervous system (CNS), in which there is destruction of myelin and nerve axons within several regions of the brain and spinal cord at different times. This results in temporary, repetitive, or sustained disruptions in nerve impulse conduction, causing symptoms such as muscular weakness, numbness, visual disturbances, or loss of control of bowel, bladder, and sexual functions. MS is a relatively common disorder: more than 250,000 Americans are affected. Women are twice as likely to have the disease as men, and European-Americans are more likely to be affected than African-Americans or Asian-Americans. Four main categories of MS are currently recognized. The *benign* variant is marked by several episodes of nervous system dysfunction, followed by complete recovery. The *primary progressive* variant is marked by rapid loss of neurological functions that do not resolve, causing severe functional impairments that worsen over time. More common than either of these types of MS are the two *relapsing-remitting* variants. In patients with these disorders, neurological deficits develop and then improve either completely or partially. In patients who achieve only partial restoration of neurological function, secondary progression of the disease may result in a gradual accumulation of visual, motor, or sensory disabilities. SYN: *insular s.* SEE: *Nursing Diagnoses Appendix.*

About half of all patients with MS become unable to work within 10 to 15 years of the first onset of symptoms. Within 25 years of the first symptoms, half of these patients cannot walk.

ETIOLOGY: The cause of the disease is unknown, although much evidence suggests that T lymphocytes that injure nerve cells and nerve sheaths play an important role, that is, that the disease has an autoimmune basis.

SYMPTOMS: Nearly a quarter of all patients with MS initially develop visual disturbances, or blindness. This condition, called optic (or "retrobulbar") neuritis, may respond to high doses of corticosteroids. Other consequences of the disease may include sudden or progressive weakness in one or more limbs, muscular spasticity, nystagmus, fatigue, tremors, gait instability, recurrent urinary tract infections (caused by bladder dysfunction), incontinence, and alterations in mood, including depression.

TREATMENT: Although there is no known cure for MS, corticosteroids, interferon-alpha, and glatiramer may be used in specific settings to reduce disability or the frequency of relapses and the progression of disease in patients with some variants of MS. Treatment should be individualized because these therapies may be expensive, ineffective in benign or primary progressive disease, and poorly tolerated by some patients. Symptomatic relief (e.g., of spasticity with muscle relaxants, or of bladder dysfunction with anticholinergic drugs) is provided as needed.

PATIENT CARE: The health care professional provides support to patients with multiple sclerosis and their families. The patient is advised to avoid fatigue, overexertion, exposure to extreme heat or cold, and stressful situations, and is encouraged to follow a regular plan of daily activity and exercise. The patient is taught about symptoms that may occur during exacerbations of the disease and the need to adapt the plan of care to changing needs, as well as about the administration of prescribed medications. Both the patient and family are encouraged to promote safety in the home and the work environment.

neural s. Sclerosis with chronic inflammation of a nerve trunk with branches.

nuclear s. An increase in the refractive index of the eye's crystalline lens, which culminates in the development of nuclear cataracts. Before the cataract fully opacifies, the patient's near vision may improve, a phenomenon known as senopia or "second sight."

progressive systemic s. ABBR: PSS. A chronic disease of unknown etiology that occurs four times as frequently in women than in men. It causes sclerosis of the skin and certain organs including the gastrointestinal tract, lungs, heart, and kidneys. The skin is taut, firm, and edematous and is firmly bound to subcutaneous tissue, which often causes limitation of the range of motion; it feels tough and leathery, may itch, and later becomes hyperpigmented. The skin changes usually precede the development of signs of visceral involvement. A limited variant, called the CREST syndrome, includes only the following findings: calcinosis, Raynaud's phenomenon, esophageal dysfunction, sclerodactyly, and telangiectasia.

TREATMENT: There is no specific therapy. General supportive therapy is indicated. A great number of drugs including corticosteroids, vasodilators, D-penicillamine, and immunosuppressive agents have been tried. Physical therapy will help maintain range of motion and muscular strength but will not influence the course of joint disease.

PROGNOSIS: The prognosis is variable and unpredictable with respect to the rate of pathologic changes.

renal s. Nephrosclerosis.

systemic s. Progressive systemic s.

tuberous s. ABBR: TS. An autosomal dominant disorder in which multiple tumors appear in the skin, brain, heart, and kidneys of affected children. Infants born with this disease may have facial angiofibromas, astrocytomas of the central nervous system, hamartomas of the retina, and other lesions, producing hydrocephalus, mental retardation, autism, and seizures.

vascular s. Atherosclerosis.

venous s. Phlebosclerosis.

scleroskeleton (sklĕr″ō-skĕl′ĕ-tŏn) [Gr. *skleros,* hard, + *skeleton,* a dried-up body] Skeletal changes resulting from ossification of fibrous structures, such as ligaments, fasciae, and tendons.

sclerostenosis (sklĕr″ō-stĕ-nō′sĭs) [″ + *stenosis,* act of narrowing] Contraction and induration of tissues, esp. those about an orifice.

s. cutanea Scleroderma.

sclerostomy (sklĕ-rŏs′tō-mē) [″ + *stoma,* mouth] The surgical formation of an opening in the sclera.

sclerotherapy (sklĕr″ō-thĕr′ă-pē) [″ + *therapeia,* treatment] The injection of irritating chemicals into vascular spaces or body cavities to harden, fill, or destroy them. Sclerotherapy has been used to manage varicose veins, hemorrhoids, esophageal varices, benign hepatic cysts, malignant pleural effusions, and intracranial aneurysms, among other diseases. A common complication of the procedure is injury to neighboring tissues. Commonly used sclerosing agents include absolute ethanol and sodium tetradecyl sulfate.

sclerothrix (sklĕr′ō-thrĭks) [″ + *thrix,* hair] Brittleness of the hair.

sclerotica (sklĕ-rŏt′ĭ-kă) [L. *scleroticus,* hard] Sclera.

sclerotic acid An amorphous, brown powder from ergot; a hemostatic and oxytocic.

sclerotic dentin Areas of dentin where the tubules have been filled by mineralization, producing a more dense, radiopaque dentin; it is often produced in response to caries, attrition, and abrasion.

scleroticectomy (sklĕ-rŏt″ĭ-sĕk′tō-mē) [″ + Gr. *ektome,* excision] Excision of a part of the sclera. SYN: *sclerectomy.*

scleroticochoroiditis (sklĕ-rŏt″ĭ-kō-kō″roy-dī′tĭs) [″ + Gr. *chorioeides,* skin-like, + *itis,* inflammation] Inflammation of sclerotic and choroid coats of the eye. SYN: *sclerochoroiditis.*

scleroticonyxis (sklĕ-rŏt″ĭ-kō-nĭk′sĭs) [″ + Gr. *nyxis,* a piercing] Surgical puncture of the sclera. SYN: *scleronyxis; scleroticopuncture.*

scleroticopuncture (sklĕ-rŏt″ĭ-kō-pŭnk′ tŭr) [″ + *punctura,* a piercing] Surgical puncture of the sclera. SYN: *scleronyxis; scleroticonyxis.*

scleroticotomy (sklĕ-rŏt″ĭ-kŏt′ō-mē) [″ + Gr. *tome,* incision] Sclerotomy.

sclerotitis (sklĕr-ō-tī′tĭs) [Gr. *skleros,* hard, + *itis,* inflammation] Inflammation of the sclera. SYN: *scleritis.*

sclerotium (sklĕ-rō′shē-ŭm) A hardened mass formed by the growth of certain fungi. The sclerotium formed by ergot on rye is of medical importance due to its toxicity.

sclerotome (sklĕr′ō-tōm) [″ + *tome,* incision] **1.** A knife used in incision of the sclera. **2.** One of a series of segmentally arranged masses of mesenchymal tissue lying on either side of the notochord. They give rise to the vertebrae and ribs.

sclerotomy (sklĕ-rŏt′ō-mē) Surgical incision of the sclera. SYN: *scleroticotomy.*

anterior s. An incision made at the angle of the anterior chamber of the eye in glaucoma.

posterior s. An incision through the sclera into the vitreous for treatment of a detached retina or removal of a foreign body.

sclerotrichia (sklĕ-rō-trĭk′ē-ă) [Gr. *sclerosis,* hard, + *thrix,* hair] Hardness and brittleness of the hair.

sclerous (sklĕr′ŭs) Hard; indurated. SYN: *sclerosal.*

scobinate (skō′bĭn-āt) [L. *scobina,* rasp] Having a rough, uneven, nodular surface.

scoleciasis (skō-lĕ-sī′ă-sĭs) [Gr. *skolex,* worm, + *-iasis,* condition] The presence of larval forms of butterflies or moths in the body.

scoleciform (skō-lĕs′ĭ-form) [″ + L. *forma,* form] Resembling a scolex.

scolecoid (skō′lĕ-koyd) [″ + *eidos,* form, shape] Resembling a worm.

scolex (skō′lĕks) *pl.* **scolices** [Gr. *skolex,* worm] The head-like segment of a tapeworm, by which it attaches itself to the wall of the intestine. Scolices usually possess hooks, suckers, or grooves (bothria) for attachment.

scoliokyphosis (skō″lē-ō-kī-fō′sĭs) [Gr. *skolios,* twisted, + *kyphosis,* humpback] A condition combining scoliosis and kyphosis.

scoliometer (skō″lē-ŏm′ĕt-ĕr) [″ + *metron,* measure] A device for measuring curves, esp. the lateral ones of the spine.

sciliorachitic (skō″lē-ō-ră-kĭt′ĭk) [″ + *rhachis,* spine] Pert. to, or afflicted with, spinal curvature from rickets.

scoliosis (skō″lē-ō′sĭs) [Gr. *skoliosis,* crookedness] A lateral curvature of the spine. It usually consists of two curves, the original abnormal curve and a compensatory curve in the opposite direction. SEE: illus.; *Nursing Diagnoses Appendix.*

TREATMENT: Scoliosis may be treated through the use of a brace to straighten the abnormal spinal curvature or with corrective orthopedic surgery (e.g., the placement of a supportive rod along the spine or spinal fusion).

PATIENT CARE: Provisions are made to assist the adolescent and family to meet the psychosocial needs associated with the illness. The patient and family are taught about treatment (cast brace, traction, electrical stimulation, or surgery), exercises, activity level, skin care, prevention of complications, and breathing exercises. When necessary, preoperative teaching is provided, including preanesthesia breathing exercises. Educational and support resources are discussed with the patient and family.

cicatricial s. Scoliosis due to fibrous scar tissue contraction resulting from necrosis.

congenital s. Scoliosis present at birth, usually the result of defective embryonic development of the spine.

coxitic s. Scoliosis in the lumbar spine caused by tilting of the pelvis in hip disease.

empyematic s. Scoliosis following empyema and retraction of one side of the chest.

functional s. Scoliosis that is caused not by actual spinal deformity but by another condition such as unequal leg lengths. The curve reduces when the other condition is ameliorated.

habit s. Scoliosis due to habitually assumed improper posture or position.

idiopathic s. Scoliosis due to unknown causes.

inflammatory s. Scoliosis due to disease of the vertebrae.

ischiatic s. Scoliosis due to hip disease.

myopathic s. Scoliosis due to weakening of the spinal muscles.

neuropathic s. A structural scoliosis caused by congenital or acquired neurological disorders.

ocular s. Scoliosis from tilting of the head because of visual defects or extraocular muscle imbalance.

osteopathic s. Scoliosis caused by bony deformity of the spine.

paralytic s. Scoliosis due to paralysis of muscles.

protective s. An acute side shifting of the lumbar spine, usually away from the side of pathology. The body is attempting to move a nerve root away from a bulging intervertebral disk herniation.

rachitic s. Scoliosis due to rickets.

sciatic s. Scoliosis due to sciatica.

static s. Scoliosis due to a difference in the length of the legs.

structural s. An irreversible lateral spinal curvature that has a fixed rotation. The vertebral bodies rotate toward the convexity of the curve; the rotation results in a posterior rib hump in the thoracic region on the convex side of the curve. In structural scoliosis, the spine does not straighten when the patient bends.

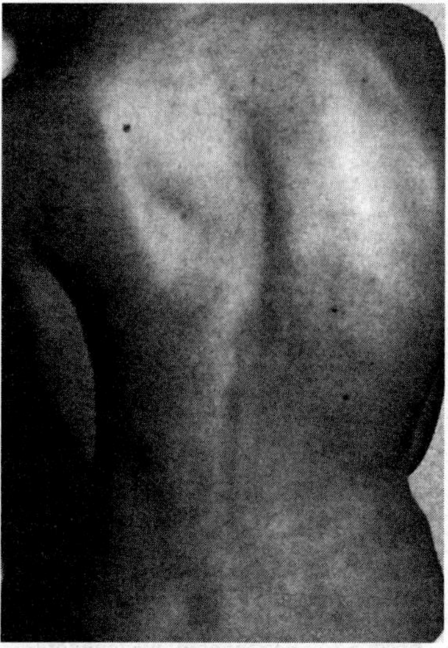

SCOLIOSIS

scoliosometry (skō″lē-ō-sŏm′ĕt-rē) [″ + *metron,* measure] Measurement of the degree of spinal curvature.

scoliotic (skō-lē-ŏt′ĭk) Suffering from, or related to, scoliosis.

scombrine (skŏm′brĭn) A protamine present in mackerel sperm.

scombroid Fish of the suborder Scombroidea, including mackerel, tuna, bonitos, albacores, and skipjacks.

scombroid fish poisoning Intoxication due to eating raw or inadequately cooked fish of the suborder Scombroidea, such as tuna and mackerel, as well as certain non-scombroid fish, including amberjack, mahimahi, and bluefish. Certain bacteria act on the fish after they are caught to produce a histamine-like toxin. Therefore, these fish should be either properly cooked and eaten shortly after being caught or refrigerated immediately.

SYMPTOMS: Nausea, vomiting, abdominal cramps, diarrhea, flushing, headache, urticaria, a burning sensation and metallic taste in the mouth, dizziness, periorbital edema, and thirst may develop 30 minutes after eating the fish and last a few hours.

TREATMENT: Antihistamines reverse many of the symptoms of the syndrome.

scoop (skoop) [ME., a ladle] A spoon-shaped surgical instrument.

bone s. A curette for scraping or removing necrosed bone or the contents of suppurative tracts.

bullet s. An instrument for dislodging bullets.

cataract s. An instrument for removing fluids or foreign growths.

ear s. A curet for removing middle ear granulations.

lithotomy s. An instrument for dislodging encysted stones or debris.

mastoid s. An instrument used in mastoid operations.

renal s. An instrument used to dislodge or remove small stones from the pelvis of a kidney.

scoparius (skō-pā′rē-ŭs) The fresh or dried tops of broom, *Cytisus scoparius.* It was used in the distant past as a diuretic and emetic.

-scope [Gr. *skopein,* to examine] Combining form, used as a suffix, meaning *to view, to examine.*

scopolamine hydrobromide (skō-pŏl′ă-mēn hī″drō-brō′mīd) The hydrobromide of alkaloids obtained from plants of the nightshade family. SYN: *hyoscine hydrobromide.*

ACTION/USES: The drug is used to prevent vertigo and motion sickness, to sedate patients, and to produce amnesia in anesthesia. Its adverse effects include confusion, hallucinations, and unwanted memory loss, which may be especially prominent in elderly patients.

transdermal s. A method of delivering scopolamine by applying a patch containing the drug to the skin. The medicine is slowly absorbed over a period of several days. It is esp. useful in treating vertigo and motion sickness. In the latter condition, the medicine is effective if applied several hours before the individual is exposed to the motion.

scopometer (skō-pŏm′ĕ-tĕr) [Gr. *skopein,* to examine, + *metron,* measure] An instrument for measuring the density of a suspension.

scopophilia (skō″pō-fĭl′ē-ă) [″ + *philein,* to love] The derivation of sexual pleasure from visual sources such as nudity and obscene pictures.

active s. Voyeurism.

passive s. Sexual pleasure derived from being observed by others.

scopophobia (skō″pō-fō′bē-ă) [″ + *phobos,* fear] An abnormal fear of being seen.

-scopy [Gr. *skopein,* to examine] Combining form meaning *examination.*

scorbutic (skor-bū′tĭk) [NL. *scorbuticus,* scurvy] Concerning or affected with scurvy.

scorbutigenic (skor-bū″tĭ-jĕn′ĭk) [LL. *scorbutus,* scurvy, + Gr. *gennan,* to produce] Something that causes scurvy.

scorbutus (skor-bū′tŭs) [LL., scurvy] Scurvy.

score (skor) **1.** A rating tool or scale to assess the level of health or the severity of an illness. SEE: *index, DMF; periodontal (Ramfjord) index.* **2.** A rating or grade as compared with a standard of other individuals, esp. in a competitive event. **3.** To mark the skin with lines in order to have landmarks available, as in plastic surgery.

Bishop's s. SEE: *Bishop's score.*

C.R.O.P. s. A critical care assessment score that measures compliance, respiratory rate, oxygenation, and pressure values.

S. for Neonatal Acute Physiology A measure of the severity of illness in patients in neonatal intensive care.

scorpion (skor'pē-ŏn) [Gr. *skorpios,* to cut off] An arthropod of the class Arachnida and order Scorpionida. It varies in length from less than 2 in. (5 cm) for the small bark scorpions of Arizona to 8 in. (20 cm) for some African scorpions. Most scorpions are nocturnal and reclusive, and are most active when the night temperatures remain above 70°F (21°C). The tail of the scorpion contains two venom glands connected to the tip of the stinger.

scorpionfish (skor'pē-ŏn-fĭsh) A family of fish with toxic spines that are found in coral reefs worldwide. Persons handling these animals may be stung or, in some instances, mortally wounded by the tissue-destructive enzymes and venoms they release. The most dangerous of the scorpionfish family is the stonefish, a well-camouflaged, bottom-dwelling fish, about the size of a chicken, with a rugged brown or gray surface and well-developed dorsal spine.

scoto- (skō'tō) Combining form meaning *darkness.*

scotodinia (skō"tō-dĭn'ē-ă) [" + *dinos,* whirling] Vertigo with black spots before the eyes and faintness of vision.

scotoma (skō-tō'mă) *pl.* **scotomata** [Gr. *skotoma,* to darken] An island-like blind spot in the visual field.

absolute s. An area in the visual field in which there is absolute blindness.

annular s. A scotomatous zone that encircles the point of fixation like a ring, not always completely closed, but leaving the fixation point intact. SYN: *ring s.*

arcuate s. An arc-shaped scotoma near the blind spot of the eye. It is caused by a nerve bundle defect on the temporal side of the optic disk.

central s. An area of depressed vision involving the point of fixation, seen in lesions of the macula.

centrocecal s. A defect in vision that is oval-shaped and includes the fixation point and the blind spot of the eye.

color s. Color blindness in a limited portion of the visual field.

eclipse s. An area of blindness in the visual field caused by looking directly at a solar eclipse.

flittering s. Scintillating s.

negative s. A scotoma not perceptible by the patient.

peripheral s. A defect in vision removed from the point of fixation of the vision.

physiological s. A blind spot caused by an absence of rods and cones where the optic nerve enters the retina.

positive s. An area in the visual field that is perceived by the patient as a dark spot.

relative s. A scotoma that causes the perception of an object to be impaired but not completely lost.

ring s. Annular s.

scintillating s. An irregular outline around a luminous patch in the visual field that occurs following mental or physical labor, eyestrain, or during a migraine.

scotometer (skō-tŏm'ĕt-ĕr) [" + *metron,* a measure] A device for detecting and measuring scotomata in the visual field.

scotometry (skō-tŏm'ĕ-trē) The locating and measurement of scotomata.

scotophobia (skō"tō-fō'bē-ă) [" + *phobos,* fear] An abnormal dread of darkness. SYN: *noctiphobia; nyctophobia.*

scotopia (skō-tō'pē-ă) [" + *ops,* eye] Adjustment of the eye for vision in dim light; the opposite of photopia. **scotopic** (-tŏp'ĭk), *adj.*

scotopsin (skō-tŏp'sĭn) The protein portion of the rods of the retina of the eye. It combines with 11-*cis*-retinal to form rhodopsin.

scout film In radiology, an x-ray film, esp. of the abdomen, for evaluating the condition of the body prior to beginning an invasive or potentially hazardous examination.

scr *scruple.*

scrape (skrāp) To remove from the surface with a scalpel or other edged instrument.

scraping (skrā'pĭng) Removal of cells, as from diseased tissue, with an edged instrument for cytologic examination. SEE: illus.

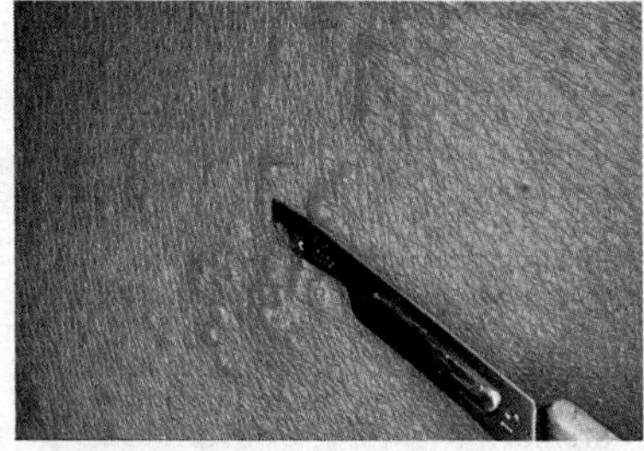

SCRAPING A BLISTER

scratch (skrăch) [ME. *cracchen,* to scratch] **1.** A mark or superficial injury produced by scraping with the nails on a rough surface. **2.** To make a thin, shallow cut with a sharp instrument. **3.** To rub the skin, esp. with the fingernails, to relieve itching. Scratching temporarily relieves itching by soothing the cutaneous nerves, but in the long run, it may worsen the condition that caused the itching. SEE: *pruritus.*

screen [O.Fr. *escren*] **1.** To determine the presence of a disease or its characteristics in a broad community or a selected group. **2.** A structure or substance used to protect, guard, or shield from a damaging influence such as x-rays, ultraviolet light, or insects. **3.** A system used to select or reject personnel. **4.** In psychiatry, the blocking of one memory with another.

intensifying s. In radiography, a paired sheet of photostimulable phosphors capable of amplifying an incoming image of x-ray photons into an image of light photons. High-speed intensifying screens are the major method of reducing patient radiation exposure.

tangent s. A simple device used in perimetry to test the central portion of the visual field. SEE: *Bjerrum's screen.*

screening **1.** Evaluating patients for diseases such as cancer, heart disease, or substance abuse before they become clinically obvious. Screening can play an important part in the early diagnosis and management of selected illnesses, which in some instances prolongs lives. SYN: *screening test.* **2.** In psychiatry, the initial examination to determine the mental status of an individual and the appropriate initial therapy.

screening test, cholesterol A preventive strategy for measuring cholesterol levels in asymptomatic people to identify those with high cholesterol (who are at risk for cardiovascular disease) and begin therapy to lower these levels. SEE: *cholesterol* for table.

screening test, multiphasic A battery of tests used to attempt to determine the presence of one or more diseases.

screw (skroo) A cylindrical fastener with a spiral groove running along its surface, often used in surgeries as an internal fixator (e.g., to attach bones to plates or prostheses).

expansion s. A mechanical device set into a removable or fixed appliance to enlarge the dental arch.

Scribner shunt [Belding Scribner, U.S. physician, b. 1921] A tube, usually made of synthetic material, used to connect an artery to a vein. It is used in patients requiring frequent venipuncture as in hemodialysis. However, the shunts may develop complications such as infection, thrombosis, and release of septic emboli.

scrobiculate (skrō-bĭk′ū-lāt) [L. *scrobiculus,* little trench] Having shallow depressions; pitted.

scrobiculus (skrō-bĭk′ū-lŭs) [L., little trench] A small groove or pit.

scrofula (skrŏf′ū-lă) [L., breeding sow] A form of extrapulmonary tuberculosis in which there is infection of the cervical lymph nodes. It is most common in children under age 15 and may be present without obvious disease in the lung. It is diagnosed with a needle biopsy and culture of the lymph nodes; a positive purified protein derivative (PPD) skin test sometimes is present. Like other forms of TB, it is treated with antitubercular drugs (e.g., isoniazid, rifampin, pyrazinamide). SEE: *lymphadenitis, tuberculous.*

scrotectomy (skrō-tĕk′tō-mē) [″ + Gr. *ektome,* excision] Excision of part of the scrotum.

scrotitis [″ + Gr. *itis,* inflammation] Inflammation of the scrotum.

scrotocele (skrō′tō-sēl) [″ + Gr. *kele,* tumor, swelling] Hernia in the scrotum.

scrotoplasty (skrō′tō-plăs″tē) [″ + Gr. *plassein,* to form] Plastic surgery on the scrotum.

scrotum (skrō′tŭm) *pl.* **scrota, -ums** [L., a bag] The pouch found in most male mammals that contains the testicles and part of the spermatic cord. Constituent parts of the scrotum are skin; a network of nonstriated muscular fibers called dartos; cremasteric, spermatic, and infundibuliform fasciae; cremasteric muscle; and tunica vaginalis. **scrotal** (-tăl), *adj.*

scrubbing [MD. *schrubben*] **1.** Washing the hands, fingernails, and forearms, including the elbows, prior to donning appropriate gowns and gloves to participate in surgery or other sterile procedures. The precise procedure to follow usually is posted in a special area where the washing is done. It typically entails scrubbing with germicidal soap and water, and using a nail brush to remove debris. **2.** Preparing the skin of the patient for surgery with an antiseptic solution.

scrub typhus An acute febrile illness, occasionally complicated by pneumonia, meningoencephalitis, respiratory distress syndrome, or septic shock, caused by *Orientia tsutsugamushi.* Generally limited to Asian and Pacific nations, the disease is transmitted to humans by the bites of infected mites and chiggers. It can be treated with tetracyclines or azithromycin. The mortality rate in untreated patients is about 1% to 4%. SYN: *tsutsugamushi disease.*

scruple (skrū′pl) [L. *scrupulus,* small, sharp stone] ABBR: scr. Twenty grains in apothecaries' weight; 1.296 g.

SCUBA *self-contained underwater breathing apparatus.*

Scultetus binder (skŭl-tē'tŭs) SEE: *binder, Scultetus.*

Scultetus position Position in which the head is low and the body is on an inclined plane.

scum (skŭm) [ME. *scume*] Slimy floating islands of bacteria or impurities on the surface of a culture; an interrupted pellicle of bacterial growth.

scurf [AS. *scurf*] A branny desquamation of the epidermis, esp. on the scalp. SEE: *dandruff.*

scurvy (skŭr'vē) [L. *scorbutus*] A disease caused by inadequate intake of ascorbic acid, whose symptoms include fatigue, skin, joint, and gum bleeding, impaired wound healing, dry skin, lower extremity edema, follicular hyperkeratosis, and coiling of body hairs. It is rare in Western nations, where it is found primarily among alcoholics, the chronically mentally ill, and the socially isolated. It can be prevented with regular consumption of fruits and vegetables, foodstuffs that provide a rich source of dietary vitamin C. SEE: illus.

infantile s. A form of scurvy that sometimes follows the prolonged use of condensed milk, sterilized milk, or proprietary foods that do not contain supplementary vitamin C.

SYMPTOMS: This condition is characterized by anemia, pseudoparalysis, thickening of the bones from subperiosteal hemorrhage, ecchymoses, nonpitting edema, and tendency toward fractures of the epiphyses. SYN: *Barlow's disease.*

rebound s. Ascorbic acid deficiency symptoms caused by discontinuation of megadoses of vitamin C.

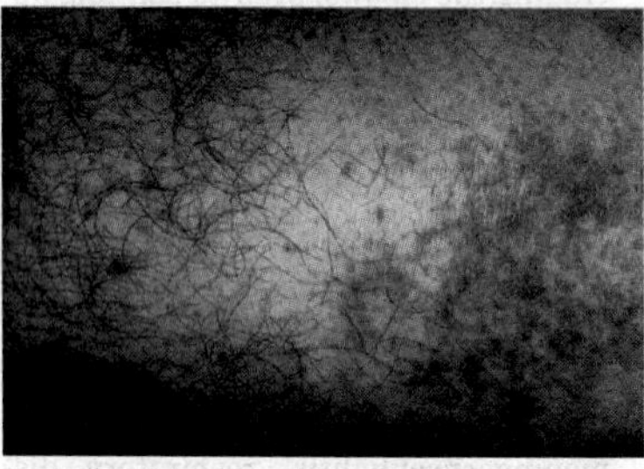

SCURVY

scute (skūt) [L. *scutum,* shield] **1.** A thin plate or scale.

scutiform (skū'tĭ-form) [" + *forma,* shape] Shield-shaped.

scutulum (skū'tū-lŭm) *pl.* **scutula** [L., a little shield] A lesion of the scalp caused by the fungus *Trichophyton schoenleinii.* The lesion appears as a yellow cup-shaped crust consisting of a dense mass of mycelia and epithelial debris. The cup faces up, and its center is pierced by the hair around which it has developed. SEE: *favus.* **scutular** (-lăr), *adj.*

scutum (skū'tŭm) [L., shield] A plate of bone resembling a shield.

scybalous (sĭb'ă-lŭs) [Gr. *skybalon,* dung] Of the nature of hard fecal matter.

scybalum (sĭb'ă-lŭm) *pl.* **scybala** A hard rounded fecal mass.

scyphoid (sī'foyd) [Gr. *skyphos,* cup, + *eidos,* form, shape] Cup-shaped.

S.D. **1.** *skin dose.* **2.** *standard deviation.*

SDA **1.** *specific dynamic action.* **2.** Abbr. for Latin *sacrodextra anterior,* the right sacroanterior fetal position.

SDMS *Society of Diagnostic Medical Sonographers.*

S.E. *standard error.*

Se Symbol for the element selenium.

sea cucumber A cylindrical marine invertebrate of the family Holothuria; some species have tentacles that contain a mild venom. Contact with the organism may produce dermatitis.

seal **1.** To close firmly. **2.** A material such as an adhesive or wax used to make an airtight closure.

border s. The edge of a denture that contacts the tissues in order to close the area under the denture to entrance by food, air, or liquids.

posterior palatal s. A seal at the posterior border of a denture.

velopharyngeal s. A seal between the oral and nasopharyngeal cavities.

sealant A substance applied to prevent leakage into or out of an area.

dental s. A resin that bonds to the etched enamel of a tooth and forms a protective coating resistant to chemical or physical breakdown. The sealant is placed in the deep pits and fissures to prevent the accumulation of debris and bacteria in cavity prone areas. Dental sealants are used in addition to fluorides to prevent caries (cavities). Also called *pit and fissure sealant.*

searcher (sĕrch'ĕr) [ME. *serchen*] An instrument for locating the opening of the ureter previous to inserting a catheter or exploring the sinuses, and esp. for detecting stones in the bladder. SYN: *sound.*

seasickness [AS. *sae,* sea, + *seocness,* illness] A form of motion sickness due to the motion of a boat. SEE: *motion sickness.*

seasonal affective disorder ABBR: SAD. A mood disorder characterized by dysphoria or depression in fall and winter, and relative mania or hypomania in the spring and summer. The disorder is more common in women than men, and in younger persons than older ones. Abnormalities of serotonin transmission in the brain have been linked to the disorder. Treatment consists of bright light exposure early in the morning during the shorter days of the year. Antidepressant medications such as fluoxetine may be helpful in treating persons who do not respond to the phototherapy.

seat The structure on which another structure rests or is supported.

basal s. Tissues in the mouth that support a denture.

elevated toilet s. Raised toilet s.

raised toilet s. A device for raising the height of a toilet to facilitate use by persons with limited strength or movement. SYN: *elevated toilet s.*

rest s. An area on which a denture or restoration rests.

Seattle foot [after the city Seattle, Washington, U.S., where it was developed] An artificial foot designed to absorb the impact of foot-to-floor contact with a dynamic elastic structure.

seatworm Pinworm.

sebaceous (sē-bā′shŭs) [L. *sebaceus,* made of tallow] Containing, or pert. to, sebum, an oily, fatty matter secreted by the sebaceous glands.

sebaceous gland An oil-secreting gland of the skin. The glands are simple or branched alveolar glands, most of which open into hair follicles. They are holocrine glands; their secretion, known as sebum, arises from the disintegration of cells filling the alveoli. Some aberrant glands are found in the cheeks or lips of the oral cavity, well separated from hair follicles. SEE: *Fordyce's disease.*

sebiparous (sē-bĭp′ă-rŭs) [″ + *parere,* to produce] Producing sebum or sebaceous matter.

sebo- Combining form meaning *fat, tallow.*

sebolite, sebolith (sĕb′ō-līt, -lĭth) [L. *sebum,* grease, tallow, + Gr. *lithos,* a stone] A concretion in a sebaceous gland.

seborrhea (sĕb-or-ē′ă) [″ + Gr. *rhoia,* flow] A disease of the sebaceous glands marked by an increase in the amount, and often an alteration of the quality, of the fats secreted by the sebaceous glands.

TREATMENT: Mild dandruff, a type of seborrhea, may be treated with a shampoo containing selenium sulfide or sulfur. Severe seborrhea is treated with a lotion or cream containing corticosteroids, rubbed into the affected areas two or three times a day.

s. capiti Seborrhea of the scalp.

s. corporis Dermatitis seborrheica.

s. faciei Seborrhea of the face.

s. furfuracea Dermatitis seborrheica.

s. nigricans Seborrhea with pigmented crusts.

s. oleosa Skin that appears shiny or oily.

s. sicca Dandruff.

seborrheic (sĕb″ō-rē′ĭk) [L. *sebum,* tallow, + Gr. *rhoia,* flow] Afflicted with or like seborrhea.

seborrheid (sĕb″ō-rē′ĭd) [″ + Gr. *rhoia,* flow] Dermatitis seborrheica.

sebum (sē′bŭm) [L., tallow] A fatty secretion of the sebaceous glands of the skin. It varies in different parts of the body. Sebum from the ears is called *cerumen;* that from the foreskin is called *smegma.*

s. palpebrale Lema.

seclusion of pupil Annular synechia.

secobarbital A barbiturate used for its sedative and hypnotic effects.

s. sodium A hypnotic and sedative drug.

secodont (sē′kō-dŏnt) [L. *secare,* to cut, + Gr. *odous,* tooth] Having molar teeth with cutting edges on the cusps.

secondary **1.** Next to or following; second in order. **2.** Produced by a primary cause.

secondary nursing care Nursing care aimed at early recognition and treatment of disease. It includes general nursing intervention and teaching of early signs of disease conditions so that prompt medical care can be obtained. SEE: *preventive nursing.*

secondary radiation X-rays produced by the interaction between primary radiation and the substance being radiated.

second cranial nerve The nerve carrying impulses for the sense of sight. It originates in the lateral geniculate body of the thalamus and travels by the optic tract and optic chiasma, where it enters the retina through the optic disk. SYN: *optic nerve.* SEE: *cranial nerve.*

second opinion An independent professional review and assessment of a patient, done to confirm, add to, or revise the diagnoses and proposed treatments of another medical professional.

secreta (sē-krē′tă) [L.] The products of secretion.

secretagogue (sē-krē′tă-gŏg) [L. *secretum,* secretion, + Gr. *agogos,* leading] **1.** That which stimulates secreting organs. **2.** An agent that causes secretion. SYN: *secretogogue.*

secrete (sē-krēt′) [L. *secretio,* separation] **1.** To separate from the blood, a living organism, or a gland. **2.** More specifically, to form a secretion.

secretin (sē-krē′tĭn) A hormone secreted by the duodenal mucosa that stimulates sodium bicarbonate secretion by the pancreas and bile secretion by the liver. It decreases gastrointestinal peristalsis and motility. SEE: *motilin.*

secretinase (sē-krē′tĭ-năs) An enzyme in blood that inactivates secretin.

secretion [L. *secretio,* separation] **1.** The making and release of substances by glands. Glandular secretions have many functions, such as digestion (bile, pepsin, stomach acid), temperature regulation (perspiration), excretion (urine), interorgan signaling (hormones), among others. **2.** The substance produced by glandular organs. If the material leaves the gland through a duct (e.g., saliva), it is called an exocrine secretion; if it enters the blood or lymph (e.g., insulin), it is called an endocrine secretion.

apocrine s. A secretion in which the apical end of a secreting cell is broken off and its contents extruded, as in the mammary gland.

external s. A secretion that passes through a duct and is discharged upon an epithelial surface, either internal or external. Also called *exocrine secretion.*

holocrine s. A secretion in which the entire cell and its contents are extruded as a part of the secretory product, as in sebaceous glands.

internal s. A secretion of the ductless glands, which, entering the bloodstream, activates other glands and organs. SYN: *hormone.* SEE: *ductless gland; endocrine; hormone.*

merocrine s. A secretion in which the product is elaborated within cells and discharged through the cell membrane, the cell itself remaining intact.

paralytic s. The continuous abundant watery secretion from a gland after section of its secretory nerves.

secretogogue (sē-krē′tō-gŏg) [L. *secretio,* separation, + Gr. *agogos,* leading] Secretagogue.

secretoinhibitory (sē-krē″tō-ĭn-hĭb′ĭ-tō″rē) Inhibiting secretion.

secretomotor (sē-krē″tō-mō′tor) Something, esp. a nerve, that stimulates secretion.

secretor (sē-krē′tor) [L. *secretio,* separation] A person who secretes ABO blood group substances into mucous secretions such as saliva, gastric juice, or semen. The secretion of such substances is sometimes used for the legal identification of individuals in violent crimes, such as rape.

secretory (sē-krē′tō-rē, sē′krē-tō″rē) Pert. to or promoting secretion; secreting.

secretory capillaries Very small canaliculi receiving secretion discharged from gland cells.

secretory fiber A peripheral motor nerve fiber that innervates glands and stimulates secretion.

sectarian (sĕk-tā′rē-ăn) [L. *sectus,* having cut] A medical practitioner who follows a dogma, tenet, or principle based on some unscientific belief.

sectile (sĕk′tĭl) [L. *sectilis*] Capable of being cut.

sectio (sĕk′shē-ō) [L., a cutting] Section or cut.

section [L. *sectio,* a cutting] **1.** Process of cutting. **2.** A division or segment of a part. SEE: *plane* for illus. **3.** A surface made by cutting.

abdominal s. Laparotomy.

cesarean s. SEE: *cesarean section.*

coronal s. Frontal s.

cross s. A section perpendicular to the long axis of an organ.

frontal s. A section dividing the body into two parts, dorsal and ventral. SYN: *coronal s.*

frozen s. A thin piece of surgically obtained tissue frozen to permit rapid examination of the specimen under the microscope. This technique is usually used while the patient is still anesthetized. The surgeon's further action (e.g., to operate further or to close the operation) is influenced by the results of this intraoperative test.

ground s. A section of bone or tooth prepared for histological study by polishing until thin enough for microscope viewing.

longitudinal s. A section parallel to the long axis of an organ.

midsagittal s. A section that divides the body into right and left halves.

paraffin s. A section of a tissue that has been infiltrated with paraffin.

perineal s. An external incision into the urethra to relieve stricture.

sagittal s. A section cut parallel to the median plane of the body.

serial s. One of the microscopic sections made and arranged in consecutive order.

vaginal s. Incision into the abdominal cavity through the vagina.

sectioning [L. *sectio,* a cutting] The slicing of thin sections of tissue for examination under the microscope. SEE: *microtome.*

ultrathin s. The cutting of sections extraordinarily thin (less than 1 μm thick), esp. for use in electron microscopy.

sector (sĕk′tor) [L., cutter] The area of a circle included between two radii and an arc.

rehab s. The location at a mass casualty incident, fire, or hazardous materials incident where rescue personnel are sent to be medically monitored, rehydrated, cooled off, or warmed, as the situation warrants.

staging s. The location near a mass casualty incident where local command and control operations are carried out.

transport s. At a mass casualty incident, the place where ambulances or helicopters, or both, are brought in to transport patients to hospitals. At the transport sector decisions are made regarding where to send patients with specialized problems, and the status of triaged patients is discussed with receiving facilities.

treatment s. The location at a mass casualty incident where patients' needs are prioritized and their injuries or illnesses are initially managed, before they are taken to a hospital.

triage s. In a mass casualty incident, the place where patients are sorted and separated according to the acuity of their illnesses or injuries, before they are transported to a treatment sector or hospital.

sectorial (sĕk-tō′rē-ăl) Having cutting edges, as teeth.

secundigravida (sē-kŭn″dĭ-grăv′ĭd-ă) [L. *secundus,* second, + *gravida,* pregnant] A woman in her second pregnancy.

secundines (sĕk′ŭn-dīnz, sĭ-kŭn′dīnz) [LL. *secundinae*] Afterbirth; the placenta and its membranes.

secundipara (sē″kŭn-dĭp′ă-ră) [L. *secundus,* second, + *parere,* to bring forth, to bear] A woman who has produced two infants at separate times that have weighed 500 g or more, regardless of their viability. SEE: *gravida; para.*

secundiparity (sē-kŭn″dĭ-păr′ĭ-tē) The condition of being a secundipara.

secure **1.** Free from danger, fear, care, or worry. **2.** Under lock and key. **3.** Stable; protected.

S.E.D. *skin erythema dose.*

sedation (sē-dā′shŭn) [L. *sedatio,* from *sedare,* to calm] **1.** The process of allaying nervous excitement. **2.** The state of being calmed.

conscious s. A minimally depressed level of consciousness during which the patient retains the ability to maintain a patent airway and respond appropriately to physical or verbal commands. This is accomplished by the use of appropriate analgesics and sedatives. This type of sedation is used for a variety of procedures including changing of wound or burn dressings and endoscopic examinations.

CAUTION: Although this method is effective, it must be used carefully to prevent loss of consciousness. The health care team must be ready to recognize and respond to complications that require airway management, intubation, and resuscitation. Drugs to reverse the effects of opioids (such as naloxone) and benzodiazepines (such as flumazenil) are used to awaken sedated patients.

---

sedative (sĕd′ă-tĭv) [L. *sedativus,* calming] **1.** Quieting. **2.** An agent that exerts a soothing or tranquilizing effect. Sedatives may be general, local, or vascular.

sedentary (sĕd′ĕn-tā′rē) [L. *sedentarius*] **1.** Sitting. **2.** Pert. to an occupation or mode of living requiring minimal physical exercise.

s. lifestyle A lifestyle involving little exercise, even of the least strenuous type. Sedentary living is associated with weight gain, obesity, type 2 diabetes mellitus, and, in many studies, an increased risk of coronary artery disease. SEE: *physical fitness; risk factor.*

sediment (sĕd′ĭ-mĕnt) [L. *sedimentum,* a settling] The substance settling at the bottom of a liquid. SEE: *precipitate.*

urinary s. Substances present in urine (i.e., bacteria, mucus, phosphates, uric acid, calcium oxalate, calcium carbonate, calcium phosphate, magnesium and ammonium phosphate; more rarely, cystine, tyrosine, xanthine, hippuric acid, hematoidin) that separate and accumulate at the bottom of a container of urine. This process may be accelerated by centrifuging the urine specimen.

sedimentation (sĕd″ĭ-mĕn-tā′shŭn) Formation or depositing of sediment.

seed (sēd) [AS. *saed*] **1.** The ripened ovule of a spermatophyte plant usually consisting of the embryo (germ) and a supply of nutrient material enclosed within the seed coats. It is a resting sporophyte. **2.** Semen. **3.** Capsule containing radon or radium for use in the treatment of cancer. **4.** To introduce microorganisms into a culture medium.

seeker, bone An ion or compound that localizes preferentially in bone (e.g., strontium).

Seessel's pouch (zā′sĕlz) [Albert Seessel, U.S. embryologist and neurologist, 1850–1910] In the embryo, a small ectodermal diverticulum of the foregut close to the buccopharyngeal membrane. It disappears in humans.

segment (sĕg′mĕnt) [L. *segmentum,* a portion] **1.** A part or section, esp. a natural one, of an organ or body. **2.** One of the serial divisions of an animal.

bronchopulmonary s. A small subdivision of the lobes of the lung.

hepatic s. A subdivision of the lobes of the liver.

interannular s. The portion of a neuron between the two nodes of Ranvier.

mesodermal s. A somite.

uterine s. One of the two functional divisions of the uterine musculature during labor. During labor the upper uterine segment forcibly contracts, becoming progressively shorter and thicker, exerting traction on the more passive lower segment, and increasing the hydrostatic pressure against the cervix. The combination of forces and traction gradually cause the lower segment to thin, resulting in cervical effacement and dilation. SEE: *physiologic retraction ring.*

segmental (sĕg-mĕn′tăl) Pert. to, resembling, or composed of segments.

segmental static reaction A postural reflex in which the movement of one extremity results in a movement in an opposite extremity.

segmentation (sĕg″mĕn-tā′shŭn) Cleavage.

segmenter A stage in the development of malarial parasites (genus *Plasmo-*

dium), in which the organism undergoes schizogony.

segregation [L. *segregare,* to separate] **1.** Setting apart, separating. **2.** In genetics, the process that takes place in the formation of germ cells (gametogenesis) in which each gamete (egg or sperm) receives only one of each pair of genes.

segregator An instrument composed of two ureteral catheters for securing urine from each kidney separately.

Séguin's signal symptom (sā-gănz′) [Edouard Séguin, French psychiatrist in U.S., 1812–1880] The involuntary contractions of the muscles just before an epileptic attack.

SeHCAT ^{75}Selenium-labeled artificial bile salt; homologue to taurocholate.

seismesthesia (sīz″měs-thē′zē-ă) [Gr. *seismos,* a shaking, + *aisthesis,* sensation] The perception of vibrations.

seizure (sē′zhūr) [O.Fr. *seisir,* to take possession of] **1.** A convulsion or other clinically detectable event caused by a sudden discharge of electrical activity in the brain. **2.** A sudden attack of pain, disease, or specific symptoms.

absence s. Seizure in which there is a sudden, brief lapse of consciousness, usually for about 2 to 10 sec. The patient (typically a child) shows a blank facial expression that may be accompanied by movements such as repeated eye-blinking or lip-smacking and minor myoclonus of the upper extremities or neck. There is no convulsion or fall. The patient resumes activity as if the seizure had not occurred. The seizure may be induced by voluntary hyperventilation for 2 to 3 min. This type of attack is characteristic of petit mal epilepsy and may recur repeatedly if it is not recognized and treated.

PATIENT CARE: The time, duration, patient's expression, and any repetitive movements occurring during the seizure are observed and documented, as is the patient's postseizure response. Prescribed medications are administered and evaluated for desired effects and adverse reactions. Support, reassurance, and education regarding the condition as well as drug actions and side effects are provided to the patient and family, and they are encouraged to discuss their feelings and concerns and to ask questions. SEE: *epilepsy*.

convulsive s. **1.** A convulsion. **2.** An attack of epilepsy. SEE: *epilepsy*.

grand mal s. SEE: Under *epilepsy*.

jacksonian s. SEE: *jacksonian epilepsy*.

petit mal s. SEE: *epilepsy*.

Seldinger technique [Sven I. Seldinger, Swedish physician, b. 1921] A method of percutaneous introduction of a catheter into a vessel. The vessel is located and a needle is inserted. Once a good blood flow is obtained, a wire is threaded through the needle well into the vessel; the needle is then removed and the catheter threaded over the wire into the vessel. The wire assists in inserting the catheter and guiding it into the appropriate vessel. Once the catheter is positioned in the desired intravascular area, the wire is removed. Sterile technique is imperative.

selection [L. *selectus,* having chosen] **1.** Choice; the process of choosing or selecting. **2.** In biology, the factors that determine the reproductive ability of a certain genotype.

artificial s. A process by which humans select desirable characteristics in animals and breed them for these phenotypes.

clonal s. **1.** The process by which T lymphocytes with receptors that react to self-antigens are destroyed in the thymus. **2.** The increase of particular B or T lymphocyte clones that multiply after recognition of a specific antigen to which the body has been previously exposed. SEE: *negative s.; clone*.

natural s. A mechanism of evolution proposed by Darwin stating that the genotypes best adapted to their environment have a tendency to survive and reproduce.

negative s. The process by which immature T lymphocytes (thymocytes) with receptors for self-antigens are destroyed in the thymus. This is part of the mechanism that prevents autoimmune diseases. SEE: *autoimmunity*.

sexual s. **1.** The choice of the gender of an offspring through methods that increase the likelihood of conceiving either a girl or a boy. **2.** A theory originated to account for differences in secondary sex characteristics between male and female animals (including humans). It assumes that individuals preferentially mate with individuals of the opposite sex who possess identifiably distinct phenotypes.

selective estrogen receptor modulator Estrogen analog.

selenium (sē-lē′nē-ŭm) [Gr. *selene,* moon] SYMB: Se. A chemical element resembling sulfur; atomic weight 78.96; atomic number 34. It is considered an essential trace element in the diet. Toxicity can occur when an excessive amount is ingested, characterized by a sour breath odor, nausea, vomiting, abdominal pain, restlessness, hypersalivation, and muscle spasms.

s. sulfide A drug used to treat dandruff and tinea versicolor.

selenoid cell Achromocyte. SYN: *crescent body*.

selenomethionine Se 75 injection (sĕl″ĕn-ō-mĕ-thī′ō-nēn) Radioactive L-selenomethionine in which the sulfur atom in the methionine has been replaced by selenium. The compound is used intravenously to investigate methionine metabolism.

self **1.** In psychology, the sum of mind and body that constitutes the identity of a person. **2.** In immunology, an individual's antigenic makeup.

self-acceptance Being realistic about oneself and at the same time comfortable with that personal assessment.

self-care **1.** A concept in Dorothea Orem's Self-Care Framework and her Theory of Self-Care referring to actions that individuals initiate and perform on their own behalf in maintaining life, health, and well-being. **2.** In rehabilitation, the subset of activities of daily living that includes eating, dressing, grooming, bathing, and toileting. SYN: *personal care.*

s.-c. deficit, feeding An impaired ability to perform or complete feeding activities. SEE: *health maintenance, altered; home maintenance management, impaired; Nursing Diagnoses Appendix.*

s.-c. deficit, bathing/hygiene Impaired ability to perform or complete bathing/hygiene activities for oneself. SEE: *health maintenance, altered; home maintenance management, impaired; Nursing Diagnoses Appendix.*

s.-c. deficit, dressing/grooming An impaired ability to perform or complete dressing and grooming activities for oneself. SEE: *health maintenance, altered; home maintenance management, impaired; Nursing Diagnoses Appendix.*

s.-c. deficit, toilet An impaired ability to perform or complete one's own toileting activities. SEE: *health maintenance, altered; home maintenance management, impaired; Nursing Diagnoses Appendix.*

Self-Care Framework A conceptual model of nursing, also known as the Self-Care Deficit Theory of Nursing, developed by Dorothea Orem. The person is a self-care agent who has a therapeutic self-care demand made up of universal, developmental, and health deviation self-care requisites. The goal of nursing is to help people to meet their therapeutic self-care demands. SEE: *Nursing Theory Appendix.*

self-concept An individual's perception of self in relation to others and the environment. SEE: *self-esteem.*

self-conscious Being aware of oneself, esp. overly aware of appearance and actions, and thus being ill at ease.

self-contained breathing apparatus ABBR: SCBA. A device that provides respiratory gases. It is used, for example, by rescue personnel, when they enter hazardous breathing environments.

self-contained underwater breathing apparatus ABBR: SCUBA. A device used by swimmers and divers that enables them to breathe underwater. The mask worn is watertight and is connected to a tank of compressed air. SEE: *bends.*

self-differentiation The differentiation of a structure or tissue due to intrinsic factors.

self-digestion Autodigestion.

self-efficacy An aspect of self-perception postulated by Albert Bandura that pertains to one's belief in his or her ability to perform a given task or behavior.

self-esteem One's personal evaluation or view of self, generally thought to influence feelings and behaviors. One's personal successes, expectations, and appraisals of the views others hold toward oneself are thought to influence this personal appraisal. SYN: *self-concept.*

chronic low s.-e. Longstanding negative feelings about self or capabilities. SEE: *situational low s.-e.; Nursing Diagnoses Appendix.*

s.-e. disturbance Negative self-evaluation/feelings about self or self-capabilities that may be directly or indirectly expressed. SEE: *Nursing Diagnoses Appendix.*

situational low s.-e. Episodic feelings about self or capabilities that develop in response to a loss or change. SEE: *chronic low s.-e.; Nursing Diagnoses Appendix.*

self-examination Inspection and palpation of a body part by the patient to screen for disease. SEE: *breast self-examination; testicle, self-examination of.*

self-governance **1.** Self-rule; local responsibility for administration and functions of an organization, even though it is part of a larger entity. **2.** A model of health care management in which the power base for decisions of patient care is decentralized. The responsibility and accountability for patient care rest directly with all levels of care providers through self-direction, self-regulation, and self-management. Advisory committees reflecting a cross section of caregivers (new graduates, experienced professionals, faculty, and managers) maintain final decision-making authority within the work setting. SEE: *shared governance.*

self-hypnosis Hypnotizing oneself.

self-insured Having personal financial responsibility for health care costs, as a result of dedicated savings or investments.

self-management Active participation by a patient in his or her own health care decisions and interventions. With the education and guidance of professional caregivers, the patient promotes his or her own optimal health or recovery.

self-medication The use of mood-altering substances, such as alcohol or opiates, in an attempt to alleviate depression, anxiety, or other psychiatric disorders.

self-mutilation, risk for A state in which an individual is at high risk to perform a deliberate act upon the self with the intent to injure, not kill, which produces immediate tissue damage to the body. SEE: *Nursing Diagnoses Appendix.*

self-pity A mental defense mechanism involving self-blame, negativism, feelings of rejection, worthlessness, hopelessness, or isolation.

self-ranging Patient-administered passive or active assistive range-of-motion exercise. Patients can be taught to prevent contractures and facilitate movement by using their unaffected extremities and by means of specific techniques. Care should be taken to prevent injury, esp. at the shoulder.

self-tolerance In immunology, the absence of an immune response to one's own antigens. SEE: *autoimmunity.*

Seligmann's disease Alpha heavy chain disease.

sellar (sĕl'ăr) Concerning the sella turcica.

sella turcica (sĕl'ă tŭr'sĭ-kă) [NL., Turkish saddle] A concavity on the superior surface of the body of the sphenoid bone that houses the pituitary gland. SEE: *empty-sella syndrome.*

Sellick's maneuver [Brian A. Sellick, contemporary Brit. anesthetist] The application of digital pressure to the cricoid cartilage in the neck in an unconscious patient to reduce gastric distention and passive regurgitation during positive pressure ventilation, and to improve visualization of the glottic opening during endotracheal intubation.

seltzer water **1.** Naturally occurring water with a high mineral and carbon dioxide content. **2.** Water that has been artificially charged with carbon dioxide.

semantics (sē-măn'tĭks) [Gr. *semantikos,* significant] The study of the meanings of words.

semen (sē'mĕn) *pl.* **semina** [L., seed] A thick, opalescent, viscid secretion discharged from the urethra of the male at the climax of sexual excitement (orgasm). Semen is the mixed product of various glands (prostate and bulbourethral) plus the spermatozoa, which, having been produced in the testicles, are stored in the seminal vesicles.

Normal values for the seminal fluid ejaculate are as follows: volume, 2 to 5 ml; pH, 7.8 to 8.0; leukocytes, absent or only an occasional one seen per high-power field; sperm count, 60 to 150 million/ml; motility, 80% or more should be motile; morphology, 80% to 90% should be normal.

frozen s. Semen stored in a bank for future use in insemination. It offers a supply of donors in small communities where it would be impossible to maintain anonymity of local donors. However, in artificial insemination the number of successful pregnancies is lower with frozen semen than with fresh.

semenarche (sē'mĕn-ăr"kē) [" + *arche,* beginning] During puberty, the beginning of the production of semen. SEE: *pubarche; thelarche.*

semenuria (sē"mĕn-ū'rē-ă) [L. *semen,* seed, + Gr. *ouron,* urine] The excretion of semen in the urine. SYN: *seminuria; spermaturia.*

semi- Prefix meaning *half.*

semicanal (sĕm"ē-kăn-ăl') [L. *semis,* half, + *canalis,* channel] A duct open on one side.

semicanalis (sĕm"ē-kă-nā'lĭs) [L., semicanal] A channel open on one side.

s. musculi tensoris tympani The semicanal of the tensor tympani muscle in the temporal bone.

s. tubae auditivae The semicanal of the auditory tube.

semicartilaginous (sĕm"ē-kăr"tĭ-lăj'ĭ-nŭs) [" + *cartilago,* gristle] Partially cartilaginous.

semicircular (sĕm"ē-sŭr'kū-lăr) [" + *circulus,* a ring] In the form of a half circle.

semicoma (sĕm"ē-kō'mă) [" + Gr. *koma,* a deep sleep] An improper term, generally used to mean *stupor* or *lethargy.*

semiconscious Half-conscious or not fully conscious.

semicrista (sĕm"ē-krĭs'tă) [L.] A small or rudimentary crest.

s. incisiva The nasal crest of the maxilla.

semidecussation (sĕm"ē-dē"kŭs-sā'shŭn) [" + *decussare,* to make an X] Incomplete crossing of nerve fibers.

semierection (sĕm"ē-ē-rĕk'shŭn) [" + *erigere,* to erect] An incomplete erection.

semiflexion (sĕm"ē-flĕk'shŭn) [" + *flexio,* bending] Halfway between flexion and extension of a limb.

semilunar (sĕm"ē-lū'năr) [L. *semis,* half, + *luna,* moon] Shaped like a crescent.

semilunar bone Crescent-shaped bone of the carpus. Also called the *lunate bone.* SYN: *semilunare.*

semilunar cusp One of the segments of the aortic valve between the left ventricle and the aorta or of the pulmonary valve between the right ventricle and the pulmonary artery.

semilunare (sĕm"ē-lū-nā'rē) [L.] Semilunar bone.

semilunar lobe A lobe on the upper surface of the cerebellum.

semiluxation (sĕm"ē-lŭk-sā'shŭn) [" + *luxatio,* dislocation] Subluxation.

semimembranosus (sĕm"ē-mĕm"brăn-ō'sŭs) [L.] A large muscle of the inner and back part of the thigh.

semimembranous (sĕm"ē-mĕm'bră-nŭs) [" + L. *membrana,* membrane] Composed partly of a membrane.

seminal (sĕm'ĭ-năl) [L. *seminalis*] Concerning the semen or seed.

seminal emission Discharge of semen.

semination (sĕm-ĭ-nā′shŭn) [L. *seminatio,* a begetting] Insemination.

artificial s. Artificial insemination.

seminiferous (sĕm-ĭn-ĭf′ĕr-ŭs) [L. *semen,* seed, + *ferre,* to produce] Producing or conducting semen, as the tubules of the testes.

seminoma (sĕm″ĭ-nō′mă) [″ + Gr. *oma,* tumor] A cancer arising from male germ cells (in the testis) that makes up about half of all testicular malignancies.

TREATMENT: Seminomas that are confined to the testes are surgically removed. Metastatic disease is treated with surgery (to remove the testis) and radiation and chemotherapy.

seminormal (sĕm″ē-nor′măl) [L. *semis,* half, + *norma,* rule] One-half the normal standard.

seminose (sĕm′ĭ-nōs) Mannose.

seminuria (sē″mĭn-ū′rē-ă) [L. *semen,* seed, + Gr. *ouron,* urine] Semen in the urine. SYN: *semenuria; spermaturia.*

semiorbicular (sĕm″ē-or-bĭk′ū-lăr) [L. *semis,* half, + *orbiculus,* a small circle] Semicircular.

semiotics (sē″mī-ŏt′ĭks) The philosophy of the function of signs and symbols in language.

semipermeable (sĕm″ē-per′mē-ă-bl) [″ + *per,* through, + *meare,* to pass] Half-permeable; said of a membrane that will allow fluids, but not the dissolved substance, to pass through it. SEE: *membrane; osmosis.*

semipronation (sĕm″ē-prō-nā′shŭn) [″ + *pronus,* prone] **1.** A semiprone position. **2.** The act of assuming a semiprone position.

semiprone (sĕm-ē-prōn′) [″ + *pronus,* prone] In a position on left side and chest, with both thighs flexed on abdomen, the right higher than the left, and left arm back. SYN: *Sims' position.*

semirecumbent (sĕm″ē-rē-kŭm′bĕnt) [″ + *recumbere,* to lie down] Reclining, but not fully recumbent.

semis (sē′mĭs) [L.] ABBR: ss. Half.

semispinalis (sĕm″ē-spī-năl′ĭs) [L.] The deep layer of muscle of the back on either side of the spinal column. It is divided into the following three parts: the semispinalis capitis, semispinalis cervicis, and semispinalis thoracis.

semisulcus (sĕm″ē-sŭl′kŭs) [L. *semis,* half, + *sulcus,* groove] A small sulcus or channel in a structure. It usually joins with another small channel to form a complete sulcus.

semisupination (sĕm″ē-sū-pĭn-ā′shŭn) [″ + *supinus,* lying on the back] A position halfway between supination and pronation.

semisupine (sĕm″ē-sū′pīn) [″ + *supinus,* lying on the back] Not completely supine.

semisynthetic (sĕm″ē-sĭn-thĕt′ĭk) [″ + Gr. *synthetikos,* synthetic] The chemical alteration of a portion of a natural substance.

semitendinosus (sĕm″ē-tĕn″dĭn-ō′sŭs) [L.] The fusiform muscle of the posterior and inner part of the thigh.

semitendinous (sĕm″ē-tĕn′dĭ-nŭs) [L. *semis,* half, + *tendinosus,* tendinous] Being partially tendinous.

Semmelweiss, Ignaz Phillip Hungarian physician, 1818–1865, the discoverer of the mode of transmission of childbed fever (puerperal sepsis) in the 19th century. Semmelweiss noted the significantly lower incidence of this condition in women who were attended by midwives who used chlorinated lime solution as a disinfectant hand rinse to prevent transfer of organisms to the birth canal during delivery.

senescence (sē-nĕs′ĕns) [L. *senescens,* growing old] **1.** The process of growing old. **2.** The period of old age.

replicative s. Hayflick's limit.

Sengstaken-Blakemore tube (sĕngz′tā-kĕn-blāk′mor) [Robert W. Sengstaken, U.S. neurosurgeon, b. 1923; Arthur H. Blakemore, U.S. surgeon, 1897–1970] A three-lumen tube used in the past to treat bleeding esophageal varices. One lumen leads to the stomach for aspiration of secretions; another leads to a balloon at the gastric end, which is used to inflate the balloon after the tube is in place; the third lumen leads to an inflatable cuff in the esophagus around a portion of the tube. This third lumen stabilizes the cuff within the esophagus, which when inflated applies pressure against the varices. Additionally, a padded stent is employed about the nares to prevent migration of the balloon cuff; external traction may also be applied.

senile (sē′nīl, sĕn′īl) [L. *senilis,* old] Pert. to growing old and the mental or physical weakness with which it is sometimes associated.

senility (sē-nĭl′ĭ-tē) [L. *senilis,* old] Mental or physical weakness that may be associated with old age.

premature s. Onset of senile characteristics before old age (e.g., in Down syndrome).

psychosis of s. Mental disorder in old age.

senium (sē′nē-ŭm) [L.] Old age, esp. its debility.

senna (sĕn′ă) [Arabic *sana*] The dried leaves of the plants *Cassia acutifolia* and *C. angustifolia;* used as a cathartic.

sennosides (sĕn′ō-sīdz) Anthraquinone glucosides present in senna that are used as cathartics.

senopia (sĕn-ō′pē-ă, sē-nō′-) [L. *senilis,* old, + Gr. *ops,* eye] Improvement in near vision of old people. Usually precedes the development of nuclear cataract. SYN: *sight, second.*

sensate (sĕn-sāt′) Perceived by the senses.

sensate focus An area, such as an erogenous zone, that is particularly sensitive to tactile stimulation.

sensation (sĕn-sā′shŭn) [L. *sensatio*] A feeling or awareness of conditions within or without the body resulting from the stimulation of sensory receptors.

cincture s. Zonesthesia.

cutaneous s. A sensation arising from the receptors of the skin.

delayed s. A sensation not experienced immediately following a stimulus.

external s. The effect upon the mind of stimuli produced from a source outside the body.

girdle s. Zonesthesia.

gnostic s. One of the more finely developed senses such as touch, tactile discrimination, position sense, and vibration.

internal s. Subjective s.

palmesthetic s. A sensation felt in the skin from vibration.

phantom s. Phantom limb pain.

primary s. A sensation that results from a direct stimulus.

proprioceptive s. Proprioception.

referred s. A sensation that seems to arise from a source other than the actual one. SYN: *reflex s.*

reflex s. Referred s.

somesthetic s. A sense; proprioception.

subjective s. A sensation that does not result from any external stimulus and is perceptible only by the subject. SYN: *internal s.*

tactile s. A sensation produced through the sense of touch.

sense, sensing (sĕns) [L. *sensus,* a feeling] **1.** To perceive through a sense organ. **2.** The general faculty by which conditions outside or inside the body are perceived. The most important of the senses are sight, hearing, smell, taste, touch and pressure, temperature, weight, resistance and tension (muscle sense), pain, position, proprioception, visceral and sexual sensations, equilibrium, and hunger and thirst. **3.** Any special faculty of sensation connected with a particular organ. **4.** Normal power of understanding. **5.** The ability of an artificial pacemaker to detect an electrically conducted signal produced by the heart, such as a P wave or QRS complex.

color s. The ability to distinguish differences in color; one of the three parts of visual function.

form s. The ability to recognize shapes; one of the three parts of visual function.

kinesthetic s. Muscular s.

light s. The ability to distinguish degrees of light intensity; one of the three parts of the visual function.

muscular s. The brain's awareness of the position of muscles, both moving and at rest; it may be conscious or unconscious. SYN: *kinesthetic s.* SEE: *proprioception.*

posture s. Proprioception.

pressure s. The ability to feel various degrees of pressure on the body surface. SYN: *baresthesia.*

proprioceptive s. Proprioception.

sixth s. A general feeling of normal functioning of the body.

space s. The sense by which people recognize objects in space, their relationship, and their dimensions.

special s. The senses of sight, touch, hearing, equilibrium, smell, and taste.

static s. The sense that makes it possible to maintain equilibrium.

stereognostic s. The ability to judge the consistency and shape of objects held in the fingers.

temperature s. The ability to detect differences of temperature.

time s. The ability to detect differences in time intervals.

tone s. The ability to distinguish between different tones.

visceral s. The subjective perception of the sensations of the internal organs.

sensibility (sĕn″sĭ-bĭl′ĭ-tē) [L. *sensibilitas*] The capacity to receive and respond to stimuli.

deep s. **1.** The sensibility existing after an area of the skin is made anesthetic. **2.** The sensation by which the position of a limb and estimation of difference in weight and tension are apparent.

palmesthetic s. The sensibility of the skin to vibration.

sensibilization (sĕn″sĭ-bĭl-ĭz-ā′shŭn) **1.** Sensitization. **2.** Production of hypersusceptibility to a foreign substance by injecting it into the body. SYN: *sensitization.*

sensible (sĕn′sĭ-bl) [L. *sensibilis,* capable of being perceived] **1.** Capable of being perceived by the senses; perceptible. **2.** Having reason.

sensiferous (sĕn-sĭf′ĕr-ŭs) [L. *sensus,* a feeling, + *ferre,* to bear] Causing, conducting, or transmitting sensations.

sensimeter (sĕn-sĭm′ĕ-tĕr) [″ + Gr. *metron,* measure] A machine for recording the degree of sensitiveness of various areas of the body.

sensitinogen (sĕn″sĭ-tĭn′ō-jĕn) [″ + Gr. *gennan,* to produce] The collective of antigens that sensitize the body.

sensitive (sĕn′sĭ-tĭv) [L. *sensitivus,* of sensation] **1.** Capable of perceiving or feeling a sensation. SYN: *sentient.* **2.** Subject to destructive action of a complement. **3.** Susceptible to suggestions, as a hypnotic. **4.** Abnormally susceptible to a substance, as a drug or foreign protein. SEE: *allergy.*

sensitivity In assessing the value of a diagnostic test, procedure, or clinical observation, the proportion of people who truly have a specific disease and are so identified by the test. SEE: *specificity, diagnostic*.

sensitivity test, antimicrobial A laboratory method of determining the susceptibility of antibiotics. The specimen obtained is cultured in various liquid dilutions or on solid media containing various concentrations of antimicrobial drugs in disks placed on the surface of the media. The disk-type test is not completely reliable. Also called *culture and sensitivity test*. SEE: illus.

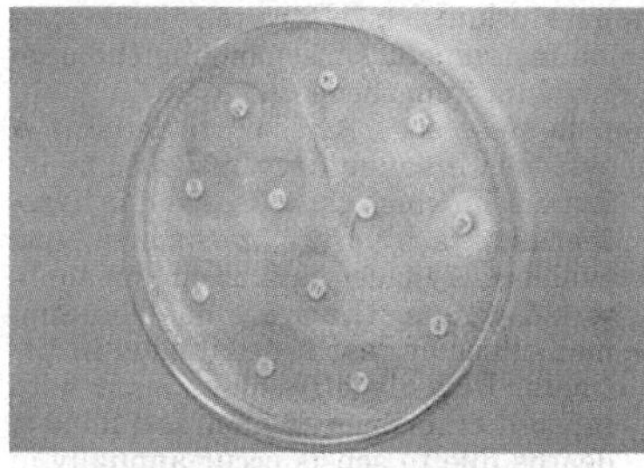

ANTIMICROBIAL SENSITIVITY TEST

Zones of inhibited bacterial growth around antibiotic disks

sensitivity training A form of group therapy in which individuals are given the opportunity to relate verbally and physically with complete candor and honesty with other members of the group. The goals of therapy are to increase self-awareness, learn constructive ways of dealing with conflicts, establish a better sense of inner direction, and relate to persons with feelings of warmth and affection.

sensitization (sěn″sĭ-tĭ-zā′shŭn) **1.** The production by B lymphocytes of specific antibodies and by T lymphocytes of specific cellular reactions to a foreign antigen. When the antigen is encountered again, an immune response occurs. SEE: *hypersensitivity*. **2.** The process of making a person susceptible to a substance by repeated injections of it. SYN: *sensibilization*.

active s. Sensitization produced by injecting an antigen into a susceptible person.

autoerythrocyte s. A syndrome characterized by the spontaneous appearance of painful ecchymoses, usually at the site of a bruise. The areas itch and burn. The condition is commonly associated with headache, nausea, vomiting, and occasionally with intracranial, genitourinary, and gastrointestinal bleeding. With few exceptions, the disorder affects women of middle age. The cause is assumed to be autosensitivity to a component of the red blood cell membrane. There is no specific therapy. SYN: *purpura, psychogenic*.

passive s. Sensitization produced in a healthy person by injecting the person with the serum from a sensitized animal or human.

protein s. Sensitization as a result of previous injection of a foreign protein into the body.

sensitized (sěn′sĭ-tīzd) Made susceptible, or immunoreactive, to an antigen.

sensitizer (sěn′sĭ-tī″zěr) [L. *sensitivus*, of sensation] In allergy and dermatology, a substance that makes the susceptible individual react to the same or other irritants.

sensitometer A calibrated instrument with an optical step wedge and light source that puts a graduated set of densities on a radiographic film; used in quality control monitoring for film processors.

sensitometry In radiography, the use of densities on an exposed and processed film to evaluate, monitor, and maintain processors, intensifying screens, film types, and exposure systems.

sensomobile (sěn″sō-mō′bĭl) [L. *sensus*, a feeling, + *mobilis*, mobile] Movement in response to a stimulus. **sensomobility,** *adj.*

sensomotor Sensorimotor.

sensor **1.** A sense organ. **2.** A device sensitive to light, heat, radiation, sound, or mechanical or other physical stimuli. These devices may be equipped to record the phenomena being detected and to sound an alarm if the value falls below or rises above a certain level.

sensoriglandular (sěn″sō-rē-glănd′dū-lăr) [L. *sensus*, a feeling, + *glandula*, little acorn] Concerning glandular secretion in reflex response to a sensation.

sensorimetabolism (sěn″sō-rē-mě-tăb′ō-lĭzm) [″ + Gr. *metaballein*, to alter, + *-ismos*, condition] Metabolic activity in response to sensory nerve stimulation.

sensorimotor (sěn″sō-rē-mō′tor) [L. *sensus*, a feeling, + *motus*, moving] Both sensory and motor. SYN: *sensomotor*.

sensorimuscular (sěn″sō-rē-mŭs′kū-lăr) [″ + *muscularis*, muscular] Muscular activity in response to a sensory stimulus.

sensorineural (sěn″sō-rē-nū′răl) [″ + *neuralis*, neural] Concerning a sensory nerve.

sensorium (sěn-sor′ē-ŭm) *pl.* **sensoriums, sensoria** [L., organ of sensation] **1.** That portion of the brain that functions as a center of sensations. **2.** The sensory apparatus of the body taken as a whole. **3.** Awareness; consciousness. **sensorial** (-sō′rē-ăl), *adj.*

sensorivasomotor (sěn″sō-rē-văs″ō-mō′tor) [L. *sensus*, a feeling, + *vas*, vessel, + *motor*, a mover] Vascular changes induced by sensory nerve stimulation.

sensory (sĕn′sō-rē) [L. *sensorius*] **1.** Conveying impulses from sense organs to the reflex or higher centers. SYN: *afferent.* **2.** Pert. to sensation.

sensory area Any area of the cerebral cortex in which sensations are perceived.

somesthetic s.a. An area in the postcentral gyrus of the parietal lobes and extending into adjacent areas in which cutaneous senses and conscious proprioceptive sense are perceived.

sensory ending A termination of an afferent nerve fiber that upon stimulation gives rise to a sensation. SEE: *receptor, sensory.*

sensory epilepsy Disturbances of sensation without convulsions.

sensory integration Skill and performance required in the development and coordination of sensory input, motor output, and sensory feedback. It includes sensory awareness, visual spatial awareness, body integration, balance, bilateral motor coordination, visuomotor integration, praxis, and other components.

sensory overload The condition in which sensory stimuli are received at a rate and intensity beyond the level that the patient can handle. This stressful situation can lead to confusion, anxiety, mental distress, and panic.

sensory/perceptual alterations (specify): visual, auditory, kinesthetic, gustatory, tactile, olfactory A state in which an individual experiences a change in the amount or patterning of incoming stimuli accompanied by a diminished, exaggerated, distorted, or impaired response to such stimuli. SEE: *Nursing Diagnoses Appendix.*

sensory registration The brain's ability to receive input and select that which will receive attention and that which will be inhibited from conscious attention.

sensory unit A single sensory neuron and all its receptors.

sensual (sĕn′shū-ăl) [L. *sensus,* a feeling] Concerning or consisting in the gratification of the senses; indulgence of the appetites; not spiritual or intellectual; carnal, worldly.

sensualism (sĕn′shū-ăl-ĭzm) The state of being sensual, in which one's actions are dominated by the emotions.

sensuous (sĕn′shū-ŭs) [L. *sensus,* a feeling] **1.** Pert. to or affecting the senses. **2.** Susceptible to influence through the senses.

sentient (sĕn′shē-ĕnt) [L. *sentiens,* perceive] Capable of perceiving sensation. SYN: *sensitive.*

sentiment (sĕn′tĭ-mĕnt) [L. *sentio,* to feel] **1.** Feeling, sensibility; any emotional attitude toward objects or subjects. **2.** Tenderness.

separation **1.** The process of disconnecting, disuniting, or severing. **2.** The purification or isolation of a chemical compound from a mixture or solution. SEE: *centrifuge; electrophoresis; iontophoresis.*

acromioclavicular s. A sprain to the acromioclavicular and coracoclavicular ligaments, commonly caused by a fall or a blow directly to the shoulder (shoulder separation).

separator [LL. *separator*] **1.** Anything that prevents two substances from mingling. **2.** Any device or instrument used for separating two substances such as cream from milk.

separatorium (sĕp″ă-rā-tō′rē-ŭm) [L.] An instrument for separating the pericranium from the skull.

sepsis (sĕp′sĭs) [Gr., putrefaction] A systemic inflammatory response to infection, in which there is fever or hypothermia, tachycardia, tachypnea, and evidence of inadequate blood flow to internal organs. The syndrome is a common cause of death in critically ill patients. Roughly 40% of patients with sepsis die; between 200,000 and 400,000 deaths due to sepsis occur annually in the U.S. Pathogenic organisms, including bacteria, mycobacteria, fungi, protozoa, and viruses, may initiate the cascade of inflammatory reactions that constitute sepsis. The number of patients with sepsis has increased significantly in the last 25 years, as a result of several factors including: the aging of the population, the increased number of patients living with immune suppressing illnesses (e.g., organ transplants), the increased number of patients living with multiple diseases, and the increased use of invasive or indwelling devices in health care, which serve as portals of entry for infection.

Complications of sepsis may include shock, organ failure (e.g., adult respiratory distress syndrome or acute renal failure), disseminated intravascular coagulation, altered mental status, jaundice, metastatic abscess formation, and multiple organ system failure.

ETIOLOGY: Sepsis results from the combined effect of a virulent infection and a powerful host response to the infection (e.g., the body's release of cytokines or chemokines such as tumor necrosis factor, nitric oxide, interleukins, and others). Infections of the lungs, abdomen, and urinary tract are implicated in sepsis more often than are infections at other body sites.

TREATMENT: The primary objectives are resuscitation of the patient, eradication of the underlying cause of infection, support of failing organ systems, and prevention of complications. Resuscitative efforts include maintaining an open airway; supporting ventilation; administering a fluid challenge; providing vasopressor drugs for persistent hypotension; and intensive care monitoring. Eradicating the underlying infection involves administering broad-spectrum antibiotics until a precise cause is identified, removing portals of infection or infected prostheses, and draining or débriding abscesses if any are present. Complications in septic patients are prevented with good supportive care: heparin to lessen the risk of venous thrombosis, skin care to prevent decubitus ulcers, enteral nutrition to prevent starvation, and aseptic technique to limit secondary hospital-acquired infections.

Experimental therapy includes the use of monoclonal antibodies designed to oppose the effects of bacterial toxins and the use of host-derived cytokines and chemokines.

CRITICAL CARE: Invasive hemodynamic monitoring in patients with sepsis typically reveals an elevated cardiac index, decreased systemic vascular resistance, decreased oxygen delivery to tissues, and decreases in mixed venous oxygen saturation. Commonly, laboratory studies in sepsis will reveal leukocytosis (or severe leukopenia), thrombocytopenia, elevated liver enzymes, hypocalcemia, hypoalbuminemia, and increases in the prothrombin time and serum creatinine level.

PATIENT CARE: Specimens of blood and body fluids are collected and cultured. Two or three consecutive blood cultures are obtained while the patient is febrile. Patient symptoms and vital signs are carefully assessed, and lungs are auscultated for normal and adventitious lung sounds. The patient's urine output is monitored for oliguria, and the patient is observed for any change in mental status. The patient's daily fluid intake and output and body weight also are measured and recorded.

An intravenous catheter is placed and prescribed antibiotic therapy is administered. The patient is given information about the therapy and assessed for desired responses and adverse effects. Antipyretics may be prescribed. Fluid and electrolyte therapy is prescribed to maintain desired balance or correct deficiencies. Oxygen is administered based on SaO_2 readings, tachypnea, and tachycardia. As soon as culture results permit, the patient's antibiotic regimen is revised to use specific drugs to which the offending organism is sensitive. After these drugs are given, serum antibiotic levels (trough and peak) may be monitored to prevent toxicity and ensure effectiveness. The patient is assessed carefully for signs of disseminated intravascular coagulation, adult respiratory distress syndrome, renal failure, heart failure, gastrointestinal ulcers, and hepatic abnormalities, any of which can complicate the clinical picture.

If septic shock occurs, oxygenation and perfusion are vigorously supported. An arterial catheter may be placed to measure blood pressure and provide access for arterial blood gas (ABG) samples. A pulmonary artery catheter may be used to monitor the patient's hemodynamic status. The health care team monitors closely for fluid overload. Nasoendotracheal intubation and mechanical ventilation may be necessary to overcome hypoxia, and ABGs are evaluated to determine FIO_2 and ventilatory volumes. If shock persists after volume expansion, vasopressor therapy may sometimes be prescribed to maintain adequate renal and brain perfusion. During vasopressor administration, central pressures and cardiac rate and rhythm are closely monitored. Metabolic acidosis may sometimes be corrected with IV bicarbonate therapy. A gram-negative endotoxin vaccine may be prescribed, as may other experimental treatments to block the rapid inflammatory process (corticosteroids, opiate antagonists, prostaglandin inhibitors, and calcium channel blockers). The patient's response is assessed, noting any adverse reactions.

A quiet and calm milieu is provided for the profoundly ill patient. Psychological support is provided. Oral hygiene is provided to prevent stomatitis, sordes, and salivary obstruction, esp. if the patient is permitted nothing by mouth. Nutritional needs are monitored, with consultations with the nutritional therapist to determine the need for enteral or parenteral nutrition. The patient's skin and joint function needs to be protected by assessing the skin and providing required care, as well as through frequent, careful repositioning, range-of-motion exercises, and correct body alignment, using supportive devices as necessary. The health care team should function as a liaison to family members, offering them emotional support and helping them to understand the patient's illness and the treatment regimen.

puerperal s. Any infection of the genital tract that occurs within 6 weeks after childbirth or abortion. Although once the greatest killer of new mothers, the incidence of postpartum infection has dropped dramatically as a result of aseptic technique during and after childbirth, and antibiotic therapy. SYN: *childbed fever*. SEE: *Nursing Diagnoses Appendix*.

SIGNS AND SYMPTOMS: Clinical findings vary with the site and type of infection. *Local:* Infections of perineal lacerations, of an episiotomy, or of the abdominal incision for cesarean delivery exhibit the classic signs of wound infections: redness, edema, ecchymosis, discharge, and interrupted approximation. *Pelvic:* Women whose infections involve the uterus, fallopian tubes, ovaries, or parametrium usually exhibit fever, chills, tachycardia, and abdominal tenderness or pain. Endometritis is accompanied by changes in the character and amount of lochia related to the causative organism; lochia may be scant or profuse, odorless or foul-smelling, colorless or bloody.

ETIOLOGY: The most common aerobic bacteria include group B streptococci and other streptococci, *Gardnerella vaginalis, Escherichia coli,* and *Staphylococcus aureus.* Infection due to group A, β hemolytic streptococci or anaerobic organisms such as *Bacteroides* or *Peptostreptococcus* are less common. Endometritis occurring late in the postpartal period usually is due to genital mycoplasmas or *Chlamydia trachomatis*.

RISK FACTORS: Conditions that predispose to postpartum infection include anemia, malnutrition, premature rupture of membranes, repeated vaginal examinations during labor, invasive procedures, surgical interventions, hemorrhage, and breaks in aseptic technique. Common modes of transmission include upward migration of vaginal bacteria, autoinfection, and contact with infected personnel or contaminated equipment.

DIAGNOSIS: The primary diagnostic criterion is a temperature of 100.4°F (38°C) occurring on any two of the first 10 days after childbirth, exclusive of the first 24 hours. Cultures of any drainage and sensitivity tests identify the causative microbe and the appropriate therapeutic antibiotic.

PATHOLOGY: In minor cases of ulceration, the vaginal tract is covered by a dirty membrane. In streptococcal and staphylococcal infections, the endometrium is smooth and the lymphatics are congested with the invading organisms. As a rule, the uterine cavity is filled with very little lochia. The uterus shows poor involution. If the infection extends farther beyond the uterus, the parametrium or cellular tissues show edema, inflammation, and in some cases purulent infiltration. Extension of the process to the veins produces infectious thrombi, which in turn produce localized abscesses in other parts of the body.

TREATMENT: Treatment includes appropriate antibiotics, incision and drainage if abscess forms, and supportive therapy.

PATIENT CARE: Puerperal infection is prevented by maintaining strict asepsis during the entire labor, delivery, and postpartum period. Preventive measures also include good prenatal nutrition; intranatal hemorrhage control; and avoidance of uterine dystocia, prolonged labor (esp. if amniotic fluid is leaking), and traumatic vaginal delivery. Fluid and electrolyte balance is maintained and unusual blood loss replaced.

The health care professional assesses for and reports suspicious clinical findings, and administers prescribed broad-spectrum antibiotics intravenously, changing to specific therapy once cultures have established sensitivity. The patient is isolated and separated from the infant while febrile, and other family members are encouraged to nurture the infant. The patient is given nutritional support, fluid intake and urinary output are measured, and care of the perineum, vaginal secretions, and breasts is provided. If surgery is required, the patient is prepared physically and psychologically for the necessary procedure and the family is given information and emotional support.

septan (sĕp′tăn) [L. *septem,* seven] Recurring every seventh day.

septate (sĕp′tāt) [L. *saeptum,* a partition] Having a dividing wall.

septectomy (sĕp-tĕk′tō-mē) [″ + Gr. *ektome,* excision] Excision of a septum, esp. the nasal septum or a part of it.

septi- Combining form meaning *seven.*

septic (sĕp′tĭk) [Gr. *septikos,* putrefying] **1.** Pert. to sepsis. **2.** Pert. to pathogenic organisms or their toxins.

septicemia (sĕp-tĭ-sē′mē-ă) [″ + *haima,* blood] The presence of pathogenic microorganisms in the blood. SEE: *sepsis; Nursing Diagnoses Appendix.* **septicemic** (-ĭk), *adj.*

septicophlebitis (sĕp″tĭ-kō-flē-bī′tĭs) [Gr. *septikos,* putrefying, + *phleps,* vein, + *itis,* inflammation] Septic inflammation of a vein.

septigravida (sĕp″tĭ-grăv′ĭ-dă) [L. *septem,* seven, + *gravida,* pregnant] A woman pregnant for the seventh time.

septimetritis (sĕp″tĭ-mē-trī′tĭs) [Gr. *septos,* putrid, + *metra,* uterus, + *itis,* inflammation] An inflammation of the uterus caused by sepsis.

septipara (sĕp-tĭp′ă-ră) [L. *septem,* seven, + *parere,* to bring forth] A woman who has had seven pregnancies, each of which produced an infant, alive or dead, weighing 500 g or more.

septivalent (sĕp-tĭ-vā′lĕnt, -tĭv′ă-lĕnt) [″ + *valere,* to be strong] Having a valence of seven or combining with or replacing seven hydrogen atoms.

septomarginal (sĕp″tō-măr′jĭ-năl) [L. *saeptum,* a partition, + *marginalis,* border] Pert. to the margin or the border of a septum.

septometer (sĕp-tŏm′ĕ-ter) [L. *saeptum,* a partition, + Gr. *metron,* measure] Calipers for measuring the width of the nasal septum.

septometer (sĕp-tŏm′ĕ-ter) [Gr. *sepsis,* putrefaction, + *metron,* measure] A device for determining bacterial contamination of air.

septonasal (sĕp-tō-nā′zăl) [L. *saeptum,* a partition, + *nasus,* nose] Concerning the nasal septum.

septoplasty (sĕp″tō-plăs′tē) [″ + Gr. *plassein,* to form] Plastic surgery of the nasal septum.

septostomy (sĕp-tŏs′tō-mē) [″ + Gr. *stoma,* mouth] Surgical formation of an opening in a septum.

amniotic s. Surgical puncturing of the membrane between twins affected by the twin oligohydramnios-polyhydramnios sequence.

balloon atrial s. The surgical enlargement of an opening between the cardiac atria for palliative relief of congestive heart failure in newborns with certain heart defects. A deflated balloon is inserted into a vein, passed through the foramen ovale, and then inflated and pulled vigorously through the atrial septum to enlarge the opening and improve oxygenation of the blood. SYN: *Rashkind procedure.*

surgical atrial s. The use of a specialized scalpel or knife to separate fused structures within the hearts of infants born with complex congenital cardiac defects.

septotome (sĕp′tō-tōm) [″ + Gr. *tome,* incision] An instrument for cutting or removing a section of the nasal septum.

septotomy (sĕp-tŏt′ō-mē) [″+ Gr. *tome,* incision] Incision of a septum, esp. the nasal septum.

septula testis The thin partition extending inward from the mediastinum testis and separating the testis into the lobuli testis.

septulum (sĕp′tū-lŭm) *pl.* **septula** [L.] A small partition or septum.

septum (sĕp′tŭm) *pl.* **septa** [L. *saeptum,* a partition] A wall dividing two cavities. **septal** (-tăl), *adj.*

atrial s. Interatrial s.

s. atriorum cordis Interatrial s.

atrioventricular s. The septum that separates the right and left atria of the heart from the respective ventricles.

crural s. Femoral s.

femoral s. Connective tissue that closes the femoral ring. SYN: *crural s.*

interatrial s. The myocardial wall between the atria of the heart.

interdental s. The bony partition across the alveolar process between adjacent teeth that forms part of the tooth sockets.

intermuscular s. **1.** A connective tissue septum that separates two muscles, esp. one from which muscles may take their origin. **2.** One of two connective tissue septa that separate the muscles of the leg into anterior, posterior, and lateral groups.

interradicular s. One of the thin bony partitions between the roots of a multirooted tooth that forms part of the walls of the tooth socket.

interventricular s. The myocardial wall between the ventricles of the heart.

lingual s. A sheet of connective tissue separating the halves of the tongue.

s. lucidum S. pellucidum.

mediastinal s. A mediastinum.

nasal s. The partition that divides the nasal cavity into two nasal fossae. The bony portion is formed by the perpendicular plate of ethmoid and the vomer bone. The cartilaginous portion is formed by septal and vomeronasal cartilages and medial crura of greater alar cartilages.

orbital s. A fibrous sheet extending partially across the anterior opening of the orbit within the eyelids.

s. pectiniforme Comblike partition that separates the corpora cavernosa.

s. pellucidum A thin, translucent, triangular sheet of nervous tissue consisting of two laminae attached to the corpus callosum above and the fornix below. It forms the medial wall and interior boundary of the lateral ventricles of the brain. SYN: *s. lucidum.*

s. primum In the embryonic heart, a septum between the right and left chambers.

rectovaginal s. The partition between the rectum and the vagina.

rectovesical s. The membranous septum between the rectum and the urinary bladder.

s. scroti The partition dividing the left and right sides of the scrotum.

ventricular s. Interventricular s.

septuplet (sĕp′tŭ-plĕt) [L. *septuplus,* sevenfold] One of seven children born from the same gestation.

sequel (sē′kwĕl) [L. *sequela,* sequel] Sequela.

sequela (sē-kwē′lă) *pl.* **sequelae** [L., sequel] A condition following and resulting from a disease.

sequence (sē′kwĕns) [L.] The order or occurrence of a series of related events.

pulse s. In magnetic resonance imaging, a series of radio waves designed to produce proton stimulation necessary to create the image.

sequential Occurring in order (i.e., one after another).

sequester (sē-kwĕs′tĕr) [L. *sequestrare,* to separate] **1.** To isolate. **2.** Sequestrum.

sequestration (sē″kwĕs-trā′shŭn) [L. *sequestratio,* a separation] **1.** The formation of sequestrum. **2.** The isolation of a patient for treatment or quarantine. **3.** Reduction of hemorrhage of the head or trunk by temporarily stopping the return of blood from the extremities by applying tourniquets to the thighs and arms. **4.** Fragment of nucleus pulposus of the intervertebral disk separating and freely floating in the spinal canal.

pulmonary s. A nonfunctioning area of the lung that receives its blood supply from the systemic circulation.

sequestrectomy (sē″kwĕs-trĕk′tō-mē) [″ + Gr. *ektome,* excision] Excision of a necrosed piece of bone. SYN: *sequestrotomy.*

sequestrotomy (sē″kwĕs-trŏt′ō-mē) [″ + Gr. *tome,* incision] Operation for removal of a sequestrum, a fragment of necrosed bone. SYN: *sequestrectomy.*

sequestrum (sē-kwĕs′trŭm) *pl.* **sequestra** [L., something set aside] A fragment of a necrosed bone that has become separated from the surrounding tissue. It is designated *primary* if the piece is entirely detached, *secondary* if it is still loosely attached, and *tertiary* if it is partially detached but still remaining in place. SYN: *sequester.* **sequestral** (-ăl), *adj.*

seralbumin (sēr-ăl-bū′mĭn) [L. *serum,* whey, + *albumen,* white of egg] Serum albumin.

serendipity (sĕr″ĕn-dĭp′ĭ-tē) The gift of finding, by chance and insight, valuable or agreeable things not sought for. In medical research, an unexpected reaction or result may produce new insights into some area totally unrelated to that which prompted the investigation.

serglycin (sĕr-gī′sĭn) An intracellular connective tissue molecule found in many different organs throughout the body.

serial (sē′rē-ăl) [L. *series,* row, chain] In numerical order, in continuity, or in sequence, as in a series.

series (sēr′ēz) [L. *series,* row, chain] **1.** Arrangement of objects in succession or in order. **2.** In electricity, batteries or mode of arranging the parts of a circuit by connecting them successively end to end to form a single path for the current. The parts so arranged are said to be "in series."

acute abdomen s. In radiology, an examination that usually includes an erect kidney, ureter, and bladder (KUB) projection, a recumbent KUB projection, and a left lateral decubitus view of the chest to assess free air, infections, or obstructions.

aliphatic s. Chemical compounds with a structure of an open chain of carbon atoms.

aromatic s. Any series of organic compounds containing the benzene ring.

erythrocytic s. The group of immature cells that develop into mature erythrocytes.

fatty s. Aliphatic series, esp. those similar to methane.

granulocytic s. The immature cells in the bone marrow that develop into mature granular leukocytes. SYN: *leukocytic s.*

homologous s. In chemistry, compounds that proceed from one to the next by some constant such as a CH_2 group.

leukocytic s. Granulocytic s.

monocytic s. The immature cells that proceed to develop into the mature monocyte.

thrombocytic s. The immature cells that proceed to develop into platelets.

upper GI s. Radiographical and fluoroscopic examinations of the stomach and duodenum after the ingestion of a contrast medium, such as barium sulfate or an iodinized glucose solution.

serine 2-amino-3-hydroxypropionic acid; an amino acid present in many proteins including casein, vitellin, and others.

serine protease inhibitor ABBR: SERPIN. Any of the compounds that inhibit platelet function and coagulation. SERPINs have been used to reduce deposition of microemboli in cases of disseminated intravascular coagulation associated with sepsis.

seriscission (sĕr-ĭ-sĕsh′ŭn) [L. *sericum,* silk, + *scindere,* to cut] The obsolete technique of dividing soft tissues with ties or ligatures.

sero- [L.] Combining form meaning *serum.*

seroalbuminuria (sē″rō-ăl-bū″mĭn-ū′rē-ă) [L. *serum,* whey, + *albumen,* white of egg, + Gr. *ouron,* urine] An old term for albuminuria (i.e., albumin in the urine).

serocolitis (sē″rō-kō-lī′tĭs) [″ + Gr. *kolon,* colon, + *itis,* inflammation] Inflammation of the serous layer of the colon. SYN: *pericolitis.*

seroconversion The development of an antibody response to an infection or vaccine, measurable in the serum.

seroculture (sē′rō-kŭl-chūr) [L. *serum,* whey, + *cultura,* tillage] A bacterial culture on blood serum.

serocystic (sē″rō-sĭs′tĭk) [″ + Gr. *kystis,* bladder, sac] Composed of cysts containing serous fluid.

serodermatosis (sē″rō-der-mă-tō′sĭs) [″ + Gr. *derma,* skin, + *osis,* condition] Skin disease with serous effusion into tissues of the epidermis.

serodiagnosis (sē″rō-dī-ăg-nō′sĭs) [″ + Gr. *dia,* through, + *gnosis,* knowledge] Diagnosis of disease based on tests of serum, esp. immunological tests.

seroenteritis (sē″rō-ĕn-tĕr-ī′tĭs) [″ + Gr. *enteron,* intestine, + *itis,* inflammation] An inflammation of the serous covering of the intestine.

seroepidemiology (sē-rō-ĕp″ĭ-dē-mē-ŏl′ō-jē) [″ + *epi,* upon, + *demos,* people, + *logos,* word, reason] Study of the epidemiology of a pathological condition by investigating the presence of a diagnostic characteristic in the serum of persons suspected of having had the particular disease being studied.

serofast (sē′rō-făst″) Serum-fast.
serofibrinous (sē″rō-fī′brĭn-ŭs) [″ + *fibra,* fiber] **1.** Composed of both serum and fibrin. **2.** Denoting a serofibrinous exudate.
serofibrous (sē″rō-fī′brŭs) [″ + *fibra,* fiber] Concerning serous and fibrous surfaces.
seroflocculation (sē″rō-flŏk″ū-lā′shŭn) [″ + *flocculus,* little tuft] Flocculation produced in serum by an antigen.
seroimmunity (sē″rō-ĭ-mū′nĭ-tē) [″ + *immunitas,* immunity] Immunity produced by the administration of an antiserum.
serologist (sē-rŏl′ō-jĭst) [″ + Gr. *logos,* word, reason] An individual trained in the science of serology.
serology (sē-rŏl′ō-jē) [″ + Gr. *logos,* word, reason] The scientific study of fluid components of the blood, esp. antigens and antibodies. **serologic, serological** (-rō-lŏj′ĭk, -rō-lŏj′ĭk-ăl), *adj.*
serolysin (sē-rŏl′ĭs-ĭn) [″ + Gr. *lysis,* dissolution] A bactericidal substance or lysin found in the blood serum.
seromembranous (sē″rō-mĕm′brăn-ŭs) [″ + *membrana,* membrane] **1.** Both serous and membranous. **2.** Relating to a serous membrane.
seromucoid Seromucous.
seromucous (sē″rō-mū′kŭs) [″ + *mucus,* mucus] Concerning a secretion that is part serous and part mucous.
seromuscular (sē″rō-mŭs′kū-lăr) [″ + *muscularis,* muscular] Concerning the serous and muscular layers of the intestinal wall.
seronegative (sē″rō-nĕg′ă-tĭv) Producing a negative reaction to serological tests.
seroperitoneum (sē″rō-pĕr″ĭ-tō-nē′ŭm) [″ + Gr. *peritonaion,* peritoneum] An obsolete term for ascites.
seropositive (sē″rō-pŏz′ĭ-tĭv) Having a positive reaction to a serological test (i.e., showing the presence of a specific antigen or antibody).
seroprevention Seroprophylaxis.
seroprognosis (sē″rō-prŏg-nō′sĭs) [″ + Gr. *pro,* before, + *gnosis,* knowledge] Prognosis of disease determined by seroreactions.
seroprophylaxis (sē″rō-prō-fī-lăks′ĭs) [″ + Gr. *prophylatikos,* guarding] Prevention of a disease by injection of serum. SYN: *seroprevention.*
seropurulent (sē″rō-pū′roo-lĕnt) [″ + *purulentus,* full of pus] Composed of serum and pus, as an exudate.
seroreaction (sē″rō-rē-ăk′shŭn) [″ + *re,* back, + *actio,* action] **1.** Any reaction taking place in or involving serum. **2.** A reaction to an injection of serum marked by rash, fever, pain, and so on.
seroresistance (sē″rō-rē-zĭs′tăns) Failure of a serum reaction to become negative or be reduced in titer following treatment.
seroresistant (sē″rō-rē-zĭs′tănt) Concerning seroresistance.
serosa (sē-rō′să) [L. *serum,* whey] A serous membrane (e.g., the peritoneum, pleura, and pericardium).
serosanguineous (sē″rō-săn-gwĭn′ē-ŭs) [L. *serum,* whey, + *sanguineus,* bloody] Containing or of the nature of serum and blood.
seroserous (sē″rō-sē′rŭs) [L. *serosus,* serous, + *serum,* whey] Pert. to two serous surfaces.
serositis (sē″rō-sī′tĭs) *pl.* **serositides** [″ + Gr. *itis,* inflammation] An inflammation of a serous membrane, such as the pleura, pericardium, or peritoneum. Serositis is one of the cardinal findings in connective tissue diseases like systemic lupus erythematosus.
serosity (sē-rŏs′ĭ-tē) [Fr. *serosite*] The quality of being serous.
serosynovial (sē″rō-sĭ-nō′vē-ăl) [L. *serum,* whey, + *synovia,* joint fluid] Concerning serous and synovial material.
serosynovitis (sē″rō-sĭn″ō-vī′tĭs) [″ + *synovia,* joint fluid, + Gr. *itis,* inflammation] Synovitis with an increase of synovial fluid.
serotherapy (sē″rō-thĕr′ă-pē) Passive immunization with antivenins—antibody-rich serum raised against toxins derived from poisonous snakes, arthropods, or other potentially deadly sources.
serotonergic neuron A neural pathway that uses serotonin as a neurotransmitter.
serotonin (sĕr″ō-tōn′ĭn) A chemical, 5-hydroxytryptamine (5-HT), found in platelets, the gastrointestinal mucosa, mast cells, carcinoid tumors, and the central nervous system. Serotonin is a vasoconstrictor, and through its action on cellular receptors, it plays important roles in intestinal motility, nausea and vomiting, sleep-wake cycles, obsessive-compulsive behaviors, depression, and eating. SEE: *carcinoid syndrome.*

s. reuptake inhibitor Any one of a class of drugs that interferes with serotonin transport, used in treating depression, obsessive-compulsive behaviors, eating disorders, and social phobias. Examples include fluoxetine (Prozac) and paroxetine (Paxil).

serotype (sē′rō-tīp) In microbiology, a microorganism determined by the kinds and combinations of constituent antigens present in the cells.
serous (sĕr′ŭs) [L. *serosus*] **1.** Having the nature of serum. **2.** Thin or watery, rather than syrupy, thick, or viscous.
serous cell A cell that secretes a thin, watery, albuminous secretion.
serous effusion The escape of serum into tissues or a body cavity.
serous exudate An exudate consisting mostly of serum.

serovaccination An injection combining serum (containing preformed antibodies, to provide immediate passive immunity) and weakened or dead microorganisms (to stimulate long-term active immunity). It may be used for unimmunized patients after rabies or tetanus exposure and for neonates born of mothers who are hepatitis B carriers.

serovar [*sero*logical *var*iation] Variants within a species defined by variation in serological reactions. SEE: *biovar; morphovar.*

serozymogenic (sē″rō-zī″mō-jĕn′ĭk) [L. *serum,* whey, + Gr. *zyme,* ferment, + *gennan,* to produce] Pert. to a serous fluid and enzymes.

serpiginous (sĕr-pĭj′ĭ-nŭs) [L. *serpere,* to creep] Creeping from one part to another.

serrate (sĕr′āt) [L. *serratus,* toothed] Dentate.

Serratia (sĕr-ā′shē-ă) [Serafino Serrati, 18th-century Italian physicist] A genus of bacteria of the family Enterobacteriaceae. It is a gram-negative rod.

S. marcescens An opportunistic bacterium that causes septicemia and pulmonary disease, esp. in immunocompromised patients, and is found in water, soil, milk, and stools. In the proper environment, the organism will grow on food and produce the red pigment prodigiosin.

serration (sĕr-ā′shŭn) [L. *serratio,* a notching] **1.** A formation with sharp projections like the teeth of a saw. **2.** A single tooth or notch in a serrated edge.

serratus muscle Any of several muscles arising from the ribs or vertebrae by separate slips.

serrefine (sār-fēn′) [Fr.] A small wire-spring forceps for compressing bleeding vessels.

serrenoeud (sār-nŭd′) [Fr. *serrer,* to squeeze, + *noeud,* knot] A device for tightening ligatures, esp. those placed on vessels in a deep cavity out of reach of the fingers.

serrulate (sĕr′ū-lāt) [L. *serrulatus*] Finely notched or serrated.

Sertoli cell (sĕr-tō′lēz) [Enrico Sertoli, Italian histologist, 1842–1910] One of the supporting elongated cells of the seminiferous tubules of the testes to which spermatids attach to be nourished until they become mature spermatozoa. Sertoli cells produce the hormone inhibin. Also called *sustentacular cell.*

serum (sē′rŭm) *pl.* **serums, sera** [L., whey] **1.** Any serous fluid, esp. the fluid that moistens the surfaces of serous membranes. **2.** The watery portion of the blood after coagulation; a fluid found when clotted blood is left standing long enough for the clot to shrink. **3.** Fluid obtained from blood that contains antibodies against a specific microorganism. It is used to provide immediate passive immunity for someone exposed to the same organism. SYN: *immune globulin.*

antitetanic s. Serum given to counteract tetanus toxin.

antitoxic s. Antitoxin.

bactericidal s. Serum having no effect on toxins but destructive to bacteria.

bacteriolytic s. Serum containing a lysin that destroys certain bacteria.

convalescent s. Serum from a person recovering from an infection, used in the past in treating others having the same disease.

foreign s. Serum from one animal injected into one of another species or into a human.

grouping s. A serum used for determining the blood group to which unknown cells belong. The grouping serums commonly used are human serums secured from donors and rabbit antiserums prepared commercially.

immune s. Serum containing antibodies for specific antigens.

polyvalent s. Serum containing antibodies to several types of the same bacterial species.

pooled s. Mixed blood serum from several persons.

pregnancy s. Blood serum from pregnant women.

pregnant mare's s. Serum derived from the blood of pregnant mares; source of hormones, esp. gonadotropins.

serum bank A laboratory or storage facility where samples of serum are kept, typically at subfreezing temperatures, for their future value in the retrospective study of important or emerging diseases. The JANUS serum bank, in Norway, has one of the largest and best organized national collections of stored serum; its specimens have been used primarily in studies of tumor markers.

serum-fast Capable of resisting the destructive forces present in serum. SYN: *serofast.*

serum glutamic-oxaloacetic transaminase ABBR: SGOT. Aspartate aminotransferase.

serum glutamic pyruvic transaminase ABBR: SGPT. Alanine aminotransferase.

serve To deliver a legal document to a person named in it. This is done formally to comply with due process of law.

service Help or assistance (e.g., for persons who are needy, sick, or injured).

servomechanism (sŭr″vō-mĕk′ă-nĭzm) In biology and physiology, a control mechanism that operates by negative or positive feedback. For example, when in the normal person the blood glucose level rises, the pancreas responds by releasing insulin, which enables the glucose to be metabolized. The level of other hormones is also regulated by this mechanism.

SES *socioeconomic status.*

sesame oil Oil obtained from the seeds of *Sesamum indicum,* used as a pharmaceutical aid and as a cooking oil.

sesamoid (sĕs′ă-moyd) [L. *sesamoides*] Resembling a grain of sesame in size or shape.

sesamoid cartilage One or more small cartilage plates present in fibrous tissue between the lateral nasal and greater alar cartilages of the nose.

sesamoiditis (sĕs″ă-moy-dī′tĭs) [″ + Gr. *itis,* inflammation] Inflammation of a sesamoid bone.

sesqui- [L.] Prefix meaning *one and one-half.*

sesquihora (sĕs″kwĭ-hō′ră) [L.] Every 1½ hr.

sessile (sĕs′l) [L. *sessilis,* low] Having no peduncle but attached directly by a broad base.

set **1.** To fix firmly in place, as to set a bone in reduction of a fracture. **2.** To allow an amalgam or plaster to harden. **3.** In psychology, a group of conditions or attitudes that favor the occurrence of a certain response. **4.** In resistance exercise, a grouping of repetitions of a specific exercise.

seta (sē′tă) *pl.* **setae** [L., bristle] A stiff, bristle-like structure. SEE: *vibrissae.*

setaceous (sē-tā′shŭs) [L. *setaceus*] Bristly, hairy; resembling a bristle.

Setchenov phenomenon [I. M. Setchenov, Russ. scientist] The more rapid recovery of a limb if the opposite limb is exercised during the rest period.

Setchenov's inhibitory centers (sĕtch′en-ŏfs) [Ivan M. Setchenov, Russian neurologist, 1829–1905] Centers in the spinal cord and medulla oblongata involved in reflex inhibition of muscular and visceral activity.

setiferous (sē-tĭf′ĕr-ŭs) [L. *seta,* bristle, + *ferre,* to bear] Having bristles.

seton (sē″tŏn) [L. *seta,* bristle] **1.** A thread or threads drawn through a fold of skin to act as a counterirritant or as a guide for instruments. **2.** A suture tied about an anal fistula to maintain drainage while fibrosis gradually obliterates the fistulous tract.

setose (sē′tōs) Having bristle-like appendages.

set-point The concept that homeostatic mechanisms maintain variables such as body temperature, body weight, blood glucose level, and hormone levels within a certain physiological range compatible with optimal function. SEE: *homeostasis.*

settlement **1.** In health insurance, payment to the policyholder for claims made against the insurance company. **2.** In liability or malpractice litigation, an agreement between disputants that satisfies the needs of both parties.

viatical s. The purchase—at a discount—of a life insurance policy from a gravely ill patient. The buyer becomes the beneficiary of the policy; the viator receives a lump sum payment before dying.

setup The arrangement of teeth on a trial denture base.

severe combined immunodeficiency disease ABBR: SCID. A syndrome marked by gross functional impairment of both humoral and cell-mediated immunity and by susceptibility to fungal, bacterial, and viral infections. Although the disorder may occur sporadically, most commonly it is inherited and transmitted as an X-linked or autosomal recessive trait. If untreated, infants rarely survive beyond one year. It is important that the disease be recognized early and that patients not be given live viral vaccines or blood transfusions. The immunologic defects may be repaired by transplantation of bone marrow or fetal liver as a source of stem cells.

Severinghaus electrode SEE: *electrode, carbon dioxide.*

Sever's disease [James W. Sever, U.S. orthopedist, 1878–1964] Apophysitis of the calcaneus in adolescent children who are actively engaged in sports. This overuse syndrome is best treated with icing, Achilles tendon stretching, anti-inflammatory medication, and rest from weight bearing. Heel lifts are usually used unless the child has pronated feet, in which case medial heel wedges are indicated.

sevoflurane (sē-vō-flū′rān) An inhaled anesthetic drug in the class of halogenated hydrocarbons.

sewage The waste water that passes through sewers. It may be composed of bodily excretions, the waste water and solid waste of residential and commercial establishments, or the solvents and other toxic wastes of industry. Bodily excretions discharged as sewage are potentially infectious and may be the source of epidemic outbreaks of diarrhea or other contagious illnesses. Other sewage components, esp. toxic oils and solvents, may pollute rivers and beaches, destroying fishing and shellfish beds.

sex [L. *sexus*] **1.** The characteristics that differentiate males and females in most plants and animals. **2.** Gender.

chromosomal s. Sex as determined by the presence of the female XX or male XY genotype in somatic cells.

morphological s. The sex of an individual as determined by the form of the external genitalia.

nuclear s. The genetic sex of an individual determined by the absence or presence of sex chromatin in the body cells, particularly white blood cells.

psychological s. The individual's self-image of his or her gender, which may be at variance with the morphological sex.

sex chromatin A mass seen within the nuclei of normal female somatic cells. According to the Lyon hypothesis, one of the two X chromosomes in each somatic cell of the female is genetically inactivated. The sex chromatin represents the inactivated X chromosome. SYN: *Barr body*.

sex clinic A clinic for the diagnosis and treatment of an individual or couple with sexual problems.

sex determination **1.** The identification of the gender of an animal or human with an ambiguous physical appearance or ambiguous genitalia. In colloquial speech, this process is sometimes referred to as "sex testing." **2.** The identification, during in vitro fertilization, of the gender of a human preimplantation embryo.

sexdigital (sĕks-dĭj'ĭ-tăl) [L. *sex,* six, + *digitus,* digit] Having six fingers and toes.

sex drive Motivation, both psychological and physiological, for behavior associated with procreation and erotic pleasure.

sexduction (sĕks-dŭk'shŭn) The process of transfer of bacterial genes from one cell to another by means of the sex factors within which they are incorporated.

sexism All of the actions and attitudes that relegate individuals of either sex to a secondary and inferior status in society.

sexivalent (sĕks"ĭ-vă'lĕnt, -ĭv'ăl-ĕnt) [" + *valere,* to be strong] Capable of combining with six atoms of hydrogen.

sex-limited The expression of a genetic character or trait in one sex only.

sex-linked A character that is controlled by genes on the sex chromosomes.

sexology [L. *sexus,* sex, + Gr. *logos,* word, reason] Scientific study of sexuality.

sextan (sĕks'tăn) [L. *sextanus,* of the sixth] Occurring every sixth day.

sex test Sex determination.

sex therapy A form of psychotherapy involving sexual guidance for partners with sexual incompatibilities or sexual dysfunction.

sextigravida (sĕks"tĭ-grăv'ĭd-ă) [L. *sextus,* six, + *gravida,* a pregnant woman] A woman pregnant for the sixth time.

sextipara (sĕks-tĭp'ă-ră) [" + *parere,* to bear a child] A woman who has had six pregnancies that produced infants of 500 g (or 20 weeks' gestation) regardless of their viability.

sextuplet (sĕks'tū-plĕt) [L. *sextus,* six] One of six children born of a single gestation.

sexual (sĕks'ū-ăl) [L. *sexualis*] **1.** Pert. to sex. **2.** Having sex.

sexual activity depressant Anything that suppresses libido, potency, or orgasmic ability. Drugs with this effect include those used to control high blood pressure or cholesterol, some contraceptives, and recreational drugs including alcohol and marijuana, which may decrease inhibitions, but impair sexual performance. Fatigue, mental depression, anxiety, excess use of tobacco products, starvation, and stress all have the potential for depressing sexual desire and activity. SEE: *sexual stimulant*.

Sexual Assault Response Team ABBR: SART. A group of health care professionals who have had special preparation in the examination of rape victims. The training includes techniques for collecting, labeling, and storing evidence so it may be used in court proceedings concerning the person accused of rape and in psychological approaches to reduce the emotional trauma. SEE: *rape*.

sexual dysfunction Inadequate enjoyment of sex, or complete failure to enjoy any form of sexual intercourse. There may be multiple causes, including lack of sexual interest or desire; impairments in sexual arousal (such as erectile function in men or vaginal lubrication or clitoral enlargement in women); inability to achieve orgasm, or to delay orgasm until one's partner is satisfied; pain during intercourse; medical or hormonal conditions that impair sexual function; substance abuse issues; or prescription drug–related problems. A careful history and physical examination will help to determine the possible pathological aspects of the various phases. Is desire absent, overactive, or is there aversion? Is arousal sufficient to maintain desire and, in men, to attain erection? Does orgasm occur, and if so, is it delayed or premature? Do the partners experience satisfaction at the completion of orgasm? Is pain present at any stage of the sexual activity?

The physical or mental factors that are involved should be treated and, when medications are responsible, alternate drugs should be substituted for those that appear to cause the disorder. SEE: *Nursing Diagnoses Appendix*.

sexual harassment Unsolicited and unprovoked mental or physical sexually oriented advances or innuendos, esp. between employers and employees. In many instances, compliance with a harasser's wishes is a condition of continued employment or advancement.

sexual health The World Health Organization has defined three elements of sexual health: a capacity to enjoy and control sexual behavior in accordance with a social and personal ethic; freedom from fear, shame, guilt, false beliefs, and other psychological factors inhibiting sexual response and impairing sexual relationships; and freedom from organic disorder, disease, and deficiencies that interfere with sexual and re-

Causative Agents of Sexually Transmitted Diseases

Organism	Associated Diseases
Bacteria	
Calymmatobacterium granulomatis	Donovanosis (granuloma inguinale)
Campylobacter species	Enteritis, proctocolitis
Chlamydia trachomatis	Genital tract infections and Reiter's syndrome
Gardnerella vaginalis	Bacterial (nonspecific) vaginosis
Group B streptococcus	Neonatal sepsis
Haemophilus ducreyi	Chancroid
Mycoplasma hominis	Postpartum fever; meningitis
Neisseria gonorrhoeae	Genital tract infections, disseminated gonococcal infection
Shigella species	Shigellosis; gay bowel syndrome
Treponema pallidum	Syphilis
Ureaplasma urealyticum	Nongonococcal urethritis
Viruses	
Cytomegalovirus	Heterophile-negative infectious mononucleosis, birth defects, protean manifestations in the immunocompromised host
Hepatitis A	Acute hepatitis
Hepatitis B	Acute and chronic hepatitis B, cirrhosis, hepatocellular carcinoma
Hepatitis C	Acute and chronic hepatitis, cirrhosis, hepatocellular carcinoma
Herpes simplex	Genital herpes, aseptic meningitis
Human herpes virus, type 8	Kaposi's sarcoma, lymphoma
Human immunodeficiency virus types 1 and 2	AIDS (acquired immunodeficiency syndrome)
Human papilloma (70 separate types)	Condyloma acuminata, cervical intraepithelial neoplasia and carcinoma, vulvar carcinoma, penile carcinoma
Human T-lymphotrophic retrovirus, type 1	Human T-cell leukemia or lymphoma
Molluscum contagiosum	Genital molluscum contagiosum
Protozoa	
Entamoeba histolytica	Amebiasis in people who have oroanal sex
Giardia lamblia	Giardiasis in people who have oroanal sex
Trichomonas vaginalis	Trichomonal vaginitis
Ectoparasites	
Phthirus pubis	Pubic lice infestation
Sarcoptes scabiei	Scabies

NOTE: Many of these diseases can be transmitted by contact that is not sexual.

productive functions. Medical studies of human sexual function and activity have provided no evidence that having attained a certain age is, of itself, reason to discontinue participating in and enjoying sexual intercourse. SEE: *sexually transmitted disease*.

sexual intercourse Any sexual union between two or more partners in which at least one partner's genitalia are stimulated. SYN: *coition; coitus; copulation*.

sexuality (sěks-ū-ăl′ĭ-tē) [L. *sexus*, sex] **1.** The state of having sex; the collective characteristics that mark the differences between the male and the female. **2.** The constitution and life of an individual as related to sex; all the dispositions related to intimacy, whether associated with the sex organs or not.

sexuality patterns, altered The state in which an individual expresses concern regarding his or her sexuality. SEE: *Nursing Diagnoses Appendix*.

sexually transmitted disease ABBR: STD. Any disease that may be acquired as a result of sexual intercourse or other intimate contact with an infected individual. A more-inclusive term than "venereal disease," STDs include disease caused by bacteria, viruses, protozoa, fungi, and ectoparasites. SEE: table; *Nursing Diagnoses Appendix*.

sexual maturity rating The order and extent of the development of a patient's primary and secondary sexual characteristics as compared with the established norms for chronological age. In both sexes, the changes leading to puberty are the result of major hormonal changes that, although somewhat variable in age of occurrence, proceed in a predictable sequence. Assessing the degree of age-related sexual maturity enables the health care provider to detect abnormalities and to provide anticipatory guidance for the patient and family. An important and easily identified development in a girl is the onset of menstruation. Physical changes in the male such as voice change, facial hair growth, and testicular and penile growth are obvious but occur over a prolonged period.

sexual preference The sexual orientation one prefers in choosing his or her sex partners.

sexual reassignment The legal, surgical, or social action or decision to assign the appropriate sexuality to an individual who has been considered previously to be of the opposite (or ambiguous) sex.

sexual stimulant Any drug (e.g., alcohol used in modest amounts) or pheromone that acts as an aphrodisiac for humans or animals.

Sézary cell [A. Sézary, Fr. dermatologist, 1880–1956] A T-cell lymphocyte, that contains an abundance of vacuoles filled with a mucopolysaccharide; present in the blood of patients with cutaneous T-cell lymphoma who develop Sézary syndrome. SEE: illus.

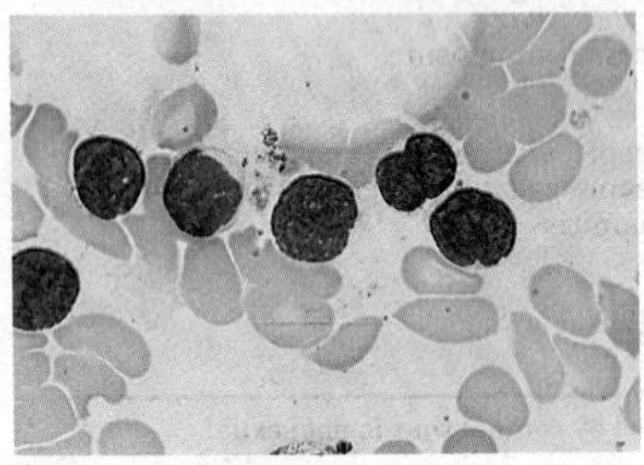

SÉZARY CELLS

In peripheral blood (×1000)

Sézary syndrome A form of cutaneous T-cell lymphoma in which there is cutaneous and systemic involvement. SEE: *cutaneous T cell lymphoma*.

SGA *small for gestational age.*

S.G.O. *Surgeon-General's Office.*

SGOT *serum glutamic-oxaloacetic transaminase.*

SGPT *serum glutamic pyruvic transaminase.*

SH *serum hepatitis.*

shadow [AS. *sceaduwe*] Achromocyte.

acoustic s. In ultrasonography, the loss of an image behind a structure that reflects sound waves.

shadow-casting A technique to increase the definition of the material being examined by use of electron microscopy. The object is sprayed from an oblique angle with a heavy metal.

shadowing In radiology, loss of the ability to visualize a body structure because of interference by another part.

shaft [AS. *sceaft*] **1.** The principal portion of any cylindrical body. **2.** The diaphysis of a long bone.

hair s. The keratinized portion of a hair that extends from a hair follicle beyond the surface of the epidermis. SEE: *hair*.

shaken-baby syndrome A syndrome seen in abused infants and children, sometimes referred to as "shaken impact syndrome" because of the accompanying impact injuries to the head. The patient has been subjected to violent, whiplash-type shaking injuries inflicted by an abuser. This may cause coma, convulsions, and increased intracranial pressure, resulting from tearing of the cerebral veins, with consequent bleeding into the subdural space. Retinal hemorrhages and bruises on the arms or trunk where the patient was forcefully grabbed are usually present.

INCIDENCE: About 50,000 cases are reported each year in the U.S. This number probably represents underreporting.

DIAGNOSIS: The presence of retinal hemorrhage, cerebral edema, and subdural hematoma—either individually or in any combination—strongly suggests the diagnosis, in the absence of other explanations for the trauma. Radiological imaging is used to identify the specific sites of injury.

PROGNOSIS: The prognosis for affected infants and children is extremely guarded. Only about 15% to 20% of them recover without sequelae, such as vision and hearing impairments, seizure disorders, cerebral palsy, and developmental disorders requiring ongoing medical, educational, and behavioral management. SEE: *battered child syndrome; child abuse*.

CAUTION: In domestic situations in which a child is abused, it is important to examine other children and infants living in the same home because about 20% of these children will have signs of physical abuse as well. That examination should be done without delay, to prevent further abuse.

---

shakes (shāks) [AS. *sceacen*] **1.** Shivering caused by a chill, esp. in intermittent fever. **2.** Colloquial term for state of tremulousness and extreme irritability often seen in chronic alcoholics. SYN: *jitters*.

shaking 1. A passive large-amplitude vibratory movement used in massage. 2. A vibratory technique used in chest physical therapy to facilitate pulmonary drainage.

shaman (shā′mŭn, shŏ′-) [Russ., ascetic] A healer (usually from a tribal or preindustrial culture) who uses non-Western practices and techniques, including faith healing, spirituality, psychological manipulation, chanting, rituals, magic, and culturally meaningful symbolism to restore health or well-being to the sick. SYN: *medicine man*. SEE: *shamanism*.

shamanism (shā′mŭn-ĭsm, shŏ′-) 1. Primitive religion of certain peoples of northern Asia who believe good and evil spirits pervade the world and can be influenced only by shamans acting as mediums. 2. Any similar form of spiritual or magical healing, such as that practiced in many tribal or preindustrial cultures.

Shanghai fever (shăng′hī) A diarrheal illness caused by *Pseudomonas* species, associated with high fever, a rose-colored spotted rash that resembles typhoid, and headache. The infection is usually contracted in the tropics.

shank (shăngk) [AS. *sceanca*] 1. Shin. 2. The tapered portion of a dental hand instrument between the handle and the blade or nub. It may be straight or angled to provide better access or leverage in its use.

shape (shāp) [AS. *sceapan*] 1. To mold to a particular form. 2. Outward form; contour.

shared decision An approach to health care decision making based on a negotiated agreement between the patient and health care professional. The success of this sharing is, of course, dependent on both the physician and patient being rational and competent.

shared governance A model of nursing management in which the staff nurse shares responsibility and accountability for patient care with the clinical agency management. Shared governance assumes a participatory style of management and aims to achieve a high quality of patient care and professional nursing practice. Shared governance differs both from self-governance and from the traditional bureaucratic model of nursing management. SEE: *self-governance*.

sharkskin A condition seen in pellagra (nicotinic acid deficiency) in which openings of sebaceous glands become plugged with a dry yellowish material.

Sharpey, William Scottish physiologist, 1802–1880.

S.'s intercrossing fibers The fibers forming the lamellae constituting the walls of the haversian canals in bone.

S.'s perforating fibers 1. The fibers extending from the periosteum into the lamellae of bone. 2. The fibers extending from the periodontal ligament into the cementum of a tooth.

sharps A colloquial term for medical articles that may cause punctures or cuts to those handling them, including all broken medical glassware, syringes, needles, scalpel blades, suture needles, and disposable razors. SEE: *medical waste; Standard and Universal Precautions Appendix*.

shear (shēr) A frictional force per unit of surface area applied parallel to the planes of any object.

sheath (shēth) [AS. *sceath*] 1. A covering structure of connective tissue, usually of an elongated part, such as the membrane covering a muscle. 2. An instrument introduced into a vessel during angiographic procedures when multiple catheter changes are anticipated. It facilitates ease of change and decreases morbidity at the puncture site.

arachnoid s. The delicate partition between the pial sheath and the dural sheath of the optic nerve.

axon s. A myelin sheath or a neurilemma. SEE: *myelin s.*

carotid s. The portion of cervical or pretracheal fascia enclosing the carotid artery, interior jugular vein, and vagus nerve.

crural s. The fascial covering of femoral vessels.

dural s. A fibrous membrane or external investment of the optic nerve.

femoral s. The fascia covering the femoral vessels.

s. of Henle SEE: *Henle's sheath*.

s. of Hertwig SEE: *Hertwig's root sheath*.

s. of Key and Retzius Henle's sheath.

lamellar s. A connective tissue sheath covering a bundle of nerve fibers. SYN: *nerve s.; perineurium*.

medullary s. An obsolete term for myelin sheath.

myelin s. Layers of the cell membrane of Schwann cells (peripheral nervous system) or oligodendrocytes (central nervous system) that wrap nerve fibers, providing electrical insulation and increasing the velocity of impulse transmission. SEE: *nerve fiber; neuron*.

nerve s. Lamellar s.

periarterial lymphoid s. The tissue composed of T lymphocytes that surrounds each arteriole in the spleen. The sheaths are attached to lymphoid follicles containing B cells and make up much of the white pulp. SEE: *spleen*.

pial s. An extension of the pia that closely invests the surface of the optic nerve.

s. of Schweigger-Seidel The thickened wall of a sheathed artery of the spleen.

root s. **1.** One of the layers of a hair follicle derived from the epidermis. It includes the outer root sheath, which is a continuation of the stratum germinativum, and the inner root sheath, which consists of three layers of cells that closely invest the root of the hair. SEE: *hair*. **2.** The epithelial covering that induces root formation in teeth. Also called *Hertwig's root sheath.*

synovial s. A double-walled tubelike bursa that encloses a tendon. It consists of an inner visceral layer lying on and adhering to a tendon and an outer parietal layer; the two layers are separated by a space filled with synovial fluid. This sheath is found esp. in the hands and feet where tendons are confined to osteofibrous canals or pass over bony surfaces.

tendon s. A dense fibrous sheath that confines a tendon to an osseous groove, converting it into an osteofibrous canal. It is found principally in the wrist and ankle. SEE: *synovial s.*

shedding [ME. *sheden,* shed] **1.** The loss of deciduous teeth. **2.** Casting off of the surface layer of the epidermis. **3.** The loss of bacteria from the skin.

Sheehan's syndrome [Harold L. Sheehan, Brit. pathologist, b. 1920] Hypopituitarism resulting from an infarct of the pituitary following postpartum shock or hemorrhage. Damage to the anterior pituitary gland causes partial to complete loss of thyroid, adrenocortical, and gonadal function.

sheep cell agglutination test ABBR: SCAT. A test for rheumatoid factor in serum. Sheep erythrocytes sensitized with rabbit antisheep erythrocyte immune globulin will be agglutinated if serum containing the rheumatoid factor is added.

sheet (shēt) [AS. *sciete,* cloth] **1.** A linen or cotton bedcovering. **2.** Something that resembles a sheet (e.g., a sheet of connective tissue).

beta s. A protein structure in which parallel layers of linked peptides are folded across each other. This structure is characteristic of amyloid proteins.

draw s. A sheet folded under a patient so that it may be withdrawn without lifting the patient. This is accomplished by turning the patient to the side of the bed to allow one side of the sheet to be removed and replaced with a clean one. The patient is then turned to the other side of the bed. The soiled sheet is removed and replaced with a clean one. In many hospitals, draw sheets have been replaced by paper and plastic pads that resemble disposable diapers.

flow s. A representation in outline or picture format of a technique or treatment.

lift s. Sheet folded under a patient over the bottom sheet to assist with moving the patient up in bed.

shelf Any shelflike structure.

dental s. SYN: *dental lamina*.

shelf-life **1.** The time a food may be kept on a store shelf and still be considered safe to eat. **2.** The length of time a substance, preparation, or medication can be kept without separation or chemical changes of its component parts.

shell A hard covering, as that for an egg or turtle.

shellac (shĕ-lăk′) A refined resinous substance obtained from plants that contain the secretions of certain insects. It is used in paints, varnishes, dry compounding, and in dentistry.

CAUTION: Some individuals may develop contact dermatitis after exposure to shellac.

shell shock A term used during World War I to designate a wide variety of psychotic and neurotic disorders associated with the stress of combat. SEE: *posttraumatic stress disorder*.

Shenton's line (shĕn′tŏnz) [Thomas Shenton, Brit. radiologist, 1872–1955] A radiographical line used to determine the relationship of the head of the femur to the acetabulum. The line follows the inferior border of the ramus of the pubic bone and continued outward follows the curve down the medial border of the neck of the femur.

shiatsu, shiatzu (shē′ăt-soo) [Chinese, finger + pressure] In traditional Japanese culture, the therapeutic application of pressure to acupuncture points.

shield (shēld) [AS. *scild,* shield] **1.** Any protecting device. **2.** In biology, a protective plate or hard outer covering.

embryonic s. The two-layered blastoderm or blastodisk from which a mammalian embryo develops. SYN: *embryonic disk.*

face s. A mask, typically made of clear plastic, that protects the mucous membranes of the eyes, nose, and mouth during patient-care procedures and activities that carry the risk of generating splashes of blood, body fluids, excretions, or secretions. SEE: *Standard and Universal Precautions Appendix.*

gonadal s. A lead device that is placed over the gonadal area to help protect it during radiation exposure.

nipple s. A cover to protect the sore nipples of a nursing woman.

shift [AS. *sciftan,* to arrange] A change in position or direction.

antigenic s. A major change in the genetic makeup of an organism, usually resulting from gene reassortment or occurring when different species share genetic material. This process may create a new pathogen against which there is no immunity in the population. Pandemic infections can result. SEE: *antigenic drift*.

chloride s. The shift of chloride ions from the plasma into the red blood cells upon the addition of carbon dioxide from the tissues, and the reverse movement when carbon dioxide is released in the lungs. It is a mechanism for maintaining constant pH of the blood.

s. to the left **1.** In hematology, an increase in the number of young polymorphonuclear leukocytes in the blood. SEE: *Arneth's classification of neutrophils.* **2.** In acid-base physiology, a left-shifted oxyhemoglobin dissociation level, indicating an increased affinity of hemoglobin for oxygen.

s. to the right In hematology, an increase in the number of older polymorphonuclear leukocytes in the blood. SEE: *Arneth's classification of neutrophils.*

shift work A staffing arrangement in which some employees work during the morning or afternoon, and others in the evening or at night. Shift work is a common method of scheduling used in many industries to maximize productivity over a 24-hr day, and in health care, where patients' needs may arise at any time of the day or night. A great number of persons work regularly at night, either on a permanent or rotating schedule. In most of these workers, adaptation to the altered work schedule is imperfect; sleep disturbances and other medical and psychosocial problems have often been found in shift workers. Among other problems, many nighttime or rotating shift workers often have family obligations during the day, which compromise their ability to obtain adequate rest before or after work.

Shiga's bacillus (shē′găs) [Kiyoshi Shiga, Japanese physician, 1870–1957] *Shigella dysenteriae.*

Shigella (shĭ-gĕl′lă) [Kiyoshi Shiga] A genus of non–lactose-fermenting, nonmotile, gram-negative rods belonging to the family Enterobacteriaceae. It contains a number of species that cause digestive disturbance ranging from mild diarrhea to a severe and often fatal dysentery. SEE: *dysentery, bacillary*.

S. boydii A species that causes acute diarrhea in humans.

S. dysenteriae A virulent form of *Shigella* responsible for severe, epidemic diarrhea.

S. flexneri A species that is a frequent cause of acute diarrhea in humans.

S. sonnei A species that is a frequent cause of bacillary dysentery.

shigellosis (shĭ″gĕl-lō′sĭs) [*Shigella* + *osis,* condition] Infection of the gastrointestinal tract, esp. the distal colon, by *Shigella*. Common symptoms include fever, bloody diarrhea, and abdominal cramps. Because *Shigella* are transmitted from person to person by contaminated feces, prevention requires thorough handwashing after toileting by toddlers, young children, and adults. The disease may also be contracted by direct oroanal contact and from food or water contaminated by sewage.

shin (shĭn) [AS. *scinu,* shin] The anterior edge of the tibia, the portion of the leg between the ankle and knee. SYN: *shank*.

saber s. A condition seen in congenital syphilis in which the anterior edge of the tibia is extremely sharp.

shingles (shĭng′lz) [L. *cingulus,* a girdle] The colloquial name of the dermatomal rash caused by *herpes zoster*. SEE: illus.; *herpes zoster*.

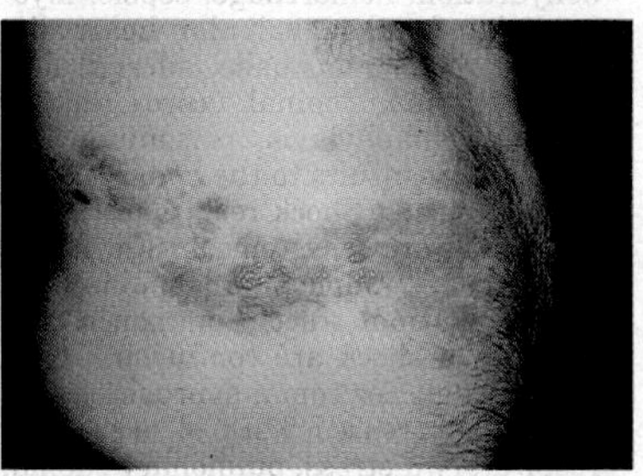

SHINGLES

shinsplints A nondescript pain in the anterior, posterior, or posterolateral compartment of the tibia. It usually follows strenuous or repetitive exercise and is often related to faulty foot mechanics such as pes planus or pes cavus. The cause may be ischemia of the muscles in the compartment, minute tears in the tissues, or partial avulsion from the periosteum of the tibial or peroneal muscles. Proper shoes and foot orthotics may help to prevent onset of the condition. A definitive diagnosis is required for proper treatment. Management may consist of ice packs, anti-inflammatory medications, decrease in the intensity of exercise (including the avoidance of hills and hard surfaces when running), and modification of footwear. SYN: *medial tibial syndrome*.

shin spots The colloquial name for necrobiosis lipoidica diabeticorum. This condition is usually, but not always, associated with diabetes. SEE: *necrobiosis lipoidica diabeticorum*.

shinrin-yoku In traditional Chinese medicine, walking and bathing in the forest to promote good health and prevent the effects of aging.

Shirodkar operation [Shirodkar, Indian physician, 1900–1971] The surgical placement of a purse-string suture around an incompetent cervical os to attempt to prevent the premature onset of labor. The suture material used for this cerclage procedure is nonabsorbable and must be removed before delivery. SEE: *cervical incompetence.*

shiver (shĭv′ĕr) [ME. *chiveren*] **1.** Involuntary increased muscle activity in response to fear, onset of fever, or exposure to cold. The activity leads to increased heat production. **2.** To tremble or shake.

shock (shŏk) [ME. *schokke*] A clinical syndrome marked by inadequate perfusion and oxygenation of cells, tissues, and organs, usually as a result of marginal or markedly lowered blood pressure. SEE: *Nursing Diagnoses Appendix.*

ETIOLOGY: Shock may be caused by dehydration, hemorrhage, sepsis, myocardial infarction, valvular heart disease, cardiac tamponade, adrenal failure, trauma, spinal cord injury, hypoxia, anaphylaxis, poisoning, and other major insults to the body.

SYMPTOMS: Shock results in failure of multiple organ systems, including the brain, heart, kidneys, lungs, skin, and gastrointestinal tract. Common consequences of shock are confusion, agitation, anxiety, or coma; syncope or presyncope; increased work of breathing; respiratory distress; pulmonary edema; decreased urinary output; and/or acute renal failure. Signs of shock include tachycardia, tachypnea, hypotension, and cool, clammy, or cyanotic skin.

TREATMENT: Attempts to restore normal blood pressure and tissue perfusion may include fluid resuscitation (in hypovolemic shock); control of hemorrhage (in shock caused by trauma or bleeding); administration of corticosteroids (in adrenal failure); pressor support (in cardiogenic or septic shock); the administration of epinephrine (in anaphylaxis); antibiotic administration with the drainage of infected foci (in sepsis); pericardiocentesis (in cardiac tamponade); transfusion; and oxygenation.

CRITICAL CARE: The shock syndrome is a serious life-endangering medical emergency and requires very careful therapy and monitoring. If the patient does not respond at once, treatment and monitoring in the best facility available (e.g., intensive care unit) is essential. It is important that the ECG; arterial and central venous blood pressures; blood gases; core and skin temperatures; pulse rate; blood volume; blood glucose; hematocrit; cardiac output; urine flow rate; and neurological status be monitored on an ongoing basis (e.g., hourly).

PATIENT CARE: Patients at risk for shock include, but are not limited to, those with severe injuries, external or suspected internal hemorrhage, profound fluid loss or sequestration (severe vomiting, diarrhea, burns), allergen exposures, sepsis, impaired left ventricular function, electrical and thermal injuries (including lightning strikes), and diabetes (if receiving supplemental insulin).

One, two, or more large-bore IV catheters are placed in the patient, and prescribed fluid therapy is initiated. External monitoring of vital signs is instituted, a pulmonary artery catheter may be placed for precise hemodynamic monitoring, and an indwelling urinary catheter is inserted to track urine output hourly. Prescribed oxygen therapy is provided; SaO_2, arterial blood gas levels (ABGs), and ventilatory function are monitored to determine the need for ventilatory support. If occult bleeding is suspected, stools and gastric fluids are tested for occult bleeding, and injured tissues and spaces are carefully assessed or imaged. The patient is maintained in a normothermic environment for comfort. Radiant warmers are useful in preventing hypothermia in patients who cannot be kept clothed or covered during assessment and treatment. The environment is kept as calm and controlled as possible. Procedures and treatments are explained to the patient in a simple, clear, easily understandable manner.

Positioning is based on the particular shock type. Although hypovolemic shock states respond best to supine positioning, or even elevation of the feet and lower legs, cardiac and anaphylactic shock states require head elevation to ease ventilatory effort. Correct body alignment should be maintained, whatever the necessary position. Oral fluids are often withheld to prevent vomiting and aspiration. Oral care and misting are provided frequently to prevent dryness, stomatitis, sordes, and salivary obstructions. The patient's sensorium is closely assessed, and sensory overload is prevented as much as possible. While providing comfort measures and emotional support, the health care professional acts as a liaison to family members or significant others, providing them with information about the patient's status and the treatment regimen. If the shock state is irreversible, the family must prepare for the patient's death; family members are encouraged to be with, talk to, and touch the patient, and social work and mental health consultations or spiritual measures may be obtained for the patient and family as determined by their beliefs and desires.

anaphylactic s. Rapidly developing,

systemic anaphylaxis that produces life-threatening vascular collapse and acute airway obstruction within minutes after exposure to an antigen. SEE: *allergy; anaphylaxis.*

ETIOLOGY: The condition is the result of a type I allergic or hypersensitivity reaction during which the allergen is absorbed into the blood directly or through the mucosa. The most common agents are bee or wasp venoms, drugs (e.g., penicillins), and radiographic contrast media. Chemical mediators released during the reaction cause constriction of the bronchial smooth muscle, vasodilation, and increased vascular permeability.

SYMPTOMS: Symptoms include acute respiratory distress, hypotension, edema, rash, tachycardia, pale cool skin, convulsions, and cyanosis. If no treatment is received, unconsciousness and death may result. Edema can be life-threatening if the larynx is involved, since air flow is obstructed with even minimal swelling.

PROGNOSIS: Death may occur if emergency treatment is not given.

PREVENTION: A history of past allergic reactions, particularly to bee stings, drugs, blood products, or contrast media, is obtained. The at-risk patient is observed for reaction during and immediately after administration of any of these agents.

PATIENT CARE: At the first sign of life-threatening respiratory distress, an airway is established, the appropriate physician is notified, and oxygen is administered by nonrebreather mask. Diphenhydramine, epinephrine, and corticosteroids are administered per protocol. Drugs should be administered intravenously if the patient is unconscious or hypotensive, and subcutaneously or intramuscularly if the patient is conscious and normotensive. Airway patency is maintained, and the patient should be observed for early signs of laryngeal edema (e.g., stridor, hoarseness, and dyspnea). Endotracheal intubation or a surgical airway may be necessary. In addition to high concentration oxygen for all patients in shock, cardiopulmonary resuscitation and defibrillation, as indicated, are initiated if the patient becomes pulseless. The patient is assessed for hypotension and shock; circulatory volume is maintained with prescribed volume expanders, and blood pressure is stabilized with prescribed vasopressors. Blood pressure, central venous pressure, and urinary output are monitored in the hospital setting. Once the initial emergency has subsided, prescribed drugs for long-term management and inhaled bronchodilators for bronchospasm may be considered. The patient is taught to identify and avoid common allergens and to recognize an allergic reaction. If a patient is unable to avoid exposure to allergens and requires medication, both patient and family are instructed in its use.

anesthesia s. Shock due to an overdose of a general anesthetic. The anesthetic should be immediately withheld and oxygen, mechanical ventilation, and vapor drugs should be given.

cardiogenic s. Failure of the heart to pump an adequate supply of blood and oxygen to body tissues. The most common cause of cardiogenic shock is acute myocardial infarction, but other causes include failure or stenosis of heart valves (e.g., aortic stenosis or mitral regurgitation), cardiomyopathies, pericardial tamponade, and sustained cardiac rhythm disturbances, among others. Cardiogenic shock is often fatal; only about 20% of affected persons survive. Its incidence has declined as the care of patients with acute myocardial infarction has incorporated thrombolytic drugs and emergency angioplasties. SEE: *Nursing Diagnoses Appendix.*

PATIENT CARE: The patient is assessed for a history of any cardiac disorder that severely decreases left ventricular function for anginal pain, dysrhythmias, urinary output, respiratory effort and rate, blood pressure, pulse, dizziness, alterations in mental status, and perfusion of the skin. Heart sounds are auscultated for a gallop rhythm, and murmurs, the lungs are checked for crackles and wheezes, and neck veins are assessed for distention.

Arterial blood gas values, electrolyte levels, and hemodynamic pressures are measured intensively. Prescribed intravenous fluids are administered via a large-bore intravenous catheter (14 G to 18 G) according to hemodynamic patterns and urine output. Oxygen is administered by face mask or artificial airway to ensure adequate tissue oxygenation. Prescribed inotropic agents and vasopressors are administered and evaluated for desired effects and any adverse reactions.

Some patients will undergo emergent cardiac catheterization, coronary angioplasty, coronary stents, bypass surgery, or placement of intra-aortic balloon pumps, tubine pumps, or ventricular assist devices. The ICU setting, special procedures, and equipment are explained to the patient and family to reduce their anxiety; a calm environment with as much privacy as possible and frequent rest periods are provided; and frequent family visits are permitted. The family is prepared for the possibility of a fatal outcome and assisted to find effective coping strategies.

compensated s. The early phase of

shock in which the body's compensatory mechanisms (e.g., increased heart rate, vasoconstriction, increased respiratory rate) are able to maintain tissue perfusion. Typically, the patient is normotensive in compensated shock.

decompensated s. The late phase of shock in which the body's compensatory mechanisms (e.g., increased heart rate, vasoconstriction, increased respiratory rate) are unable to maintain tissue perfusion. Typically, the patient is hypotensive in decompensated shock.

deferred s. Shock occurring several hours to a day after an injury or illness. SYN: *secondary s.*

distributive s. Shock in which there is a marked decrease in peripheral vascular resistance and consequent hypotension. Examples are septic shock, neurogenic shock, and anaphylactic shock.

electric s. Injury from electricity that varies according to type and strength of current and length and location of contact. Electric shocks range from trivial burns to complete charring and destruction of skin and injury to internal organs, including brain, lungs, kidneys, and heart. Approximately 1000 persons are electrocuted accidentally each year in the U.S., and 4000 persons are injured. Five percent of admissions to burn centers are related to electrical injury.

Whether or not an electric shock will cause death is influenced by the pathway the current takes through the body, the amount of current, and the skin resistance. Thus, a very small amount of electrical energy applied directly to the heart may be enough to stop it from beating, or to trigger ventricular fibrillation.

SYMPTOMS: Burns, loss of consciousness, and/or cardiac arrest are symptoms of electrical injury.

FIRST AID: Rescuers of any electrical shock victim who is unconscious should immediately call for emergency assistance. SEE: *cardiopulmonary resuscitation; electrocution; lightning safety rules; shock.*

TREATMENT: The patient should be freed carefully from the current source by first shutting off the current. Prolonged support in a critical care unit may be needed.

endotoxic s. Septic shock due to release of endotoxins by gram-negative bacteria. Endotoxins are lipopolysaccharides in the cell walls that are released during both reproduction and destruction of the bacteria. They are potent stimulators of inflammation, activating macrophages, B lymphocytes, and cytokines and producing vasodilation, increased capillary permeability, and activation of the complement and coagulation cascades. SEE: *endotoxin; septic s.*

epigastric s. Shock resulting from a blow or other trauma (surgery) in the upper abdomen.

hemorrhagic s. Shock due to loss of blood. SEE: *Nursing Diagnoses Appendix.*

hypoglycemic s. Shock produced by extremely low blood sugars (e.g., less than 40 mg/dl), usually caused by an injection of an excessive amount of insulin, failure to eat after an insulin injection, or rarely by an insulin-secreting tumor of the pancreas. Insulin-related hypoglycemic shock may be intentionally induced in the treatment of certain psychiatric conditions. SYN: *insulin s.* SEE: *hypoglycemia.*

PATIENT CARE: All unconscious patients should be treated for resumptive hypoglycemia with an injection of D_{50}. Once the patient is conscious, glucose is given by mouth to attain the desired glucose level. The rescue therapy is followed by a carbohydrate and protein snack to maintain the desired level.

The stabilized patient's immediate past history should be reviewed, looking for triggering factors. The patient and family can then be taught ways to avoid such situations in the future or to manage them before hypoglycemia again becomes this serious. If insulin levels need to be adjusted, the patient's preprandial glucose levels for the preceeding 24 hr must be reviewed. The patient and family are assisted to process the event. Their treatment actions are given positive reinforcement, correcting any errors such as inability to recognize early symptoms of insulin shock, overcorrection of insulin deficiency, or use of food products that are absorbed too slowly.

hypovolemic s. Shock occurring when there is an insufficient amount of fluid in the circulatory system. Usually, this is due to bleeding, diarrhea, or vomiting. SYN: *oligemic s.*

insulin s. Hypoglycemic s. SEE: *Nursing Diagnoses Appendix.*

irreversible s. Shock of such intensity that even heroic therapy cannot prevent death.

mental s. Shock due to emotional stress or to seeing an injury or accident. SEE: *psychic s.*

neurogenic s. A form of distributive shock due to decreased peripheral vascular resistance. Damage to either the brain or the spinal cord inhibits transmission of neural stimuli to the arteries and arterioles, which reduces vasomotor tone. The decreased peripheral resistance results in vasodilation and hypotension; cardiac output diminishes due to the altered distribution of blood volume.

oligemic s. Hypovolemic s.

protein s. Shock reaction resulting from parenteral administration of a protein.

psychic s. Shock due to excessive fear, joy, anger, grief. SEE: *mental s.*

secondary s. Deferred s.

septic s. Hypotension and inadequate blood flow to organs, as the result of sepsis (the presence of pathogens in the bloodstream). The most common organisms are gram-negative and gram-positive bacteria, but fungi and other organisms may also be responsible. Septic shock is one stage in systemic inflammatory response syndrome (SIRS). SEE: *sepsis*.

ETIOLOGY: Organisms and released endotoxins or exotoxins initiate a systemic inflammatory response. Chemical mediators of inflammation and the cell-mediated immune response (esp. tumor necrosis factor and interleukin 1) cause the physiological changes to septic shock. Initially, vasodilation, increased capillary permeability, and movement of plasma out of blood vessels produce hypovolemia and hypotension. Compensatory vasoconstriction occurs in an effort to maintain blood flow to vital organs. As sepsis progresses, secondary inflammatory mediators are released, increasing vascular endothelial damage.

Selective vasoconstriction produces tissue hypoxia and single or multiple organ dysfunction. Tissue hypoxia is increased by abnormal stimulation of the coagulation and kinin cascades in the capillaries, which produce microthrombi. Within the lung, damage to the capillary endothelium may cause adult respiratory distress syndrome. Septic shock often progresses to multiple organ dysfunction syndrome (MODS), which is the most common cause of death in surgical intensive care units.

SYMPTOMS: Confusion and other alterations of consciousness are common symptoms. Signs include hypotension, fever, tachypnea, tachycardia, decreased urinary output, and cold, clammy skin. Laboratory studies reveal acidosis and, sometimes, renal failure or coagulopathies.

TREATMENT: Empiric therapy with an extended-spectrum penicillin (e.g., ticarcillin/clavulanate, piperacillin/tazobactam) or third-generation cephalosporin (e.g., ceftriaxone), plus clindamycin or metronidazole, provide antibiotic coverage until an organism from the primary site of infection is positively identified. Intravenous fluid therapy and vasopressors such as dopamine or norepinephrine are used to stabilize blood pressure. Oxygen and other supportive interventions are used to minimize organ damage. Use of corticosteroids is not supported by research.

PATIENT CARE: Normal intensive care measures are instituted to monitor blood pressure, fluid and electrolyte balance, oxygenation, renal function, and changes in neurological status. Initially temperature and blood pressure may vary widely because of the effect of toxins on the vasculature. Assessment of progressive agitation or confusion should emphasize the possibility of hypoxia. Routine measures to reduce the risk of decubitus ulcers, muscle atrophy, and contractures are needed. Repeated teaching is necessary for family members to understand the pathology, purpose of interventions, signs of improvement, and possibility of death.

serum s. Shock occurring as part of a reaction to the injection of serum. SEE: *anaphylactic shock*.

spinal s. Immediate flaccid paralysis and loss of all sensation and reflex activity below the level of injury in acute transverse spinal cord injury. Arterial hypotension may be present in this condition.

surgical s. Shock following operations and including traumatic shock. SEE: *traumatic s.*

traumatic s. Shock due to injury or surgery. In the abdomen, it may result from hemorrhage and/or peritonitis secondary to a disrupted or perforated viscus. Additional causes of traumatic shock include the following: *Cerebral injury:* Shock from concussion of the brain secondary to cranial contusion or fracture or spontaneous hemorrhage. The shock may be evident immediately or later due to edema or delayed intracranial hemorrhage. *Chemical injury:* Shock due to physiological response to tissue injury, such as fluid mobilization, toxicity of the agent, and reflexes induced by pain due to the effect of chemicals, esp. corrosives. *Crushing injury:* Shock caused by disruption of soft tissue with release of myoglobulins, hemorrhage, and so forth, generally proportional to the extent of the injury. *Fracture (esp. open fracture):* Shock due to blood loss, fat embolism, and the physiological effects of pain. *Heart damage:* Shock caused by myocardial infarction, myocarditis, pericarditis, pericardial tamponade, or direct trauma with ensuing cardiovascular effects. *Inflammation:* Shock caused by severe sepsis, for example, peritonitis due to release of toxins affecting cardiovascular function and significant fluid mobilization.. *Intestinal obstruction:* Shock due to respiratory compromise due to distention, fluid mobilization, release of bacterial toxins, and pain. *Nerve injury:* Shock caused by injury to the area controlling respirations (e.g., high cervical cord injury) or to highly sensitive parts, such as the testicle, solar plexus, eye, and urethra, secondary to cardiovascular reflexes stimulated by pain. *Operations:* Shock that may occur even after minor operations and paracentesis or catheterization due to rapid escape of fluids resulting in abrupt alteration of intra-abdominal pressure dynamics and hemorrhage. *Perforation or rupture of viscera:* Shock resulting from acute pneumothorax, ruptured aneurysm, perforated peptic ulcer, perforation of appendicial abscess or colonic diverticulum, or ectopic pregnancy. *Strangulation:* Shock resulting from strangulated hernia, intussusception, or volvulus. *Thermal injury:* Shock caused by burn, frostbite, or heat exhaustion secondary to fluid mobilization due to the physiological effects of pain. *Torsion of viscera:* Shock caused by torsion of an ovary or a testicle secondary to the physiological effects of pain.

shoemakers' cramp A spasm of the muscles of the hand and arm occurring in shoemakers.

short bowel syndrome Inadequate absorption of ingested nutrients (especially vitamin B_{12}, macronutrients, sodium, and magnesium) resulting from a surgical procedure in which a considerable length of the intestinal tract has been removed or bypassed. Aggressive enteral nutrition or creation of an antiperistaltic segment in the remaining intestine may replace the need for partial or total parenteral nutrition in the management of this syndrome. Transplantation of the small intestine would be ideal, but as yet has limited application. SEE: *total parenteral nutrition*.

shortening Loss of bone length after a fracture, as a result of malunion or pronounced bony angulation.

shortness of breath Breathlessness.

shortsightedness (short-sīt'ĕd-nĕs) Myopia.

short stay A brief hospitalization for observation, for example, after a simple surgery, a biopsy, or a diagnostic study. The time spent in the hospital is typically limited to a few hours.

shot Injection.

shoulder (shōl'dĕr) [AS. *sculdor*] The region of the proximal humerus, clavicle, and scapula; a part of the shoulder girdle complex. SEE: *scapula*.

adhesive capsulitis of s. A condition that causes shoulder pain, with restricted movement even though there is no obvious intrinsic shoulder disease. This may follow bursitis or tendonitis of the shoulder or may be associated with systemic conditions such as chronic pulmonary disease, myocardial infarction, or diabetes mellitus. Prolonged immobility of the arm favors development of adhesive capsulitis. The condition is more common in women after age 50. It may resolve spontaneously 12 to 18 months after onset or may result in permanent restriction of movement. Treatment includes injection of glucocorticoids; use of nonsteroidal anti-inflammatory agents and physical therapy may provide symptomatic relief; early range-of-motion exercises following an injury may prevent development of the disease; manipulation of the shoulder while the patient is anesthetized may be of benefit. SYN: *frozen s.; pericapsulitis*.

dislocation of s. A condition in which the head of the humerus is displaced beyond the boundaries of the glenoid fossa. SEE: *Hill-Sachs lesion*.

ETIOLOGY: The most common cause is from trauma with the arm in external rotation with abduction, causing the head of the humerus to sublux anteriorly; a posterior subluxation may occur from a fall on an outstretched arm. An inferior dislocation may occur from poor muscle tone as with hemiplegia and from the weight of the arm pulling the humerus downward. Anterior glenohumeral dislocations are common among athletes, esp. football players.

SIGNS: A patient with a dislocated shoulder usually has a hollow in place of the normal bulge of the shoulder, as well as a slight depression at the outer end of the clavicle. Glenohumeral range of motion is restricted and such patients often cannot touch their opposite shoulder with the hand of the involved arm. Both shoulders should always be compared for symmetry.

TREATMENT/FIRST AID: An x-ray is needed to determine the type of dislocation and the presence of any fracture. If no fractures are present, one of several maneuvers can be used to reduce the humerus into the glenoid.

PATIENT CARE: Because of the potential damage to neurovascular structures as they cross the glenohumeral joint line, the vascular and neurological status of the arm and hand must be assessed. A decreased or diminished ulnar or radial pulse warrants immediate intervention and reduction of the dislocation. An anterior dislocation of the shoulder can be reduced, for example, with passive traction on the arm or by placing the patient in a supine position and medially displacing the scapula. SEE: illus.

frozen s. Adhesive capsulitis of s.

s. separation Acromioclavicular separation.

shoulder blade The scapula.

shoulder girdle The two scapulae and two clavicles attaching the bones of the upper extremities to the axial skeleton.

show (shō) [AS. *scewian*, to look at] The sanguinoserous discharge from the vagina during the first stage of labor or

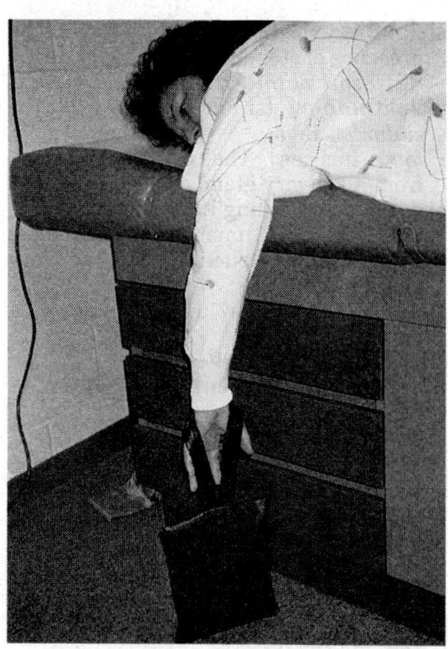

PASSIVE REDUCTION OF ANTERIOR SHOULDER DISLOCATION

just preceding menstruation. Also called *bloody show.*

bloody s. Show.

Shrapnell's membrane (shrăp′nĕls) [Henry J. Shrapnell, British anatomist, 1761–1841] A small triangular portion of the tympanic membrane lying above the malleolar folds. It is thin and lax and attached directly to the petrous bone at the tympanic notch (notch of Rivinus). SYN: *pars flaccida membranae tympani; Rivinus' ligament.*

shreds (shrĕds) [AS. *screade*] Slender strands of mucus seen in freshly voided urine, indicative of inflammation of the urinary tract or associated organs.

shrink To reduce in size.

shudder [ME. *shuddren*] A temporary convulsive tremor resulting from fright, horror, or aversion.

shunt (shŭnt) [ME. *shunten,* to avoid] **1.** To turn away from; to divert. **2.** An anomalous passage or one artificially constructed to divert flow from one main route to another. **3.** An electric conductor connecting two points in a circuit to form a parallel circuit through which a portion of the current may pass.

anatomical s. A normal or abnormal direct connection between arterial and venous circulation. An example of a normal anatomical shunt is the bronchial and thebesian vein connection.

arteriovenous s. An abnormal connection between an artery and the venous system.

cardiovascular s. An abnormal connection between the cavities of the heart or between the systemic and pulmonary vessels.

dialysis s. An arteriovenous shunt created for use during renal dialysis.

left-to-right s. The passage of blood from the left side of the heart to the right side through an abnormal opening (e.g., a septal defect).

physiological s. The route by which pulmonary blood perfuses unventilated alveoli. This process is caused by an imbalance between ventilation and perfusion.

portacaval s. Surgical creation of a connection between the portal vein and the vena cava. SYN: *postcaval s.*

postcaval s. Portacaval s.

reversed s. Right-to-left s.

right-to-left s. The movement of blood or other body fluids backward through a shunt. The shunted blood has no opportunity to become oxygenated because of failure to pass through the lungs.

Shy-Drager syndrome [George Milton Shy, U.S. neurologist, 1919–1967; G. A. Drager, U.S. physician, 1917–1967] A rare neurodegenerative disease of middle-aged or elderly persons, marked by chronic orthostatic hypotension, muscular rigidity, slow initiation of body movement, urinary incontinence, bowel dysfunction, erectile dysfunction, episodic loss of consciousness, and cardiac arrhythmias. SYN: *multiple systems atrophy.*

shyness The feeling of being timid, esp. in an unfamiliar setting or when encountering strangers. This feeling is so common that it cannot be classed as abnormal unless it interferes with activities essential to employment or interpersonal relations. Pathological shyness, in which persons avoid all kinds of social interactions because of intense psychological distress, is known as social phobia.

SI *Système International;* International System of Measurement. SEE: *SI Units Appendix.*

Si Symbol for the element silicon.

SIADH *syndrome of inappropriate antidiuretic hormone.*

siagonantritis (sī″ăg-ōn-ăn-trī′tĭs) [Gr. *siagon,* jawbone, + *antron,* cavity, + *itis,* inflammation] Inflammation of the maxillary sinus.

sialo-, sial- (sī′ă-lō) Combining form meaning *saliva.*

sialadenitis (sī″ăl-ăd″ĕ-nī′tĭs) [″ + ″ + *itis,* inflammation] Inflammation of a salivary gland. SYN: *sialitis.*

sialadenoncus (sī″ăl-ăd″ĕ-nŏng′kŭs) [″ + ″ + *onkos,* tumor] A tumor of a salivary gland.

sialagogue, sialogogue (sī-ăl′ă-gŏg, sī-ăl′ō-gŏg) [″ + *agogos,* leading] **1.** An agent increasing the flow of saliva. **2.** Producing or promoting the secretion of saliva. SYN: *ptyalagogue.*

sialectasia, sialectasis (sī″ăl-ĕk-tā′sē-ă,

sī″a-lĕk′tă-sĭs) [″ + *ektasis,* dilatation] Hypertrophy or swelling of the salivary glands.

sialemesis (sī″ăl-ĕm′ĕs-ĭs) [″ + *emein,* to vomit] The vomiting of saliva or vomiting caused by an excessive secretion of saliva.

sialic (sī-ăl′ĭk) Concerning or resembling saliva.

sialine (sī′ă-līn) [Gr. *sialon,* saliva] Concerning saliva.

sialism, sialismus (sī′ăl-ĭzm, sī-ăl-ĭz′mŭs) [″ + *-ismos,* condition] Ptyalism.

sialitis (sī″ă-lī′tĭs) [″ + *itis,* inflammation] Sialadenitis.

sialoadenitis (sī″ă-lō-ăd″ĕ-nī′tĭs) [″ + *aden,* gland, + *itis,* inflammation] Sialadenitis.

sialoadenotomy (sī″ă-lō-ăd″ĕ-nŏt′ō-mē) [″ + ″ + *tome,* incision] Incision of a salivary gland.

sialoaerophagy (sī″ă-lō-ĕr″ŏf′ă-jē) [″ + *aer,* air, + *phagein,* to eat] Constant swallowing, thus taking saliva and air into the stomach.

sialoangiectasis (sī″ă-lō-ăn″jē-ĕk′tă-sĭs) [Gr. *sialon,* saliva, + *angeion,* vessel, + *ektasis,* dilatation] Dilation of a salivary duct.

sialoangiography (sī″ă-lō-ăn″jē-ŏg′ră-fē) [″ + ″ + *graphein,* to write] Sialography.

sialoangitis, sialoangiitis (sī″ă-lō-ăn-jī′tĭs, -ăn″jē-ī′tĭs) [″ + ″ + *itis,* inflammation] Inflammation of the salivary ducts. SYN: *sialodochitis.*

sialocele (sī′ă-lō-sēl) [″ + *kele,* tumor, swelling] Cyst or tumor of a salivary gland.

sialodochitis (sī″ă-lō-dō-kī′tĭs) [″ + *doche,* receptacle, + *itis,* inflammation] Sialoangitis.

s. fibrinosa Sialodochitis with the duct obstructed by a fibrinous exudate.

sialodochoplasty (sī″ă-lō-dō′kō-plăs″tē) [″ + ″ + *plassein,* to form] Plastic surgery of a salivary gland.

sialoductitis (sī″ă-lō-dŭk-tī′tĭs) [″ + L. *ductus,* duct, + Gr. *itis,* inflammation] Inflammation of Stensen's duct.

sialogenous (sī″ă-lŏj′ĕ-nŭs) [″ + *gennan,* to produce] Forming saliva.

sialogogic (sī″ă-lō-gŏj′ĭk) Producing or promoting a secretion of saliva.

sialogram (sī-ăl′ō-grăm) [″ + *gramma,* something written] A radiograph of the ductal system of a salivary gland. A radiopaque fluid is instilled into the major duct to determine the presence or absence of calcareous deposits or other pathological changes.

sialography (sī″ă-lŏg′ră-fē) [″ + *graphein,* to write] Radiography of the salivary glands and ducts after injection of a radiopaque contrast medium. SYN: *ptyalography; sialoangiography.*

sialolith (sī-ăl′ō-lĭth) [″ + *lithos,* stone] A salivary stone.

sialolithiasis (sī″ă-lō-lĭ-thī′ă-sĭs) The presence of stones in the salivary ducts. SYN: *salivolithiasis.*

sialolithotomy (sī″ă-lō-lĭ-thŏt′ō-mē) [Gr. *sialon,* saliva, + *lithos,* stone, + *tome,* incision] The removal of a stone from a salivary gland or duct.

sialoncus (sī″ă-lŏng′kŭs) [″ + *onkos,* bulk, mass] A tumor under the tongue caused by obstruction of a salivary gland or duct.

sialorrhea (sī″ă-lō-rē′ă) [″ + *rhoia,* a flow] Ptyalism.

sialoschesis (sī″ă-lŏs′kĕ-sĭs) [″ + *schesis,* suppression] Suppression or retention of saliva.

sialosemeiology (sī″ă-lō-sē″mī-ŏl′ŏ-jē) [″ + *semeion,* sign, + *logos,* word, reason] Diagnosis based on examination of saliva.

sialosis (sī-ă-lō′sĭs) [″ + *osis,* condition] The flow of saliva.

sialostenosis (sī″ă-lō-stĕ-nō′sĭs) [″ + *stenosis,* act of narrowing] Closure of a salivary duct.

sialosyrinx (sī″ă-lō-sī′rĭnks) [″ + *syrinx,* a pipe] **1.** A fistula into the salivary gland. **2.** A syringe for washing out salivary ducts. **3.** A drainage tube for a salivary duct.

sialotic (sī″ă-lŏt′ĭk) [Gr. *sialon,* saliva] Concerning the flow of saliva.

Siamese twins (sī-ă-mēz′) [After Chang and Eng, conjoined Chinese twins in Siam, 1811–1874] Congenitally united twins. In some cases, the individuals are joined in a small area and are capable of activity, but the extent of union may be so great that survival is impossible. Nevertheless, modern surgical techniques have made it possible to separate infants who in the past would not have been expected to survive. SEE: *twin.*

sib [AS. *sibb,* kin] **1.** Sibling. **2.** A blood relative.

sibilant (sĭb′ĭ-lănt) [L. *sibilans,* hissing] Hissing or whistling, as a sound heard in a certain rale or in the formation of certain letters in speech, such as the letter "s."

sibilation Pronunciation in which the hissing sound is predominant.

sibilismus A hissing sound.

s. aurium Tinnitus.

sibilus (sĭb′ĭ-lŭs) [L. *sibilans,* hissing] A hissing rale.

sibling (sĭb′lĭng) [AS. *sibb,* kin, + *-ling,* having the quality of] One of two or more children of the same parents; a brother or sister. SYN: *sib.*

half s. A half brother or sister.

sibship Brothers and sisters of a single family.

siccant (sĭk′ănt) [L. *siccus,* dry] Siccative.

siccative (sĭk′ă-tĭv) [L. *siccativus,* drying] Drying or that which dries. SYN: *siccant.*

siccolabile (sĭk″ō-lā′bĭl) [L. *siccus,* dry, + *labilis,* unstable] Altered or destroyed by drying.

siccostabile (sĭk″ō-stā′bĭl) [″ + *stabilis,* stable] Resistant to drying.

siccus (sĭk′ŭs) [L.] Dry.

sick (sĭk) [AS *seoc,* ill] **1.** Not well. SYN: *ill.* **2.** Mentally ill or disturbed. **3.** Nauseated.

sick building syndrome An excess of work-related irritations of the skin and mucous membranes and other symptoms, including headache, fatigue, and difficulty concentrating, reported by workers in modern office buildings. The cause of this syndrome is unknown.

sicklemia (sĭk-lē′mē-ă) [AS. *sicol,* sickle, + Gr. *haima,* blood] Sickle cells in the blood.

sickling The tendency of red blood cells to be sickle-shaped. SEE: *sickle cell anemia.*

sickness [AS. *seoc,* ill] A state of being unwell. SYN: *illness.*

balloon s. Discomfort or illness due to ascent in a balloon to an altitude sufficient to cause symptoms of anoxia.

bleeding s. Hemophilia.

car s. Motion sickness.

milk s. Intoxication by fresh raw milk obtained from cows that have eaten snakeroot (*Eupatorium rugosum*). The illness is colloquially referred to as the "slows." SEE: *slows; snakeroot.*

motion s. Nausea, vomiting, pallor, profuse cold sweating, yawning, headache, and malaise due to repetitive exposure to change of body position associated with angular and linear acceleration and deceleration. This may occur in ships, aircraft, automobiles, during space travel, on swings, and even riding on a merry-go-round. The condition can occur in the absence of motion as in visualization of motion while viewing wide-screen movies. More than 90% of inexperienced ship passengers are estimated to become seasick in very rough weather conditions. Prolonged exposure to conditions that produce this motion sickness may lead to adaptation.

ETIOLOGY: Changing the rate of change of motion that acts on the labyrinth of the inner ear causes motion sickness. There may be a psychological component to the causation of motion sickness, in that some individuals may develop anxiety and motion sickness when exposed to unfamiliar modes of travel.

TREATMENT: For several hours before exposure to unaccustomed travel, persons susceptible to this condition should avoid bulky, greasy meals, particularly if there is little time to digest them before beginning the trip. Susceptible persons should be seated in the most stable part of the aircraft, boat, or vehicle and avoid head movement and reading. Anti–motion sickness medications include dimenhydrinate, diphenhydramine, meclizine, diazepam, and scopolamine. The last drug may be administered via a dermal patch applied 4 hr before exposure. If vomiting persists, the medicine may be given rectally or parenterally; IV fluids and electrolytes may be needed for replacement and maintenance of fluid-electrolyte balance.

CAUTION: Drugs used to treat motion sickness may adversely affect judgment, thinking, and motor function.

mountain s. Nausea and dyspnea caused by insufficient oxygen at high altitudes.

sea s. Sickness caused by motion of a vessel while at sea. SEE: *motion s.*

serum s. An adverse (type III hypersensitivity) immune response following administration of foreign antigens, esp. antiserum obtained from horses or other animals. Animal serum was previously used for passive immunization against rabies. Serum sickness can also occur following administration of penicillins and many other drugs. Antigen-antibody complexes form and deposit on the walls of small blood vessels, stimulating an inflammatory response that produces a pruritic rash, fever, joint pain and swelling, myalgias, and enlarged lymph nodes 7 to 14 days after exposure. Treatment consists of salicylates (such as aspirin) and antihistamines to minimize inflammation; corticosteroids may be given for severe symptoms. SEE: *hypersensitivity; Nursing Diagnoses Appendix.*

sleeping s. **1.** Encephalitis lethargica. **2.** Infection with the African trypanosome, *Trypanosoma brucei rhodesiense* or *gambiense* parasitic protozoa, introduced into the blood by the bite of a tsetse fly. The disease is marked by fever, protracted lethargy, weakness, tremors, and wasting.

space s. A transient form of motion sickness occurring in space travelers. SEE: *motion s.*

Sickness Impact Profile A standardized questionnaire designed to assess the effects of illness on function. There are 136 questions grouped into 12 categories. The categories include sleep and rest, eating, work, home management, recreation, ambulatory mobility, body care, movement, social interaction, alertness, emotional behavior, and communication. These are grouped as physical impairment, psychosocial impairment, and nonspecific.

sick sinus syndrome ABBR: SSS. Several electrocardiographical abnormalities caused by a malfunction of the sinoatrial node of the heart, in which there are episodes of tachycardia alternating with episodes of heart block or severely decreased heart rate, often with loss of consciousness. SEE: *Nursing Diagnoses Appendix.*

TREATMENT: A pacemaker should be inserted. Anticoagulant therapy may be required to prevent thromboembolism.

SICU *surgical intensive care unit.*

SID *source-to-image receptor distance.*

S.I.D. *Society for Investigative Dermatology.*

side (sīd) [AS. *side*] **1.** The left or right part of the trunk of the body. **2.** An outer portion considered as facing in a particular direction.

side effect An action or effect of a drug other than that desired. Commonly it is an undesirable effect such as nausea, headache, insomnia, rash, confusion, dizziness, or an unwanted drug-drug interaction.

side-lyer A device for positioning the patient with central nervous system dysfunction in a lateral recumbent position in order to reduce decerebrate posturing and counteract the effects of the tonic labyrinthine (supine) reflex.

side-lying position A lateral recumbent position in which the individual rests on the right or left side, usually with the knees slightly flexed. This position may be used in persons with mild forms of sleep apnea, in some patients with dysphagia, and in patients predisposed to sacral decubitus ulcers, among other conditions.

sidero- (sĭd′ĕr-ō) Combining form meaning *iron.*

sideroblast (sĭd′ĕr-ō-blăst″) [Gr. *sideros,* iron, + *blastos,* germ] A ferritin-containing normoblast in the bone marrow. Sideroblasts constitute from 20% to 90% of normoblasts in the marrow. The ferritin gives a positive Prussian-blue reaction, indicating the iron is ionized and not bound to the heme protein.

siderocyte (sĭd′ĕr-ō-sīt) [″ + *kytos,* cell] A red blood cell containing iron in a form other than hematin.

siderofibrosis (sĭd″ĕr-ō-fī-brō′sĭs) [″ + L. *fibra,* fiber, + Gr. *osis,* condition] Fibrosis associated with iron deposits.

siderogenous (sĭd″ĕr-ŏj′ĕ-nŭs) [″ + *gennan,* to produce] Producing or forming iron.

sideropenia (sĭd″ĕr-ō-pē′nē-ă) [″ + *penia,* poverty] Iron deficiency in the blood. **sideropenic,** *adj.*

siderophil (sĭd′ĕr-ō-fĭl) A cell that has an affinity for iron. **siderophilous,** *adj.*

siderophone (sĭd′ĕr-ō-fōn) A telephone-like device used to detect intraocular, iron-containing foreign bodies.

siderophore (sĭd′ĕr-ō-for) [″ + *phoros,* bearing] A macrophage that contains hemosiderin.

sideroscope (sĭd′ĕr-ō-skōp) [″ + *skopein,* to examine] An instrument for finding particles of iron in the eye.

siderosis (sĭd″ĕr-ō′sĭs) [″ + *osis,* condition] **1.** A form of pneumoconiosis resulting from inhalation of dust or fumes containing iron particles. SEE: *hemosiderosis.* **2.** The abnormal deposition or accumulation of iron in the blood or body tissues. **siderotic,** *adj.*

hepatic s. Excessive deposition of iron in the liver, a condition often found in patients with cirrhosis and hemochromatosis.

occupational s. SYN: *siderosis* (1).

s. of the central nervous system, superficial A rare neurological condition marked by bilateral sensorineural hearing loss, often with gait disturbance, cognitive impairment, and myoclonus. Excessive quantities of hemosiderin are found in the leptomeninges and subpial regions of the brain.

urinary s. Hemosiderin granules in the urine.

siderosome (sĭd″ĕr-ō-sōm′) [″ + *soma,* body] A reticulocyte in which iron-containing granules are present.

SIDS *sudden infant death syndrome.*

SIECUS *Sex Information and Education Council of the U.S.*

siemens (sē′mĕnz) A unit of conductance derived from SI units. It is the reciprocal of the resistance in ohms. SYN: *mho.*

Siemens' syndrome [Hermann Werner Siemens, German physician, 1891–1969] Harlequin fetus.

sieve (sĭv) A device consisting of a mesh with holes of uniform size. It is used to separate particles above a certain size from solutions or powders.

molecular s. A type of sieve in which the molecular material present in the gel or crystal will adsorb molecules of a certain kind and let others pass.

sievert [Rolf Maximillian Sievert, Swedish radiologist, 1896–1966] ABBR: Sv. A unit of absorbed radiation energy derived from SI units. One sievert is equal to 1 J/kg or 100 rem.

sig *signa.*

Sigault's operation (sē-gōz′) [Jean René Sigault, French obstetrician, b. 1740] Division of the symphysis pubis to facilitate childbirth by enlarging the pelvic outlet. SYN: *symphysiotomy.*

sigh [AS. *sican*] A deep inspiration followed by a slow audible expiration.

sight (sīt) [AS. *sihth*] **1.** The power or faculty of seeing. **2.** Range of sight. **3.** A thing or view seen. SYN: *vision.*

blind s. The ability to see that occurs in persons who are blind because of a brain lesion rather than damage to the eye. It is manifested by their being able to reach for and track an object. These individuals apparently do not know they can see.

day s. Night blindness.

far s. Hyperopia.
near s. Myopia.
night s. Day blindness.
old s. Presbyopia.
second s. Senopia.

sigma (sĭg′mă) The 18th letter, Σ or σ, in the Greek alphabet.

Sigma Theta Tau ABBR: STT. The international honor society of nursing, founded in 1922 by six students and one alumna of Indiana University Training School. There are 346 chapters in the U.S., Taiwan, Australia, Canada, and Korea. The national headquarters is at Indiana University in Indianapolis.

sigmatism (sĭg′mă-tĭzm) [Gr. *sigma,* letter S, + *-ismos,* condition] Excessive or defective use of "s" sounds in speech. SEE: *sibilation.*

sigmoid (sĭg′moyd) [Gr. *sigmoeides*] **1.** Shaped like the capital Greek letter sigma, Σ. **2.** Pert. to the sigmoid colon.

sigmoid colon The part of the colon that turns medially at the left iliac crest, between the descending colon and the rectum; shaped like the letter S.

sigmoidectomy (sĭg″moyd-ĕk′tō-mē) [″ + *ektome,* excision] Removal of all or part of the sigmoid colon.

sigmoiditis (sĭg″moyd-ī′tĭs) [″ + *itis,* inflammation] Inflammation of the sigmoid colon.

sigmoidopexy (sig-moy′dō-pĕk″sē) [″ + *pexis,* fixation] Fixation of the sigmoid colon by suturing it to the presacral fascia. SYN: *romanopexy.*

sigmoidoproctostomy (sĭg-moy″dō-prŏk-tŏs′tō-mē) [Gr. *sigmoeides,* shaped like Gr. letter S, + *proktos,* anus, + *stoma,* mouth] The establishment of an artificial passage by anastomosis of the sigmoid colon with the rectum.

sigmoidorectostomy (sĭg-moy″dō-rĕk-tŏs′tō-mē) [″ + L. *rectus,* straight, + Gr. *stoma,* mouth] Sigmoidoproctostomy.

sigmoidoscope (sĭg-moy′dō-skōp) [″ + *skopein,* to examine] A tubular speculum for examination of the sigmoid colon and the rectum.

flexible s. A sigmoidoscope that uses fiberoptics. This permits the tubular extension to flex, enabling the examiner to visualize a greater portion of the colon than would be possible with a rigid sigmoidoscope.

sigmoidoscopy (sĭg″moy-dŏs′kō-pē) [″ + *skopein,* to examine] Use of a sigmoidoscope to inspect the sigmoid colon.

sigmoidosigmoidostomy (sĭg-moy″dō-sĭg-moy-dŏs′tō-mē) [″ + *sigmoeides,* sigmoid, + *stoma,* mouth] Surgical creation of a connection between two segments of the sigmoid colon.

sigmoidostomy (sĭg-moyd-ŏs′tō-mē) [″ + *stoma,* mouth] Creation of an artificial anus in the sigmoid colon, that is, sigmoid colostomy.

sigmoidotomy (sĭg-moyd-ŏt′ō-mē) [″ + *tome,* incision] Incision of the sigmoid.

sigmoidovesical (sĭg-moy″dō-vĕs′ĭ-kăl) [″ + L. *vesica,* bladder] Concerning a pathological connection between the sigmoid colon and the urinary bladder secondary to malignancy, inflammatory bowel disease, or diverticulitis.

sign (sīn) [L. *signum*] **1.** Symbol or abbreviation, esp. one used in pharmacy. **2.** Any objective evidence or manifestation of an illness or disordered function of the body. Signs are apparent to observers, as opposed to symptoms, which may be obvious only to the patient. SEE: *symptom.* **3.** To use sign language to communicate.

beaten-silver skull s. The thinned, irregular appearance of the skull, as seen on x-ray examination of children with obstructive hydrocephalus.

chandelier s. Intense pelvic and lower abdominal pain brought on by palpation of the cervix. The sign points to the presence of pelvic inflammatory disease.

hair collar s. In the newborn, a ring of long, dark, coarse hair surrounding a midline nodule on the scalp. This may indicate neural tube closure defect.

jump s. During physical examination, an involuntary reaction to stimulation of a tender area or trigger point. This may take the form of wincing or sudden jerking of the part being examined, of adjacent areas, or even of the entire body. This sign should not be confused with the startle reaction seen in Jumping Frenchmen of Maine.

Levine s. Holding a clenched fist over the sternum, a characteristic gesture that individuals experiencing anginal chest pain use frequently.

objective s. In physical diagnosis, a sign that can be seen, heard, measured, or felt by the diagnostician. Finding of such sign(s) can be used to confirm or deny the diagnostician's impressions of the disease suspected of being present. SYN: *physical s.*

physical s. Objective s.

pop-eye s. A bulging of the body of the biceps brachii muscle that results from rupture of the muscle's tendon. It superficially resembles an exaggerated attempt to flex the biceps muscle.

positive s. of pregnancy Assessment findings present only during pregnancy: fetal heart tones, fetal movements felt by the examiner, and visualization by sonogram.

presumptive s. of pregnancy Signs and symptoms commonly associated with pregnancy that may be present in other conditions. SEE: *pregnancy.*

probable s. of pregnancy Objective assessment findings that strongly suggest but do not confirm pregnancy. SEE: *pregnancy.*

psoas s. Abdominal pain produced by extension of the hip. The sign indicates a retrocecal or retroperitoneal lesion.

spinnaker sail s. An outline of the thymus of a child by radiolucent lines. It is seen on chest x-ray examinations of children with pneumomediastinum.

steeple s. Narrowing of the column of subglottic air in the trachea, seen on anteroposterior radiographs of the neck in children with croup.

sunset s. Newborn assessment finding often associated with hydrocephaly; the newborn's eyes are open with the irises directed downward, resembling the sun setting below the horizon.

vital s. Those physical signs concerning functions essential to life (i.e., pulse, rate of respiration, blood pressure, and temperature). Some health care professionals consider a patient's level of pain to be a "fifth" vital sign, although this is not accepted by all parties. While all health care professionals agree that a patient's experience of pain is a critical feature of his or her adaptation to illness, the traditional vital signs are objectively measurable and verifiable, while the level of pain is considered by many to be experiential or subjective.

signa (sĭg′nă) [L.] ABBR: S or sig. A term used in writing prescriptions meaning to label the subscription according to the dose, route of administration, and frequency of medication.

signal Any form of communication that provides information. It is usually visual, verbal, or written, or it could be transmitted by electronic means (i.e., telephone, TV, radio, laser, or via optical fibers).

cellular s. A chemical released by cells and tissues to stimulate metabolic activities within those same tissues, or in other parts of the body. Neurotransmitters, hormones, peptides, cytokines, arachidonic acid derivatives, and other chemicals are all signaling molecules.

s. void A dark or blank space in a radiographic image of a fluid-filled structure. SEE: *filling d.*

signature (sĭg′nă-tūr) [L. *signatura,* to mark] **1.** The part of a prescription giving instructions to the patient. **2.** The act of writing one's name on a document to certify its validity; the written name on the document.

significance, statistical SEE: *statistical significance.*

significant (sĭg-nĭf′ĭ-kănt) Important or meaningful.

significant other A person with whom a patient has a close relationship, which may or may not include relatives or a spouse.

signing The use of sign language to communicate with hearing-impaired persons.

sign language Representing words by signs made with the position and movement of the fingers and hand. SEE: *American Sign Language.*

silencer (sī′lĕn-sĕr) A sequence of base pairs in DNA that prevents the transcription of a gene.

silent Free from noise; mute; still.

silent disease A disease that produces no clinically obvious symptoms or signs. Examples include hypertension, many forms of cancer (including small lesions of the breast and prostate cancer), and hearing loss, which may be either not noticed or denied by the individual. Many diseases begin silently, becoming obvious only when they are advanced.

silent period A period in a tendon reflex that immediately follows the contraction of the responding muscles during which the motor neurons do not respond to afferent impulses entering the reflex center.

silica (sĭl′ĭ-kă) [L. *silex,* flint] SiO_2; silicon dioxide. SEE: *silicon.*

silicate (sĭl′ĭ-kāt) [L. *silicus,* flintlike] A salt of silicic acid.

siliceous, silicious (sĭ-lĭsh′ŭs) Containing silica.

silicic (sĭl-ĭs′ĭk) Pert. to silica or silicon.

silicoanthracosis (sĭl″ĭ-kō-ăn″thră-kō′sĭs) [L. *silex,* flint, + Gr. *anthrax,* coal, + *osis,* condition] Silicosis combined with anthracosis, in coal miners.

silicofluoride (sĭl″ĭ-kō-floo′ō-rīd) A compound of silicon, fluorine, and the fluoride of a metal.

silicon (sĭl′ĭ-kŏn) [L. *silex,* flint] SYMB: Si. A nonmetallic element found in the soil; atomic weight 28.086; atomic number 14; specific gravity 2.33. Silicon makes up approx. 25% of the earth's crust, being exceeded only by oxygen. It occurs in trace amounts in skeletal structures (bones and teeth). Silicon is commonly combined with oxygen to form silicon dioxide, SiO_2, which occurs in many forms, both crystalline and amorphous. In a pure state, it forms quartz or rock crystal. It is present in many abrasive materials and is the principal constituent of glass.

silicone (sĭl′ĭ-kōn″) **1.** An organic compound in which all or part of carbon has been replaced by silicon. **2.** Any of a group of polymeric organic silicon compounds; used in adhesives, lubricants, synthetic rubber, and prostheses.

injectable s. Medical-grade silicone used in the past for breast augmentation, and currently for short-term use in retinal detachment and surgeries of the vitreous or the urethra. The more purified the silicone oils used, the better tolerated and the more biocompatible the implant application. Numerous prostheses are made of silicone and it is controversially used in breast implants. SEE: *breast implant.*

silicosiderosis (sĭl″ĭ-kō-sĭd″ĕr-ō′sĭs) [″ + Gr. *sideros,* iron, + *osis,* condition] A type of pneumonoconiosis in which the inhaled particles contain silicates and iron.

silicosis (sĭl-ĭ-kō'sĭs) [" + Gr. *osis,* condition] A form of pneumonoconiosis resulting from inhalation of silica (quartz) dust, characterized by the formation of small discrete nodules. In advanced cases, a dense fibrosis and emphysema with impairment of respiratory function may develop.

silicotic (sĭl-ĭ-kŏt'ĭk) **1.** Relating to silicosis. **2.** One affected with silicosis.

silicotuberculosis (sĭl"ĭ-kō-tū-bĕr-kū-lō'sĭs) [" + *tuberculum,* a little swelling, + Gr. *osis,* condition] Silicosis associated with pulmonary tuberculosis.

siliqua olivae (sĭl'ĭ-kwē ŏl'ĭ-vē) [L.] Fibers that appear to encircle the olive of the brain.

siliquose (sĭl'ĭ-kwōs) [L. *siliqua,* pod] Resembling a two-valve capsule or a pod.

siliquose cataract A cataract with a dry, wrinkled capsule.

siliquose desquamation Shedding of dried vesicles from the skin.

silo-filler's disease, silo-filler's syndrome A rare respiratory illness produced by exposure to nitrogen oxides that are released from fermenting organic matter in freshly filled, poorly ventilated farm silos. The silage gases produce irritation of the mouth, nose, pharynx, bronchi, and lungs, interfering with oxygenation and gas exchange. Alveolar damage and hemorrhagic pulmonary edema may result; about 20% of affected persons die of the exposure. Delayed injury to the lungs, esp. emphysema or bronchiolitis obliterans, may occur long after the initial exposure to silage gases.

PREVENTION: No one should enter a silo until 7 to 10 days after it is filled. Good ventilation above the base of a silo should be maintained during the 7- to 10-day period. The area should be fenced in, to prevent children or animals from straying into the space surrounding a silo. The blower fan should always be activated before a person enters a silo.

TREATMENT: Corticosteroid drugs, such as prednisone or methylprednisolone help prevent lung injury in patients exposed to silage gases.

silver (sĭl'vĕr) [AS. *siolfor*] SYMB: Ag. A white, soft, ductile malleable metal, its salts being widely used in medicine for their caustic, astringent, and antiseptic effects. Its atomic weight is 107.870; atomic number is 47; and specific gravity is 10.5. In dentistry, silver is used in prosthetic devices, as an alloy with copper or mercury, as silver solder, and as tapering points to obliterate root canals in the endodontic treatment of teeth. Silver nitrate has been used as a germicidal astringent with the treatment of caries, root canals, tooth sensitivity, and gingival diseases. SEE: *argyria.*

s. amalgam An alloy of silver with varying amounts of tin or copper, using mercury as a major component to produce a silvery, malleable restorative material used in dentistry. It is mixed and condensed, then placed in the space left after removal of the decayed area of the tooth, where it hardens into a solid mass that can be shaped to the desired shape. SYN: *s. filling.*

s. chloride SYMB: AgCl. An insoluble salt of silver.

colloidal s. Silver preparations in which the particles of silver or silver proteinate are suspended in the solution rather than being dissolved in it.

s. filling Silver amalgam.

s. halide The active ingredient in a radiographical film emulsion that, when exposed to electromagnetic radiation and developed, forms the image on the film.

s. nitrate $AgNO_3$; a toxic preparation made from silver. Most of its former uses have passed out of vogue, but it remains important as a germicide and local astringent. It is incompatible with aspirin and sodium chloride. SEE: *silver nitrate poisoning.*

s. nitrate, toughened A mixture of silver nitrate and silver chloride used as a caustic on wounds and granulation tissue, and in treating warts.

s. picrate A compound formerly used as an antiseptic.

s. protein A combination of silver and protein, containing from 7.5% to 8.5% (strong) silver.

s. sulfadiazine ABBR: AgSD; SSD. An antibacterial medication, commonly applied as a topical cream on burns, to promote wound healing and prevent infections with germs such as *Staphylococcus aureus* and *Pseudomonas aeruginosa.*

silverfish An insect, *Ctenolepisma longicaudata,* whose scales are often found in house dust, are antigenic, and may be a cause of childhood and adult perennial allergies and asthma. This house pest may be controlled with the use of insecticides.

silver fork deformity A deformity in the Colles' fracture of the wrist and hand resembling the curve on the back of a fork.

silver nitrate poisoning Toxicity resulting from repeated exposure to silver compounds, marked by a bluish pigmentation of the skin or occasionally of the eyes. In the past, many medications contained biologically available silver; the incidence of this intoxication now, however, is very low. SYN: *argyria.*

silybum marianum (sĭ-lē-bŭm') Milk thistle.

silymarin (sĭ-lē-măr'ĭn) Milk thistle.

simethicone (sī-mĕth'ĭ-kōn) A mixture of liquid demethylpolysiloxanes that because of its antifoaming properties is used to treat intestinal gas.

simian crease A crease on the palm of the hand, so termed because of its similarity to the transverse flexion crease found in some monkeys. Normally the palm of the hand at birth contains several flexion creases, two of which are separate and approx. transverse. When these two appear to fuse and thus form a single transverse crease, a simian crease is present. The crease may be present in a variety of developmental abnormalities including Down syndrome, rubella syndrome, Turner's syndrome, Klinefelter's syndrome, pseudohypoparathyroidism, and gonadal dysgenesis. SEE: illus.

SIMIAN AND NORMAL PALMAR CREASES

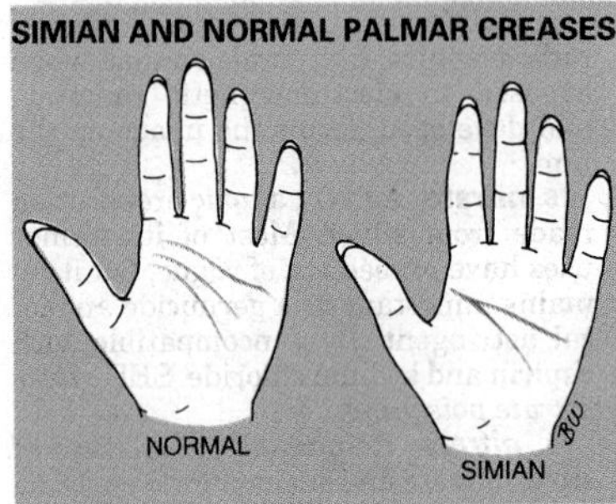

similia similibus curantur (sĭ-mĭl'ē-ă sĭ-mĭl'ĭ-bŭs kū-răn'tūr) [L., likes are cured by likes] The homeopathic doctrine that a drug producing pathological symptoms in those who are well will cure such symptoms in persons with disease. **similimum,** *adj.*

Simmonds' disease (sĭm'mŏnds) [Morris Simmonds, German physician, 1855–1925] Complete atrophy of the pituitary gland, producing loss of function of the thyroid, adrenals, and gonads, hair loss, hypotension, and cachexia. SYN: *pituitary cachexia,.*

Simon's position (zē'mŏns) [Gustav Simon, German surgeon, 1824–1876] An exaggerated lithotomy position in which the hips are somewhat elevated and the thighs are strongly abducted. It is used in operations on the vagina. SYN: *Edebohls' position.*

simple (sĭm'pl) [L. *simplex*] **1.** Not complex; not compound. **2.** A medicinal plant.

simple inflammation Inflammation without pus or other inflammatory exudates.

Simple Triage and Rapid Treatment ABBR: START. A procedure for quickly classifying injured patients according to the severity of their injuries and for treating those who are most severely injured first.

Sims' position (sĭmz) [James Marion Sims, U.S. gynecologist, 1813–1883] A semiprone position with the patient on the left side, right knee and thigh drawn well up, left arm along the patient's back, and chest inclined forward so that the patient rests on it. It is the position of choice for administering enemas because the sigmoid and descending colon are located on the left side of the body and fluid is readily accepted in this position. It is also used in curettement of the uterus, intrauterine irrigation after labor, flexible sigmoidoscopy, colonoscopy, rectal examination, and postanesthesia recovery.

simul (sī'mŭl, sĭm'ŭl) [L.] At once or at the same time; term used in signature of prescription.

simulation (sĭm-ū-lā'shŭn) [L. *simulatio,* imitation] **1.** Pretense of having a disease; feigning of illness. SEE: *malingerer; Munchausen syndrome.* **2.** The imitation of symptoms of one disease by another. **3.** A replica. **4.** An educational or technological model of an actual situation (such as cardiac arrest) that is used to train new students or to predict or estimate outcomes that may be obtainable in practice.

simulator (sĭm"ū-lā'tor) Any situation or device that imitates or re-creates a condition or situation similar to one that might be encountered by a student or trainee. Simulations are used to prepare learners for social occupational or educational roles.

Simulium (sĭ-mū'lē-ŭm) A genus of insects of the order Diptera that includes the black flies (buffalo gnats). The females are blood suckers.

S. damnosum A species that serves as the intermediate host of a filarial worm *Onchocerca volvulus.*

S. venustum A species common in North America.

simultanagnosia The failure to perceive simultaneously all the elements of a scene.

SIMV *synchronized intermittent mandatory ventilation.*

Sinapis (sĭn-ā'pĭs) [Gr. *sinapi,* mustard] A genus of plants commonly known as mustard plants.

sincipital (sĭn-sĭp'ĭ-tăl) [L. *sinciput,* half a head] Concerning the sinciput.

sinciput (sĭn'sĭp-ŭt) [L., half a head] **1.** The fore and upper part of the cranium. **2.** The upper half of the skull. SYN: *calvaria.*

Sinding-Larsen Johansson disease Anterior knee pain caused by persistent traction on an immature inferior patellar pole. There is point tenderness at the patellar-patellar tendon junction, and Osgood-Schlatter disease may be present. The adult equivalent of this disease is patellar tendinitis. This condition occurs commonly in boys 10 to 12 years of age who are actively involved in running and jumping sports. It resolves eventually but can be treated with activity modification, a patella-stabilizing knee brace, ice, and nonsteroidal anti-inflammatory drugs.

sinew (sĭn'ū) [AS. *sinu*] A tendon.

weeping s. A ganglion cyst that contains synovial fluid.

sing [L., *singulorum*] Of each; used in writing prescriptions.

singleton One of something described, esp. a single infant rather than a twin.

singultation (sĭng″gŭl-tā'shŭn) [L. *singultus,* a hiccup] Hiccupping.

singultus (sĭng-gŭl'tŭs) [L.] Hiccup.

sinister (sĭn-ĭs'tĕr) [L.] In anatomy, left; or present on the left side of the body.

sinistrad (sĭn'ĭs-trăd) [L. *sinister,* left, + *ad,* toward] Toward the left.

sinistral (sĭn'ĭs-trăl) [L.] **1.** Pert. to or showing preference for the left hand, eye, or foot in certain actions. **2.** On the left side.

sinistrality (sĭn″ĭs-trăl'ĭ-tē) Left-handedness.

sinistraural (sĭn-ĭs-traw'răl) [″ + *auris,* ear] Having better hearing with the left ear.

sinistro- (sĭn'ĭs-trō) Combining form meaning *left.*

sinistrocardia (sĭn″ĭs-trō-kăr'dē-ă) [L. *sinister,* left, + Gr. *kardia,* heart] Displacement of the heart to left of the medial line; the opposite of dextrocardia.

sinistrocerebral (sĭn″ĭs-trō-sĕr'ĕ-brăl) [″ + *cerebrum,* brain] Located in the left cerebral hemisphere.

sinistrocular (sĭn-ĭs-trŏk'ū-lar) [″ + *oculus,* eye] Having stronger vision in the left eye.

sinistrocularity (sĭn″ĭs-trŏk″ū-lăr'ĭ-tē) Condition in which the left eye is dominant.

sinistrogyration (sĭn″ĭs-trō-jī-rā'shŭn) [″ + Gr. *gyros,* a circle] Inclination to the left.

sinistromanual (sĭn″ĭs-trō-măn'ū-ăl) [″ + *manus,* hand] Left-handed.

sinistropedal (sĭn-ĭs-trŏp'ĕd-ăl) [″ + *pes,* foot] Left-footed.

sinistrotorsion (sĭn″ĭs-trō-tor'shŭn) [″ + *torsio,* a twisting] A twisting or turning toward the left.

sinistrous (sĭn'ĭs-trŭs) Awkward, clumsy, unskilled; the opposite of dextrous.

sinoatrial (sīn″ō-ā'trē-ăl) Pert. to the sinus venosus and atrium.

sinobronchitis (sī″nō-brŏng-kī'tĭs) [L. *sinus,* curve, + *bronchos,* windpipe, + Gr. *itis,* inflammation] Paranasal sinusitis with bronchitis.

sinogram (sī'nō-grăm″) [L. *sinus,* curve, + Gr. *gramma,* something written] A radiograph of a sinus tract filled with a radiopaque contrast medium to determine the range and course of the tract.

sinter (sĭn'tĕr) **1.** The calcium or silica deposits formed from water obtained from mineral springs. **2.** To reduce material to a solid form by heating without melting.

sinuous (sĭn'ū-ŭs) [L. *sinuosus,* winding] Winding; wavy; tortuous.

sinus (sī'nŭs) *pl.* **sinuses, sinus** [L., curve, hollow] **1.** A cavity within a bone. **2.** A dilated channel for venous blood. **3.** A canal or passage leading to an abscess. **4.** Any cavity having a relatively narrow opening.

accessory nasal s. paranasal s.

anal s. The saclike recesses behind the anal columns.

aortic s. **1.** The area in the wall of the aortic arch that contains pressoreceptors innervated by the vagus nerves. These receptors detect changes in blood pressure and bring about reflex changes in heart rate and arterial diameter. **2.** A dilatation of the aorta opposite the segment of the semilunar valve. SYN: *s. of Valsalva.*

basilar s. Transverse s. (2).

carotid s. The site at the base of the internal carotid artery of pressoreceptors innervated by the glossopharyngeal nerve. These receptors detect changes in blood pressure and bring about reflex changes in heart rate and arterial diameter.

s. cavernosus A large sinus from the sphenoidal fissure to the apex of the petrous portion of the temporal bone.

cerebral s. Any ventricle of the brain.

circular s. A venous sinus around the pituitary gland, communicating on each side with the cavernous sinus.

coccygeal s. A sinus in the midline of the gluteal cleft just over the coccyx.

coronary s. of heart A vein in the transverse groove between the left cardiac atrium and ventricle.

cranial s. One of the large veins between the two layers of the cranial dura mater.

dermal s. A congenital sinus tract connecting the surface of the body with the spinal canal.

draining s. An abnormal passageway leading from inside the body to the outside. This is usually due to an infectious process.

ethmoidal s. One of the air cavities in the ethmoid bone.

frontal s. An irregular cavity in the frontal bone on each side of the midline above the nasal bridge. One may be larger than the other. A duct carries secretions to the upper part of the nasal cavity.

genitourinary s. Urogenital s.

hair s. The sinus formed when hair is embedded in the skin and acts as a foreign body.

inferior longitudinal s. Inferior sagittal s.

inferior petrosal s. A large venous sinus from the cavernous sinus, running along the lower margin of the petrous portion of the temporal bone.

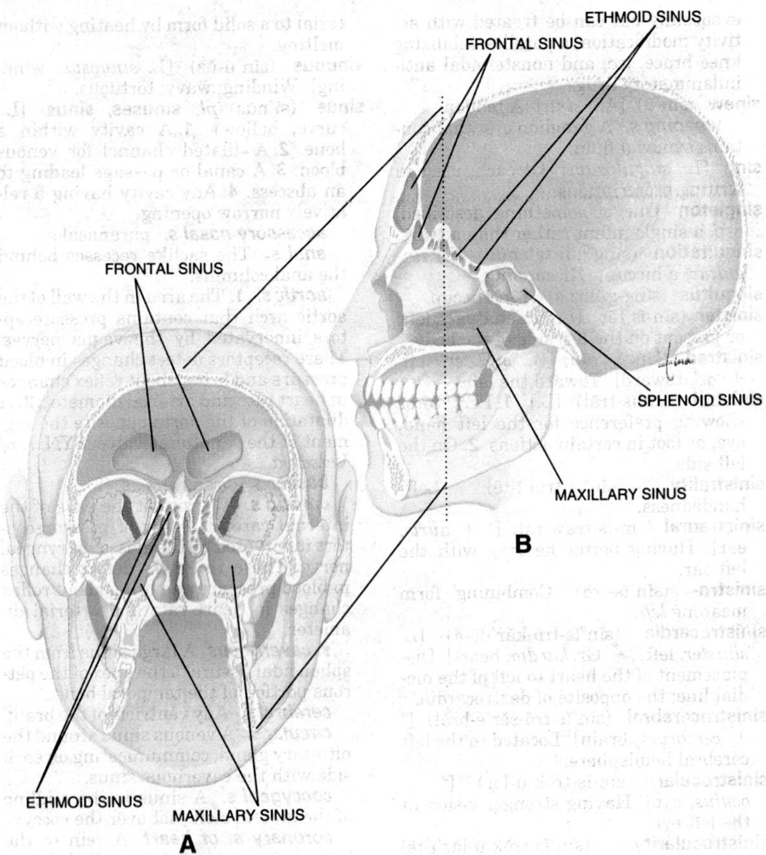

PARANASAL SINUSES

(A) anterior, (B) left lateral

inferior sagittal s. A venous sinus in the inferior margin of the falx cerebri. SYN: *inferior longitudinal s.*

intercavernous s. One of the anterior and posterior halves of the circular sinus.

lateral s. One of two large venous sinuses in the inner side of the skull passing near the mastoid antrum and emptying into the jugular vein.

lymph s. A pathway for lymph through a lymph node. SYN: *lymph channel.*

marginal s. **1.** A large venous sinus around part of the margin of the placenta. **2.** One of the small bilateral venous sinuses of the dura mater at the edge of the foramen magnum. **3.** A venous sinus around a portion of the white pulp of the spleen.

maxillary s. A cavity in the maxillary bone communicating with the middle meatus of the nasal cavity. SYN: *antrum of Highmore.*

occipital s. A small venous sinus in the attached margin of the falx cerebelli extending to the margin of the foramen magnum.

paranasal s. One of the air cavities in the frontal, maxillary, sphenoid, or ethmoid bones. The anterior group consists of the frontal, maxillary, and anterior ethmoids; the posterior group includes the posterior ethmoids and sphenoid. These sinuses develop embryologically from nasal cavities, are lined with the same type of ciliated epithelium, are filled with air, and communicate with nasal cavities through their various ostia. They lighten the skull, being lighter than dense bone, and are resonating chambers for the voice. SEE: illus.

pilonidal s. Pilonidal fistula.

pleural s. One of the spaces in the pleural sac along the lower and inferior portions of the lung that the lung does not occupy.

s. pocularis A lacuna in the prostatic part of the urethra. SYN: *s. prostaticus.*

s. prostaticus S. pocularis.

s. of the pulmonary trunk One of the dilatations in the pulmonary trunk, across from a cusp of the pulmonary valve of the heart.

s. rectus A venous sinus at the junction of the falx cerebri and the cerebellar tentorium. SYN: *straight s.*

renal s. The area in the kidney composed of the renal pelvis, renal calices, vessels, nerves, and fatty tissue.

rhomboid s. The fourth cranial ventricle.

scleral venous s. Schlemm's canal.

sigmoid s. The continuation, on both sides, of the transverse sinuses down along the posterior border of the petrous part of the temporal bone to the jugular foramen and jugular veins.

sphenoidal s. One of the air sinuses that occupy the body of the sphenoid bone and connect with the nasal cavity.

sphenoparietal s. **1.** A venous sinus uniting the cavernous sinus and a meningeal vein. **2.** The portion of the cavernous sinus below the ensiform process.

s. of spleen A large-capacity venous channel in the spleen.

straight s. S. rectus.

superior longitudinal s. Superior sagittal s.

superior petrosal s. A venous canal running in a groove in the petrous portion of the temporal bone.

superior sagittal s. A large venous sinus along the attached border of the falx cerebri from the crista galli to the internal occipital protuberance where it joins either the right or left transverse sinuses or both. SYN: *superior longitudinal s.*

tarsal s. A tunnel between the calcaneus and talus of the ankle.

tentorial s. SEE: *s. rectus.*

terminal s. A vein encircling the vascular area of the blastoderm.

transverse s. **1.** A sinus that unites the two inferior petrosal sinuses of the cranium. **2.** Venous network in the dura over the basilar process of the occipital bone. SYN: *basilar s.*

transverse s. of the dura mater One of the large, bilateral venous sinuses along the attached margin of the cerebellar tentorium. They receive the superior sagittal and straight sinuses and drain into the sigmoid sinuses and then into the jugular veins.

transverse s. of the pericardium A channel posterior to the aorta and the pulmonary trunk but in front of the atria.

tympanic s. A deep recess in the labyrinthine wall of the tympanic cavity. It opens into the fenestra of the cochlea.

urogenital s. **1.** A duct into which, in the embryo, the wolffian ducts and bladder empty; it opens into the cloaca. **2.** The common receptacle of the genital and urinary ducts. SYN: *genitourinary s.*

uterine s. One of the venous channels in the walls of the uterus during pregnancy.

uteroplacental s. One of the slanting venous channels from the placenta serving to convey the maternal blood from the intervillous lacunae back into the uterine veins.

s. of Valsalva Aortic s.

s. of venal canal The portion of the right atrium of the heart posterior, and to the left of, the crista terminalis. The inferior and superior vena caval veins empty into it.

venous s. A sinus conveying venous blood.

venous s. of the dura mater One of the large veins between the two layers of the dura mater. They reabsorb cerebrospinal fluid and drain the venous blood from the brain.

venous s. of sclera Schlemm's canal.

sinusitis (sī-nŭs-ī′tĭs) [L. *sinus,* curve, hollow, + Gr. *itis,* inflammation] Inflammation of a sinus, esp. a paranasal sinus. It may be caused by various agents, including viruses, bacteria, or allergy. Predisposing factors include inadequate drainage, which may result from presence of polyps, enlarged turbinates, or deviated septum; chronic rhinitis; general debility; or dental abscess in maxillary bone.

acute suppurative s. Purulent inflammation with pain over the facial sinuses, often accompanied by fever, chills, and headache.

TREATMENT: Therapy is conservative. Shrinkage in the nasal mucosa is useful to facilitate ventilation and drainage of the sinus. The patient should rest, force fluids, take decongestants, and apply hot packs. If inflammation is due to bacterial infection, antibiotic therapy is indicated.

allergic fungal s. Chronic nasal obstruction with symptoms that include a runny nose and postnasal discharge, that is caused by allergies to soil-based fungi (such as *Curvularia* or *Alternaria*). The condition is occasionally diagnosed in patients with an allergic history and nasal polyposis who have failed treatments for other sinus diseases. Tenacious mucus with a large number of eosinophils are often present.

chronic hyperplastic s. Polyps present in sinuses and nose and underlying osteitis of sinus walls.

TREATMENT: This condition is treated surgically. Conservative surgery involves the removal of polyps and intranasal opening into sinuses for adequate ventilation and drainage. Radical surgery would involve the complete removal of sinus mucosa through either the external or the intranasal route.

invasive fungal s. Sinus, ophthalmic, and cerebral invasion by opportunistic fungi. The disease usually occurs in immunosuppressed patients (such as diabetic or neutropenic patients) and is frequently fatal despite aggressive medical and surgical therapies. *Aspergillus, Mucor,* and *Rhizopus* are the most commonly implicated causes.

sinusoid (sī′nŭs-oyd) [″ + Gr. *eidos,* form, shape] **1.** Resembling a sinus. **2.** A large, permeable capillary, often lined with macrophages, found in organs such as the liver, spleen, bone marrow, and adrenal glands. Their permeability allows cells or large proteins to easily enter or leave the blood.

sinusoidal (sī-nŭs-oyd′ăl) Pert. to a sinusoid.

sinusoidal current Alternating induced electric current, the two strokes of which are equal.

sinusoidalization (sī″nŭ-soy″dăl-ĭ-zā′shŭn) [L. *sinus,* hollow, curve, + Gr. *eidos,* form, shape] The use of a sinusoidal current.

sinusotomy (sī-nŭs-ŏt′ō-mē) [″ + Gr. *tome,* incision] The incising of a sinus.

SiO_2 Silicon dioxide.

si op sit [L., *si opus sit*] If needed; used in writing prescriptions.

siphon (sī′fŭn) [Gr. *siphon,* tube] A tube bent at an angle to form two unequal lengths for transferring liquids from one container to another by atmospheric pressure. One container must be higher than the other for this to work.

siphonage (sī′fŭn-ĭj) Use of a siphon to drain a body cavity such as the stomach or bladder.

Siphonaptera (sī″fō-năp′tĕr-ă) [″ + *apteros,* wingless] An order of insects commonly called fleas. They are wingless, undergo complete metamorphosis, and have piercing and sucking mouth parts. The body is compressed laterally, and the legs are adapted for leaping. Fleas feed on the blood of birds and mammals. They transmit the causative organisms of several diseases (bubonic plague, endemic or murine typhus, and among rodents, tularemia) and also serve as intermediate hosts of certain tapeworms. SEE: *flea.*

Sipple syndrome [John H. Sipple, U.S. physician, b. 1930] Multiple endocrine neoplasia type IIA. SEE: *multiple endocrine neoplasia.*

sirenomelia (sī″rĕn-ŏm-ē′lē-ă) [Gr. *seiren,* mermaid, + *melos,* limb] A congenital anomaly in which the lower extremities are fused.

-sis [Gr.] Suffix meaning *condition, state.* Depending on the preceding vowel, it may appear in the form of *-asis, -esis, -iasis,* or *-osis.*

sister A term used by the British for *nurse,* esp. a senior or head nurse.

Sister Mary Joseph nodule A hard, periumbilical lymph node sometimes present when pelvic or gastrointestinal tumors have metastasized.

site [L. *situs,* place] Position or location.

active s. The active portion of a chemical substance, esp. a catalyst or enzyme, which binds to the material it is acting upon.

binding s. The particular location on a cell surface or chemical to which other chemicals bind or attach.

cleavage s. The location on a polypeptide molecule where peptide bonds are broken down by hydrolysis.

exit s. The location on the skin where an implanted device (e.g., a surgical drain) leaves the body.

implant s. The location in a jaw bone where a dental prosthesis will be or is seated.

port s. The location on the skin where a laparoscope or other device (e.g., subcutaneously implanted medicine reservoir) is inserted into the body.

primary s. The tissue of origin of a metastatic tumor.

receptor s. The particular component of a cell surface that has the ability to react with certain molecules such as proteins, or a virus.

splice s. The location on a strand of messenger RNA where the molecule can be cut and reannealed during the regulation of protein synthesis by cells.

site-specific Properties of cellular receptors that vary with their body location or milieu.

sitio-, sito- Combining form meaning *bread, made from grain, food.*

sitophobia (sī″tō-fō′bē-ă) [Gr. *sition, sitos,* food, + *phobos,* fear] Psychoneurotic abhorrence of food, or morbid dread of or repugnance to food, whether generally or only to specific dishes.

sitosterols (sī-tŏs′tĕr-ōls) A group of similar organic compounds that occur in plants. They contain the steroid nucleus, perhydrocyclopentanophenanthrene.

sitotherapy (sī″tō-thĕr′ă-pē) [″ + *therapeia,* treatment] The therapeutic use of diet and nutrition.

sitotoxin (sī″tō-tŏk′sĭn) [″ + *toxikon,* poison] Any poison developed in food, esp. one produced by bacteria growing in a cereal or grain product.

sitotoxism (sī″tō-tŏks′ĭzm) [″ + ″ + *-ismos,* condition] Poisoning by vegetable foods infested with molds or bacteria. SEE: *aflatoxin; food poisoning.*

situation **1.** A set of circumstances. **2.** The location of an entity in relation to other objects.

situs (sī′tŭs) [L.] A position.

s. inversus viscerum The abnormal relation and displacement of viscera to the opposite side of the body.

s. perversus Malposition of any visceral structure.

International System of Units (SI Units)

Basic Quantity	Basic Unit	Symbol
Length	meter	m
Mass	kilogram	kg
Time	second	s
Electric current	ampere	A
Thermodynamic temperature	kelvin	K
Luminous intensity	candela	cd
Amount of substance	mole	mol

SI units SEE: tables; *International System of Units; SI Units Appendix.*

size-up The assessment of the safety of a scene for rescuers and patients, before proceeding with the initial patient assessment.

Sjögren's syndrome ABBR: SS. An autoimmune disorder marked by decreased lacrimal and salivary secretions, resulting in dry eyes (keratoconjunctivitis sicca) and dry mouth (xerostomia). In 50% of patients it occurs alone; in the other 50% it is seen in conjunction with other autoimmune diseases, such as systemic lupus erythematosus, thyroiditis, scleroderma, and esp. rheumatoid arthritis. It occurs primarily in middle-aged women.

In Sjögren's syndrome, the lacrimal and salivary glands are destroyed by autoantibodies and T lymphocytes. Approx. 90% of patients have antiribonucleoprotein antibodies in the blood (anti-Ro or anti-La), which are considered diagnostic markers; approx. 75% also have rheumatoid factor, even if there is no evidence of rheumatoid arthritis. Patients with Sjögren's syndrome have a 40% to 60% increased risk of developing cancer of the lymph glands.

PROGNOSIS: The most common signs and symptoms are blurred vision, thick secretions, itching and burning of the eyes, decreased sense of taste, difficulty swallowing, and dry, cracked oral mucous membranes. Enlarged parotid glands, dry nasal membranes, bronchitis and pneumonitis, synovitis, vaginal dryness, superimposed *Candida* infections, and vasculitis also may occur. Patients usually have anemia, leukopenia, and an elevated erythrocyte sedimentation rate.

TREATMENT: Sjögren's syndrome can be controlled with symptomatic treatment. Careful oral hygiene, using fluoride toothpaste and mouthwash, and routine dental examinations are essential to minimize oral infection and tooth decay. Sugarless gum or candies, frequent sips of water, pilocarpine, and artificial saliva may help relieve the xerostomia. Artificial tears are effective for dry eyes, and glasses are recommended to block the wind when the patient is outside. Nonsteroidal anti-inflammatory drugs are used for joint discomfort.

skateboard **1.** A therapeutic device used for upper or lower extremity rehabilitation. It consists of a platform mounted on ball-bearing rollers. It assists the patient in making coordinated movements. **2.** A recreational device often used by children and adolescents, consisting of a long, narrow platform mounted on wheels. Skateboard use is often associated with high-energy trauma. Common injuries associated with the use of the device are fractures, traumatic brain injury, contusions, and lacerations.

skatol(e) (skăt'ōl) [Gr. *skatos,* dung] C_9H_9N; beta-methyl indole; a malodorous, solid, heterocyclic nitrogen compound found in feces, formed by protein decomposition in the intestines and giving them their odor.

skatoxyl (skă-tŏk'sĭl) A derivative of skatole.

Prefixes and Their Symbols Used to Designate Decimal Multiples and Submultiples in SI Units

Prefix	Symbol		Factor
tera	T	10^{12}	1 000 000 000 000
giga	G	10^{9}	1 000 000 000
mega	M	10^{6}	1 000 000
kilo	k	10^{3}	1 000
hecto	h	10^{2}	100
deka	da	10^{1}	10
deci	d	10^{-1}	0.1
centi	c	10^{-2}	0.01
milli	m	10^{-3}	0.001
micro	μ	10^{-6}	0.000 001
nano	n	10^{-9}	0.000 000 001
pico	p	10^{-12}	0.000 000 000 001
femto	f	10^{-15}	0.000 000 000 000 001
atto	a	10^{-18}	0.000 000 000 000 000 001

skein (skān) A continuous tangled thread.

skeletal (skĕl'ĕ-tăl) [Gr. *skeleton,* a dried-up body] Pert. to the skeleton.

skeletal muscle Muscle fibers that with few exceptions are attached to parts of the skeleton and involved primarily in movements of the parts of the body. SYN: *striated muscle; voluntary muscle.*

skeletal survey A radiographic study of the entire skeleton to look for evidence of occult fractures, multiple myeloma, metastatic tumor, or child abuse.

skeletal traction A pulling force applied directly to the bone through surgically applied pins and tongs.

PATIENT CARE: The patient in traction is placed on a firm mattress in the prescribed position. Ropes, weights, and pulleys are assessed daily for wear, chafe, and improper position. Care must be taken to keep the skin insertion points of pins and tongs clean and free of infection. Infection at insertion sites can lead to osteomyelitis. Assessing the area for odor and other signs of infection and cleansing the area and then applying prescribed medication and sterile dressing can help to prevent osteomyelitis; aseptic technique is used to perform these procedures. Daily skin inspection for signs of pressure or friction is performed, and appropriate nursing measures are instituted to alleviate any pressure or friction. Proper traction alignment should be maintained at all times and adjusted as necessary. An exercise regimen is established for the unaffected extremities. Patient complaints should be responded to without delay. Respiratory toilet is provided to prevent pulmonary complications. Analgesics are administered as prescribed. Adequate nutrition and fluid intake promote tissue healing and repair. Dietary and medical management helps to prevent constipation and fecal impaction. The affected extremity is assessed daily or more frequently if necessary for complications such as phlebitis and nerve or circulatory impairment, and the lower extremity, for footdrop. Social and diversional activities are promoted. The patient is instructed about the use of a trapeze, exercises, and activity limitations and establishes discharge plans and follow-up care.

skeletization (skĕl"ĕt-ĭ-zā'shŭn) Excessive emaciation.

skeleto- Combining form meaning *skeleton.*

skeletogenous (skĕl-ĕ-tŏj'ĕ-nŭs) [Gr. *skeleton,* a dried-up body, + *gennan,* to produce] Forming skeletal structures or tissues.

skeletology (skĕl"ĕ-tŏl'ō-jē) [" + *logos,* word, reason] The special division of anatomy and biomechanics concerned with the skeleton.

skeleton (skĕl'ĕt-ŏn) [Gr., a dried-up body] The bony framework of the body consisting of 206 bones: 80 axial or trunk and 126 of the limbs (appendicular). This number does not include teeth or sesamoid bones other than the patella. SEE: illus.; table.

appendicular s. The bones that make up the shoulder girdle, upper extremities, pelvis, and lower extremities.

axial s. Bones of the head and trunk.

cartilaginous s. The part of the skeleton formed by cartilage; in the adult, the cartilage of the ribs and joints. Cartilage is more flexible and resistant to resorption due to pressure than bone.

Skene's glands (skēns) [Alexander Johnston Chalmers Skene, Scot.-born U.S. gynecologist, 1837–1900] Glands lying just inside of and on the posterior area of the urethra in the female. If the margins of the urethra are drawn apart and the mucous membrane gently everted, the two small openings of Skene's tubules or glands, one on each side of the floor of the urethra, become visible. Trauma frequently causes a gaping of the urethra and ectropion of the mucous membrane. In acute gonorrhea, these glands are almost always infected. SYN: *paraurethral glands.*

skenitis (skē-nī'tĭs) [*Skene* + Gr. *itis,* inflammation] Inflammation of Skene's glands.

skew (skyū) [ME. *skewen,* to escape] Turned to one side; asymmetrical.

skew deviation A condition in which one eyeball is directed upward and outward, the other inward and downward.

skia- (skī'ă) [Gr.] Combining form meaning *shadow.*

skiascopy **1.** Retinoscopy. **2.** Fluoroscopy.

skill Proficiency in a specific task.

skimming In health care, the practice of a for-profit corporation entering the market, attracting the business of patients who can pay, and avoiding treating the indigent.

skin (skĭn) [Old Norse *skinn*] The organ that forms the outer surface of the body. It shields the body against infection, dehydration, and temperature changes; provides sensory information about the environment; manufactures vitamin D; and excretes salts and small amounts of urea.

Skin consists of two major divisions: the epidermis and the dermis. Depending on its location and local function, skin varies in terms of its thickness, strength, presence of hair, nails, or glands, pigmentation, vascularity, nerve supply, and keratinization. Skin may be classified as thin and hairy or thick and hairless (glabrous). Thin hairy skin covers most of the body. Glabrous skin covers the surface of the palms of the hands, soles of the feet, and

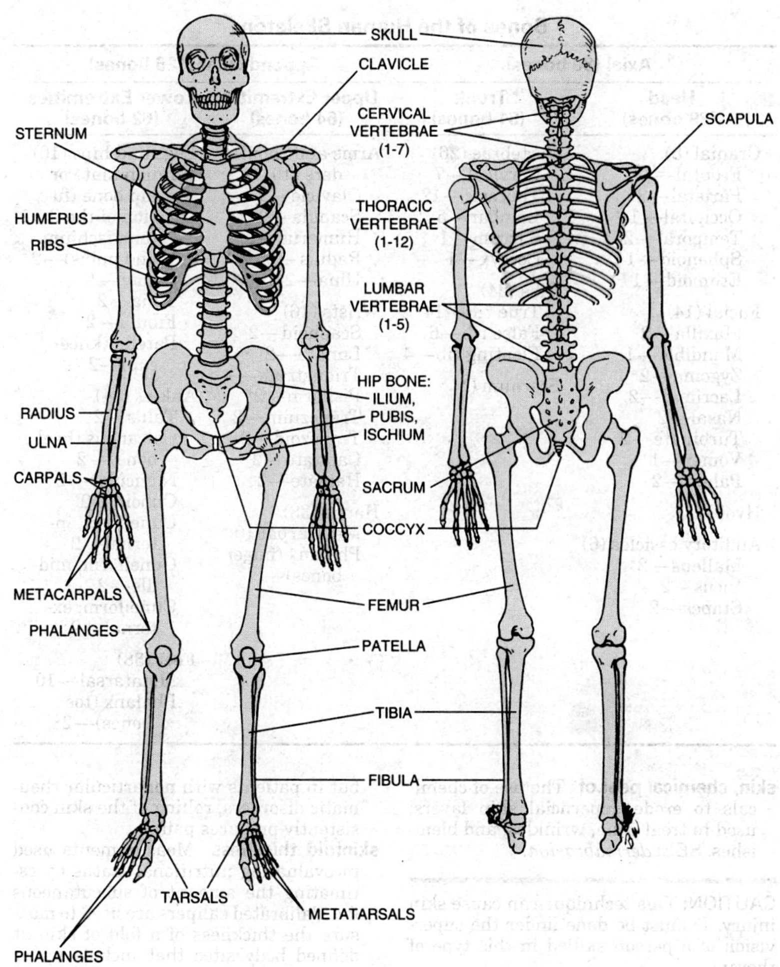

SKELETON

flexor surfaces of the digits. SEE: illus.; *hair* for illus; *burn; dermatitis; dermis; eczema; epidermis; rash.*

alligator s. Severe scaling of the skin with formation of thick plates resembling the hide of an alligator. SEE: *ichthyosis.*

artificial s. Synthetic skin, used in the treatment of burn patients.

deciduous s. Keratolysis.

elastic s. Ehlers-Danlos syndrome.

glabrous s. Skin that does not contain hair follicles, such as that over the palms and soles.

glossy s. Shiny appearance of the skin due to atrophy or injury to nerves.

hidebound s. Scleroderma.

loose s. Hypertrophy of the skin.

parchment s. Atrophy of the skin with stretching.

photoaged s. Skin changes caused by chronic sun exposure. This condition is prevented by avoiding suntanning and sunburning and has been treated with topical tretinoin and chemical peels. SYN: *photodamaged skin.* SEE: *dermatoheliosis.*

photodamaged s. Photoaged s.

piebald s. Vitiligo.

scarf s. The cuticle, epidermis; the outer layer of the skin.

sun-damaged s. Photoaged s.

true s. The corium or inner layer of the skin.

Bones of the Human Skeleton

Axial (80 bones)		Appendicular (126 bones)	
Head (29 bones)	**Trunk (51 bones)**	**Upper Extremities (64 bones)**	**Lower Extremities (62 bones)**
Cranial (8) Frontal—1 Parietal—2 Occipital—1 Temporal—2 Sphenoid—1 Ethmoid—1 Facial (14) Maxilla—2 Mandible—1 Zygoma—2 Lacrimal—2 Nasal—2 Turbinate—2 Vomer—1 Palate—2 Hyoid (1) Auditory ossicles (6) Malleus—2 Incus—2 Stapes—2	Vertebrae (26) Cervical—7 Thoracic—12 Lumbar—5 Sacrum—1 Coccyx—1 Ribs (24) True rib—14 False rib—6 Floating rib—4 Sternum (1)	Arms and shoulders (10) Clavicle—2 Scapula—2 Humerus—2 Radius—2 Ulna—2 Wrists (16) Scaphoid—2 Lunate—2 Triquetrum—2 Pisiform—2 Trapezium—2 Trapezoid—2 Capitate—2 Hamate—2 Hands (38) Metacarpal 10 Phalanx (finger bones)—	Legs and hips (10) Innominate or hip bone (fusion of the ilium, ischium, and pubis)—2 Femur—2 Tibia—2 Fibula—2 Patella (kneecap)—2 Ankles (14) Talus—2 Calcaneus (heel bone)—2 Navicular—2 Cuboid—2 Cuneiform, internal—2 Cuneiform, middle—2 Cuneiform, external—2 Feet (38) Metatarsal—10 Phalanx (toe bones)—28

skin, chemical peel of The use of chemicals to erode superficial skin layers; used to treat acne, wrinkles, and blemishes. SEE: *dermabrasion*.

CAUTION: This technique can cause skin injury. It must be done under the supervision of a person skilled in this type of therapy.

skin, tenting of A delay in the return of pinched skin to a flat position, after it has been tugged, elevated above the rest of the epidermis, and released. The return becomes progressively slower as the skin ages and subcutaneous elastic tissue decreases. It is also slowed in dehydrated persons. SEE: *dehydration*.

skin cancer A broad term that includes basal cell carcinomas, squamous cell carcinomas, and melanomas. Together, the skin cancers are the most common cancers in the U.S. They are all associated with excessive exposure to ultraviolet light (e.g., sun exposure). SEE: *basal cell c.; squamous cell c.; melanoma*.

skinfold tenderness Tenderness elicited by the examiner's rolling the skin and subcutaneous tissues over the upper border of the trapezius muscle. Normally, this produces minor discomfort, but in patients with nonarticular rheumatic disorders, rolling of the skin consistently produces pain.

skinfold thickness Measurements used in evaluating nutritional status by estimating the amount of subcutaneous fat. Calibrated calipers are used to measure the thickness of a fold of skin at defined body sites that include upper arm or triceps, subscapular region, and upper abdomen.

skin integrity, impaired A state in which an individual has altered epidermis and/or dermis. SEE: *Nursing Diagnoses Appendix*.

skin integrity, impaired, risk for A state in which an individual's skin is at risk of being adversely altered. SEE: *Nursing Diagnoses Appendix*.

skin marking The application of nontoxic, temporary paints or dyes to the skin to provide landmarks as in plastic surgery, to permit accurate alignment of wound edges at the time the skin is closed, or to align the treatment beam accurately during radiotherapy.

Skinner box (skĭn′ĕr) [Burrhus Frederic Skinner, U.S. psychologist, 1904–1990] A device used in experimental psychology in programmed learning. It is designed so that an animal that performs a desired behavior is rewarded, for example, by receiving food.

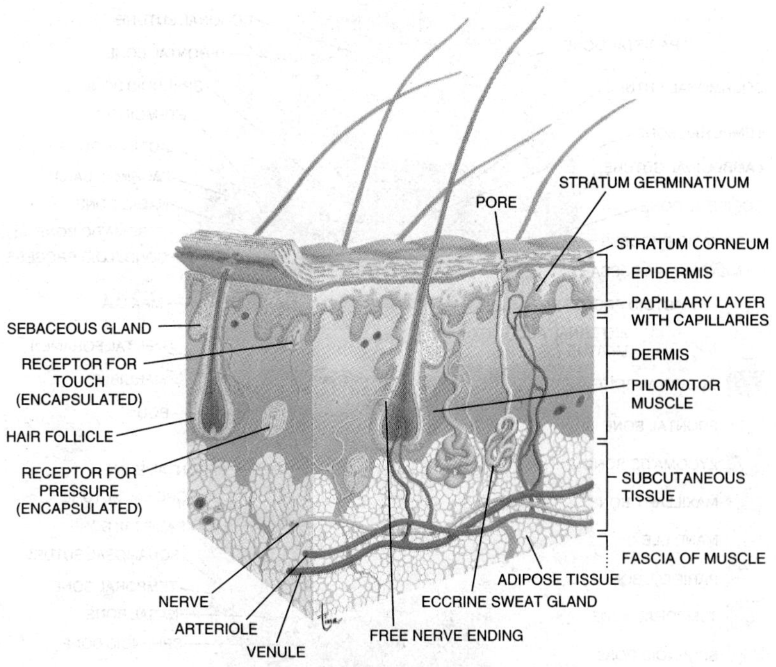

SKIN SECTION

skin popping The subcutaneous injection of illicit drugs, a practice that may result in localized abscesses, limb cellulitis, fasciitis, sepsis, or death. Injection drug users who "skin pop" may be recognized by the presence of atrophied circular lesions on the skin, usually of the forearms.

skin test Any test in which a suspected allergen is applied to the skin. A variety of tests have been developed to detect the presence of IgE antibodies to specific substances. Cutaneous tests include the *scratch test,* in which a tiny amount of dilute allergen solution is placed on 1 cm skin scratch created by a sterile needle and the *prick or puncture test,* in which a drop of allergen solution is placed on the skin and a needle prick is made in the center of the drop. These tests are performed on the back or arm and are unlikely to produce systemic anaphylaxis. For an intradermal test, approx. .01 ml of dilute solution is injected into the skin on the arm using a tuberculin syringe with a 25- to a 27-gauge needle; the patient must be monitored for an anaphylactic reaction.

The appearance of a wheal and flare 15 to 20 min after injection indicates a positive response to cutaneous or intradermal tests; the size of the wheal and intensity of erythema are graded on a scale of 1+ to 4+. Simultaneous tests assess normal skin reactivity. Histamine or another substance known to produce a wheal and flare serves as a positive control; normal saline is usually used for the negative control. Antihistamines inhibit these skin tests and must be discontinued before testing begins.

Delayed hypersensitivity tests are intradermal tests used to assess T cell–mediated responses rather than IgE-mediated responses. They are used to assess for anergy (inability to respond to common antigens) and as the basis for tuberculosis testing with PPD. The response is read 24 and 48 hr after the antigen is injected. Positive response is indicated by skin induration greater than 5 mm; a wheal and flare may occur shortly after the injection but fades within 12 hr. Corticosteroid drugs interfere with the test and should be discontinued before testing.

Patch tests are performed to identify allergens producing IgE-mediated contact dermatitis. A dilute solution of suspected allergen is applied using a patch taped to the skin. After 48 hr, the skin is inspected for a positive response marked by erythema, vesicles, or papules. Multiple tests are performed at once, usually on the back or upper arms. False-positive and false-negative reactions are common if the concentration of allergen is too high or too low.

skin tightening A loss of normal skin

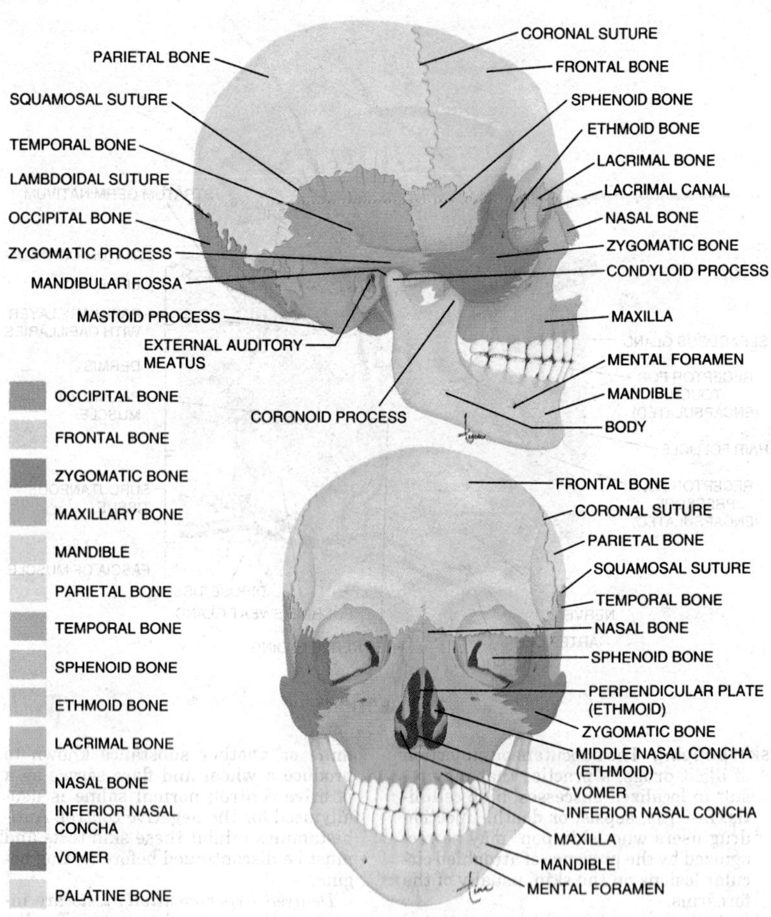

BONES OF SKULL

Right lateral and anterior views

folds and shrinkage of collagen either as a result of overly aggressive resurfacing of the skin, or as a consequence of a sclerosing disorder such as progressive systemic sclerosis.

skodaic (skō-dā′ĭk) Concerning Josef Skoda. SEE: *Skoda, Josef.*

Skoda, Josef (skō′dă) Austrian physician, 1805–1881.

S.'s crackles Bronchial crackles heard through consolidated tissue of the lungs in pneumonia.

S.'s resonance Tympanic resonance above the line of fluid in pleuritic effusion, or above consolidation in pneumonia.

skull (skŭl) [ME. *skulle,* bowl] The bony framework of the head, composed of 8 cranial bones, the 14 bones of the face, and the teeth. SYN: *calvaria; cranium.* SEE: illus.; *skeleton.*

fracture of s. Loss of the integrity of one or more bones of the cranium. A fracture is classified according to whether it is in the vault or the base but, from the point of view of treatment, a more useful classification is differentiating between a *simple fracture* (uncommon) and a *compound fracture.* When a compound fracture occurs in the vault of the skull, the bone is depressed and driven inward, possibly damaging the brain. Treatment is operative. SEE: *fracture.*

skullcap The upper round portion of the skull covering the brain. Also called *calvaria.*

slant A tube of solid culture medium that is slanted to increase the surface area of the medium; used in culturing bacteria. SYN: *slope.*

slave A device that allows the body movements to be transferred to a machine either directly or by remote control (e.g.,

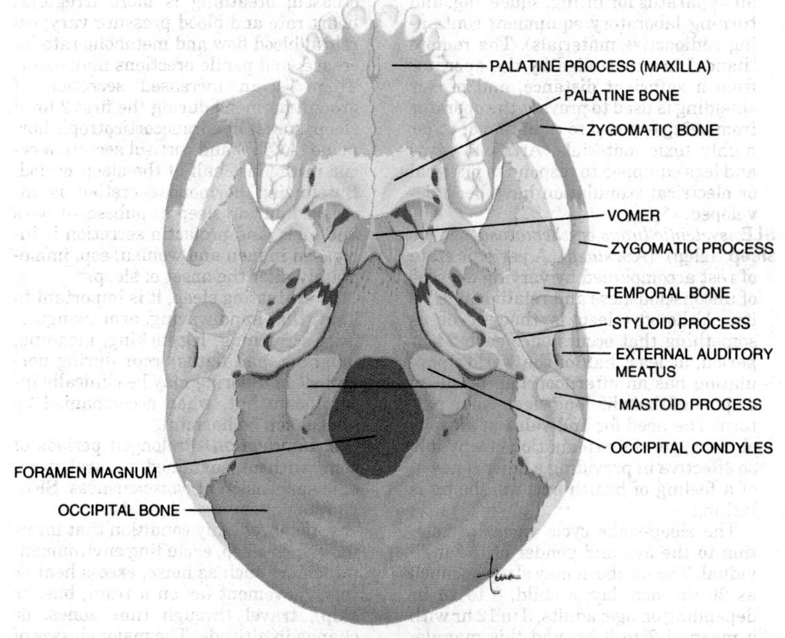

SKULL

Inferior view with mandible removed

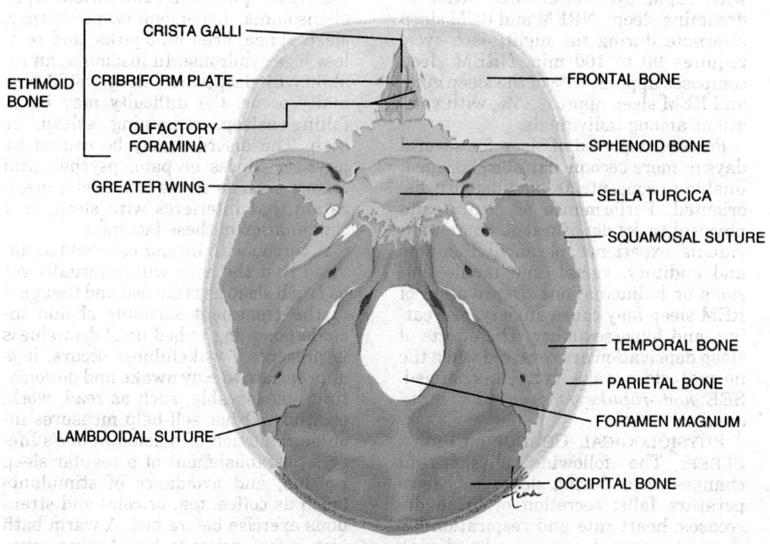

SKULL

Superior view with top of cranium removed

an apparatus for lifting, squeezing, and turning laboratory equipment containing radioactive materials). The remote "hands" are controlled by the operator from a sufficient distance, and proper shielding is used to prevent the operator from being exposed to radiation or other highly toxic materials. Artificial arms and legs equipped to respond to physical or electrical stimulation have been developed.

SLE *systemic lupus erythematosus.*

sleep (slēp) [AS. *slaep*] A periodic state of rest accompanied by varying degrees of unconsciousness and relative inactivity. Although sleep is thought of as something that occurs once each 24-hr period, at least half of the world's population has an afternoon nap or siesta as part of their lifelong sleep-wake pattern. The need for and value of sleep is obvious, yet the explanation of why it is so effective in providing a daily renewal of a feeling of health and well-being is lacking.

The sleep-wake cycle varies in relation to the age and gender of the individual. The newborn may sleep as much as 20 hr each day; a child, 8 to 14 hr depending on age; adults, 3 to 12 hr with a mean of 7 to 8 hr, and this may decrease to 6.5 hr in the elderly. Women past age 35 tend to sleep more than men. There is great individual variation in the amount and depth of sleep.

Sleep has been found to have two states: one with no rapid eye movements (NREM or synchronized sleep, which involves four stages) and one with rapid eye movements (REM or dreaming sleep). NREM and REM sleep alternate during the night; each cycle requires 90 to 100 min. NREM sleep composes approx. 75% of the sleep cycle and REM sleep approx. 25%, with variations among individuals.

Persons deprived of sleep for several days or more become irritable, fatigued, unable to concentrate, and usually disoriented. Performance of mental and physical tasks deteriorates. Some individuals experience paranoid thoughts and auditory, visual, and tactile illusions or hallucinations. Deprivation of REM sleep may cause anxiety, overeating, and hypersexuality. The effects of sleep deprivation are reversed when the normal sleep-wake cycle is resumed. SEE: *non–rapid eye movement s.; rapid eye movement s.*

PHYSIOLOGICAL CHANGES DURING SLEEP: The following physiological changes occur during sleep: body temperature falls; secretion of urine decreases; heart rate and respiration become slower and more regular during NREM sleep, then more rapid and less regular during REM sleep. During REM sleep, blood flow to the brain is increased; breathing is more irregular; heart rate and blood pressure vary; cerebral blood flow and metabolic rate increase; and penile erections may occur. There is an increased secretion of growth hormone during the first 2 hr of sleep; surges of adrenocorticotropic hormone (ACTH) and cortisol secretion occur in the last half of the sleep period. Luteinizing hormone secretion is increased during sleep in pubescent boys and girls, and prolactin secretion is increased in men and women, esp. immediately after the onset of sleep.

In evaluating sleep, it is important to know that hand waving, arm swinging, nose scratching, leg kicking, moaning, laughing, and flatus occur during normal sleep. Snoring may be clinically insignificant but, when accompanied by apnea, can be harmful.

s. deprivation Prolonged periods of time without sustained natural, periodic suspension of consciousness. SEE: *Nursing Diagnoses Appendix.*

s. disorder Any condition that interferes with sleep, excluding environmental factors such as noise, excess heat or cold, movement (as on a train, bus, or ship), travel through time zones, or change in altitude. The major classes of sleep disorders are dyssomnias, parasomnias, and sleep pattern disruption associated with medical illness. Other factors that may interfere with sleep include poor sleep hygiene, effects of drugs or alcohol, and dietary changes. SEE: *s. hygiene.*

Dyssomnias, sleep disturbances or excessive sleepiness, include various types of insomnia, hypersomnia, narcolepsy, sleep apnea, brief limb jerks, and restless legs syndrome. In insomnia, an inability to sleep when sleep would normally occur, the difficulty may be in falling asleep, remaining asleep, or both. The disorder may be caused by physical illness or pain, psychological factors such as stress or anxiety, medication that interferes with sleep, or a combination of these factors.

A person with insomnia should be advised that the body will eventually get as much sleep as is needed and that part of the treatment schedule should include not going to bed until drowsiness is present; if wakefulness occurs, it is appropriate to stay awake and do something pleasurable, such as read, work, or study. Other self-help measures include reduction of tension in one's lifestyle, establishment of a regular sleep routine, and avoidance of stimulants (such as coffee, tea, or cola) and strenuous exercise before bed. A warm bath just before going to bed relaxes tense muscles. Afternoon naps should be avoided. One should sleep in a quiet, clean, cool, dark environment. A snack or glass of warm milk prior to going to bed will do no harm, but evidence that this practice helps to induce sleep is lacking.

CAUTION: Some drugs used to treat insomnia are less rapidly biotransformed in elderly patients than in the young. These drugs have been associated with delirium, increased risk of falls and hip fractures, and excessive sedation in elderly patients.

Parasomnias include night (sleep) terrors, nightmares, sleepwalking, and disorders related to mental illness.

Factors associated with medical illness may include neurological, cerebrovascular, or endocrine disorders, infection, musculoskeletal disorders, or pulmonary disease.

s. drunkenness A condition in which one requires a long period of time to become fully alert upon awakening from deep sleep. During the transition period, the affected person may become ataxic, disoriented, or aggressive. Persons whose usual awakening sequence includes sleep drunkenness should not attempt to make decisions until they are fully alert and awake.

s. hygiene The influence of behavioral patterns or sleeping environment on the quality and quantity of sleep. Persons with insomnia not caused by a known disease may find that the following may assist in obtaining a good night's sleep: establishing a routine time to go to bed; avoiding trying to sleep; using practices that assist in going to sleep such as reading, watching television, or listening to music; sleeping in a dark room, free of noise; and avoiding caffeine and excessive food or drink before bedtime.

hypnotic s. **1.** Sleep induced by hypnotic suggestion. **2.** Sleep induced by the use of medicines classified as hypnotics.

CAUTION: Many hypnotic drugs are habit-forming.

non–rapid eye movement s. ABBR: NREM sleep. Sleep during which non–rapid eye movements occur. In NREM stage 1, the transition from wakefulness to sleep occurs. Eye movements are slow, and an electroencephalogram (EEG) shows low brain wave activity. In stage 2, EEG activity is increased, with the appearance of spikes called K complexes. Eye movement ceases in stage 3; wave frequency is reduced and amplitude increased. In stage 4, the EEG is dominated by large spikes, or delta activity. Stages 3 and 4 are considered deep sleep. SEE: *rapid eye movement s.; sleep.*

pathological s. A term used in encephalitis lethargica, in which sleep is excessive.

rapid eye movement s. ABBR: REM sleep. Sleep during which rapid eye movements occur. In REM sleep, which follows stage 4 of non–rapid eye movement (NREM) sleep, electroencephalographic activity is similar to that of NREM stage 1, and muscle paralysis occurs. SEE: *non–rapid eye movement s.; sleep.*

sleep architecture The organization of brain wave activity characteristic of each of the stages of sleep.

sleep pattern disturbance Time limited disruption of sleep (natural, periodic suspension of consciousness) amount and quality. SEE: *Nursing Diagnoses Appendix.*

sleep-phase syndrome disorder A condition in which the person sleeps well and for a normal amount of time but not at the usual bedtime hours. Those with the delayed type of syndrome may function best if they go to sleep about the time most people are awakening. Those with the advanced type of syndrome do best when they go to sleep in late afternoon or early evening and arise about midnight. When allowed to sleep at these hours, persons with this disease function normally.

sleep-wake cycle The amount of time spent asleep and awake and the cycle of that schedule from day to day.

sleepwalking Autonomic actions performed during sleep. This condition occurs mostly in children, each episode lasting less than 10 min. The eyes are open and the facial expression is blank. The patient appears to awaken, sits on the edge of the bed, and may walk or talk. Some patients may even leave the bedroom. Activity may cause trauma to the patient and others. The principal aim is to prevent injury by removing objects that could be dangerous, locking doors and windows, and preventing the person from falling down stairs. Night terrors may accompany sleepwalking. There is little or no recollection of the event the next day. Children usually outgrow this condition. SYN: *somnambulism.*

slide **1.** A thin glass plate on which an object is placed for microscopic examination. **2.** A photograph prepared so that it may be used in a film slide projector. **3.** To move along a smooth surface in continuous contact, as the movement in dentistry of the mandibular teeth toward a centric position with the teeth in contact before closing completely in occlusion.

slimy (slī′mē) [AS. *slim,* smooth] Resembling slime or a viscid substance; regarding a growth, the ability to adhere to a needle so it can be drawn out as a long thread.

sling (slĭng) [AS. *slingan*, to wind] A support for an injured upper extremity. SEE: *triangular bandage* for illus.; *bandage*.

CAUTION: Prolonged skin-to-skin contact should be avoided while a sling is in use.

clove-hitch s. A sling made by placing a clove hitch in the center of a roller bandage, fitting it to the hand, and carrying the ends over the shoulder. The sling is tied beside the neck with a square knot, making longer ends. These may be carried over and behind the shoulders, brought under each axilla, and tied over the chest.

counterbalanced s. A rehabilitation device to assist upper extremity motion; it suspends the arm by way of an overhead frame and a pulley and weight system. SYN: *suspension s.*

cravat s. A sling made by placing the center of the cravat under the wrist or forearm with the ends tied around the neck.

folded cravat s. A lower-arm sling made by placing a broad fold of cloth in position on the chest with one end over the affected shoulder and the other hanging down in front of the chest. The arm is flexed as desired across the sling. The lower end is brought up over the uninjured shoulder and secured with a knot located where it will not press on the affected shoulder.

open s. A sling made by placing the point of a triangular cloth at the tip of the elbow. The ends are brought around at the back of the neck and tied. The point should be brought forward and pinned or tied in a single knot, forming a cup to prevent the elbow from slipping out.

reversed triangular s. A sling made as follows: A triangular bandage is applied with one end over the injured shoulder, point toward the sound side, the base vertical under the injured elbow. The arm is flexed acutely over the triangle. The lower end is brought upward over the front of the arm and over the sound shoulder. The ends are pulled taut and tied over the sound shoulder. The point is pulled taut over the forearm and fixed to the anterior and posterior layers between the forearm and arm. This sling holds the elbow more acutely flexed—the weight is supported by the elbow.

simple figure-of-eight roller arm s. A sling made as follows: The arm is flexed on the chest in the desired position, then a bandage is fixed with a single turn toward the uninjured side around the arm and chest, crossing the elbow just above the external epicondyle of the humerus. A second turn is made, overlapping two thirds of the first, and the bandage is brought forward under the tip of the elbow, then upward along the flexed forearm to the root of the neck of the sound side. Then it is brought downward over the scapula, crossing the chest and arm horizontally, overlapping, turning above, and continued as in a progressive figure-of-eight.

St. John's s. A sling made by applying a triangular bandage with the point downward under the elbow, the upper end over the sound shoulder. The arm is flexed acutely on the chest. The lower end is brought under the affected arm and around the back to knot with the upper end on the sound shoulder. The point is brought up over the elbow and fastened to the base. Support is wholly for the injured shoulder.

suspension s. Counterbalanced s.

swathe arm s. A sling for support of the arm that is made as follows: The center of a folded cloth band is placed under the acutely flexed elbow. One end of the sling is then carried to the front and upward across the forearm and over the affected shoulder. Then it is brought obliquely across the back to the sound axilla. Next, the other end of the sling is brought around the front of the arm and across the body to the sound axilla, where it is pinned to the first end of the sling and then continued around the back to the part of the sling surrounding the affected elbow, where it is pinned again.

triangular s. A sling for the arm that is made with suspension from the uninjured side. The triangle is placed on the chest with one end over the sound shoulder, the point under the affected extremity, and the base folded. The injured arm is flexed outside of the triangle. The lower end is carried upward under the axilla of the injured side, back of the shoulder, and tied with the upper end behind the back. The point of the triangle is brought anteriorly and medially around the back of the elbow, and fastened to the body of the bandage. This bandage changes the point of carrying and also relieves the clavicle on the injured side of the load. SEE: *triangular bandage* for illus.

slippery elm An herbal remedy used by alternative medicine practitioners as a demulcent or as a poultice.

slit [ME. *slitte*] A narrow opening.

vestibular s. The opening between the left and right ventricular folds of the larynx.

slope **1.** An inclined plane or surface. **2.** A tube of solid culture medium that is slanted to increase the surface area of the medium; used in culturing bacteria. SYN: *slant.*

lower ridge s. The slope of the crest of the mandibular residual ridge from the third molar forward as viewed in profile.

slough (slŭf) [ME. *slughe,* a skin] **1.** Dead matter or necrosed tissue separated from living tissue or an ulceration. **2.** To separate in the form of dead or necrosed parts from living tissue. **3.** To cast off, as dead tissue. SEE: *escharotic.*

sloughing (slŭf'ĭng) The formation of a slough; separation of dead from living tissue.

slow (slō) [AS. *slaw,* dull] **1.** Mentally dull. **2.** Exhibiting retarded speed, as the pulse. **3.** Said of a morbid condition or of a fever when it is not acute.

slow-acting antirheumatic drug ABBR: SAARD. A drug used to treat rheumatoid arthritis that acts over the course of several months to improve inflammatory diseases. Some SAARDs are hydroxychloroquine, intramuscular gold preparations, D-penicillamine, methotrexate, and azathioprine.

slow-reacting substance of anaphylaxis ABBR: SRS-A. Old name given to leukotrienes C4, D4, and E4, arachidonic acid metabolites that play a significant role in the pathophysiology of asthma, causing prolonged bronchoconstriction, increased vascular permeability, increased bronchial mucous secretion, and vasoconstriction. SYN: *leukotriene.* SEE: *arachidonic acid; asthma.*

slows (slōz) A condition resulting from ingestion of plants such as snakeroot *(Eupatorium urticaefolium)* or jimmyweed *(Haplopappus heterophyllus).* It is common in domestic animals and may occur in humans as a result of ingesting the plants or, more commonly, from drinking milk or eating the meat of poisoned animals. Symptoms are weakness, anorexia, nausea and vomiting, prostration, and possibly death. SYN: *trembles.*

sludge (slŭjh) Under the Resource Conservation and Recovery Act of 1976, sludge is defined as any solid, semisolid, or liquid waste generated from a municipal, commercial, or industrial wastewater treatment plant, or air pollution control facility, or any such waste having similar characteristics or effects.

sludged blood A term formerly used to indicate blood that is abnormally viscous.

slurry (slŭr'ē) [ME. *slory*] A thin, watery mixture.

Sm Symbol for the element samarium.

SMA-12 *Sequential multiple analyzer.* A device that analyzes and records 12 blood chemistry tests on a single blood sample. The SMA-12 and other automated methods are subject to artifactual or methodological errors. A similar device, SMA-20, measures 20 different quantities.

small for gestational age ABBR: SGA. Term describing an infant whose birth weight is at or below the 10th percentile, as correlated with the number of weeks in utero on the intrauterine growth chart.

smallpox (smawl'pŏks) [AS. *smael,* tiny, + *poc,* pustule] An acute, contagious, systemic viral disease characterized by a prodromal stage during which the constitutional symptoms usually are severe, followed by an eruption that passes through the successive stages of macules, papules, vesicles, pustules, and crusts. SYN: *variola.*

This disease is considered to have been completely eradicated worldwide. Cultures of the virus are kept in only one or two research laboratories.

smear (smēr) [AS. *smerian,* to anoint] **1.** In bacteriology, material spread on a surface, as a microscopic slide or a culture medium. **2.** Material obtained from infected matter spread over solid culture media.

blood s. A drop of (anticoagulated) whole blood spread thinly on a glass microscope slide so that blood cell types can be examined, counted, and characterized. SYN: *peripheral blood s.*

Procedure:

1. The slide must be grease-free. It is cleaned with alcohol, rinsed in warm water, and wiped clean with a lint-free towel or lens paper.

2. A small drop of blood is placed on the slide; the end of another slide (spreader slide) is placed against the first slide at a 45° angle and pulled back against the drop of blood so that the drop spreads between the point of contact of the two slides. Then the spreader slide is pushed forward against the first slide; the blood will form an even, thin smear.

3. The slide is dried by waving it in the air; the slide should not be heated.

4. The blood smear is covered with Wright's stain and allowed to stand 2 min.

5. An equal amount of distilled water or buffer solution is added and mixed uniformly. It is allowed to stand 5 min.

6. The stain is gently washed off and the slide is allowed to dry.

7. If a permanent slide is desired, balsam or methacrylate and a glass cover slip are applied.

Stain: A common method is to cover the blood smear with Wright's stain. Allow to stand 2 min. Add an equal amount of distilled water or buffer solution, mixing uniformly. Let stand 5 min. Gently wash off stain. Allow to dry. If permanent slide is desired, apply balsam or methacrylate and apply a glass cover slip.

buccal s. A sample of cells taken from the mucosa lining the cheek for chromosomal studies.

Pap s. Papanicolaou test.

peripheral blood s. SYN: *blood s.*

smegma (smĕg′mă) [Gr. *smegma,* soap] Secretion of sebaceous glands, specifically, the thick, cheesy, odoriferous secretion found under the labia minora about the clitoris or under the male prepuce. **smegmatic** (-măt′ĭk), *adj.*

smegmolith (smĕg′mō-lĭth) [Gr. *smegma,* soap, + *lithos,* a stone] A calcified mass in the smegma.

smell (smĕl) [ME. *smellen,* to reek] **1.** To perceive by stimulation of the olfactory nerves. The sense of smell is a chemical sense dependent on sensory cells on the surface of the upper part of the nasal septum and the superior nasal concha. These sensory cells live for an average of 30 days and are affected by a variety of factors including age, nutritional and hormonal states, drugs, and therapeutic radiation. **2.** The property of something affecting the olfactory organs. In clinical medicine, the smell arising from the patient's body, feces, breath, urine, vagina, or clothing may provide information concerning diagnosis. The smell on a patient's clothing, for example, may be due to a toxic chemical that spilled on the clothes. A patient may attempt to alter or mask the smell of alcohol on the breath by using medicated or flavored lozenges, mouthwashes, sprays, or mints. Even though our sense of smell is relatively weak compared with that of some animals, humans have the capacity to distinguish among as many as 10,000 different odors. The inhaled substance must be volatile (i.e., capable of diffusing in air) for us to perceive it, and the volatile chemical must also be soluble in water. SEE: *odor*.

Abnormalities in the sense of smell include: *Anosmia:* A loss of the sense of smell. It may be a local and temporary condition resulting from acute and chronic rhinitis, mouth breathing, nasal polyps, dryness of the nasal mucous membrane, pollens, or very offensive odors. It may also result from disease or injury of the olfactory tract, bone disease near the olfactory nerve, disease of the nasal accessory sinuses, meningitis, or tumors or syphilis affecting the olfactory nerve. It may rarely represent a conversion disorder. Disease of one cranial hemisphere or of one nasal chamber may also account for anosmia. SYN: *anodmia; anosphrasia*.

Hyperosmia: An increased sensitivity to odors.

Kakosmia: The perception of bad odors where none exist; it may be due to head injuries or occur in hallucinations or certain psychoses. SYN: *cacosmia*.

Parosmia: A perverted sense of smell. Odors that are considered agreeable by others are perceived as being offensive, and disagreeable odors are found pleasant. SYN: *parosphresia*.

smile A facial expression that may represent pleasure, amusement, derision, or scorn. The corners of the mouth are turned up in expressions of pleasure or amusement, and the eyes usually appear to be warm and friendly.

Smith's fracture [Robert W. Smith, Irish physician, 1807–1873] A fracture of the lower end of the radius, with anterior displacement of the lower fragment.

Smith-Magenis syndrome [Ann C. M. Smith, contemporary U.S. genetics counselor; Ellen Magenis, contemporary U.S. physician] A rare form of genetic mental retardation characterized by chronic ear infections, erratic sleep patterns, head banging, picking at skin, and pulling off fingernails and toenails. There is abnormality of chromosome 17. Treatment is symptomatic.

Smith-Petersen nail [Marius N. Smith-Petersen, U.S. orthopedic surgeon, 1886–1953] A special nail that on cross-section has three flanges, used for stabilizing fractures of the neck of the femur.

Smith-Strang disease [Allan J. Smith, contemporary Brit. physician; Leonard B. Strang, Brit. physician, b. 1925] Methionine malabsorption syndrome, an autosomal recessive disease, which is associated with mental retardation, diarrhea, convulsions, phenylketonuria, and a characteristic odor of the urine. The odor is due to the absorption from the intestinal tract of fermentation products of methionine. SYN: *oasthouse urine disease*.

smog [blend of *smoke* and *fog*] Dense fog combined with smoke and other forms of air pollution.

smoke (smōk) Any suspension in the air of particles produced by combustion.

smoke inhalation injury Damage to the respiratory tract (i.e., upper airway inflammation and swelling), as a result of inhaling hot gases that may contain toxic substances. Persons exposed to gases produced by burning materials are at risk of developing acute injury to their lungs; and, depending on the composition of the smoke and the duration of the exposure, the combination of heat and gases may be lethal. Firefighters are esp. at risk from this kind of exposure. Construction and decorating materials produce a variety of volatile and irritating substances when burned. Repeated exposure to some of these gases may lead to chronic irritation of the respiratory tract. Firefighters should be aware that the appearance of smoke produced by a fire may not be a true indicator of the amount of toxic substances, including carbon monoxide, in the smoke. SEE: *carbon monoxide*.

SYMPTOMS: Patients who have suffered smoke inhalation injury may complain of dyspnea, cough, and black sputum. Stridor may be present if the upper airway is narrowed as a result of inflammation. Confusion may occur if carbon monoxide poisoning is also present.

smoker's cancer Cancer of the lip, throat, or lung caused by irritation from excessive smoking. SEE: *tobacco*.

smoking, passive The exposure of persons who do not smoke tobacco products to the toxic gases released by the burning of these products in their homes, workplaces, or recreational environments. Exposure to environmental tobacco smoke has been linked to allergies, asthma, cardiovascular diseases, lung diseases, and stroke, among other diseases and conditions. SEE: *tobacco*.

SMON *subacute myelo-optic neuropathy*.

smudging (smŭj′ĭng) A speech defect in which difficult consonants are omitted.

Sn [L. *stannun*] Symbol for the element tin.

snail [ME.] A small mollusk having a spiral shell and belonging to the class Gastropoda. Snails are important as intermediate hosts of many species of parasitic flukes.

s. fever Schistosomiasis.

snake [ME.] A reptile possessing scales and lacking limbs, external ears, and functional eyelids. In poisonous snakes, venom is produced in a poison gland, which is connected by a tube or groove to a poison fang, one of two sharp elongated teeth present in the upper jaw. In the U.S., the coral snake, copperhead, water moccasin (cottonmouth), and rattlesnake, of which there are 15 species, are poisonous. All except the coral snake belong to a group known as *pit vipers* (so-called because of the presence of a distinct pit between the eye and nostril). SEE: illus.

s. bite A puncture wound made by the fangs of a snake. All snakes should be considered poisonous, although only a few secrete enough venom to inoculate poison deeply into the tissues.

FIRST AID: The patient should be transported immediately to a medical facility equipped and staffed to handle snake bites. In the hospital, an intravenous infusion of Ringer's lactate or normal saline should be started. If the patient has actually received venom from the snake bite (only about 50% of patients have), antivenin should be administered, after first testing for sensitivity to horse serum. This should be done only if the equipment for treating anaphylaxis is available. Children require a larger dose of antivenin than adults.

A polyvalent antivenin serum for bites by pit vipers is prepared by Wyeth Lab. Inc., Radnor, PA. Antivenin for coral snake bite is also available from Wyeth. The use of antibodies to treat pit viper bites is being used experimentally.

If in doubt about the type of snake that bit the patient, one should call the nearest poison control center or the nearest large zoo. Snake antivenin information is also available from either the Arizona Poison Control Center at (520) 626-6016 or the Oklahoma Poison Control Center at (405) 271-5854.

CAUTION: Alcoholic stimulants must not be taken, and nothing should be done to increase circulation. One should not cauterize with strong acids or depend on home remedies. Tetanus prophylaxis is essential.

---

snakeroot (snāk′rūt) A toxic plant (*Eupatorium rugosum Houtt*) once thought to be useful as a remedy for snakebites. Animals that eat snakeroot get trembling disease (or the trembles), and humans who consume fresh raw milk obtained from intoxicated cows or goats develop milk sickness.

snap A sharp cracking sound.

closing s. The intense first heart sound heard in mitral stenosis.

opening s. A sharp sound of increased pitch heard in early systole. It is associated with the opening of the abnormal valve in mitral stenosis.

snapping hip Slipping of the hip joint with a snap owing to displacement over the great trochanter of a tendinous band.

snare (snār) [AS. *sneare*, noose] A device for excision of polyps or tumors by tightening wire loops around them. A snare may be connected to an electrosurgical unit, which may facilitate cutting and coagulation.

sneeze (snēz) [AS. *fneosan*, to pant] **1.** To expel air forcibly through the nose and mouth by spasmodic contraction of muscles of expiration caused by an irritation of nasal mucosa. The sneeze reflex may be produced by a great number of stimuli. Placing a foot on a cold surface will provoke a sneeze in some people, whereas looking at a bright light or sunlight will cause it in others. Firm pressure applied to the middle of the upper lip and just under the nose will sometimes prevent a sneeze that is about to occur. SEE: *photic sneezing; ptarmus*. **2.** The act of sneezing. SEE: *sternutation; sternutatory*.

Snellen, Herman (snĕl′ĕn) Dutch ophthalmologist, 1834–1908.

S.'s chart A chart imprinted with lines of black letters graduating in size from smallest on the bottom to largest on top; used for testing visual acuity.

S.'s reflex Congestion of the ear on the same side upon stimulation of the

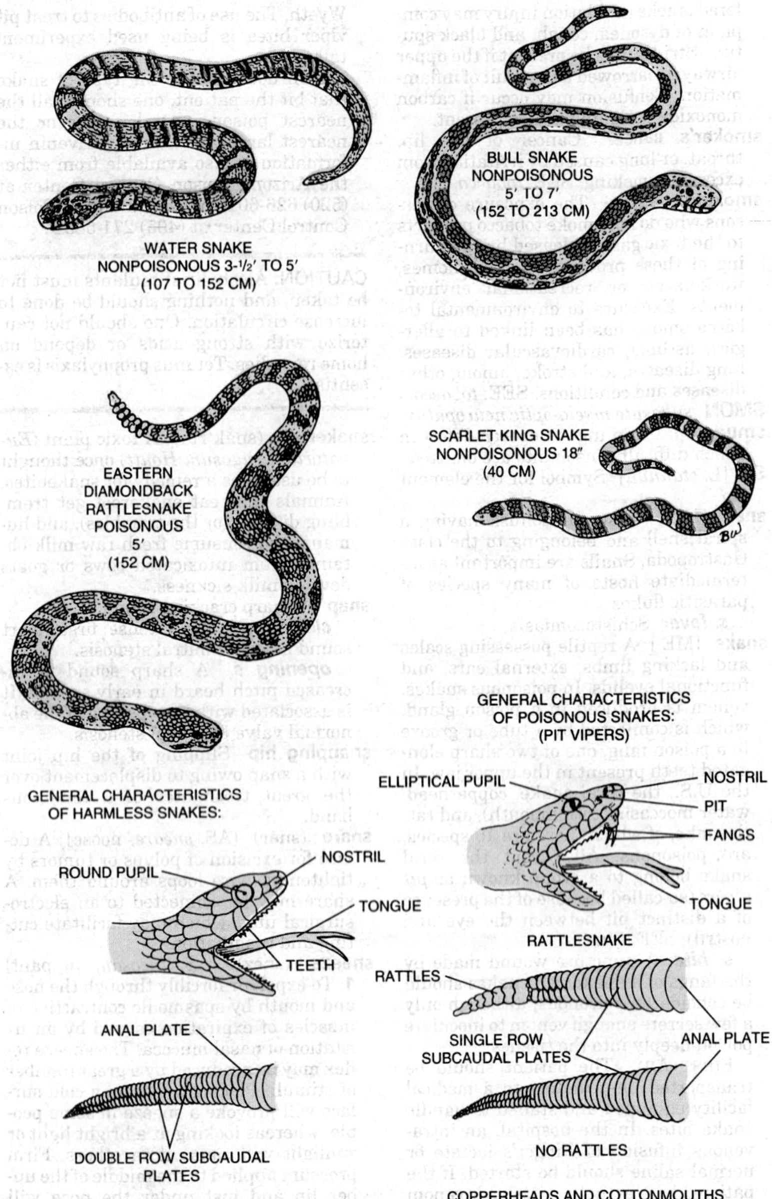

SNAKES

distal end of the divided auriculotemporal nerve. SYN: *auriculocervical nerve reflex*.

S.'s test A test for visual acuity in which the patient reads a Snellen's chart at a certain distance with one eye, then with the other eye, and then with both eyes.

sniff test A test used to detect bacterial vaginosis. The discharge from the vaginal area is swabbed, placed on a slide, and 10% KOH (potassium hydroxide) is added. The presence of a fishy odor is indicative of bacterial vaginosis.

snore (snor) [AS. *snora*] The noise produced while breathing through the mouth during sleep, caused by air passing through a narrowed upper airway. Most people snore to some extent. Snoring is of no clinical importance to the snorer unless it is prolonged, chronic, and related to other symptoms such as sleep apnea or excessive daytime sleepiness. It may be important to the snorer's partner if the snoring is so loud as to disrupt the sleep of those sharing the sleeping space. In some cases, the snoring is of such clinical or social importance that plastic or laser surgery, to remove redundant tissue in the pharynx, is indicated SYN: *stertor*. SEE: *sleep apnea*.

snow, carbon dioxide Carbon dioxide solid therapy.

SNS *Society of Neurological Surgeons.*

snuff **1.** A medicinal powder inhaled through the nose. **2.** A powdered form of tobacco inhaled through the nose or placed in the oral cavity. SYN: *smokeless tobacco*.

snuffles (snŭf'ls) [D. *snuffelen,* to snuff] Obstructed nasal breathing with discharge from the nasal mucosa, esp. in infants, chiefly in congenital syphilis.

SOAP Acronym for an organized structure for keeping progress notes in the chart. Each entry contains the date, number, and title of the patient's particular problem, followed by the SOAP headings: Subjective findings; Objective findings; Assessment, the documented analysis and conclusions concerning the findings; and Plan for further diagnostic or therapeutic action. If the patient has multiple problems, a SOAP entry on the chart is made for each problem.

soap (sōp) [AS. *sape*] A cleansing chemical compound formed by an alkali acting on a fatty acid, such as sodium stearate, $NaC_{18}H_{35}O_2$. Castile soap is made by saponifying olive oil with sodium hydroxide and contains mainly sodium oleate, $NaC_{18}H_{33}O_2$. SEE: *detergent; saponification*.

antibacterial s. A cleanser chemically altered to increase its ability to kill microorganisms.

green s. A potassium soap made by the saponification of suitable vegetable oils without the removal of glycerin.

s. liniment A solution of soap and camphor in alcohol and water; used as a stimulant and rubefacient.

soft medicinal s. A liquid soap made by saponification of vegetable oils excluding coconut oil and palm kernel oil and without removal of glycerin; used in the treatment of skin diseases. SYN: *green s.*

SOB *short of breath.*

sob [ME. *sobben,* to catch breath] **1.** To weep with convulsive movements of the chest. **2.** A cry or wail resulting from a sudden convulsive inspiration accompanied by spasmodic closure of the glottis. SEE: *sigh*.

social class **1.** Social standing or position. SYN: *socioeconomic status*. **2.** A group of people with shared culture, privilege, or position.

social interaction, impaired The state in which an individual participates in an insufficient or excessive quantity or ineffective quality of social exchange. SEE: *Nursing Diagnoses Appendix*.

social isolation Aloneness experienced by the individual and perceived as imposed by others and as a negative or threatened state. SEE: *Nursing Diagnoses Appendix*.

socialization (sō″shă-lĭ-zā'shŭn) The process of adapting an individual to the social customs of society; in the process he or she becomes an integrated member of the society.

Society for Assisted Reproductive Technology ABBR: SART. An affiliate of the American Society for Reproductive Medicine, consisting of clinics and programs that provide assisted reproductive technology. SART reports annual fertility clinic data to the Centers for Disease Control and Prevention.

socioacusis (sō″sē-ō-ă-kū'sĭs) [L. *socius,* companion, + Gr. *akoustikos,* hearing] The long-range ill effects of environmental noise on auditory acuity.

sociobiology (sō″sē-ō-bī-ŏl'ō-jē) [″ + Gr. *bios,* life, + *logos,* word, reason] Analysis of social behavior in terms of modern evolutionary theory. It is the study of the social life of animals or humans on the assumption that populations evolve and adapt to their environments in different ways, through individual learning, cultural tradition, or genetic inheritance.

socioeconomic status ABBR: SES. The relative position attained by an individual in a cultural and financial hierarchy. Differences in socioeconomic status are responsible for important disparities in the nutrition, housing, safety, and health of large groups of people. In general, the lower one's SES, the greater one's risk of malnutrition, heart disease, infectious diseases, and early mortality from all causes. Income, education, occupation, vocation, and wealth all contribute to SES.

sociogram A diagram used in group analysis and group therapy that shows patterns of relationships between participants or variables.

sociology (sō-sē-ŏl'ō-jē) [″ + *logos,* word, reason] The study of human social behavior and the origins, institutions, and functions of human groups and societies.

sociomedical Pert. to sociology and medicine, esp. the interrelationships between the two.

sociometry (sō″sē-ŏm'ĕ-trē) [″ + Gr. *metron,* measure] The science concerned with measuring social behavior.

sociopath (sō′sē-ō-păth) [″ + Gr. *pathos,* disease, suffering] An individual with antisocial personality disorder. SEE: *personality disorder, antisocial.*

sociopathy (sō″sē-ŏp′ă-thē) [″ + Gr. *pathos,* disease, suffering] The condition of being antisocial.

socket (sŏk′ĕt) [ME. *soket,* a spearhead] **1.** A hollow in a joint or part for another corresponding organ, as a bone socket or an eye socket. SEE: *acetabulum.* **2.** The proximal portion of a prosthesis, into which the stump of an amputated extremity is fitted.

alveolar s. The bony space occupied by the tooth and periodontal ligament.

dry s. Localized alveolar osteitis.

tooth s. A dental alveolus of the maxilla or mandible; a cavity that contains the root of a tooth.

soda (sō′dă) [Med. L., *barilla,* from which soda is made] **1.** A term loosely applied to various salts of sodium, esp. to caustic soda (sodium hydroxide) and baking soda (sodium bicarbonate). SEE: *sodium.* **2.** Short for soda water, which is water charged with carbon dioxide.

baking s. Sodium bicarbonate.

caustic s. Sodium hydroxide.

s. lime A white granular substance consisting of a mixture of calcium hydroxide and sodium hydroxide or potassium hydroxide, or both; used to absorb carbon dioxide. It is used as an absorbing compound in anesthesia.

s. water A solution of carbon dioxide under pressure; carbonic acid.

sodic (sō′dĭk) Relating to or containing soda or sodium.

sodio- Combining form denoting a compound containing sodium.

sodium (sō′dē-ŭm) [LL.] SYMB: Na. The most abundant cation in extracellular fluids. It is the main contributor to osmotic pressure and hydration; participates in many specialized pumps and receptors on cell membranes; and plays a fundamental part in the electrical activities of the body (e.g., nerve impulse transmission and muscular contraction).

Sodium is an inorganic metal with a strong affinity for oxygen and other nonmetallic elements. It has an atomic weight of 23; atomic number of 11; and specific gravity of 0.971. Sodium constitutes about 0.15% of the mass of the body.

The normal sodium level in serum is 135 to 145 mmol/L. A decreased level of sodium in the serum is called hyponatremia. An increased level of sodium in the serum is called hypernatremia. These conditions are not usually excesses or deficiencies of sodium per se, but rather disturbances in the body's regulation of water (i.e., a change in measured sodium concentrations usually results from water retention or water depletion and not from too little or too much sodium in the body). SYN: *natrium.*

HYPONATREMIA: Low serum sodium levels are extremely common in clinical medicine and are caused by one of the following conditions: congestive heart failure, renal failure, cirrhosis; syndrome of inappropriate antidiuretic hormone (SIADH); dehydration; thyroid or adrenal hormone dysfunction; side effects of drugs; psychogenic polydipsia; laboratory error (i.e., pseudohyponatremia). Symptoms of hyponatremia include weakness, confusion, and anorexia. If serum sodium levels drop rapidly, seizures may occur. Treatment of hyponatremia depends on the underlying cause.

HYPERNATREMIA: Elevated serum sodium levels are almost always the result of free water deficits (dehydration), and are treated with intravenous or oral replacement of water. Rarely, hypernatremia may develop after intravenous infusions of solutions with high concentrations of sodium. Symptoms of hypernatremia include thirst, orthostatic dizziness, altered mental status, and neuromuscular dysfunction.

s. acetate A chemical compound that is used to alkalize the urine and kidney dialysis solutions. It is also used as a component in many laboratory reagents, such as various buffers.

s. alginate A purified carbohydrate product extracted from certain species of seaweed. It is used as a food additive and as a pharmaceutical aid.

s. ascorbate The sodium salt of ascorbic acid, vitamin C. It may be used in a sterile solution when parenteral administration of vitamin C is required.

s. benzoate A white, odorless powder with sweet taste; used as a food preservative.

s. bicarbonate $NaHCO_3$; a white odorless powder with saline taste. It is incompatible with acids, acid salts, ammonium chloride, lime water, ephedrine hydrochloride, and iron chloride. It is used to treat acidosis (e.g., in renal failure). Orally it is used as an antacid, although its effectiveness for this purpose is questionable. Externally, it is used as a mild alkaline wash. It is also used as a component in many laboratory reagents, such as various buffers, microbiologic media, and control materials.

s. carbonate Na_2CO_3; a white crystalline powder (washing soda), used as an alkali employed chiefly in alkaline baths.

carboxymethylcellulose s. A chemical used as a pharmaceutical aid and a food additive.

s. chloride NaCl; common table salt. It is used in preparation of normal saline solution, as an emetic, and to add flavor to foods. It is incompatible with silver nitrate. In aqueous solution, sodium chloride, a neutral salt, is a strong electrolyte, being almost completely ionized. The sodium and chlorine ions are important in maintaining the proper electrolyte balance in body fluids. The kidneys regulate retention or excretion of sodium chloride in urine; aldosterone directly increases the renal reabsorption of sodium ions.

s. citrate A white granular powder, saline in taste and soluble in water. Used as an anticoagulant for blood collected for laboratory analysis or used for transfusion.

s. fluoride NaF; a white crystalline powder, saline in taste, soluble in 25 parts of water. It is added to drinking water and used in solution for local application to teeth to prevent dental caries, and it is an effective and inexpensive treatment used in the treatment of osteoporosis. SEE: *fluoridation; sodium fluoride poisoning.*

s. hydroxide NaOH; a whitish solid that is soluble in water, making a clear solution. It is an antacid and a caustic. It is used in laundry detergent and in commercial compounds used to clean sink traps, toilets, and so forth, and in the preparation of soap. It is also used as a component in any laboratory reagent that needs pH balancing. SYN: *caustic soda.*

CAUTION: Great care must be taken in handling sodium hydroxide, as it rapidly destroys organic tissues. Protective glasses should be worn while working with this chemical. If splashed in the eye, it may cause blindness.

s. hypochlorite [solution] An antiseptic used in root canal therapy. This solution is not suitable for application to wounds.

s. iodide NaI; a colorless crystalline solid that is used as an expectorant.

s. lactate [injection] Sodium salt of inactive lactic acid. In one-sixth or one-fourth molar solution, it is used intravenously to control electrolyte disturbances, esp. acidosis.

s. lauryl sulfate An anionic surface-active agent that is used as a pharmaceutical acid.

s. monofluoroacetate A toxic pesticide, once banned in the U.S., that inhibits cellular metabolism, esp. in the most metabolically active organs (i.e., brain and heart). In humans it causes arrhythmias, seizures, coma, and occasionally death. It is used commercially to kill rodents and large animals.

s. monofluorophosphate An agent suitable for topical application to teeth to prevent dental caries.

morrhuate [injection] s. The sodium salt of the fatty acids, found in cod liver oil; used as a sclerosing agent for the obliteration of varicose veins, including esophageal varices.

s. nitrite $NaNO_2$; a white crystalline powder used as an antidote for cyanide poisoning.

s. nitroprusside ABBR: SNP. An antihypertensive and powerful vasodilator used when rapid reduction in blood pressure is required.

CAUTION: Infusion of SNP at the maximum dose rate of 10 μg/kg/min should never last for more than 10 min. For treatment of overdose, SEE: *cyanide poisoning.*

s. phosphate, dibasic A chemical that is used as a cathartic.

s. phosphate P 32 [solution] A standardized preparation of radioactive phosphorus (^{32}P).

s. polystyrene sulfonate A cation-exchange resin used to remove potassium from the body.

s. propionate An antifungal compound.

s. salicylate $C_7H_5NaO_3$; a pain reliever, fever reducer, and anti-inflammatory drug.

s. sulfate A salt formerly used as a saline cathartic and diuretic. SYN: *Glauber's salt.*

s. thiosulfate A white crystalline substance used externally to remove stains of iodine and intravenously as an antidote for cyanide poisoning.

sodium fluoride poisoning A reaction to exposure to a toxic dose of sodium fluoride, a material that is normally used in dentistry or in fluoridating water supplies. Symptoms include conjunctivitis, nausea, vomiting, kidney disturbances, and interference with blood coagulation.

FIRST AID: The affected areas of the skin should be washed and the compound precipitated by addition to the wash solution of soluble calcium salts such as lime water, calcium gluconate, or calcium lactate. SEE: *Poisons and Poisoning Appendix.*

sodium modeling Titration of sodium concentrations during hemodialysis to relieve the muscle cramping, nausea, vomiting, and blood pressure fluctuations sometimes seen during the procedure.

sodokosis, sodoku (sŏd-ō-kō′sĭs) [Jap. *sodoku,* rat poison, + Gr. *osis,* condition] Rat-bite fever.

sodomist, sodomite (sŏd′ō-mĭst, -mīt) [LL. *Sodoma,* Sodom] A person who practices sodomy.

sodomy (sŏd′ō-mē) [LL. *Sodoma,* Sodom] Anal or oral intercourse.

Soemmering, Samuel T. von (sĕm′ĕr-ĭng) German anatomist, 1755–1830.

S.'s bone Marginal process of the malar (zygomatic) bone.

S.'s foramen The fovea centralis retinae.

S.'s ring An annular swelling of the periphery of the lens capsule.

S.'s spot The macula lutea of the retina.

SOFAS *Social and Occupational Functioning Assessment Scale.*

soft (sŏft) [AS. *softe*] Not hard, firm, or solid.

softening (sŏf'ĕn-ĭng) [AS.] The process of becoming soft. SYN: *malacia*.

s. of bones Osteomalacia.

s. of brain Paresis with progressive dementia. SYN: *encephalomalacia*.

soft palate The posterior portion of the roof of the mouth; it blocks the nasopharynx during swallowing. SYN: *velum palatinum*.

"soft sign" Any of a number of signs that, when considered collectively, are felt to indicate the presence of damage to the central nervous system. These signs include incoordination, visual motor difficulties, nystagmus, the presence of associated movements, and difficulties with motor control.

soft sore Chancroid.

soft venereal sore A term formerly used to indicate chancroid.

sol (sŏl, sōl) [Gr. *sole,* salt water] **1.** State of a colloid system in which the dispersion medium or solvent forms a continuous phase in which the particles of the solute are dispersed, forming a fluid mass. It is called a hydrosol if the dispersion medium is a liquid and an aerosol if a gas. SEE: *gel*. **2.** Solution.

solace An object or resource that soothes pain or mental stress. In children a teddy bear or a "security" blanket may provide solace. In later life, one's spouse, a friend, or a hobby may be a source of comfort and security.

Solanaceae (sŏl"ă-nā'sē-ē) A family of herbs, shrubs, and trees from which several important drugs such as scopolamine and belladonna are derived. The potato is one of the species.

solanaceous (sŏl"ă-nā'shŭs) Concerning the family Solanaceae.

s. glycoalkaloids ABBR: SGAa. Steroid chemicals found in plants like potatoes, tomatoes, and eggplants that may prolong the action of some anesthetics and opiates. SGAs inhibit two enzymes, butyrylcholinesterase and acetylcholinesterase, effectively decreasing the metabolism of anesthesia.

solanine (sō'lă-nēn) A poisonous narcotic alkaloid obtained from potato sprouts and tomatoes. SEE: *poisoning, potato*.

solar (sō'lăr) [L. *solaris*] Pert. to the sun or its rays.

solarium (sō-lā'rē-ŭm) [L. *solarium,* terrace] **1.** A room or porch exposed to the sun. **2.** A room designed for heliotherapy or for the application of artificial light. **3.** A day or recreational room for patients; often used as a waiting area for family or visitors.

solar plexus The celiac plexus, located behind the stomach and between the suprarenal glands and consisting of two large ganglia, the celiac and superior mesenteric ganglia, from which sympathetic fibers pass to visceral organs.

solar therapy Treatment with the sun's rays. SYN: *heliotherapy*.

solation (sō-lā'shŭn) In colloidal chemistry, the transformation of a gel into a sol.

solder (sŏd'ĕr) Any fusible alloy usually made of tin and lead but may be mostly silver or gold for use in dentistry. The alloy is applied in a molten state to build up or join metal parts.

building s. An alloy of silver with large amounts of copper used to increase the height or bulk of contact areas of dental inlays or crowns; also called *sticky solder*.

gold s. A solder alloy containing a high proportion of gold.

hard s. A solder that is used in dentistry, has a high fusion point, and is stronger and more tarnish-resistant than softer, low-melting-point solders.

soft s. A low-melting-point solder with less strength or tarnishing resistance than hard solder.

soldering The joining of two pieces of metal by use of a lower-melting-point alloy. When the melted solder cools and solidifies, it joins the parts together. Soldering is used to join many components of dental appliances or orthodontic bands and to add bulk or contours to crowns or inlays.

sole (sōl) [AS. *sole*] **1.** The underpart of the foot. SYN: *planta pedis*. **2.** The portion of a synaptic knob at the termination of a motor nerve fiber that is directly adjacent to the sarcolemma of a muscle fiber.

soleal line of tibia A line on the posterior surface of the tibia extending diagonally from below the tibial condyle to the medial border of the tibia. The soleus muscle and fascia are attached to that line.

solenoid (sō'lĕ-noyd) A coil of insulated wire in which a magnetic force is created in the long axis of the coil when an electric current flows through the wire. It may be used to activate switches.

Solenopsis invecta (sō-lĕn-ŏp'sis in-vik'-tah) The primary species of fire ant that resides in the southern U.S. Its bite can cause welts or, in some instances, generalized anaphylaxis. SEE: *fire ant bite*.

soleus (sō'lē-ŭs) [L. *solea,* sole of foot] A flat, broad muscle of the calf of the leg.

solid (sŏl'ĭd) [L. *solidus*] **1.** Not gaseous, hollow, or liquid. **2.** A substance not gaseous, liquid, or hollow.

solipsism (sŏl′ĭp-sĭzm) [L. *solus,* alone, + *ipse,* self] The theory that the self may know only its feelings and changes and there is then only subjective reality.

solitary (sŏl′ĭ-tăr-ē) [L. *solitarius,* aloneness] Alone; single or existing separately.

solitary lymph nodule One of the small spherical lymphatic nodules found in the lamina propria of the small and large intestine.

solitude Isolation; aloneness.

solo practitioner A physician, dentist, or other practitioner who practices alone rather than with a group or partner.

solubility (sŏl″ū-bĭl′ĭ-tē) [LL. *solubilis,* to loosen, dissolve] The capability of being dissolved.

aqueous s. The ability of a substance to dissolve in water. The aqueous solubility of a medication determines its ability to be compounded, administered, and absorbed.

soluble (sŏl′ū-bl) Able to be dissolved.

soluble immune response suppressor ABBR: SIRS. A lymphokine that suppresses antibody production.

solum tympani (sō′lŭm tĭm′pă-nē) [L.] The floor of the tympanic cavity.

solute (sŏl′ūt) [L. *solutus,* to loosen, dissolve] The substance that is dissolved in a solution.

solutio (sō-lū′shē-ō) [L. *solutus,* to loosen, dissolve] Solution.

solution (sō-lū′shŭn) [L. *solutus,* to loosen, dissolve] **1.** A liquid containing a dissolved substance. **2.** The process by which a solid is homogeneously mixed with a fluid, solid, or gas so that the dissolved substances cannot be distinguished from the resultant fluid. **3.** A mixture formed by dissolution of substances.

The liquid in which the substances are dissolved is called the *solvent* and the substance dissolved, the *solute.*

aqueous s. A solution containing water as the solvent.

buffer s. A solution of a weak acid and its salt (e.g., carbonic acid, sodium bicarbonate) of importance in maintaining a constant pH, esp. of the blood.

colloidal s. A solution in which the solute is suspended and not dissolved, such as gelatin or albumin.

contrast s. A solution containing a radiopaque substance. These solutions are used to facilitate x-ray examination of body cavities.

hyperbaric s. A solution with a specific gravity greater than one, or greater than the solution to which it is being compared. This is important in injecting medicines or anesthetic agents into the spinal fluid in the spinal canal.

hypertonic s. A solution having a greater osmotic pressure than that of cells or body fluids; a solution that draws water out of cells, thus inducing plasmolysis.

hypotonic s. A solution having an osmotic pressure less than that of cells or body fluids; a solution that will cause water to enter cells, thus inducing swelling and possibly lysis.

iodine s. A solution of iodine or potassium iodine used as a source of iodine.

isobaric s. A solution with a specific gravity equal to one or equal to the solution with which it is being compared. SEE: *hyperbaric s.*

isohydric s. A solution having the same hydrogen ion concentration or pH as another.

isosmotic s. A solution with the same osmotic pressure as the solution with which it is being compared.

isotonic s. A solution that has a concentration of electrolytes, nonelectrolytes, or both that will exert osmotic pressure equivalent to that of the solution with which it is being compared. Either 0.16 molar sodium chloride solution (approx. 0.95% salt in water) or 0.3 molar nonelectrolyte solution is approx. isotonic with human red blood cells.

Jessner's s. SEE: *Jessner's solution.*

Locke-Ringer's s. A buffered isotonic solution containing 9.0 g sodium chloride, 0.42 g potassium chloride, 0.24 g calcium chloride, 0.5 g sodium bicarbonate, 0.2 g magnesium chloride, 0.5 g dextrose, and distilled water to make 1000 ml.

molar s. A solution containing a gram molecular weight or mole of the reagent dissolved in 1 L (1000 ml) of solution; designated 1M.

normal s. An obsolete term for a solution in which 1 L contains 1 g equivalent of the solute. The use of this terminology is discouraged in the SI system.

normal saline s. An isotonic saline solution. SEE: *isotonic s.*

ophthalmic s. A sterile preparation suitable for instillation in the eye.

oral rehydration s. A solution used to prevent or correct dehydration due to diarrheal illnesses. The World Health Organization recommends that the solution contain 3.5 g sodium chloride; 2.9 g potassium chloride; 2.9 g trisodium citrate; and 1.5 g glucose dissolved in each liter (approx. 1 qt) of drinking water.

physiological saline s. Normal saline s.

repair s. Any solution given intravenously to treat an electrolyte or metabolic disturbance.

Ringer's s. A solution containing chlorides of sodium, calcium, and potassium. It contains 8.6 g sodium chloride, 0.3 g calcium chloride, 0.3 g potassium chloride, and sufficient distilled water to make 1 L (1000 ml).

saline s. A solution of a salt, usually sodium chloride, and distilled water. A

0.9% solution of sodium chloride is considered isotonic to the body. A normal saline solution (one having an osmolality similar to that of blood serum) consists of 0.85% salt solution, which is necessary to maintain osmotic pressure and the stimulation and regulation of muscular activity.

saturated s. A solution containing all the solute it can dissolve. This limit is called the *saturation point*.

sclerosing s. Sclerosant.

seminormal s. ABBR: 05N or N/2. A solution containing one-half of a gram equivalent weight of reagent in 1 L (1000 ml) of solution.

standard s. A solution containing a definite amount of a substance; used for comparison or analysis.

supersaturated s. A solution in which the saturation point is reached, but when heated, it is possible to dissolve more of the solute.

test s. A dissolved reagent used for a specific laboratory purpose.

Tyrode's s. A modified Ringer's solution containing, in addition, a small amount of magnesium chloride and acid and sodium phosphates.

volumetric s. A standard solution containing a definite amount of a substance in 1 L (1000 ml) of solution; used in volumetric analysis.

solv [L., *solve*] Dissolve.

solvate (sŏl′vāt) A compound formed by reaction between solvent and solute.

solvent (sŏl′vĕnt) [L. *solvens*] **1.** Producing a solution, dissolving. **2.** A liquid holding another substance in solution. **3.** A liquid that reacts with a solvent bringing it into solution.

solvent abuse Glue-sniffing.

solvolysis (sŏl-vŏl′ĭ-sĭs) A general term for reactions involving decomposition by hydrolysis, ammonolysis, and sulfolysis.

soma (sō′mă) [Gr. *soma,* body] **1.** The body as distinct from the mind. **2.** All of the body cells except the germ cells.

soman Pinacolyl methylphosphonofluoridate; an extremely toxic nerve gas.

somato-, somat- (sō′mă-tō) Combining form meaning *body.*

somatesthesia (sō″măt-ĕs-thē′zē-ă) [″ + *aisthesis,* sensation] The consciousness of the body; bodily sensation.

somatic (sō-măt′ĭk) [Gr. *soma,* body] **1.** Pert. to nonreproductive cells or tissues. **2.** Pert. to the body. **3.** Pert. to structures of the body wall, such as skeletal muscles (somatic musculature) in contrast to structures associated with the viscera, such as visceral muscles (splanchnic musculature).

somaticosplanchnic (sō-măt″ĭ-kō-splănk′nĭk) [″ + *splanchnikos,* pert. to the viscera] Somaticovisceral.

somaticovisceral (sō-măt″ĭ-kō-vĭs′ĕr-ăl) [″ + L. *viscera,* body organs] Concerning the body and the viscera.

somatization (sō″mă-tī-zā′shŭn) The process of expressing a mental condition as a disturbed bodily function.

somatization disorder A condition of recurrent and multiple somatic complaints of several years' duration for which medical attention has been sought but no physical basis for the disorder has been found. The disorder impairs social, occupational, or other forms of functioning. The age of onset is usually prior to 30. The somatic complaints may be related to virtually any organ system. If these occur in association with a general medical condition, the physical complaints must be in excess of what would be expected from the medical illness. There must be a history of pain related to at least four different sites or functions such as menstruation, sexual intercourse, or urination. There also must be a history of at least two gastrointestinal symptoms other than pain. There must be a history of at least one sexual or reproductive symptom other than pain (e.g., nausea, vomiting, bloating). In women, this may consist of irregular menses, menorrhagia, or vomiting throughout pregnancy. In men, there may be symptoms such as erectile or ejaculatory dysfunction. Both sexes may be subject to sexual indifference. And there must also be a history of at least one symptom, other than pain, that suggests a neurological condition such as impaired coordination or balance, paralysis or localized weakness, difficulty in swallowing or speaking, urinary retention, hallucinations, loss of touch or pain sensation, double vision, blindness, deafness, seizures, amnesia, and loss of consciousness other than fainting. The unexplained symptoms are not intentionally feigned or produced. SEE: *somatoform disorder*.

somatoceptors (sō-măt″ō-sĕp′tors) A term applied to proprioceptors and exteroceptors collectively.

somatochrome (sō-măt′ō-krōm) [″ + *chroma,* color] A nerve cell in which the nucleus is completely surrounded by cytoplasm.

somatocrinin Growth hormone-releasing hormone.

somatoform disorder A psychological disorder in which the physical symptoms suggest a general medical condition and are not explained by another condition such as a medication or another mental disorder. The symptoms must be clinically significant enough to impair function. A variety of conditions are included in this classification including somatization disorder, conversion disorder, pain disorder, and hypochondriasis. SEE: *Nursing Diagnoses Appendix.*

TREATMENT: The patient may benefit from reassurance, esp. when it is provided by a trusted health care professional.

somatogenic (sō″mă-tō-jĕn′ĭk) [″ + *gennan,* to produce] Originating in the body. SEE: *psychogenic.*

somatology (sō″mă-tŏl′ō-jē) [″ + *logos,* word, reason] Comparative study of structure, functions, and development of the human body.

somatome (sō′mă-tōm) [″ + *tome,* incision] **1.** A device for cutting the body of the fetus. **2.** A somite.

somatomedin Any of a group of insulin-like growth factors (somatomedin C and somatomedin A) that require growth hormone in order to exert their function of stimulating growth. These proteins are produced in the liver and other tissues.

somatometry (sō″mă-tŏm′ĕ-trē) [″ + *metron,* measure] Measurement of the body.

somatopagus (sō″mă-tŏp′ă-gŭs) [″ + *pagos,* thing fixed] A deformed twin fetus with the trunks merged.

somatopathic (sō″mă-tō-păth′ĭk) [″ + *pathos,* disease, suffering] Pert. to organic illness, as distinguished from functional illness.

somatoplasm (sō-măt′ō-plăzm) [Gr. *soma,* body, + LL. *plasma,* form, mold] The cytoplasm of all the body cells as distinguished from that of the germ cells.

somatopleural (sō″mă-tō-ploor′ăl) Concerning somatopleure.

somatopleure (sō-măt′ō-ploor) [″ + *pleura,* side] The lateral and ventral body wall of an embryo, consisting of the outer ectoderm and a layer of somatic mesoderm underlying it. It continues beyond the embryo as the amnion and chorion.

somatopsychic (sō″măt-ō-sī′kĭk) [″ + *psyche,* mind] Pert. to both body and mind.

somatopsychosis (sō″mă-tō-sī-kō′sĭs) [″ + ″ + *osis,* condition] Any psychological disorder that is a symptom of a bodily disease.

somatoschisis (sō″mă-tŏs′kĭ-sĭs) [″ + *schistos,* a splitting] A deformed fetus with a cleft in the trunk.

somatosensory evoked response ABBR: SER. Response produced by small, painless electrical stimulus administered to large sensory fibers in mixed nerves of the hand or leg. The electroencephalographical record of the character of the subsequent waves produced help to determine the functional state of the nerves involved. SEE: *brainstem auditory evoked potential; evoked response; visual evoked response.*

somatosexual (sō″mă-tō-sĕks′ū-ăl) [″ + L. *sexus,* sex] Concerning the body and sexual characteristics.

somatostatin (sō-măt′ō-stăt″ĭn) A peptide that regulates and inhibits the release of hormones by many different neuroendocrine cells in the brain, pancreas, and gastrointestinal tract. Somatostatin inhibits gastric motility and gastric acid secretion, blocks the exocrine and endocrine function of the pancreas, and inhibits the growth and release of hormones by neuroendocrine tumors. It is also used to treat variceal hemorrhage in patients with cirrhosis, and to treat pancreatitis. Octreotide is a synthetic version of somatostatin.

somatostatinoma (sō-măt′ō-stăt′ĕn-ō-mă) An islet cell tumor that secretes somatostatin.

somatotonia (sō″mă-tō-tō′nē-ă) [″ + L. *tonus,* a stretching] A personality type in which there is a predominance of physical assertiveness and activity.

somatotopic (sō″mă-tō-tŏp′ĭk) [″ + *topos,* place] Concerning the correspondence between a particular part of the body and a particular area of the brain.

somatotrophic (sō″mă-tō-trŏf′ĭk) [″ + *tropos,* a turning] **1.** Having selective attraction for or influence on body cells. **2.** Stimulating growth.

somatotrophin (sō″mă-tō-trō′fĭn) [″ + *trophe,* nourishment] Growth hormone.

somatotropic (sō″mă-tō-trŏp′ĭk) [″ + *trope,* a turn] Influencing the body or body cells.

somatotropin (sō″măt-ō-trō′pĭn) [″ + *tropos,* a turning] Human growth hormone. It increases the rate of cell division and protein synthesis in growing tissues, mobilizes stored fats, and limits glucose production.

bovine recombinant s. A growth hormone made by recombinant methods. Its use in dairy cattle to increase milk production is controversial.

somatotype (sō-măt′ō-tīp) A particular build or type of body, based on physical characteristics. SEE: *ectomorph; endomorph; mesomorph.*

somesthetic (sō-mĕs-thĕt′ĭk) Pert. to sensations and sensory structures of the body.

somesthetic area The region in the parietal lobe of the cerebral cortex in which lie the terminations of the axons of general sensory conduction pathways. This area feels and interprets the cutaneous senses and conscious proprioceptive sense.

somesthetic path General sensory conduction path leading to the cortex.

somite (sō′mīt) [Gr. *soma,* body] Embryonic blocklike segment formed on either side of the neural tube and its underlying notochord. Each somite gives rise to a muscle mass supplied by a spinal nerve and each pair gives rise to a vertebra.

somnambulism (sŏm-năm′bū-lĭzm) [L. *somnus,* sleep, + *ambulare,* to walk] Sleepwalking.

somnambulist (sŏm-năm′bū-lĭst) One who is subject to sleepwalking.
somnifacient (sŏm-nĭ-fā′shĕnt) [″ + *facere,* to make] **1.** Producing sleep. SYN: *hypnotic.* **2.** A drug producing sleep. SYN: *soporific.*
somniferous (sŏm-nĭf′ĕr-ŭs) [″ + *ferre,* to bear] Sleep-producing; pert. to that which promotes sleep.
somniloquism (sŏm-nĭl′ō-kwĭzm) [″ + ″ + *-ismos,* condition] Talking in one's sleep.
somnolence (sŏm′nō-lĕns) [L. *somnolentia,* sleepiness] Prolonged drowsiness or sleepiness. **somnolent,** *adj.*
somnolentia (sŏm″nō-lĕn′shē-ă) [L.] **1.** Drowsiness. **2.** The sleep of drunkenness in which the faculties are only partially depressed.
somnolism (sŏm′nō-lĭzm) [″ + *-ismos,* condition] The condition of being in a hypnotic trance.
Somogyi phenomenon [Michael Somogyi, U.S. biochemist, 1883–1971] In diabetes mellitus, rebound hyperglycemia following an episode of hypoglycemia caused by counterregulatory hormone release. Reduction of insulin dose will help control this condition. SEE: *dawn phenomenon; diabetes mellitus.*
sone (sōn) [L. *sonus,* sound] A unit of loudness; the loudness of a pure tone of 1000 cycles per second, 40 decibels above the listener's threshold of hearing.
sonic [L. *sonus,* sound] Pert. to sound.
sonicate (sŏn′ĭ-kāt) [L. *sonus,* sound] To expose to sound waves.
sonication (sŏn″ĭ-kā′shŭn) Exposure to high-frequency sound waves. The technique is used to destroy bacteria, hemolyze blood, and loosen substances adhering to materials such as surgical instruments.
sonic boom (sŏn′ĭk) [L. *sonus,* sound] A noise caused by shock waves from an airborne object traveling faster than the speed of sound.
sonogram (sō′nō-grăm) [L. *sonus,* sound, + Gr. *gramma,* something written] The record obtained by use of ultrasonography.
sonographer An individual professionally trained to use ultrasound, in the setting of other available clinical information, to obtain images of anatomical structures, physiological processes, and disease states for diagnostic purposes. In the U.S., professional societies of sonographers include the Society of Diagnostic Medical Sonographers and the American Society of Echocardiography. Professionally certified sonographers are credentialed by the American Registry of Diagnostic Medical Sonographers.

diagnostic medical s. One who provides patient services for those using diagnostic ultrasound under the supervision of a doctor of medicine or osteopathy.

ophthalmic s. An individual professionally trained to perform diagnostic evaluations of the eye and its diseases, including examinations for ophthalmic foreign bodies, tumors, radiation injuries, inflammatory diseases, and vascular lesions, as well as measurements of axial length (e.g., in cataract surgeries and intraocular lens implantation). In the U.S., professionally trained ophthalmic sonographers are certified in their specialty by the American Registry of Diagnostic Medical Sonographers.

sonography (sō-nŏg′ră-fē) [″ + Gr. *graphein,* to write] Ultrasonography.
sonolucent (sō″nō-loo′sĕnt) In ultrasonography, the condition of not reflecting the ultrasound waves back to their source.
sonometer (sō-nŏm′ĕ-tĕr) [″ + Gr. *metron,* a measure] A device used by dentists to cause sound for production of anesthesia.
sonorous (sō-nō′rŭs) [L.] Giving forth a loud and rounded sound.
sophomania (sŏf″ō-mā′nē-ă) [Gr. *sophos,* wise, + *mania,* madness] An unrealistic belief in one's own wisdom.
sopor (sō′por) [L.] Stupor. **soporose, soporous,** *adj.*
soporiferous (sō″pō-rĭf′ĕr-ŭs) [″ + *ferre,* to bring] Promoting sleep.
soporific (sō-pō-rĭf′ĭk) [″ + *facere,* to make] **1.** Inducing sleep. **2.** Narcotic; a drug producing sleep. SYN: *somnifacient.*
sorbefacient (sor″bē-fā′shĕnt) [L. *sorbere,* to suck up, + *facere,* to make] Causing or that which causes or promotes absorption.
sorbitol $C_6H_{14}O_6$; a crystalline alcohol present in some berries and fruits. It is used as a sweetening agent and as an excipient in formulating tablets.
sordes (sor′dēz) [L. *sordere,* to be dirty] Crusts or accumulations of food and bacteria on the teeth and about the lips.

PATIENT CARE: The nurse prevents this condition by providing frequent oral hygiene for mouth breathers, patients who cannot drink or are not permitted oral fluids, and debilitated patients. A hydrogen peroxide mouthwash (one part hydrogen peroxide to three parts water) or glycerin applied with a soft brush or sponge-stick may be used to remove crusts. Either treatment should always be followed by rinsing with clear water (mouthwashes are astringent, and glycerin dries the mucous membranes). The nurse encourages oral intake if permitted and positions the patient to discourage mouth breathing. If fluids are restricted, the patient should use a water mist or spray to moisten membranes.

sore (sor) [AS. *sar,* sore] **1.** Tender;

painful. **2.** Any type of tender or painful ulcer or lesion of the skin or mucous membrane.

bed s. Decubitus ulcer.

canker s. Aphthous ulcer.

cold s. Thin-walled blister at the junction of the mucous membranes of the mouth and lips, caused by recurrent infection with herpes simplex virus (HSV) in persons who already have antibodies to HSV. Treatment is recommended only for immunocompromised patients, who are given acyclovir. SEE: *fever blister.*

Delhi s. Cutaneous leishmaniasis.

desert s. An ulcer of the skin of the arms or legs, sometimes caused by diphtheria or staphylococci, and typically contracted in Australia or Burma.

hard s. A syphilitic chancre; primary lesion of syphilis.

jungle s. Infection of the skin or of poorly tended wounds by *Corynebacterium diphtheriae,* esp. in warm, moist, tropical climates.

Oriental s. Cutaneous leishmaniasis.

pressure s. SEE: *pressure sore.*

soft venereal s. A term formerly used to signify chancroid.

tropical s. Cutaneous leishmaniasis.

sore throat Inflammation of the tonsils, pharynx, or larynx.

quinsy s.t. Peritonsillar abscess.

septic s.t. Severe, epidemic, pseudomembranous inflammation of the fauces and tonsils caused by the hemolytic streptococcus.

streptococcal s.t. Pharyngitis caused by group A, beta-hemolytic streptococci. SEE: *scarlet fever.*

soroche Mountain sickness, chronic.

sorption (sorp'shŭn) [L. *sorbere,* to suck in] The condition of being absorbed.

s.o.s. [L., *si opus sit*] If necessary or required.

sotalol hydrochloride (sō'tă-lōl) A beta-adrenergic blocking agent.

soterenol hydrochloride (sō'tĕr'ĕ-nōl) An adrenergic medicine used as a bronchodilator.

souffle (soof'fl) [Fr. *souffler,* to puff] A soft blowing sound heard in auscultation; a bruit; an auscultatory murmur.

cardiac s. Cardiac murmur.

fetal s. A purring sound heard over the pregnant uterus and having the same rate as the fetal heartbeat. The sound is caused by blood flowing through vessels in the umbilical cord. SYN: *funic s.*

funic s. Fetal s.

placental s. The loud blowing murmur heard along the side of the uterus, caused by blood entering the dilated arteries of the uterus in the last months of pregnancy and synchronous with the maternal pulse. SYN: *uterine s.*

splenic s. The sound heard over the spleen in various diseases.

umbilical s. Fetal s.

uterine s. Placental s.

sound (sownd) [L. *sonus,* sound] **1.** Auditory sensations produced by vibrations; noise. It is measured in decibels, which is the logarithm of the intensity of sound; thus 20 d. represents not twice 10 d., but 10 times as much. Repeated exposure to excessively loud noises, esp. in certain frequencies, will cause permanent injury to the hearing. SEE: *decibel; noise; sonic boom.* **2.** A form of vibrational energy that gives rise to auditory sensations. SEE: *cochlea; ear; organ of Corti; sonic boom.* **3.** Healthy, not diseased. **4.** Heart sounds. SEE: *diastole; systole.*

absent breath s. The lack of any sound heard over the chest of the patient during auscultation.

ETIOLOGY: Absent breath sounds can be caused by a lack of breathing (apnea) or by lung disorders that block the transmission of the sounds to the surface of the chest (e.g., pneumothorax, pleural effusion).

adventitious lung s. Crackles and wheezes superimposed on the normal breath sounds; indicative of respiratory disease. Most adventitious lung sounds can be divided into continuous (wheezing) and discontinuous (crackles) according to acoustical characteristics.

anasarcous s. A moist sound heard on auscultation when the skin is edematous.

blowing s. An organic murmur as of air from an aperture expelled with moderate force.

bottle s. A noise as of fluid in a bottle. SEE: *amphoric.*

breath s. Respiratory sounds heard on auscultation of the chest. In a normal chest, they are classified as vesicular, tracheal, and bronchovesicular.

bronchial s. Sounds not heard in the normal lung but occurring in pulmonary disease, indicating infiltration and solidification of the lung.

bronchovesicular s. A mixture of bronchial and vesicular sounds.

coarse breath s. A vesicular lung sound that is lower pitched and louder than normal.

ETIOLOGY: Pneumonia, atelectasis, pulmonary edema, and other conditions may cause this type of breath sound.

cracked-pot s. A tympanic resonance heard over air cavities. This percussion sound resembles that made by striking a cracked pot.

diminished breath s. A soft, decreased, or distant vesicular lung sound as heard through a stethoscope.

ETIOLOGY: Diminished breath sounds are common in patients with poor respiratory effort, splinting, emphysema, and other lung conditions.

ejection s. Any noise made during

cardiac systole by the valves of the heart or the root of the aorta.

fetal heart s. The sound made by the fetal heart.

friction s. A sound produced by rubbing together two inflamed mucous surfaces.

heart s. The two sounds "lubb" and "dupp" heard when listening to the heart with a stethoscope. They arise from valve closure and muscular structures in the heart, and are technically called S_1 and S_2. Third and fourth heart sounds may be present in some heart diseases.

physiological s. A sound perceived when the auditory canals are closed. The sound is produced by the blood flowing through adjacent vessels.

respiratory s. Any sound heard over the lungs, bronchi, or trachea.

succussion s. A splashing sound heard over a cavity with fluid in it.

to-and-fro s. Rasping friction sounds of pericarditis.

tracheal s. A sound normally heard over the trachea or larynx.

tubular s. A sound heard over the trachea or large bronchi.

urethral s. A device suitable for use in exploring the urethra.

vesicular s. A normal breath sound heard over the entire lung during breathing.

white s. A sound made up of all audible frequencies.

sound [Fr. *sonder,* to probe] An instrument for introduction into a cavity or canal for exploration. SYN: *searcher*.

Souques' phenomenon [A. A. Souques, Fr. neurologist, 1860–1944] Finger extension on the involved side of a hemiplegic patient when the extremity is raised to a position above 90° of shoulder flexion or abduction.

source The initiator of an epidemic disease, for example, the patient who spreads an illness to others, or the location from which an epidemic spreads (e.g., a "food source," a "source of contaminated water").

Southern Blot An analytical method traditionally used in DNA analysis. After a sample of DNA fragments is separated by agarose gel electrophoresis, the fragments are transferred to a solid cellulose support by blotting. The gel is placed between a concentrated salt solution and absorbent paper. Capillary action draws the fragments onto the solid support. The support is then treated with radiolabeled DNA probes.

sowda (sou'dah) Onchocerciasis; river blindness.

soybean oil A commonly used oil obtained from the seeds of the soya plant, that is low in unsaturated fat and rich in linolenic acid, an essential fatty acid.

sp [L., *spiritus*] *spirit; species.*

spa (spă) [Spa, a Belgium resort town] A mineral spring, esp. one allegedly having healing properties.

space (spās) [L. *spatium,* space] **1.** An area, region, or segment. **2.** A cavity of the body. SYN: *spatium*. **3.** The expanse in which the solar system, stars, and galaxies exist; outside the Earth's atmosphere.

anatomical dead s. The area in the trachea, bronchi, and air passages containing air that does not reach the alveoli during inspiration and is not involved in gas exchange. SYN: *dead s.; deadspace*. SEE: *physiological dead s.*

axillary s. The axilla or space beneath the arm.

circumlental s. The space between the equator of the lens and the ciliary body.

closest speaking s. The space between the teeth during casual repetition of the sound "s." This is considered the closest relationship of the occlusal surfaces and incisal edges of the mandibular teeth to the maxillary teeth during function and rapid speech.

dead s. **1.** Anatomical dead s. **2.** The unobliterated space remaining after closure of a surgical wound. This space favors the accumulation of blood, and eventually infection.

epidural s. The space outside the dura mater of the brain and spinal cord.

extracellular s. The space between cells. It contains tissue fluid, the water derived from plasma in the adjacent capillaries. The water flows among capillaries, tissue spaces, and cells. SEE: *extracellular fluid*.

s. of Fontana Spaces in scleral meshwork in angle of the iris through which the aqueous humor passes from the anterior chamber to the canal of Schlemm.

intercostal s. The interval between ribs, filled by the intercostal muscles.

interfascial s. Tenon's space.

interglobular s. Czermak's spaces.

interpleural s. Mediastinum.

interproximal s. The space between the surfaces of adjacent teeth in the dental arch. It is divided into the septal space, gingival to the contact point of the teeth and occupied normally by the interdental papilla of the gingiva, and the embrasure, the space occlusal to the contact point of the teeth.

interradicular s. The area between the roots of a multirooted tooth, which contains an alveolar bony septum and the periodontal ligament.

intervillous s. Any area of the maternal side of the placenta where transfer of maternal oxygen, nutrients, and fetal wastes occurs.

loose s. A distensible lung interstitial tissue surrounding the acinus and terminal bronchioles.

Meckel's s. Cavum trigeminale.

mediastinal s. Mediastinum.

medullary s. The marrow-containing area of cancellous bone.

palmar s. The midpalmar and thenar spaces of the hand.

parasinoidal s. Lateral spaces in the dura mater adjacent to the superior sagittal sinus that receive meningeal and diploic veins.

perforated s. The space pierced by blood vessels at the base of the brain.

periodontal ligament s. ABBR: PDL space. A radiolucent space that appears on a dental radiograph between the tooth and the adjacent lamina dura. The space is occupied by the periodontal ligament, which lacks the density to be radiopaque.

perivascular s. The spaces within adventitia of larger blood vessels of the brain. They communicate with the subarachnoid space.

personal s. In psychiatry, an individual's personal area and the surrounding space. This space is important in interpersonal relations and in personal feelings of security and privacy.

physiological dead s. In the respiratory tract, any nonfunctional alveoli that do not receive air that participates in gas exchange. Possible causes include emphysema, pneumothorax, pneumonia, pulmonary edema, and constriction of bronchioles. SEE: *anatomical dead s.*

plantar s. One of four spaces between the fascial layers of the foot. When the foot is infected, pus may be found there.

pneumatic s. Air-containing spaces in bone, esp. those in the paranasal sinuses.

popliteal s. The space in back of the knee joint, containing the popliteal artery and vein and small sciatic and popliteal nerves.

prezonular s. The anterior portion of the posterior chamber of the eye.

Prussak's s. The space in the tympanum behind Shrapnell's membrane.

retroperitoneal s. The potential space outside the parietal peritoneum of the abdominal cavity.

retropharyngeal s. The space behind the pharynx separating prevertebral from visceral fascia. Important as a possible path for the spread of infection from oral cavity trauma downward to visceral organs of the mediastinum.

subarachnoid s. One of the spaces between the pia mater and arachnoid, containing the cerebrospinal fluid. The spaces, esp. in the cranium, are traversed by numerous trabeculae.

subdural s. Narrow space between the dura and the arachnoid.

subphrenic s. Space between the diaphragm and the abdominal organs.

suprasternal s. Triangular space immediately above the sternum between layers of deep cervical fascia.

Tenon's s. Tissue fluid space between the sclera and Tenon's capsule. SYN: *interfascial s.*

thenar s. A deep fascial space in the hand lying anterior to the adductor pollicis muscle.

tissue s. Any space within tissues not lined with epithelium and containing tissue fluid.

zonular s. Spaces within the zonule (suspensory ligament of lens). SEE: *deadspace*.

space maintainer An appliance placed within the dental arch to prevent adjacent teeth from moving into the space left by a missing tooth; it is a temporary placement until the permanent tooth erupts into the space, or until a bridge is placed to replace the missing permanent tooth.

space medicine The branch of medical science concerned with the physiological and pathological problems encountered by humans who enter the area beyond the Earth's atmosphere. Included in space medicine are investigation of effects of weightlessness (zero gravity), sensory deprivation, motion sickness, enforced inactivity during lengthy travels in space, and the heat and decelerative forces encountered at the time of reentry into the Earth's atmosphere. With prolonged flights into space, a number of medical problems have arisen, including anemia and loss of blood volume, and loss of bone and muscle mass. These changes also make adjustment to gravity after returning to earth difficult.

spacer (spā′sĕr) A hollow tube that improves the delivery of inhaled aerosols, such as beta$_2$ agonists, steroids, and other antiasthmatic drugs, to the bronchi and lungs. Spacers form a channel between metered dose inhalers and the mouth through which medicated mists can be inhaled. They improve the performance of anti-asthmatic drugs because without them, a large quantity of inhaled medications end up in the mouth, on the palate, on the buccal mucosa, or on the tongue, and fail to reach their intended target in the lower airways.

spallation (spawl-lā′shŭn) **1.** The process of breaking into very small parts. The term may be applied to gross structures or to atomic particles. **2.** The release of inert particles into the bloodstream. An example would be the splintering of bits of plastic from the pump used in hemodialysis.

span **1.** The distance from one fixed point to another, as the distance, when the hand is fully expanded, from the tip of the thumb to the tip of the little finger. **2.** A length of time. The duration of a process.

attention s. The duration of sustained concentration on a task or activity. SEE: *hyperactivity* (2); *attention deficit-hyperactivity disorder*.

digit s. A test of memory and attention. SEE: *digit span test*.

memory s. The number of words or objects one can store and recall when asked to do so. SEE: *digit span test*.

sparer (spăr′ĕr) [AS. *sparian,* to refrain] A substance destroyed by catabolism that decreases catabolic action on other substances.

nitrogen s. protein s.

protein s. Carbohydrates and fats, so designated because their presence in the diet prevents tissue proteins from being used as a source of energy.

sparganosis (spăr″gă-nō′sĭs) Infestation with a variety of Sparganum.

Sparganum (spăr′gă-nŭm) *pl.* **spargana** [Gr. *sparganon,* swathing band] The plerocercoid larva of tapeworms, esp. those of the genus *Diphyllobothrium*.

S. mansoni An elongated plerocercoid species, 3 to 14 in. (7.6 to 35 cm) in length, found in muscles and connective tissue, esp. that around the eye; common in the Far East.

S. mansonoides Species occasionally found in the U.S. in larval form.

S. proliferum Minute species infesting humans and producing acne-like nodules. It is thought to proliferate by means of budlike outgrowths.

spargosis (spăr-gō′sĭs) [Gr. *spargosis,* swelling] **1.** Distention of the female breasts with milk. **2.** Swelling or thickening of the skin. SYN: *elephantiasis*.

sparing The use of one medicine in place of another, usually to prevent side effects from high doses of the first medicine (e.g., steroid-sparing).

spasm (spăzm) [Gr. *spasmos,* convulsion] An involuntary sudden movement or muscular contraction that occurs as a result of some irritant or trauma. Spasms may be clonic (characterized by alternate contraction and relaxation) or tonic (sustained). They may involve either visceral (smooth) muscle or skeletal (striated) muscle. When contractions are strong and painful, they are called cramps. The effect depends on the part affected. Asthma is assumed to be associated with spasm of the muscular coats of smaller bronchi; renal colic to spasm of the muscular coat of the ureter.

TREATMENT: General measures to reduce tension, induce muscle relaxation, and improve circulation are needed. Specific measures include analgesics, massage, relaxation exercises, therapeutic modalities such as heat, cold, or electrotherapy, and, in some cases, gentle therapeutic exercises. Special orthopedic supports or braces are sometimes effective. For vascular spasm, chemical sympathectomy may give relief.

Bell's s. Convulsive tic of the face.

bronchial s. Bronchospasm.

carpopedal s. Involuntary muscular contraction of the hands and feet, sometimes seen in hyperventilation syndrome. It is caused by hypocalcemia and commonly encountered during hyperventilation because the lowered carbon dioxide alters the level of ionized calcium. SEE: *hyperventilation tetany*.

choreiform s. Spasmodic movements resembling chorea.

clonic s. Intermittent contractions and relaxation of muscles. SYN: *clonospasm*.

coronary s. Muscular closure of the coronary arteries, causing angina, ischemia, or myocardial infarction. SEE: *Prinzmetal's angina*.

diffuse s. An esophageal motor disorder characterized by dysphagia, odynophagia, and chest pain.

esophageal s. Intermittent inability to swallow, often associated with intense chest pain, gagging, or difficulty breathing. It can occur after swallowing cold liquids taken through a straw, or may occur in such diverse diseases as rabies, anxiety or depression, or achalasia. In most patients, it is caused by excessive motor function of the esophageal muscles.

TREATMENT: Nitrates or tricyclic antidepressants are sometimes used to treat the symptoms. Diffuse esophageal spasms can also be treated by surgical division of the esophageal muscles.

habit s. Tic.

hemifacial s. Twitching of facial muscles that usually begins in one eyelid but may generalize after many years to half of the face, or even to both sides of it. It usually results from an aneurysm of the vertebral or basilar artery or a tumor of the cerebellopontine angle. In some patients, the twitching can be treated with injections of botulinum toxin if the underlying cause is not treatable.

infantile s. Seizure activity marked by momentary flexion or extension of the neck, trunk, extremities, or any combination, with onset occurring in the first year of life. Although infantile spasms subside in late infancy, many affected children develop other types of seizure activity and may be severely retarded.

nodding s. A psychogenic condition in adults, causing nodding of the head from clonic spasms of the sternomastoid muscles. A similar nodding occurs in babies, with the head turning from side to side. SYN: *salaam convulsion*.

saltatory s. A tic of the muscles of the lower extremity, causing convulsive leaping upon attempting to stand. SEE: *Jumping Frenchmen of Maine; miryachit; palmus* (2); *Tourette's syndrome*.

tetanic s. A spasm in which contractions occur repeatedly and without interruption.

tonic s. Continued involuntary contractions.

torsion s. A spasm characterized by a turning of a part, esp. the turning of the body at the pelvis.

toxic s. Convulsions due to poison.

winking s. Blepharospasm.

spasmogen (spăz′mō-jĕn) [″ + *gennan,* to produce] Something that causes spasms or constrictions as in the bronchospasm associated with asthma.

spasmolygmus (spăz-mō-lĭg′mŭs) [″ + *lygmos,* a sob] **1.** A spasmodic hiccup. **2.** Spasmodic sobbing.

spasmolytic (spăz-mō-lĭt′ĭk) [″ + *lysis,* dissolution] Arresting spasms or that which acts as an antispasmodic.

spasmophemia (spăz-mō-fē′mē-ă) [″ + *pheme,* speech] Stuttering.

spasmophilia (spăz-mō-fĭl′ē-ă) [″ + *philein,* to love] A tendency to tetany and convulsions; almost always associated with rickets.

spasmous (spăz′mŭs) [Gr. *spasmos,* convulsion] Of the nature of a spasm.

spasmus (spăz′mŭs) [Gr. *spasmos,* convulsion] A spasm.

s. agitans Parkinson's disease.

s. bronchialis Bronchial asthma.

s. caninus Risus sardonicus.

s. coordinatus Imitative or compulsive movements, as mimic tics or festination.

s. cynicus A spasmodic contraction of the muscles on both sides of the mouth.

s. Dubini Rhythmic contractions, in rapid succession, of a group or groups of muscles, starting at an extremity or half of the face, and covering a large part or all of the body. It is usually fatal.

s. glottidis Laryngismus.

s. nictitans Blepharospasm.

s. nutans A nodding spasm in infants and young children. The eyes are also involved as manifested by rapid, pendular nystagmoid movements that may be observed in one eye. Spontaneous improvement always occurs.

spastic (spăs′tĭk) [Gr. *spastikos,* convulsive] **1.** Resembling or of the nature of spasms or convulsions. **2.** Produced by spasms. **3.** One afflicted with spasms.

spastic colon Irritable colon.

spastic gait A stiff movement of the legs while walking, usually the result of an upper motor neuron lesion and spasticity in the muscles of the lower extremity. There are several variations. Spasticity in the ankle plantar flexors results in the toes dragging or walking on the toes; spasticity in the hip adductors results in a scissoring or crossing of the legs; spasticity in the quadriceps femoris results in the knee being held rigid. If the upper extremities are involved, the arms do not swing rhythmically but are usually held still with the elbows and wrists flexed.

spastic hemiplegia Spasticity occurring in one half of the body, usually owing to a cardiovascular accident or cerebral palsy affecting only half of the brain.

spasticity (spăs-tĭs′ĭ-tē) A motor disorder that demonstrates velocity-dependent increased muscle tone, exaggerated tendon jerks, and clonus. Spasticity is the result of an upper motor neuron lesion (i.e., found in the spinal cord or brain rather than in one of the peripheral nerves).

PATIENT CARE: Spasticity can cause abnormal and variable movement patterns and restriction of range of motion.

spatial (spā′shăl) Pert. to space.

spatial discrimination The ability to perceive as separate points of contact the two blunt points of a compass when applied to the skin.

spatial localization disorder An inability to describe or to find the way even though in familiar surroundings. This neurological condition is usually due to bilateral occipitoparietal lesions of the brain.

spatial resolution In radiology, the ability to distinguish two adjacent points of similar density as being separate.

spatium (spā′shē-ŭm) *pl.* **spatia** [L.] Space.

spatula (spăch′ū-lă) [L. *spatula,* blade] An instrument for spreading or mixing semisolids. It is usually flat, thin, somewhat flexible, and shaped like a knife without a cutting edge. It may be used in blunt dissection of soft tissues (e.g., brain).

cervical s. A blade, often made of wood or plastic, with an indented tip adapted to ensure sampling during a Papanicolaou smear, of the squamous cells of the endocervix of the uterus.

eye s. A blade for separating lips of corneal wounds, arresting hemorrhage, or for making pressure.

nasal s. A device for holding mucous flaps in place or to guard against burning from cautery.

spatulate (spăch′ŭ-lāt) To mix something by use of a spatula. In dentistry, to mix or manipulate certain dental materials with a spatula to achieve a uniform, homogeneous mass.

spay, spaying (spā, spā′ĭng) [Gael. *spoth,* castrate] Surgical removal of ovaries, usually said of animals. SEE: *castration.*

SPCA *Society for the Prevention of Cruelty to Animals.*

specialist (spĕsh′ăl-ĭst) [L. *specialis*] A dentist, nurse, physician, or other health professional who has advanced education and training in one clinical area of practice such as internal medicine, pediatrics, surgery, ophthalmology, neurology, maternal and child health, or cardiology. In most specialized areas of health care, there are organizations offering qualifying examinations. When an individual meets all of the criteria of such a board, he or she is called "board certified" in that area.

specialization (spĕsh″ăl-ī-zā′shŭn) The limitation of one's practice to a particular branch of medicine, surgery, dentistry, or nursing. This is customarily done after having received postgraduate training in the area of specialization.

specialty (spĕsh′ăl-tē) The branch of medicine, surgery, dentistry, or nursing in which a specialist practices.

speciation (spē″sē-ā′shŭn) [L. *species*, a kind] The evolutionary process by which new species of living organisms are formed.

species (spē′shēz) [L. *species*, a kind] In biology, a category of classification for living organisms. This group is just below genus and is usually capable of interbreeding.

species-specific The characteristics of a species, esp. the immunological nature that differentiates that species from another.

species type The original species that served as the basis for identifying a new genus or subgenus.

specific (spĕ-sĭf′ĭk) [L. *specificus*, pert. to a kind] **1.** Referring to a remedy having a curative effect on a particular disease or symptom. **2.** Pert. to a species. **3.** Referring to a disease always caused by the same organism. **4.** Restricted, explicit; not generalized.

specific gravity ABBR: sp. gr. The weight of a substance compared with the weight of an equal volume of water. For solid and liquid materials, water is used as a standard and considered to have a specific gravity of 1.000. For gases, the weight per unit volume is compared with that of dry air at a specified temperature and usually at atmospheric pressure.

specificity (spĕ-sĭ-fĭs′ĭ-tē) The state of being specific; having a relation to a definite result or to a particular cause.

diagnostic s. For a diagnostic or screening test, the proportion of people who are truly free of a specific disease and are so identified by the test. SEE: *sensitivity*.

s. of exercise The design of exercises to stress muscles in a manner similar to the way in which they are to perform. This technique helps the muscle to meet specific demands, including speed and type of contraction, strength and endurance requirements, stabilization, and mobility activities.

specimen (spĕs′ĭ-mĕn) [L. *specere*, to look] A part of something, intended to show the kind, quality, and other characteristics of the whole. Collected urine, feces, cerebrospinal fluid, sputum, blood, skin, or tissues are all considered to be specimens.

CAUTION: Persons handling specimens of blood, body fluids, or other excretions should wear protective gloves to limit exposure to infectious agents, such as the hepatitis viruses.

The following information is important in obtaining, containing, and handling biological and forensic samples.

Sterilization of glassware: This is accomplished by the use of hot air or dry heat, boiling water, flowing steam, steam under pressure, certain gases, and germicidal chemicals.

Labels: All containers should be labeled with the names of the patient and attending physician and the room number. Labels should be placed on the container, not on the lid. Request forms, sometimes used as labels, are made up to suit the individual laboratory or hospital. Provision is made for recording necessary data as indicated, including the date the specimen was taken, the circumstances, the substances for which the examination is being performed, and any other information desired. SEE: *chain of custody*.

Time: If the required specimen cannot be furnished at once, one should note what is needed and inform the patient, supervisor, and any other caregiver who may attend the patient in one's absence.

Charting: The chart should record all specimens sent to the laboratory, when they were sent, and any other data that seem pertinent such as the appearance of the specimen or unusual occurrences while it was being obtained.

Care of specimen: The specimen should be covered immediately after it is deposited in the container. The label or request form should be checked. One should make sure that the container is intact and in no danger of spilling while in transit. Some types of specimens (e.g., blood, urine, tissues) will need special care with respect to the temperature to be maintained while they are stored or transported and the time allowed before being analyzed. SEE: *Standard and Universal Precautions Appendix*.

speckle A grainy distortion (a kind of "noise") in an ultrasonographic image.

spectacles (spĕk′tăk-lz) [L. *spectare*, to see] Glasses.

spectinomycin hydrochloride, sterile An antibiotic used primarily to treat sexually transmitted diseases.

spectral (spĕk′trăl) [L. *spectrum*, image] Concerning a spectrum.

spectro- Combining form meaning *appearance, image, form*, or *spectrum*.

spectrocolorimeter (spĕk-trō-kŭl-or-ĭm′ĕ-tĕr) [L. *spectrum,* image, + *color,* color, + Gr. *metron,* measure] A device for detecting color blindness by isolating a single spectral color.

spectrofluorometer (spĕk″trō-floo″or-ŏm′ĕ-tĕr) An instrument for measuring the degree of fluorescence.

spectrograph (spĕk′trō-grăf) [″ + Gr. *graphein,* to write] An instrument designed to photograph spectra on a sensitive photographic plate.

mass s. A device that separates ions of different masses by employing a magnetic field to deflect them as they travel along a given path.

spectrometer (spĕk-trŏm′ĕt-ĕr) [″ + Gr. *metron,* measure] A spectroscope so constructed that angular deviation of a ray of light produced by a prism or by a diffraction grating thus indicates the wavelength.

spectrometry (spĕk-trŏm′ĕ-trē) [″ + Gr. *metron,* measure] The process of determining the wavelength of light rays by use of a spectrometer.

spectrophotometer (spĕk″trō-fō-tŏm′ĕt-ĕr) [″ + Gr. *photos,* light, + *metron,* measure] A device for measuring the amount of color in a solution by comparison with the spectrum.

spectrophotometry (spĕk″trō-fō-tŏm′ĕt-rē) An estimation of coloring matter in a solution by use of the spectroscope or spectrophotometer.

spectropolarimeter (spĕk″trō-pō″lăr-ĭm′ĕ-tĕr) [″ + *polaris,* pole, + *metron,* measure] A device for measuring the rotation of light rays of a specific wavelength by passage through a translucent solid.

spectroscope (spĕk′trō-skōp) [″ + Gr. *skopein,* to examine] An instrument for separating radiant energy into its component frequencies or wavelengths by means of a prism or grating to form a spectrum for inspection.

spectroscopic (spĕk″trō-skŏp′ĭk) Concerning a spectroscope.

spectroscopy (spĕk-trŏs′kō-pē) **1.** The branch of physical science that treats the phenomena observed with the spectroscope, or those principles on which the action is based. **2.** The art of using the spectroscope.

nuclear magnetic resonance s. ABBR: NMR spectroscopy. A technique that uses the characteristic absorption of nuclei inside a strong magnetic field to identify and characterize molecules.

spectrum (spĕk′trŭm) *pl.* **spectra** [L., image] **1.** The charted band of wavelengths of electromagnetic vibrations obtained by refraction and diffraction of rays of white light. **2.** The range or breadth of a phenomenon; the distribution of values in an array.

absorption s. Spectrum recorded after light rays have passed through a substance that is capable of absorbing some of the wavelengths passing through. This spectrum is specific for various chemicals.

broad s. Referring to drugs that may be used to treat a wide variety of conditions or infections.

chromatic s. The portion of the spectrum that produces visible light. Wavelengths of about 3900 Å to 7700 Å are visible.

invisible s. The portion of the spectrum either below the red (infrared) or above the violet (ultraviolet), which is invisible to the eye, the waves being too long or too short to affect the retina. The invisible spectrum includes rays less than 3900 Å in length (ultraviolet, roentgen or x, gamma, and cosmic rays) and those exceeding 7700 Å in length (infrared, high-frequency oscillations used in short- and long-wave diathermy, radio, hertzian, and very long waves). These range in length from 7700 Å to 5,000,000 m.

narrow s. A term that refers to an antibiotic effective against only a few microorganisms.

visible s. The portion of the spectrum that is detectable by the human eye. The visible spectrum consists of the colors from red to violet with wavelengths of 3900 Å to 7700 Å.

visible electromagnetic s. The complete range of wavelengths of electromagnetic radiation.

spectrum emission **1.** In spectroscopy and fluorometry, the range of wavelengths emitted by a substance. **2.** In the case of atoms, the lines of emission.

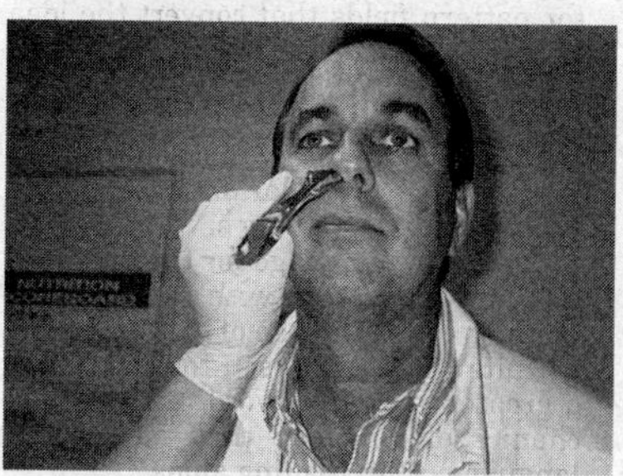

NASAL SPECULUM

speculum (spĕk′ū-lŭm) *pl.* **specula** [L., a mirror] **1.** An instrument for examination of canals or hollow organs. SEE: illus. **2.** The membrane separating the anterior cornua of lateral ventricles of the brain. SYN: *septum pellucidum.*

bivalve s. A speculum with two opposed blades that can be separated or closed. SEE: *vaginal s.*

duck-bill s. A bivalve speculum with wide blades.

ear s. A short, funnel-shaped tube, tubular or bivalve (the former being preferable), used to examine the external auditory canal and eardrum.

eye s. A device for separating the eyelids. Plated steel wire, plain, Luer's, Von Graefe's, and Steven's are the most common types.

Pedersen s. A small vaginal speculum for examining prepubertal patients or others with small vaginal orifices.

vaginal s. A speculum, usually with two opposing portions that, after being inserted, can be pushed apart, for examining the vagina and cervix. It should be warmed before use.

speech [AS. *spaec*] **1.** The verbal expression of one's thoughts. **2.** The act of uttering articulate words or sounds. **3.** Words that are spoken for the purpose of communication.

Historically, certain crude sounds are believed to have served as warnings or threats in much the same way as did facial and bodily expressions. As sounds became highly differentiated, each became associated and gradually identified with a certain idea. These word-symbols are a valuable tool in ideation, and thinking largely depends on this internal speech. Further identifications have made possible visual symbols (written language), although primitive written language was entirely unrelated to speech. The symbols were crude representations of objects.

External speech requires the coordination of the larynx, mouth, lips, chest, and abdominal muscles. These have no special innervation for speech, but the upper neurons respond to complex motor pattern fields that convert the idea into suitable motor stimuli.

aphonic s. Whispering.

ataxic s. Defective speech resulting from muscular incoordination, usually the result of cerebellar disorder.

clipped s. Scamping s.

cued s. A language for the deaf that combines lip reading with cues provided by the hands. The use of this technique permits the deaf person to understand a greater variety of words and the mechanics of language than either sign language or lip reading alone.

dyspraxia of s. In individuals with normal muscle tone and speech muscle coordination, partial loss of the ability to pronounce words consistently, resulting from injury to the central nervous system or stroke.

echo s. Echolalia.

esophageal s. In persons who have had laryngectomies, the modulation of air expelled from the esophagus to produce sound that can be used in speech. The mouth, tongue, and pharynx participate in this.

explosive s. Sudden loud sounds produced by persons with organic brain disease or mental disorders.

helium s. The altered voice produced by inhaling helium and then speaking as the helium is exhaled. The very low density of the helium causes the alteration. The intelligibility of helium speech is important, esp. to deep-water divers who transmit and unscramble verbal information using helium as a speech-enhancement medium.

interjectional s. Speech characterized by inarticulate sounds.

mirror s. Speech characterized by reversing the order of syllables of a word.

nasal s. Speech in which air from the oropharynx enters the nasopharynx, usually resulting in abnormal resonance. Emission of air through the nose, weak pressure in articulating consonants, and attempts by the patient to stifle the abnormally spoken air column are also characteristic.

paraphasic s. Speech that is fluent but may be incomprehensible. Words may have inappropriate syllables inserted, or one word may be substituted for another.

scamping s. Speech characterized by omission of consonants or syllables when unable to pronounce them. SYN: *clipped s.*

scanning s. The pronunciation of words in syllables, or slowly and hesitatingly; pauses between the syllables result in a staccato-like speech. It is a symptom of certain diseases of the cerebellum and advanced multiple sclerosis. SYN: *staccato s.*

slurring s. Slovenly articulation of letters difficult to pronounce.

staccato s. Scanning s.

telegraphic s. Nonfluent or halting speech, in which some nouns or verbs are uttered but other elements of normal sentence structure are replaced by pauses or gaps. This type of aphasia is a hallmark of Broca's aphasia.

speech abnormality Any disorder, dysfunction, or impairment of speech. Examples of speech abnormalities include expressive and receptive aphasias, dysarthrias, labialism, stammering, stuttering, word deafness, and others. *Speech failure* results in motor aphasia, in which the patient is speechless but there is no paralysis of the muscles of articulation. Although unable to express thoughts in words, the patient can still understand what he or she hears and reads.

speech delay Any disorder of childhood in the acquisition and use of spoken language.

speech and language pathologist ABBR: SLP. A health care professional trained to evaluate and treat people who have voice, speech, language, swallowing, or hearing disorders, esp. those that affect their ability to communicate or consume food.

speechreading Lip reading.

speech synthesizer An electronic device for producing speech. Activated by a keyboard, it permits persons lacking the ability to speak to communicate.

speedball Among abusers of drugs, a combination of cocaine and heroin taken intravenously.

sperm (spĕrm) [Gr. *sperma*, seed] **1.** Semen. **2.** Spermatozoa. SEE: illus.

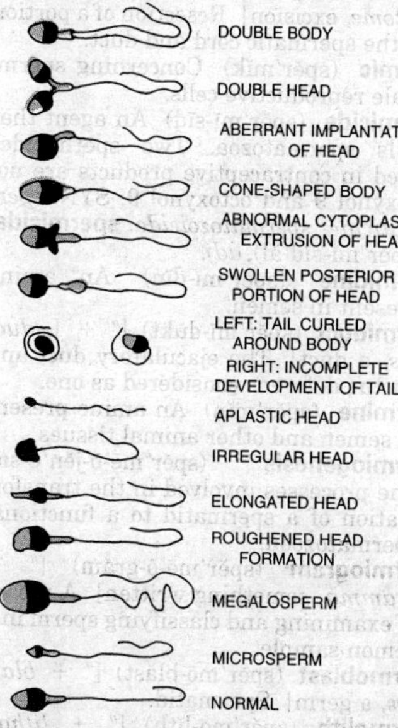

NORMAL AND ABNORMAL SPERM

sperm retrieval, posthumous Obtaining sperm from a body shortly after death, in an attempt to use the specimen to impregnate the fiancée or wife of the deceased. The sperm may be frozen for later use.

sperma- SEE: *spermato-*.

sperma (spĕr'mă) [Gr.] **1.** Semen. **2.** Spermatozoa.

spermache (spĕr'mă-kē) The age at which a boy's testes become mature (i.e., capable of producing spermatozoa).

spermacrasia (spĕr"măk-rā'zē-ă) [Gr. *sperma*, seed, + *akrasia*, bad mixture] A lack of spermatozoa in the semen. SYN: *aspermia*.

spermagglutination Agglutination of spermatozoa.

spermat- SEE: *spermato-*.

spermatemphraxis (spĕr"măt-ĕm-frăk'sĭs) [" + *emphraxis*, stoppage] An obstruction to the emission of semen.

spermatic (spĕr-măt'ĭk) [Gr. *sperma*, seed] Pert. to semen or sperm.

spermatic artery One of two long slender vessels, branches of the abdominal aorta, following each spermatic cord to the testes.

spermaticide, spermatocide (spĕrm'ăt-ĭ-sīd, spĕrm'ăt-ō-sīd) [Gr. *sperma*, seed, + L. *cidus*, kill] Spermicide. **spermaticidal** (-sīd"ăl), *adj*.

spermatic vein One of two veins draining the testes. The right one empties into the inferior vena cava, the left into the left renal vein. In the spermatic cord, each forms a dilated pampiniform plexus.

spermatid (spĕr'mă-tĭd) A cell arising by division of the secondary spermatocyte to become a spermatozoon. SYN: *spermatoblast; spermoblast*.

spermatin (spĕr'mă-tĭn) A mucilaginous substance in the semen.

spermatitis (spĕr"mă-tī'tĭs) [" + *itis*, inflammation] Inflammation of the spermatic cord or of the ductus deferens. SYN: *deferentitis; funiculitis*.

spermato-, spermat-, sperma- Combining form meaning *seed*.

spermatoblast (spĕr-măt'ō-blăst) [Gr. *sperma, spermatos*, seed, + *blastos*, germ] Spermatid.

spermatocele (spĕr-măt'ō-sēl) [" + *kele*, tumor, swelling] A cystic tumor of the epididymis containing spermatozoa.

spermatocidal (spĕr"mă-tō-sī'dăl) [" + L. *cidus*, kill] Destroying spermatozoa.

spermatocyst (spĕr-măt'ō-sĭst) [" + *kystis*, bladder] **1.** A seminal vesicle. **2.** Tumor of the epididymis containing semen. SYN: *spermatocele*.

spermatocystectomy (spĕr"măt-ō-sĭs-tĕk'tō-mē) [" + " + *ektome*, excision] Removal of the seminal vesicles.

spermatocystitis (spĕr"măt-ō-sĭs-tī'tĭs) [" + " + *itis*, inflammation] Inflammation of a seminal vesicle.

spermatocystotomy (spĕr"mă-tō-sĭs-tŏt'ō-mē) [" + " + *tome*, incision] Drainage of the seminal vesicles by use of a surgical incision into the vesicle.

spermatocytal (spĕr"mă-tō-sī'tăl) [" + *kytos*, cell] Concerning spermatocytes.

spermatocyte (spĕr-măt'ō-sīt) [" + *kytos*, cell] A cell originating from a spermatogonium that forms by division of the spermatids, which give rise to spermatozoa.

primary s. A cell arising by growth and development from a spermatogonium.

secondary s. A cell arising from a primary spermatocyte by a meiotic division. It undergoes a second meiotic division, giving rise to two spermatids with the haploid number of chromosomes.

spermatogenesis (spĕr"măt-ō-jĕn'ĕ-sĭs) [" + *genesis*, generation, birth] The formation of mature functional spermatozoa. In the process, undifferentiated spermatogonia become primary spermatocytes, each of which divides to form two secondary spermatocytes. Each of these divides to form two spermatids, which transform into functional motile spermatozoa. In the process, the chromosome number is reduced from the diploid to the haploid number. SEE: illus.; *gametogenesis; maturation; meiosis*.

spermatogenic, spermatogenous (spĕr″mă-tō-jĕn′ĭk, spĕr″mă-tŏj′ĕ-nŭs) Producing sperm.

spermatogonium (spĕr″măt-ō-gō′nē-ŭm) *pl.* **spermatogonia** [″ + *gone,* generation] A large unspecialized germ cell that in spermatogenesis gives rise to a primary spermatocyte. SYN: *spermatospore*. SEE: *spermatogenesis*.

spermatoid (spĕr′mă-toyd) [″ + *eidos,* form, shape] Resembling a spermatozoon.

spermatology (spĕr″mă-tŏl′ō-jē) [″ + *logos,* word, reason] The study of the seminal fluid.

spermatolysin (spĕr″măt-ŏl′ĭ-sĭn) [″ + *lysis,* dissolution] A lysin destroying spermatozoa.

spermatolysis (spĕr″măt-ŏl′ĭ-sĭs) [″ + *lysis,* dissolution] The dissolution or destruction of spermatozoa.

spermatolytic (spĕr″măt-ō-lĭt′ĭk) Destroying spermatozoa.

spermatopathia, spermatopathy (spĕr″mă-tō-păth′ē-ă, spĕr-mă-tŏp′ă-thē) [Gr. *spermatos,* seed, + *pathos,* disease] A disease of sperm cells or their secreting glands or ducts.

spermatophobia (spĕr″mă-tō-fō′bē-ă) [″ + *phobos,* fear] An abnormal fear of being afflicted with spermatorrhea, involuntary loss of semen.

spermatopoietic (spĕr″măt-ō-poy-ĕt′ĭk) [″ + *poiein,* to make] Promoting the formation and secretion of semen.

spermatorrhea (spĕr″mă-tō-rē′ă) [″ + *rhoia,* flow] An abnormally frequent involuntary loss of semen without orgasm.

spermatoschesis (spĕr″măt-ŏs′kĕ-sĭs) [″ + *schesis,* checking] Suppression of the semen.

spermatospore (spĕr-măt′ō-spor) [″ + *sporos,* a seed] Spermatogonium.

spermatotoxin (spĕr′mă-tō-tŏk′sĭn) [″ + *toxikon,* poison] Spermatoxin.

spermatoxin (spĕr″mă-tŏks′ĭn) [″ + *toxikon,* poison] A toxin that destroys spermatozoa. SYN: *spermatotoxin*.

spermatozoa (spĕr″măt-ō-zō′ă) Pl. of spermatozoon.

spermatozoal (spĕr″mă-tō-zō′ăl) [″ + *zoon,* life] Concerning spermatozoa.

spermatozoicide (spĕr″mă-tō-zō′ĭ-sīd) [″ + ″ + L. *cidus,* kill] Spermicide.

spermatozoon (spĕr″măt-ō-zō′ŏn) *pl.* **spermatozoa** [″ + *zoon,* life] The mature male sex or germ cell formed within the seminiferous tubules of the testes. The spermatozoon has a broad oval flattened head with a nucleus and a protoplasmic neck or middle piece and tail. It is about 51 μm long and resembles a tadpole. It has the power of self-propulsion by means of a flagellum. It develops after puberty from the spermatids in the testes in enormous quantities. The head pierces the envelope of the ovum and loses its tail when the two cells fuse. This process is called fertilization. SEE: illus.; *sperm* for illus.; *fertilization*.

spermaturia (spĕr″mă-tū′rē-ă) [″ + *ouron,* urine] Semen discharged with the urine.

spermectomy (spĕr-mĕk′tō-mē) [″ + *ektome,* excision] Resection of a portion of the spermatic cord and duct.

spermic (spĕr′mĭk) Concerning sperm, male reproductive cells.

spermicide (spĕr′mĭ-sīd) An agent that kills spermatozoa. Two spermicides used in contraceptive products are nonoxynol 9 and octoxynol 9. SYN: *spermaticide; spermatozoicide*. **spermicidal** (spĕr″mĭ-sīd′ăl), *adj.*

spermidine (spĕr′mĭ-dĭn) An amine present in semen.

spermiduct (spĕr′mĭ-dŭkt) [″ + L. *ductus,* a duct] The ejaculatory duct and ductus deferens considered as one.

spermine (spĕr′mĭn) An amine present in semen and other animal tissues.

spermiogenesis (spĕr″mē-ō-jĕn′ĕ-sĭs) The processes involved in the transformation of a spermatid to a functional spermatozoon.

spermiogram (spĕr′mē-ō-grăm) [″ + *gramma,* something written] A record of examining and classifying sperm in a semen sample.

spermoblast (spĕr′mō-blăst) [″ + *blastos,* a germ] Spermatid.

spermolith (spĕr′mō-lĭth) [″ + *lithos,* stone] A stone in the seminal vesicles or spermatic ducts.

spermolysin (spĕr-mŏl′ĭ-sĭn) A cytolysin formed following the inoculation of spermatozoa.

spermolytic (spĕr-mō-lĭt′ĭk) [″ + *lysis,* dissolution] Causing spermatozoa destruction.

spermoneuralgia (spĕr″mō-nū-răl′jē-ă) [″ + *neuron,* nerve, + *algos,* pain] Pain in the spermatic cord.

spermophlebectasia (spĕr″mō-flē″bĕk-tā′zē-ă) [″ + *phlebos,* vein, + *ektasis,* dilatation] Varicosity of the spermatic veins.

spermoplasm (spĕr′mō-plăzm) [″ + LL. *plasma,* form, mold] The cytoplasm of a male germ cell.

spermosphere (spĕr′mō-sfēr) [″ + *sphaira,* a circle] A mass of spermatids derived from spermatogonia.

spermospore (spĕr′mō-spor) [″ + *sporos,* seed] Spermatogonium.

spermotoxin (spĕr″mō-tŏk′sĭn) [″ + *toxikon,* poison] Spermatoxin.

sp. gr. *specific gravity.*

sph *spherical.*

sphacelate (sfăs′ĕl-āt) [Gr. *sphakelos,* gangrene] **1.** To develop gangrene. **2.** Gangrenous. SYN: *mortification; necrosis*.

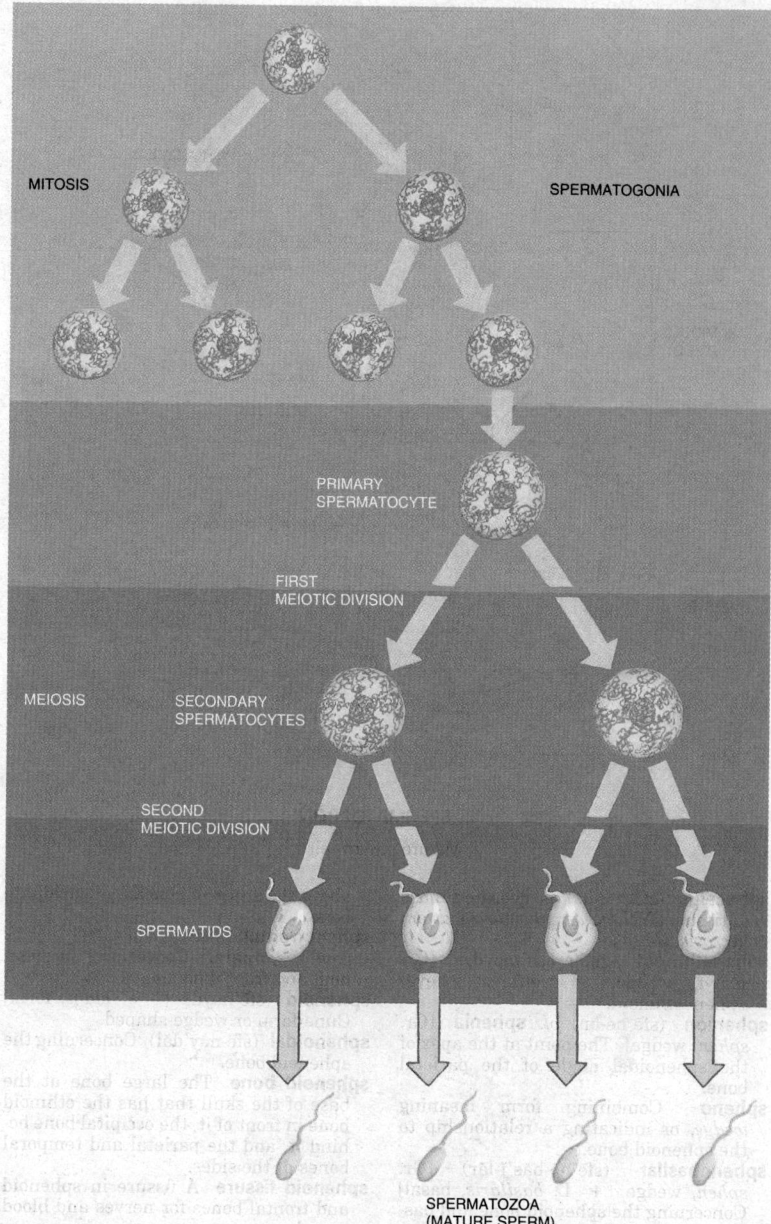

SPERMATOGENESIS

sphacelation (sfăs″ĕl-ā′shŭn) Mortification; formation of a mass of gangrenous tissue. SYN: *gangrene; necrosis*.

sphacelism (sfăs′ĕl-ĭzm) [″ + *-ismos*, condition] Condition of being affected with sphacelus or gangrene. SYN: *necrosis*.

sphaceloderma (sfăs″ĕl-ō-dĕr′mă) [″ + *derma*, skin] Gangrene of the skin. SEE: *Raynaud's disease*.

sphacelous (sfăs′ĕl-ŭs) [Gr. *sphakelos*, gangrene] Pert. to a slough or patch of gangrene. SYN: *gangrenous; necrosis; necrotic*.

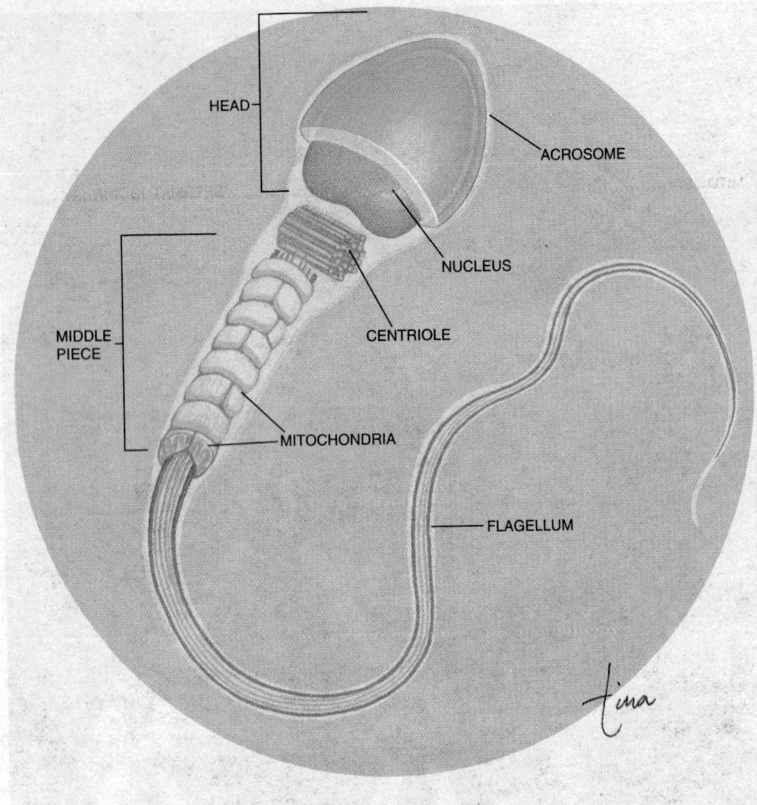

SPERMATOZOON

Mature sperm cell

sphacelus (sfăs′ĕl-ŭs) A necrosed mass of tissue. SYN: *gangrene; mortification; necrosis; slough*.

sphenethmoid (sfĕn-ĕth′moyd) [Gr. *sphen,* wedge, + *ethmos,* sieve] Sphenoethmoid.

sphenion (sfē′nē-ŏn) *pl.* **sphenia** [Gr. *sphen,* wedge] The point at the apex of the sphenoidal angle of the parietal bone.

spheno- Combining form meaning *wedge,* or indicating a relationship to the sphenoid bone.

sphenobasilar (sfē″nō-băs′ĭ-lăr) [Gr. *sphen,* wedge, + L. *basilaris,* basal] Concerning the sphenoid bone and basilar portion of the occipital bone.

sphenoccipital (sfē″nŏk-sĭp′ĭ-tăl) [″ + L. *occipitalis,* occipital] Concerning the sphenoid and occipital bones.

sphenocephalus (sfē″nō-sĕf′ă-lŭs) [″ + *kephale,* head] A deformed fetus in which the head is wedge-shaped.

sphenoethmoid (sfē″nō-ĕth′moyd) [″ + *ethmos,* sieve, + *eidos,* form, shape] Pert. to the sphenoid and ethmoid bones. SYN: *sphenethmoid*.

sphenoethmoid recess Groove back and above the superior concha, or turbinate bone.

sphenofrontal (sfē″nō-frŭn′tăl) [″ + L. *frontalis,* frontal] Concerning the sphenoid and frontal bones.

sphenoid (sfē′noyd) [″ + *eidos,* form] Cuneiform or wedge-shaped.

sphenoidal (sfē-noy′dăl) Concerning the sphenoid bone.

sphenoid bone The large bone at the base of the skull that has the ethmoid bone in front of it, the occipital bone behind it, and the parietal and temporal bones at the sides.

sphenoid fissure A fissure in sphenoid and frontal bones for nerves and blood vessels.

sphenoiditis (sfē″noy-dī′tĭs) [″ + ″ + *itis,* inflammation] **1.** Inflammation of the sphenoidal sinus. **2.** Necrosis of the sphenoid bone.

sphenoidostomy (sfē″noy-dŏs′tō-mē) [″ + ″ + *stoma,* mouth] Surgically producing an opening into the sphenoid sinus.

sphenoidotomy (sfē″noyd-ŏt′ō-mē) [″ + ″ + *tome,* incision] Incision into the sphenoid bone.

sphenomalar (sfē″nō-mā′lăr) [″ + L. *mala,* cheek] Concerning the sphenoid and malar bones.

sphenomaxillary (sfē″nō-măk′sĭ-lā-rē) [″ + L. *maxilla,* jawbone] Concerning the sphenoid bone and the maxilla.

spheno-occipital (sfē″nō-ŏk-sĭp′ĭ-tăl) [″ + L. *occipitalis,* occipital] Concerning the sphenoid and occipital bones.

sphenopalatine (sfē″nō-păl′ă-tēn) [″ + L. *palatum,* palate] Concerning the sphenoid and palatine bones.

sphenoparietal (sfē″nō-pă-rī′ĕ-tăl) [″ + L. *paries,* a wall] Concerning the sphenoid and parietal bones.

sphenorbital (sfē″nor′bĭ-tăl) [″ + L. *orbita,* track] Concerning the sphenoid bone and the orbits.

sphenosis [Gr., wedging] A condition in which the fetus becomes wedged in the pelvis.

sphenosquamosal (sfē″nō-skwā-mō′săl) [Gr. *sphen,* wedge, + L. *squamosa,* scaly] Concerning the sphenoid bone and the squamous portion of the temporal bone.

sphenotemporal (sfē″nō-tĕm′pō-răl) [″ + L. *temporalis,* temporal] Concerning the sphenoid and temporal bones.

sphenotic (sfē-nŏt′ĭk) [Gr. *sphen,* wedge, + *eidos,* form, shape] A fetal bone that becomes part of the sphenoid bone.

sphenotribe (sfē′nō-trīb) [″ + *tribein,* to crush] An instrument for breaking up the basal part of the fetal cranium.

sphenoturbinal (sfē″nō-tŭr′bĭ-năl) [″ + *turbo,* whirl] A thin curved bone anterior to each of the lesser wings of the sphenoid bone.

sphenovomerine (sfē″nō-vō′mĕr-ĭn) [″ + L. *vomer,* plowshare] Concerning the sphenoid and vomer bones.

sphenozygomatic (sfē″nō-zī″gō-măt′ĭk) [″ + *zygoma,* cheekbone] Concerning the sphenoid and zygomatic bones.

sphere (sfēr) [Gr. *sphaira,* a globe] A ball or globelike structure.

attraction s. A clear region in the cytoplasm close to the nucleus and usually containing a centriole or diplosome (a divided centriole).

segmentation s. The segmented ovum or morula.

spheresthesia (sfēr″ĕs-thē′zē-ă) [″ + *aisthesis,* sensation] An outdated term for globus hystericus.

spherical (sfĕr′ĭ-kăl) [Gr. *sphairikos*] Having the form of or pert. to a sphere. SYN: *globular*.

spherocylinder (sfē″rō-sĭl′ĭn-dĕr) [Gr. *sphaira,* globe, + *kylindros,* cylinder] A lens with a spherical surface and a cylindrical surface.

spherocyte (sfē′rō-sīt) [″ + *kytos,* cell] An erythrocyte that assumes a spheroid shape, and has no central pallor. SEE: illus.

spherocytosis (sfē″rō-sī-tō′sĭs) [″ + ″ + *osis,* condition] A condition in which erythrocytes assume a spheroid shape. It occurs in certain hemolytic anemias.

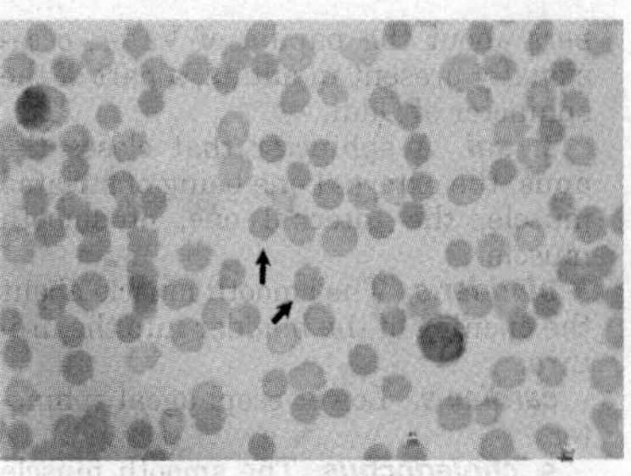

SPHEROCYTES

In peripheral blood (×400)

hereditary s. An autosomal dominant hemolytic anemia caused by a defect in the red blood cell membrane that makes the cell abnormally fragile and esp. susceptible to changes in the concentration of osmoles in the blood. Affected cells are gradually destroyed in the spleen, resulting in splenic enlargement, jaundice, and anemia, as well as a high incidence of gallstone disease. Surgical removal of the spleen prevents many of this condition's complications but carries with it a risk of postoperative immune suppression.

spheroid (sfē′royd) [″ + *eidos,* form, shape] **1.** A body shaped like a sphere. **2.** Sphere-shaped.

spheroidal (sfē-roy′dăl) Sphere-shaped.

spherolith (sfē′rō-lĭth) [″ + *lithos,* stone] A minute stone in the kidney of the newborn.

spheroma (sfē-rō′mă) [″ + *oma,* tumor] A tumor of spherical form.

spherometer (sfē-rŏm′ĕt-ĕr) [″ + *metron,* measure] A device to ascertain the curvature of a surface.

spheroplast (sfĕr′ō-plăst) In bacteriology, the cell and partial cell wall remaining after gram-negative organisms have been lysed. Spheroplasts may be formed when synthesis of the cell wall is prevented by the action of certain chemicals while cells are growing. SEE: *protoplast*.

spherospermia (sfē″rō-spĕr′mē-ă) [″ + *sperma,* seed] Round spermatozoa without tails.

spherule (sfĕr′ūl) [LL. *sphaerula,* little globe] **1.** A very small sphere. **2.** A minute granule found in the center of a centromere of a chromosome. **3.** The structures present in tissues infected with *Coccidioides immitis*. These spherules contain up to hundreds of endospores.

sphincter (sfĭngk′tĕr) [Gr. *sphinkter,* band] A circular muscle constricting an orifice. In normal tonic condition, it closes the orifice, that is, the muscle must relax to allow the orifice to open.

s. ampullae A delicate network of fibers about the papilla of Vater, occasionally present in adults, a part of the sphincter of Oddi.

s. ani A sphincter that closes the anus, the external one being of striated muscle, the internal one, of smooth muscle.

bladder s. The smooth muscle about the opening of the bladder into the urethra.

cardiac s. Lower esophageal sphincter.

s. choledochus The smooth muscle investing the common bile duct just before its junction with the pancreatic duct; a part of the sphincter of Oddi.

ileocecal s. A projection of the ileum into the cecum that acts as a sphincter. SEE: *valve, ileocecal.*

lower esophageal s. The smooth muscle around the opening of the esophagus into the stomach. SYN: *cardiac s.*

s. of Oddi A contracted region at the opening of the common bile duct into the duodenum at the papilla of Vater.

s. pancreaticus The smooth muscle encircling the pancreatic duct just before it joins the ampulla.

precapillary s. A smooth muscle cell found at the beginning of a capillary network. It regulates capillary blood flow according to the needs of the tissue. SEE: *artery* for illus.

pyloric s. The smooth muscle around the opening of the stomach into the duodenum.

sphincteral (sfĭngk′tĕr-ăl) Concerning a sphincter.

sphincteralgia (sfĭngk″tĕr-ăl′jē-ă) [Gr. *sphinkter,* band, + *algos,* pain] Pain in the sphincter ani muscles.

sphincterectomy (sfĭngk″tĕr-ĕk′tō-mē) [″ + *ektome,* excision] **1.** Excision of any sphincter muscle. **2.** Excision of part of the iris' pupillary border.

sphincteric (sfĭngk-tĕr′ĭk) Concerning a sphincter.

sphincterismus (sfĭngk″tĕr-ĭz′mŭs) [″ + *-ismos,* condition] A spasm of the sphincter ani muscles.

sphincteritis (sfĭngk″tĕr-ī′tĭs) [″ + *itis,* inflammation] Inflammation of any sphincter muscle.

sphincterolysis (sfĭngk″tĕr-ŏl′ĭ-sĭs) [″ + *lysis,* dissolution] Freeing of the iris from the cornea in anterior synechia affecting only the pupillary border.

sphincteroplasty (sfĭngk′tĕr-ō-plăs″tē) [″ + *plassein,* to form] Surgical repair of any sphincter.

sphincteroscope (sfĭngk′tĕr-ō-skōp″) [″ + *skopein,* to examine] An instrument for inspection of the anal sphincter.

sphincteroscopy (sfĭngk″tĕr-ŏs′kō-pē) Inspection of the internal anal sphincter.

sphincterotome (sfĭngk′tĕr-ō-tōm″) [″ + *tome,* incision] A surgical instrument for cutting a sphincter.

sphincterotomy (sfĭngk″tĕr-ŏt′ō-mē) [″ + *tome,* incision] The cutting of a sphincter muscle.

sphingolipid (sfĭng″gō-lĭp′ĭd) [Gr. *sphingein,* to bind, + *lipos,* fat] A lipid containing one of several long-chain bases such as sphingosine or dihydrosphingosine or bases of similar chemical structure but containing longer chains.

sphingolipidosis [″ + ″ + *osis,* condition] Any disease marked by a defective metabolism of sphingolipids. These genetically determined errors of metabolism include Sandhoff's disease, Fabry's disease, Tay-Sachs disease, Kufs' disease, Gaucher's disease, Krabbe's leukodystrophy, Niemann-Pick disease, Batten disease, and Spielmeyer-Vogt disease. They are marked by neurological deterioration, usually beginning a few months after birth and eventually leading to death except in the adult form of Gaucher's disease. These diseases can be detected by examining fluid obtained by amniocentesis.

sphingolipodystrophy (sfĭng″gō-lĭp″ō-dĭs′trō-fē) [″ + *dys,* bad, + *trophe,* nutrition] A group of diseases caused by defective sphingolipid metabolism.

sphingomyelins (sfĭng″gō-mī′ĕl-ĭns) A major group of phosphorus-containing sphingolipids. They are found primarily in nervous tissue and in lipids in the blood. They are derived from choline phosphate and a ceramide. Deficiencies in sphingomyelin manufacturing are found in many diseases. SEE: *sphingolipidosis.*

sphingosine (sfĭng′gō-sĭn) A long-chain base, $C_{18}H_{37}O_2N$, present in sphingolipids. SEE: *dihydrosphingosine; sphingolipid.*

sphygmic (sfĭg′mĭk) [Gr. *sphygmikos*] Rel. to the pulse.

sphygmo- Combining form meaning *pulse.*

sphygmobolometer (sfĭg″mō-bō-lŏm′ĕ-tĕr) [Gr. *sphygmos,* pulse, + *bolos,* mass, + *metron,* a measure] A device used to measure the force of the pulse rather than the blood pressure.

sphygmogram (sfĭg′mō-grăm) [″ + *gramma,* something written] A tracing of the pulse made by using the sphygmograph.

sphygmograph (sfĭg′mō-grăf) [″ + *graphein,* to write] Polygraph.

sphygmography (sfĭg-mŏg′ră-fē) Recording the arterial pulse by use of a polygraph.

sphygmoid (sfĭg′moyd) [Gr. *sphygmos,* pulse, + *eidos,* form, shape] Resembling the pulse.

sphygmology (sfĭg-mŏl′ō-jē) [″ + *logos,* word, reason] The scientific study of the pulse.

sphygmomanometer (sfĭg″mō-măn-ŏm′

ĕt-ĕr) [″ + *manos,* thin, + *metron,* measure] An instrument for determining arterial blood pressure indirectly. The two types are aneroid and mercury. SEE: *blood pressure.*

random-zero s. A special type of sphygmomanometer that allows the blood pressure to be taken without the observer's knowing where zero pressure is on the device. After the pressure is obtained, the mercury comes to rest at a point. The observed pressure is then corrected by subtracting the at-rest value on the device from the pressure obtained. Although this device was developed to prevent subjective bias in determining blood pressure, it is not necessarily effective in achieving this goal.

sphygmometer (sfĭg-mŏm′ĕt-ĕr) [″ + *metron,* measure] An instrument for measuring the pulse. SYN: *polygraph.*

sphygmopalpation (sfĭg″mō-păl-pā′shŭn) [″ + L. *palpatio,* palpation] Palpating the pulse.

sphygmoplethysmograph (sfĭg″mō-plĕth-ĭz′mō-grăf) [″ + *plethysmos,* to increase, + *graphein,* to write] A device that traces the pulse with its curve of fluctuation in volume.

sphygmus (sfĭg′mŭs) [Gr. *sphygmos,* pulse] A pulse or pulsation.

sphyrectomy (sfī-rĕk′tō-mē) [Gr. *sphyra,* malleus, + *ektome,* excision] Surgical excision of the malleolus of the ankle.

sphyrotomy (sfī-rŏt′ō-mē) [″ + *tome,* incision] Surgical excision of a portion of the malleolus of the ankle.

spica (spī′kă) [L., ear of grain] SEE: *bandage, spica.*

spica hip cast A cast containing the lower torso and extending to one or both lower extremities. If only one lower extremity is included, it is called a single hip spica; if two are included, it is called a double hip spica. These are used for treating pelvic and femoral fractures.

spicular (spĭk′ū-lar) [L. *spiculum,* a dart] Pert. to or resembling a spicule; dartlike.

spicule (spĭk′ūl) A small, needle-shaped body. SYN: *spiculum.*

bony s. A needle-shaped fragment of bone.

cemental s. An excementosis or pointed protuberance extending from the surface cementum of a tooth root.

spiculed red cell Crenated red blood cells with surface projections. In most instances, this is a normal variation in red cell equilibrium and is reversible. SEE: *acanthocyte.*

spiculum (spĭk′ū-lŭm) *pl.* **spicula** [L., a dart] Spicule.

spider (spī′dĕr) **1.** An arachnid, belonging to the order Araneae, class Arachnida, phylum Arthropoda. The body is divided into cephalothorax and abdomen joined by a narrow waist. A spider usually possesses four pairs of legs as well as poison fangs. It often possesses spinnerets. **2.** Anything resembling a spider in appearance.

arterial s. SEE: *spider nevus.*

s. bite Punctures of the skin and/or envenomation by the fangs of a spider. SEE: *black widow s.; brown recluse s.*

black widow s. The female of *Latrodectus mactans.* It is native to the southern U.S. but has been reported throughout the country. It is glossy black with a brilliant red or yellow spot, usually shaped like an hourglass or two triangles, on the undersurface of the abdomen. Its body measures about 1 cm and its leg spread can reach 5 cm.

The bite of a black widow spider initially produces a sensation resembling the prick of a pin and may be mistaken for a flea bite. A numbing pain usually lasts for a short time and then subsides; later the abdominal muscles become rigid and the patient becomes severely diaphoretic. Within 1/2 hr, severe abdominal cramps begin. The venom, which is neurotoxic, causes an ascending motor paralysis. Because of the extreme abdominal pain, the patient may be suspected of having an acute condition requiring abdominal surgery. Severe cases, esp. in children, can result in death; however, healthy patients usually respond to treatment, and most victims recover completely.

PATIENT CARE: Stimulant drugs should not be given to patients who have been bitten by a black widow spider. Suction is of little value as the toxin is rapidly absorbed. Symptomatic treatments include benzodiazepines and opiates. Tetanus prophylaxis should be administered. Specific antivenins may be used when envenomation has severe neurological consequences.

CAUTION: Respiratory status must be carefully monitored when morphine or a benzodiazepine is used. There is risk of acute hypersensitivity and delayed serum sickness when the antivenin *Latrodectus mactans* is used.

---

brown recluse s. *Loxosceles reclusa,* 3/8-in. (10-mm) long spider native to North America. The venom of the brown recluse spider is toxic and can be lethal. It may produce a large area of necrosis at the site of the bite.

TREATMENT: Dapsone, antivenins, and steroids are often used to treat the envenomation; however, before using dapsone, the patient should be tested for glucose-6-phosphate dehydrogenase deficiency. Tetanus prophylaxis should be administered.

spider-burst An area on the leg in which

capillaries radiate from a central point. The veins, though dilated, are not varicosities.

spider fingers Arachnodactyly.

Spielmeyer-Vogt disease [Walter Spielmeyer, Ger. neurologist, 1879–1935; Oskar Vogt, Ger. neurologist, 1870–1959] Batten disease.

spigelian line (spī-jē′lē-ăn) [Adriaan van den Spieghel, Flemish anatomist, 1578–1625] A line on the abdomen lying parallel to the median line and marking the edge of the rectus abdominis muscle. SYN: *linea semilunaris; semilunar line*.

spigelian lobe A small lobe behind the right lobe of the liver.

spike **1.** The dominant peak in the record of an action potential or electroencephalogram. **2.** The narrow vertical tracing left on an electrocardiogram by the impulse generator of an electronic pacemaker.

spikeboard An adapted device for persons with limited upper extremity or one-handed function that allows food to be held in place while it is being prepared.

spike and wave Electroencephalic evidence of grand mal seizures.

spill (spĭl) [AS. *spillan,* to squander] An overflow.

cellular s. A dissemination of cells through the lymph or the blood resulting in metastasis.

radioactive s. A release of radioactive materials into the environment. SEE: *accident, radiation*.

spillway (spĭl′way) The contour of the teeth that allows food to escape from the cusps during mastication.

spiloma, spilus (spī-lō′mă, spī′lŭs) [Gr. *spiloma, spilos,* spot] Nevus.

spina (spī′nă) *pl.* **spinae** [L., thorn] **1.** Any spinelike protuberance. **2.** The spine.

s. bifida Spina bifida cystica.

s. bifida cystica A congenital defect in the walls of the spinal canal caused by a lack of union between the laminae of the vertebrae. The lumbar portion is the section chiefly affected. The consequences of this defect may include urinary incontinence, saddle or limb anesthesia, gait disturbances, and structural changes in the pelvis. SYN: *rachischisis*.

s. bifida occulta A failure of the vertebrae to close, without hernial protrusion.

spinal (spī′năl) [L. *spinalis*] Pert. to the spine or spinal cord. SYN: *rachial; rachidial*.

spinal accessory nerve Accessory nerve.

spinal cord Part of the central nervous system, the spinal cord is an ovoid column of nerve tissue 40 to 50 cm long that extends from the medulla to the second lumbar vertebra; it is within the spinal (vertebral) canal, protected by bone and directly enclosed in the meninges. The center of the cord is gray matter in the shape of the letter H; it consists of the cell bodies and dendrites of neurons. The ventral (anterior) horns of the gray matter contain cell bodies of somatic motor neurons; the dorsal (posterior) horns contain cell bodies of interneurons. The white matter is arranged in tracts around the gray matter. It consists of myelinated axons that transmit impulses to and from the brain, or between levels of gray matter in the spinal cord, or that will leave the cord as part of peripheral nerves. The spinal cord is the pathway for sensory impulses to the brain and motor impulses from the brain; it also mediates stretch reflexes and the defecation and urination reflexes. Thirty-one pairs of spinal nerves emerge from the spinal cord and innervate the trunk and limbs. SEE: illus.

spinal cord injury, acute Acute traumatic injury of the spinal cord. Therapy for this condition includes immobilization, high doses of corticosteroids, airway maintenance, cardiovascular resuscitation, and insertion of an indwelling catheter. The use of intravenous methylprednisolone given as a bolus dose of 30 mg/kg and then a maintenance dose of 5.4 mg/kg/hr during the acute phase improves neurological recovery.

PATIENT CARE: The patient who suffers serious trauma to the spinal cord may suddenly confront many challenges to body image and functional independence, including changes in mobility, urinary and fecal continence, erectile function, skin integrity, and mood. A sensitive and caring multidisciplinary approach to rehabilitation is needed to help the client resume an active and fulfilling life.

spinal curvature Abnormal curvature of the spine, frequently constitutional in children. It may be angular, lateral (scoliosis), or anteroposterior (kyphosis, lordosis).

spinal curvature, angular Pott's disease.

spinal curvature, lateral Scoliosis.

spinal fusion Surgical immobilization of adjacent vertebrae. This procedure may be done for several conditions, including herniated disk.

spinal ganglion An enlargement on the dorsal or posterior root of a spinal nerve, composed principally of cell bodies of somatic and visceral afferent neurons. Also called *dorsal root ganglion*.

spinalgia (spī-năl′jē-ă) [L. *spina,* thorn, + Gr. *algos,* pain] Pain in a vertebra under pressure.

spinalis (spī-nā′lĭs) [L.] A muscle attached to the spinal process of a vertebra.

spinal nerve One of the nerves arising from the spinal cord: 31 pairs, consist-

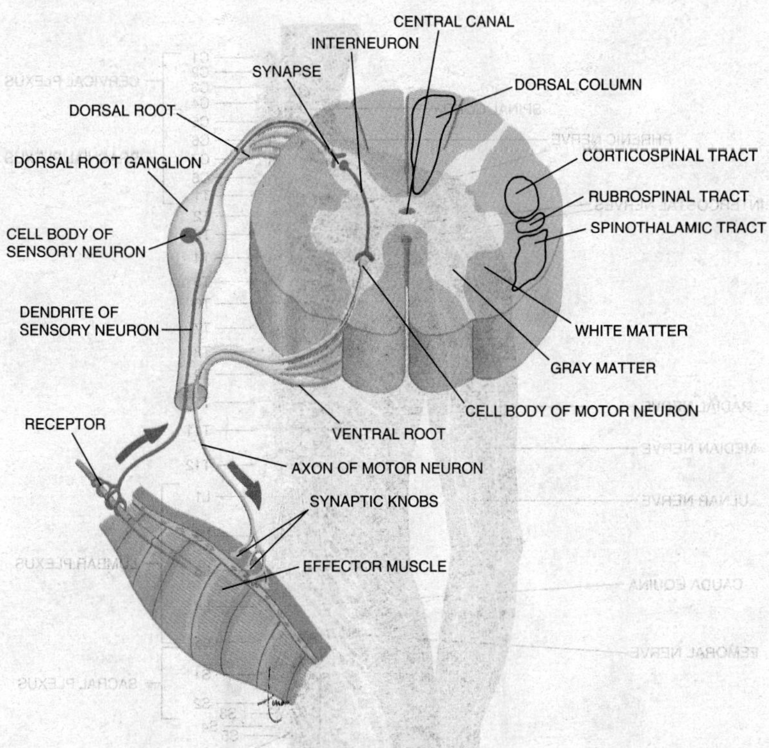

SPINAL CORD

Cross-section with nerve roots on left side and examples of tracts on right side

ing of eight cervical, 12 thoracic, five lumbar, five sacral, and one coccygeal, corresponding with the spinal vertebrae. Each spinal nerve is attached to the spinal cord by two roots: a dorsal or posterior sensory root and a ventral or anterior motor root. The former consists of afferent fibers conveying impulses to the cord; the latter of efferent fibers conveying impulses from the cord. A typical spinal nerve, on passing through the intervertebral foramen, divides into four branches, a recurrent branch, a dorsal ramus or posterior primary division, a ventral ramus or anterior primary division, and two rami communicantes (white and gray), which pass to ganglia of the sympathethic trunk. SEE: illus.

spinate (spī′nāt) Having spines or shaped like a thorn.

spindle (spĭn′dl) [AS. *spinel*] **1.** A fusiform-shaped body. **2.** The mitotic spindle, a series of microtubules formed by the centrosomes during cell division; the spindle fibers pull the new sets of chromosomes toward opposite poles of the cell.

aortic s. A dilatation of the aorta following the aortic isthmus.

enamel s. A tubular hypomineralized structure extending a short distance from the dentinoenamel junction into enamel, seen in ground sections of teeth.

muscle s. A specialized sensory fiber within a muscle that is sensitive to tension and changes in length of the muscle. The central region consists of a nuclear bag with primary or annulospiral receptor endings, and several nuclear chains with primary endings and secondary, or flower spray, endings. Each end consists of intrafusal muscle fibers innervated by gamma motor nerves. When these fibers contract, tension on the central bag and chains results in feedback to the muscle fibers outside the muscle spindle, causing them to contract.

neuromuscular s. A complex sensory nerve ending consisting of muscle fibers enclosed within a capsule and supplied by an afferent nerve fiber. It mediates proprioceptive sensations and reflexes.

neurotendinous s. A proprioceptive nerve ending found in a tendon, in muscle septa or sheaths, in muscle tissue, or at the junction of a muscle and tendon. SYN: *Golgi tendon organ*.

sleep s. Specific waves that appear in the electroencephalogram during light or early sleep.

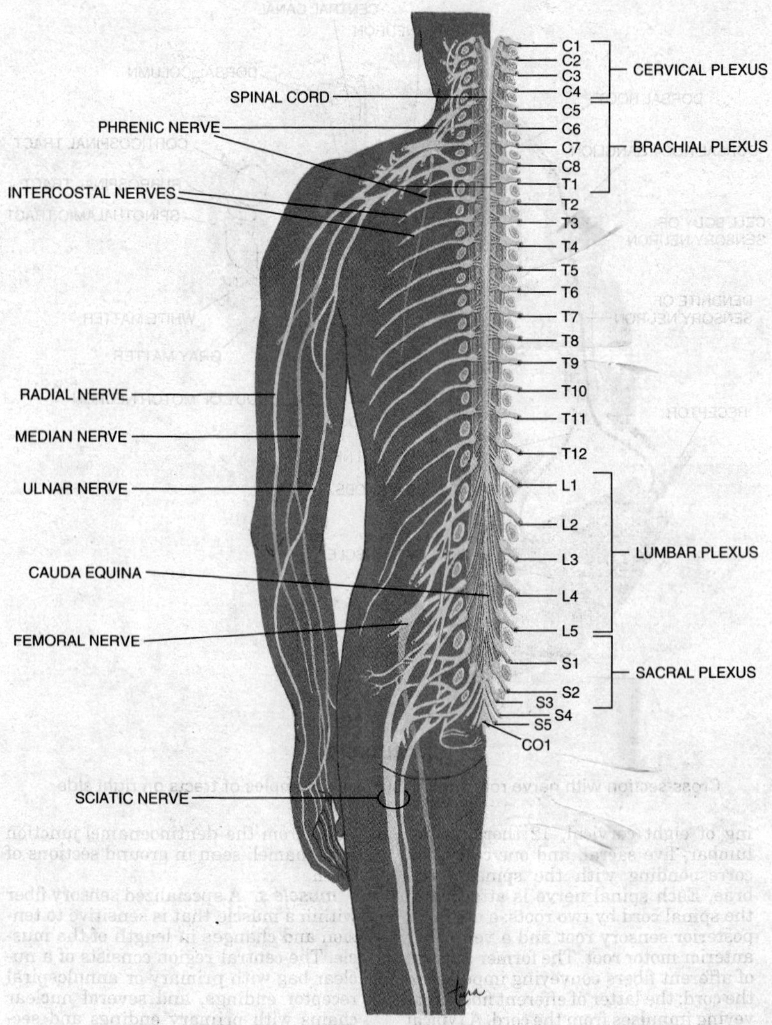

SPINAL NERVES

Left side

spine (spīn) **1.** A sharp process of bone. **2.** The spinal column, consisting of 33 vertebrae: seven cervical, 12 thoracic, five lumbar, five sacral, and four coccygeal. The bones of the sacrum and coccyx are ankylosed in adult life and counted as one each. SYN: *backbone*.

alar s. The spinous process of the sphenoid bone.

anterior nasal s. The projection formed by the anterior prolongation of the inferior border of the nasal notch of the maxilla.

bifid s. SEE: *spina bifida cystica; spina bifida occulta*.

fracture of the s. Fracture of a vertebral body or its bony prominences. SEE: *hangman's fracture; Jefferson fracture*.

TREATMENT: The patient is carefully assessed for evidence of neuromuscular compromise and other internal injuries. To prevent complications and promote healing, vests, casts, or halo devices may be used depending on the location of the fracture. A program of supervised physical therapy may be needed during recovery.

PROGNOSIS: Prognosis depends on the type of spinal fracture and associated spinal cord involvement.

frontal s. A sharp-pointed medial

process extending downward from the nasal process of the frontal bone. SYN: *nasal s.*

hemal s. That part of the hemal arch of a typical vertebra that closes it in.

Henle's s. Suprameatal s.

iliac s. One of four spines of the ilium; namely, the anterior and posterior inferior spines and the anterior and posterior superior spines.

ischial s. The spine of the ischium, a pointed eminence on its posterior border.

mandibular s. The small, tongue-shaped protuberance on the medial aspect of the mandibular ramus near the mandibular foramen, to which the sphenomandibular ligament is attached.

mental s. A small process on the inner surface of the mandible at the back of the symphysis formed of one or more small projections (genial tubercles).

nasal s. Frontal s.

neural s. The spinous process of a vertebra; the posterior projection of the neural arch.

pharyngeal s. The ridge under the basilar process of the occipital bone.

posterior nasal s. The spine formed by medial ends of the horizontal processes of the palatine bones.

s. of pubis A prominent tubercle on the upper border of the pubis.

s. of scapula An osseous plate projecting from the posterior surface of the scapula.

s. of sphenoid The spinous process of the greater sphenoid wing.

suprameatal s. A small spine at the junction of the superior and posterior walls of the external auditory meatus. SYN: *Henle's s.*

typhoid s. An acute arthritis due to infection causing spinal ankylosis during or following typhoid fever.

spinifugal (spī-nĭf′ū-găl) [L. *spina,* thorn, + *fugare,* to flee] Conducting nerve impulses away from the spinal cord.

spinipetal (spī-nĭp′ĕ-tăl) [″ + *petere,* to seek] Conducting nerve impulses toward the spinal cord.

spinnbarkeit (spĭn′băr-kīt) [Ger.] ABBR: SBK. Evaluation of the elasticity of cervical mucus used to determine time of ovulation. The cervical secretion is aspirated and placed on a slide. SBK is measured by pulling upward on the secretion with a forceps. Before ovulation, there is no elasticity. On the day of ovulation, elasticity is good, measuring 12 to 24 cm or more. The day after ovulation, elasticity diminishes. Not all women have clear-cut SBK changes. Therefore, this test is used in conjunction with other signs of ovulation. SEE: *basal temperature chart; ferning; mittelschmerz; mucorrhea.*

spinobulbar (spī″nō-bŭl′băr) [″ + Gr. *bulbos,* a bulb] Concerning the spinal cord and medulla oblongata.

spinocellular (spī″nō-sĕl′ū-lăr) [″ + *cellula,* little cell] Pert. to or like prickle cells.

spinocerebellar (spī″nō-sĕr-ĕ-bĕl′ăr) [″ + *cerebellum,* little brain] Concerning the spinal cord and cerebellum.

spinocortical (spī″nō-kor′tĭ-kăl) [″ + *cortex,* rind] Pert. to the spinal cord and cerebral cortex.

spinocostalis (spī″nō-kŏs-tā′lĭs) [″ + *costa,* rib] The combination of the superior and inferior serratus muscles.

spinoglenoid (spī″nō-glĕn′oyd) [″ + Gr. *glene,* socket, + *eidos,* form, shape] Rel. to the spine of the scapula and the glenoid cavity.

spinoglenoid ligament The ligament joining the spine of the scapula to the border of the glenoid cavity.

spinose (spī′nōs) [L. *spina,* thorn] Spinous.

spinotectal (spī″nō-tĕk′tăl) [″ + *tectum,* roof] Pert. to the spinal cord and the tectum, the dorsal portion (corpora quadrigemina) of the midbrain.

spinous (spī′nŭs) [L. *spina,* thorn] Pert. to or resembling a spine. SYN: *spinose.*

spinous point A spot over a spinous process very sensitive to pressure.

spinous process The prominence at the posterior part of each vertebra.

spintheropia (spĭn″thĕr-ō′pē-ă) [Gr. *spinther,* spark, + *ops,* eye] A sensation of sparks before the eyes. SEE: *Moore's lightning streaks.*

spiradenitis (spī″răd-ĕn-ī′tĭs) [Gr. *speira,* coil, + *aden,* gland, + *itis,* inflammation] A funiculus beginning in the coil of a sweat gland. SEE: *hidrosadenitis.*

spiradenoma (spī″răd-ĕn-ō′mă) [″ + ″ + *oma,* tumor] A benign tumor of the sweat glands. SYN: *spiroma.*

spiral (spī′răl) [L. *spiralis*] Coiling around a center like the thread of a screw.

Curschmann's s. SEE: *Curschmann's spirals.*

spiral bandage A roller bandage to be applied spirally.

spiral lamina A thin, bony plate projecting from the modiolus into the cochlear canal, dividing it into two portions, the upper scala vestibuli and lower scala tympani. Also called *lamina spiralis.*

spirillicidal (spī-rĭl″ĭ-sīd′ăl) [L. *spirillum,* coil, + *cidus,* kill] Destructive to spirochetes or spirilla.

spirillicide (spī-rĭl″ĭ-sīd) An agent that is destructive to spirilla.

spirillolysis (spī″rĭ-lŏl′ĭ-sĭs) [″ + Gr. *lysis,* dissolution] The destruction of spirilla.

spirillosis (spī-rĭl-ō′sĭs) [″ + Gr. *osis,* condition] A disease caused by the presence of spirilla in the blood.

spirillotropic (spī″rĭ-lō-trŏp′ĭk) [″ + Gr. *trope,* a turning] Having an attraction to spirilla.

spirillotropism (spī″rĭ-lŏt′rō-pĭzm) [″ + ″ + *-ismos,* condition] The ability to attract spirilla.

Spirillum (spī-rĭl′ŭm) [L., coil] A genus of spiral-shaped motile microorganisms belonging to the family Pseudomonadaceae, tribe Spirilleae. They are found in fresh water and salt water.

S. minus A species found in the blood of rats and mice; the causative agent of one form of rat-bite fever.

spirillum *pl.* **spirilla** A flagellated aerobic bacterium with an elongated spiral shape, of the genus *Spirillum.* SEE: *bacteria* for illus.

spirit (spĭr′ĭt) [L. *spiritus,* breath] **1.** A solution of essential or volatile liquid. **2.** Any distilled or volatile liquid. **3.** An alcoholic beverage. **4.** Mood; courage.

s. of ammonia A pungent solution of approx. 4% ammonium carbonate in 70% alcohol flavored with lemon, lavender, and myristica oil. It is used to elicit reflex stimulation of respiration and as smelling salts to stimulate patients who have fainted.

s. of bitter almond A mixture of oil of bitter almond, almond, and distilled water, used as a flavoring agent.

s. of camphor A mixture of camphor and alcohol, employed locally as a counterirritant.

s. of juniper A mixture of oil of juniper and alcohol.

s. of lavender A mixture of oil of lavender flowers and alcohol, used as a flavoring agent.

s. of mustard A solution of volatile oil of mustard in alcohol, used as a counterirritant.

s. of peppermint A mixture of oil of peppermint, peppermint, and alcohol, used as a carminative.

spiritual distress A crisis in faith; a disruption of belief in god, religion, or spirituality.

risk for s.d. At risk for an altered sense of harmonious connectedness with all of life and the universe in which dimensions that transcend and empower the self may be disrupted. SEE: *Nursing Diagnoses Appendix.*

spiritual well-being, enhanced, potential for The potential for personal satisfaction that may accrue to some persons as a result of religious practices or beliefs. SEE: *Nursing Diagnoses Appendix.*

spirituous (spĭr′ĭt-ū-ŭs″) [L., *spiritus,* breath] Containing alcohol.

Spirochaeta (spī″rō-kē′tă) [Gr. *speira,* coil, + *chaite,* hair] A genus of slender, spiral, motile microorganisms belonging to the family Spirochaetaceae, order Spirochaetales.

S. icterohaemorrhagiae An obsolete name for *Leptospira interrogans,* the bacterium that causes leptospirosis.

S. pallida An obsolete name for *Treponema pallidum,* the bacteria that causes syphilis.

Spirochaetales (spī″rō-kē-tā′lēs) An order of slender spiral organisms belonging to the class Scotobacteria. It includes the families Spirochaetaceae and Treponemataceae.

spirochetalytic (spī″rō-kē″tă-lĭt′ĭk) [″ + ″ + *lysis,* dissolution] Destructive to spirochetes.

spirochete (spī′rō-kēt) Any member of the order Spirochaetales. **spirochetal,** *adj.*

spirochetemia (spī″rō-kē-tē′mē-ă) [″ + *chaite,* hair, + *haima,* blood] Spirochetes in the blood.

spirocheticidal (spī″rō-kē″tĭ-sī′dăl) [″ + ″ + L. *cidus,* kill] Destructive to spirochetes.

spirocheticide (spī″rō-kē′tĭ-sīd) Anything that destroys spirochetes.

spirochetolysis (spī″rō-kē-tŏl′ĭ-sĭs) [″ + *chaite,* hair, + *lysis,* dissolution] The destruction of spirochetes by specific antibodies, chemotherapy, or lysins.

spirochetosis (spī″rō-kē-tō′sĭs) [″ + ″ + *osis,* condition] Any infection caused by spirochetes.

spirochetotic (spī″rō-kē-tŏt′ĭk) Pert. to or marked by spirochetosis.

spirocheturia (spī″rō-kē-tū′rē-ă) [Gr. *speira,* coil, + *chaite,* hair, + *ouron,* urine] Spirochetes in the urine.

spirogram (spī′rō-grăm″) [L. *spirare,* to breathe, + Gr. *gramma,* something written] A record made by a spirograph, demonstrating lung volumes and air flow.

spirograph (spī′rō-grăf) [″ + Gr. *graphein,* to write] A graphic record of respiratory movements.

spiroid (spī′royd) [Gr. *speira,* coil, + *eidos,* form, shape] Resembling a spiral.

spiroma (spī-rō′mă) [″ + *oma,* tumor] Multiple, benign, cystic epithelioma of the sweat glands. SYN: *spiradenoma.*

spirometer (spī-rŏm′ĕt-ĕr) [L. *spirare,* to breathe, + Gr. *metron,* measure] An apparatus used to measure lung volumes and airflow. The following are typical measurements made on adult patients by using the spirometer: inspiratory reserve volume: the amount that a subject can still inhale by special effort after a normal inspiration; expiratory reserve volume: the volume of air that can still be exhaled after a normal exhalation; tidal volume: the volume of air exhaled or inhaled during normal breathing; vital capacity: the maximum volume of air that can be exhaled after a maximal inhalation; forced vital capacity or forced expiratory volume: the air that can be exhaled during a maximal exhalation.

spirometry (spī-rŏm′ĕ-trē) [L. *spirare,* to breathe, + Gr. *metron,* measure] Measurement of air flow and lung volumes.

incentive s. Spirometry in which visual and vocal stimuli are given to the patient to produce maximum effort during deep breathing. Incentive spirometry is used most often in postoperative patients to prevent atelectasis.

spironolactone (spī-rō″nō-lăk′tōn) A diuretic and antihypertensive drug that blocks the action of aldosterone on the renal tubules. It acts to decrease potassium loss in the urine.

spissated (spĭs′āt-ĕd) [L. *spissatus*] Inspissated.

spissitude (spĭs′ĭ-tūd) [L. *spissitudo*] The condition of being inspissated, as a fluid thickened by evaporation almost to a solid; thickness.

spit (spĭt) [AS. *spittan*] **1.** Saliva. **2.** To expectorate spittle.

spittle [AS. *spatl*] Saliva.

splanchna (splăngk′nă) [Gr.] The viscera.

splanchnapophysis (splăngk″nă-pŏf′ĭ-sĭs) [Gr. *splanchnos,* viscus, + *apophysis,* offshoot] Any bone involved in the function of the alimentary canal, such as the lower jaw.

splanchnectopia (splăngk″nĕk-tō′pē-ă) [″ + *ektopos,* out of place] Dislocation of a viscus or of the viscera.

splanchnemphraxis (splăngk″nĕm-frăk′sĭs) [″ + *emphraxis,* stoppage] Obstruction of any internal organ, particularly the intestine.

splanchnesthesia (splăngk″nĕs-thē′zē-ă) [″ + *aisthesis,* sensation] Visceral sensation.

splanchnesthetic (splăngk″nĕs-thĕt′ĭk) Rel. to visceral consciousness or sensation.

splanchnic (splăngk′nĭk) [Gr. *splanchnikos*] Pert. to the viscera.

splanchnicectomy (splăngk″nē-sĕk′tō-mē) [Gr. *splanchnos,* viscus, + *ektome,* excision] Resection of the splanchnic nerves.

splanchnicotomy (splăngk″nĭ-kŏt′ō-mē) [″ + *tome,* incision] Section of a splanchnic nerve.

splanchnoblast (splăngk′nō-blăst) [″ + *blastos,* germ] Incipient rudiment of a viscus. SEE: *anlage; proton.*

splanchnocele (splăngk′nō-sēl) [″ + *koilos,* a cavity] That part of the coelom persisting in the adult, giving rise to the visceral cavities. SYN: *splanchnocoele.*

splanchnocele (splăngk′nō-sēl) [″ + *kele,* tumor, swelling] Protrusion of any abdominal viscus.

splanchnocoele (splăngk′nō-sēl) [″ + *koilos,* a cavity] Rudimentary embryonic cavity from which the visceral cavities arise. SYN: *splanchnocele.*

splanchnocranium (splăngk″nō-krā′nē-ŭm) [″ + *kranion,* skull] Viscerocranium.

splanchnodiastasis (splăngk″nō-dī-ăs′tă-sĭs) [″ + *diastasis,* a separation] Displacement or separation of any viscus.

splanchnography (splăngk-nŏg′ră-fē) [″ + *graphein,* to write] Examination of the viscera using fluoroscopy or transillumination.

splanchnolith (splăngk′nō-lĭth) [″ + *lithos,* stone] An outdated term for a stone in any visceral organ, such as the intestines.

splanchnology (splăngk-nŏl′ō-jē) [″ + *logos,* word, reason] The study of the viscera.

splanchnomegaly (splăngk″nō-mĕg′ă-lē) [″ + *megas,* large] Visceromegaly.

splanchnomicria (splăngk″nō-mĭk′rē-ă) [″ + *mikros,* small] The condition of having small splanchnic organs.

splanchnopathia (splăngk″nō-păth′ē-ă) [″ + *pathos,* disease, suffering] Pathological conditions of the viscera.

splanchnopleural (splăngk″nō-ploor′ăl) [″ + *pleura,* side] Concerning the splanchnopleure.

splanchnopleure (splăngk′nō-plūr) [″ + *pleura,* side] The embryonic layer formed by the union of the visceral layer of the mesoderm with the endoderm. SEE: *somatopleure.*

splanchnoptosia, splanchnoptosis (splăngk″nō-tō′sē-ă, -sĭs) [″ + *ptosis,* a dropping] Prolapse of the viscera. SYN: *enteroptosis; visceroptosis.*

splanchnosclerosis (splăngk″nō-sklĕr-ō′sĭs) [″ + *sklerosis,* to harden] A hardening of any of the viscera through overgrowth or infiltration of connective tissue.

splanchnoscopy (splăngk-nŏs′kō-pē) [″ + *skopein,* to examine] An obsolete technique of examining the viscera using x-rays or transillumination.

splanchnoskeleton (splăngk″nō-skĕl′ĕ-tŏn) [″ + *skeleton,* a dried-up body] **1.** In primitive vertebrates such as fishes, the cartilaginous or bony arches (branchial) that encircle the pharyngeal portion of the digestive tract. **2.** In higher vertebrates, the bones derived from the branchial arches, which include the maxilla, mandible, malleus, incus, stapes, hyoid bone, and cartilages of the larynx.

splanchnosomatic (splăngk″nō-sō-măt′ĭk) [″ + *soma,* body] Viscerosomatic.

splanchnotomy (splăngk-nŏt′ō-mē) [″ + *tome,* incision] Dissection of the viscera.

splanchnotribe (splăngk′nō-trīb) [″ + *tribein,* to rub] A crushing instrument formerly used to close the lumen of the intestine before surgically removing the organ.

splayfoot [ME. *splayen,* to spread out, + AS. *fot,* foot] Flatfoot.

spleen (splēn) [Gr. *splen*] A dark red, oval lymphoid organ in the upper left abdominal quadrant posterior and slightly inferior to the stomach; on the inferior side is the hilus, an indentation at which the splenic vessels and nerves enter or exit. The spleen is surrounded by an outer capsule of connective tissue from which strands of connective tissue (trabeculae) extend into the soft pulp (functional tissue), dividing the spleen into compartments.

The white pulp, composed of lymphocytes and follicles, forms sheaths around arterial vessels and collects in larger nodules containing germinal centers. The red pulp contains vascular sinuses and sinusoids with highly permeable walls, and spongelike splenic cords filled with macrophages and dendritic cells. The spleen is part of the mononuclear phagocytic system and its removal (splenectomy), though compensated for by the lymph nodes and liver, decreases immune function and may place the patient at increased risk for infection, esp. from *Streptococcus pneumoniae* and *Haemophilus influenzae*.

FUNCTION: In the embryo, the spleen forms both red and white blood cells; after birth, only lymphocytes are created except in severe anemia, when production of red blood cells may be reactivated. Blood enters via the splenic artery and passes through progressively smaller arterial vessels; foreign antigens are trapped in the white pulp, initiating proliferation of antigen-specific lymphocytes and antibodies. The arterioles terminate in the red pulp, where macrophages remove cell debris, microorganisms, and cells that are old, damaged, abnormal, or coated with antibody.

The vascular capacity of the spleen, 100 ml to 300 ml, is an average of 4% of the total blood, and the spleen may contain 30% of the total platelets. In stressful situations, sympathetic impulses stimulate constriction of the venous sinuses, forcing most of the splenic blood into circulation. If the spleen is enlarged (splenomegaly), its vascular capacity increases dramatically, and increased contact with macrophages may cause anemia, leukopenia, and thrombocytopenia. Removal of the spleen may be necessary in patients with thrombocytopenia. Many disorders cause splenomegaly, including portal hypertension (e.g., in cirrhosis), heart failure, and certain infections. Primary disorders of the spleen, however, are rare. SEE: *lymphatic system* for illus; *asplenia syndrome; germinal center*.

accessory s. Splenic tissue found outside the main bulk of the organ, usually, but not always, within the peritoneal cavity. If the patient is asymptomatic, the accessory spleen may be found only as an incidental mass on an abdominal scan; alternatively, the condition may exacerbate certain illnesses (e.g., immune thrombocytopenic purpura).

floating s. An enlarged movable spleen that is not protected by the ribs. SYN: *splenectopia*.

lardaceous s. An enlarged spleen resulting from fatty tissue. SEE: *amyloid degeneration*.

sago s. A spleen having the appearance of grains of sago.

splenadenoma (splĕn″ăd-ĕ-nō′mă) [Gr. *splen,* spleen, + *aden,* gland, + *oma,* tumor] An enlarged spleen caused by hyperplasia of its pulp.

splenalgia (splē-năl′jē-ă) [″ + *algos,* pain] Neuralgic pain in the spleen. SYN: *splenodynia*.

splenceratosis (splĕn″sĕr-ă-tō′sĭs) [″ + *keras,* horn, + *osis,* condition] Induration of the spleen.

splenectasia, splenectasis (splē″nĕk-tā′zē-ă, splē-nĕk′tă-sĭs) [″ + *ektasis,* dilatation] Enlargement of the spleen.

splenectomy (splē-nĕk′tō-mē) [″ + *ektome,* excision] **1.** Surgical removal of the spleen. Because of the importance of the spleen in the control of encapsulated bacteria in the bloodstream, all patients treated with splenectomy should be given a pneumococcal vaccine preoperatively. Children under age 10 have the highest risk of postsplenectomy sepsis. **2.** Obliteration of the spleen by trauma or illnesses (e.g., sickle cell anemia).

splenectopia, splenectopy (splē″nĕk-tō′pē-ă, -nĕk′tō-pē) [″ + *ektopos,* out of place] Floating spleen.

splenelcosis (splē″nĕl-kō′sĭs) [″ + *helkosis,* ulceration] Ulceration or abscess of the spleen.

splenemia (splē-nē′mē-ă) [Gr. *splen,* spleen, + *haima,* blood] **1.** Splenic congestion with blood. **2.** Leukemia with splenic hypertrophy.

splenemphraxis (splē″nĕm-frăk′sĭs) [″ + *emphraxis,* an obstruction] Splenic congestion.

spleneolus (splē-nē′ō-lŭs) Accessory spleen.

splenetic Splenic.

splenial (splē′nē-ăl) [Gr. *splen,* spleen] Concerning the spleen.

splenic (splĕn′ĭk) [Gr. *splenikos*] **1.** Pert. to the spleen. **2.** Suffering with chronic disease of the spleen. **3.** Surly, fretful, impatient.

splenic cord A spongelike cord in the red pulp of the spleen composed of macrophages and dendritic cells. The macrophages phagocytize pathogens, cell debris, and cells that are old, abnormal, or damaged, esp. red blood cells. Phagocytosis may be increased when the spleen is enlarged (splenomegaly).

splenic flexure Junction of transverse and descending colon, making a bend on the left side near the spleen.

splenic nodule A concentrated mass of white pulp in the spleen. SYN: *malpighian body* (2).

splenic sinus One of a series of wide vascular channels with thin walls forming an anastomosing plexus throughout red pulp of the spleen. SYN: *terminal vein.*

splenicterus (splē-nĭk′tĕr-ŭs) [Gr. *splen,* spleen, + *ikteros,* jaundice] Inflammation of the spleen associated with jaundice.

splenic vein The vein carrying blood from the spleen to the portal vein.

splenification (splē″nĭ-fĭ-kā′shŭn) [″ + L. *facere,* to make] Splenization.

spleniform (splĕn′ĭ-form) [″ + L. *forma,* form] Resembling the spleen.

splenitis (splē-nī′tĭs) [″ + *itis,* inflammation] Inflammation of the spleen, usually as a result of infection.

ETIOLOGY: Typical causes may include viral (e.g., mononucleosis), bacterial (e.g., bartonellosis, Lyme disease), or fungal (e.g., actinomycoses) infections.

splenium (splē′nē-ŭm) [Gr. *splenion,* bandage] **1.** A compress or bandage. **2.** A structure resembling a bandaged part.

s. corporis callosi The thickened posterior end of the corpus callosum.

splenius (splē′nē-ŭs) A flat muscle on either side of the back of the neck and upper thoracic area. SEE: *muscle* for illus.

splenization (splē″nī-zā′shŭn) The change in a tissue, as of the lung, when it resembles splenic tissue. SYN: *splenification.*

spleno- Combining form meaning *spleen.*

splenocele (splē′nō-sēl) [Gr. *splen,* spleen, + *kele,* tumor, swelling] **1.** A hernia of the spleen. **2.** Splenoma.

splenoceratosis (splē″nō-sĕr″ă-tō′sĭs) [″ + *keras,* horn, + *osis,* condition] Induration of the spleen.

splenocleisis (splē″nō-klī′sĭs) [″ + *kleisis,* closure] Friction on the surface of the spleen or application of gauze in order to induce the formation of fibrous tissue.

splenocolic (splē″nō-kŏl′ĭk) [″ + *kolon,* colon] Pert. to the spleen and colon or reference to a fold of peritoneum between the two viscera.

splenodynia (splē″nō-dĭn′ē-ă) [″ + *odyne,* pain] Pain in the spleen. SYN: *splenalgia.*

splenogenic, splenogenous (splē″nō-jĕn′ĭk, splē-nŏj′ĕn-ŭs) [″ + *gennan,* to produce] Originating in the spleen.

splenography (splē-nŏg′ră-fē) [″ + *graphein,* to write] **1.** A radiographic image of the spleen. **2.** A treatise on, or a description of, the spleen.

splenohepatomegaly (splē″nō-hĕp″ă-tō-mĕg′ă-lē) [Gr. *splen,* spleen, + *hepar,* liver, + *megas,* large] Enlargement of the spleen and liver.

splenoid (splē′noyd) [″ + *eidos,* form, shape] Resembling the spleen.

splenokeratosis (splē″nō-kĕr″ă-tō′sĭs) [″ + *keras,* horn, + *osis,* condition] Induration of the spleen.

splenolaparotomy (splē″nō-lăp″ă-rŏt′ō-mē) [″ + *lapara,* flank, + *tome,* incision] Incision through the abdominal wall into the spleen.

splenology (splē-nŏl′ō-jē) [″ + *logos,* word, reason] The study of functions and diseases of the spleen.

splenolymphatic (splē″nō-lĭm-făt′ĭk) [″ + L. *lympha,* lymph] Concerning the spleen and lymph nodes.

splenolysin (splē-nŏl′ĭ-sĭn) [″ + *lysis,* dissolution] An antibody that destroys splenic tissue.

splenolysis (splē-nŏl′ĭ-sĭs) Destruction of splenic tissue.

splenoma (splē-nō′mă) *pl.* **splenomas, -mata** [″ + *oma,* tumor] A tumor of the spleen. SYN: *splenocele* (2); *splenoncus.*

splenomalacia (splē″nō-mă-lā′shē-ă) [″ + *malakia,* softening] Softening of the spleen.

splenomedullary (splē″nō-mĕd′ū-lĕr″ē) [″ + L. *medulla,* marrow] Concerning the spleen and bone marrow, or originating in the spleen and bone marrow.

splenomegaly (splē″nō-mē-gā′lē, -mĕg′ă-lē) [″ + *megas,* large] Enlargement of the spleen. Causes for splenomegaly include portal hypertension, infections (such as leishmaniasis), autoimmune diseases, and blood disorders (such as some lymphomas, leukemias, and myeloproliferative disorders). It is frequently associated with anemia, leukopenia, and/or thrombocytopenia. Splenomegaly may cause a sense of discomfort in the left upper quadrant of the abdomen, particularly after eating. SEE: *spleen.*

congestive s. Enlargement of the spleen caused by various types of venous congestion: splenic vein obstruction, systemic venous congestion (e.g., due to heart failure), or hypertension from cirrhosis of the liver. Blood flow through the spleen is slowed, increasing red blood cell destruction by macrophages (hypersplenism) and resulting in focal hemorrhages. SYN: *Banti's syndrome.*

hemolytic s. Enlarged spleen associated with hemolytic anemia. The increased rigidity of red blood cell membranes results in their increased destruction as they attempt to move from splenic cords into the vascular sinuses. SEE: *spleen.*

splenometry (splē-nŏm′ĕ-trē) [″ + *metron,* measure] Determining the size of the spleen.

splenomyelogenous (splē-nō-mī″ĕ-lŏj′ĕ-nŭs) [″ + *myelos,* marrow, + *gennan,* to produce] Splenomedullary.

splenomyelomalacia (splē″nō-mī″ĕl-ō-mă-lā′shē-ă) [″ + ″ + *malakia,* softening] Abnormal softening of the spleen and bone marrow.

splenoncus (splē-nŏng′kŭs) [Gr. *splen,* spleen, + *onkos,* tumor] Splenoma.

splenonephric (splē″nō-nĕf′rĭk) [″ + *nephros,* kidney] Rel. to the spleen and kidney. SYN: *lienorenal.*

splenonephroptosis (splē″nō-nĕf″rŏp-tō′sĭs) [″ + ″ + *ptosis,* a dropping] Downward displacement of the spleen and kidney.

splenopancreatic (splē″nō-păn″krē-ăt′ĭk) [″ + *pankreas,* pancreas] Rel. to the spleen and pancreas.

splenopathy (splē-nŏp′ă-thē) [″ + *pathos,* disease, suffering] Any disorder of the spleen.

splenopexy (splē′nō-pĕk″sē) [″ + *pexis,* fixation] Artificial fixation of a movable spleen.

splenophrenic (splĕn-ō-frĕn′ĭk) [″ + *phren,* diaphragm] Concerning the spleen and diaphragm.

splenopneumonia (splē″nō-nū-mō′nē-ă) [″ + *pneumonia,* inflammation of lung] Pneumonia with splenization of the lung.

splenoportography (splē″nō-por-tŏg′ră-fē) [″ + L. *porta,* gate, + Gr. *graphein,* to write] Radiography of the spleen and portal vein after injection of a radiopaque contrast medium into the spleen.

splenoptosis (splē″nŏp-tō′sĭs) [″ + *ptosis,* a dropping] Downward displacement of the spleen.

splenorenal (splē″nō-rē′năl) Pert. to the spleen and kidney.

splenorenal shunt Anastomosis of the splenic vein to the renal vein to enable blood from the portal system to enter the general venous circulation; performed in cases of portal hypertension.

splenorrhagia (splē″nō-rā′jē-ă) [″ + *rhegnynai,* to burst forth] Hemorrhage from a ruptured spleen.

splenorrhaphy (splē-nor′ă-fē) [″ + *rhaphe,* seam, ridge] Suture of a wound of the spleen.

splenotomy (splē-nŏt′ō-mē) [″ + *tome,* incision] Incision of the spleen.

splenotoxin (splē″nō-tŏks′ĭn) [″ + *toxikon,* poison] Cytotoxin having specific action on splenic cells.

splenulus, splenunculus (splĕn′ū-lŭs) [L., a little spleen] A rudimentary or accessory spleen.

spliceosome (splī′sē-ō-sōm) A multipart ribonucleoprotein complex within the nucleus of cells that splices exons and introns from premessenger RNA during the regulation of protein synthesis.

splint (splĭnt) [MD. *splinte,* a wedge] An appliance made of bone, wood, metal, plastics, composites, or plaster of Paris, used for the fixation, union, or protection of an injured part of the body. It may be movable or immovable.

acrylic resin bite-guard s. A device fashioned to cover the incisal and occlusal surfaces of a dental arch to stabilize the teeth, treating bruxism, or facilitating proper occlusal positioning.

Agnew's s. A splint used in fractures of the patella and metacarpus.

air s. A lightweight splint used for immobilizing fractured or injured extremities. It is usually an inflatable cylinder, open at both ends, that becomes rigid when inflated, thus preventing the part confined in the cylinder from moving. SYN: *blow-up s.; inflatable s.*

CAUTION: Because of the tendency for the air cast to straighten out the limb as it is inflated, this device should not be used to immobilize joint dislocations or fractures with gross displacement.

airplane s. An appliance usually used on ambulatory patients in the treatment of fractures of the humerus. It takes its name from the elevated (abducted) position in which it holds the arm suspended away from the body.

anchor s. A splint for fracture of the jaw, with metal loops fitting over the teeth and held together by a rod.

Ashhurst's s. A bracketed splint of wire with a footpiece to cover the thigh and leg after excision of the knee joint.

Balkan s. A splint used for continuous extension in fracture of the femur.

banjo traction s. A splint made out of a steel rod bent to resemble the shape of a banjo. It provides anchor points for attachments to the fingers in the treatment of contractures and fractures of the fingers.

Bavarian s. An immovable dressing in which the plaster is applied between two layers of flannel.

blow-up s. Air s.

Bond's s. A splint used for fracture of the lower end of the radius.

Bowlby's s. A splint used for fracture of the shaft of the humerus.

box s. A splint used for fracture below the knee.

bracketed s. A splint composed of two pieces of metal or wood united by brackets.

Cabot's s. A splint composed of a metal structure placed posterior to the thigh and leg.

Carter's intranasal s. A steel bridge with wings connected by a hinge; used for operation of a depressed nasal bridge.

coaptation s. A small splint adjusted about a fractured part to prevent overriding of the fragments of bones; usually covered by a longer splint for fixation of entire section.

cylinder s. A splint constructed around an injured bone to reduce the potential for flexion contractures.

Denis Browne s. A splint used to treat talipes equinovarus (clubfoot), consisting of a curved bar attached to the soles of a pair of high-topped shoes. It is often used in late infancy and applied at bedtime. Its use generally follows casting and manipulation to reduce the deformity.

dental s. A rigid or flexible device or compound used to support, protect, or immobilize teeth that have been loosened, replanted, fractured, or subjected to surgical procedures.

dorsal blocking s. A splint constructed on the back of the hand to inhibit full extension of one or more of the finger joints and/or the wrist.

Dupuytren's s. A splint used to prevent eversion in Pott's fracture.

dynamic s. A splint that assists in movements initiated by the patient. SYN: *functional s.*

flail arm s. ABBR: FAS. An upper-extremity orthotic device used to provide support and limited function, consisting of a shoulder-operated harness, a volar supporting structure made of low-temperature thermoplastic material, and a terminal device that allows the arm to grasp or stabilize objects.

Fox's s. A splint used for a fractured clavicle.

functional s. Dynamic s.

Gibson walking s. A splint that is a modification of a Thomas splint.

Gordon's s. A side splint used for the arm and hand in Colles' fracture.

inflatable s. Air s.

Jones' nasal s. A splint used for the fracture of nasal bones.

Levis' s. A splint of perforated metal extending from below the elbow to the end of the palm; shaped to fit the arm and hand.

McIntire's s. A splint shaped like a double inclined plane, used as a posterior splint for the leg and thigh.

opponens s. A splint designed to maintain the thumb in a position to oppose the other fingers.

padded board s. A slat of wood, typically padded on one side and covered with plastic or cloth, to which an injured extremity can be fastened to immobilize it.

permanent fixed s. A nonremovable prosthesis firmly attached to an abutment used to stabilize or immobilize teeth. A fixed bridge may serve as a permanent fixed splint for such support.

static s. Any orthosis that lacks movable parts and is used for positioning, stability, protection, or support.

Stromeyer's s. A splint with two hinged sections that can be set at any angle, used esp. for the knee.

sugar tong s. A splint commonly used instead of a cast to immobilize a Colles' fracture after it has been reduced. The splint permits the affected arm to swell without being compressed within the confines of the cast, yet maintain its alignment. Follow up x-rays of the fracture are typically obtained 5 to 7 days after placement of the splint to make certain that adequate reduction of the fracture is maintained.

temporary removable s. One of a variety of splints used for temporary or intermittent support and stabilization of the teeth.

Thomas s. A long wire splint with a proximal ring. The ring fits over the lower extremity and is placed as far as it will go toward the hip. It is used in emergency treatment of femoral fracture.

Thomas' knee s. A rigid metal splint used to remove pressure of body weight from a weak knee joint by transferring weight to the ischium and perineum.

Thomas' posterior s. Thomas splint.

traction s. A splint that provides continual traction to a midshaft lower extremity fracture.

vacuum s. A negative-pressure device used to immobilize the extremities or torso after an injury. It may be used to safely transport the injured person. The splint consists of a nylon appliance filled with Styrofoam-like beads. The appliance is fitted around the injured body part and air is removed using a negative-pressure (vacuum) pump. As air is removed, the appliance conforms to the body part without straightening the limb. SEE: illus.

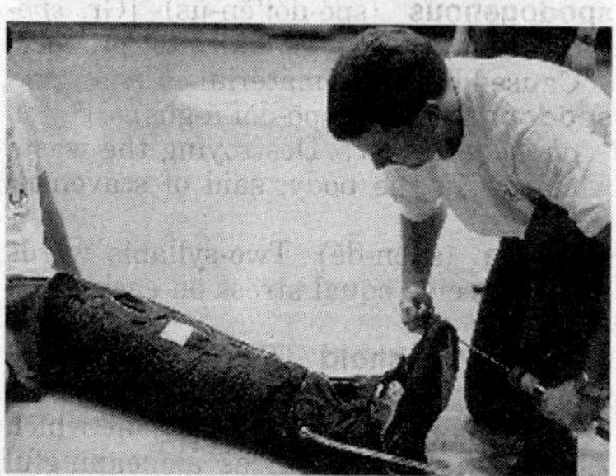

VACUUM SPLINT

CAUTION: Distal neurovascular function must be monitored after splint application. If decreased circulation or neurological involvement is noted, the splint must be loosened immediately.

Volkmann's s. A splint used for fracture of the lower extremity, consisting of a footpiece and two lateral supports.

splinter (splĭn′tĕr) [MD. *splinte*, a wedge] **1.** A fragment from a fractured bone. **2.** A slender, sharp piece of material piercing or embedded in the skin or subcutaneous tissue.

splinter hemorrhage A small linear hemorrhage under the fingernails or toenails. It may be due to subacute bacterial endocarditis.

splinting Fixation of a dislocation or fracture with a splint. Splints are also used to help support weak joints, to assist actively with functional movement, to immobilize to promote healing, and to protect from injury and deformity.

abdominal s. Involuntary tensing of abdominal muscles to protect underlying inflamed structures. Also called *rigid abdomen.*

split (splĭt) [D. *splitten,* to divide] **1.** A longitudinal fissure. **2.** Characterized by a deep fissure.

split foot Cleft foot.

split hand Cleft hand.

split pelvis Congenital failure of pubic bones to form a union at the symphysis.

splitting (splĭt′ĭng) [D. *splitten,* to divide] **1.** In chemistry, the breaking up of complex molecules into two or more simpler compounds. **2.** A defense mechanism found in some children and some patients with personality disorders, in which things are represented as being either very good (because they support one's desires or behaviors) or very bad (because they are obstructive to those desires or behaviors).

split tongue A cleft or bifid tongue resulting from developmental arrest.

SpO_2 The saturation of arterial blood with oxygen as measured by pulse oximetry, expressed as a percentage.

spodogenous (spō-dŏj′ĕn-ŭs) [Gr. *spodos,* ashes, + *gennan,* to produce] Caused by waste material.

spodophagous (spō-dŏf′ă-gŭs) [″ + *phagein,* to eat] Destroying the waste matter in the body; said of scavenger cells.

spondee (spŏn-dē) Two-syllable words that receive equal stress on each syllable.

spondee threshold [Fr., a two-syllable word with equal stress on each syllable] In audiometry, the intensity at which speech is recognized as a meaningful symbol. This is tested by presenting, through an audiometer, two-syllable words in which each symbol is accented equally. SEE: *audiometry.*

spondyl- (spŏn′dĭl) SEE: *spondylo-.*

spondylalgia (spōn″dĭl-ăl′jē-ă) [Gr. *spondylos,* vertebra, + *algos,* pain] Painful condition of a vertebra.

spondylarthritis (spŏn″dĭl-ăr-thrī′tĭs) [″ + *arthron,* joint, + *itis,* inflammation] Inflammation of the joints of the vertebrae; arthritis of the spine. SEE: *spondylitis.*

spondylarthrocace (splon″dĭl-ăr-thrŏk′ă-sē) [″ + ″ + *kake,* badness] Tuberculosis of the vertebrae. SYN: *spondylocace.*

spondylexarthrosis (spŏn″dĭl-ĕks″ăr-thrō′sĭs) [″ + *exarthrosis,* dislocation] Dislocation of a vertebra.

spondylitic (spŏn″dĭ-lĭt′ĭk) [″ + *itis,* inflammation] **1.** A person with spondylitis. **2.** Concerning spondylitis.

spondylitis (spŏn-dĭl-ī′tĭs) [″ + *itis,* inflammation] Inflammation of one or more vertebrae.

ankylosing s. ABBR: AS. A chronic progressive inflammatory disorder that, unlike other rheumatological diseases, affects men more often than women. It involves primarily the joints between articular processes, costovertebral joints, and sacroiliac joints, and occasionally, the iris or the heart valves. Bilateral sclerosis of sacroiliac joints is a diagnostic sign. Affected persons have a high incidence of a specific human leukocyte antigen (HLA-B27), which may predispose them to the disease. Changes occurring in joints are similar to those seen in rheumatoid arthritis. Ankylosis may occur, giving rise to a stiff back (poker spine). Nonsteroidal anti-inflammatory drugs and physical therapy are the primary forms of treatment. SYN: *Marie-Strümpell s.; rheumatoid s.*

s. deformans Inflammation of the vertebral joints resulting in the outgrowth of bone-like deposits on the vertebrae, which may fuse and cause rigid and distorted spine.

hypertrophic s. A condition in which bodies of vertebrae hypertrophy; it occurs in most people over 50. Bony changes such as slipping at bases and the development of bony outgrowths on articular processes occur.

Kümmell's s. A traumatic spondylitis in which symptoms do not appear until some time after the injury.

Marie-Strümpell s. Ankylosing s.

rheumatoid s. Ankylosing s.

tuberculous s. Pott's disease.

spondylizema (spŏn″dĭl-ĭ-zē′mă) [Gr. *spondylos,* vertebra, + *izema,* depression] Downward displacement of a vertebra caused by the disintegration of the one below it.

spondylo-, spondyl- Combining form meaning *vertebra.*

spondylocace (spŏn″dĭ-lŏk′ă-sē) [Gr. *spondylos,* vertebra, + *kake,* badness] Spondylarthrocace.

spondylodymus (spŏn″dĭ-lŏd′ĭ-mŭs) [″ + *didymos,* twin] Twin fetuses joined at the vertebrae.

spondylodynia (spŏn″dĭ-lō-dĭn′ē-ă) [″ + *odyne,* pain] Pain in a vertebra.

spondylolisthesis (spŏn″dĭ-lō-lĭs″thē′sĭs) [″ + *oblisthesis,* a slipping] Any forward slipping of one vertebra on the one below it. Predisposing factors include spondylolysis, degeneration, elongated pars, elongated pedicles, and birth defects in the spine such as spina bifida. SEE: *retrospondylolisthesis.*

spondylolisthetic (spŏn″dĭ-lō-lĭs-thĕt′ĭk) Concerning spondylolisthesis.

spondylolysis (spŏn″dĭ-lŏl′ĭ-sĭs) [″ + *lysis,* dissolution] The breaking down of a vertebral structure.

spondylomalacia (spŏn″dĭ-lō-mă-lā′shē-ă) [″ + *malakia,* softening] Softening of the vertebrae.

spondylopathy (spŏn″dĭl-ŏp′ă-thē) [″ + *pathos,* disease, suffering] Any disorder of the vertebrae.

spondyloptosis (spŏn″dĭ-lō-tō′sĭs) [″ + *ptosis,* a dropping] Spondylolisthesis.

spondylopyosis (spŏn″dĭ-lō″pī-ō′sĭs) [″ + *pyosis,* suppuration] Suppuration with inflammation of a vertebra.

spondyloschisis (spŏn″dĭ-lŏs′kĭ-sĭs) [″ + *schisis,* a splitting] A congenital fissure of one or more of the vertebral arches. SYN: *rhachischisis.*

spondylosis (spŏn″dĭ-lō′sĭs) [Gr. *spondylos,* vertebra, + *osis,* condition] Vertebral ankylosis.

cervical s. Degenerative arthritis, osteoarthritis, of the cervical or lumbar vertebrae and related tissues. It may cause pressure on nerve roots with subsequent pain or paresthesia in the extremities. SYN: *lumbar s.*

lumbar s. Cervical spondylosis.

rhizomelic s. Ankylosis interfering with movements of the hips and shoulders.

spondylosyndesis (spŏn″dĭ-lō-sĭn′dĕ-sĭs) [″ + *syndesis,* a binding together] Surgical formation of an ankylosis between vertebrae.

spondylotherapy (spŏn″dĭl-ō-thĕr′ă-pē) [″ + *therapeia,* treatment] Spinal therapeutics; spinal manipulation in the treatment of disease.

spondylotomy (spŏn″dĭl-ŏt′ō-mē) [″ + *tome,* incision] Removal of part of the vertebral column to correct a deformity. SYN: *rachitomy.*

spondylous (spŏn′dĭ-lŭs) [Gr. *spondylos,* vertebra] Concerning a vertebra.

sponge (spŭnj) [Gr. *sphongos,* sponge] **1.** Elastic, porous mass forming the internal skeleton of certain marine animals; or rubber or synthetic substance that resembles a sponge in properties and appearance. SYN: *spongia.* **2.** An absorbent pad made of gauze and cotton used to absorb fluids and blood in surgery or to dress wounds. **3.** Short term for sponge bath. **4.** To moisten, clean, cool, or wipe with a sponge.

abdominal s. A flat sponge from ½ to 1 in. (1.27 to 2.54 cm) thick, 3 to 6 in. (7.62 to 15.24 cm) in diameter, used as packing, to prevent closing or obstruction by intrusion of viscera, as covering to prevent tissue injury, and as absorbents.

contraceptive s. A sponge impregnated with a spermicide. It is used intravaginally during sexual intercourse as a method of contraception. SYN: *spermicidal s.* SEE: *contraceptive.*

gauze s. A sterile pad made of absorbent material. It is used during surgery.

gelatin s. A spongy substance prepared from gelatin. This nonantigenic, readily absorbable material is used esp. to stop internal bleeding (e.g., during surgery or during procedures in which blood vessels are occluded by embolization). It is sold under the trade name of Gelfoam.

spermicidal s. Contraceptive s.

sponge diver's disease Sea anemone sting.

sponge graft A sponge placed in an ulcer to cause granulation.

spongia (spŏn′jē-ă) [Gr. *sphongos,* sponge] Sponge.

spongiform (spŭn′jĭ-form) [Gr. *sphongos,* sponge, + L. *forma,* shape] Having the appearance or quality of a sponge. SYN: *spongioid.*

spongio- Combining form meaning *sponge.*

spongioblast (spŭn′jē-ō-blăst) [″ + *blastos,* germ] A cell that develops from an embryonic neural tube and serves as forerunner of ependymal cells and astrocytes.

spongioblastoma (spŭn″jē-ō-blăs-tō′mă) [″ + ″ + *oma,* tumor] A glioma of the brain derived from spongioblasts.

spongiocyte (spŭn′jē-ō-sīt″) [″ + *kytos,* cell] A neuroglial cell.

spongioid (spŭn′jē-oyd) [″ + *eidos,* form, shape] Spongiform.

spongiositis (spŭn″jē-ō-sī′tĭs) [″ + *itis,* inflammation] Inflammation of the corpus spongiosum of the urethra.

spongy (spŭn′jē) Resembling a sponge in texture.

spontaneous (spŏn-tā′nē-ŭs) [L.] Occurring unaided or without apparent cause; voluntary.

spontaneous fracture An old term for pathological fracture.

spontaneous ventilation, inability to sustain A state in which a patient is unable to maintain adequate breathing to support life. This is measured by deterioration of arterial blood gases, increased work of breathing, and decreasing energy. SEE: *Nursing Diagnoses Appendix.*

spoon [AS. *spon,* a chip] Instrument consisting of a small bowl on a handle, used in scooping out tissues or tumors, or in measuring quantities.

sporadic (spō-răd′ĭk) [Gr. *sporadikos*] Occurring irregularly, alone, or without linkage to other events. SEE: *endemic; epidemic; pandemic.*

sporangiophore (spō-răn′jē-ō-for) [Gr. *sporos,* seed, + *angeion,* vessel, + *phoros,* a bearer] In microbiology, the supporting stalk for a spore sac of certain fungi.

sporangium (spō-răn′jē-ŭm) A sac enclosing spores, seen in certain fungi.

spore (spor) [Gr. *sporos,* seed] **1.** A cell produced by fungi for reproduction. Spores may remain dormant yet viable for months. Cooking destroys spores, but pathogenic spores are usually inhaled rather than ingested. **2.** A resistant cell produced by bacteria to withstand extreme heat or cold, or dehydration; such spores may remain viable for decades. Important spore-forming bacteria include the causative agents of tetanus, botulism, and gas gangrene. The spores are heat-resistant and can survive an hour of boiling, but they can be destroyed by steam under pressure (i.e., autoclave). **3.** An airborne particle (fungal, bacterial, or derived from mosses or ferns) that may trigger an allergic response when inhaled. **4.** A stage in the life cycle of some parasitic protozoa that contains infective sporozoites.

sporicide (spor′ĭ-sīd) An agent that destroys bacterial and mold spores. Because spores are more difficult to kill than vegetative cells, a sporicide also acts as a sterilizing agent. **sporicidal** (-ăl), *adj.*

sporiferous (spor-ĭf′ĕr-ŭs) [″ + L. *ferre,* to bear] Producing spores.

spork An adapted utensil for persons with limited upper extremity function. The distal end may swivel to allow food to remain level as a result of gravitational force. The bowl end is shaped like a spoon but has modified tines, like a fork.

sporoblast (spor′ō-blăst) [″ + *blastos,* germ] The structure within the oocyst of certain parasitic protozoa (*Eimeria* and *Isospora*) that gives rise to a sporocyst and eventually a spore.

sporocyst (spor′ō-sĭst) [″ + *kystis,* sac] **1.** Any sac containing spores or reproductive cells. **2.** A sac secreted around a sporoblast by certain protozoa before spore production. **3.** A stage in the life cycle of a trematode worm usually found in the tissues of the first intermediate host, a mollusk. It develops from a miracidium and is essentially a germinal sac containing germ cells. It gives rise to daughter sporocysts or rediae.

sporogenesis (spor″ō-jĕn′ĕ-sĭs) [Gr. *sporos,* seed, + *genesis,* generation, birth] The production or formation of spores. SYN: *sporogeny; sporogony.*

sporogenic (spor″ō-jĕn′ĭk) [″ + *gennan,* to produce] Having the ability of developing into spores.

sporogenous (spor-ŏj′ĕ-nŭs) [″ + *gennan,* to produce] Concerning sporogenesis.

sporogeny (spor-ŏj′ĕ-nē) Sporogenesis.

sporogony (spor-ŏg′ō-nē) [″ + *goneia,* generation] Sporogenesis.

sporophore (spor′ō-for) [″ + *phoros,* bearing] The spore-bearing portion of an organism.

sporophyte (spor′ō-fīt) [″ + *phyton,* plant] The spore-bearing stage of a plant exhibiting alternation of generations.

sporoplasm (spor′ō-plăzm) [″ + LL. *plasma,* form, mold] The cytoplasm of spores.

Sporothrix (spor′ō-thrĭks) A genus of fungi of the family Moniliaceae; formerly called *Sporotrichum*.

S. schenckii The causative agent of sporotrichosis.

sporotrichin (spor-ŏ′trĭ-kĭn) An antigenic substance derived from *Sporothrix* organisms and used for diagnostic purposes.

sporotrichosis (spor″ō-trī-kō′sĭs) [″ + *thrix,* hair, + *osis,* condition] A chronic granulomatous infection usually of the skin and superficial lymph node, marked by the formation of abscesses, nodules, and ulcers and caused by the fungus *Sporothrix schenckii*.

Sporotrichum (spō-rŏt′rĭ-kŭm) Former name for *Sporothrix*.

Sporozoa (spor″ō-zō′ă) [″ + *zoon,* animal] A class of parasitic protozoa of the phylum Apicomplexa (apical microlobule complex), kingdom Protista. The mature forms lack a means of self-locomotion. Important genera are *Plasmodium, Toxoplasma, Cryptosporidium, Microsporidia,* and *Isospora*.

sporozoan A protozoon belonging to the group formerly called Sporozoa.

sporozoite (spor″ō-zō′īt) [″ + *zoon,* animal] An elongated sickle-shaped cell that develops from a sporoblast within the oocyst in the life cycle of malaria. Upon bursting of the oocyst within a mosquito, sporozoites are released into the body cavity and make their way to the salivary gland. They are introduced into human blood by a mosquito and almost immediately enter liver cells, where they go through two schizogonic divisions and then reenter the bloodstream and infect erythrocytes.

sport [ME. *sporten,* to divert] Mutation.

sports medicine The application of medical knowledge and science to the physiological and pathological aspects of field sports and athletics. This field includes not only prevention and treatment of injuries but also scientific investigation of training methods and practices.

sporular (spor′ū-lăr) [L. *sporula,* little spore] Concerning a spore.

sporulation (spor-ū-lā′shŭn) [L. *sporula,* little spore] **1.** The production of spores, a method of reproduction in fungi, mosses, and ferns. **2.** Bacterial production of spores, resistant forms that can withstand extremes of heat and cold, and dehydration.

spot (spŏt) [MD. *spotte*] A small surface area differing in appearance from its surroundings. SYN: *macula*.

ash-leaf s. White macules found on the trunk and extremities of persons with tuberous sclerosis.

blind s. **1.** Physiological scotoma situated 15° to the outside of the visual fixation point; the point where the optic nerve enters the eye (optic disk), a region devoid of rods and cones. SEE: *scotoma*. **2.** In psychiatry, the inability of an individual to have insight into his or her own personality.

blue s. Mongolian s.

cherry-red s. A red spot occurring on the retina in children with Tay-Sachs disease.

cold s. An area on a nuclear medicine scan in which no radioactive tracer is taken up—indicative of nonfunctioning tissue in a gland or other structure.

corneal s. Leukoma.

Fordyce's s. Ectopic sebaceous glands seen frequently as yellow spots in the oral mucosa of the cheek or lip.

genital s. The area on the nasal mucosa that tends to bleed during menstruation. SEE: *vicarious menstruation*.

hot s. An area on the surface of the skin that, when stimulated, causes a sensation of warmth.

hypnogenic s. A point on the body that, when pressed, will produce hypnosis or sleep in a susceptible person.

liver s. A popular term for pigmentary skin discolorations, usually in yellow-brown patches. SEE: *chloasma; lentigo*.

milk s. A dense area of macrophages in the omentum.

mongolian s. One of the blue or mulberry-colored spots usually located in the sacral region. It may be present at birth in Asian, American Indian, black, and Southern European infants, and usually disappears during childhood. SYN: *blue s.* SEE: illus.

rose s. Rose-colored maculae occurring on the abdomen or loins in typhoid fever.

ruby s. Senile angioma.

white s. Light-colored, elevated areas of various sizes occurring on the ventricular surface of the anterior leaflet of the mitral valve in endocarditis.

yellow s. Macula lutea retinae.

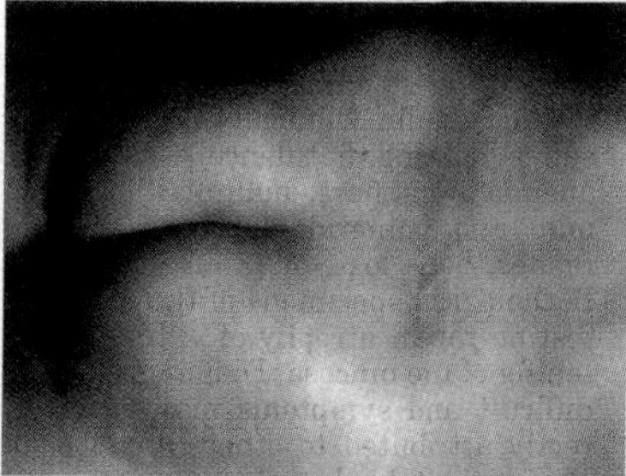

MONGOLIAN SPOTS

spotted fever General and imprecise name for various eruptive fevers including typhus, tick fever, and rickettsial fevers. SEE: *Rocky Mountain spotted fever*.

spotting The appearance of blood-tinged discharge from the vagina, usually between menstrual periods or at the onset of labor.

spp *species* (plural).

sprain (sprān) [O.Fr. *espraindre*, to wring] Trauma to ligaments that causes pain and disability depending on the degree of injury to the ligaments. In severe sprain, ligaments may be completely torn. The ankle joint is the most often sprained. SEE: *fracture; strain*.

SYMPTOMS: Pain may be accompanied by heat, discoloration, and localized swelling in the affected area. Moderate to severe sprains are marked by joint laxity, reduced range of motion, and limitation of function. When the sprained ligament is contiguous with the joint capsule (e.g., anterior talofibular ligament, medial collateral ligament), swelling occurs in the acute stage. When the sprain involves other intracapsular or extracapsular ligaments (e.g., calcaneofibular ligament, anterior cruciate ligament), swelling is slight or absent in the acute stage, and progressively increases.

DIAGNOSIS: X-ray examination is often indicated, to rule out an avulsion fracture of the ligament's attachment.

TREATMENT: The affected part should be treated initially with ice or other cooling agents to limit inflammation and hypoxic injury. Circumferential compression, in the form of an elastic wrap, should be applied to the joint, and the limb elevated to reduce swelling. Joint range of motion should be restricted to patient tolerance through the use of immobilization devices, crutches, or both. Analgesics and nonsteroidal anti-inflammatory medications may be administered for pain and swelling. In the chronic stage of the injury, massage, intermittent compression, and muscle contractions can be used to reduce swelling.

s. of ankle Trauma to the ligaments of the ankle and foot, possibly involving tendon injury, but without fracture. Sprains of the lateral ligaments (most commonly the anterior talofibular ligament) account for approx. 90% of all ankle sprains. SYN: *s.of foot*. SEE: *Nursing Diagnoses Appendix*.

TREATMENT: SEE: *sprain* for treatment.

CAUTION: Ice should not be applied directly to the foot and ankle in patients who are elderly or who have cold allergy or circulatory insufficiency.

s. of back Overstretching of the spinal ligaments, often involving the surrounding muscles and spinal structures. Small fractures of the vertebrae are often associated.

TREATMENT: Treatment includes superficial moist heat and rest. If muscle spasm is present, muscle relaxants, nonsteroidal anti-inflammatory drugs, or both, may be prescribed. After the acute symptoms have subsided, strengthening and flexibility programs are prescribed.

CAUTION: If back pain develops after acute trauma, or if the patient has a known history of cancer, the patient should not be moved until the possibility of a fracture has been ruled out. Persons with a history of back pain and fever or back pain and injection drug use should be evaluated for spinal epidural abscess.

s. of foot S. of ankle.

high ankle s. Syndesmotic ankle s.

riders' s. Sprain of the adductor longus muscles of the thigh, resulting from strain in riding horseback.

syndesmotic ankle s. Damage to the ligamentous structures of the distal tibiofibular joint, resulting from dorsiflexion or external rotation of the talus within the ankle mortise, or both, which in turn causes spreading of the joint. The distal tibiofibular syndesmosis is formed by the anterior tibiofibular ligament, the interosseous membrane, and the posterior tibiofibular ligament. SYN: *high ankle s.*

ETIOLOGY: The rate of syndesmotic ankle sprains is increased when athletes are participating on artificial surfaces, because of the increased friction between the shoe and playing surface.

SYMPTOMS: Patients may describe pain along the fibula, just superior to the lateral malleolus, that worsens during dorsiflexion or external rotation of the talus, or both.

sprain fracture The separation of a tendon or ligament from its insertion, taking with it a piece of the bone.

spray (sprā) [MD. *spraeyen,* to sprinkle] **1.** A jet of fine medicated vapor applied to a diseased part or discharged into the air. **2.** A pressurized container. SYN: *atomizer*. **3.** To discharge fluid in a fine stream.

pepper s. A chemical derived from chili peppers that irritates the eyes, mucous membranes, and bronchi. It is commonly used by law enforcement personnel against individuals to help subdue and apprehend them.

spreader (sprĕd′ĕr) **1.** An instrument for distributing something evenly over a tissue or culture plate. **2.** A bacterial culture that, as it grows, spreads over the surface of the culture medium. **3.** A surgical instrument that divides and holds apart tissues or bones.

bladder-neck s. An instrument used to expose the bladder neck and prostatic cavity while doing a retropubic prostatectomy.

root canal s. In dentistry, an instrument that is pointed and of variable diameter and taper. It is used to apply force to the material used in filling a root canal.

spreading (sprĕd′ĭng) [AS. *spraedan,* to strew] The extension of a bacterial culture on a growth medium.

spring [AS. *springan,* to jump] **1.** The season of the year that comes after winter and before summer. SYN: *vernal*. **2.** The quick movement of a body to its original position through its elasticity.

spring conjunctivitis Vernal conjunctivitis.

spring fever A feeling of lassitude, rejuvenation, or increased sex drive that affects some people in the spring.

spring finger Arrested movement of a finger in flexion or extension followed by a jerk. SYN: *trigger finger*.

spring ligament The interior calcaneonavicular ligament of the sole of the foot. It joins the calacaneus to the navicular.

spruce (sproos) Any of the evergreen coniferous trees and shrubs of the genus *Picea* (family Piceaceae), widely found in the Northern Hemisphere. Known side effects of exposure to spruce dusts (e.g., in sawmill workers) include an increased incidence of reactive airways diseases such as asthma. The gum of the spruce is used occasionally in alternative and complementary medicine as an expectorant.

sprue (sproo) [D. *sprouwe*] **1.** In dentistry, the wax, metal, or plastic used to form the aperture(s) through which molten gold or resin will pass to make a casting; also, the part of the casting that later fills the sprue hole. **2.** A disease of the intestinal tract characterized by malabsorption, weight loss, abdominal distention, bloating, diarrhea, and steatorrhea.

celiac s. Malabsorption, weight loss, and diarrhea, resulting from intolerance to dietary wheat proteins, esp. gluten and gliadin. Clinically, patients may suffer bloating, flatulence, steatorrhea, anemia, weakness, malnutrition, vitamin and mineral deficiencies, skin rashes, bone loss, or failure to thrive. Pathological specimens of the small intestine reveal atrophy of villi and flattening of the mucosa. Diagnosis may be difficult and symptoms may be incorrectly attributed to other illnesses including irritable bowel syndrome.

A life-long gluten-free diet results in virtually complete reversal of symptoms and signs (including changes in the epithelium of the bowel). SYN: *gluten-induced enteropathy; gluten-sensitive enteropathy; nontropical s.* SEE: *malabsorption syndrome.*

collagenous s. Infiltration of the small intestine by collagen fibers. Clinically, the disease is similar to severe celiac sprue. It is resistant to treatment with a gluten-free diet and immunosuppressive drugs.

nontropical s. Celiac s.

tropical s. A disease endemic in many tropical regions, marked by weakness, anemia, weight loss, steatorrhea, and malabsorption of essential nutrients. It is similar pathologically to celiac sprue, although the involvement of the small intestine is more extensive. An infectious cause is suspected. The administration of folic acid and tetracyclines for 6 to 12 months provides effective treatment.

spud (spŭd) [ME. *spudde,* short knife] Short, flattened, spadelike blade to dislodge a foreign substance.

spur [AS. *spura,* a pointed instrument] **1.** A sharp or pointed projection. **2.** A sharp horny outgrowth of the skin.

calcaneal s. An exostosis of the heel, often painful and resulting in disability.

s. cell An erythrocyte with spikes caused by a membrane deformity. Spur cells are often seen in persons with alcoholic cirrhosis and congenital abetalipoproteinemia. SEE: illus.

femoral s. A spur sometimes present on the medial and underside of the neck of the femur.

scleral s. A pointed portion of sclera that projects into the deeper part of the cornea immediately behind the canal of Schlemm at the angle of the iris.

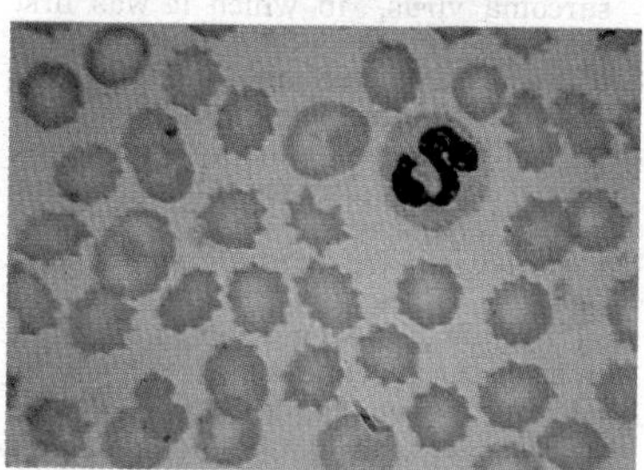

SPUR CELLS

In severe liver disease (×640)

spurious (spū'rē-ŭs) [L. *spurius*] Not true or genuine; adulterated; false.

sputum (spū'tŭm) *pl.* **sputa** [L.] Mucus expelled from the lung by coughing. It may contain a variety of materials from the respiratory tract, including in some instances cellular debris, mucus, blood, pus, caseous material, and/or microorganisms.

CONDITIONS: A wide variety of illnesses, including typical and atypical pneumonias, tuberculosis, cancers of the lungs or bronchi, reactive airway disease, and occupational diseases of the lungs, can be diagnosed with gram staining or culturing of sputum, cytological examination of sputum, or the use of special stains and microscopic techniques.

CAUTION: Sputum color or thickness cannot be relied on to diagnose any particular illness.

---

bloody s. Hemoptysis.

nummular s. Sputum laden with round, coin-shaped solids.

prune juice s. Thin, reddish, bloody sputum.

rusty s. Blood-tinged purulent sputum sometimes seen in patients with pneumococcal pneumonia.

sputum specimen A specimen of mucus from the lungs expectorated through the mouth, to identify the microorganism causing a lung infection or to identify lung cancers and/or occupational lung diseases. SEE: *postural drainage.*

PATIENT CARE: The procedure is explained to the patient. The patient should brush his or her teeth and rinse the mouth to remove food particles. Deep breathing is encouraged. Using the collection container provided, the patient is instructed to collect the specimen in the early morning before ingesting food or drink if possible. The nurse or respiratory therapist examines the specimen to differentiate between sputum and saliva, documents the characteristics (color, viscosity, odor) and volume, and records the date and time the specimen went to the laboratory and the reason for the specimen. If the patient cannot produce a specimen, the respiratory therapist can use sputum induction techniques such as heated aerosol followed by postural drainage and percussion. The airway may be suctioned with a sputum trap attached to a suction catheter in the intubated patient. The specimen should be sent to the laboratory immediately. All sputum specimens should be treated as infective until proven otherwise. Appropriate isolation procedures are used for handling specimens.

sq *subcutaneous.*

squalene (skwăl'ēn) An unsaturated carbohydrate present in shark-liver oil and some vegetable oils. It is an intermediate in the biosynthesis of cholesterol.

squama (skwā'mă) *pl.* **squamae** [L.] **1.** A thin plate of bone. **2.** A scale from the epidermis. SYN: *squame.*

squamate (skwā'māt) [L. *squama,* scale] Scaly.

squamatization (skwā"mă-tī-zā'shŭn) [L. *squama,* scale] The changing of cells into squamous cells.

squame (skwām) [L. *squama,* scale] Squama (2).

squamocellular (skwā″mō-sĕl′ū-lăr) [L. *squama,* scale, + *cellula,* little cell] Rel. to or having squamous cells.

squamofrontal (skwā″mō-frŏn′tăl) [″ + *frontalis,* frontal] Concerning the part of the frontal bone above the supraorbital arch.

squamomastoid (skwā″mō-măs′toyd) [″ + Gr. *mastos,* breast, + *eidos,* form, shape] Concerning the squamous and mastoid portions of the temporal bone.

squamo-occipital (skwā″mō-ŏk-sĭp′ĭ-tăl) [″ + *occipitalis,* occipital] Concerning the squamous portion of the occipital bone.

squamoparietal (skwā″mō-pă-rī′ĕ-tăl) [″ + *paries,* a wall] Rel. to the squamous and parietal bones.

squamopetrosal (skwā″mō-pē-trō′săl) [″ + *petrosus,* stony] Concerning the squamous and petrosal portions of the temporal bone.

squamosa (skwā-mō′să) *pl.* **squamosae** [L. scaly] **1.** The squamous part of the temporal bone. **2.** Scaly or platelike.

squamosal (skwā-mō″săl) [L. *squama,* scale] Squamous.

squamosphenoid (skwā″mō-sfē′noyd) [″ + Gr. *sphen,* wedge, + *eidos,* form, shape] Concerning the squamous portion of the temporal bone and the sphenoid bone.

squamous (skwā′mŭs) [L. *squamosus*] Scalelike.

squamous bone The upper anterior portion of temporal bone.

squamous epithelium The flat form of epithelial cells.

squamous suture The junction of the temporal and parietal bones.

squamozygomatic (sqwā″mō-zī″gō-măt′ĭk) [″ + *zygoma,* cheekbone] Concerning the squamous and zygomatic parts of the temporal bone.

square knot Double knot in which ends and standing parts are together and parallel to each other. This knot is used universally because it holds well. It is quite easy to tie but may be very difficult to untie. One should hold one end in each hand, carry the right end over the left end, and make a simple knot. Now this is reversed by carrying the left end over the right end and again tying, thus forming a simple symmetrical knot. If this is not done correctly, a false or granny knot results, a type of knot that usually slips. To untie, the knot is steadied, and one end is taken and drawn until it begins to slip out of the knot. One continues pulling in this direction until the knot slips or jumps and forms two half hitches that may be slipped off. SEE: *knot* for illus.

square lobe **1.** The quadrate lobe of the liver. **2.** A lobe on the upper surface of the cerebellum.

squarrose, squarrous (skwăr′ōs, -ŭs) [L. *squarrosus*] Scurfy or scaly; full of scabs or scales.

squatting position A position in which the person crouches with legs drawn up closely in front of, or beneath, the body; sitting on one's haunches and heels.

squeeze-bottle A bottle made of a flexible, semirigid material that can be deformed by applying hand pressure to it. It is used to contain irrigating solutions, esp. those required in ophthalmology.

squill (skwĭl) [Gr. *skilla,* a sea onion] A drug derived from a liliaceous plant. It was once popular as an expectorant and diuretic.

squint (skwĭnt) [ME. *asquint,* sidelong glance] **1.** Abnormality in which the right and left visual axes do not bear toward an objective point simultaneously. SYN: *strabismus.* **2.** To close the eyes partly, either to block out excess environmental light or to try to improve a refractive error of vision. **3.** To be unable to direct both eyes simultaneously toward a point.

convergent s. Esotropia.

divergent s. Exotropia.

external s. Exotropia.

internal s. Esotropia.

SR *sedimentation rate.*

Sr Symbol for the element strontium.

src Family of oncogenes involved in transforming normal cells to cancer cells. Src was the first transforming oncogene discovered. Proteins produced by these genes have tyrosine kinase activity. SEE: *oncogene; transformation.*

ETIOLOGY: Name comes from "Rous sarcoma virus," in which it was first found.

SRF *somatotropin releasing factor.*

sRNA *soluble ribonucleic acid.*

SRS, SRS-A *slow-reacting substance; slow-reacting substance of anaphylaxis.* SEE: *leukotriene.*

SS *saliva sample; soapsuds; sterile solution.*

ss [L. *semis,* half] One-half; *subjects,* as in ss of an experiment or clinical study.

SSD *source-skin distance.*

SSE *soapsuds enema.*

SSS *sterile saline soak.*

ST *sedimentation time.*

S.T. 37 Hexylresorcinol.

stab (stăb) [ME. *stob,* stick] **1.** To pierce with a knife. **2.** A wound produced by piercing with a knife or pointed instrument. **3.** A stab culture.

stabile (stā′bĭl) [L. *stabilis,* stable] Not moving; fixed.

stability **1.** The condition of remaining unchanged, even in the presence of forces that would normally change the state or condition (e.g., a chemical compound that remains unchanged, or a mature mental state that resists change). **2.** A measure of the ability of an aerosol to remain in suspension. This is determined by the size, type, and concentration of particles, the humidity, and the mobility of the gas in which the particles are transported.

limits of s. ABBR: LOS. The largest angle from vertical that can be maintained before balance is lost. In normal adults, the sagittal plane limit is 12 degrees and the coronal plane limit is 16 degrees.

PATIENT CARE: If the patient has decreased limits of stability, there is an increased postural response and an increased likelihood of falling.

stabilization (stā″bĭl-ī-ză′shŭn) [L. *stabilis,* stable] **1.** The act of making something, such as a body structure, chemical reaction, mood state, or disease process less variable, mobile, or volatile or more rigid. **2.** The fixation or seating of a fixed or partial denture so that it will not be displaced in function.

dynamic s. An integrated function of the neuromuscular systems requiring muscles to contract and fixate the body against fluctuating outside forces, providing postural support with fine adjustments in muscle tension. The term usually pertains to a function of the trunk, shoulder, and hip muscles and includes the lower-extremity muscles when they are functioning in a closed chain.

stable (stā′bl) **1.** Firm; steady. **2.** The structure of an atom that prevents spontaneous disintegration.

stable condition A term used in describing a patient's condition. It indicates that the patient's disease process has not changed precipitously or significantly.

Stachybotrys atra *Stachybotrys chartarum.*

Stachybotrys chartarum A mold that grows well on wood, plaster, insulation, tobacco products, and sheetrock. Inhalation of spores has been implicated in cases of fatigue, chronic headaches, and respiratory difficulties. SYN: *Stachybotrys atra.*

stachyose A nonabsorbable carbohydrate present in beans. Because the substance is not absorbed or metabolized in the small intestine, it passes into the colon where it is acted on by bacteria to form gas. This may be related to the flatus produced by eating beans.

stactometer (stăk-tŏm′ĕt-ĕr) [Gr. *staktos,* dropping, + *metron,* measure] An instrument for measuring fluid in drops.

stadiometer [Gr. stadium + meter] A device used to measure body height, esp. of children.

stadium (stā′dē-ŭm) [Gr. *stadion,* alteration] A stage or period in the progress of a disease. SYN: *stage* (1). SEE: *fastigium.*

s. sudoris The sweating stage of a paroxysm of malaria.

staff (stăf) [AS. *staef,* a stick] **1.** An instrument to be introduced into the urethra and bladder as a guide to a surgical knife. **2.** The medical, nursing, and other personnel attached to a hospital.

attending s. The group of physicians and surgeons who are in regular attendance at a hospital.

consulting s. The physicians and surgeons attached to a hospital who may be consulted by members of the attending staff.

house s. A nonspecific term for physicians, esp. interns and residents, as well as other allied health professionals employed as part of the medical care team for a hospital. These individuals are supervised by the permanent hospital staff and receive training in order to meet the requirements for licensure or certification in their specialty. SEE: *teaching hospital.*

s. of Wrisberg Prominence of the cuneiform cartilage seen in the normal larynx during examination.

stage (stāj) [O.Fr. *estage*] **1.** Period in the course of a disease or in the life history of an organism. SYN: *stadium.* **2.** The platform of a microscope on which the slide is placed.

algid s. Cold and cyanotic skin that occurs in cholera and some other diseases.

amphibolic s. The stage that intervenes between the acme of a disease and its outcome, at a time when the outcome is unknown.

asphyxial s. The preliminary stage of Asiatic cholera.

cold s. The chill or rigor of a malarial paroxysm.

defervescent s. The period in which the temperature is declining.

eruptive s. **1.** The period in which an exanthem appears. **2.** The middle stage in the pre-eruptive, eruptive, or posteruptive categorization of tooth eruption. It is characterized by root elongation and movement of the tooth mesially and toward the occlusal plane.

hot s. Febrile stage in a malarial paroxysm.

s. of invasion The period in which the causative agent is present in the body before the onset of a disease.

s. of latency The incubation period of an infectious disorder.

pre-eruptive s. The stage following infection and before the appearance of eruption.

pyrogenetic s. The stage of onset in a febrile disease.

resting s. Term sometimes used for a cell that is between mitotic divisions. It is not accurate because the cell is metabolically active and is producing a new set of chromosomes for the next division.

sweating s. The third or terminal

stage of malaria during which sweating occurs.

staggers (stăg′ĕrz) Vertigo and confusion that occur in decompression illness.

staging The process of classifying tumors, esp. malignant tumors, with respect to their degree of differentiation, to their potential for responding to therapy, and to the patient's prognosis.

stagnation (stăg-nā′shŭn) [L. *stagnans,* stagnant] **1.** Cessation of motion. **2.** Stasis.

stain (stān) [O.Fr. *desteindre,* deprive of color] **1.** Any discoloration. **2.** A pigment or dye used in coloring microscopic objects and tissues. **3.** To apply pigment to a tissue or microscopic object.

acid s. A stain in which the color-bearing ion (chromatophore) is the anion (e.g., eosin, commonly used to stain the cytoplasmic or basic elements of cells).

acid-fast s. A stain used in bacteriology, esp. for staining *Mycobacterium tuberculosis, Nocardia,* and other species. A special solution of carbolfuchsin is used, which the organism retains in spite of washing with the decolorizing agent acid alcohol. SEE: *Ziehl-Neelsen method.*

basic s. A stain in which the color-bearing ion is the cation (e.g., methylene blue, commonly used to stain the nucleic or acidic elements of cells).

Commission Certified s. A stain that has been certified by the Biological Stain Commission.

contrast s. A stain used to color one part of a tissue or cell, unaffected when another part is stained by another color.

counter s. A stain, usually a contrast stain, used after the staining of specific parts of a tissue.

dental s. A discoloration accumulating on the surface of teeth, denture, or denture base material, most often attributed to the use of tea, coffee, or tobacco. Many stains contain calcium carbon, copper, iron, nitrogen, oxygen, and sulfur. The stain may be removed by brushing, rinsing, or sonication of teeth.

differential s. In bacteriology, a stain such as Gram's stain that enables one to differentiate among different types of bacteria.

double s. A mixture of two contrasting dyes, usually an acid and a basic stain.

Giemsa s. A stain that contains azure II–eosin and azure II. It is used in staining tissues including blood cells, Negri bodies, and chromosomes.

hematoxylin-eosin s. A widely used method of staining tissues for microscopic examination. It stains the nuclei a deep blue-black and the cytoplasm pink.

intravital s. A nontoxic dye that, when introduced into an organism, selectively stains certain cells or tissues. SYN: *vital s.*

inversion s. A basic stain that, when under the influence of a mordant, acts as an acid stain.

metachromatic s. A stain with which the constituents of cells or tissues develop a color different from the stain itself.

neutral s. A combination of an acid and a basic stain.

nuclear s. A basic stain affecting nuclei.

Perl's s. SEE: *Perl's stain.*

port-wine s. Nevus flammeus.

substantive s. A stain that is directly absorbed by the tissues when they are immersed in the staining solution.

supravital s. Stain that will color living cells or tissues that have been removed from the body.

tumor s. In arteriography, an abnormally dense area in a radiographic image caused by the collection of contrast medium in the vessels. This may be a sign of neoplastic growth.

vital s. Intravital s.

Wright's s. A polychrome stain used for staining blood smears. SEE: *Wright's technique.*

staining (stān′ĭng) [O.Fr. *desteindre*] The process of impregnating a substance, esp. a tissue, with pigments so that its components may be visible under a microscope. SEE: *Wright's technique.*

stair chair A device used to transport patients capable of being moved in a sitting position up or down a staircase or through narrow and confined spaces.

staircase breaths In basic life support, the serial application of several small breaths rather than a single large-volume breath. SEE: *cardiopulmonary resuscitation.*

staircase phenomenon The effect exhibited by skeletal and heart muscle when subjected to rapidly repeated maximal stimuli following a period of rest. In the resulting series of contractions, each is greater than the preceding one until a state of maximum contraction is reached. SYN: *treppe.* SEE: *stress test.*

stalagmometer (stăl-ăg-mŏm′ĕ-tĕr) [Gr. *stalagmos,* dropping, + *metron,* a measure] An instrument for measuring the number of drops in a given amount of fluid.

stalk (stawk) [ME.] An elongated structure usually serving to attach or support an organ or structure.

belly s. The structure in an embryo that develops into the umbilical cord.

body s. A bridge of mesoderm that connects the caudal end of the embryo with the chorion. Into it grow the allantois and embryonic blood vessels, the latter forming the umbilical arteries and vein, which connect the embryo with the placenta.

cerebellar s. One of the cerebellar peduncles that connect the cerebellum with the brainstem.

infundibular s. Infundibulum (3).

optic s. The structure that connects the optic vesicle or cup to the forebrain.

yolk s. Vitelline duct.

stamina (stăm′ĭ-nă) [L., thread of the warp, thread of human life] Inherent force, constitutional energy; strength; endurance.

stammering (stăm′ĕr-ĭng) [AS. *stamerian*] Stuttering.

s. of bladder An interrupted and irregular flow of urine, with the muscles that control micturition acting spasmodically. SYN: *urinary stuttering*.

standard [O.Fr. *estandard,* marking rallying place] That which is established by custom or authority as a model, criterion, or rule.

biological s. The standardization of drugs or biological products (vitamins, hormones, antibiotics) by testing their effects on animals. It is used when chemical analysis is impossible or impracticable.

reasonable patient s. In the giving of informed consent, the amount of information that a rational patient would want before making a choice to pursue or reject a treatment or procedure.

reasonable physician s. In the giving of informed consent, the amount of information that a typical physician would provide to patients before asking that they decide to pursue or reject a treatment.

standard of care **1.** A statement of actions consistent with minimum safe professional conduct under specific conditions, as determined by professional peer organizations. **2.** In forensic medicine, a measure with which the defendant's conduct is compared to determine negligence or malpractice. **3.** The acts of omission or commission that an ordinary prudent person would have done or not done if in the defendant's position.

standard deviation ABBR: S.D. SYMB: σ. In statistics, the commonly used measure of dispersion or variability in a distribution; the square root of the variance.

standard error ABBR: S.E. A measure of variability that could be expected of a statistical constant following the taking of random samples of a given size in a particular set of observations. An important standard error is that of the difference between the means of two samples.

standard precautions SEE: under *precautions*.

standard temperature and pressure, dry ABBR: STPD. Gas volume at 0°C 760 mm Hg total pressure and partial pressure of water of zero (i.e., dry).

standing orders Orders, rules, regulations, protocols, or procedures prepared by the professional staff of a hospital or clinic and used as guidelines in the preparation and carrying out of medical and surgical procedures.

standstill A cessation of activity.

atrial s. Cessation of atrial contractions.

cardiac s. Cessation of contractions of the heart.

inspiratory s. The temporary cessation of inspiration normally following each inspiration, resulting from stimulation of proprioceptors in the alveoli of the lungs. SEE: *Hering-Breuer reflex*.

respiratory s. Cessation of respiratory movements.

ventricular s. Cessation of ventricular contractions.

stannic (stăn′ĭk) [L. *stannum,* tin] **1.** Resembling or containing tin. **2.** In chemistry, containing tetravalent tin.

stannosis The deposition of tin oxide dust in the upper or lower respiratory tract. Patients may complain of irritation of the eyes, nasal passages, and other mucous membranes. Chest x-ray examination often reveals dust deposits in the lungs, but this form of pneumoconiosis does not cause lung injury or disease.

stannous (stăn′ŭs) [L. *stannum,* tin] **1.** Resembling or containing tin. **2.** In chemistry, containing divalent tin.

stannous fluoride A fluoride compound used in toothpaste to prevent dental caries.

stannum (stăn′ŭm) [L.] Tin.

stanozolol (stăn′ō-zō-lŏl″) An anabolic steroid.

Stanton's disease Melioidosis.

stapedectomy (stā″pē-dĕk′tō-mē) [L. *stapes,* stirrup, + Gr. *ektome,* excision] Excision of the stapes to improve hearing, esp. in cases of otosclerosis. In patients with severely impaired hearing, the stapes is replaced by a prosthesis which is placed in the ear. After surgery, the patient is instructed to keep head movements to a minimum and to refrain from blowing the nose or sneezing (if possible). Subsequently, all nose blowing should be done with the mouth open, to avoid excessive pressures in the eustachian tube. Dizziness, which is common after the operation, usually resolves in a few days. The patient should not get the ear wet for at least 10 days postoperatively. For 30 days after surgery, the patient should not fly, climb to high altitudes, or be exposed to loud sounds such as those produced by a jet aircraft. Sudden movements, even in elevators, should be avoided. SEE: *Nursing Diagnoses Appendix.*

stapedial (stā-pē′dē-ăl) Rel. to the stapes.

stapediotenotomy (stā-pē″dē-ō-tĕn-ŏt′ō-mē) [″ + Gr. *tenon,* tendon, + *tome,* incision] Division of the tendon of the stapedius muscle.

stapediovestibular (stā-pē″dē-ō-vĕs-tĭb′ū-lar) [″ + *vestibulum,* an antechamber] Rel. to the stapes and vestibule of the ear.

stapedius (stā-pē′dē-ŭs) [L. *stapes,* stirrup] A small muscle of the middle ear inserted in the stapes.

stapes (stā′pēz) [L., stirrup] The ossicle in the middle ear that articulates with the incus; commonly called the *stirrup.* The footplate of the stapes fits into the oval window. SEE: *ear.*

staphylectomy (stăf″ĭ-lĕk′tō-mē) [Gr. *staphyle,* a bunch of grapes + *ektome,* excision] Staphylotomy (1).

staphyledema (stăf″ĭl-ē-dē′mă) [″ + *oidema,* swelling] Swelling of the uvula.

staphyline (stăf′ĭ-līn) [Gr. *staphyle,* a bunch of grapes] **1.** Resembling a bunch of grapes. SYN: *botryoid.* **2.** Rel. to the uvula. SYN: *uvular.*

staphylion (stăf-ĭl′ē-ŏn) [Gr., little grape] **1.** The craniometric point at the median line of the posterior border of the hard palate. **2.** Uvula.

staphylitis (stăf″ĭl-ī′tĭs) [Gr. *staphyle,* a bunch of grapes, + *itis,* inflammation] Inflammation of the uvula.

staphylo- [Gr. *staphyle,* a bunch of grapes] Combining form indicating the uvula, pert. to or resembling a bunch of grapes, or pert. to *Staphylococcus.*

staphyloangina (stăf″ĭl-ō-ăn′jĭ-nă) [″ + L. *angina,* sore throat] Sore throat due to *Staphylococcus.*

staphylococcal (stăf″ĭl-ō-kŏk′ăl) [″ + *kokkos,* berry] Pert. to or caused by staphylococci.

staphylococcal food poisoning Poisoning by food containing any one of several heat-stable enterotoxins produced by certain strains of staphylococci. When ingested, the toxin causes nausea, vomiting, diarrhea, intestinal cramps, and, in severe cases, prostration and shock. The attack usually lasts 3 to 6 hr. Fatalities are rare. Hygienic preparation techniques can prevent this form of food poisoning. Persons preparing foods should cook all foods thoroughly, refrigerate foods during storage, and wash hands before and after handling foods. Certain foods, such as meat, poultry, fish, and those containing mayonnaise, eggs, or cream, should be refrigerated and used as soon as possible.

PATIENT CARE: Patients who contract food poisoning should ingest clear fluids until abdominal pain subsides and return to a normal diet gradually. Fluid and electrolyte balance is monitored, and supportive therapy is maintained as indicated. Enteric precautions are used until evidence of infection subsides.

staphylococcemia (stăf″ĭl-ō-kŏk-sē′mē-ă) [″ + ″ + *haima,* blood] The presence of staphylococci in the blood. SYN: *staphylohemia.*

Staphylococcus (stăf″ĭl-ō-kŏk′ŭs) [Gr. *staphyle,* a bunch of grapes, + *kokkos,* berry] A genus of micrococci belonging to the family Micrococcaceae, order Eubacteriales. They are gram-positive and when cultured on agar produce white, yellow, or orange colonies. Some species are pathogenic, causing suppurative conditions and elaborating exotoxins destructive to tissues. Some produce enterotoxins and are the cause of a common type of food poisoning.

S. aureus A species of gram-positive, coagulase-positive bacteria commonly present on the skin and mucous membranes, esp. of the nose and mouth, which produce a golden-yellow pigment when cultured. These bacteria may cause suppurative conditions such as boils, carbuncles, and abscesses, as well as hospital-acquired infections, foreign body (prosthetic) infections, and life-threatening pneumonia or sepsis. Various strains of this species produce toxins, including those that cause food poisoning, staphylococcal scalded skin syndrome, and toxic shock syndrome. Some strains also produce hemolysins and staphylokinase.

S. aureus, methicillin-resistant ABBR: MRSA. A strain of *Staphylococcus aureus* resistant to anti-infective agents whose action is based on blocking penicillinase, an enzyme that inactivates penicillin. Patients with MRSA infections should be isolated and appropriate mask-gown-glove precautions used, depending on the site of the infection. SEE: *isolation; resistance, antibiotic.*

S. aureus, vancomycin-resistant ABBR: VRSA. A strain of *Staphylococcus aureus* resistant to vancomycin that may become a serious nosocomial pathogen. Strains with intermediate resistance to vancomycin (VRSA, vancomycin intermediate resistant *Staphylococcus aureus*) have caused life-threatening infections. SEE: *Standard and Universal Precautions Appendix.*

S. epidermidis A coagulase-negative species that may infect or colonize prosthetic devices and indwelling catheters. It is the most prevalent species of coagulase-negative staphylococci on skin.

S. hominis A coagulase-negative species frequently recovered from skin. It is not consistently pathogenic for humans.

S. saprophyticus A species that can cause urinary tract infections and rarely, pneumonia.

staphylococcus (stăf″ĭl-ō-kŏk′ŭs) *pl.* **staphylococci** Term applied loosely to any pathogenic micrococci. SEE: *bacteria* for illus.; *Staphylococcus.*

staphyloderma (stăf″ĭ-lō-dĕr′mă) [″ + *derma,* skin] Cutaneous infection with staphylococci.

staphylodermatitis (stăf″ĭl-ō-derm″ă-tī′tĭs) [″ + ″ + *itis,* inflammation] A dermatitis caused by staphylococci.

staphylodialysis (stăf″ĭ-lō-dī-ăl′ĭ-sĭs) [″ + *dia,* through, + *lysis,* dissolution] Relaxation or elongation of the uvula. SYN: *staphyloptosia*.

staphylohemia (stăf″ĭ-lō-hē′mē-ă) [″ + *haima,* blood] Staphylococcemia.

staphylokinase (stăf″ĭ-lō-kī′nās) An exotoxin produced by some strains of *Staphylococcus aureus* that may be used clinically as a thrombolytic drug.

staphylolysin (stăf″ĭ-lŏl′ĭ-sĭn) [″ + *lysis,* dissolution] A hemolysin produced by staphylococci.

staphyloma, staphyloma corneae (stăf″ĭl-ō′mă) [Gr.] A protrusion of the cornea or sclera of the eye. **staphylomatous,** *adj.*

anterior s. Globular enlargement of the anterior part of the eye. SYN: *keratoglobus*.

ciliary s. Staphyloma in the region of the ciliary body.

equatorial s. Staphyloma in the equatorial region of the eye.

intercalary s. Staphyloma in the region of the union of the sclera with the periphery of the iris.

partial s. Staphyloma that extends in one direction, displacing the pupil. The remainder of the cornea is clear.

posterior s. A bulging of the sclera backward.

total s. An opaque, protuberant scar found in place of the cornea. It is caused by a perforation of the cornea resulting in poor vision, increased tension, and rupture of thin scar. Treatment involves incision, excision, and ablation.

uveal s. The protrusion of any portion of the uvea through the sclera.

staphyloncus (stăf″ĭ-lŏng′kŭs) [Gr. *staphyle,* a bunch of grapes, + *onkos,* bulk, mass] A tumor or enlargement of the uvula.

staphylopharyngeus (stăf″ĭ-lō-făr-ĭn′jē-ŭs) [″ + *pharynx,* throat] Palatopharyngeus.

staphylopharyngorrhaphy (stăf″ĭ-lō-făr″ĭn-gor′ă-fē) [″ + ″ + *rhaphe,* seam, ridge] Any of several different operations on the soft palate and uvula.

staphyloplasty (stăf′ĭ-lō-plăs″tē) [″ + *plassein,* to form] Plastic surgery of the uvula or soft palate.

staphyloptosia, staphyloptosis (stăf″ĭ-lŏp-tō′sē-ă, -sĭs) [″ + *ptosis,* a dropping] Relaxation or elongation of the uvula. SYN: *staphylodialysis*.

staphylorrhaphy (stăf″ĭl-or′ă-fē) [″ + *rhaphe,* seam, ridge] Suture of a cleft palate.

staphyloschisis (stăf″ĭ-lŏs′kĭ-sĭs) [″ + *schisis,* a splitting] Cleft palate.

staphylotome (stăf′ĭ-lō-tōm) [″ + *tome,* incision] An instrument for cutting the uvula.

staphylotomy (stăf″ĭ-lŏt′ō-mē) [″+ *tome,* incision] Amputation or incision of the uvula. SYN: *staphylectomy*.

staphylotomy (stăf″ĭ-lŏt′ō-mē) [Gr. *staphyloma,* corneal protrusion, + *tome,* incision] Excision of a staphyloma.

staphylotoxin (stăf″ĭ-lō-tŏk′sĭn) [Gr. *staphyle,* a bunch of grapes, + *toxikon,* poison] A toxin elaborated by one of the staphylococci, esp. *S. aureus*. Among some of the toxins produced are an enterotoxin, a cause of food poisoning, and exotoxins, including a hemotoxin that lyses red blood cells, a dermonecrotic toxin, toxic shock syndrome toxin-1, and leukocidins.

staple food, staple Any food that supplies a substantial part, at least 25% to 35%, of the caloric requirement and is regularly consumed by a certain population.

stapling In surgery, a means of fastening tissues together by using special staples compatible with tissues. Staples are made of either titanium or an absorbable polymeric material. Numerous devices, which apply the staples in a variety of configurations, have been introduced.

gastric s. The surgical restriction of the outlet of the stomach (gastric cardia); used as a treatment for obesity in morbidly overweight patients. The procedure has many potential side effects, including esophagitis, vitamin deficiencies, and stenosis of the operative site.

surgical s. Fastening tissues to each other with a variety of applicators and staple configurations that form a binding across lacerations, wounds, incisions, or anastomoses. Stapling can usually be performed more rapidly than suturing, and therefore, may reduce anesthetic or operative time.

star [AS. *steorra*] Aster.

lens s. A starlike structure developing in the lens of the eye as a result of unequal growth of lens fibers.

s. of Verheyen Star-shaped masses of veins on the surface of the kidney. SYN: *stellate veins*.

starch [AS. *stercan*] Plant polysaccharides composed of glucose that are digestible by humans. Staple grains often comprise 50% to 58% of caloric intake. Salivary and pancreatic amylases hydrolyze starches to dextrin and maltose. These in turn are hydrolyzed to glucose, which is absorbed in the bloodstream. Glucose not immediately needed for energy is converted into glycogen and stored in the liver and muscle.

animal s. Glycogen.

corn s. Starch obtained from ordinary corn or maize (*Zea mays*). It is used as a dusting powder and an absorbent and is a constituent in many pastes and ointments. It is widely used in industry and as a food.

starch glycerite A combination of starch, benzoic acid, purified water, and glycerin; used as an emollient in formulations for external use.

stare (stār) [AS. *starian*] To gaze fixedly at anyone or anything.

Star of Life symbol The symbol designated by the Department of Transportation (DOT) to represent providers of emergency medical services (EMS). It is displayed on EMS vehicles and outside the emergency departments of hospitals. SEE: illus.

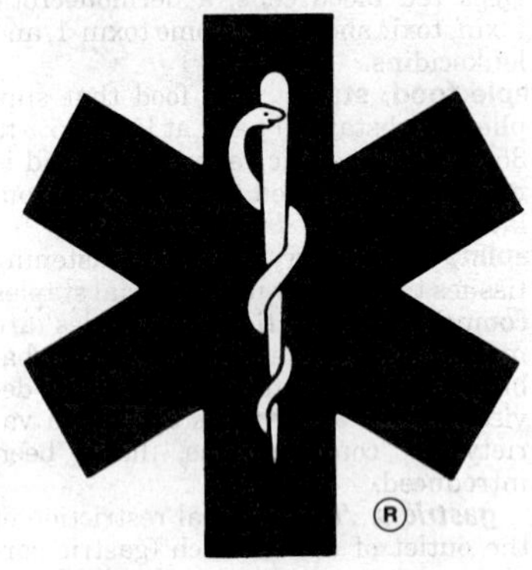

STAR OF LIFE

EMERGENCY MEDICAL CARE SYMBOL

Starling's law of heart [Ernest Henry Starling, Brit. physiologist, 1866–1927] A law that states that the force of blood ejected by the heart is determined primarily by the length of the fibers of its muscular wall (i.e., an increase in diastolic filling lengthens the fibers and increases the force of muscular contraction).

Starling's law of intestine A law stating that a stimulus within the intestine (i.e., the presence of food) initiates a band of constriction on the proximal side and relaxation on the distal side. This results in a peristaltic wave.

starter A pure culture of bacteria or other microorganism used to initiate a particular fermentation, as in the making of cheese.

star test pattern In radiography, a test to evaluate the condition of the focal spot of the x-ray tube.

starvation [AS. *steorfan*, to die] **1.** The condition of being without food for a long period of time. When everything but air and water is withheld, the sequence of events is as follows: (1) hunger, beginning about 4 hr after the last meal, accompanied by gastric contraction and general restlessness, becoming more acute periodically, esp. at times when meals were customarily taken; (2) utilization of glycogen stored in the liver and muscles; (3) utilization of stored fat; (4) loss of weight; (5) spells of nausea and diminishing acuteness of the sensation of hunger; (6) destruction of body protein. The greatest loss of weight is in the fatty tissues, spleen, and liver. **2.** The condition in which the supply of a specific food is below minimum bodily requirements, such as protein starvation. SEE: *kwashiorkor*. **3.** The condition resulting from failure of the body to digest and absorb essential foodstuffs. SEE: *deficiency disease; diet; dietetics*.

stasibasiphobia (stā″sĭ-bā″sĭ-fō′bē-ă) [Gr. *stasis*, a standing, + *basis*, step, + *phobos*, fear] The delusion of one's inability to stand or walk, or fear to make the attempt.

stasimorphia, stasimorphy (stā″sĭ-mor′fē-ă, -fē) [″ + *morphe*, form] A deformity caused by the failure to develop and grow.

stasiphobia (stā″sĭ-fō′bē-ă) [″ + *phobos*, fear] The delusion of one's inability to stand erect or hesitation to make the attempt.

stasis (stā′sĭs) [Gr. *stasis*, a standing] Stoppage of the normal flow of fluids, as of the blood or urine, or feces. SYN: *stagnation* (2).

diffusion s. Stasis with diffusion of lymph or serum.

intestinal s. Ileus.

venous s. Stasis of blood caused by venous congestion.

stat [L., *statim*] Immediately.

state [L. *status*, condition] **1.** A condition. **2.** A mode or condition of being. **3.** Status.

anxiety s. A condition marked by more or less continuous anxiety and apprehension. SEE: *neurosis, anxiety*.

central excitatory s. ABBR: CES. A condition of increased excitability in the central nervous system, esp. in the spinal cord, following an excitatory stimulus.

central inhibitory s. ABBR: CIS. A condition of decreased excitability in the central nervous system, esp. in the spinal cord, resulting from an inhibitory stimulus.

dream s. The state of diminished consciousness in which the surroundings are perceived as if in a dream.

excited s. The new state produced when energy is added to a nucleus, atom, or molecule. The energy is added by the absorption of photons or by collisions with other particles.

fatigue s. Exhaustion.

ground s. The state of the lowest energy of a system such as an atom or molecule.

locked-in s. A paralytic condition, superficially resembling coma, in which a person has no voluntary control over somatic muscles but nonetheless remains awake and alert. The locked-in state is usually the result of a lesion of the brainstem, esp. the pons. Because in some patients eye blinking is preserved, communication with locked-in patients is occasionally possible. SYN: *locked-in syndrome*. SEE: *akinetic mutism*.

persistent vegetative s. A continuing and unremitting clinical condition of complete unawareness of the environment accompanied by sleep-wake cycles with either complete or partial preservation of hypothalamic and brain-stem autonomic functions. The diagnosis is established if the condition is present for 1 month after acute or nontraumatic brain injury or has lasted for 1 month in patients with degenerative or metabolic disorders or developmental malformations.

refractory s. The condition of reduced ability to be excited just after a muscle and nerve have been stimulated.

steady s. In physiology, the condition in which energy inputs equal expended energy (e.g., in which nutrition equals metabolism); dynamic equilibrium.

statement, consensus A comprehensive summary of the opinions of a panel of experts about a particular scientific, medical, nursing, or administrative issue. Its purpose is to provide guidance to health care professionals, esp. on controversial or poorly understood aspects of care.

statement, position The official attitude assumed by a professional organization regarding an important health care topic. Position statements reflect care standards proposed by the organization and are typically updated regularly.

static (stăt′ĭk) [Gr. *statikos,* causing to stand] At rest; in equilibrium; not in motion.

static balance Static equilibrium.

static equilibrium The ability to maintain a steady position of the head and body in relation to gravity; it is integrated with the equilibrium of movement, or dynamic equilibrium. SYN: *static balance*.

static pressure The pressure existing in all points in the circulation when the heart is stopped. It provides a measure of how well the circulatory bed is filled with blood.

static reaction One of the postural reflex responses important to standing and walking. Included are local static reactions acting on individual limbs, segmental static reactions linking the extremities together, and general static reactions to the position of the head in space.

statics (stăt′ĭks) The study of matter at rest and of the forces bringing about equilibrium. SEE: *dynamics*.

statim (stăt′ĭm) [L.] ABBR: stat. Immediately; at once.

statins (stă′tĭnz) Any of the drugs from the class known as 3-hydroxy-3-methylglutaryl coenzyme A (HMG CoA) reductase inhibitors which have powerful lipid-lowering properties. The names of drugs in this class all end in "-statin." Some examples are atorvastatin, pravastatin, lovastatin, and simvastatin.

station (stā′shŭn) [L. *statio,* standing] **1.** The manner of standing. **2.** A stopping place. **3.** In obstetrics, the relationship in centimeters between the presenting part and the level of the ischial spines. SEE: *forceps*.

aid s. A site in the army for collecting the wounded in battle.

dressing s. A temporary station for soldiers wounded during combat.

rest s. A temporary relief station for the sick on a military road or railway.

stationary (stā′shŭn-ĕr-ē) [L. *stationarius,* belonging to a station] Remaining in a fixed condition.

statistical (stă-tĭs′tĭ-kăl) Pert. to statistics.

statistical significance Numerical meaningfulness; the likelihood that the results of a study are accurate, true, and valid.

statistics (stă-tĭs′tĭks) [LL. *statisticus*] The systematic collection, organization, analysis, and interpretation of numerical data pert. to any subject. SEE: *Bayes' theorem; statistical significance*.

medical s. Statistics pertinent to medical sciences, esp. data pert. to human disease.

morbidity s. Statistics pert. to sickness.

population s. Vital statistics.

vital s. Statistics dealing with births, deaths, and marriages. SYN: *population s.*

statoacoustic (stăt″ō-ă-koo′stĭk) [Gr. *statos,* placed, + *akoustikos,* acoustic] Concerning balance and hearing.

statoconia (stăt″ō-kō′nē-ă) [″ + *konos,* dust] Microscopic crystals of calcium carbonate on the hair cells of the maculae of the utricle and saccule of the middle ear. These are important in sensing the orientation to gravity. SYN: *statolith*.

statokinetic (stăt″kō-kĭn-ĕt′ĭk) [″ + *kinetikos,* moving] Pert. to reactions of the body produced by movement.

statolith (stăt′ō-lĭth) [″ + *lithos,* stone] Statoconia.

statometer (stă-tŏm′ĕt-ĕr) [″ + *metron,* a measure] An instrument for measuring the amount of abnormal protrusion of the eyeball.

statosphere (stăt′ō-sfēr) [″ + *sphaira,* a globe] Centrosome.

stature (stăt′ūr) [L. *statura*] The height of the body in a standing position.

short s. Body height at a specified

age below the level obtained at that age by 70% of the population. A number of diseases, including hormonal, nutritional, and intrauterine growth retardation, may cause this condition. It is important to determine the cause and initiate appropriate therapy as soon as possible.

tall s. Unusually great height, typically considered to be greater than 200 cm in men and 180 cm in women. This condition is usually familial and may be prevented with estrogens or testosterone, depending on gender of patient.

status (stā′tŭs) *pl.* **statuses** [L.] A state or condition.

s. asthmaticus Persistent and intractable asthma.

s. dysraphicus A condition resulting from imperfect closure of the neural tube of the embryo.

s. epilepticus Continuous seizure activity without a pause, that is, without an intervening period of normal brain function.

estrogen receptor s. The presence or absence of a receptor to the hormone estrogen on breast cancer cells. Tumors that possess receptors either to estrogen alone or to both estrogen and progesterone are more responsive to estrogen-blocking agents such as tamoxifen than are tumors that lack these receptors.

mental s. The functional state of the mind as judged by the individual's behavior, appearance, responsiveness to stimuli of all kinds, speech, memory, and judgment.

s. migrainosus Continuous or daily unilateral, throbbing, and disabling headaches that do not improve with standard therapies for migraine.

s. parathyreoprivus A condition resulting from loss of parathyroid tissue.

performance s. An assessment of the overall health and viability of a patient.

progesterone receptor s. The presence or absence of receptor to the steroid hormone progesterone on breast cancer cells. Tumors that possess receptors to estrogen, to progesterone, or to both, are more responsive to hormone-blocking agents, such as tamoxifen, than are tumors that lack these receptors.

s. raptus A state of ecstasy.

s. sternuens Continual sneezing that may be caused by transient irritation of the nasal mucosa. Treatment involves application of a topical anesthetic to the nasal mucosa.

s. verrucosus The defective development of the cerebral gyri with many small gyri. This gives a warty appearance to the surface of the brain.

statute Laws enacted by a state legislature.

statutes of limitations Federal and state laws that set maximum time limits in which lawsuits can be brought and actions, claims, or rights can be enforced. No legal action can be brought outside the time allowed by law even if the person or entity has a claim or cause of action. In medical negligence claims, the statute usually is in effect from the time the wrong occurred or from the time it was or should have been discovered. Time limitations vary from state to state.

staunch (stŏnch) [O.Fr. *estanche,* firm] To stop the flow of blood from a wound.

staurion (staw′rē-ŏn) [Gr. *stauros,* little cross] The craniometric point where the transverse palatine suture crosses the median one.

stauroplegia (staw″rō-plē′jē-ă) [″ + *plege,* stroke] Alternate hemiplegia.

stavudine (stă′vū-dēn) A nucleoside analogue reverse transcriptase inhibitor used in the treatment of HIV-1.

S.T.D. **1.** *sexually transmitted disease.* **2.** *skin test dose.*

steal (stēl) The deviation of blood flow from its normal course or rate of flow.

hand ischemic s. Deprivation of blood flow to the radial artery, after an arteriovenous access (i.e., for hemodialysis) has been surgically placed in a patient's arm. If blood flow to the hand is not restored, the limb may become cold, painful, pale, or gangrenous.

intracerebral s. The shunting of blood from ischemic to well-supplied regions of the brain, producing overperfusion of the unaffected tissue and underperfusion of the ischemic tissue.

subclavian s. SEE: *subclavian steal syndrome.*

vascular s. Steal.

steam (stēm) [AS. *steam,* vapor] **1.** The invisible vapor into which water is converted at the boiling point. **2.** The mist formed by condensation of water vapor. **3.** Any vaporous exhalation.

steam tent An obsolete device formerly used to encourage the inhalation of vapors (e.g., in respiratory diseases such as croup or cystic fibrosis).

steapsin (stē-ăp′sĭn) [Gr. *stear,* fat, + *pepsis,* digestion] Pancreatic lipase.

stearate (stē′ă-rāt) An ester or salt of stearic acid.

stearic acid (stē-ăr′ĭk) [Gr. *stear,* fat] $CH_3(CH_2)_{16}COOH$; A white, fatty acid found in solid animal fats and a few vegetable fats.

steariform (stē-ăr′ĭ-form) [″ + *forma,* shape] Resembling fat.

stearin (stē′ă-rĭn) [Gr. *stear,* fat] A white crystalline solid in animal and vegetable fats; $C_3H_5(CH_3(CH_2)_{16}COOH)_3$; any of the esters of glycerol and stearic acid, specifically glyceryl tristearate. One of the commonest fats in the body, esp. the solid ones. It breaks down into stearic acid and glycerol.

stearodermia (stē″ă-rō-dĕr′mē-ă) [″ + *derma,* skin] A disease of the sebaceous glands of the skin.

stearopten(e) (stē″ă-rŏp′tēn) [″ + *ptenos,* volatile] The more solid portion of a volatile oil as distinguished from the more fluid portion or eleoptene. Menthol and thymol are examples.

stearrhea (stē″ă-rē′ă) [Gr. *stear,* fat, + *rhoia,* flow] The excessive secretion of sebum or fat from the sebaceous glands of the skin. SYN: *seborrhea oleosa.*

steatadenoma (stē-ăt″ăd-ĕ-nō′mă) [Gr. *steatos,* fat, + *aden,* gland, + *oma,* tumor] A tumor of the sebaceous glands.

steatitis (stē″ă-tī′tĭs) [″ + *itis,* inflammation] Inflammation of adipose tissue.

steato- [Gr. *steatos,* fat] Combining form meaning *fat.* SEE: *adipo-; lipo-.*

steatocele (stē-ăt′ō-sēl, stē′ăt-ō-sēl) [″ + *kele,* tumor, swelling] Fatty tumor within the scrotum.

steatocryptosis (stē″ă-tō-krĭp-tō′sĭs) [″ + *krypte,* a sac, + *osis,* condition] Any disease of the sebaceous glands. SEE: *stearodermia.*

steatocystoma multiplex A skin disorder marked by the development of many sebaceous cysts.

steatogenous (stē″ă-tŏj′ĕn-ŭs) [Gr. *steatos,* fat, + *gennan,* to produce] **1.** Causing fatty degeneration. **2.** Producing any sebaceous gland disease.

steatolysis (stē″ă-tŏl′ĭ-sĭs) [″ + *lysis,* dissolution] **1.** The process by which fats are first emulsified and then hydrolyzed to fatty acids and glycerine preparatory to absorption. **2.** The decomposition of fat. SYN: *lipolysis.*

steatolytic (stē″ă-tō-lĭt′ĭk) Concerning steatolysis.

steatoma (stē″ă-tō′mă) [″ + *oma,* tumor] A fatty tumor. SEE: *epidermoid cyst; lipoma.*

steatomatous (stē″ă-tō′mă-tŭs) The presence of multiple sebaceous cysts.

steatonecrosis (stē″ă-tō-nē-krō′sĭs) [″ + *nekros,* corpse, + *osis,* condition] Necrosis of fatty tissue.

steatopathy (stē-ă-tŏp′ă-thē) [″ + *pathos,* disease, suffering] Disease of the sebaceous glands of the skin.

steatopygia (stē″ă-tō-pĭj′ē-ă) [″ + *pyge,* buttock] Abnormal fatness of the buttocks, occurring more frequently in women than in men.

steatorrhea (stē″ă-tō-rē′ă) [Gr. *steatos,* fat, + *rhoia,* flow] **1.** Increased secretion of fat from the sebaceous glands of the skin. SYN: *seborrhea.* **2.** Fatty stools, as seen in some malabsorption syndromes.

s. simplex Excessive secretion of the sebaceous glands of the face.

steatosis (stē″ă-tō′sĭs) [″ + *osis,* condition] **1.** Fatty degeneration. **2.** Disease of the sebaceous glands.

stegnosis (stĕg-nō′sĭs) [Gr. *stegnosis,* obstruction] **1.** Checking of a secretion or discharge. **2.** Stenosis. **3.** Constipation. **stegnotic,** *adj.*

stegnotic (stĕg-nŏt′ĭk) Bringing about stegnosis. SYN: *astringent.*

Stegomyia (stĕg″ō-mī′ē-ă) A subgenus of mosquito of the genus *Aedes,* family Culicidae, capable of transmitting many diseases to humans, including dengue, yellow fever, filariasis, and others.

Steinert's disease (stīn′ĕrts) [Hans Steinert, Ger. physician, b. 1875] A dominantly inherited disease marked by muscular wasting, decreased muscular tone, and cataracts, among other findings. SYN: *myotonia dystrophica.*

Stein-Leventhal syndrome (stīn-lĕv′ĕn-thăl) [Irving F. Stein, Sr., U.S. gynecologist, b. 1887; Michael L. Leventhal, U.S. obstetrician and gynecologist, 1901–1971] Chronic anovulation in the setting of obesity, hyperinsulinemia, type 2 diabetes mellitus, lipid abnormalities, hirsutism, infertility, and ovarian cysts. SYN: *polycystic ovary syndrome.*

Steinmann pin A metal rod used for internal fixation of the adjacent sections of a fractured bone.

Steinmann's extension (stīn′mănz) [Fritz Steinmann, Swiss surgeon, 1872–1932] Traction applied to a limb by applying weight to a pin placed through the bone at right angles to the direction of pull of the traction force.

stella [L.] Star.

s. lentis hyaloidea Posterior pole of the crystalline lens of the eye.

s. lentis iridica Anterior pole of the crystalline lens of the eye.

stellate [L. *stellatus*] Star-shaped; arranged with parts radiating from a center.

stellate bandage A bandage that is wrapped on the back, crossways.

stellate ligament One of the anterior costovertebral ligaments.

stellate reticulum The central cellular portion of the enamel organ, considered to be a nutritive store or protective covering of the developing enamel crown. SYN: *enamel pulp.*

stellate veins Star-shaped masses of veins on the surface of a kidney. SYN: *Verheyen's stars.*

stellectomy (stĕl-lĕk′tō-mē) [″ + *ektome,* excision] The surgical removal of the stellate ganglion.

Stellwag's sign (stĕl′vägs) [Carl Stellwag von Carion, Austrian oculist, 1823–1904] Widening of the palpebral aperture with absence or lessened frequency of winking, seen in Graves' disease.

stem [AS. *stemn,* tree trunk] **1.** Any stalklike structure. **2.** To derive from or originate in.

stem [ME. *stemmen*] To check, stop, or hold back.

stenion (stĕn′ē-ŏn) [Gr. *stenos,* narrow] The craniometric point at the extremities of the smallest transverse diameter in the temporal region.

steno- [Gr. *stenos,* narrow] Combining form meaning *narrow* or *short.*

stenobregmatic (stĕn″ō-brĕg-măt′ĭk) [″ + *bregma,* front of head] A term applied to a skull with narrowing of the upper and frontal portions.

stenocephaly (stĕn″ō-sĕf′ă-lē) [″ + *kephale,* head] Narrowness of the cranium in one or more diameters.

stenocompressor (stĕn″ō-kŏm-prĕs′or) [″ + L. *compressor,* that which presses together] An instrument for compressing Stensen's ducts to stop the flow of saliva.

stenopaic, stenopeic (stĕn-ŏ-pā′ĭk, -pē′ĭk) [Gr. *stenos,* narrow, + *ope,* opening] Provided with a narrow opening or slit, esp. denoting optical devices to protect against snow blindness.

stenosal (stē-nō′săl) [Gr. *stenos,* narrow] Stenotic.

stenosis (stĕ-nō′sĭs) [Gr., act of narrowing] The constriction or narrowing of a passage or orifice. SYN: *stricture.* **stenosed, stenotic,** *adj.*

ETIOLOGY: This may result from embryonic maldevelopment, hypertrophy and thickening of a sphincter muscle, inflammatory disorders, or excessive development of fibrous tissue. It may involve almost any tube or duct.

aortic s. An impairment of blood flow from the left ventricle to the aorta, as a result of aortic valve disease or obstructions just above or below the valve. Stenosis may occur congenitally or secondary to diseases that occur in adolescence or adulthood, such as rheumatic fever or fibrocalcific degeneration of the valve. SYN: *aortostenosis.* SEE: *Nursing Diagnoses Appendix.*

SYMPTOMS: Symptoms include dyspnea on exertion, fatigue, exertional syncope, angina, and palpitations. Orthopnea and paroxysmal nocturnal dyspnea are due to left ventricular failure. Peripheral edema may be present.

PHYSICAL FINDINGS: The murmur of aortic stenosis is best heard by placing the stethoscope over the base of the heart. The sound is typically described as being "diamond-shaped"; that is, it starts softly, increases in intensity, and then diminishes to a whisper. Palpation of the arteries in severe aortic stenosis may reveal a delayed and weakened pulse (e.g., at the carotids). The heart's apical impulse may be laterally and inferiorly displaced as a result of left ventricular hypertrophy.

TREATMENT: If the aortic valve area is significantly narrowed or the patient has experienced symptoms of heart failure or syncope, valvuloplasty or aortic valve replacement may be necessary.

PATIENT CARE: A history of related cardiac disorders is obtained. Cardiopulmonary function is assessed regularly by monitoring vital signs and weight, intake, and output for signs of fluid overload. The patient is monitored for chest pain, which may indicate cardiac ischemia, and the electrocardiogram evaluated for ischemic changes. Activity tolerance and fatigue are assessed.

After cardiac catheterization, the insertion site is checked according to protocol (often every 15 min for 6 hr) for signs of bleeding; the patient is assessed for chest pain, and vital signs, heart rhythm, and peripheral pulses distal to the insertion site are monitored. Problems are reported to the cardiologist.

Desired outcomes include adequate cardiopulmonary tissue perfusion and cardiac output, reduced fatigue with exertion, absence of fluid volume excess, and ability to manage the treatment regimen.

cicatricial s. Stenosis resulting from any contracted scar.

coronary artery s. A physical obstruction to the flow of blood through the epicardial arteries, usually as a result of atherosclerotic plaque.

lumbar s. Spinal s.

mitral s. ABBR: MS. Narrowing of the mitral valve orifice with obstruction of blood flow from the left atrium to the left ventricle. In most adults, previous bouts of rheumatic carditis are responsible for the lesion. Less often, MS may be present at birth (Lutembacher's disease) or it may develop as the mitral valve calcifies during aging.

The abnormality of the valve may predispose patients to infective endocarditis; to left atrial enlargement and atrial arrhythmias; or to left ventricular failure. SEE: *Nursing Diagnoses Appendix.*

pulmonary s. Narrowing of the opening into the pulmonary artery from the right cardiac ventricle.

spinal s. Narrowing of the spinal canal due to degenerative or traumatic changes in the lumbar spine. If physical therapy, back braces, or corticosteroid injections do not provide relief, surgical decompression may be helpful. SYN: *lumbar s.*

subaortic s. A congenital constriction of the aortic tract below the aortic valves. SEE: *hypertrophic cardiomyopathy.*

tricuspid s. Narrowing of the opening to the tricuspid valve.

stenostomia (stĕn″ō-stō′mē-ă) [Gr. *stenos,* narrow, + *stoma,* mouth] Narrowing of the mouth.

stenothorax (stĕn″ō-thō′răks) [″ + *thorax,* chest] An unusually narrow thorax.

Stenotrophomonas maltophilia (stĕn′ō-trō-fō-mōn″as) The current name for the bacteria previously known as *Xanthomonas maltophilia* or *Pseudomonas maltophilia.*

Stensen's duct (stĕn′sĕns) [Niels Stensen, Danish anatomist, 1638–1686] The duct leading from the parotid gland to the oral cavity.

Stensen's foramina Incisive foramina of the hard palate, transmitting anterior branches of the descending palatine vessels.

stent [Charles R. Stent, Brit. dentist, 1845–1901] **1.** Originally a compound used in making dental molds. **2.** Any material or device used to hold tissue in place, to maintain open blood vessels, or to provide a support for a graft or anastomosis while healing is taking place.

intraluminal coronary artery s. A stent made of an inert material, usually metallic, with a self-expanding mesh introduced into the coronary artery. It is used to prevent lumen closure (restenosis) following bypass surgery and to treat acute vessel closure after angioplasty.

urologic s. A biologically compatible tube inserted into the ureter or urethra to relieve or prevent urinary tract obstruction. Stents are commonly placed in the urinary tract after endoureterotomy and endopyelotomy.

step 1. To move one foot in relation to the other, as in walking. **2.** A series of rests for the foot, used for ascending or descending. **3.** A single movement or act within a sequence of behaviors necessary for completing a task.

Rönne's s. A steplike defect in the visual field.

Stephan's curve A mathematical model used to determine the impact of ingested foods on the pH of dental plaque and subsequent caries formation. Decalcification of teeth occurs when the pH in the oral cavity is less than 5.5.

DENTAL IMPLICATIONS: To reduce decalcification of tooth surfaces, patients should be encouraged to consume foods that do not result in a drop in plaque pH.

stephanion (stĕ-fā′nē-ŏn) [Gr. *stephanos,* crown] The point at the intersection of the superior temporal ridge and coronal suture.

steradian (stē-rā′dē-ăn) The unit of measurement of solid angles. It encloses an area on the surface of a sphere equal to the square of the radius of the sphere.

sterco- [L. *stercus,* dung] Combining form meaning *feces.* SEE: *scato-.*

stercobilin (stĕr″kō-bī′lĭn) [″ + *bilis,* bile] A brown pigment derived from the bile, giving the characteristic color to feces. SEE: *urobilin.*

stercobilinogen (stĕr″kō-bī-lĭn′ō-jĕn) A colorless substance derived from urobilinogen. It is present in the feces and turns brown on oxidation.

stercolith, stercorolith (stĕr′kō-lĭth) [″ + Gr. *lithos,* stone] A fecal stone.

stercoraceous (stĕr″kō-rā′shŭs) [L. *stercoraceus*] Having the nature of, pert. to, or containing feces.

stereo-, stere- Combining form meaning *solid, having three dimensions,* or *firmly established.*

stereoacuity (stĕr″ē-ō-ă-kew′ĭt-ē) The accuracy and sharpness of images acquired with binocular depth perception.

stereoagnosis (stĕr″ē-ō-ăg-nō′sĭs) [Gr. *stereos,* solid, + *a-,* not, + *gnosis,* knowledge] Astereognosis.

stereoanesthesia (stĕr″ē-ō-ăn″ĕs-thē′zē-ă) [″ + *an-,* not, + *aisthesis,* sensation] The inability to recognize objects by feeling their form.

stereoarthrolysis (stĕr″ē-ō-ăr-thrŏl′ĭ-sĭs) [″ + *arthron,* joint, + *lysis,* dissolution] The surgical formation of a movable new joint in bony ankylosis.

stereoauscultation (stĕr″ē-ō-aws″kŭl-tā′shŭn) [″ + L. *auscultare,* listen to] Auscultation by use of a two-headed stethoscope. One tube of each instrument is inserted into an ear while the other is squeezed shut by the fingers.

stereocampimeter (stĕr″ē-ō-kăm-pĭm′ĕ-tĕr) [″ + L. *campus,* field, + Gr. *metron,* measure] A device for measuring the visual field of both eyes simultaneously.

stereochemistry (stĕr″ē-ō-kĕm′ĭs-trē) That branch of chemistry dealing with atoms in their space relationship, and the effect of such a relationship on the action and effects of the molecule. **stereochemical,** *adj.*

stereocilia (stĕr″ē-ō-sĭl′ē-ă) *sing.,* **stereocilium** Nonmotile protoplasmic projections from free surfaces of cells of the ductus epididymis and ductus deferens and on the hair cells of the receptors of the inner ear.

stereoencephalotomy (stĕr″ē-ō-ĕn-sĕf″ă-lŏt′ō-mē) [″ + *enkephalos,* brain, + *tome,* incision] Surgical incision by use of stereotaxis.

stereognosis (stĕr″ē-ŏg-nō′sĭs) [″ + *gnosis,* knowledge] The ability to recognize the form of solid objects by touch.

stereogram (stĕr′ē-ō-grăm) [″ + *gramma,* something written] Stereoscopic radiographs.

stereoisomerism (stĕr″ē-ō-ī-sŏ′mĕr-ĭzm) A condition in which two or more substances may have the same empirical formula but mirror-image structural formulas.

stereology (stĕr″ē-ŏl′ō-jē) [Gr. *stereos,* solid, + *logos,* word, reason] The study of three-dimensional aspects of objects.

stereometry (stĕr″ē-ŏm′ĕ-trē) [″ + *metron,* a measure] The measurement of a solid body or the cubic contents of a hollow body.

stereo-ophthalmoscope (stĕr″ē-ō-ŏf-thăl′mō-skōp) [″ + *ophthalmos,* eye, + *skopein,* to examine] An ophthalmoscope that is designed to permit the fundus to be seen simultaneously by both eyes of the examiner.

stereo-orthopter (stĕr″ē-ō-or-thŏp′tĕr) [″ + *orthos,* straight, + *opsis,* vision] A mirror-reflecting device for the treatment of strabismus.

stereophantoscope (stĕr″ē-ō-făn′tō-skōp) [″ + *phantos,* visible, + *skopein,* to examine] A stereoscopic device with rotating disks for testing vision.

stereophorometer (stĕr″ē-ō-for-ŏm′ĕ-tĕr) [″ + *phoros,* a bearer, + *metron,* measure] A prism-refracting device for use in correcting extraocular eye muscle imbalance.

stereophotography (stĕr″ē-ō-fō-tŏg′ră-fē) [″ + *phos,* light, + *graphein,* to write] Photography that produces the effect of solidity or depth in the pictures.

stereophotomicrograph (stĕr″ē-ō-fō″tō-mī′krō-grăf) [″ + ″ + *mikros,* tiny, + *graphein,* to write] A photograph showing the solidity or depth of a microscopic subject.

stereopsis (stĕr″ē-ŏp′sĭs) [″ + *opsis,* vision] Binocular depth perception.

stereoradiography (stĕr″ē-ō-rā″dē-ŏg′ră-fē) [″ + L. *radius,* ray, + Gr. *graphein,* to write] Radiography from two slightly different angles to simulate the distance between the viewer's eyes (usually 4 in.) so that a stereoscopic effect is produced when the radiographs are viewed through a stereoscope.

stereoscope (stĕr′ē-ō-skōp) [″ + *skopein,* to examine] An instrument that creates an impression of solidity or depth of objects seen by combining images of two pictures.

stereoscopic, stereoscopical Pert. to the stereoscope or its use.

stereospecific (stĕr″ē-ō-spĕ-sĭf′ĭk) Specific for only one of the possible receptors on a cell.

stereotactic Having precise spatial coordinates, located precisely in three-dimensional space. Stereotactic techniques are used in brain surgery, breast biopsies, and other procedures in which precision is needed in identifying, cutting, or removing tissues.

stereotropism (stĕr″ē-ŏt′rō-pĭzm) [″ + *tropos,* a turning, + *-ismos,* condition] A response toward (positive stereotropism) or away from (negative stereotropism) a solid object. SYN: *thigmotropism.*

stereotypic movement disorder Motor behavior, persisting for at least 4 weeks, that is repetitive, often seemingly driven and nonfunctional to the extent that it interferes with normal activities or results in self-inflicted bodily injury sufficient to require medical treatment. The disorder cannot be accounted for by a compulsion, a tic, or hair pulling, and is not due to the effects of a substance or a general medical condition.

stereotypy (stĕr-ē-ō-tī′pē) [″ + *typos,* type] The persistent repetition of words, posture, or movement without meaning.

steric (stē′rĭk) Concerning the spatial arrangement of atoms in a chemical compound.

sterile (stĕr′ĭl) [L. *sterilis,* barren] **1.** Free from living microorganisms. Solutions that have passed through certain filters are called sterile solutions because bacteria, fungi, and their spores have been removed. However, viruses can pass through some filters, and the term sterile is incorrectly used in this context. **2.** Not fertile; unable to reproduce young. SYN: *barren.* SEE: *sterility.*

sterility (stĕr-ĭl′ĭ-tē) [L. *sterilitas,* barrenness] **1.** Freedom from contamination or colonization by living microorganisms. **2.** The inability of the female to become pregnant or for the male to impregnate a female.

When investigating sterility, both partners should be examined. A routine examination for the female includes a study of the vaginal secretions, a bimanual pelvic examination, visualization of the cervix, in some cases a test for patency of the fallopian tubes, and a record of basal body temperature. A history of pelvic disease in the female is of great importance. The male should have the seminal fluid examined for the number, motility, viability, and normality of the spermatozoa, and occasionally other tests (e.g., of testosterone levels).

TREATMENT: Treatment of sterility depends on the finding and correction of any or all causes of the condition. A high percentage of couples who have an infertility problem during the first year in which they are trying to have a child will, without treatment, produce offspring within 2 to 3 years. SEE: *embryo transfer; gamete intrafallopian transfer; fertilization, in vitro.*

absolute s. The inability to produce offspring as a result of anatomical or physiological factors that prevent production of functional germ cells, conception, or the normal development of a zygote; this type of sterility is incurable.

female s. The inability of a female to conceive. This may result from a failure to produce or transport viable ova or to sustain a pregnancy due to a congenital absence or maldevelopment of the reproductive organs. Sterility also may be secondary to endocrine disorders, infections, trauma, neoplasms, inactivation of the ovaries by irradiation, or surgical excision of the ovaries, tubes, or uterus. SEE: *infertility; gonadal dysgenesis.*

male s. The inability of a male either to produce sperm or to produce viable sperm, thereby prohibiting fertilization of the ovum. This may result from congenital factors such as cryptorchidism or maldevelopment of the testicular ducts or testis; or acquired factors, such as radiation to, or surgical removal of, the testes.

primary s. Sterility resulting from failure of the testis or ovary to produce functional germ cells.

relative s. Sterility due to causes other than a defect of the sex organs.

sterilization (stĕr″ĭl-ĭ-zā′shŭn) [L. *sterilis,* barren] **1.** The process of completely removing or destroying all microorganisms on a substance by exposure to chemical or physical agents, ionizing radiation, or by filtering gas or liquids through porous materials that remove microorganisms. A substance cannot be properly described as being partially sterile. SEE: *sterile*. **2.** The process of rendering barren. This can be accomplished by the surgical removal of the testes or ovaries (castration) or inactivation by irradiation, or by tying off or removing a portion of the reproductive ducts (ductus deferens or uterine tubes). SEE: *salpingectomy; vasectomy.*

dry heat s. Sterilization of microorganisms by subjection to high temperatures (165°C to 170°C) for 2 to 3 hr in sterilization chambers.

fractional s. Sterilization of microorganisms in which heating is done at separated intervals, so that spores can develop into bacteria and be destroyed. This is usually accomplished by subjecting organisms to free-flowing steam for 15 min for 3 or 4 successive days. SYN: *intermittent s.*

gas s. Exposure to gases such as formaldehyde or ethylene oxide that destroy microorganisms.

intermittent s. Fractional s.

laparoscopic s. Sterilization by use of a laparoscope to gain access to the fallopian tubes so they can be banded, clipped, or electrocoagulated.

steam s. Sterilization by exposure of microorganisms at 212°F (100°C) to flowing steam in an unsealed receptacle or by exposure of microorganisms to steam under pressure in an autoclave.

sterilize (stĕr′ĭ-līz) [L. *sterilis,* barren] **1.** To free from microorganisms. **2.** To make incapable of reproduction.

sterilizer (stĕr′ĭ-lī″zĕr) An oven or appliance for sterilizing.

steam s. An autoclave that sterilizes by steam under pressure at temperatures above 100°C.

sternad (stĕr′năd) [Gr. *sternon,* chest] Toward the sternum.

sternal (stĕr′năl) [Gr. *sternalis*] Rel. to the sternum or breastbone.

sternalgia (stĕr-năl′jē-ă) [Gr. *sternon,* chest, + *algos,* pain] Pain in the sternum. SYN: *sternodynia.*

sternal puncture Use of a large-bore needle to obtain a specimen of marrow from the sternum.

Sternberg-Reed cell Reed-Sternberg cell.

sternebra (stĕr′nē-bră) [″ + L. *vertebra,* vertebra] Parts of the sternum during development of the fetus.

sternen (stĕr′nĕn) [Gr. *sternon,* chest] Concerning the sternum and no other structures.

sterno- [Gr. *sternon,* chest] Combining form meaning *sternum.*

sternoclavicular (stĕr″nō-klă-vĭk′ū-lăr) [″ + L. *clavicula,* little key] Concerning the sternum and clavicle.

sternocleidal (stĕr″nō-klī″dăl) [″ + *clavis,* key] Sternoclavicular.

sternocleidomastoid (stĕr″nō-klī″dō-măs′toyd) [″ + *clavis,* key, + *mastos,* breast, + *eidos,* form, shape] One of two muscles arising from the sternum and inner part of the clavicle.

sternocostal (stĕr″nō-kŏs′tăl) [″ + L. *costa,* rib] Rel. to sternum and ribs.

sternodymia (stĕr″nō-dĭm′ē-ă) [″ + *didymos,* twin] A condition in which deformed twin fetuses are joined at the sternum. SYN: *sternopagia.*

sternodynia (stĕr″nō-dĭn′ē-ă) [″ + *odyne,* pain] Pain in the sternum. SYN: *sternalgia.*

sternohyoid (stĕr″nō-hī′oyd) [″ + *hyoeides,* U-shaped] The muscle from the medial end of the clavicle and sternum to the hyoid bone.

sternoid (stĕr′noyd) [″ + *eidos,* form, shape] Resembling the breastbone.

sternomastoid (stĕr″nō-măs′toyd) [″ + *mastos,* breast, + *eidos,* form, shape] Pert. to the sternum and mastoid process of the temporal bone.

sternomastoid region The wide area on the lateral region of the neck covered by sternocleidomastoid muscle.

sternopagia (stĕr″nō-pā′jē-ă) [″ + *pagos,* thing fixed] Sternodymia.

sternopericardial (stĕr″nō-pĕr″ĭ-kăr′dē-ăl) [″ + *peri,* around, + *kardia,* heart] Concerning the sternum and pericardium.

sternoschisis (stĕr-nŏs′kĭ-sĭs) [″ + *schisis,* a splitting] A cleft or fissured sternum.

sternothyroid (stĕr″nō-thī′royd) [″ + *thyreos,* shield, + *eidos,* form, shape] The muscle extending beneath the sternohyoid that depresses the thyroid cartilage.

sternotomy (stĕr-nŏt′ō-mē) [″ + *tome,* incision] The operation of cutting through the sternum.

sternotracheal (stĕr″nō-trā′kē-ăl) [″ + *tracheia,* trachea] Concerning the sternum and trachea.

sternotrypesis (stĕr″nō-trī-pē′sĭs) [″ + *trypesis,* a boring] Surgical perforation of the sternum.

sternovertebral (stĕr″nō-vĕr′tĕ-brăl) [″ + L. *vertebra,* vertebra] Concerning the sternum and vertebrae.

sternum (stĕr′nŭm) [L.] The narrow, flat bone in the median line of the thorax in front. It consists of three portions:

the manubrium, the body or gladiolus, and the ensiform or xiphoid process. SEE: illus.

cleft s. A congenital fissure of the sternum.

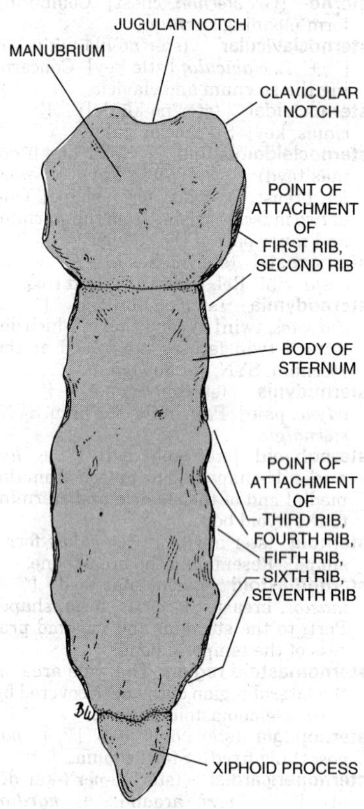

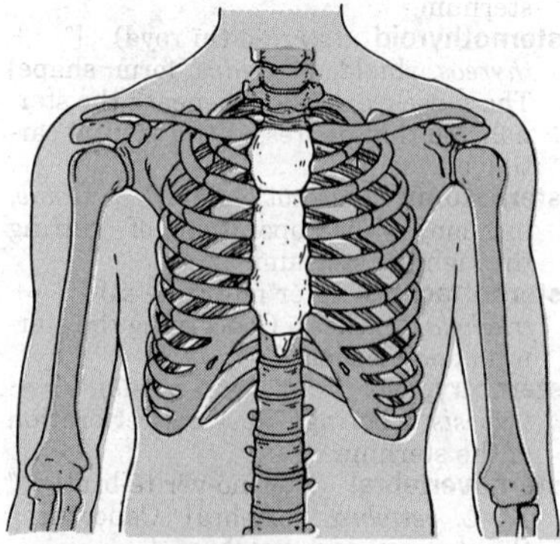

ANTERIOR VIEW

sternutament (stĕr-nū′tăm-ĕnt) [L. *sternutare,* to sneeze] A substance causing sneezing.

sternutatio (stĕr-nū-tā′shē-ō) [L.] Sneezing.

s. convulsiva Paroxysmal sneezing, as in hay fever.

sternutation (stĕr-nū-tā′shŭn) The act of sneezing.

sternutator (stĕr′nū-tā″tor) [L. *sternutatorius,* causing sneezing] An agent, such as a war gas, that induces sneezing. **sternutatory,** *adj.*

steroid (stĕr′oyd) **1.** An organic compound containing in its chemical nucleus the perhydrocyclopentanophenanthrene ring. SEE: *steroid hormone* for illus.; *perhydrocyclopentanophenanthrene.* **2.** A term applied to any one of a large group of substances chemically related to sterols, including cholesterol, D vitamins, bile acids, certain hormones, saponins, glucosides of digitalis, and certain carcinogenic substances.

steroid hormone One of the sex hormones and hormones of the adrenal cortex. SEE: illus.

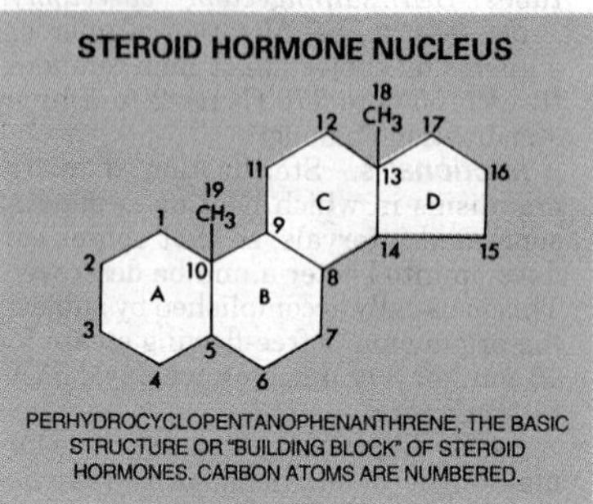

PERHYDROCYCLOPENTANOPHENANTHRENE, THE BASIC STRUCTURE OR "BUILDING BLOCK" OF STEROID HORMONES. CARBON ATOMS ARE NUMBERED.

steroid hormone therapy Treatment with intravenous, oral, inhaled, or topical adrenal hormones (or their synthetic derivatives), usually to relieve inflammatory diseases (such as asthma or chronic obstructive lung disease; arthritis or colitis; or dermatitis or eczema), or as part of a combined modality treatment for some malignancies. Common side effects of prolonged, high-dose steroid hormone therapy include alterations in the sleep-wake cycle, fluid and sodium retention, muscle weakness, thinning of the skin, cataract formation, diabetes mellitus, osteoporosis, or immune suppression. Few if any of these effects are likely to occur when steroids are given for 1- or 2-week courses of therapy.

steroidogenesis (stē-roy″dō-jĕn′ĕ-sĭs) Production of steroids.

sterol (stĕr′ōl, stĕr′ŏl) [Gr. *stereos,* solid, + L. *oleum,* oil] One of a group of substances (such as cholesterol) with a cyclic nucleus and alcohol moiety. They are found free or esterified with fatty acids (cholesterides). They are found in animals (zoosterols) or in plants (phytosterols). They are generally colorless, crystalline compounds, nonsaponifiable and soluble in certain organic solvents.

stertor (stěr′tor) [NL. *stertor,* to snore] Snoring or laborious breathing owing to obstruction of air passages in the head, seen in certain diseases such as apoplexy.

stertorous (stěr′tō-rŭs) Pert. to laborious breathing provoking a snoring sound.

stetho- [Gr. *stethos,* chest] Combining form meaning *chest.*

stethogram (stěth′ō-grăm) [″ + *gramma,* something written] A record of heart sounds. The record may be stored for later comparison with subsequent heart sounds. SYN: *phonocardiogram.*

stethomyitis, stethomyositis (stěth″ō-mī-ī′tĭs, -mī″ō-sī′tĭs) [″ + *mys,* muscle, + *itis,* inflammation] Inflammation of the muscles of the chest.

stethoparalysis (stěth″ō-pă-răl′ĭ-sĭs) [″ + *paralyein,* to disable] Paralysis of the muscles of the chest.

stethoscope (stěth′ō-skōp) [″ + *skopein,* to examine] An instrument used to transmit to the examiner's ears sounds produced in the body. It ordinarily consists of rubber tubing in a Y shape and a bell or diaphragm.

binaural s. A stethoscope designed for use with both ears.

compound s. A stethoscope in which more than one set is attached to the same fork and chest piece.

double s. A stethoscope with two earpieces and tubes.

electronic s. A stethoscope equipped to amplify electronically sounds from the body.

single s. A rigid or flexible stethoscope designed for one ear only.

stethoscopic (stěth″ō-skŏp′ĭk) Concerning or done by use of a stethoscope.

stethospasm (stěth′ō-spăzm) [″ + *spasmos,* convulsion] A spasm of the pectoral or chest muscles.

Stevens-Johnson syndrome (stē′vĕnz-jŏn′sŏn) [Albert M. Stevens, 1884–1945, Frank C. Johnson, 1894–1934, U.S. pediatricians] A systemic skin disease, probably identical to toxic epidermal necrolysis, that produces fevers and lesions of the oral, conjunctival, and vaginal mucous membranes. It is marked by a cutaneous rash that is often widespread and severe. Skin loss may lead to dehydration, infection, or death. SEE: illus.; *erythema multiforme.*

STH *somatotropic hormone.*

sthenia (sthē′nē-ă) [Gr. *sthenos,* strength] Normal or unusual strength. Opposite of asthenia. **sthenic,** *adj.*

stibialism (stĭb′ē-ăl-ĭzm) [L. *stibium,* antimony, + Gr. *-ismos,* condition] Antimony poisoning.

stibiated (stĭb′ē-āt″ĕd) [L. *stibium,* antimony] Containing antimony.

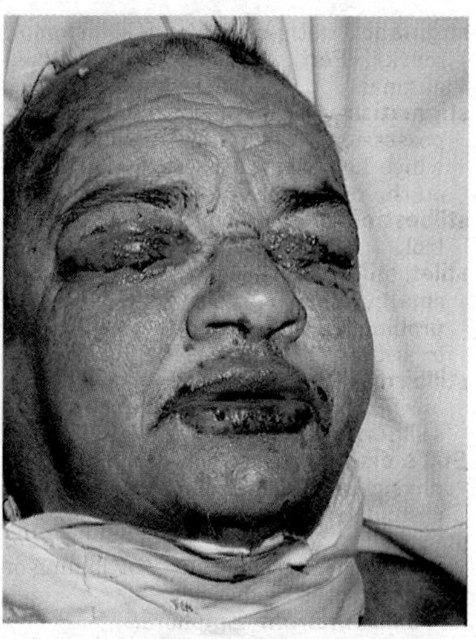

STEVENS-JOHNSON SYNDROME

stibium (stĭb′ē-ŭm) [L.] Antimony.

stibophen (stĭb′ō-fĕn) A trivalent tin compound, used in treating schistosomiasis, leishmaniasis, and granuloma inguinale.

stiff [AS. *stif*] Rigid, firm, inflexible.

stiff joint A joint with reduced mobility.

stiff man syndrome/stiff person syndrome A rare disorder of the central nervous system characterized by fluctuating but progressive muscle rigidity and spasms. The etiology is unknown but is most probably of autoimmune origin. Some cases are associated with carcinoma. Treatments may include symptomatic remedies such as baclofen, diazepam, or clonazepam, or immunological therapies such as plasma exchange or infusions of intravenous immune globulins.

stiff neck Rigidity of neck resulting from spasm of neck muscles. It is a symptom of many disorders. SYN: *torticollis; wryneck.*

stigma (stĭg′mă) *pl.* **stigmata, -mas** [Gr., mark] **1.** A mark or spot on the skin; lesions or sores of the hands and feet that resemble crucifixion wounds. **2.** The spot on the ovarian surface where rupture of a graafian follicle occurs. **3.** A social condition marked by attitudinal devaluing or demeaning of persons who, because of disfigurement or disability, are not viewed as being capable of fulfilling valued social roles.

hysterical s. Any of the peculiar marks or symptoms of hysteria, such as spots on the skin or impairment of sensory functions.

psychic s. A mental state marked by susceptibility to suggestion.

stigmata Cutaneous evidence of systemic illness.

stigmatic (stĭg-măt′ĭk) [Gr. *stigma,* mark] Pert. to or marked with a stigma.

stigmatism **1.** A condition marked by possession of stigmata. **2.** A condition in which light rays are accurately focused on the retina. SEE: *astigmatism.*

stilbestrol (stĭl-bĕs′trŏl) Diethylstilbestrol.

stilet, stilette (stī-lĕt′) [Fr. *stilette*] **1.** A small, sharp-pointed instrument for probing. **2.** A wire used to pass through or stiffen a flexible catheter.

stillbirth [AS. *stille,* quiet, + Old Norse *burdhr,* birth] The birth of a dead fetus. **stillborn,** *adj.*

Still's disease [Sir George F. Still, Brit. physician, 1868–1941] Juvenile rheumatoid arthritis.

stillicidium (stĭl″ĭ-sĭd′ē-ŭm) [L. *stilla,* drop, + *cadere,* to fall] A dribbling or flowing, drop by drop.

s. lacrimarum Epiphora.

s. narium A watery mucus discharged at the onset of coryza.

s. urinae Strangury.

stimulant (stĭm′ū-lănt) [L. *stimulans,* goading] Any agent temporarily increasing functional activity. Stimulants may be classified according to the organ upon which they act, as follows: cardiac, bronchial, gastric, cerebral, intestinal, nervous, motor, vasomotor, respiratory, and secretory. Commonly used stimulants include caffeine, low doses of ethanol, methamphetamines, and cocaine.

stimulate (stĭm′ū-lāt) [L. *stimulare,* to goad on] **1.** To increase activity of an organ or structure. **2.** To apply a stimulus.

stimulation (stĭm″ū-lā′shŭn) **1.** Irritating or invigorating action of agents on muscles, nerves, or sensory end organs by which excitation or activity in a part is evoked. **2.** A stimulus.

double simultaneous s. In the neurological examination, a test of unilateral neglect. A light touch, audible signal, or visual cue is provided to both sides of the patient at the same time (e.g., both arms, both ears, both the left and right visual fields). Failure to detect one of the stimuli suggests a lesion in the opposite side of the cerebral cortex. Double simultaneous stimulation can also be performed on one side of the body, for instance, by tapping the left arm and left side of the face at the same time. If the distal stimulus is undetected even after several trials, the patient may have an organic brain syndrome.

fetal scalp s. An assessment of fetal well-being in which the examiner reaches into the vagina and rubs the scalp of the fetus. The fetal heart rate is monitored for accelerations. If the fetal heart rate does not accelerate appropriately, further testing, such as scalp blood sampling, may be needed.

fetal (vibratory) acoustic s. ABBR: FAST. A noninvasive means of assessing fetal reactivity during labor. It typically is used as an adjunct to nonstress testing. The examiner applies an electronic source of low-frequency sound (such as an electrolarynx) firmly to the mother's abdomen over the fetal head. A reactive test is characterized by fetal heart rate accelerations or other measurable forms of increased fetal activity.

neural s. The activation or energizing of a nerve, through an external source.

stimulator (stĭm″ū-lā′tor) Something that stimulates.

long-acting thyroid s. SEE: *long-acting thyroid stimulator.*

stimulus (stĭm′ū-lŭs) *pl.* **stimuli** [L., a goad] **1.** A change of environment of sufficient intensity to evoke a response in an organism. **2.** An excitant or irritant.

adequate s. **1.** Any stimulus capable of evoking a response, that is, an environmental change possessing a certain intensity, acting for a certain length of time, and occurring at a certain rate. **2.** A stimulus capable of initiating a nerve impulse in a specific type of receptor.

chemical s. A chemical (liquid, gaseous, or solid) that is capable of evoking a response.

conditioned s. A stimulus that gives rise to a conditioned response. SEE: *reflex, conditioned.*

electric s. A stimulus resulting from initiation of or cessation of a flow of electrons as from a battery, induction coil, or generator.

homologous s. A stimulus that acts only on specific sensory end organs.

iatrotropic s. Any stimulus or event that makes a person seek or receive medical attention, such as a symptom, a physical finding, or the need for a routine or required health screening examination.

liminal s. Threshold s.

mechanical s. A stimulus produced by a physical change such as contact with objects or changes in pressure.

minimal s. Threshold s.

nociceptive s. A painful and usually injurious stimulus.

subliminal s. A stimulus that is weaker than a threshold stimulus.

thermal s. A stimulus produced by a change in skin temperature, a rise giving sensations of warmth, a fall giving sensations of coldness.

threshold s. The least or weakest stimulus that is capable of initiating a response or giving rise to a sensation. SYN: *liminal s.; minimal s.*

unconditioned s. Any stimulus that elicits an unconditioned response (i.e., a response that occurs by reflex rather than by learning).

sting [AS. *stingan*] **1.** A sharp, smarting sensation, as of a wound or astringent. **2.** A puncture wound made by a venomous barb or spine (e.g., of a marine animal or an insect). SEE: *bite*.

SYMPTOMS: Pain at the puncture site is almost universally reported. The patient may also develop local swelling, which at times is massive, and localized itch. Generalized hives, dizziness, a tight feeling in the chest, difficulty breathing, swelling of the lips and tongue, stridor, respiratory failure, hypotension, syncope, or cardiac arrest may also occur. Anaphylactic reactions such as these require prompt effective treatment.

TREATMENT: If the stinger is still present in the skin, it should be carefully removed. Ice should be applied locally, to limit inflammation at the site of the sting as well as systemic distribution of venom. Diphenhydramine (or other antihistamine) should be given by mouth or parenterally; additionally, if signs and symptoms of anaphylaxis exist, epinephrine should be administered. Corticosteroids are given to reduce the risk of delayed allergic responses. Patients who have had large local reactions or systemic reactions to stings should be referred for desensitization (immunotherapy). In this treatment, gradually increasing dilutions of venom are injected subcutaneously over weeks or months, until immunological tolerance develops.

PREVENTION: Persons with a history of anaphylactic reactions to venom should avoid exposure to the vectors (e.g., ants, bees, snakes, wasps) as much as possible. Protective clothing, such as specialized gloves or shoes, may prevent some stings. Cosmetics, perfumes, hair sprays, and bright or white clothing should be avoided to prevent attracting insects. Because foods and odors attract insects, care should be taken when cooking and eating outdoors.

bee s. Injury resulting from bee venom and causing pain, redness, and swelling. SEE: *hymenoptera s.*

caterpillar s. Irritating contact with the hairs of a butterfly or moth larva. More than 50 species of larvae possess urticating hairs that contain a toxin. Contact can cause numbness and swelling of the infected area, severe radiating pain, localized swelling, enlarged regional lymph nodes, nausea, and vomiting. Although shock and convulsions may occur, no deaths have been reported. The disease is self-limiting. The larva of the flannel moth, *Megalopyge opercularis,* known as the puss caterpillar or woolly worm, is frequently the cause of this sting, particularly in the southern U.S. The fuzz from these larvae can be transported by wind. Treatment involves local application of moist soaks and administration of antihistamines.

catfish s. A toxic and allergic reaction caused by exposure to the venom contained in venomous glands at the base of catfish fins. The stung part should be immdediately immersed in water as hot as the patient can stand for 1 hr or until the pain is controlled. Tetanus prophylaxis should be administered if needed.

hornet s. A sting from a wasp of the family Vespidae, which may cause a general urticaria. SEE: *hymenoptera s.*

hymenoptera s. Envenomation by a fire ant, bee, hornet, or wasp. The sting from any of these insects may cause localized or, in some sensitized patients, systemic allergic reactions. Stings by venomous insects are one of the most common causes of anaphylaxis found in hospital emergency departments.

scorpion s. Injury resulting from scorpion venom. The stings of most species in the U.S. seldom produce severe toxic reactions, but because of the difficulty of distinguishing one species of scorpion from another, each scorpion sting should be treated as if it had been inflicted by a species capable of delivering a very toxic dose of venom. The stings vary in severity from local tissue reactions consisting of swelling and pain at the puncture site, to systemic reactions that compromise breathing and neuromuscular function. Death may rarely occur (e.g., in very young children).

TREATMENT: For mild local reactions, cold compresses and antihistamines are sufficient. Severe reactions may need to be treated with airway management, antivenins, and intensive observation in the hospital. For the source of local antivenins, the use of which is controversial, contact the nearest poison control center.

sea anemone s. Contact with the nematocysts or stinging cells of certain species of the flower-like marine coelenterates causing severe dermatitis with chronic ulceration. In some cases, signs and symptoms of a systemic reaction develop, including headache, nausea, vomiting, sneezing, chills, fever, paralysis, delirium, seizures, anaphylaxis, cardiac arrhythmias, heart failure, pulmonary edema, and collapse. In rare cases, it is fatal. SYN: *sponge diver's disease*.

TREATMENT: When systemic changes are present, vigorous therapy is indicated for hypotension. Diazepam is administered for convulsions. An electrocardiogram should be monitored for arrhythmias. Treatment for mild stings is symptomatic; application of vinegar to the sting area may inactivate the irritating secretion. All victims should be observed for 6 to 8 hr after initial therapy for rebound phenomenon.

stingray s. Penetration of the skin by the spine of a stingray and injection of venom.

TREATMENT: This type of injury should be treated by washing the wound with copious amounts of water; seawater should be used if sterile water is unavailable. The wound, which is very painful, should be cleansed thoroughly, and all foreign material should be removed. The wound site should be soaked in hot water (113°F or 45°C) for 30 to 60 min to inactivate the venom. Surgical débridement may be necessary, and narcotics may be needed for pain. Tetanus prophylaxis may be required, depending on the patient's immunization status. The wound is either packed open or loosely sutured to provide adequate drainage. Failure to treat this sting may result in gas gangrene or tetanus.

wasp s. SEE: *hymenoptera s.*

stinger Burner.

stingray Any of the rays of the family Dasyatidae with wide pectoral fins that resemble wings. Venom glands are located in the spine running along the top of its whiplike tail; severe injuries can be inflicted if this spine penetrates the skin.

S-T interval The interval in an electrocardiogram that represents ventricular repolarization. An elevation of the S-T segment may be seen in myocardial infarction, Prinzmetal's angina, and ventricular aneurysms; depression of the S-T segment is seen in conditions such as coronary ischemia, left ventricular hypertrophy, and digitalis use. SEE: *electrocardiogram* for illus.; *QRST complex.*

stippling (stĭp′lĭng) [Dutch *stippelen,* to spot] A spotted condition (e.g., in the retina in some diseases of the eye, or in basophilic red blood cells).

gingival s. An orange-peel appearance of healthy gingiva, believed to be due to the enlargement of the underlying connective tissue papillae in response to massage and toothbrushing; the indent lies between the bulging papillae where the epithelia grow downward as rete ridges.

stirrup, stirrup bone (stĭr′ŭp) [AS. *stigrap,* a stirrup] A common name for the stapes, the third of the three bones in the middle ear. SEE: *ear.*

stitch (stĭch) [AS. *stice,* a pricking] **1.** A local, sharp, or spasmodic pain that often occurs in the side or flank of athletes. The following maneuvers may offer relief: bending forward while tightening the abdomen; breathing deeply and exhaling slowly through pursed lips; tightening the belt or pushing one's fingers into the painful area. It is advisable not to eat for 30 to 90 min before exercising, to warm up before exercising, and to work out at a lower intensity for longer periods. **2.** A single loop of suture material passed through skin or flesh by a needle, to facilitate healing of a wound.

stochastic model (stō-kăs′tĭk) [Gr. *stokastikos,* skillful in guessing] A statistical model that attempts to reproduce the sequence of events that would be expected to occur in a real-life situation. This technique has some usefulness in predicting the importance and extent of disease in a specified population.

stock (stŏk) [AS. *stocc,* tree trunk] The original individual, race, or tribe from which others have descended.

Stockholm syndrome The emotional involvement between a hostage and the person holding him or her captive. The hostage's action may be due to sympathy for the terrorist's cause, to stress, or to the need to cooperate in order to survive. This syndrome is named after the romantic involvement of a terrorist and a bank employee held hostage during a 1973 bank robbery in Stockholm.

stockinet A tubular woven material of uniform size that is open at both ends. It is used to hold bandages in place or to place uniform pressure on a leg, finger, arm, or other part of an extremity.

stocking A snug covering for the foot and leg. A stocking made of elastic material will place firm, even pressure on the extremity, which is useful in preventing thrombophlebitis of the leg in bedfast patients and in treating varicose veins. Pneumatic hose have replaced elasticized stockings in certain applications (e.g., perioperatively).

stocking aid A device for assisting persons with limited function to put on socks or stockings.

stoichiometry (stoy″kē-ŏm′ĕ-trē) [Gr. *stoicheion,* element, + *metron,* measure] The study of the mathematics of chemistry and chemical reactions; chemical calculations.

stoke (stōk) [Sir George Stokes, Brit. physicist, 1819–1903] A unit of viscosity equal to 10^{-4} m^2/sec.

Stokes-Adams syndrome (stōks-ăd′ăms) [William Stokes, Irish physician, 1804–1878; Robert Adams, Irish physician, 1791–1875] Loss of consciousness caused by a decreased flow of blood to the brain. It may be caused by any transient interference with cardiac output such as incomplete or complete heart block. The patient may be lightheaded or become completely unconscious and have brief convulsive body movements. Treatment includes basic and advanced cardiac life support measures (e.g., rescue breathing, chest compressions, administration of epinephrine, or cardiac pacing, as indicated by the patient's responses). SYN: *Adams-Stokes syndrome*.

PATIENT CARE: The patient's airway, breathing, apical and radial pulses, blood pressure, and cardiac rhythm are monitored and supported. Emergency treatment (atropine sulfate, external pacing) is provided as necessary according to prescribed protocols. The patient is prepared for cardiac pacemaker implantation; reassurance and support are provided to the patient and family, pacemaker maintenance is taught, and the patient is assisted to return to usual activities.

Stokes' law (stōks) [William Stokes] A law stating that a muscle lying above an inflamed serous or mucous membrane may be paralyzed.

Stokes' lens [George Stokes] Device used to diagnose astigmatism.

stoma (stō'mă) *pl.* **stomata, -mas** [Gr., mouth] **1.** A mouth, small opening, or pore. **2.** An artificially created opening between two passages or body cavities or between a cavity or passage and the body's surface. **3.** A minute opening between cells of certain epithelial membranes, esp. peritoneum and pleura.

stomach (stŭm'ăk) [Gr. *stomachos,* mouth] A muscular, distensible saclike portion of the alimentary tube between the esophagus and duodenum. SEE: illus.

ANATOMY: It is below the diaphragm to the right of the spleen, partly under the liver. It is composed of an upper fundus, a central body, and a distal pylorus. It has two openings: the upper cardiac orifice opens from the esophagus and is surrounded by the lower esophageal (cardiac) sphincter. The lower pyloric orifice opens into the duodenum and is surrounded by the pyloric sphincter. The wall of the stomach has four layers. The outer serous layer (visceral peritoneum) covers almost all of the organ. The muscular layer just beneath it has three layers of smooth muscle: an outer longitudinal layer, a medial circular layer, and an inner oblique layer. The submucosa is made of connective tissue that contains blood vessels. The mucosa is the lining that contains the gastric glands, simple tubular glands of columnar epithelium that secrete gastric juice. Chief cells secrete pepsinogen; parietal cells secrete hydrochloric acid and the intrinsic factor; mucus cells secrete mucus.

FUNCTION: The stomach is a reservoir that permits digestion to take place gradually; emptying of the stomach is under both hormonal and nervous control. Secretions and motility are increased by parasympathetic impulses (vagus nerves) and decreased by sympathetic impulses. The presence of food stimulates the production of the hormone gastrin, which increases the secretion of gastric juice. Protein digestion begins in the stomach; pepsin digests proteins to peptones. Hydrochloric acid converts pepsinogen to active pepsin and has little effect on unemulsified fats except those of cream. The intrinsic factor in gastric juice combines with vita-

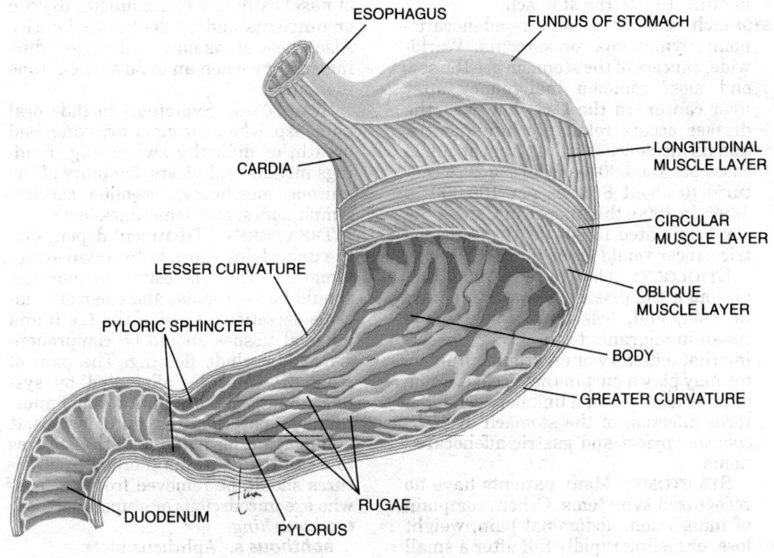

STOMACH

Anterior view, sectioned

min B_{12} (extrinsic factor) to prevent its digestion and promote its absorption in the small intestine. Little absorption takes place in the stomach because digestion has hardly begun, but water and alcohol are absorbed.

bilocular s. Hourglass s.

cardiac s. The fundus of the stomach.

cascade s. A form of hourglass stomach in which there is a constriction between the cardiac and pyloric portions. The cardiac portion fills first, and then the contents cascade into the pyloric portion.

cow horn s. A high, transversely placed stomach.

foreign bodies in the s. Accidental or intentional ingestion of materials such as coins, nails, bottle tops, marbles, and buttons. In some instances, these should be removed endoscopically (e.g., copper coins).

hourglass s. The division of the stomach (in the form of an hourglass) by a muscular constriction; often associated with gastric ulcer. SYN: *bilocular s.*

leather-bottle s. A condition of the stomach caused by hypertrophy of the stomach walls or their infiltration with malignant cells.

thoracic s. A condition in which the stomach lies above the diaphragm. This may result from an embryonic anomaly in which the stomach fails to descend, or from a hernia of the diaphragm.

water-trap s. A stomach with the pylorus situated unusually high, causing slow emptying.

stomachal (stŭm′ă-kăl) [Gr. *stomachos,* mouth] Rel. to the stomach.

stomach cancer Gastric adenocarcinoma, lymphoma, or sarcoma. Worldwide, cancers of the stomach are the second most common malignancy after liver cancer. In the U.S., however, the disease occurs relatively infrequently, and its incidence is falling from about 33 cases per 100,000 (early in the 20th century) to about 8 cases per 100,000 in 1999. In 2000, the American Cancer Society estimated 13,000 deaths from gastric cancer would occur in the U.S.

ETIOLOGY: The cause is unknown, although the disease occurs frequently in Asia, and, less frequently, among Asian immigrants to the U.S., suggesting that a dietary or environmental factor may play a part in the disease. Some studies have found a link between long-term infection of the stomach by *Helicobacter pylori* and gastric adenocarcinoma.

SYMPTOMS: Many patients have no recognized symptoms. Others complain of indigestion, abdominal pain, weight loss, or feeling rapidly full after a small meal. When cancer obstructs the pylorus, gastric dilatation, nausea, and vomiting are common complaints.

TREATMENT: Surgical removal of the stomach provides the only chance for cure.

PROGNOSIS: The likelihood that a patient will survive a gastric malignancy depends on the depth of invasion of the tumor and on whether it has spread to the lymph nodes. On average, patients live 6 to 9 months after diagnosis. Superficial cancers have the best prognosis.

stomachic (stō-măk′ĭk) **1.** Concerning the stomach. **2.** A medicine that stimulates the action of the stomach.

stomach intubation Passage of a tube into the stomach to obtain gastric contents for examination, for prophylaxis and treatment of ileus, or to remove ingested poisons.

stomal (stō′măl) [Gr. *stoma,* mouth] Concerning a stoma.

stomata Pl. of stoma.

stomatal (stō′mă-tăl) [Gr. *stoma,* mouth] Concerning stomata.

stomatic Pert. to or rel. to the mouth.

stomatitis (stō-mă-tī′tĭs) [″ + *itis,* inflammation] Inflammation of the mouth (including the lips, tongue, and mucous membranes). SEE: illus.; *noma; thrush.*

ETIOLOGY: Stomatitis may be associated with a variety of conditions including viral infections, chemical irritation, radiation therapy, mouth breathing, paralysis of nerves supplying the oral area, chemotherapy that damages or destroys the mucous membranes, adverse reactions to other medicines, or acute sun damage to the lips. The nasal and oral mucosa are esp. vulnerable to being traumatized by the use of nasal catheters to administer oxygen or nutrients and by dental appliances. Also, these areas may be damaged during surgery when an endotracheal tube is in place.

SYMPTOMS: Symptoms include oral pain, esp. when eating or drinking, bad breath, or difficulty swallowing. Findings include oral ulcers, friability of the mucous membranes, swollen cervical lymph nodes, and sometimes fever.

TREATMENT: Treatment depends on the underlying cause but is often symptomatic. The mucous membranes should be kept moist and clear of tenacious secretions. Care of the teeth and gingival tissues should be comprehensive and include flossing. The pain of stomatitis may be alleviated by systemic analgesics or application of anesthetic preparations to painful lesions. It is important for patients with dentures to clean the dentures thoroughly. Dentures should be removed from patients who are unconscious or stuporous. SEE: *toothbrushing.*

aphthous s. Aphthous ulcer.

corrosive s. Stomatitis resulting from intentional or accidental exposure to corrosive substances.

diphtheritic s. Inflammation of the oral mucosa caused by infection with *Corynebacterium diphtheriae*. SEE: *diphtheria*.

herpetic s. Stomatitis seen with primary infection with herpes simplex virus.

membranous s. Stomatitis accompanied by the formation of a false or adventitious membrane.

mercurial s. A form of stomatitis seen in those exposed to elemental mercury or mercury vapors.

mycotic s. Thrush.

simple s. Erythematous inflammation of the mouth occurring in patches on the mucous membranes.

traumatic s. Stomatitis resulting from mechanical injury as from ill-fitting dentures, sharp jagged teeth, or biting the cheek.

ulcerative s. Necrotizing ulcerative gingivitis.

vesicular s. Aphthous ulcer.

Vincent's s. Necrotizing ulcerative gingivitis.

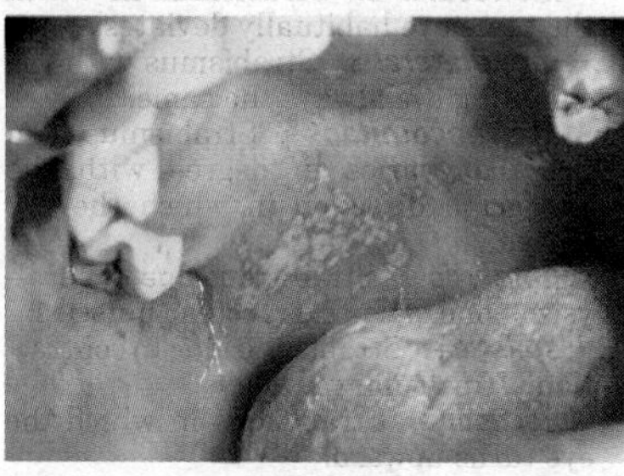

STOMATITIS

As caused by herpes simplex virus

stomato- Combining form meaning *mouth*.

stomatocyte A swollen erythrocyte with a slit-like area of central pallor that is found in hereditary stomatocytosis.

stomatocytosis, hereditary A disorder of erythrocytes usually inherited as an autosomal dominant. A membrane defect in the red blood cells permits the entry of excess sodium ions and water, causing the cells to swell. Hemolysis and anemia range from mild to severe.

stomatodynia (stō″mă-tō-dĭn′ē-ă) [Gr. *stoma,* mouth, + *odyne,* pain] Pain in the mouth.

stomatogastric (stō″mă-tō-găs′trĭk) [″ + *gaster,* belly] Concerning the stomach and mouth.

stomatognathic (stō″mă-tŏg-năth′ĭk) [″ + *gnathos,* jaw] Indicating the mouth and jaws together.

stomatologist (stō″mă-tŏl′ō-jĭst) [″ + *logos,* word, reason] A specialist in the treatment of diseases of the mouth.

stomatology (stō″mă-tŏl′ō-jē) The science of the mouth and teeth and their diseases.

stomatomalacia (stō″mă-tō-mă-lā′shē-ă) [″ + *malakia,* softening] Pathological softening of any structures of the mouth.

stomatomenia (stō″mă-tō-mē′nē-ă) [″ + *meniaia,* menses] Bleeding from the mouth at the time of menstruation.

stomatomycosis (stō″mă-tō-mī-kō′sĭs) [″ + *mykes,* fungus, + *osis,* condition] Any disease of the mouth caused by fungi.

stomatopathy (stō″mă-tŏp′ă-thē) [″ + *pathos,* disease, suffering] Any mouth disease.

stomatoplasty (stō′mă-tō-plăs″tē) [″ + *plassein,* to form] Plastic surgery or repair of the mouth.

stomatorrhagia (stō″mă-tō-rā′jē-ă) [″ + *rhegnynai,* to burst forth] Hemorrhage from the mouth or gums.

stomatosis (stō″mă-tō′sĭs) [″ + *osis,* condition] Any disease of the mouth.

stomion (stō′mē-ŏn) [Gr., dim. of *stoma,* mouth] A landmark used in physical anthropology. It is the central point in the oral fissure when the lips are together.

stomocephalus (stō″mō-sĕf′ă-lŭs) [Gr. *stoma,* mouth, + *kephale,* head] A deformed fetus with a very small head and neck.

stomodeum (stō″mō-dē′ŭm) [″ + *hodaios,* a way] An external depression lined with ectoderm and bounded by frontonasal, mandibular, and maxillary processes of the embryo. It forms the anterior portion of the oral cavity. Its floor, the pharyngeal membrane, separates the stomodeum from the foregut.

stone [AS. *stan*] **1.** Calculus. **2.** In Britain, a unit of weight, 14 lb avoirdupois.

dental s. A hemihydrate of gypsum divided into four classes according to the qualities resulting from differing methods of preparation. It is used in dentistry in the preparation of models and study casts.

gray s. A synthetic stone composed of carborundum and rubber used to polish dental restorations.

pulp s. A calcified structure present in the pulp chamber of a tooth. SYN: *denticle* (2).

red s. An abrasive stone with garnet as its main component, for polishing dental restorations.

salivary s. A calcified stone present in the ducts of salivary glands; also called *sialolith*.

stonefish A poisonous member of the scorpionfish family (*Synanceja trachynis* or *S. horrida*) that carries a deadly cell–and tissue–destructive enzyme in its spines. Divers exposed to the toxin may die within days of exposure, often after a painful and mutilating illness.

stonustoxin (stōn′us-tŏk-sĭn) A purified protein isolated from the venom of the stonefish, one of the most lethal members of the animal kingdom. The protein dissolves cells and tissues, and produces hypotension and death after it contacts animal tissues.

stool (stool) [AS. *stol,* a seat] **1.** Evacuation of the bowels. **2.** Feces.

bilious s. Yellow or yellow-brown discharges in diarrhea, becoming darker on exposure to air.

fatty s. Steatorrhea (2).

pea soup s. Liquid stools characteristic of typhoid.

rice water s. Watery serum stools with detached epithelium, as in cholera.

stool softener A substance that acts as a wetting agent and thus promotes soft malleable bowel movements. They are not laxatives and therefore are not indicated for constipation caused by decreased or absent peristaltic activity. Two examples are docusate sodium and docusate calcium.

stopcock (stŏp′kŏk) A valve that regulates the flow of fluid from a container.

stoppage (stŏp′ăj) [AS. *stoppian*] Obstruction of an organ. SEE: *cholestasia.*

storax (stō′răks) A balsam obtained from the scarred trunk of *Liquidambar orientalis.* It has been used as an expectorant. It is a component of tincture of benzoin.

storm [AS.] A sudden outburst or exacerbation of the symptoms of a disease.

thyroid s. A complication of thyrotoxicosis that, if untreated, may be life-threatening. It consists of the abrupt onset of fever, sweating, tachycardia, pulmonary edema or congestive heart failure, tremulousness, and restlessness. It is usually precipitated by infection, trauma, or a surgical emergency.

stout (stowt) [O.Fr. *estout,* bold] **1.** Having a bulky body. **2.** Strong, dark beer.

STP *standard temperature and pressure.*

STPD *standard temperature and pressure, dry.*

Str *Streptococcus.*

strabismal (stră-bĭz′măl) [Gr. *strabismos,* a squinting] Strabismic.

strabismic (stră-bĭz′mĭk) [Gr. *strabismos,* a squinting] Pert. to or afflicted with strabismus.

strabismometer (stră-bĭz-mŏm′ĕt-ĕr) [″ + *metron,* a measure] An instrument for determining the amount of strabismus.

strabismus (stră-bĭz′mŭs) [Gr. *strabismos,* a squinting] A disorder of the eye in which optic axes cannot be directed to the same object. This disorder is present in about 4% of children. The squinting eye always deviates to the same extent when the eyes are carried in different directions: *unilateral* when the same eye always deviates; *alternating* when either deviates, the other being fixed; *constant* when the squint remains permanent; *periodic* when the eyes are occasionally free from it. Strabismus can result from reduced visual acuity, unequal ocular muscle tone, or an oculomotor nerve lesion. SYN: *heterotropia; squint.* SEE: *microstrabismus.*

accommodative s. Strabismus due to disorder of ocular accommodation. SYN: *bilateral s.*

alternating s. Strabismus affecting either eye alternately.

bilateral s. Accommodative s.

concomitant s. Strabismus in which both eyes move freely but retain an unnatural relationship to each other.

convergent s. Strabismus in which the deviating eye turns inward.

divergent s. Strabismus in which the deviating eye turns outward.

horizontal s. Strabismus in which the deviation of the visual axis is in the horizontal plane.

intermittent s. Strabismus recurring at intervals.

monocular s. Strabismus in which the same eye habitually deviates.

monolateral s. Strabismus with the squinting eye always the same.

nonconcomitant s. Strabismus of an eye that varies in degree with the change in direction in which the eye moves.

paralytic s. Strabismus due to paralysis of one of the extraocular muscles.

spastic s. Strabismus due to contraction of an ocular muscle.

vertical s. Strabismus in which the eye turns upward.

Strachan syndrome [William H. W. Strachan, Brit. physician, 1857–1921] The neurological syndrome of amblyopia, painful neuropathy, and orogenital dermatitis that occurs in undernourished persons in many tropical countries. In the U.S., the syndrome occasionally is seen in alcoholic patients. Treatment is symptomatic and includes adequate nutrition. Formerly called Jamaican neuritis.

strain (strān) [AS. *streon,* offspring] **1.** A stock, said of bacteria or protozoa from a specific source and maintained in successive cultures or animal inoculation. **2.** A hereditary streak or tendency.

strain (strān) [O.Fr. *estreindere,* to draw tight] **1.** To pass through, as a filter. **2.** To injure by making too strong an effort or by excessive use. **3.** Excessive use of a part of the body so that it is injured. **4.** Trauma to the muscle or the musculotendinous unit from violent contraction or excessive forcible stretch. It may be associated with failure of the synergistic action of muscles. SEE: *sprain.* **5.** To make a great effort, as in straining to have a bowel movement. This is done by means of the Valsalva maneuver, which increases intra-abdominal pressure and helps to expel feces. **6.** Force applied per unit area. Tension, compression, or shear stress placed on a tissue leads to distortion of the structure and the release of energy.

strainer (strān′ĕr) **1.** Device used for retaining solid pieces while liquid passes through. SYN: *filter*. **2.** In river rescue, a term used to describe locations where water is moving through grating, wire mesh, or downed trees. A strainer is dangerous because victims can get caught in it or pinned up against it by the force of the moving current.

strain radiography A radiographical image taken with the involved region, usually a bone or joint, under static force or tension; used to determine if a partial tear or rupture of the ligaments has occurred. Greater than normal gaping of the joint surfaces indicates a tear. Strain radiography reveals pathological changes that might be inapparent without use of this technique. SYN: *stress radiography*.

strait (strāt) [O.Fr. *estreit*, narrow] A constricted or narrow passage.

inferior s. The lower outlet of the pelvic canal.

s. of pelvis The inferior and superior openings of the true pelvis.

superior s. The upper opening or inlet of the pelvic canal.

straitjacket A shirt with long sleeves laced on a patient and fastened to restrain the arms.

stramonium (stră-mō′nē-ŭm) [L.] The dried leaves of the toxic anticholinergic plant *Datura stramonium*. SYN: *jimson weed*.

stramonium poisoning Accidental or intentional intoxication with the dried leaves of *Datura stramonium*, a powerful anticholinergic agent (containing belladonna alkaloids) that produces atropine-like effects. Common signs and symptoms include delirium and hallucinations, tachycardia and hypertension, fever, pupillary dilation, and sometimes, seizures, coma, cardiac rhythm disturbances, or death. SEE: *atropine sulfate poisoning*.

PATIENT CARE: After the gastrointestinal tract is decontaminated with activated charcoal, stimulation of the intoxicated person should be minimized. Severely poisoned persons, e.g., those with seizures, extremely high body temperatures, or cardiac dysrhythmias may be treated with intravenous physostigmine, given slowly.

strand A single thread or fiber.

strangalesthesia (străng″găl-ĕs-thē′zē-ă) [L. *strangulare*, halter, + *aisthesis*, sensation] A girdle-like sensation of constriction. SYN: *zonesthesia*.

strangle (străng′gl) [L. *strangulare*, halter] **1.** To choke or suffocate. **2.** To be choked from compression of the trachea.

strangulation (străng″gū-lā′shŭn) [L. *strangulare*, halter] The compression or constriction of a part, as the bowel or throat, causing suspension of breathing or of the passage of contents. Congestion accompanies this condition. **strangulated,** *adj.*

internal s. The entrapment of a segment of the intestine in an internal hernia or by adhesion, or through a rent or hiatus in the diaphragm, which leads to vascular compromise with ensuing gangrene.

strangury (străng′gū-rē) [Gr. *stranx*, drop, squeezed out, + *ouron*, urine] Painful and interrupted urination in drops produced by spasmodic muscular contraction of the urethra and bladder.

strap, strapping (străp) [Gr. *strophos*, a cord] **1.** A band, as one of adhesive tape, used to hold dressings in place or to approximate surfaces of a wound. **2.** To bind with strips of adhesive tape.

stratification (străt″ĭ-fĭ-kā′shŭn) [L. *stratificare*, to arrange in layers] The act or process of arranging in layers.

stratified (străt′ĭ-fīd) [L. *stratificare*, to arrange in layers] Arranged in the form of layers.

stratified epithelium Epithelium in superimposed layers with differently shaped cells in the various layers.

stratiform (străt′ĭ-form) [L. *stratum*, layer, + *forma*, shape] Arranged in layers.

stratum (strā′tŭm, străt′ŭm) *pl.* **strata** [L.] A layer.

s. basale **1.** The innermost or deepest layer of the endometrium. **2.** S. germinativum.

s. compactum The superficial or outermost layer of the endometrium.

s. corneum The outermost horny layer of the epidermis.

s. disjunction The outermost layer of the stratum corneum, which is being shed constantly.

s. functionalis Functional layer.

s. germinativum The innermost layer of the epidermis; a row of cuboidal cells that divide to replace the rest of the epidermis as it wears away. It is part of the stratum malpighii. SYN: *s. basale* (2). SEE: *s. malpighii*.

s. granulosum A layer of cells containing deeply staining granules of keratohyalin found in the epidermis of the skin between the stratum and the stratum lucidum. SEE: *s. malpighii*.

s. lucidum The translucent layer of the epidermis between the stratum corneum and the stratum granulosum in the palms and soles.

s. malpighii The inner layer of the epidermis. It was first seen with low magnification and described in the 1600s by Marcello Malpighi. It includes both the stratum germinativum and stratum spinosum of today's nomenclature.

s. papillare The papillary layer of the corium adjacent to the epidermis.

s. reticulare The recticular layer of the corium just beneath the papillary layer.

s. spinosum The prickle cell layer, so called because of its prominent intercellular attachments. It is part of the stratum malpighii. SEE: *s. malpighii*.

s. spongiosum The middle layer of decidua of the endometrium.

s. submucosum The layer of smooth muscle fibers of the myometrium lying contiguous with the endometrium.

s. subserosum The layer of smooth muscle fibers of myometrium that lies immediately under the serous coat.

s. supravasculare The layer of circular and longitudinal muscle fibers lying between the stratum subserosum and the stratum vasculare of the endometrium.

s. vasculare The layer of smooth muscle fibers in myometrium lying between the stratum submucosum and the stratum supravasculare of the endometrium.

strawberry mark A soft, modular, vascular nevus usually present on the face or neck, occurring at birth or shortly afterward. SEE: *nevus flammeus*.

straw itch A self-limiting skin condition accompanied by itching owing to working in straw or sleeping on a straw mattress. The straw contains a mite that causes the pruritic eruption.

streak (strēk) [AS. *strica*] A line or stripe. SYN: *stria*.

angioid s. A dark streak seen in the retina that represents a defect in Bruch's membrane. It is often an age-related phenomenon but sometimes is seen in connective tissue diseases, like pseudoxanthoma elasticum, or hemoglobinopathies, such as sickle cell anemia.

gonadal s. Ovarian atrophy or aplasia; a finding in persons with Turner's syndrome.

medullary s. A deep longitudinal groove on the dorsal surface of the embryo that becomes the medullary tube.

meningitic s. A red line across the skin formed by drawing a pointed article across it; seen in meningitis and nerve center disorders.

Moore's lightning s. The subjective visual sensation of lightning-like flashes at the time of eye movements, esp. noticeable in dim or absent light. They are usually vertical and on the lateral part of the visual field. The flashes are accompanied by or followed by dark spots before the eyes. This condition is not related to significant eye disease.

primitive s. SEE: *primitive streak*.

stream (strēm) A steady flow of a liquid.

cathode s. Negatively charged electrons emitted from a cathode and accelerated in a straight line to interact with an anode. X-ray photons are then produced. SEE: *Bremsstrahlung radiation; ray, cathode*.

strength 1. Muscular power. **2.** The concentration of a solution or substance. **3.** The intensity of light, color, or sound. **4.** The ability to resist deformation, fracture, or abrasion.

breaking s. The point at which an amount of applied force breaks a material. Also called *tensile strength*.

compression s. The point at which a material loses its shape when force is applied. Also called *crushing strength*.

ego s. In classical psychoanalytical theory, the ability of the ego to maintain its various functions, the prime one of which is to perceive reality and adapt to it.

impact s. The force required to fracture a material.

shear s. The resistance of a material to force applied parallel to the plane of the material.

strephosymbolia (strĕf″ō-sĭm-bō′lē-ă) [Gr. *strephein*, to twist, + *symbolon*, symbol] **1.** Difficulty in distinguishing between letters that are similar but face in opposite directions (e.g., p-q, b-d). **2.** The perception of objects as reversed, as in a mirror.

strepitus (strĕp′ĭ-tŭs) [L.] A sound or noise, as that heard on auscultation.

strepticemia (strĕp″tĭ-sē′mē-ă) [Gr. *streptos*, twisted, + *haima*, blood] Streptococcemia.

strepto- [Gr. *streptos*, twisted] Combining form meaning *twisted*.

streptoangina (strĕp″tō-ăn′jĭ-nă) [″ + L. *angina*, quinsy] A sore throat with membranous formation caused by streptococci.

Streptobacillus moniliformis A gram-negative bacillus present in the mouths of rats, mice, and cats. It is transmitted to humans through bites or by ingestion of milk contaminated by rats. It causes one form of rat-bite fever, marked by prolonged fever, skin rash, and generalized arthritis. The infection may be treated with amoxicillin-clavulanate or doxycycline. SYN: *Haverhill fever*. SEE: *Spirillum minus*.

streptococcal (strĕp″tō-kŏk′ăl) [″ + *kokkos*, berry] Caused by or pert. to streptococci.

streptococcemia (strĕp″tō-kŏk-sē′mē-ă) [″ + ″ + *haima*, blood] Presence of streptococci in the blood, causing infection. SYN: *strepticemia*.

streptococci (strĕp″tō-kŏk′sī) Pl. of streptococcus. SEE: *Streptococcus*.

streptococcic (strĕp″tō-kŏk′sĭk) [″ + *kokkos*, berry] Resembling, produced by, or pert. to streptococci.

streptococcicosis (strĕp″tō-kŏk″sĭ-kō′sĭs) [″ + ″ + *osis*, condition] Any streptococcal infection.

streptococcolysin (strĕp″tō-kŏk-kŏl′ĭ-sĭn) [″ + ″ + *lysis,* dissolution] A hemolysin produced by streptococci. SYN: *streptocolysin; streptolysin.*

Streptococcus (strĕp″tō-kŏk′ŭs) [″ + *kokkos,* berry] ABBR: Str. A genus of bacteria belonging to the family Lactobacillaceae, tribe Streptococceae. They are gram-positive cocci occurring in chains. Most species are harmless saprophytes, but some are among the most common and dangerous pathogens of humans. They are differentiated on the basis of their reactions on blood-agar plates into three types: alpha (α), beta (β), and gamma (γ). Those of the alpha-hemolytic type partially hemolyze blood and form a greenish coloration round colonies; those of the beta-hemolytic type completely hemolyze blood and form clear zones round colonies; those of the gamma type are nonhemolytic and do not change the color of the medium. Streptococci were also classified into several immunological groups (Lancefield groups) designated by the letters A through H, and K through O. Most human infections are caused by groups A, B, D, F, G, H, K, and O. More than 55 types of group A beta-hemolytic streptococci have been identified. SEE: *rheumatic fever; scarlet fever.*

S. agalactiae A group B β-hemolytic species found in raw milk that is the leading cause of bacterial sepsis and meningitis in newborns and a major cause of endometritis and fever in postpartum women.

Infected infants develop early-onset symptoms in the first 5 days of life, including lethargy, jaundice, respiratory distress, shock, pneumonia, and anorexia. The fatality rate is 50% for very low birth weight neonates and 2% to 8% in term infants.

Infected postpartum women develop late-onset symptoms 7 days to several months after giving birth. Symptoms include sepsis, meningitis, seizures, and psychomotor retardation.

S. bovis A species found in the alimentary tract of cattle. It may cause endocarditis in humans.

S. equisimilis An organism that has been isolated from the upper respiratory tract. It may be associated with erysipelas, puerperal sepsis, pneumonia, osteomyelitis, bacteremia, and endocarditis.

S. faecalis The former name of *Enterococcus faecalis.*

S. iniae A pathogen of fish that may cause cellulitis in persons who handle affected fish and have skin abrasions.

S. mutans A species that has been implicated in dental caries initiation and bacterial endocarditis.

S. pneumoniae A species with cells that are oval or spherical, gram-positive, nonmotile, and possess a capsule. It is sometimes referred to as the pneumococcus. The species consists of strains based on capsular chemistry of which more than 80 serological types have been isolated. It is the causative agent of certain types of pneumonia, esp. lobar pneumonia, and is associated with other infectious diseases such as meningitis, conjunctivitis, endocarditis, periodontitis, septic arthritis, osteomyelitis, otitis media, septicemia, spontaneous bacterial peritonitis, and, rarely, urinary tract infections. About 40,000 people die of pneumococcal disease each year in the U.S., more than any other vaccine-preventable illness. SYN: *pneumococcus.*

S. pyogenes Any of the group A β-hemolytic streptococci causing suppurative infections. These streptococci are the causative agents of scarlet fever, erysipelas, septic sore throat, puerperal sepsis, and necrotizing fasciitis.

S. viridans A group of α-hemolytic streptococci that are normally present in the upper respiratory tract. This may produce bacterial endocarditis. *S. mitis* and *S. salivarius* are members of the viridans group. These may be normal inhabitants of the respiratory tract or be pathogenic.

streptococcus (strĕp″tō-kŏk′ŭs) *pl.* **streptococci** An organism of the genus *Streptococcus.* SEE: *bacteria* for illus.

α-hemolytic s. Streptococci that, when grown on blood-agar, produce a zone of partial hemolysis around each colony and often impart a greenish appearance to the agar. Included are *S. pneumoniae* and *S. viridans.*

β-hemolytic s. Streptococci that, when grown on blood-agar, produce complete hemolysis around each colony, indicated by a clear zone. Included are *S. pyogenes* and *S. agalactiae.*

group A s. Beta-hemolytic streptococci that consist of a number of organisms that differ in their ability to cause disease. They may be causative agents of pharyngitis, tonsillitis, otitis media, sinusitis, scarlet fever, erysipelas, cellulitis, impetigo, pneumonia, endometritis, and septicemia. In addition, group A streptococci may cause nonsuppurative sequelae, such as necrotizing fasciitis, acute rheumatic fever, and acute glomerulonephritis.

group B s. Beta-hemolytic streptococci that are a leading cause of early-onset neonatal infections and late-onset postpartal infections. In women, this is marked by urinary tract infection, chorioamnionitis, postpartum endometritis, bacteremia, and wound infections complicating cesarean section.

streptocolysin (strĕp″tō-kŏl′ĭ-sĭn) [″ + *lysis,* dissolution] A hemolysin produced by streptococci. SYN: *streptococcolysin; streptolysin.*

streptodermatitis (strĕp″tō-dĕr″mă-tī′tĭs) [″ + *derma,* skin, + *itis,* inflammation] Inflammation of the skin caused by streptococci.

streptodornase (strĕp″tō-dor′nās) One of the enzymes produced by certain strains of hemolytic streptococci. It is capable of liquefying fibrinous and purulent exudates. SEE: *streptokinase.*

streptokinase (strĕp″tō-kī′nās) An enzyme produced by certain strains of streptococci that is capable of converting plasminogen to plasmin. It is used as a clot-busting agent to help remove thrombi from arteries (e.g., in acute myocardial infarction). SEE: *reperfusion* (1).

streptokinase-streptodornase A mixture of the enzymes streptokinase and streptodornase, which are produced by hemolytic streptococci. This mixture is used topically and in body cavities to remove clotted blood and purulent material.

streptolysin (strĕp-tŏl′ĭ-sĭn) An enzyme produced by streptococci that destroys blood cells. SYN: *streptococcolysin; streptocolysin.*

s. O Streptolysin that is inactivated by oxygen.

s. S Streptolysin that is inactivated by heat or acid, but not by oxygen.

streptomycin sulfate (sterile) (strĕp″tō-mī′sĭn) An antibiotic derived from a soil microbe, *Streptomyces griseus,* used with other drugs to treat tuberculosis.

streptomycosis (strĕp″tō-mī-kō′sĭs) [″ + *mykes,* fungus, + *osis,* condition] An infection caused by microorganisms of the genus *Streptomyces.* SYN: *streptococcemia; streptosepticemia.*

streptosepticemia (strĕp″tō-sĕp″tĭ-sē′mē-ă) [″ + *septikos,* putrid, + *haima,* blood] Septicemia resulting from streptococcal infection. SYN: *streptococcemia; streptomycosis.*

stress (strĕs) [O.Fr. *estresse,* narrowness] **1.** Any physical, physiological, or psychological force that disturbs equilibrium **2.** The consequences of forces that disturb equilibrium. **3.** Force applied per unit area. In the physical sciences, stresses include forces that deform or damage materials, such as impact, shear, torsion, compression, and tension. These physical stresses are particularly important in certain branches of health care (e.g., dentistry or orthopedic surgery) and in biotechnology industries (e.g., in the design and use of prostheses, grafts, and perfusion pumps).

Physiological stresses include agents that upset homeostasis, such as infection, injury, disease, internal organ pressures, or psychic strain.

In psychology, stresses include perceptions, emotions, anxieties, and interpersonal, social, or economic events that are considered threatening to one's physical health, personal safety, or well-being. Marital discord; conflicts with others; battle, torture, or abuse; bankruptcy; incarceration; health care crises; and self-doubt are all examples of conditions that increase psychic stresses. The response of an organism or material to stress is known as adaptation. SEE: *adaptation; anxiety; fracture; homeostasis; Laplace, law of; relaxation response.*

critical incident s. One's emotional reaction to a catastrophic event such as a mass casualty incident or the death of a patient or coworker. Often such events negatively affect the well-being of health care providers.

oxidative s. The cellular damage caused by oxygen-derived free radical formation. The three most important are superoxide (O_2^-), hydrogen peroxide (H_2O_2), and hydroxyl ions; these are produced during normal metabolic processes as well as in reaction to cell injury. The extent of their damaging potential can be decreased by antioxidants. SEE: *antioxidant; free radical; superoxide; superoxide dismutase.*

shear s. shear.

stress-breaker A device incorporated into a removable denture. It is designed to relieve abutting teeth from excessive stress during chewing.

stress incontinence SEE: under *incontinence.*

stressor An agent or condition capable of producing stress.

systemic s. A stressor that produces generalized systemic responses.

topical s. Stress that causes mild inflammation or local damage.

stress radiography Strain radiography.

stress test Exercise tolerance test.

adenosine s.t. A test for coronary artery disease that uses the drug adenosine as a vasodilator, usually along with radionuclide imaging of the heart or echocardiography. The drug is used in place of physical exercise to demonstrate obstructions in the coronary arteries (e.g., in patients who cannot perform physical exercise or whose exercise testing results have been uninterpretable).

stretch (strĕch) [AS. *streccan,* extend] To draw out or extend to full length.

static s. A sustained, low-intensity lengthening of soft tissue (e.g., muscle, tendon, or joint capsule), performed to increase range of motion. The stretch force may be applied continuously for as short as 15 to 30 sec or as long as several hours.

stretcher (strĕch′er) A device for carrying the sick, injured, or dead. SYN: *ambulance cot; gurney.*

basket s. A stretcher made of metal or strong synthetic material in which a patient is placed for removal from an accident site. The stretcher may also be lifted by ropes. Also called *Stokes stretcher*.

orthopedic s. A metal stretcher that is hinged along its long axis and designed to be split so that it can be placed on both sides of the patient and then reassembled to lift the patient. SYN: *scoop s.*

pole s. A type of stretcher, also known as the Army type, composed of folding cloth or canvas supported by poles.

scoop s. Orthopedic s.

spineboard s. A type of stretcher made from a wooden board or strong synthetic material used to secure patients with spinal trauma to prevent movement and possible paralysis; also called a long backboard.

split-frame (scoop) s. A metal stretcher that can be split down the middle, slid under a patient, and reconnected.

stretching of contractures Techniques performed to increase the length of tissues that have been abnormally shortened (e.g., ligaments, muscles, or joint capsules). A slow, steady, and gradually increasing force should be used.

stretch mark Stria atrophica.

stretch receptor A proprioceptor located in a muscle or tendon that is stimulated by a stretch or pull.

stria (strī′ă) *pl.* **striae** [L., a channel] A line or band elevated above or depressed below surrounding tissue, or differing in color and texture. SYN: *streak.*

striae acusticae Horizontal white stripes on the floor of the fourth ventricle of the brain.

striae atrophica A fine pinkish-white or gray line, usually 14 cm long, seen in parts of the body where skin has been stretched; commonly seen on thighs, abdomen, and breasts of women who are or have been pregnant; in persons whose skin has been stretched by obesity, tumor, or edema; or in persons who have taken adrenocortical hormones for a prolonged period. SYN: *stretch mark.* SYN: *s. gravidarum.*

striae gravidarum S. atrophica.

striae longitudinalis lateralis One of the longitudinal bands of gray matter, slightly elevated on the upper part of the corpus callosum.

olfactory striae Three bands of fibers (lateral, intermediate, and medial) that form the roots of the olfactory tract.

striae of Retzius The benign incremental lines seen periodically in the calcified enamel of teeth.

striae terminalis A band of fibers in the roof of the inferior horn running to the floor of the body of the lateral ventricle.

striatal (strī-ā′tăl) [L. *striatus,* striped] Concerning the corpus striatum.

striate, striated (strī′āt, strī′ā-tĕd) [L. *striatus*] Striped; marked by streaks or striae.

striated artery One of the branches of the middle cerebral artery that supply the basal nuclei of the brain.

striated body Corpus striatum.

striated vein, inferior One of the branches of the basal vein that drain the corpus striatum.

striation (strī-ā′shŭn) [L. *striatus,* striped] **1.** State of being striped or streaked. **2.** Stria.

striatum (strī-ā′tŭm) [L., grooved] Corpus striatum.

stricture (strĭk′chŭr) [LL. *strictura,* contraction] A narrowing or constriction of the lumen of a tube, duct, or hollow organ such as the esophagus, ureter, or urethra. Strictures may be congenital or acquired. Acquired strictures may result from infection, trauma, fibrosis resulting from mechanical or chemical irritation, muscular spasm, or pressure from adjacent structures or tumors. They may be temporary or permanent, depending on the cause.

annular s. Ringlike obstruction of an organ involving the entire circumference of a structure.

anorectal s. A fibrotic narrowing of the anorectal canal.

bridle s. A stricture caused by a band of membrane stretched across a tube, partially occluding it.

cicatricial s. A stricture resulting from a scar or wound.

functional s. A stricture caused by muscular spasm.

impermeable s. A stricture closing the lumen of a tube or canal so that an instrument cannot pass through it.

irritable s. A stricture causing pain when an instrument is passed.

s. of the urethra Partial or complete narrowing of the urethra, occurring most commonly in men. The condition is marked by straining to pass urine, esp. at the commencement of urination. It is caused by spasm of the urethral muscle, congestion of the urethra, and fibrous formation.

stricturotomy (strĭk″chūr-ŏt′ō-mē) The operation of cutting strictures of the urethra.

stride length The length of the step taken during ambulation; useful in the assessment of a neuromuscular disease that affects only one leg.

strident (strī′dĕnt) Stridulous.

stridor (strī′dor) [L., a harsh sound] A high-pitched, harsh sound occurring during inspiration, often heard without the use of a stethoscope. It is a sign of upper airway obstruction, which may indicate the presence of a life-threatening condition (e.g., epiglottitis). The lack of stridor should never be interpreted as a sign that the upper airway is patent in the patient with signs of having difficulty breathing.

congenital laryngeal s. Stridor present at birth or occurring during the first weeks or months of life.

s. dentium The noise from grinding of the teeth. SEE: *bruxism.*

s. serraticus A sound of respiration similar to that of sawing, produced by the patient's tracheostomy tube.

stridulous (strĭd′ū-lŭs) [L. *stridulus*] Making a shrill, grating sound. SYN: *strident.*

string-of-pearls deformity Fusiform enlargement of the proximal and middle phalanges, seen in rickets.

string sign In gastrointestinal radiology, extreme narrowing of a segment of the terminal ileum (in Crohn's disease) or of the pylorus (in congenital pyloric stenosis).

string test A test used to diagnose *Giardia lamblia,* in which a string is swallowed, then removed, and examined for parasites.

striocerebellar (strī″ō-sĕr″ĕ-bĕl′ăr) [L. *striatus,* striped, + *cerebellum,* little brain] Concerning or affecting the corpus striatum and the cerebellum.

strip (strĭp) [AS. *striepan,* to plunder] To remove all contents from a hollow organ or tube, esp. by gentle pressure, as to strip the seminal vesicles.

stripper A surgical instrument used to remove veins, tendons, or the surfaces of bones.

strobila (strō-bī′lă) [Gr. *strobilos,* anything twisted up] The series of proglottids of the adult form of a tapeworm.

strobiloid (strō′bĭ-loyd) [″ + *eidos,* form] Resembling a chain of tapeworm segments.

stroboscope (strō′bō-skōp) [Gr. *strobos,* whirl, + *skopein,* to examine] A device that produces light intermittently. When the light is shown on moving or vibrating objects, the object appears to be stationary. A photograph taken at the precise time the light is flashed on the object will not be blurred.

strobovideolaryngoscopy (strō′bō-vĭd-ē-ō-lăr″ĭnj-ŏs-kō-pē) The use of a stroboscope in video recordings of diseases of the larynx and vocal cords.

stroke (strōk) [ME.] **1.** A sharp blow. **2.** To rub gently in one direction, as in massage. **3.** A gentle movement of the hand across a surface. **4.** In dentistry, a complete simple movement that is often repeated with modifications of position, strength, or speed, perhaps as a part of a continuing activity; for example, the closing stroke in mastication when the jaw closes and the teeth come together. In scaling or planing the roots of teeth, the scaling instrument is introduced carefully into the subgingival area in what is called an exploratory stroke, perhaps followed by a power stroke designed to break or dislodge encrusted calculus. This is followed by a shaving stroke, intended to smooth or plane the root surface. **5.** A sudden loss of neurological function, caused by vascular injury to the brain. Stroke is both common and deadly: 600,000 strokes occur in the U.S. each year; the disease is the third leading cause of death worldwide. Because of the long-term disability it often produces, stroke is the disease most feared by older Americans. In the U.S., 80% of strokes are caused by cerebral infarction (i.e., blockage of the carotid or intracerebral arteries by clot or atherosclerosis); intracranial hemorrhage and cerebral emboli are responsible for most other strokes. Innovations in the management of stroke (e.g., in prevention, the early use of thrombolytic drugs, vascular ultrasonography, and endarterectomy) have revolutionized the acute and the follow-up care of the stroke patient. SYN: *apoplexy; brain attack; cerebrovascular accident.* SEE: *carotid endarterectomy; intracranial hemorrhage; transient ischemic attack;* illus.

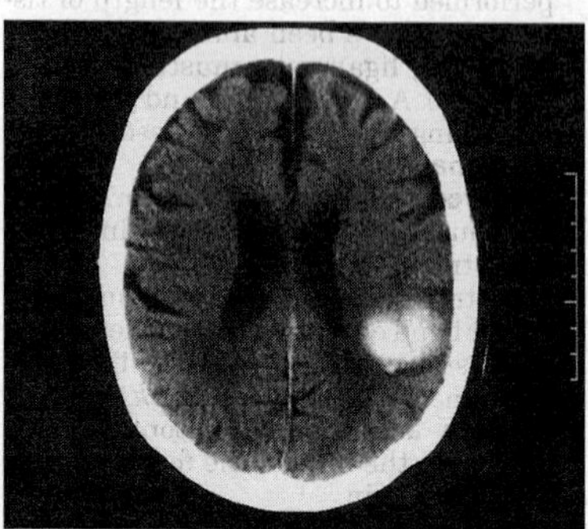

HEMORRHAGIC STROKE

Bleeding into the brain, seen on noncontrast head CT (Courtesy of Harvey Hatch, MD, Curry General Hospital)

ETIOLOGY: Risk factors for stroke include advanced age (esp. greater than 65 years), hypertension, carotid artery disease, cigarette use, hyperlipidemia, diabetes mellitus, atrial fibrillation, a history of myocardial infarction, atherosclerosis of the aortic arch, and possibly hyperhomocystinemia.

SYMPTOMS: The National Institute of Neurological Disorders and Stroke lists the following symptoms as warning signs of stroke: sudden weakness or numbness of the face, arm or leg; sudden loss of vision or dimming of vision; sudden difficulty speaking or understanding speech; sudden severe headache; and sudden falling, gait disturbance, or dizziness. In clinical practice, stroke patients often present with more than one of these symptoms (e.g., limb paralysis and aphasia; severe headache and hemibody deficits). It is also important to note that these symptoms are not specific for stroke: sudden dizziness or gait disturbance can occur as a result of intoxication with drugs or alcohol, for example, and sudden severe head pain can result from cluster headache, migraine, and many other disorders.

TREATMENT: Acute ischemic stroke can be treated with intravenous tissue plasminogen activator (TPA) if the disease is recognized in the first 90 to 180 min and intracerebral hemorrhage has been excluded with CT or MRI scanning of the brain. This form of therapy is not without risk—thrombolytic drugs can reduce long-term disability and death by 20%, but acutely triple the risk of brain hemorrhage. Hemorrhagic strokes, which have about a 50% mortality, can sometimes be treated by evacuating blood clots from the brain, or by repairing intracerebral aneurysms.

PROGNOSIS: The prognosis is directly related to the degree and length of time blood flow to the affected area of the brain is deficient or completely blocked and to the region of the brain affected by the stroke.

PATIENT CARE: *Acute phase:* The medical team, including physicians, nurses (acutely), occupational therapists, physical therapists, and speech therapists (during rehabilitation), obtain a physical and neurological status exam, to obtain baseline measurements. Focus is on maintaining appropriate life support functions and on early intervention to prevent long-term sequelae of prolonged bedrest and response to neurological changes in muscle tone and motor function. A patent airway is maintained, and adequate ventilation and oxygenation are provided. As necessary, the trachea or pharynx is suctioned gently to remove secretions. The patient is positioned in the lateral or semiprone position with the head elevated 15 to 30 degrees to decrease cerebral venous pressure. Neurological status (Glasgow Coma Scale; vital signs; pupillary responses; respiratory patterns; and sensory and motor responses to verbal, tactile, and painful stimulation) are monitored for signs of deterioration or improvement, and findings are documented on a neurological flow sheet. A history of the incident is obtained, including time frame, related past medical history (hypertension, use of anticoagulant drugs, cardiac dysrhythmias), and associated injuries. The patient is prepared for prescribed diagnostic studies, including computed tomography or magnetic resonance imaging; arteriography; and lumbar puncture.

The patient is oriented frequently and reassured with verbal and tactile contacts. The ability to speak is assessed, and if aphasia is present a consultation by a speech therapist is obtained. Bladder function is assessed; noninvasive measures are used to encourage voiding in the presence of urinary retention, voiding pattern is determined, and the incontinent patient is kept clean and dry. Use of indwelling catheters is limited because these promote urinary tract infection. Bowel function is assessed, and dietary intervention and stool softeners or laxatives as necessary are used to prevent constipation. Straining at stool or use of enemas is avoided. Fluid and electrolyte balance (intake, output, daily weight, laboratory values) is monitored and maintained. Adequate enteral or parenteral nutrition is provided as appropriate. Nursing measures are instituted to prevent complications of immobility. In consultation with occupational therapists and physical therapists, a program of positioning and mobility should be initiated, as appropriate. Examples of activities include: repositioning at least every 2 hr, maintaining correct body alignment, supporting joints to prevent flexion and rotation contractures, and providing range-of-motion exercises (passive to involved joints, active-assisted or active to uninvolved joints). Irrigation and lubrication prevent oral mucous membranes and eyes (cornea) from drying. Prescribed medical therapy is administered to decrease cerebral edema, and antihypertensives or anticoagulants are given as appropriate for etiology. The patient is observed for seizure activity, and drug therapy and safety precautions are initiated.

Rehabilitative phase: After the acute phase has subsided, the focus shifts from obtaining baseline measurements and providing necessary life support to more comprehensive rehabilitation efforts. Long-term rehabilitation goals depend on the severity of the initial stroke, the age of the patient, the presence of co-morbidities and other chronic conditions, prior functional status and ability to perform activities of daily living independently, and the family and social support systems available to the patient. When the patient is medically stable, he or she may be transferred from an acute, neurological hospital unit to a rehabilitation setting, or subacute setting. Here, the rehabilitation team collaborates with the patient and family to develop a comprehensive care plan based on realistic goals. The rehabilitation program will consist of various types of exercises, including neuromuscular retraining, motor learning and motor control, and functional activities that emphasize relearning or retraining in basic skills required for self-care. This may include instruction in the use of adaptive and supportive devices to facilitate independence in daily tasks. The goal of rehabilitation is to achieve an optimal functional outcome that will allow the patient to be discharged to the least restrictive environment. Ideally, the patient will achieve sufficient independence to return to community living, either independently or with family and community support.

All patient efforts should receive positive reinforcement. Patient communication should be a priority. Exercises, proper positioning, and supportive devices help to prevent deformities. Use of foot boards is controversial because they may increase spasticity. Quiet rest periods are provided based on the patient's response to activity. The patient should either assist with or perform own personal hygiene and establish independence in other activities of daily living. The rehabilitation team evaluates the patient's ability to feed self and continues to provide enteral feeding as necessary. A bowel and bladder retraining program is initiated, and both the patient and family receive instruction in its management. Both the patient and family are taught about the therapeutic regimen (activity and rest, diet, and medications), including desired effects and adverse reactions to report. Emotional lability is recognized and explained, and assistance is provided to help the patient deal with outbursts or inappropriate affect. The rehabilitation team assists the patient to accept deficits and disabilities, maintaining hope while establishing realistic goals. Both the patient and family should participate in available social and financial support groups and services. The patient needs help to accept residual deficits present after 6 months, because these may be permanent. Recovery and survival expectations may be influenced by the patient's age and presence of other chronic illnesses, in addition to early and later responses to stroke damage and therapies.

Specific rehabilitation efforts are complex and varied. Individualized assessments must be performed, and a plan of care designed to achieve the maximum functional outcome, based on the nature and location of the mechanism of the cerebrovascular accident.

PREVENTION: The most important strategy for reducing the incidence of stroke is to control its risk factors, especially hypertension, hyperlipidemia, and tobacco smoking. Patients who have suffered a transient ischemic attack and those with atherosclerotic thickening of the carotid arteries may prevent stroke with medical therapies (e.g., aspirin, ticlopidine, clopidogrel, or warfarin) or surgical interventions (carotid endarterectomy).

NOTE: Thrombolytic therapies and endarterectomy are most likely to prove beneficial in highly specialized treatment centers with demonstrably low complication rates.

ischemic s. A stroke due to diminished blood supply to the brain or a particular area of the brain (e.g., the lodging of an embolus from the heart in an artery of the brain).

lacunar s. A pathological change in the brain caused by diminished or lack of blood flow through one of the brain's small penetrating arteries. When this occurs, there may be no clinically detectable changes in the patient, or signs and symptoms of stroke. A group of little strokes may cause progressive dementia.

mini-s. A colloquial term for a transient ischemic attack.

paralytic s. A stroke that produces loss of muscular functions.

stroking **1.** A massage technique of moving the hand over the body surface, used to facilitate relaxation and improve flow of tissue fluids. **2.** A technique of slow tactile stimulation over the posterior primary rami, used to inhibit muscle responses and promote relaxation during neuromotor rehabilitation.

stroma (strō′mă) *pl.* **stromata** [Gr., bed covering] **1.** Foundation-supporting tissues of an organ. The opposite of parenchyma. **2.** The membranous lipid-protein framework within a red blood cell to which hemoglobin molecules are attached. **stromal, stromatic,** *adj.*

stromatolysis (strō″mă-tŏl′ĭ-sĭs) [″ + *lysis,* dissolution] Destruction of the stroma of a cell.

stromatosis (strō″mă-tō′sĭs) [″ + *osis,* condition] Presence of mesenchyma-like tissue throughout the endometrium of the uterus.

stromelysin (strō′mă-līs-ĭn) ABBR: MMP-3. Member of the matrix metalloproteinase family of enzymes that plays a major role in the degradation of proteoglycans, gelatin, and other constituents of the extracellular matrix. Two forms of stromelysin have been described, stromelysin-1 and -2. Stromelysin-1 degrades proteoglycans, gelatin, fibronectin, laminin, collagen types III, IV, IX, and X. Stromelysin-2 degrades proteoglycans, fibronectin, laminin, and collagen type IV.

Stromeyer's splint (strō′mī-ĕrz) [Georg F. L. Stromeyer, Ger. surgeon, 1804–1876] A hinged splint for a joint, which can be fixed at an angle.

Strong Interest Inventory ABBR: SII. A psychological test that traditionally measures vocational interests but also identifies personality traits. Previous versions (the original was developed in 1927) were known as the Strong Vocational Interest Bank.

Strongyloides (strŏn″jĭ-loy′dēz) A genus of roundworms that infect humans.

S. stercoralis A roundworm that causes gastrointestinal infections (primarily in persons from developing nations) and opportunistic infections (in immunosuppressed patients). It may occasionally be life-threatening. In the U.S., *S. stercoralis* is found mainly in the rural South. The ova hatch in the intestines of the host, and rod-shaped larvae are passed in the stool. In the soil, these may develop into adults and continue their life cycle or may metamorphose into filariform larvae that can infect humans. The filariform larvae enter the skin, pass through the venous system to the lungs, where they migrate upward and are swallowed. A rash or pneumonia may accompany their migration. The larvae mature in the intestine, and ova of the next generation hatch. The rod-shaped larvae may metamorphose into the filariform larvae in the intestine. These may enter the circulation, migrate to the lungs, and begin the cycle again.

Such auto-infection may be sufficient to cause overwhelming systemic infection with fever, severe abdominal pain, shock, and possibly death. Severe reactions are more likely to occur in immunosuppressed patients. The diagnosis is made by finding larvae in the patient's feces. Thiabendazole or mebendazole are the drugs of choice. Repeated courses of treatment may be required.

strongyloidosis (strŏn″jĭ-loy-dō′sĭs) [Gr. *strongylos,* compact, + *osis,* condition] Infestation with organisms of the genus *Strongyloides.*

strongylosis (strŏn″jĭ-lō′sĭs) Infestation with organisms of the genus *Strongylus.*

Strongylus (strŏn′jĭ-lŭs) A genus of parasitic nematodes.

strontium (strŏn′shē-ŭm) [Strontian, mining village in Scotland] SYMB: Sr. A dark yellow metal; atomic weight, 87.62; atomic number, 38; specific gravity, 2.6. Medically it is of interest because its radioactive isotope ^{90}Sr constitutes a radioactive hazard in fallout from atom bombs. The isotope has a half-life of 28 years and is stored in bone when ingested.

Strophanthus (strō-făn′thŭs) [Gr. *strophos,* twisted cord, + *anthos,* flower] A genus of plants yielding a poisonous, white, crystalline glucoside, previously used as a heart stimulant.

strophocephaly (strŏf″ō-sĕf′ă-lē) [″ + *kephale,* head] Distortion of the head and face resulting from a developmental anomaly.

structural (strŭk′tū-răl) [L. *structura,* structure] Pert. to organic structure.

structural integration Rolfing.

structure (strŭk′shŭr) The arrangement of the component parts of an organism.

denture-supporting s. The tissues that support a partial or complete denture.

struma (stroo′mă) [L. *struma,* a mass] Goiter.

s. aberranta A struma of the accessory thyroid glands.

cast iron s. Riedel's s.

s. lymphomatosa A rare condition involving a diffuse and extensive infiltration of the entire thyroid gland.

s. maligna Carcinoma of the thyroid gland.

s. ovarii A form of ovarian teratoma in which the mass is composed of typical thyroid follicles filled with colloid.

Riedel's s. A form of chronic thyroiditis in which the gland becomes enlarged, hard, and adherent to adjacent tissues. The follicles become atrophic and fibrosis occurs. SYN: *cast iron s.*

strumectomy (stroo-mĕk′tō-mē) [″ + *ektome,* excision] The removal of a goiter.

strumitis (stroo-mī′tĭs) [″ + Gr. *itis,* inflammation] Thyroiditis.

Strümpell's disease (strĭm′pĕlz) Strümpell-Marie disease.

Strümpell-Marie disease [Adolf G. G. von Strümpell, Ger. physician, 1853–1925; Pierre Marie, Fr. neurologist, 1853–1940] Ankylosing spondylitis.

Strümpell's sign (strĭm′pĕls) Dorsiflexion of the foot when the thigh is flexed on the abdomen. This sign may be associated with spastic paralysis of the leg.

struvite Magnesium ammonium phosphate crystals, important in health care because they cause about 15% of all kidney stones. They are formed in the urinary tract in conjunction with some bacterial infections, such as infection with *Proteus mirabilis,* and in some patients with hypercalciuria.

strychnine (strĭk′nīn, -nēn, -nĭn) [Gr. *strychnos,* nightshade] A poisonous alkaloid, used to kill rodents, that may produce nausea and vomiting, symmetrical muscle spasms, fever, muscle breakdown (rhabdomyolysis), and renal failure. It has no therapeutic usefulness but has been used as an experimental tool in neuropharmacology.

s. poisoning Toxicity produced by ingestion of strychnine.

PATIENT CARE: Overdoses should be treated with gastric decontamination (e.g., with activated charcoal) and drugs (e.g., diazepam) that limit muscular contraction. Supportive care includes intravenous hydration with alkalinization of the urine to prevent or treat the consequences of rhabdomyolysis. SEE: *Poisons and Poisoning Appendix.*

strychninism (strĭk′nĭn-ĭzm) [″ +

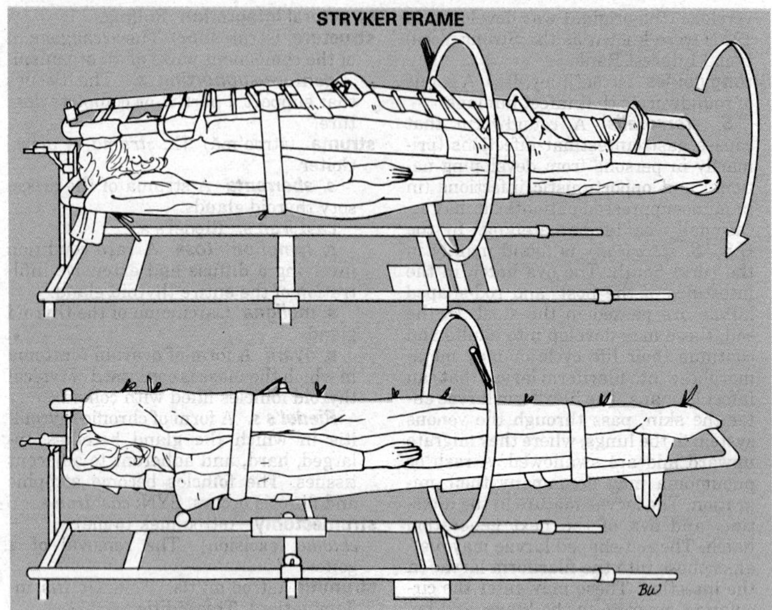

-ismos, condition] Chronic strychnine poisoning.

Stryker frame A device that supports two rectangular pieces of lightweight but strong material so that one side is on the anterior surface of the patient and the other is on the posterior surface. The patient is sandwiched firmly between the pieces of material. The device may be rotated around the patient's long axis. This permits turning the patient without his or her assistance. After a turn is completed, the uppermost portion of the frame can be moved away from the patient. SEE: illus.

Stryker's saw An electric-powered oscillating saw that cuts through bone or dense tissue with minimal damage to the underlying soft tissues.

STS *serological test for syphilis.*

STU *skin test unit.*

study, blinded In research, a study in which the subjects and/or the researchers are unaware of which group is receiving active treatment and which is receiving a placebo. Blinding reduces the potential for bias.

study, case-control An investigative technique used in epidemiology and medical research whereby cases are selected for study on the basis of the dependent variable, that is, the presence (study group) or absence (control group) of the condition or disease being investigated. Differences in the rates of the factor, trait, exposure, characteristic, or possible cause (independent variables) are then compared between the two groups. For example, a study might involve two groups of patients from the same population—one that has cancer (study group) and one that does not have cancer (control group). The smoking rates in these otherwise similar groups could then be compared to see if exposure to cigarettes differed between them. The first such study involved an investigation of chimney sweeps in England who developed cancer of the scrotum. The hypothesis was that something peculiar to their occupation led to a higher incidence of cancer than was prevalent in the general population, and indeed it was subsequently shown that soot deposits in the testicular skin (rugae) could lead to this cancer. It is important to remember that case-control studies cannot prove causation but can only suggest associations between the variables. Because this type of study is retrospective, there is no way to control for bias in the study from differential reporting between the groups, nor to match the two groups as closely as would be necessary to exclude possible confounding factors and prove cause and effect.

study, double-blinded A method of scientific investigation in which neither the subject nor the investigator knows what treatment, if any, the subject is receiving. At the completion of the experiment, the blinding is removed and data are analyzed with respect to the various treatments used. This method attempts to eliminate observer and subject bias.

study, nerve conduction ABBR: NCS. An electrodiagnostic test used to determine whether the conduction of impulses along specific nerves is normal or pathologically slowed. In the test an electrical shock is given to a nerve that controls a particular muscle. The time required for the muscle to contract and the distance the electrical stimulus has to travel along the nerve are recorded. In patients with neuropathies, the expected velocity of impulse conduction will not be met; slowing will be evident. Patients with cut or injured nerves will show maximal slowing of impulse conduction.

study, prospective A scientific investigation that collects data as they accumulate and analyzes the results after they have accrued. Prospective studies in which both the investigators and the research subjects are unaware of treatment assignments are considered among the most meaningful in health care.

study, retrospective A research project that collects data and draws conclusions from events that have already occurred.

study, role delineation ABBR: RD study. A document that describes those tasks that are critical for competent job performance, by identifying the minimum amount of knowledge and skills required to perform job-related functions. RD study results are often used to develop certification and licensing examinations in the health professions.

study, single-blinded A study in which only the subject or the investigator is unaware of which parties are receiving the active treatment.

stump The distal portion of an amputated extremity.

stun (stŭn) [O.Fr. *estoner,* a blow] To render unconscious or stupefied by a blow.

stupe (stūp) [L. *stupa,* tow] A counterirritant for topical use, prepared by adding a small amount of an irritant such as turpentine to a hot liquid.

stupor (stū′por) [L., numbness] A state of altered mental status (decreased responsiveness to one's environment) in which a person is arousable only with vigorous or unpleasant stimulation. **stuporous,** *adj.*

epileptic s. Postictal confusion or drowsiness that sometimes follows a seizure.

Sturge-Weber syndrome [William Sturge, Brit. physician, 1850–1919; Frederick Parkes Weber, Brit. physician, 1863–1962] A congenital neurocutaneous syndrome (technically a "phocomatosis") marked by port-wine nevi along the distribution of the trigeminal nerve, angiomas of leptomeninges and choroid, intracranial calcifications, mental retardation, seizures, and glaucoma. SYN: *nevoid amentia.*

stuttering (stŭt′ĕr-ĭng) [ME. *stutten,* to stutter] A disruption in the fluency of speech in which affected persons repeat letters or syllables, pause or hesitate abnormally, or fragment words when attempting to speak. The symptoms are exaggerated during times of stress, and may also be worsened by some medications, some strokes, or other diseases and conditions. Stuttering often occurs in more than one family member. SYN: *stammering.*

This condition occurs in approx. 1% to 2% of the school population. Boys are affected three or four times as often as girls. The onset is in two periods: between the ages of 2 and 4 years when speech begins and between 6 and 8 years of age when the need for language increases. It usually resolves spontaneously by adulthood.

Therapies, including relaxation techniques, hypnosis, delayed auditory feedback, and medications such as haloperidol can provide some help.

Educational materials are available from the Stuttering Foundation of America (800-992-9392) and from the American Speech-Language-Hearing Association (800-638-8255).

acquired s. The sudden appearance of stuttering in a person over age 10 with no previous history of an articulation disorder. It may occur after a stroke, after the administration of certain drugs (e.g., theophylline), as an affectation, or as a reaction to unusually stressful circumstances.

urinary s. Irregular, spasmodic urination. SYN: *stammering of bladder.*

sty, stye (stī) *pl.* **styes, sties** [AS. *stigan,* to rise] A localized inflammatory swelling of one or more of the glands of the eyelid. They are mildly tender, and may discharge some purulent fluid. SEE: *chalazion.*

SYMPTOMS: General edema of the lid, pain, and localized conjunctivitis mark the condition. As the internal sty progresses, an abscess will form that can be seen through the conjunctiva.

TREATMENT: Applying warm, moist compresses to the eyelid several times a day for 4 or 5 days usually helps the sty drain. If the sty does not resolve, it can be incised and drained surgically. SYN: *hordeolum.*

meibomian s. An inflammation of a meibomian gland.

zeisian s. An inflammation of one of the Zeis' glands.

style, stylet (stīl, stī′lĕt) [Gr. *stylos,* pillar] **1.** A slender, solid or hollow, plug of metal for making a canal permanent after operation or for stiffening or clearing a cannula or catheter. **2.** A thin probe.

styliform (stī′lĭ-form) [″ + L. *forma,* form] Long and pointed.

styloglossus (stī-lō-glŏs′ŭs) [Gr. *stylos,*

pillar, + *glossa,* tongue] A muscle connecting the tongue and styloid process that raises and retracts the tongue.

stylohyal (stī″lō-hī′ăl) [″ + *hyoeides,* hyoid] Stylohyoid.

stylohyoid (stī-lō-hī′oyd) [″ + *hyoeides,* hyoid] Pert. to the styloid process of the temporal and hyoid bones. SYN: *stylohyal.*

stylohyoideus (stī″lō-hī-oyd′ē-ŭs) A muscle having its origin on the styloid process and its insertion on the hyoid bone. It draws the hyoid bone upward and backward.

styloid (stī′loyd) [″ + *eidos,* form, shape] Resembling a stylus or pointed instrument.

styloiditis (stī″loyd-ī′tĭs) [″ + ″ + *itis,* inflammation] Inflammation of a styloid process.

stylomandibular (stī″lō-măn-dĭb′ū-lar) [″ + L. *mandibula,* lower jawbone] Concerning the styloid process of the temporal bone and mandible.

stylomastoid (stī″lō-măs′toyd) [″ + *mastos,* breast, + *eidos,* form, shape] Concerning the styloid and mastoid processes of the temporal bone.

stylopharyngeus (stī″lō-făr-ĭn′jē-ŭs) [″ + *pharynx,* throat] The muscle connecting the styloid process and the pharynx that elevates and dilates the pharynx.

stylostaphyline (stī″lō-stăf′ĭ-līn) [″ + *staphyle,* bunch of grapes] Concerning the styloid process of the temporal bone and uvula.

stylosteophyte (stī-lŏs′tē-ō-fīt) A peg-shaped outgrowth from bone.

stylus (stī′lŭs) [Gr. *stylos,* a pillar] **1.** A probe or slender wire for stiffening or clearing a canal or catheter. **2.** A pointed medicinal preparation in stick form for external application (e.g., silver nitrate). **3.** A pointed writing instrument.

stypsis (stĭp′sĭs) [Gr. *styphein,* to contract] Astringency or the use of an astringent.

styptic (stĭp′tĭk) [Gr. *styptikos,* contracting] **1.** Contracting a blood vessel; stopping a hemorrhage by astringent action. **2.** Anything that stops a hemorrhage such as alum, ferrous sulfate, or tannic acid. SYN: *astringent; hemostat.*

sub- [L. *sub,* under, below] Prefix meaning *under, beneath, in small quantity, less than normal.* SEE: *hypo-.*

subabdominal (sŭb″ăb-dŏm′ĭ-năl) [L. *sub,* under, below, + *abdomen,* abdomen] Below the abdomen.

subabdominoperitoneal (sŭb″ăb-dŏm″ĭ-nō-pĕr″ĭ-tō-nē′ăl) [″ + ″ + Gr. *peritonaion,* peritoneum] Deep to the abdominal peritoneum.

subacetate (sŭb-ăs′ĕ-tāt) [″ + *acetum,* vinegar] A basic acetate.

subacid (sŭb-ăs′ĭd) [″ + *acidus,* sour] Moderately acid.

subacromial (sŭb-ă-krō′mē-ăl) [″ + Gr. *akron,* point, + *osmos,* shoulder] Under the acromial process.

subacute (sŭb″ă-kūt′) [″ + *acutus,* sharp] Between acute and chronic, said of the course of a disease or of the healing process that develops at a moderate, rather than a slow or fast pace.

subacute myelo-optic neuropathy ABBR: SMON. A neurological disease that usually begins with abdominal pain or diarrhea, followed by sensory and motor disturbances in the lower limbs, ataxia, impaired vision, and convulsions or coma. It is reported mostly in Japan and Australia. Most patients survive, but neurological disability remains. Many of those who have the disease have a history of taking drugs of the halogenated oxyquinoline group such as clioquinol (previously called iodochlorhydroxyquin).

subanconeus (sŭb″ăn-kō′nē-ŭs) [″ + Gr. *ankon,* elbow] **1.** Below the elbow. **2.** The muscle beneath the elbow that contracts its posterior ligament.

subapical (sŭb-ăp′ĭ-kăl) [″ + *apex,* tip] Below the apex.

subaponeurotic (sŭb″ăp-ō-nū-rŏt′ĭk) [″ + Gr. *apo,* from, + *neuron,* sinew] Below an aponeurosis.

subarachnoid (sŭb″ă-răk′noyd) [″ + Gr. *arachne,* spider, + *eidos,* form, shape] Below or under the arachnoid membrane and above the pia mater of the covering of the brain and spinal cord.

subarachnoid cisternae Spaces at the base of the brain where the arachnoid becomes widely separated from the pia, giving rise to large cavities.

subarachnoid space The space between the pia mater and the arachnoid, containing the cerebrospinal fluid.

subarcuate (sŭb-ăr′kū-āt) [L. *sub,* under, below, + *arcuatus,* bowed] Slightly arched.

subarcuate fossa A depression that extends backward as a blind tunnel under the superior semicircular canal of the temporal bone.

subareolar (sŭb″ă-rē′ō-lăr) [″ + *areola,* a small space] Below the areola.

subastragalar (sŭb-ăs-trăg′ă-lăr) [″ + Gr. *astragalos,* ball of the ankle joint] An outdated term for the space beneath the ankle joint.

subastringent (sŭb″ăs-trĭn′jĕnt) [″ + *astringere,* to bind fast] Mildly astringent.

subatomic (sŭb″ă-tŏm′ĭk) [″ + Gr. *atomos,* indivisible] Less than the size of an atom.

subaural (sŭb-aw′răl) [″ + *auris,* ear] Below the ear.

subauricular (sŭb″aw-rĭk′ū-lăr) [″ + *auricula,* little ear] Below an auricle, esp. of the ear.

subaxial (sŭb-ăk′sē-ăl) [″ + *axis,* axis] Below an axis.

subaxillary (sŭb-ăk′sĭ-lĕr″ē) [″ + *axilla,* armpit] Below the axilla, or armpit.

subbrachycephalic (sŭb″brā-kē-sĕ-făl′ĭk) [″ + Gr. *brachys,* short, + *kephale,* head] Having a cephalic index of 78 to 79.

subcalcarine (sŭb-kăl′kăr-īn) [″ + *calcar,* spur] Below the calcarine sulcus of the brain.

subcapsular (sŭb-kăp′sū-lăr) [″ + *capsula,* little box] Below any capsule, esp. the capsule of the brain, or a capsular ligament.

subcarbonate (sŭb-kăr′bō-nāt) [″ + *carbo,* carbon] A basic carbonate; one having a proportion of carbonic acid radical less than the normal carbonate.

subcartilaginous (sŭb″kăr-tĭ-lăj′ĭn-ŭs) [″ + *cartilago,* gristle] **1.** Located beneath a cartilage. **2.** Cartilaginous in part.

subchondral (sŭb″kŏn′drăl) [″ + Gr. *chondros,* cartilage] Below or under a cartilage.

subchoroidal (sŭb″kō-roy′dăl) [″ + Gr. *chorioeides,* skinlike] Below the choroid.

subclass (sŭb′klăs) In taxonomy, a category between a class and an order.

subclavian (sŭb-klā′vē-ăn) [″ + *clavis,* key] Under the clavicle or collarbone. SYN: *subclavicular.*

subclavian artery The large artery at the base of the neck that supplies blood to the arm. The right subclavian artery branches from the brachiocephalic artery; the left subclavian artery branches from the aortic arch.

subclavian steal syndrome The clinical consequences of shunting blood from the vertebrobasilar artery, usually on the left side, around an occluded subclavian artery on that side, and into the left arm.

SYMPTOMS: The affected person often experiences numbness or weakness of the arm when he or she tries to use it. In some people, the diversion of blood from the brain into the arm results in signs and symptoms of brainstem ischemia or stroke, such as loss of consciousness. On physical examination, a bruit may be heard over the obstructed subclavian artery, and the blood pressure in the arm on the affected side will be lower than in the unaffected arm.

TREATMENT: The subclavian artery may be surgically bypassed or opened with angioplasty.

subclavian triangle The triangle-shaped part of the neck, formed by the clavicle and the omohyoid and sternomastoid muscles.

subclavian vein A large vein draining the arm. It unites with the internal jugular vein to form the brachiocephalic (innominate) vein.

subclavicular (sŭb″klă-vĭk′ū-lăr) [L. *sub,* under, below, + *clavicula,* little key] Subclavian.

subclavius (sŭb-klā′vē-ŭs) [″ + *clavis,* key] A tiny muscle from the first rib to the undersurface of the clavicle.

subclinical (sŭb-klĭn′ĭ-kăl) [″ + Gr. *klinikos,* pert. to a bed] Pert. to a period before the appearance of typical symptoms of a disease or to a disease or condition that does not present clinical symptoms. Mildly increased or decreased levels of thyroid hormone in the body often present subclinically.

subcollateral (sŭb-kō-lăt′ĕr-ăl) [″ + *con,* together, + *lateralis,* pert. to a side] Below the collateral fissure, indicating a cerebral convolution.

subconjunctival (sŭb″kŏn-jŭnk-tī′văl) [″ + *conjungere,* to join together] Beneath the conjunctiva.

subconsciousness (sŭb-kŏn′shŭs-nĕs) [″ + *conscius,* aware] The condition in which mental processes take place without the individual's being aware of their occurrence. SEE: *subliminal.*

subcontinuous (sŭb″kŏn-tĭn′ū-ŭs) [″ + *continere,* to hold together] Almost continuous; with periods of abatement.

subcoracoid (sŭb-kor′ă-koyd) [″ + Gr. *korakoeides,* like a crow's beak] Beneath the coracoid process.

subcortex (sŭb-kor′tĕks) [″ + *cortex,* rind] The white matter of the brain underlying the cortex.

subcortical (sŭb-kor′tĭ-kăl) Pert. to the region beneath the cerebral cortex.

subcostal (sŭb-kŏs′tăl) [″ + *costa,* rib] Beneath the ribs.

subcostalgia (sŭb″kŏs-tăl′jē-ă) [″ + ″ + Gr. *algos,* pain] Pain in the region over the subcostal nerve.

subcranial (sŭb-krā′nē-ăl) [″ + Gr. *kranion,* skull] Beneath or below the cranium.

subcrepitant (sŭb-krĕp′ĭ-tănt) [″ + *crepitare,* to rattle] Partially crepitant or crackling in character; noting a rale.

subcrureus (sŭb-kroo-rē′ŭs) [″ + *crus,* leg] A small muscle between the anterior surface of the femoral shaft and the synovial membrane of the knee joint.

subculture (sŭb-kŭl′chūr) [″ + *cultura,* tillage] **1.** To make a culture of bacteria with material derived from another culture. **2.** A relatively cohesive group of individuals living within a society, who, because of shared traditions, customs, socioeconomic status, or genetic heritage, may be predisposed to particular states of health or illness.

subcutaneous (sŭb″kū-tā′nē-ŭs) [″ + *cutis,* skin] Beneath the skin. SYN: *hypodermic.*

subcutaneous surgery An operation performed through a small opening in the skin.

subcutaneous wound A wound with only a small opening through the skin.

subcuticular (sŭb″kū-tĭk′ū-lăr) [L. *sub,* under, below, + *cuticula,* little skin] Subepidermal.

subcutis (sŭb-kū′tĭs) The layer of connective tissue beneath the skin.
subdeltoid (sŭb-dĕl′toyd) [″ + Gr. *delta,* letter d, + *eidos,* form, shape] Beneath the deltoid muscle.
subdental (sŭb-dĕn′tăl) [″ + *dens,* tooth] Beneath the teeth or a tooth.
subdermal [″ + Gr. *derma,* skin] Below the skin.
subdiaphragmatic (sŭb″dī-ă-frăg-măt′ĭk) [″ + Gr. *diaphragma,* a partition] Beneath the diaphragm. SYN: *subphrenic.*
subdorsal (sŭb-dor′săl) [″ + *dorsum,* back] Below the dorsal area.
subduct (sŭb-dŭkt′) [″ + *ducere,* to lead] To draw down.
subdural (sŭb-dū′răl) [″ + *durus,* hard] Beneath the dura mater.
subendocardial (sŭb″ĕn-dō-kăr′dē-ăl) [″ + Gr. *endon,* within, + *kardia,* heart] Below the endocardium.
subendothelial, subendothelium (sŭb″ĕn-dō-thē′lē-ăl, sŭb″ĕn-dō-thē′lē-ŭm) [″ + Gr. *endon,* within, + *thele,* nipple] Beneath the endothelium.
subependymal (sŭb″ĕp-ĕn′dĭ-măl) [″ + Gr. *ependyma,* an upper garment, wrap] Beneath the ependyma.
subepidermal (sŭb″ĕp-ĭ-dĕr′măl) [″ + Gr. *epi,* upon, + *derma,* skin] Beneath the epidermis. SYN: *subcuticular.*
subepithelial (sŭb″ĕp-ĭ-thē′lē-ăl) [″ + ″ + *thele,* nipple] Beneath the epithelium.
suberosis (sū″bĕr-ō′sĭs) [L. *suber,* cork, + Gr. *osis,* condition] Pulmonary hypersensitivity reaction in workers exposed to cork. The antigen is present in a mold in the cork.
subfamily (sŭb-făm′ĭ-lē) In taxonomy, the category between a family and a genus.
subfascial (sŭb-făsh′ē-ăl) [L. *sub,* under, below, + *fascia,* a band] Beneath a fascia.
subfebrile (sŭb-fē′brĭl) [″ + *febris,* fever] Having a mildly increased body temperature, usually considered to be less than 101°F (38.3°C).
subfertility (sŭb″fĕr-tĭl′ĭ-tē) [″ + *fertilis,* fertile] Fertility considered to be less than normal.
subflavous (sŭb-flā′vŭs) [″ + *flavus,* yellow] Yellowish.
subflavous ligament The yellowish ligament connecting the laminae of the vertebrae.
subfolium (sŭb-fō′lē-ŭm) [″ + *folium,* leaf] A leaflike division of the cerebellar folia.
subfrontal (sŭb-frŏn′tăl) [″ + *frontalis,* brow] Below a frontal convolution or lobe of the brain.
subgenus (sŭb-jē′nŭs) In taxonomy, the category between a genus and a species.
subgingival (sŭb-jĭn′jĭ-văl) [″ + *gingiva,* gum] Beneath the gingiva; rel. to a point or area apical to the margin of the free gingiva, usually within the confines of the gingival sulcus (e.g., subgingival calculus, or the subgingival margin of a restoration).
subglenoid (sŭb-glē′noyd) [″ + Gr. *glene,* socket, + *eidos,* form, shape] Below the glenoid fossa or glenoid cavity. SYN: *infraglenoid.*
subglossal (sŭb-glŏs′ăl) [″ + Gr. *glossa,* tongue] Sublingual.
subglossitis (sŭb-glŏs-sī′tĭs) [″ + ″ + *itis,* inflammation] An inflammation of the undersurface or tissues of the tongue.
subglottic (sŭb-glŏt′ĭk) [″ + Gr. *glottis,* back of tongue] Beneath the glottis.
subgranular (sŭb-grăn′ū-lăr) [″ + *granulum,* little grain] Not completely granular.
subgrondation, subgrundation (sŭb-grŏn-dā′shŭn, -grŭn-dă′shŭn) [Fr.] The depression of one fragment of a broken bone beneath the other, as of the cranium.
subhepatic (sŭb″hē-păt′ĭk) [L. *sub,* under, below, + Gr. *hepatikos,* pert. to the liver] Beneath the liver.
subhyaloid (sŭb-hī′ă-loyd) [″ + Gr. *hyalos,* glass, + *eidos,* form, shape] Located beneath the hyaloid membrane.
subhyoid (sŭb-hī′oyd) [″ + Gr. *hyoeides,* U-shaped] Beneath the hyoid bone.
subicular (sŭb-bĭk′ū-lăr) Concerning the uncinate gyrus.
subiliac (sŭb-ĭl′ē-ăk) [″ + *iliacus,* pert. to the ilium] **1.** Below the ilium. **2.** Pert. to the subilium.
subilium (sŭb-ĭl′ē-ŭm) The lowest part of the ilium.
subincision The production of a fistula of the penile urethra, which may interfere with conception. It is used for contraception by some primitive groups, esp. Australian aborigines.
subintimal (sŭb-ĭn′tĭ-măl) [″ + *intima,* innermost] Beneath the intima.
subinvolution (sŭb″ĭn-vō-lū′shŭn) [L. *sub,* under, below, + *involutio,* a turning into] Imperfect involution; incomplete return of a part to normal dimensions after physiological hypertrophy, as when the uterus fails to reduce to normal size following childbirth. SEE: *uterus.*
subjacent (sŭb-jā′sĕnt) [″ + *jacere,* to lie] Lying underneath.
subject (sŭb′jĕkt) [L. *subjectus,* brought under] **1.** A patient undergoing treatment, observation, or investigation; this includes a well person participating in a medical or scientific study. **2.** A body used for dissection. **3.** To have a liability to develop attacks of a particular disease. **4.** To submit to a procedure or to the action of another.
subjective [L. *subjectivus*] Arising from or concerned with the individual; not perceptible to an observer; the opposite of objective.

subjective symptoms A symptom of internal origin, evident only to the patient.
subjugal (sŭb-jū′găl) [L. *sub,* under, below, + *jugum,* yoke] Below the malar bone or os zygomaticum.
sublatio (sŭb-lā′shē-ō) [L.] Sublation.
s. retinae Detachment of the retina.
sublation (sŭb-lā′shŭn) [L. *sublatio,* elevation] The displacement, elevation, or removal of a part. SYN: *sublatio.*
sublesional (sŭb-lē′shŭn-ăl) [L. *sub,* under, below, + *laesio,* wound] Beneath a lesion.
sublethal (sŭb-lē′thăl) [″ + Gr. *lethe,* oblivion] Less than lethal; almost fatal.
sublethal dose A dose containing not quite enough of a toxin or noxious substance to cause death.
sublimate (sŭb′lĭ-māt) [L. *sublimare,* to elevate] **1.** A substance obtained or prepared by sublimation. **2.** To cause a solid or gas to change state without becoming a liquid during transition. For example, ice may evaporate without first becoming a liquid. **3.** An ego defense mechanism by which one converts unwanted aggressive or sexual drives into socially acceptable activities.
sublimation (sŭb″lĭ-mā′shŭn) [L. *sublimatio*] **1.** The altering of the state of a gas or solid without first changing it into a liquid. **2.** A freudian term pert. to the unconscious mental processes of ego defense whereby unwanted aggressive or sexual drives find an outlet through creative mental work.
sublime (sŭb-līm′) [L. *sublimis,* to the limit] To evaporate a substance directly from the solid into the vapor state and condense it again. For example, metallic iodine on heating does not liquefy but forms directly a violet gas.
subliminal (sŭb-lĭm′ĭn-ăl) [L. *sub,* under, below, + *limen,* threshold] **1.** Below the threshold of sensation; too weak to arouse sensation or muscular contraction. **2.** Below the normal consciousness.
subliminal self In psychoanalytical theory, part of the normal individual's personality in which mental processes function without consciousness, under normal waking conditions.
sublimis (sŭb-lī′mĭs) [L.] Near the surface.
sublingual (sŭb-lĭng′gwăl) [L. *sub,* under, below, + *lingua,* tongue] Beneath or concerning the area beneath the tongue. SYN: *subglossal.*
sublinguitis (sŭb″lĭng-gwī′tĭs) [″ + ″ + Gr. *itis,* inflammation] An inflammation of the sublingual gland.
sublobular (sŭb-lŏb′ū-lăr) [″ + *lobulus,* small lobe] Beneath a lobule.
sublumbar (sŭb-lŭm′băr) [″ + *lumbus,* loin] Below the lumbar region.
subluxation (sŭb″lŭks-ā′shŭn) [″ + *luxatio,* dislocation] **1.** A partial or incomplete dislocation. **2.** In dentistry, injury to supporting tissues that results in abnormal loosening of teeth without displacement or rotation. When loosely applied to the temporomandibular joint, subluxation refers to the relaxation or stretching of the capsule and ligaments that results in popping noises during movement or partial dislocation of the mandible forward.
submammary (sŭb-măm′ă-rē) [″ + *mamma,* breast] Below the mammary gland.
submandibular [″ + *mandibula,* lower jawbone] Beneath the mandible or lower jaw.
submandibularitis An inflammation of or mumps affecting the submandibular gland.
submarginal (sŭb-măr′jĭn-ăl) [″ + *marginalis,* border] Close to or next to a margin or border of a part. In dentistry, pert. to a deficiency in material or contour at the margin of a restoration in a tooth.
submaxillary Below the maxilla or upper jaw.
submedial, submedian (sŭb-mē′dē-ăl, -ăn) [″ + *medianus,* middle] Below or close to the middle.
submembranous (sŭb-mĕm′bră-nŭs) [″ + *membrana,* membrane] Containing partly membranous material.
submental [″ + *mentum,* chin] Under the chin.
submerge (sŭb-mĕrj′) [″ + *mergere,* to immerse] To place under water.
submerged tooth A tooth that is below the plane of occlusion; usually a deciduous tooth retained as a result of ankylosis.
submetacentric (sŭb″mĕt-ă-sĕn′trĭk) [″ + Gr. *meta,* beyond, + *kentron,* center] Concerning a chromosome in which the centromere is within the two central quarters but not precisely centrally located.
submicron [″ + Gr. *mikros,* tiny] A particle smaller than 10^{-5} cm in diameter, visible only with an ultramicroscope. SEE: *micron.*
submicroscopic [″ + ″ + *skopein,* to examine] Too minute to be seen through a microscope.
submucosa (sŭb″mū-kō′să) [L. *sub,* under, below, + *mucosus,* mucus] The layer of connective tissue below the mucosa. It may vary from areolar to quite dense irregular connective tissue and, in addition to the distributing vessels and nerves, may contain extensive deposits of fat, mucous glands, or muscle.
submucous (sŭb-mū′kŭs) [″ + *mucus,* mucus] Beneath a mucous membrane.
submucous resection Removal of tissue below the mucosa, esp. excision of cartilaginous tissue beneath the mucosal tissue of the nose.
subnasal [″ + *nasus,* nose] Under the nose. SYN: *subnasion.*

subnasale (sŭb″nā-sā′lē) [″ + *nasus,* nose] The base of the anterior nasal spine.
subnasal point The craniometric point at the base of the nasal spine.
subnasion (sŭb-nā′zē-ŏn) [″ + *nasus,* nose] Subnasal.
subneural (sŭb-nū′răl) [″ + Gr. *neuron,* nerve] Beneath the neural axis or the central nervous system.
subnormal (sŭb-nor′măl) [″ + *normalis,* accord. to pattern] Less than normal or average.
subnucleus (sŭb-nū′klē-ŭs) [″ + *nucleus,* kernel] One of the secondary nuclei into which a nucleus of the central nervous system may be divided.
suboccipital (sŭb″ŏk-sĭp′ĭ-tăl) [″ + *occiput,* back of head] Situated below the occiput or occipital bone.
suboperculum (sŭb″ō-pĕr′kū-lŭm) [″ + *operculum,* a covering] The portion of the occipital convolution overlapping the insula. SEE: *operculum.*
suboptimal (sŭb-ŏp′tĭ-măl) [″ + *optimus,* best] Less than optimum.
suborbital (sŭb-or′bĭ-tăl) [″ + *orbita,* track] Beneath the orbit.
suborder (sŭb-or′dĕr) In taxonomy, a category between an order and a family.
suboxide (sŭb-ŏk′sīdz) In a series of oxides, one that contains the smallest amount of oxygen.
subpapular (sŭb-păp′ū-lăr) [″ + *papula,* pimple] Very slightly papular, such as papules elevated scarcely more than macules.
subparietal (sŭb″pă-rī′ĕ-tăl) [″ + *paries,* a wall] Below the parietal bone or lobe.
subpatellar (sŭb″pă-tĕl′ăr) [″ + *patella,* a small pan] Beneath the patella.
subpectoral (sŭb-pĕk′tor-ăl) [″ + *pectus,* chest] Below the pectoral area; beneath the pectoral muscles.
subpeduncular (sŭb″pē-dŭn′kū-lăr) [″ + *pedunculus,* a little foot] Below a peduncle.
subpeduncular lobe A tiny lobe on the undersurface of either cerebellar hemisphere. SYN: *flocculus.*
subpelviperitoneal (sŭb-pĕl″vē-pĕr″ĭ-tō-nē′ ăl) [L. *sub,* under, below, + *pelvis,* basin, + Gr. *peritonaion,* peritoneum] Beneath the pelvic peritoneum.
subpericardial (sŭb″pĕr-ĭ-kăr′dē-ăl) [″ + Gr. *peri,* around, + *kardia,* heart] Beneath the pericardium.
subperiosteal (sŭb″pĕr-ē-ŏs′tē-ăl) [″ + ″ + *osteon,* bone] Beneath the periosteum.
subperitoneal (sŭb″pĕr-ĭ-tō-nē′ăl) [″ + Gr. *peritonaion,* peritoneum] Beneath, behind, or deep to the peritoneum. SYN: *subperitoneoabdominal.*
subperitoneoabdominal (sŭb″pĕr-ĭ-tō-nē″ō-ăb-dŏm′ĭ-năl) [″ + ″ + L. *abdomen,* belly] Subperitoneal.
subpharyngeal (sŭb″făr-ĭn′jē-ăl) [″ + Gr. *pharynx,* throat] Beneath the pharynx.
subphrenic (sŭb-frĕn′ĭk) [″ + Gr. *phren,* diaphragm] Subdiaphragmatic.
subphylum (sŭb-fī′lŭm) In taxonomy, the category between a phylum and a class.
subpial (sŭb-pī′ăl) [″ + *pia,* soft] Beneath the pia.
subplacenta (sŭb″plă-sĕn′tă) [″ + *placenta,* a flat cake] During pregnancy, the endometrium that lines the entire uterine cavity except at the site of the implanted blastocyst. SYN: *decidua parietalis.*
subpleural (sŭb-plū′răl) [″ + Gr. *pleura,* side] Beneath the pleura.
subpoena A court order that requires a person to come to court or appear at a specific time and place to give testimony. Failure to appear can result in punishment by the court.
subpoena duces tecum A process used in litigation that compels the party having control of documents, items, and materials relevant to issues in a lawsuit to produce them at a designated time and place.
subpontine (sŭb-pŏn′tĭn, -tīn) [″ + *pons,* bridge] Below the pons.
subpreputial (sŭb″prē-pū′shăl) [″ + *praeputium,* prepuce] Under the prepuce.
subpubic (sŭb-pū′bĭk) [″ + *pubes,* pubic region] Beneath the pubic arch, as a ligament, or performed beneath the pubic arch.
subpulmonary (sŭb-pŭl′mō-nā-rē) [″ + *pulmon,* lung] Below the lung.
subpyramidal (sŭb″pī-răm′ĭ-dăl) [″ + Gr. *pyramis,* a pyramid] Beneath a pyramid-shaped structure, such as the pyramids of the kidney or the pyramidal tracts of the brain.
subretinal (sŭb-rĕt′ĭ-năl) [″ + *rete,* a net] Beneath the retina.
subscapular (sŭb-skăp′ū-lăr) [″ + *scapula,* shoulder blade] Below the scapula.
subscleral (sŭb-sklē′răl) [″ + Gr. *skleros,* hard] Beneath the sclera of the eye. SYN: *subsclerotic* (1).
subsclerotic (sŭb-sklē′rŏt-ĭk) [″ + Gr. *skleros,* hard] **1.** Subscleral. **2.** Not completely sclerosed.
subscription (sŭb-skrĭp′shŭn) [L. *subscriptas,* written under] The part of a prescription that contains directions for compounding ingredients.
subserous (sŭb-sē′rŭs) [L. *sub,* under, below, + *serum,* whey] Beneath a serous membrane.
subsibilant (sŭb-sĭb′ĭ-lănt) [″ + *sibilans,* hissing] Having the sound of a muffled whistle.
subsidence (sŭb-sīd′ĕns) [L. *subsidere,* to sink down] The gradual disappearance of symptoms or manifestations of a disease.

subsistence The minimum amount of something essential for life (e.g., a subsistence diet).

subspecies (sŭb′spē-sēz) [L. *sub,* under, below, + *species,* a kind] In taxonomy, subordinate to a species.

subspinale (sŭb″spī-nā′lē) [″ + *spina,* thorn] The deepest point between the nasal spine and the crest of the maxilla.

subspinous (sŭb-spī′nŭs) [″ + *spina,* thorn] **1.** Beneath any spinous process. **2.** Anterior to or beneath the spinal column.

subspinous dislocation A dislocation with the head of the humerus resting below the spine of the scapula.

substage (sŭb′stāj) [″ + O.Fr. *estage,* position] The part of the microscope below the stage by which attachments are held in place.

substance (sŭb′stăns) [L. *substantia*] **1.** Material of which any organ or tissue is composed; matter. SYN: *substantia.* **2.** A chemical or drug. **3.** When used in a medicolegal context, a chemical with potential for abuse. A great variety of entities are included such as alcohol, nicotine, caffeine, sedatives, hypnotics, anxiolytics, illicit drugs such as cannabis, heroin, or methamphetamines. Almost any substance may be abused even though its clinical use is approved when used as prescribed.

anterior perforated s. The portion of the rhinencephalon lying immediately anterior to the optic chiasm. It is perforated by numerous small arteries.

black s. Substantia nigra.

chromophilic s. A substance found in the cytoplasm of certain cells that stains similar to chromatin with basic dyes. It includes Nissl bodies of neurons and granules in serozymogenic cells.

colloid s. Jelly-like substance in colloid degeneration.

gray s. An outdated term for the gray matter of the brain.

ground s. The matrix or intercellular substance in which the cells of an organ or tissue are embedded.

high threshold s. A substance such as glucose or sodium chloride present in the blood and excreted by the kidney only when its concentration exceeds a certain level.

ketogenic s. A substance that, in its metabolism, gives rise to ketone bodies.

low threshold s. A substance such as urea or uric acid that is excreted by the kidney from the blood almost in its entirety. It occurs in the urine in high concentrations.

medullary s. The inner part of an organ, such as a bone.

Nissl s. Nissl bodies.

posterior perforated s. A triangular area forming the floor of the interpeduncular fossa. It lies immediately behind the corpora mammillaria and contains numerous openings for blood vessels.

pressor s. A substance that elevates arterial blood pressure.

reticular s. The skein of threads present in some red blood cells. These are visible only when the cells are appropriately stained.

slow-reacting s. SEE: *slow-reacting substance of anaphylaxis.*

transmitter s. An outdated term for a neurotransmitter.

white s. White matter of the brain and spinal cord.

white s. of Schwann A nerve fiber's myelin sheath.

substance abuse A maladaptive pattern of behavior marked by the use of chemically active agents such as prescription and illicit drugs, alcohol, and tobacco. Of all deaths occurring in the U.S. each year, half are caused by substance abuse. Substance abuse is pervasive. About 33% of all Americans smoke cigarettes, 6% use illicit drugs regularly, and about 14% of all Americans are alcoholics. The consequences of substance abuse include heart disease, cancer, stroke, chronic obstructive lung disease, cirrhosis, and trauma, as well as familial, social, legal, and economic difficulties. SEE: *alcoholism; drug dependence; nicotine; tobacco;* Nursing Diagnoses Appendix.

substance dependence A cluster of cognitive, behavioral, and physiological symptoms indicating that the individual continues use of the substance despite the presence of significant substance-related problems. Patients develop a tolerance for the substance and require progressively greater amounts to elicit the effects desired. In addition, patients experience physical and psychological signs and symptoms of withdrawal if the agent is not used. SEE: *alcoholism; substance abuse.*

substance P An 11-amino acid peptide that is believed to be important as a neurotransmitter in the pain fiber system. This substance may also be important in eliciting local tissue reactions resembling inflammation. SEE: *neurotransmitter; pain.*

substandard Unable to meet a generally accepted benchmark for quality.

substantia (sŭb-stăn′shē-ă) [L.] The material of which any organ or tissue is composed; matter. SYN: *substance.*

s. alba The white matter of the brain and spinal cord.

s. cinerea The gray matter of the brain and spinal cord.

s. ferruginea The elongated mass of pigmented cells in the locus ceruleus.

s. gelatinosa The gray matter of the cord surrounding the central canal and capping the head of the posterior horns of the spinal cord.

s. grisea The gray matter of the spinal cord.

s. nigra Nuclei of the midbrain that help regulate unconscious muscle activity. SYN: *black substance; locus niger.*

s. propria membranae tympani The fibrous middle layer of the drum membrane.

substantivity The ability of tissue to absorb an active ingredient and release it slowly over a period of time.

substernal (sŭb-stĕr′năl) [L. *sub,* under, below, + Gr. *sternon,* chest] Situated beneath the sternum.

substernomastoid (sŭb-stĕr-nō-măs′toyd) [″ + ″ + Gr. *mastos,* breast, + *eidos,* form, shape] Beneath the sternomastoid muscle.

substituent One part of a molecule substituted with another atom or group.

substitute (sŭb′stĭ-tūt) Something that may be used in place of another.

blood s. An oxygen-carrying fluid that can be used in place of human blood products for transfusion therapy. Candidate substances that have been investigated for this purpose include polymerized hemoglobin and fluorinated hydrocarbons.

red blood cell s. Solutions made of specially prepared hemoglobins, perfluorocarbons, or other oxygen-carrying molecules, which may have uses in transfusion medicine.

substitution (sŭb-stĭ-tū′shŭn) [L. *substitutio,* replacing] **1.** Displacing an atom (or more than one) of an element in a compound by atoms of another element of equal valence. **2.** In psychiatry, the ego defense mechanism of turning from an obstructed desire to one whose gratification is socially acceptable. **3.** The turning from an obstructed form of behavior to a more primitive one, as a substitution neurosis. **4.** The replacement of one substance by another. **5.** In pharmacy, the replacement of one drug by another drug in dispensing. Usually a generic drug is substituted for a proprietary one. SEE: *interchange.*

substitution product A compound formed by an element or a radical replacing another element or radical in a compound.

substitutive (sŭb′stĭ-tū″tĭv) [L. *substitutivus*] Causing a change or substitution of characteristics.

substitutive therapy Treatment to overcome an inflammation of a specific character by exciting an acute nonspecific inflammation.

substrate, substratum (sŭb′strāt, sŭb-strā′tŭm) [L. *substratum,* to lie under] **1.** An underlying layer or foundation. **2.** A base, as of a pigment. **3.** The substance acted upon, as by an enzyme. SEE: *enzyme.*

substructure (sŭb′strŭk-chŭr) The underlying structure of supporting material.

subsultus (sŭb-sŭl′tŭs) [L., to leap up] Any tremor, twitching, or spasmodic movement.

s. tendinum An involuntary twitching of the muscles, esp. of those of the arms and feet, causing movement of the tendons. It is thought to be a hallmark of some febrile diseases, such as typhoid fever.

subsylvian (sŭb-sĭl′vē-ăn) Below the fissure of Sylvius.

subtarsal (sŭb-tăr′săl) [L. *sub,* under, below, + Gr. *tarsos,* a broad, flat surface] Below the tarsus.

subtentorial Located beneath the tentorium.

subterminal (sŭb-tĕr′mĭ-năl) [″ + *terminus,* a boundary] Close to the end of an extremity.

subtetanic (sŭb″tē-tăn′ĭk) [″ + Gr. *tetanikos,* suffering from tetanus] Moderately tetanic.

subthalamic (sŭb″thă-lăm′ĭk) [″ + Gr. *thalamos,* inner chamber] Located below the thalamus.

subthalamic nucleus An elliptical mass of gray matter lying in the ventral thalamus above the cerebral peduncle and rostral to the substantia nigra. It receives fibers from the globus pallidus.

subthalamus The portion of the diencephalon lying below the thalamus and above the hypothalamus. SEE: *thalamus.*

subtile, subtle (sŭb′tĭl, sŭt′l) [L. *subtilis,* fine] **1.** Very fine or delicate. **2.** Very acute. **3.** Mentally acute or crafty. **4.** Causing injury without attracting attention, as subtle poisons or early symptoms of a disease.

subtilin (sŭb′tĭl-ĭn) An antibiotic biosynthesized by *Bacillus subtilis.* This member of the lantibiotic family is effective against gram-positive organisms.

subtotal (sŭb-tō′tăl) [L. *sub,* under, below, + *totus,* all] Less than total, as partial removal of a gland.

subtraction The process by which undesired, overlying structures can be removed from a radiographical image.

subtrapezial (sŭb″tră-pē′zē-ăl) [″ + Gr. *trapezion,* a little table] Beneath the trapezius muscle.

subtribe (sŭb′trīb) In taxonomy, the category between a tribe and a genus.

subtrochanteric (sŭb″trō-kăn-tĕr′ĭk) [″ + Gr. *trochanter,* to run] Below a trochanter.

subtrochlear (sŭb-trŏk′lē-ăr) [″ + Gr. *trokhileia,* system of pulleys] Beneath the trochlea.

subtuberal (sŭb-tū′bĕr-ăl) [″ + *tuber,* a swelling] Located under a tuber.

subtympanic (sŭb-tĭm-păn′ĭk) [″ + Gr. *tympanon,* drum] Below the tympanum.

subtyping The precise identification of the genetic identity of a microorganism, often using DNA fingerprinting techniques.

subumbilical (sŭb″ŭm-bĭl′ĭ-kăl) [″ + *umbilicus,* navel] Below the umbilicus.

subumbilical space The triangular space within the body cavity below the navel.

subungual, subunguial (sŭb-ŭng′gwăl, -gwē-ăl) [″ + *unguis,* nail] Situated beneath the nail of a finger or toe.

subungual hematoma A collection of blood under the nail as a result of trauma. This condition may be treated by heating the end of a paper clip and then placing its point against the nail, which permits a small hole to be melted painlessly in the nail and allows the trapped blood to escape.

subunit In chemistry, a portion of a compound that represents a smaller part of the molecule than the remainder of the substance. SEE: *beta subunit.*

suburethral (sŭb″ū-rē′thrăl) [″ + Gr. *ourethra,* urethra] Below the urethra.

subvaginal (sŭb-văj′ĭn-ăl) [″ + *vagina,* sheath] **1.** Below the vagina. **2.** On the inner side of any tubular sheathing membrane.

subvertebral (sŭb-vĕr′tĕ-brăl) [″ + *vertebra,* vertebra] Beneath, or on the ventral side of, the vertebral column or a vertebra.

subvitrinal (sŭb-vĭt′rĭn-ăl) [″ + *vitrina,* vitreous body] Located beneath the vitreous body.

subvolution (sŭb″vō-lū′shŭn) [″ + *volutus,* turning] A method of turning over a flap surgically to prevent adhesions, particularly involving a pterygium of the eye.

subzonal (sŭb-zō′năl) Beneath a zone.

subzygomatic (sŭb″zī-gō-măt′ĭk) [″ + Gr. *zygoma,* cheekbone] Beneath the zygomatic bone.

succedaneous (sŭk″sē-dā′nē-ŭs) [L. *succedaneus,* substituting] **1.** Acting as a substitute or relating to one. **2.** In dentistry, referring to the secondary or permanent set of teeth, which follows an earlier deciduous set.

succedaneum (sŭk″sĕ-dā′nē-ŭm) [L. *succedaneus,* substituting] Something that may be used as a substitute.

succimer An oral drug (2,3-dimercaptosuccinic acid) used to remove lead from the body by chelation. It has been used for children with elevated blood levels of lead, and experimentally in adults as well. Its side effects include gastrointestinal upset, skin rashes, and elevated liver function test results. SEE: *acute lead encephalopathy; lead poisoning, acute.*

CAUTION: Use of this drug should always be accompanied by identification and removal of the source of the lead exposure.

---

succinate (sŭk′sĭ-nāt) Any salt of succinic acid.

succinylcholine chloride (sŭk″sĭ-nĭl-kō′lēn) A drug used for its neuromuscular blocking effect. It is used as an adjuvant in surgical anesthesia, and to prevent trauma in electroconvulsive shock therapy.

CAUTION: This drug should be used only by physicians who have had extensive training in its use and in a setting where facilities for respiratory and cardiovascular resuscitation are immediately available.

---

succorrhea (sŭk-kō-rē′ă) [L. *succus,* juice, + Gr. *rhoia,* flow] An unnatural increase in the secretion of any juice, esp. of a digestive fluid.

succus (sŭk′kŭs) *pl.* **succi** [L. *succus,* juice] A juice or fluid secretion.

s. entericus Intestinal juice.

s. gastricus Gastric juice.

succussion (sŭ-kŭsh′ŭn) [L. *succussio,* a shaking] The shaking of a person to detect the presence of fluid in the body cavity by listening for a splashing sound, esp. in the thorax.

suck [AS. *sucan,* to suck] **1.** To draw fluid into the mouth, as from the breast. **2.** To exhaust air from a tube and thus draw fluid from a container. **3.** That which is drawn into the mouth by sucking.

suckle To nurse at the breast.

sucralfate A medication, consisting of a complex formed from sucrose octasulfate and polyaluminum hydroxide, that is used to treat and prevent peptic ulcers and gastroesophageal reflux disease. It may be given as tablets or a slurry. Trade name is Carafate.

sucrase (sū′krās) [Fr. *sucre,* sugar] A digestive enzyme that splits cane sugar into glucose and fructose, the two being absorbed into the portal circulation. SYN: *invertase.*

sucrose (sū′krōs) [Fr. *sucre,* sugar] A dissacharide, $C_{12}H_{22}O_{11}$, obtained from sugar cane, sugar beet, and other sources. In the intestine, it is hydrolyzed to glucose and fructose by sucrase present in the intestinal juice. The monosaccharides resulting from the digestion of sucrose are absorbed by the small intestine and carried to the liver, where they may be converted to glycogen and stored if they are not needed immediately for energy.

sucrosuria (sū″krō-sū′rē-ă) [″ + Gr. *ouron,* urine] Sucrose in the urine.

suction [LL. *suctio,* sucking] The drawing of fluids or solids from a surface, using negative pressures. SEE: *aspiration.*

endotracheal s. Tracheobronchial suction.

nasogastric s. The suction of gas, fluid, and solid material from the gastrointestinal tract by use of a tube extending from the suction device to the stomach or intestines via the nasal passage. SEE: *Wangensteen tube*.

post-tussive s. The suction sound over a lung cavity heard on auscultation after a cough.

tracheobronchial s. Clearing the airways of mucus, pus, or aspirated materials to improve oxygenation and ventilation. SYN: *endotracheal s.*

PATIENT CARE: To avoid hypoxia to the lower airways, the patient must be aggressively ventilated before suctioning. During insertion of the suction tube no negative pressure is used to avoid damaging the fragile lining of the bronchi. Suction is then applied during tubal withdrawal for 15 sec or less.

suction abortion The removal of the products of conception from the uterus using a device that sucks the tissues away from the lining of the uterus.

suction biopsy A technique for obtaining tissue by use of a device that applies suction to the area from which the tissue is desired. It is used in obtaining tissue from the mucosa of the stomach and intestines.

suctorial (sŭk-tō'rē-ăl) [LL. *suctio,* sucking] **1.** Concerning sucking. **2.** Equipped for sucking.

sudamen (sū-dā'mĕn) *pl.* **sudamina** [L., sweat] A noninflammatory eruption from sweat glands marked by whitish vesicles caused by the retention of sweat in the cornified layer of the skin, appearing after profuse sweating or in certain febrile diseases.

Sudan (sū-dăn') One of a number of related biological stains for which fats have a special affinity, including Sudan II, Sudan III (G), Sudan IV, and Sudan R.

sudanophil (sū-dăn'ō-fĭl) [*sudan* + Gr. *philein,* to love] A leukocyte that stains readily with Sudan III, indicative of fatty degeneration. **sudanophilic,** *adj.*

sudanophilia (sū-dăn"ō-fĭl'ē-ă) An affinity for Sudan stains.

sudden infant death syndrome ABBR: SIDS. The sudden death of an infant younger than 1 year of age that remains unexplained after a thorough investigation, including a complete autopsy, examination of the death scene, and review of the clinical history. More than 90% of all SIDS deaths occur before the age of 6 months. SIDS is a major contributor to infant mortality in the U.S. and other industrialized nations. SYN: *crib death.*

ETIOLOGY: The causes of SIDS are still not clearly understood. Some evidence has linked SIDS to unrecognized congenital abnormalities of either the central nervous system or the electrical conduction system of the heart; to rare metabolic diseases; occult infections; unintentional injuries, or in some cases, child abuse.

RISK FACTORS: Although the cause of SIDS is unknown, some of the identified factors that increase the risk of SIDS include sleeping on the stomach; sharing a bed with an infant; maternal age less than 20 years; tobacco use in the home; and lack of prenatal care. Very low birthweight babies, babies of African-American and Native American ethnicity, and male infants have a higher rates of SIDS than other babies. More SIDS occurs during the winter months than at other times of year.

PREVENTION: Parents should attempt to remedy those risk factors listed that can be altered or prevented. The prone position for sleep should be avoided. The slogan, "Back to Sleep" was devised to remind parents that infants should be positioned on their backs when put to bed. Since the introduction of this campaign, SIDS deaths have declined by about 40%. A firm sleeping surface is recommended. Soft, plush, or bulky items, such as pillows, rolls of bedding, or cushions should not be placed in the infant's sleeping environment. These items could come into close contact with the infant's face, thereby interfering with ventilation or entrapping the infant's head and causing suffocation. Home monitoring of the infant with apnea monitors or baby listening devices provide parents with reassurance about the status of their infants, but have not been clearly proven to prevent SIDS. Parental smoking should, of course, be discouraged. SEE: *apnea; apnea alarm mattress.*

PATIENT CARE: Loss of an infant because of SIDS may produce a severe grief and guilt reaction. Thus, the family needs expert counseling in the several months after the death. A valuable source of support and information about SIDS is the Sudden Infant Death Syndrome Alliance (Phone: 1-800-221-7437; Internet: www.sidsalliance.org).

Sudeck's disease, Sudeck's atrophy (soo'dĕks) Reflex sympathetic dystrophy.

sudokeratosis (sū"dō-kĕr"ă-tō'sĭs) [L. *sudor,* sweat, + Gr. *keras,* horn, + *osis,* condition] Circumscribed horny overgrowths that obstruct the sweat ducts.

sudomotor (sū"dō-mō'tor) [" + *motor,* a mover] Pert. to stimulating the secretion of sweat; noting certain nerves.

sudor (sū'dor) [L.] Sweat.

s. cruentus Blood-tinged sweat. SYN: *hemathidrosis.*

sudoral (sū'dor-ăl) Pert. to, caused by, or marked by perspiration.

sudoresis (sū"dō-rē'sĭs) [L.] Diaphoresis.

sudoriferous (sū-dor-ĭf'ĕr-ŭs) [" + *ferre,* to bear] Conveying or producing sweat. SYN: *sudoriparous.*

sudorific (sū″dor-ĭf′ĭk) [L. *sudorificus*] **1.** Secreting or promoting the secretion of sweat. **2.** An agent that produces sweating. SYN: *diaphoretic*.

sudoriparous (sū″dor-ĭp′ă-rŭs) [L. *sudor,* sweat, + *parere,* to produce] Sudoriferous.

sue **1.** To initiate legal action. **2.** To make a petition or pleading to the court.

suet (sū′ĕt) [Fr. *sewet,* suet] A hard fat from cattle or sheep kidneys and loins, used as the base of certain ointments and as an emollient.

suffer **1.** To experience pain or distress. **2.** To be subjected to injury, loss, or damages.

suffocate (sŭf′ō-kāt) [L. *suffocare*] To impair respiration; to smother, asphyxiate.

suffocation (sŭf″ō-kā′shŭn) Deprivation of air exchange (e.g., by drowning, smothering, or other forms of airway obstruction) that produces an intense sensation of air hunger. SYN: *asphyxiation*. SEE: *asphyxia; resuscitation; unconsciousness*.

s., risk for Accentuated risk of accidental suffocation (inadequate air available for inhalation). SEE: *Nursing Diagnoses Appendix*.

suffusion (sŭ-fū′zhŭn) [L. *suffusio,* a pouring over] **1.** Extravasation. **2.** Pouring of a fluid over the body as treatment.

sugar [O.Fr. *zuchre*] A sweet-tasting, low-molecular-weight carbohydrate of the monosaccharide or disaccharide groups. Common sugars include fructose, glucose, lactose, maltose, sucrose, and xylose. Oral or parenteral administration of sugars can prevent hypoglycemia caused by insulin or oral hypoglycemic agents.

CLASSIFICATION: Sugars are classified in two ways: the number of atoms of simple sugars yielded on hydrolysis by a molecule of the given sugar and the number of carbon atoms in the molecules of the simple sugars so obtained. Therefore, glucose is a monosaccharide because it cannot be hydrolyzed to a simpler sugar; it is a hexose because it contains six carbon atoms per molecule. Sucrose is a disaccharide because on hydrolysis it yields two molecules, one of glucose and one of fructose. SEE: *carbohydrate*.

beet s. Sucrose obtained from sugar beets.

blood s. Glucose in the blood, normally 60 to 100 mg/100 ml of blood. It rises after a meal to variable levels, depending on the content of the meal, the activity level of and medications used by the consumer, and other variables. In diabetes mellitus, fasting blood sugar levels exceed 126 mg/dl. SEE: *glucose*.

cane s. Sucrose obtained from sugar cane.

fruit s. Fructose.

invert s. Mixture consisting of one molecule of glucose and one of fructose resulting from the hydrolysis of sucrose.

malt s. Maltose.

milk s. Lactose.

muscle s. Inositol; not a true sugar.

wood s. Xylose.

suggestible, suggestibility (sŭg-jĕs′tĭ-bl) Very susceptible to the opinions or suggestions of others.

suggestion (sŭg-jĕs′chŭn) [L. *suggestio*] **1.** The imparting of an idea indirectly; the act of implying. **2.** The idea so conveyed. **3.** The psychological process of having an individual adopt or accept an idea without argument or persuasion.

posthypnotic s. A suggestion made to a subject while under hypnosis. After emerging from the hypnotic state, the person may perform the suggested act.

suggestive (sŭg-jĕs′tĭv) Stimulating or pert. to suggestion.

suggestive therapeutics The practice of treating disease by hypnotic suggestions.

suicide (sū′ĭ-sīd) [L. *sui,* of oneself, + *caedere,* to kill] Intentionally causing one's own death. In the U.S., about 30,000 people commit suicide each year. Currently suicide is the ninth most common cause of death in the U.S. Suicide is much more common in persons who are elderly, chronically ill, substance abusers, or schizophrenic and those with untreated or undertreated mood disorders.

RISK FACTORS: Although suicide attempts are more frequently made by young women than any other demographic group, successful suicide is most likely to occur when attempted by older men who live alone. Older men are most likely to use truly violent means in their suicide attempts, such as shooting themselves, jumping from heights, or hanging. Other risk factors for suicide include having: a first-degree relative with a mood disorder; recurrent thoughts or discussion of suicide, esp. if a concrete plan for suicide has been contemplated; the means to commit suicide, esp. a weapon, in one's possession; a new diagnosis of a mortal illness; or uncontrolled pain caused by physical illness. Most individuals who kill themselves have consulted a health care provider in the months or weeks immediately before death, which suggests that many opportunities to intervene in the at-risk population may be missed.

PREVENTION: Health care professionals should be alert to the warning signs of suicide, such as statements indicating a desire to die or a prediction that suicide will occur. Persons contemplating suicide may be depressed, act to get their lives in order, give away possessions, have failing grades or poor work performance, adopt risk-taking behavior, or have a history of alcoholism or drug abuse.

Management of persons who are contemplating or have attempted suicide includes removal of lethal means from them and the provision of professional, social, and family support. If the patient is being treated as an outpatient, then he or she should be scheduled for specific future appointments and informed of a telephone number where help or assistance will be immediately available on a 24-hr basis. During a crisis, the patient should not be left alone even for a few minutes. For medicolegal reasons, careful and complete medical records should be kept concerning the plans and actions for management of the patient.

physician-assisted s. The prescription by a physician of a lethal dose of a medication to a patient. Physician-assisted suicide is illegal in most nations, but was legalized in the U.S. in the state of Oregon in the late 1990s. The drug most frequently used is secobarbital. SEE: *assisted suicide*.

suicide cluster An epidemic of suicides, within either a defined location or a brief period of time.

suicidology (soo″ĭ-sīd-ŏl′ō-jē) [″ + ″ + Gr. *logos,* word, reason] The science of suicide, including its cause, prediction of those susceptible, and prevention.

suit **1.** A lawsuit, legal action, or court proceeding by one party against another for damages or other legal remedies. **2.** An outer garment.

anti-G s. A garment designed to produce uniform pressure on the lower extremities and abdomen. Normally the suit is used by aviators to help prevent pooling of blood in the lower half of the body during certain flight maneuvers. The garment has also been used in treating severe forms of postural hypotension. The suit's usefulness in treating shock is questionable.

CAUTION: This garment is contraindicated in congestive heart failure, cardiogenic shock, and penetrating chest trauma.

sulcal (sŭl′kăl) [L.] Pert. to a sulcus.

sulcal artery A tiny branch of the anterior spinal artery.

sulcate, sulcated (sŭl′kāt, -ĕd) [L. *sulcatus*] Furrowed or grooved.

sulciform (sŭl′sĭ-form) [L. *sulcus,* groove, + *forma,* form] Resembling a sulcus.

sulculus (sŭl′kū-lŭs) [L.] A small sulcus.

sulcus (sŭl′kŭs) *pl.* **sulci** [L., groove] A furrow, groove, slight depression, or fissure, esp. of the brain.

alveololingual s. The space in the floor of the mouth between the base of the tongue and the alveolar ridge, on each side extending from the frenum of the tongue back to the retromolar wall.

calcarine s. A deep horizontal fissure on the medial surface of the occipital lobe of the brain.

s. centralis A fissure dividing the frontal and parietal lobes of each cerebral hemisphere. SYN: *Rolando's fissure.*

collateral s. A sulcus on the tentorial surface of the brain. It bounds the inferior lingual gyrus and is parallel to the calcarine and postcalcarine sulci.

s. cutis The ridges on the skin of the palmar surface of the fingers and toes, which comprise the fingerprints.

gingival s. The space or crevice between the free gingiva and the tooth surface. In health, the sulcus produces gingival sulcular fluid (GSF), which helps remove bacteria from the sulcus. When enlarged by disease, the gingival sulcus deepens and becomes a periodontal pocket.

hippocampal s. The sulcus on the medial side of the hippocampal gyrus.

intraparietal s. The groove that separates the inferior from the superior parietal bones and lobes.

nymphocaruncular s. The depression between the caruncula of the hymen and the labium minus.

nymphohymenal s. Trench between the labium minus and the hymen on either side.

s. precentralis An interrupted sulcus generally parallel with the fissure of Rolando and anterior to it.

s. pulmonalis A depression on either side of the vertebral column.

s. spiralis cochleae A groove between the labium tympanicum and labium vestibulare.

sulfacetamide (sŭl″fă-sĕt′ă-mīd) An antibacterial sulfonamide used for topical application to the eye, for treatment of burns and other wounds, and for vaginal infections.

sodium s. A soluble sulfonamide used in solution to treat infections of the cornea and conjunctiva.

sulfadiazine (sŭl″fă-dī′ă-zēn) A diazine derivative of sulfanilimide. It is used to treat skin infections, esp. those caused by burns, and toxoplasmosis, because it readily crosses the blood-brain barrier. A truncal, pruritic rash is a common side effect. Like other sulfur drugs, sulfadiazine carries a small but important risk of causing Stevens-Johnson syndrome.

sulfa drug Any drugs of the sulfonamide group, which possess bacteriostatic properties.

sulfamethizole (sŭl″fă-mĕth′ĭ-zōl) A sulfonamide used in treating urinary tract infections.

sulfamethoxazole (sŭl″fă-mĕth-ŏks′ă-zōl) A sulfonamide used in combination with trimethoprim to treat urinary tract infections, sinus and bronchial infections, and *Pneumocystis carinii*. A common side effect is an itchy rash appearing on the trunk about 10 days after starting therapy. The trade names of the combined product are Bactrim and Septra. SEE: *trimethoprim*.

sulfanilamide (sŭl″făn-ĭl′ă-mīd) Para-aminobenzenesulfonamide. It is a white, slightly bitter crystalline substance from coal tar, the parent of the azo dyes. Formerly it was widely used in the treatment of a number of infections, but because of its toxic reactions it has been superseded by more effective and less toxic sulfonamides.

sulfapyridine (sŭl″fă-pĭr′ĭ-dēn) A sulfonamide that is used only to treat dermatitis herpetiformis.

sodium monohydrate s. A soluble salt of sulfapyridine for intravenous use only.

sulfasalazine (sŭl″fă-săl′ă-zēn) A sulfonamide that is used to treat Crohn's disease, ulcerative colitis, and rheumatoid arthritis.

sulfatase (sŭl′fă-tās) An enzyme that hydrolyzes sulfuric acid esters.

sulfate (sŭl′fāt) [L. *sulphas*] A salt or ester of sulfuric acid.

ferrous s. An iron compound used to treat iron-deficiency anemia.

iron s. Ferrous sulfate. SEE: *copperas; copper salts* in *Poisons and Poisoning Appendix*.

magnesium s. SEE: *magnesium sulfate*.

sulfatide (sŭl′fă-tīd) Any cerebroside with a sulfate radical esterified to the galactose.

sulfhemoglobin (sŭlf″hēm-ō-glō′bĭn) Sulfmethemoglobin.

sulfhemoglobinemia (sŭlf″hēm-ō-glō″bĭn-ē′mē-ă) A persistent cyanotic condition caused by sulfhemoglobin in the blood.

sulfhydryl (sŭlf-hī′drĭl) The univalent radical, SH, of sulfur and hydrogen.

sulfide (sŭl′fīd) Any compound of sulfur with an element or base.

sulfinpyrazone (sŭl″fĭn-pī′ră-zōn) A drug used to promote excretion of uric acid in the urine.

sulfisoxazole (sŭl″fĭ-sŏk′să-zōl) A sulfonamide used to treat certain bacterial infections, esp. certain urinary tract infections.

sulfmethemoglobin (sŭlf″mĕt-hē″mō-glō′bĭn) The greenish hemoglobin compound formed when hemoglobin and hydrogen sulfide are combined. SYN: *sulfhemoglobin*.

sulfobromophthalein (sŭl″fō-brō″mō-thăl′ē-ĭn) A drug administered intravenously to test liver function; no longer commonly used.

sulfonamide Any of a group of compounds consisting of amides of sulfanilic acid derived from their parent compound sulfanilamide. They are bacteriostatic. Their action on bacteria results from interference with the functioning of enzyme systems necessary for normal metabolism, growth, and multiplication.

CAUTION: This drug and related compounds should not be used in patients with known allergies to sulfa drugs.

sulfone (sŭl′fōn) An oxidation product of sulfur compound in which the $=SO_2$ is united to two hydrocarbon radicals.

sulfonylurea One of a class of oral drugs used to control hyperglycemia in type 2 diabetes mellitus. Members of this group include tolazamide, glyburide, and glipizide.

CAUTION: Hypoglycemia may occur as a side effect of these medications if they are taken when dietary intake is limited or restricted voluntarily or during illness.

sulfourea (sŭl″fō-ū-rē′ă) Thiourea.

sulfoxide (sŭl-fŏk′sīd) The divalent radical $=SO$.

sulfur (sŭl′fŭr) [L.] SYMB: S. A pale yellow, crystalline element; atomic weight, 32.06; atomic number, 16; specific gravity, 2.07. It burns with a blue flame, producing sulfur dioxide.

Sulfur is part of some amino acids (cystine, cysteine) and is necessary for the synthesis of proteins such as insulin and keratin. The amount of sulfur (as sulfate) excreted in urine varies with the amount of protein in the diet but more or less parallels the amount of nitrogen excreted, as both are derived from protein catabolism. The S:N ratio is approx. 1:14 (i.e., for each gram of sulfur excreted, 14 g of nitrogen are excreted). The amount of sulfur excreted daily is about 1 g.

DEFICIENCY SYMPTOMS: Sulfur deficiency produces dermatitis and imperfect development of hair and nails. A deficiency of cystine or cysteine proteins in the diet inhibits growth and may be fatal. Tissue oxidation of cystine forms inorganic sulfate if the protein intake is sufficient.

s. dioxide An irritating gas used in industry to manufacture acids and as a bactericide and disinfectant. It is a major component of air pollution.

precipitated s. A form of sulfur used in various skin diseases, including scabies. Its keratolytic effect helps to make it effective in those disorders.

sublimed s. A form of sulfur used in various skin diseases. Its keratolytic effect helps to make it effective in those disorders. It is a scabicide.

sulfurated, sulfureted (sŭl′fū-rā″tĕd, -rĕt″ĕd) Combined or impregnated with sulfur.

sulfurated hydrogen Hydrogen sulfide.

sulfuric acid poisoning Injury sustained from contact with, or ingestion of, sulfuric acid (e.g., in laboratories, agriculture, or weapons manufacturing).

SYMPTOMS: Early local effects of acid injury, such as necrosis of the skin or the upper gastrointestinal tract, result from direct contact of sulfuric acid with the epithelium. The patient may complain of intense pain (e.g., in the mouth or throat). If acid contacts the eye, it may cause pain and corneal injury, sometimes resulting in blindness. Several days to 2 weeks after massive acid ingestion, perforation of internal organs may occur. When the stomach is involved, the perforation may leak acid into the mediastinum or peritoneum, causing pain, dyspnea, hypotension, tachycardia, or shock.

TREATMENT: Exposed surfaces should be promptly washed in water to dilute the concentration of acid and minimize the depth of acid penetration. If the airway is compromised, the patient should be immediately intubated and ventilated, before undergoing dilutional therapy. Neutralizing substances, such as diluted alkalies, are probably not helpful. Activated charcoal, which is helpful in many other exposures, is not useful.

Most patients who ingest significant quantities of acid will undergo upper gastrointestinal endoscopy to evaluate the extent of the acid burn. Strictures (e.g., esophageal) that develop as a result of scarring from acid burns are treated with dilation. Persons with ocular exposures need immediate ophthalmological consultation. Immediate surgery is warranted for patients with internal organ perforation. SEE: *acids* in *Poisons and Poisoning Appendix.*

CAUTION: Blind nasogastric intubation is generally contraindicated because it may damage the upper gastrointestinal tract. Gastric intubation and lavage should be performed by experienced endoscopists.

sumac (soo′măk) General term applied to several species of *Rhus.*

poison s. A type of sumac that causes a contact dermatitis. SEE: *poison sumac.*

sumatriptan (soo-mă-trĭp′tăn) A drug from the class of 5-hydroxytryptamine antagonists that can be given, either orally or by injection, to treat migraine headaches. Adverse effects include return of the headache and precipitation of angina pectoris in patients with coronary artery disease, among others.

summation (sŭm-ā′shŭn) [L. *summatio,* adding] A cumulative action or effect, as of stimuli; thus, an organ reacts to two or more weak stimuli as if they were a single strong one.

sunburn [AS. *sunne,* sun, + *bernan,* to burn] Dermatitis due to excessive exposure to the actinic rays of the sun. The rays that produce the characteristic changes in the skin are ultraviolet, between 290 and 320 nm (sunburn rays). Some people are more resistant to these rays than others, but the skin will be damaged in anyone who has sufficient exposure.

PREVENTION: Direct exposure of the skin to sunlight between 10 AM and 3 PM, when ultraviolet rays are strongest, should be avoided to minimize the risk of sunburn and skin cancer. Clothing should be worn to cover the skin or a sun-blocking agent with a sun protective factor (SPF) of 15 or more should be used (to be reapplied each hour if the person is sweating heavily).

CAUTION: Sunbathing and sunburn are risk factors for skin cancers, including basal cell carcinoma, squamous cell carcinoma, and melanoma.

TREATMENT: Cool, wet dressings may be applied to the burned area if the reaction is moderate. For severe sunburn, lukewarm baths with oatmeal or cornstarch and baking soda should be given. Aspirin or other nonsteroidal anti-inflammatory agents may reduce inflammation and pain.

Sunday morning paralysis Radial nerve palsy, sometimes the indirect result of acute alcoholism resulting from the stuporous patient lying immobile with his or her arm pressed over a projecting surface. SYN: *musculospiral paralysis; Saturday night paralysis.*

sundowning (sun′dow-nĭng) Confusion or disorientation that increases in the afternoon or evening. It is a common finding in patients with cognitive disorders (e.g., elderly persons with dementia) and tends to improve when the patient is reassured and reoriented.

sunflower eyes Slang term for the appearance of the eyes of patients with Wilson's disease. Deposits of copper around the edge of the cornea (Kayser-Fleischer rings) cause this condition.

sunglasses Eyeglasses that protect the eyes from exposure to visible as well as ultraviolet rays. For optimal eye protection outdoors, wraparound sunglasses or solar shields that block both ultraviolet A and ultraviolet B rays should be worn.

sunscreen A substance, used as a second line of defense, against damage to the skin and eyes by ultraviolet rays. It is usually applied as an ointment or cream. SEE: *photosensitivity; ultraviolet radiation.*

CAUTION: Sunscreens are much less effective in protecting against the damaging effects of the sun than avoiding midday sunlight and wearing protective clothing and headgear—these are the primary defenses against solar injury. Sunscreens should be reapplied after vigorous exercise and swimming. Some sunscreens may cause allergic or contact dermatitis.

sunscreen protective factor index In preparations (sunscreens) for protecting the skin from the sun, the ratio of the amount of exposure needed to produce a minimal erythema response with the sunscreen in place divided by the amount of exposure required to produce the same reaction without the sunscreen. This index assesses the ability of sunscreens to block (short-wavelength) ultraviolet B rays but does not measure the protective effect of sunscreens against (long-wavelength) ultraviolet A radiation. SEE: *erythema dose.*

sunstroke (sŭn′strōk) [AS. *sunne,* sun, + *strake,* a blow] Heatstroke.

suntan Darkening of the skin caused by exposure to the sun. SEE: *tanning salon; sunburn; sunscreen.*

CAUTION: A suntan predisposes exposed skin to basal cell carcinoma, squamous cell carcinoma, melanoma, and premature aging.

super- [L., over, above] Combining form meaning *above, beyond, superior.*

superabduction (soo″pĕr-ăb-dŭk′shŭn) [L. *super,* over, above, + *abducens,* drawing away] Pronounced or extreme abduction.

superacromial (soo″pĕr-ă-krō′mē-ăl) Supra-acromial.

superantigen An antigen that binds with class I major histocompatibility antigens and T-cell receptors and causes the simultaneous activation of large numbers of T cells and massive release of cytokines. Such antigens do not have to be processed by macrophages to be recognized by T cells. Exotoxins from bacteria such as staphylococci and group A streptococci act as superantigens. A superantigen known as toxic shock syndrome toxin-I causes toxic shock syndrome.

superciliary (soo″pĕr-sĭl′ē-ă-rē) [L. *supercilium,* eyebrow] Pert. to or in the region of an eyebrow. SYN: *supraciliary.*

supercilium (soo″pĕr-sĭl′ē-ŭm) *pl.* **supercilia** [L.] **1.** Eyebrow. **2.** A hair of the eyebrow.

superclass (soo′pĕr-klăs) In taxonomy, a category between a phylum and a class.

superego (soo″pĕr-ē′gō) [″ + *ego,* I; later translators of Freud's writings feel the word *uber-ich* should have been translated to over-I or upper-I and not to superego] In Freudian psychoanalytical theory, the portion of the personality associated with ethics, self-criticism, and the moral standard of the community. It is formed in infancy by the individual's adopting as his or her personal standards the values of the significant persons with whom he or she identifies. This helps to form the conscience. The superego functions to protect and to reward when the ego-ideal of behavior or thought is satisfied; and to criticize, punish, and evoke a sense of guilt when the reverse is true. In neuroses, symptoms develop when instinctual drives conflict with those dictated by the superego. SEE: *ego.*

superexcitation (soo″pĕr-ĕk″sī-tā′shŭn) [″ + *excitatio,* excitation] Excess excitement.

superextension (soo″pĕr-ĕks-tĕn′shŭn) [″ + *extensio,* extension] Hyperextension.

superfamily (soo″pĕr-făm′ĭ-lē) In taxonomy, a category between an order and a family.

superfecundation (soo″pĕr-fē″kŭn-dā′shŭn) [″ + *fecundare,* to fertilize] Successive fertilization by two or more separate instances of sexual intercourse of two or more ova formed during the same menstrual cycle. Fertilization may be by the same male or by two different males.

superfemale A female having three X chromosomes.

superfetation (soo″pĕr-fē-tā′shŭn) [″ + *fetus,* fetus] The fertilization of two ova in the same uterus at different menstrual periods within a short interval.

superficial (soo″pĕr-fĭsh′ăl) [L. *superficialis*] **1.** Pert. to or situated near the surface. **2.** Not thorough; cursory.

superficialis (soo″pĕr-fĭsh-ē-ā′lĭs) [L.] Noting a structure such as an artery, vein, or nerve that is near the surface. SYN: *superficial* (1).

superficies (soo″pĕr-fĭsh′ē-ēz) [L.] An outer surface.

superflexion (soo″pĕr-flĕk′shŭn) [L. *super,* over, above, + *flexio,* flexion] Hyperflexion.

supergenual (soo″pĕr-jĕn′ū-ăl) [″ + *genu,* knee] Above the knee.

superglue An extremely strong adhesive made of cyanoacrylate. It can be used to reapproximate the edges of a wound, without sutures.

CAUTION: This glue is quite effective in gluing skin to skin. It should not be used near the eyes, mouth, nose, labia, or other sensitive body parts.

superinduce (soo″pĕr-ĭn-dūs′) [″ + *in,* into, + *ducere,* to lead] To bring on, over, or above an already existing condition or situation.

superinfection (soo″pĕr-ĭn-fĕk′shŭn) [″ + *infectio,* a putting into] A new infection caused by an organism different from that which caused the initial infection. The microbe responsible is usually resistant to the treatment given for the initial infection.

superinvolution (soo″pĕr-ĭn-vō-lū′shŭn) [″ + *involutus,* a turning] Hyperinvolution.

superior (soo-pē′rē-or) [L. *superus,* upper] **1.** Higher than; situated above something else. **2.** Better than. **3.** One in charge of others.

superjacent (soo″pĕr-jā′sĕnt) Immediately above.

supermedial (soo″pĕr-mē′dē-ăl) [″ + *medium,* middle] Above the middle.

supermotility (soo″pĕr-mō-tĭl′ĭ-tē) [″ + *motilis,* moving] Excessive motility in any part. SYN: *hyperkinesia.*

supernatant (soo″pĕr-nā′tănt) [″ + *natare,* to float] **1.** Floating on a surface, as oil on water. **2.** The clear liquid remaining at the top after a precipitate settles. **3.** The cell-derived fluids containing chemical mediators that develop in a laboratory culture of leukocytes mixed with an antigen or mitogen stimulus. Supernatants can be assessed for the presence of monokines or lymphokines by adding them to other white blood cell cultures and measuring cell proliferation and activity.

supernate (soo′pĕr-nāt) A supernatant fluid.

supernumerary (soo″pĕr-nū′mĕr-ăr″ē) [L. *supernumerarius*] Exceeding the regular number.

supernumerary teeth More than the usual number of teeth. Extra teeth develop in approx. 2% of the population, with almost all of them being maxillary incisors or mesiodens. A cleft palate or other developmental disturbances disrupt the dental lamina and often result in palatal supernumerary teeth.

superolateral (soo″pĕr-ō-lăt′ĕr-ăl) [″ + *latus,* side] Above and to the side.

superovulation (soo″pĕr-ŏv″ū-lā′shŭn) [″ + *ovulum,* little egg] An increased frequency of ovulation or production of a greater number of ova at one time. This is usually caused by the administration of gonadotropins.

superoxide A highly reactive form of oxygen. Superoxide is produced during the normal catalytic function of certain enzymes, by the oxidation of hemoglobin to methemoglobin, and when ionizing radiation passes through water. It is also produced when granulocytes phagocytize bacteria. Superoxide is destroyed by the enzyme superoxide dismutase, which catalyzes the conversion of two molecules of superoxide anion to one molecule of oxygen and one of hydrogen peroxide. Superoxides play a part in many diseases and conditions, including, for example, central nervous system damage in amyotrophic lateral sclerosis and endothelial damage in hypertension and diabetes mellitus.

superoxide dismutase An enzyme that destroys superoxide. One form of the enzyme contains manganese and another contains copper and zinc.

superparasite (soo″pĕr-păr′ă-sīt) [″ + Gr. *para,* beside, + *sitos,* food] **1.** A parasite that lives upon another parasite. **2.** A parasite involved in superparasitism.

superparasitism (soo″pĕr-păr′ă-sī″tĭzm) [″ + ″ + *-ismos,* condition] A condition in which the host is infested or infected with a greater number of parasites than can be supported.

superphosphate (soo″pĕr-fŏs′fāt) Acid phosphate.

supersaturate To add more of a substance to a solution than can be dissolved permanently.

superscription (soo″pĕr-skrĭp′shŭn) [L. *super,* over, above, + *scriptio,* a writing] The beginning of a prescription noted by the sign ℞, signifying (L.) *recipe,* take.

supersensitive (soo″pĕr-sĕn′sĭ-tĭv) [″ + *sensitivus,* feeling] Hypersensitive.

supersoft (soo″pĕr-sŏft′) [″ + AS. *softe,* soft] Exceptionally soft; noting roentgen rays of extremely long wavelength and low penetrating power.

supersonic (soo″pĕr-sŏn′ĭk) [″ + *sonus,* sound] **1.** Ultrasonic. **2.** Used to describe speeds greater than that of sound. At sea level, in air at 0°C, the speed of sound is about 331 m, or 1087 ft per second (741 mph). **3.** A sound frequency that is greater than 20,000 cycles per second.

superstructure (soo″pĕr-strŭk′chŭr) The visible portion of a structure, esp. those parts external to the main structure.

supervenosity (soo″pĕr-vē-nŏs′ĭ-tē) Abnormally decreased oxygen in the venous blood.

supervention (soo″pĕr-vĕn′shŭn) [L. *superventio,* a coming over] The development of an additional condition as a complication to an existing disease.

supervirulent (soo″pĕr-vĭr′ū-lĕnt) [L. *super,* over, above, + *virulentus,* full of poison] More virulent than usual.

supervisor (soo′pĕr-vīz″ĕr) [L. *supervisus,* having looked over] One who directs and evaluates the performance of others. In a health care setting, the supervisor usually has the knowledge and skills to provide the same service as those being directed (e.g., the supervisor of the pharmacy, physical therapy, or maternity nursing).

supervitaminosis Hypervitaminosis.

supervoltage (soo′pĕr-vŏl″tĭj) A term applied to x-rays produced by very high voltage, usually in the megavolt range.

supinate (sū′pĭ-nāt) [L. *supinatus,* bent backward] **1.** To turn the forearm or hand so that the palm faces upward. **2.** To rotate the foot and leg outward.

supination (sū″pĭn-ā′shŭn) [L. *supinatio*] **1.** The turning of the palm or the hand anteriorly or the foot inward and upward. **2.** The act of lying flat upon the back. **3.** The condition of being on the back or having the palm of the hand facing upward or the foot turned inward and upward.

supinator (sū″pĭn-ā′tor) [L.] A muscle producing the motion of supination of the forearm.

supine (sū-pīn′) [L. *supinus,* lying on the back] **1.** Lying on the back with the face upward. **2.** A position of the hand or foot with the palm or foot facing upward; the opposite of prone.

supplement (sŭp″lĕ-mĕnt) [L. *supplementum,* an addition] **1.** An additive (e.g., something added to a food to increase its nutritive value). **2.** To add. **supplemental,** *adj.*

supplemental air Expiratory reserve volume.

support (sŭp-port′) **1.** That which assists in maintaining something in place. **2.** In dentistry, the abutting teeth, alveolar ridge, and mucosal tissues upon which the denture rests.

s. groups Groups of persons with similar concerns who meet to discuss what is known about their problems or disease. The composition and focus of support groups vary. Some groups may be comprised of patients who are experiencing or have experienced the same disorder; such groups may include family members. Discussions often center on current treatments, resources available for assistance, and what individuals can do to improve and maintain their health or adjust to their illness, handicap, or life situation. Other groups may involve those who have experienced the same psychological and emotional trauma, such as rape victims or persons who have lost a loved one. Benefits expressed by members include the knowledge that they are not alone but that others have experienced the same or similar problems and that they have learned to cope effectively.

s. hose Elastic stockings that may extend from the toes to the knee or above. These are worn by bedridden patients to provide sufficient pressure on the tissues to facilitate venous return and to help to prevent the formation of thrombi in the veins of the legs.

social s. Help given by others to provide feedback, satisfy needs, and validate one's experience. A large body of research suggests that the loss of social support is a factor in the etiology of both physical and psychological disease. Nursing practice uses social supports such as tangible materials, teaching, and intimate interactions to restore, promote, and care for patients.

suppository (sŭ-pŏz′ĭ-tō-rē) *pl.* **suppositories** [L. *suppositorium,* something placed underneath] A semisolid substance for introduction into the rectum, vagina, or urethra, where it dissolves. It often serves as a vehicle for medicines to be absorbed. It is commonly shaped like a cylinder or cone and may be made of soap, glycerinated gelatin, or cocoa butter (oil of theobroma).

PATIENT CARE: Privacy is provided. The nurse instructs the patient to retain the suppository for about 20 min for effectiveness and positions the patient appropriately. The suppository is lubricated and inserted into the appropriate orifice. For neurological rehabilitation, a rectal suppository may be used by the patient after instruction in bowel management. The nurse checks with the patient about effectiveness and notes that in the chart.

suppression (sŭ-prĕsh′ŭn) [L. *suppressio,* a pressing under] **1.** The repression of the external manifestation of a morbid condition. **2.** The complete failure of the natural production of a secretion or excretion, as distinguished from retention, in which normal secretion occurs but the discharge is retained within the organ or body. **3.** In psychoanalysis, the Freudian ego defense mechanism of conscious inhibition of an idea or desire, as distinguished from repression, which is considered an unconscious process.

active immune s. The use of agents to block an antigen-specific immune response. An example is the administration of anti-Rh antibodies (Rh_0 immune globulin) to Rh-negative mothers during the 28th week of pregnancy to prevent the formation of maternal antibodies that cause erythroblastosis fetalis in the Rh-positive newborn.

androgen s. Androgen deprivation.

appetite s. The use of drugs, biofeedback, hypnosis, cognitive therapies, or other means to regulate the desire for food and its consumption.

suppression of menses **1.** Amenorrhea in which menstruation ceases after once being established and from some cause other than hysterectomy, pregnancy, or menopause. SEE: *hypothalamic amenorrhea; pathological amenorrhea.* **2.** Any suppression of the menses.

suppressor T cells A subpopulation of T lymphocytes that slows and stops a specific immune response.

suppurant (sŭp′ū-rănt) [L. *suppurans*] **1.** Producing, tending to produce, or marked by pus formation. **2.** An agent causing pus formation.

suppurate (sŭp′ū-rāt) [L. *suppurare*] To form or generate pus.

suppuration (sŭp-ū-rā′shŭn) [L. *suppuratio*] **1.** The formation of pus. SEE: *pus*. **2.** Pus.

suppurative (sŭp′ū-rā″tĭv, -rā-tĭv) [L. *suppuratus*] **1.** Producing or associated with generation of pus. SEE: *pus; pyogenic*. **2.** An agent producing pus formation.

supra- [L.] Combining form meaning *above, beyond,* or *on the top side*.

supra-acromial (soo″pră-ă-krō′mē-ăl) [L. *supra,* above, on top, beyond, + Gr. *akron,* extremity, + *omos,* shoulder] Located above the acromion.

supra-anal (soo-pră-ā′năl) [″ + *analis,* anal] Located above the anus.

supra-auricular (soo″pră-ŏ-rĭk′ū-lăr) [″ + *auricula,* little ear] Located above the auricle.

supra-axillary (soo″pră-ăk′sĭ-lĕr″ē) [″ + *axilla,* underarm] Located above the axilla.

suprabuccal (soo″pră-bŭk′ăl) [″ + *bucca,* cheek] Located above the buccal area.

suprabulge (soo′pră-bŭlj) The part of the crown of a tooth that curves toward the occlusal surface.

supracerebellar (soo″pră-sĕr″ĕ-bĕl′ăr) [″ + *cerebellum,* little brain] Located on or above the upper surface of the cerebellum.

suprachoroid (soo″pră-kō′royd) [″ + Gr. *chorioeides,* skinlike] Situated on or above the choroid layer of the eyeball.

suprachoroidea (soo″pră-kō-roy′dē-ă) Suprachoroid lamina.

suprachoroid lamina The superficial layer of the choroid consisting of thin transparent layers, the outermost adhering to the sclera. SYN: *lamina suprachoroidea; suprachoroidea*.

supraciliary (soo″pră-sĭl′ē-ĕr″ē) [L. *supra,* above, on top, beyond, + *cilia,* eyelid] Superciliary.

supraclavicular (soo″pră-klă-vĭk′ū-lar) [″ + *clavicula,* little key] Located above the clavicle.

supraclavicular fossa A depression on either side of the neck extending down behind the clavicle.

supraclavicular point A stimulation point over the clavicle at which contraction of the arm muscles may be produced.

supracondylar (soo″pră-kŏn′dĭ-lăr) [″ + Gr. *kondylos,* knuckle] Above a condyle.

supracostal (soo″pră-kŏs′tăl) [″ + *costa,* rib] Above the ribs.

supracotyloid (soo″pră-kŏt′ĭ-loyd) [″ + Gr. *kotyloeides,* cup-shaped] Above the acetabulum.

supradiaphragmatic (soo″pră-dī″ă-frăg-măt′ĭk) [″ + Gr. *dia,* across, + *phragma,* wall] Above the diaphragm.

supraduction (soo″pră-dŭk′shŭn) [″ + *ducere,* to lead] Turning upward of the eye.

supraepicondylar (soo″pră-ĕp″ĭ-kŏn′dĭ-lăr) [″ + Gr. *epi,* upon, + *kondylos,* condyle] Located above an epicondyle.

supragingival Above the gingiva; used in reference to the location of dental restorations, bacterial plaque, or calculus on the tooth. It is often contrasted with subgingival, the gingival margin being the reference point.

supraglenoid (soo″pră-glē′noyd) [″ + Gr. *glene,* socket, + *eidos,* form, shape] Above the glenoid cavity or fossa.

supraglenoid tuberosity A rough surface of the scapula above the glenoid cavity to which is attached the long head of the biceps muscle.

supraglottic (soo″pră-glŏt′ĭk) Located above the glottis.

supraglottitis Epiglottitis.

suprahepatic (soo″pră-hē-păt′ĭk) [″ + Gr. *hepar,* liver] Located above the liver.

suprahyoid (soo″pră-hī′oyd) [″ + *hyoeides,* U-shaped] Located above the hyoid bone; denoting accessory thyroid glands within the geniohyoid muscle.

suprahyoid muscles The digastric, geniohyoid, mylohyoid, and stylohyoid muscles.

suprainguinal (soo″pră-ĭn′gwĭn-ăl) [″ + *inguinalis,* pert. to the groin] Above the groin.

supraintestinal (soo″pră-ĭn-tĕs′tĭ-năl) [″ + *intestinum,* intestine] Overlying the intestine.

supraliminal (soo″pră-lĭm′ĭ-năl) [L. *supra,* above, on top, beyond, + *limen,* threshold] **1.** Above the threshold of consciousness; conscious. **2.** Exceeding the stimulus threshold. SEE: *subliminal*.

supralumbar (soo″pră-lŭm′băr) [″ + *lumbus,* loin] Located above the lumbar region.

supramalleolar (soo″pră-mă-lē′ō-lăr) [″ + *malleolus,* little hammer] Located above either malleolus.

supramammary (soo″pră-măm′ă-rē) [″ + *mamma,* breast] Located above the breast.

supramandibular (soo″pră-măn-dĭb′ū-lăr) [″ + *mandibula,* lower jawbone] Located above the mandible.

supramarginal (soo″pră-măr′jĭn-ăl) [″ + *marginalis,* border] Located above any border.

supramarginal convolution A cerebral convolution on the lateral surface of the parietal lobe above the posterior part of the sylvian fissure.

supramastoid (soo″pră-măs′toyd) [″ + *mastos,* breast, + *eidos,* form, shape] Located above the mastoid process of the temporal bone.

supramastoid crest A ridge on the superior edge of the posterior root of the zygomatic bone. SYN: *temporal line*.

supramaxillary (soo″pră-măk′sĭ-lĕr-ē) **1.** Rel. to the upper jaw. **2.** Located above the upper jaw.

suprameatal (soo″pră-mē-ā′tăl) [″ + *meatus,* passage] Above a meatus, esp. denoting the suprameatal spine, a small bony projection at the posterosuperior margin of the external auditory meatus.

suprameatal triangle The triangular space bordered by the posterior wall of the external auditory meatus and the posterior root of the zygomatic process of the temporal bone.

supramental (soo″pră-mĕn′tăl) [L. *supra,* above, on top, beyond, + *mentum,* chin] Located above the chin.

supranasal (soo″pră-nā′zăl) [″ + *nasus,* nose] Located above the nose.

supranuclear (soo″pră-nū′klē-lăr) [″ + *nucleus,* little kernel] Concerning nerve fibers located above a nucleus in the brain.

supraoccipital (soo″pră-ŏk-sĭp′ĭ-tăl) [″ + *occiput,* back of head] Lying above or in the upper portion of the occiput.

supraocclusion (soo″pră-ŏ-kloo′zhŭn) [″ + *occlusio,* occlusion] The condition of teeth that are beyond the occlusal plane.

supraorbital (soo″pră-or′bĭ-tăl) [″ + *orbita,* track] Located above the orbit.

supraorbital neuralgia Neuralgia of the supraorbital nerve. SYN: *hemicrania* (1).

supraorbital notch A notch in the superior margin of the orbital arch for transmitting supraorbital vessels and nerve.

suprapatellar (soo″pră-pă-tĕl′ăr) [″ + *patella,* a small pan] Located above the patella.

suprapelvic (soo″pră-pĕl′vĭk) [″ + *pelvis,* basin] Located above the pelvis.

suprapontine (soo″pră-pŏn′tĭn) [″ + *pons,* bridge] Located above the pons varolii.

suprapubic (soo″pră-pū′bĭk) [″ + NL. *(os) pubis,* bone of the groin] Located above the pubic arch.

suprapubic aspiration of urine A procedure for draining the bladder when it is not possible to use a urethral catheter. The skin over the lower abdominal area is cleansed. An incision in the abdominal wall is made with a needle or trocar to gain access to the bladder. To prevent complications during the procedure, it is important to observe the following guidelines: The patient should be positioned in the marked Trendelenburg position. The bladder should be distended with 400 ml of fluid. Any previous abdominal wall incisions that may have left the bladder or bowel adherent to the scar tissue should be noted. The incision should be no more than 3 cm above the pubic symphysis. The trocar should be inserted 30 degrees toward the bladder, that is, away from the pubic symphysis (if in doubt, a small-gauge needle should be inserted for orientation); the trocar should not be placed in a vertical direction. The depth of trocar insertion should be monitored, using gentle pressure on the trocar to prevent damage to the bladder base.

CAUTION: The needle may pierce a loop of bowel that is lying over the anterior surface of the bladder.

---

suprapubic catheter A tube that permits direct urinary drainage from the bladder through the lower abdominal wall, from a surgically fashioned opening located just above the pubic symphysis. Suprapubic urinary diversion is typically (but not exclusively) used as a temporary means of decompressing the bladder when the urethra is obstructed (e.g., in children with congenital deformities of the penis or urethra, or in adults with bladder outlet obstruction). When it is used for this purpose it is considered a bridge prior to definitive surgery. SEE: *suprapubic aspiration of urine; suprapubic cystotomy.*

PATIENT CARE: The nurse observes for hemorrhage or prolonged hematuria and signs of local or systemic infection. Aseptic technique is used during dressing or equipment changes. Bladder irrigation is performed as prescribed. Medications such as analgesics, antispasmodics, and bowel stimulants are administered as prescribed. The patient's ability to micturate is evaluated. Intake and output are monitored and recorded. Fluids are forced unless otherwise restricted to ensure passage of dilute urine.

suprarenal (soo″pră-rē′năl) [L. *supra,* above, on top, beyond, + *ren,* kidney] **1.** Located above the kidney. **2.** Pert. to the gland above each kidney. SEE: *adrenal gland.*

suprarenalectomy (soo″pră-rē″năl-ĕk′tō-mē) [″ + ″ + Gr. *ektome,* excision] Adrenalectomy.

suprarenal gland An endocrine gland lying adjacent to and in a superior and medial position to the kidney. SYN: *adrenal gland.* SEE: *ACTH; Adrenalin; corticosterone; cortisone; endocrine gland; epinephrine; norepinephrine.*

suprarenalopathy (soo″pră-rē-năl-ŏp′ă-thē) [″ + ″ + Gr. *pathos,* disease, suffering] Any disorder caused by abnormal functioning of the adrenal glands.

suprascapular (soo″pră-skăp′ū-lăr) [″ + *scapula,* shoulder blade] Located above the scapula.

suprascleral (soo″pră-sklē′răl) [″ + Gr. *skleros,* hard] Located on the surface of the sclera.

suprasegmental [″ + *segmentum,* segment] Located above the segmented portion.

suprasegmental brain The cerebrum, midbrain, and cerebellum as distinguished from the segmental portion (pons and medulla oblongata).

suprasellar (soo″pră-sĕl′ăr) [″ + *sella,* saddle] Located above or over the sella turcica.

supraspinal (soo″pră-spī′năl) [″ + *spina,* thorn] Located above a spine.

supraspinous Located above any spinous process.

supraspinous fossa A groove above the spine of the scapula.

suprastapedial (soo″pră-stă-pē′dē-ăl) [″ + *stapes,* stirrup] Located above the stapes of the inner ear.

suprasternal (soo″pră-stĕr′năl) [L. *supra,* above, on top, beyond, + Gr. *sternon,* chest] Located above the sternum.

suprasylvian (soo″pră-sĭl′vē-ăn) Located above the sylvian fissure of the brain.

supratemporal (soo″pră-tĕm′pō-răl) [″ + *temporalis,* temporal] Located above the temporal bone or fossa.

supratentorial (soo″pră-tĕn-tō′rē-ăl) Located above the tentorium.

suprathoracic (soo″pră-thō-răs′ĭk) [″ + Gr. *thorax,* chest] Located above the thorax.

supratonsillar (soo″pră-tŏn′sĭ-lăr) [″ + *tonsilla,* almond] Located above the tonsil.

supratrochlear (soo″pră-trŏk′lē-ăr) [″ + *trochlea,* pulley] Located above a trochlea, esp. that of the humerus.

supratympanic (soo″pră-tĭm-păn′ĭk) [″ + *tympanon,* drum] Located above the tympanic membrane of the ear.

supravaginal (soo″pră-văj′ĭ-năl) [″ + *vagina,* sheath] Located above the vagina or any sheathing membrane.

supraventricular (soo″pră-vĕn-trĭk′ū-lăr) [″ + *ventriculus,* a little belly] Located above the ventricle, esp. the heart ventricles.

supravergence (soo″pră-vĕr′jĕns) [″ + *vergere,* to be inclined] A condition in which one eye moves upward in the vertical plane while the other does not.

supraversion (soo″pră-vĕr′zhŭn) [″ + *versio,* a turning] **1.** A turning upward. **2.** In dentistry, a tooth out of occlusal line.

sura (sū′ră) [L.] The calf of the leg; the muscular posterior portion of the lower leg.

sural (sū′răl) Rel. to the calf of the leg.

suramin sodium (soo′ră-mĭn) A urea derivative used to treat African trypanosomiasis (sleeping sickness), as well as a variety of human tumors, including renal cell carcinoma, prostate cancer, melanoma, and others.

surefooted Being able to walk or run without stumbling or falling.

surface (sŭr′fĕs) [Fr. *sur,* above, + L. *facies,* face] **1.** The exterior boundary of an object. **2.** The external or internal exposed portions of a hollow structure, as the outer or inner surfaces of the cranium or stomach. **3.** The face or faces of a structure such as a bone. **4.** The side of a tooth or the dental arch; usually named for the adjacent tissue or space. The outer or facial surface is called the labial surface of the incisors or canines, and the buccal surface of the premolars and molars. The facial surface may also be called the vestibular surface. The inner surface of each tooth is called the lingual or oral surface. Within the arch, each tooth is said to have a mesial surface, the side toward the midpoint in the front of the dental arch, and a distal surface, the side of the tooth farthest from the midpoint in the front of the dental arch. SEE: illus.

body s. **1.** The exterior of the human body, or one of its parts. **2.** The epidermis. SEE: *body surface area.*

surface tension A condition at the surface of a liquid in contact with a gas or another liquid that causes its surface to act as a stretched rubber membrane. It results from the mutual attraction of the molecules to each other, thus producing a cohesive state that causes liquids to assume a shape presenting the smallest surface area to the surrounding medium. This accounts for the spherical shape assumed by fluids, such as drops of oil or water.

surfactant (sŭr-făk′tănt) A surface-active agent that lowers surface tension (e.g., oils and various forms of detergents). Artificial surfactants may be given endotracheally to relieve respiratory distress.

modified natural s. A replacement phospholipid from a natural source with some components removed. Trade name is Survanta.

pulmonary s. A lipoprotein secreted by type II alveolar cells that decreases the surface tension of the fluid lining the alveoli, permitting expansion. Synthetic lung surfactant is available for treating patients with respiratory distress syndrome. In obstetrics, fetal production of surfactant can be stimulated by administration of a glucocorticoid 24 to 48 hr before an inevitable preterm birth. SYN: *lung surfactant.* SEE: *betamethasone; lecithin-sphingomyelin ratio.*

surfer's ear The growth of a bony area in the subcutaneous area of the ear owing to prolonged exposure to cold, as may occur in persons who participate in surfing.

surfer's knots Nodules that form on the foot, leg, or chest as a result of trauma from repetitive contact with surfboards.

surgeon (sŭr′jŭn) [L. *chirurgia*] A medical practitioner who specializes in surgery.

ghost s. Any person, esp. one not designated by the patient or not licensed to practice surgery, who replaces

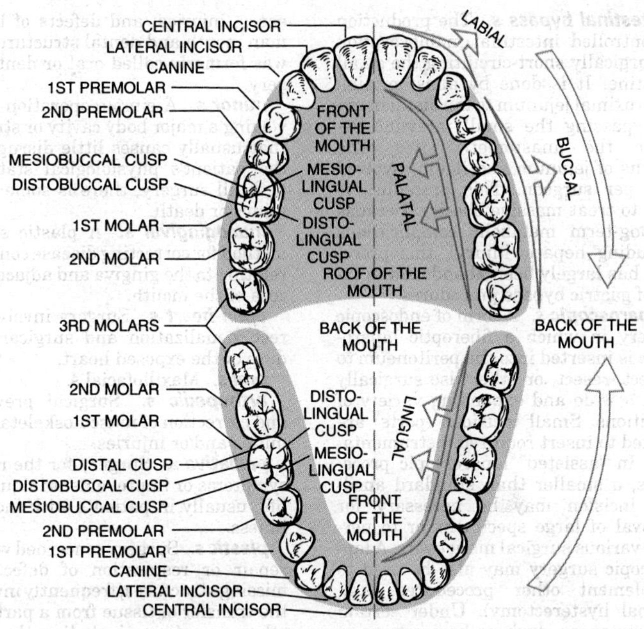

RELATIONSHIP OF DENTAL SURFACES

the patient's chosen surgeon in performing an operation, without the patient's consent. Ghosts may include surgical residents or representatives of pharmaceutical or biomedical engineering firms.

surgeon general The chief medical officer in each branch of the armed forces of the U.S. or of the U.S. Public Health Service.

surgery (sŭr′jĕr-ē) [L. *chirurgia*] **1.** The branch of medicine dealing with manual and operative procedures for correction of deformities and defects, repair of injuries, and diagnosis and cure of certain diseases. **2.** A surgeon's operating room. **3.** Treatment or work performed by a surgeon. SYN: *operation*. SEE: *Nursing Diagnoses Appendix.*

ablative s. Operation in which a part is removed or destroyed.

aesthetic s. Cosmetic surgery.

ambulatory s. Surgery done between the time the patient is admitted in the morning and the time the patient is discharged the same day. Also called *day surgery.*

aseptic s. An operative procedure carried on under sterile conditions.

aural s. Surgery of the ear.

breast conservation s. Removal of a malignant growth from the breast, and dissection of axillary lymph nodes, without mastectomy. Breast conservation surgery, popularly known as lumpectomy, is an alternative to mastectomy for patients with early stage breast cancer. Its outcomes are equivalent to those of mastectomy when used as part of a treatment plan that includes postoperative radiation therapy to the affected breast.

colorectal s. Operative procedures on the anus, rectum, or large intestine.

conservative s. Surgery in which as much as possible of a part or structure is retained. It is an alternative to radical surgery that is often equally effective.

cosmetic s. Surgery done to revise or change the texture, configuration, or relationship of contiguous structures of any feature of the human body. SYN: *aesthetic s.* SEE: *plastic s.*

exploratory s. An operation performed for diagnostic purposes, which may be extended to be a definitive procedure if necessary.

flap s. A surgical procedure in which a flap of tissue or periosteum is raised. An amputation flap is a tissue flap produced to cover the amputation stump.

image-guided s. The use of real-time computed tomography, magnetic resonance imagery, or ultrasound to place surgical instruments in precise anatomical locations (e.g., during biopsies or tissue resections). Images taken before the operation are compared with those obtained during surgery to improve the localization of tumors or vascular structures, the placement of prosthetic parts, or the identification of moving structures.

intestinal bypass s. The production of controlled intestinal malabsorption by surgically short-circuiting the small intestine. It is done by anastomosing the proximal jejunum to the distal ileum by bypassing the small intestine between the anastomotic sites. The lengths of jejunum and ileum involved vary per surgeon. This procedure is used to treat massive obesity. Because of long-term metabolic complications (including hepatic injury), this procedure has largely been abandoned in favor of gastric bypass procedures.

laparoscopic s. A form of endoscopic surgery in which a fiberoptic laparoscope is inserted into the peritoneum to inspect, resect, or otherwise surgically treat a wide and expanding variety of conditions. Small incisions (ports) are created to insert required instrumentation. In "assisted" laparoscopic procedures, a smaller than standard ancillary incision may be necessary for removal of large specimens or to perform various surgical maneuvers. A laparoscopic surgery may also be used to complement other procedures (e.g., vaginal hysterectomy). Under certain circumstances, such as hemorrhage or dense adhesions, the laparoscopic procedure cannot be completed. Operating time is longer and equipment is more expensive in laparoscopic surgery than in laparotomy, but the convalescence of patients who have undergone laparoscopic procedures is shorter and pain, nausea, vomiting, and obstipation are diminished. Operations that are commonly performed with a laparoscope include cholecystectomy, appendectomy, colonic surgery, hernia repairs (including hiatal hernias), and many gynecological surgeries. SEE: *laparoscopic laser cholecystectomy*.

lung volume reduction s. The removal of emphysematous lung tissue (esp. inelastic air spaces in the upper lobes of the lungs) to enhance the ability of the remainder of the lung to expand and contract. This procedure improves respiratory function for many patients with advanced chronic obstructive lung disease, although the long-term benefits of its use are uncertain.

major s. An operation involving a potential hazard and disruption of physiological function (e.g., entering a body cavity, excision of large tumors, amputation of a large body part, insertion of a prosthesis, open heart procedures). All surgeries are potentially dangerous and may involve a risk to life.

manipulative s. Use of manipulation in surgery or bone-setting.

maxillofacial s. The branch of dental practice and/or plastic surgery that deals with the diagnosis and the surgical and adjunctive treatment of diseases, injuries, and defects of the human mouth and dental structures. This was formerly called oral or dental surgery.

minor s. A simple operation not involving a major body cavity or structure that usually causes little disruption of the patient's physiological status. As with all surgery, there is some risk of injury or death.

mucogingival s. A plastic surgical method for correcting disease conditions relating to the gingiva and adjacent mucosa of the mouth.

open heart s. Surgery involving direct visualization and surgical procedure of the exposed heart.

oral s. Maxillofacial s.

orthopedic s. Surgical prevention and correction of musculoskeletal deformities and/or injuries.

palliative s. Surgery for the relief of symptoms or improvement in quality of life, usually in patients with incurable illness.

plastic s. Surgery concerned with the repair or restoration of defective or missing structures, frequently involving the transfer of tissue from a part to another, sometimes including the use of prosthetic materials. SEE: *cosmetic s.; tissue expansion, soft*.

radical s. An operation performed to remove a large amount of damaged or neoplastic tissue and/or adjoining areas of lymphatic drainage in an attempt to obtain complete cure. This is in contrast to conservative surgery.

reconstructive s. An operation to repair a loss or defect or to restore function.

second-look s. Surgery some months after the original operation for cancer to detect possible recurrences. Second-look procedures are also performed on a more immediate basis (e.g., within hours of the initial surgery) when vascular injuries created by the initial operation or condition are suspected. Occasionally, an endoscopic second look may be performed in lieu of an open surgical procedure.

subtotal s. An operation in which only a portion of the organ is removed, as subtotal removal of the thyroid gland.

surgery, antimicrobial prophylaxis in The use of antibiotics before, and sometimes during, procedures that are prolonged or involve potential risk of infection. This practice has been shown to prevent infectious complications in colorectal surgery, gynecological and obstetric surgeries, and some cardiac, cancer, and orthopedic procedures. The type of antibiotic administered depends on the surgical procedure. This practice is best suited to procedures involving contaminated areas or implantation of prosthetic material. SEE: *antibiotic resistance*.

surgical (sŭr′jĭ-kăl) Of the nature of or pert. to surgery.

surgical dressing A sterile protective covering of gauze or other substance applied to an operative wound.

surgical neck The constricted part of the shaft of the humerus below the tuberosities; commonly the site of fracture.

surgical resident A physician who is enrolled in a hospital-based training program to complete the requirements for board certification in a surgical specialty.

surname The family name, as distinguished from the individual's given or Christian name. In some societies, the surname is written first.

surrogate (sŭr′ō-gāt) [L. *surrogatus*, substituted] **1.** Something or someone replacing another; a substitute, esp. an emotional substitute for another. **2.** In psychoanalysis, the representation of one whose identity is concealed from conscious recognition as in a dream; a figure of importance may represent one's loved one.

sex s. A professional sex partner employed to assist persons with sexual dysfunction.

surrogate father A man who serves as a substitute father for a child's biological father. SEE: *parenting, surrogate*.

surrogate mother SEE: under *mother*.

sursumduction (sŭr″sŭm-dŭk′shŭn) [L. *sursum*, upward, + *ducere*, to lead] Elevation, as the power or act of turning an eye upward independently of the other one.

sursumvergence (sŭr″sŭm-vĕr′jĕns) [″ + *vergere*, to turn] An upward turning, as of the eyeballs.

sursumversion (sŭr″sŭm-vĕr′zhŭn) [″ + *versio*, turning] The process of turning upward; simultaneous movement of both eyes upward.

surveillance (sŭr-vāl′ăns) In health care, the monitoring of a disease, condition, epidemic, risk factor, or physiological function.

disease s. In epidemiology and public health, the identification of index patients and their contacts; the detection of outbreaks and epidemics; the determination of the incidence and demographics of an illness; and the policy-making that may prevent further spreading of a disease.

immunological s. The idea that the immune system destroys some malignant cells as they grow in the body. Support for this theory is found in research data that show tumor cells killed by natural killer cells and activated macrophages, and the presence of blocking factors against white blood cells found on tumors. SEE: *natural killer cell*.

post-marketing s. The review of adverse reactions to drugs and medical technologies that occurs after these agents are released for sale and use. Nurses, pharmacists, physicians, and other providers participate in this process by recording their observations on the adverse effects of drugs to the Food and Drug Administration, which accumulates this survey data and issues warnings to practitioners when needed. On occasion medicines or medical technologies thought to be useful are retired from the marketplace because of this reporting mechanism.

survey **1.** The study of a particular disease or condition, esp. its epidemiological aspects. **2.** In emergency care, the rapid and careful assessment of a patient's respiratory, circulatory, and neurological status. The *primary* survey focuses on the patency of a patient's airway, respiratory effort, circulation and cardiac rhythm, and neurological disability. The patient is then undressed or exposed, with environmental protection given to prevent hypothermia. In a *secondary* survey the stabilized patient is examined thoroughly for other conditions that may need prompt care.

survival Continuing to live, esp. under conditions in which death would be the expected outcome.

graft s. Persistent functioning of a transplanted organ or tissue in a recipient of that organ. Survival rates of transplanted organs are influenced by many factors, including the age and health status of both the donor and the recipient of the graft, the immunological match between the donor and the recipient, the preparation of the organ before transplantation, and the use of immunosuppressive drugs. For some organ transplantation, graft survival approximates 90%.

survivor guilt A grief reaction marked by feelings of depression, loss, or responsibility experienced by persons who have survived an event in which others have lost their lives (e.g., a war, holocaust, or epidemic illness).

susceptibility (sŭs-sĕp″tĭ-bĭl′ĭ-tē) The degree to which an individual is resistant to disease.

susceptible (sŭ-sĕp′tĭ-bl) [L. *susceptibilis*, capable of receiving] **1.** Having little resistance to a disease or foreign protein. **2.** Easily impressed or influenced.

sushi (soo′shē) A traditional Japanese food made of raw fish, usually wrapped in a soft rice shell. Some raw fish contain adults or larvae of the nematodes of the family Anisakidae. In order to prevent these organisms from infecting persons who eat raw fish, the U.S. Food and Drug Administration has directed that prior to serving, the fish must be suddenly frozen to −31°F (−34.4°C) or below for 15 hr, or held in a commercial freezer at −4°F (−20°C) for 24 hr. After that period, the fish may be thawed and served. SEE: *anisakiasis*.

sushi domain An amino acid sequence that creates a specific protein conformation in a polypeptide.

suspended (sŭs-pĕnd′ĕd) [L. *suspendere*, to hang up] **1.** Hanging. **2.** Temporarily inactive.

suspension (sŭs-pĕn′shŭn) [L. *suspensio*, a hanging] **1.** A condition of temporary cessation, as of any vital process. **2.** Treatment using a hanging support to immobilize a body part in a desired position. **3.** The state of a solid when its particles are mixed with, but not dissolved in, a fluid or another solid; also a substance in this state.

cephalic s. The supported suspension of a patient by the head to extend the vertebral column.

colloid s. A colloidal solution in which particles of the dispersed phase are relatively large. SYN: *suspensoid*.

tendon s. Fixation of a tendon. SYN: *tenodesis*.

suspensoid (sŭs-pĕn′soyd) [″ + Gr. *eidos*, form, shape] Colloid suspension.

suspensory (sŭs-pĕn′sō-rē) [L. *suspensorius*, hanging] **1.** Supporting a part, as a muscle, ligament, or bone. **2.** A structure that supports a part. **3.** A bandage or sac for supporting or compressing a part, esp. the scrotum.

suspiration (sŭs″pĭr-ā′shŭn) [L. *suspiratio*] A sigh or the act of sighing.

suspirious (sŭs-pī′rē-ŭs) [L. *suspirare*, to sigh] Breathing with apparent effort; sighing.

sustentacular (sŭs″tĕn-tăk′ū-lăr) [L. *sustentaculum*, support] Supporting; upholding.

sustentacular cell A supporting cell such as those found in the acoustic macula, organ of Corti, olfactory epithelium, taste buds, or testes. Those in the testes secrete the hormone inhibin and are also called *Sertoli cells*. SEE: *Sertoli cell*.

sustentacular fibers of Müller [Friedrich von Müller, Ger. physician, 1858–1941] Fibers forming the supporting framework of the retina.

sustentaculum (sŭs″tĕn-tăk′ū-lŭm) *pl.* **sustentacula** [L.] A supporting structure.

s. hepatis A fold of peritoneum upon which rests the right margin of the liver.

s. lienis The phrenocolic ligament that apparently supports the spleen.

s. tali A process of the calcaneum that supports part of the talus.

sutilains (soo′tĭ-lāns) Proteolytic enzymes derived from the bacterium *Bacillus subtilis*. Calculated on the dry basis, they contain not less than 2,500,000 USP casein units. They are used in ointment form to débride necrotic lesions, such as burns.

CAUTION: This product should be kept away from the eyes.

Sutton's disease (sŭt′ŏnz) [Richard L. Sutton, Sr., U.S. dermatologist, 1878–1952] Halo nevus.

Sutton's disease (sŭt′ŏnz) [Richard L. Sutton, Jr., U.S. dermatologist, b. 1908] Granuloma fissuratum.

Sutton's law A method of diagnostic reasoning that states one should look for diseases where they are most likely to be (e.g., malaria in tropical areas that harbor *Anopheles* mosquitoes; atherosclerosis in patients who are smokers, hypertensives, or diabetics). The law is attributed to Willie Sutton, a U.S. bank robber, who, when asked why he robbed banks said, "because that's where the money is."

sutura (sū-tū′ră) *pl.* **suturae** [L., a seam] **1.** Suture (1). **2.** Any kind of suture.

s. dentata A sutura with interlocking of bony processes resembling the teeth of a saw.

s. harmonia A simple apposition of two contiguous bones.

s. limbosa A beveled suture in which opposing margins fit in parallel ridges as between the parietal and frontal bones.

s. notha A false suture with ill-defined projections.

s. serrata A suture with deeper and more irregular indentations than a dental suture.

s. squamosa A suture formed by the overlapping of contiguous bones by broad beveled edges as in the suture between the squamous portion of the temporal and parietal bones.

s. vera A true suture in which no movement of united bones can occur. SEE: *synarthrosis*.

sutural (sū′tū-răl) [L. *sutura*, a seam] Rel. to a suture.

sutural joint An articulation between two cranial or facial bones.

sutural ligament Fibers that unite opposed bones forming a cranial suture.

suturation (sū″tū-rā′shŭn) The application of sutures; stitching.

suture (sū′chūr) [L. *sutura*, a seam] **1.** The line of union in an immovable articulation, as those between the skull bones; also such an articulation itself. SYN: *sutura*. SEE: *raphe; synarthrosis*. **2.** An operation in which soft tissues of the body are united by stitching them together. **3.** The thread, wire, or other material used to stitch parts of the body together. **4.** The seam or line of union formed by surgical stitches. **5.** To unite by stitching.

absorbable surgical s. A sterile strand prepared from collagen derived from healthy mammals or from a synthetic polymer. This type of suture is absorbed and thus does not need to be removed.

apposition s. The suture in the superficial layers of the skin in order to produce precise apposition of the edges.

approximation s. A deep suture for joining the deep tissues of a wound.

basilar s. The suture between the occipital bone and sphenoid bone that persists until the 16th to 18th year as the anteroposterior growth center of the base of the skull; also called *spheno-occipital synchondrosis*.

bifrontal s. The suture between the frontal and parietal bones.

biparietal s. The suture between the two parietal bones.

buried s. A suture placed so that it is completely covered by skin or other surrounding tissue.

button s. A suture in which the threads are passed through buttons or other prosthetic material on the surface and tied to prevent the suture material from cutting into the skin. SEE: *quilled s.*

catgut s. A suture material made from the sterilized submucosa of the small intestine of sheep. Eventually it is absorbed by body fluids. Treatment with chromium trioxide (chromic catgut) or other chemicals delays the absorption time.

coaptation s. A preliminarily placed suture to approximate wound edges before definitive closure.

cobbler's s. A suture in which the thread has a needle at each end.

continuous s. The closure of a wound by means of one continuous thread, usually by transfixing one edge of the wound and then the other alternately from within outward in a variety of techniques. SYN: *uninterrupted s.*

coronal s. A suture between the frontal and parietal bones. SYN: *frontoparietal s.*

cranial s. One of the sutures between the bones of the skull.

dentate s. A suture consisting of long and toothlike processes.

ethmoidofrontal s. A suture between the ethmoid and frontal bones.

ethmoidolacrimal s. A suture between the ethmoid and lacrimal bones.

ethmosphenoid s. A suture between the ethmoid and sphenoid bones.

false s. A junction of opposing bones in which fibrous union has not occurred. SYN: *sutura notha.*

figure-of-eight s. A suture shaped like the figure eight.

frontal s. An occasional suture in the frontal bone from the sagittal suture to the root of the nose. SYN: *mediofrontal s.; metopic s.*

frontolacrimal s. A suture between the frontal and lacrimal bones.

frontomalar s. A suture between the frontal and malar bones.

frontomaxillary s. Suture between the frontal bone and superior maxilla.

frontonasal s. A suture between the frontal bones and the nasal bones.

frontoparietal s. Coronal s.

frontotemporal s. A suture between the frontal and temporal bones.

glover's s. A continuous suture in which the needle is passed through the loop of the preceding stitch; more commonly referred to as a locking suture.

harmonic s. A suture in which there is simple apposition of bone.

intermaxillary s. A suture between the superior maxillae.

internasal s. A suture between the nasal bones.

interparietal s. Sagittal s.

interrupted s. A suture formed by single stitches inserted separately, the needle usually being passed through one lip of the wound from without inward and through the other from within outward.

lambdoid s. A suture between the parietal bones and the two superior borders of the occipital bone. SYN: *occipital s.; occipitoparietal s.*

longitudinal s. Sagittal s.

maxillolacrimal s. A suture between the maxilla and lacrimal bone.

mediofrontal s. Frontal s.

metopic s. Frontal s.

nasomaxillary s. A suture between the nasal bone and superior maxilla.

nonabsorbable s. A suture made from a material that is not absorbed by the body, such as silk, polymers, cotton, or wire. These sutures ultimately are removed or are placed in tissue deep to the skin where their presence will have minimal long-term consequences.

nonabsorbable surgical s. A sterile or nonsterile strand of material that is suitably resistant to the action of living mammalian fluids and tissue. This suture should be used only in those applications in which it may eventually be removed or its staying in the tissues will cause no harm.

occipital s. Lambdoid s.

occipitomastoid s. A suture between the occipital bone and the mastoid portion of the temporal bone. SYN: *temporo-occipital s.*

occipitoparietal s. Lambdoid s.

palatine s. A suture between the palatine bones.

palatine transverse s. A suture between the palatine processes and superior maxilla.

parietal s. Sagittal s.

parietomastoid s. A suture between the parietal bone and the mastoid portion of the temporal bone.

petro-occipital s. A suture between the petrous portion of the temporal bone and the occipital bone.

petrosphenoidal s. A suture between the petrous portion of the temporal bone and the ala magna of the sphenoid bone.

purse-string s. A suture entering and exiting around the periphery of a circular opening. Drawing the suture taut closes the opening.

quilled s. An interrupted suture in which a double thread is passed deep into the tissues below the bottom of the wound, the needle being so withdrawn as to leave a loop hanging from one lip of the wound and the two free ends of the thread from the other. A quill, or more commonly a piece of bougie, is passed through the loops, which are tightened upon it, and the free ends of each separate thread are tied together over a second quill. The purpose of a quilled suture is prevention of tearing when tension becomes greater. SEE: *button s.*

relaxation s. A suture that may be loosened to relieve excessive tension.

relief s. A suture used primarily in abdominal wound closures to bring large margins of the wound close together to relieve tension and to provide protection to the primary wound closure; more commonly called a retention suture. These sutures are made of heavy-grade material and are tied over wound bridges or tubes of latex to avoid injury to the wound.

right-angled s. A suture used in sewing intestine. The needle is passed in the same direction as the long axis of the incision, and the process is repeated on the opposite side of the incision, the suture being continuous.

sagittal s. A suture between the two parietal bones. SYN: *interparietal s.; longitudinal s.; parietal s.*

serrated s. An articulation by suture in which there is an interlocking of bones by small projections and indentations resembling sawlike teeth.

shotted s. A suture in which both ends of a wire or silkworm gut are passed through a perforated shot that is then compressed tightly over them in lieu of tying a knot.

silk s. A suture made of silk. It may be twisted, braided, or floss.

sphenoparietal s. The suture between the parietal bone and the ala magna of the sphenoid bone.

sphenosquamous s. An articulation of the great wing of the sphenoid with the squamous portion of the temporal bone.

sphenotemporal s. A suture between the sphenoid and temporal bones.

squamoparietal s. A suture between the parietal and squamous portions of the temporal bone.

squamosphenoidal s. A suture between the squamous portion of the temporal bone and great wing of the sphenoid bone.

squamous s. A suture between flat overlapping bones.

subcuticular s. A buried (usually) continuous suture in which the needle is passed horizontally under the epidermis into the cutis vera, emerging at the edge of the wound but beneath the skin, then in a similar manner passed through the cutis vera of the opposite side of the wound, and so on until the other angle of the wound is reached.

temporo-occipital s. Occipitomastoid s.

temporoparietal s. The suture between the temporal and parietal bones.

twisted s. A suture in which pins are passed through the opposite lips of a wound and material is wound about the pins, crossing them first at one end and then at the other in a figure-of-eight fashion, thus holding the lips of the wound firmly together.

uninterrupted s. Continuous s.

vertical mattress s. An interrupted suture in which a deep stitch is taken and the needle inserted upon the same side as that from which it emerged, and passed back through both immediate margins of the wound. The suture is then tied to the free end on the side the needle originally entered. This suture is primarily used in closing the skin.

wire s. A suture of varying gauges of metal (usually stainless steel) that may be used in a wide variety of applications, including wound closure, intestinal repair, and the repair of sternotomies.

Sv *sievert.*

SvO$_2$ *mixed venous oxygen saturation.*

swab (swăb) [Dutch *swabbe,* mop] **1.** Cotton or gauze on the end of a slender stick, used for cleansing cavities, applying remedies, or for obtaining a piece of tissue or secretion for bacteriological examination. **2.** To wipe with a swab.

test tube s. A swab for cleansing tubes.

urethral s. A slender rod for holding cotton used in examinations with the speculum, in treating ulcers, or removing secretions. The male urethral swab is a rod about 7 in. (17.8 cm) long.

uterine s. A slender flattened wire, or a plain rod or one with coarse thread on the distal end for absorbing or wiping away discharges.

swage (swāj) **1.** To shape metal, esp. around something in order to make a close fit. **2.** Fusing a suture to a needle.

swager A dental tool or device used to shape silver amalgam or gold by applying pressure from different directions simultaneously.

swallow (swăl′ō) [AS. *swelgan*] To cause or enable the passage of something from the mouth through the throat and esophagus into the stomach by muscular action. SYN: *deglutition.*

swallowed blood syndrome A condition

in which blood in an infant's stool reflects ingestion of maternal blood, either during delivery or during breastfeeding (from a bleeding nipple fissure). SEE: *APT test*.

swallowing (swăl'ō-ĭng) A complicated act, usually initiated voluntarily but always completed reflexively, whereby food is moved from the mouth through the pharynx and esophagus to the stomach. It occurs in the following three stages. SYN: *deglutition*.

In the *first stage,* food is placed on the surface of the tongue. The tip of the tongue is placed against the hard palate; then elevation of the larynx and backward movement of the tongue forces food through the isthmus of the fauces in the pharynx.

In the *second stage,* the food passes through the pharynx. This involves constriction of the walls of the pharynx, backward bending of the epiglottis, and an upward and forward movement of the larynx and trachea. This may be observed externally with the bobbing of the Adam's apple. Food is kept from entering the nasal cavity by elevation of the soft palate and from entering the larynx by closure of the glottis and backward inclination of the epiglottis. During this stage, respiratory movements are inhibited by reflex.

In the *third stage,* food moves down the esophagus and into the stomach. This movement is accomplished by momentum from the second stage, peristaltic contractions, and gravity. With the body in an upright position, liquids pass rapidly and do not require assistance from the esophagus. However, second-stage momentum and peristaltic contractions are sufficient to allow liquids to be drunk even when the head is lower than the stomach.

Difficulty in swallowing is called dysphagia. SEE: *dysphagia*.

impaired s. Abnormal functioning of the swallowing mechanism associated with deficits in oral, pharyngeal, or esophageal structure or function. SEE: *Nursing Diagnoses Appendix*.

tongue s. SEE: *tongue swallowing*.

swallow's nest Cerebral depression between the uvula and the posterior velum. SYN: *nidus hirundinis*.

Swan-Ganz catheter [Harold James Swan, U.S. physician, b. 1922; William Ganz, U.S. physician, b. 1919] A soft, flexible catheter that is inserted into the pulmonary artery of patients in shock or acute pulmonary edema to determine intracardiac pressures, oxygen saturation, and other hemodynamic parameters.

CAUTION: Its use may produce bleeding, vessel rupture, dysrhythmias, and other life-threatening complications.

---

swan-neck deformity A finger deformity marked by flexion of the distal interphalangeal joints and hyperextension of the proximal interphalangeal joints, often seen in rheumatoid arthritis.

swarming (sworm'ĭng) The spread of bacteria over a culture medium.

sway-back (swā'băk) A faulty, slouched posture in which the pelvis is shifted forward and the thorax posteriorly. Lordosis occurs in the lower lumbar spinal region; a compensating reversal to kyphosis occurs in the upper lumbar and thoracic regions.

sway, postural Forward and backward movement of the body with motion occurring around the ankle joints when the feet are fixed on the floor. Backward sway is controlled by the anterior tibialis, quadriceps, and abdominal muscles; forward sway is controlled by the gastrocnemius, hamstring, and paraspinal muscles. Patients with lesions of the dorsal and lateral columns of the central nervous system exhibit increased postural sway when they close their eyes and may fall down if they are not supported.

sweat (swĕt) [AS. *sweatan*] **1.** Perspiration. **2.** The condition of perspiring or of being made to perspire freely, as to order a sweat for a patient. **3.** To emit moisture through the skin's pores. SYN: *perspire*.

It is a colorless, slightly turbid, salty, aqueous fluid, although that from the sweat glands in the axillae, around the anus, and of the ceruminous glands has an oily consistency. It contains urea, fatty substances, and sodium chloride. This salty, watery fluid is difficult to collect without contamination with sebum. Perspiration is controlled by the sympathetic nervous system through true secretory fibers supplying sweat glands.

FUNCTION: Sweat cools the body by evaporation and rids it of what waste may be expressed through the pores of the skin. The daily amount is about a liter; this figure is subject to extreme variation according to physical activity and atmospheric conditions, and in hot conditions may be as much as 10 to 15 L in 24 hr.

bloody s. Hemathidrosis.

colliquative s. Profuse, clammy sweat.

colored s. Chromidrosis.

fetid s. Bromidrosis.

night s. Sweating during the night; it may be a symptom of many diseases including lymphomas, other cancers, and many infections.

profuse s. Hyperhidrosis.

scanty s. Anhidrosis.

sweat center One of the principal centers controlling perspiration located in the hypothalamus; secondary centers are present in the spinal cord.

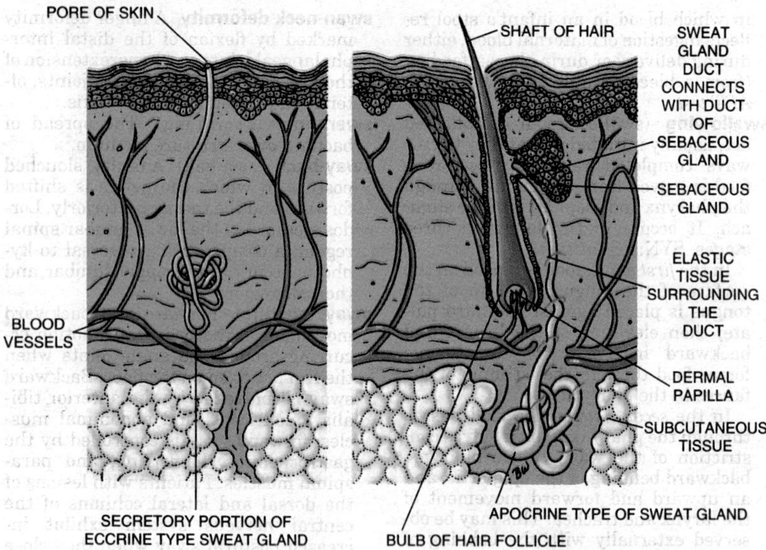

ECCRINE AND APOCRINE SWEAT GLANDS

sweat gland A simple, coiled, tubular gland found on all body surfaces except the margin of the lips, glans penis, and inner surface of the prepuce. The coiled secreting portion lies in the corium or subcutaneous portion of skin; the secretory duct follows a straight or oblique course through the dermis but becomes spiral in passing through the epidermis to its opening, a sweat pore. Most sweat glands are merocrine; those of the axilla, areola, mammary gland, labia majora, and circumanal region are apocrine. Sweat glands are most numerous on the palms of the hands and soles of the feet. SEE: illus.; *gland, apocrine; gland, eccrine.*

sweating (swĕt′ĭng) [AS. *swat,* sweat] **1.** The act of exuding sweat. **2.** Emitting sweat. **3.** Causing profuse sweat.

deficiency of s. Anhidrosis.

excessive s. Hyperhidrosis.

gustatory s. Sweating and flushing over the distribution of the auriculotemporal nerve in response to chewing.

insensible s. The evaporation of water from the skin without the production of visible sweat. This is done by the water vapor diffusing through the skin rather than being secreted by the sweat glands.

sensible s. The production of moisture on the skin by means of the secretions of the sweat glands.

urinous s. Uridrosis.

Swedish gymnastics A system of active and passive exercise of the various muscles and joints of the body without using apparatus.

sweet [AS. *swete,* sweet] **1.** Pleasing to the taste or smell. SEE: *taste.* **2.** Containing or derived from sugar. **3.** Free from excess of acid, sulfur, or corrosive salts.

Sweet's syndrome [R. D. Sweet, contemporary Brit. physician] A febrile illness with raised painful plaques on the limbs, face, and neck; neutrophilic leukocytosis; and dense neutrophilic infiltrates in the skin lesions. It responds promptly to treatment with glucocorticoids. Although the cause is unknown, the condition is often associated with the administration of drugs (such as hydralazine or sulfa drugs) and occasionally is found in persons with connective tissue diseases, hematologic malignancies, or inflammatory bowel disease.

sweetener, artificial A chemical compound, such as saccharin or aspartame, that tastes sweet, but has no available calories. These agents are used in foods and candies as sugar substitutes (e.g., for persons who are overweight or diabetic).

swelling (swĕl′ĭng) [AS. *swellan,* swollen] An abnormal transient enlargement, esp. one appearing on the surface of the body. Ice applied to the area helps to limit swelling. SEE: *edema.*

albuminous s. Cloudy s.

Calabar s. A swelling occurring in infestations by the nematode *Loa loa.* Temporary and painless, the swelling is thought to be the result of temporary sensitization. SYN: *fugitive s.*

cloudy s. A degeneration of tissues marked by a cloudy appearance, swelling, and the appearance of tiny albuminoid granules in the cells as observed with a microscope. SYN: *albuminous s.*

fugitive s. Calabar s.

glassy s. A swelling occurring in amyloid degeneration of tissues. SEE: *amyloid degeneration.*

white s. A swelling seen in tuberculous arthritis, esp. of the knee.

Swift's disease Acrodynia.

swimmer's ear A type of external otitis seen in persons immersed in water, usually during the summer months. It is typically caused by *Staphylococcus aureus* or *Pseudomonas aeruginosa* and is treated with a suspension of neomycin, polymixin B sulfate, and hydrocortisone.

swimming pool granuloma A chronic skin granuloma caused by *Mycobacterium marinum.* The lesion may develop in those who experience an abrasion of the skin while working in a home aquarium or in a marine environment. The condition is treated with clarithromycin or doxycycline.

switch (swĭch) [MD. *swijch,* bough] **1.** A device used to break or open an electrical circuit or to divert a current from one conductor to another. **2.** An assistive technology device used as an input device for a microcomputer. Types of adaptive switches include those activated by the tongue, eyelids, voice, movements of the head and trunk, and gross hand movements.

foot s. A foot-activated electrical switch that enables the operator to use both hands in the application of an electrical device (e.g., light source, electrosurgical unit, drill).

pole-changing s. A switch by which the polarity of a circuit may be reversed.

swoon [AS. *swogan,* to suffocate] To faint.

sycoma (sī-kō′mă) [Gr. *sykoma*] Condyloma.

sycosiform (sī-kō′sĭ-form) [Gr. *sykosis,* figlike disease, + L. *forma,* shape] Resembling sycosis.

sycosis (sī-kō′sĭs) [Gr. *sykosos,* figlike disease] A chronic inflammation of the hair follicles.

SYMPTOMS: The patient has inflammation of hairy areas of the body marked by an aggregation of papules and pustules, each of which is pierced by a hair. The pustules show no disposition to rupture but dry to form yellow-brown crusts. There is itching and burning. If the disease persists, it may lead to extreme destruction of hair follicles and permanent alopecia. The disease is curable with prolonged treatment and relapses do occur. *Staphylococcus aureus* and *S. epidermidis* entering through hair follicles cause the disease. Trauma and disability are predisposing factors.

s. barbae Sycosis of the beard marked by papules and pustules perforated by hairs and surrounded by infiltrated skin.

lupoid s. A pustular lesion of the hair follicles of the beard.

Sydenham's chorea (sĭd′ĕn-hămz) [Thomas Sydenham, Brit. physician, 1624–1689] A rare neurological syndrome that is associated with acute rheumatic fever, marked by dancing movements of the muscles of the trunk and extremities, anxiety and other psychological symptoms, and, occasionally, cognitive disorders. It is seen infrequently in Western societies because of the prompt and effective treatment of most cases of strep throat.

TREATMENT: Benzodiazepines, such as diazepam or lorazepam, are given to limit the choreiform movements. Penicillin or another appropriate antibiotic is given to eradicate the streptococcal infection causing the rheumatic fever.

PROGNOSIS: Recovery usually occurs within 2 to 3 months. Relapses, esp. in young women, may occur when oral contraceptives are used or during pregnancy. Other complications, such as congestive heart failure or death, may result from the carditis that accompanies rheumatic fever. SYN: *chorea minor.*

syllabic utterance (sĭ-lăb′ĭk) [Gr. *syllabikos*] A staccato accentuation of syllables, slowly but separately, observed in patients with multiple sclerosis. SYN: *scanning speech.*

syllable stumbling (sĭl′ă-bl) [Gr. *syllabe,* syllable] Hesitating utterance (dysphasia) with difficulty in pronouncing certain syllables.

syllabus (sĭl′ă-bŭs) [Gr. *syllabos,* table of contents] An abstract of a lecture or outline of a course of study or of a book.

sylvian aqueduct (sĭl′vē-ăn) [François (Franciscus del la Boë) Sylvius, Dutch anatomist, 1614–1672] A narrow canal from the third to the fourth ventricle.

sylvian artery [François Sylvius] The middle cerebral artery in the fissure of Sylvius.

sylvian fissure [François Sylvius] SEE: *fissure of Sylvius.*

sylvian line [François Sylvius] Line on exterior of the cranium, marking direction of the sylvian fissure.

sym- [Gr. *syn,* together] Combining form meaning *with, along, together with, beside.*

symballophone (sĭm-băl′ō-fōn) [″ + *ballein,* to throw, + *phone,* sound] A special stethoscope with two chest pieces. Its use assists in locating a lesion in the chest by comparing the different sounds detected by the two chest pieces.

symbion, symbiont (sĭm′bē-ŏn, -bē-ŏnt) [Gr. *syn,* together, + *bios,* life] An organism that lives with another in a state of symbiosis.

symbiosis (sĭm″bē-ō′sĭs) [Gr.] **1.** The

living together in close association of two organisms of different species. If neither organism is harmed, this is called *commensalism;* if the association is beneficial to both, *mutualism;* if one is harmed and the other benefits, *parasitism.* **2.** In psychiatry, a dependent, mutually reinforcing relationship between two persons. In a healthy context, it is characteristic of the infant-mother relationship. In an unhealthy context, it may accentuate shared depression or paranoia.

symbiote (sĭm′bī-ōt) [Gr. *syn,* together, + *bios,* life] An organism symbiotic with another.

symbiotic (sĭm″bī-ŏt′ĭk) Concerning symbiosis.

symblepharon (sĭm-blĕf′ă-rŏn) [″ + *blepharon,* eyelid] An adhesion between the conjuctivae of the lid and the eyeball, typically caused by burns with acids or bases, surgical trauma, or inadequately treated infections. The adhesions are surgically lysed to permit free movement and use of the affected eye.

symblepharopterygium (sĭm-blĕf″ă-rō-tĕr-ĭj′ē-ŭm) [″ + ″ + *pterygion,* wing] The abnormal joining of the eyelid to the eyeball.

symbol (sĭm′bŏl) [Gr. *symbolon,* a sign] **1.** An object or sign that represents an idea or quality by association, resemblance, or convention. **2.** In psychoanalytical theory, an object used as an unconscious substitute that is not connected consciously with the libido, but into which the libido is concentrated. **3.** A mark or letter representing an atom or an element in chemistry.

phallic s. An object that bears some resemblance to the penis.

symbolia (sĭm-bō′lē-ă) The ability to identify or recognize an object by the sense of touch.

symbolism (sĭm′bŏl-ĭzm) [″ + *-ismos,* condition] **1.** The unconscious substitutive expression of subconscious thoughts of sexual significance in terms recognized by the objective consciousness. **2.** An abnormal condition in which everything that occurs is interpreted as a symbol of the patient's own thoughts.

symbolization An unconscious process by which an object or idea comes to represent another object or idea on the basis of similarity or association.

symbolophobia (sĭm″bŏl-ō-fō′bē-ă) [″ + *phobos,* fear] A hesitancy in expressing oneself in words or action for fear that it may be interpreted as possessing a symbolic meaning.

symbrachydactyly (sĭm-brăk″ē-dăk′tĭ-lē) [″ + *brachys,* short, + *daktylos,* finger] The webbing of abnormally short fingers.

Syme's operation (sīmz) [James Syme, Scottish surgeon, 1799–1870] **1.** Amputation of the foot at the ankle joint with removal of the malleoli. **2.** Excision of the tongue. **3.** External urethrotomy.

symmelia (sĭm-mē′lē-ă) [Gr. *syn,* together, + *melos,* limb] Fusion of limbs.

symmelus, symelus (sĭm′ĕ-lŭs, -ē-lŭs) [″ + *melos,* limb] Sirenomelia.

symmetromania (sĭm″ĕ-trō-mā′nē-ă) [Gr. *symmetria,* symmetry, + *mania,* madness] A compulsive impulse to make symmetrical motions such as moving both arms instead of one.

symmetry (sĭm′ĕt-rē) Correspondence in shape, size, and relative position of parts on opposite sides of a body.

bilateral s. Symmetry of an organism or body whose right and left halves are mirror images of each other or in which a median longitudinal section divides the organism or body into equivalent right and left halves. SYN: *bilateralism.*

radial s. Symmetry of an organism whose parts radiate from a central axis.

sympathectomize (sĭm″pă-thĕk′tō-mīz) To perform a sympathectomy.

sympathectomy (sĭm″pă-thĕk′tō-mē) [Gr. *sympathetikos,* sympathy, + *ektome,* excision] Excision of a portion of the sympathetic division of the autonomic nervous system, used, for example, to treat refractory sweating of the palms or feet, or Raynaud's phenomenon. It may include a nerve, plexus, ganglion, or a series of ganglia of the sympathetic trunk. SYN: *sympathicectomy.*

chemical s. The use of drugs to destroy or temporarily inactivate part of the sympathetic nervous system.

periarterial s. Removal of the sheath of an artery in which sympathetic nerve fibers are located; used in trophic disturbances.

sympatheoneuritis (sĭm-păth″ē-ō-nū-rī′tĭs) [″ + *neuron,* nerve, + *itis,* inflammation] An inflammation of the sympathetic nerve.

sympathetic (sĭm″pă-thĕt′ĭk) **1.** Pert. to the sympathetic nervous system. **2.** Caused by or pert. to sympathy.

sympatheticalgia (sĭm″pă-thĕt″ĭ-kăl′jē-ă) [″ + *algos,* pain] Pain in the cervical sympathetic ganglion.

sympathetic irritation The irritation of one structure caused by irritation of a related one.

sympathetic nervous system SEE: *system, sympathetic nervous.*

sympatheticoparalytic (sĭm″pă-thĕt″ĭ-kō-păr″ă-lĭt′ĭk) [″ + *paralysis,* a loosening at the sides] Resulting from paralysis of the sympathetic nervous system.

sympatheticopathy (sĭm″pă-thĕt″ĭ-kŏp′ă-thē) [″ + *pathos,* disease, suffering] Any condition resulting from a disorder of the sympathetic nervous system.

sympathetic ophthalmia Inflammation of the uveal tract in one eye caused by a similar inflammation in the other eye.

sympatheticotonia (sĭm″pă-thĕt″ĭ-kō-tō′nē-ă) [″ + *tonos,* act of stretching, tension] A condition marked by excessive tone of the sympathetic nervous system with unusually high blood pressure, fine tremor of the hands, and insomnia; the opposite of vagotonia. It may be present in thyrotoxic patients.

sympathetic plexus One of the plexuses formed at intervals by the sympathetic nerves and ganglia.

sympathicectomy (sĭm-păth″ĭ-sĕk′tō-mē) [″ + *ektome,* excision] Sympathectomy.

sympathicolytic (sĭm-păth″ĭ-kō-lĭt′ĭk) [″ + *lytikos,* dissolving] Interfering with, opposing, inhibiting, or destroying impulses from the sympathetic nervous system. SYN: *adrenolytic; sympatholytic.*

sympathiconeuritis (sĭm-păth″ĭ-kō-nū-rī′tĭs) [″ + *neuron,* nerve, + *itis,* inflammation] An inflammation of the sympathetic nerves.

sympathicopathy (sĭm-păth″ĭ-kŏp′ă-thē) [″ + *pathos,* disease, suffering] A disease or disordered function caused by a malfunction of the autonomic nervous system.

sympathicotripsy (sĭm-păth″ĭ-kō-trĭp′sē) [″ + *tripsis,* a crushing] The crushing of a sympathetic ganglion.

sympathicotropic (sĭm-păth″ĭ-kō-trŏp′ĭk) [″ + *tropos,* a turning] Having a special affinity for the sympathetic nerve.

sympathicus (sĭm-păth′ĭ-kŭs) The sympathetic nervous system.

sympathoadrenal (sĭm″păth-ō-ă-drē′năl) [″ + L. *ad,* to, + *ren,* kidney] Concerning the sympathetic part of the autonomic nervous system and the adrenal medulla.

sympathoblastoma (sĭm″păth-ō-blăs-tō′mă) [″ + ″ + *oma,* tumor] A malignant tumor made up of sympathetic nerve cells.

sympathoglioblastoma (sĭm″păth-ō-glī″ō-blăs-tō′mă) [Gr. *sympathetikos,* sympathy, + *glia,* glue, + *blastos,* germ, + *oma,* tumor] A tumor made up primarily of sympathoblasts with scattered neuroblasts and spongioblasts.

sympathogonia (sĭm″pă-thō-gō′nē-ă) [″ + *gone,* seed] Primitive cells from which sympathetic nervous system cells are derived.

sympathogonioma (sĭm″pă-thō-gō″nē-ō′mă) [″ + ″ + *oma,* tumor] A tumor containing sympathogonia.

sympatholytic Sympathicolytic.

sympathomimetic (sĭm″pă-thō-mĭm-ĕt′ĭk) [″ + *mimetikos,* imitating] Adrenergic; producing effects resembling those resulting from stimulation of the sympathetic nervous system, such as effects following the injection of epinephrine.

sympathy (sĭm′pă-thē) [Gr. *sympatheia*] **1.** An association or feeling of closeness between individuals such that something that affects one affects the other. SEE: *empathy.* **2.** In biology, something that affects one of a paired organ influencing the other. The mechanism of this interaction is not always clearly understood.

sympexion (sĭm-pĕks′ē-ŏn) [Gr. *sympexis,* concretion] A calcified mass in certain sites such as the prostate or seminal vesicles.

symphalangism (sĭm-făl′ăn-jĭzm) [Gr. *syn,* together, + *phalanx,* closely knit row] **1.** An ankylosis of the joints of the fingers or toes. **2.** A web-fingered or web-toed condition.

symphyogenetic (sĭm″fē-ō-jĕ-nĕt′ĭk) [Gr. *syn,* together, + *phyein,* to grow, + *gennan,* to produce] Concerning the combined effect of heredity and environment upon the development and function of an organism.

symphyseal (sĭm-fĭz′ē-ăl) [Gr. *symphysis,* growing together] Pert. to symphysis.

symphyseotomy, symphysiectomy (sĭm-fĭz″ē-ŏt′ō-mē) [″ + *tome,* incision] A section of the symphysis pubis to enlarge the pelvic diameters during delivery. SYN: *pubiotomy; symphysiotomy.*

symphysion (sĭm-fĭz′ē-ŏn) [Gr. *symphysis,* growing together] The most anterior point of the alveolar process of the lower jaw.

symphysiorrhaphy (sĭm-fĭz″ē-or′ă-fē) [″ + *rhaphe,* seam, ridge] The surgical repair of a divided symphysis.

symphysiotome (sĭm-fĭz′ē-ō-tōm) [″ + *tome,* incision] An instrument for dividing a symphysis.

symphysiotomy (sĭm-fĭz″ē-ŏt′ō-mē) [″ + *tome,* incision] Symphyseotomy.

symphysis (sĭm′fĭ-sĭs) *pl.* **symphyses** [Gr., growing together] **1.** A line of fusion between two bones that are separate in early development, as symphysis of the mandible. **2.** A form of synchondrosis in which the bones are separated by a disk of fibrocartilage, as in joints between bodies of vertebrae or between pubic bones. SEE: *intervertebral disk.*

s. cartilaginosa Synchondrosis.

s. of jaw An anterior, median, vertical ridge on the outer surface of the lower jaw representing a line of union of its halves.

s. ligamentosa Syndesmosis.

s. mandibulae S. menti.

s. menti The symphysis of the chin or the ridge marking the line of union of the two halves of the mandible. SYN: *s. mandibulae.*

s. pubis The junction of the pubic bones on the midline in front; the bony eminence under the pubic hair.

symphysodactyly (sĭm″fĭ-sō-dăk′tĭ-lē) [″ + *daktylos,* finger] Syndactylism.

sympodia (sĭm-pō′dē-ă) [″ + *pous,* foot] A fusion of the lower extremities.

symporter (sĭm-por′tĕr) A membrane protein that carries two different ions or molecules in the same direction through the membrane, as in the absorption of glucose linked with that of sodium ions in the small intestine.

symptom (sĭm′tŭm, sĭmp-) [Gr. *symptoma,* occurrence] Any change in the body or its functions, as perceived by the patient. A symptom represents the subjective experience of disease. Symptoms are described by patients in their complaint or history of the present illness. By contrast, signs are the objective findings observed by health care providers during the examination of patients.

Aspects of general symptom analysis include the following: *onset:* date, manner (gradual or sudden), and precipitating factors; *characteristics:* character, location, radiation, severity, timing, aggravating or relieving factors, and associated symptoms; *course since onset:* incidence, progress, and effects of therapy.

accessory s. A minor symptom, or a nonpathognomonic one. SYN: *assident s.*

accidental s. A symptom occurring incidentally during the course of a disease but having no relationship to the disease.

assident s. Accessory s.

cardinal s. A principal symptom in the diagnosis of a disease.

concomitant s. A symptom occurring along with the essential symptoms of a disease.

constitutional s. A symptom (such as fever, malaise, loss of appetite) caused by or indicating systemic disease. SYN: *general s.*

delayed s. A symptom appearing sometime after the precipitating cause.

direct s. A symptom resulting from direct effects of the disease.

dissociation s. Anesthesia to heat, cold, and pain without loss of tactile sensibility; seen in syringomyelia.

equivocal s. A symptom that may occur in several diseases.

focal s. A symptom at a specific location.

general s. Constitutional s.

indirect s. A symptom occurring secondarily as a result of a disease.

labyrinthine s. A group of symptoms, such as tinnitus, vertigo, or nausea, indicating a disease or lesion of the inner ear.

local s. A symptom indicating the specific location of the pathological process.

negative pathognomonic s. A symptom that never occurs in a certain disease or condition; hence, its occurrence rules out the existence of that disease.

objective s. A symptom apparent to the observer. SEE: *sign* (2).

passive s. Static s.

pathognomonic s. A symptom that is unmistakably associated with a particular disease.

presenting s. The symptom that led the patient to seek medical care.

prodromal s. Prodrome.

rational s. Subjective s.

signal s. A symptom that is premonitory of an impending condition such as the aura that precedes an attack of epilepsy or migraine.

static s. A symptom pert. to the condition of a single organ or structure without reference to the remainder of the body. SYN: *passive s.*

subjective s. A symptom apparent only to the patient. SYN: *rational s.*

supratentorial s. A symptom due to psychological rather than organic causes. The term is slang and refers to symptoms with causes originating "above the tentorium cerebelli" (i.e., in the brain rather than in the body).

sympathetic s. A symptom for which there is no specific inciting cause and usually occurring at a point more or less remote from the point of disturbance. SEE: *sympathy* (1).

withdrawal s. One of the symptoms following sudden withdrawal of a substance to which a person has become addicted.

symptomatic (sĭmp″tō-măt′ĭk) [Gr. *symptomatikos*] Of the nature of or concerning a symptom.

symptomatology (sĭmp″tō-mă-tŏl′ō-jē) [Gr. *symptoma,* symptom, + *logos,* word, reason] **1.** The science of symptoms and indications. **2.** All of the symptoms of a given disease as a whole.

symptom complex Syndrome.

sympus (sĭm′pŭs) [″ + *pous,* foot] A deformed fetus fused at the lower limbs.

syn- [Gr., together] Prefix meaning *joined, together*. SEE: *con-*.

synactosis (sĭn″ăk-tō′sĭs) [Gr. *syn,* together, + L. *actio,* function, + Gr. *osis,* condition] A malformation resulting from the abnormal fusion of parts.

synadelphus (sĭn″ă-dĕl′fŭs) [″ + *adelphos,* brother] A deformed fetus with eight limbs.

synalgic (sĭn-ăl′jĭk) Pert. to or marked by referred pain.

synapse (sĭn′ăps) [Gr. *synapsis,* point of contact] The space between the junction of two neurons in a neural pathway, where the termination of the axon of one neuron comes into close proximity with the cell body or dendrites of another. The electrical impulse traveling along a presynaptic neuron to the end of its axon releases a chemical neurotransmitter that stimulates or inhibits an electrical impulse in the postsynaptic neuron; synaptic transmission is in one direction only. Synapses are susceptible to fatigue, offer a resistance to the passage of impulses, and are markedly sus-

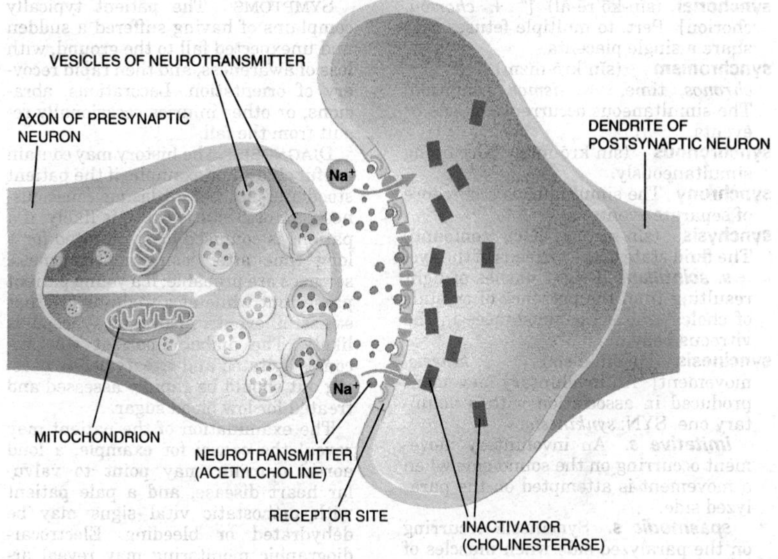

SYNAPSE

Transmission at an excitatory synapse (arrow indicates direction of impulse)

ceptible to the effects of oxygen deficiency, anesthetics, and other agents, including therapeutic drugs and toxic chemicals. SYN: *synapsis* (1). SEE: illus.

axodendritic s. The synapse between an axon of one neuron and the dendrites of another.

axodendrosomatic s. The synapse between the axon of one neuron and the dendrites and cell body of another.

axosomatic s. The synapse between the axon of one neuron and the cell body of another.

synapsis (sĭn-ăp′sĭs) [Gr., point of contact] **1.** Synapse. **2.** The process of first maturation division in gametogenesis, in which there is conjugation of pairs of homologous chromosomes forming double or bivalent chromosomes. In the resulting meiotic division, the chromosome number is reduced from the diploid to the haploid number. It is at this stage that crossing over occurs.

synaptic Pert. to a synapse or synapsis.

synaptology (sĭn″ăp-tŏl′ō-jē) [″ + *logos,* word, reason] The study of synapses.

synarthrodia (sĭn″ăr-thrō′dē-ă) [Gr. *syn,* together, + *arthron,* joint, + *eidos,* form, shape] Synarthrosis.

synarthrodial Pert. to a synarthrosis.

synarthrophysis (sĭn″ăr-thrō-fī′sĭs) [″ + *arthron,* joint, + *physis,* growth] A progressive ankylosis of joints.

synarthrosis [″ + *arthron,* joint, + *osis,* condition] A type of immovable joint with fibrous connective tissue or cartilage between the bone surfaces. Movement is absent or limited, and a joint cavity is lacking. It includes the synchondrosis, suture, and syndesmosis types of joints. SYN: *synarthrodia.*

syncanthus (sĭn-kăn′thŭs) [″ + *kanthos,* angle] An adhesion of the eyeball to the structures of the orbit.

syncephalus (sĭn-sĕf′ă-lŭs) [″ + *kephale,* head] A deformed fetus with one head, one face, and four ears.

synchilia (sĭn-kī′lē-ă) [″ + *cheilos,* lip] The congenital adhesion of the lips or atresia of the mouth.

synchiria (sĭn-kī′rē-ă) [″ + *cheir,* hand] A disorder of sensibility in which a stimulus applied to one side of the body is felt on both sides. SEE: *achiria; allochiria; dyschiria.*

synchondroseotomy (sĭn″kŏn-drō″sē-ŏt′ō-mē) [″ + *chondros,* cartilage, + *tome,* incision] An operation of cutting through the sacroiliac ligaments and closing the arch of the pubes in the congenital absence of the anterior wall of the bladder (exstrophy).

synchondrosis (sĭn″kŏn-drō′sĭs) [″ + ″ + *osis,* condition] An immovable joint having surfaces between the bones connected by cartilages. This may be temporary, in which case the cartilage eventually becomes ossified, or permanent. SYN: *symphysis cartilaginosa.*

synchondrotomy (sĭn-kŏn-drŏt′ō-mē) [″ + ″ + *tome,* incision] **1.** The division of articulating cartilage of a synchondrosis. **2.** A section of the symphysis pubis to facilitate childbirth. SYN: *symphyseotomy.*

synchorial (sĭn-kō′rē-ăl) [″ + *chorion,* chorion] Pert. to multiple fetuses that share a single placenta.

synchronism (sĭn′krō-nĭzm) [″ + *chronos,* time, + *-ismos,* condition] The simultaneous occurrence of acts or events.

synchronous (sĭn′krō-nŭs) Occurring simultaneously.

synchrony The simultaneous occurrence of separate events.

synchysis (sĭn′kĭs-ĭs) [Gr., confound] The fluid state of the vitreous of the eye.

s. scintillans Bright flashes of light resulting from the presence of crystals of cholesterol or fat substances in the vitreous body.

syncinesis (sĭn″sĭn-ē′sĭs) [″ + *kinesis,* movement] An involuntary movement produced in association with a voluntary one. SYN: *synkinesis.*

imitative s. An involuntary movement occurring on the sound side when a movement is attempted on the paralyzed side.

spasmodic s. Syncinesis occurring on the paralyzed side when muscles of the opposite side are voluntarily moved.

synciput (sĭn′sĭ-pŭt) The anterior upper half of the cranium. SYN: *sinciput.*

synclinal (sĭn-klī′năl) [Gr. *synklinein,* to lean together] Inclined in the same direction toward a point.

synclitism (sĭn′klĭt-ĭzm) [Gr. *synklinein,* to lean together, + *-ismos,* condition] Parallelism between the planes of the fetal head and those of the maternal pelvis.

synclonus (sĭn′klō-nŭs) [″ + *klonos,* turmoil] **1.** Clonic contraction of several muscles together. **2.** A disease marked by muscular spasms.

s. ballismus Paralysis agitans.

s. tremens Generalized tremor.

syncopal (sĭn′kō-păl) [Gr. *synkope,* fainting] Rel. to or marked by syncope.

syncope (sĭn′kō-pē) [Gr. *synkope,* fainting] Transient (and usually sudden) loss of consciousness, accompanied by an inability to maintain an upright posture. Syncope occurs commonly; it results in about 1% to 6% of all hospital admissions in the U.S. SEE: *coma; faint; transient ischemic attack; unconsciousness.*

ETIOLOGY: The most frequent causes of syncope are vasovagal (the common fainting spell); cardiogenic (esp. arrhythmogenic, valvular, or ischemic); orthostatic (e.g., due to dehydration or hemorrhage); and neurogenic (e.g., due to seizures). Many medications (e.g., sedatives, tranquilizers, excessive doses of insulin, and others), hypoglycemia, hyperventilation, massive pulmonary embolism, aortic dissection, atrial myxoma, carotid sinus hypersensitivity, coughing, urination, and psychiatric disease can also result in loss of consciousness.

SYMPTOMS: The patient typically complains of having suffered a sudden and unexpected fall to the ground, with loss of awareness, and then rapid recovery of orientation. Lacerations, abrasions, or other injuries occasionally result from the fall.

DIAGNOSIS: The history may contain useful clues. For example, if the patient stood up just before losing consciousness, an orthostatic cause is likely; if a patient is confused or disoriented for a long time after losing consciousness, seizures are probable; if a young patient passes out while at a wedding or other stressful event, vasovagal syncope is likely. The diabetic patient who becomes agitated and sweaty before passing out should be rapidly assessed and treated for low blood sugar.

The examination of the patient may reveal the cause; for example, a loud aortic murmur may point to valvular heart disease, and a pale patient with orthostatic vital signs may be dehydrated or bleeding. Electrocardiographic monitoring may reveal arrhythmias or evidence of ischemia. Depending on clinical circumstances, further evaluation may include carotid sinus massage, tilt-table testing, echocardiography, or psychiatric evaluation. In most cases, despite thorough evaluation, a precise diagnosis is not determined.

FIRST AID: Any individual with sudden loss of consciousness should be placed in a supine position, preferably with the head low to facilitate blood flow to the brain. At the same time, a clear airway should be ensured. Clothing must be loosened, esp. if collar is tight.

Fainting (one form of syncope) usually is of short duration and is counteracted by placing the individual supine. If recovery from fainting is not prompt and complete, a prompt assessment of airway, breathing, circulation, and cardiac rhythm is needed; assistance should be obtained and the person transported to a hospital. An individual who refuses hospital evaluation after recovering from a fainting episode should be encouraged to be examined by a physician as soon as possible.

s. anginosa Syncope occurring with anginal pain.

cardiac s. Syncope of cardiac origin as in Stokes-Adams syndrome, aortic stenosis, tachycardia, bradycardia, or myocardial infarction.

carotid sinus s. Syncope resulting from pressure on, or hypersensitivity of, the carotid sinus. It may result from turning the head to one side or from wearing too tight a collar.

cough s. Syncope occurring during a coughing spell.

defecation s. Loss of consciousness

occurring during or immediately after a bowel movement.

deglutition s. Fainting triggered by swallowing, an abnormal reflex in which stimulation of the esophagus elicits vagal motor impulses that cause bradycardia, peripheral vasodilation, and hypotension.

hysterical s. Syncope resulting from a conversion reaction.

laryngeal s. Brief unconsciousness following coughing and tickling in the throat.

local s. Numbness of a part with sudden blanching, as of the fingers; a symptom of Raynaud's disease or of local asphyxia.

micturition s. The abrupt loss of consciousness during urination. It usually occurs in men who get up at night to urinate and is mediated by an increase in vagal tone.

neurocardiogenic s. Vasodepressor syncope.

shallow water s. Loss of consciousness during diving that occurs when a diver hyperventilates, and then holds his or her breath while swimming underwater for an extended period before resurfacing. The loss of consciousness may result in drowning or near-drowning.

situational s. Loss of consciousness that occurs only in certain distinct clinical circumstances, such as after urinating, coughing, or having a bowel movement. It is sometimes associated with inadequate return of blood to the right side of the heart, Valsalva maneuver, or increased parasympathetic tone.

swallow s. Deglutition s.

tussive s. Fainting following a paroxysm of coughing. This is a rare condition in patients with chronic bronchitis. SYN: *laryngeal vertigo.*

vasodepressor s. The common fainting spell.

SYMPTOMS: The patient, who may have just experienced a stressful or emotionally upsetting event, reports a feeling of wooziness, nausea, and weakness, followed often by a feeling that darkness is closing in on him or her. A ringing in the ears may follow, along with inability to maintain an erect posture. Witnesses may report a profuse sweating or a loss of color in the face. During the event, an unusually slow pulse may be present. Several convulsive movements of the body may be noted if blood flow to the brain is inadequate, but the loss of consciousness is not accompanied by other signs of seizures, such as tongue biting, incontinence, or a prolonged postictal period of confusion.

PATIENT CARE: Placing the patient in a horizontal or Trendelenburg position restores blood flow to the heart and brain and promptly aborts the attack. A brief examination should be performed to make sure the affected person can move all extremities and facial muscles, and speak clearly and understand speech. Fluids should be administered by mouth if nausea has resolved, or by vein if the patient cannot take liquids orally and has an intravenous access in place. An electrocardiogram should be obtained or cardiac monitoring ordered if the patient has a history of cardiac disease, is elderly, or has multiple risk factors for cardiac disease or dysrhythmias. Before the patient is allowed to get up again, vital signs should be checked; if they are normal, the patient should be assisted first to a sitting position, and then to a standing position, before he or she walks independently. SYN: *vasovagal s.*

vasovagal s. Vasodepressor s.

syncretio (sĭn-krē′shē-ō) [L.] The development of adhesions between opposing inflamed surfaces.

syncytial (sĭn-sĭ′shăl) Of the nature of a syncytium.

syncytioma (sĭn″sĭt-ē-ō′mă) [″ + ″ + *oma,* tumor] A tumor of the chorion. SYN: *deciduoma.*

s. benignum A mole.

s. malignum A tumor formed of cells from the syncytium and chorion, occurring frequently after abortion or during puerperium at the site of the placenta.

syncytiotrophoblast (sĭn-sĭt″ē-ō-trō′fō-blăst) [″ + ″ + *trophe,* nourishment, + *blastos,* germ] The outer layer of cells covering the chorionic villi of the placenta. These cells are in contact with the maternal blood or decidua. SYN: *syntrophoblast.*

syncytium (sĭn-sĭt′ē-ŭm) [″ + *kytos,* cell] **1.** A multinucleated mass of protoplasm such as a striated muscle fiber. **2.** A group of cells in which the protoplasm of one cell is continuous with that of adjoining cells such as the mesenchyme cells of the embryo. SYN: *coenocyte.*

syndactylism (sĭn-dăk′tĭl-ĭzm) [″ + *daktylos,* finger, + *-ismos,* condition] A fusion of two or more toes or fingers.

syndactylous (sĭn-dăk′tĭ-lŭs) [″ + *daktylos,* finger] Concerning syndactylism.

syndectomy (sĭn-dĕk′tō-mē) [″ + *dein,* to bind, + *ektome,* excision] The excision of a circular strip of the conjunctiva around the cornea to relieve pannus. SYN: *peritomy* (1).

syndesis (sĭn-dē′sĭs) [″ + *desis,* binding] **1.** The condition of being bound together. **2.** Surgical fixation or ankylosis of a joint.

syndesmectomy (sĭn″dĕs-mĕk′tō-mē) [Gr. *syndesmos,* ligament, + *ektome,* excision] The excision of a section of a ligament.

syndesmectopia (sĭn″dĕs-mĕk-tō′pē-ă)

[″ + *ektopos,* out of place] An abnormal position of a ligament.

syndesmitis (sĭn″dĕs-mī′tĭs) [″ + *itis,* inflammation] **1.** An inflammation of a ligament or ligaments. **2.** An inflammation of the conjunctiva.

syndesmochorial (sĭn″dĕs″mō-kor′ē-ăl) Pert. to a type of placenta found in ungulates (e.g., sheep and goats) in which there is destruction of the surface layer of the uterine mucosa, thus allowing chorionic villi to come into direct contact with maternal blood vessels.

syndesmography (sĭn-dĕs-mŏg′ră-fē) [Gr. *syndesmos,* ligament, + *graphein,* to write] A treatise on the ligaments.

syndesmologia (sĭn″dĕs-mō-lō′jē-ă) [″ + *logos,* word, reason] A term concerned with the articulations of joints and their related ligaments.

syndesmology (sĭn″dĕs-mŏl′ō-jē) [″ + *logos,* word, reason] The study of the ligaments, joints, their movements, and their disorders.

syndesmoma (sĭn″dĕs-mō′mă) [″ + *oma,* tumor] A connective tissue tumor.

syndesmopexy (sĭn-dĕs′mō-pĕk″sē) [″ + *pexis,* fixation] Joining of two ligaments or fixation of a ligament in a new place, used in correction of a dislocation.

syndesmophyte (sĭn-dĕs′mō-fīt) [″ + *phyton,* plant] **1.** A bony bridge formed between adjacent vertebrae. **2.** A bony outgrowth from a ligament.

syndesmoplasty (sĭn-dĕs′mō-plăs″tē) [″ + *plassein,* to form] Plastic surgery on a ligament.

syndesmorrhaphy (sĭn″dĕs-mor′ă-fē) [″ + *rhaphe,* seam, ridge] The repair or suture of a ligament.

syndesmosis (sĭn″dĕs-mō′sĭs) *pl.* **syndesmoses** [Gr. *syndesmos,* ligament, + *osis,* condition] An articulation in which the bones are united by ligaments. SYN: *symphysis ligamentosa.*

syndesmotomy (sĭn″dĕs-mŏt′ō-mē) [″ + *tome,* incision] The surgical section of ligaments.

syndrome (sĭn′drōm) [Gr., a running together] A group of symptoms, signs, laboratory findings, and physiological disturbances that are linked by a common anatomical, biochemical, or pathological history. SEE: *disease; disorder.* **syndromic** (sĭn-drŏm′ĭk), *adj.*

acute chest s. A complication of sickle cell disease resulting from vascular occlusion or infection in the lungs and marked by chest pain, tachypnea, fever, rales and rhonchi, leukocytosis, and lobar consolidation.

Adair-Dighton s. Osteogenesis imperfecta.

adiposogenital s. Fröhlich's syndrome.

adrenogenital s. A syndrome marked by abnormally early puberty in children, overmasculinization in adults, virilism, and hirsutism, caused by the excessive production of adrenocortical hormones. SEE: *Cushing's syndrome.*

Angelman s. A rare genetic condition marked by severe mental retardation, microcephaly, and paroxysms of laughter. It is due to an abnormal chromosome 15 of maternal origin. SEE: *Prader-Willi s.*

Angelucci's s. Palpitation, excitable temperament, and vasomotor disturbance in some individuals who experience spring conjunctivitis.

antiphospholipid antibody s. A condition characterized by hypercoagulability associated with high blood levels of IgG antibodies against phospholipids, which are a major component of cell membranes. Many affected patients have a systemic autoimmune disease, such as systemic lupus erythematosus, but others present only with a history of frequent arterial and venous thrombi or pregnancy loss. Recent evidence suggests that antiphospholipid antibodies play a role in approx. 20% of strokes, esp. in patients who do not have common risk factors for stroke. Antiphospholipid antibodies include lupus anticoagulant and anticardiolipins; the presence of the latter causes these patients to test positive for syphilis.

Thromboses caused by the syndrome are treated and prevented with heparin, warfarin, corticosteroids, or, in some instances, immunosuppressant drugs such as cyclophosphamide.

CAUTION: Warfarin should not be used during pregnancy, because of the associated risk of fetal malformations.

apallic s. Persistent vegetative state.

autoimmune endocrine failure s. Polyendocrine deficiency syndromes.

Bloom's s. [David Bloom, Am. physician, b. 1892] An autosomal recessive disease, found predominantly but not exclusively in persons of Jewish ancestry, marked by chromosomal abnormalities, facial rashes, dwarfism, and a propensity to develop leukemia.

cholesterol embolization s. The systemic consequences that result from the splintering of cholesterol-containing plaques from the aorta; when this occurs fragments of cholesterol crystals may travel to and obstruct blood vessels throughout the body. The renal, mesenteric, and femoral arteries are most often affected; involvement of the cerebral vessels is unusual. This condition may arise after trauma to the aorta (e.g., during catheterization or cardiac surgery). It may produce renal failure, and ischemia or infarction of the bowel, toes, or skin. It may ultimately result in death in about half of all affected patients. There is no effective treatment.

Christ-Siemen's-Touraine s. A rare congenital disease whose hallmarks are hairlessness, inability to sweat, and dental abnormality.

cleft lip–cleft palate s. Van der Woude's syndrome.

congenital rubella s. Infection of the fetus from maternal rubella. The newborn may have severe central nervous system impairment, including deafness and mental retardation. SEE: *live rubella virus.*

cri du chat s. A hereditary congenital anomaly so named because the infant's cry resembles the cry of a cat. Characterized by mental retardation, microcephaly, dwarfism, epicanthal folds, and laryngeal defect. It is due to a deletion of the short arm of chromosome 4 or 5 of the B group.

cubital tunnel s. Medial elbow pain, hand fatigue, and sensations in the fourth and fifth fingers resulting from ulnar nerve damage in the cubital tunnel. This condition is frequently seen in athletes who throw objects.

culture bound s. A recurrent, locality-specific pattern of behavior or disease; a folk illness; an illness that affects a specific ethnic group, tribe, or society.

cumulative trauma s. Overuse syndrome.

DiGeorge s. A congenital aplasia or hypoplasia of the thymus caused by a missing gene on chromosome 22, and subsequent deficiency of competent T lymphocytes and cell-mediated immunity. Also characteristic are hypoparathyroidism and heart defects.

dumping s. A syndrome marked by sweating and weakness after eating, occurring in patients who have had gastric resections. The exact cause is unknown but rapid emptying (dumping) of the stomach contents into the small intestine is associated with the symptoms. This syndrome consists of weakness, nausea, sweating, palpitations, diarrhea, and occasionally, syncope. Eating small meals or lying down after eating may afford some relief.

dyscontrol s. A condition marked by sudden outbursts of violence or rage, associated with abnormal electrical discharges in the amygdaloid nuclear complex of the brain.

epidermal nevus s. The association of multiple cutaneous abnormalities, including multiple nevi, hemangiomas, and/or skin cancers, with scattered skeletal, neurological, urological, ophthalmic, and vascular malformations. The syndrome is sometimes transmitted to offspring by autosomal dominant inheritance.

euthyroid sick s. Any derangement in thyroid hormone blood levels in patients affected by another (usually critical) illness. The altered levels of thyroid hormones are not caused by primary thyroid dysfunction; they return to normal when the underlying illness is successfully treated.

excited skin s. The eruption of inflammatory rashes far from an initial exposure to an allergen or irritant. The syndrome can cause false-positive reactions during allergy patch testing.

familial cancer s. Any genetic predisposition to cancer that is found in several generations of a kindred. Some recognized cancer syndromes that recur in families include the multiple endocrine neoplasias (MEN), retinoblastoma, familial polyposis of the colon, and Fanconi's anemia, among others.

Fröhlich's s. A syndrome in adolescent boys marked by an increase in fat, atrophy of the genitals, and feminization owing to lesions of the pituitary and hypothalamus. SYN: *adiposogenital s.*

functional somatic s. Any of several poorly understood conditions in the group that includes multiple chemical sensitivity syndrome, sick building syndrome, repetition stress injury, chronic whiplash, chronic fatigue syndrome, irritable bowel syndrome, and fibromyalgia syndrome.

Gerstmann-Sträussler-Scheinker s. ABBR: GSS syndrome. A rare, autosomal dominant neurodegenerative disorder that may also be transmitted from person to person by infectious proteins (called prions). Clinically, the onset of symptoms and signs in midlife are related to progressive cerebellar dysfunction with ataxia, unsteadiness, incoordination, and progressive gait difficulty. The prognosis is poor and there is no specific therapy. SEE: *prion disease.*

Gradenigo's s. Paralysis of the external rectus muscle with severe temporoparietal pain and suppurative otitis media on the affected side. It is caused by an infection in the petrous portion of the temporal bone involving the sixth nerve.

hepatopulmonary s. A combination of liver disease, decreased arterial oxygen concentration, and dilatation of the blood vessels of the lung. Clinically the patient may have signs and symptoms of liver disease including gastrointestinal bleeding, esophageal varices, ascites, palmar erythema, and splenomegaly. Pulmonary signs include clubbing of the fingers, cyanosis, dyspnea, and decreased arterial oxygen concentration while in an upright position (orthodeoxia). With the exception of liver transplantation, therapy has been ineffective.

hepatorenal s. Renal failure that results from abnormal kidney perfusion, in patients with cirrhosis and ascites. Patients with HRS are typically critically ill, and have a very poor prognosis. Liver transplantation or portosystemic shunts are occasionally effective treatments.

holiday heart s. The association of cardiac arrhythmias, esp. atrial fibrillation, with binge drinking.

Horner's s. A condition marked by contracted pupils and ptosis, enophthalmos, and a dry, cool face on the affected side produced by paralysis of sympathetic nerves. It is caused by tumors in the neck, trauma, apical tuberculosis, tabes, syringomyelia, and neuritis of the cervical plexus.

HTLV-1 induced lymphoproliferative s. A disease seen in persons infected with human T-cell leukemia-lymphoma virus (HTLV-1). The clinical signs are lymphadenopathy, hepatomegaly, splenomegaly, cutaneous infiltration with neoplastic T cells, hypercalcemia, lymphocytosis, and skeletal changes. Most of these patients develop T-cell leukemia.

TREATMENT: Patients are treated with combination chemotherapy. The median duration of remission is 12 months.

hyperimmunoglobulinemia E s. An autosomal dominant disorder marked by high serum levels of IgE; eczema, mucosal candidiasis, and other cutaneous infections; pulmonary infections; retained primary dentition; scoliosis; and increased frequency of fractures.

idiopathic hyperkinetic heart s. Hyperactivity of the heart not due to a disease process. Its cause is unknown. In the past, this syndrome was referred to as neurocirculatory asthenia.

iliotibial band s. ABBR: ITB or IT band. An inflammatory overuse syndrome caused by mechanical friction between the iliotibial band and the lateral femoral condyle. It is commonly seen in distance runners and cyclists. Pain is manifested over the lateral aspect of the knee along the iliotibial band with no effusion of the knee.

impingement s. The compromise of soft tissues in the subacromial space, causing pain with overhead motions or rotational motions with an abducted arm (e.g., throwing). This syndrome is seen in repetitive overhead activities. It is treated with rotator cuff strengthening exercises, anti-inflammatory medications, and subacromial steroid injection. If conservative management fails, subacromial decompression (acromioplasty) is used.

incompetent palatal s. Incomplete or ineffective separation by the soft palate of the nasopharynx from the oropharynx, characterized by hypernasality and distortion of speech called whinolalia. This syndrome may be due to congenital or acquired defects of the palate.

irritable bowel s. ABBR: IBS. A condition marked by abdominal pain (often relieved by the passage of stool or gas); disturbances of evacuation (constipation, diarrhea, or alternating episodes of both); bloating and abdominal distention; and the passage of mucus in stools. These symptoms must be present despite the absence of anatomical, biochemical, or clinical evidence of active intestinal disease. The condition is the most common gastrointestinal complaint prompting patients to seek medical help. Its prognosis is benign. It is not associated with weight loss, fevers, or intestinal bleeding. Characteristically, although patients are symptomatic during the day, they do not have pain, bloating, distention, diarrhea, or other abdominal symptoms while sleeping. Women are typically affected more often than men; in some studies the ratio of women to men is 3:1.

ETIOLOGY: The symptoms of irritable bowel occur more often in patients who have had a history of physical or sexual abuse in childhood than in patients without such a history. Many studies have found a relationship between irritable bowel syndrome and a history of anxiety, psychological stress, or personality disorders. Physiologically, patients with IBS may have an increased or decreased rate of bowel motility.

TREATMENT: Management of IBS should begin with establishing a therapeutic physician-patient relationship and educating the patient about the benign nature of the illness and the excellent long-term prognosis. Initial recommendations are concerned with dietary modifications that may lessen the symptoms. Foods that the patient has found to cause difficulties are eliminated (dairy foods and gas-forming foods often cause symptoms). Specific symptoms can be alleviated by bulk-forming agents (e.g., psyllium), by increasing one's intake of fluids, and by engaging in increased levels of physical exercise. Low doses of antidepressant medications are sometimes helpful. Alternative therapy, including psychotherapy, hypnotherapy, imagery, and biofeedback, alone or in combination, may be effective in some patients.

DIAGNOSIS: Young patients suspected of having IBS should undergo testing to exclude other illnesses; tests should include a careful physical examination, complete blood count, metabolic panel, assessment of thyroid and liver functions; estimated sedimentation rate; and stool testing for occult blood. Patients over age 45 should also have sigmoidoscopy to rule out structural or anatomical lesions of the colon.

Jerusalem s. Jerusalem syndrome.

Kallmann's s. SEE: *Kallmann's syndrome.*

Korsakoff's s. Korsakoff's syndrome.

lactase deficiency s. Lactose intolerance.

lip-pit s. Van der Woude's syndrome.

locked-in s. Locked-in state.

long QT s. QT s.

loose cast s. Pressure sores or skin sloughing caused by the movement of an inappropriately secured cast against the underlying limb.

lupus-like s. A cluster of symptoms resembling an autoimmune disease (including arthritis, pleural or pericardial effusions, and rashes) sometimes seen in patients with widespread malignancy.

magic s. A variant of Behçet's syndrome, in which patients have mouth and genital ulcerations and inflammation of cartilage.

maxillofacial s. Maxillofacial dysostosis.

medial plica s. Patellar pain, and a feeling of instability, clicking, or locking of the knee as a result of inflammation of the medial synovial fold of the knee joint.

Moschcowitz s. Thrombotic thrombocytopenic purpura.

multiple chemical sensitivity s. ABBR: MCSS. The association of multiple physical symptoms with prolonged or recurrent exposures to low levels of environmental pollutants. Clinical research has failed to establish the precise nature of the syndrome, its causes, the functional limitations it may cause, or the best course of treatment. Many hypotheses have been suggested: some proponents of the syndrome believe that it results from allergic or immune-mediated mechanisms; skeptics have suggested that the symptoms are a form of masked depression, adverse conditioning to unusual odors, or, in some instances, a form of malingering. None of these hypotheses has been definitively proven.

myelodysplastic s. ABBR: MDS. Myelodysplasia.

numb-chin s. Loss of sensation in the area from the lower lip to the chin, caused by a lesion of the third division of the trigeminal nerve (fifth cranial nerve).

nursing-bottle s. Tooth decay that results when an infant is allowed to drink from a nursing bottle for a prolonged period. The sugar in the bottle contents promotes bacterial growth on the tooth surface.

oral allergy s. A form of contact dermatitis of the lips, tongue, or other tissues of the mouth, usually triggered by exposure to fresh fruits or vegetables.

ovarian hyperstimulation s. ABBR: OHSS. A potentially life-threatening complication that may occur in women receiving drugs to stimulate ovulation. The acute onset occurs within the first week ovulation is induced and is characterized by marked cystic ovarian enlargement, ascites, hydrothorax, arterial hypotension, tachycardia, hemoconcentration, oliguria, sodium retention, hypernatremia, and in severe cases renal failure. The condition is usually mild if the diameter of the ovary is less than 8 cm; moderate if 8 to 12 cm; and severe if greater than 12 cm.

Treatment includes symptomatic therapy to maintain circulatory function, bedrest, low-sodium diet, and diuretic therapy. The life-threatening possibility can be avoided with close monitoring and withholding of drugs if ovarian response becomes excessive.

overlap s. A rheumatological disorder with features suggestive of several kinds of connective tissue disease, but not definitively diagnostic of any single syndrome. Overlap syndromes typically have elements of systemic lupus erythematosus, rheumatoid arthritis, and progressive systemic sclerosis, among other illnesses.

Patau s. Trisomy 13.

patellofemoral pain s. Pain in the knee that occurs with exertion (e.g., walking upstairs) and is associated with stiffness after prolonged sitting and tenderness when the patella is compressed on the femoral condyle or when it is moved laterally.

Persian Gulf s. ABBR: PGS. A term used to describe a variety of symptoms experienced by veterans of the Persian Gulf war, including fatigue, loss of memory, muscle and joint pains, shortness of breath, and gastrointestinal complaints. The cause of these complaints remains obscure.

POEMS s. A rare multisystem disease characterized by the presence of polyneuropathy, organomegaly, endocrinopathy, monoclonal gammopathy, and skin changes. It often presents with osteosclerotic bone lesions associated with plasma cell dyscrasia. The cause is unknown.

post nasal drip s. ABBR: PNDS. An important cause of chronic cough, often associated with chronic or allergic rhinitis, in which nasal secretions drain via the posterior pharynx.

postcardiotomy s. Postpericardiotomy s.

postconcussion s. Traumatic brain injury.

postfall s. The inability to stand or walk without support for fear of repeating a fall. It is not associated with any physical disability and usually occurs in the elderly.

postmaturity s. A condition occurring in infants born after 42 weeks' gestation who exhibit signs of perinatal compromise related to diminished intrauterine oxygenation and nutrition secondary to placental insufficiency. During labor the fetal monitor may display late decelerations, and fetal hypoxia may result in meconium expulsion and aspiration. Characteristic assessment findings include skin desquamation and an absence of lanugo and vernix caseosa. Laboratory findings may include polycythemia and hypoglycemia. Postmature infants may also be at increased risk of cold stress due to diminished subcutaneous fat.

postmyocardial infarction s. Nonischemic chest pain, occurring after a patient has had a myocardial infarction, that typically worsens with deep breathing, improves while sitting up, and is aggravated by lying down. The patient may develop a low-grade fever, an elevated erythrocyte sedimentation rate, and elevated levels of antimyocardial antibodies. The cause is unknown. Patients usually are treated with nonsteroidal anti-inflammatory drugs or corticosteroids. A similar syndrome occurs in some patients who have undergone cardiac surgery (postpericardiotomy syndrome). SEE: *Dressler's syndrome.*

postpericardiotomy s. Fever, pericardial friction rub, and chest pain occurring several days or weeks after cardiac surgery. The syndrome appears to be an autoimmune response to damaged cardiac cells. Congestive heart failure may ensue. SYN: *postcardiotomy s.* SEE: *Postmyocardial infarction s.*

postphlebitic s. Pain and swelling in a limb, which follows about 80% of all cases of deep venous thrombosis. It is usually relieved somewhat by elevating the limb and worsened when the limb is dependent. Elastic or pressure stockings improve the symptoms for many patients.

posttachycardia s. Secondary ST and T wave changes associated with decreased filling of the coronary arteries and subsequent ischemia during tachycardia.

posttrauma s. A sustained maladaptive response to a traumatic, overwhelming event. SEE: *Nursing Diagnoses Appendix.*

Prader-Willi s. A rare congenital condition marked by genetic obesity, mental retardation, short stature, sexual infantilism, and hypotonia. The cause is an abnormal chromosome 15 of maternal origin. SEE: *Angelman s.*

QT s. A life-threatening syndrome marked by a prolonged Q-T interval combined with episodes of torsades de pointes. This condition may be congenital or may be acquired as a result of drug administration. Also called *prolonged QT interval syndrome* or *long QT syndrome.*

rape-trauma s. Sustained maladaptive response to a forced, violent sexual penetration against the victim's will and consent. SEE: *rape; Nursing Diagnoses Appendix.*

Like other posttraumatic stress disorders, this condition initially causes an acute phase of disorganization and involves a long-term reorganization of lifestyle. Sequelae may include marked changes in lifestyle and a variety of phobias.

Acute phase: Profound emotional responses mark the acute phase (i.e., fear, shame, and feelings of humiliation; self-blame and self-degradation; and anger and desire for revenge). Most commonly, rape victims exhibit crying, trembling, talkativeness, statements of disbelief, and emotogenic shock. Some may exhibit overt signs of hostility, which reflect their anger and feelings of powerlessness. Later, patient complaints of sleep pattern disturbances, gastrointestinal irritability, and genitourinary discomforts reflect physical responses to emotional trauma. Some women may appear quiet, dispassionate, and smiling; however, these behaviors should not be misinterpreted as indicating a lack of concern; rather, they may represent an avoidance reaction.

Long-term phase: Many rape victims experience one or more of the following: nightmares; chronic suspicion, inability to trust, and altered interpersonal relationships; anxiety, aversion to men, and avoidance of sex; depression; and phobias. Paradoxically, patients express feelings of guilt and shame because they feel that either they invited the attack, should have prevented the episode, or that they deserved being punished.

PATIENT CARE: The nurse exhibits empathy and understanding and ensures privacy and a quiet supportive environment. The patient is encouraged to verbalize feelings, fears, and concerns. Positive self-perception and self-esteem are promoted and supported. The nurse emphasizes that rape usually is an expression of the rapist's overwhelming feelings of psychosocial impotence and anger and that the act conveys a sense of power over others; the woman was a victim of the rapist's inability to contain a violent personal rage that is not related to her or to sex. The patient is referred to community resources (support groups).

rape-trauma s.: compound reaction A nursing diagnosis accepted at the NANDA 13th Conference (1998); forced violent sexual penetration against the victim's will and consent. The trauma syndrome that develops from this attack or attempted attack includes an acute phase of disorganization of the victim's lifestyle and a long-term process of reorganization of lifestyle. SEE: *Nursing Diagnoses Appendix.*

rape-trauma s.: silent reaction A nursing diagnosis accepted at the NANDA 13th Conference (1998); forced violent sexual penetration against the victim's will and consent. The trauma syndrome that develops from this attack or attempted attack includes an acute phase of disorganization of the victim's lifestyle and a long-term process of reorganization of lifestyle. SEE: *Nursing Diagnoses Appendix.*

refeeding s. The potentially fatal metabolic response of a starved individual to feeding, either enteral or parenteral. The correction of electrolyte imbalances is imperative before gradual refeeding to prevent hypophosphatemia, rhabdomyolysis, and other life-threatening complications.

Rendu-Osler-Weber s. Hereditary hemorrhagic telangiectasia.

risk for posttrauma s. A nursing diagnosis accepted at the NANDA 13th Conference (1998); a risk for sustained maladaptive response to a traumatic, overwhelming event. SEE: *Nursing Diagnoses Appendix.*

scimitar s. A rare congenital malformation of the heart and lungs, marked by dextroposition of the heart, a malformed right lung, abnormal connections between the right pulmonary veins and the inferior vena cava, and abnormal pulmonary arterial connections to the right lung.

sepsis s. Septic shock.

shoulder-hand s. Reflex sympathetic dystrophy.

skin-eye s. A syndrome consisting of deposits on the anterior surface of the lens and posterior cornea, and skin pigmentation. It is due to extensive medication with some of the phenothiazine-type tranquilizers.

soft-calorie s. Weight gain in persons who have undergone gastric stapling but who consume an excessive amount of calories through the consumption of liquids and/or mechanically soft foods like refined breads, cereals, ice creams, and custards, as opposed to raw fruits, vegetables, and whole grain products.

startle s. A rare, autosomal dominant neurological disorder in which affected persons have either brisk reflexes or sudden loss of consciousness with muscular rigidity when suddenly stimulated (e.g., by a loud noise or bright light). Treatment with benzodiazepines, such as clonazepam, is often beneficial.

steroid withdrawal s. The appearance of symptoms of adrenal insufficiency in persons who discontinue the use of corticosteroids after having been treated with them for a prolonged period. In those patients, adrenal function has been suppressed by exogenous hormone and the patient's adrenal glands do not provide an appropriate response when the patient has a serious infection, surgery, or an accident. This failure to respond to stress may be present for as long as a year after discontinuation of corticosteroid therapy. The syndrome may be prevented by gradual rather than abrupt withdrawal of corticosteroid therapy.

Stokes-Adams s. SEE: *Stokes-Adams syndrome.*

straight back s. An abnormally erect position of the spine, associated with pectus excavatum and functional cardiac murmurs.

superior vena cava s. A partial occlusion of the superior vena cava with resulting interference of venous blood flow from the head and neck to the heart. This emergency condition is typically caused by obstruction of the great vessels, usually by a cancer located in the mediastinum. It is marked by venous engorgement and edema of the head and neck.

supine hypotensive s. Sudden fall in blood pressure due to diminished venous return caused by compression of the vena cava by the gravid uterus when the pregnant woman rests flat on her back. The low venous return also results in decreased placental perfusion and potentially in fetal hypoxia. SYN: *vena caval s.*

symptom magnification s. A term relating to the rehabilitation of persons with work-related injuries, used in reference to behaviors that exaggerate the pain or functional limitation.

s. of inappropriate antidiuretic hormone ABBR: SIADH. A syndrome of increased ADH activity in spite of reduced plasma osmolarity. Often first suggested by a relative hyponatremia, it is most commonly associated with disorders of the central nervous system, various tumors, anxiety, pain, pneumonia, and drugs.

systemic capillary leak s. A rare disease whose hallmarks are episodes of hypotension associated with extravasation or plasma from the systemic circulation.

systemic inflammatory response s. A progressive state of systemic inflammation characterized by a white blood cell count greater than 12,000/mm^3 or less than 4000/mm^3, temperature greater than 38°C or < 36°C, tachycardia, tachypnea, and decreased blood carbon dioxide levels. SIRS can begin with any serious illness or injury involving inflammation but is most often associated with systemic infection (sepsis) caused by gram-negative bacteria. SEE: *sepsis; septic shock.*

ETIOLOGY: Lipopolysaccharide endotoxins released by gram-negative and gram-positive bacteria bind with lymphocytes and endothelial cells, stimulating a cascade of cytokine release, which produces systemic inflammation of blood vessels, tissues, and organs. Shock develops when cytokines cause vasodilation and increased vascular permeability. SIRS is one of the main causes of multiple organ dysfunction syndrome.

TREATMENT: Treatment for SIRS is focused on treating the primary cause. Multiple antibiotic therapy is required in sepsis. Supportive measures include the use of intravenous fluids and pressors, to support blood pressure, and intensive monitoring and optimization of oxygenation, ventilation, blood pressure, cardiac rhythms, serum electrolytes, and renal function.

tachybrady s. Sick sinus syndrome.

tarsal tunnel s. Neuropathy of the distal portion of the tibial nerve at the ankle caused by chronic pressure on the nerve at the point it passes through the tarsal tunnel. It causes pain in and numbness of the sole of the foot and weakness of the plantar flexion of the toes.

toxic shock s. SEE: *toxic shock syndrome.*

Turner's s. Gonadal dysgenesis.

vena caval s. Supine hypotensive s.

vulvar vestibulitis s. The presence of severe pain on pressing or touching the vestibule of the vagina or on attempted vaginal entry. Physical findings of localized erythema are limited to the mucosa of the vestibule. Although the etiology is unknown, the syndrome often develops in women who have intractable moniliasis or who are receiving long-term antibiotic therapy. No therapy, including vestibulectomy, has been 100% effective. SEE: *vulvodynia.*

Weber's s. Paralysis of the hypoglossal nerve on one side and of the oculomotor nerve on the other, with paralysis of the limbs owing to a lesion of a cerebral peduncle.

s. X The presence of four interrelated atherosclerotic risk factors: insulin resistance, hypertension, hyperlipidemia, and obesity.

synechia (sĭn-ĕk′ē-ă) *pl.* **synechiae** [Gr. *synecheia,* continuity] An adhesion of parts, esp. adhesion of the iris to the lens and cornea.

annular s. An adhesion of the iris to the lens throughout its entire pupillary margin.

anterior s. An adhesion of the iris to the cornea.

posterior s. An adhesion of the iris to the capsule of the lens.

total s. An adhesion of the entire surface of the iris to the lens.

s. vulvae Fusion of the vulvae, usually congenital.

synechotomy (sĭn″ĕk-ŏt′ō-mē) [″ + *tome,* incision] The division of a synechia or adhesion.

synechtenterotomy (sĭn″ĕk-tĕn″tĕr-ŏt′ō-mē) [″ + *enteron,* intestine, + *tome,* incision] The division of an intestinal adhesion.

synecology (sĭn″ē-kŏl′ō-jē) [Gr. *syn,* together, + *oikos,* house, + *logos,* word, reason] The study of organisms in relationship to their environment in group form.

synencephalocele (sĭn″ĕn-sĕf′ă-lō-sēl″) [″ + *enkephalos,* brain, + *kele,* tumor, swelling] An encephalocele with adhesions to adjacent structures.

syneresis (sĭn-ĕr′ĕ-sĭs) [Gr. *synairesis,* drawing together] The contraction of a gel resulting in its separation from the liquid, as a shrinkage of fibrin when blood clots.

synergetic (sĭn″ĕr-jĕt′ĭk) [Gr. *syn,* together, + *ergon,* work] Exhibiting cooperative action, said of certain muscles; working together. SYN: *synergic.*

synergia (sĭn-ĕr′jē-ă) The association and correlation of the activity of synergetic muscle groups.

synergic (sĭn-ĕr′jĭk) [″ + *ergon,* work] Rel. to or exhibiting cooperation, as certain muscles. SYN: *synergetic.*

synergist (sĭn′ĕr-jĭst) **1.** A remedy that acts to enhance the action of another. SYN: *adjuvant.* **2.** A muscle or organ functioning in cooperation with another, as the flexor muscles; the opposite of antagonist.

synergistic (sĭn″ĕr-jĭs′tĭk) **1.** Concerning synergy. **2.** Acting together.

synergy, synergism (sĭn′ĕr-jē) [Gr. *synergia*] An action of two or more agents or organs working with each other, cooperating. Their action is combined and coordinated.

synesthesia (sĭn″ĕs-thē′zē-ă) [Gr. *syn,* together, + *aisthesis,* sensation] **1.** A sensation in one area from a stimulus applied to another part. **2.** A subjective sensation of a sense other than the one being stimulated. Hearing a sound may also produce the sensation of smell. SEE: *phonism.*

s. algica Painful synesthesia.

synesthesialgia (sĭn″ĕs-thē-zē-ăl′jē-ă) [″ + ″ + *algos,* pain] A painful sensation giving rise to a subjective one of different character. SEE: *synesthesia.*

Syngamus (sĭn′gă-mŭs) A genus of nematode worms parasitic in the respiratory tract of birds and mammals.

S. laryngeus A species normally parasitic in ruminants but sometimes accidentally infesting humans.

syngamy (sĭn′gă-mē) [Gr. *syn,* together, + *gamos,* marriage] **1.** Sexual reproduction. **2.** The final stage of fertilization in which the haploid chromosome sets from the male and female gametes come together following breakdown of the pronuclear membranes to form the zygote. SYN: *sexual reproduction.*

syngeneic Descriptive of individuals or cells without detectable tissue incompatibility. Strains of mice that are inbred for a great number of generations become syngeneic. Identical twins may be syngeneic.

syngenesis (sĭn-jĕn′ĕ-sĭs) [″ + *genesis,* generation, birth] Arising from the germ cells derived from both parents, rather than from a single cell from one parent.

syngnathia (sĭn-nā′thē-ă) [″ + *gnathos,* jaw] Congenital adhesions between the jaws.

synizesis (sĭn″ĭ-zē′sĭs) [Gr. *synizesis*] **1.** An occlusion or shutting. **2.** A clumping of nuclear chromatin during the prophase of mitosis.

s. pupillae Closure of the pupil of the eye with loss of vision.

synkaryon (sĭn-kăr′ē-ŏn) [Gr. *syn,* together, + *karyon,* kernel] A nucleus resulting from fusion of two pronuclei.

synkinesis (sĭn″kĭ-nē′sĭs) [″ + *kinesis,* movement] An involuntary movement of one part occurring simultaneously with reflex or voluntary movement of another part.

imitative s. An involuntary movement in a healthy or normal muscle accompanying an attempted movement of a paralyzed muscle on the opposite side.

synnecrosis (sĭn″nĕ-krō′sĭs) [″ + *nekrosis,* state of death] The condition of association between groups or individuals that causes mutual inhibition or death.

synonym (sĭn′ō-nĭm) [Gr. *synonymon*] ABBR: syn. One of two words that have the same or very similar meaning; an additional or substitute name for the same disease, sign, symptom, or anatomical structure.

synophrys (sĭn-ŏf′rĭs) [Gr. *syn,* together, + *ophrys,* eyebrow] A condition in which the eyebrows grow across the midline.

synophthalmus (sĭn″ŏf-thăl′mŭs) [″ + *ophthalmos,* eye] Cyclops.

synopsia (sĭn′ŏp-sē-ă) [″ + *opsis,* vision] A condition in which there is a congenital fusion of the eyes.

synopsis (sĭn-ŏp′sĭs) [Gr.] A summary; a general review of the whole.

synoptophore (sĭn-ŏp′tō-for) [″ + *ops,* sight, + *phoros,* bearing] An apparatus for diagnosis and treatment of strabismus. SYN: *synoptoscope.*

synoptoscope (sĭn-ŏp′tō-skōp) [″ + ″ + *skopein,* to examine] Synoptophore.

synorchidism, synorchism (sĭn-or′kĭd-ĭzm, -kĭzm) [″ + *orchis,* testicle, + *-ismos,* condition] The union or partial fusion of the testicles.

synoscheos (sĭn-ŏs′kē-ŏs) [″ + *oscheon,* scrotum] An adhesion between the penis and scrotum.

synosteology (sĭn″ŏs-tē-ŏl′ō-jē) [″ + ″ + *logos,* word, reason] The branch of medical science concerned with joints and articulations.

synosteosis (sĭn″ŏs-tē-ō′sĭs) Synostosis.

synosteotomy (sĭn″ŏs-tē-ŏt′ō-mē) [″ + *osteon,* bone, + *tome,* incision] Dissection of joints.

synostosis (sĭn″ŏs-tō′sĭs) *pl.* **synostoses** [″ + ″ + *osis,* condition] **1.** Articulation by osseous tissue of adjacent bones. **2.** Union of separate bones by osseous tissue.

synostotic (sĭn″ŏs-tŏt′ĭk) [″ + ″ + *osis,* condition] Concerning synostosis.

synotia (sĭn-ō′shē-ă) [″ + *ous,* ear] The union of, or approximation of, the ears occurring in embryonic development, usually associated with absence of, or incomplete development of, the lower jaw.

synotus (sī-nō′tŭs) [″ + *ous,* ear] A fetus with synotia.

synovectomy (sĭn″ō-vĕk′tō-mē) [L. *synovia,* joint fluid, + Gr. *ektome,* excision] Excision of the synovial membrane.

synovia (sĭn-ō′vē-ă) [L.] Synovial fluid.

synovial (sĭn-ō′vē-ăl) Pert. to synovia, the lubricating fluid of the joints.

synovial bursa Bursa.

synovial crypt Diverticulum of a synovial membrane of a joint.

synovial cyst Accumulation of synovia in a bursa, synovial crypt, or sac of a synovial hernia, causing a tumor.

synovial fluid Clear viscid lubricating fluid of the joint, bursae, and tendon sheaths, secreted by the synovial membrane of a joint. It contains mucin, albumin, fat, and electrolytes. SYN: *synovia.* SEE: *joint, synovial.*

synovial fold One of the smooth folds of synovial membrane on the inner surface of the joint capsule. SYN: *plica, synovial.*

synovial hernia Protrusion of a portion of synovial membrane through a tear in the stratum fibrosum of a joint capsule.

synovial tendon sheath One of the sheaths that develop in osteofibrous canals through which tendons pass. Each is a double-layered tube; the space between the layers contains synovial fluid. SYN: *vagina mucosa tendinis.*

synovial villi Slender avascular processes on the free surface of a synovial membrane projecting into the joint cavity.

synovioma (sĭn″ō-vē-ō′mă) [L. *synovia,* joint fluid, + Gr. *oma,* tumor] A tumor arising from a synovial membrane.

synoviparous (sĭn″ō-vĭp′ă-rŭs) [″ + *parere,* to produce] Forming synovia.

synovitis (sĭn″ō-vī′tĭs) [″ + Gr. *itis,* inflammation] Inflammation of a synovial membrane. Inflammation may be the result of an aseptic wound, rheumatologic diseases, infections, a subcutaneous injury (contusion or sprain), irritation produced by damaged cartilage, overuse, or trauma. SEE: *Nursing Diagnoses Appendix.*

SYMPTOMS: The joint is painful, much more so on motion, esp. at night. It is swollen and tense. The condition may fluctuate. In synovitis of the knee, the patella is floated up from the condyles, and it can be readily depressed, to rise again when pressure is taken off. The part is never in full extension, as this increases the pain. Skin, which is very sensitive to pressure only at certain points, is neither thickened nor reddened. After a few days, when pain lessens and swelling diminishes as the effusion and extravasated blood are absorbed, the limb returns to its natural position, and recovery follows.

TREATMENT: The condition is managed symptomatically, restricting or avoiding range of motion that produces pain. Therapeutic treatments include cold, heat, ultrasound, and medications to reduce inflammation. Rehabilitation includes strengthening, flexibility, and neuromuscular regimens.

chronic s. Synovitis in which an undue amount of fluid remains in the cavity and the membrane itself is edematous. Prolonged inflammation causes thickening of the membrane and articular structures by plastic exudation and the formation of fibrous tissue, which increases joint dysfunction and exacerbates symptoms. The joint is weak but not esp. painful, except on pressure and sometimes not even then. Movements, esp. in extension, are restricted, and generally attended by crepitus or creaking. Symptoms are well marked when the patient has an excess accumulation of synovial fluid (the amount of fluid depends on the joint involved and also on the patient's body build). Fluid can be removed with a needle and syringe and sent to the laboratory for analysis.

dendritic s. Synovitis with villous growths developing in the sac.

detritic s. Inflammation and proliferation of the synovial tissues, esp. when occurring around foreign bodies (such as silicone joint prostheses) or loose bodies (such as fragments of cartilage or subchondral bone).

dry s. Synovitis with little or no effusion. SYN: *s. sicca.*

purulent s. Synovitis with purulent effusion within the sac.

serous s. Synovitis with nonpurulent, copious effusion.

s. sicca Dry s.

simple s. Synovitis with only slightly turbid, if not clear, effusion.

tendinous s. Inflammation of a tendon sheath. SYN: *vaginal s.*

vaginal s. Tendinous s.

vibration s. Synovitis resulting from a wound near a joint.

synovium (sĭn-ō′vē-ŭm) [L. *synovia,* joint fluid] A synovial membrane.

syntactic (sĭn-tăk′tĭk) Concerning or affecting syntax.

syntaxis (sĭn-tăk′sĭs) [″ + *taxis,* arrangement] A junction between two bones. SYN: *articulation.*

synthase Synthetase.

nitric oxide s. ABBR: NOS. An enzyme that synthesizes nitric oxide from arginine; present in the central nervous system, the lining of blood vessels, the heart, joints, some autonomic neurons, and other organs.

synthermal (sĭn-thĕr′măl) [″ + *therme,* heat] Having the same temperature.

synthesis (sĭn′thĕs-ĭs) [Gr.] In chemistry, the union of elements to produce compounds; the process of building up. In general, the process or processes involved in the formation of a complex substance from simpler molecules or compounds, as the synthesis of proteins from amino acids. Synthesis is the opposite of decomposition.

synthesize (sĭn″thĕ-sīz′) To produce by synthesis.

synthetase (sĭn′thĕ-tās) An enzyme that acts as a catalyst for joining two molecules with the loss or splitting off of a high-energy phosphate group. SYN: *ligase; synthase.*

ATP s. An enzyme that makes adenosine triphosphate from adenosine monophosphate.

synthetic (sĭn-thĕt′ĭk) [Gr. *synthetikos*] Rel. to or made by synthesis; artificially prepared.

synthorax (sĭn-thō′răks) [Gr. *syn,* together, + *thorax,* chest] Thoracopagus.

syntone (sĭn′tōn) [″ + *tonos,* act of stretching, tension] An individual whose personality indicates a stable responsiveness to the environment and its social demands. SEE: *syntonic.*

syntonic (sĭn-tŏn′ĭk) Pert. to a personality characterized by an even temperament, a normal emotional responsiveness to life situations; the opposite of schizoid. SEE: *syntone.*

syntonin (sĭn′tō-nĭn) An acid albumin formed by the action of dilute hydrochloric acid on muscle during gastric digestion.

syntoxoid (sĭn-tŏk′soyd) [Gr. *syn,* together, + *toxikon,* poison, + *eidos,* form, shape] A toxoid having the same degree of affinity for an antitoxin as that possessed by the toxin.

syntrophism (sĭn′trŏf-ĭzm) [″ + *trophe,* nourishment, + *-ismos,* condition] Stimulation of an organism to grow by mixing with or through the closeness of another strain.

syntrophoblast (sĭn-trŏf′ō-blăst) [″ + ″

+ *blastos,* germ] The outer syncytial layer of the trophoblast. SEE: *trophoblast.*

syntropic (sĭn-trŏp′ĭk) [″ + *trope,* a turn] Concerning syntropy.

syntropy (sĭn′trō-pē) [″ + *trope,* a turn] Turning or pointing in the same direction.

synulosis (sĭn″ū-lō′sĭs) [Gr. *synoulosis*] The formulation of scar tissue. **synulotic,** *adj.*

syphilid(e) (sĭf″ĭl-ĭd) *pl.* **syphilides** [Fr.] A skin eruption caused by secondary syphilis.

syphiliphobia (sĭf″ĭl-ĭ-fō′bē-ă) [″ + Gr. *phobos,* fear] Syphilophobia (1).

syphilis (sĭf′ĭ-lĭs) [*Syphilis,* shepherd having the disease in a Latin poem] A multistage infection caused by the spirochete *Treponema pallidum*. The disease is typically transmitted sexually, although a small number of congenital infections occur during pregnancy. In the U.S. the incidence of syphilis fluctuates from year to year and decade to decade. In 1998 only 7,000 cases of primary and secondary syphilis were reported to the Centers for Disease Control in Atlanta, marking a new low for the disease. The majority of cases in the U.S. are concentrated in the Southeastern states, among teenagers and young adults, illicit drug users, African-Americans, and patients with human immunodeficiency virus (HIV) infection. SYN: *lues*. SEE: illus.; *Standard and Universal Precautions Appendix*. **syphilitic,** *adj.*

Syphilis is typically passed from person to person by direct contact with skin or mucous membranes. Spirochetes readily penetrate skin and disseminate from the initial site of inoculation to regional lymph nodes, the bloodstream, and multiple other sites including the central nervous system. After an incubation period of 10 days to 2 months, a papule appears on the skin that develops into a painless ulcer ("chancre") that is characteristic of the *primary stage* of infection. The chancre and other skin lesions caused by syphilis are highly infectious. The genitals are the most common site of primary infection and chancre formation in syphilis.

In the *secondary stage* a widespread body rash appears, often with systemic symptoms such as fever, headache, lymph node swelling and malaise. Highly infectious moist, broad papules may appear in the perineum ("condyloma lata") along with shallow ulcers in the mouth ("mucous patches"). If the disease is not eradicated with antibiotics, it establishes latent infection that may cause multiple destructive changes in many organ systems years later.

In the *tertiary stage* tissue destruction in the aorta, the central nervous system, the bone, and the skin occurs. The consequences may include aortic aneurysm, meningitis, sensory and gait disturbances, dementia, optic atrophy, and many other illnesses.

SEROLOGICAL TESTS FOR SYPHILIS: Commonly used laboratory tests for syphilis do not have optimal sensitivity or specificity. Screening is usually performed with the nontreponemal rapid plasma reagin test or the Venereal Disease Research Laboratory test, either of which may yield inaccurate results. If either test result is positive, a confirmatory treponemal test with the microhemagglutination assay for antibody to *T. pallidum* immobilization, or with the fluorescent treponemal antibody absorbed, is performed. Two-stage testing increases the likelihood of obtaining an accurate diagnosis. The polymerase chain reaction test may be the most precise method of diagnosing syphilis, but it is not in common use outside research laboratories.

CAUTION: Individuals diagnosed with syphilis may have other sexually transmitted illnesses, esp. HIV infection. Public health experts recommend testing all individuals with either disease for the other.

TREATMENT: Long-acting preparations of penicillin are typically given to

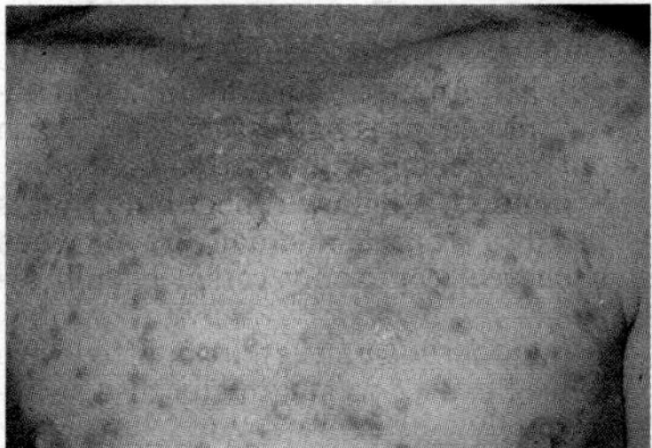

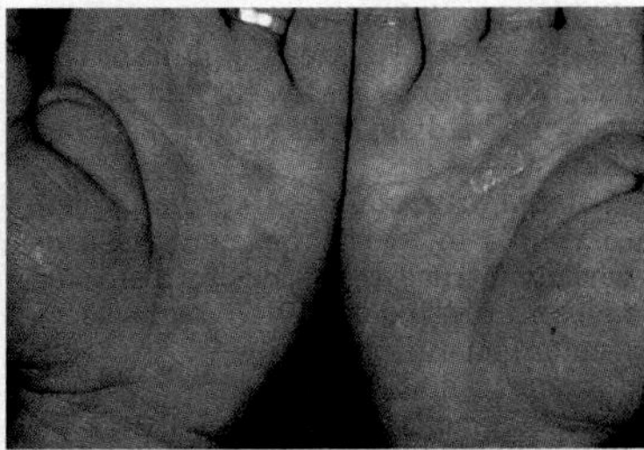

SYPHILIS

Secondary syphilitic rash on chest and palm

patients with syphilis. The duration of treatment varies depending on the stage of the disease and on whether there are comorbid illnesses, such as HIV infection, or complications, such as evidence of neurosyphilis. Doxycycline or tetracycline may be substituted in patients who are allergic to penicillin.

PATIENT CARE: The patient is taught about the illness and the importance of locating all contacts, treatment, and follow-up care. Penicillin is administered as prescribed or an alternative antibiotic is given if the patient is allergic to penicillin. The patient is referred to a public health agency to assist in identifying contacts. Preventive methods are taught, and supportive counseling is provided. Caution should be used when handling laboratory specimens. The patient should avoid sexual contact with anyone until the full course of therapy has been completed, including previous partners who have not received adequate evaluation and treatment, if indicated, for syphilis. Secretory precautions are instituted from the time the disease is suspected until 24 hr after initiation of proper antibiotic therapy. SEE: *Standard and Universal Precautions Appendix.*

cardiovascular s. Tertiary syphilis involving the heart and great blood vessels, esp. the aorta. Saccular aneurysms of the aorta and aortic insufficiency frequently result.

congenital s. Syphilis transmitted from the mother to the fetus in utero. Transplacental fetal infection may occur if a pregnant woman is not treated by the 18th week of gestation or contracts the disease later in pregnancy. SYN: *prenatal s.* SEE: *Nursing Diagnoses Appendix.*

endemic s. Chronic, nonvenereal syphilis infection of childhood. It is characterized in its early stages by mucocutaneous or membrane lesions. Later, gummas of bone and skin occur. The causative organism is *T. pallidum.* Penicillin is the treatment of choice.

extragenital s. Syphilis in which the primary chancre is located elsewhere than on genital organs.

latent s. The phase of syphilis during which symptoms are absent and the disease can be diagnosed only by serological tests.

meningovascular s. A form of neurosyphilis in which the meninges and vascular structures of the brain and spinal cord are involved. It may be localized or general.

prenatal s. Congenital s.

serological tests for s. ABBR: STS. Nonspecific blood tests for syphilis. Two general types are available: (1) Procedures that identify the presence of a nontreponemal antibody against a lipoidal agent that is generated in response to infection with *Treponema pallidum* (i.e., a reagin). These tests include the Wassermann, the Venereal Disease Research Laboratory, and the rapid plasma reagin tests. (2) An antibody-specific test, the fluorescent treponemal antibody absorption (FTA-ABS) procedure. Because of a high rate of false-positive findings by the nonspecific antibody tests, diagnosis of syphilitic infection is established by the more accurate FTA test.

visceral s. Syphilis in which visceral organs are involved.

syphilitic macule One of the small red eruptions manifested in secondary syphilis, often covering the entire body. These eruptions are associated with chancre or scar, alopecia, pain in bones, swollen glands, and sore throat.

syphiloderm, syphiloderma (sĭf′ĭl-ō-dĕrm″, sĭf″ĭl-ō-dĕr′mă) [″ + Gr. *derma,* skin] A syphilitic cutaneous disorder.

syphiloid (sĭf′ĭ-loyd) [″ + Gr. *eidos,* form, shape] Resembling syphilis.

syphilology (sĭf″ĭl-ŏl′ō-jē) The study of syphilis and its treatment.

syphiloma (sĭf″ĭl-ō′mă) [″ + Gr. *oma,* tumor] A syphilitic tumor; a gumma.

syphilomania (sĭf″ĭl-ō-mā′nē-ă) [″ + Gr. *mania,* madness] Syphilophobia (1).

syphilophobia (sĭf″ĭl-ō-fō′bē-ă) [″ + Gr. *phobos,* fear] **1.** A morbid fear of syphilis. **2.** A delusion of having syphilis.

syphilophobic (sĭf″ĭl-ō-fō′bĭk) Pert. to or affected with syphilophobia.

syphilotherapy (sĭf″ĭl-ō-thĕr′ă-pē) [″ + Gr. *therapeia,* treatment] The treatment of syphilis.

syr [L., *syrupus*] Syrup.

syrigmophonia (sĭr″ĭg-mō-fō′nē-ă) [Gr. *syrigmos,* a whistle, + *phone,* voice] **1.** A sibilant rale. **2.** A whistling sound in pronunciation of "s" due to a denture peculiarity.

syrigmus (sĭr-ĭg′mŭs) [Gr. *syrigmos,* a whistle] A subjective sound such as a hissing or ringing heard in the ears.

syringadenoma (sĭr-ĭng″ă-dē-nō′mă) [Gr. *syrinx,* pipe, + *aden,* gland, + *oma,* tumor] Tumor of a sweat gland.

syringe (sĭr-ĭnj′, sĭr′ĭng) [Gr. *syrinx,* pipe] **1.** An instrument for injecting fluids into cavities or vessels. **2.** To wash out or introduce fluid with a syringe.

hand s. A hollow rubber bulb that is fitted to a nozzle and delivers air when squeezed; commonly called a bulb syringe.

hypodermic s. A syringe, fitted with a needle, used to administer drugs subdermally.

oral s. A syringe made of plastic or glass. It is not fitted with a needle but is graduated and is used to dispense liquid medication to children. The tip is constructed to prevent its breaking in the child's mouth.

syringectomy (sĭr″ĭn-jĕk′tō-mē) [″ + *ektome,* excision] Removal of the walls of a fistula.

syringocarcinoma (sĭ-rĭng″gō-kăr″sĭ-nō′mă) [″ + *karkinos,* crab, + *oma,* tumor] Carcinoma of a sweat gland.

syringocele (sĭr-ĭn′gō-sēl) [″ + *koilia,* cavity] **1.** The central canal of the myelon or spinal cord. **2.** A form of meningomyelocele that contains a cavity in the ectopic spinal cord.

syringocystadenoma (sĭr-ĭn″gō-sĭs″tă-dĕ-nō′mă) [″ + *kystis,* bladder, sac, + *aden,* gland, + *oma,* tumor] Adenoma of the sweat glands, characterized by tiny, hard, papular formations.

syringocystoma (sĭr-ĭn″gō-sĭs-tō′mă) [″ + ″ + *oma,* tumor] A cystic tumor having its origin in ducts of the sweat gland.

syringoencephalomyelia (sĭ-rĭng″gō-ĕn-sĕf″ă-lō-mī-ē′lē-ă) [″ + *enkephalos,* brain, + *myelos,* marrow] A condition of cavities in the brain and spinal cord.

syringoid (sĭr-ĭn′goyd) [Gr. *syrinx,* pipe, + *eidos,* form, shape] Resembling a tube; fistulous.

syringoma (sĭr″ĭn-gō′mă) [″ + *oma,* tumor] A tumor of the sweat glands.

syringomeningocele (sĭr-ĭn″gō-mĕn-ĭn′gō-sēl) [″ + *meninx,* membrane, + *kele,* tumor, swelling] A meningocele that is similar to a syringomyelocele.

syringomyelia (sĭr-ĭn″gō-mī-ē′lē-ă) [″ + *myelos,* marrow] A disease of the spinal cord characterized by the development of a cyst or cavities with the cord. It usually begins at the site of a congenital malformation of the cerebellum, but sometimes results from spinal cord trauma, tumors, or after spinal cord infection. SEE: *Nursing Diagnoses Appendix.*

SYMPTOMS: Depending on the location of the syrinx, there may be pain, sensory losses, paralysis, or autonomic dysfunction.

TREATMENT: Some patients are managed conservatively. Sudden enlargement of a cavity may warrant surgical intervention with decompression of the cavity. Persistent pain may necessitate chordotomy or medullary tractotomy for relief.

syringomyelitis (sĭr-ĭn″gō-mī″ĕ-lī′tĭs) [″ + *myelos,* marrow, + *itis,* inflammation] Inflammation coincident with abnormal dilation of the central canal of the spinal cord.

syringomyelocele (sĭr-ĭn″gō-mī″ĕl-ō-sēl) [″ + ″ + *kele,* tumor, swelling] A form of spina bifida in which the cavity of the projecting portion communicates with the central canal of the spinal cord.

syringomyelus (sĭr-ĭn″gō-mī′ĕl-ŭs) An abnormal dilatation of the central canal of the spinal cord.

syringopontia (sĭr-ĭn″gō-pŏn′shē-ă) [″ + L. *pons,* bridge] Cavity formation in the pons varolii similar to syringomyelia.

syringosystrophy (sĭr-ĭn″gō-sĭs′trō-fē) [″ + *systrophe,* a twist] Twisting of the oviduct.

syringotomy (sĭr″ĭn-gŏt′ō-mē) An operation for incision of a fistula.

syrinx (sĭr′ĭnks) [Gr., pipe] **1.** A tube or pipe. **2.** A pathological cavity (cyst) in the spinal cord or brain. **3.** A fistula.

syrup (sĭr′ŭp) [L. *syrupus*] ABBR: syr. A concentrated solution of sugar in water to which specific medicinal substances are usually added. Syrups usually do not represent a very high percentage of the active drug. Some syrups are used principally to give a pleasant odor and taste to solutions.

simple s. A combination of purified water and sucrose.

syssarcosis (sĭs″ăr-kō′sĭs) [Gr. *syn,* together, + *sarkosis,* fleshy growth] The union of bones by muscles; a muscular articulation such as the hyoid and patella.

systaltic (sĭs-tăl′tĭk) [Gr. *systaltikos,* contracting] An obsolete term for pulsating.

system (sĭs′tĕm) [Gr. *systema,* a composite whole] **1.** An organized grouping of related structures or parts. **2.** A group of structures or organs related to each other and performing certain functions together (e.g., the digestive system). **3.** A group of cells or aggregations of cells that perform a particular function (e.g., the mononuclear phagocyte, and the cardiovascular, respiratory, and central nervous systems).

alimentary s. Digestive system.

cardiovascular s. The heart and blood vessels (aorta, arteries, arterioles, capillaries, venules, veins, venae cavae).

centimeter-gram-second s. ABBR: CGS. An early version of the SI units system, no longer in use.

central nervous s. ABBR: CNS. The brain and spinal cord. SEE: *brain* and *cranial nerve* for illus.

COMPOSITION: Nerve tissue that forms the brain and spinal cord consists of gray and white matter. Gray matter is made of the cell bodies of neurons, and white matter is made of the axons and dendrites of these neurons. White matter transmits impulses within the CNS.

chromaffin s. The mass of tissue forming paraganglia and medulla of suprarenal glands, which secretes epinephrine and stains readily with chromium salts. Similar tissue is found in the organs of Zuckerkandl and in the liver, testes, ovary, and heart. SYN: *chromaffin tissue.*

circulatory s. A system concerned with circulation of body fluids. It includes the cardiovascular and lymphatic systems.

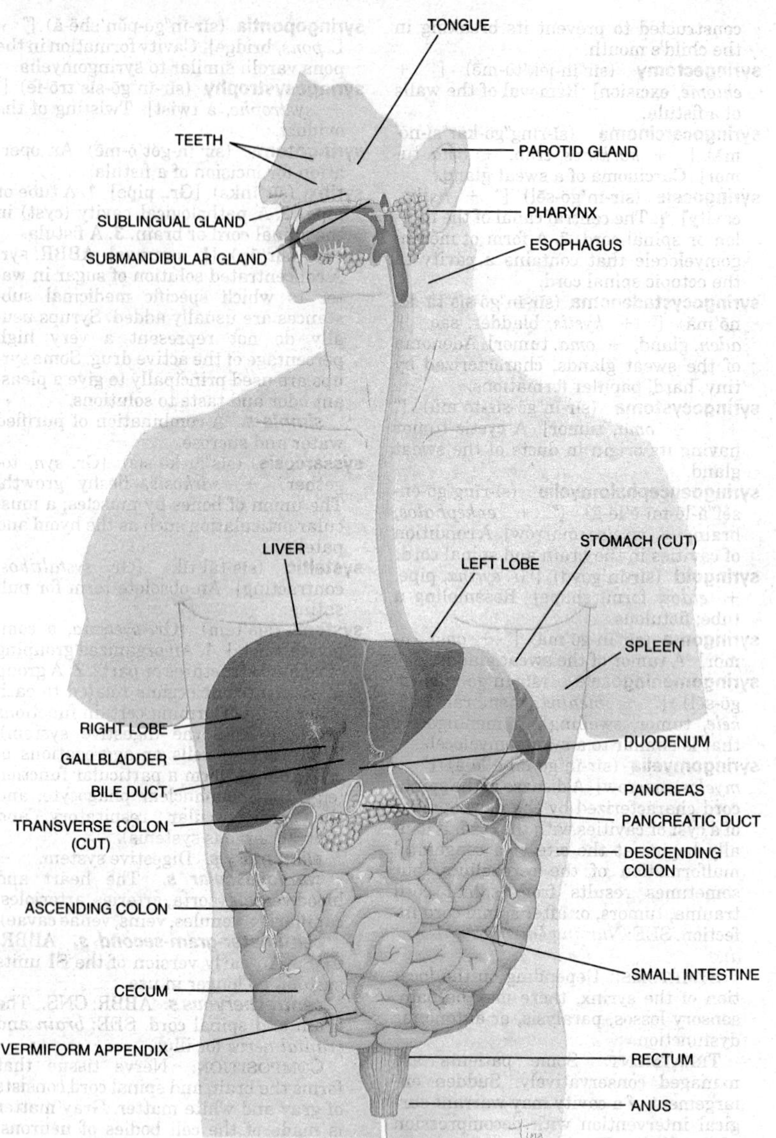

THE DIGESTIVE SYSTEM
(With spleen shown)

cytochrome transport s. The last stage in aerobic cell respiration. SYN: *electron transport c.*

digestive s. The alimentary canal (oral cavity, pharynx, esophagus, stomach, small and large intestines) and the accessory organs (teeth, tongue, salivary glands, liver, and pancreas). SEE: *digestive system; digestion;* illus.

endocrine s. The ductless glands or the glands of internal secretion, which include the pineal gland, hypothalamus, pituitary, thyroid, parathyroid, adrenal glands, ovaries, testes, and pancreas. SEE: *endocrine gland.*

enteric nervous s. The millions of nerve fibers of the alimentary tube, arranged in the submucosal and myenteric plexuses, which regulate the motility and secretions of the gastrointestinal tract. This system is connected to the central nervous system by sympathetic and parasympathetic pathways, but can function independently of the CNS.

extrapyramidal motor s. The functional system that includes all descending fibers arising in cortical and subcortical motor centers that reach the medulla and spinal cord by pathways other than recognized corticospinal tracts. The system is important in maintenance of equilibrium and muscle tone.

genital s. Reproductive s.

genitourinary s. The urinary and reproductive systems, which are anatomically adjacent in the adult and develop from the same mesodermal ridge in the embryo. In men, the urethra is part of both systems. In women, the systems are entirely separate, but infections and other diseases in one may affect the other. SEE: *genitalia* for illus.

haversian s. Architectural unit of bone consisting of a central tube (haversian canal) with alternate layers of intercellular material (matrix) surrounding it in concentric cylinders. Alternating layers of matrix and cells are called haversian lamellae.

health care s. An organized system that manages and provides treatments and preventive services for healthy, sick, and injured. Elements include physicians and their assistants, dentists and their associates, nurses and their surrogates, the various levels of diagnostic and care facilities, voluntary organizations, medical administrators including those in hospitals and government agencies, the medical insurance industry, and the pharmaceutical and medical device manufacturers. An ideal health care system would emphasize preventive medicine and encourage preventive self-care; enable access to primary care for assessment of and assistance with health problems; provide secondary or acute care involving emergency medical services and complex medical and surgical services; facilitate tertiary care for patients who need referral to facilities that provide rehabilitative services; offer respite care to allow families temporary relief from the daily tasks of caring for individuals for whom they are responsible; provide continuing supportive services for those whose mental or physical illness or disability is such that they need assistance with everyday tasks of living (e.g., home health and nursing home care); and provide hospice care for those with terminal illnesses, all at a reasonable cost.

hematopoietic s. The blood-forming tissues and organs of the body. It includes the bone marrow, spleen, and lymphatic tissue.

heterogeneous s. Any system whose components may be separated mechanically.

homogeneous s. Any system whose components cannot be separated mechanically.

hypophyseoportal s. The series of vessels that lead from the hypothalamus to the anterior lobe of the pituitary. The releasing hormones are carried to the pituitary through this system.

integumentary s. The skin and its derivatives (hair, nails) and the subcutaneous tissue.

International S. of Units ABBR: SI. The modern version of the metric system. SEE: *SI Units Appendix.*

lymphatic s. The system concerned with lymph circulation, the protection of the body against pathogens, and the establishment of immunity to certain diseases. It includes lymph vessels and lymph nodes. SEE: *lymph; lymphatic.*

metric s. A system of weights and measures based on the meter (39.37 in.) as the unit of linear measure; the kilogram as the unit of mass; and the liter (1.057 qt) as the unit of volume. SEE: Metric System and SI Units in *Units of Measurements Appendix.*

microsomal ethanol oxidizing s. ABBR: MEOS. A hepatic enzyme system that catabolizes drugs and other potentially toxic substances. Ethanol ingested in relatively small amounts is catabolized by the hepatic enzyme alcohol dehydrogenase. Whenever ingested amounts of ethanol are large enough to overcome or deplete the alcohol dehydrogenase system, the microsomal ethanol oxidizing system (MEOS) becomes the major route for ethanol catabolism. Ethanol breakdown by the MEOS is not thought to produce as much energy as alcohol dehydrogenase breakdown, resulting in less weight gain than would be expected from the ethanol calories consumed.

movement s. The physiological components that function together to produce motion at a joint or multiple body segments. The components include the support and base; modulating nerves and muscles; cardiovascular and pulmonary reserves; and cognitive-affective elements. Physical therapists, kinesiologists, and specialists in physical medicine are trained to manage the components of the movement system.

muscular s. The system that includes the skeletal muscles and their tendons. SEE: *muscle.*

needleless intravenous infusion s. A device for administering intravenous solutions that permits intravascular access without the necessity of handling a needle. These systems were developed to reduce the number of needle-stick injuries related to traditional intravenous administration of fluids. The possibility

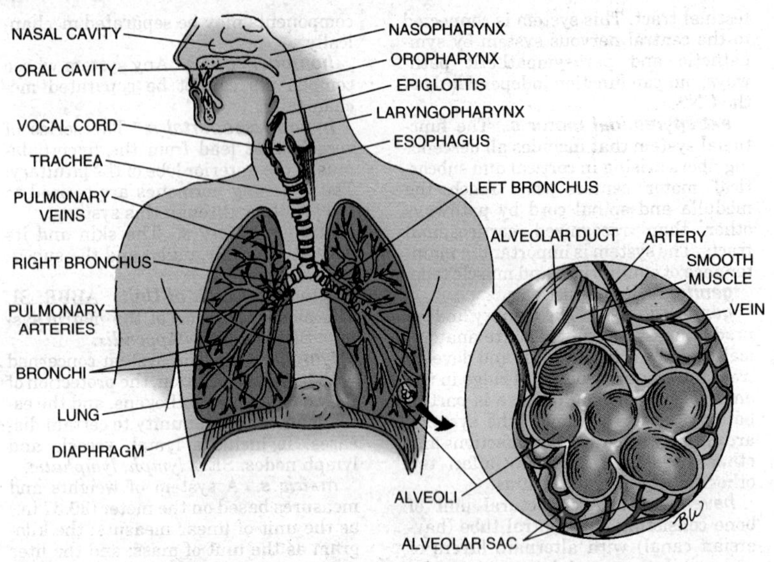

RESPIRATORY SYSTEM

(A) anterior view, (B) alveoli and pulmonary capillaries

that their use increases the patient's chance of infection is being investigated. SEE: *needle-stick injury*.

osseous s. The bony structures of the body; the skeleton. SEE: *skeleton*.

oxygen delivery s. An apparatus that provides a concentration of inhaled oxygen greater than that of room air. A *fixed-performance* oxygen delivery system provides a consistent oxygen concentration. A *variable-performance* oxygen delivery system provides an oxygen concentration that may vary with changes in the patient's breathing pattern.

peripheral nervous s. The cranial nerves and spinal nerves. SEE: *nervous system*.

portal s. A system of vessels in which blood passes through a capillary network, a large vessel, and then another capillary network before returning to the systemic circulation (e.g., the circulation of blood through the liver).

prosthetic control s. A mechanical system of cables and attachments that, used with a harness, permits the wearer of a prosthetic device to perform desired movements, such as grasping objects.

reproductive s. The gonads and their associated structures and ducts. In the female, this system includes the ovaries, uterine tubes (oviducts), uterus, vagina, and vulva. In the male, it includes the testes, efferent ducts, epididymis, ductus deferens, ejaculatory duct, urethra and accessory glands (bulbourethral, prostate, seminal vesicles), and penis. SYN: *genital s.* SEE: *female genitalia* and *male genitalia* for illus.

respiratory s. The organs involved in the interchange of gases between an organism and the atmosphere. In humans, this system consists of the air passageways and organs (nasal cavities, pharynx, larynx, trachea, and lungs, including bronchi, bronchioles, alveolar ducts, and alveoli) and the respiratory muscles. SEE: illus.; *lung* for illus.

reticuloendothelial s. ABBR: RES. Old name for the system of monocytes, macrophages, and dendritic phagocytes and antigen presenting cells found in the blood and lymphoid tissues. This system is now called the mononuclear phagocytic system. SEE: *macrophage*.

seating s. Adapted seating device.

skeletal s. The bony framework of the body. SEE: *skeleton*.

sympathetic nervous s. The thoracolumbar division of the autonomic nervous system. Preganglionic fibers originate in the thoracic and lumbar segments of the spinal cord and synapse with postganglionic neurons in the sympathetic ganglia. Most of these ganglia are in two chains lateral to the backbone, and others are within the trunk; postganglionic fibers extend to the organs innervated. Some effects of sympathetic stimulation are increased heart rate, dilation of the bronchioles, dilation of the pupils, vasoconstriction in the skin and viscera, vasodilation in the skeletal muscles, slowing of peristalsis, conversion of glycogen to glucose by the liver, and secretion of epinephrine and norephinephrine by the adrenal medulla. Sympathetic effects are general rather than specific and prepare the body to cope with stressful situations. SEE: *autonomic nervous system* for illus.; *parasympathetic nervous system.*

token economy s. Any program using positive reinforcement (operant conditioning) to teach or train desired skills or behaviors.

urinary s. The kidneys, ureters, bladder, and urethra.

urogenital s. The urinary and reproductive systems combined. SEE: *genitalia* for illus.

vaccine adverse event reporting s. ABBR: VAERS. A national surveillance system for monitoring undesirable reactions to administered vaccines.

vascular s. The system of all the blood vessels (arteries, capillaries, and veins).

vasomotor s. The part of the nervous system that controls the size of the vascular system vessels.

vegetative nervous s. An out-of-date term for the autonomic nervous system. SEE: *autonomic nervous system.*

visceral efferent s. An out-of-date term for the autonomic nervous system. SEE: *autonomic nervous system.*

systema (sĭs-tē′mă) [Gr., a composite whole] System.

systematic (sĭs″tĕ-măt′ĭk) Concerning a system or organized according to a system.

systematization (sĭs-tĕm″ă-tī-zā′shŭn) The process of organizing something according to a plan.

systemic (sĭs-tĕm′ĭk) Pert. to a whole body rather than to one of its parts; somatic.

systemic circulation The blood flow from the left ventricle through the aorta and all its branches (arteries) to the capillaries of the tissues and its return to the heart through veins and the venae cavae, which empty into the right atrium.

systemic remedy A remedy that acts on the body as a whole.

Systematized Nomenclature of Medicine ABBR: SNOMED. A systematized collection of medically useful terms published by the American College of Pathologists. The words in the collection are arranged in various fields to permit coding, computerization, sorting, and retrieval of large amounts of information from medical records.

systemoid (sĭs′tĕ-moyd) [″ + *eidos,* form, shape] **1.** Resembling a system. **2.** Pert. to tumors made up of several types of tissues.

Systems Model Neuman's systems model.

system theory, general A theory developed by Ludwig von Bertalanffy, which asserts that all living systems are open systems constantly exchanging information, matter, and energy with the environment. There are three levels of reference for systems: the system level on which one is focusing, such as a person; the suprasystems level above the focal system, such as the person's family, community, and culture; and the subsystem, that below the focal system, such as the bodily systems and the cell. The theory suggests that the treatment of people is more important than the treatment of illnesses. SEE: *holistic medicine.*

systole (sĭs′tō-lē) [Gr., contraction] Contraction of the chambers of the heart. The myocardial fibers shorten, making the chamber smaller and forcing blood out. In the cardiac cycle, atrial systole precedes ventricular systole, which pumps blood into the aorta and pulmonary artery. SEE: *diastole; murmur; presystole.*

aborted s. A premature cardiac systole in which arterial pressure is increased little if at all because of inadequate filling of ventricles resulting from shortening of the preceding diastole.

anticipated s. A systole that is aborted because it occurs before the ventricle is filled.

arterial s. The rebound or recoil of the stretched elastic walls of the arteries following ventricular systole.

atrial s. The contraction of the atria; it precedes the ventricular systole.

electrical s. The total duration of the QRST complex in an electrocardiogram; it occurs just before the mechanical systole.

premature s. Extrasystole.

ventricular s. Ventricular contraction.

systolic (sĭs-tŏl′ĭk) [Gr. *systole,* contraction] Pert. to the systole.

systolic discharge An outdated term for ejection fraction.

systolic murmur A cardiac murmur during systole.

systolic pressure Maximum blood pressure. This occurs during contraction of the ventricle. SEE: *blood pressure; diastolic pressure; pulse; pulse pressure.*

systremma (sĭs-trĕm′ă) [Gr. *systremma,* anything twisted together] A cramp in the calf of the leg, the muscles forming a hard knot.

syzygiology (sĭ-zĭj″ē-ŏl′ō-jē) [″ + *logos,* word, reason] The study of interdependence or interrelationship of the whole as opposed to that of isolated functions or separate parts. SEE: *holism.*

syzygium (sĭ-zĭj′ē-ŭm) [Gr. *syzygia,* conjunction] Fusion of two parts or structures without loss of identity of the parts. **syzygial,** *adj.*

syzygy (sĭz′ĭ-jē) Fusion of organs, each remaining distinct.

T

T *temperature; time; intraocular tension.*
t *temporal;* L. *ter,* three times.
T1, T2, etc. *first thoracic nerve, second thoracic nerve,* and so forth.
$T_{1/2}$, $t_{1/2}$ In nuclear medicine, the symbol of half-life of a radioactive substance.
T_3 *triiodothyronine.*
T_4 *thyroxine.*
T-1824 Evans blue.
T.A. *toxin-antitoxin.*
Ta Symbol for the element tantalum.
tabacosis (tăb″ă-kō′sĭs) [″ + Gr. *osis,* condition] Chronic tobacco poisoning or pneumoconiosis from inhaling tobacco dust.
tabanid (tăb′ă-nĭd) [L. *tabanus,* horsefly] A member of the dipterous family Tabanidae.
Tabanidae (tă-băn′ĭ-dē) [L. *tabanus,* horsefly] A family of insects belonging to the order Diptera. It includes horseflies, gadflies, deer flies, and mango flies, all bloodsucking insects that attack humans and other warm-blooded animals. Tabanidae is of medical importance because flies serve as vectors of the filaria worm, *Loa loa,* tularemia, and other diseases. Their bites are extremely painful and heal slowly.
Tabanus (tă-bā′nŭs) [L., horsefly] A genus of flies of the family Tabanidae.
tabardillo (tăb″ăr-dē′lyō) [Sp.] An epidemic louse-borne typhus fever occurring in parts of Mexico. SEE: *typhus.*
tabatière anatomique (tă-bă″tē-ār′ ă-nă″tō-mēk′) [Fr., anatomical snuffbox] The triangular area of the dorsum of the hand at the base of the thumb. When the thumb is extended, the tendons of the long and short extensor muscles of the thumb bound this area, which appears as a depression. When snuff was used, a small pinch could be placed in this "box" and snuffed up into the nose from that site. Tenderness in this area may be present when the navicular bone is fractured. SYN: *anatomical snuffbox.*
tabella (tă-bĕl′ă) *pl.* **tabellae** [L., tablet] A medicated mass of material formed into a small disk. SEE: *lozenge; tablet; troche.*
tabes (tā′bēz) [L., wasting disease] A gradual, progressive wasting in any chronic disease.

diabetic t. Peripheral neuritis affecting diabetics; may affect the spinal cord and simulate tabes caused by syphilis.

t. dorsalis A form of neurosyphilis, in which the dorsal roots of sensory nerves are damaged by inflammation. It causes problems in coordinating muscles for voluntary movement and ambulation (locomotor ataxia), which produce a staggering gait, absence of deep tendon reflexes (e.g., at the ankles), and loss of pain in the lower extremities, interrupted occasionally by flashes of sharp pain (lightning pains). Tabes is frequently seen in combination with the other forms of neurosyphilis, meningitis, and dementia. Physical therapy and teaching are needed to reduce the risk of falls. Penicillin G is the treatment of choice; for penicillin-allergic persons, tetracyclines are used. SYN: *locomotor ataxia.* SEE: *syphilis.*

t. ergotica Tabes resulting from the use of ergot.

t. mesenterica Emaciation and malnutrition caused by engorgement and tubercular degeneration of the mesenteric glands.

tabetic (tă-bĕt′ĭk) [L. *tabes,* wasting disease] Pert. to or afflicted with tabes.

t. foot Twisted foot in locomotor ataxia.

tabetiform (tă-bĕt′ĭ-form) [″ + *forma,* shape] Resembling or characteristic of tabes.
tablature (tăb′lă-chūr) The formation of the cranial bones into two outer hard layers and a spongy center, the diploë.
table (tā′bl) [L. *tabula,* board] **1.** A flat-topped structure, as an operating table. **2.** A thin flat plate, as of bone.

t. of the skull The inner and outer layers of a cranial bone, made of compact bone. These are separated by diploë, spongy bone that contains red bone marrow.

tilt t. A table that can be inclined or tipped over while a person is strapped to it. It is used to study patients with loss of consciousness of unknown cause.

vitreous t. The inner cranial table.

water t. The level at which rock or any underground stratum is saturated with water. This overlies an impervious stratum.

tablespoon (tā′bl-spoon) ABBR: Tbs. A rough measure, equal approx. to 15 ml of fluid. To administer a tablespoon of medicine, 15 ml of the substance should be given.
tablet (tăb′lĕt) [O.Fr. *tablete,* a small table] A small, disklike mass of medicinal powder.

buccal t. A tablet designed to be placed in the mouth and held between the cheek and gum until dissolved and absorbed through the buccal mucosa.

coated t. A type of tablet usually made by enclosing a drug in a protective shell.

compressed t. A tablet made by forcibly compressing powdered medications into the desired shape to decrease their solubility. These tablets may be very hard and not readily soluble.

dispensing t. A tablet that contains a clinically effective large amount of an active drug.

enteric-coated t. A tablet that resists digestion in gastric acid.

fluoride t. A tablet of sodium fluoride for prevention of dental caries and osteoporosis.

hypodermic t. A tablet used to form injectable solutions.

sublingual t. A small, flat, oval tablet placed beneath the tongue to permit direct absorption of the active substance.

t. triturate A tablet made by moistening the medication mixed with a powdered lactose or sucrose, and then molding it into shape and allowing the liquid to evaporate. They usually disintegrate readily.

tablier (tă-blyā′) [Fr., apron] Pudendal apron; enlarged vulvae. SEE: *Hottentot apron.*

taboo [Polynesian *tabu, tapu,* inviolable] An act, object, or social custom separated or set aside as being sacred or profane, thus forbidden for general use.

taboparalysis (tā″bō-păr-ăl′ĭ-sĭs) [L. *tabes,* wasting disease, + Gr. *paralyein,* to disable] Tabes associated concurrently with general paralysis. SYN: *taboparesis.*

taboparesis (tā″bō-păr-ē′sĭs, -păr′ĕ-sĭs) [″ + Gr. *paresis,* relaxation] Taboparalysis.

tabophobia (tā″bō-fō′bē-ă) [″ + Gr. *phobos,* fear] An unusual fear of being afflicted with tabes dorsalis (neurosyphilis).

tabular (tăb′ū-lăr) [L. *tabula,* board] **1.** Resembling a table. **2.** Set up in columns, as a tabulation.

t. bone A flat bone, or one with two compact bonelike parts with cancellous tissue between them.

tabun Ethyl *N*-dimethylphosphoramidocyanidate; an extremely toxic nerve gas.

tache (tŏsh) [Fr., spot] A colored spot or macule on the skin, as a freckle.

t. bleuâtre Macula caerulea.

t. cérébrale The red line that occurs in meningitis and other neurological disorders when a fingernail is drawn across the skin.

t. motrice The motor endplate of a striated muscle fiber.

t. noire A small round or oval ulcer covered by a black scab; the primary lesion of boutonneuse fever and rickettsialpox.

tachetic (tăk-ĕt′ĭk) [Fr. *tache,* spot] Marked by purple or reddish blue patches (taches).

tachistoscope (tă-kĭs′tō-skōp) [Gr. *tachistos,* swiftest, + *skopein,* to view] A device used to determine the speed of visual perception. The time of exposure can be adjusted so that the length of time needed for detection of the viewed object can be measured.

tachy- Combining form meaning *swift, rapid.*

tachyarrhythmia (tăk″ē-ă-rĭth′mē-ă) [Gr. *tachys,* swift, + *a,* not, + *rhythmos,* rhythm] Any cardiac rhythm disturbance in which the heart rate exceeds 100 beats per minute.

tachycardia (tăk″ē-kăr′dē-ă) [″ + *kardia,* heart] An abnormally rapid heart rate, greater than 100 beats per minute in adults. SYN: *accelerated p.*

atrial t. Rapid heart rate arising from an irritable focus in the atria, with a rate of less than 220 beats per minute.

atrioventricular reentrant t. ABBR: AVNRT. A narrow complex tachycardia that results from abnormal conduction of electrical impulses through a self-sustaining circuit in the atrioventricular node. SEE: *re-entry.*

ectopic t. A rapid heartbeat caused by stimuli arising from outside the sinoatrial node.

fetal t. A fetal heart rate faster than 160 beats per minute that persists throughout one 10-min period.

multifocal atrial t. ABBR: MAT. A cardiac arrhythmia that sometimes is confused with atrial fibrillation, because the heart rate is greater than 100 beats per minute and the ventricular response is irregular. However, in MAT p waves are clearly visible on the electrocardiogram, and they have at least three distinct shapes. MAT is seen most often in patients with poorly compensated chronic obstructive lung disease. It may resolve with management of the underlying respiratory problem.

nodal t. Tachycardia resulting from an arrhythmogenic focus in the atrioventricular node. It may be the result of digitalis therapy.

pacemaker-mediated t. A problem of dual-chamber cardiac pacemakers in which tachycardia develops due to improper functioning of the pacemaker. This can be treated by reprogramming the electronic signals to the atrium.

paroxysmal atrial t. A term formerly used for paroxysmal supraventricular tachycardia (an arrhythmia that begins and ends suddenly).

paroxysmal nodal t. Tachycardia due to increased activity of the AV junctional focus. The rate is usually from 120 to 180 beats per minute.

paroxysmal supraventricular t. ABBR: PSVT. A sporadically occurring arrhythmia with an atrial rate that is usually 160 to 200 beats per minute. It originates above the bundle of His, and typically appears on the surface electrocardiogram as a rapid, narrow-complex tachycardia. This relatively common arrhythmia may revert to sinus rhythm with rest, sedation, vagal maneuvers, or drug therapy (e.g., adenosine or verapamil).

paroxysmal ventricular t. Ventricular tachycardia beginning and ending suddenly.

polymorphic ventricular t. Torsade de pointes.

reflex t. Tachycardia resulting from stimuli outside the heart, reflexly accelerating the heart rate or depressing vagal tone.

sinus t. A rapid heart rate (over 100 beats per minute) originating in the sinoatrial node of the heart. It may be caused by fevers, exercise, dehydration, bleeding, stimulant drugs (e.g., epinephrine, aminophyline), thyrotoxicosis, or many other diseases or conditions.

TREATMENT: The underlying cause is addressed.

ventricular t. ABBR: VT. Three or more consecutive ventricular ectopic complexes (duration greater than 120 ms) occurring at a rate of 100 to 250 beats per minute. Although non-sustained VT may occasionally be well-tolerated, it often arises in hearts that have suffered ischemic damage or cardiomyopathic degeneration and may be a cause of sudden death. Non-sustained VT lasts less than 30 sec. Sustained VT lasts more than 30 sec, and is much more likely to produce loss of consciousness or other life-threatening symptoms. SEE: illus.

TREATMENT: The acute treatment of sustained VT is outlined in advanced life support protocols but may include the administration of lidocaine or other antiarrhythmic drugs, cardioversion, or defibrillation. Chronic, recurring VT may be treated with sotalol, amiodarone, or implantable cardioverter-defibrillators.

wide complex t. ABBR: WCT. An arrhythmia with a sustained rate of more than 100 beats per minute in which the surface electrocardiogram reveals QRS complexes lasting at least 120 msec. WCT is usually caused by ventricular tachycardia, although it may occasionally result from a supraventricular tachycardia whose conduction through the ventricles produces an abnormally wide QRS complex.

tachycardia-bradycardia syndrome A form of sick sinus syndrome; a group of arrhythmias produced by a defect in the sinus node impulse generation or conduction. Arrhythmias associated may include supraventricular tachycardias, atrial fibrillation, atrial flutter that alternates with sinus arrest, and sinus bradycardia.

tachycardiac (tăk″ē-kăr′dē-ăk) [Gr. *tachys,* swift, + *kardia,* heart] Pert. to or afflicted with tachycardia.

tachygastria Increased rate of contractions of the stomach.

tachylalia (tăk″ē-lā′lē-ă) [″ + *lalein,* to speak] Rapid speech.

tachyphasia (tăk″ē-fā′zē-ă) [″ + *phasis,* speech] Tachyphrasia.

tachyphrasia (tăk″ē-frā′zē-ă) [″ + *phrasis,* speech] Excessive volubility or rapidity of speech, as seen in mania and some other psychotic illnesses. SYN: *tachyphasia.*

tachyphrenia (tăk″ē-frē′nē-ă) [″ + *phren,* mind] Abnormally rapid mental activity.

tachyphylaxis (tăk″ē-fī-lăk′sĭs) [″ + *phylaxis,* protection] **1.** Rapid immunization to a toxic dose of a substance by previously injecting tiny doses of the same substance. **2.** Diminishing responsiveness to a drug after routine usage.

tachypnea (tăk″ĭp-nē′ă) [″ + *pnoia,* breath] Abnormally rapid respiration.

nervous t. An out-of-date term for panic attack. SEE: *alkalosis, respiratory; hyperventilation.*

transient t. of the newborn ABBR: TTN. A self-limited condition often affecting newborns who have experienced intrauterine hypoxia resulting from aspiration of amniotic fluid, delayed clearance of fetal lung fluid, or both. Signs of respiratory distress commonly appear within 6 hr after birth, improve within 24 to 48 hr, and resolve within 72 hours of birth, without respiratory assistance.

tachyrhythmia (tăk″ē-rĭth′mē-ă) [″ + *rhythmos,* rhythm] **1.** Tachycardia. **2.** Increase in the frequency of brain waves in electroencephalography up to 12 to 50 per second.

tachysterol (tă-kĭs′tĕ-rŏl) One of the isomers of ergosterol. It is a compound related to vitamin D.

tacrine A drug sometimes used to treat Alzheimer's disease. It does not cure the illness, but it reduces signs and symptoms of impaired thinking.

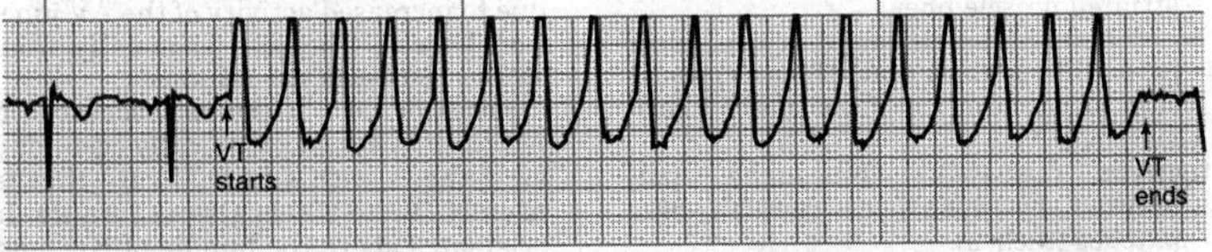

VENTRICULAR TACHYCARDIA

tacrolimus (tăk″rō-lĕ′mŭs) An immunosuppressive agent that suppresses rejection in organ transplant recipients. Trade name is Prograf.

tactile (tăk′tĭl) [L. *tactilis*] Perceptible to the touch. SYN: *tactual*.

t. defensiveness A defense reaction owing to sensitivity to being touched.

t. discrimination The ability to localize two points of pressure on the surface of the skin and to identify them as discrete sensations.

t. disk The tiny expanded end of a sensory nerve fiber found in the epidermis and in the epithelial root sheath of a hair.

t. localization An individual's ability to accurately identify the site of tactile stimulation (touch, pressure, or pain). Tactile localization is often tested in sensory evaluations following disease or trauma of the nervous system.

t. system That portion of the nervous system concerned with the sensation of touch. It includes sensory nerve endings (Meissner's corpuscles, Merkel's tactile disks, hair-root endings), afferent nerve fibers, conducting pathways in the cord and brain, and the sensory (somesthetic) area of the cerebral cortex.

taction (tăk′shŭn) [L. *tactio*] **1.** The sense of touch. **2.** Touching.

tactometer (tăk-tŏm′ĕt-ĕr) [L. *tactus,* touch, + Gr. *metron,* measure] An instrument for determining the acuity of tactile sensitiveness.

tactual (tăk′tū-ăl) [L. *tactus,* touch] Tactile.

tactus (tăk′tŭs) [L.] Touch (1).

t. eruditus A sensitivity of touch acquired by long practice.

taedium vitae (tē′dē-ŭm vē″tī) [L.] Weariness of life, with suicidal inclination.

taen-, taeni- Combining form meaning *tapeworm.* SEE: *ten-*.

Taenia (tē′nē-ă) [L., tape] A genus of tapeworms, parasitic flatworms belonging to the class Cestoda, phylum Platyhelminthes. They are elongated ribbonlike worms consisting of a scolex, usually with suckers and perhaps hooks, and a chain of segments (proglottids). Adults live as intestinal parasites of vertebrates; larvae parasitize both vertebrates and invertebrates, which are intermediate hosts. SEE: *taeniasis; tapeworm.*

T. echinococcus *Echinococcus granulosus.*

T. lata *Diphyllobothrium latum.*

T. saginata A tapeworm whose larvae live in cattle. The adult worm lives in the small intestine of humans, who acquire it by eating insufficiently cooked beef infested with the encysted larval form (cysticercus or bladderworm). Adult worms may reach a length of 15 to 20 ft (4.6 to 6.1 m) or longer. SYN: *beef tapeworm.* SEE: illus.

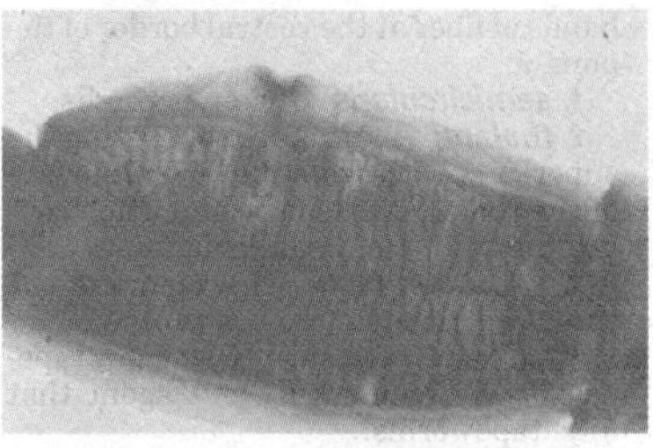

TAENIA SAGINATA

Gravid proglottid (orig. mag. ×5)

T. solium A tapeworm whose larvae live in hogs; its scolex possesses a row of hooks about the rostellum. The adult worm lives in the small intestine of humans, who acquire it by eating insufficiently cooked pork infested with the larval form. Infected pork containing the bladderworm *(Cysticercus cellulosae)* is called measly pork. The cysticerci may also develop in humans; infection occurs from self-infection with eggs from contaminated hands or by hatching of eggs liberated in the intestine. The infection is treated with niclosamide or praziquantel. SYN: *armed tapeworm; pork tapeworm.* SEE: illus.

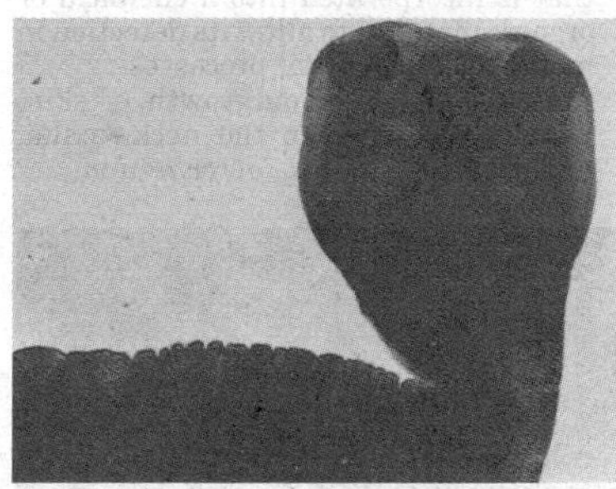

TAENIA SOLIUM

(Orig. mag. ×100)

taenia (tē′nē-ă) [L., tape] **1.** A flat band or strip of soft tissue. **2.** A tapeworm of the genus *Taenia.* SYN: *tenia.*

t. coli The three bands of smooth muscle into which the longitudinal muscle layer of the colon is gathered. They are taenia mesocolica (mesenteric insertion), taenia libera (opposite mesocolic band), and taenia omentalis (at place of attachment of omentum to transverse colon).

t. fimbriae The folded or recurved lateral edge of the fimbria to which the epithelium covering the choroid plexus of the inferior horn of the lateral ventricle is attached.

t. pontis One or two small transverse

bands of fiber at the rostral border of the pons.

t. semicircularis Stria terminalis.

t. thalami A structure separating the superior surface from the lateral surface of the thalamus, its lateral portion containing the stria medullaris.

t. ventriculi tertii The taenia of the third ventricle.

taeniacide (tē′nē-ă-sīd) [L. *taenia,* tapeworm, + *cidus,* kill] An agent that kills tapeworms.

taeniafuge (tē′nē-ă-fūj″) [″ + *fugere,* to put to flight] Tenifuge.

taeniasis (tē-nī′ă-sĭs) [″ + Gr. *-iasis,* condition] The condition of being infested with tapeworms of the genus *Taenia.* SEE: *tapeworm.*

taeniform (tē′nĭ-form) [″ + *forma,* shape] Having the structure of, or resembling, a tapeworm.

taenifuge (tē′nĭ-fūj) [″ + *fuga,* flight] Tenifuge.

taeniophobia (tē″nē-ō-fō′bē-ă) [″ + Gr. *phobos,* fear] The morbid fear of becoming infested with tapeworms.

tag **1.** A small polyp or growth. **2.** A label or tracer; or the application of a label or tracer.

hemorrhoidal t. The remaining anal skin tag from an old external hemorrhoid.

radioactive t. A radioactive isotope that is incorporated into a chemical or organic material to allow its detection in metabolic or chemical processes.

skin t. A small outgrowth of skin, usually occurring on the neck, axilla, and groin. SEE: illus.; *acrochordon.*

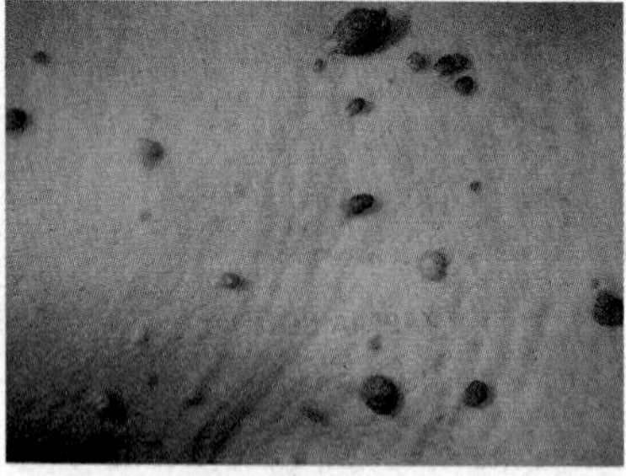

SKIN TAGS

tagging Introduction of a radioactive isotope into a molecule in order to distinguish the molecule from others without that "tag." SYN: *labeling.*

tagliacotian operation, tagliacotian flap (tă-lē-ă-kō′shē-ăn) [Gasparo Tagliacozzi, It. surgeon, 1546–1599] A plastic operation on the nose in which skin is used from another part of the body.

tai chi (tī-chē) A traditional Chinese martial art in which a series of slow controlled movements are made through various postures designed to develop flexibility, balance, strength, relaxation, and mental concentration. It is being investigated as a treatment for balance disorders.

tail (tāl) [AS. *taegel*] **1.** The long end of a structure, such as the extremity of the spinal column or the final segments of a polypeptide or nucleic acid. SEE: *cauda.* **2.** An uninterrupted extension of the insurance policy period; also called the *extended reporting endorsement.* SEE: *professional liability insurance.*

tailgut (tāl′gŭt) A transient diverticulum of the endodermal cloaca of the embryo that extends to the anal opening.

tailor's cramp An occupational syndrome marked by overuse of and spasm of the muscles of the arms and hands.

taint (tānt) [O.Fr. *teint,* color, tint] To spoil or cause putrefaction, as in tainted meat.

Takayasu's arteritis [Michishige Takayasu, Japanese physician, 1872–1938] A rare vasculitis of the aorta and its branches, marked by inflammatory changes in the large arteries. Blood flow through those arteries is limited, esp. to the arms or head of affected persons. The disease, which is found most often in young women of Japanese descent, produces symptoms such as dizziness or arm claudication. Affected individuals usually have markedly reduced blood pressures or pulses in one or both arms. SYN: *pulseless disease.*

take To be effective, as in administering a vaccine; or to be successful in grafting skin or transplanting an organ.

talalgia (tăl-ăl′jē-ă) [L. *talus,* heel, + Gr. *algos,* pain] Pain in the heel or ankle.

talar (tā′lăr) [L. *talaris,* of the ankle] Pert. to the talus, the ankle.

talar tilt test An orthopedic test used to determine the collateral stability of the ankle joint. The amount of laxity in the affected ankle is determined relative to the laxity in the uninvolved limb.

Eversion talar tilt test. The foot and ankle are maintained in the neutral position. The examiner stabilizes the distal lower leg while cupping the calcaneus with the opposite hand. The talus is then rolled outward to eversion.

This test checks the integrity of the deltoid ligament group of the medial ankle, esp. the tibiocalcaneal and tibionavicular ligaments. The mechanical block formed by the lateral malleolus limits the amount of eversion.

Inversion talar tilt test. The foot and ankle are maintained in the neutral position. The examiner stabilizes the distal lower leg while cupping the calcaneus with the opposite hand. The talus is then rolled inward to inversion.

This test checks the integrity of the lateral ligaments, specifically the calcaneofibular, anterior talofibular, and posterior talofibular ligaments (in order of involvement). The anterior talofibular ligament can be isolated through the use of the anterior drawer test.

talc (tălk) [Persian *talk*] Powdered soapstone; a soft, soapy powder; native hydrous magnesium silicate, $Mg_3Si_4O_{10}(OH)_2$, used, for example, in pleurodesis. SYN: *talcum*.

CAUTION: Talc used for industrial, cosmetic, or health products should not contain asbestos fibers.

talcosis (tăl-kō'sĭs) [Persian *talk*, talc, + Gr. *osis*, condition] A disease caused by the inhalation or implantation of talc in the body.

talcum (tălk'ŭm) [L.] Talc.

tali (tā'lī) Pl. of talus.

talipes (tăl'ĭ-pēz) [L. *talus*, ankle, + *pes*, foot] Any of several deformities of the foot, esp. those occurring congenitally; a nontraumatic deviation of the foot in the direction of one or two of the four lines of movement.

t. arcuatus Talipes in which there is an exaggerated normal arch of the foot. SYN: *t. cavus*.

t. calcaneus Talipes in which the foot is dorsiflexed and the heel alone touches the ground, causing the patient to walk on the inner side of the heel. It often follows infantile paralysis of the calf muscles.

t. cavus T. arcuatus.

t. equinovarus A combination of talipes equinus and talipes valgus. SYN: *clubfoot*.

t. equinus Talipes in which the foot is plantar flexed and the person walks on the toes.

t. percavus Talipes in which there is excessive plantar curvature.

t. valgus Talipes in which the heel and foot are turned outward.

t. varus Talipes in which the heel is turned inward from the midline of the leg.

talipomanus (tăl"ĭp-ŏm'ăn-ŭs) [L. *talus*, ankle, + *pes*, foot, + *manus*, hand] A deformity of the hand in which it is twisted out of position. SYN: *clubhand*.

tallow (tăl'ō) Fat obtained from suet, the solid fat of certain ruminants.

talocalcaneal (tā"lō-kăl-kā'nē-ăl) [" + *calcaneus*, heel bone] Pert. to the talus and calcaneus, bones of the tarsus.

talocrural (tā"lō-kroo'răl) [" + *crus*, leg] Pert. to the talus and leg bones.

talocrural articulation The ankle joint; a ginglymoid or hinge joint.

talofibular (tā"lō-fĭb'ū-lăr) [" + *fibula*, pin] Concerning the talus and fibula.

talon (tăl'ōn) [L.] The portion of the claw of a bird, esp. a bird of prey, that projects posteriorly.

t. noir Minute black areas on the heels (or less often the toes or hands) caused by repetitive injuries that produce hemorrhage into the skin.

talonavicular (tā"lō-nă-vĭk'ū-lăr) [L. *talus*, ankle, + *navicula*, boat] Concerning the talus and navicular bones. SYN: *taloscaphoid*.

talonid (tăl'ō-nĭd) [ME. *talon*, heel] The crushing region, the posterior or heel part, of a lower molar tooth.

taloscaphoid (tā"lō-skăf'oyd) [L. *talus*, ankle, + Gr. *skaphe*, skiff, + *eidos*, form, shape] Talonavicular.

talotibial (tā"lō-tĭb'ē-ăl) [" + *tibia*, shinbone] Concerning the talus and tibial.

talus (tā'lŭs) *pl.* **tali** [L., ankle] The ankle bone articulating with the tibia, fibula, calcaneus, and navicular bone; formerly called astragalus.

tambour (tăm-boor') [Fr., drum] A shallow, drum-shaped appliance used in registering information such as changes in rate or intensity of pulse, respiration, or arterial blood pressure.

Tamm-Horsfall mucoprotein [Igor Tamm, Russian-born U.S. virologist, 1922–1971; Frank L. Horsfall, Jr., U.S. physician, 1906–1971] A normal mucoprotein in the urine, produced by the ascending limb of the loop of Henle. When this protein is concentrated at low pH, it forms gel, which may protect the kidney from infection by bacteria.

tamoxifen citrate (tă-mŏks'ĭ-fĕn) An antiestrogenic drug used in treating and preventing breast cancer.

tampon (tăm'pŏn) [Fr., plug] A roll or pack made of various absorbent substances, such as cotton, rayon, wool, and gauze, used to arrest hemorrhage or absorb secretions from a wound or body cavity.

menstrual t. An absorbent material suitably shaped and prepared to provide a hygienic means of absorbing menstrual fluid in the vagina. A cord is attached and remains outside the vagina to facilitate removal. These tampons are made for self-insertion. SEE: *menstruation; sanitary napkin*.

Mikulicz's t. Mikulicz's drain.

nasal t. A soft rubber bulb dilated with compressed air, used in plugging nostrils to stop hemorrhage from the nose.

tamponade (tăm"pŏn-ăd') [Fr., plug] **1.** The act of using a tampon. SYN: *tamponage; tamponing; tamponment*. **2.** The pathological or intentional compression of a part.

balloon t. The application of pressure against a part of the body with an inflatable high-pressure balloon. Balloon tamponade was formerly used to arrest bleeding caused by esophageal varices (e.g., with a Sengstaken-Blakemore tube). Esophageal varices are more often treated with medications (such as nitrates and beta blockers), rubber banding, or the injection of sclerosing agents. SEE: *epistaxis; varicose vein*.

PATIENT CARE: After balloon insertion, vital signs, electrolyte status, and changes in hematocrit are monitored. Because the balloon prevents swallowing, fluids and tube feedings are administered as prescribed. The nurse instructs the patient to expectorate saliva and provides an emesis basin for oral secretions. Aspiration of secretions is necessary. Comatose patients require continuous drainage of the esophagus above the balloon.

cardiac t. A life-threatening condition in which elevated intrapericardial pressures impair the filling of the heart during diastole.

Tamponade may result from injuries to the heart or great vessels, or other causes of large pericardial effusions. If fluid accumulates rapidly, as little as 250 ml can create an emergency. Slow accumulation and a rise in pressure, as in pericardial effusion associated with cancer, may not produce immediate signs and symptoms because the fibrous wall of the pericardial sac can gradually stretch to accommodate as much as 1 to 2 L of fluid.

ETIOLOGY: Cardiac tamponade may be idiopathic (Dressler's syndrome) or may result from any of the following causes: effusion (in cancer, bacterial infections, tuberculosis, and, rarely, acute rheumatic fever); hemorrhage from trauma (such as gunshot or stab wounds of the chest, perforation by catheter during cardiac or central venous catheterization, or after cardiac surgery); hemorrhage from nontraumatic causes (such as rupture of the heart or great vessels, or anticoagulant therapy in a patient with pericarditis); viral, postirradiation, or idiopathic pericarditis; acute myocardial infarction; chronic renal failure; drug reaction (procainamide, hydralazine, minoxidil, isoniazid, penicillin, methysergide, and daunorubicin); or connective tissue disorders (such as rheumatoid arthritis, systemic lupus erythematosus, rheumatic fever, vasculitis, and scleroderma).

DIAGNOSIS: Cardiac tamponade is suggested by chest radiograph (slightly widened mediastinum and enlargement of the cardiac silhouette), ECG (reduced QRS amplitude, electrical alternans of the P wave, QRS complex, and T wave and generalized ST-segment elevation), and pulmonary artery pressure monitoring (increased right atrial pressure, right ventricular diastolic pressure, and central venous pressure). It is definitively diagnosed with echocardiography, or MRI or CT of the chest.

TREATMENT: Treatment is directed to relieving intrapericardial pressure and cardiac compression by removing accumulated blood or fluid. Pericardiocentesis (needle aspiration of the pericardial cavity) or surgical creation of a pericardial opening ("a window") dramatically improves systemic arterial pressure and cardiac output. In patients with malignant tamponade, a balloon-aided opening in the pericardium may be made (so-called "balloon pericardiotomy").

PATIENT CARE: The patient is assessed for a history of disorders that can cause tamponade and for symptoms such as chest pain and dyspnea. Other findings include orthopnea, diaphoresis, anxiety, restlessness, and pallor or cyanosis. The neck veins are inspected for distention; peripheral pulses are palpated for rapidity and weakness; the liver is palpated and percussed for hepatomegaly; the anterior chest wall percussed for a widening area of flatness; and the blood pressure auscultated for decreased arterial pressure, pulsus paradoxus (an abnormal inspiratory drop of greater than 15 mm Hg in systemic blood pressure), and narrow pulse pressure. Heart sounds may be muffled. A quiet heart with faint sounds usually accompanies only severe tamponade and occurs within minutes of the tamponade (as in cardiac rupture or trauma). The lungs are clear.

When these findings are apparent, the patient is transferred to intensive care immediately for hemodynamic monitoring and support. Prescribed inotropic drugs, intravenous solutions to maintain the patient's blood pressure, and oxygen are administered as necessary and prescribed.

The patient is prepared for central line insertion, pericardiocentesis, thoracotomy, or other therapeutic measures as indicated; brief explanations of procedures and expected sensations are provided; and the patient is reassured to decrease anxiety. The patient is observed for a decrease in central venous pressure and a concomitant rise in blood pressure after treatment, which indicate relief of cardiac compression.

If the patient is not acutely ill, the patient is educated about the condition, including its cause and its treatment. The importance of reporting any worsening of symptoms immediately is stressed.

nasal t. Compression of nasal blood vessels to stop bleeding. SEE: *epistaxis; nosebleed* for illus.

tamponage (tăm′pŏn-ŏj) [Fr., plug] Tamponade.

tamponing, tamponment (tăm′pŏn-ĭng, tăm-pŏn′mĕnt) Tamponade.

tandem A curved stainless steel tube inserted into the uterine canal during brachytherapy to hold radioactive sources.

tang **1.** A strong taste or flavor. **2.** A long slender projection or prong forming a part of a chisel, file, or knife. **3.** In dentistry, an apparatus for joining the rests and retainers to palatal or lingual bars of a denture.

Tangier disease (tăn-jēr′) [Tangier Island, in Chesapeake Bay, where the disease was first discovered] A rare autosomal co-dominant disease caused by familial high-density lipoprotein deficiency. Symptoms and signs include polyneuropathy, lymphadenopathy, orange-yellow discoloration of enlarged tonsillar tissue, hepatosplenomegaly, and a marked decrease in high-density lipoproteins. Cholesterol esters accumulate in various organs. There is no specific therapy.

tannin (tăn′ĭn) [Fr. *tanin*] **1.** An acid found in the bark of certain plants and trees or their products, usually from nutgall. It is found in coffee and to a greater extent in tea. **2.** Any of several substances containing tannin.

ACTION/USES: Tannin was once used as an astringent, an antidote for various poisons, and a topical hemostatic.

tanning salon A commercial establishment where patrons can expose themselves to ultraviolet light to darken their skin. Because ultraviolet light ages the skin and increases the likelihood of skin cancers, tanning salons are frowned on by dermatologists, cancer specialists, and other health care professionals. SEE: *actinic keratosis; basal cell carcinoma; melanoma; photosensitivity; squamous cell carcinoma*.

tantalum (tăn′tă-lŭm) SYMB: Ta. A rare metallic element derived from tantalite; atomic weight, 180.947; atomic number, 73. Because it is noncorrosive and malleable, it has been used to repair cranial defects, as a wire suture, and in prostheses.

tantrum, temper An explosive outburst, usually by a child, often as a result of frustration or developmental disabilities. It may resolve with a variety of parental interventions, such as behavioral modification techniques (e.g., positive reinforcement of more acceptable behaviors by the child).

Tanyoz's sign **1.** In ascites, the downward displacement of the umbilicus. **2.** In pregnancy, the upward displacement of the umbilicus.

tap (tăp) [AS. *taeppa*] To puncture or to empty a cavity of fluid. SEE: *lumbar puncture; paracentesis; thoracentesis*.

spinal t. Lumbar puncture.

tap (tăp) [O.Fr. *taper*] **1.** A light blow. **2.** An instrument used for performing a tap. **3.** An instrument used to create an internal thread.

tape (tāp) [AS. *taeppe*] **1.** A flexible, narrow strip of linen, cotton, paper, or plastic such as adhesive tape. **2.** To wrap a part with a long bandage made of adhesive or other type of material.

adhesive t. A fabric, film, or paper, one side of which is coated with an adhesive so that it remains in place when applied to the skin. In general, there are two types of backings for the adhesive material: occlusive and nonocclusive. The former prevents air from going through the backing and the latter does not. The occlusive type increases the possibility of skin irritation, so it is rarely used. SYN: *adhesive plaster*.

PATIENT CARE: To prevent skin damage, adhesive tape should be removed by carefully peeling back the tape following the direction of hair growth while the skin is held taut behind the tape removal edge or alternatively compressing the skin from the tape as it is held on gentle tension. The skin should be checked for irritation. If the adhesive material has irritated the skin, solvents may be used judiciously to assist in removal. Because some patients are allergic to certain adhesive agents, information about this type of allergy should be gathered as part of the history; other varieties of tape may be nonreactive. If the patient is intolerant of all adhesives, alternative bandage applications are used.

tapeinocephalic (tăp″ĭ-nō-sĕ-făl′ĭk) [Gr. *tapeinos,* low-lying, + *kephale,* head] Pert. to tapeinocephaly.

tapeinocephaly (tăp″ĭ-nō-sĕf′ă-lē) A flattened head in which the vertical index of the skull is less than 72.

tapetum (tă-pē′tŭm) [NL., a carpet] A layer of fibers from the corpus callosum forming the roof and lateral walls of the inferior and posterior horns of the lateral ventricles of the brain. The fibers pass to the temporal and occipital lobes.

t. choroideae T. lucidum.

t. lucidum A layer of tissue in the choroid of the eye between the vascular and capillary layers in some animals, but not in humans. This membrane reflects light shined into the animal's eyes. It produces a green reflection, readily seen in cats. SYN: *t. choroideae*.

tapeworm [AS. *taeppe,* a narrow band, + *wyrm,* worm] Any of the species of worms of the class Cestoda, phylum Platyhelminthes; all are intestinal parasites of humans and other animals. A typical tapeworm consists of a scolex, with hooks and suckers for attachment, and a series of a few to several thousand segments, or proglottids. New proglottids develop at the scolex, so that a worm is actually a linear colony of immature, mature, and gravid proglottids; adult worms range from less than an inch to 50 ft or more, depending on the species. The terminal proglottids, which contain fertilized eggs, break off and pass from the host in the feces. The eggs develop into small, hooked embryos, which, when ingested by the proper intermediate host (usually another vertebrate such as a pig), develop into encysted larvae (cysticerci) in the muscle tissue. Humans acquire tapeworm infestation by eating undercooked meat that contains the cysticerci. SEE: *Taenia.*

Species of medical importance are *Diphyllobothrium latum, Echinococcus granulosus, Hymenolepis nana, H. diminuta, Taenia saginata,* and *T. solium.* SEE: *cysticercosis; cysticercus; hydatid; taeniasis.*

SYMPTOMS: Often symptoms are absent, although abdominal discomfort, bloating, or changes in bowel habits may be present. If tapeworms are very numerous, they may cause intestinal obstruction (but this is rare). Some species of tapeworms may cause severe disease: *Echinococcus* can cause life-threatening cysts in the liver or pericardium; *Taenia solium* can encyst in the brain and cause seizures or strokelike symptoms.

armed t. *Taenia solium.*

beef t. *Taenia saginata.*

broad t. *Diphyllobothrium latum.*

dog t. *Dipylidium caninum.*

dwarf t. *Hymenolepis nana.*

fish t. *Diphyllobothrium latum.*

hydatid t. *Echinococcus granulosus.*

mouse t. *Hymenolepis nana.*

pork t. *Taenia solium.*

rat t. *Hymenolepis nana.*

unarmed t. *Taenia saginata.*

taphephobia (tăf″ĕ-fō′bē-ă) [Gr. *taphos,* grave, + *phobos,* fear] An abnormal fear of being buried alive.

taphophilia (tăf″ō-fĭl′ē-ă) [″ + *philos,* love] An abnormal attraction for graves.

Tapia syndrome (tā′pē-ă) [Antonio García Tapia, Sp. physician, 1875–1950] Paralysis of the pharynx and larynx on one side and atrophy of the tongue on the opposite side, caused by a lesion affecting the vagus (10th) and hypoglossal (12th) cranial nerves on the side in which the pharynx is affected.

tapinocephalic (tăp″ĭn-ō-sĕf-ăl′ĭk) [Gr. *tapeinos,* lying low, + *kephale,* head] Pert. to flatness of the top of the cranium.

tapinocephaly (tăp″ĭn-ō-sĕf′ă-lē) Flatness of the top of the cranium.

tapotement (tă-pōt-mŏn′) [Fr.] Percussion in massage. Techniques include beating with the clinched hand, clapping performed with the palm of the hand, hacking with the ulnar border of the hand, and punctuation with the tips of the fingers. The strength of the manipulations is an essential factor in the massage treatment, and care must be taken not to bruise the patient. As a rule, one should begin with moderate pressure, and then ascertain from the patient the appropriate level of stimulation. A lubricating lotion or cream should be used to avoid abrading the skin. SYN: *tapping* (1). SEE: *massage.*

tapping (tăp′ĭng) [O.Fr. *taper,* of imitative origin] Tapotement.

muscle t. Tapping the skin over a muscle belly to recruit more motor units and facilitate contraction.

tapping (tăp′ĭng) [AS. *taeppa,* tap] The withdrawal of fluid from a body cavity. Examples include paracentesis and thoracentesis.

tar A dark, viscid mass of complex chemicals obtained by destructive distillation of tobacco, coal, shale, and organic matter, esp. wood from pine and juniper trees.

coal t. A tar produced in the destructive distillation of bituminous coal. It is used as an ingredient in ointments for treating eczema, psoriasis, and other skin diseases.

juniper t. A material obtained from the destructive distillation of oil of the wood of the juniper tree, *Juniperus oxycedrus.* It is contained in medicines used to treat skin diseases.

tarantism (tăr′ăn-tĭzm) [*Taranto,* seaport in southern Italy, + Gr. *-ismos,* condition] A neurological disorder marked by stupor, melancholy, and uncontrollable dancing mania; popularly attributed to the bite of the tarantula. SYN: *tarentism.*

tarantula (tă-răn′tū-lă) A large venomous spider feared by many people; however, its bite is comparable in severity to a bee sting. SEE: *spider bite.*

Tardieu's spot (tăr-dyūz′) [Auguste A. Tardieu, Fr. physician, 1818–1879] One of the subpleural spots of ecchymosis following death by strangulation.

tardive (tăr′dĭv) [Fr., tardy] Characterized by lateness, esp. pert. to a disease in which the characteristic sign or symptom appears late in the course of the disease. SEE: *dyskinesia, tardive.*

tare (tār) The weight of an empty container. That weight is subtracted from the total weight of the vessel and substance added to it in order to determine the precise weight of the material added to the container.

tared A container of known and predetermined tare.

tarentism (tăr′ĕn-tĭzm) Tarantism.

target (tăr′gĕt) [O.Fr. *targette,* light shield] **1.** A structure or organ to which something is directed. **2.** The portion of the anode of an x-ray or therapeutic tube in which electrons from the filament or electron gun are focused and x-ray photons are produced; usually made of a heavy metal such as tungsten or molybdenum.

target cell An erythrocyte with a rounded

central area surrounded by a lightly stained clear ring, which in turn is surrounded by a dense ring of peripheral protoplasm. It is present in certain blood disorders. SEE: illus.

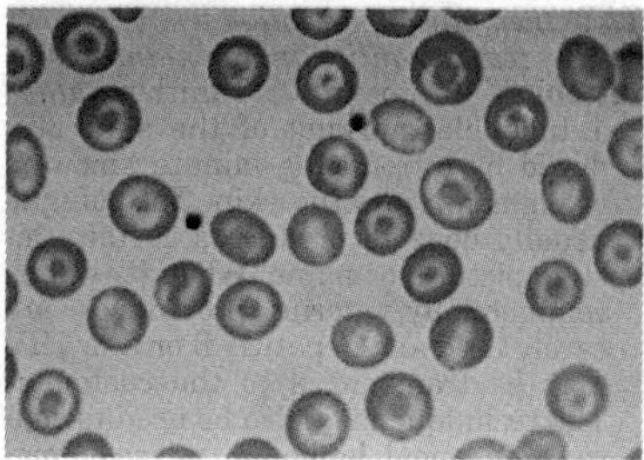

TARGET CELLS

In hemoglobin C disease (×600)

tarichatoxin (tăr″ĭk-ă-tŏk′sĭn) A neurotoxin from the *Taricha* newt.

Tarnier's sign (tăr-nē-āz′) [Etienne Stéphene Tarnier, Fr. obstetrician, 1828–1897] A sign of impending miscarriage; the disappearance of the angle between the upper and lower uterine segments in pregnancy.

tarnish Surface discoloration or reduced luster of metals owing to the effect of corrosive substances or galvanic action. In dental restorations, such action may be enhanced by accumulation of bacterial plaque.

tarsadenitis (tăr″săd-ĕn-ī′tĭs) [Gr. *tarsos,* a broad, flat surface, + *aden,* gland, + *itis,* inflammation] An inflammation of the tarsal or meibomian glands of the eyelid.

tarsal (tăr′săl) [Gr. *tarsalis*] **1.** Pert. to the tarsus or supporting plate of the eyelid. **2.** Pert. to the ankle or tarsus.

tarsal bone One of the seven bones of the ankle, hind foot, and midfoot, consisting of the talus, calcaneus, navicular, cuboid, and three cuneiform bones. SYN: *tarsale.*

tarsale (tăr-sā′lē) *pl.* **tarsalia** [L.] Tarsal bone.

tarsalgia (tăr-săl′jē-ă) [Gr. *tarsos,* a broad, flat surface, + *algos,* pain] Pain in the tarsus or ankle; it may be due to flatfoot, shortening of the Achilles tendon, or other causes.

tarsalis (tăr-sā′lĭs) [L.] One of the tarsal muscles.

tarsectomy (tar-sĕk′tō-mē) [″ + *ektome,* excision] **1.** An excision of the tarsus or a tarsal bone. **2.** The removal of the tarsal plate of an eyelid.

tarsectopia (tăr″sĕk-tō′pē-ă) A dislocation of the tarsus.

tarsitis (tăr-sī′tĭs) [″ + *itis,* inflammation] **1.** An inflammation of the tarsus of the foot. **2.** Blepharitis.

tarso- [Gr. *tarsos,* a broad, flat surface] Combining form indicating *the flat of the foot* or *the edge of the eyelid.*

tarsocheiloplasty (tăr″sō-kī′lō-plăs″tē) [″ + *cheilos,* lip, + *plassein,* to form] The plastic repair of the borders of the eyelid.

tarsoclasia, tarsoclasis (tăr″sō-klā′sē-ă, tăr-sŏk′lăs-ĭs) [″ + *klasis,* a breaking] A surgical fracture of the tarsus for the correction of clubfoot.

tarsomalacia (tăr″sō-mă-lā′sē-ă) [″ + *malakia,* a softening] The softening of the tarsal plate of the eyes.

tarsomegaly (tăr″sō-mĕg′ă-lē) [″ + *megas,* large] An enlargement of the heel bone, the calcaneus.

tarsometatarsal (tăr″sō-mĕt″ă-tăr′săl) [″ + *meta,* between, + *tarsos,* a broad, flat surface] Pert. to the tarsus and the metatarsus.

tarso-orbital (tăr″sō-or′bĭ-tăl) [″ + L. *orbita,* track] Concerning the tarsus of the eyelid and the orbit.

tarsophalangeal (tăr″sō-fă-lăn′jē-ăl) [″ + *phalanx,* closely knit row] Concerning the tarsus of the foot and the phalanges of the toes.

tarsophyma (tăr″sō-fī′mă) [″ + *phyma,* a growth] Sty(e).

tarsoplasia, tarsoplasty (tăr″sō-plā′zē-ă, tăr′sō-plăs″tē) [″ + *plassein,* to form] Blepharoplasty.

tarsoptosis (tăr″sŏp-tō′sĭs) [″ + *ptosis,* falling] Flatfoot; fallen arch of the foot.

tarsorrhaphy (tăr-sor′ă-fē) [″ + *rhaphe,* seam, ridge] Blepharorrhaphy.

tarsotarsal (tăr″sō-tăr′săl) [″ + *tarsos,* a broad, flat surface] Concerning the articulation between two rows of tarsal bones.

tarsotibial (tăr″sō-tĭb′ē-ăl) [″ + L. *tibia,* shinbone] Concerning the tarsus and the tibia.

tarsotomy (tăr-sŏt′ō-mē) [″ + *tome,* incision] **1.** An incision of the tarsal plate of an eyelid. **2.** Any surgical incision of the tarsus of the foot.

tarsus (tăr′sŭs) *pl.* **tarsi** [Gr. *tarsos,* a broad, flat surface] **1.** The ankle with its seven bones located between the bones of the lower leg and the metatarsus and forming the proximal portion of the foot. It consists of the calcaneus (os calcis), talus (astragalus), cuboid (os cuboideum), navicular (scaphoid), and first, second, and third cuneiform bones. The talus articulates with the tibia and fibula, the cuboid and cuneiform bones with the metatarsals. SEE: *foot; skeleton;* names of individual bones. **2.** A curved plate of dense white fibrous tissue forming the supporting structure of the eyelid; also called the *tarsal plate.*

t. inferior palpebrae The firm layer of connective tissue that provides internal support for the lower eyelid.

t. superior palpebrae The firm layer of connective tissue that provides internal support for the upper eyelid.

tartar [Gr. *tartaron,* dregs] **1.** An acid compound found in the juice of grapes and deposited on the sides of casks during winemaking. **2.** Dental plaque that has mineralized.

t. emetic Antimony potassium tartrate; formerly used as an emetic.

tartrate A salt of tartaric acid.

tartrazine A pyrazole aniline dye widely used to color foods, cosmetics, drugs, and textiles.

task analysis The process of dividing up an activity into components for the purposes of delineating the specific abilities needed to perform that activity. Purposeful activities require various levels of cognitive, perceptual (e.g., vision, proprioception), musculoskeletal, and neuromuscular abilities. Through understanding the abilities necessary for a specific task, practitioners are better able to develop a rehabilitation program for patients who cannot do it for themselves.

task, cancellation A type of cognitive test that measures attention by determining an individual's ability to select and mark a line through selected target letters or symbols within a larger field of many letters or symbols.

taste (tāst) [O.Fr. *taster,* to feel, to taste] **1.** To attempt to determine the flavor of a substance by touching it with the tongue. **2.** A chemical sense dependent on the sensory buds on the surface of the tongue, the nerves that innervate them, and the smell center (rhinencephalon) of the brain. The taste buds, when appropriately stimulated, produce one or a combination of the four fundamental taste sensations: sweet, bitter, sour, and salty. The sensation is influenced by the sense of smell. Information from the taste buds is carried to the brain by the facial nerve (from the anterior two thirds of the surface of the tongue) and the glossopharyngeal nerve (from the posterior third). Loss of taste may be caused by many conditions, such as bilateral disease of the facial nerve, lesions of the gustatory fibers of the glossopharyngeal nerve, or the therapeutic use of cytotoxic drugs.

The cells of the taste buds undergo continual degeneration and replacement. None survives for more than a few days.

t. area An area in the cerebral cortex at the lower end of the somesthetic area in the parietal lobe.

t. blindness An inability to taste certain substances such as phenylthiocarbamide (PTC). This inability is due to a hereditary factor that is transmitted as an autosomal recessive trait.

t. cell One of the neuroepithelial cells within a taste bud that serve as receptors for the sense of taste. Each possesses on the free surface a short taste hair that projects through the inner taste pore. SYN: *gustatory cell.*

taster (tās′tĕr) A person capable of detecting a particular substance by using the taste sense. SEE: *phenylthiocarbamide.*

TAT *thematic apperception test.*

T.A.T. *tetanus antitoxin; toxin-antitoxin.*

tattooing (tă-too′ĭng) [Tahitian *tatau*] **1.** Indelible marking of the skin produced by introducing minute amounts of pigments into the skin. Tattooing is usually done to produce a certain design, picture, or name. When it is done commercially, sterile procedures are rarely used and hepatitis B or C or HIV may be transmitted to the customer. The technique may also be used to conceal a corneal leukoma, to mask pigmented areas of skin, or to color skin to look like the areola in mammoplasty. **2.** In radiation therapy, the induction of a small amount of indelible pigment under the skin used to designate an area to be treated with radiation.

removal of t. Use of a ruby laser to "erase" the pigment in an unwanted tattoo. This usually causes no permanent skin changes.

traumatic t. Following abrasion of the skin, embedding of fine dirt particles under the superficial layers of the skin; or as a result of forceful deposit of gunpowder granules. This can be prevented by immediate removal of the particles.

taurine (taw′rĭn) $NH_2CH_2CH_2SO_3H$. A derivative of cysteine. It is present in bile, as taurocholic acid, in combination with bile acid.

taurocholate (taw″rō-kō′lāt) A salt of taurocholic acid.

taurocholemia (taw″rō-kō-lē′mē-ă) [Gr. *tauros,* a bull, + *chole,* bile, + *haima,* blood] Taurocholic acid in the blood.

taurodontism (taw″rō-dŏn′tĭzm) [″ + *odous,* tooth, + *-ismos,* condition] A condition in which the teeth have greatly enlarged and deepened pulp chambers that encroach on the roots of the teeth.

Taussig-Bing syndrome (tau′sĭg-bĭng) [Helen B. Taussig, U.S. pediatrician, 1898–1986; Richard J. Bing, U.S. surgeon, 1909–1986] A congenital deformity of the heart in which the aorta arises from the right ventricle and the pulmonary artery arises from both ventricles. An intraventricular septal defect is present.

tauto- Prefix meaning *identical.*

tautomer (taw′tō-mĕr) [″ + *meros,* a part] A chemical that is capable of tautomerism.

tautomeral, tautomeric (taw-tŏm′ĕr-ăl, -tō-mĕr′ĭk) [″ + *meros,* a part] Pert. to certain neurons that send processes to the white matter on the same side of the spinal cord.

tautomerase (taw-tŏm′ĕr-ās) [″ + ″ + *-ase,* enzyme] An enzyme that catalyzes tautomeric reactions.

tautomerism (taw-tŏm′ĕr-ĭzm) [″ + ″ + *-ismos,* condition] A phenomenon in which a chemical may be present in two forms, existing in dynamic equilibrium so that as the amount of one substance is altered, the second is changed into the other form in order to maintain the equilibrium. SEE: *isomerism.*

tautorotation (taw″tō-rō-tā′shŭn) [″ + L. *rotare,* to turn round] A change in specific rotation that occurs when a solution of certain sugars stands for a while.

taxis (tăk′sĭs) [Gr., arrangement] **1.** The manual replacement or reduction of a hernia or dislocation. **2.** The response of an organism to its environment; a turning toward (positive taxis) or away from (negative taxis) a particular stimulus. SEE: *chemotaxis.*

taxol A chemotherapeutic drug obtained from the bark of the yew tree, *Taxus brevifolia.* It is used to treat cancers of the breast, ovary, and other organs. Side effects include bone marrow suppression, neuropathy, mucositis, and hypersensitivity reactions.

taxon (tăk′sŏn) [Gr. *taxis,* arrangement] A taxonomic group.

taxonomic (tăk″sō-nŏm′ĭk) Concerning taxonomy.

taxonomy (tăks-ŏn′ō-mē) [″ + *nomos,* law] The laws and principles of classification of living organisms; also used for classification of learning objectives.

Taylor brace (tā′lĕr) [Charles Fayette Taylor, U.S. surgeon, 1827–1899] A brace with two rigid posterior oblique portions and soft straps crossed anteriorly over the chest.

Taylor, Euphemia Jane [U.S. nurse, 1878–1957] A pioneer of psychiatric nursing. She graduated from the Johns Hopkins Hospital School of Nursing in 1907 and became Director of Nursing Services at the Henry Phipps Clinic at Johns Hopkins from 1913–1919. Due to her efforts, Johns Hopkins was the first general hospital school of nursing to offer a course in psychiatric nursing. She became the Dean of the Yale School of Nursing in 1934 and served in this position until 1944. She was also a leader in the International Council of Nurses until her death.

Tay-Sachs disease [Warren Tay, Brit. physician, 1843–1927; Bernard Sachs, U.S. neurologist, 1858–1944] The most severe (and most common) of the lipid storage diseases, Tay-Sachs disease is characterized by neurological deterioration in the first year of life. It is caused by a genetic abnormality on chromosome 15, which results in the deficient manufacture of lysosomal beta-hexosaminidase A. As a result of this metabolic error, sphingolipids accumulate in the neural tissues of affected offspring. The illness is especially prominent in families of Eastern European (Ashkenazi) Jews. In this ethnic group it is carried by approximately 1 in 25 individuals. Carriers of the trait can be accurately detected by assay of hexosaminidase A. SEE: *Nursing Diagnoses Appendix; sphingolipidosis.*

SYMPTOMS: The disease is characterized by normal development until the third to sixth month of life, after which profound regression occurs. Physical findings may include cherry-red spots on the macula, and enlargement of the head in the absence of hydrocephalus. Alterations in muscle tone, an abnormal startle response (hyperacusis), blindness, social withdrawal, and mental retardation are common early signs. A vegetative state is nearly universal by the second year of life. Death may occur before age 4.

Tay's spot Cherry-red spot.

TB *tuberculosis.*

Tb Symbol for the element terbium.

t.b. *tubercle bacillus; tuberculosis.*

T bandage A bandage resembling the letter T, used for the head and the perineum.

T-bar T-shaped tubing connected to an endotracheal tube; used to deliver oxygen therapy to an intubated patient who does not require mechanical ventilation.

TBI *total body irradiation; traumatic brain injury.*

TBP *thyroxine-binding protein.*

Tbs *tablespoon.*

TBSA *total body surface area.*

3TC Lamivudine, a nucleoside analogue reverse transcriptase inhibitor used in the treatment of HIV-1 and chronic hepatitis B.

Tc Symbol for the element technetium.

T-cell growth factor Interleukin-2.

T-cell–mediated immunity Cell-mediated immunity.

T-cell receptor ABBR: TCR. One of two polypeptide chains (α or β) on the surface of T lymphocytes that recognize and bind foreign antigens. TCRs are antigen specific; their activity depends on antigen processing by macrophages or other antigen-presenting cells and the presence of major histocompatibility complex proteins to which peptides from the antigen are bound. SEE: *autoimmunity; immune response; cell, T.*

$TCID_{50}$ *tissue culture infective dose.*

TCR *T-cell receptor.*

t.d.s. L. *ter die sumendum,* to be taken three times a day.

Te Symbol for the element tellurium.

tea (tē) **1.** An infusion of a medicinal plant. **2.** The leaves of the plant *Thea chinensis* or *Camellia sinensis,* from which a beverage is made by steeping the leaves in boiling hot water.

COMPOSITION: A number of pharmacologically active ingredients including caffeine, theophyline, various antioxidants including polyphenolic compounds, and sufficient fluoride to help prevent tooth decay are present in tea. The caloric content is negligible unless sugar and/or milk is added prior to consumption. SEE: *caffeine; caffeine withdrawal.*

CAUTION: Teas should be avoided by patients with a history of oxalate-containing kidney stones.

---

black t. Tea made from leaves that have been fermented before they are dried.

green t. Tea prepared by heating leaves in open trays.

herb t. Tea made of a variety of plants, including leaves of certain flowers, herbs, barks, and grasses. Some herbs used in these teas have been demonstrated to have pharmacological properties.

Paraguay copper t. Tea, also known as yerba maté, made from the leaves and stems of *Ilex paraguayensis.* It is a stimulating drink and contains volatile oil, tannin, and caffeine.

TEAB *tetraethylammonium bromide.*

TEAC *tetraethylammonium chloride.*

tear (tār) [AS. *taer*] To separate or pull apart by force.

bucket handle t. A longitudinal tear, usually beginning in the middle of a meniscus (cartilage) of the knee.

tears (tērs) [AS. *tear*] The watery saline solution secreted continuously by the lacrimal glands. They lubricate the surfaces between the eyeball and eyelids (i.e., the conjunctiva). These are called continuous tears. Irritant tears are produced when a foreign object or substance is in the eye. SEE: *Schirmer's test.*

artificial t. A solution used to lubricate the conjunctivae.

crocodile t. Excess tear production that occurs when salivary glands are stimulated during eating. This condition may be present in patients with incomplete recovery from facial paralysis.

tease (tēz) [AS. *taesan,* to pluck] To separate a tissue into minute parts with a needle to prepare it for microscopy.

teaspoon (tē′spoon) ABBR: tsp. A household measure equal to approx. 5 ml. Teaspoons used in the home vary from 3 to 6 ml. Because household measures are not accurate, when a teaspoon dose is prescribed or ordered, 5 ml of the substance should be given.

teat (tēt) [ME. *tete,* from AS. *tit,* teat] **1.** The nipple of the mammary gland. SYN: *papilla mammae.* SEE: *nipple; breast.* **2.** Any protuberance resembling a nipple.

teatulation (tēt″ū-lā′shŭn) [AS. *tit,* teat] The development of a nipple-like elevation.

technetium (tĕk-nē′shē-ŭm) SYMB: Tc. A synthetic metallic chemical element; atomic weight, 98.9062; atomic number, 43. Radioisotopes of technetium are used in imaging studies in nuclear medicine (e.g., myocardial perfusion scans, bone scans, and V/Q scans).

technetium-99m SYMB: ^{99m}Tc. An isomer of technetium that emits gamma rays. It has a half-life of 6 hr.

technetium Tc 99m albumin aggregated injection A radioactive isotope of technetium-99m. It is used intravenously for scanning the lung.

technical (tĕk′nĭ-kăl) [Gr. *tekhnikos,* skilled] Requiring technique or special skill.

technician (tĕk-nĭsh′ăn) An individual who has the knowledge and skill required to carry out specific technical procedures. This individual usually has a diploma from a specialized school or an associate degree from college or has received training through preceptorship.

biomedical engineering t. A technician who assembles, repairs, and adapts medical equipment used for the delivery of health care and assists in the development and maintenance of these systems.

certified pulmonary function t. An individual trained to evaluate respiratory function who has passed the examination offered by the National Board for Respiratory Care.

dental t. A technician who constructs complete and partial dentures, makes orthodontic appliances, and fixes bridgework, crowns, and other dental restorations as authorized by dentists.

dialysis t. A technician who operates and maintains an artificial kidney machine following approved methods to provide dialysis treatment for patients with kidney disorders.

dietetic t. A technician who assists the food service manager and dietitian in a health care facility with planning, implementing, and evaluating food programs, and may train and supervise dietary aides.

electrocardiographical t. A technician who operates and maintains electrocardiographic machines, records the heart's electrical activity, and provides data for diagnosis and treatment of heart ailments by physicians.

electromyographical t. A technician who assists the neurologist in recording and analyzing bioelectric potentials that originate in muscle tissue. This includes the operation of various electronic devices, maintenance of electronic equipment, assisting with patient care during testing, and record keeping.

emergency medical t.—paramedic A technician who responds to medical emergency calls, evaluates the nature of the emergency, and carries out specific diagnostic measures and emergency treatment procedures under the standing orders or specific directions of a physician.

environmental health t. A technician who assists in the survey of environmental hazards and performs technical duties under professional supervision in areas such as pollution control, radiation protection, and sanitation.

histological t. A technician who works under the supervision of a pathologist in sectioning, staining, and mounting human and animal tissue and fluid for microscopic study.

medical laboratory t. A technician who performs biological and chemical tests requiring limited independent judgment or correlation competency under the supervision of a medical technologist, pathologist, or physician.

medical record t. A technician who assists the medical record administrator by coding, analyzing, and preserving patients' medical records and compiling reports, disease indices, and statistics in health care institutions.

orthopedic t. A technician who is trained in maintaining traction devices, applying traction, making casts, and applying splints.

pharmacy t. A technician who assists the pharmacist in certain activities such as medication profile reviews for drug incompatibilities, typing of prescription labels, prescription packaging, handling of purchase records, and inventory control, and may, where state law and hospital policy permit, dispense drugs to patients under the supervision of a registered pharmacist.

psychiatric t. A technician who works under the supervision of a professional in the care of mentally ill patients in a psychiatric care facility. This person assists in carrying out the prescribed treatment plan and assigned individual and group activities with patients.

respiratory therapy t. A technician who routinely treats patients requiring noncritical respiratory care and who recognizes and responds to specified respiratory emergencies.

technique (tĕk-nēk′) [Fr., Gr. *technikos*] **1.** A systematic procedure or method by which an involved or scientific task is completed. **2.** The skill in performing details of a procedure or operation. **3.** In radiology, the various technical factors that must be determined in order to produce a diagnostic radiograph, such as kilovoltage, milliamperage, time of exposure, and focal-film distance.

bisecting angle t. A dental radiographic technique that requires (1) placement of the film as close as possible to the teeth, causing the film to rest against the crown; (2) visualization of a bisector, which bisects the angle formed by the long axis of the teeth and the film; and (3) positioning of the central ray perpendicular to the bisector. The image produced is distorted in a buccolingual direction. Also called *short-cone technique*. SEE: *Cieszynski's rule*.

compensatory t. The use of modified procedures or assistive devices to enable the successful performance of tasks by persons with a disability.

enzyme-multiplied immunoassay t. ABBR: EMIT. An enzyme immunoassay based on a mixture of analyte and enzyme substrate such that no immobile phase is necessary. SEE: *enzyme i.; cloned enzyme donor i.*

forced expiration t. A type of cough that facilitates clearance of bronchial secretions while reducing the risk of bronchiolar collapse. One or two expirations are forced from average to low lung volume with an open glottis. A period of diaphragmatic breathing and relaxation follows.

minimal leak t. ABBR: MLT. A method of determining the appropriate cuff inflation volume on endotracheal tubes. Excessive cuff inflation volume may lead to necrosis of the trachea, and excessive leaking may render oxygenation and ventilation ineffective or allow aspiration of large particles from the oral cavity.

paralleling t. A dental radiographic technique that requires placement of the film parallel to the teeth and positioning of the central ray perpendicular to the teeth. The orientation of the film, teeth, and central ray produces a radiograph with minimal geometric distortion. Also called *right-angle* or *long-cone technique*.

techno- Combining form meaning *art, skill*.

technologist (tĕk″nŏl′ō-jĭst) [Gr. *techne*, art, + *logos*, word, reason] An individual specializing in the application of scientific knowledge in solving practical or theoretical problems. The knowledge and skills required for performing these functions are achieved through formal education and a period of supervised clinical practice.

blood bank t. A technologist trained to assist in all of the routine and special functions and tasks concerned with blood bank and transfusion services.

cardiovascular t. A technologist who performs a wide range of tests related to the functions and therapeutic care of the heart and lung system. These include operating and maintaining a heart-lung machine, assisting in cardiac catheterization, cardiac resuscitation, postoperative monitoring, and the care and treatment of patients who have undergone heart or lung surgery.

electroencephalographic t. A technologist who operates and maintains electroencephalographic machines.

histologic t. A technologist who performs all the functions of the histological technician, as well as more complex procedures for processing tissues, such as identifying tissue structures, cell components, and their staining characteristics, and relates them to physiological functions. He or she may also implement and test new techniques and procedures.

medical t. A technologist who works in conjunction with pathologists, physicians, and scientists in all general areas of the clinical laboratory. Independent and correlational judgments are made in a wide range of complex procedures. A medical technologist may teach and supervise laboratory personnel.

nuclear medicine t. Radiation therapy t.

radiation therapy t. ABBR: RT(T). A technologist trained to assist the radiation oncologist in the safe application of radiation for therapeutic purposes. Also called *radiation therapist*. SYN: *nuclear medicine t.*

radiological t. A technologist trained in the safe application of ionizing radiation to portions of the body to assist the physician in the diagnosis of injuries and disease. This individual may also supervise or teach others. Technology programs approved by the Joint Review Commission on Education in the Radiologic Sciences are conducted in hospitals, medical schools, and colleges with hospital affiliations.

registered pulmonary function t. An individual who has completed the pulmonary function registry examination administered by the National Board for Respiratory Care.

surgical t. A technologist who assists in providing a safe environment for surgical care and assists surgeons, nurses, and other operating room staff.

vascular t. A person skilled in obtaining and interpreting ultrasonic images from blood vessels.

technology (tĕk-nŏl′ō-jē) [″ + *logos,* word, reason] **1.** The application of scientific knowledge. **2.** The scientific knowledge used in solving or approaching practical problems and situations.

adaptive t. Assistive t.

assistive t. ABBR: AT. A device or adaptation that enables or assists persons with disability to perform everyday tasks of living. Assistive technologies are categorized by rehabilitation personnel as high technology or low technology, with the former including devices that use microprocessors. An example of a high-technology device is an environmental control unit or robotic aid. An example of a low-technology device is a reacher or a tool with a built-up handle. SYN: *adaptive t.; adaptive device.*

The Technology Related Assistance for Individuals with Disabilities Act Amendments of 1994 provide for programs that support the development, acquisition, or application of assistive technology devices or equipment to assist persons with activity limitations resulting from functional impairments.

tectocephalic (tĕk″tō-sĕ-făl′ĭk) [L. *tectum,* roof, + Gr. *kephale,* head] Concerning tectocephaly.

tectocephaly (tĕk-tō-sĕf′ăl-ē) Scaphocephalism.

tectorial (tĕk-tō′rē-ăl) [L. *tectum,* roof] Pert. to tectorium.

tectorium (tĕk-tō′rē-ŭm) *pl.* **tectoria** [L. *tectorium,* a covering] **1.** Any rooflike structure. SYN: *tectum; tegmentum; tegument.* **2.** The membrane that overhangs the receptors for hearing (hair cells) in the organ of Corti.

tectospinal (tĕk″tō-spī′năl) [L. *tectum,* roof, + *spina,* thorn] From the tectum mesencephali to the spinal cord.

tectospinal tract A tract of white fibers of the spinal cord passing from the tectum of the midbrain and going down through the medulla to the spinal cord. It begins on one side and crosses to the other.

tectum (tĕk′tŭm) [L., roof] **1.** Any structure serving as, or resembling, a roof. SYN: *tectorium; tegmentum; tegument.* **2.** The dorsal portion of the midbrain consisting of the superior and inferior colliculi (corpora quadrigemina). SYN: *tegmentum.*

t. mesencephali The roof of the midbrain, including the corpora quadrigemina.

T.E.D. *threshold erythema dose.*

teenage Adolescent.

teeth (tēth) *sing.,* **tooth** [AS. *toth,* tooth] Hard bony projections in the jaws serving as organs of mastication. Each individual has two complete sets of teeth during the life cycle. The first set of teeth an individual develops are the primary teeth. They exfoliate by age 14 and are replaced by the permanent teeth. There are 20 primary teeth and 32 permanent teeth. The permanent teeth include the following types: incisors, canines (cuspids), premolars (bicuspids), and molars. On average, a child should have 6 teeth at 1 year, 12 teeth at 18 months, 16 teeth at 2 years, and 20 teeth at 12 years. Some children are born with a few erupted teeth; in others, the teeth may not appear until 16 months. SEE: *dentition* for illus.; *tooth; plaque, dental; periodontal disease.*

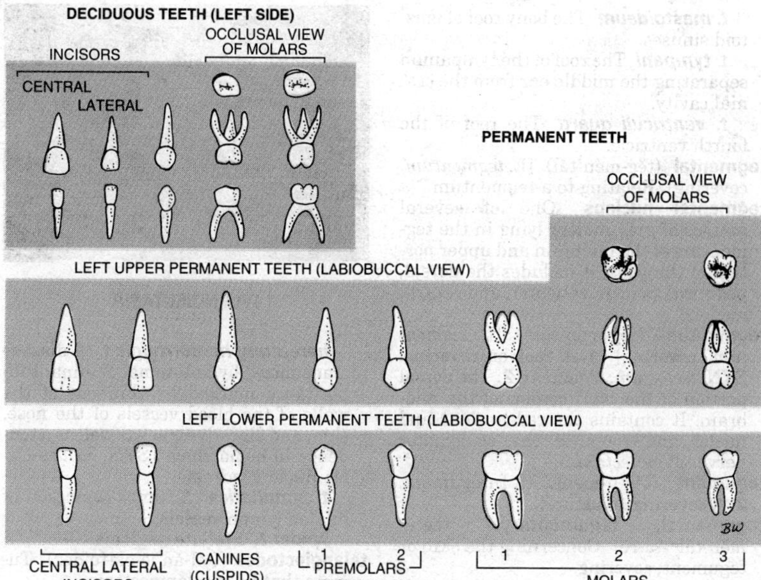

PATIENT CARE: Individuals with unusual eruption patterns should be referred to a dental professional for evaluation.

anterior t. Teeth located close to the midline of the dental arch on either side of the jaw, including the incisors and canines.

auditory t. Minute toothlike projections along the free margin of the labium vestibulare of the cochlea. SYN: *Huschke's auditory teeth.*

charting and numbering of t. The various systems developed for designating teeth in a chart system including numbers, letters, or symbols. They are not uniformly accepted. Widely used are the two-digit system of Federation Dentaire Internationale (FDI system) and the American system, which numbers the permanent teeth consecutively from the upper right third molar as #1 through the maxillary teeth to #16, and then to the left mandibular third molar as #17 and through the mandibular teeth to the right third molar as #32.

deciduous t. The 20 teeth that make up the first dentition, which are shed and replaced by the permanent teeth. SYN: *baby tooth; milk t.; temporary t.* SEE: illus.

malacotic t. Teeth that are esp. prone to decay, soft in structure and white in color.

milk t. Deciduous t.

permanent t. Teeth that develop as the second dentition, replacing the deciduous teeth. SYN: *secondary t.* SEE: *deciduous t.* for illus.

reimplantation or repair of t. The preservation and restoration of teeth dislodged or broken by trauma.

FIRST AID: If a tooth is completely knocked out of its socket by trauma or fracture, the tooth or fragment should be gently cleaned (not scrubbed), placed in clean water, and taken with the patient without delay to a dentist. For an adult who is conscious, the tooth may be replaced in the socket during transport to the dentist.

sclerotic t. Yellowish teeth that are naturally hard and highly resistant to caries.

secondary t. Permanent t.

stained t. Deep or superficial discoloration of teeth. A number of conditions cause this (e.g., exposure of the fetus to tetracycline the mother took during pregnancy or mottling caused by exposure to high levels of fluoride in drinking water). No matter what the cause, the stains may be covered by applying a resin or porcelain laminate veneer over the stain, a process called bonding. This same technique may be used to rebuild or repair chipped or cracked teeth.

temporary t. Deciduous t.

twinning of t. A dental anomaly in which two teeth are joined together.

wisdom t. The third molar teeth of the permanent dentition, which are the last to erupt.

teething (tēth′ĭng) [AS. *toth,* tooth] Eruption of the teeth. SEE: *dentition.*

tegmen (tĕg′mĕn) *pl.* **tegmina** [L. *tegmen,* covering] A structure that covers a part.

t. mastoideum The bony roof of mastoid sinuses.

t. tympani The roof of the tympanum separating the middle ear from the cranial cavity.

t. ventriculi quarti The roof of the fourth ventricle.

tegmental (tĕg-mĕn′tăl) [L. *tegmentum,* covering] Relating to a tegmentum.

tegmental nucleus One of several masses of gray matter lying in the tegmentum of the midbrain and upper portion of the pons; it includes the dorsal, pedunculopontile, reticular, and ventral nuclei.

tegmentum (tĕg-mĕn′tŭm) [L. *tegmentum,* covering] **1.** A roof or covering. SYN: *tectorium; tegument.* **2.** The dorsal portion of the cruri cerebri of the midbrain. It contains the red nucleus and nuclei and roots of the oculomotor nerve. SYN: *tectum.*

tegument (tĕg′ū-mĕnt) **1.** Integument. **2.** A covering structure.

tegumental, tegumentary (tĕg″ū-mĕn′tăl, -tă-rē) Concerning the skin or tegument; covering.

teichoic acid A polymer found in the cell wall of certain bacteria.

teichopsia (tī-kŏp′sē-ă) [Gr. *teichos,* wall, + *opsis,* vision] Zigzag lines bounding a luminous area appearing in the visual field. It causes temporary blindness in that portion of the field of vision. This condition is sometimes associated with migraine headaches or mental or physical strain. SYN: *scintillating scotoma.*

teinodynia (tī″nō-dĭn′ē-ă) [Gr. *tenon,* tendon, + *odyne,* pain] Tenodynia.

tel-, tele- **1.** Combining form meaning *end.* **2.** Combining form meaning *distant.*

tela (tē′lă) *pl.* **telae** [L. *tela,* web] Any weblike structure.

t. choroidea Part of the pia mater covering the roof of the third and fourth cerebral ventricles.

t. conjunctiva Connective tissue.

t. elastica Elastic tissue.

t. subcutanea Subcutaneous connective tissue. SYN: *superficial fascia.*

t. submucosa The submucosa of the intestine.

telalgia (tĕl-ăl′jē-ă) [Gr. *tele,* distant, + *algos,* pain] Pain felt at a distance from its stimulus. SYN: *pain, referred.*

telangiectasia, telangiectasis (tĕl-ăn″jē-ĕk-tā′zē-ă, -ĕk′tă-sĭs) [Gr. *telos,* end, + *angeion,* vessel, + *ektasis,* dilatation] A vascular lesion formed by dilatation of a group of small blood vessels. It may appear as a birthmark or become apparent in young children. It may also be caused by long-term sun exposure. Although the lesion may occur anywhere on the skin, it is seen most frequently on the face and thighs. SEE: illus. **telangiectatic,** *adj.*

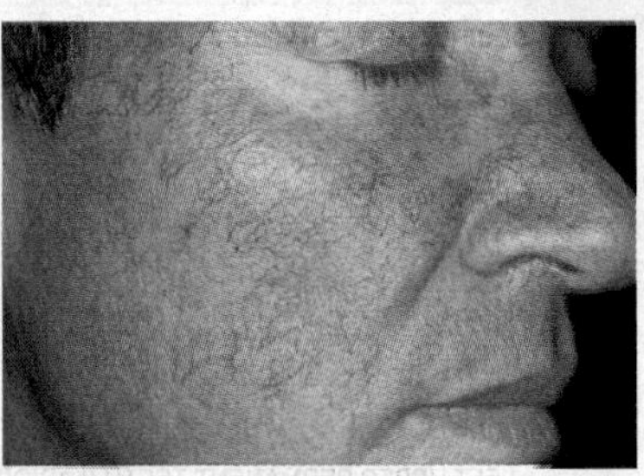

TELANGIECTASIA

hereditary hemorrhagic t. A disease transmitted by autosomal dominant inheritance marked by thinness of the walls of the blood vessels of the nose, skin, and digestive tract as well as a tendency to hemorrhage. SYN: *Rendu-Osler-Weber syndrome.*

t. lymphatica A tumor composed of dilated lymph vessels.

spider t. Stellate angioma.

telangiectodes (tĕl-ăn″jē-ĕk-tō′dēz) Tumors that have telangiectasia.

telangiitis (tĕl-ăn″jē-ī′tĭs) [″ + ″ + *itis,* inflammation] An inflammation of the capillaries.

telangioma (tĕl-ăn″jē-ō′mă) [Gr. *telos,* end, + *angeion,* vessel, + *oma,* tumor] A tumor made up of dilated capillaries or arterioles.

telangion (tĕl-ăn′jē-ŏn) [″ + *angeion,* vessel] A capillary or terminal arteriole.

telangiosis (tĕl″ăn-jē-ō′sĭs) [″ + ″ + *osis,* condition] A disease of capillary vessels.

telecanthus (tĕl″ĕ-kăn′thŭs) [Gr. *tele,* distant, + *kanthos,* corner of the eye] Increased distance between the inner canthi of the eyelids.

telecardiogram (tĕl″ĕ-kăr′dē-ō-grăm) [″ + *kardia,* heart, + *gramma,* something written] A cardiogram that records at a distance from the patient. The signal is transmitted electronically to the recording device. SYN: *telelectrocardiogram.*

telecardiography (tĕl″ĕ-kăr″dē-ŏg′ră-fē) [″ + ″ + *graphein,* to write] The process of taking telecardiograms.

telecardiophone (tĕl″ĕ-kăr′dē-ō-fōn) [″ + ″ + *phone,* voice] A stethoscope that will magnify heart sounds so they may be heard at a distance from the patient.

teleceptive (tĕl-ĕ-sĕp′tĭv) [″ + L. *ceptivus,* take] Relating to a teleceptor.

teleceptor (tĕl′ĕ-sĕp″tor) [″ + L. *ceptor,* a receiver] A distance receptor; a sense organ that responds to stimuli arising some distance from the body, such as the eye, ear, and nose. SYN: *teloceptor.*

telecurietherapy (tĕl-ĕ-kū″rē-thĕr′ă-pē) [″ + *curie,* + Gr. *therapeia,* treatment] The application of radiation therapy from a source distant from the lesion or patient.

teledendrite, teledendron (tĕl-ĕ-dĕn′drīt, -dĕn′drŏn) [Gr. *telos,* end, + *dendron,* a tree] One of the terminal processes of an axon. SYN: *telodendron.*

telediagnosis (tĕl″ĕ-dī″ăg-nō′sĭs) [Gr. *tele,* distant,+ *diagignoskein,* to discern] Diagnosis made on the basis of data transmitted electronically to the physician's location.

telediastolic (tĕl″ĕ-dī-ă-stŏl′ĭk) [Gr. *telos,* end, + *diastole,* a dilatation] Concerning the last phase of the diastole.

telefluoroscopy (tĕl″ĕ-floo″or-ŏs′kō-pē) The transmission of fluoroscopic images by electronic means.

telekinesis (tĕl″ĕ-kĭ-nē′sĭs) [″ + *kinesis,* movement] The ability to move objects by pure mental concentration. Claims of telekinetic powers are typical of patients with psychotic illnesses.

telelectrocardiogram (tĕl″ē-lĕk″trō-kăr′dē-ō-grăm) [Gr. *tele,* distant, + *elektron,* amber, + *kardia,* heart, + *gramma,* something written] Telecardiogram.

telemedicine The use of telecommunications equipment to transmit video images, x-rays and other images, electronic medical records, and laboratory results about patients from distant sites. This improves health care access and delivery to remote rural, military, or international health care facilities.

telemeter (tĕl′ĕ-mē″tĕr) [″ + *metron,* measure] An electronic device used to transmit information to a distant point.

telemetry (tĕ-lĕm′ĕ-trē) The transmission of data electronically to a distant location.

telencephalic (tĕl″ĕn-sĕf-ăl′ĭk) [Gr. *telos,* end, + *enkephalos,* brain] Pert. to the endbrain (telencephalon).

telencephalization (tĕl″ĕn-sĕf″ăl-ī-zā′shŭn) The evolutionary degree of control over functions previously mediated by lower nerve centers.

telencephalon (tĕl-ĕn-sĕf′ă-lŏn) [″ + *enkephalos,* brain] The embryonic endbrain or posterior division of the prosencephalon from which the cerebral hemispheres, corpora striata, and rhinencephalon develop.

teleneurite (tĕl″ĕ-nū′rīt) [″ + *neuron,* nerve] The branching end of an axon.

teleneuron (tĕl″ĕ-nū′rŏn) [″ + *neuron,* nerve] A nerve ending.

teleo- Combining form meaning *perfect, complete.*

teleological (tē″lē-ō-lŏj′ĭ-kăl) Concerning teleology.

teleology (tĕl-ē-ŏl′ō-jē) [Gr. *teleos,* complete, + *logos,* word, reason] **1.** The belief that everything is directed toward some final purpose. **2.** The doctrine of final causes.

teleomitosis (tĕl″ē-ō-mī-tō′sĭs) [″ + *mitos,* thread, + *osis,* condition] Completed mitosis.

teleonomy (tĕl″ē-ŏn′ō-mē) [″ + *nomos,* law] The concept that, in an organism or animal, the existence of a structure, capability, or function indicates that it had survival value. **teleonomic** (tĕl″ē-ō-nŏm′ĭk), *adj.*

teleoperator A machine or device operated by a person at a distance. Such a machine allows tasks to be done deep in the ocean or on orbiting satellites, and allows radioactive materials to be manipulated without danger of exposure to the radioactivity.

teleopsia (tĕl-ē-ŏp′sē-ă) [Gr. *tele,* distant, + *ops,* eye] A visual disorder in which objects perceived in space have excessive depth or in which close objects appear far away.

teleotherapeutics (tĕl″ē-ō-thĕr-ă-pū′tĭks) [Gr. *tele,* distant, + *therapeutikos,* treating] The use of hypnotic suggestion in the treatment of disease. SYN: *suggestive therapeutics.*

telepathy (tĕ-lĕp′ă-thē) The ability to communicate with others wordlessly, that is, by broadcasting one's thoughts or by receiving the transmitted thoughts of others. Claims of telepathic powers are typical of patients with psychoses and of some shamans. SYN: *telesthesia* (1).

teleradiogram (tĕl″ĕ-rā′dē-ō-grăm) [Gr. *tele,* distant, + L. *radius,* ray, + Gr. *gramma,* something written] An x-ray picture obtained by teleradiography.

teleradiography (tĕl″ĕ-rā-dē-ŏg′ră-fē) Radiography with the radiation source about 2 m (6½ ft) from the body. Because the rays are virtually parallel at that distance, distortion is minimized. SYN: *teleroentgenography.*

teleradiology The transmission of an x-ray image to a distant center where it may be interpreted by a radiologist.

teleradium (tĕl″ĕ-rā′dē-ŭm) A radium source distant from the area being treated.

teleroentgenogram (tĕl″ĕ-rĕnt-gĕn′ō-grăm) [″ + *roentgen* + Gr. *gramma,* something written] Teleradiogram.

teleroentgenography (tĕl″ĕ-rĕnt″gĕn-ŏg′ră-fē) [″ + ″ + Gr. *graphein,* to write] Teleradiography.

telesthesia (tĕl-ĕs-thē′zē-ă) [″ + *aisthesis,* sensation] **1.** Telepathy. **2.** Distance perception. SEE: *paranormal.*

telesystolic (tĕl″ĕ-sĭs-tŏl′ĭk) [Gr. *telos,* end, + *systole,* contraction] Pert. to the termination of cardiac systole.

teletherapy (tĕl-ĕ-thĕr′ă-pē) [Gr. *tele,* distant, + *therapeia,* treatment] Cancer treatment in which the radiation source is placed outside the body.

teletypewriter ABBR: TTY. A typewriter that may be connected to a telephone. This device permits deaf persons to communicate by sending and receiving typewritten messages.

telluric (tĕ-lūr′ĭk) [L. *tellus,* earth] Of or rel. to the earth.

tellurism (tĕl′ū-rĭzm) [″ + Gr. *-ismos,* condition] The unproven and vague concept that emanations from the earth cause disease.

tellurium (tĕl-ū′rē-ŭm) [L. *tellus,* earth] SYMB: Te. A nonmetallic element used as an electric rectifier and in coloring glass; atomic weight, 127.60; atomic number, 52; specific gravity, 6.24.

tellurium poisoning Toxicity resulting from the ingestion of tellurium, a rare form of intoxication usually resulting from an occupational exposure to tellurium. It is marked by a garlic odor of all secretions, dry skin and mouth, anorexia, nausea, drowsiness, weakness, and, in severe cases, respiratory and circulatory collapse. Treatment includes administration of saline cathartics and an increase in fluid intake. In addition, perspiration should be induced; otherwise, treatment is symptomatic.

telocentric (tĕl″ō-sĕn′trĭk) [Gr. *telos,* end, + *kentron,* center] Location of the centromere in the extreme end of the replicating chromosome so that there is only one arm on the chromosome.

teloceptor Teleceptor.

telodendron (tĕl-ō-dĕn′drŏn) [Gr. *telos,* end, + *dendron,* tree] Teledendrite.

telogen (tĕl′ō-jĕn) [″ + *genesis,* generation, birth] The resting stage of the hair growth cycle. SEE: *anagen; catagen.*

teloglia (tĕl-ŏg′lē-ă) The Schwann cells at the end of a motor nerve fiber near the neuromuscular junction.

telolecithal Concerning an egg in which the large yolk mass is concentrated at one pole.

telolemma (tĕl″ō-lĕm′mă) [″ + *lemma,* rind] The membrane of the axon terminal at a neuromuscular junction.

telomerase An enzyme that helps cells repair the damage that occurs to the end of the DNA molecule during each cycle of cell division. Without such repair, cells eventually age and die. Cancer cells have telomerases that allow infinite repair to the DNA strands, a factor that contributes to their "immortality." SEE: *telomere.*

telomere (tĕl′ō-mēr) [″ + *meros,* part] A repetitive segment of DNA found on the ends of chromosomes. With each mitotic division, parts of the telomeres of a chromosome are lost. A theory of cellular aging proposes that the telomeres act as a biological clock and that when they are depleted, the cell dies or becomes much less active.

telomeric theory of aging The progressive shortening of the end regions of chromosomes that occurs with each cell replication cycle; this loss of genetic material may serve as the clock that defines aging at the cellular level.

telophase (tĕl′ō-fāz) [″ + *phasis,* an appearance] The final phase or stage of mitosis (karyokinesis) during which reconstruction of the daughter nuclei takes place and the cytoplasm of the cell divides, giving rise to two daughter cells.

telophragma (tĕl″ō-frăg′mă) [″ + *phragmos,* a fencing in] The Z line or disk in striated muscle. SEE: *Z disk.*

telosynapsis (tĕl″ō-sĭ-năp′sĭs) [″ + *synapsis,* point of contact] End-to-end union of pairs of homologous chromosomes during gametogenesis.

TEM *triethylenemelamine.*

tempeh A wheat-soybean mold-modified and fermented food used traditionally in Asia. The quality of protein in tempeh is close to that of casein.

temper [AS. *temprian,* to mingle] The state of an individual's mood, disposition, or mind (e.g., even-tempered or foul-tempered).

temperament (tĕm′pĕr-ă-mĕnt) [L. *temperamentum,* mixture] The combination of intellectual, emotional, ethical, and physical characteristics of a specific individual.

temperance Moderation in one's thoughts and actions, esp. with respect to use of alcoholic beverages.

temperate (tĕm′pĕr-ĭt) Moderate; not excessive.

temperature (tĕm′pĕr-ă-tūr) [L. *temperatura,* proportion] The degree of hotness or coldness of a substance.

Body temperature varies with the time of day and the site of measurement. Oral temperature is usually 97.5° to 99.5°F (36° to 38°C). Daily fluctuations in an individual may be 1° or 2°F. Body temperature may be measured by a placing a thermometer in the mouth, the rectum, under the arm, in the bladder, within the chambers of the heart, or in the external auditory canal of the ear. Rectal temperature is usually from 0.5° to 1.0°F (0.28° to 0.56°C) higher than by mouth; axillary temperature is about 0.5°F (0.28°C) lower than by mouth. Oral temperature measurement may be inaccurate if performed just after the patient has ingested cold substances or has been breathing with the mouth open.

Body temperature is regulated by thermoregulatory centers in the hypothalamus that balance heat production and heat loss. Eighty-five percent of body heat is lost through the skin (radiation, conduction, sweating) and the remainder through the lungs and fecal and urinary excretions. Muscular work (including shivering) is a mechanism for raising body temperature. Elevation of temperature above normal is called fever (pyrexia), and subnormal temperature is hypothermia. Other factors that can influence body temperature are age (infants and children have a wider

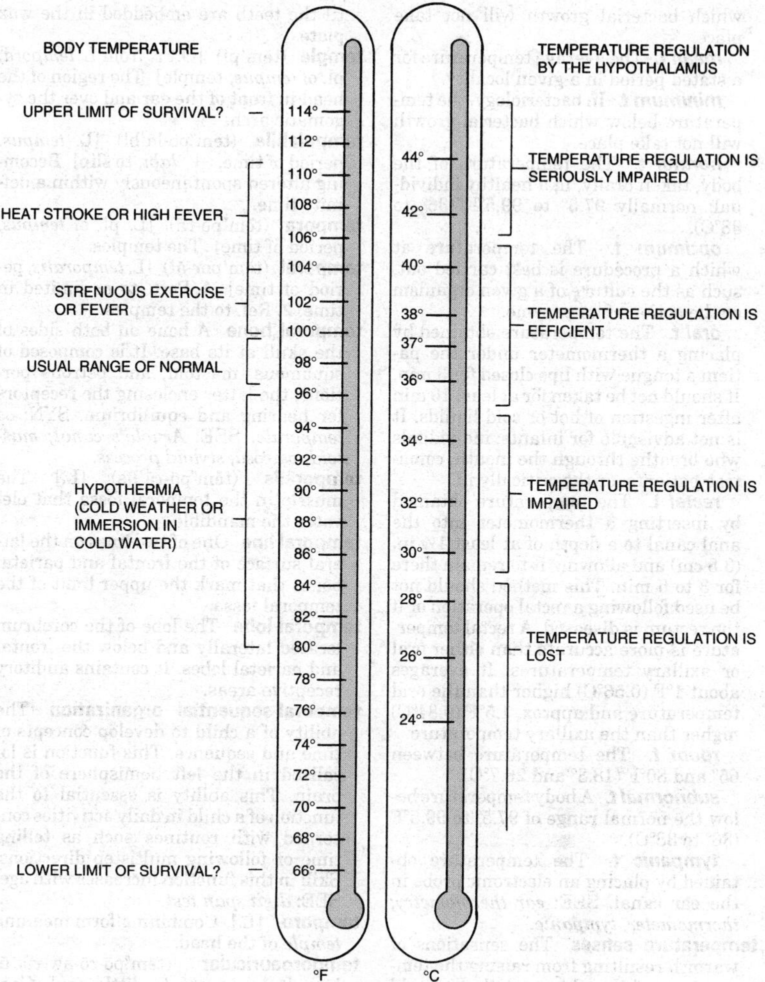

TEMPERATURE REGULATION

Effects of changes in body temperature

range of body temperature than adults, and elderly have lower body temperatures than others); menstruation cycle in women (the temperature rises in the ovulatory midcycle and remains high until menses); and exercise (temperature rises with moderate to vigorous muscular activity). SEE: illus.

absolute t. The temperature measured from absolute zero, which is −273.15°C.

ambient t. The surrounding temperature or that present in the place, site, or location indicated.

axillary t. The temperature obtained by placing a thermometer in the apex of the axilla with the arm pressed closely to the side of the body. The temperature obtained by this method is usually 0.5° to 1.0°F (0.28° to 0.56°C) lower than oral.

body t. The temperature of the body, an indicator of health and disease and one of the vital signs.

core t. The body's temperature in deep internal structures, such as the heart or bladder, as opposed to peripheral parts such as the mouth or axilla.

critical t. The temperature below which a gas may be converted to liquid form by pressure.

inverse t. A condition in which the body temperature is higher in the morning than in the evening.

maximum t. The temperature above

which bacterial growth will not take place.

mean t. The average temperature for a stated period in a given locality.

minimum t. In bacteriology, the temperature below which bacterial growth will not take place.

normal t. The temperature of the body, taken orally, in a healthy individual: normally 97.5° to 99.5°F (36° to 38°C).

optimum t. The temperature at which a procedure is best carried out, such as the culture of a given organism or the action of an enzyme.

oral t. The temperature obtained by placing a thermometer under the patient's tongue with lips closed for 3 min. It should not be taken for at least 10 min after ingestion of hot or cold liquids. It is not advisable for infants, individuals who breathe through the mouth, comatose patients, or the critically ill.

rectal t. The temperature obtained by inserting a thermometer into the anal canal to a depth of at least 1½ in. (3.8 cm) and allowing it to remain there for 3 to 5 min. This method should not be used following a rectal operation or if the rectum is diseased. A rectal temperature is more accurate than either oral or axillary temperatures. It averages about 1°F (0.56°C) higher than the oral temperature and approx. 1.5°F (0.84°C) higher than the axillary temperature.

room t. The temperature between 65° and 80°F (18.3° and 26.7°C).

subnormal t. A body temperature below the normal range of 97.5° to 99.5°F (36° to 38°C).

tympanic t. The temperature obtained by placing an electronic probe in the ear canal. SEE: *ear thermometry; thermometer, tympanic*.

temperature senses The sensations of warmth resulting from raising the temperature of the skin and that of cold aroused by lowering it. The sensation of warmth is mediated by Ruffini's corpuscles; that of cold, by the end-bulbs of Krause. These receptors are distributed so as to form cold and warm sensing spots on the skin. Afferent impulses from receptors, on reaching the thalamus, may give rise to crude uncritical temperature sensations; on being relayed to the somesthetic area of the cortex, they result in discrete and fairly well localized sensations of heat and cold. Adaptation is rapid.

template (tĕm′plāt) A pattern, mold, or form used as a guide in duplicating a shape, structure, or device.

occlusal t. A stone or metal base made from a wax occlusal registration against which artificial teeth are set in the preparation of a denture.

wax t. A wax impression of the occlusion of teeth made by closing the jaw until the teeth are embedded in the wax plate.

temple (tĕm′pl) [O.Fr. from L. *tempora,* pl. of *tempus,* temple] The region of the head in front of the ear and over the zygomatic arch.

tempolabile (tĕm″pō-lā′bl) [L. *tempus,* period of time, + *labi,* to slip] Becoming altered spontaneously within a definite time.

tempora (tĕm′pō-ră) [L. pl. of *tempus,* period of time] The temples.

temporal (tĕm′por-ăl) [L. *temporalis,* period of time] **1.** Pert. to or limited in time. **2.** Rel. to the temples.

temporal bone A bone on both sides of the skull at its base. It is composed of squamous, mastoid, and petrous portions, the latter enclosing the receptors for hearing and equilibrium. SYN: *os temporale*. SEE: *Arnold's canal; mastoid; petrosa; styloid process*.

temporalis (tĕm″pō-rā′lĭs) [L.] The muscle in the temporal fossa that elevates the mandible.

temporal line One of two lines on the lateral surface of the frontal and parietal bones that mark the upper limit of the temporal fossa.

temporal lobe The lobe of the cerebrum located laterally and below the frontal and parietal lobes. It contains auditory receptive areas.

temporal-sequential organization The ability of a child to develop concepts of time and sequence. This function is localized in the left hemisphere of the brain. This ability is essential to the function of a child in daily activities concerned with routines such as telling time or following multistep directions. Skill in this function increases with age. SEE: *digit span test*.

temporo- [L.] Combining form meaning *temple* of the head.

temporoauricular (tĕm″pō-rō-aw-rĭk′ū-lăr) [″ + *auricula,* little ear] Concerning the temples and auricular areas.

temporohyoid (tĕm″pō-rō-hī′oyd) [″ + Gr. *hyoeides,* U-shaped] Concerning the temporal and hyoid bones.

temporomalar (tĕm″pō-rō-mā′lăr) [″ + *mala,* cheek] Temporozygomatic.

temporomandibular (tĕm″pō-rō-măn-dĭb′ū-lăr) [″ + *mandibula,* lower jawbone] Pert. to the temporal and mandible bones; esp. important in dentistry because of the articulation of the bones of the temporomandibular joint.

temporomandibular joints The encapsulated, bicondylar, synovial joints between the condyles of the mandible and the temporal bones of the skull.

temporomandibular joint syndrome ABBR: TMJ syndrome. Severe pain in and about the temporomandibular joint, made worse by chewing. The syndrome is marked by limited movement of the joint and clicking sounds during chewing. Tinnitus, pain, and rarely, deafness may be present. Causes include lesions of the temporomandibular joint tissues, malocclusion, overbite, poorly fitting dentures, and tissue changes resulting in pressure on nerves. Treatments may include bite blocks worn at night, nonsteroidal anti-inflammatory drugs, local massage, or joint surgeries. SYN: *Costen's syndrome.*

temporomaxillary (tĕm″pō-rō-măk′sĭ-lĕr-ē) [″ + *maxilla,* jawbone] Pert. to the temporal and maxillary bones.

temporo-occipital (tĕm″pō-rō-ŏk-sĭp′ĭ-tăl) [″ + *occipitalis,* pert. to the occiput] Pert. to the temporal and occipital bones or their regions.

temporoparietal (tĕm″pō-rō-pă-rī′ĕ-tăl) [″ + *paries,* wall] Concerning the temporal and parietal bones.

temporopontine [″ + *pons,* bridge] Concerning or situated between the temporal lobe of the brain and the pons.

temporosphenoid (tĕm″pō-rō-sfē′noyd) [″ + Gr. *sphen,* wedge, + *eidos,* form, shape] Pert. to the temporal and sphenoid bones.

temporozygomatic (tĕm″pō-rō-zī″gō-măt′ĭk) [″ + Gr. *zygoma,* cheekbone] Concerning the temporal and zygomatic bones. SYN: *temporomalar.*

tempostabile (tĕm″pō-stā′bĭl) [L. *tempus,* time, + *stabilis,* stable] Descriptive of something, esp. a chemical compound, that remains stable with the passage of time.

ten- SEE: *taen-.*

tenacious (tĕ-nā′shŭs) [L. *tenax*] Adhering to; adhesive; retentive.

tenacity (tĕ-năs′ĭ-tē) Toughness, stubbornness, obstinacy, durability.

tenaculum (tĕn-ăk′ū-lŭm) [L., a holder] Sharp, hooklike, pointed instrument with a slender shank for grasping and holding an anatomical part.

tenalgia (tĕn-ăl′jē-ă) [Gr. *tenon,* tendon, + *algos,* pain] Tenodynia.

t. crepitans An inflammation of a tendon sheath that on movement results in a crackling sound.

Tenckhoff peritoneal dialysis catheter A large-bore, indwelling catheter used for continuous ambulatory peritoneal dialysis; it is inserted into the peritoneal cavity through the abdominal wall. SEE: *dialysis, continuous ambulatory peritoneal.*

tender loving care ABBR: TLC. The concept of administering medical and nursing care and attention to a patient in a kindly, compassionate, and humane manner.

tenderness (tĕn′dĕr-nĕs) Sensitivity to pain upon pressure.

rebound t. The production or intensification of pain when pressure that has been applied during palpation (esp. of the abdomen) is suddenly released. SEE: *Blumberg's sign.*

tendinoplasty (tĕn′dĭ-nō-plăs″tē) [″ + Gr. *plassein,* to form] Plastic surgery of tendons. SYN: *tendoplasty; tenontoplasty; tenoplasty.*

tendinosis **1.** Degeneration of a tendon from repetitive microtrauma. **2.** Collagen degeneration.

tendinosuture (tĕn″dĭn-ō-sū′tŭr) [″ + *sutura,* a seam] The suturing of a divided tendon. SYN: *tenorrhaphy.*

tendinous (tĕn′dĭ-nŭs) [L. *tendinosus*] Pert. to, composed of, or resembling tendons.

tendo- SEE: *teno-.*

tendo [L.] Tendon.

tendolysis (tĕn-dŏl′ĭ-sĭs) [″ + Gr. *lysis,* dissolution] The process of freeing a tendon from adhesions. SYN: *tenolysis.*

tendon (tĕn′dŭn) [L. *tendo,* tendon] Fibrous connective tissue serving for the attachment of muscles to bones and other parts. SYN: *sinew; tendo.*

Achilles t. The large tendon at the lower end of the gastrocnemius muscle, inserted into the calcaneus. It is the strongest and thickest tendon in the body. SYN: *calcaneal t.*

calcaneal t. Achilles t.

central t. The central portion of the diaphragm, consisting of a flat aponeurosis into which the muscle fibers of the diaphragm are inserted.

superior t. of Lockwood The portion of the fibrous ring from which the superior oblique muscle of the eye originates.

t. of Zinn The portion of the fibrous ring (annulus tendineus communis) from which the inferior rectus muscle of the eye originates.

tendon action Passive movement of a joint when a two-joint or multijoint muscle is stretched across it.

tendon cell One of the fibroblasts of white fibrous connective tissue of tendons that are arranged in parallel rows.

tendonitis, tendinitis (tĕn″dĭn-ī′tĭs) [L. *tendo,* tendon, + Gr. *itis,* inflammation] Inflammation of a tendon.

rotator cuff t. A common cause of shoulder pain, thought to be due to inflammation of the intrinsic tendons of the shoulder, esp. that of the supraspinatus. The onset usually follows injury or overuse during activities involving repeated overhead arm motions, as occurs in certain occupations (e.g., construction workers, painters) and sports (e.g., baseball, tennis, swimming).

ETIOLOGY: Individuals over age 40 are particularly susceptible because of decreased vascular supply to the rotator cuff tendons. Those who perform repeated overhead motions are also at risk.

SYMPTOMS: The patient will describe pain with overhead arm motion; on examination, the extremity may be postured for comfort; muscle strength and tone of the scapular muscles may be decreased.

TREATMENT: Conservative treatment consists of the use of moist heat and strengthening and range-of-motion exercises; if the patient does not respond to these treatment methods and loss of function is present, corticosteroid injections may be helpful. Surgery to resect the coracoacromial ligament may be indicated in persons who fail other therapies.

tendon spindle A fusiform nerve ending in a tendon.

tendoplasty (tĕn′dō-plăs″tē) [″ + Gr. *plassein,* to mold] Reparative surgery of an injured tendon. SYN: *tendinoplasty; tenontoplasty; tenoplasty.*

tendosynovitis (tĕn″dō-sĭn″ō-vī′tĭs) [″ + *synovia,* joint fluid, + Gr. *itis,* inflammation] Tenosynovitis.

tendotome (tĕn′dō-tōm) [″ + Gr. *tome,* incision] Tenotome.

tendotomy (tĕn-dŏt′ō-mē) Tenotomy.

tendovaginal (tĕn″dō-văj′ĭ-năl) [L. *tendo,* tendon, + *vagina,* sheath] Rel. to a tendon and its sheath.

tendovaginitis (tĕn″dō-văj″ĭn-ī′tĭs) [″ + ″ + Gr. *itis,* inflammation] Tenosynovitis. SYN: *tendosynovitis.*

Tenebrio (tĕ-nĕb′rē-ō) A genus of beetles including the species of *T. molitor,* which is an intermediate host of helminth parasites of vertebrates.

tenectomy [″ + *ektome,* excision] Excision of a lesion of a tendon or tendon sheath.

graduated t. Partial division of a tendon.

tenesmus (tĕ-nĕz′mŭs) [Gr. *teinesmos,* a stretching] Spasmodic contraction of anal or bladder sphincter with pain and persistent desire to empty the bowel or bladder, with involuntary ineffectual straining efforts. **tenesmic** (tĕn-ĕz′mĭk), *adj.*

teni- SEE: *taen-.*

tenia (tē′nē-ă) [L. *taenia,* tape] Taenia.

teniasis (tē-nī′ă-sĭs) [L. *taenia,* tapeworm, + Gr. *-iasis,* a condition] Presence of tapeworms in the body.

tenicide (tĕn′ĭ-sīd) [″ + *cidus,* killing] Taeniacide.

tenifuge (tĕn′ĭ-fūj) [″ + *fuga,* flight] Causing or that which causes expulsion of tapeworms.

tennis elbow A condition marked by pain over the lateral epicondyle of the humerus or the head of the radius. The pain radiates to the outer side of the arm and forearm due to injury or overuse of the extensor carpi radialis brevis or longus muscle, as may occur in playing tennis. The condition is aggravated by resisted wrist extension or forearm supination, or by a stretch force with the wrist flexed, forearm pronated, and elbow extended. Present are weakness of the wrist and difficulty in grasping objects. A reliable diagnostic sign is increased pain when the middle finger or wrist is extended against resistance. SYN: *epicondylitis, lateral humeral.*

TREATMENT: In mild cases, treatment includes immobilization by a splint or adhesive strapping, supplemented by application of cold, as well as use of nonsteroidal anti-inflammatory agents and muscle relaxants. In some patients it may be possible to decrease the pain and inflammation by applying a wide strap just below the elbow. This will alter the action of the stressed muscles in the forearm and splint the area. This strap should be worn during exercise. Injection of cortisone and local anesthetic into the painful area may be of assistance in cases that have not been helped by conservative therapy. In persistent cases, surgical intervention (often involving the resection of the extensor carpi radialis brevis tendon) may be indicated.

teno-, tendo- Combining form meaning *tendon.*

tenodesis (tĕn-ŏd′ĕ-sĭs) [Gr. *tenon,* tendon, + *desis,* a binding] **1.** Surgical fixation of a tendon. Usually a tendon is transferred from its initial point of origin to a new origin in order to restore muscle balance to a joint, to restore lost function, or to increase active power of joint motion. **2.** Closing of the fingers through tendon action of the extrinsic finger flexor muscles when they are stretched across the wrist joint during wrist extension. This mechanism is used for functional grip in the quadriplegic individual when paralysis is due to loss below the sixth cervical vertebra. SEE: *tendon action.*

tenodesis splint Orthosis fabricated to allow pinch and grasp movements through use of wrist extensors. Also called *wrist-driven flexor hinge hand splint.*

tenodynia (tĕn″ō-dĭn′ē-ă) [″ + *odyne,* pain] Pain in a tendon. SYN: *teinodynia; tenalgia; tenontodynia.*

tenofibril (tĕn′ō-fī″brĭl) [″ + *fibrilla,* little fiber] A filament in the cytoplasm of epithelial cells; part of the cytoskeleton.

tenolysis (tĕn-ŏl′ĭ-sĭs) [″ + *lysis,* dissolution] Tendolysis.

tenometer Tonometer.

tenomyoplasty (tĕn″ō-mī′ō-plăs″tē) [″ + *mys,* muscle, + *plassein,* to form] Reparative operation upon a tendon and muscle. SYN: *tenontomyoplasty.*

tenomyotomy (tĕn″ō-mī-ŏt′ō-mē) [″ + ″ + *tome,* incision] Excision of lateral portion of a tendon or muscle.

Tenon's capsule (tē′nŏns) [Jacques R. Tenon, Fr. surgeon, 1724–1816] A thin connective tissue envelope of the eyeball behind the conjunctiva.

tenonectomy (tĕn″ō-nĕk′tō-mē) [″ + *ektome,* excision] Excision of a portion of a tendon.

tenonitis (tĕn″ō-nī′tĭs) [″ + *itis,* inflammation] **1.** Inflammation of a tendon. SYN: *tendonitis.* **2.** Inflammation of Tenon's capsule.

tenonometer (tĕn″ō-nŏm′ĕ-tĕr) [Gr. *teinein,* to stretch, + *metron,* measure] A device for measuring degree of intraocular tension. SYN: *tonometer.*

Tenon's space Space between the posterior surface of the eyeball and Tenon's capsule.

tenontitis (tĕn″ŏn-tī′tĭs) [Gr. *tenontos,* tendon, + *itis,* inflammation] Tendonitis.

tenontodynia (tĕn″ŏn-tō-dĭn′ē-ă) [″ + *odyne,* pain] Tenodynia.

tenontography (tĕn″ŏn-tŏg′ră-fē) [″ + *graphein,* to write] A treatise on tendons.

tenontolemmitis (tĕn-ŏn″tō-lĕm-mī′tĭs) [″ + *lemma,* rind, + *itis,* inflammation] Tenosynovitis.

tenontology (tĕn″ŏn-tŏl′ō-jē) [″ + *logos,* word, reason] The study of tendons.

tenontomyoplasty (tĕn-ŏn″tō-mī′ō-plăs″tē) [″ + *mys,* muscle, + *plassein,* to form] Plastic surgery, including muscle and tendon repair in treatment of hernia. SYN: *myotenontoplasty; tenomyoplasty.*

tenontomyotomy (tĕn-ŏn″tō-mī-ŏt′ō-mē) [″ + ″ + *tome,* incision] Cutting of the principal tendon of a muscle with excision of the muscle in part or in whole. SYN: *myotenotomy.*

tenontoplasty (tĕn-ŏn′tō-plăs″tē) [″ + *plassein,* to form] Plastic surgery of defective or injured tendons. SYN: *tenoplasty.*

tenontothecitis (tĕn-ŏn″tō-thē-sī′tĭs) [″ + *theke,* sheath, + *itis,* inflammation] An inflammation of a tendon and its sheath. SYN: *tendosynovitis; tendovaginitis; tenosynovitis.*

t. stenosans A chronic form of tenontothecitis with narrowing of the sheath.

tenophyte (tĕn′ō-fīt) [″ + *phyton,* a growth] A cartilaginous or osseous growth on a tendon.

tenoplastic (tĕn″ō-plăs′tĭk) Concerning tenoplasty.

tenoplasty (tĕn′ō-plăs″tē) [″ + *plassein,* to form] Reparative surgery of tendons. SYN: *tendinoplasty; tenontoplasty.*

tenoreceptor (tĕn″ō-rē-sĕp′tor) [″ + L. *receptor,* receiver] Proprioceptive nerve ending in a tendon.

tenorrhaphy (tĕn-or′ă-fē) [″ + *rhaphe,* seam, ridge] Suturing of a tendon.

tenositis (tĕn″ō-sī′tĭs) [″ + *itis,* inflammation] An inflammation of a tendon. SYN: *tendonitis.*

tenostosis (tĕn″ŏs-tō′sĭs) [Gr. *tenon,* tendon, + *osteon,* bone, + *osis,* condition] Calcification of a tendon.

tenosuspension (tĕn″ō-sŭs-pĕn′shŭn) [″ + L. *suspensio,* a hanging under] In surgery, use of a tendon to support a structure.

tenosuture (tĕn″ō-sū′chūr) [″ + L. *sutura,* a seam] Suture of a partially or completely divided tendon. SYN: *tenorrhaphy.*

tenosynovectomy (tĕn″ō-sĭn″ō-vĕk′tō-mē) [″ + *synovia,* joint fluid, + Gr. *ektome,* excision] Excision of a tendon sheath.

tenosynovitis (tĕn″ō-sĭn″ō-vī′tĭs) [″ + ″ + Gr. *itis,* inflammation] An inflammation of a tendon sheath. SYN: *tendosynovitis; tendovaginitis.* SEE: *de Quervain's disease.*

de Quervain's t. SEE: *de Quervain's disease.*

t. hyperplastica Painless swelling of extensor tendons over the wrist joint.

tenotome (tĕn′ō-tōm) [″ + *tome,* incision] An instrument used for dividing a tendon. SYN: *tendotome.*

tenotomist (tĕ-nŏt′ō-mĭst) Specialist in tenotomy.

tenotomy (tĕ-nŏt′ō-mē) Surgical section of a tendon.

tenovaginitis (tĕn″ō-văj″ĭn-ī′tĭs) [″ + L. *vagina,* sheath, + Gr. *itis,* inflammation] Inflammation of a tendon sheath. SYN: *tendosynovitis; tenontothecitis; tenosynovitis.*

TENS *transcutaneous electrical nerve stimulation.*

tense (tĕns) **1.** Tight, rigid. **2.** Anxious, under mental stress.

Tensilon test A test used in the diagnosis of myasthenia gravis (MG). A short-acting anticholinesterase drug, such as edrophonium chloride or neostigmine, is injected, and the patient is observed for improved muscular strength. The patient is also observed after an injection of a placebo (e.g., saline). Improvement with the active drug, but not the placebo, is a strong indication of MG.

tensiometer (tĕn″sē-ŏm′ĕ-tĕr) [L. *tensio,* a stretching, + Gr. *metron,* measure] **1.** A device for determining the surface tension of liquids. **2.** A device used to measure the amount of force a muscle can produce. Also called *cable tensiometer.*

tension (tĕn′shŭn) [L. *tensio,* a stretching] **1.** Process or act of stretching; state of being strained or stretched. **2.** Pressure, force. **3.** Expansive force of a gas or vapor. **4.** Mental, emotional, or nervous strain.

arterial t. Tension resulting from the force exerted by the blood pressure on the walls of arteries.

arterial oxygen t. ABBR: PaO_2. The partial pressure of oxygen in the plasma of the arterial blood.

intraocular t. The pressure of the fluid within the eyeball. SEE: *tonometry.*

intravenous t. Force exerted by the blood pressure on the walls of a vein.

muscular t. Condition of a muscle in which fibers tend to shorten and thus perform work or liberate heat.

premenstrual t. Premenstrual dysphoric disorder.

surface t. Molecular property of film on surface of a liquid to resist rupture. The molecules are mutually attracted and their cohesive state presents the smallest surface area to the surrounding medium.

tissue t. The theoretical state of equilibrium between the cells of a tissue.

tension myalgia Chronic muscular pain. SEE: *fibromyalgia*.

tension of gases The partial pressure of gas in a mixture. In clinical applications this is usually measured in millimeters of mercury (mm Hg) or kilopascals (kPa).

tension suture A suture used to reduce the pull on the edges of a wound.

tensometer (tĕn-sŏm'ĕ-tĕr) [L. *tensio,* a stretching, + Gr. *metron,* measure] A device for testing the tensile strength of materials.

tensor (tĕn'sor) [L., a stretcher] Any muscle that makes a part tense.

tent (tĕnt) [O.Fr. *tente,* from L. *tenta,* stretched out] **1.** A plug of soft material used to maintain or dilate the opening to a sinus, canal, or body cavity. A variety of cylindrically shaped materials may be used. **2.** A portable covering or shelter composed of fabric.

cool mist t. An enclosure into which nebulized medications and mist are sprayed; it is used to treat croup, asthma, and other respiratory illnesses in children.

laminaria t. A plug made of *Laminaria digitata,* that is placed in the cervical canal of the uterus to dilate it.

medical t. A portable clinic erected to provide supportive care in outdoor settings, such as war zones, outdoor concerts, or marathon races.

oxygen t. A tent that can be placed over a bed for the continuous administration of oxygen and mist.

pleural t. In thoracoscopy or thoracic surgery, a mediastinal or subpleural blanket used to reinforce the suture line.

sponge t. A plug made of compressed sponge that is placed in the cervical canal to dilate it.

tentacle (tĕn'tă-k'l) A slender projection of invertebrates. It is used for prehension, tactile purposes, or feeding.

tentative (tĕn'tă-tĭv) [L. *tentativus,* feel, try] **1.** Rel. to a diagnosis subject to change because of insufficient data. **2.** Indecisive.

tenth cranial nerve Nerve supplying most of the abdominal viscera, the heart, lungs, and esophagus. SYN: *vagus nerve*. SEE: *cranial nerve*.

tentorial (tĕn-tō'rē-ăl) Pert. to a tentorium.

tentorial pressure cone Projection of a portion of the temporal lobe of the cerebrum through the incisure of the tentorium due to increased intracranial pressure.

tentorium (tĕn-tō'rē-ŭm) *pl.* **tentoria** [L., tent] A tentlike structure or part.

t. cerebelli The process of the dura mater between the cerebrum and cerebellum supporting the occipital lobes.

tepid (tĕp'ĭd) [L. *tepidus,* lukewarm] Slightly warm; lukewarm.

TEPP *tetraethylpyrophosphate.*

ter- [L., thrice] Combining form meaning *three times.*

teracurie (tĕr″ă-kū'rē) A unit of radioactivity, 10^{12} curies.

teramorphous (tĕr-ă-mor'fŭs) [Gr. *teras,* monster, + *morphe,* form] Similar to, or of the nature of, a congenitally deformed fetus, infant, or child.

teras (tĕr'ăs) *pl.* **terata** [Gr.] A severely deformed fetus.

teratic (tĕr-ăt'ĭk) [Gr. *teratikos,* monstrous] Pert. to a severely malformed fetus.

teratism (tĕr'ă-tĭzm) [Gr. *teratisma*] An anomaly or structural abnormality either inherited or acquired.

acquired t. Abnormality resulting from a prenatal environmental influence.

atresic t. Teratism in which natural openings such as the mouth or anus fail to form.

ceasmic t. Teratism in which a normal union of parts fails to occur (e.g., as in spina bifida or cleft palate).

ectogenic t. Condition in which parts are absent or defective.

ectopic t. Abnormality in which a part becomes displaced.

hypergenic t. Teratism in which a part is duplicated (e.g., polydactylism).

symphysic t. Teratism in which parts that are normally separate are fused.

terato- Combining form meaning *monster.*

teratoblastoma (tĕr″ă-tō-blăs-tō'mă) [Gr. *teratos,* monster, + *blastos,* germ, + *oma,* tumor] A tumor that contains embryonic material but that is not representative of all three germinal layers. SEE: *teratoma.*

teratocarcinoma (tĕr″ă-tō-kăr″sĭ-nō'mă) [″ + *karkinos,* cancer, + *oma,* tumor] A carcinoma that has developed from the epithelial cells of a teratoma.

teratogen (tĕr-ăt'ō-jĕn) [″ + *gennan,* to produce] Anything that adversely affects normal cellular development in the embryo or fetus. Certain chemicals,

U.S. FDA Categories for Drugs by Teratogenic or Fetotoxic Potential*

Pregnancy Category	Description	Examples
A	Medications for which no harm has been demonstrated in well-designed studies of pregnant and lactating women.	folic acid supplementation
B	Medications without known risk when used in human pregnancy or breastfeeding. Studies in laboratory animals have been performed with positive or negative results, but no demonstrable risk in pregnancy is yet known. Individual considerations of risk and benefit guide usage in patients.	acyclovir, amoxicillin/clavulanate, fluoxetine, glyburide, ranitidine
C	Medications whose use in human pregnancy or breastfeeding has not been adequately studied; risk of usage cannot be excluded but has not been proven. Individual considerations of risk and benefit guide drug usage in patients.	albuterol, hydrocodone, omeprazole, verapamil
D	Medications known to cause fetal harm when administered during pregnancy or harm to children during breastfeeding. In some specific settings the potential benefits of use may outweigh the risk.	tetracycline antibiotics
X	Medications judged to be unsafe (contraindicated) in pregnancy. Evidence of risk has accrued from clinical trials or postmarketing surveillance.	isotretinoin, thalidomide, warfarin

*All medication use during pregnancy should be carefully reviewed with health professionals experienced in reproductive pharmacology and patient care.

some therapeutic and illicit drugs, radiation, and intrauterine viral infections are known to adversely alter cellular development in the embryo or fetus. SEE: table; *mutagen*.

teratogenesis (těr″ă-tō-gĕn′ĕ-sĭs) [″ + *genesis,* generation, birth] The development of abnormal structures in an embryo.

teratogenetic (těr″ă-tō-jĕ-nĕt′ĭk) [″ + *genesis,* generation, birth] Concerning teratogenesis.

teratogenic (tĕr″ă-tō-gĕn′ĭk) Causing abnormal development of the embryo.

teratoid (tĕr′ă-toyd) [Gr. *teratos,* monster, + *eidos,* form, shape] Resembling a severely malformed fetus.

teratoid tumor Tumor of embryonic remains from all germinal layers. SYN: *teratoma.*

teratology (tĕr-ă-tŏl′ō-jē) [″ + *logos,* word, reason] Branch of science dealing with the study of congenital deformities and abnormal development. **teratologic,** *adj.*

teratoma (tĕr-ă-tō′mă) [″ + *oma,* tumor] A congenital tumor containing one or more of the three primary embryonic germ layers. Hair and teeth as well as endodermal elements may be present. SYN: *dermoid cyst*. SEE: *fetus in fetu*.

teratomatous (tĕr″ă-tō′mă-tŭs) Pert. to or resembling a teratoma.

teratophobia (tĕr″ă-tō-fō′bē-ă) [″ + *phobos,* fear] An abnormal fear of giving birth to a malformed fetus or being in contact with one.

teratosis (tĕr″ă-tō′sĭs) [″ + *osis,* condition] A deformed fetus.

teratospermia (tĕr″ă-tō-spĕr′mē-ă) [″ + *sperma,* seed] Malformed sperm in semen.

terazosin hydrochloride An antihypertensive agent, also effective in relieving symptoms of benign prostatic hypertrophy.

terbium (tĕr′bē-ŭm) SYMB: Tb. A metal of the rare earths; atomic weight, 158.9254; atomic number, 65; specific gravity, 8.272.

terbutaline sulfate A synthetic sympathomimetic amine used in treating asthma. It is a bronchodilator.

terchloride (tĕr-klō′rīd) Trichloride.

terebrant (tĕr′ĕ-brănt) Piercingly painful.

terebration (tĕr″ĕ-brā′shŭn) [L. *terebratio*] **1.** Boring; trephination. **2.** A boring pain.

teres (tĕ′rēz) [L., round] Round and smooth; cylindrical; used to describe certain muscles and ligaments.

tergal (tĕr′găl) [L. *tergum,* back] Concerning the back or dorsal surface.

tergum (tĕr′gŭm) [L.] The back.

ter in die (tĕr ĭn dē′ă) [L.] ABBR: t.i.d. Three times a day.

term [L. *terminus,* a boundary] **1.** A limit or boundary. **2.** A definite or limited period of duration such as the normal period of pregnancy, approx. nine calendar months or 38 to 42 weeks' gestation.

terminal (tĕr′mĭ-năl) [L. *terminalis*] Pert. to or placed at the end.

terminal arteriole An arteriole that has no branches but splits into capillaries.
terminal bars Minute bars of dense intercellular cement that occupy and close spaces between epithelial cells and bind them together.
terminal cancer Widespread or advanced cancer, from which recovery is not expected.
terminal device ABBR: TD. Component of an upper extremity prosthesis that substitutes for the functions of the hand. There are many types of terminal devices, some of which are designed for use with specific tools and implements. These devices are classified basically by whether or not the action of the prosthesis wearer results in opening the device (voluntary opening) or closing it (voluntary closing). SYN: *hook*.
terminal ganglia Ganglia of the parasympathetic division of the autonomic nervous system that are located in or close to their visceral effectors such as the heart or intestines.
terminal illness A final, fatal illness.

PATIENT CARE: The health care professional supports the patient and family by anticipating their loss and grief and helps the patient to deal with major concerns: pain, fear, hopelessness, dependency, disability, loss of self-esteem, and loss of pleasure. Hospice care is provided if desired and available. The patient receives caring comfort and help in adjusting to decreased quality of life to ensure that death is with dignity.

terminal infection Infection appearing in the late stage of another disease; often fatal.
terminal vein One of two veins (anterior and posterior) draining portions of the brain and emptying into the interior cerebral veins.
terminatio (tĕr″mĭ-nā′shē-ō) [L.] The termination or ending.
termination [L. *terminatio,* limiting] **1.** The distal end of a part. **2.** The cessation of anything.
terminology (tĕr-mĭ-nŏl′ō-jē) [L. *terminus,* a boundary, + Gr. *logos,* word] The vocabulary of scientific and technical terms used in specific arts, trades, or professions. SYN: *nomenclature*.
terminus (tĕr′mĭ-nŭs) [L.] An ending; a boundary.
terpene (tĕr′pēn) Any member of the family of hydrocarbons of the formula $C_{10}H_{16}$.
terpin hydrate (tĕr′pĭn hī′drāt) A white crystalline substance with a turpentine taste; made by the interaction of rectified spirits of turpentine, alcohol, and nitric acid. It is given in the form of an elixir as an expectorant.
terra (tĕr′ă) [L.] Earth; soil.

t. alba White clay.

territoriality (tĕr″ĭ-tor″ē-ăl′ĭ-tē) The tendency of animals and humans to defend a particular area or region.
terror [L. *terrere,* to frighten] Great fear.
tertian (tĕr′shŭn) [L. *tertianus,* the third] Occurring every third day; usually pert. to a form of malarial fever.
tertiary (tĕr′shē-ār-ē) [L. *tertiarius*] Third in order or stage.
tertiary alcohol Alcohol containing the trivalent group ≡COH.
tertiary care A level of medical care that would be available only in large medical care institutions. Included would be techniques and methods of therapy and diagnosis involving equipment and personnel that would not be economically feasible to have in a smaller institution because of the lack of utilization. SEE: *primary care; care, secondary medical*.
tertiary syphilis The third and most advanced stage of syphilis. SEE: under *syphilis*.
tertigravida (tĕr″shē-grăv′ĭ-dă) [″ + *gravida,* pregnant] A woman pregnant for the third time.
tertipara (tĕr-shĭp′ă-ră) [L. *tertius,* third, + *parere,* to bring forth] A woman who has had three pregnancies terminating after the 20th week of gestation or has produced three infants weighing at least 500 g, regardless of their viability.
tesla [Nikola Tesla, U.S. physicist, 1856–1943] ABBR: T. In the SI system, a measure of magnetic strength; 1 tesla equals 1 weber per square meter.
tessellated (tĕs′ĕ-lā″tĕd) [L. *tessella,* a square] Composed of little squares.
test [L. *testum,* earthen vessel] **1.** An examination. **2.** A method to determine the presence or nature of a substance or the presence of a disease. **3.** A chemical reaction. **4.** A reagent or substance used in making a test.

abduction stress t. A maneuver to assess whether a patient has suffered a ligamentous injury to the knee. With the patient's hip extended over the edge of the examining table, the examiner externally rotates the patient's lower extremity at the ankle, while providing internal rotation from the lateral border of the thigh.

acetic acid t. A test for albumin in urine. Adding a few drops of acetic acid to urine that has been boiled causes a white precipitate if albumin is present.

acetone t. A test for the presence of acetone in the urine; made by adding a few drops of sodium nitroprusside to the urine along with strong ammonia water. The presence of acetone causes the formation of a magenta ring at outline of contacts.

acromioclavicular traction t. A maneuver used to identify acromioclavicular and costoclavicular ligament sprains. As the patient sits or stands with the involved shoulder hanging in the neutral position, the clinician pulls the humerus down.

A positive test result is marked by a visible separation of the acromioclavicular joint.

Adams t. SEE: *Adams test.*

agglutination t. A widely used test in which adding an antiserum containing antibodies to cells or bacteria causes them to agglutinate. SEE: *agglutination.*

alkali denaturation t. A quantitative test for hemoglobin F (fetal hemoglobin, HbF) in the blood, which relies on the light absorbance of a mixture of saline-diluted and alkali-diluted blood. Spectrophotometry is used in this test.

Allen-Doisy t. A test to determine the amount of estrogen content in female blood serum by its reaction on secretions of mice.

apprehension t. A test of chronic joint instability. If this is present, the patient displays concern or discomfort when a joint is put in a position of risk for dislocation. There is an obvious facial display of discomfort; the patient may try to resist the maneuver by muscle contraction.

Patella: The patient lies supine with a relaxed quadriceps, and the examiner places digital pressure on the patella, attempting to locate it laterally.

Shoulder: The arm is abducted to 90° and rotated externally. With continued external rotation, the patient with an unstable shoulder complains of pain and expresses fear of dislocation.

APT t. APT test.

aptitude t. A mental or physical (or both) test designed to evaluate skill or ability to perform certain tasks or assignments.

Aschheim-Zondek t. SEE: *Zondek-Aschheim test.*

association t. A test used to determine an individual's response to word stimuli. The nature of the response and time required may provide insight into the subject's personality and previous experiences.

autohemolysis t. A test of the rate of hemolysis of sterile defibrinated whole blood incubated at 37°C. Normal cells hemolyze at a certain rate, but red blood cells from persons with certain types of disease (such as hereditary spherocytosis) hemolyze at a faster rate.

Berg balance t. SEE: *Berg balance test.*

biuret t. A test to determine the presence of proteins or urea. SYN: *biuret reaction.*

block design t. A neuropsychological test involving the placement of wooden blocks according to three-dimensional drawings. The test assesses the presence of constructional apraxia, often exhibited in patients with brain lesions.

box and block t. A standardized, timed test of manual dexterity and endurance, used in rehabilitation, in which the subject transfers small blocks from one side of a box to another.

caries activity t. Any laboratory test that measures the degree of caries activity in a dental patient. The tests may identify the number of cariogenic bacteria or the acid production from saliva samples.

carioca t. A side-shuffling, sport-specific functional test of agility and kinesthetic awareness that is used toward the end of a rehabilitation program to reintegrate athletes back into competition following lower extremity injuries. Derived from a Latin dance step, the carioca test involves the alternate stepping of one foot in front and then behind the other.

category t. One of the neuropsychological tests of abstract thinking; it assesses a patient's ability to learn strategies for sorting objects into related groups.

challenge t. Administering a substance in order to determine its ability to cause a response, esp. the giving of an antigen and observing or testing for the antibody response.

cholecystokinin-secretin t. A direct test of pancreatic function that assesses both the endocrine and exocrine functions of the pancreas. A double-lumen tube is inserted into the patient's gastrointestinal tract. One lumen samples the duodenal juices, the other removes gastric secretions. First secretin and then cholecystokinin are given to the patient intravenously; then the duodenal juices are analyzed to determine whether adequate levels of bicarbonate and trypsin are secreted. SYN: *secretin injection t.*

chromatin t. A test for genetic sex in which blood or tissue cells are examined for the presence or absence of Barr bodies.

CLO t. *Campylobacter*-like organism test; an assay to determine the presence of urea-splitting organisms in the upper gastrointestinal tract. The test is one of several used to diagnose whether or not ulcers or gastritis are caused by *Helicobacter pylori.*

clock drawing t. One of the mental status tests that assesses a person's ability to draw a complex, but frequently used, object. Persons with normal cognitive function and a normal sense of time can draw a clock face, place the hours 1 through 12 in appropriate positions, and insert the hands of the clock to demonstrate a particular time of day (e.g., "10:25"). Demented patients make several characteristic errors: the clock face may be poorly drawn; the hours may be spaced unevenly; and the hour and minute hands misplaced or left off the clock face entirely.

coin t. A test for pneumothorax. A metal coin is placed flat on the chest and struck with another coin. The chest is auscultated at the same time. If a pneumothorax is present, a sharp, metallic ringing sound is heard.

complement-fixation t. Fixation of complement in the laboratory. SEE: *complement fixation.*

concentration t. A kidney function test based on the ability of the person to produce concentrated urine under conditions that would normally cause such production, as in intentional dehydration.

confirmatory t. A test that is used to validate the results obtained by another. The confirmatory test may be more sensitive or specific but must be based on different testing principles.

conjunctival t. An outdated allergy test in which the suspected antigen is placed in the conjunctival sac; if it is allergenic for that patient, the conjunctiva becomes red and itchy and tears are produced.

cover t. A test for strabismus. The eyes are observed and the patient is asked to focus on an object. A cover is placed first over one eye and then the other. If either eye moves, strabismus is present.

creatinine clearance t. ABBR: CrCl test. A laboratory test for estimating glomerular filtration rate of the kidney. Creatinine clearance can be estimated by use of the following formula for males:

$$\frac{(140 - \text{age})(\text{body weight in kg})}{72 \times \text{serum creatinine (mg/dl)}}$$

For females, the formula is multiplied by 0.85. The normal creatinine clearance is about 125 ml/min. Lower levels reflect renal insufficiency and may influence the excretion of many drugs and toxins from the body.

Developmental T. of Visual Motor Integration A test of visual perception and motor planning requiring the copying of shapes and forms.

distance vision t. Snellen's chart.

double-blind t. A test in which neither the clinician nor the patient knows whether an active agent or a placebo (control substance) is administered. SEE: *double-blind technique.*

drop arm t. A test used to identify tears of the rotator cuff muscle group, esp. supraspinatus. With the patient sitting or standing, the fully abducted shoulder is slowly lowered to the side. In the presence of rotator cuff tears, the arm will fall uncontrollably to the side from a position of about 90 degrees of abduction.

effort-independent t. A test whose accuracy or success does not depend on patient compliance.

empty can t. An orthopedic test of the shoulder, used to determine the integrity of the supraspinatus muscle. With the patient sitting or standing, the shoulder is fully internally rotated, abducted to 90 degrees, and placed in 30 degrees of forward flexion, as if emptying a beverage can. The patient then attempts to maintain this position against resistance. Inability to hold this position, or pain while holding it, suggests pathology of the supraspinatus muscle.

fecal fat t. The measurement of the total quantity of lipids in a timed stool specimen, as a part of the evaluation of chronic diarrhea, especially when fat malabsorption is suspected. The collected feces must not be contaminated by urine or by chemicals used in toilets. High levels of fecal fat (e.g., more than 14 g/day) suggest biliary, pancreatic, or small bowel disorders.

fecal occult blood t. A screening test for disorders of the gastrointestinal tract, including cancer of the colon.

finger-to-finger t. A test for coordination of the movements of the upper extremities. The patient is asked to touch the tips of the fingers of one hand to the opposite fingertips.

finger-nose t. A test of cerebellar function wherein the patient is asked to, while keeping the eyes open, touch the nose with the finger and remove the finger, and repeat this rapidly. The test is done by using a finger of each hand successively or in concert. How fast and well this is done is recorded.

fluorescein-dilaurate t. An indirect test of pancreatic function in which fluorescein bound to dilaurate is given orally to a patient and its excretion in the urine is measured. Patients with markedly abnormal pancreatic function fail to excrete the fluorescent tracer in the urine.

Friedman t. One of the first tests for pregnancy in which the patient's urine was injected into unmated mature female rabbits; a positive reaction was indicated by formation of corpora lutea and corpora haemorrhagica. This test is no longer used.

foam stability t. Shake t.

Gaenslen's t. SEE: *Gaenslen's test.*

galactose tolerance t. A test of the ability of the liver to metabolize galactose. A standard dose of galactose is administered to the fasting patient, and the amount of galactose excreted in the urine in the next 5 hr is determined. If the liver is damaged, the galactose is not metabolized to glycogen but is instead excreted in the urine.

Godfrey's t. SEE: *Godfrey's test.*

guaiac t. A test for unseen blood in stool. SEE: *fecal occult blood t.*

hardness t. A test designed to determine the relative hardness of materials by correlating the size or depth of an indent produced by a particular instrument with a known amount of compressive force. SEE: *hardness number.*

heterophile antibody t. A laboratory test for infectious mononucleosis.

histamine t. **1.** Injection of histamine subcutaneously to stimulate gastric secretion of hydrochloric acid. **2.** A test for vasomotor headache; a histamine injection precipitates the onset of a headache in persons with this disease.

Huhner t. SEE: *Huhner test.*

human repeated patch insult t. The serial application of substances to the skin to test for reaction. The material is applied fresh to the same skin site every other day for 10 applications. Each application remains on for 48 hr. After a rest period of about 2 weeks, the test material is applied again for 48 hr to a different skin site than that originally used. This area is examined daily for the next 4 days for evidence of irritation. The test measures the ability of the test substance to cause sensitization or irritation reactions or both.

in-home t. A test done in the home to provide information about an individual's health status. Examples include tests to measure blood sugar (glucose), cholesterol, occult blood in feces, and blood pressure, as well as ovulation predictors and pregnancy tests. The materials and devices needed for in-home tests may be available over the counter (i.e., a prescription from a health care professional is not needed).

intelligence t. A test designed to assess the intelligence of an individual, used as a basis for determining intelligence quotient (IQ). Some standardized tests of intelligence are flawed and may assess achievement, experience, or sociocultural advantages rather than intelligence. SEE: *intelligence; quotient, intelligence.*

intracutaneous t. A test done by injecting an antigen intracutaneously and observing the response. SEE: *skin test.*

Kleiger t. SEE: *Kleiger test.*

lactose tolerance t. An assessment of a person's blood sugar and exhaled hydrogen level within 2 hr after drinking a loading dose of lactose (usually about 100 g of lactose for average-sized adults). People who readily digest lactose will have an increase in their blood sugar and little increase in exhaled hydrogen gas during the test. People who are unable to digest lactose will have no increase in their blood sugar (they will not be able to break down and absorb milk sugars), and the level of hydrogen they exhale will exceed 50 parts per million.

limulus amebocyte lysate t. ABBR: LAL test. A test used to detect minute quantities of bacterial endotoxins and to test for pyrogens in various materials; it is also used to detect septicemia due to gram-negative bacteria. Limulus amebocyte lysate is formed from the lysed circulating amebocytes of the horseshoe crab *(Limulus polyphemus).*

liver function t. A blood test for a specific aspect of liver metabolism. Because of the diversity of liver functions and the disorders that may affect those functions, no single test provides a reliable measure of overall liver function. The ability to excrete bile pigments is measured by determining the serum bilirubin level; the levels of serum enzymes such as the aminotransferases aspartate (AST) and alanine (ALT) may be used to assess damage to the liver cells and biliary tract obstruction or dysfunction. Levels of the serum proteins albumin and globulin and their ratio are used to judge the synthetic functions of the liver. Certain blood clotting factors are also synthesized in the liver, and abnormalities may indicate impairments in hepatic synthesis. Blood ammonia levels are elevated in some patients with either acute or chronic liver disease; marked elevations may suggest acute or chronic liver failure. SEE: *liver.*

loading t. The administration of a substance to determine the individual's ability to metabolize or excrete it. Thus, a glucose tolerance test is one form of this test.

McMurray t. A test for a torn meniscus of the knee. The examiner flexes the patient's knee completely, rotates the tibia outward, and applies a valgus force against the knee while slowly extending it. A painful click indicates a torn medial meniscus. If a click is felt when the tibia is rotated inward and a varus force is applied against the knee during extension, the lateral meniscus is torn.

Motor-Free Visual Perception T. A standardized test of visual perception that does not require motor performance.

mucin clot t. A test of synovial fluid precipitation in acetic acid, formerly used to determine whether inflammatory arthritis was present in a joint. Other tests have replaced it, such as the cell count, cultures, Gram stain, and crystal examination.

multiple-puncture t. Any skin test, but esp. a tuberculin test, in which the material is placed on the skin and multiple superficial punctures are produced under the material, thus allowing the material to enter the skin.

navicular drop t. A test used to determine hyperpronation of the foot. While the patient's foot is in a non-weight-bearing position, the examiner places a mark over the navicular tuberosity. Next, the foot is placed on the floor, again in a non-weight-bearing position, and a mark is made on a 3 × 5 index card to measure the distance between the floor and the navicular tubercle. The measure is repeated when the patient bears weight on the foot and the distance between the two marks is recorded. Inferior displacement of greater than 10 mm while bearing weight is considered hyperpronation of the foot.

neural tension t. Various assessment techniques that stretch neural tissues (meninges, nerve roots, axons, and peripheral nerves) and assess the mobility and/or length of the structures and their ability to withstand tensile forces. Positive signs may include the reproduction of symptoms, limitation of motion, or asymmetric responses. The tests include the slump test, the straight leg raise, and the upper limb tension test.

neutralization t. A test of the ability of an antibody to neutralize the effects of an antigen.

ninhydrin t. A neurological test of sensation following peripheral nerve injury; used to detect a sympathetic response as indicated by sweat.

nonstress t. ABBR: NST. An external electronic monitoring procedure to assess fetal well-being. An acceleration in fetal heart rate should be evident in response to fetal movement. *Reactive test:* Two criteria indicate satisfactory fetal status. The monitor records a minimum of two episodes of heart rate acceleration accompanying fetal movement within one 20-min period, and accelerations of 15 beats per minute persist for a minimum of 15 sec per episode. *Nonreactive test:* The monitor record does not meet either criterion for reactivity. This indicates the need for a second test within the next several hours, contraction stress testing, a fetal biophysical profile, or all three. *Inconclusive test:* The monitor records less than one acceleration in 20 min or an acceleration less than 15 bpm lasting less than 15 sec.

oral glucose tolerance t. ABBR: OGTT. A screening test for diabetes mellitus (DM), in which plasma glucose levels are measured after the patient consumes an oral glucose load. In screening patients for type 2 DM, measuring fasting plasma glucose levels generally is preferable to an OGTT because the fasting blood test is simpler, cheaper, and better tolerated by patients. An OGTT reveals type 2 DM when plasma glucose levels exceed 200 mg/dl 2 hr after drinking a 75-g glucose load. Plasma glucose levels between 140 mg/dl and 199 mg/dl suggest impaired glucose tolerance.

GESTATIONAL DIABETES MELLITUS: (GDM) In pregnancy, a modified OGTT is used to screen women with risk factors for DM (such as obesity, family history of type 2 DM, age greater than 25 years, a history of unexplained stillbirths, among others). At 24 to 28 weeks' gestation, a 50-g glucose load is given; 1-hr plasma glucose levels greater than 140 mg/dl constitute a positive screening result. Any patient having a positive test result should then undergo a 3-hr, 100-g OGTT to determine whether GDM is present. SEE: table.

Criteria for Diabetes Mellitus in Pregnancy Using the 3-hr OGTT

Time:	Glucose level exceeds:
Fasting	105 mg/dl
60 min	190 mg/dl
120 min	165 mg/dl
180 min	145 mg/dl

patch t. A skin test in which a low concentration of a presumed allergen is applied to the skin beneath an occlusive dressing. If the concentration of the agent is too high or an allergy exists to the material used in the dressing, false-positive reactions can occur because of local irritation. False-negative reactions may result if the concentration of the suspected allergen is too low. SEE: illus; *skin test.*

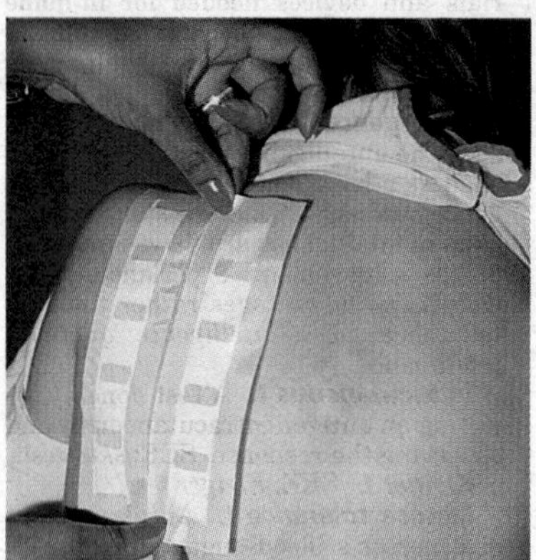

APPLYING PATCH TEST

personality t. A neuropsychiatric assessment tool, such as the Minnesota Multiphasic Personality Inventory–2, used to identify an individual's predominant emotional make-up. Personality tests measure adjustment, adventurousness, agitation, anxiety, coping styles, depression, introversion, hypochondriasis, paranoia, and other emotional variables.

pinprick t. A test for cutaneous pain receptors. A small, clean, sharp object such as a pin or needle is gently applied to the skin and the patient is asked to describe the sensation. One must be certain the patient is reporting the sensation of pain rather than that of pressure. Usually, application of the sharp object is interspersed with application of a dull object, and the patient is asked to state each time whether a sharp or dull sensation was felt. The patient is not, of course, allowed to observe the test procedure.

CAUTION: The sharp object should not penetrate the dermis, and to prevent passage of infectious material from one patient to another, the test objects should be either discarded after use or sterilized before their use on another patient.

postcoital t. In the evaluation of infertile couples, sampling of the woman's cervical mucus within two hours after male ejaculation, to determine the number of actively moving sperm in the specimen. In a favorable specimen, between 6 and 20 motile sperm should be seen per high-power microscopic field.

precipitin t. An antigen-antibody test in which a specific antigen is added to a solution. If the solution contains the antibody to that antigen, a precipitate is formed.

pregnancy t. SEE: *pregnancy test.*

prothrombin consumption t. A test for the amount of thromboplastin present in the plasma that reacts with prothrombin. This is determined by quantitating the prothrombin that remains in the serum after coagulation is complete.

provocation t. A diagnostic test in which drugs, chemicals, allergens, or physical forces are systematically administered to reproduce symptoms, in order to discover the source of a symptom or the tissue origin of a lesion. Provocation tests are used by specialists in several fields of health care, such as: allergists, to determine which of several agents may produce a patient's rhinitis, wheezing, or rash; physical therapists, to identify relationships between a patient's tissue pathology or impairment and his or her functional limitations; and cardiologists and neurologists, who use tilt table provocation tests to diagnose the cause of a patient's loss of consciousness.

psychometric t. A measurement technique used to assist in diagnosing cognitive and behavioral difficulties in infants and children. Several different tests are available.

pulp vitality t. A determination of the vitality of a tooth pulp by the application of hot, cold, or electrical stimuli. Also called *vitalometry.*

radioimmunosorbent t. ABBR: RIST. Use of radioimmunoassay to measure the immune globulin E (IgE) antibody in serum.

rapid surfactant t. Shake t.

resisted t. Assessment of muscle or nerve integrity or injury by applying an isometric force in the mid-range of muscle contraction. Mid-range is used to minimize stress on the joint and periarticular structures. The reproduction of pain and the relative strength of the tested muscles provide diagnostic information about specific injuries and functional impairments.

Rubin t. The original test for patency of the fallopian tubes by insufflation with carbon dioxide; used in investigating the cause of sterility. SYN: *tubal insufflation.*

Schiller's t. A test for detection of cancer of the cervix by painting the tissue with iodine solution; areas that contain glycogen are stained by the iodine. Those sites that do not stain, but become white or yellow, are assumed to be abnormal. Tissue is taken from those areas for microscopic examination.

scratch t. Placement of an appropriate dilution of a test material, suspected of being an allergen, in a lightly scratched area of the skin. If the material is an allergen, a wheal will develop within 15 min. The scratch test is one of three tests used for detection of IgE antibodies, esp. in patients with a history of penicillin allergy. SEE: *skin test.*

screening t. Screening.

secretin injection t. Cholecystokinin-secretin t.

Sensory Integration and Praxis T. ABBR: SIPT. A standardized battery of assessment tests to identify motor planning and sensory processing deficits in children 4 through 8 years of age. It includes 17 subtests.

serial sevens t. A test of mental status. The patient is asked to subtract 7 from 100 and to take 7 from that value and continue serially.

serologic t. Any test done on serum.

set t. A global (i.e., holistic) test of a patient's ability to make categories. It demonstrates motivation, alertness, concentration, short-term memory, and problem solving. The patient is asked to name 10 items in each of four groups: fruits, animals, colors, and towns or cities. Then the patient is asked to categorize, count, name, and remember the items listed. The test is scored by giving one point for each correctly recalled item. A maximum of 40 points is possible. Scoring less than 15 is associated with dementia; more than 25 indicates absence of dementia; and scores between 15 and 24 require further investigation to distinguish between mental changes and cultural, educational, and social factors.

shake t. A quick test to estimate fetal lung maturity. A sample of amniotic fluid is diluted with normal saline, mixed with 95% ethyl alcohol, and shaken for 30 sec. The continued presence of small foamy bubbles in the solution after 15 min confirms the presence of pulmonary surfactant. SYN: *foam stability t.; rapid surfactant t.*

sickling t. A test for the ability of red cells to sickle. The red cells are placed in an atmosphere of reduced oxygen tension. If they contain hemoglobin S, they will sickle.

slump t. A test used to assess the effects of tension on the neuromeningeal tract (e.g., in nerve root injury, meningeal irritation, meningitis, disk disease, or central nervous system tumors). The patient is directed to sit slumped forward, flexing the entire trunk. The patient's foot is dorsiflexed and the knee is then extended. Inability to extend the knee fully or production of back or leg pain symptoms, or both, are positive signs. If no positive sign is elicited, then the patient actively extends the neck, and knee extension and pain are then reassessed. Variations of this test are used to target injuries to specific spinal nerves.

standardized t. A test that has been developed empirically, has adequate norms, definite instructions for administration, and evidence of reliability and validity.

starch-iodine t. A test for the presence of starch. When an iodine solution is applied to a substance or material that contains starch, a dark blue color appears.

sulfosalicylic acid t. A test for protein in the urine.

thematic apperception t. A projective test in which the subject is shown life situations in pictures that could be interpreted in several ways. The subject is asked to provide a story of what the picture represents. The results may provide insights into the subject's personality.

three-glass t. A test to identify the site of a urinary tract infection. On awakening, the patient empties the bladder by passing urine sequentially into three test tubes (glasses). The amount of cellular debris visible to the naked eye in the glasses helps to determine whether the infection is located in the anterior urethra, posterior urethra, or prostate. If the first glass is turbid and the other two are clear, the anterior urethra is inflamed but the rest of the urinary tract is clear. If the initial specimen is clear and the second and third ones are turbid, the posterior urethra or prostate is inflamed. If only the third specimen is turbid, then only the prostate is inflamed.

tine t. A skin test for tuberculosis. The tuberculin is placed on metal tines that are barely pressed into the skin. The test is read in 48 and 72 hr. The unit is used in mass screening for tuberculosis, esp. in children. SEE: *tuberculin skin t.*

Tinetti balance t. A measurement of functional ability that incorporates observation of performance of 13 activities. The activities include sitting, rising from a chair, standing, turning, reaching up, and bending down. The rating scale is normal, adaptive, or abnormal.

tolerance t. A test of the ability of the patient or subject to endure the medicine given or exercise taken.

tourniquet t. A test used to determine pain thresholds, or alternately, capillary fragility. A blood pressure cuff is inflated sufficiently to occlude venous return. It is kept in place for a set time. The anesthetic effect, or the impact on skin integrity, is subsequently assessed. SEE: illus.

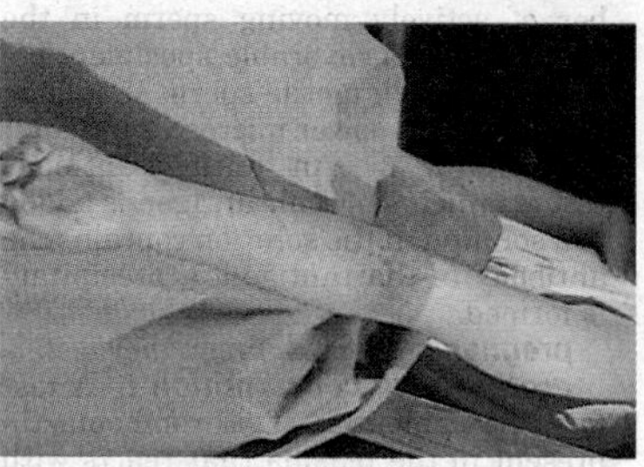

TOURNIQUET TEST

Positive test for idiopathic thrombocytopenic purpura

TPI t. *Treponema pallidum*–immobilizing test (for syphilis).

tuberculin skin t. A test to determine the presence of infection with tuberculosis (TB). A solution containing purified protein derivative of TB is injected intradermally into the arm, and the response is read 48 to 72 hr later. A 5-mm induration is considered a positive reaction if the patient has been in close contact with persons infected with TB, is infected with human immunodeficiency virus (HIV), has risk factors for HIV, or has a chest x-ray examination that suggests a history of pulmonary TB. A 10-mm induration is considered positive in people born in nations where TB is endemic, in nursing home patients, in patients with other serious illnesses, and in people of low socioeconomic status. In all other people, a 15-mm induration is considered a positive result. A positive response indicates infection but does not distinguish between active infection and that which has been controlled by the immune system or drugs. SEE: *tine t.*

tuberculin tine t. A tuberculin test performed by using a special disposable instrument that contains multiple sharp points or prongs for piercing the skin. These tines penetrate the skin and introduce the tuberculin that has been applied to them. The test is read in 48 to 72 hr.

up and go t. A timed test of lower-extremity mobility. It measures the time required to rise from a chair, walk 10 ft, turn, and return to the sitting position. Performance on this test is affected by abnormal gaits that increase the risk of falling.

urea balance t. A test of kidney function by measuring intake and output of urea.

wrinkle t. A test of sensibility following complete transection of or damage to peripheral nerves based on the characteristic sympathetic response of skin following extended immersion in water. SEE: *nerve*.

Yergason's t. SEE: *Yergason's test*.

testa (tĕs'tă) [L.] A shell.

testalgia (tĕs-tăl'jē-ă) [L. *testis,* testicle, + Gr. *algos,* pain] Pain in the testicle.

testectomy (tĕs-tĕk'tō-mē) [" + Gr. *ektome,* excision] **1.** Removal of a testicle. SYN: *castration*. **2.** Removal of a corpus quadrigeminum.

testes (tĕs'tēs) [L.] Pl. of testis.

testicle (tĕs'tĭ-kl) [L. *testiculus,* a little testis] Testis.

self-examination of t. A technique that enables a man to detect changes in the size and shape of his testicles and evaluate any tenderness. Each testicle is examined separately and in comparison with the other. The best time to perform the test is just after a warm bath or shower, when the scrotal tissue is more nearly relaxed. The man places his thumbs on the anterior surface of the testicle, supporting it with the index and middle fingers of both hands. Each testicle is gently rolled between the fingers and thumbs and carefully felt for lumps, hardness, or thickening, esp. as compared with the other testicle. The epididymis is a soft, slightly tender, tubelike body behind the testicle. Abnormal findings should be reported immediately to a health care professional.

testicond (tĕs'tĭ-kŏnd) [L. *testis,* testicle, + *condere,* to hide] The condition of having the testicles remain undescended. It is abnormal in man and in many animals.

testicular (tĕs-tĭk'ū-lăr) Rel. to a testicle.

testicular cancer, germ-cell A group of malignant diseases of the testicles that include choriocarcinomas, embryonal carcinomas, seminomas, spermatocytic seminomas, sex cord tumors, teratomas, and tumors with mixtures of several different malignant cell types.

testis (tĕs'tĭs) *pl.* **testes** [L.] The male gonad or testicle. It is one of two reproductive glands located in the scrotum that produces the male reproductive cells (spermatozoa) and the male hormones testosterone and inhibin. SEE: illus.

ANATOMY: Each is an ovoid body about 4 cm long and 2 to 2.5 cm in width and thickness, enclosed within a dense inelastic fibrous tunica albuginea. The testis is divided into numerous lobules separated by septa, each lobule containing one to three seminiferous tubules within which the spermatozoa arise. The lobules lead to straight ducts that join a plexus, the rete testis, from which 15 to 20 efferent ducts lead to the epididymis. The epididymis leads to the ductus deferens, through which sperm are conveyed to the urethra. Between the seminiferous tubules are the interstitial cells (cells of Leydig), which secrete testosterone. Within the tubules are sustentacular cells, which secrete inhibin. The testes are suspended from the body by the spermatic cord, a structure that extends from the inguinal ring to the testis and contains the ductus deferens, testicular vessels (spermatic artery, vein, lymph vessels), and nerves.

DISORDERS: Hyperfunction (hypergonadism) may cause early maturity such as large sexual organs with early functional activity and increased growth of hair. Hypofunction (hypogonadism) is indicated by undeveloped testes, absence of body hair, high-pitched voice, sterility, smooth skin, loss of sexual desire, low metabolism, and eunuchoid or eunuch body type.

descent of t. The migration of the testis from the abdominal cavity to the scrotum during fetal development.

displaced t. A testis located abnormally within the inguinal canal or pelvis.

femoral t. An inguinal testis near or over the femoral ring.

inverted t. A testis reversed in the scrotum so that the epididymis attaches to the anterior instead of the posterior part of the gland.

perineal t. A testis located in the perineal region outside the scrotum.

undescended t. Cryptorchidism.

testis compression reflex Contraction of abdominal muscles following moderate compression of a testis.

testitis (tĕs-tī'tĭs) [L. *testis,* testicle, + Gr. *itis,* inflammation] Inflammation of a testis. SEE: *orchitis*.

test meal A meal usually small and of definite quality and composition, given to aid in chemical analysis of the stomach contents or radiographical examination of the stomach.

testoid (tĕs'toyd) Resembling a testis.

testolactone (tĕs-tō-lăk'tōn) An anti-

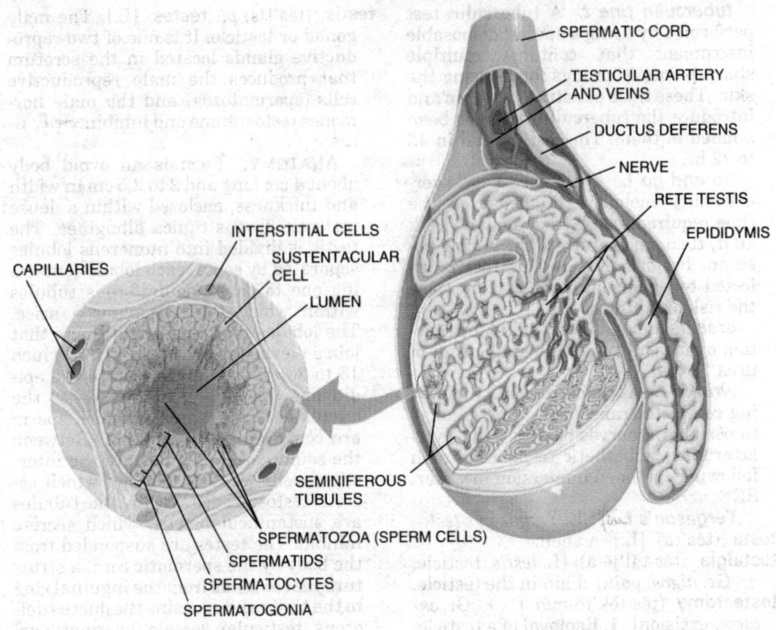

TESTIS

Midsagittal section of testis and epididymis (right), cross-section through a seminiferous tubule (left)

neoplastic agent used in treating carcinoma of the breast in postmenopausal women.

testopathy (tĕs-tŏp′ă-thē) [″ + Gr. *pathos,* disease, suffering] Any disease of the testes.

testosterone (tĕs-tŏs′tĕr-ōn) [L. *testis,* testicle] A steroid sex hormone that is responsible for the growth and development of masculine characteristics. It directly influences the maturation of male sexual organs, development of sperm within the testes, sexual drive, erectile function of the penis, and male secondary sexual characteristics (facial hair, thickened vocal cords, and pronounced musculature). In addition, it is linked to aggressive and predatory behaviors.

Testosterone is produced in the Leydig cells of the testes. It has also been synthesized for replacement therapy in men with sex hormone deficiencies (e.g., men with hypogonadal conditions such as Klinefelter's syndrome).

Testosterone adversely affects diseases of the prostate gland by sponsoring the growth of both benign hyperplasia of the gland and carcinomas of the prostate. Both of these conditions may be treated with antiandrogenic therapies. Predatory sexual behaviors also depend on testosterone and can be treated with interventions that block the effects of the hormone.

test tube baby A baby born to a mother whose ovum was removed, fertilized outside her body, and then implanted in her uterus. SEE: *gamete intrafallopian transfer; in vitro fertilization.*

test type Letters or figures of various size printed on paper. These are used in testing visual acuity.

tetanic (tĕ-tăn′ĭk) [Gr. *tetanikos*] **1.** Pert. to or producing tetanus. **2.** Any agent producing tetanic spasms.

tetanic convulsion A tonic convulsion with constant muscular contraction.

tetaniform (tĕ-tăn′ĭ-form) [Gr. *tetanos,* stretched, + L. *forma,* shape] Resembling tetanus.

tetanigenous (tĕt″ă-nĭj′ĕ-nŭs) [″ + *gennan,* to produce] Causing tetanus or tetanic spasms.

tetanism (tĕt′ă-nĭzm) [″ + *-ismos,* condition] Persistent muscular hypertonicity resembling tetanus, esp. in infants.

tetanization (tĕt″ă-nī-zā′shŭn) [Gr. *tetanos,* stretched] **1.** Production of tetanus or tetanic spasms by induction of the disease. **2.** Induction of tetanic contractions in a muscle by electrical stimuli.

tetanize (tĕt′ă-nīz) To induce tonic muscular spasms.

tetanode (tĕt′ă-nōd) [″ + *eidos,* form, shape] In tetany, the quiet period between spasms.

tetanoid paraplegia Paralysis of lower extremities due to lateral sclerosis of the spinal cord. SYN: *spastic paraplegia.*

tetanolysin (tĕt″ă-nŏl′ĭ-sĭn) A hemolytic component of the toxin produced by *Clostridium tetani,* causative organism of tetanus. It does not cause the clinical signs and symptoms of this disease.

tetanomotor (tĕt″ăn-ō-mō′tor) [″ + L. *motor,* a mover] Appliance for the production of tetanic motor spasms mechanically by electrical stimulation of a nerve.

tetanophil, tetanophilic (tĕt′ăn-ō-fĭl, tĕt″ăn-ō-fĭl′ĭk) [″ + *philein,* to love] Possessing an affinity for tetanus toxin.

tetanospasmin (tĕt″ă-nō-spăs′mĭn) [″ + *spasmos,* a convulsion] A component of the toxin produced by clostridium tetanus that causes the clinical disease state known as tetanus.

tetanus (tĕt′ă-nŭs) [Gr. *tetanos,* stretched] An acute, life-threatening illness caused by a toxin (tetanospasmin) produced in infected wounds by the bacillus *Clostridium tetani.* The disease is marked by extreme muscular rigidity, violent muscle spasms, and often, respiratory and autonomic failure. Because of proactive immunization programs in the U.S., the disease affects only 100 patients annually. In nations without effective immunization programs, the disease is exceptionally common and usually deadly. SEE: *Clostridium tetani; lockjaw; tetanolysin; tetanospasmin; trismus.*

ETIOLOGY: The responsible bacteria is most likely to proliferate in "tetanus-prone" wounds (e.g., those contaminated by soil or debris); puncture, avulsion, or bite wounds; burns; frostbite; necrotic tissues; gangrene; injection site infections; umbilical stump infections; or uterine infections. It is less likely to infect shallow wounds with cleanly cut edges. The spores of *C. tetani* germinate in the anaerobic depths of tetanus-prone injuries, producing bacteria that release tetanospasmin. This neurotoxin is carried to the central nervous system, where it blocks impulses that modulate muscle contraction. The incubation period varies from 1 or 2 days to a few months. The shorter the incubation, the more deadly the illness is likely to be.

SYMPTOMS: Unopposed muscular contraction leads to rigidity and spasticity, esp. of the muscles of the jaw, neck, back, abdomen, and esophagus. Lockjaw (also called trismus) is a hallmark of the disease, as are violent arching of the back muscles (opisthotonus), and a rigid, fixed smile (risus sardonicus). Intense muscle spasms may be triggered by noises, bright lights, attempts to swallow or eat, or other stimuli. In addition, the patient may suffer wild fluctuations in pulse, blood pressure, and respirations.

TREATMENT: Débridement may lessen the burden of toxin-producing bacteria in the wound. Muscle-relaxing drugs, like diazepam, reduce muscle spasm. Beta blockers like propranolol decrease the incidence of tachycardias and hypertension. Advanced airway and ventilatory support are best provided in an intensive care unit. Tetanus antitoxin (tetanus immune globulin) is typically administered in an attempt to provide passive immunity. Penicillin G or metronidazole is administered intravenously to stop toxin production.

PATIENT CARE: The patient is kept in a quiet, dimly lit room, where stimulation is minimized. Oral feedings are withheld to limit esophageal spasms and the aspiration of nutrients. Intravenous hydration and nutrition may be needed. A Foley catheter is placed to prevent urinary retention.

CAUTION: Recovery from tetanus does not guarantee natural immunity. Therefore, the patient should begin an immunization series before leaving the hospital.

PREVENTION: Initial immunization should begin in infancy. The toxoid should be given in three doses at 4- to 8-week intervals when the infant is 6 to 8 weeks old, and a fourth dose 6 to 12 months thereafter. A fifth dose is usually administered at 4 to 6 years of age before school entry. Tetanus toxoid is commonly given in combination with diphtheria toxoid and acellular pertussis vaccine. Active immunization with adsorbed tetanus toxoid provides protection for at least 10 years. Although it has been the practice to give a tetanus booster every 10 years, current advice is to give a single booster dose at age 50 if the individual received all 5 doses as a child. Tetanus booster vaccination should be given to patients with tetanus-prone wounds who have not received the toxoid in the past 5 years.

t. anticus Form of tetanus in which the body is bowed forward.

artificial t. Tetanus produced by a drug such as strychnine.

ascending t. Tetanus in which muscle spasms occur first in the lower part of the body and then spread upward, finally involving muscles of the head and neck.

cephalic t. A form of tetanus due to a wound of the head, esp. one near the eyebrow. It is marked by trismus, facial paralysis on one side, and pronounced dysphagia. It resembles rabies and is often fatal. SYN: *hydrophobic t.*

cerebral t. A form of tetanus produced by inoculating the brain of animals with tetanus antitoxin; it is marked by epileptiform convulsions and excitement.

chronic t. **1.** A latent infection in a healed wound, reactivated on opening the wound. **2.** A form of tetanus in which the onset and progress of the disease are slower and more prolonged and the symptoms are less severe.

cryptogenic t. Tetanus in which the site of entry of the organism is not known.

descending t. Tetanus in which muscle spasms occur first in the head and neck and later are manifested in other muscles of the body.

t. dorsalis Tetanus in which the body is bent backward.

extensor t. Tetanus that affects the extensor muscles.

hydrophobic t. Cephalic t.

idiopathic t. Tetanus that occurs without any visible lesion.

imitative t. A conversion disorder that simulates tetanus.

t. infantum T. neonatorum.

t. lateralis A form of tetanus in which the body is bent sideways.

local t. Tetanus marked by spasticity of a group of muscles near the wound. Trismus, tonic contraction of jaw muscles, is usually absent.

t. neonatorum Tetanus of very young infants, usually due to infection of the navel caused by using nonsterile technique in ligating the umbilical cord.

t. paradoxus Cephalic tetanus combined with paralysis of the facial or other cranial nerve.

postoperative t. Tetanus that follows an operation as a result of contamination of the surgical incision.

puerperal t. Tetanus that occurs following childbirth.

toxic t. Tetanus produced by overdose of strychnine.

tetanus antitoxin An antibody that develops in the blood of humans or other animals (horses) as a result of infection by the tetanus organism (*Clostridium tetani*) or inoculation with tetanus toxin or toxoid.

tetanus immune globulin A solution containing antibodies to *Clostridium tetani* obtained from human blood and used to provide passive immunity to prevent and treat tetanus infection. The prophylactic dose is 250 to 500 units injected intramuscularly (IM); the therapeutic dose is 3000 to 5000 units IM.

tetanus toxoid Tetanus toxin modified so that its toxicity is greatly reduced, while retaining its capacity to promote active immunity.

tetany (tĕt′ă-nē) [Gr. *tetanos*, stretched] A neurological disorder marked by intermittent tonic spasms that are usually paroxysmal and involve the extremities. It may occur in infants, esp. newborns in intensive care units. High-risk infants include premature newborns of diabetic mothers and those who have had perinatal asphyxia.

SYMPTOMS: The condition is marked by nervousness, irritability, and apprehension; numbness and tingling of the extremities; cramps of various muscles (particularly those of the hands, producing a typical accoucheur type of hand, such as carpopedal spasm); and extreme extension of the feet. Bilateral tonic spasms occur in the arms and legs, with the jaws involved rarely. Contractions are usually paroxysmal and are attended with pain. Sensation and mental status are normal and fever is slight or absent.

SIGNS: Characteristic diagnostic signs are Trousseau's sign, Chvostek's sign, and the peroneal sign. Prolongation of the isoelectric phase of the S-T segment of the electrocardiogram may be present with tetany that is caused by a low serum calcium level. SEE: *Chvostek's sign; hyperventilation; Trousseau's sign*.

ETIOLOGY: Causative factors are parathyroid deficiency or inadvertent operative removal of parathyroids during thyroidectomy, alkalosis, vitamin D deficiency, or hyperventilation.

PROGNOSIS: The outcome is usually favorable if the underlying cause is addressed.

alkalotic t. Tetany resulting from respiratory alkalosis, as in hyperventilation, or from metabolic alkalosis induced by excessive intake of sodium bicarbonate or excessive loss of chlorides by vomiting, gastric lavage, or suction.

duration t. Continuous contraction, esp. in degenerated muscles, in response to a continuous electric current.

epidemic t. A form of tetany occurring in Europe, esp. in the winter. It is of short duration and is seldom fatal.

gastric t. A severe form of tetany from stomach disorders accompanied by tonic, painful spasms of the extremities.

hyperventilation t. Tetany caused by continued hyperventilation.

hypocalcemic t. Tetany due to low serum calcium and high serum phosphate levels. This may be due to lack of vitamin D, factors that interfere with calcium absorption such as steatorrhea or infantile diarrhea, or defective renal excretion of phosphorus.

latent t. Tetany that requires mechanical or electrical stimulation of nerves to show characteristic signs of excitability; the opposition of manifest tetany.

manifest t. Tetany in which the characteristic symptoms such as carpopedal spasm, laryngospasm, and convulsions are present; the opposite of latent tetany.

parathyroid t. Tetany resulting from excision of the parathyroid glands or from hyposecretion of the parathyroid glands as a result of disease or disorders of the glands. SEE: *hypoparathyroidism.*

rachitic t. Tetany due to hypocalcemia accompanying vitamin D deficiency.

thyreoprival t. Tetany resulting from removal of the thyroid gland accompanied by inadvertent removal of the parathyroid glands.

tetarcone (tĕt′ăr-kōn) [Gr. *tetartos,* fourth, + *konos,* cone] The fourth or distolingual cusp of an upper premolar tooth. SYN: *tetartocone.*

tetartanopia, tetartanopsia (tĕt″ăr-tăn-ō′pē-ă, -ŏp′sē-ă) [″ + *opsis,* vision] Symmetrical blindness in the same quadrant of each visual field. SYN: *quadrantanopsia.*

tetartocone (tĕt-ăr′tō-kōn) [″ + *konos,* cone] Tetarcone.

tetra-, tetr- Combining form meaning *four.*

tetrabasic (tĕt″ră-bā′sĭk) [Gr. *tetras,* four, + *basis,* base] Having four replaceable hydrogen atoms, said of an acid or acid salt.

tetrablastic (tĕt″ră-blăs′tĭk) [″ + *blastos,* germ] Having four germinal layers: the ectoderm, endoderm, and two mesodermic layers.

tetrabrachius (tĕt″ră-brā′kē-ŭs) [″ + *brachion,* arm] A deformed fetus with four arms.

tetrabromofluorescein (tĕt″ră-brōm″ō-flū-or-ĕs′ĭn, -ē-ĭn) A dye, $C_{20}H_8Br_4O_5$, obtained from the action of bromine on fluorescein, used as a stain in microscopy. SYN: *eosin.*

tetracaine hydrochloride A local anesthetic agent used topically and by infiltration. Trade name is Pontocaine Hydrochloride.

tetrachirus (tĕt″ră-kī′rŭs) [″ + *cheir,* hand] A deformed fetus with four hands.

tetrachlorethylene (tĕt″ră-klor-ĕth′ĭ-lēn) A clear, colorless liquid with a characteristic odor, used as a solvent.

tetrachloride (tĕt″ră-klō′rīd) A radical with four atoms of chlorine.

tetracid (tĕ-trăs′ĭd) [″ + L. *acidus,* sour] **1.** Able to react with four molecules of a monoacid or two of a diacid to form a salt or ester, said of a base or alcohol. This term is disapproved by some authorities. **2.** Having four hydrogen atoms replaceable by basic atoms or radicals, said of acids.

Tetracoccus (tĕt″ră-kŏk′ŭs) [″ + *kokkos,* berry] A genus of micrococcus arranged in groups of four by division into two planes.

tetracrotic (tĕt″ră-krŏt′ĭk) [″ + *krotos,* beat] Noting a pulse or pulse tracing with four upward strokes in the descending limb of the wave.

tetracycline (tĕt″ră-sī′klēn) A bacteriostatic antibiotic used, for example, to treat acne, chlamydia, and atypical pneumonia.

CAUTION: Tetracyclines should not be given to pregnant women or young children, because they damage developing teeth and bones.

---

tetrad (tĕt′răd) [Gr. *tetras,* four] **1.** A group of four things with something in common. **2.** An element having a valence or combining power of four. **3.** A group of four similar bodies. **4.** A group of four parts, said of cells produced by division in two planes. **5.** The group of four chromosomes in prophase 1 of mitosis; the pairs of homologous chromosomes, each having two chromatids, that line up together on the spindle fibers. SEE: *meiosis* for illus.

tetradactyly (tĕt″ră-dăk′tĭ-lē) [″ + *daktylos,* finger] Having four digits on a hand or foot.

tetraethylpyrophosphate (tĕt-ră-ĕth″ĭl-pī-rō-fŏs′fāt) ABBR: TEPP. A powerful cholinesterase inhibitor used as an insecticide. It is poisonous to humans; the antidote is atropine.

tetrahydrocannabinol (tĕt″ră-hī″drō-kă-năb′ĭ-nōl) A chemical, $C_{21}H_{30}O_2$, that is the principal active component in cannabis, or marijuana.

tetrahydrozoline hydrochloride (tĕt″ră-hī-drō′zō-lēn) A vasoconstrictor agent used as a nasal decongestant and ophthalmic vasoconstrictor.

tetraiodothyronine (tĕt″ră-ī″ō-dō-thī′rō-nēn) Thyroxine.

tetralogy The combination of four symptoms or elements.

t. of Fallot A congenital anomaly of the heart consisting of pulmonary stenosis, interventricular septal defect, dextroposed aorta that receives blood from both ventricles, and hypertrophy of the right ventricle.

tetramastia, tetramazia (tĕt″ră-măs′tē-ă, tĕt″ră-mā′zē-ă) [″ + *mastos, mazos,* breast] A condition characterized by the presence of four breasts.

tetramastigote (tĕt″ră-măs′tĭ-gōt) [″ + *mastix,* lash] Having four flagella.

tetrameric, tetramerous (tĕt″ră-mĕr′ĭk, tĕt-răm′ĕr-ŭs) [″ + *meros,* a part] Having four parts.

tetranopsia (tĕt″ră-nŏp′sē-ă) [″ + *an-,* not, + *opsis,* vision] Obliteration of one quarter of the visual field.

tetraotus (tĕt″ră-ō′tŭs) [Gr. *tetras,* four, + *otos,* ear] Tetrotus.

tetraparesis (tĕt″ră-păr′ĕ-sĭs) [″ + *parienai,* to let fall] Muscular weakness of all four extremities.

tetrapeptide (tĕt″ră-pĕp′tīd) A peptide that yields four amino acids when it is hydrolyzed.

tetraplegia (tĕt″ră-plē′jē-ă) [″ + *plege,* a stroke] Quadriplegia.

tetraploid (tĕt′ră-ployd) [″ + *ploos,* a fold, + *eidos,* form, shape] **1.** Concerning tetraploidy, the state of having twice the diploid number of chromosomes. **2.** Having four sets of chromosomes.

tetrapus (tĕt′ră-pŭs) [″ + *pous,* foot] A deformed fetus having four feet.

tetrasaccharide (tĕt″ră-săk′ă-rīd) A carbohydrate composed of four monosaccharides.

tetrascelus (tĕt-răs′ē-lŭs) [″ + *skelos,* leg] A deformed fetus having four legs.

tetrasomic (tĕt-ră-sō′mĭk) [″ + *soma,* body] Possessing four instead of the usual pair of chromosomes in an otherwise diploid cell; that is, having a chromosome number of 2n + 2.

tetraster (tĕt-răs′tĕr) [″ + *aster,* star] A mitotic figure in which there are four asters instead of the usual two; occurring abnormally in mitosis.

tetrastichiasis (tĕt″ră-stĭ-kī′ă-sĭs) [″ + *stichos,* row, + *-iasis,* condition] A deformed fetus having four rows of eyelashes.

tetratomic (tĕt″ră-tŏm′ĭk) [″ + *atomos,* indivisible] Having four atoms.

tetravalent (tĕt″ră-vā′lĕnt) Having a valence or combining power of four. SYN: *quadrivalent.*

tetrodotoxin (tĕt″rō-dō-tŏks′ĭn) A powerful nerve poison found in the eggs of the California newt and in certain puffer fish in Japan. In concentrated form, it is more toxic than cyanide.

tetrotus (tĕt-rō′tŭs) [″ + *otos,* ear] A deformed fetus with two faces, four eyes, and four ears.

tetroxide (tĕ-trŏk′sīd) A chemical compound containing four oxygen atoms.

textiform (tĕks′tĭ-form) [L. *textum,* something woven, + *forma,* shape] Resembling a network, web, or mesh.

textoblastic (tĕks″tō-blăs′tĭk) [L. *textus,* tissue, + Gr. *blastos,* germ] Forming adult tissue; regenerative.

textural (tĕks′tū-răl) [L. *textura,* weaving] Concerning the texture or constitution of a tissue.

texture (tĕks′tūr) [L. *textura*] The organization of a tissue or structure.

textus (tĕks′tŭs) [L.] Tissue.

T fracture Fracture in which bone splits both longitudinally and transversely.

T-group A group of individuals who meet in training sessions to become more sensitive to themselves and others.

Th Symbol for the element thorium.

thalamencephalon (thăl″ă-mĕn-sĕf′ă-lŏn) [Gr. *thalamos,* inner chamber, + *enkephalos,* brain] The part of the diencephalon that includes the thalamus, pineal body, and geniculate bodies.

thalamic (thăl-ăm′ĭk) [Gr. *thalamos,* inner chamber] Pert. to the thalamus.

thalamic syndrome A syndrome caused by an optic thalamic lesion, with vascular lesions of the thalamus, causing disturbances of sensation and partial or complete paralysis of one side of the body. An extremely severe, sharp, boring-type pain may occur spontaneously. There also is a tendency to overrespond to a sensory stimulus and to be aware of the stimulus long after it has ceased.

thalamo- **1.** Combining form meaning *chamber.* **2.** Combining form meaning *thalamus.*

thalamocortical (thăl″ăm-ō-kor′tĭ-kăl) [″ + L. *cortex,* rind] Pert. to the thalamus and the cerebral cortex.

thalamolenticular (thăl′ăm-ō-lĕn-tĭk′ū-lăr) [″ + L. *lenticula,* lentil] Concerning the thalamus and the lenticular nucleus.

thalamotomy (thăl-ă-mŏt′ō-mē) [″ + *tome,* incision] Destruction by one of several methods of a portion of the thalamus to treat psychosis or intractable pain.

thalamus (thăl′ă-mŭs) *pl.* **thalami** [L.] The largest subdivision of the diencephalon on either side, consisting chiefly of an ovoid gray nuclear mass in the lateral wall of the third ventricle. Each consists of a number of nuclei (anterior, medial, lateral, and ventral), the medial and lateral geniculate bodies, and the pulvinar.

FUNCTION: All sensory stimuli, with the exception of olfactory, are received by the thalamus. These are associated, integrated, and then relayed through thalamocortical radiations to specific cortical areas. Impulses are also received from the cortex, hypothalamus, and corpus striatum and relayed to visceral and somatic effectors. The thalamus is also the center for appreciation of primitive uncritical sensations of pain, crude touch, and temperature.

thalassemia (thăl-ă-sē′mē-ă) [Gr. *thalassa,* sea, + *haima,* blood] A group of hereditary anemias occurring in populations bordering the Mediterranean and in Southeast Asia. Anemia is produced by either a defective production rate of the alpha or beta hemoglobin polypeptide chain or a decreased synthesis of the beta chain. Heterozygotes are usually asymptomatic. The severity in homozygotes varies according to the complexity of the inheritance pattern, but thalassemia may be fatal. SEE: *anemia, sickle cell.*

t. intermedia A chronic hemolytic anemia caused by deficient alpha chain synthesis. It is also called *hemoglobin H disease.*

t. major The homozygous form of deficient beta chain synthesis, which presents during childhood. It is characterized by fatigue, splenomegaly, severe anemia, enlargement of the heart, slight jaundice, leg ulcers, and cholelithiasis. Increased bone marrow activity causes thickening of the cranial bones and increased malar eminences. Prognosis varies; however, the younger the child when the disease appears, the more unfavorable the outcome. SYN: *Cooley's anemia.*

t. minor A mild disease produced by heterozygosity for either beta or alpha chain. It may be completely asymptomatic. It is usually revealed by chance or as a result of study of the family of an individual having thalassemia major. The prognosis is excellent.

thalassophobia (thăl-ăs″ō-fō′bē-ă) [Gr. *thalassa,* sea, + *phobos,* fear] An abnormal fear of the sea.

thalassotherapy (thăl-ăs″sō-thĕr′ă-pē) [″ + *therapeia,* treatment] Treatment of disease by living at the seaside, by sea bathing, or by sea voyages.

thalidomide (thă-lĭd′ō-mīd) A hypnotic drug that, if taken in early pregnancy, may cause severe malformation in limbs of developing fetuses. It is used in treating erythema nodosum leprosum and is being investigated as an immunosuppressive agent. It has antiangiogenetic properties in the treatment of some tumors. SEE: *phocomelia.*

CAUTION: This drug should not be administered to women of childbearing age.

thallitoxicosis (thăl″ĭ-tŏk″sĭ-kō′sĭs) Thallium poisoning. SEE: *thallium* in *Poisons and Poisoning Appendix.*

thallium (thăl′ē-ŭm) [Gr. *thallos,* a young shoot] SYMB: Tl. A metallic element. Atomic weight, 204.37; atomic number, 81; specific gravity, 11.85. Its salts may be poisonous in overdose; its radioisotope is used to assess myocardial perfusion and viability.

t. 201 A radionuclide used to diagnose ischemic heart disease. When injected at the peak of exercise during a graded exercise tolerance test, it circulates to the myocardium. Images of the heart can then be obtained to aid in the diagnosis of impaired coronary blood flow or prior myocardial infarction. SEE: *exercise tolerance test; redistribution.*

t. sulfate A chemical used as a rodenticide. It is also toxic to humans.

thallium poisoning Poisoning characterized by severe abdominal pain, vomiting, diarrhea, tremors, delirium, convulsions, paralysis, coma, and death. SYN: *thallitoxicosis; thallotoxicosis.* SEE: *Poisons and Poisoning Appendix.*

thallotoxicosis (thăl″ō-tŏk″sĭ-kō′sĭs) Thallium poisoning.

thanato- Combining form meaning *death.*

thanatobiological (thăn″ă-tō-bī-ō-lŏj′ĭ-kăl) [Gr. *thanatos,* death, + *bios,* life, + *logos,* word, reason] Rel. to the processes of life and death.

thanatognomonic (thăn″ăt-ŏg-nō-mŏn′ĭk) [″ + *gnomonikos,* knowing] Indicative of the approach of death.

thanatology (thăn″ă-tŏl′ō-jē) [Gr. *thanatos,* death, + *logos,* word, reason] The study of death.

thanatomania (thăn″ă-tō-mā′nē-ă) [″ + *mania,* madness] The condition of homicidal or suicidal mania.

thanatophidia (thăn″ă-tō-fĭd′ē-ă) [″ + *ophis,* snake] Venomous snakes.

thanatophobia (thăn″ă-tō-fō′bē-ă) [″ + *phobos,* fear] A morbid fear of death. SYN: *necrophobia.*

thanatophoric dwarfism Dwarfism caused by generalized failure of endochondral bone formation. It is characterized by a large head, a prominent forehead, hypertelorism, a saddle nose, and short limbs extending straight out from the trunk. Most of these infants die soon after birth.

Thayer-Martin medium A special medium used for growing the causative organism of gonorrhea, *Neisseria gonorrhoeae.*

theaism (thē′ă-ĭzm) [L. *thea,* tea, + Gr. *-ismos,* condition] Chronic caffeine poisoning from excessive tea drinking.

thebaine (thē-bā′ĭn) An alkaloid present in opium.

thebesian foramen (thē-bē′zē-ăn) [Adam Christian Thebesius, Ger. physician, 1686–1732] The orifice of a thebesian vein, opening into the right atrium of the heart.

thebesian valve Coronary valve.

thebesian veins Venules conveying blood from the myocardium to the atria or ventricles.

theca (thē′kă) *pl.* **thecae** [Gr. *theke,* sheath] A sheath of investing membrane.

t. cordis Pericardium that sheaths the heart.

t. folliculi The outer wall of a graafian follicle, consisting of an inner vascular layer (theca interna) and outer fibrous layer (theca externa).

thecal (thē′kăl) [Gr. *theke,* sheath] Pert. to a sheath.

thecitis (thē-sī′tĭs) [″ + *itis,* inflammation] Inflammation of the sheath of a tendon.

theco- Combining form meaning *sheath, case, receptacle.*

thecodont (thē′kō-dŏnt) [Gr. *theke,* sheath, + *odous,* tooth] Having teeth that are inserted in sockets.

thecoma (thē-kō′mă) [″ + *oma,* tumor] A tumor of the ovary usually occurring during or after menopause. It is usually benign.

thecomatosis (thē″kō-mă-tō′sĭs) [″ + ″ + *osis,* condition] Increased connective tissue in the ovary.

thecostegnosia, thecostegnosis (thē″kō-stĕg-nō′sē-ă, -nō′sĭs) [″ + *stegnosis,* a narrowing] Constriction of a tendon sheath.

thelalgia (thē-lăl′jē-ă) [Gr. *thele,* nipple, + *algos,* pain] Pain in the nipples.

thelarche (thē-lăr′kē) [″ + *arche,* beginning] The beginning of breast development at puberty. SEE: *pubarche; semenarche.*

Thelazia (thē-lā′zē-ă) [Gr. *thelazo,* to suck] A genus of nematodes that inhabit the conjunctival sac and lacrimal ducts of various species of vertebrates. Occasionally species of *Thelazia* are found in humans.

thelaziasis (thē″lā-zī′ă-sĭs) [″ + *-iasis,* condition] The condition of being infested by worms of the genus *Thelazia.*

theleplasty (thē′lĕ-plăs″tē) [Gr. *thele,* nipple, + *plassein,* to form] Plastic surgery of the nipple. SYN: *mammilliplasty.*

thelerethism (thēl-ĕr′ĕ-thĭzm) [″ + *erethisma,* stimulation] Erection of the nipple.

thelitis (thē-lī′tĭs) [″ + *itis,* inflammation] Inflammation of the nipples. SYN: *acromastitis.*

thelium (thē′lē-ŭm) *pl.* **thelia** [L.] **1.** A papilla. **2.** A nipple. **3.** A cellular layer.

theloncus (thē-lŏn′kŭs) [″ + *onkus,* bulk, mass] A tumor of a nipple.

thelophlebostemma (thē″lō-flĕb″ō-stĕm′mă) [″ + *phelps,* vein, + *stemma,* wreath] A dark or venous circle of veins about the nipple.

thelorrhagia (thē″lō-rā′jē-ă) [″ + *rhegnynai,* to burst forth] Hemorrhage from a nipple.

thelygenic (thē″lē-jĕn′ĭk) [Gr. *thelys,* female, + *gennan,* to produce] Producing only female children.

thenad (thē′năd) [Gr. *thenar,* palm, + L. *ad,* toward] Toward the palm or thenar eminence.

thenal (thē′năl) [Gr. *thenar,* palm] Pert. to the palm or thenar eminence.

thenal aspect The outer side of the palm.

thenar (thē′năr) [Gr. *thenar,* palm] **1.** The palm of the hand or sole of the foot. **2.** A fleshy eminence at the base of the thumb. **3.** Concerning the palm.

thenar cleft A fascial cleft of the palm overlying the volar surface of the adductor pollicis muscle.

thenar eminence A prominence at the base of the thumb.

thenar fascia A thin membrane covering the short muscles of the thumb.

thenar muscle The abductor or flexor muscle of the thumb.

theobromine (thē-ō-brō′mēn) [Gr. *theos,* god, + *broma,* food] A white powder obtained from *Theobroma cacao,* the plant from which chocolate is obtained. It dilates blood vessels in the heart and peripherally. It is used as a mild stimulant and as a diuretic.

theomania (thē-ō-mā′nē-ă) [Gr. *theos,* god, + *mania,* madness] Religious insanity; esp. that in which the patient thinks he or she is a deity or has divine inspiration.

theophobia (thē″ō-fō′bē-ă) [″ + *phobos,* fear] An abnormal fear of the wrath of God.

theophylline (thē-of′ĭ-lēn, -ĭn) [L. *thea,* tea, + Gr. *phyllon,* plant] A white crystalline powder used as an oral agent for reactive airway diseases such as asthma. The drug has a narrow therapeutic index, and toxicity to this agent, marked by gastrointestinal upset, tremor, cardiac arrhythmias, and other complications, is common in clinical practice. Other drugs for reactive airway diseases, such as inhaled beta-agonists and inhaled steroids, are often prescribed instead of theophylline to avoid its toxicities. SEE: *aminophylline.*

t. ethylenediamine Previously used name for aminophylline.

theorem (thē′ō-rĕm) [Gr. *theorema,* principle arrived at by speculation] A proposition that can be proved by use of logic, or by argument, from information previously accepted as being valid.

theory (thē′ō-rē) [Gr. *theoria,* speculation as opposed to practice] A statement that best explains all the available evidence on a given topic. If evidence that contradicts the theory becomes available, the theory must be abandoned, modified, or changed to incorporate it. When a theory becomes generally accepted and firmly established, it may be called a doctrine or principle.

t. of aging Any coherent set of concepts that explains the aging process at the cellular, biological, psychological, and sociological levels.

clonal selection t. of immunity The theory that precursor cell lines for lymphocytes are made up of innumerable clones with identical antigen receptors. The clones capable of reacting with "self" components (i.e., the individual's own cells) are eliminated or suppressed in the prenatal period. Those clones not eliminated or suppressed react only with specific foreign antigens that fit their receptors, leading to the proliferation of that lymphocyte cell line. Within the body, there are many different lymphocyte clones, each of which only reacts to one antigen (clonal restriction).

five elements t. A fundamental premise in traditional Chinese medicine and some branches of alternative medicine that holds that illness results from imbalances in these elements: wood, fire, earth, metal, and water. A similar concept in ancient Western and medieval medicine held that diseases resulted from imbalances in four elements: earth, air, fire, and water. SEE: *feng shui.*

germ t. The proposition that infectious diseases are caused by microorganisms.

learning t. An approach to understanding how learning comes about by applying certain laws of learning; learning represents a change in behavior that has come about as a result of practice, education, and experience.

nursing t. A theory that explores, describes, and analyzes the epistemological origins of nursing knowledge.

quantum t. The proposition that energy can be emitted in discrete quantities (quanta) and that atomic particles can exist only in certain energy states. Quanta are measured by multiplying the frequency of the radiation, v, by Planck's constant, h.

recapitulation t. The theory that during development an individual organism goes through the same progressive stages as did the species in developing from the lower to the higher forms of life; the theory that ontogeny recapitulates phylogeny.

summation t. The concept that excessive or intense stimulation of nerves will eventually produce a disagreeable sensation—the sensation of pain.

target t. A model used in radiobiology to describe cell survival from radiation. Each cell has a certain number of critical structures (targets) that must be inactivated for the cell to die. If all are inactivated, the cell will recover.

Theory of Clinical Nursing A nursing theory developed by Reva Rubin that focuses on patients' experiences of tension or stress during illness. The goal of nursing is to help patients adjust to, endure through, and usefully integrate health problem situations. SEE: *Nursing Theory Appendix.*

Theory of Cultural Care Diversity and Universality A nursing theory developed by Madeleine Leininger that focuses on diversities and universalities in human care. The goal of nursing is to provide culturally congruent care to people. SEE: *Nursing Theory Appendix.*

Theory of the Deliberative Nursing Process A nursing theory developed by Ida Jean Orlando Pelletier that focuses on how the nurse identifies patients' immediate needs for help. The goal of nursing is to identify and meet patients' immediate needs for help through use of the deliberative nursing process. SEE: *Nursing Theory Appendix.*

Theory of Health as Expanding Consciousness A nursing theory developed by Margaret Newman that proposes that all people in every situation, no matter how disordered and hopeless the situation may seem, are part of a universal process of expanding consciousness. The goal of nursing is the authentic involvement of nurse and patient in a mutual relationship of pattern recognition and augmentation. SEE: *Nursing Theory Appendix.*

Theory of Human Becoming A nursing theory developed by Rosemarie Parse that focuses on the individual's experiences of health. The goal of nursing is to respect and facilitate the quality of life as perceived by the individual and the family. SEE: *Nursing Theory Appendix.*

Theory of Human Caring A nursing theory developed by Jean Watson that focuses on the transpersonal caring relationship between nurse and patient and the caring actions or interventions used by nurses. The goal of nursing is to help individuals to gain a higher degree of harmony within the mind, body, and soul through the use of 10 nursing interventions. SEE: *Nursing Theory Appendix.*

Theory of Interpersonal Relations A nursing theory developed by Hildegard Peplau that identifies the three phases of the interpersonal process between the nurse and the patient: orientation, working, and termination. In this theory, the goal of nursing is to resolve the patient's perceived health difficulties. SEE: *Nursing Theory Appendix.*

theotherapy (thē″ō-thĕr′ă-pē) [Gr. *theos,* god, + *therapeia,* treatment] The treatment of disease by spiritual and religious methods.

thèque (tĕk) [Fr., a box] A nest of nevus cells or other cells close to the basal layer of the epidermis.

therapeutic (thĕr-ă-pū′tĭk) [Gr. *therapeutikos,* treating] **1.** Pert. to results obtained from treatment. **2.** Having medicinal or healing properties. **3.** A healing agent.

therapeutic equivalents Drugs that have the same pharmacological effects and actions in the treatment of illnesses, even though the drugs may not be chemically equivalent.

therapeutic recreation A specialized field within recreation whose specialists plan and direct recreational activities for patients recovering from physical or mental illness or who are attempting to cope with a permanent or temporary disability.

therapeutic regimen (community), ineffective management of A pattern of regulating and integrating into community processes programs for treatment of illness and the sequelae of illness that is unsatisfactory for meeting health-related goals. SEE: *Nursing Diagnoses Appendix.*

therapeutic regimen (families), ineffective management of A pattern of regulating and integrating into family processes a program for treatment of illness and the sequelae of illness that is unsatisfactory for meeting specific health needs. SEE: *Nursing Diagnoses Appendix.*

therapeutic regimen (individual), effective management of A pattern of regulating and integrating into daily living a program for treatment of illness and its sequelae that is satisfactory for meeting specific health goals. SEE: *Nursing Diagnoses Appendix.*

therapeutic regimen (individual), ineffective management of A pattern of regulating and integrating into daily living a program for treatment of illness and the sequelae of illness that is unsatisfactory for meeting specific health goals. SEE: *Nursing Diagnoses Appendix.*

therapeutics (thĕr″ă-pū′tĭks) [Gr. *therapeutike,* treatment] That branch of medicine concerned with the application of remedies and the treatment of disease. SYN: *therapy.*

therapia sterilisans magna (thĕr″ă-pē′ă stē-rĭl′ĭ-săns măg′nă) [L.] Ehrlich's method of administering a chemical agent that would destroy in one large dose all the parasites in a patient without causing serious injury to the patient.

therapist (thĕr′ă-pĭst) [Gr. *therapeia,* treatment] A person skilled in giving therapy, usually in a specific field of health care. SEE: *psychotherapist.*

certified respiratory t. ABBR: CRT. An entry-level respiratory care practitioner who has passed the examination offered by the National Board for Respiratory Care.

licensed occupational t. ABBR: LOTR; OTR/L. An occupational therapist who has met the requirements to practice in states with licensure laws governing occupational therapy. Usually, licensed therapists have been certified by the National Board for Certification in Occupational Therapy as a registered occupational therapist (OTR). Some state governments, as part of their licensure statutes, permit use of the OTR/L or LOTR designations.

occupational t. ABBR: OT. One who provides assessment and intervention to ameliorate physical and psychological deficits that interfere with the performance of activities and tasks of living.

physical t. A licensed practitioner of physical therapy who has graduated from an accredited physical therapy education program. SYN: *registered physical t.*

radiation t. Radiation therapy technologist.

registered physical t. ABBR: RPT. Physical therapist.

respiratory t. A person skilled in managing the techniques and equipment used in treating those with acute and chronic respiratory diseases.

speech t. A person skilled in assisting patients who have speech and language difficulties.

therapy (thĕr′ă-pē) [Gr. *therapeia,* treatment] Treatment.

adjuvant t. In cancer therapy, the use of another form of treatment in addition to the primary therapy. For example, chemotherapy may be the primary treatment and radiation therapy may be an adjuvant therapy.

anticoagulant t. The use of drugs, such as heparin, low-molecular-weight heparin, or warfarin, that interfere with coagulation. It is used to prevent or treat disorders, such as pulmonary embolism, that result from vascular thrombosis. SEE: *heparin; thrombosis; warfarin sodium.*

CAUTION: Anticoagulant therapy increases the risk of bleeding.

PATIENT CARE: The patient is observed closely for desired and adverse effects of anticoagulation therapy. This includes assessing the results of laboratory tests (protime, INR, aPTT) specific to the anticoagulant drug being used and assessing the patient daily for signs or symptoms of bleeding.

aquatic t. Exercises performed in or underwater for conditioning or rehabilitation (e.g., in injured athletes or patients with joint diseases).

behavior t. Techniques used to change maladaptive behaviors, based on principles of learning theory. Cigarette smoking, eating disorders, and alcohol abuse are commonly treated through behavior therapy, which may include the use of positive reinforcement, aversive conditioning, discrimination, and modeling.

biological t. Therapy with immunologically active agents.

cell t. of Niehans [Niehans, Paul] An alternative medical therapy in which cells derived from living animal tissues are injected directly into patients to bolster endocrine, immunological, and solid organ function. The technique has no proven uses and has caused serious allergic side effects in many patients.

collapse t. The production of a pneumothorax on one side to treat pulmonary tuberculosis. It allows the lung on that side to be at rest. This form of treatment was popular in the preantibiotic era, but has been superseded by newer pharmaceutical practices.

craniosacral t. A form of massage that aims to cure ailments by redirecting the flow of cerebrospinal fluid or manipulating the cranial sutures. To date it has no objective validation.

cymatic t. The therapeutic uses of music and sound.

diet t. The alteration of dietary intake to treat or prevent clinical disease. SEE: *diet*.

differentiation t. The use of medications to make cancer cells evolve into cells no longer capable of infinite replication.

electroconvulsive t. ABBR: ECT. The use of an electric shock to produce convulsions and thereby treat drug-resistant psychiatric disorders, such as some cases of major depression, bipolar disorder, suicidal ideation, and schizophrenia. SYN: *electric shock treatment; electroshock t.; shock t.; shock treatment*.

electroshock t. Electroconvulsive t.

empirical t. Use of antibiotics to treat an infection before the specific causative organism has been identified with laboratory tests.

estrogen replacement t. ABBR: ERT. Administration of estrogen to women who have a deficiency of this hormone (e.g., menopausal and postmenopausal women) and women with hypothalamic amenorrhea. Estrogen is also used as adjunctive therapy for hormone-sensitive cancers, such as prostatic cancer. SEE: *conjugated estrogen; hormone replacement therapy*.

Reported health benefits are vigorously debated. ERT is credited with retarding bone loss and lowering the risk of osteoporotic fractures. In addition, ERT relieves symptoms associated with menopause (e.g., hot flashes, diaphoresis, vaginal dryness, dyspareunia, moodiness, depression, and insomnia).

CAUTION: Women who have a history of thromboembolic disorders, current tobacco use, impaired liver function, undiagnosed vaginal bleeding, endometrial cancer, or estrogen-stimulated tumors should not receive ERT. Estrogen replacement should be used with caution in women who have a family history of breast cancer or who have diseases of the liver, kidney, or gallbladder.

fever t. Therapy involving artificially produced fever. This is accomplished by exposure to high environmental temperature or by the injection of foreign proteins.

gene t. The introduction of genetic material into cells on vehicles or vectors like viruses or plasmids. The donated genes are used to produce proteins that may combat host diseases, such as immunodeficiencies, malignancies, neurodegenerative disorders, or inflammatory diseases.

highly active antiretroviral t. ABBR: HAART. The combined use of antiviral agents from three or more classes of drugs to treat patients with human immunodeficiency virus (HIV) infection. HAART reduces the number of viruses circulating in the blood (viral load), and prolongs life and disease-free survival. Reverse transcriptase inhibitors such as azidothymidine, dideoxyinosine, and abacavir; nonnucleoside reverse transcriptase inhibitors such as delavirdine and nevirapine; and protease inhibitors such as saquinavir, ritonavir, and indinavir are used in HAART. SEE: *Acquired immunodeficiency syndrome*.

home drug infusion t. Out-of-hospital management of diseases or disorders that require intravenous administration of therapeutic agents. Patients who receive this form of therapy need to be carefully selected and trained. Their home care providers also need to be experienced in the procedures. If these qualifications are not met, the patients are at high risk for adverse events including severe infection, shock, and even death.

hormone replacement t. ABBR: HRT. The administration of supplemental conjugated estrogen and progestin to treat hormonal deficiency states; relieve menopausal vasomotor symptoms; and manage postmenopausal atrophic vaginitis. It also is used as adjunctive therapy for osteoporosis. In some but not all studies, HRT has been credited with lowering the potential risk of heart disease, colon cancer, and Alzheimer's disease. SEE: *estrogen replacement therapy*.

immunosuppressive t. Treatment with drugs that impair immune responses. SEE: *immunosuppressive agent*.

inhalation t. The administration of medicines, water vapor, gases (e.g., oxygen, carbon dioxide, or helium), or anesthetics by inhalation. The medicines usually are nebulized by using an aerosol or spray apparatus.

insulin shock t. An obsolete form of shock therapy in which a patient was deliberately made hypoglycemic with injected insulin.

life review t. A type of group therapy that encourages individuals to remember and share with others their personal life experiences, unresolved conflicts, anxieties, resentments, and guilt.

light t. Treatment with radiation from the visible spectrum.

liquid air t. The therapeutic application of air that is so cold as to be liquefied. SEE: *CO_2 therapy; cryotherapy; hypothermia*.

magnet t. The application of permanent magnets to painful regions of the human body in an attempt to alleviate chronic diseases or chronic pain. Although this form of treatment is advocated by some complementary or alternative medical practitioners, there is no evidence that it is effective.

manual t. A collection of techniques used by physical therapists, in which hand movements skillfully are applied to mobilize joints and soft tissue. These techniques may be used to alleviate pain, improve extension and motion, induce relaxation, reduce edema, and improve pulmonary and musculoskeletal function. SEE: *manipulation; joint mobilization; soft-tissue mobilization.*

milieu t. A method of psychotherapy that controls the environment of the patient to provide interpersonal contacts that will develop trust, assurance, and personal autonomy.

nonspecific t. The use of injections of foreign proteins or bacterial vaccines in the treatment of infection to stimulate general immunological responses. SEE: *specific t.*

occupational t. Therapeutic activities used to develop, regain, or maintain the skills necessary for health, productivity, and independence in everyday life. It may include the use of assistive technologies or orthotics to enhance function or prevent disability. SEE: *rehabilitation.*

opsonic t. Vaccine t.

parenteral t. A medicine or solution administered via a route other than ingestion.

photodynamic t. A method of treating cancer by using light-absorbing chemicals that are selectively retained by malignant cells. When these cells are exposed to light in the visible range, the cancer cells are killed.

physical t. ABBR: PT. The health profession responsible for management of the patient's movement system. This includes conducting an examination; alleviating impairments and functional limitation; preventing injury, impairment, functional limitation, and disability; and engaging in consultation, education, and research. Direct interventions include the appropriate use of patient education, therapeutic exercise, and physical agents such massage, thermal modalities, hydrotherapy, and electricity.

play t. The use of play, esp. with dolls and toys, to allow children to express their feelings. This may permit insight into their thought processes that could not be obtained through verbal communication.

polarity t. In alternative medicine, a massage technique aimed at healing the body by manipulating its electromagnetic currents. There is no objective validation of this method.

replacement t. The therapeutic use of a medicine to substitute for a natural substance that is either absent or diminished (e.g., insulin or thyroid hormone).

salvage t. Treatment that follows the relapse of an illness that had already been treated in standard fashion.

serum t. The use of injections of serum from immunized animals or persons in the treatment of disease. Also called *serotherapy.*

sham t. Treatment that has no known therapeutic effect. Such treatment may be employed by clinical researchers who are trying to determine whether another intervention will be more effective than doing nothing. Sham therapies are also sometimes used by people engaging in health care fraud.

shock t. Electroconvulsive t.

specific t. Administration of a remedy acting directly against the cause of a disease, as penicillin for syphilis or acyclovir for herpes simplex virus. SEE: *nonspecific t.*

speech t. The study, diagnosis, and treatment of defects and disorders of the voice and of spoken and written communication.

spiritual t. The application of spiritual knowledge in the treatment of mental and physical disorders.

substitution t. Administration of a substance that the body normally produces, such as a hormone.

transgenerational t. A type of psychotherapy that addresses long-standing patterns from at least three generations of the patient's family. This method focuses on functional and nonfunctional family processes.

vaccine t. Injection of bacteria or their products to produce active immunization against a disease. SYN: *opsonic t.*

validation t. A communication technique used for patients with moderate to late dementia in which the caregiver makes statements to the patient that demonstrate respect for the patient's feelings and beliefs. This method helps prevent argumentative and agitated behavior. In some cases, the caregiver may need to agree with the patient's statements, even though they are not true or real. It is used when reality orientation is not successful.

therapy putty The generic name for a malleable plastic material to provide resistance in various hand exercises.

therm [Gr. *therme,* heat] Term used to indicate a variety of quantities of heat. SEE: *MET.*

thermacogenesis (thĕr″mă-kō-jĕn′ĕs-ĭs) [Gr. *therme,* heat, + *genesis,* generation, birth] Production of an increase of body temperature by drug therapy or biological methods, such as, in the distant past, injection of malarial parasites.

thermal (thĕr′măl) [Gr. *therme,* heat] Pert. to heat.

thermal death point In bacteriology, the degree of heat that will kill organisms in a fluid culture in 10 min.

thermalgesia (thĕr″măl-jē′zē-ă) [″ + *algesis,* sense of pain] Pain caused by heat. SYN: *thermoalgesia.*

thermalgia (thĕr-măl′jē-ă) [″ + *algos,* pain] Neuralgia accompanied by an intense burning sensation, pain, redness, and sweating of the area involved. SYN: *causalgia.*

thermal radiation Heat radiation.

thermal sense Thermesthesia.

thermanesthesia (thĕrm″ăn-ĕs-thē′zē-ă) [″ + ″ + *aisthesis,* sensation] Thermoanesthesia.

thermatology (thĕr-mă-tŏl′ō-jē) [Gr. *therme,* heat, + *logos,* word, reason] The study of heat in the treatment of disease.

thermelometer (thĕr″mĕl-ŏm′ĕ-tĕr) [″ + *elektron,* amber, + Gr. *metron,* a measure] An electric thermometer used to indicate temperature changes too slight to be measured on an ordinary thermometer.

thermesthesia (thĕr″mĕs-thē′zē-ă) [″ + *aisthesis,* sensation] The capability of perceiving heat and cold; temperature sense. SYN: *thermal sense; thermoesthesia.*

thermesthesiometer (thĕrm″ĕs-thē-zē-ŏm′ĕt-ĕr) [″ + *aisthesis,* sensation, + *metron,* a measure] A device for determining sensibility to heat.

thermic (thĕr′mĭk) [Gr. *therme,* heat] Pert. to heat.

thermic sense The temperature sense; ability to react to heat stimuli.

thermistor (thĕr-mĭs′tor) An apparatus for quickly determining very small changes in temperature. Materials that alter their resistance to the flow of electricity as the temperature changes are used in these devices.

thermo- Combining form indicating *hot, heat.*

thermoalgesia (thĕr″mō-ăl-jē′zē-ă) [Gr. *therme,* heat, + *algesis,* sense of pain] Thermalgesia.

thermoanesthesia (thĕr″mō-ăn″ĕs-thē′zē-ă) [″ + ″ + *aisthesis,* sensation] **1.** Inability to distinguish between heat and cold. **2.** Insensibility to heat or temperature changes. SYN: *thermanesthesia.*

thermobiosis (thĕr″mō-bī-ō′sĭs) [″ + *biosis,* way of life] The ability to withstand high temperature. **thermobiotic,** *adj.*

thermocautery (thĕr″mō-kaw′tĕr-ē) **1.** Cautery by application of heat. **2.** Cauterizing iron.

thermochemistry (thĕr″mō-kĕm′ĭs-trē) The branch of science concerned with the interrelationship of heat and chemical reactions.

thermochroism (thĕr-mŏk′rō-ĭzm) [″ + *chroa,* color] Property of a substance reflecting or transmitting portions of thermal radiation and absorbing or altering others. **thermochroic,** *adj.*

thermocoagulation (thĕr″mō-kō-ăg-ū-lā′shŭn) [″ + L. *coagulatio,* clotting] The use of high-frequency currents to produce coagulation to destroy tissue.

thermocouple (thĕr′mō-kŭ″pl) [″ + L. *copula,* a bond] Thermopile.

thermocurrent (thĕr″mō-kŭr′ĕnt) An electric current produced by thermoelectric means.

thermode A device for heating or cooling a part of the body. Thermodes have been used in studying the effect on body function when the temperature of some organ or tissue is changed.

thermodiffusion (thĕr″mō-dĭ-fū′zhŭn) Increased diffusion of a substance as a result of increased heat.

thermodilution (thĕr″mō-dĭ-lū′shŭn) The use of an injected cold liquid such as sterile saline into the bloodstream and measurement of the temperature change downstream. This technique has been used to determine cardiac output.

thermoduric (thĕr″mō-dū′rĭk) [″ + L. *durus,* resistant] Thermophilic.

thermodynamics (thĕr″mō-dī-năm′ĭks) [″ + *dynamis,* power] The branch of physics concerned with laws that govern heat production, changes, and conversion into other forms of energy.

thermoelectric (thĕr″mō-ē-lĕk′trĭk) Concerning thermoelectricity.

thermoelectricity (thĕr″mō-ē-lĕk-trĭs′ĭ-tē) Electricity generated by heat.

thermoesthesia (thĕr″mō-ĕs-thē′zē-ă) [Gr. *therme,* heat, + *aisthesis,* sensation] Thermesthesia.

thermoexcitatory (thĕr″mō-ĕk-sī′tă-tor-ē) [″ + L. *excitare,* to irritate] Stimulating the production of heat in the body.

thermogenesis (thĕr″mō-jĕn′ĕ-sĭs) [″ + *genesis,* generation, birth] The production of heat, esp. in the body.

dietary t. The heat-producing response to ingesting food. For several hours after eating, the metabolic rate increases. Heat is a by-product of the digestion, absorption, and breakdown of consumed foods, and the synthesis and storage of proteins and fats. Because the calories used in the thermic response are expended, they are not stored as fat.

nonshivering t. A limited physiological response of the newborn infant to chilling. Hypothermia stimulates sympathetic catabolism of brown fat, which is not coupled with ATP formation, and therefore releases most energy in the form of heat. Brown fat is located mainly in the neck and chest of the infant. SEE: *hypothermia.*

thermograph (thĕr′mō-grăf) [″ + *graphein,* to write] A device for registering variations of heat.

thermography In medicine, the use of a

device that detects and records the heat present in very small areas of the part being studied. When multiple readings are accumulated, the relatively hot and cold spots on the body surface are revealed. The technique has been used to study blood flow and to detect cancer of the breast.

thermohyperalgesia (thĕr″mō-hī″pĕr-ăl-jē′zē-ă) [″ + *hyper,* excessive, + *algesis,* sense of pain] Unbearable pain on the application of heat.

thermohyperesthesia (thĕr″mō-hī″pĕr-ĕs-thē′zē-ă) [″ + *hyper,* excessive, + *aisthesis,* sensation] Exceptional sensitivity to heat.

thermohypesthesia (thĕr″mō-hī″pĕs-thē′zē-ă) [″ + *hypo,* below, + *aisthesis,* sensation] Diminished perception of heat.

thermoinhibitory (thĕr″mō-ĭn-hĭb′ĭ-tor″ē) [″ + L. *inhibere,* to restrain] Arresting or impeding the generation of body heat.

thermolamp (thĕr′mō-lămp) [″ + *lampe,* torch] A lamp used for providing heat.

thermology (thĕr-mŏl′ō-jē) [″ + *logos,* word, reason] The science of heat.

thermoluminescent dosimeter A monitoring device consisting of a small crystal in a container that can be attached to a patient or to a health care worker. It stores energy when struck by ionizing radiation. When heated, it will emit light proportional to the amount of radiation to which it has been exposed.

thermolysis (thĕr-mŏl′ĭ-sĭs) [″ + *lysis,* dissolution] **1.** Loss of body heat, as by evaporation. **2.** Chemical decomposition by heat.

thermolytic (thĕr″mō-lĭt′ĭk) [″ + *lytikos,* dissolving] Promoting thermolysis.

Comparative Thermometric Scale

	Celsius*	Fahrenheit
Boiling point of water	100°	212°
	90	194
	80	176
	70	158
	60	140
	50	122
	40	104
Body temperature	37°	98.6°
	30	86
	20	68
	10	50
Freezing point of water	0°	32°
	−10	14
	−20	−4

*Also called *Centigrade.*

thermomassage (thĕr″mō-mă-săzh′) Massage by use of heat.

thermometer (thĕr-mŏm′ĕ-tĕr) [″ + *metron,* measure] An instrument for indicating the degree of heat or cold. **thermometric** (thĕr″mō-mĕt′rĭk), *adj.*

alcohol t. A thermometer containing alcohol.

Celsius t. A thermometric scale generally used in scientific notation. Temperature of boiling water at sea level is 100°C and the freezing point is 0°C. SYN: *centigrade t.* SEE: tables.

centigrade t. Celsius t.

clinical t. A thermometer for measuring the body temperature. SEE: *clinical thermometry.*

differential t. A thermometer recording slight variations of temperature.

Fahrenheit t. A thermometric scale used in English-speaking countries, in which the boiling point is 212°F and the freezing point is 32°F. SEE: tables at *Celsius t.*

gas t. A thermometer filled with gas, such as air, helium, or oxygen.

Kelvin t. A thermometric scale in which absolute zero is 0°K; the freezing point of water is 273.15°K; and the boiling point of water is 373.15°K. Thus 1°K on the Kelvin scale is exactly equivalent to 1°C.

mercury t. A thermometer containing mercury for measurement of temperature. Mercury thermometers are an important source of heavy metal pollution of rivers, streams, and aquatic life.

recording t. A device with a suitable sensor that continuously monitors and records temperature.

rectal t. A thermometer that is inserted into the rectum for determining body temperature.

self-registering t. A thermometer recording variations of temperature.

spirit t. A thermometer filled with alcohol for registering low temperatures.

surface t. A thermometer for indicating the temperature of the body's surface.

tympanic t. A thermometer that determines the temperature electronically by measuring it from the tympanic membrane of the ear. SEE: *ear thermometry; temperature, tympanic.*

wet-and-dry-bulb t. A device for determining relative humidity consisting of two thermometers, the bulb of one being kept saturated with water vapor. The difference in temperatures between the two depends on relative humidity.

thermometer, disinfection of Disinfection of a thermometer with a substance that is able to kill ordinary bacteria and *Mycobacterium tuberculosis* as well as viruses. A variety of chemical solutions are used, but the effectiveness of these agents can be greatly diminished if the thermometer is not washed thoroughly before being disinfected.

Thermometric Equivalents (Celsius and Fahrenheit)

C°	F°	C°	F°	C°	F°	C°	F°
0	32	27	80.6	54	129.2	81	177.8
1	33.8	28	82.4	55	131	82	179.6
2	35.6	29	84.2	56	132.8	83	181.4
3	37.4	30	86.0	57	134.6	84	183.2
4	39.2	31	87.8	58	136.4	85	185
5	41	32	89.6	59	138.2	86	186.8
6	42.8	33	91.4	60	140	87	188.6
7	44.6	34	93.2	61	141.8	88	190.4
8	46.4	35	95	62	143.6	89	192.2
9	48.2	36	96.8	63	145.4	90	194
10	50	37	98.6	64	147.2	91	195.8
11	51.8	38	100.4	65	149	92	197.6
12	53.6	39	102.2	66	150.8	93	199.4
13	55.4	40	104	67	152.6	94	201.2
14	57.2	41	105.8	68	154.4	95	203
15	59	42	107.6	69	156.2	96	204.8
16	60.8	43	109.4	70	158	97	206.6
17	62.6	44	111.2	71	159.8	98	208.4
18	64.4	45	113	72	161.6	99	210.2
19	66.2	46	114.8	73	163.4	100	212
20	68	47	116.6	74	165.2		
21	69.8	48	118.4	75	167		
22	71.6	49	120.2	76	168.8		
23	73.4	50	122	77	170.6		
24	75.2	51	123.8	78	172.4		
25	77	52	125.6	79	174.2		
26	78.8	53	127.4	80	176		

CONVERSION: *Fahrenheit to Celsius:* Subtract 32 and multiply by 5/9. *Celsius to Fahrenheit:* Multiply by 9/5 and add 32.

thermometry (thĕr-mŏm′ĕ-trē) Measurement of temperature.

clinical t. Measurement of the temperature of warm-blooded organisms, esp. humans. The oral temperature of the healthy human body ranges between 96.6° and 100°F (35.9° and 37.8°C). During a 24-hr period, a person's body temperature may vary from 0.5° to 2.0°F (0.28° to 1.1°C). It is highest in late afternoon and lowest during sleep in the early hours of the morning. It is slightly increased by eating, exercising, and external heat, and is reduced about 1.5°F (0.8°C) during sleep. In disease, the temperature of the body deviates several degrees above or below that considered the average in healthy persons.

In acute infections such as meningitis or pneumonia, body temperature sometimes rises as high as 106° to 107°F (41.1° to 41.7°C).

Subnormal temperatures are sometimes seen in exposure, sepsis, or myxedema coma. In general, for every degree of fever the pulse rises 10 beats per minute.

thermoneurosis (thĕr″mō-nū-rō′sĭs) [Gr. *therme,* heat, + *neuron,* nerve, + *osis,* condition] Elevation of body temperature in hysteria and other nervous conditions.

thermonuclear (thĕr″mō-nū′klē-ăr) Concerning thermonuclear reactions.

thermopenetration (thĕr″mō-pĕn-ĕ-trā′shŭn) [″ + L. *penetrare,* to go within] Application of heat to the deeper tissues of the body by diathermy. SYN: *thermoradiotherapy.*

thermophilic (thĕr″mō-fĭl′ĭk) [″ + *philein,* to love] Preferring or thriving best at high temperatures, said of bacteria that thrive best at temperatures between 40° and 70°C (104° and 158°F). SYN: *thermoduric.*

thermophils (thĕr′mō-fĭlz) Organisms that grow best at elevated temperatures (i.e., 40° to 70°C).

thermophobia (thĕr″mō-fō′bē-ă) [″ + *phobos,* fear] An abnormal dread of heat.

thermophore (thĕr′mō-for) [″ + *phoros,* a bearer] An apparatus for applying heat to a part, consisting of a water heater and tubes conveying water to a coil and returning to the heater or salts that produce heat when moistened.

thermophylic (thĕr″mō-fī′lĭk) [″ + *phylake,* guard] Resistant to destruction by heat, characteristic of certain bacteria.

thermopile (thĕr′mō-pīl) [″ + L. *pila,* pile] In physical therapy, a thermoelectric battery used in measuring small variations in the degree of heat. It consists of a number of connected dissimilar metallic plates. Under the influence of heat, these plates produce an electric current. SYN: *thermocouple.*

thermoplastic (thĕr″mō-plăs′tĭk) Concerning or being softened or made malleable by heat.

thermopolypnea (thĕr″mō-pŏl-ĭp-nē′ă) [″ + *polys,* many, + *pnoia,* breath] Quickened breathing caused by high fever or increased ambient temperature.

thermoradiotherapy (thĕr″mō-rā″dē-ō-thĕr′ă-pē) [″ + L. *radius,* ray, + Gr. *therapeia,* treatment] Application of heat to the deep tissues by diathermy. SYN: *thermopenetration.*

thermoreceptor (thĕr″mō-rē-sĕp′tor) [″ + L. *receptor,* a receiver] A sensory receptor that is stimulated by a rise of body temperature.

thermoregulation (thĕr″mō-rĕg″ū-lā′shŭn) Heat regulation.

ineffective t. The state in which the individual's temperature fluctuates between hypothermia and hyperthermia. SEE: *Nursing Diagnoses Appendix.*

thermoregulatory (thĕr″mō-rĕg′ū-lă-tor″ē) Pert. to the regulation of temperature, esp. body temperature.

thermoregulatory center A center in the hypothalamus that regulates heat production and heat loss, esp. the latter, so that a normal body temperature is maintained. It is influenced by nerve impulses from cutaneous receptors and by the temperature of the blood flowing through it.

thermoresistant (thĕr″mō-rē-zĭs′tănt) [″ + L. *resistentia,* resistance] An ability to survive in relatively high temperature; characteristic of some types of bacteria.

thermostabile (thĕr″mō-stā′bĭl) [″ + L. *stabilis,* stable] Not changed or destroyed by heat.

thermostat (thĕr′mō-stăt) [″ + *statikos,* standing] An automatic device for regulating the temperature.

thermosterilization Mircrobial sterilization by use of heat.

thermotaxis (thĕr″mō-tăks′ĭs) [″ + *taxis,* arrangement] **1.** Regulation of bodily temperature. **2.** Reaction of organisms or of protoplasm in the living body to heat. **3.** The movement of certain organisms or cells toward (positive thermotaxis) or away from (negative thermotaxis) heat.

thermotherapy (thĕr″mō-thĕr′ă-pē) [″ + *therapeia,* treatment] The therapeutic application of heat. Heat may be applied locally by radiant heating devices that give off infrared rays and by conductive heating that uses hot water bottles, paraffin baths, or moist hot packs. The temperature of the body may be increased by artificial fever, by raising environmental temperature, or by preventing heat loss from the body. SEE: *heat; hyperthermia.*

thermotolerant (thĕr″mō-tŏl′ĕr-ănt) [″ + L. *tolerare,* to tolerate] Able to live normally in high temperature.

thermotonometer (thĕr″mō-tō-nŏm′ĕ-tĕr) [″ + *tonos,* tension, + *metron,* measure] A device for measuring muscle contraction caused by heat stimuli.

theroid (thē′royd) [Gr. *theriodes,* beastlike] Having animal instincts and characteristics.

thiabendazole (thī″ă-bĕn′dă-zŏl) An antihelmintic drug used in treating cutaneous larva migrans and strongyloidiasis.

thiaminase (thī-ăm′ĭ-nās) An enzyme that hydrolyzes thiamine.

thiamine hydrochloride $C_{12}H_{17}ClN_4OS \cdot HCl$; a white crystalline compound which occurs naturally or can be synthesized. It is found in a wide variety of foods including sunflower seeds, pork, whole and enriched grains, legumes, brewers yeast, and fortified baked goods. The daily requirement for adults is 1.2 mg/day for men and 1.1 mg/day for women. SYN: *vitamin B_1.*

FUNCTION: It acts as a coenzyme of carboxylases in the decarboxylation of pyruvic acid and is therefore essential for the liberation of energy and the transfer of pyruvic acid into the Krebs cycle.

DEFICIENCY SYMPTOMS: Symptoms may include fatigue, muscle tenderness and increased irritability, disturbances of extraocular movement, loss of appetite, or cardiovascular disturbances. Alcoholics are especially prone to develop thiamine deficiency. Prolonged severe deficiency (e.g., during starvation) results in beriberi.

thiamine pyrophosphate An enzyme important in carbohydrate metabolism. It is the active form of thiamine. In individuals suspected of malnutrition, administering thiamine before the infusion of glucose-containing solutions prevents brain damage (Wernicke-Korsakoff's encephalopathy). SYN: *cocarboxylase.*

thiazolidinedione (thī′ă-zō″lĭ-dēn-dī-ŏn) An oral drug that lowers blood sugars by decreasing hepatic glucose output and increasing glucose metabolism in skeletal muscles.

thienopyridines (thī-ē-nō-pĭr′ă-dēnz) Any of a group of drugs that block the aggregation of platelets. Drugs in this class are used to prevent arterial clotting, and are effective in the prevention of strokes, heart attacks, stent thromboses, and peripheral arterial disease. Examples include ticlopidine and clopidogrel. Their most common side effect is bleeding.

Thiersch's graft (tērsh′ĕz) [Karl Thiersch, Ger. surgeon, 1822–1895] A method of skin grafting using the epidermis and a portion of the dermis.

thiethylperazine maleate (thī-ĕth″ĭl-pĕr′ă-zēn) An antiemetic drug.

thigh (thī) [AS. *theoh*] The proximal portion of the lower extremity; the portion lying between the hip joint and the knee. SEE: *femur; hip; pectineus; sartorius.*

thigmesthesia (thĭg″mĕs-thē′zē-ă) [Gr. *thigma,* touch, + *aisthesis,* sensation] Sensitivity to touch.

thigmotaxis (thĭg″mō-tăks′ĭs) [″ + *taxis,* arrangement] The negative or positive response of certain motile cells to touch.

thigmotropism (thĭg-mŏt′rō-pĭzm) [″ + *tropos,* a turning, + *-ismos,* condition] The response of certain motile cells to move toward something that touches them.

thimerosal (thī-mĕr′ō-săl) An organic mercurial antiseptic used topically and as a preservative in pharmaceutical preparations.

CAUTION: Children and pregnant women should not be given immune globulin or vaccinations that use thimerosal as a preservative.

thinking Intellectual activity. Thinking includes the interpretation and ordering of symbols, learning, planning, forming ideas and opinions, organizing information, and problem solving.

abstract t. The ability to calculate, sort, categorize, conceptualize, draw conclusions, or interpret and condense complex ideas. In clinical medicine, abstract thinking is assessed by asking patients to interpret proverbs. Patients with dementia or other cognitive deficits may fail to do so, as they fail to see the relationships between similar objects and ideas.

concrete t. Thinking in simple, tangible, real, or nonidealized terms, without drawing relations between objects or concepts.

critical t. A purposeful approach to problem solving that relies on flexibility, creativity, perspective, and communication to achieve desired outcomes. Critical thinking focuses on goals rather than processes or tasks.

thin-layer chromatography ABBR: TLC. Chromatography involving the adsorption and partitioning of compounds on a thin porous solid applied as a thin layer on a glass plate or other solid support medium.

thiocyanate (thī″ō-sī′ă-nāt) Any compound containing the radical —SCN.

thiogenic (thī″ō-jĕn′ĭk) [Gr. *theion,* sulfur, + *gennan,* to produce] Able to convert hydrogen sulfide into more complex sulfur compounds, said of bacteria in the water of some mineral springs.

thioglucosidase (thī″ō-glū-kō′sĭ-dās) An enzyme that catalyzes the hydrolysis of thioglycoside to a thiol and a sugar.

thioguanine (thī″ō-gwă′nēn) An antimetabolite used in treating certain types of leukemia. It also acts as an immunosuppressant.

thiopectic, thiopexic (thī-ō-pĕk′tĭk, -pĕks′ĭk) [″ + *pexis,* fixation] Pert. to the fixation of sulfur.

thiopental sodium (thī″ō-pĕn′tăl) An ultra–short-acting barbiturate used as an adjuvant in surgical anesthesia.

thiophil, thiophilic (thī′ō-fĭl, thī″ō-fĭl′ĭk) [Gr. *theion,* sulfur, + *philein,* to love] Thriving in the presence of sulfur or its compounds, which is true of some bacteria.

thioridazine hydrochloride (thī″ō-rĭd′ă-zēn) An antipsychotic drug.

thiosulfate (thī″ō-sŭl′fāt) Any salt of thiosulfuric acid.

thiotepa (thī″ō-tē′pă) An alkylating agent that is cytotoxic. It is used in treating certain types of neoplasms.

CAUTION: Great care should be taken to prevent inhaling particles of thiotepa or exposing the skin to it.

thiothixene (thī″ō-thĭks′ēn) An antipsychotic drug.

thiourea (thī″ō-ūr-ē′ă) [Gr. *theion,* sulfur, + *ouron,* urine] H_2NCSNH_2; A colorless crystalline compound of urea in which sulfur replaces the oxygen. SYN: *sulfourea.*

thiram poisoning Toxic exposure to thiram. This may occur in those engaged either in manufacturing or applying this compound in agricultural work.

third cranial nerve Oculomotor nerve. SEE: *cranial nerve.*

third-party payer An entity (other than the patient or the health care provider) that reimburses and manages health care expenses. Third-party payers include insurance companies, governmental agencies, and employers.

third ventricle The third ventricle of the brain, a narrow cavity between the two optic thalami. It communicates anteriorly with the lateral ventricles and posteriorly, via the cerebral aqueduct of Sylvius, with the fourth ventricle. SYN: *ventriculus tertius.*

thirst [AS. *thurst*] The sensation resulting from the lack of adequate body water or desire for liquids. Excessive thirst may be an early symptom of diabetes as the kidneys excrete extra water in an effort to decrease circulating glucose levels. Thirst is common following fever, vomiting, diarrhea, bleeding, vigorous exercise, or other causes of hypovolemia or hyperosmolality. In addition, thirst may be associated with the use of diuretics, tricyclic antidepressants, and some antihistamines, among other drugs.

thixolabile (thĭk″sō-lā′bĭl) Esp. susceptible to being changed by shaking.

thixotropy (thĭks-ŏt′rō-pē) [Gr. *thixis,* a

touching, + *trope,* turning] The property of certain gels in which they liquefy when agitated and revert to a gel on standing.

thlipsencephalus (thlĭp″sĕn-sĕf′ă-lŭs) [Gr. *thlipsis,* pressure, + *enkephalos,* brain] A deformed fetus with a malformed or absent skull.

Thomas splint [Hugh Owen Thomas, Brit. orthopedic surgeon, 1834–1891] A splint originally developed to treat hip-joint disease. It is now used mainly to place traction on the leg in its long axis, in treating fractures of the upper leg. It consists of a proximal ring that fits around the upper leg and to which two long rigid slender steel rods are attached. These extend down to another smaller ring distal to the foot.

Thomas test A test used to identify hip flexor contractures. Lying supine with the legs off the end of the table, the patient flexes the knee and tries to pull the thigh to the chest. Inability to perform this maneuver or extension of the opposite knee indicates tightness of the iliopsoas or rectus femoris muscle.

Thomas-White hypothesis [Clayton Thomas, b. 1921, U.S. physician; Arthur White, b. 1925, U.S. physician] The hypothesis that there will eventually be reported a congenital abnormality in which a fetus has two umbilici.

Thompson test A test to evaluate the integrity of the Achilles tendon. The patient kneels on the examination table with the feet hanging off; the examiner squeezes the calf while observing for plantar flexion. The result is positive if there is no movement of the foot; this indicates an Achilles tendon rupture.

Thomsen's disease (tŏm′sĕnz) [Asmus Julius Thomsen, Danish physician, 1815–1896] Myotonia congenita.

thorac- SEE: *thoraco-*.

thoracalgia (thō″răk-ăl′jē-ă) [Gr. *thorakos,* chest, + *algos,* pain] Thoracic pain.

thoracectomy (thō″ră-sĕk′tō-mē) [″ + *ektome,* excision] Incision of the chest wall with resection of a portion of rib.

thoracentesis (thō″ră-sĕn-tē′sĭs) [″ + *kentesis,* a puncture] Surgical puncture of the chest wall for removal or instillation of fluids; usually done by using a large-bore needle. SYN: *pleurocentesis; thoracocentesis*.

Patient Care: Before the procedure, the patient is carefully examined and the chest x-ray and report should be obtained. The procedure should be explained to the patient and the signed consent verified. The nurse or respiratory therapist should prepare the patient for sensations that may be experienced and emphasize to the patient the importance of his or her remaining still during the procedure. Baseline vital signs should be obtained. Allergies should be identified and a sedative, if prescribed, should be administered. The patient should be positioned comfortably. The nurse or respiratory therapist should assist the physician and support the patient throughout the procedure. The patient's vital signs should be checked frequently throughout the procedure. The health care professional should assess for dizziness, faintness, tachycardia, dyspnea, chest pain, nausea, pallor or cyanosis, weakness, diaphoresis, and cough or expectoration of blood. An occlusive dressing should be applied to the puncture wound after the needle or cannula is removed. The specimen should be sent for diagnostic testing as ordered. The physician should order a postprocedure chest radiograph to detect pneumothorax and evaluate the results. Vital signs and dressing status should continue to be monitored, and the patient assessed for diminished breath sounds on the affected side, coughing or expectoration of blood, or other evidence of respiratory distress.

thoraci- SEE: *thoraco-*.

thoracic (thō-răs′ĭk) [Gr. *thorax,* chest] Pert. to the chest or thorax.

thoracic cage The bony structure surrounding the thorax, consisting of the 12 paired ribs, the thoracic vertebrae, and the sternum.

thoracic duct The main lymphatic duct, originating at the cisterna chyli in the abdomen. It passes upward through the diaphragm into the thorax, continuing upward alongside the aorta and esophagus to the neck, where it turns to the left and enters the left subclavian vein near its junction with the left internal jugular vein. It receives lymph from all parts of the body except the right side of the head, neck, and thorax and right upper extremity. SEE: *lymphatic system* for illus.

thoracic limb One of the upper extremities.

thoracicoabdominal (thō-răs″ĭ-kō-ăb-dŏm′ĭ-năl) Concerning the thorax and abdomen.

thoracicohumeral (thō-răs″ĭ-kō-hū′mĕr-ăl) Concerning the thorax and humerus.

thoracic outlet compression syndrome, thoracic outlet syndrome ABBR: TOS. A symptom complex caused by the compression of nerves and/or vessels in the neck, such as by the first rib pressing against the clavicle or entrapment of brachial nerves and vessels between the pectoralis minor muscle and the ribs. It is marked by brachial neuritis with or without vascular or vasomotor disturbance in the upper extremities. The practitioner must differentiate TOS from cervical disk lesions, osteoarthritis affecting cervical vertebrae, bursitis, brachial plexus injury, angina, lung cancer, and carpal tunnel syndrome.

thoracic squeeze A rare occurrence in divers who are skilled enough to descend approx. 80 to 100 ft (24.4 to 30.5 m) deep in water while holding their breath. The lungs become compressed sufficiently to cause rupture of alveolar capillaries. Treatment involves immediately removing the patient from the water and giving artificial respiration, preferably with an apparatus that will deliver increased oxygen concentration rather than just air.

thoracic surgery Surgery involving the rib cage and structures contained within the chest.

PATIENT CARE: *Preoperative:* Preparation involves the usual preoperative teaching, with special emphasis on breathing and coughing, incisional splinting, pain evaluation, invasive and noninvasive relief measures that will be available, and basic information about the chest drainage tube and system that will be required in most such surgeries. The health care professional should encourage the patient to voice fears and concerns, allay misapprehensions, and correct misconceptions. *Postoperative:* Vital signs and breath sounds should be monitored. Water-seal chest drainage should be maintained as prescribed, and the volume and characteristics of drainage should be monitored. The health care professional should maintain sterile impervious wound dressings; provide analgesia and comfort measures to ensure patient cooperation with respiratory toilet, exercises, and rest and activity; provide emotional support and encouragement; and provide instructions to be followed by the patient and family after discharge and follow-up care. The respiratory therapist provides mechanical ventilation in the immediate postoperative period and evaluates the patient for weaning from the ventilator.

thoraco- Combining form meaning *chest, chest wall.*

thoracoacromial (thō″ră-kō-ā-krō′mē-ăl) Concerning the thorax and acromion.

thoracocautery (thō″răk-ō-kaw′tĕr-ē) [″ + *kauterion,* branding iron] The use of cautery in breaking up pulmonary adhesions to collapse the lung.

thoracoceloschisis (thō″răk-ō-sē-lŏs′kĭ-sĭs) [Gr. *thorakos,* chest, + *koilia,* belly, + *schisis,* a splitting] A congenital fissure of the thoracic and abdominal cavities.

thoracocentesis (thō″răk-ō-sĕn-tē′sĭs) [″ + *kentesis,* a puncture] Thoracentesis.

thoracodelphus (thō″ră-kō-dĕl′fŭs) [″ + *adelphos,* brother] A deformed fetus with a single head and thorax, but four legs.

thoracodidymus (thō″ră-kō-dĭd′ĭ-mŭs) [″ + *didymos,* twin] Conjoined twins united at the thorax.

thoracodynia (thō″răk-ō-dĭn′ē-ă) [″ + *odyne,* pain] Thoracic pain.

thoracogastroschisis (thō″răk-ō-găs-trŏs′kĭ-sĭs) [″ + *gaster,* belly, + *schisis,* a splitting] A congenital fissure of the abdomen and thorax.

thoracograph (thō-răk′ō-grăf) [″ + *graphein,* to write] A device for plotting and recording the contour of the thorax and its change during inspiration and expiration.

thoracolumbar (thō″răk-ō-lŭm′bar) [″ + L. *lumbus,* loin] Pert. to the thoracic and lumbar parts of the spinal cord; denoting their ganglia and the fibers of the sympathetic nervous system.

thoracolysis (thō″răk-ŏl′ĭ-sĭs) [″ + *lysis,* dissolution] Pneumonolysis.

thoracomelus (thō″ră-kŏm′ē-lŭs) [″ + *melos,* limb] A deformed fetus with an extra leg attached to the thorax.

thoracometer (thō″ră-kŏm′ĕ-tĕr) [Gr. *thorakos,* chest, + *metron,* measure] A device for measuring the expansion of the chest.

thoracometry (thō″ră-kŏm′ĕt-rē) [″ + *metron,* measure] The measurement of the thorax.

thoracomyodynia (thō″ră-kō-mī″ō-dĭn′ē-ă) [″ + *mys,* muscle, + *odyne,* pain] Pain in the chest muscles.

thoracopagus (thō″ră-kŏp′ă-gŭs) [″ + *pagos,* fixed] Two malformed fetuses joined at the thorax.

thoracoparacephalus (thō″ră-kō-păr″ă-sĕf′ă-lŭs) [″ + *para,* beside, + *kephale,* head] Thoracopagus twins in which a rudimentary head is attached to the smaller twin.

thoracopathy (thō″răk-ŏp′ă-thē) [″ + *pathos,* disease, suffering] Any disease of the thorax, thoracic organs, or tissues.

thoracoplasty (thō′ră-kō-plăs″tē, thō-ră′kō-plăs″tē) [″ + *plassein,* to form] A plastic operation on the thorax; removal of portions of the ribs in stages to collapse diseased areas of the lung. It has been used on occasion to manage empyema or pulmonary tuberculosis, among other illnesses. SEE: *empyema.*

thoracopneumoplasty (thō″ră-kō-nū′mō-plăs-tē) [″ + *pneumon,* lung, + *plassein,* to form] Plastic surgery involving the chest and lung.

thoracoschisis (thō″ră-kŏs′kĭ-sĭs) [″ + *schisis,* a splitting] A congenital fissure of the chest wall.

thoracoscope (thō-ră′kō-skōp, -răk′ō-skōp) [″ + *skopein,* to examine] An instrument for inspection of the thoracic cavity. It has fiberoptic illumination and fiberoptic or mini TV camera visualization and is inserted through an intercostal space.

thoracoscopy (thō″ră-kŏs′kō-pē) A diagnostic examination and/or therapeutic procedure within the pleural cavity with an endoscope.

thoracostenosis (thō″ră-kō-stĕn-ō′sĭs) [″ + *stenosis,* act of narrowing] Narrowness of the thorax due to atrophy of trunk muscles.

thoracostomy (thō″răk-ŏs′tō-mē) [″ + *stoma,* mouth] Incision into the chest wall, usually followed by insertion of a tube between the pleurae and a system for draining fluid from that space.

thoracotomy (thō″răk-ŏt′ō-mē) [″ + *tome,* incision] Surgical incision of the chest wall.

thorax (thō′răks) *pl.* **thoraces, thoraxes** [Gr., chest] That part of the body between the base of the neck superiorly and the diaphragm inferiorly. SYN: *chest.* SEE: illus.

The surface of the thorax is divided into regions as follows: *Anterior surface:* supraclavicular, above the clavicles; suprasternal, above the sternum; clavicular, over the clavicles; sternal, over the sternum; mammary, the space between the third and sixth ribs on either side; inframammary, below the mammae and above the lower border of the 12th rib on either side. *Posterior surface:* scapular, over the scapulae; interscapular, between the scapulae; infrascapular, below the scapulae. *On sides:* axillary, above the sixth rib.

barrel-shaped t. A malformed chest rounded like a barrel, seen in advanced pulmonary emphysema.

bony t. The part of the skeleton that is made up of the thoracic vertebrae, 12 pairs of ribs, and the sternum.

t. paralyticus The long, flat chest of patients with constitutional visceroptosis.

Peyrot's t. A chest that has an obliquely oval deformed shape, seen with large pleural effusions.

Thorel's bundle (tō′rĕlz) [Christen Thorel, Ger. physician, 1880–1935] A muscle bundle in the heart that connects the sinoatrial and atrioventricular nodes and passes medial to the orifice of the inferior vena cava.

thorium (thō′rē-ŭm) SYMB: Th. A radioactive metallic element. Atomic weight, 232.038; atomic number, 90. At one time, it was used to outline blood vessels in radiography.

Thorn test [George W. Thorn, U.S. physician, b. 1906] An obsolete test for adrenal insufficiency involving the administration of corticotrophin, which causes a decrease in circulating eosinophils in healthy persons but not in those with adrenal insufficiency.

thoron (thō′rŏn) SYMB: Tn. A radioactive isotope of radon having a half-life of 51.5 sec; atomic weight, 220; atomic number, 86.

thought processes, altered A state in which an individual experiences a disruption in cognitive operations and activities. SEE: *Nursing Diagnoses Appendix.*

thread (thrĕd) **1.** Any thin filamentous structure (e.g., a stringy substance present in the urine in some infectious diseases of the urinary tract). **2.** Suture material.

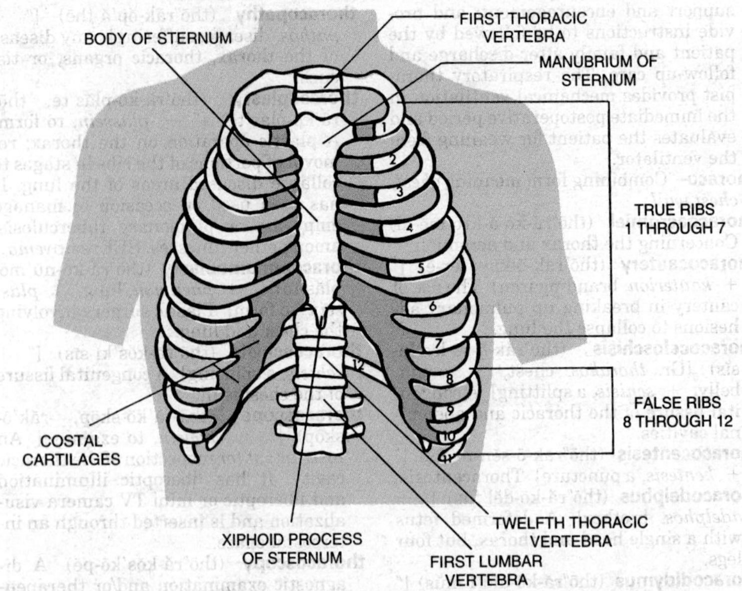

THORAX

threadworm Common name applied to the pinworm, *Enterobius vermicularis.*

three-day fever A viral disease transmitted by the sandfly, *Phlebotomus papatasii.* The disease resembles dengue but is less severe. SYN: *sandfly fever.*

thremmatology (thrĕm″ă-tŏl′ō-jē) [Gr. *thremma,* nursling, + *logos,* word, reason] Scientific breeding of plants and animals.

threonine (thrē′ō-nīn) $C_4H_9N0_3$ Alpha-amino-beta-hydroxybutyric acid. One of the essential amino acids.

threshold (thrĕsh′ōld) [AS. *therscold*] **1.** Point at which a psychological or physiological effect begins to be produced. **2.** A measure of the sensitivity of an organ or function that is obtained by finding the lowest value of the appropriate stimulus that will give the response.

absolute t. The lowest amount or intensity of a stimulus that will give rise to a sensation or a response.

acoustic reflex t. The decibel level that provokes reflex contraction of the stapedius muscle. Tests that measure the triggering of the acoustic stapedius reflex are used to determine the presence of sensorineural hearing loss.

anaerobic t. The point at which increased carbon dioxide production and minute ventilation result from increased levels of lactic acid during exercise.

auditory t. Minimum audible sound perceived.

t. of consciousness In psychoanalysis, the point at which a stimulus is just barely perceived.

differential t. The lowest limit at which two stimuli can be differentiated from each other.

erythema t. The stage of ultraviolet skin injury in which erythema of the skin due to radiation begins.

ketosis t. The lower limit at which ketone bodies (acetoacetic acid, hydroxybutyric acid, and acetone), on their accumulation in the blood, are excreted by the kidney. At that point, ketone bodies are being produced faster by the liver than the body can oxidize them.

pain t. The minimum level of stimulation of a body part that a person will perceive as being noxious or unpleasant.

renal t. The concentration at which a substance in the blood normally not excreted by the kidney begins to appear in the urine. The renal threshold for glucose is 160 to 180 mg/dl.

sensory t. The minimal stimulus for any sensory receptor that will give rise to a sensation.

t. stimulus The least or minimal stimulus that will give rise to a sensation or bring about a response such as a muscle contraction. SYN: *liminal stimulus.*

threshold dose **1.** The minimum dose that will produce an effect on the patient. **2.** Erythema dose.

threshold substance A substance present in the blood that, on being filtered through glomeruli of the kidney, is reabsorbed by the tubules up to a certain limit, that being the upper limit of the concentration of the substance in normal plasma. High-threshold substances (e.g., chlorides or glucose) are entirely or almost entirely reabsorbed. Low-threshold substances (e.g., phosphates or urea) are reabsorbed in limited quantities. No-threshold substances (e.g., creatinine sulfate) are excreted entirely.

thrifty Thriving, growing vigorously, and being healthy, esp. when assessing the health status of animals or plants.

thrill (thrĭl) [ME. *thrillen,* to pierce] **1.** An abnormal tremor accompanying a vascular or cardiac murmur felt on palpation. SYN: *fremitus.* **2.** A tingling or shivering sensation of tremulous excitement as from pain, pleasure, or horror.

aneurysmal t. A thrill felt on palpation of an aneurysm.

aortic t. A thrill perceived over the aorta or aortic valve.

arterial t. A thrill perceived over an artery.

diastolic t. A thrill perceived over the heart during ventricular diastole.

hydatid t. A peculiar tremor felt on palpation of a hydatid cyst.

presystolic t. A thrill sometimes felt over the apex of the heart preceding ventricular contraction.

systolic t. A thrill felt during systole over the precordium. Systolic thrill may be associated with aortic or pulmonary stenosis or an interventricular septal defect.

thrix Hair.

t. annulata Hair with light and dark segments alternating along the shaft.

-thrix [Gr. *thrix,* hair] A word ending indicating hair.

throat (thrōt) [AS. *throte*] **1.** The pharynx and fauces. **2.** The cavity from the arch of the palate to the glottis and superior opening of the esophagus. **3.** The anterior portion of the neck. **4.** Any narrow orifice.

throat, foreign bodies in The presence of foreign objects in the pharynx or throat. Symptoms depend somewhat on the location and size of the foreign body, and vary from simple discomfort to severe coughing and difficulty in breathing. If the airway is obstructed, suffocation occurs, resulting in unconsciousness and death.

FIRST AID: If complete airway obstruction is present, as evidenced by an inability to speak, breathe, or cough, the Heimlich maneuver should be performed. This consists of wrapping one's arms around the victim's waist from behind; making a fist with one hand and placing it against the victim's abdomen between the navel and rib cage; and clasping the fist with the free hand and pressing in with a quick, forceful upward thrust. This may be repeated several times if necessary. If the airway remains obstructed, tracheostomy will be required to save the patient's life. SEE: *Heimlich maneuver* for illus.

CAUTION: The Heimlich maneuver should not be performed unless complete airway obstruction is present. If the patient can cough, this maneuver should not be performed. In infants, extremely obese patients, and obviously pregnant patients, chest thrusts are used instead of abdominal thrusts to facilitate removal of the obstruction.

---

throb (thrŏb) [ME. *throbben,* of imitative origin] **1.** A beat or pulsation, as of the heart. **2.** To pulsate.

throbbing (thrŏb′ĭng) Pulsation.

Throckmorton's reflex (thrŏk′mor″tŭnz) [Thomas Bentley Throckmorton, U.S. neurologist, 1885–1961] The extension of the great toe and flexion of the other toes when the dorsum of the foot is percussed in the metatarsophalangeal region.

thrombase (thrŏm′bās) Thrombin.

thrombasthenia (thrŏm″băs-thē′nē-ă) [Gr. *thrombos,* clot, + *astheneia,* weakness] A hemorrhagic disorder caused by abnormal platelet function characterized by abnormal clot retraction, prolonged bleeding time, and lack of aggregation of the platelets on a blood smear.

thrombectomy (thrŏm-bĕk′tō-mē) [″ + *ektome,* excision] Surgical removal of a thrombus.

thrombi (thrŏm′bī) Pl. of thrombus.

thrombin (thrŏm′bĭn) [Gr. *thrombos,* clot] **1.** An enzyme formed in coagulating blood from prothrombin, which reacts with soluble fibrinogen converting it to fibrin, which forms the basis of a blood clot. SEE: *coagulation, blood.* **2.** A sterile protein prepared from prothrombin of bovine origin. It is used topically to control capillary oozing during surgical procedures. When used alone, it is not capable of controlling arterial bleeding.

topical t. A type of fibrin glue that may be applied locally (not injected) to a bleeding wound to stop blood loss.

thrombinogen (thrŏm-bĭn′ō-jĕn) An obsolete term for prothrombin.

thrombo- Combining form meaning *clot.*

thromboangiitis (thrŏm″bō-ăn″jē-ī′tĭs) [Gr. *thrombos,* clot, + *angeion,* vessel, + *itis,* inflammation] Inflammation of the intimal layer of a blood vessel, with clot formation. SEE: *thrombosis.*

t. obliterans Buerger's disease.

thromboarteritis (thrŏm″bō-ăr-tē-rī′tĭs) [″ + *arteria,* artery, + *itis,* inflammation] Inflammation of an artery in connection with thrombosis. SYN: *thromboendarteritis.*

thromboclasis (thrŏm-bŏk′lă-sĭs) [″ + *klasis,* a breaking] Thrombolysis.

thromboclastic (thrŏm″bō-klăs′tĭk) Thrombolytic.

thrombocyst (thrŏm′bō-sĭst) [Gr. *thrombos,* clot, + *kystis,* a sac] A membranous sac enveloping a thrombus. SYN: *thrombocystis.*

thrombocystis Thrombocyst.

thrombocyte (thrŏm′bō-sīt) [″ + *kytos,* cell] Platelet.

thrombocythemia (thrŏm″bō-sī-thē′mē-ă) [″ + ″ + *haima,* blood] An absolute increase in the number of platelets in the blood.

thrombocytocrit (thrŏm″bō-sī′tō-krĭt) [″ + ″ + *krinein,* to separate] A device for estimating the platelet content of the blood.

thrombocytolysis (thrŏm″bō-sī-tŏl′ĭ-sĭs) [″ + ″ + *lysis,* dissolution] Dissolution of thrombocytes.

thrombocytopathy (thrŏm″bō-sī-tŏp′ă-thē) [″ + ″ + *pathos,* disease, suffering] Deficient function of platelets.

thrombocytopenia (thrŏm″bō-sī″tō-pē′nē-ă) [″ + ″ + *penia,* lack] An abnormal decrease in the number of platelets. SYN: *thrombopenia.*

PATIENT CARE: The patient is watched for signs of internal hemorrhage, esp. intracranial bleeding, as well as hematuria, hematemesis, bleeding gums, abdominal distention, melena, prolonged menstruation, epistaxis, ecchymosis, petechiae, or purpura, and is handled carefully (e.g., during blood drawing) to prevent trauma and hemorrhage. Bleeding is controlled by applying pressure to bleeding sites. If arterial blood collection is necessary (i.e., for blood gases), a patient care plan should be developed in conjunction with the physician and the laboratory/blood collection staff to ensure that occult bleeding does not occur. Use of a soft toothbrush helps to prevent injury. An electric razor should be used for shaving. Platelet transfusions are administered as prescribed, and the patient is observed for chills, fever, or allergic reactions. Aspirin and other nonsteroidal anti-inflammatory agents should be avoided, because these drugs may inhibit platelet function. If splenectomy is performed, preoperative and postoperative nursing care is provided as required. The patient is encouraged to express feelings and concerns.

thrombocytopoiesis (thrŏm″bō-sī″tō-poy-ē′sĭs) [″ + ″ + *poiesis,* production] The formation of platelets.

thrombocytosis (thrŏm″bō-sī-tō′sĭs) [″

+ *kytos,* cell] An increase in the number of platelets.

thromboelastogram ABBR: TEG. A device used to determine the presence of intravascular fibrinolysis and for monitoring the effect of antifibrinolytic therapy on the formation and dissolution of clots.

thromboembolism (thrŏm″bō-ĕm′bō-lĭzm) [″ + *embolos,* thrown in, + *-ismos,* condition] An embolism; the blocking of a blood vessel by a thrombus that has become detached from its site of formation.

thromboendarterectomy (thrŏm″bō-ĕnd″ăr-tĕr-ĕk′tō-mē) [″ + *endon,* within, + *arteria,* artery, + *ektome,* excision] Surgical removal of a thrombus from an artery, and removal of the diseased intima of the artery.

thromboendarteritis (thrŏm″bō-ĕnd-ăr″tĕr-ī′tĭs) [″ + ″ + ″ + *itis,* inflammation] Thromboarteritis.

thromboendocarditis (thrŏm″bō-ĕn″dō-kăr-dī′tĭs) [″ + *endon,* within, + *kardia,* heart, + *itis,* inflammation] Formation of a clot on an inflamed surface of a heart valve.

thrombogenesis (thrŏm″bō-jĕn′ĕ-sĭs) [″ + *genesis,* generation, birth] The formation of a blood clot.

thrombogenic (thrŏm″bō-jĕn′ĭk) [″ + *gennan,* to produce] Producing or tending to produce a clot.

thromboid (thrŏm′boyd) [″ + *eidos,* form, shape] Resembling a thrombus or clot.

thrombokinase (thrŏm″bō-kĭn′ās) [″ + *kinesis,* movement] Obsolete term for the 10th blood coagulation factor (factor X) or Stuart factor.

thrombokinesis (thrŏm″bō-kĭ-nē′sĭs) [″ + *kinesis,* movement] The coagulation of the blood.

thrombolectomy Surgical removal of a blood clot.

thrombolymphangitis (thrŏm″bō-lĭm″făn-jī′tĭs) [″ + L. *lympha,* lymph, + Gr. *angeion,* vessel, + *itis,* inflammation] Inflammation of a lymphatic vessel due to obstruction by thrombus formation.

thrombolysis (thrŏm-bŏl′ĭ-sĭs) [″ + *lysis,* dissolution] The breaking up of a thrombus. SYN: *thromboclasis.*

thrombolytic (thrŏm-bō-lĭt′ĭk) Pert. to or causing the breaking up of a thrombus.

thrombomodulin (thrŏm′bō-mŏ-dū-lĭn) A protein released by the vascular endothelium. Acting in concert with other factors, it helps to prevent formation of intravascular thrombi. SEE: *endothelium.*

thrombon (thrŏm′bŏn) [Gr. *thrombos,* clot] The portion of the hematopoietic system concerned with platelet formation.

thrombopathy (thrŏm-bŏp′ă-thē) [″ + *pathos,* disease, suffering] A defect in coagulation.

thrombopenia (thrŏm-bō-pē′nē-ă) [″ + *penia,* lack] Thrombocytopenia. An abnormal decrease in the number of blood platelets.

thrombophilia (thrŏm-bō-fĭl′ē-ă) [″ + *philein,* to love] A tendency to form blood clots.

thrombophlebitis (thrŏm″bō-flē-bī′tĭs) [″ + *phleps,* vein, + *itis,* inflammation] Inflammation of a vein in conjunction with the formation of a thrombus. It usually occurs in an extremity, most frequently a leg. SEE: *deep venous thrombosis; phlebitis; Nursing Diagnoses Appendix.*

TREATMENT: Drug therapies include heparins or warfarin.

PATIENT CARE: Prevention includes identifying patients at risk and encouraging leg exercises, use of antiembolic stockings, and early ambulation to prevent venous stasis. The patient should be assessed at regular intervals for signs of inflammation, tenderness, aching, and differences in calf circumference measurements. Anticoagulants are administered as prescribed, the patient is evaluated for signs of bleeding, and coagulation results are monitored. The patient is assessed for signs of pulmonary emboli, dyspnea, tachypnea, hypotension, chest pain, changes of level of consciousness, arterial blood gas abnormalities, and electrocardiogram changes. The patient is prepared for the diagnostic procedures and medical or surgical interventions prescribed. Patients at greatest risk for thrombophlebitis are those on prolonged bedrest; those with congestive heart failure, obesity, or cancer; and people older than 65 years.

t. migrans Recurring attacks of thrombophlebitis in various sites.

postpartum iliofemoral t. Thrombophlebitis of the iliofemoral artery that occurs after childbirth.

thromboplastic (thrŏm″bō-plăs′tĭk) [″ + *plassein,* to form] Pert. to or causing acceleration of clot formation in the blood.

thromboplastid (thrŏm″bō-plăs′tĭd) A platelet.

thromboplastin (thrŏm″bō-plăs′tĭn) [″ + *plassein,* to form] Blood coagulation factor (III), a substance found in both blood and tissues. It accelerates the clotting of blood.

thromboplastinogen (thrŏm″bō-plăs-tĭn′ō-jĕn) Blood clotting factor VIII. SEE: *coagulation factor.*

thrombopoiesis (thrŏm″bō-poy-ē′sĭs) [″ + *poiesis,* production] The formation of blood platelets.

thrombopoietin ABBR: TPO. A growth factor that acts on the bone marrow to stimulate platelet production as well as the proliferation of other cell lines.

thrombosed (thrŏm′bōzd) [Gr. *thrombos,* a clot] **1.** Coagulated; clotted. **2.** Denoting a vessel containing a thrombus.

thrombosinusitis (thrŏm″bō-sī-nŭs-ī′tĭs) [″ + L. *sinus,* a curve, hollow, + Gr. *itis,* inflammation] Thrombus formation of a dural sinus in the brain.

thrombosis (thrŏm-bō′sĭs) [″ + *osis,* condition] The formation or presence of a blood clot within the vascular system. This is a life-saving process when it occurs during hemorrhage. It is a life-threatening event when it occurs at any other time because the clot can occlude a vessel and stop the blood supply to an organ or a part. The thrombus, if detached, can travel through the bloodstream and occlude a vessel at a distance from the original site; for example, a clot in the leg may break off and cause a pulmonary embolus.

ETIOLOGY: Trauma (esp. following an operation and parturition), cardiac and vascular disorders, obesity, hereditary coagulation disorders, age over 65, an excess of erythrocytes and of platelets, an overproduction of fibrinogen, and sepsis are predisposing causes.

SYMPTOMS: *Lungs:* Obstruction of the smaller vessels in the lungs causes an infarct that may be accompanied by sudden pain in the side of the chest, similar to pleurisy; also present are the spitting of blood, a pleural friction rub, and signs of consolidation. *Kidneys:* Blood appears in the urine. *Skin:* Small hemorrhagic spots may appear in the skin. *Spleen:* Pain is felt in the left upper abdomen. *Extremities:* If a large artery in one of the extremities, such as the arm, is suddenly obstructed, the part becomes cold, pale, bluish, and the pulse disappears below the obstructed site. Gangrene of the digits or of the whole limb may ensue. The same symptoms may be present with an embolism.

If the limb is swollen, one should watch for pressure sores. Burning with a hot water bottle or electric pad should be guarded against. Prolonged bedrest may be necessary, depending on the patient's condition.

TREATMENT: Pathological clots are treated with thrombolytic agents (e.g., streptokinase), antiplatelet drugs (e.g., heparins or aspirin), anticoagulants (e.g., warfarin), or platelet glycoprotein receptor antagonists (e.g., abciximab). When a thrombus or embolus is large and life threatening, surgical removal may be attempted.

cardiac t. coronary t.

coagulation t. Thrombosis due to coagulation of fibrin in a blood vessel.

coronary t. A blood clot in a coronary artery, the most common cause of a myocardial infarction (heart attack). SEE: *myocardial infarction.*

deep venous t. ABBR: DVT. A blood clot in one or more of the deep veins of the legs (the most common site), arms, pelvis, neck, axilla, or chest. The clot may damage the vein or may embolize to other organs (e.g., the heart or lungs). Such emboli are occasionally fatal. SEE: *embolism, pulmonary.*

ETIOLOGY: DVT results from one or more of the following conditions: blood stasis (e.g., bedrest); endothelial injury (e.g., after surgery or trauma); hypercoagulability (e.g., factor V Leiden, or deficiencies of antithrombin III, protein C, or protein S); congestive heart failure; estrogen use; malignancy; nephrotic syndrome; obesity; pregnancy; thrombocytosis; or many other conditions). DVT is a common occurrence among hospitalized patients, many of whom cannot walk or have one or more of the other risk factors just mentioned.

SYMPTOMS: The patient may report a dull ache or heaviness in the limb, and swelling or redness may be present, but just as often patients have vague symptoms, making clinical diagnosis unreliable.

DIAGNOSIS: Compression ultrasonography is commonly used to diagnose DVT (failure of a vein to compress is evidence of a clot within its walls). Other diagnostic techniques include impedance plethysmography and venography.

TREATMENT: Unfractionated heparin or low molecular weight heparin (LMWH) is given initially, followed by several months of therapy with an oral anticoagulant such as warfarin.

COMPLICATIONS: Pulmonary emboli are common and may compromise oxygenation or result in frank cardiac arrest. Postphlebitic syndrome, a chronic swelling and aching of the affected limb, also occurs often.

PREVENTION: In hospitalized patients and other immobilized persons, early ambulation, pneumatic compression stockings, or low doses of unfractionated heparin, LMWH, or warfarin may be given to reduce the risk of DVT.

embolic t. Thromboembolism.

hepatic vein t. An often fatal thrombotic occlusion of the hepatic veins, marked clinically by hepatomegaly, weight gain, ascites, and abdominal pain. SYN: *Budd-Chiari syndrome.*

infective t. Thrombosis in which there is bacterial infection.

marasmic t. Thrombosis due to wasting diseases.

mural t. Mural thrombus.

placental t. Thrombi in the placenta and veins of the uterus.

plate t. Thrombus formed from an accumulation of platelets.

puerperal t. Coagulation in veins following labor.

sinus t. Formation of a blood clot in a venous sinus.

traumatic t. Thrombosis due to a wound or injury of a part.

venous t. Thrombosis of a vein. SEE: *Nursing Diagnoses Appendix.*

thrombostasis (thrŏm-bŏs′tă-sĭs) [″ + *stasis,* standing still] Stasis of blood in a part, causing or caused by formation of a thrombus.

thrombosthenin (thrŏm″bō-sthē′nĭn) [″ + *sthenos,* strength] A contractile protein present in platelets. This protein is active in clot retraction.

thrombotic (thrŏm-bŏt′ĭk) [Gr. *thrombos,* clot] Related to, caused by, or of the nature of a thrombus.

thromboxane A_2 ABBR: TXA_2. An unstable compound synthesized in platelets and other cells from a prostaglandin, PGH_2. It acts to aggregate platelets, is a potent vasoconstrictor, and mediates inflammation. SEE: *eicosanoid; prostaglandin; prostanoids.*

thrombus (thrŏm′bŭs) [Gr. *thrombos*] A blood clot that obstructs a blood vessel or a cavity of the heart. Anticoagulants are used to prevent and treat this condition.

agonal t. A blood clot formed in the heart just at the time of death.

annular t. A thrombus whose circumference is attached to the walls of a vessel, while an opening still remains in the center.

antemortem t. A clot formed in the heart or large vessels before death.

ball t. A round clot in the heart, esp. in the atria.

hyaline t. A thrombus having a glassy appearance, usually occurring in smaller blood vessels.

lateral t. Mural t.

milk t. A curdled milk tumor in the female breast caused by obstruction in a lactiferous duct.

mural t. A blood clot that forms on the wall of the heart, esp. along an immobile section of the heart damaged by myocardial infarction or cardiomyopathy. Such clots may occasionally embolize, causing stroke or organ damage. SYN: *lateral t.; mural thrombosis; parietal t.*

obstructing t. A thrombus completely occluding the lumen of a vessel.

occluding t. A thrombus that completely closes the vessel.

parietal t. Mural t.

postmortem t. Blood clot formed in the heart or a large blood vessel after death.

progressive t. Propagated t.

propagated t. A thrombus that increases in size. SYN: *progressive t.*

stratified t. A thrombus composed of layers.

white t. A pale thrombus in any site; made up principally of platelets.

through-and-through drainage Irrigation and drainage of a cavity or an organ such as the bladder by placing two perforated tubes, drains, or catheters in the area. A solution is instilled through one tube, usually by continuous drip, and the other tube is attached to either straight or gravity drainage or to a suction machine.

through illumination Passage of light through the walls of an organ or cavity for medical examination. SYN: *transillumination.*

throwback 1. To reflect. SEE: *atavism.* **2.** To impair progress.

thrush (thrŭsh) [D. *troske,* rotten wood] Infection of the mucosa of the mouth caused by *Candida albicans.* In patients with healthy immune systems, it occurs when the balance of normal flora is destroyed during antibiotic therapy or following the use of corticosteroid-based inhalers, which suppress normal white blood cell function in the mouth. It is also common in patients receiving immunosuppressive therapy for organ transplants, in cancer patients, and in those with acquired immunodeficiency syndrome, in whom oral candida infection may be chronic. Occasionally healthy neonates and persons who wear dentures develop thrush.

Thrush is marked by white, raised, creamy patches found on the tongue and other oral mucosal surfaces; these patches can be easily removed. The organism is identified by a microscopic examination of these scrapings. The infection is treated with a single dose of fluconazole, with clotrimazole lozenges, or with a nystatin oral solution (which must be held in the mouth for 3 min before swallowing) for 14 days; long-term immunosuppressive therapy may be needed for patients with impaired immunity. Dentures should be soaked in an antifungal solution of nystatin. Careful handwashing is essential before doing oral care. SEE: *aphtha; candidiasis; stomatitis.*

thrust 1. To move forward suddenly and forcibly, as in tongue thrust when the tongue is pushed against the teeth or alveolar ridge at the beginning of deglutition. This may cause open bite or malformed jaws. **2.** In physical medicine, a manipulative technique in which the therapist applies a rapid movement to tear adhesions and increase flexibility of restricted joint capsules.

abdominal t. Treatment of airway obstruction that consists of inward and upward thrusts of the thumb side of a closed fist in the area between the umbilicus and the xiphoid process. If the patient is conscious, the procedure is performed from behind the person standing; if the patient is unconscious, it can be performed while kneeling beside or straddling the patient and using the heel of the hand rather than a closed fist. SEE: *Heimlich maneuver.*

subdiaphragmatic abdominal t. Treatment for patients suspected of having a complete airway obstruction. For conscious, standing adults, it consists of upward and inward thrusts of the thumb side of the rescuer's closed fist, coming from behind the victim, in the area between the umbilicus and the xiphoid process. For unconscious adults with a complete airway obstruction, the procedure is performed while kneeling alongside or straddling the victim, by using the heel of the hand to apply the inward and upward thrusts between the umbilicus and the xiphoid process. SEE: *Heimlich maneuver*.

substernal t. A palpable heaving of the chest in the substernal area. This is a physical finding detectable in some persons with right ventricular hypertrophy. SEE: *apical heave*.

thrypsis (thrĭp′sĭs) [Gr., breaking in pieces] A fracture in which the bone is splintered or crushed.

thulium (thū′lē-ŭm) SYMB: Tm. A rare metallic element found in combination with minerals; atomic weight, 168.934; atomic number, 69.

thumb (thŭm) [AS. *thuma,* thumb] The short, thick first finger on the radial side of the hand, having two phalanges and being opposable to the other four digits. SYN: *pollex*. SEE: *hand* for illus.

gamekeeper's t. Skier's t.

skier's t. An injury to the ulnar collateral ligament of the metacarpophalangeal joint of the thumb. SYN: *gamekeeper's t.*

tennis t. Calcification and inflammation of the tendon of the flexor pollicis longus muscle owing to repeated irritation and stress while playing tennis.

thumb sign Protrusion of the thumb across the palm and beyond the clenched fist; seen in Marfan's syndrome.

thumb sucking The habit of sucking one's thumb. Intermittent thumb sucking is not abnormal, but prolonged and intensive thumb sucking past the time the first permanent teeth erupt at 5 or 6 years of age can lead to a misshapen mouth and displaced teeth. If the habit persists, combined dental and psychological therapy should be instituted.

thymectomy (thī-mĕk′tō-mē) [Gr. *thymos,* mind, + *ektome,* excision] Surgical removal of the thymus gland.

thymelcosis (thī″mĕl-kō′sĭs) [″ + *helkosis,* ulceration] Ulceration of the thymus gland.

-thymia [Gr. *thymos,* mind] A word ending indicating *a state of the mind*.

thymic (thī′mĭk) [L. *thymicus*] Rel. to the thymus gland.

t. hormone Any of the hormones produced by the thymus that may help attract lymphoid stem cells to the thymus and stimulate their development into mature T lymphocytes. These hormones include thymulin, thymopoietin, and thymosin.

thymicolymphatic (thī″mĭ-kō-lĭm-făt′ĭk) Rel. to the thymus and lymph glands.

thymidine (thī′mĭ-dēn) A nucleoside present in deoxyribonucleotide. It is formed from the condensation product of thymine and deoxyribose.

thymine (thī′mĭn) $C_5N_2H_6O_2$; a pyrimidine base present in DNA (not RNA) where it is paired with adenine.

thymitis (thī-mī′tĭs) [Gr. *thymos,* mind, + *itis,* inflammation] Inflammation of the thymus gland.

thymo- **1.** Combining form meaning *thymus*. **2.** Combining form meaning *mind.*

thymocyte (thī′mō-sīt) [Gr. *thymos,* mind, + *kytos,* cell] Immature T lymphocytes that reside in the thymus. Fewer than 1% of the lymphoid stem cells that migrate to the thymus reproduce and develop into T lymphocytes capable of binding with specific antigens.

thymokesis (thī″mō-kē′sĭs) An abnormal enlargement of the thymus in the adult.

thymokinetic (thī″mō-kĭ-nĕt′ĭk) [″ + *kinesis,* movement] Stimulating the thymus gland.

thymol (thī′mōl) [Gr. *thumon,* thyme, + L. *oleum,* oil] White crystals obtained from oil of thyme; formerly used in treatment of hookworm.

t. iodide An antifungal and antibacterial agent.

thymolytic (thī-mō-lĭt′ĭk) Destructive to thymus tissue.

thymoma (thī-mō′mă) [″ + *oma,* tumor] A rare neoplasm, usually found in the anterior mediastinum and originating in the epithelial cells of the thymus. It is often associated with autoimmune diseases. Treatments may include surgical removal, radiation therapy, or chemotherapy.

thymopathy (thī-mŏp′ă-thē) A disease of the thymus.

thymopoietin (thī″mō-poy′ĕ-tĭn) A peptide hormone secreted by the thymus that helps thymocytes to mature and respond to specific antigenic stimuli.

thymoprivic (thī″mō-prĭv′ĭk) [″ + L. *privus,* deprived of] Concerning or caused by removal of the thymus.

thymosin (thī′mō-sĭn) A peptide hormone, produced in cells of the thymus and believed to play a part in T lymphocyte development.

thymotoxic (thī″mō-tŏks′ĭk) [″ + *toxikon,* poison] Poisonous to thymic tissue.

thymulin (thī′mū-lĭn) A peptide hormone, released by the thymus, with immune modulating and analgesic actions.

thymus (thī′mŭs) [Gr. *thymos*] A lymphoid organ located in the mediastinal cavity anterior to and above the heart, composed of two fused lobes each containing multiple lobules, which are roughly divided into an outer cortex and inner medulla. Immature T cells (thymocytes) make up most of the cortex and some of the medulla. The remaining cells are epithelial cells, with some macrophages. Epithelial cells in some areas of the medulla develop hard cores and are known as Hassall's corpuscles; their purpose is unknown. SEE: illus.

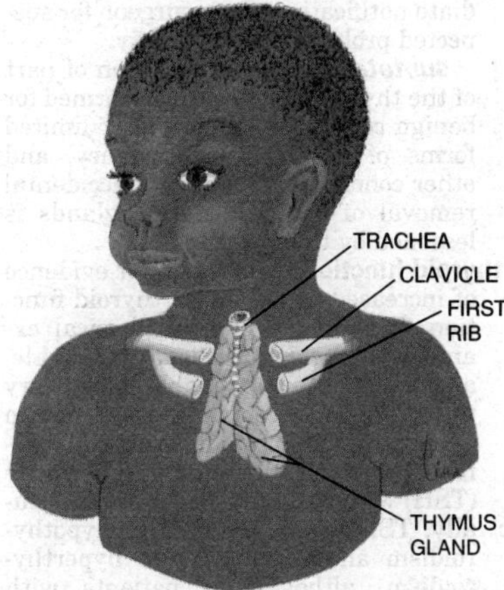

THYMUS IN A YOUNG CHILD

The thymus is the primary site for T-lymphocyte differentiation. During the prenatal period, lymphoid stem cells migrate from the bone marrow to the thymus. They fill and expand the interstitial spaces between epithelial cells and proliferate rapidly. Almost all of these immature thymocytes are destroyed, to eliminate those that would attack self-antigens. Approx. 1% of the thymocytes mature into T cells, with either a CD4 or a CD8 protein marker and receptors capable of binding with specific antigens. The mature T lymphocytes leave the thymus and migrate to the spleen, lymph nodes, and other lymphoid tissue, where they control cell-mediated immune responses.

The thymus weighs 15 g to 35 g at birth and continues to grow until puberty, when it begins to shrink and the lymphoid tissue is replaced by fibrotic tissue; only about 5 g of thymic tissue remains in adulthood. The reason for involution may be that the organ has produced enough T lymphocytes to seed the tissues of the immune system and is no longer necessary. Removal of the thymus in an adult does not cause the decrease in immune function seen when the gland is removed from children.

PATHOLOGY: Lack of a thymus or thymus hypoplasia is one component of DiGeorge syndrome, which is marked by severe lack of cell-mediated immunity. Thymic hyperplasia results from the growth of lymph follicles containing both B lymphocytes and dendritic cells. It is found in myasthenia gravis and, occasionally, in other autoimmune diseases such as Graves' disease, rheumatoid arthritis, and systemic lupus erythematosus. Thymomas, which are malignant or benign tumors of the thymus, involve only the thymic epithelial cells. Other tumors, including those associated with Hodgkin's disease and lymphomas, involve thymocytes.

accessory t. A lobule isolated from the mass of the thymus gland.

t. persistens hyperplastica Thymus persisting into adulthood, sometimes hypertrophying.

thymus dependent antigen One of the foreign antigens that require B lymphocyte stimulation by T cells before production of antibodies and memory cells can occur.

thymus independent antigen One of the foreign antigens that are capable of stimulating B cell activation and the production of antibodies without T cell interaction. Most of these antibodies fall into the IgM class. A few memory cells are created.

thymusectomy (thī″mŭs-ĕk′tō-mē) [Gr. *thymos,* mind, + *ektome,* excision] Surgical excision of the thymus.

thyr- SEE: *thyroido-.*

thyreo- [Gr. *thyreos,* shield] Combining form indicating *thyroid.*

thyreoplasia Defective functioning of the thyroid gland owing to abnormal development.

thyro- SEE: *thyroido-.*

thyroadenitis (thī″rō-ăd-ĕ-nī′tĭs) [″ + *aden,* gland, + *itis,* inflammation] Inflammation of the thyroid gland.

thyroaplasia (thī″rō-ă-plā′zē-ă) [″ + *a-,* not, + *plasis,* a molding] Imperfect development of the thyroid gland.

thyroarytenoid (thī″rō-ă-rĭt′ĕn-oyd) [″ + *arytaina,* ladle, + *eidos,* form, shape] Rel. to the thyroid and arytenoid cartilages.

thyrocalcitonin (thī″rō-kăl″sĭ-tō′nĭn) Calcitonin.

thyrocardiac (thī″rō-kăr′dē-ăk) [″ + *kardia,* heart] **1.** Pert. to the heart and thyroid gland. **2.** A person suffering from thyroid disease complicated by a heart disorder.

thyrocele (thī′rō-sēl) [″ + *kele,* tumor, swelling] Goiter.

thyrochondrotomy (thī″rō-kŏn-drŏt′ō-mē) [″ + *chondros,* cartilage, + *tome,* incision] Surgical incision of thyroid cartilage.

thyrocolloid (thī″rō-kŏl′oyd) Colloid contained in the thyroid gland.

thyrocricotomy (thī″rō-krī-kŏt′ō-mē) [″ + *krikos,* ring, + *tome,* incision] A division of the cricothyroid membrane.

thyroepiglottic (thī″rō-ĕp″ĭ-glŏt′ĭk) [″ + *epi,* upon, + *glottis,* back of tongue] Rel. to the thyroid and epiglottis.

thyroepiglottic muscle A muscle arising on the inner surface of the thyroid cartilage. It extends upward and backward and is inserted on the epiglottis. It depresses the epiglottis.

thyroepiglottideus (thī″rō-ĕp″ĭ-glŏt-ĭd′ē-ŭs) A muscle in the thyroid cartilage that depresses the epiglottis.

thyrofissure (thī″rō-fĭsh′ŭr) Surgical creation of an opening through the thyroid cartilage to expose the inside of the larynx.

thyrogenic, thyrogenous (thī-rō-jĕn′ĭk, thī-rŏj′ĕ-nŭs) [″ + *gennan,* to produce] Having its origin in the thyroid.

thyroglobulin (thī″rō-glŏb′ū-lĭn) [″ + L. *globulus,* globule] **1.** An iodine-containing glycoprotein secreted by the thyroid gland and stored within its colloid, from which thyroxine and triiodothyronine are derived. **2.** A substance obtained by the fractionation of thyroid glands from the hog, *Sus scrofa.*

thyroglossal (thī″rō-glŏs′săl) [″ + *glossa,* tongue] Pert. to the thyroid gland and the tongue.

thyroglossal duct A duct that in the embryo connects the thyroid diverticulum with the tongue. It eventually disappears, its point of origin being indicated as a pit, the foramen cecum. It sometimes persists as an anomaly.

thyrohyal (thī″rō-hī′ăl) Concerning the thyroid cartilage and the hyoid bone.

thyrohyoid (thī″rō-hī′oyd) [″ + *hyoeides,* U-shaped] Rel. to thyroid cartilage and hyoid bone.

thyroid (thī′royd) [″ + *eidos,* form, shape] **1.** An endocrine gland in the neck, anterior to and partially surrounding the thyroid cartilage and upper rings of the trachea. SEE: *thyroid gland.* **2.** The cleaned, dried, and powdered thyroid gland of animals (also known as thyroid extract). Thyroid extract is used infrequently to treat hypothyroidism and goiter because of its unpredictable potency.

thyroid- SEE: *thyroido-.*

thyroid cachexia Exophthalmic goiter. SEE: *hyperthyroidism.*

thyroid cartilage The principal cartilage of the larynx, consisting of two broad laminae united anteriorly to form a V-shaped structure. It forms a subcutaneous projection called the laryngeal prominence or Adam's apple. SEE: *thyroid gland* for illus.

thyroidea accessoria, thyroidea ima (thī-roy′dē-ă) Accessory thyroid.

thyroidectomy (thī″royd-ĕk′tō-mē) Excision of the thyroid gland. SEE: *Nursing Diagnoses Appendix.*

PATIENT CARE: *Postoperative:* In addition to standard monitoring and clinical observation, attention to airway compromise due to either hemorrhage or recurrent laryngeal nerve injury is emphasized. Signs of tetany due to parathyroid gland injury or excision and of thyroid storm must also be assessed. In the recovery room, there should be equipment for immediate airway reintubation, tracheostomy set, or both, as well as various pharmacological agents (e.g., calcium chloride, antithyroid agents, and antihypertensives). Immediate notification of the surgeon for suspected problems is mandatory.

subtotal t. Surgical excision of part of the thyroid gland, as is performed for benign conditions, equivocal or limited forms of low-grade malignancy, and other conditions. The risk of accidental removal of the parathyroid glands is lessened by this procedure.

thyroid function test A test for evidence of increased or decreased thyroid function, including a clinical physical examination, which is usually reliable, and a variety of reliable laboratory tests. The most commonly used test to assess thyroid function is the measurement of thyroid-stimulating hormone (TSH) with supersensitive assays. Usually, TSH levels are high in hypothyroidism and suppressed in hyperthyroidism, although in patients with pituitary masses this pattern may be reversed. Other thyroid function tests include measurements of free and total thyroxine (T_4) and triiodothyronine (T_3), tests of thyroid-binding globulin levels, antithyroid antibody tests, and thyroid gland radioactive iodine uptake (RAIU) measurement. Many of these test results are more difficult to interpret than are TSH results because their normal ranges may vary with pregnancy, liver disease, nutritional status, and other medical conditions. SEE: *hyperthyroidism; hypothyroidism.*

thyroid gland An endocrine gland located in the base of the neck on both sides of the lower part of the larynx and upper part of the trachea. It consists of two lateral lobes connected by an isthmus. Sometimes a third medial or pyramidal lobe extends upward from the isthmus. Histologically, it consists of a large number of closed vesicles called follicles that contain a homogeneous substance called colloid, which contains the thyroglobulin. It in turn contains various active substances such as thyroxine and triiodothyronine. Parafollicular cells secrete the hormone calcitonin. The thyroid gland is enlarged in goiter and it may pulsate due to its increased blood supply. SEE: illus.

thyroidism (thī′royd-ĭzm) A disease caused by hyperactivity of the thyroid gland.

thyroiditis (thī″royd-ī′tĭs) [″ + *eidos,* form, shape, + *itis,* inflammation] In-

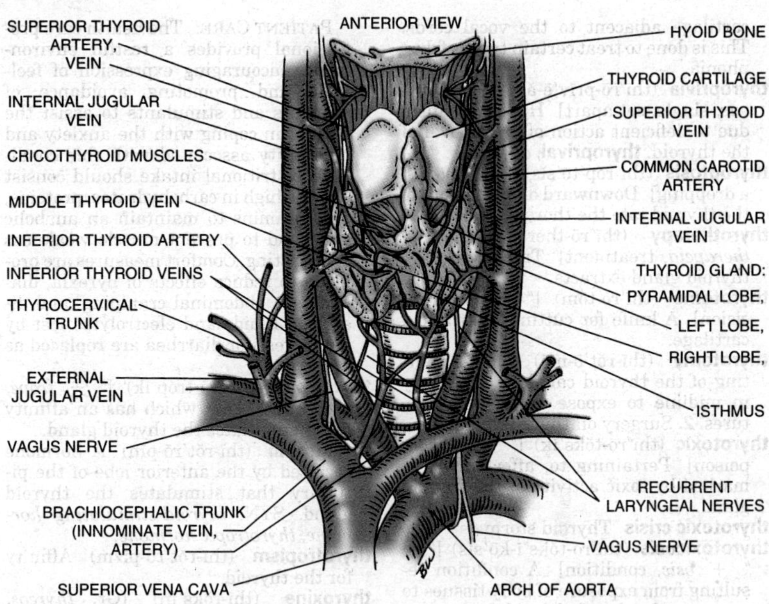

THYROID GLAND AND RELATED STRUCTURES

flammation of the thyroid gland. SEE: *struma, Riedel's*.

giant cell t. Thyroiditis characterized by the presence of giant cells, round-cell infiltration, fibrosis, and destruction of follicles.

Hashimoto's t. SEE: *Hashimoto's thyroiditis*.

Reidel's t. A rare form of thyroiditis characterized by fibrotic destruction of the thyroid gland. The fibrotic tissue extends beyond the capsule of the gland into the surrounding structures of the neck and may develop sufficiently to compress the trachea. The etiology is unknown.

thryoido-, thyroid-, thyro-, thyr- [Gr. *thyreoedes,* fr. *thyreos,* shield + *eidos,* form] Combining form meaning *thyroid gland.*

thyroidomania (thī″royd-ō-mā′nē-ă) [″ + ″ + *mania,* frenzy] A mental disorder associated with hyperthyroidism.

thyroidotomy (thī″royd-ŏt′ō-mē) [″ + ″ + *tome,* incision] Incision of the thyroid gland.

thyroidotoxin (thī″royd-ō-tŏk′sĭn) A substance that is specifically toxic for cells of the thyroid gland.

thyroid-stimulating hormone ABBR: TSH. A hormone secreted by the anterior lobe of the pituitary that stimulates the thyroid gland to secrete thyroxine and triiodothyronine. SYN: *thyrotropic hormone; thyrotropin.*

thyroid stimulating hormone-releasing factor ABBR: TSH-RF. An obsolete term for thyrotropin releasing hormone.

thyroid storm A rare but often life-threatening medical emergency resulting from untreated hyperthyroidism. It is marked by fevers, sweating, restlessness, tachycardia, congestive heart failure, shock, and cardiac arrhythmias, among other findings. It may begin when a patient with hyperthyroidism suffers a second illness (e.g., an infection), after thyroid gland surgery, or after withdrawal from antithyroid drug treatment. SYN: *thyroid crisis; thyrotoxic crisis.*

TREATMENT: Antithyroid medications (e.g., propylthiouracil), beta blockers (e.g., propranolol), high-dose steroids, and volume infusions are needed. Any secondary illness should be aggressively treated as well.

thyrolysin (thī-rŏl′ĭ-sĭn) Anything that destroys thyroid tissue.

thyrolytic (thī″rō-lĭt′ĭk) [Gr. *thyreos,* shield, + *lysis,* dissolution] Causing destruction of thyroid tissue.

thyromegaly (thī″rō-mĕg′ă-lē) [″ + *megas,* large] Enlargement of the thyroid gland.

thyroparathyroidectomy (thī″rō-păr″ă-thī″royd-ĕk′tō-mē) [″ + *para,* beside, + *thyreos,* shield, + *eidos,* form, shape, + *ektome,* excision] Surgical removal of the thyroid and parathyroid glands.

thyropathy (thī-rŏp′ă-thē) [″ + *pathos,* disease, suffering] Any disease of the thyroid.

thyroplasty A surgical procedure for altering the configuration of the thyroid cartilage adjacent to the vocal cords. This is done to treat certain types of dysphonia.

thyroprivia (thī″rō-prĭv′ē-ă) [″ + L. *privus,* single, set apart] Hypothyroidism due to deficient action of or removal of the thyroid. **thyroprival,** *adj.*

thyroptosis (thī″rŏp-tō′sĭs) [″ + *ptosis,* a dropping] Downward displacement of the thyroid into the thorax.

thyrotherapy (thī″rō-thĕr′ă-pē) [″ + *therapeia,* treatment] Treatment with thyroid gland extracts.

thyrotome (thī′rō-tōm) [″ + *tome,* incision] A knife for cutting the thyroid cartilage.

thyrotomy (thī-rŏt′ō-mē) **1.** The splitting of the thyroid cartilage anteriorly in midline to expose laryngeal structures. **2.** Surgery on the thyroid gland.

thyrotoxic (thī″rō-tŏks′ĭk) [″ + *toxikon,* poison] Pertaining to, affected by, or marked by toxic activity of the thyroid gland.

thyrotoxic crisis Thyroid storm.

thyrotoxicosis (thī″rō-tŏks″ĭ-kō′sĭs) [″ + ″ + *osis,* condition] A condition resulting from exposure of body tissues to excessive levels of thyroid hormones. This may be caused by an overactive or damaged thyroid gland or by the administration of excessive doses of thyroid hormone. SEE: *Graves' disease; hyperthyroidism; Nursing Diagnoses Appendix.*

ETIOLOGY: Graves' disease, overactive thyroid nodules, toxic multinodular goiter, thyroiditis, excessive exposure to iodine, and excessive ingestion of thyroid hormones all may cause thyrotoxicosis.

SYMPTOMS: Common symptoms include anxiety and irritability, insomnia, heat intolerance, fever, weight loss despite an increased appetite, muscular weakness, palpitations, amenorrhea or erectile dysfunction, and hyperdefecation. In the elderly, high-output congestive heart failure, atrial fibrillation, or depression may be presenting symptoms. Signs of thyrotoxicosis include tachycardia, systolic hypertension, tremor, diaphoresis, fevers, cardiac murmurs, powerful pulses, exaggerated deep tendon reflexes, lid lag, goiter, and in Graves' disease, protrusion of the eyes (exophthalmos).

TREATMENT: The treatment and prognosis depend on the underlying cause of the disease. Beta-blockers mask many of the symptoms of thyrotoxicosis, regardless of the underlying cause, and are typically administered to relieve symptoms. Patients with Graves' disease, the most common cause of thyrotoxicosis, may be treated with antithyroid drugs (e.g., methimazole), radioactive iodine ablation of the thyroid gland, or surgical removal of the thyroid gland.

PATIENT CARE: The health care professional provides a restful environment, encouraging expression of feelings, and promoting avoidance of stressors and stimulants to assist the patient in coping with the anxiety and irritability associated with this condition. Nutritional intake should consist of foods high in carbohydrates, proteins, and vitamins to maintain an anabolic state and to prevent muscle weakness and wasting. Comfort measures are provided to reduce effects of pyrexia, diaphoresis, abdominal cramping, and diarrhea. Fluids and electrolytes lost by diaphoresis or diarrhea are replaced as ordered.

thyrotropic (thī″rō-trŏp′ĭk) [″ + *trope,* a turning] That which has an affinity for or stimulates the thyroid gland.

thyrotropin (thī-rŏt′rō-pĭn) A hormone secreted by the anterior lobe of the pituitary that stimulates the thyroid gland. SYN: *thyroid-stimulating hormone; thyrotropic hormone.*

thyrotropism (thī-rŏt′rō-pĭzm) Affinity for the thyroid.

thyroxine (thī-rŏks′ĭn) [Gr. *thyreos,* shield] ABBR: T_4. One of the principal hormones secreted by the thyroid gland that increases the use of all food types for energy production and increases the rate of protein synthesis in most tissues. It is used to treat hypothyroidism. Chemically, it is 3,5,3′,5′-tetraiodothyronine. SYN: *tetraiodothyronine.* SEE: *thyroid; thyroid function test; triiodothyronine.*

Ti Symbol for the element titanium.

TIA *transient ischemic attack.*

tibia (tĭb′ē-ă) [L., *tibia,* shinbone] The inner and larger bone of the leg between the knee and the ankle; it articulates with the femur above and with the talus below.

saber-shaped t. A deformity caused by gummatous periostitis (syphilitic) in which the tibia curves outward.

t. valga A bulging of the lower legs in which the convexity is inward. SYN: *genu valgum.*

t. vara Blount's disease.

tibiad (tĭb′ē-ăd) [″ + *ad,* to] Toward the tibia.

tibial (tĭb′ē-ăl) [L. *tibialis*] Concerning the tibia.

tibialgia (tĭb″ē-ăl′jē-ă) [″ + Gr. *algos,* pain] Pain in the tibia.

tibialis (tĭb″ē-ā′lĭs) [L.] Pert. to the tibia.

tibioadductor reflex (tĭb″ē-ō-ăd-dŭk′tor) [L. *tibia,* shinbone, + *adducere,* to lead to] Adduction of either the stimulated leg or the opposite one when the tibia is percussed on the inner side.

tibiocalcanean (tĭb″ē-ō-kăl-kā′nē-ăn) Concerning the tibia and calcaneus.

tibiofemoral (tĭb″ē-ō-fĕm′or-ăl) [″ + L. *femur,* thigh] Rel. to the tibia and femur.

tibiofibular (tĭb″ē-ō-fĭb′ū-lăr) [″ + L. *fibula*, pin] Rel. to the tibia and fibula. SYN: *tibioperoneal*.

tibionavicular (tĭb″ē-ō-nă-vĭk′ū-lăr) Concerning the tibia and navicular bones. SYN: *tibioscaphoid*.

tibioperoneal (tĭb″ē-ō-pĕr″ō-nē′ăl) Tibiofibular.

tibioscaphoid (tĭb″ē-ō-skăf′oyd) Tibionavicular.

tibiotarsal (tĭb″ē-ō-tăr′săl) [″ + Gr. *tarsos*, broad, flat surface] Rel. to the tibia and tarsus.

tic (tĭk) [Fr.] A spasmodic muscular contraction, most commonly involving the face, mouth, eyes, head, neck, or shoulder muscles. The spasms may be tonic or clonic. The movement appears purposeful, is often repeated, is involuntary, and can be inhibited for a short time only to burst forth with increased severity.

Children between the ages of 5 and 10 years are esp. likely to develop tics. These tend to cease in a few weeks if they are ignored. SEE: *Tourette's syndrome*.

ETIOLOGY: In most cases, the cause is unknown. In some individuals, the tic is worsened by anxiety and nervous tension.

convulsive t. Spasm of the facial muscles supplied by the seventh cranial nerve.

t. douloureux Trigeminal neuralgia. SEE: *Nursing Diagnoses Appendix*.

facial t. Tic of the facial muscles.

habit t. Habitual repetition of a grimace or muscular action.

t. rotatoire Spasmodic torticollis in which the head and neck are forcibly rotated or turned from one side to the other.

spasmodic t. Tonic contractions and paralysis of the muscles of one or both sides of the face.

vocal t. Grunts and barking sounds that may be made by persons with Tourette's syndrome.

ticarcillin disodium, sterile (tī″kăr-sĭl′ĭn) A semisynthetic penicillin esp. effective against *Pseudomonas aeruginosa* and other gram-negative bacteria.

tick (tĭk) [ME. *tyke*] Any of the numerous bloodsucking arthropods of the order Acarida. Ixodidae is the hard tick family and Argasidae the soft. Ticks transmit many diseases to humans and animals. SEE: illus.

t. bite A wound produced by a bloodsucking tick. Adult ticks (and immature nymphs) may be vectors for infectious diseases, including Rocky Mountain spotted fever, Q fever, tularemia, borreliosis, babesiosis, ehrlichiosis, and Lyme disease. They can also produce tick paralysis, a disease that may mimic Guillain-Barré syndrome.

The bite itself may produce a localized reddened area of skin, which is typically of little importance. This area may be raised or slightly itchy. Only ticks that remain attached to the body for 16 to 24 hr are thought to transmit diseases to humans because it takes many hours for the tick to gain access to the blood supply.

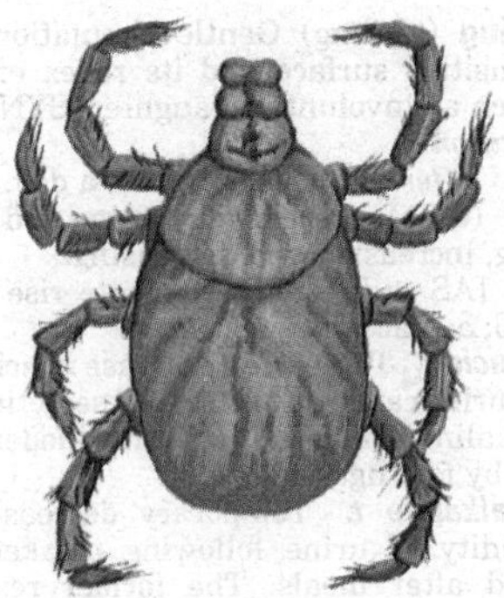

WOOD TICK
Dermacentor (×4)

FIRST AID: Ticks should be removed from the skin by taking a pair of small tweezers or forceps, grasping the tick firmly by the mouth parts, and pulling the insect directly out of the skin, leaving no body parts embedded.

CAUTION: Ticks should not be removed by burning them with matches, soaking them in petroleum jelly, or injecting the subcutaneous tissue beneath their mouth parts with lidocaine. None of these methods is effective, and some may be hazardous.

wood t. *Dermacentor andersoni*, an important North American species of tick, which causes tick paralysis and transmits causative organisms of Rocky Mountain spotted fever and tularemia. SEE: *tick* for illus.

tick-borne rickettsiosis The spotted-fever group (SFG) of tick-borne rickettsioses. Included are infections caused by the pathogenic organism *Rickettsia rickettsii*, which causes Rocky Mountain spotted fever. There are six other pathogenic SFG rickettsial species, five of which (*R. conorii, R. sibirica, R. japonica, R. australis*, and *R. africae*) are most likely to be transmitted by a tick bite. *R. akari*, which causes rickettsialpox, is transmitted to humans by mouse mites.

tickle (tĭk′l) [ME. *tikelen*] **1.** Peculiar sensation caused by titillation or touching, esp. in certain areas of the body, resulting in reflex muscular movements, laughter, or other forms of emotional expression. **2.** To arouse such a sensation by touching a surface lightly.

tickling (tĭk'lĭng) Gentle stimulation of a sensitive surface and its reflex effect, such as involuntary laughter. SYN: *titillation*.

t.i.d. L. *ter in die,* three times a day.

tidal (tī'dăl) Periodically rising and falling, increasing and decreasing.

tide [AS. *tid,* time] Alternate rise and fall; a space of time.

acid t. Temporary increase in acidity of urine caused by increased secretion of alkaline substances into the duodenum or by fasting.

alkaline t. Temporary decrease in acidity of urine following awakening and after meals. The former results from an increased rate of breathing, in which excess carbon dioxide is eliminated; the latter results from an increase of base in the blood following the secretion of HCl into gastric juice.

fat t. Increased fat in the lymph and blood after a fatty meal.

Tietze's syndrome (tēt'sĕz) [Alexander Tietze, Ger. surgeon, 1864–1927] Inflammation of the costochondral cartilages. This self-limiting disease is of unknown etiology. The pain may be confused with that of myocardial infarction. There is no specific therapy, but some relief is provided by injecting the area with local anesthetics or corticosteroids. SYN: *costochondritis*.

tigering [Gr. *tigris,* tiger] Tigerlike striped appearance of the heart muscle owing to irregular areas of fatty degeneration. This is seen in conditions that cause severe hypoxemia.

tigretier (tē-grĕt"ē-ā') [Fr.] A dancing mania or form of tarantism caused by the bite of a poisonous spider, occurring in Tigre, Ethiopia.

tigroid (tī'groyd) [Gr. *tigroeides,* tiger-spotted] Striped, spotted, or marked like a tiger.

tigroid bodies Masses of chromophil substance present in the cell bodies of neurons. SYN: *Nissl bodies*.

tigrolysis (tĭg"rŏl'ĭ-sĭs) Chromatolysis.

tilmus (tĭl'mŭs) [Gr. *tilmos,* a plucking] Carphology.

tiltometer (tĭl-tŏm'ĕ-tĕr) A device for measuring the degree of tilt of a bed or operating table; used to determine which end of the spinal canal is lower when spinal anesthesia has been given.

timbre (tĭm'bĕr, tăm'br) [Fr., a bell to be struck with a hammer] The resonance quality of a sound by which it is distinguished, other than pitch or intensity, depending on the number and character of the vibrating body's overtones.

time (tīm) [AS. *tima,* time] The interval between beginning and ending; measured duration.

backup t. In radiography, the time setting selected prior to an automated exposure, usually 150% of the anticipated total exposure time for projection.

bleeding t. The time required for blood to stop flowing from a small wound or pinprick. It is assessed using one of several techniques. Depending on the method used, the time may vary from 1 to 3 min (Duke method) or from 1 to 9 min (Ivy method). The Duke method consists of timing the cessation of bleeding after the ear lobe has received a standardized puncture. The Ivy method is done in a similar manner following puncture of the skin of the forearm. The validity of this test to predict clinically significant bleeding has been questioned.

clot retraction t. The time required following withdrawal of blood for a clot to completely contract and express the serum entrapped within the fibrin net. The normal time is about 1 hr. Clot retraction depends on the number of platelets in the specimen.

coagulation t. The time required for a small amount of blood to clot. This can be determined by collecting blood in a small test tube and noting elapsed time from the moment blood is shed to the time it coagulates.

doubling t. The length of time needed for a malignant tumor cell population to double in size.

dwell t. The length of time a therapeutic substance will be retained in the body.

intestinal transit t. The speed with which consumed food passes through the gut. It is slowed by anticholinergic agents (such as tricyclic antidepressants) and by neuropathic diseases of the stomach or intestines (e.g., diabetes mellitus). Many agents increase intestinal transit, including erythromycin and nonabsorbable laxatives.

median lethal t. The time required for the death of 50% of the individuals of an organism group that were exposed to ionizing radiation.

partial thromboplastin t. The time needed for plasma to clot after the addition of partial thromboplastin; used to test for defects of the clotting system.

prothrombin t. The time required for plasma coagulation in the formation of thrombin from prothrombin. Normal levels of calcium, thromboplastin, and other essential tissue coagulation factors are required.

reaction t. The period between application of a stimulus and the response.

setting t. The time required for a material to polymerize or harden, as in dental amalgam, cement, plaster, resin, or stone.

thermal death t. The time required to kill a bacterium at a certain temperature.

time frame The limits of time for any event or occurrence.

time inventory An assessment approach used by occupational therapists to determine a patient's perception of the value of time and its organization.

time-out A method of discipline that involves removing the child from social interaction and placing him or her in a nonstimulating location (i.e., in a chair facing a corner) for a few minutes after an unacceptable behavior has occurred.

timer (tīm'ĕr) A device for measuring, signaling, recording, or otherwise indicating elapsed time. Various forms of timers are used in radiographic, surgical, and laboratory work.

tin (tĭn) [AS.] SYMB: Sn. A metallic element used in various industries and in making certain tissue stains; atomic weight, 118.69; atomic number, 50. SEE: *tin poisoning*.

tinct *tincture*.

tinctable (tĭnk'tă-bl) Stainable.

tinction (tĭnk'shŭn) [L. *tingere*, to dye] **1.** The process of staining. **2.** A stain.

tinctorial (tĭnk-tō'rē-ăl) [L. *tinctorius*, dyeing] Rel. to staining or color.

tinctura (tĭnk-tū'ră) *pl.* **tincturae** [L., a dyeing] Tincture.

tincturation (tĭnk"tū-rā'shŭn) Making a tincture from an appropriate drug.

tincture (tĭnk'chūr) [L. *tincture*, a dyeing] An alcoholic extract of vegetable or animal substances. SYN: *tinctura*.

tincture of iodine Obsolete term for a simple alcoholic solution of iodine.

tincture of iodine poisoning Iodine poisoning.

tine A sharp, pointed prong.

tinea (tĭn'ē-ă) [L., worm] Any fungus skin disease occurring on various parts of the body. It is commonly called ringworm. SEE: *dermatomycosis*.

FINDINGS: There are two types of findings. Superficial findings are marking by scaling; slight itching; reddish or grayish patches; and dry, brittle hair that is easily extracted with the hair shaft. The deep type is characterized by flat, reddish, kerion-like tumors, the surface studded with dead or broken hairs or by gaping follicular orifices. Nodules may be broken down in the center, discharging pus through dilated follicular openings.

TREATMENT: Griseofulvin, terbinafine, or ketoconazole is given orally for all types of true trichophyton infections. Local treatment alone is of little benefit in ringworm of the scalp, nails, and in most cases the feet. Topical preparations containing fungicidal agents are useful in the treatment of tinea cruris and tinea pedis.

Personal hygiene is important in controlling these two common diseases. The use of antiseptic foot baths to control tinea pedis does not prevent spread of the infection from one person to another. Persons affected should not let others use their personal items such as clothes, towels, and sports equipment.

Tinea of the scalp, tinea capitis, is particularly resistant if due to *Microsporum audouinii*. It should not be treated topically. Systemic griseofulvin is quite effective.

t. amiantacea Sticky scaling of the scalp following infection or trauma.

t. barbae Barber's itch (2).

t. capitis A fungal infection of the scalp. It may be due to one of several types of *Microsporum* or *Trichophyton tonsurans*. SEE: illus.; *kerion*.

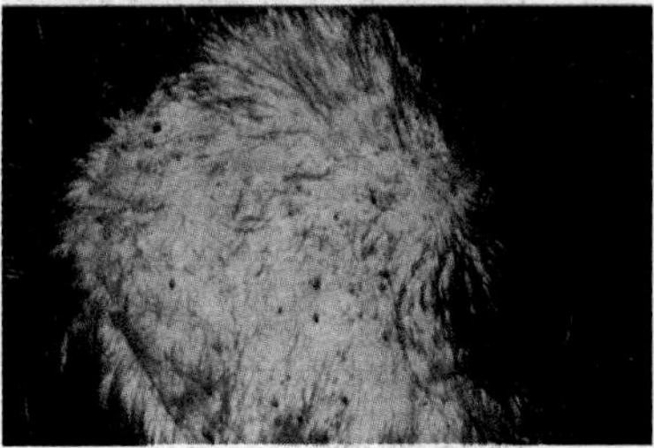

TINEA CAPITIS

t. corporis Tinea of the body. It begins with red, slightly elevated scaly patches that on examination reveal minute vesicles or papules. New patches spring from the periphery while the central portion clears. There is often considerable itching. SEE: illus.

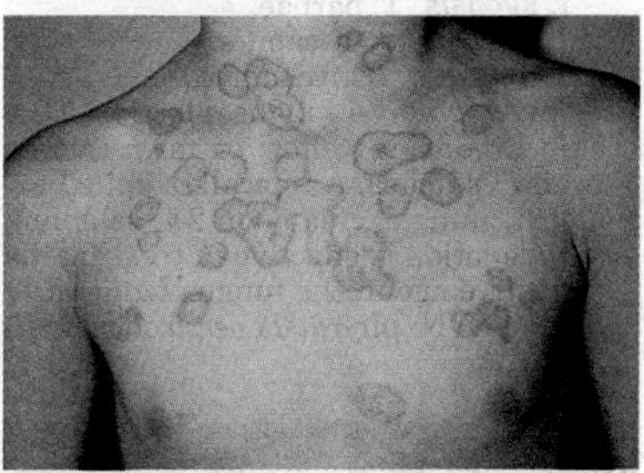

TINEA CORPORIS

t. cruris A fungus skin disease of surfaces of contact in the scrotal, crural, anal, and genital areas. Also called "jock itch." SYN: *dhobie itch*. SEE: illus.

t. imbricata Chronic tinea caused by *Trichophyton concentricum*. It is present in tropical regions. The annular lesions have scales at their periphery.

t. kerion Kerion.

t. nigra An asymptomatic superficial fungal infection that affects the skin of the palms. Caused by *Cladosporium werneckii* or *C. mansonii*, it is characterized by deeply pigmented, macular, nonscaly patches. SYN: *pityriasis nigra*.

t. nodosa Sheathlike nodular masses in the hair of the beard and mustache from growth of either *Piedraia hortae*, which causes black piedra,

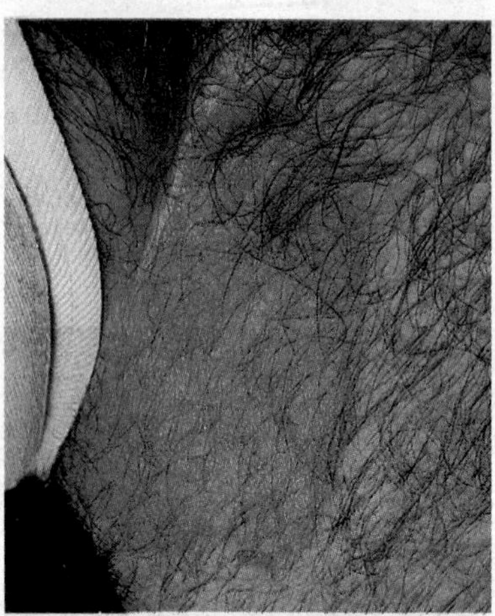

TINEA CRURIS (inner thigh)

or *Trichosporon beigelii,* which causes white piedra. The masses surround the hairs, which become brittle; hairs may be penetrated by fungus and thus split. SYN: *piedra*.

t. pedis Athlete's foot.

t. profunda A rare type of tinea characterized by indolent nodules and plaques, which may ulcerate.

t. sycosis T. barbae.

t. tonsurans T. capitis.

t. unguium Onychomycosis.

t. versicolor A fungus infection of the skin producing yellow or fawn-colored branny patches. A topically applied azole antifungal cream or 2% selenium sulfide lotion is effective in treating the causative agent, the fungus *Malassezia furfur*. SYN: *pityriasis versicolor*. SEE: illus.

TINEA VERSICOLOR (on back)

Tinel's sign (tĭn-ĕlz') [Jules Tinel, Fr. neurologist, 1879–1952] A cutaneous tingling sensation produced by pressing on or tapping the nerve trunk that has been damaged or is regenerating following trauma.

tingibility (tĭn″jĭ-bĭl'ĭ-tē) The property of being stainable.

tingible (tĭn'jĭ-bl) [L. *tingere,* to stain] Capable of being stained by a dye.

tingle (tĭng'gl) A prickling or stinging sensation that may be caused by cold or nerve injury.

tinnitus (tĭn-ī'tŭs) [L., a jingling] A subjective ringing, buzzing, tinkling, or hissing sound in the ear. For some patients, this causes only minor irritation; for others, it is disabling.

ETIOLOGY: It may be caused by impacted cerumen, myringitis, otitis media, Ménière's disease, otosclerosis, or drug toxicities (esp. salicylates and quinine).

tin poisoning Poisoning that results from exposure to organic compounds containing tin or tin arsenites. Most of the symptoms are neurological: changes in behavior, cognition, or awareness. Some toxic effects of tin are found on electroencephalographic examination.

tintometer (tĭn-tŏm'ĕ-ter) [L. *tinctus,* a dyeing, + Gr. *metron,* a measure] A scale used to determine by comparison the intensity of color of the blood or other fluid. **tintometric,** *adj.*

tintometry (tĭn-tŏm'ĕ-trē) Estimation of color by comparison with a scale of colors.

tip (tĭp) [ME.] A point or apex of a part.

tipped uterus Malposition of the uterus. In the past, this has been invoked as the cause of numerous conditions, including pelvic pain, back pain, abnormal uterine bleeding, infertility, and emotional difficulties. Simple malposition of the uterus without evidence of a specific disease condition that accounts for the malposition is felt to be harmless and virtually symptomless. It is essential therefore that individuals who have been told that a tipped uterus is the cause of their symptoms be carefully examined to attempt to find a specific organic cause for the symptoms. If in the absence of other findings a vaginal pessary relieves symptoms associated with a retrodisplaced uterus and these symptoms return when the pessary is removed, then surgical suspension of the uterus is indicated. If surgery is not acceptable to the patient, the pessary may be worn intermittently. Evidence is lacking that a tipped uterus is an important cause of pelvic pain and discomfort.

tipping (tĭp'ĭng) Angulation of a structure, such as a tooth about its long axis, the patella when it moves away from the frontal plane of the femur, or the scapula when the inferior angle moves away from the rib cage.

tiqueur (tĭ-kĕr') [Fr.] One afflicted with a tic.

tire (tīr) [AS. *teorian,* to tire] **1.** To become fatigued. **2.** To exhaust or fatigue.

tires (tīrz) Trembles.

tiring (tīr'ĭng) Fastening wire around the fragments of a bone.

tissue (tĭsh'ū) [O.Fr. *tissu,* from L. *texere,* to weave] A group or collection of similar cells and their intercellular substance that perform a particular function. Examples include epithelial, connective, muscular, and nervous tissues.

adipose t. Fat.

areolar t. A form of loose connective tissue consisting of fibroblasts in a matrix of tissue fluid and collagen and elastin fibers. Many white blood cells are present. It is found subcutaneously and beneath the epithelium of all mucous membranes. SEE: *connective t.* for illus.

bone t. Osseous t.

bronchus-associated lymphoid t. ABBR: BALT. Small sacs or follicles that contain clusters of T and B lymphocytes and macrophages lying below the mucosa of the bronchial wall; a component of the mucosal immune system that defends all mucosal surfaces against pathogens. SEE: *immune system, mucosal.*

brown adipose t. ABBR: BAT. Brown fat.

cancellous t. Spongy bone with many marrow cavities. It is present at the ends of long bones and in the interior of most flat bones.

chondroid t. Embryonic cartilage.

chordal t. Tissue of the notochord or derived from it. The nucleus pulposus is derived from the notochord.

chromaffin t. Chromaffin system.

cicatricial t. Scar.

connective t. Tissue that supports and connects other tissues and parts of the body. Connective tissue has comparatively few cells. Its bulk consists of intercellular substance or matrix, whose nature gives each type of connective tissue its particular properties. The vascular supply varies: cartilage, none; fibrous and adipose, poor; and bone, abundant. Connective tissue includes the following types: areolar, adipose, fibrous, elastic, reticular, cartilage, and bone. Blood may also be considered a connective tissue. SEE: illus.

elastic t. A form of connective tissue in which yellow elastic fibers predominate. It is found in certain ligaments, the walls of blood vessels, esp. the larger arteries, and around the alveoli of the lungs.

embryonic t. Mucous t.

endothelial t. Endothelium.

epithelial t. Epithelium.

erectile t. Spongy tissue, the spaces of which fill with blood, causing it to harden and expand. It is found in the penis, clitoris, and nipples.

fatty t. Fat.

fibrous t. Connective tissue consisting principally of collagen fibers. Also called white fibrous or dense connective tissue; may be regular (parallel fibers) or irregular.

gelatiginous t. Tissue from which gelatin may be obtained by treating it with hot water.

glandular t. A group of epithelial cells capable of producing secretions.

granulation t. The newly formed vascular and connective tissue produced in the early stages of wound healing.

hard t. In dentistry, the term used to denote any of the three calcified tissue components of the tooth: enamel, dentin, and cementum.

homologous t. Tissues that are identical in structure.

indifferent t. Tissue composed of undifferentiated cells as in embryonic tissue.

interstitial t. Connective tissue that forms a network with the cellular elements of an organ.

lymphadenoid t. Lymphoid tissue present in various sites, including the spleen and bone marrow.

lymphoid t. Collections of lymphocytes ranging from immature to mature stages of development found in lymphoid organs (e.g., thymus, spleen), in lymph nodes, and below the mucosal epithelium of the gastrointestinal, respiratory, and genitourinary tracts (e.g., tonsils, Peyer's patches).

mesenchymal t. The embryonic mesenchyme.

mucosa-associated lymphoid t. ABBR: MALT. Tissue formed by collections of T and B lymphocytes that line mucosal organs (e.g., the gastrointestinal tract or the bronchi) and protect against infection. Examples include Peyer's patches in the small intestine and colon, and lymphoid nodules in the appendix. MALT contains CD4+ and CD8+ T cells and activated B cells. They may occasionally undergo malignant transformation into lymphomas.

mucous t. Jelly-like tissue from which connective tissue is derived. SYN: *embryonic t.*

muscular t. The cells composing the muscles. *Voluntary:* Striated or skeletal muscle attached to bones or the skin. The cells are long cylinders with apparent striations and several nuclei each. *Involuntary:* Smooth or visceral muscle not under voluntary control, found mainly in the walls of hollow organs such as the stomach, intestines, arteries, veins, and uterus. The cells are small and tapered with no striations and one nucleus each. *Cardiac:* Found only in the walls of the chambers of the heart; not under voluntary control. The cells are branched, with striations and one nucleus each. SEE: *muscle.*

myeloid t. The bone marrow in which most blood cells are formed.

nerve t. The neurons and neuroglia of the nervous system.

osseous t. Connective tissue with a

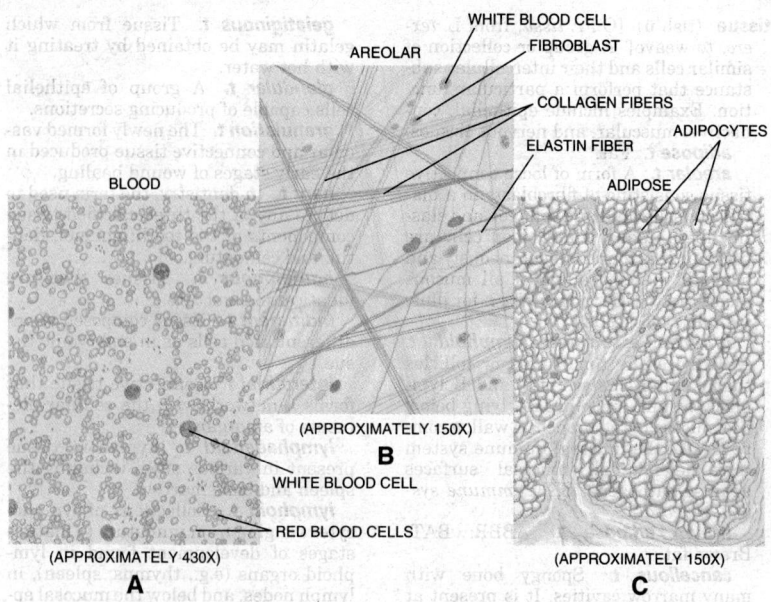

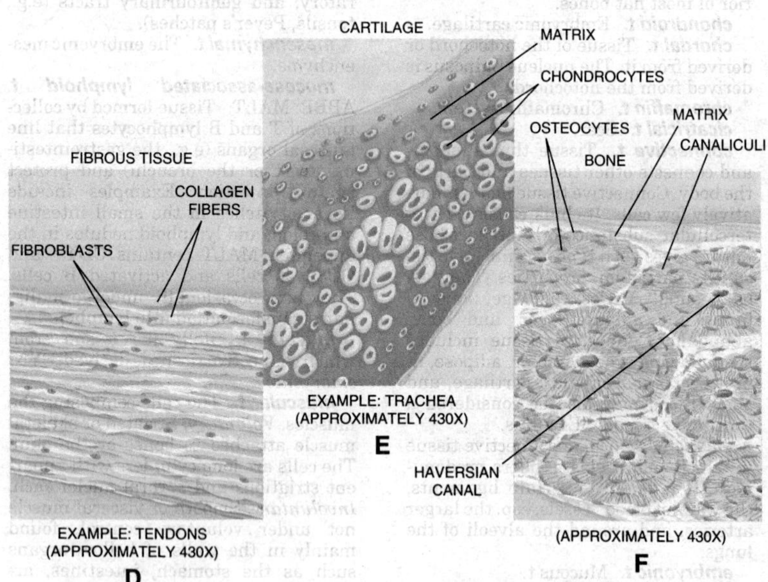

CONNECTIVE TISSUES

(A) blood, (B) areolar, (C) adipose, (D) fibrous, (E) cartilage, (F) bone

matrix of phosphate and carbonate of calcium, the minerals being two thirds of the bone's dry weight. It may be in its usual or abnormal site (i.e., in calcified tissue). SYN: *bonet.*

reticular t. A type of connective tissue consisting of delicate fibers forming interlacing networks. Fibers stain selectively with silver stains and are called argyrophil fibers. Reticular tissue supports blood cells in lymph nodes, bone marrow, and the spleen.

scar t. Scar.

sclerous t. Firm connective tissue such as bone and cartilage.

skeletal t. Bone.

splenic t. The highly vascular splenic pulp.

subcutaneous t. Areolar and adipose tissue found between the dermis and the muscles. SYN: *superficial fascia.*

tissue bank A facility for collecting, processing, and storing tissue for later transplantation. Tissue stored includes bone, skin, nerve, fascia, tendon, heart valve, dura mater, cornea, and bone marrow. These are tested for microbial pathogens and stored either in a freeze-dried or frozen state.

tissue culture Growth of tissue in vitro on artificial media for experimental research.

tissue culture ineffective dose ABBR: $TCID_{50}$. Dose that will produce a cytopathic effect in 50% of the cultures inoculated.

tissue expansion, soft A technique used in plastic surgery to expand skin prior to excising an area to achieve a more cosmetic wound closure. One or more expander balloons are inserted under the skin. The balloons are then expanded by progressively increasing the amount of saline solution in them. This is done on a weekly basis for whatever time is required to sufficiently stretch the overlying skin. After the expansion is completed, the plastic surgical procedure is performed. This permits removal of skin without having to cover the area by a skin graft. SEE: *surgery, plastic; W-plasty; Z-plasty.*

tissue factor ABBR: TF. Coagulation factor III.

tissue integrity, impaired A state in which an individual experiences damage to mucous membrane or corneal, integumentary, or subcutaneous tissue. SEE: *Nursing Diagnoses Appendix.*

tissue perfusion, altered (specify type): renal, cerebral, cardiopulmonary, gastrointestinal, peripheral The state in which an individual experiences a decrease in nutrition and oxygenation at the cellular level due to a deficit in capillary blood supply. SEE: *Nursing Diagnoses Appendix.*

tissue plasminogen activator ABBR: TPA. **1.** A natural enzyme that helps degrade blood clots by freeing plasmin from plasminogen. Plasmin in turn breaks down fibrin, the substance that forms the structural meshwork of clots. **2.** A recombinant enzyme, produced in the laboratory by *Escherichia coli,* for use in the treatment of thrombosis, esp. in myocardial infarction and ischemic stroke. Recombinant TPA is one of several thrombolytic drugs that can be given to patients during myocardial infarction (MI) to restore the flow of blood through occluded coronary arteries. Restoring perfusion keeps heart muscle from dying, reduces the damage caused by the infarction, and reduces the subsequent risk of congestive heart failure and death. It is somewhat more effective than another thrombolytic agent, streptokinase, in the treatment of very large and anterior wall myocardial infarctions. Both agents are effective in the treatment of inferior MI or smaller infarcts. The time during which TPA is safe and effective in the management of MI is 360 min. SYN: *recombinant TPA.*

Unlike streptokinase, TPA is also safe and effective in treating large ischemic strokes if the drug is given within the first 90 to 180 min after the onset of symptoms. After that period, the drug does not have demonstrable benefits.

Thrombolytic agents like TPA are also occasionally used (instead of heparins or emergency thrombolectomy) to manage life-threatening pulmonary emboli.

PATIENT CARE: The patient maintains strict bedrest throughout infusion. Additional IV access sites are initiated for adjuvant therapies or required blood studies before administering TPA. No further needle sticks should occur during therapy. The IV access site is inspected for bleeding throughout therapy, and the patient is assessed for indications of intracerebral or gastric bleeding. Heparin is administered with or after therapy as prescribed to maintain activated partial thromboplastin time at two times the patient's normal baseline. The health care professional evaluates for indications of reperfusion: sudden cessation of chest pain, early peak of creatine phosphokinase-MB enzyme (at 12 hr after injury), resolution of electrocardiographic injury current patterns, and "reperfusion dysrhythmias," including accelerated idioventricular rhythm, ventricular tachycardia, sinus bradycardia, and atrioventricular block. Mild allergic reactions to therapy (pruritus, urticaria, flushing, fever, headache, nausea, and malaise) are assessed, documented, and treated, as well as more acute reactions (bronchospasm, angioedema). If patients develop severe reactions to the drug, the infusion should be stopped and hospital protocols for emergency management of thrombolytic complications initiated.

CAUTION: Thrombolytic drugs should not be given to patients with active bleeding, a history of surgery or major trauma within the last two weeks, brain tumors, or other known risks for intracerebral hemorrhage.

---

tissue reaction The response of living tissues to altered conditions or types of restorative materials, metals, cements.

tissue typing Technique for determining the histocompatibility of tissues to be used in grafts and transplants with the recipient's tissues and cells. SEE: *transplantation*.

tissular (tĭsh′ū-lăr) Concerning living tissues.

titanium (tī-tā′nē-ŭm) [L. *titan*, the sun] SYMB: Ti. A metallic element found in combination with minerals; atomic weight, 47.90; atomic number, 22; specific gravity, 4.54. In dentistry, it is used as an alloy chiefly for appliances and implants because of its biological acceptance and resistance to corrosion.

t. dioxide A chemical used to protect the skin from the sun. It is also used in industrial applications to produce white in paints and plastics.

titer (tī′tĕr) [F. *titre*, standard] Standard of strength per volume of a volumetric test solution.

agglutination t. The highest dilution of a serum that will cause clumping (agglutination) of the bacteria being tested.

antibody t. A measure of the amount of antibody against a particular antigen present in the blood. One use is in detection of antibodies against herpes simplex and Epstein-Barr viruses. This titer is also useful in following the course of many acute infectious diseases. A rising titer usually indicates the disease is present and the body is reacting to the specific antigen.

titillation (tĭt″ĭl-ā′shŭn) [L. *titillatio*, a tickling] **1.** The act of tickling. **2.** The state of being tickled. **3.** The sensation produced by tickling.

titin An elastic protein in sarcomeres that anchors myosin filaments to the Z disks.

titrate (tī′trāt) To determine or estimate by titration.

titration (tī-trā′shŭn) [Fr. *titre*, a standard] **1.** Estimation of the concentration of a chemical solution by adding known amounts of standard reagents until alteration in color or electrical state occurs. **2.** Determination of the quantity of antibody in an antiserum.

titre Titer.

titrimetric (tī″trĭ-mĕt′rĭk) [″ + Gr. *metron*, measure] Employing the process of titration.

titrimetry (tī-trĭm′ĕ-trē) [*titration* + Gr. *metron*, measure] Analysis by titration.

titubation (tĭt″ū-bā′shŭn) [L. *titubatio*, a staggering] A coarse and backward tremor of the trunk. In patients with cerebellar disease, standing sometimes provokes this tremor.

lingual t. Stuttering.

Tl Symbol for the element thallium.

TLC **1.** *tender loving care.* **2.** *total lung capacity.* **3.** *thin-layer chromatography.*

TLD *thermoluminescent dosimeter.*

T.L.R. *tonic labyrinthine reflex.*

Tm **1.** Symbol for the element thulium. **2.** Symbol for maximal tubular excretory capacity of the kidneys.

TMJ *temporomandibular joint.*

TMP *trimethoprim.*

Tn Symbol for normal intraocular tension.

TNF *tumor necrosis factor.*

TNM classification Method of classifying malignant tumors with respect to primary *t*umor, involvement of regional lymph *n*odes, and presence or absence of *m*etastases. SEE: *cancer.*

TNT *trinitrotoluene.*

TO *old tuberculin* (also abbr. OT).

toadskin (tōd′skĭn) A condition characterized by excessive dryness, wrinkling, and scaling of skin sometimes seen in vitamin deficiencies.

toadstool (tōd′stool) Any of various fungi with an umbrella-shaped cap, esp. a poisonous mushroom.

toadstool poisoning Mushroom poisoning.

tobacco (tō-băk′ō) [Sp. *tabaco*] A plant whose leaves are cultivated, dried, and adulterated for use in smoking, chewing, and snuffing. Its scientific name is *Nicotiana tabacum*. The use of tobacco creates more preventable disability and death than the use of any other commercially available product. The tobacco leaf contains nicotine, a highly addictive alkaloid, and numerous other chemicals. During its combustion, it releases thousands of hydrocarbons into the oral, digestive, and respiratory tract of the smoker. These substances have been linked to coronary and peripheral arterial disease, emphysema, chronic bronchitis, peptic ulcer disease, and cancers of the lungs, oral cavity, and gastrointestinal tract. SEE: *risk factor; smokeless tobacco; smoking, passive.*

smokeless t. Tobacco used in the form of snuff, tobacco powder, or chewing tobacco. These products irritate the oral mucosa and gingiva, and their continued use results in an increased risk of cancer of the mouth, larynx, throat, and esophagus. Smokeless tobacco contains nicotine and is addictive. Its use is greatest among adolescents, esp. males. An estimated 1.4% to 8.8% of adults in the U.S. use smokeless tobacco products. SEE: *snuff* (2).

tobramycin (tō″bră-mī′sĭn) An aminoglycoside antibiotic used primarily to treat infections with gram-negative germs.

tocainide (tō-kāy′nīd) A lidocaine analogue used in treating ventricular arrhythmias. Trade name is Tonocard.

toco- Combining form indicating relationship to *labor* or *childbirth.*

tocodynagraph (tō″kō-dī′nă-grăf) [Gr. *tokos*, birth, + *dynamis*, power, + *graphein*, to write] A device for measuring the intensity of uterine contractions.

tocodynamometer (tō″kō-dī″năm-ŏm′ĕ-tĕr) [″ + *dynamis,* power, + *metron,* a measure] A device for estimating the force of uterine contractions in labor.

tocograph (tŏk′ō-grăf) [″ + *graphein,* to write] A device for estimating and recording the force of uterine contractions.

tocography (tō″kŏg′ră-fē) Recording the intensity of uterine contractions.

tocology (tō-kŏl′ō-jē) [″ + *logos,* word, reason] Science of parturition and obstetrics.

tocolysis (tō″kō-lī′sĭs) [″ + *lysis,* dissolution] Inhibition of uterine contractions. Drugs used for this include adrenergic agonists, magnesium sulfate, and ethanol.

tocopherol (tō-kŏf′ĕr-ŏl) [″ + *pherein,* to carry, + L. *oleum,* oil] Generic term for vitamin E (alpha-tocopherol) and a number of chemically related compounds, most of which have the biological activity of vitamin E.

tocophobia (tō″kō-fō′bē-ă) [″ + *phobos,* fear] An abnormal fear of childbirth.

tocus (tō′kŭs) [L.] Parturition; childbirth.

Todd's paralysis Transient, focal neurological deficits, occurring after a seizure, that resemble a stroke but resolve spontaneously.

toe (tō) [AS. *ta*] A digit of the foot. SYN: *digit.* SEE: *foot* for illus.

claw t. Hammertoe.

dislocation of the t. Traumatic displacement of bones of a toe. This condition is treated essentially the same as dislocation of the finger. SEE: *finger, dislocation of.*

fanning of t. Spreading of toes, esp. when the sole is stroked.

Morton's t. Metatarsalgia.

pigeon t. Walking with the toes turned inward.

turf t. A hyperextension injury of the first metatarsophalangeal (MTP) joint. Severe hyperextension also injures the plantar sesamoids and flexor tendons. The injury commonly occurs on artificial surfaces such as Astro Turf®, where the competitors wear light, flexible-soled shoes that allow MTP hyperextension on the firm surface.

webbed t. Toes joined by webs of skin.

toe clonus Contraction of the big toe caused by sudden extension of the first phalanx.

toe drop Inability to lift the toes.

toenail (tō′nāl) Unguis. SEE: *nail.*

toe reflex A reflex in which strong flexion of the great toe flexes all the muscles below the knee.

tofu (tō-foo′) Soybean curd.

Togaviridae [L. *toga,* coat, + *virus,* poison] A family of viruses that include the genus *Alphavirus.* They cause Western and Eastern equine encephalitis. Other Togaviridae include the rubiviruses (e.g., rubella virus).

toilet (toy′lĕt) [Fr. *toilette,* a little cloth] **1.** Cleansing of a wound after operation or of an obstetrical patient. **2.** An apparatus for use during defecation and urination to collect and dispose of these waste products.

toilet training Teaching a child to control urination and defecation until placed on a toilet. The bowel movements of an infant may habitually occur at the same time each day very early in life, but because the child does not have adequate neuromuscular control of bowel and bladder function until the end of the second year, it is not advisable to begin this training until then. Close to that time, placing the child on a small potty chair for a short period several times a day may allow him or her to stay dry. First the diapers are removed while the child is awake, later removed during naps and the child told he or she should be able to stay dry. This schedule may need to be interrupted for several days to a week if the child does not remain dry.

To protect the bed, a rubber sheet should be used during the training period. Training pants or "pull-ups" may help in the transition from passive to active control of toilet habits. There is no difference in ease of training between boys and girls, each taking about 3 to 6 months.

Children who are unsuccessful in remaining dry or controlling their bowels should not be punished. To do so may promote the later development of enuresis or constipation. In any event, it is neither abnormal nor harmful for training to be delayed until well into the third year of life. If not achieved by then, professional evaluation should be undertaken to detect the rare case of genitourinary or gastrointestinal abnormalities contributing to such a delay.

toko- SEE: *toco-.*

tolazamide (tŏl-ăz′ă-mīd) $C_{14}H_{21}N_3O_3S$; a first-generation oral hypoglycemic agent of the sulfonylurea class (used to lower blood sugar levels).

tolazoline hydrochloride (tŏl-ăz′ō-lēn) An alpha-adrenergic blocking agent used to produce peripheral vasodilation.

tolbutamide (tŏl-bū′tă-mīd) $C_{12}H_{18}N_2O_3S$; a first-generation oral hypoglycemic agent of the sulfonylurea class (used to lower blood sugars).

tolerance (tŏl′ĕr-ăns) [L. *tolerantia,* tolerance] Capacity for enduring a large amount of a substance (food, drug, or poison) without an adverse effect and showing a decreased sensitivity to subsequent doses of the same substance.

drug t. The progressive decrease in the effectiveness of a drug.

exercise t. The amount of physical activity that can be done under supervision before exhaustion.

glucose t. The ability of the body to absorb and use glucose.

immunological t. The state in which the immune system does not react to the body's own antigens. This is caused by mechanisms that destroy the lymphocytes with receptors to self-antigens, as they develop. Failure of these mechanisms may result in autoimmune disease.

oral t. The suppression of autoimmune or allergic responses as a result of eating antigenic material.

pain t. The degree of pain an individual can withstand.

radiation t. The level below which tissue radiation exposure will be least harmful. Some organs are less tolerant to radiation than others.

tissue t. The ability of specific tissues to withstand the effects of ionizing radiation.

tolerant Capable of enduring or withstanding drugs without experiencing ill effects.

tolerogen (tŏl′ĕr-ō-jĕn) That which causes immunological tolerance or failure of the body to react to an antigen by forming an antibody. The mechanism of formation of this specific unresponsive state is poorly understood.

tolerogenic (tŏl″ĕr-ō-jĕn′ĭk) Producing immunological tolerance.

tollwut (tŏl-voot′) [Ger.] Rabies.

tolnaftate (tŏl-năf′tāt) A synthetic antifungal agent used topically in treating various forms of tinea.

tolu balsam A balsam obtained from *Myroxylon balsamum,* used as an expectorant.

toluene A toxic hydrocarbon derived from coal tar.

toluene poisoning SEE: *benzene* in *Poisons and Poisoning Appendix.*

toluidine (tŏl-ū′ĭ-dĭn) C_7H_9N; aminotoluene, a derivative of toluene.

tomaculous neuropathy (tō-mā′cū-lŭs) [L. *tomaculum,* a kind of sausage] The presence of sausage-shaped areas of thickened myelin with secondary axon constriction in some cases of familial recurrent brachial neuropathy.

tomatine (tō′mă-tēn) A substance derived from tomato plants affected by wilt. It has antifungal action.

-tome Combining form meaning *cutting, cutting instrument.*

tomo- Combining form indicating *section, layer.*

tomogram (tō′mō-grăm) [Gr. *tome,* incision, + *gramma,* something written] The radiograph obtained during tomography.

tomograph (tō′mō-grăf) [″ + *graphein,* to write] An x-ray tube attached to a Bucky diaphragm by a rigid rod allowing rotation around a fixed point (fulcrum) during the radiographical exposure for tomography.

tomography (tō-mŏg′ră-fē) A radiographic technique that selects a level in the body and blurs out structures above and below that plane, leaving a clear image of the selected anatomy. This is accomplished by moving the x-ray tube in the opposite direction from the imaging device around a stationary fulcrum defining the plane of interest. Tube movements can be linear, curvilinear, circular, elliptical, figure eight, hypocycloidal, or trispiral. SYN: *body section radiography.*

computed t. ABBR: CT. Tomography in which transverse planes of tissue are swept by a pinpoint radiographic beam and a computerized analysis of the variance in absorption produces a precise reconstructed image of that area. This technique has a greater sensitivity in showing the relationship of structures than conventional radiography.

computerized axial t. ABBR: CAT. SEE: *magnetic resonance imaging; tomography, computed.*

electron-beam t. Ultrafast computerized t.

helical computed t. Computed tomographic (CT) images that are obtained as the CT table moves continuously during a single, held breath. Detailed evaluation of dynamic internal features is feasible with this technique. SYN: *spiral computed t.*

positron emission t. ABBR: PET. Reconstruction of brain sections by using positron-emitting radionuclides. By using several different radionuclides, researchers can measure regional cerebral blood flow, blood volume, oxygen uptake, and glucose transport and metabolism, and can locate neurotransmitter receptors. PET has been used with fludeoxyglucose F 18 to identify and localize regional lymph node metastases and to help assess response to therapy.

The images produced by PET are in colors that indicate the degree of metabolism or blood flow. The highest rates appear red, those lower appear yellow, then green, and the lowest rates appear blue. The images in various disease states may then be compared to those of normal subjects. SEE: illus.

quality computed t. ABBR: QCT. Bone densitometry performed through software algorithms on a computed tomography unit.

single photon emission computed t. ABBR: SPET, SPECT. A medical imaging method for reconstructing cross-sectional images of radiotracer distributions. SEE: *nuclear medicine scanning test; positron emission t.*

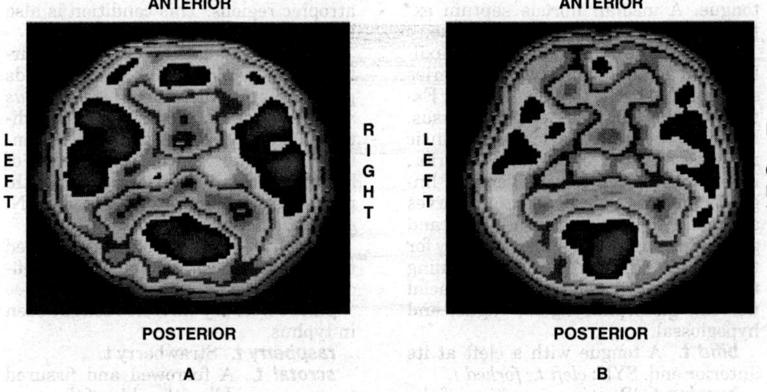

PET SCAN OF BRAIN

Transverse section in (A) normal young patient, (B) normal aging patient

spiral computed t. Helical computed t.

ultrafast computerized t. Computerized tomographic (CT) scanning that produces images by rotating the x-ray (electron) beam at targets placed around a patient, instead of moving a patient on a gantry through the scanner. The technique minimizes patient movement artifacts and decreases scanning times to about 50 to 100 msec. It is capable of providing good resolution of vascular structures, such as the aorta and the coronary arteries. SYN: *electron-beam t.*

-tomy Combining form meaning *cutting, incision.*

tonaphasia (tō″nă-fā′sē-ă) [L. *tonus,* a stretching, + *a-,* not, + *phasis,* speech] Inability to remember a tune owing to cerebral lesion.

tone (tōn) [L. *tonus,* a stretching] **1.** That state of a body or any of its organs or parts in which the functions are healthy and normal. In a more restricted sense, the resistance of muscles to passive elongation or stretch. **2.** Normal tension or responsiveness to stimuli, as of arteries or muscles, seen particularly in involuntary muscle (such as the sphincter of the urinary bladder). SYN: *tonicity* (2); *tonus.* **3.** A musical or vocal sound.

muscular t. The state of slight contraction usually present in muscles that contributes to posture and coordination; the ability of a muscle to resist a force for a considerable period without change in length.

tone deafness The inability to detect differences in musical sounds. SYN: *amusia.*

tongue (tŭng) [AS. *tunge*] A freely movable muscular organ that lies partly in the floor of the mouth and partly in the pharynx. It is the organ of taste and contributes also to chewing, swallowing, and speech. SYN: *lingua.* SEE: illus.

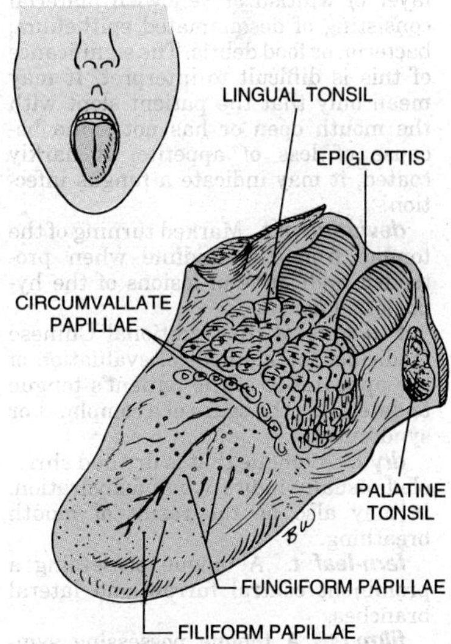

SURFACE OF TONGUE

ANATOMY: The tongue consists of a body and root and is attached by muscles to the hyoid bone below, the mandible in front, the styloid process behind, and the palate above, and by mucous membrane to the floor of the mouth, the lateral walls of the pharynx, and the epiglottis. A median fold (frenulum linguae) connects the tongue to the floor of the mouth. The surface of the tongue bears numerous papillae of three types: filiform, fungiform, and vallate. Taste buds are present on the surfaces of many of the papillae, esp. the vallate papillae. Mucous and serous glands (lingual glands) are present; their ducts open on the surface. The lingual tonsils are lymphatic tissue on the base of the tongue. A median fibrous septum extends the entire length of the tongue.

Arteries: The lingual, exterior maxillary, and ascending pharyngeal arteries supply blood to the tongue. *Muscles:* Extrinsic muscles include genioglossus, hypoglossus, and styloglossus; intrinsic muscles consist of four groups: superior, inferior, transverse, and vertical lingualis muscles. The hypoglossal nerves are motor to the tongue; the facial and glossopharyngeal nerves are sensory for taste. *Nerves:* Lingual nerve (containing fibers from trigeminal and facial nerves), glossopharyngeal, vagus, and hypoglossal.

bifid t. A tongue with a cleft at its anterior end. SYN: *cleft t.; forked t.*

burning t. Burning sensation of the tongue. SYN: *glossopyrosis.*

cleft t. Bifid t.

coated t. A tongue covered with a layer of whitish or yellowish material consisting of desquamated epithelium, bacteria, or food debris. The significance of this is difficult to interpret. It may mean only that the patient slept with the mouth open or has not eaten because of loss of appetite. If darkly coated, it may indicate a fungus infection.

deviation of t. Marked turning of the tongue from the midline when protruded, indicative of lesions of the hypoglossal nerve.

t. diagnosis In traditional Chinese medicine, the methodical evaluation of the appearance of the patient's tongue to determine the cause of a complaint or syndrome.

dry t. A tongue that is dry and shriveled, usually indicative of dehydration. It may also be the result of mouth breathing.

fern-leaf t. A tongue possessing a prominent central furrow and lateral branches.

filmy t. A tongue possessing symmetrical whitish patches.

fissured t. A tongue bearing deep furrows in its epithelium and changes in its papillae, which may be normal or may be a familial syndrome transmitted by autosomal dominant inheritance.

forked t. Bifid t.

furred t. A coated tongue on which the surface epithelium appears as a coat of white fur. It is seen in nearly all fevers. Unilateral furring may result from disturbed innervation, as in conditions affecting the second and third branches of the fifth nerve. It has been noted in neuralgia of those branches and in fractures of the skull involving the foramen rotundum. Yellow fur indicates jaundice.

geographic t. A tongue with white raised areas, normal epithelium, and atrophic regions. This condition is also known as benign migratory glossitis.

hairy t. A tongue covered with hairlike papillae entangled with threads produced by the fungi *Aspergillus niger* or *Candida albicans.* This condition is usually seen as the result of antibiotic therapy that inhibits growth of bacteria normally present in the mouth, permitting overgrowth of fungi. SYN: *glossotrichia; lingua nigra.*

magenta t. A magenta-colored tongue seen in cases of riboflavin deficiency.

parrot t. A dry shriveled tongue seen in typhus.

raspberry t. Strawberry t.

scrotal t. A furrowed and fissured tongue, resembling the skin of the scrotum.

smoker's t. Leukoplakia.

smooth t. A tongue with atrophic papillae. It is characteristic of many conditions, such as anemia and malnutrition.

strawberry t. A tongue that first has a white coat except at the tip and along the edges, with enlarged papillae standing out distinctly against the white surface. Later the white coat disappears, leaving a bright red surface. This is characteristic of scarlet fever. SYN: *raspberry t.*

trifid t. A tongue in which the anterior end is divided into three parts.

trombone t. The rapid involuntary movement of the tongue in and out.

tongue-swallowing A condition in which the tongue tends to fall backward and obstruct the openings to the larynx and esophagus. The tongue is not swallowed and the term is inaccurate; nevertheless, it is occasionally used. The condition is due to excessive flaccidity of the tongue during unconsciousness. Airway control is achieved through one of the following maneuvers: forceful elevation of the chin and extension of the head during artificial respiration, in order to open the airway; or insertion of a mechanical airway device, such as an oropharyngeal airway, to push the tongue out of the airway.

CAUTION: The rescuer should never place his or her hand inside the victim's mouth to move the tongue.

---

tongue thrust The infantile habit of pushing the tongue between the alveolar ridges or incisor teeth during the initial stages of suckling and swallowing. If this habit persists beyond infancy, it may cause anterior open occlusion, jaw deformation, or abnormal tongue function.

tongue-tie Lay term for ankyloglossia, congenital shortness of the frenulum of the tongue. The condition has been shown to have no functional significance, even for speech.

tonic (tŏn′ĭk) [Gr. *tonikos,* from *tonos,* tone] **1.** Pert. to or characterized by tension or contraction, esp. muscular tension. **2.** Restoring tone. **3.** A medicine that increases strength and tone. Tonics are subdivided according to action, such as cardiac or general.

tonicity (tō-nĭs′ĭ-tē) [Gr. *tonos,* act of stretching] **1.** Property of possessing tone, esp. muscular tone. **2.** Tone (2).

tonic labyrinthine reflex Labyrinthine righting reflex.

tonicoclonic (tŏn″ĭ-kō-klŏn′ĭk) Tonoclonic.

tonoclonic (tŏn″ō-klŏn′ĭk) [″ + *klonos,* tumult] Both tonic and clonic, said of muscular spasms. SYN: *tonicoclonic.*

tonofibril (tŏn′ō-fī″brĭl) Tenofibril.

tonogram (tō′nō-grăm) [″ + *gramma,* something written] The record produced by a tonograph.

tonograph (tō′nō-grăf) [″ + *graphein,* to write] A recording tonometer.

tonography (tō-nŏg′ră-fē) The recording of changes in intraocular pressure.

tonometer (tōn-ŏm′ĕ-tĕr) [″ + *metron,* measure] An instrument for measuring tension or pressure, esp. intraocular pressure.

Schiötz t. An instrument for measuring intraocular pressure by the degree of indentation produced by pressure on the cornea.

tonometry (tōn-ŏm′ĕ-trē) The measurement of tension of a part, as intraocular tension, used to detect glaucoma. SEE: illus.

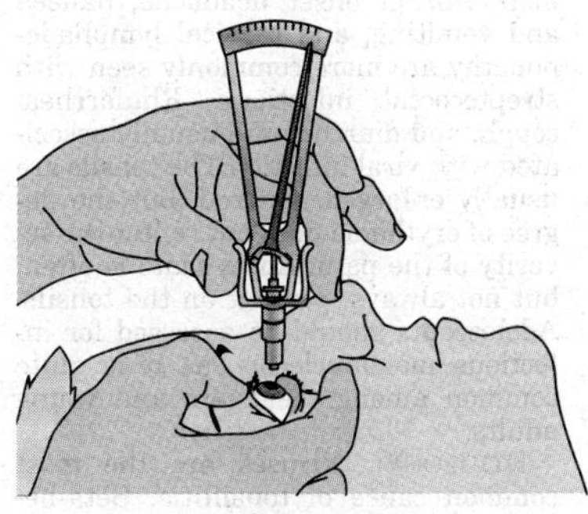

TONOMETRY

Measuring intraocular eye pressure

analytical t. A technique formerly used in blood gas analysis in which the liquid blood sample and its gas are held at equilibrium and the partial pressures of oxygen and carbon dioxide are measured.

digital t. Determining intraocular pressure by use of the fingers.

noncontact t. Determining intraocular pressure by measuring the degree of indentation of the cornea produced by a puff of air.

tonoplast (tŏn′ō-plăst) [″ + *plassein,* to form] The membrane surrounding an intracellular vacuole.

tonsil (tŏn′sĭl) [L. *tonsilla,* almond] **1.** A mass of lymphoid tissue in the mucous membranes of the pharynx and base of the tongue. The free surface of each tonsil is covered with stratified squamous epithelium that forms deep indentations, or crypts, extending into the substance of the tonsil. The palatine tonsils, pharyngeal tonsils (adenoids), and lingual tonsils form a ring of immunologically active tissue. **2.** A rounded mass on the inferior surface of the cerebellum lying lateral to the uvula.

Infection of the Tonsils: Tonsils detect and respond to pathogens entering the body through the mouth and nose. Inflammation of the tonsils (tonsillitis) occurs during upper respiratory infections caused by common viruses. Beta-hemolytic streptococci or, occasionally, *Staphylococcus aureus* infections may occur as primary infections or follow viral infections, most commonly in children and immunocompromised adults. Clinically, the patient will have enlarged, reddened, tender glands, often coated with inflammatory exudate, which may form a pseudomembrane. The tonsils may stay enlarged after multiple infections, and are sometimes surgically removed (tonsillectomy). SEE: illus.

Rheumatic fever, an autoimmune inflammatory disease, develops 2 to 3 weeks after streptococcal infections in about 3% of patients; it is believed that antibodies against streptococcal pharyngitis cross-react with antigens in the heart and joints.

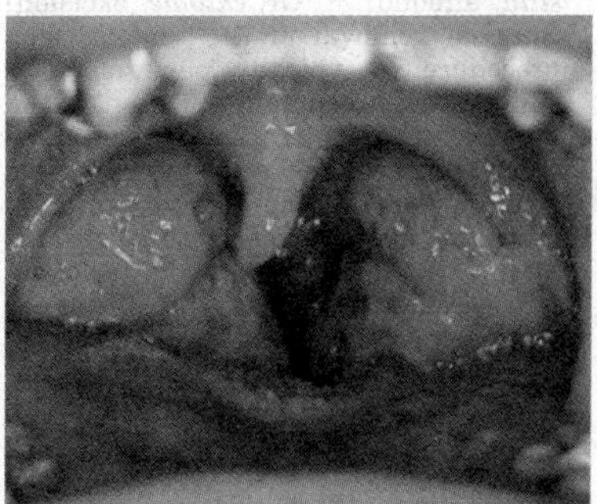

INFLAMED TONSILS

cerebellar t. One of a pair of cerebellar lobules on either side of the uvula, projecting from the inferior surface of the cerebellum.

faucial t. Palatine t.

lingual t. A mass of lymphoid tissue located in the root of the tongue.

Luschka's t. Pharyngeal t.

nasal t. Lymphoid tissue on the nasal septum.

palatine t. Two oval masses of lymphoid tissue that lie in the tonsillar fossa on each side of the oral pharynx between the glossopalatine and pharyngopalatine arches. They are commonly known as the tonsils. SYN: *faucial t.*

pharyngeal t. Lymphoid tissue on the roof of the posterior superior wall of the nasopharynx. It is commonly called adenoids. SYN: *Luschka's t.* SEE: *adenoid.*

tubal t. Lymphoid tissue located in the mucous membrane of the tube connecting the middle ear to the nasopharynx.

tonsilla (tŏn-sĭl′ă) [L.] A general anatomical term for a small, discrete, rounded mass of tissue.

tonsillar (tŏn′sĭ-lăr) Pert. to a tonsil, esp. the faucial or palatine tonsil.

tonsillar area An area composed of the palatine arch, tonsillar fossa, glossopalatine sulcus, and posterior faucial pillar.

tonsillar crypt A deep indentation into the pharyngeal surface of a tonsil. It is lined with stratified squamous epithelium.

tonsillar fossa A depression, located between the glossopalatine and pharyngopalatine arches, in which the palatine tonsil is situated.

tonsillar ring The almost complete ring of tonsillar tissue encircling the pharynx. It includes the palatine, lingual, and pharyngeal tonsils. SEE: *lymphoid ring.*

tonsillar sinus The space lying between the plica triangularis and the anterior surface of the palatine tonsil.

tonsillectomy (tŏn-sĭl-ĕk′tō-mē) [L. *tonsilla,* almond + Gr. *ektome,* excision] Surgical removal of the tonsils. This procedure is typically performed for children with recurrent infections of the throat, although it may also be used when enlarged tonsils cause obstructive sleep apnea. Whether the procedure is advisable in children with recurrent pharyngeal infections is a matter of debate. Complications of the procedure may include local bleeding, throat pain, injury to the upper airway, and aspiration pneumonia, among others. SEE: *Nursing Diagnoses Appendix.*

PATIENT CARE: *Preoperative:* The anesthetic methods and expected sensations are explained to the adult patient. For children, the anesthetic methods and hospital routines are explained in simple, nonthreatening language; the child is allowed to try on hospital garb; and the child is shown the operating and recovery rooms, as appropriate to age. Parents are encouraged to remain with the child.

Postoperative: A patent airway is maintained, and the patient is placed in a semiprone or sidelying position until he or she has fully recovered from anesthesia. Vital signs are monitored, and the patient is assessed for bleeding (excessive swallowing in a semiconscious child), restlessness, tachycardia, and pallor. After the patient's gag reflex has returned, water and nonirritating fluids are permitted by mouth. Deep breathing and turning help to prevent pulmonary complications. Ice packs are applied and analgesics administered as prescribed. Vocal rest is encouraged and the patient is instructed not to clear the throat or cough, because this may precipitate bleeding. Written discharge instructions covering use of fluids and soft diet and avoidance of overactivity are provided to the patient and family. Within 5 to 10 days postoperatively, a white scab will form in the patient's throat. The patient or family should report any bleeding, ear discomfort, or persistent fever.

tonsillitis (tŏn-sĭl-ī′tĭs) [″ + Gr. *itis,* inflammation] Inflammation of a tonsil, esp. the faucial tonsil. SEE: *Nursing Diagnoses Appendix.*

acute parenchymatous t. Tonsillitis in which the entire tonsil is affected.

acute t. Inflammation of the lymphatic tissue of the pharynx, esp. the palatine or faucial tonsils. It may occur sporadically or in epidemic form, and usually is self-limiting.

SYMPTOMS: Throat pain, esp. while swallowing, is the cardinal symptom of tonsillitis; fever and malaise are common. Abrupt onset headache, nausea and vomiting, and cervical lymphadenopathy are more commonly seen with streptococcal infections. Rhinorrhea, cough, and diarrhea are usually associated with viral infection.The tonsils are usually enlarged and red, but the degree of erythema does not reflect the severity of the pain. An exudate is often, but not always, present on the tonsils. Adolescents should be assessed for infectious mononucleosis, as it is quite common among teenagers and young adults.

ETIOLOGY: Viruses are the most common cause of tonsillitis. Beta-hemolytic streptococci infections may follow viral infections or occur as primary infections, esp. in school-aged children and immunocompromised adults (5% to 20% of cases).

TREATMENT: Viral tonsillitis is treated symptomatically. If group A beta-hemolytic streptococci infection is suspected, a throat culture is taken. Streptococcal tonsillitis must be treated with a 10-day course of oral penicillin or one intramuscular dose of long-acting benzathine penicillin to decrease the risk of rheumatic fever or glomerulonephritis. Rheumatic fever develops 2 to 3 weeks after streptococcal infections in about 3% of patients. If chronic tonsillitis occurs, the tonsils may be removed, but this operation is not as common as it was years ago. SEE: *rheumatic fever*.

follicular t. Inflammation of the follicles on the surface of the tonsil, which become filled with pus.

ulceromembranous t. Tonsillitis that ulcerates and develops a membranous film.

tonsillolith (tŏn′sĭl-ō-lĭth) [″ + Gr. *lithos,* stone] A stone within a tonsil. SYN: *amygdalolith*.

tonsillopathy (tŏn″sĭ-lŏp′ă-thē) Any disease of the tonsil.

tonsilloscopy (tŏn″sĭl-lŏs′kō-pē) [″ + Gr. *skopein,* to examine] Inspection of the tonsils.

tonsillotome (tŏn-sĭl′ō-tōm) A surgical instrument used in tonsillectomy.

tonsillotomy (tŏn″sĭl-ŏt′ō-mē) [″ + Gr. *tome,* incision] Incision of the tonsils.

tonus (tō′nŭs) [L., tension] The partial steady contraction of muscle that determines tonicity or firmness; the opposite of clonus. SYN: *tone; tonicity*.

tooth [AS. *toth*] One of the conical hard structures of the upper and lower jaws used for mastication. A tooth consists of a crown portion above the gum, a root portion embedded in a socket (alveolus) of the jaw bone, and a neck or cervical constricted region between the crown and root. The soft tissue gingiva covers the neck and root to a variable extent, depending on age and oral hygiene. The major portion of a tooth consists of dentin, which surrounds the pulp chamber in the crown and root of the tooth. Dentin is harder than bone. Enamel, the hardest tissue of the body, covers the crown. Cementum is similar to bone and covers the root, attaching the tooth to the surrounding bony socket by the periodontal ligament fibers embedded in both bone and cementum. The pulp cavity contains the dental pulp, a loose connective tissue containing many cells, nerves, and blood or lymph vessels. Each tooth has five surfaces: occlusal, mesial, distal, lingual, and facial or buccal. SEE: illus.; *dentition; teeth*.

accessional t. The permanent molar tooth that arises without deciduous predecessors in the dental arch.

anatomic t. An artificial tooth that duplicates the anatomical form of a natural tooth.

baby t. Deciduous teeth.

hypersensitive t. A tooth that is sensitive to temperature changes, sweets, or percussion. It may exhibit gingival recession, exposed root dentin, caries, or periodontal disease.

impacted t. A tooth that is unable to erupt due to adjacent teeth or malposition of the tooth.

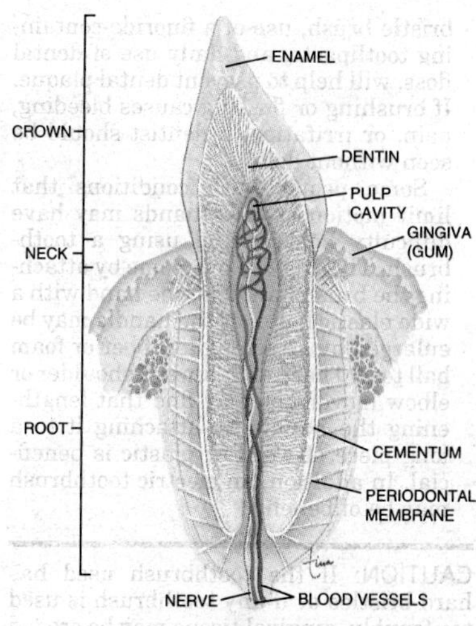

TOOTH STRUCTURE

(longitudinal section)

implanted t. An artificial tooth implanted permanently into the jaw.

t. surface The external aspect of a tooth. Each tooth has five surfaces, usually named for the adjacent tissue or space. The outer (facial) surface is called the *labial* surface for the incisors or canines, and the *buccal* surface for the premolars and molars. The inner surface of each tooth is called the *lingual* (oral) surface. Within the arch, each tooth has a *mesial* surface, the side toward the midpoint in the front of the dental arch, and a *distal* surface, the side farthest from the midpoint in the front of the dental arch. The *occlusal* surface comes in contact with a tooth in the opposing jaw.

toothache Pain in a tooth or the region about a tooth. SYN: *dentalgia; odontalgia; odontodynia*.

tooth bleaching The application of chemical bleaching agents to teeth to make them whiter.

toothbrushing The act of cleaning the teeth and gums by using a soft brush specifically designed for this purpose. The toothbrush consists of tufts of soft, synthetic fibers or natural bristles mounted in a handle that may be straight or angled for better access or brushing action. It is usually used with fluoride toothpaste (a mildly abrasive, flavored dentifrice) in a manner suggested by dentists and dental hygienists as being a suitable method for cleaning. The proper use of a toothbrush stimulates periodontal tissue. SEE: *hygiene, oral; periodontal disease; plaque, dental*.

Good oral hygiene, consisting of proper brushing of the teeth with a soft bristle brush, use of a fluoride-containing toothpaste, and daily use of dental floss, will help to prevent dental plaque. If brushing or flossing causes bleeding, pain, or irritation, a dentist should be seen without delay.

Some people with conditions that limit motion of their hands may have difficulty holding and using a toothbrush. This may be overcome by attaching the brush handle to the hand with a wide elastic band, or the handle may be enlarged by attaching a rubber or foam ball to it. Those with limited shoulder or elbow movement may find that lengthening the handle by attaching it to a long piece of wood or plastic is beneficial. In addition, an electric toothbrush may be of benefit.

CAUTION: If the toothbrush used has hard bristles or if any toothbrush is used too forcibly, gingival tissue may be eroded and damaged.

---

tooth migration, pathological Drifting or movement of teeth due to the pathological changes in areas adjacent to the moving teeth. SEE: *drift, mesial; tooth movement.*

tooth migration, physiological The natural and expected movement of teeth as growth and development occur. SEE: *drift, mesial; tooth migration, pathological; tooth movement.*

tooth movement The change in position of a tooth or teeth in the dental arch. This may be due to abnormal pressure from the tongue, pathological changes in tooth-supporting structures, malocclusion, missing teeth, or a therapeutic orthodontic procedure. Thumb sucking, if prolonged, may cause malocclusion and, eventually, displacement of teeth. SEE: *tooth migration, pathological.*

toothpaste A dentifrice used with a toothbrush to clean the exposed surfaces of teeth. It may contain mild abrasives, whiteners, deodorants, sodium bicarbonates, peroxide, or caries-preventing agents. SEE: *toothbrushing.*

toothpick Any small tapering sliver of wood or other material used to remove food debris from between the teeth. Early examples were made of gold, carved bone, or ivory.

top-, topo- Combining form meaning *place, locale.*

topagnosis (tŏp″ăg-nō′sĭs) [Gr. *topos,* place, + *a,* not, + *gnosis,* knowledge] Loss of the ability to localize the site of tactile sensations.

topalgia (tō-păl′jē-ă) [″ + *algos,* pain] Pain in a localized site.

topectomy (tō-pĕk′tō-mē) [″ + *ektome,* excision] A form of neurosurgery in which small incisions are made through the thalamofrontal tracts.

topesthesia (tŏp″ĕs-thē′zē-ă) [″ + *aisthesis,* sensation] The ability through tactile sense to determine that skin is touched. SYN: *topognosia.*

tophaceous (tō-fā′shŭs) [L. *tophaceus,* sandy] **1.** Relating to a tophus. **2.** Sandy or gritty.

tophus (tō′fŭs) *pl.* **tophi** [L., porous stone] **1.** A deposit of sodium biurate in tissues near a joint, in the ear, or in bone in gout. **2.** A salivary calculus. **3.** Tartar on the teeth.

tophyperidrosis (tŏf″ĭ-pĕr″ĭ-drō′sĭs) [Gr. *topos,* place, + *hyper,* above, + *hidros,* sweat] Excessive sweating in local areas.

topical [Gr. *topos,* place] Pert. to a definite surface area; local.

topoalgia (tō″pō-ăl′jē-ă) [″ + *algos,* pain] Localized pain, common in neurasthenia following emotional upsets.

topoanesthesia (tō″pō-ăn″ĕs-thē′zē-ă) [″ + *an-,* not, + *aisthesis,* sensation] Loss of the ability to recognize the location of a tactile sensation.

topognosia, topognosis (tō″pŏg-nō′sē-ă, -sĭs) [″ + *gnosis,* knowledge] Recognition of the location of a tactile sensation. SYN: *topesthesia.*

topographical (tŏp″ō-grăf′ĭk) [″ + *graphein,* to write] Pert. to description of special regions.

topographical anatomy A study of all the structures and their relationships in a given region (e.g., the axilla).

topography (tō-pŏg′ră-fē) Description of a part of the body.

topology (tō-pŏl′ō-jē) **1.** Topographical anatomy. **2.** In obstetrics, the relationship of the presenting fetal part to the pelvic outlet. **3.** In mathematics, the study of the properties of geographical configurations, both solid and plane.

toponarcosis (tō″pō-năr-kō′sĭs) [″ + *narkosis,* a benumbing] Local anesthesia.

toponeurosis (tō″pō-nū-rō′sĭs) [″ + *neuron,* nerve, + *osis,* condition] Neurosis of a limited area.

toponym (tŏp′ō-nĭm) The name of a region.

toponymy (tō-pŏn′ĭ-mē) [″ + *onoma,* name] Nomenclature of the regions of the body.

topophobia (tō″pō-fō′bē-ă) [″ + *phobos,* fear] A neurotic fear of being in a particular place or area.

topothermesthesiometer (tŏp″ō-thĕr″mĕs-thē-zē-ŏm′ĕ-ter) [″ + *therme,* heat, + *aisthesis,* sensation, + *metron,* measure] A device for measuring local temperature sense.

TOPV *trivalent oral polio vaccine.*

TORCH An acronym originally coined from the first letters of *T*oxoplasmosis, *R*ubella, *C*ytomegalovirus, and *H*erpesvirus type 2. Contemporary revisions describe the O as standing for *Other transplacental infections* (by human im-

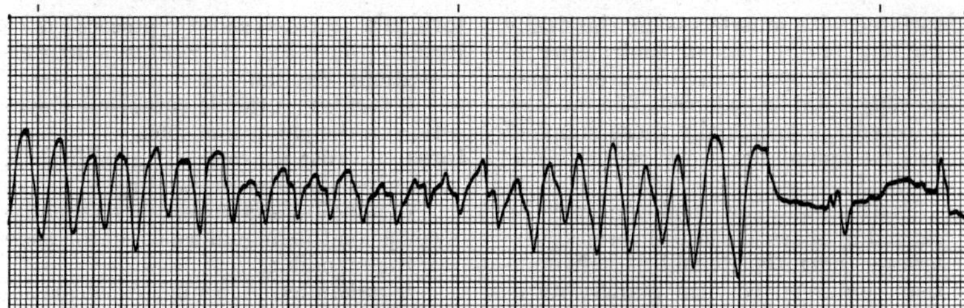

TORSADE DE POINTES
Ventricular tachycardia converting spontaneously to sinus rhythm

munodeficiency virus, hepatitis B, human parvovirus, and syphilis). TORCH infections can attack a growing embryo or fetus and cause abortion, abnormal fetal development, severe congenital anomalies, mental retardation, and fetal or neonatal death.

torcular herophili (tor′kū-lăr) The confluence of sinuses at the internal occipital protuberance of the skull.

toric (tō′rĭk) Concerning a torus.

tormina (tor′mĭn-ă) *sing.*, **tormen** [L., twistings] Intestinal colic.

torose, torous (tō′rōs, -rŭs) [L. *torosus,* full of muscle] Knobby or bulging; tubercular.

torpent (tor′pĕnt) [L. *torpens,* numbing] **1.** Medicine that modifies irritation. **2.** Not capable of functioning; dormant, apathetic, torpid.

torpid (tor′pĭd) [L. *torpidus,* numb] Not acting vigorously; sluggish.

torpidity (tor-pĭd′ĭ-tē) Sluggishness; inactivity.

torpor [L. *torpor,* numbness] Abnormal inactivity; dormancy; numbness; apathy.

t. retinae Reduced sensitivity of retina to light stimuli.

torque (tork) [L. *torquere,* to twist] **1.** A force producing rotary motion. **2.** In dentistry, the application of force to rotate a tooth around its long axis.

torr (tor) A pressure quantity equivalent to 1/760 of standard atmospheric pressure; for most practical purposes, this equals 1 mm Hg.

torrefaction (tor″ĕ-făk′shŭn) [L. *torrefactio*] Roasting or parching something, esp. a drug, to dry it.

torsade de pointes A rapid, unstable form of ventricular tachycardia in which the QRS complexes appear to twist, or shift, electrical orientation around the isoelectric line of the electrocardiogram. It often occurs as a life-threatening effect of a medication (e.g., quinidine, amiodarone, or a tricyclic antidepressant) that prolongs the Q-T interval but may also complicate congenital long Q-T syndromes. Intravenous magnesium sulfate may be used to treat this arrhythmia. SYN: *polymorphic ventricular tachycardia*. SEE: illus.

torsiometer (tor″sē-ŏm′ĕ-tĕr) A device for measuring the rotation of the eyeball around the visual axis (i.e., its anterior-posterior axis).

torsion (tor′shŭn) [L. *torsio,* a twisting] **1.** The act of twisting or the condition of being twisted. **2.** In dentistry, the state of a tooth when rotated around its long axis. **3.** Rotation of the vertical meridians of the eye.

lung t. A rare injury in which the lung rotates around its pedicle, typically after violent trauma to the chest. The injured lung can usually only be repaired with immediate surgery.

torsionometer (tor″shŭn-ŏm′ĕ-tĕr) [″ + Gr. *metron,* measure] A device for measuring the rotation of the vertebral column around the long axis.

torsive (tor′sĭv) Twisted, as in a spiral.

torsiversion (tor″sĭ-vĕr′zhŭn) Rotation of a tooth around its long axis.

torso (tor′sō) [It.] The trunk of the body.

torsoclusion (tor″sō-kloo′zhŭn) [″ + L. *occlusio,* to occlude] **1.** Acupressure in combination with torsion to stop a bleeding vessel. **2.** Malocclusion characterized by rotation of a tooth on its long axis.

tort A wrongful act or injury, committed by an entity or person against another person or another person's property, that may be pursued in civil court by the injured party. The purpose of tort law is to make amends to the injured party, primarily through monetary compensation or damages.

intentional t. An intentional wrongful act by a person or entity who means to cause harm, or who knows or is reasonably certain that harm will result from the act.

unintentional t. An unintended wrongful act against another person that produces injury or harm.

torticollar (tor″tĭ-kŏl′ăr) Concerning torticollis.

torticollis (tor″tĭ-kŏl′ĭs) [L. *tortus,* twisted, + *collum,* neck] Stiff neck associated with muscle spasm, classically causing lateral flexion contracture of the cervical spine musculature. It may be congenital or acquired. The muscles affected are principally those supplied by the spinal accessory nerve. SYN: *wryneck*.

ETIOLOGY: The condition may be caused by scars, disease of cervical vertebrae, adenitis, tonsillitis, rheumatism, enlarged cervical glands, retropharyngeal abscess, or cerebellar tumors. It may be spasmodic (clonic) or permanent (tonic). The latter type may be due to Pott's disease (tuberculosis of the spine).

congenital muscular t. Congenital fibrosis of the sternocleidomastoid muscle in the newborn, causing rotation of the infant's head to the opposite side. The condition usually becomes evident in the first 2 weeks of life. Treatments include physical therapy, or in refractory cases, surgical division of the muscle. SYN: *fibromatosis colli*.

fixed t. An abnormal position of the head owing to organic shortening of the muscles.

intermittent t. Spasmodic t.

ocular t. Torticollis from inequality in sight of the two eyes.

spasmodic t. Torticollis with recurrent but transient contractions of the muscles of the neck and esp. of the sternocleidomastoid. SYN: *intermittent t.*

TREATMENT: Botulinus toxin has been used to inhibit the spastic contractions of the affected muscles. SEE: *toxin, botulinus*.

spurious t. Torticollis from caries of the cervical vertebrae.

tortipelvis (tor″tĭ-pĕl′vĭs) [″ + *pelvis*, basin] Muscular spasms that distort the spine and hip. SYN: *dystonia musculum deformans*.

tortuous (tor′choo-ŭs) [L. *tortuosus*, fr. *torqueo*, to twist] Having many twists or turns.

torture (tor′chūr) [LL. *tortura*, a twisting] Infliction of severe mental or physical pain by various methods, usually for the purpose of coercion.

Torula (tor′ū-lă) Former name of a genus of yeastlike organisms, now called *Cryptococcus*.

toruloid (tor′ū-loyd) [L. *torulus*, a little bulge, + Gr. *eidos*, form, shape] Beaded; noting an aggregate of colonies like those seen in the budding of yeast.

toruloma (tor-ū-lō′mă) [*Torula*, old name for Cryptococcus, + *oma*, tumor] The nodular lesion of cryptococcosis (torulosis).

Torulopsis glabrata A yeast of the family Cryptococcaceae, closely related to the *Candida* species. It is usually nonpathogenic for humans but may cause serious illness in immunocompromised patients.

torulosis (tor-ū-lō′sĭs) Cryptococcosis.

torulus (tor′ū-lŭs) [L. *torulus*, a little elevation] Papilla.

t. tactiles A tactile cutaneous elevation on the palms and soles.

torus (tō′rŭs) *pl.* **tori** [L., swelling] A rounded elevation or swelling.

t. mandibularis An exostosis that develops on the lingual aspect of the body of the mandible.

t. palatinus A benign exostosis located in the midline of the hard palate. Also called *palatine protuberance*.

total allergy syndrome An outdated term for multiple chemical sensitivity syndrome.

total joint replacement Surgical removal of a diseased or injured joint and its replacement with an orthosis. SEE: *knee, replacement of; total hip replacement; Nursing Diagnoses Appendix*.

total parenteral nutrition ABBR: TPN. The intravenous provision of dextrose, amino acids, emulsified fats, trace elements, vitamins, and minerals to patients who are unable to assimilate adequate nutrition by mouth. Patients with many illnesses become malnourished if they are unable to eat a balanced diet for more than a few weeks. However, only a small percentage of these patients clearly benefit from parenteral nutritional support in clinical trials. Patients who benefit most from TPN are those at the extremes of nutritional risk (e.g., preterm or newborn infants who require surgery or the 5% of adult surgical candidates who are the most nutritionally deficient). Patients who may occasionally benefit from TPN include those with inflammatory bowel disease, radiation enteritis, bowel obstruction, and related intestinal diseases. In many other patients, the anticipated risks of malnutrition and starvation are exceeded by the potential risks of TPN, which include injury during central line placement, sepsis as a result of infectious contamination of intravenous lines, and metabolic complications (e.g., refeeding syndrome).

Patients requiring 7 to 10 days of nutritional support may benefit from the administration of parenteral nutrition through a peripheral venous catheter. This method limits the caloric intensity of TPN to about 2300 kcal/day (about 900 mOsm/kg) because more concentrated formulas cause peripheral vein inflammation. With central TPN, patients have been occasionally supported for several months with limited overt complications. The superior vena cava tolerates feedings of up to 1900 mOsm/kg. Typically, central TPN includes individually tailored amounts of dextrose, amino acids, lipids, vitamins, trace elements, heparin, insulin, and other substances. In patients with specific diseases, some nutrients may be limited, for example, sodium (in congestive heart failure), protein content (in liver failure), and potassium (in renal failure).

PATIENT CARE: The procedure is explained to the patient, and a nutritional assessment is obtained. Intake and output are monitored and recorded. The nurse assists with catheter insertion and observes for adverse effects, documents procedure and initial fluid administration, and continues to monitor fluid intake. The catheter insertion site is inspected and redressed every 25 to 48 hr; a strict aseptic technique is used for this procedure. The condition of the site and position of the catheter are documented, and the catheter is evaluated for leakage; if present, this should be reported to the physician. Electrolytes are monitored. Vitamin supplements are administered as prescribed. The patient is observed for edema and dehydration. If diarrhea or nausea occurs, the infusion rate is slowed. Urine sugar and acetone tests are performed every 6 hr, and blood sugar levels are monitored as prescribed. Daily weights are obtained. The solution should never be discontinued abruptly but tapered off with isotonic glucose administered for several hours. In the event of catheter blockage or removal, the physician should be notified immediately. Some patients recuperating from long illnesses are released from the hospital with self-administered TPN until they are able to resume eating. These patients need to be taught how to facilitate TPN use in the home.

CAUTION: The best way to obtain nutrition is usually enteral. Oral and enteral feedings preserve the integrity of the intestinal mucosa, maintain a normal pH in the stomach, prevent the entry of bacteria into the body through the walls of the gastrointestinal tract, and are less expensive than parenteral nutrition.

totipotent (tō-tĭp′ō-tĕnt) [L. *totus,* all, + *potentia,* power] In embryology, the ability of a cell or group of cells to produce all of the tissues required for development (i.e., the embryonic membranes, the embryo, and finally the fetus). **totipotency,** *adj.*

touch (tŭch) [O.Fr. *tochier*] **1.** To perceive by the tactile sense; to feel with the hands, to palpate. **2.** The sense by which pressure on the skin or mucosa is perceived; the tactile sense. **3.** Examination with the hand. SYN: *palpation.*

Various disorders may disturb or impair the tactile sense or the ability to feel normally. There are a number of words and suffixes pert. to sensation and its modifications. A few of the more important ones are as follows: algesia, -algia, anesthesia, dysesthesia, -dynia, esthesia, esthesioneurosis, hyperesthesia, paresthesia, and synesthesia.

after-t. Persistence of the sensation of touch after contact with the stimulus has ceased.

double t. Vaginal and rectal examination made at the same time.

therapeutic t. The practice of running the hands of a nurse or therapist on or above a patient's body to restore health. The practice has many exponents but no objective validation. It was originally devised in the 1970s by Dolores Kreiger, a nurse educator in New York, and its hypotheses and practices have been further explored by other prominent nursing educators, including Martha Rogers. The practice of therapeutic touch is founded on the concept that ill patients have lost contact with the flow of "life energy" and that disturbances in their personal "energy fields" can be felt and manipulated by therapists without technologies, drugs, or other standard medical therapies. The hypothesis has been disproved by direct study, which has failed to demonstrate the presence of energy fields around patients or the ability of practitioners experienced in the technique to sense the presence of patients, much less their emanations.

vaginal t. Digital examination of the vagina.

vesical t. Digital examination of the bladder.

tour de maître (toor″ dĕ mā-tr′) [Fr., the master's turn] A method of introducing a catheter or sound into the male bladder or into the uterus. This involves very carefully turning and angulating the device so as to follow the curvature of the passageway.

Tourette's syndrome, Tourette's disorder [Georges Gilles de la Tourette, Fr. neurologist, 1857–1904] A neurological disorder marked by repetitive motor and verbal tics. Affected persons may blink, jerk, grunt, clear their throats, swing their arms, grasp or clasp others, have obsessive-compulsive behaviors, or use verbal expletives uncontrollably. In some instances, people with this condition can control the urge to use these mannerisms while in public, but they may express them vigorously when alone. The condition often appears in multiple family members. It may be caused by a disorder of dopamine uptake in the basal ganglia. Dopamine-blocking drugs such as haloperidol can be used to treat this disorder. SYN: *Gilles de la Tourette's syndrome.* SEE: *tic.*

Tournay's sign (tūr-nāz′) [Auguste Tournay, Fr. ophthalmologist, 1878–1969] Dilatation of the pupil of the eye on unusually strong lateral fixation.

tourniquet (toor′nĭ-kĕt) [Fr., a turning instrument] Any constrictor used on an extremity to apply pressure over an artery and thereby control bleeding; also used to distend veins to facilitate venipuncture or intravenous injections.

Arterial hemorrhage: In emergent circumstances, the tourniquet is applied between the wound and the heart, close to the wound, placing a hard pad over the point of pressure. This should be discontinued as soon as possible and a tight bandage substituted under the loosened tourniquet. SEE: *bleeding, arterial* for table.

CAUTION: A tourniquet should never be left in place too long. Ordinarily, it should be released from 12 to 18 min after application to determine whether bleeding has ceased. If it has, the tourniquet is left loosely in place so that it may be retightened if necessary. If bleeding has not ceased, it should be retightened at once. In general, a tourniquet should not be used if steady firm pressure over the bleeding site will stop the flow. As an adjunct to surgery on extremities, a pneumatic tourniquet is applied after exsanguinating the limb with an Esmarch or similar bandage. The tourniquet is released at appropriate intervals to prevent tissue damage due to ischemia. An additional application utilizes two tourniquets or a double cuff tourniquet for retrograde intravenous nerve block (e.g., Bier block).

---

rotating t. The application of blood pressure cuffs to three extremities; used in certain types of medical emergencies, such as acute pulmonary edema, to reduce the return of blood to the heart. The patient is placed in a head-high position (Fowler's). The pressure is kept midway between systolic and diastolic. Every 10 min, the cuffs are deflated and when inflated, the previously free extremity is now used. This allows each extremity to be free of a tourniquet for 10 min out of each 40-min cycle.

NOTE: A cuff would not be applied to an extremity into which an intravenous infusion is running.

Touton cell (toot′ŏn) [Karl Touton, Ger. dermatologist, 1858–1934] A giant multinucleated cell found in lesions of xanthomatosis.

towelette (tow″ĕl-ĕt′) [ME. *towelle,* towel] A small towel.

tox- SEE: *toxi-*.

toxanemia (tŏks″ă-nē′mē-ă) [Gr. *toxikon,* poison, + *an-,* not, + *haima,* blood] Anemia due to a hemolytic toxin.

toxemia (tŏk-sē′mē-ă) [″ + Gr. *haima,* blood] Distribution throughout the body of poisonous products of bacteria growing in a focal or local site, thus producing generalized symptoms.

SYMPTOMS: The condition is marked by fever, diarrhea, vomiting, and symptoms of shock. In tetanus, the nervous system is esp. affected; in diphtheria, nerves and muscles are affected.

eclamptogenic t. Pregnancy-induced hypertension.

t. of pregnancy Previously used term for pregnancy-induced hypertension. SEE: *eclampsia; pre-eclampsia; Nursing Diagnoses Appendix.* **toxemic** (-mĭk), *adj.*

toxenzyme (tŏks-ĕn′zīm) [″ + Gr. *en,* in, + *zyme,* leaven] A poisonous enzyme.

toxi-, tox-, toxo- Combining form meaning *poison.*

toxic- SEE: *toxico-*.

toxic (tŏks′ĭk) [Gr. *toxikon,* poison] Pert. to, resembling, or caused by poison. SYN: *poisonous.*

toxicant (tŏks′ĭ-kănt) [L. *toxicans,* poisoning] **1.** Poisonous; toxic. **2.** Any poison.

toxicemic Toxemic.

toxic erythema Redness of the skin or a rash resulting from toxic agents such as drugs.

toxicide (tŏks′ĭ-sīd) [Gr. *toxikon,* poison, + L. *cidus,* kill] **1.** Destructive to toxins. **2.** A chemical antidote for poisons.

toxicity (tŏks-ĭs′ĭ-tē) The extent, quality, or degree of being poisonous.

neurobehavioral t. Alterations in attention, concentration, coordination, mood, muscle activity, neurological development, or sensation resulting from exposure to a poisonous chemical, drug, or physical agent.

toxic-nutritional optic neuropathy Bilateral visual impairment with central scotomas. This is usually associated with a toxic or nutritional disorder, such as the ingestion of methyl alcohol.

toxico-, toxic- [Gr. *toxikon,* poison] Combining form meaning *poisonous.*

Toxicodendron (tŏk″sĭ-kō-dĕn′drŏn) A genus of plants that includes poison ivy and poison oak.

toxicoderma (tŏks″ĭ-kō-dĕr′mă) [″ + *derma,* skin] Any skin disease resulting from a poison. SYN: *toxicodermatosis; toxidermitis.*

toxicodermatitis (tŏks″ĭ-kō-dĕrm-ă-tī′tĭs) [″ + ″ + *itis,* inflammation] Inflammation of the skin caused by a poison.

toxicodermatosis (tŏks″ĭ-kō-dĕrm-ă-tō′sĭs) [″ + ″ + *osis,* condition] Toxicoderma.

toxicogenic (tŏks″ĭ-kō-jĕn′ĭk) [″ + *gennan,* to produce] Caused by, or producing, a poison.

toxicoid (tŏks′ĭ-koyd) [″ + *eidos,* form, shape] Of the nature of a poison.

toxicologist (tŏks″ĭ-kŏl′ō-jĭst) [″ + *logos,* word, reason] A specialist in the field of poisons or toxins.

toxicology (tŏks″ĭ-kŏl′ō-jē) Division of medical and biological science concerned with toxic substances, their detection, their avoidance, their chemistry and pharmacological actions, and their antidotes and treatment.

toxicopathy (tŏks″ĭ-kŏp′ă-thē) [″ + *pathos,* disease, suffering] Any disease caused by a poison.

toxicophidia (tŏk″sĭ-kō-fĭd′ē-ă) [″ + Gr. *ophis,* snake] Poisonous snakes. SYN: *thanatophidia.*

toxicophobia (tŏks″ĭ-kō-fō′bē-ă) [″ + *phobos,* fear] An abnormal fear of being poisoned by any medium: food, gas, water, or drugs.

toxicosis (tŏks″ĭ-kō′sĭs) [″ + *osis,* condition] A disease resulting from poisoning.

endogenic t. A disease due to poisons generated within the body. SYN: *autointoxication.*

exogenic t. Any toxic condition resulting from a poison not generated in the body.

retention t. Toxicosis from retained products that normally are excreted shortly after formation.

toxic shock-like syndrome ABBR: TSLS. An infection in which the initial site is skin or soft tissue. This may occur in adults or children and it is readily transmitted from person to person. Typically there is a history of a minor usually nonpenetrating local trauma that within the next 1 to 3 days develops into the usual toxic shock syndrome (TSS) caused by a toxin elaborated by certain strains of *Staphylococcus aureus.* SEE: *toxic shock syndrome.*

toxic shock syndrome ABBR: TSS. A rare disorder similar to septic shock caused by an exotoxin produced by certain strains of *Staphylococcus aureus* and group A streptococci. It originally was seen in young women using vaginal tampons during menstruation, but also can complicate any staphylococcal infection in others. A similar syndrome is caused by streptococcal infections. SEE: *Nursing Diagnoses Appendix.*

SYMPTOMS: The diagnosis is made when the following criteria are met: fever of 102°F (38.9°C) or greater; diffuse, macular (flat), erythematous rash, followed in 1 or 2 weeks by peeling of the skin, particularly of the palms and soles; hypotension or orthostatic syncope; and involvement of three or more of the following organ systems: gastrointestinal (vomiting or diarrhea at the onset of illness), muscular (severe myalgia), mucous membrane (vaginal, oropharyngeal, or conjunctival) hyperemia, renal, hepatic, hematological (platelets fewer than 100,000/mm^3), and central nervous system (disorientation or alteration in consciousness without focal neurological signs when fever and hypotension are absent). Results of blood, throat, and cerebrospinal fluid cultures are usually negative. The possibility of Rocky Mountain spotted fever, leptospirosis, or rubeola should be eliminated by blood tests. The disease is fatal in approx. 5% to 15% of cases.

CAUTION: Anyone who develops these symptoms and signs should seek medical attention immediately. If a tampon is being used, it should be removed at once.

TREATMENT: Penicillinase-resistant antibiotics such as nafcillin or oxacillin do not affect the initial syndrome but may prevent its recurrence. Supportive care (intravenous fluids, pressor drugs, intensive care) is provided.

toxidermitis (tŏks″ĭ-dĕr-mī′tĭs) [″ + *derma,* skin, + *itis,* inflammation] Toxicoderma.

toxidrome (tŏk′sĭ-drōm) A specific cluster of symptoms that occurs after patients are exposed to a poisonous agent; a toxic syndrome.

toxigenic (tŏks″ĭ-jĕn′ĭk) [″ + *gennan,* to produce] Producing toxins or poisons.

toxigenicity (tŏks″ĭ-jĕn-ĭs′ĭ-tē) The virulence of a toxin-producing pathogenic organism.

toxin (tŏks′ĭn) [Gr. *toxikon,* poison] A poisonous substance of animal or plant origin. SEE: *antitoxin; hazardous material; health hazard; permissible exposure limits; phytotoxin; right-to-know law; toxoid.*

bacterial t. Poisons produced by bacteria that cause cell damage. They include exotoxins, such as those secreted by *Staphylococcus aureus* and *Corynebacterium diphtheriae,* and endotoxins, lipopolysaccharides in the cell walls of many gram-negative bacteria. Endotoxins continue to cause damage even after the bacteria are killed. SEE: *bacteria.*

botulinum t. type A A neuromuscular blocking drug used to paralyze muscles, esp. muscles in spasm. It is also used for cosmetic purposes, for example, by patients wanting to maintain a fixed facial appearance.

botulinus t. A neurotoxin that blocks acetylcholine release, produced by *Clostridium botulinum,* the causative organism for botulism. Seven types of the toxin have been identified.

dermonecrotic t. Any one of a group of different toxins that can cause necrosis of the skin. Coagulase-positive *Staphylococcus aureus* produce several such toxins. SYN: *exfoliative t.* SEE: *Kawasaki disease; scalded skin syndrome, staphylococcal; toxic shock syndrome.*

Dick t. An obsolete term for the streptococcal exotoxin that causes the fever and rash in scarlet fever. SYN: *erythrogenic t.*

diphtheria t. The specific toxin produced by *Corynebacterium diphtheriae.*

dysentery t. The exotoxin of various species of *Shigella.*

erythrogenic t. A poison, released by streptococci, associated with scarlet fever, impetigo, and poststreptococcal glomerulonephritis.

exfoliative t. Dermonecrotic toxin.

plant t. Any toxin produced by a plant; a phytotoxin.

Shiga t. An extremely poisonous compound secreted by certain enteric bacteria that causes hemorrhagic and necrotic colitis.

toxin-antitoxin (tŏks′ĭn-ăn″tĭ-tŏks′ĭn) [Gr. *toxikon,* poison, + *anti,* against, + *toxikon,* poison] ABBR: T.A.T. Diphtheria toxin with its antitoxin in a nearly neutral mixture, the diphtheria toxin being about 85% neutralized; used for immunization against diphtheria.

toxinicide (tŏks-ĭn′ĭs-īd) [″ + *cidus,* kill] That which is destructive to toxins.

toxinosis (tŏk″sĭ-nō′sĭs) [″ + Gr. *osis,* condition] Any disease or condition caused by a toxin.

toxipathy (tŏks-ĭp′ă-thē) [″ + Gr. *pathos,* disease, suffering] Any disease caused by poison.

toxiphobia (tŏks″ĭ-fō′bē-ă) [″ + Gr. *phobos,* fear] An abnormal fear of being poisoned.

toxisterol (tŏk-sĭs′tĕr-ŏl) A toxic derivative obtained by radiating ergosterol.

toxitherapy (tŏks″ĭ-thĕr′ă-pē) [″ + Gr. *therapeia,* treatment] The use of toxins in treatment of disease (e.g., the use of botulinum toxin injected locally to treat certain eye muscle imbalance conditions and to treat spasmodic torticollis).

toxituberculid (tŏks″ĭ-tū-bĕr′kū-lĭd) A skin lesion resulting from the action of a toxin produced by *Mycobacterium tuberculosis.*

toxo- SEE: *toxi-.*

toxocariasis (tŏks″ō-kār-ī′ă-sĭs) [″ + *kara,* head, + *-iasis,* condition] A self-limiting disease due to infection with nematode worms *Toxocara canis* or *T. cati.* In humans, the eggs penetrate the bowel wall and enter the circulation. Larvae may be carried to any part of the body where the blood vessel is large enough to accommodate them. They may end up in the brain, retinal vessels, liver, lung, or heart and produce myocarditis, endophthalmitis, epilepsy, or encephalitis. Diagnosis is made by immunological tests and by the presence of larvae in tissue obtained by liver biopsy. It is important that toxocariasis be considered in cases diagnosed as retinoblastoma. SYN: *visceral larva migrans.*

toxoid (tŏks′oyd) [″ + *eidos,* form, shape] A toxin that has been treated to destroy its toxicity but is still capable of inducing formation of antibodies on injection. SYN: *anatoxin.*

alum-precipitated t. Toxoid of diphtheria or tetanus precipitated with alum.

diphtheria t. Diphtheria toxin that has been altered so that it cannot cause disease but is still able to stimulate the production of antibodies (antitoxin) for active immunization; it is used in diphtheria-pertussis-tetanus vaccine.

toxolecithin (tŏks″ō-lĕs′ĭ-thĭn) [″ + *lekithos,* egg yolk] A compound of lecithin with a toxin such as certain snake venoms.

toxolysin (tŏks-ŏl′ĭ-sĭn) [″ + *lysis,* dissolution] A substance that destroys toxins. SYN: *antitoxin; toxicide.*

toxomucin (tŏks″ō-mū′sĭn) [″ + L. *mucus,* mucus] Specific toxic albuminoid from cultures of tubercle bacilli.

toxonosis (tŏks″ō-nō′sĭs) [″ + *osis,* condition] Toxicosis.

toxopeptone (tŏks″ō-pĕp′tōn) [″ + *pepton,* digesting] A protein derivative produced by action of a toxin on peptones.

toxophil(e) (tŏks′ō-fĭl, -fīl) [″ + *philein,* to love] Having a special affinity for toxins.

toxophilic (tŏk″sō-fĭl′ĭk) [″ + *philein,* to love] Concerning a toxophile.

toxophore (tŏks′ō-for) [″ + *phoros,* a bearer] The portion of a toxin that gives the toxin its poisonous qualities.

toxophorous (tŏk-sŏf′ō-rŭs) Concerning a toxophore.

toxophylaxin (tŏks″ō-fĭ-lăks′ĭn) [″ + *phylax,* guard] A substance that neutralizes bacterial toxins.

Toxoplasma (tŏks″ō-plăs′mă) A genus of protozoa.

T. gondii The causative agent of toxoplasmosis.

toxoplasmin (tŏk″sō-plăs′mĭn) An antigen obtained from mouse peritoneal fluid infected with *Toxoplasma gondii.*

toxoplasmosis (tŏks-ō-plăs-mō′sĭs) Infection with the protozoan *Toxoplasma gondii.* It usually is a recurrence of a mild infection that is subclinical in persons with normal immune systems; approx. 30% of the U.S. population have antibodies indicating they have been infected. In persons with acquired immunodeficiency syndrome (AIDS) or those receiving immunosuppressive therapy after an organ transplant, reactivation of dormant organisms may be fatal. Approx. 25% of women who become infected for the first time during pregnancy pass the infection on to the developing fetus.

ETIOLOGY/TRANSMISSION: *T. gondii* is carried by many mammals and birds, and is commonly transmitted to humans by inadequate handwashing after handling cat feces or by eating incompletely cooked pork or lamb. Once inside the intestines, the organism may spread via the blood to other organs. It is destroyed by T lymphocytes, which are not adequate in the fetus, people with AIDS, or patients receiving immunosuppressive therapy.

In 25% of fetuses, toxoplasmosis damages the heart, brain, and lungs. It also causes eye infection (chorioretinitis), which may produce blindness. In people with AIDS, toxoplasmosis is the most common cause of encephalitis; systemic disease also may occur. In immunosuppressed patients, the infection causes reactivation of latent infection in the transplanted organ. Toxoplasmosis is diagnosed by clinical presentation, brain biopsy, brain scans, and response to treatment.

SYMPTOMS: In healthy persons, primary infection may be indicated only by mild lymphadenopathy. AIDS patients with neurological involvement usually show confusion, weakness, focal neurological deficits, seizures, and decreased levels of consciousness; fever may be present.

TREATMENT: A combination of pyrimethamine, sulfadiazine, and leucovorin (folinic acid) is administered until 2 weeks after symptoms disappear; the latter helps prevent bone marrow depression. Prednisone is added to the regimen, for patients with toxoplasma meningitis or chorioretinitis. In persons with AIDS, trimethoprim/sulfamethoxazole is used for prophylaxis and sulfadiazine for suppressive therapy after acute infection. Infected pregnant women are treated with spiramycin to prevent placental infections.

Toynbee maneuver [Joseph Toynbee, Brit. physician, 1815–1866] Changing the pressure within the middle ear by swallowing or gently blowing while the nose is pinched closed and the mouth is tightly shut. This maneuver is used to "clear the ears" when quickly changing altitude, as in an airplane flight.

In some cases, the effect of this maneuver may be enhanced by tilting the head backward while it is done. This places tension on the tensor tympani muscle and opens the eustachian tubes. SEE: *Valsalva's maneuver*.

TPA *total parenteral alimentation; tissue plasminogen activator.*

T.P.I. test *Treponema pallidum immobilizing test* (for syphilis).

TPN *triphosphopyridine nucleotide; total parenteral nutrition.*

TPR *temperature, pulse, respiration.*

tr L. *tinctura,* tincture.

trabecula (tră-bĕk′ū-lă) *pl.* **trabeculae** [L., a little beam] **1.** A cord of tissue that serves as a supporting structure by forming a septum that extends into an organ from its wall or capsule. **2.** The network of osseous tissue that makes up the cancellous structure of a bone.

t. carnea cordis Any of the thick muscular tissue bands attached to the inner walls of the ventricles of the heart. SYN: *columna carnea.*

trabecular (tră-bĕk′ū-lăr) Concerning a trabecula.

trabeculate (tră-bĕk′ū-lāt) Having trabeculae.

trabeculoplasty Surgical procedure on the trabecular meshwork of the eye. This procedure is used to allow the escape of aqueous humor in the treatment of glaucoma. SEE: *glaucoma.*

trace (trās) [O.Fr. *tracier*] **1.** A very small quantity. **2.** A visible mark or sign.

primitive t. SYN: *primitive streak.*

trace element An essential element required in only very small amounts for normal function (chromium, cobalt, copper, fluoride, iodine, magnesium, manganese, selenium, and zinc).

tracer A radioactive isotope, capable of being incorporated into compounds, that when introduced into the body "tags" a specific portion of the molecule so that its course may be traced. This is used in absorption and excretion studies, in identification of intermediary products of metabolism, and in determination of distribution of various substances in the body. Radioactive carbon (^{14}C), calcium (^{42}Ca), and iodine (^{131}I) are examples of tracers commonly used. SEE: *label.*

trachea (trā′kē-ă) *pl.* **tracheae** [Gr. *tracheia,* rough] A cylindrical cartilaginous tube, 4½ in. (11.3 cm) long, from the larynx to the primary bronchi. It extends from the sixth cervical to the fifth thoracic vertebra, where it divides at a point called the carina into two bronchi, one leading to each lung. The mucosa is made of ciliated epithelium that sweeps mucus, trapped dust, and pathogens upward. SYN: *windpipe.* SEE: *bronchi.*

tracheaectasy (trā″kē-ă-ĕk′tă-sē) [Gr. *tracheia,* rough, + *ektasis,* dilatation] Dilatation of the trachea.

tracheal (trā′kē-ăl) Pert. to the trachea.

trachealgia (trā″kē-ăl′jē-ă) [″ + *algos,* pain] Pain in the trachea.

trachealis (trā″kē-ā′lĭs) [L.] A muscle composed of smooth muscle fibers that extends between the ends of the tracheal rings. Its contraction reduces the size of the lumen.

tracheal tickle A maneuver designed to elicit a reflex cough.

tracheal tugging A slight downward movement of the trachea with each inspiratory effort, resulting from descent of the diaphragm in a person with a low, flat diaphragm. This sign may also be present as a result of the proximity of an aortic aneurysm to the trachea. It should not be confused with the pulsations from a normal vessel beneath the trachea.

tracheitis (trā″kē-ī′tĭs) [Gr. *tracheia,* rough, + *itis,* inflammation] An inflammation of the trachea most often caused by infection. It may be acute or chronic and may be associated with bronchitis and laryngitis. SYN: *trachitis*.

TREATMENT: Cool mist and hydration are useful in more severe cases. Patients must be monitored for signs of airway obstruction. Antibiotics are given when bacterial infection is the cause.

PATIENT CARE: Vital signs are monitored, and the patient is assessed for fever and acute airway obstruction (croupy cough, stridor) due to the presence of inflammation and thick secretions. Humidified oxygen is administered as prescribed, and suctioning is performed as necessary to remove secretions. Antibiotics are administered as prescribed if disease-causing bacteria are present in cultures or Gram stains. If airway obstruction persists and results in respiratory failure, emergency endotracheal intubation or tracheostomy is performed. The patient is comforted to reduce anxiety.

trachelectomopexy (trā″kē-lĕk′tŏm-ō-pĕk″sē) [″ + *ektome*, excision, + *pexis*, fixation] Fixation of the uterine neck with partial excision.

trachelectomy (trā″kĕl-ĕk′tō-mē) [″ + *ektome*, excision] Amputation of the cervix uteri.

trachelematoma (trā″kĕl-ĕm″ă-tō′mă) [″ + *haima*, blood, + *oma*, tumor] A hematoma situated on the neck.

trachelism, trachelismus (trā′kĕ-lĭzm, trā-kĕ-lĭz′mŭs) [″ + *-ismos*, condition] Backward spasm of the neck, sometimes preceding an epileptic attack.

trachelitis (trā-kĕ-lī′tĭs) [″ + *itis*, inflammation] Inflammation of the mucous membrane of the cervix uteri. SYN: *cervicitis*.

trachelo- Combining form meaning *neck*.

trachelobregmatic (trā″kĕ-lō-brĕg-măt′ĭk) [Gr. *trachelos*, neck, + *bregma*, front of the head] Pert. to the neck and the bregma.

trachelocele (trăk′ĕ-lō-sēl) [″ + *kele*, tumor, swelling] Tracheocele.

trachelocyrtosis (trā″kĕ-lō-sĭr-tō′sĭs) [″ + *kyrtos*, curved, + *osis*, condition] Trachelokyphosis.

trachelocystitis (trā″kĕl-ō-sĭs-tī′tĭs) [″ + *kystis*, bladder, + *itis*, inflammation] Inflammation of the neck of the bladder.

trachelodynia (trā″kĕ-lō-dĭn′ē-ă) [″+ *odyne*, pain] Pain in the neck.

trachelokyphosis (trā″kĕl-ō-kī-fō′sĭs) [″ + *kyphosis*, humpback] Excessive anterior curvature of the cervical portion of the spine. SYN: *trachelocyrtosis*.

trachelology (trā″kĕ-lŏl′ō-jē) [″ + *logos*, word, reason] Scientific study of the neck, its diseases, and its injuries.

trachelomastoid (trā″kĕ-lō-măs′toyd) [″ + *mastos*, breast, + *eidos*, form, shape] A muscle of the neck.

trachelomyitis (trā″kĕ-lō-mī-ī′tĭs) [″ + *mys*, muscle,+ *itis*, inflammation] Inflammation of the muscles of the neck.

trachelopexy (trā′kĕl-ō-pĕks″ē) [″ + *pexis*, fixation] Surgical fixation of the cervix uteri to an adjacent part.

tracheloplasty (trā′kĕl-ō-plăs″tē) [″ + *plassein*, to form] Surgical repair or plastic surgery of the neck of the uterus.

trachelorrhaphy (trā″kĕl-or′ă-fē) [″ + *rhaphe*, seam, ridge] Suturing of a torn cervix uteri.

tracheloschisis (trā″kĕ-lŏs′kĭ-sĭs) [″ + *schisis*, a splitting] Congenital opening or fissure in the neck.

trachelotomy (trā″kĕl-ŏt′ō-mē) [″ + *tome*, incision] Incision of the cervix of the uterus.

tracheo- Combining form meaning *trachea, windpipe*.

tracheoaerocele (trā″kē-ō-ĕr′ō-sēl) [Gr. *tracheia*, rough, + *aer*, air, + *kele*, tumor, swelling] Hernia or cyst of the trachea containing air.

tracheobronchial (trā″kē-ō-brŏng′kē-ăl) Concerning the trachea and bronchus.

tracheobronchomegaly (trā″kē-ō-brŏng″kō-mĕg′ă-lē) Congenitally enlarged size of the trachea and bronchi.

tracheobronchoscopy (trā″kē-ō-brŏng-kŏs′kō-pē) [″ + *bronchos*, windpipe, + *skopein*, to examine] Inspection of the trachea and bronchi through a bronchoscope.

tracheocele (trā′kē-ō-sēl) [″ + *kele*, hernia] Protrusion of mucous membrane through the wall of the trachea. SYN: *trachelocele*.

tracheoesophageal (trā″kē-ō-ē-sŏf″ă-jē′ăl) [″ + *oisophagos*, esophagus] Pert. to the trachea and esophagus.

tracheolaryngeal (trā″kē-ō-lăr-rĭn′jē-ăl) Concerning the trachea and larynx.

tracheolaryngotomy (trā″kē-ō-lăr″ĭn-gŏt′ō-mē) [″ + *larynx*, larynx, + *tome*, incision] Incision into the larynx and trachea.

tracheomalacia (trā″kē-ō-mă-lā′shē-ă) Softening of the tracheal cartilage. It may be caused by pressure of the left pulmonary artery on the trachea.

tracheopathia, tracheopathy (trā″kē-ō-păth′ē-ă, -ŏp′ă-thē) [″ + *pathos*, disease, suffering] A disease of the trachea.

tracheopharyngeal (trā″kē-ō-făr-ĭn′jē-ăl) [″ + *pharynx*, throat] Pert. to both the trachea and the pharynx.

tracheophony (trā″kē-ŏf′ō-nē) [″ + *phone*, a sound] The sound heard over the trachea in auscultation.

tracheoplasty (trā′kē-ō-plăs″tē) [″ + *plassein*, to form] Plastic operation on the trachea.

tracheopyosis (trā″kē-ō-pī-ō′sĭs) [″ + *pyon*, pus, + *osis*, condition] Tracheitis with suppuration.

tracheorrhagia (trā″kē-ō-rā′jē-ă) [Gr.

tracheia, rough, + *rhegnynai,* to burst forth] Tracheal hemorrhage.

tracheoschisis (trā″kē-ŏs′kĭs-ĭs) [″ + *schisis,* a splitting] A fissure of the trachea.

tracheoscopy (trā″kē-ŏs′kō-pē) [″ + *skopein,* to examine] Inspection of the interior of the trachea by means of reflected light.

tracheostenosis (trā″kē-ō-stĕn-ō′sĭs) [″ + *stenosis,* act of narrowing] Contraction or narrowing of the lumen of the trachea.

tracheostoma (trā″kē-ŏs′tō-mă) Opening into the trachea, via the neck.

tracheostomize (trā″kē-ŏs′tō-mīz) To perform a tracheostomy.

tracheostomy (trā″kē-ŏs′tō-mē) [″ + *stoma,* mouth] The surgical opening of the trachea to provide and secure an open airway. This procedure may be performed in emergency situations (e.g., when there is upper airway obstruction) or electively to replace a temporary airway provided by an endotracheal tube that has been in place for more than several weeks. SEE: illus.; *tube, endotracheal.*

CAUTION: To avoid injury to the structures of the neck, tracheostomy should be performed only by skilled or well-trained health care professionals.

PATIENT CARE: Vital signs are monitored frequently after surgery. Warm, humidified oxygen is administered. The patient is placed in the semi-Fowler position to promote ease of breathing. A restful environment is provided. Communication is established by questions with simple yes and no answers, hand signals, and simple sign language and with use of a "magic slate" or an alphabet board for writing. (Written communication requires vision, hand strength, and dexterity and is often difficult or impossible for acutely ill patients.) Later, the patient is taught how to cover the tracheostomy with the cuff deflated to permit vocalization. The nurse should be alert to the patient's unmet needs and assist with these to prevent increased anxiety. Chest physiotherapy promotes aeration of the lung. Suctioning of secretions and tracheostomy care are provided as necessary. Dressing is changed frequently during the first 24 hr postoperatively, and the surgical site is observed for excessive bleeding. Coughing and deep breathing are encouraged at regular intervals. A teaching plan should cover stoma care, which includes cleansing, removing crusts, and filtering air with a suitable filter. The patient and his or her health care team should be alert for signs of infection. The patient should avoid smoking.

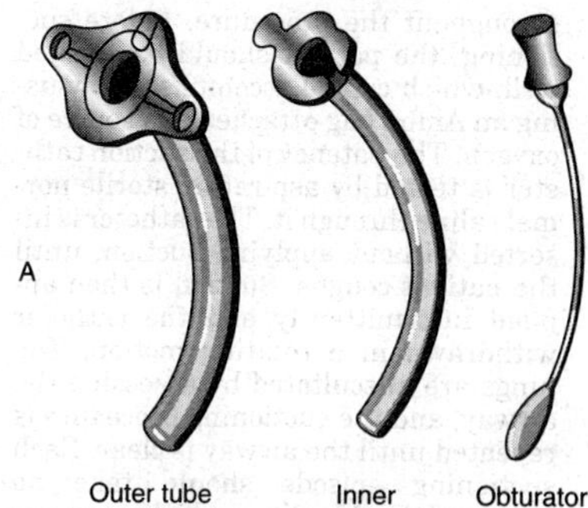

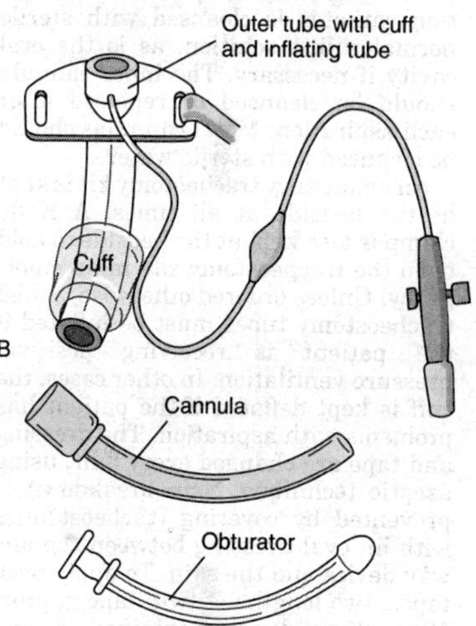

TRACHEOSTOMY TUBE

(A) Metal tube, (B) Cuffed plastic tube

Activities may be gradually increased to include noncontact sports but should not include swimming. Showering may be permitted if the patient wears a protective plastic bib or uses the hand to cover the stoma. The patient should be reassured that secretions will decrease and that taste and smell will gradually return. The importance of follow-up care with an ear, nose, and throat specialist is stressed.

mini-t. Placement of a 4 mm (about 1/6th of an inch) cannula through an incision made through the cricothyroid membrane into the trachea. This is done using local anesthesia. This type of tracheostomy is esp. useful in removing sputum retained in the tracheobronchial tree.

tracheostomy care Management of the tracheostomy wound and the airway device. The patient should be suctioned as often as necessary to remove secretions. Sterile technique is maintained throughout the procedure. Before suctioning, the patient should be aerated well, which can be accomplished by using an Ambu bag attached to a source of oxygen. The patency of the suction catheter is tested by aspirating sterile normal saline through it. The catheter is inserted without applying suction, until the patient coughs. Suction is then applied intermittently and the catheter withdrawn in a rotating motion. The lungs are auscultated by assessing the airway, and the suctioning procedure is repeated until the airway is clear. Each suctioning episode should take no longer than 15 sec, and the patient should be allowed to rest and breathe between suctioning episodes. The suction catheter is cleansed with sterile normal saline solution, as is the oral cavity if necessary. The inner cannula should be cleansed or replaced after each aspiration. Metal cannulas should be cleansed with sterile water.

An emergency tracheotomy kit is kept at the bedside at all times. A Kelly clamp is also kept at the bedside to hold open the tracheostomy site in an emergency. Unless ordered otherwise, cuffed tracheostomy tubes must be inflated if the patient is receiving positive-pressure ventilation. In other cases, the cuff is kept deflated if the patient has problems with aspiration. The dressing and tape are changed every 8 hr, using aseptic technique. Skin breakdown is prevented by covering tracheostomies with an oval dressing between the airway device and the skin. To apply neck tapes, two lengths of twill tape approx. 10 in. (25 cm) long are obtained; the end of each is folded and a slit is made 0.5 in. (1.3 cm) long about 1 in. (2.5 cm) from the fold. The slit end is slipped under the neck plate and the other end of the tape pulled through the slit. This is repeated for the other side. The tape is wrapped around the neck and secured with a square knot on the side. Neck tapes should be left in place until new tapes are attached. Tracheal secretions are cultured as ordered; their color, viscosity, amount, and abnormal odor, if any, are observed. The site is inspected daily for bleeding, hematoma formation, subcutaneous emphysema, and signs of infection. Appropriate skin care is provided. The medical care team should help alleviate the patient's anxiety and apprehension and communicate openly with the patient. The patient's response is documented.

tracheotome (trā′kē-ō-tōm) [″ + *tome,* incision] An instrument used to open the trachea.

tracheotomy (trā″kē-ŏt′ō-mē) Incision of the trachea through the skin and muscles of the neck overlying the trachea. SEE: *tracheostomy.*

trachitis (trā-kī′tĭs) [″ + *itis,* inflammation] Tracheitis.

trachoma (trā-kō′mă) [Gr., roughness] A chronic, contagious form of conjunctivitis that is one of the leading causes of blindness in the world. It is caused by *Chlamydia trachomatis,* which is endemic in Africa, India, and the Middle East and is seen also in the southwestern U.S. The disease is transmitted by flies, clothing, bedding, and hands contaminated by exudate. Over time, the inflammation is followed by scarring, which causes the cornea to become opaque. SYN: *Egyptian ophthalmia; granular conjunctivitis.* SEE: *Standard and Universal Precautions Appendix.*

Trachoma is treated with oral tetracycline or sulfonamides for 3 to 6 weeks, but reinfection in endemic areas is common. Surgery may be necessary when lid deformities occur.

brawny t. Trachoma with general lymphoid infiltration without granulation of the conjunctiva.

t. deformans Trachoma with scarring.

diffuse t. Trachoma with large granulations.

trachomatous (trăk-ō′mă-tŭs) Concerning trachoma.

trachychromatic (trā″kĭ-krō-măt′ĭk) [Gr. *trachys,* rough, + *chroma,* color] Pert. to a nucleus with very deeply staining chromatin.

trachyphonia (trā″kĭ-fō′nē-ă) [″ + *phone,* voice] Roughness or hoarseness of the voice.

tracing (trā′sĭng) **1.** A graphic record of some event that changes with time such as respiratory movements or electrical activity of the heart or brain. **2.** In dentistry, a graphic display of movements of the mandible.

contact t. An attempt to find the source of an infectious or toxic outbreak, typically through patient interviews and laboratory specimens.

tract (trăkt) [L. *tractus,* extent] **1.** A course or pathway. **2.** A group or bundle of nerve fibers within the spinal cord or brain that constitutes an anatomical and functional unit. SEE: *fasciculus.* **3.** A group of organs or parts forming a continuous pathway.

aerodigestive t. The anatomic region in the oral cavity and throat through which both air and food pass.

afferent t. Ascending t.

alimentary t. The canal or passage from the mouth to the anus. SYN: *digestive t.*

ascending t. White fibers in the spinal cord that carry nerve impulses toward the brain. SYN: *afferent t.*

biliary t. The organs and ducts that participate in the secretion, storage, and delivery of bile into the duodenum. SEE: illus.; *bile ducts; gallbladder; liver.*

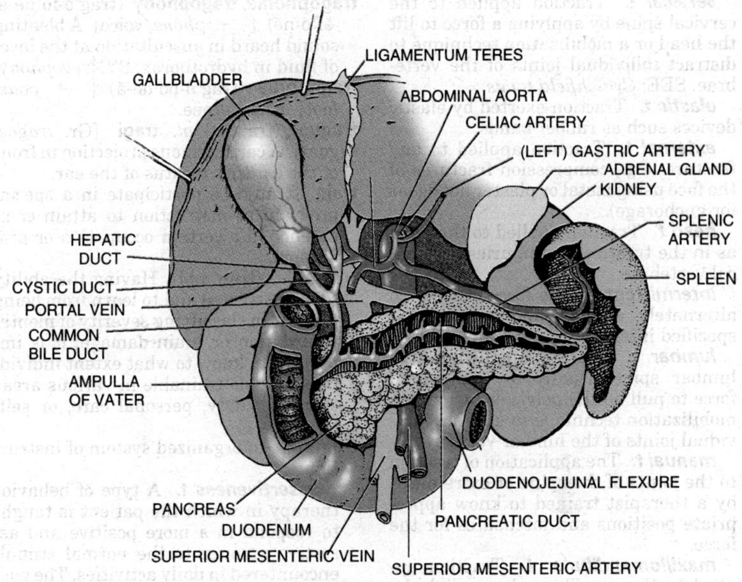

BILIARY TRACT (IN RELATION TO LIVER, PANCREAS, AND DUODENUM)

corticospinal t. Pyramidal t.

descending t. White fibers in the spinal cord that carry nerve impulses from the brain.

digestive t. Alimentary t.

dorsolateral t. A spinal cord tract superficial to the tip of the dorsal horn. It is made up of short pain and temperature fibers that are processes of neurons having their cell bodies in the dorsal root ganglion.

extrapyramidal t. SEE: *extrapyramidal motor s.*

gastrointestinal t. The stomach and intestines.

genitourinary t. The genital and urinary pathways.

iliotibial t. A thickened area of fascia lata extending from the lateral condyle of the tibia to the iliac crest.

intestinal t. The small and large intestines.

motor t. A descending pathway that conveys motor impulses from the brain to the lower portions of the spinal cord.

olfactory t. A narrow white band that extends from the olfactory bulb to the anterior perforated substance of the brain.

optic t. Fibers of the optic nerve that continue beyond the optic chiasma, most of which terminate in the lateral geniculate body of the thalamus. Some continue to the superior colliculus of the midbrain; others enter the hypothalamus and terminate in the supraoptic and medial nuclei.

pyramidal t. One of three descending tracts (lateral, ventral, ventrolateral) of the spinal cord. The tract consists of fibers arising from the giant pyramidal cells of Betz present in the motor area of the cerebral cortex. SYN: *corticospinal tract.*

respiratory t. The respiratory organs in continuity.

rubrospinal t. A descending tract of fibers arising from cell bodies located in the red nucleus of the midbrain. Fibers terminate in the gray matter of the spinal cord.

supraopticohypophyseal t. A tract consisting of fibers arising from cell bodies located in supraoptic and paraventricular nuclei of the hypothalamus and terminating in the posterior lobe of the hypophysis.

urinary t. The urinary passageway from the kidney to the outside of the body, including the pelvis of the kidney, ureter, bladder, and urethra.

uveal t. The vascular and pigmented tissues that constitute the middle coat of the eye, including the iris, ciliary body, and choroid.

tractellum (trăk-těl′ŭm) [L.] An anterior flagellum of a protozoan. It propels the cell by traction.

traction (trăk′shŭn) [L. *tractio*] The process of drawing or pulling. SEE: *Nursing Diagnoses Appendix.*

axis t. Traction in line with the long axis of a course through which a body is to be drawn.

cervical t. Traction applied to the cervical spine by applying a force to lift the head or a mobilization technique to distract individual joints of the vertebrae. SEE: *Crutchfield tongs*.

elastic t. Traction exerted by elastic devices such as rubber bands.

external t. Traction applied to any fracture (e.g., compression fractures of the face using metal or plaster headgear for anchorage).

head t. Traction applied to the head as in the treatment of injuries to cervical vertebrae.

intermittent t. The force of traction alternately applied and released at specified intervals.

lumbar t. Traction applied to the lumbar spine usually by applying a force to pull on the pelvis or by using a mobilization technique to distract individual joints of the lumbar vertebrae.

manual t. The application of traction to the joints of the spine or extremities by a therapist trained to know appropriate positions and intensities for the force.

maxillomandibular t. Traction applied to the maxilla and mandible by means of elastic or wire ligatures and interdental wiring or splints.

mechanical t. The use of a device or mechanical linkage (i.e., pulleys and weights) to apply a traction force.

sustained t. The application of a constant traction force up to ½ hr.

weight t. Traction exerted by means of weights.

tractor (trăk'tor) [L., drawer] Any device or instrument for applying traction.

tractotomy (trăk-tŏt'ō-mē) Surgical section of a fiber tract of the central nervous system. It is sometimes used for relief of intractable pain.

tractus (trăk'tŭs) *pl.* **tractus** [L.] A tract or path.

tragacanth (trăg'ă-kănth) [Gr. *tragakantha,* a goat thorn] The dried gummy exudation from the plant *Astragalus gummifer* and related species, grown in Asia. It is used in the form of mucilage, as a greaseless lubricant, and as an application for chapped skin.

tragal (trā'găl) [Gr. *tragos,* goat] Relating to the tragus.

Trager work (trā-gĕr) [Milton Trager, American physician] A form of massage therapy that involves rhythmic manipulations of the body, combined with mental gymnastics.

tragi (trā'jī) Pl. of tragus.

tragicus (trăj'ĭk-ŭs) [L.] The muscle on the outer surface of the tragus.

tragion (trăj'ē-ŏn) An anthropometric point at the upper margin of the tragus of the ear.

tragomaschalia (trăg"ō-măs-kāl'ē-ă) [Gr. *tragos,* goat, + *maschale,* the armpit] Odorous perspiration (bromidrosis) of the axilla.

tragophonia, tragophony (trăg"ō-fō'nē-ă, -ŏf'ō-nē) [" + *phone,* voice] A bleating sound heard in auscultation at the level of fluid in hydrothorax. SYN: *egophony*.

tragopodia (trăg"ō-pō'dē-ă) [" + *pous,* foot] Knock-knee.

tragus (trā'gŭs) *pl.* **tragi** [Gr. *tragos,* goat] A cartilaginous projection in front of the exterior meatus of the ear.

train (trān) To participate in a special program of instruction to attain competence in a certain occupation or profession.

trainable (trān'ă-bl) Having the ability to be instructed and to learn from being taught. In classifying severity of mental retardation or brain damage, it is important to know to what extent individuals may be trainable in various areas such as safety, personal care, or self-feeding.

training An organized system of instruction.

assertiveness t. A type of behavior therapy in which the patient is taught to respond in a more positive and assertive manner to the normal stimuli encountered in daily activities. The goal is to be able to express one's true feelings, positive or negative. Role playing in group therapy may be used to teach this to patients.

athletic t. **1.** The physical and mental conditioning program used by athletes to increase their proficiency in sports. **2.** Performing the tasks that an athletic trainer is prepared to do. SEE: *athletic trainer*.

aversive t. Aversion therapy.

habit t. The development in young children of specific behavior patterns for performing basic activities such as eating, dressing, using the toilet, and sleeping.

in-service t. Clinical education designed to inform and update staff about important ongoing projects, technologies, and therapeutic agents.

social skills t. The components of rehabilitation programs that focus on the skills necessary for effective interaction with other people.

trait (trāt) A distinguishing feature; a characteristic or property of an individual.

acquired t. A trait that is not inherited; one resulting from the effects of the environment.

inherited t. A trait due to genes transmitted through germ cells.

personality t. An enduring pattern of perceiving, communicating, and thinking about oneself, others, and the environment that is exhibited in multiple contexts. SEE: *personality disorder*.

sickle cell t. The condition of being heterozygous with respect to hemoglobin S, the gene responsible for sickle cell anemia. In people with sickle cell trait each red blood cell has one copy each of hemoglobin A and hemoglobin S. These cells will not become sickled until extremely low concentrations of oxygen occur. SEE: *hemoglobin S disease*.

trajector (tră-jĕk′tor) [L. *trajectus,* thrown across] A device for determining the approximate location of a bullet in a wound.

trance (trăns) [L. *transitus,* a passing over] A sleeplike state, as in deep hypnosis, appearing also in hysteria and in some spiritualistic mediums, with limited sensory and motor contact with the ordinary surroundings, and with subsequent amnesia of what has occurred during the state.

death t. A trance simulating death.

induced t. A trance caused by some external event such as hypnosis.

tranexamic acid An antifibrinolytic drug that is approximately 10 times as potent and with more sustained activity than aminocaproic acid. It is used to decrease bleeding time during surgical procedures. Loss of blood is decreased when this drug is used.

tranquilizer (trăn″kwĭ-līz′ĕr) [L. *tranquillus,* calm] A drug that reduces tension and anxiety. The minor tranquilizers include antihistamines (e.g., hydroxyzine), buspirone, and benzodiazepines (e.g., diazepam or alprazolam). The benzodiazepines decrease anxiety, provide sedation, and may cause dependence, tolerance, or addiction. The major tranquilizers include neuroleptic drugs such as haloperidol, fluphenazine, or risperidone. They are used to treat psychotic symptoms, such as delusions, hallucinations, and catatonia, and to manage psychotic disorders, such as schizophrenia. A prominent delayed side effect of many neuroleptic agents is the movement disorder known as tardive dyskinesia.

CAUTION: Some tranquilizers may injure the developing embryo. Therefore, before prescribing one, one should know whether it is approved for use during pregnancy, esp. early pregnancy.

---

trans- [L.] Prefix meaning *across, over, beyond, through.*

transabdominal (trăns″ăb-dŏm′ĭ-năl) Through, into, or across the abdomen or abdominal wall.

transacetylation (trăns-ăs″ĕ-tĭl-ā′shŭn) Transfer of an acetyl group (CH_3CO—) in a chemical reaction.

transaction The interaction of a person with others.

transactional analysis Psychotherapy involving role playing in an attempt to understand the relationship between the patient and the therapist and eventually that between the patient and reality.

transamidination (trăns-ăm″ĭ-dĭn-ā′shŭn) The transfer of an amidine group from one amino acid to another.

transaminase (trăns-ăm′ĭn-ās) The old term for aminotransferase.

glutamic-oxaloacetic t. Aspartate aminotransferase

glutamic-pyruvic t. Alanine aminotransferase.

transamination (trăns″ăm-ĭ-nā′shŭn) The transfer of an amino group from one compound to another or the transposition of an amino group within a single compound.

transaortic (trăns″ā-or′tĭk) Done through the aorta (e.g., a surgical procedure).

transatrial (trăns-ā′trē-ăl) Done through the atrium (e.g., a surgical procedure).

transaudient (trăns-aw′dē-ĕnt) [″ + *audire,* to hear] Permeable to sound waves.

transaxial (trăns-ăk′sē-ăl) Across the long axis of a structure or part.

transbronchial Across the bronchi or the bronchial wall.

transcalent (trăns-kā′lĕnt) [″ + *calere,* to be hot] Permeable by heat rays. SYN: *diathermal.*

transcapillary (trăns″kăp′ĭl-lă-rē) [″ + *capillaris,* relating to hair] Across the endothelial wall of a capillary.

transcapillary exchange The passage of substances between blood and tissue (interstitial) fluid.

transcervical (trăns-sĕr′vĭ-kăl) Done through the cervical os of the uterus.

transcortical (trăns-kor′tĭ-kăl) Joining two parts of the cerebral cortex.

transcortin (trăns-kor′tĭn) A corticosteroid-binding globulin.

transcriptase (trăns-krĭp′tās) A polymerase enzyme that constructs a messenger RNA molecule that is a complementary copy of the base sequence on a DNA gene. SYN: *RNA polymerase.*

transcription (trăn-skrĭp′shŭn) The first step in protein synthesis, the synthesis of a messenger RNA (mRNA) molecule that is a complementary copy of a DNA gene. This takes place in the nucleus of the cell; the mRNA then travels to the ribosomes in the cytoplasm, the site of protein synthesis.

transcutaneous Percutaneous.

transcutaneous electrical nerve stimulation ABBR: TENS. The application of mild electrical stimulation to skin electrodes placed over a painful area. It alleviates pain by interfering with transmission of painful stimuli.

transcutaneous oxygen monitoring Oximetry.

transdermal infusion system A method of delivering medicine by placing it in a special gel-like matrix that is applied to the skin. The medicine is absorbed through the skin at a fixed rate. Each application will provide medicine for from one to several days. Nitroglycerin and scopolamine are examples of medicines that have been prepared for use in this type of system. Also called *transdermal drug-delivery system.*

transducer (trăns-dū'sĕr) [L. *trans,* across, + *ducere,* to lead] A device that converts one form of energy to another. The telephone is an example. It is used in medical electronics to receive the energy produced by sound or pressure and relay it as an electrical impulse to another transducer, which can either convert the energy back into its original form or produce a record of it on a recording device.

ultrasonic t. A device used in ultrasound that sends and receives the sound wave signal.

transduction (trăns-dŭk'shŭn) A phenomenon causing genetic recombination in bacteria in which DNA is carried from one bacterium to another by a bacteriophage. SEE: *transformation.*

signal t. Biochemical conversions that is part of a process, such as the docking of hormones to receptor stimulating cellular production of specific enzymes or other proteins.

transection, transsection (trăn-sĕk'shŭn, trăns-sĕk'shŭn) [" + *sectio,* cutting] A cutting made across a long axis; a cross section.

trans fatty acid SEE: under *fatty acid.*

transfection (trans-fĕk'shŭn) The infection of bacteria by purified phage DNA.

transfer, transference (trăns'fer, trăns-fĕr'ĕns) [" + *ferre,* to bear] **1.** The mental process whereby a person transfers patterns of feelings and behavior that had previously been experienced with important figures such as parents or siblings to another person. Quite often these feelings are shifted to the caregiver. **2.** The state in which the symptoms of one area are transmitted to a similar area.

blastocyst t. An assisted reproduction technique in which a zygote created by in vitro fertilization is incubated in the laboratory to the pre-embryonic stage of the blastocyst before being placed in the uterus.

egg t. Transfer of eggs retrieved from ovarian follicles into the fallopian tubes. SEE: *gamete intrafallopian transfer.*

embryo t. An assisted reproduction technique in which eggs fertilized in the laboratory are deposited in the fallopian tubes surgically or by catheterization. SEE: *gamete intrafallopian transfer; in vitro fertilization.*

somatic cell nuclear t. In cloning, the transfer of genetic material from a differentiated, adult cell into an egg.

zygote intrafallopian t. ABBR: ZIFT. An in vitro fertilization technique in which a woman's ova are surgically removed and mixed with her partner's sperm. The resulting zygotes are placed in her fallopian tube. SEE: *embryo transfer; fertilization, in vitro; GIFT.*

transferase (trăns'fĕr-ās) An enzyme that catalyzes the transfer of atoms or groups of atoms from one chemical compound to another.

gamma glutamyl t. ABBR: GGT. An enzyme present in the liver and biliary tree that is used to diagnose liver, gallbladder, and pancreatic diseases. Elevated levels of GGT are often found in people who use drugs (such as alcohol) that are metabolized by the liver.

transfer board A device used to bridge the space between a wheelchair and a bed, toilet, or car seat. It is used to facilitate independent or assisted transferring of the patient from one of these sites to another. It is also called a *sliding board.*

transfer factor In immunology, a factor present in lymphocytes that have been sensitized to antigens, which can, in humans, be transferred to a nonsensitized recipient. As a result of this transfer, the recipient will react to the same antigen that was originally used to sensitize the lymphocytes of the donor. In humans, the factor can be transferred by injecting the recipient with either intact lymphocytes or extracts of disrupted cells.

transferrin (trăns-fĕr'rĭn) A globulin that binds and transports iron.

carbohydrate-deficient t. A globulin used imperfectly as a marker for alcohol abuse. The compound is elevated in some chronic heavy drinkers, but not in most nondrinkers.

transferring The act of moving a person with limited function from one location to another. This may be accomplished by the patient or with assistance.

transfix (trăns-fĭks') [" + *figere,* to fix] To pierce through or impale with a sharp instrument.

transfixion (trăns-fĭk'shŭn) A maneuver in performing an amputation in which a knife is passed into the soft parts and cutting is from within outward.

transforation (trăns"for-ā'shŭn) [" + *forare,* to pierce] The perforation of the fetal skull at the base in craniotomy.

transforator (trăns'for-ā"tor) An instrument for perforating the fetal skull.

transformation (trăns"for-mā'shŭn) [" + *formatio,* a forming] **1.** Change of shape or form. **2.** In oncology, the change of one tissue into another. SEE: *metastasis.* **3.** In bacterial genetics, the acquisition of bacterial DNA fragments by other bacterial cells; antibiotic resistance is often acquired this way.

transformer (trăns-form'er) [" + *formare,* to form] A stationary induction apparatus to change electrical energy at one voltage and current to electrical energy at another voltage and current through the medium of magnetic energy, without mechanical motion.

step-down t. A transformer that changes electricity to a lower voltage.

step-up t. A transformer that changes electricity to a higher voltage.

transfuse To infuse blood or blood products.

transfusion (trăns-fū′zhŭn) [″ + *fusio*, a pouring] **1.** The collection of blood or a blood component from a donor followed by its infusion into a recipient. In the U.S. in 1998, more than 12 million blood products were transfused. SEE: *blood transfusion; intraosseous infusion.* **2.** The injection of saline or other solutions into a vein for a therapeutic purpose.

autologous blood t. A procedure for collecting and storing a patient's own blood several weeks before its anticipated need by the patient. Alternatively, blood lost during a surgical procedure can be recovered from the operation site and processed for transfusion. This method of providing blood for an individual is used to prevent the transmission of disease that can occur with the use of donor blood. SEE: *blood doping; blood transfusion.*

cadaver blood t. A transfusion using blood obtained from a cadaver within a short time after death.

direct t. The transfer of blood directly from one person to another.

exchange t. The removal of a patient's blood (e.g., in sickle cell disease, thrombotic thrombocytopenic purpura, hemolytic disease of the newborn, and other illnesses) and its replacement with blood donated by others. SYN: *replacement t.*

indirect t. A transfusion of blood from a donor to a suitable storage container and then to the patient.

replacement t. Exchange t.

single unit t. The infusion of one unit of packed red blood cells.

transfusion reaction An adverse response to a transfusion caused by the presence of foreign antigens, antibodies, or cytokines. There are three basic types of true transfusion reactions, and several other complications of transfusion therapy.

Hemolytic reactions (type II hypersensitivity reactions) occur when ABO-incompatible blood is given; antibodies or complement, or both, coat blood cells, stimulating their destruction (hemolysis) by macrophages and neutrophils. These reactions occur in fewer than 1% of all blood transfusions. In acute hemolytic reactions, patients develop fever, chills, nausea, flank pain, hypotension, flushing, and hematuria within 20 min after the transfusion has begun. Delayed reactions develop 3 to 14 days later; the patient presents with fever, jaundice, and a decreased hemoglobin level. In rare cases, disseminated intravascular coagulopathy, respiratory distress syndrome, acute renal tubular necrosis, and/or death may occur.

Allergic reactions occur when patients have been sensitized to foreign antigens on proteins in the blood or plasma. A history of allergies is usually present, indicating the patient has developed immunoglobulin E antibodies to allergens. Patients develop itching and hives. Mild allergic reactions can be prevented or treated with antihistamines; the use of washed red blood cells (RBCs), which have fewer antigens, also reduces the risk of allergic reactions. Very rarely, systemic anaphylaxis occurs, as indicated by severe hypotension, and wheezing.

Febrile reactions are the result of cytokine release by leukocytes while the blood was being stored. Antipyretics are used to treat the transient fever that appears; the use of fresh blood and leukocyte-poor RBC transfusion also reduces the risk of a febrile response.

Other problems associated with blood transfusions include circulatory overload in patients with heart disease, and the transmission of infectious organisms and graft-versus-host disease, esp. in patients with immunological deficits. The ability to screen blood for antibodies to hepatitis and human immunodeficiency virus has decreased the risk of acquiring these diseases through blood transfusion; however, malaria and bacterial infections can still occasionally be transmitted if the donor is asymptomatic. The acute pulmonary edema that develops from circulatory overload can be diagnosed through the presence of rales on auscultation of the chest, severe difficulty breathing, frothy sputum, decreased oxygen saturation, and abnormal findings on chest x-ray examination. Immunosuppressed patients may receive blood that has been irradiated to prevent activation of donor leukocytes and graft-versus-host disease.

PATIENT CARE: Hemolytic blood transfusion reactions are prevented by meticulous accuracy in labeling the patient's blood sample for typing and cross-matching; double-checking the patient's name and identification number at the time of transfusion is essential. Antihistamines and antipyretics may be given to patients with a history of multiple blood transfusions, allergies, or a previous febrile transfusion reaction. Patients at risk for circulatory overload are placed in an upright position before the transfusion is started and the blood is administered very slowly; packed RBCs create less risk than whole blood, but also must be transfused over several hours.

All patients receiving blood transfusions should be monitored closely for signs of an adverse response. If a reaction occurs, the infusion is stopped immediately, but an intravenous line is kept patent with saline. A description of the patient's signs or symptoms, and the blood container and tubing, are sent to the blood bank; blood and urine samples are sent to the laboratory.

transfusion syndrome, multiple Bleeding that results from the transfusion of multiple units of blood. SEE: *posttransfusion syndrome.*

transgendered (trăns-jĕn′dĕrd) Having a gender identity or gender perception different from one's phenotypic gender.

transgenic An organism into which hereditary (i.e., genetic) material from another organism has been introduced.

transient [L. *transi,* to go by] Not lasting; of brief duration.

transient ischemic attack ABBR: TIA. A neurologic deficit, having a vascular cause, that produces stroke symptoms that resolve within 24 hr. (In practice, most TIAs resolve within an hour of onset.) Patients who have suffered a TIA have an increased risk of peripheral and coronary artery atherosclerosis, and an increased risk of subsequent heart attack and stroke. SEE: *carotid bruit; stroke.*

SYMPTOMS: TIAs and strokes have similar symptoms. These include weakness of one half of the face or half of the body, aphasia, monocular visual loss, hemibody sensory loss, or sudden loss of balance. A person who develops any of these symptoms should seek emergency medical assistance.

ETIOLOGY: TIAs usually occur in patients with underlying atherosclerosis, esp. of the carotid arteries, intracranial arteries, or the aorta. Emboli to the brain caused by atrial fibrillation, cerebrovascular vasospasm, transient episodes of hypotension, cerebral vasculitis, polycythemia vera, and other illnesses may occasionally produce TIAs.

TREATMENT: Studies involving large numbers of patients have shown that the risk of subsequent stroke in those who have suffered TIAs can be substantially reduced with antiplatelet or anticoagulant drugs (e.g., aspirin, ticlopidine, clopidogrel, or warfarin) and with drugs that control blood pressure and lipids. Carotid endarterectomy is a better option than medical therapy for stroke prevention in TIA patients with extensive carotid artery blockages, provided their surgeons have an operative mortality rate of less than 5%.

PATIENT CARE: The health care professional supports the patient and family during diagnostic procedures by explaining the procedures and expected sensations and by encouraging verbalization of feelings and concerns. Therapeutic interventions are provided, and the patient is instructed about desired effects and adverse reactions of prescribed drugs.

transiliac (trăns-ĭl′ē-ăk) [L. *trans,* across, + *iliacus,* pert. to ilium] Extending between the two ilia.

transilient (trăns-sĭl′ē-ĕnt) Jumping across or passing over as occurs when nerve fibers in the brain link nonadjacent convolutions.

transillumination (trăns″ĭl-lū″mĭ-nā′shŭn) [″ + *illuminare,* to light up] Inspection of a cavity or organ by passing a light through its walls. When pus or a lesion is present, the transmission of light is diminished or absent.

transinsular (trăns-ĭn′sū-lăr) Across the insula of the brain.

transischiac (trăns-ĭs′kē-ăk) Across or between the ischia of the pelvis.

transisthmian (trăns-ĭs′mē-ăn) Across an isthmus.

transition (trăn-zĭ′shŭn) [L. *transitio,* a going across] **1.** Passage from one state or position to another, or from one part to another part; a change in health status, roles, family, abilities, and other important areas. Transitions often require adaptations within the person, the group, or the environment and define the need for and context of nursing care. **2.** In obstetrics, the final phase of the first stage of labor. Cervical dilation is 8 to 10 cm and strong uterine contractions occur every 1.5 to 2 min and persist for 60 to 90 sec. Accompanying behavioral changes include increasing irritability and anxiety, declining coping abilities, and expressions of a strong desire for the labor to be ended immediately.

transitional (trăn-zĭsh′ŭn-ăl) Marked by or relating to change.

translation (trăns-lā′shŭn) [L. *trans,* across, + *latus,* borne] **1.** The synthesis of proteins under the direction of ribonucleic acid. **2.** To change to another place or to convert into another form.

translocation (trăns″lō-kā′shŭn) [″ + *locus,* place] **1.** The alteration of a chromosome by transfer of a portion of it either to another chromosome or to another portion of the same chromosome. The latter is called shift or intrachange. When two chromosomes interchange material, it is called reciprocal translocation. **2.** Movement of bacteria across the intestinal wall to invade the body. **3.** The linear motion of one structure across the parallel surface of another.

translucent (trăns-lū′sĕnt) [″ + *lucens,* shining] Not transparent but permitting passage of light.

transmethylase (trăns-mĕth′ĭ-lās) Methyltransferase.

transmethylation (trăns″mĕth-ĭ-lā′shŭn) The process in the metabolism of amino acids in which a methyl group is transferred from one compound to another; for example, the conversion in the body of homocysteine to methionine. In this case, the methyl group is furnished by choline or betaine.

transmigration (trănz″mī-grā′shŭn) [″ + *migrare,* to move from place to place] Wandering across or through, esp. the passage of white blood cells through capillary membranes into the tissues.

external t. Transfer of an ovum from an ovary to an opposite tube through the pelvic cavity.

internal t. Transfer of an ovum through the uterus to the opposite oviduct.

transmissible (trăns-mĭs′ă-bl) [L. *transmissio,* a sending across] Capable of being carried from a source, such as an individual, or an animal to a person, for example, an infectious disease.

transmission (trăns-mĭsh′ŭn) Transfer of anything, as a disease or hereditary characteristics.

airborne t. The spread of infectious organisms by aerosol or dust particles.

biological t. A condition in which the organism that transmits the causative agent of a disease plays an essential role in the life history of a parasite or germ.

duplex t. The passage of impulses through a nerve trunk in both directions.

horizontal t. **1.** The transfer of a disease between sexual partners. **2.** The acquisition of an infection by individuals of the same generation. SEE: *vertical t.*

mechanical t. The passive transfer of causative agents of disease, esp. by arthropods. This may be indirect, as when flies pick up organisms from excreta of humans or animals and deposit them on food, or direct, as when they pick up organisms from the body of a diseased individual and directly inoculate them into the body of another individual by bites or through open sores. SEE: *vector.*

neuromyal t. The transmission of excitation from a motor neuron to a muscle fiber at a neuromyal (myoneural) junction.

perinatal t. The transmission of an infectious illness from mother to infant during childbirth.

placental t. The transmission of substances in the mother's blood to the blood of the fetus by way of the placenta.

synaptic t. The release of a neurotransmitter by a neuron that initiates or inhibits an electrical impulse in the next neuron in the pathway.

transovarial t. The transmission of causative agents of disease to offspring following invasion of the ovary and infection of eggs; occurs in ticks and mites.

vertical t. **1.** In certain insects, transovarial passage of infection from one generation to the next. **2.** In mammals, passage of infection from the mother's body fluids to the infant either in utero, during delivery, or during the neonatal period (via breast milk).

transmission-based precautions Measures suggested by the Centers for Disease Control and Prevention to reduce the risk of airborne, droplet, and direct-contact transmission of infection in hospitals. SEE: *Standard and Universal Precautions Appendix.*

transmural (trăns-mū′răl) [L. *trans,* across, + *murus,* a wall] Across the wall of an organ or structure, as in transmural myocardial infarction, in which the tissue in the entire thickness of a portion of the cardiac wall dies.

transmutation (trăns″mū-tā′shŭn) [L. *transmutatio,* a changing across] A transformation or change, as the evolutionary change of one species into another.

transocular (trăns-ŏk′ū-lăr) [″ + *oculus,* eye] Across the eye.

transonance (trăns′ō-năns) [L. *trans,* across + *sonans,* sounding] The transmission of sounds through an organ, as heart sounds through the lungs and chest wall.

transorbital (trăns-or′bĭ-tăl) [″ + *orbita,* track] Passing through the orbit of the eye.

transovarial passage (trăns-ō-vā′rē-ăl) The passage of infectious or toxic agents into the ovary, a process that might invade and infect the oocytes.

transparent (trăns-păr′ĕnt) [″ + *parere,* to appear] **1.** Transmitting light rays so that objects are visible through the substance. **2.** Pervious to radiant energy.

transparietal (trăns″pă-rī′ĕ-tăl) [″ + *paries,* a wall] Through a parietal region or wall.

transpeptidase (trăns-pĕp′tĭ-dās) An enzyme that catalyzes the transfer of a peptide from one compound to another.

transperitoneal (trăns″pĕr-ĭ-tō-nē′ăl) Across or through the peritoneum.

transphosphorylase (trăns-fŏs-for′ĭ-lās) An enzyme that catalyzes the transfer of a phosphate group from one compound to another.

transphosphorylation (trăns-fŏs″for-ĭ-lā′shŭn) The exchange of phosphate groups from one compound to another.

transpirable (trăns-pī′ră-bl) [″ + *spirare,* to breathe] Permitting evaporation of water through living tissue.

transpiration (trăns″pī-rā′shŭn) [″ + *spirare,* to breathe] The passage of water or a vapor through a membrane. SEE: *perspiration.*

cutaneous t. The insensible evaporation of water vapor through the skin.

pulmonary t. The evaporation of water from the alveolar cells into the air in the lungs.

transpire To emit vapor through the skin or other tissues. SEE: *perspire.*

transplacental (trăns″plă-sĕn′tăl) Through the placenta, esp. penetration of the placenta by a toxin, chemical, or organism that would affect the fetus.

transplant (trăns-plănt′) [″ + *plantare,* to plant] To transfer tissue or an organ from one part to another (or one body to another) as in grafting or plastic surgery.

transplant (trăns′plănt) [″ + *plantare,* to plant] A piece of tissue or organ used in transplantation.

transplantar (trăns-plăn′tăr) [″ + *planta,* sole] Across the sole of the foot.

transplantation (trăns″plăn-tā′shŭn) **1.** The grafting of living tissue from its normal position to another site or the transplantation of an organ or tissue from one person to another. Organs and tissues that have been successfully transplanted include the heart, lung, kidney, liver, pancreas, cornea, large blood vessels, tendon, cartilage, skin, bone, and bone marrow. Brain tissue has been implanted experimentally to treat patients with Parkinson's disease. The matching of histocompatibility antigens that differentiate one person's cells from another's helps prevent rejection of donated tissues. Cyclosporine, tacrolimus, corticosteroids, monoclonal antibodies, and other immunosuppressive agents have been approx. 80% effective in preventing rejection of transplanted organs for 2 or more years. SEE: *autotransplantation; graft; heart transplantation; organ donation; renal transplantation; replantation.* **2.** In dentistry, the transfer of a tooth from one alveolus to another.

allogeneic t. Transplantation of material from a donor to another person.

autologous bone marrow t. ABBR: ABMT. The harvest, cryopreservation, and reinfusion of a patient's own bone marrow, a procedure that may be used in posttreatment marrow hypoplasia following cancer therapy. After the bone marrow is removed from the patient, it may be purged of malignant cells and then returned to the patient. Cells can be purged by using monoclonal antibodies to bind the unwanted cells, by using chemotherapy to kill cancer cells, or by using magnetic microspheres to bind to the two cells and separate them by use of a magnetic field. Purging cells by use of these methods is experimental and is not used in the majority of patients undergoing autologous transplantation. SEE: *immunomagnetic technique; magnetic microspheres.*

autologous t. Transplantation of material from one location in the body to another site.

autoplastic t. Transplantation of tissue from one part to another part of the same body. SYN: *homoplastic t.*

bone marrow t. ABBR: BMT. Transplantation of bone marrow from one individual to another. It is used in treating aplastic anemia, thalassemia and sickle cell anemia, immunodeficiency disorders, acute leukemia, chronic myelogenous leukemia, non-Hodgkin's lymphoma, Hodgkin's disease, and testicular cancer, among others.

fat t. In cosmetic surgery, the movement of adipose tissue from one body site to another to augment structure, change body contours, or reduce skin wrinkling.

hair t. A surgical procedure for placing plugs of skin containing hair follicles from one body site to another. This time-consuming technique is used to treat baldness.

heart t. Surgical transplantation of the heart from a patient who died of trauma or a disease that left the heart intact and capable of functioning in the recipient. The only absolute contraindications are uncontrollable cancer or infection, irreversible pulmonary vascular disease, or a separate life-threatening disease; in general, however, patients over 65 years, those with severe renal or liver disease, and those with a history of noncompliance with medical regimens do not receive heart transplants. The major barrier to heart transplantation is the lack of donors; the number of potential recipients is approx. 10 times the number of donors each year.

After receiving a heart transplant, continuous immunosuppression with cyclosporine, corticosteroids, or related drugs is required to prevent rejection of the donated organ. Acute episodes of rejection are treated with monoclonal antibodies (OKT3) or antilymphocyte immune globulin. Clinical signs of rejection—fatigue, dyspnea, hypotension, and extra heart sounds—are nonspecific, so biopsies are performed frequently during the first 2 years after surgery. Average patient survival is greater than 75% 1 year after the surgery, and greater than 50% after 10 years. SEE: *rejection* (2).

heteroplastic t. Transplantation of a part from one individual to another individual of the same or a closely related species.

heterotopic t. Transplantation in which the transplant is placed in a different location in the host than it had been in the donor.

homoplastic t. Autoplastic t.

homotopic t. Transplantation in which the transplant occupies the same location in the host as it had in the donor.

kidney t. Renal t.

renal t. The grafting of a kidney from a living donor or from a cadaver to an individual with renal failure. It is used as the definitive form of renal replacement for patients with kidney failure. Tissue typing for HLA antigens as well as ABO blood groups is used to decrease the likelihood of acute or chronic rejection. Family members are often the best-matched donors. In patients with diabetes mellitus, combined renal and pancreatic transplants are sometimes performed, with a very high likelihood of success. The high success rate of kidney transplants (85% to 95% at 2 years) is primarily due to immunosuppressive drugs such as corticosteroids, cyclosporine, azathioprine, or tacrolimus. Because cyclosporine is nephrotoxic, careful monitoring of serum drug levels after transplantation is required. SYN: *kidney t.* SEE: *major histocompatibility complex; suppressive immunotherapy; Nursing Diagnoses Appendix.*

small intestine t. A semi-experimental procedure in which the small intestine is replaced with a donor organ.

syngeneic t. A specific type of allogeneic transplantation of material between identical twins.

transplantation antigen The commonly used term for one of the histocompatibility antigens that cause the immune system of one individual to reject transplanted tissue.

transpleural (trăns-ploor′răl) Through the pleura.

transport Movement or transfer of substances in a biological system, esp. movement of electrolytes, nutrients, and liquids across cell membranes. Transport may occur actively, passively, or with the assistance of a carrier.

active t. The process by which a cell membrane moves molecules against a concentration or electrochemical gradient. This requires metabolic work. Potassium, for example, is maintained at high concentrations within cells, and low concentrations in extracellular fluid by active transport. Other ions actively transported are sodium, calcium, hydrogen, iron, chloride, iodide, and urate. Several sugars and the amino acids are also actively transported in the small intestine.

transportation of the injured The process of moving an injured person to a hospital or other treatment center. In serious injuries such as cranial and spinal trauma, airway compromise, and hemorrhage, the patient should be moved by properly trained support personnel with equipment to stabilize vital structures and prevent further injury. In particular, the airway should be secured, ventilation provided, circulation supported, and the spine protected from injury with specially designed appliances. It is crucial that critically injured persons receive definitive care within the first hour of their injury to optimize their chances of survival. Patients with lesser injuries whose vital signs are relatively stable may be transported by means listed here.

Carrying in arms: The patient is picked up in both arms, as the carrying of a child.

One-arm assist: The patient's arm is placed about the neck of the bearer, and the bearer's arm is placed about the patient's waist, thus assisting the patient to walk.

Chair carry, chair stretcher: Any ordinary firm chair may be used. The patient is seated on the tilted-back chair. One bearer grasps the back of the chair and the other the legs of the chair (either the front or rear, depending on the construction of the chair). Both bearers face in the same direction.

Fireman's drag: The patient's wrists are crossed and tied with a belt or rope. The bearer kneels alongside the patient, with his or her head under the patient's wrists, and walks on all fours, dragging the patient underneath.

Fireman's lift: The bearer grasps the patient's left wrist with the right hand. The bearer's head is placed under the patient's left armpit, drawing the patient's body over the bearer's left shoulder. The bearer's left arm should encircle both thighs, then lift the patient. The patient's wrist is transferred to the bearer's left hand, thus leaving one hand free to remove obstacles or to open doors.

Four-handed basket seat: Each of two bearers grasps own wrist and then grasps the partner's free wrist. The patient sits on this support.

Pack-strap carry: The patient is supported along the bearer's back. The patient's right arm is brought over the bearer's right shoulder and held by the bearer's left hand. The patient's left arm is brought over the left shoulder and held by the bearer's right hand. The patient is thus carried on the back, with the arms resembling pack straps.

Piggyback carry: The patient is supported along the bearer's back with the knees raised to the sides of the bearer's torso. This leaves the patient practically in a sitting position astride the bearer's back, with arms around the bearer's neck or trunk.

Six- or eight-person carry: This is done as the three-person carry, except three or four bearers are on each side of the patient, thus dividing the patient's weight more uniformly.

Three-handed basket seat: The bearer grasps his or her own wrist; the partner grasps the bearer's wrist and leaves one arm free for supporting the patient.

Three- or four-person carry: This is the litter-type carry used by emergency squads. Three persons kneel on one side of the patient, place their hands under the patient and lift up. The head bearer supports the patient's head and shoulders, the center bearer lifts the waist and hips, and the third bearer lifts both the lower extremities. A fourth person, if available, should help steady the patient while he or she is being lifted.

Two-handed seat: The bearers kneel on either side of the patient. Each passes one arm around the patient's back (under the armpits) and the other arm under the knees and lifts the patient carefully in a sitting position.

Wheelchair, improvised: To make this, the legs of a chair, preferably one with arms, are fastened to parallel boards and skates or casters are attached to the bottom of the boards. A footrest can be made by attaching a broom handle or stick across the parallel boards in front of the chair.

Vehicles: If an ambulance is not available, stretchers can be improvised with ropes and chairs, ladders, or poles. The patient should always be tied to the stretcher during transportation. Several bearers will be necessary to assist entering and leaving the vehicle.

transport protein One of the proteins important in transporting materials such as hormones from their site of origin to the site of cellular action and metabolism.

transpose To change places (e.g., moving the insertion of a muscle or ligament to another site).

transposition (trănz″pō-zĭ′shŭn) [L. *trans,* across, + *positio,* a placing] **1.** A transfer of position from one spot to another. SYN: *metathesis.* **2.** Displacement of an organ, esp. a viscus, to the opposite side. **3.** Transplantation of a flap of tissue without severing it entirely from its original position until it has united in the new position.

transposition of the great vessels A fetal deformity of the heart in which the aorta arises from the right ventricle and the pulmonary artery arises from the left ventricle. SEE: *dextroposition of the great vessels.*

ansposon (trănz-pō′zŏn) A genetic unit such as a DNA sequence that is transferred from one cell's genetic material to another.

trans-retinal The form of retinal created when light strikes the retina. It separates from the opsin of the photopigment (rhodopsin in rods), which is then said to be bleached. The enzyme retinal isomerase converts it back to *cis*-retinal, and the photopigment is again able to respond to light.

transsegmental (trăns″sĕg-mĕn′tăl) [″ + *segmentum,* a cutting] Extending across or beyond a segment, as of a limb.

transseptal (trăns-sĕp′tăl) [″ + *saeptum,* partition] Across a septum.

transsexual (trăns-sĕks′ū-ăl) [″ + *sexus,* sex] **1.** An individual who has an overwhelming desire to be of the opposite sex. **2.** An individual who has had his or her external sex changed by surgery.

transsexualism (trăns-sĕks′ū-ă-lĭzm) The condition of being of a certain definite sex (i.e., male or female) but feeling and acting as if a member of the opposite sex. In some instances, the desire to alter this situation leads individuals to seek medical and surgical assistance to alter anatomical characteristics so that their anatomy would more nearly match their feelings about their true sexuality. The success of this therapy is controversial.

transsexual surgery Surgical therapy for alteration of the anatomical sex of an individual whose psychological gender is not consistent with the anatomical sexual characteristics.

transsphenoidal (trăns″sfē-noy′dăl) Through or across the sphenoid bone.

transtemporal (trăns-tĕm′pō-răl) [″ + *temporalis,* pert. to a temple] Crossing the temporal lobe of the cerebrum.

transthalamic (trăns″thăl-ăm′ĭk) [″ + Gr. *thalamos,* chamber] Passing across the thalamus.

transthoracic (trăns″thō-răs′ĭk) [″ + Gr. *thorax,* chest] Across the thorax.

transthoracotomy (trăns″thō-ră-kŏt′ō-mē) [″ + Gr. *thorax,* chest, + *tome,* incision] The operation of incising across the thorax.

transthyretin ABBR: TTR. A normal serum prealbumin protein that binds and transports thyroxine (T_4).

transtracheal Across or through the trachea.

transtracheal jet insufflation The life-saving technique of ventilating a patient with a complete airway obstruction. A small catheter is placed via a cricothyroid puncture and attached to a pressure-controlled oxygen outlet via a one-way valve.

transtympanic neurectomy Surgical interruption of the parasympathetic nerve supply to the parotid and submandibular glands by bilateral sectioning of the tympanic and chorda tympani nerves. The technique was developed in the 1980s to treat excessive drooling, esp. in mentally retarded children.

transubstantiation (trăn″sŭb-stăn″shē-ā′shŭn) [″ + *substantia,* substance] The process of replacing one tissue for another.

transudate (trăns′ū-dāt) [″ + *sudare,* to sweat] The fluid that passes through a membrane, esp. that which passes through capillary walls. Compared to an exudate, a transudate has fewer cellular elements and is of a lower specific gravity.

transudation (trăns-ū-dā′shŭn) Oozing of a fluid through pores or interstices, as of a membrane.

transureteroureterostomy (trăns″ū-rē″tĕr-ō-ū-rē″tĕr-ŏs′tō-mē) Section of one ureter and joining both ends to the opposite ureter.

transurethral (trăns″ū-rē′thrăl) [″ + Gr. *ourethra,* urethra] Pert. to an operation performed through the urethra.

transurethral resection of the prostate ABBR: TUR, TURP. The removal of prostatic tissue using a device inserted through the urethra. SEE: *prostatectomy.*

transvaginal (trăns-văj′ĭn-ăl) [″ + *vagina,* sheath] Through the vagina or across its wall as in a surgical procedure.

transvector (trăns-vĕk′tor) An animal that transmits a toxin that it does not produce and by which it is itself unaffected, as when a bivalve mollusc, such as the oyster, filters viruses out of the water and transmits them to those who ingest the mollusc.

transvenous Through a vein.

transversalis (trăns″vĕr-să′lĭs) [″ + *vertere,* to turn] A structure occurring at right angles to the long axis of the body.

transversalis fascia A thin membrane forming the peritoneal surface of the transversus muscle and its aponeurosis.

transverse (trăns-vĕrs′) [L. *transversus*] Lying at right angles to the long axis of the body; crosswise.

transversectomy (trăns″vĕr-sĕk′tō-mē) [″ + Gr. *ektome,* excision] Excision of a transverse vertebral process.

transverse foramen A canal through the transverse processes of the cervical vertebrae for passage of the vertebral arteries.

transverse plane A plane that divides the body into a top and bottom portion.

transversion (trăns-vĕr′zhŭn) The eruption of a tooth at an abnormal site.

transversocostal (trăns-vĕr″sō-kŏs′tăl) Costotransverse.

transversospinalis (trăns-vĕr″sō-spī-nā′lĭs) [L. *transversus,* turned across, + *spina,* thorn] Semispinalis capitis, semispinalis cervicis.

transversourethralis (trăns-vĕr″sō-ū″rē-thrā′lĭs) The transverse fibers of the sphincter urethrae muscle.

transversus (trăns-vĕr′sŭs) [L.] **1.** Any of several small muscles. **2.** Lying across the long axis of a part or organ.

transvesical (trăns-vĕs′ĭ-kăl) Across or through the bladder.

transvestism, transvestitism (trăns-vĕst′ĭzm, -ĭ-tĭzm) [L. *trans,* across, + *vestitus,* clothed, + Gr. *-ismos,* condition] The desire to dress in the clothes of and be accepted as a member of the opposite sex.

transvestite (trăns-vĕs′tīt) An individual who practices transvestism.

Trantas' dots (trăn′tăs) [Alexios Trantas, Gr. ophthalmologist, 1867–1960] Chalky concretions of the conjunctiva around the limbus. These are associated with vernal conjunctivitis.

trap, food A space or area in or between teeth where particles of food may become lodged.

trapeze bar Triangular device suspended above a bed to facilitate transferring and positioning the patient; also called a *swivel trapeze bar.*

trapezial (tră-pē′zē-ăl) Concerning the trapezium.

trapeziform (tră-pē′zĭ-form) Shaped like a trapezoid.

trapeziometacarpal (tră-pē″zē-ō-mĕt″ă-kăr′păl) Concerning or connecting the trapezium and the metacarpus of the thumb.

trapezium (tră-pē′zē-ŭm) [Gr. *trapezion,* a little table] **1.** A four-sided, single-plane geometric figure in which none of the sides are parallel. **2.** The os trapezium, the first bone on the radial side of the distal row of the bones of the wrist. It articulates with the base of the metacarpal bone of the thumb. SYN: *multangular bone, greater.*

trapezius (tră-pē′zē-ŭs) A flat, triangular muscle covering the posterior surface of the neck and shoulder.

trapezoid (trăp′ĕ-zoyd) [Gr. *trapezoeides,* table-shaped] A four-sided figure having two parallel sides and two divergent sides.

trapezoid body A bundle of transverse fibers in the ventral portion of the tegmentum of pons. SYN: *corpus trapezoideum.*

trapezoid bone The second bone in the distal row of carpal bones. It lies between the trapezium and capitate bones. SYN: *multangular bone, lesser.*

trapezoid ligament The lateral portion of the coracoclavicular ligament.

trauma (traw′mă) *pl.* **traumata, traumas** [Gr. *trauma,* wound] **1.** A physical injury or wound caused by external force or violence. It may be self-inflicted. In the U.S., trauma is the principal cause of death between the ages of 1 and 44 years. In addition to each death from trauma, there are at least two cases of permanent disability caused by trauma. The principal types of trauma include motor vehicle accidents, falls, burns, gunshot wounds, and drowning. The majority of deaths occur in the first several hours after the event. **2.** An emotional or psychological shock that may produce disordered feelings or behavior.

birth t. **1.** Injury to the fetus during the birthing process. **2.** Otto Rank's term to describe what he considered the basic source of anxiety in human beings, the birth process. The importance of this concept is controversial.

risk for t. Accentuated risk of acci-

Revised Trauma Score (RTS)

Glasgow Coma Scale (GCS)	Systolic Blood Pressure (SBP)	Respiratory Rate (RR)	Coded Value
13–15	>89	10–29	4
9–12	76–89	>29	3
6–8	50–75	6–9	2
4–5	1–49	1–5	1
3	0	0	0

RTS = $0.9368\ GCS_c + 0.7326\ SBP_c + 0.2908\ RR_c$ coded values × Revised score coefficient

SOURCE: From Champion, HR, et al: J Trauma 29:623–629, 1989.

dental tissue injury (e.g., wound, burn, fracture). SEE: *Nursing Diagnoses Appendix.*

occlusal t. Any injury to part of the masticatory system as a result of malocclusion or occlusal dysfunction. It may be abrupt in its development in response to a restoration or ill-fitting prosthetic device, or result from years of tooth wear, drift, or faulty oral habits. It may produce adverse periodontal changes, tooth mobility or excessive wear, pain in the temporomandibular joints, or spasms and pain in the muscles of mastication.

psychic t. A painful emotional experience that may cause anxiety.

toothbrush t. Abrasion or grooving of teeth and gingival injury or recession as a result of improper brushing with a stiff-textured brush.

trauma center A regional hospital capable of providing care for critically injured patients. Available on a 24-hr basis are a surgical team, operating suite, surgical subspecialties, intensive care unit, and specialized nursing team.

Trauma Score Numerical grading system that combines the Glasgow Coma Scale and measurements of cardiopulmonary function as a gauge of severity of injury and predictor of survival after blunt trauma to the head. Each parameter is given a number (high for normal and low for impaired or absent function). Severity of injury is estimated by summing the numbers. The lowest score is 1, the highest 16. SEE: table.

traumatic (traw-măt′ĭk) [Gr. *traumatikos*] Caused by or relating to an injury.

traumatic psychosis Psychosis resulting from physical injuries or emotional shock.

traumatism (traw′mă-tĭzm) [Gr. *traumatismos*] Morbid condition of a system owing to an injury or a wound.

traumato- Combining form meaning *trauma.*

traumatology (traw-mă-tŏl′ō-jē) [Gr. *trauma,* wound, + *logos,* word, reason] The branch of surgery dealing with wounds and their care.

traumatopathy (traw″mă-tŏp′ă-thē) [″ + *pathos,* disease, suffering] Pathological state caused by trauma.

traumatophilia (traw″mă-tō-fĭl′ē-ă) [″ + *philein,* to love] The enjoyment of or unconscious desire to be traumatized, either mentally or physically. SEE: *masochism.*

traumatopnea (traw″mă-tŏp-nē′ă) [″ + *pnoia,* breath] The passage of air in and out of a wound in the chest wall.

traumatotherapy (traw″mă-tō-thĕr′ă-pē) Treatment of injury.

tray (trā) A flat surface with raised edges.

impression t. In dentistry, a U-shaped receptacle with raised edges made of metal or acrylic resin used to carry impression material and support it in contact with the surfaces to be recorded until the impression material is set or firm.

Treacher Collins syndrome [Edward Treacher Collins, Brit. ophthalmologist, 1862–1919] Mandibulofacial dysostosis.

treadmill (trĕd′mĭl) A conveyor belt for walking or running in place; the speed of movement and angle of inclination can be varied during tests of cardiopulmonary health and conditioning. SEE: *exercise tolerance test.*

treatment (trēt′mĕnt) [ME. *treten,* to handle] **1.** Medical, surgical, dental, or psychiatric management of a patient. **2.** Any specific procedure used for the cure or the amelioration of a disease or pathological condition. SEE: *therapy.*

active t. Treatment directed specifically toward cure of a disease.

causal t. Treatment directed toward removal of the cause of the disease.

conservative t. **1.** The withholding of treatments and management of disease by observation. **2.** In surgical cases, the preservation of the organ or part if at all possible with the least possible mutilation.

dental t. Any of a variety of treatments of the teeth and adjacent tissues to restore or maintain normal oral health and function.

dietetic t. Treatment of disease based on regulation of diet.

electric shock t. Electroconvulsive therapy.

empiric t. Treatment based on observation and experience rather than having a scientific basis.

expectant t. Relief of symptoms as they arise (i.e., not directed at the specific cause).

legally mandated t. Compulsory treatment; that is, treatment that is demanded by the courts. Usually, patients who are commanded to receive particular forms of treatment are prisoners, probationers, mentally ill individuals, people with certain communicable diseases (e.g., tuberculosis), or persons with a history of substance abuse.

palliative t. Treatment designed for the relief of symptoms of the disease rather than curing the disease.

preventive t. Treatment directed at the prevention of disease.

radiation t. The administration of high-energy x-ray photons, electrons, or nuclear emissions for the cure of cancer or palliation of symptoms.

rational t. Treatment based on scientific principles.

shock t. Electroconvulsive therapy.

specific t. Treatment directed at the cause of a disease.

supportive t. Special measures employed to supplement specific therapy.

symptomatic t. Treatment directed toward constitutional symptoms, such as fever, shock, and pain.

treatment plan The projected series and sequence of treatment procedures based on an individualized evaluation of what is needed to restore or improve the health and function of a patient.

tree A structure that resembles a tree.

bronchial t. The right or left primary bronchus with its branches and their terminal arborizations.

tracheobronchial t. The trachea, bronchi, and their branches.

trehalase (trē-hā′lās) An enzyme that hydrolyzes trehalose to form two molecules; D-glucose.

trehalose (trē-hā′lōs) A disaccharide of trehalase. It is also present in certain fungi.

Trematoda (trĕm″ă-tō′dă) [Gr. *trematodes,* pierced] A class of flatworms commonly called flukes belonging to the phylum Platyhelminthes. It includes two orders: Monogenea, which are external or semiexternal parasites having direct development with no asexual multiplication, and Digenea, internal parasites with asexual generation in their life cycle. The Digenea usually require two or more hosts, the hosts alternating. SEE: *fluke*.

trematode (trĕm′ă-tōd) A parasitic flatworm belonging to the class Trematoda. SEE: *cercaria; fluke*.

trematodiasis (trĕm″ă-tō-dī′ă-sĭs) Infestation with a trematode.

tremble (trĕm′bl) [O.Fr. *trembler*] **1.** An involuntary quivering or shaking. **2.** To shiver, quiver, or shake.

trembles (trĕm′blz) A condition resulting from ingestion of plants such as snakeroot *(Eupatorium urticaefolium)* or jimmyweed *(Haplopappus heterophyllus)*. The condition is common in domestic animals and may occur in humans as a result of ingesting the plants or more commonly from drinking milk or eating the meat of poisoned animals. Symptoms are weakness, anorexia, nausea and vomiting, and prostration, possibly resulting in death. In humans, the illness is called milk sickness.

tremelloid, tremellose (trĕm′ĕ-loyd, -lōs) Jelly-like.

tremetol (trĕm′ĕ-tŏl) A poisonous substance occurring in snakeroot, rayless goldenrod, and other plants that may cause trembles in animals or humans. SEE: *trembles*.

tremograph (trĕm′ō-grăf) [″ + Gr. *graphein,* to write] A device for recording tremors.

tremolabile (trē″mō-lā′bl) [″ + *labi,* to slip] Easily destroyed or inactivated by shaking; said of an enzyme.

tremophobia (trē″mō-fō′bē-ă) [″ + Gr. *phobos,* fear] An abnormal fear of trembling.

tremor (trĕm′or, trē′mor) [L. *tremor,* a shaking] **1.** A quivering, esp. a continuous quivering of a convulsive nature. **2.** An involuntary movement of a part or parts of the body resulting from alternate contractions of opposing muscles. SEE: *subsultus*.

Tremors may be classified as involuntary, static, dynamic, kinetic, or hereditary. Pathological tremors are independent of the will. The trembling may be fine or coarse, rapid or slow, and may appear on movement (intention tremor) or improve when the part is voluntarily exercised. It is often caused by organic disease; trembling may also express an emotion (e.g., fear). All abnormal tremors except palatal and ocular myoclonus disappear during sleep.

action t. Intention t.

alcoholic t. The visible tremor exhibited by alcoholics.

cerebellar t. An intention tremor of 3 to 5 Hz frequency, associated with cerebellar disease.

coarse t. A tremor in which oscillations are relatively slow.

continuous t. A tremor that resembles tremors of paralysis agitans.

enhanced physiological t. An action tremor associated with catecholamine excess (e.g., in association with anxiety, thyrotoxicosis, hypoglycemia, or alcohol withdrawal). It may occur as a side effect of drugs, such as epinephrine, caffeine, theophylline, amphetamines, levodopa, tricyclic antidepressants, lithium, and corticosteroids.

essential t. A benign tremor, usually of the head, chin, outstretched hands, and occasionally the voice, that needs to be differentiated from the tremor of parkinsonism. Essential tremor, which is made worse by anxiety or action, is usually 8 to 10 cycles per second and that of parkinsonism 4 to 5. In essential tremor, there is usually a family history but not in parkinsonism. The medicines that are effective in treating parkinsonism have no effect on essential tremor.

familial t. A tremor indistinguishable from essential tremor in its clinical manifestation. Unlike essential tremor, it is inherited as an autosomal dominant trait.

fibrillary t. A tremor caused by consecutive contractions of separate muscular fibrillae rather than of a muscle or muscles.

fine t. A rapid tremor.

flapping t. Asterixis.

forced t. A tremor continuing after voluntary motion has ceased.

Hunt's t. A tremor associated with all voluntary movements. It is present in certain cerebellar lesions.

hysterical t. A fine tremor occurring in hysteria. It may be limited to one extremity or generalized.

intention t. A tremor exhibited or intensified when attempting coordinated movements. SYN: *action t.*

intermittent t. A tremor common to paralyzed muscles in hemoplegia when attempting voluntary movement.

muscular t. Slight oscillating muscular contractions in rhythmical order.

parkinsonian t. A rest tremor esp. of the fingers and hands, that is suppressed briefly during voluntary activity. The tremor disappears during all but the lightest phases of sleep.

physiological t. A tremor occurring in normal individuals. It may be transient and occur in association with excessive physical exertion, excitement, hunger, fatigue, or other causes. SEE: *enhanced physiological t.*

rest t. A tremor present when the involved part is at rest but absent or diminished when active movements are attempted. SYN: *static t.*

senile t. A form of benign essential tremor found in individuals older than 60, marked by rapid, alternating movements of the upper extremities that occur at a frequency of about 6 cycles/sec.

static t. Rest t.

volitional t. Trembling of the limbs or of the body when making a voluntary effort. It is seen in many cerebellar diseases.

tremorgram (trĕm′or-grăm) Graphic representation of a tremor recorded on a tremograph.

tremulor (trĕm′ū-lor) A device for administering vibratory massage.

tremulous (trĕm′ū-lŭs) [L. *tremulus*] Trembling or shaking.

trench fever A febrile disease whose characteristics include headache, malaise, pain, tenderness (esp. in the shins), splenomegaly, and often a transient macular rash. The causative agent is *Bartonella quintana,* a microbe that lives only within cells; it is transmitted to people by infected body lice. The disease is rarely encountered in industrialized nations, except among the homeless; it is prevalent in many developing nations. The disease is treated with doxycycline 100 mg orally, twice a day.

trend [ME. *trenden,* to revolve] The inclination to proceed in a certain direction or at a certain rate; used to describe the prognosis or course of a symptom or disease.

Trendelenburg gait A side lurching of the trunk over the stance leg due to weakness in the gluteus medius muscle.

Trendelenburg position (trĕn-dĕl′ĕn-bŭrg) [Friedrich Trendelenburg, Ger. surgeon, 1844–1924] A position in which the patient's head is low and the body and legs are on an elevated and inclined plane. This may be accomplished by having the patient flat on a bed and elevating the foot of the bed. In this position, the abdominal organs are pushed up toward the chest by gravity. The foot of the bed may be elevated by resting it on blocks. This position is used in abdominal surgery. In treating shock, this position is usually used, but if there is an associated head injury, the head should not be kept lower than the trunk. SEE: *position* for illus.

Trendelenburg sign A pelvic drop on the side of the elevated leg when the patient stands on one leg and lifts the other. It indicates weakness or instability of the gluteus medius muscle on the stance side.

Trendelenburg test A test to evaluate the strength of the gluteus medius muscle. The examiner stands behind the patient and observes the pelvis as the patient stands on one leg and then the other. A positive result determines muscle weakness on the standing leg side when the pelvis tilts down on the opposite side.

trepan (trē-păn′) [Gr. *trypanon,* a borer] **1.** To perforate the skull. **2.** An instrument resembling a carpenter's bit for incision of the skull. SYN: *trephine.*

trepanation (trĕp″ă-nā′shŭn) [L. *trepanatio*] Surgery using a trepan.

corneal t. Keratoplasty.

trephination (trĕf″ĭn-ā′shŭn) [Fr. *trephine,* a bore] The process of cutting out a piece of bone with the trephine.

trephine (trē-fīn′) **1.** To perforate with a trephine. **2.** A cylindrical saw for cutting a circular piece of bone out of the skull. SYN: *trepan.*

trephining The process of cutting bone with a trephine.

trephocyte (trĕf′ō-sīt) [Gr. *trephein,* to feed, + *kytos,* cell] Trophocyte.

trepidant (trĕp′ĭ-dănt) [L. *trepidans,* trembling] Marked by tremor.

trepidatio (trĕp″ĭ-dā′shē-ō) [L.] Trepidation.

trepidation (trĕp″ĭ-dā′shŭn) [L. *trepidatio,* a trembling] **1.** Fear, anxiety. **2.** Trembling movement, esp. when involuntary.

Treponema (trĕp″ō-nē′mă) [Gr. *trepein,* to turn, + *nema,* thread] A genus of spirochetes, parasitic in humans, which belongs to the family Treponemataceae. They move by flexing, snapping, and bending. SEE: *bacteria* for illus.

T. carateum The causative agent of pinta, an infectious disease of the skin.

T. pallidum The causative organism of syphilis. SYN: *Spirochaeta pallida.*

T. pertenue The causative organism of yaws (frambesia).

Treponemataceae (trĕp″ō-nē″mă-tā′sē-ē) A family of spiral organisms belonging to the order Spirochaetales; includes the genera *Borrelia, Leptospira,* and *Treponema.*

treponematosis (trĕp″ō-nē-mă-tō′sĭs) Infection with *Treponema.*

treponeme (trĕp′ō-nēm) Any organism of the genus *Treponema.*

treponemiasis (trĕp″ō-nē-mī′ă-sĭs) [″ + *nema,* thread, + *-iasis,* condition] Infestation with *Treponema.*

treponemicidal (trĕp″ō-nē″mĭ-sī′dăl) [″ + ″ + L. *cidus,* to kill] Destructive to *Treponema.*

trepopnea (trĕp-ŏp′nē-ă) [″ + *pnoia,* breath] The condition of being able to breathe with less difficulty when in a certain position.

treppe Staircase phenomenon.

tretinoin (trĕt′ĭ-noyn) All-*trans*-retinoic acid. It is a keratolytic agent used topically in treating acne. Trade name is Retin-A.

TRH *thyrotropin-releasing hormone.*

tri- [Gr.] Prefix meaning *three.*

triacetate (trī-ăs′ĕ-tāt) Any acetate that contains three acetic acid groups.

triacetin (trī-ăs′ĕ-tĭn) An antifungal agent used topically, whose previously used name was glyceryl triacetate.

triacidic (trī″ă-sĭd′ĭk) Containing three acidic hydrogen ions.

triacylglycerol Triglyceride.

triad (trī′ăd) [Gr. *trias,* group of three] **1.** Any three things having something in common. **2.** A trivalent element. **3.** Trivalent.

Hutchinson's t. A syndrome characteristic of congenital syphilis consisting of notched teeth, interstitial keratitis, and eighth-nerve deafness due to meningeal involvement.

triage (trē-ăzh′) [Fr., sorting] **1.** The screening and classification of casualties to make optimal use of treatment resources and to maximize the survival and welfare of patients. **2.** Sorting patients and setting priorities for their treatment in urgent care settings, emergency rooms, clinics, hospitals, and health maintenance organizations.

Patient Care: The health care professional must obtain a brief history, perform a rapid physical assessment, determine the severity of the illness, and transfer the patient to the appropriate care setting. A quick, convenient protocol for noting each patient's condition is essential. The patient's needs may change while waiting for care—recognition of the improvement or deterioration of a patient is a dynamic and fundamental part of triage.

Most emergency triage systems rely on patient surveys. In the primary survey of the patient, the Airway, Breathing, Circulation, need for Defibrillation (or neurological Disability) are assessed and the patient is undressed or Exposed (ABCDE). Resuscitation of the patient begins immediately, based on the findings. In the secondary survey, the same elements of care are reviewed, but this time the emphasis is on assessing the effectiveness of interventions to maintain the airway, support ventilation, control hemorrhage and blood pressure, and restore normal physiology.

trial, phase 1 A clinical trial to determine the toxicity of a new drug.

trial, phase 2 A clinical trial to determine the potential effectiveness of a new drug.

trial, phase 3 A clinical trial to explore the clinical use of a new drug, esp. relative to other known effective agents.

triamcinolone (trī″ăm-sĭn′ō-lōn) A synthetic glucosteroid drug.

triamterene (trī-ăm′tĕr-ēn) A potassium-sparing diuretic drug.

triangle (trī′ăng-gl) [L. *triangulum*] A figure or area formed by three angles and three sides.

anal t. The triangle with its base between the two ischial tuberosities and its apex at the coccyx.

anterior t. of neck The space bounded by the middle line of the neck, the anterior border of the sternocleidomastoid muscle, and a line running along the lower border of the mandible and continued to the mastoid process of the temporal bone.

cephalic t. The triangle on the anteroposterior plane of the skull formed by lines joining the occiput and forehead and chin, and a line uniting the occiput and the chin.

digastric t. The triangular region of the neck. Its borders are the mandible, stylohyoid muscle, and the anterior belly of the digastric muscle.

t. of elbow The area in front of the elbow bounded by the brachioradialis and the pronator teres muscles on the sides, and with the base toward the humerus.

facial t. The triangle bounded by the lines uniting the basion and the alveolar and nasal points, and one uniting the nasal and basion.

femoral t. The triangle on the inner part of the thigh, bounded by the sartorius and adductor longus muscles and above by the inguinal ligament. SYN: *Scarpa's t.*

frontal t. The triangle bounded by the maximum frontal diameter and the lines joining its extremities and the glabella.

Hesselbach's t. The interval in the groin bounded by Poupart's ligament, the edge of the rectus muscle, and the deep epigastric artery.

inferior carotid t. The space bounded by the middle line of the neck, the sternomastoid muscle, and the anterior belly of the omohyoid muscle. SYN: *muscular t.; t. of necessity*.

inferior occipital t. The area having the bimastoid diameter for its base and the inion for its apex.

Lesser's t. The triangle bounded below by the anterior and posterior bellies of the digastric muscle and above by the hypogastric nerve.

lumbocostoabdominal t. The triangle bounded in front by the obliquus abdominis externus, above by the lower border of the serratus posterior inferior and the point of the 12th rib, behind by the outer edge of the erector spinae, and below by the obliquus abdominis internus.

muscular t. Inferior carotid t.

mylohyoid t. The triangular space formed by the mylohyoid muscle and the two bellies of the digastric muscle.

t. of necessity Inferior carotid t.

occipital t. of the neck The triangle bounded by the sternocleidomastoid, the trapezius, and the omohyoid muscles.

omoclavicular t. Subclavian t.

omohyoid t. Superior carotid t.

t. of Petit The space above the hip bone between the exterior oblique muscle, the latissimus dorsi, and the interior oblique muscle.

posterior cervical t. The triangle bounded by the upper border of the clavicle, the posterior border of the sternocleidomastoid muscle, and the anterior border of the trapezius muscle.

pubourethral t. A triangular space in the perineum bounded laterally by the ischiocavernous muscle, medially by the bulbocavernous muscle, and posteriorly by the superficial transverse perineus muscle.

Scarpa's t. Femoral t.

subclavian t. A triangular space bounded by the posterior belly of the omohyoid, the upper border of the clavicle, and the posterior margin of the sternocleidomastoid. SYN: *omoclavicular t.; supraclavicular t.*

submandibular t. The triangular region of the neck, bounded by the inferior border of the mandible, the stylohyoid muscle and the posterior belly of the digastric muscle, and the anterior belly of the digastric muscle; it is one of three triangles included in the anterior triangle of the neck. This was formerly called the submaxillary triangle.

suboccipital t. The triangle bounded by the obliquus inferior and superior muscles on two sides and the rectus capitis posterior major muscle on the third side. The floor contains the posterior arch of the atlas bone and the vertebral artery. It is covered by the semispinalis capitis muscle.

superior carotid t. The space bounded by the anterior belly of the omohyoid muscle, the posterior belly of the digastricus muscle, and the sternomastoid muscle. SYN: *omohyoid t.*

supraclavicular t. Subclavian t.

suprameatal t. The triangle slightly above and behind the exterior auditory meatus. It is bounded above by the root of the zygoma and anteriorly by the posterior wall of the exterior auditory meatus.

urogenital t. The triangle with its base formed by a line between the two ischial tuberosities and its apex just below the symphysis pubis.

vesical t. Trigone.

triangular Having three sides; shaped like a triangle. SYN: *triquetral; triquetrous*.

triangular bandage A square bandage folded diagonally. When folded, the several thicknesses can be applied to afford support. SEE: illus.; *bandage*.

triangularis (trī-ăng″gū-lā′rĭs) [L.] A muscle of the chin.

triangular ligament One of two ligaments, right and left, connecting posterior portions of the right and left lobes of the liver with corresponding portions of the diaphragm.

triangular nucleus of Schwalbe The chief or dorsal nucleus of the vestibular division of the eighth cranial nerve. It is located in the pons and occupies most of the acoustic area of the rhomboid fossa.

triangulation In qualitative research, a technique for enhancing validity by comparing information gathered from several sources. Qualitative research, meta-analysis, and related techniques are being used increasingly in the rehabilitation sciences, behavioral medicine, and clinical medicine.

Triatoma (trī-ăt′ō-mă) A genus of blood-sucking insects belonging to the order Hemiptera, family Reduviidae; com-

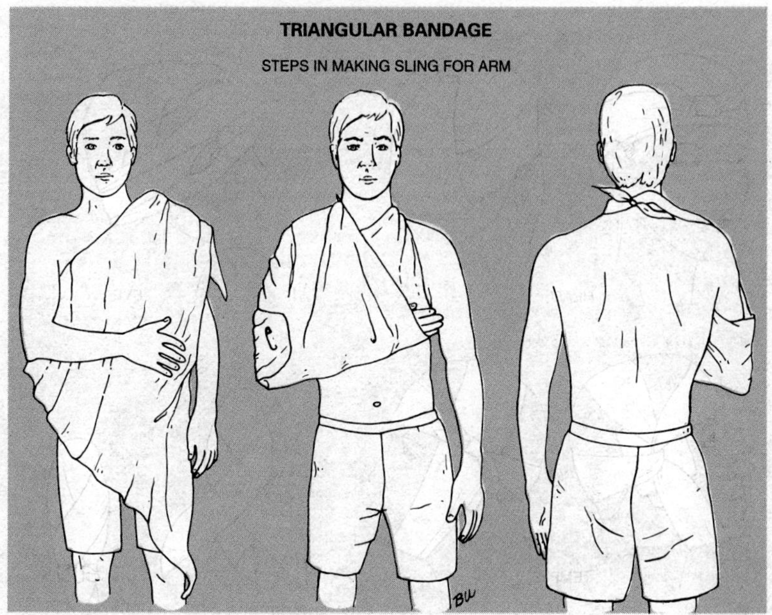

monly called cone-nosed bugs or assassin bugs. It includes the species *T. braziliensis, T. dimidiata, T. infestans, T. protracta, T. recuva, T. rubida,* and others. They are house-infesting pests and some species, esp. *T. infestans,* transmit *Trypanosoma cruzi,* the causative agent of Chagas' disease.

triatomic (trī″ă-tŏm′ĭk) Composed of three atoms.

tribade A lesbian.

tribadism (trĭb′ăd-ĭzm) [Gr. *tribein,* to rub, + *-ismos,* condition] A relationship in which women attempt to imitate heterosexual intercourse with each other.

tribasic (trī-bā′sĭk) [Gr. *treis,* three, + L. *basis,* base] Capable of neutralizing or accepting three hydrogen ions.

tribasilar (trī-băs′ĭl-ăr) [″ + L. *basilaris,* base] Having three bases.

tribasilar synostosis A condition resulting from the premature fusion of three skull bones—the occipital, sphenoid, and temporal. This results in arrested cerebral development and mental deficiency.

tribe (trīb) [L. *tribus,* division of the Roman people] In taxonomy, an occasional subdivision of a family; often equal to or below subfamily and above genus.

tribology (trĭ-bŏl′ō-jē) The study of the effect of friction on the body, esp. the articulating joints.

triboluminescence (trī″bō-lū″mĭ-nĕs′ĕns) [Gr. *tribein,* to rub, + L. *lumen,* light, + O.Fr. *escence,* continuing] Luminescence or sparks produced by friction or mechanical force applied to certain chemical crystals.

tribrachia (trī-brā′kē-ă) The condition of having three arms.

tribrachius (trī-brā′kē-ŭs) A deformed fetus, usually conjoined twins, having three arms.

tribromide (trī-brō′mīd) [Gr. *treis,* three, + *bromos,* stench] A compound having three atoms of bromine in the molecule.

TRIC Acronym for *tr*achoma and *i*nclusion *c*onjunctivitis. SEE: *Chlamydia trachomatis.*

tricarboxylic acid cycle Krebs cycle.

tricellular (trī-sĕl′ū-lăr) Three-celled.

tricephalus (trī-sĕf′ă-lŭs) [Gr. *treis,* three, + *kephale,* head] A deformed fetus having three heads.

triceps (trī′sĕps) [″ + L. *caput,* head] A muscle arising by three heads with a single insertion.

triceps brachii A muscle of the arm with three points of origin and one insertion. It extends the forearm. SEE: *arm* for illus.

triceps skin fold The thickness of the skin including subcutaneous fat as measured on the skin over the triceps muscle of the arm. Comparison of the value obtained from a patient to standard values helps to provide an estimate of body fat. It is used in assessing and documenting both malnutrition and obesity.

Tricercomonas (trī″sĕr-cŏm-ō′năs) Genus of very small protozoa considered identical to *Enteromonas.* SEE: *Enteromonas hominis.*

trich- SEE: *trichi-.*

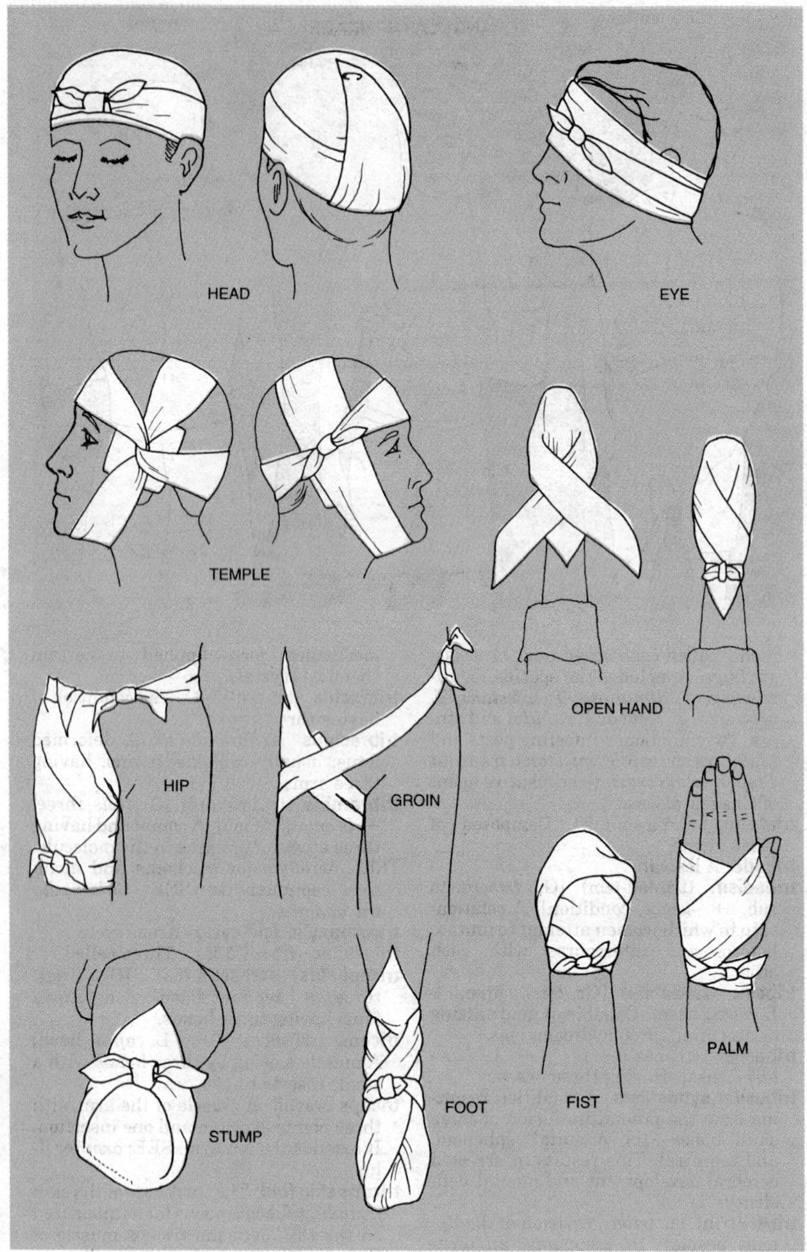

TRIANGULAR BANDAGES

trichalgia Pain caused by touching or moving the hair.

trichangiectasia, trichangiectasis (trĭk″ ăn-jē-ĕk-tā′zē-ă, -ĕk′tă-sĭs) [Gr. *thrix*, hair, + *angeion*, vessel, + *ektasis*, dilatation] Telangiectasia.

trichatrophia (trĭk″ă-trō′fē-ă) [″ + *atrophia*, atrophy] Brittleness of hair resulting from atrophy of the root.

trichi-, trich-, tricho- Combining form meaning *hair*.

trichiasis (trĭk-ī′ă-sĭs) [Gr. *thrix*, hair,

+ *-iasis,* condition] Inversion of eyelashes so that they rub against the cornea, causing a continual irritation of the eyeball. Symptoms are photophobia, lacrimation, and feeling of a foreign body in the eye. The condition is treated by epilation, electrolysis, and operation, such as correcting the underlying entropion with which this condition is usually associated.

trichilemmoma (trĭk″ĭ-lĕm-ō′mă) A benign tumor of the outer root sheath epithelium of a hair follicle.

Trichina (trĭk-ī′nă) [Gr. *trichinos,* of hair] Trichinella.

trichina (trĭ-kī′nă) *pl.* **trichinae** A larval worm of the genus *Trichinella.*

Trichinella (trĭk″ĭ-nĕl′lă) A genus of nematode worms belonging to the suborder Trichurata. They are parasitic in humans, hogs, rats, and many other mammals.

T. spiralis The species of *Trichinella* that commonly infests humans, causing trichinosis. Infection occurs when raw or improperly cooked meat, particularly pork, containing cysts is eaten. Larvae excyst in the duodenum and invade the mucosa of the small intestine, becoming adults in 5 to 7 days. After fertilization, each female deposits 1000 to 2000 larvae, which enter the blood or lymph vessels and circulate to various parts of the body where they encyst, esp. in striated muscle. SEE: illus.; *trichinosis.*

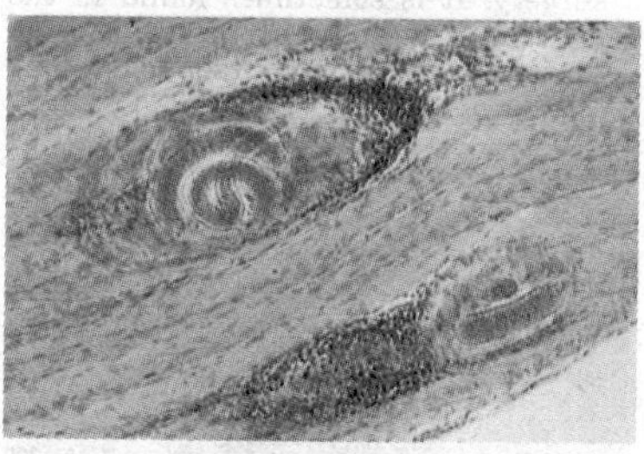

TRICHINELLA SPIRALIS

Encysted in muscle tissue (×800)

trichinellosis (trĭk″ĭ-nĕl-lō′sĭs) [Gr. *trichinos,* of hair, + *osis,* condition] Trichinosis.

trichinophobia (trĭk″ĭn-ō-fō′bē-ă) [Gr. *trichinos,* of hair, + *phobos,* fear] An abnormal fear of developing trichinosis.

trichinosis (trĭk″ĭn-ō′sĭs) [″ + *osis,* condition] Infection by the roundworm parasite *Trichinella spiralis,* resulting from consumption of undercooked pork or wild game. The organisms produce larvae in the gastrointestinal tract that move through the bloodstream and infect muscle cells, producing cysts. In the U.S. fewer than 0.5% of pigs are infected, and fewer than 40 cases of the disease are now reported annually. SYN: *trichinellosis.* SEE: *Nursing Diagnoses Appendix.*

SYMPTOMS: Occasionally, nausea, vomiting, and diarrhea may be present when the infected meat is eaten. After the larvae invade the muscles, patients have fever, muscle pain, and periorbital edema. Rarely, signs of encephalitis, myocarditis, and invasion of the diaphragm occur. After encystment, the only symptom may be vague muscular pains, which may persist for weeks. Laboratory testing reveals an increase in eosinophils circulating in the blood.

TREATMENT: Albendazole is administered for 14 days after diagnosis. Muscle pains should be relieved by analgesics. Corticosteroids are indicated for allergic reaction or central nervous system involvement. Treatment is generally symptomatic and supportive.

PROGNOSIS: The prognosis depends on the number of worms ingested. The majority of patients recover.

PREVENTION: Pork and wild game should always be cooked to an internal temperature of at least 160°F (71°C) to destroy trichinella; smoking and pickling do not destroy the organism. The meat industry advocates irradiation to ensure roundworm destruction, but this process is controversial.

PATIENT CARE: The caregiver provides support and encourages the patient to report adverse symptoms, because treatment is primarily directed at their relief. The patient should also obtain sufficient rest.

trichinous (trĭk′ĭn-ŭs) [Gr. *trichinos,* of hair] Infested with trichinae.

trichinous myositis Myositis trichinosa.

trichion (trĭk′ē-ŏn) [Gr.] The anthropometric point at which the midsagittal plane of the head intersects the hairline.

trichitis (trĭk-ī′tĭs) [Gr. *thrix,* hair, + *itis,* inflammation] Inflammation of hair follicles.

trichloride (trī-klō′rīd) A compound containing three atoms of chlorine.

trichloroacetic acid A drug used as a caustic to destroy certain types of warts, condylomata, keratoses, and hyperplastic tissue.

trichloroethylene (trī″klor-ō-ĕth′ĭl-ēn) A colorless clear volatile liquid with a specific gravity of 1.47 at 59°F (15°C). It is used as an analgesic and anesthetic agent to supplement the action of nitrous oxide. It should not be used with epinephrine.

CAUTION: This substance should not be used in a system that requires soda lime. The heat generated in this type of system by the action of carbon dioxide and the lime will break down trichloroethylene to form the toxic gas phosgene and hydrochloric acid. Also, in the presence of alkali the toxic and flammable substance dichloroacetylene is formed.

2,4,5-trichlorophenoxyacetic acid ABBR: 2,4,5-T. A widely used herbicide that contains dioxin, a toxic and undesirable contaminant.

tricho- [Gr. *thrix, trichos,* hair] SEE: *trichi-*.

trichoanesthesia (trĭk″ō-ăn″ĕs-thē′zē-ă) Loss of sensibility of the hair.

trichobacteria (trĭk″ō-băk-tē′rē-ă) [Gr. *thrix, trichos,* hair, + *bakterion,* rod] **1.** Filamentous bacteria. **2.** Bacteria possessing flagella.

trichobezoar (trĭk″ō-bē′zor) [″ + Arabic *bazahr,* protecting against poison] Hairball.

trichocardia (trĭk-ō-kăr′dē-ă) [″ + *kardia,* heart] Pericardial inflammation with elevations resembling hair. SYN: *shaggy pericardium.*

trichoclasia, trichoclasis (trĭk″ō-klā′zē-ă, -ŏk′lăs-ĭs) [″ + *klasis,* a breaking] Brittleness of the hair.

trichocryptosis (trĭk″ō-krĭp-tō′sĭs) [″ + *kryptos,* concealed] Any disease of the hair follicles.

trichocyst (trĭk′ō-sĭst) [″ + *kystis,* bladder] **1.** A cell structure derived from cytoplasm. **2.** In some single-celled organisms, a vesicle equipped with a thread that can be thrust out for the purposes of defense or attack.

Trichodectes (trĭk″ō-dĕk′tēz) [″ + *dektes,* biter] A genus of lice of the suborder Mallophaga. These lice do not bite humans.

trichoepithelioma (trĭk″ō-ĕp″ĭ-thē-lē-ō″mă) [″ + *epi,* upon, + *thele,* nipple, + *oma,* tumor] A benign skin tumor originating in the hair follicles.

trichoesthesia (trĭk″ō-ĕs-thē′zē-ă) [″ + *aisthesis,* sensation] **1.** The sensation felt when a hair is touched. **2.** A paresthesia causing a sensation of the presence of a hair on a mucous membrane or on the skin.

trichogen (trĭk′ō-jĕn) [″ + *gennan,* to produce] An agent stimulating hair growth.

trichogenous (trĭk-ŏj′ĕn-ŭs) Promoting hair growth.

trichoglossia (trĭk″ō-glŏs′ē-ă) [″ + *glossa,* tongue] Hairy condition of the tongue.

trichohyalin (trĭk″ō-hī′ă-lĭn) [″ + *hyalos,* glass] The hyaline of the hair.

trichoid (trĭk′oyd) [″ + *eidos,* form, shape] Hairlike.

trichokryptomania (trĭk″ō-krĭp″tō-mā′nē-ă) [″ + *kryptos,* hidden, + *mania,* madness] An abnormal desire to break off the hair or beard with the fingernail.

tricholith (trĭk′ō-lĭth) [″ + *lithos,* stone] **1.** A hairy nodule on the hair; seen in piedra. **2.** A calcified intestinal bezoar that contains hair.

trichology (trĭk-ŏl′ō-jē) [″ + *logos,* word, reason] The study of the hair and its care and treatment.

trichoma (trĭk-ō′mă) [Gr., hairiness] **1.** Inversion of one or more eyelashes. SYN: *entropion.* **2.** Matted, verminous, encrusted state of the hair.

trichomatosis (trĭk″ō-mă-tō′sĭs) [″ + *osis,* condition] Entangled matted hair caused by scalp fungus.

trichomatous (trĭ-kŏm′ă-tŭs) Of the nature of or affected with trichoma.

trichome (trī′kōm) [Gr. *trichoma,* a growth of hair] **1.** A hair or other appendage of the skin. **2.** A colony of blue-green algae that grows end-to-end in a chainlike fashion.

trichomegaly (trĭk″ō-mĕg′ă-lē) [Gr. *trichos,* hair, + *megas,* large] Long, coarse eyebrows.

trichomonacide (trĭk″ō-mō′nă-sīd) Anything that is lethal to trichomonads.

trichomonad (trĭk″ō-mō′năd) Related to or resembling the genus of flagellate *Trichomonas.*

Trichomonas (trĭk″ō′mō′năs) [″ + *monas,* unit] Genus of flagellate parasitic protozoa.

T. hominis A benign trichomonad found in the large intestine.

T. tenax A benign trichomonad that may be present in the mouth.

T. vaginalis A species found in the vagina that produces discharge. *T. vaginalis* is fairly common in women, esp. during pregnancy or following vaginal surgery. It is sometimes found in the male urethra and may be transmitted through sexual intercourse. SEE: illus.; *colpitis macularis.*

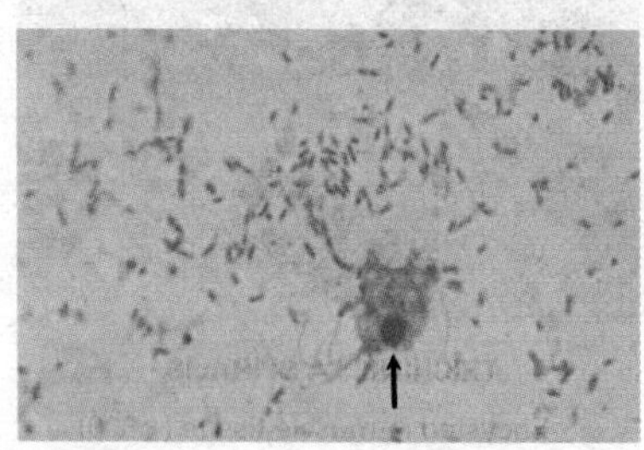

***TRICHOMONAS VAGINALIS* (arrow) AND BACTERIA IN VAGINAL SMEAR (X1000)**

SYMPTOMS: *T. vaginalis* causes persistent burning, redness, and itching of the vulvar tissue associated with a profuse vaginal discharge that may be frothy or malodorous or both. Occasionally, infection with *T. vaginalis* is asymptomatic.

TREATMENT: Metronidazole (Flagyl) is taken orally by the woman and her sexual partner. The drug is contraindicated during the first trimester of pregnancy because of potential damage to the developing fetus; clotrimazole vaginal suppositories provide symptomatic relief during the first 12 weeks of gestation.

NOTE: Alcohol should not be consumed during metronidazole therapy.

trichomoniasis (trĭk″ō-mō-nī′ă-sĭs) [″ + ″ + *-iasis,* infection] Infestation with a parasite of the genus *Trichomonas.*

trichomycosis (trĭk″ō-mī-kō′sĭs) [″ + *mykes,* fungus, + *osis,* condition] Any disease of the hair caused by a fungus.

t. axillaris An infection of the axillary region and sometimes pubic hairs caused by *Nocardia tenuis.*

t. nodosa Piedra.

trichonosis, trichonosus (trĭk-ō-nō′sĭs, -ŏn′ō-sŭs) [Gr. *trichos,* hair, + *nosos,* disease] Any disease of the hair. SYN: *trichopathy.*

trichopathophobia (trĭk″ō-păth″ō-fō′bē-ă) [″ + *pathos,* disease, suffering, + *phobos,* fear] A morbid fear of hair on the face experienced by women, or any abnormal anxiety regarding hair.

trichopathy (trĭk-ŏp′ă-thē) [″ + *pathos,* disease, suffering] Trichonosis.

trichophagia, trichophagy (trĭk-ō-fā′jē-ă, -ŏf′ă-jē) [″ + *phagein,* to eat] The habit of eating hair.

trichophobia (trĭk″ō-fō′bē-ă) [″ + *phobos,* fear] An abnormal dread of hair or of touching it.

trichophytic (trĭk″ō-fĭt′ĭk) [″ + *phyton,* plant] **1.** Relating to *Trichophyton.* **2.** Promoting hair growth.

trichophytic granulosa (trĭk″ō-fĭt′ĭk) Tinea profunda.

trichophytid (trĭ-kŏf′ĭ-tĭd) A skin disorder considered to be an allergic reaction to fungi of the genus *Trichophyton.*

trichophytin (trĭ-kŏf′ĭ-tĭn) An extract prepared from cultures of the fungi of the genus *Trichophyton;* used as an antigen for skin tests and for the treatment of certain trichophytid infections.

trichophytobezoar (trĭk-ō-fī″tō-bē′zor) [″ + *phyton,* plant, + Arabic *bazahr,* protecting against poison] A hairball found in the stomach or intestine composed of hair, vegetable fibers, and miscellaneous debris.

Trichophyton (trĭ-kŏf′ĭt-ŏn) A genus of parasitic fungi that lives in or on the skin or its appendages (hair and nails) and is the cause of various dermatomycoses and ringworm infections. Species that produce spores arranged in rows on the outside of the hair are designated ectothrix; if spores are within the hair, endothrix.

T. mentagrophytes A species, one form of which, called *granulare,* is parasitic on several mammals including horses, dogs, and rodents and can also affect humans. Another variety, called *interdigitale,* is associated with tinea pedis.

T. schoenleinii The causative agent of favus of the scalp. SEE: *favus.*

T. tonsurans The most frequent cause of ringworm of the scalp. SEE: *tinea capitis.*

T. violaceum The causative agent of some forms of ringworm of the scalp, beard, or nails.

trichophytosis (trĭk″ō-fī-tō′sĭs) [″ + *phyton,* plant, + *osis,* condition] Infestation with *Trichophyton* fungi.

trichoptilosis (trĭk″ŏp-tĭl-ō′sĭs) [″ + *ptilon,* feather, + *osis,* condition] **1.** The splitting of hairs at their ends, giving them a feather-like appearance. **2.** A disease of hair marked by development of nodules along the hair shaft, at which point it splits off.

trichoscopy (trĭk-ŏs′kō-pē) [″ + *skopein,* to examine] Inspection of the hair.

trichosiderin (trĭk″ō-sĭd′ĕr-ĭn) [″ + *sideros,* iron] An iron-containing pigment normally present in red hair.

trichosis (trī-kō′sĭs) [″ + *osis,* condition] Any disease of the hair or its abnormal growth or development in an abnormal place.

t. decolor Any abnormal coloring or lack of coloring of the hair. SYN: *canities.*

t. setosa Coarse hair.

Trichosporon (trī-kŏs′pō-rŏn) [″ + *sporos,* a seed] A genus of fungi that grows on hair and causes piedra.

T. beigelii The causative agent of white piedra. SEE: *piedra.*

trichosporosis (trĭk″ō-spō-rō′sĭs) [″ + ″ + *osis,* condition] Infestation of the hair with *Trichosporon.*

trichostasis spinulosa (trĭ-kŏs′tă-sĭs spĭn″ū-lō′să) [″ + *stasis,* a standing] A congenital condition in which the hair follicle is plugged with keratin and fine, lanugo hairs.

trichostrongyliasis (trĭk″ō-strŏn-jĭ-lī′ă-sĭs) Infestation with the intestinal parasite *Trichostrongylus;* a rare disease in the U.S.

trichostrongylosis (trĭk″ō-strŏn″jĭ-lō′sĭs) Infestation with *Trichostrongylus.*

Trichostrongylus (trĭk″ō-strŏn′jĭ-lŭs) A genus of nematode worms of the family Trichostrongylidae. These worms are of economic importance because of the damage they cause to domestic animals and birds.

Trichothecium (trĭk″ō-thē′sē-ŭm) [″ + *theke,* a box] A genus of mold fungi causing disease of the hair.

T. roseum A species of mold fungus found in certain cases of inflammation of the eardrum (mycomyringitis).

trichotillomania (trĭk″ō-tĭl″ō-mā′nē-ă) [″ + *tillein,* to pull, + *mania,* madness] The unnatural and irresistible urge to pull out one's own hair. Clomipramine has been effective in treating this condition.

trichotomous (trī-kŏt′ō-mŭs) [Gr. *tricha,* threefold, + *tome,* incision] Divided into three.

trichotomy (trī-kŏt′ō-mē) Division into three parts.

trichotoxin (trĭk″ō-tŏks′ĭn) [Gr. *trichos,* hair, + *toxikon,* poison] An antibody or cytotoxin that destroys ciliated epithelial cells.

trichotrophy (trĭ-kŏt′rō-fē) [″ + *trophe,* nourishment] Nutrition of the hair.

trichroic (trī-krō′ĭk) [Gr. *treis,* three, + *chroa,* color] Presenting three different colors when viewed along each of three different axes.

trichroism (trī′krō-ĭzm) [″ + ″ + *-ismos,* condition] Quality of showing a different color when viewed along each of three axes. SYN: *trichromatism.*

trichromatic (trī″krō-măt′ĭk) [″ + *chroma,* color] Rel. to or able to see the three primary colors; denoting normal color vision. SYN: *trichromic.*

trichromatism (trī-krō′mă-tĭzm) Trichroism.

trichromatopsia (trī″krō-mă-tŏp′sē-ă) Normal color vision.

trichromic (trī-krō′mĭk) Pert. to normal color vision or the ability to see the three primary colors. SYN: *trichromatic.*

trichuriasis (trĭk″ū-rī′ă-sĭs) [Gr. *trichos,* hair, + *oura,* tail + *-iasis,* condition] The presence of worms of the genus *Trichuris* in the colon or in the ileum.

Trichuris (trĭ-kū′rĭs) Parasitic nematode worms that belong to the class Nematoda.

T. trichiura A species of *Trichuris* that infects humans when the ova that have undergone incubation in the soil are ingested. The larvae develop into adults, which inhabit the large intestine. Symptoms of the infection include diarrhea and abdominal pain. Rectal prolapse may occur if a great number of worms are present. Mebendazole is the drug of choice; albendazole or ivermectin may be of benefit. SYN: *whipworm.* SEE: illus.

tricipital (trī-sĭp′ĭ-tăl) [Gr. *treis,* three, + L. *caput,* head] Three-headed, as the triceps muscle.

tricitrates oral solution A solution of sodium citrate, potassium citrate, and citric acid in a suitable aqueous medium. The sodium and potassium ion contents of the solution are approx. 1 mEq/ml.

tricornic, tricornute (trī-kor′nĭk) [″ + L. *cornu,* horn] Having three horns or cornua.

tricrotic (trī-krŏt′ĭk) [Gr. *trikrotos,* rowed with a triple stroke] A condition in which three accentuated waves or notches occur with each pulse.

tricrotism (trī′krŏt-ĭzm) [″ + *-ismos,* condition] The condition of being tricrotic.

tricuspid (trī-kŭs′pĭd) [Gr. *treis,* three, + L. *cuspis,* point] **1.** Pert. to the tricuspid valve. **2.** Having three points or cusps.

tricuspid area The lower portion of the body of the sternum where sounds of the right atrioventricular orifice are best heard.

tricuspid atresia Stenosis of the tricuspid valve. A fairly uncommon congenital malformation that causes cyanosis and clubbing. Symptoms include paroxysmal dyspnea and difficulty in feeding.

tricuspid murmur A murmur caused by stenosis of or regurgitation by the tricuspid valve.

tricuspid orifice Right atrioventricular cardiac aperture.

tricuspid tooth A tooth with a crown that has three cusps.

tricuspid valve SEE: under *valve.*

trident, tridentate (trī′dĕnt, trī-dĕn′tāt) [L. *tres, tria,* three, + *dens,* tooth] Having three prongs.

tridermic (trī-dĕr′mĭk) [Gr. *treis,* three, + *derma,* skin] Developed from the ectoderm, endoderm, and mesoderm.

tridermoma (trī″dĕr-mō′mă) [″ + ″ + *oma,* tumor] A teratoid growth containing all three germ layers.

trielcon (trī-ĕl′kŏn) [″ + *helkein,* to draw] An instrument with three branches for removing bullets or other foreign bodies from wounds.

triencephalus (trī″ĕn-sĕf′ă-lŭs) [″ + *enkephalos,* brain] A deformed fetus lack-

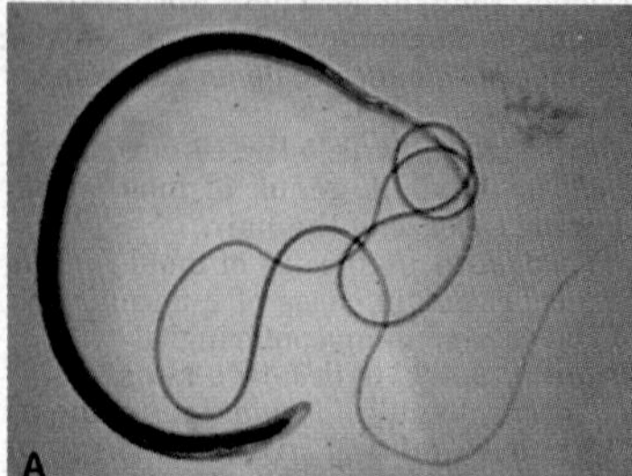

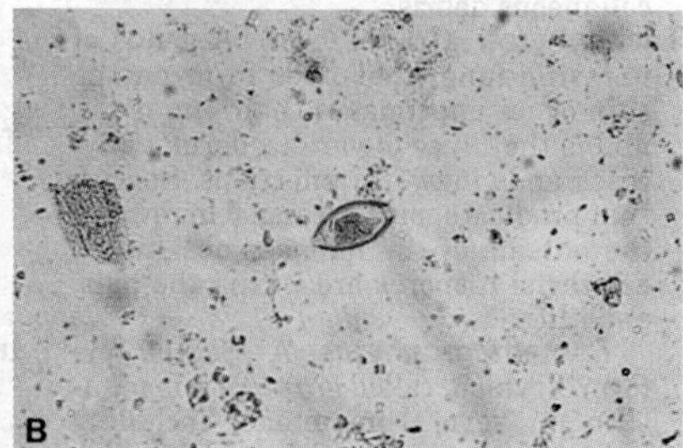

TRICHURIS TRICHIURA

(A) adult female (×4), (B) eggs in feces (×100)

ing the organs of sight, hearing, and smell.

triethylenethiophosphoramide (trī-ĕth″ĭ-lēn-thī″ō-fŏs-for′ă-mīd) Thiotepa.

trifacial (trī-fā′shăl) [L. *trifacialis*] Trigeminal.

trifid (trī-fĭd) [L. *trifidus,* split thrice] Split into three; having three clefts.

trifluoperazine hydrochloride (trī″floo-ō-păr′ă-zēn) An antipsychotic drug.

triflupromazine (trī″floo-prō′mă-zēn) An antipsychotic drug that is also used in treating nausea and vomiting.

trifurcation (trī″fŭr-kā′shŭn) [Gr. *treis,* three, + L. *furca,* fork] **1.** Division into three branches. **2.** In dentistry, the area of root division in a tooth with three roots.

trifurcation involvement The extension of periodontitis or a periodontal pocket into an area where the tooth roots divide.

trigastric (trī-găs′trĭk) [Gr. *treis,* three, + *gaster,* belly] Having three bellies, as certain muscles.

trigeminal (trī-jĕm′ĭn-ăl) [L. *tres, tria,* three, + *geminus,* twin] Pert. to the trigeminus or fifth cranial nerve.

trigeminal cough A reflex cough from irritation of the trigeminal terminations in respiratory upper passages.

trigeminal nerve The fifth cranial nerve, a large, mixed nerve arising from the pons in a large sensory root and a smaller motor root. At the junction of the roots, the semilunar gasserian ganglion gives rise to three branches. These branches are *ophthalmic,* purely sensory, from the skin of the upper part of the head, mucous membranes of the nasal cavity and sinuses, cornea, and conjunctiva; *maxillary,* purely sensory, from the dura mater, gums and teeth of the upper jaw, upper lip, and orbit; and *mandibular,* sensory fibers from the tongue, gums, and teeth of the lower jaw, skin of the cheek, lower jaw, and lip, and motor fibers supplying principally the muscles of mastication. SYN: *fifth cranial nerve.*

trigeminal pulse A pulse with a longer or shorter interval after each three beats because the third beat is an extrasystole.

trigeminus (trī-jĕm′ĭ-nŭs) Trigeminal nerve.

trigeminy (trī-jĕm′ĭ-nē) Occurring in threes, esp. three pulse beats in rapid succession.

trigenic (trī-jĕn′ĭk) [Gr. *treis,* three, + *gennan,* to produce] In genetics, a condition in which three alleles are present at any particular locus on the chromosome.

trigger (trĭg′ĕr) [D. *trekker,* something pulled] **1.** Stimulus. **2.** To initiate or start with suddenness. **3.** A chemical that initiates a function or action.

trigger action A physiological process or a pathological change initiated by a sudden stimulus.

trigger finger A state in which flexion or extension of a digit is arrested temporarily but is finally completed with a jerk. Any finger may be involved, but the ring or middle finger is most often affected. SEE: illus.

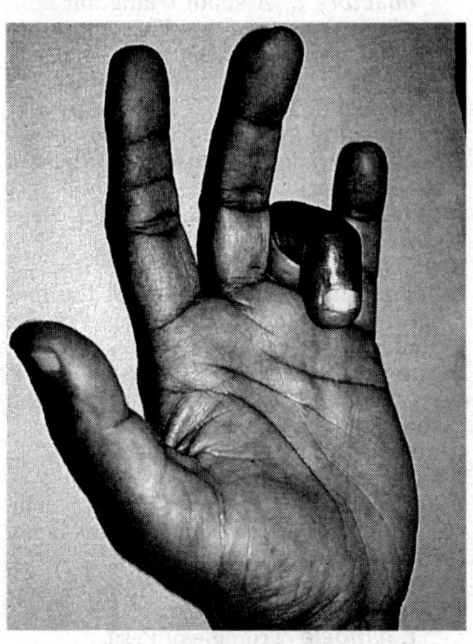

TRIGGER FINGER

Treatment: A finger splint or cortisone injection may be used to treat this condition. Surgery may be required.

trigger point, trigger zone **1.** An area of tissue that is tender when compressed and may give rise to referred pain and tenderness. **2.** An area of the cerebral cortex that, when stimulated, produces abnormal reactions similar to those in acquired epilepsy. SEE: *epileptogenic zone.*

triglyceride (trī-glĭs′ĕr-īd) Any combinations of glycerol with three of five different fatty acids. These substances, triacylglycerols, are also called neutral fats. In the blood, triglycerides are combined with proteins to form lipoproteins. The liver synthesizes lipoproteins to transport fats to other tissues, where they are a source of energy. Fat in adipose tissue is stored energy. SEE: *hyperlipoproteinemia.*

medium-chain t. Triglycerides with 8 to 10 carbon atoms. They are digested and absorbed differently than the usual dietary fats and, for that reason, have been used in treating malabsorption.

trigonal (trĭg′ō-năl) [Gr. *trigonon,* a three-cornered figure] Triangular; pert. to a trigone.

trigone (trī′gōn) A triangular space, esp. one at the base of the bladder, between the two openings of the ureters and the urethra. SYN: *t. of bladder; trigonum; vesical t.*

t. of bladder Trigone.

carotid t. The triangular area in the neck bounded by the posterior belly of the digastric muscle, the sternocleidomastoid muscle, and the midline of the neck.

olfactory t. A small triangular eminence at the root of the olfactory peduncle and anterior to the anterior perforated space of the base of the brain.

vesical t. Trigone.

trigonectomy (trī″gōn-ĕk′tō-mē) [″ + *ektome,* excision] Excision of the base of the bladder.

trigonid (trī-gō′nĭd) The first three cusps of a lower molar tooth.

trigonitis (trĭg″ō-nī′tĭs) [″ + *itis,* inflammation] Inflammation of the mucous membrane of the trigone of the bladder.

trigonocephalic (trĭ″gō-nō-sĕ-făl′ĭk) [″ + *kephale,* head] Having a head shaped like a triangle.

trigonocephalus (trĭg″ō-nō-sĕf′ă-lŭs) A fetus exhibiting trigonocephaly.

trigonocephaly (trī-gō″nō-sĕf′ă-lē) The condition of the head of the fetus being shaped like a triangle.

trigonum (trī-gō′nŭm) *pl.* **trigona** [L.] Trigone.

t. lumbale Triangle of Petit.

trihexyphenidyl hydrochloride (trī-hĕk″sē-fĕn′ĭ-dĭl) An anticholinergic drug used in treating parkinsonism.

trihybrid (trī-hī′brĭd) [Gr. *treis,* three, + L. *hybrida,* mongrel] In genetics, the offspring of a cross between two individuals differing in three unit characters.

triiniodymus (trī″ĭn-ē-ŏd′ĭ-mŭs) [″ + *inion,* nape of the neck, + *didymos,* twin] A deformed fetus with a single body and three heads joined at the occiput.

triiodothyronine (trī″ī-ō″dō-thī′rō-nēn) ABBR: T_3. One of two forms of the principal hormone secreted by the thyroid gland. Chemically it is 3,5,3′-triiodothyronine (liothyronine). SEE: *tetraiodothyronine; thyroid gland; thyroid function test; thyroxine.*

trikates A solution of potassium acetate, potassium bicarbonate, and potassium citrate; used in treating electrolyte deficiencies.

trilabe (trī′lāb) [Gr. *treis,* three, + *labe,* a handle] Three-pronged forceps for removing foreign substances from the bladder.

trilaminar (trī-lăm′ĭ-năr) Composed of three layers.

trilateral (trī-lăt′ĕr-ăl) [″ + L. *latus,* side] Concerning three sides.

trill (trĭl) [It. *trillare,* probably imitative] A tremulous sound, esp. in vocal music.

trilobate (trī-lō′bāt) [″ + *lobos,* lobe] Having three lobes.

trilocular (trī-lŏk′ū-lăr) [″ + L. *loculus,* cell] Having three compartments.

trilogy (trĭl′ō-jē) A series of three events.

trimanual (trī-măn′ū-ăl) [″ + *manualis,* by hand] Performed with three hands, as an obstetrical maneuver.

trimensual (trī-mĕn′shū-ăl) [″ + *mensualis,* monthly] Occurring every 3 months.

trimester (trī-mĕs′tĕr) A 3-month period.

first t. The first 3 months of pregnancy.

second t. The middle 3 months of pregnancy.

third t. The third and final 3 months of pregnancy.

trimethaphan camsylate (trī-mĕth′ă-făn) A ganglionic blocking agent used to diminish blood pressure in acute hypertensive crisis.

trimethoprim (trī-mĕth′ō-prĭm) An antibacterial drug usually used in combination with sulfamethoxazole; together, the drugs interfere with sequential steps in the metabolism of certain bacteria. The combination is used to treat various bacterial infections, esp. urinary tract pathogens such as *Proteus mirabilis, Escherichia coli,* and *Klebsiella* species.. The combination is used to treat *Pneumocystis carinii* pneumonia and travelers' diarrhea caused by susceptible strains of enterotoxigenic *E. coli.* The trade names of the combined product are Bactrim and Septra. SEE: *sulfamethoxazole.*

CAUTION: An important side effect of trimethoprim is renal failure. It occurs occasionally.

trimethylene (trī-mĕth′ĭ-lēn) Cyclopropane.

trimmer A device or instrument used to shape something by cutting off the material along its margin.

gingival margin t. A cutting instrument for shaping gingival contours. It has a curved and angled shaft for use either on the right or left sides and on the mesial or distal surfaces.

model t. A rotary flat grinder used to trim dental plaster or stone casts. Water keeps the cutting surface clean and obviates any dust problem as the casts are squared into proper study models.

trimorphous (trī-mor′fŭs) [″ + *morphe,* form] **1.** Having three different forms as the larva, pupa, and adult of certain insects. **2.** Having three different forms of crystals.

trinitrophenol (trī″nī-trō-fē′nōl) A yellow crystalline powder that precipitates proteins. It is used as a dye and as a reagent. SYN: *picric acid.*

trinitrotoluene (trī″nī-trō-tŏl′ū-ēn) ABBR: TNT. $C_7H_5N_3O_6$; an explosive compound.

triocephalus (trī″ō-sĕf′ă-lŭs) [″ + *kephale,* head] A deformed fetus with a rudimentary head without eyes, nose, or mouth.

triolein Olein.

triolism (trī'ō-lĭzm) Sexual activity involving two persons of one sex and one person of the opposite sex.

triophthalmos (trī"ŏf-thăl'mōs) [" + *ophthalmos,* eye] A deformed fetus with three eyes.

triopodymus (trī"ō-pŏd'ĭ-mŭs) [" + *ops,* face, + *didymos,* twin] A deformed fetus with three fused heads and three faces.

triorchid, triorchis (trī-or'kĭd, -kĭs) [" + *orchis,* testicle] A person who has three testicles.

triorchidism (trī-or'kĭd-ĭzm) [" + " + *-ismos,* condition] The condition of having three testicles.

triose (trī'ōs) A monosaccharide having three carbon atoms in its molecule.

triotus (trī-ō'tŭs) [" + *ous,* ear] A person with a third ear.

trioxsalen (trī-ŏk'să-lĕn) An agent used to promote repigmentation in vitiligo. Trade name is Trisoralen. SEE: *psoralen; vitiligo.*

trip (trĭp) A slang term used to refer to hallucinations produced by various drugs, including LSD, mescaline, and some narcotics.

tripara (trĭp'ă-ră) [L. *tres, tria,* three, + *parere,* to bear] A woman who has had three pregnancies that have lasted beyond 20 weeks or that have produced an infant of at least 500 g; also designated Para III. SYN: *tertipara.*

tripeptide (trī-pĕp'tīd) [Gr. *treis,* three, + *pepton,* digested] The product of a combination of three amino acids formed during proteolytic digestion.

triphalangia (trī"fă-lăn'jē-ă) [" + *phalanx,* closely knit row] A deformity marked by the presence of three phalanges in a thumb or great toe.

triphasic (trī-fā'sĭk) [" + *phasis,* phase] Consisting of three phases or stages, said of electric currents.

triphenylmethane (trī-fĕn"ĭl-mĕth'ān) A coal tar–derived chemical that is the basis of some dyes and stains.

Tripier's amputation (trĭp-ē-āz') [Léon Tripier, Fr. surgeon, 1842–1891] Amputation of a foot with part of the calcaneus removed.

triple (trĭp'l) [L. *triplus,* threefold] Consisting of three; threefold; treble.

triplegia (trī-plē'jē-ă) [" + *plege,* stroke] Hemiplegia with paralysis of one limb on the other side of the body.

triple response The three reactions of the skin to injury: a red reaction along the line of injury; a red area (flare or erythema) about the injury; and an elevated area (welt or wheal) resulting from localized edema.

triplet (trĭp'lĕt) [L. *triplus,* threefold] **1.** One of three children produced in one gestation and one birth. SEE: *Hellin's law.* **2.** A combination of three of a kind.

triplex (trī'plĕks, trĭp'lĕks) [Gr. *triploos,* triple] Triple; threefold.

triploblastic (trĭp"lō-blăst'ĭk) [" + *blastos,* germ] Consisting of three germ layers: ectoderm, endoderm, and mesoderm.

triploid (trĭp'loyd) Concerning triploidy.

triploidy (trĭp'loy-dē) In the human, having three sets of chromosomes.

triplokoria (trĭp"lō-kor'ē-ă) [" + *kore,* pupil] Possessing three pupillary openings in one eye.

triplopia (trĭp-lō'pē-ă) [" + *ope,* vision] A condition in which three images of the same object are seen.

tripod (trī'pŏd) [Gr. *treis,* three, + *pous,* foot] A stand having three supports, usually legs.

tripodia (trī-pō'dē-ă) Having three feet.

tripoding (trī'pŏd-ĭng) The use of three bases for support (e.g., two legs and a cane, or one leg and two crutches).

triprosopus (trī"prō-sō'pŭs) [" + *prosopon,* face] A deformed fetus with three faces.

tripsis (trĭp'sĭs) [Gr. *tripsis,* friction] **1.** The process of trituration. **2.** Massage.

-tripsy (trĭp'sē) [Gr. *tripsis,* friction] A word ending indicating intentional crushing of something.

triquetral (trī-kwē'trăl) [L. *triquetrus*] Triangular.

triquetral bone **1.** The third carpal bone in the proximal row, enumerated from the radial side. **2.** Any wormian bone. SYN: *cuneiform bone.*

triquetrous (trī-kwē'trŭs) [L. *triquetrus,* triangular] Triangular.

triquetrum (trī-kwē'trŭm) [L.] Three-cornered.

triradial, triradiate (trī-rā'dē-ăl, -āt) [Gr. *treis,* three, + L. *radiatus,* rayed] Having three rays; radiating in three directions.

triradius (trī-rā'dē-ŭs) In classifying fingerprints, the point of convergence of dermal ridges coming from three directions.

trisaccharide (trī-săk'ă-rīd) A carbohydrate that on hydrolysis yields three molecules of simple sugars (monosaccharides).

triskaidekaphobia (trĭ-skī-dĕk-ă-fō'bē-ă) [Gr. *triskaideka,* thirteen, + *phobos,* fear] Superstition concerning the number 13.

trismic (trĭz'mĭk) Concerning trismus.

trismoid (trĭz'moyd) [Gr. *trismos,* grating, + *eidos,* form, shape] **1.** Of the nature of trismus. **2.** A form of trismus nascentium; once thought to be due to pressure on the occiput during delivery.

trismus (trĭz'mŭs) [Gr. *trismos,* grating] Tonic contraction of the muscles of mastication; may occur in mouth infections, encephalitis, inflammation of salivary glands, and tetanus. SYN: *lockjaw.*

trisomic (trī-sōm'ĭk) In genetics, an individual possessing 2n+1 chromosomes, that is, one set of chromosomes contains an extra (third) chromosome. SEE: *chromosome; karyotype*.

trisomy (trī'sō-mē) In genetics, having three homologous chromosomes per cell instead of two.

t. 13 A severe developmental disorder in which a third copy of chromosome 13 is present in the cell nucleus. It is often lethal in utero. Children who survive fetal development may have severe facial, scalp, and cranial deformities, and a predisposition to leukemia. SYN: *Patau syndrome*.

t. 18 A severe, usually lethal developmental disorder in which a third copy of chromosome 18 is present in the cell nucleus. Children with trisomy 18 usually do not survive beyond the first year of life. The condition is characterized by cranial, neurological, facial, cardiac, and gastrointestinal malformations. The disease can be sometimes detected during pregnancy with ultrasound or specialized blood tests. SYN: *Edward's syndrome*.

t. 21 Down syndrome.

trisplanchnic (trī-splănk'nĭk) [Gr. *treis,* three, + *splanchna,* viscera] Pert. to the three large body cavities: cranial, thoracic, and abdominal.

tristichia (trī-stĭk'ē-ă) [" + *stichos,* row] The presence of three rows of eyelashes.

tristimania (trĭs"tĭ-mā'nē-ă) [L. *tristis,* sad, + Gr. *mania,* madness] Melancholia.

trisulcate (trī-sŭl'kāt) [L. *tres, tria,* three, + *sulcus,* groove] Having three grooves or furrows.

trisulfate (trī-sŭl'fāt) A chemical compound containing three sulfate, SO_4, groups.

trisulfide (trī-sŭl'fīd) A chemical compound containing three sulfur atoms.

tritanomalopia (trī"tă-nŏm'ă-lō-pē-ă) [Gr. *tritos,* third, + *anomalos,* irregular, + *ope,* sight] A color vision defect similar to tritanopia but less pronounced. SYN: *tritanomaly*.

tritanomaly (trī"tă-nŏm'ă-lē) Tritanomalopia.

tritanopia (trī"tă-nō'pē-ă) [Gr. *tritos,* third, + *an-,* not, + *ope,* vision] Blue blindness; color blindness in which there is a defect in the perception of blue. SEE: *color blindness*.

tritiate (trĭt'ē-āt) To treat with tritium.

tritiated thymidine ^{3}H-Tdr; a radioactively labeled nucleoside used to measure T lymphocyte proliferation in vitro. Thymidine is essential for DNA synthesis, thus the amount of ^{3}H-Tdr taken up is a general measure of the number of new lymphocytes produced.

triticeous (trĭt-ĭsh'ŭs) [L. *triticeus,* of wheat] Shaped like a grain of wheat.

t. cartilage A cartilaginous nodule in the thyrohyoid ligament.

tritium (trĭt'ē-ŭm, trĭsh'ē-ŭm) [Gr. *tritos,* third] The mass three isotope of hydrogen; triple-weight hydrogen.

triturable (trĭt'ū-ră-bl) [L. *triturare,* to pulverize] Capable of being powdered.

triturate (trĭt'ū-rāt) **1.** To reduce to a fine powder by rubbing. **2.** A finely divided substance made by rubbing.

trituration (trĭt-ū-rā'shŭn) [LL. *triturare,* to pulverize] **1.** The act of reducing to a powder. **2.** A finely ground and easily mixed powder. **3.** The mixing of dental alloy particles with mercury. Trituration may be done either manually in a mortar with a pestle or with a mechanical device. The goal of trituration is to abrade the alloy particles to facilitate the uptake of mercury.

CAUTION: Mercury compounds are toxic; care should be taken to avoid touching mercury during trituration. Inhaling mercury vapor and mercury particles produced when removing amalgam restorations also should be avoided.

---

trivalence (trĭv'ă-lĕns) Condition of being trivalent.

trivalent (trī-vā'lĕnt, trĭv'ăl-ĕnt) [Gr. *treis,* three, + L. *valens,* powerful] **1.** Combining with or replacing three hydrogen atoms. **2.** Having three components (e.g., a trivalent vaccine).

trivalve (trī'vălv) Having three valves.

trivial name A nonsystematic or semisystematic name and qualifying term used to name drugs. These names do not provide assistance in determining biological action or function of the drug. Examples are aspirin, caffeine, and belladonna.

trizonal (trī-zō'năl) Having three zones or layers.

tRNA *transfer RNA.*

trocar (trō'kăr) [Fr. *trois quarts,* three quarters] A sharply pointed surgical instrument contained in a cannula; used for aspiration or removal of fluids from cavities.

trochanter (trō-kăn'tĕr) [Gr. *trokhanter,* to run] Either of the two bony processes below the neck of the femur.

greater t. A thick process at the lateral upper end of the femur projecting upward to the union of the neck and shaft. SYN: *t. major*.

lesser t. A conical tuberosity on the medial and posterior surface of the upper end of the femur, at the junction of the shaft and neck. SYN: *t. minor*.

t. major Greater trochanter.

t. minor Lesser trochanter.

t. tertius Third trochanter.

third t. The gluteal ridge of the femur when it is unusually prominent. SYN: *T. tertius*.

trochanterian, trochanteric (trō"kăn-tē'rē-ăn, trō-kăn-tĕr'ĭk) Rel. to a trochanter.

trochanterplasty (trō-kăn′tĕr-plăs″tē) Plastic surgery of the neck of the femur.

trochantin (trō-kăn′tĭn) Trochanter minor.

trochantinian (trō″kăn-tĭn′ē-ăn) Concerning the lesser trochanter of the femur.

troche, troch (trō′kē, trōk′) [Gr. *trokhiskos,* a small wheel] A solid, discoid, or cylindrical mass consisting chiefly of medicinal powder, sugar, and mucilage. Troches are used by placing them in the mouth and allowing them to remain until, through slow solution or disintegration, their mild medication is released. SYN: *lozenge.*

trochiscus (trō-kĭs′kŭs) [L., Gr. *trochiskos,* a small disk] A medicated tablet or troche.

trochlea (trŏk′lē-ă) *pl.* **trochleae** [Gr. *trokhileia,* system of pulleys] **1.** A structure having the function of a pulley; a ring or hook through which a tendon or muscle projects. **2.** The articular smooth surface of a bone on which glides another bone.

trochlea of the elbow A surface on the distal humerus that articulates with the ulna.

trochlear (trŏk′lē-ăr) **1.** Of the nature of a pulley. **2.** Pert. to a trochlea.

trochlear fovea A depression on the orbital plate of the frontal bone for attachment of the cartilaginous pulley of the superior oblique muscle.

trochleariform (trŏk″lē-ăr′ĭ-form) Pulley-shaped.

trochlearis (trŏk″lē-ā′rĭs) [L.] The superior oblique muscle of the eye.

trochlear nerve The fourth cranial nerve, a small mixed nerve arising from the midbrain. It is both sensory and motor to the superior oblique muscle of the eye. SYN: *fourth cranial nerve.*

trochocardia (trō″kō-kăr′dē-ă) [Gr. *trokhos,* a wheel, + *kardia,* heart] Rotary displacement of the heart on its axis.

trochocephalia, trochocephaly (trō″kō-sē-fā′lē-ă, -sĕf′ă-lē) [″ + *kephale,* head] Roundheadedness, a deformity due to premature union of the frontal and parietal bones.

trochoid (trō′koyd) [Gr. *trokhos,* a wheel, + *eidos,* form, shape] Rotating or revolving, noting an articulation resembling a pivot or pulley. SEE: *joint, pivot.*

trochoides (trō-koy′dēz) A pivot or rotary joint.

Troglotrematidae (trŏg″lō-trē-măt′ĭ-dē) A family of flukes that includes *Paragonimus* (human lung fluke).

Troisier's node (trwă-zē-āz′) [Charles E. Troisier, Fr. physician, 1844–1919] Sentinel node.

trolamine (trō′lă-mēn) An alkalizing agent.

troland (trō′lănd) A unit of visual stimulation to the retina of the eye. It is equal to the illumination received per square millimeter of the pupil from a source of 1 lux brightness.

troleandomycin (trō″lē-ăn-dō-mī′sĭn) A macrolide antibacterial drug.

Trombicula (trŏm-bĭk′ū-lă) A genus of mites belonging to the Trombiculidae. The larvae, called redbugs or chiggers, cause an irritating dermatitis and rash. They may serve as vectors of various diseases.

T. akamushi A species of mites that transmits the causative agent of scrub typhus.

trombiculiasis (trŏm-bĭk″ū-lī′ă-sĭs) Infestation with Trombiculidae.

Trombiculidae (trŏm-bĭk′ū-lī″dē) A family of mites; only the genus *Trombicula* is of medical significance.

tromethamine (trō-mĕth′ă-mēn) A drug used intravenously to correct acidosis. It should not be used longer than 1 day except in life-threatening emergencies.

troph- SEE: *tropho-.*

trophectoderm (trŏf-ĕk′tō-dĕrm) [Gr. *trophe,* nourishment, + *ectoderm*] In embryology, the peripheral cells of the blastocyst that form the chorion surrounding the embryo, and eventually the placenta.

trophedema (trŏf″ĕ-dē′mă) [Gr. *trophe,* nourishment, + *oidema,* a swelling] Localized edema caused by congenital hypoplasia of lymphatic vessels or resulting secondarily from obstruction to lymph flow by external pressure. Repeated low-grade infection may also obstruct the flow of lymph.

trophic (trŏf′ĭk) [Gr. *trophikos*] Concerned with nourishment; applied particularly to a type of efferent nerves believed to control the growth and nourishment of the parts they innervate. SEE: *autotrophic.*

trophism (trŏf′ĭzm) Nutrition.

tropho-, troph- Combining form meaning *nourishment.*

trophoblast (trŏf′ō-blăst) [Gr. *trophe,* nourishment, + *blastos,* germ] The outermost layer of the developing blastocyst (blastodermic vesicle) of a mammal. It differentiates into two layers, the cytotrophoblast and syntrophoblast, the latter coming into intimate relationship with the uterine endometrium, with which it establishes nutrient relationships. SEE: *fertilization* for illus. **trophoblastic,** *adj.*

trophoblastoma (trŏf″ō-blăs-tō′mă) [″ + ″ + *oma,* tumor] A neoplasm due to excessive proliferation of chorionic epithelium. SYN: *chorioepithelioma.*

trophocyte (trŏf′ō-sīt) A cell that nourishes (e.g., Sertoli cells of the testicle, which support developing spermatozoa). SYN: *trephocyte.*

trophoneurosis (trŏf″ō-nū-rō′sĭs) [″ + *neuron,* nerve, + *osis,* condition] Any trophic disorder caused by defective function of the nerves concerned with nutrition of the part.

disseminated t. Thickening and hardening of the skin. SYN: *sclerema; scleroderma.*

facial t. Progressive facial atrophy.

muscular t. Muscular changes in connection with nervous disorders.

trophonucleus (trŏf″ō-nū′klē-ŭs) [″ + *nucleus,* kernel] Protozoan nucleus concerned with vegetative functions in metabolism and not reproduction.

trophopathia (trŏf″ō-păth′ē-ă) [″ + *pathos,* disease, suffering] **1.** Any disorder of nutrition. **2.** A trophic disease.

trophozoite (trŏf″ō-zō′īt) [″ + *zoon,* animal] A sporozoan nourished by its hosts during its growth stage.

tropia (trō′pē-ă) [Gr. *trope,* turn] Deviation of the eye or eyes away from the visual axis; observed with the eyes open and uncovered. Esotropia indicates inward or nasal deviation; exotropia, outward; hypertropia, upward; hypotropia, downward. SYN: *manifest squint; strabismus.* SEE: *-phoria.*

tropical (trŏp′ĭ-kal) [Gr. *tropikos,* turning] Pert. to the tropics.

tropical immersion foot Immersion foot.

tropical lichen Acute inflammation of the sweat glands. SYN: *Miliaria.*

tropicamide (trō-pĭk′ă-mīd) An anticholinergic drug used to produce mydriasis and cycloplegia in treating eye conditions.

-tropin [Gr. *tropos,* a turn] Combining form, used as a suffix, indicating the stimulating effect of a substance, esp. a hormone, on its target organ.

tropine (trō′pĭn) An alkaloid, $C_8H_{15}NO$, that smells like tobacco. It is present in certain plants.

tropism (trō′pĭzm) [Gr. *trope,* turn, + *-ismos,* condition] **1.** Reaction of living organisms involuntarily toward or away from light, darkness, heat, cold, or other stimuli. **2.** The involuntary response of an organism as a bending, turning, or movement toward (positive tropism) or away from (negative tropism) an external stimulus. SYN: *taxis.* SEE: *chemotropism; phototropism.*

tropocollagen (trō″pō-kŏl′ă-jĕn) [″ + *collagen*] The basic molecular unit of collagen fibrils, composed of three polypeptide chains.

tropometer (trŏp-ŏm′ĕ-ter) [″ + *metron,* measure] **1.** A device for measuring the rotation of the eyeballs. **2.** An instrument for measuring torsion in long bones.

tropomyosin (trō″pō-mī′ō-sĭn) An inhibitory protein in muscle fibers; it blocks myosin from forming cross-bridges with actin until shifted by troponin-calcium ion interaction.

troponin (trō′pō-nĭn) An inhibitory protein in muscle fibers. The action potential at the sarcolemma causes the sarcoplasmic reticulum to release calcium ions, which bond to troponin and shift tropomyosin away from the myosin-binding sites of actin, permitting contraction. SEE: *muscle* for illus.

t. I A protein that is released into the blood by damaged heart muscle (but not skeletal muscle), and therefore is a highly sensitive and specific indicator of recent myocardial infarction.

t. T A protein, found in both skeletal and cardiac muscle, that can be detected in the blood following injury to heart muscle. Assays for it can be used as rapid tests for myocardial infarction (MI). Troponin I (which is released only by heart and not by skeletal muscles) is a more specific marker for MI than troponin T.

Trotter's syndrome A unilateral neuralgia in the mandible, tongue, and ear. The causes are mandibular nerve lesions, deafness on the same side due to eustachian tube lesions, and damage to the levator palatini muscle resulting in kinesthesia of the soft palate.

trough (trŏf) A groove or channel.

focal t. A three-dimensional area within which structures are accurately reproduced on a panoramic radiograph. Positioning the patient within the focal trough is critical to producing a panoramic radiograph that clearly reproduces oral structures.

gingival t. Gingival sulcus.

synaptic t. The depression in a muscle fiber adjacent to the axon terminal of a motor neuron in a myoneural junction.

Trousseau's sign (troo-sōz′) [Armand Trousseau, Fr. physician, 1801–1867] A muscular spasm of the hand and wrist resulting from pressure applied to nerves and vessels of the upper arm. It is indicative of latent tetany, usually as a result of hypocalcemia. SEE: *tetany.*

Trousseau's spots Streaking of the skin with the fingernail, seen in meningitis and other cerebral diseases.

troy weight A system of weighing gold, silver, precious metals, and jewels in which 5760 gr equal 1 lb; 1 gr equals 0.0648 g. SEE: *Weights and Measures Appendix.*

true (troo) [AS. *treowe,* faithful] Not false; real; genuine.

true conjugate diameter of pelvic inlet True conjugate.

true pelvis The portion of the pelvis that falls below the iliopectineal line.

true ribs The seven upper ribs on each side with cartilages articulating directly with the sternum. SYN: *costa vera.* SEE: *rib.*

truncal (trŭng′kăl) [L. *truncus,* trunk] Rel. to the trunk.

truncate (trŭng′kāt) [L. *truncare,* to cut off] **1.** Having a square end as if it were cut off; lacking an apex. **2.** To shorten by amputation of a part of the entity.

truncus (trŭng′kŭs) Trunk (2).

t. arteriosus The arterial trunk from the embryonic heart.

t. brachiocephalicus The initial branch of the arch of the aorta.

t. celiacus Celiac trunk.

t. pulmonalis Pulmonary trunk.

trunk (trŭnk) [L. *truncus,* trunk] **1.** The body exclusive of the head and limbs. SYN: *torso.* **2.** The main stem of a lymphatic vessel, nerve, or blood vessel.

celiac t. The trunk arising from the abdominal aorta. Most of the blood supply for the liver, stomach, spleen, gallbladder, pancreas, and duodenum comes from this trunk. SYN: *truncus celiacus.*

lumbosacral t. Part of the fourth and all of the fifth lumbar spinal nerves. These nerves accompany part of the first, second, and third sacral nerves to form the sciatic nerve.

pulmonary t. The great vessel that arises from the right ventricle of the heart and gives rise to the right and left pulmonary arteries to the lungs. SYN: *truncus pulmonalis.*

sympathetic t. The two long chains of ganglia, connected by sympathetic nerve fibers, that extend along the vertebral column from the skull to the coccyx.

trusion (troo′zhŭn) [L. *trudere,* to show] Malposition of a tooth or teeth.

truss (trŭs) [ME. *trusse,* a bundle] **1.** A restraining device for pushing a hernia, esp. an inguinal or abdominal wall hernia, back in place. A truss is almost always a poor substitute for surgical therapy. **2.** To tie or bind as with a cord or string.

trust In the relations between health care providers and patients, reliance by both parties on the integrity and sincerity of each other, and the patient's confidence in the ability and good will of the care provider. Trust is essential in the relationship between patients and those who provide medical care for them.

truth serum One of several hypnotic drugs supposedly having the effect of causing a person on questioning to talk freely and without inhibition. In actual practice, serum is not given, but a short-acting barbiturate or benzodiazepine is given intravenously. The reliability of the information obtained is questionable.

trybutyrase An enzyme present in the stomach that digests the short-chain diglycerides of butter. SEE: *digestion.*

try-in The temporary placement of a dental restoration or device to determine its fit and comfortableness.

trypanocide (trĭp-ăn′ō-sīd) [Gr. *trypanon,* a borer, + L. *cide,* kill] **1.** Destructive to trypanosomes. **2.** An agent that kills trypanosomes. SYN: *trypanosomicide.* **trypanocidal** (trĭp″ăn-ō-sī′dăl), *adj.*

trypanolysis (trĭp-ăn-ŏl′ĭ-sĭs) [″ + *lysis,* dissolution] The dissolution of trypanosomes.

Trypanoplasma (trī″păn-ō-plăz′mă) [″ + LL. *plasma,* form, mold] A genus of protozoan parasites resembling trypanosomes.

Trypanosoma (trī″păn-ō-sō′mă) [″ + *soma,* a body] A genus of parasitic, flagellate protozoa found in the blood of many vertebrates, including humans. The protozoa are transmitted by insect vectors. SEE: illus.

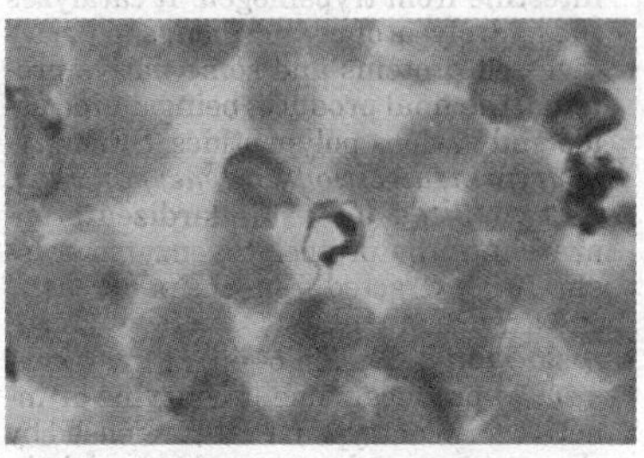

TRYPANOSOMA (center) IN BLOOD

(Orig. Mag. ×1000)

T. brucei The causative agent of trypanosomiasis in horses and other domestic animals. This organism is nonpathogenic in humans.

T. cruzi The causative agent of American trypanosomiasis (Chagas' disease). It is transmitted by blood-sucking insects (triatomids) belonging to the family Reduviidae.

T. gambiense The causative agent of African sleeping sickness. It is transmitted by the tsetse fly.

T. rhodesiense An organism parasitic in wild game and domestic animals of portions of Africa. It may cause East African sleeping sickness in humans.

trypanosome (trī′păn-ō-sōm) Any protozoan belonging to the genus Trypanosoma. **trypanosomal, trypanosomic,** *adj.*

trypanosomiasis (trī-păn″ō-sō-mī′ă-sĭs) [″ + *soma,* body, + *-iasis,* infection] Any of the several diseases occurring in humans and domestic animals caused by a species of *Trypanosoma.* SEE: *sleeping sickness.*

African t. African sleeping sickness, caused by *Trypanosoma gambiense.*

American t. A disease caused by *Trypanosoma cruzi* and transmitted by the biting reduviid bug. It is characterized by fever, lymphadenopathy, hepatosplenomegaly, and facial edema. Chronic cases may be mild or asymptomatic, or may be accompanied by myocarditis, cardiomyopathy, megaesophagus, megacolon, or death. SYN: *Chagas' disease.*

TREATMENT: Nifurtimox, available from the Centers for Disease Control and Prevention, or benzinazole is given.

trypanosomicide Trypanocide.

trypanosomid (trī-păn′ō-sō-mĭd) A skin eruption in any disease caused by a trypanosome.

tryparsamide (trĭp-ărs′ă-mĭd, -mīd) An arsenic compound containing about 25% arsenic; used chiefly in treating sleeping sickness.

trypsin (trĭp′sĭn) [Gr. *tripsis,* friction] **1.** A proteolytic enzyme formed in the intestine from trypsinogen. It catalyzes the hydrolysis of peptide bonds in partly digested proteins and some native proteins, the final products being amino acids and various polypeptides. SEE: *chymotrypsin; digestion; enzyme; pancreas.*

crystallized t. A standardized preparation of the proteolytic enzyme trypsin. It is extracted from the pancreas of the ox, *Bos taurus.*

trypsinogen (trĭp-sĭn′ō-jĕn) [″ + *gennan,* to produce] The proenzyme or inactive form of trypsin that is released by the pancreas and converted to trypsin in the intestine.

tryptic (trĭp′tĭk) Rel. to trypsin.

tryptolysis (trĭp-tŏl′ĭ-sĭs) [″ + *lysis,* dissolution] The hydrolysis of proteins or their derivatives by trypsin.

tryptone (trĭp′tōn) A peptide produced by the action of trypsin on a protein.

tryptophan (trĭp′tō-făn) $C_{11}H_{12}N_2O_2$; An essential amino acid present in high concentrations in animal and fish protein. It is necessary for normal growth and development. Tryptophan is a precursor of serotonin, a neurotransmitter in the central nervous system. In high doses, it may cause nausea, vomiting, and sedation.

tryptophanase (trĭp′tō-făn-ās) An enzyme that catalyzes the splitting of tryptophan into indole, pyruvic acid, and ammonia.

tryptophanuria (trĭp″tō-fă-nū′rē-ă) [*tryptophan* + Gr. *ouron,* urine] The presence of excessive levels of tryptophan in the urine.

T/S *thyroid:serum* (thyroid to serum iodine ratio).

T.S. *test solution; triple strength.*

T score A measure of bone density in which the mass of a patient's bones are compared with the bone mass of premenopausal women. A T score that is more than 1 standard deviation (SD) from the norm identifies bone that is osteopenic. A T score that is more than 2.5 SDs identifies osteoporosis.

TSD *target skin distance.*

tsetse fly (tsĕt′sē) [S. African] One of several species of blood-sucking flies belonging to the genus *Glossina,* order Diptera, confined to Africa south of the Sahara Desert. It is an important transmitter of trypanosomes, the causative agents of African sleeping sicknesses in humans, and nagana and other diseases of cattle and game animals. SEE: *Trypanosoma; trypanosomiasis.*

TSH *thyroid-stimulating hormone.*

TSH-RF *thyroid-stimulating hormone releasing factor.*

tsp *teaspoon.*

TSTA *tumor-specific transplantation antigen.*

tsutsugamushi disease (soot″soo-gă-moo′shĭ) [Japanese, dangerous bug] Scrub typhus.

TT *transit time* of blood through heart and lungs.

T-tube A device inserted into the biliary duct after removal of the gallbladder. It allows for drainage of the gallbladder and introduction of contrast medium for postoperative radiographical study of the bile duct.

T.U. *toxic unit; toxin unit.*

tub (tŭb) [ME. *tubbe*] **1.** A receptacle for bathing. **2.** The use of a cold bath. **3.** To treat by using a cold bath.

tuba (too′bă) [L. *tubus,* tube] Tube.

tubal (tū′băl) [L. *tubus,* tube] Pert. to a tube, esp. the fallopian tube.

tubal nephritis An obsolete term for inflammation of kidney tubules.

tubatorsion (tū″bă-tor′shŭn) [″ + *torsio,* a twisting] The twisting of an oviduct.

tubba, tubboe (tŭb′ă, -ō) Yaws that attacks the palms and soles.

tube (tūb) [L. *tubus,* a tube] A long, hollow, cylindrical structure.

auditory t. Eustachian t.

Cantor t. Intestinal decompression t.

cathode ray t. A vacuum tube with a thin window at the end opposite the cathode to allow the cathode rays to pass outside. More generally, any discharge tube in which the vacuum is fairly high.

Coolidge t. A kind of hot-cathode tube that is so highly exhausted that the residual gas plays no part in the production of the cathode stream, and that is regulated by variable heating of the cathode filament.

Crookes' t. A vacuum tube used in producing roentgen rays.

cuffed endotracheal t. An airway catheter used to provide an airway through the trachea and at the same time to prevent aspiration of foreign material into the bronchus. This is accomplished by an inflatable cuff that surrounds the tube. The cuff is inflated after the tube is placed in the trachea. SEE: illus.

drainage t. A tube that, when inserted into a cavity, facilitates removal of fluids.

endobronchial t. A double-lumen tube used in anesthesia. One tube may be used to aerate a portion of the lung, while the other is occluded to deflate the other lung or a portion of it.

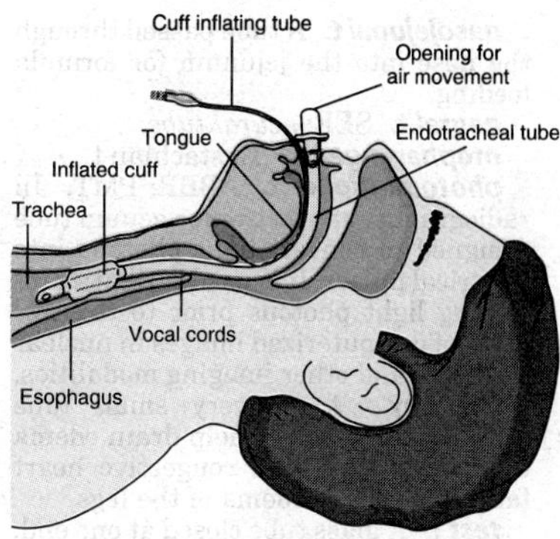

CUFFED ENDOTRACHEAL TUBE

endotracheal t. A catheter inserted into the trachea to provide or protect an airway. SYN: *intubation t.*

esophageal t. A tube inserted in the esophagus.

eustachian t. The auditory tube, extending from the middle ear to the nasopharynx, 3 to 4 cm long and lined with mucous membrane. Occlusion of the tube leads to the development of otitis media. SYN: *auditory t.; otopharyngeal t.* SEE: *politzerization.*

fallopian t. The hollow, cylindrical structure that extends laterally from the lateral angle of the fundal end of the uterus and terminates near the ovary. It conveys the ovum from the ovary to the uterus and spermatozoa from the uterus toward the ovary. Medially each tube opens into the uterus; distally, into the peritoneal cavity. Each lies in the superior border of the broad ligament of the uterus. SYN: *oviduct; uterine t.* SEE: *female genitalia* for illus; *uterus.*

ANATOMY: The narrow region near the uterus, the isthmus, continues laterally as a wider ampulla. The latter expands to form the terminal funnel-shaped infundibulum, at the bottom of which lies a small opening, the ostium, through which the ovum enters the tube. Surrounding each ostium are several finger-like processes called fimbriae extending toward the ovary. Each tube averages about 4½ in. (11.4 cm) in length and ¼ in. (6 mm) in diameter. Its wall consists of three layers: mucosa, muscular layer, and serosa. The epithelium of the mucosa consists of ciliated and nonciliated cells. The muscular layer has an inner circular and an outer longitudinal layer of smooth muscle. Ciliary action and peristalsis move the ovum or zygote toward the uterus. The serosa is connective tissue underlying the peritoneum.

fenestrated tracheostomy t. A double-cannulated tracheostomy tube that allows patients to breathe through the mouth or nose when the inner cannula is removed. The tube has an opening in the posterior wall of the outer cannula above the inflatable cuff.

fermentation t. A U-shaped tube open at one end. If gas is produced by the bacteria cultured, the level of fluid decreases in the side of the tube with the closed end.

gastrostomy t. A tube placed directly into the stomach for long-term enteral feeding. This may be done laparoscopically, with a percutaneous endoscopic gastrostomy (PEG) tube, or surgically. SEE: *percutaneous endoscopic gastrostomy.*

hot-cathode t. A vacuum tube in which the cathode is electrically heated to incandescence and in which the supply of electrons depends on the temperature of the cathode.

hot-cathode roentgen-ray t. An evacuated glass envelope, containing a positive anode and negative cathode separated by a gap, that produces x-ray photons. Electrons are supplied from a heated cathode in the form of a stream that interacts with the anode when a potential difference is placed between the anode and cathode.

intestinal t. A flexible tube, usually made of plastic or rubber, placed in the intestinal tract to aspirate gas, fluid, or solids from the stomach or intestines or to administer fluids, electrolytes, or nutrients to the patient. The tube may be passed through the nose, mouth, or anus, or through a stomach opening (e.g., gastrostomy, jejunostomy).

PATIENT CARE: When a long intestinal tube (e.g., Cantor, Miller-Abbott) is inserted, the caregiver must assist its advancement into the intestinal tract. The patient is usually placed on the right side for ½ hr, then the left side for ½ hr, and then on the back. These position changes, as well as ambulation, will facilitate movement of the tube into the intestinal tract. These maneuvers may be performed under radiographic control.

Frequent oral hygiene is needed to prevent oral ulceration because the patient usually will not be taking fluids by mouth. While the tube is in, the patient should be taught not to mouth breathe or swallow air. This enhances entry of air into the gastrointestinal tract and works counter to the principle of intestinal tubes and drainage.

intestinal decompression t. A tube placed in the intestinal tract, usually via the nose and esophagus, to relieve gas pressure produced when paralytic ileus or intestinal obstruction is present. Tubes may be plain; made of rubber, plastic, or silicone; or equipped with a mercury-filled tip to facilitate passage into the intestinal tract. The latter type is called a Cantor tube. The tubes are impregnated with a radiopaque substance to allow radiographic visualization of their location. SEE: *intestinal t.*

intubation t. Endotracheal t.

jejunostomy t. A tube placed directly into the jejunum for long-term enteral feeding. This may be done laporoscopically, with a percutaneous endoscopic jejunostomy tube, or surgically. It is not as commonly used as the gastrostomy tube.

Levin t. A tube passed via the nose into the gastrointestinal tract. A variant includes the addition of a sump channel, which helps to reduce gas build-up and excessive pressure in the upper gastrointestinal tract.

Miller-Abbott t. A double-channel intestinal tube used to relieve intestinal distention. One channel is used for aspiration or irrigation and the other channel leads to a balloon, which may be inflated with air, saline, or mercury to facilitate its passage. Inserted through a nostril, the tube is passed through the stomach into the small intestine.

nasoduodenal t. A flexible tube of silicone or a similar synthetic material, inserted through the nose into the duodenum for short-term enteral feeding. The small weight on the distal end of the tube moves the tube into place through the stomach into the duodenum. Aspiration is less likely than with a nasogastric tube. SEE: *Miller-Abbott t.*

nasogastric t. A tube inserted through the nose and extending into the stomach. It may be used for emptying the stomach of gas and liquids or for administering liquids to the patient. SEE: illus.

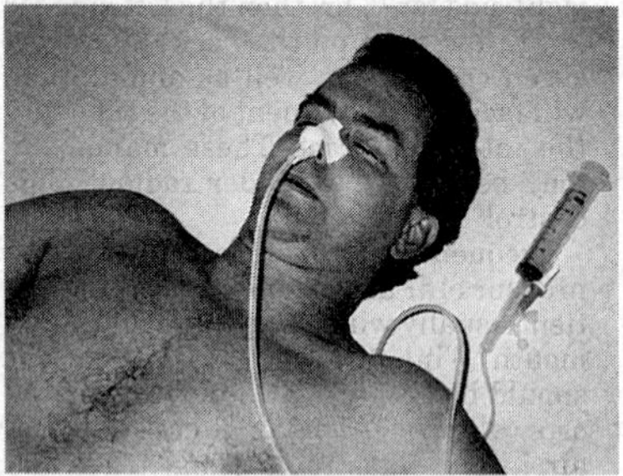

NASOGASTRIC TUBE

nasointestinal t. A long tube inserted through the nose into the stomach for decompression. The weight at the end promotes its advancement into the small intestine. The most common use is to relieve the abdominal distention associated with intestinal obstruction.

nasojejunal t. A tube passed through the nose into the jejunum for formula feeding.

neural t. SEE: *neural tube.*

otopharyngeal t. Eustachian t.

photomultiplier t. ABBR: PMT. In radiography, an electronic vacuum tube designed to convert light photons into electrical pulses. It is used to digitize incoming light photons prior to the creation of computerized images in nuclear medicine and other imaging modalities.

Southey's t. A very small tube pushed into tissue to help drain edema fluid; used in severe congestive heart failure to relieve edema of the legs.

test t. A glass tube closed at one end. It is used in chemistry to hold chemicals and materials being tested.

thoracostomy t. A tube inserted into the pleural space via the chest wall to remove air or fluid present in the space.

tracheostomy t. Tracheotomy tube.

tracheotomy t. A tube for insertion into the trachea.

transnasal t. A tube passed through the nose into the gastrointestinal tract for feeding.

uterine t. Fallopian t.

ventilation t. SEE: *grommet.*

tubectomy (too-bĕk′tō-mē) Surgical removal of all or part of a tube, esp. the fallopian tube.

tube feeding Enteral tube feeding.

tuber (tū′bĕr) *pl.* **tubera** [L., a swelling] A swelling or enlargement.

t. cinereum A part of the base of the hypothalamus bordered by the mammillary bodies, the optic chiasma, and on either side by the optic tract. It is connected by the infundibulum with the posterior lobe of the pituitary.

tubercle (tū′bĕr-kl) [L. *tuberculum,* a little swelling] **1.** A small rounded elevation or eminence on a bone. **2.** A small nodule, esp. a circumscribed solid elevation of the skin or mucous membrane. **3.** The characteristic lesion resulting from infection by tubercle bacilli. It consists typically of three parts: a central giant cell, a midzone of epithelioid cells, and a peripheral zone of nonspecific structure. SYN: *tuberculum.* SEE: *tuberculosis.*

adductor t. The tubercle of the femur to which is attached the tendon of the adductor magnus.

articular t. The tubercle at the base of the zygomatic arch to which is attached the temporomandibular ligament; it is lateral to the articular eminence of the glenoid fossa, with which it is often confused. SYN: *zygomatic t.*

condyloid t. An eminence on the mandibular condyle for the attachment of the lateral ligament of the temporomandibular joint.

deltoid t. The tubercle on the clavicle or humerus for attachment of the deltoid muscle.

dental t. A small elevation of variable size on the crown of a tooth representing a thickened area of enamel or an accessory cusp.

fibrous t. A fibrous tissue that has replaced a previously inflamed area.

genial t. The tubercle on either side of the lower jawbone.

genital t. The embryonic structure that becomes the clitoris or the penis.

Gerdy's t. SEE: *Gerdy's tubercle*.

lacrimal t. A small tubercle between the lacrimal crest and the frontal process of the maxilla.

laminated t. The cerebellar nodule.

Lisfranc's t. A tubercle on the first rib for attachment of the scalenus anterior muscle.

mental t. A small tubercle on either side of the midline of the chin.

miliary t. A small tubercle resembling a millet seed, caused by tuberculosis. SEE: *tuberculosis, miliary*.

pharyngeal t. The point of attachment of the superior pharyngeal constrictor and its fibrous raphe on the inferior surface of the basilar part of the occipital bone.

pubic t. A small projection at the lateral end of the crest of the pubic bone. The inguinal ligament attaches to it.

supraglenoid t. A rough, elevated area just above the glenoid cavity of the scapula. The long head of the biceps muscle of the arm attaches to this tubercle.

t. of the upper lip The prominence of the upper part of the vermilion border that represents the distal termination of the philtrum of the upper lip.

zygomatic t. Articular t.

tubercula (tū-bĕr′kū-lă) Pl. of tuberculum.

tubercular (tū-bĕr′kū-lăr) [L. *tuberculum,* a little swelling] Relating to or marked by nodules. SYN: *torose; tuberculate*.

tuberculate, tuberculated (tū-bĕr′kū-lāt, -lāt″ĕd) [L. *tuberculum,* a small swelling] Tubercular.

tuberculation (tū-bĕr″kū-lā′shŭn) The formation of tubercles.

tuberculid, tuberculide (tū-bĕr′kū-lĭd, -līd) [L. *tuberculum,* a little swelling] A tuberculous cutaneous eruption caused by toxins of tuberculosis. SYN: *tuberculoderma*.

follicular t. A cutaneous eruption characterized by the presence of groups of follicular lesions, esp. on the trunk.

papulonecrotic t. A form of tuberculid characterized by symmetrically distributed bluish papules, esp. on the extremities. These undergo central necrosis and, on healing, leave deep scars.

tuberculin (tū-bĕr′kū-lĭn) [L. *tuberculum,* a little swelling] A solution of purified protein derivative of tuberculosis that is injected intradermally to determine the presence of a tuberculosis infection. SEE: *tuberculin skin test*.

new t. A suspension of tubercle bacilli fragments from which the soluble materials have been removed and to which glycerin has been added.

old t. ABBR: OT. Tuberculin originally prepared by (H. H.) Robert Koch from cultures of *Mycobacterium tuberculosis*.

purified protein derivative t. ABBR: PPD. A purified tuberculin obtained by the same technique as that used for old tuberculin except a synthetic broth is used to culture the *Mycobacterium tuberculosis*.

tuberculitis (tū″bĕr-kū-lī′tĭs) Inflammation of a tubercle.

tuberculocele (tū-bĕr′kū-lō-sēl″) [″ + *kele,* tumor] Tuberculosis of the testis.

tuberculocidal (tū-bĕr″kū-lō-sī′dăl) Anything that destroys *Mycobacterium tuberculosis*.

tuberculoderma (tū-bĕr″kū-lō-dĕr′mă) [″ + Gr. *derma,* skin] Tuberculid.

tuberculofibroid (tū-bĕr″kū-lō-fī′broyd) [″ + *fibra,* fiber, + Gr. *eidos,* form, shape] Denoting fibroid degeneration of tubercles.

tuberculofibrosis (tū-bĕr″kū-lō-fī-brō′sĭs) [″ + ″ + Gr. *osis,* condition] **1.** Chronic pulmonary inflammation with formation of fibrous tissue. **2.** Interstitial pneumonia.

tuberculoid (tū-bĕr′kū-loyd) [L. *tuberculum,* a little swelling, + Gr. *eidos,* form, shape] Resembling tuberculosis or a tubercle.

tuberculoma (tū-bĕr″kū-lō′mă) [″ + Gr. *oma,* tumor] **1.** A tuberculous abscess. **2.** Any tuberculous neoplasm.

tuberculophobia (tū-bĕr″kū-lō-fō′bē-ă) [″ + Gr. *phobos,* fear] An abnormal fear of being infected with tuberculosis.

tuberculoprotein (tū-bĕr″kū-lō-prō′tē-ĭn) A protein derived from *Myobacterium tuberculosis*.

tuberculosilicosis (tū-bĕr″kū-lō-sĭl″ĭ-kō′sĭs) Silicosis and pulmonary tuberculosis at the same time.

tuberculosis (tū-bĕr″kū-lō′sĭs) [″ + Gr. *osis,* condition] ABBR: TB. An infectious disease caused by the tubercle bacillus, *Mycobacterium tuberculosis,* and characterized pathologically by inflammatory infiltrations, formation of tubercles, caseation, necrosis, abscesses, fibrosis, and calcification. It most commonly affects the respiratory system, but other parts of the body such as the gastrointestinal and genitourinary tracts, bones, joints, nervous system, lymph nodes, and skin may also become infected. Fish, amphibians, birds, and mammals (esp. cattle) are subject to the disease. Three types of the tubercle bacillus exist: human, bovine, and avian. Humans may become infected by any of the three types, but in the U.S. the human type predominates. Infection usually is acquired from contact with an infected person or an infected cow or through drinking contaminated milk. In the U.S., about 10 to 15 million persons have been infected with tuberculosis. Worldwide, about 1.7 billion people harbor the infection.

Tuberculosis usually affects the lungs, but the disease may spread to other organs including the gastrointestinal and genitourinary tracts, bones, joints, nervous system, lymph nodes, and skin. Macrophages surround the bacilli in an attempt to engulf them but cannot, producing granulomas with a soft, cheesy (caseous) core. From this state, lesions may heal by fibrosis and calcification and the disease may exist in an arrested or inactive stage. Reactivation or exacerbation of the disease or reinfection gives rise to the chronic progressive form.

The incidence of TB declined steadily from the 1950s to about 1990, when the acquired immunodeficiency syndrome epidemic, an increase in the homeless population, an increase in immigrants from endemic areas, and a decrease in public surveillance caused a resurgence of the disease. Populations at greatest risk for TB include patients with human immunodeficiency virus (HIV), Asian and other refugees, the urban homeless, alcoholics and other substance abusers, persons incarcerated in prisons and psychiatric facilities, nursing home residents, patients taking immunosuppressive drugs, and people with chronic respiratory disorders, diabetes mellitus, renal failure, or malnutrition. People from these risk groups should be assessed for TB if they develop pneumonia; all health care workers should be tested annually. SEE: illus.; *immunological therapy; tine test; tuberculin skin test; Nursing Diagnoses Appendix.*

INCUBATION PERIOD: Approx. 4 to 12 weeks will elapse between the time of infection and the time a demonstrable primary lesion or positive tuberculin skin test occurs.

SYMPTOMS: Pulmonary TB produces chronic cough, sputum production, fevers, sweats, and weight loss. TB may also cause neurological disease (meningitis), bone infections, urinary bleeding, and other symptoms if it spreads to other organs.

DIAGNOSIS: A positive tuberculin skin test indicates the patient has had a tuberculous infection; however, unless repeated tests indicate a recent change from negative, it is impossible to tell how recently the infection occurred. A presumptive diagnosis of active disease is made by finding acid-fast bacilli in stained smears from sputum or other body fluids. The diagnosis is confirmed by isolating *Mycobacterium tuberculosis* on culture or rapid nucleic acid test probes.

TREATMENT: Regimens for TB have been developed for patients depending on their HIV status, the prevalence of multidrug-resistant disease in the community, drug allergies, and drug interactions. Uncomplicated TB in the non-HIV infected patient is typically treated with a four-drug regimen for 2 months (isoniazid, rifampin, ethambutol, and pyrazinamide), followed by isoniazid and rifampin for an additional 4 months. Some experts recommend a longer course of therapy in patients co-infected with HIV. To ensure compliance and prevent the evolution of drug-resistant strains of *Mycobacteria,* directly observed therapy should be used. Multidrug-resistant TB is more difficult to treat successfully. It has a mortality rate as high as 80% and may require treatment for as long as 2 years. SEE: *multidrug resistant t.*

CAUTION: All patients with HIV should be tested for TB, and all patients with TB should be tested for HIV, because about one fourth of all patients with one disease may be infected with the other.

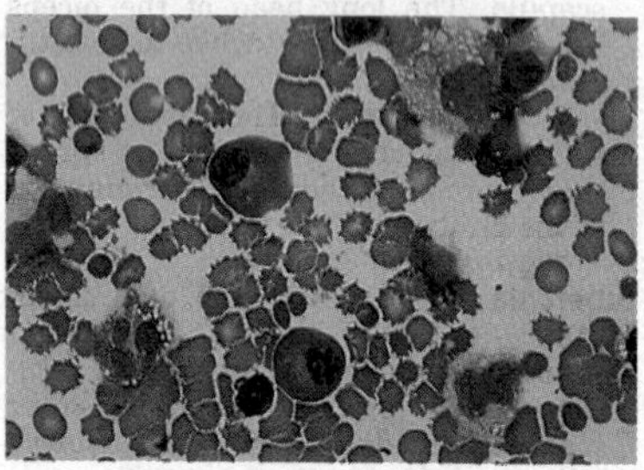

TUBERCULOSIS
Pleural fluid with plasma cells (×1000)

avian t. Tuberculosis of birds caused by *Mycobacterium avium.*

bovine t. Tuberculosis of cattle caused by *Mycobacterium bovis.*

endogenous t. Tuberculosis that reactivates after a previous infection.

exogenous t. Tuberculosis originating from a source outside the body.

hematogenous t. The spread of tuberculosis from a primary site to another site via the bloodstream.

miliary t. Tuberculosis that spreads throughout the body via the bloodstream. It may be fatal.

multidrug resistant t. ABBR: MDR-TB. *Mycobacterium tuberculosis* bacilli that are resistant to therapy with at least two standard antitubercular drugs (esp. isoniazid and rifampin, the two drugs that have formed the cornerstone of therapy for tuberculosis). MDR-TB must be treated with at least three antitubercular drugs to which the organism is presumed or proven to be sensitive.

open t. Tuberculosis in which the tubercle bacilli are present in bodily secretions that leave the body.

tuberculostatic (tū-bĕr″kū-lō-stăt′ĭk) Arresting the growth of the tubercle bacillus.

tuberculotic (tū-bĕr″kū-lŏt′ĭk) Concerning tuberculosis.

tuberculous (tū-bĕr′kū-lŭs) [L. *tuberculum,* a little swelling] Relating to or affected with tuberculosis, or conditions marked by infiltration of a specific tubercle, as opposed to the term *tubercular,* referring to a nonspecific tubercle.

tuberculum (tū-bĕr′kū-lŭm) *pl.* **tubercula** [L. *tuberculum,* a little swelling] A small knot or nodule; a tubercle.

t. acusticum The dorsal nucleus of the cochlear nerve.

t. impar A small median eminence on the floor of the embryonic oral cavity, the precursor of the tongue, though it is not a distinct part of the tongue after birth.

t. majus humeri The larger tuberosity of the humerus at the upper end of its lateral surface, giving attachment to the infraspinatus, supraspinatus, and teres minor muscles.

t. minus humeri The projection at the proximal end of the anterior humerus, providing attachment to the subscapularis muscle.

tuberosis (tū″bĕr-ō′sĭs) A condition in which nodules develop; a nonspecific term that indicates no specific disease process.

tuberositas (tū-bĕr-ŏs′ĭt-ăs) *pl.* **tuberositates** [L.] A projection, nodule, or prominence.

tuberosity (tū-bĕr-ŏs′ĭ-tē) [L. *tuberositas,* tuberosity] **1.** An elevated round process of a bone. **2.** A tubercle or nodule.

ischial t. A palpable prominence on the inferior margin of the ischium that supports a person's weight when sitting.

maxillary t. A rounded eminence on the posteroinferior surface of the maxilla that enlarges with the development and eruption of the third molar. It articulates medially with the palatine bone and laterally with the lateral pterygoid process of the sphenoid. It forms the anterior surface of the pterygopalatine fossa, including a groove for the passage of the maxillary nerve, which is anesthetized in this region for a maxillary or second-division block.

tuberous (tū′bĕr-ŭs) Pert. to tubers.

tubo- Combining form meaning *tube.*

tuboabdominal (tū″bō-ăb-dŏm′ĭn-ăl) [L. *tubus,* tube, + *abdominalis,* pert. to the abdomen] Pert. to the fallopian tubes and the abdomen.

tubocurarine chloride (tū″bō-kū-ră′rĭn klō′rīd) A drug used to produce skeletal muscle relaxation during anesthesia and convulsive states and to treat poisoning caused by black widow spider bites. Tubocurarine was originally obtained from the Indian arrow poison, curare.

CAUTION: Tubocurarine should be administered only by those who have the proper equipment and are fully capable of providing artificial ventilation, tracheal intubation, appropriate antidotes, and additional therapy in case of overdose.

---

tuboligamentous (tū″bō-lĭg-ă-mĕn′tŭs) [″ + *ligamentum,* a band] Pert. to the fallopian tube and broad ligament of the uterus.

tubo-ovarian (tū″bō-ō-vā′rē-ăn) [″ + LL. *ovarium,* ovary] Pert. to the fallopian tube and the ovary.

tubo-ovariotomy (tū″bō-ō-vā-rē-ŏt′ō-mē) [″ + LL. *ovarium,* ovary, + Gr. *tome,* incision] Excision of ovaries and oviducts.

tubo-ovaritis (tū″bō-ō″vă-rī′tĭs) [″ + ″ + Gr. *itis,* inflammation] Inflammation of the ovary and fallopian tube.

tuboperitoneal (tū″bō-pĕr-ĭ-tō-nē′ăl) [″ + Gr. *peritonaion,* peritoneum] Rel. to the fallopian tube and peritoneum.

tuboplasty (tū′bō-plăs″tē) **1.** Plastic repair of any tube. **2.** Plastic repair of a fallopian tube or tubes in an attempt to restore patency so that fertilization of the ovum may occur. SYN: *salpingoplasty.*

tuboplasty, transcervical balloon Catheterization and dilation of the fallopian tubes, a method of treating infertility in women whose fallopian tubes are occluded proximally. A balloon catheter is inserted through the cervical os of the uterus and into the fallopian tube to the point of occlusion in the tube. The balloon is then expanded by filling it with sterile saline. This dilation of the tube may restore tubal patency. SEE: *catheter, balloon; infertility.*

tuborrhea (tū-bor-rē′ă) [″ + Gr. *rhoia,* flow] Discharge from the eustachian tube.

tubotorsion (tū″bō-tor′shŭn) The act of twisting a tube.

tubotympanal (tū″bō-tĭm′pă-năl) [″ + Gr. *tympanon,* a drum] Rel. to the tympanum of the ear and the eustachian tube.

tubouterine (tū″bō-ū′tĕr-ĭn) [″ + *uterinus,* pert. to the uterus] Rel. to the fallopian tube and the uterus.

tubovaginal (tū″bō-văj′ĭ-năl) Concerning the fallopian tube and vagina.

tubular (tū′bū-lăr) [L. *tubularis,* like a tube] Rel. to or having the form of a tube or tubule.

tubule (tū′būl) [L. *tubulus,* a tubule] A small tube or canal.

collecting t. One of the small ducts that receive urine from several renal tubules, which join together to provide a passage for the urine to larger straight collecting tubules (papillary ducts of Bellini) that open into the pelvis of the kidney. SEE: *kidney* for illus.

convoluted t. of the kidney The proximal and distal convoluted tubules of the nephron that, with the loop of Henle and collecting tubule, form the renal tubule through which the glomerular filtrate passes before entering the renal pelvis. SEE: *kidney* for illus.; *nephron.*

convoluted seminiferous t. One of the tubules present in each lobe of the testes.

dentinal t. One of the very small canals in the dentin. These extend from the pulp cavity of the tooth to the enamel and are occupied by odontoblastic processes and occasional nerve filaments.

excretory t. Renal t.

galactophorous t. Lactiferous t.

Henle's t. Henle's loop.

junctional t. The short segment of a renal tubule that connects the distal convoluted tubule with the collecting tubule.

lactiferous t. One of the lactiferous ducts of the breast. It provides a channel for the milk formed in the lobes of the breast to pass to the nipple. SYN: *galactophorous t.*

mesonephric t. One of the embryonic tubules that in the female gives rise only to vestigial structures but in the male gives rise to the efferent ducts of the testes. SYN: *wolffian tubule.*

metanephritic t. One of the tubes that make up the permanent kidneys of amniotes.

renal t. The part of a nephron through which renal filtrate from the renal corpuscle flows and is changed to urine by reabsorption and secretion. The parts, in order, are the proximal convoluted tubule, the loop of Henle, the distal convoluted tubule, and collecting tubule. SYN: *excretory t.* SEE: *kidney* for illus; *nephron.*

seminiferous t. One of the very small channels of the testes in which spermatozoa develop and through which they leave the testes.

transverse t. ABBR: T-tubule. An invagination of the cell membrane of a muscle fiber that carries the action potential to the interior of the cell and the innermost sarcomeres.

uriniferous t. SEE: *renal t.*

tubulin (tū′bū-lĭn) A protein present in the microtubules of cells.

tubulization (too″bū-lī-zā′shŭn) A method of repairing severed nerves in which the nerve ends are placed in a tube of absorbable material.

tubuloalveolar Consisting of tubes and alveoli, as in a tubuloalveolar salivary gland.

tubulocyst (too′bū-lō-sĭst) The cystic dilatation of a functionless duct or canal.

tubulodermoid (tū″bū-lō-dĕr′moyd) [″ + Gr. *derma,* skin, + *eidos,* form, shape] A dermoid tumor caused by the persistent embryonic tubular structure.

tubuloracemose (too″bū-lō-răs′ĕ-mōs) Pert. to a gland that has tubular and racemose characteristics.

tubulorrhexis (too″bū-lō-rĕk′sĭs) [″ + *rhexis,* a breaking] Focal ruptures of renal tubules.

tubulus (tū′bū-lŭs) *pl.* **tubuli** [L.] A tubule.

tubus (too′bŭs) [L.] Tube.

t. digestorius The alimentary canal.

tuft A small clump, cluster, or coiled mass.

enamel t. An abnormal structure formed in the development of enamel, consisting of poorly calcified twisted rods.

malpighian t. The renal glomerulus.

tugging A dragging or pulling.

tracheal t. An indication of a thoracic aneurysm. There is a sense of downward pulling of the larynx with cardiac systole when the thyroid cartilage is gently raised between the finger and thumb.

tularemia (tū-lăr-ē′mē-ă) [*Tulare,* part of California where disease was first discovered] An acute plaguelike infectious disease caused by *Francisella tularensis* (formerly classed as *Pasteurella tularensis*). It is transmitted to humans by the bite of an infected tick or other bloodsucking insect, by direct contact with infected animals, by eating inadequately cooked meat, or by drinking water that contains the organism. Streptomycin or gentamicin is effective in treating the disease. SYN: *deer fly fever; rabbit fever.*

SYMPTOMS: The symptoms may appear from 1 to 10 days, but averaging 3 days, after infection and include headache, chilliness, vomiting, aching pains, and fever. An ulcer develops at the entry site of the bacteria, and regional lymph nodes enlarge, become painful, and may develop into abscesses. Serious cases involve pneumonia, debilitation, and an extended recovery period.

tumbu fly A species of fly belonging to the genus *Cordylobia* in Africa and the genus *Dermatobia* in tropical America. Their larvae develop in the skin of wild domesticated animals, and humans are frequently attacked.

tumefacient (tū-mĕ-fā′shĕnt) [L. *tumefaciens,* producing swelling] Producing or tending to produce swelling; swollen.

tumefaction (tū″mĕ-făk′shŭn) [L. *tumefactio,* a swelling] Intumescence.

tumentia (tū-mĕn′shē-ă) [L.] Swelling.

vasomotor t. Irregular swellings in the lower extremities associated with vasomotor disturbances.

tumescence (tū-mĕs′ĕns) **1.** A condition of being swollen or tumid. **2.** A swelling.

tumor (tū′mor) [L. *tumor,* a swelling] **1.** A swelling or enlargement; one of the four classic signs of inflammation. **2.** An abnormal mass. Growth or proliferation that is independent of neighboring tissues is a hallmark of all tumors, benign and malignant. SYN: *neoplasm.* SEE: *cancer.*

brain t. An inexact term to describe any intracranial mass—neoplastic, cystic, inflammatory (abscess), or syphilitic. SEE: illus.; *Nursing Diagnoses Appendix.*

PATIENT CARE: The patient is evaluated for neurological deficits, such as weakness, sensory losses, or disturbances of vision, speech, gait, or balance. The patient is monitored for seizure activity and for increased intracranial pressure (ICP).

If the patient is aphasic or develops dysphagia, a speech pathologist is consulted. Emotional support is provided to the patient and family as they struggle to cope with treatments, disabilities, changes in lifestyle, and end-of-life issues. The patient and family are referred to resource and support services (e.g., social service, home health care agencies, the American Cancer Society, and other such voluntary agencies).

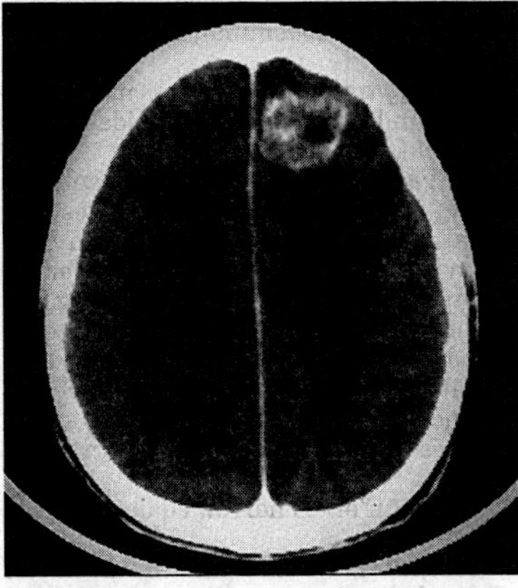

BRAIN TUMOR

brown t. A benign fibrotic mass found within the bone of patients with unchecked hyperparathyroidism. The tumor appears brown on gross examination because it contains blood and byproducts of the metabolism of hemoglobin, such as hemosiderin.

Buschke-Lowenstein t. A giant condyloma acuminata, typically found on the genitals or anus, caused by infection with papilloma virus. In men, it is almost always found under the foreskin (it is rarely reported in circumcised men). It may transform into a verrucous carcinoma and cause deep local tissue invasion.

carotid body t. A benign tumor of the carotid body.

connective tissue t. Any tumor of connective tissue such as fibroma, lipoma, chondroma, or sarcoma.

desmoid t. A tumor of fibrous connective tissue.

erectile t. A tumor composed of erectile tissue.

false t. An enlargement due to hemorrhage into tissue or extravasation of fluid into a space, rather than cancer.

fibroid t. Uterine fibroma.

giant cell t. of bone A benign or malignant tumor of bone in which the cells are multinucleated and surrounded by cellular spindle cell stroma.

giant cell t. of tendon sheath A localized nodular tenosynovitis.

granulosa cell t. An estrin-secreting neoplasm of the granulosa cells of the ovary.

granulosa-theca cell t. An estrogen-secreting tumor of the ovary made up of either granulosa or theca cells.

heterologous t. A tumor in which the tissue differs from that in which it is growing.

homologous t. A tumor in which the tissue resembles that in which it is growing.

Hürthle cell t. A benign or malignant tumor of the thyroid gland. The cells are large and acidophilic.

islet cell t. A tumor of the islets of Langerhans of the pancreas.

Klatskin t. SEE: under *Klatskin.*

Krukenberg's t. A cancer that originates in the gastrointestinal tract and spreads (metastasizes) to the ovaries.

lipoid cell t. of the ovary A masculinizing tumor of the ovary. It may be malignant.

mast cell t. A benign nodular accumulation of mast cells.

melanotic neuroectodermal t. A benign tumor of the jaw, occurring mostly during the first year of life.

mesenchymal mixed t. A tumor composed of tissue that resembles mesenchymal cells.

t. of pregnancy The abdominal swelling produced by the growing conceptus of pregnancy.

phantom t. **1.** An apparent tumor due to muscular contractions or flatus that resolves on re-examination of the patient. **2.** A mass that resembles a tumor in only one view of a chest x-ray film. On other views it either disappears or appears to be an encapsulated fluid collection.

primary t. In a patient with metastatic cancer, the lesion assumed to be the source of the metastases.

sand t. Psammoma.

turban t. Multiple cutaneous cylindromata that cover the scalp like a turban.

tumoraffin (tū′mor-ăf-ĭn) [L. *tumor,* a swelling, + *affinis,* related] Having an affinity for tumor cells.

tumor angiogenesis factor ABBR: TAF. A protein present in animal and human cancer tissue that in experimental studies appears to be essential to growth of the cancer. The substance is thought to act by stimulating the growth of new blood capillaries for supplying the tumor with nutrients and removing waste products.

tumor burden The sum of cancer cells present in the body.

tumoricidal (too″mor-ĭ-sī′dăl) Lethal to neoplastic cells.

tumorigenesis (too″mor-ĭ-jĕn′ĕ-sĭs) The production of tumors.

tumorigenic (tū″mor-ĭ-jĕn′ĭk) [″ + Gr. *genesis,* generation, birth] Forming and developing tumors.

tumor marker A substance whose presence in blood serum serves as a biochemical indicator for the possible presence of a malignancy. Examples of markers and the malignancies they may indicate are carcinoembryonic antigen for cancers of the colon, lung, breast, and ovary; beta subunit of chorionic gonadotropin for trophoblastic and testicular tumors; alpha-fetoprotein for testicular teratocarcinoma and primary hepatocellular carcinoma; and prostate-specific antigen for prostate cancer.

tumor necrosis factor ABBR: TNF. A protein mediator or cytokine released primarily by macrophages and T lymphocytes that helps regulate the immune response and some hematopoietic functions. There are two factors: alpha (TNFα), also called cachectin, produced by macrophages, and beta (TNFβ), called lymphotoxin, which is produced by activated CD4+ T cells. The functions of TNFs are very similar to those of interleukin-1. SEE: *cytokine; interleukin-1.*

tumorous (too′mor-ŭs) Tumor-like.

tumultus (tū-mŭl′tŭs) [L.] Excessive or agitated activity.

t. cordis Irregular heart action with palpitation.

t. sermonis Extreme stuttering due to a pathological cause.

Tunga (tŭng′ă) A genus of fleas of the family Hectopsyllidae.

T. penetrans A small flea common in tropical regions. It infests humans, cats, dogs, rats, pigs, and other animals and produces a severe local inflammation frequently liable to secondary infection.

tungiasis (tŭng-gī′ă-sĭs) Infestation of the skin with *Tunga penetrans.*

tungsten (tŭng′stĕn) SYMB: W (for wolfram). A metallic element; atomic weight, 183.85; atomic number, 74.

tunic (tū′nĭk) [L. *tunica,* a sheath] An investing membrane.

Bichat's t. Tunica intima.

tunica (tū′nĭ-kă) *pl.* **tunicae** [L. *tunica,* a sheath] A layer, or coat, of tissue.

t. adventitia The outermost fibroelastic layer of a blood vessel or other tubular structure. SYN: *t. externa.*

t. albuginea The white fibrous coat of the eye, testicle, ovary, or spleen.

t. conjunctiva Conjunctiva.

t. dartos The muscular, contractile tissue beneath the skin of the scrotum.

t. externa T. adventitia.

t. interna SEE: *t. intima.*

t. intima The lining of a blood vessel composed of an epithelial (endothelium) layer and the basement membrane, a subendothelial connective tissue layer, and usually an internal elastic lamina. SYN: *Bichat's tunic.*

t. media The middle layer in the wall of a blood vessel composed of circular or spiraling smooth muscle and some elastic fibers.

t. mucosa The mucous membrane lining of various structures.

t. muscularis The smooth muscle layer in the walls of organs such as the bronchi, intestines, and blood vessels.

t. serosa The membrane lining the walls of the closed body cavities and folded over the organs in those cavities, forming the outermost layer of the wall of these organs. The body cavities are the thoracic, abdominal, and pericardial cavities.

t. vaginalis The serous membrane surrounding the front and sides of the testicle.

t. vasculosa Any vascular layer.

tuning fork A device that vibrates and makes a sound when struck, and thus can be heard and felt. It is used, for example, in simple tests of hearing, including tests of air and bone conduction, and in tests of the ability to perceive vibration (e.g., from the nerves of the hand or foot). A fork that vibrates at 256 cycles/sec is suitable for use in these tests.

tunnel (tŭn′ĕl) A narrow channel or passageway.

carpal t. The canal in the wrist bounded by osteofibrous material through which the flexor tendons and the median nerve pass. SYN: *flexor t.*

flexor t. Carpal t.

inner t. The triangular canal lying between the inner and outer pillars of Corti in the organ of Corti of the inner ear.

tarsal t. The osteofibrous canal in the tarsal area bounded by the flexor retinaculum and tarsal bones. The posterior tibial vessels, tibial nerve, and flexor tendons pass through this tunnel.

TUR *transurethral resection* (of the prostate).

turbid (tŭr'bĭd) [L. *turba,* a tumult] Cloudy; not clear. SEE: *turbidity.*

turbidimeter (tŭr-bĭ-dĭm'ĕ-ter) [L. *turbidus,* disturbed, + Gr. *metron,* measure] A device for estimating the degree of turbidity of a fluid.

turbidimetry (tŭr-bĭ-dĭm'ĕ-trē) [" + Gr. *metron,* measure] Estimation of the turbidity of a liquid.

turbidity (tŭr-bĭd'ĭ-tē) [L. *turbiditas,* turbidity] Opacity due to the suspension of flaky or granular particles in a normally clear liquid.

turbinal (tŭr'bĭ-năl) [L. *turbinalis,* fr. *turbo,* a child's top] Shaped like an inverted cone.

turbinate (tŭr'bĭ-n-āt) [L. *turbinalis,* fr. *turbo,* a child's top] **1.** Shaped like an inverted cone. **2.** A coiled bone inside the nasal cavity.

turbinated (tŭr'bĭ-nā"tĕd) [L. *turbo,* whirl] Top-shaped or cone-shaped. SEE: *concha.*

turbinectomy (tŭr-bĭn-ĕk'tō-mē) [" + Gr. *ektome,* excision] Excision of a turbinated bone.

turbinoplasty (tŭr-bĭn'ō-plă-tē) Reduction of the size of the nasal turbinates. The surgery is used occasionally in the management of snoring and airflow disorders.

turbinotome (tŭr-bĭn'ō-tōm) [" + Gr. *tome,* incision] An instrument for excision of a turbinated bone.

turbinotomy (tŭr-bĭn-ŏt'ō-mē) [" + Gr. *tome,* incision] Surgical incision of a turbinated bone.

turgescence (tŭr-jĕs'ĕns) [L. *turgescens,* swelling] Swelling or enlargement of a part.

turgescent (tŭr-jĕs'ĕnt) [L. *turgescens,* swelling] Swollen; inflated.

turgid (tŭr'jĭd) [L. *turgidus,* swollen] Swollen; bloated.

turgometer (tŭr-gŏm'ĕ-tĕr) [L. *turgor,* swelling, + Gr. *metron,* measure] A device for measuring turgescence.

turgor [L., a swelling] **1.** Normal tension in a cell. **2.** Distention, swelling.

skin t. The resistance of the skin to deformation, esp. to being grasped between the fingers. In a healthy person, when the skin on the back of the hand is grasped between the fingers and released, it returns to its normal appearance either immediately or relatively slowly. The state of hydration of the skin can determine which of these reactions occurs, but age is the most important factor. As a person ages, the skin returns much more slowly to its normal position after having been pinched between the fingers. The skin over the forehead or sternum may be used when assessing turgor in elderly persons.

t. vitalis Normal fullness of the capillaries and blood vessels.

turista (tū-rēs'tă) [Sp.] One of the many names applied to travelers' diarrhea, esp. that which occurs in tourists in Mexico.

Türk's irritation cell A cell resembling a plasma cell, found in cases of severe anemia or chronic infection.

Turner's syndrome [Henry Hubert Turner, U.S. physician, 1892–1970] Gonadal dysgenesis.

turning [AS. *turnian,* to turn] **1.** Rotating to change position. **2.** Version (2).

turpentine (tŭr'pĕn-tīn) [Gr. *terebinthos,* turpentine tree] Oleoresin obtained from various species of pine trees. It is a mixture of terpenes and other hydrocarbons obtained from pine trees. It was once used in liniments and counterirritants.

turpentine poisoning Toxicity resulting usually from inhalation of turpentine. SEE: *Poisons and Poisoning Appendix.*

SYMPTOMS: Symptoms include a warm or burning sensation in the esophagus and stomach, followed by cramping, vomiting, and diarrhea. Pulse and respiration become weak, slow, and irregular. Irritation of the urinary tract and central nervous system resembles alcoholic intoxication.

FIRST AID: The airway should be secured and breathing assessed. Other therapies are supportive (intravenous fluids, oxygen, etc.).

turunda (tū-rŭn'dă) [L.] **1.** A surgical tent, drain, or tampon. **2.** A suppository.

tussal (tŭs'ăl) [L. *tussis,* cough] Tussive.

tussicular (tŭ-sĭk'ū-lăr) [L. *tussis,* cough] Pert. to a cough.

tussiculation (tŭ-sĭk"ū-lā'shŭn) A short, dry cough.

tussis (tŭs'ĭs) [L.] Cough.

tussive (tŭs'ĭv) [L. *tussis,* cough] Relating to a cough. SYN: *tussal.*

tutamen (tū-tā'mĕn) *pl.* **tutamina** [L.] Any tissue that has a protective action.

tutamina oculi The structures around the eye that protect it: the eyebrows, eyelids, and eyelashes.

T wave The portion of the electrical activity of the heart that reflects repolarization of the ventricles. SEE: *electrocardiogram; QRST complex.*

twelfth cranial nerve The hypoglossal nerve, motor to muscles of the tongue. SEE: *cranial nerve; hypoglossal nerve.*

twig The final branch of a structure such as a nerve or vessel.

twilight sleep A state of partial anesthesia and hypoconsciousness in which pain sense has been greatly reduced by the injection of morphine and scopolamine. The patient responds to pain, but afterward the memory of the pain is

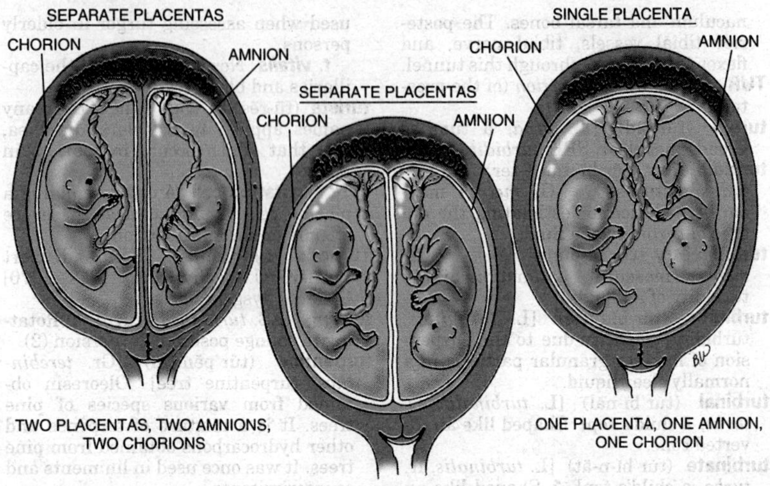

POSSIBLE RELATIONS OF FETAL MEMBRANES IN TWIN PREGNANCIES

dulled or effaced. Although once in common use as a method of analgesia for childbirth and minor surgery, twilight sleep has been replaced by more effective contemporary approaches to pain control.

twilight state A state in which consciousness is disordered and autonomic dysfunction or dissociation may occur. This may occur in epilepsy.

twin (twĭn) [AS. *twinn*] One of two children developed within the uterus at the same time from the same pregnancy. SEE: illus.; *fetus papyraceus; Hellin's law*.

INCIDENCE: Per 1000 live births, incidence rates for American whites are 1:88; for American blacks, 1:70. Generally, the rates are higher in blacks and East Indians and lower in Northern Europeans.

RESEARCH ON TWINS: Identical and fraternal twins provide a unique resource for investigating the origin and natural history of various diseases and discovering the different rates of environmental and hereditary factors in causing physical and mental disorders. Esp. important are studies that follow the course of identical twins separated shortly after birth and who then grew up in different social, economic, educational, and environmental conditions. In other research, the second-born twin was found to be at increased risk for an unfavorable outcome (e.g., need for intubation and resuscitation, lower 5-min Apgar score), even when delivered by cesarean section.

biovular t. Dizygotic t.

conjoined t. Twins that are united. SEE: *Siamese twins*.

dizygotic t. Twins from two separate ova fertilized at the same time. SYN: *biovular t.; fraternal t.*

enzygotic t. Monozygotic t.

fraternal t. Dizygotic t.

growth discordant t. The unequal growth of twins while in utero. The smaller twin is at greater risk of having congenital anomalies than is the normal birth-weight twin. SYN: *unequal t.*

identical t. Monozygotic t.

impacted t. Twins so entwined in utero as to prevent normal delivery.

interlocked t. Twins in which the neck of one becomes interlocked with the head of the other, making vaginal delivery impossible.

monozygotic t. Twins that develop from a single fertilized ovum. Monozygotic twins have the same genetic makeup and, consequently, are of the same gender and strikingly resemble each other physically, physiologically, and mentally. They develop within a common chorionic sac and have a common placenta. Each usually develops its own amnion and umbilical cord. Such twins may result from development of two inner cell masses within a blastocyst, development of two embryonic axes on a single blastoderm, or the division of a single embryonic axis into two centers. SYN: *enzygotic t.; identical t.; true t.; uniovular t.*

parasitic t. The smaller of a pair of conjoined twins, when there is a marked disparity in size.

true t. Monozygotic t.

unequal t. Growth discordant t.
uniovular t. Monozygotic t.
vanishing t. SEE: *gestation, multiple.*

twinge (twĭnj) [AS. *twengan,* to pinch] A sudden keen pain.

twinning (twĭn′ĭng) Delivery of or producing twins.

twitch (twĭch) [ME. *twicchen*] **1.** A single contraction of one muscle fiber in response to one nerve impulse. SEE: *myokymia.* **2.** To jerk convulsively.

twitching (twĭtch′ĭng) Repeated contractions of portions of muscles.

two-point discrimination test A test of cutaneous sensation involving determination of the ability of the patient to detect that the skin is being touched by two pointed objects at once. It is used to determine the degree of sensory loss following disease or trauma affecting the nervous system.

TXA$_2$ *thromboxane A$_2$.*

tybamate (tī′bă-māt) A minor tranquilizer.

tylectomy (tī-lĕk′tō-mē) [Gr. *tylos,* knot, + *ektome,* excision] Lumpectomy.

tylion (tĭl′ē-ŏn) [Gr. *tyleion,* knot] The point at the middle of the anterior edge of the optic groove.

tyloma (tī-lō′mă) [Gr. *tylos,* knot, + *oma,* tumor] A callosity.

tylosis (tī-lō′sĭs) [″ + *osis,* condition] Formation of a callus.

tyloxapol (tī-lŏks′ă-pōl) A nonionic liquid polymer of the alkyl aryl polyether alcohol type. It is a mucolytic used to reduce the viscosity of bronchopulmonary secretions.

tympan- SEE: *tympano-.*

tympanal (tĭm′păn-ăl) [Gr. *tympanon,* drum] Tympanic (1).

tympanectomy (tĭm″păn-ĕk′tō-mē) [″ + *ektome,* excision] Excision of the tympanic membrane.

tympanic (tĭm-păn′ĭk) [Gr. *tympanon,* drum] **1.** Pert. to the tympanum. SYN: *tympanal.* **2.** Resonant. SYN: *tympanitic* (2).

tympanism (tĭm′păn-ĭzm) [Gr. *tympanon,* drum, + *-ismos,* condition] Tympanites.

tympanites (tĭm-păn-ī′tēz) [Gr., distention] Distention of the abdomen or intestines due to the presence of gas. SYN: *meteorism; tympanism; tympanosis.*

tympanitic (tĭm-păn-ĭt′ĭk) **1.** Pert. to or characterized by tympanites. **2.** Tympanic (2).

tympanitis (tĭm-păn-ī′tĭs) [Gr. *tympanon,* drum, + *itis,* inflammation] Otitis media.

tympano-, tympan-, myringo-, myring- [Gr. *tympanon,* drum] Combining form meaning *tympanic membrane* or *eardrum.*

tympanocentesis (tĭm″pă-nō-sĕn-tē′sĭs) Drainage of fluid from the middle ear by using a small gauge needle to puncture the tympanic membrane. The fluid is cultured to determine the identity of any microbes that may be present.

tympanoeustachian (tĭm″pă-nō-ū-stā′kē-ăn) Concerning the tympanic cavity and eustachian tube.

tympanography Radiographic examination of the eustachian tubes and middle ear after introduction of a contrast medium.

tympanohyal (tĭm″pă-nō-hī′ăl) Concerning the tympanic cavity and hyoid arch.

tympanomalleal (tĭm″pă-nō-măl′ē-ăl) Concerning the tympanic membrane and malleus.

tympanomandibular (tĭm″pă-nō-măn-dĭb′ū-lăr) Concerning the middle ear and mandible.

tympanomastoiditis (tĭm″păn-ō-măs″toy-dī′tĭs) [″ + *mastos,* breast, + *eidos,* form, shape, + *itis,* inflammation] Inflammation of the tympanum and mastoid cells.

tympanometry (tĭm″pă-nŏm′ĕ-trē) A procedure for objective evaluation of the mobility and patency of the eardrum and for detection of middle-ear disorders and patency of the eustachian tubes. SEE: *audiometry.*

tympanoplasty (tĭm″păn-ō-plăs′tē) [″ + *plassein,* to form] Any one of several surgical procedures designed either to cure a chronic inflammatory process in the middle ear or to restore function to the sound-transmitting mechanism of the middle ear. SEE: *Nursing Diagnoses Appendix.*

tympanosclerosis (tĭm″pă-nō-sklĕ-rō′sĭs) Infiltration by hard fibrous tissue around the ossicles of the middle ear.

tympanosis (tĭm-pă-nō′sĭs) [″ + *osis,* condition] Tympanites.

tympanosquamosal (tĭm″pă-nō-skwă-mō′săl) Concerning the tympanic and squamosal portions of the temporal bone.

tympanostapedial (tĭm″pă-nō-stă-pē′dē-ăl) Concerning the tympanic cavity and stapes.

tympanostomy Myringotomy.

tympanostomy tube A tube placed through the tympanic membrane of the ear to allow ventilation of the middle ear as part of the treatment of otitis media with effusion. SYN: *grommet.* SEE: *otitis media with effusion.*

tympanotemporal (tĭm″pă-nō-tĕm′pō-răl) Concerning the tympanic cavity and area of the temporal bone.

tympanotomy (tĭm″păn-ŏt′ō-mē) [″ + *tome,* incision] Incision of the tympanic membrane. SYN: *myringotomy.*

tympanous (tĭm′păn-ŭs) [Gr. *tympanon,* a drum] Marked by abdominal distention with gas.

tympanum (tĭm′păn-ŭm) [L.; Gr. *tympanon*] The middle ear or tympanic cavity. SYN: *cavum tympani; eardrum.* SEE: *ear, middle.*

tympany (tĭm′pă-nē) **1.** Abdominal distention with gas. **2.** Tympanic resonance on percussion. It is a clear hollow note like that of a drum. It indicates a pathological condition of the lung or of a cavity.

type (tīp) [Gr. *typos,* mark] The general character of a person, disease, or substance.

asthenic t. Having a thin, flat, long-chested body build with poor muscular development.

athletic t. Having broad shoulders, a deep chest, flat abdomen, thick neck, and powerful muscular development.

blood t. Blood group.

phage t. Distinguishing subgroups of bacteria by the type of bacteriophage associated with that specific bacterium.

pyknic t. Having a rounded body, large chest, thick shoulders, broad head, thick neck, and usually short stature.

typhlectasis (tĭf-lĕk′tă-sĭs) [Gr. *typhlon,* cecum, + *ektasis,* dilatation] Cecal distention.

typhlectomy (tĭf-lĕk′tō-mē) [″ + *ektome,* excision] Excision of the cecum. SYN: *cecectomy.*

typhlenteritis (tĭf″lĕn-tĕr-ī′tĭs) [″ + *enteron,* intestine, + *itis,* inflammation] Inflammation of the cecum. SYN: *typhlitis; typhloenteritis.*

typhlitis (tĭf-lī′tĭs) [″ + *itis,* inflammation] Inflammation of the cecum. SYN: *typhlenteritis; typhloenteritis.*

typhlo- **1.** Combining form meaning *cecum.* **2.** Combining form meaning *blindness.*

typhlodicliditis (tĭf″lō-dĭk-lĭ-dī′tĭs) [″ + *diklis,* door, + *itis,* inflammation] Inflammation of the ileocecal valve.

typhloempyema (tĭf″lō-ĕm-pī-ē′mă) [″ + *en,* in, + *pyon,* pus, + *haima,* blood] An abdominal abscess following appendicitis.

typhloenteritis (tĭf″lō-ĕn-tĕr-ī′tĭs) [″ + *enteron,* intestine, + *itis,* inflammation] Inflammation of the cecum. SYN: *typhlenteritis; typhlitis.*

typhlolithiasis (tĭf″lō-lĭ-thī′ă-sĭs) [Gr. *typhlon,* cecum, + *lithos,* stone, + *-iasis,* condition] Formation of a stone in the cecum.

typhlomegaly (tĭf″lō-mĕg′ă-lē) [Gr. *typhlon,* cecum, + *megas,* large] An abnormally large cecum.

typhlon (tĭf′lŏn) [Gr.] Cecum.

typhlopexy (tĭf′lō-pĕks″ē) [Gr. *typhlon,* cecum, + *pexis,* fixation] Suturing of a movable cecum to the abdominal wall.

typhlorrhaphy (tĭf-lor′ă-fē) Surgical repair of the cecum.

typhlospasm (tĭf′lō-spăsm) Spasm of the cecum.

typhlostenosis (tĭf″lō-stĕn-ō′sĭs) [Gr. *typhlon,* cecum, + *stenosis,* act of narrowing] Stenosis or stricture of the cecum.

typhlostomy (tĭf-lŏs′tō-mē) [″ + *stoma,* mouth] Establishment of a permanent cecal fistula.

typhlotomy (tĭf-lŏt′ō-mē) [Gr. *typhlon,* cecum, + *tome,* incision] Incision of the cecum, a procedure used only in veterinary medicine.

typhloureterostomy (tĭf″lō-ū-rē″tĕr-ŏs′tō-mē) [″ + *oureter,* ureter, + *stoma,* mouth] Implantation of a ureter in the cecum.

typho- [Gr. *typhos,* fever] Combining form meaning *fever, typhoid.*

typhoid (tī′foyd) [Gr. *typhos,* fever, + *eidos,* form, shape] Resembling typhus.

typhoidal (tī-foy′dăl) Resembling typhoid.

typhoid carrier An individual who has recovered from typhoid fever but who harbors the bacteria, usually in the gallbladder or kidneys, and who excretes it in the feces or urine, respectively.

typhoid fever A severe infectious disease marked by fever and septicemia. Approx. 12.5 million cases of typhoid fever occur each year worldwide; 70% of the 400 cases in the U.S. each year are acquired during travel to developing countries in Asia, Latin America, and Africa, where the disease is endemic. SYN: *enteric fever.* SEE: *typhoid vaccine.*

SYMPTOMS: The disease is marked initially by a fever up to 104° F for about 7 days, followed by a flat, rose-colored, fleeting rash, generalized lymphadenopathy, abdominal pain, anorexia, and extreme exhaustion as the bacteria spread through the bloodstream. About 14 days after the infection begins, internal bleeding usually develops, as the result of gastrointestinal ulcers, and this may lead to hypovolemic shock. Damage to the liver and spleen is commonly seen. In approx. 10% of patients, typhoid fever is complicated by osteomyelitis, septic arthritis, or meningitis, which account for the majority of deaths.

ETIOLOGY: Typhoid fever is caused by *Salmonella typhi,* gram-negative bacteria that invade the walls of the ileum and colon and then gain access to the bloodstream. The disease is most commonly transmitted through water or food contaminated by human feces, but it can be spread also by vomitus and oral secretions during the acute stage. Unlike *S. enteritidis,* it lives only in humans. A small percentage of persons become carriers after recovering from infection.

DIFFERENTIAL DIAGNOSIS: Paratyphoid, pneumonia, dysentery, meningitis, smallpox, and appendicitis are among the differential diagnoses. Diagnostic points of value are the presence of rose spots, splenomegaly, leukopenia, the Widal serological test result, blood culture, and examination of feces for the presence of the causative organism. The best means of providing bacterial confirmation is through bone marrow culture. This method is successful even after patients have received antibiotics. SEE: *paratyphoid fever.*

TREATMENT: The disease is treated with ciprofloxacin for 10 days. Dexamethasone is administered a few minutes before antibiotics are given in patients with shock or decreased levels of consciousness. Travelers to developing countries should consider vaccination with typhoid vaccine, which is available in oral and parenteral forms. The vaccinations should be completed at least 1 week before the trip; boosters are required every 2 to 5 years, depending on the type of vaccine. The vaccinations should not be given to patients who are taking mefloquine for malaria prophylaxis. SEE: *Standard and Universal Precautions Appendix.*

PATIENT CARE: Enteric precautions (handwashing, patient handwashing, glove and gown for disposal of feces or fecally contaminated objects) are followed until three consecutive stool cultures at 24-hr intervals are negative. Drugs are administered as prescribed, and the patient is observed for signs and symptoms of complications, such as bacteremia, intestinal bleeding, and bowel perforation. During the acute phase, the temperature is monitored, and prescribed antipyretics are administered; tepid sponge baths are also provided to promote vasodilation without shivering. The incontinent patient is cleansed, and high fluid intake by mouth or IV is encouraged to maintain adequate hydration. Adequate nutrition is maintained. The caregiver explains the importance of follow-up care and examination to ensure that the patient is not a carrier. SEE: *Standard and Universal Precautions Appendix.*

typholysin (tī-fŏl'ĭ-sĭn) [" + *lysis,* dissolution] A lysin destructive to typhoid bacilli.

typhomalarial (tī"fō-mă-lā'rē-ăl) [" + It. *malaria,* bad air] Having symptoms of both typhoid and malarial fevers.

typhomania (tī-fō-mā'nē-ă) [" + *mania,* madness] An old term for febrile delirium experienced in typhoid fever or typhus.

typhopneumonia (tī"fō-nū-mō'nē-ă) [" + *pneumon,* lung, + *-ia,* condition, abnormal state] **1.** Pneumonia occurring in typhoid fever. **2.** Pneumonia with typhoid symptoms.

typhous (tī'fŭs) [Gr. *typhos,* fever] Pert. to typhus fever.

typhus (tī'fŭs) [Gr. *typhos,* fever] One of several forms of infection by rickettsial species transmitted to people by ticks and fleas. The causative microbe invades the lining of blood vessels and smooth muscle cells, causing widespread vasculitis. The most common causes of typhus are *Rickettsia prowazekii, R. typhi, and Orientia tsutsugamushi,* all of which are carried by bloodsucking insects. *R. prowazekii* causes the epidemic typhus found in crowded conditions with poor sanitation, such as refugee camps. SEE: *Nursing Diagnoses Appendix.*

SYMPTOMS: The disease may be mild, marked only by a flat rash that spreads out from the trunk and petechiae or by flu-like symptoms. In more severe cases, patients have fever, skin necrosis, and gangrene on the tips of the fingers, toes, earlobes, and penis as a result of thrombus formation in blood vessels; focal inflammation and thrombosis in organs throughout the body, including the brain, produce organ-specific signs. Rickettsial infections are diagnosed by identifying the organism through immunofluorescent staining.

TREATMENT: Typhus is treated with doxycycline for 7 days. SEE: *Standard and Universal Precautions Appendix.*

COMPLICATIONS: Bronchopneumonia occurs more frequently than lobar pneumonia. Hypostatic congestion of the lungs, nephritis, and parotid abscess also may occur.

PROGNOSIS: The prognosis is variable. Mortality may be quite high in epidemic typhus and almost nonexistent in murine typhus. Broad-spectrum antibiotics are life-saving if given early enough.

endemic t. Murine t.

epidemic t. An infectious disease caused by *Rickettsia prowazekii* and transmitted by the human body louse *(Pediculus humanus corporis).*

flea-borne t. Murine t.

Mexican t. A louse-borne epidemic typhus present in certain portions of Mexico. SYN: *tabardillo.*

mite-borne t. Scrub t.

murine t. A disease caused by *Rickettsia typhi* and occurring in nature as a mild infection of rats and transmitted from rat to rat by the rat-louse or flea. Humans may acquire it by being bitten by infected rat fleas or ingesting food contaminated by rat urine or flea feces. SYN: *endemic t.; flea-borne t.*

recrudescent t. The recurrence of epidemic typhus after the initial attack.

scrub t. A self-limited febrile disease of 2 weeks' duration caused by *Orientia tsutsugamushi* and transmitted by two species of mites (chiggers) of the genus *Thrombicula.* It occurs principally in the Pacific-Asiatic area. SYN: *mite-borne t.; tsutsugamushi disease.*

typical (tĭp'ĭ-kăl) [Gr. *typikos,* pert. to type] Having the characteristics of, pert. to, or conforming to a type, condition, or group.

typing (tīp'ĭng) Identification of type.

bacteriophage t. Determination of the subdivision of a bacterial species using a type-specific bacteriophage.

blood t. The method used to determine the antigens present on a person's blood cells.

tissue t. Determination of the histocompatibility of tissues to be used in grafts and transplants. SEE: *transplantation.*

typo- Combining form meaning *type.*

typodont A replica of the natural dentition and alveolar mucosa used in training dental students.

typoscope (tī′pō-skōp) [Gr. *typos,* type, + *skopein,* to examine] A reading aid device for patients with amblyopia or cataract.

typus (tī′pŭs) [L.] Type.

tyramine (tī′ră-mēn) An intermediate product in the conversion of tyrosine to epinephrine. Tyramine is found in most cheeses and in beer, broad bean pods, yeast, wine, and chicken liver.

CAUTION: When persons taking certain monoamine oxidase inhibitors eat these foods, they may experience severe hypertension, headache, palpitation, neck pain, and perhaps intracranial hemorrhage.

tyrannism (tĭr′ăn-ĭzm) [Gr. *tyrannos,* tyrant, + *-ismos,* condition] Sadism.

tyrogenous (tī-rŏj′ĕn-ŭs) [Gr. *tyros,* cheese, + *gennan,* to produce] Having origin in or produced by cheese.

Tyroglyphus (tī-rŏg′lĭ-fŭs) [Gr. *tyros,* cheese, + *glyphein,* to carve] A genus of sarcoptoid mites commonly known as cheese mites. They infest cheese and dried vegetable food products and occasionally infest humans, causing pruritus. This genus includes species that cause grocer's itch, vanillism, and copra itch.

tyroid (tī′royd) [″ + *eidos,* form, shape] Caseous; cheesy.

tyroma (tī-rō′mă) A tumor that contains cheeselike material.

tyromatosis (tī″rō-mă-tō′sĭs) [″ + *oma,* tumor, + *osis,* condition] Caseation (1).

tyrosinase (tī-rō′sĭn-ās) [Gr. *tyros,* cheese] An enzyme that acts on tyrosine to produce melanin.

tyrosine (tī′rō-sĭn) $C_9H_{11}NO_3$; an amino acid present in many proteins, esp. casein. It serves as a precursor of epinephrine, thyroxine, and melanin. Two vitamins, ascorbic acid and folic acid, are essential for its metabolism.

tyrosinemia (tī″rō-sĭ-nē′mē-ă) A disease of tyrosine metabolism caused by a deficiency of the enzyme tyrosine aminotransferase. In addition to an accumulation of tyrosine in the blood, mental retardation, keratitis, and dermatitis are present. Treatment consists of controlling phenylalanine and tyrosine intake.

tyrosinosis (tī″rō-sĭn-ō′sĭs) [″ + *osis,* condition] A condition resulting from faulty metabolism of tyrosine, whereby its oxidation products appear in the urine.

tyrosinuria (tī″rō-sĭn-ū′rē-ă) [″ + *ouron,* urine] Tyrosine in the urine.

tyrosis (tī-rō′sĭs) [″ + *osis,* condition] **1.** Curdling of milk. **2.** Vomiting of cheesy substance by infants. **3.** Caseation (1).

tyrosyluria (tī″rō-sĭl-ū′rē-ă) Increased tyrosine-derived products in the urine.

tyrotoxism (tī″rō-tŏks′ĭzm) [″ + *toxikon,* a poison, + *-ismos,* condition] Poisoning produced by a milk product or by cheese.

Tyrrell's fascia (tĭr′rĕlz) [Frederick Tyrrell, Brit. anatomist, 1797–1843] An ill-defined fibromuscular layer from the middle aponeurosis of the perineum, behind the prostate gland.

Tyson's gland (tī′sŭnz) [Edward Tyson, Brit. physician and anatomist, 1650–1708] One of the modified sebaceous glands located on the neck of the penis and the inner surface of the prepuce. The secretion of these glands is one of the components of smegma. SYN: *preputial gland.*

tysonitis (tī″sŏn-ī′tĭs) Inflammation of Tyson's glands.

tyvelose (tī′vĕl-ōs) A carbohydrate, 3-6-dideoxy-D-mannose, derived from certain strains of *Salmonella* and *Trichinella.*

Tzanck cell A degenerated cell from the keratin layer of the skin, disconnected from adjacent cells. It is seen in pemphigus.

Tzanck test (tsănk) [Arnault Tzanck, Russ. dermatologist in Paris, 1886–1954] The examination of cells scraped from the lower surface of a vesicle to determine the underlying disease (e.g., infection with a herpesvirus).

tzetze (sĕt′sē) Tsetse fly.

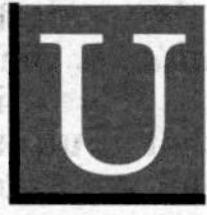

U **1.** *unit.* **2.** Symbol for the element uranium.

^{235}U Isotope of uranium with mass number 235.

UAO *upper airway obstruction.*

ubiquinol (ū-bĭk′wĭ-nŏl) Coenzyme QH_2, the reduced form of ubiquinone.

ubiquinone (ū-bĭk′wĭ-nōn) [*ubi*quitous + coenzyme *quinone*] Coenzyme Q, a lipid-soluble quinone present in virtually all cells. It collects reducing equivalents during intracellular respiration and is converted to its reduced form, ubiquinol, while involved in this process. This substance is widely used in Europe and Asia as a health food supplement for congestive heart failure and other disorders, although confirmation of its effectiveness is uncertain.

ubiquitin A small protein present in eukaryotic cells that combines with other proteins to make them susceptible to destruction. It is also important in promoting the functions of proteins that make up ribosomes.

UDP *uridine diphosphate.*

Uffelmann's test (oof′ĕl-mănz) [Jules Uffelmann, Ger. physician, 1837–1894] A test for the determination of lactic acid in gastric juice.

Uhthoff's sign (oot′hŏfs) [Wilhelm Uhthoff, Ger. ophthalmologist, 1853–1927] The nystagmus that occurs in multiple sclerosis.

ulcer (ŭl′sĕr) [L. *ulcus,* ulcer] A lesion of the skin or mucous membranes marked by inflammation, necrosis, and sloughing of damaged tissues. A wide variety of insults may produce ulcers, including trauma, caustic chemicals, intense heat or cold, arterial or venous stasis, cancers, drugs (e.g., nonsteroidal anti-inflammatory drugs), and infectious agents such as *Herpes simplex* or *Helicobacter pylori*.

amputating u. An ulcer that destroys tissue to the bone by encircling the part.

aphthous u. A lesion of the skin or mucous membranes (e.g., of the oral mucosa, conjunctiva, or genitalia). It is usually less than 0.5 cm in diameter. If it persists for longer than 2 weeks, it should be biopsied in order to rule out cancer. SYN: *aphthous stomatitis; canker sore*.

ETIOLOGY: Aphthous ulcers are found in stomatitis, Behçet's syndrome, Crohn's disease, human immunodeficiency syndrome, some cancers, and other diseases.

TREATMENT: For patients with oral ulcers, application of a topical anesthetic or a protective paste provides symptomatic relief and makes it possible to eat without pain.

atonic u. A chronic ulcer with scant tendency to heal.

callous u. A chronic ulcer with indurated, elevated edges and no granulation that heals slowly.

chronic leg u. Any long-standing, slow-to-heal ulcer of a lower extremity, esp. one caused by occlusive disease of the arteries or veins or by varicose veins.

Curling's u. A peptic ulcer that sometimes occurs following severe burns to the body; a form of stress ulcer.

Cushing's u. Stress ulcers that occur in patients with increased intracranial pressure. Cushing's ulcers may be caused by increased secretion of gastric acid as the result of vagus nerve stimulation.

denture u. An ulcer of the oral mucosa caused by irritation from wearing dentures.

duodenal u. An open sore on the mucosa of the first portion of the duodenum, most often as the result of infection with *Helicobacter pylori*. It is the most common form of peptic ulcer. SEE: *peptic ulcer*.

follicular u. A tiny ulcer originating in a lymph follicle and affecting a mucous membrane.

fungal u. **1.** An ulcer in which the granulations protrude above the edges of the wound and bleed easily. **2.** An ulcer caused by a fungus.

gastric u. An ulcer of the gastric mucosa.

ETIOLOGY: Common causes are nonsteroidal anti-inflammatory drugs, use of alcohol or tobacco, and infection with *Helicobacter pylori*. SEE: *peptic ulcer*.

Hunner's u. A painful, slow-to-heal ulcer of the urinary bladder.

indolent u. A nearly painless ulcer usually found on the leg, characterized by an indurated and elevated edge and a nongranulating base.

Meleney's u. SEE: under *Meleney*.

peptic u. SEE: under *peptic*.

perforating u. An ulcer that erodes through an organ, such as the stomach or duodenum.

phagedenic u. Tropical ulcer.

pressure u. Pressure sore.

rodent u. A basal cell carcinoma that has caused extensive local invasion and tissue destruction, esp. on the face. The usual sites are the outer angle of the eye, near the side and on the tip of the nose, and at the hairline. SYN: *Jacob's ulcer*.

serpiginous u. A creeping ulcer that heals in one part and extends to another.

simple u. A local ulcer with no severe inflammation or pain.

specific u. An ulcer caused by a specific disease, such as syphilis or lupus.

stercoral u. **1.** An ulcer caused by pressure from impacted feces. **2.** A perforating ulcer through which feces escape.

stress u. Multiple, small, shallow ulcers that form in the mucosa of the stomach or, occasionally, in the duodenum, in response to extreme physiological stressors. Stress ulcers seen in patients with shock, extensive burns, or sepsis are called Curling's ulcers and may be caused by mucosal ischemia secondary to systemic vasoconstriction. Stress ulcers that occur in patients with increased intracranial pressure (Cushing's ulcers) may be caused by increased secretion of gastric acid as the result of vagus nerve stimulation. SEE: *peptic u.*

traumatic u. An ulcer due to injury of the oral mucosa. Causes include biting, denture irritation, toothbrush injury, and sharp edges of teeth or restorations.

trophic u. An ulcer caused by the failure to supply nutrients to a part.

tropical u. **1.** An indolent ulcer, usually of a lower extremity, that occurs in persons living in hot, humid areas. The etiology may or may not be known, and it may be caused by a combination of bacterial, environmental, and nutritional factors. SYN: *phagedenic u.* **2.** The tropical sore caused by leishmaniasis.

varicose u. An ulcer, esp. of the lower extremity, associated with varicose veins.

venereal u. An ulcer caused by a sexually transmitted disease (i.e., chancre or chancroid).

venous stasis u. A poorly and slowly healing ulcer, usually located on the lower extremity above the medial malleolus. It typically is edematous, pigmented, and scarred. The skin is extremely fragile and easily injured.

ulcera Pl. of ulcus.

ulcerate (ŭl′sĕr-āt) [L. *ulcerare,* to form ulcers] To produce or become affected with an ulcer.

ulcerated (ŭl′sĕr-ā″tĕd) Of the nature of an ulcer or affected with one.

ulcerated tooth Suppuration of the alveolar periosteum with ulceration of the gum surrounding the decaying root of a tooth.

ulceration (ŭl″sĕr-ā′shŭn) A suppurative or non-healing lesion on a surface such as skin, cornea, or mucous membrane.

ulcerative (ŭl′sĕr-ā-tĭv) [L. *ulcerare,* to form ulcers] Pert. to or causing ulceration.

ulcerogangrenous (ŭl″sĕr-ō-găng′grĕ-nŭs) Rel. to an ulcer that contains gangrenous tissue.

ulcerogenic drug A medicine, such as a nonsteroidal anti-inflammatory drug, that may cause peptic ulcers.

ulceromembranous (ŭl″sĕr-ō-mĕm′brăn-ŭs) [″ + *membrana,* membrane] Pert. to ulceration and formation of a fibrous pseudomembrane.

ulcerous (ŭl′sĕr-ŭs) Pert. to or affected with an ulcer.

ulcus (ŭl′kŭs) *pl.* **ulcera** [L.] Ulcer.

ulegyria (ū″lē-jī′rē-ă) [Gr. *oule,* scar, + *gyros,* ring] A condition in which gyri of the cerebral cortex are abnormal due to scar tissue from injuries, usually occurring in early development.

ulerythema (ū-lĕr-ĭ-thē′mă) [″ + *erythema,* redness] An erythematous disorder with atrophic scar formation.

u. ophryogenes Folliculitis of the eyebrows, characterized by loss of hair and scarring.

u. sycosiforme Inflammation of the hair follicles of the beard with alopecia in the affected area.

uletomy (ū-lĕt′ō-mē) [″ + *tome,* incision] Incision of a scar to relieve tension. SYN: *cicatricotomy*.

uliginous (ū-lĭj′ĭ-nŭs) [L. *uliginosus,* wet] Muddy; slimy.

ulitis Gingivitis.

ulna (ŭl′nă) [L., elbow] The inner and larger bone of the forearm, between the wrist and the elbow, on the side opposite that of the thumb. It articulates with the head of the radius and humerus proximally, and with the radius and carpals distally.

ulnad (ŭl′năd) [″ + *ad,* to] In the direction of the ulna.

ulnar (ŭl′năr) [L. *ulna,* elbow] Rel. to the ulna, or to the nerve or artery named from it.

ulnar drift A joint abnormality at the metacarpophalangeal joints, frequently seen in rheumatoid arthritis, resulting from chronic synovitis. In this condition, the long axis of the fingers deviates in an ulnar direction with respect to the metacarpals.

ulnaris (ŭl-nā′rĭs) **1.** Ulnar. **2.** Concerning the ulna.

ulnocarpal (ŭl″nō-kăr′păl) [″ + Gr. *karpos,* wrist] Relating to the carpus and ulna, or to the ulnar side of the wrist.

ulnoradial (ŭl″nō-rā′dē-ăl) [″ + *radius,* spoke of a wheel] Rel. to the ulna and radius, as their ligaments and articulations.

ultimate (ŭl′tĭm-ĭt) [L. *ultimus,* last] Final or last.

ultimobranchial body (ŭl″tĭ-mō-brăng′kē-ăl) One of two embryonic pharyngeal pouches usually considered as rudimentary fifth pouches. They become separated from the pharynx and incorporated into the thyroid gland, where they give rise to parafollicular cells that secrete calcitonin, a hormone that lowers the blood calcium level.

ultra- [L.] Prefix meaning *beyond, excess.*

ultrabrachycephalic (ŭl″tră-brăk″ĭ-sē-făl′ĭk) [L. *ultra,* beyond, + Gr. *brachys,* short, + *kephale,* head] Having a cephalic index of 90 or more.

ultracentrifugation (ŭl″tră-sĕn-trĭf″ū-gā′shŭn) Treatment or preparation of substances by use of the ultracentrifuge.

ultracentrifuge (ŭl-tră-sĕn′trĭ-fūj) [″ + *centrum,* center, + *fugere,* to flee] A high-speed centrifuge capable of producing centrifugal forces more than 100,000 times gravity; it is used in the study of proteins, viruses, and other substances present in body fluids.

ultradian (ŭl-trā′dē-ăn) [″ + *dies,* day] Concerning biological rhythms that occur less frequently than every 24 hr.

ultrafilter (ŭl-tră-fĭl′tĕr) A filter by which colloidal particles may be separated from their dispersion medium or from crystalloids.

ultrafiltration (ŭl″tră-fĭl-trā′shŭn) [″ + *filtrum,* a filter] Filtration of a colloidal substance in which the dispersed particles, but not the liquid, are held back.

ultramicrobe (ŭl″tră-mī′krōb) [″ + Gr. *mikros,* small, + *bios,* life] A microorganism too small to be visible with an ordinary microscope.

ultramicroscope (ŭl″tră-mī′krō-skōp) [″ + ″ + *skopein,* to examine] A microscope by which objects invisible through an ordinary microscope may be seen by means of powerful side illumination. SYN: *dark-field microscope.*

ultramicroscopy (ŭl″tră-mī-krŏs′kō-pē) The use of the ultramicroscope.

ultramicrotome (ŭl″tră-mī′krō-tōm) A microtome that makes extremely thin slices of tissue.

ultrasonic (ŭl-tră-sŏn′ĭk) [″ + *sonus,* sound] Pert. to sounds of frequencies above approx. 20,000 cycles/sec, which are inaudible to the human ear. SEE: *supersonic; ultrasonography; ultrasound.*

ultrasonic cleaning The use of ultrasonic energy to sterilize objects, including medical and surgical instruments.

ultrasonics (ŭl-tră-sŏn′ĭks) The division of acoustics that studies inaudible sounds (i.e., those with frequencies greater than 20,000 cycles/sec). Biological effects may result, depending on the intensity of the beams. Heating effects are produced by beams of low intensity, paralytic effects by those of moderate intensity, and lethal effects by those of high intensity. The lethal action of ultrasonics is primarily the result, either directly or indirectly, of cavitation of tissues. Ultrasonics is used clinically for therapeutic and diagnostic purposes. In dentistry, instruments producing 29,000 cycles/sec are used in periodontal surgery, curettage, and root planing. SEE: *ultrasound.*

ultrasonogram (ŭl″tră-sŏn′ō-grăm) The image produced by use of ultrasonography.

ultrasonography (ŭl-tră-sŏn-ŏg′ră-fē) The use of ultrasound to produce an image or photograph of an organ or tissue. Ultrasonic echoes are recorded as they strike tissues of different densities.

arterial duplex u. A diagnostic procedure that helps to identify areas within arteries where blood flow is blocked or reduced. SEE: *LEAS.*

Doppler u. The shift in frequency produced when an ultrasound wave is echoed from something in motion. The use of the Doppler effect permits measuring the velocity of that which is being studied (e.g., blood flow in a vessel). SEE: illus.

gray-scale u. Use of a television scan technique to process the strength of ultrasound echoes with the strongest being registered as white and the weakest as different shades of gray.

pelvic u. Ultrasonographic visualization of the uterus, fallopian tubes, endometrium, and, in pregnant patients, the fetus. The test may be used to di-

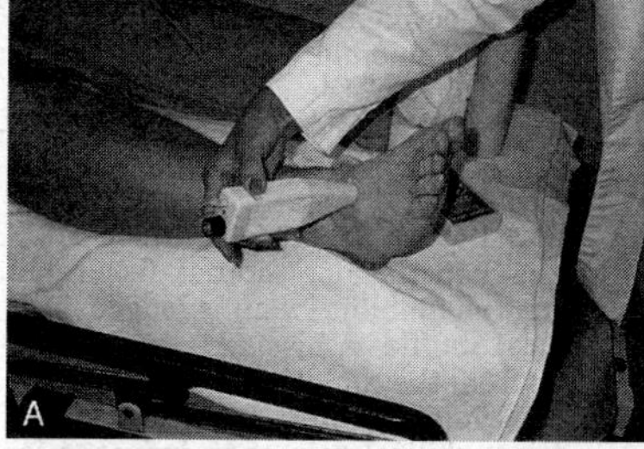

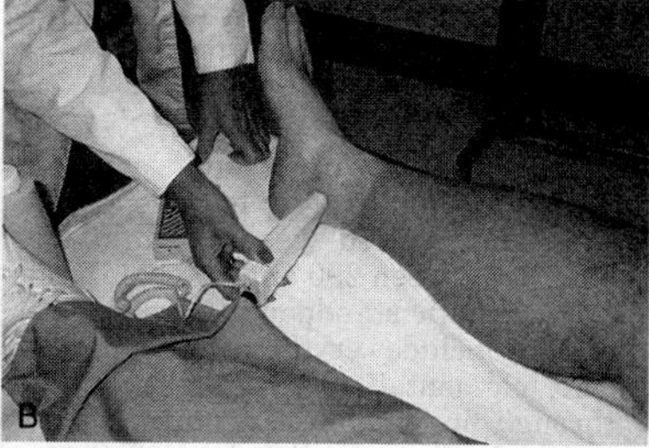

DOPPLER ULTRASONOGRAPHY

Doppler probe used on (A) dorsal pedis and (B) posterior tibial arteries

agnose ectopic pregnancy, determine multiple pregnancies, identify ovarian cysts and pelvic cancers, and visualize tubo-ovarian abscesses. To obtain the needed images, the transducer (ultrasound probe) can be placed either on the abdominal wall or within the vagina.

ultrasound Inaudible sound in the frequency range of approx. 20,000 to 10 billion (10^9) cycles/sec. Ultrasound has different velocities that differ in density and elasticity from one kind of tissue to the next. This property permits the use of ultrasound in outlining the shape of various tissues and organs in the body. In obstetrics, for example, identifying the size and position of the fetus, placenta, and umbilical cord enables estimation of gestational age, detects some fetal anomalies and fetal death, and facilitates other diagnostic procedures, such as amniocentesis. In physical therapy, the thermal effects of ultrasound are used to treat musculoskeletal injuries by warming tissue, increasing tissue extensibility, and improving local blood flow. Ultrasound is used to facilitate movement of certain medications (e.g., pain relievers) into tissue (phonophoresis). Ultrasound is also used with electric current for muscular stimulation. The diagnostic and therapeutic uses of ultrasound require special equipment. SEE: *phonophoresis; sonographer; ultrasonography.*

A-mode u. Sonographic information presented as a single line representing the time it takes for the ultrasound wave to reach the interface of a structure and reflect back to the transducer.

intravascular u. In ultrasonography, a technique for imaging intimal tissue proliferation and blood vessel blockages.

real-time u. A sonographic procedure that provides rapid, multiple images of an anatomical structure in the form of motion.

ultrastructure (ŭl′tră-strŭk″chŭr) The fine structure of tissues. It is visible only by use of electron microscopy.

ultraviolet (ŭl″tră-vī′ō-lĕt) [″ + *viola,* violet] Beyond the visible spectrum at its violet end, said of rays between the violet rays and x-rays. SEE: *infrared ray.*

ultraviolet radiation ABBR: UVR. Rays emitted by natural and artificial sources, including very hot bodies, the sun, and ionized gases with wavelengths between 290 and 400 nm. From a therapeutic standpoint, physiological effects include erythema production, skin pigmentation, antirachitic effect through production of vitamin D, bactericidal effects, and various effects on metabolism. In clinical practice, dosage is measured in terms of minimum erythema dose.

In addition to erythema, UVR can cause degenerative and neoplastic changes in the skin, retinal damage, cataracts, and modification of the immunological system of the skin.

The UVR spectrum has been described and categorized as follows:

UV-A, which includes wavelengths of 320 to 400 nm, can produce skin erythema, but the required dose is 1000 times that of UV-B.

UV-B, with the included wavelength of 290 to 320 nm, is the principal portion of the UVR spectrum that causes sunburn. A large portion of the UV-B emitted by the sun is absorbed by the ozone layer in the earth's atmosphere.

UV-C includes those wavelengths below 290 nm. These rays are completely absorbed by the ozone layer and have no role in causing pathological changes caused by exposure to sunlight.

UVR in combination with various chemical compounds may cause phototoxic or photoallergic reactions. SEE: *erythema dose; sunscreen; tanning salon.*

ultraviolet therapy Treatment with ultraviolet radiation. SEE: *heliotherapy; light therapy.*

ululation (ŭl″ū-lā′shŭn) [L. *ululare,* to howl] Howling; wailing.

umbilical (ŭm-bĭl′ĭ-kăl) [L. *umbilicus,* navel] Pert. to the umbilicus.

umbilical cord The attachment connecting the fetus with the placenta. It contains two arteries and one vein surrounded by a gelatinous substance, Wharton's jelly. The umbilical arteries carry blood from the fetus to the placenta, where nutrients are obtained and carbon dioxide and oxygen are exchanged; this oxygenated blood returns to the fetus through the umbilical vein. SEE: illus.

The umbilical cord is surgically severed after the birth of the child. To give the infant a better blood supply, the cord should not be cut or tied until the umbilical vessels have ceased pulsating. However, in preterm infants, the cord should be clamped and cut before pulsation ceases to avoid maternal-newborn transfusion and reduce the risk of hypovolemia, polycythemia, and hyperbilirubinemia.

The stump of the severed cord atrophies and leaves a depression on the abdomen of the child, called a navel or umbilicus.

umbilical fissure In the fetus, the portion of the hepatic longitudinal fissure in which the umbilical vein is lodged.

umbilical souffle A hissing sound said to arise from the umbilical cord.

umbilical vein catheter A catheter placed in the umbilical vein of an infant to facilitate administration of medicines parenterally or to do an exchange transfusion.

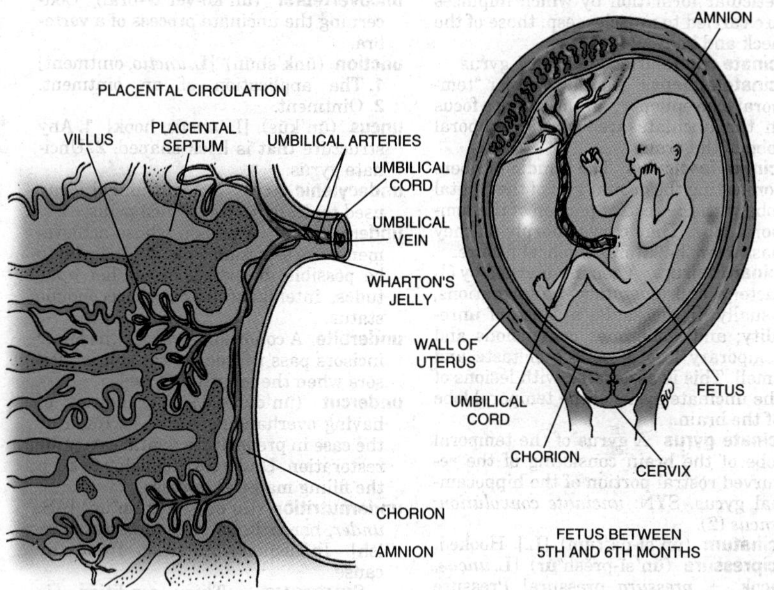

UMBILICAL CORD

umbilical vesicle That part of the embryonic yolk sac leading from the umbilicus.

umbilicate (ŭm-bĭl′ĭ-kāt) [L. *umbilicatus,* dimpled] Dimpled, pitted, or shaped like a navel. Said of the appearance of certain rashes, such as molluscum contagiosum. **umbilicated,** *adj.*

umbilication (ŭm-bĭl-ĭ-kā′shŭn) [L. *umbilicatus,* dimpled] **1.** A depression resembling a navel. **2.** Formation at the apex of a pustule or vesicle of a pit or depression.

umbilicus (ŭm-bĭ-lī′kŭs, -bĭl′ĭ-kŭs) *pl.* **umbilici** [L., a pit] A depressed point in the middle of the abdomen; the scar that marks the former attachment of the umbilical cord to the fetus. SEE: *Cullen's sign; nodule, Sister Mary Joseph; Tanyoz's sign.*

umbo (ŭm′bō) [L., boss of a shield] The projecting center of a round surface.

u. of tympanic membrane The central depressed portion of the concavity on the lateral surface of the tympanic membrane. It marks the point where the malleus is attached to the inner surface.

umbra (ŭm′bră) [L., shade, shadow] The edge of the radiographic image proper.

umbrella filter A filter placed in a blood vessel to prevent emboli from passing that point. It has been used in the vena cava to prevent emboli in the veins from reaching the lungs, but has not been proven to be clearly effective.

UMP *uridine monophosphate.*

un- [AS.] Prefix meaning *back, reversal, annulment, not.*

uncal (ŭng′kăl) Concerning the uncus of the brain.

uncal herniation Transtentorial herniation.

Uncaria tomentosa (ŭn-kă′rē-ă tō-mĕn-tō′să) A medicinal plant, known popularly as cat's claw or *uña de gato,* whose extracts include alkaloids that have effects on thinking, concentration, and sedation.

unciform, unciforme (ŭn′sĭ-form) [L. *uncus,* hook, + *forma,* shape] Uncinate.

unciform bone The hamate bone, the hook-shaped bone on the ulnar side of the distal row of the carpus. SYN: *os hamatum.*

unciform fasciculus Uncinate fasciculus.

unciform process **1.** Long thin lamina of bone from the orbital plate of the ethmoid articulating with the inferior turbinate. **2.** The hook at the anterior end of the hippocampal gyrus. **3.** The hooked end of the unciform bone.

uncinariasis (ŭn″sĭn-ă-rī′ă-sĭs) The condition of being infested with hookworms (i.e., worms of the genus *Uncinaria*).

uncinate (ŭn′sĭn-āt) [L. *uncinatus,* hooked] Hook-shaped; hooked. SYN: *unciform.*

uncinate bundle of Russell [James S. Risien Russell, Brit. physician, 1863–1939] Fibers that arise in the fastigial superior cerebellar peduncle and pass inferiorly to the vestibular nuclei and reticular formation by which impulses are carried to muscles, esp. those of the neck and body.

uncinate convolution Uncinate gyrus.

uncinate epilepsy An old term for "temporal lobe epilepsy," arising from a focus in the uncinate area of the temporal lobe of the brain.

uncinate fasciculus The bundle of fibers connecting the orbital gyri of the frontal lobe with the rostral portion of the temporal lobe. They curve sharply as they pass over the lateral cerebral fissure.

uncinate seizure A seizure marked by olfactory and gustatory hallucinations, usually disagreeable; a sense of unreality; and sometimes convulsions and temporary loss of senses of taste and smell. This is associated with lesions of the uncinate gyrus of the temporal lobe of the brain.

uncinate gyrus A gyrus of the temporal lobe of the brain consisting of the recurved rostral portion of the hippocampal gyrus. SYN: *uncinate convolution; uncus* (2).

uncinatum (ŭn″sĭ-nā′tŭm) [L.] Hooked.

uncipressure (ŭn′sĭ-prĕsh″ŭr) [L. *uncus,* hook, + *pressura,* pressure] Pressure applied with the use of a blunt hook to arrest bleeding.

uncomplemented (ŭn-kŏm′plē-mĕnt″ĕd) Not joined or associated with complement and thus inactive.

unconscious (ŭn-kŏn′shŭs) [AS. *un,* not, + L. *conscius,* aware] **1.** Insensible; lacking in awareness of the environment. SEE: *unconsciousness.* **2.** In Freudian psychiatry, that part of our personality consisting of a complex of feelings and drives of which we are unaware and that are not available to our consciousness.

collective u. One of two divisions of the unconscious, according to the unproven hypotheses of Carl Jung, the other category being personal unconscious. The personal unconscious includes all of the material stored in the unconscious that was acquired through personal experience. The collective unconscious comprises material that the species inherits. Thus, the collective unconscious would be common to all members of a society, a people, or to humankind in general. Instinct is included in the collective unconscious. SEE: *sociobiology.*

unconsciousness (ŭn-kŏn′shŭs-nĕs) [AS. *un,* not, + L. *conscius,* aware] The state of being partly or completely unaware of external stimuli. Unconsciousness occurs normally in sleep, and pathologically, in such conditions as syncope (fainting), shock, unperfused cardiac dysrhythmias, and intoxications. SEE: *coma; Glasgow Coma Scale; Nursing Diagnoses Appendix.*

unco-ossified (ŭn″kō-ŏs′ĭ-fīd) Not ossified into one bone.

uncovertebral (ŭn″kō-vĕr′tĕ-brăl) Concerning the uncinate process of a vertebra.

unction (ŭnk′shŭn) [L. *unctio,* ointment] **1.** The application of an ointment. **2.** Ointment.

uncus (ŭn′kŭs) [L. *uncus,* hook] **1.** Any structure that is hook-shaped. **2.** Uncinate gyrus.

undecylenic acid An antifungal drug used topically to treat tinea pedis.

underachiever A person whose achievements are less than what is predicted to be possible, based on his or her aptitudes, intelligence, and socioeconomic status.

underbite A condition in which the lower incisors pass in front of the upper incisors when the mouth is closed.

undercut (ŭn′dĕr-kŭt) A condition of having overhanging tissue as could be the case in preparing a dental cavity for restoration. Undercutting helps to keep the filling material in place.

undernutrition (ŭn″dĕr-nū-trĭsh′ŭn) [AS. *under,* beneath, + LL. *nutritio,* nourish] Inadequate nutrition from any cause.

SYMPTOMS: This condition is marked by loss of body weight that begins with loss of glycogen, loss of body fat, and then proceeds to loss of protein. Vitamin, mineral, and micronutrient deficiencies are also usually present. SEE: *malnutrition.*

The term undernutrition is also used to indicate reduced caloric consumption while maintaining adequate intake of all micronutrients.

undertoe (ŭn′dĕr-tō) [″ + *ta,* toe] The displacement of the great toe underneath the others.

underweight (ŭn′dĕr-wāt″) Body weight for height that is 15-20% below healthy weight; a body mass index below 19. By this standard, which is the one promoted both by the World Health Organization and the National Heart, Lung, and Blood Institute, a person who stands 5'7" tall is underweight if he or she weighs less than 120 lb.

undifferentiation (ŭn-dĭf″ĕr-ĕn-shē-ā′shŭn) [AS. *un,* not, + L. *differens,* bearing apart] An alteration in cell character to a more embryonic type or toward a malignant state. SYN: *anaplasia.*

undinism (ŭn′dĭn-ĭzm) An awakening of the libido by running water, as by urination or at the sight of urine. SEE: *urolagnia.*

undulant (ŭn′dū-lănt) [L. *undulatio,* wavy] Rising and falling like waves, or moving like them.

undulant fever (ŭn′dū-lănt) Brucellosis.

undulate (ŭn′dū-lāt) [L. *undulatio,* wavy] Wavy; having a wavy border with shallow sinuses, said of bacterial colonies.

undulation (ŭn-dū-lā′shŭn) A continuous wavelike motion or pulsation.

ung [L.] *unguentum,* ointment.

ungual (ŭng′gwăl) [L. *unguis,* nail] Pert. to or resembling the nails.

ungual phalanx The terminal phalanx of each finger and toe.

ungual tuberosity The spatula-shaped extremity of the terminal phalanx that supports the nails of fingers and toes.

unguent, unguentum (ŭng′gwĕnt) [L. *unguentum,* ointment] Ointment.

unguis (ŭng′gwĭs) *pl.* **ungues** [L., nail] **1.** A fingernail or toenail. SYN: *onyx.* **2.** The lacrimal bone. **3.** A white prominence on the floor of the posterior horn of the lateral ventricle. SYN: *hippocampus minor.*

u. incarnatus An ingrowing nail, esp. a toenail.

uni- Combining form meaning *one.* SEE: *mono-.*

uniarticular (ū″nē-ăr-tĭk′ū-lăr) [L. *unus,* one, + *articulus,* joint] Pert. to a single joint.

uniaxial (ū″nē-ăk′sē-ăl) [″ + *axis,* axis] Having a single axis.

unibasal (ū″nē-bā′săl) [″ + *basis,* base] Having a single base.

unicameral (ū″nĭ-kăm′ĕr-ăl) [″ + *camera,* vault] Having a single cavity.

unicellular (ū″nĭ-sĕl′ū-lăr) [″ + *cellula,* a little box] Having only one cell.

unicentral (ū″nĭ-sĕn′trăl) [″ + *centrum,* center] Having a single center.

uniceps (ū′nĭ-sĕps) [″ + *caput,* head] Having a single head or origin, as in muscles.

unicorn, unicornous (ū′nĭ-korn, ū-nĭ-kor′nŭs) [″ + *cornu,* horn] Having a single cornu or horn. Women with a unicornous uterus are at higher risk for repeated pregnancy loss.

unicuspid (ū″nĭ-kŭs′pĭd) Having a single cusp.

uniform Having the identical shape or form of other objects of the same class.

unigerminal (ū″nĭ-jĕr′mĭ-năl) Concerning a single ovum or germ.

uniglandular (ū″nĭ-glăn′dū-lăr) Concerning one gland.

unigravida (ū″nĭ-grăv′ĭ-dă) [″ + *gravida,* pregnant] A woman who is pregnant for the first time. SEE: *primigravida.*

unilaminar (ū″nĭ-lăm′ĭ-năr) Having a single layer.

unilateral (ū″nĭ-lăt′ĕr-ăl) [″ + *latus,* side] Affecting or occurring on only one side. SEE: *contralateral; homolateral; ipsilateral.*

unilateral neglect The state in which an individual is perceptually unaware of and inattentive to one side of the body and the immediate unilateral area that the patient visualizes. SEE: *Nursing Diagnoses Appendix.*

unilobar (ū″nĭ-lō′băr) Having a single lobe.

unilocular (ū″nĭ-lŏk′ū-lăr) [″ + *loculus,* a small space] Having only one cavity.

uninuclear (ū″nĭ-nū′klē-ăr) [″ + *nucleus,* a kernel] Having only one nucleus.

uninucleated (ū″nĭ-nū′klē-āt″ĕd) Having a single nucleus.

uniocular (ū″nē-ŏk′ū-lăr) [″ + *oculus,* eye] Pert. to or having only one eye.

union (ūn′yŭn) [L. *unio*] **1.** The act of joining two or more things into one part, or the state of being so united. **2.** Growing together of severed or broken parts, as of bones or the edges of a wound. SEE: *healing.*

secondary u. **1.** A healing by second intention with adhesion of granulating surfaces. SEE: *healing.* **2.** Operative correction of nonunion of a fracture.

vicious u. The union of the ends of a broken bone formed in such a way as to cause deformity.

unioval (ū″nē-ō′văl) [L. *unus,* one, + *ovum,* egg] Developed from one ovum, as identical twins.

uniovular (ū″nē-ŏv′ū-lăr) [″ + *ovum,* egg] Monozygotic, as in the case of twins that develop from a single ovum.

unipara (ū-nĭp′ă-ră) [″ + *parere,* to bring forth, to bear] A woman who has had one pregnancy of more than 20 weeks' duration or has produced a fetus weighing at least 500 g, regardless of the fetus's viability. SEE: *primipara.*

uniparous (ū-nĭp′ă-rŭs) [″ + *parere,* to bring forth, to bear] **1.** Giving birth to one offspring at a time. **2.** Having produced one child weighing at least 500 g or having a pregnancy lasting 20 weeks, regardless of the fetus's viability.

unipolar (ū″nĭ-pō′lăr) [″ + *polus,* pole] **1.** Having or pert. to one pole. **2.** Having a single process, as a unipolar neuron.

unipotent, unipotential (ū-nĭp′ō-tĕnt, ū″nĭ-pō-tĕn′shăl) In cell biology, committed to a single, differentiated structure and a single mode of functioning.

uniseptate (ū″nē-sĕp′tāt) Having only one septum.

unisex **1.** Lack of gender distinction by external appearance, esp. with respect to hairstyle or clothing. **2.** Suitable for use by either sex.

unit (ū′nĭt) [L. *unus,* one] ABBR: u. **1.** One of anything. **2.** A determined amount adopted as a standard of measurement.

amboceptor u. The smallest amount of amboceptor required in the presence of which a given quantity of red blood cells will be hemolyzed by an excess of complement.

angström u. ABBR: Å; A.U. An internationally adopted unit of measurement of wavelength, 1/10,000,000 mm, or 1/254,000,000 in.

antigen u. The smallest quantity of antigen required to fix one unit of complement.

antitoxin u. A unit for expressing the strength of an antitoxin. Originally, the various units were defined biologically but now are compared with a weighed standard specified by the U.S. Public Health Service and the World Health Organization.

atomic mass u. ABBR: AMU. One-twelfth of the mass of a neutral carbon atom; equal to 1.657 $\times$ 10^{-24} g.

British thermal u. ABBR: BTU. The amount of heat necessary to raise the temperature of 1 lb of water from 39°F to 40°F.

u. of capacity The capacity of a condenser that gives a difference of potential of 1 volt when charged with 1 coulomb. SYN: *curie; farad.*

cat u. The amount of drug per kilogram of body weight just sufficient to kill a cat when injected intravenously slowly and continuously.

complement u. The smallest quantity of complement required for hemolysis of a given amount of red blood cells with one amboceptor (hemolysin) unit present.

controlled cold therapy u. ABBR: CCT. A cooling jacket that simultaneously delivers cold therapy and static compression to an extremity, joint, or other body part. Water is chilled in an external container to a temperature of 45° to 55°F (7.2° to 12°C) and is then circulated through a circumferentially applied compression device. More effective than standard cold packs, CCT units are used immediately after surgery or joint injury to control swelling and reduce pain.

CAUTION: This device should not be used with patients who have known contraindications to cold application or external compression (e.g., peripheral vascular disease, Raynaud's phenomenon, advanced diabetes, or neurological insufficiency).

dental u. **1.** A masticatory unit consisting of a single tooth and its adjacent tissues. **2.** A mobile or fixed piece of equipment, usually complete with chair, light, engine, and other accessories or utilities necessary for dental examinations or operations.

electrostatic u. ABBR: ESU or ESE (from the German *elektrostatische Einheit*). Any electrical unit of measure based on the attraction or repulsion of a static charge, as distinguished from an electromagnetic unit, which is defined in terms of the attraction or repulsion of magnetic poles.

geriatric evaluation u. Geriatric evaluation and management unit.

geriatric evaluation and management u. ABBR: GEM. An in-patient unit or program devoted to the evaluation and management of the complex needs of the elderly patient. SYN: *geriatric evaluation u.*

hemolytic u. The amount of inactivated immune serum that causes complete hemolysis of 1 ml of a 5% emulsion of washed red blood cells in the presence of complement.

international u. ABBR: I.U. An internationally accepted amount of a substance. Usually this form of expressing quantity is used for fat-soluble vitamins and some hormones, enzymes, and biologicals such as vaccines. These units are defined by the International Conference for Unification of Formulae.

light u. A foot-candle, or the amount of light 1 ft from a standard candle. The ideal amount of light required for work varies with the specific type of work being done. The term *foot-candle* took the place of *candle power,* but light intensity in the International System of Units is indicated by lumen. SEE: *candela; lumen.*

Mache u. ABBR: M.u. A unit of measurement of radium emanation.

motor u. A somatic motor neuron and all the muscle cells it innervates.

mouse u. SEE: *Allen-Doisy unit.*

rat u. The greatest dilution of estrogen that will cause desquamation and cornification of the vaginal epithelium if given to a mature spayed rat in three injections, one every 4 hr. This must occur in the first day of treatment.

short-stay u. A hospital ward where patients are kept for observation or monitoring for several hours (e.g., after minor surgery or as part of a diagnostic study).

SI u. Any of the units specified by the International System of Units adopted by an International Conference of Weights and Measures in 1960 and updated since then. SEE: *SI units* for tables; *SI Units Appendix.*

terminal duct lobular u. ABBR: TDLU. The blind ending of the lactiferous duct that contains the lobule and its duct. Most benign and malignant breast lesions arise here.

Todd u. In a test of inhibition hemolysis by enzymes such as antistreptolysin O, the reciprocal of the highest dilution that inhibits hemolysis.

USP u. Any unit specified in the U.S. Pharmacopeia.

unitarian (ū-nĭ-tār′ē-ăn) [L. *unitarius*] Composed of a single unit.

unitary (ū′nĭ-tĕr-ē) Rel. to a single unit.

unit dose A dose form in which doses of medicine are prepared in individual packets. This saves time in dispensing medicines, esp. to hospitalized patients.

United Network for Organ Sharing ABBR: UNOS. An organization established in 1984 to facilitate donation of organs for possible transplantation.

Website: www.unos.org. SEE: *organ donation.*

United States Adopted Names ABBR: USAN. Dictionary of nonproprietary names, brand names, code designations, and Chemical Abstracts Service registry numbers for drugs published by the U.S. Pharmacopeial Convention, Inc. The purpose is to have nonproprietary names assigned to new drugs in accordance with established principles. SEE: *USAN and the USP Dictionary of Drug Names.*

United States Pharmacopeia A pharmacopeia issued every 5 years, but with periodic supplements, prepared under the supervision of a national committee of pharmacists, pharmacologists, physicians, chemists, biologists, and other scientific and allied personnel. The U.S. Pharmacopeia was adopted as standard in 1906. Beginning with the U.S. Pharmacopeia XIX, 1975, the National Formulary has been included in that publication.

United States Public Health Service ABBR: USPHS. An agency of the U.S. Department of Health and Human Services (HHS). Its function is to assess health care needs and promote national and international health. Included in the organization are the Centers for Disease Control and Prevention (CDC); Food and Drug Administration (FDA); Alcohol, Drug Abuse and Mental Health Administration; Agency for Toxic Substances and Disease Registry; and various USPHS regional offices.

uniterminal (ū″nĭ-tĕr′mĭn-ăl) [L. *unus,* one, + *terminus,* end] Having only one terminal.

univalence (ū″nĭ-vā′lĕns) The condition of having only one valence.

univalent (ū″nĭ-vā′lĕnt, ū-nĭv′ă-lĕnt) [″ + *valens,* to be powerful] Possessing the power of combining or replacing one atom of hydrogen. SYN: *monovalent.*

universal (ū″nĭ-vĕr′săl) [L. *universalis,* combined into one whole] General or applicable or common to all situations or conditions.

universal antidote An antidote that was once used in poisoning where the specific antidote was unknown or not available; consisting of two parts activated charcoal, one part tannic acid, and one part magnesium oxide.

CAUTION: The idea that there is a "universal antidote" for poisonings is flawed.

---

universal cuff A device fitted around the palm of the hand to permit attachment of self-care tools when normal grasp is absent. SYN: *palmar cuff.*

universal precautions Guidelines designed to protect workers with occupational exposure to bloodborne pathogens (such as HIV and hepatitis B virus). These "universal blood and body fluid precautions" (e.g., gloves, masks, and gowns), originally recommended by the Centers for Disease Control and Prevention in 1985, were mandated by the OSHA Bloodborne Pathogens Standard in 1991 for workers in all U.S. health care settings. SEE: *Standard and Universal Precautions Appendix.*

universal recipient A person belonging to blood type AB, Rh positive, whose serum will not agglutinate the cells of the other ABO blood types. Nevertheless, the recipient's blood must be tested by cross-matching before the transfusion.

unlicensed assistive personnel Persons who assist the licensed nurse in providing care to patients (formerly called nurse's aides or nursing attendants).

unmedullated (ŭn-mĕd′ū-lāt″ĕd) Unmyelinated.

unmyelinated (ŭn-mī′ĕ-lĭ-nāt″ĕd) Lacking a myelin sheath; used of neurons. SYN: *unmedullated.*

Unna's paste (oo′năz) [Paul G. Unna, Ger. dermatologist, 1850–1929] A mixture of 15% zinc oxide in a glycogelatin base.

Unna's (paste) boot A bootlike dressing of the lower extremity made of layers of gauze and Unna's paste. It is used in treating chronic ulcers of the leg.

UNOS *United Network for Organ Sharing.*

unsaturated (ŭn-săt′ū-rāt″ĕd) [AS. *un,* not, + L. *saturare,* to fill] **1.** Capable of dissolving or absorbing to a greater degree. **2.** Not combined to the greatest possible extent.

unsaturated compound An organic compound having double or triple bonds between the carbon atoms.

unsex (ŭn-sĕks′) [″ + L. *sexus,* sex] **1.** To castrate; to spay or excise the ovaries or testes. **2.** To deprive of sexual character.

unstriated (ŭn-strī′āt-ĕd) [″ + *striatus,* striped] Unstriped, as smooth muscle fiber.

Unverricht's disease, Unverricht's syndrome (oon′fĕr-ĭkts) [Heinrich Unverricht, Ger. physician, 1853–1912] A rare, fatal disease inherited as an autosomal recessive trait. It is characterized by the onset in later childhood of progressive myoclonic epilepsy, tetraplegia, and dementia. Also called *Unverricht-Lafora disease.*

upper airway obstruction ABBR: UAO. Any potentially life-threatening abnormality in which the flow of air into and out of the lungs is partially or completely blocked by such conditions as laryngeal swelling, foreign bodies, or angioedema. SEE: *cardiopulmonary resuscitation; tracheostomy.*

upper GI *upper gastrointestinal.*

upper motor neuron lesion Neurological

damage to the corticospinal or pyramidal tract in the brain or spinal cord. This lesion results in hemiplegia, paraplegia, or quadriplegia, depending on its location and extent. Clinical signs include loss of voluntary movement, spasticity, sensory loss, and pathological reflexes.

upper respiratory infection ABBR: URI. An imprecise term for almost any kind of infectious disease process involving the nasal passages, pharynx, and bronchi. The etiological agent may be bacterial or viral.

upsiloid (ŭp′sĭ-loyd) [Gr. *upsilon,* letter U, + *eidos,* form, shape] Shaped like the letter U or V.

uptake (ŭp′tāk) The absorption of nutrients, chemicals (including radioactive materials), and medicines by tissues or by an entire organism.

urachal (ū′ră-kăl) [Gr. *ourachos,* fetal urinary canal] Rel. to the urachus.

urachus (ū′ră-kŭs) [Gr. *ourachos,* fetal urinary canal] An epithelioid cord surrounded by fibrous tissue extending from the apex of the bladder to the umbilicus. In the embryo, it is continuous with the allantoic stalk; postnatally it forms the middle umbilical ligament of the bladder.

patent u. A condition in which the urachus remains as a hollow tube that connects the vertex of the bladder with the umbilicus, resulting in an umbilical urinary fistula.

uracil (ū′ră-sĭl) $C_4H_4N_2O_2$; a pyrimidine base found in RNA (not DNA) which, if paired, pairs with adenine.

uracil mustard Nitrogen mustard.

uranisconitis (ū-răn-ĭs″kōn-ī′tĭs) [Gr. *ouraniskos,* palate, + *itis,* inflammation] Inflammation of the palate.

uraniscoplasty (ū-răn-ĭs′kō-plăs″tē) [″ + *plassein,* to form] Operation for repair of a cleft palate.

uraniscorrhaphy (ū″răn-ĭs-kor′ră-fē) [″ + *rhaphe,* seam, ridge] Operation for suturing of a cleft palate. SYN: *uraniscoplasty.*

uraniscus (ū-răn-ĭs′kŭs) [Gr. *ouraniskos,* palate] The palate, or the roof of the mouth.

uranium (ū-rā′nē-ŭm) [LL., planet Uranus] SYMB: U. A radioactive element, the parent of radium and other radioelements; atomic weight, 238.029; atomic number, 92. Uranium ore contains the isotopes ^{238}U, ^{235}U, and ^{234}U.

uranoplegia (ū″ră-nō-plē′jē-ă) [″ + *plege,* stroke] Paralysis of muscles of the soft palate.

uranoschisis (ū-răn-ŏs′kĭs-ĭs) [″ + *schisis,* a splitting] Cleft palate.

uranostaphyloschisis (ū″ră-nō-stăf″ĭ-lŏs′kĭ-sĭs) Cleft of the hard and soft palates.

uranyl (ū′ră-nĭl) The bivalent uranium radical UO^{2+}. It forms salts with many acids. An example is uranyl nitrate, $UO_2(NO_3)_2$.

urapostema (ū″ră-pŏs-tē′mă) [Gr. *ouron,* urine, + *apostema,* abscess] An abscess containing urine.

uraroma (ū-ră-rō′mă) [″ + *aroma,* spice] Aromatic spicy odor of freshly voided urine.

urase (ū′rās) Urease.

urate (ū′rāt) [Gr. *ouron,* urine] The combination of uric acid with a base; a salt of uric acid.

uratemia (ū″ră-tē′mē-ă) [″ + *haima,* blood] Excessive amounts of urates, esp. sodium urate, in the blood.

uratosis (ū″ră-tō′sĭs) Any condition leading to deposition of urates in tissues.

uraturia (ū″ră-tū′rē-ă) [Gr. *ouron,* urine] Excess of urates in the urine. Uraturia is seen in some individuals with gout or renal failure. SYN: *lithuria.*

urceiform (ŭr-sē′ĭ-form) [L. *urceus,* pitcher, + *forma,* shape] Pitcher-shaped.

ur-defense(s) (ŭr″dē-fĕns′) [Ger. *ur,* ultimate, + *defense*] Basic beliefs, such as religious or scientific ones, that are thought by the individual to be essential to people's emotional well-being. These beliefs may include faith in a personal or universal God or the fundamental goodness of humankind.

urea (ū-rē′ă) [Gr. *ouron,* urine] The diamide of carbonic acid, a crystalline solid having the formula CH_4N_2O; found in blood, lymph, and urine.

It is formed in the liver from ammonia derived from the deamination of amino acids.

Urea is the chief nitrogenous constituent of urine and, along with carbon dioxide, the final product of protein metabolism in the body. In normal conditions, urea represents 80% to 90% of the total urinary nitrogen. It is odorless and colorless, appears as white prismatic crystals, and forms salts with acids. The amount of urea excreted varies directly with the amount of protein in the diet. Its excretion is increased in fever, diabetes, or increased activity of the adrenal gland, and decreased in kidney failure.

urea cycle The complex cyclic chemical reactions in some (ureotelic) animals, including humans, that produce urea from the metabolism of nitrogen-containing foods. This cycle provides a method of excreting the nitrogen produced by the metabolism of amino acids as urea. The cycle was first described by Sir Hans Krebs [1900–1981].

urea frost White flaky deposits of urea seen on the skin in patients with advanced uremia.

ureagenetic (ū-rē″ă-jĕn-ĕt′ĭk) [″ + *genesis,* generation, birth] Pert. to or producing urea.

ureametry (ū-rē-ăm′ĕt-rē) Determination of the amount of urea in urine.

urea nitrogen The nitrogen of urea (as

distinguished from nitrogen in blood proteins).

Ureaplasma urealyticum A microorganism that is usually sexually transmitted. It may cause inflammation of the urogenital tract in males and females. It has been implicated in a wide variety of infections in babies with low birth weight.

urease (ū′rē-ās) [Gr. *ouron,* urine] **1.** An enzyme that accelerates the hydrolysis of urea into carbon dioxide and ammonia. It is used in determining the amount of urea in blood or in urine. **2.** An enzyme used by certain microorganisms to facilitate their existence in otherwise inhospitable body locations.

urelcosis (ū-rĕl-kō′sĭs) [″ + *helkosis,* ulceration] Ulceration of the urinary tract.

uremia (ū-rē′mē-ă) [″ + *haima,* blood] In patients with renal failure, the intoxication caused by the body's accumulation of metabolic byproducts that are normally excreted by healthy kidneys. SEE: *azotemia; coma, uremic.* **uremic,** *adj.*

SYMPTOMS: Symptoms include nausea, vomiting, anorexia, headache, dizziness, coma, or convulsions.

ETIOLOGY: Although nitrogen-containing waste products have long been considered the principal cause of uremia, other metabolic waste products, such as glycosylated wastes and byproducts of abnormal oxidation, may actually be the most important toxins responsible for uremia.

TREATMENT: Dialysis removes many soluble waste products that accumulate in renal failure and helps to improve some conditions associated with uremia. Other uremic conditions can be partly alleviated with a protein-restricted diet, careful management of acid-base balance, and calcium and folate supplementation.

extrarenal u. Prerenal u.

prerenal u. Uremia resulting not from primary renal disease but from other conditions such as disturbances in circulation, fluid balance, or metabolism arising in other parts of the body. SYN: *extrarenal u.*

uremigenic (ū-rē″mĭ-jĕn′ĭk) [Gr. *ouron,* urine, + *haima,* blood, + *gennan,* to produce] Caused by or producing uremia.

ureogenesis (ūr″ē-ō-jĕn′ĕ-sĭs) [″ + *genesis,* generation, birth] Formation of urea.

ureotelic (ū″rē-ō-tĕl′ĭk) [*urea* + Gr. *telikos,* belonging to the completion] Concerning animals that excrete amino nitrogen in the form of urea. Included in this group are mammals. SEE: *urea cycle; uricotelic.*

uresis (ū-rē′sĭs) [Gr. *ouresis*] Urination.

ureter (ū′rĕ-ter, ū-rē′tĕr) [Gr. *oureter*] The tube that carries urine from the kidney to the bladder. It originates in the pelvis of the kidney and terminates in the posterior base of the bladder. Each kidney has one ureter measuring from 28 to 34 cm long, the right being slightly shorter than the left. The diameter varies from 1 mm to 1 cm. The wall consists of three layers: the mucosal, muscular, and fibrous layers. SEE: *kidney; urethra.*

ureteral (ū-rē′tĕr-ăl) Concerning the ureter. SYN: *ureteric.*

ureteralgia (ū″rē-tĕr-ăl′jē-ă) [″ + *algos,* pain] Pain in the ureter.

uretercystoscope (ū-rē″tĕr-sĭs′tō-skōp) [″ + *kystis,* bladder, + *skopein,* to examine] A cystoscope combined with a ureteral catheter. SYN: *ureterocystoscope.*

ureterectasis (ū-rē″tĕr-ĕk′tă-sĭs) [″ + *ektasis,* dilatation] Dilatation of the ureter.

ureterectomy (ū-rē″tĕr-ĕk′tō-mē) [″ + *ektome,* excision] Excision of a ureter.

ureteric (ū″rĕ-tĕr′ĭk) Ureteral.

ureteritis (ū-rē″tĕr-ī′tĭs) [″ + *itis,* inflammation] Inflammation of the ureters.

uretero- Combining form indicating *ureter.*

ureterocele (ū-rē′tĕr-ō-sēl) [″ + *kele,* tumor, swelling] Cystlike dilatation of the ureter near its opening into the bladder; usually a result of congenital stenosis of the ureteral orifice.

ureterocelectomy (ū-rē″tĕr-ō-sē-lĕk′tō-mē) [″ + ″ + *ektome,* excision] Surgical removal of a ureterocele.

ureterocervical (ū-rē″tĕr-ō-sĕr′vĭ-kăl) [″ + L. *cervicalis,* pert. to cervix] Concerning the ureter and the cervix uteri.

ureterocolostomy (ū-rē″tĕr-ō-kō-lŏs′tō-mē) [″ + *kolon,* colon, + *stoma,* mouth] The implantation of the ureter into the colon.

ureterocystoscope (ū-rē″tĕr-ō-sĭs′tō-skōp) [″ + ″ + *skopein,* to view] Uretercystoscope.

ureteroenterostomy (ū-rē″tĕr-ō-ĕn-tĕr-ŏs′tō-mē) [″ + *enteron,* intestine, + *stoma,* mouth] Formation of a passage between a ureter and the intestine.

ureterography (ū-rē″tĕr-ŏg′ră-fē) [″ + *graphein,* to write] Radiography of the ureter after injection of a radiopaque substance into it.

ureteroheminephrectomy (ū-rē″tĕr-ō-hĕm″ĭ-nĕ-frĕk′tō-mē) [″ + *hemi-,* half, + *nephros,* kidney, + *ektome,* excision] In cases of reduplication of the upper urinary tract on one side, surgical removal of the reduplicated portion.

ureterohydronephrosis (ū-rē″tĕr-ō-hī″drō-nĕ-frō′sĭs) [″ + *hydor,* water, + *nephros,* kidney, + *osis,* condition] Dilatation of the ureter and the pelvis of the kidney resulting from a mechanical or inflammatory obstruction in the urinary tract.

ureteroileostomy (ū-rē″tĕr-ō-ĭl″ē-ŏs′tō-mē) [″ + *ileum,* ileum, + *stoma,* mouth] Surgical anastomosis of a ureter to an isolated segment of the ileum. The ileum is connected to an abdominal stoma so that urine leaves the body via that opening.

ureterolith (ū-rē′tĕr-ō-lĭth) [″ + *lithos,* stone] A stone or calculus in the ureter.

ureterolithiasis (ū-rē″tĕr-ō-lĭth-ī′ăs-ĭs) [″ + ″ + *iasis,* condition] Development of a stone in the ureter.

ureterolithotomy (ū-rē″tĕr-ō-lĭth-ŏt′ō-mē) [″ + ″ + *tome,* incision] Surgical incision for removal of a stone from the ureter.

ureterolysis (ū-rē″tĕr-ŏl′ĭ-sĭs) [″ + *lysis,* dissolution] **1.** Rupture of a ureter. **2.** Paralysis of the ureter. **3.** The process of loosening adhesions around the ureter.

ureteroneocystostomy (ū-rē″tĕr-ō-nē″ō-sĭs-tŏs′tō-mē) [″ + *neos,* new, + *kystis,* bladder, + *stoma,* mouth] Surgical formation of a new passage between a ureter and the bladder.

ureteroneopyelostomy (ū-rē″tĕr-ō-nē″ō-pī-ĕ-lŏs′tō-mē) [″ + ″ + *pyelos,* pelvis, + *stoma,* mouth] Excision of a portion of the ureter with attachment of the severed end of the lower portion to a new aperture in the renal pelvis. SYN: *ureteropyelostomy.*

ureteronephrectomy (ū-rē″tĕr-ō-nĕf-rĕk′tō-mē) [″ + *nephros,* kidney, + *ektome,* excision] Removal of a kidney and its ureter.

ureteropelvioplasty (ū-rē″tĕr-ō-pĕl′vē-ō-plăs″tē) [Gr. *oureter,* ureter, + L. *pelvis,* basin, + Gr. *plassein,* to mold] Plastic surgery of the junction of the ureter and the pelvis of the kidney.

ureteroplasty (ū-rē′tĕr-ō-plăs″tē) [″ + *plassein,* to form] Plastic surgery of the ureter.

ureteroproctostomy (ū-rē″tĕr-ō-prŏk-tŏs′tō-mē) [″ + *proktos,* anus, + *stoma,* mouth] The formation of a passage from the ureter to the lower rectum.

ureteropyelitis (ū-rē″tĕr-ō-pī-ĕl-ī′tĭs) [″ + *pyelos,* pelvis, + *itis,* inflammation] Inflammation of the pelvis of the kidney and a ureter.

ureteropyelonephritis (ū-rē″tĕr-ō-pī″ĕl-ō-nĕf-rī′tĭs) [″ + ″ + *nephros,* kidney, + *itis,* inflammation] Inflammation of the renal pelvis and the ureter.

ureteropyeloplasty (ū-rē″tĕr-ō-pī′ĕl-ō-plăs″tē) [″ + ″ + *plassein,* to mold] Plastic surgery of the ureter and renal pelvis.

ureteropyelostomy (ū-rē″tĕr-ō-pī″ĕ-lŏs′tō-mē) [″ + ″ + *stoma,* mouth] Ureteroneopyelostomy.

ureteropyosis (ū-rē″tĕr-ō-pī-ō′sĭs) [″ + *pyon,* pus, + *osis,* condition] Suppurative inflammation within a ureter.

ureterorrhagia (ū-rē″tĕr-or-rā′jē-ă) [″ + *rhegnynai,* to burst forth] Hemorrhage from the ureter.

ureterorrhaphy (ū-rē″tĕr-or′ră-fē) [″ + *rhaphe,* seam, ridge] Suture of the ureter, as for fistula.

ureterosigmoidostomy (ū-rē″tĕr-ō-sĭg-moyd-ŏs′tō-mē) [″ + *sigma,* letter S, + *eidos,* shape, + *stoma,* mouth] Surgical implantation of the ureter into the sigmoid colon.

ureterostegnosis (ū-rē″tĕr-ō-stĕg-nō′sĭs) Stricture of a ureter.

ureterostoma (ū″rē-tĕr-ŏs′tō-mă) [Gr. *oureter,* ureter, + *stoma,* mouth] The orifice through which the ureter enters the urinary bladder.

ureterostomy (ū-rē″tĕr-ŏs′tō-mē) [″ + *stoma,* mouth] The formation of a permanent fistula for drainage of a ureter.

cutaneous u. Surgical implantation of the ureter into the skin. This allows urine to drain via the ureter to the outside of the body by going through the stoma.

ureterotomy (ū-rē″tĕr-ŏt′ō-mē) [″ + *tome,* incision] Incision or surgery of the ureter.

ureterotrigonoenterostomy (ū-rē″tĕr-ō-trī-gō″nō-ĕn″tĕr-ŏs′tō-mē) [″ + *trigonon,* three-sided figure, + *enteron,* intestine, + *stoma,* mouth] Surgical removal of the trigone of the bladder with one or both of the ureteral openings and implantation of it into the intestine.

ureteroureterostomy (ū-rē″tĕr-ō-ū-rē″tĕr-ŏs′tō-mē) [″ + ″ + *stoma,* mouth] **1.** The formation of a connection from one ureter to the other. **2.** The re-establishment of a passage between the ends of a divided ureter.

ureterouterine (ū-rē″tĕr-ō-ū′tĕr-ĭn) [″ + L. *uterus,* womb] Concerning the ureter and uterus or a fistula between them.

ureterovaginal (ū-rē″tĕr-ō-văj′ĭ-năl) [″ + L. *vagina,* sheath] Relating to a ureter and the vagina, denoting a fistula connecting them.

ureterovesicostomy (ū-rē″tĕr-ō-vĕs″ĭ-kŏs′tō-mē) [″ + ″ + Gr. *stoma,* mouth] Reimplantation of a ureter into the bladder.

urethra (ū-rē′thră) [Gr. *ourethra*] The tube for the discharge of urine extending from the bladder to the outside. In females, its orifice lies in the vestibule between the vagina and clitoris; in males, the urethra passes through the prostate gland and the penis, opening at the tip of the glans penis. In males, it serves as the passage for semen as well as urine. Its lining, the mucosa, is thrown into folds and contains the openings of the urethral glands. Surrounding the mucosa is a lamina propria containing many elastic fibers and blood vessels, outside of which is an indefinite muscular layer. SEE: *penis.*

u. muliebris The female urethra.

u. virilis The male urethra.

urethral (ū-rē′thrăl) [Gr. *ourethra,* urethra] Relating to the urethra.

urethralgia (ū-rē-thrăl′jē-ă) [″ + *algos,* pain] Pain in the urethra.

urethratresia (ū-rē″thră-trē′zē-ă) [″ + *a-,* not, + *tresis,* a perforation] Occlusion or imperforation of the urethra.

urethrectomy (ū-rē-thrĕk′tō-mē) [″ + *ektome,* excision] Surgical excision of the urethra or part of it.

urethreurynter (ū-rēth″rūr-ĭn′tĕr) [″ + *eurynein,* to dilate] An appliance for dilating the urethra.

urethrism, urethrismus (ū′rē-thrĭzm, ū″rē-thrĭz′mŭs) [″ + *-ismos,* condition] Irritability or spasm of the urethra.

urethritis (ū″rē-thrī′tĭs) [″ + *itis,* inflammation] Inflammation of the urethra.

anterior u. Inflammation of that portion of the urethra anterior to the anterior layer of the triangular ligament.

gonococcal u. Urethritis caused by *Neisseria gonorrhoeae.*

nongonococcal u. ABBR: NGU. A urethral inflammation caused by organisms other than *Neisseria gonorrhoeae.* NGU is the most common sexually transmitted disease in men. It accounts for 4 to 6 million physician visits annually. Clinically the symptoms usually develop within about 7 to 14 days but may range from 2 to 35 days. The symptoms usually include painful urination and a urethral discharge. Because of the similarity of NGU to gonococcal urethritis, the disease is diagnosed from bacteriological culture of the discharge. The two organisms most frequently associated with NGU are *Chlamydia trachomatis* and *Ureaplasma urealyticum.* Other causes include herpes simplex virus, *Trichomonas vaginalis, Haemophilus influenzae, Gardnerella vaginalis,* and *Clostridium difficile.*

TREATMENT: NGU due to *C. trachomatis* or *U. urealyticum* is treated with doxycycline or azithromycin. Appropriate antibiotics are used for other causative organisms.

nonspecific u. ABBR: NSU. Nongonococcal u.

posterior u. Inflammation of membranous and prostatic portions of the urethra.

specific u. Urethritis due to a specific organism, usually gonococcus.

urethro- [Gr. *ourethra*] Combining form meaning *urethra.*

urethrobulbar (ū-rē″thrō-bŭl′băr) Concerning the urethra and the bulbar penis.

urethrocele (ū-rē′thrō-sēl) [″ + *kele,* tumor, swelling] **1.** Pouchlike protrusion of the urethral wall in the female. **2.** Thickening of connective tissue around the urethra in the female.

urethrocystitis (ū-rē″thrō-sĭs-tī′tĭs) [″ + *kystis,* bladder, + *itis,* inflammation] Inflammation of the urethra and bladder.

urethrocystopexy (ū-rē″thrō-sĭs′tō-pĕk″sē) [″ + *kystis,* bladder, + *pexis,* fixation] Plastic surgery of the urethral-bladder junction to relieve urinary stress incontinence.

urethrograph (ū-rē′thrō-grăf) A device for recording the caliber of the urethra.

urethrography (ū-rē-thrŏg′ră-fē) [″ + *graphein,* to write] Radiography of the urethra after it has been filled with contrast medium.

voiding u. Radiographic examination of the urethra during urination after the introduction of a contrast medium.

urethrometer (ū-rē-thrŏm′ĕt-ĕr) [Gr. *ourethra,* urethra, + *metron,* measure] An instrument for measuring the diameter of the urethra or the lumen of a stricture.

urethropenile (ū-rē″thrō-pē′nīl) [″ + L. *penis,* penis] Relating to the urethra and penis.

urethroperineal (ū-rē″thrō-pĕr-ĭ-nē′ăl) [″ + *perinaion,* perineum] Rel. to the urethra and perineum.

urethroperineoscrotal (ū-rē″thrō-pĕr-ĭ-nē″ō-skrō′tăl) [″ + ″ + L. *scrotum,* a bag] Relating to the urethra, perineum, and scrotum.

urethropexy (ū-rē′thrō-pĕks-ē) [″ + Gr. *pexis,* fixation] Surgical fixation of the urethra.

urethrophraxis (ū-rē-thrō-frăks′ĭs) [″ + *phrassein,* to obstruct] Urethral obstruction.

urethroplasty (ū-rē′thrō-plăs″tē) [″ + *plassein,* to mold] Reparative surgery of the urethra.

urethroprostatic (ū-rē″thrō-prŏs-tăt′ĭk) Concerning the urethra and prostate.

urethrorectal (ū-rē″thrō-rĕk′tăl) [Gr. *ourethra,* urethra, + L. *rectus,* straight] Rel. to the urethra and rectum.

urethrorrhagia (ū-rē″thror-ā′jē-ă) [″ + *rhegnynai,* to burst forth] Hemorrhage from the urethra.

urethrorrhaphy (ū-rē-thror′ăf-ē) [″ + *rhaphe,* seam, ridge] Suture of the urethra or of a urethral fistula.

urethrorrhea (ū-rē″thror-ē′ă) [″ + *rhoia,* flow] An abnormal discharge from the urethra.

u. ex libidine The discharge of normal glandular secretions resulting from sexual stimulation, esp. that preceding sexual intercourse. SEE: *Cowper's glands.*

urethroscopy (ū-rē-thrŏs′kō-pē) An examination of the mucous membrane of the urethra with a urethroscope.

urethrospasm (ū-rē′thrō-spăzm) [″ + *spasmos,* a convulsion] Spasmodic stricture of the urethra.

urethrostenosis (ū-rē″thrō-stĕn-ō′sĭs) [″ + *stenosis,* act of narrowing] Stricture of the urethra.

urethrostomy (ū-rē-thrŏs′tō-mē) [″ + *stoma,* mouth] The formation of a permanent fistula opening into the urethra by perineal section and fixation of the membranous urethra in the perineum.

urethrotome (ū-rē′thrō-tōm) [″ + *tome,* incision] An instrument for incision of a urethral stricture.

urethrotomy (ū-rē-thrŏt′ō-mē) Incision of a urethral stricture.

urethrotrigonitis (ū-rē″thrō-trī″gō-nī′tĭs) [″ + *trigonon,* three-sided figure, + *itis,* inflammation] Inflammation of the urethra and the trigone of the bladder.

urethrovaginal (ū-rē″thrō-văj′ĭ-năl) [″ + L. *vagina,* sheath] Pert. to the urethra and vagina.

urethrovesical (ū-rē″thrō-vĕs′ĭ-kăl) [″ + L. *vesicula,* little bladder] Concerning the urethra and the bladder.

urgency A sudden, almost uncontrollable need to urinate.

urhydrosis (ūr″hī-drō′sĭs) [Gr. *ouron,* urine, + *hidros,* sweat] Excretion of urea in sweat.

URI *upper respiratory infection.*

uric (ū′rĭk) [Gr. *ourikos,* urine] Of or pert. to urine.

uric acid A crystalline acid, $C_5H_4N_4O_3$, occurring as an end product of purine metabolism. It is formed from purine bases derived from nucleic acids (DNA and RNA). It is a common constituent of urinary stones and gouty tophi. SEE: illus.

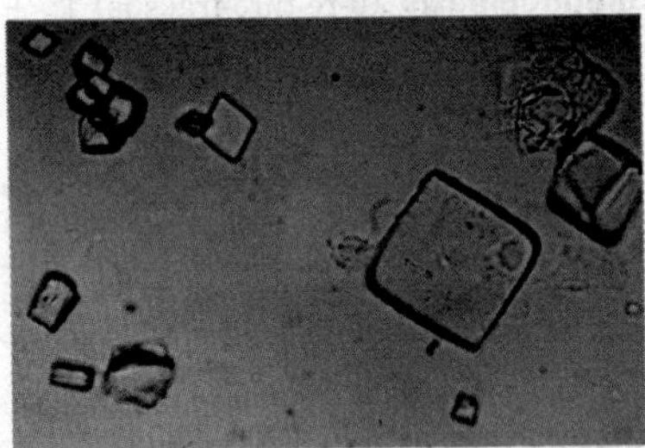

URIC ACID CRYSTALS (X400)

OUTPUT: The uric acid output should be between 0.8 and 1 g/day if the patient is on an ordinary diet. Uric acid must be excreted because it cannot be metabolized.

Increased elimination is observed after ingestion of proteins and nitrogenous foods, after exercise, after administration of cytotoxic agents, and in gout and leukemia. Decreased elimination is observed in kidney failure, lead poisoning, and in people who eat a protein-free diet.

endogenous u.a. Uric acid derived from purines undergoing metabolism from the nucleic acid of body tissues.

exogenous u.a. Uric acid derived from purines from food made up of free purines and nucleic acids. SEE: *urate; uraturia.*

uricacidemia (ū″rĭk-ăs-ĭd-ē′mē-ă) [Gr. *ourikos,* urine, + L. *acidus,* sour, + Gr. *haima,* blood] Hyperuricemia.

uricaciduria (ū″rĭk-ăs-ĭd-ū′rē-ă) [″ + ″ + Gr. *ouron,* urine] Excessive uric acid in the urine.

uricase (ū′rĭ-kāz) [″ + *-ase,* enzyme] An enzyme present in the liver and kidneys of most mammals, but not humans. This enzyme is capable of oxidizing uric acid into allantoin and carbon dioxide.

uricemia (ū-rĭ-sē′mē-ă) [″ + *haima,* blood] An obsolete term for hyperuricemia.

uricocholia (ū″rĭ-kō-kō′lē-ă) [″ + *chole,* bile] Uric acid in the bile.

uricopoiesis (ū″rĭ-kō-poy-ē′sĭs) [″ + *poiesis,* formation] Producing uric acid.

uricosuria (ū″rĭ-kō-sū′rē-ă) [″ + *ouron,* urine] The excessive excretion of uric acid in the urine.

uricosuric (ū″rĭ-kō-sū′rĭk) Potentiating the excretion of uric acid in the urine.

uricosuric agent A drug (such as probenecid) that increases the urinary excretion of uric acid, thereby reducing the concentration of uric acid in the blood. It is used to treat gout.

PATIENT CARE: The health care professional assesses the patient for a history of gastrointestinal complaints or ulceration and for drug sensitivities and drug regimens to prevent interactions. The patient should take drugs with milk or food. Fluid intake of at least 3 L /day is advised (unless contraindicated), and alkalinization of urine with sodium bicarbonate and alkaline-ash diet to prevent uric acid crystallization until serum urate levels return to normal. The patient should avoid the use of salicylates while taking probenecid; the patient may use acetaminophen for analgesia. Gastrointestinal side effects should be reported.

uricotelic (ū″rĭ-kō-tĕl′ĭk) [″ + *telikos,* belonging to the completion] Concerning animals that excrete amino nitrogen in the form of uric acid. Included in this group are birds, snakes, and lizards. SEE: *urea cycle; ureotelic.*

uricoxidase (ū″rĭk-ŏks′ĭ-dās) [″ + *oxys,* sharp, + *-ase,* enzyme] An enzyme capable of oxidizing uric acid.

uridine (ūr′ĭ-dĭn) A nucleoside that is one of the four main riboside components of ribonucleic acid. It consists of uracil and D-ribose.

u. diphosphate A uridine-containing nucleotide important in certain metabolic reactions, in which it transports sugars such as glucose and galactose.

uridrosis (ū-rĭ-drō′sĭs) [″ + *hidrosis,* a sweating] The presence of urea in the sweat. Evaporation may show white scales, the crystals of urea.

urin- SEE: *urino-*.

urinaccelerator (ū″rĭn-ăk-sĕl′ĕr-ā″tor) Musculus bulbospongiosus.

urinal (ū′rĭn-ăl) [L. *urina,* urine] **1.** A container into which one urinates. **2.** A toilet or bathroom fixture for receiving urine and flushing it away.

condom u. Condom catheter.

urinalysis (ū″rĭ-năl′ĭ-sĭs) [″ + Gr. *ana,* apart, + *lysis,* a loosening] Analysis of the urine. SEE: *urine*.

COLLECTION OF URINE: For a routine urinalysis, a voided specimen of urine in a clean container is usually sufficient. For culture, either a clean-catch or a catheterized specimen is required. For a clean-catch specimen, the individual cleanses the perineum or glans penis with soap and water or an antiseptic solution such as benzalkonium chloride before voiding. A midstream specimen of urine is then collected in a sterilized container. A catheterized specimen is obtained by passing a catheter into the bladder, using sterile technique. SEE: *suprapubic catheter*.

NOTE: A urine specimen may be obtained to test for excretion of drugs of abuse. In such cases, care must be taken to ensure that appropriate consent is obtained, and the specimen was produced by the individual and that there was no opportunity for the specimen to be diluted.

urinary (ū′rĭ-nār″ē) [L. *urina,* urine] Pert. to, secreting, or containing urine.

urinary bladder A receptacle for urine excreted by the kidneys. SEE: *bladder*.

urinary calculus A concretion formed in the urinary passages. These vary in composition but may contain urates, calcium, oxalate, calcium carbonate, phosphates, and cystine. SEE: *calculus, renal; lithotriptor*.

PATIENT CARE: The patient is encouraged to verbalize anxieties and concerns regarding severe pain. Pain relief measures are instituted as prescribed; they include analgesics, antispasmodics, and warm, moist heat. All urine is strained for stones, and any calculus is sent for laboratory analysis. If a lithotriptor is to be used, the duration of the procedure and follow-up care are explained. All diagnostic studies are explained and the patient is encouraged to verbalize fears and concerns. Urine is observed for hematuria, and voided specimens are tested for specific gravity. Vital signs are monitored; if temperature is elevated, antipyretic measures are instituted as ordered. Fluids are forced to enhance dilution of urine, and intake and output are monitored. The health care professional stays alert for complications such as infection, stasis, and retention. A catheter is inserted as ordered. Dietary management is based on the composition of the stone. If phosphate stones are present, patients should increase their intake of acid-ash foods such as cereals, eggs, meat, and cranberry and grape juices. Persons prone to uric acid stones should consume an alkaline-ash diet of green vegetables and fruits. To minimize urinary tract infections, esp. for female patients, the patient is taught proper perineal hygiene, and the need for increased fluid intake is emphasized.

urinary director appliance A hand-held, hollow, plastic device that fits over the vulva, enabling a woman to urinate while standing. The device collects urine and allows it to be directed away from the user through an outlet spout. Intended use is for women who are active outdoors and need to urinate without partially disrobing. Medically, the appliance has been found to be useful in patients who have had a radical vulvectomy.

Other devices for use by women in collecting urine are available. Some of these have the capacity to contain the specimen for disposal rather than merely redirecting the flow.

urinary diversion The surgical redirection of urine flow. SEE: *Nursing Diagnoses Appendix.*

urinary elimination, altered The state in which an individual experiences a disturbance in urine elimination. SEE: *Nursing Diagnoses Appendix.*

urinary incontinence Loss of control over urination. SEE: *incontinence; incontinence, stress urinary*.

urinary retention The state in which the individual experiences incomplete emptying of the bladder. High urethral pressure inhibits voiding until increased abdominal pressure causes urine to be involuntarily lost, or high urethral pressure inhibits complete emptying of the bladder. SEE: *Nursing Diagnoses Appendix.*

urinary stammering Temporary interruptions in voiding urine.

urinary system The organ system that includes the kidneys, ureters, bladder, and urethra. The kidneys form urine from blood plasma by filtration, reabsorption, and secretion. The formation of urine includes the excretion of waste products, but the kidneys also regulate the water and mineral content and the acid-base balance of the blood and all other body fluids. The other organs of the system are concerned with the elimination of urine after it has been formed. SEE: illus.

urinary tract Urinary system.

urinary tract infection ABBR: UTI. Infection of the kidneys, ureters, or bladder by microorganisms that either ascend from the urethra (95% of cases) or

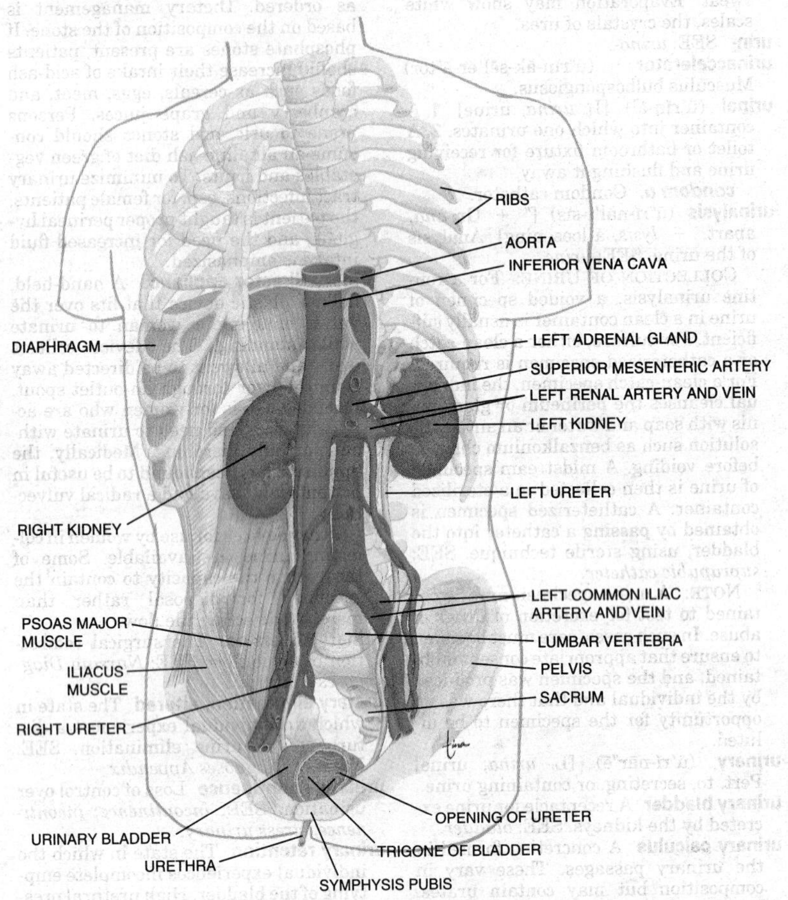

URINARY SYSTEM

that spread to the kidney from the bloodstream (5%). About 7 million American patients visit health care providers each year because of UTIs. These infections commonly occur in otherwise healthy women, men with prostatic hypertrophy or bladder outlet obstruction, children with congenital anatomical abnormalities of the urinary tract, and patients with indwelling bladder catheters. SEE: *clean-catch method; cystitis; pyelonephritis; urethritis.*

ETIOLOGY: *Escherichia coli* causes about 80% of all UTIs. In young women, *Staphylococcus saprophyticus* is also common. In men with prostate disease, enterococci are often responsible. The small remaining percentage of infections may be caused by *Klebsiella* species, *Proteus mirabilis, Staphylococcus aureus, Pseudomonas aeruginosa,* or other virulent organisms.

SYMPTOMS: The presenting symptoms of UTI vary enormously. Young patients with bladder infections may have pain with urination; urinary frequency or urgency, or both; pelvic or suprapubic discomfort; low-grade fevers; or a change in the appearance or odor of their urine. Older patients may present with fever, confusion, or coma caused by urosepsis. Patients with pyelonephritis often complain of flank pain, prostration, nausea, vomiting, and high fevers. UTI may also be asymptomatic, esp. during pregnancy. Asymptomatic UTI during pregnancy is a contributing factor to maternal pyelonephritis, or fetal prematurity and stillbirth.

DIAGNOSIS: Urinalysis and subsequent urinary culture are used to determine the presence of UTI, the culprit microorganism, and the optimal antibiotic therapy. A dipstick test may identify leukocyte esterase and nitrite in a urinary specimen, strongly suggesting a

UTI. The presence of more than 8 to 10 white blood cells per high-power field of spun urine also strongly suggests UTI, as does the presence of bacteria in an uncentrifuged urinary specimen.

TREATMENT: Sulfa drugs, nitrofurantoin, cephalosporins, or quinolones may be used for the outpatient treatment of UTIs while the results of cultures are pending. Patients sick enough to be hospitalized may also be treated with intravenous aminoglycosides, medicine to treat nausea and vomiting, and hydration. The duration of therapy and the precise antibiotics used depend on the responsible organism and the underlying condition of the patient. Patients with anatomical abnormalities of the urinary tract (e.g., children with ureteropelvic obstruction, or older men with bladder outlet obstruction) may sometimes require urological surgery.

RISK FACTORS: The following conditions predispose sexually active women to development of UTI: the use of a contraceptive diaphragm, the method of sexual intercourse (i.e., greatly prolonged or cunnilingus), and failure to void immediately following intercourse.

PREVENTION OF UTI IN YOUNG WOMEN: Fluid intake should be increased to six to eight glasses daily; the anal area should be wiped from front to back to prevent carrying bacteria to the urethral area; the bladder should be emptied shortly before and after intercourse; the genital area should be washed before intercourse; if vaginal dryness is a problem, water-soluble vaginal lubricants should be used before intercourse; a contraceptive diaphragm or sponge should not remain in the vagina longer than necessary. An alternative method of contraception should be considered. Wearing tight jeans and body suits should be avoided; pantyhose with cotton perineal panels should be worn.

PATIENT CARE: Patient teaching should emphasize self-care procedures and prevention of recurrent episodes. The medication regimen should be explained, and the patient should be aware of signs and symptoms and, when they occur, should report them promptly to the primary caregiver.

urinate (ū′rĭ-nāt) [L. *urinare,* to discharge urine] To pass urine from the bladder. SYN: *micturate*.

urination (ū″rĭ-nā′shŭn) [L. *urinatio,* a discharging of urine] The release of urine from the body. SYN: *micturition; uresis*.

DIFFERENTIAL DIAGNOSIS: Increased frequency is seen in polydipsia; polyuria; diabetes mellitus and diabetes insipidus; irritation of the bladder, urethra, or urinary meatus; diseases of the spinal cord; enlarged prostate in males; pregnancy in females; beer drinking; interstitial nephritis; use of medications (e.g., diuretics); and phimosis. Decreased frequency occurs after dehydration, sweating, diarrhea, or bleeding; and in anuria, oliguria, uremia, and anticholinergic drug use. SEE: *urine*.

urine (ū′rĭn) [L. *urina;* Gr. *ouron,* urine] The fluid and dissolved solutes (including salts and nitrogen-containing waste products) that are eliminated from the body by the kidneys. SEE: tables.

COMPOSITION: Urine consists of approx. 95% water and 5% solids. Solids amount to 30 to 70 g/L and include the following (values are in grams per 24 hr unless otherwise noted): *Organic substances:* urea (10 to 30), uric acid (0.8 to 1.0), creatine (10 to 40 mg/24 hr in men and 10 to 270 mg/24 hr in women), creatinine (15 to 25 mg/kg of body weight per day), ammonia (0.5 to 1.3). *Inorganic substances:* chlorides (110 to 250 nmol/L depending on chloride intake), calcium (0.1 to 0.2), magnesium (3 to 5 nmol/24 hr), phosphorus (0.4 to 1.3). *Osmolarity:* 0.1 to 2.5 mOsm/L.

In addition to the foregoing, many other substances may be present depending on the diet and state of health of the individual. Among component substances indicating pathological states are abnormal amounts of albumin, glucose, ketone bodies, blood, pus, casts, and bacteria. SEE: illus.

double-voided u. A urine sample voided within 30 min after the patient has emptied the bladder.

midstream specimen of u. A urinary specimen collected after the first few milliliters of urine are voided and discarded. SEE: *clean-catch method*.

residual u. Urine left in the bladder after urination, an abnormal occurrence that may accompany enlargement of the prostate. SYN: *post-void residual*.

urino-, urin- Combining form meaning *urine*. SEE: *uro-*.

urinogenital (ū″rĭ-nō-jĕn′ĭ-tăl) [″ + *genitalia,* genitals] Urogenital.

urinology (ū″rĭ-nŏl′ō-jē) Urology.

urinoma (ū″rĭ-nō′mă) [″ + Gr. *oma,* mass] A cyst containing urine.

urinometer (ū″rĭ-nŏm′ĕ-tĕr) [″ + Gr. *metron,* measure] A device, a form of hydrometer, for determining the specific gravity of urine. SEE: *hydrometer*.

urinophil (ū′rĭ-nō-fĭl) [″ + Gr. *philein,* to love] Capable of existing in the urine, such as bacteria that grow well in the urinary bladder or in urine.

urinose, urinous (ū′rĭ-nōs, ū′rĭ-nŭs) [L. *urina,* urine] Having the characteristics of or containing urine.

uriposia (ū″rĭ-pō′zē-ă) [″ + *posis,* drinking] Drinking of urine.

uro- [Gr. *ouron,* urine] Combining form meaning *urine*. SEE: *urino-*.

uroammoniac (ū″rō-ă-mō′nē-ăk) Containing urine and ammonia.

Significance of Changes in Urine

Normal	Abnormal	Significance
QUANTITY		
1000–3000 ml/day		Varies with fluid intake, food consumed, exercise, temperature, kidney function
	High (polyuria >3000 ml/day)	Diabetes insipidus, diabetes mellitus, water intoxication, chronic nephritis, diuretic use
	Low (oliguria)	Dehydration, hemorrhage, diarrhea, vomiting, urinary obstruction, or many intrinsic kidney diseases
	None (anuria)	Same as oliguria
COLOR		
Yellow to amber		Depends on concentration of urochrome pigment
	Pale	Dilute urine, diuretic effect
	Milky	Fat globules, pus, crystals
	Red	Drugs, blood or muscle pigments
	Green	Bile pigment (jaundiced patient)
	Brown-black	Toxins, hemorrhage, drugs, metabolites
HEMATURIA (blood in urine)		
0–2 RBC/high-powered field (hpf)		Normal (physiological) filtration
	3 or more RBCs/hpf	Extrarenal: urinary tract infections, cancers, or stones. Renal: infections, trauma, malignancies, glomerulopathies, polycystic kidneys
PYURIA (leukocytes in urine)		
0–9 leukocytes per hpf		
	10 or more leukocytes/hpf	Urinary tract infection, urethritis, vaginitis, urethral syndrome, pyelonephritis, and others
PROTEINURIA		
10–150 mg/day		
	30–300 mg/day of albumin	Indicative of initial glomerular leakage in diabetes mellitus or hypertension (microalbuminuria)
	>300 mg/day	Macroalbuminuria. Indicative of progressive kidney failure. Injury to glomeruli or tubulointerstitium of kidney.
	>3500 mg/day	Nephrotic range proteinuria. Evaluation may include kidney biopsy.

Table continued on following page

Significance of Changes in Urine (Continued)

SPECIFIC GRAVITY		
Normal	**Abnormal**	**Significance**
1.010–1.025		Varies with hydration
	<1.010 (Low)	Excessive fluid intake, impaired kidney concentrating ability
	>1.025 (High)	Dehydration, hemorrhage, salt-wasting, diabetes mellitus, and others

ACIDITY		
Normal	**Abnormal**	**Significance**
Acid (slight)		Diet of acid-forming foods (meats, eggs, prunes, wheat) overbalances the base-forming foods (vegetables and fruits)
	High acidity	Acidosis, diabetes mellitus, many pathological disorders (fevers, starvation)
	Alkaline	Vegetarian diet changes urea into ammonium carbonate; infection or ingestion of alkaline compounds

urobilin (ū″rō-bī′lĭn) [″ + L. *bilis,* bile] A brown pigment formed by the oxidation of urobilinogen, a decomposition product of bilirubin. Urobilin may be formed from the urobilinogen in stools or in urine after exposure to air.

urobilinemia (ū″rō-bī″lĭn-ē′mē-ă) [″ + ″ + Gr. *haima,* blood] Urobilin in the blood.

urobilinicterus (ū″rō-bī-lĭn-ĭk′tĕr-ŭs) [″ + L. *bilis,* bile, + Gr. *ikteros,* jaundice] Jaundice resulting from urobilinemia.

urobilinogen (ū″rō-bī-lĭn′ō-jĕn) [″ + ″ + Gr. *gennan,* to produce] A colorless derivative of bilirubin, from which it is formed by the action of intestinal bacteria.

urobilinogenemia (ū″rō-bī″lĭn-ō-jĕn-ē′mē-ă) [″ + ″ + ″ + *haima,* blood] Urobilinogen in the blood.

urobilinuria (ū″rō-bī″lĭn-ū′rē-ă) [″ + ″ + Gr. *ouron,* urine] Excess of urobilin in the urine.

urocele (ū′rō-sēl) [″ + *kele,* tumor, swelling] Escape of urine into the scrotum. SYN: *uroscheocele.*

urochesia (ū-rō-kē′zē-ă) [″ + *chezein,* to defecate] A discharge of urine in the feces.

urochrome (ū′rō-krōm) [″ + *chroma,* color] The pigment that gives urine its characteristic color. It is derived from urobilin.

urocyanin (ū-rō-sī′ă-nĭn) [″ + *kyanos,* blue] A blue pigment present in the urine in certain diseases.

urocyanogen (ū″rō-sī-ăn′ō-jĕn) [″ + ″ + *gennan,* to produce] A blue pigment in urine, esp. in cholera patients.

urocyanosis (ū″rō-sī-ăn-ō′sĭs) [″ + ″ + *osis,* condition] Blue discoloration of the urine; possibly due to the presence of indigo blue from oxidation of indican or to ingestion of drugs such as methylene blue. SEE: *indicanuria.*

urodynamics (ū″rō-dī-năm′ĭks) The study of the holding or storage of urine

Common Disorders of Urination

Anuria	Complete (or nearly complete) absence of urination
Diversion	Drainage of urine through a surgically constructed passage (e.g., a ureterostomy or ileal conduit)
Dysuria	Painful or difficult urination (e.g., in urethritis, urethral stricture, urinary tract infection, prostatic hyperplasia, or bladder atony)
Enuresis	Involuntary discharge of urine, esp. by children at night (bedwetting)
Incontinence	Loss of control over urination from any cause (e.g., from involuntary relaxation of urinary sphincter muscles or overflow from a full or paralyzed bladder)
Nocturia	Excessive urination at night
Oliguria	Decreased urinary output (usually less than 500 cc/day), often associated with dehydration, shock, hemorrhage, acute renal failure, or other conditions in which renal perfusion or renal output are impaired
Polyuria	Increased urinary output (usually more than 3000 ml/day), such as occurs in diabetes mellitus, diabetes insipidus, and diuresis

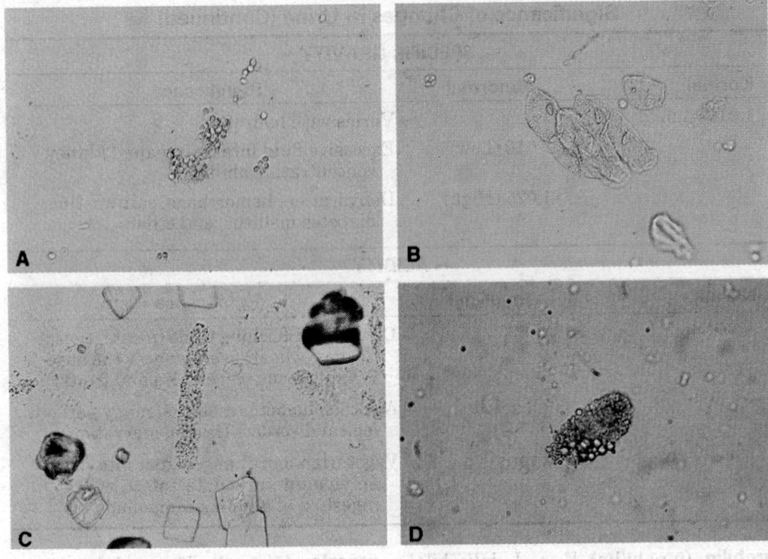

URINE

(A) white blood cells, (B) squamous epithelial cells, (C) granular cast and uric acid crystals, (D) fat body (×400)

in the bladder, the facility with which it empties, and the rate of movement of urine out of the bladder during micturition.

urodynia (ū″rō-dĭn′ē-ă) [″ + *odyne,* pain] Pain associated with urination.

uroerythrin (ū″rō-ĕr′ĭth-rĭn) [″ + *erythros,* red] A reddish pigment sometimes present in urine.

uroflavin (ū″rō-flā′vĭn) A fluorescent compound present in the urine of persons taking riboflavin.

uroflowmeter A device for recording urine flow; used to quantitate obstruction to urine flowing from the bladder.

urofuscin (ū″rō-fŭs′ĭn) [″ + L. *fuscus,* dark brown] A red-brown pigment sometimes found in samples of urine, esp. in cases of porphyrinuria.

urofuscohematin (ū″rō-fŭs″kō-hĕm′ăt-ĭn) [″ + ″ + Gr. *haima,* blood] A reddish-brown pigment in urine in some diseases.

urogastrone (ū″rō-găs′trōn) [″ + *gaster,* belly] A polypeptide present in urine that has an inhibitory effect on gastric secretion.

urogenital (ū″rō-jĕn′ĭ-tăl) [″ + L. *genitalia,* genitals] Pert. to the urinary and reproductive organs. SYN: *urinogenital.*

urogenous (ū-rŏj′ĕn-ŭs) [″ + *gennan,* to produce] **1.** Producing urine. **2.** Originating in urine.

urogram (ū′rō-grăm) [″ + *gramma,* something written] A radiograph of the urinary tract.

urography (ū-rŏg′ră-fē) [Gr. *ouron,* urine, + *graphein,* to write] Radiography of the urinary tract after the introduction of a contrast medium.

ascending u. Urography in which the radiopaque dye is injected into the bladder during cystoscopy. SYN: *cystoscopic u.; retrograde u.*

cystoscopic u. Ascending u.

descending u. Urography in which an injected dye is excreted by the kidney and studied by x-ray examination during excretion. SYN: *excretory u.; intravenous u.*

excretory u. Descending u.

intravenous u. Descending u.

retrograde u. Ascending u.

urohematin (ū″rō-hĕm′ăt-ĭn) [″ + *haima,* blood] Pigment in urine, considered as identical with hematin, that alters the color of urine in proportion to the degree of oxidation.

urohematonephrosis (ū″rō-hĕm″ă-tō-nē-frō′sĭs) [″ + ″ + *nephros,* kidney] A pathological condition of the kidney in which the pelvis is distended with blood and urine.

urohematoporphyrin (ū″rō-hĕm″ă-tō-por′fĭr-ĭn) [″ + ″ + *porphyra,* purple] Iron-free hematin in urine when intravascular hemolysis occurs.

urokinase (ū-rō-kī′nās) An enzyme obtained from human urine; used to dissolve venous thrombi and pulmonary emboli. It is administered intravenously.

urokinetic (ū″rō-kĭ-nĕt′ĭk) [″ + *kinesis,* movement] Resulting reflexly from stimulation of the urinary organs.

urolagnia (ū-rō-lăg′nē-ă) [″ + *lagneia,* lust] Sexual excitation associated with urine or urination (e.g., watching another person urinate or having another person urinate on one's own body). SEE: *undinism*.

urolith (ū'rō-lĭth) [" + *lithos,* stone] A concretion in the urine.

urolithiasis (ū"rō-lĭ-thī'ă-sĭs) [" + " + *-iasis,* condition] The formation of kidney stones. SEE: *Nursing Diagnoses Appendix.*

urolithic (ū"rō-lĭth'ĭk) Concerning kidney stones..

urological (ū-rō-lŏj'ĭk-ăl) [" + *logos,* word, reason] Pert. to urology.

urologist (ū-rŏl'ō-jĭst) A physician who specializes in the practice of urology.

urology (ū-rŏl'ō-jē) [" + *logos,* word, reason] The branch of medicine concerned with the urinary tract in both sexes and the male genital tract.

urolutein (ū-rō-lū'tē-ĭn) [" + L. *luteus,* yellow] A yellow pigment seen in the urine.

uromedulin, human The most abundant protein of renal origin in normal urine. This glycoprotein is the same protein termed Tamm-Horsfall mucoprotein. SEE: *mucoprotein, Tamm-Horsfall*.

uromelanin (ū-rō-mĕl'ăn-ĭn) [" + *melas,* black] A black pigment occurring in urine resulting from the decomposition of urochrome.

uromelus (ū-rŏm'ē-lŭs) [Gr. *oura,* tail, + *melos,* limb] A congenitally deformed fetus in which the lower extremities are fused. SYN: *sirenomelia*.

uronephrosis (ū"rō-nĕf-rō'sĭs) [" + *nephros,* kidney, + *osis,* condition] Dilatation of the renal structures from obstruction of the urinary flow; distention of the renal pelvis and tubules with urine. SYN: *hydronephrosis*.

uropathogen (ū"rō-păth'ō-jĕn) [" + *pathos,* disease, suffering, + *gennan,* to produce] A microorganism capable of causing disease of the urinary tract.

uropathy (ū-rŏp'ă-thē) Any disease affecting the urinary tract.

obstructive u. Any disease that blocks the flow of urine (e.g., prostatic hyperplasia).

uropepsin (ū"rō-pĕp'sĭn) The end product of pepsin metabolism. It is excreted in the urine.

urophein, urophaein (ū"rō-fē'ĭn) [" + *phaios,* gray] Gray pigment sometimes found in urine.

urophosphometer (ū"rō-fŏs-fŏm'ĕ-tĕr) [" + L. *phosphas,* phosphorus] A device for estimating the amount of phosphorus in the urine.

uroplania (ū"rō-plā'nē-ă) [" + *plane,* a wandering] A condition in which urine is present in or discharged from parts other than the urinary organs.

uropoiesis (ū"rō-poy-ē'sĭs) [Gr. *ouron,* urine, + *poiesis,* production] The formation of urine by the kidneys.

uropoietic (ū"rō-poy-ĕt'ĭk) [" + *poiein,* to form] Pert. to the formation of urine.

uroporphyria (ū"rō-por-fĭr'ē-ă) Porphyria in which an excess amount of uroporphyrin is excreted in the urine.

uroporphyrin (ū"rō-por'fĭ-rĭn) A red pigment present in the urine and feces in cases of porphyria; may also be present in the urine of persons taking certain drugs.

uroporphyrinogen (ū"rō-por"fĭ-rĭn'ō-jĕn) Any one of several porphyrins that are the precursors of uroporphyrins.

u. I An abnormal isomer of a precursor of protoporphyrin, which accumulates in one form of porphyria. It causes the urine to be red, the teeth to fluoresce brightly in ultraviolet light, and the skin to be abnormally sensitive to sunlight. This is observed in congenital erythropoietic porphyria.

uropsammus (ū"rō-săm'ŭs) [" + *psammos,* sand] Gravel or calcified sediment in the urine.

uropyoureter (ū"rō-pī"ō-ū-rē'tĕr) [" + " + *oureter,* ureter] Accumulation of urine and pus in the ureter.

urorrhodin (ū-rō-rō'dĭn) [" + *rhodon,* rose] A rose-colored pigment in the urine in certain infectious diseases such as typhoid fever and tuberculosis.

uroscheocele (ū-rŏs'kē-ō-sēl) [" + *oscheon,* scrotum, + *kele,* tumor, swelling] Urocele.

uroschesis (ū-rŏs'kĕs-ĭs) [" + *schesis,* a holding] **1.** Suppression of urine. **2.** Retention of urine.

uroscopy (ū-rŏs'kō-pē) [" + *skopein,* to examine] **1.** Examination of the urine. **2.** Diagnosis by examination of the urine.

urotoxin (ū"rō-tŏk'sĭn) Toxic substances in the urine.

uroureter (ū"rō-ū'rĕ-tĕr, ū"rō-ū-rē'tĕr) [" + *oureter,* ureter] Distention of the ureter with urine caused by stricture or obstruction.

uroxanthin (ū"rō-zăn'thĭn) [" + *xanthos,* yellow] Yellow pigment of the urine; an indigo-forming substance.

uroxin (ū-rŏk'sĭn) [" + *oxys,* sharp] Alloxantin, a derivative of alloxan.

ursodiol A drug used to treat biliary diseases, including gallstones and primary biliary cirrhosis. SEE: *gallstone*.

urtica (ŭr-tī'kă) *pl.* **urticae** [L., nettle] Wheal.

urticant (ŭr'tĭ-kănt) That which causes hives.

urticaria (ŭr-tĭ-kā'rē-ă) [L. *urtica,* nettle] Multiple swollen raised areas on the skin that are intensely itchy and last up to 24 hr; they may appear primarily on the chest, back, extremities, face, or scalp. SYN: *hives; nettle rash*. SEE: illus.; *allergy; angioedema*.

ETIOLOGY: Urticaria is caused by vasodilation and increased permeability of capillaries of the skin as the result of mast cell release of vasoactive mediators. The mast cell degranulation is the result of an immunoglobulin E–mediated reaction to allergens (e.g., foods, drugs, or drug additives), heat, cold, and, rarely, infections or emotions. Urticaria is a primary sign of local and systemic anaphylactic reactions. It affects people of all ages but is most common between 20 and 40 years of age. Urticaria is closely related to angioedema, which causes edema in deeper regions of the skin and subcutaneous tissue.

TREATMENT: Drugs that block histamine-1 (H_1) receptors (antihistamines) are the primary treatment for urticaria. The use of both H_1 and H_2 receptor blockers has been recommended but has not been proven more effective. Patients should avoid identified allergens. Corticosteroids are not usually used.

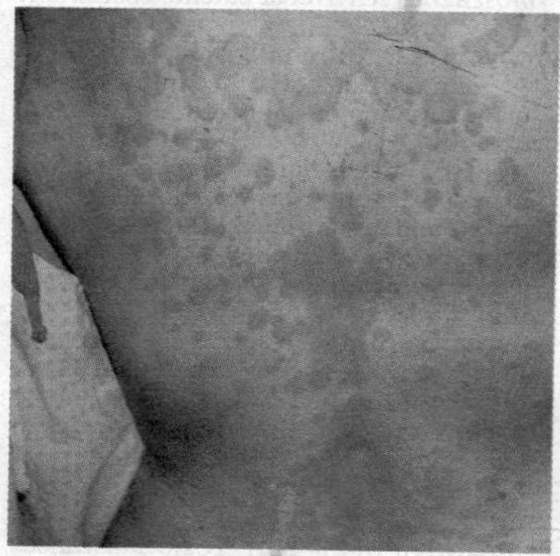

URTICARIA

aquagenic u. Urticaria caused by exposure of the skin to ordinary water.

u. bullosa Eruption of temporary vesicles with infusion of fluid under the epidermis.

cold u. Cold-induced urticarial eruption that may progress to angioedema.

u. factitia Urticaria following slight irritation of the skin.

u. gigantea Angioedema.

u. haemorrhagica Urticaria with lesions infiltrated with blood.

u. maculosa A chronic form of urticaria with red-colored lesions.

u. medicamentosa Urticaria due to certain drugs.

u. papulosa A form of urticaria in which the wheal is followed by a lingering papule that is attended by considerable itching; most commonly observed in debilitated children. SYN: *prurigo simplex*.

u. pigmentosa A form of urticaria characterized by persistent, pigmented maculopapular lesions that urticate when stroked (Darier's sign). It typically occurs in childhood. Biopsy reveals infiltration by mast cells.

pressure u. Urticaria that is produced by pressure perpendicular to the surface of the skin. The persistent red swelling appears after a delay of 1 to 4 hr.

solar u. Urticaria occurring in certain individuals following exposure to sunlight.

urticarial (ŭr″tĭ-kā′rē-ăl) [L. *urtica,* nettle] Pert. to urticaria.

urticate (ŭr′tĭ-kāt) **1.** To produce urticaria. **2.** Marked by the appearance of wheals.

urushiol (ū-roo′shē-ŏl″) [Japanese *urushi,* lac, + L. *oleum,* oil] The principal toxic irritant substance of plants such as poison ivy, which produces characteristic severe dermatitis on contact.

USAEC *U.S. Atomic Energy Commission.*

USAN *United States Adopted Names* (for drugs).

USAN and the USP Dictionary of Drug Names A dictionary of nonproprietary names, brand names, code designations, and Chemical Abstracts Service registry numbers for drugs.

USDA *United States Department of Agriculture.*

Usher's syndrome [Charles Howard Usher, Brit. ophthalmologist, 1865–1942] An autosomal recessive disorder marked by a combination of congenital sensorineural deafness and retinitis pigmentosa that results in a gradual loss of vision.

USP, U.S. Phar. *United States Pharmacopeia.*

U.S.P.H.S. *United States Public Health Service.*

USP-PRN *United States Pharmacopeia–Practitioners' Reporting Network.*

ustilaginism (ŭs-tĭl-ăj′ĭn-ĭzm) [L. *ustulatus,* scorched, + Gr. *-ismos,* condition] Poisoning resulting from eating corn infected with smut fungus, *Ustilago maydis.*

Ustilago (ŭs-tĭl-ā′gō) A moldlike fungus, *Ustilago maydis,* commonly called smut.

uta (ū′tă) American leishmaniasis.

Utah Elbow A myoelectric prosthesis that uses an electrode and microprocessors to control both the elbow and the terminal device. The system is also designed to permit a natural elbow swing during walking.

ut dict L. *ut dictum,* as directed.

utend L. *utendus,* to be used.

uter- SEE: *utero-*.

uteralgia (ū″tĕr-ăl′jē-ă) [L. *uterus,* womb, + Gr. *algos,* pain] Uterine pain.

uterectomy (ū″tĕr-ĕk′tō-mē) [″ + Gr. *ektome,* excision] Hysterectomy.

uterine (ū′tĕr-ĭn, -īn) [L. *uterinus*] Pert. to the uterus.

uterine artery Doppler velocimetry SEE: *Doppler echocardiography.*

uterine bleeding Bleeding from the uterus. Physiological bleeding via the vagina occurs in normal menstruation. Abnormal forms include excessive menstrual flow (hypermenorrhea, menorrhagia) or too frequent menstruation (polymenorrhea). Nonmenstrual bleeding is called metrorrhagia. Pseudomenstrual or withdrawal bleeding may occur following estrogen therapy. Breakthrough bleeding is the term used for intermenstrual bleeding that sometimes occurs in women who take progestational agents such as birth control pills or receive estrogen-progesterone replacement therapy. SEE: *amenorrhea; dysfunctional uterine bleeding; menstruation; Nursing Diagnoses Appendix.*

uterine gland One of the tubular glands in the endometrium.

uterine tube Fallopian tube.

utero-, uter- Combining form meaning *uterus*. SEE: *hystero-; metro-*.

uteroabdominal (ū″tĕr-ō-ăb-dŏm′ĭ-năl) [L. *uterus,* womb, + *abdomen,* belly] Pert. to both the uterus and abdomen.

uterocele (ū-tĕr′ō-sēl) [″ + Gr. *kele,* tumor, swelling] Hernia containing the uterus.

uterocervical (ū″tĕr-ō-sĕr′vĭ-kăl) [″ + *cervix,* neck] Rel. to the uterus and cervix.

uterocystostomy (ū″tĕr-ō-sĭs-tŏs′tō-mē) [″ + Gr. *kystis,* bladder, + *stoma,* mouth] The formation of a passage between the uterine cervix and the bladder.

uterofixation (ū″tĕr-ō-fĭks-ā′shŭn) [″ + *fixatio,* a fixing] Fixation of a displaced uterus.

uterography (ū″tĕr-ŏg′ră-fē) [″ + Gr. *graphein,* to write] Hysterogram.

uterolith (ū′tĕr-ō-lĭth) [″+ Gr. *lithos,* stone] A uterine stone.

uterometer (ū″tĕr-ŏm′ĕt-er) [″ + Gr. *metron,* measure] Hysterometer.

uteroovarian (ū″tĕr-ō-ō-vā′rē-ăn) [″ + LL. *ovarium,* ovary] Rel. to the uterus and ovary.

uteropexia, uteropexy (ū″tĕr-ō-pĕks′ē-ă, ū′tĕr-ō-pĕks″ē) [″ + Gr. *pexis,* fixation] Fixation of the uterus to the abdominal wall.

uteroplacental (ū″tĕr-ō-plă-sĕn′tăl) [″ + *placenta,* a flat cake] Rel. to the placenta and uterus.

uteroplasty (ū″tĕr-ō-plăs′tē) [″ + Gr. *plassein,* to form] Plastic surgery of the uterus. SYN: *metroplasty*.

uterorectal (ū″tĕr-ō-rĕk′tăl) Concerning the uterus and rectum.

uterosacral (ū″tĕr-ō-sā′krăl) [″ + *sacralis,* pert. to the sacrum] Rel. to the uterus and sacrum.

uterosalpingography (ū″tĕr-ō-săl-pĭng-ŏg′ră-fē) [″ + Gr. *salpinx,* tube, + *graphein,* to write] Radiography of the uterus and fallopian tubes after the introduction of a contrast medium. SYN: *hysterosalpingography*.

uterotomy (ū-tĕr-ŏt′ō-mē) Incision of the uterus.

uterotractor (ū″tĕr-ō-trăk′tor) [″ + *tractor,* drawer] An instrument for applying traction to the cervix uteri.

uterotubal (ū″tĕr-ō-tū′băl) [″ + *tuba,* tube] Relating to the uterus and oviducts.

uterovaginal (ū″tĕr-ō-văj′ĭ-năl) [″ + *vagina,* sheath] Rel. to the uterus and vagina.

uteroventral (ū″tĕr-ō-vĕn′trăl) Uteroabdominal.

uterovesical (ū″tĕr-ō-vĕs′ĭ-kăl) [″ + *vesica,* bladder] Rel. to the uterus and bladder.

uterus (ū′tĕr-ŭs) [L.] A reproductive organ for containing and nourishing the embryo and fetus from the time the fertilized egg is implanted to the time the fetus is born. SYN: *womb*. SEE: *genitalia, female* for illus.

ANATOMY: The uterus is a muscular, hollow, pear-shaped organ situated in the midpelvis between the sacrum and the pubic symphysis. Before childbearing, it is about 3 in. (7.5 cm) long, 2 in. (5 cm) wide, and 1 in. (2.5 cm) thick. Its upper surface is covered by peritoneum called the perimetrium, and it is supported by the pelvic diaphragm supplemented by the two broad ligaments, two round ligaments, and two uterosacral ligaments. It is usually anteflexed, or tilted forward, over the top of the urinary bladder. The upper portion of the uterus, between the openings of the fallopian tubes, is the fundus; the large central portion is the body; and the narrow lower end is the cervix, which projects into the vagina. The cavity of the uterus is widest in the fundus. The canal of the cervix is narrow, opens into the uterine cavity at the internal os, and into the vagina at the external os.

The wall of the uterus consists of the outer perimetrium, middle myometrium, and inner endometrium. The perimetrium is the visceral peritoneum that covers the uterus, except for the portion that rests on the bladder and the vaginal part of the cervix. The thick myometrium is smooth muscle that contracts for labor and delivery. The endometrium is the vascular lining that can become the placenta for nourishment of the embryo-fetus; it is thin before puberty; grows and is shed cyclically during childbearing years, and degenerates after menopause. The uterine and ovarian arteries supply blood to the uterus.

POSITIONS: *Anteflexion:* The uterus bends forward. *Anteversion:* The fundus is displaced forward toward the pubis, while the cervix is tilted up toward the sacrum. *Retroflexion:* The uterus bends backward at the junction of the body and the cervix. *Retroversion:* The uterus inclines backward with retention of the normal curve; this position is the opposite of anteversion. SEE: *hysterectomy; pregnancy.*

u. acollis A uterus without a cervix.

u. arcuatus A uterus with a depressed arched fundus.

u. bicornis A uterus in which the fundus is divided into two parts.

u. biforis A uterus in which the external os is divided into two parts by a septum.

u. bilocularis A uterus in which the cavity is divided into two parts by a partition.

bipartite u. A uterus in which the body is partially divided by a median septum.

cancer of u. A malignant neoplasm of the uterus, suggested by size, intermittent bleeding, purulent discharge, and detected by vaginal or Papanicolaou smear, or cervical or endometrial biopsy. Cancer may produce sterility, abortion, hemorrhage, or sepsis. SEE: *the Bethesda System; cervical intraepithelial neoplasia.*

u. cordiformis A heart-shaped uterus.

u. didelphys Double uterus.

u. duplex A double uterus resulting from failure of union of müllerian ducts.

fetal u. A uterus that is retarded in development and possesses an extremely long cervical canal.

fibroids of u. Uterine fibroma.

gravid u. A pregnant uterus.

u. masculinus The prostatic utricle.

u. parvicollis A normal uterus with a disproportionately small vaginal portion.

prolapse of u. A condition in which a defective pelvic floor allows the uterus or part of it to protrude out of the vagina. In first-degree uterine prolapse, the cervix uteri reaches down to the vaginal introitus. In second-degree uterine prolapse, it protrudes out from the vagina. In third-degree uterine prolapse, the entire uterus lies outside of the vagina. SYN: *descensus uteri.* SEE: *procidentia.*

SYMPTOMS: The condition is most often seen following instrumental deliveries or when the patient has been allowed to bear down during labor before the cervix is fully dilated. Frequently associated with this is a prolapse of the anterior and posterior vaginal walls, as seen in cystocele and rectocele. In the early stages, there are dragging sensations in the lower abdomen, back pain while standing and on exertion, a sensation of weight and bearing down in the perineum, and frequency of urination and incontinence of urine in cases associated with cystocele. In the later stages, a protrusion or swelling at the vulva is noticed on standing or straining, and leukorrhea is present. In procidentia, there is frequently pain on walking, an inability to urinate unless the mass is reduced, and cystitis.

ETIOLOGY: This condition may be congenital or acquired; most often, however, it is acquired. The etiological factors are congenital weakness of the uterine supports and injury to the pelvic floor or uterine supports during childbirth.

TREATMENT: The treatment depends on the age of the patient, the degree of prolapse, and the associated pathology. Abdominal surgery with fixation of the uterus is required if the prolapse is complete.

pubescent u. An adult uterus that resembles that of a prepubertal female.

rupture of u. in pregnancy SEE: under *rupture; Nursing Diagnoses Appendix.*

subinvolution of u. The lack of involution of the uterus following childbirth, manifested by a large uterus (greater than 100 g) and a continuation of lochia rubra beyond the usual time. It is caused usually by puerperal infection, overdistention of the uterus by multiple pregnancy or polyhydramnios, lack of lactation, malposition of the uterus, and retained secundines. Involution is aided by the certainty that the placenta is intact at the time of delivery and the use of ecbolics to cause uterine contraction.

tumors of u. Uterine neoplasia, which may cause sterility or abortion or obstruct labor; they may become infected or twisted on their attachments. SEE: *cancer of uterus; endometrioma; uterine fibroma.*

u. unicornis A uterus possessing only one lateral half and usually having only one uterine tube. About 20% to 30% of women who have this structural abnormality also experience repeated spontaneous abortion during early pregnancy.

utilization review Evaluation of the necessity, quality, effectiveness, or efficiency of medical services, procedures, and facilities. In regard to a hospital, the review includes appropriateness of admission, services ordered and provided, length of stay, and discharge practices.

utricle (ū′trĭk′l) [L. *utriculus,* a little bag] **1.** Any small sac. **2.** The larger of two sacs of the membranous labyrinth in the vestibule of the inner ear. It communicates with the semicircular ducts, the saccule, and the endolymphatic duct, all of which are filled with endolymph. In its wall is the macula utriculi, a sensory area with hair cells that respond to movement of otoliths as the position of the head changes. SYN: *utriculus.*

prostatic u. A small blind pouch of the urethra extending into the substance of the prostate gland. It is a remnant of the embryonic müllerian duct. SYN: *u. masculinus; u. prostaticus; uterus masculinus.*

u. of urethra The prostatic vesicle of the male.

u. of vestibule The vestibular cavity connecting with the semicircular canals.

utricular (ū-trĭk′ū-lăr) [L. *utriculus,* a little bag] **1.** Pert. to the utricle. **2.** Like a bladder.

utriculitis (ū-trĭk-ū-lī′tĭs) [″ + Gr. *itis,* inflammation] Inflammation of the utricle, that of either the vestibule or the prostate.

utriculoplasty (ū-trĭk′ū-lō-plăs″tē) [″ + Gr. *plassein,* to form] Surgical reduction of the size of the uterus by excision of a longitudinal wedge-shaped section.

utriculosaccular (ū-trĭk″ū-lō-săk′ū-lăr) [″ + *sacculus,* a small bag] Pert. to the utricle and saccule of the labyrinth.

utriculus (ū-trĭk′ū-lŭs) [L., a little bag] Utricle.

u. masculinus Prostatic utricle.

u. prostaticus Prostatic utricle.

uva-ursi An evergreen perennial shrub, *Arctostaphylos uva-ursi* (family Ericaceae)—commonly known as bearberry—whose dried leaves are used as a urinary antiseptic and diuretic. There have been few clinical trials on its effectiveness.

uvea (ū′vē-ă) [L. *uva,* grape] The highly vascular middle layer of the eyeball, immediately beneath the sclera. It consists of the iris, ciliary body, and choroid, and forms the pigmented layer.

uveal (ū′vē-ăl) Pert. to the middle layer of the eye, or uvea.

uveitic (ū-vē-ĭt′ĭk) [″ + Gr. *itis,* inflammation] Marked by or pert. to uveitis.

uveitis (ū-vē-ī′tĭs) A nonspecific term for any intraocular inflammatory disorder. The uveal tract structures—iris, ciliary body, and choroid—are usually involved, but other nonuveal parts of the eye, including the retina and cornea, may be involved.

Uveitis that is not associated with known infections or that is associated with diseases of unknown cause is termed endogenous uveitis. This is thought to be due to an autoimmune phenomenon.

TREATMENT: Corticosteroids and other immunosuppressive agents, including cyclosporine, are used in treating some causes of uveitis, but their use may make some types of uveitus worse. Short-acting cycloplegic agents such as hematropine, scopolamine, or cyclopentolate are used during therapy to prevent inflammatory adhesions (posterior synechiae) between the iris and lens.

sympathetic u. Severe, bilateral uveitis that starts as inflammation of the uveal tract of one eye resulting from a puncture wound. The injured eye is termed the "exciting eye." SEE: *sympathetic ophthalmia.*

TREATMENT: High-dose corticosteroids are often effective.

uveoparotitis (ū″vē-ō-păr-ō-tī′tĭs) [″ + Gr. *para,* beside, + *ous,* ear, + *itis,* inflammation] Inflammation of the parotid gland and uveitis.

uveoplasty (ū′vē-ō-plăs″tē) [″ + Gr. *plassein,* to form] Reparative operation of the uvea.

uveoscleritis (ū″vē-ō-sklĕr-ī′tĭs) Inflammation of the sclera in which the infection has spread from the uvea.

uviform (ū′vĭ-form) [″ + *forma,* form] Shaped like a grape.

uviofast (ū′vē-ō-făst) Uvioresistant.

uviol (ū′vē-ŏl) Glass that is unusually transparent to ultraviolet rays.

uvioresistant (ū″vē-ō-rē-zĭs′tănt) Resistant to the effects of ultraviolet radiation. SYN: *uviofast.*

uviosensitive (ū″vē-ō-sĕn′sĭ-tĭv) Sensitive to the effects of ultraviolet radiation.

uvula (ū′vū-lă) [L. *uvula,* a little grape] **1.** The free edge of the soft palate that hangs at the back of the throat above the root of the tongue; it is made of muscle, connective tissue, and mucous membrane. **2.** Any small projection.

u. of cerebellum A small lobule of the cerebellum lying on the inferior surface of the inferior vermis, anterior to the pyramis.

u. fissa A cleft uvula.

u. vermis A small, triangular elevation on the vermis of the cerebellum of the brain.

u. vesicae A median projection of mucous membrane of the urinary bladder located immediately anterior to the orifice of the urethra.

uvulaptosis (ū″vū-lăp-tō′sĭs) [″ + Gr. *ptosis,* a dropping] Uvuloptosis.

uvular (ū′vū-lăr) [L. *uvula,* little grape] Pert. to the uvula.

uvularis (ū-vū-lā′rĭs) [L.] The azygos uvulae muscle.

uvulectomy (ū″vū-lĕk′tō-mē) [″ + Gr. *ektome,* excision] Surgical removal of the uvula.

uvulitis (ū″vū-lī′tĭs) [″ + Gr. *itis,* inflammation] Inflammation of the uvula.

uvulopalatopharyngoplasty ABBR: UPPP. Plastic surgery of the oropharynx in which redundant soft palate, uvula, pillars, fauces, and sometimes posterior pharyngeal wall mucosa are removed. The procedure may be done by using laser therapy. It is usually done to correct intractable snoring or sleep apnea. SEE: *sleep disorder; snore.*

uvuloptosis (ū″vū-lŏp-tō′sĭs) [″ + Gr. *ptosis,* a dropping] A relaxed and pendulous condition of the palate. SYN: *uvulaptosis.*

U wave In the electrocardiogram, a low-amplitude deflection that follows the T wave. It is exaggerated in hypokalemia and with digitalis use, and negative in ventricular hypertrophy. SEE: *QRST complex; electrocardiogram.*

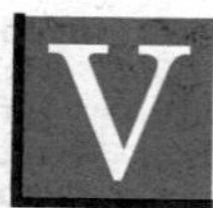

V 1. *Vibrio; vision; visual acuity.* 2. Symbol for the element vanadium.

V̇ 1. Symbol for gas flow. 2. Symbol for ventilation.

v L. *vena,* vein; *volt.*

vaccina (văk-sī′nă) Vaccinia.

vaccinable (văk-sĭn′ă-b′l) Capable of being successfully vaccinated.

vaccinal (văk′sĭn-ăl) Rel. to vaccine or to vaccination.

vaccinate (văk′sĭn-āt) [L. *vaccinus,* pert. to cows] To inoculate with vaccine to produce immunity against disease.

vaccination (văk″sĭ-nā′shŭn) [L. *vaccinus,* pert. to cows] 1. Inoculation with any vaccine or toxoid to establish resistance to a specific infectious disease. SEE: *immunization.* 2. A scar left on the skin by inoculation of a vaccine.

catch-up v. The immunization of unvaccinated children at the most convenient times (e.g., on the first day of school) rather than at the optimal time for antibody production. Because many children miss vaccines at regularly scheduled times, catch-up immunization offers unvaccinated children, their families, and the communities in which they live a second opportunity for disease prevention and control.

mass v. The use of vaccines during an outbreak of a communicable disease in an attempt to prevent an epidemic. In the U.S. mass vaccinations are sometimes carried out in schools and hospitals during meningitis or hepatitis epidemics.

vaccine (văk′sēn, văk-sēn′) [L. *vaccinus,* pert. to cows] 1. An infectious liquid that Edward Jenner (Brit. physician, 1749–1823) derived from cowpox lesions, and used to prevent and attenuate smallpox in humans. 2. Any suspension containing antigenic molecules derived from a microorganism, given to stimulate an immune response to an infectious disease. Vaccines may be made from weakened or killed microorganisms; inactivated toxins; toxoids derived from microorganisms; or immunologically active surface markers extracted or copied from microorganisms. They can be given intramuscularly, subcutaneously, intradermally, orally, or intranasally; as single agents; or in combinations. SEE: table.

The ideal vaccine should be effective, well-tolerated, easy and inexpensive to manufacture, easy to administer, and easy to store. In practice, vaccine side effects such as fevers, muscle aches, and injection site pain are common but generally mild. Adverse reactions to vaccines that should be reported include anaphylaxis, shock, seizures, active infection, and death. SEE: *immunization.*

CAUTION: Because vaccines may cause side effects, all persons who receive them should carefully review federally mandated Vaccine Information Sheets before they are immunized.

autogenous v. Bacterial vaccine prepared from lesions of the individual to be inoculated. SYN: *homologous v.*

bacterial v. A suspension of killed or attenuated bacteria; used for injection into the body to produce active immunity to the same organism.

BCG v. A preparation of a weakened live culture of bacille Calmette-Guérin, of the strain *Mycobacterium bovis.* In some countries with a high incidence of tuberculosis, it provides effective immunity against the disease, lowering the risk of infection by about 75%. A disadvantage of this vaccine is that it produces hypersensitivity to tuberculin so that skin testing for tuberculosis becomes inaccurate, esp. in the first 5 years after inoculation. The vaccine is also used as an immunomodulating treatment for some forms of cancer (e.g., bladder cancers).

cholera v. A vaccine prepared from killed *Vibrio cholerae.* It is effective for only a few months.

diphtheria v. A vaccination against *Corynebacterium diphtheriae.* SEE: *DTaP v.*

DNA v. A vaccine made by genetic engineering in which the gene that codes for an antigen is inserted into a bacterial plasmid and then injected into the host. Once inside the host, it uses the nuclear machinery of the host cell to manufacture and express the antigen. Unlike other vaccines, DNA vaccines may have the potential to induce cellular as well as humoral immune responses.

DPT v. An obsolete combination of diphtheria and tetanus toxoids and killed pertussis bacilli that is no longer given in pediatric immunizations because of the superiority of DTaP, a vaccine that contains only acellular pertussis.

DTaP v. A preparation of diphtheria and tetanus toxoids and acellular pertussis proteins. It is used to immunize children against all three infections.

Vaccines*

Name	Age Administered	Booster Schedule	Comments
BCG (bacillus of Calmette and Guérin)	In epidemic conditions, administered to infants as soon as possible after birth.	None	The only contra-indications are symptomatic human immunodeficiency virus (HIV) infection or other illnesses known to suppress immunity.
Cholera	See Comments.	Every 3 to 6 mo for those who remain in epidemic areas.	Only those traveling to countries where cholera is present need to be vaccinated. Whole cell vaccines provide partial protection for 3 to 6 mo.
DTaP (diphtheria, pertussis toxoids, and acellular pertussis)†	At 2 mo, 4 mo, 6 mo, 15–18 mo, and 4–6 yr.	Every 10 yr for tetanus and diphtheria, esp. for those over 50. Persons who have received five doses of tetanus toxoid in childhood may not need a booster until age 50.	DTaP is the preferrred vaccine for all doses in the series. (DTP is no longer used.)
Haemophilus influenzae b (Hib)‡	At 2 mo, 4 mo, 6 mo, and 12–15 mo.	None	If PRP-OMP (Pedvax-HIB) is given at 2 and 4 mo, a 6-mo dose is not required.
Hepatitis A[§]	Two doses at least 6 mo apart.	None	For use in travelers to endemic nations, individuals at occupational risk for exposure, injection drug users, men who have sex with men, patients with chronic liver diseases, and populations where outbreaks are occurring.
Hepatitis B[‖]	Hep B-1 at birth to 2 mo; Hep B-2 at 1–4 mo; Hep B-3 at 6–18 mo.	None	Individuals not vaccinated in infancy may begin the series during any visit. All health-care workers should receive the series. A 2-dose formulation is available.

Influenza	All ages.	Annually. Available intranasally.	Recommended for the elderly, health care professionals, residents of long-term care facilities, and those of any age who have chronic disease of the heart or lungs, metabolic diseases such as diabetes, or immunosuppression.
Lyme disease	Three doses at 0, 1, and 12 mo. Use is recommended in endemic areas. Experience in the young and old is limited.	Unknown	Efficacy is 60–90% after three doses.
MMR (measles [live attenuated rubeola], mumps, rubella)¶	12–15 mo. Second dose by 4–6 yr.	Unimmunized children should receive the second dose no later than 11–12 yr.	Vaccine will usually prevent measles if given within 2 days after a child has been exposed to the disease. Not given to adults. Contraindicated for those with allergy to egg or neomycin, active infection, or severe immunosuppression.
Plague	See Comments.	See Comments.	Recommended for those traveling to Southeast Asia, persons who work closely with wild rodents in plague areas, and laboratory personnel working with *Yersinia pestis* organisms.
Pneumococcal vaccine, polyvalent	Should not be given to children under age 2 or to pregnant women.	None	Vaccine is effective against the 23 most prevalent types of pneumococci. Administered to those who have an increased risk of developing pneumococcal pneumonia. Included are those who have chronic diseases, have had a splenectomy, are in chronic care facilities, or are 65 years of age or older.
Polio (IPV [inactivated poliovirus])#	At 2 mo, 4 mo, 6–18 mo, and between 4–6 yr.	None	IPV is preferred over oral polio vaccine. (Oral polio vaccine caused 8–10 cases of polio annually and was discontinued in 2000.)

Table continued on following page

Vaccines* (Continued)

Name	Age Administered	Booster Schedule	Comments
Rabies	Five doses of 1 ml are given for post-exposure prophylaxis. Three doses of 1 ml are given on days 0–7, 21, and 28 for primary prevention.	None	Primary prevention should be given to veterinarians, animal handlers, and spelunkers. Secondary prophylaxis is given after significant exposures.
Rotavirus (oral)	At 2, 3, and 4 mo.	None	Prevents childhood diarrhea and dehydration. This vaccine has been discontinued because of risk and intussusception.
Typhoid	See Comments.	See Comments.	Immunization is indicated when a person has come into contact with a known typhoid carrier, if there is an outbreak of typhoid fever, or prior to traveling to an area where typhoid is endemic.
Varicella zoster (chickenpox, shingles)**	12–18 mo	None	Susceptible children with no history of chickenpox should be immunized at 11–12 yr to prevent adult disease.
Yellow fever	See Comments.	Every 10 years.	Vaccine should be given to all persons traveling or living in areas where yellow fever is present.

SOURCE: Advisory Committee on Immunization Practices, Centers for Disease Control and Prevention, Atlanta, GA, 2000.

NOTE: On October 22, 1999, the Advisory Committee on Immunization Practice (ACIP) recommended that Rotashield (rhesus rotavirus vaccine-tetravalent [RRV-TV]), the only U.S.-licensed rotavirus vaccine, no longer be used in the U.S. (*MMWR* Vol. 48, No. 43, November 5, 1999). Parents should be reassured that children who received rotavirus vaccine before July 1999 are not now at increased risk for intussusception. Use of trade names and commercial sources is for identification only and does not constitute or imply endorsement by the Centers for Disease Control and Prevention or the U.S. Department of Health and Human Services.

*This schedule indicates the recommended ages for routine administration of licensed childhood vaccines as of November 1, 1999. Any dose not given at the recommended age should be given as a "catch-up" vaccination at any subsequent visit when indicated and feasible. Additional vaccines may be licensed and recommended during the year. Licensed combination vaccines may be used whenever any components of the combination are indicated and the vaccine's other components are not contraindicated. Providers should consult the manufacturers' package inserts for detailed recommendations.

†The fourth dose of diphtheria and tetanus toxoids and acellular pertussis vaccine (DTaP) can be administered as early as age 12 months, provided 6 months have elapsed since the third dose and the child is unlikely to return at age 15–18 months. Tetanus and diphtheria toxoids (Td) is recommended at age 11–12 years if at least 5 years have elapsed since the last dose of diphtheria and tetanus toxoids and pertussis vaccine (DTP), DTaP, or diphtheria and tetanus toxoids (DT). Subsequent routine Td boosters are recommended every 10 years.

‡Three *Haemophilus influenzae* type b (Hib) conjugate vaccines are licensed for infant use. If Hib conjugate vaccine (PRP-OMP) (PedvaxHIB or ComVax) is administered at ages 2 months and 4 months, a dose at age 6 months is not required. Because clinical studies in infants have demonstrated that using some combination products may induce a lower immune response to the Hib vaccine component, DTaP/Hib combination products should not be used for primary vaccination in infants at ages 2, 4, or 6 months unless approved by the Food and Drug Administration for these ages.

§Hepatitis A vaccine (Hep A) is recommended for use in selected states and regions. Information is available from local public health authorities and *MMWR* Vol. 48, No. RR-12, October 1, 1999.

|| Infants born to hepatitis B surface antigen (HBsAg)-negative mothers should receive the first dose of hepatitis B vaccine (Hep B) by age 2 months. The second dose should be administered at least 1 month after the first dose. The third dose should be administered at least 4 months after the first dose and at least 2 months after the second dose, but not before age 6 months. Infants born to HBsAg-positive mothers should receive Hep B and 0.5 ml hepatitis B immune globulin (HBIG) within 12 hours of birth at separate sites. The second dose is recommended at age 1–2 months and the third dose at age 6 months. Infants born to mothers whose HBsAg status is unknown should receive Hep B within 12 hours of birth. Maternal blood should be drawn at delivery to determine the mother's HBsAg status; if the HBsAg test is positive, the infant should receive HBIG as soon as possible (no later than age 1 week). All children and adolescents (through age 18 years) who have not been vaccinated against hepatitis B may begin the series during any visit. Providers should make special efforts to vaccinate children who were born in or whose parents were born in areas of the world where hepatitis B virus infection is moderately or highly endemic.

¶The second dose of measles, mumps, and rubella vaccine (MMR) is recommended routinely at age 4–6 years but may be administered during any visit, provided at least 4 weeks have elapsed since receipt of the first dose and that both doses are administered beginning at or after age 12 months. Those who previously have not received the second dose should complete the schedule no later than the routine visit to a health care provider at age 11–12 years.

#To eliminate the risk for vaccine-associated paralytic poliomyelitis (VAPP), an all-inactivated poliovirus vaccine (IPV) schedule is now recommended for routine childhood polio vaccination in the U.S. All children should receive four doses of IPV: at age 2 months, age 4 months, between ages 6 and 18 months, and between ages 4 and 6 years. Oral poliovirus vaccine (OPV) (if available) may be used only for the following special circumstances: (1) mass vaccination campaigns to control outbreaks of paralytic polio; (2) unvaccinated children who will be traveling in <4 weeks to areas where polio is endemic or epidemic; and (3) children of parents who do not accept the recommended number of vaccine injections. Children of parents who do not accept the recommended number of vaccine injections may receive OPV only for the third or fourth dose or both; in this situation, health care providers should administer OPV only after discussing the risk for VAPP with parents or caregivers. During the transition to an all-IPV schedule, recommendations for the use of remaining OPV supplies in physicians' offices and clinics have been issued by the American Academy of Pediatrics (*Pediatrics* Vol. 104, No. 6, December 1999).

**Varicella (Var) vaccine is recommended at any visit on or after the first birthday for susceptible children, that is, those who lack a reliable history of chickenpox (as judged by a health care provider) and who have not been vaccinated. Susceptible persons aged ≥13 years should receive two doses given at least 4 weeks apart.

edible v. A genetically manipulated food containing organisms or related antigens that may provide active immunity against infection. In one research trial of edible vaccines, individuals who ate an uncooked potato containing antigens from *Escherichia coli* bacteria developed antibodies against the bacteria.

v. extraimmunization The giving of excessive or repetitive doses of vaccines to children or adults, usually because of incomplete or inaccurate recordkeeping.

Haemophilus influenzae type b v. ABBR: HIB. A vaccine created by combining purified polysaccharide antigen from the *H. influenzae* bacteria and a carrier protein. It reduces the risks of childhood epiglottitis, meningitis, and other diseases caused by *H. influenzae*.

hepatitis B v. A vaccine prepared from hepatitis B protein antigen produced by genetically engineered yeast.

heterologous v. A vaccine derived from an organism different from the organism against which the vaccine is used.

homologous v. Autogenous v.

human diploid cell rabies v. ABBR: HDCV. An inactivated virus vaccine prepared from fixed rabies virus grown in human diploid cell tissue culture.

inactivated poliovirus v. An injectable vaccine made from three types of inactivated polioviruses. SYN: *Salk v.*

influenza virus v. A polyvalent vaccine containing inactivated antigenic variants of the influenza virus (types A and B either individually or combined) for annual usage. It prevents epidemic disease and the morbidity and mortality caused by influenza virus, esp. in the aged and persons with chronic illnesses. The vaccine is reformulated each year to match the strains of influenza present in the population.

killed v. A vaccine prepared from dead microorganisms. This type of vaccine is used to prevent disease caused by highly virulent microbes.

live attenuated measles (rubeola) virus v. A vaccine prepared from live strains of the measles virus. It is the preferred form except in patients who have one of the following: lymphoma, leukemia, or other generalized malignancy; radiation therapy; pregnancy; active tuberculosis; egg sensitivity; prolonged treatment with drugs that suppress the immune response (i.e., corticosteroids or antimetabolites); or administration of gamma globulin, blood, or plasma. Those persons should be given immune globulin immediately following exposure.

live measles and mumps virus v. A standardized vaccine containing attenuated measles and mumps viruses.

live measles and rubella virus v. A standardized vaccine containing attenuated measles and rubella viruses.

live measles, mumps, and rubella virus v. ABBR: MMR vaccine. A standardized vaccine containing attenuated measles, mumps, and rubella viruses.

live measles virus v. A standardized attenuated virus vaccine for use in immunizing against measles.

live oral poliovirus v. A vaccine prepared from three types of live attenuated polioviruses. In 1999, an advisory panel to the Centers for Disease Control and Prevention recommended that its routine use be discontinued. Because it contains a live, although weakened virus, it has caused 8 to 10 cases of polio each year. This risk is no longer acceptable now that the polio epidemic has been eliminated in the U.S. SYN: *Sabin v.*

live rubella virus v. An attenuated virus vaccine used to prevent rubella (German measles). All nonpregnant susceptible women of childbearing age should be provided with this vaccine to prevent fetal infection and the congenital rubella syndrome (i.e., possible fetal death, prematurity, impaired hearing, cataract, mental retardation, and other serious conditions). SEE: *rubella*.

meningococcal v. A vaccine prepared from bacterial polysaccharides from certain types of meningococci. Meningococcal polysaccharide vaccines A, C, Y, and W135 are available for preventing diseases caused by those serogroups. A vaccine for meningococcal serogroup B is not available. SEE: *meningitis, acute meningococcal*.

mumps v. A live attenuated vaccine used to prevent mumps. Its use should be governed by the same restrictions listed for live attenuated measles virus vaccine.

pertussis v. A vaccine against *Bordetella pertussis*. SEE: *DTaP v.*

plague v. A vaccine made either from a crude fraction of killed plague bacilli, *Yersinia pestis*, or synthetically from recombinant proteins. It is rarely used, except in a laboratory or for field workers in areas where plague is endemic.

polyvalent v. A vaccine produced from cultures of a number of strains of the same species.

polyvalent pneumococcal v. A vaccine that contains 23 of the known 83 pneumococcal capsular polysaccharides, and induces immunity for 3 to 5 years. This vaccine is estimated to protect against 90% of the pneumococcal types that produce serious disease in patients over 2 years of age. Children at high risk can be vaccinated at age 6 months and reinoculated at age 2 years.

The vaccine is particularly indicated in high-risk groups such as persons with sickle cell diseases, chronic debilitating disease, immunological defects, and the elderly.

PATIENT CARE: The importance of vaccinating older adults, children, and other patients at risk for pneumococcal disease is continually rising, as *Streptococcus pneumoniae* becomes more and more resistant to antibiotics.

pneumococcal 7-valent conjugate v. A pneumococcal vaccine used for active immunization of infants and toddlers. The vaccine contains antigens from 7 capsular serotypes of *Streptococcus pneumoniae*.

rabies v. A vaccine prepared from killed rabies virus used for pre-exposure immunization for persons at high occupational risk. Following a bite by a rabid animal, both the vaccine and rabies immune globulin, containing preformed antibodies, are given. SEE: *human diploid cell rabies v.; immnune globulin; rabies.*

reassortant v. A vaccine made by combining antigens from several viruses or from several strains of the same virus.

Sabin v. Live oral poliovirus v. SEE: *poliomyelitis*.

Salk v. Inactivated poliovirus v.

sensitized v. A vaccine prepared from bacteria treated with their specific immune serum.

smallpox v. A vaccine made from the lymph of cowpox vesicles obtained from healthy vaccinated bovine animals. NOTE: This vaccine is no longer used because smallpox has been eradicated worldwide.

tetanus v. A vaccine against *Clostridium tetani*. SEE: *DTaP v.*

typhoid v. One of two forms of vaccine against typhoid fever. Attenuated (weakened) live virus is used for an oral vaccine taken in four doses by adults and children over age 6; it provides protection for 5 years. This vaccine should not be given to persons taking antimicrobial drugs or to those with AIDS. A parenteral type of the vaccine, made from the capsular polysaccharide of *Salmonella typhi,* given to children at least 6 months old, requires two doses 4 weeks apart, is effective 55% to 75% of the time, and lasts 3 years.

typhus v. A sterile suspension of the killed rickettsial organism of a strain or strains of epidemic typhus rickettsiae.

varicella (chickenpox) v. A chickenpox vaccine prepared from attenuated virus. SEE: *chickenpox; herpes zoster*.

yellow fever v. A vaccine made from a live attenuated strain of yellow fever that protects against this tropical, mosquito-borne, viral hemorrhagic fever.

vaccinia (văk-sĭn′ē-ă) [L. *vaccinus,* pert. to cows] A contagious disease of cattle, produced in humans by inoculation with cowpox virus to confer immunity against smallpox. Papules form about the third day after vaccination, changing to umbilicated vesicles about the fifth day, and at the end of the first week becoming umbilicated pustules surrounded by red areolae. They dry and form scabs, which fall off about the second week, leaving a white pitted depression. SYN: *cowpox; vaccina*. SEE: *vaccination; varicella; variola*.

v. necrosum Spreading necrosis at the site of a smallpox vaccination; may be accompanied by similar necrotic areas elsewhere on the body.

vaccinia immune globulin Hyperimmune gamma globulin; the therapeutic agent of choice for dermal complications of vaccination for smallpox (i.e., eczema vaccinatum and progressive vaccinia).

NOTE: There is no longer a need for this material because smallpox has been eradicated worldwide.

vacciniform (văk-sĭn′ĭ-form) [L. *vaccinus,* pert. to cows, + *forma,* shape] Of the nature of vaccinia or cowpox.

vaccinogenous (văk″sĭn-ŏj′ĕn-ŭs) [L. *vaccinus,* pert. to cows, + Gr. *gennan,* to produce] Producing vaccine or pert. to its production.

vaccinostyle (văk-sĭn′ō-stīl) A pointed stylus used in vaccination.

vaccinotherapeutics (văk″sĭn-ō-thĕr″ă-pū′tĭks) Treatment by injection of bacterial vaccines.

vacuolar (văk′ū-ō-lăr) [L. *vacuum,* empty] Pert. to or possessing vacuoles.

vacuolar degeneration Swelling of cells with an increase in the number and size of vacuoles. SYN: *cloudy swelling*.

vacuolated (văk′ū-ō-lāt″ĕd) Possessing or containing vacuoles.

vacuolation (văk″ū-ō-lā′shŭn) Formation of vacuoles. SYN: *vacuolization*.

vacuole (văk′ū-ōl) [L. *vacuum,* empty] A membrane-bound cell organelle, which may contain water, secretions, enzymes, or the remains of ingested material.

autophagic v. A vacuole that contains recognizable fragments of the ribosomes or mitochondria.

contractile v. A cavity filled with fluid in the cytoplasm of a protozoan. The cavity is emptied by sudden contraction of its walls.

heterophagous v. A vacuole that contains substances that come from outside the cell.

plasmocrine v. A vacuole present in the cytoplasm of a secretory cell that is filled with crystalloid material.

rhagiocrine v. A vacuole present in

the cytoplasm of a secretory cell that is filled with colloid material.

vacuolization (văk″ū-ō-lĭ-zā′shŭn) [L. *vacuum*, empty] Vacuolation.

vacuum (văk′ū-ŭm) [L., empty] A space exhausted of its air content.

vacuum aspiration Evacuation of the uterine contents by means of a curet or catheter attached to a suction apparatus. The procedure is performed before the 12th week of gestation.

vacuum extractor A device for applying traction to the fetus during delivery by using a suction cup attached to the fetal head. Its use may be hazardous except in the hands of experts.

vacuum tube A vessel of insulating material (usually glass) that is sealed and has a vacuum sufficiently high to permit the free flow of electrons between the electrodes that extend into the tube from the outside. In England, it is called a vacuum valve.

vagabond's disease Discoloration of the skin caused by exposure and scratching owing to the presence of lice. SEE: *pediculosis corporis.*

vagal (vā′găl) [L. *vagus,* wandering] Pert. to the vagus nerve.

vagal attack Vasodepressor syncope.

vagi (vā′gī) Pl. of vagus.

vagin- SEE: *vagino-.*

vagina (vă-jī′nă) *pl.* **vaginae, vaginas** [L., sheath] **1.** A musculomembranous tube that forms the passageway between the cervix uteri and the vulva. **2.** A sheathlike part between the cervix and the vulva in the female mammal. SEE: illus.

ANATOMY: In the uppermost part, the cervix divides the vagina into four small vaulted cavities, called fornices: two lateral, the anterior, and the posterior. The bladder and urethra are adjacent to the anterior wall of the vagina, and the rectum is behind the posterior wall. The cavity of the vagina is a potential space; the walls are usually in contact with each other. Close to the cervix uteri the walls form a horizontal crescent shape, at the midpoint an H shape, and close to the vulva the shape of a vertical slit. The vaginal mucosa is stratified squamous epithelium that is very resistant to bacterial colonization. This lining is in folds called rugae, and the connective tissue external to it also permits stretching. The blood supply of the vagina is furnished from the inferior vesical, inferior hemorrhoidal, and uterine arteries. Except for the area close to the entrance, the vaginal tissue and mucosa contain few, if any, sensory nerve endings. The vagina is a passage for the insertion of the penis, for the reception of semen, and for the discharge of the menstrual flow. It also serves as the birth canal.

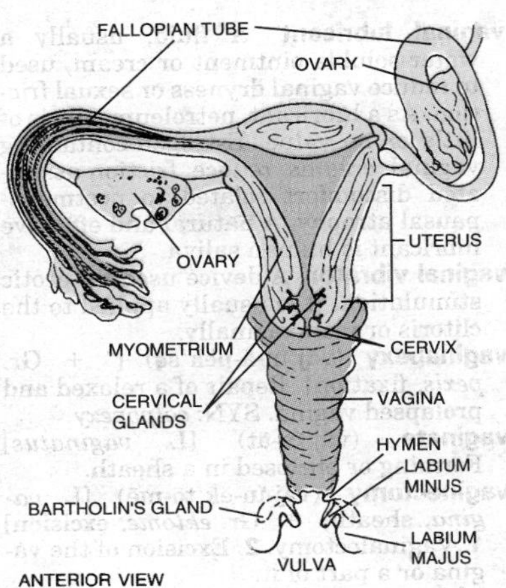

VAGINA AND OTHER FEMALE ORGANS

artificial v. A vagina constructed by plastic surgery for a patient whose vagina was removed for treatment of carcinoma or one who has congenital absence of the vagina.

bulb of v. The small erectile body on each side of the vestibule of the vagina. SEE: *vestibule of vagina.*

v. fibrosa tendinis A fibrous sheath surrounding a tendon that usually confines it to an osseous groove.

foreign bodies in v. SEE: *foreign body.*

v. masculina Prostatic utricle.

v. mucosa tendinis A synovial sheath that develops about a tendon.

septate v. A congenital condition in which the vagina is divided longitudinally into two parts. This division may be partial or complete.

vaginal (văj′ĭn-ăl) [L. *vagina,* sheath] Pert. to the vagina or to any enveloping sheath.

vaginal atrophy, postmenopausal Drying and shrinking of the vaginal tissues, related to the hormonal changes associated with menopause. Menopausal women who continue to engage in sexual intercourse during and following menopause have less vaginal atrophy than do those women who become sexually inactive. SEE: *hormone replacement therapy.*

vaginal birth after previous cesarean ABBR: VBAC. Vaginal childbirth subsequent to cesarean delivery of a previous pregnancy. The risk of uterine rupture is 1% to 2%.

vaginalectomy (văj″ĭn-ăl-ĕk′tō-mē) [″ + Gr. *ektome,* excision] Excision of the tunica vaginalis. SYN: *vaginectomy* (1).

vaginalitis (văj-ĭn-ăl-ī′tĭs) [″ + Gr. *itis,* inflammation] Inflammation of the tunica vaginalis testis.

vaginal lubricant A fluid, usually a water-soluble ointment or cream, used to reduce vaginal dryness or sexual friction. As a lubricant, petroleum jelly is of little or no value. Estrogen-containing vaginal creams reduce friction-associated discomfort related to postmenopausal atrophy. A natural and effective lubricant is human saliva.

vaginal vibrator A device used for erotic stimulation. It is usually applied to the clitoris or intravaginally.

vaginapexy (văj″ĭn-ă-pĕk′sē) [″ + Gr. *pexis,* fixation] Repair of a relaxed and prolapsed vagina. SYN: *colpopexy.*

vaginate (văj′ĭn-āt) [L. *vaginatus*] Forming or enclosed in a sheath.

vaginectomy (văj-ĭn-ĕk′tō-mē) [L. *vagina,* sheath, + Gr. *ektome,* excision] **1.** Vaginalectomy. **2.** Excision of the vagina or a part of it.

vaginismus (văj″ĭn-ĭz′mŭs) [L.] Painful spasm of the vagina from contraction of the muscles surrounding it, a condition that may interfere with coitus. SEE: *Nursing Diagnoses Appendix.*

PATIENT CARE: Patients with vaginismus need factual information and emotional support. Information about sexual concerns, practices, and responses should be geared specifically to the problem or question posed by the patient. Correcting myths and misinformation and teaching the woman about the range of normal sexual responses can be helpful. The patient should understand that the goal of instrumental dilator therapy is to gain control of the spasm. Specific information should be given about practicing relaxation techniques before dilator sessions, when one should switch from one size dilator to another, and what to do if problems occur. It helps to address a patient's emotional concerns to provide psychological support. The woman should be helped to attain security and comfort in her own sexual responses. Additional suggestions for patients may include advice about extending foreplay to increase vaginal relaxation and lubrication, as well as alternatives to dilator therapy, such as the intravaginal use of progressively heavier tampons.

vaginitis (văj-ĭn-ī′tĭs) [L. *vagina,* sheath, + Gr. *itis,* inflammation] **1.** Inflammation of a sheath. **2.** Inflammation of the vagina. SYN: *colpitis.* SEE: *sexually transmitted disease; Nursing Diagnoses Appendix.*

SYMPTOMS: The patient experiences vaginal discharge, sometimes malodorous and occasionally stained with blood; irritation or itching; increased urinary frequency; and pain during urination on examination. The vaginal mucous membrane is reddened and there may be superficial ulceration.

ETIOLOGY: This condition may be caused by microorganisms such as gonococci, chlamydiae, *Gardnerella vaginalis,* staphylococci, streptococci, spirochetes; viruses; irritation from fungal chemicals in douching; infection (candidiasis) caused by *Candida albicans;* protozoal infection (*Trichomonas vaginalis*); neoplasms of the cervix or vagina; or irritation from foreign bodies (e.g., a pessary or a retained tampon). Other rare causes are parasitic illnesses, or, in malnourished women, pellagra.

TREATMENT: Specific therapy is given as indicated. Improved perineal hygiene is emphasized by instructing in the proper method of cleaning the anus after a bowel movement, the proper use of menstrual protection materials, and the necessity of drying the vulva following urination.

PATIENT CARE: Aseptic technique is used to collect specimens. The health care provider supports the patient throughout the procedures, explaining each procedure and forewarning the patient of possible discomfort. If vaginitis is due to a sexually transmitted disease, the sexual partner should receive treatment together with the patient to prevent reinfection. Certain sexually transmitted vaginal infections are reported to local Public Health Service officials along with the patient's known sexual contacts.

v. adhaesiva Inflammation of the vagina causing adhesions between its walls.

atrophic v. Postmenopausal thinning and dryness of the vaginal epithelium related to decreased estrogen levels. SYN: *postmenopausal v.; senile v.*

Symptoms include burning and pain during intercourse. Estrogen replacement therapy, hormone replacement therapy, or application of topical estrogen restores the integrity of the vaginal epithelium and supporting tissues and relieves symptoms.

candidal v. A yeast infection caused by *Candida albicans.*

Symptoms include a thick, curdlike adherent discharge; itching; dysuria; and dyspareunia. The vulva and vagina are bright red. History usually reveals one or more risk factors: use of oral contraceptives or broad-spectrum antibiotics; immune defects; diabetes mellitus; pregnancy; or frequent douching. Diagnosis is established by the presence of hyphae and buds on a wet smear treated with 10% potassium hydroxide solution, and/or of growth of culture on Nickerson's or Sabouraud's media. Oral ketoconazole or topical applications of an imidazole (e.g., miconazole, clotrimazole, butoconazole, or ketoconazole), or both, promptly relieve symptoms and produce negative culture results after 3 to 7 days of therapy. In 20% to 30% of patients, however, infection recurs 1 month later. SYN: *moniliasis*.

***chlamydial* v.** The most common sexually transmitted vaginal infection in the U.S., caused by an obligate intracellular parasite, *Chlamydia trachomatis*. Chlamidial infection is also a major cause of pelvic inflammatory disease, tubal occlusion, infertility, ectopic pregnancy, nongonococcal urethritis, and ophthalmia neonatorum. Asymptomatic chlamydial infection has been implicated in the development of preterm labor and birth in high-risk women. Symptoms include a thin or purulent vaginal discharge, dysuria, and lower abdominal pain. Diagnosis is established by testing for specific monoclonal antibodies. Doxycycline is the drug of choice, except during pregnancy (it damages fetal bone and tooth formation). During pregnancy the infection is treated with erythromycin. SEE: *Chlamydia*.

***diphtheritic* v.** Vaginitis with membranous exudate caused by infection with *Corynebacterium diphtheriae*.

***emphysematous* v.** Vaginitis with gas-bubble formation in connective tissues.

***granular* v.** Vaginitis with cellular infiltration and enlargement of papillae.

***nonspecific* v.** A rare condition in which no particular factor or etiological agent is identifiable; a contact-related allergic response may be involved. The inflammation usually resolves spontaneously. Treatments include topical creams and ointments. SEE: *bacterial vaginosis*.

DIAGNOSIS: The diagnosis is established when clinical symptoms of vaginitis are present, but no organisms are found in laboratory specimens.

***postmenopausal* v.** Atrophic v.

***senile* v.** Atrophic v.

v. testis Inflammation of the tunica vaginalis of the testis.

***Trichomonas vaginalis* v.** An inflammation of the vagina caused by flagellate protozoa that infect the vagina, urethra, and Skene's ducts. Although the individual inflammatory response can include severe vulvar irritation and burning, dysuria, dyspareunia, and profuse, thin, "frothy," yellow-green to gray discharge, nearly 50% of infected women are asymptomatic. Sixty percent of the sexual partners of infected women share the infection. On inspection, the vulva may appear reddened and edematous. About 10% of infected women exhibit characteristic "strawberry patches" in the upper vagina and upper cervix. Diagnosis is based on seeing the highly motile organism with three to five flagella in a saline wet smear. Oral metronidazole is the organism-specific treatment. SEE: *Trichomonas*.

vagino-, vagin- [L. *vagina*, sheath] Combining form meaning *vagina*.

vaginoabdominal (văj″ĭn-ō-ăb-dŏm′ĭn-ăl) [L. *vagina*, sheath, + *abdominalis*, abdominal] Rel. to the vagina and abdomen.

vaginocele (văj′ĭn-ō-sēl) [″ + Gr. *kele*, tumor, swelling] Vaginal hernia. SYN: *colpocele*.

vaginodynia (văj″ĭn-ō-dĭn′ē-ă) [″ + Gr. *odyne*, pain] Pain in the vagina.

vaginogenic (văj″ĭn-ō-jĕn′ĭk) [″ + Gr. *gennan*, to produce] Developed from or originating in the vagina.

vaginogram (văj′ĭn-ō-grăm) [″ + *gramma*, something written] A radiograph of the vagina.

vaginography (văj-ĭn-ŏg′ră-fē) [″ + Gr. *graphein*, to write] Radiography of the vagina. This technique is useful in diagnosing ureterovaginal fistula.

vaginolabial (văj″ĭn-ō-lā′bē-ăl) [″ + *labium*, lip] Rel. to the vagina and labia.

vaginometer (văj-ĭn-ŏm′ĕ-tĕr) [″ + Gr. *metron*, measure] A device for measuring the length and expansion of the vagina.

vaginomycosis (văj″ĭn-ō-mī-kō′sĭs) [″ + Gr. *mykes*, fungus, + *osis*, condition] A fungus infection (mycosis) of the vagina.

vaginopathy (văj″ĭ-nŏp′ă-thē) [″ + Gr. *pathos*, disease, suffering] Any disease of the vagina.

vaginoperineal (văj″ĭn-ō-pĕr-ĭ-nē′ăl) [″ + Gr. *perinaion*, perineum] Rel. to the vagina and perineum.

vaginoperineoplasty Plastic surgery involving the vagina and perineum.

vaginoperineorrhaphy (văj″ĭn-ō-pĕr″ĭ-nē-or′ăf-ē) [″ + ″ + *rhaphe*, seam, ridge] Repair of a laceration involving both the perineum and vagina. SYN: *colpoperineorrhaphy*.

vaginoperineotomy (văj″ĭn-ō-pĕr″ĭn-ē-ŏt′ō-mē) [″ + ″ + *tome*, incision] Surgical incision of the vagina and perineum; usually done to facilitate childbirth. SEE: *episiotomy*.

vaginoperitoneal (văj″ĭn-ō-pĕr″ĭ-tō-nē′ăl) Rel. to the vagina and peritoneum.

vaginoplasty (vă-jī′nō-plăs″tē) [″ + Gr. *plassein*, to form] Plastic surgery on the vagina.

vaginoscope (văj′ĭn-ō-skōp) [″ + Gr. *skopein*, to examine] An instrument for inspection of the vagina. This may be a speculum or an optical instrument.

vaginoscopy (văj″ĭn-ŏs′kō-pē) Visual examination of the vagina.

vaginosis, bacterial Inflammation of the vagina and upper genital tract caused by *Gardnerella vaginalis*. The diagnosis is confirmed by characteristic "fishy" odor produced when the vaginal discharge is mixed with 10% potassium hydroxide. A wet smear reveals vaginal epithelial cells that are heavily stippled with bacteria, called clue cells. Oral metronidazole or oral clindamycin is prescribed; intravaginal metronidazole gel and intravaginal clindamycin cream also are effective. Asymptomatic bacterial vaginosis during pregnancy has been implicated in causing preterm labor. During pregnancy, treatment with metronidazole plus erythromycin reduces the rate of preterm delivery in at-risk women. SEE: *Gardnerella vaginalis vaginitis*.

vaginotome (vă-jī′nō-tōm) [″ + Gr. *tome,* incision] An instrument for making an incision in the vaginal walls.

vaginotomy (văj″ĭ-nŏt′ō-mē) [″ + Gr. *tome,* incision] Incision of the vagina.

vaginovesical (văj″ĭ-nō-vĕs′ĭ-kăl) [″ + *vesica,* bladder] Rel. to the vagina and bladder. SYN: *vesicovaginal*.

vaginovulvar (văj″ĭn-ō-vŭl′văr) [″ + *vulva,* covering] Vulvovaginal.

vagitis (vă-jī′tĭs) [L. *vagus,* wandering, + Gr. *itis,* inflammation] Inflammation of the vagal nerve.

vagitus (vă-jī′tŭs) [L. *vagire,* to squall] The first cry of a newborn.

v. uterinus The crying of a fetus while still in the uterus.

v. vaginalis The cry of an infant with its head still in the vagina.

vagolysis (vā-gŏl′ĭ-sĭs) [L. *vagus,* wandering, + Gr. *lysis,* dissolution] Surgical destruction of the vagus nerve.

vagolytic (vā″gō-lĭt′ĭk) **1.** Concerning vagolysis. **2.** An agent, surgical or chemical, that prevents function of the vagus nerve.

vagomimetic (vā″gō-mĭ-mĕt′ĭk) [″ + Gr. *mimetikos,* imitating] Resembling action caused by stimulation of the vagus nerve.

vagosympathetic (vā″gō-sĭm-pă-thĕt′ĭk) [″ + Gr. *sympathetikos,* suffering with] The cervical sympathetic and vagus nerves considered together.

vagotomy (vā-gŏt′ō-mē) [″ + Gr. *tome,* incision] Section of the vagus nerve.

medical v. Administration of drugs to prevent function of the vagus nerve.

vagotonia (vā″gō-tō′nē-ă) [″ + Gr. *tonos,* tension] Hyperirritability of the parasympathetic nervous system. SEE: *sympatheticotonia*. **vagotonic,** *adj.*

vagotropic (vā″gō-trŏp′ĭk) [″ + Gr. *tropos,* a turning] Acting on the vagus nerve.

vagotropism (vā-gŏt′rō-pĭzm) [″ + ″ + *-ismos,* condition] Affinity for the vagus nerve, as a drug.

vagovagal (vā″gō-vā′găl) Concerning reflex activity mediated entirely through the vagus nerve (i.e., via efferent and afferent impulses transmitted through the vagus nerve).

vagrant (vā′grănt) [L. *vagrans*] **1.** Wandering from place to place without a fixed home. **2.** A homeless person who wanders from place to place.

vagus (vā′gŭs) *pl.* **vagi** [L., wandering] The 10th cranial nerve; a mixed nerve that arises from the medulla and has branches to many organs. Its impulses slow the heart rate, constrict the bronchioles, and increase peristalsis and digestive secretions. SEE: illus.; *cranial nerve*.

vagus pulse Decreased heart rate caused by the slowing action of stimuli from the vagus nerve. SEE: *vagotomy; vagotonia*.

vagusstoff (vā′gŭs-stŏf) [″ + Ger. *Stoff,* substance] Acetylcholine.

valence, valency (vā′lĕns, -lĕn-sē) [L. *valens,* powerful] **1.** The property of an atom or group of atoms causing them to combine in definite proportion with other atoms or groups of atoms. Valency may be as high as 8 and is determined by the number of electrons in the outer orbit of the atom. **2.** The degree of the combining power or replacing power of an atom or group of atoms, the hydrogen atom being the unit of comparison. The number indicates how many atoms of hydrogen can unite with one atom of another element.

Valentin's ganglion (văl′ĕn-tēnz) [Gabriel Gustav Valentin, Ger. physician, 1810–1883] A small ganglion at the junction of the middle and posterior branches of the superior dental plexus.

valerian (vă-lĕhr′ē-an) A perennial herb, *Valeriana officinalis,* used by alternative and complementary medical practitioners as a sedative and sleep aid. The drug acts by inhibiting the breakdown of gamma-aminobutyric acid in the brain. Persons habituated to the use of this agent may develop tachycardia, delirium, and other symptoms of dependence and withdrawal.

valgus (văl′gŭs) [L., bowlegged] Bent or turned outward, used esp. of deformities in which the most distal anatomical part is bent outward and away from the midline of the body, as talipes valgus or hallux valgus. SEE: *knock-knee; varus*.

valid [L. *validus,* strong] Producing the desired effect; correct.

validate To ensure that the item in question is valid and correct.

validation, consensual The process of testing thoughts, emotions, and behaviors with other human beings. The desired outcome is acknowledgment of similar viewpoints and feelings.

validity (vă-lĭd′ĭ-tē) **1.** The degree to which data or results of a study are correct or true. **2.** The extent to which a situation as observed reflects the true situation.

valine (văl′ēn, vā′lēn) An amino acid, $C_5H_{11}NO_2$, derived from digestion of proteins. It is essential in the diet, esp. for normal growth in infants.

valinemia (văl″ĭ-nē′mē-ă) Increased valine in the blood.

vallate (văl′āt) [L. *vallatus,* walled] Having a rim around a depression.

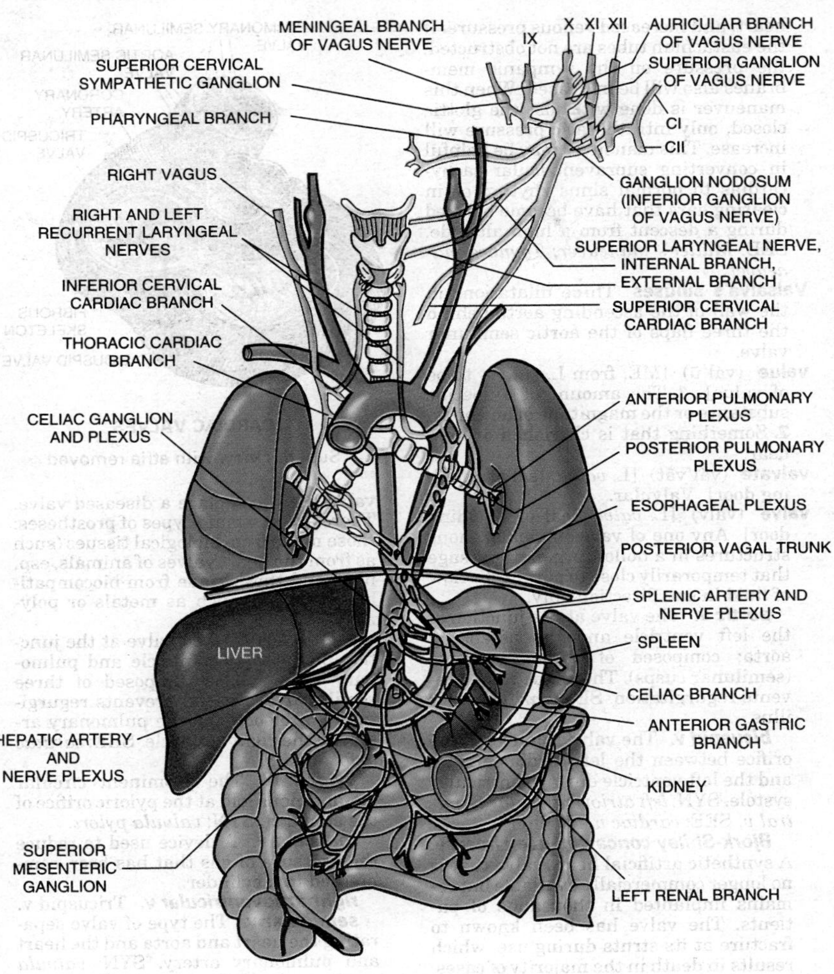

VAGUS NERVE (10TH CRANIAL)

vallate papilla A circumvallate papilla; one of a group of papillae forming a V-shaped row on the posterior dorsal surface of the tongue.

vallecula (văl-lĕk′ū-lă) [L., a depression] A depression or crevice.

v. cerebelli A deep fissure on the inferior surface of the cerebellum. SYN: *valley of cerebellum.*

v. epiglottica A depression lying lateral to the median epiglottic fold and separating it from the pharyngoepiglottic fold.

v. ovata A depression in the liver in which rests the gallbladder.

v. sylvii A depression marking the beginning of the fissure of Sylvius in the brain.

v. unguis A fold of skin in which the proximal and lateral edges of the nails are embedded.

Valleix's points (văl-lāz′) [François L. I. Valleix, Fr. physician, 1807–1855] In neuralgia, distinct painful points along the course of the affected nerve.

valley of cerebellum Vallecula cerebelli.

valley fever Coccidioidomycosis.

vallum unguis (văl′ŭm ŭng′gwĭs) The fold of skin overlapping the nail.

Valsalva's maneuver (văl-săl′văz) [Antonio Maria Valsalva, It. anatomist, 1666–1723] An attempt to forcibly exhale with the glottis, nose, and mouth closed. This maneuver causes increased intrathoracic pressure, slowing of the pulse, decreased return of blood to the heart, and increased venous pressure. If the eustachian tubes are not obstructed, the pressure on the tympanic membranes also will be increased. When this maneuver is done with just the glottis closed, only intrathoracic pressure will increase. This maneuver may be helpful in converting supraventricular tachycardias to normal sinus rhythm or in clearing ears that have become blocked during a descent from a high altitude. SEE: *Müller's maneuver; Toynbee maneuver*.

Valsalva's sinuses Three dilatations in the wall of the ascending aorta behind the three flaps of the aortic semilunar valve.

value (văl'ū) [ME. from L. *valere,* to be of value] **1.** The amount of a specific substance or the magnitude of an entity. **2.** Something that is cherished or held dear.

valvate (văl'vāt) [L. *valva,* leaf of a folding door] Valvular.

valve (vălv) [L. *valva,* leaf of a folding door] Any one of various membranous structures in a hollow organ or passage that temporarily close to permit the flow of fluid in one direction only.

aortic v. The valve at the junction of the left ventricle and the ascending aorta; composed of three segments (semilunar cusps). The aortic valve prevents regurgitation. SEE: *cardiac v.* for illus.

bicuspid v. The valve that closes the orifice between the left cardiac atrium and the left ventricle during ventricular systole. SYN: *left atrioventricular v.; mitral v.* SEE: *cardiac v.* for illus.

Bjork-Shiley concavoconvex heart v. A synthetic artificial heart valve that is no longer commercially available but remains implanted in thousands of patients. The valve has been known to fracture at its struts during use, which results in death in the majority of cases.

cardiac v. One of the four valves that prevent the backflow of blood as it passes into, through, and out of the heart. In order of the entry of the venous blood into the right atrium, they are right atrioventricular, pulmonary, left atrioventricular, and aortic. SEE: illus.

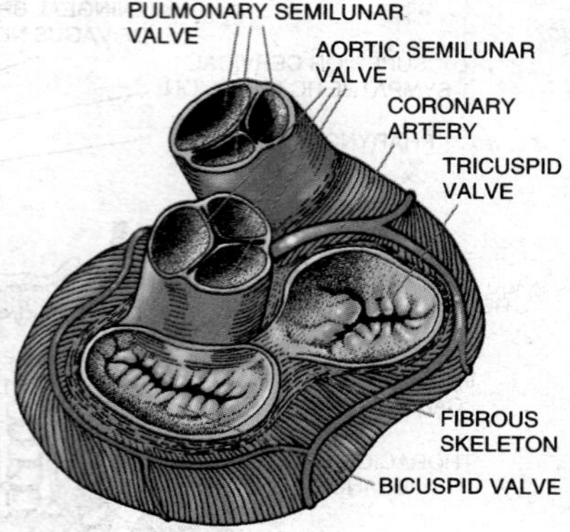

CARDIAC VALVES

Superior view with atria removed

coronary v. The coronary sinus valve at the entrance of the coronary sinus into the right atrium. SYN: *thebesian v.*

Houston's v. One of the mucosal folds of the rectum. SYN: *transverse plica of the rectum.*

ileocecal v. A projection of two membranous folds of the ileum of the small intestine into the cecum of the colon. It prevents backup of fecal material into the small intestine. SYN: *v. of Varolius; valvula coli.*

left atrioventricular v. Bicuspid v.

mitral v. Bicuspid v.

prosthetic heart v. A substitute valve used to replace a diseased valve. There are two main types of prostheses: those made from biological tissues (such as from the heart valves of animals, esp. pigs) and those made from biocompatible materials, such as metals or polymers.

pulmonary v. The valve at the junction of the right ventricle and pulmonary artery. It is composed of three semilunar cusps and prevents regurgitation of blood from the pulmonary artery to the right ventricle. SEE: *cardiac v.* for illus.

pyloric v. The prominent circular membranous fold at the pyloric orifice of the stomach. SYN: *valvula pylori.*

reducing v. A device used to reduce the pressure of gas that has been compressed in a cylinder.

right atrioventricular v. Tricuspid v.

semilunar v. The type of valve separating the heart and aorta and the heart and pulmonary artery. SYN: *valvula semilunaris.* SEE: *cardiac v.* for illus.

thebesian v. Coronary v.

tricuspid v. The valve that closes the orifice between the right cardiac atrium and right ventricle during ventricular systole. SYN: *right atrioventricular v.; valvula tricuspidalis.* SEE: *cardiac v.* for illus.

v. of Varolius Ileocecal v.

valvectomy Surgical excision of a valve, esp. a heart valve. SEE: *valvuloplasty.*

valvotomy (văl-vŏt'ō-mē) [" + Gr. *tome,* incision] Valvulotomy.

mitral balloon v. Expansion of a balloon in the orifice of a mitral valve as a means of treating mitral stenosis, instead of mitral valve replacement or commissurotomy. SYN: *valvuloplasty.*

valvula (văl'vū-lă) *pl.* **valvulae** [L., a small fold] A valve, specifically a small valve.

v. bicuspidalis Bicuspid valve.

v. coli Ileocecal valve.

v. pylori Pyloric valve.

v. semilunaris Semilunar valve.

v. tricuspidalis Tricuspid valve.

valvulae (văl′vū-lē) Pl. of valvula.

v. conniventes Circular plica.

valvular (văl′vū-lăr) [L. *valvula,* a small fold] Rel. to or having one or more valves. SYN: *valvate.*

valvulitis (văl″vū-lī′tĭs) [″ + Gr. *itis,* inflammation] Inflammation of a valve, esp. a cardiac valve.

valvuloplasty (văl′vū-lō-plăs″tē) Plastic or restorative surgery on a valve, esp. a cardiac valve.

percutaneous balloon v. The percutaneous insertion of one or more balloons across a stenotic heart valve. Inflating the balloons decreases the constriction. This technique has been used to treat mitral and/or pulmonic stenosis.

valvulotome (văl′vū-lō-tōm) [″ + Gr. *tome,* incision] An instrument for incising a valve.

valvulotomy (văl″vū-lŏt′ō-mē) The process of cutting through a valve. SYN: *valvotomy.*

vanadium (vă-nā′dē-ŭm) [*Vanadis,* a Scandinavian goddess] SYMB: V. A light gray metallic element; atomic weight, 50.941; atomic number, 23.

vanadiumism (vă-nā′dē-ŭm-ĭzm) Toxicity due to chronic exposure to vanadium. The consequences include bronchitis, pneumonitis, conjunctivitis, and anemia.

van Buren's disease (văn bū′rĕnz) [William Holme van Buren, U.S. surgeon, 1819–1883] Induration of the corpora cavernosa of the penis. SYN: *Peyronie's disease.*

vancomycin hydrochloride (văn′kō-mī″sĭn) A glycopeptide antibacterial drug used to treat infections with gram-positive organisms, such as methicillin-resistant *Staphylococcus aureus* (MRSA). It may occasionally produce exfoliative dermatitis as a side effect.

van den Bergh's test (văn″dĕn-bŭrgz′) [A. A. Hijmans van den Bergh, Dutch physician, 1869–1943] A test to detect the presence of bilirubin in blood serum or plasma.

van der Hoeve's syndrome [Jan van der Hoeve, Dutch ophthalmologist, 1878–1952] Conductive deafness caused by otosclerosis-like changes in the temporal bone. Blue sclerae and osteogenesis imperfecta are also present.

van der Waals forces [Johannes D. van der Waals, Dutch physicist, 1837–1923] The definite but weak forces of attraction between the nuclei of atoms of compounds. These forces do not result from ionic attraction, hydrogen bonding, or sharing of electrons, but rather from the motion of electrons in atoms and molecules.

Van der Woude's syndrome An autosomal dominant syndrome marked by cleft lip, palate, or both, paramedian pits of the lower lip, hypodontia, and missing second premolar teeth. SYN: *cleft lip–cleft palate syndrome; lip-pit syndrome.*

vanilla (vă-nĭl′ă) [Sp. *vainilla,* little sheath] Any one of a group of tropical orchids. The cured seed pods of *Vanilla planifolia* contain an aromatic substance, also called vanilla, that is used for flavoring.

vanillin A crystalline compound found in vanilla pods or produced synthetically; used for flavoring foods and in pharmaceuticals.

vanillism (vă-nĭl′ĭzm) Irritation of the skin, mucous membranes, and conjunctiva sometimes experienced by workers handling raw vanilla. It is caused by a mite.

vanillylmandelic acid ABBR: VMA. 3-methoxy-4-hydroxymandelic acid. Metabolic product of catecholamines representing approx. 90% of the metabolites of catecholamines epinephrine and norepinephrine. VMA's are secreted in the urine. Persons with pheochromocytoma produce excess amounts of catecholamines; thus, increased amounts of VMA are present in their urine.

vanishing twin Fetal resorption in multiple gestation.

van't Hoff's rule [Jacobus Henricus van't Hoff, Dutch chemist, 1852–1911] The rule that the speed of chemical reactions is doubled, at least, for each 10°C rise in temperature.

vapor (vā′por) [L., steam] **1.** The gaseous state of any substance. **2.** A medicinal substance for administration by inhalation.

vaporization (vā″por-ī-zā′shŭn) [L. *vapor,* steam] **1.** The conversion of a liquid or solid into vapor. **2.** Therapeutic use of a vapor.

laser v. The resection of tissue by converting it to gas with laser energy.

PATIENT CARE: SEE: *laser safety.*

vaporize (vā′por-īz) To change a material to a vapor form.

vaporizer (vā′por-ī″zer) A device for converting liquids into a vapor spray.

vaporous (vā′por-ŭs) [L. *vapor,* steam] Consisting of, pert. to, or producing vapors.

vapor-permeable membrane A membrane, usually transparent, that is permeable to oxygen and water vapor. It may be prepared with an adhesive backing that will stick only to dry skin. This type of membrane has been used in covering wounds. The membrane must be applied properly without wrinkles and changed as often as necessary to prevent excess accumulation of fluid and bacteria under it.

Vaquez's disease (vă-kāz′) [Louis Henri

Vaquez, Fr. physician, 1860–1936] Polycythemia vera.

variability (văr″ē-ă-bĭl′ĭ-tē) The ability and tendency to change.

baseline v. Fluctations in the fetal heart rate, recorded by the electronic monitor, that reflect the status of the fetal autonomic nervous system. Absence of short-term variability (beat-to-beat changes) is a sign of fetal compromise. Long-term variability (wavelike undulations) occurs normally three to five times per minute. Increased long-term variability is common during fetal sleep but may reflect prematurity, congenital abnormalities such as anencephaly, or fetal response to drugs.

heart rate v. ABBR: HRV. Spontaneous fluctuations above and below the mean heart rate. A reduced HRV is associated with an increased incidence of total mortality and cardiac events in post-myocardial infarction patients, as well as in apparently healthy individuals, esp. elderly persons.

variable (vā′rē-ă-b′l) [L. *variare*, to vary] **1.** Any changing, measurable thing. In statistics, it is often possible to measure and graph the relationship of one variable to another (e.g., height and weight in the growing child). **2.** Changing in form, structure, behavior, or physiology.

dependent v. In epidemiology and research design, the condition or disease under study or the response part of a dose-response curve. In a study measuring smoking and heart disease, for example, heart disease would be the dependent variable.

independent v. In epidemiology and research, the agent that incites a response; the stimulus (e.g., the dose part of a dose-response curve). In the smoking and heart disease study cited in the entry called *dependent variable*, smoking would be the independent variable.

variance (văr′ē-ăns) [L. *variare*, to vary] A statistical index of the degree to which measurements in a data set are different from each other or deviate from the mean; the square of the standard deviation.

variant (văr′ē-ănt) That which is different from the characteristics of the other organisms or entities in a particular classification, esp. a disease, species, or physical appearance.

variate (vā′rē-āt) Variable (2).

variation (vā″rē-ā′shŭn) Differences between individuals of a certain species or class.

continuous v. Variation in which the difference between successive groups or individuals is quite small.

meristic v. Variation in number as opposed to kind.

varication (văr″ĭ-kā′shŭn) **1.** Formation of a varix. **2.** The condition of a varicosity.

variced Concerning a varix.

varicella (văr″ĭ-sĕl′ă) [L., a tiny spot] An acute infectious disease, usually seen in children under age 15, caused by varicella-zoster virus. Its hallmark is a rash, described clinically as having a "dewdrop on a rose petal" pattern, scattered in clusters ("crops") over the trunk, face, scalp, upper extremities, and sometimes the thighs. It is transmitted mainly by respiratory droplets that contain infectious particles; direct contact with a lesion and contaminated equipment also can spread the virus. Reactivation of the virus in adults causes shingles. SYN: *chickenpox*. SEE: illus; *herpes zoster; varicella-zoster immune globulin*.

SYMPTOMS: After an incubation period of 2 to 3 weeks (usually 13 to 17 days), patients develop fever, malaise, anorexia, and lymphadenopathy, followed by the appearance of an extremely pruritic (itchy) rash that starts flat and, over time, becomes a small blister on a red base, and then eventually forms crusted scabs. All three stages of the rash may be present on the body at one time. Varicella may be transmitted to others until all lesions are crusted over.

Occasionally, for example, when it occurs in adults or immunosuppressed children, chickenpox is complicated by superimposed bacterial pneumonia, encephalitis, or thrombocytopenia. Immunization with varicella vaccine provided during infancy is designed to prevent these complications.

ETIOLOGY: Chickenpox may strike individuals of any age who have not been previously been exposed to the virus. Epidemics are most frequent in winter and spring in temperate climates.

DIFFERENTIAL DIAGNOSIS: Impetigo, dermatitis herpetiformis, herpes zoster, and furunculosis may occasionally need to be distinguished from varicella, although usually the difference is obvious.

COMPLICATIONS: Secondary infections may occur, caused by scratching, which may result in abscess formation; at times, development of erysipelas or even septicemia may result. Occasionally, lesions in the vicinity of the larynx may cause edema of the glottis and threaten the life of the patient. Encephalitis is a rare complication. Varicella may be fatal in children with leukemia or children who are taking adrenocorticosteroids.

PREVENTION: Administration of varicella-zoster immune globulin (VZIg) within 72 hr of exposure will prevent clinical varicella in susceptible, healthy children. The following conditions should alert one to the possible need for use of VZIg: immunocompromised children; newborns of mothers who develop varicella in the period 5 days before to 48 hr after delivery; postnatal exposure of newborns (esp. those who are premature) to varicella; healthy adults who are susceptible to varicella and who have been exposed; pregnant women who have no history of having had varicella and who have had significant exposure. The use of VZIg in pregnant women will not prevent fetal infection or congenital varicella syndrome. Live attenuated vaccine is now available for general use.

CAUTION: Because severe illness and death have resulted from varicella in children being treated with corticosteroids, these children should avoid exposure to varicella.

TREATMENT: Otherwise healthy affected children are treated with diphenhydramine or hydroxyzine to reduce itch and acetaminophen to reduce fever. Children at increased risk for complications and immunosuppressed adults are given varicella-zoster immune globulin as prophylaxis after exposure. If varicella infection develops in immunosuppressed persons or pregnant women in the third trimester, intravenous acyclovir is administered. Immunization with varicella vaccination is recommended for those children who have not had chickenpox and have not previously received the immunization. SEE: *Standard and Universal Precautions Appendix.*

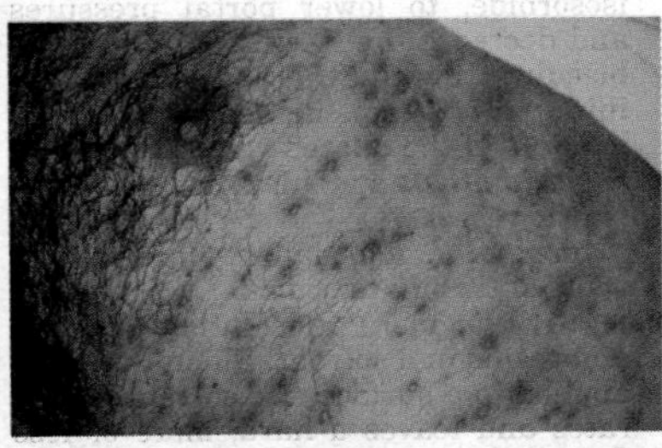

VARICELLA (CHICKENPOX)

v. gangrenosa Varicella in which necrosis occurs around the vesicles, resulting in gangrenous ulceration.

varicella-zoster immune globulin ABBR: VZIg. An immune globulin obtained from the blood of healthy persons found to have high antibody titers to varicella-zoster. SEE: *varicella.*

varicelliform (văr″ĭ-sĕl′ĭ-form) Resembling varicella. SYN: *varicelloid.*

varicelloid (văr″ĭ-sĕl′oyd) [″ + Gr. *eidos,* form, shape] Varicelliform.

varices (văr′ĭ-sēz) [L.] Pl. of varix.

variciform (văr-ĭs′ĭ-form) [L. *varix,* twisted vein, + *forma,* shape] Varicose.

varicoblepharon (văr″ĭ-kō-blĕf′ă-rŏn) [″ + Gr. *blepharon,* eyelid] Varicose tumor of the eyelid.

varicocele (văr′ĭ-kō-sēl) [″ + Gr. *kele,* tumor, swelling] Enlargement of the veins of the spermatic cord, commonly occurring above the left testicle. Varicoceles, present in more than 10% of males, are usually identified during adolescence. Male infertility has been linked to varicoceles, but a definitive causal relation has not been established. SYN: *varicole.*

SYMPTOMS: There is a dull ache along the cord and a slight dragging sensation in the groin. On examination, the vessels on the affected side of the scrotum are full, feel like a bundle of worms, and are sometimes purplish.

TREATMENT: Most varicoceles are asymptomatic and are followed conservatively. When they cause intolerable symptoms, or when they are found during the evaluation of men with infertility, they may be surgically repaired. However, there is no firm evidence that varicocele repair improves male fertility.

ovarian v. Varicosity of the veins of the ovarian or pampiniform plexus of the broad ligament.

utero-ovarian v. Varicosity of the veins of the ovarian (pampiniform) plexus and the uterine plexus of the broad ligament.

varicocelectomy (văr″ĭ-kō-sē-lĕk′tō-mē) [L. *varix,* twisted vein, + Gr. *kele,* tumor, swelling, + *ektome,* excision] Excision of a portion of the scrotal sac with ligation of the dilated veins to relieve varicocele.

varicography (văr″ĭ-kŏg′ră-fē) [″ + Gr. *graphein,* to write] Radiography of varicose veins after the injection of a contrast medium.

varicoid (văr′ĭ-koyd) [″ + Gr. *eidos,* form, shape] Resembling a varix.

varicole (văr′ĭ-kōl) Varicocele.

varicomphalus (văr″ĭ-kŏm′fă-lŭs) [″ + Gr. *omphalos,* navel] Varicose tumor of the navel.

varicophlebitis (văr″ĭ-kō-flē-bī′tĭs) [″ + Gr. *phleps,* vein, + *itis,* inflammation] Phlebitis combined with varicose veins.

varicose (văr′ĭ-kōs) [L. *varicosus,* full of dilated veins] Pert. to varices; distended, swollen, knotted veins. SYN: *variciform.*

varicose vein An enlarged, dilated superficial vein. This condition may occur in almost any part of the body but is most common in the lower extremities and in the esophagus. SEE: *Nursing Diagnoses Appendix.*

SYMPTOMS: Most varicose veins of the legs are asymptomatic, although they may be cosmetically undesirable. Esophageal varices and hemorrhoidal varices may bleed profusely. SEE: illus.

ETIOLOGY: The development of varicose veins of the legs is promoted and aggravated by pregnancy, obesity, and occupations that require prolonged standing. Esophageal varices are caused by portal hypertension that accompanies cirrhosis of the liver.

TREATMENT: In hemorrhage, elevation of the extremity and gentle but firm pressure over the wound will stop the bleeding. The patient should not be permitted to walk until the acute condition is controlled. Sclerotherapy, rubber band ligation, or octreotide may be used to control bleeding caused by hemorrhage from esophageal varices.

PATIENT CARE: The patient with lower extremity varicosities is taught to avoid anything that impedes venous return, such as wearing garters and tight girdles, crossing the legs at the knees, and prolonged sitting. After the legs have been elevated for 10 to 15 min, support hose are applied. The patient should not sit in a chair for longer than 1 hr at a time. Ambulation is encouraged for at least 5 min every hour. The patient should elevate the legs whenever possible, but no less than twice a day for 30 min each time, and should avoid prolonged standing. Signs of thrombophlebitis, a complication of varicose veins, include heat and local pain. If surgery is performed, elastic stockings or antithrombus devices are applied postoperatively and the foot of the bed is elevated above the level of the heart. Overweight patients need to lose weight. Patients with esophageal varices may be treated with oral nitrates and beta blockers and consultation with a gastroenterologist.

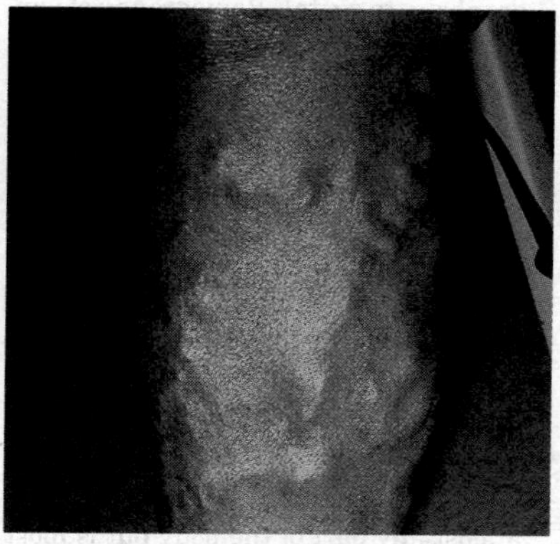

VARICOSE VEINS IN LEG

varicosis (văr″ĭ-kō′sĭs) [L.] Varicose condition of veins.

varicosity (văr″ĭ-kŏs′ĭ-tē) [L. *varix,* twisted vein] **1.** Condition of being varicose. **2.** Varix (1).

varicotomy (văr″ĭ-kŏt′ō-mē) [″ + Gr. *tome,* incision] Excision of a varicose vein.

varicula (văr-ĭk′ū-lă) [L., a tiny dilated vein] A small varix, esp. of the conjunctiva.

variety (vă-rī′ĕ-tē) [L., *varietas,* variety] A term used in classifying individuals in a subpopulation of a species.

variola (vă-rī′ō-lă) [L., pustule] Smallpox. **variolar** (-lăr), *adj.*

v. minor A mild form of smallpox with sparse rash and low-grade fever.

varix (vā′rĭks) *pl.* **varices** [L., twisted vein] **1.** A tortuous dilatation of a vein. SEE: *varicose vein.* **2.** Less commonly, dilatation of an artery or lymph vessel.

aneurysmal v. A direct communication between an artery and a varicose vein without an intervening sac.

arterial v. A varicosity or dilation of an artery.

chyle v. A varix of a lymphatic vessel that conveys chyle.

esophageal v. A tortuous dilatation of an esophageal vein, esp. in the distal portion. It results from any condition that causes portal hypertension, typically cirrhosis of the liver. SEE: *Müller's maneuver; Nursing Diagnoses Appendix.*

SYMPTOMS: If an esophageal varix bursts, massive hemorrhage occurs, and the patient may die within minutes.

TREATMENT: Medical treatment includes administration of a beta blocker, such as nadolol, with a nitrate, such as isosorbide, to lower portal pressures and decrease the likelihood of variceal bleeding. Invasive therapies include the injection of sclerosing agents or rubber banding of the dilated vein.

lymphaticus v. Dilatation of a lymphatic vessel.

turbinal v. Permanent dilatation of veins of turbinate bodies.

varnish (văr′nĭsh) A solution of gums and resins in a solvent. When these are applied to a surface, the solvent evaporates and leaves a hard, more or less flexible film. In dentistry, varnishes are used to protect sensitive tooth areas such as the pulp. SYN: *cavity v.*

cavity v. Varnish.

periodontal v. A protective coating applied to the outer tooth surface to alleviate pain and promote healing after deep scaling or curettage.

varolian (vă-rō′lē-ăn) [Costanzo Varolio (Varolius), It. anatomist, 1543–1575] Rel. to the pons varolii.

varolian bend The anterior extension of the hindgut on its ventral surface in the fetus.

varus (vā′rŭs) [L.] Bent or turned inward, used esp. of deformities in which the most distal part of the anatomy is turned toward the body's midline. There are many varus conditions. In *coxa varus,* the shaft of the femur turns inward with respect to the neck of the femur. In *genu varus,* either the femur or tibia turns inward at the knee, causing a bowlegged deformity. *Talipes varus* is a clubfooted condition in which the foot turns inward and the person walks on the outer border of the foot. SEE: *valgus.*

vas (văs) *pl.* **vasa** [L., vessel] A vessel or duct.

v. aberrans **1.** A narrow tube varying in length from 1½ to 14 in. (3.8 to 35.6 cm), occasionally found connected with the lower part of the canal of the epididymis or with the commencement of the vas deferens. **2.** A vestige of the biliary ducts sometimes found in the liver.

v. afferens An afferent vessel of a lymph node.

v. afferens glomeruli The afferent arteriole that conveys blood to the glomerulus of a renal corpuscle.

v. capillare A capillary blood vessel.

v. deferens The secretory duct of the testis, a continuation of the epididymis. This slim, muscular tube, approx. 18 in. (45.7 cm) long, transports the sperm from each testis to the ejaculatory duct, which empties into the prostatic urethra. SYN: *ductus deferens.* SEE: illus.; *genitalia* for illus.

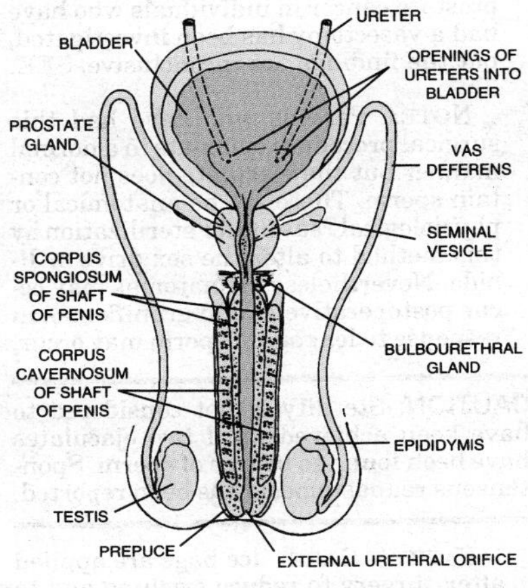

VAS DEFERENS AND OTHER MALE ORGANS

v. lymphaticum One of the vessels carrying the lymph.

v. prominens Blood vessel on the cochlea's accessory spiral ligament.

v. spirale A large blood vessel beneath the tunnel of Corti in the basilar membrane.

vasa (vā'să) [L. *vas,* vessel] Pl. of vas.

v. afferentia The lymphatic vessels entering a lymph node.

v. brevia Branches of the splenic artery going to the greater curvature of the stomach.

v. efferentia **1.** Lymphatics that leave a lymph node. **2.** The secretory ducts of the testis to the head of the epididymis.

v. praevia The blood vessels of the umbilical cord presenting before the fetus.

v. recta **1.** Tubules that become straight before entering the mediastinum testis. **2.** Capillary branches of the renal efferent arterioles, parallel to the loops of Henle.

v. vasorum Minute blood vessels that are distributed to the walls of the larger veins and arteries.

v. vorticosa Stellate veins of the choroid, carrying blood to the superior ophthalmic vein.

vasal (vā'săl) [L. *vas,* vessel] Rel. to a vas or vessel.

vasalgia (vă-săl'jē-ă) Pain in a vessel of any kind.

vascular (văs'kū-lăr) [L. *vasculum,* a small vessel] Pert. to or composed of blood vessels.

vascular endothelium The simple squamous epithelial tissue lining the blood vessels. It is a semipermeable barrier between the blood and the vascular smooth muscle, produces vasodilator chemicals, and may inhibit vasoactive substances and, in turn, produce vasodilator substances. Damage to the endothelium leads to increased production of prostaglandins and stimulates blood clotting.

vascularity (văs″kū-lăr'ĭ-tē) The state of being vascular.

vascularization (văs″kū-lăr-ī-zā'shŭn) [L. *vasculum,* a small vessel] The development of new blood vessels in a structure.

vascularize (văs'kū-lăr″īz) [L. *vasculum,* a small vessel] To become vascular by development of new blood vessels.

vascular ring A congenital abnormality in which an arterial ring encircles the trachea and esophagus. This causes signs of compression of their structures. Surgery may be required to relieve the symptoms.

vascular system The blood vessels: the arteries, capillaries, and veins. Pulmonary and systemic circulation are included.

vascular tuft One of the vascular processes on the chorion in the fetus at an early stage of development. SYN: *chorionic villi.*

vascular tumor Hemangioma.

vasculature (văs'kū-lă-tūr″) The arrangement of blood vessels in the body or any part of it, including their relationship and functions.

vasculitis (văs″kū-lī′tĭs) *pl.* **vasculitides** [″ + *itis,* inflammation] Inflammation of blood vessels. SYN: *angiitis*.

It is usually caused by direct invasion by infectious organisms, deposition of antigen-antibody immune complexes, or other immune-mediated events, radiation therapy, or trauma. Vasculitis due to immune complexes is seen in patients with systemic lupus erythematosus, rheumatoid arthritis, hepatitis B and C, serum sickness, and drug reactions. Vasculitis found in patients with inflammatory bowel disease, Wegener's granulomatosis, graft rejection, and temporal arteritis involves other immune-mediated processes. Vasculitis often affects the renal glomeruli, joints, cerebral vessels, testes, or respiratory system.

Vasculitis can affect large, medium-sized, and small blood vessels. When it is found in small blood vessels in the skin, characteristic rashes are found. Vasculitis is loosely classified by the size of the vessel involved. Takayasu's and giant cell arteritis involve large arteries, including the aorta and carotids. Polyarteritis nodosa and Kawasaki disease involve medium-sized vessels, and Wegener's granulomatosis, Henoch-Schönlein purpura, and microscopic polyangiitis involve small vessels, particularly in the kidney and respiratory tract. SEE: illus; *autoimmune disease; immune complex.*

SYMPTOMS: Although fever, pain, and malaise are common, the inflammatory changes of the blood vessels are seen primarily through the signs and symptoms associated with the organ or tissues involved. Vasculitis in superficial vessels may present as painful nodules. Inflammation of the glomerular capillaries of the kidney in small vessel vasculitis produces glomerulonephritis and decreased renal function. When blood vessels of the respiratory tract are involved, pneumonitis, sinusitis, and ulceration of the nasopharynx may result. Involvement of vessels in the heart leads to coronary artery disease and aneurysms.

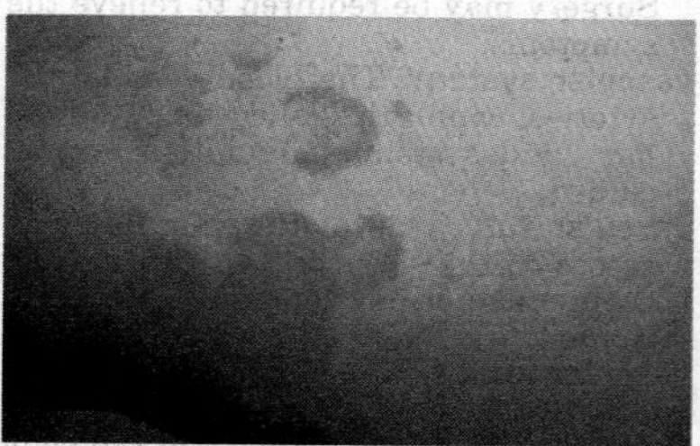

VASCULITIS

TREATMENT: Immunosuppressive therapy is used to treat most forms of autoimmune-mediated vasculitis. Vasculitis that results from infections may also be treated with antiviral or antibiotic drugs.

livedoid v. A vasculitis with blood-clotting that affects small blood vessels in the skin, esp. near the feet and ankles. The cause in most cases in unknown, but it may be associated with diseases such as antiphospholipid antibody syndrome, systemic lupus, or scleroderma.

rejection v. The inflammation that occurs when antigen-antibody complexes are deposited on the walls of small blood vessels in transplanted organs. Although the transplant rejection process is dominated by T-cell–mediated activities, antibodies also may form against the histocompatibility antigens on the transplanted organ and compromise its viability. SEE: *major histocompatibility complex.*

vasculogenesis (văs″kū-lō-jĕn′ĕ-sĭs) [″ + Gr. *genesis,* generation, birth] Development of the vascular system.

vasculomotor (văs″kū-lō-mō′tor) Vasomotor.

vasectomy (văs-ĕk′tō-mē) [L. *vas,* vessel, + Gr. *ektome,* excision] Removal of all or a segment of the vas deferens. Bilateral vasectomy is the most successful method of male contraception. The question of the possible increased risk of prostate cancer in individuals who have had a vasectomy has been investigated, but the findings are inconclusive. SEE: illus.

NOTE: Persons who have had this surgical procedure ejaculate in a normal manner but the ejaculate does not contain sperm. There are no anatomical or physiological reasons for sterilization by this method to alter the sex drive or libido. Nevertheless, hematomas may occur postoperatively, and granulomas in response to leakage of sperm may occur.

CAUTION: Sterility is not considered to have been achieved until two ejaculates have been found to be free of sperm. Spontaneous reanastomosis has been reported.

PATIENT CARE: Ice bags are applied after surgery to reduce swelling and to promote comfort. Sitz baths may promote comfort in the days immediately after the surgery. Surgery does not prevent sexually transmitted diseases.

vasectomy reversal Surgical procedure for the rejoining of the previously severed vas deferens. Although this procedure may be successful, the chance of success varies in published reports.

vasiform (văs′ĭ-form) [″ + *forma,* shape] Resembling a tubular structure or vas.

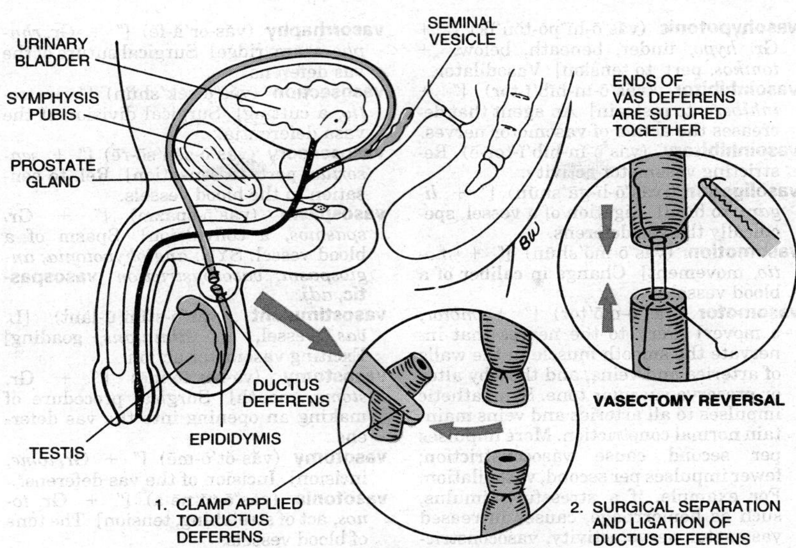

VASECTOMY AND ITS REVERSAL

vasitis (vă-sī′tĭs) Inflammation of the ductus deferens of the testicle.

vaso- [L. *vas,* vessel] Combining form meaning *vessel,* as a blood vessel.

vasoactive (văs″ō-ăk′tĭv) Affecting blood vessels.

vasoactive intestinal polypeptide ABBR: VIP. A peptide present in the mucosa of the gastrointestinal tract. One of its principal actions is to inhibit gastric acid secretion. Vasoactive intestinal polypeptide is also present in nerve fibers of the female genital tract.

vasoconstriction (văs″ō-kŏn-strĭk′shŭn) A decrease in the diameter of blood vessels, which decreases blood flow and raises blood pressure.

hypoxic pulmonary v. Narrowing of the small arterioles in the alveoli in response to hypoxia.

vasoconstrictive (văs″ō-kŏn-strĭk′tĭv) [″ + *constrictus,* bound] Causing constriction of the blood vessels.

vasoconstrictor (văs″ō-kŏn-strĭk′tor) [″ + *constrictor,* a binder] **1.** Causing constriction of the blood vessels. **2.** That which constricts or narrows the caliber of blood vessels, as a drug or a nerve.

vasodepression (văs″ō-dē-prĕsh′ŭn) [″ + *depressio,* a pressing down] Vasomotor depression or collapse.

vasodepressor (văs″ō-dē-prĕs′or) [″+ *depressor,* that which presses down] **1.** Having a depressing influence on the circulation, lowering blood pressure by dilatation of blood vessels. **2.** An agent that decreases circulation.

vasodilatation (văs″ō-dĭl-ă-tā′shŭn) [″ + *dilatare,* to enlarge] Dilatation of blood vessels, esp. small arteries and arterioles.

antidromic v. Vasodilatation resulting from stimulation of the dorsal root of a spinal nerve.

reflex v. Blood vessel dilation caused by stimulation of its dilator nerves or inhibition of its constrictor substance or nerves. This can be done by stimulating the sensory reflex arc.

vasodilation (văs″ō-dī-lā′shŭn) An increase in the diameter of blood vessels, which increases blood flow and lowers blood pressure.

vasodilative (văs″ō-dī′lā-tĭv) Causing dilation of blood vessels.

vasodilator (văs″ō-dī-lā′tor) [″ + *dilatare,* to enlarge] **1.** Causing relaxation of blood vessels. **2.** A nerve or drug that dilates blood vessels.

vasoepididymostomy (văs″ō-ĕp″ĭ-dĭd-ĭ-mŏs′tō-mē) [″ + Gr. *epi,* upon, + *didymos,* testicle, + *stoma,* mouth] The formation of a passage between the vas deferens and the epididymis.

vasofactive (văs″ō-făk′tĭv) [″ + *facere,* to make] Forming new blood vessels.

vasoganglion (văs″ō-găng′glē-ŏn) A dated term for a mesh or local network of blood vessels.

vasography (văs-ŏg′ră-fē) [″ + Gr. *graphein,* to write] Radiography of the blood vessels, usually after the injection of a contrast medium.

vasohypertonic (văs″ō-hī″pĕr-tŏn′ĭk) [″ + Gr. *hyper,* over, above, excessive, + *tonikos,* pert. to tension] Vasoconstrictor.

vasohypotonic (văs″ō-hī″pō-tŏn′ĭk) [″ + Gr. *hypo,* under, beneath, below, + *tonikos,* pert. to tension] Vasodilator.

vasoinhibitor (văs″ō-ĭn-hĭb′ĭ-tor) [″ + *inhibere,* to restrain] An agent that decreases the action of vasomotor nerves.

vasoinhibitory (văs″ō-ĭn-hĭb′ĭ-tor-ē) Restricting vasomotor activity.

vasoligation (văs″ō-lī-gā′shŭn) [″ + *ligare,* to bind] Ligation of a vessel, specifically the vas deferens.

vasomotion (văs″ō-mō′shŭn) [″ + *motio,* movement] Change in caliber of a blood vessel.

vasomotor (văs″ō-mō′tor) [″ + *motor,* a mover] Pert. to the nerves that innervate the smooth muscle in the walls of arteries and veins, and thereby alter or preserve vascular tone. Sympathetic impulses to all arteries and veins maintain normal constriction. More impulses per second cause vasoconstriction; fewer impulses per second, vasodilation. For example, if a stressful stimulus, such as hemorrhage, causes increased vasomotor nerve activity, vasoconstriction results, which limits blood loss and maintains blood pressure. SEE: *vasoconstrictor; vasodilator.*

vasomotor epilepsy Epilepsy with vasomotor changes in the skin.

vasomotor spasm Spasm of smaller arteries.

vasoneuropathy (văs″ō-nū-rŏp′ă-thē) Disease due to the combined effect of the vascular and nervous systems.

vasoneurosis (văs″ō-nū-rō′sĭs) [L. *vas,* vessel, + Gr. *neuron,* nerve, + *osis,* condition] A neurosis affecting blood vessels; a disorder of the vasomotor system.

vaso-orchidostomy (văs″ō-or″kĭd-ŏs′tō-mē) [″ + Gr. *orchis,* testicle, + *stoma,* mouth] Surgical connection of the epididymis to the severed end of the vas deferens.

vasoparesis (văs″ō-păr-ē′sĭs) [″ + Gr. *parienai,* to let fall] Partial paralysis or weakness of the vasomotor nerves.

vasopressin (văs″ō-prĕs′ĭn) Antidiuretic hormone.

vasopressin injection A sterile solution, in a suitable diluent, of material containing the polypeptide hormone having the properties of causing the contraction of vascular and other smooth muscle, and of antidiuresis.

vasopressor (văs″ō-prĕs′or) **1.** Causing contraction of the smooth muscle of arteries and arterioles. This increases resistance to the flow of blood and thus elevates blood pressure. **2.** An agent that stimulates contraction of smooth muscle of arteries and arterioles.

vasopuncture (văs′ō-pŭnk″chūr) [″ + *punctura,* prick] Puncture of the vas deferens.

vasoreflex (văs″ō-rē′flĕx) A reflex that alters the caliber of blood vessels.

vasorrhaphy (văs-or′ă-fē) [″ + Gr. *rhaphe,* seam, ridge] Surgical suture of the vas deferens.

vasosection (văs″ō-sĕk′shŭn) [″ + *sectio,* a cutting] Surgical division of the vasa deferentia.

vasosensory (văs″ŏ-sĕn′sō-rē) [″ + *sensorius,* pert. to sensation] Rel. to sensation in the blood vessels.

vasospasm (văs′ō-spăzm) [″ + Gr. *spasmos,* a convulsion] Spasm of a blood vessel. SYN: *angiohypotonia; angiospasm; vasoconstriction.* **vasospastic,** *adj.*

vasostimulant (văs″ō-stĭm′ū-lănt) [L. *vas,* vessel, + *stimulans,* goading] Exciting vasomotor action.

vasostomy (vă-sŏs′tō-mē) [″ + Gr. *stoma,* mouth] Surgical procedure of making an opening into the vas deferens.

vasotomy (văs-ŏt′ō-mē) [″ + Gr. *tome,* incision] Incision of the vas deferens.

vasotonia (văs″ō-tō′nē-ă) [″ + Gr. *tonos,* act of stretching, tension] The tone of blood vessels.

vasotonic (văs″ō-tŏn′ĭk) [″ + Gr. *tonikos,* pert. to tone] **1.** Pert. to the tone of a vessel. **2.** Causing vasotonia.

vasotrophic (văs″ō-trŏf′ĭk) [″ + Gr. *trophe,* nourishment] Concerned with the nutrition of blood vessels.

vasotropic (văs″ō-trŏp′ĭk) Affecting blood vessels.

vasovagal (văs″ō-vā′găl) Concerning the action of stimuli from the vagus nerve on blood vessels.

vasovasostomy (văs″ō-vă-sŏs′tō-mē) [″ + *vas,* vessel, + *stoma,* mouth] Rejoining of the previously severed ductus deferens of the testicle.

vasovesiculectomy (văs″o-vě-sĭk″ū-lěk′tō-mē) [″ + *vesicula,* tiny sac, + Gr. *ektome,* excision] Excision of the vas deferens and seminal vesicles.

vasovesiculitis (văs″ō-vě-sĭk″ū-lī′tĭs) [″ + *vesicula,* a tiny bladder, + Gr. *itis,* inflammation] Inflammation of the vas deferens and seminal vesicles.

vastus (văs′tŭs) [L., vast] **1.** Great, large, extensive. **2.** One of three muscles of the thigh.

Vater's ampulla (fă′tĕrz) [Abraham Vater, Ger. anatomist, 1684–1751] Former name for Vater's papilla.

Vater's corpuscles Pacinian corpuscles.

Vater's papilla The duodenal end of the drainage systems of the pancreatic and common bile ducts. Formerly called Vater's ampulla.

vault (vawlt) A part or structure resembling a dome or arched roof.

VBAC *vaginal birth after previous cesarean.*

VC *vital capacity.*

VD *venereal disease.*

VDH *valvular disease of the heart.*

VDRL *Venereal Disease Research Laboratories.*

vection (věk′shŭn) [L. *vectio,* a carrying] **1.** Transfer of disease agents by a vector from the sick to the well. **2.** Illusion of self-motion. This may be produced experimentally by having the subject seated within a drum that rotates while the subject remains stationary.

vectis (věk′tĭs) [L., pole] A curved lever for making traction on the presenting part of the fetus.

vector (věk′tor) [L., a carrier] **1.** Any force or influence that is a quantity completely specified by magnitude, direction, and sense, which can be represented by a straight line of appropriate length and direction. **2.** A carrier, usually an insect or other arthropod, that transmits the causative organisms of disease from infected to noninfected individuals, esp. one in which the organism goes through one or more stages in its life cycle. **3.** An agent such as a retrovirus that is used to introduce genetic material into the nucleus of a diseased cell in an attempt to cure a genetic illness or a malignancy.

biological v. An animal vector in which the disease-causing organism multiplies or develops prior to becoming infective for a susceptible person.

mechanical v. A vector in or upon which growth and development of the infective agent do not occur.

vectorcardiogram (věk″tor-kăr′dē-ō-grăm) [″ + Gr. *kardia,* heart, + *gramma,* something written] A graphic record of the direction and magnitude of the electrical forces of the heart's action by means of a continuous series of vector loops. Analysis of the configuration of these loops permits certain statements to be made about the state of health or diseased condition of the heart. At any moment the electrical activity of the heart can be represented as an electrical vector with a specific direction and magnitude. This is called the instantaneous cardiac vector. A series of these vectors may be established for the entire cardiac cycle. By joining the tips of these vectors with a continuous line, the vectorcardiogram loop is formed. The configuration so obtained may be projected on the frontal plane or viewed as a three-dimensional loop. Three vectorcardiogram loops are formed during each cardiac cycle—one for the electrical activity of the atrium; one for ventricular depolarization; one for ventricular repolarization.

spatial v. Depiction of the vectorcardiogram in three planes—frontal, sagittal, and horizontal.

vectorcardiography Analysis of the direction and magnitude of the electrical forces of the heart's action by a continuous series of loops (vectors) that represent the cardiac cycle.

vectorial (věk-tō′rē-ăl) [L. *vector,* a carrier] Rel. to a vector.

VEE *Venezuelan equine encephalitis.*

vegan (věj′ăn) A vegetarian who omits all animal protein from the diet.

veganism (věj′ă-nĭzm) A form of vegetarianism in which no forms of animal protein are consumed. The diet is devoid of meat, fish, poultry, eggs and dairy products.

vegetable (věj′ĕ-tă-bl) **1.** Pert. to, of the nature of, or derived from plants. **2.** A herbaceous plant, esp. one cultivated for food. **3.** The edible part or parts of plants that are used as food, including the leaves, stems, seeds and seed pods, flowers, roots, tubers, and fruits.

Vegetables are important sources of minerals and vitamins; provide bulk, which stimulates intestinal motility; and are sources of energy. Caloric value is indirectly proportional to water content. Copper is estimated at 1.2 mg/kg for leafy vegetables, and 0.7 mg/kg for nonleafy ones.

Plant and vegetable proteins individually do not contain the complete complement of essential amino acids. By combining vegetables, it is possible to obtain an adequate and balanced mixture of essential amino acids. For example, corn is low in lysine but has an adequate amount of tryptophan; beans are adequate in lysine but low in tryptophan. Although neither is a sufficient source of protein alone, in combination, they are an adequate protein source. Similarly rice and beans serve to complement the deficiencies in the other and together are a complete source of protein. SEE: *incaparina.*

All starches in vegetables must be changed to sugars before they can be absorbed. Dry heat changes starch to dextrin; heat and acid or an enzyme change dextrin to dextrose. In germinating grain, starch is changed to dextrin and dextrose. Fermented dextrose produces alcohol and carbon dioxide.

cruciferous v. A family of vegetables (including broccoli, brussels sprouts, cabbage, and cauliflower) named for their cross-shaped flowers. People who eat a diet rich in these vegetables are found to have a decreased incidence of cardiovascular diseases, strokes, and cancer, among other illnesses.

vegetal (věj′ĕ-tăl) **1.** Pert. to plants. **2.** Tropic or nutritional, esp. with reference to that part of an ovum which contains the yolk. SEE: *pole, vegetal.*

vegetarian (věj-ĕ-tā′rē-ăn) [from *vegetable,* coined 1847 by the Vegetarian Society] A person who does not eat animal flesh or, in some instances, any animal byproducts. Different approaches result in individual variation in whether fish, eggs, and/or dairy foods are accepted dietary components. Vegetarians must carefully plan their meals to ensure that they consume an adequately nutritive diet.

vegetarianism (věj-ě-tā′rē-ăn-ĭzm) [″ + Gr. *-ismos,* condition] The practice and philosophy of eating grains, nuts, vegetables and fruits, but not meats or animal flesh. Approaches to vegetarianism differ—some vegetarians eat fish, eggs, and/or dairy products, while others do not.

vegetate (věj′ě-tāt) [LL. *vegetare,* to grow] **1.** To grow luxuriantly with the production of fleshy or warty outgrowths such as a polyp. **2.** To lead a passive existence mentally or physically, or both; to do little more than eat and maintain autonomic body functions.

vegetation (věj-ě-tā′shŭn) A morbid luxurious outgrowth on any part, esp. wartlike projections made up of collections of fibrin in which are enmeshed white and red blood cells; sometimes seen on denuded areas of the endocardium covering the valves of the heart.

adenoid v. Fungus-like masses of lymphoid tissue in the nasopharynx.

vegetative (věj′ě-tā″tĭv) **1.** Having the power to grow, as plants. **2.** Functioning involuntarily. **3.** Quiescent, passive, denoting a stage of development.

vegetative state SEE: under *state.*

vegetoanimal (věj″ě-tō-ăn′ĭ-măl) Concerning plants and animals.

vehicle (vē′ĭ-kl) [L. *vehiculum,* that which carries] An inert agent that carries the active ingredient in a medicine (e.g., a syrup in liquid preparations).

veil (vāl) [L. *velum,* a covering] **1.** Any veil-like structure. **2.** A piece of the amniotic sac occasionally covering the face of a newborn infant. SYN: *caul.* **3.** Slight alteration in the voice in order to disguise it.

vein (vān) [L. *vena,* vein] A vessel carrying deoxygenated (dark red) blood to the heart, except for the pulmonary veins, which carry oxygenated blood. Veins have three coats: inner, middle, and outer. They differ from arteries in their larger capacity and greater number; also in their thinner walls, larger and more frequent anastomoses, and presence of valves that prevent backward circulation. The systemic veins consist of two sets, superficial or subcutaneous, and the deep veins, with frequent communications between the two. The former do not usually accompany an artery, as do the latter. The systemic veins may also be considered in three groups—those entering the right atrium through the superior vena cava, those through the inferior vena cava, and those through the coronary sinus. SEE: illus.; *circulation; vena.*

brachiocephalic v. The right and left veins, each formed by the union of the internal jugular with the subclavian vein.

innominate v. Brachiocephalic v.

velamen (vē-lā′měn) *pl.* **velamina** [L., veil] Any covering membrane.

v. nativum The skin covering the body.

v. vulvae Hottentot apron.

velamentous (věl″ă-měn′tŭs) Expanding like a veil, or sheet.

velamentum (věl″ă-měn′tŭm) *pl.* **velamenta** [L., a cover] A membranous covering.

velar (vē′lăr) [L. *velum,* a veil] Pert. to a velum or veil-like structure.

veliform (věl′ĭ-form) Velamentous.

vellus (věl′ŭs) [L., fleece] The fine hair present on the body after the lanugo hair of the newborn is gone.

velopharyngeal (věl″ō-fă-rĭn′jē-ăl) [L. *velum,* veil, + Gr. *pharynx,* throat] Concerning the soft palate and the pharynx.

Velpeau's bandage (věl-pōz′) [Alfred Velpeau, Fr. surgeon, 1795–1867] A special immobilizing roller bandage that incorporates the shoulder, forearm, and arm. SEE: *bandage* for illus.

Velpeau's deformity Deformity seen in Colles' fracture, in which the lower fragment is displaced backward.

velum (vē′lŭm) [L., veil] Any veil-like structure.

v. palatinum Soft palate.

vena (vē′nă) *pl.* **venae** [L.] A vein.

v. cava inferior The principal vein draining blood from the lower portion of the body. It is formed by junction of the two common iliac veins and terminates in the right atrium of the heart. SEE: *heart.*

v. cava superior The principal vein draining blood from the upper portion of the body. It is formed by the junction of the right and left brachiocephalic veins and empties into the right atrium of the heart. SEE: *heart.*

venacavography (vē″nă-kā-vŏg′ră-fē) Radiography of the vena cava during the injection of a contrast medium.

venae comitantes [L.] Two or more veins accompanying an artery. They are usually present with the deep arteries of the extremities.

venation The distribution of veins to an organ or structure.

venectasia (vē″něk-tā′zē-ă) [L. *vena,* a vein, + Gr. *ektasis,* dilation] Dilation of a vein. SYN: *phlebectasia.*

venectomy (vē-něk′tō-mē) [″ + Gr. *ektome,* excision] Phlebectomy.

veneer In dentistry, a man-made material, such as an acrylic resin, that can be bonded to the surface of a tooth. It is sometimes used for cosmetic reasons.

venene (vē-nēn′) A mixture of venoms from poisonous snakes.

venenosalivary (věn″ě-nō-săl′ĭ-věr″ē) Venomosalivary.

venenosity (věn″ě-nŏs′ĭ-tē) State of being venomous.

venenous (věn′ěn-ŭs) [L. *venenum,* poison] Poisonous.

venepuncture (vĕn′ē-pŭnk″chūr) [L. *vena,* vein, + *punctura,* a point] Venipuncture.

venereal (vē-nē′rē-ăl) [L. *venereus*] Pert. to or resulting from sexual intercourse.

venereal collar SEE: *leukoderma, syphilitic.*

venereal disease A term formerly used to describe any illness transmitted by intimate sexual contact. SEE: *Nursing Diagnoses Appendix.*

venereologist (vē-nēr″ē-ŏl′ō-jĭst) [″ + Gr. *logos,* word, reason] A doctor who specializes in the treatment of sexually transmitted diseases.

venereology (vē-nēr″ē-ŏl′ō-jē) The scientific study and treatment of sexually transmitted diseases.

venereophobia (vē-nēr″ē-ŏ-fō′bē-ă) [L.

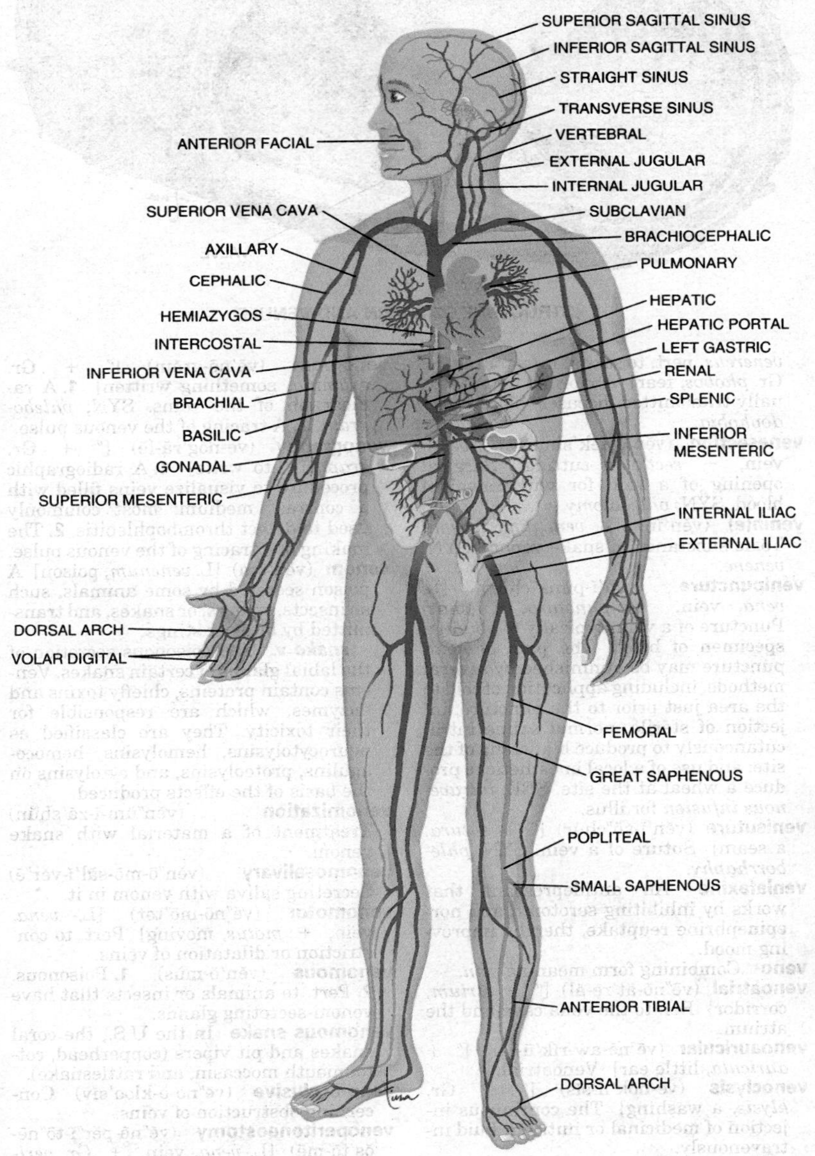

SYSTEMIC VEINS

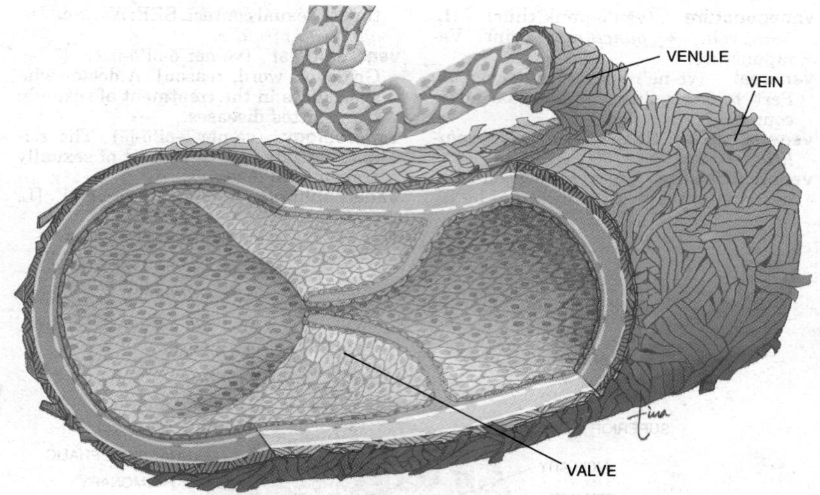

STRUCTURE OF A VEIN AND VENULE

venereus, pert. to sexual intercourse, + Gr. *phobos,* fear] Abnormal fear of sexually transmitted diseases. SYN: *cypridophobia.*

venesection (vĕn″ĕ-sĕk′shŭn) [L. *vena,* vein, + *sectio,* a cutting] Surgical opening of a vein for withdrawal of blood. SYN: *phlebotomy.*

venin(e) (vĕn′ĭn) [L. *venenum,* poison] Toxic substance in snake venom. SYN: *venene.*

venipuncture (vĕn′ĭ-pŭnk″chūr) [L. *vena,* vein, + *punctura,* a point] Puncture of a vein, typically to obtain a specimen of blood. The pain of venipuncture may be diminished by several methods, including application of cold to the area just prior to the puncture; injection of sterile, normal saline intracutaneously to produce blanching of the site; and use of a local anesthetic to produce a wheal at the site. SEE: *intravenous infusion* for illus.

venisuture (vĕn′ĭ-sū″chūr) [″ + *sutura,* a seam] Suture of a vein. SYN: *phleborrhaphy.*

venlafaxine An antidepressant that works by inhibiting serotonin and norepinephrine reuptake, thereby improving mood.

veno- Combining form meaning *vein.*

venoatrial (vē″nō-āt′rē-ăl) [″ + *atrium,* corridor] Rel. to the vena cava and the atrium.

venoauricular (vē″nō-aw-rĭk′ū-lăr) [″ + *auricula,* little ear] Venoatrial.

venoclysis (vē-nŏk′lĭ-sĭs) [″ + Gr. *klysis,* a washing] The continuous injection of medicinal or nutrient fluid intravenously.

venofibrosis (vē″nō-fī-brō′sĭs) Phlebosclerosis.

venogram (vē′nō-grăm) [″ + Gr. *gramma,* something written] **1.** A radiograph of the veins. SYN: *phlebogram.* **2.** A tracing of the venous pulse.

venography (vē-nŏg′ră-fē) [″ + Gr. *graphein,* to write] **1.** A radiographic procedure to visualize veins filled with a contrast medium; most commonly used to detect thrombophlebitis. **2.** The making of a tracing of the venous pulse.

venom (vĕn′ŏm) [L. *venenum,* poison] A poison secreted by some animals, such as insects, spiders, or snakes, and transmitted by bites or stings.

snake v. The poisonous secretion of the labial glands of certain snakes. Venoms contain proteins, chiefly toxins and enzymes, which are responsible for their toxicity. They are classified as neurocytolysins, hemolysins, hemocoagulins, proteolysins, and cytolysins on the basis of the effects produced.

venomization (vĕn″ŭm-ī-zā′shŭn) Treatment of a material with snake venom.

venomosalivary (vĕn″ō-mō-săl′ĭ-vĕr″ē) Secreting saliva with venom in it.

venomotor (vē″nō-mō′tor) [L. *vena,* vein, + *motus,* moving] Pert. to constriction or dilatation of veins.

venomous (vĕn′ō-mŭs) **1.** Poisonous. **2.** Pert. to animals or insects that have venom-secreting glands.

venomous snake In the U.S., the coral snakes and pit vipers (copperhead, cottonmouth moccasin, and rattlesnake).

veno-occlusive (vē″nō-ŏ-kloo′sĭv) Concerning obstruction of veins.

venoperitoneostomy (vē″nō-pĕr″ĭ-tō″nē-ŏs′tō-mē) [L. *vena,* vein, + Gr. *peritonaion,* peritoneum, + *stoma,* mouth] A one-way valve shunt that connects the peritoneum with the saphenous vein, permitting the escape of ascitic fluid into the venous circulation. SEE: *Le-Veen shunt*.

venosclerosis (vē″nō-sklĕ-rō′sĭs) [″ + Gr. *sklerosis,* to harden] Sclerosis of veins. SYN: *phlebosclerosis*.

venosinal (vē″nō-sī′năl) Concerning the vena cava and the right atrium of the heart.

venosity (vē-nŏs′ĭ-tē) [L. *vena,* vein] **1.** A condition in which there is an excess of venous blood in a part, causing venous congestion. **2.** Deficient aeration of venous blood.

venospasm (vē′nō-spăzm) [″ + Gr. *spasmos,* a convulsion] Contraction of a vein, which may follow infusion of a cold or irritating substance into the vein.

venostasis (vē″nō-stā′sĭs) [″ + Gr. *stasis,* standing still] The trapping of blood in an extremity by compression of veins, a method sometimes employed for reducing the amount of blood being returned to the heart.

venostat (vē′nō-stăt) [″ + Gr. *statikos,* standing] An appliance for performing venous compression.

venothrombotic (vē″nō-thrŏm-bŏt′ĭk) Having the property of inducing the formation of thrombi in veins.

venotomy (vē-nŏt′ō-mē) [″ + Gr. *tome,* incision] Incision of a vein.

venous (vē′nŭs) [L. *vena,* vein] Pert. to the veins or blood passing through them.

venous access device A specially designed catheter for use in gaining and maintaining access to the venous system. This device provides access for patients who require intravenous fluids or medications for several days or more (e.g., those having a bone marrow transplant or who are receiving long-term total parenteral nutrition). SEE: *venous port*.

venous admixture A mixture of venous and arterial blood.

venous blood The dark, poorly oxygenated blood in the veins.

venous cutdown Surgical incision in a vein to place a catheter to permit intravenous administration of fluids or drugs. It is used in patients with vascular collapse when gaining percutaneous access to the circulation is difficult; however, this procedure is usually tried only when subclavian, jugular, or femoral access cannot be established. SEE: illus.

venous hum A murmur heard on auscultation over the larger veins of the neck.

venous hyperemia Venosity (1).

venous port Part of a venous access device consisting of a subcutaneously implanted port through which medications are injected. Leading from the port is a catheter that is inserted in the cephalic, jugular, or subclavian vein. The catheter extends into the superior vena cava. The port has a self-sealing septum through which a needle is inserted to have access for administering medicines. The septum of the port is made to withstand from 1000 to 2000 punctures depending on the size needle used. Sterile technique is used each time a needle enters the port. The port permits unrestricted patient activity. Each time it is used care must be taken to be certain the line is open and that the catheter in the vein has remained in the proper position.

venous return The amount of blood returning to the atria of the heart.

venous sinus A large-capacity vessel that carries venous blood. Important venous sinuses are those of the dura mater draining the brain and those of the spleen.

venous sinus of sclera Schlemm's canal.

venovenostomy (vē″nō-vē-nŏs′tō-mē) [″ + ″ + Gr. *stoma,* mouth] The formation of an anastomosis of a vein joined to a vein.

vent (vĕnt) [O.Fr. *fente,* slit] An opening in any cavity, esp. one for excretion.

alveolar v. An opening between adjacent alveoli of the lung.

venter (vĕn′tĕr) [L., belly] **1.** A belly-shaped part. **2.** The cavity of the abdomen. **3.** The wide swelling part or belly of a muscle.

ventilation (vĕn″tĭ-lā′shŭn) [L. *ventilare,* to air] **1.** The movement of air into and out of the lungs. **2.** Circulation of fresh air in a room and withdrawal of foul air. **3.** In physiology, the amount of air inhaled per day. This can be estimated by spirometry, multiplying the tidal air by the number of respirations per day. An average figure is 10,000 L. This must not be confused with the total amount of oxygen consumed, which is on the average only 360 L/day. These volumes are more than doubled during hard physical labor.

abdominal displacement v. A noninvasive type of artificial ventilation that relies on displacement of the abdominal contents to move the patient's diaphragm.

airway pressure release v. A type of mechanical ventilation in which continuous airway pressure is intermittently released to a lower pressure.

alveolar v. The movement of air into and out of the alveoli. It is a function of the size of the tidal volume, the rate of ventilation, and the amount of deadspace present in the respiratory system. It is determined by subtracting the deadspace volume from the tidal volume and multiplying the result by the respiratory rate.

continuous positive-pressure v. A method of mechanically assisted pul-

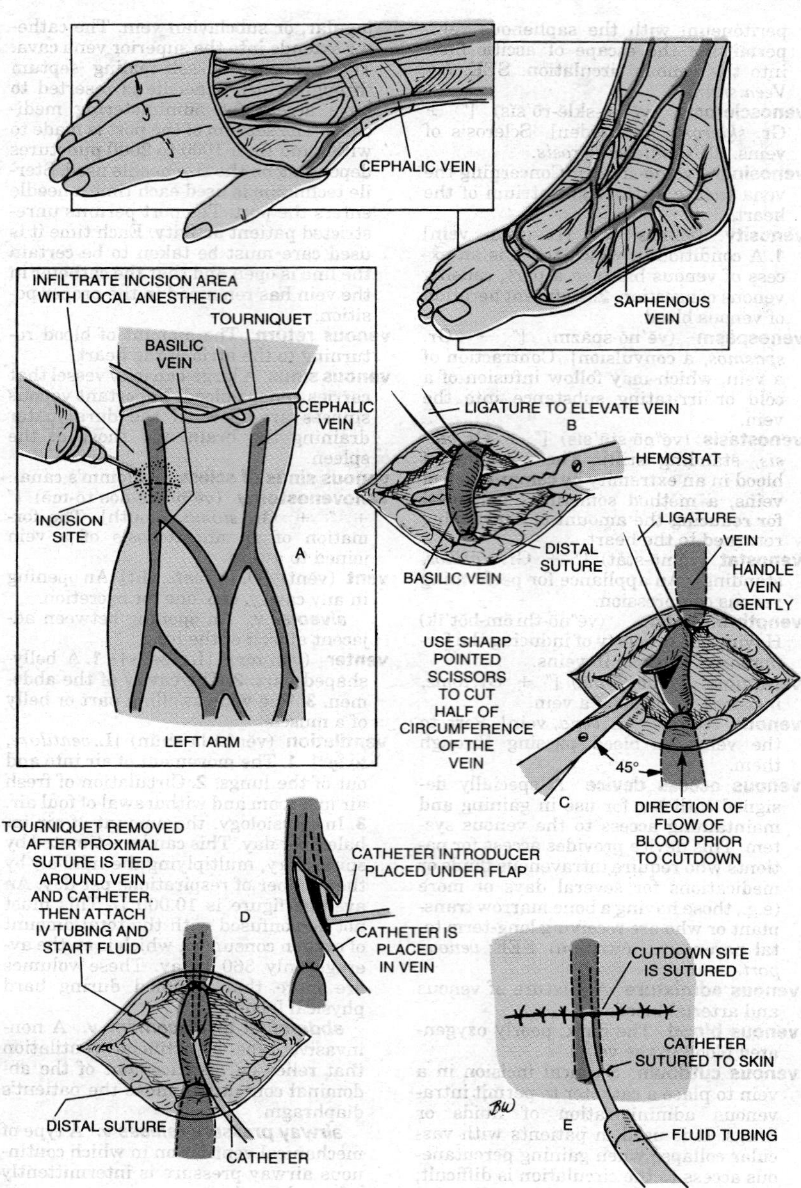

VENOUS CUTDOWN

monary ventilation. A device administers air or oxygen to the lungs under a continuous pressure that never returns to zero.

high-frequency jet v. A type of ventilation that continuously ventilates at 100 to 150 cycles/min; used in respiratory failure to provide continuous ventilation without the side effects of positive-pressure ventilation.

intermittent mandatory v. ABBR: IMV. Machine ventilation that delivers pressurized breaths at intervals while allowing for spontaneous breathing.

intermittent positive-pressure v. A mechanical method of assisting pulmonary ventilation, using a device that inflates the lungs under positive pressure. Exhalation is usually passive. SYN: *breathing, intermittent positive-pressure.*

liquid v. An experimental technique used in treating premature infants with surfactant-deficient lungs. Perfluorcarbons are used to carry oxygen to the lungs and remove carbon dioxide from them.

mandatory minute v. Ventilatory support that provides mechanical breaths when the patient's spontaneous breathing does not occur frequently enough.

maximum sustainable v. The normal maximum breathing pattern that can be maintained for 15 min (usually approx. 60% of maximum voluntary ventilation).

maximum voluntary v. The maximum amount of gas that can be ventilated into and out of the lungs in a voluntary effort in a given time, measured in liters per minute.

mechanical v. Any form of artificially supplied ventilation.

minute v. ABBR: MV. The volume of air inhaled and exhaled in 60 sec. SEE: *minute volume.*

noninvasive v. The use of airway support administered through a face ("nasal") mask instead of an endotracheal tube. Inhaled gases are given with positive end-expiratory pressure often with pressure support at a controlled rate and tidal volume. Numerous studies have shown this technique to be as effective, and better tolerated, than intubation and mechanical ventilation in selected patients with acute respiratory failure.

positive-pressure mechanical v. Mechanical ventilatory support that applies positive pressure to the airway. The objectives include improving pulmonary gas exchange, relieving acute respiratory acidosis, relieving respiratory distress, preventing and reversing atelectasis, improving pulmonary compliance, preventing further lung injury, and avoiding complications. Positive-pressure ventilation can be life saving, but complications such as toxic effects of oxygen, laryngeal injury, tracheal stenosis, alveolar injury, barotrauma, pneumonia, and psychological problems may occur. SEE: *pressure, positive end-expiratory.*

pressure support v. A type of assisted ventilation that supplements a spontaneous breath. The patient controls the frequency and the duration and flow of inspiration from the ventilator.

pulmonary v. The inspiration and expiration of air from the lungs.

synchronized intermittent mandatory v. ABBR: SIMV. Periodic assisted ventilation with positive pressure initiated by the patient and coordinated with spontaneous patient breaths. SEE: *intermittent mandatory v.*

transtracheal catheter v. An emergency procedure in which a catheter is placed percutaneously through the cricothyroid membrane and attached to a high-pressure, high-flow jet ventilator. This form of ventilation is used for patients who cannot be intubated.

ventilation coefficient The amount of air that must be respired for each liter of oxygen to be absorbed.

ventilator A mechanical device for artificial ventilation of the lungs. The mechanism may be hand operated (although this is unusual) or machine driven and automated.

automatic transport v. ABBR: ATV. A portable ventilator that can be used while transporting patients between locations. The ATV is designed for short-term use and often has volume and rate controls.

ventilator support, weaning from The act of gradually removing persons with reversible forms of respiratory failure who are receiving mechanical ventilation from that support. This may be done by alternating full ventilatory support with increasingly long periods of unassisted breathing. The timing and frequency of the weaning periods should be individualized to each patient. Usually by the time the patient can tolerate 2 hr of spontaneous breathing, ventilatory support may be discontinued. There are sophisticated tests for adequacy of oxygenation of the blood during the weaning process, but the most reliable method is information provided by the patient.

PATIENT CARE: Weaning from mechanical ventilation is done only in the stable patient in whom the acute precipitating event has been corrected. The respiratory therapist should review current arterial blood gas reports, breathing pattern, vital signs, and vital capacity before each attempt at weaning. The procedure should be described to the patient and he or she should be told what to expect and what his or her role in weaning will be. The nurse, physician, and respiratory therapist should reassure the patient that he or she will not be endangered by weaning trials or left alone during these periods. The nurse and respiratory therapist should also provide positive reinforcement regarding the patient's progress and the anticipated successful termination of support. Patient status and response to the procedure should be continuously evaluated.

ventilatory weaning response, dysfunctional ABBR: DVWR. A state in which a patient cannot adjust to lowered levels of mechanical ventilator support, which interrupts and prolongs the weaning process. SEE: *Nursing Diagnoses Appendix.*

ventouse (vĕn-toos′) [Fr.] A glass or glass-shaped vessel used in cupping.

ventrad (vĕn′trăd) [L. *venter,* belly, + *ad,* to] Toward the ventral aspect; the opposite of dorsad.

ventral (vĕn′trăl) [L. *ventralis,* pert. to the belly] Pert. to the belly; the opposite of dorsal. Hence, in quadrupeds, pert. to the lower or underneath side of the body; in humans, pert. to the anterior portion or the front side of the body.

ventralis (vĕn-trā′lĭs) [L.] Anterior, or closer to the front.

ventricle (vĕn′trĭk-l) [L. *ventriculus,* a little belly] **1.** A small cavity. **2.** Either of two lower chambers of the heart that, when filled with blood, contract to propel it into the arteries. The right ventricle forces blood into the pulmonary artery and thence into the lungs; the left pumps blood into the aorta to the rest of the body. **3.** One of the cavities of the brain filled with cerebrospinal fluid. SEE: illus.

aortic v. The left ventricle of the heart.

v. of Arantius The terminal depression of the median sulcus of the fourth ventricle of the brain.

fifth v. The cavity of the septum lucidum of the brain. It is between the two laminae of the septum lucidum.

fourth v. The cavity posterior to the pons and medulla and anterior to the cerebellum of the brain. It extends from the central canal of the upper end of the spinal cord to the aqueduct of the midbrain. Its roof is the cerebellum and the superior and inferior medullary vela. Its floor is the rhomboid fossa.

v. of larynx The space between the true and false vocal cords.

lateral v. The cavity in each cerebral hemisphere that communicates with the third ventricle through the interventricular foramen. It consists of a triangular central body and four horns, two inferior and two posterior.

left v. The cavity of the heart that receives blood from the left atrium and pumps it into the systemic circulation via the aorta.

Morgagni's v. The recess in the lateral wall on each side of the larynx between the vestibular and vocal folds.

pineal v. The pineal recess of the third ventricle of the brain.

right v. The cavity of the heart that receives blood from the right atrium and pumps it into the lungs via the pulmonary artery.

third v. The median cavity in the brain bounded by the thalamus and hypothalamus on either side, anteriorly by the optic chiasm; the floor is made up of

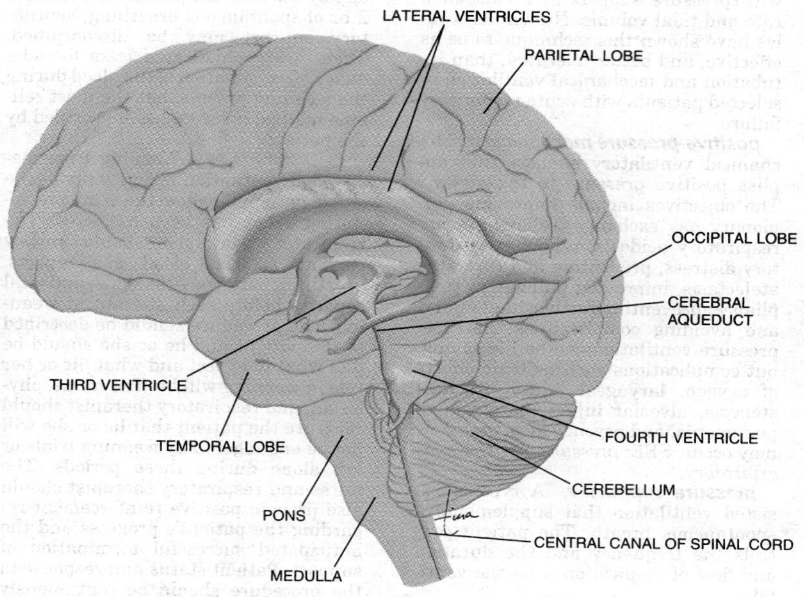

VENTRICLES OF THE BRAIN

Left lateral view

the tuber cinereum, mammillary body, the posterior perforated substance and tegmentum of the cerebral peduncle; the roof is the ependyma. Anteriorly, it communicates with the lateral ventricles, and posteriorly, with the aqueduct of the midbrain.

ventricular (vĕn-trĭk′ū-lăr) [L. *ventriculus,* a little belly] Pert. to a ventricle.

ventricular assist pumping Use of a device to temporarily replace the pumping action of a diseased or nonfunctioning heart.

ventricular compliance Distensibility or stiffness of the relaxed ventricle of the heart.

ventricular fold One of the false vocal cords or folds of mucous membrane parallel to or above the true vocal cords.

ventricular ligament A narrow band of fibrous tissue lying within each ventricular fold.

ventricular septal defect An abnormal opening in the septum between the ventricles of the heart that may produce shunting of blood from left to right, or other diseases.

ventriculitis (vĕn-trĭk″ū-lī′tĭs) [″ + Gr. *itis,* inflammation] Inflammation of a ventricle.

ventriculoatriostomy (vĕn-trĭk″ū-lō-ā″trē-ŏs′tō-mē) [″ + *atrium,* corridor, + Gr. *stoma,* mouth] Plastic surgery for the relief of hydrocephalus. Subcutaneous catheters are placed to connect a cerebral ventricle to the right atrium via the jugular vein. The catheters contain one-way valves so that cerebrospinal fluid can flow into the catheters, but blood may not flow back into the cerebral ventricle.

ventriculocisternostomy (vĕn-trĭk″ū-lō-sĭs″tĕr-nŏs′tō-mē) [″ + *cisterna,* box, chest, + Gr. *stoma,* mouth] Plastic surgery to create an opening between the ventricles of the brain and the cisterna magna.

ventriculocordectomy (vĕn-trĭk″ū-lō-kor-dĕk′tō-mē) [″ + Gr. *khorde,* cord, + *ektome,* excision] Surgery for the relief of laryngeal stenosis. The ventricular floor is removed, but the buccal processes are left in place.

ventriculogram (vĕn-trĭk′ū-lō-grăm) [″ + Gr. *gramma,* something written] **1.** A radiograph of the cerebral ventricles. **2.** Injection of a contrast medium into the cardiac ventricles during angiocardiography, in order to estimate ejection fraction and wall motion.

ventriculography (vĕn-trĭk″ū-lŏg′ră-fē) [″ + Gr. *graphein,* to write] **1.** An obsolete technique for visualizing the brain radiographically, that relied on the injection of air into the cerebrospinal fluid. It has been replaced by CT and MRI scans of the brain. **2.** Visualization of ventricles of the heart by radiograph after injection of a contrast material.

ventriculometry (vĕn-trĭk″ū-lŏm′ĕ-trē) [″ + Gr. *metron,* measure] The measurement of the intraventricular cerebral pressure.

ventriculonector (vĕn-trĭk″ū-lō-nĕk′tor) [L. *ventriculus,* a little belly, + *nector,* a joiner] Atrioventricular bundle.

ventriculopuncture (vĕn-trĭk′ū-lō-pŭnk″tūr) [″ + *punctura,* a point] The use of a needle to puncture a lateral ventricle of the brain.

ventriculoscopy (vĕn-trĭk″ū-lŏs′kō-pē) [″ + Gr. *skopein,* to examine] Examination of the ventricles of the brain with an endoscope.

ventriculostomy (vĕn-trĭk″ū-lŏs′tō-mē) [″ + Gr. *stoma,* mouth] Plastic surgery to establish communication between the floor of the third ventricle of the brain and the cisterna interpeduncularis. This is done to treat hydrocephalus.

ventriculosubarachnoid (vĕn-trĭk″ū-lō-sŭb″ă-răk′noyd) Concerning the cerebral ventricles and the subarachnoid spaces.

ventriculotomy (vĕn-trĭk″ū-lŏt′ō-mē) [″ + Gr. *tome,* incision] Surgical incision of a ventricle.

ventriculus (vĕn-trĭk′ū-lŭs) [L., a little belly] **1.** Ventricle. **2.** Stomach. **3.** A ventricle of the brain or heart.
 v. tertius Third ventricle.

ventrimeson (vĕn″trĭ-mēs′ŏn) [″ + Gr. *mesos,* middle] The median line on the ventral surface of the body.

ventripyramid (vĕn″trĭ-pĭr′ă-mĭd) [″ + Gr. *pyramis,* a pyramid] An anterior pyramid of the medulla oblongata.

ventro- Combining form meaning *abdomen* or *ventral* (anterior).

ventrodorsal (vĕn″trō-dor′săl) [″ + *dorsum,* back] In a direction from the front to the back.

ventrofixation (vĕn″trō-fĭks-ā′shŭn) [″ + *fixatio,* to fix] The suture of a displaced viscus to the abdominal wall.

ventroinguinal (vĕn″trō-ĭng′gwĭ-năl) [″ + *inguen,* groin] Concerning the ventral and inguinal regions.

ventrolateral (vĕn″trō-lăt′ĕr-ăl) [″ + *latus,* side] Both ventral and lateral.

ventromedial (vĕn″trō-mē′dē-ăl) [″ + *medianus,* median] Both ventral and medial.

ventroscopy (vĕn-trŏs′kō-pē) [L. *venter,* belly, + Gr. *skopein,* to examine] Examination of the abdominal cavity by illumination. SYN: *celioscopy.*

ventrose (vĕn′trōs) Having a swelling like a belly.

ventrosity (vĕn-trŏs′ĭ-tē) Having an enlarged belly; obesity.

ventrosuspension (vĕn″trō-sŭs-pĕn′shŭn) [″ + *suspensio,* a hanging] The fixation of a displaced uterus to the abdominal wall.

ventrotomy (vĕn-trŏt′ō-mē) [″ + Gr. *tome,* incision] Incision into the abdominal cavity. SYN: *celiotomy; laparotomy.*

ventrovesicofixation (věn″trō-věs″ĭ-kō-fĭks-ā′shŭn) [″ + L. *vesica,* bladder, + *fixare,* to fix] The suture of the uterus to the abdominal wall and bladder.

Venturi mask [Giovanni Battista Venturi, It. scientist, 1746–1822] A special mask for administering a controlled concentration of oxygen to a patient.

venturimeter (věn″tūr-ĭm′ĕ-tĕr) A device for measuring the flow of fluids through vessels.

venula (věn′ū-lă) [L., little vein] Venule.

venule (věn′ūl) [L., *venula,* little vein] A tiny vein continuous with a capillary. SYN: *venula*. SEE: *vein* for illus.

Venus, crown of A papular eruption around the hairline on the forehead caused by secondary syphilis.

Venus, mount of Mons pubis.

Venus's collar (vē′nŭs) [L., the Roman goddess of love] Pigmentation around the neck; an eruption due to syphilis.

verbigeration (věr-bĭj″ĕr-ā′shŭn) [L. *verbigerare,* to chatter] Repetition of words that are either meaningless or have no significance.

verbomania (věr″bō-mā′nē-ă) [L. *verba,* word, + Gr. *mania,* madness] The flow of talk in some forms of psychosis.

verdigris (věr″dĭ-grĭs) [O.Fr. *vert de Grece,* green of Greece] **1.** Mixture of basic copper acetates. **2.** The green-gray deposit of copper carbonate on copper and bronze vessels.

verdigris poisoning Poisoning due to ingestion of verdigris, which contains copper salts. Symptoms are identical to those caused by ingesting copper sulfate. SEE: *copper salts* in *Poisons and Poisoning Appendx.*

verdohemoglobin (věr″dō-hēm′ō-glōb″ĭn) A greenish pigment occurring as an intermediate product in the formation of bilirubin from hemoglobin.

Verga's ventricle (věr′găz) [Andrea Verga, It. neurologist, 1811–1895] A cleftlike space between the corpus callosum and the body of the fornix of the brain.

verge (věrj) An edge or margin.

anal v. The transitional area between the smooth perianal area and the hairy skin.

vergence (věr′jĕns) [L. *vergere,* to bend] A turning of one eye with reference to the other; may be horizontal (convergence or divergence) or vertical (intravergence or supravergence). SEE: *-phoria.*

Verheyen's stars (fĕr-hī′ĕns) [Philippe Verheyen, Flemish anatomist, 1648–1710] Starlike venous plexuses on the surface of the kidney below its capsule.

vermicidal (věr″mĭ-sī′dăl) [L. *vermis,* worm, + *cidus,* kill] Destroying worms parasitic in the intestines.

vermicide (věr′mĭ-sīd) **1.** Destroying worms. **2.** An agent that will kill intestinal worms.

vermicular (věr-mĭk′ū-lăr) [L. *vermicularis*] Resembling a worm.

vermiculation (věr-mĭk″ū-lā′shŭn) [L. *vermiculare,* to wriggle] A wormlike motion, as in the intestines. SEE: *peristalsis.*

vermicule (věr′mĭ-kūl) [L. *vermiculus,* a small worm] **1.** A small worm. **2.** Having a wormlike shape.

vermiculose, vermiculous (věr-mĭk′ŭ-lōs, věr-mĭk′ū-lŭs) [L. *vermicularis,* wormlike] **1.** Infested with worms or larvae. **2.** Wormlike.

vermiform (věr′mĭ-form) [L. *vermis,* worm, + *forma,* shape] Shaped like a worm.

vermiform appendix A long, narrow, worm-shaped tube connected to the cecum. It varies in length from less than 1 in. to more than 8 in. (2.5 to 20.3 cm) with an average of about 3 in. (7.6 cm). Its distal end is closed. It is lined with mucosa similar to that of the large intestine. Its inflammation is called appendicitis. The appendix contains many lymph nodules, but its function, if any, is not known. SEE: illus.

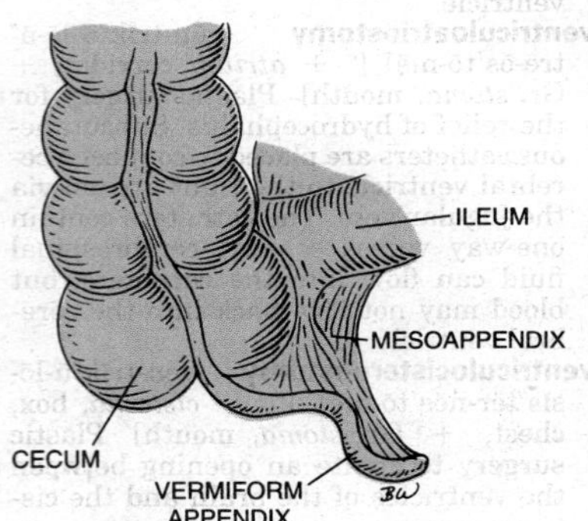

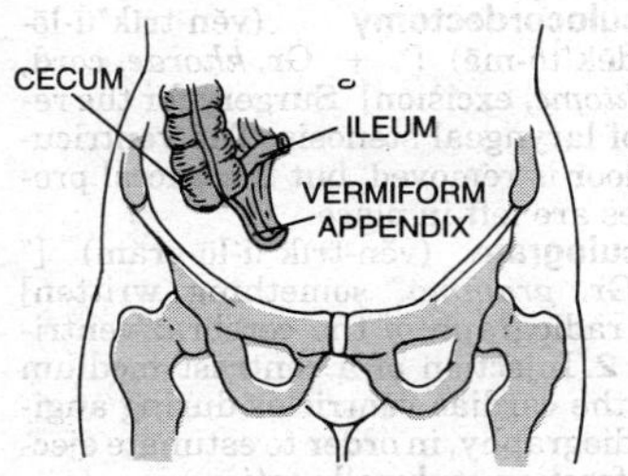

VERMIFORM APPENDIX

vermifugal (věr-mĭf′ū-găl) [″ + *fugare,* to put to flight] Expelling worms from the intestines.

vermifuge (věr′mĭ-fūj) Anthelmintic.

vermilionectomy (věr-mĭl″yŏn-ĕk′tō-mē) [″ + Gr. *ektome,* excision] Surgical removal of the vermilion border of the lip.

vermin (vĕr′mĭn) [L. *vermis,* worm] Small insects and animals such as mice, lice, or bedbugs that are annoying or cause destruction or disease.

verminal (vĕr′mĭ-năl) Concerning or caused by worms.

vermination (vĕr″mĭn-ā′shŭn) Vermin or worm infestation.

verminosis (vĕr″mĭn-ō′sĭs) [″ + Gr. *osis,* condition] Infestation with vermin.

vermiphobia (vĕr″mĭ-fō′bē-ă) [″ + Gr. *phobos,* fear] An abnormal fear of being infested with worms.

vermis (vĕr′mĭs) [L. worm] **1.** A worm. **2.** Vermis cerebelli.

v. cerebelli Median connecting lobe of the cerebellum.

inferior v. The anteroinferior portion of the vermis of the cerebellum, which includes the nodule, uvula, pyrami, and tuber.

superior v. The posterior dorsal portion of the vermis, which includes the folium, declive, culmen, and central lobule.

vernal (vĕr′năl) [L. *vernalis,* pert. to spring] Occurring in or pert. to the spring.

Vernet's syndrome (vĕr-nāz′) [Maurice Vernet, Fr. physician, b. 1887] Paralysis of the glossopharyngeal, vagus, and spinal accessory nerves on the opposite side of a lesion involving the jugular foramen.

vernix (vĕr′nĭks) [L.] Varnish.

v. caseosa A protective sebaceous deposit covering the fetus during intrauterine life, consisting of exfoliations of the outer skin layer, lanugo, and secretions of the sebaceous glands. It is most abundant in the creases and flexor surfaces. It is not necessary to remove this after the fetus is delivered. SEE: *sebum.*

verotoxin A heat-labile toxin produced by some types of *Escherichia coli.*

verruca (vĕr-roo′kă) *pl.* **verrucae** [L., wart] Wart.

v. acuminata A pointed, reddish, moist wart about the genitals and the anus. It develops near mucocutaneous junctures, forming pointed, tufted, or pedunculated pinkish or purplish projections of varying lengths and consistency. Venereal warts should be treated with topically applied podophyllum resin. SYN: *condyloma; genital wart; venereal wart.*

v. digitata A form of verruca seen on the face and scalp, possibly serving as a starting point of cutaneous horns. Several filiform projections with horny caps are formed, closely grouped on a comparatively narrow base that in turn may be separated from the skin surface by a slightly contracted neck.

v. filiformis A small threadlike growth on the neck and eyelids covered with smooth and apparently normal epidermis.

v. gyri hippocampi One of the small wartlike protuberances on the convex surface of the gyrus hippocampi.

v. plana A flat or slightly raised wart.

v. plantaris Plantar wart.

v. vulgaris The common wart, usually found on the backs of the hands and fingers; however, it may occur on any area of the skin. SEE: illus.

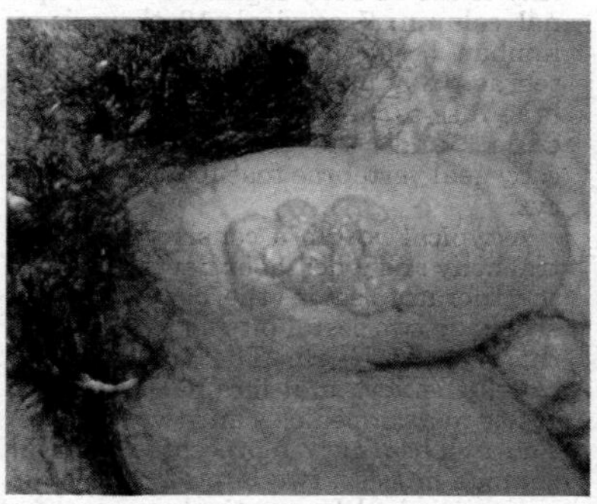

VERRUCA VULGARIS

verruciform (vĕ-roo′sĭ-form) [L. *verruca,* wart, + *forma,* shape] Wartlike.

verrucose, verrucous (vĕr′roo-kōs, vĕr-roo′kŭs) [L. *verrucosus,* wartlike] Wartlike, with raised portions.

verrucosis (vĕr″oo-kō′sĭs) [L. *verruca,* wart, + Gr. *osis,* condition] The condition of having multiple warts.

verruga peruana (vĕ-roo′gă pĕr-wăn′ă) [Sp., Peruvian wart] The eruptive second clinical stage of bartonellosis. Oroya fever is the first or febrile stage.

versicolor (vĕr′sĭ-kŏl″or) [L., of changing colors] **1.** Having many shades or colors. **2.** Changeable in color. SEE: *tinea versicolor.*

version (vĕr′zhŭn) [L. *versio,* a turning] **1.** Altering of the position of the fetus in the uterus. It may occur naturally or may be done mechanically by the physician to facilitate delivery. SEE: *conversion.* **2.** Deflection of an organ such as the uterus from its normal position.

bipolar v. Changing of the position of the fetus by combined internal and external manipulation.

cephalic v. Turning of the fetus so that the head presents.

combined v. Mechanical version by combined internal and external manipulation.

external v. Improving the presentation of an unengaged fetus by placing one's hands on the mother's abdomen and pushing, turning, or rotating the child.

internal v. Podalic v.

pelvic v. Turning a fetus from a transverse lie to a vertex (head down) presentation.

podalic v. Using two hands (one inside the uterus and one on the abdominal wall) to change a twin fetus from a breech to a vertex presentation. SYN: *internal v.*

spontaneous v. Unassisted conversion of fetal presentation by uterine muscular contractions.

vertebra (vĕr′tĕ-bră) *pl.* **vertebrae** [L.] Any of the 33 bony segments of the spinal column: 7 cervical, 12 thoracic, 5 lumbar, 5 sacral, and 4 coccygeal vertebrae. In adults, the five sacral vertebrae fuse to form a single bone, the sacrum, and the four rudimentary coccygeal vertebrae fuse to form the coccyx.

A typical vertebra consists of a ventral body and a dorsal or neural arch. In the thoracic region, the body bears on each side two costal pits for reception of the head of the rib. The arch that encloses the vertebral foramen is formed of two roots or pedicles and two laminae. The arch bears seven processes: a dorsal spinous process, two lateral transverse processes, and four articular processes (two superior and two inferior). A deep concavity, the inferior vertebral notch, on the inferior border of the arch provides a passageway for a spinal nerve. The successive vertebral foramina form the vertebral, or spinal, canal that encloses the spinal cord.

The bodies of successive vertebrae articulate with one another and are separated by intervertebral disks, disks of fibrous cartilage enclosing a central mass, the nucleus pulposus. The inferior articular processes articulate with the superior articular processes of the next succeeding vertebra in the caudal direction. Several ligaments (supraspinous, interspinous, anterior and posterior longitudinal, and the ligamenta flava) hold the vertebrae in position, yet permit a limited degree of movement. Motions of the vertebral column include forward bending (flexion), backward bending (extension), side bending (lateral flexion), and rotation. Lateral flexion and rotation motions are coupled so that whenever the vertebrae bend to the side, they also rotate and vice versa. SEE: *sacrum* for illus.

basilar v. The lowest of the lumbar vertebrae.

cervical v. One of the seven vertebrae of the neck.

coccygeal v. One of the rudimentary vertebrae of the coccyx.

v. dentata The second cervical vertebra. SYN: *axis; odontoid v.*

false v. Fixed vertebra.

fixed v. The sacral and coccygeal vertebrae that fuse to form the sacrum and coccyx.

lumbar v. One of the five vertebrae between the thoracic vertebrae and the sacrum.

v. magnum Sacrum.

odontoid v. V. dentata.

v. prominens The seventh cervical vertebra.

sacral v. One of the five fused vertebrae forming the sacrum. SEE: *sacrum* for illus.

sternal v. One of the segments of the sternum.

thoracic v. One of the 12 vertebrae that connect the ribs and form part of the posterior wall of the thorax. SEE: *spinal column* for illus.

true v. One of the vertebrae that remain unfused through life: the cervical, thoracic, and lumbar.

vertebral (vĕr′tĕ-brăl) [L. *vertebra,* vertebra] Pert. to a vertebra or the vertebral column.

vertebral groove The groove lying on either side of the spinous processes of the vertebrae.

vertebrarium (vĕr″tĕ-brā′rē-ŭm) [L.] A dated term for the vertebral column.

Vertebrata (vĕr″tĕ-brā′tă) A subphylum of the phylum Chordata characterized by possession of a segmented backbone or spinal column. It includes the following classes: Agnatha (cyclostomes), Chondrichthyes (cartilaginous fishes), Osteichthyes (bony fishes), Amphibia, Reptilia, Aves, and Mammalia. Members of this subphylum possess an axial notochord at some period of their existence.

vertebrate (vĕr′tĕ-brāt) [L. *vertebra,* vertebra] Having or resembling a vertebral column.

vertebrated (vĕr′tĕ-brāt″ĕd) Composed of jointed segments.

vertebrectomy (vĕr″tĕ-brĕk′tō-mē) [″ + Gr. *ektome,* excision] Excision of a vertebra or part of one.

vertebro- Combining form indicating *vertebra.*

vertebroarterial (vĕr″tĕ-brō-ăr-tē′rē-ăl) [″ + Gr. *arteria,* artery] Concerning the vertebral artery.

vertebrobasilar (vĕr″tĕ-brō-băs′ĭ-lăr) [″ + *basilaris,* basilar] Concerning the vertebral and basilar arteries.

vertebrochondral (vĕr″tĕ-brō-kŏn′drăl) [″ + Gr. *chondros,* cartilage] Pert. to the vertebrae and the costal cartilages.

vertebrocostal (vĕr″tĕ-brō-kŏs′tăl) [″ + *costa,* rib] Costovertebral.

vertebrofemoral (vĕr″tĕ-brō-fĕm′or-ăl) [″ + *femur,* thigh] Concerning the vertebrae and femur.

vertebroiliac (vĕr″tĕ-brō-ĭl′ē-ăk) [″ + *iliacus,* pert. to ilium] Concerning the vertebrae and ilium.

vertebromammary (vĕr″tĕ-brō-măm′mă-rē) [″ + *mamma,* breast] Pert. to the vertebral and mammary areas.

vertebroplasty (ver′tē-brō-plăs-tē) Plastic surgical repair of a vertebra.

vertebrosacral (vĕr″tĕ-brō-sā′krăl) [″ + *sacrum,* sacred] Concerning the vertebrae and sacrum.

vertebrosternal (vĕr″tĕ-brō-stĕr′năl) [″ + Gr. *sternon,* chest] Pert. to a vertebra and the sternum.

vertex (vĕr′tĕks) [L., summit] The top of the head. SYN: *corona capitis; crown.*

v. cordis The apex of the heart.

vertical (vĕr′tĭ-kăl) [L. *verticalis,* summit] **1.** Pert. to or situated at the vertex. **2.** Perpendicular to the plane of the horizon of the earth; upright.

verticalis (vĕr″tĭ-kā′lĭs) [L.] Vertical, indicating any plane that passes through the body parallel to the long axis of the body.

verticality The ability to perceive accurately the vertical position in the absence of environmental cues.

verticillate (vĕr-tĭs′ĭl-āt, -tĭs-ĭl′āt) [L. *verticillus,* a little whirl] Arranged like the spokes of a wheel or a whorl.

verticomental (vĕr″tĭ-kō-mĕn′tăl) [L. *vertex,* summit, + *mentum,* chin] Concerning the crown of the head and the chin.

vertiginous (vĕr-tĭj′ĭ-nŭs) [L. *vertiginosus,* one suffering from dizziness] Pert. to or afflicted with vertigo.

vertigo (vĕr′tĭ-gō, vĕr-tī′gō) [L. *vertigo,* a turning round] The sensation of moving around in space (subjective vertigo) or of having objects move about the person (objective vertigo). Vertigo is sometimes inaccurately used as a synonym for dizziness, lightheadedness, or giddiness. It may be caused by a variety of entities, including middle ear disease; toxic conditions such as those caused by salicylates, alcohol, or streptomycin; sunstroke; postural hypotension; or toxemia due to food poisoning or infectious diseases. SEE: *vection* (2).

PATIENT CARE: Assessment should include whether the patient experiences a sense of turning or whirling and its direction; whether it is intermittent and the time of day it occurs; whether it is associated with drugs, turning over in bed, occupation, or menses; whether it is associated with nausea and vomiting or with nystagmus and migraine. Safety measures, such as the use of siderails in bed, are instituted. The patient should ambulate gradually after a slow, assisted move from a sitting position. The call bell should be available at all times; tissues, water, and other supplies should be within easy reach; and furniture and other obstacles should be removed from the path of ambulation. The patient who has undergone ear surgery and experiences severe vertigo should be confined to bed for several days and then begin to gradually increase activity.

alternobaric v. Vertigo associated with a sudden decrease in the pressure to which the inner ear is exposed. This could occur when a scuba diver ascends quickly or when an aircraft ascends quickly. SEE: *bends.*

auditory v. Vertigo due to disease of the ear.

benign positional v. A disorder of the labyrinth of the inner ear characterized by paroxysmal vertigo and nystagmus only when the head is in a certain position or moves in a certain direction. The diagnosis is made at the bedside by moving the patient from the sitting position to recumbency with the head tilted down 30° over the end of the table and 30° to one side. This causes a paroxysm of vertigo. This test is called the Hallpike maneuver. Each episode of vertigo may last less than a minute but may recur for weeks.

central v. Vertigo caused by disease of the central nervous system.

cerebral v. Vertigo due to brain disease.

epidemic v. Vertigo that may occur in epidemic form. It is believed to be due to vestibular neuronitis.

epileptic v. Vertigo accompanying or following an epileptic attack.

essential v. Vertigo from an unknown cause.

gastric v. Vertigo associated with a gastric disturbance.

horizontal v. Vertigo that occurs while the patient is supine.

hysterical v. Vertigo accompanying hysteria.

labyrinthine v. An out-of-date term for Ménière's disease.

laryngeal v. Vertigo and fainting during a coughing spell in patients with chronic bronchitis. SYN: *laryngeal syncope.*

objective v. Vertigo in which stationary objects appear to be moving.

ocular v. Vertigo caused by disease of the eye.

organic v. Vertigo due to a brain lesion.

peripheral v. Vertigo due to disturbances in the peripheral areas of the central nervous system.

positional v. Vertigo that occurs when the head is tilted toward a specific axis. SYN: *postural v.* SEE: *benign positional v.; canalith repositioning maneuver.*

postural v. Positional vertigo.

rotary v. Subjective v.

subjective v. Vertigo in which the patient has the sensation of turning or rotating. SYN: *rotary v.*

toxic v. Vertigo caused by the presence of a toxin in the body.

vertical v. Vertigo produced by standing or by looking up or down.

vestibular v. Vertigo due to disease or malfunction of the vestibular apparatus.

verumontanitis (vĕr″ū-mŏn″tăn-ī′tĭs) [L. *veru,* spit, dart, + *montanus,* mountainous, + Gr. *itis,* inflammation] Inflammation of the verumontanum. SYN: *colliculitis.*

verumontanum (vĕr″ū-mŏn-tā′nŭm) [L. *veru,* spit, dart, + *montanus,* mountainous] An elevation on the floor of the prostatic portion of the urethra where the seminal ducts enter.

vesalianum (vĕs-ā″lē-ā′nŭm) [Andreas Vesalius, Flemish anatomist and physician, 1514–1564] One of the sesamoid bones in the tendon of origin of the gastrocnemius muscle, and another on the outer border of the foot in the angle between the cuboid and fifth metatarsal.

Vesalius, foramen of (vĕs-ā′lē-ŭs) [Andreas Vesalius] The opening in the base of the skull transmitting an emissary vein.

Vesalius, vein of The small emissary vein from the cavernous sinus passing through the foramen of Vesalius and conveying blood to the pterygoid plexus.

vesica (vĕ-sī′kă) [L.] A bladder.

v. fellea Gallbladder.

v. prostatica A minute pouch in the prostatic urethra, remnant of the müllerian duct. SYN: *utriculus prostaticus.*

v. urinaria Urinary bladder.

vesical (vĕs′ĭ-kăl) Pert. to or shaped like a bladder.

vesical reflex An inclination to urinate caused by moderate bladder distention.

vesicant (vĕs′ĭ-kănt) [L. *vesicare,* to blister] **1.** Blistering; causing or forming blisters. **2.** An agent used to produce blisters. It is much less severe in its effects than are escharotics. **3.** A blistering gas used in chemical warfare. SYN: *vesicatory.* SEE: *gas, vesicant.*

vesication (vĕs″ĭ-kā′shŭn) **1.** The process of blistering. **2.** A blister.

vesicatory (vĕs′ĭ-kă-tor″ē) Vesicant.

vesicle (vĕs′ĭ-kl) [L. *vesicula,* a little bladder] A small blister-like elevation on the skin containing serous fluid. Vesicles may vary in diameter from a few millimeters to a centimeter. They may be round, transparent, opaque, or dark elevations of the skin, sometimes containing seropurulent or bloody fluid. In sudamina, they result from sweat that cannot escape from the skin; in herpes, they are mounted on an inflammatory base, having no tendency to rupture but associated with burning pain. In herpes zoster, they follow dermatomes. In dermatitis venenata, they result from contact with poison ivy or oak and are accompanied by great itching. They are also seen in dermatitis herpetiformis or multiformis. In impetigo contagiosa, they occur, esp. in children, in discrete form, flat and umbilicated, filled with straw-colored fluid, with no tendency to break. They dry up, forming yellow crusts with little itching. They are also seen in vesicular eczema, molluscum contagiosum, miliaria (prickly heat or heat rash), chickenpox, smallpox, and scabies. SEE: illus.; *herpes; miliaria.*

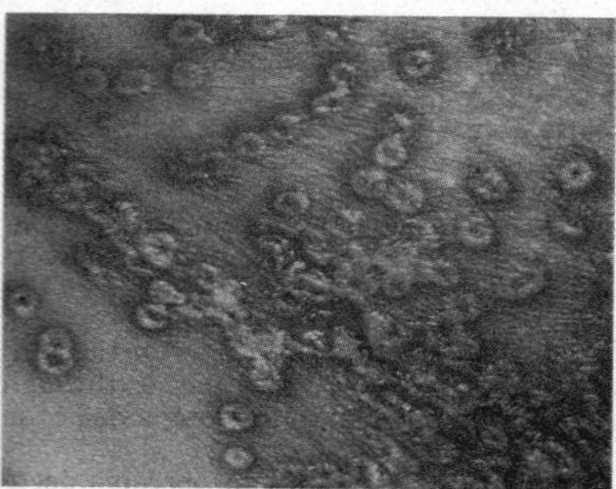

VESICLES

allantoic v. The hollow, enlarged part of the allantois, esp. in birds and reptiles.

auditory v. That portion of the cerebral vesicle from which the exterior ear is formed. SYN: *otic v.*

blastodermic v. Blastocyst.

brain v. One of the five embryonic subdivisions of the brain. SYN: *encephalic v.*

cerebral v. Brain v.

chorionic v. The outer villus-covered layer of the early embryo. It encloses the embryo, amnion, umbilical cord, and yolk stalk.

compound v. Multilocular v.

encephalic v. Brain v.

lens v. The embryonic vesicle formed from the lens pit. It develops into the lens of the eye.

multilocular v. A vesicle that contains multiple chambers.

optic v. A hollow outgrowth from the lateral aspects of the embryonic brain. The retinae and optic nerves develop from these paired vesicles.

otic v. Auditory v.

primary brain v. One of the three earliest subdivisions of the embryonic neural tube.

seminal v. One of two saccular glands below the urinary bladder in males. The duct from each joins the vas deferens on its own side to form the ejaculatory duct. The seminal vesicle produces an alkaline, fructose-rich secretion that enhances sperm motility and nourishes the sperm.

umbilical v. The portion of the embryonic yolk sac outside the body cavity.

vesico- (vĕs′ĭ-kō) Combining form meaning *bladder, vesicle.*

vesicoabdominal (vĕs″ĭ-kō-ăb-dŏm′ĭ-năl) [L. *vesica,* bladder, + *abdomen,* belly] Concerning the urinary bladder and the abdomen.

vesicocele (vĕs′ĭ-kō-sēl″) [L. *vesica,* bladder, + Gr. *kele,* tumor, swelling] Hernia of the bladder into the vagina. SYN: *cystocele.*

vesicocervical (vĕs″ĭ-kō-sĕr′vĭ-kăl) [″ + *cervix,* neck] Rel. to the urinary bladder and cervix uteri.

vesicoclysis (vĕs″ĭ-kŏk′lĭ-sĭs) [″ + Gr. *klysis,* a washing] Injection of fluid into the bladder.

vesicoenteric (vĕs″ĭ-kō-ĕn-tĕr′ĭk) [″ + Gr. *enteron,* intestine] Concerning the urinary bladder and intestine.

vesicofixation (vĕs″ĭ-kō-fĭks-ā′shŭn) [L. *vesica,* bladder, + *fixatio,* a fixing] Attachment of the uterus to the bladder or the bladder to the abdominal wall.

vesicoprostatic (vĕs″ĭ-kō-prŏs-tăt′ĭk) [″ + Gr. *prostates,* prostate] Rel. to the bladder and prostate.

vesicopubic (vĕs″ĭ-kō-pū′bĭk) [″ + NL. *(os) pubis,* bone of the groin] Pert. to the bladder and os pubis.

vesicopustule (vĕs″ĭ-kō-pŭs′tūl) [″ + *pustula,* blister] A vesicle in which pus has developed.

vesicosigmoid (vĕs″ĭ-kō-sĭg′moyd) [″ + Gr. *sigmoid,* shaped like Gr. letter σ] Concerning the urinary bladder and sigmoid colon.

vesicosigmoidostomy (vĕs″ĭ-kō-sĭg″moy-dŏs′tō-mē) [″ + ″ + *stoma,* mouth] Surgical creation of an anastomosis between the urinary bladder and sigmoid colon.

vesicospinal (vĕs″ĭ-kō-spī′năl) [″ + *spina,* thorn] Rel. to the urinary bladder and spinal cord.

vesicostomy (vĕs″ĭ-kŏs′tō-mē) [″ + Gr. *stoma,* mouth] Surgical production of an opening into the bladder.

vesicotomy (vĕs″ĭ-kŏt′ō-mē) [″ + Gr. *tome,* incision] Incision of the bladder.

vesicoumbilical (vĕs″ĭ-kō-ŭm-bĭl′ĭ-kăl) [″ + *umbilicus,* navel] Concerning the urinary bladder and umbilicus.

vesicoureteral (vĕs″ĭ-kō-ū-rē′tĕr-ăl) [″ + Gr. *oureter,* ureter] Concerning the urinary bladder and a ureter.

vesicouterine (vĕs″ĭ-kō-ū′tĕr-ĭn) [″ + *uterinus,* pert. to the womb] Pert. to the urinary bladder and uterus.

vesicouterine pouch Downward extension of the peritoneal cavity located between the bladder and uterus.

vesicouterovaginal (vĕs″ĭ-kō-ū″tĕr-ō-văj′ĭ-năl) [″ + *uterus,* womb, + *vagina,* sheath] Concerning the urinary bladder, the uterus, and the vagina.

vesicovaginal (vĕs″ĭ-kō-văj′ĭ-năl) [″ + *vagina,* sheath] Vaginovesical.

vesicovaginorectal (vĕs″ĭ-kō-văj″ĭ-nō-rĕk′tăl) [″ + *vagina,* sheath, + *rectum,* straight] Concerning the urinary bladder, vagina, and rectum.

vesicula (vĕ-sĭk′ū-lă) *pl.* **vesiculae** [L.] A small bladder or vesicle.

v. seminalis Seminal vesicle.

vesicular (vĕ-sĭk′ū-lăr) Pert. to vesicles or small blisters.

vesicular eczema Eczema accompanied by the formation of vesicles.

vesiculated (vĕ-sĭk′ū-lāt″ĕd) Having vesicles present.

vesiculation (vĕ-sĭk″ū-lā′shŭn) [L. *vesicula,* a tiny bladder] The formation of vesicles or the state of having or forming them.

vesiculectomy (vĕ-sĭk″ū-lĕk′tō-mē) [″ + Gr. *ektome,* excision] Partial or complete excision of a vesicle, particularly a seminal vesicle.

vesiculiform (vĕ-sĭk′ū-lĭ-form) [″ + *forma,* shape] Having the shape of a vesicle.

vesiculitis (vĕ-sĭk″ū-lī′tĭs) [″ + Gr. *itis,* inflammation] Inflammation of a vesicle, particularly the seminal vesicle.

vesiculobronchial (vĕ-sĭk″ū-lō-brŏng′kē-ăl) [″ + Gr. *bronchos,* windpipe] Both vesicular and bronchial.

vesiculocavernous (vĕ-sĭk″ū-lō-kăv′ĕr-nŭs) [″ + *caverna,* a hollow] Vesicular and cavernous.

vesiculogram (vĕ-sĭk′ū-lō-grăm) [″ + Gr. *gramma,* something written] A radiograph of the seminal vesicles.

vesiculography (vĕ-sĭk″ū-lŏg′ră-fē) [″ + Gr. *graphein,* to write] Radiography of the seminal vesicles after the injection of a contrast medium. This procedure has been replaced by ultrasound imaging.

vesiculopapular (vĕ-sĭk″ū-lō-păp′ū-lăr) [″ + *papula,* pimple] Composed of vesicles and papules.

vesiculopustular (vĕ-sĭk″ū-lō-pŭs′tū-lăr) [″ + *pustula,* blister] Having both vesicles and pustules.

vesiculotomy (vĕ-sĭk″ū-lŏt′ō-mē) [″ + Gr. *tome,* incision] Surgical incision into a vesicle, as a seminal vesicle.

vesiculotubular (vĕ-sĭk″ū-lō-tū′bū-lăr) [″ + *tubularis,* like a tube] Sounds from auscultation of the chest that have both vesicular and tubular qualities.

vesiculotympanic (vĕ-sĭk″ū-lō-tĭm-păn′ĭk) [″ + Gr. *tympanon,* drum] Having both vesicular and tympanic qualities.

Vespidae [L. *vespa,* wasp] Family of wasps, including paper wasps, hornets, and yellow jackets.

vessel (vĕs′ĕl) [O.Fr. from L. *vascellum,* a little vessel] A tube, duct, or canal to convey the fluids of the body. SYN: *vas.*

absorbent v.'s The lacteals and capillaries of the small intestines.

blood v. Any of the vessels carrying blood (i.e., arteries, veins, and capillaries).

chyliferous v. Lacteal (2).

collateral v. A vessel parallel to the vessel from which it arose.

great v. One of the large blood vessels entering and leaving the heart.

lacteal v. Lacteal (2).

lymphatic v. A thin-walled vessel that conveys lymph from the tissues. These vessels resemble veins in structure, possessing three layers (intima, media, and adventitia) and paired valves.

nutrient v. One of the vessels supply-

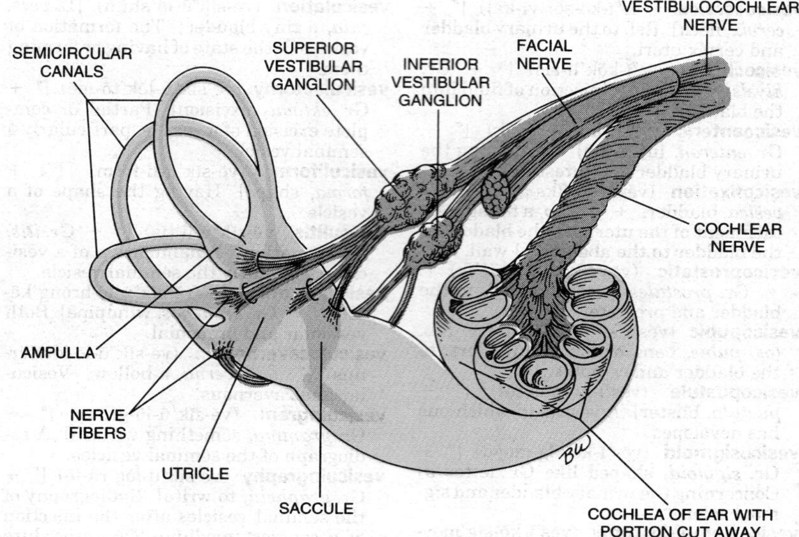

VESTIBULOCOCHLEAR NERVE (8TH CRANIAL)

ing specific areas such as the interior of bones.

radicular v. A branch of a vertebral artery supplying the cerebral nerve root.

vestibular (vĕs-tĭb′ū-lăr) [L. *vestibulum,* vestibule] Pert. to a vestibule.

vestibular bulb One of the two sacculated collections of veins, lying on either side of the vagina beneath the bulbocavernosus muscle, connected anteriorly by the pars intermedia, and through this strip of cavernous tissue communicating with the erectile tissue of the clitoris. The vestibular bulbs are the homologues of the male corpus spongiosum. Injury during labor may give rise to troublesome bleeding. SEE: *Bartholin's gland; vagina; vestibule of vagina.*

vestibular nerve A main division of the acoustic or eighth cranial nerve; arises in the vestibular ganglion and is concerned with equilibrium.

vestibule (vĕs′tĭ-būl) A small space or cavity at the beginning of a canal, such as the aortic vestibule.

aortic v. The part of the left ventricle of the heart just below the aortic valve.

buccal v. The part of the oral cavity bounded by the teeth, gingiva, and alveolar processes and laterally by the cheek.

v. of ear The middle part of the inner ear, behind the cochlea, and in front of the semicircular canals; it contains the utricle and saccule.

v. of larynx The portion of the larynx above the vocal cords.

v. of mouth The part of the oral cavity between the lips and the cheeks and between the teeth and the gums.

v. of nose The anterior part of the nostrils, containing the vibrissae.

v. of pharynx The space surrounded by the soft palate, base of the tongue, and the palatoglossal and palatopharyngeal arches.

v. of vagina An almond-shaped space between the lines of attachment of the labia minora. The clitoris is situated at the superior angle; the inferior boundary is the fourchette. The vestibule is approx. 4 to 5 cm long and 2 cm in greatest width when the labia minora are separated. Four major structures open into the vestibule: the urethra anteriorly, the vagina into the midportion, and the two secretory ducts of the glands of Bartholin laterally. The mucous membrane is stratified squamous epithelium. SEE: *Bartholin's gland; vagina; vestibular bulb.*

vestibulocochlear nerve (vĕs-tĭb″ū-lō-kŏk′lē-ăr) [L. *vestibulum,* vestibule, + Gr. *kokhlos,* land snail] The eighth cranial nerve, which emerges from the brain behind the facial nerve between the pons and medulla oblongata. It is concerned with hearing and equilibrium. SYN: *acoustic nerve.* SEE: illus.

vestibuloplasty (vĕs-tĭb′ū-lō-plăs″tē) [″ + Gr. *plassein,* to mold] Plastic surgery of the vestibule of the mouth.

vestibulotomy (vĕs-tĭb″ū-lŏt′ō-mē) [″ + Gr. *tome,* incision] Surgical incision into the vestibule of the inner ear.

vestibulourethral (věs-tĭb″ū-lō-ū-rē′thrăl) [″ + Gr. *ourethra,* urethra] Rel. to the vestibule of the vagina and urethra.

vestibulum (věs-tĭb′ū-lŭm) *pl.* **vestibula** [L.] Vestibule.

vestige (věs′tĭj) [L. *vestigium,* footstep] A small degenerate or incompletely developed structure that has been more fully developed in the embryo or in a previous stage of the species.

vestigial (věs-tĭj′ē-ăl) Of the nature of a vestige. SYN: *rudimentary.*

vestigium (věs-tĭj′ē-ŭm) *pl.* **vestigia** [L., a footstep] Vestige.

veterinarian (vĕt″ĕr-ĭ-năr′ē-ăn) One who is trained and licensed to practice veterinary medicine and surgery.

veterinary (vĕt′ĕr-ĭ-năr″ē) **1.** Pert. to animals, their diseases, and their treatment. **2.** A veterinarian.

VF *ventricular fibrillation; vocal fremitus.*

V.H. *viral hepatitis.*

via (vē′ă, vī′ă) *pl.* **viae** [L.] Any passage in the body such as nasal, intestinal, or vaginal.

viability (vī″ă-bĭl′ĭ-tē) [L. *vita,* life, + *habilis,* fit] The capacity for living, growing, developing, or surviving. It is used, for example, in reference to a premature fetus once it reaches a certain size or gestational age, or in determining the likelihood that an injured limb or transplanted organ will survive or flourish. **viable,** *adj.*

Viagra The trade name for sildenafil citrate, a medication used for erectile dysfunction. Its use is contraindicated in patients taking nitrates in any form owing to the risk of death.

vial (vī′ăl) [Gr. *phiale,* a drinking cup] A small glass bottle for medicines or chemicals.

viator (vī′ă-tŏr) An individual, usually one with a terminal illness, who sells rights to his or her insurance policy in exchange for an antemortem benefit collection.

vibex (vī′bĕks) *pl.* **vibices** [L. *vibix,* mark of a blow] A narrow linear mark of hemorrhage into the skin.

vibrapuncture (vī″bră-pŭnk′tūr) The medical use of a tattoo technique to introduce medicine into skin lesions. Multiple punctures are made into the skin by a needle that has passed through a small amount of the solution of medicine placed on the site.

vibration (vī-brā′shŭn) **1.** A to-and-fro movement. SYN: *oscillation.* **2.** Therapeutic shaking of the body, a form of massage. It consists of a quick motion of the fingers or the hand vertical to the body or use of a mechanical vibrator. Chest wall vibration is a component of pulmonary hygiene; it improves respiratory function in patients with chronic obstruction lung disease, and can be used as an adjunctive treatment for pneumonia when it is used with postural drainage.

vibrative (vĭb′ră-tĭv) **1.** Vibratory. **2.** Indicating sound produced by vibration of parts of the respiratory tract as air passes through.

vibrator (vī′brā-tor) [L. *vibrator,* a shaker] A device that produces rapid to-and-fro movements in the body or one of its parts. In health care, vibrators are used in hearing aids and middle ear implants; in pulmonary hygiene to assist in clearing secretions or to stimulate diaphragmatic movement; in patients with sexual dysfunction (e.g., patients with spinal cord injuries affecting orgasm, or other orgasmic difficulties); or in the relief of muscle contraction in some patients with neurological deficits.

whole body v. Exposure of the entire body to vibration as would occur in occupations such as truck and tractor drivers, jackhammer operators, helicopter pilots, and construction workers using various vibration-producing tools. Such exposure may produce diseases of the peripheral nerves, prostatitis, and back disorders.

vibratory (vī′bră-tō″rē) [L. *vibrator,* a shaker] Having a vibrating or oscillatory movement.

vibratory sense The ability to perceive vibrations transmitted through the skin to deep tissues; usually tested by placing a vibrating tuning fork over bony prominences.

Vibrio (vĭb′rē-ō) A genus of curved, motile, gram-negative bacilli, several of which may be pathogenic for humans.

V. cholerae The causative agent of cholera.

v. parahemolyticus A marine vibrio, a common cause of gastroenteritis involving raw or poorly cooked seafood.

V. vulnificus A gram-negative bacillus commonly found in seawater. It may cause a fulminant gangrene if it contaminates wounds or may cause a fatal septicemia if ingested by those with impaired gastric, liver, kidney, or immune function. The usual source in such cases is raw shellfish.

vibrio (vĭb′rē-ō) *pl.* **vibriones** An organism of the genus *Vibrio.* SEE: *bacteria* for illus.

vibriocidal (vĭb″rē-ō-sī′dăl) Destructive to vibrio organisms.

vibrion (vē″brē-ŏn′) [Fr.] A vibrio organism.

vibriosis (vĭb″rē-ō′sĭs) The condition of being infected with organisms of the genus *Vibrio.*

vibrissae (vī-brĭs′ē) *sing.* **vibrissa** [L. *vibrissa,* that which shakes] Stiff hairs within the nostrils at the anterior nares.

vibromassage (vī″brō-mă-săj′) A massage given by a mechanical vibrator.

vibrometer (vī-brŏm′ĕt-ĕr) [L. *vibrare,* to shake, + Gr. *metron,* measure] A device used to measure the vibratory sensation threshold. It is particularly useful in judging the progression or remission of peripheral neuropathy.

vicarious (vī-kā'rē-ŭs) [L. *vicarius,* change, alternation] Acting as a substitute; pert. to assumption of the function of one organ by another.

vicarious learning Learning through indirect experience.

vicarious respiration Increased respiration in one lung when respiration in the other is lessened or abolished.

Vicq d'Azyr's tract (vĭk dă-zērz') [Felix Vicq d'Azyr, Fr. anatomist, 1748–1794] A large myelinated bundle arising in mammillary nuclei and terminating in the anterior thalamic nuclei of the brain.

vidarabine (vī-dār'ă-bēn) An antiviral agent effective against the herpes simplex and herpes zoster–varicella viruses.

video display terminal ABBR: VDT. A terminal used in information processing (computer terminal) and entertainment (TV picture tube) that produces an image on a screen (target) by bombarding it with electrons. This causes the fluorescent material that coats the screen to emit light. The effects on workers involved with the use of VDTs have been investigated with respect to a variety of factors. There is no evidence that reproductive or visual health is impaired by working with VDTs. Those who work with VDTs may experience musculoskeletal difficulties if the workplaces are poorly designed. This may be due to the screen being positioned in a way that promotes poor posture, or the chair being of improper design. SEE: *ergonomics*.

videognosis (vĭd"ē-ŏg-nō'sĭs) [L. *videre,* to see, + Gr. *gnosis,* knowledge] Diagnosis using data and radiographic images transmitted by the use of television.

video-stroboscope A closed-circuit television recording technique used to obtain images while the field is illuminated by use of a stroboscope. Using this provides sequential views of objects in motion.

vidian artery (vĭd'ē-ăn) [Guido Guidi (L. *Vidius*), It. physician, 1500–1569] The artery passing through the pterygoid canal.

vidian canal A canal in the medial pterygoid plate of the sphenoid bone for transmission of pterygoid (vidian) vessels and nerve. SYN: *pterygoid canal*.

vidian nerve A branch from the sphenopalatine ganglion.

view box In radiology, a uniform light source used to view a radiograph.

vigil (vĭj'ĭl) [L., awake] Insomnia, wakefulness.

coma v. A delirious, drowsy state in which the patient is partially conscious and occasionally responsive to stimuli. SEE: *vigilambulism*.

vigilambulism (vĭj"ĭl-ăm'bū-lĭzm) [" + *ambulare,* to walk, + Gr. *-ismos,* condition] Automatism that occurs while the person is awake; resembles somnambulism.

vigilance (vĭj'ĭ-lăns) [L. *vigilantia,* wastefulness] The condition of being attentive, alert, and watchful.

vigintinormal (vī-jĭn"tĭ-nor'măl) [L. *viginti,* twenty, + *normal,* rule] Consisting of one twentieth of what is normal, as a solution.

vignetting In radiology, a loss in brightness and focus toward the periphery of the output phosphor during image intensification.

vigor (vĭg'or) [L.] Active force or strength of body or mind.

Villaret's syndrome (vē-lăr-āz') [Maurice Villaret, Fr. neurologist, 1877–1946] Ipsilateral paralysis of the 9th, 10th, 11th, 12th, and sometimes the 7th cranial nerves and the cervical sympathetic fibers. It is caused by a lesion in the posterior retroparotid space. The signs and symptoms include paralysis and anesthesia of the pharyngeal area with difficulty swallowing; loss of taste sensation in the posterior third of the tongue; paralysis of the vocal cords, and the sternocleidomastoid and trapezius muscles; and Horner's syndrome.

villi (vĭl'ī) [L.] Pl. of villus.

villiferous (vĭl-ĭf'ĕr-ŭs) [" + *ferre,* to bear] Having villi or tufts of hair.

villoma (vĭ-lō'mă) [L. *villus,* tuft of hair, + Gr. *oma,* tumor] A villous tumor.

villose, villous (vĭl'ōs, vĭl'ŭs) [L. *villus,* tuft of hair] Pert. to or furnished with villi or with fine hairlike extensions.

villositis (vĭl"ōs-ī'tĭs) [" + Gr. *itis,* inflammation] Inflammation of the placental villi.

villosity (vĭ-lŏs'ĭ-tē) The condition of being covered with villi.

villus (vĭl'ŭs) *pl.* **villi** [L., tuft of hair] A small fold or projection of some mucous membranes.

arachnoid v. Arachnoid granulation.

chorionic v. One of the tiny vascular projections of the chorionic surface that become vascular and help to form the placenta. SEE: *embryo* for illus.; *chorion*.

intestinal v. One of the multiple, minute projections of the intestinal mucosa into the lumen of the small intestine. These projections increase the surface area for absorption of water and nutrients; each contains a capillary network and a lacteal. SEE: illus.

synovial v. One of the thin projections of the synovial membrane into the joint cavity.

villusectomy (vĭl"ŭs-ĕk'tō-mē) [" + Gr. *ektome,* excision] Surgical removal of a synovial villus.

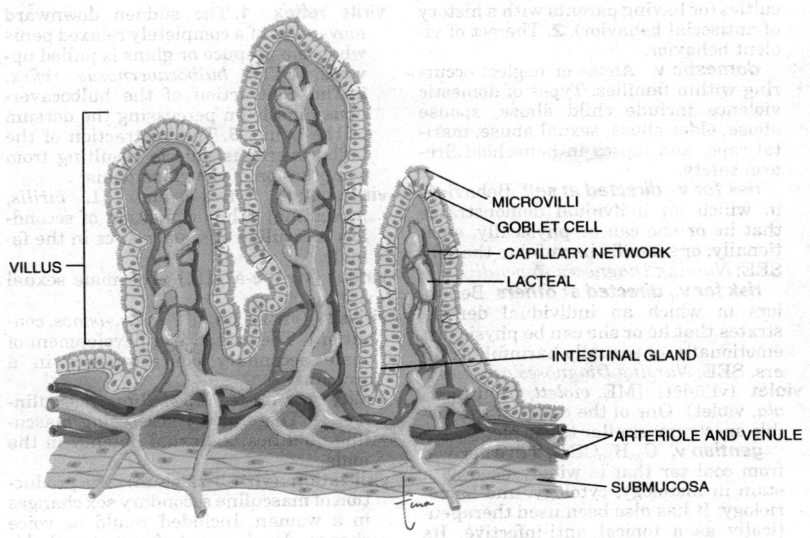

VILLI OF SMALL INTESTINE

vinblastine sulfate (vĭn-blăs′tēn) A fraction of an extract obtained from the periwinkle plant, *Vinca rosea,* a species of myrtle. It is a cytotoxic agent used in treating certain types of malignant tumors.

CAUTION: Like other cytotoxic drugs, vinblastine should be handled with barriers to protect the administrator. It must be disposed of in environmentally sound containers.

Vinca (vĭn′kă) A genus of herbs including periwinkles, from which vincristine and vinblastine are obtained.

Vincent's angina Necrotizing ulcerative gingivitis.

vincristine sulfate (vĭn-krĭs′tēn) A fraction of an extract obtained from the periwinkle plant, *Vinca rosea,* a species of myrtle. It is a cytotoxic agent used in treating certain types of malignant tumors.

CAUTION: Like other cytotoxic drugs, vincristine should be handled with barriers to protect the administrator. It must be disposed of in environmentally sound containers.

vinculum (vĭn′kū-lŭm) *pl.* **vincula** [L., to bind, tie] A uniting band or bundle. SYN: *frenulum; frenum; ligament.*

v. tendinum **1.** Slender tendinous filaments connecting the phalanges with the flexor tendons. **2.** The ringlike ligament of the ankle or wrist.

vinegar (vĭn′ĕ-găr) [ME. *vinegre,* from Fr. *vin,* wine, + *aigre,* sour] An impure solution containing 4-6% acetic acid. It is the product of fermentation of weak alcoholic solutions such as apple cider. SEE: *condiment.*

vinyl (vī′nĭl) The univalent ethenyl hydrocarbon molecule, $CH_2{=}CH{-}$.

v. chloride A vinyl radical attached to a chlorine atom, $CH_2{=}CHCl$. It is used commercially to make pipes, tubing, and plastic resin. Some individuals exposed to vinyl chloride have developed hepatic angiosarcoma.

v. cyanide A toxic liquid compound, $CH_2{=}CHCN$, used in making plastics. SYN: *acrylonitrile.*

v. ether An anesthetic agent that is virtually obsolete because it is explosive or flammable in the concentration required to produce anesthesia.

violaceous (vī″ĕ-lā′shŭs) [L. *violaceus,* violet] Having a purple discoloration, esp. of the skin.

violate (vī′ĕ-lāt″) [L. *violare,* to injure] To harm or injure a person, esp. to rape a female.

violence (vī′ō-lĕnts) [L. *violentia*] **1.** The use of force or physical compulsion to abuse or damage. Interpersonal violence among children and young adults rose to epidemic levels in the U.S. in the 1990s. Known risk factors for interpersonal violence among young people include a previous history of violence, rejection by others, academic underachievement, and parental difficulties (or having parents with a history of antisocial behavior). **2.** The act of violent behavior.

domestic v. Abuse or neglect occurring within families. Types of domestic violence include child abuse, spouse abuse, elder abuse, sexual abuse, marital rape, and lapses in household firearm safety.

risk for v., directed at self Behaviors in which an individual demonstrates that he or she can be physically, emotionally, or sexually harmful to the self. SEE: *Nursing Diagnoses Appendix.*

risk for v., directed at others Behaviors in which an individual demonstrates that he or she can be physically, emotionally, or sexually harmful to others. SEE: *Nursing Diagnoses Appendix.*

violet (vī′ō-lĕt) [ME. *violett,* from L. *viola,* violet] One of the colors of the visible spectrum; similar to purple.

gentian v. $C_{25}H_{30}ClN_3$; a dye derived from coal tar that is widely used as a stain in histology, cytology, and bacteriology. It has also been used therapeutically as a topical anti-infective. Its chemical name is hexamethylpararosaniline chloride.

violet blindness Inability to see violet tints.

viosterol (vī-ŏs′tĕr-ōl) A solution of irradiated ergosterol in vegetable oil. SYN: *calciferol.*

viper (vī′pĕr) Any venomous snake of the family Viperidae.

VIPoma [*v*asoactive *i*ntestinal *p*olypeptide + *oma,* tumor] A rare form of neuroendocrine tumor that causes watery diarrhea, hypokalemia, and achlorhydria as a result of the release of vasoactive intestinal peptide.

viraginity (vĭr″ă-jĭn′ĭ-tē) [L. *virago,* an amazon or manlike woman] A condition in which a woman believes that she should be a male even though she is aware that her body is female. SEE: *transsexual.*

viral Pert. to or caused by a virus.

viral interference The inhibition of the multiplication of one type of virus by the presence of another virus in the same cell. SEE: *interferon.*

Virchow's node Node, sentinel.

viremia (vī″rēm′ē-ă) The presence of viruses in the blood.

vires (vī′rēs) Pl. of vis.

virga [L., a rod] Penis.

virgin (vĕr′jĭn) [L. *virgo,* a maiden] **1.** A woman or man who has not had sexual intercourse. **2.** Uncontaminated; fresh; new.

virginal (vĕr′jĭn-ăl) [L. *virgo,* a maiden] Rel. to a virgin or to virginity.

virginity (vĕr-jĭn′ĭt-ē) [L. *virginitas,* maidenhood] The state of being a virgin; not having experienced sexual intercourse.

virile (vĭr′ĭl) [L. *virilis,* masculine] Masculine.

virile reflex **1.** The sudden downward movement of a completely relaxed penis when the prepuce or glans is pulled upward. SYN: *bulbocavernosus reflex.* **2.** The contraction of the bulbocavernous muscle on percussing the dorsum of the penis. **3.** The contraction of the bulbocavernous muscle resulting from compression of the glans penis.

virilescence (vĭr-ĭl-ĕs′ĕns) [L. *virilis,* masculine] The acquisition of secondary masculine characteristics in the female.

virilia (vĭr-ĭl′ē-ă) [L.] The male sexual organs.

virilism (vĭr′ĭl-ĭzm) [″ + Gr. *-ismos,* condition] The presence or development of male secondary characteristics in a woman.

virility (vĭr-ĭl′ĭ-tē) [L. *virilitas,* masculinity] **1.** The state of possessing masculine qualities. **2.** Sexual potency in the male.

virilization (vĭr″ĭ-lī-zā′shŭn) The production of masculine secondary sex changes in a woman. Included would be voice change, development of male-type baldness, clitoral enlargement, and increased growth of facial and body hair. Virilization may be caused by one of several endocrine diseases that lead to excess production of testosterone, or by the woman's taking anabolic steroids. In the latter case, this is often done to attempt to enhance muscular development.

virion (vī′rē-ŏn, vĭ′rē-ŏn) A complete virus particle; a unit of genetic material, the genome, surrounded by a protective protein coat, the capsid. Sometimes the capsid is surrounded by a lipid envelope. SEE: *capsid.*

viripotent (vī-rĭp′ō-tĕnt) [L. *viripotens*] Sexually mature, as applied to a man.

viroid A small, naked, infectious molecule of RNA. Viroids differ from viruses by the absence of a dormant phase and by genomes that are much smaller than those of known viruses.

virology (vī-rŏl′ō-jē) [L. *virus,* poison, + Gr. *logos,* word, reason] The study of viruses and viral diseases.

viropexis (vī″rō-pĕk′sĭs) [″ + Gr. *pexis,* fixation] The fixation of a virus particle to a cell. This leads to the inclusion of the virus inside the cell.

virtual (vĕr′tū-ăl) [L. *virtus,* capacity] Appearing to exist but not existing in actual fact or form.

virucidal (vĭr-ū-sī′dăl) [L. *virus,* poison, + *cidus,* to kill] Destructive of a virus.

virucide An agent that destroys or inactivates a virus, esp. a chemical substance used on living tissue.

virulence (vĭr′ū-lĕns) [LL. *virulentia,* stench] **1.** The relative power and degree of pathogenicity possessed by organisms. Properties that influence the virulence of an organism include (1) the

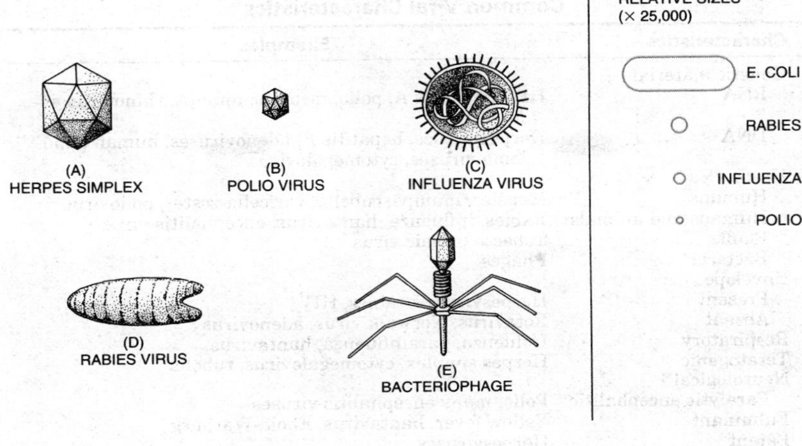

VIRUSES

strength of its adhesion molecules, which link it to the target cell; (2) its ability to secrete enzymes or exotoxins that damage target cells, or endotoxins that interfere with the body's normal regulatory systems; and (3) its ability to inhibit or evade the actions of white blood cells and their chemical mediators. SEE: *immunocompetence; immunocompromised*. **2.** The property of being virulent; venomousness, as of a disease. SEE: *attenuation*.

virulent (vĭr′ū-lĕnt) [L. *virulentus*, poison] **1.** Very poisonous. **2.** Infectious; able to overcome the host's defensive mechanism.

viruria (vīr-ūr′ē-ă) [″ + Gr. *ouron*, urine] The presence of viruses in the urine.

virus (vī′rŭs) [L., poison] A pathogen made of nucleic acid inside a protein shell, which can grow and reproduce only after infecting a host cell. More than 400 types of viruses, with a broad array of structures and pathogenic features, are known. All of them can attach to cell membranes, enter the cytoplasm, take over cellular functions, reproduce their parts, and assemble themselves into mature forms capable of infecting other cells.

Some of the most virulent agents known are viruses (e.g., the hemorrhagic fever caused by Ebola virus). Viruses are also responsible for the common cold, childhood exanthems (chickenpox, measles, rubella), latent infections (herpes simplex), some cancers or lymphomas (Epstein-Barr virus), and diseases of virtually any organ system of the body.

Viruses with envelopes have a greater ability to adhere to cell membranes and to avoid destruction by the immune system. Both the capsid and envelope have antigens (protein markers recognizable to white blood cells). Many of these antigens change frequently, so that the body is unable to create one immunoglobulin (antibody) that can neutralize both the original antigen and its replacement. The common influenza viruses have antigens that mutate or combine readily, requiring new vaccines with each mutation. The body's primary immune defenses against viruses are cytotoxic T lymphocytes, interferons, and to some extent immunoglobulins; destruction of the virus often requires destruction of the host cell.

When viruses enter a cell, they may immediately trigger a disease process or remain quiescent for many years. They damage the host cell by blocking its normal protein synthesis and using its metabolic machinery for their own reproduction. New viruses are then released either by destroying their host cell or by forming small buds that break off and infect other cells. SEE: illus.; table.

CLASSIFICATION: The 400 known viruses are classified in several ways: by genome core (RNA or DNA), host (animals, plants, or bacteria), method of reproduction (e.g., retrovirus), mode of transmission (e.g., enterovirus), and disease produced (e.g., hepatitis virus).

TREATMENT: Antiviral drugs include such agents as acyclovir (for herpes simplex); amantadine and rimantadine (for influenza A); interferons (for chronic hepatitis B and C); ribavirin (for respiratory syncytial virus and chronic hepatitis C); and lamivudine (among many others, for human immunodeficiency virus [HIV]).

arbor v. Former name for arbovirus.

Common Viral Characteristics

Characteristics	Examples
Genetic material	
RNA	HIV, hepatitis A, polio, measles, mumps, rhinovirus, influenza
DNA	Herpesviruses, hepatitis B, adenoviruses, human papilloma viruses, cytomegalovirus
Hosts	
Humans	Measles, mumps, rubella, varicella-zoster, poliovirus
Humans and animals	Rabies, influenza, hantavirus, encephalitis virus
Plants	Tobacco mosaic virus
Bacteria	Phages
Envelope	
Present	Herpesviruses, rabies, HIV
Absent	Rotavirus, Norwalk virus, adenovirus
Respiratory	Influenza, parainfluenza, hantavirus
Teratogenic	Herpes simplex, cytomegalovirus, rubella
Neurological	
Paralytic encephalitic	Polio, many encephalitis viruses
Fulminant	Yellow fever, hantavirus, Ebola-Warburg
Latent	Herpesviruses
Cancer causing	Human T-cell lymphotropic virus, hepatitis viruses, papillomavirus

attenuated v. A virus with reduced pathogenicity due to treatment or repeated passage through hosts.

B v. *Cercopithecine herpesvirus* 1.

bacterial v. Bacteriophage.

Borna disease v. A family of negative-stranded RNA viruses that infects the central nervous system of animals causing movement and behavioral disorders. It has been isolated from about 15% of both patients with schizophrenia and mental health care workers, but from only about 1% of the general population. This finding (and other associations with depression) have fueled speculation that the virus may play a part in human neuropsychiatric disorders.

chikungunya v. An alphavirus, typically found in Africa or Southeast Asia, that can be transmitted to humans by the bite of *Aedes* mosquitoes. After an incubation period of about a week, the virus produces high fevers, headache, nausea, vomiting, and severe joint pain, usually in the wrists or ankles.

coxsackie v. SEE: *coxsackievirus*.

cytomegalic v. ABBR: CMV. Cytomegalovirus.

defective v. A virus particle that, because of a lack of certain essential factors, is unable to replicate. Sometimes this can be overcome by the presence of a helper virus that provides the missing factor or factors.

EB v. Epstein-Barr virus.

enteric v. Enterovirus.

enteric cytopathogenic human orphan v. ABBR: ECHO virus. A virus that was accidentally discovered in human feces and not known to be associated with a disease, thus the name "orphan." Initially 33 ECHO virus serotypes were designated, but numbers 10 and 28 have been reclassified. Various serotypes have been associated with aseptic meningitis, encephalitis, acute upper respiratory infection, enteritis, pleurodynia, and myocarditis.

enteric orphan v. SEE: *enteric cytopathogenic human orphan v.*

filtrable v. A virus causing infectious disease, so small it retains infectivity after passing through a filter of the Berkefeld type. SEE: *filter, Berkefeld*.

fixed v. A rabies virus that was stabilized and modified but only partially attenuated by serial passage through rabbits.

GB v. type C Hepatitis G virus.

guanarito v. An arenavirus (from the Tacaribe virus group) that chronically infects rodents. It is the cause of sporadic outbreaks of Venezuelan hemorrhagic fever.

helper v. A virus that permits a defective virus present in the same cell to replicate. SEE: *defective v.*

hepatitis G v. An RNA flavivirus found in blood in about 2% of blood donors that may be transmitted by injection drug abuse, sexual contact, transfusions, and childbirth (from mother to infant). It is remotely related to Hepatitis C virus. It causes chronic viremia, but does not seem to cause hepatitis or liver damage. The effects of long-term infection are unknown. SYN: *GB virus type C*.

herpes v. Herpesviruses.

human immunodeficiency v. ABBR: HIV. SEE: *human immunodeficiency virus*.

JC v. A DNA papovavirus that

causes progressive multifocal leukoencephalopathy in immunosuppressed patients. It is carried asymptomatically by a large percentage of the population.

Junin v. An arenavirus that chronically infects rodents. It is the cause of sporadic outbreaks of Argentine hemorrhagic fever, a potentially lethal infection usually found in South America.

latent v. A virus that has the ability to infect the host, initially causing little or no evidence of illness but persisting for the lifetime of the infected individual; later on, a specific triggering mechanism may cause the virus to produce a clinically apparent disease. This occurs with herpes simplex virus that remains latent in sensory ganglia and is reactivated by trauma to the skin supplied by the distal sensory nerves associated with these ganglia. After reactivation, the virus may cause localized or generalized lesions in the affected area and the central nervous system.

lytic v. Any virus that, after infecting a cell, lyses it.

masked v. A virus that ordinarily occurs in the host in a noninfective state but is activated and demonstrated by indirect methods.

neurotropic v. A virus that reproduces in nerve tissue.

Nipah v. ABBR: NiV. A member of the family of paramyxoviruses that can cause outbreaks of encephalitis and respiratory disease in humans. It is transmitted to humans from infected swine (e.g., in slaughterhouses).

Oliveros v. An arenavirus of the Tacaribe complex of viruses that normally infects rodents in the pampas of Argentina. It may cause a fatal hemorrhagic fever in humans.

oncogenic v. Tumor virus.

orphan v. One of several viruses that initially were not thought to be associated with human illness. This group includes the enteroviruses and rhinoviruses.

parainfluenza v. One of a group of viruses that affect infants and young children. It causes respiratory infections that may be mild or may progress to pneumonia. Most infections are so mild as to be clinically inapparent.

plant v. Any virus that is pathogenic for plants.

pox v. Poxvirus.

reassortant v. A virus whose genetic material has been recombined or reshuffled so that it contains new nucleic acid sequences, new antigenic structures, and new combinations of protein products.

respiratory syncytial v. A virus that is a major cause of lower respiratory tract disease during infancy and early childhood. It induces the formation of cell masses in which the cytoplasm of group cells are connected (syncytium) in cell cultures. Attempts to develop an effective and safe vaccine have been unsuccessful so far. Because it is difficult to recognize the disease early and inapparent cases are frequent, isolation and public health measures are not adequate to control the spread of the disease. Ribavirin is the primary drug used in its treatment. The administration of high doses of respiratory syncytial virus immune globulin is an effective means of preventing lower respiratory tract infection in infants and young children at high risk for contracting this disease.

Rift Valley v. A phlebovirus that causes sporadic epidemics among both humans and animals of hemorrhagic fever, in Africa. It is transmitted by the bite of infected mosquitoes.

sandfly fever v. Any member of the group of Bunyaviruses, typically found in or near the Mediterranean Sea, that may be transmitted to humans by the bite of the *Phlebotomus* fly.

Sindbis v. An alphavirus typically found in South Africa or Oceania that is disseminated to humans by mosquitoes of the genus *Culex*. It can cause a transient febrile illness accompanied by a diffuse maculopapular rash and muscle and joint pains.

slow v. A virus that replicates and causes disease indolently. SEE: *slow v. infection*.

slow v. infection An infection caused by a virus that remains dormant in the body for a prolonged period before causing signs and symptoms of illness. Such viruses may require years to incubate before causing diseases. Examples include progressive multifocal leukoencephalopathy and subacute sclerosing panencephalitis.

street v. A rabies virus obtained from an infected animal rather than from a laboratory strain.

SV 40 v. Simian virus 40, which is a member of the papovavirus family. The virus produces sarcomas after subcutaneous inoculation into newborn hamsters.

Tacaribe complex v. A group of viruses, originally identified in South America, that cause hemorrhagic fever in humans. They are members of the arenavirus family and are typically found in rodents. One member of this group is the Sabia virus.

tumor v. A virus that causes malignant neoplasms. Viruses suspected of causing tumors in humans include Epstein-Barr virus (associated with Burkitt's lymphoma), hepatitis B virus (with hepatocellular carcinoma), papilloma virus (with carcinoma of the cervix), and human herpesvirus 8 (with Kaposi's sarcoma). SYN: *oncogenic v.*

West Nile v. An avian virus that can

be transmitted to humans by mosquitoes and may cause encephalitis ranging from mild to fatal. This emerging infection was first identified in the Western Hemisphere in the fall of 1999, when it was found to be responsible for the death of seven New Yorkers and many birds in the Bronx Zoo.

virusemia (vī″rŭs-ēm′ē-ă) [″+ Gr. *haima,* blood] Viremia.

virus shedding The release of a virus from the host.

virustatic (vīr″ŭ-stăt′ĭk) [″+ Gr. *statikos,* bringing to a standstill] Stopping the growth of viruses.

vis (vĭs) *pl.* **vires** [L., strength] Force, strength, energy, power.

viscera (vĭs′ĕr-ă) *sing.,* **viscus** [L.] Internal organs enclosed within a cavity, esp. the abdominal organs. SEE: *celosomia; evisceration; splanchnic.*

viscerad (vĭs′ĕr-ăd) [″ + *ad,* toward] Toward the viscera.

visceral (vĭs′ĕr-ăl) [L. *viscera,* body organs] **1.** Pert. to viscera. **2.** Pert. to or derived from the gill arches of vertebrates.

visceral cavity The body cavity containing the viscera.

visceral cleft One of the fissures separating the visceral arches.

visceral skeleton The pelvis, ribs, and sternum enclosing the viscera.

viscerimotor (vĭs″ĕr-ĭ-mō′tor) [″ + *motor,* mover] Visceromotor.

viscero- (vĭs′ĕr-ō) [L. *viscera,* body organs] Combining form meaning *viscera.*

viscerocranium (vĭs″ĕr-ō-krā′nē-ŭm) That portion of the skull derived from the pharyngeal arches.

viscerogenic (vĭs″ĕr-ō-jĕn′ĭk) [″ + Gr. *gennan,* to produce] Originating in the viscera.

visceroinhibitory (vĭs″ĕr-ō-ĭn-hĭb′ĭ-tō-rē) [″ + *inhibere,* to restrain] Checking the action of the viscera.

visceromegaly (vĭs″ĕr-ō-mĕg′ă-lē) [″ + Gr. *megalos,* great] Generalized enlargement of the abdominal visceral organs.

visceromotor (vĭs″ĕr-ō-mō′tor) [L. *viscera,* body organs, + *motor,* a mover] Rel. to a nerve conveying motor impulses to the viscera. SYN: *viscerimotor.*

visceromotor reflex An increase in tonus of the abdominal muscles resulting from painful stimuli originating in a viscus.

visceroparietal (vĭs″ĕr-ō-pă-rī′ĕ-tăl) [″ + *paries,* wall] Rel. to the viscera and abdominal wall.

visceroperitoneal (vĭs″ĕr-ō-pĕr″ĭ-tō-nē′ăl) [″ + Gr. *peritonaion,* peritoneum] Rel. to the abdominal viscera and peritoneum.

visceropleural (vĭs″ĕr-ō-ploo′răl) [″ + Gr. *pleura,* a side] Rel. to the thoracic viscera and pleura. SYN: *pleurovisceral.*

visceroptosis (vĭs″ĕr-ŏp-tō′sĭs) [″ + Gr. *ptosis,* a dropping] Downward displacement of a viscus.

visceroreceptors (vĭs″ĕr-ō-rē-sĕp′torz) A group of receptors that includes those located in visceral organs. Their stimulation gives rise to poorly localized and ill-defined sensations. In hollow visceral organs, they are stimulated principally by excessive contraction or by distention.

viscerosensory (vĭs″ĕr-ō-sĕn′sō-rē) [″ + *sensorius,* sensory] Pert. to sensations aroused by stimulation of visceroreceptors.

viscerosensory reflex Pain or tenderness elicited in somatic structures (skin and muscle) caused by visceral disorder. SEE: *pain, referred.*

visceroskeletal (vĭs″ĕr-ō-skĕl′ĕt-ăl) [″ + Gr. *skeleton,* a dried-up body] Rel. to the visceral skeleton.

viscerosomatic (vĭs″ĕr-ō-sō-măt′ĭk) [″ + Gr. *soma,* body] Rel. to the viscera and the body.

viscerosomatic reaction A reaction occurring in muscles of the body wall as a result of stimulation of visceroreceptors.

viscerotome (vĭs′ĕr-ō-tōm) [″ + Gr. *tome,* incision] The part of an abdominal organ that is supplied with afferent nerves from a single posterior root.

viscerotonia (vĭs″ĕr-ō-tōn′ē-ă) [″ + Gr. *tonos,* tension] Personality traits characterized by predominance of social over intellectual and physical traits. The individual is sociable and convivial, exhibits unusual appreciation of food, and loves company, affection, social support, and approval.

viscerotrophic (vĭs″ĕr-ō-trŏf′ĭk) [″ + Gr. *trophe,* nourishment] Pert. to trophic changes rel. to or associated with visceral conditions.

viscerotropic (vĭs″ĕr-ō-trŏp′ĭk) [″+ Gr. *tropos,* a turn] Primarily affecting the viscera.

viscerovisceral reaction (vĭs″ĕr-ō-vĭs′ĕr-ăl) A reaction taking place in the viscera as a result of stimulation of visceral receptors. Such reactions are usually below the level of consciousness.

viscid (vĭs′ĭd) [L. *viscum,* mistletoe, birdlime] Adhering, glutinous, sticky. In bacteriology, said of a colony that strings out by clinging to a needle when it is touched to the culture and withdrawn. The sediment rises in a coherent whirl when the liquid culture is shaken.

viscoelasticity The property of being viscous and elastic.

viscosimeter (vĭs″kŏs-ĭm′ĕ-tĕr) [LL. *viscosus,* viscous, + Gr. *metron,* measure] A device for estimating the viscosity of a fluid, esp. of blood.

viscosimetry (vĭs″kō-sĭm′ĕ-trē) Measurement of the viscosity of a substance.

viscosity (vĭs″kŏs′ĭ-tē) [LL. *viscosus,* viscous] **1.** The state of being sticky or gummy. **2.** Resistance offered by a fluid to change of form or relative position of its particles due to attraction of molecules to each other.

specific v. The internal friction of a fluid, measured by comparing the rate of flow of the liquid through a tube with that of some standard liquid, or by measuring the resistance to rotating paddles.

viscous (vĭs′kŭs) Sticky, gummy, gelatinous, with high viscosity.

viscus (vĭs′kŭs) *pl.* **viscera** [L., body organ] Any internal organ enclosed within a cavity, such as the thorax or abdomen.

visibility (vĭz″ĭ-bĭl′ĭ-tē) [L. *visibilitas*] The quality of being visible.

visible (vĭz′ĭ-bl) [L. *visibilis*] Capable of being seen.

visile (vĭz′ĭl) [L. *visum,* seeing] **1.** Pert. to vision. **2.** Readily recalling what is seen, more than that which is audible or motile.

vision (vĭzh′ŭn) [L. *visio,* a seeing] **1.** Act of viewing external objects. SYN: *sight.* SEE: *reading machine for the blind.* **2.** Sense by which light, color, form, and contrast are apprehended. **3.** An imaginary sight.

achromatic v. Complete color blindness.

artificial v. A technique, still in the experimental stage, designed to make it possible for some persons who are blind to see as a result of electrical stimulation of the retina or the connection of digital video cameras to the visual cortex of the brain.

binocular v. The visual sensation that is produced when the images perceived by each eye are fused to appear as one.

central v. Vision resulting from light falling on the fovea centralis.

day v. A condition in which one sees better during the day than at night, found in peripheral lesions of the retina such as retinitis pigmentosa. SYN: *photopic v.*

dichromatic v. A form of defective color vision in which only two of the primary colors are perceived.

double v. Diplopia.

field of v. The space within which an object can be seen while the eye remains fixed on one point. SEE: *perimetry*.

half v. Hemianopia.

indirect v. Peripheral v.

low v. A significant loss of vision that cannot be corrected medically, surgically, or with eyeglasses.

monocular v. Vision using only one eye.

multiple v. Polyopia.

night v. Ability to see when illumination is reduced. SYN: *scotopic v.*

oscillating v. Oscillopsia.

peripheral v. Vision resulting from rays falling on the retina outside of the macular field. SYN: *indirect v.*

phantom v. An experience of visual sensations following surgical removal of an eye; usually a transient condition.

photopic v. Day v.

scotopic v. Night v.

stereoscopic v. Vision in which things have the appearance of solidity and relief, as though seen in three dimensions. Binocular vision produces this effect. SYN: *stereopsis.*

tunnel v. **1.** Visual acuity that is limited to the central visual field, for example, two to three degrees of visual radius. **2.** An inability to appreciate the full scope of an issue.

v. without sight The ability of individuals who are blind and unable to perceive visual stimuli including bright light, to respond to light.

visit An encounter between a patient and a health professional that requires either the patient to travel from his or her home to the professional's usual place of practice (office visit) or vice versa (home visit).

Visiting Nurse Association A voluntary health agency that provides nursing services in the home, including health supervision, education and counseling, and maintenance of the medical regimen. Nurses and other personnel such as home health aides who are specifically trained for tasks of personal bedside care provide the services offered by the agency. These agencies originated in the visiting or district nurse service provided to the poor in their homes by voluntary agencies such as the New York City Mission, which existed in the 1870s. The first visiting nurse associations were established in Buffalo, Boston, and Philadelphia between 1886 and 1887.

visual (vĭzh′ū-ăl) [L. *visio,* a seeing] **1.** Pert. to vision. **2.** One whose learning and memorizing processes are largely of a visual nature.

visual acuity A measure of the resolving power of the eye; usually determined by one's ability to read letters of various sizes at a standard distance from the test chart. The result is expressed as a fraction. For example, 20/20 is normal vision, meaning the subject's eye has the ability to see from a distance of 20 ft (6.1 m) what the normal eye would see at that distance. Visual acuity of 20/40 means that a person sees at 20 ft (6.1 m) what the normal eye could see at 40 ft (12.2 m).

visual angle The angle between the line of sight and the extremities of the object seen.

visual axis The line of vision from the object seen through the pupil's center to the macula lutea.

visual cone The cone whose vertex is at the eye and whose generating lines touch the boundary of a visible object.

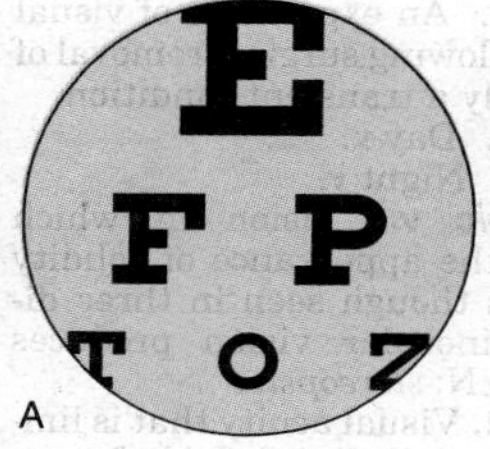

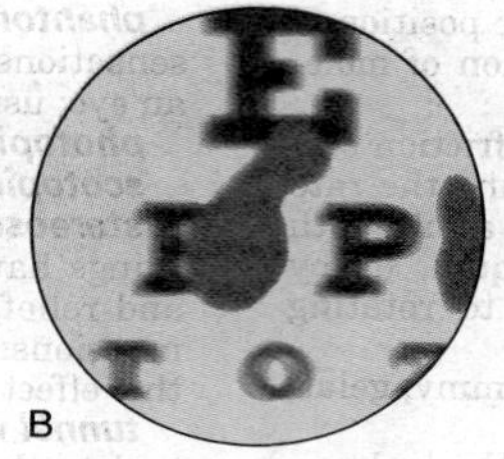

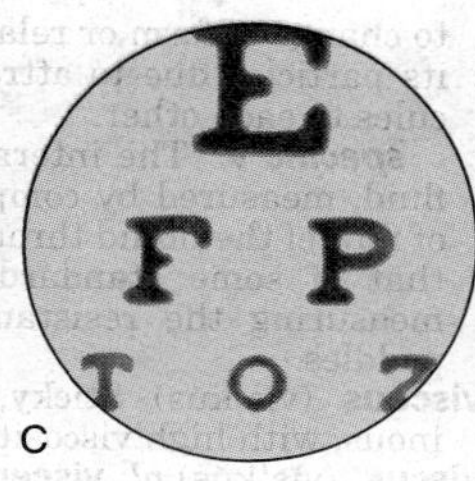

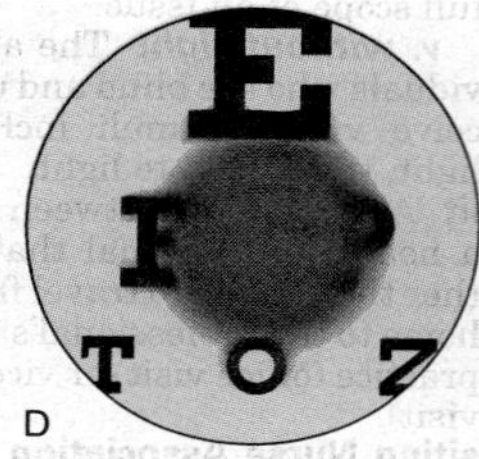

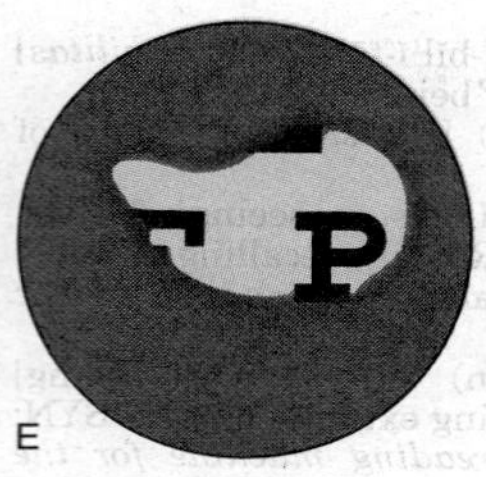

VISUAL FIELD ABNORMALITIES

(A) normal vision, (B) diabetic retinopathy, (C) cataracts, (D) macular degeneration, (E) advanced glaucoma

visual evoked response ABBR: VER. A reaction produced in response to visual stimuli. While the patient is watching a pattern projected on a screen, the electroencephalogram is recorded. The characteristics of the wave form, its latency, and the amplitude of the wave can be compared with the normal, and important information concerning the function of the visual apparatus in transmitting stimuli to the brain can be obtained. SEE: *brainstem auditory evoked potential; evoked response; somatosensory evoked response*.

visual field The area within which objects may be seen when the eye is fixed. SEE: illus; *perimetry*.

visual function Vision.

visualization (vĭzh″ū-ăl-ī-zā′shŭn) The act of viewing or sensing a picture of an object, esp. the picture of a body structure as obtained by radiographic study.

visualize (vĭzh′ū-ăl-īz) **1.** To make visible. **2.** To imagine or picture something in one's mind.

visual object agnosia Loss of the ability to visually recognize objects presented, even though some degree of ability to see is intact.

visual plane The plane in which both optic axes lie.

visual point The center of vision.

visuoauditory (vĭzh″ū-ō-aw′dĭ-tor″ē) [L. *visio,* a seeing, + *auditorius,* pert. to hearing] Rel. to sight and hearing, as connecting nerve fibers between auditory and visual centers.

visuognosis (vĭzh″ū-ŏg-nō′sĭs) [″ + Gr. *gnosis,* knowledge] The recognition and appreciation of what is seen.

visuopsychic (vĭzh″ū-ō-sī′kĭk) [″ + Gr. *psyche,* soul, mind] Both visual and psychic, applied to the cerebral area involved in perception of visual sensations.

visuosensory (vĭzh″ū-ō-sĕn′sō-rē) [L. *visio,* a seeing, + *sensorius,* sensory] Rel. to the recognition of visual impressions.

visuospatial Concerning the ability to discern spatial relationships from visual presentations.

vita glass (vī′tă-glăs) [L. *vita,* life, + AS. *glaes,* glass] Window glass containing quartz for transmitting the ultraviolet rays of sunlight.

vital (vī′tăl) [L. *vitalis,* pert. to life] **1.** Pert. to or characteristic of life. **2.** Contributing to or essential for life.

vital center Any of the centers in the medulla concerned with respiration, heart rate, or blood pressure.

vitality (vī-tăl′ĭ-tē) **1.** Animation, action. **2.** The state of being alive.

vitalometer A diagnostic device that measures the response of a nerve in the pulp of a tooth to an electrical stimulus.

vital statistics Statistics relating to births (natality), deaths (mortality), marriages, health, and disease (morbidity). Vital statistics for the U.S. are published annually by the National Center for Health Statistics of the Department of Health and Human Services.

vitamer (vī′tă-mĕr) Any one of a number of compounds that have specific vitamin activity.

vitamin (vī′tă-mĭn) [L. *vita,* life, + *amine*] An accessory but vital nutrient that serves as a coenzyme or cofactor in an essential metabolic process. Small quantities of the substance assist biological reactions such as oxidation and reduction, or the synthesis of nucleic acids, hemoglobin, clotting factors, or collagen. Vitamin deficiencies produce well-recognized syndromes (e.g., scurvy [vitamin C deficiency], or beriberi [thiamine deficiency]). Unlike proteins, carbohydrates, fats, and organic salts, vitamins are not energy sources or components of body structures. Instead, they are agents that hasten or facilitate biochemical processes involving these other organic molecules. SEE: *dietary reference intakes; mineral.*

Only vitamins A, D, and K are made within the body. The rest must be consumed in the diet. Vitamin A is formed from its precursor, carotene; vitamin D is formed by the action of ultraviolet light on the skin; and vitamin K is formed by the symbiotic action of bacteria within the intestines.

A common classification system distinguishes fat-soluble vitamins (A, D, E, and K) from water-soluble vitamins (B and C). Fat-soluble vitamins are poorly assimilated in diseases that interfere with the digestion of fat, such as steatorrhea, but accumulate in organs like the liver when taken in excess. Water-soluble vitamins are readily lost from the body in urine and sweat and are more likely to be lacking from the body than overabundant. SEE: *Vitamins Appendix.*

One's need for vitamins increases in conditions that deplete their stores from the body, such as pregnancy and lactation, alcoholism, and febrile illnesses. Some drugs block the action of specific vitamins, or create illnesses that can be prevented with vitamin supplementation. In patients taking isoniazid for tuberculosis, for example, vitamin supplementation with pyridoxine is needed to prevent peripheral neuropathy.

SYMPTOMS: Refer to the *Vitamins Appendix* for signs and symptoms of vitamin deficiency.

antiberiberi v. Vitamin B_1.

antineuritic v. Vitamin B_1.

antipellagra v. Nicotinamide.

antirachitic v. The vitamin D group.

antiscorbutic v. Vitamin C.

antixerophthalmic v. Vitamin A.

vitamin A A fat-soluble vitamin formed within the body from alpha, beta, and gamma carotene, the yellow pigments of plants. It is essential for normal growth and development, normal function and integrity of epithelial tissues, formation of visual pigment, and normal tooth and bone development. It is stored in the liver. The recommended daily requirement for adults is 1000 mg. Retinol is the form of vitamin A found in mammals. One retinol equivalent is equal to 6 mg of beta-carotene. Excessive intake of vitamin A may cause acute or chronic effects and may increase risk of developing cancer in smokers. SYN: *retinol.* SEE: *hypervitaminosis; Vitamins Appendix.*

SOURCES: Butter, butterfat in milk, egg yolks, and cod liver oil are rich sources. The vitamin is found also in liver, green leafy and yellow vegetables, prunes, pineapples, oranges, limes, and cantaloupes.

STABILITY: This vitamin resists boiling for some time if not exposed to oxidation. It is quite stable with brief exposure to heat but not with continued high temperatures (above 100°C or 212°F).

DEFICIENCY DISORDERS: A deficiency of vitamin A causes interference with growth, reduced resistance to infections, and interference with nutrition of the cornea, conjunctiva, trachea, hair follicles, and renal pelvis. Thus these tissues have an increased susceptibility to infections. Vitamin A deficiency also interferes with the ability of the eyes to adapt to darkness (night blindness) and impairs visual acuity. Children with vitamin A deficiency will experience impaired growth and development. SEE: *Bitot's spots.*

vitamin A_1 A form of vitamin A found in fish liver oils.

vitamin A_2 A compound found in the livers of freshwater fish; similar in properties to vitamin A but with different ultraviolet absorption spectra.

vitamin B complex A group of water-soluble vitamins isolated from liver, yeast, and other sources. Only grain-made yeast preserves its potency if dried. Among vitamins included are thiamine (B_1), riboflavin (B_2), niacin (nicotinic acid), pyridoxine (B_6), biotin, folic acid, and cyanocobalamin (B_{12}).

SOURCES: *Thiamine:* Whole grains, wheat embryo, brewer's yeast, legumes, nuts, egg yolk, fruits, and vegetables. *Riboflavin:* Brewer's yeast, liver, meat, esp. pork and fish, poultry, eggs, milk, and green vegetables. *Nicotinic acid:* Brewer's yeast, liver, meat, poultry, and green vegetables. *Pyridoxine:* Rice, bran, and yeast. *Folic acid:* Leafy green vegetables, organ meats, lean beef and veal, and wheat cereals. *General:* Fortified cereals, breads and baked goods are good sources of these.

ACTION/USES: The B vitamins affect growth, stimulate appetite, lactation, and the gastrointestinal, neurological, and endocrine systems; aid in prevention of marasmus; stimulate appetite; are important in metabolism of carbohydrates, including sugar; and stimulate biliary action.

Vitamin B_1, thiamine, affects growth and nutrition and carbohydrate metabolism. B_2, riboflavin, affects growth and cellular metabolism. Nicotinic acid prevents pellagra. Pyridoxine is used by patients taking the antitubercular drug, isoniazid, to prevent peripheral neuropathy.

NOTE: Prolonged use of antibiotics may destroy intestinal flora that produce some of the B vitamins. Vitamin supplementation may be required to prevent deficiencies.

STABILITY: B vitamins are stable during normal cooking, although they may be destroyed by excessive heating for 2 to 4 hours. Baking soda destroys thiamine. Riboflavin and nicotinic acid are more stable than thiamine and are not destroyed by heat or oxidation.

DEFICIENCY DISORDERS: Deficiency causes beriberi, pellagra, digestive disturbances, enlargement of the liver, disturbance of the thyroid, degeneration of sex glands, and disturbance of the nervous system. It also induces edema; affects the heart, liver, spleen, and kidneys; enlarges the adrenals; and causes dysfunction of the pituitary and salivary glands.

vitamin B_1 Thiamine, or thiamine hydrochloride. The recommended daily allowance is approx. 1.5 mg for men and 1.1 mg for women. SEE: *Vitamins Appendix*.

vitamin B_2 Riboflavin. SEE: *Vitamins Appendix*.

vitamin B_6 Pyridoxine; found in rice, bran, and yeast. Excess doses (2 to 5 g/day for months) have caused impairment of central nervous system function. SEE: *Vitamins Appendix*.

vitamin B_{12} A red crystalline substance, a cobamide, extracted from the liver, that is essential for the formation of red blood cells. Its deficiency results in pernicious anemia. It is used for prophylaxis and treatment of these and other diseases in which there is defective red cell formation. The recommended adult daily requirement is 2 μg/day. The terms vitamin B_{12} and cyanocobalamin are used interchangeably as the generic term for all of the cobamides active in humans. SYN: *cyanocobalamin*. SEE: *Vitamins Appendix*.

vitamin C Ascorbic acid, a factor necessary for formation of collagen in connective tissues and essential in maintenance of integrity of intercellular cement in many tissues, esp. capillary walls. Vitamin C deficiency leads to scurvy. SEE: *Vitamins Appendix*.

NOTE: The recommended adult daily allowance is 60 mg. Large daily doses of vitamin C have been recommended for prevention and treatment of the common cold. Although the effectiveness of vitamin C for this purpose has not been established, it is felt that the vitamin may at least decrease the severity of cold symptoms. Excess doses of vitamin C for an extended period can interfere with absorption of vitamin B_{12}, cause uricosuria, and promote formation of oxalate kidney stones.

SOURCES: Vitamin C is found in raw cabbage, young carrots, orange juice, lettuce, celery, onions, tomatoes, radishes, and green peppers. Citrus fruits and rutabagas are esp. rich in this vitamin. Strawberries are about as rich a source as tomatoes. Apples, pears, apricots, plums, peaches, and pineapples also contain vitamin C.

STABILITY: The vitamin is destroyed easily by heat in the presence of oxygen, as in open-kettle boiling. It is less affected by heat in an acid medium; otherwise, it is stable.

DEFICIENCY DISORDERS: Vitamin C deficiency causes scurvy, imperfect prenatal skeletal formation, defective teeth, pyorrhea, anorexia, and anemia. It also leads to undernutrition injury to bone, cells, and blood vessels.

vitamin D One of several vitamins having antirachitic activity. The vitamin D group, which is fat-soluble, includes D_2 (calciferol), D_3 (irradiated 7-dehydrocholesterol), D_4 (irradiated 22-dihydroergosterol), and D_5 (irradiated dehydrositosterol). It is essential in calcium and phosphorus metabolism; consequently, it is required for normal development of bones and teeth. The recommended daily allowance is 10 μg. The stability of this vitamin is not affected by oxidation; heat, unless over 100°C (212°F); or long-continued cooking. A deficiency of vitamin D causes imperfect skeletal formation, bone diseases, rickets, and caries. SEE: *Vitamins Appendix*.

SOURCES: Milk, cod liver oil, salmon and cod livers, egg yolk, and butter fat contain vitamin D. Ergosterol in the skin activated by sunlight or ultraviolet radiation possesses vitamin D potency.

ACTION/USES: Vitamin D is necessary for the absorption of calcium and phosphorus from food in the small intestine. It is called the antirachitic vitamin because its deficiency interferes with calcium and phosphorus use, which in turn causes rickets. Sun or ultraviolet radiation exposure synthesizes this vitamin in the body. Its presence is necessary for the most efficient absorption of calcium and phosphorus. It is used to treat and prevent infantile rickets, spasmophilia (infantile tetany), and softening of bone. Vitamin D is also important in normal growth and mineralization of skeleton and teeth.

Prolonged excessive doses of vitamin D (100,000 IU daily) cause hypercalcemia with anorexia, nausea, vomiting, polyuria, polydipsia, weakness, anxiety, pruritus, and altered renal function.

vitamin E Alpha-tocopherol, an essential nutrient for humans, although the exact biochemical mechanism whereby it functions in the body is unknown. Because of the amount of vitamin E present in foods, its deficiency is absent in the general population. Excessive doses (100 mg/kg/day) in low-birth-weight neonates have been implicated in the development of necrotizing enterocolitis and sepsis. The recommended adult daily allowance is 10 mg for men and 8 mg for women. SEE: *Vitamins Appendix.*

vitamin K An antihemorrhagic factor whose activity is associated with compounds derived from naphthoquinone. Vitamin K, which is fat soluble, is present in alfalfa, fats, oats, wheats, and rye; vitamin K_2, in fishmeal. Vitamin K_3 is synthesized as menadione sodium bisulfite. Vitamin K is necessary for synthesis of clotting factors VII, IX, X, and prothrombin by the liver. Its deficiency prolongs blood-clotting time and causes bleeding. Its roles in bone metabolism include its requirement for the conversion of osteocalcin to its active form and is requirement for matrix Gla-protein (MGP) function in bones, teeth and cartilage. Within the kidney, it acts to inhibit calcium oxalate stone formation. It appears to have a role in normal retinal signaling. In the newborn, the colon is sterile until food is ingested and bacteria colonize the site. Because this bacterial source of vitamin K is not immediately available, an intramuscular injection of 1 mg of water-soluble vitamin K_1 (phytonadione) is recommended for all newborns.

Large doses may cause hemolysis in persons with G6PD deficiency and in some healthy individuals. Large doses in the newborn may lead to anemia and kernicterus. The recommended adult daily allowance is 65 μg for women and 80 μg for men. SEE: *Vitamins Appendix.*

ACTION/USES: Vitamin K helps to eliminate prolonged bleeding in operations and in the biliary tract of jaundiced patients. Bile salts are necessary for its absorption.

vitamin loss Loss of vitamin content in food products as a result of oxidation or heating. Methods of preserving foods such as pickling, salting, curing, or fermenting and canning enhance vitamin loss. Vitamin C is especially labile; up to 85% is lost in commercial canning and pasteurization. Vitamin B_1 in wheat is lost through milling because the vitamin B_1 wheat embryo is removed.

vitamin supplement Any vitamin tablet or capsule containing one or more vitamins. Thus, a tablet or capsule may contain a single vitamin or many, and in some instances, a preparation will contain more than a dozen vitamins and an even greater number of minerals. The rationale for daily use of this latter type of vitamin and mineral supplement has not been established. In general, healthy adult men and healthy nonpregnant, nonlactating women consuming a normal, varied diet do not need vitamin supplements.

The difficulties of individuals choosing to treat themselves with vitamin supplements are: (1) People who take the supplements are usually already consuming an adequate diet. (2) The vitamins chosen are often not the ones inadequate in their diet. (3) The dose may be many times greater than the daily needs.

Some cardiologists, epidemiologists, and nutritionists feel that the combination of antioxidants and vitamin supplements such as vitamin C and vitamin E decreases the risk of developing heart disease. Others disagree and feel that essential nutrients should be and can be obtained from a healthy diet.

Also, excessive doses of pyridoxine (vitamin B_6) or vitamins A and D can cause toxic symptoms. SEE: *Food Guide Pyramid; vitamin C.*

vitellary (vĭt′ĕl-ā-rē) [L. *vitellus,* yolk of an egg] Vitelline.

vitellin (vī-tĕl′ĭn) A protein that can be extracted from egg yolk and contains lecithin. SEE: *nucleoprotein; ovovitellin.*

vitelline (vī-tĕl′ēn) Pert. to the yolk of an egg or the ovum.

vitelline circulation The embryonic circulation of blood to the yolk sac via the vitelline arteries and its return to general circulation through the vitelline veins.

vitelline duct The narrow duct connecting the yolk sac with the embryonic gut.

vitelline vein One of two veins conveying blood from the yolk sac.

vitellogenesis (vī″tĕl-ō-jĕn′ĕ-sĭs) The production of yolk.

vitellointestinal (vī″tĕl-ō-ĭn-tĕs′tĭn-ăl) Concerning the embryonic yolk sac and the intestinal tract.

vitellolutein (vī″tĕl-ō-lū′tē-ĭn) [L. *vitellus,* yolk, + *luteus,* yellow] A yellow pigment present in lutein.

vitellorubin (vī″tĕl-ō-rū′bĭn) [″ + *ruber,* red] A red pigment present in lutein.

vitellose (vī-tĕl′ōs) A proteose present in vitellin.

vitellus (vī-tĕl′ŭs) [L.] The yolk of an ovum, esp. the yolk of a hen's egg.

vitiation (vĭsh″ē-ā′shŭn) [L. *vitiare,* to corrupt] Injury, contamination, impairment of use or efficiency.

vitiligines (vĭt″ĭ-lĭj′ĭ-nēz) Depigmented areas of skin. SEE: *vitiligo.*

vitiliginous (vĭt″ĭ-lĭj′ĭ-nŭs) Concerning vitiligo.

vitiligo (vĭt-ĭl-ī′gō) [L.] A skin disorder characterized by the localized loss of melanocytes, with patchy loss of skin pigment. The depigmented areas, which appear most commonly on the hands, face, and genital region, are flat and pale and surrounded by normal pigmentation. Vitiligo affects all ages and races but is most noticeable in people with dark skin. The cause is unknown, but may be an autoimmune process since autoantibodies to melanocytes have been identified and vitiligo often occurs with autoimmune diseases. SYN: *leukoderma; skin, piebald.* SEE: illus.

TREATMENT: Oral and topical synthetic trioxsalen and a natural psoralen, methoxsalen, are used with exposure to long-wave ultraviolet light, but the efficacy is doubtful. The lesions may be masked by use of cosmetic preparations. Vitiliginous areas should be protected from sunburn by applying a 5% aminobenzoic acid solution or gel to the affected areas. The use of 5% fluorouracil cream applied under an occlusive dressing to the depigmented areas may cause erosion of the dermis and, after re-epithelialization, pigment may reappear.

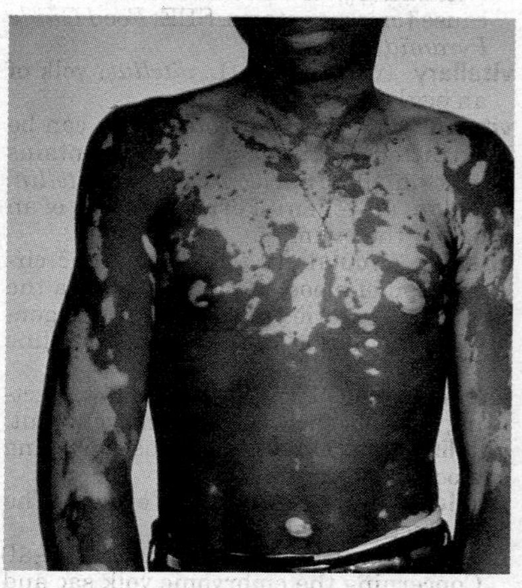

VITILIGO

v. capitis Vitiligo of the scalp with depigmentation of the hairs of the affected area.

perinevic v. Vitiligo surrounding a nevus.

vitium (vĭsh′ē-ŭm) *pl.* **vitia** [L., fault] A fault, defect, or vice.

vitrectomy (vĭ-trĕk′tō-mē) [L. *vitreus,* glassy, + Gr. *ektome,* excision] The use of a special instrument to remove the contents of the vitreous chamber and replace them with a sterile physiological saline solution.

vitreocapsulitis (vĭt″rē-ō-kăp″sū-lī′tĭs) [L. *vitreus,* glassy, + *capsula,* capsule, + Gr. *itis,* inflammation] Inflammation of the vitreous humor. SYN: *hyalitis.*

vitreodentin (vĭt″rē-ō-dĕn′tĭn) A particularly hard and brittle form of dentin.

vitreoretinal (vĭt″rē-ō-rĕt′ĭ-năl) Concerning the vitreous and the retina.

vitreous (vĭt′rē-ŭs) [L. *vitreus,* glassy] **1.** Glassy. **2.** Pert. to the vitreous body of the eye. **3.** Vitreous body.

vitrescence (vĭ-trĕs′ĕns) Becoming hard and transparent like glass.

vitreum (vĭt′rē-ŭm) Vitreous body.

vitrification The process of converting a silicate material into a smooth, viscous substance by heat. The silicate material hardens on cooling and possesses a smooth, glossy surface. In dentistry, it is related to the extensive use of ceramics, cements, and porcelains. These vary by the additive components that determine their density and refractive qualities.

vitriol (vĭt′rē-ōl) [L. *vitriolum*] A sulfate of any of various metals.

vitropression (vĭt″rō-prĕsh′ŭn) [L. *vitrum,* glass, + *pressio,* a squeezing] A method of temporarily eliminating redness of the skin caused by hyperemia by pressure with a glass slide on the skin for the purpose of studying any lesions or discolorations.

vivi- (vĭv′ĭ) [L. *vivus*] Combining form meaning *alive.*

vividiffusion (vĭv″ĭ-dĭf-ū′zhŭn) [L. *vivus,* alive, + *dis,* apart, + *fundere,* to pour] The process of removing diffusible substances from the blood of a living animal by allowing it to flow through dialyzing membranes immersed in saline solution.

vivification (vĭv″ĭ-fĭ-kā′shŭn) [″ + *facere,* to make] **1.** Trimming of the surface layer of a wound to aid the union of tissues. **2.** Transformation of protein through assimilation into the living matter of cellular organisms.

viviparity (vĭv″ĭ-păr′ĭ-tē) The ability to produce living young rather than producing young by laying an egg that hatches.

viviparous (vĭv-ĭp′ăr-ŭs) [″ + *parere,* to bring forth, to bear] Developing young within the body, the young being expelled and born alive; the opposite of oviparous.

vivisect (vĭv′ĭ-sĕkt) [L. *vivus,* alive, + *sectio,* a cutting] To dissect a living animal for experimental purposes.

vivisection (vĭv″ĭ-sĕk′shŭn) [″ + *sectio,* a cutting] Cutting of or operation on a living animal for physiological investigation and the study of disease.

vivisectionist (vĭv″ĭ-sĕk′shŭn-ĭst) One

who practices or believes in vivisection. SEE: *antivivisection*.

vivisector (vĭv-ĭs-ĕk′tor) [″ + *sector*, a cutting] One who practices vivisection.

VLDL *very low–density lipoprotein*.

Vleminckx's solution (flĕm′ĭnks) [Jean François Vleminckx, Belgian physician, 1800–1876] A solution of sulfurated lime used in various skin diseases, such as acne.

VMA *vanillylmandelic acid*.

V_{max} *maximum velocity*.

V.N.A. *Visiting Nurse Association*.

VO_2 Ventilatory oxygen extraction, a measure of the exercise capacity of a patient.

vocal (vō′kăl) [L. *vocalis*, talking] Pert. to the voice.

vocal cord Either of two thin, reedlike folds of tissue within the larynx that vibrate as air passes between them, producing sounds that are the basis of speech.

vocal cords, false The ventricular folds of the larynx.

vocal cords, true Vocal folds.

vocal folds The true vocal cords; the inferior pair of folds within the larynx; each contains a vocal ligament. They form the edges of the rima glottidis and are involved in the production of sound. SYN: *vocal cords, true*.

vocal ligament A strong band of elastic tissue lying within the vocal fold.

vocal lips Two shelflike projections of the lateral walls of the larynx. Their edges bear the vocal folds.

vocal muscle An intrinsic muscle of the larynx that pulls a vocal cord across the rima glottidis; exhaled air vibrates the vocal cords to produce sound.

vocal process The area of the arytenoid cartilage to which are attached the vocal cords.

vocal signs The indication of disease by changes in the voice.

voces (vō′sēz) [L.] Pl. of vox.

voice (voys) [L. *vox*] A sound, uttered by human beings, produced by vibration of the vocal cords.

amphoric v. Cavernous v.

v. break The sudden interruption of speech, or a sudden decrease in vocal amplitude. It is a sign of laryngeal spasm.

cavernous v. A hollow voice sound heard during auscultation of the chest, indicating a pulmonary cavity. SEE: *amphoric v.*

eunuchoid v. The characteristic high-pitched voice of a male in whom the normal sexual development has not occurred or in a male who was castrated before puberty.

voiceprint A graphical representation of the characteristics of an individual's speech pattern. Because voiceprints, like fingerprints, can be used to distinguish one person from another, the technique is useful in forensic medicine and in identifying the voices of criminal suspects.

voices (voys′ĕz) In psychiatry, verbal-auditory hallucinations expressed as being heard by the patient.

void (voyd) [O.Fr. *voider*, to empty] To evacuate the bowels or bladder.

vol *volume*.

vol% *volume percent*.

vola, volar (vō′lă, vō′lăr) [L.] Terms originally used to refer to the palm of the hand or sole of the foot. The preferred terms for reference to the palm of the hand are palmar and palmaris.

vola manus (vō′lă) Palm.

vola pedis The sole of the foot.

volaris (vō-lā′rĭs) Vola.

volatile (vŏl′ă-tĭl) [L. *volatilis*, flying] Easily vaporized or evaporated. Examples of volatile liquids are ether (boiling point, 34.5°C) and ethyl chloride (boiling point, 12.2°C).

volatilization (vŏl″ă-tĭl-ī-zā′shŭn) Conversion of a solid or liquid into a vapor.

volatilize (vŏl′ă-tĭl-īz) To vaporize a liquid or solid.

volition (vō-lĭsh′ŭn) [L. *volitio*, will] The act or power of willing or choosing.

volitional (vō-lĭsh′ŭn-ăl) Performed by volition.

Volkmann's canals (fōlk′mănz) [Alfred Wilhelm Volkmann, Ger. physiologist, 1800–1877] Vascular channels in compact bone. They are not surrounded by concentric lamellae as are the haversian canals.

Volkmann's contracture (fōlk′mănz) [Richard von Volkmann, Ger. surgeon, 1830–1889] Degeneration, contracture, fibrosis, and atrophy of a muscle resulting from injury to its blood supply; usually seen in the hand. SYN: *ischemic paralysis*.

volley (vŏl′ē) [L. *volare*, to fly] The simultaneous or nearly simultaneous discharge of a number of nerve impulses from a center within the brain or spinal cord.

volt (vōlt) [Count Alessandro Volta, It. physicist, 1745–1827] An electrical unit of pressure, the electromotive force required to produce 1 ampere of current through a resistance of 1 ohm.

voltage (vōl′tĭj) Electromotive force or difference in potential expressed in volts.

voltaic (vŏl-tā′ĭk) Concerning electricity produced by a battery.

voltaism (vŏl′tă-ĭzm) Galvanism.

voltammeter (vōlt-ăm′mē-tĕr) A device for measuring both volts and amperes.

voltammetry, anodic stripping ABBR: ASV. An analytical technique used to assay blood lead content.

voltampere (vōlt-ăm′pēr) The value obtained by multiplying volts times amperes.

voltmeter A device for measuring voltage, esp. for determining the voltage between two points of an electrical circuit.

volubility (vŏl″ū-bĭl′ĭ-tē) [L. *volubilitas,* flow of discourse] Excessive speech.

volume (vŏl′ūm) The space occupied by a substance, usually a gas or liquid. Liquid volume is expressed in liters or milliliters; gas volume in cubic centimeters.

closing v. The amount of gas remaining in the lung when the small airways close during a maximum expiratory effort. It is increased in patients with small airway disease.

compressed v. The portion of the mechanically delivered tidal volume that is not delivered to the patient owing to expansion of the ventilator circuit with pressure. Tubing with a high compliance increases the compressed volume, esp. when the tidal volume is delivered under high pressure.

expiratory reserve v. The maximal amount of air that can be forced from the lungs after normal expiration.

hospital v. The number of cases of specific conditions (e.g., stroke, acute myocardial infarction, or organ transplantation) treated at an inpatient facility. Morbidity and mortality are typically lowest in treatment centers where professional staff has the greatest clinical experience.

inspiratory reserve v. The maximal amount of air that can be inhaled after a normal inspiration.

mean corpuscular v. ABBR: MCV. The mean volume of an average erythrocyte. Normal values range from 82 to 92 cubic microns.

minute v. The volume of gas expired or inspired per minute in quiet breathing, usually measured as expired ventilation.

packed cell v. Hematocrit.

residual v. ABBR: RV. The volume of air remaining in the lungs after maximal expiration. This air is essential for continuous gas exchange.

stroke v. The amount of blood ejected by the left ventricle at each heartbeat. The amount varies with age, sex, and exercise. SYN: *systolic discharge.*

tidal v. The volume of air inspired and expired in a normal breath.

volumenometer (vŏl″ūm-nŏm′ĕ-tĕr) Volumometer.

volume percent ABBR: vol%. The number of cubic centimeters (milliliters) of a substance (usually oxygen or carbon dioxide) contained in 100 ml of another substance (e.g., blood).

volumetric (vŏl″ū-mĕt′rĭk) [L. *volumen,* a volume, + Gr. *metron,* measure] Pert. to measurement of volume.

volumometer (vŏl″ū-mŏm′ĕ-tĕr) A device for measuring volume. SYN: *volumenometer.*

voluntary (vŏl′ŭn-tĕr″ē) [L. *voluntas,* will] Pert. to or under control of the will.

voluntary health agency Any nonprofit, nongovernmental agency, governed by lay or professional individuals and organized on a national, state, or local level, whose primary purpose is health related. This term applies to agencies supported mainly by voluntary public contributions. These agencies are usually engaged in programs of service, education, and research related to a particular disability or group of diseases and disabilities; for example, the American Heart Association, American Cancer Society, National Lung Institute, and their state and local affiliates. The term can also be applied to such agencies as nonprofit hospitals, visiting nurse associations, and other local service organizations that have both lay and professional governing boards and are supported by both voluntary contributions and charges and fees for service provided.

voluntary muscle Any muscle that is normally controlled by the will. These muscles are generally attached to the skeleton and are innervated by myelinated nerves coming directly from the brain or spinal cord. Microscopically, they consist of long cylindrical fibers bearing crosswise striations. The terms voluntary, striated, and skeletal are synonymous when applied to muscle.

voluptuous (vō-lŭp′tū-ŭs) [L. *voluptas,* pleasure] **1.** Pert. to, arising from, or provoking, consciously or otherwise, sensual desire, usually applied to the female sex. **2.** Given to sensualism.

volute (vō-lūt′) [L. *volutus,* rolled] Convolute.

volvulosis (vŏl″vū-lō′sĭs) Onchocerciasis.

volvulus (vŏl′vū-lŭs) [L. *volvere,* to roll] A twisting of the bowel on itself, causing obstruction. A prolapsed mesentery is the predisposing cause. This usually occurs at the sigmoid and ileocecal areas of the intestines.

vomer (vō′mĕr) [L., plowshare] The plow-shaped bone that forms the lower and posterior portion of the nasal septum, articulating with the ethmoid, the sphenoid, the two palate bones, and the two superior maxillary bones.

vomerine (vō′mĕr-ĭn) Pert. to the vomer.

vomerobasilar (vō″mĕr-ō-băs′ĭ-lăr) Concerning the vomer and base of the skull.

vomeronasal (vō″mĕr-ō-nā′săl) Pert. to the vomer and nasal bones.

vomeronasal cartilage One of two narrow strips of cartilage lying along the anterior portion of the inferior border of the septal cartilage of the nose.

vomeronasal organ A small tubular epithelial sac lying on the anteroinferior surface of the nasal septum; rudimentary in humans. SYN: *Jacobson's organ.*

vomica (vŏm′ĭ-kă) *pl.* **vomicae** [L., ulcer] **1.** A cavity in the lungs, as from suppuration. **2.** Sudden and profuse expectoration of putrid purulent matter.

vomicose (vŏm′ĭ-kōs) Marked by many ulcers; ulcerous; purulent.

vomit (vŏm′ĭt) [L. *vomere,* to vomit] **1.** Material that is ejected from the stomach through the mouth. **2.** To eject stomach contents through the mouth. SYN: *vomitus.* SEE: *melena; nausea.*

PHYSIOLOGY: The act is usually a reflex involving the coordinated activity of both voluntary and involuntary muscles. A certain position is assumed, the glottis is closed, the diaphragm and abdominal muscles contract, and the cardiac sphincter of the stomach relaxes while antiperistaltic waves course over the duodenum, stomach, and esophagus.

bilious v. Bile forced back into the stomach and ejected with vomited matter.

black v. Vomit containing blood acted on by gastric digestion; seen in digestion conditions where blood collects in the stomach.

coffee-ground v. Vomit having the appearance and consistency of coffee grounds because of blood mixed with gastric contents. It can occur in any condition associated with hemorrhage into the stomach.

vomiting (vŏm′ĭt-ĭng) [L. *vomere,* to vomit] Ejection through the mouth of the contents of the gastrointestinal tract. Along with diarrhea and hemorrhage, vomiting is an important potential cause of dehydration. It may result from toxins, drugs, uremia, and fevers; cerebral tumors; meningitis (often unaccompanied by nausea and failing to relieve associated headache); diseases of the stomach such as ulcer, cancer, dysmotility, or dyspepsia; reflex from pregnancy, uterine or ovarian disease, irritation of the fauces, intestinal parasites, biliary colic; intestinal obstruction; motion sickness; and neurological disorders such as migraine. Vomiting may also be psychological ("psychogenic") in origin. Esophageal vomiting may result from reflux or obstruction. SYN: *emesis.* SEE: table; *bulimia; hyperemesis gravidarum.*

TREATMENT: Antinausea medicines should be taken by mouth, rectally, intramuscularly or intravenously. Fluids may be given by mouth if the patient will accept them. If vomiting continues, intravenous fluids and electrolytes will be required to replace those lost in the vomit.

PATIENT CARE: Causative factors such as drugs, food, diseases, and psychological factors are assessed and treated if possible. Frequency, amount, time, and characteristics of vomit are assessed. The patient is positioned to protect the airway and prevent aspiration, and suction equipment is available. Antiemetics are administered as prescribed. Food and fluids are withheld for several hours, and mouth care is offered. If the patient requires surgery, restriction of foods and fluids for approx. 8 hr before surgery helps to prevent vomiting. Comfort measures, such as a cool cloth applied to the face, are instituted. Serum electrolytes are monitored, and accurate intake and output records are kept to ensure proper fluid replacement. Vital signs are monitored for evidence of dehydration. The health caregiver promotes a calm environment and provides distraction.

cyclic v. Periodic and recurring attacks of vomiting occurring in patients with a nervous temperament. Continued vomiting causes metabolic alkalosis as a result of chloride loss.

SYMPTOMS: Dizziness, loss of appetite, headache, and nausea may occur. The patient then vomits about every half hour for 1 to 2 days. Great thirst, slight rise of temperature, rapid pulse, and prostration are present.

PATIENT CARE: The patient's symptoms are assessed and documented, vital signs monitored, fluid and electrolyte balance maintained, and prescribed

Causes of Vomiting

Gastrointestinal diseases	Esophageal obstruction, gastric distention, peptic ulcer disease, gastroparesis, cholecystitis, cholelithiasis, pancreatitis, intestinal obstruction, ileus
Metabolic illnesses	Hyponatremia, hypokalemia, hypercalcemia, adrenal insufficiency, uremia, ketoacidosis
Intoxications	Acetaminophen, arsenic, mercury, methanol, opiates, mescaline, food poisoning and many others
Drug side effects	Antidepressants, digitalis, erythromycin, theophyllines, many chemotherapeutic drugs for the treatment of cancer (e.g., cisplatin).
Intracranial illnesses	Migraine, meningitis, intracranial hemorrhage
Febrile illnesses	Strep throat (esp. in children), pyelonephritis, many others
Pregnancy	Hyperemesis gravidarum

medications administered to relieve headache, nausea, and vomiting. A calm, stress-free environment is provided.

dry v. Nausea and retching without vomit.

epidemic v. Sudden unexplained attacks of gastroenteritis characterized by nausea, vomiting, and sometimes diarrhea. Although not proven, the symptoms are believed to be due to a virus. Treatment is symptomatic.

induced v. The production of vomiting by administering certain types of emetics (e.g., syrup of ipecac or amorphine) or by physical stimulation of the posterior pharynx.

CAUTION: Vomiting should never be induced after patients ingest caustic chemicals or in patients who cannot protect their own airways.

---

pernicious v. Hyperemesis gravidarum.

v. of pregnancy The vomiting, esp. morning sickness, that some women experience during pregnancy.

projectile v. Ejection of vomit with great force.

psychogenic v. Occasional or persistent vomiting associated with severe emotional stress or brought on by the anticipation of stress. Each person has the potential for this reaction to emotional stress, but the threshold varies from one person to another.

stercoraceous v. Vomiting of fecal matter.

vomitus (vŏm′ĭ-tŭs) Vomit.

von Gierke disease (fŏn gēr′kĕz) [Edgar von Gierke, Ger. pathologist, 1877–1945] Glycogen storage disease type 1a. SYN: *glycogenosis; glycogen storage disease.*

von Graefe's sign (fŏn grā′fēz) [Albrecht von Graefe, Ger. ophthalmologist, 1828–1870] The failure of the eyelid to move downward promptly with the eyeball; the lid moves tardily and jerkily. This sign is seen in exophthalmic goiter.

von Hippel's disease Hippel's disease.

von Jaksch's disease [Rudolf von Jaksch-Wartenhorst, Austrian physician, 1855–1947] A symptom complex consisting of anemia, hepatosplenomegaly, and infections that are associated with a number of chronic diseases such as tuberculosis and malnutrition.

von Pirquet's test (fŏn pēr′kāz) [Clemens Peter Johann von Pirquet, Austrian pediatrician, 1874–1929] A diagnostic test for tuberculosis in which a small amount of tuberculin is applied to a scarified area of the skin of the arm. A positive reaction is seen if a pimply red eruption appears several days later at the site of inoculation. SEE: *tine test.*

von Recklinghausen's canals Recklinghausen's canals.

von Recklinghausen's disease Type 1 neurofibromatosis.

von Recklinghausen's tumor Recklinghausen's tumor.

von Willebrand's disease [Erik Adolph von Willebrand, Finnish physician, 1870–1949] A congenital bleeding disorder caused by a deficiency of coagulation factor VIII. This disease is inherited as an autosomal dominant trait. The bleeding tendency manifests at an early age, usually as epistaxis and easy bruising and, rarely, petechiae. Bleeding in the intestinal tract during surgery and excess loss of blood during menstruation are common. The symptoms decrease in severity with age and during pregnancy. The disorder is diagnosed by prolonged bleeding time and factor VIII deficiency. Treatment involves administering factor VIII 24 to 48 hr before surgery or during attacks of bleeding.

Voorhees' bag (voor′ēz) [James Ditmors Voorhees, U.S. obstetrician, 1869–1929] An inflatable rubber bag used in the distant past for dilating the cervix uteri to induce and facilitate labor.

voracious (vō-rā′shŭs) [L. *vorare,* to devour] Having an insatiable or ravenous appetite.

vortex (vor′tĕks) *pl.* **vortices** [L., a whirlpool] A structure having a spiral or whorled appearance.

coccygeal v. The region over the coccyx where lanugo hairs of the embryo come to a point.

v. of heart The region at the apex of the heart where muscle fibers of the ventricles make a tight spiral and turn inward.

v. lentis Spiral patterns on the surface of the lens owing to a concentric pattern of fiber growth.

vortices (vor′tĭ-sēz) [L.] Pl. of vortex.

v. pilorum Hair whorls as in arrangement of hairs on the scalp.

vorticose (vor′tĭk-ōs) [L. *vortices,* whirlpools] Whirling or having a whorled arrangement.

vorticose vein One of four veins (two superior and two inferior) that receive blood from all parts of the choroid of the eye. They empty into posterior ciliary and superior ophthalmic veins.

vox (vŏks) *pl.* **voces** [L.] Voice.

voyeur (voy-yĕr′) [Fr., one who sees] One who derives sexual pleasure from observing nude persons or the sexual activity of others.

voyeurism (voy′yĕr-ĭzm) The experiencing of sexual gratification by observing nude persons or the sexual activity of others.

V.R. *right vision; ventilation rate; vocal resonance.*

VRE *vancomycin-resistant enterococcus.*

V.S. *vesicular sound; vital signs; volumetric solution.*

VSD *ventricular septal defect.*

vuerometer (vū″ĕr-ŏm′ĕ-tĕr) [Fr. *vue*, sight, + Gr. *metron*, measure] An apparatus for measuring the interpupillary distance of the eyes.

vulgaris (vŭl-gā′rĭs) [L.] Ordinary, common.

vulnerable (vŭl′nĕr-ă-bl) [L. *vulnerare*, to wound] Easily injured or wounded.

vulnerant (vŭl′nĕr-ănt) **1.** Something that wounds or injures. **2.** To inflict injury.

vulnerary (vŭl′nĕr-ār″ē) **1.** Pert. to wounds. **2.** An agent, esp. a folk remedy or herb, used to promote wound healing.

Vulpian-Heidenhain-Sherrington phenomenon [Edme-Felix Alfred Vulpian, French physician, 1826–1887; Rudolph Peter Heinrich Heidenhain, Ger. physiologist, 1834–1897; Sir Charles Scott Sherrington, Brit. physiologist, 1857–1952] Contraction of denervated skeletal muscle by stimulating autonomic cholinergic fibers innervating its blood vessels.

vulsella, vulsellum (vŭl-sĕl′ă, vŭl-sĕl′ŭm) [L. *vulsella*, tweezers] A forceps with a hook on each blade.

vulva (vŭl′vă) *pl.* **vulvae** [L., covering] That portion of the female external genitalia lying posterior to the mons veneris, consisting of the labia majora, labia minora, clitoris, vestibule of the vagina, vaginal opening, Bartholin's glands. SYN: *pudendum femininum.* SEE: illus.

v. connivens Vulva in which the labia majora are in apposition.

v. hians Vulva in which the labia majora are gaping.

velamen v. An abnormally elongated clitoris.

vulval, vulvar [L. *vulva*, covering] Relating to the vulva.

vulvar dystrophy Lichen sclerosis et atrophicus.

vulvar leukoplakia Lichen sclerosis et atrophicus.

vulvectomy (vŭl-vĕk′tō-mē) [″ + Gr. *ektome*, excision] Excision of the vulva, used to manage cancers of the vulva. Surgical approaches depend on the stage of neoplasia and range from simple vulvar excision to radical vulvectomy with node dissection. SEE: *vulvar cancer.*

Patient Care: The caregiver provides emotional support, encourages questions, and meets the patient's informational needs. *Preoperative:* Care includes skin preparation, administration of prophylactic medications to prevent infection, and insertion of an indwelling catheter. The caregiver encourages the woman to verbalize her anxieties, fears, and concerns; validates her understanding of the procedure and its implications (change in body image and alterations in sexual function); and witnesses her informed consent. *Postoperative:* Care includes cleansing the wound with diluted hydrogen peroxide, rinsing with normal saline, and drying with a heat lamp, a cool-air hair dryer, or exposure

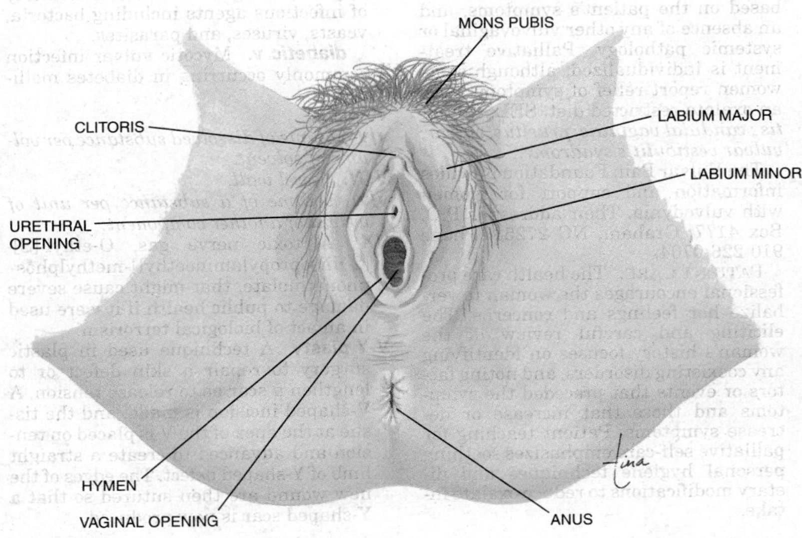

VULVA

Inferior view of the perineum

to the air three or more times daily as ordered. The caregiver positions the woman for comfort and administers analgesics as needed and ordered. Discharge teaching emphasizes meticulous wound care. The patient is advised to report bleeding, purulent discharge, or intolerable pain to the primary caregiver. After a simple vulvectomy, sexual intercourse may resume when the wound has healed.

vulvitis (vŭl-vī′tĭs) [L. *vulva,* covering, + Gr. *itis,* inflammation] Inflammation of the vulva.

acute nongonorrheal v. Vulvitis resulting from chafing of the opposed lips of the vulva or from accumulated sebaceous material around the clitoris.

follicular v. Inflammation of the hair follicles of the vulva.

gangrenous v. Necrosis and sloughing of areas of the vulva, often a complication of infectious diseases such as diphtheria, scarlatina, herpes genitalis, or typhoid fever.

leukoplakic v. Lichen sclerosis et atrophicus.

mycotic v. Vulvitis caused by various fungi, most commonly *Candida albicans.*

vulvo- Combining form meaning *covering, vulva.*

vulvocrural (vŭl″vō-kroo′răl) [L. *vulva,* covering, + *cruralis,* pert. to the leg] Rel. to the vulva and thigh.

vulvodynia [″ + *dynia,* pain] Vulvar pain; a nonspecific syndrome of unknown etiology. Common complaints include sporadic pain, dyspareunia, and pruritus. A provisional diagnosis is based on the patient's symptoms, and an absence of any other vulvovaginal or systemic pathology. Palliative treatment is individualized, although some women report relief of symptoms with an oxalate-restricted diet. SEE: *vaginitis ; candidal vaginitis; pruritus, vulvar; vulvar vestibulitis syndrome.*

The Vulvar Pain Foundation provides information and support for women with vulvodynia. Their address is P.O. Box 4177, Graham, NC 27253. Phone 910-226-0704.

PATIENT CARE: The health care professional encourages the woman to verbalize her feelings and concerns. The eliciting and careful review of the woman's history focuses on identifying any coexisting disorders, and noting factors or events that preceded the symptoms and those that increase or decrease symptoms. Patient teaching for palliative self-care emphasizes soothing personal hygiene techniques and dietary modifications to reduce oxalate intake.

PERSONAL HYGIENE: Recommendations include the use of bland bath soap, warm water rinses over the vulva after voiding, and daily lukewarm sitz baths, while avoiding the use of known common irritants such as perfumed soaps, douches, and feminine hygiene sprays, as well as spermicidal agents (e.g., jellies and creams).

DIETARY MODIFICATIONS: Avoiding foods high in oxalic acid (e.g., beets, black tea, chocolate and cocoa, dried figs, ground pepper, nuts, parsley, rhubarb, spinach, Swiss chard) and taking the over-the-counter nutritional supplement calcium citrate may help reduce symptoms associated with urination.

idiopathic v. Vulvar dysesthesia.

vulvopathy (vŭl-vŏp′ă-thē) [″ + Gr. *pathos,* disease, suffering] Any disorder of the vulva.

vulvouterine (vŭl″vō-ū′tĕr-ĭn) [″ + *uterinus,* pert. to the uterus] Rel. to the vulva and uterus.

vulvovaginal (vŭl″vō-văj′ĭ-năl) [″ + *vagina,* a sheath] Pert. to the vulva and vagina. SYN: *vaginovulvar.*

vulvovaginal gland One of the small glands on either side of the vaginal orifice. SYN: *Bartholin's gland.*

vulvovaginitis (vŭl″vō-văj″ĭ-nī′tĭs) [″ + ″ + Gr. *itis,* inflammation] Simultaneous inflammation of the vulva and vagina, or of the vulvovaginal glands. The condition may be due to chemical irritation produced by materials present in medications, tight-fitting or nonabsorbent underclothes, inadequate perineal hygiene, allergic conditions, or a variety of infectious agents including bacteria, yeasts, viruses, and parasites.

diabetic v. Mycotic vulvar infection commonly occurring in diabetes mellitus.

vv *veins.*

v/v *volume of dissolved substance per volume of solvent.*

V.W. *vessel wall.*

v/w *volume of a substance per unit of weight of another component.*

VX A toxic nerve gas, O-ethyl-[S]-[2-diisopropylaminoethyl]-methylphosphonothiolate, that might cause severe damage to public health if it were used in an act of biological terrorism.

V-Y-plasty A technique used in plastic surgery to repair a skin defect or to lengthen a scar as to release tension. A V-shaped incision is made, and the tissue at the apex of the V is placed on tension and advanced to create a straight limb of Y-shaped defect. The edges of the new wound are then sutured so that a Y-shaped scar is now produced.

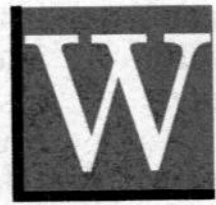

W Symbol for the element tungsten (wolfram).

w *watt; week; wife; with.*

Waardenburg syndrome [Petrus Johannes Waardenburg, Dutch ophthalmologist, 1886–1979] One of several related autosomally transmitted syndromes that may produce skin, neurological, ophthalmic, and auditory deficits.

Wachendorf's membrane (vŏk′ĕn-dorfs) [Eberhard J. Wachendorf, Dutch physician, 1703–1758] **1.** A thin membrane occluding the pupil of the embryo. **2.** The outer membrane ensheathing a cell.

wafer (wā′fĕr) [Ger. *wafel*] **1.** A thin sheet of flour paste used to enclose a medicinal dose of powder. **2.** A flat vaginal suppository.

Wagstaffe's fracture (wăg′stăfs) [William Warwick Wagstaffe, Brit. surgeon, 1843–1910] A fracture with displacement of the medial malleolus of the ankle.

waist (wāst) [ME. *wast,* growth] The small part of the human trunk between the thorax and hips.

waiting list A form of health care rationing that is used esp. in the distribution of scarce resources, such as organs for transplantation.

wakeful (wāk′fŭl) [AS. *wacian,* to be awake, + *full,* complete] Not able to sleep; sleepless.

Walcher's position (vŏl′kĕrz) [Gustav Adolf Walcher, Ger. gynecologist, 1856–1935] A position in which the patient assumes a dorsal recumbent posture with the hips at the edge of the bed and the legs hanging down.

Wald, Lillian (wăld) U.S. nurse, 1867–1940, who founded the Henry Street Settlement in New York City, one of the world's first visiting nurse associations.

Wald cycle The transformations involved in the breakdown or resynthesis of rhodopsin.

Waldenström's disease (văl′dĕn-strĕmz) [Johann Henning Waldenström, Swedish surgeon, b. 1877] Osteochondritis deformans juvenilis.

Waldeyer's gland (vŏl′dī-ĕrz) [Wilhelm von Waldeyer, Ger. anatomist, 1836–1921] A sweat gland of the eyelids; usually found most prominently in the lower lid margin.

Waldeyer's neuron The nerve cell and its processes.

Waldeyer's ring SEE: *ring, lymphoid.*

walk **1.** A method of locomotion of upright bipeds such as humans. **2.** The particular way an individual moves. SEE: *gait.*

walker A device used to assist a person in walking, esp. a person prone to falling. It consists of a stable platform made of lightweight metal tubing that is at a height that permits it to be grasped by the hands and used as support while taking a step. The walker is then moved forward and another step is taken. SEE: *crutch.*

walking [AS. *wealcan,* to roll] The act of moving on foot; advancing by steps.

impaired w. Limitation of independent movement within the environment on foot. SEE: *Nursing Diagnoses Appendix.*

walking cast A cast that allows the patient to be ambulatory.

walking system A complex device that enables patients with spinal injuries resulting in paralysis of the legs to walk. The device uses computer-controlled electrical stimulation to muscles so that walking may be accomplished. Each of these devices is made esp. for each patient, and their use is experimental.

walking wounded In military medicine, an ambulatory case.

wall [AS. *weall*] The limiting or surrounding substance or material of a cell, vessel, or cavity such as an artery, vein, chest, or bladder. In dentistry, it may refer to specific boundaries of a cavity preparation or its location within the tooth, for example, cavity walls: buccal, lingual, mesial, distal, pulpal, coronal, axial, cervical, facial, incisal, gingival, or enamel.

Wallenberg's syndrome (vŏl′ĕn-bĕrgz) [Adolf Wallenberg, Ger. physician, 1862–1949] A complex of symptoms resulting from occlusion of the posteroinferior cerebellar artery or one of its branches supplying the lower portion of the brainstem. Dysphagia, muscular weakness or paralysis, impairment of pain and temperature senses, and cerebellar dysfunction are characteristic.

wallerian degeneration (wŏl-ē′rē-ăn) [Augustus Volney Waller, Brit. physician, 1816–1870] The degeneration of a nerve fiber (axon) that has been severed from its cell body. The myelin sheath also degenerates and is transformed into a chain of lipoid droplets that stains by the Marchi method, which is used in tracing the course of injured nerve fibers. The neurilemma does not degenerate but forms a tube that directs the growth of the regenerating axon.

walleye [ME. *wawil-eghed*] **1.** An eye in which the iris is light-colored or white.

2. Leukoma or dense opacity of the cornea. 3. A squint in which both visual axes diverge. SYN: *strabismus, divergent.*

Walthard's islets, Walthard's inclusions [Max Walthard, Swiss gynecologist, 1867–1933] Nests or small cysts of embryological squamous epithelium-like cells in the superficial parts of the ovary, tubes, and uterine ligaments. They are thought to represent the beginning Brenner tumor.

wandering (wăn′dĕr-ĭng) [AS. *wandrian*] Moving about; not fixed.

wandering spleen A dislocated floating spleen.

Wangensteen tube (wăn′gĕn-stēn) [Owen H. Wangensteen, U.S. surgeon, 1898–1981] A double-lumen tube used for relieving postoperative abdominal distention, nausea, vomiting, and certain cases of mechanical bowel obstruction. It is used as an intranasal catheter in combination with a suction siphonage apparatus. SEE: *decompression.*

Warburg apparatus [Otto H. Warburg, Ger. biochemist, 1883–1970] A capillary manometer used for determining oxygen consumption and carbon dioxide production of small bits of cellular tissue. It is widely used in metabolism studies.

ward [AS. *weard,* watching over] A large room in a hospital for the care of several patients.

accident w. A ward reserved for the care of traumatic injuries.

psychiatric w. A ward in a general hospital for mentally ill patients.

Wardrop's operation Ligation of an artery for aneurysm at a distance beyond the sac.

warehousemen's itch Eczema of the hands resulting from touching irritating substances.

warfarin poisoning Poisoning caused by accidental administration of an overdose of warfarin or by the cumulative effect of repeated administration of the drug. SEE: *Poisons and Poisoning Appendix.*

TREATMENT: Vitamin K and/or fresh frozen plasma may be given as antidotes.

PATIENT CARE: The patient is instructed to observe for signs of bleeding such as epistaxis, bleeding gums, hematuria, hematochezia, hemetemesis, melena, and bleeding into the skin (ecchymosis, purpura, or petechia). The importance of regular blood tests (to assess the protime and international normalized ratio) and medical follow-up is stressed. The patient should wear or carry a medical identification tag listing the prescribed drug, dosage, frequency of administration, and physician's name and telephone number. Because many drugs interact with anticoagulants to interfere with their action, the patient should consult with the health care professional before taking new over-the-counter or prescribed medication.

warfarin potassium An anticoagulant drug.

warfarin sodium [name derived from initials of *W*isconsin *A*lumni *R*esearch *F*oundation] An anticoagulant drug. Coumadin and Panwarfin are trade names.

wart (wort) [AS. *wearte*] A circumscribed cutaneous elevation resulting from hypertrophy of the papillae and epidermis. SEE: illus.

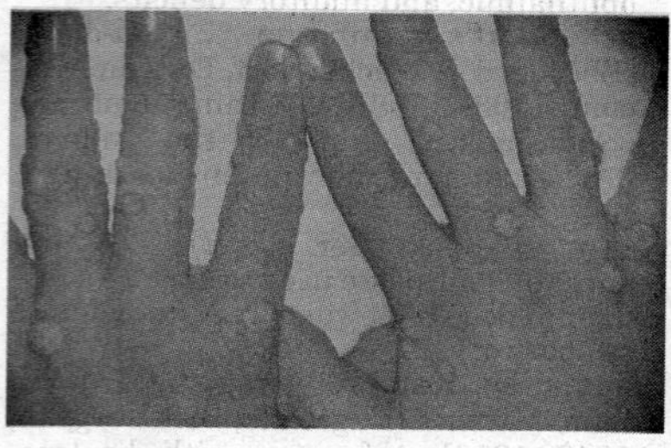

COMMON WARTS

common w. Verruca vulgaris.

genital w. A wart of the genitalia, caused by human papillomavirus (HPV). In women, these warts may be associated with cancer of the cervix. An estimated 1 million new cases of genital warts occur each year in the U.S. SYN: *venereal w.* SEE: illus.

TREATMENT: A variety of therapies, including topically applied chemicals

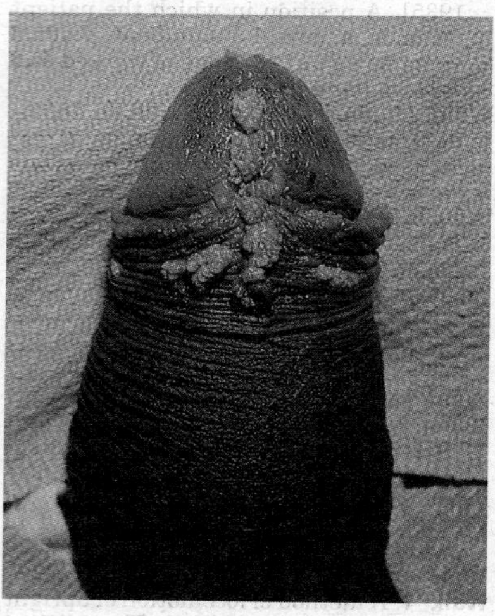

GENITAL WARTS ON PENIS

such as podophyllin, laser therapy, surgery, and recombinant interferon alfa-2a, have been used with varying degrees of success. Nevertheless, there is no completely safe and effective therapy available for genital warts.

PATIENT CARE: A history is obtained for unprotected sexual contact with a partner with known infection, a new partner, or multiple partners. Universal precautions are used to examine the patient, to collect a specimen, or to perform associated procedures. The health care professional inspects the genitalia for warts growing on the moist genital surfaces, such as the subpreputial sac, the urethral meatus, and less commonly, the penile shaft or scrotum in male patients and the vulva and vaginal and cervical wall in female patients. In both sexes, the papillomas may spread to the perineum and perianal area. These warts begin as tiny pink or red swellings and may grow as large as 4 in. (10 cm) and become pedunculated. Multiple warts have a cauliflower-like appearance. The patient usually reports no other symptoms, but a few complain of itching and pain. Infected lesions become malodorous. The patient is monitored for signs of genital cancer and for infection. A nonthreatening, nonjudgmental atmosphere is provided to encourage the patient to verbalize feelings about perceived changes in sexual behavior and body image. Sexual abstinence or condom use during intercourse is recommended until healing is complete. The patient must inform sexual partners about the risk for genital warts and the need for evaluation. The patient should be tested for human immunodeficiency virus and for other sexually transmitted diseases. Genital warts can recur and the virus can mutate, causing warts of a different strain. The patient should report for weekly treatment until all warts are removed and then schedule a checkup for 3 months after all warts have disappeared. Female patients should have a Papanicolaou test every 6 months.

plantar w. A wart on a pressure-bearing area, esp. the sole of the foot. SYN: *verruca plantaris*. SEE: illus.

seborrheic w. Seborrheic keratosis.

venereal w. Genital wart.

Warthin's tumor (wŏr′thĭns) [Aldred Warthin, U.S. pathologist, 1866–1931] A common benign tumor of the parotid gland. SYN: *papillary cystadenoma lymphomatosum*.

wash (wăsh) [AS. *wacsan*] **1.** The act of cleaning, esp. a part or all of the body. **2.** A medicinal preparation used in washing or coating.

eye w. A solution used to rinse the eyes. SYN: *collyrium*.

washerwoman's itch Eczema of the hands of laundry workers who are repeatedly exposed to harsh soaps.

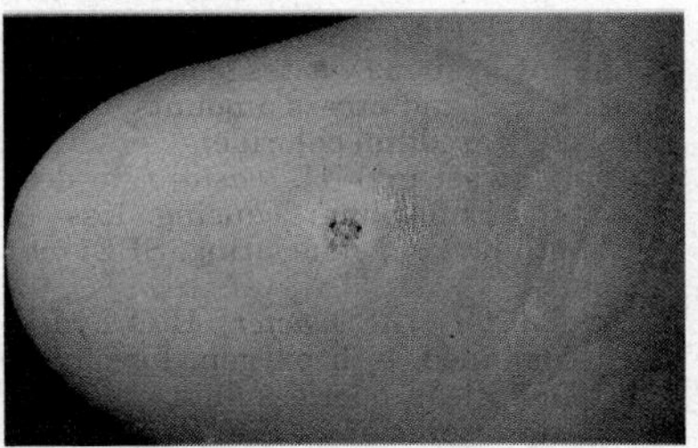

PLANTAR WART

washout, nitrogen The removal of nitrogen from the body by breathing either 100% oxygen or a combination of oxygen and helium. Although complete removal of nitrogen requires 12 hr of breathing nitrogen-free air, 2 hr may be sufficient to prevent the development of bends in aviators preparing to ascend to high altitudes.

wasp [AS. *waesp*] Term sometimes applied to all insects belonging to the suborder Apocrita, order Hymenoptera (except the Formicidae or ants), but more generally restricted to the superfamilies Scolioidea, Vespoidea, and Specoidea. Members have the base of the abdomen constricted, and females have a piercing ovipositor, which in many species is modified into a sting. Many are social, living in large colonies. Common representatives are yellow jackets and hornets.

waste (wāst) [L. *vastus*, empty] **1.** Cachexia. **2.** Loss by breaking down of bodily tissue. **3.** Excreted material no longer useful to an organism.

hazardous w. In health care, any tissues; bioproducts such as blood, surgical sponges, needles, infectious materials, human remains; toxic substances; cytotoxic drugs; chemicals; or radioactive isotopes. These materials must be clearly labeled and securely stored before disposal, to prevent them from endangering public health.

solid w. Garbage, rubbish, trash, refuse, or sludge, as well as other discarded materials produced by agricultural, community, industrial, home, medical, mining, or municipal processes. Efforts to limit the environmental impact of solid waste, from the point of production through recovery processes to disposal and recycling, are known as solid waste management.

waste products Metabolic byproducts that would be harmful if allowed to accumulate, which are removed from the body by elimination. Carbon dioxide is exhaled from the lungs; undigested food and bile pigments are eliminated by the colon. The kidneys form urine and excrete nitrogenous wastes (e.g., urea and creatinine) and excess amounts of minerals (e.g., sodium chloride).

wasting (wāst′ĭng) [L. *vastare,* to devastate] Enfeebling; causing loss of strength or size; emaciating. SEE: *marasmus.*

water (wă′tĕr) [AS. *waeter*] H_2O, hydrogen combined with oxygen, forming a tasteless, clear, odorless fluid.

Water freezes at 32°F (0°C) and boils at 212°F (100°C). It is the principal chemical constituent of the body, composing approx. 65% of the body weight of an adult male and 55% of the adult female. It is distributed within the intracellular fluid and outside of the cells in the extracellular fluid. Water is indispensable for metabolic activities within cells, as it is the medium in which chemical reactions usually take place. Outside of cells, it is the principal transporting agent of the body. The following properties of water are important to living organisms: it is almost a universal solvent; it is a medium in which acids, bases, and salts ionize, and the concentrations of these substances (electrolytes) must be and are normally regulated quite precisely by the body; it possesses a high specific heat and has a high latent heat of vaporization, important in regulation and maintenance of a constant body temperature; it possesses a high surface tension; and it is an important reacting agent and essential in all hydrolytic reactions.

Water is the principal constituent of all body fluids (blood, lymph, tissue fluid), secretions (salivary juice, gastric juice, bile, sweat), and excretory fluid (urine). Intake of water is determined principally by the sense of thirst. Excessive intake may lead to water intoxication; excessive loss to dehydration. Humans can survive for only a short time without water intake. The exact length of survival time varies with ambient temperature, moisture in available food, and amount of physical activity.

bound w. Intracellular water attached to organic molecules. It is not available for metabolic processes.

deionized w. Water that has been passed through a substance that removes cations and anions present as contaminants.

distilled w. Water that has been purified by distillation. It is used in preparing pharmaceuticals.

emergency preparation of safe drinking w. The purification of water when only unclean water is available or when the available drinking water is believed to be contaminated. One of the following methods may be used: (1) Water is strained through a filter and boiled vigorously for 30 min. (2) Three drops of alcoholic solution of iodine are added to each quart (approx. 1 L) of water. The water is then mixed well and left to stand for 30 min before using. (3) Ten drops of 1% chlorine bleach, 2 drops of 4% to 6% chlorine bleach, or 1 drop of 7% to 10% chlorine bleach is added to each quart (liter) of water. The water is then mixed well and left to stand for 30 min. If the water is cloudy to begin with, double the amount of chlorine is used.

When the water is contaminated by *Giardia* organisms, heating to 55°C (131°F) kills the protozoa (method 1). Methods 2 and 3 also kill the cysts, but more time is required. Bacteria and viruses are killed by water kept at 60°C (140°F) for 30 min.

hard w. Water that contains dissolved salts of magnesium or calcium.

heavy w. D_2O; an isotopic variety of water, esp. deuterium oxide, in which hydrogen has been displaced by its isotope, deuterium. Its properties differ from ordinary water in that heavy water has a higher freezing and boiling point and is incapable of supporting life.

w. for injection Water for parenteral use that has been distilled and sterilized. Distilled, sterilized water that is stored in sealed containers remains free of pyrogens and may be used after longer periods of storage.

lime w. Aqueous calcium hydroxide solution.

potable w. Water suitable for drinking, in that it is hygienic and free of odor, pathogenic microorganisms, and objectionable minerals.

purified w. Water that is mineral free; obtained by distillation, or deionization.

pyrogen-free w. Water that has been rendered free of fever-producing proteins (bacteria and their metabolic products). SEE: *w. for injection.*

soft w. Water that contains very little, if any, dissolved salts of magnesium or calcium.

water bed A rubber mattress partially filled with warm water (100°F or 37.8°C). It is used to prevent and treat bedsores.

water cure Hydrotherapy.

waterhammer pulse A pulse marked by a quick, powerful beat, collapsing suddenly; associated with aortic insufficiency. SYN: *Corrigan's pulse.*

Waterhouse-Friderichsen syndrome [Rupert Waterhouse, Brit. physician, 1873–1958; Carl Friderichsen, Danish physician, b. 1886] An acute adrenal insufficiency due to hemorrhage into the adrenal gland caused by meningococcal infection. SEE: *adrenal gland; meningitis, acute meningococcal.*

waters The common term for the amniotic fluid surrounding the fetus.

water syringe In dentistry, a syringe for

delivering water spray to a localized area. The flow, pressure, and temperature are controlled.

Watson-Crick helix [James Dewey Watson, U.S. biochemist, b. 1928; Francis Harry Compton Crick, Brit. biochemist, b. 1916] The double helix of DNA, named after the two scientists who established its structure. Each strand consists of nucleotides of phosphate, deoxyribose, and nitrogenous bases. The sequence of bases is the genetic code for the organism and is transmitted to new cells in mitosis or to offspring in egg and sperm. SEE: *code, triplet; deoxyribonucleic acid*.

Watson, Margaret Jean Harman A nursing educator, born 1940, who developed the Theory of Human Caring. SEE: *Nursing Theory Appendix*.

Watson-Schwartz test (wŏt′sŏn-shwărts) [Cecil J. Watson, U.S. physician, 1901–1983; Samuel Schwartz, U.S. physician, b. 1916] A test used in acute porphyria to differentiate porphobilinogen from urobilinogen.

watt [James Watt, Scottish engineer, 1736–1819] ABBR: w. A unit of electrical power. One watt is the power produced by 1 ampere of current flowing with a force or pressure (i.e., electromotive force) of 1 volt. In SI units, 1 w equals 1 J/sec. In other units, 1 w equals 1 newton m/sec. This is also equal to 0.7376 ft-lb/sec. SEE: *electromotive force*.

wattage (wŏt′ĭj) The electrical energy produced or consumed by an electrical device, expressed in watts.

wave (wāv) [ME. *wave*] **1.** A disturbance, usually orderly and predictable, observed as a moving ridge with a definable frequency and amplitude. **2.** An undulating or vibrating motion. **3.** An oscillation seen in the recording of an electrocardiogram, electroencephalogram, or other graphic record of physiological activity. SEE: illus.

***a* w.** **1.** A venous neck wave produced by atrial contraction. **2.** A component of right atrial and pulmonary artery wedge pressure tracings produced by atrial contraction. The a wave just precedes the first heart sound. It is absent in atrial fibrillation and is larger in atrioventricular dissociation and in conditions causing dilation of the right atrium.

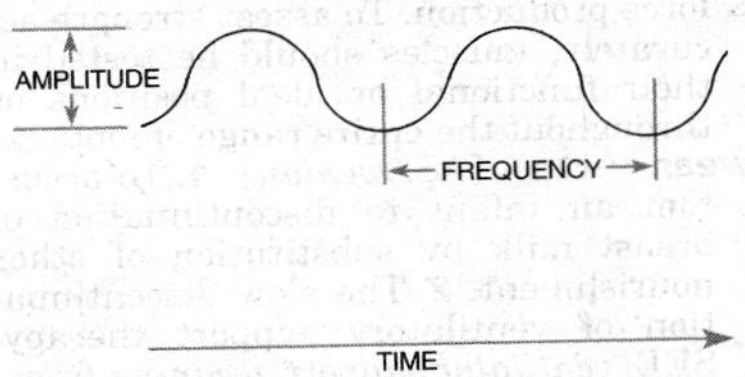

COMPONENTS OF WAVES

***alpha* w.** An electroencephalographic deflection often generated by cells in the visual cortex of the brain. SEE: *alpha rhythm*.

***beta* w.** An electroencephalographic deflection. Its frequency is between 18 and 30 Hz. SEE: *beta rhythm*.

***brain* w.** The fluctuation, usually rhythmic, of electrical impulses produced by the brain. SEE: *electroencephalography*.

***c* w.** A component of right atrial and pulmonary capillary wedge pressure waves. It reflects the closing of the tricuspid valve at the beginning of ventricular systole. An abnormal configuration is seen in increased right heart pressure and with abnormalities of the tricuspid valve.

***delta* w.** An abnormal deflection seen on the electrocardiogram in patients with pre-excitation syndromes, such as Wolff-Parkinson-White syndrome. It occurs at the take-off of the QRS complex.

***electromagnetic* w.** A wave-form produced by simultaneous oscillation of electric and magnetic fields perpendicular to each other. The direction of propagation of the wave is perpendicular to the oscillations. The following waves, in order of increasing frequency and decreasing wavelength, are electromagnetic: radio, television, microwave, infrared, visible light, ultraviolet, x-rays, and gamma rays. SEE: *electromagnetic spectrum* for table.

***excitation* w.** The wave of irritability originating in the sinoatrial node that sweeps over the conducting tissue of the heart and induces contraction of the atria and ventricles.

***F* w.** A flutter wave seen as a "saw-tooth" or "picket fence" base line on the electrocardiogram tracing of atrial flutter. F waves are caused by a re-entry electrophysiological mechanism.

***f* w.** A fibrillatory wave seen as the wavy base line on the electrocardiogram tracing of atrial fibrillation. These waves are caused by multiple ectopic foci in the atria.

***J* w.** An upwardly curving deflection of the J point of the electrocardiogram, found in patients whose body temperature is less than 32°C. This finding is one cardiac effect of hypothermia. The J wave has a particular shape; viewed from above, its surface is convex. SYN: *osborne w*.

***light* w.** An electromagnetic wave that stimulates the retina or other optical sensors.

***osborne* w.** J wave.

***P* w.** SEE: *electrocardiogram*.

***pulse* w.** The pressure wave originated by the systolic discharge of blood into the aorta. It is not due to the passage of the ejected blood but is the result of the impact being transmitted through the arterial walls. The velocity in the aorta may be as high as 500 cm/sec and as low as 0.07 cm/sec in capillaries. The speed of transmission varies with the nature of the arterial wall, increasing with age as the arteries become less resilient. Thus in arteriosclerosis, the velocity is increased over normal.

***Q* w.** A downward or negative wave of an electrocardiogram following the P wave. It is usually not prominent and may be absent without significance. New Q waves are present on the electrocardiogram after patients suffer myocardial infarction. SEE: *electrocardiogram*.

***R* w.** SEE: *electrocardiogram*.

***radio* w.** An electromagnetic wave between the frequencies of 10^{11} and 10^4 Hz.

***S* w.** SEE: *electrocardiogram*.

w. scheduling A method for assigning appointments for patients that brings several patients in to see their health care professionals at the same time (e.g., at the beginning of each hour instead of every 15 or 20 min during the hour).

***sound* w.** A vibration of a vibrating medium that, on stimulating sensory receptors of the cochlea, is capable of giving rise to a sensation of sound. In dry air, the velocity is 1087 ft (331.6 m)/sec at 0°C; in water, it is approx. four times faster than in air.

***T* w.** SEE: *electrocardiogram*.

***theta* w.** A brain wave present in the electroencephalogram. It has a frequency of about 4 to 7 Hz.

***ultrashort* w.** An arbitrary designation of radio waves of a wavelength of less than 1 m.

***ultrasonic* w.** A sound wave of greater frequency than 20 kHz. These waves do not produce sound audible to the human ear.

wavelength (wāv′lĕngth) The distance between the beginning and end of a single wave cycle, usually measured from the top of one wave to the top of the next one.

wax [AS. *weax*] **1.** A substance obtained from bees (beeswax), plants, or petroleum (paraffin). It is solid at room temperature. In medicine, a purified form, white wax, is used in making ointments and to stop bleeding from bones during surgery. **2.** Any substance with the consistency of beeswax. **3.** Earwax. SYN: *cerumen*.

***bone* w.** A nontoxic, biocompatible wax used during surgery to plug cavities in cranial bones and other bones to control bleeding.

***casting* w.** A mixture of several waxes that can be carved or formed into shapes to be cast in metal.

***dental* w.** A variety of waxes compounded for their specific properties desired for dental procedures (e.g., baseplate wax, bone wax, boxing wax, burnout wax, casting wax, inlay wax, and pattern wax).

waxing-up In dentistry, the shaping of wax around the contours of a trial denture or cast restoration.

waxy (wăks′ē) [AS. *weax,* wax] Resembling or pert. to wax.

waxy degeneration Amyloid degeneration seen in wasting diseases.

WBC *white blood cells; white blood count.*

weak (wēk) [Old Norse *veikr,* flexible] **1.** Lacking physical strength or vigor; infirm, esp. as compared with what would be the normal or usual for that individual. **2.** Dilute, as in a weak solution, or weak tea.

weakness A subjective term used by a patient to indicate a lack of strength as compared with what he or she feels is normal. The cause may be organic disease or a combination of an organic disease and a mental state. In either event, the symptom, if it is unremitting, requires careful investigation with special attention being given to determining potentially lethal causes that may be curable (e.g., cancer, anemia, certain parasitic or infectious diseases, or neurological conditions).

***positional* w.** The apparent weakness of a muscle when tested in a shortened range of motion. This is a normal phenomenon of a muscle's length-tension curve. To differentiate positional weakness from general muscle weakness, the muscle must be tested throughout its entire range of motion.

PATIENT CARE: The patient should be positioned carefully when testing for muscle force production. To assess strength accurately, muscles should be tested throughout the entire range of motion.

***stretch* w.** The apparent weakness of a muscle resulting from prolonged positioning in a lengthened position, thus shifting the muscle length-tension curve to the right; a form of positional weakness. This phenomenon is observed when the force production of the lengthened muscle is limited when it is tested in a relatively short position.

PATIENT CARE: Care must be taken in positioning when testing for muscle force production. To assess strength accurately, muscles should be tested in their functional or ideal positions or throughout the entire range of motion.

wean (wēn) [AS. *wenian*] **1.** To accustom an infant to discontinuation of breast milk by substitution of other nourishment. **2.** The slow discontinuation of ventilatory support therapy. SEE: *ventilator support, weaning from.*

weanling A young child or infant recently changed from breast to formula feeding.

weanling diarrhea Severe gastroenteritis that sometimes occurs in infants who recently have been weaned.

web A tissue or membrane extending across a space.

esophageal w. A group of thin membranous structures that include mucosal and submucosal coats across the esophagus. They may be congenital or may follow trauma, inflammation, or ulceration of the esophagus. SEE: *Plummer-Vinson syndrome.*

terminal w. A microscopic weblike network that is beneath the microvilli of intestinal absorption cells and beneath the hair cells of the inner ear.

webbed (wĕbd) [AS. *webb,* a fabric] Having a membrane or tissue connecting adjacent structures, as the toes of a duck's feet.

Weber-Christian disease (wĕb′ĕr-krĭs′chĕn) [Fredrick Parkes Weber, Brit. physician, 1863–1962; Henry A. Christian, U.S. physician, 1876–1951] Relapsing, febrile, nodular, nonsuppurative panniculitis, a generalized disorder of fat metabolism characterized by recurring episodes of fever and the development of crops of subcutaneous fatty nodules.

Weber's gland (vā′bĕrz) [Moritz I. Weber, Ger. anatomist, 1795–1875] One of the mucous glands of the tongue.

Weber's paralysis (wĕb′ĕrz) [Sir Hermann David Weber, Brit. physician, 1823–1918] Paralysis of the oculomotor nerve on one side with contralateral spastic hemiplegia. It is caused by a lesion of the crus cerebri.

Weber test [Friedrich Eugen Weber, Ger. otologist, 1823–1891] A test for unilateral deafness. A vibrating tuning fork held against the midline of the top of the head is perceived as being so located by those with equal hearing ability in the ears; to persons with unilateral conductive-type deafness, the sound will be perceived as being more pronounced on the diseased side; in persons with unilateral nerve-type deafness, the sound will be perceived as being louder in the good ear. SEE: *hearing.*

Wechsler Intelligence Scale for Children ABBR: WISC. A widely used intelligence test for children aged 5 to 16.

wedge 1. A solid object with a broad base and two sides arising from the base to intersect each other and to form an acute angle opposite the base. **2.** In radiography, a filter placed in the primary x-ray beam to vary the intensity.

step w. A device consisting of increasing thicknesses of absorber through which radiographs are taken to determine the amounts of radiation reaching the film.

wedge pressure Pulmonary artery wedge pressure.

WEE *western equine encephalomyelitis.*

WeeFIM The Functional Independence Measure adapted for children aged 6 months to 7 years. SEE: *Functional Independence Measure.*

weeping [AS. *wepan,* to lament] **1.** Shedding tears. **2.** Moist, dripping.

weeping sinew A circumscribed cystic swelling of a tendon sheath.

Wegener's granulomatosis, Wegener's syndrome [Frederich Wegener, Ger. pathologist, 1843–1917] A systemic necrotizing vasculitis marked by pneumonitis and glomerulonephritis; small and medium-sized blood vessels throughout the body may be affected. The average age of onset is 40, and the disease affects men more often than women.

ETIOLOGY: The precise etiology is unknown. Autoantibodies have been identified in the blood of approx. 90% of patients. Granulomas may be present in the lung, upper respiratory tract, and small arteries and veins. Localized or diffuse inflammatory patches are seen in the glomerular capillaries of the kidney.

SYMPTOMS: Chronic pneumonitis and glomerulonephritis are the most prominent signs; ulcerations of the nasopharyngeal mucosa also are common. Other signs and symptoms include muscle and joint pain, skin rashes, fever, and neuropathy.

TREATMENT: Suppressive immunotherapeutic drugs such as cyclophosphamide and corticosteroids are used to control the disease. Trimethoprim-sulfamethoxazole may prevent relapses. There is a 1-year, 80% mortality rate in untreated patients; when treatment is effective, patients can live normal lifespans. Those with diffuse glomerular damage may develop chronic renal failure.

Weidel reaction (vī′dĕl) [Hugo Weidel, Austrian chemist, 1849–1899] **1.** A test for the presence of xanthine bodies. **2.** A test for the presence of uric acid.

Weigert's law (vī′gĕrts) [Carl Weigert, Ger. pathologist, 1845–1904] An observation stating that loss or destruction of tissue results in an excess of new tissue during repair.

weighing, underwater Hydrodensitometry.

weight (wāt) [AS. *gewiht*] The gravitational force exerted on an object, usually by the earth. The unit of weight is the newton; 1 newton equals 0.225 lb. The difference between weight and mass is that the weight of an object varies with the force of gravity, but the mass remains the same. For example, an object weighs less on the moon than on earth because the force of gravity is less on the moon; but the object's mass is the same in both places. SEE: *mass* (3).

Many diseases cause alterations of

1983 Metropolitan Height and Weight Tables for Men and Women According to Frame, Ages 25 to 59

Men					Women				
Height (in shoes)*		Weight in Pounds (in indoor clothing)†			Height (in shoes)*		Weight in Pounds (in indoor clothing)†		
Ft.	In.	Small Frame	Medium Frame	Large Frame	Ft.	In.	Small Frame	Medium Frame	Large Frame
5	2	128–134	131–141	138–150	4	10	102–111	109–121	118–131
5	3	130–136	133–143	140–153	4	11	103–113	111–123	120–134
5	4	132–138	135–145	142–156	5	0	104–115	113–126	122–137
5	5	134–140	137–148	144–160	5	1	106–118	115–129	125–140
5	6	136–142	139–151	146–164	5	2	108–121	118–132	128–143
5	7	138–145	142–154	149–168	5	3	111–124	121–135	131–147
5	8	140–148	145–157	152–172	5	4	114–127	124–138	134–151
5	9	142–151	148–160	155–176	5	5	117–130	127–141	137–155
5	10	144–154	151–163	158–180	5	6	120–133	130–144	140–159
5	11	146–157	154–166	161–184	5	7	123–136	133–147	143–163
6	0	149–160	157–170	164–188	5	8	126–139	136–150	146–167
6	1	152–164	160–174	168–192	5	9	129–142	139–153	149–170
6	2	155–168	164–178	172–197	5	10	132–145	142–156	152–173
6	3	158–172	167–182	176–202	5	11	135–148	145–159	155–176
6	4	162–176	171–187	181–207	6	0	138–151	148–162	158–179

SOURCE OF BASIC DATA: Build Study, 1979, Society of Actuaries and Association of Life Insurance Medical Directors of America, 1980. Copyright 1983 Metropolitan Life Insurance Company. Reprinted Courtesy of Metropolitan Life Insurance Company, *Statistical Bulletin*. Copyright 1983 Metropolitan Life Insurance Company.

* Shoes with 1-in. heels.

† Indoor clothing weighing 5 lb for men and 3 lb for women.

body weight (BW), for example, BW decreases in Addison's disease, AIDS, cancer, chronic diarrhea, chronic infections, untreated type I diabetes mellitus, anorexia, lactation when prolonged, marasmus, obstruction of the pylorus or thoracic duct, starvation, tuberculosis, and peptic ulcer.

Normal weight depends on the frame of the individual. SEE: table.

apothecaries' w. SEE: *apothecaries' weights and measures.*

atomic w. ABBR: at. wt. The weight of an atom of an element compared with that of 1/12 the weight of carbon-12.

avoirdupois w. SEE: *avoirdupois measure.*

w. cycling Rapid increases and decreases in body weight. SEE: *yo-yo diet.*

equivalent w. An obsolete term for the weight of a chemical element that is equivalent to and will replace a hydrogen atom (1.008 g) in a chemical reaction.

ideal body w. ABBR: IBW. The number of pounds or kilograms a person should weigh, based on height and frame, to achieve and maintain optimal health. Several tables, such as the Metropolitan Life Height and Weight Table, show ideal body weights for men and women of varying heights. These references may be used to help set goals for patients who are underweight or overweight. SEE: *weight* for table.

molecular w. ABBR: mol. wt. The weight of a molecule attained by totaling the atomic weight of its constituent atoms. SEE: *atomic w.*

set point w. The concept that body weight is controlled by the central nervous system and set at a certain value; the value is more or less stable until something occurs to alter it. An example of resetting of the set point occurs in persons with a disturbance of hypothalamic function that interferes with the satiety and feeding centers.

usual body w. ABBR: UBW. Body weight value used to compare a person's current weight with his or her own baseline weight. The UBW may be a more realistic goal than the ideal body weight for some individuals. SEE: *ideal body w.*

w. in volume ABBR: w/v. The amount by weight of a solid substance dissolved in a measured quantity of liquid. Percent w/v expresses the number of grams of an ingredient in 100 mL of solution.

w. in weight ABBR: w/w. The amount by weight of a solid substance dissolved in a known amount (by weight) of liquid. Percent w/w expresses the number of grams of one ingredient in 100 g of solution.

weighting In radiation therapy using two opposing fields, the use of a higher dose for one of the fields.

weightlessness The condition of not being acted on by the force of gravity. It is present when astronauts travel in areas so distant from the earth, moon, or planets that the force of gravity is virtually absent.

weights and measures SEE: *Weights and Measures Appendix*.

Weil's disease (vīlz) [Adolf Weil, Ger. physician, 1848–1916] Leptospirosis caused by any one of several serotypes of *Leptospira interrogans* such as *L. icterohemorrhagica* in rats, *L. pomona* in swine, or *L. canicola* in dogs. All of these may be pathogenic for humans.

ETIOLOGY: The infection is caused by contact with infected rat urine or feces.

SYMPTOMS: Symptoms include muscular pains, fever, jaundice, and enlargement of the liver and spleen.

TREATMENT: Penicillins or tetracyclines are curative.

PREVENTION: Doxycycline may be used to prevent infection in those exposed to the spirochetes.

Weil-Felix reaction, Weil-Felix test (vīl-fā'lĭks) [Edmund Weil, Austrian bacteriologist, 1880–1922; Arthur Felix, Ger. bacteriologist, 1887–1956] The agglutination of certain *Proteus* organisms caused by the development of *Proteus* antibodies in certain rickettsial diseases.

Weir Mitchell's treatment (wēr mĭt'chĕlz) [Silas Weir Mitchell, U.S. neurologist, 1829–1914] The treatment for hysteria and neurasthenia that consisted of bedrest, massage, nourishing diet, and a change of environment.

weismannism (wīs'măn-ĭzm) [August F. L. Weismann, Ger. biologist, 1834–1914] The theory that acquired characteristics are not inherited.

Weitbrecht's foramen (vīt'brĕkts) [Josias Weitbrecht, Ger.-born Russian anatomist, 1702–1747] An opening in the articular cartilage of the shoulder joint.

Weitbrecht's ligament The oblique cord connecting the ulna and radius.

Welch's bacillus (wĕlsh'ĕz) [William Henry Welch, U.S. pathologist, 1850–1934] *Clostridium perfringens,* the causative organism of gas gangrene. SEE: *gangrene, gas*.

Wellens' syndrome The electrocardiographic (ECG) signs of impending occlusion of the left main or left anterior descending coronary artery. ECG shows an inverted symmetrical T wave with little or no associated change of the ST segment or R wave. Inversion appears principally in the V leads. The finding identifies patients who are at risk for an extensive myocardial infarction.

wellness The condition of being in good health, including the appreciation and enjoyment of health. Wellness is more than a lack of disease symptoms; it is a state of mental and physical balance and fitness.

welt [ME. *welte*] An elevation on the skin produced by a lash, blow, or allergic stimulus. The skin is unbroken and the mark is reversible.

wen (wĕn) [AS.] A cyst resulting from the retention of secretion in a sebaceous gland. One or more rounded or oval elevations, varying in size from a few millimeters to about 10 cm, appear slowly on the scalp, face, or back. They are painless, rather soft, and contain a yellow-white caseous mass. The sac and contents should be carefully dissected to prevent its recurrence. SYN: *sebaceous cyst; steatoma*. SEE: *Fordyce's disease*.

Wenckebach's period, Wenckebach's phenomenon (vĕn'kĕ-băks) [Karel F. Wenckebach, Dutch-born Aust. internist, 1864–1940] A form of incomplete heart block in which, as detected by electrocardiography, there is progressive lengthening of the P-R interval until there is no ventricular response; and then the cycle of increasing P-R intervals begins again.

Werdnig-Hoffmann disease (vĕrd'nĭg-hŏf'măn) [Guido Werdnig, Austrian neurologist, 1844–1919; Johann Hoffmann, Ger. neurologist, 1857–1919] Spinal muscular atrophy.

Werdnig-Hoffmann paralysis Infantile muscular atrophy, considered by some to be identical with amyotonia congenita.

Werdnig-Hoffmann syndrome Werdnig-Hoffmann paralysis.

Werlhof's disease (vĕrl'hŏfs) [Paul G. Werlhof, Ger. physician, 1699–1767] Idiopathic thrombocytopenic purpura.

Wermer's syndrome [Paul Wermer, U.S. physician, d. 1975] Multiple endocrine neoplasia.

Werner's syndrome (vĕr'nĕrz) [C. W. O. Werner, Ger. physician, 1879-1936] A disease in which adults age at an accelerated pace. SEE: *progeria*.

Wernicke's aphasia (vĕr'nĭ-kēz) [Karl Wernicke, Ger. neurologist, 1848–1905] An injury to the Wernicke's area in the temporal lobe of the dominant hemisphere of the brain, resulting in an inability to comprehend the spoken or written word. Visual and auditory pathways are unaffected; however, patients are unable to differentiate between words or interpret their meaning. Although patients speak fluently, they are unable to function socially because their ability to communicate effectively is impaired by a disordered speech pattern called paraphasia (i.e., inserting inappropriate syllables into words or substituting one word for another). They also may be unable to repeat spoken words. If the condition is due to a stroke, the aphasia may improve with time. The disorder is often caused by impairment of blood flow through the lower division of the left middle cerebral artery. SEE: *speech, paraphasic.*

Wernicke's center An area in the dominant hemisphere of the brain that recalls, recognizes, and interprets words and other sounds in the process of using language.

Wernicke's encephalopathy Encephalopathy associated with thiamine deficiency; usually associated with chronic alcoholism or other causes of severe malnutrition. SYN: *Wernicke's syndrome.*

Wernicke's syndrome Wernicke's encephalopathy.

Western blotting A technique for analyzing protein antigens. Initially, the antigens are separated by electrophoresis on a gel and transferred to a solid membrane by blotting. The membrane is incubated with antibodies, and then the bound antibodies are detected by enzymatic or radioactive methods. This method is used to detect small amounts of antibodies.

Weston Hurst syndrome Acute hemorrhagic leukoencephalitis.

Westphal-Edinger nucleus [Karl Westphal, Ger. neurologist, 1833–1890; Ludwig Edinger, Ger. neurologist, 1855–1918] A small group of nerve cells in the rostral portion of the nucleus of the oculomotor nerve. Efferent fibers pass to the ciliary ganglion conveying impulses destined for the intrinsic muscles of the eye.

Westphal-Strümpell pseudosclerosis (vĕst′făl-strĭm′p′l) [K. Westphal; Adolf G. G. von Strümpell, Ger. physician, 1853–1925] Wilson's disease.

wet (wĕt) [AS. *waet*] Soaked with moisture, usually water.

wet brain An increased amount of cerebrospinal fluid with edema of the meninges; may be associated with alcoholism.

wet cup A cupping glass used after scarification.

wet dream Nocturnal emission.

wet nurse A woman who breastfeeds another's child.

wet nurse phenomenon The production of milk in response to repeated stimulation of the nipples in unpregnant women who have previously been pregnant.

wet pack A form of bath given by wrapping a patient in hot or cold wet sheets, covered with a blanket, used in the distant past esp. to reduce fever.

Wetzel grid (wĕt′sĕl) [Norman C. Wetzel, U.S. pediatrician, b. 1897] A graph for use in evaluating growth and development in children aged 5 to 18 years.

Wharton's duct (hwăr′tŏnz) [Thomas Wharton, Brit. anatomist, 1614–1673] The duct of the submandibular salivary gland opening into the mouth at the side of the frenulum linguae.

Wharton's jelly A gelatinous intercellular substance consisting of primitive connective tissue of the umbilical cord. It is rich in hyaluronic acid.

wheal (hwēl) [AS. *hwele*] A more or less round and temporary elevation of the skin, white in the center with a pale-red periphery, accompanied by itching. It is seen in urticaria, insect bites, anaphylaxis, and angioneurotic edema. SYN: *pomphus.*

wheal (hwēl) [ME. *wale,* a stripe] An elongated mark or ridge. Such a ridge is produced by intradermal injection.

wheat (hwēt) [AS. *hwaete*] Any of various cereal grasses, widely cultivated for its edible grain used in making flour. Wheat preparations and pastas include macaroni, vermicelli, and noodles, which are made from flour and water, molded, dried, and slightly baked. They are easy to digest.

STRUCTURE: Wheat is composed of the husk or outer coat, which is removed before grinding; bran coats, which are removed in making white flour and contain the mineral substances; gluten, which contains the fat and protein; and starch, the center of the kernel. Refined wheat products do not include the bran and germ, which contain B complex vitamins, phosphorus, and iron.

Individuals who are gluten intolerant (e.g., persons with celiac sprue) cannot digest the protein gluten found in wheat.

wheat germ The embryo portion of wheat. It is a source of B vitamins and vitamin E.

wheat germ oil The oil expressed from the germ of the wheat seed. It is a rich source of vitamin E.

wheatstone bridge An electric circuit with two branches, each containing two resistors. These branches are joined to complete the circuit. If the resistance in three resistors is known, the resistance of the fourth and unknown one can be calculated.

wheel A disk attached through its middle to an axle that rotates. In dentistry, small wheels are attached to a handpiece or lathe, and used for polishing and shaping teeth, restorations, and appliances.

carborundum w. A cutting wheel containing silicon carbide, in variable grit sizes.

diamond w. In dentistry, a wheel that contains diamond powder or chips.

polishing w. In dentistry, a wheel made of soft material suitable for polishing teeth or restorations.

wire w. A wheel containing pieces of wire. It is used for cleaning metal surfaces.

wheelchair A type of mobility device for

personal transport. Traditional wheelchairs have a seating area positioned between two large wheels, with two smaller wheels at the front. These can be self-propelled through handrims or pushed by another person. Advances in wheelchair design have provided alternatives that accommodate obstacles and rough terrain. Lightweight, collapsible models exist, as well as models designed for racing and sports. Powered wheelchairs and scooters, driven by electric motors, can be controlled through electronic switches and enable mobility by persons with muscle weakness or even paralysis.

wheeze (hwēz) [ME. *whesen*] A continuous musical sound caused by narrowing of the lumen of a respiratory passageway. Often noted only by the use of a stethoscope, it occurs in asthma, croup, hay fever, mitral stenosis, and bronchitis. It may result from asthma, tumors, foreign body airway obstructions, bronchial spasm, pulmonary infections, emphysema and other chronic obstructive lung diseases, or pulmonary edema.

wheezing The production of whistling sounds during difficult breathing such as occurs in asthma, coryza, croup, and other respiratory disorders. SEE: *wheeze.*

whey The watery material separated from the curd of milk that has coagulated.

whinolalia (wīn″ō-lā′lē-ă) [AS. *whinan,* whine, + Gr. *lalein,* to talk] Hypernasality and distortion of speech, which occurs in incompetent palate syndrome.

whiplash injury An imprecise term for injury to the cervical vertebrae and adjacent soft tissues. It is produced by a sudden jerking or relative backward or forward acceleration of the head with respect to the vertebral column. This type of injury may occur in a vehicle that is suddenly and forcibly struck from the rear.

Whipple's disease (hwĭp′ĕlz) [George Hoyt Whipple, U.S. pathologist, 1878–1976] Intestinal lipodystrophy, characterized by abnormal skin pigmentation, fatty stools, loss of weight and strength, chronic arthritis, a distinctive lesion of the mucosa of the jejunum and ileum, and other signs of a malabsorption syndrome. This rare disease resembles idiopathic steatorrhea. SYN: *intestinal lipodystrophy.*

ETIOLOGY: It is believed that the causative organism is a gram-positive bacillus, *Tropheryma whippelii.*

TREATMENT: Intensive antibiotic therapy with procaine penicillin followed by maintenance therapy with tetracycline yields good results.

whipworm *Trichuris trichiura.*

whirlbone **1.** The patella. **2.** The head of the femur.

whiskey, whisky (hwĭs′kē) A distilled alcoholic liquor made from grain. The alcohol present is ethyl alcohol.

whisper (hwĭs′pĕr) [AS. *hwisprian*] **1.** Speech with a low, soft voice; a low, sibilant sound. **2.** To utter in a low sound.

cavernous w. Direct transmission of a whisper through a cavity in auscultation.

whistle (hwĭs′ĕl) **1.** A sound produced by pursing one's lips and blowing. **2.** A tubular device driven by wind that produces a loud and usually shrill sound.

whistling face syndrome A congenital malformation with muscle dysfunction that produces a masklike "whistling face," hypoplastic nasal bones, and clubfeet. The genetic transmission may be autosomal recessive.

white (hwīt) [AS. *hwit*] **1.** The achromatic color of maximum lightness that reflects all rays of the spectrum. **2.** The color of milk or fresh snow; opposite of black.

white cell Leukocyte.

white-damp Carbon monoxide formed in a mine following an explosion.

white of egg The albumin of an egg.

white of eye The part of the sclera visible around the iris.

white gangrene Gangrene caused by local impairments of blood flow.

whitehead (hwīt′hĕd) A closed comedo containing pale, dried sebum. SEE: *blackhead; comedo.*

white leg SEE: *phlegmasia alba dolens.*

white line Linea alba.

white lotion A combination of zinc sulfate and sulfurated potassium diluted in purified water, used in treating certain skin diseases.

white ointment An ointment containing white wax and white petrolatum.

whitepox (hwīt′pŏks) Variola minor.

whites Slang for leukorrhea.

white softening The stage of softening of any tissue in which the affected area has become white and anemic.

whitlow (hwĭt′lō) [ME. *whitflawe,* white flow] Suppurative inflammation at the end of a finger or toe. It may be deep seated, involving the bone and its periosteum, or superficial, affecting parts of the nail. SYN: *felon; panaris; paronychia; runaround.*

herpetic w. Whitlow due to herpes simplex virus. It is painful and accompanied by lymphadenopathy.

Whitmore's disease [Alfred Whitmore, Brit. surgeon, 1876–1946] Melioidosis.

WHO *World Health Organization.*

whole body counter An instrument that detects the radiation present in the entire body.

whole bowel irrigation Administration of large volumes of a nonabsorbable fluid to remove potentially hazardous contents from the gastrointestinal tract.

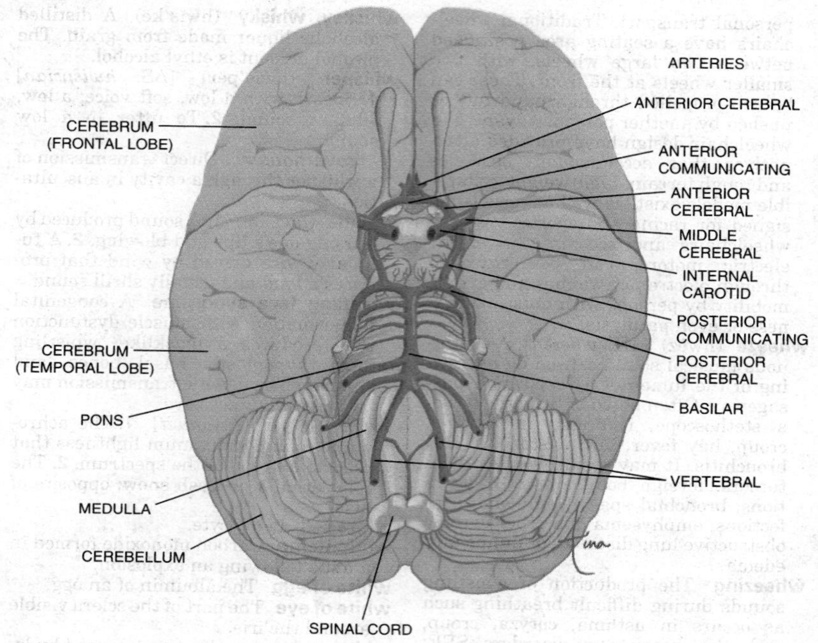

CIRCLE OF WILLIS
Inferior view of brain

The technique is used both in the preparation of some patients for bowel surgery, and in the decontamination of the gut after drug or poison overdose.

wholism Holism.

wholistic health Holistic medicine.

whoop (hoop) [AS. *hwopan,* to threaten] The sonorous and convulsive inspiratory crow following a paroxysm of whooping cough.

whooping cough Pertussis.

whorl (hwŭrl) [ME. *whorle*] **1.** A spiral arrangement of cardiac muscle fibers. SYN: *vortex.* **2.** A type of fingerprint in which the central papllary ridges turn through at least one complete circle. SEE: *fingerprint* for illus.

WIC *Special Supplementary Food Program for Women, Infants, and Children.*

Wickham's striae (wĭ'kămz strē'ă) [L. F. Wickham, Fr. dermatologist, 1861–1913] Lines that are demonstrable on the buccal mucosa in patients with lichen planus.

Widal's reaction, Widal's test (vē-dălz') [Georges Fernand Isidore Widal, Fr. physician, 1862–1929] An agglutination test for typhoid fever.

wig A covering for the head to simulate hair if the individual is bald or partially bald. Wigs may be made of hair or synthetic fibers such as acrylic. Wigs are esp. beneficial for use by patients who have lost their hair due to exposure to certain types of cytotoxic agents used in cancer chemotherapy.

wild cherry The dried bark of *Prunus serotina,* used principally in the form of syrup as a flavored vehicle for cough medicine.

will [AS.] **1.** The mental faculty used in choosing or deciding on an act or thought. **2.** The power of controlling one's actions or emotions.

Willis, Thomas (wĭl'ĭs) British anatomist, 1621–1675.

circle of W. An arterial anastomosis that encircles the optic chiasm and hypophysis, from which the principal arteries supplying the brain are derived. It receives blood from the two internal carotid arteries and the basilar artery formed by union of the two vertebral arteries. SEE: illus.

Willis' cord One of the cords crossing the superior longitudinal sinus transversely.

Wilms' tumor (vĭlmz) [Max Wilms, Ger. surgeon, 1867–1918] A rapidly developing tumor of the kidney that usually occurs in children. It is the most common renal tumor of childhood. It is associated with chromosomal deletions, esp. from chromosomes 11 and 16. In the past, the mortality from this type of cancer was extremely high; however, newer approaches to therapy have been very effective in controlling the tumor in about 90% of patients. SYN: *embryonal carcinosarcoma; nephroblastoma*. SEE: *Nursing Diagnoses Appendix*.

Wilson's disease (wĭl'sŭnz) [Samuel Alexander Kinnier Wilson, Brit. internist, 1877–1937] A hereditary syndrome transmitted as an autosomal recessive trait in which a decrease of ceruloplasmin permits accumulation of copper in various organs (brain, liver, kidney, and cornea) associated with increased intestinal absorption of copper. A pigmented ring (Kayser-Fleischer ring) at the outer margin of the cornea is pathognomonic. This syndrome is characterized by degenerative changes in the brain, cirrhosis of the liver, hemolysis, splenomegaly, tremor, muscular rigidity, involuntary movements, spastic contractures, psychic disturbances, dysphagia, and progressive weakness and emaciation. SYN: *hepatolenticular degeneration; Westphal-Strümpell pseudosclerosis*.

TREATMENT: The untreated disease is fatal. The goal is to prevent further copper accumulation in tissues by avoiding foods high in copper such as organ meats, shellfish, nuts, dried legumes, chocolate, and whole cereals. Reduction of the copper in the tissues is achieved by giving the copper binder, D-penicillamine, orally until the serum copper level returns to normal. Carefully controlled doses of this therapy will probably be required for the patient's entire lifetime. Blood cell counts and hemoglobin should be monitored every 2 weeks during the first 6 weeks of treatment. Nonsteroidal anti-inflammatory drugs or systemic corticosteroids may help to relieve symptoms.

CAUTION: The copper binder, D-penicillamine, may cause pyridoxine and iron deficiency.

Wilson-Mikity syndrome [Miriam G. Wilson, U.S. pediatrician, b. 1922; Victor G. Mikity, U.S. radiologist, b. 1919] A so-called pulmonary dysmaturity syndrome seen in premature infants. The symptoms are insidious onset of dyspnea, tachypnea, and cyanosis in the first month of life. Radiographs of the lungs reveal evidence of emphysema that develops into multicysts. Therapy is directed at the pulmonary insufficiency and cardiac failure. The death rate is about 25%.

Winckel's disease (vĭng'kĕlz) [Franz von Winckel, Ger. gynecologist, 1837–1911] A fatal disease of the newborn characterized by hematuria, jaundice, enlarged spleen, collapse, and convulsions.

windburn Erythema and irritation of the skin caused by exposure to wind. Simultaneous exposure to the sun, moisture, wind, and cold may cause a severe dermatitis.

windchill The cooling effect wind has on exposed human skin. The effect is intensified if the skin is moist or wet.

windchill factor Loss of heat from exposure of skin to wind. Heat loss is proportional to the speed of the wind. Thus, skin exposed to a wind velocity of 20 mph (32 km/hr) when the temperature is 0°F (−17.8°C) is cooled at the same rate as in still air at −46°F (−43.3°C). Similarly, when the temperature is 20°F (−6.7°C) and the wind is 10, 20, or 35 mph (16.1, 32.2, or 56.3 km/hr), the equivalent skin temperature is −4°, −18°, or −28°F (−20°, −27.8°, or −33.3°C), respectively.

The windchill factor is calculated for dry skin; skin that is wet from any cause and exposed to wind loses heat at a much higher rate. Wind blowing over wet skin can cause frostbite, even on a comfortably warm day as judged by the thermometer.

windchill index A table listing the windchill factor for various combinations of temperature and wind velocity.

window [Old Norse *vindauga*] **1.** An aperture for the admission of light or air or both. **2.** A small aperture into a cavity, esp. that of the inner ear. SYN: *fenestra*.

aortic w. In radiology, in a left anterior oblique or lateral view of the chest, a clear area bounded by the aortic arch, the bifurcation of the trachea, and the pericardial border.

beryllium w. The part of a radiographic tube through which the x-ray photons pass to the outside.

cochlear w. Round w.

w. level ABBR: WL. In computed tomography, the center of the range of gray scale in the image.

oval w. The opening from the middle ear cavity to the inner ear, over which the plate of the stapes fits; it transmits vibrations for hearing. SYN: *fenestra vestibuli*.

pericardial w. A surgically constructed drainage portal through the pericardium into the peritoneum, used for the relief of pericardial effusions or tamponade.

radiation w. A translucent lead glass window in a radiographic control booth.

radiographic w. A thinner area on the glass envelope of an x-ray tube from which x-rays are emitted toward the patient.

round w. A membrane-covered opening below the oval window. Vibrations in the inner ear cause the membrane to bulge outward, decreasing the pressure in the cochlea and preventing damage to the hair cells. SYN: *fenestra cochleae; fenestra rotunda; cochlear w.*

vestibular w. Oval window.

window w. ABBR: WW. In computed tomography, the number of shades of gray in an image.

windowing Cutting a hole in anything, such as a plaster cast, to relieve pressure on the skin or a bony area.

windpipe Trachea.

wine (wīn) [L. *vinum*, wine] **1.** Fermented juice of any fruit, usually made from grapes and containing 10% to 15% alcohol.

red w. An alcoholic beverage made from pressed grapes, which contains polyphenolic antioxidants. Consumption of red wine, not in excess of 1–2 glasses per day, is associated with reduced risk of coronary artery disease.

wineglass A fluid measure of approx. 2 fl oz (60 ml).

wine sore Slang term for a superficial infected area of the skin seen in alcoholics with poor personal hygiene; erroneously thought to be due to specific action of the wine.

wing [Old Norse *vaengi*] A structure resembling the wing of a bird, esp. the great and small wings of the sphenoid bone. SEE: *ala*.

wink [AS. *wincian*] The brief, voluntary closure of one eye. In hemiplegia, the patient may not be able to blink or close the eye on the paralyzed side without simultaneously closing the other eye. This is called *Revilliod sign* or *orbicularis sign.* SEE: *blink; Marcus Gunn syndrome*.

winking Wink.

jaw w. The involuntary simultaneous closing of the eyelid as the jaw is moved.

jaw w. syndrome The unilateral ptosis of the eye at rest, and the rapid exaggerating elevation of the lid when the mandible is either depressed or moved to the opposite side of the ptosed lid. SYN: *Marcus Gunn syndrome*.

Winslow, foramen of (wĭnz′lō) [Jacob Benignus Winslow, Danish-born Fr. anatomist, 1669–1760] Epiploic foramen.

Winslow, ligament of The oblique popliteal ligament located at the back of the knee.

Winslow, pancreas of The processus uncinatus of the pancreas.

wintergreen oil Methyl salicylate. This colorless, yellowish, or reddish liquid has a characteristic taste and odor. It is used as a flavoring substance and as a counterirritant applied topically in the form of salves, lotions, and ointments.

winter itch A mild form of eczematous dermatitis of the lower legs of elderly persons during dry periods of the year. The skin contains fine cracks and there is no erythema. Excessive skin dryness should be avoided. The skin should be rehydrated with a cream or emulsion of water in oil. SYN: *asteatotic eczema; pruritus hiemalis*.

wire (wīr) **1.** Metal drawn out into threads of varying thickness. **2.** To join fracture fragments together by use of wire.

arch w. In dentistry, application of wire around the dental arch to correct irregularities of position of the teeth and/or arch.

Kirschner w. SEE: *Kirschner wire*.

ligature w. A soft, thin wire used in orthodontics to anchor an arch wire or other dental devices.

separating w. A brass wire used in dentistry to separate teeth before banding them.

wired Slang for tense and anxious, esp. when the condition is caused by the effect of a psychoactive drug.

wiring (wīr′ĭng) Fastening bone fragments together with wire.

circumferential w. A method of treating a fractured mandible by passing wires around the bone and a splint in the oral cavity.

continuous loop w. The forming of wire loops on both mandibular and maxillary teeth to provide attachment sites for rubber bands. These are used in treating fractures of the mandible. SYN: *Stout's w.*

craniofacial suspension w. Wiring using bones not contiguous with the oral cavity for attachment of wires that lead from those bones to the fractured jaw segments.

Gilmer w. Wiring of single opposed teeth by use of wire passed circumferentially around the two teeth and the ends twisted together. The twisted ends are placed where they will not irritate adjacent soft tissues. This procedure is used to produce intermaxillary fixation.

Ivy loop w. The placement of wire around adjacent teeth to provide an attachment site for rubber bands.

perialveolar w. The use of wires to fix a splint to the mandible. The wires are passed through the alveolar process from the buccal plate to the palate.

pyriform w. Wiring using the nasal bones to stabilize a fracture of the jaw. The wires are passed through the pyriform aperture of the nasal bone and then to the segment.

silver w. Abnormal reflections of light seen on the ophthalmoscopic examination of the retina of persons with long-standing, uncontrolled hypertension.

Stout's w. Continuous loop w.

Wirsung, duct of (vēr′soong) [Johann Georg Wirsung, Ger. physician, 1600–1643] The main secretory duct of the pancreas. SYN: *pancreatic duct*.

wisdom tooth (wĭz′dŏm) The third most

distal molar on each side of the jaw. These four molars may appear as late as the 25th year or may never erupt.

Wiskott-Aldrich syndrome [Alfred Wiskott, Ger. pediatrician, 1898–1978; Robert A. Aldrich, U.S. pediatrician, b. 1917] An X-linked immune deficiency syndrome whose hallmarks are decreased resistance to infection, eczema, and thrombocytopenia. The number of T lymphocytes in the blood and lymph nodes declines, blood levels of immunoglobulin M class antibodies are reduced, and the response to many antigens is inadequate. If bone marrow transplant is unsuccessful, the patients die at a young age from infection.

withdrawal Cessation of administration of a drug, esp. a narcotic, or alcohol to which the individual has become either physiologically or psychologically addicted. Withdrawal symptoms vary with the type of drug used. Neonates may exhibit withdrawal symptoms from drugs or alcohol ingested by the mother during pregnancy. SEE: *drug addiction*.

withdrawal syndrome Irritability, autonomic hyperactivity, hallucinations, or other phenomena resulting from the withdrawal of alcohol, stimulants, or some opiates.

opiate perinatal w.s. Intrauterine hyperactivity and increased oxygen consumption associated with opiate withdrawal in infants of addicted mothers. The syndrome places infants at increased risk for meconium aspiration pneumonia and transient tachypnea.

witkop (wĭt′kŏp) [Afrikaans, white scalp] Matted crusts in the hair producing a scalplike structure; seen in South African natives.

witness A person having knowledge or information about a particular subject or event.

expert w. A qualified person who assists a judge and jury in understanding technical aspects of a lawsuit, such as breaches of the standard of care and damages or injuries sustained.

fact w. A person who has knowledge of circumstances surrounding the events of the alleged incident in a complaint or petition for damages. SYN: *material w.*

material w. Fact w.

Witzel jejunostomy [Friedrich O. Witzel, Ger. surgeon, 1865–1925] A jejunostomy created by inserting a rubber or silicone catheter into the jejunum and bringing it to the skin surface. Medication and feedings can be administered on a long-term basis. SEE: *jejunostomy*.

witzelsucht (vĭt′sĕl-zookt) [M. Jastrowitz, Ger. physician, b. 1839] A condition produced by frontal lobe lesions characterized by self-amusement from poor jokes and puns. SEE: *moria*.

primary affective w. A peculiar variety of witzelsucht characterized by teutonization of nomenclature.

Wohlfahrtia (vōl-făr′tē-ă) [Peter Wohlfahrtia, Ger. author, 1675–1726] A genus of flies parasitic in animal tissue, belonging to the family Sarcophagidae, order Diptera.

W. magnifica A species found in southeast Europe. The larvae may occur in human and animal wounds.

W. opaca A species occurring in Canada. This species commonly infests wild animals; human infants also may become infested.

W. vigil A species found in Canada and the northern United States.

wolffian body (wool′fē-ăn) [Kaspar Friedrich Wolff, Ger. anatomist, 1733–1794] Mesonephros. SEE: *embryo; paroophoron; parovarium*.

wolffian cyst A cyst lying in one of the broad ligaments of the uterus.

wolffian duct The duct in the embryo leading from the mesonephros to the cloaca. From it develop the ductus epididymis, ductus deferens, seminal vesicle, ejaculatory duct, ureter, and pelvis of the kidney. SYN: *mesonephric duct*.

wolffian tubule One of 30 to 34 tubules that develop within the mesonephros and empty into the mesonephric duct. Most are transitional, persisting for only a short time. Some persist in men as the efferent ductules of the testis; others persist only as vestigial structures. SYN: *mesonephric tubule*. SEE: *epoophoron; paradidymis; paroophoron*.

Wolff-Parkinson-White syndrome [Louis Wolff, U.S. cardiologist, 1898–1972; Sir John Parkinson, Brit. physician, 1885–1976; Paul Dudley White, U.S. cardiologist, 1886–1973] ABBR: WPW. An abnormality of cardiac rhythm that manifests as supraventricular tachycardia. The diagnosis is made by use of electrocardiography. The P-R interval is less than 0.12 sec and the QRS complex contains an initial slur, called the delta wave, that broadens the complex. SEE: *pre-excitation, ventricular*.

wolfram (wool′frăm) Tungsten.

wolfsbane (wŏlfs′bān) Common name for several species of *Aconitum*, a genus of highly toxic, hardy perennials. Also called *monkshood*. SEE: *aconite*.

Wolhynia fever Trench fever.

Wolman's disease [Moshe Wolman, Israeli physician, b. 1914] An autosomal recessive disorder in which infants develop hepatosplenomegaly, calcification of the adrenal glands, and foam cells in the bone marrow and other tissues.

woman An adult human female. SEE: *man*.

womb (woom) [AS. *wamb*] Uterus.

wood alcohol Methyl alcohol.

woodruff A low-growing, hardy perennial herb (*Galium odoratum* or *Asperula odorata*) used in alternative medicine to treat nervousness, insomnia, and cardiac irregularity. Liver damage has been reported in some patients after long-term use.

Wood's rays [Robert Williams Wood, U.S. physicist, 1868–1955] Ultraviolet rays; used to detect fluorescent materials in the skin and hair in certain disease states such as tinea capitis. The terms Wood's light and Wood's lamp have become synonymous with Wood's rays, even though these are misnomers.

wool fat Anhydrous lanolin, a fatty substance obtained from sheep's wool; used as a base for ointments. It can produce contact dermatitis in susceptible persons.

woolsorter's disease A pulmonary form of anthrax that develops in those who handle wool contaminated with *Bacillus anthracis.*

word blindness Alexia.

word salad The use of words indiscriminantly and haphazardly, that is, without logical structure or meaning. It is a finding in uncontrolled mania and schizophrenia.

work [Ger. *wirken*] **1.** A force moving a resistance. The amount of work done is the product of the force in the direction of movement times the distance the resisting object is moved. Regardless of the force applied, if the resisting object is not moved, then no work has been done. This is not to say that energy has not been expended. Work is measured in units of force times distance, or newton meters. SEE: *calorie; erg.* **2.** The job, occupation, or task one performs as a means of providing a livelihood. **3.** The effort employed to explore interpersonal or psychological issues.

social w. Provision of social services (in fields such as child welfare, criminal justice, hospital-based medicine, or mental health) and the promotion of social welfare by a professionally trained person. Social work often involves advocacy and aid for individuals who are poor, elderly, homeless, unemployed, or discriminated against in society because of gender, race, or other biases.

work of breathing ABBR: WOB. The amount of effort used to expand and contract the lungs. It is determined by lung and thorax compliance, airway resistance, and the use of accessory muscles for inspiration or forced expiration.

worker, sex An individual who engages in sexual activities in exchange for payment.

work hardening A series of conditioning exercises that an injured worker performs in a rehabilitation program. These are designed to simulate the functional tasks encountered on the job to which the individual will return.

working through In psychiatry, the combined endeavor of the patient and the therapist to understand the unconscious genesis of a symptom or mental illness.

workout In athletics, a practice or training session.

workup The process of obtaining all of the necessary data for diagnosing and treating a patient. It should be done in an orderly manner so that essential elements will not be overlooked. Included are retrieval of all previous medical and dental records, the patient's family and personal medical history, social and occupational history, physical examination, laboratory studies, x-ray examinations, and indicated diagnostic surgical procedures. The patient's workup is an ongoing process wherein all hospital personnel involved cooperate in attempting to determine the correct diagnosis and effective therapy. SEE: *charting; medical record, problem-oriented.*

World Health Organization ABBR: WHO. The United Nations agency concerned with international health and the eradication of disease.

worm (wŭrm) [AS. *wyrm*] **1.** An elongated invertebrate belonging to one of the following phyla: Platyhelminthes (flatworms); Nemathelminthes or Aschelminthes (roundworms or threadworms); Acanthocephala (spinyheaded worms); and Annelida (Annulata) (segmented worms). SYN: *helminth.* **2.** Any small, limbless, creeping animal. **3.** The median portion of the cerebellum. **4.** Any wormlike structure.

wormian bone (wŭr′mē-ăn) [Ole Worm, Danish physician, 1588–1654] One of the small, irregular bones found along the cranial sutures.

wormwood (wĕrm′wood) A toxic substance, absinthium, obtained from *Artemisia absinthium.* It was used in certain alcoholic beverages (absinthe), but because of its toxicity such use is prohibited in most countries.

worried well Persons who are healthy, but who, because of their anxiety or an imagined illness, frequent medical care facilities seeking reassurance concerning their health.

wound (woond) [AS. *wund*] A break in the continuity of body structures caused by violence, trauma, or surgery to tissues. In treating the nonsurgically created wound, tetanus prophylaxis must be considered. If not previously immunized, the patient should be given tetanus immune globulin.

abdominal w. A wound that damages the abdominal wall and intraperitoneal and extraperitoneal organs and tissues. A careful examination (often including peritoneal lavage, ultrasonography, or computed tomographic scanning of the abdomen) is necessary to determine the precise nature of the injury and the proper course of treatment. Superficial injuries may require no more than ordinary local care; immediate laparotomy may be needed, however, when major bleeding or organ damage has occurred. Intravenous fluids, blood components, antibiotics, and tetanus prophylaxis are given when necessary. Major abdominal trauma may be overlooked in comatose or otherwise critically injured patients when there is no obvious abdominal injury.

***bullet* w.** A penetrating wound caused by a missile discharged from a firearm. The extent of injury depends on the wound site and the speed and character of the bullet. SEE: *Nursing Diagnoses Appendix.*

TREATMENT: Tetanus booster injection or tetanus immune globulin and antibiotics, if indicated, should be given. An appropriate bandage should be applied. Emergency surgery may be necessary. Complications, including hemorrhage and shock, should be treated.

***contused* w.** A bruise in which the skin is not broken. It may be caused by a blunt instrument. Injury of the tissues under the skin, leaving the skin unbroken, traumatizes the soft tissue. Ruptured blood vessels underneath the skin cause discoloration. If extravasated blood becomes encapsulated, it is termed hematoma; if it is diffuse, ecchymosis. SEE: *ecchymosis; hematoma.*

TREATMENT: Cold compresses, pressure, and rest, along with elevation of the injured area, will help prevent or reduce swelling. When the acute stage is over (within 24 to 48 hr), continued rest, heat, and elevation are prescribed. Aseptic drainage may be indicated.

***crushing* w.** Trauma due to force applied to tissues so they are disrupted or compressed, but with minimal or no frank lacerations. If there is no bleeding, cold should be applied; if the wound is bleeding, application of the dressing should be followed by cold packs until the patient can be given definitive surgical treatment. If the bone is fractured, a splint should be applied.

***fishhook* w.** An injury caused by a fishhook becoming embedded in soft tissue. Deeply embedded fishhooks are difficult to remove. One should push the hook through, then cut off the barb with an instrument, and pull the remainder of the fishhook out by the route of entry. Antitetanus treatment should be given as indicated. Because these injuries often become infected, prophylactic use of a broad-spectrum antibiotic is indicated.

***gunshot* w.** ABBR: GSW. A penetrating injury from a bullet shot from a gun. At very close range, the wound may have gunpowder deposits and the skin burn marks. GSWs can crush, penetrate, stretch, cavitate, or fracture body structures. The severity of the wound may depend on the structures damaged, the velocity and caliber of the bullet, and the underlying health of the victim. SEE: *bullet.*

***lacerated* w.** Laceration.

***nonpenetrating* w.** A wound in which the surface of the skin remains intact.

***open* w.** A contusion in which the skin is also broken, such as a gunshot, incised, or lacerated wound.

***penetrating* w.** A wound in which the skin is broken and the agent causing the wound enters subcutaneous tissue or a deeplying structure or cavity.

***perforating* w.** Any wound that has breached the body wall or internal organs. The perforation may be partial or complete.

***puncture* w.** A wound made by a sharp-pointed instrument such as a dagger, ice pick, or needle. The chief danger is from thrombosis and possible release of emboli. A puncture wound usually is collapsed, which provides ideal conditions for infection. The placement of a drain, antitetanus therapy or prophylaxis, and gas gangrene prophylaxis may be required. This will depend on the nature of the instrument that caused the injury.

***subcutaneous* w.** A wound, such as contusion, that is unaccompanied by a break in the skin.

***tunnel* w.** A wound having a small entrance and exit of uniform diameter.

wound ballistics The study of the effects on the body produced by penetrating projectiles.

wound healing SEE: *healing; inflammation.*

W-plasty A technique used in plastic surgery to prevent contractures in straight-line scars. Either side of the wound edge is cut in the form of connected W's, and the edges are sutured together in a zigzag fashion. SEE: *tissue expansion, soft; Z-plasty.*

Wright's stain [James H. Wright, U.S. pathologist, 1871–1928] A combination of eosin and methylene blue used in staining blood cells to reveal malarial parasites and to differentiate white blood cells.

Wright's technique A method of staining blood smears. The following procedures are used: (1) The dried blood smear is covered with 5 to 10 drops of Wright's stain and left to stand for 1 min. (2) An equal amount of neutral distilled water is added to the stain. The diluted stain is left to stand for 3 to 10 min. A metallic sheen should appear. (3) The stain is removed by gently washing with distilled water. (4) The slide is stood on end and allowed to dry. (5) The slide is mounted in balsam or methacrylate. If staining results are good, red cells will be pink or copper, white cells will have densely stained blue nuclei, and the cytoplasmic granules will stain variously in the different types of leukocytes. SEE: *leukocyte*.

wrinkle (rĭng′kl) [AS. *gewrinclian,* to wind] **1.** A crevice, furrow, or ridge in the skin. **2.** To make creases or furrows, as in the skin by habitual frowning.

Wrisberg's cartilages The cuneiform cartilages of the larynx.

Wrisberg's ganglion (rĭs′bŭrgz) [Heinrich August Wrisberg, Ger. anatomist, 1739–1808] A ganglion of the superficial cardiac plexus, between the aortic arch and the pulmonary artery. Also called *Wrisberg's cardiac ganglion*. SYN: *cardiac ganglion*.

Wrisberg's nerve **1.** The medial brachial cutaneous nerve, a branch of the medial cord of the brachial plexus. **2.** The nervus intermedius (pars intermedia), a branch of the facial nerve lying between the motor root and the acoustic nerve.

wrist (rĭst) [AS] The joint or region between the hand and the forearm.

wrist bone One of the eight bones composing the carpus. SEE: *hand* for illus.; *skeleton*.

wrist drop A condition in which the hand is flexed at the wrist and cannot be extended; may be due to injury of the radial nerve or paralysis of the extensor muscles of the wrist and hand.

wrist unit A component of an upper-extremity prosthesis that attaches the terminal device to the forearm section and provides for pronation or supination.

writing The act of placing characters, letters, or words together for the purpose of communicating ideas.

dextrad w. Writing that progresses from left to right.

mirror w. Writing so that letters and words are reversed and appear as in a mirror.

wrongful birth, wrongful life The idea that conception would have been prevented or pregnancy would have been interrupted if the parents had been adequately informed of the possibility that the mother would give birth to a physically or mentally defective child.

wryneck (rī′nĕk) Torticollis.

w.s. *water-soluble.*

wt *weight.*

Wuchereria (voo″kĕr-ē′rē-ă) [Otto Wucherer, Ger. physician, 1820–1873] A genus of filarial worms of the class Nematoda, commonly found in the tropics.

W. bancrofti A parasitic worm that is the causative agent of elephantiasis. Adults of the species live in human lymph nodes and ducts. Females give birth to sheathed microfilariae, which remain in internal organs during the day but at night are in circulating blood, where they are sucked up by night-biting mosquitoes, in which they continue their development, becoming infective larvae in about 2 weeks. They are then passed on to humans when the mosquito bites. SYN: *Filaria bancrofti*. SEE: illus.

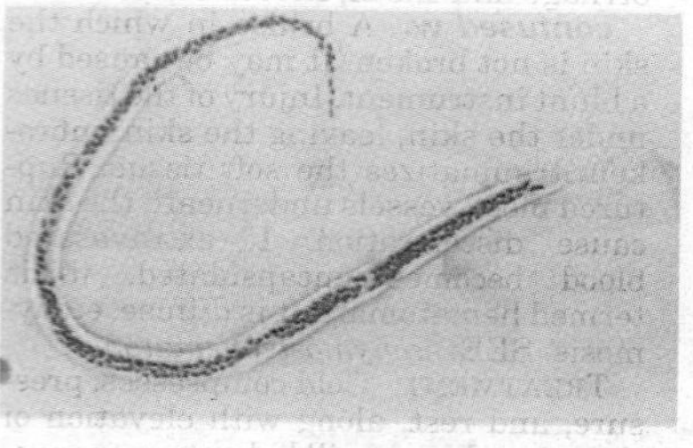

WUCHERERIA BANCROFTI

Microfilaria (×400)

W. malayi A species occurring in Southeast Asia and largely responsible for lymphangitis and elephantiasis in that region. It closely resembles *W. bancrofti*.

wuchereriasis (voo″kĕr-ē-rī′ă-sĭs) Elephantiasis.

w/v *weight in volume.*

w/w *weight in weight.*

X

X Symbol for Kienböck's unit of x-ray dose; symbol for xanthine.
xanchromatic (zăn″krō-măt′ĭk) Xanthochromic.
xanthelasma (zăn″thĕl-ăz′mă) [Gr. *xanthos,* yellow, + *elasma,* plate] A yellow, lipid-rich plaque (a xanthoma) present on the eyelids, esp. near the inner canthus. SEE: illus.

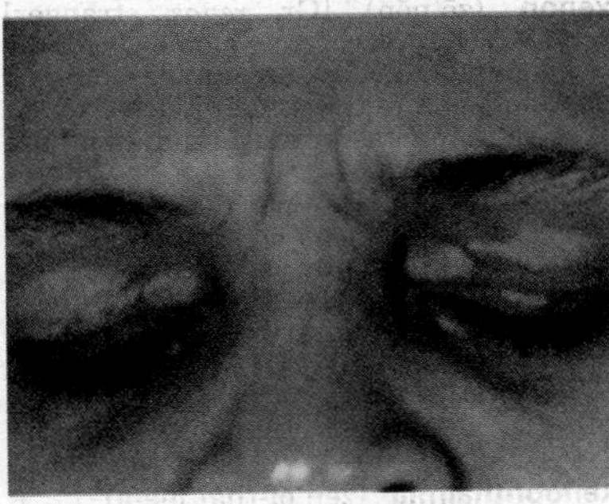

XANTHELASMA

xanthematin (zăn-thĕm′ă-tĭn) A yellow substance produced by the action of nitric acid on hematin.
xanthemia (zăn-thē′mē-ă) [″ + *haima,* blood] Carotenemia.
xanthene (zăn′thēn) A crystalline compound, $O{=}(C_6H_4)_2{=}CH_2$, from which various dyes are formed, including rhodamine and fluorescein.
xanthic (zăn′thĭk) [Gr. *xanthos,* yellow] **1.** Yellow. **2.** Pert. to xanthine.
xanthine (zăn′thĭn, -thēn) A nitrogenous compound present in muscle tissue, liver, spleen, pancreas, and other organs, and in the urine. It is formed during the degradation of adenosine monophosphate to uric acid.
dimethyl-x. Theobromine.
xanthine base A group of chemical compounds including xanthine, hypoxanthine, uric acid, and theobromine, which have a purine as their base. SYN: *purine base.*
xanthinuria, xanthiuria (zăn″thē-ū′rē-ă) The excretion of large amounts of xanthine in the urine. SYN: *xanthuria.*
xanthochromia (zăn″thō-krō′mē-ă) [″ + *chroma,* color] Yellow discoloration, as of the skin in patches or of the cerebrospinal fluid, resembling jaundice.
xanthochromic (zăn″thō-krō′mĭk) **1.** Pert. to anything yellow. **2.** Pert. to xanthochromia.
xanthocyanopia, xanthocyanopsia (zăn″thō-sī-ăn-ō′pē-ă, -ŏp′sē-ă) [Gr. *xanthos,* yellow, + *kyanos,* blue, + *opsis,* sight] A form of color blindness in which yellow and blue are distinguishable, but not red and green. SYN: *xanthokyanopy.*
xanthocyte (zăn′thō-sīt) [″ + *kytos,* cell] A cell containing yellow pigment.
xanthoderma (zăn″thō-dĕr′mă) [″ + *derma,* skin] Yellowness of the skin.
xanthodont (zăn′thō-dŏnt) [″ + *odous,* tooth] An individual who has yellow teeth.
xanthogranuloma (zăn″thō-grăn″ū-lō′mă) [″ + L. *granulum,* grain, + *oma,* tumor] A tumor having characteristics of both an infectious granuloma and a xanthoma.
juvenile x. A skin disease that may be present at birth or develop in the first months of life. Firm dome-shaped yellow, pink, or orange papules, ranging from a few millimeters to 4 cm in diameter, are usually present on the scalp, face, and upper trunk. Biopsy of these lesions reveals lipid-filled histiocytes, inflammatory cells, and Touton giant cells (multinucleated vacuolated cells with a wreath of nuclei and peripheral rim of foamy cytoplasm). The lesions regress spontaneously during the first years of life.
xanthokyanopy (zăn″thō-kī-ăn′ō-pē) [″ + *kyanos,* blue, + *opsis,* sight] Xanthocyanopia.
xanthoma (zăn-thō′mă) [Gr. *xanthos,* yellow, + *oma,* tumor] Soft, yellow skin plaques or nodules that contain deposits of lipoproteins inside histiocytes; they are esp. likely to be found on the skin of patients with hyperlipidemia.
diabetic x. A yellow fatty skin deposit associated with uncontrolled diabetes mellitus.
x. disseminatum A condition characterized by the presence of xanthomata throughout the body, esp. on the face, in tendon sheaths, and in mucous membranes. SYN: *Hand-Schüller-Christian disease.*
x. multiplex Xanthomata all over the body.
x. palpebrarum Xanthoma affecting the eyelids.
x. tuberosum A form of xanthoma that may appear on the neck, shoulders, trunk, or extremities, consisting of small elastic and yellowish nodules.
xanthomatosis (zăn″thō-mă-tō′sĭs) [″ + ″ + *osis,* condition] A condition in which there is a deposition of lipid in tis-

sues, usually accompanied by hyperlipemia. Cholesterol may accumulate in tumor nodules (xanthoma) or in individual cells, esp. histiocytes and reticuloendothelial cells.

xanthomatous (zăn-thō'mă-tŭs) Concerning xanthoma.

Xanthomonas maltophilia Former name for a gram-negative, motile, strictly aerobic bacteria of the genus *Stenotrophomonas,* family Pseudomonadaceae, that frequently cause infections related to the use of central venous catheters and in wounds, pneumonia, meningitis, endocarditis, and conjunctivitis. Infections are treated with ticarcillin, clavulanate, trimethoprim, or sulfamethoxazole. This bacterium is now known as *Stenotrophomonas maltophilia*.

xanthophose (zăn'thō-fōz) [″ + *phos,* light] Any yellow phose. SEE: *phose.*

xanthophyll (zăn'thō-fĭl) [″ + *phyllon,* leaf] A yellow pigment derived from carotene. It is present in some plants and egg yolk.

xanthoprotein (zăn″thō-prō'tē-ĭn) A yellow substance produced by heating proteins with nitric acid.

xanthopsia (zăn-thŏp'sē-ă) [″ + *opsis,* sight] A condition in which objects appear to be yellow.

xanthopsis (zăn-thŏp'sĭs) A yellow pigmentation seen in certain cancers and degenerating tissue.

xanthosis (zăn-thō'sĭs) [″ + *osis,* condition] A yellowing of the skin seen in carotenemia resulting from ingestion of excessive quantities of carrots, squash, egg yolk, and other foods containing carotenoids. The condition is usually harmless, but it may indicate an increase of lipochromes in the blood caused by other conditions such as hypothyroidism, diabetes, or a malignancy.

xanthous (zăn'thŭs) [Gr. *xanthos,* yellow] Yellow.

xanthurenic acid (zăn-thū-rēn'ĭk) An acid, $C_{10}H_7NO_4$, excreted in the urine of pyridoxine-deficient animals after they are fed tryptophan. Also called 4,8-dihydroxyquinaldic acid.

xanthuria (zăn-thū'rē-ă) [″ + *ouron,* urine] Xanthinuria.

x-disease Poisoning caused by ingestion of peanuts or peanut products contaminated with *Aspergillus flavus* or other *Aspergillus* strains that produce aflatoxin. Farm animals and humans are susceptible to this toxicosis. SYN: *aflatoxicosis*.

Xe Symbol for the element xenon.

xeno- [Gr. *xenos,* stranger] Combining form indicating *strange, foreign.*

xenobiotic (zĕn″ō-bī-ŏt'ĭk) An antibiotic not produced by the body, and thus foreign to it.

xenogeneic (zĕn″ō-jĕn-ā'ĭk) [″ + *gennan,* to produce] Obtained from a different species. Antigenically foreign.

xenogenous (zĕn-ŏj'ĕn-ŭs) [Gr. *xenos,* stranger, + *gennan,* to produce] **1.** Caused by a foreign body. **2.** Originating in the host, as a toxin resulting from stimuli applied to cells of the host.

xenograft (zĕn'ō-grăft) [″ + L. *graphium,* stylus] A surgical graft of tissue from an individual of one species to an individual of a different species. SYN: *heterograft*.

xenomenia (zĕn-ō-mē'nē-ă) [″ + *meniaia,* menses] Menstruation from a part of the body other than the uterus. SYN: *stigmata; vicarious menstruation*. SEE: *endometriosis*.

xenon (zē'nŏn) [Gr. *xenos,* stranger] SYMB: Xe. A gaseous element; atomic weight, 131.29; atomic number, 54.

xenon-133 A radioactive isotope of xenon used in photoscanning studies of the lung.

xenoparasite (zĕn″ō-păr'ă-sīt) An ectoparasite of a weakened animal, one that would not normally serve as a host.

xenophobia (zĕn″ō-fō'bē-ă) [″ + *phobos,* fear] Abnormal dread of strangers.

xenophonia (zĕn″ō-fō'nē-ă) [″ + *phone,* voice] Alteration in accent and intonation of a person's voice resulting from a speech defect.

xenophthalmia (zĕn″ŏf-thăl'mē-ă) [″ + *ophthalmia,* eye inflammation] Inflammation of the eye caused by a foreign body.

Xenopsylla (zĕn″ŏp-sĭl'ă) [″ + *psylla,* flea] A genus of fleas belonging to the family Pulicidae, order Siphonaptera.

X. cheopis The rat flea; other hosts include humans. This species is a vector for a number of pathogens including *Hymenolepis nana,* the dwarf tapeworm; *Salmonella* organisms; the causative organisms of bubonic and sylvatic plague and endemic typhus.

xenorexia (zĕn″ō-rĕk'sē-ă) [″+ *orexis,* appetite] An abnormality of appetite marked by persistent swallowing of foreign objects. SEE: *pica*.

xenotransplantation Transplantation of animal tissues or organs into humans.

xerantic (zē-răn'tĭk) [Gr. *xeros,* dry] Causing dryness. SYN: *siccant; siccative*.

xerasia (zē-rā'sē-ă) [Gr. *xeros,* dry] A disease of the hair in which there is abnormal dryness and brittleness, and eventually hair loss.

xero- Combining form meaning *dry*.

xerocheilia (zē″rō-kī'lē-ă) [″ + *cheilos,* lip] Dryness of the lips; a type of cheilitis.

xerocyte An erythrocyte that is dehydrated and appears to have "puddled" at one end, seeming half dark and half light. This type of cell is found in hereditary xerocytosis. SEE: illus.; *xerocytosis, hereditary*.

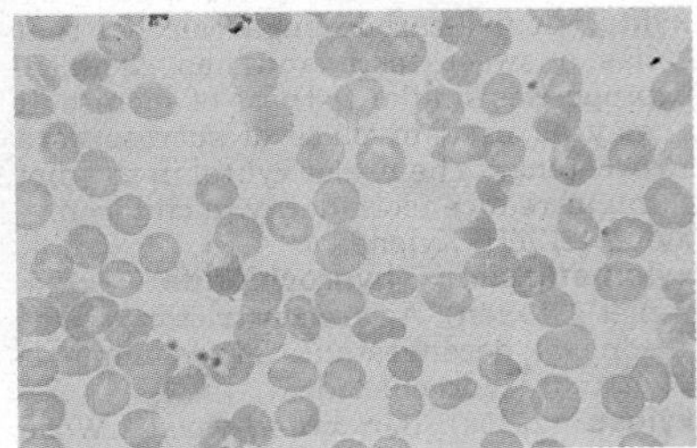

XEROCYTES

xerocytosis, hereditary A disorder of erythrocytes usually inherited as an autosomal dominant trait. A membrane defect in the red blood cells permits the loss of excess potassium ions and water, causing dehydration of the cells. Hemolysis and anemia range from mild to severe. SEE: *xerocyte* for illus.

xeroderma (zē″rō-dĕr′mă) [″ + *derma,* skin] Roughness and dryness of the skin; mild ichthyosis.

x. pigmentosum A rare, progressive, autosomal recessive, degenerative disease characterized by severe photosensitivity developing in the first years of life. There is rapid onset of erythema, bullae, pigmented macules, hypochromic spots, and telangiectasia. The skin becomes atrophic, dry, and wrinkled. A variety of benign and malignant growths appear early in life. The condition is treated symptomatically and sunlight is avoided. SYN: *Kaposi's disease; melanosis lenticularis.*

xerography (zē-rŏg′ră-fē) Xeroradiography.

xeroma (zē-rō′mă) [″ + *oma,* tumor] Xerophthalmia.

xeromammography (zē″rō-măm-mŏg′ră-fē) Xeroradiography of the breast.

xeromycteria (zē″rō-mĭk-tē′rē-ă) [″ + *mykter,* nose] Dryness of the nasal passages.

xerophthalmia (zē-rŏf-thăl′mē-ă) [″ + *ophthalmos,* eye] Conjunctival dryness with keratinization of the epithelium following chronic conjunctivitis and in disease caused by vitamin A deficiency. SYN: *xeroma; xerophthalmus.* SEE: *Schirmer's test.*

xerophthalmus (zē″rŏf-thăl′mŭs) Xerophthalmia.

xeroradiography (zē″rō-rā″dē-ŏg′ră-fē) A method of photoreproduction used in radiography. It is a dry process involving the use of metal plates covered with a powdered substance, such as selenium, electrically and evenly charged. The x-rays alter the charge of the substance to varying degrees, depending on the tissues they have traversed. This produces the image. This procedure has been replaced by film and screen mammography because of its high radiation dose.

xerosis (zē-rō′sĭs) [Gr.] Abnormal dryness of the skin, mucous membranes, or conjunctiva. SEE: illus. **xerotic,** *adj.*

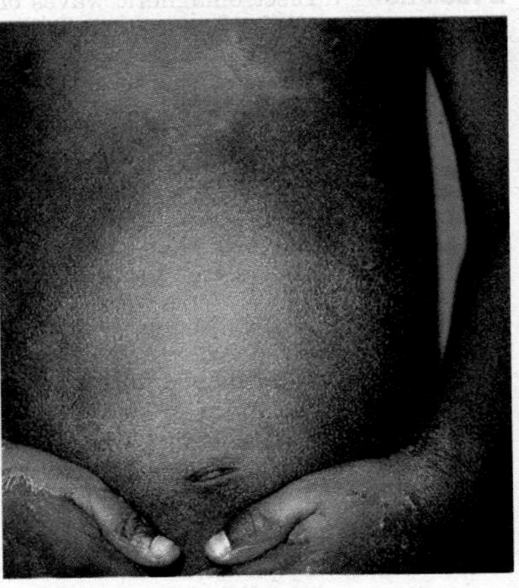

XEROSIS

xerostomia (zē″rō-stō′mē-ă) [″ + *stoma,* mouth] Dry mouth.

xerotocia (zē″rō-tō′sē-ă) [″ + *tokos,* birth] Dry labor caused by a diminished amount of amniotic fluid.

xiphi-, xipho-, xiph- Combining form meaning *sword-shaped, xiphoid.*

xiphisternum (zĭf″ĭ-stĕr′nŭm) [Gr. *xiphos,* sword, + *sternon,* chest] Xiphoid process.

xiphocostal (zĭf″ō-kŏs′tăl) [″ + L. *costa,* rib] Rel. to the xiphoid process and ribs.

xiphocostal ligament The ligament connecting the xiphoid process to the cartilage of the eighth rib.

xiphodynia (zĭf″ō-dĭn′ē-ă) [″ + *odyne,* pain] Pain in the xiphoid process.

xiphoid (zĭf′oyd) [Gr. *xiphos,* sword, + *eidos,* form, shape] Sword-shaped. SYN: *ensiform; gladiate.*

xiphoiditis (zĭf″oyd-ī′tĭs) [″ + ″ + *itis,* inflammation] Inflammation of the xiphoid process.

xiphoid process The lowest portion of the sternum; a sword-shaped cartilaginous process supported by bone. No ribs attach to the xiphoid process; however, some abdominal muscles are attached. The xiphoid process ossifies in the aged. SYN: *xiphisternum.* SEE: *sternum* for illus.

xiphopagotomy (zī-fŏp″ă-gŏt′ō-mē) Surgical separation of twins joined at the xiphoid process.

xiphopagus (zī-fŏp′ă-gŭs) [″ + *pagos,* thing fixed] Symmetrical twins joined at the xiphoid process.

X-linked Denoting characteristics that

are transmitted by genes on the X chromosome.

X-linked disorder A disease caused by genes located on the X chromosome. SEE: *choroideremia; hemophilia.*

x radiation **1.** Electromagnetic waves or energy composed of x-rays. **2.** Treatment with or exposure to x-rays.

x-ray photon An uncharged particle of energy, moving in waves produced by the interaction of high-speed electrons with a target (commonly tungsten). These particles vary from those of lower energy (1 to 0.1 A.U.), used in diagnostic imaging, to those of higher energy (0.1 to 10^{-4} A.U.), used in therapy. SYN: *roentgen ray.*

xylene (zī′lēn, zī-lēn′) A mixture of isomeric dimethylbenzenes used in making lacquers and rubber cement. SYN: *xylol.*

xylene poisoning Injury to body tissues caused by a benzene-like compound. SEE: *benzene* in *Poisons and Poisoning Appendix.*

xylenol (zī′lĕ-nŏl) General name for a series of dimethylphenols found in the pine-type coal tar disinfectants.

xylitol A five-carbon sugar alcohol that has a sweet taste and has chemical properties similar to those of sucrose. It may be used in place of sucrose as a sweetener. The use of xylitol in the diet might reduce tooth decay in children.

xylol (zī′lŏl) Xylene.

xylometazoline hydrochloride (zī″lō-mĕt″ă-zō′lēn) A vasoconstrictor used as a nasal decongestant. Trade name is Otrivin Hydrochloride.

xylose (zī′lōs) [Gr. *xylon,* wood] Wood sugar, a crystalline, nonfermentable pentose.

xylulose (zī′lū-lōs) A pentose sugar present in nature as L-xylulose. It appears in the urine in essential pentosuria and in the form of D-xylulose.

xylyl (zī′lĭl) A radical, $CH_3C_6H_4CH_2$—, formed by the removal of a hydrogen atom from xylene.

xyrospasm (zī′rō-spăzm) [Gr. *xyron,* razor, + *spasmos,* a convulsion] An occupational spasm or overuse syndrome involving the fingers and arms; seen in barbers.

xyster (zĭs′tĕr) [Gr., scraper] Raspatory.

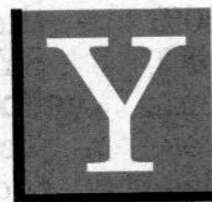

Y Symbol for the element yttrium.

Yale brace A type of head-cervical-thoracic orthosis designed to control flexion, extension and rotation of the head, and moderate restriction of lateral bending.

Yankauer suction catheter A rigid suction tip used to aspirate secretions from the oropharynx.

yard [AS. *gerd,* a rod] A measure of 3 ft or 36 in.; equal to 0.9144 m. SEE: *Weights and Measures Appendix.*

yawn (yawn) [AS. *geonian*] To open the mouth involuntarily and take a deep breath, a movement mediated by neurotransmitters in the hypothalamus and often associated with stretching.

yawning (yawn′ĭng) Deep inspiration with the mouth wide open. It is associated with drowsiness, boredom, anxiety, or fatigue, and in some animals, penile erection. SEE: *pandiculation.*

yaws (yawz) An infectious nonvenereal disease caused by a spirochete, *Treponema pertenue,* and mainly found in humid, equatorial regions. The disease is marked by fevers, joint pains, and caseating eruptions on the hands, feet, face, and external genitals. The infection is rarely, if ever, fatal but can be disfiguring and disabling. It is treated with penicillin. SYN: *frambesia; pian.*

mother y. A papilloma that is the initial lesion of yaws, occurring at the site of inoculation 3 to 4 weeks after infection. This lesion persists for several weeks or months and is painless unless there is a secondary infection. SYN: *frambesioma.*

Yb Symbol for the element ytterbium.

Y cartilage The cartilage that connects the pubis, ilium, and ischium and extends into the acetabulum.

Y-connector A glass or plastic connector that divides one incoming line into two outgoing ones.

years of life lost The number of years a person is estimated to have remained alive if the disease experienced had not intervened.

yeast (yēst) [AS. *gist*] **1.** Any of several unicellular fungi of the genera *Saccharomyces* or *Candida,* which reproduce by budding. They are capable of fermenting carbohydrates. Yeasts, esp. *Candida albicans,* may cause systemic infections as well as vaginitis and oral thrush. Yeast infections are frequently present in patients with malignant lymphomas, poorly controlled diabetes mellitus, AIDS, or other conditions causing immunocompromise. SEE: illus.; *Candida; candidiasis; fungi.* **2.** A commercial product composed of meal impregnated with living fungi, used, for example, in fermenting beer and ale and baking bread.

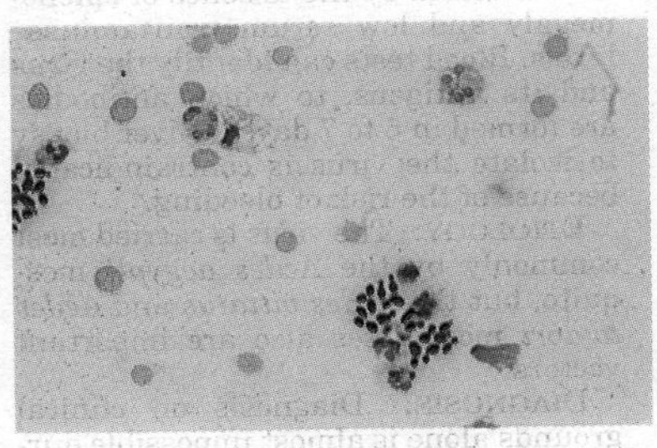

BUDDING YEAST

In peritoneal fluid (×400)

brewer's y. Yeast obtained during the brewing of beer. It may be used in the dried form as a source of vitamin B.

dried y. Dried yeast cells from strains of *Saccharomyces cerevisiae.* It is used as a source of proteins and vitamins, esp. B complex.

yellow (yĕl′ō) [AS. *geolu*] One of the primary colors resembling that of a ripe lemon.

visual y. A retinal pigment.

yellow body Corpus luteum.

yellow fever One of two forms of an acute, infectious disease caused by a flavivirus and transmitted by the *Aedes* mosquito. It is endemic in Western Africa, Brazil, and the Amazon region of South America but is no longer present in the U.S.

There are two forms of yellow fever: urban, in which the transmission cycle is mosquito to human to mosquito; and sylvan, in which the reservoir is wild primates.

Except for a few cases in Trinidad in 1954, urban yellow fever has not been reported in North or South America since 1942. Outbreaks occur in parts of Africa near rain forests.

SYMPTOMS: After a 3- to 6-day incubation period, patients develop high fever, headache, bradycardia, myalgia, oliguria, nausea, vomiting, and diarrhea. The white blood cell and thrombocyte counts are low, as is the erythrocyte sedimentation rate; serum bilirubin and transaminase are elevated. In most patients, the disease resolves in 2 to 3 days, but in approx. 20% the fever returns after an absence of 1 to 2 days and is accompanied by abdominal pain, severe diarrhea, gastrointestinal bleeding (producing a characteristic "black vomit"), anuria, and jaundice (from which the name "yellow fever" was derived) caused by liver infection. Rarely, there is progressive liver failure, renal failure, and death.

Yellow fever is distinguished from dengue by the presence of jaundice, and from malaria by the absence of splenomegaly and low serum transaminase levels. Blood tests can identify the virus and its antigens, to which antibodies are formed in 5 to 7 days. A liver biopsy to isolate the virus is contraindicated because of the risk of bleeding.

ETIOLOGY: The virus is carried most commonly by the *Aedes aegypti* mosquito, but the *Aedes vittatus* and *Aedes taylori* mosquitoes also are important vectors.

DIAGNOSIS: Diagnosis on clinical grounds alone is almost impossible during the period of infection or in atypical mild forms. Yellow fever viral antigen or antibodies may be detected during the acute phase of the illness.

PROPHYLAXIS: Preventive measures include mosquito control by screening, spraying with nontoxic insecticides, and destruction of breeding areas. Yellow fever vaccine prepared from the 17D strain is available for those who plan to travel or live in areas where the disease is endemic. The vaccine is contraindicated in the first 4 months of life and the first trimester of pregnancy.

TREATMENT: No antiviral agents are effective against the yellow fever virus. Fluids are given to maintain fluid and electrolyte balance, acetaminophen to reduce fever, and histamine blockers (e.g., ranitidine) or gastric acid pump inhibitors (e.g., omeprazole) to decrease the risk of gastrointestinal bleeding. Vitamin K is given if there is decreased production of prothrombin by the liver.

A live virus vaccine, which can be obtained only at designated vaccination centers, may be given to adults and children over age 9 months who are traveling to countries where yellow fever is endemic; the vaccine is effective for 10 years, after which a booster is required. Persons who are immunosuppressed, pregnant, or allergic to eggs should not receive the vaccine. Travelers need to determine if the country they are visiting has regulations about vaccination.

PROGNOSIS: The prognosis is grave. Mortality is 5% for natives of an area where the disease is endemic.

yellow spot **1.** The yellow nodule of the anterior end of the vocal cord. SYN: *macula flava laryngis.* **2.** The center of the retina, the point of clearest vision. SYN: *macula lutea retinae.*

yellow vision A condition in which objects seem yellow in color. SYN: *xanthopsia.*

Yergason's test A test used to identify subluxation of the long head of the biceps brachii muscle from the bicipital groove. The patient is seated, the glenohumeral joint is in the anatomical position, the elbow flexed to 90 degrees, and the forearm supinated to assume the "palm up" position. The evaluator resists the patient as the shoulder is externally rotated and the elbow flexed. A positive test result is marked by a "snapping" sensation as the long head of the biceps brachii subluxates from the bicipital groove, indicating a tear of the transverse humeral ligament.

Yersinia (yĕr-sĭn′ē-ă) [Alexandre Emil Jean Yersin, Swiss bacteriologist who worked in Paris, 1863–1943] A genus of gram-negative bacteria.

Y. enterocolitica A species of large coccobacilli that are pathogenic for humans. Clinical infections may be characterized by acute mesenteric lymphadenitis or enterocolitis. The disease may progress to a septicemic form in children, and mortality may be as high as 50%. Therapy with trimethoprim-sulfamethoxazole, aminoglycosides, tetracycline, third-generation cephalosporin, or quinolones is effective.

Y. pestis The causative organism of plague; formerly termed *Pasteurella pestis.*

Y. pseudotuberculosis A gram-negative coccoid or ovoid organism that produces pseudotuberculosis in humans.

yersiniosis (yĕr-sĭn″ē-ō′sĭs) Infection with *Yersinia* organisms.

yin-yang The Chinese symbol of presumptively opposing but complementary entities or concepts such as light-dark, male-female, and sun-moon. In traditional Chinese philosophy and medicine, the goal is to have a proper balance of such forces. SEE: illus.

-yl [Gr. *hyle,* matter, substance] Suffix signifying a radical in chemistry.

-ylene Suffix denoting a bivalent hydrocarbon radical in chemistry.

Y ligament A Y-shaped band covering the

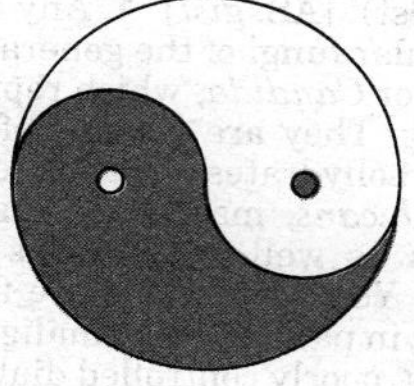

YIN-YANG

upper and anterior portions of the hip joint. Also called *iliofemoral ligament*.

yoga [Sanskrit, union] A system of traditional Hindu beliefs, rituals, and activities that aims to provide spiritual enlightenment and self-knowledge. In the Western world, the term has been associated primarily with physical postures (asanas) and coordinated, diaphragmatic breathing. Many practitioners of complementary medicine use yoga to treat chronic musculoskeletal pain, anxiety, insomnia, and other conditions.

yogurt, yoghurt (yōg′hŭrt) [Turkish] A form of curdled milk created by culturing milk with *Lactobacillus bulgaricus*. Yogurt is a source of calcium and protein that is palatable. It may be better tolerated than milk in persons with lactase deficiency. Yogurt with live cultures may also be useful for replenishing the intestinal flora that have been eliminated following a course of antibiotics. SEE: *milk*.

yohimbine (yō-hĭm′bēn) An alkaloid derived from the bark of the tree *Corynanthe yohimbi*. It is an alpha-adrenergic blocking agent that in excess causes antidiuresis, increased blood pressure, tachycardia, irritability, tremor, sweating, dizziness, nausea, and vomiting. It is used therapeutically to treat erectile dysfunction.

yoke (yōk) A tissue connecting two structures.

yolk (yōk) [AS. *geolca*] The contents of the ovum; sometimes only the nutritive portion. SYN: *vitellus*. SEE: *zona pellucida*.

y. sac In mammals, the embryonic membrane that is the site of formation of the first red blood cells and the cells that will become oogonia or spermatogonia. SEE: *embryo* for illus.

y. stalk The umbilical duct connecting the yolk sac with the embryo.

Young-Helmholtz theory (yŭng-hĕlm′hōlts) [Thomas Young, Brit. physician, 1773–1829; Hermann Ludwig Ferdinand von Helmholtz, Ger. physician, 1821–1894] The theory that color vision depends on three different sets of retinal fibers responsible for perception of red, green, and violet. The loss of red, green, or violet as color perceptive elements in the retina causes an inability to perceive a primary color or any color of which it forms a part.

youth (yooth) [AS. *geoguth*] The period between childhood and maturity. Young adulthood is between 18 and 35 years of age.

ypsiliform (ĭp-sĭl′ĭ-form) Y-shaped.

y.s. *yellow spot* of the retina.

ytterbium (ĭ-tŭr′bē-ŭm) SYMB: Yb. A rare metallic earth element used in screens in radiography; atomic weight, 173.04; atomic number, 70.

yttrium (ĭt′rē-ŭm) SYMB: Y. A metallic element; atomic weight, 88.905; atomic number, 39.

yushi Minamata disease.

Z

Z **1.** Ger. *Zuckung,* contraction. **2.** Symbol for atomic number.

z *zero; zone.*

Z-79 Committee of the American National Standards Institute A committee that develops standards for anesthetic and ventilatory equipment. The label "Z-79" signifies that a device meets the established standard.

zafirlukast (ză-fĕr-lū′k′ăst) A leukotriene inhibitor used to treat asthma. Trade name is Accolate.

Zaglas' ligament (ză′glŭs) The part of the posterior sacroiliac ligament from the posterosuperior spinous process of the ilium to the side of the sacrum.

Zahn's line (zŏnz) [Frederick W. Zahn, Ger. pathologist, 1845–1904] One of the transverse whitish marks on the free surface of a thrombus made by the edges of layered platelets.

zalcitabine (zăl-cī′tă-bēn) ABBR: ddc. A nucleoside analogue reverse transcriptase inhibitor used in the treatment of HIV-1.

Zang's space (zăngz) [Christoph B. Zang, Ger. surgeon, 1772–1835] The space between the two lower tendons of the sternomastoid muscle in the supraclavicular fossa.

Zavanelli maneuver In obstetrics, the manual return of the head of a partially born fetus with intractable shoulder dystocia to the vagina. This is followed by cesarean section.

Z disk A thin, dark disk that transversely bisects the I band (isotropic band) of a striated muscle fiber. The thin filaments, made primarily of actin, are attached to the Z disk; the area between the two Z disks is a sarcomere, the unit of contraction. SYN: *Krause's membrane; Z line.*

ZDV Zidovudine.

zea Maize or corn.

zeatin (zē′ă-tĭn) A cytotoxin that can be isolated from sweet corn.

zeaxanthin (zē″ă-zăn′thĭn) A pigmented antioxidant (a member of the carotenoid family) that is found in broccoli, corn, leafy green vegetables, and squash. Consumption of zeaxanthin-rich foods has been associated with a decreased risk of age-related macular degeneration, among other illnesses.

zein (zē′ĭn) [Gr. *zeia,* a kind of grain] A protein obtained from maize. It is deficient in tryptophan and lysine.

Zeis' gland [Eduard Zeis, Ger. ophthalmologist, 1807–1868] One of the sebaceous glands of the eyelid, close to the free edge of the lid. Each gland is associated with an eyelash. SEE: *Moll's glands.*

zeisian (zī′sē-ăn) Pert. to something originally described by Eduard Zeis.

zeitgeber [German *zeitgeber,* timekeeper] Any of the mechanisms in nature that keep internal biological clocks synchronized (entrained) with the environment. Zeitgebers can be physical, involving light or temperature (e.g., sunrise, sunset), or social, involving regular activities (e.g., consistent mealtimes).

zeitgeist [German] The spirit of the people, or trend of thought at a particular time.

zelotypia (zē″lō-tĭp′ē-ă) [Gr. *zelos,* zeal, + *typtein,* to strike] **1.** Morbid or monomaniacal zeal in the interest of any project or cause. **2.** Insane jealousy.

Zenker, Friedrich Albert von (zĕng′kĕr) German pathologist, 1825–1898.

Z.'s degeneration A glassy or waxy hyaline degeneration of skeletal muscles in acute infectious diseases, esp. in typhoid. SYN: *zenkerism.*

Z.'s diverticulum Herniation of the mucous membrane of the esophagus through a defect in the wall of the esophagus. The location is usually in the posterior hypopharyngeal wall. Small diverticuli are asymptomatic. Large ones trap food and may cause esophageal obstruction, dysphagia, or the regurgitation of food. Treatment is surgical or endoscopic.

zenkerism (zĕng′kĕr-ĭzm) Zenker's degeneration.

Zenker's fluid [Konrad Zenker, 19th-century Ger. histologist] A tissue fixative consisting of mercuric chloride, potassium dichromate, glacial acetic acid, and water. It is used to examine cells, and particularly nuclei, in detail.

zero (zē′rō) [It.] **1.** Corresponding to nothing. SYMB: 0. **2.** The point from which the graduation figures of a scale commence.

On the Celsius scale for example, zero (0°) is the temperature of melting ice. SEE: *thermometer.*

absolute z. The temperature at which all molecular motion (translational, vibrational, rotational) ceases. It is the lowest possible temperature, −273.15°C or −459.6°F; equal to zero degrees Kelvin.

limes z. SYMB: L0. The greatest amount of toxin that, when mixed with one unit of antitoxin and injected into a guinea pig weighing 250 g, will cause no local edema.

zero population growth ABBR: ZPG. The demographic equilibrium in which in a given period of time the population neither increases nor decreases, that is, the death and birth rates are equal.

zero-sum game A game in which the sum of the wins is equal to the sum of the losses. In such a game, every victory by one party results in equivalent losses by other participants.

zestocausis (zĕs″tō-kŏw′sĭs) [Gr. *zestos,* boiling hot, + *kausis,* burning] Cauterization with a tube containing heated steam.

zidovudine A reverse transcriptase inhibitor used to treat HIV infection. It was formerly called azidothymidine and is still often referred to as AZT. Trade name is Retrovir.

Ziehl-Neelsen method (zēl-nēl′sĕn) [Franz Ziehl, Ger. bacteriologist, 1857–1926; Friedrich Karl Adolf Neelsen, Ger. pathologist, 1854–1894] A method for staining *Mycobacterium tuberculosis.* A solution of carbolfuchsin is applied, which the organism retains after rinsing with acid alcohol.

Zieve's syndrome [L. Zieve, U.S. physician, b. 1915] Hyperlipidemia, jaundice, hemolytic anemia, and abdominal pain following the intake of a large amount of alcoholic beverages.

ZIFT *zygote intrafallopian transfer.*

Zim jar opener Trademarked name for a variety of devices allowing one-handed opening of bottles and jars for persons with disability.

zinc (zĭnk) [L. *zincum*] SYMB: Zn. A bluish-white, crystalline metallic element that boils at 906°C; atomic weight, 65.37; atomic number, 30; specific gravity, 7.13. It is found as a carbonate and silicate, known as calamine, and as a sulfide (blende). Dietary sources are meat, including liver; eggs; seafood; and, to a lesser extent, grain products.

FUNCTION: Zinc is an essential dietary element for animals, including humans. It is involved in most metabolic pathways. The recommended dietary intake is 12 to 15 mg of zinc daily for adults, 19 mg daily during the first 6 months of pregnancy, and 5 mg daily for infants.

DEFICIENCY SYMPTOMS: Loss of appetite, growth retardation, hypogonadism and dwarfism, skin changes, immunological abnormalities, altered rate of wound healing, and impaired taste characterize this condition. Zinc deficiency during pregnancy may lead to developmental disorders in the child.

z. acetate White, pearly crystals; used as an astringent, antiseptic, contraceptive, and copper-binding compound.

z. bacitracin SEE: *bacitracin, zinc.*

z. cadmium sulfide A fluorescent material used in radiographic screens.

z. carbonate A mild astringent used topically in dusting powders.

z. chloride A white granular powder used as an antiseptic. It is corrosive. Inhalation of zinc chloride smoke may cause damage to the airways.

z. gelatin A combination of zinc oxide, glycerin, and purified water. This smooth jelly is placed between layers of gauze dressing to serve as a protective dressing and to support varicosities. It is removed by soaking in warm water.

z. oxide A very fine white powder of zinc. It is slightly antiseptic and astringent and is used chiefly in the form of ointment containing 20% zinc oxide. SYN: *white z.*

z. oxide and eugenol Two substances that react together to produce a relatively hard mass, used in dentistry for impression material, cavity liners, sealants, temporary restorations, and cementing layers.

z. salts A bluish-white metal used to make various containers and also to galvanize iron to prevent rust. The most commonly used compounds are zinc oxide as a pigment for paints and ointments. The salts also are used as a wood preservative, in soldering, in medicine to neutralize tissue, and in dilute solutions as an astringent and emetic. SEE: *zinc phosphide poisoning.*

z. stearate A very fine smooth powder used as a nonirritating antiseptic and astringent for burns and abrasions.

z. sulfate An astringent agent used as a 0.25% solution for temporary relief of minor eye irritation.

z. undecylenate An antifungal agent used in treating fungal infection of the feet.

white z. Z. oxide.

zinc-eugenol cement A cement and protectant used in dentistry. SEE: *zinc oxide and eugenol.*

zinciferous (zĭng-kĭf′ĕr-ŭs) Containing zinc.

zinc phosphide poisoning Intoxication with zinc phosphide, a rodent killer that causes fatal lung and cardiac injury. There is no specific antidote.

Zinn's ligament (zĭnz) [Johann G. Zinn, Ger. anatomist, 1727–1759] Connective tissue giving attachment to the rectus muscles of the eyeball. SEE: *zonule of Zinn.*

zipper pull A device allowing persons with limited function to fasten zippers on clothing, esp. those in back.

zirconium (zĭr-kō′nē-ŭm) SYMB: Zr. A metallic element found only in combination; atomic weight, 91.22; atomic number, 40. It is used in corrosion-resistant alloys and as a white pigment in dental porcelain and other ceramics.

Z line Z disk.

Zn Symbol for the element zinc.

zoacanthosis (zō″ăk-ăn-thō′sĭs) Dermatitis due to foreign bodies such as bristles, hairs, or stingers from animals.

zoanthropy (zō-ăn′thrō-pē) [Gr. *zoon,* animal, + *anthropos,* man] The delusion that one is an animal.

Zollinger-Ellison syndrome [Robert M. Zollinger, 1903–1992; Edwin H. Ellison, 1918–1970, U.S. surgeons] A condition caused by neuroendocrine tumors, usually of the pancreas, which secrete excess amounts of gastrin. This stimulates the stomach to secrete great amounts of hydrochloric acid and pepsin, which in turn leads to peptic ulceration of the stomach and small intestine. About 60% of the tumors are malignant. Hyperacidity produced by the tumor can be treated with proton-pump inhibitors (such as omeprazole). Surgical removal of the tumor (called gastrinoma) may be curative.

zolpidem (zăl′pē-dĕm) A sedative/hypnotic drug for treating insomnia; it belongs to the imidazopyridine class, with similarities to the benzodiazepines. The brand name is Ambien.

zona (zō′nă) *pl.* **zonae** [L., a girdle] **1.** A band or girdle. **2.** Herpes zoster.

z. ciliaris Ciliary zone.

z. fasciculata The middle layer of the adrenal cortex. It secretes glucocorticoids, mainly cortisol.

z. glomerulosa The outer layer of the adrenal cortex. It secretes mineralocorticoids, mainly aldosterone.

z. ophthalmica Old name for herpes zoster of the area supplied by the ophthalmic nerve.

z. pellucida The inner, solid, thick, membranous envelope of the ovum. It is pierced by many radiating canals, giving it a striated appearance. SYN: *z. radiata; z. striata; membrane, vitelline.*

z. radiata Z. pellucida.

z. reticularis The inner layer of the adrenal cortex. It secretes very small amounts of androgens and estrogens.

z. striata Z. pellucida.

zonal (zō′năl) [L. *zonalis*] Pert. to a zone.

zonary (zō′năr-ē) [L. *zona,* a girdle] Pert. to or shaped like a zone.

zonary placenta Placenta arranged in the form of a broad ring around the chorion.

Zondek-Aschheim test (zŏn′dĕk-ăsh′hīm) [Bernhardt Zondek, Ger.-born Israeli obstetrician-gynecologist, 1891–1966; Selmar Aschheim, Ger. gynecologist, 1878–1965] SEE: *Aschheim-Zondek test.*

zone (zōn) [L. *zona,* a girdle] An area or belt.

cell-free z. In dentistry, an area below the odontoblastic layer of the dental pulp that has relatively few cells; also called the *zone of Weil.*

cell-rich z. The area of increased cell frequency between the cell-free zone and the central pulp of the tooth.

chemoreceptor trigger z. ABBR: CTZ. A zone in the medulla that is sensitive to certain chemical stimuli. Stimulation of this zone may produce nausea.

ciliary z. The peripheral part of the anterior surface of the iris of the eye.

cold z. In a hazardous materials incident, an unexposed area where rescue personnel wait for assignments and the command post is located, which is safe from any potential contamination.

comfort z. The range of temperature, humidity, and, when applicable, solar radiation and wind in which an individual doing work at a specified rate and in a certain specified garment is comfortable.

epileptogenic z. Any area of the brain that after stimulation produces an epileptic seizure.

erogenous z. An area of the body that may produce erotic sensations when stimulated. These areas include, but are not limited to, the breasts, lips, genital and anal regions, buttocks, and sometimes the special senses that cause sexual excitation, such as the sense of smell or taste.

H z. H band.

hot z. In a hazardous materials incident or biohazard laboratory, the area where the hazardous materials are located. This area cannot be entered without protective equipment, special permission, and specialized training.

hypnogenic z. Any area of the body that, when pressed on, induces hypnosis.

lung z. A hypothetical region of the lung defined by the relationship between the degree of alveolar ventilation and pulmonary blood flow (perfusion). Three lung zones have been identified: I, ventilation exceeds perfusion; II, ventilation and perfusion are equal; and III, perfusion exceeds ventilation. Zone I is found in the upper lung field, where gravity impedes perfusion, and zone III in the inferior portion of the lung, where gravity assists perfusion.

transitional z. The area of the lens of the eye where the epithelial capsule cells change into lens fibers.

warm z. In a hazardous materials incident, the area between the hot zone and the cold zone, where decontamination occurs. Only specialized personnel who are appropriately dressed are permitted in this location.

zonesthesia (zōn″ĕs-thē′zē-ă) [″ + *aisthesis,* sensation] A sensation, as a cord constricting the body. SYN: *girdle s.; girdle pain.*

zonifugal (zō-nĭf′ū-găl) [″ + *fugere,* to flee] Passing outward from within any zone or area.

zoning The occurrence of a stronger fixation of complement in a lesser amount of suspected serum; a phenomenon occasionally observed in diagnosing syphilis by the complement-fixation method.

zonipetal (zō-nĭp′ĕt-ăl) [″ + *petere,* to seek] Passing from outside into a zone or area of the body.

zonography A type of tomography, using a tomographic angle less than 10°, that produces an image of a larger thickness of tissue. This technique is used for kidneys or structures lacking inherent contrast.

zonoskeleton (zōn″ō-skĕl′ĕ-tŏn) The proximal bones to which limbs attach, such as the hip bone, scapula, and clavicle.

zonula (zōn′ū-lă) [L.] A small zone. SYN: *zonule.*

z. adherens The portion of the junctional complex between columnar epithelial cells below the zonula occludens where there is an intercellular space of about 200 A.U. and the cellular membranes are supported by filamentous material.

z. ciliaris The suspensory ligament of the crystalline lens. SYN: *zonule of Zinn.*

z. occludens The portion of the junctional complex between columnar epithelial cells just below the free surface where the intercellular space is obliterated. Also called *tight junction.*

zonular (zōn′ū-lăr) Pert. to a zonula.

zonular cataract A cataract with opacity limited to certain layers of the lens.

zonular fiber One of the interlacing fibers of the zonula ciliaris.

zonular space A space between the fibers of the ligaments of the lens.

zonule (zōn′ūl) [L. *zonula,* small zone] A small band or area. SYN: *zonula.*

z. of Zinn Zonula ciliaris.

zonulitis (zōn-ū-lī′tĭs) [″ + Gr. *itis,* inflammation] Inflammation of the zonule of Zinn.

zonulolysis (zŏn″ū-lŏl′ĭ-sĭs) [″ + Gr. *lysis,* dissolution] The use of enzymes to dissolve the zonula ciliaris of the eye. SYN: *zonulysis.*

zonulotomy (zŏn″ū-lŏt′ō-mē) [″ + Gr. *tome,* incision] Surgical incision of the ciliary zonule.

zonulysis (zŏn″ū-lī′sĭs) Zonulolysis.

zoo- Combining form meaning *animal, animal life.*

zoobiology (zō″ō-bī-ŏl′ō-jē) [Gr. *zoon,* animal, + *bios,* life, + *logos,* word, reason] The biology of animals.

zoochemistry (zō″ō-kĕm′ĭs-trē) Biochemistry of animals.

zooerasty (zō″ō-ĕ′răs-tē) Bestiality.

zoofulvin (zō″ō-fŭl′vĭn) A yellow pigment derived from certain animal feathers.

zoogenous (zō-ŏj′ĕn-ŭs) [″ + *gennan,* to produce] Derived or acquired from animals.

zoogeny (zō″ŏj′ĕ-nē) [″ + *gennan,* to produce] The development and evolution of animals.

zoogeography (zō″ō-jē-ŏg′ră-fē) The study of the distribution of animals on the earth.

zooglea (zō″ō-glē′ă) [″ + *gloios,* sticky] A stage in development of certain organisms in which colonies of microbes are embedded in a gelatinous matrix.

zoograft (zō′ō-grăft) [″ + L. *graphium,* stylus] A graft of tissue obtained from an animal.

zoografting (zō″ō-grăft′ĭng) The use of animal tissue in grafting on a human body.

zooid (zō′oyd) [″ + *eidos,* form, shape] **1.** Resembling an animal. **2.** A form resembling an animal; an organism produced by fission. **3.** An animal cell that can move or exist independently.

zoolagnia (zō″ō-lăg′nē-ă) [″ + *lagneia,* lust] Sexual desire for animals.

zoologist (zō-ŏl′ō-jĭst) [″ + *logos,* word, reason] A biologist who specializes in the study of animal life.

zoology (zō-ŏl′ō-jē) The science of animal life.

zoom lens A type of lens that can be adjusted to focus on near or distant objects.

zoomania (zō″ō-mā′nē-ă) [Gr. *zoon,* animal, + *mania,* madness] A morbid and excessive affection for animals.

Zoomastigophora A class of unicellular organisms within the phylum Sarcomastigophora. These organisms usually have one or more flagella, but these may be absent in some species. It includes free-living and parasitic species such as *Giardia lamblia.*

zoonosis (zō-ō-nō′sĭs) *pl.* **zoonoses** [″ + *nosos,* disease] A disease communicable from animals to humans. Over 250 organisms are known to cause zoonotic infections, of which 30 to 40 spread from pets and animals used by the blind and deaf. Immunosuppressed persons and persons who work with animals are esp. at risk of developing zoonoses.

zoonotic (zō″ō-nŏt′ĭk) Concerning zoonoses.

zooparasite (zō″ō-păr′ă-sīt) [″ + *para,* beside, + *sitos,* food] An animal parasite.

zoopathology (zō″ō-păth-ŏl′ō-jē) [″ + *pathos,* disease, + *logos,* word, reason] The science of the diseases of animals.

zoophilia The preference for obtaining sexual gratification by having intercourse or other sexual activity with animals.

zoophile (zō′ō-fīl) [″ + *philein,* to love] **1.** One who likes animals. **2.** An antivivisectionist.

zoophilism (zō-ŏf′ĭl-ĭzm) [″ + ″ +

-*ismos,* condition] An abnormal love of animals.

zoophobia (zō″ō-fō′bē-ă) [″ + *phobos,* fear] An abnormal fear of animals.

zoophyte (zō′ō-fīt) [″ + *phyton,* plant] An animal that appears plantlike; any of numerous invertebrate animals resembling plants in appearance or mode of growth.

zooplankton (zō″ō-plănk′tŏn) [″ + *planktos,* wandering] A small animal organism present in natural waters. SEE: *phytoplankton.*

zoopsia (zō-ŏp′sē-ă) [″ + *opsis,* vision] Hallucinations involving animals. SYN: *zooscopy* (1).

zoopsychology (zō″ō-sī-kŏl′ō-jē) Animal psychology.

zoosadism (zō″ō-sā′dĭzm) The act of being sadistic to animals.

zooscopy (zō-ŏs′kō-pē) [″ + *skopein,* to examine] **1.** Zoopsia. **2.** The scientific observation of animals.

zoosmosis (zō″ŏs-mō′sĭs) [Gr. *zoe,* life, + *osmos,* impulsion] Osmosis that occurs within cells.

zoospore (zō′ō-spor) [″ + *sporos,* seed] A motile asexual spore that moves by means of one or more flagella.

zoosterol (zō″ō-stē′rŏl) Any sterol derived from animals.

zootechnics (zō″ō-tĕk′nĭks) [Gr. *zoon,* animal, + *techne,* art] The complete care, management, and breeding of domestic animals.

zootic (zō-ŏt′ĭk) Concerning animals.

zootomy (zō-ŏt′ō-mē) [″ + *tome,* incision] Dissection of animals.

zootoxin (zō″ō-tŏks′ĭn) [″ + *toxikon,* poison] Any toxin or poison produced by an animal (e.g., snake venom).

zootrophic (zō″ō-trŏf′ĭk) [″ + *trophe,* nutrition] Concerning animal nutrition.

zoster (zŏs′tĕr) [Gr. *zoster,* girdle] Herpes zoster.

z. auricularis Herpes zoster of the ear.

z. ophthalmicus Herpes zoster affecting the ophthalmic nerve.

z. sine herpete Cutaneous pain of dermatomal distribution, suggestive of herpes zoster but without the typical rash of shingles. That the pain is caused by a reactivation of herpes zoster may be confirmed by antibody titer or polymerase chain reaction tests.

zosteroid (zŏs′tĕr-oyd) [″ + *eidos,* form, shape] Resembling herpes zoster.

ZPG *zero population growth.*

Z-plasty The use of a Z-shaped incision in plastic surgery to relieve tension in scar tissue. The area under tension is lengthened at the expense of the surrounding elastic tissue. SEE: illus.; *tissue expansion, soft; W-plasty.*

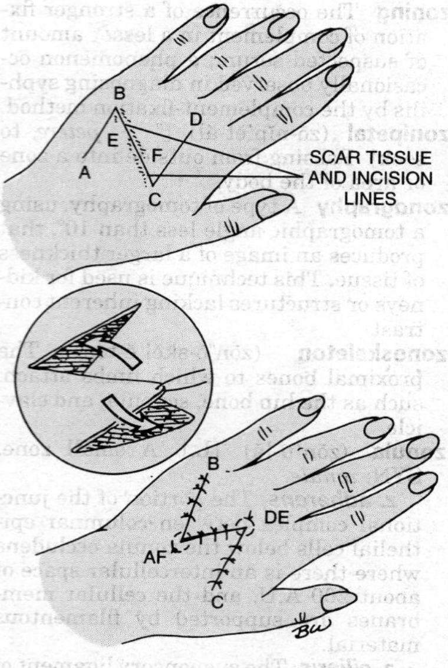

Z-PLASTY METHOD OF CORRECTING A DEFORMING SCAR

Zr Symbol for the element zirconium.

Z-track An injection technique in which the surface (skin and subcutaneous) tissues are pulled and held to one side before insertion of the needle deep into the muscle in the identified site. The medication is injected slowly, followed by a 10-sec delay; then the needle is removed, and the tissues are quickly permitted to resume their normal position. This provides a Z-shaped track, which makes it difficult for the injected irritating drug to seep back into subcutaneous tissues.

zwitterion (tsvĭt′ĕr-ī′ŏn) A dipolar ion that contains positive and negative charges of equal strength. This ion is therefore not attracted to either an anode or cathode. In a neutral solution, amino acids function as zwitterions.

zygal (zī′găl) [Gr. *zygon,* yoke] Concerning or shaped like a yoke.

zygapophyseal (zī″gă-pō-fĭz′ē-ăl) Concerning a zygapophysis.

zygapophysis (zī″gă-pŏf′ĭ-sĭs) [″ + *apo,* from, + *physis,* growth] One of the articular processes of the neural arch of a vertebra.

zygion (zĭj′ē-ŏn) *pl.* **zygia** [Gr. *zygon,* yoke] The craniometrical point on the zygoma at either end of the bizygomatic diameter.

zygocyte A dated term for zygote.

zygodactyly (zī″gō-dăk′tĭl-ē) [″ + *daktylos,* digit] Syndactylism.

zygoma (zī-gō′mă) [Gr., cheekbone]

1. The long arch that joins the zygomatic processes of the temporal and malar bones on the sides of the skull. **2.** The malar bone.

zygomatic (zī″gō-măt′ĭk) Pert. to the zygomatic bone, also called the cheekbone or malar bone.

zygomatic arch The formation, on each side of the cheeks, of the zygomatic process of each malar bone articulating with the zygomatic process of the temporal bone.

zygomatic bone The cheekbone; the bone on either side of the face below the eye. SYN: *malar bone*.

zygomaticoauricularis (zī″gō-măt″ĭ-kō-ăw-rĭk″ū-lā′rĭs) [L.] The muscle that draws the pinna of the ear forward.

zygomaticofacial (zī″gō-măt″ĭ-kō-fā′shăl) Concerning the zygomatic bone and face.

zygomaticofrontal (zī″gō-măt″ĭ-kō-frŏn′tăl) Concerning the zygomatic bone and frontal bone of the face.

zygomaticomaxillary (zī″gō-măt″ĭ-kō-măk′sĭ-lĕr″ē) Concerning the zygomatic bone and maxilla.

zygomatico-orbital (zī″gō-măt″ĭ-kō-or′bĭ-tăl) Concerning the zygomatic bone and orbit of the eye.

zygomaticosphenoid (zī″gō-măt″ĭ-kō-sfē′noyd) Concerning the zygomatic bone and sphenoid bone.

zygomaticotemporal (zī″gō-măt″ĭ-kō-tĕm′por-ăl) Concerning the zygomatic bone and temporal bone.

zygomatic process **1.** A thin projection from the temporal bone; it forms the posterior part of the zygomatic arch. **2.** The posterior projection of the zygomatic bone; forms the anterior part of the zygomatic arch.

zygomatic reflex The movement of the lower jaw toward the percussed side when the zygomatic bone is percussed.

zygomaticum (zī″gō-măt′ĭ-kŭm) [L.] Zygomatic bone.

zygomaticus (zī″gō-măt′ĭk-ŭs) [L.] A muscle that draws the upper lip upward and outward.

zygomaxillary (zī″gō-măks′ĭl-ār-ē) [Gr. *zygoma,* cheekbone, + L. *maxilla,* jawbone] Pert. to the cheekbone and upper jaw.

zygomaxillary point A craniometrical point marked at the lower end of the zygomatic suture.

Zygomycetes A class of fungi that includes those which cause mucormycosis and entomophthoramycosis.

zygomycosis Fungal infections caused by various species including those involved in mucormycosis and entomophthoramycosis.

zygon (zī′gŏn) [Gr.] The short crossbar connecting the parallel limbs of a cerebral fissure.

zygopodium (zī″gō-pō′dē-ŭm) The intermediate-distal portion of a limb, such as the ulna and radius, and the tibia and fibula.

zygosis (zī-gō′sĭs) [Gr. *zygosis,* a balancing] The sexual union of two unicellular animals.

zygosity (zī-gŏs′ĭ-tē) [Gr. *zygon,* yoke] Concerning zygosis.

zygosperm (zī′gō-spĕrm) Zygospore.

zygospore (zī′gō-spor) A spore formed by fusion of morphologically identical structures. SYN: *zygosperm*.

zygote (zī′gōt) [Gr. *zygotos,* yoked] The cell produced by the union of two gametes; the fertilized ovum. SYN: *oosperm; zygocyte*.

zygote intrafallopian transfer SEE: under *transfer*.

zygotene (zī′gō-tēn) [Gr. *zygotos,* yoked] The second stage of the prophase of the first meiotic division. During this stage, the homologous chromosomes pair side by side. SEE: *cell division*.

zygotic (zī-gŏt′ĭk) Concerning a zygote.

zygotoblast (zī-gō′tō-blăst) [″ + *blastos,* germ] Sporozoite.

zygotomere (zī-gō′tō-mēr) [″ + *meros,* part] Sporoblast.

zymase (zī′mās) [Gr. *zyme,* leaven, + *-ase,* enzyme] Any of a group of enzymes that, in the presence of oxygen, convert certain carbohydrates into carbon dioxide and water or, in the absence of oxygen, into alcohol and carbon dioxide or lactic acid. It is found in yeast, bacteria, and higher plants and animals. SEE: *enzyme, fermenting*.

zymic (zī′mĭk) Concerning enzymes.

zymogen (zī′mō-jĕn) [″ + *gennan,* to produce] A protein that becomes an enzyme. It exists in an inactive form antecedent to the active enzyme. **zymogenic,** *adj.* SYN: *proenzyme*. SEE: *pepsinogen; trypsinogen*.

zymogene (zī′mō-jēn) A microbe causing fermentation.

zymogenous (zī-mŏj′ĕ-nŭs) Zymogenic.

zymogram (zī′mō-grăm) An electrophoretic graph of the separation of the enzymes in a solution.

zymohexase (zī″mō-hĕk′sās) The enzyme involved in splitting fructose 1,6-diphosphate into dihydroxyacetone phosphate and phosphoglyceric aldehyde.

zymologist (zī-mŏl′ō-jĭst) One who specializes in the study of enzymes.

zymology (zī-mŏl′ō-jē) The science of fermentation.

zymolysis (zī-mŏl′ĭ-sĭs) [Gr. *zyme,* leaven, + *lysis,* dissolution] The changes produced by an enzyme; the action of enzymes.

zymolyte (zī′mō-līt″) Substrate.

zymolytic (zī″mō-lĭt′ĭk) [″ + *lytikos,* dissolved] Causing a reaction catalyzed by an enzyme.

Zymonema (zī″mō-nē′mă) [″ + *nema,* thread] A genus of fungi.

zymoprotein (zī″mō-prō′tē-ĭn) Any protein that also functions as an enzyme.

zymosan (zī′mō-săn) An anticomplement obtained from the walls of yeast cells.

zymose (zī′mōs) Invertase.

zymosterol (zī-mŏs′tĕr-ŏl) A sterol obtained from yeast.

zymotic (zī-mŏt′ĭk) Rel. to or produced by fermentation.

Z.Z.'Z." Symbol for increasing strengths of contraction.

Appendices

Table of Contents

Index to Appendices

APPENDIX 1
Nutrition

Appendix 1-1 Explanation of Dietary Reference Values

AI, Adequate Intake The amount of a specific nutrient needed to achieve a specific indication (e.g., to maintain bone mass).

DRI, Dietary Reference Intake A nutrient recommendation index based on the parameters specified in the Average Intake, Estimated Average Requirement, Recommended Dietary Allowance and Upper Intake values.

DRV, Daily Reference Value Standards for nutrient intake set for both macronutrient and micronutrient dietary components that lack a Recommended Dietary Allowance. The Dietary Reference Value for some nutrients represents their Upper Limit.

DV, Daily Value A dietary reference term that encompasses the Dietary Reference Value and Reference Daily Intake. It is used to calculate the labeled percent of each nutrient that a serving of the product provides.

EAR, Estimated Average Requirement The estimated intake of a nutrient that meets the nutritional needs of 50% of the individuals within a given age-gender cohort.

RDA, Recommended Dietary Allowance The amount of a specific dietary component, as established by the National Academy of Sciences, required to meet the needs of 97% of the individuals in a given age-gender cohort.

RDI, Reference Daily Intake The nutrient intake standard established by the U.S. Food and Drug Administration as a food label reference for macronutrients and micronutrients.

RNI, Recommended Nutrient Intake The Canadian nutrient intake standard.

US RDA, U.S. Recommended Daily Allowance A nutritional standard formerly promulgated by the FDA and now replaced by the Recommended Dietary Allowance.

UL, Upper Limit The maximum amount of a nutrient that can be safely consumed.

Appendix 1–2 Recommended Daily Dietary Allowances[a] (Revised 1989)

Category	Age (yr) or Condition	Weight[b] (kg)	Weight[b] (lb)	Height[b] (cm)	Height[b] (in.)	Protein (g)	Fat-Soluble Vitamins: Vitamin A (μg RE)[c]	Fat-Soluble Vitamins: Vitamin E (mg α-TE)[c]	Fat-Soluble Vitamins: Vitamin K (μg)	Water-Soluble Vitamins: Vitamin C (mg)	Minerals: Iron (mg)	Minerals: Zink (mg)	Minerals: Iodine (μg)	Minerals: Selenium (μg)
Infants	0.0–0.5	6	13	60	24	13	375	3	5	30	6	5	40	10
	0.5–1.0	9	20	71	28	14	375	4	10	35	10	5	50	15
Children	1–3	13	29	90	35	16	400	6	15	40	10	10	70	20
	4–6	20	44	112	44	24	500	7	20	45	10	10	90	20
	7–10	28	62	132	52	28	700	7	30	45	10	10	120	30
Male	11–14	45	99	157	62	45	1000	10	45	50	12	15	150	40
	15–18	66	145	176	69	59	1000	10	65	60	12	15	150	50
	19–24	72	160	177	70	58	1000	10	70	60	10	15	150	70
	25–50	79	174	176	70	63	1000	10	80	60	10	15	150	70
	5+	77	170	173	68	63	1000	10	80	60	10	15	150	70
Female	11–14	46	101	157	62	46	800	8	45	50	15	12	150	45
	15–18	55	120	163	64	44	800	8	55	60	15	12	150	50
	19–24	58	128	164	65	46	800	8	60	60	15	12	150	55
	25–50	63	138	163	64	50	800	8	65	60	15	12	150	55
	5+	65	143	160	63	50	800	8	65	60	10	12	150	55
Pregnant					60	800	10	65	70	30	15	175	65	
Lactating	1st 6 months				65	1300	12	65	95	15	19	200	75	
	2nd 6 months				62	1200	11	65	90	15	16	200	75	

The allowances, expressed as average daily intakes over time, are intended to provide for individual variations among most normal persons as they live in the United States under usual environmental stresses. Diets should be based on a variety of common foods in order to provide other nutrients for which human requirements have been less well defined.

[a] Weights and heights of reference adults are actual medians for the U.S. population of the designated age, as reported by NHANES II [second National Health and Nutrition Examination Survey]. The median weights and heights of those under 19 years of age were taken from Hamill et al. [Physical Growth: National Center for Health Statistics percentiles. Am J Clin Nutr 32:607, 1979]. The use of these figures does not imply that the height-to-weight ratios are ideal.

[b] Retinol equivalents. 1 RE 1 μg retinol or 6 μg beta-carotene.

[c] Alpha-tocopherol equivalents. 1 mg d-alpha tocopherol = 1 alpha-TE.

SOURCE: Reprinted with permission from National Research Council. Recommended Dietary Allowances, ed 10. Courtesy of the National Academy Press, Washi[illegible] DC.

Appendix 1–3 Dietary Reference Intakes: Recommended Intakes for Individuals

Life Stage Group		Calcium (mg/day)	Phosphorus (mg/day)	Magnesium (mg/day)	Vitamin D (μm/day)[a,b]	Fluoride (mg/day)	Thiamine (mg/day)	Riboflavin (mg/day)	Niacin (mg/day)[c]	Vitamin B_6 (mg/day)	Folate (μg/day)[d]	Vitamin B_{12} (μg/day)	Pantothenic Acid (mg/day)	Biotin (μg/day)	Choline (mg/day)[e]
Infants															
	0–6 months	210	100	30	5	0.01	0.2	0.3	2	0.1	65	0.4	1.7	5	125
	7–12 months	270	275	75	5	0.5	0.3	0.4	4	0.3	80	0.5	1.8	6	150
Children															
	1–3 years	500	460	80	5	0.7	0.5	0.5	6	0.5	150	0.9	2	8	200
	4–8 years	800	500	130	5	1	0.6	0.6	8	0.6	200	1.2	3	12	250
Males															
	9–13 years	1,300	1,250	240	5	2	0.9	0.9	12	1.0	300	1.8	4	20	375
	14–18 years	1,300	1,250	410	5	3	1.2	1.3	16	1.3	400	2.4	5	25	550
	19–30 years	1,000	700	400	5	4	1.2	1.3	16	1.3	400	2.4	5	30	550
	31–50 years	1,000	700	420	5	4	1.2	1.3	16	1.3	400	2.4	5	30	550
	51–70 years	1,200	700	420	10	4	1.2	1.3	16	1.7	400	2.4[f]	5	30	550
	>70 years	1,200	700	420	15	4	1.2	1.3	16	1.7	400	2.4[f]	5	30	550
Females															
	9–13 years	1,300	1,250	240	5	2	0.9	0.9	12	1.0	300	1.8	4	20	375
	14–18 years	1,300	1,250	360	5	3	1.0	1.0	14	1.2	400[g]	2.4	5	25	400
	19–30 years	1,000	700	310	5	3	1.1	1.1	14	1.3	400[g]	2.4	5	30	425
	31–50 years	1,000	700	320	5	3	1.1	1.1	14	1.3	400[g]	2.4	5	30	425
	51–70 years	1,200	700	320	10	3	1.1	1.1	14	1.5	400	2.4[f]	5	30	425
	>70 years	1,200	700	320	15	3	1.1	1.1	14	1.5	400	2.4[f]	5	30	425
Pregnancy															
	≤ 18 years	1,300	1,250	400	5	3	1.4	1.4	18	1.9	600[h]	2.6	6	30	450
	19–30 years	1,000	700	350	5	3	1.4	1.4	18	1.9	600[h]	2.6	6	30	450
	31–50 years	1,000	700	360	5	3	1.4	1.4	18	1.9	600[h]	2.6	6	30	450

Lactation														
≤ 18 years	1,300	**700**	**360**	5	3	**1.4**	**1.6**	**17**	**2.0**	**500**	**2.8**	7	35	550
19–30 years	1,000	**700**	**310**	5	3	**1.4**	**1.6**	**17**	**2.0**	**500**	**2.8**	7	35	550
31–50 years	1,000	**700**	**320**	5	3	**1.4**	**1.6**	**17**	**2.0**	**500**	**2.8**	7	35	550

[a] As cholecalciferol. 1 μg cholecalciferol = 40 IU vitamin D.
[b] In the absence of adequate exposure to sunlight.
[c] As niacin equivalents (NE). 1 mg of niacin = 60 mg of tryptophan; 0–6 months = preformed niacin (not NE).
[d] As dietary folate equivalents (DFE). 1 DFE = 1 μg food folate = 0.6 μg of folic acid from fortified food or as a supplement consumed with food = 0.5 μg of a supplement taken on an empty stomach.
[e] Although AIs have been set for choline, there are few data to assess whether a dietary supply of choline is needed at all stages of the life cycle, and it may be that the choline requirement can be met by endogenous synthesis at some of these stages.
[f] Because 10 to 30% of older people may malabsorb food-bound B_{12}, it is advisable for those older than 50 years to meet their RDA mainly by consuming foods fortified with B_{12} or a supplement containing B_{12}.
[g] In view of evidence linking folate intake with neural tube defects in the fetus, it is recommended that all women capable of becoming pregnant consume 400 μg from supplements or fortified foods in addition to intake of food folate from a varied diet.
[h] It is assumed that women will continue consuming 400 μg from supplements or fortified food until their pregnancy is confirmed and they enter prenatal care, which ordinarily occurs after the end of the periconceptional period—the critical time for formation of the neural tube.

This table presents Recommended Dietary Allowances (RDAs) in bold type and Adequate Intakes (AIs) in ordinary type followed by an asterisk (*). RDAs and AIs may both be used as goals for individual intake. RDAs are set to meet the needs of almost all (97 to 98%) individuals in a group. For healthy breastfed infants, the AI is the mean intake. The AI for other life-stage and gender groups is believed to cover needs of all individuals in the group, but lack of data or uncertainty in the data prevents being able to specify with confidence the percentage of individuals covered by this intake.

SOURCE: National Academy of Sciences.

Appendix 1–4 Dietary Reference Intakes: Tolerable Upper Intake Levels (UL[a]) for Certain Nutrients and Food Components

Life-Stage Group	*Calcium (g/day)*	*Phosphorus (g/day)*	*Magnesium (mg/day)*[b]	*Vitamin D (μg/day)*	*Fluoride (mg/day)*	*Niacin (mg/day)*[c]	*Vitamin B₆ (mg/day)*	*Folate (μg/day)*[c]	*Choline (g/day)*
0–6 months	ND[d]	ND	ND	25	0.7	ND	ND	ND	ND
7–12 months	ND	ND	ND	25	0.9	ND	ND	ND	ND
1–3 years	2.5	3	65	50	1.3	10	30	300	1.0
4–8 years	2.5	3	110	50	2.2	15	40	400	1.0
9–13 years	2.5	4	350	50	10	20	60	600	2.0
14–18 years	2.5	4	350	50	10	30	80	800	3.0
19–70 years	2.5	4	350	50	10	35	100	1,000	3.5
> 70 years	2.5	3	350	50	10	35	100	1,000	3.5
Pregnancy									
≤ 18 years	2.5	3.5	350	50	10	30	80	800	3.0
19–50 years	2.5	3.5	350	50	10	35	100	1,000	3.5
Lactation									
≤ 18 years	2.5	4	350	50	10	30	80	800	3.0
19–50 years	2.5	4	350	50	10	35	100	1,000	3.5

[a] UL = The maximum level of daily nutrient intake that is likely to pose no risk of adverse effects. Unless otherwise specified, the UL represents total intake from food, water, and supplements. Due to lack of suitable data, ULs could not be established for thiamine, riboflavin, vitamin B_{12}, pantothenic acid, and biotin. In the absence of ULs, extra caution may be warranted in consuming levels above recommended intakes.

[b] The UL for magnesium represents intake from a pharmacological agent only and does not include intake from food and water.

[c] The ULs for niacin and folate apply to synthetic forms obtained from supplements, fortified foods, or a combination of the two.

[d] ND: Not determinable due to lack of data of adverse effects in this age group and concern with regard to lack of ability to handle excess amounts. Source of intake should be from food only to prevent high levels of intake.

SOURCE: National Academy of Sciences

Appendix 1–5 Food Guide Pyramids

Food Guide Pyramid for Young Children: A Daily Guide for 2- to 6- Year Olds

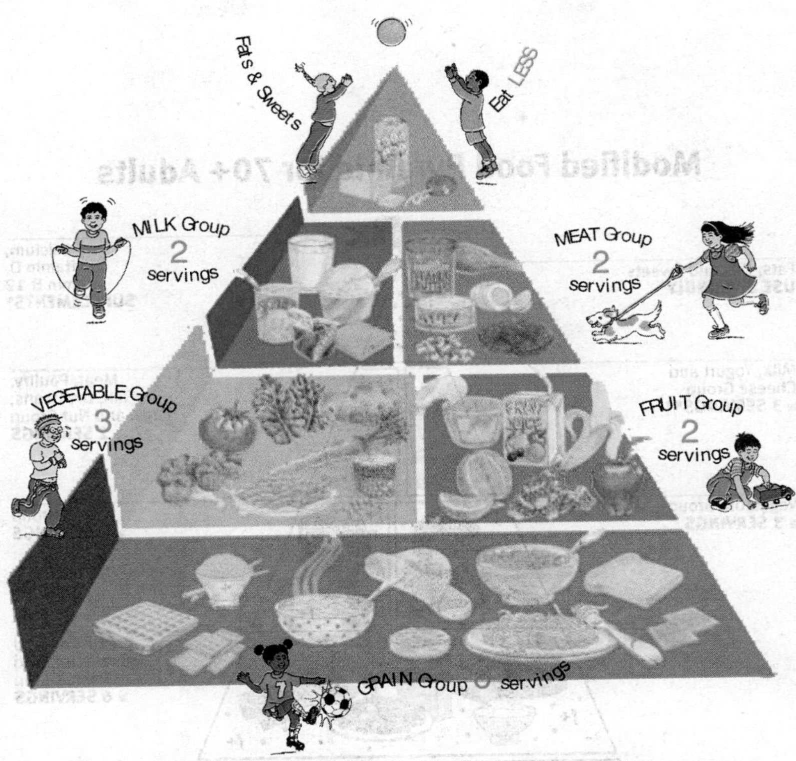
Fats & Sweets
Eat LESS
MILK Group
2
servings
MEAT Group
2
servings
VEGETABLE Group
3
servings
FRUIT Group
2
servings
GRAIN Group 6 servings

WHAT COUNTS AS ONE SERVING?

GRAIN GROUP
1 slice of bread
1/2 cup of cooked rice or pasta
1/2 cup of cooked cereal
1 ounce of ready-to-eat cereal

VEGETABLE GROUP
1/2 cup of chopped raw or cooked vegetables
1 cup of raw leafy vegetables

FRUIT GROUP
1 piece of fruit or melon wedge
3/4 cup of juice
1/2 cup of canned fruit
1/2 cup of dried fruit

MILK GROUP
1 cup of milk or yogurt
2 ounces of cheese

MEAT GROUP
2 to 3 ounces of cooked lean meat, poultry' or fish.

1/2 cup of cooked dry beans, or 1 egg counts as 1 ounce of lean meat, 2 tablespoons of peanut butter count as 1 ounce of meat.

FATS AND SWEETS
Limit calories from these

Four- to 6-year-olds can eat these serving sizes. Offer 2- to 3-year-olds less, except for milk. Two- to 6-year-old children need a total of 2 servings from the milk group each day.

SOURCE : U.S. Department of Agriculture Center for Nutrition Policy and Promotion

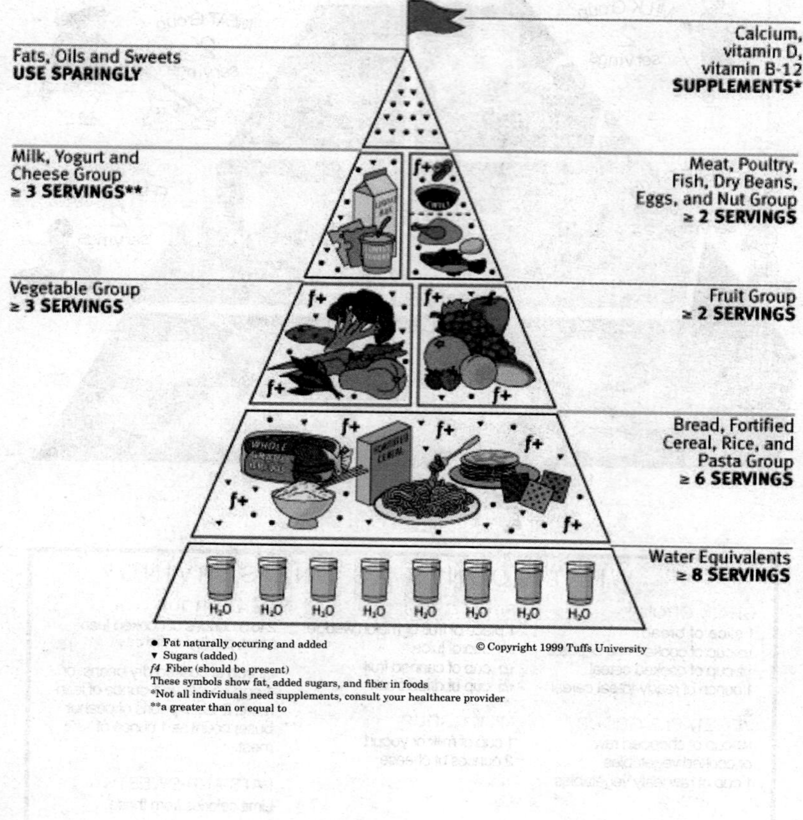
Modified Food Pyramid for 70+ Adults
Calcium, vitamin D, vitamin B-12
SUPPLEMENTS*
Fats, Oils and Sweets
USE SPARINGLY
Milk, Yogurt and Cheese Group
≥ 3 SERVINGS**
Meat, Poultry, Fish, Dry Beans, Eggs, and Nut Group
≥ 2 SERVINGS
Vegetable Group
≥ 3 SERVINGS
Fruit Group
≥ 2 SERVINGS
Bread, Fortified Cereal, Rice, and Pasta Group
≥ 6 SERVINGS
Water Equivalents
≥ 8 SERVINGS
f+
H2O
● Fat naturally occuring and added
▼ Sugars (added)
f4 Fiber (should be present)
These symbols show fat, added sugars, and fiber in foods
*Not all individuals need supplements, consult your healthcare provider
**a greater than or equal to
© Copyright 1999 Tufts University

Modified Food Pyramid for 70+ Adults: Translating Guidelines into Daily Eating

Food Group	*What's a Senior to Do Every Day*	*Best Choices (each equals one serving)*
Bread, fortified cereal, rice, and pasta	Strive for 6 servings of high-fiber, unrefined whole grains.	1 slice whole-grain bread; $\frac{1}{2}$ cup cooked brown rice; 1 oz fortified cereal
Vegetables	Munch on 3 servings of bright-colored vegetables each day—look for dark green, red, orange, and yellow (best sources of valuable nutrients).	1 cup raw spinach; $\frac{1}{2}$ cup mashed squash; $\frac{3}{4}$ cup 100% vegetable juice. NOTE: If you boil vegetables, use the cooking water (many vitamins and minerals are in it) in sauces, soups, or stews.
Fruits	Snack on 2 servings of brightly colored fruits	1 med. orange, banana, apple; $\frac{1}{2}$ cup berries; $\frac{1}{4}$ cup raisins or prunes; $\frac{3}{4}$ cup 100% juice—select juice with calcium
Milk, yogurt, and cheese	Eat 2–3 servings of low-fat or non-fat dairy foods. These are great sources of calcium and vitamin D.	1 cup low-fat milk or yogurt; $1\frac{1}{2}$ oz low-fat natural cheese. NOTE: If you have trouble digesting milk products, try lactose-free dairy products, or add lactose enzymes to milk.
Meat, poultry, fish, dried beans, (legumes), eggs, and nuts	Eat 2 servings of these high-protein foods. Fish is great—its omega-3 fatty acids have many health benefits. Beans provide fiber and nutrients as well as protein, and are less expensive than meat.	$\frac{1}{2}$ cup cooked lentils or other legumes (dried or canned); 1 egg or 2 egg whites; 2–3 oz fish, lean meat, or skinless poultry
Fats, oils, and sweets	Choose these foods sparingly. Use oils, tub margarine, and butter instead of solids (shortening, stick butter, and margarine.	1 teaspoon oil: olive, canola, peanut, safflower, sunflower, corn, cottonseed, or flaxseed

Pay Special Attention to:

Fluid. Drink 8 eight-ounce glasses per day whether you feel thirsty or not. Don't count alcohol or caffeine-containing fluids in the 8 glasses per day.

Fiber. Dietary fiber may help to relieve constipation. A symbol (f+) appears with the food groups that offer high-fiber food choices.

Supplements. It's tough to people over 70 to get enough calcium, vitamin B_{12}, and vitamin D in their diets. Take supplements of these three nutrients regularly.

SOURCE: Nutrition in Clinical Care, Vol 2, No. 3, 1999, p 186, with permission.

Appendix 1–6 Vitamins*

Vitamin	*Chief Functions*	*Results of Deficiency or Overdose*	*Characteristics*	*Good Sources*
VITAMIN A Retinol (animal sources) Carotene Beta-carotene (plant sources)	Maintains epithelial membranes; functions in infection resistance; needed to form rhodopsin; prevents night blindness; ensures proper bone growth; facilitates RNA transcription.	*Deficiency:* Increased susceptibility to infection; abnormal function of gastrointestinal, genitourinary, and respiratory tracts; skin dries, shrivels, thickens; sometimes pustule formation; xerophthalmia, a characteristic eye disease. *Overdose:* Bleeding disorders; bone decalcification; immune system stimulation; fatigue; nausea; diarrhea; dry skin; brittle nails; jaundice.	Fat soluble; stable during cooking; destroyed by heat and oxygen together; marked capacity for storage in the liver.	Liver; dark green leafy vegetables, esp. escarole, kale, and parsley; yellow-orange fruits, esp. carrots, apricots, and cantaloupe; butter or fortified margarine; milk and dairy products; meats, fish, and poultry.
VITAMIN B_1 Thiamine	Involved in carbohydrate metabolism; essential for normal nervous tissue function; acts as a coenzyme for cellular energy production.	*Deficiency:* Weakness; wasting; mental confusion; peripheral paralysis; edema; beriberi.	Water soluble; stable during most cooking; destroyed by alkali or sulfites; not stored in the body. Note: Deficiency often accompanies alcoholism.	Brewer's yeast; pork; soy milk; liver; milk; enriched or whole-grain cereals; beans; nuts.
VITAMIN B_2 Riboflavin	Acts as a coenzyme in cellular oxidation; essential to normal growth; participates in light adaptation; vital to protein metabolism; associated with functions of niacin and vitamin B_6.	Cheilosis; glossitis; dermatitis around mouth and nose; corneal reddening; light hypersensitivity.	Water soluble; alcohol soluble; stable during most cooking; destroyed by alkali; unstable in light.	Milk and dairy products; collard greens; broccoli; whole-grain or enriched breads and cereals; liver; meat, fish, and poultry; eggs; legumes.
VITAMIN B_6 Pyridoxine Pyridoxal Pyridoxamine	Used in hemoglobin synthesis; essential for metabolism of tryptophan to niacin; needed for utilization of other amino acids.	Anemias; depressed immunity; dermatitis around mouth and nose; neuritis; anorexia; nausea; vomiting.	Water soluble; alcohol soluble; inactivated by heat, sunlight, or air.	Meats; liver; cereal grains; bananas; nuts.

*See App. 1-2 for recommended daily allowances.

VITAMIN B_{12} Cyanocobalamin Hydroxycobalamin	Needed for myelin synthesis; essential for proper red blood cell development; associated with folate metabolism.	Pernicious anemia; neurological disorders.	Water soluble; alcohol soluble; unstable in hot alkaline or acid solutions	Synthesized by gastrointestinal flora; meat; yeast; milk; eggs.
VITAMIN C Ascorbic acid	Acts as an antioxidant; essential to formation of the protein collagen; facilitates iron absorption; facilitates cholesterol conversion to bile acids; essential to serotonin synthesis.	*Deficiency:* Joint tenderness; lowered resistance to infections; susceptibility to dental caries, pyorrhea, and bleeding gums; delayed wound healing; bruising; anemia; hemorrhaging; scurvy. *Overdose:* Nausea; diarrhea; hemolytic anemia; gout; kidney stones.	Water soluble; destroyed by light; heat hastens the process; lost in cooking when water is discarded; cooking loss is increased in iron or copper utensils. Stored in the body to a limited extent	Citrus fruit; strawberries; green peppers; mustard greens; cauliflower.
VITAMIN D Calciferol Ergocalciferol Cholecalciferol Calcitriol Antirachitic factor	Promotes gastrointestinal absorption of calcium and phosphorus; promotes bone and tooth mineralization; promotes renal calcium absorption; antirachitic.	*Deficiency:* Interferes with utilization of calcium and phosphorus in bone and tooth formation; irritability; weakness; rickets in young children; osteomalacia in adults. *Overdose:* Irritability; kidney stone formation; calcification of soft tissues.	Fat soluble; soluble in organic solvents; relatively stable when refrigerated; stored in liver; often associated with vitamin A.	Formed in the skin by sunlight exposure; fortified milk and dairy products; egg yolks; liver; fatty fish, esp. salmon, tuna, herring, and sardines; oysters.
VITAMIN E Alpha-tocopherol Beta-tocopherol Gamma-tocopherol	Prevents oxidative damage of lipids and cell membranes; promotes red blood cell stability.	Immune system suppression; red blood cell hemolysis.	Fat soluble; destroyed by heat; destroyed by oxidation.	Vegetable oils, esp. soybean and corn; wheat germ.
FOLATE Folacin Folic acid	Needed for normal hematopoiesis; important coenzyme for nucleic acid synthesis; facilitates fetal development for neural tube closure; functions interrelated with those of vitamin B_{12}.	*Deficiency:* Note: Neural tube defects including spina bifida and anencephalus are associated with maternal deficiency; alcohol interferes with absorption; diarrhea; glossitis; macrocytic anemia. *Overdose:* Masking of vitamin B_{12} deficiency, which may lead to nerve damage.	Slightly water soluble; destroyed by heat at low pH; loss in food stored at room temperature.	Liver; green leafy vegetables; legumes; beets; broccoli; cauliflower; citrus fruits; sweet potatoes.

Vitamins (Continued)

Vitamin	*Chief Functions*	*Results of Deficiency or Overdose*	*Characteristics*	*Good Sources*
VITAMIN K Phylloquinone (plant form) Menaquinone (bacterial form)	Regulates blood coagulation; regulates blood Ca^{++} levels.	*Deficiency:* Hemorrhagic disease; fat malabsorption can cause deficiency. *Overdose:* Kernicterus.	Fat soluble; stable to heat.	Produced by gastrointestinal flora; green leafy vegetables esp. broccoli; cauliflower; liver.
NIACIN Nicotinic acid Nicotinamide Antipellagra vitamin	Facilitates glycolysis, tissue respiration, fat synthesis, and cellular energy production.	*Deficiency:* Dermatitis; edema; diarrhea; irritability; mental confusion. *Overdose:* Flushed skin; intestinal irritation; liver damage.	Soluble in hot water and alcohol; stable during cooking; not destroyed by light, air, or alkali.	Milk; eggs; meat; legumes; whole-grain or enriched breads and cereals. Note: Also formed in the body from dietary tryptophan (amino acid).

Appendix 1–7 FDA-Approved Dietary Health Claims

Health Claim	*Requirements*	*Sample Claim*
Calcium and osteoporosis Low calcium intake is one risk factor for osteoporosis. Lifelong adequate calcium intake helps maintain bone health by increasing, as much as genetically possible, the amount of bone formed in the teens and early adult life and by helping to slow the rate of bone loss that occurs later in life.	Food or supplement must be "high" in calcium and must not contain more phosphorus than calcium. Claims must cite other risk factors; state the need for regular exercise and a healthful diet; explain that adequate calcium early in life helps reduce fracture risk later by increasing, as much as genetically possible, a person's peak bone mass; and must indicate that those at greatest risk of developing osteoporosis later in life are white and Asian teenage and young adult women who are in their bone-forming years. Claims for products with more than 400 mg of calcium per day must state that a daily intake over 2,000 mg offers no added known benefit to bone health.	*Regular exercise and a healthy diet with enough calcium help teen and young adult white and Asian women maintain good bone health and may reduce their high risk of osteoporosis later in life.*
Dietary fat and cancer Diets high in fat increase the risk of some types of cancer, such as cancers of the breast, colon, and prostate. Although scientists don't know how total fat intake affects cancer development, low-fat diets reduce the risk. Experts recommend that Americans consume 30% or less of daily calories as fat. Typical U.S. intakes are 37%.	Foods must meet criteria for "low fat." Fish and game meats must meet criteria for "extra lean." Claims may not mention specific types of fats and must use "total fat" or "fat" and "some types of cancer" or "some cancers" in discussing the nutrient-disease link.	*Development of cancer depends on many factors. A diet low in total fat may reduce the risk of some cancers.*

FDA-Approved Dietary Health Claims (Continued)

Health Claim	*Requirements*	*Sample Claim*
Dietary saturated fat and cholesterol and risk of coronary heart disease Diets high in saturated fat and cholesterol increase total and low-density (bad) blood cholesterol levels and, thus, the risk of coronary heart disease. Diets low in saturated fat and cholesterol decrease the risk. Guidelines recommend that American diets contain less than 10% of calories from saturated fat and less than 300 mg cholesterol daily. The average American adult diet has 13% saturated fat and 300 to 400 mg cholesterol a day.	Foods must meet criteria for "low saturated fat," "low cholesterol," and "low fat." Fish and game meats must meet criteria for "extra lean." Claims must use "saturated fat and cholesterol" and "coronary heart disease" or "heart disease" in discussing the nutrient-disease link.	*Although many factors affect heart disease, diets low in saturated fat and cholesterol may reduce the risk of this disease.*
Dietary soluble fiber, such as that found in whole oats and psyllium seed husk, and coronary heart disease When included in a diet low in saturated fat and cholesterol, soluble fiber may affect blood lipid levels, such as cholesterol, and thus lower the risk of heart disease. However, because soluble dietary fibers constitute a family of very heterogeneous substances that vary greatly in their effect on the risk of heart disease, FDA has determined that sources of soluble fiber for this health claim need to be considered case-by-case. To date, FDA has reviewed and authorized two sources of soluble fiber eligible for this claim: whole oats and psyllium seed husk.	Foods must meet criteria for "low saturated fat," "low cholesterol," and "low fat." Foods that contain whole oats must contain at least 0.75 g of soluble fiber per serving. Foods that contain psyllium seed husk must contain at least 1.7 g of soluble fiber per serving. The claim must specify the daily dietary intake of the soluble fiber source necessary to reduce the risk of heart disease and the contribution one serving of the product makes toward that intake level. Soluble fiber content must be stated in the nutrition label. Claims must use "soluble fiber" qualified by the name of the eligible source of soluble fiber and "heart disease" or "coronary heart disease" in discussing the nutrient-disease link. Because of the potential hazard of choking, foods containing dry or incompletely hydrated psyllium seed husk must carry a label statement telling consumers to drink adequate amounts of fluid, unless the manufacturer shows that a viscous adhesive mass is not formed when the food is exposed to fluid.	*Diets low in saturated fat and cholesterol that include 3 g of soluble fiber from whole oats per day may reduce the risk of heart disease. One serving of this whole-oats product provides [number] grams of this soluble fiber.*

Fiber-containing grain products, fruits, and vegetables and cancer Diets low in fat and rich in fiber-containing grain products, fruits, and vegetables may reduce the risk of some types of cancer. The exact role of total dietary fiber, fiber components, and other nutrients and substances in these foods is not fully understood.	Foods must meet criteria for "low fat" and, without fortification, be a "good source" of dietary fiber. Claims must not specify types of fiber and must use "fiber," "dietary fiber," or "total dietary fiber" and "some types of cancer" or "some cancers" in discussing the nutrient-disease link.	*Low-fat diets rich in fiber-containing grain products, fruits, and vegetables may reduce the risk of some types of cancer, a disease associated with many factors.*
Fruits, vegetables, and grain products that contain fiber, particularly soluble fiber, and risk of coronary heart disease Diets low in saturated fat and cholesterol and rich in fruits, vegetables, and grain products that contain fiber, particularly soluble fiber, may reduce the risk of coronary heart disease. (It is impossible to adequately distinguish the effects of fiber, including soluble fiber, from those of other food components.)	Foods must meet criteria for "low saturated fat," "low fat," and "low cholesterol." They must contain, without fortification, at least 0.6 g of soluble fiber per reference amount, and the soluble fiber content must be listed. Claims must use "fiber," "dietary fiber," "some types of dietary fiber," "some dietary fibers," or "some fibers" and "coronary heart disease" or "heart disease" in discussing the nutrient-disease link. The term "soluble fiber" may be added.	*Diets low in saturated fat and cholesterol and rich in fruits, vegetables, and grain products that contain some types of dietary fiber, particularly soluble fiber, may reduce the risk of heart disease, a disease associated with many factors.*
Folate and neural tube birth defects Defects of the neural tube occur within the first six weeks after conception, often before the pregnancy is known. The U.S. Public Health Service recommends that all women of childbearing age in the United States consume 0.4 mg (400 μg) of folic acid daily to reduce their risk of having a baby affected with spina bifida or other neural tube defects.	Foods must meet or exceed criteria for "good source" of folate—that is, at least 40 μg of folic acid per serving (at least 10% of the Daily Value). A serving of food cannot contain more than 100% of the Daily Value for vitamin A and vitamin D because of their potential risk to fetuses. Claims must use "folate," "folic acid," or "folacin" and "neural tube defects," "birth defects spina bifida or anencephaly," "birth defects of the brain or spinal cord anencephaly or spina bifida," "spina bifida and anencephaly, birth defects of the brain or spinal cord," "birth defects of the brain and spinal cord," or "brain or spinal cord birth defects" in discussing the nutrient-disease link. Folic acid content must be listed on the Nutrition Facts panel.	*Healthful diets with adequate folate may reduce a woman's risk of having a child with a brain or spinal cord birth defect.*

FDA-Approved Dietary Health Claims (Continued)

Health Claim	*Requirements*	*Sample Claim*
Fruits and vegetables and cancer Diets low in fat and rich in fruits and vegetables may reduce the risk of some cancers. Fruits and vegetables are low-fat foods and may contain fiber or vitamin A (as beta-carotene) and vitamin C. (The effects of these vitamins cannot be adequately distinguished from those of other fruit or vegetable components.)	Foods must meet criteria for "low fat" and, without fortification, be a "good source" of fiber, vitamin A, or vitamin C. Claims must characterize fruits and vegetables as foods that are low in fat and may contain dietary fiber, vitamin A, or vitamin C; characterize the food itself as a "good source" of one or more of these nutrients, which must be listed; refrain from specifying types of fatty acids; and use "total fat" or "fat," "some types of cancer" or "some cancers," and "fiber," "dietary fiber," or "total dietary fiber" in discussing the nutrient-disease link.	*Low-fat diets rich in fruits and vegetables (foods that are low in fat and may contain dietary fiber, vitamin A, or vitamin C) may reduce the risk of some types of cancer, a disease associated with many factors. Broccoli is high in vitamins A and C, and it is a good source of dietary fiber.*
Sodium and hypertension (high blood pressure) Hypertension is a risk factor for coronary heart disease and stroke deaths. The most common source of sodium is table salt. Diets low in sodium may help lower blood pressure and related risks in many people. Guidelines recommend daily sodium intakes of not more than 2,400 mg. Typical U.S. intakes are 3,000 to 6,000 mg.	Foods must meet criteria for "low sodium." Claims must use "sodium" and "high blood pressure" in discussing the nutrient-disease link.	*Diets low in sodium may reduce the risk of high blood pressure, a disease associated with many factors.*
Dietary sugar alcohol and dental caries (cavities) Eating foods high in sugar and starches between meals may promote tooth decay. Sugarless candies made with certain sugar alcohols do not.	Foods must meet the criteria for "sugar free." The sugar alcohol must be xylitol, sorbitol, mannitol, maltitol, isomalt, lactitol, hydrogenated starch hydrolysates, hydrogenated glucose syrups, erythritol, or a combination of these. When the food contains a fermentable carbohydrate, such as sugar or flour, the food must not lower plaque pH in the mouth below 5.7 while it is being eaten or up to 30 minutes afterwards. Claims must use "sugar alcohol," "sugar alcohols," or the name(s) of the sugar alcohol present and "dental caries" or "tooth decay" in discussing the nutrient-disease link. Claims must state that the sugar alcohol present "does not promote," "may reduce the risk of," "is useful in not promoting," or "is expressly for not promoting" dental caries.	Full claim: *Frequent between-meal consumption of foods high in sugars and starches promotes tooth decay. The sugar alcohols in this food do not promote tooth decay.* On small packages only: *Does not promote tooth decay.*

Appendix 1–8 FDA-Approved Terminology for Food Labels

extra lean Description of the fat content of meat, poultry, seafood, or game meat that contains less than 5 g fat, less than 2 g saturated fat, and less than 95 mg cholesterol per serving and per 100 g.

free A food or product that contains no amount of or physiologically inconsequential amounts of fat, saturated fat, cholesterol, sodium, sugar, or calories.

good source One serving of a food or product that contains 10% to 19% of the Daily Value for a particular nutrient.

healthy A food low in fat and saturated fat with limited amounts of cholesterol and sodium. Additionally, single-item foods must contain 10% or more of vitamin A, vitamin C, iron, protein, or fiber while not exceeding 360 mg sodium; meal-type products must provide 10% of 2 or 3 of these nutrients as well as not exceeding 480 mg of sodium per serving.

high A product that contains 20% or more of the Daily Value for a particular nutrient.

lean Description of the fat content of meat, poultry, seafood, or game meat that contains less than 10 g fat, less than 4.5 g saturated fat, and less than 95 mg cholesterol per serving and per 100 g.

less A food containing 25% less of a nutrient or of calories than the reference food.

light 1. A nutritionally altered product that contains either $\frac{1}{3}$ fewer calories or half the fat of the reference food. If the caloric content of the reference food is derived 50% or more from fat, then the reduction must reduce the fat by 50%. **2.** A reduction by 50% in the sodium content of a low-calorie, low-fat food.

low A food or product that can be consumed in large amounts without exceeding the Daily Value for the referenced nutrient.

more One serving of a food that contains at least 10% more of the Daily Value of a nutrient than the reference food. This 10% rule also applies to the claims of fortified, enriched, added, extra, and plus, specifically where the food has been altered to attain the increase in nutrient content.

APPENDIX 2

Integrative Therapies: Complementary and Alternative Medicine

Appendix 2–1 Herbal Medicines and Their Uses

Common Name	*Uses*	*Adverse Reactions and Contraindications*	*Interactions*	*Route/Commonly Used Doses*
aloe	**External:** Heals burns/sunburns, wounds, skin irritation; used as anti-infective agent, moisturizer. **Internal:** Used as laxative and for general healing.	Contact dermatitis, intestinal contractions. Avoid oral use in various GI conditions (i.e., obstruction, inflammation), ulcers, abdominal pain, menstruation, kidney conditions.	May increase risk associated with cardiac glycosides. Use with other K+-wasting drugs may add to hypokalemic effect of aloe.	**PO:** *Capsules*—50–200 mg daily; *gel*—30 ml t.i.d.; *tincture (1:10, 50% alcohol)* —15–60 drops. **Top:** Aloe gel can be applied liberally to affected area 3–5 times daily.
anise	Common cold, cough/bronchitis, fevers, liver and gallbladder complaints, loss of appetite.	Occasional allergic reactions (skin, respiratory, and GI). Avoid if allergy to anise exists.	Excessive doses may interfere with anticoagulants, MAO inhibitors, and hormone therapy.	**PO:** *Dried fruit*— 0.5–1 g; *essential oil*— 50–200 ml; *tea*— 3 times daily.
arnica	**External:** Used after injuries (bruises, dislocations, contusions, muscular and joint problems). Inflammation caused by insect bites.	Prolonged use on broken skin may cause edematous dermatitis with pustular formations. Eczema (long-term use). Use of higher concentrations may cause toxic skin reactions with vesicle formation and necrosis. Avoid use on broken skin; avoid if allergy to arnica and plants in Asteraceae family exists.	None known.	**Top:** Typical strength is 2 g of flower heads in 100 ml of water. For poultice, dilute tincture 3–10 times with water. For mouthwash, dilute tincture 10 times with water.
black cohosh	Premenstrual symptoms, perimenopausal and postmenopausal symptoms such as hot flashes, depression, mood swings, profuse sweating, and sleep disorders.	GI discomfort (occasionally). Avoid during pregnancy and lactation.	None known.	**PO:** *Dried root*— 0.3–2 g 3 times daily; *liquid extract (1:1, 90% alcohol)*— 0.3–2 ml. Do not use for more than 6 mo.

brewer's yeast	Common cold, cough/bronchitis, dyspepsia, eczema, acne, fevers, inflammation (oral, pharyngeal), loss of appetite, prevention of infections.	Allergic skin reactions may occur. Migraine headaches may be triggered in susceptible patients. GI gas may result from large doses. Avoid during pregnancy and lactation.	Concurrent use with MAO inhibitors can cause an increase in BP.	**PO:** 6 g of brewer's yeast daily.
camphor	**External:** Pain relief for warts, cold sores, hemorrhoids, muscular aches. Antipruritic. Inflammatory conditions of the respiratory tract. **Internal:** Circulatory regulation disorders, catarrhal diseases of the respiratory tract (internal use is unsafe and should be avoided).	Skin irritation (local effect), contact dermatitis may occasionally occur following application of oily salves with camphor. Avoid during pregnancy and lactation. Avoid if GI conditions (infectious, inflammatory) exist.	None known.	**Top:** 0.1–3% 3–4 times daily for cold sores, antipruritic agent, hemorrhoids. **Inhaln:** 1 tbsp of camphor solution per quart of water in a hot steam vaporizer or bowl up to 3 times daily.
chamomile	**External:** Inflammation of skin and mucous membranes, bacterial skin diseases including oral cavity and gums. Respiratory tract inflammation and irritation. Anogenital inflammation. **Internal:** GI spasms and inflammatory conditions.	Contact dermatitis, severe hypersensitivity reactions, anaphylaxis, vomiting. Avoid during pregnancy and lactation.	None known.	**PO:** *Dried flower heads*— 2–8 g 3 times daily; *tea*— 1 cup of tea 3–4 times daily. Tea is made by steeping 3 g of flower heads in 150 ml of boiling water for 10 min. *Liquid extract*— 1–4 ml 3 times daily.
comfrey	**External:** Bruises and sprains.	No adverse reactions known. Avoid during pregnancy and lactation. Do not use on broken or abraded skin.	None known.	**Top:** 5–20% comfrey ointment. Use should be limited to 10 days.
dill	Dyspepsia, fever, colds, cough, bronchitis, digestive aid.	Contact dermatitis. No contraindications known.	None known.	**PO:** *Dill seeds*— 3 g; *dill oil*— 100–300 mg/day.

Herbal Medicines and Their Uses (Continued)

Common Name	*Uses*	*Adverse Reactions and Contraindications*	*Interactions*	*Route/Commonly Used Doses*
echinacea	Cold remedy, cough and bronchitis, fevers, wounds and burns, inflammation of the mouth and pharynx.	Tingling sensation on tongue, nausea, vomiting, allergic reaction, fever. Avoid if multiple sclerosis, leukoses, collagenoses, AIDS, or tuberculosis is present; avoid if hypersensitivity and cross-sensitivity exist in patients allergic to sunflower seeds; avoid during pregnancy and lactation.	May possibly interfere with immunosuppressant agents because of its immunostimulant activity.	**PO:** *Fluid extract*— 1–2 ml t.i.d.; *solid form (6.5:1)*— 300 mg t.i.d.. Should not be used for more than 8 weeks at a time.
eucalyptus	Cough/bronchitis, rheumatism, catarrhs of the respiratory tract.	Nausea, vomiting, and diarrhea may occur after ingestion of eucalyptus (rare). Avoid if severe liver disease, GI tract and bile duct inflammation, hypotension, kidney inflammation are present.	Induction of liver enzymes, which may increase the metabolism of other drugs.	**PO:** *Eucalyptus oil*—300–600 mg/day. **Top:** *Eucalyptus oil (5–20%) in vegetable oil or semisolid preparations,* used for local application by diluting 30 ml of oil in 500 ml of lukewarm water.
fennel	Dyspepsias, catarrhs of the respiratory tract.	Allergic reactions (skin and respiratory tract) have been reported. Avoid during pregnancy and lactation.	None known.	**PO:** *Dried fruit / seed*— 5–7 g/day; *tea*— 1 cup daily. Tea is made by steeping 1–2 g of ground seed/fruit in 150 ml boiling water for 10 min and then straining.
feverfew	Prophylaxis of migraine headaches, fever, arthritis.	Dizziness, heartburn, indigestion, inflammation (lips, mouth, tongue), light-headedness, mouth ulceration, and weight gain. Allergic contact dermatitis (reported with many species of feverfew). Avoid during pregnancy and lactation.	May inhibit platelet activity (avoid use with warfarin or other anticoagulants).	**PO:** 50–125 mg of freeze-dried leaf per day with food.

garlic	Reduction of BP and serum cholesterol level.	GI irritation (rare), allergic reactions, alters intestinal flora. No contraindications known when used in normal amounts.	Decreases platelet aggregation (may affect warfarin and other anticoagulant therapy).	**PO:** One clove of fresh garlic 1–2 times daily.
ginger	Prevention and treatment of nausea and vomiting associated with motion sickness. Prevention of postoperative nausea and vomiting. May be used for dyspepsia, flatulence, and relief of joint pain in rheumatoid arthritis.	Minor heartburn, dermatitis. Avoid during pregnancy and lactation (if using amounts larger than those typically found in food); avoid if gallstones exist. Use cautiously in patients with increased risk of bleeding or diabetes.	**Natural Product–Drug:** may theoretically increase risk of bleeding when used with anticoagulants and antiplatelet agents. **Natural Product–Natural Product:** may theoretically increase risk of bleeding when used with other herbs that have anticoagulant or antiplatelet activities.	**PO:** 1000 mg ginger taken 3–60 min before travel for motion sickness or before surgery.
ginkgo	Symptomatic relief of organic brain dysfunction (dementia syndromes, short-term memory deficits, inability to concentrate, depression), Intermittent claudication, Vertigo and tinnitus of vascular origin.	Dizziness, headache, upset stomach, allergic skin reaction, palpitations. Avoid if hypersensitivity exists; avoid during pregnancy and lactation.	**Natural Product–Drug:** theoretically may potentiate effects of antiplatelet agents and MAO inhibitors. **Natural Product–Natural Product:** may increase risk of bleeding when used with other herbs with antiplatelet effects (some include angelica, arnica, chamomile, feverfew, garlic, ginger, and licorice).	**PO:** *native dry extract*— 120–240 mg in 2 or 3 doses for organic brain syndromes; 120–160 mg. in 2 or 3 doses for intermittent claudication, vertigo, and tinnitus.

Herbal Medicines and Their Uses (Continued)

Common Name	*Uses*	*Adverse Reactions and Contraindications*	*Interactions*	*Route/Commonly Used Doses*
ginseng	Improving physical stamina, general tonic to energize during times of fatigue and inability to concentrate, sedative, sleep aid, antidepressant, diabetes.	Depression, dizziness, headaches, insomnia, hypertension, tachycardia, amenorrhea, vaginal bleeding, skin eruptions, estrogen-like effects, mastalgia, Stevens-Johnson syndrome. Avoid during pregnancy and lactation; avoid if manic-depressive disorders or psychosis exists.	**Natural Product–Food:** may potentiate effects of caffeine in coffee or tea. **Natural Product–Drug:** may decrease anticoagulant activity of warfarin. Avoid concomitant use with warfarin, heparin, aspirin, and NSAIDs. May interfere with phenelzine treatment and cause headache, tremulousness, and manic episodes. May potentiate the toxic effects of corticosteroids. **Natural Product–Natural Product:** may increase risk of bleeding when used with herbs that have antiplatelet or anticoagulant activities.	**PO:** *capsule*— 200–600 mg/day; *root powder*— 0.6–3 g 1–3 times daily.
goldenseal	Infections of the mucous membranes (bacterial and fungal), conjunctivitis, and GI infections associated with diarrhea, cirrhosis, gallbladder inflammation, and cancer. Topically used to treat eczema, acne, itching.	CNS stimulant, hallucinations, occasionally delirium, nausea, vomiting, constipation, ulceration (vaginal use), may affect production of B vitamins in colon. Avoid during pregnancy and lactation; avoid if hypertension exists.	**Natural Product–Drug:** May theoretically interfere with antacids, sucralfate, and H_2 antagonists. May interfere with antihypertensive agents and anticoagulants. May have additive effects when used concurrently with other drugs with sedative properties. **Natural Product–Natural Product:** concurrent use with herbs that have sedative properties may potentiate sedative effects.	**PO:** *dried root and rhizone*— 0.5–1 g t.i.d.; *liquid extract*—(1:1 in 60% ethanol)— 0.3–1 ml t.i.d.; *tincture*—(1:10 in 60% ethanol)— 2–4 ml t.i.d. **Top:** used as mouthwash 3–4 times daily.

hawthorne	Hypertension, mild to moderate CHF, angina, spasmolytic, sedative.	Agitation, dizziness, headache, sedation (high dose), sleeplessness, hypotension (high dose), palpitations, nausea. Avoid during pregnancy.	**Natural Product–Drug:** increases vitamin C utilization in body, may inhibit metabolism of ACE inhibitor, potentiates effect of cardiac glycosides, concurrent use with other coronary vasodilators (theophylline, caffeine, epinephrine) may potentiate vasodilatory effects, may have additive CNS depressant effect when used with other CNS depressants. **Natural Product–Natural Product:** additive effect with other cardiac glycoside–containing herbs (digitalis leaf, black hellebore, oleander leaf).	**PO:** *Hawthorn fluid extract (1:1 in 25% alcohol)*— 0.5–1 ml t.i.d.; *hawthorn fruit tincture (1:5 in 45% alcohol)*— 1–2 ml t.i.d.; *dried hawthorn berries*— 300–1000 mg t.i.d.
kava-kava	Anxiety, stress, restlessness, insomnia, mild muscle aches and pains.	Dizziness, headache, sedation, sensory disturbances, pupil dilation, visual accommodation disorders, gastrointestinal complaints, allergic skin reactions, yellow discoloration of skin, pellagroid dermopathy, weight loss, ataxia, muscle weakness. Avoid during pregnancy and lactation; avoid if endogenous depression exists. Do not give to children under 12 yr of age.	**Natural Product–Drug:** additive effect when used with alprazolam. Potentiates effect of CNS depressants (ethanol, barbiturates, benzodiazepines), has decreased the effectiveness of levodopa in a few cases. May have additive effects with antiplatelet agents and MAO inhibitors. **Natural Product–Natural Product:** May have additive sedative effects when used with other herbs with sedative properties.	**PO:** *dried kava root extract*— 100–250 mg for antianxiety; *kavalactones*— 180–210 mg for insomnia.

Herbal Medicines and Their Uses (Continued)

Common Name	Uses	Adverse Reactions and Contraindications	Interactions	Route/Commonly Used Doses
ma-huang	Asthma, hay fever, colds, weight-loss aid.	Increased BP and heart rate, insomnia, motor restlessness, headaches, nausea, vomiting, anxiety. Avoid during pregnancy and lactation. Avoid if heart disease, hypertension, diabetes, hyperthyroidism, or BPH is present.	Potentiates sympathomimetic effects of antihypertensives, antidepressants, MAO inhibitors, and caffeine.	**PO:** *Ephedra*— 15–30 mg of 2–3 times daily; *crude herb*— 500–1000 mg 2–3 times daily.
milk thistle	Cirrhosis, chronic hepatitis, gallstones, psoriasis.	Mild laxative, mild allergic reaction. Avoid during pregnancy and lactation.	None known.	**PO:** *Extract (70%)*—200–400; *dried fruit/seed*—12–15 g/day; *tea*—3–4 times daily 30 min before meals. Tea is prepared by steeping and 3–5 g of crushed fruit/seed in 150 ml of boiling water for 10 min and then straining.
mugwort	GI ailments (colic, diarrhea, constipation), worm infestations, persistent vomiting, hysteria, epilepsy, menstrual problems and irregular periods; as a sedative.	Allergic reactions. Avoid during pregnancy and lactation.	None known.	**PO:** *Tincture*—5 ml 30 min before bedtime or 1–4 ml up to 3 times daily.
nettle	Urinary tract infections, kidney and bladder stones. Supportive therapy for rheumatic ailments.	Allergic reactions (rare). Avoid during pregnancy and lactation.	None known.	**PO:** *Tea*—1 cup up to 3 times daily with adequate fluid intake. Tea is made by steeping 1.5–5 g of nettle in 150 ml of boiling water for 10 min and then straining. *Dried extract (7:1)*—770 mg twice daily; *liquid extract (1:1, 25% alcohol)*—3–4 ml 3 times daily. **Top:** *Tincture (1:10)* for external use.

oak bark	External: Inflammatory skin disease. Internal: diarrhea (nonspecific, acute), mild inflammation of oral and pharyngeal regions and genital and anal areas.	GI disturbances, kidney damage, liver necrosis. Avoid during pregnancy and lactation. Avoid oak bark baths if weeping eczema, large areas of skin damage, febrile or infectious disease, cardiac insufficiency is present.	May reduce or inhibit the absorption of alkaloids and other alkaline drugs.	**PO:** For diarrhea, 1 cup of tea up to 3 times daily for 3–4 days. Tea is made by steeping 1 g coarsely ground bark in 150 ml of boiling water and then straining. **Top:** For rinses, compresses, gargles, use 20 g bark in 1 liter of water. For baths, use 5 g bark in 1 liter of water and add to bath water. Topical use should be limited to 2–3 week.
pennyroyal	External: Skin diseases. Internal: Digestive disorders, liver and gallbladder disorders, gout, colds, and increased urinary frequency.	Abortifacent in high doses. Hepatotoxicity (use not recommended because of hepatoxicity). Avoid during pregnancy and lactation.	None known.	Use not recommended because of toxicity.
peppermint	Colds, coughs, inflammation of mouth and pharynx, GI cramps and as an antiflatulent and antipyretic agent. The oil is used topically for myalgias, toothaches, pruritus, urticaria and as an anti-infective agent.	Heartburn when taken orally. Allergic reactions (headache and flushing). External use may cause skin irritation and contact dermatitis. In small children and babies, the oil may cause bronchial spasms and collapse when applied to their facial, nasal, or chest areas. Avoid during pregnancy and lactation. Avoid use of oil on infants/small children. Avoid if hypersensitivity to peppermint exists. Avoid if bile duct obstruction, severe liver disease, or gallbladder inflammation is present.	Gastric acid–blocking drugs.	**PO:** *Peppermint oil*—0.2–0.4 ml 3 times daily in diluted preparation; *capsules*—1–2 capsules 3 times daily (0.2 ml/capsule). **Top:** 5–20% peppermint oil in oily preparations, 5–10% in aqueous/ethanol preparations, 1–5% in nasal preparations. To apply, rub small amount on affected skin areas. **Inhaln:** 3–4 drops of oil placed in hot water and inhaled. Inhalation contraindicated in children.

Herbal Medicines and Their Uses (Continued)

Common Name	Uses	Adverse Reactions and Contraindications	Interactions	Route/Commonly Used Doses
psyllium	Constipation, diarrhea, lowering serum cholesterol	Flatulence, abdominal distention, esophageal/bowel obstruction if not taken with water/fluid. Allergic reactions. Avoid if fecal impaction, GI tract obstruction or narrowing is present.	Interferes with absorption of other drugs taken simultaneously.	**PO:** 3.5 g 1–3 times daily of the seed husk taken with adequate fluids.
Saint John's wort	Management of mild to moderate depression. Externally used for inflammation of the skin, blunt injuries, wounds, and burns.	Dizziness, restlessness, sleep disturbances, hypertension, abdominal pain, bloating, constipation, dry mouth, feeling of fullness, flatulence, nausea, vomiting, allergic skin reactions, phototoxicity. Avoid during pregnancy and lactation. Do not give to children.	Concurrent use with alcohol or other antidepressants may increase the risk of adverse reactions. Concurrent use with indinavir may significantly reduce blood concentrations of indinavir.	**PO:** *hypericum extract*— 300 mg t.i.d. for depression. **Top:** *hypericin*—0.2–1 mg daily.
saw palmetto	Urination problems in BPH, irritable bladder.	Headaches, stomach problems (rare). Avoid during pregnancy and lactation; avoid if breast cancer exists.	Oral contraceptives and hormone therapy (possible).	**PO:** *Dried berry*—0.5–1 g of dried berry three times daily; *tea*—1 cup of tea 3 times daily. Tea is made by steeping 0.5–1 g of dried berry in 150 ml of boiling water for 10 min and then straining. *Saw palmetto extracts with 80–90% fatty acids*—160 mg twice daily.

spruce	Colds, cough, bronchitis, fevers, inflammation of the mouth and pharynx.	May worsen bronchial spasms. Avoid during pregnancy and lactation. Avoid if asthma or whooping cough exists. Avoid baths with spruce if extensive skin damage, acute skin diseases, fevers, infectious diseases, or cardiac insufficiency is present.	None known.	**PO:** *Fresh shoots*—5–6 g/per day. *Essential oil*—given as 4 drops in water or with sugar 3 times daily. **Top:** 200–300 g of shoots boiled in 1 liter of water; steep for 5 min, strain, and add to full bath. **Inhaln:** Inhale 2 g of oil in hot water several times daily.
uva-ursi	Urinary tract infections.	Nausea, vomiting, GI upset, hepatotoxicity, high toxic doses (30–100 g of uva-ursi) can cause death. Avoid during pregnancy and lactation. Avoid if kidney disorders or GI irritable disorders exist. Do not give to children.	Use with urine-acidifying drugs may reduce the efficacy of uva-ursi.	**PO:** 1 cup of tea up to 4 times daily. Tea is made by steeping 3 g of dried leaf in 150 ml cold water for 12–24 hr and then straining. This herb should not be used for more than 1 week at a time, no more than 5 times a year.
valerian	Restlessness, sleeping disorders due to nervous conditions.	Morning drowsiness, headaches, excitability, insomnia. Avoid during pregnancy and lactation.	Use with alcohol and other sedatives may potentiate sedative effects	**PO:** *Extract (0.8% valeric acid)*—150–300 mg 30 min before bedtime. *Tea*—1 cup 1–3 times daily. Tea is made by steeping 2–3 g of root in 150 ml of boiling water for 10 min and then straining.
woodruff	Nervousness, sleeplessness, hysteria, cardiac irregularity.	Headache, stupor (high doses). Liver damage (reversible) may occur with long-term use in susceptible patients. Avoid during pregnancy and lactation.	None known.	**PO:** 1 cup of tea once a day, shortly before bedtime. Tea is made with 2 teaspoonfuls (1.8 g) in one glass of water.

BPH: benign prostatic hyperplasia; Inhaln: Inhalation; PO: by mouth; PSA: prostate-specific antigen; Top: topical.

*NOTE: Instruct patient to consult health care professional before taking any prescription or OTC medications concurrently with any of these herbal products. The purity, safety, and effectiveness of many herbal remedies remains untested and unproven.

SOURCE: Deglin, JH and Vallerand, AH: Davis's Drug Guide for Nurses, F.A. Davis, Philadelphia, 2000.

Appendix 2–2 Forms of Herbal Preparations

bath A form of hydrotherapy. Immerse the full body in a bath with 500 ml or 1 pint of infusion or decoction. The full-strength herbal infusion or decoction is used for foot or hand baths.

capsule or pill Powdered herbs may be enclosed in gelatin capsules or pressed into a hard pill. The powder can also be rolled into a pill with bread or cream cheese. This is one of the most common ways herbs are supplied and used.

compress A clean cloth is soaked in an herbal infusion or decoction and applied over injured or inflamed areas. Also called a fomentation.

crude herb The fresh or dried herb in an unprocessed form. Measurements are expressed by weight.

decoction An aqueous preparation of hard and woody herbs, which are made soluble by simmering in almost boiling water for 30 minutes or more. If the active ingredients are volatile oils, it is important to cover the pan to prevent vaporization. The decoction is then strained while hot and either stored or consumed as needed.

essential oils Volatile oils, usually mixtures of a variety of odoriferous organic compounds of plants.

extract Concentrated form of natural products obtained by treating crude herb with solvent and then discarding the solvent to result in a fluid extract, solid extract, powdered extract, or tincture. Strength is expressed as the ratio of the concentration of the crude herb to the extract (e.g., 5:1 means five parts crude herb is concentrated in 1 part extract, and 1:2 means one part of extract is comparable to 0.5 parts herb).

fluid extract Concentrated tinctures with a strength of one part solvent to one part herb.

fomentation A clean cloth is soaked in an herbal infusion or decoction and applied over injured or inflamed areas.

infusion The preferred method used for soft plant parts such as leaves, flowers, or green stems, an infusion is prepared just like making a tea. In the case of volatile oils or heat-sensitive ingredients, soaking in water or milk for 6 to 12 hours in a sealed earthenware pot makes a cold infusion.

liniment Usually a mixture of herbs and alcohol or vinegar to be applied topically over muscles and ligaments.

lozenge Dissolvable tablet often used for upper respiratory and throat problems. They are made by combining a powdered herb with sugar and viscous jelly obtained from either an edible gum or mucilaginous plant.

ointment An herb or mixture of herbs in a semi-solid mixture such as petroleum jelly. This is applied externally for injuries or inflammation. If made with volatile oils, it can even be used as a respiratory anticatarrhal. Also known as a salve.

powdered extract A solid extract which has been dried to a powder.

poultice A raw or mashed herb applied directly to the body or wrapped in cheesecloth or other clean cloth. They are used either hot or cold for bruises, inflammation, spasm, and pain.

salve An herb or mixture of herbs in a semi-solid mixture such as petroleum jelly. This is applied externally for injuries or inflammation. If made with volatile oils, it can even be used as a respiratory anticatarrhal.

tincture An alcohol-based preparation. Alcohol is a better solvent than water for many plant ingredients, so mixing herbs in alcohol such as vodka or wine with a specific water/alcohol ratio is a common method of extraction. The mixture is soaked for about 2 weeks. Then the herbs are strained out and the liquid is saved in a dark, well-stoppered bottle. These preparations are much stronger volume-for-volume than infusions or decoctions. Strengths are typically 1:5 to 1:10.

tea Made by steeping herbs in hot water (The same as an *Infusion*). Place 1 tsp dried herb or 2 to 3 tsp fresh herb into 1 cup (250 ml) hot or boiling water. Steep for 5 to 15 minutes. For larger quantities, use 1 oz (30 g) of herb in 1 pint (500 ml) of hot water. Bruise or powder seeds before making an infusion or tea. The shelf life of these bioactive fluids is short, even in the refrigerator. Discard them after 8 to 12 hours.

SOURCE: Sierpina, VS: Integrative Health Care: Complementary and Alternative Therapies for the Whole Person, FA Davis, Philadelphia, 2000.

Appendix 2–3 Premises of Mind-Body Medicine

Mind and body are simply two aspects of a whole individual. The mind is no less medically real and significant than the body.
Every person has self-healing abilities.
Each person is unique, and must be responded to as such. To be most effective, the treatment program must be individualized for each person.
Each person is an integration of physical, psychological, intellectual, and spiritual aspects. All aspects are equally important. All must be addressed in the approach to health.
Patients' healing abilities are strongly affected by their expectations and beliefs. The expectations, attitudes, beliefs, and words of practitioners strongly influence the expectations of their patients.
Mainline medicine does not have a monopoly on the search for health.
Patients need to be actively involved in their own healing and in the decision making concerning their treatments.

SOURCE: Reprinted from Mind-Body Medicine: A Clinician's Guide to Psychoneuroimmunology, Watkins, A, p. 99, 1997, by permission of the publisher Churchill Livingstone.

Appendix 2–4 Websites for Complementary and Alternative Medicines

This list of Web sites, though not exhaustive, is intended to provide general sources of useful information on complementary and alternative medical therapies. Many of these Web sites provide links to information on specific therapies and medical conditions. Inclusion of a Web site on this list does not imply endorsement of the information contained on that site.

Alternative Health News Online
www.altmedicine.com

Alternative Link, LLC (information on billing codes)
www.alternativelink.com

Alternative Medicine Homepage, Falk Library of the Health Sciences, University of Pittsburgh
www.pitt.edu/cbw/altm.html

American Association of Naturopathic Physicians
www.naturopathic.org

American Chiropractic Association
www.amerchiro.org

American Holistic Medical Association
www.holisticmedicine.org

American Osteopathic Association
www.am-osteo-assn.org

The Ardell Wellness Report
www.yourhealth.com

Ask Dr. Weil
www.pathfinder.com/drweil

Biotecnoquimica (Venezuela–Spanish language)
www.biotecnoquimica.com

Children's Hospital, Boston: Center for Holistic Pediatric Education and Research (CHPER)
www.childrenshospital.org/holistic

Choices for Health
www.choicesforhealth.com

Columbia-Presbyterian Med Center: The Richard and Hinda Rosenthal Center for Complementary and Alternative Medicine
www.cpmcnet.columbia.edu/dept/rosenthal/

Complementary and Alternative Medicine Program at Stanford University (CAMPS)
www.scrdp.stanford.edu/camps.html

Duke's Phytochemical and Ethnobotanical Database
www.ars-grin.gov/duke

Fetzer Institute (a nonprofit organization promoting the study of the spiritual elements of life)
http://www.fetzer.org

Getwell (Australia)
www.getwell.com.au

Global Health 2000 (10 languages)
www.globalhealth2000.com

Harvard Medical School–General Medical Conditions
www.bidmc.harvard.edu/medicine/camr

Healthfinder
healthfinder.com

HerbalGram (American Botanical Council)
www.herbalgram.org

HerbMed
www.amfoundation.org/herbmed.htm

Herb Research Foundation
www.herbs.org

Holistic Medicine Interest Group (Oregon Health Sciences University)
www.ohsu.edu/ohmig

Longwood Herbal Task Force
www.mcp.edu/herbal

McMaster University (Hamilton, Ontario) Alternative Medicine Health Care Information Resources
www-hsl.mcmaster.ca/tomflem/altmed.html

Medical College of Wisconsin: Alternative Medicine Resources
www.intmed.mcw.edu/gimcme/altmed.html

MEDLINE (U.S. National Library of Medicine)
www.nlm.nih.gov

National Council for Reliable Health Information (NCRHI)
www.ncahf.org

National Health Information Center (NHIC)
www.nhic-nt.health.org

National Institutes of Health, National Center for CAM
nccam.nih.gov

Natural Healthline
www.naturalhealthvillage.com

Nurse Healers–Professional Associates International
www.therapeutic-touch.org

Office of Dietary Supplements (National Institutes of Health): The International Bibliographic Information on Dietary Supplements (IBIDS)
odp.od.nih.gov/ods/databases/ibids.html

Quackwatch
www.quackwatch.com

Tufts University Nutrition Navigator
www.navigator.tufts.edu

University of Texas Medical Branch Alternative and Integrative Healthcare Program
www.atc.utmb.edu/altmed

University of Virginia Center for the Study of Complementary and Alternative Therapies (CSCAT)
www.nursing.virginia.edu/centers/altther.html

University of Washington Medicinal Herb Garden
www.nnlm.nlm.nih.gov/pnr/uwmhg/index.html

WebMD Self-Care Advisor
www.mywebmd.com

WholeHealthMD
www.wholehealthmd.com

Appendix 2–5 Alternative Therapies for Anxiety

Therapy	*Best Evidence**	*Probably Useful* †	*Least Evidence*‡
Herbals	Valerian (150–300 mg t.i.d.; 1–3 ml of tincture t.i.d.); kava-kava (45–70 mg kavalactones t.i.d.); Saint John's Wort (300 mg t.i.d.).	Chamomile; hops; oats (oat straw); passion flower; peppermint; skullcap.	Aromatherapy.
Diet and Nutrition/Lifestyle	High potency multivitamin; exercise; eliminate caffeine, alcohol, tobacco, sugar.	Flaxseed oil (1 T/day); magnesium; (200–300 mg t.i.d.); niacinamide (500 mg q.i.d.); phosphatidyl choline (4g t.i.d.).	
Mind-Body Interventions	Biofeedback; cognitive-behavioral therapy; deep breathing; group therapy; hypnotherapy; meditation; relaxation response; spiritual healing.	Dance; music; qi gong; tai chi; yoga.	
Bioelectromagnetic Therapies	Craniostimulation; energy healing.		Electrosleep.
Alternative Systems of Care	Acupuncture; ayurveda.	*Homeopathic:* gelsemium 30C t.i.d.–q.i.d.; argentum nitricum 6C t.i.d.–q.i.d.; ignatia amara 6C t.i.d.–q.i.d.	
Hands-On Healing Techniques	Massage.	Chiropractic.	Craniosacral therapy.

* Therapies with the highest degree of scientific support for efficacy and safety.
† Therapies that are often helpful but that do not have the highest degree of supporting evidence for efficacy and safety.
‡ Therapies that may be useful but that have limited scientific evidence for efficacy and safety.
NOTE: C denotes the number of times that a substance is diluted at a ratio of 1:100.
SOURCE: Sierpina, VS: Integrative Health Care: Complementary and Alternative Therapies for the Whole Person, FA Davis, Philadelphia, 2000.

Appendix 2–6 Alternative Therapies for Arthritis

Therapy	*Best Evidence**	*Probably Useful†*	*Least Evidence‡*
Herbals	Boswellia (150–400 mg t.i.d.); capsaicin (topically); ginger concentrate (500 mg t.i.d.).	White willow (60–120 mg/day salicin; 1–2 ml t.i.d. tincture).	Aromatherapy; devil's claw; horsetail; sea cucumber; yucca.
Diet and Nutrition/Lifestyle	Weight loss; exercise; vitamin C (500–1000 mg t.i.d.); vitamin E (400–800 IU/day).	Vitamin B_3 (niacinamide): (1–3 g/day), check liver enzymes; boron 6 mg/day; omega-3 fatty acids (fish oil) 3 g/day.	Eliminate solanine from diet (found in nightshade plants: tomatoes, white potatoes, peppers [except black pepper], eggplant, tobacco); copper bracelet or supplement; D-phenylalanine; pantothenic acid; zinc.
Mind-Body Interventions	Cognitive-behavioral therapy.	Biofeedback; qi gong; relaxation; social support; tai chi; yoga.	Guided imagery; meditation; music.
Pharmacological and Biological Treatments	Glucosamine sulfate (500 mg t.i.d. or as single dose); S-adenosyl-L-methionine (SAMe) (400 mg t.i.d.).	Chondroitin sulfate (400 mg t.i.d.).	DMSO; chelation therapy; shark and bovine cartilage.
Bioelectromagnetic Therapies		Static magnet therapy; pulsed electromagnetic fields; TENS.	
Alternative Systems of Care	Acupuncture; acupressure; ayurveda; traditional Chinese medicine.		Homeopathy: *Gout:* nux vomica 6C; belladonna 6C; calcarea 6C; colchicum 6C. *Osteoarthritis:* Rhus toxicodendron 6C t.i.d. for 2 weeks; ledum 6C q.i.d. for 2 weeks; *belladonna* 6C qd for 2 weeks; *Apis millifica* 6C t.i.d. for 2 weeks. *Rheumatoid arthritis:* Rhus toxicodendron 6C for 2 weeks; bryonia 6C q.i.d. for 2 weeks; ruta graveolens 6C q.i.d. for 2 weeks; pulsatilla 30C t.i.d. for 2 weeks; arnica ointments and gels.
Hands-On Healing Techniques	Physical therapy.	Massage; chiropractic; osteopathy.	Craniosacral therapy; rolfing.

* Therapies with the highest degree of scientific support for efficacy and safety.
† Therapies that are often helpful but that do not have the highest degree of supporting evidence for efficacy and safety.
‡ Therapies that may be useful but that have limited scientific evidence for efficacy and safety.
NOTE: C denotes the number of times that a substance is diluted at a ratio of 1:100.
SOURCE: Sierpina, VS: Integrative Health Care: Complementary and Alternative Therapies for the Whole Person, FA Davis, Philadelphia, 2000.

Appendix 2–7 Alternative Therapies for Asthma

Therapy	*Best Evidence**	*Probably Useful†*	*Least Evidence‡*
Herbals	Atropa belladona; capsaicin; ephedra sinensis (12.5–25 mg t.i.d.); quercetin (400 mg ac t.i.d.); glycyrrhiza glabra (1–2 g t.i.d. powdered root; 2–4 ml t.i.d. extract; 250–500 mg dry powdered extract t.i.d.); grape seed extract (50–100 mg t.i.d.); guaiac wood (guafenisin 600 mg b.i.d.).	Ginkgo biloba (60 mg b.i.d.); tylophora asthmatica (200 mg b.i.d.).	Coleus forskohli (50 mg t.i.d.); lobelia inflata; coltsfoot (potentially toxic).
Diet and Nutrition/Lifestyle	Avoid sulfites, aspirin, tartrazine, biogenic amines; environmental control; vitamin C (10–30 mg/kg/day in divided doses).	Carotenes (25,000–50,000 IU/d); essential fatty acids (fish oils, omega-3 fatty acids); magnesium (200–400 mg t.i.d.); vitamin E (200–400 IU/d); zinc (15–30 mg/d); food allergy identification & avoidance (milk, egg, wheat); green tea (*Camellia sinensis*); onions, garlic; reduced sodium intake.	Treat hypochlorhydria; probiotics; selenium (200 μg/day); vitamin B_6 (if on theophylline: 25–50 mg b.i.d.); vitamin B_{12} (sulfite-sensitive children: 1000 μg/d or IM weekly).
Mind-Body Interventions		Biofeedback; hypnosis; yoga breathing techniques.	Treat depression; stress management.
Pharmacological and Biological Treatments			Anti-*Candida* diet; DHEA.
Bioelectromagnetic Therapies			Electrical stimulation.
Alternative Systems		Acupuncture; African herbs; ayurvedic herbals; Chinese herbals; homeopathy.	
Hands-On Healing Techniques	Massage.		Chiropractic; osteopathy

* Therapies with the highest degree of scientific support for efficacy and safety.
† Therapies that are often helpful but that do not have the highest degree of supporting evidence for efficacy and safety.
‡ Therapies that may be useful but that have limited scientific evidence for efficacy and safety.
SOURCE: Sierpina, VS: Integrative Health Care: Complementary and Alternative Therapies for the Whole Person, FA Davis, Philadelphia, 2000.

Appendix 2–8 Alternative Therapies for Cancer Prevention and Treatment

Therapy	*Best Evidence**	*Probably Useful†*	*Least Evidence‡*
Herbals		Mistletoe (bladder); yew (paclitaxol), (breast); hoxsey; astragalus membranaceus; polysaccharide krestin; chlorella; PC SPES; capsaicin.	Chaparral (toxic); Pau d'arco; essiac tea; evening primrose oil.
Diet and Nutrition/Lifestyle		Mushrooms: maitake, shiitake (colon), enokitake.	Whole grain barley; macrobiotic diet; Gerson diet; Hippocrates wheat grass diet; Livingston-Wheeler; Kelley-Gonzales nutritional programs; vitamins A, C, E (controversial).
Mind-Body Interventions		Getting rid of anger, negative emotions; support groups (breast); group therapy (melanoma); stress management; treatment of depression, feelings of helplessness, hopelessness; encouraging a fighting spirit; imagery, biofeedback, hypnosis, meditation; yoga, qi gong; spiritual approaches, prayer, faith healing.	Intuitive, psychic approaches.
Pharmacological and Biological Treatments			Antineoplastins (brain); shark cartilage; bovine tracheal cartilage; hydrazine (cachexia, lung); ozone therapy, hydrogen peroxide; Livingston therapy; immunoaugmentive therapies; melatonin.
Bioelectromagnetic Therapies			Nordenstrom electrical stimulation; therapeutic touch.

Alternative Systems of Care		Acupuncture, acupressure, moxibustion for relief of pain, nausea, side effects of cancer treatment.	Chinese herbal remedies; ayurveda; *Homeopathy:* gelsemium 6C (anxiety) 2–3×; ipecac 30C (nausea) 3–4× q 15–30 min; nux vomica (nausea/vomiting) 6C t.i.d.–q.i.d. for 1–2 days; cadmium; sulfuricum 30C (vomiting, exhaustion) t.i.d. for 1–2 days.
Hands-On Healing Techniques		Massage and gentle manipulation for pain control, immunostimulation, relaxation.	Laying on of hands.

* Therapies with the highest degree of scientific support for efficacy and safety.
† Therapies that are often helpful but that do not have the highest degree of supporting evidence for efficacy and safety.
‡ Therapies that may be useful but that have limited scientific evidence for efficacy and safety.

NOTE: C denotes the number of times that a substance is diluted at a ratio of 1:100.
SOURCE: Sierpina, VS: Integrative Health Care: Complementary and Alternative Therapies for the Whole Person, FA Davis, Philadelphia, 2000.

Appendix 2–9 Alternative Therapies for Congestive Heart Failure

Therapy	*Best Evidence**	*Probably Useful*†	*Least Evidence*‡
Herbals	Hawthorn (80–300 mg b.i.d., tincture 4–5 ml t.i.d.).		Cinnamon (2–3 mg/day, tincture 2–3 ml t.i.d.).
Diet and Nutrition/Lifestyle	Coenzyme Q10 (30–100 mg t.i.d.); magnesium (300 mg/day); thiamine (20–100 mg/day).	Carnitine (500 mg b.i.d.–t.i.d.); taurine (3–6 g/day).	L-Arginine (1500 mg–12 g/day).
Mind-Body Interventions	Relaxation and stress management; screen and treatment for depression; guided imagery.	Cognitive-behavioral therapy; social support; anger/hostility management; meditation; tai chi; yoga.	

* Therapies with the highest degree of scientific support for efficacy and safety.
† Therapies that are often helpful but that do not have the highest degree of supporting evidence for efficacy and safety.
‡ Therapies that may be useful but that have limited scientific evidence for efficacy and safety.
SOURCE: Sierpina, VS: Integrative Health Care: Complementary and Alternative Therapies for the Whole Person, FA Davis, Philadelphia, 2000.

Appendix 2–10 Alternative Therapies for Coronary Artery Disease

Therapy	*Best Evidence**	*Probably Useful†*	*Least Evidence‡*
Herbals		Ginkgo biloba (40 mg t.i.d.); garlic (900 mg/day or 1 clove); curcumin (400 mg t.i.d.); green tea (3–5C/day).	Khella (250–300 mg/day); eutherococcus (Siberian ginseng) (2–3 g/day); gugulipid (25 mg/t.i.d.)—lipid-lowering agent.
Diet and Nutrition/Lifestyle	Exercise; eliminate tobacco, caffeine, alcohol; low-fat diet/dietary antioxidants; ornish program; vegeterian diets; vitamin C (1 g/day); vitamin E (400–800 IU/day); vitamin B_6(50–100 mg/day); vitamin B_{12} (800 μg/day); folic acid (800 μg/day).	Resveratrol (red wine) and other bioflavonoids; consumption of nuts; selenium (100–200 μg/day); pantethine (300 mg t.i.d.).	Evening primrose oil (3–6 g/day).
Mind-Body Interventions	Relaxation and stress management; screen and treat for depression; guided imagery.	Cognitive-behavioral therapy; social support; anger/hostility management; meditation; tai chi; yoga.	
Pharmacological and Biological Treatments			Chelation therapy.
Alternative Systems of Care		Acupuncture; traditional Chinese medicine; ayurveda	

*Therapies with the highest degree of scientific support for efficacy and safety.
†Therapies that are often helpful but that do not have the highest degree of supporting evidence for efficacy and safety.
‡Therapies that may be useful but that have limited scientific evidence for efficacy and safety.
NOTE: C denotes the number of times that substance is diluted at a ratio of 1:100.
SOURCE: Sierpina, VS: Integrative Health Care: Complementary and Alternative Therapies for the Whole Person, FA Davis, Philadelphia, 2000.

Appendix 2–11 Alternative Therapies for Depression

Therapy	*Best Evidence**	*Probably Useful †*	*Least Evidence‡*
Herbals	Saint John's Wort (300 mg t.i.d., 0.3% hypericin).	Ginkgo biloba (80mg t.i.d.) in elderly.	Saint John's Wort and 5-HTP in combination; damiana; yohimbe; aromatherapy
Diet and Nutrition/Lifestyle	Exercise; relaxation, stress reduction; thiamine (1–10 mg/d); niacin (500–1000 mg b.i.d.); pyridoxine (50–100 mg/d); folic acid (800 μg/d); vitamin B_{12} (800 μg/d); vitamin C (500-1000 mg t.i.d.).	S-adenosyl-L-methionine (SAMe) (200mg b.i.d.–400 mg q.i.d.). *Avoid in bipolar disorder.* 5-HT (hydroxytryptophan) (100–200 mg t.i.d.); flaxseed oil (1T/day); iron replacement; vitamin E (200–400 IU/day).	Inositol; phenylalanine; phosphatidylserine; tyrosine; detect and treat food allergy; restrict caffeine and sugar.
Mind-Body Interventions	Cognitive-behavioral therapy; spiritual approaches, prayer.	Tai chi; qi gong; hypnosis; meditation; biofeedback.	
Pharmacological and Biological Treatments			DHEA; neural therapy
Bioelectromagnetic Therapies	Light therapy (for seasonal affective disorder).	Magnetic brain stimulation; energy healing.	
Alternative Systems of Care	Acupuncture.	Ayurveda.	Homeopathy (not commonly used except for postpartum depression): *Each t.i.d. for 2 weeks:* sepia 30C; ignatia 30C; pulsatilla 30C; natrum muriatricum 30C.
Hands-On Healing Techniques	Massage.	Craniosacral therapy.	

* Therapies with the highest degree of scientific support for efficacy and safety.
† Therapies that are often helpful but that do not have the highest degree of supporting evidence for efficacy and safety.
‡ Therapies that may be useful but that have limited scientific evidence for efficacy and safety.
NOTE: C denotes the number of times that a substance is diluted at a ratio of 1:100.
SOURCE: Sierpina, VS: Integrative Health Care: Complementary and Alternative Therapies for the Whole Person, FA Davis, Philadelphia, 2000.

Appendix 2–12 Alternative Therapies for Diabetes

Therapy	*Best Evidence**	*Probably Useful†*	*Least Evidence‡*
Herbals		*Atremsia herba alba;* bilberry (*Vaccinium myrtillus*) (retinopathy): 80–160 mg t.i.d.; bitter melon (*Momordica charantia*): 30–60 ml of juice/day; coccinia indica; gymnema sylvestre: 200 mg b.i.d.; ginkgo biloba (retinopathy, neuropathy, and vascular complications): 40 mg t.i.d.; garlic; green tea (*Camellia sinensis*) 2C/day; *Trigonella foenum-graecum*.	Artichoke; dandelion leaves; eleutherococcus; fenugreek (*Trigonella foenum-graecum*): 50 g/day defatted seed powder; ginseng 100 mg t.i.d.; glucomannan; guar gum; horehound; juniper; lavender; myrrh; neem; primrose oil (neuropathy); salt bush (*Atriplex halimu*); silymarin (cirrhosis in diabetes); Spanish needles (*Bidens pilosa*); tragacanth; yellow bells (*Tecoma stans*).
Diet and Nutrition/Lifestyle	Regular exercise; weight loss; diet high in fiber, low in simple sugars and fats; Pritikin diet; Ornish diet.	Alpha-lipoic acid; biotin (type 1 and type 2 DM): 9–16 mg/day; chromium (200 μg/day); essential fatty acids (cold-water fish, 480 mg/day; gamma linoleic acid, 1 T/day flaxseed oil); magnesium (300–500 mg/day); onion; potassium (dietary); vitamin C (2 g/day in divided dosess); vitamin B_3 (prevention of new-onset type 1: 25 mg/kg/day); inositol hexaniacinate (hyperlipidemia): 500–1000 mg/day; vitamin B_6 (neuropathy): 50–100 mg/day; vitamin B_{12} (neuropathy): 1000–3000 μg /day p.o. or 1000 μg/wk IM; vitamin E (800–900 IU/day); zinc (30 mg/day).	Flavonoids (dietary, 1–2/day); manganese (30 mg/day).

Alternative Therapies for Diabetes (Continued)

Therapy	*Best Evidence**	*Probably Useful†*	*Least Evidence‡*
Mind-Body Interventions	Self-care, personal locus of control and responsibility.	Biofeedback; reduction of threat of DM (adolescents); relaxation therapy; social support; spiritual approaches; yoga.	Treatment of depression; qi gong.
Bioelectromagnetic Therapies		Therapeutic touch.	Electrical stimulation.
Alternative Systems of Care		Acupuncture (neuropathy); traditional Chinese medicine.	Ayurveda; curanderismo herbalism.
Hands-On Healing Techniques			Massage.

* Therapies with the highest degree of scientific support for efficacy and safety.
† Therapies that are often helpful but that do not have the highest degree of supporting evidence for efficacy and safety.
‡ Therapies that may be useful but that have limited scientific evidence for efficacy and safety.
SOURCE: Sierpina, VS: Integrative Health Care: Complementary and Alternative Therapies for the Whole Person, FA Davis, Philadelphia, 2000.

Appendix 2–13 Alternative Therapies for Gastroesophageal Reflux Disease

Therapy	*Best Evidence**	*Probably Useful†*	*Least Evidence‡*
Herbals	Deglycyrrhizinated licorice (DGL), 380-760 mg t.i.d./ac.	Caraway; lemon balm; raspberry tea; white wine (increases gastric emptying).	Oregon grape, yellow dock, wormwood.
Diet and Nutrition/Lifestyle	Lactase (for those with lactose intolerance); lipase (pancreatic insufficiency); weight loss; small meals; don't lie down for 2 hr after a meal; elevate head of bed 6 in; avoid foods that promote reflux, like alcohol, tobacco, caffeine, onions, spicy foods, peppermint.		Proteolytic enzymes; vitamin A up to 25,000 IU/day; vitamin C 500 mg t.i.d.; vitamin E 100 IU t.i.d.; zinc 20 mg/day.
Alternative Systems of Care		Acupuncture; ayurveda.	*Homeopathy:* bryonia 6C q 30 min for 2 hr; carbo vegetabilis 6C q 30 min for 2 hr; lycopodium 6C q 30 min for 2 hr; nux vomica 6C q 30 min for 2 hr.
Hands-on Healing Techniques		Osteopathic manipulation.	

* Therapies with the highest degree of scientific support for efficacy and safety.
† Therapies that are often helpful but that do not have the highest degree of supporting evidence for efficacy and safety.
‡ Therapies that may be useful but that have limited scientific evidence for efficacy and safety.

NOTE: C denotes the number of times that a substance is diluted at a ratio of 1:100.
SOURCE: Sierpina, VS: Integrative Health Care: Complementary and Alternative Therapies for the Whole Person, FA Davis, Philadelphia, 2000.

Appendix 2–14 Alternative Therapies for Gastrointestinal Problems

Therapy	*Best Evidence**	*Probably Useful†*	*Least Evidence‡*
Herbals	Aloe (constipation), 30 ml t.i.d.; cascara (constipation), tea from 1 tsp. bark b.i.d., 1 ml tincture b.i.d.; deglycyrrhizinated licorice (DGL) (peptic ulcer disease [PUD]), 380–760 mg t.i.d./ac; peppermint (indigestion), 0.2 ml–0.4 ml enteric coated oil b.i.d.–t.i.d./ac; senna (constipation).	Aloe (heartburn), 30 ml t.i.d.; bilberry (diarrhea); boldo (cholagogue, indigestion); caraway; chamomile (antispasmodic, colic, PUD) 2–3 g/day, 3–5 ml tincture t.i.d., as tea t.i.d.–q.i.d.; ginger (nausea), 500 mg t.i.d.; goldenseal (diarrhea) 500 mg t.i.d., use with caution; fennel (colic, antispasmodic), tea 1 cup t.i.d.; 600-mg caps t.i.d., for infants, 2 tsp seeds t.i.d.; garlic (antispasmodic), up to 3 g b.i.d.; lemon balm; marijuana (nausea); raspberry tea; sage (antispasmodic); white wine (increases gastric emptying).	Bitters (indigestion): barberry, dandelion; Oregon grape, yellow dock, wormwood; butcher's broom (hemorrhoids); horse chestnut (hemorrhoids).
Diet and Nutrition/Lifestyle	Lactase (for those with lactose intolerance); lipase (pancreatic insufficiency).	Bismuth (PUD), 240 mg subcitrate b.i.d./ac, subsalicylate 500 mg q.i.d./ac; cabbage (PUD), 1 L juice daily, effects possibly due to glutamine content; charcoal (excess gas); lactobacillus acidophilus (diarrhea, antibiotic-induced diarrhea).	Betaine HCl (low stomach acidity); flavonoids (PUD), 500 mg t.i.d.; proteolytic enzymes; yogurt (antibiotic-induced diarrhea); vitamin A up to 25,000 IU/day; vitamin C 500 mg t.i.d.; vitamin E 100 IU t.i.d.; zinc 30 mg/day.
Mind-Body Interventions	Depression (functional bowel complaints), detect and treat; exercise (constipation); psychotherapy; stress management (PUD).		

Alternative Systems of Care	Acupuncture (nausea); acupressure (nausea); ayurveda.	Homeopathy: *Colic:* cuprum metallicum 6C t.i.d.–q.i.d.; chamomile 6C t.i.d. for 3–4 days; colocynthis 30C t.i.d.; nux vomica 6C q 15 min until vomiting ceases; belladonna 6C q 1 hr for up to 6 doses; bryonia 6C q 1 hr for up to 6 doses. *Constipation:* nux vomica 6C t.i.d. for 10 days; sepia 30C: 3 doses in 24 hr once a month; sulfur 6C t.i.d. up to 10 days. *Diarrhea:* arsenicum album 6C q 30 min for up to 6 doses, then t.i.d.; argentum nitricum 6C q 1 hr up to 6 doses; podophyllum 30C t.i.d.–q.i.d. for 2 days; pulsatilla 6C q 2 hr for up to 6 doses; sulfur 6C q 1 hr up to 6 doses, then t.i.d. *Hemorrhoids:* hamamelis 6C t.i.d. for 3 days; calcarea fluorica 6C t.i.d.–q.i.d. for 3–4 days; arnica 30C q.i.d. for 2–3 days; aesculus; hippocastanum 30C t.i.d. for 3 days. *Heartburn, indigestion, and gas:* nux vomica 6C q 30 min for 2 hr; carbo vegetabilis 6C q 30 min for 2 hr; lycopodium 6C 2–3 times after meals; natrum phosphoricum 6C q 30 min for 2 hr; arsenicum album 6C q 1 hr up to 6 doses, then t.i.d.

* Therapies with the highest degree of scientific support for efficacy and safety.
† Therapies that are often helpful but that do not have the highest degree of supporting evidence for efficacy and safety.
‡ Therapies that may be useful but that have limited scientific evidence for efficacy and safety.

NOTE: C denotes the number of times that a substance is diluted at a ratio of 1:100.
SOURCE: Sierpina, VS: Integrative Health Care: Complementary and Alternative Therapies for the Whole Person, FA Davis, Philadelphia, 2000.

Appendix 2–15 Alternative Therapies for Migraine Headache

Therapy	*Best Evidence**	*Probably Useful†*	*Least Evidence‡*
Herbals	Feverfew 0.25-0.5 mg, parthenolide b.i.d.	Ginger 4–6 g/day, 1.5–3 ml tincture t.i.d., 500 mg q.i.d. dried ginger, also treats nausea; ginkgo biloba 40–60 mg t.i.d.	Capsaicin intranasal; yucca.
Diet and Nutrition/Lifestyle	Vitamin B_2 (riboflavin) 400 mg/day for at least 3–4 months.	Magnesium 250–400 mg t.i.d., especially for premenstrual migraine and those with low Mg levels; calcium 800 mg/day; vitamin D 400 IU/day; avoid dietary amines, which provoke migraine: chocolate, cheese, beer, red wine; food allergy: detect and eliminate most common allergenic foods: dairy, wheat, chocolate, eggs; use elimination diet; vitamin B_{12} 25 mg t.i.d.	Fish oil, EPA/DHA; S-adenosyl-L-methionine (SAMe) 400 mg q.i.d., gradually increase dose from 200 mg b.i.d. to 400 mg q.i.d. over 3 weeks; 5-hydroxytryptophan (5-HTP) 100–200 mg t.i.d.
Mind-Body Interventions	Relaxation therapy; biofeedback.	Guided imagery; meditation; stress management; tai chi; therapeutic touch; yoga.	
Bioelectromagnetic			Energy healing; magnets; TENS.
Alternative Systems of Care		Acupuncture; traditional Chinese medicine; ayurveda.	Homeopathy: belladonna 6C q 30 min for 1.5; hrs; bryonia 6C q 30 min for 1.5; hrs; gelsemium 30C q 30 min for 1.5; hrs; kali bichromicum 6C q 1 hr up to 6 doses, then t.i.d.
Hands-On Healing Techniques			Chiropractic.

* Therapies with the highest degree of scientific support for efficacy and safety.
† Therapies that are often helpful but that do not have the highest degree of supporting evidence for efficacy and safety.
‡ Therapies that may be useful but that have limited scientific evidence for efficacy and safety.
NOTE: C denotes the number of times that a substance is diluted at a ratio of 1:100.
SOURCE: Sierpina, VS: Integrative Health Care: Complementary and Alternative Therapies for the Whole Person, FA Davis, Philadelphia, 2000.

Appendix 2–16 Alternative Therapies for Tension Headache

Therapy	*Best Evidence**	*Probably Useful†*	*Least Evidence‡*
Diet and Nutrition/Lifestyle		Magnesium 250 mg b.i.d.–t.i.d.	
Mind-Body Interventions	Relaxation therapy; biofeedback; cognitive therapy.	Guided imagery; meditation; progressive muscle relaxation; stress management; tai chi; therapeutic touch; yoga.	
Bioelectromagnetic Therapies			Energy healing; magnets; TENS.
Alternative Systems of Care		Acupuncture; traditional Chinese medicine; ayurveda.	Homeopathy: belladonna 6C q 30 min for $1\frac{1}{2}$ hrs; bryonia 6C q 30 min for $1\frac{1}{2}$ hrs; gelsemium 30C q 30 min for $1\frac{1}{2}$ hrs; kali bichromicum 6C q 1 hr up to 6 doses, then t.i.d.
Hands on Healing			Chiropractic.

*Therapies with the highest degree of scientific support for efficacy and safety.
†Therapies that are often helpful but that do not have the highest degree of supporting evidence for efficacy and safety.
‡Therapies that may be useful but that have limited scientific evidence for efficacy and safety.
NOTE: C denotes the number of times that a substance is diluted at a ratio of 1:100.
SOURCE: Sierpina, VS: Integrative Health Care: Complementary and Alternative Therapies for the Whole Person, FA Davis, Philadelphia, 2000.

Appendix 2–17 Alternative Therapies for Hepatitis

Therapy	*Best Evidence**	*Probably Useful†*	*Least Evidence‡*
Herbals	Milk thistle (hepatitis, cirrhosis), 70–140 mg t.i.d.	Artichoke; *Astragalus membranaceus* caraway; glycyrrhizin, licorice root <100 mg/day, 1 g root t.i.d., higher doses affect electrolytes, BP; goldenseal 500 mg t.i.d., use with caution; lemon balm; raspberry tea; turmeric, 250–500 mg b.i.d.	Oregon grape, yellow dock, wormwood; evening primrose oil (alcoholic liver disease); Sho-Saiko-to (TJ-9); Compound 861; *Phyllanthus amafus*.
Diet and Nutrition/Lifestyle			Proteolytic enzymes; vitamin A up to 25,000 IU/day; vitamin C 500 mg t.i.d.; vitamin E 100 IU t.i.d.; zinc 20 mg/day.
Mind-Body Interventions	Psychotherapy.		
Alternative Systems of Care		Ayurveda.	

* Therapies with the highest degree of scientific support for efficacy and safety.
† Therapies that are often helpful but that do not have the highest degree of supporting evidence for efficacy and safety.
‡ Therapies that may be useful but that have limited scientific evidence for efficacy and safety.
SOURCE: Sierpina, VS: Integrative Health Care: Complementary and Alternative Therapies for the Whole Person, FA Davis, Philadelphia, 2000.

Appendix 2–18 Alternative Therapies for Hypercholesterolemia

Therapy	*Best Evidence**	*Probably Useful†*	*Least Evidence‡*
Herbals	Garlic 1–4 cloves/day, tabs 300 mg t.i.d. (4000–5000 μg of allicin), tincture 2–4 ml t.i.d.; Guggul 500 mg tab t.i.d. (5–10% guggelsterones or total of 25 mg t.i.d.); psyllium 5–10 g/day; Chinese red yeast rice (cholestin) (*Monascus purpureus*), two 600-mg capsules b.i.d..	Artichoke 320 mg of std extract t.i.d.; avocado; barley; evening primrose oil; flax seeds 20 g/day, 1 T flaxseed oil daily; glucomannan; pectin; plantain.	Fenugreek 5–20 g with meals t.i.d. or 15–90 g once daily with a meal; fo-ti 3–5 g/day as tea t.i.d., 500-mg tabs, up to 5 tabs t.i.d.; ginseng; proanthocyanidins (grape seed extract, pine bark); wild yam 2–3 ml tincture t.i.d., 1–2 tabs t.i.d.; yogurt.
Diet and Nutrition/Lifestyle	Exercise; 5–7 servings/day fruits and vegetables (source of bioflavonoids and beta carotene); fiber; Mediterranean diet; quit smoking; soy protein 30 g/day; vegetarian diet; very low-fat diet (Ornish); vitamin B_3 (niacin) up to 3 g/day (potential hepatoxicity); weight loss.	Calcium 800–1000 mg/day; coenzyme Q10 100–200 mg/day; fish intake (EPA/DHA omega-3 oils); inositol hexaniacinate 500–1000 mg t.i.d.; olive and canola oil; Pritikin program; reduce intake of refined sugars; reduce caffeine intake; red wine or other form of alcohol 1–2 drinks/day; selenium 200 mg/day; vitamin B_5 (pantothenic acid) 300 mg b.i.d.–t.i.d. esp. for diabetics, hypertriglyceridemia; vitamin C 100–1000 mg/day; vitamin E 100–800 IU/day.	Beta-sitosterol; brewer's yeast 2 T/day carnitine 1–4 g/day; chitosan 3–6 g/day; chromium 200 mg/day; green tea 3C/day; lecithin; magnesium 400 mg/day; mushrooms: shiitake, maitake; oats; octacosanol; vitamins B_6 (pyridoxine) 50 mg/day; B_9 (folic acid) 400 mg/day; B_{12} (cyanocobalamin) 1000 mg/day (may lower homocysteine levels, alone or together); quercetin >35 mg/day (apples, onion, black tea); safflower oil.
Mind-Body Interventions		Modifying type A behavior, stress reduction, reducing hostility, time urgency, competitiveness; reducing chronic arousal; improving sleep pattern; relaxation therapy.	Meditation; qi gong.
Pharmacological and Biological Treatments			Chelation therapy.
Alternative Systems of Care		Ayurveda; traditional Chinese medicine.	

*Therapies with the highest degree of scientific support for efficacy and safety.
†Therapies that are often helpful but that do not have the highest degree of supporting evidence for efficacy and safety.
‡Therapies that may be useful but that have limited scientific evidence for efficacy and safety.

NOTE: C denotes the number of times that a substance is diluted at a ratio of 1:100.
SOURCE: Sierpina, VS: Integrative Health Care: Complementary and Alternative Therapies for the Whole Person, FA Davis, Philadelphia, 2000.

Appendix 2–19 Alternative Therapies for Hypertension

Therapy	*Best Evidence**	*Probably Useful*†	*Least Evidence*‡
Herbals		Garlic; hawthorn.	Ginseng, 1 g dried root/day; guar gum, 5 g t.i.d.; yellow root; yucca.
Diet and Nutrition/Lifestyle	DASH diet; fiber; aerobic exercise; potassium in diet; quit smoking; reduce caffeine; low sodium; weight loss.	Vegetarian diet; CoQ10, 50 mg b.i.d.; alcohol intake <3 drinks/day; calcium, 800–1500 mg/day; magnesium, 350–500 mg/day (esp. if taking diuretics); fish oil, EPA/DHA, omega-3 fatty acids >3 g/day.	Check for heavy metals such as lead; reduce sugar intake; vitamin C; chitosan; arginine, 2 g t.i.d.
Mind-Body Interventions		Anger prevention or management; anxiety reduction (men); guided imagery; meditation; music therapy; religious attendance; social support; stress management; tai chi; yoga.	
Pharmacological and Biological Treatments			Chelation therapy.
Alternative Systems of Care		Ayurveda; traditional Chinese medicine.	Homeopathy.

* Therapies with the highest degree of scientific support for efficacy and safety.
† Therapies that are often helpful but that do not have the highest degree of supporting evidence for efficacy and safety.
‡ Therapies that may be useful but that have limited scientific evidence for efficacy and safety.
SOURCE: Sierpina, VS: Integrative Health Care: Complementary and Alternative Therapies for the Whole Person, FA Davis, Philadelphia, 2000.

Appendix 2–20 Alternative Therapies for Irritable Bowel Syndrome

Therapy	Best Evidence*	Probably Useful†	Least Evidence‡
Herbals	Peppermint, 0.2 ml–0.4 ml enteric-coated oil b.i.d.–t.i.d./ac	Caraway; chamomile, 2–3 g/day; 3–5 ml tincture t.i.d., as tea t.i.d.–q.i.d.; fennel (colic antispasmodic), tea 1 cup t.i.d., 600 mg caps t.i.d., for infants 2 tsp seeds t.i.d.; garlic (antispasmodic), up to 3 g b.i.d.; lemon balm; raspberry tea; sage (antispasmodic).	Oregon grape, yellow, dock, wormwood.
Diet and Nutrition/Lifestyle	Lactase (for those with lactose intolerance); lipase (pancreatic insufficiency); fiber; food allergy: identify and eliminate if present; dairy and grain most common factors.	Charcoal (excess gas); lactobacillus acidophilus; refined sugar: reduce amount in diet.	Proteolytic enzymes; vitamin A up to 25,000 IU/day; vitamin C 500 mg t.i.d.; vitamin E 100 IU t.i.d.; zinc 20 mg/day.
Mind-Body Interventions	Cognitive behavioral therapy; depression (functional bowel complaints), detect and treat; exercise; hypnotherapy; biofeedback; progressive muscle relaxation; psychotherapy; stress management.		
Alternative Systems of Care		Traditional Chinese medicine herbals; acupuncture; ayurveda.	Homeopathy: (follow label dosages) argentum nitricum; asa foetida; colocynthis; lillium tigrinum; lycopodium; natrum carbonicum; nux vomica; podophyllum; sulfur.

* Therapies with the highest degree of scientific support for efficacy and safety.
† Therapies that are often helpful but that do not have the highest degree of supporting evidence for efficacy and safety.
‡ Therapies that may be useful but that have limited scientific evidence for efficacy and safety.
SOURCE: Sierpina, VS: Integrative Health Care: Complementary and Alternative Therapies for the Whole Person, FA Davis, Philadelphia, 2000.

Appendix 2–21 Alternative Therapies for Musculoskeletal Problems

Therapy	*Best Evidence**	*Probably Useful†*	*Least Evidence‡*
Herbals	Arnica ointment/gel (topical); tiger balm; white willow (salicylate).	*Topical agents for wound and tissue healing, pain:* aescin (horse chestnut); aloe gel; angelica; calendula; comfrey; echinacea; Saint. John's wort oil; tea tree; witch hazel; wintergreen oil; curcumin (anti-inflammatory)	*Tissue and wound healing:* cat's claw; gotu kola; aromatherapy: lavender, camphor, eucalyptus, chamomile, rosemary. *Athletic performance enhancement:* Asian ginseng, eleuthero; guarana.
Diet and Nutrition/Lifestyle	Stretching, conditioning, warm-up to prevent injuries; bioflavonoids: citrus 900–1800 mg/day (improves healing time of injuries); enzymes: bromelain 500 MCU q.i.d. (proteolytic, anti-inflammatory).	Calcium 800–1000 mg/day (bone, muscle injury); magnesium 300 mg t.i.d. (muscle spasm, injury); vitamin C 400–3000 mg/day (connective tissue support, muscle damage); vitamin E 400–1200 IU/day (muscle damage), topically for scars; eliminate food allergy (may worsen inflammation).	*Tissue / Wound Healing:* vitamin A; copper, manganese, silicon, zinc; chondroitin sulfate; glucosamine sulfate; arginine, glutamine, L-carnitine. *Bursitis:* vitamin B_{12} 1000 μg q.d. for 2–4 wk IM or subcutaneously. *Fibromyalgia:* vitamin B_1 10–100 mg/day; magnesium 300–600 mg/day; vitamin E 100–300 IU/day; D, L-phenylalanine 500–700 mg t.i.d. (for pain). *Enhancing athletic performance:* antioxidants, B complex vitamins, chromium, zinc, iron, magnesium, branched-chain amino acids, carnitine, pyruvate whey protein, leucine, inosine, ornithine, ornithinine alpha-ketoglutarate, glutamine, creatine, gamma oryzanol, medium-chain triglycerides.

Mind-Body Interventions	Regular exercise, stretching; tai chi; yoga.	Biofeedback; guided imagery; hypnosis; music therapy; qi gong; relaxation therapy; spiritual interventions.	
Pharmacological and Biological Treatments			Hydrotherapy (add essential oils, Epsom salts); spa therapy; DMSO topically.
Bioelectromagnetic Therapies	TENS unit.	Energy medicine; healing touch; reiki; therapeutic touch.	Hyperbaric oxygen; light therapy; magnet therapy.
Alternative Systems of Care		Acupuncture; acupressure; traditional Chinese medicine: cupping; ayurveda: massage, oil, herbal techniques.	Homeopathy: *Broken bone support:* arnica 30C q 15–30 min for 2 hr, then t.i.d. for 2 days; ruta graveolens 6C t.i.d. for 2–3 days. *Sprains and injuries:* arnica 30C t.i.d.–q.i.d. for 2–3 days; Ruta graveolens 6C t.i.d. for 2–3 days; Ledum 30C t.i.d. for 2-3 days. *Bursitis:* Rhus toxicodendron 6C t.i.d.–q.i.d. for 3–4 days; Ruta graveolens 6C t.i.d. for 3–4 days; belladonna 6C t.i.d.–q.i.d. for 1–2 days.
Hands-On Healing Techniques		Craniosacral; feldenkrais; rolfing; trager.	Chiropractic; massage; osteopathy.

* Therapies with the highest degree of scientific support for efficacy and safety.
† Therapies that are often helpful but that do not have the highest degree of supporting evidence for efficacy and safety.
‡ Therapies that may be useful but that have limited scientific evidence for efficacy and safety.
NOTE: C denotes the number of times that a substance is diluted at a ratio of 1:100.
SOURCE: Sierpina, VS: Integrative Health Care: Complementary and Alternative Therapies for the Whole Person, FA Davis, Philadelphia, 2000.

APPENDIX 3

Normal Reference Laboratory Values

BLOOD, PLASMA, OR SERUM VALUES

Determination	Reference Range: Conventional	Reference Range: SI	Minimal ml Required*	Note
Acetoacetate plus acetone	Negative		1-B	
Aldolase	1.3–8.2 U/L	22–137 nmol · sec^{-1}/L	2-S	Use unhemolyzed serum
Ammonia	12–55 μmol/L	12–55 μmol/L	2-B	Collect in heparinized tube; deliver *immediately* packed in ice
Amylase	4–25 units/ml	4–25 arb. unit	1-S	
Ascorbic acid	0.4–1.5 mg/100 ml	23–85 μmol/L	7-B	Collect in heparinized tube before any food is given
Bilirubin	Direct: up to 0.4 mg/100 ml Total: up to 1.0 mg/100 ml	Up to 7 μmol/L Up to 17 μmol/L	1-S	
Blood volume	8.5–9.0% of body weight in kg	80–85 ml/kg		
Calcium	8.5–10.5 mg/100 ml (slightly higher in children)	2.1–2.6 mmol/L	1-S	
Carbamazepine	4.0–12.0 μg/ml	17–51 μmol/L		
Carbon dioxide content	24–30 mEq/L	24–30 mmol/L	1-S	Fill tube to top
Carbon monoxide	Less than 5% of total hemoglobin		3-B	Fill tube to top
Carotenoids	0.8–4.0 μg/ml	1.5–7.4 μmol/L	3-S	Vitamin A may be done on same specimen
Ceruloplasmin	27–37 mg/100 ml	1.8–2.5 μmol/L	2-S	
Chloramphenicol	10–20 μg/ml	31–62 μmol/L	0.2-S	
Chloride	100–106 mEq/L	100–106 mmol/L	1-S	
CK isoenzymes	5% MB or less		0.2-S	
Copper	Total: 100–200 μg/100 ml	16–31 μmol/L	1-S	
Creatine kinase (CK)	Female: 10–79 U/L Male: 17–148 U/L	167–1317 nmol · sec^{-1}/L 283–2467 nmol · sec^{-1}/L	1-S	
Creatinine	0.6–1.5 mg/100 ml	53–133 μmol/L	1-S	
Ethanol	0 mg/100 ml	0 mmol/L	2-B	Collect in oxalate and refrigerate

Glucose	Fasting: 70–110 mg/100 ml	3.9–5.6 mmol/L	1-P	Collect with oxalate-fluoride mixture
Iron	50–150 μg/100 ml (higher in males)	9.0–26.9 μmol/L	1-S	
Iron-binding capacity	250–410 μg/100 ml	44.8–73.4 μmol/L	1-S	
Lactic acid	0.6–1.8 mEq/L	0.6–1.8 mmol/L	2-B	Collect with oxalate-fluoride mixture; deliver immediately packed in ice
Lactic dehydrogenase	45–90 U/L	750–1500 nmol · sec^{-1}/L	1-S	Unsuitable if hemolyzed
Lead	50 μg/100 ml or less	Up to 2.4 μmol/L	2-B	Collect with oxalate-fluoride mixture
Lipase	2 units/ml or less	Up to 2 arb. unit	1-S	
Lipids				
Cholesterol	<200 mg/dl	<5.18 mmol/L	1-S	Fasting
Triglycerides	40–150 mg/100 ml	0.4–1.5 g/L	1-S	Fasting
Lipoprotein electrophoresis (LEP)			2-S	Fasting, do not freeze serum
Lithium	0.6–1.2 mEq/L	0.6–1.2 nmol/L	1–S	
Magnesium	1.5–2.0 mEq/L	0.8–1.3 mmol/L	1-S	
5′ Nucleotidase	1–11 U/L	17–183 nmol · sec^{-1}/L	1-S	
Osmolality	280–296 mOsm/kg water	280–296 mmol/kg	1-S	
Oxygen saturation (arterial)	96–100%	0.96–1.00	3-B	Deliver in sealed heparinized syringe packed in ice
PCO_2	35–45 mm Hg	4.7–6.0 kPa	2-B	Collect and deliver in sealed heparinized syringe
pH	7.35–7.45	Same	2-B	Collect without stasis in sealed heparinized syringe; deliver packed in ice
PO_2	75–100 mm Hg (dependent on age) while breathing room air Above 500 mm Hg while on 100% O_2	10.0–13.3 kPa	2-B	
Phenobarbital	15–50 μg/ml	65–215 μmol/L	1-S	
Phenytoin (Dilantin)	10–20 μg/ml	20–80 μmol/L	1-S	

BLOOD, PLASMA, OR SERUM VALUES (Continued)

Determination	Reference Range: Conventional	Reference Range: SI	Minimal ml Required*	Note
Phosphatase (acid)	Male–Total: 0.13–0.63 sigma U/ml Female–Total: 0.01–0.56 sigma U/ml Prostatic: 0–0.05 Fishman-Lerner U/100 ml	36–175 nmol · sec^{-1}/L 2.8–156 nmol · sec^{-1}/L	1-S	Must always be drawn just before analysis or stored as frozen serum; avoid hemolysis
Phosphatase (alkaline)	13–39 U/L, infants and adolescents up to 104 U/L	217–650 nmol · sec^{-1}/L, up to 1.26 μmol/L	1-S	
Phosphorus (inorganic)	3.0–4.5 mg/100 ml (infants in first year up to 6.0 mg/100 ml)	1.0–1.5 mmol/L	1-S	
Potassium	3.5–5.0 mEq/L	3.5–5.0 mmol/L	1-S	Serum must be separated promptly from cells
Primidone (Mysoline)	4–12 μg/ml	18–55 μmol/L	1-S	
Procainamide	4–10 μg/ml	17–42 μmol/L	1-S	
Protein: Total	6.0–8.4 g/100 ml	60–84 g/L	1-S	
Albumin	3.5–5.0 g/100 ml	35–50 g/L	1-S	
Globulin	2.3–3.5 g/100 ml	23–35 g/L		Globulin equals total protein minus albumin
Electrophoresis	(% of total protein)		1-S	Quantitation by densitometry
Albumin	52–68			
Globulin:				
$Alpha_1$	4.2–7.2			
$Alpha_2$	6.8–12			
Beta	9.3–15			
Gamma	13–23			
Pyruvic acid	0–0.11 mEq/L	0–0.11 mmol/L	2-B	Collect with oxalate fluoride. Deliver immediately packed in ice
Quinidine	1.2–4.0 μg/ml	3.7–12.3 μmol/L	1-S	

Salicylate:	0		2-P	
Therapeutic	20–25 mg/100 ml; 25–30 mg/100 ml to age 10 yr 3 hr post dose	1.4–1.8 mmol/L 1.8–2.2 mmol/L		
Sodium	135–145 mEq/L	135–145 mmol/L	1-S	
Sulfonamide	5–15 mg/100 ml		2-P	
Transaminase, aspartate aminotransferase	7–27 U/L	117–450 nmol · sec^{-1}/L	1-S	
Transaminase, alanine aminotransferase	1–21 U/L	17–350 nmol · sec^{-1}/L	1-S	
Urea nitrogen (BUN)	8–25 mg/100 ml	2.9–8.9 mmol/L	1-S	
Uric acid	3.0–7.0 mg/100 ml	0.18–0.42 mmol/L	1-S	
Vitamin A	0.15–0.6 μg/ml	0.5–2.1 μmol/L	3-S	

URINE VALUES

Determination	Reference Range: Conventional	Reference Range: SI	Minimal ml Required*	Note
Acetone plus acetoacetate (quantitative)	0	0 mg/L	2 ml	
Amylase	24–76 units/ml	24–76 arb. unit		
Calcium	300 mg/day or less	7.5 mmol/day or less	24-hr specimen	Collect in special bottle with 10 ml of concentrated HCl
Catecholamines	Epinephrine: under 20 μg/day	<109 nmol/day	24-hr specimen	Should be collected with 10 ml of concentrated HCl (pH should be between 2.0 and 3.0)
	Norepinephrine: under 100 μg/day	<590 nmol/day		
Chorionic gonadotropin	0	0 arb. unit	1st morning void	
Copper	0–100 μg/day	0–1.6 μmol/day	24-hr specimen	

URINE VALUES (Continued)

Determination	Reference Range: Conventional	Reference Range: SI	Minimal ml Required*	Note
Coproporphyrin	50–250 μg/day	80–380 nmol/day	24-hr specimen	Collect with 5 g of sodium carbonate
	Children under 80 lb (36 kg): 0–75 μg/day	0–115 nmol/day		
Creatine	Under 100 mg/day or less than 6% of creatinine. In pregnancy: up to 12%. In children under 1 yr: may equal creatinine. In older children: up to 30% of creatinine.	<0.75 mmol/day	24-hr specimen	Also order creatinine
Creatinine	15–25 mg/kg of body weight/day	0.13–0.22 mmol · kg^{-1}/day	24-hr specimen	
Cystine or cysteine	0	0	10 ml	Qualitative
Hemoglobin and myoglobin	0		Freshly voided sample	Chemical examination with benzidine
5–Hydroxyindoleacetic acid	2–9 mg/day (women lower than men)	10–45 μmol/day	24-hr specimen	Collect with 10 ml of concentrated HCl
Lead	0.08μg/ml or 120 μg/day or less	0.39μmol/L or less	24-hr specimen	
Phosphorus (inorganic)	Varies with intake; average, 1 g/day	32 mmol/day	24-hr specimen	Collect with 10 ml of concentrated HCl
Porphobilinogen	0	0	10 ml	Use freshly voided urine
Protein:				
Quantitative	<150 mg/24 hr	<0.15 g/day	24-hr specimen	

Determination	Conventional	SI	Minimal ml Required*	Note
Steroids:				
17–Ketosteroids (per day)	Age / Male / Female 10 / 1–4 mg / 1–4 mg 20 / 6–21 / 4–16 30 / 8–26 / 4–14 50 / 5–18 / 3–9 70 / 2–10 / 1–7	3–14 μmol / 3–14 μmol 21–73 / 14–56 28–90 / 14–49 17–62 / 10–31 7–35 / 3–24	24-hr specimen	Not valid if patient is receiving meprobamate
17–Hydroxysteroids	3–8 mg/day (women lower than men)	8–22 μmol/day as tetrahydrocortisol	24-hr specimen	Keep cold; chlorpromazine and related drugs interfere with assay
Sugar:				
Quantitative glucose	0	0 mmol/L	24-hr or other timed specimen	
Urobilinogen	Up to 1.0 Ehrlich U	To 1.0 arb. unit	2-hr sample (1–3 P.M.)	
Uroporphyrin	0–30 μg/day	<36 nmol/day	Coproporphyrin	
Vanillylmandelic acid (VMA)	Up to 9 mg/24 hr	Up to 45 μmol/day	24-hr specimen	Collect as for catecholamines

SPECIAL ENDOCRINE TESTS

Steroid Hormones

Determination	Reference Range: Conventional	Reference Range: SI	Minimal ml Required*	Note
Aldosterone	Excretion: 5–19 μg/24 hr	14–53 nmol/day	5/day	Keep specimen cold
	Supine: 48±29 pg/ml	133±80 pmol/L	3-S, P	Fasting, at rest, 210-mEq sodium diet
	Upright (2 hr): 65± 23 pg/ml	180±64 pmol/L		Upright, 2 hr, 210-mEq sodium diet

SPECIAL ENDOCRINE TESTS (Continued)

Steroid Hormones

Determination	Reference Range: Conventional	Reference Range: SI	Minimal ml Required*	Note
	Supine: 107±45 pg/ml	279±125 pmol/L		Fasting, at rest, 110-mEq sodium diet
	Upright (2 hr): 239±123 pg/ml	663±341 pmol/L		Upright, 2 hr, 110-mEq sodium diet
	Supine: 175±75 pg/ml	485±208 pmol/L		Fasting, at rest, 10-mEq sodium diet
	Upright (2 hr): 532±228 pg/ml	1476±632 pmol/L		Upright, 2 hr, 10–mEq sodium diet
Cortisol	8 A.M.: 5–25 μg/100 ml	0.14–0.69 μmol/L	1-P	Fasting
	8 P.M.: Below 10 μg/100 ml	0–0.28 μmol/L	1-P	At rest
	4-hr ACTH test: 30–45 μg/100 ml	0.83–1.24 μmol/L	1-P	20 U ACTH, IV per 4 hr
	Overnight suppression test: Below 5 μg/100 ml	0.14 nmol/L	1-P	8 a.m. sample after 0.5 mg dexamethasone by mouth at midnight
	Excretion: 20–70 μg/24 hr	55–193 nmol/day	2/day	Keep specimen cold
Dehydroepiandrosterone (DHEA)	Male: 0.5–5.5 ng/ml	1.7–19 nmol/L	2-S, P	
	Female			
	1.4–8.0 ng/ml	4.9–28 nmol/L		Adult
	0.3–4.5 ng/ml	1.0–15.6 nmol/L		Postmenopausal

Dehydroepiandrosterone sulfate (DHEA–S)	Male		2-S, P	
	151–446 µg/100 ml	3.9–11.4 µgmol/L		
	Female			
	84–433 µg/100 ml	2.2–11.1 µmol/L		Adult
	1.7–177 µg/100 ml	0.04–4.5 µmol/L		Postmenopausal
11–Deoxycortisol	Responsive		1-P	8 a.m. sample, preceded by 4.5 g of metyrapone by mouth per 24 hr or by single dose of 2.5 g by mouth at midnight
	Over 7.5 µg/100 ml	>0.22 µmol/L		
Estradiol	Male: <50 pg/ml	<184 pmol/L	5-S, P	
	Female: 23–361 pg/ml	84–1325 pmol/L		Adult
	<30 pg/ml	<110 pmol/L		Postmenopausal
	<20 pg/ml	<73 pmol/L		Prepubertal
Progesterone	Male: <1.0 ng/ml	<3.2 nmol/L	5-S, P	
	Female			
	0.2–0.6 ng/ml	0.6–1.9 nmol/L		Follicular phase
	0.3–3.5 ng/ml	0.95–11 nmol/L		Midcycle peak
	6.5–32.2 ng/ml	21–102 nmol/L		Postovulatory
Testosterone	Adult male:		1-P	a.m. sample
	300–1100 ng/100 ml	10.4–38.1 nmol/L		
	Adolescent male:			
	Over 100 ng/100 ml	>3.5 nmol/L		
	Female			
	25–90 ng/100 ml	0.87–3.12 nmol/L		
Unbound testosterone	Adult male:		2-P	a.m. sample
	3.06–24.0 ng/100 ml	106–832 pmol/L		
	Adult female:			
	0.09–1.28 ng/100 ml	3.1–44.4 pmol/L		

Polypeptide Hormones

Determination	Reference Range: Conventional	Reference Range: SI	Minimal ml Required*	Note
Adrenocorticotropin (ACTH)	15–70 pg/ml	3.3–15.4 pmol/L	5-P	Place specimen on ice and send promptly to laboratory. Use EDTA tube only.
Alpha subunit	<0.5–2.5 ng/ml	<0.4–2.0 nmol/L	2-S	Adult male or female
	<0.5–5.0 ng/ml	<0.4–4.0 nmol/L		Postmenopausal female
Calcitonin	Male: 0–14 pg/ml	0–4.1 pmol/L	5-S	Test done only on known or suspected cases of medullary carcinoma of the thyroid
	Female: 0–28 pg/ml	0–8.2 pmol/L		
	>100 pg/ml in medullary carcinoma	>29.3 pmol/L		
Follicle-stimulating hormone (FSH)	Male 3–18 mU/ml	3–18 arb. unit	5-S, P	Same sample may be used for LH
	Female: 4.6–22.4 mU/ml	4.6–22.4 arb. unit		Pre- or postovulatory
	13–41 mU/ml	13–41 arb. unit		Midcycle peak
	30–170 mU/ml	30–170 arb. unit		Postmenopausal
Growth hormone	Below 5 ng/ml	<233 pmol/L	1-S	Fasting, at rest
	Children: Over 10 ng/ml	>465 pmol/L		After exercise
	Male: Below 5 ng/ml	<233 pmol/L		
	Female: Up to 30 ng/ml	0–1395 pmol/L		
	Male: Below 5 ng/ml	<233 pmol/L		After glucose load
	Female: Below 5 ng/ml	<233 pmol/L		
Insulin	6–26 μU/ml	43–187 pmol/L	1-S	Fasting
	Below 20 μU/ml	<144 pmol/L		During hypoglycemia
	Up to 150 μU/ml	0–1078 pmol/L		After glucose load
Luteinizing hormone (LH)	Male: 3–18 mU/ml	3–18 arb. unit	5-S, P	Same sample may be used for FSH
	Female:			
	2.4–34.5 mU/ml	2.4–34.5 arb. unit		Pre- or postovulatory
	43–187 mU/ml	43–187 arb. unit		Midcycle peak
	30–150 mU/ml	30–150 arb. unit		Postmenopausal
Parathyroid hormone	<25 pg/ml	<2.94 pmol/L	5-P	Keep blood on ice, or plasma frozen, if it is to be sent any distance; a.m. sample

Prolactin	2–15 ng/ml	0.08–6.0 nmol/L	2-S	
Renin activity	Supine:		4-P	EDTA tubes, on ice, normal diet
	1.1±0.8 ng/ml/hr	0.9±0.6 nmol/L/hr		
	Upright:			
	1.9±1.7 ng/ml/hr	1.5±1.3 nmol/L/hr		
	Supine:			Low-sodium diet
	2.7±1.8 ng/ml/hr	2.1±1.4 nmol/L/hr		
	Upright:			
	6.6±2.5 ng/ml/hr	5.1±1.9 nmol/L/hr		Low-sodium diet
	Diuretics:			
	10.0±3.7 ng/ml/hr	7.7±2.9 nmol/L/hr		
Somatomedin C (Sm–C, IGF–1)	0.08–2.8 U/ml	0.08–2.8 arb. unit	2-P	EDTA plasma prepubertal
	0.9–5.9 U/ml	0.9–5.9 arb. unit		During puberty
	0.34–1.9 U/ml	0.34–1.9 arb. unit		Adult males
	0.45–2.2 U/ml	0.45–2.2 arb. unit		Adult females

Thyroid Hormones

Determination	Reference Range: Conventional	Reference Range: SI	Minimal ml Required*	Note
Thyroid-stimulating hormone (TSH)	0.5–5.0 μU/ml	0.5–5.0 arb. unit	2-S	
Thyroxine-binding globulin capacity	15–25 μg T_4/100 ml	193–322 nmol/L	2-S	
Total triiodothyronine (T_3)	75–195 ng/100 ml	1.16–3.00 nmol/L	2-S	
Reverse triiodothyronine (rT_3)	13–53 ng/ml	0.2–0.8 nmol/L	2-S	
Total thyroxine by RIA (T_4)	4–12 μg/100 ml	52–154 nmol/L	1-S	
T_3 resin uptake	25–35%	0.25–0.35	2-S	
Free thyroxine index (FT_4I)	1–4		2-S	

VITAMIN D DERIVATIVES

Determination	Reference Range: Conventional	Reference Range: SI	Minimal ml Required*	Note
1,25-Dihydroxy–vitamin D	26–65 pg/ml	62–155 pmol/L	1-S	
25-Hydroxy–vitamin D	8–55 ng/ml	19.4–137 nmol/L	1-S	

HEMATOLOGIC VALUES

Determination	Reference Range: Conventional	Reference Range: SI	Minimal ml Required*	Note
Coagulation factors				
Factor I (fibrinogen)	0.15–0.35 g/100 ml	4.0–10.0 μmol/L	4.5-P	Collect in Vacutainer containing sodium citrate
Factor II (prothrombin)	60–140%	0.60–1.40	4.5-P	Collect in plastic tubes with 3.8% sodium citrate
Factor V (accelerator globulin)	60–140%	0.60–1.40	4.5-P	Collect as in factor II
Factor VII–X (proconvertin-Stuart)	70–130%	0.70–1.30	4.5-P	Collect as in factor II
Factor X (Stuart factor)	70–130%	0.70–1.30	4.5-P	Collect as in factor II
Factor VIII (antihemophilic globulin)	50–200%	0.50–2.0	4.5-P	Collect as in factor II
Factor IX (plasma thromboplastic cofactor)	60–140%	0.60–1.40	4.5-P	Collect as in factor II
Factor XI (plasma thromboplastic antecedent)	60–140%	0.60–1.40	4.5-P	Collect as in factor II
Factor XII (Hageman factor)	60–140%	0.60–1.40	4.5-P	Collect as in factor II
Coagulation screening tests:				
Bleeding time (Simplate)	3–9.5 min	180–570 sec		
Prothrombin time	Less than 2-sec deviation from control	Less than 2-sec deviation from control	4.5-P	Collect in Vacutainer containing 3.8% sodium citrate
Partial thromboplastin time (activated)	25–38 sec	25–38 sec	4.5-P	Collect in Vacutainer containing 3.8% sodium citrate
Whole-blood clot lysis	No clot lysis in 24 hr	0/day	2.0-whole blood	Collect in sterile tube and incubate at 37°C

Test	Conventional	SI units	Volume/specimen	Notes
Fibrinolytic studies:				
Euglobin lysis	No lysis in 2 hr	0/2 hr	4.5-P	Collect as in factor II
Fibrinogen split products	Negative reaction at >1:4 dilution	0 (at 1:4 dilution)	4.5-S	Collect in special tube containing thrombin and epsilon aminocaproic acid
Thrombin time	Control ±5 sec	Control ± 5 sec	4.5-P	Collect as in factor II
"Complete" blood count:				
Hematocrit	Male: 45–52% Female: 37–48%	Male: 0.45–0.52 Female: 0.37–0.48	1-B	Use EDTA as anticoagulant; the seven listed tests are performed automatically on the Ortho ELT 800, which directly determines cell counts, hemoglobin (as the cyanmethemoglobin derivative), and MCV and computes hematocrit, MCH, and MCHC
Hemoglobin	Male: 13–18 g/100 ml Female: 12–16 g/100 ml	Male: 8.1–11.2 mmol/L Female: 7.4–9.9 mmol/L		
Leukocyte count	4,300–10,800/mm^3	4.3–10.8 × 10^9/L		
Erythrocyte count	4.2–5.9 million/mm^3	4.2–5.9 × 10^{12}/L		
Mean corpuscular volume (MCV)	86–98 μm^3/cell	86–98 fl		
Mean corpuscular hemoglobin (MCH)	27–32 pg/RBC	1.7–2.0 pg/cell		
Mean corpuscular hemoglobin concentration (MCHC)	32–36%	0.32–0.36		
Erythrocyte sedimentation rate	Male: 1–13 mm/hr Female: 1–20 mm/hr	Male: 1–13 mm/hr Female: 1–20 mm/hr	5-B	Use EDTA as anticoagulant
Erythrocyte enzymes				
Glucose-6-phosphate dehydrogenase	5–15 U/g Hb	5–15 U/g	9-B	Use special anticoagulant (ACD solution)
Pyruvate kinase	13–17 U/g Hb	13–17 U/g	8-B	Use special anticoagulant (ACD solution)
Ferritin (serum)				
Iron deficiency	0–12 ng/ml 13–20 Borderline	0–4.8 nmol/L 5.2–8 nmol/L Borderline		
Iron excess	>400 ng/L	>160 nmol/L		
Folic acid				
Normal	>3.3 ng/ml	>7.3 nmol/L	1-S	
Borderline	2.5–3.2 ng/ml	5.75–7.39 nmol/L	1-S	
Haptoglobin	40–336 mg/100 ml	0.4–3.36 g/L	1-S	

HEMATOLOGIC VALUES (Continued)

Determination	Reference Range: *Conventional*	Reference Range: *SI*	*Minimal ml Required**	*Note*
Hemoglobin studies:				
Electrophoresis for abnormal hemoglobin			5-B	Collect with anticoagulant
Electrophoresis for:				
A_2 hemoglobin	3.0%	0.015–0.035	5-B	Use oxalate as anticoagulant
Borderline	0.3–3.5%	0.03–0.035		
Hemoglobin F (fetal hemoglobin)	Less than 2%	<0.02	5-B	Collect with anticoagulant
Hemoglobin, met- and sulf-	0	0	5-B	Use heparin as anticoagulant
Serum hemoglobin	2–3 mg/100 ml	1.2–1.9 μmol/L	2-S	
Thermolabile hemoglobin	0	0	1-B	Any anticoagulant
Lupus anticoagulant	0	0	4.5-P	Collect as in factor II
LE (lupus erythematosus) preparation:				
Method I	0	0	5-B	Use heparin as anticoagulant
Method II	0	0	5-B	Use defibrinated blood
Leukocyte alkaline phosphatase:			20-Isolated blood leukocytes	Special handling of blood necessary
Qualitative method	Males: 33–188 U Females (off contraceptive pill): 30–160 U	33–188 U 30–160 U	Smear-B	
Muramidase	Serum, 3–7 μg/ml Urine, 0–2 μg/ml	3–7 mg/L 0–2 μg/L	1-S 1-U	
Osmotic fragility of erythrocytes	Increased if hemolysis occurs in over 0.5% NaCl; decreased if hemolysis is incomplete in 0.3% NaCl		5-B	Use heparin as anticoagulant
Peroxide hemolysis	Less than 10%	0.10	6-B	Use EDTA as anticoagulant

Platelet count	150,000–350,000/mm^3	150–350 x 10^9/L	0.5-B	Use EDTA as anticoagulant; counts are performed on Clay Adams Ultraflow; when counts are low, results are confirmed by hand counting
Platelet function tests:				
Clot retraction	50–100%/2 hr	0.50–1.00/2 hr	4.5-P	Collect as in factor II
Platelet aggregation	Full response to ADP, epinephrine, and collagen	1.0	18-P	Collect as in factor II
Platelet factor 3	33–57 sec	33–57 sec	4.5-P	Collect as in factor II
Reticulocyte count	0.5–2.5% red cells	0.005–0.025	0.1-B	
Vitamin B_{12}	205–876 pg/ml	150–674 pmol/L	12-S	
Borderline	140–204 pg/ml	102.6–149 pmol/L		

CEREBROSPINAL FLUID VALUES

Determination	Reference Range		Minimal ml Required*	Note
	Conventional	*SI*		
Bilirubin	0	0	2	
Cell count	0–5 mononuclear cells		0.5	
Chloride	120–130 mEq/L	120–130 mmol/L	0.5	
Colloidal gold	0000000000–0001222111	Same	0.1	
Albumin	Mean: 29.5 mg/100 ml	0.295 g/L	2.5	
	±2 SD: 11–48 mg/100 ml	±2 SD: 0.11–0.48		
IgG	Mean: 4.3 mg/100 ml	0.043 g/L		
	±2 SD: 0–8.6 mg/100 ml	±2 SD: –0.086		
Glucose	50–75 mg/100 ml	2.8–4.2 mmol/L	0.5	
Pressure (initial)	70–180 mm of water	70–180 arb. unit		
Protein:				
Lumbar	15–45 mg/100 ml	0.15–0.45 g/L	1	
Cisternal	15–25 mg/100 ml	0.15–0.25 g/L	1	
Ventricular	5–15 mg/100 ml	0.05–0.15 g/L	1	

MISCELLANEOUS VALUES

Determination	Reference Range: Conventional	Reference Range: SI	Minimal ml Required*	Note
Carcinoembryonic antigen (CEA)	0–2.5 ng/ml	0–2.5 μg/L	20-P	Must be sent on ice
Chylous fluid				Use fresh specimen
Digitoxin	17±6 ng/ml	22±7.8 nmol/L	1-S	Medication with digitoxin or digitalis
Digoxin	1.2±0.4 ng/ml	1.54±0.5 nmol/L	1-S	Medication with digoxin 0.25 mg per day
	1.5±0.4 ng/ml	1.92±0.5 nmol/L	1-S	Medication with digoxin 0.5 mg per day
Duodenal drainage				pH should be in proper range with minimal amount of gastric juice
pH (urine)	5–7	5–7		
Gastric analysis	Basal:			
	Females: 2.0±1.8 mEq/hr	0.6±0.5 μmol/sec		
	Males: 3.0±2.0 mEq/hr	0.8±0.6 μmol/sec		
	Maximal (after histalog or gastrin)			
	Females: 16±5 mEq/hr	4.4±1.4 μmol/sec		
	Males: 23±5 mEq/hr	6.4±1.4 μmol/sec		
Gastrin-I	0–200 pg/ml	0–95 pmol/L	4-P	Heparinized sample
Immunologic tests:				
Alpha-fetoprotein	Undetectable in normal adults		2-S	
Alpha-1-antitrypsin	85–213 mg/100 ml	0.85–2.13 g/L	10-B	
Rheumatoid factor	<60 IU/ml		10 ml clotted blood	Fasting sample preferred
Antinuclear antibodies	Negative at a 1:8 dilution of serum		2-S	Send to laboratory promptly
Anti-DNA antibodies	Negative at a 1:10 dilution of serum		2-S	

Antibodies to Sm and RNP (ENA)	None detected		10 ml clotted blood	
Antibodies to SS-A (Ro) and SS-B (La)	None detected		10 ml clotted blood	
Autoantibodies to:				
Thyroid colloid and microsomal antigens	Negative at a 1:10 dilution of serum		2-S	Low titers in some elderly normal women
Gastric parietal cells	Negative at a 1:20 dilution of serum		2-S	
Smooth muscle	Negative at a 1:20 dilution of serum		2-S	
Mitochondria	Negative at a 1:20 dilution of serum		2-S	
Interstitial cells of the testes	Negative at a 1:10 dilution of serum		2-S	
Skeletal muscle	Negative at a 1:60 dilution of serum		2-S	
Adrenal gland	Negative at a 1:10 dilution of serum		2-S	
Bence Jones Protein	No Bence Jones protein detected in a 50-fold concentrate of urine		50-U	
Complement, total hemolytic	150–250 U/ml		10-B	Must be sent on ice
Cryoprecipitable proteins	None detected	0 arb. unit	10-S	Collect and transport at 37°C
C3	Range, 83–177 mg/100 ml	0.83–1.77 g/L	2-S	
C4	Range, 15–45 mg/100 ml	0.15–0.45 g/L	2-S	
Factor B	12–30 mg/100 ml		5 ml clotted blood	
C1 esterase inhibitor	13.2–24 mg/100 ml		5 ml of clotted blood	
Hemoglobin A_{1c}	3.8–6.4%	0.038–0.064	5-P	Send EDTA tube on ice promptly to laboratory
Hypersensitivity pneumonitis screen	No antibodies to those antigens assayed		5 ml clotted blood	
Immunoglobulins:				
IgG	639–1349 mg/100 ml	6.39–13.49 g/L	2-S	
IgA	70–312 mg/100 ml	0.7–3.12 g/L	2-S	

MISCELLANEOUS VALUES (Continued)

Determination	Reference Range: *Conventional*	Reference Range: *SI*	*Minimal ml Required**	*Note*
IgM	86–352 mg/100 ml	0.86–3.52 g/L	2-S	
Viscosity	1.4–1.8 relative viscosity units		10-B	Expressed as the relative viscosity of serum compared with water
Iontophoresis	Children: 0–40 mEq sodium/L Adults 0–60 mEq sodium/L	0–40 mmol/L 0–60 mmol/L		Value given in terms of sodium
Propranolol (includes bioactive 4-OH metabolite)	100–300 ng/ml	386–1158 nmol/L	1-S	Obtain blood sample 4 hr after last dose of beta-blocking agent
Stool fat	Less than 5 g in 24 hr or less than 4.0% of measured fat intake in 3-day period	<5 g/day	24-hr or 3-day specimen	
Stool nitrogen	Less than 2 g/day or 10% of urinary nitrogen	<2 g/day	24-hr or 3-day specimen	
Synovial fluid:				
Glucose	Not less than 20 mg/100 ml lower than simultaneously drawn blood sugar	Blood glucose	ml of fresh fluid	Collect with oxalate–fluoride mixture
D-Xylose absorption	5–8 g/5 hr in urine; 40 mg per 100 ml in blood 2 hr after ingestion of 25 g of D-Xylose	33–53 mmol/day 2.7 mmol/L	5-U 5-B	For directions see Benson et al.: N Engl J Med 256:335, 1957

* Abbreviations used: SI, Système International d'Unités; P, plasma; S, serum; B, blood; and U, urine.

SOURCE: Adapted from Scully, Robert E. (ed): Case Records of the Massachusetts General Hospital, New England Journal of Medicine, vol. 314, pp. 39–49, January 2, 1986, with permission.

APPENDIX 4

Prefixes, Suffixes, and Combining Forms

a-, an-. Without; away from; not.
ab-, abs-. From; away from; absent.
abdomin-, abdomino. Abdomen.
abs-. SEE: *ab-*.
acanth-, acantho-. Thorn; spine.
acous-, acoust-, acousto-. Hearing.
acro-. Extremity; top; extreme point.
actin-, actino-. Ray; some form of radiation.
ad-. Adherence; increase; toward.
-ad. Toward; in the direction of.
aden-, adeno-. Gland.
adip-, adipo-. Fat.
adren-, adreno-. Adrenal glands.
adrenal-, adrenalo-. Adrenal glands.
-aemia. Blood.
aer-, aero-. Air or gas.
-aesthesia, aesthesio-. SEE: *-esthesia*.
-agogue. An agent that promotes the expulsion of a specific substance.
-agra. Sudden severe pain.
-al. Relating to (e.g., abdominal, intestinal). In chemistry, an aldehyde.
-algesia, -algia. Suffering; pain.
algi-. Pain.
all-. SEE: *allo-*.
allo-, all-. Other.
amb-, ambi-. Both; on both sides; around; about.
amph-, amphi-, ampho-. Both; on both sides; on all sides; double; around; about.
an-. SEE: *a-*.
ana-, an-. Up; against; back.
andro-. Man; male; masculine.
angi-, angio-. Blood or lymph vessels.
aniso-. Unequal; asymmetrical; dissimilar.
ankyl-, ankylo-. Crooked; bent; fusion or growing together of parts.
ante-. Before.
antero-. Anterior; front; before.
anthropo-. Human beings; human life.
ant-, anti-. Against.
antr-, antro-. Antrum.
apo-. From; derived from; separated from; opposed.
arch-, arche-, archi-. First; principal; beginning; original.
arteri-, arterio-. Artery.
arthr-, arthro-. Joint.
-ase. Enzyme.
-asis, -esis, -iasis, -isis, -sis. Condition; pathological state.
astro-. Star; star-shaped.
atelo-. Imperfect; incomplete.
ather-, athero-. Fatty plaque.
atmo-. Steam; vapor.
atreto-. Absence of an opening.
aut-, auto-. Self.
axio-. Axis; the long axis of a tooth.
axo-. Axis; axon.
bacteri-, bacterio-. Bacteria; bacterium.
balan-, balano-. Glans clitoridis; glans penis.
bar-, baro-. Weight; pressure.
basi-, basio-. Base; foundation.
bi-, bis-. Two; double; twice.
bili-. Bile
bio-. Life.
bis-. SEE: *bi-*.
blast-, -blast. Germ; bud; embryonic state of development.
blenn-, blenno-. Mucus.
blephar-, blepharo-. Eyelid.
brachio-. Arm.
brachy-. Short.
brady-. Slow.
brom-, bromo-. Bromine.
bronch-, bronchi-, broncho-. Airway.
bronchiol-, bronchiolo-. Bronchiole.
cac-, caci-, caco-. Bad; ill.
carcin-, carcino-. Cancer.
cardi-, cardio-. Heart.
carpo-. Carpus.
cary-, caryo-. SEE: *kary-*.
cat-, cata-, cath-, kat-, kata-. Down; downward; destructive; against; according to.
cath-. SEE: *cat-*.
cel-, celo-. **1.** Tumor; hernia. **2.** Cavity.
-cele. Tumor; swelling; hernia.
cent-. Hundred.
cephal-, cephalo-. Head.
cervic-, cervico-. Neck; the neck of an organ.
cheil-, cheilo. SEE: *chil-*.
chil-, chilo-. Lip; lips.
chol-, chole-. Bile; gall.
cholangi-, cholangio-. Bile vessel.
cholecyst-, cholecysto-. Gallbladder.
choledoch-, choledocho-. Bile duct.
chondr-, chondro-. Cartilage.
chrom-, chromo-. Color.
-cide. Causing death.
cine-. Movement.
circum-. Around.
-cle, -cule. Little (e.g., molecule, corpuscle).
cleid-, cleido-. Clavicle.
co-, com-, con-. Together.
colp-, colpo-. SEE: *kolp-*.
contra-. Against; opposite.
crani-, cranio-. Skull; cranium.
cry-, cryo-. Cold.
cyan-, cyano-. Blue.
cycl-, cyclo-. Circular; cyclical; ciliary body of the eye.
cyst-, cysto-, -cyst. Cyst; urinary bladder.
cyt-, cyto-, -cyte. Cell.
dacry-. Tears.
dactyl-, dactylo. Finger; toe.
de-. From; down; not.

dec-, deca-. Ten.
deci-. One tenth.
demi-. Half.
dent-, denti-, dento-. Teeth.
derm-, derma-, dermato-, dermo-. Skin.
deuter-, deutero-, deuto-. Second; secondary.
dextro-. Right.
di-. Double; twice; two; apart from.
dia-. Through; between; asunder.
dipla-, diplo-. Double; twin.
dis-. Negative; double; twice; apart; absence of.
dors-, dorsi-, dorso-. Back.
duoden-, duodeno-. Duodenum.
-dynia. Pain.
dys-. Difficult; bad; painful.
ec-, ecto-. Out; on the outside.
-ectomy. Excision.
ectro-. Congenital absence of a part.
ef-, es-, ex-, exo-. Out.
electr-, electro-. Electricity.
-emesis. Vomiting.
-emia. Blood.
en-. In; into.
enantio-. Opposite.
end-, endo-. Within.
ent-, ento-. Within; inside.
enter-, entero-. Intestine.
ep-, epi-. Upon; over; at; in addition to; after.
erythr-, erythro-. Red.
-esis. SEE: *-asis.*
esophag-, esophago-. Esophagus.
-esthesia. Sensation.
etio-. Causation.
eu-. Well; good; healthy; normal.
eury-. Broad.
ex-. Out; away from; completely.
exo-. Out; outside of; without.
extra-. Outside of; in addition; beyond.
-facient. Causing; making happen.
-ferous. Producing.
ferri-, ferro-. Iron.
fibro-. Fibers; fibrous tissues.
fluo-. Flow.
fore-. Before; in front of.
-form. Form.
-fuge. To expel; to drive away; fleeing.
galact-, galacto-. Milk.
gam-, gamo-. Marriage; sexual union.
gaster-, gastero-, gastr-, gastro-. Stomach.
gen-. Producing; forming.
-gen, -gene, -genesis, -genetic, -genic. Producing; forming.
genito-. Organs of reproduction.
gero-. Old age.
giga-. Billion.
gingiv-, gingivo-. Gums (of the mouth).
gloss-, glosso-. Tongue.
gluc-, gluco-, glyc-, glyco-. Sugar; glycerol or similar substance.
gnath-, gnatho-. Jaw; cheek.
-gog, -gogue. To make flow.
gon-, gono-. Semen; seed; genitals; offspring.
-gram. A tracing; a mark.
-graph. Instrument used to make a drawing or record.
-graphy. Writing; record.
gyn-, gyne-, gyneco-, gyno-. Woman; female.
gyro-. Circle; spiral; ring.
hem-, hema-, hemato-, hemo-. Blood.
hemi-. Half.
hepat-, hepato-. Liver.
heredo-. Heredity.
heter-, hetero-. Other; different.
hex-, hexa-. Six.
histo-. Tissue.
hol-, holo-. Complete; entire; homogeneous.
homeo-. Likeness; resemblance; constant unchanging state.
homo-. Same; likeness.
hydra-, hydro-, hydr-. Water.
hyo-. Hyoid bone.
hyp-, hyph-, hypo-. Less than; below or under; beneath; deficient.
hyper-. Above; excessive; beyond.
hypno-. Sleep; hypnosis.
hyster-, hystero-. Uterus.
-ia. Condition, esp. an abnormal state.
-iasis. SEE: *asis.*
-iatric. Medicine; medical profession; physicians.
-ic. Pertaining to; relating to.
ichthyo-. Fish.
-id. Secondary skin eruption distant from primary infection site.
ideo-. Mental images.
idio-. Individual; distinct.
ileo-. Ileum.
ilio-. Ilium; flank.
im-. SEE: *in-*. Used before b,m, or p.
in-. In; inside; within; intensive action; negative.
infra-. Below; under; beneath; inferior to; after.
inter-. Between; in the midst.
intra-, intro-. Within; in; into.
ipsi-. Same; self.
irid-, irido-. Iris.
ischio-. Ischium.
-isis. SEE: *-asis.*
-ism. Condition; theory.
iso-. Equal.
-ite. 1. Of the nature of. **2.** In chemistry, a salt of an acid with the termination *-ous.*
-itis. Inflammation of.
-ize. To treat by special method.
jejuno-. Jejunum.
juxta-. Close proximity.
kary-, karyo-, cary-, caryo-. Nucleus; nut.
kat-, kata-. SEE: *cat-.*
kera-, kerato-. Horny substance; cornea.
kilo-. Thousand.
kinesi-, kino-, -kinesis. Movement
klepto-. To steal.
kolp-, kolpo-, colp-, colpo-. Vagina.

kypho-. Humped.
kysth-, kystho-. Vagina.
lact-. Milk.
laparo-. Flank; abdominal wall.
laryng-, laryngo-. Larynx.
latero-. Side.
leio-. Smooth.
lepido-. Flakes; scales.
lepto-. Thin; fine; slight; delicate.
leuk-, leuko-, leuc-. White; white corpuscle.
linguo-. Tongue.
lip-, lipo-. Fat.
-lite, -lith, lith-, litho-. Stone; calculus.
-logia, -logy. Science of; study of.
lumbo-. Loins.
lyo-. Loosen; dissolve.
-lysis. 1. Loosen; dissolve. **2.** In medicine, reduction of; relief from.
macr-, macro-. Large; long.
mal-. Ill; bad; poor.
mamm-, mammo-. Breast.
-mania. Frenzy; madness.
mast-, masto-. Breast.
med-, medi-, medio-. Middle.
mega-, megal-, megalo-. Large; of great size.
-megalia, -megaly. Enlargement of a body part.
meio-, mio-. Less; smaller.
melan-, melano-. Black.
mening-, meningo-. Meninges.
mes-, meso-. 1. Middle. **2.** In anatomy, the mesentery. **3.** In medicine, secondary; partial.
mesio-. Toward the middle.
meta-. 1. Change; transformation; next in a series. **2.** In chemistry, the 1,3 position of benzene derivatives.
metacarp-, metacarpo-. Metacarpus (bones of the hand).
-meter. Measure.
metr-, metra-, metro-. Uterus.
micr-, micro-. Small.
mio-. SEE: *meio-*.
mon-, mono-. Single; one.
muc-, muci-, muco-, myxa-, myxo-. Mucus.
multi-. Many; much.
musculo-, my-, myo-. Muscle.
my-, myo-. SEE: *musculo-*.
myc-, myco-. Fungus.
myel-, myelo-. Spinal cord; bone marrow.
myring-, myringo-. Tympanic membrane, eardrum.
myx-, myxo-. SEE: *muc-*.
nano-. 1. One billionth. **2.** Dwarfism (nanism).
narco-. Numbness; stupor.
naso-. Nose.
necr-, necro-. Death; necrosis.
neo-. New; recent.
nephr-, nephra-, nephro-. Kidney.
neur-, neuri-, neuro-. Nerve; nervous system.
nitr-, nitro-. Nitrogen.
non-. No.
normo-. Normal; usual.
noso-. Disease.
noto-. The back.
nucleo-. Nucleus.
nyct-, nycto-. Night; darkness.
ob-. Against.
occipit-, occipito-. Occiput.
octa-, octo-. Eight.
oculo-. Eye.
-ode, -oid. Form; shape; resemblance.
odont-, odonto-. Tooth; teeth.
-odynia, odyno-. Pain.
-oid. SEE: *-ode*.
oleo-. Oil.
olig-, oligo-. Few; small.
-ology. Science of; study of.
-oma. Tumor.
omo-. Shoulder.
omphal-, omphalo-. Navel.
onco-. Tumor; swelling; mass.
onych-, onycho-. Fingernails; toenails.
oo-, ovi-, ovo-. Egg; ovum.
oophor-, oophoro-, oophoron-. Ovary.
ophthalm-, ophthalmo-. Eye.
-opia. Vision.
opisth-, opistho-. Backward.
optico-, opto-. Eye; vision.
orchi-, orchid-, orchido-. Testicle.
oro-. Mouth.
orth-, ortho-. Straight; correct; normal; in proper order.
os-. Mouth; bone.
oscheo-. Scrotum.
-ose. 1. Carbohydrate. **2.** Primary alteration of a protein.
-osis. Condition; status, process; abnormal increase.
osmo-. 1. Odor; smell. **2.** Impulse. **3.** Osmosis.
oste-, osteo-. Bone.
-ostomosis, -ostomy, -stomosis, -stomy. A created mouth or outlet.
ot-, oto-. Ear.
-otomy. Cutting.
-ous. 1. Possessing; full of. **2.** Pertaining to.
ovi-, ovo-. SEE: *oo-*.
ox-. Oxygen.
oxy-. 1. Sharp; keen; acute; acid; pungent. **2.** Oxygen in a compound. **3.** Hydroxyl group.
pach-, pachy-. Thick.
-pagus. Twins joined at a specific site (e.g., craniopagus).
pali-, palin-. Recurrence; repetition.
pan-. All; entire.
pant-, panto-. All or the whole of something.
papulo-. Pimple; papule.
para-, -para. 1. Prefix: near; alongside of; departure from normal. **2.** Suffix: Bearing offspring.
path-, patho-, -path, -pathic, -pathy. Disease; suffering.
ped-, pedi-, pedo-. Foot.
pedia-. Child.
-penia. Decrease from normal; deficiency.
pent-, penta-. Five.

per-. Throughout; through; utterly; intense.
peri-. Around; about.
perineo-. Perineum.
peritoneo-. Peritoneum.
pero-. Deformed.
petro-. Stone; the petrous portion of the temporal bone.
-pexy. Fixation, usually surgical.
phaco-. Lens of the eye.
phag-, phago-. Eating; ingestion; devouring.
phalang-, phalango-. Phalanges (bones of fingers and toes).
phall-. Penis.
pharmaco-. Drug; medicine.
pharyng-, pharyngo-. Pharynx.
-phil, -philia, -philic. Love for; tendency toward; craving for.
phlebo-. Vein.
-phobia. Abnormal fear or aversion.
phono-. Sound; voice.
-phoresis. Transmission.
-phoria. In ophthalmology, a turning with reference to the visual axis.
photo-. Light.
phren-, phreno-, -phrenia. Mind; diaphragm.
-phylaxis. Protection.
physico-. Physical; natural.
physio-. Rel. to nature.
physo-. Air; gas.
phyt-, phyto-. Plant; something that grows.
pico-. One trillionth.
picr-, picro-. Bitter.
-piesis. Pressure.
pimel-, pimelo-. Fat.
plagio-. Slanting; oblique.
-plasia. Growth; cellular proliferation.
plasm-, -plasm. 1. Prefix: Living substance or tissue. **2.** Suffix: To mold.
-plastic. Molded; indicates restoration of lost or badly formed features.
platy-. Broad.
-plegia. Paralysis; stroke.
pleur-, pleuro-. Pleura; side; rib.
-ploid. Chromosome pairs of a specific number.
plur-, pluri-. Several; more.
pneo-. Breath; breathing.
pneum-, pneuma-, pneumato-. Air; gas; respiration.
pneumo-, pneumono-. Air; lung.
pod-, podo-. Foot.
-poiesis, -poietic. Production; formation.
polio-. Gray matter of the nervous system.
poly-. Much; many.
post-. After.
postero-. Posterior; behind; toward the back.
-praxis. 1. Act; activity. **2.** Practice; use.
pre-. Before; in front of.
presby-. Old age.
pro-. Before; in behalf of.
proct-, procto-. Anus; rectum.
proso-. Forward, anterior.
prostat-, prostato-. Prostate gland.
proto-. 1. First. **2.** In chemistry, the lowest of a series of compounds with the same elements.
pseud-, pseudo-. False.
psych-, psycho-. Mind; mental processes.
psychro-. Cold.
pubio-, pubo-. Pubic bone or region.
pulmo-. Lung.
py-, pyo-. Pus.
pycn-, pycno-, pykn-, pykno-. Dense; thick; compact; frequent.
pyelo-. Pelvis.
pyg-, pygo-. Buttocks.
pykn-, pykno-. SEE: *pycn-*.
pyle-. Orifice, esp. of the portal vein.
pyloro-. Gatekeeper; applied to the pylorus.
pyreto-. Fever.
pyro-. Heat; fire.
quadr-, quadri-. Four.
quinqu-. Five.
rachi-, rachio-. Spine.
radio-. 1. Radiant energy; a radioactive substance. **2.** In chemistry, a radioactive isotope.
re-. Back; again.
recto-. Straight; rectum.
ren-, reno-. Kidney.
reticulo-. Reticulum.
retro-. Backward; back; behind.
rhabdo-. Rod.
rheo-, -(r)rhea. Current; stream; to flow; to discharge.
rhino-. Nose.
rhizo-. Root.
rhodo-. Red.
roseo-. Rose-colored.
-(r)rhage, -(r)rhagia. Rupture; profuse fluid discharge.
-(r)rhaphy. A suturing or stitching.
-(r)rhexis. Rupture of a specific body part.
sacchar- saccharo-. Sugar.
sacro-. Sacrum.
salping-, salpingo-. Auditory tube; fallopian tube.
sapro-. Putrid; rotten.
sarco-. Flesh.
scapho-. Boat-shaped; scaphoid.
scapulo-. Shoulder.
scato-. Dung; fecal matter.
schisto-. Split; cleft.
schizo-. Division.
scirrho-. Hard; hard tumor or scirrhus.
sclero-. Hard; relating to the sclera.
-sclerosis. Dryness; hardness.
-scope. Instrument for viewing or examining (includes other methods of examination).
-scopy. Examination.
scoto-. Darkness.
sebo-. Fatty substance.
semi-. Half.
septi-. Seven.
sero-. Serum.
sesqui-. One and one half.
sial-, sialo-. Saliva.
sidero-. Iron; steel.

-sis. SEE: *-asis.*
sitio-, sito-. Bread; made from grain; food.
skeleto-. Skeleton.
skia-. Shadow.
sodio-. Sodium.
somat-, somato-. Body.
spectro-. Appearance; image; form; spectrum.
sperma-, spermat-, spermato-. Sperm; spermatozoa.
spheno-. Wedge; sphenoid bone.
sphygmo-. Pulse.
spleno-. Spleen.
spondyl-, spondylo-. Vertebra.
spongio-. Spongelike.
staphylo-. Uvula; bunch of grapes; *Staphylococcus.*
steato-. Fat.
steno-. Narrow; short.
sterco-. Feces.
stere-, stereo-. Three dimensions.
sterno-. Sternum.
stetho-. Chest.
stomato-. Mouth.
-stomosis, -stomy. SEE: *-ostomosis.*
strepto-. Twisted.
sub-. Under; beneath; in small quantity; less than normal.
super-. Above; beyond; superior.
supra-. Above; beyond; on top.
sym-. With; together with; along; beside.
syn-. Joined; together.
tachy-. Swift; rapid.
taen-, taeni-, ten-, teni-. Tapeworm.
tarso-. Flat of the foot; edge of the eyelid.
tauto-. Same.
techno-. Art; skill.
tel-, tele-. 1. End. **2.** Distant.
teleo-. Perfect; complete.
temporo-. Temples of the head.
ten-, teni-. SEE: *taen-.*
tendo-, teno-. Tendon.
ter-. Three.
tera-. One trillionth.
terato-. Severely malformed fetus.
tetra-. Four.
thalamo-. Chamber; part of the brain where a nerve originates; thalamus.
thanato-. Death.
theco-. Sheath; case; receptacle.
thermo-. Hot; heat.
thio-. Sulfur.
thorac-, thoraci-, thoraco-. Chest; chest wall.
thrombo-. Blood clot; thrombus.
thymo-. 1. Thymus. **2.** Soul; emotions.
thy-, thyro-. Thyroid gland; oblong; shield.
thyroid-, thyroido-. Thyroid gland.
toco-. Childbirth.
-tome. Cutting instrument.
tomo-. Section; layer.
-tomy. Cutting operation; excision.
top-, topo-. Place; locale.
tox-, toxi-, toxico-, toxo-, -toxic. Toxin; poison; toxic.
trachelo-. Neck.
tracheo-. Trachea; windpipe.
trans-. Across; over; beyond; through.
traumato-. Trauma.
tri-. Three.
trich-, trichi-, tricho-. Hair.
troph-, tropho-, -trophic. Nourishment.
-tropin. Stimulation of a target organ by a substance, esp. a hormone.
tubo-. Tube.
tympan-, tympano-. Eardrum; tympanum.
typhlo-. 1. Cecum. **2.** Blindness.
typho-. Fever; typhoid.
ulo-. Scar; scarring.
ultra-. Beyond; excess.
uni-. One.
uretero-. Ureter.
urethro-. Urethra.
-uria. Urine.
urin-, urino, uro-. Urine.
uter-, utero-. Uterus.
vagin-, vagino-. Vagina.
vaso-. Vessel (e.g., blood vessel).
veno-. Vein.
ventro-, ventr-, ventri-. Abdomen; anterior surface of the body.
vertebro-. Vertebra; vertebrae.
vesico-. Bladder; vesicle.
viscero-. Viscera.
vulvo-. Covering; vulva.
xanth-. Yellow.
xeno-. Strange; foreign.
xero-. Dry.
xiph-, xiphi-, xipho-. Xiphoid cartilage.
zoo-. Animal; animal life.

APPENDIX 5
Latin and Greek Nomenclature

Appendix 5–1 English with Latin and Greek Equivalents

acid. Acidum.
ague. Febris.
and. Et.
arm. Brachium. Gr., brachion.
artery. Arteria.
attachment. Adhesio.
back. Tergum; dorsum.
backbone. Spina.
backward. Retro.
bath. Balneum.
beef. Bubula.
belly. Venter; abdomen.
bend. Flexus.
bile. Bilis. Gr., chole.
bladder. Vesica.
bleed. Fluere.
blind. Caecus.
blister. Pustula vesicatorium.
bloat. Tumere.
blood. Sanguis. Gr., haima.
blood vessel. Vena.
body. Corpus. Gr., soma.
boiling up. Effervescens.
bone. Os. Gr., osteon.
bony. Osseus.
bowels. Intestina; viscera.
bowlegged. Valgus.
brain. Cerebrum. Gr., enkephalos.
breach. Ruptura.
breast. Mamma. Gr., mastos.
breath. Halitus.
bubble. Pustula.
bulb. Bulbus.
buttock. Clunis. Gr.,gloutos.
calcareous. Calci similis.
canal. Canalis.
cartilage. Cartilago. Gr., chondros.
catarrh. Coryza.
cavity. Caverna.
change. Mutatio.
chest. Thorax. Gr., thorax.
chin. Mentum. Gr., geneion.
choke. Strangulare.
clavicle. Clavicula.
congestion. Conglobatio.
consumption. Phthisis, pulmonaria.
convulsion. Convulsio.
cord. Corda.
corn. Callus-clavus.
cornea. Cornu. Gr., keras.
costive. Astrictus.
cough. Tussio.
countenance. Vultus.
cramp. Spasmus.
crisis. Dies crisimus.
cup. Poculum.
cure. Sanare.
curvature. Curvatura.
cuticle. Cuticula.
daily. Diurnus.
dandruff. Furfures capitis.
day. Dies.
dead. Mortuus; defunctus.
deadly. Lethalis.
deafness. Surditas.
decompose. Desolvere.
dental. Dentalis.
depression. Depressio.
digestive. Digestorius; pepticus.
dilute. Diluere.
discharge. Eluvies; effluens.
disease. Morbus.
dorsal. Dorsalis.
dose. Potio.
dram. Drachma.
drink. Bibere; potis.
dropsy. Hydrops; opis.
drug. Medicamentum.
duct. Ductus.
dysentery. Dysenteria.
ear. Auris. Gr., ous.
eat. Edere. Gr., phagos.
egg. Ovum.
elbow. Cubitum. Gr., ankon.
embryo. Partus immaturus.
emission. Emissio.
entrails. Viscera.
epidemic. Epidemus.
epilepsy. Morbus comitalis; epilepsia.
epileptic. Epilepticus.
erection. Erectio.
erotic. Amatorius.
eunuch. Eunuchus.
every. Omnis.
excrement. Excrementum.
excretion. Excrementum; excretio.
exhalation. Exhalatio.
exhale. Exhalare.
expel. Expellere.
expire. Expirare.
external. Externus.
extract. Extractum.
eye. Oculus. Gr., ophthalmos.
eyeball. Pupula.
eyebrow. Supercilium.
eyelid. Palpebra.
eyetooth. Dens caninus.
face. Facies.
faculty. Facultas.
faint. Collabi.
fat. Adeps. Gr., lipos.
feature. Lineomentum.
febrile. Febriculosus.
fecundity. Fecunditas.
feel. Tactus.
fever. Febris.
film. Membranula.
filter. Percolare.

finger. Digitus. Gr., daktylos.
fistula. Fistula putris.
fit. Accessus.
flesh. Carnis. Gr., sarx.
fluid. Fluidus.
food. Cibus.
foot. Pes, pedis. Gr., pous.
forearm. Brachium.
forehead. Frons.
freckle. Lentigo.
gall. Bilis.
gangrene. Gangraena.
gargle. Gargarizein.
gland. Glandula.
gleet. Ichor.
gout. Morbus articularis; (in feet) podagra.
grain. Granum.
gravel. Calculus.
grinder tooth. Dens maxillaris.
gullet. Gula.
gum. Gingiva.
gut. Intestinum.
hair. Capillus. Gr., thrix.
half. Dimidius.
hand. Manus. Gr., cheir.
harelip. Labrum fissum.
haunch. Clunis.
head. Caput. Gr., kephale.
heal. Sanare.
healer. Medicus.
healing. Salutaris.
health. Sanitas.
healthful. Salutaris; saluber.
healthy. Sanus.
hear. Audire.
hearing. Auditio; (sense of) auditus.
heart. Cor. Gr., kardia.
heartburn. Redundatio stomachi.
heat. Calor.
hectic. Hecticus.
heel. Calx, talus.
hirsute. Hirsutus.
homeopathic. Homeopathicus.
hysterics. Hysteria.
illness. Morbus.
incisor. Dens acutus.
infant. Infans; puerilis.
infect. Inficere.
infectious. Contagiosus.
infirm. Infirmus; debilis.
inflammation. Inflammatio; (of lungs) inflammatio pulmonaria.
injection. Injectio.
insane. Insanus.
intellect. Intellectus.
intercourse. Congressus.
internal. Intestinus.
intestine. Intestinum. Gr., enteron.
itch. Scabies.
itching. Pruritus.
jaw. Maxilla.
joint. Artus. Gr., arthron.
jugular vein. Vena jugularis.
kidney. Ren. Gr., nephros.
knee. Genu. Gr., gonu.
kneepan. Patella.
knuckle. Condylus.
labor. Partus.
labyrinth. Labyrinthus.
lacerate. Lacerare.
larynx. Guttur.
lateral. Lateralis.
leech. Sanguisuga.
leg. Tibia.
leprosy. Lepra.
ligament. Ligamentum. Gr., syndesmos.
ligature. Ligatura.
limb. Membrum.
lime. Calx.
listen. Auscultare.
liver. Jecur. Gr., hepar.
livid. Lividus.
loin. Lumbus. Gr., lapara.
looseness. Laxitas.
lotion. Lotio.
lukewarm. Tepidus.
lung. Pulmo. Gr., pneumon.
lymph. Lympha.
mad. Insanus.
malady. Morbus.
male. Masculinus.
malignant. Malignus.
maternity. Conditio matris.
medicated. Medicatus.
medicine. (Remedy) Medicamentum.
milk. Lac.
mind. Animus.
mix. Miscere.
mixture. Mistura.
moist. Humidus.
molar. Dens molaris.
month. Mensis.
monthly. Menstruus.
morbid. Morbidus.
mouth. Os. Gr., stoma.
mucous. Mucosus.
muscle. Musculus. Gr., mys.
mustard. Sinapis.
nail. Unguis.
navel. Umbilicus. Gr., omphalos.
neck. Cervix; collum. Gr., trachelos.
nerve. Nervus. Gr., neuron.
nipple. Papilla.
no, none. Nullus.
normal. Normalis.
nose. Nasus. Gr., rhis.
nostril. Naris.
not. Non.
nourish. Nutrire.
nourishment. Alimentus.
now. Nunc.
nudity. Nudatio.
nurse. Nutrix.
obesity. Obesitas.
ocular. Ocularis.
oculist. Ocularis medicus.
oil. Oleum.
ointment. Unguentum.
operator. Manus curatio.
opiate. Medicamemtum somnificum.
optics. Optica.
orifice. Foramen.
pain. Dolor.
palate. Palatum.

palm. Palma.
parasite. Parasitus.
part. Pars.
patient. Patiens.
pectoral. Pectoralis.
pedal. Pedale.
phlegm. Pituita.
pill. Pilus.
pimple. Pustula.
plaster. Emplastrum.
poison. Venenum.
poultice. Cataplasma.
powder. Pulvis.
pregnant. Gravida.
prepare. Parare.
prescribe. Praescribere.
prescription. Praescriptum.
puberty. Pubertas.
pubic bone. Os pubis. Gr., pecten.
pulverize. Pulverare.
pupil. Pupilla.
purgative. Purgativus.
putrid. Putridus.
quinsy. Cynanche; angina.
rash. Exanthema.
recover. Convalescere.
recumbent. Recumbens.
recur. Recurrere.
redness. Rubor.
remedy. Remedium.
respiration. Respiratio.
rheum. Fluxio.
rib. Costa.
rigid. Rigidus.
ringing. Tinnitus.
rupture. Hernia.
saliva. Sputum.
sallow. Salix.
salt. Sal.
salve. Unguentum.
sane. Sanus.
scab. Scabies.
scalp. Pericranium.
scaly. Squamosus.
scar. Cicatrix.
sciatica. Ischias.
scruple. Scrupulum.
seed. Semen.
senile. Senilis.
serum. Sanguinis pars equosa.
sheath. Vagina.
shin. Tibia.
shock. Concussio; (of electricity) ictus electricus.
short. Brevis.
shoulder. Humerus. Gr., omos.
shoulder blade. Scapula.
shudder. Tremor.
sick. Aegrotus.
side. Latus.
sinew. Nervus.
skeleton. Gr., skeleton.
skin. Cutis. Gr., derma.
skull. Cranium. Gr., kranion.
sleep. Somnus.
smallpox. Variola.
smell. Odoratus.
soap. Sapo.
socket. Cavum.
soft. Mollis.
solid. Solidus.
solution. Dilutum.
soporific. Soporus.
sore. Ulcus.
spasm. Spasmus.
spinal. Dorsalis; spinalis.
spine. Spina.
spirit. Spiritus.
spittle. Sputum.
spleen. Lien.
spoon. Cochleare.
sprain. Luxatio.
stomach. Stomachus. Gr., gaster.
stone. Calculus.
stricture. Strictura.
sugar. Saccharum.
suture. Sutura.
swallow. Glutire.
sweat. Sudor. Gr., hidros.
symptom. Symptoma.
system. Systema.
tail. Cauda.
take. Sumere.
tapeworm. Taenia.
taste. Gustatus.
tear. Lacrima.
teeth. Dentes.
tendon. Tendo. Gr., tenon.
testicle. Testis. Gr., orchis.
thigh. Femur.
throat. Fauces. Gr., pharynx.
throb. Palpitare.
thumb. Pollex.
tongue. Lingua. Gr., glossa.
tonsil. Tonsilla.
tooth. Dens. Gr., odous.
troche. Trochiscus.
tube. Tuba.
twin. Geminus.
twitching. Subsultus.
ulcer. Ulcus.
unless. Nisi.
urine. Urina.
uterine. Uterinus.
vaccine. Vaccinum.
vagina. Vagina. Gr., kolpos.
valve. Valvula.
vein. Vena. Gr., phleps.
vertebra. Vertebra. Gr., spondylos.
vessel. Vas.
wash. Lavare.
water. Aqua.
wax. Cera.
waxed dressing. Ceratum.
weary. Lassus.
wet. Humidus.
windpipe. Arteria aspera.
wine. Vinum.
woman. Femina.
womb. Uterus. Gr., hystera.
worm. Vermis.
wound. Vulnus.
wrist. Carpus. Gr., karpos.
yolk. Luteum.

COLORS

black. Niger; nigra; nigrum.
blue. Caeruleus; cyaneus; lividus.
brown. Fulvus.
crimson. Coccum; coccineus.
gray. Cinereus.
green. Viridis.
lemon. Citreus.
pink. Rosaceus.
purple. Purpura; purpureus.
red. Ruber.
scarlet. Coccineus.
violet. Violaceus.
white. Albus.
yellow. Flavus; luteus; croceus.

QUALITIES

bitter. Acerbus.
chill. Friguscolum.
cold. Frigidus.
dry. Aridus.
dull. Stupidus; hebes.
faintness. Languor.
fat. Obesus; pinguis.
heat. Calor; ardor; fervor.
heavy. Gravis; ponderosus.
hot. Calidus; fervens; candens.
light. Levis.
liquid. Liquidus.
moist. Humidus; uvidus.
sharp. Acutus.
short. Brevis.
sour. Acidus.
sweet. Dulcis.
tall. Longus; celsus; procerus.
thick. Densus.
thin. Tenuis; macer.
warm. Calidus.
warmth. Calor.
weary. Lassus; languidus; fatigatus.
wet. Humidus.

METALS

copper. Cuprum; cuprinus.
gold. Aurum; aureus.
iron. Ferrum; ferreus.
silver. Argentum; argenteus.
tin. Stannum; plumbum album.

TIME

afternoon. Post meridiem.
age. Aetas; maturus; adultus; impubis.
autumn. Autumnus.
birth. Partus; natales.
breakfast. Prandium.
child. Infans; puer; filius.
daily. Diurnus.
date. Status diei.
dawn. Prima lux.
day. Dies.
death. Mors.
dinner. Cena.
evening. Vesper.
hour. Hora.
infant. Infans.
maturity. Maturitas; aetas matura.
meal. Epulae.
midnight. Media nox.
midsummer. Media aestas.
moment. Punctum.
month. Mens.
monthly. Menstruus.
morning. Matutinum.
night. Nox, noctis.
noon. Meridies.
old. Antiquus.
puberty. Pubertas.
second. Secundum.
spring. Ver; veris.
summer. Aestas.
sunrise. Solis ortus.
sunset. Solis occasus.
supper. Cena.
time. Tempus.
winter. Hiems; hiemis.
year. Annus.
young. Parvus; infans.
youth. Adolescentia.

NUMERALS (ROMAN)

SEE: *Roman Numerals Appendix*

Appendix 5–2 Greek Alphabet

Name of Letter	*Capital*	*Lower-case*	*Trans-literation*	*Name of Letter*	*Capital*	*Lower-case*	*Trans-literation*
alpha	Α	α	a	xi	Ξ	ξ	x
beta	Β	ϐ or β	b	omicron	Ο	ο	o short
gamma	Γ	γ	g	pi	Π	π	p
delta	Δ	δ	d	rho	Ρ	ρ	r
epsilon	Ε	ϵ	e short	sigma	Σ	σ or ς	s
zeta	Ζ	ζ	z	tau	Τ	τ	t
eta	Η	η	e long	upsilon	ϒ	υ	y
theta	Θ	θ	th	phi	Φ	ϕ or φ	f
iota	Ι	ι	i	chi	Χ	χ	ch as in German "echt"
kappa	Κ	κ	k, c				
lambda	Λ	λ	l				
mu	Μ	μ	m	psi	Ψ	ψ	ps
nu	Ν	ν	n	omega	Ω	ω	o long

Appendix 5–3 Roman Numerals

A line placed over a letter increases its value one thousand times.

1	I	6	VI	11	XI	40	XL	90	XC	5000	$\overline{V}$
2	II	7	VII	12	XII	50	L	100	C	10,000	$\overline{X}$
3	III	8	VIII	15	XV	60	LX	500	D	100,000	$\overline{C}$
4	IV	9	IX	20	XX	70	LXX	1000	M	1,000,000	$\overline{M}$
5	V	10	X	30	XXX	80	LXXX	2000	MM		

APPENDIX 6
Medical Abbreviations

A	accommodation; acetum; angström unit; anode; anterior
a	artery
$\bar{a}$	before
A_2	aortic second sound
aa	of each; arteries
abd	abdominal/abdomen
ABG	arterial blood gas
ABO	three basic blood groups
AC	alternating current; air conduction; axiocervical; adrenal cortex
a.c.	before a meal
acc.	accommodation
ACE	angiotensin-converting enzyme
ACh	acetylcholine
ACLS	advanced cardiac life support
ACTH	adrenocorticotropic hormone
AD	advance directive
ad	to; up to
add.	add
ADH	antidiuretic hormone
ADHD	attention deficit-hyperactivity disorder
ADL	activities of daily living
ad lib.	freely; as desired
admov.	apply
ad sat.	to saturation
AF	atrial fibrillation
AFB	acid-fast bacillus
AFP	alpha-fetoprotein
A/G; A-G ratio	albumin/globulin ratio
Ag	silver; antigen
$AgNO_3$	silver nitrate
ah	hypermetropic astigmatism
AHF	antihemophilic factor
AI	aortic incompetence
AICD	automatic implantable cardiac defibrillator
AIDS	acquired immunodeficiency syndrome
AK	above the knee
Al	aluminum
Alb	albumin
ALS	amyotrophic lateral sclerosis
ALT	alanine aminotransferase
alt. dieb.	every other day
alt. hor.	every other hour
alt. noc.	every other night
AM	morning
Am	mixed astigmatism
a.m.a.	against medical advice
AMI	acute myocardial infarction
amp	ampule; amputation
ANA	antinuclear antibody
anat	anatomy or anatomic
ant.	anterior
A.P.	anteroposterior
A-P	anterior-posterior
A & P	auscultation and percussion
ap	before dinner
AQ, aq	water
aq. dest.	distilled water
aq. frig.	cold water
ARC	AIDS-related complex
ARDS	acute respiratory distress syndrome
ARMD	age-related macular degeneration
AS	ankylosing spondylitis; aortic stenosis; auris sinistra (left ear)
As.	astigmatism
ASCVD	atherosclerotic cardiovascular disease
ASD	atrial septal defect
AsH	hypermetropic astigmatism
AsM	myopic astigmatism
AST	aspartate aminotransferase
Ast	astigmatism
at. wt.	atomic weight
Au	gold
A-V; AV; A/V	arteriovenous; atrioventricular
av.	avoirdupois
B	boron; bacillus
Ba	barium
BAC	blood alcohol concentration
BBB	blood-brain barrier
BBT	basal body temperature
BCLS	basic cardiac life support
BE	barium enema
Be	beryllium
Bi	bismuth
bib.	drink
b.i.d.	twice a day
b.i.n.	twice a night
BK	below the knee
BM	bowel movement
BMR	basal metabolic rate
bol.	pill
BP	blood pressure
B.P.	British Pharmacopeia
BPH	benign prostatic hyperplasia
bpm	beats per minute
BSA	body surface area
BSE	breast self-examination
BUN	blood urea nitrogen
BW	birth weight
Bx	biopsy
C	Calorie (kilocalorie); Celsius
c	calorie (small calorie)
$\bar{c}$	with

ca. about; approximately
CABG coronary artery bypass graft
$CaCO_3$ calcium carbonate
CAD coronary artery disease
CAH chronic active hepatitis
Cal large calorie
C&S culture and sensitivity
CAP let (the patient) take
cap. a capsule
cath. catheter
CBC complete blood count
CC chief complaint
cc cubic centimeter
CCl_4 carbon tetrachloride
CCU coronary care unit; critical care unit
CDC Centers for Disease Control and Prevention
CF cystic fibrosis; Christmas factor
cg centigram
CHD congenital heart disease; coronary heart disease
ChE cholinesterase
CHF congestive heart failure
CI cardiac index
Ci curie
CIS carcinoma in situ
CK creatine kinase
Cl chlorine
cm centimeter
c.m.s. to be taken tomorrow morning
CMV cytomegalovirus
c.n. tomorrow night
CNS central nervous system
c.n.s. to be taken tomorrow night
CO carbon monoxide; cardiac output
CO_2 carbon dioxide
Co cobalt
c/o complains of
COLD chronic obstructive lung disease
comp. compound; compounded of
COPD chronic obstructive pulmonary disease
CP cerebral palsy; cleft palate
CPAP continuous positive airway pressure
CPC clinicopathologic conference
CPD cephalopelvic disproportion
CPR cardiopulmonary resuscitation
CR crown-rump length; conditioned reflex
CS cesarean section
CSF cerebrospinal fluid
CT computed tomography
Cu copper
CV cardiovascular
CVA cerebrovascular accident; costovertebral angle
CVP central venous pressure
CVS chronic villi sampling
CXR chest X-ray
D diopter; dose
d density; right
/d per day
D and C dilatation and curettage
dB decibel
DC direct current; doctor of chiropractic
dc discontinue
det. let it be given
DIC disseminated intravascular coagulation
dieb. alt. every other day
dieb. tert. every third day
DJD degenerative joint disease
dil. dilute; diluted
dim. halved
DKA diabetic ketoacidosis
dl deciliter
DM diabetes mellitus
DNA deoxyribonucleic acid
DNR do not resuscitate
DOA dead on arrival
DOB date of birth
DOE dyspnea on exertion
DPT diphtheria-pertussis-tetanus (vaccine)
dr. dram
DRG diagnosis-related group
DT's delirium tremens
DTR deep tendon reflex
dur. dolor while pain lasts
Dx diagnosis
D5W dextrose 5% in water
E eye; *Escherichia*
EBV Epstein-Barr virus
ECF extended care facility; extracellular fluid
ECG electrocardiogram, electrocardiograph
ECHO echocardiography
ECMO extracorporeal membrane oxygenation
ECT electroconvulsive therapy
ED emergency department; effective dose; erythema dose; erectile dysfunction
EDD estimated date of delivery (formerly EDC: estimated date of confinement)
EEG electroencephalogram
EENT eye, ear, nose, and throat
EKG electrocardiogram; electrocardiograph
ELISA enzyme-linked immunosorbent assay
elix. elixir
Em emmetropia
EMG electromyogram
EMS emergency medical service
ENT ear, nose and throat
EOM extraocular muscles
ER Emergency Room
ESR erythrocyte sedimentation rate

ESRD	end-stage renal disease
EST	electroshock therapy
F	Fahrenheit
f	female
FA	fatty acid
FD	fatal dose; focal distance
Fe	iron
FEV	forced expiratory volume
Fld	fluid
fl. dr.	fluidram
fl. oz.	fluidounce
FP	family practice
FSH	follicle-stimulating hormone
FTT	failure to thrive
FUO	fever of unknown origin
g, gm	gram
garg	a gargle
GB	gallbladder
GC	gonococcus or gonorrheal
GDM	gestational diabetes mellitus
GERD	gastroesophageal reflux disease
GFR	glomerular filtration rate
GH	growth hormone
GI	gastrointestinal
GP	general practitioner
gr	grain
grad	by degrees
GRAS	generally recognized as safe
GSW	gunshot wound
GTT	glucose tolerance test
Gtt, gtt	drops
GU	genitourinary
guttat.	drop by drop
GYN	gynecology
G6PD	glucose-6-phosphate dehydrogenase
H	hydrogen
H^+	hydrogen ion
h, hr	hour
HAV	hepatitis A virus
HBV	hepatitis B virus
HCG	human chorionic gonadotropin
HCT	hematocrit
HCV	hepatitis C virus
HD	hearing distance
HDL	high-density lipoprotein
HEENT	head, eye, ear, nose, and throat
Hg	mercury
hgb	hemoglobin
Hib	*haemophilus influenzae* type B
HIV	human immunodeficiency virus
h/o	history of
H_2O	water
H_2O_2	hydrogen peroxide
hor. decub.	bedtime
hor. som, h.s.	bedtime
HPI	history of present illness
HR	heart rate
HSV	herpes simplex virus
HTN	hypertension
HTLV-III	human T lymphotropic virus type III
hx, Hx	history
Hy	hyperopia
Hz	hertz (cycles per second)
I	iodine
^{131}I	radioactive isotope of iodine (atomic weight 131)
^{132}I	radioactive isotope of iodine (atomic weight 132)
I & O	intake and output
IBW	ideal body weight
IC	inspiratory capacity
ICP	intracranial pressure
ICS	intercostal space
ICSH	interstitial cell-stimulating hormone
ICU	intensive care unit
Id.	the same
IDDM	insulin-dependent diabetes mellitus
Ig	immunoglobulin
IM	intramuscular
in d.	daily
INF	interferon
inj.	injection
instill.	instillation
IOP	intraocular pressure
IPPB	intermittent positive pressure breathing
IQ	intelligence quotient
IRV	inspiratory reserve volume
I.U.	international unit
IUCD	intrauterine contraceptive device
IUD	intrauterine device
IUFD	intrauterine fetal death
IV	intravenous
IVP	intravenous pyelogram
J	joule
JRA	juvenile rheumatoid arthritis
K	potassium
kg	kilogram
KI	potassium iodine
KUB	kidney, ureter, and bladder
kv	kilovolt
KVO	keep vein open
L	liter
L & D	labor and delivery
lab.	laboratory
lat.	lateral
lb.	pound
LBW	low birth weight
LD_{50}	lethal dose, median
LDL	low-density lipoprotein
lmp	lower extremity; lupus erythematosus
LGA	large for gestational age
LH	luteinizing hormone
Li	lithium
lig	ligament
liq.	liquid; fluid
LLE	left lower extremity

LLL left lower lobe
LLQ left lower quadrant
lmp last menstrual period
LOC level/loss of consciousness
LP lumbar puncture
LR lactated Ringer's
LTD lowest tolerated dose
LUE left upper extremity
LUL left upper lobe
LUQ left upper quadrant
LV left ventricle
LVH left ventricular hypertrophy
M master; medicine; molar; thousand; muscle
m male; meter; minim; mole; meta
MA mental age
man. prim. first thing in the morning
MAP mean arterial pressure
MBD minimal brain dysfunction
mc; mCi millicurie
mcg microgram
MCH mean corpuscular hemoglobin
MCHC mean corpuscular hemoglobin concentration
MCV mean corpuscular volume
MD muscular dystrophy
MDI metered-dose inhaler
MED minimum effective dose
mEq milliequivalent
mEq/L milliequivalent per liter
ME ratio myeloid/erythroid ratio
Mg magnesium
mg milligram
MI myocardial infarction
MID minimum infective dose
mist. a mixture
ml milliliter
MLD minimum lethal dose
MM mucous membrane
mm millimeter
mm Hg millimeters of mercury
mMol millimole
MMR measles-mumps-rubella (vaccine)
Mn manganese
mol. wt. molecular weight
mor. dict. as directed
mor. sol. as accustomed
MPC maximum permitted concentration
MPN most probable number
mr milliroentgen
MRA magnetic resonance angiography
MRI magnetic resonance imaging
MS mitral stenosis; multiple sclerosis
mV millivolt
MVA motor vehicle accident
MW molecular weight
My myopia

μEq microequivalent
μg microgram
N nitrogen
n nerve
N/A not applicable
Na sodium
NAD acute distress
n.b. note well
nCi nanocurie
NG, ng nasogastric
NH_3 ammonia
Ni nickel
NICU neonatal intensive care unit
NIDDM noninsulin-dependent diabetes mellitus
NIH National Institutes of Health
NKA no known allergies
NMR nuclear magnetic resonance
nn nerves
noct. in the night
noct. maneq. night and morning
non rep; n.r. do not repeat
NPN nonprotein nitrogen
n.p.o. nothing by mouth
NRC normal retinal correspondence
NS normal saline
NSAID nonsteroidal anti-inflammatory drug
NSR normal sinus rhythm
N&V, N/V nausea and vomiting
O pint
O_2 oxygen
OB obstetrics
OC oral contraceptive
O.D. right eye
ol. oil
om. mane vel noc. every morning or night
omn. hor. every hour
omn. noct. every night
OOB out of bed
OPD outpatient department
OR operating room
ORIF open reduction and internal fixation
O.S. left eye
os mouth
OT occupational therapy
OTC over-the-counter
OU each eye
oz ounce
P, p melting point
$\bar{p}$ after
P_2 pulmonic second sound
P-A;PA; pa posteroanterior; pulmonary artery
PABA para-aminobenzoic acid
PALS pediatric advanced life support
Pap test Papanicolaou smear
part. vic in divided doses
Pb lead
PBI protein-bound iodine
p.c. after meals
PCA patient-controlled analgesia

P_{CO_2}	carbon dioxide pressure
PCP	*Pneumocystis carinii* pneumonia; primary care physician; primary care provider
PCWP	pulmonary capillary wedge pressure
PD	interpupillary distance
pd	prism diopter; pupillary distance
PDA	patent ductus arteriosus
PDR	*Physician's Desk Reference*
PE	physical examination
PEEP	positive end expiratory pressure
PEFR	peak expiratory flow rate
PEG	percutaneous endoscopic gastrostomy
per	through or by
PERRLA	pupils equal, regular, react to light and accommodation
PET	positron emission tomography
pH	hydrogen ion concentration
Pharm; Phar.	pharmacy
PI	present illness; previous illness
PICC	peripherally inserted central catheter
PID	pelvic inflammatory disease
pil.	pill
PKU	phenylketonuria
PM	afternoon/evening
PMH	past medical history
PMI	point of maximal impulse
PMN	polymorphonuclear neutrophil leukocytes
PMS	premenstrual syndrome
PND	paroxysmal nocturnal dyspnea
PNH	paroxysmal nocturnal hemoglobinuria
PO; p.o.	orally (per os)
post.	posterior
PPD	purified protein derivative (TB test)
ppm	parts per million
p.r.	through the rectum
p.r.n.	as needed
pro time/PT	prothrombin time
PSA	prostate-specific antigen
PT	prothrombin time; physical therapy
Pt	platinum; patient
pt	pint
PTT	partial thromboplastin time
Pu	plutonium
p.v.	through the vagina
PVC	premature ventricular contraction
q	every
q.d.	every day
q.h.	every hour
q.2h.	every 2 hours
q.3h.	every 3 hours
q.4h.	every four hours
q.i.d	four times a day
q.l.	as much as wanted
qns	quantity not sufficient
q.o.d	every other day
q.p.	as much as desired
q.s.	as much as needed
qt	quart
quotid.	daily
q.v.	as much as you please
RA	rheumatoid arthritis
Ra	radium
rad	radiation absorbed dose
RAI	radioactive iodine
RAIU	radioactive iodine uptake
RBC	red blood cell; red blood count
RDA	recommended daily/dietary allowance
RDS	respiratory distress syndrome
RE	right eye
Re	rhenium
REM	rapid eye movements
Rh	symbol of rhesus factor; symbol for rhodium
RHD	rheumatic heart disease
RLE	right lower extremity
RLL	right lower lobe
RLQ	right lower quadrant
RML	right middle lobe of lung
Rn	radon
RNA	ribonucleic acid
R/O	rule out
ROM	range of motion
ROS	review of systems
RPM	revolutions per minute
RQ	respiratory quotient
RR	recovery room; respiratory rate
RT	radiation therapy; respiratory therapy
R/T	related to
RUE	right upper extremity
RUL	right upper lobe
RUQ	right upper quadrant
S	mark
$\bar{s}$	without
S.	sacral
S-A; S/A; SA	sinoatrial
SB	small bowel
Sb	antimony
SC, sc, s.c.	subcutaneous(ly)
S.D.	standard deviation
S.E.	standard error
Se	selenium
Sed rate	sedimentation rate
semih.	half an hour
SGA	small for gestational age
SI	international system of units (stroke index)
Si	silicon
SIDS	sudden infant death syndrome
Sig.	write on label
SLE	systemic lupus erythematosus

SLP speech-language pathology
Sn tin
SNF skilled nursing facility
SOB shortness of breath
sol solution, dissolved
s.o.s. if necessary
S/P no change after
sp. gr. specific gravity
sph spherical
spt. spirit
s.q. subcutaneous(ly)
Sr strontium
ss a half
SSS sick sinus syndrome
st. let it (them) stand
Staph *Staphylococcus*
stat. immediately
STD sexually transmitted disease
Strep *Streptococcus*
STS serologic test for syphilis
STU skin test unit
SV stroke volume; supraventricular
Sx symptoms
syr. syrup
T temperature
T_3 triiodothyronine
T_4 thyroxine
TA toxin-antitoxin
Ta tantalum
TAH total abdominal hysterectomy
T&A tonsillectomy and adenoidectomy
TAT thematic apperception test
T.A.T. toxin-antitoxin
TB tuberculin; tuberculosis; tubercle bacillus
Tb terbium
t.d.s. to be taken three times daily
Te tellurium; tetanus
TENS transcutaneous electrical nerve stimulation
Th thorium
TIA transient ischemic attack
TIBC total iron-binding capacity
t.i.d. three times a day
t.i.n. three times a night
tinct., tr tincture
Tl thallium
TLC, tlc tender loving care; thin layer chromatography; total lung capacity
TM tympanic membrane
TMJ temporomandibular joint
TNT trinitrotoluene
TNTM too numerous to mention
top. topically
TPI *Treponema pallidum* immobilization test for syphilis
TPN total parenteral nutrition
TPR temperature, pulse, and respiration
trit. triturate or grind
TSD time since death
TSE testicular self-examination
TSH thyroid-stimulating hormone
TUR transurethral resection
TURP transurethral resection of the prostate
Tx treatment
U uranium; unit
UA urinalysis
UE upper extremity
UHF ultrahigh frequency
ult. praes. the last ordered
Umb; umb umbilicus
ung. ointment
URI upper respiratory infection
US ultrasonic
USAN United States Adopted Name
USP United States Pharmacopeia
ut. dict. as directed
UTI urinary tract infection
UV ultraviolet
v vein
VA visual acuity
VC vital capacity
VD venereal disease
VDRL Venereal Disease Research Laboratories
Vf field of vision
VLBW very low birth weight
VLDL very low density lipoprotein
VMA vanillylmandelic acid
vol. volume
vol. % volume percent
VS volumetric solution; vesicular sound; vital signs
VSD ventricular septal defect
vv veins
VZIG varicella zoster immune globulin
W tungsten
w watt
WBC white blood cell; white blood count
WDWN well developed, well nourished
WF/BF white female/black female
WH well hydrated
WM/BM white male/black male
WN well-nourished
WNL within normal limits
wt. weight
w/v. weight in volume
x multiplied by
yo years old
yr year
Z atomic number
Zn zinc

APPENDIX 7
Symbols

♏	Minim
℈	Scruple
ʒ	Dram
fʒ	Fluidram
℥	Ounce
f℥	Fluidounce
O	Pint
℔	Pound
℞	Recipe (L. take)
M	Misce (L. mix)
$\overline{aa}$	Of each
A, Å, AU	angström unit
C-1, C-2, etc.	Complement
c, $\bar{c}$	cum (L. with)
Δ	Change; heat
E_0	Electroaffinity
F_1	First filial generation
F_2	Second filial generation
mμ	Millimicron, nanometer
μg	Microgram
mEq	Milliequivalent
mg	Milligram
mg%	Milligrams percent; milligrams per 100 ml
QO_2	Oxygen consumption
m-	Meta-
o-	Ortho-
p-	Para-
$\bar{p}$	After
PO_2	Partial pressure of oxygen
PCO_2	Partial pressure of carbon dioxide
$\bar{s}$	Without
$\overline{ss}$, ss	[L. semis]. One half
μm	Micrometer
μ	Micron (former term for micrometer)
μμ	Micromicron

+	Plus; excess; acid reaction; positive
−	Minus; deficiency; alkaline reaction; negative
±	Plus or minus; either positive or negative; indefinite
#	Number; following a number, pounds
÷	Divided by
×	Multiplied by; magnification
/	Divided by
=	Equals
≈	Approximately equal
>	Greater than; from which is derived
<	Less than; derived from
≮	Not less than
≯	Not greater than
≦	Equal to or less than
≧	Equal to or greater than
≠	Not equal to
$\sqrt{}$	Root; square root; radical
$\sqrt[2]{}$	Square root
$\sqrt[3]{}$	Cube root
∞	Infinity
:	Ratio; "is to"
::	Equality between ratios, "as"
∴	Therefore
°	Degree
%	Percent
π	3.1416—ratio of circumference of a circle to its diameter
□, ♂	Male
○, ♀	Female
⇌	Denotes a reversible reaction
n	Subscripted n indicates the number of the molecules can vary from two to greater
↑	Increase
↓	Decrease

APPENDIX 8
Units of Measurement (Including SI Units)

Appendix 8–1 Scientific Notation

Sometimes it is necessary to use very large and very small numbers. These can best be indicated and handled in calculations by use of scientific notation, which is to say by use of exponents. Use of scientific notation requires writing the number so that it is the result of multiplying some whole number power of 10 by a number between 1 and 10. Examples are:

$$1234 = 1.234 \times 10^3$$

$$0.01234 = 1.234 \times \frac{1}{100} = 1.234 \times 10^{-2}$$

$$0.001234 = 1.234 \times \frac{1}{1000} = 1.234 \times 10^{-3}$$

To convert a number to its equivalent in scientific notation:

Place the decimal point to the right of the first non-zero digit. This will now be a number between 1 and 9.

Multiply this number by a power of 10, the exponent of which is equal to the number of places the decimal point was moved. The exponent is positive if the decimal point was moved to the left, and negative if it was moved to the right. For example:

$$\frac{1{,}234{,}000.0 \times 0.000072}{6000.0} = \frac{1.234 \times 10^6 \times 7.2 \times 10^{-5}}{6.0 \times 10^3}$$

Now, by simply adding or subtracting the exponents of ten, and remembering that moving an exponent from the denominator of the fraction to the numerator changes its sign,

$$= \frac{1.234 \times 10^6 \times 10^{-5} \times 10^{-3} \times 7.2}{6} = \frac{1.234 \times 10^{-2} \times 7.2}{6}$$

Now, dividing by 6,

$$= 1.234 \times 10^{-2} \times 1.2 = 1.4808 \times 10^{-2} = \frac{1.4808}{100} = 0.014808$$

The last operation changed 1.4808×10^{-2} into the final value, 0.014808, which is not expressed in scientific notation.

Appendix 8–2 SI Units (Système International d'Unités or International System of Units)

This system includes two types of units important in clinical medicine. The *base units* are shown in the first table, derived units in the second table, and derived units with special names in the third table.

SI BASE UNITS

Quantity	*Name*	*Symbol*
Length	meter	m
Mass	kilogram	kg
Time	second	s
Electric current	ampere	A
Temperature	kelvin	K
Luminous intensity	candela	cd
Amount of a substance	mole	mol

SOME SI DERIVED UNITS

Quantity	Name of Derived Unit	Symbol
Area	square meter	m^2
Volume	cubic meter	m^3
Speed, velocity	meter per second	m/s
Acceleration	meter per second squared	m/s^2
Mass density	kilogram per cubic meter	kg/m^3
Concentration of a substance	mole per cubic meter	mol/m^3
Specific volume	cubic meter per kilogram	m^3/kg
Luminescence	candela per square meter	cd/m^2

SI DERIVED UNITS WITH SPECIAL NAMES

Quantity	Name	Symbol	Expressed in Terms of Other Units
Frequency	hertz	Hz	s^{-1}
Force	newton	N	$kg{\cdot}m{\cdot}s^{-2}$ or $kg{\cdot}m/s^2$
Pressure	pascal	Pa	$N{\cdot}m^{-2}$ or N/m^2
Energy, work, amount of heat	joule	J	$kg{\cdot}m^2{\cdot}s^{-2}$ or $N{\cdot}m$
Power	watt	W	J·s or J/s
Quantity of electricity	coulomb	C	A·s
Electromotive force	volt	V	W/A
Capacitance	farad	F	C/V
Electrical resistance	ohm	Ω	V/a
Conductance	siemens	S	A/V
Inductance	henry	H	Wϕ/A
Illuminance	lux	lx	ln/m^2
Absorbed (radiation) dose	gray	Gy	J/kg
Dose equivalent (radiation)	sievert	Sv	J/kg
Activity (radiation)	becquerel	Bq	s^{-1}

PREFIXES AND MULTIPLES USED IN SI

Prefix	Symbol	Power	Multiple or Portion of a Multiple
tera	T	10^{12}	1,000,000,000,000.
giga	G	10^9	1,000,000,000.
mega	M	10^6	1,000,000.
kilo	k	10^3	1,000.
hecto	h	10^2	100.
deca	da	10^1	10.
unity			1.
deci	d	10^{-1}	0.1
centi	c	10^{-2}	0.01
milli	m	10^{-3}	0.001
micro	μ	10^{-6}	0.000001
nano	n	10^{-9}	0.000000001
pico	p	10^{-12}	0.000000000001
femto	f	10^{-15}	0.000000000000001
atto	a	10^{-18}	0.000000000000000001

Appendix 8–3 Metric System

MASSES

Table		Grams		Grains
1 Kilogram	=	1000.0	=	15,432.35
1 Hectogram	=	100.0	=	1,543.23
1 Decagram	=	10.0	=	154.323
1 Gram	=	1.0	=	15.432

MASSES (Continued)

Table		Grams		Grains
1 Decigram	=	0.1	=	1.5432
1 Centigram	=	0.01	=	0.15432
1 Milligram	=	0.001	=	0.01543
1 Microgram	=	10^{-6}	=	15.432×10^{-6}
1 Nanogram	=	10^{-9}	=	15.432×10^{-9}
1 Picogram	=	10^{-12}	=	15.432×10^{-12}
1 Femtogram	=	10^{-15}	=	15.432×10^{-15}
1 Attogram	=	10^{-18}	=	15.432×10^{-18}

Arabic numbers are used with masses and measures, as 10 g, or 3 ml, etc. Portions of masses and measures are usually expressed decimally. 10^{-1} indicates 0.1; 10^{-6} = 0.000001; etc. SEE: *Scientific Notation Appendix*.

Appendix 8–4 Weights and Measures

Arabic numerals are used with masses and measures, as 10 g, or 3 ml, etc. Portions of masses and measures are usually expressed decimally. For practical purposes, 1 cm^3 (cubic centimeter) is equivalent to 1 ml (milliliter) and 1 drop (gtt.) of water is equivalent to a minim (m).

LENGTH

Millimeters (mm)	*Centimeters (cm)*	*Inches (in)*	*Feet (ft)*	*Yards (yd)*	*Meters (m)*
1.0	0.1	0.03937	0.00328	0.0011	0.001
10.0	1.0	0.3937	0.03281	0.0109	0.01
25.4	2.54	1.0	0.0833	0.0278	0.0254
304.8	30.48	12.0	1.0	0.333	0.3048
914.40	91.44	36.0	3.0	1.0	0.9144
1000.0	100.0	39.37	3.2808	1.0936	1.0

1 μm = 1 micrometer = 0.001 millimeter. 1 mm = 100 μm.
1 km = 1 kilometer = 1000 meters = 0.62137 statute mile.
1 statute mile = 5280 feet = 1.609 kilometers.
1 nautical mile = 6076.042 feet = 1852.276 meters.

VOLUME (FLUID)

Milliliters (ml)	*US Fluidrams (fʒ)*	*Cubic Inches (in.³)*	*U.S. Fluidounces (f℥)*	*U.S. Fluid Quarts (qt)*	*Liters (L)*
1.0	0.2705	0.061	0.03381	0.00106	0.001
3.697	1.0	0.226	0.125	0.00391	0.00369
16.3866	4.4329	1.0	0.5541	0.0173	0.01639
29.573	8.0	1.8047	1.0	0.03125	0.02957
946.332	256.0	57.75	32.0	1.0	0.9463
1000.0	270.52	61.025	33.815	1.0567	1.0

1 gallon = 4 quarts = 8 pints = 3.785 liters.
1 pint = 473.16 ml.

WEIGHT

Grains (gr)	*Grams (g)*	*Apothecaries' Ounces (f℥)*	*Avoirdupois Pounds (lb)*	*Kilograms (kg)*
1.0	0.0648	0.00208	0.0001429	0.000065
15.432	1.0	0.03215	0.002205	0.001
480.0	31.1	1.0	0.06855	0.0311
7000.0	453.5924	14.583	1.0	0.45359
15432.358	1000.0	32.15	2.2046	1.0

1 microgram (μg) = 0.001 milligram.
1 mg = 1 milligram = 0.001 g; 1000 mg = 1 g.

APOTHECARIES' WEIGHT

20 grains = 1 scruple
8 drams = 1 ounce
3 scruples = 1 dram
12 ounces = 1 pound

AVOIRDUPOIS WEIGHT

27.343 grains = 1 dram
16 ounces = 1 pound
2000 pounds = 1 short ton
1 oz troy = 480 grains
1 lb troy = 5760 grains
16 drams = 1 ounce
100 pounds = 1 hundredweight
2240 pounds = 1 long ton
1 oz avoirdupois = 437.5 grains
1 lb avoirdupois = 7000 grains

CIRCULAR MEASURE

60 seconds = 1 minute
90 degrees = 1 quadrant
60 minutes = 1 degree
4 quadrants = 360 degrees = circle

CUBIC MEASURE

1728 cubic inches = 1 cubic foot
2150.42 cubic inches = 1 standard bushel
1 cubic foot = about four fifths of a bushel
27 cubic feet = 1 cubic yard
268.8 cubic inches = 1 dry (U.S.) gallon
128 cubic feet = 1 cord (wood)

DRY MEASURE

2 pints = 1 quart
8 quarts = 1 peck
4 pecks = 1 bushel

LIQUID MEASURE

16 ounces = 1 pint
1000 milliliters = 1 liter
4 gills = 1 pint
4 quarts = 1 gallon
31.5 gallons = 1 barrel (U.S.)
2 pints = 1 quart
2 barrels = 1 hogshead (U.S.)
1 quart = 946.35 milliliters
1 liter = 1.0566 quart

Barrels and hogsheads vary in size. A U.S. gallon is equal to 0.8327 British gallon; therefore, a British gallon is equal to 1.201 U.S. gallons. 1 liter is equal to 1.0567 quarts.

LINEAR MEASURE

1 inch = 2.54 centimeters
12 inches = 1 foot
1 statute mile = 5280 feet
40 rods = 1 furlong
3 feet = 1 yard
3 statute miles = 1 statute league
8 furlongs = 1 statute mile
5.5 yards = 1 rod
1 nautical mile = 6076.042 feet

TROY WEIGHT

24 grains = 1 pennyweight
20 pennyweights = 1 ounce
12 ounces = 1 pound

Used for weighing gold, silver, and jewels.

HOUSEHOLD MEASURES AND WEIGHTS

Approximate Equivalents: 60 gtt. = 1 teaspoonful = 5 ml = 60 minims = 60 grains = 1 dram = $\frac{1}{8}$ ounce

1 teaspoon = $\frac{1}{8}$ fl. oz; 1 dram
3 teaspoons = 1 tablespoon
1 tablespoon = $\frac{1}{2}$ fl. oz; 4 drams
16 teaspoons (liquid) = 1 cup
12 tablespoons (dry) = 1 cup
1 cup = 8 fl. oz
1 tumbler or glass = 8 fl. oz; $\frac{1}{2}$ pint

---

* Household measures are not precise. For instance, a household tsp will hold from 3 to 5 ml of liquid. Therefore, household equivalents should not be substituted for medication prescribed by the physician.

NOTE: Traditionally, the word "weights" is used in these tables, but "masses" is the correct term.

Appendix 8–5 Conversion Rules and Factors

To convert units of one system into the other, multiply the number of units in column I by the equivalent factor opposite that unit in column II.

WEIGHT

1 attogram	=	15.432 × 10^{-18} grains
1 femtogram	=	15.432 × 10^{-15} grains
1 picogram	=	15.432 × 10^{-12} grains
1 nanogram	=	15.432 × 10^{-9} grains
1 microgram	=	15.432 × 10^{-6} grains
1 milligram	=	0.015432 grain
1 centigram	=	0.15432 grain
1 decigram	=	1.5432 grains
1 decagram	=	154.323 grains
1 hectogram	=	1543.23 grains
1 gram	=	15.432 grains
1 gram	=	0.25720 apothecaries' dram
1 gram	=	0.03527 avoirdupois ounce
1 gram	=	0.03215 apothecaries' or troy ounce
1 kilogram	=	35.274 avoirdupois ounces
1 kilogram	=	32.151 apothecaries' or troy ounces
1 kilogram	=	2.2046 avoirdupois pounds
1 grain	=	64.7989 milligrams
1 grain	=	0.0648 gram
1 apothecaries' dram	=	3.8879 grams
1 avoirdupois ounce	=	28.3495 grams
1 apothecaries' or troy ounce	=	31.1035 grams
1 avoirdupois pound	=	453.5924 grams

VOLUME (AIR OR GAS)

1 cubic centimeter (cm^3)	=	0.06102 cubic inch
1 cubic meter (m^3)	=	35.314 cubic feet
1 cubic meter	=	1.3079 cubic yard
1 cubic inch ($in.^3$)	=	16.3872 cubic centimeters
1 cubic foot (ft^3)	=	0.02832 cubic meter

CAPACITY (FLUID OR LIQUID)

1 milliliter	=	16.23 minims
1 milliliter	=	0.2705 fluidram
1 milliliter	=	0.0338 fluidounce
1 liter	=	33.8148 fluidounces
1 liter	=	2.1134 pints
1 liter	=	1.0567 quart
1 liter	=	0.2642 gallon
1 fluidram	=	3.697 milliliters
1 fluidounce	=	29.573 milliliters
1 pint	=	473.1765 milliliters
1 quart	=	946.353 milliliters
1 gallon	=	3.785 liters

TIME

1 millisecond = one thousandth (0.001) of a second
1 second = 1/60 of a minute
1 minute = 1/60 of an hour
1 hour = 1/24 of a day

TEMPERATURE

Given a temperature on the Fahrenheit scale, to convert it to degrees Celsius, subtract 32 and multiply by 5/9. Given a temperature on the Celsius scale; to convert it to degrees Fahrenheit, multiply by 9/5 and add 32. Degrees Celsius are equivalent to degrees Centigrade.

* SEE: *thermometer, Celsius* for table

PRESSURE

TO OBTAIN	MULTIPLY	BY
lb/sq in.	atmospheres	14.696
lb/sq in.	in. of water	0.03609
lb/sq in.	ft of water	0.4335
lb/sq in.	in. of mercury	0.4912
lb/sq in.	kg/sq meter	0.00142
lb/sq in.	kg/sq cm	14.22
lb/sq in.	cm of mercury	0.1934
lb/sq ft	atmospheres	2116.8
lb/sq ft	in. of water	5.204
lb/sq ft	ft of water	62.48
lb/sq ft	in. of mercury	70.727
lb/sq ft	cm of mercury	27.845
lb/sq ft	kg/sq meter	0.20482
lb/cu in.	g/ml	0.03613
lb/cu ft	lb/cu in.	1728.0
lb/cu ft	gm/ml	62.428
lb/U.S. gal	gm/L	8.345
in. of water	in. of mercury	13.60
in. of water	cm of mercury	5.3543
ft of water	atmospheres	33.95
ft of water	lb/sq in.	2.307
ft of water	kg/sq meter	0.00328
ft of water	in. of mercury	1.133
ft of water	cm of mercury	0.4461
atmospheres	ft of water	0.02947
atmospheres	in. of mercury	0.03342
atmospheres	kg/sq cm	0.9678
bars	atmospheres	1.0133
in. of mercury	atmospheres	29.921
in. of mercury	lb/sq in.	2.036
mm of mercury	atmospheres	760.0
g/ml	lb/cu in.	27.68
g/sq cm	kg/sq meter	0.1
kg/sq meter	lb/sq in.	703.1
kg/sq meter	in. of water	25.40
kg/sq meter	in. of mercury	345.32
kg/sq meter	cm of mercury	135.95
kg/sq meter	atmospheres	10332.0
kg/sq cm	atmospheres	1.0332

FLOW RATE

TO OBTAIN	MULTIPLY	BY
cu ft/hr	cc/min	0.00212
cu ft/hr	L/min	2.12
L/min	cu ft/hr	0.472

PARTS PER MILLION

Conversion of parts per million (ppm) to percent:
1 ppm = 0.0001%, 10 ppm = 0.001%, 100 ppm = 0.01%, 1000 ppm = 0.1%, 10,000 ppm = 1%, etc.

ENERGY

1 foot pound = 1.35582 joule
1 joule = 0.2389 Calorie (kilocalorie)
1 Calorie (kilocalorie) = 1000 calories = 4184 joules
A large Calorie, or kilocalorie, is always written with a capital C.

pH

The pH scale is simply a series of numbers stating where a given solution would stand in a series of solutions arranged according to acidity or alkalinity. At one extreme (high pH) lies a highly alkaline solution, which may be made by dissolving 4 g of sodium hydroxide in water to make a liter of solution; at the other extreme (low pH) is an acid solution containing 3.65 g of hydrogen chloride per liter of water. Halfway between lies purified water, which is neutral. All other solutions can be arranged on this scale, and their acidity or alkalinity can be stated by giving the numbers that indicate their relative positions. If the pH of a certain solution is 5.3, it falls between gastric juice and urine on the above scale, is moderately acid, and will turn litmus red.

Tenth-normal HCl	−1.00	Litmus is red in this acid range
Gastric juice	1.4	
Urine	*6.0	
Water	7.00	— Neutral
Blood	7.35–7.45	Litmus is blue in this alkaline range.
Bile	*7.5	
Pancreatic juice	8.5	
Tenth-normal NaOH	13.00	

* These body fluids vary rather widely in pH; typical figures have been used for simplicity. Urine samples obtained from healthy individuals may have pHs anywhere between 4.7 and 8.0.

APPENDIX 9
Phobias

Fear of	Condition
Air	Aerophobia
Animals	Zoophobia
Anything new	Neophobia
Bacilli	Bacillophobia
Bearing a deformed child	Teratophobia
Bees	Apiphobia, melissophobia
Being buried alive	Taphephobia
Birds	Ornithophobia
Blood	Hematophobia, hemophobia
Blushing	Ereuthrophobia
Brain disease	Meningitophobia
Bridges (crossing of)	Gephyrophobia
Cats	Ailurophobia, galeophobia
Change or novelty	Kainophobia
Childbirth	Tocophobia
Choking	Pnigophobia
Cold or something cold	Psychrophobia
Color(s)	Chromatophobia, chromophobia
Confinement	Claustrophobia
Contamination or infection	Molysmophobia
Corpses	Necrophobia
Crowds	Ochlophobia
Dampness	Hygrophobia
Darkness	Nyctophobia, scotophobia
Dawn	Eosophobia
Daylight	Phengophobia
Death	Thanatophobia
Definite, specific disease	Monopathophobia
Deformity	Dysmorphophobia
Depth	Bathophobia
Developing a phobia	Phobophobia
Dirt	Mysophobia, rupophobia
Disease	Nosophobia, pathophobia
Dogs	Cynophobia
Dolls	Pediophobia
Drafts	Anemophobia
Dust	Amathophobia
Eating	Phagophobia
Electricity	Electrophobia
Emptiness	Kenophobia, cenophobia
Error	Hamartophobia
Everything	Panphobia, panophobia, pantophobia
Excrement	Coprophobia
Eyes	Ommatophobia
Failure	Kakorrhaphiophobia
Fatigue	Kopophobia
Feathers	Pteronophobia
Fever	Pyrexeophobia
Filth	Mysophobia
Filth or odor, personal	Automysophobia
Fire	Pyrophobia
Fish	Ichthyophobia
Floods	Antlophobia
Fog	Homichlophobia
Food	Cibophobia, sitophobia
Forest	Hylophobia
Frogs	Batrachophobia
Ghosts	Phasmophobia
Girls	Parthenophobia
Glare of light	Photaugiaphobia
Glass	Crystallophobia, hyalophobia
God	Theophobia
Gravity	Barophobia
Hair	Trichopathophobia
Heat	Thermophobia
Height	Acrophobia
Hell	Hadephobia, stygiophobia
Heredity and hereditary disease	Patroiophobia
High objects or being on tall buildings	Batophobia
House, being in a	Domatophobia, oikophobia
Ideas	Ideophobia
Injury	Traumatophobia
Innovation	Neophobia
Insane, becoming	Maniaphobia
Insects	Acarophobia, entomophobia
Jealousy	Zelophobia
Justice	Dikephobia
Knife or pointed objects	Aichmophobia
Large objects	Megalophobia
Left	Levophobia
Light	Photophobia
Lightning	Astraphobia, astrapophobia, keraunophobia
Locked in, being	Clithrophobia
Looked at, being	Scopophobia
Machinery	Mechanophobia
Many things	Polyphobia
Marriage	Gamophobia
Medicine	Pharmacophobia
Men	Androphobia
Metals	Metallophobia

Phobias (Continued)

Fear of	*Condition*	*Fear of*	*Condition*
Mice	Musophobia	Sin	Hamartophobia
Mirror and seeing oneself in	Eisoptrophobia, spectrophobia	Sinning	Peccatiphobia
Missiles	Ballistophobia	Sitting	Thaasophobia
Moisture	Hygrophobia	Sitting down	Kathisophobia
Money	Chrematophobia	Skin of animals	Doraphobia
Motion	Kinesophobia	Skin disease	Dermatosiophobia
Myths	Mythophobia	Skin lesion	Dermatophobia
Naked body	Gymnophobia	Sleep	Hypnophobia
Name, hearing a certain	Onomatophobia	Small objects	Microphobia, microbiophobia
Needles	Belonephobia	Smothering	Pnigerophobia
Neglect or omission of duty	Paralipophobia	Snake	Ophidiophobia
Night	Noctiphobia, nyctophobia	Snow	Chionophobia
Northern lights	Auroraphobia	Solitude or being alone	Eremophobia
Novelty	Kainophobia	Sounds	Acousticophobia
Odor	Olfactophobia, osmophobia, osphresiophobia	Sourness	Acerophobia
Odor, personal	Bromidrosiphobia	Speaking, talking	Lalophobia
Open space	Agoraphobia	Spider	Arachnophobia
Overwork	Ponophobia	Stairs	Climacophobia
Pain	Algophobia, odynophobia	Standing up	Stasiphobia
Parasites	Parasitophobia	Standing or walking	Stasibasiphobia
People	Anthropophobia	Stars	Siderophobia
Place	Topophobia	Stealing	Kleptophobia
Pleasure	Hedonophobia	Stories	Mythophobia
Pointed objects	Aichmophobia	Strangers	Xenophobia
Poison	Iophobia, toxicophobia	Street	Agyiophobia
Poverty	Peniaphobia	String	Linonophobia
Precipices	Cremnophobia	Sunlight	Heliophobia
Punishment	Poinephobia	Symbolism	Symbolophobia
Rabies	Cynophobia, lyssophobia	Syphilis	Syphilophobia
Railroad or train	Siderodromophobia	Tapeworms	Taeniophobia
Rain or rain storm	Ombrophobia	Taste	Geumaphobia
Rectum	Proctophobia	Teeth	Odontophobia
Red	Erythrophobia	Thinking	Phronemophobia
Responsibility	Hypengyophobia	Thunder	Astraphobia, brontophobia
Returning home	Nostophobia	Time	Chronophobia
Right	Dextrophobia	Touched, being	Haphephobia, haptephobia
River	Potamophobia	Travel	Hodophobia
Robbers	Harpaxophobia	Trembling	Tremophobia
Rod or instrument of punishment	Rhabdophobia	Trichinosis	Trichinophobia
Ruin	Atephobia	Tuberculosis	Phthisiophobia, tuberculophobia
Sacred things	Hierophobia	Vaccination	Vaccinophobia
Scabies	Scabiphobia	Vehicle, being in	Amaxophobia
School	School phobia	Venereal disease	Cypridophobia
Scratches or being scratched	Amychophobia	Voice, one's own	Phonophobia
Sea	Thalassophobia	Void	Kenophobia
Self	Autophobia	Vomiting	Emetophobia
Semen, loss of	Spermatophobia	Walking	Basiphobia
Sex	Genophobia	Water	Hydrophobia
Sexual intercourse	Coitophobia	Weakness	Asthenophobia
Shock	Hormephobia	Wind	Anemophobia
		Women	Gynephobia
		Words, hearing certain	Onomatophobia
		Work	Ergasiophobia
		Writing	Graphophobia

SOURCE: Adapted from Campbell, R.J.: Psychiatric Dictionary, ed 5. Oxford University Press, N.Y., 1981.

APPENDIX 10
Manual Alphabet

A	H	O	V
B	I	P	W
C	J	Q	X
D	K	R	Y
E	L	S	Z
F	M	T	
G	N	U	

APPENDIX 11

The Interpreter in Three Languages

Basic Medical Diagnosis and Treatment in English, Spanish, and French

TABLE OF CONTENTS

INTRODUCTION

When attempting to communicate with a patient whose language is foreign to you, it is important to establish that while you may be able to say a few words in his or her language you will not be able to understand the patient's replies. The patient may need to use signs in replying. The following paragraphs are given for your convenience in explaining your language difficulty to the patient.

English

Hello. I want to help you. I do not speak (English) but will use this book to ask you some questions. I will not be able to understand your spoken answers. Please respond by shaking your head or raising one finger to indicate "no"; nod your head or raise two fingers to indicate "yes."

Spanish

Translation

Saludos. Quiero ayudarlo. Yo no hablo español, pero voy a usar este libro para hacerle algunas preguntas. No voy a poder entender sus respuestas; por eso haga el favor de contestar, negando con la cabeza o levantando un dedo para indicar "no" y afirmando con la cabeza o levantando dos dedos para indicar "sí."

Phonetic

Sah-loo'dohs. Ki-air'oh ah-joo-dar'loh. Joh noh ah'bloh es'panyohl, pair'oh voy ah oo-sawr' es'tay lee'broh pahr'ah ahsair'lay ahl-goo'nahs pray-goon'tahs. Noh voy ah poh-dair' en-ten-dair' soos res-poo-es'tahs; pore es-soh ah'gah el fah-vohr' day kohn-tes-tahr', naygahn'doh kohn lah kah-bay'thah oh layvahn-tahn'doh oon day'doh pahr'ah een-dee-kahr' noh ee ah-feer-mahn'doh kohn lah kah-bay'thah oh lay-vahntahn'doh dohs day'dohs pahr'a een-deekahr' see.

French

Translation	Phonetic
Bonjour. Je veux bien vous aider. Je ne parle pas français mais tout en me servant de ce livre je vais vous poser des questions. Je ne comprendrai pas ce que vous dites en français. Je vous en prie, pour répondre: pour indiquer "non", secouez la tête ou levez un seul doigt; pour indiquer "oui", faites un signe de tête ou levez deux doigts.	Bon-zhoor'. Zheh veh bih-ehn' vooz ay-day'. Zheh neh parl pah frahn-say' may toot ahn meh sehr-vahn' d' seh lee'vrah zheh vay voo poh-say' day kehs-tih-on'. Zheh neh kahm-prahn'dry pah seh keh voo deet ahn frahn-say'. Zheh vooz ahn pree, por ray-pahn'drah; por ahn-dee-kay nohn, seh-kway' lah teht oo leh-vay' oon sool dwoit; por ahn-dee-kay wee', fayt oon seen deh teht oo leh-vay' duh dwoit.

GENERAL

Basic Questions and Replies

English	*Spanish*	*French*
Good morning.	Buenos días.	Bonjour.
My name is . . . I am a (nurse, physician, social worker, psychologist, etc.).	Me llamo . . . soy (enfermera, médico, trabador social, psicólogo, etc.)	Je m'appelle . . . Je suis (infirmière, médecin, assistante sociale, psychologue, etc.)
What is your name?	¿Cómo se llama?	Quel est votre nom?
How old are you?	¿Cuántos años tiene?	Quel âge avez-vous?
Do you understand me?	¿Me entiende?	Me comprenez-vous?
Answer only . . .	Contestesolamente . . .	Répondez seulement . . .
Yes No	Sí No	Oui Non
What do you say?	¿Qué dice?	Que dites-vous?
Speak slower.	Hable más despacio.	Parlez plus lentement.
Say it once again.	Repítalo, por favor.	Répétez ça.
Don't be afraid.	No tenga miedo.	N'ayez pas peur.
Try to recollect.	Trate de recordar.	Cherchez à vous rappeler.
You cannot remember?	¿No recuerda?	Vous ne vous en souvenez pas?
Come to my office.	Venga a mi oficina.	Venez à mon bureau.
Please remove all your clothes and put on this gown.	Por favor, quítese la ropa y póngase esta bata.	S'il vous plaît, déshabillez-vous et mettez cette robe.
You will?	¿Ud. quiere?Ud.—Usted.	Vous voulez bien?
You will not?	¿No quiere Ud.?	Vous ne voulez pas?
You don't know?	¿No sabe?	Vous ne savez pas?
Is it impossible?	¿Es imposible?	C'est impossible?
It is necessary.	Es necesario.	C'est necéssaire.
That is right.	Está bien.	C'est bien.
Show me . . .	Enséñeme . . .	Montrez-moi . . .
Here There	Aquí Allí	Ici Là
Which side?	¿En qué lado?	Quel côté?
Since when?	¿Desde cuándo?	Depuis quand?
Right	Derecha	A droite
Left	Izquierda	A gauche
More or less	Más o menos	Plus ou moins
How long?	¿Cuánto tiempo?	Combien de temps?
Not much	No mucho	Pas beaucoup
Try again.	Trate otra vez.	Essayez encore une fois.
Never	Nunca	Jamais
Never mind.	Olvídelo.	Ça ne fait rien.
That will do.	Suficiente.	Ça suffit.
About how much daily?	¿Más o menos qué cantidad diaramente?	A peu près combien par jour?

English	Spanish	French
Seasons		
Spring	Primavera	Printemps
Summer	Verano	Été
Autumn	Otoño	Automne
Winter	Invierno	Hiver
Months		
January	Enero	Janvier
February	Febrero	Février
March	Marzo	Mars
April	Abril	Avril
May	Mayo	Mai
June	Junio	Juin
July	Julio	Juillet
August	Agosto	Août
September	Septiembre	Septembre
October	Octubre	Octobre
November	Noviembre	Novembre
December	Diciembre	Décembre
Days of the Week		
Sunday	Domingo	Dimanche
Monday	Lunes	Lundi
Tuesday	Martes	Mardi
Wednesday	Miércoles	Mercredi
Thursday	Jueves	Jeudi
Friday	Viernes	Vendredi
Saturday	Sábado	Samedi
Numbers and Time		
One	Uno	Un
Two	Dos	Deux
Three	Tres	Trois
Four	Cuatro	Quatre
Five	Cinco	Cinq
Six	Seis	Six
Seven	Siete	Sept
Eight	Ocho	Huit
Nine	Nueve	Neuf
Ten	Diez	Dix
Twenty	Veinte	Vingt
Thirty	Treinta	Trente
Forty	Cuarenta	Quarante
Fifty	Cincuenta	Cinquante
Sixty	Sesenta	Soixante
Seventy	Setenta	Soixante-dix
At 10:00	A las diez	A dix heures
At 2:30	A las dos y media	A deux heures et demie
Early in the morning	Temprano por la mañana	De bon matin
In the daytime	En el día	Pendant la journée
At noon	Al mediodía	A midi
At bedtime	Al acostarse	A l'heure de se coucher
At night	Por la noche	Le soir
With meals	Con las comidas	Avec les repas
Before meals	Antes de las comidas	Avant les repas
After meals	Después de las comidas	Après les repas
Today	Hoy	Aujourd'hui
Tomorrow	Mañana	Demain
Every day	Todos los días	Chaque jour
Every other day	Cada dos días	Tous les deux jours
Every hour	Cada hora	Chaque heure

English	*Spanish*	*French*
How long have you felt this way?	¿Desde cuándo se siente así?	Depuis quand vous sentez-vous comme ça?
It came all of a sudden?	¿Vino de repente?	Ça vous est arrivé tout à coup?
For how many days or weeks?	¿Cuántos días o semanas?	Depuis combien de jours ou semaines?
Do they come every day?	¿Los tiene todos los días?	Ça vous gêne tous les jours?
At the same hour?	¿A la misma hora?	A la même heure?
At intervals?	¿De vez en cuando?	De temps à autre?
It will be too late.	Será demasiado tarde.	Çe sera trop tard.

Colors

English	Spanish	French
Black	Negro	Noir
Blue	Azul	Bleu
Green	Verde	Vert
Pink	Rosado	Rose
Red	Rojo	Rouge
White	Blanco	Blanc
Yellow	Amarillo	Jaune

Parts of Body

English	Spanish	French
In the abdomen	En el vientre	Dans l'abdomen
The ankle	El tobillo	La cheville
The arm	El brazo	Le bras
The back	La espalda	Le dos
The bones	Los huesos	Les os
The chest	El pecho	La poitrine
The ears	Los	Les oreilles
The elbow	El codo	Le coude
The eye	El ojo	L'oeil
The foot	El pie	Le pied
The gums	Las encías	Les gencives
The hand	La mano	La main
The head	La cabeza	La tête
The heart	El corazón	Le coeur
The leg	La pierna	La jambe
The liver	El hígado	Le foie
The lungs	Los pulmones	Les poumons
The mouth	La boca	La bouche
The muscles	Los músculos	Les muscles
The neck	El cuello	Le cou
The nerves	Los nervios	Les nerfs
The nose	La nariz	Le nez
The penis	El pene	Le pénis
The perineum	El perineo	Le périnée
The rectal area	La parte rectal	La partie rectale
The ribs	Las costillas	Les côtes
The shoulder blades	Las paletillas	Les omoplates
The side	El flanco	Le côté
The skin	La piel	La peau
The skull	El cráneo	Le crâne
The stomach	El estómago	L'estomac
The teeth	Los dientes	Les dents
The temples	Las sienes	Les tempes
The thigh	El muslo	La cuisse
The throat	La garganta	La gorge
The thumb	El dedo pulgar	Le pouce
The tongue	La lengua	La langue
The wrist	La muñeca	Le poignet
The vagina	La vagina	Le vagin

English	Spanish	French

HISTORY

Family

English	Spanish	French
Are you married?	¿Es Ud. casado?	Etes-vous marié?
A widower?	¿Viudo?	Veuf?
A widow?	¿Viuda?	Veuve?
Do you have children?	¿Tiene Ud. hijos?	Avez-vous des enfants?
Are they still living?	¿Viven todavía?	Sont-ils encore vivants?
Do you have any sisters?	¿Tiene hermanas?	Avez-vous des soeurs?
Do you have any brothers?	¿Tiene hermanos?	Avez-vous des frères?
Of what did your mother die?	¿De qué murió su madre?	De quoi est morte votre mère?
And your father?	¿Y su padre?	Et votre père?
Your grandfather?	¿Su abuelo?	Votre grand-père?
Your grandmother?	¿Su abuela?	Votre grand-mère?

General

English	Spanish	French
Do you have . . . ?	¿Tiene . . . ?	Avez-vous . . . ?
Have you ever had . . . ?	¿Ha tenido . . . ?	Avez-vous jamais eu . . . ?
Chills	Escalofrios	Les frissons
Dizziness	El vértigo	Le vertige
Shortness of breath	Corto de aliento	Essoufflement
Night sweats	Sudores de noche	Transpiration dans la nuit
An attack of fever	Un ataque de calentura	Une attaque de fièvre
Toothache	Dolor de muelas	Mal aux dents
Hemorrhage	Hemorragia	Hémorragie
Hoarseness	Ronquera	Enrouement
Nosebleeds	Hemorragia por la nariz	Saignements de nez
Unusual vaginal bleeding	Hemorragia vaginal fuera de los períodos	Du saignement vaginal anormal
When did you last have a period?	¿Cuándo tuvo Ud. su última menstruación?	Quand avez-vous eu vos règles pour la dernière fois?
Are you menopausal?	¿Padece de la menopausia?	Passez-vous par la ménopause?
Are you on hormone therapy?	¿Sigue un tratamiento hormonal?	Faites-vous un traitment hormonal?
Do you take birth control pills?	¿Toma. Ud. píldoras anticonceptivas?	Est-ce que vous prenez des médicaments anticonceptionnels?
How many pregnancies (abortions or miscarriages) have you had?	¿Cuántos embarazos (abortos, abortos involuntarios) ha tenido Ud.?	Combien de grossesses (avortements, fausses couches) avez-vous eu?
How many living children do you have? What are their ages?	¿Cuántos hijos vivos tiene Ud.? ¿Cuántos años de edad tienen?	Combien d'enfants vivants avez-vous? Quel âge ont-ils?
Any difficulties in pregnancies? Deliveries?	¿Dificultades con el embarazo? ¿En el parto?	Des difficultés avec la grossesse? Avec l'accouchement?
Do you have any sexual difficulties?	¿Tiene problemas sexuales?	Avez-vous des problèmes sexuels?

Work History

English	Spanish	French
What work do you do?	¿Cuál es su ocupación?	Quelle est votre profession?
Is it heavy physical work?	¿Es un trabajo corporal pesado?	Est-ce que c'est un travail physiquement fatigant?
What work have you done?	¿Qué trabajo ha hecho?	A quoi avez-vous travaillé?

English	*Spanish*	*French*

Diseases

English	Spanish	French
What diseases have you had?	¿Qué enfermedades ha tenido?	Quelles maladies avez-vous eu?
What type of allergy (types of allergies) do you have?	¿Qué clase de alergia tiene Ud.?	Quelle sorte d'allergie avez-vous?
What is the reaction?	¿Cuál es la reacción?	Quelle est la réaction?
What is the treatment?	¿Cuál es el tratamiento?	Quel est le traitement?
Anemia	Anemia	L'anémie
Bleeding tendency	Tendencia a sangrar	Une tendance à saigner
Bowel problems	Problemas de vientre (evacuación)	Problèmes au ventre (évacuation)
Broken bones	Huesos partidos	Des os cassés
Cancer	Cáncer	Le cancer
Chicken pox	Varicela	La varicelle
Diabetes	Diabetes	Le diabète
Diphtheria	Difteria	La diphthérie
German measles	Rubéola	Rubéole
Gonorrhea	Gonorrea	La gonorrhée
Heart disease	Enfermedad del corazón	Une maladie de coeur
High blood pressure	Presión sanguínea elevada	La tension artérielle trop élevée
HIV (AIDS)	HIV (SIDA)	HIV (SIDA)
Influenza	Gripe (influenza)	La grippe
Injuries	Daños	Blessures
Lead poisoning	Envenenamiento con plomo	Empoisonnement causé par le plomb
Liver disease	Enfermedad del hígado	Une maladie de foie
Malaria	Malaria (paludismo)	La malaria
Measles	Sarampión	La rougeole
Mental disease	Enfermedades mentales	Une maladie mentale
Mumps	Paperas	Les oreillons
Nervous disease	Enfermedades nerviosas	Une maladie nerveuse
Pleurisy	Pleuresía	Une pleurésie
Pneumonia	Pulmonía	Pneumonie
Rheumatic fever	Reumatismo (fiebre reumática)	La fièvre rhumatismale
Rheumatism	Reumatismo	Le rhumatisme
Scarlet fever	Escarlatina	La fièvre scarlatine
Seizures	Ataques	Des crises
Skin rashes	Erupciones de la piel	Eruptions de la peau
Smallpox	Viruela	La variole
Syphilis	Sífilis	La syphilis
Tuberculosis	Tuberculosis	Tuberculose
Typhoid fever	Tifoidea	La fièvre typhoide
What immunizations have you had?	¿Qué inmunizaciones ha tenido Ud.?	Quelles immunisations avez-vous eu?

EXAMINATION

General

English	Spanish	French
How do you feel?	¿Cómo se siente?	Comment vous sentez-vous?
Good	Bien	Bien
Bad	Mal	Mal
Let me look at . . . ; listen to your heart/lungs.	Déjeme reconocerle el corazón/los pulmones.	Permettez-moi de vous examiner le coeur/les poumons.
Let me feel your pulse.	Déjeme tomarle el pulso.	Permettez-moi de vous tâter le pouls.
Let me check your temperature.	Déjeme tomarle la temperatura.	Permettez-moi de vous prendre la température.
Whisper: one, two, three.	Repita en voz baja: uno, dos, tres.	Dites tout bas: un, deux, trois.

English	*Spanish*	*French*
Say it out loud.	Dígalo en voz alta.	Dites-le à voix haute.
Sit down.	Siéntese.	Asseyez-vous.
Stand up.	Levántese.	Levez-vous.
Walk a little way.	Ande algunos pasos.	Faites quelques pas.
Turn back and come this way.	Dé la vuelta y regrese por aquí.	Faites demi-tour et revenez par ici.
Do you feel like falling?	¿Le parece que se va a caer?	Vous sentez vous comme si vous allez tomber?
Do you feel dizzy?	¿Tiene Ud. vértigo?	Avez-vous le vertige?
Are you tired?	¿Está Ud. cansado?	Êtes vous fatigué?
Do you exercise? What type? How often? How long?	¿Hace ejercicio? ¿De qué tipo? ¿Con qué frecuencia? ¿Por cuánto tiempo?	Prenez-vous de l'exercice? De quelle sorte? Combien de fois? Pour combien de temps?
Do you sleep well?	¿Duerme Ud. bien?	Dormez-vous bien?
Do you wake up feeling rested?	¿Se despierta Ud. descansado(a)?	Vous réveillez-vous bien reposé(e)?
Do you have any difficulty in breathing?	¿Tiene dificultad para respirar?	Avez-vous du mal à respirer?
Have you lost weight?	¿Ha perdido Ud. peso?	Avez-vous maigri?
How long have you had this skin rash?	¿Desde cuándo tiene Ud. esta erupción en la piel?	Depuis quand avez-vous cette éruption sur la peau?
Are you usually (now) cold?	¿Tiene Ud. frío usualmente (ahora)?	Avez-vous froid d'habitude (maintenant)?
Are you usually (now) warm?	¿Tiene Ud. calor usualmente (ahora)?	Avez-vous chaud d'habitude (maintenant)?
Can you swallow easily?	¿Puede Ud. tragar facilmente?	Pouvez-vous avaler facilement?
Have you a good appetite?	¿Tiene Ud. buen apetito?	Avez-vous bon appétit?
Are you thirsty?	¿Tiene sed?	Avez-vous soif?
Do you feel weak?	¿Se siente Ud. débil?	Vous sentez-vous faible?
Had you been drinking alcohol? Have you been drinking alcohol?	¿Había tomado Ud. alcohol? ¿Ha tomado Ud. alcohol?	Aviez-vous bu de l'alcool? Avez-vous bu de l'alcool?
Do you drink wine? Beer? Whisky? Gin? Rum? Vodka? Something else?	¿Toma Ud. vino? ¿Cerveza, whisky, gin, ron, vodka? ¿Otra cosa?	Buvez-vous du vin? Bière, whisky, gin, rhum, vodka? Quelque chose d'autre?
Are you a drinking person?	¿Toma Ud. bebidas alcohólicas normalmente?	Buvez-vous de l'alcool d'habitude?
How much do you drink at one time?	¿Cuánto toma Ud. cada vez?	Combien buvez-vous chaque fois?
How often do you drink? Every day? On weekends?	¿Con qué frecuencia toma Ud.? ¿Cada día? ¿El fin de semana?	Combien de fois buvez-vous? Tous les jours? Le weekend?
Do you smoke tobacco? Cigarettes? Pipe? Cigars?	¿Fuma Ud. tobaco? ¿Cigarrillos? ¿Pipa? ¿Cigarros?	Fumez-vous le tabac? Cigarettes? Pipe? Cigares?
How many do you smoke per day?	¿Cuántos fuma Ud. al día?	Combien fumez-vous par jour?
For how many years?	¿Por cuántos años?	Depuis combien d'années?
Do you inhale?	¿Traga Ud. el humo?	Avalez-vous la fumée?
Do you use caffeine? What beverages?	¿Usa Ud. la cafeína? ¿Qué bebidas?	Prenez-vous de la caféine? Quelles boissons?
How much/how frequently?	¿Cuántas/con qué frecuencia?	Combien/combien de fois?
What drugs do you take (prescriptions, over-the-counter, street)?	¿Qué medicinas/drogas toma Ud. (recetas, sin-recetas, droga de la calle)?	Quels médicaments/drogues prenez-vous (ordonnances, sans-ordonnance, drogues de la rue)?

English	*Spanish*	*French*
Are you nervous?	¿Está Ud. nervioso?	Etes-vous nerveux?
When were you first taken sick?	¿Cuándo le empezó esta enfermedad?	Quand êtes-vous tombé malade d'abord?
How did this illness begin?	¿Cómo empezó esta enfermedad?	Comment cette maladie a-t-elle commencé?
Did you take anything for it?	¿Tomó algo para mejorarla?	Avez-vous pris quelque chose pour cela?
Have you taken the (any) medicine?	¿Ha tomado Ud. la (alguna) medicina?	Avez-vous pris du (quelque) médicament?
Did it (the medicine) help?	¿Le ayudó (la medicina)?	Il vous a fait du bien (le médicament)?
Did a dog bite you?	¿Le mordió un perro?	Est-ce qu'un chien vous a mordu?
Did an insect sting you?	¿Le picó un insecto?	Un insecte vous a piqué?
Did you prick yourself with a pin?	¿Se ha pinchado con un alfiler?	Vous êtes-vous piqué avec une épingle?
Did you burn yourself?	¿Se quemó?	Vous êtes-vous brûlé?
Did you twist your ankle?	¿Se torció Ud. el tobillo?	Vous êtes-vous tordu la cheville?

Pain

English	*Spanish*	*French*
Have you any pain?	¿Tiene dolor?	Avez-vous mal quelque part?
Show me where it hurts.	Enséñeme donde le duele.	Montrez-moi où vous avez mal.
Does it move to another area?	¿Se mueve para otra parte?	Cela se déplace à un autre endroit?
What did you feel in the beginning?	¿Qué sentía cuando empezó?	Qu'avez-vous senti au commencement?
Sharp pain	Dolor agudo	Elancement
Shooting pains	Dolores agudos	Des élancements
Dull pain	Dolor sordo	Douleur sourde
Heavy aching pain	Dolor continuo fuerte	Grosse et vive douleur
Is the pain always there?	¿Le duele constantemente?	Ça vous fait mal continuellement?
Does it come and go?	¿Se va y vuelve?	Ça s'en va et revient?
How bad is the pain now? usually?	¿Cuánto le duele ahora? ¿Usualmente?	Combien de mal avez-vous maintenant? D'habitude?
Small/little	Un poco/muy poco	Un peu/très peu
Very bad	Muchísimo	Beaucoup
In between	Así, así	Entre les deux
Does anything make it worse?	¿Hay algo que lo hace peor?	Quelque chose le rend pire?
Does anything make it better/easier?	¿Hay algo que lo hace mejor/más fácil?	Quelque chose le rend mieux/plus facile?
Is the pain better since the medicine I gave you?	¿El dolor está mejor con la medicina que le di?	La douleur va mieux depuis le médicament que je vous ai donné?
A little better? A lot?	¿Un poco mejor? ¿Mucho mejor?	Un peu mieux? Beaucoup mieux?

Head

English	*Spanish*	*French*
How does your head feel?	¿Cómo siente la cabeza?	Comment va votre tête?
Can you remember things that happened?	¿Puede Ud. recordar lo que le ha pasado?	Pouvez-vous vous souvenir de ce qui s'est passé?
Can you remember what you did today? day? Last month/year? Many years ago?	¿Puede Ud. recordar lo que hizo hoy? ¿Ayer? ¿El mes/año pasado? ¿Muchos años atrás?	Pouvez-vous vous souvenir de ce que vous avez fait aujourd'hui? Hier? Le mois dernier? L'année dernière? Il y a beaucoup d'années?
Have you any pain in the head?	¿Le duele la cabeza?	Avez-vous mal à la tête?

English	Spanish	French
Did you fall?	¿Se cayó?	Etes-vous tombé?
How did you fall?	¿Cómo se cayó?	Comment êtes-vous tombé?
Did you faint?	¿Se desmayó?	Vous êtes-vous évanoui?
Have you ever had fainting spells?	¿Ha tenido desmayos alguna vez?	Avez-vous jamais eu des évanouissements?
Do you feel dizzy?	¿Tiene Ud. vértigo?	Avez-vous le vertige?
	Ears	
Do you have ringing in the ears?	¿Le pitan los oídos?	Avez-vous des bourdonnements d'oreilles?
Can you hear me speaking? [Examiner then repeats more loudly and more softly.] [Examiner should look for discharge from ears rather than ask about it.]	¿Puede Ud. oírme cuando hablo?	Pouvez-vous m'entendre quand je parle?
	Eyes	
Do you wear eyeglasses? Contact lenses? What type?	¿Usa Ud. anteojos? ¿Lentes de contacto? ¿Qué tipo?	Portez-vous des lunettes? Des verres de contact? Quelle sorte?
When did you last have your eyes examined?	¿Cuándo fue la última vez que le examinaron los ojos?	Quand est-ce que vous vous êtes fait examiner les yeux la dernière fois?
Look up.	Mire para arriba.	Regardez en haut.
Look down.	Mire para abajo.	Regardez en bas.
Look toward your nose.	Mire la nariz.	Regardez le nez.
Look at me.	Míreme.	Regardez-moi.
Can you see what is on the wall?	¿Puede ver lo que está en la pared?	Pouvez-vous voir ce qu'il y a contre le mur?
Can you see it now?	¿Puede verlo ahora?	Le voyez-vous maintenant?
And now?	¿Y ahora?	Et maintenant?
What is it?	¿Qué es esto?	Qu'est-ce que c'est?
Tell me what number it is.	Dígame qué número es éste.	Dites-moi quel est le numéro.
Tell me what letter it is.	Dígame qué letra es ésta.	Dites-moi quelle est la lettre.
Can you see clearly?	¿Puede ver claramente?	Pouvez-vous voir clairement?
Better at a distance?	¿Mejor a cierta distancia?	Mieux à distance?
(Can you see) better at close range?	¿Puede Ud. ver mejor de cerca?	Pouvez-vous voir mieux de près?
Is your vision cloudy? Blurred? Double?	¿Tiene Ud. la vista velada? ¿Borrosa? ¿Doble?	Avez-vous la vue trouble? Voilée? Double?
Do you see haloes/rings around things?	¿Ve Ud. halos/anillos alrededor de las cosas?	Voyez-vous des halos/ronds autour des choses?
Do you see flashing lights?	¿Ve Ud. destellos?	Voyez-vous des lumières à éclats?
Does light (sun) bother your eyes?	¿La luz (el sol) le molesta los ojos?	La lumière (le soleil) vous gêne les yeux?
Do(es) your eye(s) hurt? Sting? Burn? Itch?	¿Le duele(n) el ojo (los ojos)? ¿Le pica(n)? ¿Está(n) irritado(s)? ¿Le arde(n)?	Avez-vous mal à l'oeil (aux yeux)? Cela pique, brûle, démange?
Can you read?	¿Puede Ud. leer?	Pouvez-vous lire?
Can you read a newspaper/newsprint?	¿Puede Ud. leer el periódico?	Pouvez-vous lire le journal?

English	*Spanish*	*French*
Do your eyes water a good deal?	¿Le lagrimean mucho los ojos?	Est-ce que les yeux vous coulent beaucoup?
Can't you open your eye?	¿No puede abrir el ojo?	Ne pouvez-vous pas ouvrir l'oeil?
Did anything get into your eye?	¿Le entró algo en el ojo?	Est-ce que quelque chose est entré dans l'oeil?
Does the eyeball feel as if it were swollen?	¿Le parece que el ojo está hinchado?	L'oeil vous semble-t-il gonflé?
Wear this patch (shield) on your eye [give time frame].	Use Ud. este parche en el ojo.	Mettez-vous ce couvre-oeil.
It would harm your eyes.	Le haría daño a los ojos.	Cela vous abîmerait les yeux.
How long has your eyesight been failing?	¿Desde cuándo ha bajado su vista?	Depuis quand diminue votre vue?
	Nose, Throat, and Mouth	
How long have you been hoarse?	¿Desde cuando está Ud. ronco(a)?	Depuis quand êtes-vous enroué(e)?
Can you breathe through your nose?	¿Puede Ud. respirar por la nariz?	Pouvez-vous réspirer par le nez?
Can you breathe through each nostril?	¿Puede Ud. respirar por cada ventana de la nariz?	Pouvez-vous réspirer par chaque narine?
Open your mouth.	Abra la boca.	Ouvrez la bouche.
Can you swallow easily?	¿Puede Ud. tragar facilmente?	Pouvez-vous avaler facilement?
Does it hurt you to open your mouth?	¿Le duele al abrir la boca?	Ouvrir la bouche vous fait-il mal?
Do you go to (have you been to) a dentist?	¿Consulta Ud. (ha consultado) a un dentista?	Consultez-vous (avez-vous consulté) un OW
Do you go regularly? When was the last time?	¿Lo consulta regularmente? ¿Cuándo fue la última vez?	Vous le consultez regulièrement? Quand a été la dernière fois?
Do you brush your teeth?	¿Se lava Ud. los dientes?	Vous lavez-vous les dents?
Do you floss?	¿Usa Ud. hilo dental?	Utilizez-vous le fil dentaire?
Do you wear dentures?	¿Usa Ud. dentadura postiza?	Portez-vous des dentiers?
Please remove your denture(s).	Por favor, quítese la(s) dentadura(s).	S'il vous plaît, enlevez le(s) dentier(s).
Take a deep breath.	Respire profundamente.	Respirez profondément.
Cough.	Tosa.	Toussez.
Cough again.	Tosa otra vez.	Toussez encore une fois.
How long have you had this cough?	¿Desde cuándo tiene la tos?	Depuis quand avez-vous la toux?
Is it worse at night? In the morning?	¿Está peor por la noche? ¿Por la mañana?	C'est pire dans la nuit? Pendant le matin?
Do you expectorate much?	¿Escupe mucho?	Crachez-vous beaucoup?
What is the color of your expectorations?	¿De qué color es el esputo?	De quelle couleur sont vos crachats?
Does your tongue feel swollen?	¿Siente Ud. la lengua hinchada?	Est-ce que la langue vous paraît gonflée?
Do you have a sore throat?	¿Le duele la garganta?	Avez-vous mal à la gorge?
Does it hurt to swallow?	¿Le duele al tragar?	Ça vous fait mal quand vous avaler?
	Upper Extremities	
Let me see your hand.	Enséñeme la mano.	Montrez-moi la main.
Grasp my hand.	Apriete mi mano.	Serrez-moi la main.
Squeeze (my hand) harder.	Apriete Ud. (mi mano) más fuerte.	Serrez-moi (la main) plus fort.

English	Spanish	French
Can you not do it better than that?	¿No puede hacerlo más fuerte?	Vous ne pouvez pas serrer plus fort que cela?
Your arm feels paralyzed?	¿Parece que el brazo está paralizado?	Est-ce que le bras vous paraît paralysé?
Raise your arm.	Levante el brazo.	Levez le bras.
Raise it more.	Más alto.	Plus haut.
Now the other.	Ahora el otro.	Maintenant l'autre.
Hold both arms out in front of you and push against my hand.	Extienda los brazos delante de Ud. y empuje contra mi mano.	Tendez vos bras devant vous et poussez contre ma main.
Your arm feels weak?	¿El brazo le parece débil?	Le bras vous semble faible?
How long have you had no strength in your arm?	¿Desde cuándo no tiene fuerza en el brazo?	Depuis quand vous n'avez pas de force dans le bras?
Had you been sleeping on your arm?	¿Ha dormido encima del brazo?	Vous êtes-vous endormi sur le bras?

Cardiopulmonary

English	Spanish	French
Do you experience a rapid (irregular) heartbeat?	¿Siente el latido del corazón rápido (irregular)?	Eprouvez-vous le battement du coeur rapide (irrégulier)?
Do you have pain in your chest? Your jaw? Your arm?	¿Le duele el pecho? ¿La mandíbula? ¿El brazo?	Avez-vous mal à la poitrine? A la mâchoire? Au bras?
Do you get short of breath? With exertion?	¿Se le corta la respiración? ¿Después de un esfuerzo?	Vous vous essoufflez? Après de l'effort?
Do you breathe more easily sitting upright?	¿Respira mejor cuando está sentado?	Respirez-vous mieux quand vous êtes assis?
How many pillows do you need to sleep?	¿Cuántas almohadas necesita Ud. para dormir?	Vous avez besoin de combien d'oreillers pour dormir?
Does it hurt you to breathe?	¿Le duele cuando respira?	Vous avez mal quand vous respirez?
Do you breathe in dust or chemicals at home? At work?	¿Respira Ud. polvos o productos químicos en casa? ¿En el trabajo?	Respirez-vous des poussières ou des produits chimiques chez vous? Au travail?
Do you cough up mucus (phlegm/sputum)?	¿Tose mocos (flema/esputo)?	Toussez-vous gras (flegme/crachats)?
What is the color of your sputum?	¿De qué color es el esputo?	De quelle couleur sont les crachats?
[Examiner should demonstrate any desired motion for patient.]		

Gastrointestinal

English	Spanish	French
Do you have stomach cramps?	¿Tiene calambres en el estómago?	Avez-vous des crampes de l'estomac?
How long has your tongue been that color?	¿Desde cuándo tiene la lengua de ese color?	Depuis quand votre langue a-t-elle cette couleur?
Have you a pain in the pit of your stomach?	¿Tiene dolor en la boca del estómago?	Est-ce que ça vous fait mal dans le creux de l'estomac?
Does eating make you vomit?	¿El comer le hace vomitar?	Rendez-vous ce que vous mangez?
Are you constipated?	¿Está estreñido?	Etes-vous constipé?
Do you have diarrhea?	¿Tiene diarrea?	Avez-vous la diarrhée?
Do you pass any blood?	¿Con sangre?	Y-a-t-il du sang?
Do you belch gas?	¿Eructa Ud. (gases)?	Eructez-vous (des gaz)?
Do you have burning pain (indigestion)?	¿Padece Ud. de la rescoldera (indigestión)?	Avez-vous des brûlures d'estomac (indigestions)?

English	*Spanish*	*French*
What have you been eating? How much? How often?	¿Qué come? ¿Cuánto? ¿Con qué frecuencia?	Qu'est-ce que vous mangez? Combien? Combien de fois?
Are your stools formed? Soft? Hard? Liquid?	¿Cómo son sus evacuaciones de vientre? ¿Sueltas? ¿Duras? ¿Líquidas?	Comment sont vos évacuations de ventre? Molles? Dures? Liquides?
When do you usually have a bowel movement?	¿Cuándo evacúa el vientre usualmente?	Quand évacuez-vous le ventre d'habitude?
Do you pass gas?	¿Suelta gases del vientre?	Lâchez-vous des gaz du ventre?
Do you pass stools involuntarily?	¿Evacúa el vientre sin querer?	Evacuez-vous le ventre involontairement?
Do you feel nauseated (sick to your stomach)?	¿Tiene náuseas (asco grande)?	Avez-vous la nausée (mal au coeur)?
Have you been vomiting? How long? How many times?	¿Ha vomitado? ¿Desde cuándo? ¿Cuántas veces?	Avez-vous vomi? Depuis quand? Combien de fois?
What does the vomitus look like?	¿A qué se parece el vómito?	A quoi ressemble le vomissement?
Is the vomitus (or stool) brown? Black?	¿Es de color café el vómito (o la evacuación)? ¿Negro?	Le vomissement est brun (ou la selle)? Noir?

Genitourinary

English	*Spanish*	*French*
Have you any difficulty passing water?	¿Tiene dificultad en orinar?	Avez-vous de la difficulté à uriner?
Do you pass water involuntarily?	¿Orina sin querer?	Urinez-vous involontairement?
Are any of your limbs swollen?	¿Están hinchados algunos de sus miembros?	Avez-vous des membres gonflés?
How long have they been swollen like this?	¿Desde cuándo estan hinchados así?	Depuis quand sont-ils gonflés comme ça?
Were they ever swollen before?	¿Han estado hinchados alguna vez antes?	Ont-ils jamais été gonflés autrefois?
What color is your urine? Is it clear?	¿De qué color es su orina? ¿Clara?	De quelle couleur est votre urine? Claire?
Do you have any burning when you urinate?	¿Le arde al orinar?	Cela brûle quand vous urinez?
Do you have vaginal itching? Burning? Discharge?	¿Tiene irritación vaginal? ¿Sensaciones ardientes? ¿Derrames?	Avez-vous de l'irritation vaginale? Sensations de chaleur? Ecoulements?
What does the discharge look like?	¿A qué se parece el derrame?	A quoi ressemblent les écoulements?
Do your breasts hurt?	¿Le duelen los senos?	Avez-vous mal aux seins?
Are there any lumps?	¿Hay alguna masa?	Il y a des grosseurs?
Is there any discharge from the nipples?	¿Hay derrame de los pezones?	Les bouts des seins écoulent?
Were they ever swollen before?	¿Han estado hinchados antes?	Ils ont été gonflés avant?
Have you ever breastfed? Are you breastfeeding?	¿Ha criado al pecho alguna vez? ¿Cría al pecho ahora?	Avez-vous allaité un enfant? Vous allaitez maintenant?

Back and Lower Extremities

English	*Spanish*	*French*
Is your movement limited in any way?	¿Está Ud. limitado para moverse de alguna forma?	Etes-vous limité pour vous déplacer de quelque manière?
Do your legs/feet hurt? Feel cold? Numb?	¿Le duelen las piernas/los pies? ¿Sensación de frío? ¿Entumecidas/entumecidos?	Avez-vous mal aux jambes/aux pieds? Sensation de froid? Engourdies/engourdis?

English	Spanish	French
Do you have pins and needles?	¿Tiene sensaciones de pinchazos?	Eprouvez-vous des fourmillements?
Is the pain/symptom worse when you walk?	¿El dolor/síntoma está peor cuando Ud. anda?	La douleur/le symptôme est pire quand vous marchez?
Is it eased when you stop walking?	¿Se alivia cuando deja de andar?	Ça se calme quand vous arrêtez de marcher?
Raise your right leg (your left leg) (both legs).	Levante su pierna derecha (su pierna izquierda) (las dos piernas).	Levez la jambe droite (la jambe gauche) (les deux jambes).
Bend your knees.	Doble las rodillas.	Pliez les genoux.
Wiggle your toes.	Mueva los dedos (de pie).	Remuez les doigts (de pied).
Do you have back pain? Where?	¿Le duele la espalda? ¿Dónde?	Avez-vous mal au dos? Oú?
Bend forward at the waist.	Inclínese hacia adelante.	Penchez-vous en avant.
Bend from side to side. [Examiner should demonstrate desired motion for patient.]	Inclínese de lado en lado.	Penchez-vous d'un côté à l'autre.
I need to check other pulses in your legs.	Necesito tomarle otros pulsos en sus piernas.	J'ai besoin de vous tâter d'autres pouls dans vos jambes.

TREATMENT

General

English	Spanish	French
It is nothing serious.	No es nada grave.	Ce n'est rien de grave.
You will get better.	Ud. se mejorará.	Vous vous remettrez.
You will need to follow these directions.	Tiene Ud. que seguir estas instrucciones.	Vous devez suivre ces indications.
You will need to take this medicine until it is finished.	Tiene Ud. que tomar esta medicina hasta que se le acabe.	Il faut prendre ce médicament jusqu'à le terminer.
You will need to take this treatment until your doctor (nurse) tells you to stop.	Tiene Ud. que seguir este tratamiento hasta que el médico (la enfermera) diga que lo deje.	Vous devez suivre ce traitement jusqu'à ce que le médecin (l'infirmière) vous dise de l'arrêter.
Take a bath.	Tome un baño.	Prenez un bain.
A sponge bath.	Un baño de esponja.	Un bain à l'éponge.
An oatmeal bath.	Un baño de harina de avena.	Un bain de farine d'avoine.
A cornmeal bath.	Un baño de harina de maíz.	Un bain de farine de maïs.
Soak in warm water (for 20 minutes three times a day for the next week). [Length and duration of treatment are specified.]	Báñese en agua caliente (por 20 minutos tres veces al día durante la semana que viene).	Baignez-vous dans de l'eau chaude (pour 20 minutes trois fois par jour pendant la semaine prochaine).
Apply ice (for 20 minutes of every hour for the next 2 days). [Length and duration of treatment are specified.]	Ponga hielo (por 20 minutos de cada hora durante los 2 próximos días).	Mettez de la glace (pour 20 minutes de chaque heure pendant les 2 jours suivants).
Wash the wound with . . .	Lave la herida con . . .	Lavez la blessure avec . . .
Apply a bandage to . . .	Ponga un vendaje a . . .	Mettez un bandage à . . .
Keep the bandage dry and clean.	Mantenga el vendaje limpio y seco.	Gardez le bandage propre et sec.
Wash your hands thoroughly before and after treatment (caring for the wound/applying drops).	Lávese las manos completamente antes y después del tratamiento (cuidando la herida/aplicando gotas).	Lavez-vous les mains complètement avant et après le traitement (soignant la blessure/applicant les gouttes).

English	Spanish	French
Apply ointment (lotion/cream/powder).	Aplíquese ungüento (loción, crema, polvos).	Appliquez un onguent (lotion, crème, poudre).
Keep very quiet.	Estése muy quieto.	Restez tranquille.
You must not speak.	No debe hablar.	Vous ne devez pas parler.
Swallow small pieces of ice.	Trague pedacitos de hielo.	Avalez de petits morceaux de glace.
	Diet	
In a few days you may eat food.	Dentro de algunos días podrá comer.	Après quelques jours vous pouvez prendre de la nourriture.
You will need to eat a special (high-protein/low-fat/diabetic) diet.	Tiene que estar a una dieta de (alta proteína/baja grasa/diabética).	Vous devez suivre un régime de (haute protéine/basses graisses/diabétique).
You may eat . . .	Puede comer . . .	Vous pouvez manger . . .
Soft foods only.	Solamente comida blanda.	Seulement de la nourriture molle.
Your regular diet when your symptoms are gone.	Su dieta normal cuando terminados sus síntomas.	Votre régime normal quand vos symptômes seront terminés.
You may drink . . .	Puede tomar . . .	Vous pouvez boire . . .
Water	Agua	De l'eau
Clear liquids (tea, bouillon, Jell-O)	Líquidos claros (té, caldo, Jell-O)	Liquides clares (thé, bouillon, Jell-O)
All liquids including milk and juices	Todo líquido, inclusive leche y jugo	Toute liquide, lait et jus y compris
No caffeine (coffee, tea, chocolate, cola)	Ninguna cafeína (café, té, chocolate, cola)	Pas de caféine (café, thé, chocolat, cola)
Only decaffeinated drinks	Unicamente bebidas descafeínadas	Seulement les boissons décaféinées
	Surgery	
You will need an operation on your . . . (to remove . . .)	Tendrá Ud. que operarse en su . . . (para quitarle . . .)	Il faut que l'on vous fasse une opération (pour enlever votre . . .)
You will need tests before the operation (blood tests, chest radiograph, electrocardiogram).	Tendrá que hacerse análisis antes de la operación (análisis de sangre, radiografía del pecho, electrocardiograma).	Il faut que l'on vous fasse des analyses avant l'opération (analyse du sang, radiographie de la poitrine, electrocardiogramme).
[Examiner explains nature of tests and tells patient when and where they will be given.]		
You will be in the hospital for [length of time].	Ud. estará en el hospital por [cuanto tiempo].	Vous resterez à l'hôpital pour [combien de temps].
[Examiner tells patient when and where the surgery will take place.]		
	Medication (use with Numbers and Time)	
I will give you something for that.	Le daré algo para eso.	Je vous donnerai quelque chose pour cela.
I will leave a prescription.	Le dejaré una receta.	Je laisserai une ordonnance.
Use it as directed [give dosing intervals] until it is gone (until you are told to stop).	Tómelo según indicado [intervalo de dósis] hasta terminarlo (hasta que se le diga dejarlo).	Prenez-le [intervalle de dose] jusqu'au bout (jusqu'à ce que l'on vous dise d'arrêter).

English	Spanish	French
Take 1 teaspoonful three times daily (in water).	Tome 1 cucharadita tres veces al día, con agua.	Prenez-en une cuillerée à café trois fois par jour (avec de l'eau).
Take 1 tablespoonful.	Tome una cucharada.	Prenez-en une cuillerée à soupe.
Mix in [amount] of water (juice) and drink the entire amount.	Mescle en [cantidad] de agua (jugo) y beba lo todo.	Mélangez avec [quantité] d'eau jus) et buvez le tout.
Gargle.	Haga gárgaras.	Gargarissez-vous.
Inject the drug into your abdomen (arm, leg, buttock, muscle tissue).	Inyéctese la medicina en el abdomen (el brazo, la pierna, la nalga, el tejido muscular).	Faites-vous une piqûre du médicament dans l'abdomen (le bras, la jambe, la fesse, le tissu musculaire).
Insert the suppository into your rectum (vagina).	Métase el supositorio en el recto (la vagina).	Mettez le suppositoire dans votre rectum (votre vagin).
A pill	Una píldora	Une pilule
Do not crush the tablet (open the capsule).	No aplaste el comprimido (no abra la cápsula).	N'écrasez pas le comprimé (n'ouvrez pas la capsule).
Drop [number of drops] into the right (left) eye.	Vierta [número de gotas] en el ojo derecho (izquierdo).	Versez [nombre de gouttes] dans l'oeil droit (gauche).
Drop [number of drops] into each eye.	Vierta [número de gotas] en cada ojo.	Versez [nombre de gouttes] dans chaque oeil.
Who is available to assist you at home? With medications? With diet?	¿Quién está disponible en su casa para atenderle a Ud.? ¿Con las medicinas? ¿Con la dieta?	Qui est disponible chez vous pour vous aider? Avec les médicaments? Avec le régime?
Who is available to transport you to the doctor (hospital) (home)?	¿Quién está disponible para llevarle al médico (hospital) (a casa)?	Qui est disponible pour vous conduire au médecin (à l'hôpital) (chez vous)?

NURSING CARE CONCERNS

English	Spanish	French
Do you need to pass water?	¿Necesita Ud. orinar?	Avez-vous besoin d'uriner?
Do you need to have a bowel movement?	¿Necesita Ud. evacuar el vientre?	Avez-vous besoin d'évacuer le ventre?
Do you need a drink of water?	¿Necesita Ud. tomar agua?	Avez-vous besoin de prendre de l'eau?
Do you need your mouth rinsed?	¿Necesita que le limpien la boca?	Avez-vous besoin de vous faire rincer la bouche?
Do you need something to eat?	¿Necesita Ud. algo de comer?	Avez-vous besoin de manger quelque chose?
Do you need your position changed?	¿Necesita que le cambien de posición?	Avez-vous besoin de vous faire changer de position?
Do you need medicine for pain?	¿Necesita medicina contra el dolor?	Avez-vous besoin d'un médicament pour la douleur?
You will be getting oxygen.	Le van a poner oxígeno.	On va vous donner de l'oxigène.
You will be getting a breathing treatment.	Le van a dar un tratamiento de respiración.	On va vous donner un traitement de respiration.
You will be getting intravenous fluid.	Le van a dar un flúido intravenoso.	On va vous donner un fluide intraveineux.
You will be getting a bland diet.	Le van a poner una dieta blanda.	On va vous mettre au régime simple.
You will be getting an injection.	Le van a dar una inyección.	On va vous faire une piqûre.

APPENDIX 12
Medical Emergencies

Appendix 12–1 Poisons and Poisoning

Substances	*Pathology*	*Symptoms*	*Emergency Measures*	*Comments*
Acetaminophen	Production of toxic intermediate metabolite that cannot be detoxified due to glutathione depletion.	Phase 1 (0–24 hr): Sometimes asymptomatic—anorexia, nausea, vomiting. Phase 2 (24–48 hr): GI symptoms resolve; hepatotoxicity is subclinical, but liver function tests and coagulation tests are abnormal. If liver damage is significant, patient may progress to phase 3. Phase 3 (48–96 hr): Problems due to severe hepatic compromise—bleeding disorders, hypoglycemia, hepatic encephalopathy. Phase 4 (96 hr): Recovery period. Laboratory values return to normal and symptoms resolve.	Gastric lavage. Toxicity is unlikely at a dose <140 mg/kg. For significant serum levels of acetaminophen, acetylcysteine can be administered orally in a loading dose followed by a maintenance regimen.	In general, patients require hospitalization for observation and supportive treatment. Hepatic failure can occur several days after the ingestion, and renal complications or failure can also develop. Most patients recover fully without further sequelae. In some instances, hepatic failure may require transplantation.
Acids Acetic Hydrochloric Nitric Phosphoric Sulfuric Any other strong acid	Immediate destruction and necrosis with eschar formation of mucous membranes and tissues on contact.	Burning pain on contact with mucous membranes of the mouth and throat, dysphagia, abdominal pain, nausea, hematemesis, thirst, esophageal or gastric perforation, shock, death.	Establishment of airway patency, aggressive volume resuscitation, radiographic evaluation of damage, irrigation of exposed tissues. Surgical intervention may be required.	Permanent damage to the esophagus and stomach can result in chronic dysphagia and stricture formation.

Poisons and Poisoning (Continued)

Substance	*Pathology*	*Symptoms*	*Emergency Measures*	*Comments*
Alkalis	Irreversible destruction and liquefactive tissue necrosis that penetrates beyond surface contact with alkali.	Immediate burning and blistering of tissue on contact; severe pain of mouth, esophagus, and chest; esophageal or gastric perforation; pancreatitis; hematemesis; shock; death.	Establishment of airway patency, aggressive volume resuscitation, radiographic evaluation of damage, irrigation of exposed tissues. Surgical intervention may be required.	Permanent damage to the esophagus and stomach can result in chronic dysphagia, stricture formation, and necrosis of tissue.
Ammonia and ammonium hydroxide	Tissue destruction due to alkaline injury on contact with mucous membranes. Degree of destruction depends on alkalinity of product and amount and length of exposure.	Burning of mouth and throat, chest pain, esophageal and gastric damage, hematemesis. Inhalation of gas can cause coughing, bronchospasm, and pulmonary edema.	Airway protection if needed, supplemental humidified oxygen and bronchodilators for inhalation exposures, moderate amounts of water or milk to dilute ingestion, analgesics for pain. Additional procedures may be required to assess extent of tissue injury.	Most significant damage is seen with intentional massive ingestions or occupational exposures to concentrated strengths of ammonia. Most accidental exposures to household strength products resolve without residual damage.
Amphetamines and amphetamine-like agents	Excessive stimulation of the CNS and of peripheral alpha and beta receptor sites.	Excitement, restlessness, tremors, hyperactive reflexes, nausea, vomiting, diarrhea, palpitations, arrhythmias, hypertension, hyperthermia, dehydration, mydriasis, agitation, seizures, coma, death.	Supportive care including airway maintenance and cardiac monitoring; administration of activated charcoal and a cathartic; cooling measures for hyperthermia; benzodiazepines for seizures; vasodilators and beta-adrenergic blockers.	Toxicity can occur with slightly higher than therapeutic doses. Tolerance can readily develop with repeated use.

Antidepressants: selective serotonin reuptake inhibitors (SSRI) Fluoxetine Paroxetine Sertraline	CNS depression, excessive stimulation of serotonin receptors.	Serotonin syndrome: hypomania, confusion, myoclonus, diaphoresis, hyperreflexia, tremor, hyperthermia, agitation, restlessness, insomnia, nausea, vomiting, drowsiness, ataxia, coma.	Maintenance of airway, breathing, and circulation; gastric decontamination with activated charcoal or whole-bowel irrigation; cooling measures. The serotonin antagonists cyproheptadine and methysergide have reportedly been used with success.	These agents are considered relatively safe, even in overdoses. As a class, the SSRIs do cause the anticholinergic effects seen with cyclic antidepressants. However, they are less toxic in excessive doses.
Antidepressants: cyclic Amitriptyline Amoxapine Clomipramine Desipramine Doxepin Imipramine Nortriptyline Protriptyline	Toxic cardiovascular and CNS effects secondary to anticholinergic activity, inhibited reuptake of neurotransmitters, peripheral alpha-adrenergic blockade, alteration of cardiac cells resulting in conduction disturbances.	Confusion, dizziness, altered mental status (lethargy to coma), hypotension, tachycardia, hyperthermia, mydriasis, dry mucous membranes, prolonged QRS complex, cardiac dysrhythmias, seizures.	Cardiac monitoring; gastric decontamination with activated charcoal and cathartic or whole-bowel irrigation. Alkalinization of the urine with bicarbonate-containing solutions.	Death can occur within a few hours of an overdose.
Antihistamines: sedating (major classes) Alkylamines Ethanolamines Ethylenediamines Phenothiazines Piperazines	Excessive central and peripheral anticholinergic effects.	Lethargy, agitation, confusion, miosis, tachycardia, hyperthermia, decreased GI motility, hypotension, respiratory depression, ataxia, stupor, seizures, dysrhythmias, coma, circulatory collapse, death.	Maintenance of airway, breathing, circulation, and fluids for hypotension; gastric decontamination by activated charcoal with cathartic or whole-bowel irrigation. For massive ingestion or if patient is sedated, intubation and gastric lavage followed by activated charcoal and cathartic; IV physostigmine for anticholinergic toxicity; benzodiazepines for seizures.	Most ingestions are complex to manage because many antihistamines are commercially available in combination with various analgesics and decongestants. With early intervention, most overdoses have excellent outcomes without sequelae. Some newer antihistamines have a minimal CNS effect.

Poisons and Poisoning (Continued)

Substance	*Pathology*	*Symptoms*	*Emergency Measures*	*Comments*
Arsenic and arsenic salts	Disruption of enzymatic reactions that are essential for cellular metabolism; possible phosphate replacement or interaction with sulfhydryl groups.	Nausea, vomiting, hemorrhagic gastritis, severe watery diarrhea, dehydration, pulmonary edema, hypotension, delirium, encephalopathy, arrhythmias, convulsions, shock, death. Symptoms may have delayed onset.	Aggressive fluid replacement, activated charcoal or gastric lavage for larger ingestions, dimercaprol (BAL) 3–5 mg/kg IM every 4–6 hr for symptomatic patients.	Toxicity depends on the type of arsenic, amount involved, and route of exposure. Systemic toxicity can result from percutaneous absorption. Arsenic is a carcinogenic agent.
Aspirin —SEE: *salicylates*				
Atropine and anticholinergic agents	Acetylcholine blockade at muscarinic receptor sites; affects exocrine glands and cardiac tissue.	Dry mouth and burning pain in throat, thirst, blurred vision, mydriasis, dry, hot, flushed skin, hyperpyrexia, tachycardia, palpitations, restlessness, excitement, confusion, convulsions, delirium; rarely, death.	Airway maintenance and ventilation assistance, gastric lavage, activated charcoal and cathartic, diazepam for sedation and control of convulsions, physostigmine 0.5–1 mg IV for severe atropine toxicity, cooling measures for hyperthermia.	Classes of drugs that possess anticholinergic activity include antihistamines, antipsychotics, antispasmodics, cyclic antidepressants, and skeletal muscle relaxants. Atropine in ophthalmic preparations may be toxic to infants/young children.
Barbiturates Amobarbital Aprobarbital Butabarbital Mephobarbital Methohexital Pentobarbital Phenobarbital Secobarbital Talbutal Thiopental	Depressed neuronal activity of the brain, hypotension caused by depression of central sympathetic tone, inhibition of cardiac contractility.	Drowsiness, confusion, ataxia, vertigo, slurred speech, shallow respiration and pulse, headache, stupor, hypotension, areflexia, cyanosis, hypothermia, cardiovascular collapse, respiratory arrest, death.	Airway maintenance and ventilation assistance, treatment of hypotension, gastric lavage, activated charcoal and cathartic, alkalinization of urine to enhance phenobarbital elimination, hemoperfusion for severe toxicity.	Severity of toxicity depends on the agent ingested.

Benzene Xylene Toluene	Irritation of mucous membranes and airway caused by agents and their metabolites, CNS depression, myocardial effects resulting in conduction disturbances.	Burning sensation of mouth and stomach, nausea, vomiting, chest pain, cough, headache, pneumonitis (if inhaled), vertigo, ataxia, confusion, stupor, ventricular dysrhythmias, convulsions, coma, respiratory failure, death.	Airway maintenance and ventilation assistance, activated charcoal and cathartic, therapy for arrhythmias and seizures. Gastric lavage within 30 min is useful for larger ingestions.	Chronic exposure can result in permanent renal damage, bone marrow suppression, and neuropsychological damage.
Benzodiazepines Alprazolam Chlordiazepoxide Clonazepam Clorazepate Diazepam Estazolam Flurazepam Lorazepam Midazolam Oxazepam Prazepam Quazepam Temazepam Triazolam	Generalized CNS depressant effects caused by enhanced activity of gamma-aminobutyric acid, an inhibitory neurotransmitter.	Confusion, dizziness, somnolence, ataxia, hypotension, coma, respiratory depression, cardiovascular depression.	Airway maintenance and ventilation assistance, gastric lavage, activated charcoal and cathartic, flumazenil IV administered and repeated to reverse unconsciousness or respiratory depression, fluids and vasopressors for hypotension.	Generally considered safe, even in high doses. Fatalities are rare and usually due to coingestions with other CNS depressants.
Boric acid and borate salts	Exact mechanism of toxicity unknown.	Headache, nausea, vomiting (vomitus may be blue green), fever, oliguria or anuria, diarrhea, stomach pain, lethargy, restlessness, distinctive erythroderma, tremor, convulsions, renal and hepatic injury or failure, cyanosis, coma, shock with vascular collapse, death.	Airway maintenance and ventilatory assistance. Treat convulsions with benzodiazepines. Activated charcoal is not effective. Hemodialysis may sometimes be needed for large ingestions (e.g., more than 12 g).	Reports of toxicity from boric acid ingestions and exposures has declined in recent years due to decreased use as an irrigant and antiseptic agent.

Poisons and Poisoning (Continued)

Substance	*Pathology*	*Symptoms*	*Emergency Measures*	*Comments*
Botulinum toxin	Potent neurotoxicity produced by *Clostridium botulinum;* prevents release of acetylcholine by irreversibly binding to cholinergic nerve terminals.	Nausea, vomiting, occasional diarrhea, dysphagia, diplopia, loss of visual acuity and pupillary reflexes, profuse sweating, rapid and weak pulse, death usually caused by respiratory failure. Symptoms may present up to a week after ingestion.	Airway maintenance and ventilatory assistance, as needed. Trivalent botulism antitoxin may be administered in severe overdoses to bind free toxin, although its use often causes hypersensitivity reactions.	Even with excellent supportive care, recovery may take months to years. Common long-term sequelae include dysgeusia, dry mouth, dyspepsia, constipation, tachycardia, arthralgias, and fatigue. Botulinum antitoxin is available from the local health department or the CDC [(404) 329-2888].
Cadmium salts or fumes	Diverse multisystemic toxicities that are not clearly understood.	Nausea, vomiting, diarrhea, abdominal cramps, salivation, gastritis, headache, vertigo, exhaustion, collapse, acute renal failure, chemical pneumonitis with pulmonary edema on inhalation, death.	Gastric lavage and catharsis, with chelating agents such as EDTA, may be useful in some acute exposures. Inhalation may require ventilatory support.	Long-term effects vary with duration and severity of exposure. Renal function may be affected. Chronic exposures have resulted in osteomalacia, emphysema, and increased risk of lung or prostrate cancer.

Calcium channel blockers Myocardial and vascular effects Bepridil Diltiazem Verapamil Primarily vascular effects Amlodipine Felodipine Isradipine Nicardipine Nifedipine	Prevention of calcium entry into cells, resulting in decreased myocardium contractility, blockade of AV and SA nodes, and peripheral vasodilation.	Nausea, vomiting, dizziness, headache, confusion, stupor, hyperglycemia, hypotension, bradycardia, metabolic acidosis, cardiac conduction disturbances, seizures, coma, death.	Maintenance of airway, breathing, and circulation; fluids and vasopressors for hypotension; gastric lavage and cathartic; multiple-dose activated charcoal; whole-bowel irrigation; calcium chloride or calcium gluconate for hypotension and bradydysrhythmias, atropine or isoproterenol for bradycardia.	Intentional overdoses of calcium channel blockers are life threatening and often fatal despite aggressive management.
Camphor	CNS stimulant with toxic effects; underlying mechanism is not known.	Burning of mouth and throat, nausea, vomiting, headache, CNS hyperactivity followed by CNS depression, vertigo, liver function abnormalities, delirium, tremor, convulsions, apnea, coma, death from respiratory arrest secondary to status epilepticus.	Airway maintenance, gastric lavage with copious amounts of fluid, activated charcoal and cathartic, benzodiazepines for seizures.	Fatalities have been reported with 1- or 2-g doses; however, most exposures can be effectively managed and resolved without residual complications.
Carbon monoxide	Hemoglobin binding preventing delivery of oxygen to cells; has significantly greater affinity for hemoglobin than oxygen.	Mild headache, dyspnea with moderate exertion, irritability, fatigue, nausea, vomiting, confusion, ataxia, syncope, convulsions, death from respiratory arrest.	100% oxygen by face mask or endotracheal tube, IV fluids, cardiac monitoring, hyperbaric oxygen for significant exposures.	Residual effects can include dementia, psychosis, paralysis, peripheral neuropathy, and parkinsonism.

Poisons and Poisoning (Continued)

Substance	*Pathology*	*Symptoms*	*Emergency Measures*	*Comments*
Carbon tetrachloride	Metabolites cause renal and hepatic toxicity; potent CNS depressant effects.	Nausea, vomiting, abdominal pain, headache, confusion, drowsiness, coma, renal and hepatic failure. Death is caused by respiratory arrest, circulatory collapse, or ventricular fibrillation.	Airway maintenance and ventilation assistance, gastric lavage, activated charcoal and cathartic, acetylcysteine to decrease effects of intermediate metabolite.	Toxicity from inhalation can be severe; small ingestions (<10 ml) can be fatal.
Chlorate salts	Potent oxidative properties that destroy red blood cells; toxicity to kidneys are due to direct effects and hemolysis.	Abdominal pain, nausea, vomiting, diarrhea, methemoglobinemia, intravascular hemolysis, delirium, coagulopathy, coma, convulsions, cyanosis, renal failure, death.	Gastric lavage and activated charcoal, methylene blue for mild toxicities, hemodialysis to remove toxin. Sodium thiosulfate IV has been used to inactivate the chlorate ion, with inconsistent results.	In some instances, exchange transfusions have been advocated to reverse effects of poisoning.
Chlorinated compounds Chlorine Chlorine gas Sodium hypochlorite	Corrosive effect on contact with mucous membranes.	Immediate burning of mouth and throat, coughing, choking, bronchospasm, chest and abdominal pain, stridor, pulmonary edema, esophageal burns.	For inhalation, humidified supplemental oxygen and bronchodilators; for dilute ingestions, water or milk; for concentrated ingestions, gastric lavage and endoscopic evaluation.	Esophageal damage can result in stricture formation.

Chlorinated hydrocarbon pesticides Aldrin Chlordane DDT (chlorophenothane) Dieldrin Heptachlor Lindane Thiodan Toxaphene	Direct toxicity to neuronal axons, interfering with transmission; affects myocardium stability resulting in arrhythmias.	Vomiting, headache, fatigue, tremors, ataxia, weakness, confusion, seizures, respiratory depression, arrhythmias, coma. In agents other than DDT, seizure may be first sign of toxicity.	Maintenance of airway, breathing, circulation; activated charcoal and cathartic; lavage for large ingestions; multiple-dose activated charcoal and cholestyramine to enhance removal; appropriate therapy for seizures and arrhythmias.	These agents can be absorbed transdermally and by inhalation. Toxicity and outcomes vary.
Cocaine	CNS stimulation and inhibition of neuronal uptake of catecholamines, depressed conduction, and myocardial contractility.	Anxiety, agitation, delirium, hypertension, tachycardia, hyperthermia, diaphoresis, tremor, mydriasis, flushing, seizures, ECG abnormalities, areflexia, coma, death.	Airway maintenance and ventilatory assistance, cardiac monitoring, activated charcoal or whole-bowel irrigation for ingestion, benzodiazepines, cooling measures.	Cocaine continues to be a popular drug of abuse and a high number of fatalities continue to be reported each year.
Copper salts	Mucous membrane irritation, multisystemic toxicities with salts. Elemental copper is poorly absorbed and causes little toxicity.	Pain in mouth, esophagus, and stomach; abdominal pain; vomiting; gastroenteritis; shock; hepatic and renal injury; hemolysis; seizures; coma; death.	Fluid replacement and pressors, whole-bowel irrigation; dimercaprol and penicillamine for large ingestions.	Long-term copper exposures have resulted in liver fibrosis, cirrhosis, and renal dysfunction.
Cyanide	Nonspecific inhibition of enzyme systems; binds to cytochrome oxidase of cells, blocking oxygen use.	Nausea, vomiting, abdominal pain, almond odor of breath, headache, dyspnea, agitation, confusion, syncope, convulsions, lethargy, coma, cardiovascular collapse, death. Onset of symptoms is abrupt.	Oxygen and assisted ventilation, if needed; gastric lavage, activated charcoal, and cathartic; inhalation of amyl nitrite pearls until antidote is available. Antidote kit contains amyl and sodium nitrites and sodium thiosulfate. The administration of vitamin B_{12} may be helpful.	Delayed neurological sequelae including dystonias and parkinsonism have been reported following acute cyanide poisoning.

Poisons and Poisoning (Continued)

Substance	*Pathology*	*Symptoms*	*Emergency Measures*	*Comments*
Digoxin and digitalis	Excessive excitability and automaticity of myocardium resulting in conduction disturbances and dysrhythmias; AV block.	Anorexia, nausea, vomiting, diarrhea, headache, fatigue, weakness, drowsiness, electrolyte disturbances, confusion, delirium, visual disturbances, dysrhythmias, bradycardia, AV block, death from ventricular fibrillation.	Cardiac monitoring, activated charcoal, digoxin-specific antibody fragments (Fab) for severe toxicity, lidocaine or phenytoin for ventricular irritability. Correct electrolyte abnormalities, such as hypokalemia, immediately.	Most poisonings result from ingestion of prescribed digoxin, esp. in patients with renal failure, hypokalemia, or advanced age.
Dinitrophenol and pentachlorophenol	Uncoupling of oxidative phosphorylation in mitochondria, hypermetabolic state and lactic acid production. Dinitrophenol oxidizes hemoglobin to methemoglobin.	Fatigue, thirst, nausea, vomiting, abdominal pain, sweating, flushing, restlessness, excitement, hyperthermia, tachycardia, hyperpnea, metabolic acidosis, cyanosis, seizures, coma, death from respiratory or circulatory failure.	Maintenance of airway, breathing, circulation; activated charcoal and cathartic; gastric lavage for large ingestions; methylene blue IV; fluid replacement; benzodiazepines; cooling measures.	Ingestion of 1–3 g of these agents can be lethal. Many accidental transdermal poisonings have been reported.
Ergotamines or ergot alkaloids	Central sympatholytic effects: serotonin release and interference with neuronal uptake. Peripherally, may act as a partial alpha-adrenergic agonist or an antagonist at adrenergic, dopaminergic, and tryptaminergic receptors.	Nausea, vomiting, dizziness, diarrhea, headache, thirst, weak pulse, tingling and numbness of extremities, dyspnea, hallucinations, blood pressure changes, hemorrhagic vesiculations, paresthesias, peripheral ischemia, convulsions, loss of consciousness, gangrene.	Protect the airway, and provide ventilatory assistance as needed. Give multiple doses of activated charcoal to enhance drug elimination. Provide benzodiazepines to control seizures. Use nitroglycerin, heparin, or thrombolytics for organ ischemia.	Outcome is based on route and amount of ingestion.

Ethanol	CNS depression; effects can be additive when combined with other CNS depressants.	Impaired motor coordination, slurred speech, inebriation, ataxia, peripheral vasodilation, rapid pulse, nausea, vomiting, drowsiness, stupor, coma, peripheral vascular collapse, hypotension, tachycardia, hypothermia, death from respiratory or circulatory failure.	Provide intravenous fluids, esp. with dextrose, to prevent hypoglycemia. Give patient thiamine. Provide other supportive measures, including airway control and ventilation, external warming, and prophylaxis against alcohol withdrawal symptoms as indicated.	Ethanol is often coingested with other toxic substances in suicide attempts; emergency treatment may vary depending on other substances ingested.
Ethylene glycol	Metabolism to oxalic, glyoxylic, and glycolic acids; conversion to lactate, increasing the lactic acid level; calcium oxalate crystal formation and deposition in tissues; metabolite toxicity to kidneys, CNS, and lungs.	Nausea, vomiting, excitability, hypotension, abdominal cramps, weakness, metabolic acidosis, ataxia, vertigo, arrhythmias, stupor, coma, death from respiratory or renal failure with uremia.	Maintain airway, breathing, and circulation. Provide ethanol, folic acid, 4-methylpyrazole, pyridoxine, and thiamine. Hemodialysis will remove ethylene glycol from the blood in cases of severe toxicity.	Outcomes vary; in general, comatose patients have a poor prognosis.
Fluoride salts	Direct metabolic and cytotoxic effects; multiple adverse effects from calcium and magnesium binding.	Salivation, thirst, nausea, abdominal pain, vomiting, diarrhea, muscle weakness, hypocalcemia, hyperkalemia, tetanic contractions, death due to vascular collapse and shock.	Maintenance of airway, breathing, circulation; cardiac monitoring; calcium salts; for severe toxicity, IV calcium chloride; therapy for electrolyte disturbances.	Degree of toxicity depends on salt solubility and the amount of elemental fluoride ingested. Pediatric toxicities are often caused by fluorinated toothpaste ingestions.

Poisons and Poisoning (Continued)

Substance	*Pathology*	*Symptoms*	*Emergency Measures*	*Comments*
Hydrogen sulfide gas	Inhibition of oxidative phosphorylation enzymes, potent inhibition of cytochrome oxidase. Exposure results in cellular hypoxia.	Irritated mucous membranes, conjunctivitis, headache, nausea, vomiting, weakness, bradycardia, hypotension, dyspnea, rapid loss of consciousness with larger exposure, pulmonary edema, cyanosis, convulsions, coma, death due to cardiac or respiratory arrest.	High-flow oxygen, advanced cardiac life support as indicated, sodium nitrite, blood pressure monitoring, hyperbaric oxygen if available. Methemoglobin level should be recorded 30 min after infusion.	If patient is immediately removed from the exposure, recovery may be rapid and complete. More severe exposures have resulted in permanent neurologic changes and myocardial ischemia.
Ipecac syrup or fluid extract	Cardiac and neuromuscular toxicity with systemic absorption; toxicities are seen with chronic and prolonged use.	Vomiting, diarrhea, lethargy, irritability, hypothermia, hypotonia, dehydration, gastritis, seizures, cardiac toxicity, neuromuscular toxicity, shock, death.	Activated charcoal or gastric lavage for large ingestions, fluid replacement, correction of electrolyte abnormalities, cardiac monitoring, therapy for arrhythmias.	Chronic exposures are reported in patients with eating disorders; cases of toxicity secondary to Munchausen's syndrome by proxy have also been documented.
Iron salts	Several mechanisms: direct corrosive effects on GI mucosa, hepatocellular toxicity, cardiovascular compromise, metabolic acidosis. Neurological manifestations are caused by hypoperfusion, metabolic acidosis, and hepatic compromise.	Nausea, vomiting, severe gastroenteritis, hematemesis, diarrhea, tachypnea, tachycardia, hypotension, lethargy, cyanosis, convulsions, coma, shock, or death.	Use gastric lavage or whole-bowel irrigation to remove tablets from the gastrointestinal tract. Intravenous deferoxamine is used as an iron-chelating agent.	Patients with systemic complications require hospital admission, constant monitoring, and supportive care until resolution. Late complications (2–8 wk) include GI stricture and obstruction. Toxicity is unlikely at a dose <20 mg/kg.

Isopropanol Isopropyl alcohol Rubbing alcohol	Potent CNS depressant metabolized to acetone; may contribute to CNS depression.	Nausea, vomiting, abdominal pain, hypotension, ataxia, areflexia, inebriation, muscle weakness, ketonemia, ketonuria, respiratory depression, hemorrhagic tracheobronchitis, myocardial depression, coma, death.	Maintain airway and provide ventilatory support when neurological depression is present. Do not induce emesis. Irrigate the GI tract after recent ingestions. Use Hemodialysis for near-fatal overdoses.	A majority of cases resolve without sequelae.
Lead and lead salts	Heavy metal interaction with sulfhydryl groups and interference with action of numerous enzymes, interference with heme production and survival of red blood cells. Chronic exposure can cause irreversible CNS and developmental effects.	Abdominal pain, vomiting, lethargy, behavioral changes, ataxia, arthralgias, abdominal or renal colic, anemia, acute encephalopathy, seizures, coma, death.	Use whole-bowel irrigation to empty the GI tract shortly after oral ingestions. Chelating agents that remove lead from the blood include Calcium Disodium Versenate, dimercaprol and related compounds, and D-penicillamine. Seizures are treated with benzodiazepines.	Chronic exposure to lead can produce developmental, renal, and neuropsychiatric effects, esp. in children. Blood lead levels and erythrocyte protoporphyrin levels are used to gauge the effect of treatment.
Lithium	Lithium often produces cellular disturbances in the central nervous system, kidneys, and gastrointestinal tract. This is probably due to its effects on cell membrane ion transport, as well as its effects on cAMP.	Nausea, vomiting, diarrhea, fine resting tremor, lethargy, confusion, tremors, ataxia, ECG abnormalities, profound weakness, muscle fasciculations, hyperreflexia, clonus, stupor, seizures, acute renal failure, coma, death.	Maintain the airway and provide assisted ventilation to patients who are comatose or difficult to arouse. For acute ingestions use gastric lavage or whole bowel irrigation. Activated charcoal is ineffective because it does not bind to metals. Hemodialysis is used to clear lithium from the body in life-threatening intoxications.	Chronic or acute-on-chronic overdoses are more life threatening than acute poisonings. Chronic exposure permits intracellular accumulation. In acute poisonings, most lithium remains in the extracellular fluid for many hours, causing toxicity.

Poisons and Poisoning (Continued)

Substance	*Pathology*	*Symptoms*	*Emergency Measures*	*Comments*
Mercuric salts	Reaction with carboxyl, sulfhydryl, phosphoryl, and amide groups; interference with enzyme and cellular functions; toxicity involving multiple organ systems.	Burning of mouth and throat, thirst, abdominal pain, nausea, corrosive gastroenteritis, hematemesis, diarrhea, dehydration, shock, acute tubular necrosis. Neurological symptoms such as tremor, irritability and other personality changes, and depression are common.	The patient should be treated with oxygen and the gastrointestinal tract decontaminated (e.g., with whole-bowel irrigation). Chelating agents such as dimercaprol, dimercaptosuccinic acid, or D-penicillamine, should be given to bind and remove mercury from the body.	Doses of 1–4 g of mercuric chloride can be fatal. Chronic poisonings have resulted in neurological abnormalities, renal dysfunction, and gastrointestinal symptoms.
Methanol	Metabolism to formaldehyde and formic acid.	Latent period (24–72 hr) before development of symptoms, dizziness, inebriation, blurred vision, headache, nausea, vomiting, abdominal pain, delirium, visual disturbances that may progress to blindness, weak and rapid pulse, shallow respirations, cyanosis, coma, metabolic acidosis, respiratory failure, death.	Activated charcoal for recent ingestion, ethanol IV or orally to inhibit toxic metabolites, hemodialysis in severe cases, aggressive management of metabolic acidosis. Folic acid and 4-methylpyrazole can be used as antidotes.	Visual impairment, optic atrophy, and blindness are due to effects of formic acid on the optic nerve.

Mushrooms containing muscarine *Amanita muscaria* (fly agaric) *Amanita panterina* (panther) *Clitocybe dealbata* (sweater) *Clitocybe dilatata* *Clitocybe illudens* Most *Inocybe* species	Peripheral cholinergic effect due to muscarine; stimulation of autonomic nervous system.	Lacrimation, diaphoresis, salivation, abdominal cramps, vomiting, loss of bowel and bladder control.	Gastric decontamination (with activated charcoal or whole-bowel irrigation) may remove recently ingested mushrooms from the GI tract and prevent absorption. Patients with fulminant hepatic failure will need intensive care and possible referral for liver transplantation.	Identification of ingested mushroom may help guide therapy if uneaten mushroom samples are available for analysis. Patients afflicted with fulminant liver failure have a high risk of death if a donor liver is not available.
Mushrooms containing cyclopeptides *Amanita phalloides* (death cap) *Amanita tennifolia* *Amanita virosa* (destroying angels) *Galerina autumnalis* *Galerina marginata* *Galerina venenata* *Lepiota helveola* *Lepiota josserandii*	Cytotoxicity of cyclopeptides (phallotoxins, amatoxins, virotoxins), cellular insult causing hepatic, renal, GI, and CNS damage.	Phase 1 (6–12 hr): Nausea, abdominal pain, vomiting, watery diarrhea, thirst. Phase 2 (12–24 hr): Symptomatic improvement, elevated hepatic enzymes. Phase 3 (1–6 days): Restlessness, delirium, hallucinations, hematuria, gastroenteritis, pancreatitis, hypoglycemia, shock, acute renal failure, jaundice, hepatic coma, death.	Gastric lavage and multiple-dose activated charcoal every 2–4 hr, activated charcoal hemoperfusion, fluid and electrolyte resuscitation, hepatic transplantation in fulminant hepatic failure.	Cyclopeptide-containing mushrooms are responsible for most mushroom fatalities in North America. Toxic cyclopeptides are heat stable, insoluble in water, and not affected by drying.
Naphthalene	Metabolism to numerous by-products including alpha-napthol, a potent hemolytic agent.	Fever, nausea, vomiting, abdominal pain, diarrhea, lethargy, seizures, hemolysis, pallor, jaundice, cyanosis.	Gastric lavage for larger ingestions, activated charcoal and cathartic, IV hydration and urinary alkalinization, transfusions for hemolysis.	Hemolysis is acute and severe in patients with glucose-6-phosphate dehydrogenase deficiency. Naphthalene is used in mothballs and toilet bowl cleaners, but less toxic agents are available.

Poisons and Poisoning (Continued)

Substance	*Pathology*	*Symptoms*	*Emergency Measures*	*Comments*
Nicotine	Binding to cholinergic nicotine receptors; toxicity due to sympathetic and parasympathetic stimulation followed by ganglionic and neuromuscular blockade.	Nausea, vomiting, abdominal pain, headache, salivation, diarrhea, hyperpnea, diaphoresis, tachycardia, hypertension, pallor, agitation, tremor, ataxia, confusion, dysrhythmias, hypotension, shock, muscle paralysis, coma, death.	Maintenance of airway, breathing, circulation; multiple-dose activated charcoal and cathartic for large oral ingestions; lavage for large, recent liquid ingestions; thorough washing of exposed skin; therapy for seizures, hypertension, hypotension, and arrhythmias.	Because most commercial sources of nicotine are not concentrated, a majority of exposures cause mild toxicity and resolve without complications.
Nitroglycerines, nitrates, nitrites	Vasodilation causing hypotension. Nitrites are potent oxidizing agents that cause methemoglobinemia.	Headache, hypotension, skin flushing, nausea, methemoglobinemia, cyanosis, symptoms of cardiac ischemia or cerebrovascular disease, seizures secondary to hypotension.	Gastric decontamination (e.g., with activated charcoal or whole-bowel irrigation) may remove recently ingested pills from the GI tract and prevent absorption. Other supportive care includes the use of intravenous fluids, anticonvulsant medication, hemodialysis, or therapies for GI bleeding (if needed).	Most cases can be managed successfully with early, aggressive interventions.

Nonsteroidal anti-inflammatory agents Ibuprofen Ketoprofen Naproxen and many others	Inhibition of prostacyclin and prostaglandin E_2 production resulting in acute renal failure.	Nausea, vomiting, gastrointestinal distress and bleeding, tinnitus, metabolic acidosis, CNS depression, respiratory depression, mild hepatic toxicity, acute renal failure, seizures.	Gastric decontamination with activated charcoal, gastric lavage and activated charcoal for those needing intubation; multiple-dose activated charcoal for severe toxicity or ingestion of agents with long half-lives; therapy for seizures.	Baseline renal and hepatic function should be assessed. Most toxic exposures to this class of agents are successfully treated and resolve fully without residual sequelae.
Opioids and Opiates Codeine Fentanyl Heroin Morphine Methadone and other synthetic opioids	Excessive stimulation of CNS opiate receptors causing sedation and respiratory failure.	Drowsiness, nausea, dysphoria, bradypnea, miosis, hypothermia, respiratory depression, hypotension, bradycardia, weak pulse, coma, apnea, death.	The airway should be secured and ventilatory assistance provided to comatose or apneic patients. Naloxone, naltrexone, or nalmefene can be given as an antidote. Gastric decontamination (e.g., with activated charcoal or whole-bowel irrigation) may remove recently ingested pills.	Antidotes are useful in reversing effects of the opiates, but administration may precipitate severe withdrawal symptoms. The effects of naloxone are short-term. The drug may need to be given repeatedly or by intravenous infusion to prevent repeated episodes of respiratory depression or coma.
Oxalic acid and oxalate salts	Corrosion of tissues on contact; precipitation with calcium to form insoluble deposits throughout organs, causing systemic damage.	Irrigation of mouth and esophagus, vomiting, weakness, shock, tetany, convulsions, cardiac arrest, death. Inhalation can cause pneumonitis and pulmonary edema.	Calcium chloride, calcium gluconate, or calcium carbonate to precipitate oxalate; flushing and lavage with copious amounts of water; IV calcium chloride or calcium gluconate for symptomatic hypocalcemia; maintenance of high urine output; therapy for seizures and arrhythmias.	Ingestions of 5–15 g of oxalic acid have resulted in death.

Poisons and Poisoning (Continued)

Substance	*Pathology*	*Symptoms*	*Emergency Measures*	*Comments*
Parathion and other organophosphates	Acetylcholinesterase inhibition, resulting in excessive acetylcholine stimulation of muscarinic and nicotinic receptors.	Nausea, vomiting, diarrhea, abdominal pain, tremor, muscle fasciculations, excessive salivation and sweating, dehydration, bradycardia, weakness, shock, death usually caused by respiratory paralysis.	Maintain airway and clear secretions. Provide assistance with ventilation. Decontaminate exposed skin and remove soaked clothing. Decontaminate the GI tract. Use atropine and/or pralidoxime for anticholinergic crises. Give diazepam or related drugs for seizures, and standard antiarrhythmic protocols for ventricular rhythm disturbances.	Toxicity depends on the relative toxicity of the organophosphate and the quantity involved.
Phenol	Corrosive injury to skin, eyes, and respiratory tract; protein denaturation and coagulation necrosis.	Vomiting, diarrhea, gastrointestinal injury, agitation, confusion, seizures, hypotension, shock, coma, respiratory failure, death.	Multiple-dose activated charcoal and cathartic; washing of exposed areas; benzodiazepines for seizures. Low molecular weight polyethylene glycol has been used for gastric decontamination and topical exposures. If corrosion has occurred, tube passage may cause rupture.	Corrosive burns of the skin and mucous membranes and GI perforation can occur. Esophageal stricture and renal failure rarely occur.

Phenothiazines and neuroleptics	Prominent cardiovascular and CNS effects; toxicity due to inhibitory effects of dopaminergic, cholinergic, alpha-adrenergic, histaminic, and seritonergic receptors.	Sedation, somnolence, stupor, dry mouth, tachycardia, labile blood pressure, hypothermia or hyperthermia, dysrhythmias, extrapyramidal symptoms, coma, NMS, seizures, cardiac arrest, death, akathisias.	Maintain airway and provide ventilatory and circulatory support if necessary. Decontaminate the GI tract. Follow standard ACLS protocols for managing cardiac rhythm disturbances. Give diphenhydramine or benztropine for dystonias. Bromocryptine, benzodiazepines, and/or dantrolene may be helpful in NMS.	Although death from neuroleptic overdose is rare, NMS may be fatal in 20% or more of affected patients.
Phosphorus and phosphides	Local irritation and tissue burns; direct toxic effect to myocardium and vessels; hepatic, renal, and GI damage due to latent systemic toxicity.	Painful burns to mucous membranes and skin on contact, nausea, vomitus and diarrhea with garlicky odor, jaundice, metabolic derangements, dysrhythmias, coma, shock, seizures, hepatic or renal failure, cardiac arrest. Inhalation can cause pneumonitis and pulmonary edema.	Maintenance of airway, breathing, circulation; endoscopy to assess GI burns; cautious gastric lavage with hydrogen peroxide or potassium permanganate, followed by activated charcoal and mineral oil cathartic; fluid replacement and correction of electrolyte imbalance.	After acute effects from ingestion, a symptom-free period of a few weeks may be followed by a stage of systemic toxicity involving the liver, kidneys, heart, CNS, and GI tract.
Salicylates Aspirin Salicylate salts	Effect on multiple organ systems, metabolic derangement. Effects are due to stimulation of respiratory center, intracellular uncoupling of oxidative phosphorylation, and alteration of platelet function.	Nausea, vomiting, agitation, hyperthermia, lethargy, hyperglycemia or hypoglycemia, hyperpnea, tachypnea, tinnitus, hemorrhagic gastritis, delirium, stupor, acid-base disturbances, electrolyte imbalance, cerebral edema, convulsions, cardiovascular collapse.	Maintenance of airway, breathing, circulation; lavage for several hours; multiple-dose activated charcoal; urinary alkalinization; correction of acid-base and fluid-electrolyte abnormalities; hemodialysis for severe toxicity or deteriorating condition.	The prognosis of patients suffering from an acute toxic ingestion can be assessed on the basis of serum levels obtained within 6 hr of ingestion.

Poisons and Poisoning (Continued)

Substance	*Pathology*	*Symptoms*	*Emergency Measures*	*Comments*
Strychnine	Competitive antagonism of glycine at postsynaptic spinal cord motor neuron.	Muscle twitching, extensor spasm, opisthotonos, trismus or facial grimacing, seizures, medullary paralysis, death. Symptoms occur within 20 min.	Gastric lavage and activated charcoal, dark and quiet environment, benzodiazepines or neuromuscular blockade, mechanical ventilation.	Poisonings are rare since commercial use in rodenticides has decreased. Most exposures result in death. The approximate fatal dose for a child is 15 mg; for an adult, 5–10 mg/kg.
Thallium salts	Combination with mitochondrial sulfhydryl groups, interference with oxidative phosphorylation.	Nausea, vomiting, abdominal pain, hematemesis, bloody diarrhea, headache, alopecia, hematuria, proteinuria, elevated hepatic enzymes, lethargy, tremors, ataxia, delirium, seizures, coma, death.	Syrup of ipecac or gastric lavage; activated charcoal with sorbitol; fluid, electrolyte, and glucose treatment to prevent shock; benzodiazepines for seizures. Hemoperfusion and hemodialysis may be moderately successful.	Alopecia and Mee's sign, single white transverse lines on the nails 2–3 weeks postexposure, are common diagnostic features. Long-term neurological impairment can occur.

Theophylline —SEE: *xanthine derivatives*				
Xanthine derivatives Aminophylline Caffeine Theophylline	Antagonism of adenosine activity and release of catecholamines; in high doses, phosphodiesterase inhibition. Toxic effects are secondary to smooth muscle relaxation, peripheral vasodilation, myocardial stimulation, and CNS excitation.	Nausea, protracted vomiting, hypotension, respiratory alkalosis, metabolic acidosis, hypokalemia, tachycardia, hypercalcemia, ventricular dysrhythmias, seizures, death due to cardiovascular collapse.	Decontaminate the GI tract (with activated charcoal or whole-bowel irrigation). For deteriorating conditions or severe intoxications, charcoal hemoperfusion enhances removal of the drug. Treat seizures with benzodiazepines or barbiturates, and cardiac rhythm disturbances with standard ACLS protocols. Monitor theophylline levels several times a day.	Eliminate drugs that increase theopylline levels, such as erythromycins or related antibiotics, cimetidine, estrogens, or allopurinol. Consider use of safer drugs for obstructive lung diseases, such as albuterol or other inhaled medications.
Warfarin and related anticoagulant compounds	Inhibition of vitamin K 2,3-epoxide reductase and quinone reductase activity (these are necessary to activate vitamin K, which is essential in coagulation).	Fatigue, hematuria, nosebleeds, ecchymoses, GI hemorrhage, hypotension, intracranial hemorrhage, hemorrhagic shock, death (rare).	Decontaminate the GI tract (for recent ingestions only). Hold warfarin if the protime is slightly elevated and no bleeding is present. Give vitamin K for markedly prolonged protimes, or fresh frozen plasma for life-threatening bleeding.	Most accidental ingestions resolve without further sequelae. Intentional ingestions or delay in seeking treatment may result in severe coagulopathy. Symptomatic patients require hospitalization and aggressive therapy to prevent hemorrhage.

AV = atrioventricular; BAL = British anti-lewisite; CNS = central nervous system; ECG = electrocardiogram; EDTA = ethylenediamenetetra-acetic acid; GI = gastrointestinal; NMS = neuroleptic malignant syndrome; PT = prothrombin time; SA = sinoatrial.

Appendix 12–2 Substances Generally Nontoxic When Ingested*

Adhesives	Lipstick
Barium sulfate	Magnesium silicate (antacid)
Bathtub toys (floating)	Matches
Blackboard chalk (calcium carbonate)	Methylcellulose
Bromide salts	Mineral oil (if not aspirated)
Candles (insect-repellent type may be toxic)	Modeling clay
Carbowax (polyethylene glycol)	Oxide salts
Carboxymethylcellulose (dehydrating material packed with drugs, film, etc.)	Paraffin, chlorinated
Castor oil	Pencil lead (graphite)
Cetyl alcohol	Pepper, black (except inhaled in mass)
Chloride salts	Petrolatum (Vaseline)
Contraceptives	Play-Doh®
Crayons (children's: marked A.P., C.P., or C.S. 130–46)	Polyethylene glycols
Detergents, anionic and nonionic	Polyethylene glycol stearate
Dichloral (herbicide)	Polysorbate (Tweens®)
Dry cell battery	Putty
Glycerol	Red oil (turkey-red oil, sulfated castor oil)
Glyceryl monostearate	Shaving cream
Graphite	Silica (silicon dioxide)
Gums (acacia, agar, ghatti, etc.)	Spermaceti
Hormones	Stearic acid
Ink (amount in one ballpoint pen)	Sweetening agents
Iodide salts	Talc (except when inhaled)
Kaolin	Tallow
Lanolin	Thermometer fluid (including liquid mercury)
Lauric acid	Titanium oxide
Linoleic acid	Triacetin (glyceryl triacetate)
Linseed oil (not boiled)	Vitamins, children's multiple (with or without iron)
	Vitamins, multiple without iron

* This table is intended only as a guide; substances may be present in combination with phenol, petroleum, distillate vehicles, or other toxic chemicals. A poison control center should be consulted for up-to-date information.

SOURCE: The Merck Manual, Ed. 17, Merck & Co. Inc., 1999, with permission.

Appendix 12–3 Emergency Situations

Medical Emergency	*Underlying Causes*	*Findings*	*Treatment*
Acute myocardial infarction (MI, AMI)	Most heart attacks are caused by the rupture of a plaque in the wall of the coronary artery that results in the blockage of blood flow and the death of myocardial tissue. Risk factors often present include tobacco use, hypertension, hypercholesterolemia, diabetes mellitus, or family history of heart disease. Men and postmenopausal women are at greater risk than premenopausal women. Modification of risk factors lowers the risk for disease.	Usually, tightness, pressure, heaviness, or burning in the chest. Pain may radiate to the neck, jaw, back, or arms. Often the patient feels short of breath. Palpitations, nausea, and vomiting may occur. Breath sounds may have crackles, indicating congestive heart failure. A new heart murmur may be present. Pulses may become thready. Skin may be pale and clammy. A 12-lead ECG may show evidence of an MI (up to 40% of patients may have a nondiagnostic ECG initially). Cardiac enzymes, such as creatine kinase and troponins, may be elevated when the patient presents for care, or may rise to diagnostic levels during the first 24 hours.	Oxygen, aspirin, beta blockers, nitrates, morphine, heparin, glycoprotein IIB/IIIA antagonists, thrombolytic (clot-busting) drugs, and ACE inhibitors may be used acutely. Cardiac monitoring, an oximeter, and automatic blood pressure monitors are used to identify changes in hemodynamic and respiratory status. Angioplasty may be used to open the blocked blood vessel. Other treatments may depend on the presentation (e.g., the patient in shock may be treated with pressors); the patient in full cardiac arrest is treated with standard life support protocols.
Airway obstruction	Complete or partial obstruction of the oropharynx or nasopharynx, larynx, or trachea, with impairment of gas exchange, caused by foreign bodies, anatomical abnormalities, allergic reactions, infection, or trauma.	Signs of respiratory distress or choking are often present. The patient appears agitated, may grasp at his or her throat, appear cyanotic, or make labored, ineffective efforts to breathe. Loss of consciousness may occur if the obstruction is not relieved within a few minutes.	Foreign body airway obstruction is treated using the Heimlich maneuver in adults and back blows and chest thrusts in infants and children. Endotracheal intubation or cricothyroidotomy, along with mechanical ventilation, may be lifesaving interventions.

Emergency Situations (Continued)

Medical Emergency	*Underlying Causes*	*Findings*	*Treatment*
Angina pectoris	Inadequate supply of oxygen to the myocardium when oxygen demand exceeds supply. Unstable angina, marked by more frequent attacks, pain with less exertion or at rest, reduced response to nitroglycerin, or more severe episodes may indicate a progression in the patient's coronary artery disease and a higher risk for MI. Stable angina is discomfort typical of the patient's usual pattern.	Similar to MI. Chest discomfort typically resolves in less than 15 min, and improves with nitroglycerin and rest. There may be evidence of ischemia on a 12-lead ECG. Cardiac enzymes will not demonstrate the characteristic pattern of an MI.	Oxygen, nitroglycerin, and aspirin are the initial therapies. Heparin is used in unstable angina when there are no contraindications. Generally the patient with unstable or new-onset angina will require risk assessment, either in the hospital or as an outpatient. Cardiac catheterization, to define the patient's coronary anatomy, is usually performed.
Asthma	Episodic bronchospasm, caused by exposure to allergens (such as pollens), smoke, pollutants, cold air, exercise, or other triggers of airway inflammation.	Difficulty breathing, wheezing, and chest tightness. Patients are often able to identify the triggering event. They may report that their inhalers are not providing adequate relief. Physical findings include tachycardia and labored breathing. Patient may be frightened, agitated, or, in the final stages of a severe attack, sleepy. Lung sounds have a prolonged expiratory phase. The most common sound will be wheezes. In severe cases there may be no lung sounds.	Emergency treatment includes the administration of supplemental oxygen and bronchodilators such as albuterol, sometimes in combination with ipratropium. Epinephrine may be injected subcutaneously in severe cases. Oral or intravenous steroids are helpful in reducing the return of symptoms once the acute attack has been aborted. Severe cases may require intubation.

Chronic Obstructive Pulmonary Disease (COPD), exacerbation of	An acute or gradual worsening of pulmonary function in patients with chronic lung disease, typically brought on by a viral or bacterial infection, or by congestive heart failure, allergies, pulmonary emboli, or the rupture of an emphysematous bleb at the margins of the lung.	Patients typically report increased shortness of breath, cough, sputum production, and fevers, and appear to labor more than usual to breathe. Tachypnea, tachycardia, and hypoxemia or carbon dioxide retention are often present. Breath sounds may be distant, or wheezing may be present.	Oxygen is supplied (e.g., at 1 L/min), but careful monitoring of blood gases may be needed to avoid decreasing a patient's drive to breathe. Bronchodilators such as albuterol and ipratropium are given by inhalation. Corticosteroids and antibiotics are often administered. Theophylline may be used in low doses or with careful monitoring by some patients.
Cold-induced soft tissue injury (frostnip, chilblain, frostbite)	*Frostnip:* superficial, reversible injury caused by ice crystal formation on the surface of the skin. *Chilblain:* superficial injury caused by exposure to cold, humid air. Tissue does not freeze. *Frostbite:* destruction of tissue by freezing. The extent of tissue loss reflects the duration of cold exposure and the magnitude of temperature depression.	*Frostnip:* usually, paresthesias, pain, and numbness. *Chilblain:* redness, itching, numbness, burning, and pain. *Frostbite:* similar to chilblain. Frostbitten skin may be waxy and white or mottled and cyanotic. The frozen part will have no sensation. Surrounding tissue may be painful and tender. As the tissue thaws its appearance changes. In partial-thickness frostbite the skin becomes red and warm. Blisters containing clear fluid may appear. In full-thickness frostbite the blisters contain a bloody fluid. There is no sensation in full-thickness frostbite.	Initial treatment involves removing the patient from the cold environment. Concomitant hypothermia is a hazard. The frozen parts should not be rewarmed if there is danger of refreezing. Rapid rewarming should be performed by soaking the injured part in warm water (42°C). Rubbing or other manipulation of frozen tissue may worsen the injury. Further treatment may be needed for more serious injuries.

Emergency Situations (Continued)

Medical Emergency	*Underlying Causes*	*Findings*	*Treatment*
Congestive heart failure (CHF)	An impairment in the ability of the heart to move blood into the systemic circulation, either because of damage to heart muscle (e.g., example after a heart attack), failure of the heart muscle to relax properly, pericardial restriction, valvular heart disease, or other causes.	Most patients are winded with exertion, and some are short of breath at rest. Many cannot lie flat in bed at night because the supine position makes them breathless. Lower extremity and sacral swelling are common physical findings, along with ascites, liver enlargement, and elevated jugular veins. Crackles or wheezes may be heard in the lung bases or throughout the lungs in left ventricular CHF. The patient is often hypoxemic. Chest x-rays may show an enlarged heart with fluffy infiltrates near the hila.	Oxygen, potent diuretics, morphine sulfate, nitroglycerin, and ACE inhibitors may be used to manage CHF or acute pulmonary edema as long as the patient is not hypotensive. Hypotensive patients may be treated with dobutamine, combinations of dopamine and nitroprusside, or other drugs and interventions.
Gastrointestinal (GI) bleeding	Upper gastrointestinal bleeding often results from esophagitis, esophageal tears, gastritis, peptic ulcer disease, esophageal varices, or vascular malformations. Lower GI bleeding typically is caused by hemorrhoids, anal fissures, diverticuli, vascular malformations, or cancers.	The rapidly bleeding patient may present in shock (i.e., dizzy on arising, hypotensive, tachycardic, cool, clammy, diaphoretic, and confused). Bleeding from the upper GI tract often reveals itself when the patient vomits bright red blood or digested blood that resembles coffee grounds. Occasionally, bleeding from the upper tract is so vigorous that it causes the loss of bright red blood from the rectum. Usually, however, this is a finding in lower GI bleeding. Digested blood that is expelled in the feces is typically black and tarry (melenic).	Significant blood loss will require intravenous fluids and possibly blood transfusions. A cause of the bleeding must be sought.

Hyperglycemia	Elevated blood sugars are usually caused by impairments in glucose metabolism (type 1 or type 2 diabetes mellitus, gestational diabetes mellitus, or drugs or infections that temporarily predispose patients to high blood sugars). In diabetic patients, sudden elevations of blood sugar are typically the result of the failure to maintain a careful dietary and medical regimen, the taking of medications (such as corticosteroids), or a serious infection.	Patients often report thirst, frequent urination, increased appetite, and increased consumption of fluids. Those who become dehydrated may be dizzy when they get up from a bed or chair. Blood chemistries typically reveal a blood glucose of more than 200 mg/dl, and glucose is present in the urine.	Fluids are administered by mouth (if possible) and intravenously. Insulin or oral hypoglycemic agents are given.
Hyperthermia (heat cramps, heat exhaustion, heatstroke)	Inability of the body to cope with heat stress resulting from excessive heat production or decreased heat loss. *Heat cramps:* muscle cramps and fatigue accompanied by water and mild salt depletion. *Heat exhaustion:* serious dehydration with water and electrolyte depletion. Patients maintain thermoregulatory control. Heat exhaustion may progress to *heatstroke,* characterized by thermoregulatory failure and profound dehydration.	The person with heat cramps complains of painful muscle spasms. There is a history of recent exertion in a hot environment. The patient has been sweating profusely with inadequate or hypotonic fluid replacement. The patient with heat exhaustion has also been sweating in a hot environment. Symptoms include thirst, weakness, fatigue, vomiting, and anorexia. The skin is cool and clammy. Body temperature may be normal or subnormal. The heatstroke victim will have an altered mental status and will be tachycardic, hypotensive, hyperthermic, and tachypneic. Signs of dehydration will be present.	First aid begins with removal of the patient from the hot environment. Heat cramp victims are treated with an oral or intravenous fluid and electrolyte solution. Heat exhaustion is treated by intravenous fluids. Patients with severe dehydration may require more than 4 L of IV fluid. Patients with heatstroke require rapid cooling. Many techniques are available, but evaporation with water is practical and effective. The patient may be sprayed with water and fanned until the core temperature is about 38.5°C. Cooling beyond this may cause overshoot hypothermia. IV fluid resuscitation as for heat exhaustion is also needed.

Emergency Situations (Continued)

Medical Emergency	*Underlying Causes*	*Findings*	*Treatment*
Hypoglycemia	The most frequent causes are an excessive dose of insulin or an oral hypoglycemic agent, or inadequate food intake by a diabetic patient treated with those drugs (e.g., during an illness that causes anorexia, nausea, or vomiting). Low blood sugars deprive the brain and other organs of the glucose they need for normal metabolism.	Mental status may vary from confused to agitated to unconscious. The patient is often sweaty, tremulous, and tachycardic. Occasionally, hypoglycemia may mimic strokes or seizures.	Glucose or dextrose should be given immediately—intravenously if the patient is unable to safely eat, orally if the patient is conscious and sufficiently oriented. One mg of glucagon, administered by intramuscular injection, is an alternative. Blood sugar levels should be tested with a glucometer. Hospitalization may be necessary if the patient has taken an overdose of long-acting insulin or an oral antihyperglycemic agent.
Hypothermia	Core temperature less than 35°C (95°F), caused by decreased heat production, increased heat loss, or impaired temperature regulation. Exposure to cold or wet conditions, sepsis, or profound hypothyroidism may be predisposing conditions. Central nervous system, cardiovascular, and respiratory systems are impaired when the temperature is below 35°C.	Lethargy, confusion, and fatigue in mild cases. Heart rate and respiratory rate may be increased. As hypothermia worsens, the patient stops shivering. Heart rate, blood pressure, and respirations slow. The patient eventually loses consciousness. Respirations and pulses may be difficult to detect.	Cold or wet clothing should be removed. The patient should be rewarmed. Warm blankets, warm oxygen, and warm IV fluids may be used. An accurate core temperature must be recorded, if possible. Temperatures less than 32°C may require more aggressive rewarming techniques, such as gastric lavage, peritoneal lavage, hemodialysis, or cardiopulmonary bypass. If pulses are absent, cardiopulmonary resuscitation is indicated.

Seizure	An abnormal electrical discharge by central nervous system neurons that produces autonomic, behavioral, motor, or sensory abnormalities. Seizures may result from structural diseases of the brain (e.g., arteriovenous malformations, strokes, trauma, or tumors), from metabolic disorders (e.g., severe electrolyte disorders, low blood sugars, renal failure, or hypoxia), or from drugs (or drug or alcohol withdrawal).	During a generalized motor seizure, the patient is unconscious and has repetitive back-and-forth movements of the upper and lower extremities. Patients may bite the tongue, lose control of the bowels or bladder, or injure themselves when they fall. After the seizure, there is usually a period of gradual and progressive return to normal consciousness, which may take 30 to 60 min. Some patients may have a brief period of focal paralysis after the event.	During the seizure, the patient should be guarded against injury. This may involve helping the patient to the floor and moving furniture out of the way. Supplemental oxygen should be given. Objects should not be inserted into the patient's mouth—an obstructed airway may result. The patient cannot swallow the tongue. Medications such as diazepam or phenytoin may be used. Most seizure patients will require some investigation into the cause of the seizure. In patients with a history of prior seizures, this may include checking blood levels of antiseizure medications. Patients with first-time seizures may need a more extensive evaluation, including a CT scan, an EEG, blood work, and a lumbar puncture.
Stroke (cerebrovascular accident)	Inadequate blood flow to an area of the brain causing tissue death. In thrombotic stroke, blood vessels narrowed by atherosclerosis limit delivery of oxygenated blood to the brain or a portion of it. In embolic stroke, clots travel from other areas of the body to block cerebral vessels. Hemorrhagic stroke results from bleeding caused by hypertension or rupture of cerebral aneurysms.	Patients often present with weakness or numbness on one side of the body or the face; with speech disturbances; or with confusion, clumsiness, difficulty walking, loss of consciousness, or coma.	Oxygen is administered and cardiac monitoring is begun. A computed tomographic (CT) scan of the brain is used to rule out a hemorrhage as a cause of new neurological deficits. Tissue plasminogen activator (a thrombolytic, or "clot-busting" drug) may be given to patients who present in the first 3 hr of nonhemorrhagic stroke.

Emergency Situations (Continued)

Medical Emergency	*Underlying Causes*	*Findings*	*Treatment*
Thermal burns	*First- and second-degree burns:* partial-thickness injuries involving only the epidermis or the epidermis and dermis. *Third-degree burns:* full-thickness injuries involving the deeper tissues. Burns impair the skin's ability to prevent heat and water loss. Burned skin is not an effective barrier to injection. Severity depends on the character and temperature of the agent, the duration of exposure, and the type of skin injured.	*First-degree burns:* red and painful. *Second-degree burns:* red, painful, and weeping. These burns heal without scarring. *Third-degree burns:* may be white or charred. The subcutaneous nerves have been destroyed; thus there is no pain. Surrounding areas are painful. Full-thickness burns heal poorly, leaving a scar.	The first step is to stop the burning process. Oxygen should be administered if there has been smoke inhalation. Jewelry and clothing should be removed in anticipation of swelling. Sterile sheets or dressings should be applied to the burned areas.
Transient ischemic attack (TIA)	See *Stroke*.	Symptoms and signs are similar to those of a stroke, but usually last less than 1 or 2 hr.	Patients with TIAs are treated with antiplatelet therapies, such as aspirin or clopidogrel, and are evaluated with electrocardiographic monitoring (e.g., to rule out atrial fibrillation), CT scans of the head (to rule out small strokes), and carotid ultrasonography (to determine whether the patient has a surgically correctable stenosis of the carotid arteries).

APPENDIX 13
Computer Glossary

AI *artificial intelligence.*
ALT *alternate.*
alternate ABBR: ALT. A board key that, when depressed in conjunction with other keys, sends a code to the computer instructing it to perform an operation.
American Standard Code for Information Interchange SEE: *ASCII.*
America Online A popular Internet service and content provider.
AOL *America Online.*
application A software package or program that performs a set of tasks (e.g., word processing, graphics, spreadsheet).
artificial intelligence ABBR: AI. The ability of a computer or other machine to simulate intelligent thought or behavior.
ASCII *American Standard Code for Information Interchange;* a basic format for storing and transferring text-based materials from one computer or software package to another.
attribute A characteristic of an electronic file (e.g., read only, system, hidden).
audio Sounds produced by computers equipped with sound cards and speakers (beyond simple beeps that can occur without a sound card). Computer audio can include text-to-speech translation used by disabled people to communicate.
streaming a. The transmission of a continuous stream of audio data (over the Internet or other network connection) that is buffered and then played through appropriate media player software. The effect is similar to a radio broadcast received by the computer.
autoexec.bat A file used by DOS on IBM-type computers on start-up to discover instructions that should be executed automatically. Installation programs of many software packages modify this file to facilitate the operation of the computer.
axis Either of the two lines on a bar or line graph that act as the scale. The horizontal line is the X axis; the vertical line is the Y axis. Line graph format is often used to record the length of hospital stays.
backup A copy of a file, program, or disk made to prevent loss of data.
bandwidth The speed or capacity of the electronic connection of a network or modem, expressed in bits per second—that is, kilobits per second (Kbps) or megabits per second (Mbps).
basic input/output system ABBR: BIOS. Information stored on a chip that determines how data are channeled into and out of the computer through the central processing unit chip. SEE: *central processing unit.*
bat *batch file.*
batch file SEE: under *file.*
battery A chip that maintains information relating to the configuration of the computer. It contains essential origination and setup information and is maintained by a battery.
baud One pulse per second.
b. rate The speed of data transmission via a modem, expressed in kilobits per second. Higher baud rates indicate faster transmission.
BBS *bulletin board service.*
benchmark A standard against which machine-operating parameters are compared. It is used to test the speed of a computer and its processor.
binary system A number system to "base" the system used by all microcomputers. All of the information placed into a computer is in binary form, that is, numbers made up of zeros and ones (0 and 1). In this system each "place" in a binary number represents a power of 2 (i.e., the number of times 2 is to be multiplied by itself).
BIOS *basic input/output system.*
bit Abbreviation for *binary digit.* Computers work with binary numbers (bytes) made up of zeros and ones (0 and 1). A bit is one digit in a binary number. SEE: *binary system; byte.*
bitmap A graphic image stored as a pattern of dots. Some graphic image files are referred to as bitmap images; such files are identified by the extension *.bmp.*
bits per second ABBR: bps. The number of bits transmitted in a second. SEE: *bit.*
board SEE: *circuit board; clipboard; motherboard.*
boilerplate Text that has been prepared in one document and stored for use in others. Boilerplating is convenient for forms, headings, contract language, and paragraphs of standard text used frequently in various documents.
bookmark **1.** A method of marking a particular place in a document so that you can find it easily. **2.** A method of saving a Web address (URL) to a personal list of often used sites in a Web browser.
boot To start or restart a computer. All information stored in random access memory is erased, and the machine executes all initiation instructions.
cold b. Initiation of a machine system by turning the computer off and then on again.
hot b. Reinitiation of a program or machine system without turning off the main power switch. This is done most often by the concurrent pressing of the control, alternate, and delete (CTRL-ALT-DEL) keys. Also called *warm boot.*

bps *bits per second.*

broadband Relating to a high-speed, high-bandwidth connection to the Internet (e.g., ISDN, cable modem, or DSL).

browser A program that allows navigation through the resources of the World Wide Web. The two best known Web browsers are Netscape Navigator and Microsoft's Internet Explorer, but there are others, such as Oracle, Mosaic, and Opera.

Web b. A program that provides an interface to the World Wide Web.

buffer A temporary storage area of computer memory that holds data until it can be processed (e.g., by a printer).

bug A fault in a program instruction that causes malfunction of the computer or program.

bulletin board service ABBR: BBS. A computer messaging system, accessed by modem, that allows users to post messages to an electronic "bulletin board," join in newsgroup discussions, and exchange files.

byte A unit of data usually composed of eight bits. It takes one byte to represent an ASCII character. SEE: *binary system*; *bit*.

cable A flexible set of metal wires or glass fibers encased in a protective sheath used to connect computers into a network or to an Internet service provider.

coaxial c. A two-wire cable consisting of a central conducting core, an insulating layer, a braided external conducting layer, and a protective sheath used to connect computers in Ethernet networks or, via cable modem, to a cable TV system's connection to the Internet.

cache A method of storing data in a section of temporary random access memory. This method is used for storing instructions to a hard disk or video card to facilitate processing speed.

CAD *computer-assisted design.*

card A hard plastic, sometimes glass-reinforced, board on which all circuit components are mounted and electrically "wired" to each other by printed copper paths. Numerous types of boards provide graphics representation, color capability, boost of storage capacity, and other features to a computer. SYN: *circuit board.*

graphics c. A circuit board enabling display of graphic images.

network interface c. ABBR: NIC. A circuit board card placed into a slot in a computer to allow it to be connected to a local area network.

sound c. A circuit board that permits the computer to produce sound effects or text recognition in a multimedia package.

video c. A plug-in board that determines proper operation of the monitor.

carriage return ABBR: CR. The key that indicates the decision to accept and perform a command or enter recently typed information. Until CR is used, entered data can be altered or the entire command canceled. Also called *ENTER.*

cartridge **1.** An insertable device containing data or program information; often used with central processing units or laser printers to extend memory capacity. **2.** An insert for an inkjet or laser printer or office copier containing toner.

cathode ray tube ABBR: CRT. Technical term for a monitor or screen.

CD-ROM *compact disk, read-only memory.*

central processing unit ABBR: CPU. The basic box or cabinet containing all of a computer's circuit boards. Sometimes only the single main chip on a circuit board (e.g., the Pentium III chip) is known as the CPU.

chat room An online "gathering place" where individuals can communicate with others in real time.

Check Disk ABBR: CHKDSK. A program built into MS-DOS, permitting a quick examination of the hard disk drive to make sure files are stored properly and ready to use.

chip An integrated circuit. Complete electronic subsystems or operating systems can be included in a single chip.

CHKDSK *Check Disk.*

circuit board Card. SEE: *motherboard.*

click Use of the left, middle, or right button of a mouse to initiate an action. This is equivalent to hitting the ENTER or ESCAPE key or initiating other functions of the keyboard. "Double click" is the rapid succession of two clicks on a mouse button at a specified location.

client In a local area network hookup, a computer that draws its information or uses the resources of a server. A client may have access to all or only some server resources (e.g., a program or a printer), depending on the decisions made by the system administrator. SEE: *server*.

clipboard A temporary storage file that holds recently cut, copied, or deleted information for later retrieval. The data may be restored in either the source document or in a new location. Clipboards are widely used in GUI applications for transfer of data to another file in the same or a different application.

cold boot SEE: under *boot*.

command An instruction issued to the computer for execution of a specific task.

communications port SEE: under *port*.

communications protocol A standard way in which one computer communicates with others or with other terminals. Protocols are usually established and selected by system managers. Names include XMODEM and KERMIT. All such protocols are software driven and mostly unseen to the casual modem user.

compact disk, read-only memory ABBR: CD-ROM. A storage medium that uses a laser beam to retrieve binary data encoded on the surface of the disk. A writable CD-

ROM (CD-R) and a rewritable CD-ROM (CD-RW) can be written to as well as read from.

compatibility The ability of one computer to run a program generated on or written for another.

COM port SEE: under *port*.

compressed file SEE: under *file*.

computer An electronic device for storing and retrieving numerical or textual data and for processing and analyzing numerical or mathematical data. In medicine and the biological sciences, the use of computers has made it possible to store and retrieve quantities of data that would require an inordinate amount of space if stored in conventional files.

laptop c. A lightweight, portable computer that is usually battery-operated. SEE: *notebook*.

mainframe c. A major computer installation requiring one or more large cabinets. Mainframe computers are fixed in place.

personal c. ABBR: PC. Microcomputer.

computer-assisted design ABBR: CAD. The use of computer systems to assist in designing two- or three-dimensional objects. Application may occur in plastic surgery or in orthopedics to design replacement parts, such as an artificial hip.

config.sys A file prepared by the user to tell the machine what devices to use. It is loaded automatically on start-up.

configuration The manner in which hardware and software are programmed and arranged to operate a system or network.

console ABBR: CON. A monitor or screen.

control ABBR: CTRL. One of the special keys on an IBM-type computer. Depressing it in conjunction with another key or keys generates a different set of commands or characters.

control-alternate-delete ABBR: Ctrl-Alt-Del. Three keys that, if struck simultaneously, will reboot the computer. SEE: *hot boot*.

controller A special card or a part of a hard drive. It translates the signals coming from the central processing unit into physical motion of the read-write head, as well as its read-write functions.

conversion The changing of data or a file into a format different from the one in which it was generated.

cookie Coded information about a computer user's personal preferences and Internet habits that are stored on the user's computer by a Web site so that content can be customized to the user. Cookies are increasingly used by Web marketers and advertisers to build user profiles.

CPU *central processing unit*.

crash A sudden and unexpected program termination that may cause a computer to cease operating or to "hang up" and require a reboot. SEE: *hang-up*.

CRT *cathode ray tube*.

Ctrl *control* (key).

Ctrl-Alt-Del *control-alternate-delete* (keys).

cursor On a computer monitor screen the flashing line, square, or rectangle that moves each time a key is struck and indicates where the next keystroke will appear.

data (Pl. of datum) Information. Data units in order of increasing size are bit, byte, word, line, paragraph, and page. Data may be alphabetical, numerical, or graphic, and may be manipulated with all conventional mathematical functions.

d. security **1.** The automatic prevention of updates to the same file by more than one operator at one time. **2.** The automatic prevention of unauthorized use or theft of information in a computer.

d. transfer The moving of information from one machine to another, as through a hard-wire direct connection, a local area network, an intermediate telephone link, or infrared ports.

database A collection of data, either numerical or textual, that has been keyed in and stored on disk or another storage medium. A database is usually created in a specific format, allowing easy insertion of future additions and sorting of information according to identified categories or sequences.

default An automatic choice made by a computer program unless another choice is specified by the user.

default drive SEE: under *drive*.

defragment To rearrange computer data using a special program that stores all files in contiguous sectors. With continual storage changes (removal of old and addition of new material), segments of one file can be scattered over the disk, which is then said to be "fragmented." This slows retrieval and causes extra wear on the drive.

desktop publishing ABBR: DTP. The computerized production of documents ready for duplication.

destination drive SEE: under *drive*.

diagnostics The use of a special program to check the inner workings of a computer. The technician can find every bit stored and its location, as well as critical machine parameters, peripherals, and procedures.

dialogue box In Windows and similar programs, a menu of choices offered in a graphic area indicating that a specific response is required for the program to proceed.

digital camera A device that records and stores photographs in computer files rather than on film. These files can be stored in the camera or on various storage media (e.g., a diskette) and downloaded to a computer for electronic manipulation before being printed out or sent to another computer.

digital radiography Radiography using computerized imaging instead of conventional film or screen imaging.

digital subscriber line ABBR: DSL. A high-speed connection to the Internet using conventional copper telephone wires.

DIR *directory.*

directory ABBR: DIR. A listing of all the filenames in a specified location or sublocation of a disk.

root d. The top-level directory of a formatted disk (e.g., C:\). SEE: *subdirectory.*

disk A round plastic or metal platter coated with a magnetic medium and used for data storage.

backup d. 1. A precautionary or safety disk used to duplicate information from a master disk. Backup disks are usually used for archiving or storage and to preserve data if the master disk is lost or damaged. 2. A set of disks to which all of the information on a hard disk drive or floppy disks will be copied for safe storage and retrieval in case the original data are no longer usable.

d. capacity The number of bytes that can be stored on a disk.

destination d. The disk to which information is transferred from the source disk. SEE: *source disk.*

digital versatile d. ABBR: DVD. A format identical in physical size to a CD-ROM disk but having much greater storage capacity. A DVD can store audio, video, and other information on two layers on each of its two sides, up to about 17 gigabytes of data, compared with 600 megabytes on a CD-ROM disk. DVDs can be read only by a DVD drive. Also called *digital video disk.*

digital video d. ABBR: DVD. *digital versatile disk.*

d. drive SEE: *drive.*

floppy d. A thin, flexible plastic platter inside a protective covering. SYN: *diskette.*

hard d. A nonremovable set of platters sealed in an airtight metal case within the central processing unit. A hard disk rotates and reacts much faster than a floppy disk drive.

source d. The disk from which data are copied to the destination disk. SEE: *destination disk.*

virtual d. A section of the computer's random access memory that functions like a hard disk drive. The advantage is that data transfer is much faster than with a mechanical drive. The disadvantage is that the data exist in the virtual memory only while the computer is turned on and must be saved to a permanent storage medium before it is turned off. Also called *virtual memory.*

diskette SEE: *floppy disk.*

disk operating system ABBR: DOS. A basic set of files and commands that control the computer's operation, such as input/output control or data management.

display A visual image of numbers, letters, and graphic characters on a monitor screen.

distance learning Coursework completed at a site remote from the educational institution that sponsored or developed it, usually via the Internet.

document Any body of text that is typed and stored in a file.

documentation Manuals, instruction books, and programs or help menus that provide guidance to a user.

DOS *disk operating system.*

download To transfer and save a program or data from a computer at a remote location. SEE: *upload.*

drag To move an item from one location to another by clicking on it, holding down the left mouse button, and repositioning it until the desired location has been reached.

drive The mechanism that rotates a disk (or the platters in a hard disk drive), reading and writing data in the process. Also called *disk drive.*

CD-R d. A drive that uses a laser to read data on CD-ROM and CD-R disks and which can also write information to blank CD-R disks.

CD-ROM d. A drive that uses a laser to read data from CD-ROM and CD-R disks.

CD-RW d. A drive that uses a laser to read data from CD-ROM, CD-R, and CD-RW disks or to write to blank CD-R and CD-RW disks. The CD-RW drive can also erase CD-RW disks so that they can be reused.

default d. The disk drive automatically used by the computer for data storage and retrieval unless the user specifies otherwise. Usually the default drive is designated by the letter "C."

destination d. The drive to which data to be stored are sent.

disk d. Drive.

DVD-ROM d. A mechanism that uses a laser to read data from DVD disks but that can also read CD-ROM and CD-R disks.

logical d. Partition.

removable hard d. ABBR: removable HD. A hard disk drive with interchangeable modules that can be moved from one computer to another.

tape d. A high-speed storage medium to receive and hold data from a computer. It is used primarily as a backup device so that data lost or damaged on the machine's hard disk drive can be restored if needed.

zip d. A device that functions like a hard drive in providing fast data access but that has the portability of a floppy disk. Zip disks come in 100-megabyte and 250-megabyte storage capacities.

driver A piece of software that tells a computer with a specific operating system how to control and use a piece of hardware attached to it (e.g., a printer). Drivers may be provided with the operating system or the peripheral hardware and are frequently improved and updated to allow greater functionality or compatibility.

DSL *digital subscriber line.*
DTP *desktop publishing.*
DVD *digital versatile disk; digital video disk.*
e-mail **1.** To send a message electronically. **2.** A method of sending and receiving messages electronically over a network. SEE: *Internet.*
e-mail *electronic mail.*
encryption The use of mathematical algorithms to encode data so that it can be kept private.
Enter A key that is the official "do it" command. Before this key is pressed, issued instructions can usually be changed or canceled. Also called *carriage return.*
error message A message appearing on the screen that indicates a problem with either the hardware or a software application. Most error messages may be interpreted by consulting the appropriate manual. Some error messages require interpretation by a technician.
Esc *escape* (key).
escape The key marked "ESC" on the top row of the keyboard. It is usually used to exit a specific activity within a program or to return to a menu.
Ethernet A major protocol and hardware for a local area network.
.exe An extension used to indicate an executable file.
executable file SEE: under *file.*
Extensible Markup Language ABBR: XML. A formal method of coding structured documents for the World Wide Web; a subset of SGML (Standard Generalized Markup Language).
extension The three letters following the period at the end of a filename (e.g., .doc, .exe, or .tif).
external A peripheral item, such as a modem or CD-ROM drive, that is outside the computer cabinet. It has its own power supply and must be connected by cables.
eye-gaze communicator An electronic (assistive) device that allows a person to control a computer by eye movement directed toward the screen or other connected device.
fax modem SEE: under *modem.*
file A collection of data, computer instructions, or text that is stored as a single unit.

batch f. ABBR: bat. A file that completes more than one task (e.g., autoexec.bat).

compressed f. A file that has been processed by a software routine to take up less space on a disk. Special software must be used for compressing and decompressing such files. Also called *zipped file.* SEE: *PKZIP/PKUNZIP.*

executable f. A type of file that can be processed (or executed) by the computer without further translation. It is usually the file that makes a program operate.

hidden f. A file that is not normally listed in a directory. It is not meant to be modified by a user.

filename **1.** A name assigned to a computer file that enables the user to identify and retrieve that file later. **2.** A program that can be initiated by typing the name.
firewall A combination of security software and hardware that prevents access to proprietary information or private data by unauthorized users.
font The typeface, type size, and type style of a document. Fonts are easily changed in most word processing packages.
footer In desktop publishing, text repeated at the bottom of each page. SEE: *header.*
format **1.** To install the primary divisions and structure required for storage and retrieval on a new disk. All new disks must be formatted by the user unless preformatted by the manufacturer. **2.** The structural arrangement (sectors and tracks) of a disk.

file f. The organization or structure of a computer file, often specific to individual applications. There are many different file formats, denoted by the DOS-derived three-letter file extensions (e.g., .doc). Some programs can interpret many different file formats; others may be able to use only their own proprietary native format.

Tagged Image File f. ABBR: TIFF. A common graphic image format employing the file extension *.tif.*

freeze SEE: *hang-up.*
function key On a computer keyboard any of several keys whose designation begins with the letter "F." Alone or in conjunction with the Alt or Shift key, a function key executes many different, often programmable, routines. On most keyboards, function keys are found on the top row.
GANTT chart A graphic, annotated representation of a project, used for scheduling. It shows when tasks are to be started and finished, and the crews assigned to each component of the work.
garbage in, garbage out ABBR: GIGO. An expression indicating that flawed input will lead to flawed or useless output.
gateway A system that translates information between two otherwise incompatible segments of a network. A network composed of MacIntosh and Wintel computer segments requires a gateway, often in the form of a Windows NT server, to translate data between the two segments.
GIF *Graphical Interface Format.*
gigabyte A storage capacity of a billion bytes (or 1000 megabytes), used in hard-drive data storage.
GIGO *garbage in, garbage out.*
gopher A network resource client-server feature within the Internet. It is designed like a menu so that users can select areas of interest, avoiding the need for complex searching. Once the selection has been made, the gopher facilitates connection to the selected topic.
Graphical Interface Format ABBR: GIF. A bit-mapped file that sends instructions to a

computer about what to do with each pixel of a graphic image (e.g., on, off, highlighted, color); a trademark of CompuServe.

graphics card SEE: under *card*.

graphical user interface ABBR: GUI (pronounced "gooey"). Software that employs an arrangement of graphics, icons, and menus to allow user-friendly interaction with a computer program. Examples include Windows and OS/2.

groupware Software designed for use by more than one individual. It is used by groups of people working on a single project and sharing the same or similar data.

GUI *graphical user interface*.

hacker A person who gains unauthorized access to, and sometimes damages, computer networks.

hang-up A nonoperational condition, in which the computer does not respond to any keystroke. When the computer "hangs up" (i.e., crashes or freezes), it is necessary to reboot the computer. SEE: *boot*.

hardware The central processing unit, monitor, keyboard, printer, and any add-on circuit boards or other devices installed in or connected to the computer.

hard-wire Connection by wire rather than by radio waves to interrelate two or more computers in a network.

header In desktop publishing, text repeated at the top of each page. SEE: *footer*.

hertz ABBR: Hz. A unit of frequency equal to 1 cycle/sec; in computer terminology, usually used to judge the relative speed of a machine.

hidden file SEE: under *file*.

home page The opening screen on a World Wide Web site, usually intended to welcome visitors, provide general information, and provide links to other pages at that Web site or to other sites. SEE: *browser*; *Hypertext Markup Language*; *Internet*; *uniform resource locator*.

hot boot SEE: under *boot*.

hot key A keystroke or combination of keystrokes, used in conjunction with a memory-resident program, that brings up the program on the screen. Using the Esc (Escape) key usually closes the program.

hot swap Replacement of a hardware device, such as a hard drive or CD-ROM drive, with a similar device without first turning off the power to the computer.

HTML *Hypertext Markup Language*.

HTTP *Hypertext Transfer Protocol*.

hypertext A system of help screens interconnected in layers. Each lower or higher layer is accessible by clicking on a key word or icon. Hypertext is used in developing teaching-learning packages, Internet content, and other applications. SEE: *Hypertext Markup Language*.

Hypertext Markup Language ABBR: HTML. A set of codes added to content intended for display on the World Wide Web. The codes, also called *markup* or *tags*, allow links to be made with graphic files, compressed video or sound files, or text on the same or another Web page. SEE: *hypertext*.

Hypertext Transfer Protocol ABBR: HTTP. A set of rules for exchanging text and multimedia files on the World Wide Web. This protocol allows a computer to request and receive files from the Web server on which those files are stored.

Hz *hertz*.

icon A small symbol on the screen that corresponds to a program and is interactive with the user. Clicking on the icon will start the program or execute a specific function using the program.

immunization registry A computerized system that stores information about the vaccinations that particular persons have received. The registry can be used to ensure that required immunizations are obtained but that excessive immunization is avoided.

import To bring material from a different source into a working program; most often done with text, spreadsheets, pictures, and symbols.

informatics A combination of information science and computer; the study of the transformation of data into information and information into knowledge.

medical i. The application of information science and computer technology to all aspects of medical knowledge, practice, and management, including medical education and research.

nursing i. The application of computer science, information science, and nursing science in the management and processing of nursing data, information, and knowledge to support the practice of clinical nursing and the delivery of patient care.

input and output ABBR: I/O. The transfer of data between the central processing unit and its peripherals.

insert To place a letter, number, or graphics character between two others. Text is usually typed in Insert mode. Pressing the Insert (or Ins) toggle key changes the mode to that of overwriting, in which the new text replaces the existing text as it is typed in. Pressing Insert again changes the mode from overwriting back to inserting.

Integrated Services Digital Network ABBR: ISDN. A higher bandwidth connection to an Internet service provider via telephone wires than is possible with a conventional telephone connection. An ISDN adapter is used instead of a modem to connect to the computer.

interactive Relating to two-way communication in a computer application (i.e., the program waits for user input and performs tasks responsively).

interface A connection among devices or software packages that allows compatibility or performance of a desired function. A modem is a telephone interface.

small computer system i. ABBR: SCSI. A hardware interface that allows for the connections of up to seven peripherals daisy-chained to the computer via an SCSI (pronounced "scuzzy") port or SCSI host adapter card.

internal Relating to equipment enclosed within the main computer.

Internet A worldwide linkage of computers designed to facilitate communication and information exchange. Features include the World Wide Web, electronic mail, newsgroups, bulletin boards, special interest groups, and file downloads to personal computers. Participation includes universities, corporations, governments, agencies, and individuals. SEE: *home page; uniform resource locator*.

Internet service provider ABBR: ISP. A company that provides Internet access, e-mail accounts, access to newsgroups, and sometimes Web site design and hosting services.

intranet An organization's internal client-server network, which functions like an internal internet with its own home page and network resources. Though an intranet may be accessed via the Internet, it is not a public site and is available only to registered users with the proper user ID and password.

I/O *input and output.*

ISDN *Integrated Services Digital Network.*

ISP *Internet service provider.*

joystick A device for video computer games that moves the onscreen pointer left and right or up and down.

JPEG *Joint Photographic Experts Group,* the developers of the popular standard for compressing digitized still images into the graphics file type denoted by the file extension *.jpg* (pronounced "JAY-peg").

justification Text alignment at the left or right margin or both. Many word processing programs have automatic justification capability that may be selected through a dialogue box.

keypad A secondary grouping of keys to the right of the typewriter keyboard similar to that of an adding machine. It contains numbers and several special keys, such as directional arrows. SYN: *numberpad.*

label In a spreadsheet, text made up of alphabetical characters, as opposed to *value,* which is numerical.

LAN *local area network.*

landscape A page orientation in which the long dimension is horizontal. SEE: *orientation*; *portrait*.

laptop computer SEE: under *computer*.

laser printer SEE: under *printer*.

LCD *liquid crystal display.*

LCD panel A computer peripheral used with an overhead projector to display computer data onto a liquid crystal display screen for presentations.

LISTSERV® A list management software in which the e-mail subscription list is maintained on a server and automatically distributes e-mail messages to members of the group. Thousands of listservs exist, covering various topics, including health care subjects such as nursing, health professionals, occupational therapy, depression, and many others. One directory of listservs is found at www.liszt.com.

liquid crystal display ABBR: LCD. A computer screen technology in which liquid crystals and polarized light, rather than an electron beam and a cathode ray tube, are used to display information. LCD screens were first used on laptop computers but are now available for desktop models. LCD screens emit less radiation, have no screen flicker, and take up less desk space than conventional CRT monitors.

login The process of attaching an outlying computer (a client) to a server electronically. To obtain access to the local area network, the user must provide a name and password. SEE: *client*; *logout*; *server*.

logout The process of ending a local area network session. SEE: *login*.

low-radiation monitor SEE: under *monitor*.

M, MB *megabyte.*

Massachusetts General Hospital Utility Multi-Programming System ABBR: MUMPS. A programming language designed to handle complex data, such as patient records.

Mbps *Megabits per second,* used to measure the speed at which data are transmitted on most networks.

MEDLINE An online database provided by the U.S. National Library of Medicine of more than 11 million abstracts and references to articles in biomedical journals from 1966 to the present. MEDLINE*plus* offers consumer health information. Both databases are located at www.nlm.nih.gov.

megabyte ABBR: M, MB. A measure of computer data storage capacity equal to roughly 1 million bytes (or exactly 1,048,576 bytes).

memory The basic volatile memory space, or random access memory (RAM) area, where unsaved data are processed by programs before being committed to hard storage. All changes made to RAM and not saved to a disk are lost when the computer is turned off.

random access m. ABBR: RAM. The segment of central processing unit internal memory available to the user for programs, data manipulation, and storage. RAM can be changed as often as desired. All changes made to RAM are lost when the computer is turned off. SEE: *memory*.

read-only m. ABBR: ROM. The portion of a computer's memory that contains permanent instructions as opposed to random access memory. ROM is not lost when the computer is turned off. ROM information is programmed into an on-board chip.

m. upgrade The addition of memory chips to provide more space for data and programs. It is important to use the type of memory specified for a particular brand and model of computer.

menu-driven Relating to a programming technique that permits the user to make all required choices from a list shown on the monitor. Selecting appropriate numbers or letters from the menu will help lead the user through necessary commands.

microcomputer A computer in which all equipment fits on a desk and is readily transportable to another location. SYN: *personal computer.*

MIDI *Musical Instrument Digital Interface.*

MIDI sequencer A program that plays or records songs in the form of musical instrument digital interface (MIDI) files.

minicomputer A computer with size and computing capacity between those of a mainframe computer and a microcomputer. The central processing unit is usually a floor model cabinet with hard disk drives of gigabyte capacity. A minicomputer may be moved if necessary.

modem An internal or external device that allows data to be transmitted via telephone or cable lines. SEE: *fax modem*; *baud rate.*

cable m. A type of modem that connects a computer to an Internet Service Provider through a cable television system's cable. Cable modems can provide high bandwidth, which means faster downloading of data.

fax m. An external device or internal board that plugs into a personal computer, permitting the receipt and transmission of data across telephone lines. It may connect to fax machine or another fax modem.

monitor A viewing screen, similar to a television screen, connected to a computer to enable entering and reading of text, graphics, and data.

low-radiation m. A monitor designed for minimum emission of electromagnetic energy into the atmosphere.

Mosaic A World Wide Web client server developed by the National Center for Supercomputing Applications at the University of Illinois. A graphic user interface, it allows users to navigate easily through the Internet and to access hypertext documents relating to the designated search area. SEE: *browser.*

motherboard A computer's primary circuit board, containing the main central processing unit chip. All other boards, controllers, and some peripherals are plugged into the motherboard, from which they derive their power and instructions.

mouse A hand-manipulated device that generates electrical signals in relation to its motion and position. Signals interpreted by the central processing unit reflect corresponding motion of a cursor, arrow, or other indicator on the monitor screen. Clicking a mouse button sends a specific instruction to an application.

MP3 A format for compressed audio files, used for downloading music files from the Internet and for storing music on certain portable music players.

MPG A file format similar to JPG but used for the compression of video instead of still images.

MS-DOS *Microsoft disk operating system.* SEE: *disk operating system.*

multimedia The production of sound, animation, full-motion video, or a combination of these for learning or entertainment. CD-ROM encyclopedias, game packages, and other applications make full use of multimedia. The personal computer requires a sound card, a CD-ROM, and speakers.

multitasking The use of several programs on a computer at the same time.

MUMPS *Massachusetts General Hospital Utility Multi-Programming System* (language).

Musical Instrument Digital Interface ABBR: MIDI. A board that causes the computer to play music by converting computer information into analog signals that are processed by audio circuits. Information needed to play a song is stored in a MIDI file. Keyboards attached to computers use a MIDI interface.

network A series of computers or databases connected by communication lines.

local area n. ABBR: LAN. A system of two or more computers, hard-wired to each other, in the same office or building. Special cables are required, but no telephone is involved. SEE: *wide area network.*

wide area n. ABBR: WAN. A system in which computers are linked by long-distance communication equipment, such as telephone lines or satellite dishes, over a large geographical area. The Internet is an example of a WAN. SEE: *local area network.*

network hub A box where cables from two or more computers are connected to form a local area network.

newsgroup An electronic bulletin board on the Internet devoted to a particular topic. Newsgroups are organized into subject categories, such as comp (computer), sci (science), and misc (miscellaneous), and then further subcategorized. Some newsgroups are controlled by a moderator who selects which of the submitted entries will be posted to the group.

NIC *network interface card.*

notebook A lightweight computer very similar to a laptop but smaller and lighter (about 4 lb).

Novell A major vendor of local area networks. It uses its own operating system, distinct from DOS.

numberpad Keypad.
Num Lock A keyboard toggle key that forces all the calculator keys into numerical mode, so that arrows and other motion keys are no longer operational. Pressing Num Lock again switches back to arrow key functions.
OCR *optical character reader; optical character recognition.*
optical character reader ABBR: OCR. A device used for optical character recognition.
optical character recognition ABBR: OCR. Software that reads printed or handwritten text and transforms it into characters suitable for computer processing. OCR software is used with a scanner.
orientation The position of the long dimension of a page—vertical (portrait) or horizontal (landscape).
OS/2 A graphical user interface developed by IBM Corporation to run on personal computers. It is a multiprocessing operating system that can run native programs as well as programs designed for Windows and DOS.
palette The collection of colors available in a graphics package.
parameter A value that can be added to customize a command to perform a specific task. If a parameter is not specified by the user, a predetermined parameter (default) is used.
partition Any of several divisions of a large hard disk drive. Although physically part of the actual drive (e.g., C:), a partition is assigned a different letter (D:, E:) and functions as a separate unit. SYN: *logical drive.*
password An identification code or name that allows a user access to a network, a computer, a computer program, or a computer-related service such as a bulletin board. Passwords are effective in protecting word processing files.
PC *personal computer.*
PCMCIA slot A slot usually found on the outside of a laptop computer to allow peripherals such as a network interface card to connect the computer to a network.
Pentium A trademark for a series of microprocessors manufactured by Intel Corp.; the successor to Intel's 80486 series of computer chips.
peripheral Any piece of hardware added to the basic computer (central processing unit, monitor, keyboard). Major peripherals include the printer, external modem, joystick, mouse, sound speakers, external CD-ROMs, scanners, Zip drives, and Webcams.
pixel Abbreviation for *picture element;* the smallest area on the screen that can be turned on or off. The greater the number of pixels, the sharper the definition of alphanumeric characters or graphic representations. Hundreds of thousands of pixels are often necessary to create a useful graphic image.
PKZIP/PKUNZIP A form of file compression (PKZIP) and uncompression (PKUNZIP). SEE: *compressed file.*
plotter Equipment that uses one or more drawing pens to generate a graphic or pictorial image on paper.
plug-in An addition to a software package (as a Web browser) in order to add functionality (e.g., streaming audio).
pocket LAN A connector between a computer and a telephone that makes it possible to hook a remote portable or laptop computer to the server at home base. SEE: *local area network.*
port An input-output connection through which data flow can be directed.

COM p. *communications port.*

communications p. ABBR: COM port. A device used for output to any device that responds to data. Typical devices connected to COM ports are the modem and the mouse.

printer p. The port designated to receive the data output and route it to a printer. Possibilities are LPT1, LPT2, LPT3, and PRN (equivalent to LPT1). Most printers are connected to LPT1. Devices such as Zip drives and scanners may also be connected to LPT1.

portrait A page orientation in which the short dimension is horizontal. SEE: *landscape; orientation.*
printer A keyless device that physically prints output data from a computer; also called a *line printer.*

inkjet p. A printer that generates characters by using ink cartridges and directing minute sprays of ink onto the paper. This type of printer produces high-quality color and black-and-white output.

laser p. A printer capable of very high quality type and photographic resolution. It uses toner and a laser beam to fabricate the image on plain paper.

line p. SEE: *printer.*

printer port SEE: under *port.*
prompt A standard symbol that appears onscreen, indicating that the computer is ready to receive commands. The most common is the C: prompt, which indicates that a command may be executed directly to the C: drive.
RAM *random access memory.*
random access memory SEE: under *memory.*
read-only memory SEE: under *memory.*
remote access A mode in which a user can control unattended terminals in another location.
resolution The degree of detail, measured in dots per inch, that a monitor, scanner, printer, or fax machine can create in an image. Typical values range from 75 × 75 (very coarse) to 1280 × 1024 (fine).

restore To retrieve data from a backup source (e.g., tape, disk) and replace it on the computer's hard drive. SEE: *backup*.
ROM *read-only memory*.
root directory SEE: under *directory*.
save To send information to a permanent storage medium such as a disk.
Scandisk A program built into newer versions of Windows that checks for and attempts to repair missing or damaged files or damage to disks. Scandisk is usually set to run automatically on start-up after the computer has been shut down improperly.
scanner Equipment that reads characters or graphic material on a page and converts them into a computer file.
screen saver Any moving pattern that prevents burning of the screen phosphor by keeping the same material from remaining onscreen too long. It is usually activated by a timer after a few minutes of screen inactivity and is released by any keystroke.
SCSI *small computer systems interface*.
search engine Software that facilitates the identification and retrieval of specified information, as from a database or the World Wide Web.
server The source of data, programs, and other resources for the client computers in a client-server local area network. There may be multiple servers on a network managing specialized functions, such as e-mail or access to specific files.
setup **1.** Preparation of the computer system for operation. **2.** The command used to install many Windows applications.
SGML *Standard Generalized Markup Language*.
shareware Software that a user can obtain on a trial basis. Programs are available on disks from commercial sources for a fee or may be downloaded free from a bulletin board service.
Shift A board key that capitalizes all letters or accesses the characters above the numbers. It also provides alternate responses for the function keys (F1 to F12) and some other keys.
SIG *special-interest group*.
software Programs written for the computer (e.g., word processing, data processing, graphics, utilities, spreadsheets, games).
sound card SEE: under *card*.
special-interest group ABBR: SIG. Computer users who share a common focus. Segments of bulletin board service networks, Internet chat groups, and other such facilities are devoted to the use of SIGs.
spreadsheet A program that presents columns of numerical data; used in accounting and other administrative settings. It allows sorting of entered data and, through formulas, the modification of related cells.
SQL *Structured Query Language*.
Standard Generalized Markup Language ABBR: SGML. An international, formal, platform- and application-independent method of encoding the structure of a document to facilitate exchange or reuse of the data. The markup consists of codes, or tags, applied to specific elements in the document content.
storage A method of retaining data, text, or graphics by preserving the information on larger disk drives (hard drives) within the computer or on removable (floppy) disks. Information may be transferred from one computer to another by using data stored on removable disks.
primary s. The location where data and programs are kept during processing.
secondary s. The location of space not being used to store data and programs during processing.
Structured Query Language ABBR: SQL. A high-level language that permits almost ordinary, sentence-like expressions by the user.
subdirectory A directory that branches off from the root directory (e.g., C:\subdir).
surge protector A device that protects a computer from damage caused by sudden increases in electrical power.
telecommunication The transmission of data over telephone lines. SEE: *modem*.
terminal A work station, usually consisting of a keyboard and monitor, with no storage device (i.e., hard disk). The terminal relies on a network server for its files and program.
dumb t. A work station that does not have storage facilities. It relies on a remote server for input and storage.
TIFF *Tagged Image File Format*.
trackball A point-and-click device, similar to a mouse. The ball, placed at the top, is the only moving part. It is rotated by hand in any direction to move the cursor onscreen.
typeface The design of type. Two broad categories are serif and sans serif. Serif faces vary in stroke thickness and include a thin line (finial) at the end of each stroke. A typical example is Times Roman, the typeface used in most newspapers. Sans serif (without serif) type has no thickness variation and no finials. Helvetica, most often seen in headings, is typical. SEE: *font*.
type size The height and width of type, expressed in points. There are 12 points per pica and 72 points per inch. Newspaper type size is generally nine points. SEE: *font*.
type style Any variation within the same typeface family. There are four variations: normal (roman), italic, bold, and bold italic. Normal type is generally straight up and down, italic type is slanted, and bold type has a heavier body. SEE: *font*.
uniform resource locator ABBR: URL. An address uniquely identifying a resource or page on the World Wide Web. URLs are

frequently written in a format such as *http: //www.tabers.com*. Also called *web page address*.

uninterruptible power supply ABBR: UPS. A device that uses a battery to power a computer when the primary power supply is interrupted or fails and also protects the computer against power surges. If the primary power supply is lost, the battery power will keep the computer running long enough to allow computer data to be saved and the computer to be properly shut down.

upload To transfer data from one computer to another at a remote site. Files that the user has prepared may be uploaded to a bulletin board or other appropriate site. SEE: *download*.

UPS *uninterruptible power supply.*

URL *uniform resource locator.*

utility program A program that facilitates and speeds the operation of a computer.

value A number or numerical symbol in a spreadsheet. SEE: *label*.

vaporware A derogatory nickname for computer software that is always on the verge of coming to market but never does.

video The computer monitor display, or the output to it.

streaming v. The transmission of a continuous stream of video data in real time over the Internet or other network connection via appropriate media player software. The effect is similar to a television broadcast played through the computer, though the size and clarity of the image depends on the speed and quality of the network connection.

virtual disk SEE: under *disk*.

virus A flaw deliberately introduced into a program to cause humorous, annoying, or destructive results. The most severe result is a disk crash, in which all data and programs are lost. Most viruses are transmitted by programs downloaded with e-mail, from the Internet, or from copying and sharing disks. Programs and devices are available to spot viruses and eliminate them before they activate, multiply across the system, and cause major damage. Computers should have antivirus software installed as soon as they are purchased and it should be updated frequently, as new viruses are introduced constantly.

voice recognition The capacity of a computer to transform spoken input into electronic signals that it can process as an instruction or translate into typed words.

WAN *wide area network.*

warm boot SEE: *hot boot.*

Webcam A video camera connected to a computer, used for video conferences and transmission of still images and video over the World Wide Web.

Webcast The transmission of a live or recorded audio or video program over the World Wide Web.

Web portal A Web page (frequently a home page) offering specialized content, such as stock market or weather information, Web-based e-mail, a search engine, and links to news stories. Examples include MSN, Yahoo, and Netscape and may include customizable, personalized versions through the use of cookies.

wide area network ABBR: WAN. A system in which computers are linked over a large area. This system may extend over several cities or even countries.

Windows A graphic user interface that depends on icons and a mouse for program manipulation, selection, and start-up, rather than conventional, keyed-in DOS commands.

word wrap The automatic movement of text to the next line when the end of a line is reached. Use of the return key is not necessary.

World Wide Web ABBR: WWW. An extremely large set of hypertext resources (pages) found within the Internet. Web pages can be located by conducting a search on the Internet or by directly entering the universal resource locator (web page address). This resource is growing rapidly each year and can provide a wealth of information to researchers. SEE: *Internet*.

worm A type of computer virus that replicates and consumes computer resources, downgrading the computer's performance.

write protect To safeguard information on a diskette and prevent the overwriting of old material with new material. The square notch on the floppy disk is blocked, thereby preventing writing to the disk. Data on a protected disk can be read and used but not altered.

WYSIWYG Acronym for "What You See Is What You Get" (pronounced "wizzywig"), relating to a program in which the printed output mimics exactly what is shown on the screen.

XML *Extensible Markup Language.*

zip drive SEE: under *drive*.

zipped file SEE: *compressed file*.

APPENDIX 14
Health Care Resource Organizations

Appendix 14–1 Resource Organizations in the United States

AIDS

American Red Cross
National Headquarters
AIDS Education Program
Jefferson Park
8111 Gatehouse Road
Falls Church, VA 22042
(703) 206-7130
Fax (703) 206-8143
www.redcross.org/hss/HIVAIDS

CDC National AIDS Clearinghouse
Publication Ordering Department
P.O. Box 6003
Rockville, MD 20840-6003
(800) 458-5231
(800) 243-7012 (Deaf access)
www.cdcnpin.org

CDC National AIDS Hot Line
P.O. Box 13827
Research Triangle Park, NC 27709
(800) 342-AIDS
(800) 344-7432 (Spanish)
(800) 243-7889 (Deaf access)

National Association of People with AIDS
1413 K Street NW
Washington, DC 20005
(202) 898-0414
Fax (202) 898-0435
www.napwa.org

National Hospice and Palliative Care Organization
1700 Diagonal Road, Suite 300
Alexandria, VA 22314
(703) 243-5900
www.nho.org

ALCOHOLISM

SEE: *Substance Abuse*

ALZHEIMER'S DISEASE

Alzheimer's Association
919 N. Michigan Avenue, Suite 1100
Chicago, IL 60611-16176
(312) 335-8700
(800) 272-3900
Fax (312) 335-1110
www.alz.org

ARTHRITIS

National Arthritis Foundation
1330 West Peachtree Street
Atlanta, Georgia 30309
(800) 283-7800
www.arthritis.org

ASTHMA AND ALLERGY

SEE: *Respiratory Disorders*

BLINDNESS

SEE: *Visual Impairment*

BURNS

American Burn Association
National Headquarters Office
625 N. Michigan Avenue, Suite 1530
Chicago, IL 60611
www.ameriburn.org

National Burn Victim Foundation
246A Madisonville Road
P. O. Box 409
Basking Ridge, NJ 07920
(908) 953-9091
Fax (908) 953-9099
www.nbvf.org

CANCER

American Cancer Society
1599 Clifton Road NE
Atlanta, GA 30329-4251
(800) ACS-2345
(404) 320-3333
www.cancer.org

The Leukemia & Lymphoma Society of America
600 3rd Avenue
New York, NY 10016
(212) 573-8484
(800) 955-4LSA
www.leukemia.org

National Cancer Institute
Public Inquiries Office
Building 31, Room 10A03
31 Center Drive, MSC 2580
Bethesda, MD 20892-2580
(301) 435-3848
(800) 4-CANCER
www.nci.nih.gov

R. A. Bloch Cancer Foundation
4435 Main Street
Kansas City, MO 64111
(816) 932-8453
(800) 433-0464
Fax (816) 931-7486
www.blochcancer.org

CEREBRAL PALSY

United Cerebral Palsy Associations
1660 L Street NW, Suite 700
Washington, DC 20036
(800) USA-5UCP
(202) 973-7143
Fax (202) 776-0414
www.ucpa.org

CYSTIC FIBROSIS

SEE: *Respiratory Disorders*

DEAFNESS

SEE: *Hearing Impairment*

DEPRESSION

SEE: *Mental Health*

DIABETES

American Diabetes Association
ATTN: Customer Service
1701 North Beauregard Street
Alexandria, VA 22311
(800) DIABETES
www.diabetes.org

Juvenile Diabetes Foundation International
120 Wall Street
New York, NY 10005
(800) JDF-CURE
(212) 785-9500
Fax (212) 785-9595
www.jdf.org

DISABILITY

Job Accommodation Network
West Virginia University
P.O. Box 6080
Morgantown, WV 26506-6080
(800) 526-7234 (V/TTY)
http://janweb.icdi.wvu.edu

National Rehabilitation Information Center
8455 Colesville Road, Suite 935
Silver Spring, MD 20919-3319
(301) 588-9284
(800) 346-2742
www.naric.com

DIVING ACCIDENTS

Divers Alert Network
The Peter B. Bennett Center
6 West Colony Place
Durham, NC 27705
(800) 446-2671
Fax (919) 490-6630
www.diversalertnetwork.org

DOWN SYNDROME

National Down Syndrome Society
666 Broadway
New York, NY 10012
(800) 221-4602
Fax (212) 979-2873
www.ndss.org

DRUG ABUSE

SEE: *Substance Abuse*

DYSLEXIA

Orton Dyslexia Society
Chester Bldg., Suite 382
860 LaSalle Road
Baltimore, MD 21286-2044
(800) 222-3123
Fax (410) 321-5069
www.selu.edu/Academics/Education/TEC/orton.htm

EATING DISORDERS

National Association of Anorexia Nervosa and Associated Disorders
Box 7
Highland Park, IL 60035
(708) 831-3438
Fax (847) 433-4632
www.anad.org

ELDERLY

American Association of Retired Persons
601 E Street NW
Washington, DC 20049
(800) 424-3410
www.aarp.org

American Geriatric Society
The Empire State Building
350 Fifth Avenue, Suite 801
New York, NY 10118
(212) 308-1414
Fax (212) 832-8646
www.americangeriatrics.org

Gerontological Society of America
1030 15th Street NW, Suite 250
Washington, DC 20005
(202) 842-1275
www.geron.org

EMERGENCY RESPONSE SYSTEM

Lifeline Systems, Inc.
111 Lawrence Street
Framingham, MA 01702-8156
(508) 988-1000
www.lifelinesys.com

EPILEPSY

Epilepsy Foundation of America
4351 Garden City Drive
Landover, MD 20785
(800) EFA-1000
Fax (301) 577-4941
www.efa.org

GASTROINTESTINAL

Crohn's and Colitis Foundation of America
386 Park Avenue S.
New York, NY 10016-8804
(800) 932-2423
Fax (212) 779-4098
www.ccfa.org

GRIEF COUNSELING

American Association of Retired Persons
601 E Street NW
Washington, DC 20049
(202) 434-2260
www.aarp.org/griefandloss

The Compassionate Friends
Box 3696
Oak Brook, IL 60522-3696
(630) 990-0010
www.compassionatefriends.org

National Catholic Ministry to the Bereaved
28700 Euclid Avenue
Cleveland, OH 44092
(440) 943-3480
www.griefwork.org

PetFriends
P.O. Box 131
Moorestown, NJ 08057-0131
(800) 404-PETS

HEARING IMPAIRMENT

Alexander Graham Bell Association for the Deaf
3417 Volta Place NW
Washington, DC 20007
(202) 337-5220
Fax (202) 337-8314
www.agbell.org

Better Hearing Institute
515 King Street, Suite 420
Alexandria, VA 22314
(800) EAR WELL
Fax (703) 684-3394
www.betterhearing.org

International Hearing Society
16880 Middlebelt Road, Suite 4
Livonia, MI 48154
(734) 522-7200
Fax (734) 522-0200
www.hearingihs.org

National Association of the Deaf
814 Thayer Avenue
Silver Spring, MD 20910
(301) 587-1788
Fax (301) 587-1791
www.nad.org

HEART DISEASE

American Heart Association
7272 Greenville Avenue
Dallas, TX 75231-4596
(800) 242-8721
www.americanheart.org

Mended Hearts
7272 Greenville Avenue
Dallas, TX 75231-4596
(800) AHAUSA1
www.mendedhearts.org

National Heart Savers Association
9140 W. Dodge Road
Omaha, NE 68114
(402) 398-1993
www.heartsavers.org

HEMOPHILIA

National Hemophilia Foundation
116 West 32nd Street, 11th Floor
New York, NY 10001
(212) 328-3700
(800) 42-HANDI
Fax (212) 328-3777
www.hemophilia.org

KIDNEY DISEASE

American Kidney Fund
6110 Executive Blvd., Suite 1010
Rockville, MD 20852
(800) 638-8299
Fax (301) 881-0898
www.akfinc.org

National Kidney Foundation
30 E. 33rd Street, Suite 1100
New York, NY 10016
(800) 622-9010
Fax (212) 689-9261
www.kidney.org

LIVER DISEASE

American Liver Foundation
75 Maiden Lane, Suite 603
New York, NY 10038
1-800-GO LIVER
www.liverfoundation.org

LUNG DISEASES

SEE: *Respiratory Disorders*

LUPUS ERYTHEMATOSUS

Lupus Foundation of America
1300 Piccard Drive, Suite 200
Rockville, MD 20850-4303
(301) 670-9292
(800) 558-0121
www.lupus.org/lupus

MENTAL HEALTH

Anxiety Disorders Association of America
11900 Parklawn Drive, Suite 100
Rockville, MD 20852
(301) 231-9350
Fax (301) 231-7392
www.adaa.org

Depression and Related Affective Disorders
600 N. Wolfe Street
Baltimore, MD 21287-7381
(410) 955-4647
www.med.jhu.edu/drada

National Depressive and Manic-Depressive Association
730 N. Franklin Street, Suite 501
Chicago, IL 60610
(312) 642-0049
Fax (312) 642-7243
www.ndmda.org

National Mental Health Association
1021 Prince Street
Alexandria, VA 22314-2971
(703) 684-7722
Fax (703) 684-5968
(800) 969-NMHA
www.nmha.org

NEUROLOGICAL DISORDERS

Amyotrophic Lateral Sclerosis Association
27001 Agoura Road, Suite 150
Calabasas Hills, CA 91301-5104
(800) 782-4747
www.alsa.org

Multiple Sclerosis Foundation
6350 N. Andrews Avenue
Fort Lauderdale, FL 33309
(800) 441-7055
www.msfacts.org

Muscular Dystrophy Association
3300 E. Sunrise Drive
Tucson, AZ 85718
(800) 572-1717
(602) 529-2000
www.mdausa.org

National Multiple Sclerosis Society
733 3rd Avenue, 6th Floor
New York, NY 10017
(212) 986-3240
(800) FIGHT-MS
www.nmss.org

Norris MDA/ALS Center
Robert G. Miller, M.D.
California Pacific Medical Center
2324 Sacramento Street, Suite 150
San Francisco, CA 94115
(415) 923-3604
Fax (415) 923-6567
www.mdausa.org/clinics/alsserv.html

ORGAN DONATION

Living Bank
4545 Post Oak Place, Suite 315
Houston, TX 77027
(800) 528-2971
www.livingbank.org

United Network for Organ Sharing
1100 Boulders Pkwy, Suite 500
P.O. Box 13770
Richmond, VA 23225
(888) TXINFO1
www.unos.org

PAIN

American Chronic Pain Association
P.O. Box 850
Rocklin, CA 95677
(916) 632-0922
Fax (916) 632-3208
www.theacpa.org

International Association for the Study of Pain
909 NE 43rd Street, Suite 306
Seattle, WA 98105-6020
(206) 547-6409
Fax (206) 547-1703
www.halcyon.com/iasp

PARKINSON'S DISEASE

National Parkinson Foundation
1501 N.W. 9th Avenue
Bob Hope Road
Miami, FL 33136-1494
(800) 327-4545
(305) 243-4403
www.parkinson.org

Parkinson's Disease Foundation, Inc.
William Black Medical Building
Columbia-Presbyterian Medical Center
710 W. 168th Street
New York NY 10032-9982
(212) 923-4700
(800) 457-6676
www.parkinsons-foundation.org

PESTICIDES

National Pesticide Telecommunication Network
Oregon State University
333 Weniger
Corvallis, OR 97331-6502
(800) 858-7378
Fax (541) 737-0761
www.ace.orst.edu/info/nptn

RARE DISORDERS

National Organization for Rare Disorders
P.O. Box 9823
New Fairfield, CT 16812
(800) 999-6673
Fax (203) 746-6481
www.rarediseases.org

RESPIRATORY DISORDERS

American Lung Association
1740 Broadway
New York, NY 10019
(212) 315-8700
(800) LUNG-USA
www.lungusa.org

Asthma and Allergy Foundation of America
1233 20th Street, NW, Suite 402
Washington, DC 20036
(800) 7-ASTHMA (727-8462)
Fax (202) 466-8940
www.aafa.org

Cystic Fibrosis Foundation
6931 Arlington Road, No. 200
Bethesda, MD 20814
(800) 344-4823
www.cff.org

REYE'S SYNDROME

National Reye's Syndrome Foundation
426 N. Lewis Street
Bryan, OH 43506
(800) 233-7393
www.bright.net/reyessyn

SICKLE CELL ANEMIA

Sickle Cell Disease Association of America, Inc.
200 Corporate Pointe, Suite 495
Culver City, CA 90230-7633
(800) 421-8453
Fax (310) 215-3722
www.sicklecelldisease.org

SPINA BIFIDA

Spina Bifida Association of America
4590 MacArthur Blvd. NW, Suite 250
Washington, DC 20007
(202) 944-3285
(800) 621-3141
Fax (202) 944-3295
www.sbaa.org

SPINAL CORD INJURY

National Spinal Cord Injury Association
8701 Georgia Avenue, Suite 500
Silver Spring, Maryland 20910
(800) 962-9629
Fax (301) 588-9414
www.spinalcord.org

SUBSTANCE ABUSE

Alcoholics Anonymous
P.O. Box 459, Grand Central Station
New York, NY 10163
(212) 870-3400
www.aa.org

Cottage Program International
57 W. South Temple, Suite 420
Salt Lake City, UT 84101-1511
(800) 752-6100

National Families in Action
Century Plaza II
2957 Clairmont Road, Suite 150
Atlanta, GA 30329
(404) 248-9676
Fax (404) 248-1312
www.emory.edu/NFIA

SUICIDE

American Association of Suicidology
4201 Connecticut Avenue NW, Suite 408
Washington, DC 20008
(202) 237-2280
www.suicidology.org

American Foundation for Suicide Prevention
120 Wall Street, 22nd floor
New York, NY 10005
(212) 363-3500
www.afsp.org

TAY-SACHS DISEASE

National Foundation for Jewish Genetic Diseases
250 Park Avenue, Suite 1000
New York, NY 10177
(212) 371-1030
www.nfjgd.org

VISUAL IMPAIRMENT

American Foundation for the Blind
11 Penn Plaza, Suite 300
New York, NY 10001
(212) 502-7600
www.afb.org

Lighthouse National Center for Education
111 E. 59th Street
New York, NY 10022
(212) 821-9200
(800) 334-5497
TTY (212) 821-9713
www.lighthouse.org

National Association for Visually Handicapped
22 W. 21st Street
New York, NY 10010
(212) 889-3141
Fax (212) 727-2931
www.navh.org

Recording for the Blind and Dyslexic
20 Roszel Road
Princeton, NJ 08540
(800) 803-7201
www.rfbd.org

Appendix 14–2 Resource Organizations in Canada

AIDS

AIDS Committee of Ottawa
207 Queens Street, 4th Floor
Ottawa, Ontario K1P 6E5
(613) 238-5014
www.ncf.ca/aids

Canadian Public Health Association
1565 Carling Avenue, Suite 400
Ottawa, ON K1Z 8R1
(877) 999-7740
(613) 725-3434
Fax (613) 725-1205
www.cpha.ca

ALZHEIMER'S DISEASE

Alzheimer Society of Canada
20 Eglinton Ave. W., Suite 1200
Toronto, Ontario M4R 1K8
(416) 488-8772
Fax (416) 488-3778
www.alzheimer.ca

ARTHRITIS

The Arthritis Society
393 University Avenue, Suite 1700
Toronto, Ontario M5G 1E6
(416) 979-7228
Fax (416) 979-8366
www.arthritis.ca

BIRTH DEFECTS

AboutFace
99 Crowns Lane, 4th Floor
Toronto, Ontario M5R 3P4
(800) 665-FACE (3223)
www.abtface.ca

CANCER

Canadian Cancer Society
National Office
10 Alcorn Avenue, Suite 200
Toronto, Ontario M4V 3B1
(416) 961-7223
Fax (416) 961-4189
www.cancer.ca

DIABETES

Canadian Diabetes Association
15 Toronto Street, Suite 800
Toronto, Ontario M5C 2E3
(416) 363-3373
(800) BANTING
www.diabetes.ca

EATING DISORDERS

National Eating Disorders Information Centre
College Wing, 1-211
200 Elizabeth Street
Toronto, Ontario M5G-2C4
(416) 340-4156
Fax (416) 340-4736
www.nedic.on.ca

HEARING IMPAIRMENT

Canadian Association of the Deaf
251 Bank Street, Suite 203
Ottawa, Ontario K2P 1X3 Canada
(613) 565-2882
Fax (613) 565-1207
www.cad.ca

HEART DISEASE

Canadian Adult Congenital Heart Network
The Toronto Hospital
200 Elizabeth Street, EN 12-213

Toronto, Ontario M5G 2C4
(416) 977-5096
Fax (416) 340-5014
www.cachnet.org

Canadian Cardiovascular Society
360 Victoria Avenue, Room 401
Westmont, Quebec H3Z 2N4
(514) 482-3407
(514) 482-6574
www.ccs.ca

HEMOPHILIA

World Federation of Hemophilia
1425 René Lévesque Boulevard West, Suite 1010
Montreal, Quebec H3G 1T7
(514) 875-7944
Fax (514) 875-8916
www.wfh.org

KIDNEY

Kidney Foundation of Canada
2300 René LeVesque Blvd.
Montreal, Quebec H3H 2R5
(514) 938-4515
(800) 565-4515
Fax (514) 938-4757
www.kidney.ca

LIVER

Canadian Liver Foundation
National Office
365 Bloor Street E, Ste. 200
Toronto, Ontario M4W 3L4
(416) 964-1953
(800) 563-5483
Fax (416) 964-0024
www.liver.ca

MENTAL HEALTH

Canadian Mental Health Association
2160 Yonge Street
Toronto, Ontario M4S 2Z3
(416) 484-7750
Fax (416) 484-4617
www.cmha.ca

NEUROLOGICAL DISORDERS

ALS Society of Canada
265 Yorkland Boulevard, Suite 300
Toronto, Ontario M2J 1S5
(416) 497-2267
Fax (416) 497-1256
www.als.ca

Canadian Association of Friedreich's Ataxia
5620, rue C.A. Jobin
Montreal, Quebec H1P 1H8
(514) 321-8684
www.cam.org/acaf

ORGAN DONATION

M.O.R.E. of Ontario
984 Bay Street, Ste. 503
Toronto, Ontario M5S 2A5
(416) 921-1130
(800) 263-2833

REPRODUCTIVE DISORDERS

Canadian Pelvic Inflammatory Disease Society
802-1170 Pendrell
Vancouver, British Columbia V6J 4L6
(604) 684-5704

Infertility Awareness Association of Canada
406 - One Nicholas Street
Ottawa, Ontario K1N 7B7 Canada
(613) 244-7222
Fax (613) 244-8908
www.iaac.ca

RESPIRATORY DISORDERS

Lung Association
Three Raymond Street
Ottawa, Ontario K1R 1A3
(613) 230-4200
Fax (613) 230-5210
www.on.lung.ca

VISUAL IMPAIRMENT

Canadian Council of the Blind
405-396 Cooper Street
Ottawa, Ontario K2P 2H7
(613) 567-0311

WEB-BASED RESOURCES

Inclusion of a website on this list does not imply endorsement of the information contained on that site.

HealthAnswers.com
www.healthanswers.com

Healtheon/WebMD
www.webmd.com

InteliHealth
www.intelihealth.com

Mayo Clinic Health Oasis
www.mayohealth.com

APPENDIX 15
Professional Designations and Titles in the Health Sciences

AARCF American Association for Respiratory Care Fellow
ACCE ASPO (American Society for Psychoprophylaxis in Obstetrics) Certified Childbirth Educator
ANP Adult Nurse Practitioner
AOCN American Oncology Certified Nurse
ARNP Advanced Registered Nurse Practitioner
ARRT American Registry of Radiologic Technologists
ART Accredited Record Technologist
ATC Athletic Trainer, Certified
BC Bachelor of Surgery
BCh Bachelor of Surgery
BM Bachelor of Medicine
BS Bachelor of Science; Bachelor of Surgery
BSN Bachelor of Science in Nursing
CAPA Certified Ambulatory Post-Anesthesia Nurse
CARN Certified Addiction Registered Nurse
CB Bachelor of Surgery
CCCN Certified Continence Care Nurse
CCM Certified Case Manager
CCP Certified Clinical Perfusionist
CCRN Certified Critical Care Registered Nurse
CDA Certified Dental Assistant
CDE Certified Diabetes Educator
CEN Certified Emergency Nurse
CETN Certified Enterostomal Therapy Nurse
CFNP Certified Family Nurse Practitioner
CFRN Certified Flight Registered Nurse
CGN Certified Gastroenterology Nurse
CGRN Certified Gastroenterology Registered Nurse
CGT Certified Gastroenterology Technician
ChB Bachelor of Surgery
ChD Doctor of Surgery
CHN Certified Hemodialysis Nurse
CIC Certified Infection Control Nurse
CLA Certified Laboratory Assistant
CLPNI Certified Licensed Practitioner Nursing, Intravenous
CLS Clinical Laboratory Specialist
CLT Certified Laboratory Technician; Clinical Laboratory Technician
CMA-A Certified Medical Assistant, Administrative
CMA-C Certified Medical Assistant, Clinical
CNA Certified Nursing Assistant; Certified in Nursing Administration
CNAA Certified in Nursing Administration, Advanced
CNDLTC Certified Nursing Director of Long-Term Care
CNM Certified Nurse Midwife
CNMT Certified Nuclear Medical Technologist
CNN Certified Nephrology Nurse
CNOR Certified Nurse, Operating Room
CNP Community Nurse Practitioner
CNRN Certified Neuroscience Registered Nurse
CNS Clinical Nurse Specialist
CNSN Certified Nutrition Support Nurse
COCN Certified Ostomy Care Nurse
COHN Certified Occupational Health Nurse
COHN-S Certified Occupational Health Nurse—Specialty
CORLN Certified Otorhinolaryngology Nurse
CORN Certified Operating Room Nurse
COTA Certified Occupational Therapy Assistant
CPAN Certified Post-Anesthesia Nurse
CPDN Certified Peritoneal Dialysis Nurse
CPN Certified Pediatric Nurse
CPNP Certified Pediatric Nurse Practitioner
CPON Certified Pediatric Oncology Nurse
CPSN Certified Plastic Surgical Nurse
CRNA Certified Registered Nurse Anesthetist
CRNFA Certified Registered Nurse, First Assistant
CRNH Certified Registered Hospice Nurse
CRNI Certified Registered Nurse, Intravenous

CRNO Certified Registered Nurse, Ophthalmology
CRRN Certified Rehabilitation Registered Nurse
CRTT Certified Respiratory Therapy Technician
CSN Certified School Nurse
CST Certified Surgical Technologist
CURN Certified Urology Registered Nurse
CWCN Certified Wound Care Nurse
DC Doctor of Chiropractic
DCh Doctor of Surgery
DDS Doctor of Dental Surgery
DM Doctor of Medicine
DMD Doctor of Dental Medicine
DME Doctor of Medical Education
DMSc Doctor of Medical Science
DMV Doctor of Veterinary Medicine
DN Doctor of Nursing
DNE Doctor of Nursing Education
DNS Doctor of Nursing Science
DNSc Doctor of Nursing Science
DO Doctor of Osteopathy; Doctor of Ophthalmology
DP Doctor of Pharmacy
DPH Doctor of Public Health
DPhil Doctor of Philosophy
DPHN Doctor of Public Health Nursing
DPM Doctor of Podiatric Medicine
DrPH Doctor of Public Health
DS Doctor of Science
DSc Doctor of Science
DSW Doctor of Social Work
DVM Doctor of Veterinary Medicine
DVMS Doctor of Veterinary Medicine and Surgery
EdD Doctor of Education
EMT-B Emergency Medical Technician—Basic
EMT-D Emergency Medical Technician—Defibrillation
EMT-I Emergency Medical Technician—Intermediate
EMT-P Emergency Medical Technician—Paramedic
FAAAI Fellow of the American Academy of Allergy and Immunology
FAAFP Fellow of the American Academy of Family Physicians
FAAN Fellow of the American Academy of Neurology
FAAN Fellow of the American Academy of Nursing
FAAO Fellow of the American Academy of Ophthalmology
FAAO Fellow of the American Academy of Osteopathy
FAAOS Fellow of the American Academy of Orthopedic Surgeons
FAAP Fellow of the American Academy of Pediatrics
FACC Fellow of the American College of Cardiology
FACCP Fellow of the American College of Chest Physicians
FACE Fellow of the American College of Endocrinology
FACEP Fellow of the American College of Emergency Physicians
FACOG Fellow of the American College of Obstetrics and Gynecology
FACP Fellow of the American College of Physicians
FACS Fellow of the American College of Surgeons
FACSM Fellow of the American College of Sports Medicine
FAOTA Fellow of the American Occupational Therapy Association
FAPHA Fellow of the American Public Health Association
FCPS Fellow of the College of Physicians and Surgeons
FFA Fellow of the Faculty of Anaesthetists
FFARCS Fellow of the Faculty of Anaesthetists of the Royal College of Surgeons
FICC Fellow of the International College of Chiropractors
FNAAOM Fellow of the National Academy of Acupuncture and Oriental Medicine
FNP Family Nurse Practitioner
FP Family Practitioner
FRCGP Fellow of the Royal College of General Practitioners
FRCOG Fellow of the Royal College of Obstetricians and Gynaecologists
FRCP Fellow of the Royal College of Physicians
FRCPC Fellow of the Royal College of Physicians of Canada
FRCR Fellow of the Royal College of Radiologists
FRCS Fellow of the Royal College of Surgeons
FRCSC Fellow of the Royal College of Surgeons of Canada
FRCVS Fellow of the Royal College of Veterinary Surgeons
FRS Fellow of the Royal Society
GNP Gerontological Nurse Practitioner
GPN General Pediatric Nurse
HT Histologic Technician/ Histologic Technologist

LAT Licensed Athletic Trainer
LATC Licensed Athletic Trainer, Certified
LPN Licensed Practical Nurse
LVN Licensed Visiting Nurse; Licensed Vocational Nurse
MB Bachelor of Medicine
MBBS Bachelor of Medicine; Bachelor of Surgery
MCh Master of Surgery
MD Doctor of Medicine
ME Medical Examiner
MEd Master of Education
MPH Master of Public Health
MPharm Master in Pharmacy
MRCP Member of the Royal College of Physicians
MRCS Member of the Royal College of Surgeons
MRL Medical Records Librarian
MS Master of Science; Master of Surgery
MSc Master of Surgery
MSN Master of Science in Nursing
MSurg Master of Surgery
MT Medical Technologist
MTA Medical Technologist Assistant
MT-(ASCP) Medical Technologist (American Society of Clinical Pathologists)
ND Doctor of Naturopathy
NMT Nurse Massage Therapist; Nursing Massage Therapist
NP Nurse Practitioner
NREMT-P National Registry of Emergency Medical Technician—Paramedics
OCN Oncology Certified Nurse
OD Doctor of Optometry
ONC Orthopedic Nurse Certified
OT Occupational Therapist
OT-C Occupational Therapist (Canada)
OTL Occupational Therapist, Licensed
OTR Registered Occupational Therapist
PA Physician Assistant
PA-C Physician Assistant Certified
PD Doctor of Pharmacy
PharmD Doctor of Pharmacy
PharmG Graduate in Pharmacy
PhD Doctor of Philosophy
PNP Pediatric Nurse Practitioner
PT Physical Therapist
RD Registered Dietitian
RDA Registered Dental Assistant
RDCS Registered Diagnostic Cardiac Sonographer
RDH Registered Dental Hygienist
RDMS Registered Diagnostic Medical Sonographer
R EEG T Radiologic Electro-encephalography Technologist
R EP T Registered Evoked Potentials Technologist
RMA Registered Medical Assistant
RN Registered Nurse
RNA Registered Nurse Anesthetist
RNC Registered Nurse Certified (OB/GYN and Neonatal)
RPh Registered Pharmacist
RPT Registered Physical Therapist
RRA Registered Record Administrator
RRT Registered Respiratory Therapist
RT Radiologic Technologist; Respiratory Therapist
RT(N) Nuclear Medicine Technologist
RT(R) Technologist in Diagnostic Radiology
RTR Registered Recreational Therapist
RT(T) Radiation Therapy Technologist
RVT Registered Vascular Technologist
ScD Doctor of Science
SCT Specialist in Cytotechnology
SM Master of Surgery
VMD Veterinary Medical Doctor

APPENDIX 16
Documentation System Definitions

ALERT. A charting system used primarily in long-term care in which the patient's chart is tagged to indicate that special charting procedures/precautions need to be initiated and followed for a specified time.

CBE. Acronym for *C*harting *B*y *E*xception, a system for documentation that eliminates the need to chart repetitious findings and tasks. The health care provider uses specially designed admission history and flow sheets that highlight important findings and trends. Only significant findings or exceptions to established standards of care and protocols are documented in the progress notes.

CLINICAL PROGRESSION. A critical path that has been enhanced by the addition of (1) nursing diagnosis, (2) intermediate and discharge goals, and (3) variance tracking. This type of plan is usually used for longer hospital stays not requiring critical care.

CORE. A documentation system designed to support the nursing process. Key elements include database, care plans, flow sheets, progress notes, and discharge summaries. Progress notes use a three-column format and are organized using patient *D*atabase; *A*ction of the health care provider; and *E*valuation of patient outcome.

CRITICAL PATH. A cause-and-effect grid that outlines usual interventions by health care providers against a timeline for a case type (diagnosis-related group) or otherwise defined homogeneous patient population. This type of plan is usually used in cases requiring critical care.

DAR. Acronym for the organizing structure for writing progress notes using Focus Charting©. Each Focus entry includes *D*atabase describing the current patient condition; *A*ction taken by the health care provider; and patient *R*esponse or outcome to the intervention.

FACT. Acronym for a documentation system including these key elements: *F*lowsheets for specific patient populations; standardized *A*ssessment parameters printed on the chart form; *C*oncise integrated progress notes; and *T*imely entries by health care providers at the time care is given.

FOCUS CHARTING©. Trademark title for a three-column format for organizing the progress notes in the patient record. The FOCUS column serves as an index. The body of the note is organized by identifying the DATAbase describing the current patient condition; ACTION taken by the health care provider; and patient RESPONSE to or outcome of the intervention.

PIE. Acronym for a process-oriented documentation system. The progress notes in the patient record use (P) to define the particular *P*roblem; (I) to document *I*ntervention; and (E) to *E*valuate the patient outcome. PIE charting integrates care planning with progress notes.

POMR. Acronym for *P*roblem-*O*riented *M*edical *R*ecord, a method of establishing and maintaining the patient's medical record so that problems are clearly stated. These data are kept in the front of the chart and are evaluated as frequently as indicated with respect to recording changes in the patient's problems as well as progress made in solving the problems. Use of this system may bring a degree of comprehensiveness to total patient care that might not be possible with conventional medical records.

SOAP. Acronym for an organized structure for keeping progress notes in the chart. Each entry contains the date, number, and title of the patient's particular problem, followed by the SOAP headings: *S*ubjective findings; *O*bjective findings; *A*ssessment, the documented analysis and conclusions concerning the findings; and *P*lan for further diagnostic or therapeutic action. If the patient has multiple problems, a SOAP entry on the chart is made for each problem.

SOAPIER. Adds to the SOAP headings listed above: documentation of *I*ntervention implemented to solve the identified problem; *E*valuation of the effectiveness of the intervention; and care plan *R*evisions indicated.

VARIANCE. A task or outcome that does not occur as described or within the time frame identified on a critical path or clinical progression.

APPENDIX 17
Standard and Universal Precautions

Appendix 17–1 Standard Precautions (CDC Isolation Precautions)

BACKGROUND AND SUMMARY

In January 1996, the Centers for Disease Control and Prevention (CDC) issued new guidelines for isolation precautions in hospitals. The guidelines, based on the latest epidemiologic information on transmission of infection in hospitals, are intended primarily for use in acute-care hospitals, although some of the recommendations may be applicable to subacute-care or extended-care facilities. The recommendations are not intended for use in day care, well care, or domiciliary care programs.

The revised guidelines contain two tiers of precautions. In the first, and most important, tier are those precautions designed for the care of all patients in hospitals regardless of their diagnosis or presumed infection status. Implementation of these "Standard Precautions" is the primary strategy for successful nosocomial infection control. In the second tier are precautions designed only for the care of specified patients. These additional "Transmission-Based Precautions" are used for patients known or suspected to be infected or colonized with epidemiologically important pathogens that can be transmitted by airborne or droplet transmission or by contact with dry skin or contaminated surfaces.

Standard Precautions synthesize the major features of Universal (Blood and Body Fluid) Precautions (designed to reduce the risk of transmission of bloodborne pathogens) and Body Substance Isolation (designed to reduce the risk of transmission of pathogens from moist body substances). Standard Precautions apply to (1) blood; (2) all body fluids, secretions, and excretions *except sweat*, regardless of whether they contain visible blood; (3) nonintact skin; and (4) mucous membranes. Standard Precautions are designed to reduce the risk of transmission of both recognized and unrecognized sources of infection in hospitals.

Transmission-Based Precautions are designed for patients documented or suspected to be infected or colonized with highly transmissible or epidemiologically important pathogens for which additional precautions beyond Standard Precautions are needed to interrupt transmission in hospitals. There are three types of Transmission-Based Precautions: *Airborne Precautions, Droplet Precautions,* and *Contact Precautions*. They may be combined for diseases that have multiple routes of transmission. When used either singly or in combination, they are to be used in addition to Standard Precautions.

Airborne Precautions are designed to reduce the risk of airborne transmission of infectious agents. Airborne transmission occurs by dissemination of either airborne droplet nuclei (small-particle residue [5 microns or smaller in size] of evaporated droplets that may remain suspended in the air for long periods of time) or dust particles containing the infectious agent. Microorganisms carried in this manner can be dispersed widely by air currents and may become inhaled by or deposited on a susceptible host within the same room or over a longer distance from the source patient, depending on environmental factors; therefore, special air handling and ventilation are required to prevent airborne transmission. Examples of diseases spread by airborne droplet nuclei include measles, varicella (including disseminated zoster), and tuberculosis.

Droplet Precautions are designed to reduce the risk of droplet transmission of infectious agents. Droplet transmission involves contact of the conjunctivae or the mucous membranes of the nose or mouth of a susceptible person with large-particle droplets (larger than 5 microns in size) containing microorganisms generated from a person who has a clinical disease or who is a carrier of the microorganism. Droplets are generated from the source person primarily during coughing, sneezing, or talking and during the performance of certain procedures such as suctioning and bronchoscopy. Transmission via large-particle droplets requires close contact between source and recipient persons, because droplets do not remain suspended in the air and generally travel only short distances, usually 3 ft or less, through the air. Because droplets do not remain suspended in the air, special air handling and ventilation are not required to prevent droplet transmission.

Examples of illnesses spread by large-particle droplets include invasive *Haemophilus influenzae* type B disease (including meningitis, pneumonia, epiglottitis, and sepsis); invasive *Neisseria meningitidis* disease (including meningitis, pneumonia, and sepsis); diphtheria (pharyngeal); mycoplasma pneumonia; pertussis; pneumonic plague; streptococcal pharyngitis, pneumonia, or scarlet fever in infants and young children; adenovirus influenza; mumps; parvovirus B19; and rubella.

Contact Precautions are designed to reduce the risk of transmission of epidemiologically important microorganisms by direct or indirect contact. Direct-contact transmission involves skin-to-skin contact and physical transfer of microorganisms to a susceptible host from an infected or colonized person, such as occurs when personnel turn patients, bathe patients, or perform other patient-care activities that require physical contact. Direct-contact transmission can also occur between two patients (e.g., by hand contact), with one serving as the source of infectious microorganisms and the other as a susceptible host. Indirect-contact transmission involves contact of a susceptible host with a contaminated intermediate object, usually inanimate, in the patient's environment.

Examples of illnesses spread by direct contact include gastrointestinal, respiratory, skin, or wound infections or colonization with multidrug-resistant bacteria judged by the infection control program (based on current state, regional, or national recommendations) to be of special clinical and epidemiologic significance; enteric infections with a low infectious dose or prolonged environmental survival, including *Clostridium difficile*; for diapered or incontinent patients: enterohemorrhagic *Escherichia coli* O157:H7, *Shigella*, hepatitis A, or rotavirus; respiratory syncytial virus, parainfluenza virus, or enteroviral infections in infants and young children; viral/hemorrhagic conjunctivitis; viral hemorrhagic infections (Ebola, Lassa, or Marburg); and skin infections that are highly contagious or that may occur on dry skin, including:

Diphtheria (cutaneous)
Herpes simplex virus (neonatal or mucocutaneous)
Impetigo
Major (noncontained) abscesses, cellulitis, or decubiti
Pediculosis
Scabies
Staphylococcal furunculosis in infants and young children
Zoster (disseminated or in the immunocompromised host)

STANDARD PRECAUTIONS

Use the following Standard Precautions, or the equivalent, for the care of all patients.

- **Handwashing:**
  1. Wash hands after touching blood, body fluids, secretions, excretions, and contaminated items, whether or not gloves are worn. Wash hands immediately after gloves are removed, between patient contacts, and when otherwise indicated to avoid transfer of microorganisms to other patients or environments. It may be necessary to wash hands between tasks and procedures on the same patient to prevent cross-contamination of different body sites.
  2. Use a plain (nonantimicrobial) soap for routine handwashing.
  3. Use an antimicrobial agent or a waterless antiseptic agent for specific circumstances (e.g., control of outbreaks or hyperendemic infections), as defined by the infection control program. (SEE: Contact Precautions for additional recommendations on using antimicrobial and antiseptic agents.)
- **Gloves:** Wear gloves (clean, nonsterile gloves are adequate) when touching blood, body fluids, secretions, excretions, and contaminated items. Put on clean gloves just before touching mucous membranes and nonintact skin. Change gloves between tasks and procedures on the same patient after contact with material that may contain a high concentration of microorganisms. Remove gloves promptly after use, before touching noncontaminated items and environmental surfaces, and before going to another patient, and wash hands immediately to avoid transfer of microorganisms to other patients or environments.
- **Mask, Eye Protection, Face Shield:** Wear a mask and eye protection or a face shield to protect mucous membranes of the eyes, nose, and mouth during procedures and patient-care activities that are likely to generate splashes or sprays of blood, body fluids, secretions, and excretions.
- **Gown:** Wear a gown (a clean, nonsterile gown is adequate) to protect skin and to prevent soiling of clothing during procedures and patient-care activities that are likely to generate splashes or sprays of blood, body fluids, secretions, or excretions. Select a gown that is appropriate for the activity and amount of fluid likely to be encountered. Remove a soiled gown as promptly as possible, and wash hands to avoid transfer of microorganisms to other patients or environments.
- **Patient-Care Equipment:** Handle used patient-care equipment soiled with blood, body fluids, secretions, and excretions in a manner that prevents skin and mucous membrane exposures, contamination of clothing, and transfer of microorganisms to other patients and environments. Ensure that reusable equipment is not used for the

care of another patient until it has been cleaned and reprocessed appropriately. Ensure that single-use items are discarded properly.

- **Environmental Control:** Ensure that the hospital has adequate procedures for the routine care, cleaning, and disinfection of environmental surfaces, beds, bedrails, bedside equipment, and other frequently touched surfaces, and ensure that these procedures are being followed.
- **Linen:** Handle, transport, and process used linen soiled with blood, body fluids, secretions, and excretions in a manner that prevents skin and mucous membrane exposures and contamination of clothing, and that avoids transfer of microorganisms to other patients and environments.
- **Occupational Health and Bloodborne Pathogens:**
  1. Take care to prevent injuries when using needles, scalpels, and other sharp instruments or devices; when handling sharp instruments after procedures; when cleaning used instruments; and when disposing of used needles. Never recap used needles, or otherwise manipulate them using both hands, or use any other technique that involves directing the point of a needle toward any part of the body; rather, use either a one-handed "scoop" technique or a mechanical device designed for holding the needle sheath. Do not remove used needles from disposable syringes by hand, and do not bend, break, or otherwise manipulate used needle by hand. Place used disposable syringes and needles, scalpel blades, and other sharp items in appropriate puncture-resistant containers, which are located as close as practical to the area in which the items were used, and place reusable syringes and needles in a puncture-resistant container for transport to the reprocessing area.
  2. Use mouthpieces, resuscitation bags, or other ventilation devices as an alternative to mouth-to-mouth resuscitation methods in areas where the need for resuscitation is predictable.
- **Patient Placement:** Place a patient who contaminates the environment or who does not (or cannot be expected to) assist in maintaining appropriate hygiene or environmental control in a private room. If a private room is not available, consult with infection control professionals regarding patient placement or other alternatives.

TRANSMISSION-BASED PRECAUTIONS

Airborne Precautions

In addition to Standard Precautions, use Airborne Precautions, or the equivalent, for patients known or suspected to be infected with microorganisms transmitted by airborne droplet nuclei (small-particle residue [5 microns or smaller in size] of evaporated droplets containing microorganisms that remain suspended in the air and that can be dispersed widely by air currents within a room or over a long distance).

- **Patient Placement:** Place the patient in a private room that has (1) monitored negative air pressure in relation to the surrounding areas, (2) 6–12 air changes per hour, and (3) appropriate discharge of air outdoors or monitored high-efficiency filtration of room air before the air is circulated to other areas in the hospital. Keep the room door closed and the patient in the room. When a private room is not available, place the patient in a room with a patient who has active infection with the same microorganism unless otherwise recommended, but with no other infection. When a private room is not available and cohorting is not desirable, consultation with infection control professionals is advised before patient placement.
- **Respiratory Protection:** Wear respiratory protection when entering the room of a patient with known or suspected infectious pulmonary tuberculosis. Susceptible persons should not enter the room of patients known or suspected to have measles (rubeola) or varicella (chickenpox) if other immune caregivers are available. If susceptible persons must enter the room of a patient known or suspected to have measles or varicella, they should wear respiratory protection. Persons immune to measles or varicella need not wear respiratory protection.
- **Patient Transport:** Limit the movement and transport of the patient from the room to essential purposes only. If transport or movement is necessary, minimize patient dispersal of droplet nuclei by placing a surgical mask on the patient, if possible.

Additional Precautions for Preventing Transmission of Tuberculosis

Consult CDC "Guidelines for Preventing the Transmission of Tuberculosis in Health-Care Facilities"[1] for additional prevention strategies.

Droplet Precautions

In addition to Standard Precautions, use Droplet Precautions, or the equivalent, for a patient known or suspected to be infected with microorganisms transmitted by droplets (large-particle droplets [larger than 5 microns in size] that can be generated during coughing, sneezing, talking, or the performance of procedures).

- **Patient Placement:** Place the patient in a private room. When a private room is not available, place the patient in a room with a patient(s) who has active infection with the same microorganism but with no other infection (cohorting). When a private room is not available and cohorting is not achievable, maintain spatial separation of at least 3 ft between the infected patient and other patients and visitors. Special air handling and ventilation are not necessary, and the door may remain open.
- **Mask:** In addition to standard precautions, wear a mask when working within 3 ft of the patient. (Logistically, some hospitals may want to implement the wearing of a mask to enter the room.)
- **Patient Transport:** Limit the movement and transport of the patient from the room to essential purposes only. If transport or movement is necessary, minimize patient dispersal of droplets by masking the patient, if possible.

Contact Precautions

In addition to Standard Precautions, use Contact Precautions, or the equivalent, for specified patients known or suspected to be infected or colonized with epidemiologically important microorganisms that can be transmitted by direct contact with the patient (hand or skin-to-skin contact that occurs when performing patient-care activities that require touching the patient's dry skin) or indirect contact (touching) with environmental surfaces or patient-care items in the patient's environment

- **Patient Placement:** Place the patient in a private room. When a private room is not available, place the patient in a room with a patient(s) who has active infection with the same microorganism but with no other infection (cohorting). When a private room is not available and cohorting is not achievable, consider the epidemiology of the microorganism and the patient population when determining patient placement. Consultation with infection control professionals is advised before patient placement.
- **Gloves and Handwashing:** In addition to wearing gloves as outlined under Standard Precautions, wear gloves (clean, nonsterile gloves are adequate) when entering the room. During the course of providing care for a patient, change gloves after having contact with infective material that may contain high concentrations of microorganisms (fecal material and wound drainage). Remove gloves before leaving the patient's environment and wash hands immediately with an antimicrobial agent or a waterless antiseptic agent. After glove removal and handwashing, ensure that hands do not touch potentially contaminated environmental surfaces or items in the patient's room to avoid transfer of microorganisms to other patients or environments.
- **Gown:** In addition to wearing a gown as outlined under Standard Precautions, wear a gown (a clean, nonsterile gown is adequate) when entering the room if you anticipate that your clothing will have substantial contact with the patient, environmental surfaces, or items in the patient's room, or if the patient is incontinent or has diarrhea, an ileostomy, a colostomy, or wound drainage not contained by a dressing. Remove the gown before leaving the patient's environment. After gown removal, ensure that clothing does not contact potentially contaminated environmental surfaces to avoid transfer of microorganisms to other patients or environments.
- **Patient Transport:** Limit the movement and transport of the patient from the room to essential purposes only. If the patient is transported out of the room, ensure that precautions are maintained to minimize the risk of transmission of microorganisms to other patients and contamination of environmental surfaces or equipment.
- **Patient-Care Equipment:** When possible, dedicate the use of noncritical patient-care equipment to a single patient (or cohort of patients infected or colonized with the pathogen requiring precautions) to avoid sharing between patients. If use of common equipment or items is unavoidable, then adequately clean and disinfect them before use for another patient.

Additional Precautions for Preventing the Spread of Vancomycin Resistance

Consult the Hospital Infection Control Practices Advisory Committee report on preventing the spread of vancomycin resistance for additional prevention strategies.[2]

---

[1] Centers for Disease Control and Prevention. Guidelines for preventing the transmission of tuberculosis in health-care facilities, 1994. *MMWR* 1994; 43 (RR-13):1–132, and *Federal Register* 1994; 59 (208):54242–54303.

[2] Hospital Infection Control Practices Advisory Committee. Recommendations for preventing the spread of vancomycin resistance. *Amer J Infect Control* 1995; 23:87–94, *Infect Control Hosp Epidemiol* 1995; 16:105–113, and *MMWR* 1995; 44 (NO. RR-12):1–13.

SOURCE: Adapted from Garner, JS, Hospital Infection Control Practices Advisory Committee. Guidelines for isolation precautions in hospitals. Infect Control Hosp Epidemiol 1996; 17:53–80.

Appendix 17–2 OSHA Bloodborne Pathogens Standard

WHO IS COVERED?

The Occupational Safety and Health Administration (OSHA) standard protects employees who may be occupationally exposed to blood and other potential infectious materials, which includes but is not limited to physicians, physician's assistants, nurses, nurse practitioners, and other health care employees in clinics and physicians' offices; employees of clinical and diagnostic laboratories; housekeepers in health care and other facilities; personnel in hospital laundries or commercial laundries that service health care or public safety institutions; tissue bank personnel; employees in blood banks and plasma centers who collect, transport, and test blood; freestanding clinic employees (e.g., hemodialysis clinics, urgent care clinics, health maintenance organization (HMO) clinics, and family planning clinics); employees in clinics in industrial, educational, and correctional facilities (e.g., those who collect blood and clean and dress wounds); employees designated to provide emergency first aid; dentists, dental hygienists, dental assistants, and dental laboratory technicians; staff of institutions for the developmentally disabled; hospice employees; home health care workers; staff of nursing homes and long-term care facilities; employees of funeral homes and mortuaries; HIV and HBV research laboratory and production facility workers; employees handling regulated waste; custodial workers required to clean up contaminated sharps or spills of blood or OPIM; medical equipment service and repair personnel; emergency medical technicians, paramedics, and other emergency medical service providers; fire fighters, law enforcement personnel, and correctional officers (employees in the private sector, the federal government, or a state or local government in a state that has an OSHA-approved state plan); maintenance workers, such as plumbers, in health care facilities and employees of substance abuse clinics.

Blood means human blood, blood products, or blood components (plasma, platelets, and serosanguineous fluids, [e.g., exudates from wounds]. Also included are medications derived from blood, such as immune globulins, albumin, and factors 8 and 9). Other potentially infectious materials include human body fluids such as saliva in dental procedures; semen; vaginal secretions; cerebrospinal, synovial, pleural, pericardial, peritoneal, and amniotic fluids; body fluids visibly contaminated with blood; unfixed human tissues or organs; HIV-containing cell or tissue cultures; and HIV- or HBV-containing culture media or other solutions.

Occupational exposure means a "reasonably anticipated skin, eye, mucous membrane, or parenteral contact [human bites that break the skin, which are most likely to occur in violent situations such as may be encountered by prison personnel and police and in emergency rooms or psychiatric wards] with blood or other potentially infectious materials that may result from the performance of the employee's duties." (The term *reasonably anticipated contact* includes the potential for contact as well as actual contact with blood or other potentially infectious material [OPIM]. Lack of history of blood exposures among designated first aid personnel of a particular manufacturing site, for instance, does not preclude coverage. *Reasonably anticipated contact* includes, among others, contact with blood or OPIM, including regulated waste, as well as incidents of needlesticks. For example, a compliance officer may document incidents in which an employee observes uncapped needles or contacts other regulated waste in order to substantiate occupational exposure.)

Federal OSHA authority extends to all private sector employers with one or more employees, as well as federal civilian employees. In addition, many states administer their own occupational safety and health programs through plans approved under section 18(b) of the OSH Act. These plans must adopt standards and enforce requirements that are at least as effective as federal requirements. Of the current 25 state plan states and territories, 23 cover the private and public (state and local governments) sectors and 2 cover the public sector only.

Determining occupational exposure and instituting control methods and work practices appropriate for specific job assignments are key requirements of the standard. The required written exposure control plan and methods of compliance show how employee exposure can be minimized or eliminated.

THE EXPOSURE CONTROL PLAN

A written exposure control plan is necessary for the safety and health of workers. At a minimum, the plan must include the following:

- Identify job classifications where there is exposure to blood or other potentially infectious materials.
- Explain the protective measures currently in effect in the acute care facility and/or a schedule and methods of compliance to be implemented, including hepatitis B

vaccination and post-exposure follow-up procedures; how hazards are communicated to employees; personal protective equipment; housekeeping; and recordkeeping.
- Establish procedures for evaluating the circumstances of an exposure incident.

The schedule of how and when the provisions of the standard will be implemented may be a simple calendar with brief notations describing the compliance methods, an annotated copy of the standard, or a part of another document, such as the infection control plan.

The written exposure control plan must be available to workers and OSHA representatives and updated at least annually or whenever changes in procedures create new occupational exposures.

WHO HAS OCCUPATIONAL EXPOSURE?

The exposure determination must be based on the definition of occupational exposure **without regard to personal protective clothing and equipment.** Exposure determination begins by reviewing job classifications of employees within the work environment and then making a list divided into two groups: job classifications in which **all** of the employees have occupational exposure, and those classifications in which **some** of the employees have occupational exposure.

Where **all** employees are occupationally exposed, it is not necessary to list specific work tasks. Some examples include phlebotomists, lab technicians, physicians, nurses, nurse's aides, surgical technicians, and emergency room personnel.

Where only **some** of the employees have exposure, specific tasks and procedures causing exposure must be listed. Examples include ward clerks or secretaries who occasionally handle blood or infectious specimens, and housekeeping staff who may be exposed to contaminated objects and/or environments some of the time.

When employees with occupational exposure have been identified, the next step is to communicate the hazards of the exposure to the employees.

COMMUNICATING HAZARDS TO EMPLOYEES

The initial training for current employees must be scheduled within 90 days of the effective date of the bloodborne pathogens standard, at no cost to the employee, and during working hours.[1] Training also is required for new workers at the time of their initial assignment to tasks with occupational exposure or when job tasks change, causing occupational exposure, and annually thereafter.

Training sessions must be comprehensive in nature, including information on bloodborne pathogens (While hepatitis B virus and HIV are specifically identified in the standard, the term includes any pathogenic microorganism that is present in human blood or other potentially infectious materials and can infect and cause disease in persons who are exposed to blood containing the pathogen. Pathogenic microorganisms can also cause diseases such as hepatitis C, malaria, syphilis, babesiosis, brucellosis, leptospirosis, arboviral infections, relapsing fever, Creutzfeldt-Jakob disease, adult T-cell leukemia/lymphoma [caused by HTLV-I], HTLV-I associated myelopathy, diseases associated with HTLV-II, and viral hemorrhagic fever.) as well as on OSHA regulations and the employer's exposure control plan. The person conducting the training must be knowledgeable in the subject matter as it relates to acute care facilities.

Specifically, the training program must do the following:

1. Explain the regulatory text and make a copy of the regulatory text accessible.
2. Explain the epidemiology and symptoms of bloodborne diseases.
3. Explain the modes of transmission of bloodborne pathogens.
4. Explain the employer's written exposure control plan.
5. Describe the methods to control transmission of HBV and HIV.
6. Explain how to recognize occupational exposure.
7. Inform workers about the availability of free hepatitis B vaccinations, vaccine efficacy, safety, benefits, and administration.
8. Explain the emergency procedures for and reporting of exposure incidents.
9. Inform workers of the post-exposure evaluation and follow-up available from health care professionals.
10. Describe how to select, use, remove, handle, decontaminate, and dispose of personal protective clothing and equipment.
11. Explain the use and limitations of safe work practices, engineering controls (controls that isolate or remove the bloodborne pathogens hazard from the workplace. Examples include needleless devices, shielded needle devices, blunt needles, plastic capillary tubes), and personal protective equipment.
12. Explain the use of labels, signs, and color coding required by the standard.
13. Provide a question-and-answer session on training.

In addition to communicating hazards to employees and providing training to identify and control hazards, other preventive measures also must be taken to ensure employee protection.

PREVENTIVE MEASURES

Preventive measures such as hepatitis B vaccination, universal precautions, engineering controls, safe work practices, personal protective equipment, and housekeeping measures help reduce the risks of occupational exposure.

Hepatitis B Vaccination

The hepatitis B vaccination series must be made available within 10 working days of initial assignment to every employee who has occupational exposure. The hepatitis B vaccination must be made available without cost to the employee, at a reasonable time and place for the employee, by a licensed health care professional,[2] and according to recommendations of the U.S. Public Health Service, including routine booster doses.[3]

The health care professional designated by the employer to implement this part of the standard must be provided with a copy of the bloodborne pathogens standard. The health care professional must provide the employer with a written opinion stating whether the hepatitis B vaccination is indicated for the employee and whether the employee has received such vaccination.

Employers are not required to offer hepatitis B vaccination (a) to employees who have previously completed the hepatitis B vaccination series, (b) when immunity is confirmed through antibody testing, or (c) if vaccine is contraindicated for medical reasons. Participation in a prescreening program is not a prerequisite for receiving hepatitis B vaccination. Employees who decline the vaccination may request and obtain it at a later date, if they continue to be exposed. Employees who decline to accept the hepatitis B vaccination must sign a declination form, indicating that they were offered the vaccination but refused it.

For more information, refer to *Immunization of Health-Care Workers: Recommendations of ACIP and HICPAC*, Vol. 46, No RR-18, MMWR, 1997.

Universal Precautions

The single most important measure to control transmission of HBV and HIV is to treat all human blood and other potentially infectious materials (Coverage under this definition also extends to blood and tissues of experimental animals who are infected with HIV or HBV.) AS IF THEY WERE infectious for HBV and HIV. Application of this approach is referred to as "universal precautions." *Blood and certain body fluids from all acute care patients should be considered as potentially infectious materials.*[4] These fluids cause *contamination*, defined in the standard as "the presence or the reasonably anticipated presence of blood or other potentially infectious materials on an item or surface."

Alternative concepts in infection control are called Body Substance Isolation (BSI) and Standard Precautions. These methods define all body fluids and substances as infectious. These methods incorporate not only the fluids and materials covered by this standard but expands coverage to include all body fluids and substances.

These concepts are acceptable alternatives to universal precautions, provided that facilities utilizing them adhere to all other provisions of this standard.

METHODS OF CONTROL

Engineering and Work Practice Controls

Engineering and work practice controls are the primary methods used to control the transmission of HBV and HIV in acute care facilities. Engineering controls isolate or remove the hazard from employees and are used in conjunction with work practices. Personal protective equipment also shall be used when occupational exposure to bloodborne pathogens remains even after instituting these controls. Engineering controls must be examined and maintained, or replaced, on a scheduled basis. Some engineering controls that apply to acute care facilities and are required by the standard include the following:

1. Use puncture-resistant, leak-proof containers, color-coded red or labeled, according to the standard (SEE: table) to discard contaminated items like needles, broken glass, scalpels, or other items that could cause a cut or puncture wound.
2. Use puncture-resistant, leak-proof containers, color-coded red or labeled to store contaminated reusable sharps until they are properly reprocessed.
3. Store and process reusable contaminated sharps in a way that ensures safe

handling. For example, use a mechanical device to retrieve used instruments from soaking pans in decontamination areas.

4. Use puncture-resistant, leak-proof containers to collect, handle, process, store, transport, or ship blood specimens and potentially infectious materials. Label these specimens if shipped outside the facility. Labeling is not required when specimens are handled by employees trained to use universal precautions with all specimens and when these specimens are kept within the facility.

Similarly, work practice controls reduce the likelihood of exposure by altering the manner in which the task is performed. All procedures shall minimize splashing, spraying, splattering, and generation of droplets. Work practice requirements include the following:

1. Wash hands when gloves are removed and as soon as possible after contact with blood or other potentially infectious materials.
2. Provide and make available a mechanism for immediate eye irrigation, in the event of an exposure incident.
3. Do not bend, recap, or remove contaminated needles unless required to do so by specific medical procedures or the employer can demonstrate that no alternative is feasible. In these instances, use mechanical means such as forceps or a one-handed technique to recap or remove contaminated needles.
4. Do not shear or break contaminated needles.
5. Discard contaminated needles and sharp instruments in puncture-resistant, leak-proof, red or biohazard-labeled containers[5] that are accessible, maintained upright, and not allowed to be overfilled.
6. Do not eat, drink, smoke, apply cosmetics, or handle contact lenses in areas of potential occupational exposure. (NOTE: use of hand lotions is acceptable.)
7. Do not store food or drink in refrigerators or on shelves where blood or potentially infectious materials are present.
8. Use red, or affix biohazard labels to, containers to store, transport, or ship blood or other potentially infectious materials, such as lab specimens. (SEE: figure)
9. Do not use mouth pipetting to suction blood or other potentially infectious materials; **it is prohibited.**

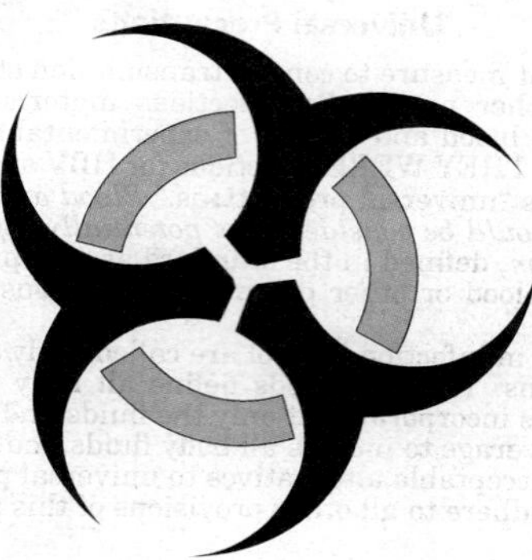

BIOHAZARD SYMBOL

Additional Information on Engineering Controls

Effective Engineering Controls. ECRI: www.healthcare.ecri.org/site/whatsnew/press.releases/980724hdneedle.html; ECRI (formerly Emergency Care Research Institute), designated as an evidence-based practice center by the Agency for Healthcare Research and Quality, is a nonprofit international health services research organization. This web site discusses the June 1998 issue of ECRI's Health Devices, which evaluated 19 needlestick-prevention devices, and provides information on how to obtain this document.

Food and Drug Administration (FDA) Safety Alert: Needlestick and Other Risks from Hypodermic Needles on Secondary IV Administration Sets-Piggyback and Intermittent IV. www.fda.gov/cdrh/safety.html; Warns of the risk of needlestick injuries from the use of hypodermic needles as a connection between two pieces of intravenous (IV) equipment. Describes characteristics of devices which have the potential to decrease the risk of needlestick injuries.

International Health Care Worker Safety Center, University of Virginia. www.people.virginia.edu/epinet/products.html; Features a list of safety devices with manufacturers and specific product names.

National Institute for Occupational Safety and Health (NIOSH) Sharps Disposal Containers. www.cdc.gov/niosh/sharps1.html; Features information on selecting, evaluating, and using sharps disposal containers.

Occupational Safety and Health Administration (OSHA) Glass Capillary Tubes: Joint Safety Advisory About Potential Risks. www.oshaslc.gov/OshDoc/Interpdata/I19990222.html; Describes safer alternatives to conventional glass capillary tubes.

Occupational Safety and Health Administration (OSHA) Needlestick Injuries. www.osha-slc.gov/SLTC/needlestick/index.html; Features recent news, recognition, evaluation, controls, compliance, and links to information on effective engineering controls.

Safety Sharp Device Contract. www.va.gov/vasafety/osh-issues/needlesafety/safetysharpcontracts.htm; Features safety sharp devices on contract with the U.S. Department of Veterans Affairs (VA).

SHARPS Injury Control Program. www.ohb.org/sharps.htm; Established by Senate Bill 2005 to study sharps injuries in hospitals, skilled nursing facilities, and home health agencies in California. Features a beta version of Safety Enhanced Device Database Listing by Manufacturer.

Training for Development of Innovative Control Technologies (TDICT) Project. www.tdict.org/criteria.html; Features safety feature evaluation forms for specific devices.

Personal Protective Equipment

In addition to instituting engineering and work practice controls, the standard requires that appropriate personal protective equipment be used to reduce worker risk of exposure. Personal protective equipment is specialized clothing or equipment used by employees to protect against direct exposure to blood or other potentially infectious materials. Protective equipment must not allow blood or other potentially infectious materials to pass through to workers' clothing, skin, or mucous membranes. Such equipment includes, but is not limited to, gloves, gowns, laboratory coats, face shields or masks, eye protection, and resuscitator devices. Hypoallergenic gloves, glove liners, powderless gloves, or other similar alternatives must be readily available and accessible at no cost to those employees who are allergic to the gloves normally provided.

The employer is responsible for providing, maintaining, laundering, disposing, replacing, and assuring the proper use of personal protective equipment. The employer is responsible for ensuring that workers have access to the protective equipment, at no cost, including proper sizes and types that take allergic conditions into consideration.

An employee may temporarily and briefly decline to wear personal protective equipment **under rare and extraordinary circumstances** and when, in the employee's professional judgment, it prevents the delivery of health care or public safety services or poses an increased or life-threatening hazard to employees. In general, **appropriate personal protective equipment is expected to be used whenever occupational exposure may occur.**

The employer also must ensure that employees observe the following precautions for safely handling and using personal protective equipment:

1. Remove all personal protective equipment immediately following contamination and upon leaving the work area, and place in an appropriately designated area or container for storing, washing, decontaminating, or discarding.
2. Wear appropriate gloves when contact with blood, mucous membranes, non-intact skin (skin with dermatitis, hangnails, cuts, abrasions, chafing, acne, etc.), or potentially infectious materials is anticipated; when performing vascular access procedures;[6] and when handling or touching contaminated items or surfaces.
3. Provide hypoallergenic gloves, liners, or powderless gloves or other alternatives to employees who need them.
4. Replace disposable, single-use gloves as soon as possible when contaminated, or if torn, punctured, or barrier function is compromised.
5. Do not reuse disposable (single-use) gloves.
6. Decontaminate reusable (utility) gloves after each use and discard if they show signs of cracking, peeling, tearing, puncturing, deteriorating, or failing to provide a protective barrier.
7. Use full face shields or face masks with eye protection, goggles, or eyeglasses with side shields when splashes of blood and other bodily fluids may occur and when contamination of the eyes, nose, or mouth can be anticipated (e.g., during invasive and surgical procedures).
8. Also wear surgical caps or hoods and/or shoe covers or boots when gross contamination may occur, such as during surgery and autopsy procedures.

Remember: The selection of appropriate personal protective equipment depends on the quantity and type of exposure expected.

Housekeeping Procedures

Equipment

The employer must ensure a clean and sanitary workplace. Contaminated work surfaces must be decontaminated with a disinfectant upon completion of procedures or when contaminated by splashes, spills, or contact with blood, other potentially infectious materials, and at the end of the work shift. Surfaces and equipment protected with plastic wrap, foil, or other nonabsorbent materials must be inspected frequently for contamination; and these protective coverings must be changed when found to be contaminated.

Waste cans and pails must be inspected and decontaminated on a regularly scheduled basis. Broken glass should be cleaned up with a brush or tongs; never pick up broken glass with hands, even when wearing gloves.

Waste

Waste removed from the facility is regulated by local and state laws. Special precautions are necessary when disposing of contaminated sharps and other contaminated waste, and include the following:

1. Dispose of contaminated sharps in closable, puncture-resistant, leak-proof, red or biohazard-labeled containers (SEE: table)
2. Place other regulated waste[7] in closable, leak-proof, red or biohazard-labeled bags or containers. If outside contamination of the regulated waste container occurs, place it in a second container that is closable, leak-proof, and appropriately labeled.

Labeling Requirements

Item	*No Label Needed If Universal Precautions Are Used and Specific Use of Container is Known to All Employees*		*Biohazard Label*		*Red Container*
Regulated waste container (e.g., contaminated sharps container			X	or	X
Reusable contaminated sharps container (e.g., surgical instruments soaking in a tray)			X	or	X
Refrigerator/freezer holding blood or other potentially infectious material			X		
Containers used for storage, transport, or shipping of blood			X	or	X
Blood/blood products for clinical use	X				
Individual specimen containers of blood or other potentially infectious materials remaining in facility	X	or	X	or	X
Contaminated equipment needing service (e.g., dialysis equipment, suction apparatus)			X Plus a label specifying where the contamination exists		
Specimens and regulated waste shipped from the primary facility to another facility for service or disposal			X	or	X
Contaminated laundry	*	or	X	or	X
Contaminated laundry sent to another facility that does not use universal precautions			X	or	X

*Alternative labeling or color coding is sufficient if it permits all employees to recognize containers as requiring compliance with universal precautions.

Laundry

Laundering contaminated articles, including employee lab coats and uniforms meant to function as personal protective equipment, is the responsibility of the employer. Contaminated laundry shall be handled as little as possible with minimum agitation. This can be accomplished through the use of a washer and dryer in a designated area on-site, or the contaminated items can be sent to a commercial laundry. The following requirements should be met with respect to contaminated laundry:

1. Bag contaminated laundry as soon as it is removed and store in a designated area or container.
2. Use red laundry bags or those marked with the biohazard symbol unless universal precautions are in effect in the facility and all employees recognize the bags as contaminated and have been trained in handling the bags.
3. Clearly mark laundry sent off-site for cleaning, by placing it in red bags or bags clearly marked with the orange biohazard symbol; and use leak-proof bags to prevent soak-through.
4. Wear gloves or other protective equipment when handling contaminated laundry.

WHAT TO DO IF AN EXPOSURE INCIDENT OCCURS

An exposure incident is the specific eye, mouth or other mucous membrane, non-intact skin, or parenteral contact with blood or other potentially infectious materials that results from the performance of an employee's duties. An example of an exposure incident would be a puncture from a contaminated sharp.

The employer is responsible for establishing the procedure for evaluating exposure incidents.

When evaluating an exposure incident, immediate assessment and confidentiality are critical issues. Employees should immediately report exposure incidents to enable timely medical evaluation and follow-up by a health care professional as well as a prompt request by the employer for testing of the source individual's blood for HIV and HBV. The "source individual" is any patient whose blood or body fluids are the source of an exposure incident to the employee.

At the time of the exposure incident, the exposed employee must be directed to a health care professional. The employer must provide the health care professional with a copy of the bloodborne pathogens standard; a description of the employee's job duties as they relate to the incident; a report of the specific exposure, including route of exposure; relevant employee medical records, including hepatitis B vaccination status; and results of the source individual's blood tests, if available. At that time, a baseline blood sample should be drawn from the employee, if he/she consents. If the employee elects to delay HIV testing of the sample, the health care professional must preserve the employee's blood sample for at least 90 days.[8]

Testing the source individual's blood does not need to be repeated if the source individual is known to be infectious for HIV or HBV; and testing cannot be done in most states without written consent.[9] The results of the source individual's blood tests are confidential. As soon as possible, however, the test results of the source individual's blood must be made available to the exposed employee through consultation with the health care professional.

Following post-exposure evaluation, the health care professional will provide a written opinion to the employer. This opinion is limited to a statement that the employee has been informed of the results of the evaluation and told of the need, if any, for any further evaluation or treatment. The employer must provide a copy of the written opinion to the employee within 15 days. This is the only information shared with the employer following an exposure incident; all other employee medical records are confidential.

All evaluations and follow-up must be available at no cost to the employee and at a reasonable time and place, performed by or under the supervision of a licensed physician or another licensed health care professional, such as a nurse practitioner, and according to recommendations of the U.S. Public Health Service guidelines current at the time of the evaluation and procedure. In addition, all laboratory tests must be conducted by an accredited laboratory and at no cost to the employee.

RECORDKEEPING

There are two types of records required by the bloodborne pathogens standard: medical and training.

A medical record must be established for each employee with occupational exposure. **This record is confidential and separate from other personnel records.** This record may be kept on-site or may be retained by the health care professional who provides services to employees. The medical record contains the employee's name, social security number, hepatitis B vaccination status, including the dates of vaccination, and the written opinion of the health care professional regarding the hepatitis B vaccination. If an occupational exposure occurs, reports are added to the medical record to document the incident and the results of testing following the incident. The post-evaluation written opinion of the health care professional is also part of the medical record. The medical record also must document what information has been provided to the health care provider. Medical records must be maintained 30 years past the last date of employment of the employee.

Emphasis is on confidentiality of medical records. No medical record or part of a medical record should be disclosed without direct, written consent of the employee or as required by law.

Training records document each training session and are to be kept for 3 years. Training records must include the date, content outline, trainer's name and qualifications, and names and job titles of all persons attending the training sessions.

If the employer ceases to do business, medical and training records are transferred to the successor employer. If there is no successor employer, the employer must notify the Director of the National Institute for Occupational Safety and Health, U.S. Department of Health and Human Services, for specific directions regarding disposition of the records at least 3 months prior to disposal.

Upon request, both medical and training records must be made available to the Assistant Secretary of Labor of Occupational Safety and Health. Training records must be available to employees upon request. Medical records can be obtained by the employee or anyone having the employee's written consent.

Additional recordkeeping is required for employers with 11 or more employees (SEE OSHA's "Recordkeeping Guidelines for Occupational Injuries and Illnesses" for more information.)

OTHER SOURCES OF OSHA ASSISTANCE

Consultation Programs

Consultation assistance is available to employers who want help in establishing and maintaining a safe and healthful workplace. Largely funded by OSHA, the service is provided at no cost to the employer. Primarily developed for smaller employers with more hazardous operations, the consultation service is delivered by state government agencies or universities employing professional safety consultants and health consultants. Comprehensive assistance includes an appraisal of all mechanical, physical work practice, and environmental hazards of the workplace and all aspects of the employer's present job safety and health program. No penalties are proposed or citations issued for hazards identified by the consultant.

Voluntary Protection Programs

Voluntary protection programs (VPPs) and on-site consultation services, when coupled with an effective enforcement program, expand worker protection to help meet the goals of the OSH Act. The three VPPs—Star, Merit, and Demonstration—are designed to recognize outstanding achievement by companies that have successfully incorporated comprehensive safety and health programs into their total management system. They motivate others to achieve excellent safety and health results in the same outstanding way, and they establish a cooperative relationship between employers, employees, and OSHA.

Employee Training

All employees who have occupational exposure to bloodborne pathogens should receive training on the epidemiology, symptoms, and transmission of bloodborne pathogen diseases. In addition, the training program covers, at a minimum, the following elements:

- a copy and explanation of the standard
- an explanation of our Engineering Control Plan and how to obtain a copy
- an explanation of methods to recognize tasks and other activities that may involve exposure to blood and other potentially infectious materials, including what constitutes an exposure incident
- an explanation of the use and limitations of engineering controls, work practices, and personal protective equipment (PPE)
- an explanation of the types, uses, location, removal, handling, decontamination, and disposal of PPE
- an explanation of the basis for PPE selection
- information on the hepatitis B vaccine, including information on its efficacy, safety,

method of administration, the benefits of being vaccinated, and that the vaccine will be offered free of charge

- information on the appropriate actions to take and persons to contact in an emergency involving blood or OPIM
- an explanation of the procedure to follow if an exposure incident occurs, including the method of reporting the incident and the medical follow-up that will be made available
- information on the post-exposure evaluation and follow-up that the employer is required to provide for the employee following an exposure incident
- an explanation of the signs and labels and/or color coding required by the standard and used at this facility
- an opportunity for interactive questions and answers with the person conducting the training session.

For more information on grants, and training and education, contact the OSHA Training Institute, Office of Training and Education, 1555 Time Drive, Des Plaines, IL 60018, (708) 297-4810.

For more information on AIDS, contact the Centers for Disease Control National AIDS Clearinghouse, (800) 458-5231.

---

[1] Employees who received training in the year preceding the effective date of the standard need only receive training pertaining to any provisions not already included.

[2] Licensed health care professional is a person whose legally permitted scope of practice allows him or her to perform independently the activities required under paragraph (f) of the standard regarding hepatitis B vaccination and post-exposure and follow-up.

[3] Health care professionals can call the Centers for Disease Control disease information hotline (404) 332-4555, extension 234, for updated information on hepatitis B vaccination.

[4] See also: "Recommendations for Prevention of HIV Transmission in Health-Care Settings," *MMWR* (36) 2S: August 21,1987.

[5] Biohazard labeling requires a fluorescent orange or orange-red label with the biological hazard symbol as well as the word **Biohazard** in contrasting color affixed to the bag or container.

[6] Phlebotomists in volunteer blood donation centers are exempt in certain circumstances. See section (d)(3)(ix)(D) of the standard for specific details.

[7] Liquid or semiliquid blood or other potentially infectious materials; items contaminated with these fluids and materials, which could release these substances in a liquid or semiliquid state, if compressed; items caked with dried blood or other potentially infectious materials that are capable of releasing these materials during handling; contaminated sharps; and pathological and microbiological wastes containing blood or other potentially infectious materials.

[8] If, during this time, the employee elects to have the baseline sample tested, testing shall be performed as soon as feasible.

[9] If consent is not obtained, the employer must show that legally required consent could not be obtained. Where consent is not required by law, the source individual's blood, if available, should be tested and the results documented.

NOTE: Osha References for hepatitis C and HIV: *Occupational Exposure to Bloodborne Pathogens OSHA Instruction,* Field Inspection Manual; The current CDC recommendation for HCV is found in *Recommendations for Prevention and Disease Control of Hepatitis C virus (HCV) Infection and HCV-Related Chronic Disease*, vol 47, no RR-19, 1998, www.cdc.gov/epo/mmwr/preview/mwrhtml/00055154.htm; The most current HIV post-exposure follow-up recommendations for an exposure incident made applicable by the bloodborne pathogens standard are found in the CDC Morbidity and Mortality Weekly Report: *Public Health Service Guidelines for the Management of Health-Care Worker Exposures to HIV and Recommendations for Postexposure Prophylaxis,* vol 47, no. RR-7, 1998, www.cdc.gov/epo/mmwr/preview/mmwrhtml/00052722.htm

SOURCE: Bloodborne Pathogens and Acute Care Facilities (OSHA 3128), Occupational Safety and Health Administration, Washington, DC, 1992.

Nursing Appendix

APPENDIX N-1
Nursing Organizations

Appendix N1-1 Nursing Organizations in the United States

Academy of Medical-Surgical Nurses
E. Holly Ave., Box 56, Pitman, NJ 08071; (856) 257-2323, Fax (856) 589–7463
www.amsn@inurse.com

Air & Surface Transport Nurses Association (National Flight Nurses Association)
915 Lee Street, Des Plaines, IL 60016-6569; (847) 460-1170, Fax (847) 460-4001, (800) 897-NFNA(6362)
www.nfna.org

American Academy of Ambulatory Nursing Administration
E. Holly Ave., Box 56, Pitman, NJ 08071; (856) 582-9617, Fax (856) 589–7463
www.aaacn.inurse.com

American Academy of Nurse Practitioners
Box 12846, Austin, TX 78711; (623) 376–9467, Fax (623) 376-0369
www.aanp.org

American Academy of Nursing
600 Maryland Avenue, SW Suite 100 West Washington, DC 20024-2571; (202) 651-7238, Fax (202) 554-2641
www.ana.org/aan

American Assembly for Men in Nursing
11 Cornell Road, Latham, NY 12110; (518) 782-9400, Ext. 346
www.aamn.org

American Association of Critical-Care Nurses
101 Columbia, Aliso Viejo, CA 92656; (800) 899-2226 or (949) 362-2000
www.aacn.org

American Association of Diabetes Educators
100 West Monroe Street, Fourth Floor, Chicago, IL 60603-1901; (312) 424-2426
www.aadenet.org

American Association of Legal Nurse Consultants
4700 W. Lake Avenue, Glenview, IL 60025; (877) 402-2562, Fax (847) 375-6313
www.aalnc.org

American Association of Neuroscience Nurses
4700 W. Lake Avenue, Glenview, IL 60025-1485; (847) 375-4733, (888) 557-2266, Fax (847) 375-6333
www.aann.org

American Association of Nurse Anesthetists
222 South Prospect Avenue, Park Ridge, IL 60068-4001; (847) 692-7050, Fax (847) 692-6968
www.aana.com

American Association of Occupational Health Nurses
222 South Prospect Avenue, Park Ridge, IL 60068-4001; (847) 692-7050, Fax (847) 692-6968
www.aaohn.org

American Association of Spinal Cord Injury Nurses
75–20 Astoria Blvd., Jackson Heights, NY 11370-1178; (718) 803-3782
www.aascin.org

American Board of Perianesthesia Nursing Certification
475 Riverside Drive, 7th Floor, New York, NY 10115-0089; (800) 6ABPANC, Fax (212) 367-4256
www.cpancapa.org

American College of Nurse-Midwives
818 Connecticut Avenue NW, Suite 900, Washington, DC 20006;(202) 728-9860, Fax (202) 728-9897
www.acnm.org

American Licensed Practical Nurses Association
1090 Vermont Ave. NW, Suite 1200, Washington, DC 20005; (202) 682-5800

American Nephrology Nurses' Association
E. Holly Ave., Box 56, Pitman, NJ 08071; (888) 600-ANNA, (856) 256-2320 Fax: (856) 589-7463
www.anna.inurse.com

American Nurses Association
600 Maryland Ave. SW, Suite 100 West, Washington, DC 20024-2571; (202) 651-7000
www.ana.org

American Nurses' Foundation
600 Maryland Ave SW, Ste. 100 West, Washington, DC 20024; (202) 651-7227
www.nursingworld.org/anf

American Organization of Nurse Executives
One N. Franklin, 34th Fl., Chicago, IL 60606; (312) 422-4503
www.aone.org

American Psychiatric Nurses Association
1200 19th St. NW, Ste. 300, Washington, DC 20036; (202) 857-1133; Fax (202) 857–1102
www.apna.org

American Society of Ophthalmic Registered Nurses, Inc.
Box 193030, San Francisco, CA 94119; (415) 561-8513

American Society of Peri-Anesthesia Nurses
10 Melrose Avenue, Suite 110, Cherry Hill, NJ 08003-3696; (856) 616-9600, Fax (856) 616-9601
www.aspan.org

American Society of Plastic and Reconstructive Surgical Nurses
E. Holly Ave., Box 56, Pitman, NJ 08071; (609) 256-2340, Fax (609) 589-7463
www.asprsn.org

American Thoracic Society, Section on Nursing
1749 Broadway, New York, NY 10019; (212) 315-8700, Fax (212) 315-6498

American Urological Association, Inc.
1120 North Charles Street Baltimore, MD 21201; (410) 727-1100, Fax (410) 223-4370
www.auanet.org

Assembly of Hospital Schools of Nursing
American Hospital Association, Center for Nursing, 840 N. Lake Shore Dr., Chicago, IL 60611; (312) 280-6432

Association of Pediatric Oncology Nurses
5700 Old Orchard Rd., Skokie, IL 60077; (708) 966-3723
www.apon.org

Association of Peri-Operative Registered Nurses
2170 S. Parker Road, Suite 300 Denver, CO 80231-5711; (303) 755-6300
www.aorn.org

Association of Rehabilitation Nurses
4700 W. Lake Ave., Glenview, IL 60025-1485; (847) 375-4710
www.rehabnurse.org

Association of Women's Health, Obstetric, and Neonatal Nurses
700 14th St. NW, Ste. 600, Washington, DC 20005-2019; (202) 662-1600
www.awhonn.org

Baromedical Nurses Association
P.O. Box 24113, Halthrope, MD 21227
www.hyperbaricnurses.org

Commission on Graduates of Foreign Nursing Schools
3600 Market St., Suite 400, Philadelphia, PA 19104; (215) 349-8767, Fax (215) 662-0425
www.cgfns.org

Dermatology Nurses Association
E. Holly Ave., Box 56, Pitman, NJ 08071; (609) 582-1915
www.dna.inurse.com

Emergency Nurses Association
915 Lee Street, Des Plaines, IL 60016-6569; (800) 900-9659, Fax (847) 460-4001
www.ena.org

Federation for Accessible Nursing Education and Licensure
Box 1418, Lewisburg, WV 24901; (304) 645-4357

Frontier Nursing Service
100 Wendover Rd., Wendover, KY 41775; (606) 672-2317
www.frontiernursing.org

International Flying Nurses Association
c/o Terri A. Sinkowski, R.N., Box 561218, Harwood Heights, IL 60656

Intravenous Nurses Society
Fresh Pond Sq., 10 Fawcett St., Cambridge, MA 02138; (617) 441-3008, Fax (617) 441-3009
www.ins1.org

National Association of Hispanic Nurses
1501 16th St. NW, Washington, DC 20036; (202) 387-2477
www.nahnhq.org

National Association of Orthopaedic Nurse
E. Holly Ave., Box 56, Pitman, NJ 08071; (856) 256-2310, Fax (856) 589-7463
www.naon.inurse.com

National Association of Pediatric Nurse Associates and Practitioners
1101 Kings Hwy. N., #206, Cherry Hill, NJ 08034; (609) 667-1773, Fax (856) 667-7187
www.napnap.org

National Association of Physician Nurses
900 S. Washington St., #G-13, Falls Church, VA 22046; (703) 237-8616

National Association of Registered Nurses
11508 Allecingie Pky., Ste. C, Richmond, VA 23235; (804) 794-6513

National Association of School Nurses
163 U.S. Route #1, P.O. Box 1300, Scarborough, ME 04070-1300; 207-883-2117, Fax (207) 883-2683
www.nasn.org

National Black Nurses Association, Inc.
8630 Fenton Street, Suite 330, Silver Spring, MD 20910-3803; (301) 589-3200, Fax (301) 589-3223
www.nbna.org

National Certification Corporation for the Obstetric, Gynecologic, and Neonatal Specialties
P.O. Box 11082 Chicago, IL 60611-0082; (312) 951-0207, Fax 1-800-367-5613
www.nccnet.org

National Council of State Boards of Nursing, Inc.
676 N. St. Clair St., Ste. 550, Chicago, IL 60611; (312) 787-6555
www.ncsbn.org

National Federation of Licensed Practical Nurses, Inc.
1418 Aversboro Rd., Garner, NC 27529-4547; (919) 779-0046 or (800) 948-2511, Fax (919) 779-5642
www.nflpn.org

National Gerontological Nursing Association
7794 Grow Drive, Pensacola, FL 32514; (850) 473-1174, Fax (850) 484-8762
www.ngna.org

National League for Nursing
61 Broadway, New York, NY 10006; (800) 669-1656 or (212) 363-5555, Fax (212) 812-0393
www.nln.org

National Nurses Society on Addictions
4101 Lake Boone Trl., Ste. 201, Raleigh, NC 27607; (919) 783-5871, Fax (919) 787-4916
www.nnsa.org

National Organization for Associate Degree Nursing
11250 Roger Bacon Dr., Ste. 8, Reston, VA 22090-5202; 703) 437-4377, Fax (703) 435-4390
www.noadn.org

National Student Nurses' Association
555 W. 57th St., Ste. 1327, New York, NY 10019; (212) 581-2211, Fax (212) 581-2368
www.nsna.org

North American Nursing Diagnosis Association
1211 Locust St., Philadelphia, PA 19107; (215) 545-8105 or (800) 647-9002
www.nanda.org

Nurses Organization of Veterans Affairs (NOVA)
1726 M Street, N.W. Suite 1101, Washington, DC 20036; Fax (202) 833-1577
www.vanurse.org

Oncology Nursing Society
501 Holiday Dr., Pittsburgh, PA 15220; (412) 921-7373
www.ons.org

Respiratory Nursing Society
7794 Grow Drive, Pensacola, FL 32514; (850) 474-8869, Fax (850) 484-8762

Society of Gastroenterology Nurses and Associates
401 N. Michigan Ave., Chicago, IL 60611-4267; (800) 245-7462, Fax (312) 527-6658
www.sgna.org

Society of Otorhinolaryngology and Head/Neck Nurses
116 Canal St., Ste. A, New Smyrna Beach, FL 32168; (904) 428-1695, Fax (904) 423-7566
www.sohnnurse.com

Society for Vascular Nursing
7794 Grow Drive, Pensacola, FL 32414; (888) 536-4SVN (4786), (850) 474-6963, Fax (850) 484-8762
www.svnnet.org

Visiting Nurse Associations of America
11 Beacon Street, Suite 910, Boston, MA 02108; (617) 523-4042, Fax (617) 227-4843
www.vnaa.org

Wound, Ostomy, and Continence Nurses
1550 South Coast Highway, Suite #201, Laguna Beach, CA 92651; (888) 224-WOCN, Fax (949) 376-3456
www.wocn.org

Appendix N1-2 Nursing Organizations in Canada

NATIONAL ORGANIZATIONS

Aboriginal Nurses Association of Canada
12 Sterling Avenue, 3rd Floor, Ottawa ON K1Y 1P8; (613) 724-4677, Fax (613) 724-4718
www.anac.ca

Academy of Canadian Executive Nurses
418 Balliol, Toronto ON M4S1E2; (416) 489-9234, Fax (416) 785-2501

Academy of Chief Executive Nurses of Teaching Hospitals
Director of Nursing, Saint John Regional Hospital, Box 2100, Saint John, New Brunswick E2L 4L2; (506) 648-6369

Association of Women's Health, Obstetric and Neonatal Nurses - Canada (AWHONN)
851 Falcon Blvd., Burlington ON L7T 3B5; (905) 521-2100 ext 76443, Fax (905) 577-0471
www.awhonn.org/section/canada

Canadian Association of Advanced Practice Nurses
Clinical Nurse Specialist, Acute Gerontology c/o HP C321, Vancouver Hospital & Health Sciences Center, 855 West 10 Avenue, Vancouver BC V5Z 1M9; (604) 875-5666 ext. 61759, Fax (604) 875-5441

Canadian Association of Apheresis Nurses
5 Playdell Court, Etobicoke ON M9V 1G4; (416) 946-4688, Fax (416) 946-4693

Canadian Association of Burn Nurses
48 Strath Lane, Dartmouth NS B2X 1Z3; (902) 474-0300, Fax (902) 473-7583

Canadian Association of Critical Care Nurses
P.O. Box 25322, London, On N6C 6B1; (519) 652-1989, Fax (519) 652-5545
www.caccn.ca

Canadian Association for Enterostomal Therapy
6139 Voyageur Drive, Orleans ON K1C 2X5; (613) 824-7115, Fax (613) 824-5419
www.caet.ca

Canadian Association for the History of Nursing
32 Citadel Pass, Cresent N.W. Calgary AB T3G 3V1; Tel/Fax (403) 289-3194
www.ualberta.ca/~hibberd/cahn_achn

Canadian Association of Nephrology Nurses and Technicians
Suite 322, 336 Yonge Street Barrie Ontario L4N 4C8 (705) 720-2819, Fax (705) 720-1451
www.cannt.ca

Canadian Association of Neuroscience Nurses
1602 Summer Street, S.W., Calgary AB T3C 2J6; (403) 209-8350, Fax (403) 209-8340
www.cann.ca

Canadian Association of Nurses in AIDS Care
Ottawa Hospital–General Site, 501 Smyth Road, Ottawa ON K1H 8L6
www.canac.org

Canadian Association of Nurses in Hemophilia Care
Sudbury & NorthEastern Ontario Hemophilia Program, 41 Ramsay Lake Road, Sudbury ON P3E 5J1; (705) 522-2200 ext. 3264, Fax (705) 523-7077
email: eparadis@hrsrh.on.ca

Canadian Association of Nurses in Independent Practice
1017 - 3240 66 Avenue, SW, Calgary, AB T3E 6M5; (403) 240-2368, Fax (403) 242-7241

Canadian Association of Nurses in Oncology
Regional Operations/Cancer Care Leader, Fraser Valley Cancer Centre, Surrey BC V3V 1Z2; (604) 930-4020, Fax (604) 930-4049

Canadian Association for Nursing Research
P.O. Box 20242 Steinbach MB R0A 1T1 (204) 326-3417

Canadian Council of Cardiovascular Nurses
96 Strathaven Circle SW Calgary AB T3H 2E9 (403) 670-2399, Fax (403) 670-2314
www.hsf.ab.ca/cccn

Canadian Diabetes Association, Professional Health Workers Section
15 Toronto St. Ste. #800, Toronto, ON M5C 2E3; (416) 363-3373, 1-800-BANTING
www.diabetes.ca

Canadian Federation of Mental Health Nurses
195 Kirk Drive Thornhill On L3T 3LT
www.iciweb.com/cfmhn

Canadian Federation of Nurses' Union
2841 Riverside Drive, Ottawa ON K1V 8X7; (613) 526-4661, Fax (613) 526-1023
www.nursesunions.ca

Canadian Gerontological Nursing Association
CGNA Professional Services, c/o South Granville Business Services, 101-1001 West Broadway, Dept, 370 Vancouver, B.C. V6H 4E4, Canada
www.cgna.ca

Canadian Holistic Nurses Association
787 Chaparral Place, Kamloops BC V2C 6E7; (250) 374-3508, Fax (250) 374-3581

Canadian Intravenous Nurses Association
18 Wynford Drive, Suite 516, North York ON M3C 3S2; (416) 445-4516, Fax (416) 445-4513
www.web.idirect.com/csotcina/

Canadian Nurses Association
50 Driveway, Ottawa ON K2P 1E2; (613) 237-2133, Fax (613) 237-3520
www.can-nurses.ca

Canadian Nurses Foundation
50 Driveway, Ottawa ON K2P 1E2; (613) 237-2133, Fax (613) 237-3720
can-nurses.ca/cnf

Canadian Nurses Protective Society
50 Driveway, Ottawa ON K2P 1E2; (800) 267-3390 or (613) 237-2092, Fax (613) 237-6300
www.cnps.ca

Canadian Nurses Respiratory Society
Faculty of Nurses 3rd floor, Clinical Sciences Bldg., University of Alberta, Edmonton, AB T6G 2G3; (613) 747-6776, Fax (613) 747-7430

Canadian Nursing Coalition for Immunization
Newfoundland Dept. of Health, P.O. Box 8700, Confederation Building, St. John's NF A1V 4J6; (709) 729-5019, Fax (709) 729-5824

Canadian Nursing Students Association
c/o Canadian Association of University Schools of Nursing, 325 350 Alberta Street, Ottawa ON K1R 1B1; (613) 563-1236, Fax (613) 653-7739
www.cnsa.ca

Canadian Occupational Health Nurses Association
Workplace Health, Safety and Compensation Commission, 146-148 Forest Road, P.O. Box 9000, St. John's NF A1A 3B8; (709) 778-1030, Fax (709) 778-1564

Canadian Orthopaedic Nurses Association
National CONA President, Terry Kane, 3534 Colonel Talbot Road, London, Ontario N6P 1H1; (519) 652-6727, Fax (519) 657-3375
www.nursing.ucalgary.ca/cona

Canadian Pediatric Nurses Association
1043 Town Line, R.R #1, Acton, ON L7J2L7; (519) 758-8228, Fax (905) 878-7092

Canadian Society of Gastroenterology Nurses and Associates
546 Kanmarr Crescent, Burlington ON L7L 4R7; (905) 632-4110, Fax (905) 634-0323
www.csgna.com

Canadian Society of Opthalmic Registered Nurses
c/o VH - University of British Columbia Eye Care Center, 2550 Willow Street, Vancouver BC V5Z 3N8; (604) 734-2693

COACH
Nursing Informatics Special Interest Group, 1807-110 Erskine Avenue, Toronto ON M4P 1Y4; (416) 484-1563

Community Health Nurses Association of Canada
106 Bellavista Drive, Dartmouth NS B2W 2X7; (902) 481- 5828, Fax (902) 481-5803

Community and Hospital Infection Control Association—Canada
P.O. Box 46125, RPO Westdale Winnipeg, MB, R3R 3S3 (204) 897-5990, Fax (204) 895-9595
www.chica.org

National Emergency Nurses' Affiliation
114 LaPierre Crescent, Dartmouth NS B2W 5C9; (902) 461-1897, Fax (902) 465-8470
www.nena.ca

Nurses Christian Fellowship Committee of Canada
318 West 19 Avenue, Vancouver, BC V5Y 2B7; (604) 872-1234

Nursing Sisters Association of Canada
164 Beechwood Avenue North York ON M2L 1K1; (416) 447-6843

Operating Room Nurses Association of Canada
R.R. #1 Crapaud PE C0A 1J0; (902) 658-2937, Fax (902) 658-2126
www.ornac.ca

Urology Nurses of Canada
Clinical Nurse Educator, D Main Surgery, Ottawa Civic Hospital, 1053 Carling Avenue, Ottawa ON K1Y 4E9; (613) 798-5555 ext. 3945
www.unc.org

PROVINCIAL AND TERRITORIAL ASSOCIATIONS

Alberta Association of Registered Nurses
11620–168 St., Edmonton, Alberta T5M 4A6; 1-800-252-9392, Fax (780) 452-3276
www.nurses.ab.ca

Association of Registered Nurses of Newfoundland
55 Military Rd., Box 6116, St. John's, Newfoundland A1C 5X8; (709) 753-6040

Association of Registered Nurses of Prince Edward Island
Box 1838, Charlottetown, Prince Edward Island C1A 7N5; (902) 368-3764, Fax (902) 628-1430
For information on registration/licensure in Quebec, contact l'Ordre des infirmières et infirmiers du Quebec, 4200 ouest, boul. Dorchester, Montreal, Quebec H3Z 1V4; (800) 363-6048; (514) 935-2501

Manitoba Association of Registered Nurses
647 Broadway, Winnipeg, Manitoba R3C 0X2; (204) 774-3477
www.marn.mb.ca

Northwest Territories Registered Nurses Association
Box 2757, Yellowknife, Northwest Territories X1A 2R1; (867) 873-2745, Fax (867) 873-2336
www.nwtrna.com

Nurses Association of New Brunswick
165 Regent St., Fredericton, New Brunswick E3B 3W5; (506) 458-8731, (800) 442-4417, Fax (506) 459-2838
www.nanb.nb.ca

Registered Nurses Association of British Columbia
2855 Arbutus St., Vancouver, British Columbia V6J 3Y8; (604) 736-7331, Fax (604) 738-2272
www.rnabc.bc.ca

Registered Nurses' Association of Nova Scotia
Suite 600, Barrington Tower Scotia Square, 1894 Barrington Street Halifax, Nova Scotia B3J 2A8; (902) 491-9744, (800) 565-9744, Fax (902) 491-9510
www.rnans.ns.ca

Registered Nurses Association of Ontario
438 University Avenue, Ste 1600, Toronto, Ontario M5G 2K8; (416) 599-1925, (800) 268-7199, Fax (416) 599-1926
www.rnao.org
For information on registration/licensure in Ontario, contact College of Nurses of Ontario, 101 Davenport Rd., Toronto, Ontario M5R 3P1; (800) 387-5526; (416) 928-0900.

Saskatchewan Registered Nurses Association
2066 Retallack St., Regina, Saskatchewan S4T 2K2; (306) 757-4643
www.srna.org

United Nurses of Alberta (Nurses Union) (Provincial Office)
#900, 10611 - 98 Avenue Edmonton, Alberta T5K 2P7; (780) 425-1025, Fax (780) 426-2093
www.una.ab.ca

United Nurses of Alberta (Nurses Union) (Southern Alberta Regional Office)
#505, 700 - 6th Avenue, SW Calgary, Alberta T2P 0T8; (403) 237-2377, Fax (403) 263-2908
www.una.ab.ca

Yukon Registered Nurses Association
Suite 14, 1114 - 1 Avenue, Whitehorse YT Y1A 1A3; (867) 667 4062, Fax: (867) 668 5123

SOURCE: Encyclopedia of Associations, ed 30 (Gale Research Co., Detroit, 1996); Canadian Nurses Association, Ottawa, Ontario.

APPENDIX N-2
Conceptual Models and Theories of Nursing

Jacqueline Fawcett, PhD, FAAN

Appendix N2-1 The Forerunners

FLORENCE NIGHTINGALE'S NOTES ON NURSING

Overview

Nightingale maintained that *every* woman is a nurse because every woman, at one time or another in her life, has charge of the personal health of someone. Nightingale equated knowledge of nursing with knowledge of sanitation. The focus of nursing knowledge was how to keep the body free from disease or in such a condition that it could recover from disease. According to Nightingale, nursing ought to signify the proper use of fresh air, light, warmth, cleanliness, quiet, and the proper selection and administration of diet—all at the least expense of vital power to the patient. That is, she maintained that the purpose of nursing was to put patients in the best condition for nature to act upon them.

Implications for Nursing Practice

Nursing practice encompasses care of both well and sick people. Nursing actions focus on both patients and their environments. Thirteen "hints" provided the boundaries of nursing practice:

1. **Ventilation and warming**—the nurse must be concerned first with keeping the air that patients breathe as pure as the external air, without chilling them.
2. **Health of houses**—attention to pure air, pure water, efficient drainage, cleanliness, and light will secure the health of houses.
3. **Petty management**—all the results of good nursing may be negated by one defect: not knowing how to manage what you do when you are there and what shall be done when you are not there.
4. **Noise**—unnecessary noise, or noise that creates an expectation in the mind, is that which hurts patients. Anything that wakes patients suddenly out of their sleep will invariably put them into a state of greater excitement and do them more serious and lasting mischief than any continuous noise, however loud.
5. **Variety**—the nerves of the sick suffer from seeing the same walls, the same ceiling, the same surroundings during a long confinement to one or two rooms. The majority of cheerful cases is to be found among those patients who are not confined to one room, whatever their suffering, and the majority of depressed cases will be seen among those subjected to a long monotony of objects about them.
6. **Taking food**—the nurse should be conscious of patients' diets and remember how much food each patient has had and ought to have each day.
7. **What food?**—to watch for the opinions the patient's stomach gives, rather than to read "analyses of foods," is the business of all those who have to decide what the patient should eat.
8. **Bed and bedding**—the patient should have a clean bed every 12 hours. The bed should be narrow, so that the patient does not feel "out of humanity's reach." The bed should not be so high that the patient cannot easily get in and out of it. The bed should be in the lightest spot in the room, preferably near a window. Pillows should be used to support the back below the breathing apparatus, to allow shoulders room to fall back, and to support the head without throwing it forward.
9. **Light**—with the sick, second only to their need of fresh air is their need of light. Light, especially direct sunlight, has a purifying effect upon the air of a room.
10. **Cleanliness of rooms and walls**—the greater part of nursing consists in preserving cleanliness. The inside air can be kept clean only by excessive care to rid rooms and their furnishings of the organic matter and dust with which they become saturated. Without cleanliness, you cannot have all the effects of ventilation; without ventilation, you can have no thorough cleanliness.
11. **Personal cleanliness**—nurses should always remember that if they allow patients to remain unwashed or to remain in clothing saturated with perspiration or other excretion, they are interfering injuriously with the natural processes of health just as much as if they were to give their patients a dose of slow poison.

12. **Chattering hopes and advices**—there is scarcely a greater worry which invalids have to endure than the incurable hopes of their friends. All friends, visitors, and attendants of the sick should avoid the practice of attempting to cheer the sick by making light of their danger and by exaggerating their probabilities of recovery.
13. **Observation of the sick**—the most important practical lesson nurses can learn is what to observe, how to observe, which symptoms indicate improvement, which indicate the reverse, which are important, which are not, and which are the evidence of neglect and what kind of neglect.

Implications for Nursing Education

Nightingale's primary contribution to nursing education was her belief that nursing schools should be administratively and economically independent from hospitals, even though the training could take place in the hospital. The purpose of nursing education was to teach the theoretical and practical knowledge underlying physician's orders. Knowledge of the 13 "hints" for nursing practice was considered an essential part of the training of every nurse.

Reference

Nightingale, F. (1859). *Notes on nursing: What it is, and what it is not.* London: Harrison and Sons. [Commemorative edition printed by J. B. Lippincott Company, Philadelphia, 1992]

VIRGINIA HENDERSON'S DEFINITION OF NURSING

Overview

The unique function of the nurse is to help individuals, sick or well, to perform those activities contributing to health or its recovery (or to peaceful death) that they would perform unaided if they had the necessary strength, will, or knowledge, and to do this in such a way as to help them gain independence as soon as possible.

Implications for Nursing Practice

The practice of nursing requires nurses to know and understand patients by putting themselves in the place of the patients. Nurses should not take at face value everything that patients say, but rather should interact with patients to ascertain their true feelings. *Basic nursing care* involves helping the patient perform the following activities unaided:

1. Breathe normally.
2. Eat and drink adequately.
3. Eliminate body wastes.
4. Move and maintain desirable postures.
5. Sleep and rest.
6. Select suitable clothes and dress and undress.
7. Maintain body temperature within normal range by adjusting clothing and modifying the environment.
8. Keep the body clean and well groomed and protect the integument.
9. Avoid dangers in the environment and avoid injuring others.
10. Communicate with others in expressing emotions, needs, fears, or opinions.
11. Worship according to one's faith.
12. Work in such a way that there is a sense of accomplishment.
13. Play or participate in various forms of recreation.
14. Learn, discover, or satisfy the curiosity that leads to normal development and health and use the available health facilities.

Implications for Nursing Education

Henderson's definition of nursing identifies an area of health and human welfare in which the nurse is an expert and independent practitioner. This kind of nursing requires a liberal education within a college or university, with grounding in the physical, biological, and social sciences and ability to use analytic processes. The professional aspects of the curriculum should focus on the nurse's major function of supplementing patients when they need strength, will, or knowledge in performing daily activities or in carrying out prescribed therapy, with emphasis on the individualization of patient care.

Reference

Henderson, V. (1966). *The nature of nursing. A definition and its implications for practice, research, and education.* New York: Macmillan.

Appendix N2-2 Conceptual Models

A conceptual model is defined as a set of relatively abstract and general concepts that address the phenomena of central interest to a discipline, the propositions that broadly describe those concepts, and the propositions that state relatively abstract and general relations between two or more of the concepts. Conceptual models of nursing, which also are referred to as conceptual frameworks, conceptual systems, and paradigms, provide distinctive frames of reference for thinking about people, their environments, their health, and nursing.

DOROTHY JOHNSON'S BEHAVIORAL SYSTEM MODEL

Overview

Focus is on the person as a behavioral system, made up of all the patterned, repetitive, and purposeful ways of behavior that characterize life. Seven subsystems carry out specialized tasks or functions needed to maintain the integrity of the whole behavioral system and to manage its relationship to the environment:

1. **Attachment or affiliative**—function is the security needed for survival as well as social inclusion, intimacy, and formation and maintenance of social bonds.
2. **Dependency**—function is the succoring behavior that calls for a response of nurturance as well as approval, attention or recognition, and physical assistance.
3. **Ingestive subsystem**—function is appetite satisfaction in terms of when, how, what, how much, and under what conditions the individual eats, all of which is governed by social and psychological considerations as well as biological requirements for food and fluids.
4. **Eliminative**—function is elimination in terms of when, how, and under what conditions the individual eliminates wastes.
5. **Sexual**—functions are procreation and gratification, with regard to behaviors dependent upon the individual's biological sex and gender role identity, including but not limited to courting and mating.
6. **Aggressive**—function is protection and preservation of self and society.
7. **Achievement**—function is mastery or control of some aspect of self or environment, with regard to intellectual, physical, creative, mechanical, social, and care-taking (of children, partner, home) skills.

The *structure* of each subsystem includes four elements:

1. **Drive or goal**—the motivation for behavior.
2. **Set**—the individual's predisposition to act in certain ways to fulfill the function of the subsystem.
3. **Choice**—the individual's total behavioral repertoire for fulfilling subsystem functions, which encompasses the scope of action alternatives from which the person can choose.
4. **Action**—the individual's actual behavior in a situation. Action is the only structural element that can be observed directly; all other elements must be inferred from the individual's actual behavior and from the consequences of that behavior.

Three *functional requirements* are needed by each subsystem to fulfill its functions:

1. **Protection** from noxious influences with which the system cannot cope.
2. **Nurturance** through the input of appropriate supplies from the environment.
3. **Stimulation** to enhance growth and prevent stagnation.

Implications for Nursing Practice

Nursing practice is directed toward restoration, maintenance, or attainment of behavioral system balance and dynamic stability at the highest possible level for the individual. Johnson's practice methodology, which is called the Nursing Diagnostic and Treatment Process, encompasses four steps:

1. **Determination of the existence of a problem** The nurse obtains past and present family and individual behavioral system histories by means of interviews, structured and unstructured observations, and objective methodologies. The nurse obtains data about the nature of behavioral system functioning in terms of the efficiency and effectiveness with which the client's goals are obtained. The nurse obtains data to determine the degree to which the behavior is purposeful, orderly, and predictable. The nurse interviews the client and family to determine the condition of the subsystem structural components and uses the obtained data to: make inferences about drive strength, direction, and value; make inferences about the solidity and specificity of the set; make inferences about the range of behavior patterns available to the client; make inferences about the usual behavior in a given situation. The nurse assesses and compares the client's behavior with the following in-

dices for behavioral system balance and stability: the behavior is succeeding to achieve the consequences sought; effective motor, expressive, or social skills are evident; the behavior is purposeful; the behavior is orderly; the behavior is predictable; the amount of energy expended to achieve desired goals is acceptable; the behavior reflects appropriate choices; the client is sufficiently satisfied with the behavior; the nurse makes inferences about the organization, interaction, and integration of the subsystems.

2. **Diagnostic classification of problems** *Internal Subsystem Problems* are present when: functional requirements are not met; inconsistency or disharmony among the structural components of subsystems is evident; the behavior is inappropriate in the ambient culture. *Intersystem Problems* are present when: the entire behavioral system is dominated by one or two subsystems; a conflict exists between two or more subsystems.
3. **Management of nursing problems** The general goals of action are to: restore, maintain, or attain the client's behavioral system balance and stability; help the client to achieve a more optimum level of balance and functioning when this is possible and desired. The nurse determines what nursing is to accomplish on behalf of the behavioral system by determining who makes the judgment regarding the acceptable level of behavioral system balance and stability. The nurse identifies the value system of the nursing profession as well as his or her own explicit value system.

   The nurse negotiates with the client to select a type of treatment: The nurse temporarily *Imposes External Regulatory or Control Mechanisms* by: setting limits for behavior by either permissive or inhibitory means; inhibiting ineffective behavioral responses; assisting the client to acquire new responses; reinforcing appropriate behaviors. The nurse *Repairs Damaged Structural Components* in the desirable direction by: reducing drive strength by changing attitudes; redirecting goal by changing attitudes; altering set by instruction or counseling; adding choices by teaching new skills. The nurse *Fulfills Functional Requirements* of the subsystems by: protecting the client from overwhelming noxious influences; supplying adequate nurturance through an appropriate input of essential supplies; providing stimulation to enhance growth and to inhibit stagnation. The nurse negotiates the treatment modality with the client by: establishing a contract with the client; helping the client to understand the meaning of the nursing diagnosis and the proposed treatment. If the diagnosis and/or proposed treatment is rejected, the nurse continues to negotiate with the client until agreement is reached.
4. **Evaluation of Behavioral System Balance and Stability** The nurse compares the client's behavior after treatment to indices of behavioral system balance and stability.

Implications for Nursing Education

Education for nursing practice requires a thorough grounding in the natural and social sciences, with emphasis on the genetic, neurological, and endocrine bases of behavior; psychological and social mechanisms for the regulation and control of behavior; social learning theories; and motivational structures and processes. The professional aspects of the curriculum focus on study of the behavioral system as a whole and as a composite of subsystems; pathophysiology; the clinical sciences of nursing and medicine; and the health care system.

References

Johnson, D. E. (1980). The behavioral system model for nursing. In J. P. Riehl & C. Roy, *Conceptual models for nursing practice* (2nd ed., pp. 207–216). New York: Appleton-Century-Crofts.

Johnson, D. E. (1990). The behavioral system model for nursing. In M. E. Parker (Ed.), *Nursing theories in practice* (pp. 23–32). New York: National League for Nursing.

IMOGENE KING'S GENERAL SYSTEMS FRAMEWORK

Overview

Focus is on the continuing ability of individuals to meet their basic needs so that they may function in their socially defined roles, and on individuals' interactions within three open, dynamic, interacting systems.

1. **Personal systems** are individuals, who are regarded as rational, sentient, social beings. Concepts related to the personal system are:
   Perception—a process of organizing, interpreting, and transforming information from sense data and memory that gives meaning to one's experience, represents one's image of reality, and influences one's behavior.
   Self—a composite of thoughts and feelings that constitute a person's awareness of individual existence, of who and what he or she is.

Growth and development—cellular, molecular, and behavioral changes in human beings that are a function of genetic endowment, meaningful and satisfying experiences, and an environment conducive to helping individuals move toward maturity.

Body image—a person's perceptions of his or her body.

Time—the duration between the occurrence of one event and the occurrence of another event.

Space—the physical area called territory that exists in all directions.

Learning—gaining knowledge.

2. **Interpersonal systems** are composed of two, three, or more individuals interacting in a given situation. The concepts associated with this system are:

   Interactions—the acts of two or more persons in mutual presence; a sequence of verbal and nonverbal behaviors that are goal directed.

   Communication—the vehicle by which human relations are developed and maintained; encompasses intrapersonal, interpersonal, verbal, and nonverbal communication.

   Transaction—a process of interaction in which human beings communicate with the environment to achieve goals that are valued; goal-directed human behaviors.

   Role—a set of behaviors expected of a person occupying a position in a social system.

   Stress—a dynamic state whereby a human being interacts with the environment to maintain balance for growth, development, and performance, involving an exchange of energy and information between the person and the environment for regulation and control of stressors.

   Coping—a way of dealing with stress.

3. **Social systems** are organized boundary systems of social roles, behaviors, and practices developed to maintain values and the mechanisms to regulate the practices and roles. The concepts related to social systems are:

   Organization—composed of human beings with prescribed roles and positions who use resources to accomplish personal and organizational goals.

   Authority—a transactional process characterized by active, reciprocal relations in which members' values, backgrounds, and perceptions play a role in defining, validating, and accepting the authority of individuals within an organization.

   Power—the process whereby one or more persons influence other persons in a situation.

   Status—the position of an individual in a group or a group in relation to other groups in an organization.

   Decision making—a dynamic and systematic process by which goal-directed choice of perceived alternatives is made and acted upon by individuals or groups to answer a question and attain a goal.

   Control—being in charge.

Implications for Nursing Practice

Nursing practice is directed toward helping individuals maintain their health so they can function in their roles. King's practice methodology, which is the essence of the Theory of Goal Attainment, is called the Interaction-Transaction Process.

1. **Assessment phase**

   Perception The nurse and the client meet in some nursing situation and perceive each other. Accuracy of perception will depend upon verifying the nurse's inferences with the client. The nurse can use the Goal-Oriented Nursing Record (GONR) throughout the assessment phase.

   Judgment The nurse and the client make mental judgments about the other.

   Action The nurse and the client take some mental action.

   Reaction The nurse and the client mentally react to each one's perceptions of the other.

2. **Disturbance** is the *diagnosis phase* of the interaction-transaction process. The nurse and the client communicate and interact, and the nurse identifies the client's concerns, problems, and disturbances in health. The nurse conducts a nursing history to determine the client's activities of daily living, using the Criterion-Referenced Measure of Goal Attainment Tool (CRMGAT); roles; environmental stressors; perceptions; and values, learning needs, and goals. The nurse records the data from the nursing history on the GONR, the medical history and physical examination data, results of laboratory tests and x-ray examination, and information gathered from other health professionals and the client's family members on the GONR. The nurse also records diagnoses on the GONR.

3. **Planning phase**

   Mutual Goal Setting The nurse and the client interact purposefully to set mutually agreed on goals. The nurse interacts with family members if the client cannot verbally participate in goal setting. Mutual goal setting is based on the nurse's assessment of the client's concerns, problems, and disturbances in health; the nurse's and client's perceptions of the interference; and the nurse's sharing of information with the client and his or her family to help the client attain the goals identified. The nurse records the goals on the GONR.

Exploration of Means to Achieve Goals The nurse and the client interact purposefully to explore the means to achieve the mutually set goals.

Agreement on Means to Achieve Goals The nurse and the client interact purposefully to agree on the means to achieve the mutually set goals. The nurse records the nursing orders with regard to the means to achieve goals on the GONR.

4. **Transaction** is the *implementation phase* of the interaction-transaction process. Transaction refers to the valuational components of the interaction. The nurse and the client carry out the measures agreed upon to achieve the mutually set goals. The nurse can use the GONR flow sheet and progress notes to record the implementation of measures used to achieve goals.
5. **Attainment of Goals** is the *evaluation phase* of the interaction-transaction process. The nurse and the client identify the outcome of the interaction-transaction process. The outcome is expressed in terms of the client's state of health, or ability to function in social roles. The nurse and the client make a decision with regard to whether the goal was attained and, if necessary, determine why the goal was not attained. The nurse can use the CRMGAT to record the outcome and the GONR to record the discharge summary.

Implications for Nursing Education

The General Systems Framework and the theory of goal attainment lead to a focus on the dynamic interaction of the nurse-client dyad. This focus, in turn, leads to emphasis on nursing student behavior as well as client behavior. The concepts related to the personal, interpersonal, and social systems serve as the theoretical content for nursing courses in associate degree, baccalaureate, and master's nursing programs. The theoretical knowledge is used by students in learning experiences involving concrete nursing situations.

References

King, I. M. (1981). *A theory for nursing. Systems, concepts, process.* New York: Wiley. [Reissued 1990. Albany, NY: Delmar.]

King, I. M. (1986). *Curriculum and instruction in nursing.* Norwalk, CT: Appleton-Century-Crofts.

King, I.M. (1992). King's theory of goal attainment. *Nursing Science Quarterly,* 5, 19–26.

King, I.M. (1997). King's theory of goal attainment in practice. *Nursing Science Quarterly,* 10, 180–185.

MYRA LEVINE'S CONSERVATION MODEL

Overview

Focus is on conservation of the person's wholeness. Adaptation is the process by which people maintain their wholeness or integrity as they respond to environmental challenges and become congruent with the environment. Sources of challenges are:

1. **Perceptual environment**—encompasses that part of the environment to which individuals respond with their sense organs.
2. **Operational environment**—includes those aspects of the environment that are not directly perceived, such as radiation, odorless and colorless pollutants, and microorganisms.
3. **Conceptual environment**—the environment of language, ideas, symbols, concepts, and invention.

Individuals respond to the environment by means of four integrated processes:

1. *Fight-or-flight mechanism*
2. *Inflammatory-immune* response
3. *Stress* response
4. *Perceptual awareness*—includes the basic orienting, haptic, auditory, visual, and taste-smell systems.

Implications for Nursing Practice

Nursing practice is directed toward promoting wholeness for all people, well or sick. Patients are partners or participants in nursing care and are temporarily dependent on the nurse. The nurse's goal is to end the dependence as quickly as possible. Levine's practice methodology is a nursing process directed toward conservation, which is defined as "keeping together," and consists of three steps:

1. **Trophicognosis**—formulation of a nursing care judgment arrived at by the scientific method. The nurse observes and collects data that will influence nursing practice rather than medical practice. The nurse uses appropriate assessment tools derived from the Conservation Model and data to establish an objective and scientific rationale for nursing practice. The nurse fully understands his or her role in medical and paramedical prescriptions and the basis for the prescribed medical regimen. The nurse consults with the physician to share information and clarify nursing decisions. The nurse understands the basis for the prescribed paramedical regimen and determines the nursing processes required by medical and paramedical treatment. The nurse assesses the patient's *Conservation of Energy* by determining his or her ability to perform necessary activities without producing excessive fatigue. The nurse assesses the patient's *Conservation of Structural Integrity* by determining his or her physical functioning. The nurse assesses the patient's *Conservation of Personal Integrity* by determining his or her moral and ethical values and life experiences. The nurse assesses the patient's *Conservation of Social Integrity* by taking the patient's family members, friends, and conceptual environment into account. The nurse understands the basis for implementation of the nursing care plan, including principles of nursing science, and how to adapt nursing techniques to the unique cluster of needs demonstrated in the individual patient. The nurse identifies the provocative facts within the data collected, that is, the data that provoke attention on the basis of knowledge of the situation. The provocative facts provide the basis for an hypothesis, or trophicognosis.
2. **Intervention/Action**—test of the hypothesis. The nurse implements the nursing care plan within the structure of administrative policy, availability of equipment, and established standards of nursing. The nurse accurately records and transmits evaluation of the patient's response to implementation of the nursing care plan and identifies the general type of nursing intervention required:
   Therapeutic—when nursing intervention influences adaptation favorably or toward renewed social well-being.
   Supportive—when nursing intervention cannot alter the course of the adaptation and can only maintain the status quo or fail to halt a downward course.
   Intervention is structured according to four conservation principles:
   Principle of conservation of energy—balancing the patient's energy output and energy input to avoid excessive fatigue.
   Principle of conservation of structural integrity—focusing attention on healing by maintaining or restoring the structure of the body through prevention of physical breakdown and promotion of healing.
   Principle of conservation of personal integrity—maintaining or restoring the individual patient's sense of identity, self-worth and acknowledgment of uniqueness.
   Principle of conservation of social integrity—acknowledging patients as social beings and helping them to preserve their places in family, community, and society.
3. **Evaluation of Intervention/Action**—the nurse's evaluation of the effects of the intervention/action. The nurse evaluates the effects of intervention and revises the trophicognosis as necessary. An indicator of the success of nursing interventions is the patient's organismic response.

Implications for Nursing Education

Education focuses on understanding both the person and the environment, with emphasis placed on processes by which the person adapts to environmental challenges. Theoretical and clinical knowledge related to the four conservation principles provides the structure for nursing courses. Students are prepared for the practice of holistic nursing and for lifelong learning.

References

Levine, M. E. (1973). *Introduction to clinical nursing* (2nd ed.). Philadelphia: F. A. Davis.

Levine M. E. (1996). The conservation principles: A retrospective. *Nursing Science Quarterly,* 9, 38–41.

Schaefer, K. M., & Pond, J. B. (Eds.). (1991). *Levine's conservation model: A framework for nursing practice.* Philadelphia: F. A. Davis.

BETTY NEUMAN'S SYSTEMS MODEL

Overview

Focus is on the wellness of the client system in relation to environmental stress and reactions to stress. The client system, which can be an individual, a family or other group, or a community, is a composite of five interrelated variables:

1. **Physiological variables**—bodily structure and function.
2. **Psychological variables**—mental processes and relationships.
3. **Sociocultural variables**—social and cultural functions.
4. **Developmental variables**—developmental processes of life.
5. **Spiritual variables**—aspects of spirituality on a continuum from complete unawareness or denial to a consciously developed high level of spiritual understanding.

The client system is depicted as a central core, which is a basic structure of survival factors common to the species, surrounded by three types of concentric rings:

1. **Flexible line of defense**—the outermost ring; a protective buffer for the client's normal or stable state that prevents invasion of stressors and keeps the client system free from stressor reactions or symptomatology.
2. **Normal line of defense**—lies between the flexible line of defense and the lines of resistance; represents the client system's normal or usual wellness state.
3. **Lines of resistance**—the innermost concentric rings; involuntarily activated when a stressor invades the normal line of defense. They attempt to stabilize the client system and foster a return to the normal line of defense. If they are effective, the system can reconstitute; if ineffective, death may ensue.

Environment is defined as "all internal and external factors or influences surrounding the client system":

1. **Internal environment**—"all forces or interactive influences internal to or contained solely within the boundaries of the defined client system"; the source of *intrapersonal stressors.*
2. **External environment**—all forces or interaction influences external to or existing outside the defined client system; the source of *interpersonal and extrapersonal stressors.*
3. **Created environment**—subconsciously developed by the client as a symbolic expression of system wholeness. It supersedes and encompasses the internal and external environments, and functions as a subjective safety mechanism that may block the true reality of the environment and the health experience.

Implications for Nursing Practice

Nursing practice is directed toward facilitating optimal wellness through retention, attainment, or maintenance of client system stability. Neuman's practice methodology is the Neuman Systems Model Nursing Process Format, which encompasses three steps:

1. **Nursing diagnosis**—formulated on the basis of assessment of the variables and lines of defense and resistance making up the client system.
2. **Nursing goals**—negotiated with the client for desired prescriptive changes to correct variances from wellness.
3. **Nursing outcomes** The nurse implements nursing interventions through the use of one or more of the three prevention-as-intervention modalities.

   Primary Prevention as Intervention—nursing actions to retain system stability are implemented by: preventing stressor invasion; providing resources to retain or strengthen existing client/client system strengths; supporting positive coping and functioning; desensitizing existing or possible noxious stressors; motivating the client/client system toward wellness; coordinating and integrating interdisciplinary theories and epidemiological input; educating or reeducating the client/client system; using stress as a positive intervention strategy.

   Secondary Prevention as Intervention—nursing actions to attain system stability are implemented by: protecting the client/client system's basic structure; mobilizing and optimizing the client/client system's internal and external resources to attain stability and energy conservation; facilitating purposeful manipulation of stressors and reactions to stressors; motivating, educating, and involving the client/client system in mutual establishment of health care goals; facilitating appropriate treatment and intervention measures; supporting positive factors toward wellnesss; promoting advocacy by coordination and integration; providing primary preventive intervention as required.

   Tertiary Prevention as Intervention—nursing actions to maintain system stability are implemented by: attaining and maintaining the highest possible level of client/client system wellness and stability during reconstitution; educating, reeducating, and/or reorienting the client/client system as needed; supporting the client/client system toward appropriate goals; coordinating and integrating health services resources; providing primary and/or secondary preventive intervention as required. The nurse evaluates the outcome goals by: confirming attainment of outcome goals with the client/client system; reformulating goals as necessary with the client/client system. The nurse and client/client system set intermediate and long-range goals for subsequent nursing action that are structured in relation to short-term goal outcomes. The nurse uses the Neuman Systems Model Assessment and Intervention Tool, the Neuman Systems Model Nursing Diagnosis Taxonomy, and any other relevant clinical tools to guide collection of data and facilitate documentation of nursing diagnoses, nursing goals, and nursing outcomes.

Implications for Nursing Education

The model is an appropriate curriculum guide for all levels of nursing education. The components of the model serve as curriculum content, including the five variable areas (physiological, psychological, sociocultural, developmental, spiritual), the three categories of stressors (intrapersonal, interpersonal, extrapersonal), and the three prevention-as-intervention modalities (primary, secondary, tertiary).

References

Lowry, L. (Ed.). (1998). *The Neuman systems model and nursing education: Teaching strategies and outcomes.* Indianapolis: Sigma Theta Tau International Center for Nursing Press.

Neuman, B. (1995). *The Neuman systems model* (3rd ed.). Norwalk, CT: Appleton and Lange.

DOROTHEA OREM'S SELF-CARE FRAMEWORK

Overview

Focus is on patients' deliberate actions to meet their own and dependent others' therapeutic self-care demands and nurses' deliberate actions to implement nursing systems designed to assist individuals and multiperson units who have limitations in their abilities to provide continuing and therapeutic self-care or care of dependent others. The concepts of Orem's conceptual model are:

1. **Self-care**—behavior directed by individuals to themselves or their environments to regulate factors that affect their own development and functioning in the interests of life, health, or well-being.
2. **Self-care agency**—a complex capability of maturing and mature individuals to determine the presence and characteristics of specific requirements for regulating their own functioning and development, make judgments and decisions about what to do, and perform care measures to meet specific self-care requisites. The person's ability to perform self-care is influenced by 10 *power components:*
   - Ability to maintain attention and exercise requisite vigilance with respect to self as self-care agent and internal and external conditions and factors significant for self-care.
   - Controlled use of available physical energy that is sufficient for the initiation and continuation of self-care operations.
   - Ability to control the position of the body and its parts in the execution of the movements required for the initiation and completion of self-care operations.
   - Ability to reason within a self-care frame of reference.
   - Motivation (i.e., goal orientations for self-care that are in accord with its characteristics and its meaning for life, health, and well-being).
   - Ability to make decisions about care of self and to operationalize these decisions.
   - Ability to acquire technical knowledge about self-care from authoritative sources, to retain it, and to operationalize it.
   - A repertoire of cognitive, perceptual, manipulative, communication, and interpersonal skills adapted to the performance of self-care operations.
   - Ability to order discrete self-care actions or action systems into relationships with prior and subsequent actions toward the final achievement of regulatory goals of self-care.
   - Ability to consistently perform self-care operations, integrating them with relevant aspects of personal, family, and community living.

   The person's ability to perform self-care as well as the kind and amount of self-care required are influenced by 10 internal and external factors called *basic conditioning factors:*
   - Age
   - Gender
   - Developmental state
   - Health state
   - Sociocultural orientation
   - Health care system factors; for example, medical diagnostic and treatment modalities
   - Family system factors

Patterns of living including activities regularly engaged in
Environmental factors
Resource availability and adequacy

3. **Therapeutic self-care demand**—the action demand on individuals to meet three types of self-care requisites:
   Universal self-care requisites—actions that need to be performed to maintain life processes, the integrity of human structure and function, and general well-being.
   Developmental self-care requisites—actions that need to be performed in relation to human developmental processes, conditions, and events and in relation to events that may adversely affect development.
   Health deviation self-care requisites—actions that need to be performed in relation to genetic and constitutional defects, human structural and functional deviations and their effects, and medical diagnostic and treatment measures prescribed or performed by physicians.
4. **Self-care deficit**—the relationship of inadequacy between self-care agency and the therapeutic self-care demand.
5. **Nursing agency**—a complex property or attribute that enables nurses to know and help others to know their therapeutic self-care demands, meet their therapeutic self-care demands, and regulate the exercise or development of their self-care agency.
6. **Nursing system**—a series of coordinated deliberate practical actions performed by nurses and patients directed toward meeting the patient's therapeutic self-care demand and protecting and regulating the exercise or development of the patient's self-care agency.

Implications for Nursing Practice

Nursing practice is directed toward helping people to meet their own and their dependent others' therapeutic self-care demands. Orem's practice methodology encompasses the Professional-Technologic Operations of Nursing Practice:

1. **Case Management Operations**—The nurse uses a case management approach to control, direct, and check each of the nursing diagnostic, prescriptive, regulatory, and control operations. The nurse maintains an overview of the interrelationships between the social, interpersonal, and professional-technologic systems of nursing. The nursing history and other appropriate tools are used for collection and documentation of information and measurement of the quality of nursing. The nurse records appropriate information in the patient's chart and records progress notes as appropriate.
2. **Diagnostic Operations**—The nurse identifies the unit of service for nursing practice as an individual, an individual member of a multiperson unit, or a multiperson unit. The nurse determines why the person needs nursing in collaboration with the patient or family and with continued review of decisions by the patient or family. The nurse collects demographic data about the patient and information about the nature and boundaries of the patient's health care situation and nursing's jurisdiction within those boundaries. The nurse calculates the person's present and future therapeutic self-care demand and determines the person's self-care agency or dependent-care agency. The nurse identifies the influence of power components and basic conditioning factors on the exercise and operability of self-care or dependent-care agency.

   The nurse determines whether the person should be helped to refrain from self-care actions or dependent-care actions for therapeutic purposes and whether the person should be helped to protect already developed self-care or dependent-care capabilities for therapeutic purposes. The nurse determines the person's potential for self-care or dependent-care agency in the future by: identifying the person's ability to increase or deepen self-care or dependent-care knowledge; identifying the person's ability to learn techniques of care; identifying the person's willingness to engage in self-care or dependent-care; identifying the person's ability to effectively and consistently incorporate essential self-care or dependent-care measures into daily living.

   The nurse calculates the self-care deficit or dependent-care deficit by: determining the qualitative or quantitative inadequacy of self-care agency or dependent-care agency in relation to the calculated therapeutic self-care demand; determining the nature of and reasons for the existence of the self-care deficit or dependent-care deficit; specifying the extent of the self-care deficit or dependent-care deficit as complete or partial.

   The nurse states the nursing diagnosis for the individual or a multiperson unit within the context of four levels:
   Level 1: Focuses on health and well-being, with emphasis on the relationship of self-care and self-care management to the overall life situation.
   Level 2: Deals with the relationship between the therapeutic self-care demand and self-care agency.
   Level 3: Expresses the relationship of the action demand by particular self-care

requisites to particular self-care operations as influenced by the power components.

Level 4: Expresses the influence of the basic conditioning factors on the therapeutic self-care demand and self-care agency.

3. **Prescriptive Operations**—The nurse specifies the means to be used and all measures needed to meet the therapeutic self-care demand, in collaboration with the patient or family. The nurse specifies the roles to be played by the nurse(s), patient, and dependent-care agent(s) in meeting the therapeutic self-care demand and in regulating the patient's exercise or development of self- or dependent-care agency, in collaboration with the patient or family.
4. **Regulatory Operations: Design of Nursing Systems for Performance of Regulatory Operations**—The nurse designs a *nursing system*, which is a series of coordinated deliberate practical actions performed by the nurse and the patient directed toward meeting the patient's therapeutic self-care demand and protecting and regulating the exercise or development of the patient's self- or dependent-care agency, in collaboration with the patient or family.

The nursing system includes one or more *methods of helping*, which are sequential series of actions that will overcome or compensate for the health-associated limitations of patients to regulate their own or their dependents' functioning and development.

The selection of the appropriate nursing system is based on the answer to the question of who can or should perform self-care actions, and the determination of the patient's role (no role, some role) in the production and management of self-care. The *wholly compensatory nursing system* is selected when the patient cannot or should not perform any self-care actions, and thus the nurse must perform them. The *partly compensatory nursing system* is selected when the patient can perform some, but not all, self-care actions. The *supportive-educative nursing system* is selected when the patient can and should perform all self-care actions. A single patient may require one or a sequential combination of the three types of nursing systems. All three nursing systems are most appropriately used with individuals. Multiperson units usually require combinations of the partly compensatory and supportive-educative nursing systems, although it is possible that such multiperson units as families or residence groups would need wholly compensatory nursing systems under some circumstances.

Wholly compensatory nursing system—The nurse accomplishes the patient's therapeutic self-care, compensates for the patient's inability to engage in self-care, and supports and protects the patient. The nurse selects wholly compensatory nursing system subtype 1 for persons unable to engage in any form of deliberate action, including persons who are unable to control their position and movement in space; are unresponsive to stimuli or responsive to internal and external stimuli only through hearing and feeling; are unable to monitor the environment and convey information to others because of loss of motor ability.

The nurse selects the following *method of helping*: Acting for or doing for the patient.

The nurse selects *wholly compensatory nursing system subtype* 2 for persons who are aware and who may be able to make observations, judgments, and decisions about self-care and other matters but cannot or should not perform actions requiring ambulation and manipulative movements.

The nurse selects one or more of the following *methods of helping:* providing a developmental environment; acting for or doing for the patient; supporting the patient psychologically; guiding the patient; teaching the patient.

The nurse selects *wholly compensatory nursing system subtype 3* for persons who are unable to attend to themselves and make reasoned judgments and decisions about self-care and other matters but who can be ambulatory and may be able to perform some measures of self-care with continuous guidance and supervision.

The nurse selects one or more of the following *methods of helping:* providing a developmental environment; guiding the patient; providing support for the patient; acting for or doing for the patient.

Partly compensatory nursing system—The nurse performs some self-care measures for the patient, compensates for self-care limitations of the patient, assists the patient as required, and regulates the patient's self-care agency; the patient performs some self-care measures, regulates self-care agency, and accepts care and assistance from the nurse.

When the nurse selects *partly compensatory nursing system subtype 1*, the patient performs universal measures of self-care and the nurse performs medically prescribed measures and some universal self-care measures. The nurse selects one or more of the following *methods of helping: acting for or doing for the patient; guiding the patient; supporting the patient; providing a developmental environment; teaching the patient.*

When the nurse selects *partly compensatory nursing system subtype 2*, the patient learns to perform some new care measures. The nurse selects one or more of the following *methods of helping:* acting for or doing for the patient; guiding the patient; supporting the patient; providing a developmental environment; teaching the patient.

Supportive-educative nursing system—The nurse regulates the exercise and development of the patient's self-care agency or dependent-care agency; the patient accomplishes self-care or dependent-care and regulates the exercise and development of self-care agency or dependent-care agency.

The nurse selects *supportive-educative nursing system subtype 1* if the patient can perform care measures, and the appropriate methods of helping are guiding the patient and supporting the patient. The nurse selects *supportive-educative nursing system subtype 2* if the patient can perform care measures and the appropriate method of helping is teaching the patient. The nurse selects *supportive-educative nursing system subtype 3* if the patient can perform care measures and the appropriate method of helping is providing a developmental environment. The nurse selects *supportive-educative nursing system subtype 4* if the patient is competent in self-care and the appropriate method of helping is guiding the patient periodically.

5. **Regulatory Operations: Planning for Regulatory Operations**—The nurse specifies what is needed to produce the nursing system(s) selected for the patient.
6. **Regulatory Operations: Production of Regulatory Care**—Nursing systems are produced by means of the actions of nurses and patients during nurse-patient encounters. The nurse produces and manages the designated nursing system(s) and method(s) of helping for as long as the patient's self-care deficit or dependent-care deficit exists. The nurse provides the following direct nursing care operations:

   Performs and regulates self-care or dependent-care tasks for patients or assists patients with their performance of self- or dependent-care tasks.

   Coordinates self- or dependent-care task performance so that a unified system of care is produced and coordinated with other components of health care.

   Helps patients, their families, and others bring about systems of daily living for patients that support the accomplishment of self-care or dependent-care and are, at the same time, satisifying in relation to patients' interests, talents, and goals.

   Guides, directs, and supports patients in their exercise of, or in the withholding of the exercise of, their self-care agency or dependent-care agency.

   Stimulates patients' interests in self-care or dependent-care by raising questions and promoting discussions of care problems and issues when conditions permit.

   Is available to patients at times when questions are likely to arise.

   Supports and guides patients in learning activities and provides cues for learning as well as instructional sessions.

   Supports and guides patients as they experience illness or disability and the effects of medical care measures and as they experience the need to engage in new measures of self-care or change their ways of meeting ongoing self-care requisites.

   The nurse carries out the following decision-making operations regarding the continuation of or need for changes in direct nursing care:

   Monitors and assists patients to monitor themselves to determine if self-care or dependent-care measures were performed and to determine the effects of self-care or dependent-care, the results of efforts to regulate the exercise or development of self-care agency or dependent-care agency, and the sufficiency and efficiency of nursing action directed to these ends.

   Makes judgments about the sufficiency and efficiency of self-care or dependent-care, the regulation of the exercise or development of self-care agency or dependent-care, and nursing assistance.

   Makes judgments about the meaning of the results derived from nurses' performance when monitoring patients and judging outcomes of self-care or dependent-care for the well-being of patients. Makes or recommends adjustments in the nursing care system through changes in nurse and patient roles.
7. **Control Operations**—The nurse performs control operations concurrently with or separate from the production of regulatory care. The nurse makes observations and evaluates the nursing system to determine whether:

   The nursing system that was designed is actually produced.

   There is a fit between the current prescription for nursing and the nursing system that is being produced.

   Regulation of the patient's functioning is being achieved through performance of care measures to meet the patient's therapeutic self-care demand.

   Exercise of the patient's self-care agency or dependent-care agency is being properly regulated.

   Developmental change is in process and is adequate.

The patient is adjusting to any declining powers to engage in self-care or dependent-care.

Implications for Nursing Education

The Self-Care Framework provides a body of knowledge that can be used for curriculum development. The focus of both undergraduate and graduate nursing curricula is on components of self-care, self-care agency, self-care deficits, nursing agency, and nursing systems. Education for clinical skills emphasizes the methods of helping.

Reference

Orem, D. E. (1995). *Nursing: Concepts of practice* (5th ed.). St. Louis: Mosby.

MARTHA ROGERS' SCIENCE OF UNITARY HUMAN BEINGS

Overview

Focus is on unitary, irreducible human beings and their environments. The four basic concepts are:

1. **Energy fields**—irreducible, indivisible, pandimensional unitary human beings and environments that are identified by pattern and manifesting characteristics that are specific to the whole and cannot be predicted from knowledge of the parts. Human and environmental energy fields are integral with each other.
2. **Openness**—a characteristic of human and environmental energy fields; energy fields are continuously and completely open.
3. **Pattern**—the distinguishing characteristic of an energy field. Pattern is perceived as a single wave that gives identity to the field. Each human field pattern is unique and is integral with its own unique environmental field pattern. Pattern is an abstraction that cannot be seen; what are seen or experienced are manifestations of field pattern.
4. **Pandimensionality**—a nonlinear domain without spatial or temporal attributes.

The three principles of homeodynamics, which describe the nature of human and environmental energy fields, are:

1. **Resonancy**—asserts that human and environmental fields are identified by wave patterns that manifest continuous change from lower to higher frequencies.
2. **Helicy**—asserts that human and environmental field patterns are continuous, innovative, and unpredictable, and are characterized by increasing diversity.
3. **Integrality**—emphasizes the continuous mutual human field and environmental field process.

Implications for Nursing Practice

Nursing practice is directed toward promoting the health and well-being of all persons, wherever they are. Rogers' practice methodology, which is called the Health Patterning Practice Method, encompasses the following phases:

1. **Pattern Manifestation Knowing—Assesment**—The continuous process of apprehending and identifying manifestations of the human energy field and environmental energy field patterns that relate to current health events. The nurse uses one or more Science of Unitary Human Beings–based research instruments or clinical tools to guide application and documentation of the practice methodology. The nurse acts with pandimensional authenticity, that is, with a demeanor of genuineness, trustworthiness, and knowledgeable caring. The nurse focuses on the client as a unified whole (a unitary human being) and participates in individualized nursing by looking at each client and determining the range of behaviors that are normal for him or her. The nurse always takes diversity among clients into account, for that diversity has distinct implications for what will be done and how it will be done. The nurse comes to know human energy field pattern and environmental energy field pattern through manifestations of that pattern in the form of the client's experiences, perceptions, and expressions. The nurse attends to expressions of experiences and perceptions in such forms as the client's verbal responses, responses to questionnaires, and personal ways of living and relating. The nurse collects such relevant pattern information as the client's sensations, thoughts, feelings, awareness, imagination, memory, introspective insights, intuitive apprehensions, recurring themes and issues that pervade the client's life, metaphors, visualizations, images, nutrition, work and play, exercise, substance use, sleep/wake cycles, safety, decelerated/accelerated field rhythms, space-time shifts, interpersonal networks, and professional health care access and use.
2. **Voluntary Mutual Patterning**—The continuous process whereby the nurse, with

the client, patterns the environmental energy field to promote harmony related to the health events. The nurse facilitates the client's actualization of potentials for health and well-being. The nurse has no investment in the client's changing in a particular way. The nurse does not attempt to change anyone to conform to arbitrary health ideals. Rather, the nurse enhances the client's efforts to actualize health potentials from his or her point of view. The nurse helps to create an environment where healing conditions are optimal and invites the client to heal him- or herself as the nurse and the client participate in various health patterning modalities. The nurse uses many different modes of health patterning, including such noninvasive modalities as therapeutic touch; imagery; meditation; relaxation; balancing activity and rest; unconditional love; attitudes of hope, humor, and upbeat moods; the use of sound, color, and motion; health education; wellness counseling; nutrition counseling; meaningful presence; meaningful dialogue; affirmations (expressions of intentionality); bibliotherapy; journal keeping; esthetic experiences of art, poetry, and nature; collaborative advocacy; and computer-based virtual reality. The nurse recognizes that both noninvasive modalities and technology are simply tools used to apply knowledge in practice.

3. **Pattern Manifestation Knowing—Evaluation**—The nurse evaluates voluntary mutual patterning by means of pattern manifestation knowing. The nurse monitors and collects additional pattern information as it unfolds during voluntary mutual patterning, and nurse considers the pattern information within the context of continually emerging health patterning goals affirmed by the client.

Implications for Nursing Education

Education for nursing practice requires a commitment to lifelong learning. Education for professional nursing occurs at the baccalaureate, masters, and doctoral levels in college and university settings. The purpose of professional nursing educational programs is to provide the knowledge and tools necessary for nursing practice. The liberal arts and sciences are a predominant component of the curriculum. The principles of resonancy, helicy, and integrality represent the major integrating concepts of the nursing courses.

References

Barret, E. A. M. (1998). A Rogerian practic methodology for health patterning. *Nursing Science Quarterly*, 11, 136–138.

Cowling, W. R. III. (1997). Pattern appreciation: The unitary science/practice of reaching for essence. In M. Madrid (Ed.), *Patterns of Rogerian knowing* (pp. 129–142). New York: National League for Nursing Press.

Madrid, M., & Barrett, E. A. M. (Eds.). (1994). *Rogers' scientific art of nursing practice.* New York: National League for Nursing.

Rogers, M. E. (1990). Nursing: Science of unitary, irreducible, human beings: Update 1990. In E. A. M. Barrett (Ed.), *Visions of Rogers' science-based nursing* (pp. 5–11). New York: National League for Nursing.

Rogers, M. E. (1992). Nursing science and the space age. *Nursing Science Quarterly*, 5, 27–34.

CALLISTA ROY'S ADAPTATION MODEL

Overview

Focuses on the responses of the human adaptive system, which can be an individual or a group, to a constantly changing environment. Adaptation is the central feature of the model. Problems in adaptation arise when the adaptive system is unable to cope with or respond to constantly changing stimuli from the internal and external environments in a manner that maintains the integrity of the system. Environmental stimuli are categorized as:

1. **Focal**—the stimuli most immediately confronting the person.
2. **Contextual**—the contributing factors in the situation.
3. **Residual**—other unknown factors that may influence the situation. When the factors making up residual stimuli become known, they are considered focal or contextual stimuli.

Adaptation occurs through two types of innate or acquired coping mechanisms used to respond to changing environmental stimuli:

1. **Regulator coping subsystem**—for individuals; receives input from the external environment and from changes in the individual's internal state and processes the changes through neural-chemical-endocrine channels to produce responses.
2. **Cognator coping subsystem**—for individuals; also receives input from external

and internal stimuli that involve psychological, social, physical, and physiological factors, including regulator subsystem outputs. These stimuli then are processed through cognitive/emotive pathways, including perceptual/information processing, learning, judgment, and emotion.

3. **Stabilizer subsytem control process**—for groups; involves the established structures, values, and daily activities used by a group to accomplish its primary purpose and contribute to common purposes of society.
4. **Innovator Subsystem control process**—pertains to humans in groups; involves the structures and processes necessary for change and growth in human social systems.

Responses take place in four modes for individuals and groups:

1. **Physiological/physical mode**
   Physiological mode—for individuals; concerned with basic needs requisite to maintaining the physical and physiological integrity of the individual human system. It encompasses oxygenation; nutrition; elimination; activity and rest; protection; senses; fluid, electrolyte, and acid-base balance; neurologic function; and endocrine function. The basic underlying need is physiologic integrity.
   Physical mode—for groups; pertains to the manner in which the collective human adaptive system manifests adaptation relative to basic operating resources, that is, participants, physical facilities, and fiscal resources. The basic underlying need is resource adequacy, or wholeness achieved by adapting to change in physical resource needs.
2. **Self-concept mode**
   Self-concept mode—for the individual; addresses the composite of beliefs and feelings that a person holds about him- or herself at a given time. The basic underlying need is psychic and spiritual integrity, the need to know who one is so that one can be or exist with a sense of unity, meaning, and purposefulness in the universe. The Physical Self refers to the individual's appraisal of his or her own physical being, including physical attributes, functioning, sexuality, health and illness states, and appearance; includes the components of body sensation and body image. The Personal Self refers to the individual's appraisal of his or her own characteristics, expectations, values, and worth, including self-consistency, self-ideal, and the moral-ethical-spiritual self.
   Group identity mode—for groups; addresses shared relations, goals, and values, which create a social milieu and culture, a group self-image, and coresponsibility for goal achievement. Identity integrity is the underlying need, which implies the honesty, soundness, and completeness of the group members' identification with the group and involves the process of sharing identity and goals. This mode encompasses Interpersonal Relationships, Group Self-Image, Social Milieu, and Group Culture.
3. **Role function mode**—for the individual, focuses on the roles that the individual occupies in society. The basic underlying need is social integrity, the need to know who one is in relation to others so that one can act. For the group, focuses on the action components associated with group infrastructure that are designed to contribute to the accomplishment of the group's mission, or the tasks or functions associated with the group. The basic underlying need is role clarity, the need to understand and commit to fulfill expected tasks, so that the group can achieve common goals.
4. **Interdependence mode**—behavior pertaining to interdependent relationships of individuals and groups. The basic underlying need is relational integrity, the feeling of security in nurturing relationships. For the individual, focuses on interactions related to the giving and receiving of love, respect, and value, and encompasses Affectional Adequacy, Developmental Adequacy, Resource Adequacy, Significant Others, and Support Systems. For the group, pertains to the social context in which the group operates including both private and public contacts both within the group and with those outside the group, and encompasses Affectional Adequacy, Developmental Adequacy, Resource Adequacy, Context, Infrastructure, and Resources.

The four modes are interrelated. Responses in any one mode may have an effect on or act as a stimulus in one or all of the other modes. Responses in each mode are judged as either:

1. **Adaptive**—promote the goals of human adaptive system, including survival, growth, reproduction, and mastery.
2. **Ineffective**—those that do not contribute to the goals of the human adaptive system.

Implications for Nursing Practice

Nursing practice is directed toward promoting adaptation in each of the four response modes, thereby contributing to the person's health, quality of life, and dying with dignity. Roy's practice methodology is the Roy Adaptation Model Nursing Process, which encompasses six steps:

1. **Assessment of behavior**—The nurse systematically gathers data about the behavior of the human adaptive system and judges the current state of adaptation in each adaptive mode.

   The nurse uses one or more of the Roy Adaptation Model–based research instruments or clinical tools to guide application and documentation of the practice methodology and systematically gathers data about observable and nonobservable behaviors for each aspect of the four adaptive modes, focusing on the individual or the group of interest. The nurse gathers behavioral data by means of observation, objective measurement, and purposeful interviews.

   The nurse, in collaboration with the human adaptive system of interest, makes a tentative judgment about behaviors in each adaptive mode. Behaviors are tentatively judged as adaptive or ineffective responses, using the criteria of the human adaptive system's individualized goals and comparison of the behaviors with norms signifying adaptation. If norms are not available, the nurse considers adaptation difficulty as pronounced regulator activity with cognator ineffectiveness for individuals, or pronounced stabilizer activity with innovator ineffectiveness for groups. The nurse sets priorities for further assessment, taking the goals of adaptation into account.

   The first priority is behaviors that threaten the survival of the individual, family, group, or community. The second priority is behaviors that affect the growth of the individual, family, group, or community. The third priority is behaviors that affect the continuation of the human race or of society. The fourth priority is behaviors that affect the attainment of full potential for the individual or group.
2. **Assessment of stimuli**—The nurse recognizes that stimuli must be amenable to independent nurse functions. Consequently, factors such as medical diagnoses and medical treatments are not considered stimuli because those factors cannot be independently managed by nurses.

   The nurse identifies the internal and external focal and contextual stimuli that are influencing the behaviors of particular interest. The nurse recognizes that residual stimuli typically are present and attempts to confirm the presence of those stimuli by asking the human adaptive system about other stimuli and/or by recourse to theoretical or experiential knowledge. When residual stimuli finally are identified, they are classified as contextual or focal stimuli. The nurse identifies the internal stimulus of the adaptation level, and determines whether it reflects integrated, compensatory, or compromised life processes.

   In situations where all behaviors are judged as adaptive responses, assessment of stimuli focuses on identifying potential threats to adaptation. The nurse identifies stimuli by means of observation, objective measurement, and purposeful interviews.

   The nurse validates perceptions and thoughts about relevant stimuli with the human adaptive system of interest, using Orlando's deliberative nursing process:

   The nurse shares perceptions and thoughts about relevant stimuli with the human adaptive system.

   The nurse asks if those are the relevant stimuli.

   The human adaptive system confirms or does not confirm the identified stimuli as relevant.

   If the stimuli are not confirmed as relevant, the nurse and the human adaptive system discuss their perceptions of the situation until agreement about relevant stimuli is reached.
3. **Nursing diagnosis**—The nurse uses a process of judgment to make a statement conveying the adaptation status of the human adaptive system of interest. The nursing diagnosis is a statement that identifies the behaviors of interest together with the most relevant influencing stimuli. The nurse uses one of three different approaches to state the nursing diagnosis:

   Behaviors are stated within each adaptive mode and with their most relevant influencing stimuli.

   A summary label for behaviors in each adaptive mode with relevant stimuli is used.

   A label that summarizes a behavioral pattern across adaptive modes that is affected by the same stimuli is used.

   The nurse may link the Roy Adaptation Model–based nursing diagnosis with a relevant diagnosis from the taxonomy of the North American Nursing Diagnosis Association (NANDA). The nurse assigns a priority to each nursing diagnosis—the first priority is behaviors that threaten the survival of the individual, family, group, or community; the second priority is behaviors that affect the growth of the individual, family, group, or community; the third priority is behaviors that affect the continuation of the human race or of society; the fourth priority is behaviors that affect the attainment of full potential for the individual or group.

4. **Goal setting**—The nurse articulates a clear statement of the behavioral outcomes in response to nursing provided to the human adaptive system. The nurse actively involves the human adaptive system in the formation of behavioral goals if possible. The nurse states goals as specific short-term and long-term behavioral outcomes of nursing intervention. The goal statement designates the behavior of interest, the way in which the behavior will change, and the time frame for attainment of the goal. Goals may be stated for ineffective behaviors that are to be changed to adaptive behaviors and also for adaptive behaviors that should be maintained or enhanced.
5. **Nursing intervention**—The nurse selects and implements nursing approaches that have a high probability of changing stimuli or strengthening adaptive processes. Nursing intervention is the management of stimuli. The nurse manages the focal stimulus first if possible, and then manages the contextual stimuli. The nurse uses the McDonald and Harms nursing judgment method, in collaboration with the human adaptive system, to select a nursing intervention:
   - Alternative approaches to management of stimuli are listed, along with the consequences of management of each stimulus.
   - The probability (high, moderate, low) for each consequence is determined.
   - The value of the outcomes of each approach is designated as desirable or undesirable.

   The options are shared with the human adaptive system. The nursing intervention with the highest probability of reaching the valued goal is selected. The nurse determines and implements the steps that will manage the stimulus appropriately.
6. **Evaluation**—The nurse judges the effectiveness of nursing interventions in relation to the behaviors of the human adaptive system. The nurse systematically reassesses observable and nonobservable behaviors for each aspect of the four adaptive modes. The nurse gathers the behavioral data by means of observation, objective measurement, and purposeful interviews. The nurse uses the following criteria to judge the effectiveness of nursing intervention:
   - The goal was attained.
   - The human adaptive system manifests behavior stated in the goals.
   - The human adaptive system demonstrates a positive response to the stimuli that frees energy for responses to other stimuli.

   If the criteria for nursing intervention effectiveness are met, and if there is no threat that the behavior will become ineffective again, then that behavior may be deleted from nursing concern. If, however, the criteria are not met, the nurse must determine what went wrong. Possibilities are:
   - The goals were unrealistic or unacceptable to the human adaptive system.
   - The assessment data were inaccurate or incomplete.
   - The selected nursing intervention approaches were not implemented properly.

   The nurse then returns to Assessment of Behaviors to closely examine behaviors that continue to be ineffective and to try to further understand the situation. The end result of the Roy Adaptation Model Nursing Process is an update of the nursing care plan.

Implications for Nursing Education

The model is an appropriate curriculum guide for diploma, associate degree, baccalaureate degree, and master's degree nursing education programs. Curriculum content is based on the components of the conceptual model. The vertical strands of the curriculum focus on theory and practice. The theory strand encompasses content on the adapting person, health/illness, and stress/disruption. The practice strand emphasizes nursing management of environmental stimuli. The horizontal strands include the nursing process and student adaptation and leadership.

Reference

Roy, C., & Andrews, H. A. (1999). *The Roy Adaptation Model* (2nd ed.) Stamford, CT: Appleton and Lange.

Appendix N2-3 Nursing Theory

A theory is defined as one or more relatively concrete and specific concepts that are derived from a conceptual model, the propositions that narrowly describe those concepts, and the propositions that state relatively concrete and specific relations between two or more of the concepts. Grand theories are rather broad in scope. They are made up of concepts and propositions that are less abstract and general than the concepts and propositions of a conceptual model but are not as concrete and specific as the concepts and propositions of a middle-range theory. Middle-range theories are narrower in scope than grand theories. They are made up of a limited number of concepts and propositions that are written at a relatively concrete and specific level.

MADELEINE LEININGER'S THEORY OF CULTURAL CARE DIVERSITY AND UNIVERSALITY

Overview

A grand theory focusing on the discovery of human care diversities and universalities and ways to provide culturally congruent care to people. The concepts of the theory are:

1. **Care**—abstract and concrete phenomena related to assisting, supporting, or enabling experiences or behaviors toward or for others with evident or anticipated needs to ameliorate or improve a human condition or lifeway.
2. **Caring**—the actions and activities directed toward assisting, supporting, or enabling another individual or group with evident or anticipated needs to ameliorate or improve a human condition or lifeway or to face death.
3. **Culture**—the learned, shared, and transmitted values, beliefs, norms, and lifeways of a particular group that guide thinking, decisions, and actions in patterned ways; encompasses several cultural and social structure dimensions: technological factors, religious and philosophical factors, kinship and social factors, political and legal factors, economic factors, educational factors, and cultural values and lifeways.
4. **Language**—word usages, symbols, and meanings about care.
5. **Ethnohistory**—past facts, events, instances, experiences of individuals, groups, cultures, and institutions that are primarily people centered (ethno) and which describe, explain, and interpret human lifeways within particular cultural contexts and over short or long periods of time.
6. **Environmental context**—the totality of an event, situation, or particular experiences that give meaning to human expressions, interpretations, and social interactions in particular physical, ecological, sociopolitical, and/or cultural settings.
7. **Health**—a state of well-being that is culturally defined, valued, and practiced, and which reflects the ability of individuals (or groups) to perform their daily role activities in culturally expressed, beneficial, and patterned lifeways.
8. **Worldview**—the way people tend to look out on the world or their universe to form a picture of or a value stance about their life or the world around them.
9. **Cultural care**—the subjectively and objectively transmitted values, beliefs, and patterned lifeways that assist, support, or enable another individual or group to maintain well-being and health, to improve his or her human condition and lifeway, to deal with illness, handicaps, or death. The two dimensions are:
   Cultural care diversity—the variabilities and/or differences in meanings, patterns, values, lifeways, or symbols of care within or between collectivities that are related to assistive, supportive, or enabling human care expressions.
   Cultural care universality—the common, similar, or dominant uniform care meanings, patterns, values, lifeways, or symbols that are manifest among many cultures and reflect assistive, supportive, facilitative, or enabling ways to help people.
10. **Care systems**—the values, norms, and structural features of an organization designed for serving people's health needs, concerns, or conditions. The two types of care systems are:
   Generic lay care system—traditional or local indigenous health care or cure practices that have special meanings and uses to heal or assist people, which are generally offered in familiar home or community environmental contexts with their local practitioners.
   Professional health care system—professional care or cure services offered by diverse health personnel who have been prepared through formal professional programs of study in special educational institutions.
11. **Cultural-congruent nursing care**—cognitively based assistive, supportive, facilitative, or enabling acts or decisions that are tailored to fit with individual, group, or institutional cultural values, beliefs, and lifeways in order to provide or support meaningful, beneficial, and satisfying health care or well-being services. The three modes of cultural-congruent nursing care are:
   Cultural care preservation or maintenance—assistive, supportive, facilitative, or enabling professional actions and decisions that help people of a particular culture to retain and/or preserve relevant care values so that they can maintain their well-being, recover from illness, or face handicaps and/or death.
   Cultural care accommodation or negotiation—assistive, supportive, facilitative, or enabling creative professional actions and decisions that help people of a designated culture to adapt to, or to negotiate with, others for a beneficial or satisfying health outcome with professional care providers.
   Cultural care repatterning or restructuring—assistive, supportive, facilitative, or enabling professional actions and decisions that help clients reorder, change, or greatly modify their lifeways for a new, different and beneficial health care pattern while respecting the clients' cultural values and beliefs

and still providing a beneficial or healthier lifeway than before the changes were coestablished with the clients.

Implications for Nursing Practice

Nursing practice is directed toward improving and providing culturally congruent care to people. A practice methodology for the Theory of Culture Care Diversity and Universality is as follows:

Goals of Nursing Practice are: to improve and to provide culturally congruent care to people that is beneficial, will fit with, and be useful to the client, family, or culture group healthy lifeways; to provide culturally congruent nursing care in order to improve or offer a different kind of nursing care service to people of diverse or similar cultures.

Clients include individuals, families, subcultures, groups, communities, and institutions.

Culturalogical Assessment The nurse maintains a holistic or total view of the client's world by using the Sunrise Model and Enablers to guide assessment of cultural beliefs, values, and lifeways.

The nurse is aware that the client may belong to a subculture or special group that maintains its own values and beliefs that differ from the values and beliefs of the dominant culture. The nurse shows a genuine interest in the client and learns from and maintains respect for the client. The nurse asks open-ended questions and maintains the role of an active listener, learner, and reflector. The nurse shares professional knowledge only if the client asks about such knowledge.

The nurse begins the assessment with such questions as: What would you like to share with me today about your experiences or beliefs, to help you keep well? Are there some special ideas or ways you would like nurses to care for you? The nurse gives attention to clients' gender differences, communication modes, special language terms, interpersonal relationships, and use of space and foods.

Nursing Judgments, Decisions, and Actions Nursing practice requires the coparticipation of nurses and clients working together to identify, plan, implement, and evaluate the appropriate mode(s) of cultural-congruent nursing care. Nursing decisions and actions encompass: Assisting, Supporting, Facilitating, and Enabling Nurse and client select one or more mode of cultural-congruent nursing care:

Cultural Care Preservation or Maintenance—used when professional decisions and actions are needed to help clients of a designated culture to retain and/or preserve relevant care values so that they can maintain their well-being, recover from illness, or face handicaps and/or death.

Cultural Care Accommodation or Negotiation—used when professional actions and decisions are needed to help clients of a designated culture to adapt to, or to negotiate with, others for a beneficial or satisfying health outcome with professional care providers.

Cultural Care Repatterning or Restructuring—used when professional actions and decisions are needed to help clients of a designated culture to reorder, change, or greatly modify their lifeways for a new, different, and beneficial health care pattern while respecting the clients' cultural values and beliefs and still providing a beneficial or healthier lifeway than before the changes were coestablished with the clients.

Clinical Protocols Specific nursing practices or clinical protocols are derived from the findings of research guided by the Theory of Culture Care Diversity and Universality. The research findings are used to develop protocols for cultural-congruent care that blends with the particular cultural values, beliefs, and lifeways of the client, and is assessed to be beneficial, satisfying, and meaningful to the client.

Implications for Nursing Education

Professional nursing care, learned in formal educational programs, builds upon the generic care given by naturalistic lay and folk care givers. The curriculum emphasizes transcultural nursing knowledge, with formal study about different cultures in the world, as well as culture-universal and culture-specific health care needs of people and nursing care practices. Transcultural nurse generalists are prepared at the baccalaureate level for the general use of transcultural nursing concepts, principles, and practices. Transcultural nurse specialists, who are prepared at the doctoral level, have in-depth understanding of a few cultures and can function as field practitioners, teachers, researchers, or consultants. Certification is awarded by the Transcultural Nursing Society to nurses who have educational preparation in transcultural nursing or the equivalent and who demonstrate basic clinical competence in transcultural nursing.

Reference

Leininger, M. M. (Ed.). (1991). *Culture care diversity and universality: A theory of nursing*. New York: National League for Nursing.

NEWMAN'S THEORY OF HEALTH AS EXPANDING CONSCIOUSNESS

Overview

A grand theory focusing on health as the expansion of consciousness, with emphasis on the idea that every person in every situation, no matter how disordered and hopeless the situation may seem, is part of the universal process of expanding consciousness. The concepts of the theory are:

1. **Consciousness**—the informational capacity of human beings, that is, the ability of humans to interact with their environments. Consciousness encompasses interconnected cognitive and affective awareness, physiochemical maintenance including the nervous and endocrine systems, growth processes, the immune system, and the genetic code. Consciousness can be seen in the quantity and quality of the interaction between human beings and their environments. The process of life is toward higher levels of consciousness; sometimes this process is smooth, pleasant, harmonious; other times it is difficult and disharmonious, as in disease.
2. **Pattern**—a fundamental attribute of all there is that gives unity in diversity; information that depicts the whole; relatedness. People are identified by their pattern. The evolution of expanding consciousness is seen in the pattern of movement-space-time. Pattern is manifested as exchanging, communicating, relating, valuing, choosing, moving, perceiving, feeling, and knowing. Pattern encompasses three dimensions—Movement-Space-Time, Rhythm, and Diversity:
   - **Movement**—an essential property of matter; a means of communicating; the means whereby one perceives reality becomes aware of self; the natural condition of life.
   - **Space**—encompasses personal space, inner space, and life space as dimensions of space relevant to the individual, and territoriality, shared space, and distancing as dimensions relevant to the family.
   - **Time**—the amount of time perceived to be passing (subjective time); clock time (objective time).
   - **Rhythm**—basic to movement; the rhythm of movement is an integrating experience.
   - **Diversity**—seen in the parts.

Implications for Nursing Practice

Nursing practice is directed toward facilitating pattern recognition by connecting with the client in an authentic way, and assisting the client to discover new rules for a higher level of organization or consciousness. Newman's Research as Praxis Protocol is a research/practice methodology. The phenomenon of interest is the process of expanding consciousness.

The Interview The meeting of the nurse and the study participant/client occurs when there is a mutual attraction via congruent patterns, i.e., interpenetration of the two fields. The nurse and study participant/client enter into a partnership, with the mutual goal of participating in an authentic relationship, trusting that in the process of its unfolding, both will emerge at a higher level of consciousness.

Development of the Narrative: Pattern Recognition The nurse selects the statements deemed most important to the study participant/client and arranges the key segments of the data in chronological order to highlight the most significant events and persons. The data remain the same except in the order of presentation. Natural breaks where a pattern shift occurs are noted and form the basis of the sequential patterns. Recognition of the pattern of the whole, made up of segments of the study participant/client's relationships over time, will emerge for the nurse. The nurse then transmutes the narrative into a simple diagram of the sequential pattern configurations.

Follow-Up: Pattern Recognition The nurse conducts a second interview with the study participant/client to share the diagram or other visual portrayal of the pattern. The nurse does not interpret the diagram. Rather, it is used simply to illustrate the study participant/ client's story in graphic form, which tends to accentuate the contrasts and repetitions in relationships over time. The mutual viewing of the graphic form is an opportunity for the study participant/client to confirm and clarify or revise the story being portrayed. The mutual viewing also is an opportunity for the nurse to clarify any aspect of the story about which he or she has any doubt.

The nature of the pattern of person-environment interaction will begin to emerge in terms of energy flow (e.g., blocked, diffuse, disorganized, repetitive, or whatever descriptors and metaphors come to mind to describe the pattern). The study participant/client may express signs that pattern recognition is occurring (or already has occurred in the interval following the first interview) as the nurse and study participant/client reflect together on the study participant/client's life pattern. If no signs of pattern recognition occur, the nurse and study participant/client may want to proceed with additional reflections in subsequent interviews until no further insight is reached.

Sometimes, no signs of pattern recognition emerge, and if so, that characterizes the pattern for that person. It is not to be forced.

Application of Theory of Health as Expanding Conciousness The nurse undertakes more intense analysis of the data in light of the Theory of Health as Expanding Consciousness after the interviews are completed. The nurse evaluates the nature of the sequential patterns of interaction in terms of quality and complexity and interprets the patterns according to the study participant/client's position on Young's spectrum of consciousness. The sequential patterns represent presentational construing or relationships. Any similarities of pattern among a group of study participants/clients having a similar experience may be designated by themes and stated in propositional form.

Implications for Nursing Education

Education for nursing should be the professional doctoral degree, the Doctor of Nursing (ND), which requires a strong arts and sciences background as pre-professional education. Students and practicing nurses who plan to use the Theory of Health as Expanding Consciousness have to be prepared for personal transformation in the way that they view the world and nursing.

Reference

Newman, M. A. (1994). *Health as expanding consciousness* (2nd ed.). New York: National League for Nursing.

IDA JEAN ORLANDO'S THEORY OF THE DELIBERATIVE NURSING PROCESS OVERVIEW

Overview

A middle-range predictive theory focusing on an interpersonal process that is directed toward facilitating identification of the nature of the patient's distress and his or her immediate needs for help. The concepts of the theory are:

1. **Patient's behavior**—behavior observed by the nurse in an immediate nurse-patient situation. The two dimensions are:
   Need for help—a requirement of the patient that, if supplied, relieves or diminishes immediate distress or improves immediate sense of adequacy or well-being.
   Improvement—an increase in patients' mental and physical health, their well-being, and their sense of adequacy. The need for help and improvement can be expressed in both nonverbal and verbal forms. Visual manifestations of nonverbal behavior include such motor activities as eating, walking, twitching, and trembling, as well as such physiological forms as urinating, defecating, temperature and blood pressure readings, respiratory rate, and skin color. Vocal forms of nonverbal behavior—nonverbal behavior that is heard—include crying, moaning, laughing, coughing, sneezing, sighing, yelling, screaming, groaning, and singing. Verbal behavior refers to what a patient says, including complaints, requests, questions, refusals, demands, and comments or statements.
2. **Nurse's reaction**—the nurse's nonobservable response to the patient's behavior. The three dimensions are:
   Perception—physical stimulation of any one of the five senses by the patient's behavior.
   Thought—an idea that occurs in the nurse's mind.
   Feeling—a state of mind inclining the nurse toward or against a perception, thought, or action; occurs in response to the nurse's perceptions and thoughts.
3. **Nurse's activity**—the observable actions taken by nurses in response to their reactions, including instructions, suggestions, directions, explanations, information, requests, and questions directed toward the patient; making decisions for the patient; handling the patient's body; administering medications or treatments; and changing the patient's immediate environment. The two dimensions of nurse's activity are:
   Automatic nursing process—actions decided on by the nurse for reasons other than the patient's immediate need.
   Deliberative nursing process (process discipline)—a specific set of nurse behaviors or actions directed toward the patient's behavior that ascertain or meet the patient's immediate needs for help.

Implications for Nursing Practice

Nursing practice is directed toward identifying and meeting the patient's immediate needs for help through use of Orlando's Practice Methodology.

1. **Observations** encompass any and all information pertaining to a patient that the nurse acquires while on duty.
2. **Direct Observations** are the nurse's reaction to the patient's behavior. Direct observations are any perception, thought, or feeling the nurse has from her own experience of the patient's behavior at any or several moments in time.
3. **Indirect Observations** consist of any information that is derived from a source other than the patient. This information pertains to, but is not directly derived from, the patient.
4. **Actions** are carried out with or for the patient.
5. **Nurse's Activity: Deliberative Nursing Process** The process used to share and validate the nurse's direct and indirect observations is the Deliberative Nursing Process. Clinical protocols contain the specific requirements for the Deliberative Nursing Process. The nurse may express and explore any aspect of his or her reaction to the patient's behavior—perception, thought, or feeling. If exploration of one aspect of the nurse's reaction does not result in identification of the patient's need for help, then another aspect of the reaction can be explored. If exploration of all aspects of the nurse's reaction does not yield a verbal response from the patient, then the nurse may use negative expressions to demonstrate continued interest in the patient behavior and to give the patient permission to respond with his or her own negative reaction. Examples of negative expressions by the nurse are: Is it that you don't think I'll understand? Am I wrong? It looked like that procedure was very painful, and you didn't say a word about it.
6. **Direct Help** The nurse meets the patient's need directly when the patient is unable to meet his or her own need and when the activity is confined to the nurse-patient contact.
7. **Indirect Help** The nurse meets the patient's need indirectly when the activity extends to arranging the services of a person, agency, or resource that the patient cannot contact by himself or herself.
8. **Reporting** The nurse receives reports about the patient's behavior from other nurses, and from other health professionals. The nurse reports his or her observations of the patient's behavior to other nurses and other health professionals.
9. **Recording** The nurse records the nursing process, including: the nurse's perception of or about the patient; the nurse's thought and/or feeling about the perception; what the nurse said and/or did to, with, or for the patient.

Implications for Nursing Education

Students should be trained in the use of the deliberative nursing process for all person-to-person contacts. The purpose of training is to change the nurse's activity from personal and automatic to disciplined and professional. Training is facilitated by use of process recordings that include perceptions of or about the patient, thoughts and/or feelings about the perception, and what was said and/or done to, with, or for the patient. The process discipline can be successfully taught in 6 to 12 weeks.

References

Orlando, I. J. (1961). *The dynamic nurse-patient relationship: Function, process and principles.* New York: G. P. Putnam's Sons. [Reprinted 1990, New York: National League for Nursing]

Orlando, I. J. (1972). *The discipline and teaching of nursing process: An evaluative study.* New York: G. P. Putnam's Sons.

ROSEMARIE PARSE'S THEORY OF HUMAN BECOMING

Overview

A grand theory focusing on human experiences of participation with the universe in the cocreation of health. The concepts of the theory are:

1. **Human becoming**—a unitary construct referring to the human being's living health.
2. **Meaning**—the linguistic and imagined content of something and the interpretation that one gives to something.
3. **Rhythmicity**—the cadent, paradoxical patterning of the human-universe mutual process.
4. **Transcendence**—reaching beyond with possibles—the hopes and dreams envisioned in multidimensional experiences [and] powering the originating of transforming.
5. **Imaging**—reflective/prereflective coming to know the explicit/tacit all-at-once.
6. **Valuing**—confirming/not confirming cherished beliefs in light of a personal world view.
7. **Languaging**—signifying valued images through speaking/being silent and moving/being still.
8. **Revealing/Concealing**—disclosing/not disclosing all-at-once.

9. **Enabling/Limiting**—living the opportunities/restrictions present in all choosings all-at-once.
10. **Connecting/Separating**—being with and apart from others, ideas, objects, and situations all-at-once.
11. **Powering**—the pushing/resisting process of affirming/not affirming being in light of nonbeing.
12. **Originating**—inventing new ways of conforming/nonconforming in the certainty/uncertainty of living.
13. **Transforming**—shifting the view of the familiar/unfamiliar, the changing of change in coconstituting anew in a deliberate way.

The three major principles of the theory of human becoming are:

1. **Structuring meaning multidimensionally is cocreating reality through the languaging of valuing and imaging**—means that humans construct what is real for them from choices made at many realms of the universe.
2. **Cocreating rhythmical patterns of relating is living the paradoxical unity of revealing-concealing and enabling-limiting while connecting-separating**—means that humans live in rhythm with the universe coconstituting patterns of relating.
3. **Cotranscending with the possibles is powering unique ways of originating in the process of transforming**—means that humans forge unique paths with shifting perspectives as a different light is cast on the familiar.

Implications for Nursing Practice

Nursing practice is directed toward respecting the quality of life as perceived by the person and the family. The practice methodology is as follows:

Principle 1: Structuring meaning multidimensionally. *Illuminating Meaning:* explicating what was, is, and will be. *Explicating:* making clear what is appearing now through languaging.

Principle 2: Cocreating rhythmical patterns. *Synchronizing rhythms:* dwelling with the pitch, yaw, and roll of the human-universe process. *Dwelling with:* immersing with the flow of connecting/separating.

Principle 3: *Mobilizing transcendence:* moving beyond the meaning moment with what is not-yet. *Moving beyond:* propelling with envisioned possibles of transforming.

Contexts of nursing Nurse-person situations and nurse-group situations. Participants include children and adults. Locations include homes, shelters, health care centers, parish halls, all departments of hospitals and clinics, rehabilitation centers, offices, and other milieus where nurses are with people.

Goal of discipline of nursing is quality of life from the person's, family's, and community's perspective.

Goal of the human becoming nurse is to be truly present with people as they enhance their quality of lives.

True presence is a special way of "being with" in which the nurse is attentive to moment-to-moment changes in meaning as she or he bears witness to the person's or groups's own living of value priorities.

Coming-to-be Present is an all-at-once gentling down and lifting up. True presence begins in the coming-to-be-present moments of preparation and attention. Preparation involves: an emptying to be available to bear witness to the other or others; being flexible, not fixed but gracefully present from one's center; dwelling with the universe at the moment, considering the attentive presence about to be. Attention involves focusing on the moment at hand for immersion.

Face-to-face discussions Nurse and person engage in dialogue. Conversation may be through discussion in general or through interpretations of stories, films, drawings, photographs, music, metaphors, poetry, rhythmic movements, and other expressions.

Silent immersion A process of the quiet that does not refrain from sending and receiving messages. A chosen way of becoming in the human-universe process lived in the rhythm of speaking–being silent, moving–being still as valued images incarnate meaning. True presence without words.

Lingering presence Recalling a moment through a lingering presence that arises after an immediate engagement. A reflective-prereflective "abiding with" attended to through glimpses of the other person, idea, object, or situation.

Ways of Changing Health Patterns in True Presence Creative Imagining Picturing, by seeing, hearing, and feeling, what a situation might be like if lived in a different way.

Affirming Personal Becoming Uncovering preferred personal health patterns by critically thinking about how or who one is.

Glimpsing the paradoxical Changing one's view of a situation by recognizing incongruities in that situation.

Implications for Nursing Education

Course content flows from the three principles of the theory. Clinical courses emphasize the knowledge and skills requisite to the application of the practice methodology. Graduate education builds on baccalaureate education and prepares specialists who concentrate on creating and testing concepts of the theory of human becoming.

References

Parse, R. R. (1992). Human becoming: Parse's theory of nursing. *Nursing Science Quarterly,* 5, 35–42.

Parse, R. R. (Ed.). (1995). *Illuminations: The human becoming theory in practice and research.* New York: National League for Nursing.

Parse, R. R. (1998). *The human becoming school of thought: A perspective for nurses and other health care professionals.* Thousand Oaks, CA: Sage.

HILDEGARD PEPLAU'S THEORY OF INTERPERSONAL RELATIONS

Overview

A middle-range descriptive theory focusing on the phases of the interpersonal process that occurs when an ill person and a nurse come together to resolve a difficulty felt in relation to health. The one concept of the theory is nurse-patient relationship, which is an interpersonal process made up of four components—two persons, the professional expertise of the nurse, and the client's problem or need for which expert nursing services are sought, and which has three discernible phases; one phase has two subphases:

1. **Orientation**—the phase in which the nurse first identifies herself by name and professional status and states the purpose, nature, and time available for the patient; the phase during which the nurse conveys professional interest and receptivity to the patient, begins to know the patient as a person, obtains essential information about the patient's health condition, and sets the tone for further interactions.
2. **Working**—the phase in which the major course occurs. The two subphases are:
   - **Identification**—the subphase during which the patient learns how to make use of the nurse-patient relationship.
   - **Exploitation**—the subphase during which the patient makes full use of available professional services.
3. **Termination**—the phase in which the work accomplished is summarized and closure occurs.

Implications for Nursing Practice

Nursing practice is directed toward promoting favorable changes in patients, which is accomplished through the nurse-patient relationship. Within that relationship, the nurse's major function is to study the interpersonal relations between the patient/client and others. Peplau's clinical methodology, which can be used for both nursing practice and nursing research is as follows:

Observation—Purpose is the identification, clarification, and verification of impressions about the interactive drama, of the pushes and pulls in the relationship between nurse and patient, as they occur.

Participant observation—Nurse's Behavior includes observation of the nurse's words, voice tones, body language, and other gestural messages. Patient's Behavior includes observation of the patient's words, voice tones, body language, and other gestural messages.

Interpersonal phenomena include observation of what goes on between the patient and the nurse.

Reframing empathic linkages occurs when the nurse's and/or the patient's ability to feel in self the emotions experienced by the other person in the same situation is converted to verbal communications by the nurse asking: What are you feeling right now?

Communication aims are the selection of symbols or concepts that convey both the reference, or meaning in the mind of the individual, and referent, the object or actions symbolized in the concept; and the wish to struggle toward the development of common understanding for words between two or more people.

Interpersonal techniques are verbal interventions used by nurses during nurse-patient relationships aimed at accomplishing problem resolution and competence development in patients.

Recording is the written record of the communication between nurse and patient, that is, the data collected through participant observation and reframing of empathic linkages. The aim is to capture the exact wording of the interaction between the nurse and the patient.

Data analysis focuses on testing the nurse's hypotheses, which are formulated from first impressions or hunches about the patient.

Phases of the nurse-patient relationship: Identify the phase of nurse-patient relationship in which communication occurred: orientation phase; working phase; identification subphase; exploitation subphase; termination phase.

Roles: Identify the roles taken by the nurse and the patient in each phase of the nurse-patient relationship.

Relations: Identify the connections, linkages, ties, and bonds that go on or went on between a patient and others, including family, friends, staff, or the nurse. Analyze the relations to identify their nature, origin, function, and mode.

Pattern integrations: Identify the patterns of the interpersonal relation between two or more people which together link or bind them and which enable the people to transform energy into patterns of action that bring satisfaction or security in the face of a recurring problem. Determine the type of pattern integration: complementary—the behavior of one person fits with and thereby complements the behavior of the other person; mutual—the same or similar behaviors are used by both persons; alternating—different behaviors used by two persons alternate between the two persons; antagonistic—the behaviors of the two persons do not fit but the relationship continues.

Implications for Nursing Education

Nursing is an educative instrument, a maturing force, that aims to promote forward movement of personality in the direction of creative, constructive, productive, personal, and community living. The task of each school of nursing is the fullest development of the nurse as a person who is aware of how he or she functions in a situation and as a person who wants to nurse patients in a helpful way.

References

Peplau, H. E. (1952). *Interpersonal relations in nursing.* New York: G. P. Putnam's Sons. [Reprinted 1991. New York: Springer]

Peplau, H. E. (1992). Interpersonal relations: A theoretical framework for application in nursing practice. *Nursing Science Quarterly, 5,* 13–18.

Peplau, H. E. (1997). Peplau's theory of interpersonal relations. *Nursing Science Quarterly, 10,* 162–167.

REVA RUBIN'S THEORY OF CLINICAL NURSING

Overview

A grand theory focusing on patients as persons undergoing subjectively involved experiences of varying degrees of tension or stress in a health problem situation. The major concepts are the situation of the patient and nursing care. Statements related to the patient situation and nursing care are:

1. Nursing care is dependent on the best estimate available of the situation of the patient.
2. Nursing care exists in a one-to-one relationship with the patient.
3. The relationship of nursing care to the situation of the patient is an ever-changing process of interaction.
4. The situation of the patient is expressed as a fraction or ratio that reflects the level or intensity of nursing care required.
   - If the situation for the patient is relatively insignificant, one that the patient can cope with quite well, then nursing care probably need not go beyond careful assessment.
   - If the situation for the patient is overwhelming, nursing care may have to encompass a whole series of activities to reduce the effects of the situation or reinforce the capacities of the patient in coping with the situation.
5. Situations within the sphere of proper nursing concern are fluid.

Implications for Nursing Practice

Nursing practice is directed toward helping the patient adjust to, endure through, and usefully integrate the health problem situation in its many ramifications through the phenomenon of *situational fluidity*, which characterizes nursing care in terms of:

1. **Time**—nursing operates within the immediate present; patient needs and behavior have an immediacy if not an urgency.
2. **Definition or diagnostic sets**—nursing diagnoses are based on the definition of capacities and limitations of the persons who are patients in relation to the situations in which they find themselves.
3. **Actions**—nursing actions are primarily directed toward helping the patient realign observations and expectations into a better "fit" with each other; nursing conveys a message to patients about themselves in their immediate situations.

Implications for Nursing Education

Education for nursing practice and nursing research emphasizes learning the naturalistic method of observation of patients in action, involved in a natural situation and setting. The learners typically are graduate students in nursing. The nurse-observer is viewed as an identifiable and functional part of the setting, as well as a helpful adjunct in the situation. The student is trained to observe while providing nursing care for the patient in a particular situation and to then record the entire nurse-patient interaction. The recorded observation serves as a database for evaluation of the quality and adequacy of nursing care as well as for generation of new theories.

References

Rubin, R. (1968). A theory of clinical nursing. *Nursing Research, 17,* 210–212.
Rubin, R. (1984). *Maternal identity and the maternal experience.* New York: Springer.

JEAN WATSON'S THEORY OF HUMAN CARING

Overview

A middle-range explanatory theory focusing on the human component of caring and the moment-to-moment encounters between the one who is caring and the one who is being cared for, especially the caring activities performed by nurses as they interact with others. The concepts of the theory are:

1. **Transpersonal caring**—human-to-human connectedness, whereby each person is touched by the human center of the other; a special kind of relationship involving a high regard for the whole person and his or her being-in-the world. The concept transpersonal caring relationship encompasses three dimensions:
   - *Self*—transpersonal-mindbodyspirit oneness, an embodied self, and an embodied spirit.
   - *Phenomenal field*—the totality of human experience, one's being-in-the-world.
   - *Intersubjectivity*—refers to an intersubjective human-to-human relationship in which the person of the nurse affects and is affected by the person of the other, both of whom are fully present in the moment and feel a union with the other.
2. **Caring occasion/caring moment**—The coming together of nurse and other(s), which involves action and choice both by the nurse and the other. The moment of coming together in a caring occasion presents them with the opportunity to decide how to be in the relationship—what to do with the moment.
3. **Caring (healing) consciousness**—A holographic dynamic that is manifest within a field of consciousness, and which exists through time and space and is dominant over physical illness.
4. **Carative factors**—those aspects of nursing that actually potentiate therapeutic healing processes for both the one caring and the one being cared for. The 10 carative factors are:
   - Forming a humanistic/altruistic system of values
   - Enabling and sustaining faith/hope
   - Being sensitive to self and others
   - Developing a helping/trusting, caring relationship
   - Promoting and accepting the expression of positive and negative feelings and emotions
   - Engaging in creative, individualized problem-solving caring processes
   - Promoting transpersonal teaching/learning
   - Attending to supportive, protective, and/or corrective mental, physical, societal, and spiritual environments
   - Assisting with gratification of basic human needs while preserving human dignity and wholeness
   - Allowing for, and being open to, existential/phenomenological/spiritual dimensions of caring and healing that cannot be fully explained scientifically through modern Western medicine

Implications for Nursing Practice

Nursing practice is directed toward helping persons gain a higher degree of harmony within the mind, body, and soul, which generates self-knowledge, self-reverence, self-healing, and self-care processes while increasing diversity, which is pursued through use of the 10 carative factors.

Implications for Nursing Education

Professional nursing education should be at the postbaccalaureate level of the Doctorate of Nursing (N.D.). The nature of human life is the subject matter of nursing. The curriculum acknowledges caring as a moral ideal and incorporates philosophical theories of human caring, health, and healing. Core areas of content are the humanities, social-biomedical science, and human caring content and process. Courses should use art, music, literature, poetry, drama, and movement to facilitate understanding of responses to health and illness as well as to new caring-healing modalities.

References

Watson, J. (1985). *Nursing: Human science and human care. A theory of nursing.* Norwalk, CT: Appleton-Century-Crofts. [Reprinted 1988. New York: National League for Nursing]

Watson, J. (1996). Watson's theory of transpersonal caring. In P. Hinton Walker and B. Neuman. (Eds.), *Blueprint for use of nursing models* (pp. 141–184). New York: NLN Press.

Watson, J (1997). The theory of human caring: Retrospective and prospective. *Nursing Science Quarterly, 10,* 49–52.

SOURCE: Adapted from overviews written by Jacqueline Fawcett for the videotape series, *The Nurse Theorists: Portraits of Excellence*, produced by Studio Three, Samuel Merritt College of Nursing, Oakland, CA, and funded by the Helene Fuld Health Trust (1987–1990); from Fawcett, J. (1993). *Analysis and evaluation of nursing theories.* Philadelphia: F. A. Davis; and from Fawcett, J. (1995). *Analysis and evaluation of conceptual models of nursing* (3rd ed.). Philadelphia: F. A. Davis.

APPENDIX N-3

Nursing Interventions Classification System

Intervention Labels and Definitions

Abuse Protection Support—Identification of high-risk dependent relationships and actions to prevent further infliction of physical or emotional harm

Abuse Protection Support: Child—Identification of high-risk, dependent child relationships and actions to prevent possible or further infliction of physical, sexual, or emotional harm or neglect of basic necessities of life

Abuse Protection Support: Domestic Partner—Identification of high-risk, dependent domestic relationships and actions to prevent possible or further infliction of physical, sexual, or emotional harm or exploitation of a domestic partner

Abuse Protection Support: Elder—Identification of high-risk, dependent elder relationships and actions to prevent possible or further infliction of physical, sexual, or emotional harm; neglect of basic necessities of life; or exploitation

Abuse Protection Support: Religious—Identification of high-risk, controlling religious relationships and actions to prevent infliction of physical, sexual, or emotional harm and/or exploitation

Acid-Base Management—Promotion of acid-base balance and prevention of complications resulting from acid-base imbalance

Acid-Base Management: Metabolic Acidosis—Promotion of acid-base balance and prevention of complications resulting from serum HCO_3 levels lower than desired

Acid-Base Management: Metabolic Alkalosis—Promotion of acid-base balance and prevention of complications resulting from serum HCO_3 levels higher than desired

Acid-Base Management: Respiratory Acidosis—Promotion of acid-base balance and prevention of complications resulting from serum PCO_2 levels higher than desired

Acid-Base Management: Respiratory Alkalosis—Promotion of acid-base balance and prevention of complications resulting from serum PCO_2 levels lower than desired

Acid-Base Monitoring—Collection and analysis of patient data to regulate acid-base balance

Active Listening—Attending closely to and attaching significance to a patient's verbal and nonverbal messages

Activity Therapy—Prescription of and assistance with specific physical, cognitive, social, and spiritual activities to increase the range, frequency, or duration of an individual's (or group's) activity

Acupressure—Application of firm, sustained pressure to special points on the body to decrease pain, produce relaxation, and prevent or reduce nausea

Admission Care—Facilitating entry of a patient into a health care facility

Airway Insertion and Stabilization—Insertion or assisting with insertion and stabilization of an artificial airway

Airway Management—Facilitation of patency of air passages

Airway Suctioning—Removal of airway secretions by inserting a suction catheter into the patient's oral airway and/or trachea

Allergy Management—Identification, treatment, and prevention of allergic responses to food, medications, insect bites, contrast material, blood, or other substances

Amnioinfusion—Infusion of fluid into the uterus during labor to relieve umbilical cord compression or to dilute meconium-stained fluid

Amputation Care—Promotion of physical and psychological healing after amputation of a body part

Analgesic Administration—Use of pharmacologic agents to reduce or eliminate pain

Analgesic Administration: Intraspinal—Administration of pharmacologic agents into the epidural or intrathecal space to reduce or eliminate pain

Anaphylaxis Management—Promotion of adequate ventilation and tissue perfusion for a patient with a severe allergic (antigen-antibody) reaction

Anesthesia Administration— Preparation for and administration of anesthetic agents and monitoring of patient responsiveness during administration

Anger Control Assistance—Facilitation of the expression of anger in an adaptive nonviolent manner

Animal-Assisted Therapy—Purposeful use of animals to provide affection, attention, diversion, and relaxation

Anticipatory Guidance—Preparation of patient for an anticipated developmental and/or situational crisis

Anxiety Reduction—Minimizing apprehension, dread, foreboding, or uneasiness related to an unidentified source of anticipated danger

Area Restriction—Limitation of patient mobility to a specified area for purposes of safety or behavior management

Art Therapy—Facilitation of communication through drawings or other art forms

Artificial Airway Management—Maintenance of endotracheal and tracheostomy tubes and preventing complications associated with their use

Aspiration Precautions—Prevention or minimization of risk factors in the patient at risk for aspiration

Assertiveness Training—Assistance with the effective expression of feelings, needs, and ideas while respecting the rights of others

Attachment Promotion—Facilitation of the development of the parent-infant relationship

Autogenic Training—Assisting with self-suggestions about feelings of heaviness and warmth for the purpose of inducing relaxation

Autotransfusion—Collecting and reinfusing blood which has been lost intraoperatively or postoperatively from clean wounds

Bathing—Cleaning of the body for the purposes of relaxation, cleanliness, and healing

Bed Rest Care—Promotion of comfort and safety and prevention of complications for a patient unable to get out of bed

Bedside Laboratory Testing—Performance of laboratory tests at the bedside or point of care

Behavior Management—Helping a patient to manage negative behavior

Behavior Management: Overactivity/Inattention—Provision of a therapeutic milieu which safely accommodates the patient's attention deficit and/or overactivity while promoting optimal function

Behavior Management: Self-Harm—Assisting the patient to decrease or eliminate self-mutilating or self-abusive behaviors

Behavior Management: Sexual—Delineation and prevention of socially unacceptable sexual behaviors

Behavior Modification—Promotion of a behavior change

Behavior Modification: Social Skills—Assisting the patient to develop or improve interpersonal social skills

Bibliotherapy—Use of literature to enhance the expression of feelings and the gaining of insight

Biofeedback—Assisting the patient to modify a body function using feedback from instrumentation

Birthing—Delivery of a baby

Bladder Irrigation—Instillation of a solution into the bladder to provide cleansing or medication

Bleeding Precautions—Reduction of stimuli that may induce bleeding or hemorrhage in at-risk patients

Bleeding Reduction—Limitation of the loss of blood volume during an episode of bleeding

Bleeding Reduction: Antepartum Uterus—Limitation of the amount of blood loss from the pregnant uterus during third trimester of pregnancy

Bleeding Reduction: Gastrointestinal—Limitation of the amount of blood loss from the upper and lower gastrointestinal tract and related complications

Bleeding Reduction: Nasal—Limitation of the amount of blood loss from the nasal cavity

Bleeding Reduction: Postpartum Uterus—Limitation of the amount of blood loss from the postpartum uterus

Bleeding Reduction: Wound—Limitation of the blood loss from a wound that may be a result of trauma, incisions, or placement of a tube or catheter

Blood Products Administration—Administration of blood or blood products and monitoring of patient's response

Body Image Enhancement—Improving a patient's conscious and unconscious perceptions and attitudes toward his/her body

Body Mechanics Promotion—Facilitating the use of posture and movement in daily activities to prevent fatigue and musculoskeletal strain or injury

Bottle Feeding—Preparation and administration of fluids to an infant via a bottle

Bowel Incontinence Care—Promotion of bowel continence and maintenance of perianal skin integrity

Bowel Incontinence Care: Encopresis—Promotion of bowel continence in children

Bowel Irrigation—Instillation of a substance into the lower gastrointestinal tract

Bowel Management—Establishment and maintenance of a regular pattern of bowel elimination

Bowel Training—Assisting the patient to train the bowel to evacuate at specific intervals

Breast Examination—Inspection and palpation of the breasts and related areas

Breastfeeding Assistance—Preparing a new mother to breastfeed her infant

Calming Technique—Reducing anxiety in patient experiencing acute distress

Cardiac Care—Limitation of complications resulting from an imbalance between myocardial oxygen supply and demand for a patient with symptoms of impaired cardiac function

Cardiac Care: Acute—Limitation of complications for a patient recently experiencing an episode of an imbalance between myocardial oxygen supply and demand resulting in impaired cardiac function

Cardiac Care: Rehabilitative—Promotion of maximum functional activity level for a patient who has suffered an episode of impaired cardiac function which resulted from an imbalance between myocardial oxygen supply and demand

Cardiac Precautions—Prevention of an acute episode of impaired cardiac function by minimizing myocardial oxygen consumption or increasing myocardial oxygen supply

Caregiver Support—Provision of the necessary information, advocacy, and support to facilitate primary patient care by someone other than a health care professional

Case Management—Coordinating care and advocating for specified individuals and patient populations across settings to reduce cost, reduce resource use, improve quality of health care, and achieve desired outcomes

Cast Care: Maintenance—Care of a cast after the drying period

Cast Care: Wet—Care of a new cast during the drying period

Cerebral Edema Management—Limitation of secondary cerebral injury resulting from swelling of brain tissue

Cerebral Perfusion Promotion—Promotion of adequate perfusion and limitation of complications for a patient experiencing or at risk for inadequate cerebral perfusion

Cesarean Section Care—Preparation and support of patient delivering a baby by cesarean section

Chemotherapy Management—Assisting the patient and family to understand the action and minimize side effects of antineoplastic agents

Chest Physiotherapy—Assisting the patient to move airway secretions from peripheral airways to more central airways for expectoration and/or suctioning

Childbirth Preparation—Providing information and support to facilitate childbirth and to enhance the ability of an individual to develop and perform the role of parent

Circulatory Care: Arterial Insufficiency—Promotion of arterial circulation

Circulatory Care: Mechanical Assist Device—Temporary support of the circulation through the use of mechanical devices or pumps

Circulatory Care: Venous Insufficiency—Promotion of venous circulation

Circulatory Precautions—Protection of a localized area with limited perfusion

Code Management—Coordination of emergency measures to sustain life

Cognitive Restructuring—Challenging a patient to alter distorted thought patterns and view self and the world more realistically

Cognitive Stimulation—Promotion of awareness and comprehension of surroundings by utilization of planned stimuli

Communicable Disease Management—Working with a community to decrease and manage the incidence and prevalence of contagious diseases in a specific population

Communication Enhancement: Hearing Deficit—Assistance in accepting and learning alternate methods for living with diminished hearing

Communication Enhancement: Speech Deficit—Assistance in accepting and learning alternate methods for living with impaired speech

Communication Enhancement: Visual Deficit—Assistance in accepting and learning alternate methods for living with diminished vision

Community Disaster Preparedness—Preparing for an effective response to a large-scale disaster

Community Health Development—Facilitating members of a community to identify a community's health concerns, mobilize resources, and implement solutions

Complex Relationship Building—Establishing a therapeutic relationship with a patient who has difficulty interacting with others

Conflict Mediation—Facilitation of constructive dialogue between opposing parties with a goal of resolving disputes in a mutually acceptable manner

Conscious Sedation—Administration of sedatives, monitoring of the patient's response, and provision of necessary physiological support during a diagnostic or therapeutic procedure

Constipation/Impaction Management—Prevention and alleviation of constipation/impaction

Consultation—Using expert knowledge to work with those who seek help in problem-solving to enable individuals, families, groups or agencies to achieve identified goals

Contact Lens Care—Prevention of eye injury and lens damage by proper use of contact lenses

Controlled Substance Checking—Promoting appropriate use and maintaining security of controlled substances

Coping Enhancement—Assisting a patient to adapt to perceived stressors, changes, or threats which interfere with meeting life demands and roles

Cost Containment—Management and facilitation of efficient and effective use of resources

Cough Enhancement—Promotion of deep inhalation by the patient with subsequent generation of high intrathoracic pressures and compression of underlying lung parenchyma for the forceful expulsion of air

Counseling—Use of an interactive helping process focusing on the needs, problems, or feelings of the patient and significant others to enhance or support coping, problem-solving, and interpersonal relationships

Crisis Intervention—Use of short-term counseling to help the patient cope with a crisis and resume a state of functioning comparable to or better than the pre-crisis state

Critical Path Development—Constructing and using a timed sequence of patient care activities to enhance desired patient outcomes in a cost-efficient manner

Culture Brokerage—The deliberate use of culturally competent strategies to bridge or mediate between the patient's culture and the biomedical health care system

Cutaneous Stimulation—Stimulation of the skin and underlying tissues for the purpose of decreasing undesirable signs and symptoms such as pain, muscle spasm, or inflammation

Decision-Making Support—Providing information and support for a patient who is making a decision regarding health care

Delegation—Transfer of responsibility for the performance of patient care while retaining accountability for the outcome

Delirium Management—Provision of a safe and therapeutic environment for the patient who is experiencing an acute confusional state

Delusion Management—Promoting the comfort, safety, and reality orientation of a patient experiencing false, fixed beliefs that have little or no basis in reality

Dementia Management—Provision of a modified environment for the patient who is experiencing a chronic confusional state

Developmental Care—Structuring the environment and providing care in response to the behavioral cues and states of the preterm infant

Developmental Enhancement: Adolescent—Facilitating optimal physical, cognitive, social, and emotional growth of individuals during the transition from childhood to adulthood

Developmental Enhancement: Child—Facilitating or teaching parents/caregivers to facilitate the optimal gross motor, fine motor, language, cognitive, social, and emotional growth of preschool and school-aged children

Diarrhea Management—Prevention and alleviation of diarrhea

Diet Staging—Instituting required diet restrictions with subsequent progression of diet as tolerated

Discharge Planning—Preparation for moving a patient from one level of care to another within or outside the current health care agency

Distraction—Purposeful focusing of attention away from undesirable sensations

Documentation—Recording of pertinent patient data in a clinical record

Dressing—Choosing, putting on, and removing clothes for a person who cannot do this for self

Dying Care—Promotion of physical comfort and psychological peace in the final phase of life

Dysreflexia Management—Prevention and elimination of stimuli which cause hyperactive reflexes and inappropriate autonomic responses in a patient with a cervical or high thoracic cord lesion

Dysrhythmia Management—Preventing, recognizing, and facilitating treatment of abnormal cardiac rhythms

Ear Care—Prevention or minimization of threats to ear or hearing

Eating Disorders Management—Prevention and treatment of severe diet restriction and over exercising or binging and purging of food and fluids

Electrolyte Management—Promotion of electrolyte balance and prevention of complications resulting from abnormal or undesired serum electrolyte levels

Electrolyte Management: Hypercalcemia—Promotion of calcium balance and prevention of complications resulting from serum calcium levels higher than desired

Electrolyte Management: Hyperkalemia—Promotion of potassium balance and prevention of complications resulting from serum potassium levels higher than desired

Electrolyte Management: Hypermagnesemia—Promotion of magnesium balance and prevention of complications resulting from serum magnesium levels higher than desired

Electrolyte Management: Hypernatremia—Promotion of sodium balance and prevention of complications resulting from serum sodium levels higher than desired

Electrolyte Management: Hyperphosphatemia—Promotion of phosphate balance and prevention of complications resulting from serum phosphate levels higher than desired

Electrolyte Management: Hypocalcemia—Promotion of calcium balance and prevention of complications resulting from serum calcium levels lower than desired

Electrolyte Management: Hypokalemia—Promotion of potassium balance and prevention of complications resulting from serum potassium levels lower than desired

Electrolyte Management: Hypomagnesemia—Promotion of magnesium balance and prevention of complications resulting from serum magnesium levels lower than desired

Electrolyte Management: Hyponatremia—Promotion of sodium balance and prevention of complications resulting from serum sodium levels lower than desired

Electrolyte Management: Hypophosphatemia—Promotion of phosphate balance and prevention of complications resulting from serum phosphate levels lower than desired

Electrolyte Monitoring—Collection and analysis of patient data to regulate electrolyte balance

Electronic Fetal Monitoring: Antepartum—Electronic evaluation of fetal heart rate response to movement, external stimuli, or uterine contractions during antepartal testing

Electronic Fetal Monitoring: Intrapartum—Electronic evaluation of fetal heart rate response to uterine contractions during intrapartal care

Elopement Precautions—Minimizing the risk of a patient leaving a treatment setting without authorization when departure presents a threat to the safety of patient or others

Embolus Care: Peripheral—Limitation of complications for a patient experiencing, or at risk for, occlusion of peripheral circulation

Embolus Care: Pulmonary—Limitation of complications for a patient experiencing, or at risk for, occlusion of pulmonary circulation

Embolus Precautions—Reduction of the risk of an embolus in a patient with thrombi or at risk for developing thrombus formation

Emergency Care—Providing life-saving measures in life-threatening situations

Emergency Cart Checking—Systematic review of the contents of an emergency cart at established time intervals

Emotional Support—Provision of reassurance, acceptance, and encouragement during times of stress

Endotracheal Extubation—Purposeful removal of the endotracheal tube from the nasopharyngeal or oropharyngeal airway

Energy Management—Regulating energy use to treat or prevent fatigue and optimize function

Enteral Tube Feeding—Delivering nutrients and water through a gastrointestinal tube

Environmental Management—Manipulation of the patient's surroundings for therapeutic benefit

Environmental Management: Attachment Process—Manipulation of the patient's surroundings to facilitate the development of the parent-infant relationship

Environmental Management: Comfort—Manipulation of the patient's surroundings for promotion of optimal comfort

Environmental Management: Community—Monitoring and influencing the direction of the physical, social, cultural, economic, and political conditions that affect the health of groups and communities

Environmental Management: Home Preparation—Preparing the home for safe and effective delivery of care

Environmental Management: Safety—Monitoring and manipulation of the physical environment to promote safety

Environmental Management: Violence Prevention—Monitoring and manipulation of the physical environment to decrease the potential for violent behavior directed toward self, others, or environment

Environmental Management: Worker Safety—Monitoring and manipulating of the worksite environment to promote safety and health of workers

Environmental Risk Protection—Preventing and detecting disease and injury in populations at risk from environmental hazards

Examination Assistance—Providing assistance to the patient and another health care provider during a procedure or exam

Exercise Promotion—Facilitation of regular physical exercise to maintain or advance to a higher level of fitness and health

Exercise Promotion: Strength Training—Facilitating regular resistive muscle training to maintain or increase muscle strength

Exercise Promotion: Stretching—Facilitation of systematic slow-stretch-hold muscle exercises to induce relaxation, prepare muscles/joints for more vigorous exercise, or to increase or maintain body flexibility

Exercise Therapy: Ambulation—Promotion and assistance with walking to maintain or restore autonomic and voluntary body functions during treatment and recovery from illness or injury

Exercise Therapy: Balance—Use of specific activities, postures, and movements to maintain, enhance, or restore balance

Exercise Therapy: Joint Mobility—Use of active or passive body movement to maintain or restore joint flexibility

Exercise Therapy: Muscle Control—Use of specific activity or exercise protocols to enhance or restore controlled body movement

Eye Care—Prevention or minimization of threats to eye or visual integrity

Fall Prevention—Instituting special precautions with patient at risk for injury from falling

Family Integrity Promotion—Promotion of family cohesion and unity

Family Integrity Promotion: Childbearing Family—Facilitation of the growth of individuals or families who are adding an infant to the family unit

Family Involvement Promotion—Facilitating family participation in the emotional and physical care of the patient

Family Mobilization—Utilization of family strengths to influence patient's health in a positive direction

Family Planning: Contraception—Facilitation of pregnancy prevention by providing information about the physiology of reproduction and methods to control conception

Family Planning: Infertility—Management, education, and support of the patient and significant other undergoing evaluation and treatment for infertility

Family Planning: Unplanned Pregnancy—Facilitation of decision-making regarding pregnancy outcome

Family Process Maintenance—Minimization of family process disruption effects

Family Support—Promotion of family values, interests, and goals

Family Therapy—Assisting family members to move their family toward a more productive way of living

Feeding—Providing nutritional intake for patient who is unable to feed self

Fertility Preservation—Providing information, counseling, and treatment that facilitate reproductive health and the ability to conceive

Fever Treatment—Management of a patient with hyperpyrexia caused by nonenvironmental factors

Financial Resource Assistance—Assisting an individual/family to secure and manage finances to meet health care needs

Fire-Setting Precautions—Prevention of fire-setting behaviors

First Aid—Providing initial care of a minor injury

Fiscal Resource Management—Procuring and directing the use of financial resources to ensure the development and continuation of programs and services

Flatulence Reduction—Prevention of flatus formation and facilitation of passage of excessive gas

Fluid Management—Promotion of fluid balance and prevention of complications resulting from abnormal or undesired fluid levels

Fluid Monitoring—Collection and analysis of patient data to regulate fluid balance

Fluid Resuscitation—Administering prescribed intravenous fluids rapidly

Fluid/Electrolyte Management—Regulation and prevention of complications from altered fluid and/or electrolyte levels

Foot Care—Cleansing and inspecting the feet for the purposes of relaxation, cleanliness, and healthy skin

Forgiveness Facilitation—Assisting an individual to forgive and/or experience forgiveness in relationship with self, others, and higher power

Gastrointestinal Intubation—Insertion of a tube into the gastrointestinal tract

Genetic Counseling—Use of an interactive helping process focusing on assisting an individual, family, or group, manifesting or at risk for developing or transmitting a birth defect or genetic condition, to cope

Grief Work Facilitation—Assistance with the resolution of a significant loss

Grief Work Facilitation: Perinatal Death—Assistance with the resolution of a perinatal loss

Guilt Work Facilitation—Helping another to cope with painful feelings of responsibility, actual or perceived

Hair Care—Promotion of neat, clean, attractive hair

Hallucination Management—Promoting the safety, comfort, and reality orientation of a patient experiencing hallucinations

Health Care Information Exchange—Providing patient care information to health professionals in other agencies

Health Education—Developing and providing instruction and learning experiences to facilitate voluntary adaptation of behavior conducive to health in individuals, families, groups, or communities

Health Policy Monitoring—Surveillance and influence of government and organization regulations, rules, and standards that affect nursing systems and practices to ensure quality care of patients

Health Screening—Detecting health risks or problems by means of history, examination, and other procedures

Health System Guidance—Facilitating a patient's location and use of appropriate health services

Heat Exposure Treatment—Management of patient overcome by heat due to excessive environmental heat exposure

Heat/Cold Application—Stimulation of the skin and underlying tissues with heat or cold for the purpose of decreasing pain, muscle spasms, or inflammation

Hemodialysis Therapy—Management of extracorporeal passage of the patient's blood through a dialyzer

Hemodynamic Regulation—Optimization of heart rate, preload, afterload, and contractility

Hemofiltration Therapy—Cleansing of acutely ill patient's blood via a hemofilter controlled by the patient's hydrostatic pressure

Hemorrhage Control—Reduction or elimination of rapid and excessive blood loss

High-Risk Pregnancy Care—Identification and management of a high-risk pregnancy to promote healthy outcomes for mother and baby

Home Maintenance Assistance—Helping the patient/family to maintain the home as a clean, safe, and pleasant place to live

Hope Instillation—Facilitation of the development of a positive outlook in a given situation

Humor—Facilitating the patient to perceive, appreciate, and express what is funny, amusing, or ludicrous in order to establish relationships, relieve tension, release anger, facilitate learning, or cope with painful feelings

Hyperglycemia Management—Preventing and treating above-normal blood glucose levels

Hypervolemia Management—Reduction in extracellular and/or intracellular fluid volume and prevention of complications in a patient who is fluid overloaded

Hypnosis—Assisting a patient to induce an altered state of consciousness to create an acute awareness and a directed focus experience

Hypoglycemia Management—Preventing and treating low blood glucose levels

Hypothermia Treatment—Rewarming and surveillance of a patient whose core body temperature is below 35°C

Hypovolemia Management—Expansion of intravascular fluid volume in a patient who is volume depleted

Immunization/Vaccination Management—Monitoring immunization status, facilitating access to immunizations, and provision of immunizations to prevent communicable disease

Impulse Control Training—Assisting the patient to mediate impulsive behavior through application of problem-solving strategies to social and interpersonal situations

Incident Reporting—Written and verbal reporting of any event in the process of patient care that is inconsistent with desired patient outcomes or routine operations of the health care facility

Incision Site Care—Cleansing, monitoring, and promotion of healing in a wound that is closed with sutures, clips, or staples

Infant Care—Provision of developmentally appropriate family-centered care to the child under 1 year of age

Infection Control—Minimizing the acquisition and transmission of infectious agents

Infection Control: Intraoperative—Preventing nosocomial infection in the operating room

Infection Protection—Prevention and early detection of infection in a patient at risk

Insurance Authorization—Assisting the patient and provider to secure payment for health services or equipment from a third party

Intracranial Pressure (ICP) Monitoring—Measurement and interpretation of patient data to regulate intracranial pressure

Intrapartal Care—Monitoring and management of stages one and two of the birth process

Intrapartal Care: High-Risk Delivery—Assisting vaginal birth of multiple or malpositioned fetuses

Intravenous (IV) Insertion—Insertion of a needle into a peripheral vein for the purpose of administering fluids, blood, or medications

Intravenous (IV) Therapy—Administration and monitoring of intravenous fluids and medications

Invasive Hemodynamic Monitoring—Measurement and interpretation of invasive hemodynamic parameters to determine cardiovascular function and regulate therapy as appropriate

Kangaroo Care—Promoting closeness between parent and physiologically stable preterm infant by preparing the parent and providing the environment for skin-to-skin contact

Labor Induction—Initiation or augmentation of labor by mechanical or pharmacological methods

Labor Suppression—Controlling uterine contractions prior to 37 weeks of gestation to prevent preterm birth

Laboratory Data Interpretation—Critical analysis of patient laboratory data in order to assist with clinical decision-making

Lactation Counseling—Use of an interactive helping process to assist in maintenance of successful breastfeeding

Lactation Suppression—Facilitating the cessation of milk production and minimizing breast engorgement after giving birth

Laser Precautions—Limiting the risk of injury to the patient related to use of a laser

Latex Precautions—Reducing the risk of systemic reaction to latex

Learning Facilitation—Promoting the ability to process and comprehend information

Learning Readiness Enhancement—Improving the ability and willingness to receive information

Leech Therapy—Application of medicinal leeches to help drain replanted or transplanted tissue engorged with venous blood

Limit Setting—Establishing the parameters of desirable and acceptable patient behavior

Malignant Hyperthermia Precautions—Prevention or reduction of hypermetabolic response to pharmacological agents used during surgery

Mechanical Ventilation—Use of an artificial device to assist a patient to breathe

Mechanical Ventilatory Weaning—Assisting the patient to breathe without the aid of a mechanical ventilator

Medication Administration—Preparing, giving, and evaluating the effectiveness of prescription and nonprescription drugs

Medication Administration: Ear—Preparing and instilling otic medications

Medication Administration: Enteral—Delivering medications through an intestinal tube

Medication Administration: Epidural—Preparing and administering medications via the epidural route

Medication Administration: Eye—Preparing and instilling ophthalmic medications

Medication Administration: Inhalation—Preparing and administering inhaled medications

Medication Administration: Interpleural—Administration of medication through an interpleural catheter for reduction of pain

Medication Administration: Intradermal—Preparing and giving medications via the intradermal route

Medication Administration: Intramuscular (IM)—Preparing and giving medications via the intramuscular route

Medication Administration: Intraosseous—Insertion of a needle through the bone cortex into the medullary cavity for the purpose of short-term, emergency administration of fluid, blood, or medication

Medication Administration: Intravenous (IV)—Preparing and giving medications via the intravenous route

Medication Administration: Oral—Preparing and giving medications by mouth and monitoring patient responsiveness

Medication Administration: Rectal—Preparing and inserting rectal suppositories

Medication Administration: Skin—Preparing and applying medications to the skin

Medication Administration: Subcutaneous—Preparing and giving medications via the subcutaneous route

Medication Administration: Vaginal—Preparing and inserting vaginal medications

Medication Administration: Ventricular Reservoir—Administration and monitoring of medication through an indwelling catheter into the lateral ventricle

Medication Management—Facilitation of safe and effective use of prescription and over-the-counter drugs

Medication Prescribing—Prescribing medication for a health problem

Meditation Facilitation—Facilitating a person to alter his/her level of awareness by focusing specifically on an image or thought

Memory Training—Facilitation of memory

Milieu Therapy—Use of people, resources, and events in the patient's immediate environment to promote optimal psychosocial functioning

Mood Management—Providing for safety, stabilization, recovery, and maintenance of a patient who is experiencing dysfunctionally depressed mood or elevated mood

Multidisciplinary Care Conference—Planning and evaluating patient care with health professionals from other disciplines

Music Therapy—Using music to help achieve a specific change in behavior, feeling, or physiology

Mutual Goal Setting—Collaborating with patient to identify and prioritize care goals, then developing a plan for achieving those goals

Nail Care—Promotion of clean, neat, attractive nails and prevention of skin lesions related to improper care of nails

Nausea Management—Prevention and alleviation of nausea

Neurologic Monitoring—Collection and analysis of patient data to prevent or minimize neurological complications

Newborn Care—Management of neonate during the transition to extrauterine life and subsequent period of stabilization

Newborn Monitoring—Measurement and interpretation of physiologic status of the neonate the first 24 hours after delivery

Nonnutritive Sucking—Provision of sucking opportunities for the infant

Normalization Promotion—Assisting parents and other family members of children with chronic illnesses or disabilities in providing normal life experiences for their children and families

Nutrition Management—Assisting with or providing a balanced dietary intake of foods and fluids

Nutrition Therapy—Administration of food and fluids to support metabolic processes of a patient who is malnourished or at high risk for becoming malnourished

Nutritional Counseling—Use of an interactive helping process focusing on the need for diet modification

Nutritional Monitoring—Collection and analysis of patient data to prevent or minimize malnourishment

Oral Health Maintenance—Maintenance and promotion of oral hygiene and dental health for the patient at risk for developing oral or dental lesions

Oral Health Promotion—Promotion of oral hygiene and dental care for a patient with normal oral and dental health

Oral Health Restoration—Promotion of healing for a patient who has an oral mucosa or dental lesion

Order Transcription—Transferring information from order sheets to the nursing patient care planning and documentation system

Organ Procurement—Guiding families through the donation process to ensure timely retrieval of vital organs and tissue for transplant

Ostomy Care—Maintenance of elimination through a stoma and care of surrounding tissue

Oxygen Therapy—Administration of oxygen and monitoring of its effectiveness

Pain Management—Alleviation of pain or a reduction in pain to a level of comfort that is acceptable to the patient

Parent Education: Adolescent—Assisting parents to understand and help their adolescent children

Parent Education: Childrearing Family—Assisting parents to understand and promote the physical, psychological, and social growth and development of their toddler, preschool, or school-aged child/children

Parent Education: Infant—Instruction on nurturing and physical care needed during the first year of life

Parenting Promotion—Providing parenting information, support and coordination of comprehensive services to high-risk families

Pass Facilitation—Arranging a leave for a patient from a health care facility

Patient Contracting—Negotiating an agreement with a patient that reinforces a specific behavior change

Patient-Controlled Analgesia (PCA) Assistance—Facilitating patient control of analgesic administration and regulation

Patient Rights Protection—Protection of health care rights of a patient, especially a minor, incapacitated, or incompetent patient unable to make decisions

Peer Review—Systematic evaluation of a peer's performance compared with professional standards of practice

Pelvic Muscle Exercise—Strengthening and training the levator ani and urogenital muscles through voluntary, repetitive contraction to decrease stress, urge or mixed types of urinary incontinence

Perineal Care—Maintenance of perineal skin integrity and relief of perineal discomfort

Peripheral Sensation Management—Prevention or minimization of injury or discomfort in the patient with altered sensation

Peripherally Inserted Central (PIC) Catheter Care—Insertion and maintenance of a peripherally inserted central catheter

Peritoneal Dialysis Therapy—Administration and monitoring of dialysis solution into and out of the peritoneal cavity

Pessary Management—Placement and monitoring of a vaginal device for treating stress urinary incontinence, uterine retroversion, genital prolapse, or incompetent cervix

Phlebotomy: Arterial Blood Sample—Obtaining a blood sample from an uncannulated artery to assess oxygen and carbon dioxide levels and acid-base balance

Phlebotomy: Blood Unit Acquisition—Procuring blood and blood products from donors

Phlebotomy: Venous Blood Sample—Removal of a sample of venous blood from an uncannulated vein

Phototherapy: Neonate—Use of light therapy to reduce bilirubin levels in newborn infants

Physical Restraint—Application, monitoring, and removal of mechanical restraining devices or manual restraints which are used to limit physical mobility of a patient

Physician Support—Collaborating with physicians to provide quality patient care

Pneumatic Tourniquet Precautions—Applying a pneumatic tourniquet while minimizing the potential for patient injury from use of the device

Positioning—Deliberative placement of the patient or a body part to promote physiological and/or psychological well-being

Positioning: Intraoperative—Moving the patient or body part to promote surgical exposure while reducing the risk of discomfort and complications

Positioning: Neurologic—Achievement of optimal, appropriate body alignment for the patient experiencing or at risk for spinal cord injury or vertebrae irritability

Positioning: Wheelchair—Placement of a patient in a properly selected wheelchair to enhance comfort, promote skin integrity, and foster independence

Postanesthesia Care—Monitoring and management of the patient who has recently undergone general or regional anesthesia

Postmortem Care—Providing physical care of the body of an expired patient and support for the family viewing the body

Postpartal Care—Monitoring and management of the patient who has recently given birth

Preceptor: Employee—Assisting and supporting a new or transferred employee through a planned orientation to a specific clinical area

Preceptor: Student—Assisting and supporting learning experiences for a student

Preconception Counseling—Screening and providing information and support to individuals of childbearing age before pregnancy to promote health and reduce risks

Pregnancy Termination Care—Management of the physical and psychological needs of the woman undergoing a spontaneous or elective abortion

Prenatal Care—Monitoring and management of patient during pregnancy to prevent complications of pregnancy and promote a healthy outcome for both mother and infant

Preoperative Coordination—Facilitating preadmission diagnostic testing and preparation of the surgical patient

Preparatory Sensory Information—Describing in concrete and objective terms the typical sensory experiences and events associated with an upcoming stressful health care procedure/treatment

Presence—Being with another, both physically and psychologically, during times of need

Pressure Management—Minimizing pressure to body parts

Pressure Ulcer Care—Facilitation of healing in pressure ulcers

Pressure Ulcer Prevention—Prevention of pressure ulcers for a patient at high risk for developing them

Product Evaluation—Determining the effectiveness of new products or equipment

Program Development—Planning, implementing, and evaluating a coordinated set of activities designed to enhance wellness, or to prevent, reduce, or eliminate one or more health problems for a group or community

Progressive Muscle Relaxation—Facilitating the tensing and releasing of successive muscle groups while attending to the resulting differences in sensation

Prompted Voiding—Promotion of urinary continence through the use of timed verbal toileting reminders and positive social feedback for successful toileting

Prosthesis Care—Care of a removable appliance worn by a patient and the prevention of complications associated with its use

Pruritus Management—Preventing and treating itching

Quality Monitoring—Systematic collection and analysis of an organization's quality indicators for the purpose of improving patient care

Radiation Therapy Management—Assisting the patient to understand and minimize the side effects of radiation treatments

Rape-Trauma Treatment—Provision of emotional and physical support immediately following a reported rape

Reality Orientation—Promotion of patient's awareness of personal identity, time, and environment

Recreation Therapy—Purposeful use of recreation to promote relaxation and enhancement of social skills

Rectal Prolapse Management—Prevention and/or manual reduction of rectal prolapse

Referral—Arrangement for services by another care provider or agency

Religious Addiction Prevention—Prevention of a self-imposed controlling religious lifestyle

Religious Ritual Enhancement—Facilitating participation religious practices

Reminiscence Therapy—Using the recall of past events, feelings, and thoughts to facilitate pleasure, quality of life, or adaptation to present circumstances

Reproductive Technology Management—Assisting a patient through the steps of complex infertility treatment

Research Data Collection—Collecting research data

Resiliency Promotion—Assisting individuals, families, and communities in development, use, and strengthening of protective factors to be used in coping with environmental and societal stressors

Respiratory Monitoring—Collection and analysis of patient data to ensure airway patency and adequate gas exchange

Respite Care—Provision of short-term care to provide relief for family caregiver

Resuscitation—Administering emergency measures to sustain life

Resuscitation: Fetus—Administering emergency measures to improve placental perfusion or correct fetal acid-base status

Resuscitation: Neonate—Administering emergency measures to support newborn adaptation to extrauterine life

Risk Identification—Analysis of potential risk factors, determination of health risks, and prioritization of risk reduction strategies for an individual or group

Risk Identification: Childbearing Family—Identification of an individual or family likely to experience difficulties in parenting and prioritization of strategies to prevent parenting problems

Risk Identification: Genetic—Identification and analysis of potential genetic risk factors in an individual, family, or group

Role Enhancement—Assisting a patient, significant other, and/or family to improve relationships by clarifying and supplementing specific role behaviors

Seclusion—Solitary containment in a fully protective environment with close surveillance by nursing staff for purposes of safety or behavior management

Security Enhancement—Intensifying a patient's sense of physical and psychological safety

Seizure Management—Care of a patient during a seizure and the postictal state

Seizure Precautions—Prevention or minimization of potential injuries sustained by a patient with a known seizure disorder

Self-Awareness Enhancement—Assisting a patient to explore and understand his/her thoughts, feelings, motivations, and behaviors

Self-Care Assistance—Assisting another to perform activities of daily living

Self-Care Assistance: Bathing/Hygiene—Assisting patient to perform personal hygiene

Self-Care Assistance: Dressing/Grooming—Assisting patient with clothes and makeup

Self-Care Assistance: Feeding—Assisting a person to eat

Self-Care Assistance: Toileting—Assisting another with elimination

Self-Esteem Enhancement—Assisting a patient to increase his/her personal judgment of self-worth

Self-Modification Assistance—Reinforcement of self-directed change initiated by the patient to achieve personally important goals

Self-Responsibility Facilitation—Encouraging a patient to assume more responsibility for own behavior

Sexual Counseling—Use of an interactive helping process focusing on the need to make adjustments in sexual practice or to enhance coping with a sexual event/disorder

Shift Report—Exchanging essential patient care information with other nursing staff at change of shift

Shock Management—Facilitation of the delivery of oxygen and nutrients to systemic tissue with removal of cellular waste products in a patient with severely altered tissue perfusion

Shock Management: Cardiac—Promotion of adequate tissue perfusion for a patient with severely compromised pumping function of the heart

Shock Management: Vasogenic—Promotion of adequate tissue perfusion for a patient with severe loss of vascular tone

Shock Management: Volume—Promotion of adequate tissue perfusion for a patient with severely compromised intravascular volume

Shock Prevention—Detecting and treating a patient at risk for impending shock

Sibling Support—Assisting a sibling to cope with a brother's or sister's illness/chronic condition/disability

Simple Guided Imagery—Purposeful use of imagination to achieve relaxation and/or direct attention away from undesirable sensations

Simple Massage—Stimulation of the skin and underlying tissues with varying degrees of hand pressure to decrease pain, produce relaxation, and/or improve circulation

Simple Relaxation Therapy—Use of techniques to encourage and elicit relaxation for the purpose of decreasing undesirable signs and symptoms such as pain, muscle tension, or anxiety

Skin Care: Topical Treatments—Application of topical substances or manipulation of devices to promote skin integrity and minimize skin breakdown

Skin Surveillance—Collection and analysis of patient data to maintain skin and mucous membrane integrity

Sleep Enhancement—Facilitation of regular sleep/wake cycles

Smoking Cessation Assistance—Helping another to stop smoking

Socialization Enhancement—Facilitation of another person's ability to interact with others

Specimen Management—Obtaining, preparing, and preserving a specimen for a laboratory test

Spiritual Growth Facilitation—Facilitation of growth in patient's capacity to identify, connect with, and call upon the source of meaning, purpose, comfort, strength, and hope in his/her life

Spiritual Support—Assisting the patient to feel balance and connection with a greater power

Splinting—Stabilization, immobilization, and/or protection of an injured body part with a supportive appliance

Sports-Injury Prevention: Youth—Reduce the risk of sport-related injury in young athletes

Staff Development—Developing, maintaining, and monitoring competence of staff

Staff Supervision—Facilitating the delivery of high-quality patient care by others

Subarachnoid Hemorrhage Precautions—Reduction of internal and external stimuli or stressors to minimize risk of rebleeding prior to aneurysm surgery

Substance Use Prevention—Prevention of an alcoholic or drug use lifestyle
Substance Use Treatment—Supportive care of patient/family members with physical and psychosocial problems associated with the use of alcohol or drugs
Substance Use Treatment: Alcohol Withdrawal—Care of the patient experiencing sudden cessation of alcohol consumption
Substance Use Treatment: Drug Withdrawal—Care of a patient experiencing drug detoxification
Substance Use Treatment: Overdose—Monitoring, treatment, and emotional support of a patient who has ingested prescription or over-the-counter drugs beyond the therapeutic range
Suicide Prevention—Reducing risk of self-inflicted harm with intent to end life
Supply Management—Ensuring acquisition and maintenance of appropriate items for providing patient care
Support Group—Use of a group environment to provide emotional support and health-related information for members
Support System Enhancement—Facilitation of support to patient by family, friends, and community
Surgical Assistance—Assisting the surgeon/dentist with operative procedures and care of the surgical patient
Surgical Precautions—Minimizing the potential for iatrogenic injury to the patient related to a surgical procedure
Surgical Preparation—Providing care to a patient immediately prior to surgery and verification of required procedures/tests and documentation in the clinical record
Surveillance—Purposeful and ongoing acquisition, interpretation, and synthesis of patient data for clinical decision-making
Surveillance: Community—Purposeful and ongoing acquisition, interpretation, and synthesis of data for decision-making in the community
Surveillance: Late Pregnancy—Purposeful and ongoing acquisition, interpretation, and synthesis of maternal-fetal data for treatment, observation, or admission
Surveillance: Remote Electronic—Purposeful and ongoing acquisition of patient data via electronic modalities (telephone, video, conferencing, e-mail) from distant locations as well as interpretation and synthesis of patient data for clinical decision-making with individuals or populations
Surveillance: Safety—Purposeful and ongoing collection and analysis of information about the patient and the environment for use in promoting and maintaining patient safety
Sustenance Support—Helping a needy individual/family to locate food, clothing, or shelter
Suturing—Approximating edges of a wound using sterile suture material and a needle
Swallowing Therapy—Facilitating swallowing and preventing complications of impaired swallowing
Teaching: Disease Process—Assisting the patient to understand information related to a specific disease process
Teaching: Group—Development, implementation, and evaluation of a patient-teaching program for a group of individuals experiencing the same health condition
Teaching: Individual—Planning, implementation, and evaluation of a teaching program designed to address a patient's particular needs
Teaching: Infant Nutrition—Instruction on nutrition and feeding practices during the first year of life
Teaching: Infant Safety—Instruction on safety during first year of life
Teaching: Preoperative—Assisting a patient to understand and mentally prepare for surgery and the postoperative recovery period
Teaching: Prescribed Activity/Exercise—Preparing a patient to achieve and/or maintain a prescribed level of activity
Teaching: Prescribed Diet—Preparing a patient to correctly follow a prescribed diet
Teaching: Prescribed Medication—Preparing a patient to safely take prescribed medications and monitor for their effects
Teaching: Procedure/Treatment—Preparing a patient to understand and mentally prepare for a prescribed procedure or treatment
Teaching: Psychomotor Skill—Preparing a patient to perform a psychomotor skill
Teaching: Safe Sex—Providing instruction concerning sexual protection during sexual activity
Teaching: Sexuality—Assisting individuals to understand physical and psychosocial dimensions of sexual growth and development
Teaching: Toddler Nutrition—Instruction on nutrition and feeding practices during the second and third years of life
Teaching: Toddler Safety—Instruction on safety during the second and third years of life
Technology Management—Use of technical equipment and devices to monitor patient condition or sustain life
Telephone Consultation—Eliciting patient's concerns, listening, and providing support, information, or teaching in response to patient's stated concerns, over the telephone
Telephone Follow-up—Providing results of testing or evaluating patient's response and determining potential for problems as a result of previous treatment, examination, or testing, over the telephone
Temperature Regulation—Attaining and/or maintaining body temperature within a normal range
Temperature Regulation: Intraoperative—Attaining and/or maintaining desired intraoperative body temperature
Therapeutic Play—Purposeful and directive use of toys and other materials to as-

sist children in communicating their perception and knowledge of their world and to help in gaining mastery of their environment

Therapeutic Touch—Attuning to the universal healing field, seeking to act as an instrument for healing influence, and using the natural sensitivity of the hands to gently focus and direct the intervention process

Therapy Group—Application of psychotherapeutic techniques to a group, including the utilization of interactions between members of the group

Total Parenteral Nutrition (TPN) Administration—Preparation and delivery of nutrients intravenously and monitoring of patient responsiveness

Touch—Providing comfort and communication through purposeful tactile contact

Traction/Immobilization Care—Management of a patient who has traction and/or a stabilizing device to immobilize and stabilize a body part

Transcutaneous Electrical Nerve Stimulation (TENS)—Stimulation of skin and underlying tissues with controlled, low-voltage electrical vibration via electrodes

Transport—Moving a patient from one location to another

Triage: Disaster—Establishing priorities of patient care for urgent treatment while allocating scarce resources

Triage: Emergency Center—Establishing priorities and initiating treatment for patients in an emergency center

Triage: Telephone—Determining the nature and urgency of a problem(s) and providing directions for the level of care required, over the telephone

Truth Telling—Use of whole truth, partial truth, or decision delay to promote the patient's self-determination and well-being

Tube Care—Management of a patient with an external drainage device exiting the body

Tube Care: Chest—Management of a patient with an external water-seal drainage device exiting the chest cavity

Tube Care: Gastrointestinal—Management of a patient with a gastrointestinal tube

Tube Care: Umbilical Line—Management of a newborn with an umbilical catheter

Tube Care: Urinary—Management of a patient with urinary drainage equipment

Tube Care: Ventriculostomy/Lumbar Drain—Management of a patient with an external cerebrospinal fluid drainage system

Ultrasonography: Limited Obstetric—Performance of ultrasound exams to determine ovarian, uterine, or fetal status

Unilateral Neglect Management—Protecting and safely reintegrating the affected part of the body while helping the patient adapt to disturbed perceptual abilities

Urinary Bladder Training—Improving bladder function for those with urge incontinence by increasing the bladder's ability to hold urine and the patient's ability to suppress urination

Urinary Catheterization—Insertion of a catheter into the bladder for temporary or permanent drainage of urine

Urinary Catheterization: Intermittent—Regular periodic use of a catheter to empty the bladder

Urinary Elimination Management—Maintenance of an optimum urinary elimination pattern

Urinary Habit Training—Establishing a predictable pattern of bladder emptying to prevent incontinence for persons with limited cognitive ability who have urge, stress, or functional incontinence

Urinary Incontinence Care—Assistance in promoting continence and maintaining perineal skin integrity

Urinary Incontinence Care: Enuresis—Promotion of urinary continence in children

Urinary Retention Care—Assistance in relieving bladder distention

Values Clarification—Assisting another to clarify her/his own values in order to facilitate effective decision-making

Vehicle Safety Promotion—Assisting individuals, families, and communities to increase awareness of measures to reduce unintentional injuries in motorized and non-motorized vehicles

Venous Access Devices (VAD) Maintenance—Management of the patient with prolonged venous access via tunneled and non-tunneled (percutaneous) catheters, and implanted ports

Ventilation Assistance—Promotion of an optimal spontaneous breathing pattern that maximizes oxygen and carbon dioxide exchange in the lungs

Visitation Facilitation—Promoting beneficial visits by family and friends

Vital Signs Monitoring—Collection and analysis of cardiovascular, respiratory, and body temperature data to determine and prevent complications

Vomiting Management—Prevention and alleviation of vomiting

Weight Gain Assistance—Facilitating gain of body weight

Weight Management—Facilitating maintenance of optimal body weight and percent body fat

Weight Reduction Assistance—Facilitating loss of weight and/or body fat

Wound Care—Prevention of wound complications and promotion of wound healing

Wound Care: Closed Drainage—Maintenance of a pressure drainage system at the wound site

Wound Irrigation—Flushing of an open wound to cleanse and remove debris and excessive drainage

SOURCE: McCloskey, JC and Bulecheck, GM: Nursing Interventions Classification, ed. 3, Mosby, Philadelphia, 1999, with permission.

APPENDIX N-4
Nursing Outcomes Classification System
Outcome Labels and Definitions

Abuse Cessation—Evidence that the victim is no longer abused

Abuse Protection—Protection of self or dependent others from abuse

Abuse Recovery: Emotional—Healing of psychological injuries due to abuse

Abuse Recovery: Financial—Regaining monetary and legal control or benefits following financial exploitation

Abuse Recovery: Physical—Healing of physical injuries due to abuse

Abuse Recovery: Sexual—Healing following sexual abuse or exploitation

Abusive Behavior Self-Control—Self-restraint of own behaviors to avoid abuse and neglect of dependents or significant others

Acceptance: Health Status—Reconciliation to health circumstances

Activity Tolerance—Responses to energy-consuming body movements involved in required or desired daily activities

Adherence Behavior—Self-initiated action taken to promote wellness, recovery, and rehabilitation

Aggression Control—Self-restraint of assaultive, combative, or destructive behavior toward others

Ambulation: Walking—Ability to walk from place to place

Ambulation: Wheelchair—Ability to move from place to place in a wheelchair

Anxiety Control—Personal actions to eliminate or reduce feelings of apprehension and tension from an unidentifiable source

Aspiration Control—Personal actions to prevent the passage of fluid and solid particles into the lung

Asthma Control—Personal actions to reverse inflammatory condition resulting in bronchial constriction of the airways

Balance—Ability to maintain body equilibrium

Blood Glucose Control—Extent to which plasma glucose levels are maintained in expected range

Blood Transfusion Reaction Control—Extent to which complications of blood transfusions are minimized

Body Image—Positive perception of own appearance and body functions

Body Positioning: Self-Initiated—Ability to change own body positions

Bone Healing—The extent to which cells and tissues have regenerated following bone injury

Bowel Continence—Control of passage of stool from the bowel

Bowel Elimination—Ability of the gastrointestinal tract to form and evacuate stool effectively

Breastfeeding Establishment: Infant—Proper attachment of an infant to and sucking from the mother's breast for nourishment during the first 2 to 3 weeks

Breastfeeding Establishment: Maternal—Maternal establishment of proper attachment of an infant to and sucking from the breast for nourishment during the first 2 to 3 weeks

Breastfeeding Maintenance—Continued nourishment of an infant through breastfeeding

Breastfeeding Weaning—Process leading to the eventual discontinuation of breastfeeding

Cardiac Pump Effectiveness—Extent to which blood is ejected from the left ventricle per minute to support systemic perfusion pressure

Caregiver Adaptation to Patient Institutionalization—Family caregiver adaptation of role when the care recipient is transferred outside the home

Caregiver Emotional Health—Feelings, attitudes, and emotions of a family care provider while caring for a family member or significant other over an extended period of time

Caregiver Home Care Readiness—Preparedness to assume responsibility for the health care of a family member or significant other in the home

Caregiver Lifestyle Disruption—Disturbances in the lifestyle of a family member due to caregiving

Caregiver-Patient Relationship—Positive interactions and connections between the caregiver and care recipient

Caregiver Performance: Direct Care—Provision by family care provider of appropriate personal and health care for a family member or significant other

Caregiver Performance: Indirect Care—Arrangement and oversight of appropriate care for a family member or significant other by family care provider

Caregiver Physical Health—Physical well-being of a family care provider while caring for a family member or significant other over an extended period of time

Caregiver Stressors—The extent of biopsychosocial pressure on a family care provider caring for a family member or significant other over an extended period of time

Caregiver Well-Being—Primary care provider's satisfaction with health and life circumstances

Caregiving Endurance Potential—Factors that promote family care provider continuance over an extended period of time

Child Adaptation to Hospitalization—Child's adaptive response to hospitalization

Child Development: 2 months—Milestones of physical, cognitive, and psychosocial progression by 2 months of age

Child Development: 4 months—Milestones of physical, cognitive, and psychosocial progression by 4 months of age

Child Development: 6 months—Milestones of physical, cognitive, and psychosocial progression by 6 months of age

Child Development: 12 months—Milestones of physical, cognitive, and psychosocial progression by 12 months of age

Child Development: 2 years—Milestones of physical, cognitive, and psychosocial progression by 2 years of age

Child Development: 3 years—Milestones of physical, cognitive, and psychosocial progression by 3 years of age

Child Development: 4 years—Milestones of physical, cognitive, and psychosocial progression by 4 years of age

Child Development: 5 years—Milestones of physical, cognitive, and psychosocial progression by 5 years of age

Child Development: Middle Childhood (6–11 years)—Milestones of physical, cognitive, and psychosocial progression between 6 and 11 years of age

Child Development: Adolescence (12–17 years)—Milestones of physical, cognitive, and psychosocial progression between 12 and 17 years of age

Circulation Status—Extent to which blood flows unobstructed, unidirectionally, and at an appropriate pressure through large vessels of the systemic and pulmonary circuits

Coagulation Status—Extent to which blood clots within expected period of time

Cognitive Ability—Ability to execute complex mental processes

Cognitive Orientation—Ability to identify person, place, and time

Comfort Level—Feelings of physical and psychological ease

Communication Ability—Ability to receive, interpret, and express spoken, written, and nonverbal messages

Communication: Expressive Ability—Ability to express and interpret verbal and/or nonverbal messages

Communication: Receptive Ability—Ability to receive and interpret verbal and/or nonverbal messages

Community Competence—The ability of a community to collectively problem-solve to achieve goals

Community Health Status—The general state of well-being of a community or population

Community Health: Immunity—Resistance of a group to the invasion and spread of an infectious agent

Community Risk Control: Chronic Disease—Community actions to reduce the risk of chronic diseases and related complications

Community Risk Control: Communicable Disease—Community actions to eliminate or reduce the spread of infectious agents (bacteria, fungi, parasites, and viruses) that threaten public health

Community Risk Control: Lead Exposure—Community actions to reduce lead exposure and poisoning

Compliance Behavior—Actions taken on the basis of professional advice to promote wellness, recovery, and rehabilitation

Concentration—Ability to focus on a specific stimulus

Coping—Actions to manage stressors that tax an individual's resources

Decision Making—Ability to choose between two or more alternatives

Depression Control—Personal actions to minimize melancholy and maintain interest in life events

Depression Level—Severity of melancholic mood and loss of interest in life events

Dialysis Access Integrity—The extent to which a dialysis access site is functional and free of inflammation

Dignified Dying—Maintaining personal control and comfort with the approaching end of life

Distorted Thought Control—Self-restraint of disruption in perception, thought processes, and thought content

Electrolyte & Acid/Base Balance—Balance of the electrolytes and non-electrolytes in the intracellular and extracellular compartments of the body

Endurance—Extent that energy enables a person to sustain activity

Energy Conservation—Extent of active management of energy to initiate and sustain activity

Family Coping—Family actions to manage stressors that tax family resources

Family Environment: Internal—Social climate as characterized by family member relationships and goals

Family Functioning—Ability of the family to meet the needs of its members through developmental transitions

Family Health Status—Overall health status and social competence of family unit

Family Integrity—Extent that family members' behaviors collectively demonstrate cohesion, strength, and emotional bonding

Family Normalization—Ability of the family to develop and maintain routines and management strategies that contribute to optimal functioning when a member has a chronic illness or disability

Family Participation in Professional Care—Family involvement in decision-making, delivery, and evaluation of care provided by health care personnel

Fear Control—Personal actions to eliminate or reduce disabling feelings of alarm aroused by an identifiable source

Fetal Status: Antepartum—Conditions indicative of fetal physical well-being from conception to the onset of labor

Fetal Status: Intrapartum—Conditions and behaviors indicative of fetal well-being from onset of labor to delivery

Fluid Balance—Balance of water in the intracellular and extracellular compartments of the body

Grief Resolution—Adjustment to actual or impending loss

Growth—A normal increase in body size and weight

Health Beliefs—Personal convictions that influence health behaviors

Health Beliefs: Perceived Ability to Perform—Personal conviction that one can carry out a given health behavior

Health Beliefs: Perceived Control—Personal conviction that one can influence a health outcome

Health Beliefs: Perceived Resources—Personal conviction that one has adequate means to carry out a health behavior

Health Beliefs: Perceived Threat—Personal conviction that a health problem is serious and has potential negative consequences for lifestyle

Health Orientation—Personal view of health and health behaviors as priorities

Health Promoting Behavior—Actions to sustain or increase wellness

Health Seeking Behavior—Actions to promote optimal wellness, recovery, and rehabilitation

Hearing Compensation Behavior—Actions to identify, monitor, and compensate for hearing loss

Hope—Presence of internal state of optimism that is personally satisfying and life-supporting

Hydration—Amount of water in the intracellular and extracellular compartments of the body

Identity—Ability to distinguish between self and non-self and to characterize one's essence

Immobility Consequences: Physiological—Extent of compromise in physiological functioning due to impaired physical mobility

Immobility Consequences: Psycho-Cognitive—Extent of compromise in psycho-cognitive functioning due to impaired physical mobility

Immune Hypersensitivity Control—Extent to which inappropriate immune responses are suppressed

Immune Status—Adequacy of natural and acquired appropriately targeted resistance to internal and external antigens

Immunization Behavior—Actions to obtain immunization to prevent a communicable disease

Impulse Control—Self-restraint of compulsive or impulsive behaviors

Infection Status—Presence and extent of infection

Information Processing—Ability to acquire, organize, and use information

Joint Movement: Active—Range of motion of joints with self-initiated movement

Joint Movement: Passive—Range of motion of joints with assisted movement

Knowledge: Breastfeeding—Extent of understanding conveyed about lactation and nourishment of infant through breastfeeding

Knowledge: Child Safety—Extent of understanding conveyed about safely caring for a child

Knowledge: Conception Prevention—Extent of understanding conveyed about pregnancy prevention

Knowledge: Diabetes Management—Extent of understanding conveyed about diabetes mellitus and its control

Knowledge: Diet—Extent of understanding conveyed about diet

Knowledge: Disease Process—Extent of understanding conveyed about a specific disease process

Knowledge: Energy Conservation—Extent of understanding conveyed about energy conservation techniques

Knowledge: Fertility Promotion—Extent of understanding conveyed about fertility testing and the conditions that affect conception

Knowledge: Health Behaviors—Extent of understanding conveyed about the promotion and protection of health

Knowledge: Health Promotion—Extent of understanding of information needed to obtain and maintain optimal health

Knowledge: Health Resources—Extent of understanding conveyed about health care resources

Knowledge: Illness Care—Extent of understanding of illness-related information needed to achieve and maintain optimal health

Knowledge: Infant Care—Extent of understanding conveyed about caring for a baby up to 12 months

Knowledge: Infection Control—Extent of understanding conveyed about prevention and control of infection

Knowledge: Labor and Delivery—Extent of understanding conveyed about labor and delivery

Knowledge: Maternal-Child Health—Extent of understanding of information needed to achieve and maintain optimal health of a mother and child

Knowledge: Medication—Extent of understanding conveyed about the safe use of medication

Knowledge: Personal Safety—Extent of understanding conveyed about preventing unintentional injuries

Knowledge: Postpartum—Extent of understanding conveyed about maternal health following delivery

Knowledge: Preconception—Extent of understanding conveyed about maternal health prior to conception to ensure a healthy pregnancy

Knowledge: Pregnancy—Extent of understanding conveyed about maintenance of a healthy pregnancy and prevention of complications

Knowledge: Prescribed Activity—Extent of understanding conveyed about prescribed activity and exercise

Knowledge: Sexual Functioning—Extent of understanding conveyed about sexual development and responsible sexual practices

Knowledge: Substance Use Control—Extent of understanding conveyed about managing substance use safely

Knowledge: Treatment Procedure(s)—Extent of understanding conveyed about procedure(s) required as part of a treatment regimen

Knowledge: Treatment Regimen—Extent of understanding conveyed about a specific treatment regimen

Leisure Participation—Use of restful or relaxing activities as needed to promote well-being

Loneliness—The extent of emotional, social, or existential isolation response

Maternal Status: Antepartum—Conditions and behaviors indicative of maternal well-being from conception to the onset of labor

Maternal Status: Intrapartum—Conditions and behaviors indicative of maternal well-being from onset of labor to delivery

Maternal Status: Postpartum—Conditions and behaviors indicative of maternal well-being from delivery of placenta to completion of involution

Medication Response—Therapeutic and adverse effects of prescribed medication

Memory—Ability to cognitively retrieve and report previously stored information

Mobility Level—Ability to move purposefully

Mood Equilibrium—Appropriate adjustment of prevailing emotional tone in response to circumstances

Muscle Function—Adequacy of muscle contraction needed for movement

Neglect Recovery—Healing following the cessation of substandard care

Neurological Status—Extent to which the peripheral and central nervous systems receive, process, and respond to internal and external stimuli

Neurological Status: Autonomic—Extent to which the autonomic nervous system coordinates visceral function

Neurological Status: Central Motor Control—Extent to which skeletal muscle activity (body movement) is coordinated by the central nervous system

Neurological Status: Consciousness—Extent to which an individual arouses, orients, and attends to the environment

Neurological Status: Cranial Sensory/Motor Function—Extent to which cranial nerves convey sensory and motor information

Neurological Status: Spinal Sensory/Motor Function—Extent to which spinal nerves convey sensory and motor information

Newborn Adaptation—Adaptation to the extrauterine environment by a physiologically mature newborn during the first 28 days

Nutritional Status—Extent to which nutrients are available to meet metabolic needs

Nutritional Status: Biochemical Measures—Body fluid components and chemical indices of nutritional status

Nutritional Status: Body Mass—Congruence of body weight, muscle, and fat to height, frame, and gender

Nutritional Status: Energy—Extent to which nutrients provide cellular energy

Nutritional Status: Food and Fluid Intake—Amount of food and fluid taken into the body over a 24-hour period

Nutritional Status: Nutrient Intake—Adequacy of nutrients taken into the body

Oral Health—Condition of the mouth, teeth, gums, and tongue

Pain Control—Personal actions to control pain

Pain: Disruptive Effects—Observed or reported disruptive effects of pain on emotions and behavior

Pain Level—Severity of reported or demonstrated pain

Pain: Psychological Response—Cognitive and emotional responses to physical pain

Parent-Infant Attachment—Behaviors that demonstrate an enduring affectionate bond between a parent and infant

Parenting—Provision of an environment that promotes optimum growth and development of dependent children

Parenting: Social Safety—Parental actions to avoid social relationships that might cause harm or injury

Participation: Health Care Decisions—Personal involvement in selecting and evaluating health care options

Physical Aging Status—Physical changes that commonly occur with adult aging

Physical Fitness—Ability to perform physical activities with vigor

Physical Maturation: Female—Normal physical changes in the female that occur with the transition from childhood to adulthood

Physical Maturation: Male—Normal physical changes in the male that occur with the transition from childhood to adulthood

Play Participation—Use of activities as needed for enjoyment, entertainment, and development by children

Prenatal Health Behavior—Personal actions to promote a healthy pregnancy

Preterm Infant Organization—Extrauterine integration of physiologic and behavioral function by the infant born 24 to 37 (term) weeks gestation

Psychomotor Energy—Ability to maintain ADLs, nutrition, and personal safety

Psychosocial Adjustment: Life Change—Psychosocial adaptation of an individual to a life change

Quality of Life—An individual's expressed satisfaction with current life circumstances

Respiratory Status: Airway Patency—Extent to which the tracheobronchial passages remain open

Respiratory Status: Gas Exchange—Alveolar exchange of CO_2 or O_2 to maintain arterial blood gas concentrations

Respiratory Status: Ventilation—Movement of air in and out of the lungs

Rest—Extent and pattern of diminished activity for mental and physical rejuvenation

Risk Control—Actions to eliminate or reduce actual, personal, and modifiable health threats

Risk Control: Alcohol Use—Actions to eliminate or reduce alcohol use that poses a threat to health

Risk Control: Cancer—Actions to reduce or detect the possibility of cancer

Risk Control: Cardiovascular Health—Actions to eliminate or reduce threats to cardiovascular health

Risk Control: Drug Use—Actions to eliminate or reduce drug use that poses a threat to health

Risk Control: Hearing Impairment—Actions to eliminate or reduce the possibility of altered hearing function

Risk Control: Sexually Transmitted Diseases (STD)—Actions to eliminate or reduce behaviors associated with sexually transmitted disease

Risk Control: Tobacco Use—Actions to eliminate or reduce tobacco use

Risk Control: Unintended Pregnancy—Actions to reduce the possibility of unintended pregnancy

Risk Control: Visual Impairment—Actions to eliminate or reduce the possibility of altered visual function

Risk Detection—Actions taken to identify personal health threats

Role Performance—Congruence of an individual's role behavior with role expectations

Safety Behavior: Fall Prevention—Individual or caregiver actions to minimize risk factors that might precipitate falls

Safety Behavior: Home Physical Environment—Individual or caregiver actions to minimize environmental factors that might cause physical harm or injury in the home

Safety Behavior: Personal—Individual or caregiver efforts to control behaviors that might cause physical injury

Safety Status: Falls Occurrence—Number of falls in the past week

Safety Status: Physical Injury—Severity of injuries from accidents and trauma

Self-Care: Activities of Daily Living (ADL)—Ability to perform the most basic physical tasks and personal care activities

Self-Care: Bathing—Ability to cleanse own body

Self-Care: Dressing—Ability to dress self

Self-Care: Eating—Ability to prepare and ingest food

Self-Care: Grooming—Ability to maintain kempt appearance

Self-Care: Hygiene—Ability to maintain own hygiene

Self-Care: Instrumental Activities of Daily Living (IADL)—Ability to perform activities needed to function in the home or community

Self-Care: Non-Parenteral Medication—Ability to administer oral and topical medications to meet therapeutic goals

Self-Care: Oral Hygiene—Ability to care for own mouth and teeth

Self-Care: Parenteral Medication—Ability to administer parenteral medications to meet therapeutic goals

Self-Care: Toileting—Ability to toilet self

Self-Direction of Care—Directing others to assist with or perform physical tasks, personal care, and activities needed to function in the home or the community

Self-Esteem—Personal judgment of self-worth

Self-Mutilation Restraint—Ability to refrain from intentional self-inflicted injury (non-lethal)

Sensory Function: Cutaneous—Extent to which stimulation of the skin is sensed in an impaired area

Sensory Function: Hearing—Extent to which sounds are sensed, with or without assistive devices

Sensory Function: Proprioception—Extent to which the position and movement of the head and body are sensed

Sensory Function: Taste and Smell—Extent to which chemicals inhaled or dissolved in saliva are sensed

Sensory Function: Vision—Extent to which visual images are sensed, with or without assistive devices

Sexual Functioning—Integration of physical, socioemotional, and intellectual aspects of sexual expression

Sexual Identity: Acceptance—Acknowledgment and acceptance of own sexual identity

Skeletal Function—The functional ability of the bones to support the body and facilitate movement

Sleep—Extent and pattern of natural periodic suspension of consciousness during which the body is restored

Social Interaction Skills—An individual's use of effective interaction behaviors

Social Involvement—Frequency of an individual's social interactions with persons, groups, or organizations

Social Support—Perceived availability and actual provision of reliable assistance from other persons

Spiritual Well-Being—Personal expressions of connectedness with self, others, higher power, all life, nature, and the universe that transcend and empower the self

Substance Addiction Consequences—Compromise in health status and social functioning due to substance addiction

Suffering Level—Severity of anguish associated with a distressing symptom, injury, or loss with potential long-term effects

Suicide Self-Restraint—Ability to refrain from gestures and attempts at killing self

Swallowing Status—Extent of safe passage of fluids and/or solids from the mouth to the stomach

Swallowing Status: Esophageal Phase—Adequacy of the passage of fluids and/or solids from the pharynx to the stomach

Swallowing Status: Oral Phase—Adequacy of preparation, containment, and posteriorly movement of fluids and/or solids in the mouth for swallowing

Swallowing Status: Pharyngeal Phase—Adequacy of the passage of fluids and/or solids from the mouth to the esophagus

Symptom Control—Personal actions to minimize perceived adverse changes in physical and emotional functioning

Symptom Severity—Extent of perceived adverse changes in physical, emotional, and social functioning

Symptom Severity: Perimenopause—Extent of symptoms caused by declining hormonal levels

Symptom Severity: Premenstrual Syndrome (PMS)—Extent of symptoms caused by cyclic hormonal fluctuations

Systemic Toxin Clearance: Dialysis—Extent to which toxins are cleared from the body with peritoneal or hemodialysis

Thermoregulation—Balance among heat production, heat gain, and heat loss

Thermoregulation: Neonate—Balance among heat production, heat gain, and heat loss during the neonatal period

Tissue Integrity: Skin and Mucous Membranes—Structural intactness and normal physiological function of skin and mucous membranes

Tissue Perfusion: Abdominal Organs—Extent to which blood flows through the small vessels of the abdominal viscera and maintains organ function

Tissue Perfusion: Cardiac—Extent to which blood flows through the coronary vasculature and maintains heart function

Tissue Perfusion: Cerebral—Extent to which blood flows through the cerebral vasculature and maintains brain function

Tissue Perfusion: Peripheral—Extent to which blood flows through the small vessels of the extremities and maintains tissue function

Tissue Perfusion: Pulmonary—Extent to which blood flows through intact pulmonary vasculature with appropriate pressure and volume, perfusing alveoli/capillary unit

Transfer Performance—Ability to change body locations

Treatment Behavior: Illness or Injury—Personal actions to palliate or eliminate pathology

Urinary Continence—Control of the elimination of urine

Urinary Elimination—Ability of the urinary system to filter wastes, conserve solutes, and to collect and discharge urine in a healthy pattern

Vision Compensation Behavior—Actions to compensate for visual impairment

Vital Signs Status—Temperature, pulse, respiration, and blood pressure within expected range for the individual

Weight Control—Personal actions resulting in achievement and maintenance of optimum body weight for health

Well-Being—An individual's expressed satisfaction with health status

Will to Live—Desire, determination, and effort to survive

Wound Healing: Primary Intention—The extent to which cells and tissues have regenerated following intentional closure

Wound Healing: Secondary Intention—The extent to which cells and tissues in an open wound have regenerated

SOURCE: Johnson, M, Maas, ML, and Moorhead, S: Nursing Outcomes Classification, ed 2, Mosby, Philadelphia, 1999, with permission.

APPENDIX N-5
Home Health Care Classification (HHCC) System

HOME HEALTH CARE CLASSIFICATION NURSING COMPONENTS

Activity Cluster of elements that involve the use of energy in carrying out bodily functions.

Bowel Elimination Cluster of elements that involve the gastrointestinal system.

Cardiac Cluster of elements that involve the heart, blood vessels, and circulatory system.

Cognitive Cluster of elements involving the mental and cerebral processes.

Coping Cluster of elements that involve the ability to deal with responsibilities, problems, or difficulties.

Fluid Volume Cluster of elements that involve liquid consumption.

Health Behavior Cluster of elements that involve actions to sustain, maintain, or regain health.

Medication Cluster of elements that involve medicinal substances.

Metabolic Cluster of elements that involve the endocrine and immunological processes.

Nutritional Cluster of elements that involve the intake of food and nutrients.

Physical Regulation Cluster of elements that involve bodily processes.

Respiratory Cluster of elements that involve breathing and the pulmonary system.

Role Relationship Cluster of elements involving interpersonal, work, social, and sexual interactions.

Safety Cluster of elements that involve prevention of injury, danger, or loss.

Self-care Cluster of elements that involve the ability to carry out activities to maintain oneself.

Self-concept Cluster of elements that involve an individual's mental image of oneself.

Sensory Cluster of elements that involve senses.

Skin Integrity Cluster of elements that involve the mucous membrane, corneal, integumentary, and subcutaneous structures of the body.

Tissue Perfusion Cluster of elements that involve the oxygenation of tissues.

Urinary Elimination Cluster of elements that involve the genitourinary system.

HOME HEALTH CARE CLASSIFICATION OF NURSING DIAGNOSES*

activities of daily living (ADLs) alteration: Change or modification of ability to maintain oneself.

activity alteration: Change or modification in energy used by the body.

activity intolerance: Incapacity to carry out physiological or psychological daily activities.

activity intolerance risk: Increased chance of an incapacity to carry out physiological or psychological daily activities.

acute pain: Physical suffering or distress; to hurt.

adjustment impairment: Inadequate adaptation to condition or change in health status.

airway clearance impairment: Inability to clear secretions/obstructions in airway.

anticipatory grieving: Feeling great sorrow before the event or loss.

anxiety: Feeling of distress or apprehension whose source is unknown.

aspiration risk: Increased chance of material into trachea-bronchial passages.

auditory alteration: Diminished ability to hear.

bathing/hygiene deficit: Impaired ability to cleanse oneself.

blood pressure alteration: Change in the systolic or diastolic pressure.

body image disturbance: Imbalance in the perception of the way one's body looks.

body nutrition deficit: Less than adequate intake or absorption of food or nutrients.

body nutrition deficit risk: Increased chance of less than adequate intake or absorption of food or nutrients.

body nutrition excess: More than adequate intake or absorption of food or nutrients.

body nutrition excess risk: Increased chance of more than adequate intake or absorption of food or nutrients.

bowel elimination alteration: Change or modification of the gastrointestinal system.

bowel incontinence: Involuntary defecation.

breastfeeding impairment: Diminished ability to nourish infant at the breast.

breathing pattern impairment: Inadequate inhalation or exhalation.

cardiac output alteration: Change or modification in the pumping action of the heart.

cardiovascular alteration: Change or modification of the heart or blood vessels.

cerebral alteration: Change or modification of thought processes or mentation.

chronic low self-esteem disturbance: Persistent negative evaluation of oneself.

chronic pain: Pain that continues for longer than expected.

colonic constipation: Infrequent or difficult passage of hard, dry feces.

comfort alteration: Change or modification in sensation that is distressing.

communication impairment: Diminished ability to exchange thoughts, opinions, or information.

compromised family coping: Inability of family to function optimally.
decisional conflict: Struggle related to determining a course of action.
defensive coping: Self-protective strategies to guard against threats to self.
denial: Attempt to reduce anxiety by refusal to accept thoughts, feelings, or facts.
diarrhea: Abnormal frequency and fluidity of feces.
disabled family coping: Dysfunctional ability of family to function.
disuse syndrome: Group of symptoms related to effects of immobility.
diversional activity deficit: Lack of interest or engagement in leisure activities.
dressing/grooming deficit: Impaired ability to clothe and groom oneself.
dying process: Physical and behavioral responses associated with death.
dysfunctional grieving: Prolonged feeling of great sorrow.
dysreflexia: Life-threatening inhibited sympathetic response to a noxious stimuli in a person with a spinal cord injury at T7 or above.
endocrine alteration: Change or modification of internal secretions or hormones.
family coping impairment: Inadequate family response to problems or difficulties.
family processes alteration: Change or modification of usual functioning of a related group.
fatigue: Exhaustion that interferes with physical and mental activities.
fear: Feeling of dread or distress whose cause can be identified.
fecal impaction: Feces wedged in intestine.
feeding deficit: Impaired ability to feed oneself.
fluid volume alteration: Change or modification in bodily fluid.
fluid volume deficit: Dehydration.
fluid volume deficit risk: Increased chance of dehydration.
fluid volume excess: Fluid retention, overload, or edema.
fluid volume excess risk: Increased chance of fluid retention, overload, or edema.
functional urinary incontinence: Involuntary, unpredictable passage of urine.
gas exchange impairment: Imbalance of oxygen and carbon dioxide transfer between lung and vascular system.
gastrointestinal alteration: Change or modification of the stomach or intestines.
grieving: Feeling of great sorrow.
growth and development alteration: Change or modification in norms for age.
gustatory alteration: Diminished ability to taste.
health maintenance alteration: Change or modification in ability to manage health-related needs.
health-seeking behavior alteration: Change or modification of actions needed to improve health state.
home maintenance alteration: Inability to sustain a safe, healthy environment.
hopelessness: Feeling of despair or futility and passive abandonment.
hyperthermia: Abnormal high body temperature.
hypothermia: Subnormal low body temperature.
immunologic alteration: Change or modification of the immune system.
individual coping impairment: Inadequate personal response to problems or difficulties.
infection risk: Increased change of contamination with disease-producing germs.
infection unspecified: Unknown contamination with disease-producing germs.
injury risk: Increased chance of danger or loss.
instrumental activities of daily living (IADLs) alteration: Change or modification of more complex activities than those needed to maintain oneself.
kinesthetic alteration: Diminished ability to move.
knowledge deficit: Lack of information, understanding, or comprehension.
knowledge deficit of diagnostic test: Lack of information on tests to identify disease or assess health condition.
knowledge deficit of dietary regimen: Lack of information on the prescribed food or fluid intake.
knowledge deficit of disease process: Lack of information on the morbidity, course, or treatment of the health condition.
knowledge deficit of fluid volume: Lack of information on fluid volume intake requirements.
knowledge deficit of medication regimen: Lack of information on prescribed regulated course of medicinal substances.
knowledge deficit of safety precautions: Lack of information on measures to prevent injury, danger, or loss.
knowledge deficit of therapeutic regimen: Lack of information on regulated course of treating disease.
meaningfulness alteration: Change or modification of the ability to see the significance, purpose, or value in something.
medication risk: Increased chance of negative response to medicinal substance.
musculoskeletal alteration: Change or modification of the muscles, bones, or support structures.
noncompliance: Failure to follow therapeutic recommendations.
noncompliance of diagnostic test: Failure to follow therapeutic recommendations on tests to identify disease or assess health condition.
noncompliance of dietary regimen: Failure to follow the prescribed food or fluid intake.
noncompliance of fluid volume: Failure to follow fluid volume intake requirements.
noncompliance of medication regimen: Failure to follow prescribed regulated course of medicinal substances.

noncompliance of safety precautions: Failure to follow measures to prevent injury, danger, or loss.

noncompliance of therapeutic regimen: Failure to follow regulated course of treating disease.

nutrition alteration: Change or modification of food or nutrients.

olfactory alteration: Diminished ability to smell.

oral mucous membranes impairment: Diminished ability to maintain the tissues of the oral cavity.

parental role conflict: Struggle with parental position and responsibilities.

parenting alteration: Change or modification of nurturing figure's ability to promote growth and development of infant/child.

perceived constipation: Belief and treatment of infrequent or difficult passage of feces without cause.

peripheral alteration: Change or modification in vascularization of the extremities.

personal identity disturbance: Imbalance in the ability to distinguish between the self and the nonself.

physical mobility impairment: Diminished ability to perform independent movement.

physical regulation alteration: Change or modification of somatic control.

poisoning risk: Exposure to or ingestion of dangerous products.

polypharmacy: Use of two or more drugs together.

post-trauma response: Sustained behavior related to a traumatic event.

powerlessness: Feeling of helplessness, or inability to act.

protection alteration: Change or modification of the ability to guard against internal or external threats to the body.

rape trauma syndrome: Group of symptoms related to a forced sexual act.

respiration alteration: Change or modification in breathing.

reflex urinary incontinence: Involuntary passage of urine occurring at predictable intervals.

renal alteration: Change or modification in the kidneys.

role performance alteration: Change or modification of carrying out responsibilities.

self-care deficit: Impaired ability to maintain oneself.

self-concept alteration: Change or modification of ability to maintain one's image of self.

sensory perceptual alteration: Change in modification in the response to stimuli.

sexual dysfunction: Deleterious change in sex response.

sexuality patterns alteration: Change or modification of person's sexual response.

situational self-esteem disturbance: Negative evaluation of oneself in response to a loss or change.

skin integrity impairment: Diminished ability to maintain the integument.

skin integrity impairment risk: Increased chance of skin breakdown.

skin incision: Cutting of the integument.

sleep pattern disturbance: Imbalance in the normal sleep/wake cycle.

social interaction alteration: Inadequate quantity or quality of personal relations.

social isolation: State of aloneness, lack of interaction with others.

socialization alteration: Change or modification of personal identity.

spiritual distress: Anguish related to the spirit or soul.

spiritual state alteration: Change or modification of the spirit or soul.

stress urinary incontinence: Loss of urine occurring with increased abdominal pressure.

suffocation risk: Inadequate air for breathing.

swallowing impairment: Inability to move food from mouth to stomach.

tactile alteration: Diminished ability to feel.

thermoregulation impairment: Fluctuation of temperature between hypothermia and hyperthermia.

tissue integrity alteration: A change or modification in the mucous membrane, corneal, integumentary, or subcutaneous structures.

tissue perfusion alteration: A change or modification in the oxygenation of tissues.

toileting deficit: Impaired ability to urinate or defecate for oneself.

total urinary incontinence: Continuous and unpredictable loss of urine.

thought processes alteration: Change or modification in cognitive processes.

trauma risk: Accidental tissue injury.

unilateral neglect: Lack of awareness of one side of the body.

unspecified constipation: Other forms of abnormal feces or difficult passage of feces.

unspecified pain: Pain that is difficult to pinpoint.

urinary elimination alteration: A change or modification in the excretion of the waste matter of the kidneys.

urinary retention: Incomplete emptying of the bladder.

urge urinary incontinence: Involuntary passage of urine following a sense of urgency to void.

verbal impairment: Diminished ability to exchange thoughts, opinions, or information through speech.

violence risk: Increased chance of harming self or others.

visual alteration: A diminished ability to see.

HOME HEALTH CARE CLASSIFICATION OF NURSING INTERVENTIONS

abuse control: Actions to manage situations to avoid, detect, or minimize harm.

activities of daily living: Personal activities to maintain oneself.
activity care: Actions performed to carry out physiological daily activities.
adult day care: Actions to manage the provision of a day program for adults in a specific location.
allergic reaction care: Actions to reduce symptoms or precautions to reduce allergic reactions.
ambulation therapy: Actions to promote walking.
assistive device therapy: Actions to manage the use of products to aid in caring for oneself.
bedbound care: Actions performed to manage an individual confined to bed.
behavior care: Actions performed to manage observable responses to internal and external stimuli.
bereavement support: Actions to provide comfort to the family/friends of the person who died.
bill of rights: Statements related to entitlement during an episode of illness.
bladder care: Actions performed to manage urinary drainage problems.
bladder instillation: Actions to pour liquid in a catheter.
bladder training: Actions to provide instruction on the care of urinary drainage problems.
blood pressure: Actions to measure the diastolic and systolic pressure of the blood.
blood specimen analysis: Actions performed to collect and/or examine a sample of blood.
bowel care: Actions performed to maintain or restore functioning of the bowel.
bowel training: Actions to provide instruction on bowel elimination.
breathing exercises: Actions to provide instruction on respiratory or lung exertion.
cardiac care: Actions performed to manage changes in the heart or blood vessels.
cardiac rehabilitation: Actions taken to restore cardiac health.
cast care: Actions performed to manage a rigid dressing.
cataract care: Actions performed to control cataract conditions.
chemotherapy care: Actions performed to administer and monitor antineoplastic agents.
chest physiotherapy: Exercises to provide postural drainage of the lungs.
comfort care: Actions performed to enhance or improve well-being.
communication care: Actions performed to exchange verbal information.
community special programs: Actions to manage the provision of advice or instruction about a special community program resources.
compliance care: Actions performed to encourage conformity with therapeutic recommendations.
compliance with diet: Actions to encourage conformity with food or fluid intake.
compliance with fluid volume: Actions to encourage conformity to therapeutic intake of liquids.
compliance with medical regimen: Actions to encourage conformity to physician's plan of care.
compliance with medication regime: Actions to encourage conformity to follow prescribed course of medicinal substances.
compliance with safety precautions: Actions to encourage conformity with measures to protect self or others from injury, danger, or loss.
compliance with therapeutic regime: Actions to encourage conformity with the health team's plan of care.
coping support: Actions to sustain a person's dealing with responsibilities, problems, or difficulties.
counseling service: Actions to provide advice or instruction to help another.
decubitus care: Actions performed to prevent, detect, and treat skin integrity breakdown caused by pressure. Stage 1: actions performed to prevent skin breakdown. Stage 2: actions performed to manage tissue breakdown. Stage 3: actions performed to manage skin destruction. Stage 4: actions performed to manage open wounds.
denture care: Actions performed to manage artificial teeth.
diabetic care: Actions performed to control diabetic conditions.
dialysis care: Actions performed in the care and management of dialysis treatment.
disimpaction: Actions to manually remove feces.
drainage tube care: Actions performed to control drainage from tubes.
dressing change: Actions performed to remove and replace new bandage(s) to a wound.
dying/death measures: Actions performed to manage the dying process.
ear care: Actions performed to manage ear problems.
edema control: Actions to manage excess fluid in tissue.
emergency care: Actions performed to manage a sudden, unexpected occurrence.
emotional support: Actions to sustain a positive affective state.
enema: Actions performed to administer fluid rectally.
energy conservation: Actions taken to preserve energy.
enteral/parenteral feeding: Actions to provide nourishment through intravenous or gastrointestinal routes.
environmental safety: Precautions recommended to prevent or reduce environmental injury.
equipment safety: Precautions recommended to prevent or reduce equipment injury.
eye care: Actions performed to manage eye problems.
feeding technique: Actions using special measures to provide nourishment.

fluid therapy: Actions to provide liquid volume intake.
foot care: Actions performed to manage foot problems.
fracture care: Actions performed to manage broken bones.
funeral arrangements: Actions performed to manage preparatory measures for burial.
gastrostomy/nasogastric tube care: Actions performed to control gastrostomy/nasogastric drainage tubes.
gastrostomy/nasogastric tube insertion: Actions performed in the placement of a gastrostomy/nasogastric drainage tube.
gastrostomy/nasogastric tube irrigation: Actions performed to flush or wash out a gastrostomy/nasogastric tube.
health history: Actions to obtain information about past illness and health status.
health promotion: Actions performed to encourage behaviors to enhance health state.
hearing aid care: Actions performed to manage a hearing aid.
home health aide service: Actions performed to manage the provision of home care services by a home health aide.
home situation analysis: Analysis of living environment.
hospice: Actions to manage the provision of offering and/or providing care for terminally ill persons.
hydration status: Actions to manage the state of fluid balance.
immobilizer care: Actions to manage a splint, cast, or prescribed bed rest.
incision care: Actions performed to manage a surgical wound.
individual safety: Precautions to reduce individual injury.
infection control: Actions performed to manage communicable illness.
infusion care: Actions performed to manage solution given via vein.
inhalation therapy: Actions performed to manage breathing treatments.
injection administration: Actions performed to dispense a medication by a hypodermic.
instrumental activities of daily living (IADL): Complex activities performed to manage basic life skills.
insulin injection: Actions performed to manage a hypodermic administration of insulin.
intake/output: Actions performed to measure the amount of fluids/food and excretion of waste.
interpersonal dynamics analysis: Analysis of driving forces in a relationship between people.
intravenous care: Actions performed to manage the infusion.
meals-on-wheels: Actions performed to manage the provision of community program of meals delivered to the home.
medical regime orders: Actions performed to manage the physician's plan of treatment.
medical social worker service: Actions performed to provide advice or instruction by medical social worker.
medication actions: Activities related to management or monitoring of medicinal substances.
medication administration: Actions performed to manage the dispensing of prescribed drugs.
medication prefill preparation: Activities to ensure the continued supply of prescribed drugs.
medication side effects: Actions performed to control untoward reactions or conditions to prescribed drugs.
mental health care: Actions taken to promote emotional well-being.
mental health history: Actions to obtain information about past and present emotional well-being.
mental health promotion: Actions to encourage or further emotional well-being.
mental health screening: Actions performed to systematically examine the emotional well-being.
mental health treatment: Actions to manage protocols used to treat emotional problems.
mobility therapy: Actions performed to advise and instruct on mobility deficits.
mouth care: Actions performed to manage oral cavity
nurse specialist service: Actions to obtain advice or instruction by advanced nurse specialists or nurse practitioners.
nurse care coordination: Actions performed to synthesize all plans of care.
nursing contact: Actions to communicate with another nurse.
nursing status report: Actions performed to document condition by nurse.
nutrition care: Actions performed to manage food and nutrients.
occupational therapist service: Actions performed to provide advice or instruction by occupational therapist.
ostomy care: Actions performed to manage an artificial opening which removes waste products.
ostomy irrigation: Actions performed to flush or wash out of an ostomy.
other ancillary service: Actions performed to provide duties performed by other ancillary caregivers.
other community special program: Actions performed to manage the provision of advice or instruction for a specific community program resource.
other professional service: Actions performed to manage the duties performed by other professional caregivers.
other specimen analysis: Actions performed to collect and/or examine a sample of body tissue or fluid.
oxygen therapy care: Actions performed to manage administration of oxygen treatment.

pacemaker care Actions performed to manage an electronic device that provides a normal heartbeat.
pain control Actions performed to manage responses to injury or damage.
perineal care: Actions performed to manage perineal problems.
personal care: Actions performed to care for oneself.
physical examination: Actions performed to observe somatic events.
physical health care: Actions performed to manage somatic problems.
physical measurements: Actions performed to conduct procedures to evaluate somatic events.
physical therapist service: Actions performed to obtain advice or instruction by physical therapist.
physician contact: Actions performed to communicate with a physician.
physician status report: Actions performed to document condition by physician.
positioning therapy: Process to manage changes in body position.
professional/ancillary services: Actions performed to manage the duties performed by health team members.
psychosocial analysis: Study of psychological and social factors.
pulse: Actions performed to measure rhythmical beats of the heart.
radiation therapy care: Actions performed to administer and monitor radiation therapy.
range of motion: Actions performed to manage the active or passive exercises to maintain joint function.
reality orientation: Actions to promote the ability to locate oneself in the environment.
regular diet: Actions to manage ingestion of food and nutrients from established nutrition standards.
rehabilitation care: Actions performed to restore physical functioning.
rehabilitation exercise: Activities to promote physical functioning.
respiration: Actions performed to measure the function of breathing.
respiratory care: Actions taken to manage pulmonary hygiene.
safety precautions: Advance measures to avoid injury, danger, or harm.
skin breakdown control: Actions performed to manage tissue integrity problems.
skin care: Actions performed to manage the integument.
sleep pattern control: Actions performed to manage the sleep/wake cycle.
special diet: Actions to manage ingestion of food and nutrients prescribed for a specific purpose.
specimen analysis: Actions performed to manage the collection and/or examination of a bodily specimen.
speech therapist service: Actions performed to provide advice or instruction by a speech therapist.
spiritual comfort: Actions performed to console, restore, or promote spiritual health.
stool specimen analysis: Actions performed to collect and/or examine a sample of feces.
stress control: Actions performed to manage the physiological response of the body to a stimulus.
temperature: Actions performed to measure body temperature.
terminal care: Actions performed in the period of time surrounding death.
tracheostomy care: Actions performed to manage a tracheostomy.
transfer care: Actions performed to assist in moving from one place to another.
universal precautions: Practices to prevent spread of infection and infectious diseases.
urinary catheter care: Actions performed to manage a urinary catheter.
urinary catheter insertion: Actions performed to place a urinary catheter in bladder.
urinary catheter irrigation: Actions performed to flush out a urinary catheter.
urine specimen analysis: Actions performed to collect and/or examine a sample of urine.
venous catheter care: Actions performed to manage infusion equipment.
ventilator care: Actions performed to manage and monitor a ventilator.
violence control: Actions performed to manage behaviors which may cause harm to oneself or others.
vital signs: Actions performed to measure temperature, pulse, respiration, and blood pressure.
vitamin B_{12} injection: Actions performed to administer a hypodermic of Vitamin B_{12}.
wax removal: Actions performed to remove cerumen from ear.
weight control: Actions to manage obesity or debilitation.
wound care: Actions performed to manage open skin areas.

---

*Adapted from NANDA: Taxonomy 1: revised 1990
Terminology Modifications and definitions made in collaboration with Sheila M. Sparks, D.N.Sc., R.N., C.S. Assistant Professor, Georgetown University.
SOURCE: The Home Health Care Classification System (HHCC) has been developed by Virginia K. Saba, Ed.D., R.N., F.A.A.N., Clinical Associate Professor, Georgetown University School of Nursing. This information is in the public domain and not copyrighted by F.A. Davis Company. Used with permission.

APPENDIX N-6
Omaha System

The Omaha System is a research-based, comprehensive taxonomy that consists of the Problem Classification Scheme, the Intervention Scheme, and the Problem Rating Scale for Outcomes. Work on the Omaha System began in 1970 at the Visiting Nurse Association of Omaha (NE). Nurses from that agency and seven other test sites throughout the United States participated in four federally funded research projects between 1975 and 1993. The number and type of practice, education, and research sites that are adopting the Omaha System nationally and internationally are increasing dramatically. Numerous publications are available that describe the development, components, automation, and use of the Omaha System.

PROBLEM CLASSIFICATION SCHEME: An orderly, nonexhaustive, mutually exclusive, client-focused taxonomy of domains, modifiers, problems, and signs/symptoms addressed by nurses and other professionals. The four domains represent priority areas of professional and client health-related concerns. Each of the 40 problems may be referenced as health promotion, potential, or deficit/impairment/actual as well as individual or family. Actual problems are described by a cluster of signs and symptoms. As an open system of language and codes, the Problem Classification Scheme is used as a comprehensive method for collecting, sorting, classifying, documenting, and analyzing client data.

INTERVENTION SCHEME: An organized framework designed to address specific client problems or nursing diagnoses and consisting of three levels of nursing actions or activities. Four broad categories of interventions are further delineated by targets or objects of nursing action and by client-specific information generated by the nurse or other professional. Because the Intervention Scheme is the basis for planning and intervening, it enables professionals to describe and communicate their practice including improving, maintaining, or restoring health and preventing illness.

PROBLEM RATING SCALE FOR OUTCOMES: A five-point, Likert-type scale for measuring the entire range of severity for the concepts of knowledge, behavior, and status. Each of the three subscales is a continuum providing an evaluation framework for examining problem-specific client ratings at regular or predictable times. Suggested times include admission, specific interim points, and dismissal. The ratings are a guide for the nurse or other professional as client care is planned and provided; the ratings offer a method to monitor client progress throughout the period of service.

DOMAINS AND PROBLEMS OF THE PROBLEM CLASSIFICATION SCHEME

Domain I. Environmental:

The material resources, physical surrounding, and substances both internal and external to the client, home neighborhood, and broader community: appears at the first level of the Problem Classification Scheme.

01. Income
02. Sanitation
03. Residence
04. Neighborhood/workplace safety
05. Other

Domain II. Psychosocial:

Patterns of behavior, communication, relationships, and development; appears at the first level of the Problem Classification Scheme.

06. Communication with community resources
07. Social contact
08. Role change
09. Interpersonal relationship
10. Spirituality
11. Grief
12. Emotional stability
13. Human sexuality
14. Caretaking/parenting
15. Neglected child/adult
16. Abused child/adult
17. Growth and development
18. Other

Domain III. Physiological:

Functional status of processes that maintain life; appears at the first level of the Problem Classification Scheme.

19. Hearing
20. Vision
21. Speech and language
22. Dentition
23. Cognition
24. Pain
25. Consciousness
26. Integument
27. Neuro-musculo-skeletal function
28. Respiration
29. Circulation
30. Digestion-hydration
31. Bowel function
32. Genitourinary function
33. Antepartum/postpartum
34. Other

Domain IV Health-Related Behaviors: Activities that maintain or promote wellness, promote recovery, or maximize rehabilitation potential; appears at the first level of the Problem Classification Scheme.

35. Nutrition
36. Sleep and rest patterns
37. Physical activity
38. Personal hygiene
39. Substance use
40. Family planning
41. Health care supervision
42. Prescribed medication regimen
43. Technical procedure
44. Other

CATEGORIES AND TARGETS OF THE INTERVENTION SCHEME

I. Health Teaching, Guidance, and Counseling
Health teaching, guidance, and counseling are activities that range from giving information, anticipating client problems, encouraging client action and responsibility for self-care and coping, to assisting with decision making and problem solving. The overlapping concepts occur on a continuum with the variation due to the client's self-direction capabilities.

II. Treatments and Procedures
Treatments and procedures are technical activities directed toward preventing signs and symptoms, identifying risk factors and early signs and symptoms, and decreasing or alleviating signs and symptoms.

III. Case Management
Case management includes activities of coordination, advocacy, and referral. These activities involve facilitating service delivery on behalf of the client, communicating with health and human service providers, promoting assertive client communication, and guiding the client toward use of appropriate community resources.

IV. Surveillance
Surveillance includes activities of detection, measurement, critical analysis, and monitoring to indicate client status in relation to a given condition or phenomenon.

01. Anatomy/physiology
02. Behavior modification
03. Bladder care
04. Bonding
05. Bowel care
06. Bronchial hygiene
07. Cardiac care
08. Caretaking/parenting skills
09. Cast care
10. Communication
11. Coping skills
12. Day care/respite
13. Discipline
14. Dressing change/wound care
15. Durable medical equipment

16. Education
17. Employment
18. Environment
19. Exercises
20. Family planning
21. Feeding procedures
22. Finances
23. Food
24. Gait training
25. Growth/development
26. Homemaking
27. Housing
28. Interaction
29. Lab findings
30. Legal system
31. Medical/dental care
32. Medication action/side effects
33. Medication administration
34. Medication set-up
35. Mobility/transfers
36. Nursing care, supplementary
37. Nutrition
38. Nutritionist
39. Ostomy care
40. Other community resource
41. Personal care
42. Positioning
43. Rehabilitation
44. Relaxation/breathing techniques
45. Rest/sleep
46. Safety
47. Screening
48. Sickness/injury case
49. Signs/symptoms—mental/emotional
50. Signs/symptoms—physical
51. Skin care
52. Social work/counseling
53. Specimen collection
54. Spiritual care
55. Stimulation/nurturance
56. Stress management
57. Substance use
58. Supplies
59. Support group
60. Support system
61. Transportation
62. Wellness
63. Other

PROBLEM RATING SCALE FOR OUTCOMES

Concept	*1*	*2*	*3*	*4*	*5*
Knowledge: the ability of the client to remember and interpret information	No knowledge	Minimal knowledge	Basic knowledge	Adequate knowledge	Superior knowledge
Behavior: the observable responses, actions, or activities of the client fitting the occasion or purpose	Not appropriate	Rarely appropriate	Inconsistently appropriate	Usually appropriate	Consistently appropriate
Status: the condition of the client in relation to objective and subjective defining characteristics	Extreme signs/symptoms	Severe signs/symptoms	Moderate signs/symptoms	Minimal signs/symptoms	No signs/symptoms

References

Martin, K. S. (1999, Winter). The Omaha System: Past, present, and future. *On-line Journal of Nursing Informatics [on-line],* 3(1), 1–16. Available: http://cac.psu.edu/dxm12/ojni.htm

Martin, K. S., Norris, J. (1996, October). The Omaha System: A model for describing practice. *Holistic Nursing Practice,* 11(1), 75–83.

Martin, K. S., Scheet, N. J. (1992). *The Omaha System: Applications for Community Health Nursing*. Philadelphia: Saunders.

Martin, K. S., Scheet N. J. (1992). *The Omaha System: A pocket guide for community health nursing*. Philadelphia: Saunders.

APPENDIX N-7

Nursing Diagnoses*

Quick View of Contents

Appendices N7–1 and N7–2 Organize all approved NANDA nursing diagnoses by two nursing models: Gordon's Functional Health Patterns and Doenges & Moorhouse's Diagnostic Divisions. The use of a nursing model as a framework helps to organize the data needed to identify and validate nursing diagnoses.

Appendix N7–3 Lists the most recently approved NANDA nursing diagnoses for quick reference.

Appendix N7–4 Provides a guide to choosing appropriate nursing diagnoses by alphabetically listing almost 300 diseases/disorders with their commonly associated nursing diagnoses. Each of the listed diseases/disorders has been cross-referenced from its position in the body of the dictionary. The nursing diagnoses are written in the form of patient problem statements, also known as PES format (Problem, Etiology, Signs/Symptoms). The phrases "may be related to" and "possibly evidenced by" in the patient problem statements serve to help one individualize the care for the specific patient situations. A "risk for" diagnosis is not evidenced by signs and symptoms, as the problem has not occurred and nursing interventions are directed at prevention. Because the patient's health status is perpetual and ongoing, other nursing diagnoses may be appropriate based on changing patient situations. To identify other applicable nursing diagnoses, check Appendix N7–1, then turn to Appendix N7–5 to test and validate your choices.

Appendix N7–5 Details the NANDA-approved diagnoses through the 14th Conference in alphabetical order with their associated etiology [Related/Risk Factors] and signs and symptoms [Defining Characteristics]. This specific focus on assessment data/evaluation criteria helps you complete the validation process.

---

*Adapted from North American Nursing Diagnosis Association (1999). NANDA Nursing Diagnoses: Definitions and Classification 1999–2000. Philadelphia: NANDA.

Appendix N7–1 Gordon's Functional Health Patterns

HEALTH PERCEPTION—HEALTH MANAGEMENT PATTERN

- Energy Field Disturbance
- Environmental Interpretation Syndrome, impaired
- Falls, risk for
- Health Maintenance, altered
- Health-Seeking Behaviors (specify)
- Infection, risk for
- Injury, risk for
- Latex Allergy
- Latex Allergy, risk for
- Noncompliance (specify) [compliance, altered]
- Perioperative Positioning Injury, risk for
- Poisoning, risk for
- Protection, altered
- Recovery, delayed surgical
- Suffocation, risk for
- Suicide, risk for
- Therapeutic Regimen (Community), ineffective management of
- Therapeutic Regimen (Families), ineffective management of
- Therapeutic Regimen (Individual), effective management of
- Therapeutic Regimen (Individual), ineffective management of
- Trauma, risk for
- Wandering (specify sporadic or continual)

NUTRITIONAL—METABOLIC PATTERN

- Aspiration, risk for
- Body Temperature, altered, risk for
- Breastfeeding, effective
- Breastfeeding, ineffective
- Breastfeeding, interrupted
- Dentition, altered
- Fluid Volume Deficit [active loss]
- Fluid Volume Deficit [regulatory failure]
- Fluid Volume Deficit, risk for
- Fluid Volume Excess
- Fluid Volume Imbalance, risk for
- Infant Feeding Pattern, ineffective
- Nausea
- Nutrition: altered, less than body requirements
- Nutrition: altered, more than body requirements
- Nutrition: altered, risk for more than body requirements
- Oral Mucous Membrane, altered
- Skin Integrity, impaired
- Skin Integrity, impaired, risk for
- Swallowing, impaired
- Thermoregulation, ineffective
- Tissue Integrity, impaired

ELIMINATION PATTERN

- Bowel Incontinence
- Constipation
- Constipation, perceived
- Constipation, risk for
- Diarrhea
- Failure to Thrive, Adult
- Growth, risk for altered
- Hyperthermia
- Hypothermia
- Incontinence, functional
- Incontinence, reflex
- Incontinence, stress
- Incontinence, total
- Incontinence, urge
- Urinary Elimination, altered
- Urinary Retention [acute/chronic]

ACTIVITY—EXERCISE PATTERN

- Activity Intolerance [specify level]
- Activity Intolerance, risk for
- Airway Clearance, ineffective
- Breathing Pattern, ineffective
- Cardiac Output, decreased
- Development, Altered, risk for
- Disorganized Infant Behavior
- Disorganized Infant Behavior, risk for
- Disuse Syndrome, risk for
- Diversional Activity Deficit
- Dysreflexia
- Dysreflexia, Autonomic, risk for
- Enhanced Organized Infant Behavior, potential for
- Fatigue
- Gas Exchange, impaired
- Growth and Development, altered
- Home Maintenance Management, impaired
- Injury, Preoperative Positioning, risk for
- Mobility, Bed, impaired
- Mobility, Wheelchair, impaired
- Peripheral Neurovascular Dysfunction, risk for
- Physical Mobility, impaired
- Self-Care Deficit [specify level]: feeding, bathing/hygiene, dressing/ grooming, toileting
- Spontaneous Ventilation, inability to sustain
- Tissue Perfusion, altered (specify): cerebral, cardiopulmonary, renal, gastrointestinal, peripheral
- Ventilatory Weaning Response, dysfunctional (DVWR)
- Walking, impaired
- Wheelchair Transfer Ability, impaired

SLEEP—REST PATTERN

- Sleep Deprivation
- Sleep Pattern Disturbance

COGNITIVE—PERCEPTUAL PATTERN

- Adaptive Capacity: intracranial, decreased
- Confusion, Acute
- Confusion, Chronic
- Decisional Conflict

Knowledge Deficit [learning need] (specify)
Memory, impaired
Pain
Pain, acute
Pain, chronic
Sensory/Perceptual Alterations (specify): visual, auditory, kinesthetic, gustatory, tactile, olfactory
Thought Processes, altered
Unilateral Neglect

SELF-PERCEPTION—SELF-CONCEPT PATTERN
Anxiety [Mild, Moderate, Severe, Panic]
Anxiety, Death
Body Image Disturbance
Fear
Hopelessness
Loneliness, risk for
Personal Identity Disturbance
Powerlessness
Powerlessness, risk for
Self-Esteem, chronic low
Self-Esteem Disturbance
Self-Esteem, situational low
Self-Esteem, situational low, risk for
Self-Mutilation
Self-Mutilation, risk for

ROLE—RELATIONSHIP PATTERN
Caregiver Role Strain
Caregiver Role Strain, risk for
Communication, impaired, verbal
Family process, altered: alcoholism [substance abuse]
Family processes, altered
Grieving, anticipatory
Grieving, dysfunctional
Parental Role Conflict
Parent/Infant/Child Attachment, altered, risk for
Parenting, altered
Parenting, altered, risk for
Relocation Stress Syndrome
Relocation Stress Syndrome, risk for
Role Performance, altered
Social Interaction, impaired
Social Isolation
Sorrow, Chronic
Violence, Directed at Others, risk for
Violence, Self-Directed, risk for

SEXUALITY—REPRODUCTIVE PATTERN
Rape-Trauma Syndrome [specify]
Rape-Trauma Syndrome: compound reaction
Rape-Trauma Syndrome: silent reaction
Sexual Dysfunction
Sexuality Patterns, altered

COPING—STRESS TOLERANCE PATTERN
Adjustment, impaired
Community Coping, Enhanced, potential for
Community Coping, ineffective
Coping, defensive
Coping, individual, ineffective
Denial, ineffective
Family Coping, ineffective: compromised
Family Coping, ineffective: disabling
Family Coping: potential for growth
Post-Trauma Response [specify stage]
Post-Trauma Syndrome, risk for
Violence, Directed at Others, risk for
Violence, Self-directed, risk for

VALUE—BELIEF PATTERN
Spiritual Distress (distress of the human spirit)
Spiritual Distress, risk for
Spiritual Well-Being, enhanced, potential for

NOTE: Information appearing in brackets has been added to clarify and facilitate the use of nursing diagnoses.
SOURCE: Adapted from Gordon, M: Manual of Nursing Diagnosis, 1995–1996. St. Louis, Mosby-Year Book, Inc., 1995.

Appendix N7–2 Doenges & Moorhouse's Diagnostic Divisions

ACTIVITY/REST
Activity Intolerance [specify level]
Activity Intolerance, risk for
Disuse Syndrome, risk for
Diversional Activity Deficit
Fatigue
Mobility, Bed, impaired
Mobility, Wheelchair, impaired
Sleep Deprivation
Sleep Pattern Disturbance
Transfer ability, impaired
Walking, impaired

CIRCULATION
Adaptive Capacity: intracranial, decreased
Cardiac Output, decreased
[Autonomic] Dysreflexia
Dysreflexia, Autonomic, risk for
Tissue Perfusion, altered (specify): cerebral, cardiopulmonary, renal, gastrointestinal, peripheral

EGO INTEGRITY
Adjustment, impaired
Anxiety [Mild, Moderate, Severe, Panic]

Anxiety, death
Body Image Disturbance
Coping, defensive
Coping, individual, ineffective
Decisional Conflict
Denial, ineffective
Energy Field Disturbance
Fear
Grieving, anticipatory
Grieving, dysfunctional
Hopelessness
Personal Identity Disturbance
Post-Trauma Syndrome
Post-Trauma Syndrome, risk for
Powerlessness
Powerlessness, risk for
Rape-Trauma Syndrome [specify]
Rape-Trauma Syndrome: compound reaction
Rape-Trauma Syndrome: silent reaction
Relocation Stress Syndrome
Relocation Stress Syndrome, risk for
Self-Esteem, chronic low
Self-Esteem Disturbance
Self-Esteem, situational low
Self-Esteem, situational low, risk for
Sorrow, Chronic
Spiritual Distress (distress of the human spirit)
Spiritual Distress, risk for
Spiritual Well-Being, enhanced, potential for

ELIMINATION
Bowel Incontinence
Constipation
Constipation, perceived
Constipation, risk for
Diarrhea
Incontinence, functional
Incontinence, reflex
Incontinence, stress
Incontinence, total
Incontinence, urge
Incontinence urge, risk for
Urinary Elimination, altered patterns of
Urinary Retention [acute/chronic]

FOOD/FLUID
Breastfeeding, effective
Breastfeeding, ineffective
Breastfeeding, interrupted
Dentition, altered
Failure to Thrive, Adult
Fluid Volume Deficit [hyper/hypotonic]
Fluid Volume Deficit [isotonic]
Fluid Volume Deficit, risk for
Fluid Volume Excess
Infant Feeding Pattern, ineffective
Nutrition: altered, less than body requirements
Nutrition: altered, more than body requirements
Nutrition: altered, risk for more than body requirements
Oral Mucous Membrane, altered
Swallowing, impaired

HYGIENE
Self-Care Deficit [specify level]: feeding, bathing/hygiene, dressing/grooming, toileting

NEUROSENSORY
Confusion, acute
Confusion, chronic
Disorganized Infant Behavior
Disorganized Infant Behavior, risk for
Enhanced Organized Infant Behavior, potential for
Memory, impaired
Peripheral Neurovascular Dysfunction, risk for
Sensory/Perceptual Alterations (specify): visual, auditory, kinesthetic, gustatory, tactile, olfactory
Thought Processes, altered
Unilateral Neglect

PAIN/DISCOMFORT
Pain [acute]
Pain, chronic

RESPIRATION
Airway Clearance, ineffective
Aspiration, risk for
Breathing Pattern, ineffective
Gas Exchange, impaired
Spontaneous Ventilation, inability to sustain
Ventilatory Weaning Response, dysfunctional (DVWR)

SAFETY
Body Temperature, altered, risk for
Environmental Interpretation Syndrome, impaired
Falls, risk for
Health Maintenance, altered
Home Maintenance Management, impaired
Hyperthermia
Hypothermia
Infection, risk for
Injury, risk for
Latex Allergy
Latex Allergy, risk for
Perioperative Positioning Injury, risk for
Physical Mobility, impaired
Poisoning, risk for
Protection, altered
Self-Mutilation
Self-Mutilation, risk for
Skin Integrity, impaired
Skin Integrity, impaired, risk for
Suffocation, risk for
Suicide, risk for
Surgical Recovery, Delayed
Thermoregulation, ineffective
Tissue Integrity, impaired
Trauma, risk for
Violence, [actual/] risk for, directed at others
Violence, [actual/] risk for, self-directed

SEXUALITY [Component of Ego Integrity and Social Interaction]
- Sexual Dysfunction
- Sexuality Patterns, altered

SOCIAL INTERACTION
- Caregiver Role Strain
- Caregiver Role Strain, risk for
- Communication, impaired, verbal
- Community Coping, enhanced, potential for
- Community Coping, ineffective
- Family Coping, ineffective: compromised
- Family Coping, ineffective: disabling
- Family Coping: potential for growth
- Family Process, altered: alcoholism [substance abuse]
- Family Processes, altered
- Loneliness, risk for
- Parental Role Conflict
- Parent/Infant/Child Attachment, altered, risk for
- Parenting, altered
- Parenting, altered, risk for
- Role Performance, altered
- Social Interaction, impaired
- Social Isolation

TEACHING/LEARNING
- Growth and Development, altered
- Health-Seeking Behaviors (specify)
- Knowledge Deficit [learning need] (specify)
- Noncompliance (specify) [compliance, altered]
- Therapeutic Regimen (Community), ineffective management of
- Therapeutic Regimen (Families), ineffective management of
- Therapeutic Regimen (Individual), effective management of
- Therapeutic Regimen (Individual), ineffective management of

SOURCE: Adapted from Doenges, M. E., and Moorhouse, M. F.: Nurse's Pocket Guide: Nursing Diagnoses with Interventions, ed. 5, F. A. Davis, Philadelphia, 1995, with permission.

Appendix N7–3 Nursing Diagnoses Approved at the 14th NANDA Conference

NANDA 14th Conference, 2000 (Approved)

- Falls, risk for
- Parent-Infant Attachment, risk for insecure
- Powerlessness, risk for
- Relocation Stress Syndrome, risk for
- Self-Esteem, risk for situational low
- Self-Mutilation
- Suicide, risk for
- Wandering (specify sporadic or continual)

Appendix N7–4 Nursing Diagnoses Grouped by Diseases/Disorders

abortion, spontaneous

Fluid volume deficit [isotonic] may be related to excessive blood loss, possibly evidenced by decreased pulse volume and pressure, delayed capillary refill, or changes in sensorium.

Spiritual Distress, risk for: risk factors may include need to adhere to personal religious beliefs/practices, blame for loss directed at self or God.

Knowledge deficit [Learning Need] regarding cause of abortion, self-care, contraception/future pregnancy may be related to lack of familiarity with new self/health-care needs, sources for support, possibly evidenced by requests for information and statement of concern/misconceptions, development of preventable complications.

Grieving [expected] related to perinatal loss, possibly evidenced by crying, expressions of sorrow, or changes in eating habits/sleep patterns.

Sexuality patterns, risk for altered: risk factors may include increasing fear of pregnancy and/or repeat loss, impaired relationship with significant other(s), self-doubt regarding own femininity.

abruptio placentae

Fluid volume deficit [isotonic] may be related to excessive blood loss, possibly evidenced by hypotension, increased heart rate, decreased pulse volume and pressure, delayed capillary refill, or changes in sensorium.

Fear related to threat of death (perceived or actual) to fetus/self, possibly evidenced by verbalization of specific concerns, increased tension, sympathetic stimulation.

Pain, [acute] may be related to collection of blood between uterine wall and placenta, possibly evidenced by verbal reports, abdominal guarding, muscle tension, or alterations in vital signs.

Gas exchange, impaired fetal may be related to altered uteroplacental oxygen transfer, possibly evidenced by alterations in fetal heart rate and movement.

abscess, brain (acute)

Pain [acute] may be related to inflammation, edema of tissues, possibly evidenced by reports of headache, restlessness, irritability, and moaning.

Hyperthermia, risk for: risk factors may include inflammatory process/hypermetabolic state and dehydration.

Confusion, acute may be related to physiologic changes (e.g., cerebral edema/altered perfusion, fever), possibly evidenced by fluctuation in cognition/level of consciousness, increased agitation/restlessness, hallucinations.

Suffocation/Trauma, risk for: risk factors may include development of clonic/tonic muscle activity and changes in consciousness (seizure activity).

achalasia

Swallowing, impaired may be related to neuromuscular impairment, possibly evidenced by observed difficulty in swallowing or regurgitation.

Nutrition: altered, less than body requirements may be related to inability and/or reluctance to ingest adequate nutrients to meet metabolic demands/nutritional needs, possibly evidenced by reported/observed inadequate intake, weight loss, and pale conjunctiva and mucous membranes.

Pain [acute] may be related to spasm of the lower esophageal sphincter, possibly evidenced by reports of substernal pressure, recurrent heartburn, or gastric fullness (gas pains).

Anxiety [specify level]/Fear may be related to recurrent pain, choking sensation, altered health status, possibly evidenced by verbalizations of distress, apprehension, restlessness, or insomnia.

Aspiration, risk for: risk factors may include regurgitation/spillover of esophageal contents.

Knowledge deficit [Learning Need] regarding condition, prognosis, self-care, and treatment needs may be related to lack of familiarity with pathology and treatment of condition, possibly evidenced by requests for information, statement of concern, or development of preventable complications.

acidosis, metabolic

Refer to *diabetic ketoacidosis*.

acute respiratory distress syndrome (ARDS)

Airway Clearance, ineffective may be related to loss of ciliary action, increased amount and viscosity of secretions, and increased airway resistance, possibly evidenced by presence of dyspnea, changes in depth/rate of respiration, use of accessory muscles for breathing, wheezes/crackles, cough with or without sputum production.

Gas Exchange, impaired may be related to changes in pulmonary capillary permeability with edema formation, alveolar hypoventilation and collapse, with intrapulmonary shunting; possibly evidenced by tachypnea, use of accessory muscles, cyanosis, hypoxia per arterial blood gases (ABGs)/oximetry; anxiety and changes in mentation.

Fluid Volume, risk for deficit: risk factors may include active loss from diuretic use and restricted intake.

Cardiac Output, risk for decreased: risk factors may include alteration in preload (hypovolemia, vascular pooling, diuretic therapy, and increased intrathoracic pressure/use of ventilator/positive end-expiratory pressure, PEEP).

Anxiety [specify level]/Fear may be related to physiologic factors (effects of hypoxemia); situational crisis, change in health status/threat of death; possibly evidenced by increased tension, apprehension, restlessness, focus on self, and sympathetic stimulation.

Injury, risk for barotrauma: risk factors may include increased airway pressure associated with mechanical ventilation (PEEP).

Addison's disease

Fluid Volume deficit [hypotonic] may be related to vomiting, diarrhea, increased renal

losses, possibly evidenced by delayed capillary refill, poor skin turgor, dry mucous membranes, report of thirst.
Cardiac Output, decreased may be related to hypovolemia and altered electrical conduction (dysrhythmias) and/or diminished cardiac muscle mass, possibly evidenced by alterations in vital signs, changes in mentation, and irregular pulse or pulse deficit.
Fatigue may be related to decreased metabolic energy production, altered body chemistry (fluid, electrolyte, and glucose imbalance), possibly evidenced by unremitting overwhelming lack of energy, inability to maintain usual routines, decreased performance, impaired ability to concentrate, lethargy, and disinterest in surroundings.
Body Image Disturbance may be related to changes in skin pigmentation and mucous membranes, loss of axillary/pubic hair, possibly evidenced by verbalization of negative feelings about body and decreased social involvement.
Mobility, risk for impaired physical: risk factors may include neuromuscular impairment (muscle wasting/weakness) and dizziness/syncope.
Nutrition: altered, less than body requirements may be related to glucocorticoid deficiency; abnormal fat, protein, and carbohydrate metabolism; nausea, vomiting, anorexia, possibly evidenced by weight loss, muscle wasting, abdominal cramps, diarrhea, and severe hypoglycemia.
Home Maintenance Management, risk for impaired: risk factors may include effects of disease process, impaired cognitive functioning, and inadequate support systems.

adenoidectomy

Anxiety [specify level]/Fear may be related to separation from supportive others, unfamiliar surroundings, and perceived threat of injury/abandonment, possibly evidenced by crying, apprehension, trembling, and sympathetic stimulation (pupil dilation, increased heart rate).
Airway Clearance, risk for ineffective: risk factors may include sedation, collection of secretions/blood in oropharynx, and vomiting.
Fluid Volume, risk for deficit: risk factors may include operative trauma to highly vascular site/hemorrhage.
Pain [acute] may be related to physical trauma to oronasopharynx, presence of packing, possibly evidenced by restlessness, crying, and facial mask of pain.

adrenalectomy

Tissue Perfusion, altered (specify) may be related to hypovolemia and vascular pooling (vasodilation), possibly evidenced by diminished pulse, pallor/cyanosis, hypotension, and changes in mentation.
Infection, risk for: risk factors may include inadequate primary defenses (incision, traumatized tissues), suppressed inflammatory response, invasive procedures.
Knowledge deficit [Learning Need] regarding condition, prognosis, self-care and treatment needs may be related to unfamiliarity with long-term therapy requirements, possibly evidenced by request for information and statement of concern/misconceptions.

adult respiratory distress syndrome (ARDS)

Refer to *acute respiratory distress syndrome*

affective disorder

Refer to *bipolar disorder* and *depressive disorders, major depression*.

AIDS (acquired immunodeficiency syndrome)

Infection, risk for progression to sepsis/onset of new opportunistic infection: risk factors may include depressed immune system, use of antimicrobial agents, inadequate primary defenses; broken skin, traumatized tissue; malnutrition, and chronic disease processes.
Fluid Volume, risk for deficit: risk factors may include excessive losses: copious diarrhea, profuse sweating, vomiting, hypermetabolic state or fever; and restriction intake (nausea, anorexia; lethargy).
Pain [acute]/chronic may be related to tissue inflammation/destruction: infections, internal/external cutaneous lesions, rectal excoriation, malignancies, necrosis, peripheral neuropathies, myalgias, and arthralgias, possibly evidenced by verbal reports, self-focusing/narrowed focus, alteration in muscle tone, paresthesias, paralysis, guarding behaviors, changes in vital signs (acute), autonomic responses, and restlessness.
Nutrition: altered, less than body requirements may be related to altered ability to ingest, digest, and/or absorb nutrients (nausea/vomiting, hyperactive gag reflex, intestinal disturbances); increased metabolic activity/nutritional needs (fever, infection), possibly evidenced by weight loss, decreased subcutaneous fat/muscle mass; lack of interest in food/aversion to eating, altered taste sensation; abdominal cramping, hyperactive bowel sounds, diarrhea, sore and inflamed buccal cavity.

Fatigue may be related to decreased metabolic energy production, increased energy requirements (hypermetabolic state), overwhelming psychological/emotional demands; altered body chemistry (side effects of medication, chemotherapy), possibly evidenced by unremitting/overwhelming lack of energy, inability to maintain usual routines, decreased performance; impaired ability to concentrate, lethargy/restlessness, and disinterest in surroundings.

Protection, altered may be related to chronic disease affecting immune and neurological systems, inadequate nutrition, drug therapies, possibly evidenced by deficient immunity, impaired healing, neurosensory alterations, maladaptive stress response, fatigue, anorexia, disorientation.

Social isolation may be related to changes in physical appearance/mental status, state of wellness, perceptions of unacceptable social or sexual behavior/values, physical isolation, phobic fear of others (transmission of disease); possibly evidenced by expressed feelings of aloneness/rejection, absence of supportive significant other(s)—(SOSs), and withdrawal from usual activities.

Thought Processes, altered/Confusion, chronic: may be related to physiologic changes (hypoxemia, central nervous system [CNS] infection by HIV, brain malignancies, and/or disseminated systemic opportunistic infection); altered drug metabolism/excretion, accumulation of toxic elements (renal failure, severe electrolyte imbalance, hepatic insufficiency), possibly evidenced by clinical evidence of organic impairment, altered attention span, distractibility, memory deficit, disorientation, cognitive dissonance, delusional thinking, impaired ability to make decisions/problem solve, inability to follow complex commands/mental tasks, loss of impulse control and altered personality.

aldosteronism, primary

Fluid Volume deficit [isotonic] may be related to increased urinary losses, possibly evidenced by dry mucous membranes, poor skin turgor, dilute urine, excessive thirst, weight loss.

Mobility impaired physical may be related to neuromuscular impairment, weakness, and pain, possibly evidenced by impaired coordination, decreased muscle strength, paralysis, and positive Chvostek's and Trousseau's signs.

Cardiac Output, risk for decreased: risk factors may include hypovolemia and altered electrical conduction/dysrhythmias.

Alzheimer's disease

(Also refer to *dementia, presenile / senile*)

Injury/Trauma, risk for: risk factors may include inability to recognize/identify danger in environment, disorientation, confusion, impaired judgment, weakness, muscular incoordination, balancing difficulties, and altered perception.

Confusion, chronic related to physiological changes (neuronal degeneration); possibly evidenced by inaccurate interpretation of/response to stimuli, progressive/long-standing cognitive impairment, short-term memory deficit, impaired socialization, altered personality, and clinical evidence of organic impairment.

Sensory/Perceptual alterations: (specify) may be related to altered sensory reception, transmission, and/or integration (neurologic disease/deficit), socially restricted environment (homebound/institutionalized), sleep deprivation possibly evidenced by changes in usual response to stimuli, change in problem-solving abilities, exaggerated emotional responses (anxiety, paranoia, hallucinations), inability to tell position of body parts, diminished/altered sense of taste.

Sleep Pattern disturbance may be related to sensory impairment, changes in activity patterns, psychological stress (neurologic impairment), possibly evidenced by wakefulness, disorientation (day/night reversal); increased aimless wandering, inability to identify need/time for sleeping, changes in behavior/performance, lethargy; dark circles under eyes and frequent yawning.

Health maintenance, altered may be related to deterioration affecting ability in all areas including coordination/communication, cognitive impairment; ineffective individual/family coping, possibly evidenced by reported or observed inability to take responsibility for meeting basic health practices, lack of equipment/financial or other resources, and impairment of personal support system.

Family coping, ineffective: compromised/Caregiver Role Strain may be related to family disorganization, role changes, family/caregiver isolation, long-term illness/complexity and amount of homecare needs exhausting supportive/financial capabilities of family member(s), lack of respite; possibly evidenced by verbalizations of frustrations in dealing with day-to-day care, reports of conflict, feelings of depression, expressed anger/guilt directed toward patient, and withdrawal from interaction with patient/social contacts.

Relocation Stress Syndrome, risk for: risk factors may include little or no preparation for transfer to a new setting, changes in daily routine, sensory impairment, physical deterioration, separation from support systems.

amputation

Tissue Perfusion, risk for altered: peripheral: risk factors may include reduced arterial/venous blood flow; tissue edema, hematoma formation; hypovolemia.

Pain [acute] may be related to tissue and nerve trauma, psychological impact of loss of body part, possibly evidenced by reports of incisional/phantom pain, guarding/protective behavior, narrowed/self-focus, and autonomic responses.

Mobility, impaired physical may be related to loss of limb (primarily lower extremity), altered sense of balance, pain/discomfort, possibly evidenced by reluctance to attempt movement, impaired coordination; decreased muscle strength, control, and mass.

Body Image disturbance may be related to loss of a body part, possibly evidenced by verbalization of feelings of powerlessness, grief, preoccupation with loss, and unwillingness to look at/touch stump.

amyotrophic lateral sclerosis (ALS)

Mobility, impaired physical may be related to muscle wasting/weakness, possibly evidenced by impaired coordination, limited range of motion, and impaired purposeful movement.

Breathing Pattern, ineffective/Spontaneous Ventilation, inability to sustain may be related to neuromuscular impairment, decreased energy, fatigue, tracheobronchial obstruction, possibly evidenced by shortness of breath, fremitus, respiratory depth changes, and reduced vital capacity.

Swallowing, impaired may be related to muscle wasting and fatigue, possibly evidenced by recurrent coughing/choking and signs of aspiration.

Powerlessness [specify level] may be related to chronic/debilitating nature of illness, lack of control over outcome, possibly evidenced by expressions of frustration about inability to care for self and depression over physical deterioration.

Grieving, anticipatory may be related to perceived potential loss of self/physiopsychosocial well-being, possibly evidenced by sorrow, choked feelings, expression of distress, changes in eating habits/sleeping patterns, and altered communication patterns/libido.

Communication, impaired verbal may be related to physical barrier (neuromuscular impairment), possibly evidenced by impaired articulation, inability to speak in sentences, and use of nonverbal cues (changes in facial expression).

Caregiver Role Strain, risk for: risk factors may include illness severity of care receiver, complexity and amount of home-care needs, duration of caregiving required, caregiver is spouse, family/caregiver isolation, lack of respite/recreation for caregiver.

anemia

Activity Intolerance may be related to imbalance between oxygen supply (delivery) and demand, possibly evidenced by reports of fatigue and weakness, abnormal heart rate or blood pressure (BP) response, decreased exercise/activity level, and exertional discomfort or dyspnea.

Nutrition: altered, less than body requirements may be related to failure to ingest/inability to digest food or absorb nutrients necessary for formation of normal red blood cells (RBCs); possibly evidenced by weight loss/weight below normal for age, height, body build; decreased triceps skinfold measurement, changes in gums/oral mucous membranes; decreased tolerance for activity, weakness, and loss of muscle tone.

Knowledge deficit [Learning Need] regarding condition, prognosis, self-care and treatment needs may be related to inadequate understanding or misinterpretation of dietary/physiologic needs, possibly evidenced by inadequate dietary intake, request for information, and development of preventable complications.

anemia, sickle cell

Gas Exchange, impaired may be related to decreased oxygen-carrying capacity of blood, reduced RBC life span, abnormal RBC structure, increased blood viscosity, predisposition to bacterial pneumonia/pulmonary infarcts, possibly evidenced by dyspnea, use of accessory muscles, cyanosis/signs of hypoxia, tachycardia, changes in mentation, and restlessness.

Tissue Perfusion, altered: (specify) may be related to stasis, vaso-occlusive nature of sickling, inflammatory response, atrioventricular (AV) shunts in pulmonary and peripheral circulation, myocardial damage (small infarcts, iron deposits, fibrosis), possibly evidenced by signs and symptoms dependent on system involved, for example, renal: decreased specific gravity and pale urine in face of dehydration; cerebral: paralysis and visual disturbances; peripheral: distal ischemia, tissue infarctions, ulcerations, bone pain; cardiopulmonary: angina, palpitations.

Pain [acute]/chronic may be related to intravascular sickling with localized vascular stasis, occlusion, infarction/necrosis, deprivation of oxygen and nutrients, accumulation of noxious metabolites, possibly evidenced by reports of localized, generalized, or migratory joint and/or abdominal/back pain; guarding and distraction behaviors (moaning, crying, restlessness), facial grimacing, narrowed focus, and autonomic responses.

Knowledge deficit [Learning Need] regarding disease process, genetic factors, prognosis, self-care and treatment needs may be related to lack of exposure/recall, misinterpretation of information, unfamiliarity with resources, possibly evidenced by questions, statement of concern/misconceptions, exacerbation of condition, inadequate follow-through of therapy instructions, and development of preventable complications.

Growth and Development, altered may be related to effects of physical condition, possibly evidenced by altered physical growth and delay/difficulty performing skills typical of age group.

Family Coping, ineffective: compromised may be related to chronic nature of disease/disability, family disorganization, presence of other crises/situations impacting significant person/parent, lifestyle restrictions, possibly evidenced by significant person/parent expressing preoccupation with own reaction and displaying protective behavior disproportionate to patient's ability or need for autonomy.

angina pectoris

Pain [acute] may be related to decreased myocardial blood flow, increased cardiac workload/oxygen consumption, possibly evidenced by verbal reports, narrowed focus, distraction behaviors (restlessness, moaning), and autonomic responses (diaphoresis, changes in vital signs).

Cardiac Output, decreased may be related to inotropic changes (transient/prolonged myocardial ischemia, effects of medications), alterations in rate/rhythm and electrical conduction, possibly evidenced by changes in hemodynamic readings, dyspnea, restlessness, decreased tolerance for activity, fatigue, diminished peripheral pulses, cool/pale skin, changes in mental status, and continued chest pain.

Anxiety [specify level] may be related to situational crises, change in health status and/or threat of death, negative self-talk possibly evidenced by verbalized apprehension, facial tension, extraneous movements, and focus on self.

Activity Intolerance may be related to imbalance between oxygen supply and demand, possibly evidenced by exertional dyspnea, abnormal pulse/BP response to activity, and electrocardiogram (ECG) changes.

Knowledge deficit [Learning Need] regarding condition, prognosis, self-care and treatment needs may be related to lack of exposure, inaccurate/misinterpretation of information, possibly evidenced by questions, request for information, statement of concern, and inaccurate follow-through of instructions.

Adjustment, risk for impaired: risk factors may include condition requiring long-term therapy/change in lifestyle, assault to self-concept, and altered locus of control.

anorexia nervosa

Nutrition: altered, less than body requirements may be related to psychological restrictions of food intake and/or excessive activity, self-induced vomiting, laxative abuse, possibly evidenced by weight loss, poor skin turgor/muscle tone, denial of hunger, unusual hoarding or handling of food, amenorrhea, electrolyte imbalance, cardiac irregularities, hypotension.

Fluid Volume, risk for deficit: risk factors may include inadequate intake of food and liquids, chronic/excessive laxative or diuretic use, self-induced vomiting.

Thought Processes, altered may be related to severe malnutrition/electrolyte imbalance, psychological conflicts; possibly evidenced by impaired ability to make decisions, problem-solve, non–reality-based verbalizations, ideas of reference, altered sleep patterns, altered attention span/distractibility; perceptual disturbances with failure to recognize hunger, fatigue, anxiety, and depression.

Body Image disturbance/Self-esteem, chronic low may be related to altered perception of body, perceived loss of control in some aspect of life, unmet dependency needs, personal vulnerability, dysfunctional family system, possibly evidenced by negative feelings, distorted view of body, use of denial, feeling powerless to prevent/make changes, expressions of shame/guilt, overly conforming, dependent on others' opinions.

Family Processes, altered may be related to ambivalent family relationships and ways of transacting issues of control, situational/maturational crises possibly evidenced by enmeshed family, dissonance among family members, family developmental tasks not being met, family members acting as enablers.

anxiety disorder, generalized

Anxiety [specify level]/Powerlessness may be related to real or perceived threat to physical integrity or self-concept (may or may not be able to identify the threat), unconscious conflict about essential values/beliefs and goals of life, unmet needs, negative self-talk, possibly evidenced by sympathetic stimulation, extraneous movements (foot shuffling, hand/arm fidgeting, rocking movements, restlessness), persistent feelings of apprehension and uneasiness, a general anxious feeling that patient has difficulty alleviating, poor eye contact, focus on self, impaired functioning, free-floating anxiety, and nonparticipation in decision making.

Coping, Individual, ineffective may be related to level of anxiety being experienced by the patient, personal vulnerability; unmet expectations/unrealistic perceptions, inadequate coping methods and/or support systems possibly evidenced by verbalization of inability to cope/problem-solve, excessive compulsive behaviors (e.g. smoking, drinking), and emotional/muscle tension, alteration in societal participation, high rate of accidents.

Sleep pattern disturbance may be related to psychological stress, repetitive thoughts, possibly evidenced by reports of difficulty in falling asleep/awakening earlier or later than desired, reports of not feeling rested, dark circles under eyes, and frequent yawning.

Family Coping, ineffective: risk for compromised: risk factors may include inadequate/incorrect information or understanding by a primary person, temporary family disorganization and role changes, prolonged disability that exhausts the supportive capacity of significant other(s).

Social Interaction, impaired/Social Isolation may be related to low self-concept, inadequate personal resources, misinterpretation of internal/external stimuli, hypervigilance possibly evidenced by discomfort in social situations, withdrawal from or reported change in pattern of interactions, dysfunctional interactions; expressed feelings of difference from others; sad, dull affect.

aortic stenosis

Cardiac Output, decreased may be related to structural changes of heart valve, left ventricular outflow obstruction, alteration of afterload (increased left ventricular end-diastolic pressure and systemic vascular resistance—SVR), alteration in preload/increased atrial pressure and venous congestion, alteration in electrical conduction, possibly evidenced by fatigue, dyspnea, changes in vital signs/hemodynamic parameters, and syncope.

Gas Exchange, risk for impaired: risk factors may include alveolar-capillary membrane changes/congestion.

Pain [acute], risk for: risk factors may include episodic ischemia of myocardial tissues and stretching of left atrium.

Activity intolerance may be related to imbalance between oxygen supply and demand (decreased/fixed cardiac output), possibly evidenced by exertional dyspnea, reported fatigue/weakness, and abnormal blood pressure or ECG changes/dysrhythmias in response to activity.

appendicitis

Pain [acute] may be related to distention of intestinal tissues by inflammation, possibly evidenced by verbal reports, guarding behavior, narrowed focus, and autonomic responses (diaphoresis, changes in vital signs).

Fluid Volume, risk for deficit: risk factors may include nausea, vomiting, anorexia, and hypermetabolic state.

Infection, risk for: risk factors may include release of pathogenic organisms into peritoneal cavity.

arrhythmia, cardiac

Refer to *dysrhythmia, cardiac*.

arthritis, juvenile rheumatoid

(also refer to *arthritis, rheumatoid*)

Development, risk for altered: risk factors may include effects of physical disability and required therapy.

Social Isolation, risk for: risk factors may include delay in accomplishing developmental task, altered state of wellness, and changes in physical appearance.

arthritis, rheumatoid

Pain, [acute]/chronic may be related to accumulation of fluid/inflammatory process, degeneration of joint, and deformity, possibly evidenced by verbal reports, narrowed focus, guarding/protective behaviors, and physical and social withdrawal.

Mobility, impaired physical, may be related to musculoskeletal deformity, pain/discomfort, decreased muscle strength, possibly evidenced by limited range of motion, impaired coordination, reluctance to attempt movement, and decreased muscle strength/control and mass.

Self-Care deficit [specify] may be related to musculoskeletal impairment, decreased strength/endurance and range of motion, pain on movement, possibly evidenced by inability to manage activities of daily living (ADLs).

Body Image disturbance/Role Performance, altered may be related to change in body structure/function, impaired mobility/ability to perform usual tasks, focus on past strength/function/appearance, possibly evidenced by negative self-talk, feeling of helplessness, change in lifestyle/physical abilities, dependence on others for assistance, decreased social involvement.

arthroplasty

Infection, risk for: risk factors may include breach of primary defenses (surgical incision), stasis of body fluids at operative site, and altered inflammatory response.

Fluid Volume, risk for deficit: risk factors may include surgical procedure/trauma to vascular area.

Mobility, impaired physical may be related to decreased strength, pain, musculoskeletal changes, possibly evidenced by impaired coordination and reluctance to attempt movement.

Pain [acute] may be related to tissue trauma, local edema, possibly evidenced by verbal reports, narrowed focus, guarded movement, and autonomic responses (diaphoresis, changes in vital signs).

arthroscopy

Knowledge deficit [Learning Need] regarding procedure/outcomes and self-care needs may be related to unfamiliarity with information/resources, misinterpretations, possibly evidenced by questions and requests for information, misconceptions.

asthma

(also refer to *emphysema*)

Airway clearance, ineffective may be related to increased production/retained pulmonary secretions, bronchospasm, decreased energy/fatigue, possibly evidenced by wheezing, difficulty breathing, changes in depth/rate of respirations, use of accessory muscles, and persistent ineffective cough with or without sputum production.

Gas exchange, impaired may be related to altered delivery of inspired oxygen/air trapping, possibly evidenced by dyspnea, restlessness, reduced tolerance for activity, cyanosis, and changes in ABGs and vital signs.

Anxiety [specify level] may be related to perceived threat of death, possibly evidenced by apprehension, fearful expression, and extraneous movements.

Activity Intolerance may be related to imbalance between oxygen supply and demand, possibly evidenced by fatigue and exertional dyspnea.

athlete's foot

Skin Integrity, impaired may be related to fungal invasion, humidity, secretions, possibly evidenced by disruption of skin surface, reports of painful itching.

Infection, risk for spread: risk factors may include multiple breaks in skin, exposure to moist/warm environment.

autistic disorder

Social Interaction, impaired may be related to abnormal response to sensory input/inadequate sensory stimulation, organic brain dysfunction; delayed development of secure attachment/trust, lack of intuitive skills to comprehend and accurately respond to social cues, disturbance in self-concept, possibly evidenced by lack of responsiveness to others, lack of eye contact or facial responsiveness, treating persons as objects, lack of awareness of feelings in others, indifference/aversion to comfort, affection, or physical contact; failure to develop cooperative social play and peer friendships in childhood.

Communication, impaired verbal may be related to inability to trust others, withdrawal into self, organic brain dysfunction, abnormal interpretation/response to and/or inadequate sensory stimulation, possibly evidenced by lack of interactive communication mode, no use of gestures or spoken language, absent or abnormal nonverbal communication; lack of eye contact or facial expression; peculiar patterns of speech (form, content, or speech production), and impaired ability to initiate or sustain conversation despite adequate speech.

Self-Mutilation, risk for: risk factors may include organic brain dysfunction, inability to trust others, disturbance in self-concept, inadequate sensory stimulation or abnormal response to sensory input (sensory overload); history of physical, emotional, or sexual abuse; and response to demands of therapy, realization of severity of condition.

Personal Identity disturbance may be related to organic brain dysfunction, lack of development of trust, maternal deprivation, fixation at presymbiotic phase of development, possibly evidenced by lack of awareness of the feelings or existence of others, increased anxiety resulting from physical contact with others, absent or impaired imitation of others, repeating what others say, persistent preoccupation with parts of objects, obsessive attachment to objects, marked distress over changes in environment; autocratic/ritualistic behaviors, self-touching, rocking, swaying.

Family coping, ineffective: compromised/disabling may be related to family members unable to express feelings; excessive guilt, anger, or blaming among family members regarding child's condition; ambivalent or dissonant family relationships, prolonged coping with problem exhausting supportive ability of family members, possibly evidenced by denial of existence or severity of disturbed behaviors, preoccupation with personal emotional reaction to situation, rationalization that problem will be outgrown, attempts to intervene with child are achieving increasingly ineffective results, family withdraws from or becomes overly protective of child.

battered child syndrome

Trauma, risk for: risk factors may include dependent position in relationship(s), vulnerability (e.g., congenital problems/chronic illness), history of previous abuse/neglect, lack/nonuse of support systems by caregiver(s).

Family Processes/Parenting, altered may be related to poor role model/identity, unrealistic expectations, presence of stressors, and lack of support, possibly evidenced by verbalization of negative feelings, inappropriate caretaking behaviors, and evidence of physical/psychological trauma to child.

Self-Esteem, chronic low may be related to deprivation and negative feedback of family members, personal vulnerability, feelings of abandonment, possibly evidenced by lack of eye contact, withdrawal from social contacts, discounting own needs, nonassertive/passive, indecisive, or overly conforming behaviors.

Post-Trauma Syndrome may be related to sustained/recurrent physical or emotional abuse; possibly evidenced by acting-out behavior, development of phobias, poor impulse control, and emotional numbness.

Coping, Individual, ineffective may be related to situational or maturational crisis, overwhelming threat to self, personal vulnerability, inadequate support systems, possibly evidenced by verbalized concern about ability to deal with current situation, chronic worry, anxiety, depression, poor self-esteem, inability to problem-solve, high illness rate, destructive behavior toward self/others.

benign prostatic hypertrophy

Urinary Retention [acute/chronic] may be related to mechanical obstruction (enlarged prostate), decompensation of detrusor musculature, inability of bladder to contract adequately, possibly evidenced by frequency, hesitancy, inability to empty bladder completely, incontinence/dribbling, bladder distention, residual urine.

Pain [acute] may be related to mucosal irritation, bladder distention, colic, urinary infection, and radiation therapy, possibly evidenced by reports (bladder/rectal spasm), narrowed focus, altered muscle tone, grimacing, distraction behaviors, restlessness, and autonomic responses.

Fluid Volume, risk for deficit: risk factors may include postobstructive diuresis, endocrine/electrolyte imbalances.

Fear/Anxiety [specify level] may be related to change in health status (possibility of surgical procedure/malignancy); embarrassment/loss of dignity associated with genital exposure before, during, and after treatment, and concern about sexual ability, possibly evidenced by increased tension, apprehension, worry, expressed concerns regarding perceived changes, and fear of unspecified consequences.

bipolar disorder

Violence, risk for directed at others: risk factors may include irritability, impulsive behavior; delusional thinking; angry response when ideas are refuted or wishes denied; manic excitement, with possible indicators of threatening body language/verbalizations, increased motor activity, overt and aggressive acts; and hostility.

Nutrition: altered, less than body requirements may be related to inadequate intake in relation to metabolic expenditures, possibly evidenced by body weight 20% or more below ideal weight, observed inadequate intake, inattention to mealtimes, and distraction from task of eating; laboratory evidence of nutritional deficits/imbalances.

Poisoning, risk for lithium toxicity: risk factors may include narrow therapeutic range of drug, patient's ability (or lack of) to follow through with medication regimen and monitoring, and denial of need for information/therapy.

Sleep Pattern disturbance may be related to psychological stress, lack of recognition of fatigue/need to sleep, hyperactivity, possibly evidenced by denial of need to sleep, interrupted nighttime sleep, one or more nights without sleep, changes in behavior and performance, increasing irritability/restlessness, and dark circles under eyes.

Sensory/Perceptual alterations; (specify) [overload] may be related to decrease in sensory threshold, endogenous chemical alteration, psychological stress, sleep deprivation, possibly evidenced by increased distractibility and agitation, anxiety, disorientation, poor concentration, auditory/visual hallucination, bizarre thinking, and motor incoordination.

Family Processes, altered may be related to situational crises (illness, economics, change in roles); euphoric mood and grandiose ideas/actions of patient, manipulative behavior and limit-testing, patient's refusal to accept responsibility for own actions, possibly evidenced by statements of difficulty coping with situation, lack of adaptation to change or not dealing constructively with illness; ineffective family decision-making process, failure to send and to receive clear messages, and inappropriate boundary maintenance.

borderline personality disorder

Violence, risk for directed at self/others/Self-Mutilation: risk factors may include use of projection as a major defense mechanism, pervasive problems with negative transference, feelings of guilt/need to "punish" self, distorted sense of self, inability to cope with increased psychological or physiological tension in a healthy manner.

Anxiety [severe to panic] may be related to unconscious conflicts (experience of extreme stress), perceived threat to self-concept, unmet needs, possibly evidenced by easy frustration and feelings of hurt, abuse of alcohol/other drugs, transient psychotic symptoms and performance of self-mutilating acts.

Self-Esteem, chronic low/Personal Identity disturbance may be related to lack of positive feedback, unmet dependency needs, retarded ego development/fixation at an earlier level of development, possibly evidenced by difficulty identifying self or defining self-boundaries, feelings of depersonalization, extreme mood changes, lack of tolerance of rejection or being alone, unhappiness with self, striking out at others, performance of ritualistic self-damaging acts, and belief that punishing self is necessary.

Social isolation may be related to immature interests, unaccepted social behavior, inadequate personal resources, and inability to engage in satisfying personal relationships, possibly evidenced by alternating clinging and distancing behaviors, difficulty meeting expectations of others, experiencing feelings of difference from others, expressing interests inappropriate to developmental age, and exhibiting behavior unaccepted by dominant cultural group.

brain tumor

Pain [acute] may be related to pressure on brain tissues, possibly evidenced by reports of headache, facial mask of pain, narrowed focus, and autonomic responses (changes in vital signs).

Thought Processes, altered may be related to altered circulation to and/or destruction of brain tissue, possibly evidenced by memory loss, personality changes, impaired ability to make decisions/conceptualize, and inaccurate interpretation of environment.

Sensory/Perceptual alterations (specify) may be related to compression/displacement of brain tissue, disruption of neuronal conduction, possibly evidenced by changes in visual acuity, alterations in sense of balance/gait disturbance, and paresthesia.

Fluid Volume, risk for deficit: risk factors may include recurrent vomiting from irritation of vagal center in medulla, and decreased intake.

Self-Care deficit [specify] may be related to sensory/neuromuscular impairment interfering with ability to perform tasks, possibly evidenced by unkempt/disheveled appearance, body odor, and verbalization/observation of inability to perform activities of daily living.

bronchitis

Airway Clearance, ineffective may be related to excessive, thickened mucous secretions, possibly evidenced by presence of rhonchi, tachypnea, and ineffective cough.

Activity Intolerance [specific level] may be related to imbalance between oxygen supply and demand, possibly evidenced by reports of fatigue, dyspnea, and abnormal vital sign response to activity.

Pain [acute] may be related to localized inflammation, persistent cough, aching associated with fever, possibly evidenced by reports of discomfort, distraction behavior, and facial mask of pain.

bronchopneumonia
(also refer to *bronchitis*)

Airway Clearance, ineffective may be related to tracheal bronchial inflammation, edema formation, increased sputum production, pleuritic pain, decreased energy, fatigue, possibly evidenced by changes in rate/depth of respirations, abnormal breath sounds, use of accessory muscles, dyspnea, cyanosis, effective/ineffective cough—with or without sputum production.

Gas Exchange, impaired may be related to inflammatory process, collection of secretions affecting oxygen exchange across alveolar membrane, and hypoventilation, possibly evidenced by restlessness/changes in mentation, dyspnea, tachycardia, pallor, cyanosis, and ABGs/oximetry evidence of hypoxia.

Infection, risk for spread: risk factors may include decreased ciliary action, stasis of secretions, presence of existing infection.

burn (dependent on type, degree, and severity of the injury)

Fluid Volume, risk for deficit: risk factors may include loss of fluids through wounds, capillary damage and evaporation, hypermetabolic state, insufficient intake, hemorrhagic losses.

Airway Clearance, risk for ineffective: risk factors may include mucosal edema and loss of ciliary action (smoke inhalation), direct upper air-way injury by flame, steam, chemicals.

Infection, risk for: risk factors may include loss of protective dermal barrier, traumatized/necrotic tissue, decreased hemoglobin, suppressed inflammatory response, environmental exposure/invasive procedures.

Pain [acute]/chronic may be related to destruction of/trauma to tissue and nerves, edema formation, and manipulation of impaired tissues, possibly evidenced by verbal reports, narrowed focus, distraction and guarding behaviors, facial mask of pain, and autonomic responses (changes in vital signs).

Nutrition: altered, risk for less than body requirements: risk factors may include hypermetabolic state in response to burn injury/stress, inadequate intake, protein catabolism.

Post-Trauma Syndrome may be related to life-threatening event, possibly evidenced by reexperiencing the event, repetitive dreams/nightmares, psychic/emotional numbness, and sleep disturbance.

Protection, altered may be related to extremes of age, inadequate nutrition, anemia, impaired immune system, possibly evidenced by impaired healing, deficient immunity, fatigue, anorexia.

Diversional Activity deficit may be related to long-term hospitalization, frequent lengthy treatments, and physical limitations, possibly evidenced by expressions of boredom, restlessness, withdrawal, and requests for something to do.

Development, risk for altered: risk factors may include effects of physical disability, separation from significant other(s), and environmental deficiencies.

bursitis

Pain [acute]/chronic may be related to inflammation of affected joint, possibly evidenced by verbal reports, guarding behavior, and narrowed focus.

Mobility, impaired physical may be related to inflammation and swelling of joint, and pain, possibly evidenced by diminished range of motion, reluctance to attempt movement, and imposed restriction of movement by medical treatment.

calculus, urinary

Pain [acute] may be related to increased frequency/force of ureteral contractions, tissue trauma and edema formation, possibly evidenced by reports of sudden, severe, colicky pains; guarding and distraction behaviors and autonomic responses.

Urinary Elimination, altered may be related to stimulation of the bladder by calculi, renal or ureteral irritation, mechanical obstruction of urinary flow, inflammation possibly evidenced by urgency and frequency; oliguria (retention); hematuria.

Infection, risk for: risk factors may include stasis of urine.

Knowledge deficit [Learning Need] regarding condition, prognosis, self-care and treatment needs may be related to lack of exposure/recall and information misinterpretation, possibly evidenced by requests for information, statements of concern, and recurrence/development of preventable complications.

cancer

(also refer to *chemotherapy*)

Fear/Anxiety, death may be related to situational crises, threat to/change in health/socioeconomic status, role functioning, interaction patterns; threat of death, separation from family, interpersonal transmission of feelings, possibly evidenced by expressed concerns, feelings of inadequacy/helplessness, insomnia; increased tension, restlessness, focus on self, sympathetic stimulation.

Grieving, anticipatory may be related to potential loss of physiologic well-being (body part/function), perceived separation from significant other(s)/lifestyle (death), possibly evidenced by anger, sadness, withdrawal, choked feelings, changes in eating/sleep patterns, activity level, libido, and communication patterns.

Pain [acute]/chronic may be related to the disease process (compression of nerve tissue, infiltration of nerves or their vascular supply, obstruction of a nerve pathway, inflammation), or side effects of therapeutic agents, possibly evidenced by verbal reports, self-focusing/narrowed focus, alteration in muscle tone, facial mask of pain, distraction/guarding behaviors, autonomic responses, and restlessness.

Fatigue may be related to decreased metabolic energy production, increased energy requirements (hypermetabolic state), overwhelming psychological/emotional demands, and altered body chemistry (side effects of medications, chemotherapy), possibly evidenced by unremitting/overwhelming lack of energy, inability to maintain usual routines, decreased performance, impaired ability to concentrate, lethargy/listlessness, and lack of interest in surroundings.

Home Maintenance Management, impaired may be related to debilitation, lack of resources, and/or inadequate support systems, possibly evidenced by verbalization of problem, request for assistance, and lack of necessary equipment or aids.

Family Coping, ineffective: compromised/disabling may be related to chronic nature of disease and disability, ongoing treatment needs, parental supervision, and lifestyle restrictions, possibly evidenced by expression of denial/despair, depression, and protective behavior disproportionate to patient's abilities or need for autonomy.

Family Coping: potential for growth may be related to the fact that the individual's needs are being sufficiently gratified and adaptive tasks effectively addressed, enabling goals of self-actualization to surface, possibly evidenced by verbalizations of impact of crisis on own values, priorities, goals, or relationships.

cardiac surgery

Anxiety [specify level]/Fear may be related to change in health status and threat to self-concept/of death, possibly evidenced by sympathetic stimulation, increased tension, and apprehension.

Cardiac Output, risk for decreased: risk factors may include decreased preload (hypovolemia), depressed myocardial contractility, changes in SVR (afterload), and alterations in electrical conduction (dysrhythmias).

Fluid Volume deficit [isotonic] may be related to intraoperative bleeding with inadequate blood replacement; bleeding related to insufficient heparin reversal, fibrinolysis, or platelet destruction; or volume depletion effects of intraoperative/postoperative diuretic therapy, possibly evidenced by increased pulse rate, decreased pulse volume/pressure, decreased urine output, hemoconcentration.

Gas Exchange, risk for impaired: risk factors may include alveolar-capillary membrane changes (atelectasis), intestinal edema, inadequate function or premature discontinuation of chest tubes, and diminished oxygen-carrying capacity of the blood.

Pain [acute]/[Discomfort] may be related to tissue inflammation/trauma, edema formation, intraoperative nerve trauma, and myocardial ischemia, possibly evidenced by reports of incisional discomfort/pain in chest and donor site; paresthesia/pain in hand, arm, shoulder, anxiety, restlessness, irritability; distraction behaviors, and autonomic responses.

Skin/Tissue Integrity, impaired related to mechanical trauma (surgical incisions, puncture wounds) and edema evidenced by disruption of skin surface/tissues.

care, long-term

(also refer to *condition requiring / contributing to need for facility placement*)

Anxiety [specify level]/Fear may be related to change in health status, role functioning, interaction patterns, socioeconomic status, environment; unmet needs, recent life changes, and loss of friends/significant other(s), possibly evidenced by apprehension, restlessness, insomnia, repetitive questioning, pacing, purposeless activity, expressed concern regarding changes in life events, and focus on self.

Grieving, anticipatory may be related to perceived/actual or potential loss of physiopsychosocial well-being, personal possessions, and significant other(s); as well as cultural beliefs about aging/debilitation, possibly evidenced by denial of feelings, depression, sorrow, guilt; alterations in activity level, sleep patterns, eating habits, and libido.

Poisoning, risk for drug toxicity: risk factors may include effects of aging (reduced metabolism, impaired circulation, precarious physiologic balance, presence of multiple diseases/organ involvement), and use of multiple prescribed/OTC drugs.

Thought Processes, altered may be related to physiological changes of aging (loss of cells and brain atrophy, decreased blood supply); altered sensory input, pain, effects of medications, and psychological conflicts (disrupted life pattern), possibly evidenced by slower reaction times, memory loss, altered attention span, disorientation, inability to follow, altered sleep patterns, and personality changes.

Sleep Pattern disturbance may be related to internal factors (illness, psychological stress, inactivity) and external factors (environmental changes, facility routines), possibly evidenced by reports of difficulty in falling asleep/not feeling rested, interrupted sleep/awakening earlier than desired; change in behavior/performance, increasing irritability, and listlessness.

Sexuality Patterns, risk for altered: risk factors may include biopsychosocial alteration of sexuality; interference in psychological/physical well-being, self-image, and lack of privacy/significant other.

Relocation Stress Syndrome, risk for: risk factors may include multiple losses, feeling of powerlessness, lack of/inappropriate use of support system, changes in psychosocial/physical health status.

carpal tunnel syndrome

Pain [acute]/chronic may be related to pressure on median nerve, possibly evidenced by verbal reports, reluctance to use affected extremity, guarding behaviors, expressed fear of reinjury, altered ability to continue previous activities.

Mobility, impaired physical may be related to neuromuscular impairment and pain, possibly evidenced by decreased hand strength, weakness, limited range of motion, and reluctance to attempt movement.

Peripheral Neurovascular risk for dysfunction: risks include mechanical compression (e.g., brace, repetitive tasks/motions), immobilization.

Knowledge deficit [Learning Need] regarding condition, prognosis and treatment/safety needs may be related to lack of exposure/recall, information misinterpretation, possibly evidenced by questions, statements of concern, request for information, inaccurate follow-through of instructions/development of preventable complications.

cast

(also refer to *fractures*)

Peripheral Neurovascular risk for dysfunction: risk factors may include presence of fracture(s), mechanical compression (cast), tissue trauma, immobilization, vascular obstruction.

Skin Integrity, risk for impaired: risk factors may include pressure of cast, moisture/debris under cast, objects inserted under cast to relieve itching, and/or altered sensation/circulation.

Self-Care deficit [specify] may be related to impaired ability to perform self-care tasks, possibly evidenced by statements of need for assistance and observed difficulty in performing activities of daily living.

cataract

Sensory/Perceptual alterations: visual may be related to altered sensory reception/status of sense organs, and therapeutically restricted environment (surgical procedure, patching), possibly evidenced by diminished acuity, visual distortions, and change in usual response to stimuli.

Trauma, risk for: risk factors may include poor vision, reduced hand/eye coordination.

Anxiety [specify level]/Fear may be related to alteration in visual acuity, threat of permanent loss of vision/independence, possibly evidenced by expressed concerns, apprehension, and feelings of uncertainty.

Knowledge deficit [Learning Need] regarding ways of coping with altered abilities, therapy choices, lifestyle changes may be related to lack of exposure/recall, misinterpretation, or cognitive limitations, possibly evidenced by requests for information, statement of concern, inaccurate follow-through of instructions/development of preventable complications.

cat scratch disease

Pain [acute] may be related to effects of circulating toxins (fever, headache, and lymphadenitis), possibly evidenced by verbal reports, guarding behavior, and autonomic response (changes in vital signs).

Hyperthermia may be related to inflammatory process, possibly evidenced by increased body temperature, flushed warm skin, tachypnea, and tachycardia.

cerebrovascular accident

Tissue Perfusion, altered: cerebral may be related to interruption of blood flow (occlusive disorder, hemorrhage, cerebral vasospasm/edema), possibly evidenced by altered level of consciousness, changes in vital signs, changes in motor/sensory responses, restlessness, memory loss; sensory, language, intellectual, and emotional deficits.

Mobility, impaired physical may be related to neuromuscular involvement (weakness, paresthesia, flaccid/hypotonic paralysis, spastic paralysis), perceptual/cognitive impairment, possibly evidenced by inability to purposefully move involved body parts/limited range of motion; impaired coordination, and/or decreased muscle strength/control.

Communication, impaired verbal [and/or written] may be related to impaired cerebral circulation, neuromuscular impairment, loss of facial/oral muscle tone and control; generalized weakness/fatigue, possibly evidenced by impaired articulation, does not/cannot speak (dysarthria); inability to modulate speech, find and/or name words, identify objects and/or inability to comprehend written/spoken language; inability to produce written communication.

Self-Care Deficit [specify] may be related to neuromuscular impairment, decreased strength/endurance, loss of muscle control/coordination, perceptual/cognitive impairment, pain/discomfort, and depression, possibly evidenced by stated/observed inability to perform ADLs, requests for assistance, disheveled appearance, and incontinence.

Swallowing, risk for impaired: risk factors may include muscle paralysis and perceptual impairment.

Unilateral Neglect, risk for: risk factors may include sensory loss of part of visual field with perceptual loss of corresponding body segment.
Home Maintenance Management, impaired may be related to condition of individual family member, insufficient finances/family organization or planning, unfamiliarity with resources, and inadequate support systems, possibly evidenced by members expressing difficulty in managing home in a comfortable manner/requesting assistance with home maintenance, disorderly surroundings, and overtaxed family members.
Self-Esteem situational low/Body Image disturbance/Role performance, altered may be related to biophysical, psychosocial, and cognitive/perceptual changes, possibly evidenced by actual change in structure and/or function, change in usual patterns of responsibility/physical capacity to resume role; and verbal/nonverbal response to actual or perceived change.

cesarean birth, unplanned
Knowledge deficit [Learning Need] regarding underlying procedure, pathophysiology, and self-care needs may be related to incomplete/inadequate information, possibly evidenced by request for information, verbalization of concerns/misconceptions and inappropriate/exaggerated behavior.
Anxiety [specify level] may be related to actual/perceived threat to mother/fetus, emotional threat to self-esteem, unmet needs/expectations, and interpersonal transmission, possibly evidenced by increased tension, apprehension, feelings of inadequacy, sympathetic stimulation, and narrowed focus, restlessness.
Self-Esteem, risk for situational low: risk factors may include perceived "failure" at life event.
Pain [acute], risk for: risk factors may include increased/prolonged contractions, psychological reaction.
Infection, risk for: risk factors may include invasive procedures, rupture of amniotic membranes, break in skin, decreased hemoglobin, exposure to pathogens.

chemotherapy
(also refer to *cancer*)
Fluid volume, risk for deficit: risk factors may include gastrointestinal losses (vomiting), interference with adequate intake (stomatitis/anorexia), losses through abnormal routes (indwelling tubes, wounds, fistulas), and hypermetabolic state.
Nutrition: altered, less than body requirements may be related to inability to ingest adequate nutrients (nausea, stomatitis, and fatigue), hypermetabolic state, possibly evidenced by weight loss (wasting), aversion to eating, reported altered taste sensation, sore, inflamed buccal cavity; diarrhea and/or constipation.
Oral Mucous Membrane, altered may be related to side effects of therapeutic agents/radiation, dehydration, and malnutrition, possibly evidenced by ulcerations, leukoplakia, decreased salivation, and reports of pain.
Body Image disturbance may be related to anatomical/structural changes; loss of hair and weight, possibly evidenced by negative feelings about body, preoccupation with change, feelings of helplessness/hopelessness, and change in social involvement.
Protection, altered may be related to inadequate nutrition, drug therapy/radiation, abnormal blood profile, disease state (cancer), possibly evidenced by impaired healing, deficient immunity, anorexia, fatigue.

cholecystectomy
Pain [acute] may be related to interruption in skin/tissue layers with mechanical closure (sutures/staples) and invasive procedures (including T-tube/nasogastric—NG—tube), possibly evidenced by verbal reports, guarding/distraction behaviors, and autonomic responses (changes in vital signs).
Breathing Pattern, ineffective may be related to decreased lung expansion (pain and muscle weakness), decreased energy/fatigue, ineffective cough, possibly evidenced by fremitus, tachypnea, and decreased respiratory depth/vital capacity.
Fluid Volume, risk for deficit: risk factors may include vomiting/NG aspiration, medically restricted intake, altered coagulation.

cholelithiasis
Pain, [acute] may be related to inflammation and distortion of tissues, ductal spasm, possibly evidenced by verbal reports, guarding/distraction behaviors, and autonomic responses (changes in vital signs).
Nutrition: altered, less than body requirements may be related to inability to ingest/absorb adequate nutrients (food intolerance/pain, nausea/vomiting, anorexia), possibly evidenced by aversion to food/decreased intake and weight loss.
Knowledge deficit [Learning Need] regarding pathophysiology, therapy choices, and self-care needs may be related to lack of information, misinterpretation, possibly evidenced by verbalization of concerns, questions, and recurrence of condition.

chronic obstructive pulmonary disease

Gas Exchange, impaired may be related to altered oxygen delivery (obstruction of airways by secretions/bronchospasm, air-trapping) and alveoli destruction, possibly evidenced by dyspnea, restlessness, confusion, abnormal ABG values, and reduced tolerance for activity.

Airway Clearance, ineffective may be related to bronchospasm, increased production of tenacious secretions, retained secretions, and decreased energy/fatigue, possibly evidenced by presence of wheezes, crackles, tachypnea, dyspnea, changes in depth of respirations, use of accessory muscles, cough (persistent), and chest x-ray findings.

Activity Intolerance may be related to imbalance between oxygen supply and demand, and generalized weakness, possibly evidenced by verbal reports of fatigue, exertional dyspnea, and abnormal vital sign response.

Nutrition: altered, less than body requirements may be related to inability to ingest adequate nutrients (dyspnea, fatigue, medication side effects, sputum production, anorexia), possibly evidenced by weight loss, reported altered taste sensation, decreased muscle mass/subcutaneous fat, poor muscle tone, and aversion to eating/lack of interest in food.

Infection, risk for: risk factors may include decreased ciliary action, stasis of secretions, and debilitated state/malnutrition.

cirrhosis

(Also refer to *Substance dependence / abuse rehabilitation*; *hepatitis, acute viral*)

Nutrition: altered, less than body requirements may be related to inability to ingest/absorb nutrients (anorexia, nausea, indigestion, early satiety), abnormal bowel function, impaired storage of vitamins, possibly evidenced by aversion to eating, observed lack of intake, muscle wasting, weight loss, and imbalances in nutritional studies.

Fluid Volume excess may be related to compromised regulatory mechanism (e.g., syndrome of inappropriate antidiuretic hormone—SIADH, decreased plasma proteins/malnutrition) and excess sodium/fluid intake, possibly evidenced by generalized or abdominal edema, weight gain, dyspnea, BP changes, positive hepatojugular reflex, change in mentation, altered electrolytes, changes in urine specific gravity, and pleural effusion.

Skin Integrity, risk for impaired: risk factors may include altered circulation/metabolic state, poor skin turgor, skeletal prominence, and presence of edema/ascites, accumulation of bile salts in skin.

Confusion, risk for acute: risk factors may include alcohol abuse, increased serum ammonia level, and inability of liver to detoxify certain enzymes/drugs.

Self-Esteem disturbance/Body image disturbance may be related to biophysical changes/altered physical appearance, uncertainty of prognosis, changes in role function, personal vulnerability, self-destructive behavior (alcohol-induced disease), possibly evidenced by verbalization of changes in lifestyle, fear of rejection/reaction of others, negative feelings about body/abilities, and feelings of helplessness/hopelessness/powerlessness.

Injury, risk for hemorrhage: risk factors may include abnormal blood profile (altered clotting factors), portal hypertension/development of esophageal varices.

cocaine hydrochloride poisoning, acute

(Also refer to *substance dependence / abuse rehabilitation*)

Breathing pattern, ineffective may be related to pharmacological effects on respiratory center of the brain, possibly evidenced by tachypnea, altered depth of respiration, shortness of breath, and abnormal ABGs.

Cardiac Output, risk for decreased: risk factors may include drug effect on myocardium (degree dependent on drug purity/quality used), alterations in electrical rate/rhythm/conduction, preexisting myocardiopathy.

Nutrition: altered, less than body requirements may be related to anorexia, insufficient/inappropriate use of financial resources, possibly evidenced by reported inadequate intake, weight loss/less than normal weight gain; lack of interest in food, poor muscle tone, signs/laboratory evidence of vitamin deficiencies.

Infection, risk for: risk factors may include injection techniques, impurities of drugs; localized trauma/nasal septum damage, malnutrition, altered immune state.

Coping, Individual, ineffective may be related to personal vulnerability, negative role modeling, inadequate support systems; ineffective/inadequate coping skills with substitution of drug, possibly evidenced by use of harmful substance, despite evidence of undesirable consequences.

Sensory/Perceptual alterations (specify) may be related to exogenous chemical, altered sensory reception/transmission/integration (hallucination), altered status of sense organs, possibly evidenced by responding to internal stimuli from hallucinatory experiences, bizarre thinking, anxiety/panic changes in sensory acuity (sense of smell/taste).

coccidioidomycosis (San Joaquin/Valley Fever)

Pain [acute] may be related to inflammation, possibly evidenced by verbal reports, distraction behaviors, and narrowed focus.

Fatigue may be related to decreased energy production; states of discomfort, possibly evidenced by reports of overwhelming lack of energy, inability to maintain usual routine, emotional lability/irritability, impaired ability to concentrate, and decreased endurance/libido.

Knowledge deficit [Learning Need] regarding nature/course of disease, therapy and self-care needs may be related to lack of information, possibly evidenced by statements of concern and questions.

colitis, ulcerative

Diarrhea may be related to inflammation or malabsorption of the bowel, presence of toxins and/or segmental narrowing of the lumen, possibly evidenced by increased bowel sounds/peristalsis, urgency, frequent/watery stools (acute phase), changes in stool color, and abdominal pain/cramping.

Pain [acute]/chronic may be related to inflammation of the intestines/hyperperistalsis and anal/rectal irritation, possibly evidenced by verbal reports, guarding/distraction behaviors.

Fluid Volume, risk for deficit: risk factors may include continued gastrointestinal losses (diarrhea, vomiting, capillary plasma loss), altered intake, hypermetabolic state.

Nutrition: altered, less than body requirements may be related to altered intake/absorption of nutrients (medically restricted intake, fear that eating may cause diarrhea) and hypermetabolic state, possibly evidenced by weight loss, decreased subcutaneous fat/muscle mass, poor muscle tone, hyperactive bowel sounds, steatorrhea, pale conjunctiva and mucous membranes, and aversion to eating.

Coping, Individual, ineffective may be related to chronic nature and indefinite outcome of disease, multiple stressors (repeated over time), personal vulnerability, severe pain, inadequate sleep, lack of/ineffective support systems, possibly evidenced by verbalization of inability to cope, discouragement, anxiety; preoccupation with physical self, chronic worry, emotional tension; depression, and recurrent exacerbation of symptoms.

Powerlessness, risk for: risk factors may include unresolved dependency conflicts, feelings of insecurity/resentment, repression of anger and aggressive feelings, lacking a sense of control in stressful situations, sacrificing own wishes for others, and retreat from aggression or frustration.

colostomy

Skin Integrity, risk for impaired: risk factors may include absence of sphincter at stoma and chemical irritation from caustic bowel contents, reaction to product/removal of adhesive, and improperly fitting appliance.

Diarrhea/Constipation, risk for: risk factors may include interruption/alteration of normal bowel function (placement of ostomy), changes in dietary/fluid intake, and effects of medication.

Knowledge deficit [Learning Need] regarding changes in physiologic function and self-care/treatment needs may be related to lack of exposure/recall, information misinterpretation, possibly evidenced by questions, statement of concern, and inaccurate follow-through of instruction/development of preventable complications.

Body Image disturbance may be related to biophysical changes (presence of stoma; loss of control of bowel elimination) and psychosocial factors (altered body structure, disease process/associated treatment regimen, e.g., cancer, colitis), possibly evidenced by verbalization of change in perception of self, negative feelings about body, fear of rejection/reaction of others, not touching/looking at stoma, and refusal to participate in care.

Social Interaction, impaired may be related to fear of embarrassing situation secondary to altered bowel control with loss of contents, odor, possibly evidenced by reduced participation and verbalized/observed discomfort in social situations.

Sexual dysfunction, risk for: risk factors may include altered body structure/function, radical resection/treatment procedures, vulnerability/psychological concern about response of significant other(s), and disruption of sexual response pattern (e.g., erection difficulty).

coma, diabetic

Refer to *diabetic ketoacidosis*.

concussion of the brain

Pain [acute] may be related to trauma to/edema of cerebral tissue, possibly evidenced by reports of headache, guarding/distraction behaviors, and narrowed focus.

Fluid Volume, risk for deficit: risk factors may include vomiting, decreased intake, and hypermetabolic state (fever).

Thought Processes, risk for altered: risk factors may include trauma to/edema of cerebral tissue.

Knowledge deficit [Learning Need] regarding condition, treatment/safety needs, and potential complications may be related to lack of recall, misinterpretation, cognitive limitation, possibly evidenced by questions/statement of concerns, development of preventable complications.

Conn's syndrome

Refer to *aldosteronism, primary*.

constipation

Constipation may be related to weak abdominal musculature, gastrointestinal obstructive lesions, pain on defecation, diagnostic procedures, pregnancy, possibly evidenced by change in character/frequency of stools, feeling of abdominal/rectal fullness or pressure, changes in bowel sounds, abdominal distention.

Pain [acute] may be related to abdominal fullness/pressure, straining to defecate, and trauma to delicate tissues, possibly evidenced by verbal reports, reluctance to defecate, and distraction behaviors.

Knowledge deficit [Learning Need] regarding dietary needs, bowel function, and medication effect may be related to lack of information/misconceptions, possibly evidenced by development of problem and verbalization of concerns/questions.

coronary artery bypass surgery

Cardiac Output, risk for decreased: risk factors may include decreased myocardial contractility, diminished circulating volume (preload), alterations in electrical conduction, and increased SVR (afterload).

Pain [acute] may be related to direct chest tissue/bone trauma, invasive tubes/lines, donor site incision, tissue inflammation/edema formation, intraoperative nerve trauma, possibly evidenced by verbal reports, autonomic responses (changes in vital signs), and distraction behaviors/restlessness, irritability.

Sensory/Perceptual alterations (specify) may be related to restricted environment (postoperative/acute), sleep deprivation, effects of medications, continuous environmental sounds/activities, and psychological stress of procedure, possibly evidenced by disorientation, alterations in behavior, exaggerated emotional responses, and visual/auditory distortions.

Role Performance, altered may be related to situational crises (dependency role)/recuperative process, uncertainty about future, possibly evidenced by delay/alteration in physical capacity to resume role, change in usual role or responsibility change in self/others' perception of role.

Crohn's disease

(also refer to *colitis, ulcerative*)

Nutrition: altered, less than body requirements may be related to intestinal pain after eating; and decreased transit time through bowel, possibly evidenced by weight loss, aversion to eating, and observed lack of intake.

Diarrhea may be related to inflammation of small intestines, presence of toxins, particularly dietary intake, possibly evidenced by hyperactive bowel sounds, cramping, and frequent loose liquid stools.

Knowledge deficit [Learning Need] regarding condition, nutritional needs, and prevention of recurrence may be related to insufficient information/misinterpretation, unfamiliarity with resources, possibly evidenced by statements of concern/questions, inaccurate follow-through of instructions, and development of preventable complications/exacerbation of condition.

croup

Airway Clearance, ineffective may be related to presence of thick, tenacious mucus and swelling/spasms of the epiglottis, possibly evidenced by harsh/brassy cough, tachypnea, use of accessory breathing muscles, and presence of wheezes.

Fluid Volume deficit [isotonic] may be related to decreased ability/aversion to swallowing, presence of fever, and increased respiratory losses, possibly evidenced by dry mucous membranes, poor skin turgor, and scanty/concentrated urine.

croup, membranous

(also refer to *croup*)

Suffocation, risk for: risk factors may include inflammation of larynx with formation of false membrane.

Anxiety [specify level]/Fear may be related to change in environment, perceived threat to self (difficulty breathing), and transmission of anxiety of adults, possibly evidenced by restlessness, facial tension, glancing about, and sympathetic stimulation.

Cushing's syndrome

Fluid Volume, risk for excess: risk factors may include compromised regulatory mechanism (fluid/sodium retention).

Infection, risk for: risk factors may include immunosuppressed inflammatory response, skin and capillary fragility, and negative nitrogen balance.

Nutrition: altered, less than body requirements may be related to inability to utilize nutrients (disturbance of carbohydrate metabolism), possibly evidenced by decreased muscle mass and increased resistance to insulin.

Self-care deficit [specify] may be related to muscle wasting, generalized weakness, fatigue, and demineralization of bones, possibly evidenced by statements of/observed inability to complete or perform ADLs.

Body Image disturbance may be related to change in structure/appearance (effects of disease process, drug therapy), possibly evidenced by negative feelings about body, feelings of helplessness, and changes in social involvement.

Sexual dysfunction may be related to loss of libido, impotence, and cessation of menses, possibly evidenced by verbalization of concerns and/or dissatisfaction with and alteration in relationship with significant other.

Trauma, risk for fractures: risk factors may include increased protein breakdown, negative protein balance, demineralization of bones.

cystic fibrosis

Airway clearance, ineffective may be related to excessive production of thick mucus and decreased ciliary action, possibly evidenced by abnormal breath sounds, ineffective cough, cyanosis, and altered respiratory rate/depth.

Infection, risk for: risk factors may include stasis of respiratory secretions and development of atelectasis.

Nutrition: altered, less than body requirements may be related to impaired digestive process and absorption of nutrients, possibly evidenced by failure to gain weight, muscle wasting, and retarded physical growth.

Knowledge deficit [Learning Need] regarding pathophysiology of condition, medical management, and available community resources may be related to insufficient information/misconceptions, possibly evidenced by statements of concern, questions; inaccurate follow-through of instructions, development of preventable complications.

Family Coping, ineffective: compromised may be related to chronic nature of disease and disability, inadequate/incorrect information or understanding by a primary person, and possibly evidenced by significant person attempting assistive or supportive behaviors with less than satisfactory results, protective behavior disproportionate to patient's abilities or need for autonomy.

cystitis

Pain [acute] may be related to inflammation and bladder spasms, possibly evidenced by verbal reports, distraction behaviors, and narrowed focus.

Urinary elimination, altered may be related to inflammation/irritation of bladder, possibly evidenced by frequency, nocturia, and dysuria.

Knowledge deficit [Learning Need] regarding condition, treatment, and prevention of recurrence may be related to inadequate information/misconceptions, possibly evidenced by statements of concern and questions; recurrent infections.

cytomegalic inclusion disease

Refer to *herpes*.

dehiscence (abdominal)

Skin integrity, impaired may be related to altered circulation, altered nutritional state (obesity/malnutrition), and physical stress on incision, possibly evidenced by poor/delayed wound healing and disruption of skin surface/wound closure.

Infection, risk for: risk factors may include inadequate primary defenses (separation of incision, traumatized intestines, environmental exposure).

Tissue integrity, risk for impaired: risk factors may include exposure of abdominal contents to external environment.

Fear/Anxiety [severe] may be related to crises, perceived threat of death, possibly evidenced by fearfulness, restless behaviors, and sympathetic stimulation.

Knowledge deficit [Learning Need] regarding condition/prognosis and treatment needs may be related to lack of information/recall and misinterpretation of information, possibly evidenced by development of preventable complication, requests for information, and statement of concern.

dehydration

Fluid volume deficit [specify] may be related to etiology as defined by specific situation, possibly evidenced by dry mucous membranes, poor skin turgor, decreased pulse volume/pressure, and thirst.

Oral Mucous Membrane, risk for altered: risk factors may include dehydration and decreased salivation.

Knowledge deficit [Learning Need] regarding fluid needs may be related to lack of information/misinterpretation, possibly evidenced by questions, statement of concern, and inadequate follow-through of instructions/development of preventable complications.

delirium tremens (acute alcohol withdrawal)

Anxiety [severe/panic]/Fear may be related to cessation of alcohol intake/physiological withdrawal, threat to self-concept, perceived threat of death, possibly evidenced by increased tension, apprehension, fear of unspecified consequences; identifies object of fear.

Sensory/Perceptual alterations (specify) may be related to exogenous(alcohol consumption/sudden cessation)/endogenous (electrolyte imbalance, elevated ammonia and blood urea nitrogen—BUN) chemical alterations, sleep deprivation, and psychological stress, possibly evidenced by disorientation, restlessness, irritability, exaggerated emotional responses, bizarre thinking and visual and auditory distortions/hallucinations.

Cardiac Output, risk for decreased: risk factors may include direct effect of alcohol on heart muscle, altered SVR, presence of dysrhythmias.

Trauma, risk for: risk factors may include alterations in balance, reduced muscle coordination, cognitive impairment, and involuntary clonic/tonic muscle activity.

Nutrition: altered, less than body requirements may be related to poor dietary intake, effects of alcohol on organs involved in digestion, interference with absorption/metabolism of nutrients and amino acids, possibly evidenced by reports of inadequate food intake, altered taste sensation, lack of interest in food, debilitated state, decreased subcutaneous fat/muscle mass, signs of mineral/electrolyte deficiency, including abnormal laboratory findings.

dementia, presenile/senile

(also refer to *Alzheimer's disease*)

Memory, impaired may be related to neurological disturbances, possibly evidenced by observed experiences of forgetting, inability to determine if a behavior was performed, inability to perform previously learned skills, inability to recall factual information or recent/past events.

Fear may be related to decreases in functional abilities, public disclosure of disabilities, further mental/physical deterioration possibly evidenced by social isolation, apprehension, irritability, defensiveness, suspiciousness, aggressive behavior.

Self-Care deficit [specify] may be related to cognitive decline, physical limitations, frustration over loss of independence, depression, possibly evidenced by impaired ability to perform ADLs.

Trauma, risk for: risk factors may include changes in muscle coordination/balance, impaired judgment, seizure activity.

Caregiver Role Strain, risk for: risk factors may include illness severity of care receiver, duration of caregiving required, care receiver exhibiting deviant/bizarre behavior; family/caregiver isolation, lack of respite/recreation, spouse is caregiver.

depressive disorders, major depression, dysthymia

Violence, risk for self-directed: risk factors may include depressed mood and feeling of worthlessness and hopelessness.

Anxiety [moderate to severe]/Thought Processes, altered may be related to psychological conflicts, unconscious conflict about essential values/goals of life, unmet needs, threat to self-concept, sleep deprivation, interpersonal transmission/contagion, possibly evidenced by reports of nervousness or fearfulness, feelings of inadequacy; agitation, angry/tearful outbursts, rambling/discoordinated speech, restlessness, hand rubbing or wringing, tremulousness; poor memory/concentration, decreased ability to grasp ideas, inability to follow/impaired ability to make decisions, numerous/repetitious physical complaints without organic cause, ideas of reference, hallucinations/delusions.

Sleep Pattern disturbance may be related to biochemical alterations (decreased serotonin), unresolved fears and anxieties, and inactivity, possibly evidenced by difficulty in falling/remaining asleep, early morning awakening/awakening later than desired, reports of not feeling rested, and physical signs (e.g., dark circles under eyes, excessive yawning); hypersomnia (using sleep as an escape).

Social Isolation/Social Interaction, impaired may be related to alterations in mental status/thought processes (depressed mood), inadequate personal resources, decreased energy/inertia, difficulty engaging in satisfying personal relationships, feelings of worthlessness/low self-concept, inadequacy in or absence of significant purpose in life, and knowledge/skill deficit about social interactions, possibly evidenced by decreased involvement with others, expressed feelings of difference from others, remaining in home/room/bed, refusing invitations/suggestions of social involvement, and dysfunctional interaction with peers, family, and/or others.

Family Processes, altered may be related to situational crises of illness of family member with change in roles/responsibilities, developmental crises (e.g., loss of family member/relationship), possibly evidenced by statements of difficulty coping with situation, family system not meeting needs of its members, difficulty accepting or receiving help appropriately, ineffective family decision-making process, and failure to send and to receive clear messages.

Injury, risk for [effects of electroconvulsive therapy (ECT)]: risk factors may include effects of therapy on the cardiovascular, respiratory, musculoskeletal, and nervous systems; and pharmacological effects of anesthesia.

dermatitis seborrheica

Skin integrity, impaired may be related to chronic inflammatory condition of the skin, possibly evidenced by disruption of skin surface with dry or moist scales, yellowish crusts, erythema, and fissures.

diabetes mellitus

Knowledge deficit [Learning Need] regarding disease process/treatment and individual care needs may be related to unfamiliarity with information/lack of recall, misinterpretation, possibly evidenced by requests for information, statements of concern/misconceptions, inadequate follow-through of instructions, and development of preventable complications.

Nutrition: altered, less than body requirements may be related to inability to utilize nutrients (imbalance between intake and utilization of glucose) to meet metabolic needs, possibly evidenced by change in weight, muscle weakness, increased thirst/urination, and hyperglycemia.

Adjustment, risk for impaired: risk factors may include all-encompassing change in lifestyle, self-concept requiring lifelong adherence to therapeutic regimen and internal/altered locus of control.

Infection, risk for: risk factors may include decreased leukocytic function, circulatory changes, and delayed healing.

Sensory/Perceptual, risk for alterations (specify): risk factors may include endogenous chemical alteration (glucose/insulin and/or electrolyte imbalance).

Family Coping, ineffective: compromised may be related to inadequate or incorrect information or understanding by primary person(s), other situational/developmental crises or situations the significant person(s) may be facing, lifelong condition requiring behavioral changes impacting family, possibly evidenced by family expressions of confusion about what to do, verbalizations that they are having difficulty coping with situation; family does not meet physical/emotional needs of its members; significant other(s) preoccupied with personal reaction (e.g., guilt, fear), display protective behavior disproportionate (too little/too much) to patient's abilities or need for autonomy.

diabetic ketoacidosis

Fluid Volume deficit [specify] may be related to hyperosmolar urinary losses, gastric losses, and inadequate intake, possibly evidenced by increased urinary output/dilute urine, reports of weakness, thirst; sudden weight loss, hypotension, tachycardia, delayed capillary refill, dry mucous membranes, poor skin turgor.

Nutrition: altered, less than body requirements that may be related to inadequate utilization of nutrients (insulin deficiency), decreased oral intake, hypermetabolic state, possibly evidenced by recent weight loss, reports of weakness, lack of interest in food, gastric fullness/abdominal pain, and increased ketones, imbalance between glucose/insulin levels.

Fatigue may be related to decreased metabolic energy production, altered body chemistry (insufficient insulin), increased energy demands (hypermetabolic state/infection), possibly evidenced by overwhelming lack of energy, inability to maintain usual routines, decreased performance, impaired ability to concentrate, listlessness.

Infection, risk for: risk factors may include high glucose levels, decreased leukocyte function, stasis of body fluids, invasive procedures, alteration in circulation/perfusion.

dialysis, general

(also refer to *dialysis, peritoneal*; *hemodialysis*)

Nutrition: altered, less than body requirements may be related to inadequate ingestion of nutrients (dietary restrictions, anorexia, nausea/vomiting, stomatitis), loss of peptides and amino acids (building blocks for proteins) during procedure, possibly evidenced by reported inadequate intake, aversion to eating, altered taste sensation, poor muscle tone/weakness, sore/inflamed buccal cavity, pale conjunctiva/mucous membranes.

Grieving, anticipatory may be related to actual or perceived loss, chronic and/or fatal illness, and thwarted grieving response to a loss, possibly evidenced by verbal expression of distress/unresolved issues, denial of loss; altered eating habits, sleep and dream patterns, activity levels, libido; crying, labile affect; feelings of sorrow, guilt, and anger.

Body Image disturbance/Self-Esteem, situational low may be related to situational crisis and chronic illness with changes in usual roles/body image, possibly evidenced by verbalization of changes in lifestyle, focus on past function, negative feelings about body, feelings of helplessness/powerlessness, extension of body boundary to incorporate environmental objects (e.g., dialysis setup), change in social involvement, overdependence on others for care, not taking responsibility for self-care/lack of follow-through, and self-destructive behavior.

Self-Care deficit [specify] may be related to perceptual/cognitive impairment (accumulated toxins); intolerance to activity, decreased strength and endurance; pain/discomfort, possibly evidenced by reported inability to perform ADLs, disheveled/unkempt appearance, strong body odor.

Powerlessness may be related to illness-related regimen and health care environment, possibly evidenced by verbal expression of having no control, depression over physical deterioration, nonparticipation in care, anger, and passivity.

Family Coping, ineffective: compromised/disabling may be related to inadequate or incorrect information or understanding by a primary person, temporary family disorganization and role changes, patient providing little support in turn for the primary person, and prolonged disease/disability progression that exhausts the supportive capacity of significant persons, possibly evidenced by expressions of concern or reports about response of significant other(s)/family to patient's health problem, preoccupation of significant other(s) with own personal reactions, display of intolerance/rejection, and protective behavior disproportionate (too little or too much) to patient's abilities or need for autonomy.

dialysis, peritoneal
(also refer to *dialysis, general*)

Fluid Volume, risk for excess: risk factors may include inadequate osmotic gradient of dialysate, fluid retention (dialysate drainage problems/inappropriate osmotic gradient of solution, bowel distention), excessive PO/IV intake.

Trauma, risk for: risk factors may include improper placement during insertion or manipulation of catheter.

Pain [acute] may be related to procedural factors (catheter irritation, improper catheter placement), presence of edema/abdominal distention, inflammation, or infection, rapid infusion/infusion of cold or acidic dialysate, possibly evidenced by verbal reports, guarding/distraction behaviors, and self-focus.

Infection, risk for peritonitis: risk factors may include contamination of catheter/infusion system, skin contaminants, sterile peritonitis (response to composition of dialysate).

Breathing Pattern, risk for ineffective: risk factors may include increased abdominal pressure with restricted diaphragmatic excursion, rapid infusion of dialysate, pain/discomfort, inflammatory process (e.g., atelectasis/pneumonia).

diarrhea

Knowledge deficit [Learning Need] regarding causative/contributing factors and therapeutic needs may be related to lack of information/misconceptions, possibly evidenced by statements of concern, questions, and development of preventable complications.

Fluid Volume, risk for deficit: risk factors may include excessive losses through gastrointestinal tract, altered intake.

Pain [acute] may be related to abdominal cramping and irritation/excoriation of skin, possibly evidenced by verbal reports, facial grimacing, and autonomic responses.

Skin Integrity, impaired may be related to effects of excretions on delicate tissues, possibly evidenced by reports of discomfort and disruption of skin surface/destruction of skin layers.

digitalis poisoning

Cardiac Output, decreased may be related to altered myocardial contractility/electrical conduction, properties of digitalis (long half-life and narrow therapeutic range), concurrent medications, age/general health status and electrolyte/acid-base balance, possibly evidenced by changes in rate/rhythm/conduction (development/worsening of dysrhythmias), changes in mentation, worsening of heart failure, elevated serum drug levels.

Fluid Volume, risk for deficit/excess: risk factors may include excessive losses from vomiting/diarrhea, decreased intake/nausea, decreased plasma proteins, malnutrition, continued use of diuretics; excess sodium/fluid retention.

Knowledge deficit [Learning Need] regarding condition/therapy and self-care needs may be related to information misinterpretation and lack of recall, possibly evidenced by inaccurate follow-through of instructions and development of preventable complications.

Thought Processes, risk for altered: risk factors may include physiologic effects of toxicity/reduced cerebral perfusion.

dilation and curettage **(D and C)**

(also refer to *abortion, spontaneous*)

Knowledge deficit [Learning Need] regarding surgical procedure, possible postprocedural complications, and therapeutic needs may be related to lack of exposure/unfamiliarity with information, possibly evidenced by requests for information and statements of concern/misconceptions.

Disruptive behavior disorder (childhood, adolescence) **(Conduct disorder)**

Violence, risk for directed at self/others: risk factors may include retarded ego development, antisocial character, poor impulse control, dysfunctional family system, loss of significant relationships, history of suicidal/acting-out behaviors.

Coping, defensive may be related to inadequate coping strategies, maturational crisis, multiple life changes/losses, lack of control of impulsive actions, and personal vulnerability, possibly evidenced by inappropriate use of defense mechanisms, inability to meet role expectations, poor self-esteem, failure to assume responsibility for own actions, hypersensitivity to slight or criticism, and excessive smoking/drinking/drug use.

Thought Processes, altered may be related to physiological changes, lack of appropriate psychological conflict, biochemical changes, as evidenced by tendency to interpret the intentions/actions of others as blaming and hostile; deficits in problem-solving skills, with physical aggression the solution most often chosen.

Self-Esteem, chronic low may be related to life choices perpetuating failure, personal vulnerability, possibly evidenced by self-negating verbalizations, anger, rejection of positive feedback, frequent lack of success in life events.

Family Coping, ineffective: compromised/disabling may be related to excessive guilt, anger, or blaming among family members regarding child's behavior; parental inconsistencies; disagreements regarding discipline, limit setting, and approaches; and exhaustion of parental resources (prolonged coping with disruptive child), possibly evidenced by unrealistic parental expectations, rejection or overprotection of child; and exaggerated expressions of anger, disappointment, or despair regarding child's behavior or ability to improve or change.

Social Interaction, impaired may be related to retarded ego development, developmental state (adolescence), lack of social skills, low self-concept, dysfunctional family system, and neurological impairment, possibly evidenced by dysfunctional interaction with others (difficulty waiting turn in games or group situations, not seeming to listen to what is being said), difficulty playing quietly and maintaining attention to task or play activity, often shifting from one activity to another and interrupting or intruding on others.

disseminated intravascular coagulation **(DIC)**

Fluid Volume, risk for deficit: risk factors may include failure of regulatory mechanism (coagulation process) and active loss/hemorrhage.

Tissue perfusion, altered (specify) may be related to alteration of arterial/venous flow (microemboli throughout circulatory system and hypovolemia), possibly evidenced by changes in respiratory rate and depth, changes in mentation, decreased urinary output, and development of acral cyanosis/focal gangrene.

Gas Exchange, risk for impaired: risk factors may include reduced oxygen-carrying capacity, development of acidosis, fibrin deposition in microcirculation, and ischemic damage of lung parenchyma.

Pain [acute] may be related to bleeding into joints/muscles, with hematoma formation, and ischemic tissues with areas of acral cyanosis/focal gangrene, possibly evidenced by verbal reports, narrowed focus, alteration in muscle tone, guarding/distraction behaviors, restlessness, autonomic responses.

dissociative disorders

Anxiety [severe/panic]/Fear may be related to maladaptation of ineffective coping continuing from early life, unconscious conflict(s), threat to self-concept, unmet needs, or phobic stimulus, possibly evidenced by maladaptive response to stress (e.g., dissociating self/fragmentation of the personality), increased tension, feelings of inadequacy, and focus on self, projection of personal perceptions onto the environment.

Violence, risk for directed at self/others: risk factors may include dissociative state/conflicting personalities, depressed mood, panic states, and suicidal/homicidal behaviors.

Personal Identity disturbance may be related to psychological conflicts (dissociative state), childhood trauma/abuse, threat to physical integrity/self-concept, and underdeveloped ego, possibly evidenced by alteration in perception or experience of self, loss of one's own sense of reality/the external world, poorly differentiated ego boundaries, confusion about sense of self, purpose or direction in life; memory loss, presence of more than one personality within the individual.

Family Coping, ineffective: compromised may be related to multiple stressors repeated over time, prolonged progression of disorder that exhausts the supportive capacity of significant person(s), family disorganization and role changes, high-risk family situation possibly evidenced by family/SOs describing inadequate understanding or knowledge that interferes with assistive or supportive behaviors; relationship/marital conflict.

diverticulitis

Pain [acute] may be related to inflammation of intestinal mucosa, abdominal cramping, and presence of fever/chills, possibly evidenced by verbal reports, guarding/distraction behaviors, autonomic responses, and narrowed focus.

Diarrhea/Constipation may be related to altered structure/function and presence of inflammation, possibly evidenced by signs and symptoms dependent on specific problem (e.g., increase/decrease in frequency of stools and change in consistency).

Knowledge deficit [Learning Need] regarding disease process, potential complications, therapeutic and self-care needs may be related to lack of information/misconceptions, possibly evidenced by statements of concern, request for information, and development of preventable complications.

Powerlessness, risk for: risk factors may include chronic nature of disease process with recurrent episodes despite cooperation with medical regimen.

Down syndrome
(also refer to *mental retardation*)

Growth and development, altered may be related to effects of physical/mental disability, possibly evidenced by altered physical growth; delay/inability in performing skills and self-care/self-control activities appropriate for age.

Trauma, risk for: risk factors may include cognitive difficulties and poor muscle tone/coordination, weakness.

Nutrition: altered, less than body requirements may be related to poor muscle tone and protruding tongue, possibly evidenced by weak and ineffective sucking/swallowing and observed lack of adequate intake with weight loss/failure to gain.

Family Processes, altered may be related to situational/maturational crisis requiring incorporation of new skills into family dynamics, possibly evidenced by confusion about what to do, verbalized difficulty coping with situation, unexamined family myths.

Grieving, risk for dysfunctional: risk factors may include loss of "the perfect child," chronic condition requiring long-term care, and unresolved feelings.

Parent/Infant/Child Attachment, risk for altered: risk factors may include ill infant/child who is unable to effectively initiate parental contact due to altered behavioral organization, inability of parents to meet the personal needs.

Social isolation, risk for: risk factors may include withdrawal from usual social interactions and activities, assumption of total child care, and becoming overindulgent/overprotective.

drug overdose, acute (depressants)
(Also refer to *substance dependence/abuse rehabilitation*)

Breathing Pattern, ineffective/Gas Exchange, impaired may be related to neuromuscular impairment/CNS depression, decreased lung expansion, possibly evidenced by changes in respirations, cyanosis, and abnormal ABGs.

Trauma/Suffocation/Poisoning, risk for: risk factors may include CNS depression/agitation, hypersensitivity to the drug(s), psychological stress.

Violence, risk for directed at self/others: risk factors may include suicidal behaviors, toxic reactions to drug(s).

Infection, risk for: risk factors may include drug injection techniques, impurities in injected drugs, localized trauma; malnutrition, altered immune state.

Duchenne's muscular dystrophy

Mobility, impaired physical may be related to musculoskeletal impairment/weakness, possibly evidenced by decreased muscle strength, control, and mass; limited range of motion; and impaired coordination.

Growth and Development, altered may be related to effects of physical disability, possibly evidenced by altered physical growth and altered ability to perform self-care/self-control activities appropriate to age.

Nutrition: altered, risk for more than body requirements: risk factors may include sedentary lifestyle and dysfunctional eating patterns.

Family Coping, ineffective: compromised may be related to situational crisis/emotional conflicts around issues about hereditary nature of condition and prolonged disease/disability that exhausts supportive capacity of family members, possibly evidenced by preoccupation with personal reactions regarding disability and displaying protective behavior disproportionate (too little/too much) to patient's abilities/need for autonomy.

dysmenorrhea

Pain [acute] may be related to exaggerated uterine contractility, possibly evidenced by verbal reports, guarding/distraction behaviors, narrowed focus, and autonomic responses (changes in vital signs).

Activity intolerance, risk for: risk factors may include severity of pain and presence of secondary symptoms (nausea, vomiting, syncope, chills), depression.

Coping, Individual, ineffective may be related to chronic, recurrent nature of problem; anticipatory anxiety, and inadequate coping methods, possibly evidenced by muscular tension, headaches, general irritability, chronic depression, and verbalization of inability to cope, report of poor self-concept.

dysrhythmia, cardiac

Cardiac Output, risk for decreased: risk factors may include altered electrical conduction and reduced myocardial contractility.

Anxiety [specify level] may be related to perceived threat of death, possibly evidenced by increased tension, apprehension, and expressed concerns.

Knowledge deficit [Learning Need] regarding medical condition/therapy needs may be related to lack of information/misinterpretation and unfamiliarity with information resources, possibly evidenced by questions, statement of misconception, failure to improve on previous regimen, and development of preventable complications.

Activity Intolerance, risk for: risk factors may include imbalance between myocardial oxygen supply and demand, and cardiac depressant effects of certain drugs (beta blockers, antidysrhythmics).

Poisoning, risk for digitalis toxicity: risk factors may include limited range of therapeutic effectiveness, lack of education/proper precautions, reduced vision/cognitive limitations.

eclampsia

Refer to *pregnancy-induced hypertension*.

ectopic pregnancy (tubal)

(Also refer to *abortion, spontaneous*)

Pain [acute] may be related to distention/rupture of fallopian tube, possibly evidenced by reports, guarding/distraction behaviors, facial mask of pain, and autonomic responses (diaphoresis, changes in vital signs).

Fluid volume risk for deficit: risk factors may include hemorrhagic losses and decreased/restricted intake.

Anxiety [specify level]/Fear may be related to threat of death and possible loss of ability to conceive, possibly evidenced by increased tension, apprehension, sympathetic stimulation, restlessness, and focus on self.

eczema (dermatitis)

Pain [discomfort] may be related to cutaneous inflammation and irritation, possibly evidenced by verbal reports, irritability, and scratching.

Infection, risk for: risk factors may include broken skin and tissue trauma.

Social isolation may be related to alterations in physical appearance, possibly evidenced by expressed feelings of rejection and decreased interaction with peers.

edema, pulmonary

Fluid Volume excess may be related to decreased cardiac functioning, excessive fluid/sodium intake, possibly evidenced by dyspnea, presence of crackles (rales), pulmonary congestion on x-ray, restlessness, anxiety, and increased central venous pressure (CVP)/pulmonary pressures.

Gas Exchange, impaired may be related to altered blood flow and decreased alveolar/capillary exchange (fluid collection/shifts into interstitial space/alveoli), possibly evidenced by hypoxia, restlessness, and confusion.

Anxiety [specify level]/Fear may be related to perceived threat of death (inability to breathe), possibly evidenced by responses ranging from apprehension to panic state, restlessness, and focus on self.

emphysema

Gas Exchange, impaired may be related to alveolar capillary membrane changes/destruction, possibly evidenced by dyspnea, restlessness, changes in mentation, abnormal ABG values.

Airway Clearance, ineffective may be related to increased production/retained tenacious secretions, decreased energy level, and muscle wasting, possibly evidenced by abnormal breath sounds (rhonchi), ineffective cough, changes in rate/depth of respirations, and dyspnea.

Activity intolerance may be related to imbalance between oxygen supply and demand, possibly evidenced by reports of fatigue/weakness, exertional dyspnea, and abnormal vital sign response to activity.

Nutrition: altered, less than body requirements may be related to inability to ingest food (shortness of breath, anorexia, generalized weakness, medication side effects), possibly evidenced by lack of interest in food, reported altered taste, loss of muscle mass and tone, fatigue, and weight loss.

Infection, risk for: risk factors may include inadequate primary defenses (stasis of body fluids, decreased ciliary action), chronic disease process, and malnutrition.

Powerlessness may be related to illness-related regimen and health care environment, possibly evidenced by verbal expression of having no control, depression over physical deterioration, nonparticipation in therapeutic regimen; anger, and passivity.

encephalitis

Tissue Perfusion, risk for altered: cerebral: risk factors may include cerebral edema altering/interrupting cerebral arterial/venous blood flow, hypovolemia, exchange problems at cellular level (acidosis).

Hyperthermia may be related to increased metabolic rate, illness, and dehydration, possibly evidenced by increased body temperature, flushed/warm skin, and increased pulse and respiratory rates.

Pain [acute] may be related to inflammation/irritation of the brain and cerebral edema, possibly evidenced by verbal reports of headache, photophobia, distraction behaviors, restlessness, and autonomic response (changes in vital signs).

Trauma/Suffocation, risk for: risk factors may include restlessness, clonic/tonic activity, altered sensorium, cognitive impairment; generalized weakness, ataxia, vertigo.

endocarditis

Cardiac Output, risk for decreased: risk factors may include inflammation of lining of heart and structural change in valve leaflets.

Anxiety [specify level] may be related to change in health status and threat of death, possibly evidenced by apprehension, expressed concerns, and focus on self.

Pain [acute] may be related to generalized inflammatory process and effects of embolic phenomena, possibly evidenced by reports, narrowed focus, distraction behaviors, and autonomic responses (changes in vital signs).

Activity Intolerance, risk for: risk factors may include imbalance between oxygen supply and demand, debilitating condition.

Tissue Perfusion, risk for altered (specify): risk factors may include embolic interruption of arterial flow (embolization of thrombi/valvular vegetations).

endometriosis

Pain [acute]/chronic may be related to pressure of concealed bleeding/formation of adhesions, possibly evidenced by verbal reports (pain between/with menstruation), guarding/distraction behaviors, and narrowed focus.

Sexual dysfunction may be related to pain secondary to presence of adhesions, possibly evidenced by verbalization of problem, and altered relationship with partner.

Knowledge deficit [Learning Need] regarding pathophysiology of condition and therapy needs may be related to lack of information/misinterpretations, possibly evidenced by statements of concern and misconceptions.

enteritis

Refer to *colitis, ulcerative*; *Crohn's disease*.

epididymitis

Pain [acute] may be related to inflammation, edema formation, and tension on the spermatic cord, possibly evidenced by verbal reports, guarding/distraction behaviors (restlessness), and autonomic responses (changes in vital signs).

Infection, risk for spread: risk factors may include presence of inflammation/infectious process, insufficient knowledge to avoid spread of infection.

Knowledge deficit [Learning Need] regarding pathophysiology, outcome, and self-care needs may be related to lack of information/misinterpretations, possibly evidenced by statements of concern, misconceptions, and questions.

epilepsy

Knowledge deficit [Learning Need] regarding condition and medication control may be related to lack of information/misinterpretations, scarce financial resources, possibly evidenced by questions, statements of concern/misconceptions, incorrect use of anticonvulsant medication, recurrent episodes/uncontrolled seizures.

Self-Esteem/Personal Identity disturbance may be related to perceived neurological functional change/weakness, perception of being out of control, stigma associated with condition, possibly evidenced by negative feelings about "brain"/self, change in social involvement, feelings of helplessness, and preoccupation with perceived change or loss.

Social Interaction, impaired may be related to unpredictable nature of condition and self-concept disturbance, possibly evidenced by decreased self-assurance, verbalization of concern, discomfort in social situations, inability to receive/communicate a satisfying sense of belonging/caring, and withdrawal from social contacts/activities.

Trauma/Suffocation, risk for: risk factors may include weakness, balancing difficulties, cognitive limitations/altered consciousness, loss of large- or small-scale muscle coordination (during seizure).

failure to thrive

Nutrition: altered, less than body requirements may be related to inability to ingest/digest/absorb nutrients (defects in organ function/metabolism, genetic factors), physical deprivation/psychosocial factors), possibly evidenced by lack of appropriate weight gain/weight loss, poor muscle tone, pale conjunctiva, and laboratory tests reflecting nutritional deficiency.

Growth and Development, altered may be related to inadequate caretaking (physical/emotional neglect or abuse); indifference, inconsistent responsiveness, multiple caretakers; environmental and stimulation deficiencies, possibly evidenced by altered physical growth, flat affect, listlessness, decreased response; delay or difficulty in performing skills or self-control activities appropriate for age group.

Parenting, risk for altered: risk factors may include lack of knowledge, inadequate bonding, unrealistic expectations for self/infant, and lack of appropriate response of child to relationship.

Knowledge deficit [Learning Need] regarding pathophysiology of condition, nutritional needs, growth/development expectations, and parenting skills may be related to lack of information/misinformation or misinterpretation, possibly evidenced by verbalization of concerns, questions, misconceptions; and development of preventable complications.

fetal alcohol syndrome

Injury, risk for CNS damage: risk factors may include external chemical factors (alcohol intake by mother), placental insufficiency, fetal drug withdrawal in utero/postpartum and prematurity.

Infant behavior, disorganized may be related to prematurity, environmental overstimulation, lack of containment/boundaries, possibly evidenced by change from baseline physiological measures; tremors, startles, twitches, hyperextension of arms/legs, deficient self-regulatory behaviors, deficient response to visual/auditory stimuli.

Parenting, risk for altered: risk factors may include mental and/or physical illness, inability of mother to assume the overwhelming task of unselfish giving and nurturing, presence of stressors (financial/legal problems), lack of available or ineffective role model, interruption of bonding process, lack of appropriate response of child to relationship.

Coping, Individual, ineffective (mother) may be related to personal vulnerability, low self-esteem, inadequate coping skills, and multiple stressors (repeated over period of time), possibly evidenced by inability to meet basic needs/fulfill role expectations/problem solve, and excessive use of drug(s).

Family Processes, altered: alcoholism may be related to lack of/insufficient support from others, mother's drug problem and treatment status, together with poor coping skills, lack of family stability/overinvolvement of parents with children and multigenerational addictive behaviors, possibly evidenced by abandonment, rejection, neglectful relationships with family members, and decisions and actions by family that are detrimental.

fetal demise

Grieving [expected] may be related to death of fetus/infant (wanted or unwanted), possibly evidenced by verbal expression of distress, anger, loss; crying; alteration in eating habits or sleep pattern.

Self-Esteem, situational low may be related to perceived "failure" at a life event, possibly evidenced by negative self-appraisal in response to life event in a person with a previous positive self-evaluation, verbalization of negative feelings about the self (helplessness, uselessness), difficulty making decisions.

Spiritual Distress, risk for: risk factors may include loss of loved one, low self-esteem, poor relationships, challenged belief and value system (birth is supposed to be the beginning of life, not of death) and intense suffering.

fractures
(also refer to *casts*; *traction*)
Trauma, risk for additional injury: risk factors may include loss of skeletal integrity/ movement of skeletal fragments, use of traction apparatus, and so on.
Pain [acute] may be related to muscle spasms, movement of bone fragments, tissue trauma/edema, traction/immobility device, stress and anxiety, possibly evidenced by verbal reports, distraction behaviors, self-focusing/narrowed focus, facial mask of pain, guarding/protective behavior, alteration in muscle tone, and autonomic responses (changes in vital signs).
Peripheral Neurovascular risk for dysfunction: risk factors may include reduction/interruption of blood flow (direct vascular injury, tissue trauma, excessive edema, thrombus formation, hypovolemia).
Mobility, impaired physical may be related to neuromuscular/skeletal impairment, pain/ discomfort, restrictive therapies (bedrest, extremity immobilization), and psychological immobility, possibly evidenced by inability to purposefully move within the physical environment, imposed restrictions, reluctance to attempt movement, limited range of motion, and decreased muscle strength/control.
Gas Exchange, risk for impaired: risk factors may include altered blood flow, blood/fat emboli, alveolar/capillary membrane changes (interstitial/pulmonary edema, congestion).
Knowledge deficit [Learning Need] regarding healing process, therapy requirements, potential complications, and self-care needs may be related to lack of exposure, misinterpretation of information, possibly evidenced by statements of concern, questions, and misconceptions.

frostbite
Tissue integrity, impaired may be related to altered circulation and thermal injury, possibly evidenced by damaged/destroyed tissue.
Pain [acute] may be related to diminished circulation with tissue ischemia/necrosis and edema formation, possibly evidenced by reports, guarding/distraction behaviors, narrowed focus, and autonomic responses (changes in vital signs).
Infection, risk for: risk factors may include traumatized tissue/tissue destruction, altered circulation, and compromised immune response in affected area.

gallstone
Refer to *cholelithiasis*.

gangrene, dry
Tissue Perfusion, altered: peripheral may be related to interruption in arterial flow, possibly evidenced by cool skin temperature, change in color (black), atrophy of affected part, and presence of pain.
Pain [acute] may be related to tissue hypoxia and necrotic process, possibly evidenced by reports, guarding/distraction behaviors, narrowed focus, and autonomic responses (changes in vital signs).

gas, lung irritant
Airway clearance, ineffective may be related to irritation/inflammation of airway, possibly evidenced by marked cough, abnormal breath sounds (wheezes), dyspnea, and tachypnea.
Gas Exchange, risk for impaired: risk factors may include irritation/inflammation of alveolar membrane (dependent on type of agent and length of exposure).
Anxiety [specify level] may be related to change in health status and threat of death, possibly evidenced by verbalizations, increased tension, apprehension, and sympathetic stimulation.

gastritis, acute
Pain [acute] may be related to irritation/inflammation of gastric mucosa, possibly evidenced by verbal reports, guarding/distraction behaviors, and autonomic responses (changes in vital signs).
Fluid Volume, risk for deficit: risk factors may include excessive losses through vomiting and diarrhea, continued bleeding, reluctance to ingest/restrictions of oral intake.

gastritis, chronic
Nutrition: altered, risk for less than body requirements: risk factors may include inability to ingest adequate nutrients (prolonged nausea/vomiting, anorexia, epigastric pain).
Knowledge deficit [Learning Need] regarding pathophysiology, psychological factors,

therapy needs, and potential complications may be related to lack of information/misinterpretation, possibly evidenced by verbalization of concerns, questions, misconceptions, and continuation of problem.

gastroenteritis
Refer to *gastritis, chronic; enteritis*.

gender identity disorder **(For individuals experiencing persistent and marked distress regarding uncertainty about issues relating to personal identity, e.g., sexual orientation and behavior.)**

Anxiety [specify level] may be related to unconscious/conscious conflicts about essential values/beliefs (ego-dystonic gender identification), threat to self-concept, unmet needs, possibly evidenced by increased tension, helplessness, hopelessness, feelings of inadequacy, uncertainty, insomnia, focus on self, and impaired daily functioning.

Role Performance, altered/Personal Identity disturbance may be related to crisis in development in which person has difficulty knowing/accepting to which sex he or she belongs or is attracted, sense of discomfort and inappropriateness about anatomic sex characteristics, possibly evidenced by confusion about sense of self, purpose or direction in life, sexual identification/preference, verbalization of desire to be/insistence that person is the opposite sex, change in self-perception of role, and conflict in roles.

Sexuality Patterns, altered may be related to ineffective or absent role models and conflict with sexual orientation and/or preferences, lack of/impaired relationship with an significant other, possibly evidenced by verbalizations of discomfort with sexual orientation/role and lack of information about human sexuality.

Family Coping, ineffective: risk for compromised/disabling: risk factors may include inadequate/incorrect information or understanding, significant other unable to perceive or to act effectively in regard to patient's needs, temporary family disorganization and role changes, and patient providing little support in turn for primary person.

Family Coping: potential for growth may be related to individual's basic needs being sufficiently gratified and adaptive tasks effectively addressed to enable goals of self-actualization to surface, possibly evidenced by family member(s)' attempts to describe growth/impact of crisis on own values, priorities, goals, or relationships; family member(s) is moving in direction of health-promoting and enriching lifestyle that supports patient's search for self; and choosing experiences that optimize wellness.

glaucoma

Sensory/Perceptual alterations: visual may be related to altered sensory reception and altered status of sense organ (increased intraocular pressure/atrophy of optic nerve head), possibly evidenced by progressive loss of visual field.

Anxiety [specify level] may be related to change in health status, presence of pain, possibility/reality of loss of vision, unmet needs, and negative self-talk, possibly evidenced by apprehension, uncertainty, and expressed concern regarding changes in life event.

glomerulonephritis

Fluid Volume excess may be related to failure of regulatory mechanism (inflammation of glomerular membrane inhibiting filtration), possibly evidenced by weight gain, edema/anasarca, intake greater than output, and blood pressure changes.

Pain [acute] may be related to effects of circulating toxins and edema/distention of renal capsule, possibly evidenced by verbal reports, guarding/distraction behaviors, and autonomic responses (changes in vital signs).

Nutrition: altered, less than body requirements may be related to anorexia and dietary restrictions, possibly evidenced by aversion to eating, reported altered taste, weight loss, and decreased intake.

Diversional Activity deficit may be related to treatment modality/restrictions, fatigue, and malaise, possibly evidenced by statements of boredom, restlessness, and irritability.

Growth, risk for altered: risk factors may include infection, malnutrition, chronic illness.

gonorrhea
(also refer to *sexually transmitted disease—STD*)

Infection, risk for dissemination/bacteremia: risk factors may include presence of infectious process in highly vascular area and lack of recognition of disease process.

Pain [acute] may be related to irritation/inflammation of mucosa and effects of circulating toxins, possibly evidenced by verbal reports of genital or pharyngeal irritation, perineal/pelvic pain, guarding/distraction behaviors.

Knowledge deficit [Learning Need] regarding disease cause/transmission, therapy, and self-care needs may be related to lack of information/misinterpretation, denial of exposure, possibly evidenced by statements of concern, questions, misconceptions, and inaccurate follow-through of instructions/development of preventable complications.

gout

Pain [acute] may be related to inflammation of joint(s), possibly evidenced by verbal reports, guarding/distraction behaviors, and autonomic responses (changes in vital signs).

Mobility, impaired physical may be related to joint pain/edema, possibly evidenced by reluctance to attempt movement, limited range of motion, and therapeutic restriction of movement.

Knowledge deficit [Learning Need] regarding cause, treatment, and prevention of condition may be related to lack of information/misinterpretation, possibly evidenced by statements of concern, questions, misconceptions, and inaccurate follow-through of instructions.

Guillain-Barré syndrome (acute polyneuritis)

Breathing Pattern/Airway clearance, risk for ineffective: risk factors may include weakness/paralysis of respiratory muscles, impaired gag/swallow reflexes, decreased energy/fatigue.

Sensory/Perceptual alterations (specify) may be related to altered sensory reception/transmission/integration (altered status of sense organs, sleep deprivation), therapeutically restricted environment, endogenous chemical alterations (electrolyte imbalance, hypoxia), and psychological stress, possibly evidenced by reported or observed change in usual response to stimuli, altered communication patterns, and measured change in sensory acuity and motor coordination.

Mobility, impaired physical may be related to neuromuscular impairment, pain/discomfort, possibly evidenced by impaired coordination, partial/complete paralysis, decreased muscle strength/control.

Anxiety [specify level]/Fear may be related to situational crisis, change in health status/threat of death, possibly evidenced by increased tension, restlessness, helplessness, apprehension, uncertainty, fearfulness, focus on self, and sympathetic stimulation.

Disuse Syndrome, risk for: risk factors include paralysis and pain.

hay fever

Pain [Discomfort] may be related to irritation/inflammation of upper airway mucous membranes and conjunctiva, possibly evidenced by verbal reports, irritability, and restlessness.

Knowledge deficit [Learning Need] regarding underlying cause, appropriate therapy, and required lifestyle changes may be related to lack of information, possibly evidenced by statements of concern, questions, and misconceptions.

heart failure, congestive

Cardiac Output, decreased may be related to altered myocardial contractility/inotropic changes; alterations in rate, rhythm, and electrical conduction; and structural changes (valvular defects, ventricular aneurysm), possibly evidenced by tachycardia/dysrhythmias, changes in blood pressure, extra heart sounds, decreased urine output, diminished peripheral pulses, cool/ashen skin, orthopnea, crackles; dependent/generalized edema and chest pain.

Fluid Volume, excess may be related to reduced glomerular filtration rate/increased ADH production, and sodium/water retention, possibly evidenced by orthopnea and abnormal breath sounds, S_3 heart sound, jugular vein distention, positive hepatojugular reflex, weight gain, hypertension, oliguria, generalized edema.

Gas Exchange, risk for impaired risk factors may include alveolar-capillary membrane changes (fluid collection/shifts into interstitial space/alveoli).

Activity intolerance may be related to imbalance between oxygen supply/demand, generalized weakness, and prolonged bedrest/sedentary lifestyle, possibly evidenced by reported/observed weakness, fatigue; changes in vital signs, presence of dysrhythmias; dyspnea, pallor, and diaphoresis.

Knowledge deficit [Learning Need] regarding cardiac function/disease process, therapy and self-care needs may be related to lack of information/misinterpretation, possibly evidenced by questions, statements of concern/misconceptions; development of preventable complications or exacerbations of condition.

heatstroke

Hyperthermia may be related to prolonged exposure to hot environment/vigorous activity with failure of regulating mechanism of the body, possibly evidenced by high body temperature (greater than 105°F/40.6°C), flushed/hot skin, tachycardia, and seizure activity.

Cardiac Output, decreased may be related to functional stress of hypermetabolic state, altered circulating volume/venous return, and direct myocardial damage secondary to hyperthermia, possibly evidenced by decreased peripheral pulses, dysrhythmias/tachycardia, and changes in mentation.

hemodialysis
(also refer to *dialysis, general*)
Injury, risk for loss of vascular access: risk factors may include clotting/thrombosis, infection, disconnection/hemorrhage.
Fluid Volume, risk for deficit: risk factors may include excessive fluid losses/shifts via ultrafiltration, hemorrhage (altered coagulation/disconnection of shunt), and fluid restrictions.
Fluid volume, risk for excess: risk factors may include excessive fluid intake; rapid IV, blood/plasma expanders/saline given to support BP during procedure.
Protection, altered may be related to chronic disease state, drug therapy, abnormal blood profile, inadequate nutrition, possibly evidenced by altered clotting, impaired healing, deficient immunity, fatigue, anorexia.

hemophilia
Fluid Volume, risk for deficit: risk factors may include impaired coagulation/hemorrhagic losses.
Pain, risk for [acute]/chronic: risk factors may include nerve compression from hematomas, nerve damage or hemorrhage into joint space.
Mobility, risk for impaired physical: risk factors may include joint hemorrhage, swelling, degenerative changes, and muscle atrophy.
Protection, altered may be related to abnormal blood profile, possibly evidenced by altered clotting.
Family Coping, ineffective: compromised may be related to prolonged nature of condition that exhausts the supportive capacity of significant person(s), possibly evidenced by protective behaviors disproportionate to patient's abilities/need for autonomy.

hemorrhoidectomy
Pain [acute] may be related to edema/swelling and tissue trauma, possibly evidenced by verbal reports, guarding/distraction behaviors, focus on self, and autonomic responses (changes in vital signs).
Urinary Retention, risk for: risk factors may include perineal trauma, edema/swelling, and pain.
Knowledge deficit [Learning Need] regarding therapeutic treatment and potential complications may be related to lack of information/misconceptions, possibly evidenced by statements of concern and questions.

hemorrhoids
Pain [acute] may be related to inflammation and edema of prolapsed varices, possibly evidenced by verbal reports, and guarding/distraction behaviors.
Constipation may be related to pain on defecation and reluctance to defecate, possibly evidenced by frequency, less than usual pattern and hard, formed stools.

hemothorax
(also refer to *pneumothorax*)
Trauma/Suffocation, risk for: risk factors may include concurrent disease/injury process, dependence on external device (chest drainage system), and lack of safety education/precautions.
Anxiety [specify level] may be related to change in health status and threat of death, possibly evidenced by increased tension, restlessness, expressed concern, sympathetic stimulation, and focus on self.

hepatitis, acute viral
Fatigue may be related to decreased metabolic energy production and altered body chemistry, possibly evidenced by reports of lack of energy/inability to maintain usual routines, decreased performance, and increased physical complaints.
Nutrition: altered, less than body requirements may be related to inability to ingest adequate nutrients (nausea, vomiting, anorexia); hypermetabolic state, altered absorption and metabolism, possibly evidenced by aversion to eating/lack of interest in food, altered taste sensation, observed lack of intake, and weight loss.
Pain [acute]/[Discomfort] may be related to inflammation and swelling of the liver, arthralgias, urticarial eruptions, and pruritus, possibly evidenced by verbal reports, guarding/distraction behaviors, focus on self, and autonomic responses (changes in vital signs).
Infection, risk for: risk factors may include inadequate secondary defenses and immunosuppression, malnutrition, insufficient knowledge to avoid exposure to pathogens/spread to others.
Skin/Tissue Integrity, risk for impaired: risk factors may include bile salt accumulation in the tissues.

Home Maintenance Management, risk for impaired: risk factors may include debilitating effects of disease process and inadequate support systems (family, financial, role model).
Knowledge deficit [Learning Need] regarding disease process/transmission, treatment needs, and future expectations may be related to lack of information/recall, misinterpretation, unfamiliarity with resources, possibly evidenced by questions, statements of concerns/misconceptions, inaccurate follow-through of instructions, and development of preventable complications.

hernia, hiatal
Pain, chronic may be related to regurgitation of acidic gastric contents, possibly evidenced by verbal reports, facial grimacing, and focus on self.
Knowledge deficit [Learning Need] regarding pathophysiology, prevention of complications and self-care needs may be related to lack of information/misconceptions, possibly evidenced by statements of concern, questions, and recurrence of condition.

herniation of nucleus pulposus (ruptured intervertebral disk)
Pain [acute]/chronic may be related to nerve compression/irritation and muscle spasms, possibly evidenced by verbal reports, guarding/distraction behaviors, preoccupation with pain, self/narrowed focus, and autonomic responses (changes in vital signs when pain is acute), altered muscle tone/function, changes in eating/sleeping patterns and libido, physical/social withdrawal.
Mobility, impaired physical may be related to pain (muscle spasms), therapeutic restrictions (e.g., bedrest, traction/braces), muscular impairment, and depression, possibly evidenced by reports of pain on movement, reluctance to attempt/difficulty with purposeful movement, decreased muscle strength, impaired coordination, and limited range of motion.
Diversional Activity deficit may be related to length of recuperation period and therapy restrictions, physical limitations, pain and depression, possibly evidenced by statements of boredom, disinterest, "nothing to do," and restlessness, irritability, withdrawal.

herpes, herpes simplex
Pain [acute] may be related to presence of localized inflammation and open lesions, possibly evidenced by verbal reports, distraction behaviors, and restlessness.
Infection, risk for secondary: risk factors may include broken/traumatized tissue, altered immune response, and untreated infection/treatment failure.
Sexuality Patterns, risk for altered: risk factors may include lack of knowledge, values conflict, and/or fear of transmitting the disease.

herpes zoster (shingles)
Pain [acute] may be related to inflammation/local lesions along sensory nerve(s), possibly evidenced by verbal reports, guarding/distraction behaviors, narrowed focus, and autonomic responses (changes in vital signs).
Knowledge deficit [Learning Need] regarding pathophysiology, therapeutic needs, and potential complications may be related to lack of information/misinterpretation, possibly evidenced by statements of concern, questions, and misconceptions.

HIV positive
(also refer to *AIDS*)
Adjustment, impaired may be related to life-threatening, stigmatizing condition/disease; assault to self-esteem, altered locus of control, inadequate support systems, incomplete grieving, medication side effects (fatigue/depression), possibly evidenced by verbalization of nonacceptance/denial of diagnosis, nonexistent or unsuccessful involvement in problem solving/goal setting; extended period of shock and disbelief or anger; lack of future-oriented thinking.
Knowledge deficit [Learning Need] regarding disease, prognosis, and treatment needs may be related to lack of exposure/recall, information misinterpretation, unfamiliarity with information resources, or cognitive limitation, possibly evidenced by statements of misconception/request for information, inappropriate/exaggerated behaviors (hostile, agitated, hysterical, apathetic), inaccurate follow-through of instructions/development of preventable complications.

Hodgkin's disease
(also refer to *cancer*; *chemotherapy*)
Anxiety [specify level]/Fear may be related to threat to self-concept and threat of death, possibly evidenced by apprehension, insomnia, focus on self, and increased tension.
Knowledge deficit [Learning Need] regarding diagnosis, pathophysiology, treatment, and prognosis may be related to lack of information/misinterpretation, possibly evidenced by statements of concern, questions, and misconceptions.
Pain [acute/Discomfort] may be related to manifestations of inflammatory response (fe-

ver, chills, night sweats) and pruritus, possibly evidenced by verbal reports, distraction behaviors, and focus on self.
Breathing Pattern/Airway Clearance, risk for ineffective: risk factors may include tracheobronchial obstruction (enlarged mediastinal nodes and/or airway edema).

hydrocephalus
Tissue Perfusion, altered: cerebral may be related to decreased arterial/venous blood flow (compression of brain tissue), possibly evidenced by changes in mentation, restlessness, irritability, reports of headache, pupillary changes, and changes in vital signs.
Sensory/Perceptual alterations: visual may be related to pressure on sensory/motor nerves, possibly evidenced by reports of double vision, development of strabismus, nystagmus, pupillary changes, and optic atrophy.
Mobility, risk for impaired physical: risk factors may include neuromuscular impairment, decreased muscle strength, and impaired coordination.
Adaptive Capacity: Intracranial, risk for decreased: risk factors may include brain injury, changes in perfusion pressure/intracranial pressure.
Infection, risk for: risk factors may include invasive procedure/presence of shunt.
Knowledge deficit [Learning Need] regarding condition, prognosis, and long-term therapy needs/medical follow-up may be related to lack of information/misperceptions, possibly evidenced by questions, statements of concern, request for information, and inaccurate follow-through of instruction/development of preventable complications.

hyperbilirubinemia
Injury, risk for CNS involvement: risk factors may include prematurity, hemolytic disease, asphyxia, acidosis, hyponatremia, and hypoglycemia.
Injury, risk for effects of treatment: risk factors may include physical properties of phototherapy and effects on body regulatory mechanisms, invasive procedure (exchange transfusion), abnormal blood profile, chemical imbalances.
Knowledge deficit [Learning Need] regarding condition, prognosis, treatment/safety needs may be related to lack of exposure/recall and information misinterpretation, possibly evidenced by questions, statement of concern, and inaccurate follow-through of instructions/development of preventable complications.

hyperemesis gravidarum
Fluid Volume deficit [isotonic] may be related to excessive gastric losses and reduced intake, possibly evidenced by dry mucous membranes, decreased/concentrated urine, decreased pulse volume and pressure, thirst, and hemoconcentration.
Nutrition: altered, less than body requirements may be related to inability to ingest/digest/absorb nutrients (prolonged vomiting), possibly evidenced by reported inadequate food intake, lack of interest in food/aversion to eating, and weight loss.
Coping, Individual, risk for ineffective: risk factors may include situational/maturational crisis (pregnancy, change in health status, projected role changes, concern about outcome).

hypertension
Knowledge deficit [Learning Need] regarding condition, therapeutic regimen, and potential complications may be related to lack of information/recall, misinterpretation, cognitive limitations, and/or denial of diagnosis, possibly evidenced by statements of concern/questions, and misconceptions, inaccurate follow-through of instructions, and lack of BP control.
Adjustment, impaired may be related to condition requiring change in lifestyle, altered locus of control, and absence of feelings/denial of illness, possibly evidenced by verbalization of nonacceptance of health status change and lack of movement toward independence.
Sexual dysfunction, risk for: risk factors may include side effects of medication.
Cardiac Output, risk for decreased: risk factors may include increased afterload (vasoconstriction), fluid shifts/hypovolemia, myocardial ischemia, ventricular hypertrophy/rigidity.
Pain [acute] may be related to increased cerebrovascular pressure, possibly evidenced by verbal reports (throbbing pain located in suboccipital region, present on awakening and disappearing spontaneously after being up and about), reluctance to move head, avoidance of bright lights and noise, or increased muscle tension.

hyperthyroidism
(also refer to *thyrotoxicosis*)
Fatigue may be related to hypermetabolic imbalance with increased energy requirements, irritability of CNS, and altered body chemistry, possibly evidenced by verbalization of overwhelming lack of energy to maintain usual routine, decreased performance, emotional lability/irritability, and impaired ability to concentrate.

Anxiety [specify level] may be related to increased stimulation of the CNS (hypermetabolic state, pseudocatecholamine effect of thyroid hormones), possibly evidenced by increased feelings of apprehension, overexcited/distressed, irritability/emotional lability, shakiness, restless movements, or tremors.
Nutrition: altered, risk for less than body requirements: risk factors may include inability to ingest adequate nutrients for hypermetabolic rate/constant activity, impaired absorption of nutrients (vomiting/diarrhea), hyperglycemia/ relative insulin insufficiency.
Tissue Integrity, risk for impaired: risk factors may include altered protective mechanisms of eye related to periorbital edema, reduced ability to blink, eye discomfort/ dryness, and development of corneal abrasion/ulceration.

hypoglycemia
Thought Processes, altered may be related to inadequate glucose for cellular brain function and effects of endogenous hormone activity, possibly evidenced by irritability, changes in mentation, memory loss, altered attention span, and emotional lability.
Nutrition: altered, risk for less than body requirements: risk factors may include inadequate glucose metabolism and imbalance of glucose/insulin levels.
Knowledge deficit [Learning Need] regarding pathophysiology of condition and therapy/ self-care needs may be related to lack of information/recall, misinterpretations, possibly evidenced by development of hypoglycemia and statements of questions/misconceptions.

hypoparathyroidism (acute)
Injury, risk for: risk factors may include neuromuscular excitability/tetany and formation of renal stones.
Pain [acute] may be related to recurrent muscle spasms and alteration in reflexes, possibly evidenced by verbal reports, distraction behaviors, and narrowed focus.
Airway Clearance, risk for ineffective: risk factors may include spasm of the laryngeal muscles.
Anxiety [specify level] may be related to threat to, or change in, health status, physiological responses.

hypothermia (systemic)
(also refer to *frostbite*)
Hypothermia may be related to exposure to cold environment, inadequate clothing, age extremes (very young/elderly), damage to hypothalamus, consumption of alcohol/medications causing vasodilation, possibly evidenced by reduction in body temperature below normal range, shivering, cool skin, pallor.
Knowledge deficit [Learning Need] regarding risk factors, treatment needs, and prognosis may be related to lack of information/recall, misinterpretation, possibly evidenced by statements of concerns/misconceptions, occurrence of problem, and development of complications.

hypothyroidism
(Also refer to *myxedema*)
Mobility, impaired physical may be related to weakness, fatigue, muscle aches, altered reflexes, and mucin deposits in joints and interstitial spaces, possibly evidenced by decreased muscle strength/control and impaired coordination.
Fatigue may be related to decreased metabolic energy production, possibly evidenced by verbalization of unremitting/overwhelming lack of energy, inability to maintain usual routines, impaired ability to concentrate, decreased libido, irritability, listlessness, decreased performance, increase in physical complaints.
Sensory/Perceptual alterations (specify) may be related to mucin deposits and nerve compression, possibly evidenced by paresthesias of hands and feet or decreased hearing.
Constipation may be related to decreased peristalsis/physical activity, possibly evidenced by frequency less than usual pattern, decreased bowel sounds, hard dry stools, and development of fecal impaction.

hysterectomy
Pain [acute] may be related to tissue trauma/abdominal incision, edema/hematoma formation, possibly evidenced by verbal reports, guarding/distraction behaviors, and autonomic responses (changes in vital signs).
Urinary Elimination, altered/Urinary Retention, [acute] risk for: risk factors may include mechanical trauma, surgical manipulation, presence of localized edema/hematoma, or nerve trauma with temporary bladder atony.
Sexuality Patterns, altered/Sexual dysfunction, risk for: risk factors may include concerns regarding altered body function/structure, perceived changes in femininity, changes in hormone levels, loss of libido, and changes in sexual response pattern.

ileocolitis
Refer to *colitis, ulcerative*.

ileostomy
Refer to *colostomy*.

ileus
Pain [acute] may be related to distention/edema and ischemia of intestinal tissue, possibly evidenced by verbal reports, guarding/distraction behaviors, narrowed focus, and autonomic responses (changes in vital signs).
Diarrhea/Constipation may be related to presence of obstruction/changes in peristalsis, possibly evidenced by changes in frequency and consistency or absence of stool, alterations in bowel sounds, presence of pain, and cramping.
Fluid Volume, risk for deficit: risk factors may include increased intestinal losses (vomiting and diarrhea) and decreased intake.

impetigo
Skin integrity, impaired may be related to presence of infectious process and pruritus, possibly evidenced by open/crusted lesions.
Pain [acute] may be related to inflammation and pruritus, possibly evidenced by verbal reports, distraction behaviors, and self-focusing.
Infection, risk for secondary infection: risk factors may include broken skin, traumatized tissue, altered immune response, and virulence/contagious nature of causative organism.
Infection, risk for transmission: risk factors may include virulent nature of causative organism, insufficient knowledge to prevent infection of others.

influenza
Pain [Discomfort] may be related to inflammation and effects of circulating toxins, possibly evidenced by verbal reports, distraction behaviors, and narrowed focus.
Fluid Volume, risk for deficit: risk factors may include excessive gastric losses, hypermetabolic state, and altered intake.
Hyperthermia may be related to effects of circulating toxins and dehydration, possibly evidenced by increased body temperature, warm/flushed skin, and tachycardia.
Breathing, risk for ineffective: risk factors may include response to infectious process, decreased energy/fatigue.

insulin shock
Refer to *hypoglycemia*.

intestinal obstruction
Refer to *ileus*.

Kawasaki disease
Hyperthermia may be related to increased metabolic rate and dehydration, possibly evidenced by increased body temperature greater than normal range, flushed skin, increased respiratory rate, and tachycardia.
Pain [acute] may be related to inflammation and edema/swelling of tissues, possibly evidenced by verbal reports, restlessness, guarding behaviors, and narrowed focus.
Skin Integrity, impaired may be related to inflammatory process, altered circulation, and edema formation, possibly evidenced by disruption of skin surface including macular rash and desquamation.
Oral Mucous Membranes, altered may be related to inflammatory process, dehydration, and mouth breathing, possibly evidenced by pain, hyperemia, and fissures of lips.
Cardiac Output, risk for decreased: risk factors may include structural changes/inflammation of coronary arteries and alterations in rate/rhythm or conduction.

labor, induced/augmented
Knowledge deficit [Learning Need] regarding procedure, treatment needs, and possible outcomes may be related to lack of exposure/recall, information misinterpretation, and unfamiliarity with information resources, possibly evidenced by questions, statements of concern/misconception, and exaggerated behaviors.
Injury, risk for maternal risk factors may include adverse effects/response to therapeutic interventions.
Gas Exchange, risk for impaired fetal: risk factors may include altered placental perfusion/cord prolapse.
Pain [acute] may be related to altered characteristics of chemically stimulated contractions, psychological concerns, possibly evidenced by verbal reports, increased muscle tone, distraction/guarding behaviors, and narrowed focus.

labor, preterm

Activity Intolerance may be related to muscle/cellular hypersensitivity, possibly evidenced by continued uterine contractions/irritability.

Poisoning, risk for: risk factors may include dose-related toxic/side effects of tocolytics.

Injury, risk for fetal: risk factors may include delivery of premature/immature infant.

Anxiety [specify level] may be related to situational crisis, perceived or actual threats to self/fetus and inadequate time to prepare for labor, possibly evidenced by increased tension, restlessness, expressions of concern, and autonomic responses (changes in vital signs).

Knowledge deficit [Learning Need] regarding preterm labor treatment needs and prognosis may be related to lack of information and misinterpretation, possibly evidenced by questions, statements of concern, misconceptions, inaccurate follow-through of instruction, and development of preventable complications.

labor, stage I (active phase)

Pain [acute/Discomfort] may be related to contraction-related hypoxia, dilation of tissues, and pressure on adjacent structures, combined with stimulation of both parasympathetic and sympathetic nerve endings, possibly evidenced by verbal reports, guarding/distraction behaviors (restlessness), muscle tension, and narrowed focus.

Urinary Elimination, altered may be related to altered intake/dehydration, fluid shifts, hormonal changes, hemorrhage, severe intrapartal hypertension, mechanical compression of bladder, and effects of regional anesthesia, possibly evidenced by changes in amount/frequency of voiding, urinary retention, slowed progression of labor, and reduced sensation.

Coping, Individual/Couple, risk for ineffective: risk factors may include situational crises, personal vulnerability, use of ineffective coping mechanisms, inadequate support systems, and pain.

labor, stage II (expulsion)

Pain [acute] may be related to strong uterine contractions, tissue stretching/dilation, and compression of nerves by presenting part of the fetus, and bladder distention, possibly evidenced by verbalizations, facial grimacing, guarding/distraction behaviors (restlessness), narrowed focus, and autonomic responses (diaphoresis).

Cardiac Output, altered [fluctuation] may be related to changes in SVR, fluctuations in venous return (repeated/prolonged Valsalva's maneuvers, effects of anesthesia/medications, dorsal recumbent position occluding the inferior vena cava and partially obstructing the aorta), possibly evidenced by decreased venous return, changes in vital signs (BP, pulse), urinary output, or fetal bradycardia.

Gas Exchange, risk for impaired fetal: risk factors may include mechanical compression of head/cord, maternal position/prolonged labor affecting placental perfusion, and effects of maternal anesthesia, hyperventilation.

Skin/Tissue Integrity, risk for impaired: risk factors may include untoward stretching/lacerations of delicate tissues (precipitous labor, hypertonic contractile pattern, adolescence, large fetus) and application of forceps.

Fatigue, risk for: risk factors may include pregnancy, stress, anxiety, sleep deprivation, increased physical exertion, anemia, humidity/temperature, lights.

laminectomy (lumbar)

Tissue Perfusion, altered (specify): may be related to diminished/interrupted blood flow (dressing, edema/hematoma formation), hypovolemia, possibly evidenced by paresthesia, numbness; decreased range of motion, muscle strength.

Trauma, risk for spinal: risk factors may include temporary weakness of spinal column, balancing difficulties, changes in muscle tone/coordination.

Pain [acute] may be related to traumatized tissues, localized inflammation, and edema, possibly evidenced by altered muscle tone, verbal reports, and distraction/guarding behaviors, autonomic changes.

Mobility, impaired physical may be related to imposed therapeutic restrictions, neuromuscular impairment, and pain, possibly evidenced by limited range of motion, decreased muscle strength/control, impaired coordination, and reluctance to attempt movement.

Urinary Retention, risk for [acute]: risk factors may include pain and swelling in operative area and reduced mobility/restrictions of position.

laryngectomy

(also refer to *cancer*; *chemotherapy*)

Airway Clearance, ineffective may be related to partial/total removal of the glottis, temporary or permanent change to neck breathing, edema formation, and copious/thick secretions, possibly evidenced by dyspnea/difficulty breathing, changes in rate/

depth of respiration, use of accessory respiratory muscles, weak/ineffective cough, abnormal breath sounds, and cyanosis.

Skin/Tissue Integrity, impaired may be related to surgical removal of tissues/grafting, effects of radiation or chemotherapeutic agents, altered circulation/reduced blood supply, compromised nutritional status, edema formation, and pooling/continuous drainage of secretions, possibly evidenced by disruption of skin/tissue surface and destruction of skin/tissue layers.

Oral Mucous Membranes, altered may be related to dehydration/absence of oral intake, poor/inadequate oral hygiene, pathological condition (oral cancer), mechanical trauma (oral surgery), decreased saliva production, difficulty swallowing and pooling/drooling of secretions, and nutritional deficits, possibly evidenced by xerostomia (dry mouth), oral discomfort, thick/mucoid saliva, decreased saliva production, dry and crusted/coated tongue, inflamed lips, absent teeth/gums, poor dental health, and halitosis.

Communication, impaired verbal may be related to anatomic deficit (removal of vocal cords), physical barrier (tracheostomy tube), and required voice rest, possibly evidenced by inability to speak, change in vocal characteristics, and impaired articulation.

Aspiration, risk for: risk factors include impaired swallowing, facial/neck surgery, presence of tracheostomy/feeding tube.

laryngitis

Refer to *croup*.

lead poisoning, acute

(also refer to *lead poisoning, chronic*)

Trauma, risk for: risk factors may include loss of coordination, altered level of consciousness, clonic or tonic muscle activity, neurologic damage.

Fluid Volume, risk for deficit: risk factors may include excessive vomiting, diarrhea, or decreased intake.

Knowledge deficit [Learning Need] regarding sources of lead and prevention of poisoning may be related to lack of information/misinterpretation, possibly evidenced by statements of concern, questions, and misconceptions.

lead poisoning, chronic

(also refer to *lead poisoning, acute*)

Nutrition: altered, less than body requirements may be related to decreased intake (chemically induced changes in the gastrointestinal tract), possibly evidenced by anorexia, abdominal discomfort, reported metallic taste, and weight loss.

Thought Processes, altered may be related to deposition of lead in CNS and brain tissue, possibly evidenced by personality changes, learning disabilities, and impaired ability to conceptualize and reason.

Pain, chronic may be related to deposition of lead in soft tissues and bone, possibly evidenced by verbal reports, distraction behaviors, and focus on self.

leukemia, acute

(also refer to *chemotherapy*)

Infection, risk for: risk factors may include inadequate secondary defenses (alterations in mature white blood cells, increased number of immature lymphocytes, immunosuppression and bone marrow suppression), invasive procedures, and malnutrition.

Anxiety [specify level]/Fear may be related to change in health status, threat of death, and situational crisis, possibly evidenced by sympathetic stimulation, apprehension, feelings of helplessness, focus on self, and insomnia.

Activity Intolerance may be related to reduced energy stores, increased metabolic rate, imbalance between oxygen supply and demand, or therapeutic restrictions (bedrest)/effect of drug therapy, possibly evidenced by generalized weakness, reports of fatigue and exertional dyspnea; abnormal heart rate or BP response.

Pain [acute] may be related to physical agents (infiltration of tissues/organs/CNS, expanding bone marrow) and chemical agents (antileukemic treatments), possibly evidenced by verbal reports (abdominal discomfort, arthralgia, bone pain, headache); distraction behaviors, narrowed focus, and autonomic responses (changes in vital signs).

Fluid Volume, risk for deficit: risk factors may include excessive losses (vomiting, hemorrhage, diarrhea), decreased intake (nausea, anorexia), increased fluid need (hypermetabolic state/fever), predisposition for kidney stone formation/tumor lysis syndrome.

long-term care

Refer to *care, long-term*.

lupus erythematosus, systemic (SLE)

Fatigue may be related to inadequate energy production/increased energy requirements (chronic inflammation), overwhelming psychological or emotional demands, states of discomfort, and altered body chemistry (including effects of drug therapy), possibly evidenced by reports of unremitting and overwhelming lack of energy/inability to maintain usual routines, decreased performance, lethargy, and decreased libido.

Pain [acute] may be related to widespread inflammatory process affecting connective tissues, blood vessels, serosal surfaces, and mucous membranes, possibly evidenced by verbal reports, guarding/distraction behaviors, self-focusing, and autonomic responses (changes in vital signs).

Skin/Tissue integrity, impaired may be related to chronic inflammation, edema formation, and altered circulation, possibly evidenced by presence of skin rash/lesions, ulcerations of mucous membranes, and photosensitivity.

Body Image disturbance may be related to presence of chronic condition with rash, lesions, ulcers, purpura, mottled erythema of hands, alopecia, loss of strength, and altered body function, possibly evidenced by hiding body parts, negative feelings about body, feelings of helplessness, and change in social involvement.

Lyme disease

Pain [acute]/chronic may be related to systemic effects of toxins, presence of rash, urticaria, and joint swelling/inflammation, possibly evidenced by verbal reports, guarding behavior, autonomic responses, and narrowed focus.

Fatigue may be related to increased energy requirements, altered body chemistry, and states of discomfort evidenced by reports of overwhelming lack of energy/inability to maintain usual routines, decreased performance, lethargy, and malaise.

Cardiac Output, risk for decreased risk factors may include alteration in rate/rhythm/conduction.

Mallory-Weiss syndrome
(also refer to *achalasia*)

Fluid Volume, risk for deficit: risk factors may include excessive vascular losses, presence of vomiting, and reduced intake.

Knowledge deficit [Learning Need] regarding causes, treatment, and prevention of condition may be related to lack of information/misinterpretation, possibly evidenced by statements of concern, questions, and recurrence of problem.

mastectomy

Skin/Tissue Integrity, impaired may be related to surgical removal of skin/tissue, altered circulation, drainage, presence of edema, changes in skin elasticity/sensation, and tissue destruction (radiation), possibly evidenced by disruption of skin surface and destruction of skin layers/subcutaneous tissues.

Mobility, impaired physical may be related to neuromuscular impairment, pain, and edema formation, possibly evidenced by reluctance to attempt movement, limited range of motion, and decreased muscle mass/strength.

Self-Care deficit, bathing/dressing may be related to temporary loss/altered action of one or both arms, possibly evidenced by statements of inability to perform/complete self-care tasks.

Body Image disturbance may be related to loss of body part denoting femininity, possibly evidenced by not looking at/touching area, negative feelings about body, preoccupation with loss, and change in social involvement/relationship.

mastitis

Pain [acute] may be related to erythema and edema of breast tissues, possibly evidenced by verbal reports, guarding/distraction behaviors, self-focusing, autonomic responses (changes in vital signs).

Infection, risk for spread/abscess formation: risk factors may include traumatized tissues, stasis of fluids, and insufficient knowledge to prevent complications.

Knowledge deficit [Learning Need] regarding pathophysiology, treatment, and prevention may be related to lack of information/misinterpretation, possibly evidenced by statements of concern, questions, and misconceptions.

Breastfeeding, risk for ineffective: risk factors may include inability to feed on affected side/interruption in breastfeeding.

mastoidectomy

Infection, risk for spread: risk factors may include preexisting infection, surgical trauma, and stasis of body fluids in close proximity to brain.

Pain [acute] may be related to inflammation, tissue trauma, and edema formation, possibly evidenced by verbal reports, distraction behaviors, restlessness, self-focusing, and autonomic responses (changes in vital signs).

Sensory/Perceptual alterations: auditory may be related to presence of surgical packing, edema, and surgical disturbance of middle ear structures, possibly evidenced by reported/tested hearing loss in affected ear.

measles

Pain [acute] may be related to inflammation of mucous membranes, conjunctiva, and presence of extensive skin rash with pruritus, possibly evidenced by verbal reports, distraction behaviors, self-focusing, and autonomic responses (changes in vital signs).

Hyperthermia may be related to presence of viral toxins and inflammatory response, possibly evidenced by increased body temperature, flushed/warm skin, and tachycardia.

Infection, risk for secondary: risk factors may include altered immune response and traumatized dermal tissues.

Knowledge deficit [Learning Need] regarding condition, transmission, and possible complications may be related to lack of information/misinterpretation, possibly evidenced by statements of concern, questions, misconceptions, and development of preventable complications.

meningitis, acute meningococcal

Infection, risk for spread: risk factors may include hematogenous dissemination of pathogen, stasis of body fluids, suppressed inflammatory response (medication-induced), and exposure of others to pathogens.

Tissue Perfusion, risk for altered: cerebral: risk factors may include cerebral edema altering/interrupting cerebral arterial/venous blood flow, hypovolemia, exchange problems at cellular level (acidosis).

Hyperthermia may be related to infectious process (increased metabolic rate) and dehydration, possibly evidenced by increased body temperature, warm/flushed skin, and tachycardia.

Pain [acute] may be related to inflammation/irritation of the meninges with spasm of extensor muscles (neck, shoulders, and back), possibly evidenced by verbal reports, guarding/distraction behaviors, narrowed focus, and autonomic responses (changes in vital signs).

Trauma/Suffocation, risk for: risk factors may include alterations in level of consciousness, possible development of clonic/tonic muscle activity (seizures), and generalized weakness/prostration, ataxia, vertigo.

meniscectomy

Walking, impaired may be related to pain, joint instability, and imposed medical restrictions of movement, possibly evidenced by impaired ability to move about environment as needed/desired.

Knowledge deficit [Learning Need] regarding postoperative expectations, prevention of complications, and self-care needs may be related to lack of information, possibly evidenced by statements of concern, questions, and misconceptions.

mental retardation
(also refer to *Down syndrome*)

Communication, impaired verbal may be related to developmental delay/impairment of cognitive and motor abilities, possibly evidenced by impaired articulation, difficulty with phonation, and inability to modulate speech/find appropriate words (dependent on degree of retardation).

Self-Care deficit, risk for [specify]: risk factors may include impaired cognitive ability and motor skills.

Nutrition: altered, risk for more than body requirements: risk factors may include decreased metabolic rate coupled with impaired cognitive development, dysfunctional eating patterns, and sedentary activity level.

Social Interaction, impaired may be related to impaired thought processes, communication barriers, and knowledge/skill deficit about ways to enhance mutuality, possibly evidenced by dysfunctional interactions with peers, family, and/or significant other(s), and verbalized/observed discomfort in social situation.

Family Coping, ineffective: compromised may be related to chronic nature of condition and degree of disability that exhausts supportive capacity of significant other(s), other situational or developmental crises or situations the significant other may be facing, unrealistic expectations of significant other, possibly evidenced by preoccupation of significant other with personal reaction, significant other withdraws or enters into limited interaction with individual, protective behavior disproportionate (too much or too little) to patient's abilities or need for autonomy.

Home Maintenance Management, impaired may be related to impaired cognitive functioning, insufficient finances/family organization or planning, lack of knowledge, and inadequate support systems, possibly evidenced by requests for assistance, expression

of difficulty in maintaining home, disorderly surroundings, and overtaxed family members.
Sexual dysfunction, risk for: risk factors may include biopsychosocial alteration of sexuality, ineffectual/absent role models, misinformation/lack of knowledge, lack of significant other(s), and lack of appropriate behavior control.

mitral stenosis
Activity intolerance may be related to imbalance between oxygen supply and demand, possibly evidenced by reports of fatigue, weakness, exertional dyspnea, and tachycardia.
Gas Exchange, impaired may be related to altered blood flow, possibly evidenced by restlessness, hypoxia, and cyanosis (orthopnea/paroxysmal nocturnal dyspnea).
Cardiac Output, decreased may be related to impeded blood flow as evidenced by jugular vein distention, peripheral/dependent edema, orthopnea/paroxysmal nocturnal dyspnea.
Knowledge deficit [Learning Need] regarding pathophysiology, therapeutic needs, and potential complications may be related to lack of information/recall, misinterpretation, possibly evidenced by statements of concern, questions, inaccurate follow-through of instructions, and development of preventable complications.

mononucleosis, infectious
Fatigue may be related to decreased energy production, states of discomfort, and increased energy requirements (inflammatory process), possibly evidenced by reports of overwhelming lack of energy, inability to maintain usual routines, lethargy, and malaise.
Pain [Discomfort] may be related to inflammation of lymphoid and organ tissues, irritation of oropharyngeal mucous membranes, and effects of circulating toxins, possibly evidenced by verbal reports, distraction behaviors, and self-focusing.
Hyperthermia may be related to inflammatory process, possibly evidenced by increased body temperature, warm/flushed skin, and tachycardia.
Knowledge deficit [Learning Need] regarding disease transmission, self-care needs, medical therapy, and potential complications may be related to lack of information/misinterpretation, possibly evidenced by statements of concern, misconceptions, and inaccurate follow-through of instructions.

mood disorders
Refer to *depressive disorders*.

multiple personality
Refer to *dissociative disorders*.

multiple sclerosis
Fatigue may be related to decreased energy production/increased energy requirements to perform activities, psychological/emotional demands, pain/discomfort, medication side effects, possibly evidenced by verbalization of overwhelming lack of energy, inability to maintain usual routine, decreased performance, impaired ability to concentrate, increase in physical complaints.
Sensory/Perceptual alterations: visual, kinesthetic, tactile may be related to delayed/interrupted neuronal transmission, possibly evidenced by impaired vision, diplopia, disturbance of vibratory or position sense, paresthesias, numbness, and blunting of sensation.
Mobility, impaired physical may be related to neuromuscular impairment, discomfort/pain, sensoriperceptual impairments, decreased muscle strength, control and/or mass, deconditioning, as evidenced by limited ability to perform motor skills, limited range of motion, gait changes/postural instability.
Powerlessness/Hopelessness may be related to illness-related regimen and lifestyle of helplessness, possibly evidenced by verbal expressions of having no control or influence over the situation, depression over physical deterioration that occurs despite patient compliance with regimen, nonparticipation in care or decision making when opportunities are provided, passivity, decreased verbalization/affect.
Home Maintenance Management, impaired may be related to effects of debilitating disease, impaired cognitive and/or emotional functioning, insufficient finances, and inadequate support systems, possibly evidenced by reported difficulty, observed disorderly surroundings, and poor hygienic conditions.
Family Coping, ineffective: compromised/disabling may be related to situational crises/temporary family disorganization and role changes, patient providing little support in turn for significant other(s), prolonged disease/disability progression that exhausts the supportive capacity of significant other(s), feelings of guilt, anxiety, hostility, despair, and highly ambivalent family relationships, possibly evidenced by patient ex-

pressing/confirming concern or report about significant other(s)' response to patient's illness, significant other(s) preoccupied with own personal reactions, intolerance, abandonment, neglectful care of the patient, and distortion of reality regarding patient's illness.

mumps

Pain [acute] may be related to presence of inflammation, circulating toxins, and enlargement of salivary glands, possibly evidenced by verbal reports, guarding/distraction behaviors, self-focusing, and autonomic responses (changes in vital signs).

Hyperthermia may be related to inflammatory process (increased metabolic rate), and dehydration, possibly evidenced by increased body temperature, warm/flushed skin, and tachycardia.

Fluid Volume, risk for deficit: risk factors may include hypermetabolic state and painful swallowing with decreased intake.

muscular dystrophy (Duchenne's)

(Refer to *Duchenne's muscular dystrophy*)

myasthenia gravis

Breathing pattern/Airway Clearance, ineffective may be related to neuromuscular weakness and decreased energy/fatigue, possibly evidenced by dyspnea, changes in rate/depth of respiration, ineffective cough, and adventitious breath sounds.

Communication, impaired verbal may be related to neuromuscular weakness, fatigue, and physical barrier (intubation), possibly evidenced by facial weakness, impaired articulation, hoarseness, and inability to speak.

Swallowing, impaired may be related to neuromuscular impairment of laryngeal/pharyngeal muscles and muscular fatigue, possibly evidenced by reported/observed difficulty swallowing, coughing/choking, and evidence of aspiration.

Anxiety [specify level]/Fear may be related to situational crisis, threat to self-concept, change in health/socioeconomic status or role function, separation from support systems, lack of knowledge, and inability to communicate, possibly evidenced by expressed concerns, increased tension, restlessness, apprehension, sympathetic stimulation, crying, focus on self, uncooperative behavior, withdrawal, anger, and noncommunication.

Knowledge deficit [Learning Need] regarding drug therapy, potential for crisis (myasthenic or cholinergic) and self-care management may be related to inadequate information/misinterpretation, possibly evidenced by statements of concern, questions, and misconceptions; development of preventable complications.

Mobility, impaired physical may be related to neuromuscular impairment, possibly evidenced by reports of progressive fatigability with repetitive/prolonged muscle use, impaired coordination, and decreased muscle strength/control.

Sensory/Perceptual alterations: visual may be related to neuromuscular impairment, possibly evidenced by visual distortions (diplopia) and motor incoordination.

myocardial infarction

(also refer to *myocarditis*)

Pain [acute] may be related to ischemia of myocardial tissue, possibly evidenced by verbal reports, guarding/distraction behaviors (restlessness), facial mask of pain, self-focusing, and autonomic responses (diaphoresis, changes in vital signs).

Anxiety [specify level]/Fear may be related to threat of death, threat of change of health status/role functioning and lifestyle, interpersonal transmission/contagion, possibly evidenced by increased tension, fearful attitude, apprehension, expressed concerns/uncertainty, restlessness, sympathetic stimulation, and somatic complaints.

Cardiac Output, risk for decreased: risk factors may include changes in rate and electrical conduction, reduced preload, increased systemic vascular resistance, and altered muscle contractility/depressant effects of some medications, infarcted/dyskinetic muscle, structural defects.

myocarditis

(Refer to *myocardial infarction*)

Activity intolerance may be related to imbalance in oxygen supply and demand (myocardial inflammation/damage), cardiac depressant effects of certain drugs, and enforced bedrest, possibly evidenced by reports of fatigue, exertional dyspnea, tachycardia/palpitations in response to activity, ECG changes/dysrhythmias, and generalized weakness.

Cardiac Output, risk for decreased: risk factors may include degeneration of cardiac muscle.

Knowledge deficit [Learning Need] regarding pathophysiology of condition/outcomes, treatment, and self-care needs/lifestyle changes may be related to lack of information/

misinterpretation, possibly evidenced by statements of concern, misconceptions, inaccurate follow-through of instructions, and development of preventable complications.

myringotomy
Refer to *mastoidectomy*.

myxedema
(also refer to *hypothyroidism*)
Body Image disturbance may be related to change in structure/function (loss of hair/thickening of skin, masklike facial expression, enlarged tongue, menstrual and reproductive disturbances), possibly evidenced by negative feelings about body, feelings of helplessness, and change in social involvement.
Nutrition: altered, more than body requirements may be related to decreased metabolic rate and activity level, possibly evidenced by weight gain greater than ideal for height and frame.
Cardiac Output, risk for decreased: risk factors may include altered electrical conduction and myocardial contractility.

neonate, normal newborn
Gas Exchange, risk for impaired: risk factors may include prenatal or intrapartal stressors, excess production of mucus, or cold stress.
Body Temperature, risk for altered: risk factors may include large body surface in relation to mass, limited amounts of insulating subcutaneous fat, nonrenewable sources of brown fat and few white fat stores, thin epidermis with close proximity of blood vessels to the skin, inability to shiver, and movement from a warm uterine environment to a much cooler environment.
Parent/Infant attachment, risk for altered: risk factors may include developmental transition (gain of a family member); anxiety associated with the parent role, or lack of privacy (intrusive family/visitors).
Nutrition: altered, risk for less than body requirements: risk factors may include rapid metabolic rate, high caloric requirement, increased insensible water losses through pulmonary and cutaneous routes, fatigue, and a potential for inadequate or depleted glucose stores.
Infection, risk for: risk factors may include inadequate secondary defenses (inadequate acquired immunity, e.g., deficiency of neutrophils and specific immunoglobulins) and inadequate primary defenses (e.g., environmental exposure, broken skin, traumatized tissues, decreased ciliary action).

neonate, premature newborn
Gas Exchange, impaired may be related to alveolar-capillary membrane changes (inadequate surfactant levels), altered blood flow (immaturity of pulmonary arteriole musculature), altered oxygen supply (immaturity of central nervous system and neuromuscular system, tracheobronchial obstruction), altered oxygen-carrying capacity of blood (anemia), and cold stress, possibly evidenced by respiratory difficulties, inadequate oxygenation of tissues, and acidemia.
Breathing Pattern, ineffective may be related to immaturity of the respiratory center, poor positioning, drug-related depression, metabolic imbalances, or decreased energy/fatigue, possibly evidenced by dyspnea, tachypnea, periods of apnea, nasal flaring/use of accessory muscles, cyanosis, abnormal ABGs, and tachycardia.
Thermoregulation, risk for ineffective: risk factors may include immature CNS development (temperature regulation center), decreased ratio of body mass to surface area, decreased subcutaneous fat, limited brown fat stores, inability to shiver or sweat, poor metabolic reserves, muted response to hypothermia, and frequent medical/nursing manipulations and interventions.
Fluid Volume, risk for deficit: risk factors may include extremes of age and weight, excessive fluid losses (thin skin, lack of insulating fat, increased environmental temperature, immature kidney/failure to concentrate urine).
Infant Behavior, risk for disorganized: risk factors may include prematurity (immature central nervous system, hypoxia), lack of containment/boundaries, pain, or overstimulation, separation from parents.

nephrectomy
Pain [acute] may be related to surgical tissue trauma with mechanical closure (suture), possibly evidenced by verbal reports, guarding/distraction behaviors, self-focusing, and autonomic responses (changes in vital signs).
Fluid Volume, risk for deficit: risk factors may include excessive vascular losses and restricted intake.
Breathing Pattern, ineffective may be related to incisional pain with decreased lung

expansion, possibly evidenced by tachypnea, fremitus, changes in respiratory depth/chest expansion, and changes in ABGs.

Constipation may be related to reduced dietary intake, decreased mobility, gastrointestinal obstructions (paralytic ileus), and incisional pain with defecation, possibly evidenced by decreased bowel sounds, reduced frequency/amount of stool, and hard/formed stool.

nephrotic syndrome

Fluid Volume, excess may be related to compromised regulatory mechanism with changes in hydrostatic/oncotic vascular pressure and increased activation of the renin-angiotensin-aldosterone system, possibly evidenced by edema/anasarca, effusions/ascites, weight gain, intake greater than output, and blood pressure changes.

Nutrition: altered, less than body requirements may be related to excessive protein losses and inability to ingest adequate nutrients (anorexia), possibly evidenced by weight loss/muscle wasting (may be difficult to assess due to edema), lack of interest in food, and observed inadequate intake.

Infection, risk for: risk factors may include chronic disease and steroidal suppression of inflammatory responses.

Skin integrity, risk for impaired: risk factors may include presence of edema and activity restrictions.

neuralgia, trigeminal

Pain [acute] may be related to neuromuscular impairment with sudden violent muscle spasm, possibly evidenced by verbal reports, guarding/distraction behaviors, self-focusing, and autonomic responses (changes in vital signs).

Knowledge deficit [Learning Need] regarding control of recurrent episodes, medical therapies, and self-care needs may be related to lack of information/recall and misinterpretation, possibly evidenced by statements of concern, questions, and exacerbation of condition.

neuritis

Pain [acute]/chronic may be related to nerve damage usually associated with a degenerative process, possibly evidenced by verbal reports, guarding/distraction behaviors, self-focusing, and autonomic responses (changes in vital signs).

Knowledge deficit [Learning Need] regarding underlying causative factors, treatment, and prevention may be related to lack of information/misinterpretation, possibly evidenced by statements of concern, questions, and misconceptions.

obesity

Nutrition: altered, more than body requirements may be related to excessive intake in relation to metabolic needs, possibly evidenced by weight 20% greater than ideal for height and frame, sedentary activity level, reported/observed dysfunctional eating patterns, and excess body fat by triceps skinfold/other measurements.

Body Image disturbance/Self-Esteem, chronic low may be related to view of self in contrast with societal values, family/subculture encouragement of overeating; control, sex, and love issues; possibly evidenced by negative feelings about body, fear of rejection/reaction of others, feelings of hopelessness/powerlessness, and lack of follow-through with treatment plan.

Activity Intolerance may be related to imbalance between oxygen supply and demand, and sedentary lifestyle, possibly evidenced by fatigue or weakness, exertional discomfort, and abnormal heart rate/blood pressure response.

Social Interaction, impaired may be related to verbalized/observed discomfort in social situations, self-concept disturbance, possibly evidenced by reluctance to participate in social gatherings, verbalization of a sense of discomfort with others, feeling of rejection, absence of/ineffective supportive significant other(s).

osteoarthritis (degenerative joint disease)

Refer to *arthritis, rheumatoid* (Although this is a degenerative process versus the inflammatory process of rheumatoid arthritis, nursing concerns are the same.)

osteomyelitis

Pain [acute] may be related to inflammation and tissue necrosis, possibly evidenced by verbal reports, guarding/distraction behaviors, self-focus, and autonomic responses (changes in vital signs).

Hyperthermia may be related to increased metabolic rate and infectious process, possibly evidenced by increased body temperature and warm/flushed skin.

Tissue Perfusion, altered: bone may be related to inflammatory reaction with thrombosis of vessels, destruction of tissue, edema, and abscess formation, possibly evidenced by bone necrosis, continuation of infectious process, and delayed healing.

Walking, risk for impaired: risk factors may include inflammation and tissue necrosis, pain, joint instability.
Knowledge deficit [Learning Need] regarding pathophysiology of condition, long-term therapy needs, activity restriction, and prevention of complications may be related to lack of information/misinterpretation, possibly evidenced by statements of concern, questions and misconceptions, and inaccurate follow-through of instructions.

osteoporosis
Trauma, risk for: risk factors may include loss of bone density/integrity, increasing risk of fracture with minimal or no stress.
Pain [acute]/chronic may be related to vertebral compression on spinal nerve/muscles/ligaments, spontaneous fractures, possibly evidenced by verbal reports, guarding/distraction behaviors, self-focus, and changes in sleep pattern.
Mobility, impaired physical may be related to pain and musculoskeletal impairment, possibly evidenced by limited range of motion, reluctance to attempt movement/expressed fear of reinjury, and imposed restrictions/limitations.

palsy, cerebral (spastic hemiplegia)
Mobility, impaired physical may be related to muscular weakness/hypertonicity, increased deep tendon reflexes, tendency to contractures, and underdevelopment of affected limbs, possibly evidenced by decreased muscle strength, control, mass, limited range of motion, and impaired coordination.
Family Coping, ineffective: compromised may be related to permanent nature of condition, situational crisis, emotional conflicts/temporary family disorganization, and incomplete information/understanding of patient's needs, possibly evidenced by verbalized anxiety/guilt regarding patient's disability, inadequate understanding and knowledge base, and displaying protective behaviors disproportionate (too little/too much) to patient's abilities or need for autonomy.
Growth and Development, altered may be related to effects of physical disability, possibly evidenced by altered physical growth, delay or difficulty in performing skills (motor, social, expressive), and altered ability to perform self-care/self-control activities appropriate to age.

pancreatitis
Pain [acute] may be related to obstruction of pancreatic/biliary ducts, chemical contamination of peritoneal surfaces by pancreatic exudate/autodigestion, extension of inflammation to the retroperitoneal nerve plexus, possibly evidenced by verbal reports, guarding/distraction behaviors, self-focus, grimacing, autonomic responses (changes in vital signs), and alteration in muscle tone.
Fluid Volume, risk for deficit: risk factors may include excessive gastric losses (vomiting, nasogastric suctioning), increase in size of vascular bed (vasodilation, effects of kinins), third-space fluid transudation, ascites formation, alteration of clotting process, hemorrhage.
Nutrition: altered, less than body requirements may be related to vomiting, decreased oral intake as well as altered ability to digest nutrients (loss of digestive enzymes/insulin), possibly evidenced by reported inadequate food intake, aversion to eating, reported altered taste sensation, weight loss, and reduced muscle mass.
Infection, risk for: risk factors may include inadequate primary defenses (stasis of body fluids, altered peristalsis, change in pH secretions), immunosuppression, nutritional deficiencies, tissue destruction, and chronic disease.

paranoid disorders
Violence, risk for directed at others/self: risk factors may include perceived threats of danger, paranoid delusions, and increased feelings of anxiety.
Anxiety [severe] may be related to inability to trust (has not mastered tasks of trust versus mistrust), possibly evidenced by rigid delusional system (serves to provide relief from stress that justifies the delusion), frightened of other people and own hostility.
Powerlessness may be related to feelings of inadequacy, lifestyle of helplessness, maladaptive interpersonal interactions (e.g., misuse of power, force; abusive relationships), sense of severely impaired self-esteem, and belief that individual has no control over situation(s), possibly evidenced by use of paranoid delusions, use of aggressive behavior to compensate, and expressions of recognition of damage paranoia has caused self and others.
Thought Processes, altered may be related to psychological conflicts, increased anxiety, and fear, possibly evidenced by difficulties in the process and character of thought, interference with the ability to think clearly and logically, delusions, or fragmentation and autistic thinking.

Family Coping, ineffective: compromised may be related to temporary or sustained family disorganization/role changes, prolonged progression of condition that exhausts the supportive capacity of significant other(s), possibly evidenced by family system not meeting physical/emotional/spiritual needs of its members, inability to express or to accept wide range of feelings, inappropriate boundary maintenance; significant other(s) describes preoccupation with personal reactions.

paraplegia

(also refer to *quadriplegia*)

Transfer Ability, impaired may be related to loss of muscle function/control, injury to upper extremity joints (overuse).

Sensory/Perceptual alterations: kinesthetic, tactile may be related to neurologic deficit with loss of sensory reception and transmission, psychological stress, possibly evidenced by reported/measured change in sensory acuity and loss of usual response to stimuli.

Incontinence, reflex/Urinary Elimination, altered may be related to loss of nerve conduction above the level of the reflex arc, possibly evidenced by lack of awareness of bladder filling/fullness, absence of urge to void, and uninhibited bladder contraction, urinary tract infections, kidney stone formation.

Body Image disturbance/Role Performance, altered may be related to loss of body functions, change in physical ability to resume role, perceived loss of self/identity, possibly evidenced by negative feelings about body/self, feelings of helplessness/powerlessness, delay in taking responsibility for self-care/participation in therapy, and change in social involvement.

Sexual dysfunction may be related to loss of sensation, altered function, vulnerability, possibly evidenced by seeking of confirmation of desirability, verbalization of concern, and alteration in relationship with significant other, and change in interest in self/others.

parathyroidectomy

Pain [acute] may be related to presence of surgical incision and effects of calcium imbalance (bone pain, tetany), possibly evidenced by verbal reports, guarding/distraction behaviors, self-focus, and autonomic responses (changes in vital signs).

Fluid Volume, risk for excess: risk factors may include preoperative renal involvement, stress-induced release of ADH, and changing calcium/electrolyte levels.

Airway Clearance, risk for ineffective: risk factors may include edema formation and laryngeal nerve damage.

Knowledge deficit [Learning Need] regarding postoperative care/complications and long-term needs may be related to lack of information/recall, misinterpretation, possibly evidenced by statements of concern, questions, and misconceptions.

Parkinson's disease

Walking, impaired may be related to neuromuscular impairment (muscle weakness, tremors, bradykinesia) and musculoskeletal impairment (joint rigidity), possibly evidenced by inability to move about the environment as desired, increased occurrence of falls.

Swallowing, impaired may be related to neuromuscular impairment/muscle weakness, possibly evidenced by reported/observed difficulty in swallowing, drooling, evidence of aspiration (choking, coughing).

Communication, impaired verbal may be related to muscle weakness and incoordination, possibly evidenced by impaired articulation, difficulty with phonation, and changes in rhythm and intonation.

Caregiver Role Strain may be related to illness severity of care receiver, psychological/cognitive problems in care receiver, caregiver is spouse, duration of caregiving required, lack of respite/recreation for caregiver, possibly evidenced by feeling stressed, depressed, worried; lack of resources/support, family conflict.

pelvic inflammatory disease

Infection, risk for spread: risk factors may include presence of infectious process in highly vascular pelvic structures, delay in seeking treatment.

Pain [acute] may be related to inflammation, edema, and congestion of reproductive/pelvic tissues, possibly evidenced by verbal reports, guarding/distraction behaviors, self-focus, and autonomic responses (changes in vital signs).

Hyperthermia may be related to inflammatory process/hypermetabolic state, possibly evidenced by increased body temperature, warm/flushed skin, and tachycardia.

Self-Esteem, risk for situational low: risk factors may include perceived stigma of physical condition (infection of reproductive system).

Knowledge deficit [Learning Need] regarding cause/complications of condition, therapy needs, and transmission of disease to others may be related to lack of information/

misinterpretation, possibly evidenced by statements of concern, questions, misconceptions, and development of preventable complications.

periarteritis nodosa
Refer to *polyarteritis (nodosa)*.

pericarditis
Pain [acute] may be related to inflammation and presence of effusion, possibly evidenced by verbal reports, guarding/distraction behaviors, self-focus, and autonomic responses (changes in vital signs).
Activity Intolerance may be related to imbalance between oxygen supply and demand (restriction of cardiac filling/ventricular contraction, reduced cardiac output), possibly evidenced by reports of weakness/fatigue, exertional dyspnea, abnormal heart rate or blood pressure response, and signs of congestive heart failure.
Cardiac Output, risk for decreased: risk factors may include accumulation of fluid (effusion) restricting cardiac filling/contractility.
Anxiety [specify level] may be related to change in health status and perceived threat of death, possibly evidenced by increased tension, apprehension, restlessness, and expressed concerns.

peripheral vascular disease (atherosclerosis)
Tissue Perfusion, altered: peripheral may be related to reduction or interruption of arterial/venous blood flow, possibly evidenced by changes in skin temperature/color, lack of hair growth, blood pressure/pulse changes in extremity, presence of bruits, and reports of claudication.
Activity Intolerance may be related to imbalance between oxygen supply and demand, possibly evidenced by reports of muscle fatigue/weakness and exertional discomfort (claudication).
Skin Tissue Integrity, risk for impaired: risk factors may include altered circulation with decreased sensation and impaired healing.

peritonitis
Infection, risk for spread/septicemia: risk factors may include inadequate primary defenses (broken skin, traumatized tissue, altered peristalsis), inadequate secondary defenses (immunosuppression), and invasive procedures.
Fluid Volume deficit [mixed] may be related to fluid shifts from extracellular, intravascular, and interstitial compartments into intestines and/or peritoneal space, excessive gastric losses (vomiting, diarrhea, nasogastric suction), hypermetabolic state, and restricted intake, possibly evidenced by dry mucous membranes, poor skin turgor, delayed capillary refill, weak peripheral pulses, diminished urinary output, dark/concentrated urine, hypotension, and tachycardia.
Pain [acute] may be related to chemical irritation of parietal peritoneum, trauma to tissues, accumulation of fluid in abdominal/peritoneal cavity, possibly evidenced by verbal reports, muscle guarding/rebound tenderness, distraction behaviors, facial mask of pain, self-focus, autonomic responses (changes in vital signs).
Nutrition: altered, risk for less than body requirements: risk factors may include nausea/vomiting, intestinal dysfunction, metabolic abnormalities, or increased metabolic needs.

pheochromocytoma
Anxiety [specify level] may be related to excessive physiologic (hormonal) stimulation of the sympathetic nervous system, situational crises, threat to/change in health status, possibly evidenced by apprehension, shakiness, restlessness, focus on self, fearfulness, diaphoresis, and sense of impending doom.
Fluid Volume deficit [mixed] may be related to excessive gastric losses (vomiting/diarrhea), hypermetabolic state, diaphoresis, and hyperosmolar diuresis, possibly evidenced by hemoconcentration, dry mucous membranes, poor skin turgor, thirst, and weight loss.
Cardiac Output, decreased/Tissue Perfusion, altered (specify) may be related to altered preload/decreased blood volume, altered systemic vascular resistance, and increased sympathetic activity (excessive secretion of catecholamines), possibly evidenced by cool/clammy skin, change in blood pressure (hypertension/postural hypotension), visual disturbances, severe headache, and angina.
Knowledge deficit [Learning Need] regarding pathophysiology of condition, outcome, preoperative and postoperative care needs may be related to lack of information/recall, possibly evidenced by statements of concern, questions, and misconceptions.

phlebitis
Refer to *thrombophlebitis*.

phobia
(also refer to *anxiety disorder, generalized*)

Fear may be related to learned irrational response to natural or innate origins (phobic stimulus), unfounded morbid dread of a seemingly harmless object/situation, possibly evidenced by sympathetic stimulation and reactions ranging from apprehension to panic, withdrawal from/total avoidance of situations that place individual in contact with feared object.

Social Interaction, impaired may be related to intense fear of encountering feared object/activity or situation and anticipated loss of control, possibly evidenced by reported change of style/pattern of interaction, discomfort in social situations, and avoidance of phobic stimulus.

placenta previa

Fluid Volume, risk for deficit: risk factors may include excessive vascular losses (vessel damage and inadequate vasoconstriction).

Gas Exchange, impaired fetal may be related to altered blood flow, altered carrying capacity of blood (maternal anemia), and decreased surface area of gas exchange at site of placental attachment, possibly evidenced by changes in fetal heart rate/activity and release of meconium.

Fear may be related to threat of death (perceived or actual) to self or fetus, possibly evidenced by verbalization of specific concerns, increased tension, sympathetic stimulation.

Diversional Activity, risk for deficit: risk factors may include imposed activity restrictions/bedrest.

pleurisy

Pain [acute] may be related to inflammation/irritation of the parietal pleura, possibly evidenced by verbal reports, guarding/distraction behaviors, self-focus, and autonomic responses (changes in vital signs).

Breathing Pattern, ineffective may be related to pain on inspiration, possibly evidenced by decreased respiratory depth, tachypnea, and dyspnea.

Infection, risk for pneumonia: risk factors may include stasis of pulmonary secretions, decreased lung expansion, and ineffective cough.

pneumonia

Refer to *bronchitis*; *bronchopneumonia*.

pneumothorax
(also refer to *hemothorax*)

Breathing Pattern, ineffective may be related to decreased lung expansion (fluid/air accumulation), musculoskeletal impairment, pain, inflammatory process, possibly evidenced by dyspnea, tachypnea, altered chest excursion, respiratory depth changes, use of accessory muscles/nasal flaring, cough, cyanosis, and abnormal ABGs.

Cardiac Output, risk for decreased: risk factors may include compression/displacement of cardiac structures.

Pain [acute] may be related to irritation of nerve endings within pleural space by foreign object (chest tube), possibly evidenced by verbal reports, guarding/distraction behaviors, self-focus, and autonomic responses (changes in vital signs).

polyarteritis (nodosa)

Tissue Perfusion, altered (specify) may be related to reduction/interruption of blood flow, possibly evidenced by organ tissue infarctions, changes in organ function, and development of organic psychosis.

Hyperthermia may be related to widespread inflammatory process, possibly evidenced by increased body temperature and warm/flushed skin.

Pain [acute] may be related to inflammation, tissue ischemia, and necrosis of affected area, possibly evidenced by verbal reports, guarding/distraction behaviors, self-focus, and autonomic responses (changes in vital signs).

Grieving, anticipatory may be related to perceived loss of self, possibly evidenced by expressions of sorrow and anger, altered sleep and/or eating patterns, and changes in activity level or libido.

polycythemia vera

Activity Intolerance may be related to imbalance between oxygen supply and demand, possibly evidenced by reports of fatigue/weakness.

Tissue Perfusion, altered (specify) may be related to reduction/interruption of arterial/venous blood flow (insufficiency, thrombosis, or hemorrhage), possibly evidenced by pain in affected area, impaired mental ability, visual disturbances, and color changes of skin/mucous membranes.

polyradiculitis
Refer to *Guillain-Barré syndrome*.

postoperative recovery period
Breathing Pattern, ineffective may be related to neuromuscular and perceptual/cognitive impairment, decreased lung expansion/energy, and tracheobronchial obstruction, possibly evidenced by changes in respiratory rate and depth, reduced vital capacity, apnea, cyanosis, and noisy respirations.
Body Temperature, risk for altered: risk factors may include exposure to cool environment, effect of medications/anesthetic agents, extremes of age/weight, and dehydration.
Sensory/Perceptual alterations (specify)/Thought Processes, altered may be related to chemical alteration (use of pharmaceutical agents, hypoxia), therapeutically restricted environment, excessive sensory stimuli and physiologic stress, possibly evidenced by changes in usual response to stimuli, motor incoordination, impaired ability to concentrate, reason, and make decisions; and disorientation to person, place, and time.
Fluid Volume, risk for deficit: risk factors may include restriction of oral intake, loss of fluid through abnormal routes (indwelling tubes, drains), normal routes (vomiting, loss of vascular integrity, changes in clotting ability), and extremes of age and weight.
Pain [acute] may be related to disruption of skin, tissue, and muscle integrity, musculoskeletal/bone trauma, and presence of tubes and drains, possibly evidenced by verbal reports, alteration in muscle tone, facial mask of pain, distraction/guarding behaviors, narrowed focus, and autonomic responses.
Skin/Tissue Integrity, impaired may be related to mechanical interruption of skin/tissues, altered circulation, effects of medication, accumulation of drainage, and altered metabolic state, possibly evidenced by disruption of skin surface/layers and tissues.
Infection, risk for: risk factors may include broken skin, traumatized tissues, stasis of body fluids, presence of pathogens/contaminants, environmental exposure, and invasive procedures.

postpartal period
Parent/Infant Attachment/Parenting, risk for altered: risk factors may include lack of support between/from significant other(s), ineffective or no role model, anxiety associated with the parental role, unrealistic expectations, presence of stressors (e.g., financial, housing, employment).
Fluid Volume, risk for deficit: risk factors may include excessive blood loss during delivery, reduced intake/inadequate replacement, nausea/vomiting, increased urine output, and insensible losses.
Pain [acute]/Discomfort may be related to tissue trauma/edema, muscle contractions, bladder fullness, and physical/psychological exhaustion, possibly evidenced by reports of cramping (afterpains), self-focusing, alteration in muscle tone, distraction behavior, and autonomic responses (changes in vital signs).
Urinary Elimination, altered may be related to hormonal effects (fluid shifts/continued elevation in renal plasma flow), mechanical trauma/tissue edema, and effects of medication/anesthesia, possibly evidenced by frequency, dysuria, urgency, incontinence, or retention.
Constipation may be related to decreased muscle tone associated with diastasis recti, prenatal effects of progesterone, dehydration, excess analgesia or anesthesia, pain (hemorrhoids, episiotomy, or perineal tenderness), prelabor diarrhea, and lack of intake, possibly evidenced by frequency less than usual pattern, hard-formed stool, straining at stool, decreased bowel sounds, and abdominal distention.
Sleep Pattern disturbance may be related to pain/discomfort, intense exhilaration/excitement, anxiety, exhausting process of labor/delivery, and needs/demands of family members, possibly evidenced by verbal reports of difficulty in falling asleep/not feeling well-rested, interrupted sleep, frequent yawning, irritability, or dark circles under eyes.

post-traumatic stress disorder
Post-Trauma Syndrome related to having experienced a traumatic life event, possibly evidenced by reexperiencing of the event, somatic reactions, psychic/emotional numbness, altered lifestyle, impaired sleep, self-destructive behaviors, difficulty with interpersonal relationships, development of phobia, poor impulse control/irritability, and explosiveness.
Violence, risk for directed at others: risk factors may include a startle reaction, an intrusive memory causing a sudden acting-out of a feeling as if the event were occurring; use of alcohol/other drugs to ward off painful effects and produce psychic numbing, breaking through the rage that has been walled off, response to intense anxiety or panic state, and loss of control.

Coping, Individual, ineffective may be related to personal vulnerability, inadequate support system, unrealistic perceptions, unmet expectations, overwhelming threat to self, and multiple stressors repeated over period of time, possibly evidenced by verbalization of inability to cope or difficulty asking for help, muscular tension/headaches, chronic worry, and emotional tension.

Grieving, dysfunctional may be related to actual/perceived object loss (loss of self as seen before the traumatic incident occurred as well as other losses incurred in/after the incident), loss of physiopsychosocial well-being, thwarted grieving response to a loss, and lack of resolution of previous grieving responses, possibly evidenced by verbal expression of distress at loss, anger, sadness, labile affect, alterations in eating habits, sleep/dream patterns, libido; reliving of past experiences, expression of guilt, and alterations in concentration.

Family Processes, altered may be related to situational crisis, failure to master developmental transitions, possibly evidenced by expressions of confusion about what to do and that family is having difficulty coping, family system not meeting physical/emotional/spiritual needs of its members, not adapting to change or dealing with traumatic experience constructively, and ineffective family decision-making process.

pregnancy (prenatal period)

Nutrition: altered, risk for less than body requirements: risk factors may include changes in appetite, insufficient intake (nausea/vomiting, inadequate financial resources and nutritional knowledge); meeting increased metabolic demands (increased thyroid activity associated with the growth of fetal and maternal tissues).

[Discomfort]/Pain [acute] may be related to hormonal influences, physical changes, possibly evidenced by verbal reports (nausea, breast changes, leg cramps, hemorrhoids, nasal stuffiness), alteration in muscle tone, restlessness, and autonomic responses (changes in vital signs).

Injury, risk for fetal: risk factors may include environmental/hereditary factors and problems of maternal well-being that directly affect the developing fetus (e.g., malnutrition, substance use).

Cardiac Output, [maximally compensated] may be related to increased fluid volume/maximal cardiac effort and hormonal effects of progesterone and relaxin (that place the patient at risk for hypertension and/or circulatory failure), and changes in peripheral resistance (afterload), possibly evidenced by variations in blood pressure and pulse, syncopal episodes, or presence of pathological edema.

Family Coping: potential for growth may be related to situational/maturational crisis with anticipated changes in family structure/roles, needs sufficiently met and adaptive tasks effectively addressed to enable goals of self-actualization to surface, as evidenced by movement toward health-promoting and enriching lifestyle, choosing experiences that optimize pregnancy experience/wellness.

Constipation, risk for: risk factors may include changes in dietary/fluid intake, smooth muscle relaxation, decreased peristalsis, and effects of medications (e.g., iron).

Fatigue/Sleep Pattern disturbance may be related to increased carbohydrate metabolism, altered body chemistry, increased energy requirements to perform activities of daily living, discomfort, anxiety, inactivity, possibly evidenced by reports of overwhelming lack of energy/inability to maintain usual routines, difficulty falling asleep/not feeling well-rested, interrupted sleep, irritability, lethargy, and frequent yawning.

Role Performance, risk for altered: risk factors may include maturational crisis, developmental level, history of maladaptive coping, or absence of support systems.

Knowledge deficit [Learning Need] regarding normal physiological/psychological changes and self-care needs may be related to lack of information/recall and misinterpretation of normal physiological/psychological changes and their impact on the client/family, possibly evidenced by questions, statements of concern, misconceptions, and inaccurate follow-through of instructions/development of preventable complications.

pregnancy, adolescent

(also refer to *pregnancy, prenatal period*)

Family Processes, altered may be related to situational/developmental transition (economic, change in roles/gain of a family member), possibly evidenced by family expressing confusion about what to do, unable to meet physical/emotional/spiritual needs of the members, family inability to adapt to change or to deal with traumatic experience constructively, does not demonstrate respect for individuality and autonomy of its members, ineffective family decision-making process, and inappropriate boundary maintenance.

Social isolation may be related to alterations in physical appearance, perceived unacceptable social behavior, restricted social sphere, stage of adolescence, and interference with accomplishing developmental tasks, possibly evidenced by expressions of feelings of aloneness/rejection/difference from others, uncommunicative, withdrawn, no eye contact, seeking to be alone, unacceptable behavior, and absence of supportive significant other(s).

Body Image/Self-Esteem disturbance may be related to situational/maturational crisis, biophysical changes, and fear of failure at life events, absence of support systems, possibly evidenced by self-negating verbalizations, expressions of shame/guilt, fear of rejection/reaction of others, hypersensitivity to criticism, and lack of follow-through/nonparticipation in prenatal care.

Knowledge deficit [Learning Need] regarding pregnancy, developmental/individual needs, future expectations may be related to lack of exposure, information misinterpretation, unfamiliarity with information resources, lack of interest in learning, possibly evidenced by questions, statements of concern/misconception, sense of vulnerability/denial of reality, inaccurate follow-through of instruction, and development of preventable complications.

Parenting, risk for altered: may be related to chronological age/developmental stage, unmet social/emotional/maturational needs of parenting figures, unrealistic expectation of self/infant/partner, ineffective role model/social support, lack of role identity, and presence of stressors (e.g., financial, social).

pregnancy-induced hypertension **(pre-eclampsia)**

Fluid Volume deficit [isotonic] may be related to a plasma protein loss, decreasing plasma colloid osmotic pressure allowing fluid shifts out of vascular compartment, possibly evidenced by edema formation, sudden weight gain, hemoconcentration, nausea/vomiting, epigastric pain, headaches, visual changes, decreased urine output.

Cardiac Output, decreased may be related to hypovolemia/decreased venous return, increased SVR, possibly evidenced by variations in blood pressure/hemodynamic readings, edema, shortness of breath, change in mental status.

Tissue Perfusion, altered: [uteroplacental] may be related to vasospasm of spiral arteries and relative hypovolemia, possibly evidenced by changes in fetal heart rate/activity, reduced weight gain, and premature delivery/fetal demise.

Knowledge deficit [Learning Need] regarding pathophysiology of condition, therapy, self-care/nutritional needs, and potential complications may be related to lack of information/recall, misinterpretation, possibly evidenced by statements of concern, questions, misconceptions, inaccurate follow-through of instructions/development of preventable complications.

premenstrual tension syndrome **(PMS)**

Pain/chronic/[acute] may be related to cyclic changes in female hormones affecting other systems (e.g., vascular congestion/spasms), vitamin deficiency, fluid retention, possibly evidenced by increased tension, apprehension, jitteriness, verbal reports, distraction behaviors, somatic complaints, self-focusing, physical and social withdrawal.

Fluid Volume excess may be related to abnormal alterations of hormonal levels, possibly evidenced by edema formation, weight gain, and periodic changes in emotional status/irritability.

Anxiety [specify level] may be related to cyclic changes in female hormones affecting other systems, possibly evidenced by feelings of inability to cope/loss of control, depersonalization, increased tension, apprehension, jitteriness, somatic complaints, and impaired functioning.

Knowledge deficit [Learning Need] regarding pathophysiology of condition and self-care/treatment needs may be related to lack of information/misinterpretation, possibly evidenced by statements of concern, questions, misconceptions, and continuation of condition, exacerbating symptoms.

pressure ulcer or sore
(also refer to *ulcer, decubitus*)

Tissue Perfusion, altered: peripheral may be related to reduced/interrupted blood flow, possibly evidenced by presence of inflamed, necrotic lesion.

Knowledge deficit [Learning Need] regarding cause/prevention of condition and potential complications may be related to lack of information/misinterpretation, possibly evidenced by statements of concern, questions, misconceptions, and inaccurate follow-through of instructions.

preterm labor
Refer to *labor, preterm*.

prostatectomy

Urinary Elimination, altered may be related to mechanical obstruction (blood clots, edema, trauma, surgical procedure, pressure/irritation of catheter/balloon), and loss of bladder tone, possibly evidenced by dysuria, frequency, dribbling, incontinence, retention, bladder fullness, suprapubic discomfort.

Fluid Volume, risk for deficit: risk factors may include trauma to highly vascular area with excessive vascular losses, restricted intake, postobstructive diuresis.

Pain [acute] may be related to irritation of bladder mucosa and tissue trauma/edema, possibly evidenced by verbal reports (bladder spasms), distraction behaviors, self-focus, and autonomic responses (changes in vital signs).

Body Image disturbance may be related to perceived threat of altered body/sexual function, possibly evidenced by preoccupation with change/loss, negative feelings about body, and statements of concern regarding functioning.

Sexual dysfunction, risk for: risk factors may include situational crisis (incontinence, leakage of urine after catheter removal, involvement of genital area) and threat to self-concept/change in health status.

pruritus

Pain [acute] may be related to cutaneous hyperesthesia and inflammation, possibly evidenced by verbal reports, distraction behaviors, and self-focus.

Skin Integrity, risk for impaired: risk factors may include mechanical trauma (scratching) and development of vesicles/bullae that may rupture.

psoriasis

Skin Integrity, impaired may be related to increased epidermal cell proliferation and absence of normal protective skin layers, possibly evidenced by scaling papules and plaques.

Body Image disturbance may be related to cosmetically unsightly skin lesions, possibly evidenced by hiding affected body part, negative feelings about body, feelings of helplessness, and change in social involvement.

pulmonary embolus

Breathing Pattern, ineffective may be related to tracheobronchial obstruction (inflammation, copious secretions or active bleeding), decreased lung expansion, inflammatory process, possibly evidenced by changes in depth and/or rate of respiration, dyspnea/use of accessory muscles, altered chest excursion, abnormal breath sounds (crackles, wheezes), and cough (with or without sputum production).

Gas Exchange, impaired may be related to altered blood flow to alveoli or to major portions of the lung, alveolar-capillary membrane changes (atelectasis, airway/alveolar collapse, pulmonary edema/effusion, excessive secretions/active bleeding), possibly evidenced by profound dyspnea, restlessness, apprehension, somnolence, cyanosis, and changes in ABGs/pulse oximetry (hypoxemia and hypercapnia).

Tissue Perfusion, altered: cardiopulmonary may be related to interruption of blood flow (arterial/venous), exchange problems at alveolar level or at tissue level (acidotic shifting of the oxyhemoglobin curve), possibly evidenced by radiology/laboratory evidence of ventilation/perfusion mismatch, dyspnea, and central cyanosis.

Fear/Anxiety [specify level] may be related to severe dyspnea/inability to breathe normally, perceived threat of death, threat to/change in health status, physiological response to hypoxemia/acidosis, and concern regarding unknown outcome of situation, possibly evidenced by restlessness, irritability, withdrawal or attack behavior, sympathetic stimulation (cardiovascular excitation, pupil dilation, sweating, vomiting, diarrhea), crying, voice quivering, and impending sense of doom.

purpura, idiopathic thrombocytopenic

Protection, altered may be related to abnormal blood profile, drug therapy (corticosteroids or immunosuppressive agents), possibly evidenced by altered clotting, fatigue, deficient immunity.

Activity Intolerance may be related to decreased oxygen-carrying capacity/imbalance between oxygen supply and demand, possibly evidenced by reports of fatigue/weakness.

Knowledge deficit [Learning Need] regarding therapy choices, outcomes, and self-care needs may be related to lack of information/misinterpretation, possibly evidenced by statements of concern, questions, and misconceptions.

pyelonephritis

Pain [acute] may be related to acute inflammation of renal tissues, possibly evidenced by verbal reports, guarding/distraction behaviors, self-focus, and autonomic responses (changes in vital signs).

Hyperthermia may be related to inflammatory process/increased metabolic rate, possibly evidenced by increase in body temperature, warm/flushed skin, tachycardia, and chills.

Urinary Elimination, altered may be related to inflammation/irritation of bladder mucosa, possibly evidenced by dysuria, urgency, and frequency.

Knowledge deficit [Learning Need] regarding therapy needs and prevention may be related to lack of information/misinterpretation, possibly evidenced by statements of concern, questions, misconceptions, and recurrence of condition.

quadriplegia

(also refer to *paraplegia*)

Breathing Pattern, ineffective may be related to neuromuscular impairment (diaphragm and intercostal muscle function), reflex abdominal spasms, gastric distention, possibly evidenced by decreased respiratory depth, dyspnea, cyanosis, and abnormal ABGs.

Trauma, risk for additional spinal injury: risk factors may include temporary weakness/instability of spinal column.

Grieving, anticipatory may be related to perceived loss of self, anticipated alterations in lifestyle and expectations, and limitation of future options/choices, possibly evidenced by expressions of distress, anger, sorrow; choked feelings; and changes in eating habits, sleep, and communication patterns.

Self-Care deficit: total related to neuromuscular impairment, evidenced by inability to perform self-care tasks.

Mobility, impaired bed/wheelchair may be related to loss of muscle function/control.

Autonomic Dysreflexia, risk for: risk factors may include altered nerve function (spinal cord injury at T6 or above), bladder/bowel/skin stimulation (tactile, pain, thermal).

Home Maintenance Management, impaired may be related to permanent effects of injury, inadequate/absent support systems and finances, and lack of familiarity with resources, possibly evidenced by expressions of difficulties, requests for information and assistance, outstanding debts/financial crisis, and lack of necessary aides and equipment.

rape

Knowledge deficit [Learning Need] regarding required medical/legal procedures, prophylactic treatment for individual concerns (STDs, pregnancy), community resources/supports may be related to lack of information, possibly evidenced by statements of concern, questions, misconceptions, and exacerbation of symptoms.

Rape-Trauma syndrome (acute phase) related to actual or attempted sexual penetration without consent, possibly evidenced by wide range of emotional reactions, including anxiety, fear, anger, embarrassment, and multisystem physical complaints.

Tissue Integrity, risk for impaired: risk factors may include forceful sexual penetration and trauma to fragile tissues.

Coping, Individual, ineffective may be related to personal vulnerability, unmet expectations, unrealistic perception, inadequate support systems/coping methods, multiple stressors repeated over time, overwhelming threat to self, possibly evidenced by verbalizations of inability to cope or difficulty asking for help, muscular tension/headaches, emotional tension, chronic worry.

Sexual dysfunction may be related to biopsychosocial alteration of sexuality (stress of post-trauma response), vulnerability, loss of sexual desire, impaired relationship with significant other, possibly evidenced by alteration in achieving sexual satisfaction, change in interest in self/others, preoccupation with self.

Raynaud's phenomenon

Pain [acute]/chronic may be related to vasospasm/altered perfusion of affected tissues and ischemia/destruction of tissues, possibly evidenced by verbal reports, guarding of affected parts, guarding of affected parts, self-focusing, and restlessness.

Tissue Perfusion, altered, peripheral may be related to periodic reduction of arterial blood flow to affected areas, possibly evidenced by pallor, cyanosis, coolness, numbness, paresthesia, slow healing of lesions.

Knowledge deficit [Learning Need] regarding pathophysiology of the condition, potential for complications, therapy/self-care needs may be related to lack of information/misinterpretation, possibly evidenced by statements of concern, questions, and misconceptions; development of preventable complications.

reflex sympathetic dystrophy (RSD)

Pain [acute]/chronic may be related to continued nerve stimulation, possibly evidenced by verbal reports, distraction/guarding behaviors, narrowed focus, changes in sleep patterns, and altered ability to continue previous activities.

Tissue Perfusion, altered: peripheral may be related to reduction of arterial blood flow (arteriole vasoconstriction), possibly evidenced by reports of pain, decreased skin temperature and pallor, diminished arterial pulsations, and tissue swelling.

Sensory/Perceptual alteration: tactile may be related to altered sensory reception (neurologic deficit, pain), possibly evidenced by change in usual response to stimuli/abnormal sensitivity of touch, physiologic anxiety, and irritability.

Role Performance, risk for altered: risk factors may include situational crisis, chronic disability, debilitating pain.
Family Coping, risk for ineffective: compromised: risk factors may include temporary family disorganization and role changes and prolonged disability that exhausts the supportive capacity of significant other(s).

renal failure, acute
Fluid Volume excess may be related to compromised regulatory mechanisms (decreased kidney function), possibly evidenced by weight gain, edema/anasarca, intake greater than output, venous congestion, changes in BP/CVP, and altered electrolyte levels.
Nutrition: altered, less than body requirements may be related to inability to ingest/digest adequate nutrients (anorexia, nausea/vomiting, ulcerations of oral mucosa, and increased metabolic needs) in addition to therapeutic dietary restrictions, possibly evidenced by lack of interest in food/aversion to eating, observed inadequate intake, weight loss, loss of muscle mass.
Infection, risk for: risk factors may include depression of immunological defenses, invasive procedures/devices, and changes in dietary intake/malnutrition.
Thought Processes, altered may be related to accumulation of toxic waste products and altered cerebral perfusion, possibly evidenced by disorientation, changes in recent memory, apathy, and episodic obtundation.

renal transplantation
Fluid Volume, risk for excess: risk factors may include compromised regulatory mechanism (implantation of new kidney requiring adjustment period for optimal functioning).
Body Image disturbance may be related to failure and subsequent replacement of body part and medication-induced changes in appearance, possibly evidenced by preoccupation with loss/change, negative feelings about body, and focus on past strength/function.
Fear may be related to potential for transplant rejection/failure and threat of death, possibly evidenced by increased tension, apprehension, concentration on source, and verbalizations of concern.
Infection, risk for: risk factors may include broken skin/traumatized tissue, stasis of body fluids, immunosuppression, invasive procedures, nutritional deficits, and chronic disease.
Coping, Individual/Family risk for ineffective: risk factors may include situational crises, family disorganization and role changes, prolonged disease exhausting supportive capacity of significant other/family, therapeutic restrictions/long-term therapy needs.

respiratory distress syndrome (premature infant)
(also refer to *neonate, premature newborn*)
Gas Exchange, impaired may be related to alveolar/capillary membrane changes (inadequate surfactant levels), altered oxygen supply (tracheobronchial obstruction, atelectasis), altered blood flow (immaturity of pulmonary arteriole musculature), altered oxygen-carrying capacity of blood (anemia), and cold stress, possibly evidenced by tachypnea, use of accessory muscles/retractions, expiratory grunting, pallor or cyanosis, abnormal ABGs, and tachycardia.
Spontaneous Ventilation, inability to sustain may be related to respiratory muscle fatigue and metabolic factors, possibly evidenced by dyspnea, increased metabolic rate, restlessness, use of accessory muscles, and abnormal ABGs.
Infection, risk for: risk factors may include inadequate primary defenses (decreased ciliary action, stasis of body fluids, traumatized tissues), inadequate secondary defenses (deficiency of neutrophils and specific immunoglobulins), invasive procedures, and malnutrition (absence of nutrient stores, increased metabolic demands).
Tissue Perfusion, risk for altered: gastrointestinal: risk factors may include persistent fetal circulation and exchange problems.
Parent/Infant Attachment, risk for altered: risk factors may include premature/ill infant who is unable to effectively initiate parental contact (altered behavioral organization), separation, physical barriers, anxiety associated with the parental role/demands of infant.

retinal detachment
Sensory/Perceptual alterations: visual related to decreased sensory reception, possibly evidenced by visual distortions, decreased visual field, and changes in visual acuity.
Knowledge deficit [Learning Need] regarding therapy, prognosis, and self-care needs may be related to lack of information/misconceptions, possibly evidenced by statements of concern and questions.
Home Maintenance Management, risk for impaired: risk factors may include visual limitations/activity/restrictions.

Reye's syndrome

Fluid Volume deficit [isotonic] may be related to failure of regulatory mechanism (diabetes insipidus), excessive gastric losses (pernicious vomiting), and altered intake, possibly evidenced by increased/dilute urine output, sudden weight loss, decreased venous filling, dry mucous membranes, decreased skin turgor, hypotension, and tachycardia.

Tissue Perfusion, altered: cerebral may be related to diminished arterial/venous blood flow and hypovolemia, possibly evidenced by memory loss, altered consciousness, and restlessness/agitation.

Trauma, risk for: risk factors may include generalized weakness, reduced coordination, and cognitive deficits.

Breathing Pattern, ineffective may be related to decreased energy and fatigue, cognitive impairment, tracheobronchial obstruction, and inflammatory process (aspiration pneumonia), possibly evidenced by tachypnea, abnormal ABGs, cough, and use of accessory muscles.

rheumatic fever

Pain [acute] may be related to migratory inflammation of joints, possibly evidenced by verbal reports, guarding/distraction behaviors, self-focus, and autonomic responses (changes in vital signs).

Hyperthermia may be related to inflammatory process/hypermetabolic state, possibly evidenced by increased body temperature, warm/flushed skin, and tachycardia.

Activity Intolerance may be related to generalized weakness, joint pain, and medical restrictions/bedrest, possibly evidenced by reports of fatigue, exertional discomfort, and abnormal heart rate in response to activity.

Cardiac Output, risk for decreased: risk factors may include cardiac inflammation/enlargement and altered contractility.

rickets (osteomalacia)

Growth and Development, altered may be related to dietary deficiencies/indiscretions, malabsorption syndrome, and lack of exposure to sunlight, possibly evidenced by altered physical growth and delay or difficulty in performing motor skills typical for age.

Knowledge deficit [Learning Need] regarding cause, pathophysiology, therapy needs and prevention may be related to lack of information, possibly evidenced by statements of concern, questions, misconceptions, and inaccurate follow-through of instructions.

ringworm, tinea
(also refer to *athlete's foot*)

Skin Integrity, impaired may be related to fungal infection of the dermis, possibly evidenced by disruption of skin surfaces/presence of lesions.

Knowledge deficit [Learning Need] regarding infectious nature, therapy, and self-care needs may be related to lack of information/misinformation, possibly evidenced by statements of concern, questions, and recurrence/spread.

rubella

Pain [acute/Discomfort] may be related to inflammatory effects of viral infection and presence of desquamating rash, possibly evidenced by verbal reports, distraction behaviors/restlessness.

Knowledge deficit [Learning Need] regarding contagious nature, possible complications, and self-care needs may be related to lack of information/misinterpretations, possibly evidenced by statements of concern, questions, and inaccurate follow-through of instructions.

scabies

Skin Integrity, impaired may be related to presence of invasive parasite and development of pruritus, possibly evidenced by disruption of skin surface and inflammation.

Knowledge deficit [Learning Need] regarding communicable nature, possible complications, therapy, and self-care needs may be related to lack of information/misinterpretation, possibly evidenced by questions and statements of concern about spread to others.

scarlet fever

Hyperthermia may be related to effects of circulating toxins, possibly evidenced by increased body temperature, warm/flushed skin, and tachycardia.

Pain [Discomfort] may be related to inflammation of mucous membranes and effects of circulating toxins (malaise, fever), possibly evidenced by verbal reports, distraction behaviors, guarding (decreased swallowing), and self-focus.

Fluid Volume, risk for deficit: risk factors may include hypermetabolic state (hyperthermia) and reduced intake.

schizophrenia (schizophrenic disorders)

Thought Process, altered may be related to disintegration of thinking processes, impaired judgment, presence of psychological conflicts, disintegrated ego-boundaries, sleep disturbance, ambivalence, and concomitant dependence, possibly evidenced by impaired ability to reason/problem solve, inappropriate affect, presence of delusional system, command hallucinations, obsessions, ideas of reference, cognitive dissonance.

Social Isolation may be related to alterations in mental status, mistrust of others/delusional thinking, unacceptable social behaviors, inadequate personal resources, and inability to engage in satisfying personal relationships, possibly evidenced by difficulty in establishing relationships with others; dull affect, uncommunicative/withdrawn behavior, seeking to be alone, inadequate/absent significant purpose in life, and expression of feelings of rejection.

Health Maintenance/Home Maintenance Management, altered may be related to impaired cognitive/emotional functioning, altered ability to make deliberate and thoughtful judgments, altered communication, and lack/inappropriate use of material resources, possibly evidenced by inability to take responsibility for meeting basic health practices in any or all functional areas and demonstrated lack of adaptive behaviors to internal or external environmental changes, disorderly surroundings, accumulation of dirt/unwashed clothes, repeated hygienic disorders.

Violence, risk for directed at self/others: risk factors may include disturbances of thinking/feeling (depression, paranoia, suicidal ideation), lack of development of trust and appropriate interpersonal relationships, catatonic/manic excitement, toxic reactions to drugs (alcohol).

Coping, Individual, ineffective may be related to personal vulnerability, inadequate support system(s), unrealistic perceptions, inadequate coping methods, and disintegration of thought processes, possibly evidenced by impaired judgment/cognition and perception, diminished problem-solving/decision-making capacities, poor self-concept, chronic anxiety, depression, inability to perform role expectations, and alteration in social participation.

Family Processes, altered/ Family Coping, ineffective: disabling may be related to ambivalent family system/relationships, changes of roles, and difficulty of family member in coping effectively with patient's maladaptive behaviors, possibly evidenced by deterioration in family functioning, ineffective family decision-making process, difficulty relating to each other, patient's expression of despair at family's lack of reaction/involvement, neglectful relationships with patient, extreme distortion regarding patient's health problem including denial about its existence/severity or prolonged overconcern.

Self-Care deficit [specify] may be related to perceptual and cognitive impairment, immobility (withdrawal/isolation and decreased psychomotor activity), and side effects of psychotropic medications, possibly evidenced by inability or difficulty in areas of feeding self, keeping body clean, dressing appropriately, toileting self, and/or changes in bowel/bladder elimination.

sciatica

Pain [acute]/chronic may be related to peripheral nerve root compression, possibly evidenced by verbal reports, guarding/distraction behaviors, and self-focus.

Mobility, impaired physical may be related to neurologic pain and muscular involvement, possibly evidenced by reluctance to attempt movement and decreased muscle strength/mass.

scleroderma

(also refer to *lupus erythematosus, systemic—SLE*)

Mobility, impaired physical may be related to musculoskeletal impairment and associated pain, possibly evidenced by decreased strength, decreased range of motion, and reluctance to attempt movement.

Tissue Perfusion, altered (specify) may be related to reduced arterial blood flow (arteriolar vasoconstriction), possibly evidenced by changes in skin temperature/color, ulcer formation, and changes in organ function (cardiopulmonary, gastrointestinal, renal).

Nutrition: altered, less than body requirements may be related to inability to ingest/digest/absorb adequate nutrients (sclerosis of the tissues rendering mouth immobile, decreased peristalsis of esophagus/small intestines, atrophy of smooth muscle of colon), possibly evidenced by weight loss, decreased intake/food and reported/observed difficulty swallowing.

Adjustment, impaired may be related to disability requiring change in lifestyle, inadequate support systems, assault to self-concept, and altered locus of control, possibly evidenced by verbalization of nonacceptance of health status change and lack of movement toward independence/future-oriented thinking.

Body Image disturbance may be related to skin changes with induration, atrophy, and fibrosis, loss of hair, and skin and muscle contractures, possibly evidenced by verbalization of negative feelings about body, focus on past strength/function or appearance, fear of rejection/reaction by others, hiding body part, and change in social involvement.

scoliosis

Body Image disturbance may be related to altered body structure, use of therapeutic device(s), and activity restrictions, possibly evidenced by negative feelings about body, change in social involvement, and preoccupation with situation or refusal to acknowledge problem.

Knowledge deficit [Learning Need] regarding pathophysiology of condition, therapy needs and possible outcomes may be related to lack of information/misinterpretation, possibly evidenced by statements of concern, questions, misconceptions, and inaccurate follow-through of instructions.

Adjustment, impaired may be related to lack of comprehension of long-term consequences of behavior, possibly evidenced by failure to adhere to treatment regimen/keep appointments and evidence of failure to improve.

sepsis, puerperal
(also refer to *septicemia*)

Infection, risk for spread/septic shock: risk factors may include presence of infection, broken skin, and/or traumatized tissues, rupture of amniotic membranes, high vascularity of involved area, stasis of body fluids, invasive procedures, and/or increased environmental exposure, chronic disease (e.g., diabetes, anemia, malnutrition), altered immune response, and untoward effect of medications (e.g., opportunistic/secondary infection).

Hyperthermia may be related to inflammatory process/hypermetabolic state, possibly evidenced by increase in body temperature, warm/flushed skin, and tachycardia.

Parent/Infant Attachment, risk for altered: risk factors may include interruption in bonding process, physical illness, perceived threat to own survival.

Tissue Perfusion, risk for altered: peripheral: risk factors may include interruption/reduction of blood flow (presence of infectious thrombi).

septicemia
(also refer to *sepsis, puerperal*)

Tissue Perfusion, altered (specify) may be related to changes in arterial/venous blood flow (selective vasoconstriction, presence of microemboli) and hypovolemia, possibly evidenced by changes in skin temperature/color, changes in blood/pulse pressure; changes in sensorium, and decreased urinary output.

Fluid Volume, risk for deficit: risk factors may include marked increase in vascular compartment/massive vasodilation, vascular shifts to interstitial space, and reduced intake.

Cardiac Output, risk for decreased: risk factors may include decreased preload (venous return and circulating volume), altered afterload (increased SVR), negative inotropic effects of hypoxia, complement activation, and lysosomal hydrolase.

serum sickness

Pain [acute] may be related to inflammation of the joints and skin eruptions, possibly evidenced by verbal reports, guarding/distraction behaviors, and self-focus.

Knowledge deficit [Learning Need] regarding nature of condition, treatment needs, potential complications, and prevention of recurrence may be related to lack of information/misinterpretation, possibly evidenced by statements of concern, questions, misconceptions, and inaccurate follow-through of instructions.

sexually transmitted disease (STD)

Infection, risk for transmission: risk factors may include contagious nature of infecting agent and insufficient knowledge to avoid exposure to/transmission of pathogens.

Skin/Tissue Integrity, impaired may be related to invasion of/irritation by pathogenic organism(s), possibly evidenced by disruptions of skin/tissue and inflammation of mucous membranes.

Knowledge deficit [Learning Need] regarding condition, prognosis/complications, therapy needs, and transmission may be related to lack of information/misinterpretation, lack of interest in learning, possibly evidenced by statements of concern, questions, misconceptions, inaccurate follow-through of instructions, and development of preventable complications.

shock
(also refer to *shock, cardiogenic*; *shock, hemorrhagic/hypovolemic*)
Tissue Perfusion, altered (specify) may be related to changes in circulating volume and/or vascular tone, possibly evidenced by changes in skin color/temperature and pulse pressure, reduced blood pressure, changes in mentation, and decreased urinary output.
Anxiety [specify level] may be related to change in health status and threat of death, possibly evidenced by increased tension, apprehension, sympathetic stimulation, restlessness, and expressions of concern.

shock, cardiogenic
(also refer to *shock*)
Cardiac Output, decreased may be related to structural damage, decreased myocardial contractility, and presence of dysrhythmias, possibly evidenced by ECG changes, variations in hemodynamic readings, jugular vein distention, cold/clammy skin, diminished peripheral pulses, and decreased urinary output.

shock, hemorrhagic/hypovolemic
(also refer to *shock*)
Fluid Volume deficit [isotonic] may be related to excessive vascular loss, inadequate intake/replacement, possibly evidenced by hypotension, tachycardia, decreased pulse volume and pressure, change in mentation, and decreased/concentrated urine.

shock, septic
(Refer to *septicemia*)

sick sinus syndrome
(Also refer to *dysrhythmia, cardiac*)
Cardiac Output, decreased may be related to alterations in rate, rhythm, and electrical conduction, possibly evidenced by ECG evidence of dysrhythmias, reports of palpitations/weakness, changes in mentation/consciousness, and syncope.
Trauma, risk for: risk factors may include changes in cerebral perfusion with altered consciousness/loss of balance.

snow blindness
Sensory/Perceptual alterations: visual may be related to altered status of sense organ (irritation of the conjunctiva, hyperemia), possibly evidenced by intolerance to light (photophobia) and decreased/loss of visual acuity.
Pain [acute] may be related to irritation/vascular congestion of the conjunctiva, possibly evidenced by verbal reports, guarding/distraction behaviors, and self-focus.
Anxiety [specify level] may be related to situational crisis and threat to/change in health status, possibly evidenced by increased tension, apprehension, uncertainty, worry, restlessness, and focus on self.

somatoform disorders
Coping, Individual, ineffective may be related to severe level of anxiety that is repressed, personal vulnerability, unmet dependency needs, fixation in earlier level of development, retarded ego development, and inadequate coping skills, possibly evidenced by verbalized inability to cope/problem-solve, high illness rate, multiple somatic complaints of several years' duration, decreased functioning in social/occupational settings, narcissistic tendencies with total focus on self/physical symptoms, demanding behaviors, history of "doctor shopping" and refusal to attend therapeutic activities.
Pain, chronic may be related to severe level of repressed anxiety, low self-concept, unmet dependency needs, history of self or loved one having experienced a serious illness, possibly evidenced by verbal reports of severe/prolonged pain, guarded movement/protective behaviors, facial mask of pain, fear of reinjury, altered ability to continue previous activities, social withdrawal, demands for therapy/medication.
Sensory/Perceptual alterations (specify) may be related to psychological stress (narrowed perceptual fields, expression of stress as physical problems/deficits), poor quality of sleep, presence of chronic pain, possibly evidenced by reported change in voluntary motor or sensory function (paralysis, anosmia, aphonia, deafness, blindness, loss of touch or pain sensation), la belle indifference (lack of concern over functional loss).
Social Interaction, impaired may be related to inability to engage in satisfying personal relationships, preoccupation with self and physical symptoms, altered state of wellness, chronic pain, and rejection by others, possibly evidenced by preoccupation with own thoughts, sad/dull affect, absence of supportive significant other(s), uncommunicative/withdrawn behavior, lack of eye contact, and seeking to be alone.

sprain of ankle or foot

Pain [acute] may be related to trauma to/swelling in joint, possibly evidenced by verbal reports, guarding/distraction behaviors, self-focusing, and autonomic responses (changes in vital signs).

Walking, impaired may be related to musculoskeletal injury, pain, and therapeutic restrictions, possibly evidenced by reluctance to attempt movement, inability to move about environment easily.

stapedectomy

Trauma, risk for: risk factors may include increased middle-ear pressure with displacement of prosthesis and balancing difficulties/dizziness.

Infection, risk for: risk factors may include surgically traumatized tissue, invasive procedures, and environmental exposure to upper respiratory infections.

Pain [acute] may be related to surgical trauma, edema formation, and presence of packing, possibly evidenced by verbal reports, guarding/distraction behaviors, and self-focus.

substance dependency/abuse rehabilitation (following acute detoxification)
(also refer to *drug overdose*)

Denial/Coping, Individual, ineffective may be related to personal vulnerability, difficulty handling new situations, learned response patterns, cultural factors, personal/family value systems, possibly evidenced by lack of acceptance that drug use is causing the present situation, use of manipulation to avoid responsibility for self, altered social patterns/participation, impaired adaptive behavior and problem-solving skills, employment difficulties, financial affairs in disarray, and decreased ability to handle stress of recent events.

Powerlessness may be related to substance addiction with/without periods of abstinence, episodic compulsive indulgence, attempts at recovery, and lifestyle of helplessness, possibly evidenced by ineffective recovery attempts, statements of inability to stop behavior/requests for help, continuous/constant thinking about drug and/or obtaining drug, alteration in personal/occupational and social life.

Nutrition: altered, less than body requirements may be related to insufficient dietary intake to meet metabolic needs for psychological/physiological/economic reasons, possibly evidenced by weight less than normal for height/body build, decreased subcutaneous fat/muscle mass, reported altered taste sensation, lack of interest in food, poor muscle tone, sore/inflamed buccal cavity, laboratory evidence of protein/vitamin deficiencies.

Sexual dysfunction may be related to altered body function (neurologic damage and debilitating effects of drug use), changes in appearance, possibly evidenced by progressive interference with sexual functioning, a significant degree of testicular atrophy, gynecomastia, impotence/decreased sperm counts in men; and loss of body hair, thin/soft skin, spider angiomas, and amenorrhea/increase in miscarriages in women.

Family Processes, altered: alcoholism (substance abuse) may be related to abuse/history of alcoholism/drug use, inadequate coping skills/lack of problem-solving skills, genetic predisposition/biochemical influences, possibly evidenced by feelings of anger/frustration/responsibility for alcoholic's behavior, suppressed rage, shame/embarrassment, repressed emotions, guilt, vulnerability; disturbed family dynamics/deterioration in family relationships, family denial/rationalization, closed communication systems, triangulating family relationships, manipulation, blaming, enabling to maintain substance use, inability to accept/receive help.

surgery, general
(also refer to *postoperative recovery period*)

Knowledge deficit [Learning Need] regarding surgical procedure/expectation, postoperative routines/therapy, and self-care needs may be related to lack of information/misinterpretation, possibly evidenced by statements of concern, questions, and misconceptions.

Anxiety [specify level]/Fear may be related to situational crisis, unfamiliarity with environment, change in health status/ threat of death and separation from usual support systems, possibly evidenced by increased tension, apprehension, decreased self-assurance, fear of unspecific consequences, focus on self, sympathetic stimulation, and restlessness.

Perioperative Positioning Injury, risk for: risk factors may include disorientation, immobilization, muscle weakness, obesity/edema.

Breathing Pattern, risk for ineffective: risk factors may include chemically induced muscular relaxation, perception/cognitive impairment, decreased energy.

Fluid Volume, risk for deficit: risk factors may include preoperative fluid deprivation, blood loss, and excessive gastrointestinal losses (vomiting/gastric suction).

synovitis (knee)

Pain [acute] may be related to inflammation of synovial membrane of the joint with effusion, possibly evidenced by verbal reports, guarding/distraction behaviors, self-focus, and autonomic responses (changes in vital signs).

Walking, impaired may be related to pain and decreased strength of joint, possibly evidenced by reluctance to attempt movement, inability to move about environment as desired.

syphilis, congenital

(also refer to *sexually transmitted disease—STD*)

Pain [acute] may be related to inflammatory process, edema formation, and development of skin lesions, possibly evidenced by irritability/crying that may be increased with movement of extremities and autonomic responses (changes in vital signs).

Skin/Tissue Integrity, impaired may be related to exposure to pathogens during vaginal delivery, possibly evidenced by disruption of skin surfaces and rhinitis.

Growth and Development, altered may be related to effect of infectious process, possibly evidenced by altered physical growth and delay or difficulty performing skills typical of age group.

Knowledge deficit [Learning Need] regarding pathophysiology of condition, transmissibility, therapy needs, expected outcomes, and potential complications may be related to caretaker/parental lack of information, misinterpretation, possibly evidenced by statements of concern, questions, and misconceptions.

syringomyelia

Sensory/Perceptual alterations (specify) may be related to altered sensory perception (neurologic lesion), possibly evidenced by change in usual response to stimuli and motor incoordination.

Anxiety [specify level]/Fear may be related to change in health status, threat of change in role functioning and socioeconomic status, and threat to self-concept, possibly evidenced by increased tension, apprehension, uncertainty, focus on self, and expressed concerns.

Mobility, impaired physical may be related to neuromuscular and sensory impairment, possibly evidenced by decreased muscle strength, control, and mass and impaired coordination.

Self-Care deficit [specify] may be related to neuromuscular and sensory impairments, possibly evidenced by statement of inability to perform care tasks.

Tay-Sachs disease

Growth and Development, altered may be related to effects of physical condition, possibly evidenced by altered physical growth, loss of/failure to acquire skills typical of age, flat affect, and decreased responses.

Sensory/Perceptual alterations: visual may be related to neurologic deterioration of optic nerve, possibly evidenced by loss of visual acuity.

Grieving, anticipatory [family] may be related to expected eventual loss of infant/child, possibly evidenced by expressions of distress, denial, guilt, anger, and sorrow; choked feelings; changes in sleep/eating habits; and altered libido.

Powerlessness [family] may be related to absence of therapeutic interventions for progressive/fatal disease, possibly evidenced by verbal expressions of having no control over situation/outcome and depression over physical/mental deterioration.

Spiritual Distress, risk for: risk factors may include challenged belief and value system by presence of fatal condition with racial/religious connotations and intense suffering.

Family Coping, ineffective: compromised may be related to situational crisis, temporary preoccupation with managing emotional conflicts and personal suffering, family disorganization, and prolonged/progressive disease, possibly evidenced by preoccupation with personal reactions, expressed concern about reactions of other family members, inadequate support of one another, and altered communication patterns.

thrombophlebitis

Tissue Perfusion, altered: peripheral may be related to interruption of venous blood flow, venous stasis, possibly evidenced by changes in skin color/temperature over affected area, development of edema, pain, diminished peripheral pulses, slow capillary refill.

Pain [acute/discomfort] may be related to vascular inflammation/irritation and edema formation (accumulation of lactic acid), possibly evidenced by verbal reports, guarding/distraction behaviors, and self-focus.

Mobility, risk for impaired physical: risk factors may include pain and discomfort and restrictive therapies/safety precautions.

Knowledge deficit [Learning Need] regarding pathophysiology of condition, therapy/self-care needs, and risk of embolization may be related to lack of information/misinterpretation, possibly evidenced by statements of concern, questions, inaccurate follow-through of instructions, and development of preventable complications.

thrombosis, venous
Refer to *thrombophlebitis*.

thyroidectomy
(also refer to *hyperthyroidism*; *hypoparathyroidism*; *hypothyroidism*)
Airway Clearance, risk for ineffective: risk factors may include hematoma/edema formation with tracheal obstruction, laryngeal spasms.
Communication, impaired verbal may be related to tissue edema, pain/discomfort, and vocal cord injury/laryngeal nerve damage, possibly evidenced by impaired articulation, does not/cannot speak, and use of nonverbal cues/gestures.
Injury, risk for tetany: risk factors may include chemical imbalance/excessive CNS stimulation.
Trauma, risk for head/neck: risk factors may include loss of muscle control/support and position of suture line.
Pain [acute] may be related to presence of surgical incision/manipulation of tissues/muscles, postoperative edema, possibly evidenced by verbal reports, guarding/distraction behaviors, narrowed focus, and autonomic responses (changes in vital signs).

thyrotoxicosis
(also refer to *hyperthyroidism*)
Cardiac Output, risk for decreased: risk factors may include uncontrolled hypermetabolic state increasing cardiac workload, changes in venous return and SVR; and alterations in rate, rhythm, and electrical conduction.
Anxiety [specify level] may be related to physiological factors/CNS stimulation (hypermetabolic state and pseudocatecholamine effect of thyroid hormones), possibly evidenced by increased feelings of apprehension, shakiness, loss of control, panic, changes in cognition, distortion of environmental stimuli, extraneous movements, restlessness, and tremors.
Thought Processes, risk for altered: risk factors may include physiologic changes (increased CNS stimulation/accelerated mental activity), and altered sleep patterns.
Knowledge deficit [Learning Need] regarding condition, treatment needs, and potential for complications/crisis situation may be related to lack of information/recall, misinterpretation, possibly evidenced by statements of concern, questions, misconceptions; and inaccurate follow-through of instructions.

tic douloureux
Refer to *neuralgia, trigeminal*.

tonsillectomy
Refer to *adenoidectomy*.

tonsillitis
Pain [acute] may be related to inflammation of tonsils and effects of circulating toxins, possibly evidenced by verbal reports, guarding/distraction behaviors, reluctance/refusal to swallow, self-focus, and autonomic responses (changes in vital signs).
Hyperthermia may be related to presence of inflammatory process/hypermetabolic state and dehydration, possibly evidenced by increased body temperature, warm/flushed skin, and tachycardia.
Knowledge deficit [Learning Need] regardless cause/transmission, treatment needs, and potential complications may be related to lack of information/misinterpretation, possibly evidenced by statements of concern, questions, inaccurate follow-through of instructions, and recurrence of condition.

total joint replacement
Infection, risk for: risk factors may include inadequate primary defenses (broken skin, exposure of joint), inadequate secondary defenses/immunosuppression (long-term corticosteroid use), invasive procedures/surgical manipulation, implantation of foreign body, and decreased mobility.
Mobility, impaired physical may be related to pain and discomfort, musculoskeletal impairment, and surgery/restrictive therapies, possibly evidenced by reluctance to attempt movement, difficulty purposefully moving within the physical environment, reports of pain/discomfort on movement, limited range of motion, and decreased muscle strength/control.
Tissue Perfusion, risk for altered: peripheral: risk factors may include reduced arterial/venous blood flow, direct trauma to blood vessels, tissue edema, improper location/dislocation of prosthesis, and hypovolemia.

Pain [acute] may be related to physical agents (traumatized tissues/surgical intervention, degeneration of joints, muscle spasms) and psychological factors (anxiety, advanced age), possibly evidenced by verbal reports, guarding/distraction behaviors, self-focus, and autonomic responses (changes in vital signs).

toxemia of pregnancy

Refer to *pregnancy-induced hypertension*.

toxic shock syndrome

(also refer to *septicemia*)

Hyperthermia may be related to inflammatory process/hypermetabolic state and dehydration, possibly evidenced by increased body temperature, warm/flushed skin, and tachycardia.

Fluid Volume deficit [isotonic] may be related to increased gastric losses (diarrhea, vomiting), fever/hypermetabolic state, and decreased intake, possibly evidenced by dry mucous membranes, increased pulse, hypotension, delayed venous filling, decreased/concentrated urine, and hemoconcentration.

Pain [acute] may be related to inflammatory process, effects of circulating toxins, and skin disruptions, possibly evidenced by verbal reports, guarding/distraction behaviors, self-focus, and autonomic responses (changes in vital signs).

Skin/Tissue Integrity, impaired may be related to effects of circulating toxins and dehydration, possibly evidenced by development of desquamating rash, hyperemia, and inflammation of mucous membranes.

traction

(also refer to *casts*; *fractures*)

Pain [acute] may be related to direct trauma to tissue/bone, muscle spasms, movement of bone fragments, edema, injury to soft tissue, traction/immobility device, anxiety, possibly evidenced by verbal reports, guarding/distraction behaviors, self-focus, alteration in muscle tone, and autonomic responses (changes in vital signs).

Mobility, impaired physical may be related to neuromuscular/skeletal impairment, pain, psychological immobility, and therapeutic restrictions of movement, possibly evidenced by limited range of motion, inability to move purposefully in environment, reluctance to attempt movement, and decreased muscle strength/control.

Infection, risk for: risk factors may include invasive procedures (including insertion of foreign body through skin/bone), presence of traumatized tissue, and reduced activity with stasis of body fluids.

Diversional Activity deficit may be related to length of hospitalization/therapeutic intervention and environmental lack of usual activity, possibly evidenced by statements of boredom, restlessness, and irritability.

trichinosis

Pain [acute] may be related to parasitic invasion of muscle tissues, edema of upper eyelids, small localized hemorrhages, and development of urticaria, possibly evidenced by verbal reports, guarding/distraction behaviors (restlessness), and autonomic responses (changes in vital signs).

Fluid Volume deficit [isotonic] may be related to hypermetabolic state (fever, diaphoresis); excessive gastric losses (vomiting, diarrhea); and decreased intake/difficulty swallowing, possibly evidenced by dry mucous membranes, decreased skin turgor, hypotension, decreased venous filling, decreased/concentrated urine, and hemoconcentration.

Breathing Pattern, ineffective may be related to myositis of the diaphragm and intercostal muscles, possibly evidenced by resulting changes in respiratory depth, tachypnea, dyspnea, and abnormal ABGs.

Knowledge deficit [Learning Need] regarding cause/prevention of condition, therapy needs, and possible complications may be related to lack of information, misinterpretation, possibly evidenced by statements of concern, questions, and misconceptions.

tuberculosis (pulmonary)

Infection, risk for spread/reactivation: risk factors may include inadequate primary defenses (decreased ciliary action/stasis of secretions, tissue destruction/extension of infection), lowered resistance/suppressed inflammatory response, malnutrition, environmental exposure, insufficient knowledge to avoid exposure to pathogens, or inadequate therapeutic intervention.

Airway Clearance, ineffective may be related to thick, viscous, or bloody secretions; fatigue/poor cough effort, and tracheal/pharyngeal edema, possibly evidenced by abnormal respiratory rate, rhythm, and depth; adventitious breath sounds (rhonchi, wheezes), stridor, and dyspnea.

Gas Exchange, risk for impaired: risk factors may include decrease in effective lung surface, atelectasis, destruction of alveolar-capillary membrane, bronchial edema; thick, viscous secretions.
Activity Intolerance may be related to imbalance between oxygen supply and demand, possibly evidenced by reports of fatigue, weakness, and exertional dyspnea.
Nutrition: altered, less than body requirements may be related to inability to ingest adequate nutrients (anorexia, effects of drug therapy, fatigue, insufficient financial resources), possibly evidenced by weight loss, reported lack of interest in food/altered taste sensation, and poor muscle tone.
Therapeutic Regimen: Individual risk for ineffective management: risk factors may include complexity of therapeutic regimen, economic difficulties, family patterns of health care, perceived seriousness/benefits (especially during remission), side effects of therapy.

tympanoplasty
Refer to *stapedectomy*.

typhus (tick-borne fever/Rocky Mountain spotted fever)
Hyperthermia may be related to generalized inflammatory process (vasculitis), possibly evidenced by increased body temperature, warm/flushed skin, and tachycardia.
Pain [acute] may be related to generalized vasculitis and edema formation, possibly evidenced by verbal reports, guarding/distraction behaviors, self-focus, and autonomic responses (changes in vital signs).
Tissue Perfusion, altered (specify) may be related to reduction/interruption of blood flow (generalized vasculitis/thrombi formation), possibly evidenced by reports of headache/abdominal pain, changes in mentation, and areas of peripheral ulceration/necrosis.

ulcer, decubitus
Skin/Tissue Integrity, impaired may be related to altered circulation, nutritional deficit, fluid imbalance, impaired physical mobility, irritation of body excretions/secretions, and sensory impairments, evidenced by tissue damage/destruction.
Pain [acute] may be related to destruction of protective skin layers and exposure of nerves, possibly evidenced by verbal reports, distraction behaviors, and self-focus.
Infection, risk for: risk factors may include broken/traumatized tissue, increased environmental exposure, and nutritional deficits.

ulcer, peptic (acute)
Fluid Volume deficit [isotonic] may be related to vascular losses (hemorrhage), possibly evidenced by hypotension, tachycardia, delayed capillary refill, changes in mentation, restlessness, concentrated/decreased urine, pallor, diaphoresis, and hemoconcentration.
Tissue Perfusion, risk for altered (specify): risk factors may include hypovolemia.
Fear/Anxiety [specify level] may be related to change in health status and threat of death, possibly evidenced by increased tension, restlessness, irritability, fearfulness, trembling, tachycardia, diaphoresis, lack of eye contact, focus on self, verbalization of concerns, withdrawal, and panic or attack behavior.
Pain [acute] may be related to caustic irritation/destruction of gastric tissues, possibly evidenced by verbal reports, distraction behaviors, self-focus, and autonomic responses (changes in vital signs).
Knowledge deficit [Learning Need] regarding condition, therapy/self-care needs, and potential complications may be related to lack of information/recall, misinterpretation, possibly evidenced by statements of concern, questions, misconceptions; inaccurate follow-through of instructions, and development of preventable complications/recurrence of condition.

unconsciousness (coma)
Suffocation, risk for: risk factors may include cognitive impairment/loss of protective reflexes and purposeful movement.
Fluid Volume, risk for deficit/Nutrition: altered, risk for less than body requirements: risk factors may include inability to ingest food/fluids, increased needs/hypermetabolic state.
Self-Care deficit, total may be related to cognitive impairment and absence of purposeful activity, evidenced by inability to perform ADLs..
Tissue Perfusion, risk for altered: cerebral: risk factors may include reduced or interrupted arterial/venous blood flow (direct injury, edema formation, space-occupying lesions), metabolic alterations, effects of drug/alcohol overdose, hypoxia/anoxia.
Infection, risk for: risk factors may include stasis of body fluids (oral, pulmonary, urinary), invasive procedures, and nutritional deficits.

urinary diversion

Skin Integrity, risk for impaired: risk factors may include absence of sphincter at stoma, character/flow of urine from stoma, reaction to product/chemicals, and improperly fitting appliance or removal of adhesive.

Body Image disturbance, related factors may include biophysical factors (presence of stoma, loss of control of urine flow), and psychosocial factors (altered body structure, disease process/associated treatment regimen, such as cancer), possibly evidenced by verbalization of change in body image, fear of rejection/reaction of others, negative feelings about body, not touching/looking at stoma, refusal to participate in care.

Pain [acute] may be related to physical factors (disruption of skin/tissues, presence of incisions/drains), biological factors (activity of disease process, such as cancer, trauma), and psychological factors (fear, anxiety), possibly evidenced by verbal reports, self-focusing, guarding/distraction behaviors, restlessness, and autonomic responses (changes in vital signs).

Urinary elimination, altered may be related to surgical diversion, tissue trauma, and postoperative edema, possibly evidenced by loss of continence, changes in amount and character of urine, and urinary retention.

urolithiasis (urinary calculi)

Pain [acute] may be related to distention, trauma, and edema formation in sensitive tissue or cellular ischemia, possibly evidenced by verbal reports, guarding/distraction behaviors, self-focus, and autonomic responses (changes in vital signs).

Urinary Elimination, altered may be related to edema formation and irritation/inflammation of ureteral and bladder tissues, possibly evidenced by urgency, frequency, retention, and hematuria.

Fluid Volume, risk for deficit: risk factors may include stimulation of renal-intestinal reflexes causing nausea, vomiting, and diarrhea; changes in urinary output, postoperative diuresis; and decreased intake.

uterine bleeding, abnormal

Anxiety [specify level] may be related to perceived change in health status and unknown etiology, possibly evidenced by apprehension, uncertainty, fear of unspecified consequences, expressed concerns, and focus on self.

Activity intolerance may be related to imbalance between oxygen supply and demand/decreased oxygen-carrying capacity of blood (anemia), possibly evidenced by reports of fatigue/weakness.

uterus, rupture of, in pregnancy

Fluid Volume deficit [isotonic] may be related to excessive vascular losses, possibly evidenced by hypotension, increased pulse rate, decreased venous filling, and decreased urine output.

Cardiac Output, decreased may be related to decreased preload (hypovolemia), possibly evidenced by cold/clammy skin, decreased peripheral pulses, variations in hemodynamic readings, tachycardia, and cyanosis.

Pain [acute] may be related to tissue trauma and irritation of accumulating blood, possibly evidenced by verbal reports, guarding/distraction behaviors, self-focus, and autonomic responses (changes in vital signs).

Anxiety [specify level] may be related to threat of death of self/fetus, interpersonal contagion, physiological response (release of catecholamines), possibly evidenced by fearful/scared affect, sympathetic stimulation, stated fear of unspecified consequences, and expressed concerns.

vaginismus

Pain [acute] may be related to muscle spasm and hyperesthesia of the nerve supply to vaginal mucous membrane, possibly evidenced by verbal reports, distraction behaviors, and self-focus.

Sexual dysfunction may be related to physical and/or psychological alteration in function (severe spasms of vaginal muscles), possibly evidenced by verbalization of problem, inability to achieve desired satisfaction, and alteration in relationship with significant other.

vaginitis

Tissue Integrity, impaired may be related to irritation/inflammation and mechanical trauma (scratching) of sensitive tissues, possibly evidenced by damaged/destroyed tissue, presence of lesions.

Pain [acute] may be related to localized inflammation and tissue trauma, possibly evidenced by verbal reports, distraction behaviors, and self-focus.

Knowledge deficit [Learning Need] regarding hygienic/therapy needs and sexual behaviors/transmission of organisms may be related to lack of information/misinterpretation, possibly evidenced by statements of concern, questions, and misconceptions.

varices, esophageal
(also refer to *ulcer, peptic [acute]*)
Fluid Volume deficit [isotonic] may be related to excessive vascular loss, reduced intake, and gastric losses (vomiting), possibly evidenced by hypotension, tachycardia, decreased venous filling, and decreased/concentrated urine.
Anxiety [specify level]/Fear may be related to change in health status and threat of death, possibly evidenced by increased tension/apprehension, sympathetic stimulation, restlessness, focus on self, and expressed concerns.

varicose veins
Pain, chronic may be related to venous insufficiency and stasis, possibly evidenced by verbal reports.
Body Image disturbance may be related to change in structure (presence of enlarged, discolored, tortuous superficial leg veins), possibly evidenced by hiding affected parts and negative feelings about body.
Skin/Tissue Integrity, risk for impaired: risk factors may include altered circulation/venous stasis and edema formation.

venereal disease
Refer to *sexually transmitted disease—STD.*

Wilms' tumor
(also refer to *cancer*; *chemotherapy*)
Anxiety [specify level]/Fear may be related to change in environment and interaction patterns with family members and threat of death with family transmission and contagion of concerns, possibly evidenced by fearful/scared affect, distress, crying, insomnia, and sympathetic stimulation.
Injury, risk for: risk factors may include nature of tumor (vascular, mushy with very thin covering) with increased danger of metastasis when manipulated.
Family Processes, altered may be related to situational crisis of life-threatening illness, possibly evidenced by a family system that has difficulty meeting physical, emotional, and spiritual needs of its members, and inability to deal with traumatic experience effectively.
Diversional Activity deficit may be related to environmental lack of age-appropriate activity (including activity restrictions) and length of hospitalization/treatment, possibly evidenced by restlessness, crying, lethargy, and acting-out behavior.

wound, bullet **(depends on site and speed/character of bullet)**
Fluid Volume, risk for deficit: risk factors may include excessive vascular losses, altered intake/restrictions.
Pain [acute] may be related to destruction of tissue (including organ and musculoskeletal), surgical repair, and therapeutic interventions, possibly evidenced by verbal reports, guarding/distraction behaviors, self-focus, and autonomic responses (changes in vital signs).
Tissue Integrity, impaired may be related to mechanical factors (yaw of projectile and muzzle blast), possibly evidenced by damaged or destroyed tissue.
Infection, risk for: risk factors may include tissue destruction and increased environmental exposure, invasive procedures, and decreased hemoglobin.
Post-Trauma Syndrome, risk for: risk factors may include nature of incident (catastrophic accident, assault, suicide attempt) and possibly injury/death of other(s) involved.

Appendix N7–5 Nursing Diagnoses Through the 14th NANDA Conference in Alphabetical Order

Information appearing in brackets has been added by the authors to clarify and facilitate the use of nursing diagnoses.

A "RISK FOR" diagnosis is *not* evidenced by signs and symptoms, because the problem has not yet occurred, and nursing interventions are directed at prevention. Therefore, *risk* factors that are present are noted instead.

New nursing diagnoses from the NANDA 14th Conference (2000) appear in Appendix N7–3.

ACTIVITY INTOLERANCE [SPECIFY LEVEL]

Diagnostic Division: Activity/Rest

Definition: A state in which an individual has insufficient physiological or psychological energy to endure or complete required or desired daily activities.

RELATED FACTORS

Generalized weakness; Sedentary lifestyle; Imbalance between oxygen supply and demand; Bedrest or immobility; [Cognitive deficits/emotional status; secondary to underlying disease process/depression]; [Pain, vertigo, extreme stress]

DEFINING CHARACTERISTICS

Subjective

Report of fatigue or weakness; Exertional discomfort or dyspnea; [Verbalizes no desire and/or lack of interest in activity]

Objective

Abnormal heart rate or blood pressure response to activity; Electrocardiographic changes reflecting dysrhythmias or ischemia; [Pallor, cyanosis]

ACTIVITY INTOLERANCE, RISK FOR

Diagnostic Division: Activity/Rest

Definition: A state in which an individual is at risk of experiencing insufficient physiologic or psychologic energy to endure or complete required or desired daily activities.

RISK FACTORS

History of previous intolerance; Presence of circulatory/respiratory problems; Deconditioned status; Inexperience with the activity; [Diagnosis of progressive disease state/debilitating condition such as cancer, multiple sclerosis; extensive surgical procedures]; [Verbalized reluctance/inability to perform expected activity]

ADAPTIVE CAPACITY: INTRACRANIAL, DECREASED

Diagnostic Division: Circulation

Definition: A clinical state in which intracranial fluid dynamic mechanisms that normally compensate for increases in intracranial volumes are compromised, resulting in repeated disproportionate increases in intracranial pressure (ICP) in response to a variety of noxious and non-noxious stimuli.

RELATED FACTORS

Brain injuries; Sustained increase in ICP equal to 10 to 15 mm Hg; Decreased cerebral perfusion pressure less than or equal to 50 to 60 mm Hg; Systemic hypotension with intracranial hypertension

DEFINING CHARACTERISTICS

Objective

Repeated increases in ICP of greater than 10 mm Hg for more than 5 min following a variety of external stimuli; Disproportionate increases in ICP following single environmental or nursing maneuver stimulus; Elevated P2 ICP waveform; Volume pressure response test variation (volume-pressure ratio greater than 2, pressure equals volume index less than 10); Baseline ICP equal to or greater than 10 mm Hg; Wide-amplitude ICP waveform [Altered level of consciousness—coma]; [Changes in vital signs, cardiac rhythm]

ADJUSTMENT, IMPAIRED

Diagnostic Division: Ego Integrity

Definition: Inability to modify life style/behavior in a manner consistent with a change in health status.

RELATED FACTORS

Disability or health status change requiring change in life style; Multiple stressors; intense emotional state; Low state of optimism; negative attitudes toward health behavior; lack of motivation to change behaviors; Failure to intend to change behavior; Absence of social support for changed beliefs and practices; [Physical and/or learning disability]

DEFINING CHARACTERISTICS

Subjective
Denial of health status change; Failure to achieve optimal sense of control

Objective
Failure to take actions that would prevent further health problems; Demonstration of non-acceptance of health status change

AIRWAY CLEARANCE, INEFFECTIVE

Diagnostic Division: Respiration

Definition: Inability to clear secretions or obstructions from the respiratory tract to maintain a clear airway.

RELATED FACTORS
Environmental
Smoking; smoke inhalation; second-hand smoke.

Obstructed Airway
Airway spasm; retained secretions; excessive mucus; presence of artificial airway; foreign body in airway; secretions in the bronchi; exudate in the alveoli

Physiological
Neuromuscular dysfunction; hyperplasia of the bronchial walls; chronic obstructive pulmonary disease; infection; asthma; allergic airways

DEFINING CHARACTERISTICS

Subjective
Dyspnea

Objective
Diminished or adventitious breath sounds (rales, crackles, rhonchi, wheezes); Cough, ineffective or absent; sputum; Changes in respiratory rate and rhythm; Difficulty vocalizing; Wide-eyed; restlessness; Orthopnea; Cyanosis

ANXIETY

Diagnostic Division: Ego Integrity

Definition: A vague uneasy feeling of discomfort or dread accompanied by an autonomic response; the source is often nonspecific or unknown to the individual; a feeling of apprehension caused by anticipation of danger. It is an altering signal that warns of impending danger and enables the individual to take measures to deal with threat.

RELATED FACTORS
Unconscious conflict about essential [beliefs]/goals and values of life; Situational/maturational crises; Stress; Familial association/heredity; Interpersonal transmission/contagion; Threat to self-concept [perceived or actual]; [unconscious conflict]; Threat of death [perceived or actual]; Threat to or change in health status [progressive/debilitating disease, terminal illness], interaction patterns, role function/status, environment [safety], economic status; Unmet needs; Exposure to toxins; Substance abuse; [Positive or negative self talk]; [Physiological factors, such as hyperthyroidism, pheochromocytoma, drug therapy including steroids, and so on]

DEFINING CHARACTERISTICS

Subjective
Behavioral
Expressed concerns due to change in life events

Affective
Regretful; scared; rattled; overexcited; painful and persistent increased helplessness; uncertainty; increased wariness; focus on self; feelings of inadequacy; fearful; distressed; apprehension; anxious; jittery; [sense of impending doom]; [hopelessness]

Cognitive
Fear of unspecific consequences; awareness of physiologic symptoms

Physiological
Shakiness; worried; regretful; dry mouth (sympathetic); tingling in extremities (parasympathetic); heart pounding (sympathetic); nausea (parasympathetic); abdominal pain (parasympathetic); diarrhea (parasympathetic); urinary hesitancy (parasympa-

thetic); urinary frequency (parasympathetic); faintness (parasympathetic); weakness (sympathetic); decreased pulse (parasympathetic); respiratory difficulties (sympathetic); fatigue (parasympathetic); sleep disturbance (parasympathetic); [chest, back, neck pain]

Objective
Behavioral
Poor eye contact; glancing about; scanning and vigilance; extraneous movement (e.g., foot shuffling, hand/arm movements); fidgeting; restlessness; diminished productivity; [crying/tearfulness]; [pacing/purposeless activity]; [immobility]

Affective
Increased wariness; focus on self; irritability; overexcited; anguish; painful and persistent increased helplessness

Physiological
Voice quivering; trembling/hand tremors; increased tension; facial tension; increased pulse; increased perspiration; cardiovascular excitation (sympathetic); facial flushing (sympathetic); superficial vasoconstriction (sympathetic); increased blood pressure (sympathetic); twitching (sympathetic); increased reflexes (sympathetic); urinary urgency (parasympathetic); decreased blood pressure (parasympathetic); insomnia; anorexia (sympathetic); increased respiration (sympathetic)

Cognitive
Preoccupation; impaired attention; difficult concentrating; forgetfulness; diminished ability to problem-solve; diminished learning ability; rumination; tendency to blame others; blocking of thought; confusion; decreased perceptual field.

ANXIETY, DEATH

Diagnostic Division: Ego Integrity

Definition: The apprehension, worry, or fear related to death or dying.

RELATED FACTORS
To be developed by NANDA

DEFINING CHARACTERISTICS

Subjective
Fear of: developing terminal illness, the process of dying, loss of physical and/or mental abilities when dying, premature death because it prevents the accomplishment of important life goals, leaving family alone after death, delayed demise; Negative death images or unpleasant thought about any event related to death or dying; anticipated pain related to dying; Powerlessness related to dying; total loss of control over any apect of one's own death; Worrying about the impact of one's own death on significant others, being the cause of other's grief and suffering; Concerns of overworking the caregiver as terminal illness incapacitates itself; Concern about meeting one's creator or feeling doubtful about the existence of a god or higher being; Denial of one's own mortality or impending death

Objective
Deep sadness; (refer to nursing diagnosis Grieving, anticipatory)

ASPIRATION, RISK FOR

Diagnostic Division: Respiration

Definition: The state in which an individual is at risk for entry of gastrointestinal secretions, oropharyngeal sections, [or exogenous food] or solids or fluids into tracheobronchial passages [due to dysfunction or absence of normal protective mechanisms].

RISK FACTORS
Reduced level of consciousness; Depressed cough and gag reflexes; Presence of tracheostomy or endotracheal tube; [Overinflated tracheostomy/endotracheal tube cuff]; [Inadequate tracheostomy/endotracheal tube cuff inflation]; [Presence of] gastrointestinal tubes; Tube feedings/medication administration; Situation hindering elevation of upper body [weakness, paralysis]; Increased intragastric pressure; Increased gastric residual; Decreased gastrointestinal motility; Delaying gastric emptying; Impaired swallowing [owing to inability of the epiglottis and true vocal cords to move to close off trachea]; Facial/oral/neck surgery or trauma; Wired jaws; Incomplete lower esophageal sphincter [hiatal hernia or other esophageal disease affecting stomach valve function]

BODY IMAGE DISTURBANCE

Diagnostic Division: Ego Integrity

Definition: Confusion in mental picture of one's physical self.

RELATED FACTORS

Biophysical illness; trauma or injury; surgery [mutilation pregnancy]; illness treatment [change caused by biochemical agents (drugs), dependence on machine]; Pyschosocial; Cognitive/perceptual; developmental changes; Cultural or spiritual; [Significance of body part or functioning with regard to age, sex, developmental level, or basic human needs]; [Maturational changes]

DEFINING CHARACTERISTICS

Subjective

Verbalization of feelings/perception that reflect an altered view of one's body in appearance, structure, or function; change in lifestyle; Fear of rejection or of reaction by others; Focus on past strength, function, or appearance; Negative feelings about body (e.g., feelings of helplessness, hopelessness, or powerlessness); [depersonalization/grandiosity]; Preoccupation with change or loss; Refusal to verify actual change; Emphasis on remaining strengths, heightened achievement; Personalization of part or loss by name; Depersonalization of part or loss by impersonal pronouns

Objective

Missing body part; Actual change in structure and/or function; Nonverbal response to acutual or perceived change in structure and/or function; behaviors of avoidance, monitoring, or acknowledgment of one's body; Not looking at/not touching body part; Trauma to nonfunctioning part; Change in ability to estimate spatial relationshp of body to environment; Extension of body boundary to incorporate environmental objects; Hiding or overexposing body part (intentional or unintentional); Change in social involvement; [Aggression; low frustration tolerance level]

BODY TEMPERATURE, RISK FOR ALTERED

Diagnostic Division: Safety

Definition: The state in which the individual is at risk for failure to maintain body temperature within normal range.

RISK FACTORS

Extremes of age; Extremes of weight; Exposure to cold/cool or warm/hot environments; Dehydration; Inactivity or vigorous activity; Medications causing vasoconstriction/vasodilation, altered metabolic rate, sedation, [use or overdose of certain drugs or exposure to anesthesia]; Inappropriate clothing for environmental temperature; Illness or trauma affecting temperature regulation; [e.g., infections, systemic or localized; neoplasms, tumors, collagen/vascular disease]

BOWEL INCONTINENCE

Diagnostic Division: Elimination

Definition: Change in normal bowel habits characterized by involuntary passage of stool.

RELATED FACTORS

Self-care deficit—toileting; impaired cognition; immobility; environmental factors (e.g., inaccessible bathroom); Dietary habits; medications; laxative abuse; Stress; Incomplete emptying of bowel; impaction; chronic diarrhea; General decline in muscle tone; abnormally high abdominal or intestinal pressure; Impaired reservoir capacity; Rectal sphincter abnormality; loss of rectal sphincter control; upper/lower motor nerve damage

DEFINING CHARACTERISTICS

Subjective

Recognizes rectal fullness but reports inability to expel formed stool; Urgency; Inability to delay defecation; Self-report of inability to feel rectal fullness

Objective

Constant dribbling of soft stool; Fecal odor; Fecal staining of clothing and/or bedding; Red perianal skin; Inability to recognize/inattention to urge to defecate

BREASTFEEDING, EFFECTIVE

Diagnostic Division: Food / Fluid

Definition: The state in which a mother-infant dyad/family exhibits adequate proficiency and satisfaction with breastfeeding process.

RELATED FACTORS
Basic breastfeeding knowledge; Normal breast structure; Normal infant oral structure; Infant gestational age greater than 34 weeks; Support sources [available]; Maternal confidence

DEFINING CHARACTERISTICS

Subjective
Maternal verbalization of satisfaction with the breastfeeding process

Objective
Mother able to position infant at breast to promote a successful latch-on response; Infant is content after feedings; Regular and sustained sucking at the breast (8 to 10 times/24 hours); Appropriate infant weight patterns for age; Effective mother/infant communication pattern (infant cues, maternal interpretation and response); Signs and/or symptoms of oxytocin release (let-down or milk ejection reflex); Adequate infant elimination patterns for age; [soft stools; more than 6 wet diapers per day of unconcentrated urine]; Eagerness of infant to nurse

BREASTFEEDING, INEFFECTIVE

Diagnostic Division: Food / Fluid

Definition: The state in which a mother, infant, or child experiences dissatisfaction or difficulty with the breastfeeding process.

RELATED FACTORS
Prematurity; Infant anomaly; Poor infant sucking reflex; Infant receiving [numerous or repeated] supplemental feedings with artificial nipple; Maternal anxiety or ambivalence; Knowledge deficit; Previous history of breastfeeding failure; Interruption in breastfeeding; Nonsupportive partner/family; Maternal breast anomaly; Previous breast surgery [painful nipples/breat engorgement]

DEFINING CHARACTERISTICS

Subjective
Unsatisfactory breastfeeding process; Persistence of sore nipples beyond the first week of breastfeeding; Insufficient emptying of each breast per feeding; Actual or perceived inadequate milk supply

Objective
Observable signs of inadequate infant intake [decrease in number of wet diapers, inappropriate weight loss or inadequate gain]; Nonsustained or insufficient opportunity for suckling at the breast; Infant inability [failure] to attach on to maternal breast correctly; Infant arching and crying at the breasts; resistant latching on; Infant exhibiting fussiness and crying within the first hour after breastfeeding; Unresponsive to other comfort measures; No observable signs of oxytocin release

BREASTFEEDING, INTERRUPTED

Diagnostic Division: Food / Fluid

Definition: A break in the continuity of the breastfeeding process as a result of inability or inadvisability to put a baby to breast for feeding.

RELATED FACTORS
Maternal or infant illness; Prematurity; Maternal employment; Contraindications to breastfeeding (e.g., drugs, true breast milk jaundice); Need to abruptly wean infant

DEFINING CHARACTERISTICS

Subjective
Infant does not receive nourishment at the breast for some or all of feedings; Maternal desire to maintain lactation and provide (or eventually provide) her breast milk for her infant's nutritional needs; Lack of knowledge regarding expression and storage of breast milk

Objective
Separation of mother and infant

BREATHING PATTERN, INEFFECTIVE

Diagnostic Division: Respiration

Definition: Inspiration and/or expiration that does not provide adequate ventilation.

RELATED FACTORS

Neuromuscular dysfunction; spinal cord injury; neurological immaturity; Musculoskeletal impairment; bony/chest wall deformity; Anxiety; Pain; Perception/cognitive impairment; Decreased energy/fatigue; respiratory muscle fatigue; Body position; obesity; Hyperventilation; hypoventilation syndrome; [alteration of patient's normal O_2 : CO_2 ratio (e.g, O_2 therapy in COPD)]

DEFINING CHARACTERISTICS

Subjective

Shortness of breath

Objective

Dyspnea; orthopnea; respiratory rate (adults [ages 14 or greater] <11 or [>] 24, infants <25 or [>]60, ages 1–4 <20 or >30, ages 5–14 <15 or >25); depth of breathing (adults VT 500 ml at rest, infants 6–8 ml/kilo); Timing ratio; prolonged expiration phases; pursed lip breathing; Decreased minute ventilation; vital capacity; Decreased inspiratory/expiratory pressure; Use of accessory muscles to breathe; assumption of 3-point position; Altered chest excursion; [paradoxical breathing patterns]; Nasal flaring [grunting]; Increased anterior-posterior diameter

CARDIAC OUTPUT, DECREASED

Diagnostic Division: Circulation

Definition: A state in which the blood pumped by the heart is inadequate to meet the metabolic demands of the body.

NOTE: In a hypermetabolic state, although cardiac output may be within normal range, it may still be inadequate to meet the needs of the body's tissues. Cardiac output and tissue perfusion are interrelated, although there are differences. When cardiac output is decreased, tissue perfusion problems will develop; however, tissue perfusion problems can exist without decreased cardiac output.

RELATED FACTORS

To be developed by NANDA (Mechanical: Alteration in preload [e.g., decreased venous return, altered myocardial contractility]; afterload [e.g., alteration in systemic vascular resistance]; inotropic changes in heart. Electrical: Alterations in rate, rhythm, conduction. Structural [e.g., ventricular-septal rupture, ventricular aneurysm, papillary muscle rupture, valvular disease.])

NOTE: These factors were identified when this diagnosis was originally accepted and have been retained here to assist the user until NANDA completes its work.

DEFINING CHARACTERISTICS

Subjective

Fatigue; Dyspnea; Orthopnea/PND; Chest pain, [angina]; [syncope; vertigo]

Objective

Variations in blood pressure readings; decreased CO by thermodilution method; Ejection fraction <40%; Color changes, skin [and mucous membranes (cyanosis, pallor)]; Cold, clammy skin; Decreased peripheral pulses; Increased heart rate; S_3 or S_4, [gallop rhythm]; [Dys]arrhythmias, electrocardiogram (ECG) changes; Jugular vein distention (JVD); Oliguria; [anuria]; Rales [crackles]; wheezing; [frothy sputum]; cough; Restlessness; Weight gain; edema; Elevated pulmonary artery pressures; Increased respiratory rate; use of accessory muscles; Abnormal chest x-ray (pulmonary vascular cognition); Abnormal chest x-ray (pulmonary vascular congestion); Abnormal cardiac enzymes; Mixed venous O_2 (SaO_2); Altered mental status

CAREGIVER ROLE STRAIN

Diagnostic Division: Social Interaction

Definition: A caregiver's felt difficulty in performing the family caregiver role.

RELATED FACTORS
Physiological
Illness severity of the care receiver; Addiction or codependency of care receiver; Discharge of family member with significant home care needs [e.g., premature birth, congenital defect]; Caregiver health impairment; Unpredictable illness course or instability in the care receiver's health; Increasing care needs and/or dependency

Individual
Illness chronicity; Instability of care receiver's health; Problem behaviors; Psychological or cognitive problems in care receiver

Roles and Relationships
Unrealistic expectations of caregiver by care receiver; Change in relationship; History of marginal family coping, family dysfunction

Caregiver
Ongoing changes in activities; amount of activities; Unpredictability of care situation; 24 hour care responsibility; Inability to fulfill one's own or other's expectations; unrealistic expectations of self; Marginal caregiver's coping patterns; Addiction or codependency; psychological or cognitive problems

Situational
Presence of abuse or violence; Inadequate physical environment for providing care (e.g., housing, transportation, community services, equipment); Family/caregiver isolation; Inexperience with caregiving; Caregiver's competing role commitments; Complexity/amount of caregiving tasks

Social
Alienation from family, friends, and coworkers; Insufficient recreation

Resources
Insufficient information, finances; Inadequate transportation, equipment for providing care, community services; Lack of support from significant others, respite resources, recreational resources; Caregiver is not developmentally ready for caregiver role

NOTE: The presence of this problem may encompass other numerous problems/high-risk concerns such as Diversional Activity deficit; Sleep Pattern disturbance; Fatigue; Anxiety; Coping, Individual, ineffective; Decisional Conflict; Denial, ineffective; Grieving, anticpatory/[actual]; Hopelessness; Powerlessness; Spiritual distress; Health Maintenance, altered; Home Maintenance Management, impaired; Sexuality Patterns, altered; Family Coping: potential for growth; Family Processes, altered; Social Isolation. Careful attention to data gathering will identify and clarify the client's specific needs, which can then be coordinated under this single diagnostic label.

DEFINING CHARACTERISTICS
Subjective
Apprehension about possible institutionalization of care receiver, the future regarding care receiver's health and the caregiver's ability to provide care, care receiver's care when caregiver is ill or deceased; Altered caregiving activities; Altered caregiver health status (e.g., hypertension, cardiovascular disease, diabetes, headaches, gastrointestinal upset, weight change, rash); [Care receiver reports problems with care]

Objective
Difficulty performing required activities; Inability to complete caregiving tasks; Preoccupation with care routine; [Disorderly surroundings, tasks not done (e.g., bills unpaid)]

NOTE: [Although objective characteristics were not included in the NANDA diagnosis, if caregiver is in a state of denial, subjective statements may not be made by caregiver; however, statements of care receiver and observations of family members and/or other health care providers may indicate presence of problem.]

CAREGIVER ROLE STRAIN, RISK FOR

Diagnostic Division: Social Interaction

Definition: A caregiver is vulnerable for felt difficulty in performing the family caregiver role.

RISK FACTORS
Pathophysiological
Illness severity of the care receiver; Addiction or codependency; Premature birth/Congenital defect; Discharge of family member with significant home care needs; Caregiver health impairment; Unpredictable illness course or instability in the care re-

ceiver's health; Caregiver is female; Psychological or cognitive problems in care receiver

Developmental
Caregiver is not developmentally ready for caregiver role (e.g., young adult needing to provide care for a middle-aged parent); Developmental delay or retardation of the care receiver or caregiver

Psychological
Marginal family adaptation or dysfunction prior to the caregiving situation; Marginal caregiver's coping patterns; Past history of poor relationship between caregiver and care receiver; Care receiver exhibits deviant, bizarre behavior; Caregiver is spouse

Situational
Presence of abuse or violence; Presence of situational stressors that normally affect families, such as significant loss, disaster, or crisis, poverty or economic vulnerability, major life events (e.g., birth, hospitalization, leaving home, returning home, marriage, divorce, [change in] employment, retirement, death); Duration of caregiving required; Inadequate physical environment for providing care (e.g., housing, transportation, community services, equipment); Family/caregiver isolation; Lack of respite and recreation for caregiver; Inexperience with caregiving; Caregiver's competing role commitments; Complexity/amount of caregiving tasks

COMMUNICATION, IMPAIRED VERBAL

Diagnostic Division: Social Interaction

Definition: The state in which an individual experiences a decreased, delayed, or absent ability to receive, process, transmit, and use a system of symbols; anything that has meaning, i.e., transmits meaning.

RELATED FACTORS
Decrease in circulation to brain, brain tumor; Anatomic deficit (e.g., cleft palate, alteration of the neuromuscular visual system, auditory system, or phonatory apparatus); Difference related to developmental age; Physical barrier (tracheostomy, intubation); Physiological conditions [e.g., dyspnea]; alteration of central nervous system; weakening of musculoskeletal system; Psychological barriers (e.g., psychosis, lack of stimuli); emotional conditions [depression, panic, anger[; stress; Environmental barriers; Cultural difference; Lack of information; Side effects of medication; Alteration of self-esteem or self-concept; Altered perceptions; Absence of significant others

DEFINING CHARACTERISTICS
Subjective
[Reports of difficulty expressing self]

Objective
Unable to speak dominant language; Speaks or verbalizes with difficulty; Does not or cannot speak; Disorientation in the three spheres of time, space, person; Stuttering; slurring; Dyspnea; Difficulty forming words or sentences (e.g., aphonia, dyslalia, dysarthria); Difficulty expressing thought verbally (e.g., aphasia, dysphasia, apraxia, dyslexia); Inappropriate verbalization (incessant, loose association of ideas, flight of ideas); Difficulty in comprehending and maintaining the usual communicating pattern; Absence of eye contact or difficulty in selective attending; partial or total visual deficit; Inability or difficulty in use of facial or body expressions; Willful refusal to speak [Inability to modulate speech]; [Message inappropriate to content]; [Use of nonverbal cues (e.g., pleading eyes, gestures, turning away)]; [Frustration, anger, hostility]

COMMUNITY COPING, INEFFECTIVE

Diagnostic Division: Social Interaction

Definition: A pattern of community activities for adaption and problem solving that is unsatisfactory for meeting the demands or needs of the community. [Community is defined as "a group of people with a common identity or perspective, occupying space during a given period of time, and functioning through a social system to meet its needs within a larger social environment."]

RELATED FACTORS
Deficits in social support services and resources; Inadequate resources for problem solving; Ineffective or non-existent community systems (e.g., lack of emergency medical

system, transportation system, or disaster planning systems); Natural or man-made disasters

DEFINING CHARACTERISTICS

Subjective

Community does not meet its own expectations; Expressed vulnerability; community powerlessness; Stressors perceived as excessive

Objective

Deficits of community participation; Excessive community conflicts; High illness rates; Increased social problems (e.g., homicides, vandalism, arson, terrorism, robbery, infanticide, abuse, divorce, unemployment, poverty, militancy, mental illness)

COMMUNITY COPING, POTENTIAL FOR ENHANCED

Diagnostic Division: Social Interaction

Definition: A pattern of community activities for adaptation and problem solving that is satisfactory for meeting the demands or needs of the community but can be improved for management of current and future problems/stressors.

RELATED FACTORS

Social supports available; Resources available for problem solving; Community has a sense of power to manage stressors

DEFINING CHARACTERISTICS

Subjective

Agreement that community is responsible for stress management

Objective

Deficits in one or more characteristics that indicate effective coping; Active planning by community for predicted stressors; Active problem solving by community when faced with issues; Positive communication among community members; Positive communication between community/aggregates and larger community; Programs available for recreation and relaxation; Resources sufficient for managing stressors

CONFUSION, ACUTE

Diagnostic Division: Neurosensory

Definition: The abrupt onset of a cluster of global, transient changes and disturbances in attention, cognition, psychomotor activity level of consciousness, and/or sleep/wake cycle.

RELATED FACTORS

Over 60 years of age; Dementia; Alcohol abuse, drug abuse; Delirium [including febrile epilepticum (following or instead of an epileptic attack), toxic and traumatic]; [Medication reaction/interaction; anesthesia/surgery; metabolic imbalances]; [Exacerbation of a chronic illness, hypoxemia]; [Severe pain]; [Sleep deprivation]

NOTE: Although no time frame is presented to aid in differentiating acute from chronic confusion, the definition of chronic confusion identifies an irreversible state. Therefore, our belief is that acute confusion is potentially reversible.

DEFINING CHARACTERISTICS

Subjective

Hallucinations [Visual/auditory]; [Exaggerated emotional responses]

Objective

Fluctuation in cognition; Fluctuation in sleep/wake cycle; Fluctuation in level of consciousness; Fluctuation in psychomotor activity [tremors, body movement]; Increased agitation or restlessness; Misperceptions [inappropriate responses]; Lack of motivation to initiate and/or follow through with goal-directed or purposeful behavior

CONFUSION, CHRONIC

Diagnostic Division: Neurosensory

Definition: An irreversible, long-standing, and/or progressive deterioration of intellect and personality characterized by decreased ability to interpret environmental stimuli, decreased capacity for intellectual thought processes, and manifested by disturbances of memory, orientation, and behavior.

RELATED FACTORS

Alzheimer's disease [dementia of Alzheimer's type]; Korsakoff's psychosis; Multi-infarct dementia; Cerebrovascular accident; Head injury

DEFINING CHARACTERISTICS

Objective

Clinical evidence of organic impairment; Altered interpretation/response to stimuli; Progressive/long-standing cognitive impairment; No change in level of consciousness; Impaired socialization; Impaired memory (short term, long term); Altered personality

CONSTIPATION

Diagnostic Division: Elimination

Definition: A decrease in a person's normal frequency of defecation accompanied by difficult or incomplete passage of stool and/or passage of excessively hard, dry stool.

RELATED FACTORS

Functional

Irregular defecation habits; inadequate toileting, (e.g., timeliness, positioning for defecation, privacy); Insufficient physical activity; abdominal muscle weakness; Recent environmental changes; Habitual denial/ignoring of urge to defecate

Psychological

Emotional stress; depression; mental confusion

Pharmacological

Antilipemic agents; laxative overdose; calcium carbonate; aluminum-containing antacids; nonsteroidal anti-inflammatory agents; opiates; anticholinergics; diuretics; iron salts; phenothiazines; sedatives; sympathomimetics; bismuth salts; antidepressants; calcium channel blockers

Mechanical

Hemorrhoids; pregnancy; obesity; Rectal abscess or ulcer; anal fissures; prolapse; anal strictures; rectocele; Prostate enlargement; postsurgical obstruction; Neurological impairment; megacolon (Hirschsprung's disease); tumors; Electrolyte imbalance

Physiological

Poor eating habits; change in usual foods and eating patterns; insufficient fiber intake; insufficient fluid intake; dehydration; Inadequate dentition or oral hygiene; Decreased motility of gastrointestinal tract

DEFINING CHARACTERISTICS

Subjective

Change in bowel pattern; unable to pass stool; decreased frequency; decreased volume of stool; Change in usual foods and eating patterns; increased abdominal pressure; feeling of rectal fullness or pressure; Abdominal pain; pain with defecation; nausea and /or vomiting; headache; indigestion; generalized fatigue

Objective

Dry, hard, formed stool; Straining with defecation; Hypoactive or hyperactive bowel sounds; change in abdominal growling (borborygmi); Distended abdomen; abdominal tenderness with or without palpable muscle resistance; Percussed abdominal dullness; Presence of soft paste-like stool in rectum; oozing liquid stool; bright red blood with stool; dark or black or tarry stool; Severe flatus; anorexia; Atypical presentations in older adults (e.g., change in mental status, urinary incontinence, unexplained falls, elevated body temperature)

CONSTIPATION, PERCEIVED

Diagnostic Division: Elimination

Definition: The state in which an individual makes a self-diagnosis of constipation and ensures a daily bowel movement through abuse of laxatives, enemas, and suppositories.

RELATED FACTORS

Cultural/family health beliefs; Faulty appraisal; Impaired thought processes; [Long-term expectations/habits]

DEFINING CHARACTERISTICS

Subjective

Expectation of a daily bowel movement with the resulting overuse of laxatives, enemas, and suppositories; Expected passage of stool at same time every day

RISK OF CONSTIPATION

Diagnostic Division: Elimination

Definition: At risk for a decrease in a person's normal frequency of defecation accompanied by difficult or incomplete passage of stool and/or passage of excessively hard, dry stool.

RISK FACTORS

Functional

Irregular defecation habits; inadequate toileting (e.g., timeliness, positioning for defecation, privacy); Insufficient physical activity; abdominal muscle weakness; Recent environmental changes; Habitual denial/ignoring of urge to defecate

Psychological

Emotional stress; mental confusion; depression

Physiological

Change in usual foods and eating patterns; insufficient fiber/fluid intake; dehydration; poor eating habits; Inadequate dentition or oral hygiene; Decreased motility of gastrointestinal tract

Pharmacological

Phenothiazines; nonsteroidal anti-inflammatory agents; sedatives; aluminum-containing antacids; laxative overuse; iron salts; anticholinergics; antidepressants; anticonvulsants; antilipemic agents; calcium channel blockers; calcium carbonate; diuretics; sympathomimetics; opiates; bismuth salts

Mechanical

Hemorrhoids; pregnancy; obesity; Rectal abscess or ulcer; anal stricture; anal fissures; prolapse; rectocele; Prostate enlargement; postsurgical obstruction; Neurological impairment; megacolon (Hirschsprung's disease); tumors; Electrolyte imbalance

COPING, DEFENSIVE

Diagnostic Division: Ego Integrity

Definition: The state in which an individual repeatedly projects falsely positive self-evaluation based on a self-protective pattern which defends against underlying perceived threats to positive self-regard.

RELATED FACTORS

To be developed by NANDA; [Refer to ND Coping, Individual, ineffective]

DEFINING CHARACTERISTICS

Subjective

Denial of obvious problems/weaknesses; Projection of blame/responsibility; Rationalizes failures; Hypersensitive to slight/criticism; Grandiosity; [Refuses or rejects assistance]

Objective

Superior attitude toward others; Difficulty establishing/maintaining relationships [avoidance of intimacy]; Hostile laughter or ridicule of others [aggressive behavior]; Difficulty in reality-testing perceptions; Lack of follow-through or participation in treatment or therapy; [Attention-seeking behavior]

COPING, INDIVIDUAL, INEFFECTIVE

Diagnostic Division: Ego Integrity

Definition: Inability to form a valid appraisal of the stressors, inadequate choices of practiced responses, and/or inability to use available resources.

RELATED FACTORS

Situational/maturational crises; High degree of threat; Inadequate opportunity to prepare for stressor; disturbance in pattern of appraisal of threat; Inadequate level of confidence in ability to cope/perception of control; uncertainty; Inadequate resources available; inadequate social support created by characteristics of relationships; Disturbance in pattern of tension release; inability to conserve adaptive energies; Gender differences in coping strategies; [Work overload, no vacations, too many deadlines; little or no exercise]; [Impairment of nervous system; cognitive/sensory/perceptual impairment, memory loss]; [Severe/chronic pain]

DEFINING CHARACTERISTICS

Subjective

Verbalization of inability to cope or inability to ask for help; Sleep disturbance; fatigue; Abuse of chemical agents; [Reports of muscular/emotional tension, lack of appetite]

Lack of goal-directed behavior/resolution of problem including: inability to attend, difficulty with organizing information, [lack of assertive behavior]; Use of forms of coping that impede adaptive behavior [including inappropriate use of defense mechanisms, verbal manipulation]; Inadequate problem solving; Inability to meet role expectations/basic needs; Decreased use of social supports; Poor concentration; Change in usual communication patterns; High illness rate [including high blood pressure, ulcers, irritable bowel, frequent headaches/neckaches]; Risk taking; Destructive behavior toward self or others [including overeating, excessive smoking/drinking, overuse of prescribed/over the counter medications; illicit drug use]; [Behavioral changes (e.g., impatience, frustration, irritability, discouragement)]

DECISIONAL CONFLICT (Specify)

Diagnostic Division: Ego Integrity

Definition: The state of uncertainty about course of action to be taken when choice among competing actions involves risk, loss, or challenge to personal life values.

RELATED FACTORS

Unclear personal values/beliefs; perceived threat to value system; Lack of experience or interference with decision making; Lack of relevant information, multiple or divergent sources of information; Support system deficit; [Age, developmental state]; [Family system, sociocultural factors]; [Cognitive, emotional, behavioral level of functioning]

DEFINING CHARACTERISTICS

Subjective

Verbalized uncertainty about choices or of undesired consequences of alternative actions being considered; Verbalized feelings of distress or questioning personal values and beliefs while attempting a decision

Objective

Vacillation between alternative choices; delayed decision-making; Self-focusing; Physical signs of distress or tension (increased heart rate, increased muscle tension, restlessness, and so on)

DENIAL, INEFFECTIVE

Diagnostic Division: Ego Integrity

Definition: The state of a conscious or unconscious attempt to disavow the knowledge or meaning of an event to reduce anxiety/fear to the detriment of health.

RELATED FACTORS

To be developed by NANDA: [Personal vulnerability; unmet self-needs]; [Presence of overwhelming anxiety-producing feelings/situation; reality factors that are consciously intolerable]; [Fear of consequences, negative past experiences]; [Learned response patterns (e.g., avoidance)]; [Cultural factors, personal/family value systems]

DEFINING CHARACTERISTICS

Subjective

Minimizes symptoms; displaces source of symptoms to other organs; Unable to admit impact of disease on life pattern; Displaces fear of impact of the condition; Does not admit fear of death or invalidism

Objective

Delays seeking or refuses health care attention to the detriment of health; Does not perceive personal relevance of symptoms or danger; Makes dismissive gestures or comments when speaking of distressing events; Displays inappropriate affect; Uses home remedies (self-treatment) to relieve symptoms

DENTITION, ALTERED

Diagnostic Division: Food / Fluid

Definition: Disruption in tooth development/eruption patterns or structural integrity of individual teeth.

RELATED FACTORS

Dietary habits; nutritional deficits; Selected prescription medications; chronic use of tobacco, coffee or tea, red wine; Ineffective oral hygiene, sensitivity to heat or cold; chronic vomiting; Lack of knowledge regarding dental health; excessive use of abrasive cleaning agents/intake of fluorides; Barriers to self-care; access or economic barriers to professional care; Genetic predisposition; premature loss of primary teeth; bruxism; [Traumatic injury/surgical intervention]

DEFINING CHARACTERISTICS

Subjective
Toothache

Objective
Halitosis; Tooth enamel discoloration; erosion of enamel; excessive plaque; Worn down or abraded teeth; crown or root caries; tooth fracture(s); loose teeth; missing teeth or complete absence; Premature loss of primary teeth; incomplete eruption for age (may be primary or permanent teeth); Excessive calculus; Malocclusion or tooth misalignment; asymmetrical facial expression

DEVELOPMENT, RISK FOR ALTERED

Diagnostic Division: Teaching / Learning

Definition: At risk for delay of 25% or more in one or more of the areas of social or self-regulatory behavior, or cognitive, language, gross or fine motor skills.

RISK FACTORS

Prenatal
Maternal age <15 or [>]35 years; Unplanned or unwanted pregnancy; lack of, late, or poor prenatal care; Inadequate nutrition; illiteracy; poverty; Genetic or endocrine disorders; substance abuse; infections

Individual
Prematurity; congenital or genetic disorders; Vision/hearing impairment or frequent otitis media; Failure to thrive, inadequate nutrition; chronic illness; Brain damage (e.g., hemorrhage in postnatal period, shaken baby, abuse, accident); seizures; Positive drug screening test; substance abuse; Lead poisoning; chemotherapy; radiation therapy; Foster or adopted child; Behavior disorders; Technology-dependent; Natural disaster

Environmental
Poverty; Violence

Caregiver
Abuse; Mental illness; Mental retardation or severe learning disability

DIARRHEA

Diagnostic Division: Elimination

Definition: Passage of loose, unformed stools.

RELATED FACTORS

Psychological
High stress levels and anxiety

Situational
Laxative/alcohol abuse; toxins; contaminants; Adverse effects of medications; radiation; Tube feedings; Travel

Physiological
Inflammation; irritation; Malabsorption; Infectious processes; parasites

DEFINING CHARACTERISTICS

Subjective
Abdominal pain; Urgency; cramping

Objective
Hyperactive bowel sounds; At least 3 loose or liquid stools per day

DISORGANIZED INFANT BEHAVIOR

Diagnostic Division: Neurosensory

Definition: Disintegrated physiological and neurobehavioral responses to the environment.

RELATED FACTORS

Prenatal

Congenital or genetic disorders; teratogenic exposure; [exposure to drugs]

Postnatal

Prematurity; oral/motor problems; feeding intolerance; malnutrition; Invasive/painful procedures

Individual

Gestational/postconceptual age; immature neurological system; Illness; [infection]; [hypoxia/birth asphyxia].

Environmental

Physical environment inappropriateness; Sensory inappropriateness/overstimulation/deprivation; [Lack of containment/boundaries]

Caregiver

Cue misreading/cue knowledge deficit; Environmental stimulation contribution

DEFINING CHARACTERISTICS

Objective

Regulatory Problems

Inability to inhibit [e.g., locking in—inability to look away from stimulus]; irritability

State-Organization System

Active-awake (fussy, worried gaze); quiet-awake (staring, gaze aversion); Diffuse/unclear sleep, state oscillation; Irritable or panicky crying

Attention-Interaction System

Abnormal response to sensory stimuli (e.g., difficult to soothe, inability to sustain alert status)

Motor System

Increased, decreased, or limp tone; Finger splay, fisting or hands to face; hyperextension of arms and legs; Tremors, startles, twitches; jittery, jerky, uncoordinated movement; Altered primitive reflexes

Physiological

Bradycardia, tachycardia, or arrhythmias; Pale, cyanotic, mottled, or flushed color; Bradypnea, tachypnea, apnea; "Time-out signals" (e.g., gaze, grasp, hiccough, cough, sneeze, sigh, slack jaw, open mouth, tongue thrust); Oximeter desaturation; Feeding intolerances (aspiration or emesis)

DISORGANIZED INFANT BEHAVIOR, RISK FOR

Diagnostic Division: Neurosensory

Definition: Risk for alteration in integration and modulation of the physiologic and behavioral systems of functioning (i.e., autonomic, motor, state, organizational, self-regulatory, and attentional-interactional systems).

RISK FACTORS

Pain; Oral/motor problems; Environmental overstimulation; Lack of containment/boundaries; Invasive/painful procedures; Prematurity; [immaturity of the central nervous system; generic problems that alter neurologic and/or physiologic functioning conditions resulting in hypoxia and/or birth asphyxia]; [Malnutrition; infection; drug addiction]; [Environmental events or conditions such as separation from parent, exposure to loud noise, excessive handling, bright lights]

DISUSE SYNDROME, RISK FOR

Diagnostic Division: Activity/Rest

Definition: A state in which an individual is at risk for deterioration of body systems as the result of prescribed or unavoidable musculoskeletal inactivity.

NOTE: NANDA identifies complications from immobility can include pressure ulcer, constipation, stasis of pulmonary secretions, thrombosis, urinary tract infection/retention, decreased strength/endurance, orthostatic hypotension, decreased range of joint motion, disorientation, body image disturbance, and powerlessness.

RISK FACTORS
Severe pain, [chronic pain]; Paralysis [other neuromuscular impairment]; Mechanical or prescribed immobilization; Altered level of consciousness [chronic physical or mental illness]

DIVERSIONAL ACTIVITY DEFICIT

Diagnostic Division: Activity / Rest

Definition: The state in which an individual experiences a decreased stimulation from (or interest or engagement in) recreational or leisure activities.

NOTE: Internal/external factors that may or may not be beyond the individual's control.

RELATED FACTORS
Environmental lack of diversional activity as in long-term hospitalization; frequent, lengthy treatments, [home-bound]; [Physical limitations, bedridden, fatigue, pain]; [Situational, developmental problem, lack of sources]; [Psychologic condition, such as depression]

DEFINING CHARACTERISTICS

Subjective
Patient's statement regarding the following: Boredom; wish there were something to do, to read, etc.; Usual hobbies cannot be undertaken in hospital [home or other care setting]; [Changes in abilities/physical limitations]

Objective
[Flat affect, disinterested, inattentiveness]; [Restlessness; crying]; [Lethargy; withdrawal]; [Hostility]; [Overeating or lack of interest in eating; weight loss or gain]

DYSREFLEXIA

Diagnostic Division: Circulation

Definition: The state in which an individual with a spinal cord injury at T7 or above experiences a life-threatening uninhibited sympathetic response of the nervous system to a noxious stimulus.

RELATED FACTORS
Bladder or bowel distention [catheter insertion, obstruction, irrigation]; Skin irritation; Lack of patient and caregiver knowledge; [Sexual excitation]; [Environmental temperature extremes]

DEFINING CHARACTERISTICS
Individual with spinal cord injury (T-7 or above) with:

Subjective
Headache (a diffuse pain in different portions of the head and not confined to any nerve distribution area); Paresthesia; chilling; blurred vision; chest pain; metallic taste in mouth; nasal congestion

Objective
Paroxysmal hypertension (sudden periodic elevated blood pressure where systolic pressure is over 140 mm Hg and diastolic is above 90 mm Hg); Bradycardia or tachycardia (pulse rate of less than 60 or over 100 beats per minute); Diaphoresis (above the injury); red splotches on skin (above the injury); pallor (below the injury); Horner's syndrome (contraction of the pupil, partial ptosis of the eyelid, enophthalmos and sometimes loss of sweating over the affected side of the face); conjunctival congestion; Pilomotor reflex (gooseflesh formation when skin is cooled)

DYSREFLEXIA, RISK FOR AUTONOMIC

Diagnostic Division: Circulation

Definition: A lifelong threatening uninhibited response of the sympathetic nervous system for an individual with a spinal cord injury or lesion at T8 or above, and having recovered from spinal shock.

RISK FACTORS
Cardiac/Pulmonary Problems: pulmonary emboli; Gastrointestinal Problems: distention; constipation; enemas; stimulation (e.g., digital, instrumentation, surgery); gastrointestinal system pathology; gastric ulcers; esophageal reflux; Neurological Problems: painful or irritating stimuli below the level of injury; Regulatory Problems: temperature fluctuations [internal/environmental]; Reproductive [And Sexuality] Problems: menstruation, sexual intercourse, ejaculation; Integumentary Problems: cutaneous stimulations (e.g., pressure ulcer, ingrown toenail, dressings, burns, rash); heterotrophic bone; Situational Problems: positioning; range of motion exercises; pregnancy; labor and delivery; drug reactions (e.g., decongestants, sympathomimetics, vasoconstrictors, narcotic withdrawal); constrictive clothing; fractures; deep vein thrombosis; ovarian cyst; surgical procedures; Urological Problems: bladder distention; spasm; instrumentation; infection; urethritis; epididymitis

ENERGY FIELD DISTURBANCE

Diagnostic Division: Ego Integrity

Definition: A disruption of the flow of energy [aura] surrounding a person's being that results in a disharmony of the body, mind, and/or spirit.

RELATED FACTORS
To be developed by NANDA: [Block in energy field]; [Depression]; [Increased state of anxiety]; [Impaired immune system]; [Pain]

DEFINING CHARACTERISTICS
Objective
Temperature change (warmth/coolness); Visual changes (image/color); Disruption of the field (vacant/hole/spike/bulge); Movement (wave/spike/tingling/dense/flowing); Sounds (tone/words)

ENHANCED ORGANIZED INFANT BEHAVIOR, POTENTIAL FOR

Diagnostic Division: Neurosensory

Definition: A pattern of modulation of the physiologic and behavioral systems of functioning of an infant (i.e., autonomic, motor, state, organizational, self-regulatory, and attentional-interactional systems) that is satisfactory but that can be improved, resulting in higher levels of integration in response to environmental stimuli.

RELATED FACTORS
Prematurity; Pain

DEFINING CHARACTERISTICS
Objective
Stable physiologic measures; Definite sleep-wake states; Use of some self-regulatory behaviors; Response to visual/auditory stimuli

ENVIRONMENTAL INTERPRETATION SYNDROME, IMPAIRED

Diagnostic Division: Safety

Definition: Consistent lack of orientation to person, place, time, or circumstances over more than 3 to 6 months, necessitating a protective environment.

RELATED FACTORS
Dementia (Alzheimer's disease, multi-infarct dementia, Pick's disease, AIDS dementia); Parkinson's disease; Huntington's disease; Depression; Alcoholism

DEFINING CHARACTERISTICS
Subjective
[Loss of occupation or social function from memory decline]

Objective
Consistent disorientation in known and unknown environments; Chronic confusional states; Inability to follow simple directions, instructions; Inability to reason, to con-

centrate; slow in responding to questions; Loss of occupation or social function from memory decline

FAILURE TO THRIVE, ADULT

Diagnostic Division: Food / Fluid

Definition: A progressive functional deterioration of a physical and cognitive nature; the individual's ability to live with multisystem diseases, cope with ensuing problems, and manage his/her care is remarkably diminished.

RELATED FACTORS

Depression; apathy; Fatigue [Major disease/degenerative condition]; [Aging process]

DEFINING CHARACTERISTICS

Subjective

States does not have an appetite, not hungry, or "I don't want to eat"; Expresses loss of interest in pleasurable outlets, such as food, sex, work, friends, family, hobbies, or entertainment; Difficulty performing simple self-care tasks; Altered mood state—expresses feelings of sadness, being low in spirit; Verbalizes desire for death

Objective

Inadequate nutritional intake–eating less than body requirements; consumes minimal to none of food at most meals (i.e., consumes less than 75% of normal requirements at each or most meals); anorexia–does not eat meals when offered; Weight loss (decreased body mass from base line weight)–5% unintentional weight loss in 1 month, 10% unintentional weight loss in 6 months; Physical decline (decline in bodily function)–evidence of fatigue, dehydration, incontinence of bowel and bladder; Cognitive decline (decline in mental processing)–as evidenced by problems with responding appropriately to environmental stimuli, demonstrates difficulty in reasoning, decision making, judgment, memory and concentration, decreased perception; Apathy as evidenced by lack of observable feeling or emotion in terms of normal activities of daily living and environment; Decreased participation in activities of daily living that the older person once enjoyed; self-care deficit–no longer looks after or takes charge of physical cleanliness or appearance; neglects home environment and/or financial responsibilities; Decreased social skills/social withdrawal–noticeable decrease from usual past behavior in attempts to form or participate in cooperative and interdependent relationships (e.g., decreased verbal communication with staff, family, friends); Frequent exacerbations of chronic health problems such as pneumonia or urinary tract infections

FALLS, RISK FOR

Diagnostic Division: Safety

Definition: Increased susceptibility to falling that may cause physical harm.

DEFINING CHARACTERISTICS

To be developed by NANDA

FAMILY COPING, INEFFECTIVE: COMPROMISED

Diagnostic Division: Social Interaction

Definition: A usually supportive primary person (family member or close friend [significant other]) is providing insufficient, ineffective, or compromised support, comfort, assistance, or encouragement that may be needed by the client to manage or master adaptive tasks related to his or her health challenge.

RELATED FACTORS

Inadequate or incorrect information or understanding by a primary person; Temporary preoccupation by a significant person who is trying to manage emotional conflicts and personal suffering and is unable to perceive or to act effectively in regard to client's needs; Temporary family disorganization and role changes; Other situational or developmental crises or situations the significant person may be facing; Little support provided by client, in turn, for the primary person; Prolonged disease or disability progression that exhausts the supportive capacity of significant people; [Unrealistic expectations of patient/significant other(s) or each other]; [Lack of mutual decision-making skills]; [Diverse coalitions of family members]

DEFINING CHARACTERISTICS

Subjective

Client expresses or confirms a concern or complaint about significant other's response to his or her health problem; Significant person describes preoccupation with personal reaction (e.g., fear, anticipatory grief, guilt, anxiety) to client's illness/disability, or other situational or developmental crises; Significant person describes or confirms an inadequate understanding or knowledge base that interferes with effective assistive or supportive behaviors

Objective

Significant person attempts assistive or supportive behaviors with less than satisfactory results; Significant person withdraws or enters into limited or temporary personal communication with client at time of need; Significant person displays protective behavior disproportionate (too little or too much) to client's abilities or need for autonomy; [Significant person displays sudden outbursts of emotions/shows emotional lability or interferes with necessary nursing/medical interventions]

FAMILY COPING, INEFFECTIVE: DISABLING

Diagnostic Division: Social Interaction

Definition: The behavior of a significant person (family member or other primary person) that disables his or her own capacities and the client's capacity to effectively address tasks essential to either person's adaptation to the health challenge.

RELATED FACTORS

Significant person with chronically unexpressed feelings of guilt, anxiety, hostility, despair, etc.; Dissonant discrepancy of coping styles being used to deal with the adaptive tasks by the significant person and client or among significant people; Highly ambivalent family relationships; Arbitrary handling of a family's resistance to treatment that tends to solidify defensiveness as it fails to deal adequately with underlying anxiety; [High-risk family situations, such as single or adolescent parent, abusive relationship, substance abuse, acute/chronic disabilities, member with terminal illness]

DEFINING CHARACTERISTICS

Subjective

[Expresses despair regarding family reactions/lack of involvement]

Objective

Intolerance; rejection, abandonment; desertion; Psychosomaticism; Agitation, depression, aggression, hostility; Taking on illness signs of client; Neglectful relationships with other family members; Carrying on usual routines disregarding client's needs; Neglectful care of the client in regard to basic human needs and/or illness treatment; Distortion of reality regarding the health problem, including extreme denial about its existence or severity; Decisions and actions by family that are detrimental to economic or social well-being; Impaired restructuring of a meaningful life for self, impaired individualization, prolonged overconcern for client; Client's development of helpless, inactive dependence

FAMILY COPING: POTENTIAL FOR GROWTH

Diagnostic Division: Social Interaction

Definition: Effective managing of adaptive tasks by family member involved with the health challenge who now is exhibiting desire and readiness for enhanced health and growth in regard to self and in relation to the client.

RELATED FACTORS

Needs sufficiently gratified and adaptive tasks effectively addressed to enable goals of self-actualization to surface; [Developmental stage, situational crises/supports]

DEFINING CHARACTERISTICS

Subjective

Family member attempting to describe growth impact of crisis on his/her own values, priorities, goals, or relationships; Individual expresses interest in making contact on a one-to-one basis or on a mutual-aid group basis with another person who has experienced a similar situation

Objective
Family member is moving in direction of health-promoting and enriching lifestyle that supports and monitors maturational processes, audits and negotiates treatment programs, and generally chooses experiences that optimize wellness

FAMILY PROCESSES, ALTERED

Diagnostic Division: Social Interaction

Definition: A change in family relationships and/or functioning.

RELATED FACTORS
Situational transition and/or crises [e.g., economic, change in roles, illness, trauma, disabling/expensive treatments]; Developmental transition and/or crisis [e.g., loss or gain of a family member, adolescence, leaving home for college]; Shift in health status of a family member; Family roles shift; power shift of family members; Modification in family finances, social status; Informal or formal interaction with community

DEFINING CHARACTERISTICS
Subjective
Changes in: power alliances; satisfaction with family; expressions of conflict with family; effectiveness in completing assigned tasks; stress-reduction behaviors; expressions of conflict with and/or isolation from community resources; somatic complaints; [Family expresses confusion about what to do; verbalizes they are having difficulty responding to change]

Objective
Changes in: assigned tasks; participation in problem solving/decision making; communication patterns; mutual support; availability for emotional support/affective responsiveness and intimacy; patterns and rituals

FAMILY PROCESS, ALTERED: ALCOHOLISM [SUBSTANCE ABUSE]

Diagnostic Division: Social Interaction

Definition: The state in which the psychosocial, spiritual, and physiologic functions of the family unit are chronically disorganized, leading to conflict, denial of problems, resistance to change, ineffective problem-solving, and a series of self-perpetuating crises.

RELATED FACTORS
Abuse of alcohol; resistance to treatment; Family history of alcoholism; Inadequate coping skills; addictive personality; lack of problem-solving skills; Biochemical influences; genetic predisposition

DEFINING CHARACTERISTICS
Subjective
Feelings
Anxiety/tension/distress; decreased self-esteem/worthlessness; lingering resentment; Anger/suppressed rage; frustration; shame/embarrassment; hurt; unhappiness; guilt; Emotional isolation/Loneliness; powerlessness; insecurity; hopelessness; rejection; Responsibility for alcoholic's behavior; vulnerability; mistrust; Depression; hostility; fear; confusion; dissatisfaction; loss; repressed emotions; Being different from other people; misunderstood; Emotional control by others; being unloved; lack of identity; Abandonment; confused love and pity; moodiness; failure

Roles and Relationships
Family denial; deterioration in family relationships/disturbed family dynamics; ineffective spouse communication/marital problems; intimacy dysfunction; Altered role function/disruption of family roles; inconsistent parenting/low perception of parental support; chronic family problems; Lack of skills necessary for relationships; lack of cohesiveness; disrupted family rituals; Family unable to meet security needs of its members; Pattern of rejection; economic problems; neglected obligations

Objective
Roles and Relationships
Closed communication systems; Triangulating family relationships; reduced ability of

family members to relate to each other for mutual growth and maturation; Family does not demonstrate respect for individuality and autonomy of its members

Behaviors

Expression of anger inappropriately; difficulty with intimate relationships; impaired communication; ineffective problem-solving skills; inability to meet emotional needs of its members; manipulation; dependency; criticizing; broken promises; rationalization/denial of problems; Refusal to get help/inability to accept and receive help appropriately; blaming; Loss of control of drinking; enabling to maintain drinking [substance abuse]; alcohol [substance] abuse; inadequate understanding or knowledge of alcoholism [substance abuse]; Inability to meet spiritual needs of its members; Inability to express or accept wide range of feelings; orientation toward tension relief rather than achievement of goals; escalating conflict; Lying; contradictory, paradoxical communication; lack of dealing with conflict; harsh self-judgment; isolation; difficulty having fun; self-blaming; unresolved grief; Controlling communication/power struggles; seeking approval and affirmation; Lack of reliability; disturbances in academic performance in children; disturbances in concentration; chaos; failure to accomplish current or past developmental tasks/difficulty with life cycle transitions; Verbal abuse of spouse or parent; agitation; diminished physical contact; Family special occasions are alcohol-centered; nicotine addiction; inability to adapt to change; immaturity; stress-related physical illnesses; inability to deal with traumatic experiences constructively; substance abuse other than alcohol

FATIGUE

Diagnostic Division: Activity/Rest

Definition: An overwhelming sustained sense of exhaustion and decreased capacity for physical and mental work at usual level.

RELATED FACTORS

Psychological

Stress; anxiety; boring lifestyle; depression

Environmental

Noise; lights; humidity; temperature

Situational

Occupation; negative life events

Physiological

Increased physical exertion; sleep deprivation; Pregnancy; disease states; malnutrition; anemia; Poor physical condition; [Altered body chemistry (e.g., medications, drug withdrawal, chemotherapy)]

DEFINING CHARACTERISTICS

Subjective

Verbalization of an unremitting and overwhelming lack of energy; inability to maintain usual routines/level of physical activity; Perceived need for additional energy to accomplish routine tasks; increase in rest requirements; Tired; inability to restore energy even after sleep; Feelings of guilt for not keeping up with responsibilities; Compromised libido; Increase in physical complaints

Objective

Lethargic or listless; drowsy; Compromised concentration; Disinterest in surroundings/introspection; Decreased performance, [accident-prone]

FEAR

Diagnostic Division: Ego Integrity

Definition: Fear is anxiety caused by consciously recognized and realistic danger. It is a perceived threat, real or imagined. Operationally, fear is the presence of immediate feeling of apprehension and fright; source known and specific; subjective responses that act as energizers but cannot be observed; and objective signs that are the result of the transformation of energy into relief behaviors and responses.

RELATED FACTORS

Natural/innate origins; innate releasers; Knowledge deficit; discrepancy; language barrier; Environmental stimuli; sensory impairment; Physical/social conditions; separation from support system in potentially stressful situation [e.g., hospitalization, treatments]; Phobic stimulus or phobia; fear for others; ideas; learned response; classical conditioning

DEFINING CHARACTERISTICS

Subjective

Ability to identify object of fear; focus on "it" out there; Apprehension; frightened; worry; alarm; Increased tension; Panicky; terrified; dread; afraid; horror; [Associated physical symptoms, nausea, "heart beating fast," and so on]

Objective

Immediate response to object of fear; Attack/fight behavior–aggressive; Flight behavior–withdrawal; Wide-eyed, increased alertness, concentration on the source; Increased tension; wariness; jittery; Decreased self-assurance; impulsiveness; Increased heart rate; Bed wetting

FLUID VOLUME DEFICIT [HYPER/HYPOTONIC]

Diagnostic Division: Food / Fluid

Definition: The state in which an individual experiences vascular, cellular, or intracellular dehydration (in excess of needs or replacement capabilities owing to active loss).

RELATED FACTORS

[Hypertonic dehydration: uncontrolled diabetes mellitus/insipidus, HHNC increased risk of hypertonic fluids/IV therapy, inability to respond to thirst reflex/inadequate free water supplementation (high-osmolarity enteral feeding formulas), renal insufficiency failure]; [Hypotonic dehydration: chronic illness/malnutrition, excessive use of hypotonic IV solutions (e.g., D_5W), renal insufficiency]

DEFINING CHARACTERISTICS

Subjective

[Reports of fatigue, nervousness, Exhaustion]; [Thirst]

Objective

[Increased urine output, dilute urine (initially) and/or decreased output/oliguria]; [Weight loss]; [Decreased venous filling]; [Hypotension (postural)]; [Increased pulse rate; decreased pulse volume and pressure]; [Decreased skin turgor]; [Change in mental status (e.g., confusion)]; [Increased body temperature]; [Dry skin/ mucous membranes]; [Hemoconcentration; altered serum sodium]

FLUID VOLUME DEFICIT [ISOTONIC]

Diagnostic Division: Food / Fluid

Definition: The state in which an individual experiences decreased intravascular, interstitial and/or intracellular fluid. This refers to dehydration, water loss alone without change in sodium.

NOTE: This diagnosis has been structured to address isotonic dehydration (hypovolemia) excluding states in which changes in sodium occur. For patient needs related to dehydration associated with alterations in sodium, refer to [Fluid deficit hyper/hypotonic].

RELATED FACTORS

Active fluid volume loss [e.g., hemorrhage, gastric intubation, diarrhea, wounds; abdominal cancer; burns; fistulas; ascites (third spacing); use of hyperosmotic radiopaque contrast agents]; Failure of regulatory mechanisms [e.g., fever/thermoregulatory response; renal tubule damage]

DEFINING CHARACTERISTICS

Subjective

Thirst; Weakness

Objective

Decreased urine output; Increased urine concentration; Decreased venous filling; Decreased pulse volume and pressure; Sudden weight loss (except in third spacing);

Elevated Hct; Decreased blood pressure; increased pulse rate/body temperature; Decreased skin/tongue turgor, dry skin/mucous membranes; Change in mental state; [Weight gain/edema (third spacing)]

FLUID VOLUME DEFICIT, RISK FOR

Diagnostic Division: Foood / Fluid

Definition: The state in which an individual is at risk of experiencing vascular, cellular, or intracellular dehydration.

RISK FACTORS

Extremes of age and weight; Loss of fluid through abnormal routes (e.g., indwelling tubes); Knowledge deficiency related to fluid volume; Factors influencing fluid needs (e.g., hypermetabolic states); Medications (e.g., diuretics); Excessive losses through normal routes (e.g., diarrhea); Deviations affecting access to, intake of, or absorption of fluids (e.g., physical immobility)

FLUID VOLUME EXCESS

Diagnostic Division: Food / Fluid

Definition: The state in which an individual experiences increased isotonic fluid retention.

RELATED FACTORS

Compromised regulatory mechanism [e.g., SIADH or decreased plasma proteins as found in conditions such as malnutrition, draining fistulas, burns, organ failure]; Excess fluid intake; Excess sodium intake; [Drug therapies, such as chlorpropamide, tolbutamide, vincristine, triptylines, carbamazepine]

DEFINING CHARACTERISTICS

Subjective

Shortness of breath, orthopnea; Anxiety

Objective

Edema, pleural effusion, anasarca; weight gain over short period; Intake exceeds output; oliguria; Abnormal breath sounds (rales or crackles); dyspnea; Decreased hemoglobin, hematocrit; Increased central venous pressure; jugular vein distention; positive hepatojugular reflex; S_3 heart sound; Pulmonary congestion; pulmonary artery pressure changes; change is respiratory pattern; Blood pressure changes; Change in mental status; restlessness; Specific gravity changes; Azotemia, altered electrolytes

FLUID VOLUME IMBALANCE, RISK FOR

Diagnostic Division: Food / Fluid

Definition: A risk of a decrease, an increase, or a rapid shift from one to the other of intravascular, interstitial, and/or intracellular fluid. This refers to the loss or excess or to the other of intravascular, interstitial, and/or intracellular fluid. This refers to the loss or excess or both of body fluids or replacement fluids.

RISK FACTORS

Scheduled for major invasive procedures [Rapid/sustained loss (e.g., hemorrhage, burns, fistulas)]; [Rapid fluid replacement]; Other risk factors to be determined

GAS EXCHANGE, IMPAIRED

Diagnostic Division: Respiration

Definition: Excess or deficit in oxygenation and/or carbon dioxide elimination at the alveolar-capillary membrane. [This may be an entity of its own but also may be an end result of other pathology with an interrelatedness between airway clearance and/or breathing pattern problems.]

RELATED FACTORS

Ventilation perfusion imbalance [as in the following: altered blood flow (e.g., pulmonary embolus, increased vascular resistance), vasospasm, heart failure, hypovolemic shock]; Alveolar-capillary membrane changes (e.g., acute adult respiratory distress syndrome); chronic conditions such as restrictive/obstructive lung disease, pneumoconiosis, respiratory depressant drugs, brain injury, asbestosis/silicosis; [Altered oxygen supply (e.g., altitude sickness)]; [Altered oxygen-carrying capacity of blood (e.g., sickle cell/other anemia, carbon monoxide poisoning)]

DEFINING CHARACTERISTICS

Subjective
Dyspnea; Visual disturbances; Headache upon awakening; [sense of impending doom]

Objective
Confusion; [decreased mental acuity]; Restlessness, irritability, [agitation]; Somnolence, [lethargy]; Abnormal arterial blood gases/pH; hypoxia/hypoxemia; hypercapnia/hypercarbia; decreased carbon dioxide; Cyanosis (in neonates only); abnormal skin color (pale, dusky); Abnormal rate, rhythm, depth of breathing; nasal flaring; Tachycardia [development of dysrhythmias]; Diaphoresis; [polycythemia]

GRIEVING, ANTICIPATORY

Diagnostic Division: Ego Integrity

Definition: Intellectual and emotional responses and behaviors by which individuals, families, communities work through the process of modifying self-concept based on the perception of potential loss.

NOTE: May be a healthy response requiring interventions of support and information-giving.

RELATED FACTORS
To be developed by NANDA; [Perceived potential loss of significant other, physiological/psychosocial well-being (body part/function, social role), lifestyle/personal possessions]

DEFINING CHARACTERISTICS

Subjective
Sorrow; guilt; anger, [choked feelings]; Denial of potential loss; denial of the significance of the loss; Expression of distress at potential loss, [ambivalence, sense of unreality]; bargaining; Alterations in activity level, eating habits, sleep patterns, dream patterns, libido

Objective
Potential loss of significant object [personal/self, job/position, developmental stage/abilities, health, body part/function]; Altered communication patterns; Difficulty taking on new or different roles; Resolution of grief prior to the reality of loss [Altered affect]; [Crying]; [Social isolation, withdrawal]

GRIEVING, DYSFUNCTIONAL

Diagnostic Division: Ego Integrity

Definition: Extended, unsuccessful use of intellectual and emotional responses by which individuals, families, communities attempt to work through the process of modifying self-concept based on the perception of potential loss.

NOTE: Although NANDA now defines this diagnosis in terms of a potential loss (which is addressed in anticipatory grieving), the authors also view dysfunctional grieving as a response to a loss that has already occurred.

RELATED FACTORS
Actual or perceived object loss (object loss is used in the broadest sense)—objects may include people, possessions, a job, status, home, ideals, parts and processes of the body [e.g., amputation, paralysis, chronic/terminal illness]; [Thwarted grieving response to a loss]; [Lack of resolution of previous grieving response]; [Absence of anticipatory grieving]

DEFINING CHARACTERISTICS

Subjective
Expression of distress at loss; denial of loss; Expression of guilt, anger, sadness, unresolved issues; [hopelessness]; Idealization of lost object; Reliving of past experiences with little or no reduction (diminishment) of intensity of the grief; Alterations in eat-

ing habits, sleep and dream patterns, activity level, libido, concentration and/or pursuits of tasks

Objective
Onset or exacerbation of somatic or psychosomatic responses; Crying; labile affect; Difficulty in expressing loss; Prolonged interference with life functioning; developmental regression; Repetitive use of ineffectual behaviors associated with attempts to reinvest in relationships; [Withdrawal, isolation]

GROWTH AND DEVELOPMENT, ALTERED

Diagnostic Division: Teaching/Learning

Definition: The state in which an individual demonstrates deviations in norms from his/her age group.

RELATED FACTORS
Inadequate caretaking , [physical/emotional neglect/abuse]; Indifference, inconsistent responsiveness, multiple caretakers; Separation from significant others; Environmental and stimulation deficiencies; Effects of physical disability [handicapping condition]; Prescribed dependence [insufficient expectations for self-care]; [Physical/ emotional illness, chronic, traumatic (e.g., chronic inflammatory disease, pituitary tumors, impaired nutrition/metabolism, greater-than-normal energy requirements; prolonged/painful treatments; prolonged/repeated hospitilizations]; [Sexual abuse]; [Substance use/abuse including anabolic steroids]

DEFINING CHARACTERISTICS

Subjective
Inability to perform self-care or self-control activities appropriate for age

Objective
Delay or difficulty in performing skills (motor, social, or expressive) typical of age group; [Loss of previously acquired skills; precocious or accelerated skill attainment; Altered physical growth; Flat affect, listlessness, decreased responses; [Sleep disturbances, negative mood/response]

GROWTH, RISK FOR ALTERED

Diagnostic Division: Teaching/Learning

Definition: At risk for growth above the 97th percentile or below the 3rd percentile for age, crossing two percentile channels; disproportionate growth.

RISK FACTORS
Prenatal
Congenital/genetic disorders [e.g., dysfunction of endocrine gland, tumors]; Maternal nutrition; multiple gestation; Substance use/abuse; teratogen exposure

Individual
Organic and inorganic factors; Prematurity; Malnutrition; caregiver and/or individual maladaptive feeding behaviors; insatiable appetite; anorexia; [impaired metabolism, greater-than-normal energy requirements]; Infection; chronic illness [e.g., chronic inflammatory diseases]; Substance [use]/abuse [including anabolic steroids]

Environmental
Deprivation; poverty; Violence; natural disasters; Teratogen; lead poisoning

Caregiver
Abuse; Mental illness/retardation, severe learning disability

HEALTH MAINTENANCE, ALTERED

Diagnostic Division: Safety

Definition: Inability to identify, manage, and/or seek out help to maintain health. [This diagnosis contains components of other nursing diagnoses. We recommend subsuming health maintenance interventions under the "basic" nursing diagnosis when a single causative factor is identified (e.g., Knowledge Deficit; Communication, impaired verbal; Thought Processes, altered; Individual/Family Coping, ineffective; Growth and Development, altered).]

RELATED FACTORS

Lack of or significant alteration in communication skills (written, verbal, and/or gestural); Unachieved developmental tasks; Lack of ability to make deliberate and thoughtful judgments; Perceptual or cognitive impairment (complete or partial lack of gross and/or fine motor skills); Ineffective individual coping; dysfunctional grieving; disabling spiritual distress; Lack of material resource; Ineffective family coping; [Lack of psychosocial supports]

DEFINING CHARACTERISTICS

Subjective

Expressed interest in improving health behaviors; Reported lack of equipment, financial and/or other resources; impairment of personal support systems; Reported inability to take the responsibility for meeting basic health practices in any or all functional pattern areas; [Reported compulsive behaviors]

Objective

Demonstrated lack of knowledge regarding basic health practices; Observed inability to take the responsibility for meeting basic health practices in any or all functional pattern areas; history of lack of health-seeking behavior; Demonstrated lack of adaptive behaviors to internal or external environmental changes; Observed impairment of personal support system; lack of equipment, financial and/or other resources; [Observed compulsive behaviors]

HEALTH-SEEKING BEHAVIORS (SPECIFY)

Diagnostic Division: Teaching/Learning

Definition: A state in which an individual in stable health is actively seeking ways to alter personal health habits and/or the environment in order to move toward higher level of health.

RELATED FACTORS

[Situation/maturation occurrence precipitating concern about current health status]

DEFINING CHARACTERISTICS

Subjective

Expressed desire to seek a higher level of wellness; Expressed desire for increased control of health practice; Expression of concern about current environmental conditions on health status; Stated unfamiliarity with wellness community resources; [Expressed desire to modify codependent behaviors]

Objective

Observed desire to seek a higher level of wellness; Observed desire for increased control of health practice; Demonstrated or observed lack of knowledge in health promotion behaviors, unfamiliarity with wellness community resources

HOME MAINTENANCE MANAGEMENT, IMPAIRED

Diagnostic Division: Safety

Definition: Inability to independently maintain a safe, growth-promoting immediate environment.

RELATED FACTORS

Individual/family member disease or injury; Insufficient family organization or planning; Insufficient finances; Impaired cognitive or emotional functioning; Lack of role modeling; Unfamiliarity with neighborhood resources; Lack of knowledge; Inadequate support systems

DEFINING CHARACTERISTICS

Subjective

Household members express difficulty in maintaining their home in a comfortable [safe] fashion; Household requests assistance with home maintenance; Household members describe outstanding debts or financial crises

Objective

Accumulation of dirt, food or hygienic wastes; Unwashed or unavailable cooking equipment, clothes, or linen; Overtaxed family members (e.g., exhausted, anxious); Repeated hygienic disorders, infestations, or infections; Disorderly surroundings; offensive odors; Inappropriate household temperature; Lack of necessary equipment or aids; Presence of vermin or rodents

HOPELESSNESS

Diagnostic Division: Ego Integrity

Definition: A subjective state in which an individual sees limited or no alternatives or personal choices available and is unable to mobilize energy on own behalf.

RELATED FACTORS

Prolonged activity restriction, creating isolation; Failing or deteriorating physiologic condition; Long-term stress; abandonment; Lost belief in transcendent values/God

DEFINING CHARACTERISTICS

Subjective

Verbal cues (despondent content, "I can't," sighing); [believes things will not change/problems will always be there]

Objective

Passivity, decreased verbalization; Decreased affect; Lack of initiative; Decreased response to stimuli [depressed cognitive functions, problems with decisions, thought processes; regression]; Turning away from speaker; closing eyes; shrugging in response to speaker; Decreased appetite, increased/decreased sleep; Lack of involvement in care/passively allowing care; [Withdrawal from environs]; [Lack of involvement/interest in significant other(s) (children, spouse)]; [Angry outbursts]

HYPERTHERMIA

Diagnostic Division: Safety

Definition: A state in which an individual's body temperature is elevated above his/her normal range.

RELATED FACTORS

Exposure to hot environment; inappropriate clothing; Vigorous activity; dehydration; Medications/anesthesia; Increased metabolic rate, illness or trauma; Inability or decreased ability to perspire

DEFINING CHARACTERISTICS

Subjective

[Headache]

Objective

Flushed skin, warm to touch; Increase in body temperature above normal range; Increased respiratory rate, tachycardia; [Unstable blood pressure]; Seizures/convulsions; [Muscle rigidity/fasciculations]; [Confusion]

HYPOTHERMIA

Diagnostic Division: Safety

Definition: The state in which an individual's body temperature is reduced below normal range.

RELATED FACTORS

Exposure to cool or cold environment [prolonged exposure (e.g., homeless), immersion in cold water/near drowning, induced hypothermia/cardiopulmonary bypass]; Inadequate clothing; Evaporation from skin in cool environment; Inability or decreased ability to shiver; Aging [or very young]; [Debilitating] illness or trauma, damage to hypothalamus; Malnutrition; Decreased metabolic rate; Inactivity; Consumption of alcohol; Medications[/drug overdose] causing vasodilation

DEFINING CHARACTERISTICS

Objective

Reduction in body temperature below normal range; Shivering; Cool skin; Pallor; Slow capillary refill; Cyanotic nail beds; Hypertension; Tachycardia; Piloerection; [Core temperature 95°F/35°C: increased respirations, poor judgment, shivering]; [Core temperature 95° to 93.2°F/35° to 34°C: bradycardia or tachycardia, myocardial irritability/dysrhythmias, muscle rigidity, shivering, lethargic/confused, decreased coordination];

[Core temperature 93.2° to 86°F/34° to 30°C: hypoventilation, bradycardia, generalized rigidity, metabolic acidosis, coma]; [Core temperature 86°F/30°C: no apparent vital signs, heart rate unresponsive to drug therapy, comatose, cyanotic, dilated pupils, apneic, areflexic, no shivering (appears dead)]

INCONTINENCE, FUNCTIONAL URINARY

Diagnostic Division: Elimination

Definition: Inability of usually continent person to reach toilet in time to avoid unintentional loss of urine.

RELATED FACTORS

Altered environmental factors [e.g., poor lighting or inability to locate bathroom]; impaired vision/cognition; neuromuscular limitations; weakened supporting pelvic structures; psychological factors; [reluctance to use call light or bedpan]; [increased urine production]

DEFINING CHARACTERISTICS

Subjective

Senses need to void; [voiding in large amounts]

Objective

Loss of urine before reaching toilet; amount of time required to reach toilet exceeds length of time between sensing urge and uncontrolled voiding; able to completely empty bladder; may only be incontinent in early morning

INCONTINENCE, REFLEX URINARY

Diagnostic Division: Elimination

Definition: An involuntary loss of urine at somewhat predictable intervals when a specific bladder volume is reached.

RELATED FACTORS

Tissue damage from radiation cystitis, inflammatory bladder conditions, or radical pelvic surgery; neurological impairment above level of sacral micturition center or pontine micturition center

DEFINING CHARACTERISTICS

Subjective

No sensation of bladder fullness/urge to void/voiding; sensation to urge without voluntary inhibition of bladder contraction; sensations associated with full bladder such as sweating, restlessness, and abdominal discomfort

Objective

Predictable pattern of voiding; unable to cognitively inhibit or initiate voiding; complete emptying with [brain] lesion above pontine micturition center; incomplete emptying with [spinal cord] lesion above sacral micturition center

INCONTINENCE, STRESS

Diagnostic Division: Elimination

Definition: The state in which an individual experiences a loss of urine of less than 50 ml occurring with increased abdominal pressure.

RELATED FACTORS

Degenerative changes in pelvic muscles and structural supports associated with increased age [e.g., poor closure of urethral sphincter, estrogen deficiency]; High intra-abdominal pressure (e.g., obesity, gravid uterus); Incompetent bladder outlet; Overdistention between voidings; Weak pelvic muscles and structural supports [e.g., straining with chronic constipation]; [Neural degeneration, vascular deficits, surgery, radiation therapy]

DEFINING CHARACTERISTICS

Subjective

Reported dribbling with increased abdominal pressure [e.g., coughing, sneezing, lifting, impact aerobics, changing position]; Urinary urgency/frequency (more often than every 2 hours)

Objective
Observed dribbling with increased abdominal pressure

INCONTINENCE, TOTAL

Diagnostic Division: Elimination

Definition: The state in which an individual experiences a continuous and unpredictable loss of urine.

RELATED FACTORS
Neuropathy preventing transmission of reflex [signals to the reflex arc] indicating bladder fullness; Neurologic dysfunction causing triggering of micturition at unpredictable times [e.g., cerebral lesions]; Independent contraction of detrusor reflex due to surgery; Trauma or disease affecting spinal cord nerves [destruction of sensory or motor neurons below the injury level]; Anatomic (fistula)

DEFINING CHARACTERISTICS
Subjective
Constant flow of urine occurs at unpredictable times without distention or uninhibited bladder contractions/spasm; Nocturia; Lack of perineal or bladder filling awareness; Unawareness of incontinence

Objective
Unsuccessful incontinence refractory treatments

INCONTINENCE, URGE

Diagnostic Division: Elimination

Definition: The state in which an individual experiences involuntary passage of urine occurring soon after a strong sense of urgency to void.

RELATED FACTORS
Decreased bladder capacity (e.g., history of pelvic inflammatory disease, abdominal surgeries, indwelling urinary catheter); Irritation of bladder stretch receptors causing spasm (e.g., bladder infection [atrophic urethritis, vaginitis]); alcohol; caffeine; increased fluids; increased urine concentration; overdistention of bladder; [Medication use, such as diuretics, sedatives, anticholinergic agents]; [Constipation/stool impaction]; [Restricted mobility; psychological disorder such as depression, change in mentation/confusional state (e.g., stroke, dementia, Parkinson's disease)]

DEFINING CHARACTERISTICS
Subjective
Urinary urgency; Frequency (voiding more often than every 2 hours); Bladder contracture/spasm; Nocturia (more than two times per night)

Objective
Inability to reach toilet in time; Voiding in small amounts (less than 100 ml) or in large amounts (more than 550 ml)

INCONTINENCE, RISK FOR URINARY URGE

Diagnostic Division: Elimination

Definition: Risk for involuntary loss of urine associated with a sudden, strong sensation or urinary urgency.

RISK FACTORS
Effects of medications, caffeine, alcohol; Detrusor hyperreflexia from cystitis, urethritis, tumors, renal calculi; Central nervous system disorders above pontine micturition center; detrusor muscle instability with impaired contractility; involuntary sphincter relaxation; Ineffective toileting habits; Small bladder capacity

INFANT FEEDING PATTERN, INEFFECTIVE

Diagnostic Division: Food/Fluid

Definition: A state in which an infant demonstrates an impaired ability to suck or coordinate the suck-swallow response.

RELATED FACTORS
Prematurity; Neurological impairment/delay; Oral hypersensitivity; Prolonged NPO; Anatomic abnormality

DEFINING CHARACTERISTICS

Subjective
[Caregiver reports infant is unable to initiate or sustain an effective suck]

Objective
Inability to initiate or sustain an effective suck; Inability to coordinate sucking, swallowing, and breathing

INFECTION, RISK FOR

Diagnostic Division: Safety

Definition: The state in which an individual is at increased risk for being invaded by pathogenic organisms.

RISK FACTORS
Inadequate primary defenses (broken skin, traumatized tissue, decrease of ciliary action, stasis of body fluids, change in pH secretions, altered peristalsis); Inadequate secondary defenses (e.g., decreased hemoglobin, leukopenia, suppressed inflammatory response) and immunosuppression; Inadequate acquired immunity; tissue destruction and increased environmental exposure; invasive procedures; Chronic disease, malnutrition, trauma; Pharmaceutical agents [including antibiotic therapy]; Rupture of amniotic membranes; Insufficient knowledge to avoid exposure to pathogens

INJURY, RISK FOR

Diagnostic Division: Safety

Definition: A state in which the individual is at risk of injury as a result of environmental conditions interacting with the individual's adaptive and defensive resources.

NOTE: The potential for injury differs from individual to individual, and situation to situation. It is our belief that the environment is not safe, and there is no way to list everything that might present a danger to someone. Rather, we believe nurses have the responsibility to educate people throughout their life cycles to live safely in their environment.

RISK FACTORS

Internal
Biochemical, regulatory function: (sensory, integrative, effector dysfunction; tissue hypoxia), immune/autoimmune dysfunction; malnutrition; abnormal blood profile, (leukocytosis/leukopenia; altered clotting factors; thrombocytopenia; sickle cell, thalassemia; decreased hemoglobin); Physical (broken skin, altered mobility); development age; (physiologic, psychosocial); Psychologic (affective, orientation)

External
Biologic: (immunization level of community, microorganism); Chemical pollutants, poisons, drugs, pharmaceutical agents, alcohol, caffeine, nicotine, preservatives, cosmetics, and dyes, nutrients (vitamins, food types); Physical (design, structure, and arrangement of community, building and/or equipment); mode of transport/transportation; People/provider (nosocomial agent; staffing patterns; cognitive, affective, and psychomotor factors)

KNOWLEDGE DEFICIT [LEARNING NEED] (SPECIFY)

Diagnostic Division: Teaching/Learning

Definition: Absence or deficiency of cognitive information related to specific topic. [Lack of specific information necessary for patient/significant other(s) to make informed choices regarding condition/lifestyle changes.]

RELATED FACTORS
Lack of exposure; Information misinterpretation; Unfamiliarity with information resources; Lack of recall; Cognitive limitation; Lack of interest in learning; [Patient's request for no information]; [Inaccurate/incomplete information presented]

DEFINING CHARACTERISTICS

Subjective
Verbalization of the problem; [Statements reflecting misconceptions]; [Request for information]

Objective
Inaccurate follow-through of instruction; Inadequate performance of test; Inappropriate or exaggerated behaviors (e.g., hysterical, hostile, agitated, apathetic); [Development of preventable complication]

LATEX ALLERGY RESPONSE

Diagnostic Division: Safety

Definition: An allergic response to natural latex rubber products.

RELATED FACTORS
No immune mechanism response [although this is true of irritant and allergic contact dermatitis, type I/immediate reaction is a true allergic response]

DEFINING CHARACTERISTICS
Type I Reactions
Immediate [hypersensitivity; IgE-mediated reaction]

Type IV Reactions [chemical and delayed-type hypersensitivity]
Eczema; irritation; reaction to additives causes discomfort (e.g., [exposure to chemicals used in manufacture of latex] thirams, carbamates); redness; delayed onset (hours)

Irritant [contact dermatitis] Reactions
Erythema; [dry, crusty, hard bumps]; chapped or cracked skin; blisters

LATEX ALLERGY RESPONSE, RISK FOR

Diagnostic Division: Safety

Definition: At risk for allergic response to natural latex rubber products.

RISK FACTORS
History of reactions to latex (e.g., balloons, condoms, gloves); allergies to bananas, avocados, tropical fruits, kiwi, chestnuts, poinsettia plants; History of allergies and asthma; Professions with daily exposure to latex (e.g., medicine, nursing, dentistry); Conditions needing continuous or intermittent catheterization; Multiple surgical procedures, especially from infancy (e.g., spina bifida)

LONELINESS, RISK FOR

Diagnostic Division: Social Interaction

Definition: A subjective state in which an individual is at risk of experiencing vague dysphoria.

RISK FACTORS
Affectional deprivation; Physical isolation; Cathectic deprivation; Social isolation

MEMORY, IMPAIRED

Diagnostic Division: Neurosensory

Definition: The state in which an individual experiences the inability to remember or recall bits of information or behavioral skills. Impaired memory may be attributed to pathophysiologic or situational causes that are either temporary or permanent.

RELATED FACTORS
Acute or chronic hypoxia; Anemia; Decreased cardiac output; Fluid and electrolyte imbalance [e.g., brain injury/concussion]; Neurological disturbances; Excessive environmental disturbances; [manic state, fugue, traumatic event]; [Substance use/abuse; effects of medications]; [Age]

DEFINING CHARACTERISTICS

Subjective

Reported experiences of forgetting; Inability to recall recent or past events, factual information [or familiar persons, places, items]

Objective

Observed experiences of forgetting; Inability to determine if a behavior was performed; Inability to learn or retain new skills or information; Inability to perform a previously learned skill; Forget to perform a behavior at a scheduled time

MOBILITY, IMPAIRED BED

Diagnostic Division: Safety

Definition: Limitation of independent movement from one bed position to another.

RELATED FACTORS

To be developed by NANDA; [/neuromuscular impairment]; [Pain/discomfort]

DEFINING CHARACTERISTICS

Subjective

[Reported difficulty performing activities]

Objective

Impaired ability to: turn side to side; move from supine to sitting or sitting to supine position; "scoot" or reposition self in bed; move from supine to prone or prone to supine position; move from supine to long sitting or long sitting to supine position

MOBILITY, IMPAIRED PHYSICAL

Diagnostic Division: Safety

Definition: A limitation in independent, purposeful physical movement of the body or of one or more extremities.

RELATED FACTORS

Sedentary lifestyle or disuse or deconditioning; limited cardiovascular endurance; Decreased muscle strength, control and/or mass; joint stiffness or contractures; loss of integrity of bone structures; Intolerance to activity/decreased strength and endurance; Pain/discomfort; Neuromuscular/musculoskeletal impairment; Sensoriperceptual/cognitive impairment; developmental delay; Depressive mood state or anxiety; Selective or generalized malnutrition; altered cellular metabolism; body mass index above 75th age-appropriate percentile; Lack of knowledge regarding value of physical activity; cultural beliefs regarding age appropriate activity; lack of physical or social environmental supports; Prescribed movement restrictions; medications; Reluctance to initiate movement

DEFINING CHARACTERISTICS

Subjective

[Report of pain/discomfort on movement]

Objective

Limited range of motion; limited ability to perform gross/fine motor skills; difficulty turning; Slowed movement; uncoordinated or jerky movements, decreased [*sic*] reaction time; Gait changes (e.g., decreased walk, speed, difficulty initiating gait, small steps, shuffles feet, exaggerated lateral postural sway); Postural instability during performance of routine Activities of Daily Living; Movement-induced shortness of breath; Engages in substitutions for movement (e.g., increased attention to other's activity, controlling behavior, focus on pre-illness/disability activity)

MOBILITY, IMPAIRED WHEELCHAIR

Diagnostic Division: Safety

Definition: Limitation of independent operation of wheelchair within environment.

RELATED FACTORS

To be developed by NANDA

DEFINING CHARACTERISTICS
Impaired ability to operate manual or power wheelchair on even or uneven surface, on an incline or decline, on curbs

NAUSEA

Diagnostic Division: Food/Fluid

Definition: An unpleasant, wave-like sensation in the back of the throat, epigastrium, or throughout the abdomen that may or may not lead to vomiting.

RELATED FACTORS
Post-surgical anesthesia; Stimulation of neuropharmacological mechanisms; chemotherapy; [radiation therapy]; Irritation to the gastrointestinal system

DEFINING CHARACTERISTICS

Subjective
Reports "nausea" or "sick to stomach"

Objective
Usually precedes vomiting, but may be experienced after vomiting or when vomiting does not occur; Accompanied by swallowing movements affected by skeletal muscles; pallor, cold and clammy skin, increased salivation, tachycardia, gastric stasis, and diarrhea

NONCOMPLIANCE [COMPLIANCE, ALTERED] (SPECIFY)

Diagnostic Division: Teaching/Learning

Definition: The extent to which a person's and/or caregiver's behavior coincides or fails to coincide with a health-promoting or therapeutic plan agreed upon by the person (and/or family, and/or community) and health care professional. In the presence of an agreed-upon health-promoting or therapeutic plan, person's or caregiver's behavior may be fully or partially adherent or nonadherent and may lead to clinically effective, partially effective, or ineffective outcomes.

NOTE: Noncompliance is a term that may create a negative situation for patient and caregiver that may foster difficulties in resolving the causative factors. As patients have a right to refuse therapy, we see this as a situation in which the professional need is to accept the patient's point of view/behavior/choice(s) and to work together to find alternate means to meet original and/or revised goals.

RELATED FACTORS

Health Care Plan
Duration; Significant others; cost; intensity; complexity

Individual factors
Personal and developmental abilities; knowledge and skills relevant to the regimen behavior; motivational forces; Individual's value system; health beliefs; cultural influences, spiritual values; [Altered thought processes such as depression, paranoia]; [Difficulty changing behavior, as in addictions]; [Issues of secondary gain]

Health System
Individual health coverage; financial flexibility of plan; credibility of provider; Client-provider relationships; provider continuity and regular follow-up; provider reimbursement of teaching and follow-up; communication and teaching skills of the provider; Access and convenience of care; satisfaction with care

Network
Involvement of members in health plan; social value regarding plan; Perceived beliefs of significant other's communication and teaching skills; [Altered thought processes such as depression, paranoia]; [Difficulty changing behavior, as in addictions]; [Issues of secondary gain]

DEFINING CHARACTERISTICS

Subjective
Statements by patient or significant other(s) [e.g., does not perceive illness/risk to be serious, does not believe in efficacy of therapy, unwilling to follow treatment regimen or accept side effects/limitations]

Objective
Behavior indicative of failure to adhere (by direct observation); Objective tests (physiologic measures, detection of markers); Failure to progress; Evidence of development

of complications/exacerbation of symptoms; Failure to keep appointments; [Inability to set or to attain mutual goals]; [Denial]

NUTRITION: ALTERED, LESS THAN BODY REQUIREMENTS

Diagnostic Division: Food/Fluid

Definition: The state in which an individual experiences an intake of nutrients insufficient to meet metabolic needs.

RELATED FACTORS

Inability to ingest or to digest food or to absorb nutrients because of biologic, psychologic, or economic factors; [Increased metabolic demands (e.g., burns)]; [Lack of information, misinformation, misconception]

DEFINING CHARACTERISTICS

Subjective

Reported inadequate food intake less than RDA; Reported lack of food; Aversion to eating; satiety immediately after ingesting food; reported altered taste sensation; Abdominal pain with or without pathologic conditions; abdominal cramping; Lack of interest in food; perceived inability to ingest food; Lack of information; misinformation, misconceptions [NOTE: The authors view this as a related factor rather than a defining characteristic]

Objective

Body weight 20% or more under ideal [for height and frame]; Loss of weight with adequate food intake; Evidence of lack of [available] food; Weakness of muscles required for swallowing or mastication; Sore, inflamed buccal cavity; Poor muscle tone; Capillary fragility; Hyperactive bowel sounds; Diarrhea and/or steatorrhea; Pale conjunctiva and mucous membranes; Excessive loss of hair [or increased growth of hair on body (lanugo)]; [cessation of menses]; [Decreased subcutaneous fat/muscle mass]; [Abnormal laboratory studies (e.g., decreased albumin, total proteins; iron deficiency; electrolyte imbalances)]

NUTRITION: ALTERED, MORE THAN BODY REQUIREMENTS

Diagnostic Division: Food/Fluid

Definition: The state in which an individual is experiencing an intake of nutrients which exceeds metabolic needs.

RELATED FACTORS

Excessive intake in relationship to metabolic need

NOTE: Underlying cause is often complex and may be difficult to diagnose/treat

DEFINING CHARACTERISTICS

Subjective

Reported dysfunctional eating patterns: Pairing food with other activities; Eating in response to external cues such as time of day, social situation; Concentrating food intake at end of day; Eating in response to internal cues other than hunger (e.g., anxiety); Sedentary activity level

Objective

Weight 20% over ideal for height and frame [obese]; Triceps skinfold greater than 15 mm in men and 25 mm in women; Weight 10% over ideal for height and frame [overweight]; Observed dysfunctional eating patterns [as noted in Subjective]; [Percentage of body fat greater than 22% for trim women and 15% for trim men]

NUTRITION: ALTERED, RISK FOR MORE THAN BODY REQUIREMENTS

Diagnostic Division: Food/Fluid

Definition: The state in which an individual is at risk of experiencing an intake of nutrients that exceeds metabolic needs.

RISK FACTORS

Reported/observed obesity in one or both parents [/spouse; hereditary predisposition]; Rapid transition across growth percentiles in infants or children [adolescents]; Reported use of solid food as major food source before 5 months of age; Reported/observed higher baseline weight at beginning of each pregnancy [frequent, closely spaced pregnancies]; Dysfunctional eating patterns: pairing food with other activities, eating in response to external cues such as time of day or social situation, concentrating food intake at end of day, eating in response to internal cues other than hunger (e.g., anxiety); Observed use of food as reward or comfort measure; [Frequent/repeated dieting]; [Socially/culturally isolated; lacking other outlets]; [Alteration in usual activity patterns/sedentary lifestyle]; [Alteration in usual coping patterns]; [Majority of foods consumed are concentrated, high-calorie sources/fat]; [Significant/sudden decline in financial resources; lower socioeconomic status]

ORAL MUCOUS MEMBRANE, ALTERED

Diagnostic Division: Food/Fluid

Definition: Disruptions of the lips and soft tissue of the oral cavity.

RELATED FACTORS

Pathological conditions—oral cavity (radiation to head or neck); cleft lip or palate; loss of supportive structures; Trauma; Mechanical (e.g., ill-fitting dentures, braces, tubes [endotracheal/nasogastric], surgery in oral cavity); Chemical (e.g., alcohol, tobacco, acidic foods, regular use of inhalers); Chemotherapy; immunosuppression/compromised; decreased platelets; infection; radiation therapy; Dehydration; malnutrition or vitamin deficiency; NPO for more than 24 hours; Lack of/impaired or decreased salivation; mouth breathing; Ineffective oral hygiene; barriers to oral self-care/professional care; Medication side effects; Stress; depression; Diminished hormone levels (women); aging-related loss of connective, adipose, or bone tissue

DEFINING CHARACTERISTICS

Subjective

Xerostomia (dry mouth); Oral pain/discomfort; Self-report of bad/diminished or absent taste; difficulty eating or swallowing

Objective

Coated tongue; smooth atrophic, sensitive tongue; geographic tongue; Gingival or mucosal pallor; Stomatitis; hyperemia; bleeding gingival hyperplasia; macroplasia; vesicles, nodules, or papules; White patches/plaques, spongy patches or white curd-like exudate; oral lesions or ulcers; fissures, cheilitis; desquamation; mucosal denudation; Edema; Halitosis, [carious teeth]; Gingival recession, pockets deeper than 4 mm; Purulent drainage or exudates; presence of pathogens; Enlarged tonsils beyond what is developmentally appropriate; Red or bluish masses (e.g., hemangiomas); Difficult speech

PAIN, [ACUTE]

Diagnostic Division: Pain/Discomfort

Definition: An unpleasant sensory and emotional experience arising from actual or potential tissue damage or described in terms of such damage (International Association for the Study of Pain); sudden or slow onset of any intensity from mild to severe with an anticipated or predictable end and a duration of less than 6 months.

RELATED FACTORS

Injuring agents (biological, chemical, physical, psychological)

DEFINING CHARACTERISTICS

Subjective

Verbal or coded report; [may be less from patients under 40, men, and some cultural groups]; Changes in appetite and eating; [Pain unrelieved and/or increased beyond tolerance]

Objective

Guarded/protected behavior; antalgic position/gestures; Facial mask; sleep disturbance (eyes lack luster, "hecohe [beaten] look," fixed or scattered movement, grimace); Expressive behavior (restlessness, moaning, crying, vigilance, irritability, sighing); Distraction behavior (pacing, seeking out other people and/or activities, repetitive activities); Autonomic alteration in muscle tone (may span from listless [flaccid] to rigid); Autonomic responses (diaphoresis, blood pressure, respiration and pulse changes, pupillary dilation); Self-focusing; Narrowed focus (altered time perception, impaired thought process, reduced interaction with people and environment); [Fear/panic]

PAIN, CHRONIC

Diagnostic Division: Pain/Comfort

Definition: An unpleasant sensory and emotional experience arising from actual or potential tissue damage or described in terms of such damage (International Association for the Study of Pain); sudden or slow onset of any intensity from mild to severe, constant or recurring without anticipated or predictable end and a duration of greater than 6 months.

NOTE: [Pain is a signal that something is wrong. Chronic pain can be recurrent and periodically disabling (e.g., migraine headaches) or may be unremitting. While chronic pain syndrome includes various learned behaviors, psychologic factors become the primary contribution to impairment. It is a complex entity, combining elements from other nursing diagnoses (e.g., Powerlessness; Diversional Activity deficit; Family Processes, altered; Self-care deficit, and Disuse syndrome).]

RELATED FACTORS
Chronic physical/psychosocial disability

DEFINING CHARACTERISTICS
Subjective
Verbal or coded report; Fear of reinjury; Altered ability to continue previous activities; Changes in sleep patterns; fatigue; [Changes in appetite]; [Preoccupation with pain]; [Desperately seeks alternative solutions/therapies for relief/control of pain]

Objective
Observed evidence of: protective/guarding behavior; facial mask; irritability; self-focusing; restlessness; depression; Reduced interaction with people; Anorexia, weight changes; Atrophy of involved muscle group; Sympathetic mediated responses (temperature, cold, changes of body position, hypersensitivity)

PARENT/INFANT/CHILD ATTACHMENT, ALTERED, RISK FOR

Diagnostic Division: Social Interaction

Definition: Disruption of the interactive process between parent/significant other and infant that fosters the development of a protective and nurturing reciprocal relationship.

RISK FACTORS
Inability of parents to meet the personal needs; Anxiety associated with the parent role; Substance abuse; Premature infant, ill infant/child who is unable to effectively initiate parental contact due to altered behavioral organization; Separation; physical barriers; Lack of privacy; [Parents who themselves experienced altered attachment]; [Uncertainty of paternity; conception as a result of rape/sexual abuse]; [Difficult pregnancy and/or birth (actual or perceived)]

PARENT-INFANT ATTACHMENT, RISK FOR INSECURE

Diagnostic Division: Social Interaction

Definition: Risk for disruption of the interactive process between parent (or significant other person) and infant that fosters the development of a protective and nurturing reciprocal environment.

DEFINING CHARACTERISTICS
To be developed by NANDA.

PARENTAL ROLE CONFLICT

Diagnostic Division: Social Interaction

Definition: The state in which a parent experiences role confusion and conflict in response to crisis.

RELATED FACTORS
Separation from child due to chronic illness [/disability]; Intimidation with invasive or restrictive modalities (e.g., isolation, intubation), specialized care centers, policies; Home care of a child with special needs (e.g., apnea monitoring, postural drainage,

hyperalimentation); Change in marital status; Interruptions of family life due to home care regimen (treatments, caregiver's lack of respite)

DEFINING CHARACTERISTICS

Subjective

Parent(s) express concerns/feelings of inadequacy to provide for child's physical and emotional needs during hospitalization or in the home; Parent(s) express concerns about changes in parental role, family functioning, family communication, family health; Parent(s) express concern about perceived loss of control over decisions relating to their child; Parent(s) verbalize feelings of guilt, anger, fear, anxiety, and/or frustration about effect of child's illness on family process

Objective

Demonstrated disruption in caretaking routines; Reluctance to participate in usual caretaking activities, even with encouragement and support; Demonstrated feelings of guilt, anger, fear, anxiety, and/or frustration about effect of child's illness on family process

PARENTING, ALTERED

Diagnostic Division: Social Interaction

Definition: Inability of the primary caretaker to create an environment that promotes the optimum growth and development of the child. (It is important to state as a preface to this diagnosis that adjustment to parenting in general is a normal maturational process that elicits nursing behaviors of prevention of potential problems and health promotion.)

RELATED FACTORS

Social

Presence of stress (e.g., financial, legal, recent crisis, cultural move [e.g., from another country/cultural group within same country]); unemployment or job problems; financial difficulties; relocations; poor home environments; Lack of family cohesiveness; marital conflict, declining satisfaction; change in family unit; Role strain or overload; single parent; father of child not involved; Unplanned or unwanted pregnancy; lack of, or poor, parental role model; low self-esteem; Low socioeconomic class; poverty; lack of resources, access to resources, social support networks, transportation; Inadequate child care arrangements; lack of value of parenthood; inability to put child's needs before own; Poor problem-solving skills; maladaptive coping strategies; Social isolation; History of being abusive/being abused; legal difficulties

Knowledge

Lack of knowledge about child health maintenance, parenting skills, child development; inability to recognize and act on infant cues; Unrealistic expectation for self, infant, partner; limited cognitive functioning; Low educational level or attainment; lack of cognitive readiness for parenthood; Poor communication skills; Preference for physical punishment

Physiological

Physical illness

Infant or Child

Premature birth; multiple births; unplanned or unwanted child; not gender desired; Illness; prolonged separation from parent/separation at birth; Difficult temperament; lack of goodness of fit (temperament) with parental expectations; Handicapping condition or developmental delay; altered perceptual abilities; attention deficit hyperactivity disorder

Psychological

Young age, especially adolescent; Lack of, or late, prenatal care; difficult labor and/or delivery; multiple births; high number or closely spaced pregnancies; Sleep deprivation or disruption; depression; Separation from infant/child; History of substance abuse or dependencies; Disability; history of mental illness

DEFINING CHARACTERISTICS

Subjective

Parental

Statements of inability to meet child's needs; cannot control child; Negative statements about child; Verbalization of role inadequacy frustration

Objective
Infant or Child
Frequent accidents/illness; failure to thrive; Poor academic performance/cognitive development; Poor social competence; behavioral disorders; Incidence of physical and psychological trauma or abuse; Lack of attachment; separation anxiety; Runaway

Parental
Maternal-child interaction deficit; poor parent-child interaction; little cuddling; insecure or lack of attachment to infant; Inadequate child health maintenance; unsafe home environment; inappropriate visual, tactile, auditory stimulation; Poor or inappropriate caretaking skills; inconsistent care/behavior management; Inflexibility to meet needs of child, situation; High punitiveness; rejection or hostility to child; child abuse; child neglect; abandonment

PARENTING, RISK FOR ALTERED

Diagnostic Division: Social Interaction

Definition: Risk for inability of the primary caretaker to create, maintain, or regain an environment that promotes the optimum growth and development of the child. (It is important to state as a preface to this diagnosis that adjustment to parenting in general is a normal maturational process that elicits nursing behaviors of prevention of potential problems and health promotion.)

RISK FACTORS

NOTE: Lack of role identity; lack of available role model, ineffective role model

Social
Stress [e.g., financial, legal, recent crisis, cultural move (e.g., from another country/cultural group in same country)]; unemployment or job problems; financial difficulties; relocations; poor home environments; Lack of family cohesiveness; marital conflict, declining satisfaction; change in family unit; Role strain/overload; single parents; father or child not involved; Unplanned or unwanted pregnancy; lack of, or poor, parental role model; low self-esteem; Low socioeconomic class; poverty; lack of [resources], access to resources, social support networks, transportation; inadequate child care arrangements; lack of value of parenthood; inability to put child's needs before own; Poor problem-solving skills; maladaptive coping strategies; Social isolation; History of being abusive/being abused; legal difficulties

Knowledge
Lack of knowledge about child health maintenance, parenting skills, child development; inability to recognize and act on infant cues; Unrealistic expectations of child; Low educational level or attainment; low cognitive functioning; lack of cognitive readiness for parenthood; Poor communication skills; Preference for physical punishment

Physiological
Physical illness

Infant or child
Premature birth; multiple births; unplanned or unwanted child; not gender desired; Illness; prolonged separation from parent/separation at birth; Difficult temperament; lack of goodness of fit (temperament) with parental expectations; Handicapping condition or developmental delay; altered perceptual abilities; attention deficit hyperactivity disorder

Psychological
Young age, especially adolescent; Lack of, or late, prenatal care; difficult labor and/or delivery; multiple births; high number or closely spaced pregnancies; Sleep deprivation or disruption; depression; Separation from infant/child; History of substance abuse or dependence; Disability; history of mental illness

PERIOPERATIVE POSITIONING INJURY, RISK FOR

Diagnostic Division: Safety

Definition: A state in which the client is at risk for injury as a result of the environmental conditions found in the perioperative setting.

RISK FACTORS

Disorientation; sensory/perceptual disturbances due to anesthesia; Immobilization; muscle weakness; [pre-existing musculoskeletal conditions]; Obesity; Emaciation; Edema; [Elderly]

PERIPHERAL NEUROVASCULAR RISK FOR DYSFUNCTION

Diagnostic Division: Neurosensory

Definition: A state in which an individual is at risk of experiencing a disruption in circulation, sensation, or motion of an extremity.

RISK FACTORS

Fractures; Mechanical compression (e.g., tourniquet, cast, brace, dressing, or restraint); Orthopedic surgery; trauma; Immobilization; Burns; Vascular obstruction

PERSONAL IDENTITY DISTURBANCE

Diagnostic Division: Ego Integrity

Definition: Inability to distinguish between self and nonself.

RELATED FACTORS

To be developed by NANDA: [Organic brain syndrome]; [Poor ego differentiation, as in schizophrenia]; [Panic/dissociative states]; [Biochemical body change]

DEFINING CHARACTERISTICS

(To be developed by NANDA)

Subjective

[Confusion about sense of self, purpose or direction in life, sexual identification/preference]

Objective

[Difficulty in making decisions]; [Poorly differentiated ego boundaries]; [See ND Anxiety, panic, for additional characteristics]

POISONING, RISK FOR

Diagnostic Division: Safety

Definition: Accentuated risk of accidental exposure to or ingestion of drugs or dangerous products in doses sufficient to cause poisoning [/or the adverse effects of prescribed medication/drug use].

RISK FACTORS

Internal (individual)

Reduced vision; Lack of safety or drug education; Lack of proper precaution [unsafe habits, disregard for safety measures, lack of supervision]; Insufficient finances; Verbalization of occupational setting without adequate safeguards; Cognitive or emotional difficulties [behavioral]; [Age (e.g., young child, elderly)]; [Chronic disease state, disability]; [Cultural or religious beliefs/practices]

External (Environmental)

Large supplies of drugs in house; Medicines stored in unlocked cabinets accessible to children or confused persons; Availability of illicit drugs potentially contaminated by poisonous additives; Flaking, peeling paint or plaster in presence of young children; Dangerous products placed or stored within the reach of children or confused persons; Unprotected contact with heavy metals or chemicals; Paint, lacquer, etc., in poorly ventilated areas or without effective protection; Chemical contamination of food and water; Presence of poisonous vegetation; Presence of atmospheric pollutants, [proximity to industrial chemicals/pattern of prevailing winds]; [Therapeutic margin of safety of specific drugs (e.g., therapeutic versus toxic level, half-life, method of uptake and degradation in body, adequacy of organ function)]; [Use of multiple herbal supplements or megadosing]

POST-TRAUMA SYNDROME

Diagnostic Division: Ego Integrity

Definition: A sustained maladaptive response to a traumatic, overwhelming event.

RELATED FACTORS

Events outside the range of usual human experience; Serious threat or injury to self or loved ones; serious accidents; industrial and motor vehicle accidents; Physical and psychosocial abuse; rape; Witnessing mutilation, violent death, or other horrors; tragic occurrence involving multiple deaths; Natural disasters and/or man-made disasters; sudden destruction of one's home or community; epidemics; Wars; military combat; being held prisoner of war or criminal victimization (torture)

DEFINING CHARACTERISTICS

Subjective

Intrusive thoughts/dreams; flashbacks; nightmares; Palpitations; headaches; [loss of interest in usual activities, loss of feeling of intimacy/sexuality]; Hopelessness; shame; [excessive verbalization of the traumatic event, verbalization of survival guilt or guilt about behavior required for survival]; Gastric irritability; [changes in appetite; sleep disturbance/insomnia; chronic fatigue/easy fatigability]

Objective

Anxiety; fear; Hypervigilant; exaggerated startle response; neurosensory irritability; irritability; Grief; guilt; Difficulty in concentrating; depression; Anger and/or rage; aggression; Avoidance; repression; alienation; denial; detachment; psychogenic amnesia; numbing; Altered mood states; [poor impulse control/irritability and explosiveness]; panic attacks; horror; Substance abuse; compulsive behavior; Enuresis (in children); [Difficulty with interpersonal relationships; dependence on others; work/school failure]

POST-TRAUMA SYNDROME, RISK FOR

Diagnostic Division: Ego Integrity

Definition: A risk for sustained maladaptive response to a traumatic, overwhelming event.

RISK FACTORS

Occupation (e.g., police, fire, rescue, corrections, emergency room staff, mental health [and their family members]); Perception of event; exaggerated sense of responsibility; diminished ego strength; Survivor's role in the event; Inadequate social support; nonsupportive environment; displacement from home; Duration of the event

POWERLESSNESS [SPECIFY LEVEL]

Diagnostic Division: Ego Integrity

Definition: Perception that one's own action will not significantly affect an outcome; a perceived lack of control over a current situation or immediate happening.

RELATED FACTORS

Health care environment [e.g., loss of privacy, personal possessions, control over therapies]; Interpersonal interaction [e.g., misuse of power, force; abusive relationships]; Illness-related regimen [e.g., chronic/debilitating conditions]; Lifestyle of helplessness [e.g., repeated failures, dependency]

DEFINING CHARACTERISTICS

Subjective

Severe

Verbal expressions of having no control or influence over situation, outcome, or self-care; Depression over physical deterioration that occurs despite patient compliance with regimens

Moderate

Expressions of dissatisfaction and frustration over inability to perform previous tasks and/or activities; Expression of doubt regarding role performance; Reluctance to express true feelings, fear of alienation from caregivers

Low

Expressions of uncertainty about fluctuating energy levels

Objective

Severe

Apathy [withdrawal, resignation, crying]; [Anger]

Moderate

Does not monitor progress; Nonparticipation in care or decision making when opportunities are provided; Dependence on others that may result in irritability, resentment, anger, and guilt; Inability to seek information regarding care; Does not defend self-care practices when challenged

Low
Passivity

POWERLESSNESS, RISK FOR

Diagnostic Division: Ego Integrity

Definition: Risk for perceived lack of control over situation and/or ability to significantly affect an outcome.

DEFINING CHARACTERISTICS
To be developed by NANDA.

PROTECTION, ALTERED

Diagnostic Division: Safety

Definition: The state in which an individual experiences a decrease in the ability to guard the self from internal or external threats such as illness or injury.

RELATED FACTORS
Extremes of age; Inadequate nutrition; Alcohol abuse; Abnormal blood profiles (leukopenia, thrombocytopenia, anemia, coagulation); Drug therapies (antineoplastic, corticosteroid, immune, anticoagulant, thrombolytic); Treatments (surgery, radiation); Diseases, such as cancer and immune disorders

DEFINING CHARACTERISTICS
Subjective
Neurosensory alterations; Chilling; Itching; Insomnia; fatigue; weakness; Anorexia

Objective
Deficient immunity; Impaired healing; altered clotting; Maladaptive stress response; Perspiring [inappropriate]; Dyspnea; cough; Restlessness; immobility; Disorientation; Pressure sores

[NOTE: The purpose of this diagnosis seems to be to combine multiple diagnoses under a single heading for ease of planning care when a number of variables may be present. Outcomes/evaluation criteria and interventions are specifically tied to individual related factors that are present, such as: Extremes of age: Concerns may include body temperature/thermoregulation or thought process/sensory-perceptual alterations, as well as risk for trauma, suffocation, or poisoning; and fluid volume imbalances; Inadequate nutrition: Brings up issues of nutrition, less than body requirements; infection, altered thought processes, trauma, ineffective coping, and altered family processes; Alcohol abuse: May be situational or chronic with problems ranging from ineffective breathing patterns, decreased cardiac output, and fluid volume deficit to nutritional problems, infection, trauma, altered thought processes, and coping/family process difficulties; Abnormal blood profile: Suggests possibility of fluid volume deficit, decreased tissue perfusion, impaired gas exchange, activity intolerance, or risk for infection; Drug therapies, treatments, and disease concerns: Would include risk for infection, fluid volume imbalances, altered skin/tissue integrity, pain, nutritional problems, fatigue, and emotional responses. It is suggested that the user refer to specific nursing diagnoses based on identified related factors and individual concerns for this patient in order to find appropriate outcomes and interventions.]

RAPE-TRAUMA SYNDROME

Diagnostic Division: Ego Integrity

Definition: Sustained maladaptive response to a forced, violent sexual penetration against the victim's will and consent. (The trauma syndrome that develops from this attack or attempted attack includes an acute phase of disorganization of the victim's lifestyle and a long-term process of reorganization of lifestyle.)

NOTE: Although attacks are most often directed toward women, men also may be victims.

RELATED FACTORS
NOTE: Rape [actual/attempted forced sexual penetration]

DEFINING CHARACTERISTICS

Subjective

Loss of self-esteem; helplessness; powerlessness; Nightmare and sleep disturbances; Change in relationships; sexual dysfunction

Objective

Physical trauma (e.g., bruising, tissue irritation); muscle tension and/or spasms; Confusion; disorganization; inability to make decisions; Agitation; hyperalertness; aggression; Mood swings; vulnerability; dependence; depression; Substance abuse; suicide attempts; Denial; phobias; dissociative disorders

RAPE-TRAUMA SYNDROME: COMPOUND REACTION

Diagnostic Division: Ego Integrity

Definition: Forced violent sexual penetration against the victim's will and consent. The trauma syndrome that develops from this attack or attempted attack includes an acute phase of disorganization of the victim's lifestyle and a long-term process of reorganization of lifestyle.

RELATED FACTORS

To be developed by NANDA

DEFINING CHARACTERISTICS

Acute Phase

Emotional reaction (e.g., anger, embarrassment, fear of physical violence and death, humiliation, self-blame, thoughts of revenge); Multiple physical symptoms (e.g., gastrointestinal irritability, genitourinary discomfort, muscle tension, sleep pattern disturbance); Reactivated symptoms of such previous conditions (i.e., physical/psychiatric illness, reliance on alcohol and/or drugs)

Long-Term Phase

Change in lifestyles (e.g., changing residence, dealing with repetitive nightmares and phobias, seeking family/social network support)

RAPE-TRAUMA SYNDROME: SILENT REACTION

Diagnostic Division: Ego Integrity

Definition: Forced violent sexual penetration against the victim's will and consent. The trauma syndrome that develops from this attack or attempted attack includes an acute phase of disorganization of the victim's lifestyle and a long-term process of reorganization of lifestyle.

RELATED FACTORS

To be developed by NANDA

DEFINING CHARACTERISTICS

Abrupt changes in relationships with men; Increase in nightmares; Increased anxiety during interview (i.e., blocking of associations, long periods of silence, minor stuttering, physical distress); Pronounced changes in sexual behavior; Sudden onset of phobic reactions; No verbalization of the occurrence of rape

RECOVERY, DELAYED SURGICAL

Diagnostic Division: Pain/Discomfort

Definition: An extension of the number of postoperative days required for individuals to initiate and perform on their own behalf activities that maintain life, health, and well-being.

RELATED FACTORS

To be developed by NANDA

DEFINING CHARACTERISTICS

Subjective

Perception more time is needed to recover; report of pain/discomfort; fatigue; loss of appetite with or without nausea; postpones resumption of work/employment activities

Objective
Evidence of interrupted healing of surgical area (e.g., red, indurated, draining, immobile); difficulty in moving about; requires help to complete self-care

RELOCATION STRESS SYNDROME

Diagnostic Division: Ego Integrity

Definition: Physiologic and/or psychological disturbances as a result of transfer from one environment to another.

RELATED FACTORS
Past, concurrent, and recent losses; losses involved with decision to move; Feeling of powerlessness; Lack of adequate support system; Little or no preparation for the impending move; Moderate to high degree of environmental change; History and types of previous transfers; Impaired psychosocial health status; Decreased physical health status

DEFINING CHARACTERISTICS

Subjective
Anxiety; Apprehension; Depression; Loneliness; Verbalization of unwillingness to relocate; Sleep disturbance; Change in eating habits; Gastrointestinal disturbances; Insecurity; Lack of trust; Unfavorable comparison of post-transfer/pre-transfer staff; Verbalization of being concerned/upset [angry] about transfer

Objective
Change in environment/location; Increased confusion (elderly population) [/cognitively impaired]; Increased (frequency of) verbalization of needs; Dependency; Sad affect; Vigilance; Weight change; Withdrawal; Hostile behavior/outbursts

RELOCATION STRESS SYNDROME, RISK FOR

Diagnostic Division: Ego Integrity

Definition: Risk for maladaptive response to transfer from one environment to another.

DEFINING CHARACTERISTICS
To be developed by NANDA.

ROLE PERFORMANCE, ALTERED

Diagnostic Division: Social Interaction

Definition: The patterns of behavior and self-expression do not match the environmental context, norms, and expectations. [There is a typology of roles: sociopersonal (friendship, family, marital, parenting, community), home management, intimacy (sexuality, relationship building), leisure/exercise/recreation, self-management, socialization (developmental transitions), community contributor, and religious.]

RELATED FACTORS

Social
Inadequate role socialization (e.g., role model, expectations, responsibilities); Young age, developmental level; Lack of resources; low socioeconomic status; poverty; Stress and conflict; job schedule demands; Family conflict; domestic violence; Inadequate support system; lack of rewards; Inadequate or inappropriate linkage with the health care system

Knowledge
Lack of knowledge about role/role skills; lack of or inadequate role model; Inadequate role preparation (e.g., role transition, skill, rehearsal, validation); lack of opportunity for role rehearsal; Education attainment level; developmental transitions; Role transition; unrealistic role expectations

Physiological
Health alterations (e.g., physical health, body image, self-esteem, mental health, psychosocial health, cognition, learning style, neurological health); low self-esteem; pain; fatigue; depression; Substance abuse; Inadequate/inappropriate linkage with health care system

DEFINING CHARACTERISTICS

Subjective

Altered role perceptions/change in self-perception of role/usual patterns of responsibility/capacity to resume role/other's perception of role; inadequate opportunities for role enactment; role dissatisfaction; overload; denial; discrimination [by others]; powerlessness

Objective

Inadequate knowledge; inadequate role competency and skills; inadequate adaptation to change or transition; inappropriate developmental expectations; inadequate confidence; inadequate motivation; inadequate self-management; inadequate coping; inadequate opportunities/external support for role enhancement; role strain; role conflict; role confusion; role ambivalence; [failure to assume role]; uncertainty; anxiety or depression; pessimistic; domestic violence; harassment; system conflict

SELF-CARE DEFICIT, FEEDING

Diagnostic Division: Hygiene

Definition: An impaired ability to perform or complete feeding activities.

RELATED FACTORS

Weakness or tiredness; Severe anxiety; Neuromuscular impairment; Pain; discomfort; Perceptual or cognitive impairment; Environmental barriers; Decreased or lack of motivation; Musculoskeletal impairments

DEFINING CHARACTERISTICS

Inability to prepare food for ingestion, open containers; Inability to handle utensils, get food onto utensil safely, bring food from a receptacle to the mouth; Inability to manipulate food in mouth, chew/swallow food; Inability to pick up cup or glass; Inability to use assistive device; Inability to complete a meal; Inability to ingest food in a socially acceptable manner

SELF-CARE DEFICIT, BATHING/HYGIENE

Diagnostic Division: Hygiene

Definition: Impaired ability to perform or complete bathing/hygiene activities for oneself.

RISK FACTORS

Discomfort

RELATED FACTORS

Decreased or lack of motivation; weakness and tiredness; Severe anxiety; Inadequate to perceive body part or spatial relationship; Perceptual or cognitive impairment; Pain; Neuromuscular/musculoskeletal impairment; Environmental barriers

DEFINING CHARACTERISTICS

Inability to get bath supplies; Inability to wash body or body parts; Inability to obtain or get to water source, regulate temperature or flow of bath water; Inability to get in and out of bathroom [tub]; Inability to dry body

SELF-CARE DEFICIT, DRESSING/GROOMING

Diagnostic Division: Hygiene

Definition: An impaired ability to perform or complete dressing and grooming activities for oneself.

RELATED FACTORS

Weakness or tiredness; decreased or lack of motivation; Pain; discomfort; Severe anxiety; Perceptual or cognitive impairment neuromuscular/musculoskeletal impairment; Environmental barriers

DEFINING CHARACTERISTICS

Inability to choose clothing, pick up clothing, use assistive devices; Impaired ability/inability to put on or take off necessary items of clothing on upper/lower body; put on socks/shoes; Impaired ability to obtain or replace articles of clothing, fasten clothing, use zippers; Inability to maintain appearance at a satisfactory level

SELF-CARE DEFICIT, TOILET

Diagnostic Division: Hygiene

Definition: An impaired ability to perform or complete own toileting activities.

RELATED FACTORS

Environmental barriers; Weakness or tiredness; decreased or lack of motivation; Severe anxiety; Impaired mobility status; Impaired transfer ability; Neuromuscular/musculoskeletal impairment; Pain; Perceptual or cognitive impairment

DEFINING CHARACTERISTICS

Inability to manipulate clothing; Unable to carry out proper toilet hygiene; Unable to sit on or rise from toilet or commode; Unable to get to toilet or commode; Unable to flush toilet or [empty] commode

SELF-ESTEEM, CHRONIC LOW

Diagnostic Division: Ego Integrity

Definition: Long-standing negative self-evaluation/feelings about self or self-capabilities.

RELATED FACTORS

To be developed by NANDA: [Fixation in earlier level of development]; [Continual negative evaluation of self/capabilities from childhood]; [Personal vulnerability]; [Life choices perpetuating failure; ineffective social/occupational functioning]; [Feelings of abandonment by significant other; willingness to tolerate possibly life-threatening domestic violence]; [Chronic physical/psychiatric conditions; antisocial behaviors]

DEFINING CHARACTERISTICS

Subjective

(Long-standing or chronic:) Self-negating verbalization; Expressions of shame and guilt; Evaluates self as unable to deal with events; Rationalizes away/rejects positive feedback and exaggerates negative feedback about self.

Objective

Hesitant to try new things/situations (long-standing or chronic); Frequent lack of success in work and other life events; Overly conforming, dependent on others' opinions; Lack of eye contact; Nonassertive/passive; indecisive; Excessively seeks reassurance

SELF-ESTEEM DISTURBANCE

Diagnostic Division: Ego Integrity

Definition: Negative self-evaluation/feelings about self or self-capabilities that may be directly or indirectly expressed. [Self-esteem is a human need for survival.]

RELATED FACTORS

To be developed by NANDA: [Unsatisfactory parent-child relationship]; [Unrealistic expectations (on the part of self and others)]; [Unmet dependency needs]; [Absent, erratic, or inconsistent parental discipline]; [Dysfunctional family system]; [Child/sexual abuse or neglect]; [Underdeveloped ego and punitive superego, retarded ego development]; [Negative role models]; [Disorganized or chaotic environments]; [Extreme poverty]; [Lack of positive feedback, repeated negative feedback resulting in diminished self-worth]; [Perceived/numerous failures (learned helplessness); "Failure" at life events (e.g., loss of job, divorce, relationship problems)]; [Impaired cognitive fostering negative view of self]; [Aging]

DEFINING CHARACTERISTICS

Subjective

Self-negating verbalization; Evaluates self as unable to deal with events; Expressions of shame/guilt; Rationalizes away/rejects positive feedback and exaggerates negative feedback about self

Objective

Hesitant to try new things/situations; Hypersensitive to slight or criticism; Denial of problems obvious to others; Projection of blame/responsibility for problems; Rationalizing personal failures; [Inability to accept positive reinforcement]; [Lack of eye contact]; [Not taking responsibility for self-care (self-neglect)]; [Lack of follow-through]; [Nonparticipation in therapy]; [Self-destructive behavior; accident prone]

[NOTE: Taxonomically this diagnosis is a broad category that has been subdivided into situational low and chronic low. When initial assessment reveals this diagnosis, further evaluation is required to determine the patient's specific needs.]

SELF-ESTEEM, SITUATIONAL LOW

Diagnostic Division: Ego Integrity

Definition: Negative self-evaluation/feelings about self that develop in response to a loss or change in an individual who previously had a positive self-evaluation.

RELATED FACTORS

To be developed by NANDA: ["Failure" at life event (e.g., loss of job, relationship problems, divorce]; [Feelings of abandonment by significant other]; [Maturational transitions, adolescence, aging]; [Perceived loss of control in some aspect of life]; [Loss of health status/body part/independent functioning]; [Memory deficits/cognitive impairment]; [Loss of capability for effective verbal communication]

DEFINING CHARACTERISTICS

Subjective

Episodic occurrence of negative self-appraisal in response to life events in a person with previous positive self-evaluation; Verbalization of negative feelings about the self (e.g., helplessness, uselessness); Expressions of shame/guilt; Evaluates self as unable to handle situations/events

Objective

Self-negating verbalizations; Difficulty making decisions

SELF-ESTEEM, SITUATIONAL LOW, RISK FOR

Diagnostic Division: Ego Integrity

Definition: Risk for developing a negative perception of self-worth in response to a current situation. (specify situation)

DEFINING CHARACTERISTICS

To be developed by NANDA.

SELF-MUTILATION

Diagnostic Division: Safety

Definition: Deliberate, self-injurious behavior causing tissue damage with the intent of causing nonfatal injury to attain relief of tension.

DEFINING CHARACTERISTICS

To be developed by NANDA.

SELF-MUTILATION, RISK FOR

Diagnostic Division: Safety

Definition: A state in which the individual is at risk to perform an act upon the self to injure, not kill, which produces tissue damage and tension relief.

RISK FACTORS

Groups at Risk

Clients with borderline personality disorder, especially females 16 to 25 years of age; Clients in psychotic state—frequently males in young adulthood; Emotionally disturbed and/or battered children; [Clients with organic conditions, e.g.,] mental retardation and autism, [encephalitis, Tourette's syndrome, acute intoxication, Addison's disease]; Clients with a history of self-injury; Clients with a history of physical, emotional, or sexual abuse

Inability to cope with increased psychological-physiologic tension in a healthy manner; Feelings of depression, rejection, self-hatred, separation anxiety, guilt, and depersonalization; Fluctuating emotions; Command hallucinations; Need for sensory stimuli; Parental emotional deprivation; Dysfunctional family; [Difficulty achieving adolescent task of separation]

SENSORY/PERCEPTUAL ALTERATIONS (SPECIFY): VISUAL, AUDITORY, KINESTHETIC, GUSTATORY, TACTILE, OLFACTORY

Diagnostic Division: Neurosensory

Definition: A state in which an individual experiences a change in the amount or patterning of incoming stimuli accompanied by a diminished, exaggerated, distorted or impaired response to such stimuli.

RELATED FACTORS

Excessive/insufficient environmental stimuli; [Therapeutically restricted environments (e.g., isolation, intensive care, bedrest, traction, confining illnesses, incubator)]; [Socially restricted environment (e.g., institutionalization, homebound, aging, chronic/terminal illness, infant deprivation); stigmatized (e.g., mentally ill/retarded/handicapped); bereaved]; [Excessive noise level such as work environment, patient's immediate environment (ICU with support machinery and the like)]; Altered sensory reception, transmission, and/or integration; [Neurological disease, trauma, or deficit]; [Altered status of sense organs]; [Inability to communicate, understand, speak, or respond]; [Sleep deprivation]; [Pain, (phantom limb)]; Biochemical imbalances; Electrolyte imbalance; [elevated BUN, elevated ammonia, hypoxia], [drugs, (e.g., stimulants or depressants, mind-altering drugs)]; Psychological stress [narrowed perceptual fields caused by anxiety]; Altered sensory perception

DEFINING CHARACTERISTICS

Subjective

Reported change in sensory acuity [e.g., photosensitivity, hypoesthesias, diminished/altered sense of taste, inability to tell position of body parts (proprioception), visual/auditory distortions]; [Distortion of pain (e.g., exaggerated, lack of)]

Objective

Measured change in sensory acuity; Change in usual response to stimuli, [rapid mood swings, exaggerated emotional responses, anxiety/panic state, motor incoordination, altered sense of balance/falls (e.g., Ménière's syndrome)]; Change in problem-solving abilities; poor concentration; Disoriented in time, in place, or with people; Altered communication patterns; Change in behavior pattern; Restlessness; irritability; Hallucinations; [illusions]; [bizarre thinking]

SEXUAL DYSFUNCTION

Diagnostic Division: Sexuality

Definition: The state in which an individual experiences a change in sexual function that is viewed as unsatisfying, unrewarding, or inadequate.

RELATED FACTORS

Biopsychosocial alteration of sexuality: Ineffectual or absent role models; Lack of significant other; Vulnerability; Misinformation or lack of knowledge; Physical/psychosocial abuse (e.g., harmful relationships); Values conflict; Lack of privacy; Altered body structure or function (pregnancy, recent childbirth, drugs, surgery, anomalies, disease process, trauma, [paraplegia/quadriplegia], radiation, [effects of aging])

DEFINING CHARACTERISTICS

Subjective

Verbalization of problem [e.g., loss of sexual desire, disruption of sexual response patterns such as premature ejaculation, dyspareunia, vaginismus]; Actual or perceived limitation imposed by disease and/or therapy; Inability to achieve desired satisfaction; Alterations in achieving perceived sex role; Conflicts involving values; Alterations in achieving sexual satisfaction; Seeking of confirmation of desirability

Objective

Alteration in relationship with significant other; Change of interest in self and others

SEXUALITY PATTERNS, ALTERED

Diagnostic Division: Sexuality

Definition: The state in which an individual expresses concern regarding his/her sexuality.

RELATED FACTORS

Knowledge/skill deficit about alternative responses to health-related transitions, altered body function or structure, illness or medical [treatment]; Lack of privacy; Impaired relationship with a significant other; Lack of significant other; Ineffective or absent role models; Conflicts with sexual orientation or variant preferences; Fear of pregnancy or of acquiring a sexually transmitted disease

DEFINING CHARACTERISTICS

Subjective

Reported difficulties, limitations, or changes in sexual behaviors or activities; [Expressions of feeling of alienation, loneliness, loss, powerlessness, anger]

SKIN INTEGRITY, IMPAIRED

Diagnostic Division: Safety

Definition: A state in which an individual has altered epidermis and/or dermis. [The integumentary system is the largest multifunctional organ of the body.]

RELATED FACTORS

External

Hyperthermia or hypothermia; Chemical substance; radiation; medications; Physical immobilization; Humidity; moisture [excretions/secretions]; Altered fluid status; Mechanical factors (e.g., shearing forces, pressure, restraint), [trauma (e.g., injury/surgery); Extremes in age

Internal

Altered nutritional state (e.g., obesity, emaciation); altered metabolic state, pigmentation, circulation, sensation; Skeletal prominence; alterations in turgor (changes in elasticity); Developmental factors; Immunological deficit; [Psychogenic]

DEFINING CHARACTERISTICS

Subjective

[Reports of itching, pain, numbness of affected/surrounding area]

Objective

Disruption of skin surface (epidermis); Destruction of skin layers (dermis); Invasion of body structures

SKIN INTEGRITY, IMPAIRED, RISK FOR

Diagnostic Division: Safety

Definition: A state in which an individual's skin is at risk of being adversely altered.

RISK FACTORS

External

Chemical substance; radiation; Hypothermia or hyperthermia; Physical immobilization; Excretions and/or secretions; humidity; moisture; Mechanical factors (e.g., shearing forces, pressure, restraint); Extremes of age

Internal

Medication; Alterations in nutritional state (e.g., obesity, emaciation); alterations in metabolic state, circulation, sensation, pigmentation; Skeletal prominence; alterations in skin turgor (changes in elasticity); [presence of edema]; Developmental factors; Psychogenetic; Immunologic

SLEEP DEPRIVATION

Diagnostic Division: Activity/Rest

Definition: Prolonged periods of time without sustained natural, periodic suspension of relative unconsciousness [consciousness].

RELATED FACTORS

Sustained environmental stimulation; sustained unfamiliar or uncomfortable sleep environment; sustained circadian asynchrony; Inadequate daytime activity; aging-related sleep stage shifts; nonsleep-inducing parenting practices; Sustained inadequate sleep hygiene; prolonged use of pharmacologic or dietary antisoporifics; Prolonged physical/psychological discomfort; periodic limb movement (e.g., restless leg syndrome, nocturnal myoclonus); sleep-related enuresis; sleep-related painful erections; Nightmares; sleep walking; sleep terror; Sleep apnea; Sundowner's syndrome; dementia; Idiopathic central nervous system hypersomnolence; narcolepsy; familial sleep paralysis

DEFINING CHARACTERISTICS

Subjective

Daytime drowsiness; decreased ability to function; Malaise; tiredness; lethargy; Anxious; Perceptual disorders (e.g., disturbed body sensation, delusions, feeling afloat); heightened sensitivity to pain

Objective

Restlessness; irritability; Inability to concentrate; slowed reaction; Listlessness; apathy; Mild, fleeting nystagmus; hand tremors; Acute confusion; transient paranoia; agitated or combative; hallucinations

SLEEP PATTERN DISTURBANCE

Diagnostic Division: Activity/Rest

Definition: Time-limited disruption of sleep (natural, periodic suspension of consciousness) amount and quality.

RELATED FACTORS

Psychological

Daytime activity pattern; fatigue; dietary; body temperature; Social schedule inconsistent with chronotype; shift work; daylight/darkness exposure; Frequently changing sleep-wake schedule/travel across time zones; circadian asynchrony; Childhood onset; aging-related sleep shifts; periodic gender-related hormonal shifts; Inadequate sleep hygiene; maladaptive conditioned wakefulness; Ruminative pre-sleep thoughts; anticipation; thinking about home; Preoccupation with trying to sleep; fear of insomnia; Biochemical agents; medications; sustained use of anti-sleep agents; Temperament; loneliness; grief; anxiety; fear; boredom; depression; Separation from significant others; loss of sleep partner, life change; Delayed or advanced sleep phase syndrome

Environmental

Excessive stimulation; noise; lightning; ambient temperature; humidity; noxious odors; Unfamiliar sleep furnishings; Privacy control; sleep partner; Nurse for therapeutics, monitoring, lab tests; other-generated awakening; Physical restraint; Lack of sleep

Parental

Mother's sleep-wake pattern/emotional support; Parent-infant interaction

Physiological

Position; wet; fever; Gastroesophageal reflux; nausea; Shortness of breath; stasis of secretions; Urinary urgency

DEFINING CHARACTERISTICS

Subjective

Verbal complaints [reports] of difficulty falling asleep/not feeling well rested; dissatisfaction with sleep; Sleep onset greater than 30 minutes; Three or more nighttime awakenings; prolonged awakenings; Awakening earlier or later than desired; early morning insomnia; Decreased ability to function; [falling asleep during activities]

Objective

Less than age-normed total sleep time; Increased proportion of Stage 1 sleep; Decreased proportion of Stages 3 and 4 sleep (e.g., hyporesponsiveness, excess sleepiness, decreased motivation); Decreased proportion of REM sleep (e.g., REM rebound, hyperactivity, emotional lability, agitation and impulsivity, atypical polysomnographic features); Sleep maintenance insomnia; Self-induced impairment of normal pattern; [Changes in behavior and performance (increasing irritability, disorientation, listlessness, restlessness, lethargy)]; [Physical signs (mild fleeting nystagmus, ptosis of eyelid, slight hand tremor, expressionless face, dark circles under eyes, changes in posture, frequent yawning)]

SOCIAL INTERACTION, IMPAIRED

Diagnostic Division: Social Interaction

Definition: The state in which an individual participates in an insufficient or excessive quantity or ineffective quality of social exchange.

RELATED FACTORS

Knowledge/skill deficit about ways to enhance mutuality; Communication barriers [including head injury, stroke, other neurologic conditions affecting ability to communicate]; Self-concept disturbance; Absence of available significant others or peers;

Limited physical mobility [e.g., neuromuscular disease]; Therapeutic isolation; Sociocultural dissonance; Environmental barriers; Altered thought processes

DEFINING CHARACTERISTICS

Subjective

Verbalized discomfort in social situations; Verbalized inability to receive or communicate a satisfying sense of belonging, caring, interest, or shared history; Family report of change of style or pattern of interaction

Objective

Observed discomfort in social situations; Observed inability to receive or communicate a satisfying sense of belonging, caring, interest, or shared history; Observed use of unsuccessful social interaction behaviors; Dysfunctional interaction with peers, family, and/or others

SOCIAL ISOLATION

Diagnostic Division: Social Interaction

Definition: Aloneness experienced by the individual and perceived as imposed by others and as a negative or threatened state.

RISK FACTORS

Factors contributing to the absence of satisfying personal relationships, such as the following: Delay in accomplishing developmental tasks; Alterations in mental status; Altered state of wellness; Immature interests; Alterations in physical appearance; Unaccepted social behavior/values; Inadequate personal resources; Inability to engage in satisfying personal relationships; [Traumatic incidents or events causing physical and/or emotional pain]

DEFINING CHARACTERISTICS

Subjective

Expresses feeling of aloneness imposed by others; Expresses values acceptable to subculture, but unable to accept values of dominant culture; Inability to meet expectations of others; Expresses feelings of rejection; Experiences feelings of difference from others; Inadequacy in or absence of significant purpose in life; Expresses interests inappropriate to developmental age/stage; Insecurity in public

Objective

Absence of supportive significant other(s)—family, friends, group; Sad, dull affect; Inappropriate or immature interests/activities for developmental age/stage; Hostility projected in voice, behavior; Evidence of physical/mental handicap or altered state of wellness; Uncommunicative, withdrawn; no eye contact; Preoccupation with own thoughts; repetitive, meaningless actions; Seeking to be alone or exists in subculture; Shows behavior unaccepted by dominant cultural group

SORROW, CHRONIC

Diagnostic Division: Ego Integrity

Definition: A cyclical, recurring and potentially progressive pattern of pervasive sadness that is experienced by a client (parent or caregiver, or individual with chronic illness or disability) in response to continual loss, throughout the trajectory of an illness or disability.

RELATED FACTORS

Death of a loved one; Person experiences chronic physical or mental illness or disability such as: mental retardation, multiple sclerosis, prematurity, spina bifida or other birth defects, chronic mental illness, infertility, cancer, Parkinson's disease; person experiences one or more trigger events (e.g., crises in management of the illness, crises related to developmental stages and missed opportunities or milestones that bring comparisons with developmental, social, or personal norms); Unending caregiving as a constant reminder of loss

DEFINING CHARACTERISTICS

Subjective

Expresses one or more of the following feelings: anger, being misunderstood, confusion, depression, disappointment, emptiness, fear, frustration, guilt/self-blame, helplessness, hopelessness, loneliness, low self-esteem, recurring loss, overwhelmed; Client expresses periodic, recurrent feelings of sadness

Objective
Feelings that vary in intensity, are periodic, may progress and intensify over time, and may interfere with the client's ability to reach his/her highest level of personal and social well-being

SPIRITUAL DISTRESS (DISTRESS OF THE HUMAN SPIRIT)

Diagnostic Division: Ego Integrity

Definition: Disruption in the life principle that pervades a person's entire being and that integrates and transcends one's biologic and psychosocial nature.

RELATED FACTORS
Separation from religious and cultural ties; Challenged belief and value system (e.g., result of moral or ethical implications of therapy or result of intense suffering)

DEFINING CHARACTERISTICS

Subjective
Expresses concern with meaning of life/death and/or belief systems; Verbalizes inner conflict about beliefs; concern about relationship with deity; [does not experience that God is forgiving]; Angry toward God [as defined by the person]; Displacement of anger toward religious representatives; Questions meaning of suffering; Questions meaning of own existence; Questions moral/ethical implications of therapeutic regimen; Seeks spiritual assistance; Unable [or chooses not] to participate in usual religious practices; Description of nightmares/sleep disturbances; [Regards illness as punishment]; [Unable to accept self; engages in self-blame]; [Describes somatic symptoms]

Objective
Alteration in behavior/mood evidenced by anger, crying, withdrawal, preoccupation, anxiety, hostility, apathy, etc.; Gallows humor

SPIRITUAL DISTRESS, RISK FOR

Diagnostic Division: Ego Integrity

Definition: At risk for an altered sense of harmonious connectedness with all of life and the universe in which dimensions that transcend and empower the self may be disrupted.

RISK FACTORS
Physical or psychological stress; energy-consuming anxiety; physical/mental illness; situation/maturational losses; low self-esteem; blocks to self-love; poor relationships; inability to forgive; substance abuse; natural disasters

SPIRITUAL WELL-BEING, ENHANCED, POTENTIAL FOR

Diagnostic Division: Ego Integrity

Definition: Spiritual well-being is the process of an individual's developing/unfolding of mystery through harmonious interconnectedness that springs from inner strengths. [The ability to invest meaning, value, and purpose in life that gives harmony, peace, and contentment. This provides for life-affirming relationships with deity, self, community, and environment.]

RELATED FACTORS
To be developed by NANDA

DEFINING CHARACTERISTICS

Subjective
Inner strengths: sense of awareness, self-consciousness, sacred source, unifying force, inner core, and transcendence; Unfolding mystery: one's experience about life's purpose and meaning, mystery, uncertainty, and struggles; Harmonious interconnectedness: relatedness, connectedness, harmony with self, others, higher power/God, and the environment

SPONTANEOUS VENTILATION, INABILITY TO SUSTAIN

Diagnostic Division: Respiration

Definition: A state in which the response pattern of decreased energy reserves results in an individual's inability to maintain breathing adequate to support life.

RELATED FACTORS

Metabolic factors; [hypermetabolic state (e.g., infection), nutritional deficits/depletion of energy stores]; Respiratory muscle fatigue; [Airway size/resistance; problems with secretion management]

DEFINING CHARACTERISTICS

Subjective

Dyspnea; Apprehension

Objective

Increased metabolic rate; Increased heart rate; Increased restlessness; Decreased cooperation; Increased use of accessory muscles; Decreased tidal volume; Decreased PO_2; Decreased SaO_2; Increased PCO_2

SUFFOCATION, RISK FOR

Diagnostic Division: Safety

Definition: Accentuated risk of accidental suffocation (inadequate air available for inhalation).

RISK FACTORS

Internal (individual)

Reduced olfactory sensation; Reduced motor abilities; Lack of safety education, precautions; Cognitive or emotional difficulties [e.g., altered consciousness/mentation]; Disease or injury process

External (environmental)

Pillow/propped bottle placed in an infant's crib; Pacifier hung around infant's head; Children playing with plastic bags or inserting small objects into their mouths or noses; Children left unattended in bathtubs or pools; Discarded or unused refrigerators or freezers without removed doors; Vehicle warming in closed garage [/faulty exhaust system]; Use of fuel-burning heaters not vented to outside; Household gas leaks; Smoking in bed; Low-strung clothesline; Eating of large mouthfuls [or pieces] of food

SUICIDE, RISK FOR

Diagnostic Division: Safety

Definition: Risk for self-inflicted, life-threatening injury.

DEFINING CHARACTERISTICS

To be developed by NANDA.

SWALLOWING, IMPAIRED

Diagnostic Division: Food/Fluid

Definition: Abnormal functioning of the swallowing mechanism associated with deficits in oral, pharyngeal, or esophageal structure or function.

RELATED FACTORS

Congenital Deficits

Upper airway anomalies; mechanical obstruction (e.g., edema, tracheostomy tube, tumor); history of tube feeding; Neuromuscular impairment (e.g., decreased or absent gag reflex, decreased strength or excursion of muscles involved in mastication, perceptual impairment, facial paralysis); conditions with significant hypotonia; cranial nerve involvement; Respiratory disorders; congenital heart disease; Behavioral feeding problems; self injurious behavior; Failure to thrive on protein energy malnutrition

Neurological Problems

External/internal traumas; acquired anatomic defects; Nasal or nasopharyngeal cavity defects; Oral cavity or oropharynx abnormalities; Upper airway/laryngeal anomalies; tracheal, laryngeal, esophageal defects; Gastroesophageal reflux disease; achalasia; Premature infants; traumatic head injury; developmental delay; cerebral palsy

DEFINING CHARACTERISTICS

Subjective

Esophageal Phase Impairment

Complaints [reports] of "something stuck"; odynophagia; Food refusal or volume limiting; Heartburn or epigastric pain; Nighttime coughing or awakening

Objective

Oral Phase Impairment

Weak suck resulting in inefficient nippling; Slow bolus formation; lack of tongue action to form bolus; premature entry of bolus; Incomplete lip closure; food pushed out of/falls from mouth; Lack of chewing; Coughing, choking, gagging before a swallow; Piecemeal deglutition; abnormality in oral phase of swallow study; Inability to clear oral cavity; pooling in lateral sulci; nasal reflux; sialorrhea or drooling; Long meals with little consumption

Pharyngeal Phase Impairment

Food refusal; Altered head positions; delayed/multiple swallows; inadequate laryngeal elevation; abnormality in pharyngeal phase by swallow study; Choking, coughing, or gagging; nasal reflux; gurgly voice quality; Unexplained fevers; recurrent pulmonary infections

Esophageal Phase Impairment

Observed evidence of difficulty in swallowing (e.g., stasis of food in oral cavity, coughing/choking); abnormality in esophageal phase by swallow study; Hyperextension of head, arching during or after meals; Repetitive swallowing or ruminating; bruxism; Unexplained irritability surrounding mealtime; Acidic smelling breath; regurgitation of gastric contents or wet burps; vomitus on pillow; vomiting; hematemesis

THERAPEUTIC REGIMEN (COMMUNITY), INEFFECTIVE MANAGEMENT OF

Diagnostic Division: Teaching/Learning

Definition: A pattern of regulating and integrating into community processes programs for treatment of illness and the sequelae of illness that are unsatisfactory for meeting health-related goals.

RELATED FACTORS

To be developed by NANDA: [Lack of safety for community members]; [Economic insecurity]; [Health care not available]; [Unhealthy environment]; [Education not available for all community members]; [Does not possess means to meet human needs for recognition, fellowship, security, and membership]

DEFINING CHARACTERISTICS

Subjective

[Community members/agencies verbalize inability to meet therapeutic needs of all members]; [Community members/agencies verbalize overburdening of resources for meeting therapeutic needs of all members]

Objective

Deficits in persons and programs to be accountable for illness care of aggregates; Deficits in advocates for aggregates; Deficit in community activities for [primary medical care/prevention]/secondary and tertiary prevention; Illness symptoms above the norm expected for the number and type of population; unexpected acceleration of illness(es); Number of health care resources insufficient[/unavailable] for the incidence or prevalence of illness(es); [Deficits in community for collaboration and development of coalitions to address programs for treatment of illness and the sequelae of illness]

THERAPEUTIC REGIMEN (FAMILIES), INEFFECTIVE MANAGEMENT OF

Diagnostic Division: Teaching/Learning

Definition: A pattern of regulating and integrating into family processes a program for treatment of illness and the sequelae of illness that is unsatisfactory for meeting specific health needs.

RELATED FACTORS

Complexity of health care system; Complexity of therapeutic regimen; Decisional conflicts; Economic difficulties; Excessive demands made on individual or family; Family conflict

DEFINING CHARACTERISTICS

Subjective

Verbalized difficulty with regulation/integration of one or more effects or prevention of complication; [inability to manage treatment regimen]; Verbalized desire to manage the treatment of illness and prevention of sequelae; Verbalizes that family did not take action to reduce risk factors for progression of illness and sequelae

Objective

Inappropriate family activities for meeting the goals of a treatment or prevention program; Acceleration (expected or unexpected) of illness symptoms of a family member; Lack of attention to illness and its sequelae

THERAPEUTIC REGIMEN (INDIVIDUAL), EFFECTIVE MANAGEMENT OF

Diagnostic Division: Teaching/Learning

Definition: A pattern of regulating and integrating into daily living a program for treatment of illness and its sequelae that is satisfactory for meeting specific health goals.

RELATED FACTORS

NOTE: To be developed by NANDA; [Complexity of health care management; therapeutic regimen]; [Added demands made on individual or family]; [Adequate social supports]

DEFINING CHARACTERISTICS

Subjective

Verbalized desire to manage the treatment of illness and prevention of sequelae; Verbalized intent to reduce risk factors for progression of illness and sequelae

Objective

Appropriate choices of daily activities for meeting the goals of a treatment or prevention program; Illness symptoms are within a normal range of expectation

THERAPEUTIC REGIMEN (INDIVIDUAL), INEFFECTIVE MANAGEMENT OF

Diagnostic Division: Teaching/Learning

Definition: A pattern of regulating and integrating into daily living a program for treatment of illness and the sequelae of illness that is unsatisfactory for meeting specific health goals.

RELATED FACTORS

Complexity of health care system/ therapeutic regimen; Decisional conflicts; Economic difficulties; Excessive demands made on individual or family; Family conflicts; Family patterns of health care; Inadequate number and types of cues to action; Knowledge deficits; Mistrust of regimen and/or health care personnel; Perceived seriousness/susceptibility/barriers/benefits; Powerlessness; Social support deficits

DEFINING CHARACTERISTICS

Subjective

Verbalized desire to manage the treatment of illness and prevention of sequelae; Verbalized difficulty with regulation/integration of one or more prescribed regimens for treatment of illness and its effects or prevention of complications; Verbalized that did not take action to include treatment regimens in daily routines/reduce risk factors for progression of illness and sequelae

Objective

Choice of daily living ineffective for meeting the goals of a treatment or prevention program; Acceleration (expected or unexpected) of illness symptoms

THERMOREGULATION, INEFFECTIVE

Diagnostic Division: Safety

Definition: The state in which the individual's temperature fluctuates between hypothermia and hyperthermia.

RELATED FACTORS
Trauma or illness [e.g., cerebral edema, cerebrovascular accident, intracranial surgery, or head injury]; Immaturity, aging [e.g., loss/absence of brown adipose tissue]; Fluctuating environmental temperature; [Changes in hypothalamic tissue, causing alterations in emission of thermosensitive cells and regulation of heat loss/production]; [Changes in level/action of thyroxine and catecholamines]; [Changes in metabolic rate/activity]; [Chemical reactions in contracting muscles]

DEFINING CHARACTERISTICS
Objective
Fluctuations in body temperature above or below the normal range; Tachycardia; Reduction in body temperature below normal rate; cool skin; pallor (moderate); shivering (mild); piloerection; cyanotic; nailbeds; slow capillary refill; hypertension

THOUGHT PROCESSES, ALTERED

Diagnostic Division: Neurosensory

Definition: A state in which an individual experiences a disruption in cognitive operations and activities.

RELATED FACTORS
To be developed by NANDA: [Physiologic changes, aging, hypoxia, head injury, malnutrition, infections]; [Biochemical changes, medications, substance abuse]; [Sleep deprivation]; [Psychological conflicts, emotional changes, mental disorders]

DEFINING CHARACTERISTICS
Subjective
[Ideas of reference, hallucinations, delusions]

Objective
Inaccurate interpretation of environment; Inappropriate/nonreality-based thinking; Memory deficit/problems [disorientation to time, place, person, circumstances, and events, loss of short-term/remote memory]; Hypervigilance/hypovigilance; Cognitive dissonance, [decreased ability to grasp ideas, make decisions, problem-solve, use abstract reasoning or conceptualize, calculate; disordered thought sequencing]; Distractibility [altered attention span]; Egocentricity; [Confabulation]; [Inappropriate social behavior]

TISSUE INTEGRITY, IMPAIRED

Diagnostic Division: Safety

Definition: A state in which an individual experiences damage to mucous membrane, corneal, integumentary, or subcutaneous tissues.

RELATED FACTORS
Altered circulation; nutritional deficit or excess; [metabolic, endocrine dysfunction]; fluid deficit/excess; knowledge deficit; impaired physical mobility; irritants, chemical (including body excretions, secretions, medications); radiation (including therapeutic radiation); thermal (temperature extremes); mechanical (e.g., pressure, shear, friction); [infection]

DEFINING CHARACTERISTICS
Objective
Damaged or destroyed tissue (e.g., cornea, mucous membrane, integumentary, or subcutaneous)

TISSUE PERFUSION, ALTERED (SPECIFY TYPE): RENAL, CEREBRAL, CARDIOPULMONARY, GASTROINTESTINAL, PERIPHERAL

Diagnostic Division: Circulation

Definition: A decrease in oxygen resulting in the failure to nourish the tissues at the capillary level. [Tissue perfusion problems can exist without decreased cardiac output; however, there may be a relationship between cardiac output and tissue perfusion.]

RELATED FACTORS
Interruption of flow—arterial, venous; Exchange problems; Hypervolemia, hypovole-

mia; Mechanical reduction of venous and/or arterial blood flow; Decreased hemoglobin concentration in blood; Altered affinity of hemoglobin for oxygen; enzyme poisoning; Impaired transport of the oxygen across alveolar and/or capillary membrane; Mismatch of ventilation with blood flow; Hypoventilation

DEFINING CHARACTERISTICS

Renal

Objective: Altered blood pressure outside of acceptable parameters; Oliguria or anuria; hematuria; Arterial pulsations; bruits; Elevation in BUN/Creatinine ratio

Cerebral

Objective: Altered mental status; speech abnormalities; Behavioral changes; [restlessness]; changes in motor response; extremity weakness or paralysis; Changes in pupillary reactions; Difficulty in swallowing

Cardiopulmonary

Subjective: Chest pain; Dyspnea; Sense of "impending doom"; *Objective:* Dysrhythmias; Capillary refill greater than 3 sec; Altered respiratory rate outside of acceptable parameters; Use of accessory muscles; nasal flaring; chest retraction; Bronchospasms; Abnormal arterial blood gases; [Hemoptysis]

Gastrointestinal

Subjective: Nausea; Abdominal pain or tenderness; *Objective:* Hypoactive or absent bowel sounds; Abdominal distention; [Melena]

Peripheral

Subjective: Claudication; *Objective:* Altered skin characteristics (hair, nails, moisture); Skin temperature changes; Skin discolorations; skin color diminished; color pale on elevation, color does not return on lowering leg; Altered sensations; Blood pressure changes in extremities; weak or absent pulses; Edema; Slow healing of lesions; Positive Homans' sign

TRANSFER ABILITY, IMPAIRED

Diagnostic Division: Safety

Definition: Limitation of independent movement between two nearby surfaces.

RELATED FACTORS

To be developed by NANDA; [Conditions that result in poor muscle tone]; [Cognitive impairment]; [Fractures, trauma, spinal cord injury]

DEFINING CHARACTERISTICS

Impaired ability to transfer: from bed to chair and chair to bed, chair to car or car to chair, chair to floor or floor to chair, standing to floor or floor to standing, on or off a toilet or commode, in and out of tub or shower, between uneven levels

TRAUMA, RISK FOR

Diagnostic Division: Safety

Definition: Accentuated risk of accidental tissue injury (e.g., wound, burn, fracture).

RISK FACTORS

Internal (individual)

Weakness; Balancing difficulties; Reduced large, or small, muscle coordination, hand/eye coordination; Poor vision; Reduced temperature and/or tactile sensation; Lack of safety education/precautions; Insufficient finances to purchase safety equipment or to effect repairs; Cognitive or emotional difficulties; History of previous trauma

External (environmental) [includes but is not limited to:]

Slippery floors (e.g., wet or highly waxed); unanchored rug; litter or liquid spills on floors or stairways; snow or ice collected on stairs, walkways); Bathtub without hand grip or antislip equipment; Use of unsteady ladder or chairs; Obstructed passageways; entering unlighted rooms; Unsturdy or absent stair rails; children playing without gates at top of stairs; Unanchored electric wires; High beds; inappropriate call-for-aid mechanisms for bedresting client; Unsafe window protection in homes with young children; Pot handles facing toward front of stove; bathing in very hot water (e.g., unsupervised bathing of young children); Potential igniting of gas leaks; delayed lighting of gas burner or oven; Unscreened fires or heaters; wearing of plastic aprons or flowing clothing around open flame; highly flammable children's toys or clothing;

Smoking in bed or near oxygen; grease waste collected on stoves; Children playing with matches, candles, cigarettes; Playing with fireworks or gunpowder; guns or ammunition stored unlocked. Experimenting with chemical or gasoline; inadequately stored combustibles or corrosives (e.g., matches, oily rags, lye; contact with acids or alkalkis); Overloaded fuse boxes; faulty electrical plugs, frayed wires, or defective appliances; overloaded electrical outlets; Exposure to dangerous machinery; contact with rapidly moving machinery, industrial belts, or pulleys; Sliding on coarse bed linen or struggling within bed [/chair] restraints; Contact with intense cold; overexposure to sun, sun lamps, radiotherapy; Use of thin or worn-out pot holders [or mitts]; Use of cracked dishware glasses; Knives stored uncovered; children playing with sharp-edged toys; Large icicles hanging from roof; High-crime neighborhood and vulnerable clients; Driving a mechanically unsafe vehicle; driving at excessive speeds; driving without the necessary visual aids; Driving after partaking of alcoholic beverages or [other] drugs; Children riding in the front seat of car, nonuse or misuse of seat restraints/[unrestrained infant/child riding in car]; Misuse [or nonuse] of necessary headgear for motorized cyclists or young children carried on adult bicycles; Unsafe road or road-crossing conditions playing or working near vehicle pathways (e.g., driveways, lanes, railroad tracks)

UNILATERAL NEGLECT

Diagnostic Division: Neurosensory

Definition: The state in which an individual is perceptually unaware of and inattentive to one side of the body [and the immediate unilateral territory/space].

RELATED FACTORS

Effects of disturbed perceptual abilities (e.g., [homonymous] hemianopsia, one-sided blindness; [or visual inattention]); neurologic illness or trauma; [Impaired cerebral blood flow]

DEFINING CHARACTERISTICS

Subjective

[Reports feeling that part does not belong to own self]

Objective

Consistent inattention to stimuli on an affected side; Inadequate self-care [inability to satisfactorily perform activities of daily living]; [Lack of] Positioning and/or safety precautions in regard to the affected side; Does not look toward affected side; Leaves food on plate on the affected side; [Does not touch affected side]; [Failure to use the affected side of the body without being reminded to do so]

URINARY ELIMINATION, ALTERED PATTERNS OF

Diagnostic Division: Elimination

Definition: The state in which an individual experiences a disturbance in urine elimination.

RELATED FACTORS

Multiple causality, including: sensory motor impairment; anatomical obstruction; urinary tract infection; [mechanical trauma; surgical diversion; fluid/volume states; psychogenic factors]

DEFINING CHARACTERISTICS

Subjective

Frequency; urgency; Hesitancy; Dysuria; Nocturia; [enuresis]

Objective

Incontinence; Retention

URINARY RETENTION [ACUTE/CHRONIC]

Diagnostic Division: Elimination

Definition: The state in which the individual experiences incomplete emptying of the bladder. [High urethral pressure inhibits voiding until increased abdominal pressure causes urine to be involuntarily lost, or high urethral pressure inhibits timely/complete emptying of bladder.]

RELATED FACTORS

High urethral pressure caused by weak [/absent] detrusor; Inhibition of reflex arc; Strong sphincter; Blockage [e.g., BPH, perineal swelling]; [Habituation of reflex arc]; [Use of medications with side effect of retention (e.g., atropine, belladonna, psychotropics, antihistamines, opiates)]; [Infections]; [Neurologic diseases/trauma]

DEFINING CHARACTERISTICS

Subjective

Sensation of bladder fullness; Dribbling; Dysuria

Objective

Bladder distention; Small, frequent voiding or absence of urine output; Residual urine [150 ml or more]; Overflow incontinence; [Reduced stream]

VENTILATORY WEANING RESPONSE, DYSFUNCTIONAL (DVWR)

Diagnostic Division: Respiration

Definition: A state in which a patient cannot adjust to lowered levels of mechanical ventilator support, which interrupts and prolongs the weaning process.

RELATED FACTORS

Physical

Ineffective airway clearance; Sleep pattern disturbance; Inadequate nutrition; Uncontrolled pain or discomfort; [Muscle weakness/fatigue, inability to control respiratory muscles; immobility]

Psychological

Knowledge deficit of the weaning process, patient role; Patient-perceived inefficacy about the ability to wean; Decreased motivation; Decreased self-esteem; Anxiety (moderate, severe); fear; insufficient trust in the nurse; Hopelessness; Powerlessness; [Unprepared for weaning attempt]

Situational

Uncontrolled episodic energy demands or problems; Inappropriate pacing of diminished ventilator support; Inadequate social support; Adverse environment (noisy, active environment, negative events in the room, low nurse-patient ratio, extended nurse absence from bedside, unfamiliar nursing staff); History of ventilator dependence 1 week; History of multiple unsuccessful weaning attempts

DEFINING CHARACTERISTICS

Responds to lowered levels of mechanical ventilator support with:

Mild DVWR

Subjective

Expressed feelings of increased need for oxygen, breathing discomfort, fatigue, warmth; Queries about possible machine malfunction

Objective

Restlessness; Slight increased respiratory rate from baseline; Increased concentration on breathing

Moderate DVWR

Subjective

Apprehension

Objective

Slight increase from baseline blood pressure <20 mm Hg; Slight increase from baseline heart rate <20 beats/min; Baseline increase in respiratory rate <5 breaths/min; Hypervigilance to activities; Inability to respond to coaching/cooperate; Diaphoresis; Eye widening, "wide-eyed look"; Decreased air entry on auscultation; Color changes: pale, slight cyanosis; Slight respiratory accessory muscle use

Severe DVWR

Objective

Agitation; Deterioration in arterial blood gases from current baseline; Increase from baseline blood pressure >20 mm Hg; Increase from baseline heart rate >20 beats/min; Respiratory rate increases significantly from baseline; Profuse diaphoresis; Full respiratory accessory muscle use; Shallow, gasping breaths; Paradoxical abdominal breathing; Discoordinated breathing with the ventilator; Decreased level of consciousness; Adventitious breath sounds, audible airway secretions; Cyanosis

VIOLENCE, [ACTUAL]/RISK FOR DIRECTED AT OTHERS

Diagnostic Division: Safety

Definition: Behaviors in which an individual demonstrates that he/she can be physically, emotionally, and/or sexually harmful to others.

RISK FACTORS

History of violence: against others (e.g., hitting, kicking, scratching, biting or spitting, throwing objects at someone; attempted rape, rape, sexual molestation, urinating/defecating on a person); Threats (e.g, verbal threats against property/person, social threats, cursing, threatening notes/letters or gestures, sexual threats); Antisocial behavior (e.g., stealing, insistent borrowing, insistent demands for privileges, insistent interruption of meetings; refusal to eat or take medication, ignoring instructions); Indirect (e.g., tearing off clothes, urinating/defecating on floor, stamping feet, temper tantrum; running in corridors, yelling, writing on walls, ripping objects off walls, throwing objects, breaking a window, slamming doors; sexual advances)

OTHER FACTORS

Neurological impairment (e.g., positive ECG, CT, or MRI; head trauma; positive neurological findings; seizure disorders, [temporal lobe epilepsy]); Cognitive impairment (e.g., learning disabilities, attention deficit disorder, decreased intellectual functioning); [organic brain syndrome]; History of childhood abuse/witnessing family violence, [negative role modeling]; cruelty to animals; firesetting; Prenatal and perinatal complications/abnormalities; History of drug/alcohol abuse; pathological intoxication, [toxic reaction to medication]; Psychotic symptomatology (e.g, auditory, visual, command hallucinations; paranoid delusions; loose, rambling, or illogical thought processes); [panic states; rate reactions; catatonic/manic excitement]; Motor vehicle offenses (e.g., frequent traffic violations, use of motor vehicle to release anger); Suicidal behavior, impulsivity; availability and/or possession of weapon(s); Body language: rigid posture, clenching of fists and jaw, hyperactivity, pacing, breathlessness, threatening stances; [Hormonal imbalance (e.g., premenstrual syndrome, postpartal depression/psychosis)]; [Expressed intent/desire to harm others directly or indirectly]; [Almost continuous thoughts of violence]

VIOLENCE, [ACTUAL]/RISK FOR SELF-DIRECTED

Diagnostic Division: Safety

Definition: Behaviors in which an individual demonstrates that he/she can be physically, emotionally, and/or sexually harmful to self.

RISK FACTORS

Age 15–19, over 45; Marital status (single, widowed, divorced) ; Employment (unemployed, recent job loss/failure); occupation (executive, administrator, owner of business, professional, semiskilled worker); Conflictual interpersonal relationships; Family background (chaotic or conflictual, history of suicide); Sexual orientation: bisexual (active), homosexual (inactive); Physical health (hypochondriac, chronic or terminal illness); Mental health (severe depression, psychosis, severe personality disorder, alcoholism or drug abuse); Emotional status (hopelessness, despair [lifting of depressed mood]; increased anxiety, panic, anger, hostility); history of multiple suicide attempts; suicidal ideation (frequent, intense, prolonged); suicide plan (clear and specific; lethality: method and availability of destructive means); Personal resources (poor achievement, poor insight, affect unavailable and poorly controlled); Social resources (poor rapport, socially isolated, unresponsive family); Verbal clues (e.g., talking about death, "better off without me," asking questions about lethal dosages of drugs; Behavioral clues (e.g., writing forlorn love notes, directing angry messages at a significant other who has rejected the person, giving away personal items, taking out a large life insurance policy); Persons who engage in autoerotic sexual acts [e.g., asphyxiation]

WALKING, IMPAIRED

Diagnostic Division: Safety

Definition: Limitation of independent movement within the environment on foot.

RELATED FACTORS

To be developed by NANDA; [Condition affecting muscles/joints impairing ability to walk]

DEFINING CHARACTERISTICS
Impaired ability to walk required distances, walk on an incline/decline, or on on uneven surfaces, to navigate curbs, climb stairs

WANDERING (Specify sporadic or continual)

Diagnostic Division: Safety

Definition: Locomotion (with dementia or brain injury) characterized by its frequency and persistence: course appears to be meandering, aimless, or repetitive; frequently incongruent with boundaries, limits, or obstacles; impaired navigational ability.

DEFINING CHARACTERISTICS
To be developed by NANDA.